New Jersey

FOLIOMED
PHYSICIAN DIRECTORY
NEW JERSEY

TWENTY-SECOND EDITION

2020

FolioMed

297 North Street
Suite 212
Hyannis, MA 02601

Tel: (508) 862-8200
Tollfree: 1-(800) 223-2233
Fax: (508) 862-8210

Email: CustomerService@FolioMed.com
Website: www.FolioMed.com

FOLIOMED PHYSICIAN DIRECTORY OF NEW JERSEY,
22ND EDITION 2020-$100
Also Publishing FolioMed Physician Directories
- Massachusetts
- Connecticut and Rhode Island
- Maine, New Hampshire and Vermont
- New York City and Long Island
- New York Upstate
- Ohio
- Pennsylvania

FolioMed

FolioMed
Expert Provider Databases

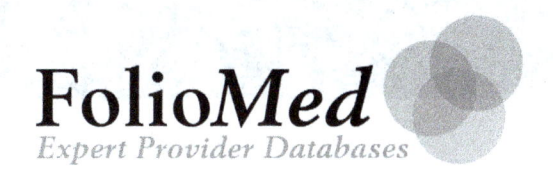

FOR REFERENCE ONLY

FOLIO*MED* PHYSICIAN DIRECTORY
New Jersey
With Group Practices
2020

New Jersey Directory 2020
Physician Directory with Group Practices 20th Edition
Copyright 2020 FolioMed, Inc.
ISBN 978-1506-908-92-2
January 2020
Published and Distributed by
First Edition Design Publishing, Inc.
P.O. Box 17646, Sarasota, FL 34276-3217
www.firsteditiondesignpublishing.com

© 2020 Folio*Med* Inc.

Every reasonable effort has been made to assure the accuracy of the information contained herein, including compilation and direct verification of all data with persons and sources deemed reliable, the accuracy of which is not guaranteed. Inquiries regarding information in the Directory, as well as additions or corrections, will be gratefully received. All rights reserved. No portion of this Directory may be duplicated or reproduced in any matter whatsoever without the written permission of the Publisher.

FolioMed... Information To Rely On

40 years of experience that you can trust. Folio's proprietary physician information is up-to-date, verified and meets your needs for accuracy.

Order by phone or over the Web!

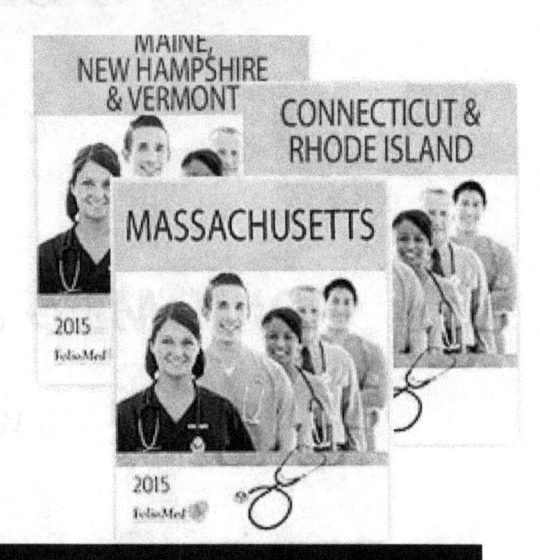

THE #1 SOURCE FOR COMPREHENSIVE, ACCURATE PHYSICIAN INFORMATION

FOLIO*MED*'S PRINTED PHYSICIAN DIRECTORIES 2020 :

MASSACHUSETTS	43rd EDITION	$100
CONNECTICUT & RHODE ISLAND	38th EDITION	$100
MAINE, NEW HAMPSHIRE & VERMONT	28th EDITION	$100
NEW ENGLAND SET (3 VOLUMES)		$250
MASSACHUSETTS DIRECTORY OF CHIROPRACTORS, PODIATRISTS, DENTISTS & OPTOMETRISTS 2019		$75
NEW YORK CITY	20th EDITIONS	$100
NEW YORK UPSTATE	22nd EDITIONS	$100
NEW YORK STATE SET (2 VOLUMES)		$150
NEW JERSEY	22nd EDITION	$100

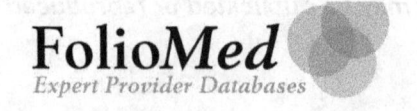

FolioMed
Expert Provider Databases

297 North Street • Suite 212 • Hyannis, MA 02601
Phone: (800) 223-2233 • Fax: (508) 862-8210
Email: customerservice@foliomed.com • www.foliomed.com

FolioMed
Expert Provider Databases

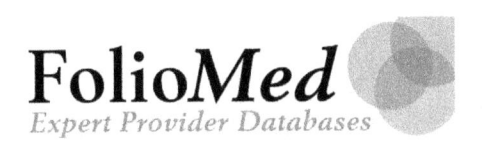

Dear Valued Customer:

Welcome to the new **FolioMed Physician Directory** for 2020!
nine
Welcome to the latest edition of the **FolioMed Physician Directory** for New Jersey 2020 twenty-second edition. As we have for almost 40 years, with this and other Directories, FolioMed continues to address a fundamental need in the medical and other communities for comprehensive, accurate and detailed data about healthcare providers and their practices.

FolioMed's databases are developed from a combination of public, semi-public, and proprietary data sources which, combined with specialized verification processes and software, result in information about healthcare practitioners that is unavailable from any other source. The uniqueness of Folio publications also derives from the integration in one volume of a healthcare provider's multiple practice addresses, practice types and names; telephone and fax numbers; specialties; hospital affiliations; E-Mail addresses; and Websites.

The 2020 editions of **FolioMed Physician Directories** include newly licensed physicians as well as thousands of changes in practice addresses and other contact and location information. Equally important are the healthcare providers that are excluded from the Directory due to retirement, relocation, non renewal of license or other non practicing statuses.

According to some industry estimates, 50-70% of provider records in health plans and healthcare institutions contain data errors or omissions. In addition to the important issues of quality impacting clinical communications, the direct cost of errors because of misidentification of providers, re-submission of healthcare claims, and reimbursement payment delays has been estimated to exceed $20 billion annually.*

This Directory was developed after research and correspondence with current Folio customers. Our goal is to provide our customers with a Directory that meaningfully assists them in efficiently accomplishing the transactions and data requirements necessary in today's healthcare environment. Our mission continues to be to provide the most up-to-date and functional information on healthcare providers and to achieve that mission we depend on and welcome your suggestions and comments.

Sincerely,

Paul G. Rooker

Paul G. Rooker
President and Publisher

* Log on to www.foliomed.com and access FolioMed's 'Analyzer' to estimate the cost of Provider Data errors to your organization

Folio Is
Internet Service

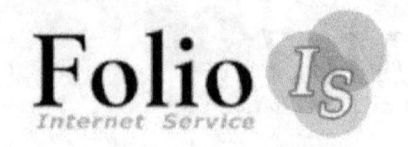

FolioMed Internet Access

**Current and real time
Provider information!
Just a mouse click away!**

'Cloud based' Internet access to the most comprehensive, up-to-date database of physicians and healthcare facilities!

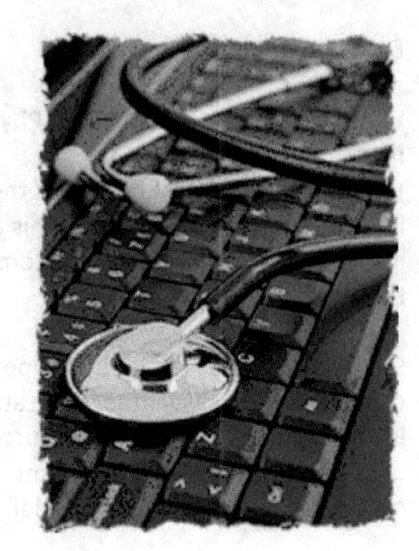

Folio Internet Service is an online subscription service that provides real-time access via the Internet to the FolioMed Database of Physicians and Healthcare Facilities.

Complete Provider & Healthcare Facility Information Including NPIs
- Physicians
- Nurse Practitioners and Physician Assistants

Individual or enterprise wide access

Updated Daily

Query by name, town or specialty.

Provider Rosters for Individual Groups

Copy & Paste critical information as needed.

Doc_Finder service for FolioMed Provider Searches

Visit us at www.Foliomed.com for a demo
Call at 508-862-8200♦800/223-2233
E-mail: customerservice@foliomed.com

Introduction

Listing Guide.. 9
Code Tables..
    Medical Specialities.. 11
    Medical Schools.. 15
    Hospitals... 22

Physicians

Section 1 Physicians Aphabetically with Practice Addresses, Medical School and Specialties.............................. 25
Section 2 Physicians by Town and Primary Medical Specialty... 553
Section 3 Physicians by Primary Medical Specialty and Town...647

Group Practices and Clinics

Section 4 Physician Rosters of Group Practices and Clinics Alphabetically by Town and Facility Name.............739

FolioMed
Expert Provider Databases

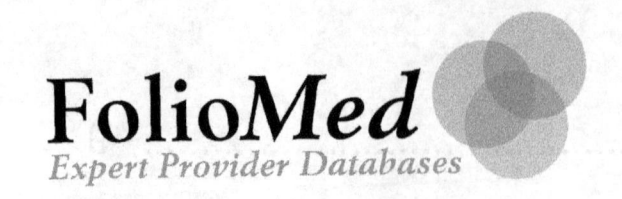

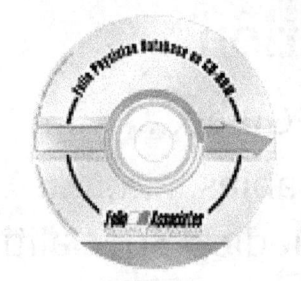

297 North Street Hyannis MA 02601 www.foliomed.com

Folio*Med* CD-ROM Applications

- Complete Census of all Practicing Physicians in the Geography
- Available as Single workstation or Networked application
- Available with built-in Query tool
    - Data-individual records
        - multiple practice addresses with phone/fax (prioritized)
        - mailing addresses if different from practice address
        - multiple medical specialties (prioritized)
        - Unique identifiers: NPI, UPIN, Board Licensure number
        - Hospital affiliations
        - email addresses (partial)
- Query Tool
    - Search criteria

        Physicians

Doctor Name	Specialty	County
Town/Distance	State	Zip/Distance
Zipcode Range	MedSchool	Facility type
Facility name	Street Address	Hospital Affil
UPIN	Language	Phone/fax

        Facilities

Facility name	Number Docs	Town
Facility type	Street Address	Town/Distance
State	Zip/Distance	Zipcode Range
Phone/fax		

        Downloadable *
        Text, dbf, xls or XML formats
        Editable
        Edits can be added by Customer or
        Email edits to FolioMed

* Standard single user CD has 2000 record download limitation

Listing Guide

Section 1 Physicians Alphabetically with Practice Addresses

Lists all Physicians Alphabetically by Name, MD/DO, NPI and medical specialty codes (3), medical school and year of graduation, hospital affiliation codes, practice addresses (3), telephone, fax numbers, and e-mail

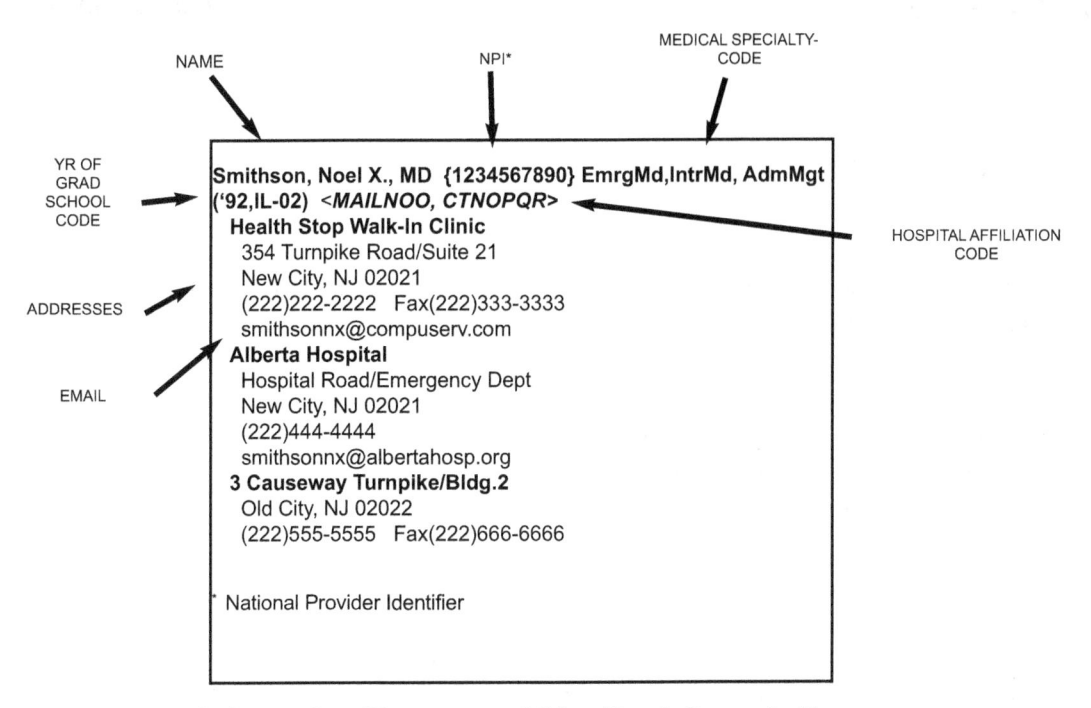

- **NAME** → Smithson, Noel X., MD
- **NPI*** → {1234567890}
- **MEDICAL SPECIALTY-CODE** → EmrgMd, IntrMd, AdmMgt
- **YR OF GRAD SCHOOL CODE** → ('92, IL-02)
- **HOSPITAL AFFILIATION CODE** → <MAILNOO, CTNOPQR>
- **ADDRESSES**:
  - Health Stop Walk-In Clinic
    354 Turnpike Road/Suite 21
    New City, NJ 02021
    (222)222-2222 Fax(222)333-3333
  - **EMAIL**: smithsonnx@compuserv.com
  - Alberta Hospital
    Hospital Road/Emergency Dept
    New City, NJ 02021
    (222)444-4444
    smithsonnx@albertahosp.org
  - 3 Causeway Turnpike/Bldg.2
    Old City, NJ 02022
    (222)555-5555 Fax(222)666-6666

*National Provider Identifier

Section 2 Physicians by Town and Medical Specialty

Lists all practicing Physicians first by Town alphabetically and then by Medical Specialty and Name (primary practice location and primary medical specialty)

Section 3 Physicians by Medical Specialty and Town

Lists all practicing Physicians in first by Medical Specialty and then by Town (primary medical specialty and primary practice location)

Section 4 Group Practices and Clinics Alphabetically by Town with Physician Rosters

Physician Rosters of all Group Practices and Clinics first by town and then by name of facility (with address, phone/fax) and finally by Physician Name

FolioMed
Expert Provider Databases

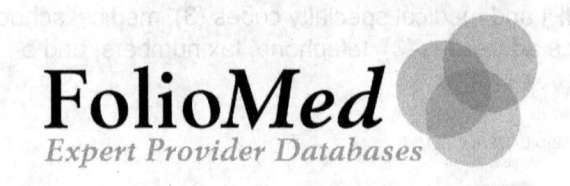

297 North Street/Suite 212
Hyannis, MA 02601
508-862-8200   fax: 508-862-8210
www.foliomed.com

Folio*Med* Data Services and Applications

Database Cleansing
- Matching of Legacy Database to FolioMed Master file
- Identification of missing information, duplications, and inactive records
- Reconciliation of data variances
- Return files in Customer format

Interactive Data Exchanges
- Changed records to FolioMed for validation
- Return file includes FolioMed data edits
- Client provider file synchronized with FolioMed Master File

Data Licensing
- Complete Census of all Practicing Physicians in the Geography
- Periodic updates – changed records only or complete database
- Available as Single workstation or networked application
- Available as Raw Data or with built in Query tool
- multiple practice addresses (prioritized)
- mailing addresses if different than practice address
- multiple medical specialties (prioritized)
- multiple identifiers: NPI, UPIN, Board Licensure #, (optional DEA)
- Hospital affiliations
- email addresses (partial)
- Available in dbf, xls, xlsx, or text formats

CD-ROM Query tool
All Physicians in a geography
Search criteria:

Physicians

Doctor Name	Specialty	County
Town/Distance	State	Zip/Distance
Zipcode Range	MedSchool	Facility type
Facility name	Street Address	Hospital Affil
UPIN	Language	Phone/fax

Facilities

Facility name	Number Docs	Facility Name
Facility type	Street Address	Town/Distance
State	Zip/Distance	Zipcode Range
Phone/fax		

Download limits based on License : Text, dbf, xls or XML formats

FolioMed IS-Cloud based internet access
- All Physicians, NPs and PAs for a geography
- Updated daily
- Single or enterprise-wide password access
- Physician rosters for individual Groups and other Healthcare Facilities
- NPI and UPINs
- Read only access with limited print functions

Code Tables: Medical Specialties

Code	Medical Specialty	Taxonomy
Acpntr	Acupuncture	
Addctn	Internal Med-Addiction Medicine	207RA0401X
AdmMgt	Administration/Medical Management	
AdolMd	Adolescent Medicine	2080A0000X
AeroMd	Aerospace Medicine	2083A0100X
AlcSub	Alcoholism/Substance Abuse	
Algylmmn	Allergy & Immunology	207K00000X
AllmCLIm	Allergy& Immun-Clinical &Lab Immun	207KI0005X
Allrgy	Allergy	207KA0200X
AltHol	Holistic Medicine	
AltnMd	Alternative Medicine	
AnesAddM	Anesthesiology- Addiction Medicine	207LA0401X
AnesCrCr	Anesthesiology : Critical Care Med	207LC0200X
AnesHPC	Anesthesiology : Hospice & Palliative	207LA0401X
AnesPain	Anesthesiology : Pain Medicine	207LP2900X
Anesth	Anesthesiology	207L00000X
Bariat	Bariatrics/Weight Control	
BhvrMd	Behavioral Medicine	
BldBnk	Bloodbanking	207ZB0001X
BrnEso	Broncho-Esophagology	
CarAne	Cardiac Anesthesia	
CarEch	Echo Cardiology	
CarEle	Electro-Cardiography	
CarNuc	Nuclear Cardiology	207UN0901X
Catrct	Cataract	
CdvDis	Cardiovascular Disease	207RC0000X
ClCdEl	Clinical Cardiac Electrophysiology	207RC0001X
ClNrPh	Clinical Neurophysiology	2084N0600X
ClinDM	Clinical Decision Making	
ClnGnt	Clinical Genetics	207SG0201X
ClnPhm	Clinical Pharmacology	208U00000X
CmptMd	Computer Medicine	
CritCr	Critical Care Medicine	207RC0200X
CrnExD	Cornea/External Disease	
CybrMd	Cyber Medicine	
DerHar	Hair Transplant/Restoration	
DerImm	Clinical & Lab Derm Immunolog	207NI0002X
DerMOH	MOHS (Micrographic Skin Cancer Srg)	207ND0101X
Dermat	Dermatology	207N00000X
Diagns	Diagnostic Lab Immunology	
DrmtPthy	Dermatology : Dermatopathology	207ND0900X
Elecen	Electroencephalography	
Elecmy	Electromyography	
EmrgEMed	Emergency Medical Services	207PE0004X
EmrgHPC	Emergency Med-Hospice & Palliative	207PH0002X
EmrgMTxy	Emerg Medicine-Medical Toxicology	207PT0002X
EmrgMd	Emergency Medicine	207P00000X
EmrgPedr	Emerg Medicine-Pediatric	207PP0204X
EmrgSptM	Emergency Medicine -Sports Medicine	207PS0010X
EmrgUHyM	Undersea & Hyperbaric Medicine	207PE0005X
EnDbMt	Endocrinology/Diabetes/Metabolism	207RE0101X
EnvnMd	Environmental Medicine	
Epdmlg	Epidemiology	
Eplpsy	Epilepsy	
FamMAdMd	Family Med-Adolescent Medicine	207QA0000X
FamMAddM	Family Med-Addiction Medicine	207QA0401X
FamMAdlt	Family Med-Adult Medicine	207QA0505X
FamMBari	Family Med-Bariatric Medicine	207QB0002X
FamMGrtc	Family Med-Geriatric Medicine	207QG0300X
FamMHPC	Family Med-Hospice & Palliative	207QH0002X
FamMSlpM	Family Med-Sleep Medicine	
FamMSptM	Family Med-Sports Medicine	207QS0010X
FamMed	Family Medicine	207Q00000X
FamThp	Family Therapy	
FrtInf	Fertility/Infertility	
GPrvMd	General Preventive Medicine	2083P0500X
Gastrn	Gastroenterology	207RG0100X
GenPrc	General Practice	208D00000X
Glacma	Glaucoma	
GnetBM	Biochemical/Molecular Genetics	
GnetCy	Clinical Cytogenetics	207SC0300X
GnetMd	Medical Genetics	207SG0205X
GntMCBCh	Medical Genetics-Clinical Biochem	207SG0202X
GntMCMol	Medical Genetics-Clinical Molecular	207SG0203X
GntMMPty	Medical Gentics-Mole Genetic Pthlgy	207SM0001X
Grtrcs	Geriatrics	207RG0300X
GynOnc	Gynecological Oncology	207VX0201X
Gyneco	Gynecology	207VG0400X
Hdache	Headache	
Hemato	Hematology	207RH0000X
Hepato	Hepatology	207RI0008X
HivAid	HIV/Acquired Immune Deficiency	
Hmpthy	Homeopathy	
Hypnss	Hypnosis	
Hypten	Hypertension	
ImmAsm	Asthma	
ImmCLa	Clinical & Laboratory Immunology	207RI0001X
Immuno	Immunology	
IndpMdEx	Independent Medical Examiner	202C00000X
InfDis	Infectious Disease	207RI0200X
InsrMd	Insurance Medicine	
IntCrd	Interventional Cardiology	207RI0011X
IntHos	Hospitalist	208M00000X
IntMAImm	Internal Med-Allergy & Immunology	207RA0201X
IntMAdMd	Internal Med-Adolescent Medicine	207RA0000X
IntMBari	Internal Med-Bariatric Medicine	207RB0002X
IntMHPC	Internal Med-Hospice & Palliative	207RH0002X
IntMSlpd	Internal Med-Sleep Medicine	207RS0012X
IntMTrHp	Internal Med-Transplant Hepatology	207RT0003X
IntrMd	Internal Medicine	207R00000X
IntrSptM	Internal Med-Sports Medicine	207RS0010X
LeglMd	Legal Medicine	209800000X
Lryngo	Laryngology	
MRImag	Magnetic Resonance Imaging	207RM1200X
MedCom	Medical Education & Communication	
MedEth	Medical Ethics	
MedMcb	Medical Microbiology	207ZM0300X
MedOnc	Medical Oncology	207RX0202X
MtFtMd	Maternal & Fetal Medicine	207VM0101X
Nephro	Nephrology	207RN0300X
NeuBeh	Behavioral Neurology	
NeuMSptM	Neuromusculoskeletal-Sports Med	204C00000X
NeuMus	Neuromusculoskeletal Med & OMM	204D00000X
Neutgy	Neurotology	
NnPnMd	Neonatal-Perinatal Medicine	2080N0001X
NrlgAddM	Psychiatry&Nrolgy-Addctn Med	2084A0401X
NrlgDNIm	Psychiatry&Nrolgy-Diagnostic NeuroImg	2084D0003X
NrlgHPC	Psychiatry&Nrolgy-Hospice & Palliative	2084H0002X
NrlgMusM	Psychiatry&Nrolgy-Neuromuscular Med	2084N0008X
NrlgPain	Psychiatry&Nrolgy-Pain Medicine	2084P2900X
NrlgSpec	Psychiatry&Nrolgy-Special Qual	2084N0402X
NrlgSptM	Psychiatry&Nrolgy-Sports Medicine	2084S0010X
NroChl	Child (Pediatric) Neurology	
NroCrCr	Neurocritical Care	2084A2900X
NrolDis	Neurodevelopmental Disorders	
Nrolgy	Neurology	2084N0400X
NuclIVVi	Nuclear Medicine-InVivo&Vitro	207UN0903X
NuclImg	Nuclear Imaging and Therapy	207UN0902X
NuclMd	Nuclear Medicine	207U00000X
Nutrtn	Nutrition	
ObGyBari	Obstetrics & Gynecigy-Bariatric Medicine	207VB0002X
ObGyCrCr	Obstetrics & Gynecigy-Critical Care	207VC0200X
ObGyHPC	Obstetrics & Gynecigy-Hospice & Palliative	207VH0002X
ObsGyn	Obstetrics & Gynecology	207V00000X
Obstet	Obstetrics	207VX0000X
OccIns	Occupational Medical Insurance	
OccpMd	Occupational Medicine	2083X0100X
OncHem	Hematology Oncology	207RH0003X
OncNeu	Neuro-Oncology	
OncOcu	Ocular Oncology	
Onclgy	Oncology	
OphNeu	Neuro-Ophthalmology	
OphSrgPl	Opthalmic Plastic & Reconst Surgery	207WX0200X
Ophthl	Ophthalmology	207W00000X
OpthCrn	Cornea and External Diseases Specialst	207WX0120X
OrtHKn	Total Hip/Knee Replacement	
OrtOst	Osteoporosis	
OrtSHand	Orthopedic-Hand Surgery	207XS0106X
OrtSpn	Spinal Cord Injury Medicine	2081P0004X
OrtTrm	Orthopedic Trauma	207XX0801X
Ortped	Orthopedics	
OstMed	Osteopathic Medicine	
OtgyAlgy	Otolaryngology-Otolaryngic Allergy	207YX0602X
OtgyFPlS	Otolaryngology/Facial Pls Surgery	207YX0905X
OtgyFPls	Otolaryngology-Facial Pls Surgery	207YS0123X
OtgyPSHN	Otolaryngology-Pls Srgy Head Neck	207YX0007X
OtgySlpd	Otolaryngology-Sleep Medicine	207YS0012X
OthrSp	Other Specialty	
Otlryg	Otolaryngology	207Y00000X
Otolgy	Otology	207YX0901X
PainInvt	Pain Medicine-Interventional	208VP0014X
PainMd	Pain Medicine	208VP0000X
PallCr	Palliative Care	
PedAlg	Pediatric Allergy	2080P0201X
PedAne	Pediatric Anesthesia	
PedChAbs	Pediatric Child Abuse	
PedCrC	Pediatric Critical Care	2080P0203X
PedCrd	Pediatric Cardiology	2080P0202X
PedDrm	Pediatric Dermatology	207NP0225X
PedDvl	Developmental Pediatrics	2080P0006X
PedEmg	Pediatric Emergency Medicine	2080P0204X
PedEnd	Pediatric Endocrinology	2080P0205X
PedGst	Pediatric Gastroenterology	2080P0206X
PedGyn	Pediatric Gynecology	
PedHem	Pediatric Hematology Oncology	2080P0207X
PedInf	Pediatric Infectious Diseases	2080P0208X
PedNph	Pediatric Nephrology	2080P0210X
PedNrD	Pediatric Neurodevelopment	2080P0008X

Code Tables: Medical Specialties

Code	Medical Specialty	Taxonomy	Code	Medical Specialty	Taxonomy
PedOnc	Pediatric Oncology		SrgFPl	Facial Plastic Surgery	
PedOph	Pediatric Ophthalmology		SrgFPlvc	Female Pelvic Medicine & Surgery	2088F0040X
PedOrt	Pediatric Orthopedics		SrgGst	Gastrointestinal Surgery	
PedOto	Pediatric Otolaryngology	207YP0228X	SrgGyn	Gynecological Surgery	
PedPth	Pediatric Pathology	207ZP0213X	SrgHdN	Head & Neck Surgery	
PedPul	Pediatric Pulmonology	2080P0214X	SrgHnd	Hand Surgery	2086S0105X
PedRad	Pediatric Radiology	2085P0229X	SrgHPC	Surgery-Hospice & Palliative	2086H0002X
PedrCLIm	Pediatrics-Clin & Lab Immunology	2080I0007X	SrgLap	Laparoscopic Surgery	
PedReh	Pediatric Rehabilitation	2081P0010X	SrgLsr	Laser Surgery	
PedRhm	Pediatric Rheumatology	2080P0216X	SrgMcr	Microsurgery	
PedrHPC	Pediatrics-Hospice & Palliative	2080H0002X	SrgNro	Neurological Surgery	207T00000X
PedrSlpd	Pediatrics-Sleep Medicine	2080S0012X	SrgO&M	Oral & Maxillofacial Surgery	204E00000X
PedrTrHp	Pediatrics-Transplant Hepatology	2080T0004X	SrgOARec	Orthopedic Surgery-Adult Recnstrct	207XS0114X
PedSpM	Pediatric Sports Medicine	2080S0010X	SrgOnc	Oncological Surgery	2086X0206X
PedSrg	Pediatric Surgery	2086S0120X	SrgOrb	Orbital Reconstructive Surgery	
PedUro	Pediatric Urology		SrgOrt	Orthopedic Surgery	207X00000X
PedrMTxy	Pediatrics-Medical Toxicology	2080T0002X	SrgPHand	Plastic Surgery-Hand	2082S0105X
Pedtrc	Pediatrics	208000000X	SrgPlstc	Plastic Surgery	208200000X
Phlebgy	Phlebology	202K00000X	SrgPrV	Peripheral Vascular Surgery	
PhyMHPC	Physical Med & Rehab-Hospice & Palliative	2081H0002X	SrgRec	Plastic and Reconstructive Surgery	2086S0122X
PhyMNMus	Physical Med & Rehab-Neuromuscular Med	2081N0008X	SrgRef	Refractive Surgery	
PhyMPain	Physical Med & Rehab-Pain Medicine	2081P2900X	SrgShr	Shoulder Surgery	
PhyMSptM	Physical Med & Rehab-Sports Medicin	2081S0010X	SrgSpn	Spinal Surgery	207XS0117X
PhysMd	Physical Medicine & Rehabilitation	208100000X	SrgThr	Thoracic Surgery	208G00000X
PlsSHNck	Plastic Surgery-Head and Neck	2082S0099X	SrgTpl	Transplant Surgery & Medicine	204F00000X
PrvMMTxy	Preventive Med-Medical Toxicology	2083T0002X	SrgTrm	Trauma Surgery	2086S0127X
PrvSpt	Preventive Sports Medicine	2083S0010X	SrgUro	Urological Surgery	
PssoMd	Psychosomatic Medicine		SrgVas	Vascular Surgery	2086S0129X
PsyAdd	Addiction Psychiatry	2084P0802X	Surgry	Surgery (General)	208600000X
PsyAdt	Adult Psychiatry		TrpPst	Tropical Disease/Parasitology	
PsyCAd	Child & Adolescent Psychiatry	2084P0804X	Txclgy	Toxicology	
PsyCom	Community Psychiatry		Ultsnd	Ultrasound	2085U0001X
PsyFor	Forensic Psychiatry	2084F0202X	UndsMd	Preventive Medicine-Undersea&Hypbri	2083P0011X
PsyGrp	Group Psychiatry		UrgtCr	Urgent Care	
PsyGrt	Geriatric Psychiatry	2084P0805X	UroGyn	Urogynecology	
PsyNro	Neuro-Psychiatry	2084P0005X	UroNro	Neuro-Urology	
PsySex	Sexual Dysfunction		Urolgy	Urology	208800000X
Psychy	Psychiatry	2084P0800X	UtlRQA	Utilization Rvw/Quality Assurance	
Psynls	Psychoanalysis		VasDis	Vascular Disease	
Psyphm	Psychopharmacology		VasNeu	Vascular Neurology	2084V0102X
Psythp	Psychotherapy		VitRet	Vitreous and Retina	
PthACl	Anatomic/Clinical Pathology	207ZP0102X	WundCr	Wound Care	
PthAna	Anatomic Pathology	207ZP0101X			
PthBst	Breast Pathology				
PthChm	Chemical Pathology	207ZP0104X			
PthClLab	Clinical Pathology/Lab Medicine	207ZP0105X			
PthCln	Clinical Pathology	207ZP0105X			
PthCyt	Cytopathology	207ZC0500X			
PthDrm	Dermatopathology	207ZD0900X			
PthFor	Forensic Pathology	207ZF0201X			
PthGyn	Gynecological Pathology				
PthHem	Hematopathology	207ZH0000X			
PthImm	Immunopathology	207ZI0100X			
PthNro	Neuropathology	207ZN0500X			
PthRso	Radioisotopic Pathology				
Pthlgy	Pathology				
PthyMGen	Pathology-Molecular Genetic	207ZP0007X			
PubHth	Public Health	2083P0901X			
PulCCr	Pulmonary Critical Care				
PulDis	Pulmonary Disease	207RP1001X			
RadBdl	Body Imaging Radiology	2085B0100X			
RadDia	Diagnostic Radiology	2085R0202X			
RadHPC	Radiology-Hospice & Palliative	2085H0002X			
RadMam	Mammography				
RadNro	Neurological Radiology	2085N0700X			
RadNuc	Nuclear Diagnostic Radiology	2085N0904X			
RadOnc	Radiation Oncology	2085R0001X			
RadPhy	Radiological Physics	2085R0205X			
RadThp	Therapeutic Radiology	2085R0203X			
RadV&I	Vascular & Interventional Radiology	2085R0204X			
Radiol	Radiology				
Rheuma	Rheumatology	207RR0500X			
Rhinol	Rhinology				
RprEnd	Reproductive Endocrinology	207VE0102X			
Rserch	Research				
SlpDis	Sleep Disorders Medicine				
SprtMd	Sports Medicine	207XX0005X			
SrgAbd	Abdominal Surgery				
SrgArt	Arthroscopic Surgery				
SrgBrtc	Bariatric Surgery				
SrgBst	Breast Surgery				
SrgC&R	Colon & Rectal Surgery	208C00000X			
SrgCTh	Cardiothoracic Surgery				
SrgCdv	Cardiovascular Surgery				
SrgCrC	Surgical Critical Care	2086S0102X			
SrgCsm	Cosmetic Surgery				
SrgDer	Dermatologic Surgery	207NS0135X			
SrgEnd	Endoscopic Surgery				
SrgFAk	Foot & Ankle Surgery	207XX0004X			

Code Tables: Medical Specialties by Category

Category / Specialty	Code
Adm/Medical Management	**AdmMgt**
Clinical Decision Making	ClinDM
Computer Medicine	CmptMd
Cyber Medicine	ybrMd
Insurance Medicine	InsrMd
Legal Medicine	LeglMd
Medical Education & Communication	MedCom
Medical Ethics	MedEth
Occupational Medical Insurance	OccIns
Utilization Rvw/Quality Assurance	UtlRQA
Allergy & Immunology	**AlgyImmn**
Allergy	Allrgy
Allergy& Immun-Clinical &Lab	AllmCLIm
Asthma	ImmAsm
Diagnostic Lab Immunology	Diagns
Immunology	Immuno
Alternative Medicine	**AltnMd**
Acupuncture	Acpntr
Holistic Medicine	AltHol
Homeopathy	Hmpthy
Anesthesiology	**Anesth**
Addiction Medicine	AnesAddM
Cardiac Anesthesia	CarAne
Critical Care Medicine	AnesCrCr
Hospice & Palliative Care	AnesHPC
Pain Medicine	AnesPain
Cardiovascular Disease	**CdvDis**
Clinical Cardiac Electrophysiology	ClCdEl
Echo Cardiology	CarEch
Electro-Cardiography	CarEle
Hypertension	Hypten
Interventional Cardiology	IntCrd
Nuclear Cardiology	CarNuc
Clinical Pharmacology	**ClnPhm**
Toxicology	Txclgy
Dermatology	**Dermat**
Clinical & Lab Derm Immunolog	DerImm
Dermatopathology	DrmtPthy
Hair Transplant/Restoration	DerHar
MOHS (Micrographic Skin Cancer Srg)	DerMOH
Surgery	SrgDer
Emergency Medicine	**EmrgMd**
Hospice & Palliative	EmrgHPC
Medical Toxicology	EmrgMTxy
Pediatrics	EmrgPedr
Emergency Medical Services	EmrgEMed
Sports Medicine	EmrgSptM
Undersea & Hyperbaric Medicine	EmrgUHyM
Family Medicine	**FamMed**
Family Med-Addiction Medicine	Fam MAddM
Family Med-Adolescent Medicine	Fam MAdMd
Family Med-Adult Medicine	FamMAdlt
Family Med-Bariatric Medicine	FamMBari
Family Med-Geriatric Medicine	FamMGrtc
Family Med-Hospice & Palliative	FamMHPC
Family Med-Sleep Medicine	FamM-SlpM
Family Med-Sports Medicine	FamMSptM
General Practice	**GenPrc**
Independent Medical Examiner	
Independent Medical Examiner	IndpMdEx
Internal Medicine	**IntrMd**
Addiction Medicine	Addctn
Adolescent Medicine	IntMAdMd
Allergy & Immunology	IntMAImm
Bariatrics/Weight Control	IntMBari
Clinical & Laboratory Immunology	ImmCLa
Critical Care Medicine	CritCr
Endocrinology/Diabetes/Metabolism	EnDbMt
Environmental Medicine	EnvnMd
Gastroenterology	Gastrn
Geriatrics	Grtrcs
Hematology	Hemato
Hepatology	Hepato
Hospice & Palliative Care	IntMHPC
Hospitalist	IntHos
Infectious Disease	InfDis
Nephrology	Nephro
Nutrition	Nutrtn
Rheumatology	Rheuma
Sleep Medicine	IntMSlpd
Sports Medicine	IntrSptM
Transplant Hepatology	IntMTrHp
Urgent Care	UrgtCr
Wound Care	WundCr
Medical Genetics	**GnetMd**
Biochemical/Molecular Genetics	GnetBM
Clinical Biochemistry	GntMCBCh
Clinical Cytogenetics	GnetCy
Clinical Genetics	ClnGnt

Category / Specialty	Code
Clinical Molecular	GntMCMol
Molecular Genetic Pthlgy	GntMMPty
Neurology	**Nrolgy**
Behavioral Neurology	NeuBeh
Clinical Neurophysiology	ClNrPh
Electroencephalography	Elecen
Electromyography	Elecmy
Epilepsy	Eplpsy
Headache	Hdache
Neurocritical Care	NroCrCr
Neurodevelopmental Disorders	NrolDis
Neuromusculoskeletal Med OMM	NeuMus
Neuromusculoskeletal-Sports Med	NeuMSptM
Sleep Disorders Medicine	SlpDis
Vascular Neurology	VasNeu
Nuclear Medicine	**NuclMd**
Nuclear Imaging and Therapy	NucImg
Nuclear Medicine-InVivo&Vitro	NuclVVi
Obstetrics & Gynecology	**ObsGyn**
Bariatric Medicine	ObGyBari
Critical Care	ObGyCrCr
Fertility/Infertility	FrtInf
Gynecology	Gyneco
Hospice & Palliative Medicine	ObGyHPC
Maternal & Fetal Medicine	MtFtMd
Obstetrics	Obstet
Reproductive Endocrinology	RprEnd
Oncology	**Onclgy**
Gynecological Oncology	GynOnc
Hematology Oncology	OncHem
Medical Oncology	MedOnc
Neuro-Oncology	OncNeu
Ocular Oncology	OncOcu
Ophthalmology	**Ophthl**
Cataract	Catrct
Cornea/External Disease	CrnExD
Cornea/External Disease Specialist	OpthCrn
Glaucoma	Glacma
Neuro-Ophthalmology	OphNeu
Refractive Surgery	SrgRef
Vitreous and Retina	VitRet
Orthopedics	**Ortped**
Foot & Ankle Surgery	SrgFAk
Head & Neck Surgery	SrgHdN
Orthopedic-Hand Surgery	OrtSHand
Orthopedic Surgery	SrgOrt
Orthopedic Surgery-Adult Recnstrct	SrgOARec
Orthopedic Trauma	OrtTrm
Osteoporosis	OrtOst
Shoulder Surgery	SrgShr
Spinal Cord Injury Medicine	OrtSpn
Spinal Surgery	SrgSpn
Sports Medicine	SprtMd
Total Hip/Knee Replacement	OrtHKn
Osteopathic Medicine	**OstMed**
Other Specialty	**OthrSp**
Otolaryngology	**Otlryg**
Broncho-Esophagology	BrnEso
Facial Plastic Surgery	OtgyFPls
Laryngology	Lryngo
Neurotology	Neutgy
Otolaryngolic Allergy	OtgyAlgy
Otolaryngology/Facial Pls Surgery	OtgyFPlS
Otology	Otolgy
Plastic Surgery Head Neck	OtgyPSHN
Rhinology	Rhinol
Sleep Medicine	OtgySlpd
Pain Medicine	**PainMd**
Pain Medicine-Interventional	PainInvt
Palliative Care	PallCr
Pathology	**Pthlgy**
Anatomic Pathology	PthAna
Anatomic/Clinical Pathology	PthACl
Bloodbanking	BldBnk
Breast Pathology	PthBst
Chemical Pathology	PthChm
Clinical Pathology	PthCln
Clinical Path-Laboratory Med	PthClLab
Cytopathology	PthCyt
Dermatopathology	PthDrm
Forensic Pathology	PthFor
Gynecological Pathology	PthGyn
Hematopathology	PthHem
Immunopathology	PthImm
Medical Microbiology	MedMcb
Molecular Genetics	PthyMGen
Neuropathology	PthNro
Radioisotopic Pathology	PthRso
Pediatrics	**Pedtrc**
Adolescent Medicine	AdolMd
Allergy	PedAlg
Anesthesia	PedAne

Category / Specialty	Code
Cardiology	PedCrd
Child Abuse	PedChAbs
Child (Pediatric) Neurology	NroChl
Clinical & Lab Immunology	PedrCLIm
Critical Care	PedCrC
Dermatology	PedDrm
Developmental Pediatrics	PedDvl
Emergency Medicine	PedEmg
Endocrinology	PedEnd
Gastroenterology	PedGst
Gynecology	PedGyn
Hematology Oncology	PedHem
Hospice & Palliative Care	PedrHPC
Infectious Diseases	PedInf
Medical Toxicology	PedrMTxy
Neonatal-Perinatal Medicine	NnPnMd
Nephrology	PedNph
Neurodevelopment	PedNrD
Oncology	PedOnc
Ophthalmology	PedOph
Orthopedics	PedOrt
Otolaryngology	PedOto
Pathology	PedPth
Pulmonology	PedPul
Radiology	PedRad
Rehabilitation	PedReh
Rheumatology	PedRhm
Sleep Medicine	PedrSlpd
Sports Medicine	PedSpM
Surgery	PedSrg
Transplant Hepatology	PedrTrHp
Urology	PedUro
Phlebology	**Phlebgy**
Physical Medicine & Rehabilitation	**PhysMd**
Hospice & Palliative Care	PhyMHPC
Neuromuscular Medicine	PhyMNMus
Pain Medicine	PhyMPain
Sports Medicine	PhyMSptM
Preventive Medicine	**GPrvMd**
Aerospace Medicine	AeroMd
Epidemiology	Epdmlg
HIV/Acquired Immune Deficiency	HivAid
Occupational Medicine	OccpMd
Medical Toxicology	PrvMMTxy
Undersea&Hyperbaric Med	UndsMd
Preventive Sports Medicine	PrvSpt
Public Health	PubHth
Tropical Disease/Parasitology	TrpPst
Psychiatry & Neurology	**PsyNro**
Addiction Psychiatry	PsyAdd
Adult Psychiatry	PsyAdt
Alcoholism/Substance Abuse	AlcSub
Behavioral Medicine	BhvrMd
Child & Adolescent Psychiatry	PsyCAd
Community Psychiatry	PsyCom
Diagnostic NeuroImaging	NrlgDNIm
Family Therapy	FamThp
Forensic Psychiatry	PsyFor
Geriatric Psychiatry	PsyGrt
Group Psychiatry	PsyGrp
Hospice & Palliative Care	NrlgHPC
Hypnosis	Hypnss
Neuromuscular Medicine	NrlgMusM
Psychiatry	Psychy
Psychiatry&Nrolgy-Addctn Med	NrlgAddM
Pain Medicine	NrlgPain
Psychiatry&Nrolgy-Special Qual	NrlgSpec
Sports Medicine	NrlgSptM
Psychoanalysis	Psynls
Psychopharmacology	Psyphm
Psychosomatic Medicine	PssoMd
Psychotherapy	Psythp
Sexual Dysfunction	PsySex
Pulmonary Disease	**PulDis**
Pulmonary Critical Care	PulCCr
Radiology	**Radiol**
Body Imaging Radiology	RadBdI
Diagnostic Radiology	RadDia
Hospice & Palliative Care	RadHPC
Magnetic Resonance Imaging	MRImag
Mammography	RadMam
Neurological Radiology	RadNro
Nuclear Diagnostic Radiology	RadNuc
Radiation Oncology	RadOnc
Radiological Physics	RadThp
Ultrasound	Ultsnd
Vascular & Interventional Radiology	RadV&I
Research	**Rserch**
Surgery	**Surgry**
Abdominal Surgery	SrgAbd
Arthroscopic Surgery	SrgArt
Breast Surgery	SrgBst

Code Tables: Medical Specialties by Category

Cardiothoracic Surgery	SrgCTh
Cardiovascular Surgery	SrgCdv
Colon & Rectal Surgery	SrgC&R
Cosmetic Surgery	SrgCsm
Endoscopic Surgery	SrgEnd
Facial Plastic Surgery	SrgFPl
Female Pelvic Medicine & Surgery	SrgFPlvc
Gastrointestinal Surgery	SrgGst
Gynecological Surgery	SrgGyn
Hand Surgery	SrgHnd
Hospice & Palliative Care	SrgHPC
Laparoscopic Surgery	SrgLap
Laser Surgery	SrgLsr
Microsurgery	SrgMcr
Neurological Surgery	SrgNro
Oncological Surgery	SrgOnc
Oral & Maxillofacial Surgery	SrgO&M
Orbital Reconstructive Surgery	SrgOrb
Peripheral Vascular Surgery	SrgPrV
Plastic Surgery	SrgPlstc
Plastic Surgery-Hand	SrgPHand
Plastic Surgery-Head and Neck	PlsSHNck
Reconstructive Surgery	SrgRec
Surgical Critical Care	SrgCrC
Thoracic Surgery	SrgThr
Transplant Surgery & Medicine	SrgTpl
Trauma Surgery	SrgTrm
Urological Surgery	SrgUro
Vascular Surgery	SrgVas
Urology	**Urolgy**
Neuro-Urology	UroNro
Urogynecology	UroGyn
Vascular Disease	**VasDis**

Medical School Codes

AB01	University of Alberta, Edmonton, Alberta, Canada
AB02	University of Calgary Faculty of Medicine, Calgary, Alberta, Canada
AL02	University of Alabama School of Medicine, Birmingham, Alabama
AL06	University of South Alabama School of Medicine, Mobile, Alabama
AR01	University of Arkansas School of Medicine, Little Rock, Arkansas
AZ01	University of Arizona College of Medicine, Tucson, Arizona
AZ02	Arizona College of Osteopathic Medicine, Glendale, Arizona
AZ03	A.T. Still University of Osteopathic MEdicine, Mesa, Arizona
BC01	University of British Columbia Faculty of Medicine, Vancouver, Canada
CA02	University of California San Francisco, School of Medicine, San Francisco, CA
CA06	University of Southern California, Keck School of Medicine, Los Angeles, California
CA11	Stanford University School of Medicine, Palo Alto, California
CA12	Loma Linda University School of Medicine, Loma Linda, California
CA14	University of California Los Angeles, School of Medicine, Los Angeles, California
CA15	University of California Irvine, School of Medicine, Irvine, California
CA18	University of California - San Diego School of Medicine, La Jolla, CA
CA19	University of California Davis, School of Medicine, Davis, California
CA21	Charles R. Drew University of Medicine & Science, Los Angeles, CA
CA22	Western University of Health Sciences, College of Osteopathic Medicine of the Pacific, Pomona, California
CA23	Touro University College of Osteopathic Medicine, San Francisco, CA
CO02	University of Colorado School of Medicine, Denver, Colorado
CT01	Yale University School of Medicine, New Haven, Connecticut
CT02	University of Connecticut School of Medicine, Farmington, Connecticut
DC01	George Washington University School of Medicine, Washington, D.C.
DC02	Georgetown University School of Medicine, Washington, D.C.
DC03	Howard University College of Medicine, Washington, D.C.
FL01	Florida State University - Tallahassee, College of Medicine, Tallahassee, Florida
FL02	University of Miami School of Medicine, Miami, Florida
FL03	University of Florida College of Medicine, Gainesville, Florida
FL04	University of South Florida College of Medicine, Tampa, Florida
FL05	Florida International University College of Medicine, Miami, Florida
FL06	Florida Atlantic Charles E. Schmidt College of Medicine, Boca Raton, FL
FL75	Nova SE Univ. College of Osteopathic Medicine, Fort Lauderdale, Florida
GA01	Medical College of Georgia, Augusta, Georgia
GA05	Emory University School of Medicine, Atlanta, Georgia
GA21	Morehouse School of Medicine, Atlanta, Georgia
GA22	Mercer University School of Medicine, Macon, Georgia
HI01	University of Hawaii School of Medicine, Honolulu, Hawaii
IA02	University of Iowa College of Medicine, Iowa City, Iowa
IA75	Des Moines University, College of Osteopathic Medicine, Des Moines, IA
IL01	Rush Medical College, Chicago, Illinois
IL02	University of Chicago, Pritzker School of Medicine, Chicago, Illinois
IL04	Hahnemann Medical College & Hospital, Chicago, Illinois
IL05	Chicago College of Medicine & Surgery, Chicago, Illinois
IL06	Feinberg School of Medicine at Northwestern University, Chicago, Illinois
IL09	Northwestern University Women's Medical School, Chicago, Illinois
IL11	University of Illinois, College of Medicine, Chicago, Chicago, Illinois
IL14	University of Illinois, College of Medicine, Urbana-Champaign, Urbana-Champaign, Illinois
IL42	Chicago Med School / Rosalind Franklin Univ of Hlth Sc (Finch), North Chicago, IL
IL43	Loyola University Chicago, Maywood, Illinois
IL45	Southern Illinois University School of Medicine, Springfield, Illinois
IL76	Chicago College of Osteopathic Medicine/Midwestern University, Downers Grove, Illinois
IN20	Indiana University School of Medicine, Indianapolis, Indiana
KS02	University of Kansas School of Medicine, Kansas City, Kansas
KY01	Kentucky School of Medicine, Louisville, Kentucky
KY02	University of Louisville School of Medicine, Louisville, Kentucky
KY12	University of Kentucky College of Medicine, Lexington, Kentucky
LA01	Tulane University School of Medicine, New Orleans, Louisiana
LA05	Louisiana State University, New Orleans, Louisiana
LA06	Louisiana State University, Shreveport, Louisiana
MA01	Harvard Medical School, Boston, Massachusetts
MA05	Boston University School of Medicine, Boston, Massachusetts
MA06	College of Physicians & Surgeons, Boston, Massachusetts
MA07	Tufts University School of Medicine, Boston, Massachusetts
MA16	University of Massachusetts Medical School, Worcester, Massachusetts
MD01	University of Maryland School of Medicine, Baltimore, Maryland
MD07	Johns Hopkins University School of Medicine, Baltimore, Maryland
MD12	Uniformed Services University of Health Sciences, Bethesda, Maryland
ME75	University of New England College of Osteopathic Medicine, Biddeford, Maine
MI01	University of Michigan Medical School, Ann Arbor, Michigan
MI07	Wayne State University School of Medicine, Detroit, Michigan
MI12	Michigan State University College of Osteopathic Medicine, East Lansing, Michigan
MI20	Michigan State University College of Human Medicine, East Lansing, MI
MN04	University of Minnesota Medical School, Minneapolis, Minnesota
MN07	University of Minnesota School of Medicine, Duluth, Minnesota
MN08	Mayo Medical School, Rochester, Minnesota
MO02	Washington University School of Medicine, St. Louis, Missouri
MO03	University of Missouri School of Medicine, Columbia, Missouri
MO07	St. Louis College of Physicians & Surgeons, St. Louis, Missouri
MO34	St. Louis University School of Medicine, St. Louis, Missouri
MO44	Kansas City University of Physicians & Surgeons, Kansas City, Missouri
MO46	University of Missouri School of Medicine, Kansas City, Missouri
MO78	Kansas City Univ of Med & Biosciences College Osteopathic Med, Kansas City, MO
MO79	Kirksville College of Osteopathic Medicine, Kirksville, Missouri
MS01	University of Mississippi School of Medicine, Jackson, Mississippi
MT01	University of Manitoba, Winnipeg, Manitoba, Canada
NC01	University of North Carolina School of Medicine, Chapel Hill, NC
NC05	Wake Forest University School of Medicine, Winston-Salem, NC
NC07	Duke University School of Medicine, Durham, North Carolina
NC08	Brody School of Medicine at East Carolina University, Greenville, NC
ND01	University of North Dakota School of Medicine, Grand Forks, ND
NE05	University of Nebraska College of Medicine, Omaha, Nebraska
NE06	Creighton University School of Medicine, Omaha, Nebraska
NF01	Memorial University of Newfoundland, St. Johns, Newfoundland, Canada
NH01	Dartmouth Medical School, Hanover, New Hampshire
NH02	The Audrey and Theodor Geisel School of Medicine at Dartmouth, Hanover, NH
NJ02	Robert Wood Johnson Medical School, University of Medicine & Dentistry of New Jersey, Camden, New Jersey
NJ03	UMDNJ, Stratford, New Jersey Medical School, Stratford, New Jersey
NJ05	UMDNJ, Newark, New Jersey Medical School, Newark, New Jersey
NJ06	UMDNJ, R.W. Johnson Medical School, Piscataway/New Brunswick, NJ
NJ15	UMDNJ, Jersey City, New Jersey Medical School, Jersey City, NJ
NJ75	UMDNJ, School of Osteopathic Medicine, Stratford, New Jersey
NM01	University of New Mexico School of Medicine, Albuquerque, New Mexico
NS01	Dalhousie University, Halifax, Nova Scotia, Canada
NV01	University of Nevada School of Medical Sciences, Reno, Nevada
NY01	Columbia University College of Physicians & Surgeons, New York, NY
NY03	Albany Medical College, Albany, New York
NY06	SUNY at Buffalo School of Medicine, Buffalo, New York
NY08	SUNY College of Medicine, Brooklyn, New York
NY09	New York Medical College, Valhalla, New York
NY10	Bellevue Hospital Medical College, New York, New York
NY15	SUNY Upstate Medical University, Syracuse, New York
NY19	New York University School of Medicine, New York, New York
NY20	Cornell University Medical College, New York, New York
NY45	University of Rochester School of Medicine and Dentistry, Rochester, NYk
NY46	Albert Einstein College of Medicine - Yeshiva University, Bronx, New York
NY47	Mount Sinai School of Medicine, New York, New York
NY48	SUNY at Stony Brook School of Medicine, Stony Brook, New York
NY49	Zucker School of Medicine at Hofstra/Northwell, Hempstead, New York
NY75	New York College of Osteopathic Medicine of the NY Institute of Technology, Old Westbury, New York
NY76	Touro College of Osteopathic Medicine, New York, New York
OH01	Medical College of Ohio, Cincinnati, Ohio
OH06	Case Western Reserve University School of Medicine, Cleveland, Ohio
OH08	Cincinnati College of Medicine & Surgery, Cincinnati, Ohio
OH40	Ohio State University College of Medicine, Columbus, Ohio
OH41	University of Cincinnati College of Medicine, Cincinnati, Ohio
OH43	Medical University of Ohio at Toledo, Toledo, Ohio
OH44	Northeast Ohio Medical University, Rootstown, Ohio
OH45	Wright State University Boonshoft School of Medicine, Dayton, Ohio
OH53	University of Toledo College of Medicine and Life Sciences, Toledo, OH
OH75	Ohio University College of Osteopathic Medicine, Athens, Ohio
OK01	University of Oklahoma College of Medicine, Oklahoma City, Oklahoma
OK05	Oral Roberts University School of Medicine, Tulsa, Oklahoma
OK79	Oklahoma State Univ. College of Osteopathic Medicine and Surgery, Tulsa, OK
ON01	University of Toronto Faculty of Medicine, Toronto, Ontario, Canada
ON02	Toronto School of Medicine, Toronto, Ontario, Canada
ON05	Queens University Faculty of Medicine, Kingston, Ontario, Canada
ON06	University of Western Ontario Faculty of Medicine, London, Ontario, Canada
ON09	University of Ottawa Faculty of Medicine, Ottawa, Ontario, Canada
ON10	McMaster University School of Medicine, Hamilton, Ontario, Canada
OR02	Oregon Health Sciences University School of Medicine, Portland, Oregon
PA01	University of Pennsylvania School of Medicine, Philadelphia, PA
PA02	Jefferson Medical College of Thomas Jefferson Univ, Philadelphia, PA
PA07	Medical College of Pennsylvania, Philadelphia, Pennsylvania
PA09	Drexel Univ (Formerly Hahnemann Univ Med Col of PA), Philadelphia, PA
PA12	University of Pittsburgh School of Medicine, Pittsburgh, Pennsylvania
PA13	Temple University School of Medicine, Philadelphia, Pennsylvania
PA14	Pennsylvania State University College of Medicine, Hershey, PA
PA77	Philadelphia College of Osteopathic Medicine, Philadelphia, PA
PA78	Lake Erie College of Osteopathic Medicine, Erie, Pennsylvania
QU01	McGill University Faculty of Medicine, Montreal, Quebec, Canada
QU02	University of Montreal Faculty of Medicine, Montreal, Quebec, Canada
QU03	Laval University Faculty of Medicine, Quebec, Canada

Medical School Codes

QU06	University of Sherbrooke Faculty of Medicine, Sherbrooke, Quebec, Canada
RI01	Brown University School of Medicine (Warren Alpert), Providence, RI
SC01	Medical University of South Carolina College of Medicine, Charleston, SC
SC04	University of South Carolina Medical School, Columbia, South Carolina
SD01	University of South Dakota School of Medicine, Vermillon, South Dakota
SK01	University of Saskatchewan College of Medicine, Saskatoon, Saskatchewan, Canada
TN05	Vanderbilt University School of Medicine, Nashville, Tennessee
TN06	University of Tennessee Memphis College of Medicine, Memphis, TN
TN07	Meharry Medical College School of Medicine, Nashville, Tennessee
TN20	East Tennessee State University (James H. Quillen) School of Medicine, Johnson City, Tennessee
TN21	LMU-DeBusk College of Osteopathic Medicine, Cumberland Gap, TN
TX01	Medical School at Galveston, University of Texas, Galveston, Texas
TX02	University of Texas Medical Branch, Galveston, Texas
TX04	Baylor College of Medicine, Houston, Texas
TX12	University of Texas Southwestern Medical School, Dallas, Texas
TX13	University of Texas Medical School, San Antonio, San Antonio, Texas
TX14	University of Texas Medical School, Houston, Houston, Texas
TX15	Texas Tech University School of Medicine, Lubbock, Texas
TX16	Texas A & M University College of Medicine, College Station, Texas
TX17	Texas College of Osteopathic Medicine, University of North Texas, Denton, Texas
TX78	Texas College of Osteopathic Medicine, Fort Worth, Texas
UT01	University of Utah College of Medicine, Salt Lake City, Utah
VA01	University of Virginia School of Medicine, Charlottesville, Virginia
VA04	Medical College of Virginia Commonwealth University, Richmond, VA
VA07	Eastern Virginia Medical School, Norfolk, Virginia
VA75	Edward Via Virginia College of Osteopathic Medicine, Blacksburg, VA
VT02	University of Vermont College of Medicine, Burlington, Vermont
WA04	University of Washington School of Medicine, Seattle, Washington
WI05	University of Wisconsin Medical School, Madison, Wisconsin
WI06	Medical College of Wisconsin, Milwaukee, Wisconsin
WV01	West Virginia University School of Medicine, Morgantown, West Virginia
WV02	Marshall University Medical School, Huntington, West Virginia
WV75	West Virginia School of Osteopathic Medicine, Lewisburg, West Virginia
AFG01	Avicenna State Medical Instute O'Kabu, Afghanistan
AFG03	Kabul University, Afghanistan
ALB01	Fakulteti i Mjekesise, Universiteti i Tiranes, Albania
ALG01	University of Algiers Medical School, Algeria
ALG02	Institut des Sciences Medicales, Universite D' Alger, Algeria
ANT02	American University of Antigua, St. John's, Antigua
ANTI	Antigua
ARG01	Universidad De Buenos Aires, Argentina
ARG02	Universidad Nacional De Cordoba, Argentina
ARG03	Universidad Nacional De La Plata, Argentina
ARG06	Universidad Nacional De Cuyo, Argentina
ARG08	Universidad Catolica De Cordoba, Argentina
ARG09	Universidad Nacional de Rosario, Argentina
ARG10	Universidad Del Salvador, Buenos Aires, Argentina
ARG13	Favaloro University School of Medicine, Buenos Aires, Argentina
ARM27	Yerevan State Medical Institute, Armenia
AST01	University of Adelaide, Australia
AST02	University of Melbourne, Australia
AST03	University of Sydney, Australia
AST06	University of Western Australia, Australia
AST07	University of Queensland, Ipswich, Australia
AST08	Monash University, Australia
AST09	University of New South Wales, Australia
AST10	University of Tasmania, Australia
AST11	Flinders University of South Australia, Australia
AUS01	Karl Franzens Universitat Graz, Austria
AUS02	Leopold Franzens Universitat Innsbruck, Austria
AUS03	University of Graz, Graz, Austria
AUS04	University Innsbruck, Innsbruck, Austria
AUS07	Universitat Vienna, Austria
AUS08	Universitat Wien, Austria
AZE01	Azerbaijan Medical Institute, Baku, Azerbaijan
BAH01	Arabian Gulf University, Nanama, Bahrain
BAN02	Dhaka Medical College, University of Dhaka, Bangladesh
BAN03	University of Chittagong, Bangladesh
BAN04	Sylhet MAG Osmani Medical College, University of Chittagong, Bangladesh
BAN05	Shere Bangla Medical College, Bangladesh
BAN06	Sir Salimullah Medical College, Bangladesh
BAN07	Mymensingh Medical College, Bangladesh
BANG	Bangladesh
BAR01	University of the West Indies, Barbados
BEL02	Faulteit der Geneeskunde, Universiteit Gent, Belgium
BEL03	Universite De Liege, Belgium
BEL04	Universite Catholique De Louvain, Belgium
BEL06	Fakulteit der Geneeskunde, Katholieke Universiteit Leuven, Belgium
BEL07	Faculte de Medicine et de Pharmacie, Universite Libre de Bruxelles, Belgium
BEL11	Faculteit Der Wetenschappen, Universitaire Instelling Antwerpen Belgium
BEL12	Vrije University, Brussel, Belgium
BLA01	Grodno Medical Institute, Grodno, Belarus
BLA02	Belarusian State Medical University (formerly Minsk Medical Institute), Minsk, Belarus
BLA46	Vitebskij Medical Institute, Belarus
BLZ01	Central America Health Science University, Belize
BLZ02	Saint Matthews University, Belize
BOL01	Universidad Mayor De San Andres, Bolivia
BOL02	Universidad Mayor, Real Y Pontificia De San Francisco Xavier De Chuquisaca, Bolivia
BOS01	Univerzitet U Sarajevo, Bosnia
BRA02	Universidade Federal Do Rio Grande Do Sul, Porto Alegre, Brazil
BRA04	Universidade De Sao Paulo, Brazil
BRA08	Ecs de Med Fund Tech-Educ Souza Marques, Rio de Janeiro, Brazil
BRA09	Faculdade de Medicina de Ribeirao Preto, Universidade De Sao Paulo, Brazil
BRA11	Curso de Medicina e Odontologia, Universidade Federal Do Parana, Brazil
BRA12	Universidade Federal de Santa Catarina, Brazil
BRA13	Universidade Federal Do Ceara, Brazil
BRA15	Escola Paulista De Medicina, Brazil
BRA16	Faculdade de Medicina de Sorocaba, Pontificia Universidade Catolica De Sao Paulo, Brazil
BRA17	Centro de Ciencias da Saude, Curso de Medicina, Universidade Federal de Pernambuco, Brazil
BRA18	Faculty of Health Sciences Medical Program, University of Brasilia, Brazil
BRA19	Curso de Medicina, Pontificia Universidade Catolica do Parana, Brazil
BRA20	Esc de Publica, Salvador, Bahia, Brazil
BRA21	Faculdade of Medicine, Rio de Janeiro State University, Brazil
BRA22	Faculdade de Medicinade Vassouras, Universidade Severino Sombra, Brazil
BRA24	Universidade Estadual de Campinas, Brazil
BRA28	Escola De Medicina-Santa Casa De Misericordia De Vitoria/Emescam, Brazil
BRA32	Universidade Federal de Minas Gerais, Brazil
BRA37	Faculty de Cien Medicine de Santos, Santos, Brazil
BRA40	Universidade Federal Fluminense, Brazil
BRA43	Pontificia Univ Catol Do Rio Grande Do Sul, Fac Med, Porto Alegre, Brazil
BRA44	Universidade Federal do Rio de Janeiro, Brazil
BRA45	Universidade Gama Filho, Brazil
BRA49	Universidade de Passo Fundo, Brazil
BRA53	Fund University de Uberlandia, Uberlandia, Brazil
BRA60	University do Estado do Rio de Janeiro, Rio de Janeiro, Brazil
BRA64	University Federal da Paraiba, Joao Pessoa, Brazil
BRA65	Guanabara State University, Brazil
BUL01	Higher Medical Institute, Sofia, Bulgaria
BUL02	Sofia University, Bulgaria
BUL03	Higher Medical Institute, Plovdiv, Bulgaria
BUL04	Higher Medical Institute, Varna, Bulgaria
BUR01	University of Rangoon, Rangoon, Burma
BUR02	University of Mandalay, Burma
BOR03	Institute of Medicine II, Mingaladon, Birma
BUR04	Institute of Medicine I, Yangon, Burma
BWI01	American University of the Caribbean, British West Indies
CHI01	Universidad De Chile, Chile
CHI02	Universidad Catolica De Chile, Chile
CHI04	Universidad De Concepcion, Chile
CHN03	Beijing Union Medical College, China
CHN04	Soochow University, China
CHN07	Hunan Medical University, Changsha, China
CHN08	Anhui Medical College, Hefei, China
CHN09	Second Shanghai Medical College- St. Johns, China
CHN14	Beng Bu Medical College, Bengbu, China
CHN15	Norman Bethune Medical College, Jilin University, Changchun, China
CHN16	National Shanghai Medical College, China
CHN17	West China University of Medical Sciences, China
CHN18	Binzhou Medical College, Binzhou, Shandong, China
CHN19	Capital Medical College (Peking Union Medical College), Beijing (Peking), China
CHN1I	Beijing Second Medical College, Capital Institute, Beijing, China
CHN1J	Shandong Medical University, Jinan, Shandong, China
CHN1K	Suzhou Medical College, Suzhou, Jiangsu, China
CHN1N	Medical Center of Fudan University, Shanghai, China
CHN1R	Xi'an Jiaotong University School of Medicine, Shaanxi, China
CHN21	Sun Yat-Sen University of Medical Sciences, China
CHN23	Chinese Medical University, Shenyang Medical College, Shenyang, China
CHN25	Chongqing Medical University, Chongqing, China
CHN27	Dalian Medical College, Dali, China
CHN2A	Second Military Medical University, Shanghai, China
CHN2B	Third Military Medical University, Chongqing, China
CHN2G	Weifang Medical University, Weifang City, China

Medical School Codes

CHN34	First Military Medical University, Faculty of Medicine, Guangdong, China
CHN38	First Shanghai Medical College, China
CHN39	Beijing University College of Medicine, China
CHN3B	Tianjin Medical College, Tianjin (Tientsin), China
CHN3C	Wuhan University Medical College, Hupeh, China
CHN40	Shanghai Second Medical College, China
CHN41	Wuhan Medical College, China
CHN42	Harbin Medical University, China
CHN43	Fourth Military University, Shaanxi, China
CHN45	Fujian Medical College, Fuzhou, China
CHN4A	Shanghai First Medical College (Nat Shanghai Med Coll), Shanghai, China
CHN4C	Xian Medical College, Xian, China
CHN4D	Zhejiang Medical University (Chekiang Prov), Hangzhou, China
CHN50	Kunming Medical College, China
CHN57	Beijing Medical University, China
CHN58	Guangzhou College of Traditional Chinese Medicine, China
CHN59	Tongji Medical University, China
CHN61	Xuzhou Medical College, Xuzhou, China
CHN62	Nanjing Univ Medical College, China
CHN63	China Medical University in Shenyang, China
CHN64	Fujian Medical School, China
CHN65	Norman Bethune Medical College, Jilin University, China
CHN67	Qingdao Medical College, Qingdao, Shandong, China
CHN68	Henan College of Traditional Chinese Medicine, Zhengshou, Henan, China
CHN6D	Jinan University Medical College, Guangzhou, China
CHN74	Huabei Medical College for the Coal Industry, Tangshan, Hebei, China
CHN78	Inner Mongolia Medical College, Hohhot, China
CHN81	Jiangxi Medical College (Kiangsi Medical College), Nanchang, Jiangxi, China
CHN82	Jilin Medical College, Jilin, China
CHN88	Liaoning College of Traditional Chinese Medicine, Shenyang, Liaoning, China
CHN8A	Shanxi Medical College, Taiyuan, China
CHN8D	Guangxi Youjiang Medical College of Nationalities, Baise, Guanxi, China
CHN92	Nanjing Medical College (Nanking Railing Med Col), Nantong, China
CHN9B	Wannan Medical College, Wuhu, China
CHN9D	Guangzhou Medical College, Guangzhou, China
CMR01	Centre Universitaire des Sciences de la Sante, Universite de Yaounde, Cameroon
COL01	Universidad Nacional De Colombia, Colombia
COL03	Universidad De Antioquia, Colombia
COL05	Universidad Javeriana, Colombia
COL06	Universidad Del Valle, Division de Ciencias de la Salud, Colombia
COL07	Escuela Nacional de Medicina Juan N.Corpas, Colombia
COL08	Colegio Mayor de Nuestra Senora del Rosario, Colombia
COL09	Universidad Industrial De Santander, Division de Ciencias de la Salud, Colombia
COL10	Universidad Pontificia Bolivariana, Colombia
COL11	Universidad Metropolitana, Colombia
COL12	Colombian School Of Medicine, Colombia
COL13	University del Cauca, Popayan, Colombia
COL14	Programa de Medicina, Universidad Del Norte, Colombia
COL15	Inst De Ciencias De La Salud, Medelli, Colombia
COL16	University Libre de Colombia, Barranquilla, Colombia
COL19	University El Bosque, Esc Medicine Colombiana, Santa Fe De Bogota, Colombia
COL22	University Libre, Cali, Colombia
COL25	Pontificia University Javeriana, Bogota, Colombia
COL26	Universidad Autonoma de Bucaramanga, Columbia
COS01	Universidad De Costa Rica, Costa Rica
COS02	Universidad Autonoma De Centro America, Costa Rica
CRO01	University of Zagreb, Croatia
CUB02	Instituto Superior De Ciencias Medicas De Camaguey, Cuba
CUB06	Institute Sup de Cien Medicine de La Habana, Habana, Cuba
CUB07	Institute Sup de Cien Medicine de Santiago de Cuba, Santiagode Cuba
CZE01	Charles University, Prague, Czechoslovakia
CZE02	Charles University, Czech Republic
CZE03	Komensky University, Czechoslovakia
CZE04	Masaryk University, Czechoslovakia
CZE05	Palacky University, Czechoslovakia
CZE06	Safarikova University, Czechoslovakia
CZE07	JE Purkyne Faculty of Medicine, Mararykova University, Brno Czechoslovakia
CZE15	University Komenskeho, Bratislava, Czechoslovakia
CZE17	University Pavla Jozefa Safarika, Kosice, Czechoslovakia
DEN01	University of Copenhagen, Denmark
DEN03	University of Aarhus, Faculty of Medicine, Denmark
DMN01	Ross University, Dominica
DOM01	Universidad Autonoma De Santo Domingo, Dominican Republic
DOM02	Universidad Central Del Este, Dominican Republic
DOM04	Escuela de Medicina, Universidad Nacional Pedro Henriquez Urena Dominican Republic
DOM08	Universidad Tecnologica de Santiago, Dominican Republic
DOM09	Facultad de Ciencies de la Salud, Pontificia Universidad Catolica Madre Y Maestra,Dominican Republic
DOM10	Universidad Tecnologica de Santiago UTESA, Dominican Republic
DOM11	Intstitute Tech de Santo Domingo (INTEC), Santo Domingo Dominican Republic
DOM13	University Auto de Santo Domingo, Santo Domingo, Dominican Republic
DOM14	University Catolic Madre Maestra (UCMM), Santiago de las Caballeros, Dominican Republic
DOM15	University del Este (UCE), Pedro de Macoris, Dominican Republic
DOM18	University Iberoamericana (UNIBE), Santo Domingo, Dominican Republic
DOM20	University Nac Pedro Henriquez Urena, Santo Domingo Dominican Republic
DOM22	All Saints University School of Medicine, Roseau, Dominica
ECU01	University Central del Ecuador, Esc de Med, Fac de Cien Med, Quito, Ecuador
ECU03	University Catol de Santiago de Guayaquil, Fac de Med, Guayaquil, Ecuador
ECU04	University de Cuenca, Fac de Cien Med, Cuenca, Ecuador
ECU05	University de Guayaquil, Fac de Cien Med, Guayaquil, Ecuador
EGY03	Kasr El Aini Faculty of Medicine, University of Cairo, Egypt
EGY04	Ain Shams University, Egypt
EGY05	University of Alexandria, Egypt
EGY07	University of Assiut, Egypt
EGY08	Tanta University, Egypt
EGY09	Mansoura University, Faculty of Medicine, Egypt
EGY10	Zagazig University, Egypt
EGY12	Ibrahim Pasha University, Cairo, Egypt
EGY13	Menoufia University, Shibin El Kom, Egypt
EGY17	October 6th University Faculty of Medicine, Giza, Egypt
ELS01	Universidad de El Salvador, El Salvador
ELS03	University Evangelica, San Salvador, El Salvador
ENG01	University of Birmingham, England
ENG02	University of Bristol, England
ENG03	School of Clinical Medicine, University of Cambridge, England
ENG04	University of Newcastle-Upon-Tyne, England
ENG05	University of Leeds, England
ENG06	University of Liverpool, England
ENG07	The Westminister Medical College, University of London, England
ENG08	University of Manchester, England
ENG09	Medical School, Oxford University, England
ENG10	The Medical School, University of Sheffield, England
ENG11	University of Southampton, England
ENG12	Imperial College School of Medicine at St. Mary's, England
ENG13	University of Nottingham Medical School, England
ENG14	Charing Cross & Westminster Medical School, England
ENG15	Reg Qual England Conjoint Board, London, England
ENG16	Royal Free Hospital School of Medicine, University of London, England
ENG17	St. Bartholomew's Hospital Medical College, University of London England
ENG18	George's Hospital Medical School, University of London, England
ENG19	United Medical and Dental Schools of Guy's and St. Thomas' Hospitals, England
ENG22	University of Leicester, Leicester, England
ENG23	Kings College School of Medicine, University of London, England
ENG24	London Hospital Medical College, University of London, England
ENG25	University of London, London, England
ENG26	Middlesex Hospital Medical School, University London, England
ENG28	University of Sheffield, Sheffield, England
ENG29	St. George's, University of London, England
ENGL	England
EST01	University of Tartu, Estonia
ETH01	Addis Ababa University, Ethiopia
ETH02	Gondar College of Medicine, Gondar, Ethiopia
ETH03	Jimma Health Science Institute, Jimma, Ethiopia
FIN02	University of Helsinki, Finland
FIN03	Turun Yliopisto, University of Turku, Finland
FRA01	Faculte de Medecine de Bordeaux, Universite De Bordeaux II, France
FRA02	Faculte de Medecine de Lille, Universite De Lille II, France
FRA04	Faculte de Medecine de Montpellier, Universite De Montpellier I, France
FRA05	Faculte de Medecine de Nancy, Universite De Nancy I, France
FRA07	Universite Paul Sabatier,Toulouse III, France
FRA08	University de Louis Pasteur, U.E.R. Sci Med, Strasbourg, France
FRA10	UFR de Medicine Xavier Bichat, University of Paris VII, Paris, France
FRA11	Faculte de Medecine d' Aix- Marseille, Universite D' Aix- Marseille II, France
FRA12	Faculte de Medecine de Caen, Universite De Caen, France
FRA19	Universite de Pierre et Marie Curie, France
FRA22	Universite Scientifique et Medicale-Grenoble I, France
FRA23	Universite de Saint-Etienne, France
FRA24	Universite Rene Descartes, France
FRA29	University De Lyon 1, UFR de Medicine Laennec, Lyon, France
FRA30	U.E.R. de Medicine, University of Nice, France
FRA33	Universite de Paris (Saint-Antoine), Paris, France
FRA39	University de Peirre et Marie Curie (Paris VI), Paris, France
FRA88	University de Paris, France

Medical School Codes

GCY01	St. Matthew's University School of Medicine, Grand Cayman
GEO01	Aieti Highest Medical School, Tbilisi, Georgia
GEO02	Tbilisi Medical Institute, Tbilisi, Georgia
GER01	Freie Universitat Berlin (Now Charite - Universitatsmedizin Berlin) Germany
GER02	Rheinische Friedrich Wilhelms Universitat Bonn, Germany
GER03	Schlesische-Friedrich-Wilhelms University, Germany
GER04	Friedrich-Alexander-University, Germany
GER05	Albert-Ludwigs Universitat Freiburg, Germany
GER06	Fachbereich Humanmedizin, Justus-Liebig Universitat, Germany
GER07	Georg-August Universitat, Germany
GER09	Martin Luther Universitat Halle- Wittenberg, Germany
GER10	Ruprecht- Karls- Universitat, Germany
GER11	Friedrich-Schiller-Universitat Jena, Germany
GER12	Christian-Albrechts-Universitat of Kiel, Germany
GER14	Universitat of Leipzig, Germany
GER15	Philipps-Universitat Marburg, Germany
GER16	Ludwig-Maximilians-Universitat Munchen, Germany
GER17	Universitat Rostock, Germany
GER19	Eberhard-Karls Universitat Tubingen, Germany
GER20	Julius-Maximilians-Universitat, Wurzburg, Germany
GER21	Universitat Hamburg, Germany
GER22	Universitat Zu Koln, Germany
GER23	Frankfurt Medical School, Johann Wolfgang Goethe Universitat Germany
GER24	Westfalische Wilhelms Universitat Munster, Germany
GER25	Heinrich Heine University Dusseldorf, Med Fak, Germany
GER30	Humboldt-Universitat Zu Berlin (Now Charite - Universitatsmedizin Berlin) Germany
GER32	Johannes-Gutenberg Universitat Mainz, Germany
GER34	Universitat Des Saarlandes, Germany
GER36	Karl-Marx University, Leipzig, Germany
GER37	Medizinische Hochschule Hannover, Germany
GER39	Rhein Westfalenisch-Westfal Universitat, Germany
GER42	Universitat Ulm, Germany
GER43	Rheinisch Westfalische Technische Hochschule Aachen, Germany
GER44	Christian-Albrechts Universitat, Germany
GER46	Ruprecht-Karls-Universitat Heidelberg, Germany
GER48	Friedrich-Alexander-Universitat Erlangen-Nurnberg, Germany
GER53	Tech University, Munchen, Munich, Germany
GER54	University Hamburg, Hamburg, Germany
GER55	University Koln, Koln (Cologne), Germany
GER56	University Regensburg, Regensburg, Germany
GER58	University Witten-Herdecke, Herdecke, Germany
GER59	University Ulm, Ulm, Germany
GERM	Germany
GHA01	University of Ghana Medical School, Ghana
GHA02	University of Science and Tech, Kumasi, Ghana
GRE01	University of Athens, Greece
GRE02	University of Crete, Heraklion, Greece
GRE03	Aristotle University of Thessaloniki, Greece
GRE04	University of Ioannina, Greece
GRE05	University of Patras, Greece
GRN01	St. Georges University School of Medicine, Grenada
GUA02	Universidad De San Carlos De Guatemala, Guatemala
GUA03	Francisco Marroquin University, Guatemala
HAI01	Faculte de Medecine et de Pharmacie, University of Haiti, Haiti
HKO01	University of Hong Kong, Hong Kong
HON01	Universidad Nacional Autonoma De Honduras, Honduras
HUN01	Debrecen Medical College, Debrecen, Hungary
HUN03	Semmelweis Medical College, Peter Pazmany University, Budapest Hungary
HUN04	Medical University of Debrecen, Hungary
HUN05	Szeged Medical College, Szeged, Hungary
HUN06	Semmelweis Medical University, Semmelweis Orvostudomanyi Egyetem Hungary
HUN07	Medical University of Pecs, Hungary
HUN08	Albert Szent-Gyorgyt University of Medicine, Hungary
ICE01	University of Iceland, Iceland
INA00	Indira Gandhi Medical College, India
INA01	Goa Medical College, Goa University, India
INA02	University Colleges of Medicine, University of Calcutta, India
INA03	Punjab University, India
INA04	Madras Medical College, University of Madras, India
INA05	King George's Medical College, University of Lucknow, India
INA06	Maharishi Dayanand University, India
INA07	Amritsar Medical College, India
INA08	Christian Medical College, Tamil Nadu Dr. Mgr. Medical University, Madras, India
INA09	Government Medical College, University of Mysore, India
INA11	Rangaraya Medical College, Andhra University, India
INA12	Sarojni Najdu Medical College, Agra University, India
INA13	S C B Medical College, Utkal University, India
INA14	Banaras Hindu University, India
INA15	N H L Municipal Medical College, Gujarat University, India
INA16	Gandhi Medical College, Osmania University, India
INA18	Gauhati Medical College, Gauhati University, India lege, Gauhati University, India
INA1C	PSG Institute of Medical Science. Bharathiar University, TN, India
INA1D	Somaiya Medical College, University of Mumbai, Chembur, BombayIndia
INA1F	JLN Medical College, Aligarh Muslim University, India
INA1H	Government Medical College, Patiala, India
INA1K	Calcutta National Medical College, Univ Of Calcutta, Calcutta, India
INA1L	Rangaraya Medical College, Vijayayawada University Health Science, India
INA1M	Mahatma Gandhi Institute of Medical Science, Nagpur University, Wardha, India
INA1N	Mahatma Gandhi Mission's MC, Bombay University, New Bombay Maharashitra, India
INA1P	Terna Medical School, University Mumbai, New Bombay, India
INA1Q	N K P Salve Institute of Medical Sciences, Nagpur Univ, Nagpur, India
INA1S	Kamineni Institute of Medical Sciences (KIMS), India
INA1U	Guntur Medical College, Andhra Pradesh, India
INA1X	Dr S N Medical College, Rajasthan University, India
INA1Y	Darbhanga Medical College, LN Mithila University, Laheriassarai, India
INA1Z	Armed Forces Medical College, University of Poona, India
INA20	BJ Medical College, Gujarat University, India
INA21	Baroda University, India
INA22	Sri Krishna Medical College, Bihar University, India
INA23	Maulana Azad Medical College, University of Delhi, India
INA24	Byramjee Jeejeebhoy Medical College, University of Poona, India
INA25	V S S Medical College, India
INA26	Government Medical College, Nagpur University, India
INA27	Gajra Raja Medical College, Vikram University, India
INA28	Mysore Medical College, Mysore University, Mysore, India
INA29	Gandhi Medical College, Bhopal University, India
INA2A	JL Nehru Medical College, Karnataka University, Belgaum, India
INA2B	MP Shah Medical College, Saurashtra University, Jamnagar, India
INA2C	Rajah Muthiah Medical College, Annamalai University, Annamalainagar, India
INA2D	Sri Devaraj URS Medical College, Bangalore University, Tamaka, Kolar, India
INA2E	Trichur Medical College, Calcut University, Kerala, India
INA2H	Santosh Medical College, Uttar Pradesh, India
INA2X	Kilpauk Medical College, University of Madras, India
INA2Y	Deccan College of Medical Science, Osmania University, Hyderabad, India
INA2Z	Dr Vaishampayan Medical College, Shivaji University, India
INA2f	Dr. Panjabrao Deshmukh Memorial Medical College, Amravati, India
INA30	All India Institute of Medical Sciences, Ansari Nagar, New Delhi, India
INA31	M.G.M. Medical College (Mahatma Gandhi Mem MC), India
INA32	Ravindra Nath Tagore Medical College, Rajasthan University, India
INA33	Mahatma Gandhi Medical College, Ranchi University, India
INA34	TD Medical College, University of Kerala, India
INA35	Karnatak Medical College, Karnatak University Dharwad, India
INA36	Government Medical College, Kashmir University, India
INA37	Medical College, Bangalore University, India
INA38	Kurnool Medical College, Sri Venkateswara University, India
INA39	Kakatiya Medical College, Osmania University, India
INA3A	JLN Medical College, Ravi Shankar University, Raipur, India
INA3B	N D M V P Samaj's Medical College, Poona University, Maharashtra, India
INA3C	Rajendra Medical College, Ranchi University, Ranchi, India
INA3D	Sri Ramachandra Medical College and Res Inst, Madras University, Porur, India
INA3X	Tirunelveli Medical College, Madurai University, India
INA3Y	Dr Ambedkar Medical College, Bangalore University, Karnataka, India
INA3Z	Mahatma Gandhi College, Wardha University, India
INA41	Guru Nanak Medical College, Guru Nanak University, India
INA43	Netaji Subhash Chandra Bose Medical College, India
INA44	Al-Ameen Medical College, Karnatak University, Bijapur, India
INA46	Krishna Institute of Medical Science, Shivaji University, India
INA47	Madurai Medical College, India
INA48	Andhra Medical College, Andhra University, Visakhapatnam, India
INA49	Nalanda Medical College, Magadh University, India
INA4A	Kewpegowda Institute of Medical Science, Bangalore, India
INA4D	Sri Venkatesvara University Medical College, Tirupati, India
INA4E	Government Medical College, Chandigarh University, Chandigarh, Punjab, India
INA4X	BJ Medical College, University of Pune, Pune, India
INA4Y	Dr P Deshmukh Mem Medical College, Amravati University, Maharashtra, India
INA4Z	Maharaja Krishna Chandra Gajapati Medical College, India
INA51	Himachal Pradesh University, India
INA53	South Gujarat University, India
INA54	JLN Medical College, Aligarh Muslim University, Aligarh, India
INA55	Silchar Medical College, Gauhati University, India
INA56	University of Calicut, India
INA57	Gajra Raja Medical College, Jiwaji University, India
INA59	Assam Medical College, University of Dibrugarh, India

Medical School Codes

INA5A	LLRM Medical College, Meerut University, Meerut, India
INA5B	Osmania Medical College, Osmania University, Hyderabad, India
INA5C	Rural Medical College, Pravara University, India
INA5D	Deccan College of Medical Sciences, Vijaywada Univ
INA5E	Kolkata Medical College and Hospital, Kolkata, India
INA5X	B S Medical College, India
INA5Y	Dr DY Patil Medical College, Shivaji University, Kilhapur, India
INA5Z	Guru Govind Singh Medical College, Punjab University, India
INA62	Guntur Medical College, Andhra University, India
INA65	Topiwala National Medical College, University of Bombay (Mumbai), India
INA66	Jawaharlal Institute of Post-Graduate Medical Education & Research (JIPMER), Pondicherry, India
INA67	Grant Medical College, University of Bombay (Mumbai), India
INA68	Bangalore Medical College, Bangalore, Karnataka, India
INA69	Seth G. S. Medical College, Bombay, India
INA6A	Miraj Medical College, Shivaji University, Miraj, India
INA6Y	Goa Medical College, University of Bombay, Panaji, India
INA6Z	Dayanand Medical College, Punjab University, India
INA70	Kasturba Medical College Manipal, Manipal Acad Higher Ed., Manipal, India
INA71	MP Shah Medical College, Gujarat University, India
INA72	Lady Hardinge Medical College, University of Delhi, India
INA74	M.G.M Medical College (Mahatma Gandhi Mem MC), Indore, India
INA75	Mahadevappa Rampure Medical College, Gulbarga, India
INA76	Trivandrum Medical College, Kerala University, India
INA77	Stanley Medical College, University of Madras, India
INA78	Christian Medical College, Vellore, India
INA79	Christian Medical College, Punjab University, Ludhiana, India
INA7B	Patna Medical College, Patna University, India
INA7C	Siddartha Medical College, Vijayawada, India
INA7X	Calcutta Medical College, Calcutta University, India
INA7Y	GSVM Medical College, Kanpur University, Kanpur, India
INA7Z	Bide Assoc Medical College, Karnataka University, Bijapur Karnataka, India
INA80	Bharati Vidyapeeth's Medical College, Pune University, Pune, India
INA81	Coimbatore Medical College, University of Madras, India
INA82	Government Medical College, Punjab University, India
INA83	Gandhi Medical College. Univ Health School, Vijayawada, Hyderabad, India
INA84	Chingleput Medical College, Madras University, India
INA85	Thanjavur Medical College, Madras University, India
INA86	Nilratan Sircar Medical College, Calcutta University, India
INA87	Lokmanya Tilak Mun Medical College, Bombay University, India
INA88	Rajendra Medical College, Bihar University, India
INA89	R G Kar Medical College, Calcutta University, India
INA8B	Pramukhswami Medical College, Sardar Patel University, Karamsad Gujarat, India
INA8C	Sri Siddartha Medical College, Bangalore University, Tumkur, Karnataka, India
INA8Y	Guntur Medical College, Nagarjuna University, Guntur, India
INA8Z	Sardar Patel Medical College, Rajasthan University, India
INA92	University College of Medical Sciences, University of Delhi, India
INA93	Jammu University, India
INA94	St Johns Medical College, Bangalore University, India
INA95	JLN Medical College, Rajasthan University, India
INA96	M S Ramaiah Medical College, Bangalore, India
INA97	JJM Medical College, Mysore University, India
INA98	Kottayam College, Kerala University, India
INA9A	Kasturba Medical College, Mysore University, India
INA9B	Sawai Man Singh Medical College, Rajasthan University, India
INA9C	Mahadevappa Rampure Medical College, India
INA9D	Kurnool Medical College, Vijayawada Univ Hlth Sci, Kurnool, AP, India
INA9F	Kasturba Medical College, Mangalore University, India
INA9Q	Maharashtra Institute of Medical Sciences, India
INA9R	King Edward College Univ. of Punjab, India
INA9S	Kilpauk Medical College, University of Chennai, Chennai, India
INA9U	Government Medical College Bhavnagar, Bhavnagar, India
INA9V	Gandhi Medical College, Secunderabad, India
INA9W	Chennai Medical College, TemilNadu, India
INA9X	Calicut University Medical College, Calicut, India
INA9Y	Jawaharial Nehru Medical College, University of Rajasthan, Ajmar Rajasthan, India
INA9Z	Kempegowda Institute of Medical Sciences, India
INAZ6	JLN Medical College, Ravi Shankar University, India
IND21	University of Udayana, Denpasar, Bali, Indonesia
INDI	India
IRA01	University of Tehran, Iran
IRA03	Isfahan University of Medical Sciences, Iran
IRA04	Pahlavi University, Iran
IRA05	Tabriz University of Medical Sciences, Iran
IRA06	Ferdowsi University of Mashhad, Iran
IRA08	Shahid Beheshti University, Tehran, Iran
IRA09	Shiraz University, Iran
IRA14	Iran Medical Center (Imperial Center of Iran), Tehran, Iran
IRA15	Iran University of Medical Science, Tehran, Iran
IRA16	Islamic Azad University, Tehran Medical Unit, Tehran, Iran
IRA18	Kerman University of Medical Science, Kerman, Iran
IRA25	Guilan University of Medical Sciences, Rasht, Iran
IRA26	Qazvin University of Medical Sciences, Iran
IRAN	Iran
IRE01	Queens University of Belfast, Ireland
IRE02	University College Cork, National University of Ireland, Ireland
IRE03	University of Dublin, Trinity College, Ireland
IRE04	Royal College of Surgeons in Ireland, Ireland
IRE05	University College Dublin, Ireland
IRE06	National University of Ireland, Galway, Ireland
IRE12	University College Dublin, National University of Ireland, Ireland
IRQ01	Baghdad Medical College, University of Baghdad, Iraq
IRQ02	University of Mosul, Iraq
IRQ04	University of AL-Mustansiriyah Medical College, Baghdad, Iraq
ISR01	Hadassah Medical School, Hebrew University, Israel
ISR02	Sackler School of Medicine, Tel-Aviv University, Israel
ISR04	Israel Institute of Technology, Israel
ISR05	Ben Gurion University, Israel
ISR06	Technion-Israel Institute of Tech, Fac of Medicine, Haifa, Israel
ISR07	Al-Quds University, Israel
ITA01	Universita Degli Studi di Bologna, Italy
ITA03	Universita Degli Studi di Milano, Italy
ITA04	Universita Di Catania, Italy
ITA05	University Catholic de Sacro Cuore (Agostino Gemelli), Roma, Italy
ITA06	Universita Degli Studi di Florence, Italy
ITA07	Universita Degli Studi di Genova, Italy
ITA08	Universita Degli Studi De Messina, Italy
ITA10	Faculta Clinica Odontoiatrica, Universita Di Napoli, Italy
ITA12	Universita Degli Studi di Palermo, Italy
ITA14	Clinica Odontoiatrica, Policlinico San Matteo, Universita Degli Studi Di Pavia, Italy
ITA15	Universita Degli Studi Di Perugia, Italy
ITA16	Universita Di Pisa, Facolta di Medicina e Chirurgia, Italy
ITA17	Universita di Roma (La Sapienza), Italy
ITA19	Universita Degli Studi Di Siena, Italy
ITA22	Universita Degli Studi Di Padova, Italy
ITA23	Universita Cattolica Sacrocuoro di Milano, Italy
ITA24	Universita Degli Studi Di Torino, Italy
ITA26	Libera Universita Degli Studi G D' Annunzio Cheiti, Italy
ITA28	University di Napoli II, Naples, Italy
ITA30	University di Roma-Tor Vergata, Roma, Italy
ITA31	University di Trieste, Trieste, Italy
ITA32	University di Verona, Verona, Italy
ITA33	Facolta Di Medicina E Chirurgia, Universita Di Napoli, Italy
JAP01	Kyoto Imperial University, Japan
JAP05	Chiba University, Japan
JAP18	Tokyo Women's Medical College, Japan
JAP20	Keio University, Japan
JAP25	Nihon University, Japan
JAP29	Toho University, Japan
JAP30	Fijita-Gakuen University, Aichi, Japan
JAP36	Hokkaido University, Japan
JAP38	Fukushima Medical College, Japan
JAP39	Tokyo Medical and Dental University, Japan
JAP41	Kyoto Prefectural University of Medicine, Japan
JAP42	Shinshu University, Japan
JAP53	St. Marianna University, School of Medicine, Japan
JAP55	Yamaguchi University School of Medicine, Japan
JAP78	Saga Medical College, Saga, Japan
JAP82	Tokai University, Kanagawa, Japan
JAP84	Tsukuba Faculty of Medicine, Ibaraki, Japan
JAP86	Yamagata University, Yamagata, Japan
JAP89	University of Tokyo, Japan
JMA01	University of the West Indies, Jamaica
JOR01	University of Jordan, Jordan
JOR02	Jordan University of Science and Technology, Irbid, Jordan
KEN01	College of Health Sciences, University of Nairobi, Kenya
KOR01	Yonsei University College of Medicine, Yonsei University, Korea
KOR03	Ewha Womens University, Korea
KOR04	Seoul National University, Korea
KOR05	Korea University, Korea
KOR06	Catholic University Medical College, Korea
KOR09	Kyungpook National University, Korea
KOR11	Kyunghee University, Korea
KOR13	Chung - Ang University, Korea
KOR14	Chonnam University Medical School, Chonnam National University, Korea
KOR15	Hanyang University, Korea
KOR25	Dankook University Medical School, Cheonan, South Korea
KUW01	Kuwait University, Kuwait
LAT01	University of Latvia, Latvia
LAT02	Medical Academy of Latvia, Latvia
LAT03	Riszkij Medical Insititue, Riga, Latvia
LEB01	Saint Joseph University, Lebanon

Medical School Codes

LEB03	American University of Beirut, Lebanon
LEB04	L'Universite Libanaise, Lebanon
LEB05	Medical School of Peres (Lebanese University College of Medicine), Beirut, Lebanon
LEB06	University of Balamand, Lebanon
LEB07	Holy Spirit University of Kaslik, Juniyah, Lebanon
LIB01	A.M. Dogliotti College of Medicine, University of Liberia, Liberia
LIT02	Kaunas Medical Academy, Lithuania
LIT41	Vilnius University, Lithuania
LIY02	Al-Fateh University, Libya
MAC02	Cyril & Methodius Medical School, University of Cyril, Skopje, Macedonia
MAL01	University of Malaya, Malaysia
MEX02	Universidad Autonoma De Nuevo Leon, Mexico
MEX03	Universidad Autonoma De Guadalajara, Mexico
MEX04	Universidad Autonoma De San Luis Potosi, Mexico
MEX06	Universidad Autonoma De Yucatan, Mexico
MEX10	University Auonoma de San Luis Potosi, Mexico
MEX14	UAG School of Medicine, Universidad Autonoma De Guadalajara, Mexico
MEX22	Universidad Autonoma De Chihuahua, Mexico
MEX27	Universidad La Salle, Mexico
MEX29	Universidad Autonoma De Ciudad Juarez, Mexico
MEX34	Universidad del Noreste, Tampico, Mexico
MEX37	Division de Ciencias Biologicas de La Salud, Universidad Autonoma Metropolitana, Mexico
MEX39	Instituto de Ciencias de la Salud, Universidad Autonoma Del Estado De Mexico, Mexico
MEX40	Universidad Anahuac, Mexico
MEX41	Universidad Nacional Autonoma De Mexico, Tlanepatta, Mexico
MEX47	University Auto de Sinaloa, Culiacan, Mexico
MEX54	University de Mexico, American del Norte, Cuidad Reynosa, Mexico
MEX55	University de Monterrey, Monterrey, Mexico
MEX61	University Nac Auto De Mexico. Esc Nac de Est Prof, DF, Mexico
MEX62	Univ Nac Auto de Mexico, Mexico City, Mexico
MEX64	Fac de Med Dr. Ignacio Chavez, Morelia, Michoacan, Mexico
MEX65	Ignacio A. Santos School of Medicine, Monterrey, Mexico
MEX66	Universidad Panamericana, Mexico City, Mexico
MEXI	Mexico
MLT01	University of Malta , Medical School, Malta
MNT01	American University of the Caribbean, Montserrat
MOL01	State Medical & Pharm University Nicolae Testemitanu, Chisinau, Moldova
MOL02	Kishinev State Medical Institute, Kishinev, Moldova
MOR01	University Hassan II, Casablanca, Morocco
MYA01	University of Rangoon, Myanmar
MYA03	Institute of Medicine II, Mingaladon, Myanmar
MYA04	Institute of Medicine I, Yangon, Myanmar
NEP01	Tribhuvan University, Kathmandu, Nepal
NEP02	Manipal College of Medical Sciences, Pokhara, Nepal
NEP03	B.P. Koirala Institute of Health Sciences, Ghopa, Nepal
NEP04	Nepal Medical College Pvt. Ltd (NMC), Nepal
NEPA	Nepal
NET01	Universiteit Van Amsterdam, Netherlands
NET02	Faculteit der Geneeskunde, Rijksuniversiteit Groningen, Netherlands
NET03	Rijksuniversiteit Leiden, Netherlands
NET06	University Limburg, Maastricht, Natherlands
NET08	Faculteit der Geneeskunde, Erasmus Universiteit, Netherlands
NET09	Saba University School of Medicine, Netherlands Antilles
NET10	Vrije University, Armsterdam, Netherlands
NET12	University of Sint Eustatius, Sint Eustatius, Netherlands Antilles
NEW02	University of Auckland, New Zealand
NEW03	University of Otago, New Zealand
NIG01	University of Ibadan, Nigeria
NIG02	University of Nigeria, Nigeria
NIG03	University of Lagos, Nigeria
NIG07	University of Benin, Benin City, Nigeria
NIG09	Nnamdi Azikiwe University, College of Health Science, Nnewi, Nigeria
NIG10	Ogun State University, Ogun, Nigeria
NIG11	University of Benin, Benin City, Nigeria
NIG12	University of Calabar, Calabar, Nigeria
NIG15	University of Port Harcourt, Port Harcourt, Nigeria
NOR01	Universitetet I Oslo, Norway
NSK01	Grace University, Cades Bay, Nevis
OMA01	Sultan Qaboos University, Al Khod, Muscat, Saltanate of Oman
PAK01	King Edward Medical University (KEMU), Pakistan
PAK02	University of The Punjab, Pakistan
PAK04	Liaquat Medical University, University of Sind, Pakistan
PAK06	Ayub Medical College, University of Peshawar, Pakistan
PAK08	Fatima Jinnah Medical College for Women, Lahore, Pakistan
PAK10	Nishtar Medical College, Bahauddin Zakariya University, Pakistan
PAK11	Dow Medical College, University of Karachi, Pakistan
PAK12	Sind (Sindh) Medical College, University of Karachi, Pakistan
PAK13	Quaid E Azim Medical College, Islamia University, Pakistan
PAK14	Aga Khan University Medical College, Pakistan
PAK15	Allama Iqbal Medical College, University of Punjab, Pakistan
PAK18	Khyber Medical College, University of Peshawar, Pakistan
PAK19	Army Medical College, Quaid-I-Azam University, Rawalpindi, Pakistan
PAK20	Rawalpindi Medical College, Pakistan
PAK21	Bagai Medical & Dental College, University of Karachi, Karachi, Pakistan
PAK24	Punjab Medical College, University of Punjab, Faisalabad, Pakistan
PAK26	Baqai Medical University, Karachi, Pakistan
PAKI	Pakistan
PAN01	Universidad De Panama, Panama
PAR01	Universidad Nacional De Asuncion, Paraguay
PER01	Universidad Nacional Mayor De San Marcos De Lima, Peru
PER02	Universidad Nacional De San Agustin, Peru
PER04	Fac de Med Alberto Hurtado, Universidad Peruana Cayetano Heredia, Peru
PER05	National University of Trujillo, Peru
PER09	University Catolica de Santa Maria, Faculity de Medicine Humana Arequipa, Peru
PER10	University San Martin de Porres, Lima, Peru
PER11	Cayetano Heredia University Medical School, Peru
PHI01	University of Santo Tomas, Philippines
PHI02	University of The Philippines, Manila, Philippines
PHI07	MCU College of Medicine, Manila Central University, Philippines
PHI08	Far Eastern University, Philippines
PHI09	University of the East, Ramon Magsaysay Memorial Medical Center, Philippines
PHI10	Cebu Institute of Medicine, Philippines
PHI11	Southwestern University, Philippines
PHI13	Western Visayas State University, Philippines
PHI15	St. Louis University, Philippines
PHI17	General Emilio Aguinaldo College, Philippines
PHI18	Cebu Doctors College of Medicine, Philippines
PHI22	Fatima College of Medicine, Philippines
PHI24	Emilo Aguinaldo College of Medicine, Dasmarinas, Philippines
PHI26	Matias Aznar Memorial Medical College, Southwestern University Cebu City, Philippines
PHI28	Remedios T Romualdez Medical Foundation, Tacloban City, Philippines
PHI29	University of Philippines, Tacloban City, Philippines
PHI30	University of City of Manila, Manila, Philippines
PHI32	De La Salle University, Cavite, Philippines
PHI33	St. Luke's College of Medicine - William H. Quasha Memorial, Philippines
POL02	Uniwersytet Jagiellonski, Poland
POL03	Akademia Medyczna W Warszawie, Poland
POL04	Medical Academy of Poznan, Poland
POL05	Akad Medicine (Kolernika), Krakow, Poland
POL06	Akademia Medyczna W Lublinie, Poland
POL08	Akademie Medyczna W Wroclawiu, Poland
POL09	Akademia Medyczna W Lodzi, Poland
POL10	Slaska Adak Med Im Ludwika Warynskiego, Poland
POL11	Pomeranian Medical Academy, Poland
POL12	Karola Marcinkowski Akad Medicine, Poznan, Poland
POL13	Akademia Medyczna W Gdasku, Poland
POL14	Akademia Medyczna W Bialymstoku, Poland
POL15	Akademia Medyczna Im Mikolaja Kopernika W Krakowie, Poland
POL16	Military Medical Academy, Lodz, Poland
POL19	Medical University of Silesia, Katowice, Poland
POL77	Academy of Medicine of Bydgoszcz, Bydgoszcz, Poland
POR01	Universidade De Coimbra, Portugal
POR02	Universidade De Lisboa, Faculdade de Medicina de Lisboa, Portugal
POR03	Universidade De Porto, Port Codox, Portugal
POR04	Universidade Nova De Lisboa, Faculdade de Ciencias Medicas, Portugal
PRO01	University of Puerto Rico School of Medicine, Puerto Rico
PRO02	Ponce School of Medicine, Puerto Rico
PRO03	Universidad Central del Caribe, Puerto Rico
QAT01	Weill Cornell Medical College in Qatar, Qatar
ROM01	Universitatea De Medicina Si Farmacie (Carol Davila) BucharestRomania
ROM02	Universitatea De Medicina Si Farmacie (Gr.T. Popa) Iasi, Romania
ROM04	Universitatea De Medicina Si Farmacie Tirgu-Mures, Romania
ROM05	Universitatea De Medicina Si Farmacie Timisoara, Romania
ROM06	Universitatea De Medicina Si Farmacie Cluj-Napoca, Cluj, Romania
ROM09	Institute of Medicine & Pharmacy in Bucharest, Bucharest, Romania
ROM11	Iuliu Hatieganu University of Medicine & Pharmacy, Romania
ROM12	Titu Maiorescu University, Bucharest, Romania
ROMA	Romania
RUS01	First St. Petersburg Medical Institute, Russia
RUS02	Altajski Medical Institute, Barnaul, Russia
RUS03	Kazan State Medical Institute, Russia
RUS05	Nizhni Novgorod State Medical Academy, Nizhni Novgorod, Russia
RUS06	First Moscow Order of Lenin Medical Institute, Russia
RUS07	Russian State Medical University (RSMU), Moscow, Russia
RUS08	Tomskij Medicinskij Institut, Russia
RUS09	Amur State University, University of Blagoveshchensk, Blagoveshchensk, Russia
RUS10	Celjabinsk Medical Institute, Celjabinsk, Russia
RUS11	Saratovskij Medicinskij Institut, Russia
RUS15	Second Moscow Medical Institute, Russia
RUS16	Omsk State Medical Institute, Russia
RUS23	Tbilisi Medical Institute, Russia

Medical School Codes

RUS25	Lvov Institute of Medicine, Russia
RUS26	Izhevsk Medical Institute, Ustinov (Izhevsk), Russia
RUS27	State Medical Institute of Yerevan Armenian, Russia
RUS32	Krasnoyarsk Medical Institute, Krasnoyarsk, Russia
RUS33	Kubanskil Medical Institute, Krasnodar, Russia
RUS34	Rostovskij Medicinskij Institut, Russia
RUS35	Kishinev Medical Institute, Russia
RUS37	Novosibirskij Medicinskij Institut, Russia
RUS38	Kazakh Medical Institute, Russia
RUS39	Orenburgskaya Medicinskay Academia, Russia
RUS40	Kuibyshev Medical Institute, Kuibyshev, Russia
RUS41	Military Medical Academy, SM Kirov School, St Petersburg (Leningrad), Russia
RUS42	Molotov Medical Institute, Perm, Russia
RUS44	Moscow Medical Institute (Min of Health), Moscow, Russia
RUS45	Astrakhanskij Medicinskij Institut, Russia
RUS47	Byelorussia Medical Institute, Russia
RUS48	Doneckij Medical Institute, Russia
RUS52	Zaporzskij Medical Institute, Russia
RUS53	Sverdlovsk Medical Institute, Russia
RUS54	St. Petersburg State Pediatric Medical Academy, Russia
RUS55	Petrozavodsk University, Petrozavodsk, Russia
RUS56	Rjazan Medical Institute, Rjazan, Russia
RUS59	St. Petersburg I. I. Mechnikov State Medical Academy, Russia
RUS60	Smolenskij Medicinskij Institut, Russia
RUS61	Volgogradskij Medicinskij Institut, Russia
RUS62	Tajik State Medical Institute, Russia
RUS63	Samara State Medical University, Russia
RUS65	Kemerovskij Medicinskij Institut, Russia
RUS72	Mediciniskij Fakultet, Chuvash Universitet I.N. Ulyanov, Russia
RUS73	Bashkirskij Medicinskij Institut, Russia
RUS74	Permskij Medicinskij Institut, Russia
RUS75	Kurskij Medicinskij Institut, The Kursk State Medical University, Russia
RUS76	Patrice Lumumba People's Friendship University, Russia
RUS77	Moscow State University, Russia
RUS79	Moscow Medical Stomatology Institute, Moscow, Russia
RUS80	St. Petersburg State Pavlov Medical University, St. Petersburg, Russia
RUS81	I. M. Sechenov Moscow Medical Academy, Russia
RUS82	Tver State Medical Academy, Tver, Russia
RUS84	Northern State Medical University, Arkhangelsk, Russia
RUSS	Rush Medical College, Russia
SAF01	University of the Witwatersrand, South Africa
SAF02	University of Cape Town, South Africa
SAF03	University of Pretoria, South Africa
SAF04	University of Stellenbosch, South Africa
SAF05	University of Natal, South Africa
SAU01	King Saud University (Univ Riyadh), Riyadh, Saudi Arabia
SAU02	King Faisal University, Saudi Arabia
SAU03	King Abdulaziz University, Saudi Arabia
SAU04	King Saud University, Abha, Sauda Arabia
SAUD	Saudi Arabia
SCO03	University of Edinburgh, Scotland
SCO05	University of Glasgow, Scotland
SCO06	University of Dundee, Dundee, Scotland
SCO17	University of Aberdeen, Scotland
SEN02	St. Christopher's College of Medicine, Dakar, Senegal
SER01	Univerzitet U Pristini, Serbia
SER03	Univerzitet U Beogradu, Serbia
SIN02	National University of Singapore, Singapore
SLO01	Medicinska Fakulteta, Univerza V Ljublani, Ljubljani, Slovenia
SLO02	Comenius University, Slovakia
SLU01	Spartan Health Sciences University, St. Lucia
SLV01	Univerza V Ljublani, Slovenia
SPA01	Universidad De Barcelona, Spain
SPA02	University of Seville, Spain
SPA04	Universidad Autonoma De Madrid, Spain
SPA06	Universidad De Zaragoza, Spain
SPA07	University de Alcala de Henares, Alcala de Henares, Spain
SPA08	Universidad De Valencia, Spain
SPA11	Universidad de Navarra, Spain
SPA12	Universidad Complutense De Madrid, Spain
SPA15	Universidad Autonoma De Barcelona, Spain
SPA16	Universidad De Cordoba, Spain
SPA17	Universidad De Malaga, Spain
SPA18	Universidad De Murcia, Spain
SPA21	University de Pais Vasco (Auto de Bilboa), Bilboa, Spain
SPA23	Faculty of Medicine, Universidad De Navarra, Spain
SPA24	University de Santander, Santander, Spain
SPA25	University Rovira I Virgil, Reus (Tarragona), Spain
SPA26	University de Cadiz, Cadiz, Spain
SPA27	University De Lisboa, Faculty of Medicine, Lisboa, Spain
SPAI	Spain
SRI01	University of Colombo, Sri Lanka
SRI02	University of Peradeniya, Sri Lanka
SRI05	North Colombo Private Medical College, Ragama, Sir Lanka
SRIL	Sri Lanka
STM01	American University of the Caribbean, St. Maarten
SUD01	University of Khartoum, Sudan
SUD02	University of Gezira, Wad Medani, Sudan
SUD04	Omdurman Medical School, Omdurman, Sudan
SUR01	Anton De Kom Universiteit Van Suriname, Suriname
SWE01	Lund University, Sweden
SWE02	Karolinska Institute, Sweden
SWE03	Uppsala Universitet, Sweden
SWE04	Goteborg University, Sweden
SWE05	UMEA University, Sweden
SWI01	Universitat Basel, Switzerland
SWI02	University of Bern, Switzerland
SWI04	Universite De Geneve, Switzerland
SWI05	Universite De Lausanne, Switzerland
SWI07	Universitat Zurich, Switzerland
SYR01	Damascus University, Syria
SYR02	University of Aleppo, Syria
SYR03	University of Tichreen (Univ Latakia), Latakia, Syria
TAI01	National Defense Medical Ctr, Taipei, Taiwan
TAI02	National Taiwan University College of Medicine, Taipei, Taiwan
TAI03	Shihezi Medical College, Shihezi, Xinjiang Upper Auto Reg, Taiwan
TAI04	Kaohsiung Medical University, Taiwan
TAI05	Taipei Medical University, Taiwan
TAI06	China Medical College, Taichung, Taiwan
TAI07	Chung Shan Medical & Dental College, Taiwan
TAI08	College of Medicine, National Taiwan University, Taiwan
TAI09	National Yang-Ming University, Taiwan
TAIW	Taiwan
THA02	Khon Kaen University, Khon Kaen, Thailand
THA03	Siriraj Hospital, Mahidol University, Thailand
THA04	Chiang Mai University, Thailand
THA05	Ramathibodi Hospital, Mahidol University, Thailand
THA08	Srinakharinwirot University, Bangkok, Thailand
THA66	Phramongkutklao Medical College, Bangkok, Thailand
TRI01	University of the West Indies, St. Augustine, Trinidad
TUN01	Universite Des Sciences Et De Medecine De Tunis, Tunisia
TUR01	Istanbul Universitesi, Turkey
TUR03	Ankara Universitesi, Turkey
TUR04	Hacettepe Universitesi, Turkey
TUR05	Ege Universitesi, Turkey
TUR07	Marmara Universitesi, Istanbul, Turkey
TUR09	Cukurova University, Adana, Turkey
TUR16	Istanbul University (Cerrahpasa), Istanbul, Turkey
TUR18	Selcuk University, Meram Faculty of Medicine, Konya, Turkey
TUR20	Uludag University (Istanbul and Bursa Univ), Bursa, Turkey
TURK	Turkey
UGA01	Makerere University, Uganda
UGA02	Kigezi Int'l School of Medicine, Uganda
UKR01	Chernovtsy State University, Ukraine
UKR04	Karazin Kharkiv National University, Kharkiv, Ukraine
UKR05	Kiev Medical Institute, Ukraine
UKR06	Uzhgorod University Medical Faculity, Uzhgorod, Ukraine
UKR11	Donetsk Medical Institute, Donetsk, Ukraine
UKR12	Odessa Medical Institute, Ukraine
UKR13	Crimean Medical Institute, Ukraine
UKR15	Zaporozskij Medical Institute, Zaporoze, Ukraine
UKR18	National Pirogov Memorial Medical University, Vinnitsa, Ukraine
UKR25	Lviv State Medical Institute, Ukraine
UKR28	Ternopil Medical Institute, Ukraine
UKR30	Ivano-Frankovskij Medicinskij Institut, Ukraine
UKR32	Kharkiv National Medical University (KNMU), Ukraine
URU01	Universidad De La Republica, Uruguay
UZB01	Andizhan Medical Institute, Andizhan, Uzbekistan
UZB02	Samarkand Medical Institute, Samarkand, Uzbekistan

Code Table: Hosptals

Code	Name	State
CT-ALLIANCE	AllianceTreatment Center, Inc.	CT
CT-BRADMEM	The Hospital of Central CT Bradley Memorial Campus	CT
CT-BRIDGPRT	Bridgeport Hospital	CT
CT-BRISTOL	Bristol Hospital	CT
CT-DANBURY	Danbury Hospital	CT
CT-GRENWCH	Greenwich Hospital	CT
CT-HALLBRK	St. Vincent's Behavioral Health Services	CT
CT-HARTFRD	Hartford Hospital	CT
CT-HOSPECL	Hospital for Special Care	CT
CT-MIDDLSX	Middlesex Hospital	CT
CT-NORWALK	Norwalk Hospital	CT
CT-STAMFDH	Stamford Hospital	CT
CT-STMARY	St. Mary's Hospital	CT
CT-STVNCNT	St. Vincent's Medical Center	CT
CT-WATRBRY	Waterbury Hospital	CT
CT-YALENHH	Yale-New Haven Hospital	CT
ME-CALAIS	Calais Regional Hospital	ME
ME-DOWNEAST	Down East Community Hospital	ME
ME-EASTMAIN	Eastern Maine Medical Center	ME
NH-ANDROSGN	Androscoggin Valley Hospital	NH
NH-CAPITHS	Capital Health/Capital Region Health Services	NH
NH-DRTMTHMC	Dartmouth-Hitchcock Medical Center	NH
NH-EXETER	Exeter Hospital Inc	NH
NH-MONADNK	Monadnock Community Hospital	NH
NJ-ACMCITY	AtlantiCare Regional Medical Center/City Campus	NJ
NJ-ACMCMAIN	AtlantiCare Regional Medical Center/Mainland	NJ
NJ-ANCPSYCH	Ancora Psychiatric Hospital	NJ
NJ-ANNKLEIN	Ann Klein Forensic Center	NJ
NJ-ATLANCHS	Atlanticare Health System	NJ
NJ-ATLANTHS	Atlantic Health System	NJ
NJ-BACHARCH	Bacharach Institute for Rehabilitation	NJ
NJ-BAYONNE	Bayonne Medical Center	NJ
NJ-BAYSHORE	Bayshore Community Hospital	NJ
NJ-BERGNMC	Bergen Regional Medical Center	NJ
NJ-BURDTMLN	Cape Regional Medical Center	NJ
NJ-CAPITLHS	Capital Health System	NJ
NJ-CARONEBA	CareOne at Raritan Bay	NJ
NJ-CARRIER	Carrier Clinic	NJ
NJ-CENTRAST	CentraState Medical Center	NJ
NJ-CHDNWBTH	Children's Hospital of NJ at Newark Beth Israel MC	NJ
NJ-CHILTON	Chilton Memorial Hospital	NJ
NJ-CHLSMT	Children's Specialized Hospital	NJ
NJ-CHLSOCEN	Children's Specialized Hospital-Ocean	NJ
NJ-CHOSHUDC	Children's Hospital of Hudson County	NJ
NJ-CHRIST	Christ Hospital	NJ
NJ-CHSFULD	Capital Health System/Fuld Campus	NJ
NJ-CHSMRCER	Capital Health System/Mercer Campus	NJ
NJ-CLARMAAS	Clara Maass Medical Center	NJ
NJ-COMMED	Community Medical Center	NJ
NJ-COOPRUMC	Cooper University Hospital	NJ
NJ-DEBRAHLC	Deborah Heart and Lung Center	NJ
NJ-EASTORNG	East Orange General Hospital	NJ
NJ-ENGLWOOD	Englewood Hospital and Medical Center	NJ
NJ-ESSEXCO	Essex County Hospital Center	NJ
NJ-GRYSTPSY	Greystone Park Psychiatric Hospital	NJ
NJ-HACKNSK	Hackensack University Medical Center	NJ
NJ-HAGEDORN	Hagedorn Psychiatric Hospital	NJ
NJ-HAMPTBHC	Hampton Behavioral Health Center	NJ
NJ-HCKTSTWN	Hackettstown Regional Medical Center	NJ
NJ-HCMEADPS	Hudson County Meadowview Psychiatric Hospital	NJ
NJ-HLTHSRE	HealthSouth Rehabilitation Hospital of New Jersey	NJ
NJ-HOBUNIMC	Hoboken University Medical Center	NJ
NJ-HOLYNAME	Holy Name Hospital	NJ
NJ-HUNTRDN	Hunterdon Medical Center	NJ
NJ-JFKJHNSN	JFK Johnson Rehabilitation Institute	NJ
NJ-JFKMED	JFK Medical Center	NJ
NJ-JRSYCITY	Jersey City Medical Center	NJ
NJ-JRSYSHMC	Jersey Shore University Medical Center	NJ
NJ-KENEDYHS	Kennedy Health System	NJ
NJ-KIMBALL	Kimball Medical Center	NJ
NJ-KMHCHRRY	Kennedy Health System/Cherry Hill Campus	NJ
NJ-KMHSTRAT	Kennedy Memorial Hospital-University Medical Ctr	NJ
NJ-KMHTURNV	Kennedy Health Systems/Washington Township	NJ
NJ-KNDRMRRS	Kindred Hospital New Jersey-Morris County	NJ
NJ-KSLRSADB	Kessler Institute for Rehabilitation	NJ
NJ-KSLRWELK	Kessler Institute for Rehabilitation Welkind Facility	NJ
NJ-KSLRWEST	Kessler Institute for Rehabilitation West Orange	NJ
NJ-LIBERTY	Liberty Rehabilitation Institute	NJ
NJ-LIBTYHCS	Liberty Health Care System	NJ
NJ-LOURDEHS	Lourdes Health System	NJ
NJ-LOURDMED	Lourdes Medical Center of Burlington County	NJ
NJ-MATHENY	The Matheny School and Hospital	NJ
NJ-MEADWLND	Meadowlands Hospital Medical Center	NJ
NJ-MEDIPLEX	Marlton Rehabilitation Hospital	NJ
NJ-MEMSALEM	Memorial Hospital of Salem County	NJ
NJ-MERIDNHS	Meridian Health System	NJ
NJ-MMHKEMBL	Morristown Memorial Hospital/Mt. Kemble Division	NJ
NJ-MONMOUTH	Monmouth Medical Center	NJ
NJ-MORRISTN	Morristown Medical Center	NJ
NJ-MTCARMEL	Mt. Carmel Guild/ Behavioral Health System	NJ
NJ-MTNSIDE	HackensackUMC Mountainside	NJ
NJ-NWRKBETH	Newark Beth Israel Medical Center	NJ
NJ-NWTNMEM	Newton Medical Center	NJ
NJ-OCEANMC	Ocean Medical Center	NJ
NJ-OURLADY	Our Lady of Lourdes Medical Center	NJ
NJ-OVERLOOK	Overlook Medical Center	NJ
NJ-PALISADE	Palisades Medical Center	NJ
NJ-RAMAPO	Ramapo Ridge Psychiatric Hospital	NJ
NJ-RBAYOLDB	Raritan Bay Medical Center/Old Bridge Division	NJ
NJ-RBAYPERT	Raritan Bay Medical Center/Perth Amboy Division	NJ
NJ-RHBHSPSJ	The Rehabilitation Hospital of South Jersey	NJ
NJ-RHBHTNTN	The Rehabilitation Hospital of Tinton Falls	NJ
NJ-RIVERVW	Riverview Medical Center	NJ
NJ-RUNNELLS	Runnells Specialized Hospital of Union County	NJ
NJ-RWJHLTS	Robert Wood Johnson Health System	NJ
NJ-RWJUBRUN	Robert Wood Johnson University Hospital	NJ
NJ-RWJUHAM	Robert Wood Johnson University Hospital Hamilton	NJ
NJ-RWJURAH	Robert Wood Johnson University Hospital at Rahway	NJ
NJ-SELSPNNJ	Select Specialty Hospital-Northeast New Jersey	NJ
NJ-SHOREMEM	Shore Memorial Hospital	NJ
NJ-SHOREREH	Shore Rehabilitation Institute	NJ
NJ-SJERSYHS	South Jersey Health System	NJ
NJ-SJHREGMC	SJH Regional Medical Center	NJ
NJ-SJRSYELM	SJH Elmer Hospital	NJ
NJ-SOCEANCO	Southern Ocean County Medical Center	NJ
NJ-SOLARIHS	Solaris Health System	NJ
NJ-SOMERSET	Somerset Medical Center	NJ
NJ-SPCLKIMB	Specialty Hospital at Kimball	NJ
NJ-SPCLMONM	Specialty Hospital at Monmouth	NJ
NJ-STBARBHC	St. Barnabas Behavioral Health Center	NJ
NJ-STBARBHS	St. Barnabas Health Care System	NJ
NJ-STBARNMC	St. Barnabas Medical Center	NJ
NJ-STCLRBOO	St. Clare's Hospital-Boonton	NJ
NJ-STCLRDEN	St. Clare's Hospital-Denville Campus	NJ
NJ-STCLRDOV	St. Clare's Hospital-Dover	NJ
NJ-STCLRSUS	Saint Clare's Hospital-Sussex	NJ
NJ-STFRNMED	St. Francis Medical Center	NJ
NJ-STJOSHCS	St. Joseph's Health Care System	NJ
NJ-STJOSHOS	St. Joseph's Regional Medical Center	NJ
NJ-STLAWRN	St. Lawrence Rehabilitation Center	NJ
NJ-STMICHL	Saint Michael's Medical Center	NJ
NJ-STMRYPAS	St. Mary's Hospital	NJ
NJ-STPETER	St. Peter's University Hospital	NJ
NJ-SUMOAKSH	Summit Oaks Hospital	NJ
NJ-TRENTPSY	Trenton Psychiatric Hospital	NJ
NJ-TRINIJSC	Trinitas Regional Medical Center-Jersey Street	NJ
NJ-TRININPC	Trinitas Regional Medical Center-New Point Campus	NJ
NJ-TRINIWSC	Trinitas Regional Medical Center-Williamson Street	NJ
NJ-UMDNJ	University Hospital	NJ
NJ-UNDRWD	Inspira Health (Underwood-Memorial Hospital)	NJ
NJ-UNIVBHC	University Behavioral Health Care	NJ
NJ-UNVMCPRN	University Medical Center of Princeton at Plainsboro	NJ
NJ-VAEASTOR	VA New Jersey Health Care System-East Orange	NJ
NJ-VALLEY	The Valley Hospital	NJ
NJ-VALLEYHS	Valley Health System	NJ
NJ-VALYONS	VA New Jersey Health Care System at Lyons	NJ
NJ-VANJHCS	VA New Jersey Health Care System	NJ
NJ-VIRTBERL	Virtua Berlin	NJ
NJ-VIRTMARL	Virtua Marlton	NJ
NJ-VIRTMHBC	Virtua Memorial	NJ
NJ-VIRTUAHS	Virtua Health System	NJ
NJ-VIRTVOOR	Virtua Voorhees	NJ
NJ-WARREN	Warren Hospital	NJ
NJ-WAYNEGEN	St. Joseph's Wayne Hospital	NJ
NJ-WESTHDSN	West Hudson Division of Clara Maass Medical Center	NJ
NJ-WOODBRDG	Woodbridge Developmental Center	NJ
NY-ALBANY	Albany Medical Center Hospital	NY
NY-ARDNHILL	Orange Regional Medical Center	NY
NY-BENEDCTN	HealthAlliance Hospital-Mary's Ave Campus	NY
NY-BETHKING	Mount Sinai-Beth Israel Brooklyn	NY
NY-BETHPETR	Mount Sinai Beth Israel	NY
NY-BLVUENYU	Bellevue Hospital Center-NYU Medical Center	NY
NY-BONSECRS	Bon Secours Community Hospital	NY
NY-BRKLNDWN	The Brooklyn Hospital Center/Downtown Campus	NY
NY-BRNXLCON	Bronx-Lebanon Hospital Center/Concourse Division	NY
NY-BRNXLFUL	Bronx-Lebanon Hospital Center/Fulton Division	NY
NY-BRNXVAMC	James J. Peters VA Medical Center	NY
NY-BROOKDAL	Brookdale University Hospital and Medical Center	NY
NY-CABRINI	Cabrini Medical Center	NY
NY-CHLDCOPR	Morgan Stanley Children's Hosp-Columbia Pres/ NY	NY
NY-CHMONTEF	The Children's Hospital at Montefiore	NY
NY-CMCSTMRY	Saint Vincent Catholic Med Ctrs- St. Mary's Brooklyn	NY
NY-CMCSTVNY	St. Vincent Hospital & Medical Center of New York	NY
NY-CMCSTVSI	Richmond University Medical Center	NY
NY-CMNTYMEM	Community Memorial Hospital, Inc.	NY
NY-CONEYISL	Coney Island Hospital	NY
NY-CROUSE	Crouse Hospital	NY
NY-DCTRSTAT	Staten Island University Hospital/Concord Site	NY
NY-ELMHRST	Elmhurst Hospital Center	NY
NY-FLUSHNG	Flushing Hospital Medical Center	NY
NY-FRANKLIN	Franklin Hospital-North Shore/LIJ Health System	NY
NY-GDSAMMC	Good Samaritan Hospital Medical Center	NY
NY-GOODSAM	Good Samaritan Hospital	NY
NY-HARLEM	Harlem Hospital Center	NY

Code Table: Hospitals

Code	Hospital	State
NY-HELNHAYS	Helen Hayes Hospital	NY
NY-HIGHLND	Highland Hospital	NY
NY-JACOBIMC	Jacobi Medical Center	NY
NY-JAMAICA	Jamaica Hospital Medical Center	NY
NY-JTORTHO	NYU Langone Medical Center-Hospital Joint Diseases	NY
NY-KINGSCO	Kings County Hospital Center	NY
NY-KINGSTON	HealthAlliance Hospital-Broadway Campus	NY
NY-KNGBKJEW	Kingsbrook Jewish Medical Center	NY
NY-LDYLORDS	Our Lady of Lourdes Memorial Hospital, Inc.	NY
NY-LDYMRCY	Montefiore Medical Center-North Division	NY
NY-LENOXHLL	North Shore/LIJ Lenox Hill Hospital	NY
NY-LICOLLGE	Suny Downstate at Long Island College Hospital	NY
NY-LIJEWSH	Long Island Jewish Medical Center	NY
NY-LINCOLN	Lincoln Medical & Mental Health Center	NY
NY-LUTHERN	Lutheran Medical Center	NY
NY-MAIMONMC	Maimonides Medical Center	NY
NY-MANHEYE	Manhattan Eye, Ear & Throat Hospital	NY
NY-MARGRTVL	Margaretville Hospital	NY
NY-METHODST	The New York Methodist Hospital	NY
NY-METROHOS	Metropolitan Hospital Center	NY
NY-MNTFMOSE	Montefiore Medical Center-Moses Division	NY
NY-MNTFWEIL	Montefiore Medical Center-Weiler Einstein Division	NY
NY-MRCYRKVL	Mercy Medical Center-Rockville Center	NY
NY-MTSINAI	The Mount Sinai Hospital	NY
NY-MTSINYHS	Mount Sinai/NYU Health System	NY
NY-MTSNAIQN	The Mount Sinai Hospital of Queens	NY
NY-MTVERNON	Montefiore Mount Vernon	NY
NY-NASSAUMC	Nassau University Medical Center	NY
NY-NRTHCBRX	North Central Bronx Hospital	NY
NY-NRTHGEN	North General Hospital	NY
NY-NSUHFORS	Forest Hills Hospital-North Shore-LIJ Health System	NY
NY-NSUHMANH	North Shore University Hospital-NS/LIJ Health Sys	NY
NY-NYACKHOS	Nyack Hospital	NY
NY-NYCOMBRK	New York Community Hospital of Brooklyn	NY
NY-NYEYEINF	New York Eye & Ear Infirmary of Mount Sinai	NY
NY-NYHQUEEN	New York-Presbyterian/Queens	NY
NY-NYPRESHS	New York Presbyterian Healthcare System	NY
NY-NYUDWNTN	New York Presbyterian/Lower Manhattan Hospital	NY
NY-NYURUSK	NYU Medical Center-Rusk Institute of Rehab Med	NY
NY-NYUTISCH	Tisch Hospital-NYU Langone Medical Center	NY
NY-PENINSUL	Peninsula Hospital Center	NY
NY-PHELPMEM	Phelps Memorial Hospital Center	NY
NY-PRSBALLN	New York Presbyterian Hospital/The Allen Hospital	NY
NY-PRSBCOLU	New York Presbyterian Hospital/Columbia Univ Med	NY
NY-PRSBWEIL	New York Presbyterian Hospital/ Weill Cornell Med	NY
NY-PRSBWEST	New York Presbyterian Hosp-Payne Whitney Westch	NY
NY-PUTNAMHC	Putnam Hospital Center	NY
NY-RCKCHPSY	Rockland Children's Psychiatric Center	NY
NY-ROCKLPSY	Rockland Psychiatric Center	NY
NY-SAMARIMC	Samaritan Medical Center	NY
NY-SCHNCHIL	Cohen Children's Medical Center of New York	NY
NY-SLOANKET	Memorial Sloan-Kettering Cancer Center	NY
NY-SLRLUKES	Mount Sinai St. Luke's	NY
NY-SLRRSVLT	Mount Sinai Roosevelt	NY
NY-SOUTHAMP	Southampton Hospital	NY
NY-SOUTHNAS	South Nassau Communities Hospital	NY
NY-SOUTHPSY	South Beach Psychiatric Center	NY
NY-SPCLSURG	Hospital for Special Surgery	NY
NY-SSWESTCH	Montefiore New Rochelle	NY
NY-STANTHNY	St. Anthony Community Hospital	NY
NY-STATNRTH	Staten Island University Hospital/North Site	NY
NY-STATNSTH	Staten Island University Hospital/South Site	NY
NY-STBARNAB	SBH Health System	NY
NY-STCLARE	Ellis Hospital/McClellan Campus	NY
NY-STFRNCIS	MidHudson Regional Hospital of Westchester MedCtr	NY
NY-STJOSHHC	St. Joseph's Hospital Health Center	NY
NY-STLAWPSY	St. Lawrence Psychiatric Center	NY
NY-STONYBRK	Stony Brook University Hospital	NY
NY-STPETERS	St. Peter's Hospital	NY
NY-STRNGMEM	Strong Memorial Hospital-Univ of Rochester Med Ctr	NY
NY-SUMMTPRK	Summit Park Hospital	NY
NY-SUNYBRKL	University Hospital of Brooklyn/SUNY	NY
NY-UHSBINGH	United Health Services -Binghamton General Hospital	NY
NY-UNTYPKRG	Unity Health System/Unity Hospital	NY
NY-UPSTSYRA	Upstate University Hospital	NY
NY-VABRKLYN	VA New York Harbor Health Care System-Brooklyn	NY
NY-VAHARBOR	VA New York Harbor Health Care System-New York	NY
NY-VANORTH	Veterans Affairs Medical Center Northport	NY
NY-VASSAR	Vassar Brothers Medical Center	NY
NY-VIAROCHS	Rochester General Hospital	NY
NY-VICTORY	Victory Memorial Hospital	NY
NY-WESTCHMC	Westchester Medical Center	NY
NY-WESTCHSQ	Montefiore- Westchester Square Medical Center	NY
NY-WHITEPLN	White Plains Hospital Center	NY
NY-WINTHROP	Winthrop University Hospital	NY
NY-WOODHULL	Woodhull Medical & Mental Health Center	NY
NY-WYCKOFF	Wyckoff Heights Medical Center	NY
NY-YONKRSGH	St. John's Riverside Hospital-ParkCare Pavilion	NY
OH-CHLDHOSP	Cincinnati Children's Hospital Medical Center	OH
OH-CLERMONT	Mercy Hospital Clermont	OH
OH-FHNRTHSD	Northside Medical Center	OH
OH-OSUMEDC	Ohio State University Medical Center	OH
OH-UNIVCINC	University of Cincinnati Medical Center	OH
PA-ABINGTON	Abington Memorial Hospital	PA
PA-ARHBUCKS	Aria Health - Bucks County Campus	PA
PA-ARHTRRDL	Aria Health-Torresdale Campus	PA
PA-BRYNMAWR	Bryn Mawr Hospital	PA
PA-CARLSLE	Carlisle Regional Medical Center	PA
PA-CHESTRCT	The Chester County Hospital	PA
PA-CHILDHOS	The Children's Hospital of Philadelphia	PA
PA-CHLHSPIT	Children's Hospital of Pittsburgh of UPMC	PA
PA-CHOPHIL	The Children's Hospital of Philadelphia	PA
PA-CHSTNHIL	Chestnut Hill Hospital	PA
PA-CROZER	Crozer Chester Medical Center	PA
PA-DUBOIS	Dubois Regional Medical Center	PA
PA-EASTON	Easton Hospital	PA
PA-ENSTEIN	Albert Einstein Medical Center	PA
PA-EPHRATA	Ephrata Community Hospital	PA
PA-FOXCAN	Fox Chase Cancer Center	PA
PA-FRIENDS	Friends Hospital	PA
PA-GRNDVIEW	Grand View Hospital	PA
PA-GSNGER	Geisinger Medical Center	PA
PA-GSNGWYVL	Geisinger Wyoming Valley	PA
PA-HHNMANN	Hahnemann University Hospital	PA
PA-HLYRDMER	Holy Redemer Hospital & Medical Center	PA
PA-JEANES	Jeanes Hospital	PA
PA-JRSYSHOR	Jersey Shore Hospital	PA
PA-LHVLYCED	Lehigh Valley Hospital Cedar Crest	PA
PA-LNKNAU	Lankenau Medical Center	PA
PA-LWBUCK	Lower Bucks Hospital	PA
PA-MGWMNS	Magee-Womens Hospital of UPMC	PA
PA-MIDVLY	Mid Valley Hospital	PA
PA-MRCYFTZG	Mercy Fitzgerald Hospital	PA
PA-MRCYPHIL	Mercy Philadelphia Hospital	PA
PA-MRCYSUB	Mercy Suburban Hospital	PA
PA-NZRTH	Nazareth Hospital	PA
PA-PENNHOSP	Pennsylvania Hospital	PA
PA-PNPRSBYT	Penn Presbyterian Medical Center	PA
PA-PNRTTNHS	Penn Medicine at Rittenhouse	PA
PA-PNSTHRSH	Penn State Hershey Medical Center	PA
PA-POCONO	Pocono Medical Center	PA
PA-READING	The Reading Hospital and Medical Center	PA
PA-RIDDLE	Riddle Memorial Hospital	PA
PA-RXBRGH	Roxborough Memorial Hospital	PA
PA-SCRDHRT	Sacred Heart Hospital	PA
PA-STCHRIS	St. Christopher's Hospital for Children	PA
PA-STJOBERN	St. Joseph Medical Center - Bern Township	PA
PA-STJORDNG	St. Joseph Medical Center	PA
PA-STLKBTHL	St. Luke's Hospital & Health Network - Bethlehem	PA
PA-STMARY	St. Mary Medical Center	PA
PA-TAYLOR	Taylor Hospital	PA
PA-TJCNTR	Thomas Jefferson University Hospital-Center City	PA
PA-TJFMETHD	Thomas Jefferson Univ Hosp/Methodist Hospital	PA
PA-TJHSP	Thomas Jefferson University Hospital	PA
PA-TMPCHLD	Temple University Children's Medical Center	PA
PA-TMPHOSP	Temple University Hospital	PA
PA-UPMCBDFD	UPMC Bedford Memorial	PA
PA-UPMCMRCY	UPMC Mercy Hospital	PA
PA-UPMCPHL	Hospital of the University of Pennsylvania	PA
PA-UPMCPRES	UPMC Presbyterian Hospital	PA
PA-VAPHIL	Philadelphia VA Medical Center	PA
PA-WARRNGEN	Warren General Hospital	PA
PA-WILLPORT	Williamsport Hospital Medical Center	PA
PA-WILLSEYE	Wills Eye Institute	PA
PA-WPSYCH	Western Psychiatric Institute and Clinic of UPMC	PA
PA-YORK	York Hospital	PA
RI-MEMHOSRI	Memorial Hospital of Rhode Island	RI
RI-MIRIAM	The Miriam Hospital	RI
RI-RIHOSPTL	Rhode Island Hospital	RI
RI-SJFATIMA	St. Joseph's Health Serv of R. I./Our Lady of Fatima	RI
VT-FAHCMCHV	University of Vermont Medical Center	VT
VT-SPRNGFLD	Springfield Hospital	VT

Section 1 Physicians by Name

Physicians Alphabetically by Name with Practice Addresses, Medical School and Specialties

New Jersey
Section 1

Physicians Alphabetically by Name with Practice Addresses, Medical School and Specialties

Physicians by Name and Address

Aamir, Tajwar, MD {1598069692} Pedtrc(87,PAK20)
+ Lotus Medical Center
40 Fuld Street/Suite 307   Trenton, NJ 08638   (609)278-9700   Fax (609)278-9744

Aaron, Bernard M., MD {1962475566} Gastrn, IntrMd(69,NY08)<NJ-JRSYSHMC, NJ-OCEANMC>
+ Atlantic Coast Gastroenterology
1640 Route 88 West/Suite 202   Brick, NJ 08724   (732)458-8300   Fax (732)458-8529
+ Atlantic Coast Gastroenterology
1944 Corlies Avenue/Suite 205   Neptune, NJ 07753   (732)458-8300   Fax (732)776-8059
+ RWJ Gastro & Hepatology
125 Paterson Street/CAB 5100B   New Brunswick, NJ 08724   (732)235-6994   Fax (732)235-7792

Aaron, Michael R., DO {1336129071} CdvDis, IntrMd(86,NY75)<NJ-JRSYSHMC, NJ-COMMED>
+ Shore Heart Group, P.A.
1820 State Route 33/Suite 4-B   Neptune, NJ 07753   (732)776-8500   Fax (732)776-8946
+ Shore Heart Group, P.A.
35 Beaverson Boulevard/Suite 9-B   Brick, NJ 08723   (732)776-8500   Fax (732)262-4317
+ Shore Heart Group, P.A.
9 Mule Road/Suite E-3   Toms River, NJ 07753   (732)281-1101   Fax (732)281-1105

Aarons, William, Jr., MD {1972551240} SrgC&R, SrgVas, Surgry(69,PA09)<NJ-ACMCITY, NJ-ACMCMAIN>
+ AtlantiCare Regional Medical Center/City Campus
1925 Pacific Avenue/Surgery   Atlantic City, NJ 08401   (609)345-4000
+ AtlantiCare Regional Med Ctr/Mainland
65 West Jimmie Leeds Road/Surgery   Pomona, NJ 08240   (609)652-1000

Aasmaa, Sirike T., DO {1861549925} IntrMd(88,NJ75)<NJ-MORRISTN>
+ 170 Changebridge Road/Suite D-1
Montville, NJ 07045   (973)575-5150   Fax (973)575-5271

Abadi, Bilal, MD {1104168814} Anesth
+ Newark Beth Israel Pulmonary Critical Care
201 Lyons Avenue   Newark, NJ 07112   (201)655-5712

Abadir, John Sobhi, MD {1891937298} Anesth(05,DC02)
+ 408 Digaetano Terrace
West Orange, NJ 07052

Abass-Shereef, Jeneba, MD {1679960942} EmrgMd
+ Jersey City Medical Center Emergency
355 Grand Street   Jersey City, NJ 07302   (201)915-2200

Abbas, Muhammad Ali, MD {1396955951} Psychy, PsyAdd(99,PAK10)
+ Jersey Shore Psychiatric Services
4 Calloway Street/Apt. 302   Howell, NJ 07731   (848)482-7764
+ 1011 Bond Street
Asbury Park, NJ 07712   (732)869-2768

Abbas, Shahida M., MD {1023104098} IntrMd(82,PAK11)
+ 1530 Route 88/Suite B
Brick, NJ 08724   (732)836-0500   Fax (732)836-0502

Abbasi, Arshia, MD {1366756553} Nephro, IntrMd
+ New Bridge Medical Center
230 East Ridgewood Avenue/Nephrology   Paramus, NJ 07652   (201)967-4000

Abbasi, Danish P., MD {1629466610} IntHos<NJ-ACMCITY>
+ AtlantiCare Regional Medical Center/City Campus
1925 Pacific Avenue   Atlantic City, NJ 08401   (609)652-1000

Abbasi, Faheem A., MD {1710047295} PhyMPain, PainMd, IntrMd(88,PAK15)
+ New Jersey Pain Spine & Sports Associates
2050 Route 27/Suite 105   North Brunswick, NJ 08902   (732)565-3777   Fax (732)746-0223
+ New Jersey Pain Spine & Sports Associates
601 Ewing Street/Suite C-3   Princeton, NJ 08540   (732)565-3777   Fax (732)746-0223
+ New Jersey Pain Spine & Sports Associates
1255 Whitehorse Mercerville Rd   Hamilton, NJ 08902   (609)688-6866   Fax (732)746-0223

Abbasi, Muhammad Rashid, MD {1245349638} MedOnc, IntrMd, Hemato(90,PAK11)<NJ-MORRISTN>
+ Oncology & Hematology Specialists, PA
23 Pocono Road/Suite 100   Denville, NJ 07834   (973)316-1701   Fax (973)316-1708
+ Oncology & Hematology Specialists, PA
100 Madison Avenue/Suite C3402   Morristown, NJ 07960   (973)316-1701   Fax (973)267-2550

Abbasi, Naheed R., MD {1487851390} Dermat(03,CA02)
+ Summit Medical Group-Berkeley Heights Campus
1 Diamond Hill Road   Berkeley Heights, NJ 07922   (908)273-4300   Fax (908)790-6576

Abbasi, Shahed, MD {1477810752} IntrMd<NJ-UMDNJ>
+ University Hospital
150 Bergen Street/H245   Newark, NJ 07103   (973)972-5672   Fax (973)972-0365

Abbasi, Tareef M., MD {1427139617} EmrgMd, IntrMd(83,JOR01)<NJ-STJOSHOS>
+ Abbasi Medical Group
1300 Main Avenue/Suite 2-D   Clifton, NJ 07011   (973)928-5500

Abbassi, Saeed R., MD {1114926664} Pedtrc(72,IRQ01)<NJ-HACKNSK, NJ-PALISADE>
+ 7827 Bergenline Avenue
North Bergen, NJ 07047   (201)868-1950   Fax (201)868-5844

Abbassi, Samih R., MD {1750380358} EmrgMd, IntrMd(71,IRAQ)
+ 372 Valley Road
West Orange, NJ 07052   (973)669-0010   Fax (973)736-8355
Sabbassi@aol.com

Abbate, Kariann Ferguson, MD {1548429582} CdvDis, IntrMd(07,PA02)<NJ-VALLEY>
+ The Valley Hospital
223 North Van Dien Avenue/Cardiology   Ridgewood, NJ 07450   (201)447-2014

Abbate, Marc Anthony, MD {1316911845} Dermat(98,NJ06)<NJ-MTNSIDE>
+ The Dermatology Group, P.C.
60 Pompton Avenue   Verona, NJ 07044   (973)571-2121   Fax (973)571-2126
marcabbate@yahoo.com
+ The Dermatology Group, P.C.
44 Route 23 North/Suite 213   Riverdale, NJ 07457   (973)571-2121   Fax (973)839-5751
+ The Dermatology Group, P.C.
30 West Century Road/Suite 320   Paramus, NJ 07044   (973)571-2121   Fax (201)986-0702

Abbate, Maribel, MD {1871769489} Psychy(99,NJ06)
+ 300 Main Street/#508
Madison, NJ 07940   (973)847-2120   Fax (973)847-2121

Abbey, Genevieve Nguyen, MD {1962678474} RadDia
+ Hackensack Radiology Group, P.A.
30 Prospect Avenue   Hackensack, NJ 07601   (201)996-2200   Fax (201)336-8451

Abbott-Fiedler, Vicky L., MD {1881673903} NnPnMd, Pedtrc, IntrMd(80,PA07)<NJ-SJHREGMC>
+ SJH Regional Medical Center
1505 West Sherman Avenue/MSO-Box 104   Vineland, NJ 08360   (856)641-8100   Fax (856)641-7650

Abboud, Somaya M., MD {1326089004} IntrMd(86,IRAQ)
+ 15 Oak Terrace
West Orange, NJ 07052   (973)736-0687   Fax (973)325-0427
+ Center for Advanced Medicine
623 Eagle Rock Avenue/Suite 1   West Orange, NJ 07052   (973)736-2100

Abboushi, Hilal Amer-Omar, MD {1548378029} IntrMd, EmrgMd(77,SPA03)
+ 482 North 12th Street
Newark, NJ 07107   (973)484-5887

Abbud, Ziad A., MD {1740373489} IntrMd, CdvDis, IntCrd(91,LEB03)<NJ-BAYSHORE, NJ-JRSYSHMC>
+ American Heart Center PC
1900 Corlies Avenue State Rout   Neptune, NJ 07753   (732)663-1123   Fax (732)663-1179
+ One Bethany Road/Bldg. 6 Suite 97
Hazlet, NJ 07730   (732)663-1123   Fax (732)847-3261

Abdeen, Yazan M., MD {1679983605} CritCr
+ St. Michael's Medical Center
111 Central Avenue   Newark, NJ 07102   (973)877-5485

Abdel Fatgah, Nail S., MD {1124071782} PulDis, IntrMd(84,JOR01)
+ Belmont Medical Center
276 Prospect Street   East Orange, NJ 07017   (973)678-8001   Fax (973)678-2121
+ Belmont Medical Center
303 Belmont Avenue   Belleville, NJ 07109   (973)678-8001   Fax (973)751-8757

Abdel-Megid, Ahmed Mahmoud, MD {1134313745} Rheuma, IntrMd(95,EGY03)
+ Rheumatology Center New Jersey
27 Monroe Street   Bridgewater, NJ 08807   (908)722-5380   Fax (908)685-7501
+ 144 Elizabeth Avenue
Iselin, NJ 08830   (908)722-5380   Fax (908)685-7501

Abdelaal, Hany Mohamed, DO {1083764831}(93,NY75)
+ 20 Aberdeen Drive
Old Bridge, NJ 08857   (732)605-1615

Abdelaal, Sameh M., MD {1770855652} IntrMd(88,EGY05)
+ Internal Medicine Faculty Practice
101 Old Short Hills Road/Suite 106   West Orange, NJ 07052   (973)322-6256   Fax (973)322-6241

Abdelfadil, Ahmed Aly, MD {1023072709} SlpDis, PulDis, IntrMd(88,EGY03)<NY-DCTRSTAT, NJ-RIVERVW>
+ North East Insomnia & Sleep Medicine
68 White Street   Red Bank, NJ 07701   (732)936-0009
info@neinsomniasleepmedicine.com

Abdelhadi, Samir I., DO {1689858011} PulCCr(05,NY75)
+ Advanced Cardiovascular Interventions, PA
20 Prospect Avenue/Suite 615   Hackensack, NJ 07601   (201)265-5700   Fax (551)996-0774

Abdelhak, Yaakov Eliezer, MD {1730156803} ObsGyn, MtFtMd(93,NY08)<NJ-HACKNSK>
+ Integrative Obstetrics
358 Beech Street   Hackensack, NJ 07601   (201)487-8600   Fax (201)487-8601
+ Integrative Obstetrics
21 McWilliams Place   Jersey City, NJ 07302   (201)487-8600   Fax (844)886-6072

Abdeljawad, Mohammad R., MD {1487917365} IntHos<NJ-VIRTVOOR>
+ Virtua Voorhees
100 Bowman Drive   Voorhees, NJ 08043   (856)247-2594   Fax (856)247-2597

Abdelmalek, Mark A., MD {1972543155} Dermat(02)
+ Dermatology Associates of South Jersey
715 Fellowship Road/Suite B   Mount Laurel, NJ 08054   (856)206-0201   Fax (856)206-0209

Abdelmalek, Moheb S., MD {1699776179} IntrMd, EmrgMd(78,EGY04)<NJ-RWJUBRUN, NJ-STPETER>
+ Drs. Abdelmalek and Habib
E5 Brier Hill Court   East Brunswick, NJ 08816   (732)698-1331   Fax (732)698-1379

Abdelmessieh, Nawal I., MD {1194990887} IntrMd(73,EGY16)
+ 16 Emerald Road
Robbinsville, NJ 08691

Abdelrahman, Badreldin, MD {1538428677}
+ Jersey City Medical Center NICU
355 Grand Street   Jersey City, NJ 07302   (201)915-2330   Fax (201)915-2705

Abdelshahed, Mina, MD {1447577457}
+ Union County Orthopaedic Group
210 West St. Georges Avenue/PO Box 330   Linden, NJ 07036   (908)486-1111   Fax (908)583-1034

Abdelshahid, Mounir Y., MD {1780872838} IntrMd(83,EGY05)<NJ-CLARMAAS>
+ SM Medical, LLC
135 Bloomfield Avenue   Bloomfield, NJ 07003   (862)213-0033   Fax (862)213-0037

Abdi, Zahra Jabeen, MD {1912907460} IntrMd(97,INA7A)
+ 100 Day Place/Suite 104/Wick Plaza 1
Edison, NJ 08817   (732)572-2233   Fax (732)572-2365

Abdo-Matkiwsky, May D., DO {1306887708} IntrMd, OncHem(00,NY75)<NJ-NWTNMEM>
+ Premier Health Associates
89 Sparta Avenue/Suite 130   Sparta, NJ 07871   (973)726-0005   Fax (973)726-4668

Abdollahi, Hamid, MD {1467640565} Surgry
+ The Plastic Surgery Ctr of NJ & Manhat
535 Sycamore Avenue   Shrewsbury, NJ 07702   (732)741-0970   Fax (732)747-2606

Abdu Nafi, Saladin A., MD {1124359864} FamMed(78,NJ06)
+ Essex County Correctional Facility
354 Doremus Avenue/Assistant   Newark, NJ 07105   (973)274-7500   Fax (973)274-6996
Pemgchick06@optonline.com

Abdul Shafi, Samya B., MD {1992813398} InfDis, IntrMd(82,JOR01)
+ 1524 Route 23 North
Butler, NJ 07405   (973)692-9773

Abdulghani, Ahsan Arshad, MD {1881670891} Grtrcs, IntrMd(95,EGY03)<NJ-KMHTURNV>
+ Turnersville Internal Medicine & Geriatrics
4991 Route 42/Suite 8   Turnersville, NJ 08012   (856)740-9777   Fax (856)740-9990

Abdulla, Heba M., MD {1104024405} Dermat(05,NY08)<NY-VABRKLYN>
+ Medical & Cosmetic Dermatology Associates
841 Franklin Avenue/Suite 4   Franklin Lakes, NJ 07417   (201)644-0228   Fax (201)644-0229

Abdullah, Muhammad, MD {1265446405} IntrMd(88,PAK12)<NJ-NWRKBETH, NJ-STMICHL>
+ 239 Lafayette Street/Suite A
Newark, NJ 07105   (973)690-5555   Fax (973)690-5559

Abdulmasih, Yousef H., MD {1942221205} Pedtrc(85,ROMA)<NJ-STJOSHOS>
+ Totowa Pediatric Group, P.A.
290 Union Boulevard/Suite 2   Totowa, NJ 07512   (973)595-0600   Fax (973)595-0206
+ Totowa Pediatric Group, P.A.
400 West Blackwell Street   Dover, NJ 07801   (973)595-0600   Fax (973)989-3651

Abdulmassih, Sami, MD {1760777270} FamMed
+ North Jersey Health PA
502 Hamburg Turnpike/Suite 108   Wayne, NJ 07470   (973)942-5224   Fax (973)942-7443

Physicians by Name and Address

Abdy, Victor A., MD {1164446795} IntrMd(74,ITA17)<NJ-WAYNE-GEN>
+ 510 Hamburg Turnpike/Suite 201
Wayne, NJ 07470   (973)790-3232   Fax (973)942-8848

Abe, Minako, MD {1578635249} EmrgMd(98,NY48)<NY-SLRRSVLT>
+ EmCare
425 Jack Martin Boulevard   Brick, NJ 08724   (732)840-3380

Abed, Mary T., MD {1134185432} CdvDis, IntrMd(84,CA02)<NJ-CHILTON>
+ Total Cardiology Care
120 Franklin Street   Jersey City, NJ 07307   (201)216-9791   Fax (201)216-1362
+ Total Cardiology Care
2035 Hamburg Pike/Suite L   Wayne, NJ 07470   (201)216-9791   Fax (973)248-3455
+ Total Cardiology Care
150 Warren Street   Jersey City, NJ 07307   (201)216-9791   Fax (201)216-1362

Abedin, Naheed, MD {1922055870} Pedtrc, NnPnMd(90,BAN02)<NJ-CHSMRCER>
+ Capital Health System/Mercer Campus
446 Bellevue Avenue   Trenton, NJ 08618   (609)394-4000   Fax (609)394-4385

Abel, Carter Grant, MD {1558347229} SrgDer, DerMOH, SrgCsm(91,DC02)<NJ-HUNTRDN, NY-PRSBCOLU>
+ Abel Dermatology/Concourse at Beaverbrook
1465 State Route 31 South   Annandale, NJ 08801   (908)735-5100   Fax (908)735-0004
jeenadir@yahoo.com

Abel, David Michael, DO {1629362850}
+ Garden State Infectious Diseases Associates, P.A.
709 Haddonfield Berlin Road   Voorhees, NJ 08043   (856)566-3190   Fax (856)783-2193
davidab@pcom.edu

Abel, Mark, MD {1023082534} Dermat(70,NY03)
+ 465b Laurel Brook Drive
Brick, NJ 08724   (732)458-4075

Abel Boenerjous, Rebakah Sumalin, MD {1205161197} IntrMd
+ Salem Medical Group
95 Woodstown Road/Suite B   Swedesboro, NJ 08085   (856)832-4359   Fax (856)832-4381

Abeles, Gwen Dee, MD {1447222625} Dermat(93,NY47)
+ 236 Grand Avenue
Park Ridge, NJ 07656

Abella, Tara M., MD {1104051242} ObsGyn
+ West Essex Ob/Gyn Associates
200 South Orange Avenue/Suite 290   Livingston, NJ 07039   (973)740-1330   Fax (973)740-8998

Abella-Ramirez, Katherine, MD {1649624560} IntHos
+ AtlantiCare Hospitalist Program
1925 Pacific Avenue/8th Floor   Atlantic City, NJ 08401   (609)441-8146   Fax (609)441-8002

Abellana, Juan C., MD {1497796023} IntrMd(65,PHI08)
+ Princeton Health Medical & Surgical Associates
2 Centre Drive/Suite 200   Monroe, NJ 08831   (609)395-2470   Fax (609)860-5288
+ Princeton HealthCare Medical Associates
11 Centre Drive/Suite A   Monroe Township, NJ 08831   (609)395-2470   Fax (609)860-5288

Abellana, Victoria D., MD {1336157635} IntrMd
+ Princeton Health Medical & Surgical Associates
2 Centre Drive/Suite 200   Monroe, NJ 08831   (609)395-2470   Fax (609)860-5288
+ Princeton Medicine
5 Plainsboro Road/Suite 300   Plainsboro, NJ 08536   (609)395-2470   Fax (609)853-7271

Abello Poblete, Maria Veronica Roman, MD {1366694416} Dermat(98,PHI01)
+ Poblete Dermatology
1601 Whitehorse-Mercerville Rd/Suite 2   Trenton, NJ 08619   (609)838-9040   Fax (609)838-9042

Abelow, Gerald G., MD {1578669099} Grtrcs, IntrMd(72,PA02)<NJ-VIRTMARL>
+ Cooper Physicians
1210 Brace Road/Suite 102   Cherry Hill, NJ 08034   (856)428-6616   Fax (856)428-4823

Abels, Jane I., MD {1275825887} Pedtrc(70,NY46)<NJ-NWRKBETH>
+ Newark Department of Health and Human Services
110 William Street   Newark, NJ 07102   (973)733-5300

Abels, Robert I., MD {1366734972} Allrgy, IntrMd(70,NY46)
+ 422 Linden Avenue
Westfield, NJ 07090   (908)654-7142

Abenante, Frank Andrew, MD {1730273418} Psychy(92,NJ06)<NJ-JRSYSHMC>
+ Jersey Shore Psychiatric Associates
3535 Route 66/Building 5/Suite D   Neptune, NJ 07753   (732)643-4350
cabenante@aol.com

Abend, David S., DO {1609806454} FamMed, OstMed, OthrSp(89,MO79)<NJ-VALLEY>
+ 550 Kinderkamack Road/Suite 203
Oradell, NJ 07649   (201)599-4100   Fax (201)599-4101

Abend, Paul J., DO {1922165349} PhysMd, FamMed(87,NJ75)
+ Consultants in Rehabilitation and Pain Medicine
16 Mount Bethel Road/Suite 322   Warren, NJ 07059   (908)226-1300   Fax (732)255-2164
+ Consultants in Rehabilitation and Pain Medicine
3830 Park Avenue/Suite 205   Edison, NJ 08820   (908)226-1300   Fax (908)226-1301

Aberbach, Eric Steven, MD {1679574982} Anesth, PainMd(90,OH41)<NJ-CHILTON>
+ Chilton Medical Center
97 West Parkway/Pain Mgmt/Anest   Pompton Plains, NJ 07444   (973)831-5140   Fax (973)831-5318

Abergel, Glen, MD {1093743924} InfDis
+ Rutgers- New Jersey Medical School
185 South Orange Avenue/InfectDis   Newark, NJ 07103   (805)389-1553
eabergel@yahoo.com

Aberger, Kate, MD {1821266719} EmrgMd(04,NJ05)<NJ-STJOSHOS>
+ St Joseph's Medical Center Emergency
703 Main Street   Paterson, NJ 07503   (973)754-2240   Fax (973)754-2249

Abesh, Daniel C., DO {1154301638} FamMed(82,ME75)<NJ-KMH-TURNV, NJ-VIRTBERL>
+ Jefferson Health Primary & Specialty Care
1A Regulus Drive   Turnersville, NJ 08012   (844)542-2273

Abesh, Jesse Susan, DO {1487067674} FamMGrtc
+ New Jersey Institute for Successful Aging
42 East Laurel Road/Suite 1800   Stratford, NJ 08084   (856)566-6843   Fax (856)566-6419

Abeshaus, Lisa Ellen, MD {1134194624} ObsGyn(90,NH01)
+ The Rubino Ob/Gyn Group
101 Old Short Hills Road/Suite 101   West Orange, NJ 07052   (973)736-1100   Fax (973)736-1834
+ The Rubino Ob/Gyn Group
33 Overlook Road   Summit, NJ 07901   (908)522-4558
+ The Rubino Ob/Gyn Group
731 Broadway   Bayonne, NJ 07052   (201)339-3300

Abessi, Hossein, MD {1841353794} Surgry(64,IRAN)
+ 502 Hamburg Turnpike/Suite 102
Wayne, NJ 07470   (973)595-7646   Fax (973)595-0141
+ St. Joseph's Regional Medical Center
703 Main Street   Paterson, NJ 07503   (973)754-2000

Abessi, Mitra, MD {1164502183} IntrMd(02,GRN01)
+ Whitehouse Station Family Medicine
263 Main Street/PO Box 128   Whitehouse Station, NJ 08889   (908)534-2249   Fax (908)534-6634

Abeysinghe, Manisha G., MD {1306807045} ObsGyn(00,OH40)
+ Advanced Obstetrics & Gynecology, LLC
4 Walter E. Foran Boulevard/Suite 302   Flemington, NJ 08822   (908)806-0080   Fax (908)806-8570
+ Advanced Obstetrics & Gynecology, LLC
1390 Route 22 West/Suite 104   Lebanon, NJ 08833   (908)806-0080   Fax (908)437-1227
+ Advanced Obstetrics & Gynecology, LLC
1100 Wescott Drive   Flemington, NJ 08822   (908)788-6488

Abich, Georgina, MD {1598775579} Pedtrc(68,SPA12)
+ 1024 East Jersey Street
Elizabeth, NJ 07201   (908)353-5920   Fax (908)353-3557

Abidi, Mutahir Ali, MD {1598780033} IntrMd, Rheuma(00,DMN01)
+ 206 Jack Martin Blvd./Suite C2
Brick, NJ 08724   (732)840-8402   Fax (732)840-8407

Abidi, Saiyid Manzoor, MD {1508816729} Nrolgy(64,INA05)<NJ-VIRTMARL, NJ-VIRTVOOR>
+ Neurological Regional Associates
504 Route 38 East   Maple Shade, NJ 08052   (856)866-0466   Fax (856)727-1483

Abiuso, Patrick D., Jr., MD {1700821873} IntrMd(75,NJ05)<NJ-VIRTMARL, NJ-VIRTVOOR>
+ Virtua Internal Medicine-Marlton
601 Route 73 North/Suite 101   Marlton, NJ 08053   (856)429-1910   Fax (856)396-0848

Abkari, Shashikala, MD {1831281799} Psychy(74,INA5B)<NY-SUMMTPRK>
+ 65 North Maple Avenue
Ridgewood, NJ 07450   (201)612-5222

Abkin, Alexander, MD {1770564742} Surgry, SrgLap, Barlat(86,RUSS)<NJ-MORRISTN, NJ-STBARNMC>
+ Advanced Laparoscopic Surgeons of Morris
83 Hanover Road/Suite 190   Florham Park, NJ 07932   (973)410-9700   Fax (973)410-9703
+ JFK for Life
98 James Street/Suite 212   Edison, NJ 08820   (732)343-7484

Abkin, Arkadiy, MD {1316928666} Anesth(90,RUS54)<NJ-MORRISTN>
+ Morristown Medical Center
100 Madison Avenue/Anesthesiology   Morristown, NJ 07962   (973)971-5000   Fax (201)943-8733

Ablaza, Valerie J., MD {1780798298} SrgPlstc(89,PA07)<NJ-STBARNMC>
+ Plastic Surgery Group
37 North Fullerton Avenue   Montclair, NJ 07042   (973)233-1933   Fax (973)233-1934

Abo, Marc N., MD {1003877267} Surgry(75,NY46)<NJ-WARREN>
+ 100 Coventry Drive
Phillipsburg, NJ 08865   (908)859-0034   Fax (908)859-3918

Abo, Stephen Michael, DO {1891717708} OncHem, IntrMd(01,ME75)<NJ-STMICHL>
+ St. Michael's Medical Center
111 Central Avenue/Hema Oncology   Newark, NJ 07102   (973)877-2829   Fax (973)877-2964

Aboody, Linda R., MD {1821177312} RadMam, Radiol, RadDia(85,NY01)<NY-SLOANKET>
+ Memorial Sloan-Kettering Cancer Center Basking Ridge
136 Mountain View Boulevard   Basking Ridge, NJ 07920   (908)542-3200   Fax (908)542-3220

Aboody, Ronald S., MD {1235109976} RadNro, RadDia(84,NY47)<NJ-STMRYPAS>
+ Diagnostic Radiology Associates of Northfield
772 Northfield Avenue   West Orange, NJ 07052   (973)325-0002   Fax (973)325-8140
+ Diagnostic Radiology Associates of Clifton
1339 Broad Street   Clifton, NJ 07013   (973)325-0002   Fax (973)778-4846
+ Diagnostic Radiology Associates of Cranford
25 South Union Avenue   Cranford, NJ 07052   (908)709-1323   Fax (908)709-1329

Abou Jaoude, Dany M., MD {1831334689} Grtrcs, IntHos(01,LEB05)<NY-STATNRTH, NH-LAKESREG>
+ Chilton Medical Center
97 West Parkway   Pompton Plains, NJ 07444   (973)831-5000

Abou-Rayan, Mohamed Magdy, MD {1639356447} PulDis<NJ-COOPRUMC>
+ Cooper University Hospital
One Cooper Plaza/Drrnce 222   Camden, NJ 08103   (856)842-3150   Fax (856)968-8418

Abou-Taleb, Ahmed K., MD {1962432799} Anesth, Otlryg, Rserch(65,EGY05)<NJ-CLARMAAS, NY-MNTFMOSE>
+ Clara Maass Medical Center
1 Clara Maass Drive/Hyperbaric Ctr   Belleville, NJ 07109   (973)450-2000

Aboujaoude, Rania Nassif, MD {1801839667} InfDis, IntrMd(99,LEB01)<NJ-DEBRAHLC>
+ Deborah Heart and Lung Center
200 Trenton Road/Inf Disease   Browns Mills, NJ 08015   (609)677-1046   Fax (609)677-1306

Abouzgheib, Wissam B., MD {1841246451} IntrMd
+ 3 Cooper Plaza/Suite 312
Camden, NJ 08103

Abraham, Alice, MD {1083857213} EnDbMt
+ Bergen Medical Alliance, P.A.
180 Engle Street   Englewood, NJ 07631   (201)567-2050   Fax (201)568-8936

Abraham, Aney M., MD {1275637720} IntrMd, PallCr(01,PA13)<NJ-COOPRUMC>
+ Cooper University Hospital
One Cooper Plaza/Dorrance 222   Camden, NJ 08103   (856)342-3150   Fax (856)968-8573

Abraham, Daniel J., MD {1861436867} Pedtrc, GenPrc(80,NJ05)<NJ-STPETER, NJ-RWJUBRUN>
+ Somerset Pediatric Group PA
155 Union Avenue   Bridgewater, NJ 08807   (908)725-1802   Fax (908)203-8825
+ Somerset Pediatric Group PA
2345 Lamington Road/Suite 101   Bedminster, NJ 07921   (908)725-1802   Fax (908)470-2845

Abraham, David, DO {1538597166} FamMed
+ 1301 South Lincoln Avenue/Apt 814
Vineland, NJ 08361   (856)405-1405   Fax (973)707-8084

Abraham, James V., MD {1770754632} CritCr, IntrMd, PulDis(80,INDI)<NJ-HOBUNIMC>
+ 124 Gregory Avenue/Suite 301
Passaic, NJ 07055   (973)777-8121   Fax (973)777-3622

Abraham, Maninder Arneja, MD {1194731414} IntrMd(91,INA70)
+ Emergency Medical Offices
651 West Mount Pleasant Avenue   Livingston, NJ 07039   (973)740-9396   Fax (973)251-1165

Abraham, Mark Barry, DO {1780603159} FamMed
+ Capital Health System/Fuld Campus
750 Brunswick Avenue   Trenton, NJ 08638   (609)815-7091

Abraham, Mathew John, MD {1083818512} PhysMd(06,MI07)<NY-BASSETT>
+ 3747 Church Road/Suite 110
Mount Laurel, NJ 08054

Physicians by Name and Address

Abraham, Rini S., MD {1285893321} Gastrn(NY03
 + Gastroenterology Associates of New Jersey
  88 Park Street Montclair, NJ 07042 (973)233-9559 Fax (973)233-9660
 + Gastroenterology Associates of New Jersey
  246 Hamburg Turnpike/Suite 203 Wayne, NJ 07470 (973)233-9559 Fax (862)336-9987

Abraham, Ruby, MD {1083620124} Psychy, IntrMd(87,INDI)
 + Center for Family Guidance, PC
  765 East Route 70/Building A-101 Marlton, NJ 08053 (856)797-4800 Fax (856)810-0110
 + Central Jersey Beharioral Health, LLC
  216 North Avenue East Cranford, NJ 07016 (856)797-4800 Fax (908)272-7502

Abraham, Shawn George, MD {1184940108} Rheuma
 + Arthritis, Rheumatic & Back Disease Associates
  2309 East Evesham Road/Suite 101 Voorhees, NJ 08043 (856)424-5005 Fax (856)424-4716

Abraham, Thanaa Nelly K., MD {1568442424} IntrMd(97,GRN01)
 + 882 Commons Way/Suite H
  Toms River, NJ 08755 (732)818-0808

Abraham, Vinod J., MD {1992793418} IntrMd(91,INDI)
 + Associates in Integrative Medicine
  27 Mountain Boulevard/Suite 9 Warren, NJ 07059 (908)769-9600 Fax (908)769-9610

Abrahim, Mena, DO {1457645707} OtgyFPIS(11,NY75)
 + ENT & Allergy Associates-Bridgewater
  245 US Highway 22/3rd Fl/Suite 300 Bridgewater, NJ 08807 (908)722-1022 Fax (908)722-2040

Abramov, Ronnen, DO {1508987892} AnesPain
 + Princeton Medicine
  5 Plainsboro Road/Suite 300 Plainsboro, NJ 08536 (609)853-7272 Fax (609)853-7271

Abramovici, Mirel I., MD {1215961958} IntrMd, Nephro, Hypten(85,BEL03)<NJ-ENGLWOOD, NJ-HACKNSK>
 + Drs. Abramovici, Jan & Zelkowitz
  140 Grand Avenue/Suite B Englewood, NJ 07631 (201)567-5787 Fax (201)567-7652

Abramowicz, Apolonia E., MD {1427127646} Anesth(75,POLA)
 + New Jersey Anesthesia Associates, P.C.
  252 Columbia Turnpike/PO Box 0037 Florham Park, NJ 07932 (973)660-9334 Fax (973)660-9779

Abramowitz, Jodi S., DO {1619985744} GenPrc, IntrMd, FamMAdlt(82,NJ75)<NJ-ACMCITY, NJ-SHOREMEM>
 + 210 New Road/Suite 11
  Linwood, NJ 08221 (609)927-6100
 + AtlantiCare Regional Medical Center/City Campus
  1925 Pacific Avenue Atlantic City, NJ 08401 (609)345-4000
 + Shore Memorial Hospital
  1 East New York Avenue Somers Point, NJ 08221 (609)653-3500

Abramowitz, Joel, MD {1356429377} Urolgy(76,MEXI)<NJ-CHRIST, NJ-PALISADE>
 + 142 Palisade Avenue/Suite 101
  Jersey City, NJ 07306 (201)656-4104 Fax (201)656-9178 Jabramowitz@yahoo.com

Abramowitz, Richard Michael, MD {1609856434} IntrMd, OccpMd(88,NJ06)<NJ-JRSYSHMC>
 + Jersey Shore University Medical Center
  1945 Route 33/Medicine Neptune, NJ 07753 (732)776-4302 Fax (732)776-4719
 + Hackensack Meridian Medical Group
  19 Davis Avenue/5th-6th Floor Neptune, NJ 07753 (732)776-4302 Fax (732)897-3997

Abrams, Jeffrey A., MD {1174582076} Gastrn, IntrMd(89,NY15)
 + South Jersey Endoscopy Center
  26 East Red Bank Avenue Woodbury, NJ 08096 (856)848-4464 Fax (856)848-8706

Abrams, Jeffrey Stuart, MD {1386658011} SrgOrt(80,NY15)<NJ-VANJHCS>
 + Princeton Orthopaedic Associates, P.A.
  325 Princeton Avenue Princeton, NJ 08540 (609)924-8131 Fax (609)924-8532
 + Princeton Orthopaedic Associates, P.A.
  11 Centre Drive Jamesburg, NJ 08831 (609)655-4848

Abrams, Jonathan Todd, MD {1780663054} Anesth(86,PA14)
 + Summit Anesthesia Associates, P.A.
  33 Overlook Road/Suite 311 Summit, NJ 07901 (908)598-1500 Fax (908)598-0197

Abrams, Laura Morrell, MD {1275794646}
 + 36 Dorset Lane
  Short Hills, NJ 07078 (973)379-2082

Abrams, Lawrence M., MD {1356596485} CarAne, IntrMd, CarEch(72,KS02)<NJ-HACKNSK>
 + 30 Second Street/Suite 104
  Hackensack, NJ 07601 (201)343-2768
 + Hackensack University MC-Anesthesia Dept
  30 Prospect Avenue/Room 2703 Hackensack, NJ 07601 (201)343-2768 Fax (201)996-3962

Abrams, Russell I., MD {1114956505} Nrolgy(91,ISR02)<NJ-KMHCHRRY, NJ-KMHSTRAT>
 + Neurology Associates & Ctr Pain
  1030 North Kings Highway/Suite 200B Cherry Hill, NJ 08034 (856)482-0030 Fax (856)779-7787
 + Neurology Pain Associates
  222 New Road/Central Park East Linwood, NJ 08221 (856)482-0030 Fax (609)601-6009

Abrams, Stephen Joel, MD {1831103324} Otlryg, Otolgy, SrgHdN(70,NY03)<NJ-MTNSIDE, NJ-CHILTON>
 + ENT & Allergy Associates, LLP
  1211 Hamburg Turnpike/Suite 205 Wayne, NJ 07470 (973)633-0808 Fax (973)633-8811 SABRAMS@entallergy.com

Abramson, David L., MD {1720046139} SrgPlstc, Surgry(88,NY19)<NJ-ENGLWOOD, NJ-HOLYNAME>
 + Dermatology Center
  363 Grand Avenue Englewood, NJ 07631 (201)568-6977 Fax (201)568-7567

Abramson, Jennifer Leigh, MD {1972707388} Psychy, PsyCAd(97,NY47)
 + 511 Valley Street/Suite 201
  Maplewood, NJ 07040 (973)275-5333 Fax (973)275-9233

Abramson, Marla Lyn, MD {1801884309} IntrMd(99,DC01)<NJ-OVERLOOK, NJ-MORRISTN>
 + Summit Medical Group-Berkeley Heights Campus
  1 Diamond Hill Road Berkeley Heights, NJ 07922 (908)273-4300 Fax (908)228-3617
 + Summit Medical Group
  560 Springfield Avenue Westfield, NJ 07090 (908)228-3610

Abrar, Dimir, MD {1205178365} PhysMd
 + Aspen Medical Associates, P.A.
  1 DeGraw Square Teaneck, NJ 07666 (201)928-0200 Fax (201)928-0820

Abrar, Samar, MD {1043236698} Psychy(91,PAK11)
 + 288 Leonard Place
  Paramus, NJ 07652

Abrarova, Nazima M., MD {1487850319} ObsGyn, IntrMd(95,UZB44)
 + Neighborhood Health Center Plainfield
  1700-58 Myrtle Avenue Plainfield, NJ 07063 (908)753-6401

Abreu, Arnaldo J., MD {1275629297} Pedtrc, PedEmg, IntrMd(88,WIND)<NJ-STPETER>
 + St. Peter's University Hospital
  254 Easton Avenue/Pediatrics New Brunswick, NJ 08901 (732)339-7444 Fax (732)745-2994 AAbreu1754@aol.com

Abreu, Paul, MD {1952388001} Pedtrc, IntrMd(83,DOM01)
 + 107 Monmouth Road
  West Long Branch, NJ 07764 (732)544-0400 Fax (732)544-0045
 + 530 Prospect Avenue
  Little Silver, NJ 07739 (732)747-9400

Abrina, Vanessa Mae S., MD {1649577495}
 + Drs. Abrina & Tsai
  319 Main Street/Suite B4 Keansburg, NJ 07734 (908)209-0485 Fax (732)787-0270 vanabrina@gmail.com

Abrutyn, David Alan, MD {1679534903} SrgOrt, SprtMd<NJ-SOMERSET>
 + Summit Medical Group
  34 Mountain Boulevard/Building B Warren, NJ 07059 (908)769-0100 Fax (908)769-8927
 + Orthopedic and Sports Medicine at SMG
  215 Union Avenue/Suite B Bridgewater, NJ 08807 (908)769-0100 Fax (908)685-8009

Absatz, Michael G., MD {1518001072} SrgOrt, SrgOARec(82,NY01)
 + Shore Orthopaedic Group
  1255 Route 70/Suite 11S Lakewood, NJ 08701 (732)942-2300 Fax (732)942-2311

Absin, Martini Perez, MD {1518960400} Anesth(86,PHI13)<NJ-SHOREMEM>
 + Shore Memorial Hospital
  1 East New York Avenue/Anesthesiology Somers Point, NJ 08244 (609)653-3500
 + Access Surgery Center
  3205 Fire Road/Suite 3 Egg Harbor, NJ 08234 (609)407-1113

Abu Al Rub, Dana M., MD {1063753051} IntrMd
 + Drs. Abu Al Rub and Abusido
  65 River Road/Suite 208 Nutley, NJ 07110

Abu Khraybeh, Wafa Said, MD {1093763856} Pedtrc, AdolMd(81,LEB03)<NJ-STJOSHOS>
 + Willowbrook Pediatrics
  57 Willowbrook Boulevard/Suite 421 Wayne, NJ 07470 (973)754-4025 Fax (973)754-4044

Abubakar, Ahmed B., MD {1609272871} IntrMd(08,INA70)
 + Drs. Abubakar and Abubakar
  452 Central Avenue Jersey City, NJ 07307 (201)222-0821 Fax (201)222-1018

Abubakar, Shaik, MD {1578558847} FamMed(80,INDI)<NJ-CHRIST, NJ-HOBUNIMC>
 + Drs. Abubakar and Abubakar
  452 Central Avenue Jersey City, NJ 07307 (201)222-0821 Fax (201)222-1018

Abubakar, Tunku Abdul R., MD {1275571515} Psychy(87,PHI02)<NJ-STBARBHC>
 + St. Barnabas Behavioral Health Center
  1691 US Highway 9 Toms River, NJ 08755 (800)300-0628

Abud, Ariel F., MD {1215975917} SrgNro(65,MEXI)<NJ-CHSFULD, NJ-CHSMRCER>
 + Trenton Neurological Surgeons Associates, P.A.
  3100 Princeton Pike/Building 1/Suite A Lawrenceville, NJ 08648 (609)219-0280 Fax (609)771-1237

Abud-Ortega, Alfredo Ramon, MD {1639115819} Surgry, SrgVas(70,MEX62)<NJ-CAPITLHS, NJ-CHSFULD>
 + Advanced Surgical Associates of New Jersey
  40 Fuld Street/Suite 403 Trenton, NJ 08638 (609)537-6000 Fax (609)537-6002

Abujudeh, Hani H., MD {1992793756} RadDia, NuclMd, Radiol(95,NJ05)<NJ-COOPRUMC>
 + Cooper University Hospital
  One Cooper Plaza/B-23 Camden, NJ 08103 (856)342-2380 Fax (856)365-0472

Abulaimoun, Bdair Matar, III, MD {1790717239} NnPnMd, Pedtrc(83,JOR01)<NY-NYACKHOS, NY-NSUHMANH>
 + 930 Clifton Avenue/Suite 103
  Clifton, NJ 07013 (973)767-2188

Abusido, Islam K., MD {1780967646}
 + Drs. Abu Al Rub and Abusido
  65 River Road/Suite 208 Nutley, NJ 07110

Abutabikh, Nael Abdelsalam, MD {1235120155} IntrMd(88,YEM02)
 + Passaic Medical Center
  362 Monroe Street Passaic, NJ 07055 (973)777-3222

Accardi, Kimberly Lynn Zambito, MD {1306038880} SrgOrt, IntrMd(02,PA09)
 + Mercer-Bucks Orthopaedics PC
  3120 Princeton Pike Lawrenceville, NJ 08648 (609)896-0444 Fax (609)896-1055
 + Mercer-Bucks Orthopaedics, P.C.
  2501 Kuser Road Hamilton, NJ 08691 (609)896-0444 Fax (609)587-4349

Accurso, Charles A., MD {1710963533} Gastrn, IntrMd(84,NJ05)<NJ-SOMERSET>
 + Digestive HealthCare Center
  511 Courtyard Drive/Building 500 Hillsborough, NJ 08844 (908)218-9222 Fax (908)218-9818

Accurso, Daniela, MD {1306229000} FamMed
 + Martinsville Family Practice
  1973 Washington Valley Road Martinsville, NJ 08836 (732)560-9225 Fax (732)560-8095

Acevedo, Rhina A., MD {1396833943} FamMed
 + Family Medicine at Monument Square
  317 George Street New Brunswick, NJ 08901 (732)235-8993 Fax (732)246-7317
 + Catholic Charities Primary Care Clinic
  271 Smith Street Perth Amboy, NJ 08861 (732)826-9160

Acevedo Beltran, Edrik Josue, MD {1427478353} IntrMd
 + Hackensack Medical Center-Internal Medicine
  30 Prospect Avenue/4 Main/Rm 4621 Hackensack, NJ 07601 (551)996-2000 Fax (551)996-0543

Achaibar, Rajendra, MD {1649225939} Radiol, RadDia(88,NY15)<NJ-STJOSHOS>
 + Medical Park Imaging
  330 Ratzer Road/Suite 6-A Wayne, NJ 07470 (973)696-5770 Fax (973)633-1204

Achakzai, Basit Khan, MD {1780903278} RadV&I<PA-RPCKER>
 + University Hospital Emergency Medicine
  150 Bergen Street/level C Newark, NJ 07103 (973)972-5188 Fax (973)972-2307

Achar, Ashwini, MD {1871910992} Pedtrc
 + Skylands Pediatrics
  328-A Sparta Avenue Sparta, NJ 07871 (973)729-2197 Fax (973)729-3653

Achar, Pankaja B.S., MD {1003876186} CritCr, IntrMd, PulDis(82,INA37)<NJ-OVERLOOK, NJ-EASTORNG>
 + Drs. Mehta and Achar
  707 South Orange Avenue South Orange, NJ 07079 (973)762-4746 Fax (973)762-6862
 + Drs. Mehta and Achar
  194 Clinton Avenue Newark, NJ 07108 (973)762-4746 Fax (973)230-0883

Acharya, Prasad G., MD {1295783785} Nephro, IntrMd(98,PA12)<NJ-LOURDMED, NJ-VIRTMHBC>
 + The Center for Kidney Care
  1261 Route 38/Suite A Hainesport, NJ 08036 (856)222-1975 Fax (856)222-0721

Physicians by Name and Address

Acharya, Rashmi, MD {1871538405} ObsGyn(87,INA29)
+ Care first OBGYN Group LLC
  1555 Ruth Road/Suite 5 North Brunswick, NJ 08902
  (732)398-3939   Fax (732)398-0909
+ Care first OBGYN Group LLC
  666 Plainsboro Road/Suite 432 Plainsboro, NJ 08536
  (732)398-3939   Fax (732)398-0909
+ Piscataway Somerset Ob/Gyn Group, LLP
  9 Clyde Road/Suite 101 Somerset, NJ 08902 (732)246-2280

Acharya, Saurav, MD {1841614252} IntrMd
+ 1034 Kennedy Boulevard/Apt B9
  Bayonne, NJ 07002 (201)401-7263

Achebe, Chidi Reuben, MD {1841558806}<NJ-NWRKBETH>
+ Newark Beth Israel Medical Center
  201 Lyons Avenue Newark, NJ 07112 (973)926-7040

Achebe, George E., MD {1114953528} IntrMd(81,NIG03)<NJ-CAPITLHS, NJ-CHSFULD>
+ 1846 Burlington Mount Holly Rd
  Mount Holly, NJ 08060

Acholonu, Emeka Joseph, MD {1598944076} Surgry
+ Virtua Surgical Group, PA
  1935 Route 70 East Cherry Hill, NJ 08003 (856)428-7700 Fax (856)424-9120

Acierno, Lynne J., MD {1184844045} IntrMd(81,NY08)<NJ-JRSYCITY>
+ Metropolitan Family Health Network
  935 Garfield Avenue Jersey City, NJ 07304 (201)478-5800 Fax (201)475-5814

Ackad, Alexandre V., MD {1649261454} IntrMd, Nephro(64,EGY03)<NJ-VALLEY, NJ-HACKNSK>
+ Bergen Hypertension & Renal Associates PA
  44 Godwin Avenue/Suite 301 Midland Park, NJ 07432
  (201)447-0013   Fax (201)447-0438
+ Bergen Hypertension & Renal Associates PA
  20 Prospect Avenue/Suite 709 Hackensack, NJ 07601
  (201)447-0013   Fax (201)678-1072

Ackad, Viviane Bichara, MD {1134149909} IntrMd(82,EGY04)
+ Newark PrimeCare
  337 Bloomfield Avenue Newark, NJ 07107 (973)497-2424 Fax (973)497-2448

Ackerman, Anika Jahn, MD {1326307877} Urolgy
+ Adult & Pediatric Urology Group PA
  261 James Street/Suite 1-A Morristown, NJ 07960
  (973)539-0333   Fax (973)539-8909

Ackerman, Melville J., MD {1598707580} Gastrn(80,MEXI)<NJ-COOPRUMC, NJ-VIRTUAHS>
+ Drs. Ackerman & Turnier
  501 Haddon Avenue/Suite 9 Haddonfield, NJ 08033
  (856)428-6024   Fax (856)216-1558
+ Drs. Ackerman & Turnier
  2301 Evesham Road/Suite 401 Voorhees, NJ 08043
  (856)428-6024   Fax (856)216-1558

Ackerman, Randy B., MD {1205893807} Urolgy(87,NJ05)<NJ-OURLADY, NJ-UNDRWD>
+ New Jersey Urology, LLC
  2401 East Evesham Road/Suite F Voorhees, NJ 08043
  (856)673-1600   Fax (856)988-0636
+ Delaware Valley Urology LLC
  17 West Red Bank Avenue/Suite 303 Woodbury, NJ 08096
  (856)673-1600   Fax (856)985-4583
+ Center for Urologic Care PA
  485 Williamstown-New Freedom R Sicklerville, NJ 08043
  (856)237-8035   Fax (856)237-8039

Ackerman, Stacey Lynn, MD {1508868498} Ophthl(81,NY06)<NJ-LOURDMED>
+ Philadelphia Eye Associates
  1113 Hospital Drive/Suite 302 Willingboro, NJ 08046
  (609)871-1112

Acocella, Michael A., DO {1770575037} IntrMd(91,PA77)
+ 138 Westfield Avenue/Suite 5
  Clark, NJ 07066 (732)381-5565 Fax (732)381-5222

Acosta, Katiusca A., MD {1922304609}(10,NET09)<NY-METHODST>
+ Passaic Pediatrics II PA
  913 Main Avenue Passaic, NJ 07055 (973)458-8000
+ Passaic Pediatrics II PC
  93 Market Street Passaic, NJ 07055 (973)458-8000 Fax (973)458-8338

Acosta, Ramon, MD {1174668834} Pedtrc, FamMed(82,DOM01)
+ 2 Leonard Avenue
  Camden, NJ 08105 (856)756-0010   Fax (856)756-0011
  racostamd@msn.com

Acosta, Regis Francisco, MD {1366523011} Psychy, PsyFor(93,DOM01)
+ 104 Independence Boulevard
  Sicklerville, NJ 08081

Acosta, Robert G., MD {1508809823} RadDia, Radiol(86,NY20)
+ Essex Imaging Associates
  5 Franklin Avenue/Suite 510 Belleville, NJ 07109
  (973)751-2011   Fax (973)751-4456

Acosta Baez, Giancarlo, MD {1609155969} IntrMd, IntHos
+ 111 Madison Avenue/Suite 408
  Morristown, NJ 07960 (973)971-6957

Acquavella, Anthony Peter, MD {1710935366} AdolMd, Pedtrc(83,DC02)
+ Cooper Peds/Children's Regional Ctr
  3 Cooper Plaza/Suite 200 Camden, NJ 08103 (856)342-2472 Fax (856)368-8297

Acquaviva, Joseph F., MD {1912054420} Psychy(82,MEXI)<NJ-HACKNSK>
+ Psychiatric Associates
  218 State Route 17 North/Suite 13 Rochelle Park, NJ 07662
  (201)488-6543   Fax (201)488-6916

Acunto, Brian Anthony, DO {1093921041} EmrgMd(05,PA77)<NJ-ACMCITY>
+ AtlantiCare Regional Medical Center/City Campus
  1925 Pacific Avenue/EmergMed/8th Fl Atlantic City, NJ 08401 (609)345-4000

Adabala, Ramesh, MD {1902898596} IntrMd, PulCCr, SlpDis(93,INA8Y)
+ Associates in Pulmonary and Internal Medicine
  35-37 Progress Street/Suite A-5 Edison, NJ 08820
  (908)668-7791   Fax (908)668-7792
+ Associates in Pulmonary and Internal Medicine
  200 Perrine Road/Suite 227 Old Bridge, NJ 08857

Adair, Robert Aton, MD {1457467862} FamMed, IntrMd, PubHth(69,DC03)<NJ-HOLYNAME>
+ Drs. Coleman & Adair
  222 Cedar Lane/Suite 111 Teaneck, NJ 07666 (201)836-7970   Fax (201)836-7973
+ Drs. Coleman & Adair
  211 60th Street West New York, NJ 07093 (201)836-7970 Fax (201)868-7185

Adal, Adefris Y., MD {1669728622}<NJ-JRSYCITY>
+ Jersey City Medical Center
  355 Grand Street Jersey City, NJ 07304 (917)474-6499
  adefris.adal@yahoo.com

Adam, Abir Moustafa, MD {1326018003} Anesth(92,EGY05)<NJ-TRINIWSC>
+ Trinitas Regional Medical Center-Williamson Street
  225 Williamson Street/Anesthesiology Elizabeth, NJ 07207
  (908)994-5000

Adam, Stephanie Paige, DO {1447459292} SrgOrt(04,NY75)<NY-ARDNHILL, NY-CGHHERMN>
+ Summit Medical Group Orthopedics and Sports Medicine
  140 Park Avenue/2nd Floor/2nd Fl Florham Park, NJ 07932
  (973)404-9800   Fax (973)267-7295

Adamczyk, Rebekah Katherine, DO {1275777609} IntrMd(06,PA77)
+ Family first Urgent Care & Walk in Medical
  1910 State Route 35 Oakhurst, NJ 07755 (732)531-0100 Fax (732)531-0144

Adamidis, Ananea, MD {1235139957} Nephro, IntrMd(00,NY09)<NJ-HOLYNAME, NJ-VALLEY>
+ Renal Medicine Associates PA
  302 Union Street Hackensack, NJ 07601 (201)646-0414 Fax (201)646-0365
+ Renal Medicine Associates PA
  400 Franklin Turnpike/Suite 208 Mahwah, NJ 07430 (201)825-3322
+ Renal Medicine Associates PA
  718 Teaneck Road Teaneck, NJ 07601 (201)833-3223

Adamoli, Donna Janine, MD {1104880871} IntrMd(92,CO02)<NJ-VALLEY>
+ Summit Medical Group
  75 East Northfield Road Livingston, NJ 07039 (973)436-1400   Fax (908)673-7336

Adams, Andrea Garcia, MD {1730391244} PulDis, PulCCr, IntrMd(05,NJ05)<NJ-LOURDMED>
+ Lourdes Medical Center of Burlington County
  218 Sunset Road/Suite A/Pulm Disease Willingboro, NJ 08046 (609)835-3056 Fax (609)835-3061

Adams, Angela, MD {1225096423} Nrolgy(94,DC02)
+ 117 Kinderkamack Road/Suite 102
  River Edge, NJ 07661 (201)968-1825   Fax (201)968-1827

Adams, John M., MD {1134194053} Surgry, EmrgEMed(93,NY19)<NJ-MORRISTN>
+ Morristown Medical Center
  100 Madison Avenue Morristown, NJ 07962 (973)971-5000

Adams, Mark Robert, MD {1922257799} SrgOrt(06,NY08)
+ UMDNJ Orthopaedics
  140 Bergen Street Newark, NJ 07103

Adams, William B., DO {1083812705} PulCCr, IntrMd(06,PA77)<NJ-ACMCITY>
+ Shore Physicians Group
  18 West New York Avenue Somers Point, NJ 08244
  (609)926-1450   Fax (609)926-8419
+ AtlantiCare Regional Medical Center/City Campus
  1925 Pacific Avenue/Pulm Crtcl Care Atlantic City, NJ 08401 (609)345-4000

Adams, William D., MD {1376522839} SrgBst, Surgry(89,NY01)<NJ-JRSYSHMC>
+ 2100 Corlies Avenue/Suite 1
  Neptune, NJ 07753 (732)988-5444   Fax (732)988-3066

Adamski, Jamie Justin, DO {1902003528} EmrgMd<NJ-TRINIWSC>
+ Trinitas Regional Medical Center-Williamson Street
  225 Williamson Street/Emergency Elizabeth, NJ 07207
  (908)994-5000

Adamson, Susanne R. M., MD {1679646012} ObsGyn(87,SWE03)
+ Ob-Gyn Specialists
  157 Route 73 Voorhees, NJ 08043 (856)874-1114   Fax (856)874-9555

Adarkwa, Agnes, MD {1982012639} IntHos<NJ-COOPRUMC>
+ Cooper University Hospital
  One Cooper Plaza Camden, NJ 08103 (856)342-2000

Adbou, Andrew Kamal, MD {1730592551}
+ Meadowlands Hospital Medical Center
  55 Meadowlands Parkway Secaucus, NJ 07096 (201)392-3100   Fax (201)392-3068

Addis, David J., MD {1770656068} GenPrc(69,PA02)<NJ-LOURDMED>
+ 334 Farnsworth Avenue
  Bordentown, NJ 08505 (609)298-1823   Fax (609)298-9363

Addis, Diana Medina, MD {1235241597} SrgBst, Surgry, IntrMd(96,NJ05)<NJ-STMICHL, NJ-OVERLOOK>
+ Summit Medical Group-Berkeley Heights Campus
  1 Diamond Hill Road Berkeley Heights, NJ 07922
  (908)277-8770   Fax (908)790-6576
+ Summit Breast Care, LLC.
  649 Morris Avenue Springfield, NJ 07081 (908)277-8770 Fax (973)258-1153

Addis, Michael Downes, MD {1275525743} SrgVas(99,NJ05)<NJ-CLARMAAS, NJ-MTNSIDE>
+ The Cardiovascular Care Group
  25 East Willow Street Millburn, NJ 07041 (973)921-9600
+ The Cardiovascular Care Group
  433 Central Avenue Westfield, NJ 07090 (973)921-9600 (908)490-1698

Adeaga, Oyedolapo O., MD {1013324490}
+ 659b Mapleview Drive
  Old Bridge, NJ 08857 (732)416-8746
  aadeaga@yahoo.com

Adedokun, Emmanuel Adekunle, MD {1417158767} FamMed
+ St. Joseph's Family Medicine @ Clifton
  1135 Broad Street/Suite 201 Clifton, NJ 07013 (973)754-4100   Fax (973)472-9062

Adefowokan, Rotanna I., MD {1417220146} ObsGyn(07,GRN01)<NJ-JFKMED>
+ JFK Medical Center
  65 James Street/Ob/Gyn Edison, NJ 08820 (732)321-7000

Adel, Nourihan, MD {1134171556} Grtrcs, IntrMd(73,TURK)<NJ-BERGNMC>
+ New Bridge Medical Center
  230 East Ridgewood Avenue/Suite 6-2 Paramus, NJ 07652
  (201)225-4700   Fax (201)261-4702

Adel, Tymaz, MD {1326429614} Psychy<NJ-BERGNMC>
+ New Bridge Medical Center
  230 East Ridgewood Avenue Paramus, NJ 07652
  (201)753-8132

Adelberg, David Eli, MD {1619075694} MedOnc, IntrMd(02,MA07)
+ AtlantiCare Cancer Institute
  2500 English Creek Avenue/Building 400 Egg Harbor Township, NJ 08234 (609)677-7777   Fax (609)677-7727

Adelekan, Tahira Gittens, MD {1801968599} Pedtrc(99,TX13)<PA-CHOPHIL>
+ CHOP Pediatric & Adolescent Specialty Care Center
  4009 Black Horse Pike Mays Landing, NJ 08330 (609)677-7895   Fax (609)677-7835
+ CHOP Pediatric & Adolescent Specialty Care Center
  1012 Laurel Oak Road Voorhees, NJ 08043 (609)677-7895 Fax (856)435-0091

Adelizzi, Angela M., DO {1356314751} IntrMd(88,PA77)
+ Coastal Health Care
  1314 Hooper Avenue/Building B Toms River, NJ 08753
  (732)349-4994   Fax (732)341-1717

Adelizzi, Raymond A., DO {1770684169} Rheuma, IntrMd(73,PA77)<NJ-KMHSTRAT, NJ-UNDRWD>
+ 215 East Laurel Road/Suite 101
  Stratford, NJ 08084 (856)782-9757   Fax (856)782-9224
+ 17 West Red Bank Avenue/Suite 201
  Woodbury, NJ 08096 (856)845-1818

Physicians by Name and Address

Adelman, Marc R., MD {1588745772} CritCr, IntrMd, PulDis(77,MEX03)<NJ-STMICHL>
+ 268 MLK Jr. Boulevard
  Newark, NJ 07102 (973)877-5090
+ 467 Mt. Prospect Avenue
  Newark, NJ 07104 (973)483-9900
+ Pope John Paul II Pavilion at St. Mary's Life Center
  135 South Center Street Orange, NJ 07102 (973)266-3000 Fax (973)266-3094

Adelsohn, Lawrence G., MD {1619944923} FrtInf, ObsGyn, Gyneco(67,IL42)<NJ-HACKNSK>
+ 140 Prospect Avenue/Suite 11
  Hackensack, NJ 07601 (201)342-4220 Fax (201)342-4219

Adem, Patricia V., MD {1417282286} PthAcl
+ Rutgers- New Jersey Medical School
  185 South Orange Avenue/MSB C579 Newark, NJ 07103 (973)972-4520

Adenwalla, Humaira Naseem, MD {1043474349} Rheuma, IntrMd(01,PAK11)
+ Arthritis & Osteoporosis Associates, P.A.
  4247 US Highway 9/Building 1 Freehold, NJ 07728 (732)780-7650 Fax (732)780-8817
+ Arthritis & Osteoporosis Associates, P.A.
  150 Route 37 West Ste A2/Suite A2 Toms River, NJ 08755 (732)780-7650 Fax (732)414-6003

Adeola, Yetunde, MD {1033314299} Psychy
+ 225 Millburn Avenue/Suite 210
  Millburn, NJ 07041 (973)494-4614

Adeoti, Adekunle G., MD {1740259639} IntrMd, Gastrn(88,NIGE)
+ 2 Korwell Circle
  West Orange, NJ 07052 (973)731-1602

Aderholdt, David Gabriel, DO {1487081030}<NJ-SJHREGMC>
+ Drs. Aderholdt and Akrout
  3 Elizabeth Street Millville, NJ 08332 (856)641-6272
+ SJH Regional Medical Center
  1505 West Sherman Avenue Vineland, NJ 08360 (856)503-6885

Aderibigbe, Adedayo Olubunmi, MD {1528226842} FamMed, IntrMd(06,DMN01)
+ 629 Amboy Avenue/Suite 109
  Edison, NJ 08837 (732)486-3365 Fax (732)486-3367
+ Henry J. Austin Health Center
  321 North Warren Street Trenton, NJ 08618 (732)486-3365 Fax (609)392-4827

Ades, Nathan Albert, MD {1528085438} Anesth(94,NY08)
+ Red Bank Anesthesia, LLC
  1 Riverview Plaza Red Bank, NJ 07701 (732)530-2255 Fax (732)450-2620

Adessa, Kenneth J., MD {1750348520} IntrMd(95,NJ05)<NJ-CLARMAAS, NJ-STBARNMC>
+ 3699 Route 46 East
  Parsippany, NJ 07054 (973)794-6081 Fax (973)827-7413
  kadessa@gmail.com

Adetunji, Babatunde A., MD {1326131699} Psychy, PsyFor, Addctn(87,NIG05)
+ 508a Lippincott Drive
  Marlton, NJ 08053
+ Pinnacle Behavioral Health Institute
  851 Route 73 North/Suite C Marlton, NJ 08053 Fax (856)267-5824

Adewunmi, Kafilat, DO {1134326010} FamMed(05,NY75)<NJ-NWRKBETH>
+ 20 N Woodbury Turnersville Rd
  Blackwood, NJ 08012 (856)374-6856 Fax (856)374-6896
+ JRMC at Dayton Street Elementary School
  226 Dayton Street Newark, NJ 07114 (856)374-6856 Fax (973)824-5652

Adeyeri, Ayotunde Olubukola, MD {1184869737} Surgry(95,NIG01)
+ 668 North Beers Street/Suite 103
  Holmdel, NJ 07733 (732)217-3897 Fax (732)739-9094

Adibe, Livinus, MD {1588046494} IntrMd
+ St. Michael's Medical Center
  111 Central Avenue Newark, NJ 07102 (973)877-5000

Adibe, Sebastian O., MD {1568494961} SrgOrt(71,NIGE)
+ 142 Palisade Avenue
  Jersey City, NJ 07306 (201)792-1555 Fax (201)792-1030

Adibi, Baback, MD {1164491346} CdvDis, IntrMd(99,PA12)
+ Bergen Cardiology Associates
  292 Columbia Avenue Fort Lee, NJ 07024 (201)224-0050 Fax (201)224-6061
+ Bergen Cardiology Associates
  400 Frank W. Burr Boulevard Teaneck, NJ 07666 (201)224-0050 Fax (201)692-3263

Adigun, Akeem Segun, MD {1841601788} ObsGyn<NJ-STPETER>
+ St. Peter's University Hospital
  254 Easton Avenue New Brunswick, NJ 08901 (732)745-8600

Adigun, Jennifer Olubusola, MD {1811162894} IntrMd(94,NIG07)<NJ-SHOREMEM>
+ Shore Hospitalists Associates
  100 Medical Center Way Somers Point, NJ 08244

  (609)653-3500 Fax (609)926-4799
+ Shore Memorial Hospital
  1 East New York Avenue/IntMed Somers Point, NJ 08244 (609)653-3500

Adija, Akinyi, MD {1265427884} Pedtrc(98,NY47)<OH-UNVH-CLEV>
+ Newark Beth Israel Medical Center
  201 Lyons Avenue Newark, NJ 07112 (973)926-7000

Adin, David R., DO {1134117211} PhysMd, PainMd(00,NY75)<NY-NYURUSK>
+ Health East Medical Center
  54 South Dean Street Englewood, NJ 07631 (201)871-4000

Adinaro, David Joseph, MD {1114039849} EmrgMd(00,NJ05)<NJ-STJOSHOS>
+ St Joseph's Medical Center Emergency
  703 Main Street Paterson, NJ 07503 (973)754-2222 Fax (973)754-2249

Adkins, Luz Stella, MD {1417011404} Psychy(86,DOM08)<NJ-ANCPSYCH>
+ Ancora Psychiatric Hospital
  301 Spring Garden Road Hammonton, NJ 08037 (609)561-1700

Adkisson, Gregory Hugh, MD {1184621047} Anesth(78,AZ01)
+ St. Joseph's Regional Medical Center Anesthesia
  703 Main Street Paterson, NJ 07503 (973)754-2323 Fax (973)977-9455

Adkoli, Sujnani, MD {1639139124} Anesth, PainMd(90,INA5B)<NJ-VALLEY>
+ The Valley Hospital
  223 North Van Dien Avenue/Anesth Ridgewood, NJ 07450 (201)447-8000

Adlakha, Anupama, MD {1649301474} IntrMd(01,GRN01)
+ 707 South Orange Avenue
  South Orange, NJ 07079 (973)761-6111 Fax (973)761-4990

Adler, Bernard H., MD {1881660876} Pedtrc, IntrMd(75,FRAN)<NJ-JRSYSHMC>
+ Northern Ocean County Medical Associates
  10 Neptune Boulevard/Suite 201 Neptune, NJ 07753 (732)455-8559 Fax (732)774-1394

Adler, Daniel G., MD {1548384209} Nrolgy, Pedtrc, NroChl(75,NY46)<NJ-VALLEY>
+ 25 Rockwood Place/Suite 110
  Englewood, NJ 07631 (201)894-1551 Fax (212)504-8100

Adler, Eric David, MD {1477699601} CdvDis, IntrMd(00,MA05)
+ 301 Church Street
  Aberdeen, NJ 07747 (732)583-1616 Fax (732)583-3085

Adler, Joel S., MD {1679655930} Grtrcs, IntrMd(84,GRN01)<NJ-HACKNSK, NJ-ENGLWOOD>
+ Aspen Medical Associates, P.A.
  1 DeGraw Square Teaneck, NJ 07666 (201)928-0200 Fax (201)928-0820
+ Hackensack University Medical Center
  30 Prospect Avenue Hackensack, NJ 07601 (201)996-2000

Adler, Kenneth R., MD {1922096916} IntrMd, OncHem(73,NY03)
+ Hematology-Oncology Associates of Northern NJ
  100 Madison Avenue/PO Box 1089 Morristown, NJ 07962 (973)538-5210 Fax (973)644-9657
+ The Heart Group, PA
  654 Broadway Bayonne, NJ 07002 (973)538-5210 Fax (201)243-9998

Adler, Michele L., MD {1962511527} Psychy(90,NJ05)<NJ-VAEASTOR>
+ VA New Jersey Health Care System-East Orange Campus
  385 Tremont Avenue East Orange, NJ 07018 (973)676-1000

Adler, Scott L., MD {1194804443} IntrMd(80,NY08)<NJ-CHSFULD>
+ Lawrence Medical Associates PA
  2999 Princeton Pike Lawrenceville, NJ 08648 (609)882-2299 Fax (609)538-8230

Adler, Uri Seth, MD {1346238334} IntrMd, PhysMd(97,NJ05)<NJ-KSLRSADB>
+ Kessler Institute for Rehabilitation
  300 Market Street Saddle Brook, NJ 07663 (201)368-6043 Fax (201)368-6135

Adler, Zachary G., MD {1235227695} IntrMd, PhysMd, WundCr(79,MEXI)<NJ-HOLYNAME>
+ 1001 Haddon Place
  Teaneck, NJ 07666

Adly, Marina, MD {1861951584} PhysMd
+ 300 Corporate Center Drive
  Manalapan, NJ 07726 (732)761-0088

Admani, Ariff, MD {1770554263} InfDis, IntrMd(92,GRN01)<NJ-STMICHL, NJ-CLARMAAS>
+ 77 Newark Avenue/Suite 2
  Belleville, NJ 07109 (201)261-4838 Fax (201)205-1871

Admani, Irfan Mohamed, MD {1043228588} CdvDis, IntrMd(96,GRN01)
+ Cross Country Cardiology
  103 River Road/2nd Floor Edgewater, NJ 07020 (201)941-8100 Fax (201)941-2899

Adolfsen, Stephen Erik, MD {1790993228} SrgOrt(03,NJ06)
+ Pediatric Orthopedic Associates, P.A.
  585 Cranbury Road/Suite A East Brunswick, NJ 08816 (732)390-1160 Fax (732)390-8449
+ Pediatric Orthopedic Associates, P.A.
  3700 State Route 33 Neptune, NJ 07753 (732)390-1160 Fax (732)897-4205

Adriance, Lori N., DO {1104223452}
+ 3457 St Martins Road/Apt 2108
  Pennsauken, NJ 08109 (732)687-8102
  adriance-lori@cooperhealth.edu

Adu-Amankwa, Bernice Abrafi, MD {1356543300} ObsGyn(OH41
+ WomenÆs Health Partners, Cliffside Park
  574 Anderson Avenue Cliffside Park, NJ 07010 (201)943-4884 Fax (201)943-4839
  bernicea2@yahoo.com

Adumala, Pradeep, MD {1770983272} Pedtrc
+ Southern Jersey Family Medical Centers, Inc.
  600 Pemberton-Browns Mills Rd Pemberton, NJ 08068 (609)894-1100 Fax (609)894-1110
+ Southern Jersey Family Medical Centers Inc.
  1125 Atlantic Avenue Atlantic City, NJ 08401 (609)894-1100 Fax (609)348-1157

Adunuthula-Jonnalagadda, Hema, MD {1699783258} ObsGyn(97,INA83)
+ Physicians of Southern New Jersey
  525 South State Street/Suite 6 Elmer, NJ 08318 (856)363-1210 Fax (856)363-1211

Adusumilli, Padmashree S., MD {1902855968} PhysMd(91,INA2X)<NJ-RHBHTNTN, NJ-MONMOUTH>
+ HealthSouth Rehabilitation Hospital of New Jersey
  14 Hospital Drive Toms River, NJ 08755 (732)505-5123 Fax (732)818-4843

Advani, Sonoo Kishu, MD {1982669123} IntrMd, EnDbMt(84,INA69)<NJ-STBARNMC>
+ 315 East Northfield Road/Suite 1 C
  Livingston, NJ 07039 (973)992-4433 Fax (973)992-1313

Afacan, Yusuf Erkan, MD {1376625905} IntrMd, InfDis(87,TUR01)<NY-WOODHULL>
+ 122 Morningside Road
  Paramus, NJ 07652

Affel, Marjorie E., MD {1003043209} FamMed(09,PA09)
+ Complete Care Family Medicine
  75 West Red Bank Avenue Woodbury, NJ 08096 (856)853-2055 Fax (856)848-2879

Affortunato, Joseph, DO {1902064199}(06,PA78)<NJ-STJOSHOS>
+ St Joseph's Medical Center Emergency
  703 Main Street Paterson, NJ 07503 (973)754-2240 Fax (973)754-2249

Afiniwala, Swara, MD {1760775506} IntrMd
+ Apogee Medical Group of New Jersey
  425 Jack Martin Boulevard Brick, NJ 08724 (732)836-4817 Fax (732)836-4818

Afonja, Olubunmi Olutoyin, MD {1194719492} Pedtrc, PedHem(90,NIG01)
+ 77 West Haledon Avenue
  Haledon, NJ 07508

Afonja, Richards A., MD {1255300141} OncHem(87,NIG01)
+ Colfax Oncology/Fast Med
  476 Colfax Avenue Clifton, NJ 07013 (973)594-7977 Fax (973)594-9983
+ Colfax Oncology/Fast Med
  680 Broadway/Suite 100 Paterson, NJ 07514 (973)594-7977

Afonso, Tania A., DO {1417210394} EmrgMd
+ St. Michael's Medical Center
  111 Central Avenue Newark, NJ 07102 (908)670-5614

Afran, Joyce G., MD {1487731113} FamMed(87,PA02)
+ Family Medicine at Monument Square
  317 George Street New Brunswick, NJ 08901 (732)235-8993 Fax (732)246-7317

Afridi, Shariq A., MD {1467436170} Gastrn, IntrMd(86,PAK11)<NJ-RWJUHAM>
+ Hamilton Gastroenterology Group, PC
  1374 Whitehorse Hamilton Squar Trenton, NJ 08690 (609)586-1319 Fax (609)586-1468

Aftab, Ghulam Mustafa, MD {1275987463}<NJ-STPETER>
+ St. Peter's University Hospital
  254 Easton Avenue New Brunswick, NJ 08901 (732)745-8600 Fax (904)639-2015

Aftab, Saba, MD {1760674287} Otlryg
+ Advocare ENT Specialty Center
  88 South Lakeview Drive/Building 1 Gibbsboro, NJ 08026 (856)435-9100 Fax (856)435-9112

Aftel, Scott, MD {1790847028} Psychy(86,MEXI)<NJ-BAYONNE>
+ 28 East 32nd Street
  Bayonne, NJ 07002 (201)437-9711 Fax (201)437-9111

Physicians by Name and Address

Afzal, Saba, MD {1508265620} Psychy
+ University Behavioral HealthCare
183 South Orange Avenue   Newark, NJ 07103   (917)374-5093

Agadi, Smitha G., MD {1902970502} IntHos<NJ-CHILTON>
+ Chilton Medical Center
97 West Parkway   Pompton Plains, NJ 07444   (973)831-5000

Agar, Monica T., MD {1790711497} ObsGyn(95,NY03)
+ Penn Medicine Department of Ob/Gyn - Medford
103 Old Marlton Pike/Suite 101   Medford, NJ 08055
+ Pinelands Obstetrics and Gynecology
1617 Route 38   Mount Holly, NJ 08060   Fax (609)261-8622

Agaronin, Igor F., MD {1295797215} IntrMd(01,DMN01)
+ Overlook Medical Center
99 Beauvoir Avenue/PO Box 210   Summit, NJ 07902   (908)522-2000
+ 53 Westgate Drive
Annandale, NJ 08801

Agarwal, Amit, MD {1427097211} IntrMd(01,DMN01)
+ 67 East Ridgewood Avenue/Suite C
Paramus, NJ 07652   (201)483-9188   Fax (201)483-9189
Amit97agarwal@gmail.com

Agarwal, Anil, MD {1497704373} Gastrn, IntrMd(79,INDI)
+ 905 Allwood Road/Suite 101
Clifton, NJ 07012   (973)546-4242   Fax (973)546-7639
anilagarwal@yahoo.com

Agarwal, Arvind Kumar, MD {1992776264} CdvDis, IntrMd(76,INA23)<NJ-VALLEY, NY-NYACKHOS>
+ Bergen Heart Center
85 Chestnut Ridge Road/Suite 111   Montvale, NJ 07645   (201)444-9913   Fax (201)444-6158

Agarwal, Ashish Madanlal, MD {1821174483} CdvDis, IntrMd(98,INA20)
+ Mercer Bucks Cardiology
One Union Street/Suite 101   Robbinsville, NJ 08691   (609)890-7292   Fax (609)890-7292

Agarwal, Ashoke, MD {1780649608} CdvDis, IntrMd(71,INDI)
+ 680 Broadway/Suite 116B
Paterson, NJ 07514   (973)684-8617   Fax (973)523-6037

Agarwal, Kishan C., MD {1205990280} PedCrd, OthrSp, Pedtrc(69,INA57)<NJ-CHLSMT, NJ-DEBRAHLC>
+ Drs. Agarwal & Agarwal
450 Plainfield Road   Edison, NJ 08820   (732)494-9500
+ Children's Specialized Hospital
150 New Providence Road   Mountainside, NJ 07092   (908)233-3720

Agarwal, Kunal, MD {1932497773}
+ 29 Geiger Lane
Warren, NJ 07059   (917)459-7336
kunal36@gmail.com

Agarwal, Meenoo, MD {1023075991} Anesth(79,INA05)
+ 905 Allwood Road
Clifton, NJ 07012   Fax (973)546-7639

Agarwal, Nalini, MD {1619072824} Pedtrc(66,INDI)
+ Kids Koncept Pediatrics, PA
1555 Ruth Road/Suite 4   North Brunswick, NJ 08902

Agarwal, Ravi, MD {1801830468} Pedtrc, NnPnMd(85,INA1Z)<NJ-STPETER, NJ-HUNTRDN>
+ 25 Biggs Place
Flemington, NJ 08822

Agarwal, Sangeeta, MD {1790756062} IntrMd(87,INA23)<NJ-RBAYOLDB, NJ-RWJUBRUN>
+ Coastal Medical Group
3 Hospital Plaza/Suite 315   Old Bridge, NJ 08857   (732)360-1500   Fax (732)360-4148

Agarwal, Saurabh, MD {1134292329} Urolgy(99,MA05)
+ 258 Cedar Street
Cedar Grove, NJ 07009
+ Urology Group PA
4 Godwin Avenue   Midland Park, NJ 07432   Fax (201)444-7228

Agarwal, Shilpa R., MD {1750647343} Dermat(12,DC01)
+ Affiliated Dermatologists
182 South Street/Suite 1   Morristown, NJ 07960   (973)267-0300   Fax (973)695-1480

Agarwal, Smita, MD {1982675633} Dermat(00,OH06)
+ Dermatology Center of New Jersey
745 US Highway 206/Suite 102   Bridgewater, NJ 08807   (908)393-9755   Fax (908)393-9757

Agarwal, Sudhir Kumar, MD {1215006275} Gastrn, IntrMd(83,INDI)<NJ-NWTNMEM, NJ-HCKTSTWN>
+ 89 Sparta Avenue/Suite 204
Sparta, NJ 07871   (973)729-2283

Agarwal, Sumitra, MD {1972673812} GenPrc
+ 24 Paris Avenue
Edison, NJ 08820   (732)635-9776   Fax (732)635-9776

Agarwal, Sushma, MD {1821016197} PhysMd(74,INA57)<NJ-RWJUBRUN, NJ-RWJURAH>
+ Drs. Agarwal & Agarwal
450 Plainfield Road   Edison, NJ 08820   (732)494-9500

Agarwala, Ajay Kumar, MD {1366415465} CdvDis, IntrMd(94,IL11)
+ 906 Oak Tree Road/Suite J
South Plainfield, NJ 07080   (908)769-9900   Fax (908)769-9999

Agarwala, Atul K., MD {1427133586} Ophthl(87,PHI08)
+ Health Excel PC
906 Oak Tree Road   South Plainfield, NJ 07080   (973)424-0776

Agathis, Allyson, MD {1487748513} Pedtrc, AdolMd(88,NJ05)
+ 395 Main Street
Bedminster, NJ 07921   (908)719-2626   Fax (908)719-2671

Agbasi, Nwogo Nnunwa, MD {1740279744} ObsGyn, IntrMd(82,NIG02)
+ Southern Jersey Family Medical Centers, Inc.
860 South White Horse Pike/Building A   Hammonton, NJ 08037   (609)567-0200   Fax (609)567-3492

Agbessi, Denise M., MD {1669527800} IntrMd, AdolMd, IntMAdMd<NJ-CHILTON>
+ Chilton Medical Center
97 West Parkway/IntMed   Pompton Plains, NJ 07444   (973)831-5120   Fax (973)831-5342

Agbodza, Kwami D., MD {1831190172} IntrMd(83,GHA02)<NJ-STFRNMED>
+ St. Francis Medical Center
601 Hamilton Avenue   Trenton, NJ 08629   (609)599-5000

Agcopra, Annabel, DO {1013364769} FamMed
+ Patient first Urgent Care
641 US Highway Route 130   Hamilton, NJ 08691   (609)568-9383   Fax (609)568-9384

Ager, Mary Ann Michelle, MD {1467581892} Psychy(80,PA13)
+ 1930 East Route 70/Suite Q-11
Cherry Hill, NJ 08003   (856)751-8333   Fax (856)751-3438

Ager, Steven A., MD {1841465044} Psychy(72,PA02)
+ The Lawyer Stress Center
1930 Marlton Pike/Suite Q20   Cherry Hill, NJ 08003   (856)751-1444

Agesen, Thomas, MD {1497782940} PhysMd(97,NJ05)<NJ-STMICHL>
+ Premier Health Associates
532 Lafayette Road/Suite 100   Sparta, NJ 07871   (973)383-3730   Fax (973)383-2285
+ New Jersey Sports Medicine
197 Ridgedale Avenue/Suite 210   Cedar Knolls, NJ 07927   (973)383-3730   Fax (973)998-8302
+ Pain Management Center
11 Overlook Road/MAC 11 Suite B110   Summit, NJ 07871   (908)522-2808   Fax (908)522-6123

Aggarwal, Aarti, MD {1104192988}
+ Inspira Health Network
509 North Broad Street   Woodbury, NJ 08096   (856)853-2056   Fax (856)686-5218

Aggarwal, Aradhana, MD {1003160623} IntrMd<NJ-NWTNMEM>
+ Newton Medical Center
175 High Street   Newton, NJ 07860   (973)383-2121

Aggarwal, Arvind Kumar, DO {1942229455} IntrMd, IntHos(00,NY75)<NJ-STCLRDEN, NJ-STCLRDOV>
+ St. Clare's Hospital-Denville Campus
25 Pocono Road/IntMed   Denville, NJ 07834   (973)625-6000
+ 400 West Blackwell Street
Dover, NJ 07801   (973)537-3905

Aggarwal, Gaurav, MD {1184113359}<NJ-JRSYCITY>
+ Jersey City Medical Center
355 Grand Street   Jersey City, NJ 07304   (201)915-2000

Aggarwal, Mukta, MD {1235458258} Anesth(95,INA41)
+ 77 Park Avenue/Apt 1513
Hoboken, NJ 07030

Aggarwal, Rashi, MD {1154514909} Psychy, PssoMd(97,INA93)
+ University Behavioral HealthCare
183 South Orange Avenue/PO Box 1709   Newark, NJ 07103

Aggarwal, Roopali, MD {1932249240} Pedtrc(95,INA02)
+ Wexford Pediatrics
1 Wexford Drive   Monmouth Junction, NJ 08852   (732)274-1332   Fax (732)274-1069

Aggarwal, Vinod K., MD {1023075363} PulDis, IntrMd, CritCr(83,INDI)<NJ-BAYSHORE, NJ-RIVERVW>
+ 721 North Beers Street/Suite 1-C
Holmdel, NJ 07733   (732)264-1678   Fax (732)264-0071

Aggrey, Gloria Kangachie, MD {1588839286} InfDis
+ Infectious Disease Physicians PA
1001 Briggs Road/Suite 250   Mount Laurel, NJ 08054   (856)866-7466   Fax (856)866-9088

Aghabi, Hanna Najib, MD {1306831557} FamMed(98,DMN01)
+ AFC Urgent Care Lyndhurst
560 New York Avenue   Lyndhurst, NJ 07071   (201)831-8125   Fax (201)345-4536

Aghai, Zubairul Hasan, MD {1023104411} Pedtrc, NnPnMd(84,INDI)<NJ-COOPRUMC>
+ Cooper Neonatology
One Cooper Plaza   Camden, NJ 08103   (856)342-2265   Fax (856)342-8007

+ The Children's Regional Hospital at Cooper Univ Hosp
One Cooper Plaza/Neonatal   Camden, NJ 08103   (856)342-2000
+ Cooper Peds/Children's Regional Ctr
3 Cooper Plaza/Suite 200   Camden, NJ 08103   (856)342-2472   Fax (856)368-8297

Agia, Gary A., DO {1154408516} PulDis, IntrMd(75,PA77)<NJ-KMHTURNV, NJ-UNDRWD>
+ Jefferson Health Primary & Specialty Care
1A Regulus Drive   Turnersville, NJ 08012   (856)553-6904   Fax (856)589-3913

Agis, Harry, MD {1760452064} Surgry, IntrMd(81,ARG10)<NJ-MORRISTN, NJ-STCLRDEN>
+ Vein Institute of New Jersey
95 Madison Avenue/Suite 109   Morristown, NJ 07960   (973)759-9000   Fax (973)759-2487
+ Vein Institute of New Jersey
532 Lafayette Road   Sparta, NJ 07871
+ Vein Institute of New Jersey
788 Broad Street/US Highway 35   Shrewsbury, NJ 07960

Agnelli, Michael Robert, MD {1548503451} IntrMd
+ St Joseph's Medical Ctr Internal Med
703 Main Street   Paterson, NJ 07503   (973)754-2000   Fax (973)754-3776

Agnello, Jennifer T., DO {1447292396} ObsGyn(91,IA75)<NJ-MORRISTN>
+ Lifeline Medical Associates, LLC
16 Pocono Road/Suite 105   Denville, NJ 07834   (973)831-2777   Fax (973)831-2780

Ago, Aileen Hope, MD {1285942839} Pedtrc(99,PHI21)
+ 1301 South Lincoln Avenue/Apt 814
Vineland, NJ 08361

Agopian, Raffi E., MD {1770584583} SrgC&R, Surgry, IntrMd(83,BULG)<NJ-CHILTON, NJ-VALLEY>
+ North Jersey Colon & Rectal Surgery Associates, LLC.
85 Harristown Road   Glen Rock, NJ 07452   (201)689-9100   Fax (201)689-9108
+ North Jersey Colon & Rectal Surgery Associates, LLC.
191 Hamburg Turnpike   Pompton Lakes, NJ 07442   (201)689-9100   Fax (973)839-2301
+ Valley Medical Group Colorectal Surgery
1124 East Ridgewood Avenue/Suite 202   Ridgewood, NJ 07452   (201)689-9100   Fax (201)689-9108

Agpaoa, Ulysses V., MD {1457419202} IntrMd, InfDis(80,PHI01)<NJ-CLARMAAS, NJ-BAYONNE>
+ 564 Broadway/1st Floor
Bayonne, NJ 07002   (201)858-2220   Fax (201)603-1167
ulyssesvagpaoamdpc@gmail.com

Agrawal, Annie, DO {1043565393}
+ 523 Third Street/2nd Floor
Union City, NJ 07087   (201)223-0030

Agrawal, Apurv, MD {1639188766} MedOnc, IntrMd(01,INA75)<NJ-COMMED, NJ-KIMBALL>
+ NJ Hematology & Oncology Associates
1608 Route 88 West/Suite 250   Brick, NJ 08724   (732)840-8880   Fax (732)840-3939

Agrawal, Neil, MD {1366416398} FamMed(95,NJ06)<NJ-CENTRAST>
+ Howell Primary Care, P.C.
1001 Route 9 North/Suite 105   Howell, NJ 07731   (732)625-1100   Fax (732)625-1110

Agrawal, Nidhi, MD {1245246982} FamMed(97,ENG25)
+ Henry J. Austin Health Center
321 North Warren Street   Trenton, NJ 08618   (609)278-5900   Fax (609)695-3532

Agrawal, Nina, MD {1972557411} Pedtrc(91,NJ05)<NJ-HACKNSK>
+ Hackensack University Medical Center
30 Prospect Avenue   Hackensack, NJ 07601   (201)336-8694

Agrawal, Rekha, MD {1073638797} IntrMd(89,INA32)<NJ-OVERLOOK, NJ-MORRISTN>
+ AMS Medical LLC
5 Mountain Boulevard/Suite 3   Warren, NJ 07059   (908)222-9004   Fax (800)206-9179
Rekha.a@att.net

Agrawal, Stuti Shah, MD {1154395192} IntrMd(93,INDI)<NJ-CENTRAST>
+ Howell Primary Care, P.C.
1001 Route 9 North/Suite 105   Howell, NJ 07731   (732)625-1100   Fax (732)625-1110

Agrawal, Trishala R., MD {1457627697}<NJ-NWRKBETH>
+ Newark Beth Israel Medical Center
201 Lyons Avenue   Newark, NJ 07112   (973)926-7300

Agres, Mildred D., MD {1598795577} Anesth(74,PHI01)<NJ-STMRYPAS>
+ St. Mary's Hospital
350 Boulevard   Passaic, NJ 07055   (973)365-4300   Fax (973)779-7385

Agress, Harry, Jr., MD {1841273117} RadDia, NuclMd, Rad-Nuc(72,MA07)<NJ-HACKNSK>
 + Hackensack University Medical Center
  30 Prospect Avenue/Radiology   Hackensack, NJ 07601
  (201)996-2254   Fax (201)336-8451
 + New Century Imaging at Oradell
  555 Kinderkamack Road   Oradell, NJ 07649   (201)996-2254
  Fax (201)599-8333
 + The Imaging Center
  30 South Newman Street   Hackensack, NJ 07601
  (201)488-1188   Fax (201)488-5244

Agresti, James V., DO {1306931837} Nephro, IntrMd(80,MO79)
 + 609 Kenilworth Boulevard
  Kenilworth, NJ 07033   (908)272-0777   Fax (908)272-6064

Agresti, James V., III, MD {1255389813} IntrMd(99,GRN01)
 + Drs. Agresti and Agresti
  181 Franklin Avenue/Suite 201   Nutley, NJ 07110
  (973)284-0777   Fax (973)284-1530

Agresti, James V., Sr., DO {1578511135} FamMed, IntrMd(68,MO79)<NJ-CLARMAAS, NJ-MTNSIDE>
 + Drs. Agresti and Agresti
  181 Franklin Avenue/Suite 201   Nutley, NJ 07110
  (973)284-0777   Fax (973)284-1530

Agresti, Robert J., DO {1619155710} SrgPlstc, SrgHnd(83,MO79)<NJ-CLARMAAS>
 + 47 Bloomfield Avenue
  Caldwell, NJ 07006   (973)228-1010   Fax (973)228-1717
 + 609 Boulevard
  Kenilworth, NJ 07033   (973)228-1010   Fax (908)272-6064

Agri, Robyn F., MD {1669554713} PhysMd(85,NY15)<NJ-STLAWRN>
 + St. Lawrence Rehabilitation Center
  2381 Lawrenceville Road   Lawrenceville, NJ 08648
  (609)896-9500   Fax (609)896-4107

Agrin, Richard Joel, MD {1316982689} EnDbMt, IntrMd(71,PA01)
 + Drs. Agrin & Shulman
  245 Union Avenue/Suite 2B   Bridgewater, NJ 08807
  (908)231-1311   Fax (908)231-1324
 + Drs. Agrin and Shulman
  78 Easton Avenue   New Brunswick, NJ 08901   (908)231-1311   Fax (732)545-1063

Aguayo-Figueroa, Lourdes, MD {1376718551} PedEnd, Pedtrc(02,PRO04)
 + Passaic Pediatrics PA
  298 Passaic Street   Passaic, NJ 07055   (973)249-8100   Fax (973)249-8110

Aguh, Chikezie J., MD {1407876261} ObsGyn(83,GRN01)<NJ-SOMERSET, NJ-STPETER>
 + Franklin Women Care, PA
  605 Franklin Boulevard/Suite 3   Somerset, NJ 08873
  (732)220-0001   Fax (732)220-9656

Aguila, Helen A., MD {1386718740} Pedtrc, PedPul(74,PHIL)<NJ-UMDNJ>
 + University Hospital-Doctors Office Center
  90 Bergen Street/DOC 5100/Pedi   Newark, NJ 07103
  (973)972-5779   Fax (973)972-5895

Aguilar, Francis, MD {1437602893} Psychy
 + Cooper Psychiatric Associates
  3 Cooper Plaza/Suite 307   Camden, NJ 08103   (856)342-2328   Fax (856)541-6137

Aguilar, Hector David, Jr., MD {1699902296} Pedtrc<NJ-UMDNJ>
 + University Hospital
  150 Bergen Street/Uh-h245   Newark, NJ 07103   (973)972-5672

Aguilar, Raul F., MD {1619911906} ObsGyn(83,PRO02)<NJ-HOBUNIMC, NJ-MEADWLND>
 + 129 Washington Street/Suite 200
  Hoboken, NJ 07030   (201)798-4044   Fax (201)798-3358

Aguirre, Frank J., MD {1144344672} Radiol(79,SPA06)
 + Aguirre Imaging
  195 Lafayette Street   Newark, NJ 07105   (973)465-3044

Aguirre-Masecampo, Alfe G., MD {1851501282} Psychy(65,PHI01)
 + South Jersey Behavioral Health Resources - Stratford
  1 Colby Avenue/Suite 5   Stratford, NJ 08084   (856)541-1700   Fax (856)346-3627

Agzamova, Gulnoza, MD {1184915936}
 + 199 Jonathan Dayton Court
  Princeton, NJ 08540   (609)497-0210
  gulnoza75@hotmail.com

Ahad, Antwan B., MD {1083729917} ClNrPh, Elecen, Elecmj(77,SYRI)<NJ-CHRIST, NJ-MEADWLND>
 + 1265 Paterson Plank Road/suite 3E
  Secaucus, NJ 07094   (201)863-6101   Fax (201)863-7777

Ahkami, Behzad, MD {1649469321} Psychy, Addctn, Psythp(69,IRAN)<NJ-CHILTON, NJ-STMRYPAS>
 + 506 Hamburg Turnpike/Suite 103
  Wayne, NJ 07470   (973)471-5444   Fax (973)778-0848

Ahkami, Rosaline N., MD {1265449334} Dermat(94,NJ05)
 + Dermatology Associates-Warren
  122 Mount Bethel Road   Warren, NJ 07059   (908)756-7999   Fax (908)756-8017

Ahkami, Shahrokh, MD {1740237197} ObsGyn(64,IRAN)
 + Ahkami Medical Group PA
  110 Passaic Avenue   Passaic, NJ 07055   (973)471-9585
  Fax (973)471-8534
  mirassiran@aol.com

Ahlawat, Stuti, MD {1073801742} RadOnc
 + MD Anderson Cancer Center at Cooper
  2 Cooper Plaza   Camden, NJ 08103   (856)735-6119   Fax (856)735-6467
 + Shore Radiation Oncology, LLC
  1 Riverview Plaza   Red Bank, NJ 07701   (856)735-6119
  Fax (732)836-4036
 + Shore Radiation Oncology, LLC
  425 Jack Martin Boulevard   Brick, NJ 08103   (732)836-4109
  Fax (732)836-4036

Ahlawat, Sushil K., MD {1760568455} IntrMd, Gastrn(86,INA7P)<NJ-UMDNJ>
 + UMDNJ Division of Gastroenterology & Hepatology
  90 Bergen Street/DOC 2100   Newark, NJ 07103   (973)972-2343   Fax (973)972-0752
  ahlawasu@umdnj.edu
 + University Hospital
  150 Bergen Street/Medicine   Newark, NJ 07103   (973)972-4300

Ahlborn, Heidi, MD {1588063002}
 + 310 Glenwood Road
  Ridgewood, NJ 07450   (201)445-1764

Ahlborn, Thomas N., MD {1801883277} Surgry(80,NY01)<NJ-VALLEY>
 + Valley Medical Group General Surgery
  385 South Maple Avenue/Suite 202   Glen Rock, NJ 07452
  (201)444-5757   Fax (201)444-0184

Ahmad, Adeel, MD {1912108044} Psychy
 + Lourdes Medical Associates
  500 Grove Street/Suite 100   Haddon Heights, NJ 08035
  (201)567-2277   Fax (201)567-7506
 + Physical Medicine & Rehabilitation Center, PA
  1530 Palisade Avenue   Fort Lee, NJ 07024   (201)567-2277
  Fax (201)363-8873

Ahmad, Ahsanuddin, MD {1962529388} ClCdEl, CdvDis, IntrMd(05,NJ15)<MA-NEMEDCEN>
 + Total Cardiology Care
  120 Franklin Street   Jersey City, NJ 07307   (201)216-9791
  Fax (201)216-1362

Ahmad, Ali, MD {1336425057} CdvDis(05,GRN01)
 + Summit Medical Group
  6 Brighton Road/2 FL   Clifton, NJ 07012   (973)777-7911
  Fax (973)777-5403
 + Summit Medical Group
  31-00 Broadway   Fair Lawn, NJ 07410   (973)777-7911
  Fax (201)796-7020

Ahmad, Arlene, MD {1669552881} Ophthl(74,NJ05)<NJ-STCLRDEN, NJ-STCLRBOO>
 + Lakeland Eye Care, PA
  223 West Main Street   Boonton, NJ 07005   (973)263-2080
  Fax (973)263-3727

Ahmad, Attiya, MD {1710354931}<NJ-VALLEY>
 + The Valley Hospital
  223 North Van Dien Avenue   Ridgewood, NJ 07450
  (201)447-8500

Ahmad, Christopher S., MD {1598795445} SrgOrt, Surgry(94,NY19)<NY-PRSBWEIL, NJ-PALISADE>
 + Columbia Grand Orthopaedics
  500 Grand Avenue/Suite 101   Englewood, NJ 07631
  (201)569-0440   Fax (201)569-4949

Ahmad, Fuad A., MD {1750350120} GenPrc, IntrMd(79,JORD)<NJ-WAYNEGEN, NJ-CHILTON>
 + 191 Hamburg Pike/Suite 2A
  Pompton Lakes, NJ 07442   (973)831-6557   Fax (973)831-6552

Ahmad, Idrees, MD {1164533527} Anesth(77,PAKI)
 + New Jersey Anesthesia Associates, P.C.
  252 Columbia Turnpike/PO Box 0037   Florham Park, NJ 07932   (973)660-9334   Fax (973)660-9779
 + Short Hills Surgery Center
  187 Millburn Avenue/Suite 101/Anesth   Millburn, NJ 07041
  (973)660-9334   Fax (973)671-0557

Ahmad, Imtiaz, MD {1720146384} Pthlgy, PthAcl(70,PAK11)<NJ-HOBUNIMC>
 + Hoboken University Medical Center
  308 Willow Avenue/Path   Hoboken, NJ 07030   (201)418-1000   Fax (201)418-1983

Ahmad, Iqbal, MD {1689856718} SrgOrt(66,PAKI)
 + 45 Academy Street/Suite 203
  Newark, NJ 07102   (973)643-5900   Fax (973)643-3171

Ahmad, Israr, MD {1669796702} IntHos, IntrMd(99,PAK06)<NJ-ACMCITY>
 + AtlantiCare Regional Medical Center/City Campus
  1925 Pacific Avenue/Hospitalist   Atlantic City, NJ 08401
  (609)441-8146

Ahmad, Kaleem U., MD {1629065982} IntrMd, OncHem, Hemato(90,PAK11)<NJ-BURDTMLN, NJ-ACMCMAIN>
 + Hope Community Cancer Center LLC
  210 South Shore Road/Suite 106-A   Marmora, NJ 08223
  (609)390-7888   Fax (609)390-2614

Ahmad, Khalid Mehmood, MD {1023001252} InfDis, IntrMd(95,PAK01)<NJ-RIVERVW>
 + Riverview Medical Center
  1 Riverview Plaza/Inf Disease   Red Bank, NJ 07701
  (732)530-2421

Ahmad, Maliha, MD {1902067952} IntrMd, Hepato(04,SENE)<NJ-UMDNJ>
 + St. Joseph's Regional Medical Center
  703 Main Street   Paterson, NJ 07503   (973)754-2315

Ahmad, Mehmood R., MD {1730178203} CdvDis, IntrMd(67,PAKI)
 + 356 Route 46
  Mountain Lakes, NJ 07046

Ahmad, Mir M., MD {1285735860} Nephro, IntrMd(95,PAK01)
 + Nephrological Associates, P.A.
  83 Hanover Road/Suite 290   Florham Park, NJ 07932
  (973)736-2212   Fax (973)736-2989
 + Nephrological Associates PA
  206 Belleville Avenue   Bloomfield, NJ 07003   (973)736-2212   Fax (973)259-0396

Ahmad, Mir S., MD {1649336264} IntrMd, PulDis(87,PAK15)<NJ-RWJUBRUN, NJ-STPETER>
 + 1950 Route 27/Suite F
  North Brunswick, NJ 08902   (732)422-8440   Fax (732)422-8404

Ahmad, Muhammad A., MD {1164500823} CdvDis, IntrMd(71,PAK01)<NJ-BAYONNE, NJ-CHRIST>
 + 2440 John F. Kennedy Boulevard
  Jersey City, NJ 07304   (201)433-3316   Fax (201)432-4965

Ahmad, Nadir, MD {1396969549} Surgry
 + Cooper Surgical Associates
  3 Cooper Plaza/Suite 403   Camden, NJ 08103   (810)814-2229   Fax (856)541-5379
  nadirahmad@hotmail.com

Ahmad, Naheed Kaleem, MD {1790974756} IntrMd, IntHos<NJ-ACMCITY>
 + AtlantiCare Hospitalist Program
  1925 Pacific Avenue/8th Floor   Atlantic City, NJ 08401
  (609)441-8146

Ahmad, Nasir Mahmood, MD {1598730186} InfDis, IntrMd(95,PAK01)
 + Meridian Medical Associates-Infectious Disease
  1 Riverview Plaza/Suite 2 West   Red Bank, NJ 07701
  (732)530-2421

Ahmad, Nauman, MD {1952441438} IntrMd(00,DMN01)<NJ-RIVERVW>
 + Hospital Medicine Associates
  157 Broad Street/Suite 317   Red Bank, NJ 07701
  (732)530-2960   Fax (732)530-7446

Ahmad, Nausher, MD {1245291996} IntrMd(01,DMN01)<NJ-NWRKBETH, NJ-STBARNMC>
 + 196 West Shirley Avenue
  Edison, NJ 08820   (973)203-3509   Fax (201)436-2962
 + St. Barnabas Health Care Center
  95 Old Short Hills Road/Internal Med   West Orange, NJ 07052   (973)203-3509   Fax (973)322-4416

Ahmad, Nazish, MD {1295098903}<NJ-CHSFULD>
 + Capital Health System/Fuld Campus
  750 Brunswick Avenue   Trenton, NJ 08638   (609)394-6031

Ahmad, Nina, MD {1124339023} FamMed(07,IL42)
 + 1 Peak Lane
  Hillsborough, NJ 08844

Ahmad, Omar Syed, MD {1043531254}<NJ-CHSFULD>
 + Capital Health System/Fuld Campus
  750 Brunswick Avenue   Trenton, NJ 08638   (609)394-6031
  Fax (609)394-6028

Ahmad, Raheela, MD {1336205020} Psychy(73,PAK08)<NJ-CLARMAAS>
 + Clara Maass Medical Center
  1 Clara Maass Drive/Psych   Belleville, NJ 07109   (973)450-2000

Ahmad, Sajida Ghani, MD {1205842499} Anesth(70,PAK10)<NJ-CHSFULD, NJ-CHSMRCER>
 + Trenton Anesthesiology Associates, PA
  One Capital Way/Second Floor   Pennington, NJ 08534
  (609)396-4700   Fax (609)396-4900

Ahmad, Sarfaraz, MD {1427064617} Surgry(64,PAK11)<NJ-CHSFULD, NJ-RWJUHAM>
 + Advanced Surgical Associates of New Jersey
  40 Fuld Street/Suite 403   Trenton, NJ 08638   (609)537-6000   Fax (609)537-6002
 + Robert Wood Johnson University Hospital at Hamilton
  1 Hamilton Health Place/Surgery   Hamilton, NJ 08690
  (609)213-1630

Physicians by Name and Address

Ahmad, Syed S., MD {1629162177} Gastrn, IntrMd(72,PAKI)<NJ-CHSFULD, NJ-RWJUHAM>
+ Ahmad Syed S MD PA
183 Franklin Corner Road   Lawrenceville, NJ 08648   (609)896-0622   Fax (609)896-0069
+ Drs. Ahmad and Lou
1607 South Broad Street   Trenton, NJ 08610   (609)393-1870

Ahmad, Tanveer, MD {1962464495} CdvDis, IntrMd, CarNuc(82,PAK01)<NJ-JRSYSHMC, NJ-OCEANMC>
+ Cardiology Associates of Ocean County PA
495 Jack Martin Boulevard/Suite 2   Brick, NJ 08724   (732)458-7575   Fax (732)458-0874
+ Cardiology Associates of Ocean County PA
500 River Avenue/Suite 220   Lakewood, NJ 08701   (732)458-7575   Fax (732)458-0874
+ Cardiology Associates of Ocean County PA
9 Hospital Drive/Suite B8   Toms River, NJ 08724   (732)349-8899   Fax (732)458-0874

Ahmad, Umer Farooq, MD {1265698591}<NJ-TRINIWSC>
+ Trinitas Regional Medical Center-Williamson Street
225 Williamson Street   Elizabeth, NJ 07207   (908)994-5000
umerfahmad@gmail.com

Ahmad, Usman Fayyaz, DO {1558676692} PhyMPain, PhysMd
+ 575 Easton Avenue/Apt 9 F
Somerset, NJ 08873   (850)832-8772
ufahmad@gmail.com

Ahmad, Yasir Jamal, MD {1275570509} FamMed, Psychy(98,SLU01)<NJ-HACKNSK>
+ Hackensack University Medical Center
30 Prospect Avenue   Hackensack, NJ 07601   (201)996-2000

Ahmadi, Cyrus, MD {1912901950} Pedtrc(67,IRAN)<NJ-STMRY-PAS>
+ 53 Passaic Avenue
Passaic, NJ 07055   (973)471-4440   Fax (973)471-4681
Doctor@CyrusAhmadiMD.com

Ahmadi, David, MD {1225039464} Otlryg, Otolgy(68,IRAN)
+ 222 Easton Avenue
New Brunswick, NJ 08901   (732)828-6404   Fax (732)846-8035

Ahmed, Aisha I., MD {1639434833} Psychy, Nrolgy(64,BAN02)
+ 9 Washburne Avenue
Berlin, NJ 08009

Ahmed, Ameer Nizam, MD {1356751838} FamMSptM(14,DMN01)
+ CityMD Union Urgent Care
2317 Center Island Route 22   Union, NJ 07083   (201)354-1951   Fax (201)354-1952

Ahmed, Amina A., MD {1255409751} IntrMd(01,DOM18)<NJ-OVERLOOK, NJ-MORRISTN>
+ 2440 Kennedy Boulevard
Jersey City, NJ 07304   (201)433-3316   Fax (201)433-4448
+ Summit Medical Group-Berkeley Heights Campus
1 Diamond Hill Road   Berkeley Heights, NJ 07922   (201)433-3316   Fax (908)790-6576

Ahmed, Asad, DO {1477972867} IntrMd<NJ-PALISADE>
+ Palisades Medical Center
7600 River Road   North Bergen, NJ 07047   (630)476-2343

Ahmed, Asma Talukder, DO {1225023682} IntrMd(00,NY75)<NJ-EASTORNG>
+ Laskin Internal Medcine
400 Grove Road/PO Box 37   Thorofare, NJ 08086   (856)845-8010

Ahmed, Atif Khalid, MD {1184981789} OrtTrm
+ Rothman Institute
1225 Whitehorse Mercerville Ro   Mercerville, NJ 08619   (800)321-9999   Fax (609)581-1212

Ahmed, Essam Abdelfattah, MD {1710969886} Pthlgy, PthACl(79,EGY03)<NJ-CHILTON>
+ Chilton Medical Center
97 West Parkway/Path   Pompton Plains, NJ 07444   (973)831-5000

Ahmed, Farooque, MD {1164424982} IntrMd(90,BAN06)
+ Memorial Hospital of Salem County
310 Woodstown Road   Salem, NJ 08079   (856)935-1000

Ahmed, Fauzia Mosarrat, MD {1730179953} IntrMd(89,INA3C)
+ Urgent Health Care Center
719 Route 22 West   North Plainfield, NJ 07060   (908)561-4300   Fax (908)561-4340

Ahmed, Ilyas, MD {1497761589} IntrMd(70,PAK01)<NJ-SJER-SYHS>
+ 217 Laurel Heights Drive
Bridgeton, NJ 08302   (856)451-4150   Fax (856)451-2645

Ahmed, Irfan Haroon, MD {1700022043} OrtSHand, SrgOrt(01,PAK11)
+ UMDNJ Dept of Orthopaedics
90 Bergen Street/DOC 1200   Jersey City, NJ 07305   (973)972-2150

Ahmed, Kamran, MD {1982631776} Pedtrc, NnPnMd(91,PAK11)<NJ-ACMCMAIN>
+ AtlantiCare Regional Med Ctr/Mainland
65 West Jimmie Leeds Road/NeoPeri   Pomona, NJ 08240   (609)652-1000

Ahmed, Lubna, MD {1821157231} IntrMd(74,PAK01)
+ 1700 Whitehorse Ham Road/Suite B4
Trenton, NJ 08690   (609)581-7555   Fax (609)584-9115

Ahmed, Mehvish, DO {1477990794} EmrgMd
+ Rowan University-School of Osteopathic Medicine
1 Medical Center Drive   Stratford, NJ 08084   (856)346-7985

Ahmed, Munir, MD {1639267875} SrgOrt, IntrMd(70,PAK01)<NJ-COMMED, NJ-KIMBALL>
+ Ultimed HealthCare PC
50 Franklin Lane   Manalapan, NJ 07726   (732)972-1267   Fax (732)972-1026

Ahmed, Mutahar, MD {1760451827} Urolgy(97,NY15)<NJ-HACKNSK, NJ-STMRYPAS>
+ New Jersey Center for Prostate Cancer & Urology
255 West Spring Valley Avenue   Maywood, NJ 07607   (201)487-8866   Fax (201)487-2602
+ New Jersey Center for Prostate Cancer & Urology
200 South Orange Avenue/Suite 228   Livingston, NJ 07039   (201)487-8866   Fax (973)322-0135

Ahmed, Naseer, MD {1982062667} IntHos<NJ-JRSYSHMC>
+ Jersey Shore University Medical Center
1945 Route 33/Medicine   Neptune, NJ 07753   (732)775-5500

Ahmed, Nasim, MD {1841266780} SrgCrC, Surgry(87,PAK11)<NJ-JRSYSHMC>
+ Jersey Shore University Medical Center
1945 Route 33/Surgery   Neptune, NJ 07753   (732)776-4747

Ahmed, Omar Zikri, MD {1609154640}
+ Atlantic Shore Surgical Associates
478 Brick Boulevard   Brick, NJ 08723   (732)701-4848   Fax (732)701-1244

Ahmed, Sabeen, MD {1619362225} IntrMd<NJ-MTNSIDE>
+ Hackensack UMC Mountainside
1 Bay Avenue   Montclair, NJ 07042   (973)429-6196   Fax (973)429-6575

Ahmed, Sadia, MD {1225223464} IntrMd
+ Advance Hospital Care @ Somerset Medical Center
110 Rehill Avenue   Somerville, NJ 08876   (908)429-5833   Fax (908)203-5970

Ahmed, Safi U., MD {1184849739} IntrMd, CdvDis(99,DMN01)<NJ-OURLADY, NJ-VIRTUAHS>
+ Associated Cardiovascular Consultants, PA
2 Sindoni Lane   Hammonton, NJ 08037   (609)561-8500   Fax (856)567-0432

Ahmed, Saira N., MD {1437325768} IntrMd(05,DMN01)<NJ-TRINIWSC>
+ Trinitas Regional Medical Center-Williamson Street
225 Williamson Street/IntMed   Elizabeth, NJ 07207   (908)994-5000

Ahmed, Shahida Y., MD {1780695882} PthACl<NJ-VAEASTOR>
+ VA New Jersey Health Care System-East Orange Campus
385 Tremont Avenue/Pathology   East Orange, NJ 07018   (973)676-1000

Ahmed, Shaikh Sultan, MD {1750316287} CdvDis, IntrMd(63,PAK11)<NJ-UMDNJ, NJ-BERGNMC>
+ University Hospital-Doctors Office Center
90 Bergen Street/Cardio/3500   Newark, NJ 07103   (973)972-2573   Fax (973)972-4695

Ahmed, Subhan, MD {1982830329} Nephro
+ Nephrology Associates PA
870 Palisade Avenue/Suite 202   Teaneck, NJ 07666   (201)836-0897   Fax (201)836-8042

Ahmed, Suhel Hussain, MD {1801042072} IntrMd(05,DMN01)
+ Dr Suhel Hussain Ahmed and Assoc
92 Summit Avenue   Hackensack, NJ 07601   (201)342-0066   Fax (201)342-0079

Ahmed, Sujood, MD {1932120615} CdvDis, IntrMd, Elecen(89,PAK15)
+ Med-Com Health Services, P.A.
258 North New Road   Pleasantville, NJ 08232   (609)646-4064   Fax (609)272-8526

Ahmed, Syed F., MD {1821022799} IntrMd(92,PAKI)<NJ-SOMERSET>
+ MEDEMERGE
1005 North Washington Avenue   Green Brook, NJ 08812   (732)968-8900   Fax (732)968-4609

Ahmed, Umrana, MD {1700885506} Nephro, IntrMd(81,MEX22)<NJ-CHRIST, NJ-BAYONNE>
+ Drs. Ahmed, Haddad & Batwara
26 Greenville Avenue   Jersey City, NJ 07305   (201)333-8222   Fax (201)333-0095
+ Bayonne Medical Center
29th Street at Avenue E/Nephrology   Bayonne, NJ 07002   (201)858-5000
+ Christ Hospital
176 Palisade Avenue/Nephrology   Jersey City, NJ 07305   (201)795-8200

Ahmed, Zaib, DO {1255711875} EmrgMd
+ St Joseph's Medical Center Emergency
703 Main Street   Paterson, NJ 07503   (973)754-2000   Fax (973)754-2249

Ahmed-Flowers, Tunizia, MD {1326219023} FamMed, IntrMd(01,SLU01)
+ Valley Health Medical Group
759 Hamburg Turnpike   Wayne, NJ 07470   (973)709-0099   Fax (973)709-0201

Ahn, Joe Kyuhyun, MD {1750557310} CdvDis
+ Medicor Cardiology
225 Jackson Street   Bridgewater, NJ 08807   (908)526-8668   Fax (908)231-6781
Ahnjoe@aol.com
+ Medicor Cardiology PA
331 US Highway 206/Suite 1A   Hillsborough, NJ 08844   (908)526-8668   Fax (908)431-0808

Ahn, Paul Michael, DO {1609934298} FamMed(93,NY75)<NJ-JFKMED, NJ-RWJURAH>
+ Oak Tree Family Practice LLC
173 Essex Avenue/Suite 101   Metuchen, NJ 08840   (732)321-5100   Fax (732)321-5252

Ahr, Lawrence M., MD {1144244294} Pedtrc(83,DOM02)<NJ-LOURDMED>
+ CHOP Primary Care Mount Laurel
3201 Marne Highway   Mount Laurel, NJ 08054   (856)829-5545   Fax (856)829-9268

Ahrens, John C., MD {1568443646} InfDis, IntrMd(87,PA13)<NJ-SJERSYHS, NJ-SJHREGMC>
+ Cumberland Internal Medicine
1450 East Chestnut Avenue   Vineland, NJ 08361   (856)794-8700   Fax (856)794-2752

Ahsan, Abu M., MD {1316994437} IntrMd(87,BAN02)<NJ-SJHREGMC>
+ 57 Wesley Road
Hillsborough, NJ 08844

Ahsan, Ambreen, MD {1811022940} Pedtrc(97,PAK11)
+ S&A Pediatrics
192 Parsippany Road   Parsippany, NJ 07054   (973)794-3170

Ahsan, Shagufta, MD {1003059866} IntrMd(00,BAN02)
+ St. Joseph's Regional Medical Center
703 Main Street   Paterson, NJ 07503   (973)754-2000

Ahsan, Syed Nadeem, MD {1043262751} Anesth(89,PAK11)<NJ-VIRTVOOR, NJ-KENEDYHS>
+ Advanced Pain Consultants, P.A.
326 Route 73   Voorhees, NJ 08043   (856)489-9822   Fax (856)489-9877
+ Advanced Pain Consultants, P.A.
120 Madison Avenue/Suite D   Mount Holly, NJ 08060   (609)267-1707
+ 23 Periwinkle Drive
Mount Laurel, NJ 08043

Ahuja, Kavita Bala, DO {1255592515} IntrMd, Nephro(02,NY75)
+ Hypertension & Nephrology Specialists, LLC
2 Research Way/Suite 301   Monroe, NJ 08831   (732)521-0800   Fax (732)521-0833
+ Hypertension & Nephrology Specialists, LLC
49 Veronica Avenue/Suite 104   Somerset, NJ 08873   (732)521-0800   Fax (732)521-0833
+ Hypertension & Nephrology Specialists, LLC
601 Ewing Street/Suite C-7   Princeton, NJ 08831   (732)521-0800   Fax (732)521-0833

Ahuja, Kishore Kanayalal, MD {1548237167} Allrgy, IntrMd, Pthlgy(73,INA1Z)<NJ-WAYNEGEN>
+ 1031 McBride Avenue/Suite C-204
Little Falls, NJ 07424   (973)785-0060   Fax (973)785-1408
kishore50@yahoo.com
+ 1 Woodbridge Center/Suite 400
Woodbridge, NJ 07095   (973)785-0060   Fax (732)636-3669

Ahuja, Naveen K., MD {1780834630} SrgPlstc(MI01
+ Plastic Surgery Arts of of New Jersey
409 Joyce Kilmer Ave./Suite 210   New Brunswick, NJ 08901   (732)418-0709   Fax (732)418-0747

Ahuja, Pouja Artee, DO {1306273669}
+ Lantern Hill Retirement Community
535 Mountain Avenue   New Providence, NJ 07974   (908)673-7157   Fax (855)865-3168
+ NHCAC Health Center at West New York
5301 Broadway   West New York, NJ 07093   (201)866-9320

Ahuja, Rakesh, MD {1578797270} IntrMd(98,INA30)
+ 175 High Street
Newton, NJ 07860   (732)824-7888
+ 9 Winans Avenue
Piscataway, NJ 08854

Ahuja, Yogesh, MD {1851331219} EmrgMd(02,IL06)
+ Emergency Physician Associates, P.A.
307 South Evergreen Avenue/PO Box 298   Woodbury, NJ 08096   (856)848-3817   Fax (856)848-1431

Physicians by Name and Address

Aiden, Kanwardeep Singh, MD {1336109875} IntrMd(92,INA23)
+ Premier Internal Medicine Associates
55 Brunswick Woods Drive   East Brunswick, NJ 08816
(732)254-4474   Fax (732)254-4475

Aiello, Kathleen Kuykendall, MD {1841262631} Pedtrc, IntrMd(02,PA02)<PA-STMARY, PA-LWBUCK>
+ Southern Jersey Medical Center
651 High Street   Burlington City, NJ 08016   (609)386-0775
Fax (609)386-4372

Aiello, Stephen Anthony, MD {1831100825} Grtrcs, IntrMd(78,PA13)
+ Capital Health Primary Care-Hamilton
1445 Whitehorse-Mercerville Rd   Hamilton, NJ 08619
(609)587-6661   Fax (609)587-8503

Aiken, Robert Dennis, MD {1851372981} Nrolgy, IntrMd(76,MI07)
+ 195 Little Albany Street/Suite 5501-A
New Brunswick, NJ 08903   (732)235-7464   Fax (732)235-6797

Aikins, James K., Jr., MD {1346337839} ObsGyn, Gyneco, GynOnc(85,PA07)<NJ-COOPRUMC, NJ-ACMCITY>
+ Cooper Gynecologic Oncology Associates
900 Centennial Boulevard/Suite F   Voorhees, NJ 08043
(856)325-6644   Fax (856)325-6643
rauch-kathleen@cooperhealth.edu
+ Women's Care Center
3 Cooper Plaza/Suite 301   Camden, NJ 08103   (856)325-6644   Fax (856)968-8575
+ Cooper Ob/Gyn
3 Cooper Plaza/Suite 300   Camden, NJ 08043   (856)342-2186   Fax (856)968-8575

Aikman, Noelle M., MD {1821057522} ObsGyn(88,NJ06)<NJ-JRSYSHMC>
+ Hackensack Meridian Medical Group Ob/Gyn, Wall
1924 Route 35/Suite 5   Wall, NJ 07719   (732)974-8404
Fax (732)974-8904
+ Hackensack Meridian Medical Group Ob/Gyn, Jackson
27 South Cooks Bridge Road/Suite 2-19   Jackson, NJ 08527
(732)974-8404   Fax (732)987-5766
+ Hackensack Meridian Medical Group Ob/Gyn, Neptune
1828 West Lake Avenue   Neptune, NJ 07719   (732)869-5700   Fax (732)776-4892

Ainslie, William, Jr., MD {1447364203} ObsGyn(75,NY47)
+ Obstetrical & Gynecological Group of Metuchen, PA
73 Amboy Avenue   Metuchen, NJ 08840   (732)548-0698
Fax (732)548-3087

Airapetian, Karine V., MD {1952593816} Psychy(87,ARM27)<NJ-BERGNMC>
+ New Bridge Medical Center
230 East Ridgewood Avenue/Psych   Paramus, NJ 07652
(201)967-4000
+ Bergen Psychiatrists, Inc
217 1st Street/Suite 2-C   Ho Ho Kus, NJ 07423

Airen, Anshul, MD {1720255474} Anesth, IntrMd(01,NY15)<NJ-UNVMCPRN>
+ University Medical Center of Princeton at Plainsboro
One Plainsboro Road/Anesth   Plainsboro, NJ 08536
(609)497-4000

Airen, Priya, MD {1083801146} IntrMd(03,INA7P)<NJ-VIRTMHBC, NJ-VIRTUAHS>
+ Virtua Marlton Hospital
90 Brick Road/Internal Med   Marlton, NJ 08053   (856)355-6730   Fax (856)355-6731
+ Virtua Memorial
175 Madison Avenue/Internal Med   Mount Holly, NJ 08060
(609)267-0700
+ Virtua Marlton Hospitalist Group
94 Brock Road/Suite 302   Marlton, NJ 08053   (856)355-6730

Airood, Moumina, MD {1831150671} Rheuma, IntrMd(89,SYR01)
+ Amana Medical Group
871 McBride Avenue   West Paterson, NJ 07424   (973)569-4488   Fax (973)565-4743

Aisenberg, Javier E., MD {1053364000} PedEnd(87,ARG01)<NJ-HACKNSK>
+ Hackensack University Medical Center
30 Prospect Avenue/PediEndocrin   Hackensack, NJ 07601
(201)996-2000

Aisner, Joseph, MD {1649328410} IntrMd, MedOnc(70,MI07)<NJ-RWJUBRUN>
+ Rutgers Cancer Institute of New Jersey
195 Little Albany Street/PO Box 2681   New Brunswick, NJ 08903   (732)235-7401   Fax (732)235-6797

Aisner, Seena C., MD {1205859410} PthAna, PthCln, PthCyt(73,DC01)<NJ-UMDNJ>
+ University Hospital
150 Bergen Street/Antmc Pthlgy   Newark, NJ 07103
(973)972-4520

Aita, Daren J., MD {1154327146} SrgOrt(92,PA09)<NJ-CAPITLHS, NJ-CHSFULD>
+ Trenton Orthopaedic Group
1225 Whitehorse Mercerville Rd   Trenton, NJ 08619

(609)581-2200   Fax (609)581-1212
+ Trenton Orthopaedic Group
116 Washington Crossing Road   Pennington, NJ 08534
(609)581-2200   Fax (609)581-1212

Aita, Wendy F., MD {1023206653}
+ University Hospital-SOM Department of Psychiatry
2250 Chapel Avenue West/Suite 100   Cherry Hill, NJ 08002
(856)482-9000   Fax (856)482-1159

Aitchison, Samantha H., MD {1447405758} SrgTpl<NJ-STBARNMC>
+ St. Barnabas Medical Center
94 Old Short Hills Road   Livingston, NJ 07039   (646)456-4381

Aitken, Robert J., DO {1285726893} FamMed(81,PA77)<NJ-OURLADY>
+ Advocare Sicklerville Internal Med
485 Williamstown Road   Sicklerville, NJ 08081   (856)237-8100   Fax (856)237-8042

Ajay, Rajasree, MD {1942257787} OncHem, IntrMd(91,INDI)<NJ-ACMCITY, NJ-SHOREMEM>
+ Premier Oncology, LLC.
54 West Jimmie Leeds Road/Suite 11   Galloway, NJ 08205
(609)748-1001   Fax (609)748-1002
+ Cancer and Blood Disorders Care
54 West Jimmie Leeds Road   Galloway, NJ 08205
(609)748-1001   Fax (609)404-9967

Ajeena, Zainab, MD {1679832091}
+ Kintiroglou Pediatrics
1500 Pleasant Valley Way/Suite 301   West Orange, NJ 07052   (916)969-0980   Fax (973)243-1227
zainab5_18@yahoo.com

Ajemian, Ara Antranik, MD {1154359727} FamMed(94,LEB03)
+ Valley Medical Group of Montvale
85 Chestnut Ridge Road/Suite 111   Montvale, NJ 07645
(201)930-1700   Fax (201)930-0705

Aji, Janah I., MD {1629164918} CdvDis, IntrMd, IntCrd(79,NY47)<NJ-DEBRAHLC, NJ-ACMCMAIN>
+ The Cooper Hospital System-Univ Hospital
3 Cooper Plaza/Suite 215   Camden, NJ 08103   (856)342-2439
+ University Cardiology
3 Cooper Plaza/Room 311   Camden, NJ 08103   (856)342-2034
+ Cooper Cardiology Associates
900 Centennial Boulevard   Voorhees, NJ 08043   (856)325-6700   Fax (856)325-6702

Aji, Wissam, MD {1902237910} GenPrc
+ 139 Buckingham Way
Mount Laurel, NJ 08054   (856)220-5421

Ajmal, Muhammad Suleman, MD {1184873234}<NJ-NWRKBETH>
+ Newark Beth Israel Medical Center
201 Lyons Avenue   Newark, NJ 07112   (973)926-7000

Ajmal, Muhammad Zafar, MD {1932149747} Anesth(93,PAK10)<NJ-VIRTMHBC>
+ Burlington Anesthesia Associates
120 Madison Ave/Suite E/PO Box 174   Mount Holly, NJ 08060   (609)261-1660   Fax (609)261-1779

Akbaripanahi, Sepideh, MD {1083032304} Nrolgy
+ Bergen Neurology Consultants
25 Rockwood Place/Suite 110   Englewood, NJ 07631
(201)894-5805   Fax (201)894-1956

Akers, Stephen M., MD {1033205323} PulDis, IntrMd, CritCrt(81,PA01)<NJ-COOPRUMC>
+ Cooper University Medical Center/Camden
3 Cooper Plaza   Camden, NJ 08103   (856)342-2000   Fax (856)342-7832
+ The Cooper Health System at Voorhees
900 Centennial Boulevard/Suite K   Voorhees, NJ 08043
(856)325-6789

Akhigbe, Kelvin Osagie, DO {1952613051} CdvDis
+ Associated Cardiovascular Consultants-Lourdes
1 Brace Road/Suite C & F   Cherry Hill, NJ 08034   (856)755-1173   Fax (856)428-5748

Akhigbe, Omoikhefe Gbemisola, MD {1932336005} ObsGyn<NJ-HCKTSTWN>
+ Women's Health at Hackettstown
108 Bilby Road/Suite 305   Hackettstown, NJ 07840
(908)813-8877   Fax (908)813-9984

Akhtar, Amana Lalarukh, MD {1154553113}
+ Radiology Associates of Ridgewood, P.A.
20 Franklin Turnpike   Waldwick, NJ 07463   (201)445-8822
Fax (201)447-5053
+ 7 Lynch Road
Voorhees, NJ 08043   (856)304-6151

Akhtar, Fahad Malik, MD {1083960124}
+ 30 Saddle Court
Monroe Township, NJ 08831   (732)521-8203
fahadakhtar4@gmail.com

Akhtar, Rabia, MD {1184030959} Nephro<NJ-RWJUBRUN>
+ RWJ University Hospital New Brunswick
One Robert Wood Johnson Place   New Brunswick, NJ 08901
(732)828-3000

Akhtar, Reza Yasin, MD {1629195748} Gastrn, IntrMd(04,MA07)
+ Shore Gastroenterology Associates, P.C.
1907 Highway 35/Suite 1   Oakhurst, NJ 07755   (732)517-0060   Fax (732)548-7408
reza.akhtar@mssm.edu
+ Shore Gastroenterology Associates, P.C.
1907 Highway 35/Suite 1   Oakhurst, NJ 07755   (732)517-0060   Fax (732)548-7408
+ Shore Gastroenterology Associates, P.C.
233 Middle Road   Hazlet, NJ 07755   (732)361-2476

Akhtar, Ruhi, MD {1407014871} IntHos<NJ-HOLYNAME>
+ Holy Name Hospital
718 Teaneck Road   Teaneck, NJ 07666   (201)833-3000

Akhtar, Shahnaz, MD {1619912102} IntrMd(88,PAK24)
+ Dr. Shahnaz Akhtar and Associates
16 East 29th Street   Bayonne, NJ 07002   (201)339-1685
Fax (201)339-2557

Akhtar, Shuaib A., MD {1639174030} Anesth(86,PAK24)<NJ-STMICHL>
+ St. Joseph's Regional Medical Center Anesthesia
703 Main Street   Paterson, NJ 07503   (973)754-2323   Fax (973)977-9455

Akhtar, Syeda Shahnaz, MD {1134215155} Psychy(91,PAK11)
+ Preferred Behavioral Health of New Jersey
700 Airport Road   Lakewood, NJ 08701   (732)367-4700
Fax (732)364-2253

Akhtar, Tanveer, MD {1609025691}
+ 45 Tudor Court
Marlton, NJ 08053   (646)469-7923

Akhtar, Umair Wasim, MD {1104098102}
+ 2151 Route 35 East/Apt 705
Cherry Hill, NJ 08002

Akhter, Rowsonara, MD {1477844421} Grtrcs, IntrMd(94,BAN05)
+ Osborn Family Health Center
1601 Haddon Road/Geriatrics   Camden, NJ 08103
(856)757-3700   Fax (856)365-7972

Akhter, Shafinaz, MD {1710040431} InfDis, IntrMd(04,PA01)
+ 350 Station Avenue
Haddonfield, NJ 08033

Akhter, Waseem, MD {1437100070} NnPnMd<PA-STLKBTHL>
+ Robert Wood Johnson University Hospital
51 French Street/MEB-234B/Suite 303   New Brunswick, NJ 08903   (732)235-5192

Akinli, Timur C., MD {1710195391} Psychy
+ Center for Family Guidance, PC
765 East Route 70/Building A-101   Marlton, NJ 08053
(856)355-8883   Fax (856)810-0110

Akinronbi, Bolanle O., MD {1912290602}
+ 2101 Orchard Terrace
Linden, NJ 07036   (908)265-0576
bakinronbi@gmail.com

Akinruli, Omowunmi Praise, MD {1689805418} FamMed
+ Southern Jersey Family Medical
238 East Broadway   Salem, NJ 08079   (856)935-7711   Fax (856)935-9123

Akinyemi, Michael Omobolaji, MD {1639305923} RadV&I<NJ-OURLADY>
+ Our Lady of Lourdes Medical Center
1600 Haddon Avenue   Camden, NJ 08103   (856)757-3500

Akkapeddi, Nirmala G., MD {1588767628} IntrMd(80,INDI)<NJ-MORRISTN>
+ Summit Medical Group
477 Route 10 East/Suite 204   Randolph, NJ 07869
(862)260-3020

Akmal, Amer, MD {1164405510} Pthlgy, BldBnk(86,PAK20)<NJ-STJOSHOS, NJ-WAYNEGEN>
+ St. Joseph's Regional Medical Center
703 Main Street/Pathology   Paterson, NJ 07503   (973)754-2000   Fax (973)754-3649

Akpalu, Daniel, MD {1770676033} Pedtrc(96,UKR15)<NJ-HOBUNIMC, NJ-HACKNSK>
+ Hoboken University Medical Center
308 Willow Avenue/Hospitalist   Hoboken, NJ 07030
(201)418-1000
+ Riverside Medical Group
714 Tenth Street/Suite 2   Secaucus, NJ 07094   (201)418-1000   Fax (201)865-0015

Akrout, Eddie, MD {1013371632} FamMed
+ Drs. Aderholdt and Akrout
3 Elizabeth Street   Millville, NJ 08332   (856)641-6272

Akrout, Hafedh, MD {1194735860} PhysMd(72,FRA19)
+ Kresson View Center
28 Sheffield Drive   Moorestown, NJ 08057   (856)608-7897
Fax (856)608-3153

Akrout, Tarak, MD {1073523742} PhysMd(80,FRAN)
+ Pennsville Sports Medicine & Rehabilitation Center
270 South Broadway/PO Box 35   Pennsville, NJ 08070
(856)678-5449   Fax (856)678-3153

Physicians by Name and Address

Aksman, Scott S., MD {1992886816} Ophthl(71,IL06)<NJ-CENTRAST, NJ-MONMOUTH>
+ Millennium Eye Care, LLC
500 West Main Street   Freehold, NJ 07728   (732)462-8707
Fax (732)462-1296
+ Millennium Eye Care, LLC
Route 130 & Princeton Road   Hightstown, NJ 08520
(732)462-8707   Fax (609)448-4197
+ Millennium Eye Care, LLC
515 Brick Boulevard/Suite G   Brick, NJ 07728   (732)920-3800   Fax (732)920-5351

Akthar, Morium, MD {1184941197}<NJ-UMDNJ>
+ University Hospital
150 Bergen Street   Newark, NJ 07103   (973)972-6056
Morium.Akthar@tampabay.rr.com

Akturk, Elvin, DO {1871804773} Pedtrc
+ Drs. Banschick, Concepcion & Stein
2500 Lemoine Avenue/Suite 200   Fort Lee, NJ 07024
(201)592-9210   Fax (201)592-6539

Akula, Devender Nagarajan, MD {1285613133} CdvDis, IntrMd(93,INA5B)
+ Associated Cardiovascular Consultants-Lourdes
1 Brace Road/Suite C & F   Cherry Hill, NJ 08034   (856)428-4100   Fax (856)428-5748

Akyar, Selma Ender, MD {1407866759} IntrMd(84,TUR16)<NJ-STBARNMC>
+ 61 Brunswick Woods Drive
East Brunswick, NJ 08816   (732)254-1057
+ Medicus Medical Associates LLC
561 Cranbury Street/Suite M   East Brunswick, NJ 08816
(732)254-1057   Fax (732)651-3144

Al Akshar, Ammar, MD {1447660022}
+ Jersey Shore University Medical Center
1945 Route 33   Neptune, NJ 07753   (732)775-5500

Al Asad, Manar M., MD {1245531680} CritCr
+ 250 Old Hook Road
Westwood, NJ 07675   (201)647-7806

Al Asha, Mohammad H., MD {1225114440} IntrMd, Gastrn(72,SYRI)<NJ-JRSYSHMC>
+ 1930 Highway 35
Wall, NJ 07719   (732)449-2212   Fax (732)974-9888

Al Dulaimi, Hamsa A., MD {1457446056} PthAcl(83,IRQ01)<NJ-OVERLOOK>
+ Overlook Medical Center
99 Beauvoir Avenue/PO Box 210   Summit, NJ 07902
(908)522-2000

Al Haddawi, Anwar, MD {1295822153} Pedtrc(88,IRAQ)<NJ-HACKNSK, NJ-HOLYNAME>
+ Riverside Medical Group
714 Tenth Street/Suite 2   Secaucus, NJ 07094   (201)863-3346   Fax (201)865-0015
+ Riverside Pediatric Group
4201 New York Avenue   Union City, NJ 07087   (201)863-3346   Fax (201)601-9516

Al Haj, Rany Samir, MD {1174649966} Rheuma(99,LEB01)<NJ-JRSYSHMC>
+ Shore Arthritis & Rheumatism Associates
1500 Allaire Avenue/Suite 203 B   Ocean, NJ 07712
(732)660-0011   Fax (732)660-0012
info@shoreara.com

Al Hilli, Rula Ahmed, MD {1154320315} FamMed(90,IRAQ)<NJ-MEMSALEM>
+ 20 Hunters Creek Circle
Mullica Hill, NJ 08062   (856)467-5370   Fax (856)467-8625

Al Kana, Randah, MD {1821048554} Hemato, PthAcl, Pthlgy(84,SYRI)<NJ-COMMED, NJ-KIMBALL>
+ Community Medical Center
99 Route 37 West   Toms River, NJ 08755   (732)240-8237

Al Kawi, Ammar, MD {1376741553} Nrolgy(98,SYR01)
+ Center for Neurological Surgery UMDNJ
90 Bergen Street/DOC 8100   Newark, NJ 07103   (973)972-7852   Fax (973)972-2333

Al Khan, Abdulla Mohammed, MD {1346296076} ObsGyn(95,GRN01)
+ Hackensack University Medical Center
30 Prospect Avenue/Box 73   Hackensack, NJ 07601
(551)996-2453   Fax (201)678-9189

Al Obaidi, Nawar, MD {1437511219}<NJ-NWRKBETH>
+ Newark Beth Israel Medical Center
201 Lyons Avenue   Newark, NJ 07112   (973)926-7425

Al Rabi, Kamal H., MD {1073714424} IntrMd(00,JOR01)
+ 165 Overmount Avenue/Apt E
Little Falls, NJ 07424

Al Shawwaf, Ahmed, MD {1619321098}<NJ-HACKNSK>
+ Hackensack University Medical Center
30 Prospect Avenue   Hackensack, NJ 07601   (551)996-2000

Al Tamsheh, Raniah, MD {1750328829} IntrMd<NJ-UMDNJ>
+ University Hospital
150 Bergen Street/H-245   Newark, NJ 07103   (973)972-4300

Al Ustwani, Omar, MD {1275769978} IntrMd(07,SYR01)
+ Southern Oncology Hematology Associates
1505 West Sherman Avenue/Suite 101   Vineland, NJ 08360
(856)696-9550   Fax (856)691-1686

Al-Bezem, Rim, MD {1629076625} CdvDis, CarNuc, IntrMd(90,SYR01)<NJ-RWJUHAM, NJ-STFRNMED>
+ Mercer Bucks Cardiology
3140 Princeton Pike/2nd Floor   Lawrenceville, NJ 08648
(609)250-4104   Fax (609)978-4860
+ Capital Health Primary Care Columbus
23203 Columbus Road/Suite 1   Columbus, NJ 08022
(609)250-4104   Fax (603)303-4451

Al-Ola, Ziyad, MD {1295756401} FamMed(92,SYR01)
+ Valley Medical Group
140 Franklin Turnpike/Suite 6-A   Waldwick, NJ 07463
(201)447-3603   Fax (201)447-5184

Al-Qassab, Usama, MD {1861779761} Urolgy
+ University Urology Associates of New Jersey
1374 Whitehorse Hamilton Sq/Suite 101   Hamilton, NJ 08690   (609)581-5900   Fax (609)581-5901

Al-Salem, Salim Suliaman, MD {1689756017} Psychy(71,PAK01)
+ 490 Forest Avenue
Paramus, NJ 07652

Al-Shrouf, Amal Ali, MD {1649249509} IntrMd, PulDis(91,JOR01)<NJ-STJOSHOS>
+ Paterson Community Clinic
355 21st Avenue   Paterson, NJ 07501   (973)523-9090
Fax (973)523-5222
AQEL@aol.com
+ Paterson Community Clinic
1300 Main Avenue/Suite 3 D   Clifton, NJ 07011   (973)685-9922

Alade, Ibijoke Adenrele, MD {1487683397} IntrMd(91,NIG01)<NJ-CHILTON>
+ Erickson Health Medical Group
1 Cedar Crest Village Drive   Pompton Plains, NJ 07444
(973)831-3540   Fax (973)831-3503

Aladjem, Asher, MD {1760544084} Psychy(80,ITA03)<NY-BLVUENYU>
+ 1 East Park Drive/Suite 5
Paterson, NJ 07504   (973)279-9063   Fax (973)278-1448
georgia.montouris@bmc.org

Alaigh, Poonam Lata, MD {1326142860} IntrMd(85,INA72)
+ 89 Old Smalleytown Road
Warren, NJ 07059   (908)222-2665

Alam, Abu S., MD {1235189507} ObsGyn(72,BANG)
+ 779 Springfield Avenue
Summit, NJ 07901   (908)273-5907   Fax (908)277-2421

Alam, Mahmood, MD {1679593875} CdvDis, IntrMd, IntCrd(83,PAK15)
+ Jersey Heart Center, LLC.
616 Amboy Avenue   Woodbridge, NJ 07095   (732)636-6262   Fax (732)636-8313

Alam, Parvez, MD {1740397181} IntrMd(85,BAN06)
+ 395 Danforth Avenue/Suite 1
Jersey City, NJ 07305   (201)332-4600

Alam, Rozana R., MD {1518932706} Psychy(75,BAN02)<NJ-OVERLOOK>
+ Overlook Medical Center
99 Beauvoir Avenue/PO Box 210   Summit, NJ 07902
(908)522-2000

Alam, Shumaila, MD {1851732143} FamMed<NJ-NWTNMEM>
+ Newton Medical Center
175 High Street   Newton, NJ 07860   (973)579-8321

Alam, Syed Fahim, MD {1023083953} Psychy(87,PAK12)<NJ-MORRISTN>
+ Morristown Medical Center
100 Madison Avenue/Box 60/Psych   Morristown, NJ 07962
(973)971-5000

Alamia, Peter Anthony, DO {1750307104} EmrgMd(00,NJ75)<NJ-MORRISTN>
+ Morristown Medical Center
100 Madison Avenue/EmrgMed   Morristown, NJ 07962
(973)971-5000

Aland, Kristen, MD {1871904482} ObsGyn
+ Healthy Woman Ob/Gyn
312 Professional View Drive   Freehold, NJ 07728
(732)431-1616   Fax (732)866-7962

Alapatt, Michael F., MD {1639401250} SrgOrt(06,MA05)<NY-SLRRSVLT>
+ New Jersey Spine Center
40 Main Street   Chatham, NJ 07928   (973)635-0800   Fax (973)635-6254

Alario, Frank C., MD {1194740225} IntrMd(84,MEX14)<NJ-JRSYSHMC, NJ-COMMED>
+ Frank C. Alario MD Inc
355 Route 9/Suite 2   Bayville, NJ 08721   (732)269-0001
Fax (732)269-9636
+ Frank C. Alario MD Inc
1220 Route 70 West   Whiting, NJ 08759   (732)350-3784
+ Medical Associates of Marlboro PC
32 North Main Street   Marlboro, NJ 08721   (732)462-4100

Fax (732)462-3798

Alban, Alvaro, MD {1356361778} EmrgMd(01,NY46)<NJ-PALISADE>
+ Palisades Medical Center
7600 River Road/Emergency   North Bergen, NJ 07047
(201)854-5100

Albana, Fouad S., MD {1750326211} IntrMd, Nephro(73,EGYP)<NJ-BAYSHORE, NJ-RBAYOLDB>
+ 2080 Route 35
Holmdel, NJ 07733   (732)706-7200   Fax (732)706-7222

Albanese, Anthony C., MD {1538269998} AdolMd, Pedtrc(85,MEXI)<NJ-STBARNMC, NJ-OVERLOOK>
+ Drs. Albanese and Vecchio
20 Valley Street   South Orange, NJ 07079   (973)762-2606
Fax (973)762-4515

Albanese, Joseph J., DO {1306850599} Nephro, IntrMd(89,IA75)<NJ-KIMBALL, NJ-SOCEANCO>
+ Jersey Coast Nephrology & Hypertension Associates
1541 Route 88/Suite A   Brick, NJ 08724   (732)836-3200
Fax (732)836-3201

Albano, Jenna, DO {1912499278}<NJ-STJOSHOS>
+ St. Joseph's Regional Medical Center
703 Main Street   Paterson, NJ 07503   (973)754-2000

Albassam, Hassan, MD {1801230248} IntHos<NJ-NWTNMEM>
+ Newton Medical Center
175 High Street   Newton, NJ 07860   (973)383-2121

Alber, George C., MD {1386688547} SrgOrt, SprtMd, IntrMd(90,NJ05)<NJ-ACMCMAIN, NJ-SHOREMEM>
+ Shore Orthopedic University Associates
24 Macarthur Boulevard/First Floor   Somers Point, NJ
08244   (609)927-1991   Fax (609)927-4203

Alberaqdar, Enis, MD {1528276615} PulDis
+ Pulmonary & Critical Care Associates
378 Belmont Avenue   Haledon, NJ 07508   (973)925-4850
Fax (973)925-4851

Alberici, Anna, DO {1184650848} FamMed(88,NJ75)
+ Community Health Care, Inc.
319 Landis Avenue/Suites A & B   Vineland, NJ 08360
(856)691-1300   Fax (856)696-0344
+ Community Health Care, Inc.
70 Cohansey Street   Bridgeton, NJ 08302   (856)691-3300
Fax (856)451-0029
+ Community Health Care Inc
335 North Delsea Drive/Route 47   Glassboro, NJ 08360
(856)863-5720

Alberino-Catapano, Amanda, MD {1558774687} EmrgMd<NJ-MTNSIDE>
+ Hackensack UMC Mountainside
1 Bay Avenue   Montclair, NJ 07042   (973)429-6200

Albert, Arthur S., MD {1972588853} RadDia, RadNuc(78,PA14)<NJ-HACKNSK>
+ New Century Imaging at Oradell
555 Kinderkamack Road   Oradell, NJ 07649   (201)599-1311
Fax (201)599-8333
+ The Imaging Center
30 South Newman Street   Hackensack, NJ 07601
(201)599-1311   Fax (201)488-5244
+ Hackensack Radiology Group, P.A.
30 Prospect Avenue   Hackensack, NJ 07649   (201)996-2200   Fax (201)336-8451

Albert Puleo, Anthony M., MD {1265478101} FamMed(83,OH06)<NJ-VIRTMHBC>
+ Dr. Albert Puleo and Assoc
155 Route 70   Medford, NJ 08055   (609)654-9100   Fax (609)654-8503

Alberta, Francis Gerard, MD {1821065863} SrgOrt, SprtMd(97,NJ05)
+ 266 Harristown Road/Suite 100
Glen Rock, NJ 07452   (201)493-8990   Fax (201)493-8933

Alberta, James David, MD {1922037258} IntrMd(96,ITA01)
+ Shore Road & New York Avenue
Somers Point, NJ 08244   (609)652-2494   Fax (609)748-0585

Alberti, Kathryn P., MD {1043377997} IntrMd(83,DC02)<NJ-MORRISTN>
+ 261 James Street
Morristown, NJ 07960   (973)898-9558   Fax (973)898-4754

Alberto, Kezia Jasmina Ribeiro, MD {1073721809} IntrMd(01,INA6Y)
+ Nephrological Associates, P.A.
83 Hanover Road/Suite 290   Florham Park, NJ 07932
(973)736-2212   Fax (973)736-2989

Alberto, Priscilla Magsalin, MD {1376551275} IntrMd(71,PHI01)
+ Alberto Medical Associates PA
25 Mule Road/Unit A-3   Toms River, NJ 08755   (732)240-0404   Fax (732)244-3555

Alberto, Renato D., MD {1245245109} IntrMd(71,PHI01)
+ Alberto Medical Associates PA
25 Mule Road/Unit A-3   Toms River, NJ 08755   (732)240-0404   Fax (732)244-3555

Physicians by Name and Address

Albicocco, Nicholas S., MD {1447274766} Gastrn(82,KY07)
+ 195 Route 46 West/Suite 203
Mine Hill, NJ 07803 (973)366-7330 Fax (973)989-0508

Albornoz, Louise A., MD {1043355381} Rheuma, IntrMd(79,MEX14)<NJ-PALISADE>
+ 1011 Clifton Avenue
Clifton, NJ 07013 (973)778-6611 Fax (973)473-8434

Alburquerque, Lucrecia A., MD {1922077817} IntrMd(70,DOMI)
+ 412 Park Avenue
Paterson, NJ 07504 (973)684-1302 Fax (973)684-0144

Alcala, Ramon L., Jr., MD {1275863524} ObsGyn(63,PHI09)<NJ-VALLEY>
+ 442 East Saddle River Road
Upper Saddle River, NJ 07458 (201)315-9359

Alcantara, Solomon V., MD {1033111869} EmrgMd(63,PHI07)<NJ-CHILTON>
+ Chilton Medical Center
97 West Parkway/Emerg Medicine Pompton Plains, NJ 07444 (973)831-5446

Alcasid, Lino M., MD {1346334547} RadDia, Radiol(69,PHIL)<NJ-OCEANMC>
+ Ocean Medical Center
425 Jack Martin Boulevard/Radiology Brick, NJ 08723 (732)840-2200 Fax (732)974-8820

Alcasid, Ninfa A., MD {1740471580} FamMed<NJ-OCEANMC>
+ Total Patient Care LLC
459 Jack Martin Boulevard Brick, NJ 08724 (732)785-1000 Fax (732)785-1222
+ Total Patient Care
2401 Route 35 Manasquan, NJ 08736 (732)785-1000 Fax (732)292-9633

Alcasid, Patrick J., MD {1184654931} PulCCr, CritCr, IntrMd(01,PHI01)<NJ-OCEANMC, NJ-COMMED>
+ Ocean Pulmonary Associates PA
457 Jack Martin Boulevard/Suite 4 Brick, NJ 08724 (732)840-4200 Fax (732)840-6444
+ Ocean Pulmonary Associates PA
3 Plaza Drive/Suite 2 Toms River, NJ 08757 (732)840-4200 Fax (732)505-9296
+ Ocean Pulmonary Associates PA
70 Lacey Road/Irish Branch Mall Whiting, NJ 08724 (732)350-4777

Alcera, Eric Cortez, MD {1912054024} PsyCAd, Psychy(99,PHI15)
+ Booker Behavioral Health Center
661 Shrewsbury Avenue Shrewsbury, NJ 07702 (732)345-3400 Fax (732)345-3401

Alcera, Lloyd C., MD {1184854259} Psychy(01,PHI15)
+ 106 Centre Boulevard/Suite G
Marlton, NJ 08053 (856)797-2810 Fax (856)797-2811

Alcera, Roanna Espino, MD {1992960991} FamMed(01,PHI15)<NJ-VIRTMHBC>
+ Epstein Internal Medicine
2906 Route 130 North Delran, NJ 08075 (856)764-4115 Fax (856)764-4116

Alcid, David V., MD {1851342380} InfDis, IntrMd(67,PHI01)<NJ-RWJUBRUN, NJ-STPETER>
+ RWJ University Hospital New Brunswick
One Robert Wood Johnson Place New Brunswick, NJ 08901 (732)828-3000

Alcid, Jess Gerald, MD {1235179896} SprtMd, SrgOrt(97,NY03)<NJ-COMMED, NJ-HLTHSRE>
+ Ocean Orthopedic Associates, P.A.
530 Lakehurst Road/Suite 1 Toms River, NJ 08755 (732)349-8454 Fax (732)341-0259

Alcorta, Carlos E., MD {1407843907} CdvDis, IntrMd(68,PER01)<NJ-HOBUNIMC, NJ-CHRIST>
+ 1009 79th Street
North Bergen, NJ 07047 (201)869-3737 Fax (201)869-4437
Alcorta@aol.com

Aldaia, Lillian, MD {1912167297} IntrMd<NJ-MORRISTN>
+ Morristown Medical Center
100 Madison Avenue/Internal Med Morristown, NJ 07962 (973)971-5000

Alday, Arnold M., MD {1659346203} IntrMd(92,PHI01)<NJ-HACKNSK>
+ United Medical, P.C.
533 Lexington Avenue Clifton, NJ 07011 (973)546-6844 Fax (973)546-7707
+ United Medical, P.C.
988 Broadway/Suite 201 Bayonne, NJ 07002 (973)546-6844 Fax (201)339-6333

Alday, Geronima G., MD {1174788467} FamMed, FamMGrtc(05,GRN01)
+ New Jersey Institute for Successful Aging
42 East Laurel Road/Suite 1800 Stratford, NJ 08084 (856)566-6843 Fax (856)566-6781

Aldea, Dyana Luz, MD {1740450261} PhysMd(97,NY01)
+ 86 Woodbury Road
Edison, NJ 08820 (732)494-0054 Fax (732)494-0054

Alder, Edward A., MD {1487749420} IntrMd(82,NIG01)<NJ-CHSFULD>
+ Dr. Alder and Associates
1177 Park Avenue Plainfield, NJ 07060 (908)222-0600 Fax (908)222-0599

Alderson, Skip Michael, MD {1669521803} RadDia
+ Radiology Affiliates of Central New Jersey, P.A.
2501 Kuser Road Hamilton, NJ 08691 (609)585-8800 (609)585-1825

Alejandro, Jason Robert, MD {1043219348} EmrgMd(00,NJ05)<NJ-MTNSIDE>
+ Hackensack UMC Mountainside
1 Bay Avenue/EmrgMed Montclair, NJ 07042 (973)429-6000

Alekseyeva, Irina, MD {1093719478} Anesth(99,NY08)<NJ-BAYONNE>
+ Bayonne Medical Center
29th Street at Avenue E/Anesth Bayonne, NJ 07002 (201)858-5000

Alemany, Carlos A., MD {1396825055} NnPnMd, Pedtrc(87,PRO02)<NJ-MONMOUTH, NJ-RIVERVW>
+ Pediatrix Medical Group
255 Third Avenue Long Branch, NJ 07740 (732)222-7006
+ Monmouth Medical Center
300 Second Avenue/Neonatology Long Branch, NJ 07740 (732)222-5200

Alemu, Kidist, MD {1528077120} Pedtrc<NJ-RWJUBRUN>
+ University Medical Group Pediatrics
125 Paterson Street/MEB 3rd Fl New Brunswick, NJ 08903 (732)235-7044 Fax (732)235-9340
+ RWJ University Hospital Somerset
110 Rehill Avenue Somerville, NJ 08876 (732)235-7044 Fax (908)231-6194

Alemu, Yohannes, DO {1346473923} IntrMd
+ Rowan University-School of Osteopathic Medicine
1 Medical Center Drive Stratford, NJ 08084 (856)566-7121

Alenick, D. Scott, MD {1639138316} PedCrd(84,NJ05)<NJ-NWRKBETH>
+ North Jersey Pediatric Cardiology PC
520 North Wood Avenue Linden, NJ 07036 (908)624-0444 Fax (201)497-6256
+ North Jersey Pediatric Cardiology PC
635 Market Street Newark, NJ 07105 (908)624-0444 Fax (201)497-6256
+ 333 Old Hook Road/Suite 101
Westwood, NJ 07036 (201)497-6255 Fax (201)497-6256

Ales, Kathy L., MD {1689711517} IntrMd(78,CT01)<NJ-UNVMCPRN>
+ 620 Cranbury Road/Suite 90
East Brunswick, NJ 08816

Aleskerov, Fuad Y., MD {1730565490}
+ 440 Cambridge Road
Ridgewood, NJ 07450 (404)353-8944
fredaleskerov@gmail.com

Alessi, Paul J., DO {1942208046} InfDis, IntrMd(77,IA75)
+ Kennedy Health Alliance
457 Haddonfield Road/Suite 110 Cherry Hill, NJ 08002 (856)406-4091 Fax (856)406-4570

Alessio, Maryann, DO {1750499257} IntrMd, Pedtrc(94,NY75)<NJ-CLARMAAS>
+ 349 Passaic Avenue
Nutley, NJ 07110 (973)667-8889

Alexander, Andrea Hope, MD {1922000520} Pedtrc(01,ISR02)
+ Drs. Gruenwald & Comandatore
90 Millburn Avenue/Suite 101 Millburn, NJ 07041 (973)378-7990 Fax (973)378-7991

Alexander, Frederick, Jr., MD {1982773545} PedSrg, IntrMd(77,NY01)<NJ-HACKNSK>
+ 140 Route 17 North/Suite 321
Paramus, NJ 07652 (201)225-9700 Fax (201)225-0031

Alexander, James B., MD {1649366956} SrgVas, Surgry(80,PA01)
+ Cooper Surgical Associates
3 Cooper Plaza/Suite 411 Camden, NJ 08103 (856)342-2151 Fax (856)365-1180
+ Cooper Surgical Associates
6017 Main Street Voorhees, NJ 08043 (856)325-6516
+ Cooper Surgical Associates
110 Marter Avenue/Suite 402 Moorestown, NJ 08103 (856)234-7073 Fax (856)866-9846

Alexander, Karen Elizabeth, MD {1386007722} IntrMd<NJ-ACMCITY>
+ AtlantiCare Regional Medical Center/City Campus
1925 Pacific Avenue Atlantic City, NJ 08401 (609)345-5000

Alexander, Leah M., MD {1013052059} Pedtrc(97,MI20)<NJ-VALLEY, NJ-CHILTON>
+ PediatriCare Associates
20-20 Fair Lawn Avenue Fair Lawn, NJ 07410 (201)791-4545 Fax (201)791-3765

Alexander, Mark P., MD {1316097223} IntrMd(83,EGY05)<NJ-ACMCITY>
+ AtlantiCare Special Care Center
1401 Atlantic Avenue/Suite 2500 Atlantic City, NJ 08401 (609)572-8800

Alexander, Nicholas, MD {1972508240} SrgOrt, SrgOARec, OthrSp(88,NJ05)<NJ-VALLEY, NJ-CHILTON>
+ 400 Franklin Turnpike/Suite 100
Mahwah, NJ 07430 (201)818-4344 Fax (201)818-2710
+ 6 Brighton Road/Suite 108
Clifton, NJ 07013 (201)818-4344 Fax (201)818-2710

Alexander, Robert Francis, MD {1285688309} PulDis(85,MO07)
+ Associates in Pulmonary Medicine, PA
16 Pocono Road/Suite 217 Denville, NJ 07834 (973)625-5651
+ Associates in Pulmonary Medicine, PA
765 State Highway 10 East Randolph, NJ 07869 (973)625-5651 Fax (973)366-6385

Alexandrova, Marina Alexandrovna, MD {1073687240} IntrMd(90,RUS06)<NJ-MTNSIDE>
+ 460 Franklin Avenue/Suite A 2
Nutley, NJ 07110 (973)667-8640 Fax (973)667-0401

Alexeeva, Aissa Timofeyevna, MD {1093799876} Nrolgy(88,RUS33)<NJ-UNVMCPRN, NJ-CHSFULD>
+ Lawrenceville Neurology Center, PA
3131 Princeton Pike Lawrenceville, NJ 08648 (609)896-1701 Fax (609)896-3735

Alexescu, Adina N., MD {1174511059} IntrMd(80,ROMA)<NJ-NWRKBETH>
+ 443 East Westfield Avenue
Roselle Park, NJ 07204 (908)241-8141

Alexianu, Maria E., MD {1235109059} Nrolgy(89,ROM01)<NJ-OVERLOOK, NY-BLVUENYU>
+ Overlook Medical Center
99 Beauvoir Avenue/PO Box 210 Summit, NJ 07902 (908)522-2000
+ Summit Neurology Consulting PC
507 Westfield Avenue Westfield, NJ 07090 (908)522-2000 Fax (908)232-2247
+ Summit Neurology Consulting, PC.
33 Overlook Road/Suite 401 Summit, NJ 07902 (908)273-9000 Fax (908)273-9022

Alfakir, Maria, MD {1790993897} PulCCr
+ Pulmonary & Critical Care Associates
378 Belmont Avenue Haledon, NJ 07508 (973)925-4850 Fax (973)925-4851

Alfaro, Abraham, DO {1962573923} PhysMd, SprtMd(92,ME75)<NJ-BACHARCH, NJ-ACMCITY>
+ Bacharach Institute for Rehabilitation
61 West Jimmie Leeds Road Pomona, NJ 08240 (609)748-5380 Fax (609)652-8749
aaalfaro@bacharach.org

Alfie, Marcos E., MD {1285691634} PedGst
+ Meridian Medical Group - Faculty Practice
61 Davis Avenue/Suite 1 Neptune, NJ 07753 (732)776-4860 Fax (732)776-4867
+ 3 Lucerne Drive
Lakewood, NJ 08701
+ Meridian Obstetrics amd Gynecology Associates PC
19 Davis Avenue/Fl 1 Neptune, NJ 07753 (732)897-7944 Fax (732)922-8264

Alfonso, Carlos Roel Villegas, MD {1801864061} CdvDis(93,PHI01)<NJ-STMICHL, NJ-HACKNSK>
+ Bart De Gregorio MD, LLC.
946 Bloomfield Avenue Glen Ridge, NJ 07028 (973)743-1121 Fax (973)743-2627

Alfonso, Flores, MD {1629180930} PthAcl, PthCyt(87,NY46)<NJ-MORRISTN, NJ-OVERLOOK>
+ 79 Cross Road
Cedar Knolls, NJ 07927
+ Morristown Pathology Associates
100 The American Road/Suite 118 Morris Plains, NJ 07950 (973)867-7298

Alfonso, Jesus Roberto, MD {1649266925} IntrMd(86,NY19)<NJ-CHRIST>
+ 4800 Park Avenue
Weehawken, NJ 07086 (201)330-8747 Fax (201)330-8947
Jramd@comcast.net

Alfonzo, Joann, MD {1316990310} Pedtrc(91,PA02)<NJ-HACKNSK>
+ Pediatric Associates
444 Neptune Boulevard/Suite 4 Neptune, NJ 07753 (732)774-4332 Fax (732)774-4077

Algazy, Jeffrey Ian, MD {1770759359} IntrMd(96,CT01)
+ 92 Edgemere Road
Livingston, NJ 07039 (973)342-7556 Fax (973)549-1562

Alhadeff, Ilan, MD {1124072194} IntrMd(02,DMN01)<NJ-SOCEANCO>
+ Southern Ocean County Medical Center
1140 Route 72 West/Internal Med Manahawkin, NJ 08050 (609)978-3331 Fax (609)978-3113

Physicians by Name and Address

Alhamrawy, Ismail A., MD {1306011101} PhysMd, NuclMd, IntrMd(89,EGY08)<NJ-CLARMAAS>
+ Center for Advanced Pain Management & Rehabilitation
249 Bridge Street/Building G   Metuchen, NJ 08840   (732)516-1060   Fax (732)516-1015
+ Garden State Pain Control Center, P.A.
1117 Route 46 East/Suite 201   Clifton, NJ 07013   (732)516-1060   Fax (973)777-0304

Ali, Adil, MD {1730213240} PhysMd, PhyMSptM(05,NJ05)
+ Performance Spine & Sports Medicine
4056 Quakerbridge Road/Suite 111   Lawrenceville, NJ 08648   (609)588-8600   Fax (609)588-8602

Ali, Amy G., MD {1033413422} IntrMd(08,NY09)<NJ-RWJUBRUN>
+ Hackensack University Medical Group Emerson
452 Old Hook Road/2nd Floor/2nd Fl   Emerson, NJ 07630   (201)666-3900   Fax (201)261-0505

Ali, Ayoola O., MD {1912951542} SrgTrm, Surgry(90,NIG01)<NJ-ACMCITY>
+ AtlantiCare Regional Medical Center/City Campus
1925 Pacific Avenue/Trauma Unit   Atlantic City, NJ 08401   (609)345-4000

Ali, Fatima, DO {1013366368} IntrMd
+ SOM - Department of Internal Medicine
42 East Laurel Road/Suite 3100   Stratford, NJ 08084   (856)566-2753   Fax (856)566-6906

Ali, Majid, MD {1659446789} GPrvMd, PthAcl, FamMed(64,PAKI)
+ Institute of Preventive Medicine
95 East Main Street/Suite 106   Denville, NJ 07834   (973)586-4111   Fax (973)586-8466

Ali, Meer S., MD {1982624300} EmrgMd, IntrMd(78,INA39)<NJ-PALISADE>
+ Palisades Emergency Consultants
7600 River Road   North Bergen, NJ 07047   (201)854-5100

Ali, Mohsin, MD {1093912909} Nrolgy(83,PAK11)
+ Mohsin Ali MD LLC
1132 Park Avenue   Plainfield, NJ 07060   (732)494-7725   Fax (732)494-5619

Ali, Nadeem Yousaf, MD {1922374750}<NJ-NWRKBETH>
+ Newark Beth Israel Medical Center
201 Lyons Avenue   Newark, NJ 07112   (973)502-0501

Ali, Nadia Dawn, MD {1922386317}
+ One John F Kennedy Boulevard/Apt 55f
Somerset, NJ 08873   (603)219-4118

Ali, Nadia Yousaf, MD {1487828861} IntrMd(02,PAK20)<NJ-OVERLOOK>
+ Overlook Medical Center
99 Beauvoir Avenue/PO Box 210   Summit, NJ 07902   (908)522-2000

Ali, Nicole Mrytle, MD {1841516069} IntrMd, Nephro(05,NY48)<NY-NSUHMANH>
+ Hackensack University Medical Center
360 Essex Street/Suite 401   Hackensack, NJ 07601   (201)996-2608   Fax (201)498-0148

Ali, Rana Y., MD {1619083177} PulDis, IntrMd(95,INA29)<NY-MTSINYHS>
+ Shore Pulmonary PA
301 Bingham Avenue/Suite B   Ocean, NJ 07712   (732)775-9075   Fax (732)775-1212
+ Shore Pulmonary PA
1608 Route 88/Suite 117   Brick, NJ 08724   (732)575-1100
+ Shore Pulmonary PA
2640 Highway 70/Building 6-A   Manasquan, NJ 07712   (732)528-5900   Fax (732)528-0887

Ali, Rayshma, DO {1932134285} EmrgMd, EmrgEMed(01,CA22)
+ Holmdel Health Center
670 North Beers Street   Holmdel, NJ 07733   (732)226-5552   Fax (732)757-0824

Ali, Rehan Basharat, MD {1144527011} Anesth(10,GCY01)<NY-MTSINAI, NY-MTSINYHS>
+ Spine Institute of North America
300A Princeon Hightstown Road   East Windsor, NJ 08520   (609)337-6496   Fax (609)371-9110
+ Spine Institute of North America
777 East Route 70   Evesham, NJ 08053   (609)337-6496   Fax (609)371-9110
+ Spine Institute of North America
385 Cranbury Road   East Brunswick, NJ 08520   (609)337-6496   Fax (609)371-9110

Ali, Sabia, MD {1740482959}
+ Overlook Family Medicine
33 Overlook Road/Suite 103   Summit, NJ 07901   (908)522-5700   Fax (908)273-8014
+ Carepoint Health
10 Exchange Place   Jersey City, NJ 07302   (201)884-5329

Ali, Sadia Y., MD {1922366897} IntrMd(11,GCY01)
+ RWJ University Hospital New Brunswick
One Robert Wood Johnson Place   New Brunswick, NJ 08901   (732)828-3000

Ali, Salma, MD {1639199722} NnPnMd, Pedtrc(81,PAKI)<NJ-UMDNJ>
+ University Hospital
150 Bergen Street/Neonatology   Newark, NJ 07103   (973)972-2637   Fax (973)972-7158

Ali, Sara Inayet, MD {1467628255} IntrMd, Grtrcs(03,PAK11)
+ Reliance Medical Group, LLC
25 Scotch Road/Suite A   Ewing, NJ 08628   (609)771-0404

Ali, Syed A., MD {1457469702} Psychy(82,INA5B)
+ Capital Health System/Fuld Campus
750 Brunswick Avenue   Trenton, NJ 08638   (609)815-7829   Fax (609)815-7814

Ali, Syed Asim, MD {1417148644} Psychy
+ 2333 Whitehorse Mercerville Rd
Trenton, NJ 08619   (732)773-2152   Fax (609)586-1851

Ali, Tahera, DO {1316104466} FamMed
+ Riverside Medical Group
714 Tenth Street/Suite 2   Secaucus, NJ 07094   (201)863-3346   Fax (201)865-0015

Ali, Tuba Muhammad, MD {1952662223} IntrMd
+ Kennedy Hospitalist Office
2201 Chapel Avenue West   Cherry Hill, NJ 08002   (856)513-4124   Fax (856)302-5932
+ Lisa A. Rink Family Medicine, LLC.
217 White Horse Pike   Haddon Heights, NJ 08035   (856)513-4124   Fax (856)672-9111

Ali, Umer, MD {1609435650}
+ Clinical Research Laboratories, Inc.
371 Hoes Lane   Piscataway, NJ 08854   (732)595-2444   Fax (732)562-1586

Aliaga, Julie M., MD {1144372889} Pedtrc(03,RI01)<NJ-HACKNSK, NJ-HOLYNAME>
+ NHCAC Health Center at West New York
5301 Broadway   West New York, NJ 07093   (201)866-9320
+ Riverside Medical Group
714 Tenth Street/Suite 2   Secaucus, NJ 07094   (201)866-9320   Fax (201)865-0015

Alias, Mathew N., DO {1508027574} Nrolgy(08,NY75)<MA-LAHEYCMC, MA-LAHEYCNS>
+ Neuroscience Center of Northern New Jersey
310 Madison Avenue   Morristown, NJ 07960   (973)285-1446   Fax (973)605-8854

Alias, Vineetha Ann, DO {1023335643} Pedtrc<PA-STCHRIS>
+ Watchung Pediatrics
76 Stirling Road/Suite 201   Warren, NJ 07059   (908)755-5437   Fax (908)755-6905

Aliasgharpour, Farzin M., MD {1881708212} CdvDis, IntrMd(88,GRNA)
+ 1139 Raritan Road
Clark, NJ 07066   (732)815-1333   Fax (732)815-0574

Aliferova, Tatyana N., MD {1235149766} IntrMd, FamMed(93,UKR14)
+ Dorfner Family Medicine
309 West Broad Street   Burlington, NJ 08016   (609)387-2142   Fax (609)387-2757

Alikhan, Ghousia, MD {1801275383}<NJ-ACMCITY>
+ AtlantiCare Regional Medical Center/City Campus
1925 Pacific Avenue/MedEdu   Atlantic City, NJ 08401   (609)441-8990

Alikhan, Salma, MD {1124082839} Pedtrc(97,PAK02)
+ Gloucester County Pediatrics
849 Cooper Street   Deptford, NJ 08096   (856)848-6346   Fax (856)848-5734

Alimam, Ammar, MD {1770542946} IntrMd, PulCCr, PulDis(88,SYR01)<NJ-KENEDYHS, NJ-OURLADY>
+ Pulmonary & Sleep Associates of SJ, LLC.
750 Route 73 South/Suite 401   Marlton, NJ 08053   (856)375-1288   Fax (856)375-2325   aalimam@pennjerseypulmonary.com
+ Pulmonary & Sleep Associates of SJ, LLC.
120 Carnie Boulevard/Suite 3   Voorhees, NJ 08043   (856)375-1288   Fax (856)325-4364
+ Pulmonary & Sleep Associates of SJ, LLC.
107 Berlin Road   Cherry Hill, NJ 08053   (856)429-1800   Fax (856)429-1081

Alino, Anne Marie G., MD {1669417523} Ophthl(92,NY48)
+ Ridgewood Ophthalmology PC
1200 East Ridgewood Avenue   Ridgewood, NJ 07450   (201)612-0044   Fax (201)612-9446

Aliparo, Madolene A., MD {1417004078} Pedtrc, NnPnMd(82,PHI10)<NJ-UMDNJ>
+ University Hospital-Doctors Office Center
90 Bergen Street/DOC 5100/Pedi   Newark, NJ 07103   (973)972-5779   Fax (973)972-5895
+ University Pediatric Group
90 Bergen Street/DOC 4300   Newark, NJ 07103   (973)972-7111   Fax (973)397-2901

Alistar, Angela Tatiana, MD {1831349745} Gastrn, Onclgy(ROM05)
+ Atlantic Surgical Oncology
100 Madison Avenue   Morristown, NJ 07960   (973)971-7111   Fax (973)397-2901

Alivisatos, Maria Regina, MD {1124360086} IntrMd, InfDis(80,GRE01)
+ 389 Terhune Road
Princeton, NJ 08540

Alizade, Azer, MD {1275562472} ObsGyn(93,RUS81)<NJ-HACKNSK>
+ Hackensack University Medical Center
30 Prospect Avenue   Hackensack, NJ 07601   (201)996-2000

Alizadeh, Parvin, MD {1730109919} Pedtrc(88,IRA24)<NJ-CHSM-RCER>
+ 445 Whitehorse Avenue/Suite 204
Trenton, NJ 08610   (609)585-1234   Fax (609)585-1070
+ Capital Health System/Mercer Campus
446 Bellevue Avenue   Trenton, NJ 08618   (609)394-4000

Aljian, John M., MD {1447268636} Ophthl, CrnExD(91,NJ05)<NY-NYEYEINF>
+ 630 Palisade Avenue
Englewood Cliffs, NJ 07632   (201)503-0302   Fax (201)503-0309   johndryeye@aol.com

Alken, Jeffrey, MD {1861472342} IntrMd(86,NY08)<NJ-UNDRWD>
+ Frank & Edith Scarpa Regional Cancer
1505 West Sherman Avenu/Suite B   Vineland, NJ 08360   (856)641-8635   Fax (856)641-8636
+ Virtua Marlton Hospital
90 Brick Road   Marlton, NJ 08053   (856)355-6000
+ Virtua Memorial
175 Madison Avenue   Mount Holly, NJ 08360   (609)267-0700

Alkon, Joseph David, MD {1891984589} SrgPlstc(00,MA05)<NJ-TRINIWSC>
+ 515 North Wood Avenue/Suite 201
Linden, NJ 07036   (908)289-6888   Fax (908)354-0888

Alla, Nivedita R., MD {1316071087} IntrMd(98,INA28)<NJ-OVERLOOK>
+ Overlook Medical Center
99 Beauvoir Avenue/PO Box 210   Summit, NJ 07902   (908)522-5000

Alladin, Irfan Ahmad, MD {1174536114} PhysMd, PhyMPain(98,GRN01)
+ Union Medical, LLC
2182 Morris Avenue   Union, NJ 07083   (908)851-2666
+ 15 West Second Street
Bound Brook, NJ 08805

Allagadda, Bharathi R., MD {1760696280} IntrMd(04,NET12)<NJ-STBARNMC>
+ St. Barnabas Medical Center
94 Old Short Hills Road   Livingston, NJ 07039   (973)322-5252

Allahverdi, Ilya Michael, MD {1093718975} Anesth(92,NY48)<NJ-SHOREMEM>
+ Shore Memorial Hospital
1 East New York Avenue/Anesthesiology   Somers Point, NJ 08244   (609)653-3500

Allam, Bharat Reddy, DO {1780001891} IntrMd<NJ-MORRISTN>
+ Morristown Medical Center
100 Madison Avenue   Morristown, NJ 07962   (973)971-5000

Allam, Naveen Reddy, MD {1790051191} IntrMd
+ Drs. Allam and Allam
73 Park Street/3rd Floor   Montclair, NJ 07042   (973)746-0595   Fax (973)746-1848

Allam, Reddy B., MD {1437117827} IntrMd(78,INDI)<NJ-MTNSIDE>
+ Drs. Allam and Allam
73 Park Street/3rd Floor   Montclair, NJ 07042   (973)746-0595   Fax (973)746-1848

Alland, David, MD {1164591871} InfDis, IntrMd(84,NY01)<NJ-UMDNJ>
+ University Hospital
150 Bergen Street   Newark, NJ 07103   (973)972-2179   Fax (973)972-6804

Allegar, Nancy E., MD {1750387494} IntrMd, PulDis(89,NJ05)<NJ-RWJUBRUN, NJ-STPETER>
+ Alatae Medical, LLC.
390 Amwell Road/Suite 501/Building 5   Hillsborough, NJ 08844   (908)281-1077   Fax (908)281-1081

Allegra, Donald T., MD {1659347649} InfDis, IntrMd(74,MA01)<NJ-STCLRDEN, NJ-MORRISTN>
+ ID Associates PA/dba ID Care
765 Route 10 East/Suite 201   Randolph, NJ 07869   (973)989-0068   Fax (973)361-8955
+ ID Associates PA/dba ID Care
8 Saddle Road   Cedar Knolls, NJ 07927   (973)989-0068   Fax (973)993-5953

Allegra, Edward Charles, II, MD {1588665913} IntrMd, Rheuma(88,MEXI)<NJ-BAYSHORE, NJ-RIVERVW>
+ Allegra Arthritis Associates
282 Broad Street   Red Bank, NJ 07701   (732)842-3600   Fax (732)842-3665
+ 115 Clark Street
Hazlet, NJ 07730   (732)739-1400

Physicians by Name and Address

Allegra, John R., MD {1467496067} EmrgMd, FamMed(74,FL02)<NJ-MORRISTN>
+ Morristown Medical Center
100 Madison Avenue   Morristown, NJ 07962   (973)971-5000

Allegra, Marshall P., MD {1740364256} SrgOrt(82,MEXI)<NJ-RIVERVW>
+ 879 Poole Avenue
Hazlet, NJ 07730   (732)888-8388

Allen, Ashleigh, MD {1881838407} PthHem<NJ-COOPRUMC>
+ Cooper University Hospital
One Cooper Plaza   Camden, NJ 08103   (856)968-7317

Allen, Lisa Rachel, MD {1932360823} Surgry
+ Mountain View Surgical Assocaites
2 Capital Way/Suite 505   Pennington, NJ 08534   (609)537-6700   Fax (609)537-6717
+ Capital Health Medical
2 Capital Way/Suite 356   Pennington, NJ 08534   (609)537-6700   Fax (609)537-6002

Allen, Luzmary, DO {1619951506} IntrMd(90,NJ75)
+ NJ VA/James J Howard Outpatient Clinic
970 Route 70 West   Brick, NJ 08724   (732)836-6009   Fax (732)836-6015

Allen, Mureen Cressida, MD {1992767198} IntrMd(89,JMA01)
+ PO Box 1929
Linden, NJ 07036

Allen, Robert Andrew, MD {1346376845} Dermat(96,NJ05)
+ Dermatology Physicians of South Jersey, P.A.
112 White Horse Pike   Haddon Heights, NJ 08035   (856)546-5353   Fax (856)546-8711

Allen Artiglere, Kara D., DO {1063607406} PhyMPain(03,NY75)
+ 384 Shunpike Road
Chatham, NJ 07928   (973)377-0702   Fax (973)377-0217

Allen Steinfeld, Isabel, MD {1457398661} Psychy(96,NY08)<NJ-UNIVBHC>
+ University Behavioral HealthCare
183 South Orange Avenue   Newark, NJ 07103   (973)972-5430   Fax (973)972-7173

Allenby, Kent Stewart, MD {1396016960} IntrMd, Grtrcs, OthrSp(78,DC01)
+ Kyowa Pharmaceutical
212 Carnegie Center/Suite 101/Research   Princeton, NJ 08540   (609)919-1100   Fax (609)919-1111

Allende, Jenys, MD {1013171362} Psychy(04,DC02)
+ Center for Family Guidance, PC
765 East Route 70/Building A-101   Marlton, NJ 08053   (856)797-4800   Fax (856)810-0110

Allert, Jesse William, MD {1336452473}(10,NY09)
+ Restoration Orthopaedics
113 West Essex Street/Suite 201   Maywood, NJ 07607   (201)226-0145   Fax (201)226-0147

Alley, Evan Wayne, MD {1497726947} OncHem
+ Penn Medicine at Cherry Hill
409 Route 70 East   Cherry Hill, NJ 08034   (856)429-1519

Alli, Kemi A., MD {1124033881} Pedtrc(95,NJ06)<NJ-CHSFULD, NJ-CHSMRCER>
+ Henry J. Austin Health Center
321 North Warren Street   Trenton, NJ 08618   (609)278-5913   Fax (609)695-3532

Alli, Padmavathy, DO {1891869483} Surgry(91,NJ75)<NJ-MTNSIDE, NJ-CLARMAAS>
+ 467 Mt. Prospect Avenue
Newark, NJ 07104   (973)483-9900
+ 557 Broad Street/Suite 22
Bloomfield, NJ 07003   (973)429-9844

Alloteh, Rose Sitsofe, MD {1336103050} Anesth(91,GHA01)<NJ-RBAYPERT>
+ Robert Wood Johnson-UMDNJ Anesthesia Group
125 Paterson Street/CAB 3100   New Brunswick, NJ 08901   (732)937-8841   Fax (732)418-8492

Alloy, Andrew Marc, DO {1275533036} Gastrn, IntrMd(78,PA77)
+ Advanced GI
2301 Evesham Road/Pav 800/Suite 110   Voorhees, NJ 08043   (856)772-1600   Fax (856)772-9031
+ Rancocas Anesthesiology, PA
151 Fries Mill Road/Suite 202   Turnersville, NJ 08012   (856)772-1600   Fax (856)228-7252

Allred, Charles Cameron, MD {1437310810} PulDis, IntrMd(08,GRN01)<NY-LENOXHLL>
+ Virtua Pulmonology - Moorestown
110 Marter Avenue   Moorestown, NJ 08057   (856)235-4656   Fax (856)235-4786
+ Virtua Pulmonology - Marlton
141 Route 70/Suite B   Marlton, NJ 08053   (856)235-4656   Fax (856)596-0837

Allu, Sridevi, MD {1982762183} IntrMd, Grtrcs(96,INA48)
+ Hem Care Medical Clinic
6 Agnes Court   Monroe Township, NJ 08831   (609)409-6767   Fax (609)409-6776

Allusson, Valerie R.C., MD {1154386688} IntrMd(94,FRA36)<NJ-MORRISTN>
+ Hackensack UMC Mountainside
1 Bay Avenue   Montclair, NJ 07042   (973)429-6048   Fax (973)429-6575

Almallah, Omar F., MD {1376528364} Ophthl(85,PA13)<NJ-COMMED>
+ Susskind & Almallah Eye Associates, P.A.
20 Mule Road/Focus Center   Toms River, NJ 08755   (732)349-5622   Fax (732)349-5625

Almanzar, Raul, MD {1164491585} Pedtrc(92,DOM01)
+ Passaic Pediatrics II PA
913 Main Avenue   Passaic, NJ 07055   (973)458-8000
+ Passaic Pediatrics II PC
93 Market Street   Passaic, NJ 07055   (973)458-8000   Fax

Almashat, Salwan Jafar, MD {1235366840} Pthlgy
+ Capital Medical Center Hopewell Pathology
Two Capital Way/Pthlgy   Pennington, NJ 08534   (800)637-2374

Almazan, Gerald C., MD {1851655476} Pedtrc, IntrMd(09)<NJ-JRSYSHMC, NJ-OCEANMC>
+ Pediatric Care Physicians, LLC
2211 Route 88/Suite 2-A   Brick, NJ 08724   (732)899-0008   Fax (732)899-0447

Almazan-Atienza, Helen, MD {1306815642} Pedtrc(66,PHIL)
+ 1812 Corlies Avenue
Neptune, NJ 07753   (732)988-3336

Almeida, Frank Gerard, MD {1518979541} IntrMd(98,GRN01)<NJ-JRSYSHMC>
+ Sea Girt Medical Associates
235 Route 71   Manasquan, NJ 08736   (732)223-4300   Fax (732)223-5273

Almeida, Laila M., MD {1730108754} Dermat, IntrMd(83,MI01)<NY-PRSBCOLU>
+ Dermatology Associates of Morris PA
199 Baldwin Road   Parsippany, NJ 07054   (973)335-2560   Fax (973)335-9421

Almeida, Vinita Maria, MD {1366548083} Pedtrc, EmrgMd(86,MI01)<NJ-MORRISTN>
+ Morristown Medical Center
100 Madison Avenue   Morristown, NJ 07962   (973)971-5000

Almendral, Jesus Leandro Gestuvo, MD {1346408689} IntrMd(92,PHI02)
+ Robert Wood Johnson Transplant Associates, P.A.
10 Plum Street/7th Floor   New Brunswick, NJ 08901   (732)253-3340   Fax (732)253-3476

Almendras, Nole E., MD {1649203498} Surgry(71,PHIL)<NJ-ACM-CITY, NJ-ACMCMAIN>
+ AtlantiCare Regional Medical Center/City Campus
1925 Pacific Avenue/Surgery   Atlantic City, NJ 08401   (609)345-4000
+ AtlantiCare Regional Med Ctr/Mainland
65 West Jimmie Leeds Road   Pomona, NJ 08240   (609)652-1000

Almentero, Felix Antonio, MD {1992738546} PhysMd, IntrMd(86,PRO03)
+ Jersey Rehab, P.A.
15 Newark Avenue/Suite 1   Belleville, NJ 07109   (973)844-9220   Fax (973)844-9221

Almodovar, Astrid Teresa, MD {1376660068} FamMed(88,DOM04)<NJ-STMICHL>
+ Forest Hill Family Health Associates, P.A.
465 Mount Prospect Avenue   Newark, NJ 07104   (973)483-3640   Fax (973)483-4895

Alnakeeb, Mohammed M., MD {1407262397} ObsGyn
+ 991 Main Street/Unit 2 B
Paterson, NJ 07503   (973)807-2727   Fax (973)807-1931

Alnuaimi, Raya Omer, DO {1548402548} ObsGyn(05,NY75)<NJ-HACKNSK, NJ-STJOSHOS>
+ Aim Obstetrics and Gynecology Medical Group
397 Haledon Avenue/Suite 101   Haledon, NJ 07508   (973)949-3422   Fax (973)949-3423

Alobeidy, Salaam T., MD {1760573513} PulCCr, IntrMd, PthAna(83,IRAQ)<NJ-ACMCMAIN, NJ-ACMCITY>
+ 54 West Jimmie Leeds Road/Suites 4 & 5
Galloway, NJ 08205   (609)404-0056   Fax (609)404-0506

Aloi, Joseph M., MD {1285895235} Anesth(04,PA02)<NJ-VALLEY>
+ Bergen Anesthesia Group, P.C.
500 West Main Street/Suite 16   Wyckoff, NJ 07481   (201)847-9320   Fax (201)847-0059
+ The Valley Hospital
223 North Van Dien Avenue/Anesth   Ridgewood, NJ 07450   (201)447-8000

Aloisio, Denise, MD {1780643296} PedDvl, Pedtrc, PedNrD(90,NY06)<NJ-JRSYSHMC>
+ Jersey Shore Child Evaluation Center
81-04 Davis Avenue   Neptune, NJ 07753   (732)776-4178   Fax (732)776-4946

Alonso, Jose A., MD {1699751685} PhysMd(83,NY01)<NY-PRSB-COLU>
+ Physical Medicine & Rehabilitation Center
500 Grand Avenue/1st Floor   Englewood, NJ 07631   (201)567-2277   Fax (201)567-7506

Alonzo-Chafart, Lorena D., DO {1912998592} FamMed(93,NY75)<NJ-OCEANMC>
+ Total Patient Care
2401 Route 35   Manasquan, NJ 08736   (732)292-9222   Fax (732)292-9633
+ Total Patient Care LLC
459 Jack Martin Boulevard   Brick, NJ 08724   (732)292-9222   Fax (732)785-1222

Alpert, Deborah R., MD {1124150834} Rheuma, IntrMd(01,NY19)<NJ-JRSYSHMC>
+ Hackensack Meridian Medical Group
19 Davis Avenue/5th-6th Floor/Rheumat   Neptune, NJ 07753   (732)897-3985   Fax (732)897-3982
+ Jersey Shore University Medical Center
1945 Route 33/AcademicOffice   Neptune, NJ 07753   (732)776-4420

Alpert, Michael Charles, MD {1730291691} Psychy, IntrMd(69,CA15)
+ 340 Diamond Spring Road/PO Box 1163
Denville, NJ 07834   (917)628-1741   Fax (212)308-7941

Alpert, Mitchel B., MD {1831166529} PedCrd(82,NJ05)<NJ-JRSYSHMC>
+ Alpert Zales & Castro Pediatric Cardiology, PA
1623 Route 88/Suite A/PO Box 1719   Brick, NJ 08723   (732)458-9666   Fax (732)458-0840
sjlesser@alpertzalescastro.com
+ Alpert Zales & Castro Pediatric Cardiology, PA
2 Apple Farm Road/PO Box 4176   Middletown, NJ 07748   (732)458-9666   Fax (732)458-0840

Alshafie, Tarek Ahmed, MD {1336182641} Surgry(80,EGY03)<NJ-VALLEY>
+ Vascular & Endovascular Associates of NJ
One West Ridgewood Avenue/Suite 106   Paramus, NJ 07652   (201)389-3700   Fax (201)670-6725

Alsheikh, Suhail N., MD {1639175367} NnPnMd, Pedtrc(72,IRAQ)<NJ-JRSYCITY, NJ-MEADWLND>
+ Children's Hospital of Hudson County
355 Grand Street   Jersey City, NJ 07302   (201)915-2330   Fax (201)915-2705
+ RWJ University Hospital Somerset
110 Rehill Avenue/Neontlgy   Somerville, NJ 08876   (201)915-2330   Fax (908)704-2730

Alspach, Charlotte A., MD {1396960464} EmrgMd, GenPrc, EmrgEMed(78,VA07)
+ 2355 Ocean Drive
Avalon, NJ 08202   (609)967-3800

Alt, Elaine R., MD {1235386582} PthACl(87,NY19)
+ Quest Diagnostics Inc.
1 Malcolm Avenue/Path   Teterboro, NJ 07608   (201)393-5000   Fax (201)393-6127

Altamura, Richard H., MD {1891722625} EmrgMd(94,NJ06)<NJ-VIRTMHBC>
+ Virtua Memorial
175 Madison Avenue/EmrgMed   Mount Holly, NJ 08060   (609)267-0700   Fax (609)914-6067

Altamuro, Christopher R., DO {1841287539} FamMed(89,PA77)<NJ-VIRTVOOR, NJ-VIRTMARL>
+ AtlantiCare Urgent Care Center
2500 English Creek Avenue   Egg Harbor Township, NJ 08234   (609)407-2273

Altema, Reynald, MD {1548238892} IntrMd(80,NY08)<NJ-NWRK-BETH, NJ-STBARNMC>
+ Dr. Reynald Altema
1395 Clinton Avenue   Irvington, NJ 07111   (973)399-1002   Fax (973)375-4837

Alter, Mark David, MD {1730263617} Psychy, Pedtrc, PsyCAd(99,PA12)
+ Center for Family Guidance, PC
765 East Route 70/Building A-101   Marlton, NJ 08053   (856)983-3900   Fax (856)810-0110

Alter, Robert S., MD {1306805460} IntrMd, MedOnc, OncHem(88,IL42)<NJ-CHILTON, NJ-HACKNSK>
+ John Theurer Cancer Center - HUMC
92 Second Street   Hackensack, NJ 07601   (201)996-5072   Fax (551)996-0719
+ Regional Cancer Care Center
7650 River Road/2nd Floor   North Bergen, NJ 07047   (212)464-0008

Alterman, Michael Adam, DO {1174834626} Ophthl(10,PA77)
+ Freehold Ophthalmology, LLC
20 Hospital Drive   Toms River, NJ 08755   (732)349-7167   Fax (732)505-4322
+ Freehold Ophthalmology, LLC
509 Stillwells Corner Road/Suite E-5   Freehold, NJ 07728   (732)349-7167   Fax (732)431-3312
+ Freehold Ophthalmology, LLC
202 Jack Martin Boulevard   Brick, NJ 08755   (732)458-5700   Fax (732)458-0693

Physicians by Name and Address

Alteveer, Janet G., MD {1376639690} EmrgMd(77,PA02)<NJ-COOPRUMC, NJ-CENTRAST>
+ CentraState Medical Center
901 West Main Street/EmergMed   Freehold, NJ 07728   (732)431-2000

Althoff, Marilyn F., MD {1013966217} EmrgMd(86,MD01)<NJ-MORRISTN>
+ Morristown Medical Center
100 Madison Avenue/EmergMed   Morristown, NJ 07962   (800)290-5309   Fax (803)434-4354

Altimore, David, MD {1609816750} CdvDis, IntrMd(94,NJ03)<NJ-DEBRAHLC>
+ Deborah Heart and Lung Center
200 Trenton Road   Browns Mills, NJ 08015   (609)893-6611   Fax (609)735-0175

Altin, Robert S., MD {1528008778} RadDia(77,DC02)<NJ-ATLANTHS, NJ-SHOREMEM>
+ Atlantic Medical Imaging, LLC.
72 West Jimmie Leeds Road   Galloway, NJ 08205   (609)677-9729   Fax (609)653-8764
+ Atlantic Medical Imaging, LLC.
401 Bethel Road   Somers Point, NJ 08244   (609)677-9729
+ Atlantic Medical Imaging, LLC.
421 Route 9 North   Cape May Court House, NJ 08205   (609)463-9500   Fax (609)465-0918

Altman, Brian, MD {1649347451} Ophthl, PedOph(69,CT01)<NJ-BURDTMLN, NJ-SHOREMEM>
+ Children's Eye Care
315 Route 9 South   Cape May Court House, NJ 08210   (609)465-7500   Fax (609)398-9725
+ Children's Eye Care
1300 Asbury Avenue   Ocean City, NJ 08226   (609)465-7500   Fax (609)398-9725

Altman, Daniel Winston, MD {1619918828} IntrMd, FamMed(94,PA09)
+ Altman and Gerety Family Medical Association
188 Fries Mill Road/Suite E-3   Turnersville, NJ 08012   (856)629-7006   Fax (856)629-0077   Dwa415@aol.com

Altman, Rachel S., MD {1235236357} Dermat
+ Northeast Regional Epilepsy Group
290 Madison Avenue/Building 5 2nd FL   Morristown, NJ 07960   (201)343-6676
+ Morristown Dermatology
290 Madison Avenue/Bldg 5   Morristown, NJ 07960   (973)538-7171

Altman, Robert Gil, MD {1023119542} SrgPlstc, Surgry(97,GRN01)<NJ-MORRISTN>
+ Altman Aesthetic Center
570 Sylvan Avenue   Englewood Cliffs, NJ 07632   (201)569-3334   Fax (201)569-3321

Altman, Wayne J., MD {1710964390} SrgHnd, SrgOrt(78,NJ06)<NJ-CHRIST, NJ-MTNSIDE>
+ 85 Orient Way
Rutherford, NJ 07070   (201)438-5888   Fax (201)438-6825

Altmann, Dory Bert, MD {1114954005} CdvDis, IntrMd(86,CT01)<NY-PRSBWEIL>
+ Cardiology Associates of New Brunswick
593 Cranbury Road/Suite 2   East Brunswick, NJ 08816   (732)390-3333   Fax (732)390-9244

Altobelli, Anthony, III, MD {1003843905} IntrMd, CdvDis(97,DC02)<NJ-RWJUBRUN, NJ-STPETER>
+ Cardiology Associates of New Brunswick
593 Cranbury Road/Suite 2   East Brunswick, NJ 08816   (732)390-3333   Fax (732)390-9244
+ 3 Executive Drive
Somerset, NJ 08873   (718)288-0310

Altomare, Corrado J., MD {1275707663} ObsGyn(80,ITAL)<NJ-HUNTRDN>
+ Affiliates in Obstetrics & Gynecology, P.A.
111 Route 31/Suite 121 2nd FL Bldg B   Flemington, NJ 08822   (908)782-2825   Fax (908)782-0196
+ Affiliates in Obstetrics & Gynecology, P.A.
99 Grayrock Road/Second Floor   Clinton, NJ 08809   (908)782-2825   Fax (908)730-8504
+ Affiliates in Obstetrics & Gynecology, P.A.
431 Highway 22 East   Whitehouse, NJ 08822   (908)823-1600   Fax (908)823-1640

Altongy, Joseph F., MD {1053367417} PedOrt, SrgOrt(80,NJ05)<NJ-OVERLOOK>
+ 33 Overlook Road/Suite 202
Summit, NJ 07901   (908)273-8340   Fax (908)273-1553

Altschul, Dorothea, MD {1740323138} Nrolgy(01,AUS07)
+ St. Joseph's Medical Center Neurosurgery
703 Main Street   Paterson, NJ 07503   (973)754-2463
+ Neurosurgeons of New Jersey
1200 East Ridgewood Avenue   Ridgewood, NJ 07450   (201)824-6131

Altshuler, Elena, MD {1679502587} Pedtrc(77,RUSS)
+ Medical Pediatrics Associates
256 Bunn Drive/Suite 3 A   Princeton, NJ 08540   Fax (609)683-7958

Altszuler, Henry M., MD {1104818186} CdvDis(82,NY19)<NJ-MORRISTN>
+ MedDiag Assocs/Central NJ Cardiology
1511 Park Avenue/Suite 2   South Plainfield, NJ 07080   (908)756-4438   Fax (908)756-9160

Altura, Rachel Allison, MD {1215933908} OncHem, Pedtrc, PthHem(92,MO02)<RI-RIHOSPTL>
+ Merck and Company Incorporated
126 East Lincoln Avenue   Rahway, NJ 07065   (732)574-4000

Alturk, Najib M., MD {1023034774} CdvDis(87,SYR02)
+ 508 Lakehurst Road/Suite 2 B
Toms River, NJ 08755   (732)281-6101   Fax (732)281-6116

Alturk, Souhir, MD {1316024888} Pedtrc(86,SYR01)
+ 9 Hospital Drive/Suite 7-B
Toms River, NJ 08755   (732)818-9955   Fax (732)818-9960

Altzman, Elana F., MD {1033194576} Pedtrc(94,NY08)<NY-SUNY-BRKL, NY-STONYBRK>
+ JFK Neurosciences Institute
65 James Street/Second Floor   Edison, NJ 08818   (732)321-7010   Fax (732)906-4906

Aluri-Vallabhaneni, Bhanu Sri, MD {1881681476} Radiol, RadDia, RadNro(88,INA7C)<NJ-STJOSHOS>
+ St. Joseph's Regional Medical Center
703 Main Street/Radiology   Paterson, NJ 07503   (973)754-2000

Aluya, Nelson Oke, MD {1942457916} IntrMd(98,NIG04)
+ 1026 Fairview Place
Hillside, NJ 07205

Alva, Suraj, MD {1588821292}
+ Associated Colon & Rectal Surgeons PA
3900 Park Avenue/Suite 101   Edison, NJ 08820   (732)494-6640   Fax (732)549-8204

Alvarado, Mark U., MD {1821090663} Psychy, PsyAdd, NrlgAddM(83,PA09)<NJ-MTCARMEL, NJ-STMICHL>
+ Mt. Carmel Guild/ Behavioral Health System
1160 Raymond Boulevard/Psych   Newark, NJ 07102   (973)596-4190

Alvarado-Rosario, Yilda Limary, MD {1922244169} Pedtrc(08,PRO02)<NJ-JFKMED>
+ Building Blocks Pediatric Group
415 Harrison Avenue   Westfield, NJ 07090   (862)955-3183   Fax (862)955-1389

Alvarez, Bethzaida, MD {1801009741} GenPrc, IntrMd(83,DOM02)
+ 345 Somerset Street
North Plainfield, NJ 07060   (908)753-9739   Fax (908)753-9831

Alvarez, Enrique F., MD {1891860938} Surgry(72,ELS01)<NJ-CHSMRCER, NJ-RWJUHAM>
+ 123 Franklin Corner Road/Suite 204
Lawrenceville, NJ 08648   (609)896-1433   Fax (609)896-2171

Alvarez, Manuel, MD {1194759282} ObsGyn, MtFtMd(81,DOMI)<NJ-HACKNSK, NJ-HOBUNIMC>
+ Hackensack Univ. Maternal Fetal Med
20 Prospect Avenue/Suite 601   Hackensack, NJ 07601   (201)996-2765   Fax (201)487-8516   malvarez@humed.com
+ Hackensack University Medical Center
30 Prospect Avenue/Ob-Gyn   Hackensack, NJ 07601   (201)996-2765   Fax (201)996-2475

Alvarez, Maria T., MD {1750508149} Pedtrc, PedEmg(90,NJ05)<NJ-UMDNJ>
+ University Hospital
150 Bergen Street/PdtrcEmergency   Newark, NJ 07103   (973)972-4300   Fax (973)972-5965
+ University Hospital-New Jersey Medical School
30 Bergen Street/Rm 205   Newark, NJ 07107   (973)972-4511

Alvarez, Marie Emma B., MD {1295916815} Pedtrc(93,PHI01)
+ 1455 Main Avenue
Clifton, NJ 07011   (862)225-9852

Alvarez, Reinaldo G., MD {1003971367} Psychy(63,SPA22)<NJ-RWJURAH>
+ Martin P. Mayer, MD PC
1503 Saint Georges Avenue   Colonia, NJ 07067   (732)382-1300   Fax (732)382-6923

Alvarez Perez, Jesus Rafael, MD {1003009473} ObsGyn(00,PRO03)<NJ-UMDNJ>
+ Hackensack University Medical Center
30 Prospect Avenue   Hackensack, NJ 07601   (551)996-2453   susomd@yahoo.com

Alvarez-Prieto, Maria R., MD {1477754893} Nrolgy, NroChl(79,SPA05)
+ Neurology Center
41-51 Wilson Avenue/Suite 2-D   Newark, NJ 07105   (973)589-1554   Fax (973)589-4079

Alvarez-Segovia, Lucia M., MD {1447274196} IntrMd, PulCCr, PulDis(85,MEX02)
+ Cross Country Cardiology
103 River Road/2nd Floor   Edgewater, NJ 07020   (201)941-9952   Fax (201)941-2899

Alvaro, Joseph M., MD {1548290885} ObsGyn, Gyneco(80,NJ06)<NJ-STPETER, NJ-RWJUHAM>
+ 7 Cedar Grove Lane/Suite 34
Somerset, NJ 08873   (732)271-0800   Fax (732)271-4099

Alves, Eric M., DO {1427020346} RadNro(93,IA75)<NJ-SJHREGMC>
+ SJH Regional Medical Center
1505 West Sherman Avenue   Vineland, NJ 08360   (856)641-8000

Alves, Lennox, MD {1922113109} Surgry(86,NY06)
+ Drs. Alves & Johnson
470 Prospect Avenue/Suite 200   West Orange, NJ 07052   (973)243-0290   Fax (973)243-1863

Alvi, Afshan Khadija, MD {1104158567} CdvDis
+ Hamilton Cardiology Associates
2073 Klockner Road   Hamilton, NJ 08690   (609)584-1212   Fax (609)584-0103

Alweiss, Gary S., MD {1609838986} Nrolgy(88,NY47)<NJ-ENGLWOOD, NJ-HACKNSK>
+ Bergen Neurology Consultants
25 Rockwood Place/Suite 110   Englewood, NJ 07631   (201)894-5805   Fax (201)894-1956   ggamd@optonline.net

Aly, Mahmoud H., MD {1699791459} OncHem, IntrMd(87,WIND)<NY-CMCSTVSI, NJ-BAYSHORE>
+ Aly Internal Medicine/Hematology Oncology
883 Poole Avenue/Suite 4   Hazlet, NJ 07730   (732)203-9500   Fax (732)203-0851

Aly, Sayed Raafat M., MD {1174680722} Pedtrc(77,EGY03)<NJ-MEADWLND, NJ-BAYONNE>
+ 451 Broadway
Bayonne, NJ 07002   (201)471-7790   Fax (201)471-7789

Alzadon, Ricardo, MD {1164571444} Surgry(66,PHI01)
+ 50 Union Avenue/Suite 604
Irvington, NJ 07111   (973)371-8300   Fax (973)374-2936

Alziadet, Moayyad Radi Barham, MD {1699182717} IntrMd
+ St Joseph's Medical Ctr Internal Med
703 Main Street/5th Fl   Paterson, NJ 07503   (973)754-2000

Amadasu-Kest, Helen E., MD {1508803420} Pedtrc, PedInf(92,NIG07)<NJ-CLARMAAS>
+ St. Joseph's Pediatrics DePaul Center
11 Getty Avenue/2nd Floor   Paterson, NJ 07503   (973)754-3729

Amadi, Mariette Yvonne, MD {1093977019} IntHos, IntrMd(98,NIG09)<NJ-SOMERSET, NJ-HACKNSK>
+ RWJ University Hospital Somerset
110 Rehill Avenue/Hospitalist   Somerville, NJ 08876   (908)927-8780
+ Hackensack Medical Center-Internal Medicine
30 Prospect Avenue/4 Main/Rm 4621   Hackensack, NJ 07601   (908)927-8780   Fax (551)996-0536

Amadi, Nkechinyere, MD {1609036599} ObsGyn(03,KS02)<NJ-COOPRUMC>
+ Mercer Ob/Gyn Associates at Mercer
446 Bellevue Avenue   Trenton, NJ 08618   (609)394-4111   Fax (609)394-4070

Amadio, Thomas J., DO {1720033996} EmrgMd<NJ-WARREN>
+ Warren Hospital
185 Roseberry Street   Phillipsburg, NJ 08865   (908)859-6700   Fax (908)853-6812

Amaefuna, Stephen C., MD {1205842408} Pedtrc, EmrgEmed(83,GRN01)
+ 4 Faas Court
West Orange, NJ 07052   (973)715-2688   Fax (973)324-9725
+ Total Support Medical Group
40 Union Avenue/Suite 301   Irvington, NJ 07111   (973)373-0903
+ Maan Pediatric Associates Inc
75 Clifton Avenue   Clifton, NJ 07052   (973)546-6400

Amalfitano, Christopher, MD {1144268442} EmrgMd(93,NY15)
+ 15 Riverside Drive
Basking Ridge, NJ 07920   (908)719-1352

Aman, Chaudhry S., MD {1619054137} IntrMd, PulCCr, CritCr(84,PAK20)
+ 550 Summit Avenue/Suite 205
Jersey City, NJ 07306   (201)217-3222

Amankwaah, Ajoa O., DO {1184933293} FamMed, IntrMd
+ Medford Family Practice
152 Himmelein Road/Suite 100   Medford, NJ 08055   (609)654-7117   Fax (609)654-8555

Amara, Shobha, MD {1871512095} Pedtrc(80,INDI)<NJ-STPETER>
+ St. Peter's University Hospital
254 Easton Avenue/Pediatrics   New Brunswick, NJ 08901   (732)745-8600   Fax (732)828-8929

Amara, Sreenivasrao, MD {1538369418} IntrMd, AlgyImmn(72,INA5B)<NY-LUTHERN>
+ Center for Asthma & Allergy
B2 Cornwall Drive East Brunswick, NJ 08816 (732)257-4008 Fax (732)257-1958

Amarnani, Sukhdev, MD {1346279494} Pedtrc, FamMAdM(94,GRN01)
+ 64 South Main Street
Manville, NJ 08835 (908)685-8000 Fax (908)685-8000

Amato, Christopher, DO {1639251903} Pedtrc(99,NJ75)<NJ-KMH-TURNV, NJ-VIRTVOOR>
+ Dr. G. Lee Lerch and Associates
63 North Lakeview Drive/Suite 202 Gibbsboro, NJ 08026 (856)435-6000 Fax (856)782-1667
camato@aap.net
+ Dr. G. Lee Lerch and Associates
239 Hurffville Crosskeys Road Sewell, NJ 08080 (856)435-6000 Fax (856)728-0808

Amato, Christopher Scott, MD {1407897721} Pedtrc, EmrgMd(94,MD01)<NJ-MORRISTN>
+ Morristown Medical Center
100 Madison Avenue Morristown, NJ 07962 (973)971-5000

Amato, Indira L., MD {1841385424} Pedtrc(00,NJ05)<NJ-RWJUBRUN>
+ RWJ University Hospital New Brunswick
One Robert Wood Johnson Place New Brunswick, NJ 08901 (732)235-7883 Fax (732)235-6609
+ University Medical Group Pediatrics
125 Paterson Street/MEB 3rd Fl New Brunswick, NJ 08903 (732)235-7883 Fax (732)235-6609

Amato, James L., Jr., MD {1720033426} CdvDis, IntCrd, IntrMd(91,NJ05)<NJ-CLARMAAS>
+ James L. Amato Jr, MD, PA
276 Prospect Street East Orange, NJ 07017 (973)751-8400 Fax (973)678-0309
+ James L. Amato Jr, MD, PA
946 Bloomfield avenue Glen Ridge, NJ 07028 (973)751-8400 Fax (973)733-2627

Amato, John Paul, MD {1457487407} SrgRec, SrgO&M(02,NY47)<NJ-STBARNMC>
+ The Amato Center for Plastic Reconstructive Surgery
101 Old Short Hills Road/Penthouse 2 West Orange, NJ 07052 (973)736-1714 Fax (973)325-3487
info@theamatocenter.com
+ The Amato Center for Plastic Reconstructive Surgery
33 Clinton Road/Suite 101 West Caldwell, NJ 07006 (973)736-1714 Fax (973)325-3487

Ambalu, Naomi, DO {1174870034}<NJ-UNIVBHC>
+ Children's Hospital Outpatient Center
266 King George Road/Suite G Warren, NJ 07059 (908)647-8847
+ University Behavioral Health Care
671 Hoes Lane/PO Box 1392 Piscataway, NJ 08855 (732)235-4433

Ambalu, Oren, MD {1649618026} Anesth
+ Robert Wood Johnson-UMDNJ Anesthesia Group
125 Paterson Street/CAB 3100 New Brunswick, NJ 08901 (732)235-7827 Fax (732)235-6131

Ambarus, Tatiana, MD {1326174715} ObsGyn<NJ-NWRKBETH>
+ Newark Beth Israel Medical Center
201 Lyons Avenue Newark, NJ 07112 (973)926-7000

Ambrose, Gunaseelan, MD {1841290517} Surgry(82,INA78)<NY-WESTCHMC>
+ Surgical Associates of Central NJ
30 Rehill Avenue/Suite 3300 Somerville, NJ 08876 (908)927-8994 Fax (908)927-8995

Ambrose, John F., MD {1760587851} SrgOrt(72,NJ05)<NJ-WAYNEGEN, NJ-STJOSHOS>
+ Elite Orthopedics & Sports Medicine, P.A.
1035 Route 46 East/Suite G-2 Clifton, NJ 07013 (973)928-2062
+ Totowa Physicians and Surgeons
426 Union Boulevard Totowa, NJ 07512 (973)928-2062 Fax (973)595-8501
+ Wayne Surgical Center, LLC.
1176 Hamburg Pike Wayne, NJ 07013 (973)709-1900 Fax (973)709-1901

Ambrosio, George Joseph, MD {1669564431} IntrMd(79,NJ05)<NJ-MTNSIDE, NJ-CLARMAAS>
+ first Care Medical Group
750 Valley Brook Avenue Lyndhurst, NJ 07071 (201)896-0900 Fax (201)896-2726
+ first Care Medical Group
50 Pompton Avenue Verona, NJ 07044 (201)896-0900 Fax (973)857-7034

Ambrosio, Patrick M., DO {1295765675} Allrgy, Pedtrc(97,NJ75)<NJ-STPETER>
+ ENT & Allergy Associates, LLP
485 Route 1 South/Bld B/Suite 350 Iselin, NJ 08830 (732)549-3934 Fax (732)549-7250

+ ENT & Allergy Associates, LLP
3663 Route 9 North/Suite102 Old Bridge, NJ 08857 (732)549-3934 Fax (732)707-3850
+ Dr. Ambrosio's Practice
1160 Kennedy Boulevard/Apt 3 Bayonne, NJ 08830 (201)436-1922 Fax (201)436-8110

Ameen, Abdul Aleem, MD {1457317844} CdvDis, IntrMd(88,INA9D)
+ Liberty Medical Associates
377 Jersey Avenue/Suite 470 Jersey City, NJ 07302 (201)918-2239 Fax (201)918-2243

Ameen, Naureen W., MD {1285710574} Pedtrc(89,PAK11)<NJ-HACKNSK, NJ-HOLYNAME>
+ Future Pediatric Group
240 Eighth Street Prospect Park, NJ 07508 (973)942-2131

Amegadzie, Richard Koku, MD {1033226931} IntrMd(94,GHA01)
+ Prompt Medical Care
636 Easton Avenue Somerset, NJ 08873 (732)220-8811 Fax (732)220-1300

Amer, Adel M., MD {1609953439} Pedtrc(79,EGY04)
+ Drs. Amer and Prasad
777 White Horse Pike/Suite E Hammonton, NJ 08037 (609)567-0608 Fax (609)567-1295

Amer, Yousef A., MD {1023109451} ObsGyn(74,EGYP)<NJ-BAYSHORE, NJ-CENTRAST>
+ Amer Ob-Gyn Associates
900 West Main Street/Suite 3 Freehold, NJ 07728 (732)294-5600

Amerson, Afriye Rochelle, MD {1952305229} ObsGyn, IntrMd(97,DC01)
+ 300 Gorge Road/P.O. Box 6106
Cliffside Park, NJ 07010 (646)325-3993

Ames, Elliot L., DO {1457394603} SrgHnd, SrgOrt, OrtSHand(74,IA75)<NJ-KMHCHRRY, NJ-KMHSTRAT>
+ New Jersey Hand Center
1878 Route 70/Suite 5 Cherry Hill, NJ 08034 (856)751-6464 Fax (856)751-1719
+ New Jersey Hand Center
202B Kings Way West Sewell, NJ 08080 (856)751-6464 Fax (856)751-1719

Ames-Bobila, Deborah, MD {1104922707} Anesth(73,PHIL)<NJ-STJOSHOS>
+ Michael I. Baruch Plastic Surgery Associates
1037 Route 46 East/Suite 103 Clifton, NJ 07013 (973)773-1973 Fax (973)773-4824

Amesur, Kiran Bhagwan, MD {1104900778} Ophthl(95,NY09)<NJ-VALLEY>
+ 85 South Maple Avenue
Ridgewood, NJ 07450 (201)447-2700

Amico, Frank Joseph, Jr., DO {1497091904} CdvDis(10,PA77)
+ Deborah Heart and Lung Center
200 Trenton Road Browns Mills, NJ 08015 (516)644-7169
frankam325@gmail.com

Amiel, Elizabeth A., MD {1871616987} Psychy, PsyCAd(88,ISR02)
+ 32 Washington Avenue/Suite 7
Tenafly, NJ 07670 (201)569-2257 Fax (201)569-2294

Amin, Alpesh Jashvant, MD {1972540797} IntrMd(00,GRN01)
+ 355 Henry Street
Orange, NJ 07050 (973)672-0352 Fax (973)672-3393

Amin, Anila P., MD {1043240823} IntrMd(81,INDI)<NJ-SHOREMEM>
+ Center for Primary Health Care/Wellness
222 New Road/Suite 101 Linwood, NJ 08221 (609)927-7070

Amin, Darshana Patel, DO {1407901382} Nrolgy, SlpDis, Psychy(04,ME75)
+ Shore Neurology, P.A.
633 Route 37 West Toms River, NJ 08755 (732)240-4787 Fax (732)240-3114

Amin, Deepak K., MD {1659372829} IntrMd(89,INA15)<NY-CMC-STMRY, NJ-PALISADE>
+ 4522 Kennedy Boulevard
Union City, NJ 07087 (201)863-1797 Fax (201)863-6117
deepmd@aol.com

Amin, Devendra Kanaiyalal, MD {1760452973} IntrMd, CdvDis(75,INA65)<NJ-WARREN>
+ 39 Roseberry Street
Phillipsburg, NJ 08865 (908)859-0789

Amin, Girish S., MD {1720171731} Hemato, IntrMd, MedOnc(87,INA53)<NJ-COMMED, NJ-KIMBALL>
+ NJ Hematology & Oncology Associates
1608 Route 88 West/Suite 250 Brick, NJ 08724 (732)840-8880 Fax (732)840-3939
+ NJ Hematology & Oncology Associates
508 Lakehurst Road/Suite 1B Toms River, NJ 08755 (732)840-8880 Fax (732)244-1955

Amin, Haris Irfan, MD {1013910942} VitRet, Ophthl(92,NY15)<NJ-COMMED>
+ Ocean County Retina, P.C.
780 Route 37 West/Suite 200 Toms River, NJ 08755 (732)797-1855 Fax (732)797-1856

Amin, Jashvant S., MD {1922116268} Hemato, IntrMd, OncHem(68,INDI)<NJ-CLARMAAS, NJ-STBARNMC>
+ 355 Henry Street
Orange, NJ 07050 (856)672-0352 Fax (973)672-3393
+ J.S. Amin MD, PA
181 Franklin Avenue/Suite 302 Nutley, NJ 07110 (973)235-1300

Amin, Naeem Muhammad, MD {1659326833} IntrMd, Nephro(87,PAK01)<NJ-SJHREGMC>
+ Cooper University Hospital
One Cooper Plaza Camden, NJ 08103 (856)342-2000
+ Kidney & Hypertension Specialists PA
215 Laurel Heights Drive Bridgeton, NJ 08302 (856)342-2000 Fax (856)455-6106

Amin, Parul S., MD {1316000540} IntrMd(84,INDI)<NJ-EASTORNG>
+ 906-N Fifth Street/Unit C101
Newark, NJ 07107

Amin, Pinakin B., MD {1215014246} EmrgMd, IntrMd, SprtMd(82,INDI)<NJ-ANCPSYCH>
+ Ancora Psychiatric Hospital
301 Spring Garden Road Hammonton, NJ 08037 (609)561-1700

Amin, Prakash P., MD {1750452744} Psychy, PsyAdd(82,INA21)
+ 2211 Whitehorse Mercerville Rd
Trenton, NJ 08619 (609)587-2255 Fax (609)587-7255

Amin, Ritesh A., MD {1689916108} Psychy
+ University Psychiatric Associates
183 South Orange Avenue/E-F Levels Newark, NJ 07103 (973)972-4670 Fax (973)972-2979

Amin, Sabina, MD {1336379270}
+ Cooper Perinatology Associates
3 Cooper Plaza/Suite 502 Camden, NJ 08103 (856)342-2380 Fax (856)968-8499

Amin, Samirlal Ramanlal, MD {1811987928} FamMed(79,INA70)
+ 9245 Kennedy Boulevard
North Bergen, NJ 07047 (201)863-6844 Fax (201)854-0050

Amin, Sejal J., MD {1013337443} ObsGyn
+ 7213 Wessex Place
Princeton, NJ 08540 (732)309-6965

Amin, Shilpa K., MD {1184860678} EmrgMd
+ 166 Winthrop Road
Edison, NJ 08817

Amin, Vishnubhai M., MD {1346286051} Surgry(65,INA20)<NJ-HACKNSK, NJ-VALLEY>
+ 333 Old Hook Road/Suite 105
Westwood, NJ 07675 (201)358-0611 Fax (201)722-0291

Amir, Saba, MD {1154572436} IntrMd<NJ-STPETER>
+ St. Peter's Family Health
123 How Lane New Brunswick, NJ 08901 (732)745-8600 Fax (732)729-0869
+ St. Peter's University Hospital
254 Easton Avenue/Internal Med New Brunswick, NJ 08901 (732)745-8600

Amir, Sabah H., MD {1649305236} Pedtrc(72,IRQ01)<NJ-ACMC-MAIN, NJ-ACMCITY>
+ Mainland Pediatric Association
741 South Second Avenue/Suite B Galloway, NJ 08205 (609)748-8500 Fax (609)748-6700

Amirata, Edwin A., MD {1437227600} Surgry(90,MA07)
+ Amirata Surgical Group
5 Franklin Avenue/Suite 406 Belleville, NJ 07109 (973)759-4499

Amistoso, Aldrin Calingacion, MD {1457683518}<NJ-VIRTMHBC>
+ Virtua Memorial
175 Madison Avenue Mount Holly, NJ 08060 (609)267-0700

Amitie, Daniel Dean, MD {1891770939} AnesCrCr, Anesth(01,IN20)<NJ-JRSYSHMC>
+ Jersey Shore University Medical Center
1945 Route 33/Anesth Neptune, NJ 07753 (732)775-5500

Amjad, Maqsood, MD {1881631398} IntrMd, Hemato, MedOnc(89,PAK01)<NJ-SOMERSET, NJ-JFKMED>
+ Regional Cancer Care Specialists
34-36 Progress Street/Suite B-2 Edison, NJ 08820 (908)757-9696 Fax (908)757-9721

Amor, Jorge Hernan, MD {1972687341} Pedtrc, IntrMd(81,SPA12)<NJ-CHILTON>
+ Chilton Medical Center
97 West Parkway/PediatricClinic Pompton Plains, NJ 07444 (973)831-5120 Fax (973)831-5342

Amorapanth, Vanna R., MD {1578775029} PedDvl, Pedtrc(73,THA03)
+ 3 Bridge Street
Metuchen, NJ 08840 (732)603-9050 Fax (732)603-9075

Amores, Edward Daniel, MD {1093973109} EmrgMd<NJ-VALLEY>
+ University Emergency Medicine
125 Paterson Street/MEB 104 New Brunswick, NJ 08901 (732)235-8717 Fax (732)235-7379

Physicians by Name and Address

Amorosa, Judith K., MD {1235111584} RadDia(70,NJ05)<NJ-RWJUBRUN>
+ University Radiology Group, P.C.
483 Cranbury Road   East Brunswick, NJ 08816   (732)235-7721   Fax (732)390-5383
+ University Radiology Group, P.C.
10 Plum Street   New Brunswick, NJ 08901   (732)235-7721   Fax (732)249-1208
+ University Radiology Group, P.C.
579A Cranbury Road   East Brunswick, NJ 08816   (732)390-0040   Fax (732)390-1856

Amorosa, Louis F., MD {1265519383} EnDbMt, IntrMd(69,NJ05)<NJ-RWJUBRUN>
+ University Medical Group - General Internal Medicine
125 Paterson Street/Suite 5100A   New Brunswick, NJ 08903   (732)235-7219   Fax (732)235-8610
+ RWJ University Hospital New Brunswick
One Robert Wood Johnson Place   New Brunswick, NJ 08901   (732)235-7219   Fax (732)235-6527

Amoroso, Michael Louis, MD {1598794158} Anesth, PainMd, PainInvt(81,NJ05)<PA-JRSYSHOR>
+ 193 West Sylvania Avenue
Neptune City, NJ 07753   (732)897-0200

Amoroso, Michael Luke, MD {1265518260} RadDia(91,NJ06)
+ 401 Sylvan Avenue
Englewood Cliffs, NJ 07632   (201)541-5401   Fax (201)541-5400

Amoruso, Daniel Robert, MD {1528386380} IntCrd
+ Atlantic Cardiology Group LLP
8 Tempe Wick Road/Suite 300   Mendham, NJ 07945   (973)543-2288   Fax (973)543-0637

Amoruso, Robert C., MD {1518069301} PulDis, CritCr, IntrMd(75,ITA01)<NJ-STJOSHOS>
+ St. Joseph's Regional Medical Center
703 Main Street/Medicine   Paterson, NJ 07503   (973)754-2476

Ampadu, Akua A., MD {1144581570} IntrMd(12,OH40)<NJ-MORRISTN>
+ IPC The Hospitalist Company
55 Madison Avenue/Suite 310   Morristown, NJ 07960   (973)971-9910   Fax (973)998-4237

Amponsah, Akwasi Peprah, MD {1750645982} AnesPain, Anesth(08,NJ06)
+ 1 Richmond Street/Suite 3001
New Brunswick, NJ 08901   (732)253-7057   Fax (732)253-7057

Amponsah, Michael Kwesi, MD {1518233899} CdvDis<NJ-NWRKBETH>
+ Newark Beth Israel Medical Center
201 Lyons Avenue/Medicine   Newark, NJ 07112   (973)926-7425

Amrick, Thomas J., MD {1538182050} Gastrn, IntrMd(85,PA02)
+ Westfield Associates in Internal Medicine/Gastro
512 East Broad Street   Westfield, NJ 07090   (908)232-6151   Fax (908)232-1920

Amrien, John R., MD {1497757173} FamMed(81,DOMI)<NJ-MEMSALEM>
+ Drs Amrien and Amrien
4 Bypass Road/Suite 201   Salem, NJ 08079   (856)935-0066   Fax (856)935-7247

Amui, Jewel Naakarley, MD {1538142120} RprEnd, FrtInf, Obs-Gyn(97,NJ06)
+ Cooper Institute for Reproductive Hormonal Disorders
17000 Commerce Parkway/Suite C   Mount Laurel, NJ 08054   (856)751-5575   Fax (856)751-7289

Amuluru, Jaladurga P., MD {1093826216} IntrMd, Grtrcs(72,INA8Y)
+ Veterans Affairs Clinic
385 Prospect Avenue   Hackensack, NJ 07601   (201)487-1390

Amuluru, Krishna, MD {1245473594} RadV&I, RadDia(08,IL06)
+ Center for Neurological Surgery UMDNJ
90 Bergen Street/DOC 8100   Newark, NJ 07103   (973)972-7605   Fax (973)972-2333

Amuluru, Prabhakara, MD {1184629511} Anesth, IntrMd(71,INDI)<NJ-STMICHL>
+ St. Michael's Medical Center
268 MLK Jr. Boulevard/Anesthesia   Newark, NJ 07102   (973)877-5032   Fax (973)877-5231
+ St. Michael's Medical Center
111 Central Avenue/Anesthesia   Newark, NJ 07102   (973)877-5032   Fax (973)877-5231

An, Jane J., MD {1326354929} RadDia
+ Hackensack Radiology Group, P.A.
30 Prospect Avenue   Hackensack, NJ 07601   (551)996-2200   Fax (201)489-2812

Anam, Khalid Sadrul, MD {1669882452}
+ Riverside Medical Group
714 Tenth Street/Suite 2   Secaucus, NJ 07094   (201)863-3346   Fax (201)865-0015
drkanam@riversidemedgroup.com

Anam, Sadrul, MD {1801982459} Pedtrc(79,BAN02)<NJ-MEADWLND, NJ-STJOSHOS>
+ Riverside Pediatric Group
4201 New York Avenue   Union City, NJ 07087   (201)601-9515   Fax (201)601-9516
+ Riverside Medical Group
714 Tenth Street/Suite 2   Secaucus, NJ 07094   (201)601-9515   Fax (201)865-0015

Anama, Luzminda M., MD {1487647202} IntrMd, Nephro(66,PHI05)
+ 1163 Route 37 West
Toms River, NJ 08755   (732)244-7555   Fax (732)505-4353

Anan, Elinor M., MD {1730177759} PhysMd(91,PA13)<NJ-KSLR-WEST>
+ Kessler Institute for Rehabilitation West Orange
1199 Pleasant Valley Way   West Orange, NJ 07052   (973)731-3600

Anana, Michael Calulo, MD {1447410493} EmrgMd, IntrMd(05,NJ05)<NJ-UMDNJ>
+ University Hospital
150 Bergen Street/WL Suite M219   Newark, NJ 07103   (973)972-5128

Anand, Ashish, MD {1538329610} Psychy, PsyCAd(08,MA05)
+ 61 North Maple Avenue/Suite 101-B
Ridgewood, NJ 07450   (201)701-2961

Anand, Kapil, MD {1912393281} IntrMd
+ RWJ Hospital Internal Medicine
One Robert Wood Johnson Place/MEB 486   New Brunswick, NJ 08901   (407)756-2150   Fax (732)235-7427

Anand, Neha, MD {1477810836}
+ 88 Morgan Street/Apt 3909
Jersey City, NJ 07302   (516)236-4882
neha23anand@yahoo.com

Anand, Neil, MD {1508271149} RadDia<NJ-MORRISTN>
+ Morristown Medical Center
100 Madison Avenue   Morristown, NJ 07962   (973)971-5000

Anand, Rishi Dev, MD {1457599300} EnDbMt, IntrMd(06,NY03)<PA-TAYLOR>
+ Endocrinology Associates
1 Brace Road/Suite B   Cherry Hill, NJ 08034   (856)234-0645   Fax (856)234-0498

Anand Chawla, Jagjit K., MD {1568462695} PthACl, Pthlgy, Pth-Cln(68,INA72)<NJ-VIRTMHBC, NJ-VIRTUAHS>
+ Virtua Memorial
175 Madison Avenue/Path   Mount Holly, NJ 08060   (609)267-0700

Anandakrishnan, Rajashree, MD {1861562688} IntrMd, InfDis(97,INA19)
+ 2087 Klockner Road
Trenton, NJ 08690   Fax (609)838-0689

Anandarangam, Thiruvengadam, MD {1427014224} IntrMd, PulDis, SrgC&R(88,INA2X)<NJ-NWRKBETH>
+ Newark Beth Israel Medical Center
201 Lyons Avenue/Pulmonary Dis   Newark, NJ 07112   (973)926-6347   Fax (973)923-5688
thiruvengadam_anandarangam@rabiaawanmd.com

Ananian, Christopher Lee, MD {1639311822} RadDia(04,NJ05)<NJ-UNVMCPRN>
+ Princeton Radiology Associates, P.A.
419 North Harrison Street   Princeton, NJ 08540   (609)921-3345   Fax (609)683-8847
+ Princeton Radiology Associates, P.A.
3674 Route 27   Kendall Park, NJ 08824   (609)921-3345   Fax (732)821-6675

Anannab, Kevin C., MD {1578587127} Anesth(02,NY48)<NJ-HACKNSK>
+ 43 Mayer Drive
Clifton, NJ 07012
+ Red Bank Anesthesia, LLC
1 Riverview Plaza   Red Bank, NJ 07701   Fax (732)450-2620

Anantharaman, Priya, MD {1518991843} Nephro, IntrMd(98,INA3D)<NJ-JRSYSHMC, NJ-OCEANMC>
+ Jersey Coast Nephrology & Hypertension Associates
1008 Commons Way/Suite G   Toms River, NJ 08755   (732)818-0700   Fax (732)818-0730
+ Jersey Coast Nephrology & Hypertension Associates
1541 Route 88/Suite A   Brick, NJ 08724   (732)818-0700   Fax (732)836-3201

Anapolle, David M., MD {1013007418} SrgOrt, SprtMd(88,NJ05)<NJ-BURDTMLN, NJ-SHOREMEM>
+ Court House Surgery Center
106 Courthouse South Dennis Rd   Cape May, NJ 08204   (609)465-0300   Fax (609)465-8771
+ Pace Orthopedics & Sports Medicine
547 New Road   Somers Point, NJ 08244   (609)465-0300   Fax (609)927-1616

Anastasi, Lawrence J., DO {1760489538} FamMed(76,PA77)<NJ-SHOREMEM>
+ The Medical Center of Margate
9501 Ventnor Avenue   Margate, NJ 08402   (609)823-6161   Fax (856)823-3413

Anastasiades, Athos C., MD {1366483174} CdvDis, IntrMd(70,GRE01)<NJ-WESTHDSN, NJ-CLARMAAS>
+ North Arlington Cardiology Associates
62 Ridge Road   North Arlington, NJ 07031   (201)991-8565   Fax (201)991-2408

Ancevska Taneva, Natasa, MD {1275773434} Anesth(93,MAC02)
+ Bayonne Medical Center
29th Street at Avenue E   Bayonne, NJ 07002   (201)858-5000

Anchipolovsky, Natalia, DO {1982725024} IntrMd, EnDbMt(02,NY75)
+ Drs. Anchipolovsky and Garger
77 Prospect Avenue/Suite 1 K   Hackensack, NJ 07601   (201)820-3596   Fax (201)322-2170

Andalft, Anthony C., MD {1255390902} Anesth(91,NJ03)<NJ-KMHSTRAT>
+ Rancocas Anesthesiology, PA
700 Route 130 North/Suite 203   Cinnaminson, NJ 08077   (856)829-9345   Fax (856)829-3605

Andavolu, Rao Hanumanth, MD {1104862028} Pthlgy, BldBnk(74,INA16)<NJ-UNVMCPRN>
+ University Medical Center of Princeton at Plainsboro
One Plainsboro Road/Pathology   Plainsboro, NJ 08536   (609)497-4351
+ Sai Inpatient Resources LLC
3626 US Highway 1   Princeton, NJ 08540   (609)497-4351   Fax (609)452-7577

Andavolu, Vani B., MD {1710910039} PhysMd(79,INDI)<NJ-UN-VMCPRN>
+ University Medical Center of Princeton at Plainsboro
One Plainsboro Road/PhysMed/Rehab   Plainsboro, NJ 08536   (609)497-4000
+ Community Medical Center
99 Route 37 West   Toms River, NJ 08755   (609)497-4000   Fax (732)557-2271

Anderson, Christine H., DO {1548359003} FamMed, Grtrcs, FamMGrtc(88,PA77)<NJ-ANCPSYCH>
+ Ancora Psychiatric Hospital
301 Spring Garden Road   Hammonton, NJ 08037   (609)561-1700   Fax (609)567-7272

Anderson, Daniel Parker, MD {1699066738} Pedtrc
+ Tenafly Pediatrics, PA
32 Franklin Street   Tenafly, NJ 07670   (201)569-2400   Fax (201)569-6081

Anderson, James Thomas, MD {1851754154} IntrMd<NJ-MORRISTN>
+ Morristown Medical Center
100 Madison Avenue   Morristown, NJ 07962   (973)971-5000

Anderson, Jeffrey Dale, MD {1841257268} Surgry, SrgTrm(85,PA13)<NJ-ACMCITY>
+ AtlantiCare Regional Medical Center/City Campus
1925 Pacific Avenue/Trauma Unit   Atlantic City, NJ 08401   (609)345-4000

Anderson, Nicole Andrea, MD {1497833164} Pedtrc, IntrMd(99,NY03)<NJ-HOLYNAME, NJ-VALLEY>
+ The Valley Hospital
223 North Van Dien Avenue/Pediatrics   Ridgewood, NJ 07450   (201)447-8388   Fax (201)447-8616

Anderson, Patrick St. George, MD {1376548925} GynOnc, Gyneco(88,NJ05)
+ Center for Gynecologic Oncology & Women's Health
120 Irvington Avenue   South Orange, NJ 07079   (973)762-7270   Fax (973)762-1980

Anderson, Richard Callis Eldon, MD {1811062094} SrgNro, Surgry(97,MD07)
+ Neurosurgeons of New Jersey
200 South Orange Avenue/Suite 116   Livingston, NJ 07039   (973)718-9919

Anderson, Terry M., MD {1770592891} PedCrd, Pedtrc(78,NY15)<PA-CHILDHOS>
+ CHOP Pediatric & Adolescent Specialty Care Center
1012 Laurel Oak Road   Voorhees, NJ 08043   (856)783-0287   Fax (856)783-0657
anderson@email.chop.edu
+ CHOP Specialty Care Center at Virtua
200 Bowman Drive/2 FL/Suite D-260   Voorhees, NJ 08043   (267)425-5400

Anderson-Wright, Phyllis, DO {1548341613} FamMed(93,NJ75)
+ Doctors MediCenter
835 Roosevelt Avenue/Plaza 12/Suite 4A   Carteret, NJ 07008   (732)969-2240   Fax (732)969-2152

Andrade, Jose G., MD {1649425083} IntHos(05,ECU03)
+ Hospital Medicine Associates
157 Broad Street/Suite 317   Red Bank, NJ 07701   (732)530-2960   Fax (732)530-7446

Andrade, Peter, DO {1417287707} Surgry
+ Concentra Medical Centers
375 McCarter Highway   Newark, NJ 07114   (973)643-8601   Fax (973)643-8609

Physicians by Name and Address

Arerangaiah, Ramya B., MD {1205003704} IntrMd, IntHos(00,INA68)<NJ-VIRTMARL>
+ Virtua Hospitalist Group Marlton
  90 Brick Road   Marlton, NJ 08053   (856)355-6011

Argeros, Olga, MD {1619202645} ObsGyn
+ Ocean Health Initiatives, Inc.
  301 Lakehurst Road   Toms River, NJ 08755   (732)552-0377   Fax (732)552-0378
+ Ocean Health Initiatives, Inc.
  101 Second Street   Lakewood, NJ 08701   (732)552-0377   Fax (732)363-6656

Arginteanu, Marc S., MD {1972570588} SrgNro(93,PA01)<NJ-ENGLWOOD, NY-MTSINYHS>
+ Metropolitan Neurosurgery Associates, PA
  309 Engle Street/Suite 6   Englewood, NJ 07631   (201)569-7737   Fax (201)569-1494

Argiroff, Alexandra Louise, MD {1508122086} Surgry
+ Summit Medical Group Florham Park Campus
  150 Park Avenue   Florham Park, NJ 07932   (973)404-9980   Fax (855)307-9476

Ariaratnam, Lemuel S., MD {1326040890} RadOnc, Radiol(68,SRIL)<NJ-VIRTMHBC>
+ Virtua Memorial
  175 Madison Avenue   Mount Holly, NJ 08060   (609)261-7074   Fax (609)261-4180

Ariaratnam, Nikki Sanghera, MD {1285885236} RadDia, Radiol, IntrMd(04,RI01)
+ South Jersey Radiology Associates, P.A.
  748 Kings Highway   West Deptford, NJ 08096   (856)848-4998   Fax (856)686-7344
+ South Jersey Radiology Associates
  1307 White Horse Road/Suite A-102   Voorhees, NJ 08043   (856)848-4998   Fax (856)232-9139
+ South Jersey Radiology Associates, P.A.
  100 Carnie Boulevard/Suite B-5   Voorhees, NJ 08096   (856)751-0123   Fax (856)751-0535

Arias, Ana L., MD {1528140084} EmrgMd, IntrMd(94,IL02)<NJ-MTNSIDE>
+ Hackensack UMC Mountainside
  1 Bay Avenue/Emerg Med   Montclair, NJ 07042   (973)429-6200

Arias, Carlos, MD {1376953232} PhysMd
+ Physical Medicine & Rehabilitation Center
  500 Grand Avenue/1st Floor   Englewood, NJ 07631   (201)567-2277   Fax (201)567-7506

Arias, Paul J., MD {1255482022} IntrMd(86,MEX03)
+ 390 New York Avenue
  Newark, NJ 07105   (973)344-3518   Fax (973)344-1167
  Paul07105@aol.com

Arias Garau, Jessica, MD {1720272479} Ortped
+ Advanced Orthopedics & Sports Medicine Institute
  301 Professional View Drive   Freehold, NJ 07728   (939)642-1214   Fax (732)720-2556
  sinq09@yahoo.com

Aridi, Imad M., MD {1760432215} IntrMd, FamMed(76,RUSS)<NJ-ACMCMAIN>
+ 76 West Jimmie Leeds Road/Suite 301
  Galloway, NJ 08205   (609)652-9111   Fax (609)652-1283

Arief, Melissa Suen, MD {1124338264}
+ 470 Longhill Road
  Gillette, NJ 07933   (718)270-8995

Arif, Faizan Ghulam, MD {1780061903}
+ Jersey Shore University Medical Center
  1945 Route 33   Neptune, NJ 07753   (732)776-4510   Fax (732)776-2328

Arif, Orooj, MD {1841605623} IntrMd
+ Summit Medical Group-Berkeley Heights Campus
  1 Diamond Hill Road   Berkeley Heights, NJ 07922   (908)273-4300   Fax (908)790-6576

Aristizabal, Michelle Anne, MD {1568760536} ObsGyn(07,AZ01)
+ Wombkeepers
  109 Valley Road   Montclair, NJ 07042   (973)655-9662   Fax (973)655-9665
  staff@wombkeepers.com

Aristy, Sary Mariell, MD {1922312628} IntrMd
+ Rheumatology Associates of North Jersey, PA
  1415 Queen Anne Road   Teaneck, NJ 07666   (201)837-7788   Fax (201)837-2077
+ Rheumatology Associates of North Jersey, PA
  420 Grand Avenue   Englewood, NJ 07631   (201)837-7788   Fax (201)837-2077
+ Rheumatology Associates of North Jersey, PA
  8305A Bergenline Avenue   North Bergen, NJ 07666   (201)837-7788   Fax (201)837-2077

Ariyaprakai, Navin, MD {1639438013} EmrgEMed
+ Newark Beth Israel Medical Center Emergency Medicine
  201 Lyons Avenue   Newark, NJ 07112   (973)926-6671   Fax (973)282-0562

Arjona, Romel A., MD {1386730802} IntrMd(94,PAN01)<NJ-RBAYPERT>
+ 400 State Street/Suite 2
  Perth Amboy, NJ 08861   (732)442-6020   Fax (732)442-1995

Arjun, Seeta, DO {1669401535} EmrgMd(00,PA77)
+ InFocus Urgent Care
  64 Princeton Hightstown Road   West Windsor, NJ 08550   (609)979-9700   Fax (609)799-7808

Ark, Jon Wong Tze-Jen, MD {1871513176} OthrSp, SrgHnd, SrgOrt(87,NJ06)<NJ-VANJHCS>
+ Princeton Orthopaedic Associates, P.A.
  325 Princeton Avenue   Princeton, NJ 08540   (609)924-8131   Fax (609)924-8532
+ Princeton Orthopaedic Associates, P.A.
  11 Centre Drive   Jamesburg, NJ 08831   (609)655-4848

Arkebauer, Matthew Robert, DO {1801148697}
+ Arthritis & Rheumatology Assoc of South Jersey
  2848 South Delsea Drive/Suite 2-C   Vineland, NJ 08360   (614)327-4968   Fax (856)794-3058
  mattarkebauer@gmail.com

Arkoulakis, Nolis Stamatis, MD {1487605689} SrgPlstc(97,NY45)
+ 98 James Street/Suite 304
  Edison, NJ 08820   (732)549-8008   Fax (732)205-1525
  info@plastic-surgery.md

Arlen, Harold, MD {1730185216} Otlryg, Otolgy(60,SWIT)<NJ-JFKMED>
+ Ear Nose & Throat Group of Central NJ
  2124 Oak Tree Road/2nd floor   Edison, NJ 08820   (732)205-1311   Fax (732)205-9648

Arlinghaus, Frank H., Jr., MD {1528056793} PulDis, IntrMd, FamMed(74,NY01)<NJ-MONMOUTH, NJ-RIVERVW>
+ Monmouth Pulmonary Associates
  655 Shrewsbury Avenue/Suite 209   Shrewsbury, NJ 07702   (732)747-1180   Fax (732)747-1468

Arluck, David Lawrence, MD {1508963240} CdvDis, IntrMd(75,PA01)<NJ-SHOREMEM, NJ-ACMCMAIN>
+ Shore Memorial Hospital
  1 East New York Avenue/Cardiology   Somers Point, NJ 08244   (609)365-3100   Fax (609)365-3165
+ Penn Medicine Somers Point
  155 Brighton Avenue/Second Floor   Somers Point, NJ 08244   (609)365-3100   Fax (609)653-1460

Armanious, Adel Youssef, MD {1417920695} IntrMd(65,EGYP)<NJ-EASTORNG>
+ Abbas Shehadeh Cardiology & Internal Medicine
  443 Northfield Avenue/Suite 301   West Orange, NJ 07052   (973)731-0203   Fax (973)731-0017

Armao, Michael Edward, MD {1528159381} Anesth(92,NJ06)
+ James Street Anesthesia
  102 James Street/Suite 103   Edison, NJ 08820   (732)494-1444   Fax (732)494-7052

Armas, Holger Giovanny, MD {1659539633} IntrMd(92,ECU05)<NJ-RBAYPERT>
+ Best Medical Care New Jersey
  2911 Summit Avenue/Suite 105   Union City, NJ 07087   (551)482-7254   Fax (201)223-5745
+ Jewish Renaissance Medical Center
  275 Hobart Street   Perth Amboy, NJ 08861   (551)482-7254   Fax (732)376-0139

Armas-Loughran, Barbara Janine, MD {1154408284} IntrMd(97,VA01)
+ University Medical Group - General Internal Medicine
  125 Paterson Street/Suite 5100A   New Brunswick, NJ 08903   (732)235-6968   Fax (732)235-8935

Armbrecht, Kimberley T., MD {1609018167} Anesth(06,PA13)<PA-TMPHOSP>
+ New Jersey Ambulatory Anesthesia Consultants, LLC
  55 Schanck Road/Suite 8-A   Freehold, NJ 07728   (732)431-9544   Fax (732)431-9313

Armbruster, Edward John, DO {1043439417} OrtSHand(02,PA77)<PA-LWBUCK>
+ Mercer-Bucks Orthopaedics, P.C.
  2501 Kuser Road   Hamilton, NJ 08691   (609)896-0444   Fax (609)587-4349
+ Mercer-Bucks Orthopaedics PC
  3120 Princeton Pike   Lawrenceville, NJ 08648   (609)896-0444   Fax (609)896-1055

Armbruster, Thomas C., MD {1558334698} FamMed(95,NJ05)<NJ-MONMOUTH>
+ EMedical Urgent Care
  2 Kings Highway   Middletown, NJ 07748   (732)957-0707   Fax (732)957-9852

Armenti, Lawrence A., MD {1982672101} IntrMd(77,NJ05)<NJ-NWRKBETH>
+ 18 Wilson Avenue
  Newark, NJ 07105   (973)589-7811   Fax (973)589-4156

Armento, Michael, MD {1255307633} PhysMd, PedReh(88,NJ05)<NJ-CHLSMT, NJ-CHLSOCEN>
+ Children's Specialized Hospital
  150 New Providence Road   Mountainside, NJ 07092   (908)301-5416   Fax (908)301-5456
+ Children's Specialized Hospital-Ocean
  94 Stevens Road   Toms River, NJ 08755   (732)914-1100

Armour, Renee Palmyra, MD {1093864779} Surgry, IntrMd(99,PA01)<NJ-RIVERVW>
+ Advanced Breast Surgery LLC
  98 James Street/Suite 202   Edison, NJ 08820   (732)744-5550   Fax (732)744-5517

Armstead, Valerie Elizabeth, MD {1407880529} Anesth
+ St. Joseph's Regional Medical Center Anesthesia
  703 Main Street/Anesth   Paterson, NJ 07503   (973)754-2323   Fax (973)977-9455

Armstrong, Aileen S., MD {1114046430} Anesth<NJ-MORRISTN>
+ Morristown Medical Center
  100 Madison Avenue   Morristown, NJ 07962   (973)971-5000

Armstrong, James M., MD {1003850207} Anesth, AnesPain(87,NJ05)<NJ-OURLADY>
+ Our Lady of Lourdes Medical Center
  1600 Haddon Avenue/Anesthesiology   Camden, NJ 08103   (856)757-3836

Armstrong, Joshua Stephen, DO {1225325343} PhysMd
+ Rothman Institute - Egg Harbor Township
  2500 English Creek Avenue/Bldg 1300   Egg Harbor Township, NJ 08234   (609)677-6060   Fax (609)677-6061

Armstrong, Lisa Kay, MD {1942481536} EmrgMd(04,NJ05)<NJ-MORRISTN>
+ Morristown Medical Center
  100 Madison Avenue/EmrgMed   Morristown, NJ 07962   (973)971-5000

Armstrong, Patrick Andrew, MD Anesth(05,IL06)<NJ-MORRISTN>
+ Morristown Medical Center
  100 Madison Avenue   Morristown, NJ 07962   (973)971-5000

Armstrong-Coben, Anne Helen, MD {1912116955} Pedtrc(89,NY01)
+ CHOP Pediatric & Adolescent Specialty Care Center
  1012 Laurel Oak Road   Voorhees, NJ 08043   (856)435-1300   Fax (856)435-0091

Arnaldez, Fernanda Ierne, MD {1205046224}
+ 421 Mills Court
  Florham Park, NJ 07932   (862)778-8309
  farnaldez@gmail.com

Arnaud-Turner, Denise Marie, MD {1477650489} Pedtrc(93,CA02)<NJ-LOURDMED, NJ-VIRTMHBC>
+ Kids first
  2006 Salem Road   Burlington, NJ 08016   (609)877-1500   Fax (609)877-4262

Arnette, Esther Elizabeth, MD {1851408942} Anesth<NJ-STFRNMED>
+ St. Francis Medical Center
  601 Hamilton Avenue/Anesth   Trenton, NJ 08629   (609)599-5000

Arno, Joseph P., MD {1649347139} SrgCsm, Dermat(63,GERM)
+ 10 Auer Court
  East Brunswick, NJ 08816   (732)390-8888   Fax (732)390-8997

Arno, Louis J., MD {1720185978} CritCr, IntrMd, PulDis(86,GRN01)<NJ-SOMERSET>
+ 3322 Route 22/Suite 605
  Branchburg, NJ 08876   (908)428-7530   Fax (908)428-7529
+ Respacare
  489 Union Avenue   Bridgewater, NJ 08807   (908)428-7530   Fax (732)356-9959

Arnofsky, Adam Garrett, MD {1245301332} Surgry, SrgThr, SrgCTh(98,PA01)<NJ-ENGLWOOD>
+ Englewood Cardiac Surgery Associates
  350 Engle Street   Englewood, NJ 07631   (201)894-3636
+ Heart and Vascular Institute at EHMC
  350 Engle Street/Suite 1000   Englewood, NJ 07631   (201)894-3636

Arnold, Monica A., DO {1053337683} PedSpM, Pedtrc, IntrMd(95,NJ75)
+ Advanced Urology Associates, P.C.
  1600 Saint Georges Avenue/Suite 111   Rahway, NJ 07065   (732)388-2422   Fax (732)388-1706

Arnold, Robert B., MD {1306943816} Nephro, IntrMd(76,ITAL)<NJ-COMMED, NJ-KIMBALL>
+ Hypertension and Kidney Group
  9 Hospital Drive/Suite 16   Toms River, NJ 08755   (732)341-2211   Fax (732)505-8229

Arnold, Thomas Bradley, DO {1497043558} Surgry
+ Rowan University-School of Osteopathic Medicine
  1 Medical Center Drive   Stratford, NJ 08084   (856)566-6746

Arnouk, Munzer M., MD {1841271939} IntrMd(78,SYRI)<NJ-CHILTON>
+ North Jersey Health PA
  502 Hamburg Turnpike/Suite 108   Wayne, NJ 07470   (973)942-5224   Fax (973)942-7443

Arnous, Nidal, MD {1841508157} IntrMd<NJ-MEMSALEM>
+ Memorial Hospital of Salem County
  310 Woodstown Road   Salem, NJ 08079   (856)935-1000   Fax (856)935-9659

Anzalone, Anthony, MD {1124071857} ObsGyn(79,MEX03)<NJ-NWTNMEM>
+ 203 Dietz Street
Cranford, NJ 07016

Apelian, Ara Z., MD {1679687073} EnDbMt, IntrMd(81,LEBA)<NJ-SOMERSET, NJ-RWJUBRUN>
+ Eck, Apelian & Mathews
1056 Stelton Road   Piscataway, NJ 08854   (732)463-0303
Fax (732)463-2289

Apfel, Howard D., MD {1134102205} Pedtrc, PedCrd(89,NY08)<NY-CHLDCOPR, NJ-MMHKEMBL>
+ Pediatric Cardiology at The Valley Hospital
205 Robin Road/Suite 100   Paramus, NJ 07652   (201)599-0026   Fax (201)986-1160

Aphale, Abhishek N., MD {1437300993} Dermat
+ Dr. Warmuth Skin Care Center
420 Front Street   Elmer, NJ 08318   (856)358-1500

Apinis, Andrey, MD {1013999150} Anesth(92,LAT02)<NJ-STJOSHOS>
+ St. Joseph's Regional Medical Center Anesthesia
703 Main Street   Paterson, NJ 07503   (973)754-2323   Fax (973)977-9455
+ St. Joseph's Regional Medical Center
703 Main Street/Anesth   Paterson, NJ 07503   (973)754-2000

Aplin, Kara Stanig, MD {1124063771} IntrMd(03,NC01)<NJ-COOPRUMC>
+ Cooper University Hospital
One Cooper Plaza/Hospitalist   Camden, NJ 08103   (856)342-3150   Fax (856)968-8418

Apolito, Renato A., MD {1457570731} CdvDis<NJ-JRSYSHMC, NJ-COMMED>
+ Shore Heart Group, P.A.
35 Beaverson Boulevard/Suite 9-B   Brick, NJ 08723   (732)262-4262   Fax (732)262-4317
+ Shore Heart Group, P.A.
1820 State Route 33/Suite 4-B   Neptune, NJ 07753   (732)262-4262   Fax (732)776-8946
+ Shore Heart Group, P.A.
555 Iron Bridge Road/Suite 15   Freehold, NJ 08723   (732)308-0774   Fax (732)333-1366

Aponte, Emilia Laura, DO {1073930186} FamMed
+ Concentra Medical Centers
595 Division Street   Elizabeth, NJ 07201   (908)289-5646   Fax (908)351-1099

Aponte, Sandra Leonora, MD {1164622684} PthACl, PthCyt, IntrMd(88,PRO03)
+ Histopathology Services, LLC.
535 East Crescent Avenue   Ramsey, NJ 07446   (201)661-7280   Fax (201)661-7297
+ Inform Diagnostics
825 Rahway Avenue   Union, NJ 07083   (201)661-7280   Fax (732)901-1555
+ Quest Diagnostics Inc.
1 Malcolm Avenue   Teterboro, NJ 07446   (201)393-5000   Fax (201)393-6127

Appel, Burton Eliot, MD {1790731925} PedHem, Pedtrc(90,IL02)<NJ-HACKNSK>
+ Tomorrow's Children's Inst/HUMC
30 Prospect Avenue/WFAN - PC 116   Hackensack, NJ 07601   (201)996-5437   Fax (201)487-7340
bappel@humed.com

Appelboom, Geoffrey, MD {1508224064} SrgNro
+ St. Joseph's Medical Center Neurosurgery
703 Main Street   Paterson, NJ 07503   (973)754-2463

Appiah, Evangeline Animah, MD {1306037791} IntHos, IntrMd(11,GHA01)<NJ-KSLRWEST>
+ Kessler Institute for Rehabilitation West Orange
1199 Pleasant Valley Way   West Orange, NJ 07052   (973)867-6565

Applbaum, Yaakov N., MD {1356386650} RadDia, RadNro, RadV&I(80,NY46)<NJ-CHSFULD, NJ-CHSMRCER>
+ Capital Health System/Fuld Campus
750 Brunswick Avenue/Radiology   Trenton, NJ 08638   (609)394-6000
yapplbaum@chsnj.org

Apple, Jerry S., MD {1447258041} RadDia, Radiol(78,NC05)<NJ-VIRTUAHS, NJ-VIRTMHBC>
+ South Jersey Radiology Associates, P.A.
100 Carnie Boulevard/Suite B-5   Voorhees, NJ 08043   (856)751-0123   Fax (856)751-0535
+ South Jersey Radiology Associates, P.A.
901 Route 168/Suites 301-305   Turnersville, NJ 08012   (856)751-0123   Fax (856)227-8537
+ South Jersey Radiology Associates, P.A.
315 Route 70 East/Suite 2   Cherry Hill, NJ 08043   (856)428-4344   Fax (856)428-0356

Applebaum, Eric S., MD {1336137272} Allrgy(87,NY46)<NJ-MORRISTN>
+ Allergic & Asthmatic Comprehensive Care of NJ PA
3799 Route 46 East/Suite 205   Parsippany, NJ 07054   (973)335-1700   Fax (973)335-4711

+ Allergic & Asthmatic Comprehensive Care of NJ PA
1033 Clifton Avenue   Clifton, NJ 07013   (973)470-8990

Applebaum, Steven Lee, DO {1770353968} FamMed(00,PA78)
+ AtlantiCare Family Medicine
210 South Shore Road/Suite 201   Marmora, NJ 08223   (609)407-2273   Fax (609)390-2753

Applebaum-Farkas, Paige S., MD {1265445563} Dermat, IntrMd(89,NY46)<NJ-VALLEY>
+ Advanced Dermatology, P.C.
1200 East Ridgewood Avenue   Ridgewood, NJ 07450   (201)493-1717   Fax (201)493-1009

Appulingam, Anbuchelvi, MD {1285705947} Pedtrc(75,INDI)<NJ-MONMOUTH, NJ-RIVERVW>
+ TLC Pediatrics
20 White Road/Suite D   Shrewsbury, NJ 07702   (732)741-3400   Fax (732)741-3104

Apter, Jeffrey T., MD {1568509495} Psychy(74,SAFR)
+ Global Medical Institutes, LLC
256 Bunn Drive/Suite 6 Woodslands Bldg   Princeton, NJ 08540   (609)921-3555   Fax (609)921-3620

Apuzzio, Joseph J., MD {1164514642} MtFtMd, ObsGyn(73,NJ05)<NJ-UMDNJ>
+ University Hospital
150 Bergen Street/Maternal/Fetal   Newark, NJ 07103   (973)972-5557   Fax (973)972-4274
+ University Physician Associates
140 Bergen Street/ACC Level C   Newark, NJ 07103   (973)972-5557   Fax (973)972-2739

Aqeel, Iram, MD {1811262330}
+ 50 Christopher Columbus Drive/Apt 2502
Jersey City, NJ 07302   (334)498-0912
iram.aqeel@gmail.com

Aqel, Mahmoud Bader, MD {1821067786} IntrMd, WundCr, VasDis(80,JOR01)<NJ-STJOSHOS>
+ Paterson Community Clinic
355 21st Avenue   Paterson, NJ 07501   (973)523-9090   Fax (973)523-5222
Aqel@aol.com
+ Paterson Community Clinic
1300 Main Avenue/Suite 3 D   Clifton, NJ 07011   (973)685-9922

Aquilino, Gaetano J., DO {1740253871} IntrMd, PulDis(81,MO78)<NJ-JRSYSHMC>
+ 2401 Lincoln Avenue
Wall Township, NJ 07719

Aquilino, Linda Kristine, DO {1770685414} IntrMd(99,PA77)<NJ-UNDRWD>
+ 1652 Cooper Street
Deptford, NJ 08096   (856)227-8611   Fax (856)227-5716

Aquilio, Ernest J., DO {1053353995} FamMed(67,MO79)
+ 41 Grandview Plaza
Caldwell, NJ 07006   (973)335-3230   Fax (973)335-7335

Aquino, Christine E., MD {1134143928} IntrMd(99,PHI32)
+ Summit Medical Group
31-00 Broadway   Fair Lawn, NJ 07410   (201)796-2255   Fax (201)796-7020

Aquino, Rainier, MD {1396718862} Surgry, SrgVas(95,NY09)<NJ-JRSYSHMC>
+ Jersey Coast Vascular Associates
425 Jack Martin Boulevard/Suite 2   Brick, NJ 08724   (732)202-1500   Fax (732)202-1058

Arabi, Mona Najib, MD {1841209590} Anesth(82,LEB01)
+ Hypertension & Nephrology Specialists, LLC
2 Research Way/Suite 301   Monroe, NJ 08831   (732)521-0800   Fax (732)521-0833

Arabi, Nida, MD {1194957639} Nephro<NY-KALBUFLO>
+ Hypertension & Nephrology Specialists, LLC
2 Research Way/Suite 301   Monroe, NJ 08831   (732)521-0800   Fax (732)521-0833

Aragona, James, MD {1831281385} SrgOrt(76,BELG)
+ IGEA Brain & Spine
1057 Commerce Avenue   Union, NJ 07083   (908)688-8800   Fax (908)688-2377

Aragones, Linnie A., MD {1205923489} Pedtrc(71,PHI02)<NJ-NWRKBETH, NJ-STBARNMC>
+ 2130 Millburn Avenue/Suite C-5
Maplewood, NJ 07040   (973)763-3444

Arams, Ronald S., MD {1801883137} Radiol, RadV&I(85,NY20)<NJ-VALLEY>
+ Radiology Associates of Ridgewood, P.A.
20 Franklin Turnpike   Waldwick, NJ 07463   (201)445-8822   Fax (201)447-5053

Aranas, Rae Ronald, MD {1861580367} PainInvt
+ Atlantic Spine Care, LLC.
1921 Oak Tree Road/Suite 103   Edison, NJ 08820   (732)494-1655   Fax (732)494-1255

Aranguren-Decastro, Yolanda S., MD {1770584278} IntrMd(88,MEX14)<NJ-RBAYPERT>
+ Raritan Bay Medical Center/Perth Amboy Division
530 New Brunswick Avenue/Internal Med   Perth Amboy, NJ 08861   (732)442-3700

Aranoff, Joanne Rachel, MD {1164488664} Pedtrc, IntrMd(01,NY46)<NJ-ENGLWOOD, NJ-HACKNSK>
+ Tenafly Pediatrics, PA
301 Bridge Plaza North   Fort Lee, NJ 07024   (201)592-8787   Fax (201)592-6350

Arapurakal, Rajiv, MD {1437568318} IntrMd<NJ-COOPRUMC>
+ Cooper University Hospital
One Cooper Plaza   Camden, NJ 08103   (856)342-2000

Aras, Rohit S., DO {1750401915} IntrMd(03,MO79)<NJ-RWJUBRUN>
+ RWJ University Hospital New Brunswick
One Robert Wood Johnson Place   New Brunswick, NJ 08901   (732)828-3000

Araujo, Martin A., MD {1992963169} FamMed
+ 628 Ripley Place
Westfield, NJ 07090

Arbes, Spiros M., MD {1215943592} IntrMd, Nephro(82,PHI02)<NJ-MONMOUTH, NJ-RIVERVW>
+ Hypertension & Nephrology Association, PA
6 Industrial Way West/Suite B   Eatontown, NJ 07724   (732)460-1200   Fax (732)460-1211

Arbit, David Lewis, MD {1497812788} Rheuma, IntrMd(87,NJ05)<NJ-VALLEY>
+ Summit Medical Group
31-00 Broadway   Fair Lawn, NJ 07410   (201)625-1732   Fax (201)796-7020

Arbour, Robert M., MD {1649227018} Surgry, SrgBst(65,NJ05)<NJ-BAYSHORE, NJ-RIVERVW>
+ Matawan Medical Associates
213 Main Street   Matawan, NJ 07747   (732)566-2363   Fax (732)566-0502

Arcaro, Maria Anna C., MD {1992141626} Pedtrc
+ East Windsor Pediatric Group
300B Princeton Hightstown/Suite 201   Hightstown, NJ 08520   (609)448-7300   Fax (609)448-8022

Arcaro, Mark E., MD {1881861102} IntrMd(05,NJ05)<NJ-UNVMCPRN, NJ-RWJUHAM>
+ Capital Health Primary Care-Hamilton
1445 Whitehorse-Mercerville Rd   Hamilton, NJ 08619   (609)587-6661   Fax (609)587-8503
+ Capital Health Primary Care
2330 Route 33/Suite 107   Robbinsville, NJ 08691   (609)587-6661   Fax (609)303-4401

Arcaro, Michael Steven, MD {1801070867} IntrMd(05,NJ05)<NJ-UNVMCPRN>
+ Capital Health Primary Care
2330 Route 33/Suite 107   Robbinsville, NJ 08691   (609)303-4400   Fax (609)303-4401

Archer, Jonathan Mckee, MD {1205879525} Ortped, SprtMd, SrgOrt(90,NY01)<NJ-ENGLWOOD, NJ-HOLYNAME>
+ North Jersey Orthopaedic Specialists
106 Grand Avenue   Englewood, NJ 07631   (201)608-0100   Fax (201)608-0104
+ North Jersey Orthopaedic Specialists
730 Palisade Avenue   Teaneck, NJ 07666   (201)608-0100   Fax (201)530-0003
+ North Jersey Orthopaedic Specialists
15 Vervalen Street   Closter, NJ 07631   (201)784-6800   Fax (201)784-6801

Archila, Arturo Plinio, MD {1669565826} Psychy(81,COL24)<NJ-HACKNSK>
+ Bergen Psychiatric Associates
765 Teaneck Road   Teaneck, NJ 07666   (201)833-7933

Arcot, Karthikeyan Mohanram, MD {1205194941} VasNeu(06,INA94)
+ Interventional Neuro Associates, LLC
777 Terrace Avenue/Suite 401   Hasbrouck Heights, NJ 07604   (201)387-1957   Fax (201)351-0656

Ardise, Patricia Marie, MD {1770526550} ObsGyn(00,NY48)<NY-STONYBRK>
+ Advanced Obstetrics & Gynecology, LLC
4 Walter E. Foran Boulevard/Suite 302   Flemington, NJ 08822   (908)806-0080   Fax (908)806-8570

Ardito, Michael F., MD {1235244609} IntrMd(87,GRNA)
+ Valley Health Medical Group
72 Hamburg Turnpike   Riverdale, NJ 07457   (973)835-7290   Fax (973)835-0696

Ardolino, Joseph M., MD {1275759516} IntrMd(86,ITAL)<NJ-CLARMAAS, NJ-STBARNMC>
+ Medical first of NY & NJ
5 Franklin Avenue/Suite 501   Belleville, NJ 07109   (973)751-4477   Fax (973)751-4444

Arefeen, Samrana, MD {1760929392} FamMed
+ Urgent Care of New Jersey
2090 Route 27   Edison, NJ 08817   (732)662-5650   Fax (732)662-5651

Arena, Mario J., MD {1306931233} SrgOrt, SrgSpn(79,DC02)
+ 17 White Horse Pike/Suite 3
Haddon Heights, NJ 08035   (856)310-0002   Fax (856)310-0003

Physicians by Name and Address

Ankamah, Andrew K., MD {1518151414} PhysMd(02,PA13)
+ 1543 State Route 27/Suite 12
  Somerset, NJ 08873   (732)249-9400   Fax (732)249-9500
+ 390 Willowbrook Drive
  North Brunswick, NJ 08902

Anmuth, Craig Jeffrey, DO {1407927478} PhysMd, PainMd, OrtSpn(89,PA77)<NJ-BACHARCH, NJ-ACMCITY>
+ Bacharach Institute for Rehabilitation
  61 West Jimmie Leeds Road   Pomona, NJ 08240   (609)748-5380   Fax (609)652-8749
  craiga@bacharach.org

Annadanam, Varalakshmi, MD {1528061751} Anesth, PainMd(87,INDI)
+ 33 Bush Road
  Denville, NJ 07834   (973)394-1465
+ Wayne Surgical Center, LLC.
  1176 Hamburg Pike   Wayne, NJ 07470   (973)394-1465   Fax (973)709-1901

Annam, Raghuveer, MD {1386735850} IntrMd(79,INDI)<NJ-WARREN>
+ 461 Corliss Avenue
  Phillipsburg, NJ 08865   (908)859-5872   Fax (908)859-1747

Annamaneni, Padmaja Sarki, MD {1205914520} PsyGrt, Psychy(93,INA7C)<NJ-UNIVBHC>
+ Raritan Bay Mental Health Center
  570 Lee Street   Perth Amboy, NJ 08861   (732)442-1666   Fax (732)442-9512

Annavajjula, Madhavi L., MD {1336264282} IntrMd(95,INA4D)
+ Rockaway Family Medicine Associates
  333 Mount Hope Avenue   Rockaway, NJ 07866   (973)895-6601   Fax (973)895-5324

Anne, Madhurima, MD {1326287624} OncHem, IntrMd(07,NY15)
+ Atlantic Hematology Oncology Associates, L.L.C.
  1707 Atlantic Avenue   Manasquan, NJ 08736   (732)528-0760   Fax (732)528-0764

Anne, Sreelatha, MD {1093888059} FamMed
+ Howell Jackson Medical Center
  4764 Route 9 South   Howell, NJ 07731   (732)370-3563

Annese, Christian P., MD {1902005093} RadDia(02,NJ06)<MA-BIDMCEST>
+ New Jersey Imaging Network of Rutherford
  69 Orient Way   Rutherford, NJ 07070   (201)933-5666   Fax (201)933-5662

Annitto, William J., MD {1275660003} Psychy, VasNeu(74,NJ05)<NJ-NWRKBETH>
+ Newark Beth Israel Medical Center
  201 Lyons Avenue   Newark, NJ 07112   (973)926-7000

Annunziato, Paula Winter, MD PedInf, Pedtrc(88,TX13)
+ Merck and Company Incorporated
  1 Merck Drive/PO Box 100   Whitehouse Station, NJ 08889   (908)423-1000

Anolik, Kenneth Jay, MD {1134197254} IntrMd(75,NY06)
+ 320 Raritan Avenue/Suite 205
  Highland Park, NJ 08904   (732)985-6901   Fax (732)985-6931

Ansari, Huma Naz, MD {1225337058} IntrMd
+ RWJ University Hospital Somerset
  110 Rehill Avenue   Somerville, NJ 08876   (814)913-1232

Ansari, Safeer A., DO {1538367727} Psychy
+ 4 Saddlebury Court
  Mount Laurel, NJ 08054
+ Pinnacle Behavioral Health Institute
  851 Route 73 North/Suite C   Marlton, NJ 08053   Fax (856)267-5824

Ansay, Editha Santillan, MD {1326127101} Pedtrc(77,PHI07)<NJ-JRSYCITY>
+ Newport Medical Associates
  610 Washington Boulevard   Jersey City, NJ 07310   (201)222-1266
+ Total Care Pediatrics in Jersey City
  550 Newark Avenue/Suite 200   Jersey City, NJ 07306   (201)222-1266   Fax (201)795-4999

Anscher, Richard M., MD {1215088869} ObsGyn(71,NY06)<NJ-HCKTSTWN>
+ Obstetrics and Gynecology Associates
  616 Willow Grove Street   Hackettstown, NJ 07840   (908)852-3443   Fax (908)852-0349

Anselmi, Gregory D., MD {1477697761} Nrolgy(88,ITAL)
+ Hudson Neurosciences PC
  142 Palisade Avenue/Suite 205   Jersey City, NJ 07306   (201)798-2453   Fax (201)216-9211
+ Hudson Neurosciences, PC
  605 Broadway   Bayonne, NJ 07002   (201)798-2453   Fax (201)339-6536

Anshelevich, Irina, MD {1235176462} IntrMd(81,LAT02)<NJ-HACKNSK, NJ-VALLEY>
+ Forest HealthCare Associates, PC
  277 Forest Avenue/Suite 200   Paramus, NJ 07652   (201)986-1881   Fax (201)986-1871

Anshelevich, Michael, MD {1851396444} IntrMd, CdvDis(88,LAT02)<NJ-VALLEY, NJ-HACKNSK>
+ Westwood Cardiology Associates PA
  333 Old Hook Road/Suite 200   Westwood, NJ 07675   (201)664-0201   Fax (201)666-7970

Antario, Joseph Michael, MD {1154321800} Urolgy, IntrMd(86,NY08)<PA-EASTON>
+ 388 Memorial Parkway
  Phillipsburg, NJ 08865   (908)387-9207   Fax (908)387-9311

Antebi, Morris E., MD {1578532404} Anesth, PainMd(78,SYR02)<NJ-ACMCITY>
+ Pain Specialist, P.A.
  1907 New Road   Northfield, NJ 08225   (609)645-8884   Fax (609)645-9780

Antebi, Yael Jennifer, MD {1467680207} ObsGyn<NJ-CLARMAAS>
+ Lifecycles OBGYN
  81 Northfield Avenue/Suite 201   West Orange, NJ 07052   (973)731-9088   Fax (973)731-6196
+ Clara Maass Medical Center
  1 Clara Maass Drive   Belleville, NJ 07109   (973)450-2145

Anter, Afaf A., DO {1003237769} IntHos(11,NY75)<NJ-COOPRUMC>
+ Cooper Perinatology Associates
  3 Cooper Plaza/Suite 502   Camden, NJ 08103   (856)356-4935   Fax (856)968-8499
+ Cooper University Hospital
  One Cooper Plaza/Dorrance 222   Camden, NJ 08103   (856)356-4935   Fax (856)968-8418

Anthony, AnnGene G, MD {1306829239} FamMed(98,NJ05)<NJ-MMHKEMBL>
+ Forest Hill Family Health Associates, P.A.
  465 Mount Prospect Avenue   Newark, NJ 07104   (973)936-0205   Fax (973)483-4895
  dranngene@gmail.com

Anthony, Michele M., MD {1720006133} IntrMd(85,NJ06)
+ Woodbine Development Center/NJ Human Services
  1175 Dehirsch Avenue   Woodbine, NJ 08270   (609)861-2164   Fax (609)861-2494

Anthony, William P., MD {1770526790} PhysMd(87,NY06)<NJ-OURLADY, NJ-VIRTMARL>
+ Associated Physiatrists of Southern New Jersey
  1600 Haddon Avenue/Room R-122   Camden, NJ 08103   (856)757-3878   Fax (856)757-3760
+ Associated Physiatrists of Southern New Jersey
  175 Madison Avenue   Mount Holly, NJ 08060   (856)757-3878   Fax (856)757-3760

Anthony Wilson, Avril Dawn, MD {1467517334} FamMed(90,TN07)<NY-JAMAICA>
+ Valley Health Medical Group
  1114 Goffle Road/Suite 103   Hawthorne, NJ 07506   (973)423-1364   Fax (973)423-0980

Antinori, Charles H., MD {1831187780} SrgThr, Srgry, SrgVas(73,MA01)<NJ-SJHREGMC, NJ-SJRSYELM>
+ Inspira Medical Group Surgical Associates
  1102 East Chestnut Avenue   Vineland, NJ 08360   (856)213-6375   Fax (856)575-4986

Antler, Arthur S., MD {1962164776} Gastrn, IntrMd(75,NY09)<NJ-VALLEY>
+ 400 Franklin Turnpike/Suite 212
  Mahwah, NJ 07430   (201)825-0091   Fax (201)825-8242

Antohina, Alena, MD {1891956652} Psychy(91,MOL01)
+ GenPsych
  981 Route 22 West   Bridgewater, NJ 08807   (551)996-4450   Fax (551)996-5729
  info@genpsych.com

Antoine, Alycia N., MD {1609882588} IntrMd(02,NY48)<NJ-VANJHCS>
+ VA New Jersey Health Care System-East Orange Campus
  385 Tremont Avenue/Internal Med   East Orange, NJ 07018   (973)676-1000
  alycia.antoine@va.gov

Antoine, Roland, MD {1902814478} IntrMd(86,HAI01)<NJ-EASTORNG>
+ 827 South Orange Avenue
  East Orange, NJ 07018   (973)674-9100   Fax (973)674-4007
  Rolanti@yahoo.com

Antoine, Wilson, MD {1043320559} IntrMd(79,HAI01)<NJ-STBARNMC>
+ 52 Underwood Street
  Newark, NJ 07106   (973)372-4937   Fax (973)372-4937

Antolin, Eleanor Banzon, MD {1285846071} Psychy(90,PHIL)
+ 33 Crabapple Lane
  Franklin Park, NJ 08823

Anton, John, MD {1780603613} CdvDis, IntrMd(84,POL03)<NJ-NWRKBETH, NJ-VIRTMARL>
+ 340 East Northfield Road/Suite 1A
  Livingston, NJ 07039   (973)994-2088   Fax (973)994-1126
  Jantonmd@aol.com

Anton, Joseph G., MD {1396831814} IntrMd(86,NJ05)
+ Emergency Medical Offices
  651 West Mount Pleasant Avenue   Livingston, NJ 07039   (973)740-9396   Fax (973)251-1165
+ One Hillside Place
  Cranford, NJ 07016

Antonacci, Mark Darryl, MD {1659349363} SrgOrt, SrgSpn, IntrMd(92,DC02)<NJ-STPETER>
+ Institute for Spine & Scoliosis, P.A.
  3100 Princeton Pike/Building 1   Lawrenceville, NJ 08648   (609)912-1500   Fax (609)912-1600
  iss9121500@yahoo.com

Antonelli, William M., DO {1609890193} IntrMd(85,PA77)<NJ-OURLADY, NJ-KMHCHRRY>
+ Exel-Med Inc.
  100 Springdale Road/Suite A3   Cherry Hill, NJ 08003   (856)651-1400   Fax (856)651-1401

Antoniadis, Ileana, MD {1699752634} IntrMd, Rheuma(83,ROMA)<NJ-JRSYSHMC>
+ 207 Route 71
  Spring Lake, NJ 07762   (732)359-7232   Fax (732)359-7233

Antonio, Edsel, DO {1265790752} ObsGyn<NJ-NWRKBETH>
+ RejuV Aesthetic Gynecology
  285 Durham Avenue/Suite 1A, Bldg. 6   South Plainfield, NJ 07080   (732)504-6917
+ Center for Gynecologic Oncology & Women's Health
  120 Irvington Avenue   South Orange, NJ 07079   (732)504-6917   Fax (973)762-1980
+ Center for Gynecologic Oncology & Women's Health
  98 James Street/Suite 101   Edison, NJ 07080   (732)515-9477

Antonio, Excelsis O., MD {1477571073} NnPnMd, Pedtrc(72,PHIL)<NJ-CHDNWBTH>
+ Children's Hospital of New Jersey
  201 Lyons Avenue/Osborne Terrace   Newark, NJ 07112   (973)926-7203   Fax (973)926-2332

Antonio, Patrick, MD {1548524838} FamMed
+ Patient first Urgent Care
  630 Mantua Pike   Woodbury, NJ 08096   (856)812-2220   Fax (856)812-2221

Antonopoulou, Marianna, MD {1588826796} EnDbMt, IntrMd(05,GRE03)<NJ-BAYSHORE, NJ-RIVERVW>
+ Northern Monmouth County Medical Associates
  100 Commons Way/Suite 150   Holmdel, NJ 07733   (732)450-2940   Fax (732)450-2942

Antonowicz, Michelle, MD {1780683128} EmrgMd(96,NJ05)<NJ-MTNSIDE>
+ Hackensack UMC Mountainside
  1 Bay Avenue/EmergMed   Montclair, NJ 07042   (973)429-6000

Antonucci, Lawrence Charles, MD {1083684914} CdvDis(84,ITAL)
+ Lawrence Charles Antonucci MD LLC
  415 Route 24/Suite E   Chester, NJ 07930   (908)879-1500   Fax (908)879-1515

Antony, Kristine Brinda, DO {1295148716} Pedtrc<NJ-MORRISTN>
+ Morristown Medical Center
  100 Madison Avenue   Morristown, NJ 07962   (973)971-

Antoun, Saad S., MD {1386655348} Urolgy(64,EGYP)<NJ-BAYSHORE, NJ-RIVERVW>
+ Urology Care Alliance
  733 North Beers Street/Suite L-6   Holmdel, NJ 07733   (732)739-2200   Fax (732)739-8988

Anukwuem, Chidi I., MD {1487719753} IntrMd(83,NIG05)<NJ-NWRKBETH, NJ-STBARNMC>
+ 1182 Stuyvesant Avenue
  Irvington, NJ 07111   (973)399-2600   Fax (973)399-5252

Anwar, David M., DO {1609196377}<NJ-DEBRAHLC>
+ Deborah Heart and Lung Center
  200 Trenton Road   Browns Mills, NJ 08015   (609)621-2080
  stmina@hotmail.com

Anwar, Khurram, MD {1619211745} IntrMd<NJ-MORRISTN>
+ Morristown Medical Center
  100 Madison Avenue   Morristown, NJ 07962   (973)971-5316

Anwar, Muhammad Usman, MD {1528047578} NnPnMd, Pedtrc, Anesth(87,PAK15)<NJ-OURLADY, NJ-SJERSYHS>
+ Our Lady of Lourdes Medical Center
  1600 Haddon Avenue/Neonatology   Camden, NJ 08103   (856)757-3500

Anwar, Mujahid, MD {1558325761} NnPnMd, Pedtrc(70,PAKI)<NJ-STPETER, NJ-HUNTRDN>
+ St. Peter's University Hospital
  254 Easton Avenue   New Brunswick, NJ 08901   (908)745-8523   Fax (908)249-6306
+ Hunterdon Medical Center
  2100 Wescott Drive/Neonatology   Flemington, NJ 08822   (908)788-6100

Anwunah-Okoye, Ifeoma Juliet, MD {1568659662} Psychy(86,NIG02)
+ University Behavioral HealthCare - UMDNJ
  Box 863/Whittlesey Road   Trenton, NJ 08625   (609)341-3093   Fax (609)341-9380

Anyanwu, Justina U., MD {1124034806} Pedtrc(85,NIGE)<NJ-NWRKBETH>
+ 1182 Stuyvesant Avenue
  Irvington, NJ 07111   (973)399-0571   Fax (973)399-1555

Andraws, Richard Zaki, MD {1649447269} CdvDis, IntrMd
  + MedDiag Assocs/Central NJ Cardiology
    1511 Park Avenue/Suite 2 South Plainfield, NJ 07080
    (908)756-4438 Fax (908)756-9160
  + Medical Diagnostic Associates, P.A.
    MAC, 11 Overlook Road/Suite 100 Summit, NJ 07901
    (908)756-4438 Fax (908)273-3125
Andre, Oswald, MD {1689736688} GenPrc, FamMed(73,HAI01)
  + 74 Drake Road
    Somerset, NJ 08873 (732)828-8085
Andreescu, Aurora C., MD {1912047754} IntrMd(93,GRNA)<NJ-HACKNSK, NJ-HOLYNAME>
  + HackensackUMG Lodi
    116 Terrace Avenue Lodi, NJ 07644 (973)473-3896 Fax (973)473-3896
Andrei, Valeriu E., MD {1932255247} Surgry(87,ROM05)<NY-MTSINAI>
  + 200 South Orange Avenue/Suite 123
    Livingston, NJ 07039 (973)322-7265 Fax (973)322-7254
Andrejko, Constance Gasda, DO {1275507238} Pedtrc, NnPnMd(01,PA77)
  + On-Site Neonatal Partners
    1000 Haddonfield-Berlin Road/Suite 210 Voorhees, NJ 08043 (856)782-2212 Fax (856)782-2213
Andreoli, Nina Needleman, MD {1013232248} IntrMd
  + Overlook Hospital-Dvpmt Disabilities
    1000 Galloping Hill Road Union, NJ 07083 (908)598-6655 Fax (908)686-8374
Andrew, Constantine T., MD {1992754063} SrgVas, Surgry(83,VA07)<NJ-OURLADY, NJ-VIRTUAHS>
  + Virtua Surgical Group, PA
    1935 Route 70 East Cherry Hill, NJ 08003 (856)428-7700 Fax (856)424-9120
Andrew, Mark S., MD {1093896771} Ophthl(81,PA02)
  + W. Reed Kindermann, M.D. and Associates
    3001 Chapel Avenue West/Suite 200 Cherry Hill, NJ 08002 (856)667-3937 Fax (856)667-0661
Andrews, Alan D., MD {1104990035} Dermat(72,VA01)<NY-PRSB-COLU>
  + Psoriasis Treatment Center
    500 Piermont Road Closter, NJ 07624 (201)767-0501 Fax (201)767-7904
  + Psoriasis Treatment Center
    595 Chestnut Ridge Road Woodcliff Lake, NJ 07677 (201)476-0602
Andrews, Jaime Lynn, DO {1497041412} FamMed(11,NJ75)
  + Woodbury Primary and Specialty Care
    159 South Broad Street Woodbury, NJ 08096 (844)542-2273 Fax (856)384-0218
  + Rowan University-School of Osteopathic Medicine
    1 Medical Center Drive Stratford, NJ 08084 (856)566-6707
Andrews, Paul Matthew, MD {1669440251} CdvDis, IntrMd(94,NY08)<NJ-HOLYNAME>
  + Bergen Cardiology Associates
    292 Columbia Avenue Fort Lee, NJ 07024 (201)224-0050 Fax (201)224-6061
  + Bergen Cardiology Associates
    400 Frank W. Burr Boulevard Teaneck, NJ 07666 (201)224-0050 Fax (201)692-3263
Andrews, Roji Zacharia, MD {1417014523} Pedtrc(92,INA78)<NJ-SHOREMEM, NJ-ATLANCHS>
  + Med for Kids
    322 Shore Road Somers Point, NJ 08244 (609)927-1353
Andrews, Tatyana, MD {1538350277} ObsGyn, IntrMd(02,GRN01)<NJ-MONMOUTH>
  + 74 Route 9 North/Suite 4
    Englishtown, NJ 07726 (732)254-8900 Fax (732)254-8902
Andrews, Waverly Stanford, IV, MD {1225120207} Psychy(75,PA01)
  + Trenton Psychiatric Hospital
    Sullivan Way/PO Box 7600 West Trenton, NJ 08628 (609)633-1500
Andreyev, Nina Vaskina, MD {1386655082} IntrMd(85,RUS33)<NJ-CHSFULD>
  + Henry J. Austin Health Center
    321 North Warren Street Trenton, NJ 08618 (609)278-5900 Fax (609)695-3532
Andrin, Margaret, MD {1851345029} ObsGyn(93,PA14)<NJ-SOMERSET>
  + 3322 Route 22/Building 13/Suite 1302
    Branchburg, NJ 08876 (908)526-0700 Fax (908)526-9988
Andriulli, John A., DO {1225063324} CdvDis, IntrMd(92,NJ75)<NJ-KMHSTRAT, NJ-KMHTURNV>
  + Southern New Jersey Cardiac Care Specialists
    1020 Laurel Oak Road/Suite 102 Voorhees, NJ 08043 (856)435-8842 Fax (856)435-8665
  + Cooper University Hospital
    One Cooper Plaza/Cardiology Camden, NJ 08103 (856)435-8842 Fax (856)435-6301

Andron, Richard I., MD {1811977762} IntrMd, Rheuma(74,PA13)<NJ-ENGLWOOD, NJ-HOLYNAME>
  + 154 Engle Street
    Englewood, NJ 07631 (201)871-1515 Fax (201)871-9683
Andronaco, John T., MD {1124095690} SrgOrt(72,MEXI)<NJ-HACKNSK>
  + 779 Albemarle Street
    Wyckoff, NJ 07481
  + Hackensack University Medical Center
    30 Prospect Avenue/Orthopedic Srg Hackensack, NJ 07601 (201)996-2000
Andronaco, Raymond B., MD {1790867026} Urolgy(76,MEX03)<NJ-ENGLWOOD, NJ-HOLYNAME>
  + Urologic Specialties PA
    177 North Dean Street/Suite 305 Englewood, NJ 07631 (201)569-7777 Fax (201)569-6861
  + Urologic Specialties PA
    6045 Kennedy Boulevard North Bergen, NJ 07047 (201)569-7777 Fax (201)569-6861
Anekstein, Carol B., MD {1427112945} PsyGrt, Psychy(80,NY09)<NJ-STBARNMC>
  + 375 Walnut Street
    Livingston, NJ 07039 (973)535-8408 Fax (973)535-8414
Anello, Tiziana, MD {1295740686} Pedtrc(94,NJ05)<NJ-STBARNMC>
  + Roseland Pediatrics
    556 Eagle Rock Avenue/Suite 106 Roseland, NJ 07068 (973)228-9190 Fax (973)228-0730
Anemelu, Ignatius I., MD {1952757619} IntrMd(72,NIG01)
  + American Physician Services/Hudson HealthCare
    679 Montgomery Street Jersey City, NJ 07306 (201)433-6500 Fax (201)433-8010
Anene, Okechukwu P., MD {1134129570} CritCr, Pedtrc(83,NIGE)
  + JFK Neurosciences Institute
    65 James Street/Second Floor Edison, NJ 08818 (732)321-7950 Fax (732)906-4906
Ang, Brian Christopher Uy, MD {1538327598} Surgry, SrgPlstc, IntrMd(03,PHI01)
  + 46 Bayberry Drive
    Somerset, NJ 08873 (732)993-3401
Ang, Dexter Ong, MD {1679788228} Pedtrc(02,PHI32)
  + CHOP Care Network at Virtua Voorhees Hospital
    100 Bowman Drive Voorhees, NJ 08043 (856)325-3000 Fax (609)261-5842
Angamuthu, Akilandanayaki, MD {1457649071} IntrMd(08,INA47)
  + 501 Zion Road/Suite 1718
    Egg Harbor Township, NJ 08234 (609)927-8067 Fax (609)927-8127
Angel, Juliette, MD {1003148818} CdvDis, IntrMd(79,MEX14)<PA-MIDVLY>
  + 13 Quaker Road
    Princeton Junction, NJ 08550 (609)799-5659 Fax (609)799-5659
Angelastro, David B., MD {1710948583} EmrgMd(95,PA02)<NJ-SHOREMEM>
  + Bayfront Emergency Physicians, P.A.
    1 East New York Avenue Somers Point, NJ 08244 (609)653-3519 Fax (609)653-3247
Angeli, Daniel, MD {1326417916} IntrMd<NJ-NWRKBETH>
  + Newark Beth Israel Medical Center
    201 Lyons Avenue Newark, NJ 07112 (800)843-2384
Angeli, Stephen J., MD {1922007707} CdvDis, IntrMd, IntCrd(81,NY08)<NJ-HACKNSK, NJ-HOLYNAME>
  + Cardiovascular Associates of Teaneck
    954 Teaneck Road Teaneck, NJ 07666 (201)833-2300 Fax (201)833-7600
Angello, Philip Joseph, MD {1083601934} FamMed, IntrMd(96,NJ06)<NJ-JRSYSHMC, NJ-KIMBALL>
  + Family Practice of CentraState
    281 Route 34/Suite 813 Colts Neck, NJ 07722 (732)431-2620 Fax (732)431-3707
  + Family Practice of CentraState
    479 Newman Springs Rd/Suite A-101 Marlboro, NJ 07746 (732)780-1601
Angelo, Mark, MD {1144319682} IntrMd(98,PA13)<NJ-COOPRUMC>
  + Cooper Physician Offices
    900 Centennial Boulevard Voorhees, NJ 08043 (856)325-6770 Fax (856)673-4300
Angelo, Melanie Elissa, DO {1881632024} EmrgMd(98,NJ75)<NJ-KMHSTRAT>
  + Kennedy Memorial Hospital-University Medical Center
    18 East Laurel Road/EmergMed Stratford, NJ 08084 (856)346-6000
Angelo, Sharon A., DO {1811991458} IntrMd(89,PA77)<NJ-RIVERVW>
  + 180 Avenue At The Common/Suite 6
    Shrewsbury, NJ 07702 (732)380-9000 Fax (732)380-9232

Angi, Priya, MD {1639376361} IntrMd, Grtrcs(93,INA48)<NJ-MONMOUTH>
  + Monmouth Medical Center
    300 Second Avenue/Geriatrics Long Branch, NJ 07740 (732)923-7550 Fax (732)923-7553
Angioletti, Lee Mitchell, MD {1881693059} Ophthl, VitRet, IntrMd(89,NY09)<NY-NYEYEINF, NJ-HACKNSK>
  + Retina Specialists of New Jersey
    330 South Street/Suite 1 Morristown, NJ 07960 (973)871-2020 Fax (973)871-2000
  + Retina Specialists of New Jersey
    422 Conventry Drive/2nd Floor Phillipsburg, NJ 08865 (973)871-2020 Fax (973)871-2000
  + Retina Specialists of New Jersey
    500 Willow Grove Street/Suite 2 Hackettstown, NJ 07960 (973)871-2020 Fax (973)871-2000
Angioletti, Louis Scott, MD {1760481030} Ophthl, VitRet(86,DC02)<NY-NYEYEINF, NJ-HACKNSK>
  + Ocean Eye Institute
    601 Route 37 West Toms River, NJ 08755 (732)244-4400 Fax (732)505-2171
Angioletti, Louis V., Jr., MD {1528067832} Ophthl, VitRet(66,NY09)<NY-NYEYEINF>
  + Retina Center of New Jersey
    1086 Teaneck Road/Suite 2a Teaneck, NJ 07666 (201)871-3414 Fax (201)871-4830
Anglade, Claudia, MD {1972865772} FamMed(09,NJ02)
  + New Jersey Family Practice Center (NJFPC)
    90 Bergen Street/DOC 300/Lower Level Newark, NJ 07103 (973)972-2111 Fax (973)972-2754
Angrist, Richard Clay, MD {1063441756} Ophthl(79,NY03)<NJ-OCEANMC, NJ-KIMBALL>
  + Cataract & Laser Institute, P.A.
    1527 Route 27/Suite 2600 Somerset, NJ 08873 (732)246-1050 Fax (732)846-1440
    rangrist@hotmail.com
  + 3810 River Road
    Point Pleasant Beach, NJ 08742 (732)892-5603
  + 26 Throckmorton Lane
    Old Bridge, NJ 08873 (732)679-9800
Anhalt, Henry, DO {1437181690} PedEnd(88,NY75)<NJ-STBARNMC, NJ-NWRKBETH>
  + St. Barnabas Ambulatory Care Center
    200 South Orange Avenue Livingston, NJ 07039 (973)322-7600 Fax (973)322-7685
Ani, Abdul Nasser, MD {1275679805} SrgOrt(84,LEBA)<NJ-BAYSHORE, NJ-RBAYOLDB>
  + Ani Orthopaedic Group
    1 Bethany Road/Bldg. 2 Suite 21 Hazlet, NJ 07730 (732)264-8282 Fax (732)264-8131
  + Ani Orthopaedic Group
    200 Perrine Road/Suite 220 Old Bridge, NJ 08857 (732)264-8282 Fax (732)264-8131
  + Ani Orthopaedic Group
    714 Route 35 South Middletown, NJ 07730 (732)264-8282 Fax (732)264-8131
Ani, Mohamad Salim, MD {1134517121} CdvDis, IntrMd(87,SYR03)
  + Ani Orthopaedic Group
    1 Bethany Road/Bldg. 2 Suite 21 Hazlet, NJ 07730 (732)264-8282 Fax (732)264-8131
Anicette, Lionel, Jr., MD {1346425188} IntrMd(94,NJ05)
  + 407 Vose Avenue
    South Orange, NJ 07079 (973)762-3399
Anido, Rosary Kristine Isidro, MD {1033423579} Pedtrc
  + PediatriCare Associates
    20-20 Fair Lawn Avenue Fair Lawn, NJ 07410 (201)791-4545 Fax (201)791-3765
Anim, Candy Kyewaa, MD {1972763548} Psychy, PhyMSptM(07,NJ06)<PA-ABINGTON>
  + 125 Patterson Street
    New Brunswick, NJ 08901 (609)955-4626
Anisetti, Vimlesh K., MD {1902803455} Anesth(91,INA29)<NJ-MONMOUTH>
  + Monmouth Medical Center
    300 Second Avenue/Anesthesiology Long Branch, NJ 07740 (732)222-5200
Anisman, Paul C., MD {1427149715} Pedtrc(80,DC01)<NJ-ACMC-ITY, NJ-ACMCMAIN>
  + AtlantiCare/Dupont Children's Health Program
    2500 English Creek Avenue Egg Harbor Township, NJ 08234 (609)641-3700 Fax (609)641-3652
Anjaria, Devashish Jayant, MD {1609806686} Surgry(97,MD01)<NJ-UMDNJ>
  + University Hospital-Doctors Office Center
    90 Bergen Street/DOC 7100/Surgry Newark, NJ 07103 (973)972-2400 Fax (973)972-6803
Anjutgi, Rajyashree, MD {1811979388} Anesth(89,INDI)
  + Morris Anesthesia Group, PA
    3799 Route 46/Suite 211 Parsippany, NJ 07054 (973)335-1122 Fax (973)335-1448

Physicians by Name and Address

Aroesty, Jeffrey H., MD {1780633131} Otlryg, SlpDis(88,NY08)<NJ-STCLRDOV, NJ-STCLRDEN>
+ Drs. Aroesty and Lin
400 Valley Road/Suite 105   Mount Arlington, NJ 07856   (973)770-7101   Fax (973)770-7108

Arole, Adebola Oyedele, MD {1740370758} Anesth(86,NIG03)<PA-TMPHOSP>
+ AtlantiCare Anesthesiology
65 West Jimmie Leeds Road   Pomona, NJ 08240   (609)748-7597

Arole, Chidinma Nwanmgbede Aloz, MD {1366519738} ObsGyn(96,CT01)
+ Advocare Magness-Stafford Ob-Gyn Associates
1810 Haddonfield Berlin Road   Cherry Hill, NJ 08003   (856)795-3313   Fax (856)354-8780
+ Advocare Magness-Stafford Ob-Gyn Associates
802 Liberty Place   Sicklerville, NJ 08081   (856)795-3313   Fax (856)740-4411

Aron, Jesse H., MD {1124341573} PedAne
+ 35 Winter Lane
Watchung, NJ 07069

Aronoff, Benjamin W., MD {1922075878} IntrMd, Nephro(99,NY46)
+ Nephrology Associates PA
870 Palisade Avenue/Suite 202   Teaneck, NJ 07666   (201)836-0897   Fax (201)836-8042

Aronova, Yelena, DO {1336384296} Anesth<NJ-STJOSHOS>
+ St. Joseph's Regional Medical Center Anesthesia
703 Main Street   Paterson, NJ 07503   (973)754-2323   Fax (973)977-9455

Aronow, Phillip Z., MD {1164423406} Surgry, IntrMd(63,PA02)
+ NaltrexZone, LLC.
1 South Centre Street/Suite 201   Merchantville, NJ 08109   (856)663-4447   Fax (856)488-6380

Aronowitz, Jeffrey S., DO {1639326960} Psychy(05,PA77)
+ University Hospital-SOM Department of Psychiatry
2250 Chapel Avenue West/Suite 100   Cherry Hill, NJ 08002   (856)482-9000   Fax (856)482-1159

Aronsky, Adam M., MD {1114993946} Pedtrc, FamMed(96,NJ06)<NJ-CHLSMT, NJ-NWRKBETH>
+ Children's Specialized Hospital
150 New Providence Road   Mountainside, NJ 07092   (908)233-3720   Fax (908)301-5456

Aronsky, Amy J., DO {1881686376} SlpDis, PulDis, IntrMd(93,PA77)
+ 3 Roseland Court
Princeton Junction, NJ 08550

Aronson, Scott Logan, MD {1285655274} Gastrn, IntrMd(02,NJ06)
+ Digestive Disease Center of New Jersey, LLC
33 Clyde Road/Suite 102   Somerset, NJ 08873   (732)873-9200   Fax (732)873-1699

Aronwald, Bruce Alan, DO {1154375467} FamMed(86,NJ75)<NJ-MORRISTN>
+ Summit Medical Group
95 Madison Avenue   Morristown, NJ 07960   (973)285-7610

Arora, Deepinder Kaur, MD {1821036922} IntrMd(95,INA07)<NJ-BAYSHORE, NJ-RIVERVW>
+ 200 White Road/Suite 209
Little Silver, NJ 07739   (908)731-1981   Fax (732)530-0043

Arora, Jasmine Kaur, MD {1548327257} IntrMd(97,INA07)
+ 321 North Warren Street
Trenton, NJ 08618   (609)278-5950   Fax (609)695-3532

Arora, Pradeep, MD {1366466476} Psychy(85,INA27)
+ 5101 Buttonwood Court
Monmouth Junction, NJ 08852

Arora, Ranjana, MD {1912196023} ObsGyn(96,INA12)
+ JFK Medical Center
65 James Street/Ob/Gyn   Edison, NJ 08820   (732)839-9341

Arora, Sanjay Kumar, MD {1619282175} IntrMd(96,INA70)<PA-POCONO>
+ Select Specialty Hospital-Northeast New Jersey
96 Parkway/Internal Med   Rochelle Park, NJ 07662   (201)221-2351

Arora, Tanisha, MD {1588898951} EmrgMd<NJ-OVERLOOK>
+ Overlook Medical Center
99 Beauvoir Avenue/PO Box 210   Summit, NJ 07902   (856)686-4306

Arora-Khera, Shruti, MD {1376884569} IntrMd
+ JFK Hospitalists
98 James Street/Suite 208   Edison, NJ 08818   (908)731-1981   Fax (732)862-1171

Arpayoglou, Beatriz Cassanello, MD {1275602906} Pedtrc, PedEmg(74,URU02)<NJ-UMDNJ, NY-BETHPETR>
+ University Hospital
150 Bergen Street   Newark, NJ 07103   (973)972-4300   Fax (973)972-5965
b_cassanello@hotmail.com

Arredondo, Mario Gaston, MD {1285652164} RadDia, Radiol, NuclMd(94,PA14)<NJ-CENTRAST>
+ Freehold Radiology Group
901 West Main Street   Freehold, NJ 07728   (732)462-4844

Arrigo, Richard J., DO {1669677811} Hepato, IntrMd(07,NY75)<NJ-UMDNJ>
+ Hunterdon Gastroenterology Associates, P.A.
1100 Wescott Drive/Suite 206-207   Flemington, NJ 08822   (908)483-4000   Fax (908)788-5090
+ Hunterdon Gastroenterology Associates, P.A.
135 West End Avenue/Suite 204   Somerville, NJ 08876   (908)483-4000   Fax (908)788-5090
+ University Hospital
150 Bergen Street/Hepatlgy   Newark, NJ 08822   (973)972-4300

Arrow Articolo, Amy Beth, DO {1356324255} ObsGyn(98,PA77)<NJ-OURLADY, NJ-VIRTMHBC>
+ Wegh Under
2301 Evesham Road/Suite 505   Voorhees, NJ 08043   (856)861-6320   Fax (856)888-2640

Arroyo, Louis, MD {1538114103} Psychy(83,DOMI)<NJ-STJOSHOS>
+ St. Joseph's Regional Medical Center
703 Main Street/Psychiatry   Paterson, NJ 07503   (973)754-2830
+ St. Joseph Medical Center Mental Health Clinic
56 Hamilton Street   Paterson, NJ 07505   (973)754-4755

Arroyo, Zuleika A., MD {1316993397} Psychy(80,DOM01)<NJ-HACKNSK>
+ Quest Adult Outpatient Psychiatry
60 Second Street/Suite 1   Hackensack, NJ 07601   (201)996-5950   Fax (201)996-5994

Arrunategui, Jose M., MD {1215037270} ObsGyn(78,PERU)
+ 717 Westfield Avenue
Elizabeth, NJ 07208   (908)353-7500   Fax (908)353-8590

Arsenescu, Razvan Ioan Paul, MD {1477560316} Gastrn, IntrMd(94,ROM04)<OH-OSUMEDC>
+ Atlantic Digestive Health
435 South Street/Suite 205   Morristown, NJ 07960   (973)971-7507

Arshad, Aysha, MD {1710964960} IntrMd, CdvDis, ClCdEl(95,PAK14)
+ Valley Medical Group-Electrophysiology & Cardiology
223 North Van Dien Avenue   Ridgewood, NJ 07450   (201)432-7837   Fax (201)432-7830

Arshad, Haroon, MD {1942694419} FamMed
+ 346 Route 46
Rockaway, NJ 07866   (973)627-4870   Fax (973)627-4908

Arslan, Asima, MD {1912171448} PthACl, PthHem(00,PAK01)
+ Pathology Associates of Princeton
One Plainsboro Road   Plainsboro, NJ 08536   (609)853-6800   Fax (609)853-6801
+ RWJ University Pathology
125 Paterson Street/MEB 212   New Brunswick, NJ 08901   (732)235-8120

Arteta, Pablo A., MD {1053331579} IntrMd, Grtrcs(82,ECUA)
+ 426-57th Street
West New York, NJ 07093   (201)869-6000
Parteta@optonline.net

Arthur, Kiersten Westrol, MD {1558446765} FamMed, SprtMd(97,PA09)
+ St. Christopher Care at Washington Township
405 Hurffville-Cross Keys Road   Sewell, NJ 08080   (856)582-0644   Fax (856)582-0622
+ St. Christopher's Marlton Orthopedics
4 Greentree Centre   Marlton, NJ 08053

Articolo, Glenn Anthony, MD {1366462780} Radiol, NuclMd, RadDia(95,PA02)<NJ-OURLADY>
+ Our Lady of Lourdes Medical Center
1600 Haddon Avenue/Radiology   Camden, NJ 08103   (856)757-3500

Artinian, Agop, MD {1861406746} IntrMd(82,ROMA)<NJ-HACKNSK, NJ-HOLYNAME>
+ 477 Bergen Boulevard
Ridgefield, NJ 07657   (201)945-6319   Fax (201)967-8443

Arturi, Frank C., MD {1659344075} Catrct, Glacma, Ophthl(77,ITAL)<NJ-HOLYNAME>
+ 559 Anderson Avenue
Cliffside Park, NJ 07010   (201)945-4600   Fax (201)945-9163
Arturieye@nac.net

Artymyshyn, Renee L., MD {1730254822} PthCyt, PthACl(83,PA07)<NJ-RWJUBRUN>
+ RWJ University Pathology
125 Paterson Street/MEB 212   New Brunswick, NJ 08901   (732)418-8076   Fax (732)418-8445

Arumugam, Dena G., MD {1831401553}
+ UH- Robert Wood Johnson Med
125 Paterson Street/MEB 596   New Brunswick, NJ 08901   (732)235-7674

Arumugam, Maheswari, MD {1942666300} Pedtrc
+ Pediatric and Adolescent Associates of Central NJ
100 Perrine Road   Old Bridge, NJ 08857   (732)316-0900   Fax (732)316-0499

Arun, Aparna, MD {1295973782} Pedtrc, IntrMd(03,INA1M)<NJ-RWJUBRUN>
+ RWJ University Medical Group/Somerset Pediatrics
1 Worlds Fair Drive/Suite 1   Somerset, NJ 08873   (732)743-5437   Fax (732)564-0212

Aruna, Pasalai N., MD {1487697744} Otlryg(69,INDI)
+ Ear Nose & Throat Group of Central NJ
2124 Oak Tree Road/2nd floor   Edison, NJ 08820   (732)205-1311   Fax (732)205-9648
+ Princeton Eye and Ear
2999 Princeton Pike/2 FL   Lawrenceville, NJ 08648   (732)205-1311   Fax (609)403-8852
+ Princeton Eye and Ear
5 Plainsboro Road/Suite 510   Plainsboro, NJ 08820   (609)403-8840   Fax (609)403-8852

Arunachalam, Muthu R., MD {1457497356} Grtrcs, IntrMd(93,INDI)<NJ-STBARNMC>
+ Geriatric & Primary Care Center
22 Old Short Hills Road/Suite 110   Livingston, NJ 07039   (973)994-0899   Fax (973)994-0866

Arvanitis, Michael L., MD {1144243684} SrgC&R, Surgry(82,PA09)<NJ-MONMOUTH, NJ-RIVERVW>
+ Specialty Surgical Associates
10 Industrial Way East/Suite 104   Eatontown, NJ 07724   (732)389-1331   Fax (732)542-8587

Arvary, Gary J., MD {1801863790} FamMed(80,NJ05)<NJ-NWTN-MEM>
+ Skylands Medical Group PA
210 Route 94   Columbia, NJ 07832   (908)362-9285   Fax (908)362-7756

Arya, Adarsh Vir, MD {1457323008} IntrMd, IntHos(82,INA06)<NJ-RWJUBRUN>
+ Foot and Ankle Care Associates
216 Stelton Road/Suite E3   Piscataway, NJ 08854   (732)529-5960   Fax (732)968-4703
piscataway@njfootdoctors.com

Arya, Rajiv, MD {1770659971} EmrgMd(99,NJ05)<NJ-RWJUBRUN>
+ University Emergency Medicine
125 Paterson Street/MEB 104   New Brunswick, NJ 08901   (732)235-8717   Fax (732)235-7379
+ RWJ University Hospital New Brunswick
One Robert Wood Johnson Place   New Brunswick, NJ 08901   (732)828-3000

Arya, Vinay, MD {1376565127} Psychy
+ 25 Cedar Avenue
South Amboy, NJ 08879

Aryal, Sunita, MD {1740498054} Pedtrc(92,BAN01)
+ 53 Passaic Avenue/1st Fl
Passaic, NJ 07055   (732)640-6421
+ Clara Maass Medical Center
1 Clara Maass Drive   Belleville, NJ 07109   (732)640-6421   Fax (973)844-4780

Arzola, Nydia, MD {1679538045} Anesth(99,NY45)
+ Summit Anesthesia Associates PA
99 Beauvoir Avenue   Summit, NJ 07901   (908)598-1500

Asaad, Imad, MD {1669725057}
+ Vascular Epicenter
7000 Boulevard East   Guttenberg, NJ 07093   (734)716-4038   Fax (201)861-9977
imadasaad86@gmail.com

Asaadi, Mokhtar, MD {1831250919} SrgPlstc, Surgry(73,IRAN)<NJ-MORRISTN>
+ Aesthetic Plastic Surgery Center
101 Old Short Hills Road/Suite 501   West Orange, NJ 07052   (973)731-2000   Fax (973)731-8656

Asamoah, Francis E., MD {1912933417} Anesth(74,GHAN)<NJ-JRSYCITY>
+ Jersey City Medical Center
355 Grand Street   Jersey City, NJ 07304   (201)915-2000   Fax (201)871-0619
Fasamoah@aol.com

Asbell, Sucha Order, MD {1770699605} RadOnc, RadThp, IntrMd(66,PA07)<NJ-COOPRUMC>
+ Cooper University Hospital
One Cooper Plaza   Camden, NJ 08103   (856)365-8504   Fax (856)365-8504

Asemota, Emiola O., MD {1518916584} Pedtrc, AdolMd(87,NIGE)<NJ-ACMCMAIN>
+ Ventnor Pediatric Center, LLC
6601 Ventnor Avenue/Suite 14   Ventnor City, NJ 08406   (609)487-6507   Fax (609)487-6508

Asfour, Mervet, MD {1952515546} FamMed(03,SLU01)<NJ-JRSYCITY>
+ AMG Primary Care at Totowa
650 Union Boulevard/Unit 16   Totowa, NJ 07512   (908)938-5200   Fax (908)938-5190
+ Horizon Health Center
714 Bergen Avenue   Jersey City, NJ 07306   (201)451-6300
+ Horizon Health Center/Family Medicine
412 Summit Avenue   Jersey City, NJ 07512   (201)963-5774   Fax (201)963-8274

Physicians by Name and Address

Asghar, Fatima, MD {1174629083} FamMed(84,PAKI)<NJ-COMMED, NJ-KIMBALL>
+ Hypertension and Kidney Group
9 Hospital Drive/Suite 16   Toms River, NJ 08755   (732)341-2211   Fax (732)505-8229

Asghar, Sheba, MD {1780865758} IntrMd, EnDbMt(PAK14)
+ AtlantiCare Regional Medical Center/City Campus
1925 Pacific Avenue   Atlantic City, NJ 08401   (609)407-2277   Fax (609)677-7280

Asghar, Syed Amir, MD {1356406631} PulDis, CritCr(86,PAK20)
+ 40 Fuld Street
Trenton, NJ 08638   (609)656-1245

Ash, Carol E., DO {1750484341} PulDis, IntrMd, SlpDis
+ RWJ University Hospital New Brunswick
One Robert Wood Johnson Place   New Brunswick, NJ 08901   (732)828-3000
+ RWJ Neurosciences
33 East Front Street   Red Bank, NJ 07701

Ashby, John Wilson, MD {1740229046} PhysMd(86,PA13)
+ Washington Medical, P.A.
100 Heritage Valley Drive/Suite 2   Sewell, NJ 08080   (856)582-6100   Fax (856)582-0397

Ashfaq, Mohammad, MD {1689690414} Psychy(79,PAK01)<NJ-ACMCMAIN>
+ AtlantiCare Regional Med Ctr/Mainland
65 West Jimmie Leeds Road/Psych   Pomona, NJ 08240   (609)652-1000

Ashinoff, Robin, MD {1811956600} Dermat, SrgDer(85,NY19)<NJ-HACKNSK>
+ 360 Essex Street/Suite 201
Hackensack, NJ 07601   (201)336-8660   Fax (201)336-8669
rashinoffmd@aol.com
+ Hackensack University Medical Center
20 Prospect Avenue/Suite 912   Hackensack, NJ 07601   (201)996-5922

Ashinoff, Russell Lee, MD {1831152719} SrgPlstc, Surgry(99,NY15)
+ The Plastic Surgery Ctr of NJ & Manhat
535 Sycamore Avenue   Shrewsbury, NJ 07702   (732)741-0970   Fax (732)747-2606

Ashinsky, Douglas S., MD {1932175361} IntrMd(84,NY19)<NJ-OVERLOOK>
+ RWJPE Warren Internal Medicine
31 Mountain Boulevard/Suite J   Warren, NJ 07059   (908)685-2505   Fax (908)753-3987

Ashir, Zainab A., MD {1831488170}<NJ-NWRKBETH>
+ Newark Beth Israel Medical Center
201 Lyons Avenue   Newark, NJ 07112   (847)637-6190
zainab.ashir@apogeephysicians.com

Ashkanazy, Mitchel, MD {1548255631} Ophthl(76,IL42)<NJ-CHILTON>
+ 170 Kinnelon Road/Suite 27
Kinnelon, NJ 07405   (973)838-1211   Fax (973)283-1281
mitchel123@prodigy.net

Ashkar, Michael George, MD {1699826420} SrgPlstc, Surgry(64,NJ05)
+ 44 Monmouth Road
Eatontown, NJ 07724   (732)389-0500   Fax (732)389-2877

Ashok, Manjula, MD {1518923309} IntrMd(94,INA85)<NJ-MONMOUTH>
+ Hypertension & Nephrology Association, PA
6 Industrial Way West/Suite B   Eatontown, NJ 07724   (732)460-1200   Fax (732)460-1211

Ashok, Viswanath K., MD {1528107646} Surgry, SrgVas(72,INDI)<NJ-CENTRAST, NJ-RBAYOLDB>
+ Central Jersey Surgical Associates
495 Iron Bridge Road/Suite 3   Freehold, NJ 07728   (732)845-0222   Fax (732)845-1002

Ashong, Emmanuel F., MD {1225016363} Pedtrc(74,GHA01)<NJ-OURLADY>
+ Our Lady of Lourdes Medical Center
1600 Haddon Avenue/Pediatrics   Camden, NJ 08103   (856)968-6534

Ashraf, Afia, MD {1225490964} IntrMd<NJ-ACMCITY>
+ AtlantiCare Regional Medical Center/City Campus
1925 Pacific Avenue   Atlantic City, NJ 08401   (609)441-8074

Ashraf, Azima F., MD {1376577403} Psychy(93,BAN07)<NJ-UNIVBHC>
+ University Behavioral Health Care
4326 Route 1 North   Monmouth Junction, NJ 08852   (732)235-5910   Fax (732)235-5644
+ University Behavioral Health Care
303 George Street/Suite 200   New Brunswick, NJ 08901   (732)235-5910   Fax (732)235-6187

Ashraf, Azra Abida, MD {1134393986} Surgry, SrgPlstc(04,RI01)<MA-STELIZAB>
+ The Plastic Surgery Ctr of NJ & Manhat
535 Sycamore Avenue   Shrewsbury, NJ 07702   (732)741-0970   Fax (732)747-2606

Ashraf, Humaira, MD {1225397433} PhysMd
+ University Hospital-Doctors Office Center
90 Bergen Street/DOC 3203   Newark, NJ 07103   (973)972-7085
+ Rutgers-Department of Physical Med
183 South Orange Ave/Suite F-1555   Newark, NJ 07101   (973)972-3606

Ashraf, Imran, MD {1134446529}
+ Hudson Pro Orthopaedics and Sports Medicine
1320 Adams Street/Unit D-E   Hoboken, NJ 07030   (201)308-6622   Fax (646)661-2599
+ Surgical Associates of Hudson County, P.A.
330 Grand Street/Suite 100   Hoboken, NJ 07030   (201)308-6622

Ashraf, Mohammad, MD {1922303189} Psychy, PsyGrt(86,PAK04)<NY-STLAWPSY>
+ Camden County Health Services Center
425 Woodbury Turnersville Rd   Blackwood, NJ 08012   (856)374-6895   Fax (856)374-6896

Ashraf, Nomaan, MD {1104957976} SrgSpn, SrgOrt(02,MA07)
+ Comprehensive Spine Care, PA
260 Old Hook Road/Suite 400   Emerson, NJ 07630   (201)634-1811   Fax (201)634-7526
nomaan.ashraf@gmail.com

Ashraf, Shehzana, MD {1497848774} IntrMd(89,PAK15)<NJ-SOMERSET>
+ Advance Hospital Care @ Somerset Medical Center
110 Rehill Avenue   Somerville, NJ 08876   (908)429-5833   Fax (908)203-5970

Ashraf, Waseem, MD {1952394389} Anesth(94,PAK20)
+ 701 Surrey Lane
Franklin Lakes, NJ 07417

Ashton, Jennifer Lee, MD {1972601649} ObsGyn(00,NY01)
+ Women Physicians Ob-Gyn Associates
300 Grand Avenue/Suite 102   Englewood, NJ 07631   (201)569-5151   Fax (201)569-9193

Ashton, Julie A., MD {1538171319} Pedtrc(87,NJ05)<NJ-MORRISTN>
+ Franklin Pediatrics, PA
91 South Jefferson Road/Suite 200   Whippany, NJ 07981   (973)538-6116   Fax (973)538-3712

Ashtyani Asl, Fariborz, MD {1891762555} CritCr, IntrMd, PulDis(81,IRA24)<NJ-HACKNSK>
+ Hackensack Sleep & Pulmonary Center
170 Prospect Avenue/Suite 20   Hackensack, NJ 07601   (201)996-0232   Fax (201)996-0095

Ashtyani Asl, Hormoz, MD {1982634952} CritCr, IntrMd, PulDis(70,IRA01)<NJ-HACKNSK>
+ Hackensack Sleep & Pulmonary at The Medical Center
20 Prospect Avenue/Suite 615   South Hackensack, NJ 07606   (201)488-1884   Fax (201)996-0242
+ Hackensack University Medical Center
30 Prospect Avenue/3-St. John   Hackensack, NJ 07601   (201)996-2000

Asiegbu, Benedict E., MD {1669502035} NnPnMd(90,NIG02)
+ 65 West Jimmie Leeds Road/Pedtrcs
Pomona, NJ 08240

Asif, Arif, MD {1598709941} IntrMd, Nephro(88,PAK02)
+ Hackensack Meridian Medical Group
19 Davis Avenue/5th-6th Floor   Neptune, NJ 07753   (732)897-3990   Fax (732)897-3997

Asif, Mohammad, MD {1912954413} CdvDis, IntCrd(86,PAK11)<NJ-NWRKBETH, NJ-BAYONNE>
+ Newark Beth Israel Medical Center
201 Lyons Avenue/Cardiology   Newark, NJ 07112   (973)926-7000   Fax (973)923-8599
+ Bayonne Medical Center
29th Street at Avenue E/Cardiology   Bayonne, NJ 07002   (201)858-5000

Asimolowo, Olabisi Omolara, MD {1871768929} Anesth<PA-PNSTHRSH>
+ Summit Medical Group
140 Park Avenue/3rd Floor   Florham Park, NJ 07932   (973)718-5800   Fax (973)743-0777

Askari, Samieh, MD {1629467386}
+ 376 Hamilton Street/Unit D
Somerset, NJ 08873   (443)554-8552
samieh68@aol.com

Askenase, Alan David, MD {1033141320} CdvDis, IntrMd(79,NY08)
+ Penn Medicine at Cherry Hill
1400 East Route 70/Cardiology   Cherry Hill, NJ 08034
+ Penn Medicine Willingboro
200 Campbell Drive/Twr Ctr/Suite 115   Willingboro, NJ 08046

Askia, Gyasi Abena, DO {1851567473} ObsGyn
+ Osborn Family Health Center
1601 Haddon Road   Camden, NJ 08103   (856)757-3700   Fax (856)365-7972

Askin, Matthew Peter, MD {1871780528} Gastrn, IntrMd(96,NY47)<NJ-MORRISTN>
+ Affiliates in Gastroenterology, P.A.
101 Old Short Hills Road/Suite 217   West Orange, NJ 07052   (973)731-4600   Fax (973)731-1477

Aslam, Fazila, MD {1316139561} InfDis, IntrMd(99,PAK11)<NJ-LOURDMED>
+ ID Associates PA/dba ID Care
765 Route 10 East/Suite 201   Randolph, NJ 07869   (973)989-0068   Fax (973)361-8955
+ ID Associates PA/dba ID Care
8 Saddle Road   Cedar Knolls, NJ 07927   (973)989-0068   Fax (973)993-5953

Aslam, Hafiz Muhammad, MD {1740761915} IntrMd<NJ-STFRNMED>
+ St. Francis Medical Center
601 Hamilton Avenue   Trenton, NJ 08629   (609)599-5000

Aslam, Masood, MD {1295719672} Psychy, PsyCAd(91,PAK12)
+ Camden County Health Services Center
20 N Woodbury-Turnersville Rd   Blackwood, NJ 08012   (856)374-4600   Fax (856)374-6436

Aslam, Tahseen N., MD {1295737021} IntrMd(80,PAK12)
+ 17 Webster Street
Nutley, NJ 07110

Aslami, Brian A., MD {1528173994} Psychy(93,NY20)<NY-PRSBCOLU>
+ 163 Engle Street/Building 2
Englewood, NJ 07631

Asnani, Sunil, MD {1669574281} IntrMd, EnDbMt, Grtrcs(96,INA23)<NJ-JRSYSHMC>
+ Jersey Shore University Medical Center
1945 Route 33/Medicine   Neptune, NJ 07753   (732)775-5500
+ Hackensack Meridian Medical Group
19 Davis Avenue/5th-6th Floor   Neptune, NJ 07753   (732)775-5500   Fax (732)897-3982

Asnes, Russell S., MD {1477518363} Pedtrc, IntrMd(63,MA07)<NJ-HACKNSK, NJ-ENGLWOOD>
+ Tenafly Pediatrics, PA
32 Franklin Street   Tenafly, NJ 07670   (201)569-2400   Fax (201)569-6081
+ Tenafly Pediatrics, PA
26 Park Place   Paramus, NJ 07652   (201)569-2400   Fax (201)261-8413

Asokan, Nalini, MD {1235100389} IntrMd(85,INDI)<NJ-MORRISTN>
+ Family Health Center
200 South Street/Suite 4   Morristown, NJ 07960   (973)889-6800

Asokan, Rengaswamy, MD {1639196256} IntrMd(79,INDI)<NJ-CHILTON>
+ 14 Oak Ridge Road/Suite A
Newfoundland, NJ 07435   (973)697-3311   Fax (973)208-8976
+ 183 Illinois Avenue
Paterson, NJ 07503   (973)523-3400

Aspen, Otter Q., MD {1356316020} Dermat(03,MA01)<MA-BOSTMC, MA-NEMEDCEN>
+ North Jersey Dermatology Center
35 Green Pond Road   Rockaway, NJ 07866   (973)625-0600   Fax (973)625-0336

Asper, Ronald Frank, MD {1306904941} InfDis, IntrMd(72,PA13)
+ 24 Phillips Road
Hainesport, NJ 08036

Asprec, Claro M., MD {1720022999} Pedtrc(88,PHIL)<NJ-RBAYOLDB, NJ-STPETER>
+ Dr. Claro Asprec Pediatrics LLC
3099 Highway 516/Suite C   Old Bridge, NJ 08857   (732)679-8200   Fax (732)679-8201
asprecpediatrics@gmail.com

Asrar, Rohail, MD {1356596761}(02,PAK26)<RI-SJFATIMA, NJ-STBARNMC>
+ North Brunswick Medical Associates
986 Shoppes Boulevard   North Brunswick, NJ 08902   (732)497-5000   Fax (732)497-5001
+ RWJ University Hospital New Brunswick
One Robert Wood Johnson Place   New Brunswick, NJ 08901   (732)828-3000

Asroff, Scott Wayne, MD {1790736924} Urolgy(86,PA13)<NJ-LOURDMED, NJ-VIRTMHBC>
+ New Jersey Urology
243 Route 130/Suite 100   Bordentown, NJ 08505   Fax (856)252-1100
+ New Jersey Urology
15000 Midlantic Drive/Suite 100   Mount Laurel, NJ 08054   Fax (856)985-4582
+ New Jersey Urology
911 Sunset Road   Willingboro, NJ 08505

Assad, Albert, MD {1053419093} Otlryg(93,CT01)<NJ-STPETER>
+ St. Peter's University Hospital
254 Easton Avenue/Otolaryngology   New Brunswick, NJ 08901   (732)745-8600   Fax (732)249-5284

Assad, Eveline N., MD {1952310658} ObsGyn, IntrMd(72,EGYP)<NJ-STPETER, NJ-RWJUHAM>
+ Ladies' Choice Ob-Gyn
314 Chris Gaupp Drive/Suite 101   Galloway, NJ 08205   (609)404-1400   Fax (609)404-1430
evelineassad@gmail.com

Assadi-Khansari, Mitra, MD {1205917952} Nrolgy, ClNrPh, NroChl(90,IRAN)
+ Capital Institute for Neurosciences
2 Capital Way/Suite 456   Pennington, NJ 08534   (609)537-7300   Fax (609)537-7301

Assaleh, Marwan David, MD {1518066000} IntrMd(79,SYR01)<NJ-HOBUNIMC, NJ-CHRIST>
+ 591 Summit Avenue/Suite 205
Jersey City, NJ 07306   (201)653-9115   Fax (201)653-8119

Assemu, Belen F., MD {1558923995} FamMed
+ JFK Hartwyck at Oak Tree
2048 Oak Tree Road   Edison, NJ 08820   (732)906-2460   Fax (732)372-9217

Assiamah, Andrew Aboagye, MD {1205839180} Anesth(00,NJ06)<NJ-SHOREMEM>
+ Rancocas Anesthesiology, PA
700 Route 130 North/Suite 203   Cinnaminson, NJ 08077   (856)829-9345   Fax (856)829-3605

Assina, Rachid, MD {1770744872} SrgNro(08,DMN01)
+ 5 Haggerty Drive
West Orange, NJ 07052

Assing, Elizabeth J., MD {1700095544} NnPnMd, Pedtrc(85,WIND)<NJ-JRSYSHMC>
+ Meridian Medical Group - Faculty Practice
61 Davis Avenue/Suite 1   Neptune, NJ 07753   (732)776-4524   Fax (732)776-4639
+ Meridian Medical Group - Faculty Practice
61 Davis Avenue/Suite 1   Neptune, NJ 07753   (732)776-4524   Fax (732)776-4867

Asslo, Fady, MD {1659653723}
+ St. Michael's Medical Center
111 Central Avenue   Newark, NJ 07102   (973)877-5000

Ast, Michael Paul, MD {1427204106} SrgOrt
+ Mercer-Bucks Orthopaedics PC
3120 Princeton Pike   Lawrenceville, NJ 08648   (609)896-0444   Fax (609)587-4349
+ Mercer-Bucks Orthopaedics, P.C.
2501 Kuser Road   Hamilton, NJ 08691   (609)896-0444   Fax (609)587-4349

Asta, Charles Francis, MD {1245314806} Nrolgy, IntrMd(97,ISR06)<NJ-VALLEY>
+ Bergen Medical Associates
466 Old Hook Road/Suite 1   Emerson, NJ 07630   (201)967-8221   Fax (201)967-0340
+ Sovereign Medical Group
85 Harristown Road/Suite 104   Glen Rock, NJ 07452   (201)967-8221   Fax (201)857-2541

Asthana, Jyothi, MD {1982704904} IntrMd(83,INA5B)<NJ-MONMOUTH>
+ 398 Brookdale Avenue
Long Branch, NJ 07740

Astiz, Donna J., MD {1003864265} IntrMd(78,NE06)<NJ-MORRISTN>
+ Family Health Center
200 South Street/Suite 4   Morristown, NJ 07960   (973)889-6800
+ Morristown Medical Center
100 Madison Avenue   Morristown, NJ 07962   (973)971-5000

Asulin, Yitzhack, MD {1073752556} ObsGyn(04,GRN01)<NJ-ENGLWOOD, NJ-HACKNSK>
+ Contemporary Women's Health, P.C.
106 Grand Avenue/Suite 450   Englewood, NJ 07631   (201)308-5591   Fax (201)908-5592
Asulinmd@gmail.com
+ Contemporary Women's Health, P.C.
20 Prospect Avenue/Suite 719   Hackensack, NJ 07601   (201)308-5591   Fax (201)308-5591

Ata, Hadia M., MD {1932120896} PthACl, BldBnk(74,EGY05)
+ PLUS Diagnostics
1200 River Avenue/Suite 10   Lakewood, NJ 08701   (732)901-7575   Fax (732)901-1555

Ata, Mohammad, MD {1215220819} IntrMd
+ Drs. Deka and Ata
2090 State Route 27/Suite 101   North Brunswick, NJ 08902   (732)979-0035   Fax (908)829-4408

Atabek, Umur M., MD {1285707554} Surgry(80,MD01)<NJ-COOPRUMC>
+ Cooper Surgical Associates
3 Cooper Plaza/Suite 411   Camden, NJ 08103   (856)342-2270   Fax (856)365-1180
+ The Cooper Health System at Voorhees
900 Centennial Boulevard/Suite G   Voorhees, NJ 08043   (856)325-6565

Atalla, Sara N., DO {1831352848} PhysMd, IntrMd
+ Summit Medical Group-Berkeley Heights Campus
1 Diamond Hill Road   Berkeley Heights, NJ 07922   (908)273-4300   Fax (908)790-6576

Atallah, Judy, DO {1538396346} RadDia<NY-NASSAUMC>
+ Coastal Imaging, LLC
79 Route 37 West/Suite 103   Toms River, NJ 08755   (732)678-0087   Fax (732)276-2325
+ Ocean Medical Center
425 Jack Martin Boulevard/Radiology   Brick, NJ 08723   (732)678-0087   Fax (732)836-4047

Atherley, Trevor H., MD {1710080114} CdvDis, IntrMd, IntCrd(71,JMAC)<NJ-NWRKBETH>
+ Newark Beth Israel Medical Center
201 Lyons Avenue   Newark, NJ 07112   (973)926-7323   Fax (973)705-3096

Athwal, Barinder D., MD {1699762674} Ophthl(82,NJ05)
+ Athwal Eye Associates, PC
14 Mule Road/Suite 1   Toms River, NJ 08755   (732)286-0900   Fax (732)244-6063
athwaleye@aol.com
+ Athwal Eye Associates, PC
550 Route 530   Whiting, NJ 08759   (732)286-0900   Fax (732)350-0093
+ Middletown Eye Care
565 Highway 35   Red Bank, NJ 08755   (732)747-4443   Fax (732)747-4439

Athwal, Harjit S., MD {1396732491} CrnExD, Ophthl(86,NJ06)<NJ-COMMED>
+ Athwal Eye Associates, PC
14 Mule Road/Suite 1   Toms River, NJ 08755   (732)286-0900   Fax (732)244-6063

Athwal, Lisa M., MD {1043576630} Ophthl(12,NJ05)
+ Athwal Eye Associates, PC
14 Mule Road/Suite 1   Toms River, NJ 08755   (732)286-0900   Fax (732)244-6063

Atienza, Kristen A., DO {1891764130} Pedtrc(96,ME75)<NJ-JRSYSHMC, NJ-MONMOUTH>
+ 1812 Corlies Avenue
Neptune, NJ 07753   (732)988-3336   Fax (732)776-8668
+ Neptune Pediatrics
1812 State Route 33   Neptune, NJ 07753   (732)988-3336   Fax (732)776-8668

Atienza-Cartnick, Kimberly A., MD {1881653848} Grtrcs, IntrMd(02,NET09)<NJ-JRSYSHMC>
+ 1812 Corlies Avenue
Neptune, NJ 07753   (732)988-3336   Fax (732)776-8668

Atik, Teddy Labib, MD {1487648309} SrgHnd(93,NY19)<NJ-BAYSHORE, NJ-CENTRAST>
+ Central Jersey Hand Surgery
2 Industrial Way West   Eatontown, NJ 07724   (732)542-4477   Fax (732)935-0355
+ Central Jersey Hand Surgery
535 Iron Bridge Road   Freehold, NJ 07728   (732)542-4477   Fax (732)431-4770
+ Central Jersey Hand Surgery
780 Route 37 West/Suite 140   Toms River, NJ 07724   (732)286-9000   Fax (732)240-0036

Atiya, Christina, MD {1760800445}<NJ-ENGLWOOD>
+ Englewood Hospital and Medical Center
350 Engle Street   Englewood, NJ 07631   (973)396-6156

Atkin, Michael Joshua, MD {1518127760} EmrgMd(04,ISR02)<NY-LDYMRCY>
+ Raritan Bay Medical Center/Perth Amboy Division
530 New Brunswick Avenue   Perth Amboy, NJ 08861   (732)442-3700

Atkin, Stuart R., MD {1538235213} Anesth, IntrMd(90,GRN01)
+ Ultimed HealthCare PC
50 Franklin Lane   Manalapan, NJ 07726   (732)972-1267   Fax (732)972-1026
isleepinnj@yahoo.com

Atkin, Suzanne H., MD {1285669721} EmrgMd, IntrMd(79,NJ05)<NJ-UMDNJ>
+ University Hospital
150 Bergen Street   Newark, NJ 07103   (201)456-5129

Atkinson, James Q., III, MD {1881671444} Grtrcs, IntrMd(79,NJ05)<NJ-VIRTMHBC, NJ-VIRTMARL>
+ Atkinson Internal Medicine, PA
180 Tuckerton Road/Suite 1   Medford, NJ 08055   (856)797-9229   Fax (856)797-9919

Atkinson, Monica, MD {1447405972} FamMed, IntrMd(02,ROM06)<NJ-COOPRUMC>
+ 2301 Woodlynne Avenue
Woodlynne, NJ 08107   (856)968-7970   Fax (856)968-7975

Atkuri, Rajeshwari Venkata, MD {1699750463} IntrMd, Ophthl(86,INA62)<NJ-COOPRUMC>
+ The Cooper Hospital System-Univ Hospital
3 Cooper Plaza/Suite 215   Camden, NJ 08103   (856)342-2439

Atlas, Arthur B., MD {1578534376} Pedtrc, PedPul, PulDis(82,MEXI)<NJ-MORRISTN, NJ-OVERLOOK>
+ Pediatric Pulmonology
100 Madison Avenue   Morristown, NJ 07960   (973)971-4242   Fax (973)290-7360

Atlas, Gayle, DO {1598849424} Anesth, FamMed(89,NY75)<NY-NASSAUMC>
+ PO Box 261
Middletown, NJ 07748

Atlas, Glen Mark, MD {1295895894} Anesth, CritCr(89,PA09)<NJ-UMDNJ>
+ University Hospital
150 Bergen Street/Level E/Anesth   Newark, NJ 07103   (973)972-5787   Fax (973)972-4172

Atlas, Ian, MD {1285634352} Urolgy(84,NY47)
+ Adult & Pediatric Urology Group PA
261 James Street/Suite 1-A   Morristown, NJ 07960   (973)539-0333   Fax (973)539-8909

Atlas, Orin Keith, MD {1528034469} SrgOrt, SrgSpn(96,NJ06)
+ 201 Creek Crossing Boulevard
Hainesport, NJ 08036   (609)261-5800   Fax (609)261-5801

Atoot, Adam, MD {1265844872}
+ 935 River Road
Edgewater, NJ 07020   (201)228-1844

Attanasio, Michael J., DO {1174593958} FamMed(93,PA77)
+ Point Plaza Family Practice
565 Egg Harbor Road   Sewell, NJ 08080

Attardi, Diane Martha, MD {1346269651} Pedtrc, NnPnMd(93,PA09)<NJ-RIVERVW>
+ Pediatrix Medical Group
255 Third Avenue   Long Branch, NJ 07740   (732)222-7006

Attas, Lewis M., MD {1437102571} Hemato, IntrMd, MedOnc(82,NY47)<NJ-ENGLWOOD, NJ-HOLYNAME>
+ Forte Schleider & Attas MD PA
350 Engle Street/Berrie Building/1 FL   Englewood, NJ 07631   (201)568-5250   Fax (201)568-5358

Atthota, Vakula Devi, MD {1821276015} IntrMd(02,INA7C)
+ Cumberland Internal Medicine
1450 East Chestnut Avenue   Vineland, NJ 08361   (856)794-8700   Fax (856)794-2752

Atti, Sukhshant Kaur, MD {1306272141}<NJ-NWRKBETH>
+ Newark Beth Israel Medical Center
201 Lyons Avenue/D11   Newark, NJ 07112   (973)926-7240

Attia, Ahmed Farouk, DO {1669538740} Surgry(01,NY75)<NJ-SJHREGMC, NJ-SJRSYELM>
+ ESA South Jersey Bariatrics, P.A.
2950 College Drive/Suite 1B   Vineland, NJ 08360   (856)362-5259   Fax (856)405-6978

Attia, Tamer A., MD {1699931386} Anesth<NJ-SJHREGMC>
+ SJH Regional Medical Center
1505 West Sherman Avenue   Vineland, NJ 08360   (856)363-1000

Attiya, Rafael, MD {1326037540} Surgry(92,NJ05)<NJ-BURDTMLN>
+ 15 Village Drive/PO Box 59
Cape May Court House, NJ 08210   (609)463-8887   Fax (609)463-1116

Au, Alexander F., MD {1386821700} SrgPlstc
+ Virtua Primary Care
401 Young Avenue/Suite 260   Moorestown, NJ 08057   (856)291-8920   Fax (856)291-8922

Au, Sonoa Ho Yee, MD {1720374507} Dermat, IntrMd(MO02)
+ Advanced Dermatology, P.C.
1200 East Ridgewood Avenue   Ridgewood, NJ 07450   (201)493-1717   Fax (201)493-1009

Auciello, Antonella, MD {1629064043} IntrMd(96,NJ05)<NJ-OVERLOOK, NJ-MORRISTN>
+ Medical Center Partners
653 Willow Grove Street/Suite 2100   Hackettstown, NJ 07840   (908)441-1352   Fax (908)441-1361

Audett, John Robert, MD {1609872878}<NJ-OVERLOOK>
+ Overlook Medical Center
99 Beauvoir Avenue/PO Box 210   Summit, NJ 07902   (908)522-5254
john.audett@atlantichealth.org

Audia, Pat Frank, MD {1780757336} Nephro
+ North Jersey Nephrology Associates PA
246 Hamburg Turnpike/Suite 207   Wayne, NJ 07470   (973)653-3366   Fax (973)653-3365

Audu, Paul Bulus, MD {1336167311} Anesth(87,NIG04)
+ 1807 Glassboro Crosskeys Road
Williamstown, NJ 08094

Physicians by Name and Address

Auerbach, Donald, MD {1225036866} PulDis, IntrMd(65,OH41)<NJ-VIRTBERL>
+ Pulmonary & Sleep Associates of SJ, LLC.
750 Route 73 South/Suite 401   Marlton, NJ 08053   (856)375-1288   Fax (856)375-2325
dauerbach@pennjerseypulmonary.com
+ Pulmonary & Sleep Associates of SJ, LLC.
107 Berlin Road   Cherry Hill, NJ 08034   (856)375-1288   Fax (856)429-1081

Auerbach, Jason M, MD {1336112648} SrgO&M(NY19
+ Riverside Oral Surgery
130 Kinderkamack Road/Suite 204   River Edge, NJ 07661   (201)487-6565
+ Riverside Oral Surgery
333 Old Hook Road/Suite 100   Westwood, NJ 07675   (201)664-2324

Aueron, Fred M., MD {1407897622} CdvDis, IntrMd(77,PA01)<NJ-BAYONNE, NJ-NWRKBETH>
+ The Heart Group, PA
161 Millburn Avenue   Millburn, NJ 07041   (973)467-4220   Fax (973)467-9889
+ Summit Medical Group-Berkeley Heights Campus
1 Diamond Hill Road   Berkeley Heights, NJ 07922   (973)467-4220   Fax (908)790-6576
+ Summit Medical Group
75 East Northfield Road   Livingston, NJ 07041   (973)436-1330   Fax (973)533-1924

Aufiero, Patrick V., MD {1649295270} InfDis, IntrMd(84,GRN01)<NJ-CHSMRCER, NJ-CHSFULD>
+ Drs. Rosenbaum & Aufiero
2085 Klockner Road   Hamilton, NJ 08690   (609)587-4122   Fax (609)588-5922
+ Capital Health System/Mercer Campus
446 Bellevue Avenue   Trenton, NJ 08618   (609)394-4000
+ Capital Health System/Fuld Campus
750 Brunswick Avenue   Trenton, NJ 08690   (609)394-6000

August, David A., MD {1881776482} SrgOnc, Nutrtn(80,CT01)<NJ-RWJUBRUN>
+ Rutgers Cancer Institute of New Jersey
195 Little Albany Street/PO Box 2681   New Brunswick, NJ 08903   (732)235-7701   Fax (732)235-6797
augustda@umdnj.edu

August, Elizabeth, MD {1841519204} FamMed(09,ANT02)
+ Riverside Medical Group
10 First Street   Hackensack, NJ 07601   (201)968-5345   Fax (201)968-5349
elizabethaugustmd@gmail.com
+ Riverside Medical Group
200 Main Street   Ridgefield Park, NJ 07660   (201)968-5345   Fax (201)870-6098
+ Riverside Medical Group
6045 Kennedy Boulevard/Suite A   North Bergen, NJ 07601   (201)861-4443   Fax (201)861-0941

Augustin, Jeffrey Franck, MD {1578653754} SrgOrt(98,PA13)
+ Augustin Orthopedics
526 Broadway   Bayonne, NJ 07002   (201)437-9700   Fax (201)437-9705
+ Augustin Orthopedics
299 Glenwood Avenue/2nd Floor   Bloomfield, NJ 07003   (201)437-9700   Fax (973)680-4205

Auld, Clara Stringer, MD {1578556866} Grtrcs(00,MA16)
+ 31 Oakwood Avenue/Apt 2
Montclair, NJ 07043

Auletta, Maria, MD {1497798581} FamMed(81,NY01)
+ 23-25 South Main Street/Suite 2
Manville, NJ 08835   (908)243-0088   Fax (908)243-0089

Aupperle, Peter M., MD {1033291208} Psychy, PsyGrt(86,NY01)<NJ-UNIVBHC>
+ University Behavioral Health Care
667 Hoes Lane   Piscataway, NJ 08854

Aurand, Lisa Ann, MD {1922096619} EnDbMt(00,NJ05)
+ 55 Corporate Drive
Bridgewater, NJ 08807

Auriemma, John A., DO {1144269655} FamMed(96,NJ75)
+ 95 Queens Drive South
Little Silver, NJ 07739

Aurilio, Joseph P., MD {1518995067} IntrMd, InfDis(73,DC03)
+ 1881 Oak Tree Road
Edison, NJ 08820   (732)494-3325

Aurora, Nadia, MD {1215427778} ObsGyn
+ University Medical Group/OBGYN
125 Paterson Street/2nd Floor   New Brunswick, NJ 08901   (732)235-6375   Fax (732)235-6627

Aurori, Brian F., MD {1689649733} SrgOrt(77,NJ05)
+ Advanced Musculoskeletal Center
131 Madison Avenue/Suite 130   Morristown, NJ 07960   (973)538-8336   Fax (973)538-8307

Aurori, Kevin C., MD {1639144132} SrgOrt(79,PA13)
+ Advanced Musculoskeletal Center
131 Madison Avenue/Suite 130   Morristown, NJ 07960   (973)538-8336   Fax (973)538-8307

Ausaf, Sadaf, MD {1548573439} IntHos<NJ-COOPRUMC>
+ Cooper University Hospital
One Cooper Plaza/Hospitalist   Camden, NJ 08103   (856)342-3150

Austin, Kimberlee Kunze, MD {1265485650} ObsGyn(99,CT02)<NJ-MORRISTN, NJ-STCLRDEN>
+ Women's Care Source
111 Madison Avenue/Suite 308   Morristown, NJ 07960   (973)285-0400   Fax (973)285-9848

Austria, Jocelyn R., MD {1760482350} NnPnMd, Pedtrc(80,PHI09)
+ On-Site Neonatal Partners
1000 Haddonfield-Berlin Road/Suite 210   Voorhees, NJ 08043   (856)782-2212   Fax (856)782-2213

Autotte, Denise L., MD {1902903370} FamMed(79,RI01)
+ 3200 Route 94/PO Box 299
Hamburg, NJ 07419   (973)827-4422   Fax (973)827-1893

Auyeung, Valerie Y., MD {1043329246} Pedtrc, PedEnd(99,MA07)<NJ-HACKNSK>
+ Hackensack University Medical Center
30 Prospect Avenue/Pedi Endo   Hackensack, NJ 07601   (201)996-2000

Avagliano, Margaret C., MD {1114021524} RadDia, Radiol, Rad-Mam(94,PA02)<NJ-ACMCITY, NJ-SHOREMEM>
+ Atlantic Medical Imaging, LLC.
72 West Jimmie Leeds Road   Galloway, NJ 08205   (609)677-9729   Fax (609)653-8764
+ Atlantic Medical Imaging, LLC.
401 Bethel Road   Somers Point, NJ 08244   (609)677-9729
+ Atlantic Medical Imaging, LLC.
421 Route 9 North   Cape May Court House, NJ 08205   (609)463-9500   Fax (609)465-0918

Avagyan, Igor Zhorzhiko, MD {1326057548} IntrMd(96,RUS79)<NY-BRKLNDWN>
+ 397 Ski Trail
Kinnelon, NJ 07405   (917)494-8226   Fax (212)426-1409

Avallone, Jennifer Mary, DO {1588800429} Pedtrc, NroChl(07,NY75)<MA-CHILDRN>
+ St. Barnabas Institute of Neurology & Neurosurgery
200 South Orange Avenue/Suite 101   Livingston, NJ 07039   (973)322-7580   Fax (973)322-7505

Avallone, Nicholas J., MD {1790823755} SrgOrt, SprtMd, SrgHnd(01,NJ02)
+ Atlantic Orthopedic Institute
111 Madison Avenue/Suite 400   Morristown, NJ 07960   (973)984-0404   Fax (973)984-2516
+ Hillcrest Colorectal Associates
755 Memorial Parkway   Phillipsburg, NJ 08865   (973)984-0404   Fax (908)859-2794

Avancha, Amarnath, MD {1740457571} IntrMd, CdvDis(82,INDI)
+ 124 Gregory Avenue/Suite 102
Passaic, NJ 07055   (973)777-1132   Fax (973)458-9850

Avanesova, Natalya Oleg, MD {1902891583} IntrMd, EmrgMd(87,UZB44)<NJ-STJOSHOS>
+ 193 Route 9 South/Suite 1-D
Manalapan, NJ 07726   (732)677-2505   Fax (732)677-2506
+ St. Joseph's Regional Medical Center
703 Main Street/EmergMed   Paterson, NJ 07503   (973)754-2000

Avella, David Paul, MD {1134127111} Anesth(89,PA09)
+ West Jersey Anesthesia Associates
102-E Center Boulevard   Marlton, NJ 08053   (856)988-6250   Fax (856)988-6270

Avella, Douglas George, MD {1437200672} PedOrt, SrgOrt(79,MEXI)<NJ-HACKNSK, NJ-VALLEY>
+ North Jersey Pediatric Orthopedics PA
140 Chestnut Street/Suite 201   Ridgewood, NJ 07450   (201)612-9988   Fax (201)445-9050
Douglas.avella@verizon.net

Avellino, Carmine, DO {1275705402} Anesth<NJ-SHOREMEM>
+ Shore Memorial Hospital
1 East New York Avenue/Anesthesia   Somers Point, NJ 08244   (609)653-3640

Avelluto, Giovanni Domenico, DO {1700228939}
+ SOM - Department of Internal Medicine
42 East Laurel Road/Suite 3100   Stratford, NJ 08084   (856)566-6477   Fax (856)566-6906

Avendano, Graciano Gary F., MD {1104999705} CdvDis, IntCrd, IntrMd(83)<NJ-RWJUBRUN, NJ-STPETER>
+ Cardio Intervent of Ctrl Jersey
465 Cranbury Road/Suite 201   East Brunswick, NJ 08816   (732)613-1988   Fax (732)651-7734

Aventurado, Tito O., MD {1336175090} Anesth(67,PHIL)<NJ-JRSYCITY>
+ Jersey City Medical Center
355 Grand Street/Anesth   Jersey City, NJ 07304   (201)915-2000   Fax (201)871-0619

Averill, Allison M., MD {1306834486} PhysMd(88,NJ06)<NJ-KSLR-WEST>
+ Kessler Institute for Rehabilitation West Orange
1199 Pleasant Valley Way   West Orange, NJ 07052   (973)731-3600

Aversa, Jeffrey Martin, MD {1992850887} IntrMd(89,PA09)<NJ-BURDTMLN>
+ Cape Regional Medical Center
2 Stone Harbor Boulevard   Cape May Court House, NJ 08210   (609)463-2000

Aversa, Thaddeus Massimo, DO {1417915968} FamMed(94,ME75)<NJ-WARREN>
+ Kaleidoscope Medical Associates
410 Coventry Drive   Phillipsburg, NJ 08865   (908)454-9902   Fax (908)454-9905

Avery, William Bradford, MD {1245559459} Anesth<NJ-HOBUNIMC>
+ Hoboken University Medical Center
308 Willow Avenue/Anesth   Hoboken, NJ 07030   (201)418-1000

Aves, Cindy, MD {1811301005} ObsGyn(10,GRN01)<NJ-COOPRUMC>
+ CAMCare Health Corporation
817 Federal Street/Suite 300   Camden, NJ 08103   (856)583-2415   Fax (856)541-4611

Avetian, Garo Charles, DO {1013936400} IntrMd(89,PA77)
+ South Jersey Health & Wellness Center
1919 Greentree Road   Cherry Hill, NJ 08003   (856)761-8100   Fax (856)761-8107

Avezzano, Eric S., MD {1578591814} IntrMd, Gastrn(85,NY48)<NJ-VALLEY>
+ Bergen Medical Associates
466 Old Hook Road/Suite 1   Emerson, NJ 07630   (201)967-8221   Fax (201)967-0340
+ Bergen Medical Associates
1 West Ridgewood Avenue/Suite 301   Paramus, NJ 07652   (201)967-8221   Fax (201)445-4296

Avhad, Prajakta Vasant, MD {1861709156} AnesPain, IntrMd(03,INA4Y)
+ New Jersey Pain Spine & Sports Associates
2050 Route 27/Suite 105   North Brunswick, NJ 08902   (732)565-3777   Fax (732)746-0223
+ New Jersey Pain Spine & Sports Associates
601 Ewing Street/Suite C-3   Princeton, NJ 08540   (732)565-3777   Fax (732)746-0223
+ New Jersey Pain Spine & Sports Associates
1255 Whitehorse Mercerville Rd   Hamilton, NJ 08902   (609)688-6866   Fax (732)746-0223

Avins, Laurence R., MD {1902133432} IntrMd, Ophthl
+ 1301 Barclay Boulevard
Princeton, NJ 08540
lravins@aol.com

Aviv, Abraham, MD {1154462687} PedNph, Pedtrc(72,NY15)<NJ-UMDNJ>
+ University Hospital
150 Bergen Street/Pdtc Nephrology   Newark, NJ 07103   (973)972-2637

Avondstondt, Andrea Mithai, MD {1821358839} ObsGyn
+ Urogynecology & Reconstructive Pelvic Surgery
435 South Street/Suite 370   Morristown, NJ 07960   (973)071-7267

Avram, Ari Jason, MD {1750524682} EmrgMd<NJ-HACKNSK>
+ Hackensack University Medical Center
30 Prospect Avenue/EmergTrauma   Hackensack, NJ 07601   (914)462-1965

Avva, Usha R., MD {1538102710} Pedtrc, PedEmg, EmrgPedr(87,INA39)<NJ-HACKNSK>
+ Hackensack Univ Medical Center Pediatric Emerg Room
30 Prospect Avenue   Hackensack, NJ 07601   (201)996-5430   Fax (201)996-3676
+ Hackensack University Medical Center
30 Prospect Avenue/PediEmrg   Hackensack, NJ 07601   (201)996-5430   Fax (201)928-1967

Awad, Ahmed Sayed, MD {1396774626} Anesth(86,EGY04)<NJ-JRSYCITY>
+ Jersey City Medical Center
355 Grand Street/Anesthesiology   Jersey City, NJ 07304   (201)915-2000

Awad, Aida Fahmy, MD {1073683033} RadDia(81,EGY04)
+ 17 Th Street
Ridgefield Park, NJ 07660   (201)641-1747

Awad, Maher Bekheet, MD {1134106677} Psychy, PsyCAd, IntrMd(89,EGY05)
+ 1130 Highway 34
Aberdeen, NJ 07747   (732)591-9100   Fax (732)219-0814

Awad, Mona S., MD {1356405419} IntrMd, PulDis, CritCr(89,EGY05)<NJ-BAYSHORE, NJ-RIVERVW>
+ Drs. Awad and Hozayen
1 Bethany Road/Building 6   Hazlet, NJ 07730   (732)264-5005   Fax (732)264-1843

Awad, Nadia Amal, MD {1205065695} Surgry(09,NY45)
+ Cooper Surgical Associates
3 Cooper Plaza/Suite 403   Camden, NJ 08103   (856)342-2151   Fax (856)541-5379

Physicians by Name and Address

Awad, Safwat M., MD {1184668980} Urolgy, SrgUro(73,EGY03)<NJ-STJOSHOS, NJ-WAYNEGEN>
+ 599 Broadway/Suite 1-H
Paterson, NJ 07514   (973)345-1443
+ St. Joseph's Regional Medical Center
703 Main Street/Surgery   Paterson, NJ 07503   (973)754-2000

Awad, Sahar Fathi, MD {1114957909} Psychy(92,EGY05)
+ 1130 Highway 34
Aberdeen, NJ 07747   (732)970-6100

Awan, Omar Q., MD {1376819243} IntrMd
+ 42 Highview Drive
Woodbridge, NJ 07095   (732)397-6000

Awan, Rabia S., MD {1477618866} FamMed, Pedtrc(84,MEX34)<NJ-NWRKBETH, NJ-JFKMED>
+ 1503 Saint Georges Avenue/Suite 101
Colonia, NJ 07067   (732)499-9449   Fax (732)499-9505

Awan, Razia S., MD {1366428567} IntrMd(87,MEX34)<NJ-RBAYPERT, NJ-JFKMED>
+ 850 B Woodbridge Center Drive
Woodbridge, NJ 07095   (732)636-6366   Fax (732)750-4117
+ Center for Geriatric Health Care
156 Lyons Avenue   Newark, NJ 07112   (732)636-6366   Fax (973)923-6599

Awasthi, Ashish, MD {1033146618} CdvDis, IntCrd, IntrMd(92,INA92)
+ Heart Specialists/Central Jersey
901 West Main Street/Suite 205   Freehold, NJ 07728   (732)866-0800   Fax (732)463-6082

Awomolo, Adeola, MD {1013406818} Obstet
+ University Medical Group/OBGYN
125 Paterson Street/2nd Floor   New Brunswick, NJ 08901   (718)909-4661   Fax (732)235-6627

Awsare, Monica B., MD {1811940091} IntrMd, Gastrn(99,DC02)<NJ-DEBRAHLC, NJ-VIRTMHBC>
+ Gastroenterology Consultants of South Jersey
693 Main Street/Suite 2   Lumberton, NJ 08048   (609)265-1700   Fax (609)265-9005
+ Burlington County Endoscopy Center
140 Mount Holly Bypass/Unit 5   Lumberton, NJ 08048   (609)267-1555

Axelrod, Alexander, MD {1306934690} SrgCrC, SrgTrm, Surgry(85,MEXI)<NJ-COOPRUMC, NJ-ACMCITY>
+ Cooper University Hospital
One Cooper Plaza/CriticalCare   Camden, NJ 08103   (856)342-2000
+ Cooper Surgical Associates
3 Cooper Plaza/Suite 411   Camden, NJ 08103   (856)342-2000   Fax (856)365-1180

Axelrad, Paul R., MD {1689765620} IntrMd(85,GRNA)<NJ-KIMBALL, NJ-CENTRAST>
+ Drs. Axelrad & Zuckerbrod
4774 Route 9 South   Howell, NJ 07731   (732)363-6222   Fax (732)363-9203

Axelrod, Alyson Fincke, DO {1225272735} PhysMd, IntrMd(09,PA77)
+ Rothman Institute - Egg Harbor Township
2500 English Creek Avenue/Bldg 1300   Egg Harbor Township, NJ 08234   (609)677-6060   Fax (609)677-7000
+ Reconstructive Orthopedics, P.A.
401 Young Avenue/Suite 245   Moorestown, NJ 08057   (609)677-6060   Fax (609)267-9457

Axelrod, Howard Ian, MD {1093705014} SrgThr, Surgry(82,NY19)<NY-WESTCHMC, NJ-ACMCMAIN>
+ Cardiac Surgery Group PC
65 Jimmie Leeds Road   Pomona, NJ 08240   (609)748-7089   Fax (609)652-3460

Axelrod, Randi Allison, MD {1598711822} NnPnMd, Pedtrc(87,NY47)<NJ-CHSMRCER>
+ Capital Health System/Mercer Campus
446 Bellevue Avenue   Trenton, NJ 08618   (609)394-4144

Axelrod Malagold, Sara H., MD {1114412033} AlgyImmn
+ ENT & Allergy Associates
B-3 Cornwall Drive   East Brunswick, NJ 08816   (732)238-0300   Fax (732)238-4066

Axilrod, Andrew Charles, MD {1417903733} Urolgy(82,OH06)
+ Jersey Urology Group
403 Bethel Road   Somers Point, NJ 08244   (609)927-8746   Fax (609)601-1406

Ayad, Lydia, MD {1548623788} IntrMd<NJ-COMMED>
+ Community Medical Center
99 Route 37 West   Toms River, NJ 08755   (732)266-0553

Ayala, Omar, MD {1952573867} Psychy
+ Cooper Psychiatric Associates
3 Cooper Plaza/Suite 307   Camden, NJ 08103   (856)342-2328   Fax (856)541-6137

Ayangade, Tolulope, MD {1942630611} IntrMd<NJ-STPETER>
+ St. Peter's University Hospital
254 Easton Avenue   New Brunswick, NJ 08901   (732)745-8600

Aydin, Emmanuel A., MD {1174524045} IntrMd(86,TUR01)<NJ-WAYNEGEN, NJ-CHILTON>
+ Wayne Primary Care, P.A.
508 Hamburg Turnpike/Suite 102   Wayne, NJ 07470   (973)595-0096   Fax (973)595-6414

Aydin, Nebil Bill, MD {1073776589} Surgry, SrgPlstc, SrgRec(00,NY09)<NJ-HOLYNAME, NY-WESTCHMC>
+ Aydin Plastic Surgery PA
149 North Route 17/Suite 200   Paramus, NJ 07652   (201)345-0100   Fax (201)345-0333

Aydin, Steve M., DO {1104099910} PhysMd, PainMd(05,NJ75)
+ Kayal Orthopaedic Center, P.C.
784 Franklin Avenue/Suite 250   Franklin Lakes, NJ 07417   (844)281-1783   Fax (201)560-0712

Ayeni, Ahisu I., MD {1023050366} Pedtrc(82,NIG05)<NJ-HACKNSK, NY-STBARNAB>
+ Maan Pediatric Associates Inc
75 Clifton Avenue   Clifton, NJ 07011   (973)546-6400
+ Hackensack University Medical Center
30 Prospect Avenue/Pedi   Hackensack, NJ 07601   (201)996-2000

Ayeni, Eniola Teju, DO {1750627519} FamMed, IntrMd(12,PA77)<NJ-PALISADE>
+ Palisades Medical Center
7600 River Road   North Bergen, NJ 07047   (201)966-7975

Ayer, Uma, MD {1215183330} PthAcl, PthCyt(71,INA72)
+ Quest Diagnostics Inc.
1 Malcolm Avenue   Teterboro, NJ 07608   (201)393-5000   Fax (201)393-6127

Ayers, Charletta A., MD {1669483475} ObsGyn(89,PA13)<NJ-RWJUBRUN>
+ UH- Robert Wood Johnson Med
125 Paterson Street/CAB-OB/GYN   New Brunswick, NJ 08901   (732)235-6979   Fax (732)235-7349
+ University Medical Group/OBGYN
125 Paterson Street/2nd Floor   New Brunswick, NJ 08901   (732)235-6979   Fax (732)235-6627
+ RWJ University Hospital New Brunswick
One Robert Wood Johnson Place   New Brunswick, NJ 08901   (732)828-3000

Aygen, Kadri M., MD {1497723092} Pedtrc(92,TUR20)<NJ-MORRISTN>
+ Advocare Aygen Pediatrics and Adult Care
530 East Main Street   Chester, NJ 07930   (908)879-4300   Fax (908)879-8956

Aygen, Zehra Zeynep, MD {1760450266} Pedtrc(90,TURK)<NJ-MORRISTN>
+ Advocare Aygen Pediatrics and Adult Care
530 East Main Street   Chester, NJ 07930   (908)879-4300   Fax (908)879-8956

Ayodeji, Olutope O., MD {1972714004} Pedtrc(05,PA09)
+ Eastside Pediatrics
625 Broadway/1st Floor   Paterson, NJ 07514   (973)523-1102   Fax (973)523-7309

Ayoub, Hanan, MD {1225499569}
+ 14 Tindall Road
Middletown, NJ 07748   (732)671-3464   Fax (732)671-3444

Ayoub, Kasem, MD {1083964720} IntrMd
+ Valley Medical Group
470 North Franklin Turnpike   Ramsey, NJ 07446   (201)327-8765   Fax (201)327-8496

Ayoub, Samia B., MD {1376833848} Pedtrc(80,EGY08)<NJ-RIVERVW, NJ-BAYSHORE>
+ Ayoub Pediatrics PA
2080 Highway 35   Holmdel, NJ 07733   (732)671-0011   Fax (732)671-2564

Ayre, Kelly Anne Bianco, MD {1336438969}
+ IPC The Hospitalist Company
55 Madison Avenue/Suite 310   Morristown, NJ 07960   (973)993-9536   Fax (973)998-4237

Ayres, Brandon Daniel, MD {1710985460} Ophthl(00,NJ06)
+ Ophthalmic Partners of New Jersey
775 Route 70 East/Elmwood/Suite F 180   Marlton, NJ 08053   (856)596-1601   Fax (856)983-0396

Ayres, Julie Clarke, MD {1396708137} Pedtrc(99,NJ06)<NJ-NWRKBETH, NJ-UMDNJ>
+ Advocare South Jersey Pediatrics Cherry Hill
1949 Route 70 East/Suite 1 & 2   Cherry Hill, NJ 08003   (856)424-6050   Fax (856)424-2943
+ Advocare South Jersey Pediatrics Collingswood
204 White Horse Pike   Collingswood, NJ 08107   (856)424-6050   Fax (856)424-2943
+ Advocare Township Pediatrics
123 Egg Harbor Road   Sewell, NJ 08003   (856)227-5437   Fax (856)227-5890

Ayres, Ronald E., DO {1891765210} ObsGyn(68,PA77)<NJ-VIRTVOOR, NJ-JFKMED>
+ University Doctors
570 Egg Harbor Road/Suite C-2   Sewell, NJ 08080   (856)218-0300   Fax (856)589-9487
+ University Doctors-Ob Gyn
42 East Laurel Road/Suite 3500   Stratford, NJ 08084   (856)218-0300   Fax (856)566-6026

Ayub, Ayesha N., MD {1174887756}
+ 547 Oakridge Avenue
Plainfield, NJ 07063   (732)239-2405
ayeshaayub1@hotmail.com

Ayub, Muhammad G., MD {1710941836} IntrMd(89,PAKI)<NJ-NWRKBETH>
+ Newark Beth Israel Medical Center
201 Lyons Avenue/Suite L 4   Newark, NJ 07112   (973)926-7472   Fax (973)923-8063

Ayub, Nudrat F., MD {1346430774} IntrMd(99,PAK11)
+ 166 Lyons Avenue
Newark, NJ 07112   (973)926-3444   Fax (973)926-3934

Ayyad, Mina N., MD {1134622665} ObsGyn<NJ-MORRISTN>
+ Morristown Medical Center
100 Madison Avenue   Morristown, NJ 07962   (973)971-5000

Ayyagari, Kalavathi, MD {1851383798} ObsGyn(68,INA8Y)<NJ-STBARNMC>
+ 7 Lenape Road
Short Hills, NJ 07078   (973)761-8500   Fax (973)761-8910

Ayyagari, Kamalakar R., MD {1508858440} Surgry(68,INA83)<NJ-NWRKBETH>
+ 7 Lenapes Road
Short Hills, NJ 07078   (973)761-8500   Fax (973)761-8910

Ayyala, Manasa, MD {1255691234} IntrMd<NJ-UMDNJ>
+ University Hospital
150 Bergen Street/Suite H-245   Newark, NJ 07103   (973)972-5672

Ayyanathan, Karpukaras, MD {1083714273} Pedtrc(75,INA47)<NJ-JFKMED, NJ-TRINIWSC>
+ Linden Pediatric Group
517 Rahway Avenue   Elizabeth, NJ 07202   (908)527-1247   Fax (908)354-8822

Azam, Muhammad, MD {1407048135} FamMed
+ Princeton Health Medical & Surgical Associates
401 Ridge Road/Suite 6   Dayton, NJ 08810   (732)329-4800   Fax (732)329-0445

Azar, Jihad Elias, MD {1932737086} ObsGyn, FamMed<NJ-STJOSHOS>
+ St. Joseph's Regional Medical Center
703 Main Street/OB/GYN   Paterson, NJ 07503   (973)754-2700

Azar, Omar Philip, MD {1265737100} PthAcl, PthFor(05,GRN01)<NY-BLVUENYU>
+ Middlesex County-Medical Examiner
1490 Livingston Avenue/Suite 800   North Brunswick, NJ 08902   (732)745-3190   Fax (732)745-3491

Azaro, Katherine Frankel, MD {1770542821} Pedtrc, AdolMd(96,RI01)
+ New Jersey Labor Department
22 South Clinton Avenue   Trenton, NJ 08608   (609)292-0607

Azer, Amal W., MD {1629007919} PhysMd(75,EGY03)<NJ-BAYSHORE>
+ 8 Windswept Road
Holmdel, NJ 07733

Azer, Andrew Elia, MD {1235387507} Otlryg(NJ02<NJ-RBAYOLDB, NJ-JFKMED>
+ ENT & Allergy Associates, LLP
3663 Route 9 North/Suite102   Old Bridge, NJ 08857   (732)679-7575   Fax (732)707-3850
+ ENT & Allergy Associates, LLP
485 Route 1 South/Bld B/Suite 350   Iselin, NJ 08830   (732)679-7575   Fax (732)549-7250

Azer, George S., MD {1184776387} FamMed(75,EGYP)<NJ-JFKMED>
+ H 14 Brier Hill Court
East Brunswick, NJ 08816   (732)254-8804   Fax (732)254-8801

Azer, Wael A., DO {1841588241}<NJ-STJOSHOS>
+ St. Joseph's Regional Medical Center
703 Main Street   Paterson, NJ 07503   (973)754-2918

Azhak, Sameer Anor, MD {1073672085} IntrMd, CdvDis(02,GRN01)
+ Cardiology Consultants
246 Hamburg Turnpike/Suite 201   Wayne, NJ 07470   (973)942-1141   Fax (973)942-1250

Azhar, Sana H., MD {1508264896} IntrMd
+ Medical Care Associates
137 Mountain Avenue   Hackettstown, NJ 07840   (908)852-1887   Fax (908)852-0614

Physicians by Name and Address

Azhar, Sarwat, MD {1518050871} Pedtrc(84,PAKI)<NJ-JFKMED>
+ All Pediatric Care, P.A.
179 Main Street   Woodbridge, NJ 07095   (732)634-3388   Fax (732)634-9055
Sarwat0211@aol.com
+ Pediatric Care PA
984 Route 9 South/Suite 3   Parlin, NJ 08859   (732)634-3388   Fax (732)727-1887
+ Pediatric Care P.A.
3342 Kennedy Boulevard   Jersey City, NJ 07095   (201)653-8999   Fax (201)653-4477

Aziz, Khalid M., MD {1821320276} Pedtrc
+ Urgent Care of New Jersey
2090 Route 27   Edison, NJ 08817   (732)662-5650   Fax (732)662-5651

Aziz, Rania, MD {1922335298} Anesth
+ Rutgers- New Jersey Medical School
185 South Orange Avenue/MSB E538   Newark, NJ 07103   (973)972-5007   Fax (973)972-0582

Aziz, Shahid Rahim, MD {1356303044} SrgO&M(99,NY01)
+ University Hospital-Doctors Office Center
90 Bergen Street/Suite 7700   Newark, NJ 07103   (973)972-2444

Azizi, Azin, MD {1437240991} Pedtrc(96,IRA10)
+ Hackensack Pediatrics
177 Summit Avenue   Hackensack, NJ 07601   (201)487-8222   Fax (201)487-2126

Azmi Ghadimi, Hooman, MD {1245389931} SrgNro(99,NY09)
+ North Jersey Brain and Surgical
680 Kinderkamack Road/Suite 300   Oradell, NJ 07649   (201)342-2550   Fax (201)342-7171

Azmy, Sherin, MD {1295069680}<NJ-STJOSHOS>
+ St. Joseph's Regional Medical Center
703 Main Street   Paterson, NJ 07503   (973)754-2000

Aznavoorian, Martin Peter, MD {1073662102} Anesth(00,AST11)
+ Progressive Diagnostic Imaging
44 Route 23 North   Riverdale, NJ 07457   (973)839-5004   Fax (973)839-5006

Azoulai, Jonathan Guy, MD {1013150044} EmrgMd<NJ-TRINI-WSC>
+ Trinitas Regional Medical Center-Williamson Street
225 Williamson Street   Elizabeth, NJ 07207   (908)994-5000

Azu, Michelle C., MD {1316105711} Surgry, SrgOnc, IntrMd(03,MO03)<NJ-CHILTON>
+ Chilton Medical Center
97 West Parkway/Surgery   Pompton Plains, NJ 07444   (973)831-5056   Fax (973)907-1084

Azu, Wilhelmina Dedo, DO {1164639217} ObsGyn
+ North Dover Ob-Gyn Associates
222 Oak Avenue/3rd Floor/Suite 301   Toms River, NJ 08753   (732)914-1919   Fax (732)914-0210

Azzam, Moh'D Hazem K., MD {1902185135}
+ St. Joseph Medical Center Surgery
703 Main Street   Paterson, NJ 07503   (973)754-2476
+ St. Michael's Medical Center
111 Central Avenue   Newark, NJ 07102   (732)997-9135

Azzariti, John, Jr., MD {1972541787} Anesth(92,NJ05)<NJ-VALLEY>
+ The Valley Hospital
223 North Van Dien Avenue   Ridgewood, NJ 07450   (201)447-8000

Babalola, Gbolagade Olanrewaju, DO {1952301681} ObsGyn(00,NJ75)<NJ-SJHREGMC>
+ Drs. Babalola and Giyanani
1601 North 2nd Street/Suite C1   Millville, NJ 08332   (856)691-3145   Fax (856)691-0625

Babalola, Ronke Latifatu, MD {1487936712} Psychy, PsyCAd(02,DOM18)
+ University Medical Group/UMDNJ
125 Paterson Street/Suite 2200   New Brunswick, NJ 08901   (732)235-7647   Fax (732)235-7617

Babar, Jawad, MD {1336300516}<NJ-ACMCITY>
+ AtlantiCare Regional Medical Center/City Campus
1925 Pacific Avenue   Atlantic City, NJ 08401   (609)441-8960

Babaria, Bhavikaben Bhavin, MD {1912227414} IntrMd
+ 110 Magnolia Road
Iselin, NJ 08830   (732)906-1384

Babayants, Alexander R., MD {1194779371} Psychy(78,RUS57)<NJ-CLARMAAS, NJ-STMICHL>
+ St. Michael's Medical Center
111 Central Avenue/Floor 8   Newark, NJ 07102   (973)465-2681   Fax (973)218-1868

Babayev, Lily L., MD {1851307136} IntrMd(85,AZE01)<NJ-OCEANMC>
+ Brick Town Medical
34 Lanes Mill Road   Brick, NJ 08724   (732)458-0300   Fax (732)458-8449

Babbar, Puneet, MD {1992776827} FamMed, IntrMd(97,DMN01)<NJ-NWRKBETH, NJ-RBAYPERT>
+ JRMC at Dayton Street Elementary School
25 Dayton Street   Newark, NJ 07114   (973)679-7709   Fax (973)824-5652
+ JRMC at Malcolm X Shabazz High School
80 Johnson Avenue   Newark, NJ 07108   (973)679-7709   Fax (973)623-8938
+ JRMC at Pace Health Center
415 Fayette Street   Perth Amboy, NJ 07114   (732)324-0500   Fax (732)324-0529

Babcock, Karen R., MD {1548280159} Pedtrc(93,NJ06)
+ St. Peter's Adult Family Health Center
123 How Lane   New Brunswick, NJ 08901   (732)745-8600   Fax (732)745-2344

Babeendran, Shan, DO {1528379062} FamMed, PhysMd(10,PA77)<NY-NYUTISCH>
+ Physical Medicine & Rehabilitation Center
500 Grand Avenue/1st Floor   Englewood, NJ 07631   (201)567-2277   Fax (201)567-7506

Babiak, Eugenia T., MD {1568400752} IntrMd, PulDis(72,POL03)<NJ-COMMED, NJ-KIMBALL>
+ 1163 Route 37 West
Toms River, NJ 08755   (732)505-0100   Fax (732)505-6680

Babich, Jay Paul, MD {1275862732} IntrMd, Gastrn(04,ISR06)<NJ-VALLEYHS>
+ Gastrointestinal Associates PA
140 Chestnut Street/Suite 300   Ridgewood, NJ 07450   (201)444-2600   Fax (201)444-9471

Babin, Elizabeth Ann, MD {1518924133} ObsGyn, UroGyn(99,AZ01)<NJ-KENEDYHS, NJ-VIRTUAHS>
+ New Jersey Urology, LLC
2401 East Evesham Road/Suite F   Voorhees, NJ 08043   (856)374-1377   Fax (856)374-2177
urogyngirl@gmail.com

Babineau, Shannon Elizabeth, MD {1538370630} Nrolgy, Pedtrc(06,NJ06)<NJ-MORRISTN>
+ Morristown Medical Center
100 Madison Avenue/Box 24   Morristown, NJ 07962   (973)971-5700   Fax (973)290-7417

Babott, Doreen, MD {1982634861} OncHem, MedOnc, IntrMd(70,NY15)<NJ-UNVMCPRN>
+ Princeton Medicine
5 Plainsboro Road/Suite 300/Lambert   Plainsboro, NJ 08536   (609)853-7272   Fax (609)430-7159
+ University Medical Center of Princeton at Plainsboro
One Plainsboro Road/2nd Floor   Plainsboro, NJ 08536   (609)853-7272   Fax (609)853-7271

Babu, Sarath, MD {1992744767} IntrMd(91,INDI)<NJ-CENTRAST, NJ-KIMBALL>
+ Medcenter
608 North High Street   Millville, NJ 08332   (856)825-8080

Babury, Rahima A., MD {1699718478} PthACl, PthCyt(81,AFG03)<NJ-HOLYNAME>
+ Holy Name Hospital
718 Teaneck Road/Pathology   Teaneck, NJ 07666   (201)833-3021   Fax (201)833-3758

Baby, Benesa, MD {1528491024} IntHos<NJ-ACMCITY>
+ AtlantiCare Regional Medical Center/City Campus
1925 Pacific Avenue   Atlantic City, NJ 08401   (609)441-8146

Bacal, Diana Ioanna, MD {1265846539} IntrMd<NJ-KMHSTRAT>
+ Kennedy Memorial Hospital-University Medical Center
18 East Laurel Road   Stratford, NJ 08084   (856)513-4124

Bacani, Victor O., MD {1932181351} CdvDis, IntrMd(80,PHIL)
+ 19 Mule Road/C7
Toms River, NJ 08755   (732)557-4488   Fax (732)557-4617

Bacarro, Arnold S., MD {1649259250} IntrMd(94,GRN01)<NJ-SHOREMEM>
+ 5429 Harding Highway/Suite 301
Mays Landing, NJ 08330   (609)625-4430   Fax (609)625-4436
Arnoldbacarro@aol.com

Bacchus, Bebi Samantha, MD {1689606915} Pedtrc(94,NJ06)<NJ-KMHTURNV>
+ Advocare Woolwich Pediatrics
300 Lexington Road/Suite 200   Woolwich Township, NJ 08085   (856)241-2111   Fax (856)241-2243

Bach, John R., MD {1295749422} PhysMd(76,NJ05)<NJ-UMDNJ>
+ University Hospital
150 Bergen Street/PhysMd/Rehab   Newark, NJ 07103   (973)972-7195   Fax (973)972-5725
bachjr@umdnj.edu
+ Rutgers-Department of Physical Med
183 South Orange Ave/Suite F-1555   Newark, NJ 07101   (973)972-3606

Bach, Mark A., MD {1225283310} PedEnd, EnDbMt, Rserch(85,TX04)
+ Merck and Company Incorporated
126 East Lincoln Avenue   Rahway, NJ 07065   (732)574-4000

Bach, Matt, MD {1639143951} CdvDis, IntCrd, IntrMd(84,NJ05)<NJ-JRSYSHMC, NJ-CENTRAST>
+ Monmouth Cardiology Associates, LLC
11 Meridian Road   Eatontown, NJ 07724   (732)663-0300   Fax (732)663-0301
+ Monmouth Cardiology Associates, LLC
222 Schanck Road/Suite 104   Freehold, NJ 07728   (732)663-0300   Fax (732)431-1712

Bach, Nancy, MD {1477571115} Nephro, IntrMd, Gastrn(84,NY06)<NY-MTSINAI>
+ Recanti/Miller Transplantation Institute-Eatontown
10 Industrial Way Easy/Suite 101   Eatontown, NJ 07724   (212)241-0034   Fax (212)289-7738

Bach, Richard Tae, MD {1386744167} PhysMd(96,NJ05)<NJ-MTN-SIDE, NJ-STBARNMC>
+ North Atlantic Rehab Medicine
799 Bloomfield Avenue/Suite 303   Verona, NJ 07044   (973)857-7800   Fax (973)857-7822

Bach, Tami L., MD {1306887245} IntrMd, Hemato(98,PA02)<NJ-UNDRWD, NJ-SJRSYELM>
+ The Minniti Center for Medical Oncology & Hematology
174 Democrat Road   Mickleton, NJ 08056   (856)423-0754

Bacha, David M., DO {1629179007} Pedtrc(78,PA77)<NJ-ENGLWOOD, NJ-HACKNSK>
+ 340 Tenafly Road
Tenafly, NJ 07670   (201)569-4477   Fax (201)569-7196

Bachar, Jean A., MD {1437318334} PhysMd, IntrMd(07,NY06)<NJ-MMHKEMBL>
+ Morristown Memorial Hospital/Mt. Kemble Division
95 Mount Kemble Avenue/Phys Rehab   Morristown, NJ 07960   (973)796-3600

Bacharach, Moshe, MD {1710943931} CdvDis, IntrMd(77,ISR06)
+ Ocean Cardiology
1166 River Avenue   Lakewood, NJ 08701   (732)905-4142   Fax (732)905-4160

Bachman, Daniel, MD {1811263791}
+ Morristown Cardiology Associates, P.A.
435 South Street/Suite 100   Morristown, NJ 07960   (973)267-3944   Fax (973)455-0399

Bachman, Jodie Ann, DO {1952697070} Ortped(11,NJ75)
+ Center for Orthopaedics
1500 Pleasant Valley Way/Suite 101   West Orange, NJ 07052   (973)669-5600   Fax (973)669-0269

Bachman, Joyce Adele, MD {1144402314} OccpMd, IntrMd(77,CO02)
+ Prudential Financial
290 West Mount Pleasant Avenue   Livingston, NJ 07039   (973)992-6363

Bachman, Michael Craig, MD {1699728832} Pedtrc(98,ISR02)<NJ-CHDNWBTH, NJ-NWRKBETH>
+ Children's Hospital of New Jersey
201 Lyons Avenue/Osborne Terrace   Newark, NJ 07112   (973)926-7000   Fax (610)617-6280

Bachmann, Gloria A., MD {1336214535} ObsGyn, IntrMd(74,PA01)<NJ-STPETER, NJ-RWJUBRUN>
+ UMDNJ OBGYN
125 Paterson Street/Suite 4200   New Brunswick, NJ 08901   (732)235-6600   Fax (732)235-6650
+ UMDNJ RWJ Clinical Genetics
125 Paterson Street/Suite 4200   New Brunswick, NJ 08901   (732)235-6600   Fax (732)235-6650
+ UMDNJ RWJ Maternal Fetal Medicine
125 Paterson Street/Suite 4200   New Brunswick, NJ 08901   (732)235-6600   Fax (732)235-6564

Bachrach, Stacey R., MD {1508936428} FamMed, GenPrc, IntrMd(81,PA12)<NJ-HUNTRDN>
+ Cornerstone Family Practice
9100 Wescott Drive/Suite 103   Flemington, NJ 08822   (908)788-6473   Fax (908)948-1046

Back, Lyle M., MD {1639172679} SrgPlstc, Surgry(84,NJ06)<NJ-KMHCHRRY>
+ Cosmetic Surgery Center of Cherry Hill
1942 Route 70 East   Cherry Hill, NJ 08003   (856)751-7550   Fax (856)751-7544
info@lylemback.md
+ Cosmetic Skin Care Specialists of Cherry Hill
1944 Route 70 East   Cherry Hill, NJ 08003   (856)751-7550   Fax (856)751-7544
+ Centennial Surgical Center LLC
502 Centennial Boulevard/Suite 1   Voorhees, NJ 08003   (856)874-0790

Back, Norman A., MD {1528055266} ObsGyn(84,ISRA)<NJ-CENTRAST>
+ Back, Seigel & Goldstein, MD, PA
501 Iron Bridge Road   Freehold, NJ 07728   (732)431-1807   Fax (732)409-2777
nback@optonline.net

Back, Steven Marc, MD {1376572875} Anesth(99,IL06)<NJ-UNVMCPRN>
+ Anesthesia Consultnts of NJ/Nova Pain
285 Davidson Avenue/Suite 204   Somerset, NJ 08873   (732)271-1400   Fax (732)271-3544

Physicians by Name and Address

Backal, Marc Ira, MD {1922057231} AdolMd, Pedtrc(92,VA04)<NJ-VIRTUAHS, NJ-VIRTMARL>
+ Advocare Laurel Pediatrics
269 Fish Pond Road   Sewell, NJ 08080   (856)863-9999   Fax (856)863-9666
+ Advocare Greentree Pediatrics
127 Church Road/Suite 800   Marlton, NJ 08053   (856)863-9999   Fax (856)988-9499

Backus, Yolanda Alicia, MD {1417185224} FamMed
+ McGuire Air Force Base/Acute Health Care Clinic
3458 Neely Road   Trenton, NJ 08641   (609)754-9068   Fax (609)754-9015

Bacon, Shoshana, MD {1457791428}
+ Chemed Family Health Center
1771 Madison Avenue   Lakewood, NJ 08701   (732)364-2144   Fax (732)364-3559

Bada, Laureto, Jr., MD {1861408593} Anesth(76,PHIL)<NJ-CLARMAAS>
+ Clara Maass Medical Center
1 Clara Maass Drive/Anesthesiology   Belleville, NJ 07109   (973)450-2000

Badach, Mark J., MD {1801891239} Anesth, PainMd(83,ITA17)<NJ-STJOSHOS>
+ St. Joseph's Regional Medical Center
703 Main Street/Anesth   Paterson, NJ 07503   (973)754-2000   Fax (973)977-9455

Badalamenti, Stephanie Silos, MD {1730273368} Dermat(96,PA02)
+ Center for Dermatology PA
128 Columbia Turnpike/Suite 200   Florham Park, NJ 07932   (973)736-9535   Fax (973)736-2607

Badami, Chirag Dilip, MD {1407001175} SrgThr<NY-GOODSAM>
+ St. Joseph Medical Center Surgery
703 Main Street   Paterson, NJ 07503   (973)754-2486

Badami, Geeta D., MD {1720057144} Pedtrc, AdolMd(73,INDI)<NJ-BAYSHORE, NJ-RIVERVW>
+ 601 Lloyd Road
Matawan, NJ 07747   (732)290-9192

Baddi, Anoosha, DO {1235519505} Pedtrc
+ University Medical Group Pediatrics
125 Paterson Street/MEB 3rd Fl   New Brunswick, NJ 08903   (732)235-7883   Fax (732)235-7345

Baddoo, Andrew O., MD {1881653608} IntrMd, Nephro(98,NJ06)
+ Pierre Medical Group LLC
745 Northfield Avenue   West Orange, NJ 07052   (973)731-3800   Fax (973)731-3881

Baddoura, Rashid Joseph, MD {1962451872} EmrgMd, IntrMd, PulDis(74,LEBA)<NJ-VALLEY>
+ Valley Emergency Room Associates
61 North Maple Avenue/Suite 302   Ridgewood, NJ 07450   (201)447-8318   Fax (201)689-9210
+ The Valley Hospital
223 North Van Dien Avenue/EmergMed   Ridgewood, NJ 07450   (201)447-8318   Fax (201)689-9210

Baddoura, Walid J., MD {1043253578} Gastrn, IntrMd(76,LEBA)<NJ-STJOSHOS>
+ 716 Broad Street
Clifton, NJ 07013   (973)777-7733   Fax (973)777-0669

Bade, Harry, III, MD {1508843624} SprtMd, SrgOrt(76,PA02)<NJ-RIVERVW, NJ-MONMOUTH>
+ Professional Orthopaedic Associates
776 Shrewsbury Avenue/Suite 201   Tinton Falls, NJ 07724   (732)530-4949   Fax (732)530-3618
+ Professional Orthopaedic Associates
1430 Hooper Avenue/Suite 101   Toms River, NJ 08753   (732)530-4949   Fax (732)349-7722
+ Professional Orthopaedic Associates
303 West Main Street   Freehold, NJ 07728   (732)530-4949   Fax (732)577-0036

Bader, Christopher William, DO {1447406913} FamMed, IntHos
+ Hospital Medicine Associates
157 Broad Street/Suite 317   Red Bank, NJ 07701   (732)530-2960   Fax (732)530-7446

Badillo, Arthur, MD {1770635484} IntrMd(83,DOMI)<NJ-CLARMAAS, NJ-MONMOUTH>
+ 643-645 Mt. Prospect Avenue
Newark, NJ 07104   (973)484-5607   Fax (973)484-6958

Badin, Diane, MD {1750772539} IntrMd
+ Drs. Badin, De Silva, and Perera
1947 Kennedy Boulevard   Jersey City, NJ 07305   (201)433-4848   Fax (201)946-9292

Badin, Michel S., MD {1750305389} IntrMd, OncHem(72,SYRI)<NJ-CHRIST>
+ Drs. Badin, De Silva, and Perera
1947 Kennedy Boulevard   Jersey City, NJ 07305   (201)433-4848   Fax (201)946-9292

Badin, Simon, MD {1467699405} OncHem
+ Drs. Badin, De Silva, and Perera
1947 Kennedy Boulevard   Jersey City, NJ 07305   (201)433-4848   Fax (201)360-0159

Badolato, Joseph Nunzio, DO {1922394576} IntHos, IntrMd(FL75<NJ-KMHTURNV>
+ Kennedy Health Systems/Washington Township Campus
435 Hurffville-Cross Keys Road   Turnersville, NJ 08012   (856)582-2500
+ 900 Medical Center Drive/Suite 211
Sewell, NJ 08080   (856)582-2500   Fax (856)218-5664

Badolato, Kevin Arthur, MD {1104137686} Pedtrc(07,PA13)<MASTLUKES>
+ CAMCare Health Corporation
817 Federal Street/Suite 300   Camden, NJ 08103   (856)583-2415   Fax (856)541-4611

Badr, Amel Afifi, MD {1528262904} Psychy(92,EGY03)<NJ-BERGNMC, NJ-STJOSHOS>
+ 50 Market Street/Suite 2
Saddle Brook, NJ 07663   (201)257-8091

Badr, Samer, MD {1215191556} IntrMd<NJ-COOPRUMC>
+ Cooper University Hospital
One Cooper Plaza/Dorrance 222   Camden, NJ 08103   (856)342-3150   Fax (856)968-8418

Badri, Ahmad, DO {1790047959} SprtMd
+ One Oak Medical
342 Hamburg Turnpike/Suite 202   Wayne, NJ 07470   (973)870-0777

Badri, M. Maher Ahmad, MD {1982785085} IntrMd(78,SYR02)<NJ-PALISADE, NJ-MEADWLND>
+ Ridgefield Medical Services LLC
8915 Bergenwood Avenue/Suite 3   North Bergen, NJ 07047   (201)295-1616   Fax (201)295-0032
maherbadrimd@aol.com

Bae, Hyun, MD {1649602509}<NJ-ENGLWOOD>
+ Englewood Hospital and Medical Center
350 Engle Street   Englewood, NJ 07631   (201)894-3000

Bae, Samuel Y., MD {1760443139} Gastrn, Hepato, IntrMd(94,NY08)<NJ-HUNTRDN>
+ Hunterdon Gastroenterology Associates, P.A.
1100 Wescott Drive/Suite 206-207   Flemington, NJ 08822   (908)483-4000   Fax (908)788-5090
+ Hunterdon Gastroenterology Associates, P.A.
135 West End Avenue/Suite 204   Somerville, NJ 08876   (908)483-4000   Fax (908)788-5090

Baek, Jennie Hyojin, MD {1215139480}
+ 244 Spruce Street
Haddonfield, NJ 08033   (215)200-3943
jennie.h.baek@gmail.com

Baer, Aryeh Zvi, MD {1104863976} IntrMd, Pedtrc, PedInf(97,NJ05)<NJ-HACKNSK, NJ-UMDNJ>
+ Hackensack University Medical Center
30 Prospect Avenue   Hackensack, NJ 07601   (201)996-2000

Baerga, Edgardo, MD {1912957895} PhysMd(96,PRO02)<NJ-RHBHTNTN, NJ-OCEANMC>
+ The Rehab Hosp of Tinton Falls
2 Centre Plaza   Tinton Falls, NJ 07724   (732)460-5360   Fax (732)460-7442

Baez, Juan Carlos, MD {1073505061} InfDis, IntrMd(91,COL08)
+ Medical Diagnostic Associates PA
525 Central Avenue/Suite D   Westfield, NJ 07090   (908)232-5333   Fax (908)389-1933
+ Medical Diagnostic Associates, P.A.
1801 East Second Street/Suite 1   Scotch Plains, NJ 07076   (908)232-5333   Fax (908)322-0191
+ Millburn Family Practice
425 Essex Street   Millburn, NJ 07090   (973)379-3051

Baez, Rafael M., MD {1750459582} Psychy
+ 2250 Chapel Avenue
Cherry Hill, NJ 08002   Fax (856)482-1159

Baffo, Aileen, MD {1457840365} ObsGyn<NJ-RWJUBRUN>
+ RWJ University Hospital New Brunswick
One Robert Wood Johnson Place   New Brunswick, NJ 08901   (732)828-3000

Bagade, Vivek Laxman, MD {1760650394} CdvDis, IntrMd(81,INA69)
+ Hackensack University Medical Group Emerson
452 Old Hook Road/2nd Floor   Emerson, NJ 07630   (201)666-3900   Fax (201)261-0505

Bagan, Stanley L., MD {1790739621} IntrMd(72,MEX14)<NJ-MEMSALEM>
+ Internal Medicine Associates
201 Laurel Heights Drive/Suite 201   Bridgeton, NJ 08302   (856)455-4800   Fax (856)455-0650

Bagaria, Surendra K., MD {1346232105} CdvDis, CritCr, IntrMd(79,INA49)
+ South Jersey Heart Group
539 Egg Harbor Road/Suite 1   Sewell, NJ 08080   (856)589-0300   Fax (856)589-1753
+ South Jersey Heart Group
181 West Whitehorse Pike/Suite 201   Berlin, NJ 08009   (856)589-0300   Fax (856)768-3371

Bagay, Leslie, MD {1265712038} PhysMd<NJ-JFKJHNSN>
+ JFK Johnson Rehabilitation Institute
65 James Street   Edison, NJ 08818   (732)321-7070   Fax (732)321-7330

Bagchi, Sonali, MD {1841363181} IntrMd(87,INA56)<NJ-ANCPSYCH>
+ Ancora Psychiatric Hospital
301 Spring Garden Road/InternalMed   Hammonton, NJ 08037   (609)561-1700   Fax (609)567-7318

Bagchi, Sudarshan, MD {1942360243} Psychy, PsyGrt(84,INDI)<NJ-ANCPSYCH>
+ Ancora Psychiatric Hospital
301 Spring Garden Road   Hammonton, NJ 08037   (609)561-1700

Bageac, Michael, MD {1811984701} CdvDis, IntrMd(82,ROMA)
+ Toms River Cardiology Associates, LLP.
780 Route 37 West/Suite 310   Toms River, NJ 08755   (732)240-0599   Fax (732)240-3039

Bagel, Jerry, MD {1992772156} Dermat(81,NY47)
+ Windsor Dermatology
59 One Mile Road Extension/Suite G   East Windsor, NJ 08520   (609)443-4500   Fax (609)426-0530

Bagga, Harpreet Kaur, MD {1972682938} FamMed(99,INA03)
+ Hillsborough Medical Associates
349 US Highway 206 South   Hillsborough, NJ 08844
+ Lakeview Medical Associates
125 US Highway 46   Budd Lake, NJ 07828   Fax (973)691-1198

Baghal, Eyad Y., MD {1093763039} Gastrn, IntrMd(87,IRAQ)<NJ-TRINIWSC, NJ-STJOSHOS>
+ Millenium Gastroenterology, P.C.
397 Haledon Avenue/Suite 103   Haledon, NJ 07508   (973)782-4872   Fax (973)782-4873
+ Millenium Gastroenterology, P.C.
695 Chestnut Street   Union, NJ 07083   (973)782-4872   Fax (973)782-4873

Baghal, Imad Y., MD {1972526606} SrgOrt(75,IRAQ)<NJ-PALISADE>
+ 7500 Kennedy Boulevard
North Bergen, NJ 07047   (201)662-8455   Fax (201)868-1905

Bagherian, Sharareh, DO {1912961582} ObsGyn(93,NY75)
+ Womens Health Care Associates of Sussex County
135 Newton Sparta Road/Suite 201   Newton, NJ 07860   (973)383-8555   Fax (973)383-8424
+ Womens Health Care Associates of Sussex County
123 Route 94/Suite 200   Vernon, NJ 07462   (973)383-8555   Fax (973)827-4441

Bagley, Michael P., MD {1790703486} Dermat(82,NJ06)
+ Dermatology Associates-Warren
122 Mount Bethel Road   Warren, NJ 07059   (908)756-7999   Fax (908)756-8017

Bagloo, Melissa Bahareh, MD {1407016108} Surgry(04,FL03)<NY-PRSBCOLU, NJ-VALLEY>
+ Ctr for Metabolic & Weight Loss Surgry
579 Franklin Turnpike   Ridgewood, NJ 07450   (201)251-3480

Bagnell, James P., MD {1437190782} EmrgMd(78,DC02)<NJ-SOCEANCO>
+ Urgent Care Now
712 East Bay Avenue/Suite 22-B   Manahawkin, NJ 08050   (609)978-0242   Fax (609)978-0241

Bagner, Ronald J., MD {1285790600} Surgry(74,MO34)<NJ-RWJUBRUN>
+ 8B Auer Court/Williamsburg Commons
East Brunswick, NJ 08816   (732)390-0073

Bahadur, Kandy, MD {1548792898} Pedtrc
+ University Medical Group Pediatrics
125 Paterson Street/MEB 3rd Fl   New Brunswick, NJ 08903   (732)235-7883   Fax (732)235-7345

Bahal, Vishal, DO {1831122704} IntrMd, CdvDis(93,PA77)
+ 4 Burton Lane/Suite 100
Mullica Hill, NJ 08062   (856)241-3838   Fax (856)241-3849

Baher, Ali Masih, DO {1972160885} FamMed
+ SJH Medical Center Family Medicine
1505 West Sherman Avenue   Vineland, NJ 08360   (856)641-8000

Bahler, Alan S., MD {1891772893} CdvDis, IntrMd(71,NY20)
+ 201 South Livingston Avenue/Suite 2F
Livingston, NJ 07039   (973)535-9292   Fax (973)535-9293

Bahler, Emily Susan, DO {1346229598} IntrMd, Grtrcs(00,NY75)
+ 201 South Livingston Avenue/Suite 2F
Livingston, NJ 07039   (973)535-9294   Fax (973)535-9293

Bahora, Masuma, MD {1912303033} ObsGyn
+ Cooper University Hospital OBGYN
3 Cooper Plaza/Suite 221   Camden, NJ 08103   (314)369-4045   Fax (856)968-8575

Bahramipour, Phillip F., MD {1154356798} RadNro, RadBdI(90,NJ05)
+ Robert and Audrey Luckow Pavilion
One Valley Health Plaza/Ste B 2010   Paramus, NJ 07652   (201)634-5590   Fax (201)986-4705

Physicians by Name and Address

Bahrampour, Ladan Haghighatjoo, MD {1003877622} IntrMd(94,IRA01)<NJ-STJOSHOS>
+ St. Joseph's Regional Medical Center
  703 Main Street   Paterson, NJ 07503   (973)754-2000
+ The Valley Hospital
  223 North Van Dien Avenue   Ridgewood, NJ 07450   (201)447-8000

Bai, Flora, MD {1740250141} IntrMd(93,CHN4A)<NJ-RIVERVW>
+ Arthritis & Rheumatism Institute
  2163 Oak Tree Road/Suite 103   Edison, NJ 08820
  (908)754-4900   Fax (908)754-4901

Bai, Sammy S., MD {1386716579} IntrMd
+ 2486 Fifth Street
  Fort Lee, NJ 07024

Baig, Khadija, MD {1063404432} IntrMd(93,PAK11)
+ 950 Stanton Avenue/2nd Floor
  Elizabeth, NJ 07208

Baig, Nadeem A., MD {1770682668} Gastrn, Hepato, IntrMd(95,PA02)<NJ-JRSYSHMC>
+ Monmouth Gastroenterology
  142 Route 35   Eatontown, NJ 07724   (732)389-5004   Fax (732)389-1850

Baig, Rifaqat, MD {1194046490} FamMed(07,GRN01)
+ Manalapan Urgent Care
  120 Craig Road   Manalapan, NJ 07726   (732)414-2991   Fax (732)414-2995

Baig, Sumeera Akhtar, MD {1124076617} IntrMd(94,VA04)
+ RWJ Medical Associates
  3100 Quakerbridge Road/Suite 28   Hamilton, NJ 08619
  (609)245-7430   Fax (609)245-7432

Baig, Zahid Imran, MD {1356325088} IntrMd, Gastrn(88,PAK10)<NJ-RWJUHAM, NJ-STFRNMED>
+ Hamilton Gastroenterology Group, PC
  1374 Whitehorse Hamilton Squar   Trenton, NJ 08690
  (609)586-1319   Fax (609)586-1468

Baigel, Colin, MD {1578689089} OccpMd, FamMed, GPrvMd(74,SAF02)
+ Bristol-Myers Squibb Co. - Occupational Health
  Route 206 & Provinceline Road   Princeton, NJ 08543
  (609)252-4000

Baik, Seoung W., MD {1902877327} Gastrn, IntrMd(79,KOR04)<NJ-JFKMED, NJ-RWJURAH>
+ Gastroenterology Associates of Central Jersey, PA
  1921 Oak Tree Road/Suite 101   Edison, NJ 08820
  (732)744-9090   Fax (732)744-1592
+ SW Baikm MD PA
  1608 Lemoine Avenue   Fort Lee, NJ 07024   (732)744-9090   Fax (201)482-0664

Bailey, Aisha Donine, DO {1750645255} Pedtrc<NJ-KMHSTRAT>
+ Advocare Marlton Pediatrics
  525 Route 73 South   Marlton, NJ 08053   (856)596-3434   Fax (856)596-9110

Bailey, James William, DO {1912226788} PhysMd(10,PA77)
+ University Pain Care Center
  42 East Laurel Road/Suite 1700   Stratford, NJ 08084
  (856)566-7010   Fax (856)566-6956

Bailey, Keneisha Renata, MD {1376817528}<NJ-NWRKBETH>
+ Newark Beth Israel Medical Center
  201 Lyons Avenue/Suite C4   Newark, NJ 07112   (973)926-7828

Bailey, Philip Daniel, Jr., DO {1538149810} Anesth, PedAne(97,ME75)
+ CHOP Pediatric & Adolescent Specialty Care Center
  1012 Laurel Oak Road   Voorhees, NJ 08043   (856)435-1300   Fax (856)435-0091

Bailon, Amy R., MD {1326397803} Pedtrc, AdolMd(63,PHI29)
+ 21 Woodbine Road
  Florham Park, NJ 07932   (973)966-1446   Fax (973)966-1446

Bain, Francis Jerome-Xavier, MD {1174537898} FamMed, Grtrcs(79,NJ05)<NJ-CHILTON>
+ Alps Family Physicians
  1500 Alps Road   Wayne, NJ 07470   (973)628-8500   Fax (973)628-7944

Bains, Ashish P. S., MD {1215078415} PthACl
+ 1945 Highway 33
  Neptune, NJ 07753

Bains, Yatinder, MD {1205908118} Gastrn(87,NJ06)<NJ-CLARMAAS, NJ-EASTORNG>
+ 116 Millburn Avenue/Suite 214
  Millburn, NJ 07041   (973)346-2121   Fax (973)467-0150

Baione, William A., MD {1871804211}<NJ-RWJUBRUN>
+ University Orthopaedic Associates, LLC.
  Two Worlds Fair Drive   Somerset, NJ 08873   (732)979-2115   Fax (732)564-9032
+ RWJ University Hospital New Brunswick
  One Robert Wood Johnson Place   New Brunswick, NJ 08901
  (732)979-2115   Fax (732)938-5680

Baird, Cynthia Marlo, MD {1902928435} AlcSub, PubHth, OccpMd(88,TX16)
+ Growth and Recovery Services
  2001 Lincoln Drive West/Suiet A   Marlton, NJ 08053
  (856)663-3000   Fax (856)488-2277

Baird, Evan Oliver, MD {1114151396} SrgOrt(09,SC01)
+ Comprehensive Spine Care, PA
  260 Old Hook Road/Suite 400   Emerson, NJ 07630
  (201)634-1811   Fax (201)634-9170

Baird, James Few, IV, DO {1548497621} EmrgMd(09,PA77)<NJ-KMHTURNV>
+ Emergency Physician Associates, P.A.
  307 South Evergreen Avenue/PO Box 298   Woodbury, NJ 08096   (856)848-3817   Fax (856)848-1431
+ Kennedy Health Systems/Washington Township Campus
  435 Hurffville-Cross Keys Road   Turnersville, NJ 08012   (856)582-2816

Baird, Jamila, MD {1629368352} FamMed<NJ-HUNTRDN>
+ Hunterdon Medical Center
  2100 Wescott Drive/Room 547   Flemington, NJ 08822
  (908)237-5486   Fax (908)237-5488
+ Hunterdon Family Medicine
  250 Route 28/Suite 100   Bridgewater, NJ 08807   (908)237-5486   Fax (908)237-4136

Bais, Pammi T., MD {1326264185} InfDis(82,DOM03)
+ 25 Zev Court
  Monmouth Junction, NJ 08852   (732)398-1800   Fax (732)398-1844

Bais, Rajney Monica, MD {1366413494} IntrMd(94,GRN01)<NJ-RIVERVW, NJ-MONMOUTH>
+ Matawan Medical Associates
  213 Main Street   Matawan, NJ 07747   (732)566-2363   Fax (732)566-0502

Baiser, Dennis Miles, MD {1770548927} Pedtrc, AdolMd(78,NY09)<NJ-CHSFULD>
+ Hamilton Pediatric Associates
  3 Hamilton Health Place/Suite A   Hamilton, NJ 08690
  (609)581-4480   Fax (609)581-5222

Baisre-De Leon, Ada, MD {1407015373} PthyMGen
+ Rutgers- New Jersey Medical School
  185 South Orange Avenue/MSB C557   Newark, NJ 07103
  (973)972-7167

Baja Quizon, Maria Cecilia, MD {1245346584} NnPnMd(94,PHI09)<NJ-NWRKBETH, NJ-JRSYCITY>
+ Newark Beth Israel Medical Center
  201 Lyons Avenue/C-9   Newark, NJ 07112   (973)926-7203   Fax (973)926-2332

Bajaj, Jasmeet Singh, MD {1588614887} IntrMd, CritCr(98,DMN01)<NJ-COOPRUMC>
+ Cooper University Medical Center/Camden
  3 Cooper Plaza   Camden, NJ 08103   (856)342-2000
+ Respiratory & Sleep Specialists, LLC.
  3546 State Route 27   Kendall Park, NJ 08824   (856)342-2000   Fax (877)632-3456

Bajaj, Jasmine, MD {1285992875} FamMed
+ Lourdes Medical Associates
  200 Campbell Drive/Suite 102   Willingboro, NJ 08046
  (609)877-4545   Fax (609)877-5129

Bajaj, Nikki, MD {1467893917} IntrMd
+ 260 Prospect Avenue/Apt 163
  Hackensack, NJ 07601   (862)250-2271

Bajor-Dattilo, Ewa Beata, MD {1851596613} PainMd<NJ-STBARNMC>
+ St. Barnabas Medical Center
  94 Old Short Hills Road   Livingston, NJ 07039   (973)322-5000

Bajpai, Enakshi, DO {1720034218} IntrMd, CdvDis(95,NJ75)<NJ-UNDRWD, NJ-OURLADY>
+ Owens Vergari Unwala Cardiology Associates PC
  17 West Red Bank Avenue/Suite 306   Woodbury, NJ 08096
  (856)845-6807   Fax (856)845-3760

Bajwa, Ghulam Murtaza, MD {1073713814} PsyAdd(92,PAK15)
+ 122 Plane Street/Apt 4G
  Boonton, NJ 07005

Bajwa, Khalid Maqsood, MD {1306914320} Psychy, PsyGrt(88,PAK04)<NJ-ANCPSYCH>
+ Ancora Psychiatric Hospital
  301 Spring Garden Road   Hammonton, NJ 08037
  (609)561-1700

Bajwa, Mohammad Ayub, MD {1720162951} Gastrn, IntrMd(67,PAK01)<NJ-CLARMAAS, NJ-STMICHL>
+ 14 Washington Street
  Bloomfield, NJ 07003   (973)429-0601   Fax (973)429-3305

Bajwa, Ravneet Singh, MD {1578926945} IntHos
+ Hackensack Univ Medical Center Hospitalists
  30 Prospect Avenue   Hackensack, NJ 07601   (551)996-1548

Bak, Yury, DO {1285834655} SrgVas, Surgry(07,PA77)
+ Virtua Surgical Group, PA
  1935 Route 70 East   Cherry Hill, NJ 08003   (856)428-7700   Fax (856)424-9120

Bakal, Keren, MD {1760657878}
+ 632 Jersey Avenue/Apt 3
  Jersey City, NJ 07302   (973)951-3774
  keren53@gmail.com

Bakare, Olubunmi, MD {1841510450} NnPnMd, Pedtrc(08,MA05)<NJ-RWJUBRUN>
+ RWJ University Hospital New Brunswick
  One Robert Wood Johnson Place   New Brunswick, NJ 08901
  (732)828-3000

Baker, Alon Elie, DO {1033163928} Pedtrc(98,FL75)<NJ-CHSMRCER, NJ-RWJUHAM>
+ Advocare Woolwich Pediatrics
  300 Lexington Road/Suite 200   Woolwich Township, NJ 08085   (856)241-2111   Fax (856)241-2243

Baker, Azzam A., MD {1669575973} Pedtrc(72,EGYP)<NJ-MEADWLND, NJ-HACKNSK>
+ Riverside Medical Group
  714 Tenth Street/Suite 2   Secaucus, NJ 07094   (201)863-3346   Fax (201)865-0015
+ Riverside Medical Group
  714 Tenth Street/Suite 2   Secaucus, NJ 07094   (201)863-3346   Fax (201)865-0015

Baker, Charles D., DO {1184788549}
+ Perth Amboy Anesthesiology PC
  530 New Brunswick Avenue   Perth Amboy, NJ 08861
  (732)324-4855
+ 141 Magee Court
  East Brunswick, NJ 08816   (570)721-0621

Baker, Donald J., MD {1922101351} Dermat, PedDrm(89,NJ02)<NJ-COOPRUMC>
+ Center for Integrative Dermatology
  146 Lakeview Drive/Suite 202   Gibbsboro, NJ 08026
  (856)782-8688   Fax (856)782-8227
  drzenderm@verizon.net

Baker, Elizabeth Anne, MD {1225090210} PhysMd, IntrMd(89,NY01)
+ Spine Center
  106 Grand Avenue/Suite 220   Englewood, NJ 07631
  (201)503-1900   Fax (201)503-1901

Baker, Iyad, MD {1730341322} Pedtrc, FamMed(08,ANTI)
+ Riverside Medical Group
  200 Main Street   Ridgefield Park, NJ 07660   (201)870-6099   Fax (201)870-6098
+ Riverside Medical Group
  714 Tenth Street/Suite 2   Secaucus, NJ 07094   (201)870-6099   Fax (201)865-0015
+ Hoboken University Medical Center
  308 Willow Avenue   Hoboken, NJ 07660   (201)418-1000

Baker, Janice E., MD {1841216181} FamMed(86,IL42)<NJ-OVERLOOK>
+ Chatham Family Practice Associates
  492 Main Street   Chatham, NJ 07928   (973)635-2432   Fax (973)635-6169

Baker, John C., MD {1740396316} SrgOrt, SrgHnd, IntrMd(72,MO34)<NJ-ACMCMAIN, NJ-ACMCITY>
+ Rothman Institute - Egg Harbor Township
  2500 English Creek Avenue/Bldg 1300   Egg Harbor Township, NJ 08234   (609)677-7002   Fax (609)677-7000

Baker, Michelle Rapacon, MD {1164453049} Anesth(04,KS02)
+ Morris Anesthesia Group, PA
  3799 Route 46/Suite 211   Parsippany, NJ 07054   (973)335-1122   Fax (973)335-1448

Baker, Noel M., MD {1598055543}
+ AtlantiCare Behav Hlth/Hartford
  13 North Hartford Avenue   Atlantic City, NJ 08401
  (609)348-1161

Baker, Omar A., MD {1609037670} Pedtrc(08,DC01)<NY-NYUTISCH>
+ Riverside Pediatric Group
  46 Essex Street   Jersey City, NJ 07302   (201)360-2228
+ Riverside Pediatric Group
  1111 Hudson Street   Hoboken, NJ 07030   (201)360-2228   Fax (201)942-9321

Baker, Robert Charles, MD {1063410306} IntrMd(74,VA04)<NJ-UNDRWD>
+ 75 Wynnewood Drive
  Voorhees, NJ 08043   (609)352-2012   Fax (856)489-1420

Baker, Stephen R., MD {1063501849} Radiol, RadDia(68,NY46)<NJ-UMDNJ>
+ University Hospital
  150 Bergen Street/Rad/ C320   Newark, NJ 07103
  (973)972-5188   Fax (973)972-7428
  bakersa@umdnj.edu

Bakerywala, Suhalia, MD {1073883229} EnDbMt
+ 199 Engle Street
  Englewood, NJ 07631   (914)255-1333

Bakhos, Abdel M., MD {1225144405} SrgHnd, SrgOrt(66,SYRI)<NJ-BAYSHORE>
+ 1145 Bordentown Avenue
  Parlin, NJ 08859   (732)727-7374   Fax (732)727-6275

Bakhos, Lisa Lovas, MD {1902932767} Pedtrc(04,NJ05)
+ EmCare
  1945 Route 33   Neptune, NJ 07753   (732)776-4510   Fax (732)776-2329

Bakhos, Nader Anthony, MD {1487861373} SrgOrt, SrgOARec(04,NJ05)<NJ-RIVERVW>
  + Orthopaedic Sports Medicine
    80 Oak Hill Road   Red Bank, NJ 07701   (732)741-2313   Fax (732)741-7154

Bakhru, Ritika, MD {1972765139}
  + Paul Phillips Eye & Surgery Center
    64 Walmart Plaza   Clinton, NJ 08809   (908)735-4100   Fax (908)735-7494
  + Paul Phillips Eye & Surgery Center
    6 Minneakoning Road/Suite B   Flemington, NJ 08822   (908)735-4100   Fax (908)968-3239
  + Paul Phillips Eye & Surgery Center
    1 Monroe Street   Bridgewater, NJ 08809   (908)526-4588   Fax (908)231-6718

Bakhshi, Aditya, MD {1538544366} IntrMd<NJ-COOPRUMC>
  + Cooper University Hospital
    One Cooper Plaza   Camden, NJ 08103   (856)342-2000

Baklajian, Robert, MD {1255300588} CdvDis, IntrMd(82,ROMA)<NJ-VALLEY, NJ-ENGLWOOD>
  + 1 Sears Drive/3rd Floor
    Paramus, NJ 07652   (201)265-8282   Fax (201)265-8680

Bakosi, Ebube A., MD {1578714507} SrgTpl
  + Drs. Potter and Bakosi
    287 Boulevard/Suite 1/PO Box 367   Pompton Plains, NJ 07444   (973)839-7400   Fax (973)831-4911

Bakosi, Emily Halldorson, DO {1487004792}<NJ-CLARMAAS>
  + Clara Maass Medical Center
    1 Clara Maass Drive   Belleville, NJ 07109   (973)450-2000

Bakr, Mohamed Mokhtar, MD {1215273818} IntHos<NJ-ACMC-ITY>
  + AtlantiCare Regional Medical Center/City Campus
    1925 Pacific Avenue/Hospitalist   Atlantic City, NJ 08401   (609)569-1000

Bakshiyev, Yuliya, MD {1609947340} Pedtrc(88,RUS18)<NJ-CENTRAST>
  + Academy Pediatrics
    25 Kilmer Road/Building 3/Suite 217   Morganville, NJ 07751   (732)617-8888   Fax (732)617-8880

Bakun, Walter Michael, MD {1093912539} EmrgMd, NeuM-SptM(83,GRN01)<NJ-RWJURAH>
  + 59 Koch Avenue
    Morris Plains, NJ 07950   (973)539-1800   Fax (973)889-8789
  + Robert Wood Johnson University Hospital at Rahway
    865 Stone Street/EmrgMed   Rahway, NJ 07065   (732)381-4200

Bal, Aswine Kumar, MD {1275502957} Pedtrc, PedInf(82,INA13)<NJ-JRSYSHMC>
  + Meridian Obstetrics amd Gynecology Associates PC
    19 Davis Avenue/Fl 1   Neptune, NJ 07753   (732)897-7944   Fax (732)922-8264
  + Jersey Shore University Medical Center
    1945 Route 33/Pediatrics   Neptune, NJ 07753   (732)775-5500

Balacco, Leonard M., MD {1417994120} FamMed(79,MEX14)<NJ-HOBUNIMC>
  + Hoboken Family Practice
    108 Washington Street   Hoboken, NJ 07030   (201)656-5688   Fax (201)656-8975

Balachandar, Sadana, MD {1528262359} Pedtrc, PedEnd(07,NY08)
  + New Jersey Pain Institute
    125 Paterson Street/CAB 6100   New Brunswick, NJ 08901   (732)235-6230   Fax (732)235-5002

Balaguru, Duraisamy, MD {1154382703} Pedtrc, PedCrd, OthrSp(87,INA85)<NJ-CHDNWBTH>
  + Children's Hospital of New Jersey
    201 Lyons Avenue/Osborne Terrace   Newark, NJ 07112   (973)926-4000

Balaji, Mini, MD {1578765863} IntrMd<NJ-STCLRDOV>
  + St. Clare's Hospital-Dover
    400 West Blackwell Street   Dover, NJ 07801   (973)989-3000

Balakrishna, Shruthi, MD {1316262256} Anesth
  + Morris Anesthesia Group, PA
    3799 Route 46/Suite 211   Parsippany, NJ 07054   (973)335-1122   Fax (973)335-1448

Balakrishnan, Beena S., MD {1417065061} PhysMd(94,INA1L)
  + 223 North Van Dien Avenue
    Ridgewood, NJ 07450   (201)690-6122
  + Primary Care NJ
    370 Grand Avenue/Suite 102   Englewood, NJ 07631   (201)690-6122   Fax (201)816-1265

Balakumar, Kalavathy, MD {1780671370} RadDia(77,INA04)<NJ-STJOSHOS>
  + St. Joseph's Regional Medical Center
    703 Main Street/Radiology   Paterson, NJ 07503   (973)754-2000

Balani, Anil R., MD {1972729098} IntrMd, Gastrn(02,NY94)<NJ-RWJUBRUN>
  + Capital Health Medical Center Hopewell
    Two Capital Way/Suite 380   Pennington, NJ 08534   (609)537-5000   Fax (609)537-5050
  + RWJ University Hospital New Brunswick
    One Robert Wood Johnson Place   New Brunswick, NJ 08901   (732)828-3000

Balani, Bindu Anand, MD {1063489243} IntrMd, InfDis(94,INDI)<NJ-HACKNSK>
  + Center for Infectious Diseases
    20 Prospect Avenue/Suite 507   Hackensack, NJ 07601   (201)487-4088   Fax (201)489-8930

Balar, Bhavesh Vasant, MD {1134113376} MedOnc, Hemato, IntrMd(98,FL04)<NJ-CENTRAST>
  + Cancer Specialists of New Jersey
    326 Professional View Drive   Freehold, NJ 07728   (732)683-0900   Fax (732)683-0909
    balarb@hotmail.com

Balaraman, Vasanthi, MD {1154688851}
  + 115 Old Short Hills Road/Apt 357
    West Orange, NJ 07052

Balashov, Konstantin E., MD {1083789556} Nrolgy(83,RUS15)<NJ-RWJUBRUN>
  + University Hospital-RWJMS Neurology
    125 Paterson Street/Suite 4100-6100   New Brunswick, NJ 08901   (732)235-7733   Fax (732)235-7041

Balasingham, Chithra, MD {1457307878} IntrMd(95,GRN01)<NJ-HACKNSK>
  + Hackensack University Medical Center
    30 Prospect Avenue/FacultyPractice   Hackensack, NJ 07601   (201)996-2000

Balasubramanian, Kanchana, MD {1780626143} IntrMd(93,INA2X)<NJ-STJOSHOS>
  + 221 Kearny Avenue
    Kearny, NJ 07032   (201)893-2939   Fax (201)460-0770

Balasundaram, Anusuya, MD {1053487439} Psychy(01,NJ06)
  + Hampton Behavioral Health Center
    650 Rancocas Road   Westampton, NJ 08060   (609)267-7000   Fax (609)518-2150

Balatsky, Igor, MD {1437159670}<NJ-DEBRAHLC>
  + Deborah Heart and Lung Center
    200 Trenton Road   Browns Mills, NJ 08015   (609)893-1200   ibalit@live.com

Balazs, Peter, MD {1891948303} ObsGyn<NJ-STJOSHOS>
  + St. Joseph's Regional Medical Center
    703 Main Street   Paterson, NJ 07503   (973)754-3343
  + St. Joseph's DePaul Center ObsGyn
    11 Getty Avenue   Paterson, NJ 07503   (973)754-4200

Balboul, Elsaid A., MD {1467421339} IntrMd(82,EGYP)<NJ-CHILTON>
  + Drs. Raouf and Balboul
    508 Hamburg Turnpike/Suite 201   Wayne, NJ 07470   (973)942-1340   Fax (973)942-1360
  + Drs. Raouf and Balboul
    55 Skyline Drive/Suite 204   Ringwood, NJ 07456   (973)942-1340   Fax (973)962-0640

Balbuena, Silera Mercedes, MD {1447780614}
  + Morristown Medical Center
    100 Madison Avenue   Morristown, NJ 07962   (973)971-5000

Baldassare, Jack Lawrence, MD {1225070121} RadDia, Radiol(74,NY15)<NY-WESTCHSQ>
  + Englewood Imaging Center
    680 Kinderkamack Road/Suite 101   Oradell, NJ 07649   Fax (201)871-8697

Baldi, Daniela J., MD {1245235399} IntrMd(91,ITAL)<NJ-MONMOUTH>
  + West Park Medical, LLC.
    100 Highway 36/Suite 2-K   West Long Branch, NJ 07764   (732)531-5600   Fax (732)660-6504

Baldino, Anna Rita, DO {1922168756} Pedtrc(82,PA77)
  + 24 Harrowgate Drive
    Cherry Hill, NJ 08003

Baldomero, Anita C., MD {1215960133} Pedtrc(73,PHI09)<NJ-STBARNMC>
  + St. Barnabas Medical Center
    94 Old Short Hills Road/Pediatrics   Livingston, NJ 07039   (973)322-5000   Fax (973)322-8833

Baldonado, Ricardo T., MD {1538292818} Radiol, RadDia(65,PHI01)<NJ-MEADWLND>
  + North Jersey Imaging
    307 60th Street   West New York, NJ 07093   (201)854-1200   Fax (201)854-3333

Baldwin, Keith Douglas, MD {1255491825} SrgOrt(NJ02<PA-CHILDHOS, PA-PENNHOSP>
  + CHOP Specialty Care Center at Virtua
    200 Bowman Drive/2 FL/Suite D-260   Voorhees, NJ 08043   (267)425-5400

Baldwin, Kimberly Staton, MD {1164487096} ObsGyn(97,MI01)
  + University Medical Group/OBGYN
    125 Paterson Street/2nd Floor   New Brunswick, NJ 08901   (732)235-6600   Fax (732)235-6627

Bale, Asha G., MD {1912090085} Surgry(95,NJ05)<NJ-UMDNJ>
  + University Hospital-Doctors Office Center
    90 Bergen Street/DOC 7200/Surgry   Newark, NJ 07103   (973)972-2540   Fax (973)972-2407

Baler, Carleton E., MD {1780640573} Surgry(85,OH01)<NJ-STPETER>
  + St. Peter's University Hospital
    254 Easton Avenue/Surgery   New Brunswick, NJ 08901   (732)745-8600   Fax (732)249-5284

Balgowan, Dennis, MD {1790781813} RadDia, Radiol, IntrMd(80,NJ05)<NJ-RWJUHAM>
  + Princeton Radiology Associates, P.A.
    3674 Route 27   Kendall Park, NJ 08824   (732)821-5563   Fax (732)821-6675
  + Quakerbridge Radiology Associates
    8 Quakerbridge Plaza/Building 8   Mercerville, NJ 08619   (732)821-5563   Fax (609)689-6067
  + Quakerbridge Radiology MRI Center at Lawrenceville
    21 Lawrenceville-Pennington Rd   Lawrenceville, NJ 08824   (609)895-1500   Fax (609)895-2647

Bali, Chhaya, MD {1326095472} PedCrd, Pedtrc(71,INDI)<NJ-DEBRAHLC>
  + 25 Gemini Lane
    Manalapan, NJ 07726   (732)409-6949   Fax (732)409-6949

Balica, Adrian Claudiu, MD {1720198096} ObsGyn, IntrMd(93,ROM05)<NJ-RWJUBRUN>
  + University Medical Group/OBGYN
    125 Paterson Street/2nd Floor   New Brunswick, NJ 08901   (732)235-6600   Fax (732)235-6627

Baliga, Arvind B., MD {1902855869} PhysMd(89,NY48)<NJ-ACM-CITY, NJ-ACMCMAIN>
  + Mid Atlantic Rehabilitation Associates PA
    611 New Road   Northfield, NJ 08225   (609)641-2581   Fax (609)641-6901

Baliga, Ravi, MD {1487699633} PsyAdd, PsyFor, PsyGrt(71,INA37)<NJ-NWTNMEM, NJ-STCLRBOO>
  + in Health Associates
    15 State Route 15   Lafayette, NJ 07848   (973)579-6700   Fax (973)579-6830
    baliga@aol.com

Balija, Tara M., MD {1518284579}<NJ-RWJUBRUN>
  + RWJ University Hospital New Brunswick
    One Robert Wood Johnson Place   New Brunswick, NJ 08901   (732)235-7674   Fax (732)235-8372

Balinski, Beth A., DO {1528033669} FamMed, IntrMd(92,NY75)<NJ-RWJUBRUN, NJ-STPETER>
  + RWJPE Old Bridge Family Medicine
    2107 Highway 516   Old Bridge, NJ 08857   (732)952-0626   Fax (732)463-6071

Balint, Elizabeth A., MD {1265520555} IntrMd(78,NY09)
  + Central Jersey Internal Medicine
    92 East Main Street/Suite 201   Somerville, NJ 08876   (908)722-7990   Fax (908)575-7930

Ball, Omega Devora, MD {1154687374} IntrMd
  + Capital Health Medical Group
    One Capital Way   Pennington, NJ 08534   (609)303-4000

Ball, Robert David, DO {1841454477} Anesth(05,FL75)<NY-UPST-SYRA>
  + 14 Willow Avenue
    Peapack, NJ 07977

Ball, Roberta R., DO {1730309386} Psychy, PsyGrt(80,PA77)
  + University Hospital-SOM Department of Psychiatry
    2250 Chapel Avenue West/Suite 100   Cherry Hill, NJ 08002   (856)482-9000   Fax (856)482-1159
  + New Jersey Institute for Successful Aging
    42 East Laurel Road/Suite 1800   Stratford, NJ 08084   (856)482-9000   Fax (856)566-6781

Ballal, Raj Sadananda, MD {1386645638} ClCdEl, IntrMd(82,INDI)<NJ-DEBRAHLC, NJ-JFKMED>
  + PrimeCare Medical Group
    98 James Street/Suite 300   Edison, NJ 08820   (732)548-2523   Fax (732)549-8827

Ballan, Douglas Arnold, MD {1508893199} FamMed(90,NY48)
  + House Calls of New Jersey
    PO Box 122   Scotch Plains, NJ 07076   (908)279-3477   Fax (908)345-6111
    NJdocB@gmail.com

Ballance, Cathleen M., MD {1760451488} Pedtrc(93,NJ05)<NJ-JRSYSHMC>
  + Jersey Shore University Medical Center
    1945 Route 33/Pedi   Neptune, NJ 07753   (732)776-4267   Fax (732)776-3161

Ballaro, Joseph, MD {1700971041} IntrMd(88,WIND)<NJ-STBARNMC>
  + 2933 Vauxhall Road/Suite 28
    Vauxhall, NJ 07088   (908)687-1520   Fax (908)687-1989

Ballas, Christopher Thomas, MD {1700809076} FamMed(93,PA01)
  + South Cumberland Medical Associates
    215 Back Neck Road   Bridgeton, NJ 08302   (856)451-4414   Fax (856)451-2052

Physicians by Name and Address

Ballem, Arunajyoth, MD {1356424162} Pedtrc(73,INDI)
+ Drs. Ballem and Jadhav
715 Broadway   Paterson, NJ 07514   (973)279-2294   Fax (973)279-7341

Ballem, Naveen, MD {1306971874} Surgry(00,WIN01)
+ Ballem Surgical
230 Sherman Avenue/Suite C   Glen Ridge, NJ 07028 (973)744-8585   Fax (973)748-5990

Ballem, Ramamohana V., MD {1699858571} SrgVas, Surgry(73,INDI)
+ Ballem Surgical
230 Sherman Avenue/Suite C   Glen Ridge, NJ 07028 (973)744-8585   Fax (973)748-5990

Ballesteros, Alberto F., MD {1972527430} PsyCAd, Psychy(82,DOM02)<NJ-STBARBHC, NJ-KIMBALL>
+ St. Barnabas Behavioral Health Center
1691 US Highway 9   Toms River, NJ 08755   (800)300-0628

Ballet, Frederick L., MD {1902990443} SrgHnd, SrgOrt(76,NY09)
+ Hand Surgery & Rehabilitation Center of New Jersey
5000 Sagemore Drive/Suite 103   Marlton, NJ 08053 (856)983-4263   Fax (856)983-9362
+ Hand Surgery & Rehabilitation Center of New Jersey
608 North Broad Street/Suite 200   Woodbury, NJ 08096 (856)983-4263   Fax (856)845-8422

Ballon, Gianna, MD {1891108676}<NJ-COOPRUMC>
+ Cooper University Hospital
One Cooper Plaza   Camden, NJ 08103   (856)342-2506 Fax (856)968-8806

Balmir, Sacha, DO {1255438131} IntrMd, Nephro(02,NY75)<NJ-HOLYNAME>
+ Teaneck Hospitalists, PA
718 Teaneck Road   Teaneck, NJ 07666   (201)530-7931 Fax (201)227-6207
sacha.balmir@mountsinai.org

Baloch, Rafia Q., MD {1144589490} Pedtrc<NJ-JRSYSHMC>
+ University Medical Center of Princeton at Plainsboro
One Plainsboro Road   Plainsboro, NJ 08536   (609)853-6500

Balog, Joshua David, MD {1508824566} IntrMd, CdvDis, ClCdEl(03,NY46)
+ Cardio Intervent of Ctrl Jersey
465 Cranbury Road/Suite 201   East Brunswick, NJ 08816 (732)613-1988   Fax (732)651-7734

Balogun, Evelyn Kemi, MD {1043348048} OccpMd, IntrMd(99,PA02)
+ 1038 East Chestnut Street
Vineland, NJ 08360   (609)330-4717
dayo_08051@yahoo.com

Balonze, Karen T., MD {1023360203} IntrMd(14,NJ06)<NJ-RWJUBRUN>
+ Summit Medical Group
31-00 Broadway   Fair Lawn, NJ 07410   (201)796-2255 Fax (201)796-7020

Balsama, Louis H., DO {1861462939} Surgry(99,NJ75)
+ University Hospital -SOM University Doctors Surgeons
42 East Laurel Road/Suite 2500-2600   Stratford, NJ 08084 (856)566-2700   Fax (856)566-6873

Balsara, Zarine Rohinton, MD {1083872493} Urolgy
+ Urology for Children, LLC
200 Bowman Drive/Suite E-360   Voorhees, NJ 08043 (856)751-7880   Fax (856)751-9113

Baltaytis, Viktor, MD {1932187085} Anesth(89,UKR05)
+ Englewood Anesthesiology
350 Engle Street   Englewood, NJ 07631   (201)894-3238 Fax (201)894-0585

Baltazar, Romulo Z., MD {1740476464} RadDia<NJ-STJOSHOS>
+ St. Joseph's Regional Medical Center
703 Main Street/Radiology   Paterson, NJ 07503   (973)754-2000

Baltuch, Gordon Hirsh, MD {1932144094} SrgNro(86,QU01)
+ Penn Neurosurgery
409 Route 70 East   Cherry Hill, NJ 08034

Baluyot, Helen M., MD {1164425625} Pedtrc, IntrMd(85,PHI01)<NJ-STJOSHOS>
+ St. Joseph's Pediatrics DePaul Center
11 Getty Avenue/2nd Floor   Paterson, NJ 07503   (973)754-2727

Balzani, Henry H., MD {1295772168} ObsGyn(79,PHI09)<NJ-STMRYPAS, NJ-STJOSHOS>
+ 1117 Route 48 East
Clifton, NJ 07013   (973)777-5819   Fax (973)777-1078

Balzer, Frederick J., MD {1710294210} Anesth(04,NJ06)<NJ-NWT-NMEM>
+ 7 Githens Lane
Lumberton, NJ 08048
+ Newton Medical Center
175 High Street/Anesthesia   Newton, NJ 07860   (973)383-2121

Bamberger, Philip David, MD {1750319174} Acpntr, Anesth, PainMd(81,MI20)<NY-SLRRSVLT>
+ Garden State Surgical Center, L.L.C.
28-06 Broadway   Fair Lawn, NJ 07410   (201)475-8940 Fax (201)475-8944

Bambhroliya, Grishma, MD {1588059513} IntrMd
+ Mountainside Medical Group
123 Highland Avenue/Suite 201   Glen Ridge, NJ 07028 (973)748-9246   Fax (973)748-8755

Bamboat, Zubin Mickey, MD {1891821567} SrgOnc
+ Summit Medical Group Orthopedics and Sports Medicine
140 Park Avenue/2nd Floor   Florham Park, NJ 07932 (973)404-9980   Fax (855)307-9476
+ Summit Medical Group-Berkeley Heights Campus
1 Diamond Hill Road   Berkeley Heights, NJ 07922 (973)404-9980   Fax (908)790-6576
+ Summit Medical Group Florham Park Campus
150 Park Avenue   Florham Park, NJ 07932   (973)404-9980

Bamdas, Lawrence Marc, MD {1104922087} IntrMd(82,DOM03)
+ 12 Pine Terrace
Wayne, NJ 07470

Banayat, Geronimo, Jr., MD {1376620500} IntrMd, Nephro(79,PHIL)
+ 29 Broadway
Clark, NJ 07066   (732)574-1887   Fax (732)574-2858

Banbahji, Salim, MD {1740508563} Radiol
+ University Radiology Group, P.C.
483 Cranbury Road   East Brunswick, NJ 08816   (732)390-0040   Fax (732)390-1856

Bancroft, James Alan, MD {1073687216} FamMed(98,PA07)
+ 2 Hamilton Health Place
Hamilton, NJ 08690
+ RWJ Medical Associates
3100 Quakerbridge Road/Suite 28   Hamilton, NJ 08619 Fax (609)245-7432

Band, Ricard Louis, MD {1659470722} PainMd, SrgOrt, Surgry(71,NY08)
+ Medical Pain Management LLC
2070 Springdale Road/Suite 200   Cherry Hill, NJ 08003 (856)433-8267

Banda, Pragati, MD {1649567298} IntHos(04,INA83)
+ Summit Medical Group-Berkeley Heights Campus
1 Diamond Hill Road   Berkeley Heights, NJ 07922 (908)273-4300   Fax (908)790-6576

Bandari, Savitra M., MD {1306005038} NroChl, Pedtrc<NJ-JFKMED>
+ JFK Medical Center
65 James Street/Neurology   Edison, NJ 08820   (732)321-7010   Fax (732)632-1584

Bandola, David Matthew, MD {1487827408} AnesPain(02,PA01)<NY-PRSBCOLU>
+ 601 Hamburg Turnpike/Suite 204
Wayne, NJ 07470   (862)248-0668   Fax (862)248-0669

Bandola, Krystin Ann, MD {1407876212} SrgO&M(97,CT02)
+ 202 Towne Centre Drive
Hillsborough, NJ 08844   (908)359-1067   Fax (908)359-6467

Bandu, Bhanumathi, MD {1851327845} IntrMd(89,INDI)
+ 14 Witmer Way
Robbinsville, NJ 08691

Bandy, Caryn Kay, DO {1851301618} FamMed(98,NJ75)<NJ-VIRTVOOR, NJ-KMHTURNV>
+ Advocare Family Medicine Associates Mt. Laurel
3115 Route 38/Suite 200B   Mount Laurel, NJ 08054 (856)231-9666   Fax (856)231-7543
+ Advocare Family Medicine Associates Williamstown
979 North Black Horse Pike   Williamstown, NJ 08094 (856)231-9666   Fax (856)629-0281
+ Advocare Family Medicine Associates Vineland
602 West Sherman Avenue/Suite B   Vineland, NJ 08054 (856)692-8484   Fax (856)896-3059

Bane, Susan H., MD {1750942231} IntrMd(74,DC01)<NJ-ACMCITY>
+ AtlantiCare Regional Medical Center/City Campus
1925 Pacific Avenue/CorporateAdmin   Atlantic City, NJ 08401   (609)345-4000

Banerjee, Indrani, DO {1275899015} IntrMd(12,AZ02)
+ Atlantic Medical Group Primary Care at Pompton Lakes
17 Wanaque Avenue   Pompton Lakes, NJ 07442   (973)617-1750   Fax (973)617-1751

Banerjee, Trina D., MD {1003042490} Nephro
+ 60 Louis Avenue
Middlesex, NJ 08846

Banfield, Kimberly Ann, DO {1154581635} EmrgMd(05,IA75)<NJ-BURDTMLN>
+ Cape Regional Medical Center
2 Stone Harbor Boulevard/Emerg Med   Cape May Court House, NJ 08210   (609)463-2139

Bang, Byung, MD {1285722140} IntrMd(73,KOR04)<NJ-CHSFULD, NJ-UNVMCPRN>
+ B. Bang, M.D., P.A.
9 Schalks Crossing Road/Suite 720   Plainsboro, NJ 08536 (609)799-4644   (609)799-4614

Bangalore, Ramamurthy L., MD {1659309227} IntrMd, PulDis(78,INDI)
+ Medical Care Associates
1740 Oak Tree Road/Suite B   Edison, NJ 08820   (732)494-5000   Fax (732)494-6698

Bangia, Neha, MD {1053648311} IntrMd<NJ-NWRKBETH>
+ 707 South Orange Avenue
South Orange, NJ 07079   (973)761-6883   Fax (973)761-4990

Banigo, Samuel, MD {1063503555} IntMAdMd(88,BUL04)
+ Hudson Physicians Associates
40 Union Avenue/Suite 204   Irvington, NJ 07111 (973)416-6981   Fax (973)375-5766
sbanigo@hotmail.com
+ Hudson Physicians Associates
700 Plaza Drive/Harmon Meadows   Secaucus, NJ 07096 (973)416-6981   Fax (201)866-1393

Banka, Puja, MD {1003076787} PedCrd, CarEch(02,CA11)<MA-CHILDRN>
+ Merck and Company Incorporated
126 East Lincoln Avenue   Rahway, NJ 07065   (732)594-2789

Banker, Gopika H., DO {1649460189} Nephro(05,NJ75)<NJ-KMHSTRAT, NJ-KMHCHRRY>
+ Nephrology & Hypertension Associates of New Jersey
201 Laurel Oak Road/Suite B   Voorhees, NJ 08043 (856)566-5478   Fax (856)566-9561

Banker, Piyush, MD {1306126958} RadDia<NY-LIJEWSH>
+ Capital Health System/Fuld Campus
750 Brunswick Avenue/Imaging   Trenton, NJ 08638 (609)815-7532

Banker, Sarika, MD {1639330855} Dermat, IntrMd(08,NY46)
+ Princeton Dermatology Associates
208 Bunn Drive/Suite 1-E   Princeton, NJ 08540   (609)683-4999   Fax (609)683-0298

Banker, Shobhana, MD {1619382959} IntrMd
+ 135 Marmora Road
Parsippany, NJ 07054   (973)216-1282

Bankole, Gawu Kamara, MD {1679836183} FamMed(10,MEX03)
+ MedExpress Urgent Care Runnemede
165 South Black Horse Pike   Runnemede, NJ 08078 (856)939-1658   Fax (856)939-1647

Bankole, Omolabake O., MD {1447697834} FamMed
+ 2330 Route 33
Robbinsville, NJ 08691   (609)303-4400   Fax (609)303-4401

Banks, Frank M., DO {1700908662} GenPrc, FamMed(75,PA77)
+ 744 Erial Road
Blackwood, NJ 08012   (856)228-3641   Fax (856)228-4906

Banks, Gerald, MD {1942540877} EmrgMd
+ Capital Health Family Health Center
433 Bellevue Avenue/4th Floor   Trenton, NJ 08618 (609)815-2671   Fax (609)815-7178

Banks, Judy L., MD {1932124070} ObsGyn(75,TN07)<NJ-MORRISTN>
+ 256 Columbia Turnpike/Suite 212
Florham Park, NJ 07932   (973)377-3374   Fax (973)377-1286

Bannerji, Rajat, MD {1942361209} OncHem, IntrMd(95,NY20)
+ Rutgers Cancer Institute of New Jersey
195 Little Albany Street/PO Box 2681   New Brunswick, NJ 08903   (732)235-7996   Fax (732)235-6797

Bannerman, Kenneth S., MD {1619969623} CdvDis, IntrMd(75,NY09)
+ Summit Medical Group Cardiology
62 South Fullerton Avenue   Montclair, NJ 07042   (973)746-8585   Fax (973)746-0088
+ Summit Medical Group
75 East Northfield Road   Livingston, NJ 07039   (973)746-8585   Fax (908)673-7336
+ Essex Heart Group LLC
1310 Broad Street   Bloomfield, NJ 07042   (973)338-0800 Fax (973)338-1140

Bannett, Gregg A., DO {1720097157} Ophthl(85,NJ75)<NJ-KMHCHRRY>
+ Kennedy Health System/Cherry Hill Campus
2201 Chapel Avenue West   Cherry Hill, NJ 08002 (856)488-6550   Fax (856)488-6513

Bannon, John T., MD {1467420042} SrgOrt(77,NJ05)<NJ-SHOREMEM>
+ 141 Shore Road
Somers Point, NJ 08244   (609)653-9377   Fax (609)926-0476

Bansal, Aditya Rakesh, MD {1720064546} PulDis, IntrMd(96,INA1Z)
+ Atlantic Pulmonary & Critical Care Associates, P.A.
741 South Second Avenue/Suite A   Galloway, NJ 08205 (609)748-7300   Fax (609)748-7919

Bansal, Meenakshi, MD {1942630769} PthAna<NJ-ACMCITY>
+ AtlantiCare Regional Medical Center/City Campus
1925 Pacific Avenue   Atlantic City, NJ 08401   (585)922-4121   Fax (585)922-4128

Bansal, Mukta, MD {1992938765} Grtrcs
+ PowerBack Rehabilitation
113 Route 73   Voorhees, NJ 08043   (856)809-3500

Bansal, Nivedita, MD {1033180880} IntrMd(95,INA9A)
+ 412 Summit Avenue
  Jersey City, NJ 07306

Bansal, Sonia, MD {1467682617} EmrgMd
+ 93 Hidden Lake Drive
  North Brunswick, NJ 08902

Bansal, Sudha, MD {1487602686} IntrMd(85,INDI)<NJ-LOURDMED, NJ-KMHTURNV>
+ Lourdes Medical Center of Burlington County
  218 Sunset Road/Suite A   Willingboro, NJ 08046   (609)835-5240
+ Kennedy Health Systems/Washington Township Campus
  435 Hurffville-Cross Keys Road   Turnersville, NJ 08012
  (609)835-5240   Fax (856)566-6906
+ Kennedy Health System/Cherry Hill Campus
  2201 Chapel Avenue West/Internal Med   Cherry Hill, NJ 08046   (856)488-6500   Fax (856)566-6906

Bansal, Vivek, MD {1831369701} EnDbMt, IntHos, IntrMd(02,INA60)
+ Center for Endocrine Health
  1738 Route 31 North/Suite 108   Clinton, NJ 08809
  (908)735-3981   Fax (908)735-3981

Banschick, Harry, MD {1881613073} Pedtrc(77,MEX14)<NJ-HOLYNAME, NJ-ENGLWOOD>
+ Drs. Banschick, Concepcion & Stein
  2500 Lemoine Avenue/Suite 200   Fort Lee, NJ 07024
  (201)592-9210   Fax (201)592-6539

Bansil, Noel Lumanog, MD {1952484388} Pedtrc(89,PHI09)<NJ-HACKNSK, NJ-HOLYNAME>
+ Riverside Medical Group
  714 Tenth Street/Suite 2   Secaucus, NJ 07094   (201)863-3346   Fax (201)865-0015
+ Riverside ENT Pediatric Group
  324 Palisade Avenue/2nd Floor   Jersey City, NJ 07307
  (201)863-3346   Fax (201)386-2343

Bansil, Rakesh K., MD {1811982499} Psychy, PsyAdd, PsyGrt(78,INDI)<NJ-UMDNJ>
+ University Psychiatric Associates
  183 South Orange Avenue/E-F Levels   Newark, NJ 07103
  (973)972-2977   Fax (973)972-2979

Bansilal, Sameer, MD {1396864328} IntrMd, CdvDis(01,INA69)<NY-MTSINAI>
+ Bayer HealthCare
  100 Bayer Boulevard   Whippany, NJ 07981   (862)404-3000

Bantz, Eric W., MD {1124172598} Allrgy, Pedtrc(77,NY06)
+ Cornerstone Asthma and Allergy Associates
  103 Old Marlton Pike/Suite 211   Medford, NJ 08055
  (609)953-7500   Fax (609)953-9085

Banu, Dana R., MD {1356366124} IntrMd(88,ROMA)
+ Denville Associates of Internal Medicine
  16 Pocono Road/Suite 317   Denville, NJ 07834   (973)627-2650   Fax (973)627-8383

Banu, Nazifa, MD {1861562662} IntrMd, Nephro(87,BAN01)
+ North Jersey Nephrology Associates PA
  246 Hamburg Turnpike/Suite 207   Wayne, NJ 07470
  (973)653-3366   Fax (973)653-3365

Banzon, Felipe T., MD {1629022298} NnPnMd, Pedtrc(77,PHIL)<NJ-CHSMRCER>
+ Capital Health System/Mercer Campus
  446 Bellevue Avenue   Trenton, NJ 08618   (609)394-4144
  Fax (609)394-4351

Banzon, Manuel T., MD {1194809095} SrgOrt, NeuMSptM, IntrMd(73,PHIL)<NJ-CENTRAST>
+ Advanced Orthopedics & Sports Medicine Institute
  301 Professional View Drive   Freehold, NJ 07728
  (732)720-6415   Fax (732)720-2554
+ 312 Applegarth Road/Suite 100
  Monroe, NJ 08831

Banzuelo Rio, Margie R., MD {1255773248} IntHos
+ 2412 Route 71/Apt 7f\F
  Spring Lake, NJ 07762

Baorto, Elizabeth P., MD {1760453468} Pedtrc, PedInf(96,NY08)<NJ-MORRISTN>
+ Morristown Medical Center
  100 Madison Avenue/Box 107/Pedi   Morristown, NJ 07962
  (973)971-5000
+ Respiratory Center for Children
  100 Madison Avenue   Morristown, NJ 07962

Bapat, Ashok R., MD {1518960384} Hemato, IntrMd, MedOnc(73,INDI)<NJ-KENEDYHS, NJ-VIRTUAHS>
+ Comprehensive Cancer & Hematology Specialists, P.C.
  705 White Horse Road   Voorhees, NJ 08043   (856)435-1777   Fax (856)435-0696
+ Comprehensive Cancer & Hematology Specialists, P.C.
  17 West Red Bank Avenue/Suite 202   Woodbury, NJ 08096
  (856)435-1777   Fax (856)848-2958
+ Comprehensive Cancer & Hematology Specialists, P.C.
  900 Medical Center Drive/Suite 200   Sewell, NJ 08043
  (856)582-0550   Fax (856)582-7640

Bapineedu, Kuchipudi, MD {1801853031} SrgVas, Surgry, Gastrn(69,INA11)<NJ-VALLEY>
+ 15-01 Broadway/Suite 22
  Fair Lawn, NJ 07410   (201)796-4848   Fax (201)797-7992

Bapineedu, Radhika Kuchipudi, MD {1841450590} PhysMd, OrtSpn(00,INA97)<NJ-KSLRWEST>
+ Kessler Institute for Rehabilitation West Orange
  1199 Pleasant Valley Way   West Orange, NJ 07052
  (973)731-3600

Baptist, Gladwyn D., MD {1255390944} CdvDis, IntrMd(76,INA94)
+ 10 Magnolia Avenue
  Bridgeton, NJ 08302   (856)455-2222   Fax (856)455-6541

Baptist, Justin Peter, MD {1982095758}
+ 22 Dellmead Drive
  Livingston, NJ 07039   (973)941-4475
+ AtlantiCare Regional Medical Center/City Campus
  1925 Pacific Avenue   Atlantic City, NJ 08401   (609)345-4000

Baptist, Selwyn J., MD {1184705956} PthAcl(70,INDI)<NJ-STBARNMC>
+ St. Barnabas Medical Center
  94 Old Short Hills Road/Path   Livingston, NJ 07039
  (973)322-5763
  sbaptist@sbhcs.com

Baptiste, Nicole Bernadette, MD {1417103789} ObsGyn(03,DMN01)
+ Nicole Bernadette Baptiste MD PC
  95 Martin Luther King Jr Drive/OB/GYN   Jersey City, NJ 07305   (551)200-9570   Fax (551)200-9773
  Nikkimd123@hotmail.com

Baqui, Huma, MD {1225328701} Nrolgy
+ Monmouth Ocean Neurology
  1944 State Route 33/Suite 206   Neptune, NJ 07753
  (732)774-8282   Fax (732)774-4407
+ Monmouth Ocean Neurology
  190 Jack Martin Boulevard/Building B-3   Brick, NJ 08724
  (732)774-8282   Fax (732)785-0116

Baquiran, Henry M., MD {1093863508} FamMed(78,PHIL)<NJ-CHILTON>
+ Health first Immediate Medical Care
  1900 Union Valley Road   Hewitt, NJ 07421   (973)728-5930
  Fax (973)728-0809

Bar, Vandna Prasad, MD {1881836815} RadDia, Radiol(03,NJ05)<NJ-STJOSHOS>
+ Imaging Subspecialists of North Jersey LLC
  703 Main Street   Paterson, NJ 07503   (973)754-2645
+ St. Joseph's Regional MedCtr-Ambulatory Imaging Ctr
  1135 Broad Street/3rd Floor/Suite 4   Clifton, NJ 07013
  (973)569-6300

Bar Eli, Howard Y., MD {1063775039}
+ 14 Eardley Road
  Edison, NJ 08817   (732)501-4679
  chaimbareli@gmail.com

Bar-Eli, Rebecca, MD {1568978757} Otlryg
+ Drs. Samadi and Bar-Eli
  10 Forest Avenue/Suite 100   Paramus, NJ 07652   (201)996-1505   Fax (201)996-1605

Barabas, Cynthia, MD {1912054362} Pedtrc(89,IL02)
+ Ocean Breastfeeding Medicine
  3350 State Route 138 West/Suite 117   Wall Township, NJ 07719   (732)280-3334   Fax (732)556-0008

Barabas, Ronald E., MD {1003809609} NroChl, ClnGnt, PedNrD(86,NJ02)
+ Child Neurology Associates PA
  3350 Highway 138 West/Suite 117   Wall, NJ 07719
  (732)556-0200   Fax (732)556-0008

Barai, Jayant H., MD {1447294178} CdvDis, IntrMd(76,INDI)<NJ-EASTORNG, NJ-NWRKBETH>
+ 345 Henry Street/Suite103
  Orange, NJ 07050   (973)678-5700   Fax (973)414-0963

Barakat, Raja, MD {1174586341} Pedtrc(73,SYRI)<NJ-BAYSHORE, NJ-RIVERVW>
+ SAMRA Pediatrics
  300 Perrine Road/Suite 331   Old Bridge, NJ 08857
  (732)727-8800   Fax (732)727-0955
+ SAMRA Pediatrics
  733 North Beers Street/Suite L-5   Holmdel, NJ 07733
  (732)727-8800   Fax (732)727-0955

Baraldi, Raymond Lawrence, Jr., MD {1770671075} RadDia, Radiol, IntrMd(68,INA48)<NJ-COOPRUMC>
+ Cooper University Hospital
  One Cooper Plaza/Radiology   Camden, NJ 08103
  (856)342-2382   Fax (856)365-0472

Baran, Natalia, MD {1992122147} IntrMd<NJ-NWRKBETH>
+ Newark Beth Israel Medical Center
  201 Lyons Avenue   Newark, NJ 07112   (973)926-7425

Baranetsky, Adrian Andrew, MD {1013015288} RadDia(79,MEX14)
+ Hudson River Radiology
  547 Summit Avenue   Jersey City, NJ 07306   (201)656-5050
  Fax (201)656-0689

Baranetsky, Nicholas G., MD {1093808164} EnDbMt, IntrMd(74,NY09)<NJ-STMICHL, NJ-CLARMAAS>
+ 111 Central Avenue
  Newark, NJ 07102   (973)877-5185   Fax (973)877-5210
+ 312 Belleville Turnpike
  North Arlington, NJ 07031   (201)997-5522

Baranowski, Katherine, MD {1255479580} Pedtrc, PedEmg(84,NJ05)<NJ-UMDNJ>
+ University Hospital
  150 Bergen Street/PediEmrgMed   Newark, NJ 07103
  (973)972-5129   Fax (973)972-5965

Baranski, Gregg Michael, MD {1447410014}
+ Virtua Medford Surgical Group
  212 Creek Crossing Boulevard   Hainesport, NJ 08036
  (609)267-1004   Fax (609)267-1044

Barasch, Jeffrey P., MD {1700866001} PulDis, SlpDis, IntrMd(79,NY19)<NJ-VALLEY>
+ Better Breathing
  140 Chestnut Street/Suite 200   Ridgewood, NJ 07450
  (201)447-3866   Fax (201)652-1332
  betterbreathing.ck@gmail.com

Barasch, Susan A., MD {1578556437} Pedtrc(89,NY08)<NJ-OVERLOOK, NJ-STBARNMC>
+ Watchung Pediatrics
  76 Stirling Road/Suite 201   Warren, NJ 07059   (908)755-5437   Fax (908)755-6905
+ Watchung Pediatrics
  346 South Avenue/Suite 3   Fanwood, NJ 07023   (908)755-5437   Fax (908)889-0047
+ Watchung Pediatrics
  225 Millburn Avenue/Suite 301   Millburn, NJ 07059
  (973)376-7337   Fax (973)218-6647

Barash, Craig Ross, MD {1245288190} IntrMd, Gastrn(91,NY47)<NJ-VIRTMHBC>
+ The Gastroenterology Group, PA
  103 Old Marlton Pike/Suite 102   Medford, NJ 08055
  (609)953-3440   Fax (609)996-4002
+ The Gastroenterology Group, PA
  15000 Midlantic Drive/Suite 110   Mount Laurel, NJ 08054
  (609)953-3440   Fax (856)996-4002

Baratta, Andrea, DO {1124080619} Dermat(00,NJ75)<NJ-WAYNEGEN, NJ-VALLEY>
+ Macaione and Papa Dermatology Associates
  707 White Horse Road/Suite C-103   Voorhees, NJ 08043
  (856)627-1900   Fax (856)627-6907

Baratta, James A., MD {1013950930} Anesth(88,NJ05)<NJ-RWJURAH>
+ 19 Thistle Lane
  Warren, NJ 07059   (732)205-8250   Fax (732)205-8258

Baratta, Jerry M., DO {1881666147} Anesth(89,NJ75)<NJ-HACKNSK>
+ Hackensack University Medical Center
  30 Prospect Avenue/Anesthesiology   Hackensack, NJ 07601
  (201)996-2000   Fax (201)488-6769

Baratta, Joseph B., MD {1871681163} SrgVas, Surgry(81,WIND)<NJ-STMRYPAS, NJ-CHILTON>
+ General & Vascular Surgical Assocs
  905 Allwood Road/Suite 204   Clifton, NJ 07012   (973)778-6676   Fax (973)778-2666
+ General & Vascular Surgical Assocs
  28 Jackson Avenue   Pompton Plains, NJ 07444   (973)839-2800
+ General & Vascular Surgical Assocs
  61 Beaver Brook Road   Lincoln Park, NJ 07012   (973)686-0420   Fax (973)778-2666

Barb, Herman T., MD {1225117682} Psychy(82,MEXI)
+ Drs. Barb & Patel
  901 Route 168/Suite 101   Turnersville, NJ 08012   (856)228-7577   Fax (856)228-0534

Barba, Jose P., MD {1427072446} RadOnc(72,PHI10)<NJ-MTNSIDE>
+ Hackensack UMC Mountainside
  1 Bay Avenue/RadOnc   Montclair, NJ 07042   (973)429-6096   Fax (973)429-6749
  JOSE.BARBA@mountainsidehosp.com

Barba, Vincent J., MD {1134139876} IntrMd, Rserch(93,NJ05)<NJ-UMDNJ>
+ University Hospital
  150 Bergen Street   Newark, NJ 07103   (973)972-3400
  Fax (973)972-6646

Barbalinardo, Joseph P., MD {1942350418} Surgry(78,MEXI)<NJ-BAYSHORE, NJ-SOCEANCO>
+ Strafford Surgical Specialists, P.A.
  1100 Route 72 West/Suite 303   Manahawkin, NJ 08050
  (609)978-3325   Fax (609)978-3123
+ Monmouth Surgical Specialists
  727 North Beers Street   Holmdel, NJ 07733   (609)978-3325
  Fax (732)290-7067

Barbalinardo, Robert J., MD {1942350426} Surgry(82,NJ05)<NJ-MTNSIDE, NJ-STMICHL>
+ Monmouth Surgical Specialists
  123 Highland Avenue/Suite 202   Glen Ridge, NJ 07028
  (973)429-7600   Fax (973)429-7602

Physicians by Name and Address

Barbara Mijares, Diego, MD {1134522634} ObsGyn
+ Metropolitan Family Health Network
935 Garfield Avenue   Jersey City, NJ 07304   (201)478-5800   Fax (201)478-5814

Barbarito, Edward Joseph, MD {1174503148} IntrMd, Gastrn(97,NJ05)<NJ-MORRISTN, NJ-STCLRDEN>
+ Morris County Gastroenterology Associates
16 Pocono Road/Suite 201   Denville, NJ 07834   (973)627-4430   Fax (973)586-2336
+ Chambers Center
435 South Street/Suite 160   Morristown, NJ 07960   (973)971-6301

Barbella, Joseph D., DO {1659317857} Anesth, PainMd, Anes-Pain(89,IL76)<NJ-OCEANMC, NJ-SHOREMEM>
+ Trilogy Pain Associates
2106 New Road/Suite D6   Linwood, NJ 08221   (609)927-1188   Fax (609)927-5515
+ Ocean Medical Center
425 Jack Martin Boulevard/Anesth   Brick, NJ 08723   (732)840-2200

Barber, Kevin G., DO {1861461196} IntrMd(78,PA77)<NJ-SJERSYHS, NJ-KMHCHRRY>
+ Cumberland Nephrology Associates, PA
1318 South Main Road   Vineland, NJ 08360   (856)205-9900   Fax (856)205-0041

Barber, Locke W., DO {1437191376} Radiol, RadDia, RadBdI(83,PA77)<NJ-KMHCHRRY>
+ Radiology Associates of New Jersey
2201 Chapel Avenue West/Suite 106   Cherry Hill, NJ 08002   (856)488-6844   Fax (856)488-6507

Barber, Matthew, MD {1083025456}
+ Covance, Inc
210 Carnegie Centre/2nd Floor   Princeton, NJ 08540   (609)936-5684

Barber, Nathaniel A., MD {1093849630} CdvDis, IntrMd(78,NY06)<NJ-JRSYCITY>
+ Drs. Barber and Dizon
377 Jersey Avenue/Suite 460   Jersey City, NJ 07302   (201)332-4110   Fax (201)332-4122

Barbera, Frank T., MD {1164478004} IntrMd, Rheuma(78,ITAL)<NJ-CLARMAAS, NJ-HOBUNIMC>
+ 68 Ridge Road
North Arlington, NJ 07031   (201)998-7333   Fax (201)998-5715

Barbier, Andrea, DO {1497816631} IntrMd(92,PA77)<NJ-CLARMAAS>
+ 135 Bloomfield Avenue
Bloomfield, NJ 07003   (973)743-9744   Fax (973)743-9745

Barbieri, Louise T., MD {1437130093} Anesth(78,NY06)<NJ-MORRISTN>
+ Anesthesia Associates of Morristown
264 South Street/Suite 2A   Morristown, NJ 07960   (973)631-8119
+ Anesthesia Associates
100 Madison Avenue   Morristown, NJ 07960   (973)631-8119   Fax (973)631-8120

Barbour, Worth L., MD {1013216134}
+ 1 Richmond Street/Apt 4009
New Brunswick, NJ 08901   (720)877-1780   wbarbour@peds.uab.edu

Barbuto, Joseph, MD {1629154075} Psychy, OthrSp(78,NY46)<NY-PRSBWEIL, NY-SLOANKET>
+ 61 North Maple Avenue/Suite 303-A
Ridgewood, NJ 07450   (201)560-0290

Barcas, Peter P., DO {1407838972} Nrolgy, VasNeu, IntrMd(86,NJ75)<NJ-JRSYSHMC, NJ-OCEANMC>
+ Monmouth Ocean Neurology
190 Jack Martin Boulevard/Building B-3   Brick, NJ 08724   (732)785-0114   Fax (732)785-0116
+ Monmouth Ocean Neurology
1944 State Route 33/Suite 206   Neptune, NJ 07753   (732)785-0114   Fax (732)774-4407

Bardeguez, Arlene D., MD {1790879641} MtFtMd, ObsGyn(81,PRO01)<NJ-HACKNSK>
+ University Physician Associates
140 Bergen Street/ACC Level C   Newark, NJ 07103   (973)972-2700   Fax (973)972-2739

Baredes, Soly, MD {1306915038} SrgHdN, OtIryg, Lryngo(76,NY01)<NJ-UMDNJ, NJ-STBARNMC>
+ University Hospital-Doctors Office Center
90 Bergen Street/DOC-7200   Newark, NJ 07103   (973)972-2400   Fax (973)972-2988
+ University Hospital
150 Bergen Street/ENT   Newark, NJ 07103   (973)972-4181

Bareket, Yaron, MD {1376548719} CdvDis, IntrMd(87,ASTL)<NJ-PALISADE, NJ-ENGLWOOD>
+ Cross Country Cardiology
103 River Road/2nd Floor   Edgewater, NJ 07020   (201)941-8100   Fax (201)941-2899
+ Cross Country Cardiology
38 Meadowlands Parkway   Secaucus, NJ 07094   (201)866-5151

Baretto, Luigi U., MD {1619361011} FamMed
+ Atlantic Care Physician Group
201 West Avenue   Ocean City, NJ 08226   (609)391-7500   Fax (609)391-0963

Barg, Vadim A., MD {1669558565} Anesth(86,RUS65)
+ Morris Anesthesia Group, PA
3799 Route 46/Suite 211   Parsippany, NJ 07054   (973)335-1122   Fax (973)335-1448

Barger Amsalem, Hamutal, MD {1447818281} IntrMd
+ 54 Norman Place
Tenafly, NJ 07670   (201)289-3937

Barghash, Claudia N., MD {1487761185} Gastrn, IntrMd(97,LEB04)<NJ-SOMERSET>
+ Digestive HealthCare Center
511 Courtyard Drive/Building 500   Hillsborough, NJ 08844   (908)218-9222   Fax (908)218-9818

Bari, Fazal, MD {1407965775} OncHem(90,PAK11)<NJ-MORRISTN, NJ-STCLRDEN>
+ Oncology & Hematology Specialists, PA
23 Pocono Road/Suite 100   Denville, NJ 07834   (973)316-1701   Fax (973)316-1708
+ Oncology & Hematology Specialists, PA
100 Madison Avenue/Suite C3402   Morristown, NJ 07960   (973)316-1701   Fax (973)267-2550

Bari, Mohammad Minhaj, MD {1093821696} Psychy(80,INDI)<NJ-TRENTPSY>
+ Trenton Psychiatric Hospital
Sullivan Way/PO Box 7600   West Trenton, NJ 08628   (609)633-1500

Bariana, Christopher Michael, DO {1992092662}
+ Kings Way Primary Care
100 Kings Way East/Suite D2   Sewell, NJ 08080   (844)542-2273   Fax (856)218-4808
+ Washington Township Thoracic Surgery
400 Medical Center Drive/Suite F   Sewell, NJ 08080   (844)542-2273   Fax (856)716-6659

Barilari, Rafael, MD {1689640393} Pedtrc, PedHem(86,ARG01)<NJ-STJOSHOS>
+ St Joseph's Medical Pedicatic EmerMed
703 Main Street   Paterson, NJ 07503   (973)754-4901

Barile, David Robert, MD {1063461283} IntrMd(95,VA07)
+ University Medical Center of Princeton at Plainsboro
One Plainsboro Road   Plainsboro, NJ 08536   (609)497-4000
+ 253 Witherspoon Street
Princeton, NJ 08540

Barisciano, Lisa, MD {1265401699} Allrgy, Pedtrc, PedAlg(98,NJ06)<NJ-MORRISTN>
+ 15 James Street
Florham Park, NJ 07932   (973)503-0600   Fax (973)503-0424

Barker, William Robert, MD {1396927364} FamMed, Surgry(06,PA13)
+ 9 Greenvale Road
Moorestown, NJ 08057

Barlapudi, Shalini Rao, MD {1225225691}<NJ-CHSFULD>
+ Capital Health System/Fuld Campus
750 Brunswick Avenue   Trenton, NJ 08638   (609)394-6000

Barlis, Cara J., MD {1356486518} FamMed(86,ON05)
+ Princeton Sports & Family Medicine
3131 Princeton Pike   Lawrenceville, NJ 08648   (609)896-9190   Fax (609)896-3555
+ College of New Jersey Student Health Services
2000 Pennington Road/Eickhoff 107   Ewing, NJ 08628   (609)896-9190   Fax (609)637-5131

Barlow, Jonathan David, MD {1215192273} SrgOrt
+ Rothman Institute
999 Route 73 North/3rd Fl   Marlton, NJ 08053   (856)821-6360   Fax (856)821-6359

Barmakian, Joseph T., MD {1427106830} SrgHnd, SrgOrt(84,NJ06)<NJ-OVERLOOK, NJ-JFKMED>
+ Summit Medical Group
574 Springfield Avenue   Westfield, NJ 07090   (908)232-7797   Fax (908)232-0540

Barn, Kulpreet S., MD {1699064600} CdvDis, CarEch(05,INA6Z)
+ Mercer Bucks Cardiology
One Union Street/Suite 101   Robbinsville, NJ 08691   (609)890-6677   Fax (609)890-7292

Barnard, Nicola J., MD {1336214428} PthACl(75,ENG25)<NJ-RWJUBRUN>
+ RWJ University Hospital New Brunswick
One Robert Wood Johnson Place   New Brunswick, NJ 08901   (732)828-3000

Barnas, Matthew Edward, MD {1285609206} Psychy, PsyGrt, IntrMd(00,NJ05)<NJ-VAEASTOR>
+ NJ Memory & Behavioral Care
14 Ridgedale Avenue/Suite 103   Cedar Knolls, NJ 07927   (973)295-6335   Fax (862)204-3456
+ NJ Memory & Behavioral Care
195 Mountain Avenue   Springfield, NJ 07081   (973)295-6335   Fax (862)204-3456

Barnea, Eytan R., MD {1316055932} ObsGyn, RprEnd(76,ITAL)<NJ-COOPRUMC, NJ-OURLADY>
+ CAMCare Health Corporation
2610 Federal Street   Camden, NJ 08104   (856)635-0212
+ Cooper University Medical Center/Camden
3 Cooper Plaza/ObsGyn/Ste. 104   Camden, NJ 08103   (856)635-0212   Fax (856)429-7414
+ Delaware Institute of Fertility & Genetics
Route 73/Suite 2001 F   Marlton, NJ 08104   (856)988-0072

Barnes, Dora Pinky, MD {1538190756} IntrMd(78,TN07)
+ PO Box 123
Orange, NJ 07051   (973)677-2285   Barnesdp@verizon.net

Barnes, Jaime Jude, DO {1780633776} PulCCr, CritCr, IntrMd(00,PA77)<NJ-KMHTURNV>
+ Kennedy Health Systems/Washington Township Campus
435 Hurffville-Cross Keys Road   Turnersville, NJ 08012   (856)582-3100

Barnes, Stacey Ann, DO {1871765073} EmrgMd(04,NY75)<NJ-STJOSHOS>
+ St Joseph's Medical Center Emergency
703 Main Street   Paterson, NJ 07503   (973)754-2240   Fax (973)754-2249

Barnes, Stephanie A., MD {1073711511} Psychy(03,STM01)<NJ-BERGNMC, NJ-STJOSHOS>
+ 93 West Palisade Avenue
Englewood, NJ 07631   (201)567-0500   Fax (201)567-9335
+ High Focus Center
40 Eisenhower Drive   Paramus, NJ 07652   (201)567-0500   Fax (201)843-1117
+ Vantage Health System
93 West Palisade Avenue   Englewood, NJ 07631   (201)567-0500   Fax (201)567-9335

Barnes, Tanganyika A., DO {1649405275} IntrMd<NJ-ENGLWOOD>
+ Englewood Hospital and Medical Center
350 Engle Street/Internal Med   Englewood, NJ 07631   (201)894-3135

Barnes, Thomas L., MD {1629005798} SrgVas, Surgry(74,PHI01)
+ Virtua Medford Surgical Group
212 Creek Crossing Boulevard   Hainesport, NJ 08036   (609)267-1004   Fax (609)267-1044

Barness, Michael, MD {1730478991} Psychy<NJ-CLARMAAS>
+ Clara Maass Medical Center
1 Clara Maass Drive   Belleville, NJ 07109   (973)450-2111

Barnett, Jordan B., MD {1477518298} EmrgMd(93,NY15)<NJ-VIRTVOOR>
+ Virtua Voorhees
100 Bowman Drive/EmrgMed   Voorhees, NJ 08043   (856)247-3000
+ Emergency Physician Associates, P.A.
307 South Evergreen Avenue/PO Box 298   Woodbury, NJ 08096   (856)247-3000   Fax (856)848-1431

Barnett, Rebecca L., MD {1497276695} ObsGyn
+ Hackensack Meridian Medical Group Ob/Gyn, Freehold
3499 Route 9 North/Suite 2B   Freehold, NJ 07728   (732)577-1199   Fax (732)577-8922

Barnett, Richard, DO {1073020269}
+ 2 Delwick Lane
New Providence, NJ 07974   (908)721-6083

Barnett, Sharon Elizabeth, MD {1992760193} Pedtrc(95,NY15)<NJ-VIRTMARL>
+ Advocare The Farm Pediatrics
975 Tuckerton Road/Suite 100   Marlton, NJ 08053   (856)983-6190   Fax (856)983-3805
+ Advocare The Farm Pediatrics
1001 Laurel Oak Boulevard/Suite B   Voorhees, NJ 08043   (856)983-6190   Fax (856)782-7404

Barnickel, Paul W., MD {1669449476} IntrMd(83,GRN01)
+ RWJBH Primary Care Eatontown
145 Wyckoff Road/Suite 301   Eatontown, NJ 07724   (732)222-0180   Fax (732)935-1590
+ Monmouth Medical Group, P.C.
223 Monmouth Road   West Long Branch, NJ 07764   (732)222-0180   Fax (732)229-4562

Barnish, Michael J., DO {1659358679} InfDis(85,IL76)
+ Garden State Infectious Diseases Associates, P.A.
709 Haddonfield Berlin Road   Voorhees, NJ 08043   (856)566-3190   Fax (856)566-1904
+ Garden State Infectious Disease Associates
570 Egg Harbor Road/Suite B-5   Sewell, NJ 08080   (856)566-3190   Fax (856)566-1904

Barnum, Kimberly Ann, DO {1730573007} FamMed
+ Summit Medical Group
202 Elmer Street   Westfield, NJ 07090   (908)228-3675   Fax (908)654-1053

Barofsky, Jonathan M., MD {1962446690} Ophthl, VitRet(91,NY47)<NJ-RIVERVW>
+ Retina Care Center
1255 Highway 70/Suite 31N   Lakewood, NJ 08701   (732)920-4700   Fax (732)920-6800

Barofsky, Kenneth D., MD {1457465080} IntrMd, PulDis, CritCr(87,PHI22)<NJ-CENTRAST, NJ-KIMBALL>
+ Monmouth Ocean Pulmonary Medicine
901 West Main Street/Suite 160   Freehold, NJ 07728   (732)577-0600   Fax (732)577-6332
+ 312 Applegarth Road
Monroe Township, NJ 08831

Baron, Ann R., MD {1346479649} Psychy(04,NJ05)
+ 79 John Place
Bergenfield, NJ 07621

Baron, Harvey L., MD {1841323136} SrgOrt(71,NY03)<NJ-SOMERSET>
+ 103 Omni Drive
Somerville, NJ 08876   (908)874-4556   Fax (908)359-6813

Baron, Jeremy Lawrence, MD {1801090667} Anesth, AnesPain
+ Anesthesia Consultnts of NJ/Nova Pain
285 Davidson Avenue/Suite 204   Somerset, NJ 08873   (732)271-1400   Fax (732)271-3543

Baron, Joseph, MD {1851572481} RadOnc(92,NJ05)<NJ-BAYONNE>
+ Bayonne Medical Center
29th Street at Avenue E/Rad/Oncology   Bayonne, NJ 07002   (201)858-5000

Baron, Leah, MD {1427098904} Anesth(78,LATV)<NJ-VIRTMHBC>
+ Virtua Memorial
175 Madison Avenue   Mount Holly, NJ 08060   (609)267-0700
+ Burlington Anesthesia Associates
120 Madison Ave/Suite E/PO Box 174   Mount Holly, NJ 08060   (609)267-0700   Fax (609)261-1779

Baron, Michelle A., MD {1861463812} EnDbMt(83,DC03)
+ 106 Skyline Drive
Morristown, NJ 07960

Baron, Phillip, MD {1942210786} CdvDis, IntrMd(78,NJ06)<NJ-RWJUBRUN, NJ-STPETER>
+ Raritan Bay Cardiology
7 Centre Dtrive/Suite 13   Monroe Township, NJ 08831   (609)655-8860   Fax (609)655-8065

Baron-Gabriel, Icynth M., MD {1104063064} PthAcl(88,PHI01)
+ Ocean County Medical Lab
525 Route 70   Brick, NJ 08723   (732)920-1772   Fax (732)920-6171

Barone, Allison, MD {1710987086} RadV&I, RadDia(93,NY47)<NJ-HOBUNIMC, NJ-UMDNJ>
+ Hoboken University Medical Center
308 Willow Avenue/Radiology   Hoboken, NJ 07030   (201)418-1000   Fax (201)418-1822
alliebar18@yahoo.com
+ University Hospital
150 Bergen Street/Radiology   Newark, NJ 07103   (973)972-4300

Barone, Catherine Ann, DO {1568676989} FamMed, GenPrc, IntrMd(84,PA77)
+ University Doctors Family Practice
100 Centruy Parkway/Suite 140   Mount Laurel, NJ 08054   (856)667-9051   Fax (856)667-9054

Barone, Christopher J., DO {1518996941} IntrMd, FamMed(77,PA77)<NJ-KENEDYHS, NJ-KMHTURNV>
+ 1 Somerdale Square
Somerdale, NJ 08083   Fax (856)661-5162
+ Kennedy Health System
1099 White Horse Road   Voorhees, NJ 08043   Fax (856)566-5277
+ Kennedy Health Systems/Washington Township Campus
435 Hurffville-Cross Keys Road   Turnersville, NJ 08083   (856)582-2500

Barone, Cynthia A., DO {1699762591} RadDia, Radiol, NuclMd(92,NJ75)<NJ-KIMBALL, NJ-MONMOUTH>
+ Monmouth Medical Center
300 Second Avenue/Radiology   Long Branch, NJ 07740   (732)923-7700   Fax (732)923-7710
+ St. Barnabas Health Care System
99 Highway 37 West/Comm Medical Center   Toms River, NJ 08755   (732)557-8151

Barone, Donald A., DO {1396933768} Nrolgy, OthrSp(74,PA77)<NJ-KMHSTRAT>
+ University Doctors-Ob Gyn
42 East Laurel Road/Suite 3500   Stratford, NJ 08084   (856)566-6406   Fax (856)566-6026
+ Kennedy Memorial Hospital-University Medical Center
18 East Laurel Road/Neurology   Stratford, NJ 08084   (856)784-6800

Barone, Frank Anthony, MD {1891724332} Anesth(85,ITAL)
+ EmCare
425 Jack Martin Boulevard   Brick, NJ 08724   (732)840-3376
+ Morris Anesthesia Group, PA
3799 Route 46/Suite 211   Parsippany, NJ 07054   (732)840-3376   Fax (973)335-1448

Barone, Gregory John, DO {1104016187} EnDbMt, IntrMd(05,NJ75)
+ Cherry Hill Primary and Specialty Care
457 Haddonfield Road/Suite 110   Cherry Hill, NJ 08002

(844)542-2273   Fax (856)406-4570
Barone, Joseph G., MD {1871662676} PedUro, Urolgy, IntrMd(87,NJ06)<NJ-RWJUBRUN, NJ-HUNTRDN>
+ UH- Robert Wood Johnson Med
125 Paterson Street/MEB 588   New Brunswick, NJ 08901   (732)235-8853   Fax (732)235-8959

Barone, Luciano V., MD {1972601862} Pedtrc(78,NY20)<NY-STANTHNY>
+ Herbert Kania Pediatric Center
1900 Union Valley Road   Hewitt, NJ 07421   (973)728-4480   Fax (973)728-4375

Barone, Paul, DO {1124004346} CdvDis, IntrMd(93,NY75)<NJ-MORRISTN>
+ Barone & Catania Cardiovascular
786 Mountain Boulevard/Suite 200   Watchung, NJ 07069   (908)754-0975   Fax (908)754-0260

Barone, Robert Gerard, MD {1467486530} Ophthl, VitRet(88,DC02)<NJ-NWTNMEM>
+ Eye Physicians of Sussex County
183 High Street/Suite 2200   Newton, NJ 07860   (973)383-6345   Fax (973)383-0032

Barone, Stephen Robert, MD {1699701425} Anesth(01,FL02)
+ PO Box 3722
Princeton, NJ 08540

Baronia-White, Bernadette, MD {1609142728}
+ Mountainside Family Practice Associates
799 Bloomfield Avenue/Suite 201   Verona, NJ 07044   (973)746-7050   Fax (973)857-2831

Barot, Prayag, MD {1366463077} Surgry(00,NJ06)<NJ-RBAYPERT, NJ-RBAYOLDB>
+ AstraHealth Urgent & Primary Care
1100 Centennial Avenue/Suite 104   Piscataway, NJ 08854   (732)981-1111   Fax (732)981-1113

Barr, Gary Alan, MD {1982730701} Anesth, PainMd(70,PA12)<NJ-MTNSIDE>
+ Hackensack UMC Mountainside
1 Bay Avenue/Anesthesia   Montclair, NJ 07042   (973)429-6000   Fax (845)357-5777

Barr, James E., MD {1417971482} FamMed(83,PA09)<NJ-HUNTRDN>
+ Pleasant Run Family Physicians
925 US Highway 202   Neshanic Station, NJ 08853   (908)788-9468   Fax (908)788-5720

Barr, Jerome Ian, MD {1396914867} Rheuma, IntrMd(02,NY08)
+ Barr Medical Limited Liability Company
17-15 Maple Avenue/Suite 2   Fair Lawn, NJ 07410   (201)677-8759   Fax (201)654-7489

Barr, Larry Allen, DO {1689610958} FamMed(03,NJ75)
+ Family Practice of Moorestown
728 Marne Highway/Suite B   Moorestown, NJ 08057   (856)235-6600   Fax (856)235-6610

Barr, Lawrence I., DO {1790859460} SrgOrt(87,PA77)
+ Garden State Orthopedics & Sports Medicine
455 Route 70 West   Cherry Hill, NJ 08002   (609)616-2999   Fax (856)616-1437

Barr, Stuart A., MD {1992700579} CdvDis, IntrMd(87,NY19)<NJ-HACKNSK>
+ Westwood Cardiology Associates PA
333 Old Hook Road/Suite 200   Westwood, NJ 07675   (201)664-0201   Fax (201)666-7970

Barravecchio, Anthony John, DO {1114996477} FamMed, Grtrcs(95,PA77)<NJ-WAYNEGEN, NJ-VALLEY>
+ Allied Medical Associates
510 Hamburg Turnpike   Wayne, NJ 07470   (973)942-6005   Fax (973)442-6009

Barrera-Tolentino, Felicisima, MD {1205956703} Pedtrc, NnPnMd(69,PHI30)<NJ-HOBUNIMC, NJ-CHRIST>
+ 3524 Kennedy Boulevard
Jersey City, NJ 07307   (201)792-3022   Fax (201)653-4458

Barrese, James C., MD {1386938843} SrgNro
+ Capital Health System/Fuld Campus
750 Brunswick Avenue/Surgery/Neuro   Trenton, NJ 08638   (941)685-7724
jamesbarresemd@gmail.com

Barrese, James I., MD {1295984953} PedOto(06,IL11)
+ Cooper University Neurosurgery
Three Cooper Plaza/Suite 400   Camden, NJ 08103   (856)968-7965

Barresi, Joseph A., MD {1508867268} ObsGyn, IntrMd(73,NJ05)<NJ-OVERLOOK, NJ-MORRISTN>
+ Summit Medical Group
890 New Mountain Avenue   New Providence, NJ 07974   (908)277-8601

Barrett, Anna Mariya, MD {1205824356} Nrolgy(91,NY19)<NJ-KSLRWEST>
+ Kessler Institute for Rehabilitation West Orange
1199 Pleasant Valley Way   West Orange, NJ 07052   (973)731-3600

Barrett, Bryan Richard, DO {1649430109} FamMed, SprtMd(07,PA77)
+ AtlantiCare Urgent Care Center
2500 English Creek Avenue   Egg Harbor Township, NJ 08234

(609)407-2273
+ AtlantiCare Urgent Care Center
459 Route 9 South   Little Egg Harbor, NJ 08087   (609)407-2273   Fax (609)296-5735

Barrett, Michael P., DO {1851334841} SrgOrt(01,PA77)
+ Orthopedic & Neurosurgical Specialists, LLC.
807 Haddon Avenue/Suite 1   Haddonfield, NJ 08033   (856)795-9222   Fax (856)795-0026

Barrett, Theodore, MD {1679583322} ObsGyn(92,NY46)<NJ-UMDNJ>
+ University Physician Associates
140 Bergen Street/ACC Level C   Newark, NJ 07103   (973)972-2700   Fax (973)972-2739

Barrett, Thomas Arthur, MD {1427047646} SrgOrt(94,NJ05)<NJ-SHOREMEM, NJ-BURDTMLN>
+ Shore Orthopedic University Associates
24 Macarthur Boulevard/First Floor   Somers Point, NJ 08244   (609)927-1991   Fax (609)927-4203
+ Shore Orthopedic University Associates
9 Stites Avenue   Cape May Court House, NJ 08210   (609)927-1991   Fax (609)927-4203

Barrett Carnes, Joy-Lynne, MD {1467723262} FamMed, Grtrcs, IntrMd(10,DMN01)
+ Capital Health Family Health Center
433 Bellevue Avenue/4th Floor   Trenton, NJ 08618   (609)278-5900   Fax (609)392-8639
+ JFK Medical Center
65 James Street   Edison, NJ 08820   (732)321-7493

Barricella, Robert Louis, DO {1518008960} PedEmg, Pedtrc(84,NJ75)<NJ-UMDNJ>
+ University Hospital
150 Bergen Street/PdtrcEmergency   Newark, NJ 07103   (973)972-4300   Fax (973)972-5965

Barrientos, Monica, MD {1356620447} IntrMd
+ Cardio-Med Services
3196 Kennedy Boulevard/3rd Floor   Union City, NJ 07087   (201)974-0077

Barrington, Dorrie-Susan Adele, MD {1184679557} IntrMd(99,NY45)<NJ-COOPRUMC>
+ Cooper University Hospital
One Cooper Plaza/Dorrance/Ste222   Camden, NJ 08103   (856)342-2000

Barrios, Tomas J., MD {1023181468} Pedtrc(75,SPAI)<NJ-HOBUNIMC>
+ 311 33rd Street
Union City, NJ 07087   (201)863-4782

Barrison, Adam F., MD {1669473328} Gastrn, IntrMd(95,NY19)<NJ-OVERLOOK, NJ-MORRISTN>
+ Summit Medical Group-Berkeley Heights Campus
1 Diamond Hill Road/4 FL/Gastro   Berkeley Heights, NJ 07922   (908)277-8940   Fax (908)673-7140

Barritta, Domenica Maria, MD {1063428878} Gastrn, IntrMd(93,ITA08)
+ 18 Oliver Street
Newark, NJ 07102   (973)645-0000   Fax (973)645-0001

Barrows, Frank P., IV, DO {1427025535} Pedtrc, PedEnd(99,NJ75)<NJ-MONMOUTH>
+ Drs. Barrows and Ostrow
180 Avenue at the Common/Suite 7B   Shrewsbury, NJ 07702   (732)935-7143   Fax (732)935-7245
+ Monmouth Medical Group, P.C.
1 Route 70   Lakewood, NJ 08701   (732)935-7143   Fax (732)901-0199

Barrucco, Robert John, DO {1346408747} CdvDis
+ Virtua Cardiology Group
2309 East Evesham Road/Suites 201-202   Voorhees, NJ 08043   (856)325-5400   Fax (856)325-5416

Barry, Kevin M., MD {1144202268} Anesth(87,NJ05)<NJ-MORRISTN>
+ Anesthesia Associates
100 Madison Avenue   Morristown, NJ 07960   (973)631-8119   Fax (973)631-8120
+ Anesthesia Associates of Morristown
264 South Street/Suite 2A   Morristown, NJ 07960   (973)631-8119

Barry, Kevin P., MD {1235131707} Radiol, RadDia(89,PA02)
+ Larchmont Medical Imaging
204-210 Ark Road/LMC 1-2   Mount Laurel, NJ 08054   (856)778-8860   Fax (609)261-4180

Barry, Peter Francis, DO {1609844828} IntrMd(99,NY75)
+ Sports Extra
67 Walnut Avenue/Suite 202B   Clark, NJ 07066   (732)388-7300   Fax (732)388-1330

Barry, Therese Maria, MD {1952359960} FamMed(96,PA77)
+ 833 Lacey Road/Suite 6
Forked River, NJ 08731   (609)242-6700   Fax (609)242-6701

Barsanti, Patricia L., DO {1699859371} IntrMd(01,PA77)
+ Internal Medicine Associates of Union PC
154 Mount Bethel Road/Bld B   Warren, NJ 07059   (908)755-5400   Fax (908)755-6979
Info@barsantimedical.com

Physicians by Name and Address

Barsbay, Dunay, MD {1013396977}<NJ-HOBUNIMC>
+ Hoboken University Medical Center
308 Willow Avenue   Hoboken, NJ 07030   (201)418-3126

Barshay, Veniamin, MD {1801802962} RadDia(03,NY45)<NJ-COOPRUMC>
+ Cooper University Hospital
One Cooper Plaza/Radiology   Camden, NJ 08103   (856)342-2380   Fax (856)365-0472

Barshikar, Surendra Shrikrishna, MD {1366684920} PhysMd<NJ-SHOREREH>
+ Shore Rehabilitation Institute
425 Jack Martin Boulevard   Brick, NJ 08724   (732)836-4500

Barsky, Aron Alan, MD {1023273703} CdvDis, IntrMd, CarEch(05,NY08)<NJ-TRINIJSC, NJ-TRININPC>
+ 4 Ethel Road/Suite 405-B
Edison, NJ 08817   (732)287-0255   Fax (732)287-0355

Barsky, Carol, MD {1811939655} EmrgMd
+ Hackensack University Medical Center
30 Prospect Avenue   Hackensack, NJ 07601   (201)996-2000

Barsky, Robert I., DO {1982641288} Urolgy(81,PA77)<NJ-KMHTURNV>
+ Delaware Valley Urology LLC
570 Egg Harbor Road/Suite A-1   Sewell, NJ 08080   (856)582-9645   Fax (856)985-4583
+ New Jersey Urology, LLC
2401 East Evesham Road/Suite F   Voorhees, NJ 08043   (856)582-9645   Fax (856)988-0636

Barsoom, Raafat S., MD {1750525432} EmrgMd, Surgry(95,EGY03)
+ JFK Medical Center
65 James Street   Edison, NJ 08820   (732)321-7605   Fax (732)744-5614

Barsoum, Sylviana S., MD {1841343688} Anesth(89,NY08)<NJ-RWJUBRUN>
+ Robert Wood Johnson-UMDNJ Anesthesia Group
125 Paterson Street/CAB 3100   New Brunswick, NJ 08901   (732)235-7827   Fax (732)235-6131

Barter, Cindy Monette, MD {1275565475} FamMed
+ Phillips Barber Family Health Center
72 Alexander Avenue   Lambertville, NJ 08530   (609)397-3535   Fax (609)397-0301

Barth, Holli Ami, MD {1245432210} Anesth(07,PA09)
+ Cape Regional Medical Center
2 Stone Harbor Boulevard   Cape May Court House, NJ 08210   (609)463-2498

Barth, Jay Allan, MD {1851537146} PedGst, Pedtrc(89,PA01)
+ 550 Warwick Avenue
Teaneck, NJ 07666

Barth, Michael, MD {1750306411} Rheuma(83,DMN01)<NJ-MORRISTN>
+ Rockaway Family Medicine Associates
333 Mount Hope Avenue   Rockaway, NJ 07866   (973)895-6601   Fax (973)895-5324
+ Internal Medicine Faculty Associates
435 South Street/Suite 210   Morristown, NJ 07960   (973)895-6601   Fax (973)290-7675

Barth, Nadine, MD {1205085214} Surgry
+ Cooper Surgical Associates
3 Cooper Plaza/Suite 411   Camden, NJ 08103   (856)342-2270   Fax (856)365-1180
+ Cooper University Physician Trauma Center
One Cooper Plaza   Camden, NJ 08103   (856)342-3014

Barthelemy, Markintosh, MD {1720247901} EmrgMd(05,NJ06)
+ 73 East Parsonage Way
Manalapan, NJ 07726
+ Community Medical Center
99 Route 37 West   Toms River, NJ 08755   (732)818-3882

Bartimus, Holly A., MD {1558373753} EmrgMd(06,WA04)
+ Cooper University Hospital
One Cooper Plaza   Camden, NJ 08103   (856)356-4935

Bartiss, Mark J., MD {1043432925} FamMed(86,MEXI)<NJ-SOCEANCO>
+ Institute for Complementary & Alternative Medicine
63 Lacey Road/Unit C   Whiting, NJ 08759   (609)978-9002   admin@icamnj.com

Bartky, Eric Jay, MD {1023233426} PsyCAd(84,NY09)<NY-PRSBCOLU>
+ Bartky HealthCare Center, LLC
513 West Mount Pleasant Avenue   Livingston, NJ 07039   (973)533-1195   Fax (973)533-1305
+ Adolescent Medicine of MMH
100 Madison Avenue   Morristown, NJ 07960   (973)971-4330

Bartlett, Jacqueline A., MD {1952468134} Psychy, PsyCAd, Pedtrc(71,OH41)<NJ-UMDNJ>
+ University Psychiatric Associates
183 South Orange Avenue/E-F Levels   Newark, NJ 07103   (973)972-2977   Fax (973)972-2979

Bartley-Chin, Dellareece M., MD {1154456580} PhysMd(92,NY08)
+ Bartley HealthCare Nursing and Rehabilitation
175 Bartley Road   Jackson, NJ 08527   (732)370-4700   Fax (732)370-8872

Bartock, Jason Lee, MD {1316176043}<NJ-STPETER>
+ Cooper University Hospital
One Cooper Plaza   Camden, NJ 08103   (856)342-2000

Bartolozzi, Arthur Robert, MD {1710921887} SprtMd, SrgArt<PA-PENNHOSP>
+ Aria 3B Orthopaedics, P.C.
1400 East Route 70/Second Floor   Cherry Hill, NJ 08034

Barton, Keith A., DO {1154326619} Anesth(99,PA77)<NJ-MERIDNHS>
+ Robert Wood Johnson-UMDNJ Anesthesia Group
1140 Route 72 West   Manahawkin, NJ 08050   (609)978-8900

Barton, Loucia C., MD {1538103866} RadDia(86,NY19)<NJ-MORRISTN>
+ Hirsch & Ratakonda MD, PA
290 Madison Avenue/Suite 4   Morristown, NJ 07960   (973)538-8181   Fax (973)538-6565

Barton, William W., MD {1710024641} IntrMd, PulDis, CritCr(89,TN05)
+ Princeton Medical Group, P.A.
419 North Harrison Street   Princeton, NJ 08540   (609)924-9300   Fax (609)924-6552
+ Princeton Medical Group PA
2 Research Way/Bldg 2/Suite 302   Monroe Township, NJ 08831   (609)924-9300   Fax (609)655-7466

Bartov, David Nir, MD {1467616664} IntrMd(05,ISR02)<CT-YALENHH>
+ Associates in Cardiovascular Disease, LLC
571 Central Avenue/Suite 115   New Providence, NJ 07974   (908)464-2000   Fax (908)464-1332

Barua, Aruna, MD {1609940121} IntrMd(94,BAN02)
+ 218 Taylor Road
Paramus, NJ 07652

Baruch, Edward M., MD {1801096284} Psychy, PsyGrt(85,NY08)
+ Psychiatric & Addiction Serv of So NJ
813 East Gate Drive   Mount Laurel, NJ 08054   (856)273-8364   Fax (856)273-6408

Baruch, Howard Michael, MD {1023025236} SrgOrt(85,DC02)<NJ-HACKNSK, NJ-BERGNMC>
+ Premier Orthopaedics and Sports Medicine, P.C.
3196 Kennedy Boulevard/Third Floor   Union City, NJ 07087   (201)770-1600   Fax (201)770-1010
+ Premier Orthopaedics and Sports Medicine, PC
663 Palisade Avenue/Suite 302   Cliffside Park, NJ 07010   (201)770-1600   Fax (201)943-7308
+ Premier Orthopaedics and Sports Medicine, P.C.
111 Galway Place   Teaneck, NJ 07087   (201)833-9500   Fax (201)862-0095

Baruch, Michael I., MD {1336189604} SrgPlstc, Surgry(77,NY46)
+ Michael I. Baruch Plastic Surgery Associates
1037 Route 46 East/Suite 103   Clifton, NJ 07013   (973)773-1973   Fax (973)773-4824

Baruchin, Mitchell Alan, MD {1013973916} CdvDis, IntrMd(84,NY47)<NJ-CHRIST>
+ Total Cardiology Care
120 Franklin Street   Jersey City, NJ 07307   (201)216-9791   Fax (201)216-1362
+ Total Cardiology Care
2035 Hamburg Pike/Suite L   Wayne, NJ 07470   (201)216-9791   Fax (973)248-3455

Baruffi, Seth L., MD {1881897916} EmrgMd
+ 1799 Ferrari Drive
Vineland, NJ 08361

Barzaga, Ricardo A., MD {1922044759} IntrMd, InfDis(80,PHIL)<NJ-ACMCITY>
+ AtlantiCare Clinical Associates
16 South Ohio Avenue   Atlantic City, NJ 08401   (609)441-2104
+ AtlantiCare Regional Medical Center/City Campus
1925 Pacific Avenue   Atlantic City, NJ 08401   (609)345-4000

Barzel, Eyal, MD {1073572020} RadDia, RadV&I, Radiol(85,NY01)<NJ-COOPRUMC>
+ American Access Care
207 South Kings Highway/Suite 2   Cherry Hill, NJ 08034   (856)616-8600   Fax (856)616-8601

Basak, Jayati, MD {1720155518} Anesth(79,INA1K)
+ Fort Lee Surgery Center
1608 Lemoine Avenue/Suite 101   Fort Lee, NJ 07024   (201)346-1112   Fax (201)346-1885

Basak, Sandip, MD {1619950490} RadNro, RadDia(96,NY19)<NJ-STPETER, NJ-RWJUBRUN>
+ University Radiology Group, P.C.
579A Cranbury Road   East Brunswick, NJ 08816   (732)390-0040   Fax (732)390-1856

Basalaev, Misha, MD {1144268137} IntrMd(87,NJ06)<NJ-RWJUBRUN, NJ-STPETER>
+ 561 Cranbury Road
East Brunswick, NJ 08816   (732)390-7400   Fax (732)390-1900

Basara, Matthew, Jr., MD {1972602191} IntrMd(88,NJ05)<NJ-VIRTMHBC, NJ-RWJUHAM>
+ Delran Internal Medicine
5045 Route 130 South/Suite E   Delran, NJ 08075   (856)764-2525   Fax (856)764-6344

Bascara, Daniel, MD {1154488237} IntrMd, Psychy, PsyCAd(94,PHI15)<NJ-UMDNJ>
+ University Psychiatric Associates
183 South Orange Avenue/E-F Levels   Newark, NJ 07103   (973)972-2977   Fax (973)972-2979

Bascelli, Lynda Marie, MD {1558350215} FamMed(97,NY03)
+ West Street Health Center
519 West Street   Camden, NJ 08103   (856)968-2320   Fax (856)968-2317

Basch, David B., MD {1053322354} SrgOrt, SrgSpn(89,NJ05)<NJ-STCLRDEN, NJ-STCLRDOV>
+ Spine & Orthopedic Center of New Jersey
90 Sparta Avenue   Sparta, NJ 07871   (973)726-9500   Fax (973)726-8218
staff@drbasch.com
+ Spine & Orthopedic Center of New Jersey
590 Newark Avenue   Jersey City, NJ 07306   (973)726-9500   Fax (973)726-8218
+ Spine & Orthopedic Center of New Jersey
635 Broadway   Paterson, NJ 07871   (973)726-9500   Fax (973)726-8218

Baseluos, Cindy Rosemary Adly, MD {1679769715} EmrgMd(07,NJ06)<NY-CMCSTVSI>
+ Emergency Medical Associates of NJ, P.A.
3 Century Drive   Parsippany, NJ 07054   (973)740-0607   Fax (973)740-9895

Baseman, Debra L., MD {1114008430} ObsGyn(90,PA13)<NJ-UNVMCPRN>
+ Princeton Medical Group, P.A.
419 North Harrison Street   Princeton, NJ 08540   (609)924-9300   Fax (609)924-6552
+ Princeton Medical Group PA
2 Research Way/Bldg 2/Suite 302   Monroe Township, NJ 08831   (609)924-9300   Fax (609)655-7466

Bash, Howard Lee, MD {1871756874} PsyCAd(03,PA09)<NJ-MORRISTN>
+ Morristown Medical Center
100 Madison Avenue/Psych   Morristown, NJ 07962   (973)971-5000   Fax (973)290-8349

Bash, Lisa Taub, MD {1295909190} RadDia(02,PA13)
+ Montclair Radiology
20 High Street   Nutley, NJ 07110   (973)284-0020   Fax (973)284-6310

Bash, Robin Ellen, MD {1730225210} PhysMd(93,NY08)
+ Ani Orthopaedic Group
1 Bethany Road/Bldg. 2 Suite 21   Hazlet, NJ 07730   (732)264-8282   Fax (732)264-8131
+ Ani Orthopaedic Group
200 Perrine Road/Suite 220   Old Bridge, NJ 08857   (732)264-8282   Fax (732)264-8131

Bashir, Asif, MD {1104021054} SrgNro, IntrMd(95,PAK01)<NJ-JFKMED>
+ JFK Neurosciences Institute
65 James Street/Second Floor   Edison, NJ 08818   (732)321-7010   Fax (732)632-1584
+ JFK Medical Center
65 James Street/Surgery/Neuro   Edison, NJ 08820   (732)321-7010   Fax (732)632-1584

Bashline, Benjamin R., DO {1982947966} Dermat
+ The Dermatology Group, P.C.
88 Park Avenue/Suite 2 A   Nutley, NJ 07110   (973)571-2121

Basi, Seema, MD {1497793202} Nephro, IntrMd(99,IL06)
+ Princeton Hypertension-Nephrology
88 Princeton Hightstown Road/Suite 203   Princeton Junction, NJ 08550   (609)750-7330   Fax (609)750-7336

Basilious, Manal, MD {1023039773} Anesth
+ 4 Winchester Drive
East Brunswick, NJ 08816

Basilone, Joseph, MD {1518995588} IntrMd, PhysMd(88,ITAL)<NJ-RIVERVW>
+ Center for Physical Medicine and Rehabilitation
30 North Main Street   Marlboro, NJ 07746   (732)761-0500
+ Center for Physical Medicine and Rehabilitation
776 Shrewsbury Avenue/Suite 203   Tinton Falls, NJ 07724   (732)761-0500   Fax (732)219-6526

Basista, Michael P., MD {1639112501} FamMed(77,NJ06)<NJ-MTNSIDE>
+ ImmediCenter/Bloomfield
557 Broad Street   Bloomfield, NJ 07003   (973)680-8300   Fax (973)743-5601
+ ImmediCenter/Clifton
1355 Broad Street   Clifton, NJ 07013   (973)680-8300   Fax (973)778-2268
+ ImmediCenter/Totowa
500 Union Boulevard   Totowa, NJ 07003   (973)790-0090   Fax (973)790-6070

Basit, Nauman A., MD {1700151701} Pedtrc
+ Bayonne Medical Care LLC
415 Avenel Street/Suite A   Avenel, NJ 07001   (732)750-1180   Fax (732)750-1182

Basius, Joseph T., DO {1952474934} Anesth(88,ME75)<NJ-STBARNMC>
+ New Jersey Anesthesia Associates, P.C.
252 Columbia Turnpike/PO Box 0037   Florham Park, NJ 07932   (973)660-9334   Fax (973)660-9779

Basius, Maureen, DO {1033110002} Pthlgy, PthACl(88,NJ75)<NJ-HUNTRDN>
+ Hunterdon Medical Center
2100 Wescott Drive/Pathology   Flemington, NJ 08822   (908)788-6100   Fax (908)237-2334

Baskerville, Renee E., DO {1376769372} Pedtrc, AdolMd(82,NJ75)<NJ-NWRKBETH>
+ Comprehensive Care Center
297 16th Avenue   Newark, NJ 07103   (973)485-3300   Fax (973)485-0226

Baskies, Arnold M., MD {1326049693} SrgVas, Surgry(75,MA05)
+ Rancocas Valley Surgical Associates PA
1000 Salem Road/Suite A   Willingboro, NJ 08046   (609)877-1737   Fax (609)877-1589

Baskies, Michael Ari, MD {1992721617} SrgOrt, OrtSHand, SrgHnd(02,NY19)
+ Atlantic Orthopedic Institute
111 Madison Avenue/Suite 400   Morristown, NJ 07960   (908)340-4800   Fax (908)340-4801

Baskin, Jonathan Jay, MD {1639136757} SrgNro, SrgSpn(92,MD07)<NJ-MORRISTN, NJ-ATLANTHS>
+ Atlantic Neurosurgical Specialists
310 Madison Avenue/Suite 300   Morristown, NJ 07960   (973)285-7800   Fax (973)285-7839

Baskin, Stuart E., MD {1043240104} IntrMd, Nephro(64,MO34)<NJ-UMDNJ, NJ-EASTORNG>
+ Rutgers- New Jersey Medical School
185 South Orange Avenue   Newark, NJ 07103   (973)972-4300
+ 225 Millburn Avenue
Millburn, NJ 07041   (973)972-4300   Fax (973)218-1801

Basralian, Kevin R., MD {1851392252} Urolgy, IntrMd(79,MEX14)<NJ-HACKNSK, NJ-HOLYNAME>
+ HUMC Faculty Practice
360 Essex Street/Suite 403   Hackensack, NJ 07601   (201)336-8090   Fax (201)336-8221

Basri, William E., MD {1992778948} Gastrn, IntrMd(88,NY47)<NJ-JRSYSHMC, NJ-OCEANMC>
+ Atlantic Coast Gastroenterology
1944 Corlies Avenue/Suite 205   Neptune, NJ 07753   (732)776-9300   Fax (732)776-8059
+ Atlantic Coast Gastroenterology
1640 Route 88 West/Suite 202   Brick, NJ 08724   (732)776-9300   Fax (732)458-8529

Bass, Irina, MD {1346212156} Pedtrc(90,BLA01)<NJ-VALLEY, NJ-HACKNSK>
+ KidKare Medical P.A.
15-01 Broadway/Suite 36   Fair Lawn, NJ 07410   (201)773-6171   Fax (201)773-4845
Irinabass13@yahoo.com

Bass, Jon Lawrence, MD {1407857659} IntrMd, PulDis, CritCr(97,NY09)<NJ-OVERLOOK, NJ-MORRISTN>
+ Summit Medical Group-Berkeley Heights Campus
1 Diamond Hill Road   Berkeley Heights, NJ 07922   (908)273-4300   Fax (908)277-8927

Bassan, Matthew Evan, DO {1881019594} SprtMd
+ Garden State Orthopaedic Associates, P.A.
28-04 Broadway   Fair Lawn, NJ 07410   (201)791-4434   Fax (201)791-9377

Bassani, Luigi, MD {1275737991} SrgNro, Surgry(06,DC02)
+ Rutgers NJ School of Medicine Neurology
90 Bergen Street/DOC 5200   Newark, NJ 07103   (973)972-9502   Fax (973)972-5059
+ Neurosurgeons of New Jersey
200 South Orange Avenue/Suite 116   Livingston, NJ 07039   (973)718-9919

Bassil, Ghassan G., MD {1154483436} PthACl(72,SYR01)<NJ-STMRYPAS>
+ St. Mary's Hospital
350 Boulevard   Passaic, NJ 07055   (973)365-4300   Fax (973)473-3367

Basta, Janette A., MD {1134137177} Pedtrc(86,EGY04)<NJ-STJOSHOS, NJ-WAYNEGEN>
+ 1035 Route 46 East/Suite G1
Clifton, NJ 07013   (973)249-9620   Fax (973)249-9621
mzbasta@hotmail.com

Basta, Magdy Z., MD {1366458689} Pedtrc(81,EGYP)<NJ-WAYNEGEN, NJ-STJOSHOS>
+ 1035 Route 46 East/Suite G1
Clifton, NJ 07013   (973)249-9620   Fax (973)249-9621
mzbasta@hotmail.com

Bastianelli, Milo, DO {1811937048} Otlryg, SrgOrt(92,NJ75)<NJ-CHRIST>
+ Associated Ear Nose & Throat Physicians
505 Chestnut Street   Roselle Park, NJ 07204   (908)241-0200   Fax (908)241-0445
+ Associated Ear Nose & Throat Physicians
778 Kennedy Boulevard   Bayonne, NJ 07002   (908)241-0200   Fax (201)829-1821

Bastidas, Jaime Adolfo, MD {1992807705} SrgPlstc, IntrMd(94,NJ05)
+ 244 Roseberry Street/Suite 5
Phillipsburg, NJ 08865   (908)454-1704   Fax (908)454-1706

Bastien, Arnaud, MD {1619065927} IntrMd(85,WIND)
+ Cooper Physicians
1210 Brace Road/Suite 102   Cherry Hill, NJ 08034   (856)428-6616   Fax (856)428-4823

Bastien, Linda, MD {1346280542} FamMed, IntrMd(00,NJ06)
+ Neighborhood Health Center Plainfield
1700-58 Myrtle Avenue   Plainfield, NJ 07060   (908)753-6401   Fax (908)226-6743

Bastien, Maria Altagrace, MD {1942305107} PhysMd(86,HAI01)
+ CareOne at Moorestown
895 Westfield Avenue   Moorestown, NJ 08057   (856)914-0444   Fax (856)914-0445

Bastien, Pascale, MD {1598792566} Pedtrc, AdolMd(91,NY09)<NJ-VIRTMHBC, NJ-LOURDMED>
+ Pediatric & Adolescent Medicine of Delran
8008 Route 130 North/Suite 204   Delran, NJ 08075   (856)824-0099   Fax (856)824-0088

Baston, Kaitlan, MD {1639464696} FamMed
+ The Cooper Hospital System-Univ Hospital
3 Cooper Plaza/Suite 215   Camden, NJ 08103   (856)342-2439

Basu, Mihir Kumar, MD {1548358690} CdvDis, IntrMd(63,INDI)<NJ-HOLYNAME>
+ General Clinic
7511 Bergenline Avenue   North Bergen, NJ 07047   (201)868-0257   Fax (201)868-0642

Basu, Sebika, MD {1932142775} Pedtrc(72,INA02)
+ Neighborhood Health Center Plainfield
1700-58 Myrtle Avenue/Pediatrics   Plainfield, NJ 07060   (908)753-6401   Fax (908)226-6743

Baszak, Sylvia, MD {1407958606} PedEmg, Pedtrc(03,POL02)<NJ-RWJUBRUN>
+ University Medical Group Pediatrics
125 Paterson Street/MEB 3rd Fl   New Brunswick, NJ 08903   (732)235-7893   Fax (732)235-9340

Batacchi, Zona Olivia, MD {1629352869} EnDbMt
+ Summit Medical Group-Berkeley Heights Campus
1 Diamond Hill Road   Berkeley Heights, NJ 07922   (908)277-8667   Fax (908)277-8707
+ Summit Medical Group
890 New Mountain Avenue   New Providence, NJ 07974   (908)277-8601

Batarseh, Hani Elias Salim, MD {1114907557} IntrMd(77,RUS01)
+ Batarseh Walk in Medical Center
540 Bordentown Avenue/Suite 2100   South Amboy, NJ 08879   (732)721-1500   Fax (732)721-1599

Batchelor, Christopher D., Jr., MD {1417215468} IntrMd
+ Summit Medical Group
31-00 Broadway   Fair Lawn, NJ 07410   (201)796-2255   Fax (201)796-7020
+ Summit Medical Group
6 Brighton Road/2 FL   Clifton, NJ 07012   (201)796-2255   Fax (973)777-5403

Batchu, Bharathi, MD {1316198252} RadDia(02,INA68)<NJ-COMMED>
+ Community Medical Center
99 Route 37 West/Radiology   Toms River, NJ 08755   (732)557-8151   Fax (732)505-0325
+ Coastal Imaging, LLC
79 Route 37 West/Suite 103   Toms River, NJ 08755   (732)557-8151   Fax (732)276-2325

Bathini, Manjula, DO {1508011719} Nrolgy, ClNrPh(94,IA75)
+ Atlantic Sleep & Pulmonary Associates
300 Madison Avenue/Suite 201   Madison, NJ 07940   (973)822-2772   Fax (973)822-2773

Batista, Jose, MD {1912055039} Pedtrc(00,DOM21)
+ Batista Pediatrics
156 Market Street   Paterson, NJ 07505   (973)742-7720   Fax (973)742-7722
Batistapediatrics@yahoo.com

Batra, Chhaya, MD {1659464667} Pedtrc, IntrMd(03,NJ06)<NJ-STBARNMC, NJ-OVERLOOK>
+ Millburn Pediatrics PA
159 Millburn Avenue   Millburn, NJ 07041   (973)912-0155   Fax (973)912-8714

Batra, Lina S., MD {1104918077} IntrMd, Nephro(73,INA07)<NJ-JFKMED, NJ-RWJURAH>
+ Prudent Med Associates LLC
220 Bridge Str at Bridge Point   Metuchen, NJ 08840   (732)548-2500   Fax (732)549-7070

Batra, Norman Mohan, MD {1275604076} PhysMd(66,INA58)<NJ-JFKMED, NJ-RWJURAH>
+ Prudent Medical Associates
220 Bridge Street/Building E   Metuchen, NJ 08840   (732)548-2500   Fax (732)549-7070
+ JFK Medical Center
65 James Street/Attending/PM&R   Edison, NJ 08820   (732)321-7000
+ Robert Wood Johnson University Hospital at Rahway
865 Stone Street/Attending/PM&R   Rahway, NJ 08840   (732)381-4200

Batra, Sonal, MD {1023202439} Psychy
+ Princetown House Behavioral Health
615 Hope Road/1B, 2nd flr.   Eatontown, NJ 07724   (848)208-2600   Fax (848)208-2601

Batsides, George Pete, MD {1992874705} SrgThr, Surgry(97,GRN01)<NJ-RWJUBRUN, NJ-STFRNMED>
+ UMDNJ RWJ CardioThoracic Surgery
125 Paterson Street/Suite 4100   New Brunswick, NJ 08901   (732)235-7800   Fax (732)235-7013
batsidgp@umdnj.edu

Batt, Gerald E., MD {1861568578} Ophthl(77,IL42)<NJ-HUNTRDN>
+ 121 Route 31/Suite 200
Flemington, NJ 08822   (908)788-2010   Fax (908)788-8492
Battmanoole@yahoo.com
+ Hunterdon Medical Center
2100 Wescott Drive   Flemington, NJ 08822   (908)788-6100

Batta, Sanjay, MD {1669693552} IntrMd(91,INDI)
+ Central Jersey Primary Care Associates
240 Williamson Street   Elizabeth, NJ 07202   (908)351-4608   Fax (908)436-9299
Epcsbatta@gmail.com

Battista, Carl J., MD {1386700987} Pedtrc(85,GRN01)<NJ-ENGLWOOD, NJ-HOLYNAME>
+ 680 Kinderkamack Road/Suite 301
Oradell, NJ 07649   (201)634-1004   Fax (201)634-1028

Battle, Karen Marie, DO {1891029088}<NJ-HOBUNIMC>
+ Hoboken University Medical Center
308 Willow Avenue   Hoboken, NJ 07030   (412)884-8990   Fax (412)884-8989

Batwara, Ruchika, MD {1164500146} Nephro, IntrMd(03,INA30)<NJ-NWRKBETH>
+ 1818 JFK Boulevard
Jersey City, NJ 07305   (201)333-8222   Fax (201)333-0095

Bauberger, Charles Joseph, MD {1053382101} FamMed, IntrMd(99,GRN01)
+ 1721 Brooklyn Avenue
Whiting, NJ 08759   (908)910-5804
+ Walson Air Force Medical Facility
5250 New Jersey Avenue   Fort Dix, NJ 08640

Bauer, Brian J., MD {1932110970} SrgOrt(81,NY08)<NJ-HACKNSK, NJ-HOLYNAME>
+ Eastern Orthopedic Associates
222 Cedar Lane/Suite 120   Teaneck, NJ 07666   (201)836-5332   Fax (201)836-4002

Bauer, Christel Janet, MD {1104852151} Radiol, RadNro, RadDia(88,NY20)
+ Fair Lawn Diagnostic Imaging
19-04 Fair Lawn Avenue   Fair Lawn, NJ 07410   (201)794-3132   Fax (201)794-6291

Bauer, Christopher Joseph, MD {1154614576}
+ Physicians for Women
330 Ratzer Road/Suite 7   Wayne, NJ 07470   (973)694-2222   Fax (973)694-7664

Bauer, Francis Douglas, MD {1275609885} IntrMd(78,MEX03)
+ Care Point Health Associates
1225 McBride Avenue/Suite 200   Little Falls, NJ 07424   (973)256-5557   Fax (973)256-5036
fdbauermd@gmail.com

Bauer, Hans Henry, Jr., MD {1972582245} CdvDis, IntCrd, IntrMd(89,NY09)<NJ-OURLADY, NJ-VIRTUAHS>
+ Associated Cardiovascular Consultants-Lourdes
1 Brace Road/Suite C & F   Cherry Hill, NJ 08034   (856)428-4100   Fax (856)428-4058

Bauer-Sheldon, Melissa Ann, DO {1114931011} FamMed(99,NJ75)
+ Advocare Grove Family Medical Associates
132 Grove Street/Suite A   Haddonfield, NJ 08033   (856)354-2211   Fax (856)354-6181

Baum, Howard B., MD {1558301176} Gastrn, IntrMd(77,NY20)
+ Summit Medical Group
6 Brighton Road/2 FL   Clifton, NJ 07012   (973)777-7911   Fax (973)777-5403

Baum, Jonathan D., MD {1760421978} ObsGyn, Obstet, IntrMd(95,PA09)<NJ-CENTRAST, NJ-JRSYSHMC>
+ Hackensack Meridian Medical Group Ob/Gyn, Freehold
3499 Route 9 North/Suite 2B   Freehold, NJ 07728   (732)577-1199   Fax (732)577-8922

Physicians by Name and Address

Baum, Mark L., MD {1689672941} RadDia, Radiol, IntrMd(82,NY47)
  + South Jersey Radiology Associates, P.A.
    100 Carnie Boulevard/Suite B-5   Voorhees, NJ 08043   (856)374-4031   Fax (856)232-9139
  + South Jersey Radiology Associates, P.A.
    748 Kings Highway   West Deptford, NJ 08096   (856)374-4031   Fax (856)853-7362
  + South Jersey Radiology Associates, P.A.
    Severan Profess Mews/Suite 105   Sewell, NJ 08043   (856)848-4998   Fax (856)589-6142

Baum, Michael Jay, DO {1376694786} FamMed(83,NJ75)<NJ-RWJURAH>
  + 908 Oak Tree Road/Suite K
    South Plainfield, NJ 07080   (908)757-6660   Fax (908)757-5332

Baum, Raymond M., MD {1508890864} PsyFor, Psychy(86,MEX34)<NJ-UNIVBHC>
  + 445 Brick Boulevard/Suite 206
    Brick, NJ 08723   (732)903-7186   Fax (732)903-7187

Baum, Richard D., MD {1891838983} Urolgy(81,LA01)<NJ-VALLEY>
  + Urology Group PA
    4 Godwin Avenue   Midland Park, NJ 07432   (201)444-7070   Fax (201)444-7228

Bauman, David C., MD {1518944784} FamMed, SprtMd(77,PA02)<NJ-MEMSALEM>
  + Woodstown Family Practice
    125 East Avenue/Suite C   Woodstown, NJ 08098   (856)769-2800   Fax (856)769-4256

Bauman, Gregory A., MD {1023225117} Anesth(06,GRN01)<CT-YALENHH>
  + St. Joseph's Regional Medical Center Anesthesia
    703 Main Street   Paterson, NJ 07503   (973)754-2323   Fax (973)977-9455

Bauman, Jeffrey Michael, MD {1447240718} IntrMd, EnDbMt(01,NJ05)<NJ-OVERLOOK, NJ-MORRISTN>
  + Summit Medical Group-Berkeley Heights Campus
    1 Diamond Hill Road   Berkeley Heights, NJ 07922   (908)277-8667   Fax (908)277-8707

Bauman, Susan M., MD {1407820475} FamMed, Grtrcs(79,PA01)<NJ-HUNTRDN>
  + Delaware Valley Family Health Center
    200 Frenchtown Road   Milford, NJ 08848   (908)995-2251   Fax (908)995-2036

Baumann, Brigitte Monika, MD {1598853814} EmrgMd(95,NY20)<NJ-COOPRUMC>
  + Cooper University Hospital
    One Cooper Plaza/EmergMed   Camden, NJ 08103   (856)342-2000

Baumann, John C., MD {1619917507} RadOnc, Radiol(77,DC03)<NJ-UNVMCPRN, NJ-CENTRAST>
  + University Medical Center of Princeton at Plainsboro
    One Plainsboro Road/Radiology   Plainsboro, NJ 08536   (609)497-4304   Fax (609)497-4306
  + Princeton Radiation Oncology Center
    9 Centre Drive/Suite 115   Jamesburg, NJ 08831   (609)497-4304   Fax (609)655-5725
  + Hunterdon Regional Cancer Ctr
    2100 Wescott Drive   Flemington, NJ 08536   (908)788-6461   Fax (908)788-6412

Baumgarten, Steven S., MD {1528038114} CritCr, IntrMd, PulDis(82,NY19)
  + Pulmonary & Sleep Associates of SJ, LLC.
    107 Berlin Road   Cherry Hill, NJ 08034   (856)429-1800   Fax (856)429-1081
  + Pulmonary & Sleep Associates of SJ, LLC.
    750 Route 73 South/Suite 401   Marlton, NJ 08053   (856)429-1800   Fax (856)375-2325
  + Pulmonary & Sleep Associates of SJ, LLC.
    811 Sunset Road/Suite 201   Burlington, NJ 08034   (609)298-1776   Fax (609)531-2391

Baumlin, Thomas, Jr., MD {1427041862} Pedtrc(67,PA09)<NJ-MONMOUTH, NJ-RIVERVW>
  + Matawan Surgical Associates
    717 North Beers Street/Suite 1-E   Holmdel, NJ 07733   (732)847-3300   Fax (732)739-5295

Bautista, Amelia B., MD {1760460703} NnPnMd, Pedtrc(74,PHI01)<NJ-OURLADY, NJ-ACMCITY>
  + Our Lady of Lourdes Medical Center
    1600 Haddon Avenue/Neo-Peri Med   Camden, NJ 08103   (856)757-3500

Bautista, Eduardo R., MD {1265405880} NnPnMd, Pedtrc(87,PHIL)<NJ-JRSYSHMC>
  + Meridian Medical Group - Faculty Practice
    61 Davis Avenue/Suite 1   Neptune, NJ 07753   (732)776-4860   Fax (732)776-4867
  + Meridian Medical Group - Faculty Practice
    61 Davis Avenue/Suite 1   Neptune, NJ 07753   (732)776-4860   Fax (732)776-4639

Bautista, Jocelyn B., MD {1326013368} Pedtrc(87)<NJ-JRSYSHMC, NJ-RIVERVW>
  + Colts Neck Pediatrics
    26 State Highway 34/Suite 208   Colts Neck, NJ 07722   (732)683-0099

Bautista, Lucien Santiago, DO {1982663480} FamMed(96,NJ75)<NJ-WARREN>
  + Village Medical Center
    207 Strykers Road   Phillipsburg, NJ 08865   (908)859-6568   Fax (908)859-6697

Bautista-Seares, Jessica M., MD {1053587998} IntrMd(79,PHI01)
  + Drs. Seares and Bautista-Seares
    35 Beaverson Boulevard/Building 7   Brick, NJ 08723   (732)262-2400   Fax (732)262-3883

Bauza, Alain Michael, MD {1619234077} Ophthl
  + The New Jersey Eye Center
    1 North Washington Avenue   Bergenfield, NJ 07621   (201)384-7333   Fax (201)384-2564

Bavuso, Nicole T., MD {1255667184}
  + Penn Medicine at Woodbury Heights
    1006 Mantua Pike   Woodbury Heights, NJ 08097   (609)472-0346   Fax (856)845-0535

Bawa, Radhika, MD {1538555115} IntrMd
  + The Heart Center of The Oranges
    310 Central Avenue/Suite 102   East Orange, NJ 07018   (973)395-1550   Fax (973)395-1556

Baxi, Naimish, MD {1073834321} PhyMPain
  + Cardio Metabolic Institute
    51 Veronica Avenue   Somerset, NJ 08873   (732)846-7000   Fax (732)846-7001

Baxi, Namrata, MD {1699181206}<NJ-COOPRUMC>
  + Cooper University Hospital
    One Cooper Plaza   Camden, NJ 08103   (856)342-2000

Baxi, Nilay Manojkumar, MD {1447420245} Pedtrc(04,TN20)
  + Drs. Sell and Baxi
    507 4th Avenue   Asbury Park, NJ 07712   (732)774-5600

Baxley, Maureen Elizabeth, MD {1407868276} Pedtrc, IntrMd(94,MD01)<NJ-MORRISTN>
  + Florham Park Pediatrics
    195 Columbia Turnpike/Suite 105   Florham Park, NJ 07932   (973)437-8300   Fax (973)845-2883

Baxt, Rebecca D., MD {1417913245} Dermat(96,PA01)<NJ-VALLEY>
  + BAXT CosMedical NJ
    351 Evelyn Street/Suite 201   Paramus, NJ 07652   (201)265-1300   Fax (201)265-3737

Baxt, Saida H., MD {1417919051} Dermat(66,NY19)<NJ-VALLEY>
  + BAXT CosMedical NJ
    351 Evelyn Street/Suite 201   Paramus, NJ 07652   (201)265-1300   Fax (201)265-3737

Baxt, Sherwood A., MD {1952368334} SrgPlstc, Surgry(66,NY19)<NJ-VALLEY>
  + BAXT CosMedical NJ
    351 Evelyn Street/Suite 201   Paramus, NJ 07652   (201)265-1300   Fax (201)265-3737

Baxter, John D., MD {1508954835} InfDis, IntrMd(85,PA14)<NJ-COOPRUMC>
  + EIP Clinic/Early Intervention Program (HIV/AIDS)
    3 Cooper Plaza/Suite 513   Camden, NJ 08103   (856)963-3715   Fax (856)342-7832
  + Cooper University Hospital
    One Cooper Plaza/InfDis   Camden, NJ 08103   (856)342-2000

Baxter, Louis E., MD {1962527051} Addctn, IntrMd(78,PA13)
  + Medical Society of New Jersey
    2 Princess Road   Lawrenceville, NJ 08648   (609)896-1766   info@msnj.org

Bayard-McNeeley, Marise, MD {1134370398} PthACl, PthHem(82,HAI01)
  + Quest Diagnostics Inc.
    1 Malcolm Avenue   Teterboro, NJ 07608   (201)393-5051   Fax (210)462-4772

Baydar, Garbis, MD {1669438388} Pedtrc(82,AUS08)<NJ-ENGLWOOD, NJ-HOLYNAME>
  + Drs. Baydar, Davidson & Tung
    370 Grand Avenue/Suite 203   Englewood, NJ 07631   (201)568-3262   Fax (201)569-2634

Baydin, Jeffrey A., MD {1487737110} SrgOrt(69,MA07)
  + The Orthopedic Group, P.A.
    261 James Street/Suite 3-F   Morristown, NJ 07960   (973)538-0029   Fax (973)538-4957
  + The Orthopedic Group, P.A.
    50 Cherry Hill Road   Parsippany, NJ 07054   (973)538-0029   Fax (973)263-3243

Baye, Heather Marie, DO {1578874962}
  + Rowan University-School of Osteopathic Medicine
    1 Medical Center Drive   Stratford, NJ 08084   (856)566-6708

Bayer, Deborah D., DO {1821072604} InfDis(89,NY75)<NJ-ACMC-MAIN, NJ-ACMCITY>
  + 1401 Atlantic Avenue/Suite 2200
    Atlantic City, NJ 08401   (609)441-2104   Fax (609)441-2140

Bayes, Lorna B., MD {1518068782} IntrMd(72,PHI01)<NJ-TRIN-INPC, NJ-STMICHL>
  + 236 East Westfield Avenue/Suite 6
    Roselle Park, NJ 07204   (908)243-3343   Fax (908)245-3344   Lbayesmd@pol.net

Bayly, Robert, MD {1932304524} CritCr, IntrMd(79,NJ05)
  + JFK Medical Center - Muhlenberg Campus
    Park Avenue & Randolph Road   Plainfield, NJ 07061   (908)668-2000   Fax (908)668-3149
  + JFK Medical Center
    65 James Street   Edison, NJ 08820   (908)668-2000   Fax (732)767-2976

Baynes, Jason R., MD {1720279243}
  + Health East Medical Center
    54 South Dean Street   Englewood, NJ 07631   (201)871-4000

Bazargan Lari, Hamed, MD {1437384062} Ophthl
  + Summit Medical Group-Berkeley Heights Campus
    1 Diamond Hill Road/Ophthamology   Berkeley Heights, NJ 07922   (908)273-4300   Fax (908)277-8694

Bazerbashi, Ammar, MD {1205885704} IntrMd<NJ-BAYSHORE>
  + Medical Arts Center
    950 Route 35   Middletown, NJ 07748   (732)888-0017   Fax (732)888-0097

Bazergui, Christopher, DO {1710365432} IntHos<NJ-COOPRUMC>
  + Cooper University Hospital
    One Cooper Plaza   Camden, NJ 08103   (856)342-3150

Bazzini, Robert M., MD {1164402814} SrgHnd, SrgOrt(87,NY09)<NJ-CHILTON, NJ-NWTNMEM>
  + Orthopaedic Hand Specialists
    1777 Hamburg Turnpike/Suite 203   Wayne, NJ 07470   (973)839-8700   Fax (973)839-1681
  + 280 Newton-Sparta Road
    Newton, NJ 07860   (973)383-3838
  + Wayne Surgical Center, LLC.
    1176 Hamburg Pike   Wayne, NJ 07470   (973)709-1900   Fax (973)709-1901

Bea, Vivian Jolley, MD {1003127366} Surgry
  + MD Anderson Cancer Center at Cooper
    2 Cooper Plaza   Camden, NJ 08103   (855)632-2667

Beach, Robert J., MD {1376543033} PthACl, Pthlgy(75,MD01)<NJ-SHOREMEM>
  + Coastal Clinical Pathologists
    1 East New York Avenue/PO Box 337   Somers Point, NJ 08244   (609)926-9056   Fax (609)926-9056

Beachler, Kent J., MD {1558467456} Dermat(73,NE05)<NJ-HUNTRDN>
  + 170 Highway 31
    Flemington, NJ 08822   (908)788-1802   Fax (908)788-0049
  + 18 Wiilson Avenue
    Newark, NJ 07105   (908)788-1802

Beagin, Erinn Elizabeth, MD {1619924388} FamMGrtc, Grtrcs(01,NY09)
  + Windsor Regional Medical Associates, LLC
    300A Princeton-Hightstown Road   East Windsor, NJ 08520   (609)490-0095   Fax (609)490-0091
  + Saint Peter's Physician Associates
    294 Applegarth Road   Monroe Township, NJ 08831   (609)409-1363

Beal, Jeffrey M., MD {1801891437} IntrMd(84,MEXI)<NJ-JRSYSHMC>
  + 108 South Main Street/Suite 6
    Ocean Grove, NJ 07756   (732)776-8473   Fax (732)869-9160

Beamer, Andrew D., MD {1326049487} CdvDis(82,MD07)<NJ-OVERLOOK, NJ-MORRISTN>
  + Summit Medical Group-Berkeley Heights Campus
    1 Diamond Hill Road   Berkeley Heights, NJ 07922   (908)273-4300   Fax (908)790-6524

Beams, Lynsey Marie, DO {1982967121} ObsGyn
  + Premier Women's Health of South Jersey
    34 Colson Lane   Mullica Hill, NJ 08062   (856)223-8930

Beams, Michael E., DO {1184692261} FamMed, FamMSptM(72,IA75)
  + Summit Medical Group
    67 Walnut Avenue/Suite 202   Clark, NJ 07066   (732)388-7300   Fax (732)388-1330

Bean, David E., MD {1568494391} Anesth(75,PA09)<NJ-OCEANMC>
  + Ocean Medical Center
    425 Jack Martin Boulevard   Brick, NJ 08723   (732)840-2200

Bear, John G., MD {1114972163} FamMed(75,MEXI)
  + Family Practice Associates of Cumberland County, PC
    230 Laurel Heights Drive   Bridgeton, NJ 08302   (856)451-9595   Fax (609)451-1832

Bear, Michelle H., DO {1508894494} FamMed(02,NJ75)
  + Family Practice Associates of Cumberland County, PC
    230 Laurel Heights Drive   Bridgeton, NJ 08302   (856)451-9595   Fax (609)451-1832

Beattie, James Ray, III, MD {1922037704} CdvDis, IntrMd(90,NY45)<NJ-UNVMCPRN>
+ Princeton Interventional Cardiology
800 Bunn Drive/Suite 101   Princeton, NJ 08540   (609)921-2800   Fax (609)921-3499

Beaty, Patrick D., MD {1851480180} IntrMd, Gastrn(83,NJ05)<NJ-JRSYCITY>
+ Metropolitan Family Health Network
935 Garfield Avenue   Jersey City, NJ 07304   (201)478-5803   Fax (201)478-5814
pbeaty@metropolitan.org

Beaubrun, Esira Jaimie, MD {1013076062}
+ People Care Institute
323 Belleville Avenue/Floor 2   Bloomfield, NJ 07003   (973)842-4272   Fax (732)997-3022
+ 234 Aldene Road
Roselle, NJ 07203   (347)232-7272

Beauchamp, Donald P., MD {1114904661} FamMed(00,PA13)
+ Prospect Medical Offices, LLC
301 Godwin Avenue   Midland Park, NJ 07432   (201)444-4526   Fax (201)301-1313

Beauchamp, Jeffrey Thomas, MD {1316046824} ObsGyn(91,PA02)
+ Lifeline Medical Associates, LLC
67 Walnut Avenue/Suite 101   Clark, NJ 07066   (732)381-0121   Fax (732)381-0105
+ Qualcare Medi-Center, P.A.
2 Lincoln Highway/Suite 411   Edison, NJ 08820   (732)381-0121   Fax (732)396-9222

Beauregard, Louanne M., MD {1376547786} CdvDis, IntrMd, ClCdEl(80,PA07)<NJ-CENTRAST>
+ Heart Specialists/Central Jersey
901 West Main Street/Suite 205   Freehold, NJ 07728   (732)866-0800   Fax (732)463-6082

Beaver, Andrew Bradley, MD {1336356021} SrgOrt, Surgry(04,PA02)<PA-ENSTEIN>
+ Cooper Bone and Joint Institute
401 South Kings Highway/Suite 3-A   Cherry Hill, NJ 08003   (856)673-4914   Fax (856)325-6678
+ Cooper Bone and Joint Institute
900 Centennial Boulevard   Voorhees, NJ 08043   (856)673-4914   Fax (856)325-6678

Beaver, Ryan, DO {1568849156}<NJ-SJHREGMC>
+ SJH Regional Medical Center
1505 West Sherman Avenue   Vineland, NJ 08360   (856)641-8000

Bebawy, Niveen, MD {1659711919} Nephro, IntrMd(00,EGY12)
+ Hudson Essex Nephrology
510 31st Street   Union City, NJ 07087   (201)866-3322   Fax (201)866-2289
+ Hudson Essex Nephrology
123 Highland Avenue/Suite G-2   Glen Ridge, NJ 07028   (201)866-3322   Fax (973)866-2289

Bebawy, Sam T., MD {1396717971} IntrMd, PulDis, SlpDis(76,EGYP)<NJ-BAYSHORE, NJ-RIVERVW>
+ Central Jersey Pulmonary & Medical Associates
719 North Beers Street/Suites 2E-2F   Holmdel, NJ 07733   (732)264-1001   Fax (732)264-4495

Becan, Arthur Frank, Jr., MD {1336362078} SrgOrt, OccpMd(74,NJ06)
+ NJ Transit Medical Services
1431 Doughty Road   Egg Harbor Township, NJ 08234   (609)407-2427   Fax (609)407-2429
+ NJ Transit Medical Services
350 Newton Avenue   Camden, NJ 08103   (609)407-2427   Fax (856)968-3982

Becher, John W., DO {1932155140} EmrgMd(70,PA77)<NJ-ACMCITY, NJ-ACMCMAIN>
+ AtlantiCare Regional Medical Center/City Campus
1925 Pacific Avenue   Atlantic City, NJ 08401   (609)345-4000

Bechler, Jeffrey R., MD {1811992746} SrgOrt, SprtMd, IntrMd(87,NY09)<NJ-STPETER, NJ-RWJUBRUN>
+ University Orthopaedic Associates, LLC.
211 North Harrison Street   Princeton, NJ 08540   (609)683-7800   Fax (609)683-7875
+ University Orthopaedic Associates, LLC.
Two Worlds Fair Drive   Somerset, NJ 08873   (609)683-7800   Fax (732)564-9032

Bechmann, Samuel, MD {1174941090}<NJ-CHSFULD>
+ Capital Health System/Fuld Campus
750 Brunswick Avenue   Trenton, NJ 08638   (609)394-6000

Bechtel, David S., MD {1427091560} FamMed, IntrMd(87,PA13)<NJ-VIRTMARL, NJ-VIRTMHBC>
+ Advocare Heritage Family Medicine
703 East Main Street/Suite 9   Moorestown, NJ 08057   (856)235-0501   Fax (856)235-0601

Becker, Adam Scott, MD {1801060058} SrgOrt(02,NY15)<NJ-ENGLWOOD, NJ-HOLYNAME>
+ Englewood Orthopedic Associates
401 South Van Brunt Street   Englewood, NJ 07631   (201)569-2770   Fax (201)569-1774

Becker, Alyssa Gelmann, MD {1023187143} IntrMd, ClnPhm(95,PA02)
+ Saddle River Medical Group
82 East Allendale Road/Suite 3-A   Saddle River, NJ 07458   (201)825-3933   Fax (201)236-1460

Becker, Andrew B., DO {1164498606} FamMed(00,NJ75)<NJ-MORRISTN>
+ Blair Medical Associates PA
261 James Street/Suite 2A   Morristown, NJ 07960   (973)539-2468   Fax (973)539-7699

Becker, Andrew Nacholas, DO {1851379549} Nrolgy(78,IA75)
+ 28 Sullivan Drive
West Orange, NJ 07052

Becker, Daniel G., MD {1316975220} Otlryg, OtgyFPlS(81,ISRA)<NJ-KMHSTRAT>
+ Becker Nose & Sinus Center, LLC.
570 Egg Harbor Road   Sewell, NJ 08080   (856)589-6673   Fax (856)589-3443
beckermailbox@aol.com
+ Becker ENT
2 Princess Road/Suite East   Lawrenceville, NJ 08648   (856)589-6673   Fax (610)303-5164

Becker, George L., III, MD {1861430001} EmrgMd(94,PA02)<NJ-VALLEY>
+ The Valley Hospital
223 North Van Dien Avenue/EmergMed   Ridgewood, NJ 07450   (201)447-8000

Becker, Jason M., DO {1801177878} PulDis, SlpDis(11,NY75)
+ Jefferson Health New Jersey Cancer Center
900 Medical Center Drive/Suite 205   Sewell, NJ 08080   (844)542-2273
+ Kennedy Health Systems/Washington Township Campus
435 Hurffville-Cross Keys Road   Turnersville, NJ 08012   (856)582-2500

Becker, Jeffrey M., MD {1699720656} Urolgy(90,RI01)<NJ-LOURDMED, NJ-VIRTMHBC>
+ New Jersey Urology
15000 Midlantic Drive/Suite 100   Mount Laurel, NJ 08054   (856)252-1000   Fax (856)985-4582
+ New Jersey Urology
243 Route 130/Suite 100   Bordentown, NJ 08505   Fax (856)252-1100
+ New Jersey Urology
911 Sunset Road   Willingboro, NJ 08054

Becker, Murray David, MD {1306829924} NuclMd, RadDia, Rad-Nuc(93,NY20)<NJ-STPETER, NJ-RWJUBRUN>
+ University Radiology Group, P.C.
483 Cranbury Road   East Brunswick, NJ 08816   (732)390-0030   Fax (732)390-5383
+ University Radiology Group, P.C.
10 Plum Street   New Brunswick, NJ 08901   (732)390-0030   Fax (732)249-1208
+ University Radiology Group, P.C.
105 Raider Boulevard/Suite 101   Hillsborough, NJ 08816   (908)359-9331   Fax (908)359-9273

Becker, Robert J., MD {1942360664} Psychy(80,WI06)<NJ-GRYSTPSY>
+ Greystone Park Psychiatric Hospital
59 Koch Avenue   Morris Plains, NJ 07950   (973)538-1800   Fax (973)889-8789

Becker, Samuel Scott, MD {1083837108} Otlryg(02,CA02)
+ Becker Nose & Sinus Center, LLC.
2301 East Evesham Road/Suite 306   Voorhees, NJ 08043   (856)772-1617   Fax (856)770-0069
+ Becker ENT
2 Princess Road/Suite East   Lawrenceville, NJ 08648   (856)772-1617   Fax (610)303-5164

Becker, Stephen A., MD {1699770081} Surgry, SrgTrm, SrgCrC(76,ITAL)<NJ-JRSYSHMC>
+ 111 Princeton Avenue
Brick, NJ 08724   Fax (732)202-6584

Becker, Steven Eric, MD {1679587323} Pedtrc(99,NY08)<NY-MAIMONMC>
+ West Englewood Pediatrics
629 West Englewood Avenue   Teaneck, NJ 07666   (201)836-4777   Fax (201)606-4210
Westenglewoodpeds@gmail.com

Becker, Steven I., MD {1851472690} Surgry(75,BEL07)<NJ-WAYNEGEN>
+ The Surgery Center
33-00 Broadway/Suite 204   Fair Lawn, NJ 07410   (201)797-3040   Fax (201)797-9284
surgery3@earthlink.net

Becker, William D., MD {1336355858} Psychy, PsyCAd(87,ISRA)
+ William D. Becker MD and Associates
589 Franklin Turnpike/Suite 11   Ridgewood, NJ 07450   (201)670-4075

Beckerman, William, MD {1275976946} SrgVas
+ UMDNJ RWJ Vascular Surgery Group
125 Paterson Street/Suite 4100   New Brunswick, NJ 08901   (732)235-7816   Fax (732)235-8538

Beckman, Harvey S., MD {1093782302} Gastrn(75,SPA15)<NJ-STCLRSUS, NY-STANTHNY>
+ 2 Hamburg Avenue
Sussex, NJ 07461   (973)875-3100   Fax (973)875-3115

Beckwith, Anna Malia, MD {1619140415} PedDvl<NJ-CHLSMT>
+ Children's Specialized Hospital
150 New Providence Road   Mountainside, NJ 07092   (908)233-3720

Beckwith-Fickas, Katherine A., MD {1518100239} Pedtrc
+ Meridian Medical Group - Faculty Practice
61 Davis Avenue/Suite 1   Neptune, NJ 07753   (732)776-4860   Fax (732)776-4867
kbeckwi3@jhmi.edu
+ Meridian Obstetrics amd Gynecology Associates PC
19 Davis Avenue/Fl 1   Neptune, NJ 07753   (732)776-4860   Fax (732)922-8264

Becz, Grace E., MD {1841209285} PedPul, Pedtrc(86,POLA)<NJ-HACKNSK>
+ Rutherford Pediatrics
338 Union Avenue/Suite 2   Rutherford, NJ 07070   (201)842-0501   Fax (201)842-9190

Bedi, Ashish, MD {1528261443} Surgry<NJ-VIRTUAHS, NJ-OURLADY>
+ Virtua Surgical Group, PA
1935 Route 70 East   Cherry Hill, NJ 08003   (856)428-7700   Fax (856)424-9120

Bedi, Sukhjeet Singh, MD {1184124976}
+ Overlook Medical Center
99 Beauvoir Avenue/PO Box 210   Summit, NJ 07902   (908)522-2000

Bedigian, Martin Peter, MD {1336524263} NuclMd, IntrMd
+ 25 West Northfield Road
Livingston, NJ 07039   (973)873-6482

Bednar, John M., MD {1750318325} SrgHnd, SrgMcr, SrgOrt(81,PA01)
+ South Jersey Hand Center
1888 Marlton Pike East/Suite E-F-G   Cherry Hill, NJ 08003   (856)489-5634   Fax (856)489-5631
+ Wills Eye Surgery Center in Cherry Hill
408 Route 70 East   Cherry Hill, NJ 08034   (856)489-5634   Fax (856)429-7555
+ AtlantiCare Surgical Center
2500 English Creek Avenue   Egg Harbor Township, NJ 08003   (609)407-2200   Fax (609)407-2250

Bednar, Myron Emil, MD {1235127622} OncHem(93,NJ06)<NJ-HUNTRDN>
+ Hunterdon Regional Cancer Ctr
2100 Wescott Drive   Flemington, NJ 08822   (908)788-6461   Fax (908)788-6412

Bednarz, Przemyslaw Jerzy, MD {1205147139}<NJ-UMDNJ>
+ University Hospital
150 Bergen Street/Room I-248   Newark, NJ 07103   (973)972-6056

Bedrosian, Andrea Stephanie, MD {1033395728} Surgry(06,NY19)
+ Advanced Laparoscopic Associates
81 Route 4 West/Suite 401/35 Plaza   Paramus, NJ 07652   (201)646-1121   Fax (201)646-1110

Bee, Kim Donaldson, MD {1366495871} EmrgMd(99,NJ06)<NJ-WARREN>
+ Warren Hospital
185 Roseberry Street/Emergency   Phillipsburg, NJ 08865   (908)859-6767   Fax (908)859-6812

Beebe, Kathleen Sue, MD {1306877485} SrgOrt(99,NY01)<NJ-UMDNJ>
+ UMDNJ Dept of Orthopaedics
90 Bergen Street/DOC 1200   Jersey City, NJ 07305   (973)972-2150

Beecher, George, MD {1073574059} Otlryg(66,BEL04)<NJ-OVERLOOK>
+ 65 Mountain Boulevard/Suite 208
Warren, NJ 07059   (732)764-9494   Fax (732)764-9496

Beede, Michael S., MD {1215933098} IntrMd, Rheuma(80,NY46)<NJ-CHSMRCER, NJ-CHSFULD>
+ Ann Klein Forensic Center
1609 Stuyvesant Avenue/PO Box 7717   West Trenton, NJ 08628   (609)633-6351   Fax (609)633-2969
+ Medical Associates of Lawrenceville
3131 Princeton Pike/Building 6C   Lawrenceville, NJ 08648   (609)633-6351   Fax (609)896-1402

Beelitz, John Darren, MD {1003249566} AnesPain
+ Cooper University Medical Center/Camden
3 Cooper Plaza/Suite 314   Camden, NJ 08103   (856)963-6770

Beenstock, Steven Marc, DO {1043250707} FamMed(98,IA75)
+ Mahwah Medical
10 Franklin Turnpike   Mahwah, NJ 07430   (201)529-0033   Fax (201)529-5913

Physicians by Name and Address

Beggs, Donald James, MD {1699749119} IntrMd, InfDis(93,GRN01)<NJ-HOLYNAME>
+ Drs. Johnson and Beggs
   5 Franklin Avenue/Suite 103   Belleville, NJ 07109   (973)751-3399

Beggs, Nancy H., MD {1407945272} IntrMd(86,PA13)<NJ-COOPRUMC>
+ Cooper Physician Offices
   900 Centennial Boulevard   Voorhees, NJ 08043   (856)325-6770   Fax (856)673-4300
+ The Cooper Health System at Voorhees
   900 Centennial Boulevard   Voorhees, NJ 08043   (856)325-6500

Begleiter, David A., MD {1790893808} Radiol, RadBdI(86,NY15)<NJ-SHOREMEM, NJ-ACMCITY>
+ Atlantic Medical Imaging, LLC.
   72 West Jimmie Leeds Road   Galloway, NJ 08205   (609)677-9729   Fax (609)653-8764
+ Atlantic Medical Imaging, LLC.
   401 Bethel Road   Somers Point, NJ 08244   (609)677-9729
+ Atlantic Medical Imaging, LLC.
   421 Route 9 North   Cape May Court House, NJ 08205   (609)463-9500   Fax (609)465-0918

Behar, Lonny J., MD {1265522460} Psychy, PsyCAd(83,NY06)<NJ-MORRISTN, NJ-MMHKEMBL>
+ 7 Union Place
   Summit, NJ 07901   (908)273-9525   Fax (908)273-0436

Behar, Robert David, MD {1174525067} Ophthl(78,PA01)
+ Philadelphia Eye Associates
   1113 Hospital Drive/Suite 302   Willingboro, NJ 08046   (609)871-1112

Behar, Roger, MD {1386685303} IntrMd, Nrolgy(80,NY09)<NJ-RWJHLTS>
+ Princeton & Rutgers Neurology
   77 Veronica Avenue/Suite 102   Somerset, NJ 08873   (732)246-1311   Fax (732)246-3089
+ University Behavioral HealthCare
   183 South Orange Avenue   Newark, NJ 07103
+ Princeton & Rutgers Neurology
   9 Centre Drive/Suite 130   Monroe Township, NJ 08873   (609)395-7615   Fax (609)395-1885

Behbakht, Mojgan, MD {1104802438} Pedtrc(86,OH40)<NJ-MORRISTN, NJ-OVERLOOK>
+ 29 Columbia Turnpike/Suite 201
   Florham Park, NJ 07932   (973)410-0422   Fax (973)410-1057

Beheshtian, Azadeh, MD {1508136276} IntCrd
+ 630 East Palisade Avenue
   Englewood Cliffs, NJ 07632   (201)855-8492   Fax (855)256-1093

Behin, Babak, MD {1205931466} Otlryg(99,NJ05)<NJ-CHRIST>
+ 142 Palisade Avenue/Suite 207
   Jersey City, NJ 07306   (201)659-4706   Fax (201)659-4707   bbehin@hotmail.com
+ Christ Hospital
   176 Palisade Avenue   Jersey City, NJ 07306   (201)795-8200

Behin, Fereidoon, MD {1003911934} Otlryg, Hdache, OthrSp(67,IRAN)<NJ-PALISADE, NY-MTSINAI>
+ 142 Palisade Avenue/Suite 207
   Jersey City, NJ 07306   (201)659-4706   Fax (201)659-4707
+ Palisades Medical Center
   7600 River Road/Surgery/ENT   North Bergen, NJ 07047   (201)854-5000

Behl, Nitin, MD {1235423807} Nephro, IntrMd(03,UKR12)
+ Regional Nephrology Associates
   510 Jackson Avenue   Northfield, NJ 08225   (609)383-0200   Fax (609)383-8352

Behling, Kathryn C., MD {1750583308} Pthlgy
+ Cooper University Pathology
   3 Cooper Plaza   Camden, NJ 08103   (856)342-2506   behling-kathryn@cooperhealth.edu

Behman, Daisy M., MD {1780694166} IntrMd, EnDbMt(84,EGYP)
+ Drs. Behman & Sidhom
   48 Pulaski Avenue   Carteret, NJ 07008   (732)541-8848   Fax (732)541-1451

Behman, Haidy Mankarios, MD {1568447241} Nrolgy, Eplpsy, Elecen(87,EGYP)<NJ-JFKMED, NJ-RBAYPERT>
+ 48 Pulaski Avenue
   Carteret, NJ 07008   (732)541-0340   Fax (732)541-1451

Behman, Tamer Abdelmonam, MD {1730257619} IntrMd
+ 243 Pershing Avenue
   Carteret, NJ 07008   (732)541-7600   Fax (732)541-1380

Behme, Renee Maria, MD {1932238912} Pedtrc
+ Capital Health System/Hopewell
   One Capital Way   Pennington, NJ 08534   (609)394-4000

Behnam, Amir Babak, MD {1447215678} SrgPlstc, SrgHnd(98,NY47)
+ Cooper Orthopaedics
   2 Plaza Drive/Suite 202   Sewell, NJ 08080   (856)270-4150   Fax (856)270-4012

+ Cooper Surgical Associates
   6017 Main Street   Voorhees, NJ 08043   (856)325-6516
+ Cooper Surgical Associates
   3 Cooper Plaza/Suite 411   Camden, NJ 08080   (856)342-2270   Fax (856)365-1180

Behnam, Kazem, MD {1942266978} ObsGyn, GynOnc(66,IRA01)<NJ-VALLEY>
+ Ridgewood Gynecologic Associates
   317 Franklin Avenue   Ridgewood, NJ 07450   (201)447-1620   Fax (201)447-4977
+ 376 Hamburg Turnpike
   Wayne, NJ 07470   (973)595-5355

Behnam, Melody S., MD {1467418459} ObsGyn(01,DMN01)
+ Ridgewood Gynecologic Associates
   317 Franklin Avenue   Ridgewood, NJ 07450   (201)447-1620   Fax (201)447-4977

Behnam, Nadereh, MD {1326074568} ObsGyn(96,NJ02)<NJ-STJOSHOS, NJ-WAYNEGEN>
+ 502 Hamburg Turnpike/Suite 103
   Wayne, NJ 07470   (973)790-7090   Fax (973)790-6807

Beidleman, Danielle Melissa, MD {1811038854} ObsGyn(02,DC03)<NJ-STJOSHOS>
+ St. Joseph's Regional Medical Center
   703 Main Street/Ob/Gyn   Paterson, NJ 07503   (973)754-2000

Beim, Daniel S., MD {1144302985} ObsGyn(81,NJ05)<NJ-STPETER, NJ-SOMERSET>
+ Brunswick-Hills Ob/Gyn, PA
   620 Cranbury Road/Suite LL90   East Brunswick, NJ 08816   (732)257-0081   Fax (732)613-4845
+ Brunswick-Hills Ob/Gyn, PA
   751 Route 206/2nd Floor   Hillsborough, NJ 08844   (732)257-0081   Fax (908)725-2132

Beim, Robert B., MD {1144286543} ObsGyn(89,NY08)<NJ-STPETER>
+ St. Peter's University Hospital
   254 Easton Avenue/Ob/Gyn   New Brunswick, NJ 08901   (732)745-8600
+ Access Obstetrics and Gynecology
   190 Greenbrook Road   North Plainfield, NJ 07060   (732)745-8600   Fax (908)756-2525
+ Cares Surgicenter, LLC.
   240 Easton Avenue   New Brunswick, NJ 08901   (732)565-5400   Fax (732)296-8677

Beirne, Mary F., MD {1881782662} Psychy, PsyCAd, PsyFor(88,NJ06)
+ 75 Abe Voorhees Drive
   Manasquan, NJ 08736   (732)223-3590   Fax (732)223-3591

Beiro, Cristobal Andres, MD {1710116835}
+ Garden State Bone & Joint Specialists
   1000 Route 9 North/Suite 306   Woodbridge, NJ 07095   (732)283-2663   Fax (732)283-2661

Beiter, Kyle Aaron, MD {1902079858} ObsGyn(04,OH40)
+ Gianna Center for Women's Health & Fertility
   222 Easton Avenue/MOB 4th Floor   New Brunswick, NJ 08901   (732)565-5490   Fax (732)792-3038

Beitman, Robert G., MD {1972538288} Gastrn, IntrMd, Grtrcs(75,NY19)<NJ-BURDTMLN, NJ-SHOREMEM>
+ Robert Beitman MD PA
   15 Village Drive/PO Box 70   Cape May Court House, NJ 08210   (609)465-2112   Fax (609)463-0921

Beizem, Joanna, MD {1649402082} Pedtrc
+ 29 Barbara Terrace
   Middletown, NJ 07748

Bejaran, Juan E., MD {1184730632} IntrMd(88,DOM04)
+ Southern Jersey Family Medical Centers, Inc.
   860 South White Horse Pike/Building A   Hammonton, NJ 08037   (609)567-0200   Fax (609)567-3492

Beke, Theodore J., MD {1225083124} Anesth(80,NJ05)<NJ-VALLEY>
+ The Valley Hospital
   223 North Van Dien Avenue   Ridgewood, NJ 07450   (201)447-8350

Bekele, Wondwessen, MD {1356317028} PedHem, Pedtrc(72,ETH01)<NJ-NWRKBETH, NJ-CHDNWBTH>
+ Newark Beth Israel Medical Center
   201 Lyons Avenue/Pedi Hema/Onco   Newark, NJ 07112   (973)926-7161   Fax (973)282-0395
+ Children's Hospital of New Jersey
   201 Lyons Avenue/Osborne Terrace   Newark, NJ 07112   (973)926-4000

Bekes, Carolyn E., MD {1184713950} CritCr, IntrMd, Nephro(72,PA02)<NJ-COOPRUMC>
+ Cooper University Hospital
   One Cooper Plaza   Camden, NJ 08103   (856)342-2000   bekes@umdnj.edu

Bekhit, Mariam, MD {1952330060} PsyCAd, Psychy(95,EGY05)<NJ-UMDNJ>
+ Psychiatric Care Associates
   735 State Route 18   East Brunswick, NJ 08816   (732)257-4100

Bekhit, Maximilian M., DO {1760820294}
+ 106 Longstone Drive
   Cherry Hill, NJ 08003   (720)839-0301   maximilian.bekhit@gmail.com

Bekker, Yana, MD {1427595701} Psychy
+ Veterans Affairs Department Outpatient Clinic
   654 East Jersey Street   Elizabeth, NJ 07206   (908)994-5000   Fax (908)994-0131

Belafsky, Robert B., MD {1881692895} Otlryg, Otolgy, IntrMd(73,NY08)<NJ-LOURDMED, NJ-VIRTMARL>
+ Advanced ENT - Voorhees
   200 Bowman Drive/Suite D-285   Voorhees, NJ 08043   (856)602-4000   Fax (856)346-0757
+ Advanced ENT - Willingboro
   1113 Hospital Drive/Suite 103   Willingboro, NJ 08046   (856)602-4000   Fax (609)871-0508

Belani, Puneet B., MD {1992023089} Radiol(10,NY06)<NJ-JFKMED>
+ Advanced Medical Imaging of Old Bridge
   3548 Route 9   Old Bridge, NJ 08857   (732)970-0420   Fax (732)970-0517
+ Edison Imaging Associates at JFK
   60 James Street   Edison, NJ 08820   (732)970-0420   Fax (732)318-3883

Belani, Suresh G., MD {1538233242} Allrgy, IntrMd(80,INDI)
+ Allergy and Asthma Centers
   50 Union Avenue/Suite 301   Irvington, NJ 07111   (973)372-0528   Fax (973)372-0094   Surbel@aol.com

Belardi, Chris A., MD {1629146303} EmrgMd, GenPrc, EmrgEMed(83,PA13)<NJ-UNVMCPRN>
+ University Medical Center of Princeton at Plainsboro
   One Plainsboro Road   Plainsboro, NJ 08536   (609)497-4000

Belardinelli, Cecilia Del Carmen, MD {1194982900}
+ 73 New England Avenue/Apt D
   Summit, NJ 07901

Belazi, Misa T., MD {1407911464} ObsGyn(05,MA05)<NJ-LOURDMED, NJ-VIRTMHBC>
+ Advocare Burlington County Obstetrics & Gynecology
   1000 Salem Road/Suite B   Willingboro, NJ 08046   (609)871-2060   Fax (609)871-3535
+ Advocare Burlington County Obstetrics & Gynecology
   45b Homestead Drive/Homestead Plaza   Columbus, NJ 08022   (609)871-2060   Fax (609)871-3535
+ Burlington County Ob-Gyn
   8008 Route 130 N/Suite 320   Delran, NJ 08046   (856)764-0002   Fax (856)764-0103

BelCastro, Peter Joseph, MD {1689644361} Anesth, IntrMd(88,NY45)<NY-PRSBWEIL>
+ Summit Anesthesia Associates, P.A.
   33 Overlook Road/Suite 311   Summit, NJ 07901   (908)598-1500   Fax (908)598-0197

Belder, Olga, DO {1225072515} FamMed(99,NY75)<NJ-BAYSHORE>
+ 69 Route 516
   Old Bridge, NJ 08857   (732)264-1163   Fax (732)264-3580

Belecanech, George A., MD {1376691626} AlgyImmn, IntrMd(87,PA07)<NJ-COMMED, NJ-VIRTMHBC>
+ Allergic Disease Associates, PC - Forked River
   1044 Lacey Road/suite 9   Forked River, NJ 08731   (609)693-5317   Fax (609)693-0351
+ Allergic Disease Associates, PC - Hamilton
   8 Quakerbridge Plaza/Suite E   Hamilton, NJ 08619   (609)693-5317   Fax (609)689-3555

Belen, Kristin Marietta O., MD {1730402561} RadDia
+ Memorial Sloan Kettering Monmouth
   480 Red Hill Road/Radiology   Middletown, NJ 07748

Belenker, Stuart Lawrence, MD {1124106463} Psychy(88,MD01)
+ University Behavioral HealthCare
   183 South Orange Avenue   Newark, NJ 07103

Belete, Senayit Girma, MD {1851328181} IntrMd(93,INA72)
+ 3101 Boardwalk/Towe 1 Suite 3201
   Atlantic City, NJ 08401   (609)289-8429

Belfar, Alexandra, MD {1366700916} Anesth
+ 370 River Road/Apt L
   Nutley, NJ 07110   (908)659-6788

Belfer, Robert A., MD {1639120116} PedEmg, Pedtrc(87,PA01)<NJ-VIRTVOOR>
+ Virtua Voorhees
   100 Bowman Drive/PediEmrg   Voorhees, NJ 08043   (856)247-3000   Fax (856)325-3157

Belinsky, Tatyana, MD {1902990229} Psychy(73,UKR12)
+ South Jersey Behavioral Health Resources - Stratford
   1 Colby Avenue/Suite 5   Stratford, NJ 08084   (856)361-2712   Fax (856)346-3627   tbelinsky@sjbhr.org
+ South Jersey Behavioral Health Resources
   400 Market Street/Box 1990   Camden, NJ 08101   (856)361-2700

Physicians by Name and Address

Belitsis, Kenneth, MD {1427157155} Gastrn(96,NJ05)<NJ-SOCEANCO>
+ Monmouth Gastroenterology
  142 Route 35   Eatontown, NJ 07724   (732)389-5004   Fax (732)389-1850

Belkin, Sardana, MD {1932139631} ObsGyn(99,NY48)<NJ-RIVERVW, NJ-MONMOUTH>
+ Sunrise Obstetrics & Gynecology
  831 Tennent Road   Manalapan, NJ 07726   (732)972-4200   Fax (732)333-4643

Belkina, Yelena, MD {1326561754} ObsGyn
+ Advanced Obstetrics & Gynecology, LLC
  4 Walter E. Foran Boulevard/Suite 302   Flemington, NJ 08822   (908)806-0080   Fax (908)806-8570

Bell, Alvin, MD {1013987866} Nephro, IntrMd(78,PA13)<NJ-MTNSIDE, NJ-STJOSHOS>
+ 129 Grove Street
  Montclair, NJ 07042   (973)783-6110   Fax (973)744-7385
  bellfacp@verizon.net

Bell, Denise Marie, MD {1912931452} Pedtrc(01,NJ05)<NJ-VIRTMHBC>
+ Advocare Pedi Phys of Burlington Co
  693 Main Street/PO Box 367   Lumberton, NJ 08048   (609)261-4058   Fax (609)261-8381
+ Advocare Pedi Phys of Burlington Co
  204 Ark Road/Suite 209   Mount Laurel, NJ 08054   (609)261-4058   Fax (856)234-9402

Bell, Kameno L, MD {1982666285} EmrgMd, FamMSptM(01,IL11)<NJ-HACKNSK>
+ Hackensack University Medical Center
  30 Prospect Avenue   Hackensack, NJ 07601   (201)996-4614   Fax (201)996-4239

Bell, Kevin E., MD {1639293244} IntrMd(75,NY01)
+ 10 Mountain Boulevard
  Warren, NJ 07059   (908)226-9000   Fax (908)226-5654
+ Box 420/Millbrook Road
  New Vernon, NJ 07976   (973)539-1264

Bell, Michael Henry, MD {1740323237} Psychy(80,NJ05)<NJ-CARRIER>
+ Drs. Bell and Mason-Bell
  51 Upper Montclair Plaza/Suite 14   Upper Montclair, NJ 07043   (973)746-9615   Fax (973)316-1920

Bell, Robert Lawrence, MD {1982640207} Surgry, SrgGst(95,TX16)<CT-YALENHH>
+ Summit Medical Group
  1 Diamond Hill Road/Bensley Pav/2 FL   Berkeley, NJ 07922   (908)277-8950   Fax (908)673-7350

Bell, Theresa A., MD {1013002369} Psychy(93,PA02)
+ 310 Chris Gaupp Drive/Suite 105
  Galloway, NJ 08205   (609)652-4040   Fax (609)652-5340

Bell-Gresham, Garrett, MD {1194138560} Pedtrc
+ Rutgers- New Jersey Medical School
  185 South Orange Avenue/MSB F603   Newark, NJ 07103   (914)772-2086

Belladonna, Joseph A., MD {1871594937} Gastrn, IntrMd(69,NY20)<NJ-OVERLOOK, NJ-MORRISTN>
+ Summit Medical Group-Berkeley Heights Campus
  1 Diamond Hill Road   Berkeley Heights, NJ 07922   (908)277-8940   Fax (908)790-6524

Bellamy, James E., DO {1962477828} GenPrc, OccpMd(82,MO78)<NJ-STCLRDOV>
+ St. Clare's Hospital-Dover
  400 West Blackwell Street   Dover, NJ 07801   (973)989-3015   Fax (973)989-3306

Bellapianta, Joseph Michael, MD {1588823165} SrgOrt(04,NY03)<CT-STAMFDH, CT-GRENWCH>
+ Kayal Orthopaedic Center, P.C.
  784 Franklin Avenue/Suite 200   Franklin Lakes, NJ 07417   (844)281-1783   Fax (201)560-0712

Bellapianta, Karen Marie, MD {1447407960} PedOto(04,NY03)
+ Sovereign Northern Jersey ENT
  85 Harristown Road/Suite 105   Glen Rock, NJ 07452   (201)455-2900   Fax (201)703-0390

Bellardini, Angelo G., MD {1780680876} Grtrcs, IntrMd(79,ITAL)
+ Care Point Health Associates
  1225 McBride Avenue/Suite 200   Little Falls, NJ 07424   (973)256-5557   Fax (973)256-5036

Bellavia, Thomas S., MD {1750347449} FamMed(65,ITAL)<NJ-HACKNSK>
+ Heights Medical Associates
  288 Boulevard   Hasbrouck Heights, NJ 07604   (201)288-6781   Fax (201)288-2734

Belli, Albert J., Jr., DO {1184631012} IntrMd, PulDis(80,PA77)
+ South Jersey Chest Diseases
  107 Vine Street   Hammonton, NJ 08037   (609)561-7666   Fax (609)561-8347

Bellias, Jay Peter, DO {1194721746} Psychy(94,NJ75)
+ New Point Behavioral Health Care
  404 Tatum Street   Woodbury, NJ 08096   (856)845-8050   Fax (856)845-0688

Bellifemine, Morris, MD {1801960059} IntrMd, PulDis(83,MEXI)<NJ-MEADWLND, NJ-HOBUNIMC>
+ 106 Centre Avenue
  Secaucus, NJ 07094   (201)864-4505   Fax (201)864-8782
+ 209 60th Street/Unit 1
  West New York, NJ 07093

Bellin, Harvey Jay, MD {1710966957} PthACl(65,PA02)<PA-TJFMETHD>
+ 68 Crooked Lane
  Cherry Hill, NJ 08034

Bellingham, Charles E., MD {1245213123} Urolgy(66,NJ05)<NJ-JRSYSHMC, NJ-OCEANMC>
+ Coastal Urology Associates
  814 River Avenue   Lakewood, NJ 08701   (732)370-2250   Fax (732)901-9119

Bellish, Jenna H., MD {1427293083} ObsGyn
+ 1259 Route 46 East/Bldg 3
  Parsippany, NJ 07054

Bello, John J., MD {1174508725} Surgry(84,WIND)<NJ-HUNTRDN>
+ Hunterdon Surgical Associates
  1100 Wescott Drive/Suite 302   Flemington, NJ 08822   (908)788-6464   Fax (908)788-6459

Bello, Joseph M., MD {1841274818} Surgry(86,DC01)<NJ-HUNTRDN>
+ Hunterdon Surgical Associates
  1100 Wescott Drive/Suite 302   Flemington, NJ 08822   (908)788-6464   Fax (908)788-6459

Bello, Mary R., MD {1376637413} FamMed(84,WIND)<NJ-VALLEY>
+ 400 Franklin Turnpike/Suite 106
  Mahwah, NJ 07430   (201)327-3333   Fax (201)327-2575

Bellomo, Alyse Rosemarie, MD {1700890837} Gastrn, IntrMd(89,NY03)
+ Bergen Medical Associates
  466 Old Hook Road/Suite 1   Emerson, NJ 07630   (201)967-8221   Fax (201)967-0340
+ Bergen Medical Associates
  1 West Ridgewood Avenue/Suite 301   Paramus, NJ 07652   (201)967-8221   Fax (201)445-4296

Bellomo, Spartaco, MD {1790779833} InfDis, IntrMd(78,ITAL)<NJ-CHRIST, NJ-HOBUNIMC>
+ 142 Palisades Avenue/Suite 209
  Jersey City, NJ 07306   (201)653-8336   Fax (201)653-6697

Bellows, Aaron, MD {1689964546} Gastrn
+ Princeton Gastroenterology Associates, P.A.
  731 Alexander Road/Suite 100   Princeton, NJ 08540   (609)924-1422   Fax (609)924-7473

Belluscio, Roland L., MD {1477523314} CdvDis, CritCr, IntrMd(78,MEX03)<NJ-BAYSHORE, NJ-RIVERVW>
+ Cardiac Care Center
  21 North Gilbert Street   Tinton Falls, NJ 07701   (732)741-7400   Fax (732)741-4775

Belnekar, Rudrani K., MD {1225393382} Pedtrc
+ 255 Parsonage Road
  Edison, NJ 08837   (732)762-8799

Beloff, Michelle Lauren, DO {1942382148} ObsGyn(97,PA77)
+ Valley Medical Group Ob/Gyn in Fairlawn
  5-22 Saddle River Road   Fair Lawn, NJ 07410   (201)796-2025   Fax (201)796-0787

Belov, Khatuna Topadze, MD {1881699528} FamMed, IntrMd(90,GEO02)
+ Katy Belov, M.D.
  127 Union Street/Suite 102   Ridgewood, NJ 07450   (201)857-0066   Fax (201)857-5038
+ Drs. Belov & Dunn
  61 Crescent Avenue   Waldwick, NJ 07463   (201)857-0066   Fax (201)857-0453

Belsh, Jerry M., MD {1396810867} Nrolgy, ClNrPh(75,PA02)<NJ-RWJUBRUN>
+ UH- Robert Wood Johnson Med
  125 Paterson Street/6th Floor   New Brunswick, NJ 08901   (732)235-7733   Fax (732)235-7041

Belsh, Yitzhak, MD {1184824690} Anesth(04,NJ05)<NJ-MONMOUTH>
+ Monmouth Medical Center
  300 Second Avenue/Anesthesia   Long Branch, NJ 07740   (732)923-6980   Fax (732)923-6977

Belsky, Martin Karl, DO {1093809238} EnDbMt, IntrMd(84,PA77)<NJ-VIRTMARL, NJ-UNDRWD>
+ 100 Brick Road/Suite 108
  Marlton, NJ 08053   (856)810-7337   Fax (856)810-7917
+ Martin K. Belsky DO PC
  608 North Broad Street/Suite 201   Woodbury, NJ 08096   (856)384-9239

Belt, Gary Harvey, MD {1699707422} IntrMd, Nrolgy(81,NY47)<CT-ROCKVLLE, CT-STFRNCMP>
+ Atlantic Neuroscience Institute at Overlook Hospital
  99 Beauvoir Avenue   Summit, NJ 07901   (908)522-6142   Fax (908)522-6147

Belt, Steven D., MD {1700957479} FamMed(75,MEX14)<NJ-STBARNMC>
+ Drs. Scalea & Belt
  100 Northfield Avenue   West Orange, NJ 07052   (973)731-1535   Fax (973)731-5782

Beltzer, Blair Richard, MD {1073635421} FamMed(85,OH44)<NJ-CHILTON, NJ-VALLEY>
+ 2025 Hamburg Turnpike/Suite D
  Wayne, NJ 07470   (973)831-0006   Fax (973)839-0084
  Beltzermd@aol.com

Beluch, Brian Walter, DO {1811142508} EnDbMt, IntrMd(08,PA77)<NJ-KMHTURNV>
+ Jefferson Health Primary & Specialty Care
  1A Regulus Drive   Turnersville, NJ 08012   (844)542-2273

Belz, Marek, MD {1073732699} NrlgAddM(00,POL12)<NJ-SUMOAKSH>
+ Summit Oaks Hospital
  19 Prospect Street/Psychiatry   Summit, NJ 07901   (908)277-9722

Bembo, Shirley Abad, MD {1023041472} EnDbMt, IntrMd(97,PHI09)<NJ-STPETER, NJ-RWJUBRUN>
+ Endocrinology Associates of Princeton, LLC
  256 Bunn Drive/Suite D   Princeton, NJ 08540   (609)924-4433   Fax (609)924-4423
+ Endocrinology Associates of Princeton, LLC
  168 Franklin Corner Road   Lawrenceville, NJ 08648   (609)924-4433   Fax (609)896-0079

Ben, Sheeba, MD {1518967959} Pedtrc(00,MNT01)<NJ-JFKMED, NJ-HACKNSK>
+ Riverside Medical Group
  714 Tenth Street/Suite 2   Secaucus, NJ 07094   (201)863-3346   Fax (201)865-0015

Ben Yishay, Ari, MD {1073577052} SrgOrt, SrgSpn, IntrMd(87,PA12)<NJ-ENGLWOOD, NJ-HACKNSK>
+ Comprehensive Spine Care, PA
  260 Old Hook Road/Suite 400   Emerson, NJ 07630   (201)634-1811   Fax (201)634-9170
  ariby123@gmail.com
+ Comprehensive Spine Care, PA
  28-04 Broadway   Fair Lawn, NJ 07410   (201)634-1811   Fax (201)634-9170

Ben-Jacob, Talia K., MD {1477891760} AnesCrCr, Anesth, IntrMd(07,VT02)<NJ-COOPRUMC>
+ Cooper University Medical Center/Camden
  3 Cooper Plaza/Suite 500   Camden, NJ 08103   (856)356-4935
+ Cooper Anesthesia Associates
  One Cooper Plaza/Suite 294-B   Camden, NJ 08103   (856)356-4935   Fax (856)968-8326

Ben-Meir, Ron Simon, DO {1366637423} PhyMPain, PhyMSptM(07,CA23)
+ The Spine & Sports Health Center
  739 Bloomfield Street/Suite 1   Hoboken, NJ 07030   (201)533-9200   Fax (201)533-9299
+ The Spine & Sports Health Center
  129 Newark Avenue   Jersey City, NJ 07302   (201)533-9200   Fax (201)533-9299

Ben-Menachem, Tamir, MD {1538246509} Gastrn(88,ISR05)
+ Summit Medical Group-Berkeley Heights Campus
  1 Diamond Hill Road   Berkeley Heights, NJ 07922   (908)273-4300   Fax (908)790-6576
+ UH- Robert Wood Johnson Med
  125 Paterson Street   New Brunswick, NJ 08901   (732)828-3000

Benalcazar-Puga, Luis Marcelo, MD {1801878269} IntrMd(00,PRO02)
+ 310 Morris Avenue/Suite 301
  Elizabeth, NJ 07208   (908)353-3626   Fax (908)353-3625

Benaur, Irina V., MD {1477656783} Psychy(82,RUS06)<NJ-UNVMCPRN>
+ Princeton House Behavioral Health - Princeton
  905 Herrontown Road   Princeton, NJ 08540   (609)497-3300   Fax (609)497-3370

Bencosme, Pablo, MD {1982712865} IntrMd(75,DOM01)<NJ-RBAYPERT>
+ 287 Rector Street
  Perth Amboy, NJ 08861

Bendala, Preeti, MD {1427304815} FamMed
+ Tatem Brown Family Practice
  2225 East Evesham Road/Suite 101   Voorhees, NJ 08043   (856)795-4330   Fax (856)325-3704

Bender, Michelle Anne, MD {1184625279} AdolMd, Pedtrc(92,NY46)<NJ-OVERLOOK, NJ-MORRISTN>
+ Summit Medical Group-Berkeley Heights Campus
  1 Diamond Hill Road   Berkeley Heights, NJ 07922   (908)273-4300   Fax (908)790-6524
+ Summit Medical Group
  85 Woodland Road   Short Hills, NJ 07078   (908)273-4300   Fax (973)921-0669

Physicians by Name and Address

Bendesky, Brad S., MD {1255369716} EmrgMd, IntrMd(97,NJ06)<PA-MRCYPHIL>
+ Cooper University Hospital
One Cooper Plaza/Emerg Med   Camden, NJ 08103   (856)342-2627
+ Cooper Urgent Care
318 South. White Horse Pike   Audubon, NJ 08106

Bendich, David M., MD {1225205222} Pedtrc, IntrMd(75,NY06)
+ 143 Highview Drive
Woodbridge, NJ 07095   (732)636-1335   Fax (732)636-1335

Benecki, Theresa R., MD {1003895418} ObsGyn, Gyneco(78,PA02)<NJ-OCEANMC>
+ Pineland Associates PA
1608 Route 88/Suite 208   Brick, NJ 08724   (732)458-7878   Fax (732)840-6378

Benedetti, Robert C., MD {1417973595} Pthlgy, PthAcl(87,GRN01)<NJ-CLARMAAS, NJ-NWRKBETH>
+ Clara Maass Medical Center
1 Clara Maass Drive/Pathology   Belleville, NJ 07109   (973)450-2000   Fax (973)844-4976

Benedetto, Dominick A., MD {1730246257} Ophthl(75,FL03)<NJ-MORRISTN, NJ-BAYONNE>
+ Eye MD Associates PC
111 Madison Avenue/Suite 301   Morristown, NJ 07960   (973)984-9798
+ Eye MD Associates PC
124 Avenue B   Bayonne, NJ 07002   (201)436-1150
+ Eye Institute of Essex, PA
5 Franklin Avenue/Suite 209   Belleville, NJ 07960   (973)751-6060   Fax (973)450-1464

Benerofe, Bruce Michael, MD {1356559579} Ophthl(79,NY06)
+ 447 State Route 10/Suite 4
Randolph, NJ 07869   (973)361-5440   Fax (973)361-9277

Benett, Jodi A., DO {1154351724} ObsGyn, FamMed(87,NJ75)<NJ-OURLADY, NJ-KENEDYHS>
+ Center for Specialized Gynecology
1930 State Highway 70 East   Cherry Hill, NJ 08003   (856)424-8091   Fax (856)424-0704

Benevenia, Joseph, MD {1710911102} SrgOrt(84,NJ05)<NJ-HACKNSK, NJ-RWJUBRUN>
+ North Jersey Orthopaedic Institute
90 Bergen Street/DOC 1200   Newark, NJ 07101   (973)972-2153   Fax (973)972-2155
+ North Jersey Orthopedic Institute
20 Prospect Avenue/Suite 901   Hackensack, NJ 07601   (973)972-2153   Fax (201)820-1661
+ UMDNJ Dept of Orthopaedics
90 Bergen Street/DOC 1200   Jersey City, NJ 07101   (973)972-2150

Benevento, Barbara Therese, MD {1083603815} PhysMd(88,NY03)<NJ-KSLRWELK>
+ Kessler Institute for Rehabilitation West Orange
1199 Pleasant Valley Way   West Orange, NJ 07052   (973)731-3600

Benezra-Obeiter, Rita Beth, MD {1316907785} Pedtrc, PedNrD(78,MA05)<NJ-HACKNSK>
+ Rutgers- New Jersey Medical School
185 South Orange Avenue   Newark, NJ 07103   (973)972-4300
+ Hackensack University Medical Center
30 Prospect Avenue/Conslnt/DevPed   Hackensack, NJ 07601   (201)996-2000

Bengali, Sakina H., MD {1003841123} Psychy(67,PAK08)
+ Ocean Mental Health Services, Inc.
160 Atlantic City Boulevard   Bayville, NJ 08721   (732)349-5550   Fax (732)349-0841

Benigno, Robert A., MD {1194725549} CdvDis, IntrMd(80,PA12)
+ Hunterdon Cardiovascular Associates
1100 Wescott Drive/Suite G-3   Flemington, NJ 08822   (908)788-6471   Fax (908)788-6460
+ Hunterdon Cardiovascular Associates
1738 Route 31/Suite 210   Clinton, NJ 08809   (908)788-6471   Fax (908)823-9211

Benincasa, Peter J., MD {1326117078} Allrgy, IntrMd, IntMAImm(90,ITAL)<NJ-STMRYPAS, NJ-OVERLOOK>
+ Consultants in Asthma, Allergy and Immunology
22 Shaw Street   Garfield, NJ 07026   (973)478-5550   Fax (973)478-2290
+ Consultants in Asthma, Allergy and Immunology
67 Walnut Avenue   Clark, NJ 07066   (732)381-4634

Benisch, Barry M., MD {1033291109} PthAcl, Pthlgy, BldBnk(67,NY06)<NJ-RWJURAH>
+ Robert Wood Johnson University Hospital at Rahway
865 Stone Street/Path   Rahway, NJ 07065   (732)381-4200   Fax (732)499-6122

Benitez, Jose L., MD {1942322300} Psychy(66,NICA)
+ 346 Farview Avenue
Paramus, NJ 07652

Benitez, Olga, MD {1275741209} IntrMd, FamMed(81,PA01)<NJ-PALISADE, NJ-HOBUNIMC>
+ Trinity Family Practice
411 43rd Street/Main Floor   Union City, NJ 07087   (201)766-0377   Fax (201)540-9175

Benitez, Ronald Patrick, MD {1730146820} SrgNro(94,DC02)<NJ-MORRISTN, NJ-ATLANTHS>
+ Atlantic Neurosurgical Specialists
310 Madison Avenue/Suite 300   Morristown, NJ 07960   (973)285-7800   Fax (973)285-7839

Benito, Carlos W., MD {1487610952} MtFtMd, ObsGyn, IntrMd(90,NJ06)<NJ-MORRISTN, NJ-OVERLOOK>
+ Maternal Fetal Medicine of Practice Associates
11 Overlook Road/Suite LL 102   Summit, NJ 07901   (908)522-3846   Fax (908)522-5557

Benito Herrero, Maria I., MD {1568557510} EnDbMt(93,SPA18)
+ Princeton Integral Endocrinology
20 Nassau Street/Suite 208   Princeton, NJ 08542   (609)649-3161
mbenito@princetonintegralendocrinology.com

Beniwal, Jagbir S., MD {1134229172} Surgry, SrgVas(74,INDI)<NJ-CHILTON>
+ 508 Hamburg Turnpike/Suite 205
Wayne, NJ 07470   (973)956-0800   Fax (973)956-1885
+ 539 Clifton Avenue
Clifton, NJ 07011   (973)956-0800

Benjamin, Beth L., MD {1699728790} Pedtrc, NnPnMd(90,NJ06)<NJ-VALLEY>
+ The Valley Hospital
223 North Van Dien Avenue/Pediatrics   Ridgewood, NJ 07450   (201)447-8000

Benjamin, Charles David, DO {1982635447} ObsGyn(74,PA77)
+ Cherry Hill Women's Center
502 Kings Highway North   Cherry Hill, NJ 08034   (856)667-5910   Fax (856)667-8304
chwc@aol.com

Benjelloun, Hind, MD {1053577437} Psychy
+ Center for Family Guidance, PC
765 East Route 70/Building A-101   Marlton, NJ 08053   (856)983-3900   Fax (856)810-0110

Benke, Michael T., MD {1649432261} SrgOrt
+ Active Orthopaedics & Sports Medicine
440 Old Hook Road   Emerson, NJ 07630   (201)358-0707   Fax (201)358-9777
+ Active Orthopaedics & Sports Medicine
25 Prospect Avenue   Hackensack, NJ 07601   (201)358-0707   Fax (201)343-7410

Benn, Howard A., MD {1841364965} MedOnc, OncHem(89,CHN21)
+ Colfax Oncology/Fast Med
476 Colfax Avenue   Clifton, NJ 07013   (973)594-7977
+ Colfax Oncology/Fast Med
680 Broadway/Suite 100   Paterson, NJ 07514   (973)594-7977

Bennett, Amanda Erin, MD {1376754911} Pedtrc, PedDvl<PA-CHILDHOS>
+ CHOP Pediatric & Adolescent Specialty Care Center
1012 Laurel Oak Road   Voorhees, NJ 08043   (856)435-1300   Fax (856)435-0091

Bennett, Bruce Kevin, MD {1770518441} ObsGyn(90,VA01)
+ Comprehensive Women's Healthcare
220 Hamburg Turnpike/Suite 21   Wayne, NJ 07470   (973)790-8090   Fax (973)790-3198

Bennett, Douglas P., DO {1710903497} InfDis, IntrMd(01,NJ75)
+ IPC The Hospitalist Company
220 Ridgedale Avenue/Suite C-2   Florham Park, NJ 07932   (973)538-5844   Fax (973)267-0181

Bennett, Harvey S., MD {1285609495} NroChl, Pedtrc, NrlgSpec(75,NY46)<NJ-OVERLOOK>
+ Overlook Medical Center
99 Beauvour Avenue/PO Box 210   Summit, NJ 07902   (908)522-2000

Bennett, Robert Harris, DO {1487716957} Psychy(85,NJ75)<NJ-NWRKBETH>
+ Newark Beth Israel Medical Center
201 Lyons Avenue/Psychiatry   Newark, NJ 07112   (973)926-7000

Bennett, Robert J., MD {1225102346} Psychy(81,MONT)
+ CPC Behavioral HealthCare
1088 Highway 34   Aberdeen, NJ 07747   (732)290-1700   Fax (732)290-0040

Bennett, William Roderic, DO {1003179318} IntrMd
+ 100 Lexington Road/Bldg. 100
Swedesboro, NJ 08085   (856)467-7360
+ Family Practice Associates
188 Fries Mill Road/Suite N3   Turnersville, NJ 08012   (856)467-7360   Fax (856)875-8494

Bennett-Phillips, Fay L., MD {1659321842} Ophthl, VitRet, IntrMd(88,NY08)<NY-MANHEYE, NJ-RWJUBRUN>
+ Phillips Eye Consultants
1440 How Lane   North Brunswick, NJ 08902   (732)422-8400   Fax (732)422-8444

Benoff, Brian Alan, MD {1518021716} IntrMd, PulDis, CritCr(94,NY46)<NY-LIJEWSH>
+ S. L. Silverstein MD LLC
180 North Dean Street   Englewood, NJ 07631   (201)871-8366   Fax (201)871-8356

Benoff, Lane Jeffrey, MD {1073581997} IntrMd, CdvDis(90,NY47)
+ Cardiovascular Consultants of North Jersey
777 Terrace Avenue   Hasbrouck Heights, NJ 07604   (201)288-4252   Fax (201)288-7172

Benoy, Leena, MD {1407185838} Pedtrc
+ Drs. Sonavane and Benoy
1503 Saint Georges Avenue/Suite 205   Colonia, NJ 07067   (732)382-8111   Fax (732)381-0292

Bensimhon, Miriam H., MD {1326375130} Psychy(01,NY19)
+ BSD Nephrology & Hypertension
360 Essex Street/Suite 304   Hackensack, NJ 07601   (201)646-0110   Fax (201)646-0219

Benson, Brian Eric, MD {1336312420} Otlryg(03,NY01)<NJ-HACKNSK>
+ Hackensack University Medical Center
20 Prospect Avenue/Suite 613   Hackensack, NJ 07601   (551)996-2750   Fax (551)228-7606
+ 95 Glenwood Road
Englewood, NJ 07631   (201)735-0253

Benson, Douglas N., MD {1841204450} Surgry(71,NJ06)<NJ-HACKNSK, NJ-HOLYNAME>
+ North Jersey Surgical Specialists
83 Summit Avenue   Hackensack, NJ 07601   (201)646-0010   Fax (201)646-0600
Dbenson@ptd.net

Benson, Ellen, MD {1871603027} EmrgMd, IntrMd(79,NJ05)<NJ-STJOSHOS, NJ-NWTNMEM>
+ Newton Medical Center
175 High Street/Emerg Med   Newton, NJ 07860   (973)579-8500   Fax (973)383-1461

Benson, Jay Robert, DO {1578881884} FamMed(07,IL76)
+ The Center for Nutritional Medicine
4 Walter E. Foran Boulevard/Suite 409   Flemington, NJ 08822   (908)237-0200   Fax (908)237-0210

Benson, Michael, MD {1952720369}
+ Urology Consultants
36 Newark Avenue/Suite 200   Belleville, NJ 07109   (973)759-6180   Fax (973)759-2006

Benson, Payam, MD {1457539850} Nephro<NJ-VIRTMHBC>
+ 81 Maiden Lane
Bergenfield, NJ 07621

Benson, Peter Kurt, MD {1447264577} Anesth<NJ-HOLYNAME>
+ Holy Name Hospital
718 Teaneck Road/Anesth   Teaneck, NJ 07666   (201)833-7149
farzan2@yahoo.com

Benstock, Alan D., MD {1063450997} Pedtrc(64,DC02)<NJ-VALLEY>
+ Chestnut Ridge Pediatrics
595 Chestnut Ridge Road   Woodcliff Lake, NJ 07677   (201)391-2020   Fax (201)391-0265

Bentley, James David, MD {1184673634} PthAcl, PthCyt, IntrMd(89,OH06)<OH-EMHREGNL>
+ Inform Diagnostics
825 Rahway Avenue   Union, NJ 07083   (732)901-7575   Fax (732)901-1555

Bentley, Katherine Saltstein, MD {1245493675}
+ 30 Undercliff Terrace
West Orange, NJ 07052   (609)915-6695

Bentley, William Earl, IV, DO {1295053171} Anesth, IntrMd<NJ-HUNTRDN>
+ Hunterdon Anesthesia Associates
2100 Wescott Drive   Flemington, NJ 08822   (908)788-6181   Fax (908)788-6145

Bentolila, Eric Y., MD {1487726675} ObsGyn(84,FRA11)<NJ-VALLEY>
+ Dr. Eric Y. Bentolila and Assoc
615 Franklin Turnpike   Ridgewood, NJ 07450   (201)447-1700   Fax (201)447-9386

Benton, Marc L., MD {1003817156} CritCr, IntrMd, PulDis(82,NY47)<NJ-MORRISTN, NJ-OVERLOOK>
+ Atlantic Sleep & Pulmonary Associates
300 Madison Avenue/Suite 201   Madison, NJ 07940   (973)822-2772   Fax (973)822-2773

Bentsianov, Sari, MD {1487941779} AdolMd
+ UMDNJ Adolescent Medicine
90 Bergen Street/Suite 4600   Newark, NJ 07103   (800)249-7750

Benvenuti, Eve S., MD {1427141688} IntrMd(84,NY09)<NJ-OVERLOOK>
+ Community Health Center at Vauxhall
3 Farrington Street   Vauxhall, NJ 07088   (908)598-7950   Fax (908)686-1163

Benz, Michael, MD {1548352438} CdvDis, IntCrd, IntrMd(92,INA5B)
+ Advanced Cardiac Care
142 Palisade Avenue/Suite 215   Jersey City, NJ 07306   (201)222-1170   Fax (201)222-1159
michaelbenzmd@yahoo.com

Physicians by Name and Address

Benzel, Irwin Zachary, DO {1841586914}
+ Pedimedica PA
870 Palisade Avenue/Suite 201   Teaneck, NJ 07666   (973)809-8769   Fax (201)692-9219
irwin.benzel@gmail.com

Beppel, Elaine B., MD {1740259696} FamMed(93,PA13)
+ Virtua Family Medicine of Washington Township
239 Hurffville Crosskeys Road   Sewell, NJ 08080   (856)341-8181   Fax (856)341-8180

Bera, Dilipkumar M., MD {1700823853} IntrMd(81,INDI)<NJ-WARREN>
+ 39 Roseberry Street/Suite B
Phillipsburg, NJ 08865   (908)859-5323   Fax (908)859-5325

Berardi, Richard, Jr., DO {1245244987} IntrMd(90,NY75)
+ Peak Medical
492 Springfield Avenue   Berkeley Heights, NJ 07922   (908)665-0770   Fax (908)665-0006

Berberian, Brian, MD {1861422586} Gastrn, IntrMd(01,MEX14)<NJ-VIRTMHBC>
+ LMA Gastroenterology Associates
63 Kresson Road/Suite 104   Cherry Hill, NJ 08034   (856)751-7420   Fax (856)424-3113

Berberian, Derek Bruce, MD {1346597200} <NJ-UNIVBHC>
+ University Behavioral Health Care
671 Hoes Lane/PO Box 1392   Piscataway, NJ 08855   (732)235-4433

Berberian, Robert A., MD {1942411194} FamMed(01,MEX03)
+ PRP & MediSpa
639 Teaneck Road   Teaneck, NJ 07666   (201)815-5950   Fax (201)751-5458

Berberian, Wayne S., MD {1962591735} SrgOrt, SrgFAk(91,PA07)<NJ-CHILTON, NJ-HACKNSK>
+ North Jersey Orthopaedic Institute
90 Bergen Street/DOC 1200   Newark, NJ 07101   (973)972-2184   Fax (973)972-9367

Berberich, Matthew Robert, MD {1851320436} Anesth, CarAne, PainInvt(00,GRN01)
+ Jersey Shore Anesthesiology Associates
1945 Route 33/PO Box 397   Neptune, NJ 07754   (732)922-3308   Fax (732)897-0263

Bercik, Michael J., MD {1548364169} SrgOrt(76,DC02)<NJ-TRINI-JSC, NJ-TRININPC>
+ 711 Westminster Avenue
Elizabeth, NJ 07208   (908)353-0353   Fax (908)353-0365

Bercik, Robert J., MD {1386754349} SrgOrt(79,DC02)
+ Robert J. Bercik MD
1445 Raritan Road   Clark, NJ 07066   (908)272-5300   Fax (908)272-1177

Berdini, Jeffrey L., MD {1760450357} Urolgy(73,NJ05)<NJ-HACKNSK>
+ 92 Kinderkamack Road
Woodcliff Lake, NJ 07677   (201)391-1515   Fax (201)391-7502

Berdy, Jack M., MD {1215999115} IntrMd(93,NY47)<NJ-HACKNSK, NJ-WAYNEGEN>
+ Internal Medicine PA
155 Cedar Lane   Teaneck, NJ 07666   (201)836-4248   Fax (201)836-5420

Beredjiklian, Pedro Kirkor, MD {1114955689} SrgOrt(NY01<NJ-ATLANTHS>
+ Rothman Institute - Voorhees
443 Laurel Oak Road   Voorhees, NJ 08043   (856)821-6360

Beresford, Dianne Walker, MD {1083671234} IntrMd(83,GRNA)<NJ-CLARMAAS, NJ-STBARNMC>
+ Belmont Medical Center
303 Belmont Avenue   Belleville, NJ 07109   (973)751-4818   Fax (973)751-4886

Berg, Bruce R., MD {1336211820} Ophthl(67,MI01)<NJ-JRSYSHMC, NJ-MONMOUTH>
+ Eye Diagnostic Center
3333 Fairmont Avenue   Asbury Park, NJ 07712   (732)988-4000   Fax (732)988-9502
+ Eye Diagnostic Center
525 Route 70   Brick, NJ 08723   (732)988-4000   Fax (732)477-1444

Berg, David Adam, MD {1124286604} SrgC&R, Surgry(01,MA07)<NJ-KMHCHRRY, NJ-KMHTURNV>
+ Advocare Associates in General Surgery
2201 Chapel Avenue West/Suite 100   Cherry Hill, NJ 08002   (856)665-2017   Fax (856)488-6769

Berg, Howard M., MD {1639272289} Otlryg, SrgFPl, SrgHdN(80,NY19)<NY-NYUDWNTN, NJ-STBARNMC>
+ Specialists in Otolaryngology
101 Old Short Hills Road/Suite 520   West Orange, NJ 07052   (973)731-5400   Fax (973)669-0805
Drheshy@aol.com
+ Short Hills Surgery Center
187 Millburn Avenue/Suite 101   Millburn, NJ 07041   (973)731-5400   Fax (973)671-0557

Berg, Jodi Liebman, MD {1225032683} Pedtrc(01,PA13)
+ Kids first
2006 Salem Road   Burlington, NJ 08016   (609)877-1500   Fax (609)877-4262

Berg, Kevin James, MD {1124285176} FamMed, Grtrcs<NJ-CENTRAST>
+ Mountainside Family Practice Associates
799 Bloomfield Avenue/Suite 201   Verona, NJ 07044   (973)746-7050   Fax (973)857-2831

Bergam, Miro Nicholas, Jr., MD {1104901420} Anesth(92,MA05)<NJ-STBARNMC>
+ New Jersey Anesthesia Associates, P.C.
252 Columbia Turnpike/PO Box 0037   Florham Park, NJ 07932   (973)660-9334   Fax (973)660-9779

Bergen, Blair A., MD {1881775658} ObsGyn(84,NJ05)<NJ-ACMCITY, NJ-SHOREMEM>
+ Pavilion Ob/Gyn AtlantiCare
443 Shore Road/Suite 101   Somers Point, NJ 08244   (609)677-7211   Fax (609)611-7210

Bergen, Robert L., MD {1275785784} Ophthl(68,KY12)<NJ-HACKNSK>
+ Retina Associates of New Jersey, P.A.
628 Cedar Lane   Teaneck, NJ 07666   (201)837-7300   Fax (201)836-6426

Berger, Bruce J., MD {1942301528} Dermat(70,MA07)
+ 278 Franklin Avenue
Princeton, NJ 08540   (609)924-6600   Fax (609)683-4437
gary_mustard@yahoo.com

Berger, Daniel A., DO {1902879091} ObsGyn(96,NJ75)<NJ-WARREN>
+ Phillipsburg Ob/Gyn Associates
700 Coventry Drive   Phillipsburg, NJ 08865   (908)454-4666

Berger, Eric, MD {1508892282} Psychy(81,DMN01)<NJ-KIMBALL>
+ Kimball Medical Center
600 River Avenue/Psychiatry   Lakewood, NJ 08701   (732)363-1900

Berger, Gary, MD {1740259019} FamMed(73,NJ05)<NJ-MORRISTN>
+ Madison Family Practice
8 Shunpike Road   Madison, NJ 07940   (973)377-2610   Fax (973)377-2345

Berger, Glen W., MD {1285697201} IntrMd(89,NJ02)<NJ-VALLEY>
+ 110 Warren Avenue/Suite 5
Ho Ho Kus, NJ 07423   (201)444-9405   Fax (201)444-9408

Berger, Howard M., MD {1780654095} SrgVas, Surgry(75,NY09)<NJ-OCEANMC>
+ 147 Route 37 West
Toms River, NJ 08755   (732)505-9227   Fax (732)505-0228

Berger, Jay Steven, MD {1922268200} Anesth(03,NJ05)<NJ-UMDNJ>
+ Rutgers- New Jersey Medical School
185 South Orange Avenue   Newark, NJ 07103   (973)972-4300

Berger, John L., MD {1215999784} SrgOrt(77,MEXI)<NJ-VALLEY>
+ Orthopedic Associates
15-01 Broadway/Suite 20   Fair Lawn, NJ 07410   (201)794-6008   Fax (201)794-6190

Berger, Lance Seth, MD {1689679490} CdvDis, IntrMd(90,NY15)<NJ-COMMED, NJ-KIMBALL>
+ Monmouth Cardiology Associates, LLC
11 Meridian Road   Eatontown, NJ 07724   (732)663-0300   Fax (732)663-0301
+ Monmouth Cardiology Associates, LLC
222 Schanck Road/Suite 104   Freehold, NJ 07728   (732)663-0300   Fax (732)431-1712

Berger, Mark J., MD {1700816253} Radiol, RadDia(83,NY09)<NJ-HOBUNIMC>
+ Hoboken Medical Imaging
2 Hudson Place   Hoboken, NJ 07030   (201)418-0040   Fax (201)418-0903

Berger, Richard P., MD {1154340008} EmrgMd, FamMed(77,NY45)<NJ-SOMERSET>
+ Emergency Medical Associates of NJ, P.A.
3 Century Drive   Parsippany, NJ 07054   (973)740-0607   Fax (973)740-9895

Berger, Richard S., MD {1588612378} Dermat(65,MI01)<NJ-RWJUBRUN, NJ-UNVMCPRN>
+ Princeton Dermatology Associates
1950 State Route 27/Suite A   North Brunswick, NJ 08902   (732)297-8866   Fax (732)821-0626

Berger, Robert B., MD {1215978788} RadDia, RadNuc(78,PA02)
+ Princeton Radiology Associates, P.A.
419 North Harrison Street   Princeton, NJ 08540   (609)921-3345   Fax (609)683-8847
+ Princeton Radiology Associates, P.A.
9 Centre Drive   Jamesburg, NJ 08831   (609)921-3345   Fax (609)655-4016
+ Princeton Radiology Associates, P.A.
3674 Route 27   Kendall Park, NJ 08540   (732)821-5563   Fax (732)821-6675

Bergh, Paul Akos, MD {1639103468} ObsGyn, RprEnd(83,NJ06)<NJ-MORRISTN, NJ-STBARNMC>
+ Reproductive Medicine Associates of New Jersey
111 Madison Avenue/Suite 100   Morristown, NJ 07962   (973)971-4600   Fax (973)290-8371

+ Reproductive Medicine Associates of New Jersey
475 Prospect Avenue/Suite 101   West Orange, NJ 07052   (973)971-4600   Fax (973)290-8370
+ Reproductive Medicine Associates of New Jersey
25 Rockwood Place   Englewood, NJ 07962   (201)569-7773   Fax (201)569-8143

Berghaus, Jean E., MD {1457410888} Pedtrc(97,NJ06)<NJ-JRSYSHMC>
+ Chemed Family Health Center
1771 Madison Avenue   Lakewood, NJ 08701   (732)364-2144   Fax (732)364-3559

Bergknoff, Hugh, MD {1346300753} ObsGyn(81,FL02)<NJ-STPETER>
+ Womens Health first
114 Stanhope Street   Princeton, NJ 08540   (609)683-7979   Fax (609)683-1972
+ Cares Surgicenter, LLC.
240 Easton Avenue   New Brunswick, NJ 08901   (609)683-7979   Fax (732)296-8677

Bergman, Benjamin Ryan, MD {1679770366} IntrMd, CdvDis(06,MA07)
+ Cardiology Associates of Sussex County LLP
222 High Street/Suite 205   Newton, NJ 07860   (973)579-2100   Fax (973)579-6638

Bergman, Justin A., MD {1487726048} Otlryg, Otolgy(69,PA09)
+ 640 North Broad Street
Elizabeth, NJ 07208   (908)289-7272   Fax (908)354-0888

Bergman, Kerry S., MD {1346211174} PedSrg, Surgry(82,NY03)<NJ-OVERLOOK>
+ Overlook Medical Center
99 Beauvoir Avenue/PO Box 210   Summit, NJ 07902   (908)522-3523   Fax (908)522-3525

Bergmann, Steven Robert, MD {1972588515} CdvDis, IntrMd(85,MO02)<CT-UCONNJDH>
+ Penn Medicine Princeton Medicine Phys
5 Plainsboro Road/Suite 350   Plainsboro, NJ 08536   (609)853-7220   Fax (609)853-7271

Bergquist, Harveen Bal, MD {1265727622} EmrgMd
+ Cooper Univerisry Emergency Physicians
One Cooper Plaza/Keleman 152   Camden, NJ 08103   (856)342-2351   Fax (856)968-8272

Beri, Gagan D., MD {1578785838} Gastrn, IntrMd(01,NJ05)<NJ-UMDNJ>
+ Dr. Howard N. Guss & Dr. Gagan D. Beri
3200 Sunset Avenue/Suite 208   Ocean, NJ 07712   (732)775-9000   Fax (732)775-6660

Beri, Kavita, MD {1548391832} IntrMd(03,INA1N)
+ 3200 Sunset Avenue/Suite 107
Ocean, NJ 07712   (732)455-8118   Fax (732)455-8120

Beri, Samarth, MD {1669654372} IntrMd<NY-VABRKLYN>
+ Englewood Hospital and Medical Center
350 Engle Street   Englewood, NJ 07631   (201)894-3000

Berin, Inna, MD {1457473522} RprEnd, ObsGyn(03,NY47)
+ Fertility Institute of New Jersey
400 Old Hook Road/Suite 2-3   Westwood, NJ 07675   (201)666-4200

Bering, Thomas Gerard, MD {1700878477} Anesth<PA-MEMYORK>
+ Montclair Anesthesia Associates PC
185 Fairfield Avenue/Suite 2A   West Caldwell, NJ 07006   (973)226-1230   Fax (973)226-1232

Berinson, Howard S., MD {1053313528} Radiol(67,PA13)
+ Radiology Associates of Burlington County
1295 Route 38 West/PO Box 479   Hainesport, NJ 08036   (609)261-7017   Fax (609)261-4180

Berio-Dorta, Raul Luis, MD {1225268444} IntHos<NJ-VIRTVOOR>
+ Virtua Voorhees
100 Bowman Drive   Voorhees, NJ 08043   (856)247-2594   Fax (856)247-2597

Berk, Scott Phillip Reed, MD {1356317523} FamMed, IntrMd(96,NJ05)<NJ-HUNTRDN>
+ Hunterdon Integrative Physicians
33B Rupell Road   Hampton, NJ 08827   (908)238-0077   Fax (908)238-0057
hipmanager@gmail.com

Berk, Seth Howard, MD {1326073677} Onclgy, OncHem(94,NY01)
+ Hematology Oncology Associates PA
175 Madison Avenue/4th Floor   Mount Holly, NJ 08060   (609)702-1900   Fax (609)702-8455

Berkel, Reyhan, MD {1265630180} IntrMd(07,MI20)
+ 1300 Main Avenue/Suite 2-A
Clifton, NJ 07011   (973)340-0160   Fax (201)270-5112
info@berkelmd.com

Berkman, Avrill R., MD {1083700124} SrgOrt(81,MA05)
+ 1140 Bloomfield Avenue/Suite 106
West Caldwell, NJ 07006   (973)228-3668   Fax (973)227-6061

Berkman, Douglas S., MD {1811154362} Urolgy, Surgry(04,NJ06)
+ New Jersey Urology
15000 Midlantic Drive/Suite 100   Mount Laurel, NJ 08054   (856)252-1000   Fax (856)985-4582

Physicians by Name and Address

Berkman, Steven R., MD {1174529820} ObsGyn(71,NY08)<NJ-RBAYPERT>
+ Bay Obstetrics & Gynecology
  740 US Highway 1 North   Iselin, NJ 08830   (732)362-3840
  (732)362-3850

Berkovich, Vladimir, MD {1205806015} IntrMd, FamMed(95,DMN01)
+ Center for Aesthetic and Integrative Medicine
  2399 Highway 34/Building A5   Manasquan, NJ 08736
  (732)528-5533   Fax (732)528-0360

Berkowitz, David A., MD {1134224579} IntrMd(63,NY09)<NJ-SOMERSET>
+ 373 East Main Street
  Somerville, NJ 08876   (908)725-6113

Berkowitz, Gregg S., MD {1922095041} SrgOrt, IntrMd(86,NY15)<NJ-CENTRAST>
+ Advanced Orthopedics & Sports Medicine Institute
  301 Professional View Drive   Freehold, NJ 07728
  (732)720-2555   Fax (732)720-2556

Berkowitz, Irwin H., MD {1538106158} Pedtrc(72,NY08)<NJ-VALLEY>
+ Chestnut Ridge Pediatrics
  595 Chestnut Ridge Road   Woodcliff Lake, NJ 07677
  (201)391-2020   Fax (201)391-0265

Berkowitz, Richard H., MD {1104832492} EnDbMt, IntrMd(70,NY08)<NJ-CHILTON>
+ Atlantic Medical Group
  2025 Hamburg Turnpike/Suite D   Wayne, NJ 07470
  (973)839-5070   Fax (973)839-0084

Berkowitz, Robert, MD {1659310506} Psychy, PsyFor, PsyCAd(67,MO03)<NJ-COMMED, NJ-OCEANMC>
+ 448 Lakehurst Road
  Toms River, NJ 08755   (732)244-6066   Fax (732)244-3144
  robertberkowitz9@yahoo.com

Berkowitz, Robert Lester, MD {1437817973} CdvDis, GenPrc, IntrMd(84,CT01)<NJ-HACKNSK>
+ Hackensack University Medical Center
  20 Prospect Avenue/Cardiology   Hackensack, NJ 07601
  (551)996-4849   Fax (551)996-5703

Berkowitz, Rosalind M., MD {1720259237} IntrMd, MedOnc, Hemato(74,NY15)<NJ-LOURDMED>
+ 242 Hedgewood Road
  Moorestown, NJ 08057   (856)235-6533   Fax (856)235-6533

Berkowitz, Stewart A., MD {1720058258} RadOnc, Radiol(87,FL02)<NJ-BAYSHORE, NJ-CHILTON>
+ Shore Point Radiation Oncology
  900 Route 70   Lakewood, NJ 08701   (732)901-7333   Fax (732)370-1294

Berlanga Mineto, Alfredys R., MD {1669718698}<NJ-HOBUNIMC>
+ Hoboken University Medical Center
  308 Willow Avenue   Hoboken, NJ 07030   (201)418-3127

Berlet, Anthony C., MD {1184691594} SrgPlstc, SrgRec(86,NJ05)<NJ-CHILTON>
+ 908 Pompton Avenue/Suite A1
  Cedar Grove, NJ 07009   (973)233-1933   Fax (973)233-1934

Berlin, Ana, MD {1215175435} Surgry, IntrMd(07,NY47)<NJ-UMDNJ>
+ University Hospital-Doctors Office Center
  90 Bergen Street/Suite 7100   Newark, NJ 07103   (973)972-2400   Fax (973)972-2988

Berlin, Burgess L., MD {1740268655} SrgOrt(73,NJ05)
+ 125 Prospect Street
  South Orange, NJ 07079   (973)761-7755   Fax (973)761-0706

Berlin, Daniel, MD {1356508741} Nrolgy, NeuMus, IntrMd(06,NJ05)<NY-PRSBWEIL>
+ Neurology Group of Bergen County
  1200 East Ridgewood Avenue   Ridgewood, NJ 07450
  (201)444-0868   Fax (201)493-0797

Berlin, Fred, MD {1346408937} RadDia(07,GRN01)
+ Imaging Subspecialists of North Jersey LLC
  703 Main Street   Paterson, NJ 07503   (973)754-2645

Berlin, Melissa Gail, MD {1992029110} FamMed(07,ON09)
+ Montclair Family Practice
  230 Sherman Avenue/Suite A   Glen Ridge, NJ 07028
  (973)743-2321   Fax (973)259-0600

Berlin, Paul J., MD {1346244282} AlgyImmn, Pedtrc(85,PA02)<NJ-SJERSYHS, NJ-KENEDYHS>
+ All Allergy and Asthma Care
  188 Fries Mill Road/Suite A-1   Turnersville, NJ 08012
  (856)262-9200   Fax (856)728-6027

Berlin, Ross D., MD {1013088095} PhysMd(91,NY09)<NJ-BACHARCH, NJ-ACMCITY>
+ Bacharach Institute for Rehabilitation
  61 West Jimmie Leeds Road/Physiatry   Pomona, NJ 08240
  (609)748-5380   Fax (609)652-8749
  rossb@bacharach.org

Berlin, William H., DO {1396881447} FamMed, IntrMd(85,CA22)<NJ-VIRTMHBC>
+ AtlantiCare Urgent Care Center
  459 Route 9 South   Little Egg Harbor, NJ 08087   (609)296-4014   Fax (609)296-5735

Berliner, Brett, MD {1871948752}<NJ-HACKNSK>
+ Hackensack University Medical Center
  30 Prospect Avenue   Hackensack, NJ 07601   (551)996-2000

Berman, Adam Jay, MD {1689628935} Urolgy(01,NY19)<NJ-STCLRDEN, NJ-STCLRDOV>
+ Garden State Urology
  282 US Highway 46   Denville, NJ 07834   (973)895-6636
  Fax (973)895-5327

Berman, Barry M., MD {1003997545} Pedtrc(89,MEXI)<NJ-UNDRWD>
+ Salem Medical Group
  4 Bypass Road/Suite 101   Salem, NJ 08079   (856)935-3582   Fax (856)935-4382

Berman, David M., MD {1851729602} PthACI(99,TX12)
+ Bristol-Myers Squibb Co. - Occupational Health
  Route 206 & Provinceline Road   Princeton, NJ 08543
  (609)252-4087

Berman, Dean Adam, DO {1902998727} EmrgMd(97,NJ75)<NJ-STCLRDEN>
+ St. Clare's Hospital-Denville Campus
  25 Pocono Road/EmergMed   Denville, NJ 07834   (973)625-6000   Fax (973)989-3092

Berman, Eric David, DO {1326004185} Pedtrc(86,PA77)<NJ-VIRTMARL>
+ Advocare The Farm Pediatrics
  975 Tuckerton Road/Suite 100   Marlton, NJ 08053
  (856)983-6190   Fax (856)983-3805
+ Advocare The Farm Pediatrics
  1001 Laurel Oak Boulevard/Suite B   Voorhees, NJ 08043
  (856)983-6190   Fax (856)782-7404

Berman, Erika Jacobs, MD {1346405057} Radiol(02,NY19)<NJ-OVERLOOK, NJ-MORRISTN>
+ Summit Medical Group-Berkeley Heights Campus
  1 Diamond Hill Road   Berkeley Heights, NJ 07922
  (908)273-4300   Fax (908)277-8874
+ Summit Radiological Associates, PA
  1811 Springfield Avenue   New Providence, NJ 07974
  (908)522-9111

Berman, Gail O., MD {1427389402} CdvDis
+ Schering-Plough Research Global Clinical Development
  2015 Galloping Hill Road   Kenilworth, NJ 07033   (908)298-4000   Fax (908)740-4610

Berman, Gary K., MD {1609981281} CdvDis, IntrMd(79,NY20)
+ 1500 Pleasant Valley Way/Suite 207
  West Orange, NJ 07052   (973)669-0202   Fax (973)669-0046

Berman, Howard L., MD {1376570861} RadDia, NuclMd, Radiol(72,NY03)<NJ-HOLYNAME, NJ-TRINIWSC>
+ Holy Name Hospital
  718 Teaneck Road/Radiology   Teaneck, NJ 07666
  (201)833-3000

Berman, Jeffrey A., MD {1336175256} PsyAdd, PsyAdt, PainMd(77,NY15)
+ 1296 Pennington Road
  Teaneck, NJ 07666   (201)394-7491

Berman, Lawrence J., MD {1083673297} IntrMd, Nephro(63,MA01)<NJ-VALLEY>
+ Radburn Medical Associates
  20-20 Fair Lawn Avenue/Suite 104   Fair Lawn, NJ 07410
  (201)703-0202   Fax (201)703-1231

Berman, Lee B., MD {1548277601} IntrMd, PulDis(73,NY08)<NJ-CHILTON>
+ 330 Ratzer Road/Suite 4
  Wayne, NJ 07470   (973)628-7900   Fax (973)633-0772

Berman, Mark, MD {1659348381} SprtMd, SrgOrt(81,NY47)<NJ-HACKNSK, NJ-HOLYNAME>
+ 920 Main Street/Suite 2
  Hackensack, NJ 07601   (201)489-8250   Fax (201)489-2933

Berman, Samantha, MD {1639616543} EmrgMd
+ Robert Wood Johnson Emergency Medicine
  One Robert Wood Johnson Place/MEB 104   New Brunswick, NJ 08901   (732)235-4296

Berman, Stefanie L., MD {1235211376} Anesth(86,NY48)<NJ-RWJUBRUN>
+ Robert Wood Johnson-UMDNJ Anesthesia Group
  125 Paterson Street/CAB 3100   New Brunswick, NJ 08901
  (732)235-7827   Fax (732)235-6131

Berman, Mordechai, MD {1710069851} Anesth(87,NJ06)<NJ-RWJUBRUN>
+ Robert Wood Johnson-UMDNJ Anesthesia Group
  125 Paterson Street/CAB 3100   New Brunswick, NJ 08901
  (732)235-7827   Fax (732)235-6131
+ Robert Wood Johnson-UMDNJ Anesthesia Group
  1140 Route 72 West   Manahawkin, NJ 08050   (609)978-8900

Bermingham, John, DO {1700847910} IntrMd, PulDis(85,NJ75)<NJ-COOPRUMC, NJ-KENEDYHS>
+ Pulmonary & Sleep Associates of SJ, LLC.
  750 Route 73 South/Suite 401   Marlton, NJ 08053
  (856)375-1288   Fax (856)375-2325
  jbermingham@pennjerseypulmonary.com
+ Pulmonary & Sleep Associates of SJ, LLC.
  120 Carnie Boulevard/Suite 3   Voorhees, NJ 08043
  (856)375-1288   Fax (856)325-4364
+ Pulmonary & Sleep Associates of SJ, LLC.
  107 Berlin Road   Cherry Hill, NJ 08053   (856)429-1800
  Fax (856)429-1081

Bermudez, Juan D., MD {1982676722} Anesth(81,PRO03)<NJ-KIMBALL>
+ Kimball Medical Center
  600 River Avenue/Anesthesiology   Lakewood, NJ 08701
  (732)363-5689

Berna, Renee Ann, MD {1124176524} IntrMd(96,PA02)
+ Delran Internal Medicine
  5045 Route 130 South/Suite E   Delran, NJ 08075
  (856)764-2525   Fax (856)764-6344

Berna, Ronald A., MD {1952345845} IntrMd(89,PA02)<NJ-VIRTMHBC>
+ Alliance Internal Medicine at Lenola
  509 South Lenola Road/Suite 3   Moorestown, NJ 08057
  (856)234-2722   Fax (856)234-7746

Berna, William J., MD {1629012521} IntrMd(85,NJ06)<NJ-VIRTMHBC>
+ Alliance Internal Medicine at Lenola
  509 South Lenola Road/Suite 3   Moorestown, NJ 08057
  (856)234-2722   Fax (856)234-7746

Bernabe, Maria Joyce Row Guerrero, MD {1528203809} FamMed, Dermat(81,PHI19)
+ Dermatology Associates of Central NJ
  3548 Route 9   Old Bridge, NJ 08857   (732)679-6300
+ Dermatology Associates of Central New Jersey
  250 South Street   Freehold, NJ 07728   (732)679-6300
  Fax (732)679-9566

Bernacki, Carolyn Green, DO {1811128499} PsyCAd(09,PA77)
+ Drenk Behavioral Health Center
  795 Woodlane Road/Suite 301   Mount Holly, NJ 08060
  (609)267-1377   Fax (609)265-9268

Bernadotte, Myrvine, MD {1154534337} EmrgMd<NJ-HACKNSK>
+ Hackensack University Medical Center
  30 Prospect Avenue   Hackensack, NJ 07601   (201)996-2000

Bernal, Ileana, MD {1992770705} Psychy, PsyCAd(85,DOM02)<NJ-CHLSMT, NJ-CHLSOCEN>
+ Children's Specialized Hospital
  150 New Providence Road   Mountainside, NJ 07092
  (908)233-3720
+ Children's Specialized Hospital-Ocean
  94 Stevens Road   Toms River, NJ 08755   (732)914-1100

Bernal, Raymond Mark, MD {1073776761} Urolgy(CA19
+ Jersey Urology Group
  403 Bethel Road   Somers Point, NJ 08244   (609)927-8746
  Fax (609)601-1406

Bernard, John Marley, MD {1568400869} EmrgMd(96,PA02)<NJ-COMMED>
+ Community Medical Center
  99 Route 37 West/Emerg Medicine   Toms River, NJ 08755
  (732)557-8000

Bernard, John V., MD {1003820465} FamMed(86,DOMI)<NJ-WARREN>
+ 526 Water Street
  Belvidere, NJ 07823   (908)475-4601   Fax (908)475-4590

Bernard, Marie G., MD {1710057625} FamMed(89,NJ06)<NJ-HUNTRDN>
+ Hunterdon Family Physicians
  111 State Route 31/Suite 111   Flemington, NJ 08822
  (908)284-9880   Fax (908)782-4316

Bernard-Roberts, Lynikka, MD {1316343205} ObsGyn
+ Amer Ob-Gyn Associates
  900 West Main Street/Suite 3   Freehold, NJ 07728
  (732)308-2255

Bernardi, Bridget Dolores, DO {1598795932} Radiol, RadDia(00,NJ75)<NJ-SJHREGMC>
+ SJH Regional Medical Center
  1505 West Sherman Avenue   Vineland, NJ 08360
  (856)641-8000

Bernardin, Ronald Maurice, III, MD {1164409819} Dermat, IntrMd(02,PA09)
+ Macaione and Papa Dermatology Associates
  707 White Horse Road/Suite C-103   Voorhees, NJ 08043
  (856)627-1900   Fax (856)627-6907

Bernardini, Brad Joseph, MD {1710961107} SrgOrt(99,IL01)<NJ-SJERSYHS, NJ-VIRTMARL>
  + Reconstructive Orthopedics
    994 West Sherman Avenue   Vineland, NJ 08360   (609)267-9400   Fax (609)267-9457
  + Orthopedic Specialty Group
    239 Hurffville-Crosskeys Road   Sewell, NJ 08080   (609)267-9400   Fax (856)629-2265
Bernardini, Joseph P., MD {1134128580} SrgOrt(75,IL01)<NJ-SJERSYHS>
  + Reconstructive Orthopedics
    994 West Sherman Avenue   Vineland, NJ 08360   (609)267-9400   Fax (609)267-9457
Bernardo, Dennis N., MD {1649338971} FamMed(87,PHIL)<NJ-VALLEY>
  + Heart & Vascular Associates of Northern Jersey
    22-18 Broadway/Suite 201   Fair Lawn, NJ 07410   (201)475-5050   Fax (201)475-5522
  + H&V Associates MD Partners of Englewood
    50 South Franklin Turnpike/3rd Floor   Ramsey, NJ 07446   (201)475-5050   Fax (201)934-6217
Bernardo, Gregory, MD {1801136759} IntrMd<NJ-ACMCITY>
  + AtlantiCare Regional Medical Center/City Campus
    1925 Pacific Avenue   Atlantic City, NJ 08401   (609)652-1000
Bernardo, Salvatore, Jr., MD {1770550147} FamMed(93,NJ05)<NJ-CENTRAST>
  + Drs. Bernardo & Leonard
    4255 US Highway 9/Suite B   Freehold, NJ 07728   (732)683-9897   Fax (732)683-9674
Bernhard, Peter Howard, MD {1679579197} Urolgy, SrgUro(86,MI20)<NJ-COOPRUMC>
  + Cooper Surgical Associates
    3 Cooper Plaza/Suite 403   Camden, NJ 08103   (856)342-2439   Fax (856)968-8457
  + 66 East Avenue
    Woodstown, NJ 08098   (856)342-2439   Fax (856)935-6772
  + Cooper Surgical Care at Marlton
    127 Church Road   Marlton, NJ 08103   (856)817-3000   Fax (856)817-3023
Bernhardt, Jarrid, DO {1104023852} EmrgMd
  + 168 Tavistock
    Cherry Hill, NJ 08034
Bernheim, Joshua William, MD {1255375374} Surgry, SrgVas(97,NY46)<NJ-VALLEY>
  + NJ Endovascular Therapeutics
    1124 East Ridgewood Avenue/Suite 104   Ridgewood, NJ 07450   (201)444-5353
Bernheim, Oren Elias, MD {1639338783} Gastrn, IntrMd(08,NY46)
  + Gastroenterology Associates of New Jersey
    227 Hamburg Turnpike   Pompton Lakes, NJ 07442   (862)336-9988   Fax (862)336-9987
  + Gastroenterology Associates of New Jersey
    246 Hamburg Turnpike/Suite 203   Wayne, NJ 07470   (862)336-9988   Fax (862)336-9987
Bernier, Jean Ciara, MD {1417334418} FamMed
  + The Doctor's Office New Jersey Urgent Care
    85 Godwin Avenue   Midland Park, NJ 07432   (201)857-8400   Fax (201)857-8406
Bernik, Thomas R., MD {1366486441} SrgVas, Surgry(94,DC01)
  + Englewood Hospital and Medical Center
    350 Engle Street/2nd Floor   Englewood, NJ 07631   (201)894-3689
Bernstein, Adam Douglas, MD {1780643882} SrgOrt, SprtMd(97,DC02)<NJ-VALLEY, NJ-STJOSHOS>
  + Garden State Orthopaedic Associates, P.A.
    28-04 Broadway   Fair Lawn, NJ 07410   (201)791-4434   Fax (201)791-9377
  + Garden State Orthopaedic Associates, P.A.
    400 Franklin Turnpike/Suite 112   Mahwah, NJ 07430   (201)791-4434   Fax (201)825-9727
  + Garden State Orthopaedic Associates, P.A.
    33-41 Newark Street   Hoboken, NJ 07410   (201)876-5300   Fax (201)876-5305
Bernstein, Andrew Jay, MD {1346458833} Urolgy(01,IL42)
  + Premier Urology Group, LLC
    275 Orchard Street   Westfield, NJ 07090   (908)654-5100   Fax (908)789-8755
  + Premier Urology Group, LLC
    570 South Avenue East/Building A   Cranford, NJ 07016   (908)654-5100   Fax (908)497-1633
  + Premier Urology Group, LLC
    776 East Third Avenue   Roselle Park, NJ 07090   (908)241-5268   Fax (908)241-8755
Bernstein, Andrew Mitchell, DO {1669490975} IntrMd, Hemato, MedOnc(99,NY75)<NJ-CHILTON>
  + Chilton Medical Center
    97 West Parkway   Pompton Plains, NJ 07444   (973)831-5000

Bernstein, Barbara A., MD {1861414922} Pedtrc(87,NJ05)
  + CHOP Primary Care Mount Laurel
    3201 Marne Highway   Mount Laurel, NJ 08054   (856)829-5545   Fax (856)829-9268
Bernstein, Jay M., MD {1053314955} PedOph(80,IL06)<NJ-MORRISTN, NJ-HACKNSK>
  + Paul Phillips Eye & Surgery Center
    64 Walmart Plaza   Clinton, NJ 08809   (908)735-4100   Fax (908)730-0185
  + Paul Phillips Eye & Surgery Center
    6 Minneakoning Road/Suite B   Flemington, NJ 08822   (908)735-4100   Fax (908)968-3239
  + Paul Phillips Eye & Surgery Center
    1 Monroe Street   Bridgewater, NJ 08809   (908)526-4588   Fax (908)231-6718
Bernstein, Michael Ari, MD {1619192515} EmrgMd, IntrMd(97,NY46)
  + Robert Wood Johnson University Hospital at Rahway
    865 Stone Street/Emergency   Rahway, NJ 07065   (732)499-6100
  + Emergency Medical Offices
    651 West Mount Pleasant Avenue   Livingston, NJ 07039   (732)499-6100   Fax (973)251-1165
Bernstein, Michael H., MD {1073540613} Surgry(64,NY19)<NJ-CHILTON, NJ-WAYNEGEN>
  + Drs. Douyon & Bernstein
    220 Hamburg Turnpike/Suite 11   Wayne, NJ 07470   (973)942-4941   Fax (973)942-4259
  + 1395 Route 23 South
    Butler, NJ 07405   (973)838-8555
Bernstein, Michael R., MD {1679530273} Urolgy(94,PA01)<NJ-UNDRWD, NJ-OURLADY>
  + New Jersey Urology, LLC
    2401 East Evesham Road/Suite F   Voorhees, NJ 08043   (856)673-1600   Fax (856)988-0636
  + Delaware Valley Urology LLC
    17 West Red Bank Avenue/Suite 303   Woodbury, NJ 08096   (856)673-1600   Fax (856)985-4583
  + 502 Centennial Boulevard/Suite 2
    Voorhees, NJ 08043   (856)751-7772
Bernstein, Sambra H., MD {1063455137} ObsGyn(81,MEXI)<NJ-STPETER>
  + Somerset Ob-Gyn Associates
    215 Union Avenue/Suite A   Bridgewater, NJ 08807   (908)722-2900   Fax (908)722-1856
  + Somerset Ob-Gyn Associates
    1 New Amwell Road   Hillsborough, NJ 08844   (908)874-5900
  + Cares Surgicenter, LLC.
    240 Easton Avenue   New Brunswick, NJ 08807   (732)565-5400   Fax (732)296-8677
Bernstein, Stacy-Arlyn L, MD {1205917812} Pedtrc(01,IL42)
  + Summit Medical Group Pediatrics at Westfield
    592B Springfield Avenue   Westfield, NJ 07090   (908)233-8860   Fax (908)654-7728
Bernstein, Stanley F., MD {1881668325} IntrMd(72,NJ05)<NJ-CHILTON>
  + Wedgewood Primary Care Wedgewood Plaza
    1055 Hamburg Turnpike/Suite 200   Wayne, NJ 07470   (973)248-1440   Fax (973)248-1448
  + Physicians Health Alliance
    1777 Hamburg Turnpike/Suite 205   Wayne, NJ 07470   (973)248-1440   Fax (973)248-1448
Bernstein, William R., MD {1598779696} Pedtrc(89,NY20)
  + St. Peters Pediatric Faculty
    123 How Lane   New Brunswick, NJ 08901   (732)745-8419
Berrizbeitia, Luis Daniel, MD {1285684290} Surgry, SrgThr(76,VEN04)<MA-BRIGWMN>
  + 253 Witherspoon Street/Suite F
    Princeton, NJ 08540   (609)430-8484   Fax (609)430-9405
Berry, Sally Ann, MD {1881832129}
  + 25 Tamarack Road
    Somerset, NJ 08873   (609)865-6816
    sberry1004@hotmail.com
Berry, Tymara Bernadette, MD {1083823454} PedEnd(03,NJ05)<NJ-MORRISTN>
  + Morristown Medical Center
    100 Madison Avenue   Morristown, NJ 07962   (973)971-4340   Fax (973)290-7367
Bersalona, Holly Abate, MD {1669500492} IntrMd(96,NJ05)
  + Seaview Medical Associates
    511 Sea Girt Avenue   Sea Girt, NJ 08750   (732)282-9000   Fax (732)282-9144
Bersalona, Louis Michael, MD {1851429682} IntrMd(96,NJ05)
  + Seaview Medical Associates
    511 Sea Girt Avenue   Sea Girt, NJ 08750   (732)282-9000   Fax (732)282-9144
Bershad, Joshua Marin, MD {1407934474} IntrMd(01,NJ05)<NJ-RWJUBRUN>
  + RWJ University Hospital New Brunswick
    One Robert Wood Johnson Place   New Brunswick, NJ 08901   (732)828-3000

Berson, Casey Lee, MD {1538452230}
  + CENTRA Comprehensive Psychotherapy
    5000 Sagemore Drive/Suite 205   Marlton, NJ 08053   (856)983-3866   Fax (856)985-8148
Bertagnolli, John F., Jr., DO {1295715787} OstMed, GenPrc, FamMed(83,NJ75)
  + Hammonton Family Medicine Center
    373 South White Horse Pike   Hammonton, NJ 08037   (609)704-0185   Fax (609)704-0195
Bertel, James R., MD {1851459432} FamMed(81,DOM03)
  + Kings Way Primary Care
    100 Kings Way East/Suite D2   Sewell, NJ 08080   (844)542-2273   Fax (856)218-4808
Berth, Ulrike, MD {1487852398} Anesth
  + 375 Engle Street
    Englewood, NJ 07631
Bertha, Nicholas A., DO {1598749020} Surgry, SrgLap, Bariat(90,NJ75)<NJ-MORRISTN, NJ-STBARNMC>
  + Advanced Laparoscopic Surgeons of Morris
    83 Hanover Road/Suite 190   Florham Park, NJ 07932   (973)410-9700   Fax (973)410-9703
Bertolino, Laura, DO {1083975858} EmrgMd
  + SJ Emergency Physician, PA
    175 Madison Avenue   Mount Holly, NJ 08060   (609)914-6000   Fax (609)261-5842
Bertolucci, Alessandra, MD {1174528996} Ophthl(88,ITA16)<NY-NYEYEINF, NJ-CLARMAAS>
  + Associated Eye Physicians, P.A.
    1033 Clifton Avenue/Suite 107   Clifton, NJ 07013   (973)472-6405   Fax (973)472-4832
Bertrand, Jesse Lyle, MD {1750744504}<NJ-HACKNSK>
  + Hackensack University Medical Center
    30 Prospect Avenue   Hackensack, NJ 07601   (551)996-1548
Bery, Seema, MD {1871526632} IntrMd(91,INA87)
  + IPC The Hospitalist Company
    55 Madison Avenue/Suite 310   Morristown, NJ 07960   (973)993-9536   Fax (973)998-4237
Bery, Sumita, MD {1841245230} Pedtrc, Anesth(97,NJ05)<NJ-OVERLOOK>
  + Hunterdon Anesthesia Associates
    2100 Wescott Drive   Flemington, NJ 08822   (908)788-6181   Fax (908)788-6145
Besedina, Liliya, MD {1326102609} Dermat(92,UKR25)
  + Better Skin Dermatology, LLC
    100 Town Square/Suite 409   Jersey City, NJ 07310   (201)626-4040   Fax (201)626-4041
  + 849 Avenue C
    Bayonne, NJ 07002
Beshara, Raafat Henry, MD {1932133923} Anesth(80,EGY04)<NJ-RWJUHAM>
  + Hamilton Anesthesia Associates
    2119 Highway 33/Suite B   Trenton, NJ 08690   (609)581-5303   Fax (609)631-6839
Besingi, Cecile Ewane, MD {1407115041} Pedtrc
  + Capital Emergency Physicians & Associates
    One Capital Way   Pennington, NJ 08534   (609)303-4000
Bessen, Deborah Lynn, MD {1093830978} FamMed(99,NJ05)
  + Visiting Physician Services
    23 Main Street/Suite D1   Holmdel, NJ 07733   (732)571-1000   Fax (732)571-1156
Besser, Richard Eric, MD {1386861938} Pedtrc(86,PA01)
  + 19 Oxford Street
    Montclair, NJ 07042
Besserman, Eva B., DO {1184826661} CritCr, IntrMd(85,IA75)<NJ-SOMERSET>
  + RWJ University Hospital Somerset
    110 Rehill Avenue   Somerville, NJ 08876   (908)685-2200
Bessette, Michael John, MD {1437171766} EmrgMd(95,ISR02)
  + 29 East 29th Street
    Bayonne, NJ 07002   (201)858-5258
Betancourt, Javier E., DO {1487973491} EmrgMd<NJ-RWJUHAM>
  + Robert Wood Johnson University Hospital at Hamilton
    1 Hamilton Health Place   Hamilton, NJ 08690   (856)686-4306
Betesh, Naomi Gold, DO {1417158908} PhysMd(05,NY75)
  + Union County Orthopaedic Group
    210 West St. Georges Avenue/PO Box 330   Linden, NJ 07036   (908)486-1111   Fax (908)583-1034
Bethala, Nalini, MD {1710940234} PhysMd(79,INDI)<NJ-VALLEY, NJ-HOLYNAME>
  + Drs. Bethala & Bethala
    466 Old Hook Road/Suite 9   Emerson, NJ 07630   (201)261-1005   Fax (201)261-4208
Bethala, Vivian K., MD {1235191800} Gastrn, IntrMd(76,INDI)<NJ-VALLEY, NJ-HOLYNAME>
  + Drs. Bethala & Bethala
    466 Old Hook Road/Suite 9   Emerson, NJ 07630   (201)261-1005   Fax (201)261-4208

Physicians by Name and Address

Bethel, Colin A. I., MD {1871528943} Surgry, PedSrg(87,NY01)<NJ-STJOSHOS, NJ-UMDNJ>
+ Pediatric Surgery Group
2130 Millburn Avenue   Maplewood, NJ 07040   (973)313-3115   Fax (973)313-3188

Bethencourt, Guillermo F., MD {1952321465} IntrMd(84,MEX03)
+ 3 Hospital Plaza/Suite 303
Old Bridge, NJ 08857   (732)360-1600   Fax (732)360-1601

Betia, Reuben, MD {1659502870} Anesth(68,PHIL)<NJ-MEM-SALEM>
+ 227 Nevada Avenue
Williamstown, NJ 08094

Betsy, Michael, MD {1508954496} SrgOrt(00,NH01)
+ 595 Chestnut Ridge Road/Suite 8
Woodcliff Lake, NJ 07677   (201)391-1133   Fax (201)391-3039

Betta, Joanne, MD {1215989850} Anesth(77,NJ06)<NJ-ENGLWOOD>
+ Englewood Anesthesiology
350 Engle Street   Englewood, NJ 07631   (201)894-3238   Fax (201)871-0619

Betz, Randal Roberts, MD {1851369979} SrgOrt, OrtSpn, IntrMd(77,PA13)
+ Institute for Spine & Scoliosis, P.A.
3100 Princeton Pike/Building 1   Lawrenceville, NJ 08648   (609)912-1500   Fax (609)912-1601

Beute, Bernard John, MD {1598700437} RadDia, IntrMd(85,NJ06)
+ Diagnostic Radiology Associates of Morristown
355 Madison Avenue/Abbey Building   Morristown, NJ 07960   (973)829-0308   Fax (973)539-2946
+ Diagnostic Radiology Associates of Morris-Sussex
121 Center Grove Road/Unit 7   Randolph, NJ 07869   (973)829-0308   Fax (973)989-5208
+ Diagnostic Radiology Associates of Northfield
772 Northfield Avenue   West Orange, NJ 07960   (973)325-0002   Fax (973)325-8140

Beutel, Jonathan A., MD {1780757377} Anesth(91,NJ05)<NJ-JRSYSHMC>
+ 38 Virginia Avenue
Manasquan, NJ 08736

Bevacqua, Alejandro, MD {1487670865} Ophthl(94,NY09)
+ Essex Eye Physicians, LLC
195 Fairfield Avenue/Suite 4B   West Caldwell, NJ 07006   (973)228-4990   Fax (973)228-4464
abevacqua@hotmail.com
+ Essex Eye Physicians, LLC
213 Park Street   Montclair, NJ 07042   (973)228-4990   Fax (973)744-1233

Bewtra, Madhuri, MD {1447358700} ObsGyn(00,NE06)<NJ-ENGLWOOD>
+ Comprehensive Women's Care
401A South Van Brunt Street/Suite 405   Englewood, NJ 07631   (201)871-4346   Fax (201)871-5953

Bey, Omar M., MD {1083760441} PulDis, SrgC&R, CritCr(83,NJ05)<NJ-NWRKBETH>
+ 2040 Millburn Avenue/Suite 403
Maplewood, NJ 07040   (973)761-6761   Fax (973)761-6763
+ Newark Beth Israel Medical Center
201 Lyons Avenue/Pulmonary Dis   Newark, NJ 07112   (973)761-6761   Fax (973)761-6763

Beyer, Mark William, DO {1396181137} Ophthl(10,NJ75)
+ Beyer Eye Associates
395 Highway 33   Mercerville, NJ 08619   (609)586-0273   Fax (609)586-7018

Beyerl, Brian David, MD {1104883297} SrgNro(80,MD07)<NJ-ATLANTHS, NJ-OVERLOOK>
+ Summit Medical Group-Berkeley Heights Campus
1 Diamond Hill Road/Bensley/3 FL   Berkeley Heights, NJ 07922   (908)277-8646   Fax (908)790-6576
+ Morristown Memorial Hospital/Mt. Kemble Division
95 Mount Kemble Avenue/Neuro Surg   Morristown, NJ 07960   (973)971-4758
+ Overlook Medical Center
99 Beauvoir Avenue/PO Box 210   Summit, NJ 07922   (908)522-2000

Beyus, Christopher Michael, MD {1568661254} Anesth
+ James Street Anesthesia
102 James Street/Suite 103   Edison, NJ 08820   (732)494-1444   Fax (732)494-7052

Bezozo, Richard Craig, MD {1245233543} IntrMd(83,GRN01)<NJ-JFKMED, NJ-MEADWLND>
+ Care Station Medical Group
328 West St. Georges Avenue   Linden, NJ 07036   (908)925-2273   Fax (908)925-2235
+ Care Station Medical Group
456 Prospect Avenue   West Orange, NJ 07052   (908)925-2273   Fax (973)731-9881

Bezpalko, Lynn E., DO {1356417570} Otlryg(92,PA77)
+ Southern Ocean Otolaryngology PA
77 Nautilus Drive   Manahawkin, NJ 08050   (609)597-0321   Fax (609)597-0014

Bezpalko, Orest, DO {1649347295} Otlryg(90,IA75)
+ Southern Ocean Otolaryngology PA
77 Nautilus Drive   Manahawkin, NJ 08050   (609)597-0321   Fax (609)597-0014

Bezwada, Hari Prasad, MD {1861426835} SrgOrt(93,NY03)<PA-PENNHOSP>
+ Princeton Orthopaedic Associates, P.A.
325 Princeton Avenue   Princeton, NJ 08540   (609)924-8131   Fax (609)924-8532

Bezzek, Mark S., MD {1902862949} IntrMd(84,GRN01)
+ 6 Teaberry Drive
Medford, NJ 08055

Bhagat, Anilchandra I., MD {1114001211} Anesth, IntrMd(87,WIND)<NJ-VIRTMHBC>
+ Virtua Memorial
175 Madison Avenue/Anesthesia   Mount Holly, NJ 08060   (609)261-1600   Fax (609)261-4454

Bhagat, Mahesh H., MD {1013918531} CritCr, IntrMd, PulDis(87,WIND)<NJ-RBAYPERT, NJ-RBAYOLDB>
+ JFK Medical Center
65 James Street   Edison, NJ 08820   (732)321-7000

Bhagat, Neelakshi, MD {1609894559} Ophthl(94,NY48)
+ University Hospital-New Jersey Medical School
30 Bergen Street/Ophthalmology   Newark, NJ 07107   (973)972-4511

Bhagat, Neha, DO {1669817052} ObsGyn<NJ-NWRKBETH>
+ Newark Beth Israel Medical Center
201 Lyons Avenue   Newark, NJ 07112   (978)495-1560

Bhagat, Nitesh N., MD {1902014749} RadDia(03,MI07)
+ Regional Diagnostic Imaging Center
1505 West Sherman Avenue   Vineland, NJ 08360   (856)641-7937   Fax (856)641-7681

Bhagat, Sanjay, MD {1518998160} Gastrn, IntrMd(85,INA23)<NJ-OCEANMC>
+ 101 Prospect Street/Suite 213
Lakewood, NJ 08701   (732)367-2244

Bhagavathi, Sharathkumar M., MD {1396951661} PthHem
+ RWJ University Pathology
125 Paterson Street/MEB 212   New Brunswick, NJ 08901   (732)418-8047   Fax (732)418-8445

Bhagia, Pooja R., MD {1255587457} Pedtrc, PedHem(05,INA1D)
+ St. Joseph Medical Center Pediatric Hematology/Onc
703 Main Street   Paterson, NJ 07503   (973)754-3230

Bhagwat, Gauri S., MD {1174806665} Pedtrc
+ 1802 Oak Tree Road
Edison, NJ 08820   (732)570-6572

Bhakey, Girija G., MD {1184646754} IntrMd(96,INA26)
+ Menlo Park Medical Group PA
111 James Street   Edison, NJ 08820   (732)549-2299   Fax (732)549-2262

Bhalakia, Niraj, MD {1841426558} RadDia
+ Radiology Affiliates of Central New Jersey, P.A.
2501 Kuser Road   Hamilton, NJ 08691   (609)585-8800   Fax (609)585-1825

Bhalla, Anshu, MD {1366502163} FamMGrtc, FamMed
+ Princeton Health Medical & Surgical Associates
2 Centre Drive/Suite 200   Monroe, NJ 08831   (609)395-2470   Fax (609)860-5288

Bhalla, Meenu Gogia, MD {1689860199} IntrMd, IntHos
+ JFK Hospitalists
98 James Street/Suite 208   Edison, NJ 08818   (908)731-1981   Fax (908)213-6618

Bhalla, Ravinder N., MD {1841214566} PsyCAd, Psychy(82,INDI)<NJ-RAMAPO, NJ-UMDNJ>
+ 65 North Maple Avenue
Ridgewood, NJ 07450   (201)652-4999   Fax (973)471-1630
bhallar@pol.net
+ Mental Health Clinic of Passaic
111 Lexington Avenue   Passaic, NJ 07055   (973)471-8006
+ Bergen Wellness Associates
784 Franklin Avenue   Franklin Lakes, NJ 07450   (201)652-4999

Bhalla, Rohit, DO {1962604819} IntrMd, InfDis(01,NY75)<NJ-UNVMCPRN>
+ ID Associates PA/dba ID Care
105 Raider Boulevard/Suite 101   Hillsborough, NJ 08844   (908)281-0221   Fax (908)281-0940
+ ID Associates PA/dba ID Care
81 Veronica Avenue/Suite 203   Somerset, NJ 08873   (908)281-0221   Fax (732)729-0924
+ ID Associates PA/dba ID Care
10 Forrestal Road South/Suite 203   Princeton, NJ 08844   (609)759-2750   Fax (609)919-9700

Bhalla, Saranga, DO {1154543023} PsyCAd, Psychy(02,NY75)
+ 20 Nassau Street/Suite 121-122
Princeton, NJ 08542   (732)991-2826

Bhalodia, Amit Maganlal, DO {1982692083} FamMed(97,NJ75)<NJ-VIRTMHBC, NJ-KMHSTRAT>
+ Virtua Family Health Center
1000 Atlantic Avenue   Camden, NJ 08104   (856)246-3542   Fax (856)246-3528
+ Alliance for Better Care, PC/Mount Holly Division
1613 Route 38   Lumberton, NJ 08048   (856)246-3542   Fax (609)261-5507

Bhalodia, Manish V., MD {1396760609} IntrMd, CdvDis(92,INDI)<NJ-MTNSIDE>
+ North Jersey Cardiovascular Consultants
329 Belleville Avenue   Bloomfield, NJ 07003   (973)748-3800   Fax (973)748-3540

Bhambri, Ankur, DO {1417374414} FamMed(14,NY75)
+ Morristown Medical Center
100 Madison Avenue   Morristown, NJ 07962   (973)971-5000

Bhambri, Malanie Mathur, DO {1215294046}
+ Pediatric Specialties PA
90 Prospect Avenue/Suite 1-A   Hackensack, NJ 07601   (201)342-4001   Fax (201)342-9569

Bhambri, Neha Madhok, MD {1740511740} AlgyImmn, Pedtrc(04,NJ03)
+ 1 Woodbridge Center/Suite 245
Woodbridge, NJ 07095   (732)636-6622   Fax (718)816-1467

Bhamidipati, Anita, MD {1134582067} EmrgMd
+ Cooper Univerisry Emergency Physicians
One Cooper Plaza   Camden, NJ 08103   (856)342-2627   Fax (856)968-8272

Bhamidipati, Aparna, MD {1710967039} Pedtrc, AdolMd(97,INA23)
+ Edison Pediatrics
1802 Oak Tree Road/Suite 101   Edison, NJ 08820   (732)548-3210   Fax (906)548-3966

Bhandari, Bhavik M., MD {1679763890} IntrMd(04,NJ02)
+ Bergen Medical Associates
466 Old Hook Road/Suite 1   Emerson, NJ 07630   (201)967-8221   Fax (201)967-0340

Bhandari, Pankaj Kumar, MD {1508920836} Psychy(00,NJ05)
+ 395 Grand Street
Jersey City, NJ 07302   (201)915-2835
+ Community Psychiatric Institute
49 South Munn Avenue   East Orange, NJ 07017   (973)673-3342

Bhandari, Sheetal B., DO {1205093168}
+ 279 Janine Way
Bridgewater, NJ 08807   (732)666-8244
spatel02@nyit.edu

Bhandari, Tarun, MD {1194920637} Surgry, IntrMd(95,INA74)<NJ-JRSYSHMC, NJ-OCEANMC>
+ Atlantic Shore Surgical Associates
478 Brick Boulevard   Brick, NJ 08723   (732)701-4848   Fax (732)701-1244
+ Atlantic Shore Surgical Associates
67 Riverwood/Building 2   Toms River, NJ 08755   (732)701-4848   Fax (732)557-3518

Bhandarkar, Anjali, MD {1700879954} InsrMd, IntrMd(00,NY19)
+ RWJ Medical Associates
3100 Quakerbridge Road/Suite 28   Hamilton, NJ 08619   (609)245-7430   Fax (609)245-7432
bhanda01@yahoo.com

Bhandutia, Amit Ketan, MD {1396016705} SrgOrt
+ MidJersey Orthopaedics PA
1081 US Highway 22   Bridgewater, NJ 08807   (908)782-0600

Bharam, Srino, MD {1104828805} SrgOrt(94,NJ05)
+ Srino Bharam MD PC
541 Cedar Hill Avenue   Wyckoff, NJ 07481   (201)904-2121   Fax (201)904-2125

Bharatia, Nikita, DO {1720584170} EmrgMd
+ St. Michael's Medical Center
111 Central Avenue   Newark, NJ 07102   (973)877-5000

Bharatiya, Purabi, MD {1639140577} Psychy(71,INA7X)<NJ-TRININPC, NJ-TRINIWSC>
+ Trinitas Regional Medical Center-New Point Campus
655 East Jersey Street/Psych   Elizabeth, NJ 07206   (908)994-5000
Pbharitya@trinitas.org

Bhargava, Abha, MD {1477560324} InfDis, IntrMd(84,INA9B)<NJ-RBAYOLDB, NJ-BAYSHORE>
+ 21 Exeter Drive
Marlboro, NJ 07746   (732)316-5100
bhargava60@yahoo.com

Bhargava, Hema P., MD {1578572590} PedCrd, Pedtrc(81,INDI)<NJ-SHOREMEM>
+ Children's Hospital of Phila Cardio
1040 Laurel Oak Road/Suite 1   Voorhees, NJ 08043   (856)783-0287   Fax (856)783-0657
+ CHOP Pediatric & Adolescent Specialty Care Center
1012 Laurel Oak Road   Voorhees, NJ 08043   (856)783-0287   Fax (856)435-0091
+ CHOP Specialty Care Center at Virtua
200 Bowman Drive/2 FL/Suite D-260   Voorhees, NJ 08043   (267)425-5400

Bhargava, Ruta Manish, MD {1912107137} IntrMd(00,INA80)
+ 144 Grant Avenue
New Providence, NJ 07974

Bhargava, Sandeep, MD {1437109741} Gastrn, IntrMd(91,INA92)<NJ-STPETER>
+ St. Peter's University Hospital
254 Easton Avenue/Gastro   New Brunswick, NJ 08901   (732)745-8600

Bharucha, Dilip I., MD {1427081736} ObsGyn(77,INA15)<NJ-STPETER, NJ-RWJUBRUN>
+ Premier Ob-Gyn Associates, Inc.
5-B Auer Court   East Brunswick, NJ 08816   (732)651-4142   Fax (732)651-5950
+ Premier Ob-Gyn Associates, Inc.
1527 Route 27 South/Suite 1400   Somerset, NJ 08873   (732)651-4142   Fax (732)246-9910

Bhashyam, Vinod Rao, MD {1801831532} Psychy(79,INA83)
+ 35 Beaverson Boulevard/Suite 1-D
Brick, NJ 08723   (732)920-7933

Bhasin, Atul, MD {1619989639} IntrMd(98,INA69)
+ Drs. Bhasin & Patel
1001 West Main Street/Suite A   Freehold, NJ 07728   (732)637-8444   Fax (732)637-8440
drbhasin@mdslimnj.com

Bhasin, Yasmin, MD {1144268749} Allrgy, AlgyImmn(71,INA23)<MA-ARDHILL, NJ-VALLEY>
+ Allergy & Asthma Care
27 South Franklin Turnpike   Ramsey, NJ 07446   (201)934-9393   Fax (201)934-9394

Bhaskar, Vatsala R., MD {1306884879} Pedtrc, EmrgMd, AdolMd(89,INA2X)<NJ-CENTRAST>
+ 57 Schanck Road/Suite C
Freehold, NJ 07728   (732)431-9202   Fax (732)431-9205

Bhaskara, Jayshree A., MD {1790771228} IntrMd(90,INDI)<NJ-SOMERSET>
+ Ahmad A. Mur MD PA
503 Omni Drive   Hillsborough, NJ 08844   (908)595-1199   Fax (866)889-3643

Bhaskarabhatla, Krishna Venkata M., MD {1689621849} FamMed(81,INA48)
+ St. Joseph's Family Medicine @ Clifton
1135 Broad Street/Suite 201   Clifton, NJ 07013   (973)754-4100   Fax (973)472-9062

Bhaskarapandit, Savitha, MD {1790988244}<NJ-STPETER>
+ St. Peter's University Hospital
254 Easton Avenue   New Brunswick, NJ 08901   (732)745-8600

Bhat, Geetha K. G., MD {1700119963} EnDbMt(89,INA28)<NJ-COOPRUMC>
+ Cooper Endocrinology Associates
1210 Brace Road/Suite 107   Cherry Hill, NJ 08034   (856)795-3597   Fax (856)795-7590
+ The Cooper Hospital System-Univ Hospital
3 Cooper Plaza/Suite 215   Camden, NJ 08103   (856)342-2439

Bhat, Haimavathi, DO {1861625741}
+ Rutgers- New Jersey Medical School
185 South Orange Avenue/MSB L-689   Newark, NJ 07103   (973)972-7837
hb112@njms.rutgers.edu

Bhat, Sushanth K., MD {1396941126} Nrolgy, ClNrPh, VasNeu(00,INA70)<NJ-JFKMED>
+ JFK Medical Center
65 James Street   Edison, NJ 08820   (732)321-7010   Fax (732)744-5873

Bhat, Vishwanath, MD {1003898438} NnPnMd, Pedtrc(89,INA94)
+ The Children's Regional Hospital at Cooper Univ Hosp
One Cooper Plaza   Camden, NJ 08103   (856)342-2265   Fax (856)342-8007
+ Cooper Neonatology
One Cooper Plaza   Camden, NJ 08103   (856)342-2265   Fax (856)342-8007

Bhate, Chinmoy, MD {1609194174} Dermat(10,NJ05)
+ Advanced Dermatology, Laser, and MOHS Surgery Center
240 East Grove Street   Westfield, NJ 07090   (908)232-6446   Fax (908)232-6447

Bhate, Soniya, MD {1730294190} FamMed(03)
+ VA New Jersey Health Care System-East Orange Campus
385 Tremont Avenue   East Orange, NJ 07018   (973)676-1000
+ NHCAC Health Center at North Bergen
1116 43rd Street   North Bergen, NJ 07047   (973)676-1000   Fax (201)330-2638

Bhatia, Anum, MD {1750819850}<NJ-COOPRUMC>
+ Cooper University Hospital
One Cooper Plaza   Camden, NJ 08103   (856)342-2000

Bhatia, Divya V., MD {1891892907} IntrMd, CdvDis(99,GRN01)<NJ-NWRKBETH>
+ Newark Beth Israel Medical Center
201 Lyons Avenue   Newark, NJ 07112   (973)926-7000

Bhatia, Hemlata, MD {1801811310} FamMed(63,INA7B)<NJ-CLARMAAS>
+ 332 Bloomfield Avenue
Bloomfield, NJ 07003   (973)748-5111   Fax (973)748-5703

Bhatia, Irvinder, MD {1518189133} FamMed, IntrMd(96,ON01)<NJ-SOMERSET>
+ AFC Urgent Care South Plainfield
907 Oak Tree Avenue/Suite H   South Plainfield, NJ 07080   (908)222-3500

Bhatia, Jyoti Kamlesh, MD {1881651727} Gastrn, IntrMd(94,INA65)<NJ-CHSMRCER>
+ Mercer Gastroenterology
2 Capital Way/Suite 487   Pennington, NJ 08534   (609)818-1900   Fax (609)818-1908

Bhatia, Malini P., MD {1992760441} Psychy, PsyCAd(65,INA69)
+ Drs. Luhana, Dhirmalani & Patel
239 Baldwin Road/Suite 108   Parsippany, NJ 07054   (973)334-2265   Fax (973)335-9091

Bhatia, Nidhi, MD {1083703227}
+ 143 Morgan Street/Unit 5c
Jersey City, NJ 07302

Bhatia, Nina Prakash, MD {1295960706} Gyneco(05,DMN01)
+ Princeton Urogynecology
10 Forrestal Road South/Suite 205   Princeton, NJ 08540   (609)924-2230   Fax (609)924-5006

Bhatia, Nita, DO {1477873339} PsyCAd<NJ-MORRISTN>
+ Morristown Medical Center
100 Madison Avenue/Psychy   Morristown, NJ 07962   (973)971-5366

Bhatia, Rubina, MD {1942387360} Pedtrc(01,INA20)<NY-RCKCH-PSY>
+ 463 Livingston Street/Suite 204
Norwood, NJ 07648

Bhatia, Taruna, MD {1336371681} Gastrn
+ Gastroenterology Medical Associates PA
142 Palisades Avenue/Suite 201   Jersey City, NJ 07307   (201)795-8596   Fax (201)792-7812
tbtb11@gmail.com

Bhatiya, Savji L., MD {1457321804} Psychy(72,INDI)<NJ-JRSYSHMC, NJ-OCEANMC>
+ 17 Megan Drive
Little Silver, NJ 07739

Bhatnagar, Divya Sambandan, MD {1134480791} Dermat
+ Cosmetic & Dermatologic Surgery Associates, LLC
719 North Beers Street/Suite 2-G   Holmdel, NJ 07733   (732)739-3223   Fax (732)739-3225

Bhatnagar, Ramil S., MD {1225017775} SrgOrt, SrgSpn(95,IL06)<NJ-JRSYSHMC>
+ Orthopaedic Institute of Central Jersey
2315A Highway 34/Suite D   Manasquan, NJ 08736   (732)974-2653   Fax (732)449-4271
+ Orthopaedic Institute of Central Jersey
365 Broad Street   Red Bank, NJ 07701   (732)974-2653   Fax (732)933-1444
+ Orthopaedic Institute of Central Jersey
226 Highway 37 West/Suite 203   Toms River, NJ 08736   (732)240-6060   Fax (732)240-5329

Bhatnagar, Swati Varma, MD {1184668972} RadDia(96,NY20)
+ St. Barnabas Ambulatory Care Center
200 South Orange Avenue   Livingston, NJ 07039   (973)322-7700

Bhatnagar, Tanuj, MD {1205918679} PulDis, IntrMd, CritCr(00,DMN01)
+ The Spine & Sports Health Center
129 Newark Avenue   Jersey City, NJ 07302   (201)533-9200   Fax (201)533-9299
Tanuj.Bhatnagar@att.net

Bhatnagar, Vibhay, MD {1679507347} CdvDis, IntrMd(73,INDI)<NJ-BAYSHORE>
+ Associates in Cardiology and Internal Medicine
530 Green Street   Iselin, NJ 08830   (732)283-0440   Fax (732)283-8943

Bhatt, Advay G., MD {1598713737} ClCdEl, CdvDis(03,NY46)
+ Valley Medical Group-Electrophysiology & Cardiology
223 North Van Dien Avenue   Ridgewood, NJ 07450   (617)467-5596   Fax (201)432-7830
advaybhatt@outlook.com
+ Valley Medical Group-Electrophysiology
970 Linwood Avenue/Suite 102   Ridgewood, NJ 07450   (617)467-5596   Fax (201)432-7830

Bhatt, Harish K., MD {1114922002} PhysMd(78,INA21)<NJ-JFKMED, NJ-RWJURAH>
+ JFK Med Ctr -Physical Medicine & Rehab
4 Progress Street/Suite A-9   Edison, NJ 08820   (908)769-1101   Fax (908)663-2634
harishkb@aol.com
+ Robert Wood Johnson University Hospital at Rahway
865 Stone Street/Attending   Rahway, NJ 07065   (732)381-4200
+ RWJ University Hospital New Brunswick
One Robert Wood Johnson Place   New Brunswick, NJ 08820   (732)828-3000

Bhatt, Komal Gopalbhai, MD {1760619241} FamMed, IntrMd(07,INA15)<NJ-RWJUBRUN>
+ Family Medicine at Monument Square
317 George Street   New Brunswick, NJ 08901   (732)235-8993   Fax (732)246-7317
+ RWJ University Hospital New Brunswick
One Robert Wood Johnson Place   New Brunswick, NJ 08901   (732)235-8993   Fax (732)235-8313

Bhatt, Mahesh, MD {1881018166}<NJ-JRSYCITY>
+ Jersey City Medical Center
355 Grand Street   Jersey City, NJ 07304   (201)915-2000
mountains008@hotmail.com

Bhatt, Meeta Hasmukh, MD {1174764807} Nrolgy, ClNrPh(85,INA67)
+ University Medical Professionals LLC
240 Williamson Street/Suite 300   Elizabeth, NJ 07202

Bhatt, Nikhil Yeshavantray, MD {1013962562} IntrMd(80,INA20)<NJ-KIMBALL, NJ-CENTRAST>
+ Kimball Medical Center
600 River Avenue/Medicine   Lakewood, NJ 08701   (732)363-1900

Bhatt, Pranay Janardan, MD {1952381287} IntrMd(00,DMN01)
+ Newport Medical Associates
610 Washington Boulevard   Jersey City, NJ 07310   (201)222-1266
+ Columbus Urgent Care
350 Bloomfield Avenue/Suite 1   Bloomfield, NJ 07003   (201)222-1266   Fax (973)748-6985
+ Union Family Medicine
2300 Vauxhall Road   Union, NJ 07310   (908)688-4424

Bhatt, Raunaq Dushyantkumar, MD {1871824888} IntHos<NJ-MORRISTN>
+ Overlook Medical Center
99 Beauvoir Avenue/PO Box 210   Summit, NJ 07902   (908)522-2000   Fax (973)290-8325
+ Morristown Medical Center
100 Madison Avenue   Morristown, NJ 07962   (973)971-5000

Bhatt, Rupal S., MD {1104830272} IntrMd(96,INDI)
+ Drs. Bhatt and Bhatt
271 Route 46 West/Suite 105   Fairfield, NJ 07004   (973)575-8644   Fax (973)575-8677

Bhatt, Shirish Vinayak, MD {1982694741} IntrMd(94,WI06)<NJ-MTNSIDE>
+ Drs. Bhatt and Bhatt
271 Route 46 West/Suite 105   Fairfield, NJ 07004   (973)575-8644   Fax (973)575-8677

Bhatt, Trigun R., MD {1811927759} IntrMd, Grtrcs(95,INA8B)
+ 12 Village Drive
Voorhees, NJ 08043

Bhatt, Uday N., MD {1033147483} PhysMd(94,INA20)<NJ-KIMBALL, NJ-COMMED>
+ New Jersey Spine & Pain Center
2111 Klockner Road   Hamilton, NJ 08690   (609)587-6070   Fax (609)587-6010

Bhatt, Usha Praful, MD {1124004494} PsyCAd, Psychy(67,INA5B)<NJ-UMDNJ>
+ University Psychiatric Associates
183 South Orange Avenue/E-F Levels   Newark, NJ 07103   (973)972-2977   Fax (973)972-2979
+ 535 Sycamore Avenue
Shrewsbury, NJ 07702   (732)747-4556

Bhattacharjee, Dulal, MD {1043540172} EnDbMt
+ 1319 St. Georges Avenue/Suite 214
Rahway, NJ 07065   (570)236-0200

Bhattacharjee, Pradip, MD {1124351747} PthDrm, PthAcl, IntrMd(98,MNT01)
+ PLUS Diagnostics
1200 River Avenue/Suite 10   Lakewood, NJ 08701   (732)901-7575   Fax (732)901-1555

Bhattacharjee, Roopali, MD {1598845653} ObsGyn(74,INDI)<NJ-CHSMRCER, NJ-RWJUHAM>
+ Mercer Ob/Gyn, PA
638 Lawrence Road   Lawrenceville, NJ 08648   (609)883-8200   Fax (609)530-1881
womandoctor@yahoo.com

Bhattacharya, Ashish Kumar, MD {1467427807} SrgPlstc, Otlryg(90,NJ05)<NJ-BAYSHORE, NJ-CENTRAST>
+ Plastic Surgery PLUS
55 Schanck Road/Suite A-4   Freehold, NJ 07728   (732)683-1033   Fax (732)683-2477
Tracy@plasticsurgeryplus.net

Bhattacharya, Prianka, MD {1407264153} OncHem<NJ-COOPRUMC>
+ Cooper University Hospital
One Cooper Plaza   Camden, NJ 08103   (856)342-2000

Bhattacharyya, Adity, MD {1538192257} FamMed(81,INDI)<NJ-HOBUNIMC>
+ JFK Family Practice Group
65 James Street   Edison, NJ 08818   (732)321-7487   Fax (732)906-4927

Physicians by Name and Address

hattacharyya, Nishith, MD {1003854092} PedCrd, Surgry(84,INA7X)<NJ-UMDNJ, NJ-HACKNSK>
+ Pediatric Surgery Group
2130 Millburn Avenue   Maplewood, NJ 07040   (973)313-3115   Fax (973)313-3188
+ St. Barnabas Ambulatory Care Center
200 South Orange Avenue   Livingston, NJ 07039   (973)322-7000

Bhattacharyya, Pritish K., MD {1144258872} PthAcl(75,INDI)<NJ-HACKNSK>
+ Hackensack University Medical Center
30 Prospect Avenue/Pathology   Hackensack, NJ 07601   (201)996-2000

Bhattacharyya, Shibani S., MD {1285703157} Anesth
+ 6 Roosevelt Boulevard
North Caldwell, NJ 07006

Bhatti, Habib Arshad, MD {1487071056} IntrMd<NJ-STFRNMED>
+ St. Francis Medical Center
601 Hamilton Avenue/Medicine   Trenton, NJ 08629   (609)599-5061   Fax (609)599-6232

Bhatti, Hamza Dastigir, DO {1043598352} Dermat
+ Robert Wood Johnson Dermatology
1 World's Fair Drive   Somerset, NJ 08873   (732)235-7765   Fax (732)235-6568

Bhatti, Jamil M., MD {1124071428} Psychy(79,PAK10)<PA-FRIENDS, NJ-ANCPSYCH>
+ Ancora Psychiatric Hospital
301 Spring Garden Road   Hammonton, NJ 08037   (609)561-1700

Bhatti, Mohammad Azeem, MD {1093788101} Urolgy, SrgUro, IntrMd(92,AB01)
+ Crescent Urological Care
1205 Easton Avenue/Suite 201   Somerset, NJ 08873   (732)325-0050   Fax (732)325-0071

Bhatti, Waseem Alam, MD {1578779310} RadV&I, RadDia(06,NJ05)<NJ-OVERLOOK>
+ Overlook Medical Center
99 Beauvoir Avenue/PO Box 210   Summit, NJ 07902   (908)522-7334

Bhatty, Anis A., MD {1285668871} PedHem, Pedtrc(72,INDI)
+ Pedimedica, P.A.
18 Railroad Avenue/Suite 103   Rochelle Park, NJ 07662   (201)291-2323   Fax (201)291-2328
+ Pedimedica PA
810 Abbott Boulevard/Suite 101   Fort Lee, NJ 07024   (201)291-2323   Fax (201)224-4045

Bhavnani, Anita S., MD {1801965769} EmrgMd(87,PA09)<NJ-STPETER>
+ St. Peter's University Hospital
254 Easton Avenue/EmrgMed   New Brunswick, NJ 08901   (732)745-8600   Fax (732)418-1320

Bhavsar, Jignesh, MD {1093832404} CdvDis, IntrMd(04,NJ05)
+ Penn Medicine at Cherry Hill
1400 East Route 70/Cardiology   Cherry Hill, NJ 08034
+ Penn Medicine at Woodbury Heights
1006 Mantua Pike   Woodbury Heights, NJ 08097   Fax (856)845-0535

Bhavsar, Sejal Makvana, MD {1689952418}<NY-MTSINAI>
+ Hackensack Univ Medical Center Pediatric Emerg Room
30 Prospect Avenue   Hackensack, NJ 07601   (201)996-5430   Fax (201)996-3676

Bhavsar, Vaishali, MD {1972667467} Anesth(02,GRN01)<NJ-MEADWLND>
+ Meadowlands Hospital Medical Center
55 Meadowlands Parkway/Anesth   Secaucus, NJ 07096   (201)392-3100

Bhawsar, Nilaya Babu, DO {1265507461} Nrolgy(02,NY75)
+ Summit Medical Group
315 East Northfield Road/Suite 1-E   Livingston, NJ 07039   (973)535-3200   Fax (973)535-1450

Bhayana, Suverta, MD {1417151010} Nephro
+ 20 Prospect Avenue/Suite 404
Hackensack, NJ 07601

Bhayani, Parimal S., MD {1902872666} ObsGyn, Gyneco(68,INA65)<NJ-NWTNMEM>
+ 55 Newton-Sparta Road
Newton, NJ 07860   (973)383-0900   Fax (973)383-0558

Bhende, Sudhir S., MD {1073546495} IntrMd, MedOnc(71,INA70)<NJ-MMHKEMBL, NJ-MORRISTN>
+ Morristown Memorial Hospital/Mt. Kemble Division
95 Mount Kemble Avenue   Morristown, NJ 07960   (973)971-4465   Fax (973)267-3144

Bhendwal, Sanjay, MD {1770519944} IntrMd(84)
+ Cumberland Medical Associates
1206 West Sherman Avenue   Vineland, NJ 08360   (856)691-8444   Fax (856)691-8325
sbhendwal@aol.com

Bhimani, Chandni, DO {1770920746} RadDia<NJ-COOPRUMC>
+ Cooper University Hospital
One Cooper Plaza/Suite B23   Camden, NJ 08103   (856)342-2588

Bhimani, Siddharth D., MD {1376975870} IntrMd
+ Kennedy Family Health Center
445 Hurffville Crosskeys Road   Sewell, NJ 08080   (856)262-1900
+ 3024 Fifth Street
Voorhees, NJ 08043   (609)870-0354

Bhiro, Peter Rajendra, DO {1245296771} IntrMd(93,NY75)<NJ-COMMED, NJ-SOCEANCO>
+ 949 West Lacey Road/Suite C4
Forked River, NJ 08731   (609)693-8690   Fax (609)693-8691

Bhise, Vikram V., MD {1700047594} ClNrPh
+ Child Health Institute of New Jersey
89 French Street/Suite 2300   New Brunswick, NJ 08901   (732)235-7875   Fax (732)235-8766

Bhogal, Jasmeet Singh, MD {1295980969} FamMed, IntrMd(04,INA79)<NJ-VIRTBERL, NJ-VIRTMARL>
+ Virtua Express Urgent Care
401 Young Avenue/Suite 180   Moorestown, NJ 08057   (856)291-8600   Fax (856)291-8615
dr_jsbhogal@yahoo.com
+ Virtua Immediate Care Center
239 Hurffville Crosskeys Road   Sewell, NJ 08080   (856)291-8600   Fax (856)341-8215
+ Virtua Express Urgent Care-Voorhees
158 Route 73   Voorhees, NJ 08057   (856)247-7230   Fax (856)246-7231

Bhojwani, Amit N., DO {1477986420} Otlryg
+ Coastal Ear Nose and Throat LLC
1301 Route 72/Suite 340   Manahawkin, NJ 08050   (732)280-7855   Fax (732)280-7815
+ 708 Gregorys Way
Voorhees, NJ 08043   (908)963-3159

Bhoori, Nafisa Y., MD {1811979941} IntrMd(82,PAK12)<NJ-RIVERVW>
+ Integrated Medical Alliance/IMA Medical Care Center
30 Shrewsbury Plaza   Shrewsbury, NJ 07702   (732)542-0002   Fax (732)542-2992

Bhowmick, Tanaya, MD {1821389206} InfDis, IntrMd<NJ-RWJUBRUN>
+ Rutgers RWJ Allergy, Immunology and Infectious Group
125 Paterson Street   New Brunswick, NJ 08901   (732)235-7060

Bhuskute, Bela Hemant, MD {1760429690} IntrMd(91,INA69)
+ Shore Primary Care
1944 Corlies Avenue/Suite 103   Neptune, NJ 07753   (732)774-2336   Fax (732)774-2337

Bhuyan, Ruprekha, MD {1669405833} Psychy(78,INDI)<NJ-ACMCITY, NJ-ACMCMAIN>
+ AtlantiCare Behavioral Health/Cornerstone
6010 Black Horse Pike   Egg Harbor Township, NJ 08234   (609)646-5142   Fax (609)646-8715
+ AtlantiCare Behavioral Health/Providence House
12 North Providence Avenue   Atlantic City, NJ 08401   (609)348-1468

Bialecki, Rosemarie, DO {1467681015} FamMed
+ West Street Health Center
519 West Street   Camden, NJ 08103   (856)968-2320   Fax (856)968-2317

Bialo, Darren Andrew, MD {1104186196} RadDia(11,FL02)
+ Larchmont Medical Imaging
219 Sunset Road   Willingboro, NJ 08046   (609)835-6540   Fax (609)835-6544

Bialy, Grace B., MD {1427002351} IntrMd(79,POL08)<NJ-RWJUBRUN>
+ Princeton Hypertension-Nephrology
88 Princeton Hightstown Road/Suite 203   Princeton Junction, NJ 08550   (609)750-7330   Fax (609)750-7336

Bialy, Ted, MD {1801852058} CdvDis, Hypten(78,POLA)<NJ-HUNTRDN>
+ Hunterdon Cardiovascular Associates
1100 Wescott Drive/Suite G-3   Flemington, NJ 08822   (908)788-6471   Fax (908)788-6460
+ Hunterdon Cardiovascular Associates
1738 Route 31/Suite 210   Clinton, NJ 08809   (908)788-6471   Fax (908)823-9211

Bianchi, Glen Michael, MD {1780636019} Ophthl(99,NY48)
+ Westwood Ophthalmology Associates
300 Fairview Avenue/PO Box 698   Westwood, NJ 07675   (201)666-4014   Fax (201)664-4754
glenbianchi@hotmail.com

Bianco, Brian A., DO {1093957094} RadV&I(03,FL75)
+ 540 Eagelbrook Drive
Moorestown, NJ 08057

Bichay, Yostina Montasser, MD {1134567050}
+ Complete Care Family Medicine
75 West Red Bank Avenue   Woodbury, NJ 08096   (856)853-2055   Fax (856)848-2879

Bickenbach, Kai Asa, MD {1295976389} Surgry(02,MI07)
+ Atlantic Surgical Oncology
100 Madison Avenue   Morristown, NJ 07960   (973)971-7111   Fax (973)397-2901

+ Atlantic Surgical Oncology
99 Beauvoir Street   Summit, NJ 07901   (973)971-7111   Fax (908)598-2392

Bickerton, Michael W., MD {1518941202} Urolgy, IntrMd(79,PA02)<NJ-RIVERVW, NJ-BAYSHORE>
+ Urology Associates, P.A.
595 Shrewsbury Avenue/Suite 103   Shrewsbury, NJ 07702   (732)741-5923   Fax (732)741-2759

Biczak, Ernest S., MD {1699955245} EmrgMd(77,NJ06)<NJ-STBARNMC>
+ St. Barnabas Health Care Center
95 Old Short Hills Road   West Orange, NJ 07052   (973)322-4033   Fax (973)322-4416
ebiczak@sbhcs.com

Bid, Champa V., MD {1295743425} PhysMd(70,INA65)<NJ-STBARNMC, NJ-STMICHL>
+ 3 Yale Court
Livingston, NJ 07039   (973)533-0709
champavel@hotmail.com

Bidabadi, Bobak, MD {1548206048} Pedtrc(01,NY09)
+ East Windsor Pediatric Group
300B Princeton Hightstown/Suite 201   Hightstown, NJ 08520   (609)448-7300   Fax (609)448-8022

Bidic, Sean Michael, MD {1730124256} SrgPHand
+ Sean Michael Bidic MD
199 Mullica Hill Road   Mullica Hill, NJ 08062
+ American Surgical Arts
2950 College Drive/Suite 2-H   Vineland, NJ 08360   Fax (856)362-8903

Bidigare, Susan Ann, MD {1396737342} FamMed(95,MI07)
+ 1930 East Route 70/Suite J-52
Cherry Hill, NJ 08003

Biehl, Michael, MD {1104904101} IntrMd, CdvDis, ClCdEl(86,GRN01)<NJ-STJOSHOS, NJ-CHILTON>
+ Cardiology Consultants
246 Hamburg Turnpike/Suite 201   Wayne, NJ 07470   (973)942-1141   Fax (973)942-1250
+ Clifton Urgent and Primary Care
721 Clifton Avenue/Suite 2A   Clifton, NJ 07013   (973)942-1141   Fax (973)779-7906

Bieler, Bert Michael, MD {1659361079} FamMed
+ Cooper Endocrinology Associates
1210 Brace Road/Suite 107   Cherry Hill, NJ 08034   (856)795-3597   Fax (856)795-7590

Bieler, Harvey Phillip, MD {1336123934} Pedtrc, PedPul(90,QU01)<NJ-MORRISTN, NJ-OVERLOOK>
+ Morristown Medical Center
100 Madison Avenue/Goryeb   Morristown, NJ 07962   (973)971-5000
+ The Valerie Fund Children's Ctr/Goryeb
100 Madison Avenue/Simon 2/Suite 107   Morristown, NJ 07962   (973)971-5161

Bielory, Leonard, MD {1154352987} Allrgy, Diagns, IntrMd(80,NJ05)<NJ-UMDNJ>
+ 400 Mountain Avenue
Springfield, NJ 07081   (973)912-9817   Fax (973)376-6167

Bien-Aime, Michel J., MD {1225084411} Psychy, PsyCAd(79,HAI01)
+ 4 Sheffield Drive
Moorestown, NJ 08057

Bienenfeld, Scott I., MD {1023049939} Psychy, PsyFor(97,PA09)
+ Park West Associates
33 Plymouth Street/Suite 104   Montclair, NJ 07042   (973)509-1444   Fax (973)509-1446

Biener, Alexander, MD {1760671416} Gastrn, IntrMd(82,NY47)
+ 595 Chestnut Ridge Road/Suite 6
Woodcliff Lake, NJ 07677   (201)505-9595   Fax (201)505-9474
AlexBienerWebMD@gmail.com

Biener, Robert, MD {1780784892} Pedtrc(77,ISRA)<NJ-RWJUBRUN, NJ-STPETER>
+ Highland Park Pediatrics
85 Raritan Avenue   Highland Park, NJ 08904   (732)246-0202   Fax (732)246-8334

Bienstock, Alan Marc, MD {1811900426} SrgPlstc, SrgCsm(98,NC07)
+ 638 Lawrence Road
Lawrenceville, NJ 08648   (917)257-7560   Fax (609)530-1881

Bienstock, Jeffrey Marc, MD {1992760904} Pedtrc(83,MEX14)<NJ-VALLEY, NJ-CHILTON>
+ PediatriCare Associates
20-20 Fair Lawn Avenue   Fair Lawn, NJ 07410   (201)791-4545   Fax (201)791-3765
+ PediatriCare Associates
400 Franklin Turnpike   Mahwah, NJ 07430   (201)791-4545   Fax (201)529-1596
+ PediatriCare Associates
901 Route 23 South   Pompton Plains, NJ 07410   (973)831-4545   Fax (973)831-1527

Bier, Martin M., MD {1013982545} Psychy(67,MEXI)<NJ-RIVERVW>
+ 167 Avenue at the Common/Suite 10
Shrewsbury, NJ 07702   (732)842-0830

Bier, Rachel Elizabeth, MD {1902128325} EnDbMt
+ Endocrinology Consultants P.C.
229 Engle Street   Englewood, NJ 07631   (201)567-8999   Fax (201)567-5385

Bier, Steven Jeffrey, MD {1912952102} RadDia(82,NY47)
+ University Radiology Group, P.C.
483 Cranbury Road   East Brunswick, NJ 08816   (732)390-0030   Fax (732)390-5383
+ University Radiology Group, P.C.
579A Cranbury Road   East Brunswick, NJ 08816   (732)390-0030   Fax (732)390-1856

Bierl, Charlene, MD {1528123627} Pthlgy, BldBnk(05,MA05)
+ Cooper University Hospital
One Cooper Plaza/P037   Camden, NJ 08103   (856)361-1639

Bierman, Edward W., MD {1043280928} Pedtrc(71,NY08)
+ The University Doctors - UMDNJ -SOM
570 Egg Harbor Road/Suite C-2   Sewell, NJ 08080   (856)218-0300   Fax (856)589-5082

Bierman-Dear, Nancy A., MD {1689698813} FamMed(88,PA02)
+ Patient first Urgent Care
630 Mantua Pike   Woodbury, NJ 08096   (856)812-2220   Fax (856)812-2221

Biermann Flynn, Dana Lynn, DO {1265697429} Pedtrc(04,NJ75)<NJ-UNDRWD, NJ-SJRSYELM>
+ Advocare Woodbury Pediatrics
1050 Mantua Pike/Suite 200   Wenonah, NJ 08090   (856)853-0848   Fax (856)853-1889

Biernat, Matthew Mateusz, MD {1689061020} FamMed
+ PASE HealthCare, PC
225 Millburn Avenue/Suite 303   Millburn, NJ 07041   (973)912-7273   Fax (973)912-7275

Biester, Robert J., MD {1760449367} Urolgy(82,PA02)<NJ-VIRTVOOR, NJ-OURLADY>
+ Delaware Valley Urology LLC
63 Kresson Road/Suite 103   Cherry Hill, NJ 08034   (856)427-9004   Fax (856)267-2499
+ New Jersey Urology LLC
2090 Springdale Road/Suite D   Cherry Hill, NJ 08003   (856)427-9004   Fax (856)985-9908
+ New Jersey Urology, LLC
2401 East Evesham Road/Suite F   Voorhees, NJ 08034   (856)673-1600   Fax (856)988-0636

Bigelsen, Stephen J., MD {1780611574} Allrgy, IntMAImm(87,IL42)<NJ-HCKTSTWN>
+ Allergy & Arthritis Associates PA
600 Mount Pleasant Avenue/Suite C   Dover, NJ 07801   (973)989-0500   Fax (973)989-5046

Biggs, Danielle Deluca, MD {1598159444} EmrgMd
+ Morristown Medical Center Emergency Medicine
100 Madison Avenue   Morristown, NJ 07960   (973)971-5000

Bigornia, Edgar G., MD {1639116973} Gastrn, IntrMd(87,NY08)
+ Gastroenterologists of Ocean County
477 Lakehurst Road   Toms River, NJ 08755   (732)349-4422   Fax (732)349-5087

Bigos, David, MD {1891785879} PedCrC, Pedtrc, PedEmg(82,PA09)<NJ-VIRTVOOR>
+ Virtua Voorhees
100 Bowman Drive/PICU   Voorhees, NJ 08043   (856)247-3991   Fax (856)247-3922

Bijlani, Mona V., MD {1518054931} Psychy, PsyGrt(87,INA2X)<NJ-RWJUBRUN, NJ-UNIVBHC>
+ UH-University Behavioral Hlth
100 Metroplex Drive/Suite 200   Edison, NJ 08817   (732)235-8400   Fax (732)235-8395

Bikkina, Mahesh, MD {1205856002} CdvDis, IntrMd(83,INA62)<NJ-STJOSHOS, NJ-VALLEY>
+ Heart & Vascular Associates of Northern Jersey
22-18 Broadway/Suite 201   Fair Lawn, NJ 07410   (201)475-5050   Fax (201)475-5522

Bikoff, David J., MD {1861543662} SrgPlstc(73,NY08)<NJ-HACKNSK>
+ 146 Route 17 North/3rd Floor
Hackensack, NJ 07601   (201)488-8584   Fax (201)488-7572

Bilal, Yasmin, MD {1699932061}<NJ-TRINIWSC>
+ Trinitas Regional Medical Center-Williamson Street
225 Williamson Street   Elizabeth, NJ 07207   (862)684-1089
dr.yasmin.bilal@gmail.com

Bilaniuk, Jaroslaw W., MD {1295700417} Surgry, EmrgMd(95,NY48)<NJ-MORRISTN>
+ Morristown Medical Center
100 Madison Avenue/Surgery   Morristown, NJ 07962   (973)971-5000

Bilbao, Michelle Cifone, DO {1770899163} ObsGyn
+ Cooper Ob/Gyn
3 Cooper Plaza/Suite 300   Camden, NJ 08103   (800)826-6737   Fax (856)968-8575

Bilbraut, Krista Gayle, MD {1487856316} EmrgMd(03,MEX03)<NJ-HACKNSK>
+ Hackensack Medical Center Emergency Medicine
30 Prospect Avenue/Main 3619   Hackensack, NJ 07601   (201)996-4614   Fax (201)968-1866

Bilek, Alena, MD {1114974474} GenPrc(70,CZE01)
+ 130 Overlook Avenue
Hackensack, NJ 07601   (201)487-5944   Fax (201)487-5944
Bi300@aol.com

Bilenker, James D., MD {1649210568} EmrgMd, IntrMd(78,MEXI)<NJ-OVERLOOK>
+ Overlook Medical Center
99 Beauvoir Avenue/PO Box 210/EmergMed   Summit, NJ 07902   (908)522-2000   Fax (908)522-0227

Bilenker, Michael Evan, DO {1609974906} PedAne, Anesth(01,FL75)
+ Summit Medical Group-Berkeley Heights Campus
1 Diamond Hill Road   Berkeley Heights, NJ 07922   (908)277-8872   Fax (908)673-7382

Bilenki, Natalie I., MD {1912965153} ObsGyn(79,NJ05)<NJ-STJOSHOS>
+ St. Joseph's Family Health Center
21 Market Street   Paterson, NJ 07501   (973)754-4200   Fax (973)754-4201
+ St. Joseph's DePaul Center ObsGyn
11 Getty Avenue   Paterson, NJ 07503   (973)754-4200

Bilgrami, Sajad Syed, DO {1649278623} Anesth(98,NJ75)
+ West Jersey Anesthesia Associates
102-E Center Boulevard   Marlton, NJ 08053   (856)988-6250   Fax (856)988-6270

Bilinski, Robyn T., MD {1689880841} ObsGyn
+ Hackensack University Medical Group Westwood
250 Old Hook Road   Westwood, NJ 07675   (201)781-1750   Fax (201)781-1753

Bilkis, Michael Ross, MD {1235166349} Dermat, SrgDer(86,IL42)
+ North Jersey Dermatology Center
7 Oak Ridge Road/Suite 3   Newfoundland, NJ 07435   (973)208-8110   Fax (973)208-8106
+ The Dermatology Group, P.C.
60 Pompton Avenue   Verona, NJ 07044   (973)208-8110   Fax (973)571-2126
+ The Dermatology Group, P.C.
44 Route 23 North/Suite 213   Riverdale, NJ 07435   (973)571-2121   Fax (973)839-5751

Biller, Jeanette Marie, DO {1578505178} FamMed(96,NJ75)<NJ-VALLEY>
+ Allied Medical Associates
510 Hamburg Turnpike   Wayne, NJ 07470   (973)942-6005   Fax (973)442-6009

Billig, Janelle Elisabeth, MD {1841532223} FamMed
+ 30 Meadow Drive
Little Falls, NJ 07424   (628)485-8602

Bills, Thomas K., MD {1932105947} SrgOrt(80,PA02)<NJ-CHS-FULD, NJ-CHSMRCER>
+ Mercer-Bucks Orthopaedics PC
3120 Princeton Pike   Lawrenceville, NJ 08648   (609)896-0444   Fax (609)896-1055
+ Mercer-Bucks Orthopaedics, P.C.
2501 Kuser Road   Hamilton, NJ 08691   (609)896-0444   Fax (609)587-4349

Bilof, Michael Louis, MD {1891723136} Surgry, SrgVas(90,NJ05)<NJ-OVERLOOK, NJ-STBARNMC>
+ Garden State Bariatrics and Wellness Center LLC
225 Millburn Avenue/Suite 204   Millburn, NJ 07041   (973)218-1990   Fax (973)629-1274

Bilusic, Marijo, MD {1184884090} IntrMd(96,CRO01)<NJ-TRINI-WSC>
+ Trinitas Regional Medical Center-Williamson Street
225 Williamson Street/IntMed   Elizabeth, NJ 07207   (908)994-5000

Bimonte, Michael J., MD {1639152937} ObsGyn, IntrMd(77,NJ05)<NJ-MEADWLND>
+ New Margaret Hague Women's Health Institute
377 Jersey Avenue/Suite 220   Jersey City, NJ 07302   (201)309-2380   Fax (201)309-2381

Binas, Constantine George, MD {1427066257} ObsGyn(95,NY47)<NJ-ENGLWOOD, NJ-HOLYNAME>
+ Ob-Gyn Associates of Englewood
177 North Dean Street/Suite 208   Englewood, NJ 07631   (201)569-0200   Fax (201)569-8287

Binder, Michael, MD {1033105663} Anesth, AnesPain(78,RUS32)
+ 140 North Route 17/Suite 204
Paramus, NJ 07652   (201)880-6161   Fax (201)540-2552

Binenbaum, Gil, MD {1316073174} Ophthl, IntrMd(PA01<PA-CHILDHOS>
+ CHOP Pediatric & Adolescent Specialty Care Center
1012 Laurel Oak Road/Ophthalmology   Voorhees, NJ 08043   (856)435-5100   Fax (856)435-0091

Binenbaum, Steve Z., MD {1497861371} CdvDis, IntrMd(82,NY46)<NJ-VAEASTOR>
+ VA New Jersey Health Care System-East Orange Campus
385 Tremont Avenue   East Orange, NJ 07018   (973)676-1000

Binenbaum, Steven J., MD {1366628281} Surgry(01,GRN01)
+ Specialty Surgical Associates
10 Industrial Way East/Suite 104   Eatontown, NJ 07724   (732)389-1331   Fax (732)542-8587

Binetti, Richard G., MD {1427023357} ObsGyn(75,NJ05)<NJ-ST-BARNMC, NJ-MTNSIDE>
+ 616 Bloomfield Avenue/Suite 2B
West Caldwell, NJ 07006   (973)226-2200   Fax (973)226-7533
+ Short Hills Surgery Center
187 Millburn Avenue/Suite 101   Millburn, NJ 07041   (973)226-2200   Fax (973)671-0557

Bingham, Jemel M., MD {1447426689} ObGyCrCr
+ Bergen Ob-Gyn Associates, PA
130 Kinderkamack Road/Suite 300   River Edge, NJ 07661   (201)489-2727   Fax (201)489-5040

Bingham, Johna P., MD {1801825682} EmrgMd(81,PA02)<NJ-VIRTVOOR>
+ Virtua Voorhees
100 Bowman Drive/EmergMed   Voorhees, NJ 08043   (856)247-3000

Bingham, Richard F., MD {1073533493} EmrgMd(81,MEX14)<NJ-PALISADE>
+ Palisades Medical Center
7600 River Road/EmrgMed   North Bergen, NJ 07047   (201)854-5000

Binns, Joseph F., MD {1326049511} Gastrn, IntrMd(87,NJ06)<NJ-RIVERVW>
+ Red Bank Gastroenterology Associates PA
365 Broad Street/Suite 1-E   Red Bank, NJ 07701   (732)842-4294   Fax (732)548-7408

Binsol, Ricardo Q., MD {1891701504} PthACl(83,PHIL)
+ 9 Audobon Road
Livingston, NJ 07039

Biondi, David M., DO {1629068713} Nrolgy, PainMd(85,ME75)
+ Ortho-McNeil Janssen Scientific Affairs, LLC
1000 Route 202/PO Box 300   Raritan, NJ 08869   (908)927-6479
dbiondi@its.jnj.com

Biondi, Robert J., DO {1558361675} PthACl, Pthlgy(72,PA77)<NJ-VIRTMHBC, NJ-VIRTVOOR>
+ Virtua Memorial
175 Madison Avenue/Path   Mount Holly, NJ 08060   (609)267-0700

Biran, Noa, MD {1023277910} OncHem, IntrMd(08,DC01)<NY-MTSINAI>
+ John Theurer Cancer Center - HUMC
92 Second Street   Hackensack, NJ 07601   (201)996-5900   Fax (201)996-9246
+ Regional Cancer Care Associates LLC
100 First Street   Hackensack, NJ 07601   (201)996-5900   Fax (551)995-8578

Birch, Thomas M., MD {1447342647} InfDis, IntrMd(83,WI05)<NJ-HOLYNAME, NJ-ENGLWOOD>
+ Institute for Clinical Research - Holy Name Hospital
718 Teaneck Road   Teaneck, NJ 07666   (201)833-7274   Fax (201)833-7243

Bird, Charrell Moyo, MD {1184701369} NnPnMd, Pedtrc, IntrMd(PA13
+ Pediatrix Medical Group
1505 West Sherman Avenue/MSO-Box 104   Vineland, NJ 08360   (856)845-0100   Fax (856)641-7647
+ Inspira Health Network
509 North Broad Street/Pediatrics   Woodbury, NJ 08096   (856)845-0100   Fax (856)853-7468

Bird, Dorothy Waterbury, MD {1225361967} Surgry(06,NY09)<MA-BOSTMC>
+ Cooper Surgical Associates
3 Cooper Plaza/Suite 403   Camden, NJ 08103   (856)342-3113   Fax (856)541-5379

Bird, Joanna Marie, MD {1720202658} Psychy(02,DC01)
+ 268 Green Village Road/Suite 3
Green Village, NJ 07935   (973)822-0222

Birdi, Anil, MD {1598022873} Ophthl
+ Susskind & Almallah Eye Associates, P.A.
20 Mule Road/Focus Center   Toms River, NJ 08755   (732)349-5622   Fax (732)349-5625

Birger, Yelena, DO {1376598136} IntMAdMd, IntrMd(00,NY75)
+ 300 Craig Road/Suite 208
Manalapan, NJ 07726   (732)333-0062   Fax (732)333-0004

Biria, Nazila, MD {1114986379} IntrMd
+ The Park Medical Group
24 Elm Street   Harrington Park, NJ 07640   (201)784-0123   Fax (201)784-0065

Birkenfeld, Arie, MD {1588748669} RprEnd, ObsGyn(79,ISR01)
+ Diamond Institute for Infertility & Menopause
89 Millburn Avenue   Millburn, NJ 07041   (973)761-5600   Fax (973)761-5100
daniellee@diamondinstitute.com

Physicians by Name and Address

Birmingham, Karen Lesley, MD {1851483010} SrgPlstc, SrgCsm(91,PA09)<NJ-SHOREMEM, NJ-ACMCITY>
+ Aesthetic Horizons Plastic Surgery
110 Roosevelt Boulevard/Suite 2 B   Marmora, NJ 08223   (609)390-2404   Fax (609)390-2644

Birmingham, Mary Catherine, MD {1801070180} PedEmg, Pedtrc(99,NY47)
+ 119 Gordonhurst Avenue
Montclair, NJ 07043   (646)573-6538

Birnbaum, Glenn Alan, MD {1679517395} EmrgMd(86,PA02)<NJ-STBARNMC, NJ-MORRISTN>
+ St. Barnabas Medical Center
94 Old Short Hills Road   Livingston, NJ 07039   (973)322-5000

Birnbaum, Joseph G., MD {1669417788} EnDbMt, IntrMd(73,PA09)<NJ-COMMED>
+ Toms River Wellness Center
10 Kettle Creek Road   Toms River, NJ 08753   (732)255-8880   Fax (732)255-8885

Birnhak, Stefani, MD {1588083281} Pedtrc
+ Valley Pediatric Associates, P.A.
201 East Franklin Turnpike   Ho Ho Kus, NJ 07423   (201)652-1888   Fax (201)652-6485

Birotte Sanchez, Maria J., MD {1841326162} FamMed(88,MEX61)
+ Faith Family Health Care
400 West Front Street/Suite B   Plainfield, NJ 07060   (908)822-9700   Fax (908)822-9701
+ Neighborhood Health Center Plainfield
1700-58 Myrtle Avenue   Plainfield, NJ 07060   (908)822-9700   Fax (908)226-6743

Bisberg, Dorothy Stein, MD {1407860406} PedPul, Pedtrc, IntrMd(72,NY20)<NJ-CHDNWBTH, NJ-STBARNMC>
+ Children's Hospital of NJ Ped Cntr @ West Orange
375 Mount Pleasant Avenue/Suite 105   West Orange, NJ 07052   (973)322-6900   Fax (973)322-6999

Bischoff, Stephen M., MD {1386968501}<NJ-UNIVBHC>
+ University Behavioral Health Care
671 Hoes Lane/PO Box 1392   Piscataway, NJ 08855   (732)235-4433

Bisen, Viwek Singh, DO {1760493787} Psychy(06,ME75)
+ University Medical Group/UMDNJ
125 Paterson Street/Suite 2200   New Brunswick, NJ 08901   (732)235-7647   Fax (732)235-7677

Bishara, Christine, MD {1902990112} IntrMd(94,EGY03)<NJ-VAEASTOR, NY-BRNXVAMC>
+ VA New Jersey Health Care System-East Orange Campus
385 Tremont Avenue/Medicine   East Orange, NJ 07018   (973)676-1000

Bishburg, Eliahu, MD {1912089236} InfDis(80,ISRA)<NJ-NWRK-BETH>
+ Newark Beth Israel Medical Center
201 Lyons Avenue/Infectious Dis   Newark, NJ 07112   (973)926-5212   Fax (973)926-8182

Bishop, Douglas Scott, MD {1437354883} FamMed, Ophthl(83,CA12)<PA-TJCNTR>
+ Zufall Health Center
18 West Blackwell Street   Dover, NJ 07801   (973)328-9100   Fax (973)328-6517

Bisignano Delvecchio, Maria, MD {1700834744} IntrMd(81,NJ05)<NJ-CLARMAAS>
+ The Internet Medical Group, P.C.
181 Franklin Avenue/Suite 204   Nutley, NJ 07110   (973)667-8117   Fax (973)667-6642

Bisk, Bradley A., DO {1861417693} FamMed(88,PA77)
+ Ballys Atlantic City
Park Place and Boardwalk   Atlantic City, NJ 08401   (609)340-2914   Fax (609)345-3426

Bispo, Luciano Jose, MD {1144206384} ObsGyn(98,GRN01)<NJ-SJERSYHS>
+ 2950 College Drive/Suite 2F
Vineland, NJ 08360   (856)205-0606   Fax (856)205-0044

Bissinger, Craig L., MD {1083607865} ObsGyn(82,OH40)<NJ-MORRISTN>
+ Lifeline Medical Associates, LLC
50 Cherry Hill Road/Suite 303   Parsippany, NJ 07054   (973)335-8500   Fax (973)335-8429

Biswal, Rajiv, MD {1679578801} RadV&I, Radiol, RadDia(92,NJ06)<NJ-JRSYSHMC>
+ University Radiology Group
2100 Route 33/Neptune City Med Bld   Neptune, NJ 07753   (732)776-4121   Fax (732)776-4071
+ University Radiology Group, P.C.
3822 River Road   Point Pleasant Beach, NJ 08742   (732)776-4121   Fax (732)892-1202
+ University Radiology Group
900 West Main Street   Freehold, NJ 07728   (732)462-1900   Fax (732)462-1848

Biswas, Anjali, MD {1932146438} NnPnMd, Pedtrc(68,INA30)<NJ-JRSYCITY, NJ-MEADWLND>
+ High Risk Pregnancy Center of New Jersey PC
908 Oak Tree Road/Suite M & N   South Plainfield, NJ 07080   (908)753-5771   Fax (908)753-2473

+ 24 Quail Run
Warren, NJ 07059

Bitan, Fabien David, MD {1609816479} SrgOrt, SrgSpn, PedOrt(85,FRA35)<NY-BETHPETR>
+ Advanced Spine Surgery Center
855 Lehigh Avenue   Union, NJ 07083   (908)557-9420   Fax (908)557-9438

Bitar, Maria Teresa, MD {1093756688} ObsGyn(85,COL25)<NJ-STJOSHOS>
+ 547 Union Boulevard
Totowa, NJ 07512   (973)790-4430   Fax (973)790-5260

Bitar, Souad Youssef, DO {1619170404} EmrgMd(06,PA78)<NJ-STMICHL>
+ St. Michael's Medical Center
268 MLK Jr. Boulevard/Emerg Med   Newark, NJ 07102   (973)877-5500

Bitner, Bozena Wanda, MD {1609878438} IntrMd(83,POL03)
+ Internal Medicine Practice LLC
312 Belleville Turnpike/Suite 1 C   North Arlington, NJ 07031   (201)997-4040   Fax (201)997-4040

Bitterman, Jason, MD {1023466455} PhysMd
+ Rutgers-Department of Physical Med
183 South Orange Ave/Suite F-1555   Newark, NJ 07101   (973)972-3606

Bittman, Sara Cuccio, MD {1740570860}
+ Hackensack Hospital Obs/Gyn
30 Prospect Avenue/4E-90   Hackensack, NJ 07601   (917)969-1637

Blaber, Reginald J., MD {1174502462} CdvDis, IntrMd(89,PA09)<NJ-OURLADY, NJ-COOPRUMC>
+ LMA CardioThoracic Surgical Services
1 Brace Road/Suite C   Cherry Hill, NJ 08034   (856)470-9029   Fax (856)796-9391
+ Blaber Cardiology at Lourdes Medical Assoc.
500 Grove Street/Suite 200   Haddon Heights, NJ 08035   (856)470-9029   Fax (856)428-2986

Black, Aislinn Denise, DO {1730321084} EmrgMd<NJ-UMDNJ>
+ University Hospital
150 Bergen Street   Newark, NJ 07103   (973)910-3654

Black, Ellen M., MD {1164594735} IntrMd(79,MA05)<NJ-BAYONNE>
+ 1061 Avenue C/Suite 1
Bayonne, NJ 07002   (201)858-0800   Fax (201)858-3367

Black, Eric M., MD {1982863338} SrgOrt, SprtMd
+ Summit Medical Group Orthopedics and Sports Medicine
140 Park Avenue/2nd Floor   Florham Park, NJ 07932   (973)404-9980   Fax (973)267-7295
+ Summit Medical Group
574 Springfield Avenue   Westfield, NJ 07090   (973)404-9980   Fax (908)232-0540

Blackburn, Lisa D., MD {1538127345} Psychy, NrlgAddM(00,VA01)
+ 1101 Kings Highway North/Suite 208
Cherry Hill, NJ 08034   (856)428-1477

Blackinton, Charles H., MD {1871560029} Psychy(73,NY01)<NJ-ENGLWOOD, NJ-BURDTMLN>
+ 303 Court House/S. Dennis Road
Cape May Court House, NJ 08210   (609)465-0018

Blackman, Bonnie E., MD {1780752253} Anesth, IntrMd(83,NY03)<NJ-ENGLWOOD>
+ 1 Frick Drive
Demarest, NJ 07627   (845)406-1347   Fax (973)506-1954

Blackman, Gurvan E., MD {1215099833} RadDia
+ Radiology Affiliates of Central New Jersey, P.A.
2501 Kuser Road   Hamilton, NJ 08691   (609)585-8800   Fax (609)585-1825

Blackman, Jeffrey D., MD {1538117908} Pedtrc(89,PA09)<NJ-VIRTVOOR, NJ-VIRTUAHS>
+ Advocare Marlton Pediatrics
525 Route 73 South   Marlton, NJ 08053   (856)596-3434   Fax (856)596-9110
+ Advocare Hammonton Pediatrics
856 South Whitehorse Pike   Hammonton, NJ 08037   (856)596-3434   Fax (609)704-8849
+ Advocare Township Pediatrics
123 Egg Harbor Road   Sewell, NJ 08053   (856)227-5437   Fax (856)227-5890

Blackman, Ryan Graham, DO {1275792038} Pedtrc, IntrMd(PA77<PA-STCHRIS>
+ Bethany Pediatrics PA
1 Bethany Road/Building 5/Suite 65   Hazlet, NJ 07730   (732)264-0700   Fax (732)264-1414

Blacksin, Marcia F., MD {1457386344} RadDia(84,NY19)<NJ-UMDNJ>
+ University Hospital
150 Bergen Street   Newark, NJ 07103   (973)972-4300   Fax (973)972-2307

Blackwell, Kathryn V., DO {1144489683} Psychy(94,PA77)
+ PO Box 60
Strathmere, NJ 08248

Blackwell, Lauren M., MD {1982921888}
+ University Hospital Medicine
150 Bergen Street/Room I-248   Newark, NJ 07103   (973)972-6056   Fax (973)972-3129

Blackwell, Martin, DO {1356330534} Dermat(88,NJ75)<NJ-NWTNMEM, NJ-HCKTSTWN>
+ Associated Dermatology
136 Woodside Avenue   Newton, NJ 07860   (973)300-0555   Fax (973)300-0052
+ 653 Willow Grove Street/Suite 2700
Hackettstown, NJ 07840   (908)852-9600

Blackwood, Margaret Michele, MD {1396839502} OthrSp, Surgry(88,SC01)<NJ-STMICHL>
+ 200 South Orange Avenue/Suite 102
Livingston, NJ 07039   (973)322-7020   Fax (973)322-7039

Blades, Frederick C., MD {1053372284} Ophthl, IntrMd(69,DC01)<NJ-RIVERVW>
+ Del Negro and Senft Eye Associates, PC
152 Broad Street   Red Bank, NJ 07701   (732)747-7725   Fax (732)741-7930
ipopfcb@gmail.com

Blady, David, MD {1053386144} Nrolgy(83,NY08)<NJ-MTNSIDE, NJ-CLARMAAS>
+ Neurological Consultants
230 Sherman Avenue/Suite K   Glen Ridge, NJ 07028   (973)743-9555   Fax (973)743-7663
+ Neurological Consultants
1100 Clifton Avenue   Clifton, NJ 07013   (973)743-9555   Fax (973)743-7663

Blady, Joseph A., MD {1639323702} Anesth(74,NY15)<NJ-VALLEY>
+ 714 Butternut Drive
Franklin Lakes, NJ 07417

Blair, Brian J., DO {1841587565} Gastrn(11,PA77)
+ Woodbury Primary and Specialty Care
159 South Broad Street   Woodbury, NJ 08096   (844)542-2273   Fax (856)384-0218
+ Kennedy Health Alliance
188 Fries Mill Road/Suite N-1   Turnersville, NJ 08012   (844)542-2273   Fax (856)783-2273

Blair, Michael A., MD {1487820502} Pedtrc(05,MD01)<NJ-VIRTUAHS>
+ Advocare Haddon Pediatric Group
119 White Horse Pike   Haddon Heights, NJ 08035   (856)547-7300   Fax (856)547-4573

Blaivas, Allen J., DO {1104830397} IntrMd, PulCCr, CritCr(99,NY75)<NJ-VAEASTOR>
+ VA New Jersey Health Care System-East Orange Campus
385 Tremont Avenue   East Orange, NJ 07018   (973)676-1000

Blake, John R., MD {1982705877} Psychy(79,SAF02)
+ Cedar Glen Professional Association
170 Cold Soil Road   Princeton, NJ 08540   (609)896-1122   Fax (609)896-2688

Blake, Michael Laurence, MD {1417111493} IntrMd(06,DMN01)
+ 600 River Avenue
Lakewood, NJ 08701   (732)942-5721   Fax (732)942-5723

Blakeslee, Samantha, DO {1497070353}<NJ-VIRTVOOR>
+ Virtua Voorhees
100 Bowman Drive   Voorhees, NJ 08043   (856)247-3000

Blanc, Phillip Garven, MD {1548418577} EmrgMd
+ InFocus Urgent Care
64 Princeton Hightstown Road   West Windsor, NJ 08550   (609)799-7009   Fax (609)799-7808

Blanch, Tanya Malka, MD {1730383530} IntrMd(06,MNT01)
+ Holy Name Hospital
718 Teaneck Road   Teaneck, NJ 07666   (973)594-6650   Fax (201)833-7231

Blanchard, Jenny Ann, DO {1245207901} Psychy(94,WV75)<NJ-NWTNMEM>
+ Total Spectrum Health P.C.
171 Woodport Road   Sparta, NJ 07871   (973)726-3001   Fax (973)726-3002
drblanch@blanchmail.com
+ Atlantic Behavioral Health at Newton Medical Center
175 High Street   Newton, NJ 07860   (973)726-3001   Fax (973)383-9309

Blanchfield, Patrick Thomas, MD {1942224886} Anesth(00,DMN01)
+ Morris Anesthesia Group, PA
3799 Route 46/Suite 211   Parsippany, NJ 07054   (973)335-1122   Fax (973)335-1448

Blanco, Fiona Rose Pasternack, MD {1194768002} Dermat(02,PA02)
+ Ravits Margaret MD & Associates
130 Kinderkamack Road/Suite 205   River Edge, NJ 07661   (201)692-0800   Fax (201)488-1582

Blanco, Renato J., MD {1518936046} IntrMd(77,PHIL)<NJ-STMRYPAS>
+ 539 Clifton Avenue
Clifton, NJ 07013   (973)472-1878   Fax (973)472-5900

Blank, Andrew Jay, DO {1184720542} GenPrc(87,PA77)
+ Sunset Road Medical Associates
911 Sunset Road   Burlington, NJ 08016   (609)387-8787   Fax (609)386-8640
Ajb1@comcast.net

Blank, Benjamin I., DO {1891786455} FamMed(93,PA77)<NJ-OURLADY, NJ-VIRTVOOR>
+ 1300 Black Horse Pike
Glendora, NJ 08029   (856)939-2828

Blank, Ellen, MD {1033282900} Dermat(75,NY47)<NY-MTSINYHS, NJ-BAYONNE>
+ Hudson-Richmond Dermatology, PA
333 Avenue C   Bayonne, NJ 07002   (201)858-4800

Blank, Howard L., MD {1992763999} SrgOrt(70,NY01)
+ Associates in Orthopedic Surgery
120 Millburn Avenue/Suite 103   Millburn, NJ 07041   (973)467-1212   Fax (973)467-1216

Blank, Jacqueline P., DO {1477524213} ObsGyn, Obstet(01,NY75)<NJ-MORRISTN, NJ-MTNSIDE>
+ Women first Ob Gyn
95 Madison Avenue/Suite 204   Morristown, NJ 07960   (973)239-3865   Fax (973)239-3056

Blank, Jonathan Dirk, MD {1366511412} Anesth, PedAne, Pedtrc(90,NY08)<NJ-STBARNMC, NJ-NWRKBETH>
+ New Jersey Anesthesia Associates, P.C.
252 Columbia Turnpike/PO Box 0037   Florham Park, NJ 07932   (973)660-9334   Fax (973)660-9779

Blank, Kenneth Robert, MD {1205864964} RadOnc(92,NY46)<NJ-CLARMAAS>
+ Clara Maass Medical Center
1 Clara Maass Drive/RadOnc   Belleville, NJ 07109   (973)450-2000
+ Sovereign Oncology, LLC
20 Woodridge Avenue   Hackensack, NJ 07601   (973)450-2000   Fax (201)880-7585
+ Sovereign Oncology, LLC.
631 Grand Street   Jersey City, NJ 07109   (201)942-3999   Fax (201)942-3998

Blank, Peter Bradley, DO {1790737377} SrgOrt(00,NY75)<NJ-MORRISTN>
+ New Jersey Ctr for Orthop Sports Med
150 North Finley Avenue   Basking Ridge, NJ 07920   (908)340-4266   Fax (908)340-4269

Blank, Robert R., MD {1548265754} Gastrn, IntrMd(81,GRNA)<NJ-BAYSHORE, NJ-CENTRAST>
+ Middlesex Monmouth Gastroenterology
222 Schanck Road/Suite 302   Freehold, NJ 07728   (732)577-1999   Fax (732)845-5356
+ Middlesex Monmouth Gastroenterology
723 North Beers Street   Holmdel, NJ 07733   (732)264-4253

Blank, Susan Berman, MD {1841319662} Psychy(83,NY48)
+ Psychiatry Associates
1109 Amboy Avenue   Edison, NJ 08837   (732)549-2220   Fax (732)603-0673

Blanks, Mary Susan, MD {1952637993} ObsGyn(79,DC03)
+ 601 Route 206/Suite 26-354
Hillsborough, NJ 08844

Blankstein, Kenneth B., MD {1184612566} Hemato, MedOnc, IntrMd(84,NY09)<NJ-HUNTRDN>
+ Hunterdon Regional Cancer Ctr
2100 Wescott Drive   Flemington, NJ 08822   (908)788-6461   Fax (908)788-6412

Blaszka, Frederick M., MD {1598778326} IntrMd(72,NJ05)
+ Veterans Affairs Department Outpatient Clinic
654 East Jersey Street   Elizabeth, NJ 07206   (908)994-0120   Fax (908)994-0131

Blaszka, Matthew Christopher, MD {1962632083} IntHos<NY-MNTFMOSE>
+ Park Medical Group
1555 Center Avenue/2nd Fl   Fort Lee, NJ 07024   (201)510-0200   Fax (201)482-8198

Blatt, Kenneth B., MD {1326078320} RadDia, RadBdI, IntrMd(96,NY47)<NY-STATNRTH>
+ Millburn Medical Imaging
2130 Millburn Avenue/Suite A-8   Maplewood, NJ 07040   (973)912-0404   Fax (973)912-0444

Blau, Howard, MD {1164476495} CdvDis(88,NY08)
+ 1950 Route 27/Suite H
North Brunswick, NJ 08902   (732)422-2300   Fax (732)422-3141
howard.blau@princetonderm.com

Blaustein, Daniel Alberto, MD {1861410540} Nephro(84,ARG06)
+ 15 Stanford Place
Montclair, NJ 07042

Blaustein, Howard Stuart, MD {1760470264} IntrMd, PulDis, CritCr(92,NY19)<NJ-OVERLOOK, NJ-MORRISTN>
+ Summit Medical Group
85 Woodland Road   Short Hills, NJ 07078   (973)379-4496   Fax (973)921-0669
+ Summit Medical Group-Berkeley Heights Campus
1 Diamond Hill Road   Berkeley Heights, NJ 07922

(973)379-4496   Fax (908)790-6576

Blaustein, Silvia Adelina, MD {1508827338} AdolMd, Pedtrc(90,ARG09)<NJ-STJOSHOS>
+ St. Joseph's Pediatrics DePaul Center
11 Getty Avenue/2nd Floor   Paterson, NJ 07503   (973)754-4690

Blazar, Eric Pollack, MD {1861758211} EmrgMd<NJ-SJHREGMC>
+ SJH Regional Medical Center
1505 West Sherman Avenue   Vineland, NJ 08360   (856)686-4319

Bleazey, Scott Thomas, MD {1144525973} SrgFAk
+ MidJersey Orthopaedics, P.A.
8100 Westcott Drive/Suite 101   Flemington, NJ 08822   (908)782-0600   Fax (908)782-7575

Blecher, Mark Howard, MD {1356343248} Ophthl(82,NY46)
+ TLC Kremer Cherry Hill LASIK
1800 Chapel Avenue West/Suite 100   Cherry Hill, NJ 08002
+ Wills Eye Surgery Center in Cherry Hill
408 Route 70 East   Cherry Hill, NJ 08034   Fax (856)429-7555

Blecherman, Sarah W., MD {1548236060} Pedtrc(93,PA07)<NJ-CHILTON>
+ Advocare Pediatric Arts
1403 Route 23 South   Butler, NJ 07405   (973)283-2200   Fax (973)283-0406
+ Advocare Pediatric Arts
1777 Hamburg Turnpike/Suite 103   Wayne, NJ 07470   (973)283-2200   Fax (973)283-0406

Blechman, Adam Brandon, MD {1578908018} Dermat
+ 63 Church Street/Suite 102
Flemington, NJ 08822   (908)237-4124

Blechman, Andrew Neal, MD {1841266921} ObsGyn, UroGyn(89,NY19)<NJ-JRSYSHMC>
+ Jersey Shore University Medical Center
1945 Route 33/Obs/Gyn   Neptune, NJ 07753   (732)775-5500

Blechner, Michael Scott, MD {1437485174} PedPul, Pedtrc(08,ISR02)<NJ-STJOSHOS>
+ St. Joseph's Regional Medical Center
703 Main Street/Pulmonary   Paterson, NJ 07503   (973)754-2550   Fax (973)754-2548

Blecker, David L., MD {1245249473} IntrMd, Nephro, GPrvMd(73,MA07)<NJ-KSLRSADB, NJ-ACMCITY>
+ Regional Nephrology Associates
510 Jackson Avenue   Northfield, NJ 08225   (609)383-0200   Fax (609)383-8352

Bleeker, David Paul, MD {1023195237} IntrMd(80,NY08)
+ St. Joseph's Family Health Center
21 Market Street   Paterson, NJ 07501   (973)754-4200   Fax (973)754-4201

Bleich, David, MD {1790719193} EnDbMt, IntrMd(83,NY09)<NJ-UMDNJ>
+ The University Hospital
90 Bergen Street/EndoDiabMt   Newark, NJ 07103   (973)972-5185   Fax (973)972-7339

Bleicher, Robert H., MD {1467442426} Gastrn, IntrMd(78,NY01)<NJ-CHILTON>
+ North Jersey Gastroenterology & Endoscopy Center
1825 State Route 23 South   Wayne, NJ 07470   (973)633-1484   Fax (973)633-7980

Bleiman, Michael I., MD {1821086463} Pedtrc(93,PA13)<NJ-JRSYSHMC>
+ Meridian Pediatrics - Manahawkin
1100 Route 72 West/Suite 306B   Manahawkin, NJ 08050   (609)978-3910   Fax (609)978-3912

Bleiweiss, Warren J., MD {1548208838} Anesth, PainMd(83,NY19)<NJ-WESTHDSN>
+ West Hudson Division of Clara Maass Medical Center
206 Bergen Avenue/Anesthesiology   Kearny, NJ 07032   (201)955-7000
+ Warren J. Bleiweiss MD PA
29 Smull Avenue   Caldwell, NJ 07006   (201)955-7000   Fax (973)403-0102

Blevins, Graig E., DO {1679718563}<NJ-COOPRUMC>
+ Cooper University Hospital
One Cooper Plaza   Camden, NJ 08103   (856)342-2000

Blick, Michael D., MD {1740250380} CdvDis(82,DC01)<NJ-MORRISTN>
+ Lakeland Cardiology Center, P.A.
415 Boulevard   Mountain Lakes, NJ 07046   (973)334-7700   Fax (973)402-5847
+ Lakeland Cardiology Center PA
765 State Route 10/Suite 4   Randolph, NJ 07869   (973)989-2566

Blintsovskiy, Sergey, MD {1538459235} IntrMd<NJ-UMDNJ>
+ University Hospital
150 Bergen Street/Medi/Rm I-248   Newark, NJ 07103   (973)972-6056

Bliss, Mary J., MD {1124071535} EmrgMd(01,RI01)<NJ-HUNTRDN, NJ-OVERLOOK>
+ Hunterdon Medical Center
2100 Wescott Drive/EmrgMed   Flemington, NJ 08822

(908)788-6100
+ Overlook Medical Center
99 Beauvoir Avenue/PO Box 210/EmrgMed   Summit, NJ 07902   (908)522-2000

Blitstein, Jeffrey, MD {1538367396} Urolgy(01,NY08)<NJ-OVERLOOK, NJ-MORRISTN>
+ Summit Medical Group-Berkeley Heights Campus
1 Diamond Hill Road   Berkeley Heights, NJ 07922   (908)273-4300   Fax (908)790-6576

Blitz, Lawrence R., MD {1275596389} CdvDis, IntCrd, IntrMd(90,NY19)<NJ-CHILTON, NJ-MORRISTN>
+ Cardiology Associates of North Jersey
242 West Parkway   Pompton Plains, NJ 07444   (973)831-7455   Fax (973)831-7585

Blitz-Shabbir, Karen M., DO {1275562894} Nrolgy, IntrMd, Psychy(89,NY75)<NY-NSUHGCOV>
+ MS Center at Holy Name Hospital
718 Teaneck Road   Teaneck, NJ 07666   (201)837-0727   Fax (201)837-8504

Blloshmi, Kledia, MD {1962820365} FamMGrtc
+ Geriatric Assessment Center
435 South Street/Suite 390   Morristown, NJ 07960   (973)971-7022

Bloch, Andrea J., DO {1487790705} Psychy(91,PA77)
+ 1201 New Road/Suite 331
Linwood, NJ 08221
+ Woodbine Development Center/NJ Human Services
1175 Dehirsch Avenue   Woodbine, NJ 08270   Fax (609)861-2494

Bloch, Jay L., MD {1790717114} Urolgy(79,MA05)
+ Urological Specialists of Southern New Jersey
2301 Evesham Road/Suite 508   Voorhees, NJ 08043   (856)651-0500   Fax (856)651-0700

Bloch, Paul Jacob, MD {1548688674} Urolgy
+ Hunterdon Urological Associates
1 Wescott Drive/Suite 101   Flemington, NJ 08822   (908)782-0019   Fax (908)237-4132

Block, Deborah C., MD {1205055241} Pedtrc(66,IL02)<NJ-MORRISTN>
+ 32 Bradwahl Drive
Morristown, NJ 07960   (973)267-1875

Block, Michael, MD {1346222858} Anesth(94,NJ06)<NJ-HACKNSK>
+ Hackensack University Medical Center
30 Prospect Avenue/Anesthesiology   Hackensack, NJ 07601   (201)996-2419   Fax (201)488-6769
mblock@humed.com

Block, William Paul, DO {1477591774} EmrgMd(00,NJ75)<NJ-VIRTVOOR>
+ Virtua Voorhees
100 Bowman Drive/EmrgMed   Voorhees, NJ 08043   (856)247-3000
+ Emergency Physician Associates, P.A.
307 South Evergreen Avenue/PO Box 298   Woodbury, NJ 08096   (856)247-3000   Fax (856)848-1431

Blom, Thomas Robert, MD {1932304599} IntrMd, OncHem(02,NJ06)<NJ-UNVMCPRN>
+ Princeton Medical Group, P.A.
419 North Harrison Street   Princeton, NJ 08540   (609)924-9300   Fax (609)924-6552
+ Princeton Medical Group, P.A.
3 Liberty Street   Plainsboro, NJ 08536   (609)924-9300
+ University Medical Center of Princeton at Plainsboro
One Plainsboro Road/Attending   Plainsboro, NJ 08540   (609)497-4000

Blome, Mary, MD {1780637140} Otlryg(80,NY15)
+ 516 Knickerbocker Road
Cresskill, NJ 07626   (201)567-3898   Fax (201)567-4164

Blondo, Dennis L., MD {1235233495} Ophthl(73,VA04)<NJ-RBAYOLDB>
+ World Class LASIK
28 Throckmorton Lane   Old Bridge, NJ 08857   (732)679-6100   Fax (732)673-6703

Blonstein, Jeffrey D., MD {1497864458} RadDia(78,NY03)
+ South Mountain Imaging
120 Millburn Avenue   Millburn, NJ 07041   (973)376-0900   Fax (973)376-0010
+ Imaging Center at Morristown
95 Madison Avenue/Suite 107   Morristown, NJ 07960   (973)376-0900   Fax (973)984-1190

Blood, David King, MD {1457436909} CdvDis(66,NY01)<NY-PRSBCOLU, NJ-ENGLWOOD>
+ 163 Engle Street/Bldg 1-C
Englewood, NJ 07631   (201)569-3313   Fax (201)569-8703
+ Heart and Vascular Institute at EHMC
350 Engle Street/Suite 1000   Englewood, NJ 07631   (201)894-3636

Bloom, Allison Jill, DO {1811150675} ObsGyn(FL75
+ PennCare for Women
409 Route 70 East   Cherry Hill, NJ 08034   (856)795-0587

Physicians by Name and Address

Bloom, Tamir, MD {1164594784} PedOrt, SrgOrt(01,NY47)<NJ-CHRIST>
+ Advocare The Orthopedic Center
218 Ridgedale Avenue/Suite 104   Cedar Knolls, NJ 07927   (973)538-7700   Fax (973)538-9478

Bloomer, Courtney, DO {1730341413}<NJ-MORRISTN>
+ Morristown Medical Center
100 Madison Avenue   Morristown, NJ 07962   (973)971-5000

Bloomfield, Adam S., MD {1003854811} Pedtrc, IntrMd(97,NJ05)<NJ-VALLEY>
+ Chestnut Ridge Pediatrics
595 Chestnut Ridge Road   Woodcliff Lake, NJ 07677   (201)391-2020   Fax (201)391-0265
adam41@gmail.com

Bloomfield, Stephen M., MD {1265432603} SrgNro(80,NJ06)
+ JFK Neurosciences Institute
65 James Street/Second Floor   Edison, NJ 08818   (732)321-7010   Fax (732)632-1584
SBloomfield@solarishs.org

Bloomstein, Larry Z., MD {1548469406} SrgOrt(04,PA13)<NJ-COOPRUMC>
+ Mid Atlantic Orthopedic Associates LLP
557 Cranbury Road/Suite 10   East Brunswick, NJ 08816   (732)238-8800   Fax (732)238-8246

Bloor, James J., DO {1407899826} Radiol(99,NJ75)
+ South Jersey Radiology Associates, P.A.
100 Carnie Boulevard/Suite B-5   Voorhees, NJ 08043   (856)751-0123   Fax (856)751-0535
+ South Jersey Radiology Associates, P.A.
6650 Browning Road/Suite M14   Pennsauken, NJ 08109   (856)751-0123   Fax (856)661-0686
+ South Jersey Radiology Associates, P.A.
315 Route 70 East/Suite B   Cherry Hill, NJ 08043   (856)428-4344   Fax (856)428-0356

Blum, Christopher, DO {1609238005}<NJ-MORRISTN>
+ Morristown Medical Center
100 Madison Avenue   Morristown, NJ 07962   (973)971-5000

Blum, Jay R., MD {1013074988} Allrgy, IntrMd, IntMAImm(74,PA01)<NJ-STPETER, NJ-RWJUBRUN>
+ 85 Raritan Avenue
Highland Park, NJ 08904   (732)846-7861   Fax (732)846-2553

Blum, Karl Richard, MD {1154361285} SprtMd, SrgOrt(90,NJ05)
+ Ocean Orthopedic Associates, P.A.
530 Lakehurst Road/Suite 1   Toms River, NJ 08755   (732)349-8454   Fax (732)341-0259

Blum, Lawrence D., MD {1881851970} Psychy, Psynls(81,PA01)
+ One Mall Drive/Suite 920
Cherry Hill, NJ 08002   (856)779-7911

Blum, Mark A., MD {1134216526} CdvDis, IntCrd(83,NY47)
+ Cardiology Associates of Morristown
95 Madison Avenue/Suite 10A   Morristown, NJ 07960   (973)889-9001   Fax (973)889-9051

Blum, Paul A., MD {1386646016} IntrMd(75,NY08)
+ 69 State Highway 27
Edison, NJ 08820   (732)494-3220   Fax (732)494-5057

Blum, Richard Howard, MD {1093862914} ObsGyn, IntrMd(70,NJ05)<NJ-OVERLOOK>
+ 1457 Raritan Road
Clark, NJ 07066   (908)654-1166   Fax (908)654-5723
+ JFK Medical Center
65 James Street   Edison, NJ 08820   (908)654-1166   Fax (732)906-4927

Blumberg, Darren Reich, MD {1902813272} IntrMd, Gastrn(96,GRN01)
+ Summit Medical Group
140 Park Avenue/3rd Floor   Florham Park, NJ 07932   (973)401-0500
+ Atlantic Gastroenterology Summit Medical Group
65 Ridgedale Avenue   Cedar Knolls, NJ 07927   (973)401-0500   Fax (973)401-9306

Blumberg, Edwin D., MD {1235121229} CdvDis, IntrMd(68,NY01)<NJ-JFKMED, NJ-OVERLOOK>
+ MedDiag Assocs/Central NJ Cardiology
1511 Park Avenue/Suite 2   South Plainfield, NJ 07080   (908)756-4438   Fax (908)756-9160

Blumberg, Scott, MD {1104897339} Rheuma, IntrMd(76,MA05)<NJ-COMMED>
+ 1749 Hooper Avenue/Suite 103
Toms River, NJ 08753   (732)255-3911   Fax (732)255-0084

Blume, Jessica Wanda, MD {1295938579} AlgyImmn, IntrMd(02,NJ02)<NJ-VALLEY>
+ 85 Harristown Road/Suite 102
Glen Rock, NJ 07452   (201)855-8491

Blume, Jonathan Erik, MD {1013952084} Dermat(02,NJ06)
+ Westwood Dermatology
390 Old Hook Road   Westwood, NJ 07675   (201)666-9550   Fax (201)666-1251

Blumenfeld, Daniel J., MD {1700994134} Anesth(97,NH01)
+ 12 Maple Street
Chatham, NJ 07928

Blumenfrucht, Marvin J., MD {1689688046} Urolgy(78,GA01)<NJ-VAEASTOR>
+ VA New Jersey Health Care System-East Orange Campus
385 Tremont Avenue   East Orange, NJ 07018   (973)676-1000   Fax (212)580-0672

Blumenthal, Andrew Michael, DO {1962426338} FamMed(97,NJ75)<NJ-VIRTMHBC, NJ-KMHSTRAT>
+ Family Practice Associates of Voorhees
805 Cooper Road/Suite 3   Voorhees, NJ 08043   (856)751-1777   Fax (856)751-8090

Blumenthal, Beth A., MD {1558453373} RadDia
+ South Jersey Radiology Associates, P.A.
100 Carnie Boulevard/Suite B-5   Voorhees, NJ 08043   (856)751-0123   Fax (856)751-0535
+ South Jersey Radiology Associates, P.A.
6650 Browning Road/Suite M14   Pennsauken, NJ 08109   (856)751-0123   Fax (856)661-0686
+ South Jersey Radiology Associates, P.A.
315 Route 70 East/Suite B   Cherry Hill, NJ 08043   (856)428-4344   Fax (856)428-0356

Blumenthal, David C., MD {1992790125} Anesth(91,NY19)
+ 421 Adams Street/Suite 11
Hoboken, NJ 07030

Blumenthal, Neil C., MD {1265489215} ObsGyn(83,GRN01)
+ Phillipsburg Ob/Gyn Associates
700 Coventry Drive   Phillipsburg, NJ 08865   (908)454-4666   Fax (908)454-2332

Boak, Joseph G., MD {1013984087} CdvDis, IntrMd(70,PA01)<NJ-JRSYSHMC, NJ-CENTRAST>
+ Monmouth Cardiology Associates, LLC
11 Meridian Road   Eatontown, NJ 07724   (732)663-0300   Fax (732)663-0301
+ Monmouth Cardiology Associates, LLC.
2102 Corlies Avenue/State Highway 33   Neptune, NJ 07753   (732)663-0300   Fax (732)774-9148

Boak, Joseph G., Jr., MD {1629075064} IntrMd(95,NJ05)<NJ-RIVERVW>
+ Riverview Medical Associates, PA
4 Hartford Drive/Suite 1   Tinton Falls, NJ 07701   (732)741-3600   Fax (732)741-6079
+ Chapin Hill at Red Bank
100 Chapin Avenue   Red Bank, NJ 07701   (732)741-3600   Fax (732)842-8269

Boakye, Naana Agyeiwah, MD {1598961013} Dermat, SrgDer(04,PA13)
+ Bergen Dermatology, LLC
140 Sylvan Avenue/Suite 305   Englewood Cliffs, NJ 07632   (201)567-7546   Fax (201)585-1007
info@bergenderm.com

Boamah, Kwaku Osafo-Mensah, MD {1154413029} ObsGyn(84,GHA01)<NJ-CHRIST>
+ 1921 Kennedy Boulevard
Jersey City, NJ 07305   (201)333-8800   Fax (201)333-8585
Kb5662@aol.com

Boateng, Akwasi Afriyie, MD {1144541996}
+ Genito-Urinary Surgeons of New Jersey
579-A Cranbury Road/Suite 104   East Brunswick, NJ 08816   (646)667-6337   Fax (732)390-8555
boatenai@ucmail.uc.edu

Bobb-Mckoy, Marion Y., MD {1184709206} FamMed(91,NY48)<NY-MNTFWEIL, NY-MNTFMOSE>
+ NHCAC Health Center at Jersey City
324 Palisade Avenue   Jersey City, NJ 07306   (201)459-8888   Fax (201)459-8872
+ Ideal Family Health, PC
335A Main Street   Hackensack, NJ 07601   (201)459-8888   Fax (201)342-5454

Bobella, Stephen K., MD {1992807556} IntrMd(83,NY01)<NJ-OVERLOOK, NJ-STBARNMC>
+ Summit Medical Group
34 Mountain Boulevard   Warren, NJ 07059   (908)561-8600   Fax (908)561-7265

Bober, Craig, DO {1639583990} FamMed(14,PA77)
+ Inspira Medical Group
660 Woodbury Glassboro Road/Suite 26   Sewell, NJ 08080   (856)415-6868   Fax (856)464-1855

Bober, Mitchell C., DO {1902805013} FamMed(83,PA77)<NJ-MEMSALEM>
+ Salem Medical Group - Pennsville
181 North Broadway/Suite 3   Pennsville, NJ 08070   (856)678-9002   Fax (856)678-4027

Bobila, Alexis C., MD {1245213271} SrgVas, Surgry(73,PHI09)
+ 1037 US Highway 46/Suite 204
Clifton, NJ 07013   (973)471-8852
+ St. Joseph Medical Center Surgery
703 Main Street/Regan R1094   Paterson, NJ 07503   (973)754-4305

Bobila, Ramon T., MD {1710977160} AlgyImmn, Pedtrc(76,PHIL)<NJ-CHSMRCER>
+ 3379 Quakerbridge Road
Trenton, NJ 08619   (609)584-8880   Fax (609)584-9067

Bobila, Wilbur C., MD {1386745289} SrgVas, Surgry(74,PHI01)<NJ-VIRTMHBC>
+ Virtua Medford Surgical Group
212 Creek Crossing Boulevard   Hainesport, NJ 08036   (609)267-1004   Fax (856)222-4616

Bobrin, Bradford David, MD {1255365367} Psychy(95,PA09)
+ Cooper University Medical Center/Camden
3 Cooper Plaza   Camden, NJ 08103   (856)342-2328

Bobrow, Michael L., MD {1912147067} Radiol<NJ-OURLADY>
+ Our Lady of Lourdes Medical Center
1600 Haddon Avenue   Camden, NJ 08103   (856)757-3500

Bocage, Jean P., MD {1083789010} SrgThr(84,NJ06)
+ New Jersey Thoracic Group
35 Clyde Road/Suite 104   Somerset, NJ 08873   (732)247-3002   Fax (732)846-3819
+ New Jersey Thoracic Group
901 West Main Street/MAB Suite 106   Freehold, NJ 07728   (732)247-3002
+ The Cardio-Thoracic Surgical Group PA
12 Stults Road/Suite 123   Dayton, NJ 08873   (732)230-3272   Fax (732)230-3309

Boccia Liang, Claire G., MD {1376637702} CdvDis(00,NY20)<NJ-OVERLOOK, NJ-MORRISTN>
+ Claire G. Boccia Liang MD PA
100 Madison Avenue   Morristown, NJ 07962   (973)971-8900   Fax (973)898-1670
bocciamd@gmail.com

Bochenski, Jacek P., MD {1629037525} Pedtrc(95,POL02)<NJ-SJHREGMC>
+ 142 Covered Bridge Court
Sewell, NJ 08080
+ SJH Regional Medical Center
1505 West Sherman Avenue   Vineland, NJ 08360   (856)641-8000
+ Virtua Voorhees
100 Bowman Drive   Voorhees, NJ 08080   (856)247-3000

Bochner, Ronnie Z., MD {1689692782} ObsGyn(81,NY47)<NJ-RWJUBRUN>
+ Robert Wood Johnson Ob-Gyn Associates
50 Franklin Lane/Suite 203   Manalapan, NJ 07726   (732)536-7110   Fax (732)536-7118
+ Robert Wood Johnson Ob-Gyn Associates
3270 State Route 27/Suite 2200   Kendall Park, NJ 08824   (732)536-7110   Fax (732)422-4526
+ Robert Wood Johnson Ob-Gyn Associates
525 Route 70/Suite B-11   Lakewood, NJ 07726   (732)905-6466   Fax (732)905-6467

Bock, David Andrew, DO {1679505424} FamMed, OstMed(99,NJ75)<NJ-HUNTRDN>
+ Charm Aesthetics
6 East Main Street   Clinton, NJ 08809   (908)763-6753
charmaesthetics@gmail.com

Bock, Robert T., Jr., MD {1245251891} FamMed(95,NY48)<NJ-CHILTON>
+ Wedgewood Primary Care
1055 Hamburg Turnpike/Suite 300   Wayne, NJ 07470   (973)904-1177   Fax (973)904-1166

Bodagala, Hima, MD {1821408329} IntHos<NJ-SJHREGMC>
+ SJH Regional Medical Center
1505 West Sherman Avenue   Vineland, NJ 08360   (856)845-0100   Fax (302)651-4945

Bodala, Durga Rani, MD {1750341392} IntHos, IntrMd(99,INA83)<NJ-MONMOUTH>
+ Monmouth Medical Center
300 Second Avenue/Hospitalist   Long Branch, NJ 07740   (732)222-5200

**Bodapati, Leena, MD {1619173242}(03,INA75)<NJ-STPETER>
+ Neighborhood Health Center Plainfield
1700-58 Myrtle Avenue   Plainfield, NJ 07060   (908)753-6401   Fax (908)226-6743

Bodin, Nathan Daniel, MD {1881855955} SrgOrt(07,PA0)
+ Orthopedic & Neurosurgical Specialists, LLC.
807 Haddon Avenue/Suite 1   Haddonfield, NJ 08033   (856)795-9222   Fax (856)795-0026

Bodiwala, Brijesh Shreyas, DO {1518109834} Nephro, IntrMd(04,PA77)
+ Haddon Renal Medical Specialists
401 Kings Highway South/Suite 5   Cherry Hill, NJ 08034   (856)428-8992   Fax (856)428-9614

Bodnar, Aleksander J., MD {1417095118} ObsGyn(79,POLA)<NJ-TRINIWSC, NJ-OVERLOOK>
+ 930 North Wood Avenue
Linden, NJ 07036   (908)925-7400   Fax (908)925-7474
+ 905 Allwood Road/Suite 206
Clifton, NJ 07012   (908)925-7400   Fax (973)778-7009

Bodner, Arnold H., MD {1174621866} Anesth, Pedtrc(71,NY46)<NJ-HCKTSTWN>
+ 609 West South Orange Avenue/Apt 4K
South Orange, NJ 07079

Bodner, Bradley A., DO {1366614406} PhysMd
+ 582 Franklin Avenue
Nutley, NJ 07110

Bodner, Leonard, MD {1083696223} RadDia, RadV&I(77,NY09)<NJ-STPETER, NJ-RWJUBRUN>
+ University Radiology Group, P.C.
483 Cranbury Road   East Brunswick, NJ 08816   (732)390-0030   Fax (732)390-5383
+ University Radiology Group, P.C.
10 Plum Street   New Brunswick, NJ 08901   (732)390-0030   Fax (732)249-1208
+ University Radiology Group, P.C.
75 Veronica Avenue   Somerset, NJ 08816   (732)246-0060   Fax (732)246-4188

Bodofsky, Elliot B., MD {1619066339} PhysMd(84,PA13)<NJ-COOPRUMC>
+ Cooper PM & R Assocs
1101 North Kings Highway/Suite 100   Cherry Hill, NJ 08034   (856)414-6112   Fax (856)414-6121
+ Cooper University Medical Center/Camden
3 Cooper Plaza   Camden, NJ 08103   (856)342-2000
+ Cooper PM & R Assocs
One Cooper Plaza/Suite 550   Camden, NJ 08034   (856)342-2040   Fax (856)968-8311

Boesler, Iza Marzanna, MD {1366449795} IntrMd(86,POL03)<NJ-RIVERVW>
+ Riverview Medical Associates, PA
4 Hartford Drive/Suite 1   Tinton Falls, NJ 07701   (732)741-3600   Fax (732)741-3603

Boffard, Daryl K., MD {1497763874} ObsGyn, Gyneco(81,NJ05)<NJ-STBARNMC, NJ-OVERLOOK>
+ Union & Cranford Ob/Gyn & Infertility Group
1323 Stuyvesant Avenue   Union, NJ 07083   (908)686-4334   Fax (908)686-1744
+ Union & Cranford Ob/Gyn & Infertility Group
118 South Avenue East   Cranford, NJ 07016   (908)276-7333
+ Union & Cranford Ob/Gyn & Infertility Group
349 Valley Street   South Orange, NJ 07083   (973)763-4334

Bogacki, Gwen M., MD {1609145663} Pedtrc(83,VT02)<NJ-CHSFULD, NJ-CHSMRCER>
+ Hamilton Pediatric Associates
3 Hamilton Health Place/Suite A   Hamilton, NJ 08690   (609)581-4480   Fax (609)581-5222
+ University Pediatric Associates PA
317 Cleveland Avenue   Highland Park, NJ 08904   (609)581-4480   Fax (732)249-7827

Bogdan, Joseph P., MD {1730161084} SrgOrt(92,DC02)
+ Brielle Orthopedics PA
457 Jack Martin Boulevard   Brick, NJ 08724   (732)840-7500   Fax (732)840-2088
+ Brielle Orthopedics PA
823 Lacey Road   Forked River, NJ 08731   (732)840-7500   Fax (732)840-2088
+ Brielle Orthopedics PA
1301 Route 72 West   Manahawkin, NJ 08724   (609)971-7616   Fax (609)971-7639

Bogdan, Sergey Valentinovich, MD {1700894110} PhysMd, PhyM-Pain, SprtMd(87,RUS11)<NJ-BAYSHORE, NJ-RIVERVW>
+ Bogdan Pain Management Services
112 Professional View Drive/Bld 100   Freehold, NJ 07728   (732)577-9126   Fax (732)577-9127
+ Bogdan Pain Management
200 Perrine Road/Suite 224   Old Bridge, NJ 08857   (732)577-9126   Fax (732)553-1215

Boghdady, Maged W., MD {1548208531} ObsGyn, IntrMd(80,EGYP)
+ St. Joseph's Family Health Center
21 Market Street/OB/GYN   Paterson, NJ 07501   (973)754-4200   Fax (973)754-2725
+ St. Joseph's DePaul Center ObsGyn
11 Getty Avenue   Paterson, NJ 07503   (973)754-4200

Boghossian, Jack, MD {1083666010} IntrMd, InfDis(84,GRNA)<NJ-STMICHL, NJ-CLARMAAS>
+ St. Michael's Medical Center
268 MLK Jr. Boulevard   Newark, NJ 07102   (973)751-3399

Bogomol, Adam Russell, MD {1750366019} RadDia, RadBdI(97,ISR02)<NJ-HACKNSK>
+ Hackensack University Medical Center
30 Prospect Avenue/DiagnosticRad   Hackensack, NJ 07601   (201)996-2000   Fax (201)489-2812
+ Hackensack Radiology Group, P.A.
30 Prospect Avenue   Hackensack, NJ 07601   (201)996-2000   Fax (201)336-8451

Boguslavsky, David, MD {1114080231} FamMed, Acpntr(03,NJ06)<NJ-SOMERSET>
+ Premier Medical Acupuncture
757 Route 202/206   Bridgewater, NJ 08807   (908)450-7002   Fax (732)832-2601

Bogusz, Katie L., MD {1447425632} IntrMd
+ Drs. Bogusz & Weiss
44 State Route 23 North/Suite 6   Riverdale, NJ 07457   (973)248-9199   Fax (973)248-9299

Bohm, Steven A., MD {1154395341} Gastrn, IntrMd(73,NY08)<NJ-CENTRAST>
+ Central Jersey Gastroenterology Associates PA
535 Iron Bridge Road/Suite 12   Freehold, NJ 07728   (732)780-4224   Fax (732)780-5044

Bohnert, Katherine Ann, DO {1235440140} ObsGyn
+ A Woman's Place
34 Sycamore Avenue   Little Silver, NJ 07739   (732)747-9310   Fax (732)747-9320

Bohrer, Michael K., MD {1942230339} RprEnd, ObsGyn(81,NY08)<NJ-STPETER, NJ-MORRISTN>
+ Reproductive Medicine Associates of New Jersey
140 Allen Road   Basking Ridge, NJ 07920   (908)604-7800   Fax (973)290-8370
+ Reproductive Medicine Associates of New Jersey
81 Veronica Avenue/Suite 101   Somerset, NJ 08873   (908)604-7800   Fax (732)220-1164

Boiano, Maria Anna, MD {1366618266} PhysMd
+ Rehabilitation Specialists of New Jersey
505 Goffle Road/Suite 3   Ridgewood, NJ 07450   (201)447-4772   Fax (201)447-4277

Boiardo, Richard A., MD {1659308310} SrgOrt(79,NY09)<NJ-HOBUNIMC, NJ-STMICHL>
+ Cross County Orthopaedics
769 Northfield Avenue/Suite LL20   West Orange, NJ 07052   (973)669-9595   Fax (973)669-1050

Boim, Marilynn Dora, MD {1306801568} Pedtrc, AdolMd(82,GA05)<NJ-CHSFULD>
+ Hamilton Pediatric Associates
3 Hamilton Health Place/Suite A   Hamilton, NJ 08690   (609)581-4480   Fax (609)581-5222

Boja, Conrado A., III, MD {1255399408} FamMed(80,PHI10)
+ Drs. Boja & Boja
1150 Teaneck Road   Teaneck, NJ 07666   (201)833-9000   Fax (201)833-9510

Boja, Michael Conrad, DO {1811254980} FamMed
+ Drs. Boja & Boja
1150 Teaneck Road   Teaneck, NJ 07666   (201)833-9000   Fax (201)833-9510

Bojarski, Michael H., DO {1649216938} OccpMd, IntrMd(80,PA77)
+ American Work Care
1125 North Delsea Drive/PO Box 736   Glassboro, NJ 08028   (856)218-7600   Fax (856)218-7800   havana80@aol.com

Bojito-Marrero, Lizza Marie, MD {1336442532} IntrMd, Hepato(07,NY09)
+ UMDNJ Division of Gastroenterology & Hepatology
90 Bergen Street/DOC 2100   Newark, NJ 07103   (973)972-5252   Fax (973)972-0752

Bojko, Thomas, MD {1679631337} PedCrC, Pedtrc(85,ITAL)
+ UH- RWJ Medical School
One Robert Wood Johnson Place   New Brunswick, NJ 08903   (732)235-5600

Bokhari, Naimat U., MD {1235222522} Pedtrc(84,PAKI)<NJ-MEADWLND, NJ-HACKNSK>
+ Riverside Medical Group
714 Tenth Street/Suite 2   Secaucus, NJ 07094   (201)863-3346   Fax (201)865-0015
+ Riverside ENT Pediatric Group
324 Palisade Avenue/2nd Floor   Jersey City, NJ 07307   (201)863-3346   Fax (201)386-2343

Bokhari, Shafaq, MD {1932336559}
+ Drs. Rana & Roowala
40 Fuld Street/Suite 302   Trenton, NJ 08638   (609)393-0067   Fax (609)393-4943

Bokhari, Tahira M., MD {1619075009} Allrgy, PedInf, Pedtrc(74,PAKI)<NJ-STJOSHOS, NJ-WAYNEGEN>
+ Allergy Consultants of Elizabeth
17-15 Maple Avenue/Suite 110   Fair Lawn, NJ 07410   (201)703-4665   Fax (201)703-9097

Bokkala Pinniniti, Shaila, DO {1487816344} Nrolgy(04,NJ75)
+ Woodbury Neurology Associates
17 West Red Bank Avenue/Suite 204   Woodbury, NJ 08096   (856)853-1133   Fax (856)845-5405

Bolanowski, Paul J., MD {1407846587} SrgThr, Surgry(65,NJ05)<NJ-UMDNJ>
+ 105 Denman Road
Cranford, NJ 07016   (908)352-8110

Bolarinwa, Isiaka A., MD {1467403196} Psychy, PsyCAd, Addctn(94,DOM02)<NJ-ACMCMAIN>
+ 141 South Black Horse Pike
Blackwood, NJ 08012   (856)227-0306
+ St. Remi Behavioral Health
750 Route 73 South/Suite 106   Marlton, NJ 08053   (856)227-0306   Fax (856)396-9917

Bolarinwa, Oladayo, MD {1609193507} Nephro
+ Shore Nephrology, P.A.
2100 Corlies Avenue/Suite 15   Neptune, NJ 07753   (732)988-8228   Fax (732)774-1528
+ Shore Nephrology, P.A.
1000 West Main Street/Suite 3   Freehold, NJ 07728   (732)988-8228   Fax (732)414-1591
+ Shore Nephrology, PA
27 South Cookbridge Road/Suite 211   Jackson, NJ 07753   (732)987-5990   Fax (732)987-5994

Bolich, Christopher W., DO {1861592347} IntrMd(93,PA77)<NJ-SHOREMEM>
+ 18 Clover Hill Circle
Egg Harbor Township, NJ 08234   (609)653-3100   Fax (609)653-3155

Bolisetti, Sreedevi, MD {1497786123} IntrMd(97,INA9D)<NJ-KMHTURNV>
+ SOM - Department of Internal Medicine
42 East Laurel Road/Suite 3100   Stratford, NJ 08084   (856)566-6845   Fax (856)566-6342
+ Kennedy Health Systems/Washington Township Campus
435 Hurffville-Cross Keys Road   Turnersville, NJ 08012   (856)582-2500

Bolkus, Kelly Ann, DO {1043530678} Anesth(06,NJ75)<NJ-COOPRUMC>
+ Cooper University Hospital
One Cooper Plaza   Camden, NJ 08103   (856)342-2425   Fax (856)968-8239

Bollampally, Indira, MD {1609856913} IntrMd, PulDis(75,INA83)<NJ-JRSYSHMC>
+ 1540 Highway 138/Suite 208
Wall, NJ 07719   (732)681-9045   Fax (732)681-9494

Bollard, David A., DO {1831185768} FamMed(86,NJ75)<NJ-NWTNMEM>
+ Premier Health Associates
89 Sparta Avenue/Suite 100   Sparta, NJ 07871   (973)729-2121   Fax (973)729-3454
+ Premier Health Associates
272 Route 206 North   Andover, NJ 07821   (973)729-2121   Fax (973)729-3238

Bollu, Janardhan, MD {1952370819} Gastrn(78,INDI)
+ 32 Hine Street/Suite 10
Paterson, NJ 07503   (973)754-9600   Fax (973)754-9700
+ 1819 Oak Tree Road
Edison, NJ 08820   (973)754-9600   Fax (908)662-7082

Bolo, Peter M., MD {1649284639} Psychy(85,NY01)<NJ-SUMOAKSH>
+ Summit Oaks Hospital
19 Prospect Street   Summit, NJ 07901   (908)522-7000   Peter.bolo@ahsys.org

Bolognese, Ronald J., MD {1689662645} ObsGyn(63,PA01)<NJ-VIRTVOOR, NJ-ACMCITY>
+ Virtua Voorhees
100 Bowman Drive/Ob/Gyn   Voorhees, NJ 08043   (856)325-3328   Fax (856)325-3276
+ Virtua Family Health Center
1000 Atlantic Avenue   Camden, NJ 08104   (856)325-3328   Fax (856)246-3528

Bolona, Leopold J., MD {1700043049} Psychy<NJ-TRININPC>
+ Trinitas Regional Medical Center-New Point Campus
655 East Jersey Street/Psychiatry   Elizabeth, NJ 07206   (908)994-5000

Bona, Marzena M., MD {1710951074} NnPnMd, Pedtrc(87,POLA)<NJ-JRSYSHMC, NJ-RIVERVW>
+ On-Site Neonatal Partners
1000 Haddonfield-Berlin Road/Suite 210   Voorhees, NJ 08043   (856)782-2212   Fax (856)782-2213

Bonaker, Laura J., MD {1528078797} Pedtrc(78,PA07)
+ 211 Belhaven Avenue
Linwood, NJ 08221

Bonala, Savithri Bai, MD {1083699409} Allrgy(73,INA5B)
+ Center for Asthma & Allergy
18 North Third Avenue   Highland Park, NJ 08904   (732)545-0094   Fax (732)545-4087
+ Center for Asthma & Allergy
300 Hudson Street   Hoboken, NJ 07030   (732)545-0094   Fax (201)792-5320
+ Center for Asthma & Allergy
90 Milbum Avenue/Suite 200   Maplewood, NJ 08904   (973)763-5787   Fax (973)763-8568

Bonamo, John F., MD {1760656714} ObsGyn(77,NJ05)<NJ-STBARNMC>
+ St. Barnabas Medical Center
94 Old Short Hills Road   Livingston, NJ 07039   (973)322-5000

Bonanno, Bruce B., MD {1275576290} EmrgMd(83,GRNA)<NJ-HCKTSTWN>
+ Hackettstown Regional Medical Center
651 Willow Grove Street/Emerg Med   Hackettstown, NJ 07840   (908)850-6800

Bonaparte, Philip M., MD {1679634737} IntrMd(86,GRN01)
+ 218 N Broad Street
Trenton, NJ 08608   (609)599-4000   Fax (609)599-4001

Bonaventura, Lisa M., MD {1497850895} IntrMd(86,OH41)<NJ-MORRISTN>
+ 2345 Lamington Road/Suite 104
Bedminster, NJ 07921   (908)781-9661   Fax (908)781-2106

Physicians by Name and Address

Bonazinga, Thomas P., MD {1912041252} Nrolgy(85,NY08)<NJ-BAYSHORE, NJ-CENTRAST>
+ 1000 West Main Street/Suite 1
Freehold, NJ 07728 (732)303-1144

Bond, Laura R., MD {1407852726} RadThp, RadOnc, IntrMd(87,PA02)<NJ-SOMERSET>
+ Steeplechase Cancer Center
30 Rehill Avenue/Suite 1100 Somerville, NJ 08876 (908)927-8777
+ University Radiology, PA
239 Route 22 East/Suite 302 Green Brook, NJ 08812 (908)927-8777 Fax (732)968-8096
+ Bridgewater Imaging Center-Associated Radiologists
201 Union Avenue/Building 2/Suite G Bridgewater, NJ 08876 (908)725-1291 Fax (908)725-8335

Bond, Sheila A., MD {1609884337} SrgPlstc, SrgCsm(87,NY01)<NJ-MTNSIDE, NJ-CLARMAAS>
+ 39 South Fullerton Avenue/3rd Floor
Montclair, NJ 07042 (973)509-0007 Fax (973)509-0733
BondMD@aol.com

Bonder, Irvin Mark, MD {1740257732} Urolgy(81,MEXI)<NJ-STCLRDEN, NJ-HCKTSTWN>
+ Garden State Urology
282 US Highway 46 Denville, NJ 07834 (973)895-6636 Fax (973)895-5327
+ Associates in Pediatric & Adult Urology
20 Commerce Boulevard/Suite D Succasunna, NJ 07876 (973)895-6636 Fax (973)927-6831
+ Associates in Pediatric & Adult Urology
653 Willow Grove Street Hackettstown, NJ 07834 (908)684-4670

Boneparth, Alexis D., MD {1528232394} Pedtrc(05,NY47)
+ University Hospital-RWJ Medical School
89 French Street/Pedi Rheuma New Brunswick, NJ 08901 (732)828-3000

Bones, Victoria Mary, MD {1285054122} Otlryg(DC02
+ Coastal Ear Nose and Throat LLC
1301 Route 72/Suite 340 Manahawkin, NJ 08050 (732)280-7855 Fax (732)280-7815

Bonett, Anthony W., MD {1427059914} IntrMd, FamMed(88,PA09)<NJ-UNDRWD>
+ Drs. Bonett & Butler
50 Cooper Street Woodbury, NJ 08096 (856)848-8081 Fax (856)848-1577

Bonett, Deirdre Maria, MD {1851314223} Pedtrc(90,PA13)
+ Kids first
2006 Salem Road Burlington, NJ 08016 (609)877-1500 Fax (609)877-4262

Bongiovanni, Denise A., DO {1396738738} Nrolgy(90,NY75)<NJ-STCLRDEN, NJ-STCLRDOV>
+ Central Morris Neurology
170 East Main Street/Suite 6 Rockaway, NJ 07866 (973)625-8888 Fax (973)625-7877

Boni, Christopher M., DO {1023111507} IntrMd, PulDis(90,NJ75)
+ Summit Medical Group-Berkeley Heights Campus
1 Diamond Hill Road/Wittman Ste D Berkeley Heights, NJ 07922 (908)277-8683 Fax (908)790-6576

Bonier, Bruce S., DO {1336140920} Radiol, GenPrc(78,PA77)
+ 110 Croft Court
Hainesport, NJ 08036

Bonifield, Eric M., MD {1497771950} ObsGyn(85,GRN01)<NJ-SJHREGMC>
+ Cumberland Ob-Gyn PA
1102 East Chestnut Avenue Vineland, NJ 08360 (856)696-4484 Fax (856)690-1352
+ Cumberland Ob-Gyn, PA
2950 College Drive/Suite 2G Vineland, NJ 08360 (856)696-4484 Fax (856)696-1694

Bonilla, Mary Ann, MD {1316999154} PedHem, Pedtrc(81,IL43)<NJ-STJOSHOS>
+ St. Joseph's Children's Hospital
703 Main Street/Peds Hem/Onc Paterson, NJ 07503 (973)754-2500

Bonilla, Melissa Diaz, MD {1922106087} Pedtrc(01,NJ06)
+ 28 Deepwater Circle
Manalapan, NJ 07726

Bonilla Guerrero, Ruben, MD {1417514811} GntMCBCh
+ Admera Medical Lab
126 Corporate Boulevard/Suite D South Plainfield, NJ 07080 (908)222-0533

Bonitz, Joyce A., MD {1922242247} Surgry
+ 136 Heckel Street
Belleville, NJ 07109

Bonitz, Robert Paul, Jr., MD {1104182716} Urolgy, SrgUro(12,NJ05)
+ Urology Associates, P.A.
595 Shrewsbury Avenue/Suite 103 Shrewsbury, NJ 07702 (732)741-5923 Fax (732)741-2759
+ University Hospital
150 Bergen Street/Suite E-401 Newark, NJ 07103 (973)972-5682

Bonk, Rosemarie A., MD {1679506729} IntrMd(91,NJ06)
+ 3701 Cricket Circle
Edison, NJ 08820

Bonne, Stephanie Lynn, MD {1225294507} SrgCrC
+ Rutgers- New Jersey Medical School
185 South Orange Avenue/MSB G584 Newark, NJ 07103 (973)972-5016

Bonner, Francis John, Jr., MD {1548320328} PhysMd(70,IRE03)<NJ-RHBHSPSJ>
+ The Rehabilitation Hospital of South Jersey
1237 West Sherman Avenue Vineland, NJ 08360 (856)696-7100

Bonner, James M., DO {1235158361} EmrgMd, FamMed(86,PA77)<NJ-UNDRWD>
+ Inspira Health Network
509 North Broad Street Woodbury, NJ 08096 (856)853-2001

Bonnet, Jean-Paul, DO {1154397214} FamMed(81,PA77)
+ Skylands Medical Group PA
174 Edison Road Lake Hopatcong, NJ 07849 (973)663-1300 Fax (973)663-2848

Bonney, David Raymond, DO {1548476385} IntrMd, Dermat(98,NY75)<NJ-BAYSHORE, NJ-JRSYSHMC>
+ The Dermatology Group, P.C.
60 Pompton Avenue Verona, NJ 07044 (973)571-2121 Fax (973)571-2126
+ The Dermatology Group, P.C.
44 Route 23 North/Suite 213 Riverdale, NJ 07457 (973)571-2121 Fax (973)839-5751
+ The Dermatology Group, P.C.
30 West Century Road/Suite 320 Paramus, NJ 07044 (973)571-2121 Fax (201)986-0702

Bonomini, Luigi Vittorio, MD {1992771349} Nephro, IntrMd(85,ITA13)
+ Modern Nephrology & Transplant, LLC
767 Northfield Avenue West Orange, NJ 07052 (973)419-0417 Fax (862)766-5904

Bonsell, Joshua W., MD {1295939676} Anesth, PainMd(02,PA13)<NJ-STBARNMC>
+ New Jersey Anesthesia Associates, P.C.
252 Columbia Turnpike/PO Box 0037 Florham Park, NJ 07932 (973)660-9334 Fax (973)660-9779

Bontempo, Carl Peter, MD {1386645901} Ophthl(79,PA09)<NJ-MONMOUTH>
+ Atlantic Eye Physicians
279 Third Avenue/Suite 204 Long Branch, NJ 07740 (732)222-7373 Fax (732)571-9212
+ Atlantic Eye Physicians
180 White Road/Suite 202 Little Silver, NJ 07739 (732)222-7373 Fax (732)219-9557
+ Atlantic Eye Physicians
100 Commons Way/Suite 230 Holmdel, NJ 07740 (732)671-4060

Bontemps, Serge L., MD {1538240817} Radiol(65,HAIT)<NJ-STJOSHOS>
+ C. Dicovsky Medical Group LLC
681 Broadway Paterson, NJ 07514 (973)278-1000 Fax (973)278-1709

Bonvicino, Marie Louise, MD {1407891609} ObsGyn(92,GRN01)<NJ-COMMED>
+ North Dover Ob-Gyn Associates
222 Oak Avenue/3rd Floor/Suite 301 Toms River, NJ 08753 (732)914-1919 Fax (732)914-0725
+ North Dover Ob-Gyn Associates
442 Lacey Road Forked River, NJ 08731 (732)914-1919 Fax (609)971-9712
+ North Dover Ob-Gyn Associates
214 Jack Martin Boulevard/Building D-3 Brick, NJ 08753 (732)840-3900 Fax (732)840-9270

Bonvicino, Nicholas G., MD Surgry, AdmMgt(79,NY09)
+ 9 Sturms Place
Park Ridge, NJ 07656

Bookbinder, Ronald L., MD {1326144585} EmrgMd(81,MEXI)
+ Christ Hospital
176 Palisade Avenue Jersey City, NJ 07306 (973)740-0607

Booker, Larnie J., MD {1730279563} Pedtrc, AdolMd(98,MA07)
+ Mid Jersey Pediatrics
33 Brunswick Woods Drive East Brunswick, NJ 08816 (732)257-4330 Fax (732)257-1177

Boomsma, Joan D., MD PulcCr, IntrMd(83,MI01)<NJ-ATLANTHS>
+ Atlantic Health System
475 South Street Morristown, NJ 07960 (973)971-7043

Boor, Sonya H., MD {1114970878} Pedtrc(92,CZEC)<NJ-CHSFULD, NJ-CHSMRCER>
+ Advocare Garden State Pediatrics
2133 Highway 33 Trenton, NJ 08690 (609)581-5100 Fax (609)581-5134

Boorstein, Jerry, DO {1376644252} GenPrc, FamMed(73,PA77)
+ 55-77 Schanck Road/Suite B-13
Freehold, NJ 07728 (732)462-9355 Fax (732)462-9474

Boorujy, Dean P., DO {1790745180} FamMed, FamMAdlt(93,PA77)<NY-STBARNAB, NJ-MORRISTN>
+ Northfield Medical Associates
65 East Northfield Road Livingston, NJ 07039 (973)422-9595 Fax (973)422-9390
+ Summit Medical Group
75 East Northfield Road Livingston, NJ 07039 (973)422-9595 Fax (908)673-7336

Booth, Robert Emrey, Jr., MD {1932140266} SrgOrt(71,PA01)
+ Aria 3B Orthopaedics, P.C.
1400 East Route 70/Second Floor Cherry Hill, NJ 08034

Boothe, Deniece Tamara, DO {1881824548} PallCr, EmrgMd<NJ-STJOSHOS>
+ St. Joseph's Regional Medical Center
703 Main Street/Palliative Med Paterson, NJ 07503 (973)754-2842

Boozan, James A., MD {1548205545} Otlryg(87,OH40)<NJ-CHSFULD, NJ-CHSMRCER>
+ 3131 Princeton Pike
Lawrenceville, NJ 08648 (609)844-9661 Fax (609)844-9664

Boozan, John M., MD {1265436174} Ophthl(83,OH41)
+ 33 Overlook Road/Suite 407
Summit, NJ 07901 (908)277-1166 Fax (908)277-0141 Jboozan@comcast.net
+ 776 East Third Avenue
Roselle, NJ 07203 (908)277-1166 Fax (908)298-0172

Boradia, Chirag N., DO {1093970923} EnDbMt
+ Nambi Endocrine Associates LLC
22 Old Short Hills Road/Suite 201 Livingston, NJ 07039 (973)535-8870 Fax (973)535-8818

Borai, Nasser Eldien, MD {1427031681} OncHem(81,EGY03)<NJ-ACMCITY>
+ Cancer and Blood Disorders Care
54 West Jimmie Leeds Road Galloway, NJ 08205 (609)404-9966 Fax (609)404-9967
+ Premier Oncology, LLC.
54 West Jimmie Leeds Road/Suite 11 Galloway, NJ 08205 (609)404-9966 Fax (609)748-1002

Boral, Andrew S., MD {1922082098} Anesth(71,POL08)<NJ-HACKNSK, NJ-HOBUNIMC>
+ Hackensack Anesthesiology Associates
140 Prospect Avenue/Suite 8 Hackensack, NJ 07601 (201)488-0066 Fax (201)488-6769
+ Hackensack University MC-Anesthesia Dept
30 Prospect Avenue/Room 2703 Hackensack, NJ 07601 (201)488-0066 Fax (201)996-3962

Borao, Frank J., MD {1558383117} Surgry(94,NJ05)<NJ-MONMOUTH, NJ-RIVERVW>
+ Specialty Surgical Associates
10 Industrial Way East/Suite 104 Eatontown, NJ 07724 (732)389-1331 Fax (732)542-8587

Borbon-Reyes, Araceli O., MD {1487749040} PthAcl, PthCyt(73,PHIL)
+ Drs. Reyes & Narvaez
135 Bloomfield Avenue/Suite B Bloomfield, NJ 07003 (973)743-3556 Fax (973)743-3895

Bordan, Dennis Lawrence, MD {1164487559} Surgry(70,NY06)
+ St. Joseph Medical Center Surgery
703 Main Street Paterson, NJ 07503 (973)754-2470

Borden, Doris Rita, MD {1407965395} Psychy, PsyCAd(80,NY46)
+ 3501 Boardwalk/Apt. A105
Atlantic City, NJ 08401

Borden, Victor, MD {1043274384} ObsGyn(69,PA09)<NJ-HACKNSK, NJ-ENGLWOOD>
+ Grand Ob-Gyn, P.A.
100 State Street/Suite 1A Teaneck, NJ 07666 (201)871-1766 Fax (201)871-1391
vicobgynmd@aol.com

Bordia, Sonal, MD {1346421781} MedOnc, Hemato, IntrMd<NY-BRKLNDWN>
+ 2130 Millburn Avnue
Maplewood, NJ 07040 (201)936-6032

Bordieri, Joseph Anthony, DO {1033135793} GenPrc, FamMed(01,NJ75)<NJ-RWJUBRUN, NJ-UNVMCPRN>
+ Garden State Heart Care, P.C.
333 Forsgate Drive/Suite 205 Jamesburg, NJ 08831 (732)521-1210 Fax (732)521-1239

Borensztein, Alejandra Giselle, MD {1699909556} EnDbMt(08,ARG11)
+ Endocrinology Consultants P.C.
229 Engle Street Englewood, NJ 07631 (201)567-8999 Fax (201)567-5201

Boretz, Robert Stephen, MD {1992709760} SrgOrt, SrgHnd, OrtS-Hand(93,NY08)<NJ-MORRISTN>
+ Summit Medical Group
34 Mountain Boulevard/Building B Warren, NJ 07059 (908)769-0100 Fax (908)769-8927
+ Orthopedic and Sports Medicine at SMG
215 Union Avenue/Suite B Bridgewater, NJ 08807 (908)769-0100 Fax (908)685-8009

Borgatti, Richard J., MD {1871589952} SrgOrt(80,VA04)<NJ-OCEANMC>
+ Shore Shoulder Surgery
1430 Hooper Avenue/Suite 202   Toms River, NJ 08753
(732)244-4544   Fax (732)244-4545

Borgen, Ruth E., MD {1871533695} Pedtrc, PedEmg(86,NY47)<NJ-HACKNSK>
+ Hackensack Univ Medical Center Pediatric Emerg Room
30 Prospect Avenue   Hackensack, NJ 07601   (201)996-5430   Fax (201)996-3676
+ Hackensack University Medical Center
30 Prospect Avenue/Pediatric ER   Hackensack, NJ 07601
(201)996-2000

Borger, Caryn Beth, MD {1669569414} EnDbMt(98,NJ06)
+ The Endocrine Center
15 James Street/Suite 2   Florham Park, NJ 07932
(973)377-6868   Fax (973)377-6822
Info@DRBorger.com

Borgersen, Rudolph H., DO {1063568020} CdvDis, IntrMd(71,PA77)<NJ-CENTRAST>
+ 501 Stillwells Corner Road
Freehold, NJ 07728   (732)780-3330   Fax (732)780-4385
borgensens@yahoo.com

Borghini, Margarita, MD {1194802736} IntrMd(97,PA14)<NJ-CHRIST>
+ 550 Newark Avenue
Jersey City, NJ 07306   (201)222-9935   Fax (201)222-7935
borghinimd@aol.com

Borham, Amanda Ahmed Fouad, MD {1013184001} IntrMd, Rheuma(95,EGY03)
+ UMDNJ RWJ Rheumatology
125 Paterson Street/MEB 474   New Brunswick, NJ 08903
(732)235-6525   Fax (732)235-6526

Boris, Walter J., DO {1184671885} SrgCdv, SrgThr, Surgry(85,PA77)<NJ-DEBRAHLC>
+ Deborah Heart and Lung Center
200 Trenton Road/Surgery/Thorac   Browns Mills, NJ 08015
(609)893-6611   Fax (609)893-1213

Boriss, Michael N., DO {1255375085} CdvDis, IntrMd, CritCr(81,MO78)<NJ-BURDTMLN>
+ Cape Regional Physicians Associates-Cardiology
217 North Main Street/Suite 205   Cape May Court House, NJ 08210   (609)463-5440   Fax (609)463-9888

Borja, Manuel L., MD {1578504205} ObsGyn(77,PHIL)
+ 201 Palisades Avenue
Jersey City, NJ 07306   (201)792-3612

Borja, Susan V., MD {1629015342} Psychy, PsyCAd(76,PHIL)
+ 316 Lenox Avenue/Suite 2B
Westfield, NJ 07090   (908)233-7903   Fax (908)233-7905

Borkar, Sunita A., MD {1083989107} NuclMd
+ 10 Overlook Road/Apt 43
Summit, NJ 07901
+ Summit Medical Group-Berkeley Heights Campus
1 Diamond Hill Road   Berkeley Heights, NJ 07922   Fax (908)790-6576

Borker, Sonia V., DO {1053748236} IntHos<NJ-CHRIST>
+ Christ Hospital
176 Palisade Avenue   Jersey City, NJ 07306   (201)795-8201
Fax (201)795-8278

Borkowska, Alina, MD {1851546352} FamMed(03,POL12)
+ 1050 Galloping Hill Road/Suite 204
Union, NJ 07083   (908)258-7985   Fax (908)258-7986
+ AFC Urgent Care Lyndhurst
560 New York Avenue   Lyndhurst, NJ 07071   (908)258-7985   Fax (201)345-4536

Borkowski, Douglas Joseph, MD {1285769851} GenPrc, SprtMd(86,NJ05)<NJ-CHILTON>
+ AFC Urgent Care Paramus
67 East Ridgewood Avenue   Paramus, NJ 07652   (201)899-4765
+ The Gem Medical Group
51 State Route 23/Suite 210   Haskell, NJ 07420   (973)831-5705

Bornstein, Marc Andrew, DO {1245308576} EmrgMd(00,NJ75)<NJ-STPETER>
+ St Joseph's Medical Center Emergency
703 Main Street   Paterson, NJ 07503   (973)754-2240   Fax (973)754-2249

Borodulin, Boris, MD {1770646358} PsyAdt, PsyGrt, Psychy(84,RUSS)<NJ-RBAYPERT, NJ-NWTNMEM>
+ 180 Tices Lane/Suite 101
East Brunswick, NJ 08816   (732)247-1040   Fax (732)247-1041

Borofsky, Karen Esther, MD {1710991526} RadOnc(00,NY48)<NJ-CLARMAAS>
+ Clara Maass Medical Center
1 Clara Maass Drive/RadOnc   Belleville, NJ 07109
(973)450-2000

Borole, Swapna M., MD {1295986289} Pedtrc
+ RWJ University Hospital New Brunswick
One Robert Wood Johnson Place   New Brunswick, NJ 08901
(732)235-5709   Fax (732)235-6102

Borow, Leslie Bennett, MD {1336128487} Anesth(98,NJ05)<NJ-ENGLWOOD>
+ Englewood Hospital and Medical Center
350 Engle Street   Englewood, NJ 07631   (201)894-3000
Fax (201)871-0619

Borowski, Michelle, DO {1902027790} InfDis
+ 443 Northfield Avenue/Suite 306
West Orange, NJ 07052

Borowski, Walter J., MD {1912090168} IntrMd(82,POL03)
+ Drs. Borowski & Kibilska-Borowski
812 North Wood Avenue/Suite 101   Linden, NJ 07036
(908)486-3366

Borowsky, Larry M., MD {1174506729} IntrMd, Gastrn(80,PA09)<NJ-KMHTURNV>
+ Philadelphia Gastroenterology Group, P.C.
570 Egg Harbor Road/Suite A-2   Sewell, NJ 08080
(856)218-1410   Fax (856)218-0193

Borra, Gayatri D., MD {1972676112} IntrMd(00,INA4D)<NJ-COOPRUMC>
+ Cooper University Hospital
One Cooper Plaza   Camden, NJ 08103   (856)342-2000

Borromeo, Rita Gonzalez, MD {1366474942} ObsGyn(92,IL11)
+ Penn Medicine at Cherry Hill
409 Route 70 East   Cherry Hill, NJ 08034   (856)795-0587
Fax (856)795-0689

Borromeo, Virginia, MD {1972649333} Pedtrc(68,PHI01)<NJ-STPETER, NJ-RBAYOLDB>
+ 25 Briarwood Drive
Matawan, NJ 07747

Borrus, Stephen W., MD {1619980307} IntrMd(73,NJ05)<NJ-CHS-FULD>
+ Lawrence Medical Associates PA
2999 Princeton Pike   Lawrenceville, NJ 08648   (609)882-2299   Fax (609)538-8230

Borthwick, James Malcolm, MD {1366655052} Psychy(99,PA02)
+ 166 Bunn Drive
Princeton, NJ 08540   (609)688-9800   Fax (609)921-8355

Bortnichak, Paula M., MD {1326200106} PsyFor, Psychy, IntrMd(76,PA01)
+ 310 Ocean Avenue North/Unit 13
Long Branch, NJ 07740

Bortnik, Kristy E., MD {1376748780} Psychy
+ Northeast Regional Epilepsy Group
20 Prospect Avenue/Suite 800   Hackensack, NJ 07601
(201)343-6676   Fax (201)343-6689

Bortniker, David Leonard, MD {1033156286} Otlryg, SrgCsm, SrgHdN(80,NY46)<NJ-SOMERSET>
+ Ear, Nose & Throat Care, P.C.
242 East Main Street   Somerville, NJ 08876   (908)704-9696
Fax (908)704-0097
+ Raritan Valley Surgery Center
100 Franklin Square Drive/Suite 100   Somerset, NJ 08873
(908)704-9696   Fax (732)560-5999

Borton, Miriam A., MD {1275639601} Psychy(75,MEXI)
+ American Institute for Counseling
1952 US Highway 22/Suite 102   Bound Brook, NJ 08805
(732)469-6444   Fax (732)469-6445
dr.borton@hotmail.com

Boruchoff, Susan E., MD {1659459626} InfDis, IntrMd(82,NY01)<NJ-RWJUBRUN>
+ Rutgers RWJ Allergy, Immunology and Infectious Group
125 Paterson Street   New Brunswick, NJ 08901   (732)235-7060

Boruchow, Scott D., MD {1891775755} RadDia, Radiol(94,NY09)<NJ-JFKMED>
+ Edison Radiology Group, P.A.
65 James Street   Edison, NJ 08820   (732)321-7917   Fax (732)737-2968
+ JFK Medical Center
65 James Street/Radiology   Edison, NJ 08820   (732)321-7000

Boruta, Andrew Michael, DO {1972771772} Anesth(07,MI12)
+ 54 Moore Avenue
Waldwick, NJ 07463

Boscamp, Jeffrey R., MD {1477563286} PedInf, Pedtrc(81,NY09)<NJ-HACKNSK, NJ-HOLYNAME>
+ Joseph M. Sanzari ChildrenÆs Hospital
30 Prospect Avenue/Pediatrics   Hackensack, NJ 07602
(201)996-2000
+ Hackensack University Medical Center
30 Prospect Avenue/Pediatrics   Hackensack, NJ 07601
(201)996-2000   Fax (201)996-9815
+ Pediatric Infectious Disease/Hackensack Univ Med Ctr
30 Prospect Avenue   Hackensack, NJ 07602   (201)996-5308   Fax (201)996-9815

Bose, Konika Paul, MD {1336470228} IntrMd, Gastrn
+ Summit Medical Group
1 Diamond Hill Road/Bensley Pav/2 FL   Berkeley, NJ 07922
(908)277-8700   Fax (908)288-7993

Physicians by Name and Address

Bosin, Corey S., MD {1912051970} ObsGyn, Gyneco(88,GRNA)<NJ-STPETER, NJ-SOMERSET>
+ Central Jersey Women's Health Associates, PC
1 Robertson Drive/Suite 25   Bedminster, NJ 07921
(908)532-0788   Fax (908)532-0787

Bosompem, Daryl Ama, MD {1205217569} EmrgMd
+ Hackensack Medical Center Emergency Medicine
30 Prospect Avenue/Main 3619   Hackensack, NJ 07601
(551)996-2331   Fax (201)968-1866

Boss, David T., MD {1194877589} Gastrn, IntrMd(85,MA16)<NJ-OCEANMC>
+ Ocean Medical Center
425 Jack Martin Boulevard/Gastro   Brick, NJ 08723
(732)840-2200

Boss, William K., Jr., MD {1598769317} SrgCsm, SrgMcr, SrgHnd(75,NJ05)<NJ-HACKNSK, NJ-VALLEY>
+ Sidney Rabinowitz & William K. Boss M.D., P.A.
305 North Route 17/Suite 3-100A   Paramus, NJ 07652
(201)967-1100   Fax (201)967-9300

Bosscher, James Reed, MD {1265522627} GynOnc(79,MI07)
+ Meridian Obstetrics amd Gynecology Associates PC
19 Davis Avenue/Fl 1   Neptune, NJ 07753   (570)336-2689
Fax (732)922-8264
james.bosscher@gmail.com
+ Hackensack Meridian Health Gyn Oncology
1 Riverview Plaza   Red Bank, NJ 07701   (570)336-2689
Fax (732)268-8474

Bosworth, Eric, MD {1154327013} RadDia, RadNuc(91,CT02)<NJ-STFRNMED>
+ Radiology Affiliates of Central New Jersey, P.A.
2501 Kuser Road   Hamilton, NJ 08691   (609)585-8800
Fax (609)585-1825
+ Radiology Affiliates of Central New Jersey, P.A.
3120 Princeton Pike   Lawrenceville, NJ 08648   (609)585-8800   Fax (609)219-0439

Botea, Andrei, MD {1609920842} Anesth, CritCr, CarAne(92,RUS35)<NJ-UMDNJ>
+ University Hospital
150 Bergen Street/Anesth   Newark, NJ 07103   (973)972-5254   Fax (973)972-4172

Botros, Carolyn, DO {1003243361} ObsGyn<NJ-MORRISTN>
+ Morristown Medical Center
100 Madison Avenue   Morristown, NJ 07962   (973)971-5233

Botros, Lamia Kamel, MD {1366536682} Psychy(88,EGY03)<NY-ROCKLPSY>
+ 589 Franklin Turnpike
Ridgewood, NJ 07450   (201)956-1422

Botros, Nashed G., MD {1689793275} Gastrn, IntrMd(80,EGY08)<NJ-STPETER>
+ 37 Brunswick Woods Drive
East Brunswick, NJ 08816   (732)967-9595   Fax (732)967-0711
+ Cares Surgicenter, LLC.
240 Easton Avenue   New Brunswick, NJ 08901   (732)967-9595   Fax (732)296-8677

Botrous, Suzanne W., MD {1992861116} Pedtrc(84,EGY04)<NJ-ST-BARNMC, NJ-NWRKBETH>
+ Mediterranean Pediatrics
185 Central Avenue/Suite 308   East Orange, NJ 07018
(973)678-3776   Fax (973)678-6065
centralpediatrics@msn.com

Botti, Anthony C., MD {1598787640} Hemato, MedOnc, IntrMd(82,SPA11)<NJ-STBARNMC>
+ Livingston Subspecialty Group, P.A.
349 East Northfield Road/Suite 200   Livingston, NJ 07039
(973)597-0900   Fax (973)597-0910

Botti, Carla G., DO {1396963401} FamMed(97,MO79)
+ Johnson & Johnson
1 Johnson & Johnson/EmpHlth Rm5G32   New Brunswick, NJ 08933   (732)524-3000   Fax (732)828-5493

Bottiglieri, Thomas S., DO {1669496469} SprtMd, FamMed(04,NJ75)
+ Columbia Grand Orthopaedics
500 Grand Avenue/Suite 101   Englewood, NJ 07631
(201)569-0440   Fax (201)569-4949

Botu, Devi Prasad, MD {1841440096} IntHos<NJ-OCEANMC>
+ Ocean Medical Center
425 Jack Martin Boulevard   Brick, NJ 08723   (480)543-7004
Fax (480)393-2989
deviprasad.botu@apogeephysicians.com

Botvinov, Mikhail A., DO {1760685622} Surgry
+ Advanced Laparoscopic Surgeons of Morris
83 Hanover Road/Suite 190   Florham Park, NJ 07932
(973)410-9700   Fax (973)410-9703
+ JFK for Life
98 James Street/Suite 212   Edison, NJ 08820   (732)343-7484

Physicians by Name and Address

Botwin, Clifford A., DO {1689673352} SrgOrt(71,MO78)<NJ-OVERLOOK>
+ Associated Orthopaedics
  1000 Galloping Hill Road,/Suite 202   Union, NJ 07083   (908)964-6600   Fax (908)364-1025
+ Associated Orthopaedics
  654 Broadway   Bayonne, NJ 07002   (908)964-6600   Fax (201)436-8110

Boucard, Herve C., MD {1891674718} IntrMd, Gastrn(00,PA01)
+ Hamilton Gastroenterology Group, PC
  1374 Whitehorse Hamilton Squar   Trenton, NJ 08690   (609)586-1319   Fax (609)586-1468

Boucher, Gregory M., DO {1295990042} Surgry
+ 7300 River Road
  North Bergen, NJ 07047

Boucree, Thaddeus Stanice, MD {1942464417}
+ The Plastic Surgery Ctr of NJ & Manhat
  535 Sycamore Avenue   Shrewsbury, NJ 07702   (732)741-0970   Fax (732)747-2606

Boudwin, James E., MD {1467597922} FamMed(80,NJ06)<NJ-RWJUBRUN, NJ-STPETER>
+ RWJPE Dayton Medical Group
  12 Stults Road/Suite 121   Dayton, NJ 08810   (732)329-8600   Fax (609)395-7519

Bouffard, John Paul, MD {1306801931} PthNro(90,MD12)<NJ-OVERLOOK, NJ-MORRISTN>
+ Overlook Medical Center
  99 Beauvoir Avenue/PO Box 210   Summit, NJ 07902   (908)522-2000

Bough, Irvin David, Jr., MD {1598710899} Otlryg, IntrMd(89,PA02)<NJ-VALLEY>
+ ENT & Allergy Associates, LLP
  690 Kinderkamack Road/Suite 101   Oradell, NJ 07649   (201)722-9850   Fax (201)722-9851
  dbough@entandallergy.com

Bouillon, Louis R., MD {1730274473} SrgOrt(79,QU03)
+ Orthopedic Associates of West Jersey
  600 Mount Pleasant Avenue/Suite A   Dover, NJ 07801   (973)989-0888   Fax (973)989-0885

Boujaoude, Ziad C., MD {1619954286} PulDis
+ Three Cooper Plaza/Suite 312
  Camden, NJ 08103

Boukiia, Marina, MD {1588667711} Anesth(85,RUS06)<NJ-STMRYPAS>
+ St. Mary's Hospital
  350 Boulevard   Passaic, NJ 07055   (973)365-4300

Boulghassoul-Pietrzykows, Nadia, MD {1346401528} IntrMd(96,POL03)
+ Pathlink, LLC
  66 West Gilbert Street/Suite 100   Tinton Falls, NJ 07701   (732)212-0060   Fax (732)212-0061
+ 1901 North Olden Avenue/Suite 29
  Ewing, NJ 08618   (609)882-1686

Boulos, Mona, MD {1043316565} Pedtrc(84,EGY04)<NJ-CHRIST>
+ 2780 Kennedy Boulevard
  Jersey City, NJ 07306   (201)239-7777   Fax (201)239-0070

Boulos, Nader, MD {1518971456} EmrgMd, EmrgEMed(98,NJ06)<NJ-STJOSHOS>
+ St Joseph's Medical Center Emergency
  703 Main Street   Paterson, NJ 07503   (973)754-2240   Fax (973)754-2249

Boulware, Jason Peter, DO {1013211168} EmrgMd(08,NY75)<RI-SJFATIMA>
+ Emergency Medical Associates of NJ, P.A.
  3 Century Drive   Parsippany, NJ 07054   (877)692-4665   Fax (973)740-9895
  jasonboulware@hotmail.com

Bourne, Jeffrey Alan, MD {1457311920} Pedtrc(74,MO34)<NJ-CHRIST, NJ-CLARMAAS>
+ Bourne Pediatrics
  431 60th Street   West New York, NJ 07093   (201)854-0303   Fax (201)854-0982

Boutros, Maged T., MD {1497785281} IntrMd(03,NET09)<NJ-MTNSIDE>
+ Prevention Clinics of New Jersey
  1033 Route 46/Suite G-1   Clifton, NJ 07013   (973)777-3711

Boutsikaris, Amy Shah, MD {1407017064}<NJ-STPETER>
+ St. Peter's University Hospital
  254 Easton Avenue   New Brunswick, NJ 08901   (732)745-8600

Boutsikaris, Daniel Gregory, MD {1922267822} EmrgMd
+ Robert Wood Johnson Emergency Medicine
  One Robert Wood Johnson Place/MEB 104   New Brunswick, NJ 08901   (973)461-9664

Bouyea, Michelle Marie, MD {1124001797} Anesth(92,NY03)
+ Robert Wood Johnson-UMDNJ Anesthesia Group
  1140 Route 72 West   Manahawkin, NJ 08050   (609)978-8900

Bouzane, Gayten Carroll, MD {1770806200} PhysMd(89,NY47)
+ Studio 39 West Medical Spa
  39 Littleton Road   Parsippany, NJ 07054   (973)334-0014   Fax (973)334-0155
+ 45 Briarcliff Road
  Mountain Lakes, NJ 07046

Bove, Joseph, DO {1972943652} EmrgMd<NJ-WAYNEGEN>
+ St. Joseph's Wayne Hospital
  224 Hamburg Turnpike   Wayne, NJ 07470   (973)956-3333

Bowe, John A., MD {1861597221} SrgOrt(76,NY01)
+ Pediatric Orthopedic Associates, P.A.
  585 Cranbury Road/Suite A   East Brunswick, NJ 08816   (732)390-1160   Fax (732)390-8449
+ Pediatric Orthopedic Associates, P.A.
  3700 State Route 33   Neptune, NJ 07753   (732)390-1160   Fax (732)897-4205

Bowen, Frank Winslow, III, MD {1467496612} Surgry, SrgCTh, CdvDis(96,PA01)
+ Cooper Surgical Associates
  3 Cooper Plaza/Suite 411   Camden, NJ 08103   (856)342-2270   Fax (856)365-1180

Bowen, Jay E., DO {1821625370} PhysMd, SprtMd(94,NY75)
+ New Jersey Sports Medicine
  197 Ridgedale Avenue/Suite 210   Cedar Knolls, NJ 07927   (973)998-8301   Fax (973)998-8302

Bowen, Zakia Dele, MD {1982937931} IntrMd
+ Apogee Physicians
  201 Lyons Avenue   Newark, NJ 07112   (973)926-2164   Fax (973)391-8524

Bowers, Andrea Legath, MD {1831259753} SrgOrt, SprtMd(04,TN05)
+ Burlington County Orthopaedic Specialists, PA
  204 Ark Road/Suite 105   Mount Laurel, NJ 08054   (856)235-7080   Fax (856)273-6384

Bowers, Charles, Jr., MD {1659373926} SrgOrt(79,NJ05)<NJ-STBARNMC>
+ 312 Briant Park Drive
  Springfield, NJ 07081

Bowers, Gabriela W., MD {1316996853} IntrMd(00,NJ06)
+ Windsor Regional Medical Associates, LLC
  300A Princeton-Hightstown Road   East Windsor, NJ 08520   (609)490-0095   Fax (609)490-0091

Bowers, Geoffrey David, MD {1740496991} ObsGyn
+ Garden State Obstetrics and Gynecological Associates
  2401 Evesham Road/Suite A   Voorhees, NJ 08043   (856)424-3323   Fax (856)424-4994

Bowers, Mamie Sue, MD {1124014402} ObsGyn(85,NJ06)<NJ-HUNTRDN>
+ All Women's Healthcare
  1100 Wescott Drive/Suite 105   Flemington, NJ 08822   (908)788-6469   Fax (908)788-6483

Bowers, Steven Richard, DO {1548436884} FamMed
+ Shore Physicians Group
  2605 Shore Road   Northfield, NJ 08225   (609)365-5300   Fax (609)365-5301

Bowers Pepe, Jessica Sue, DO {1699988212} FamMed, EmrgMd(00,NJ75)
+ 400 North Church Street
  Moorestown, NJ 08057   (609)410-3078

Bowie, Lester J., MD {1912914599} Anesth(86,NJ06)<NJ-LOURDMED>
+ Rancocas Anesthesiology, PA
  700 Route 130 North/Suite 203   Cinnaminson, NJ 08077   (856)829-9345   Fax (856)829-3605

Bowman, Cynthia L., MD {1962566869} PthACl, Pthlgy(74,TN05)
+ VA New Jersey Health Care System-East Orange Campus
  385 Tremont Avenue   East Orange, NJ 07018   (774)254-0746

Boxer, Andrew Scott, MD {1225294499} Gastrn, IntrMd(07,NJ02)
+ Gastroenterology Associates of New Jersey
  1011 Clifton Avenue   Clifton, NJ 07013   (973)471-8200   Fax (973)471-3032
+ Gastroenterology Associates of New Jersey
  71 Union Avenue/Suite 210   Rutherford, NJ 07070   (973)471-8200   Fax (201)896-0863

Boxer, Douglas C., MD {1063456754} RadDia(92,NY46)
+ Toms River X-Ray
  154 Highway 37 West   Toms River, NJ 08753   (732)244-0777   Fax (732)244-0428

Boxman, Jeffrey R., DO {1376548172} Nrolgy(92,IA75)<NJ-SHOREMEM>
+ Neurology Institute South Jersey
  436 Chris Gaupp Drive/Suite 104   Galloway, NJ 08205   (609)748-6696   Fax (609)748-6693

Boyajian, Robert Wayne, MD {1174547426} IntrMd(82,MEX03)<NJ-HACKNSK, NJ-CHRIST>
+ Robert Wayne Boyajian MD PA
  255 Route 3 East/Suite 203   Secaucus, NJ 07094   (201)865-3100   Fax (201)865-8311

Boyajian, Stephen S., DO {1073547311} AnesPain, Anesth(84,IL76)<NJ-VIRTVOOR, NJ-KENEDYHS>
+ Advanced Pain Consultants, P.A.
  326 Route 73   Voorhees, NJ 08043   (856)489-9822   Fax (856)489-9877
+ Advanced Pain Consultants, P.A.
  120 Madison Avenue/Suite D   Mount Holly, NJ 08060   (609)267-1707
+ Advanced Pain Consultants, P.A.
  1401 Whitehorse Mercerville Rd   Hamilton, NJ 08043   (609)528-8888   Fax (609)584-5151

Boyan, William P., MD {1679568877} Grtrcs, IntrMd(83,GRNA)<NJ-OCEANMC>
+ Shore Medical Group
  1640 Highway 88/Suite 203   Brick, NJ 08724   (732)458-7777   Fax (732)263-9470

Boyarsky, Yael, MD {1528290897} Pedtrc(06,NY46)
+ North Jersey Pediatrics
  17-10 Fair Lawn Avenue   Fair Lawn, NJ 07410   (201)794-8585   Fax (201)703-9889

Boyd, Linda, DO {1316969132} FamMed(84,NJ75)<NJ-UMDNJ, NJ-RWJUBRUN>
+ The University Doctors - UMDNJ -SOM
  570 Egg Harbor Road/Suite C-2   Sewell, NJ 08080   (856)218-0300   Fax (856)589-5082
+ New Jersey Family Practice Center (NJFPC)
  90 Bergen Street/DOC 300/Lower Level   Newark, NJ 07103   (856)218-0300   Fax (973)972-2754
+ University Hospital-Doctors Office Center
  90 Bergen Street   Newark, NJ 08080   (973)972-2500

Boyd, Marvin T., MD {1417095126} Nephro, IntrMd(74,NY06)
+ 791 14th Avenue
  Paterson, NJ 07504

Boyd, Robert D., DO {1548474257} FamMed, GenPrc(74,IA75)<NJ-JFKMED>
+ Woodbridge Medical Group PA
  270 Main Street   Woodbridge, NJ 07095   (732)636-5252   Fax (732)636-5452

Boyd-Woschinko, Gillian Susanne, MD {1639336175} IntrMd, EnDbMt(07,PA02)
+ Valley Medical Group-Endocrinology
  947 Linwood Avenue/Suite 1W   Ridgewood, NJ 07450   (201)444-5552   Fax (201)444-4490

Boye-Nolan, Melinda L., DO {1760438626} EmrgMd(94,NJ75)<NJ-SOCEANCO>
+ Southern Ocean County Medical Center
  1140 Route 72 West/EMCARE   Manahawkin, NJ 08050   (609)978-8900
  mbtangle@aol.com

Boylan, Edward F., MD {1144286105} IntrMd, EmrgMd(87,GRN01)<NJ-CHRIST>
+ Midtown Primary Care LLC
  550 Newark Avenue/Suite 308   Jersey City, NJ 07306   (201)656-2300   Fax (201)656-2390

Boyle, Elizabeth Anne, DO {1336220300} ObsGyn, Gyneco(86,NJ75)<NJ-STJOSHOS>
+ Clifton Ob/Gyn
  1033 Route 46 East/Suite 102   Clifton, NJ 07013   (973)779-7979   Fax (973)779-7970

Boyle, Jay Owen, MD {1427030667} Otlryg(90,AZ01)<NY-SLOAN-KET>
+ Memorial Sloan-Kettering Cancer Center Basking Ridge
  136 Mountain View Boulevard   Basking Ridge, NJ 07920   (908)542-3000   Fax (908)542-3220

Boyle, Maria Pilar T., MD {1083758775} Pedtrc(88,PHI01)
+ 260 Chestnut Street/2 FL
  Newark, NJ 07105   (973)578-4745

Boynton, Christopher J., MD {1265433536} Surgry(82,NJ06)
+ Surgical Specialists of New Jersey
  668 Main Street/Suite 4   Lumberton, NJ 08048   (609)267-7050   Fax (609)267-7065

Bozdogan, Ulas, MD {1417112731} ObsGyn(97,TUR01)
+ 140 Prospect Avenue/Suite 15
  Hackensack, NJ 07601   (201)880-6181   Fax (201)880-6184

Bozic, Vladimir Stefan, MD {1871798777} SrgOrt
+ Orthopedic & Neurosurgical Specialists, LLC.
  807 Haddon Avenue/Suite 1   Haddonfield, NJ 08033   (856)795-9222   Fax (856)795-0026

Brabson, Thomas A., DO {1356397590} EmrgMd, EmrgEMed(89,PA77)<NJ-ACMCITY>
+ Medical Associates of North Jersey PA
  525 Wanaque Avenue   Pompton Lakes, NJ 07442   (973)839-3333   Fax (973)839-0580

Brabston, Timothy B., MD {1184607863} IntrMd, Grtrcs(95,NJ05)<NJ-CHILTON>
+ Medical Associates of North Jersey PA
  525 Wanaque Avenue   Pompton Lakes, NJ 07442   (973)839-3333   Fax (973)839-0580

Brachman, Gwen O., MD {1174737985} IntrMd, OccpMd, Rheuma(82,MA05)
+ University Hospital-Doctors Office Center
  90 Bergen Street/4600 DOC   Newark, NJ 07103   (973)972-2900   Fax (973)972-2904
  brachmgo@umdnj.edu

Bracilovic, Ana, MD {1598944258} PhysMd
+ Princeton Spine and Joint Center
601 Ewing Street/Suite A-2 Princeton, NJ 08540
(609)454-0760   Fax (609)454-0761

Brackenrich, Justin, DO {1669852729}<NJ-PALISADE>
+ Palisades Medical Center
7600 River Road North Bergen, NJ 07047 (201)854-5000

Brackett, Valerie A., MD {1992964738} IntrMd, OccpMd(81,GER16)
+ 6 Stewart Road
Short Hills, NJ 07078 (973)376-5036

Brackin, Phillip Snowden, Jr., MD {1598754640} Urolgy(98,PA01)<NJ-RWJBURUN>
+ Urology Care Alliance
2105 Klockner Road Hamilton, NJ 08690 (609)588-0770 Fax (609)588-0454

Bradish, Glen Edward, MD {1275584526} SprtMd, SrgOrt(95,NJ05)<NJ-NWTNMEM>
+ Andover Orthopaedic Surgery & Sports
280 Newton-Sparta Road/Suite 4 Newton, NJ 07860
(973)579-7443 Fax (973)579-5628
+ Andover Orthopaedic Surgery & Sports
452 Route 206 Montague, NJ 07827 (973)579-7443 Fax (973)293-7581

Bradley, Douglas D., MD {1740280148} SrgOrt, SrgSpn(81,NY15)
+ The Back Institute
700 Rahway Avenue/Suite A-14 Union, NJ 07083
(908)688-1999 Fax (908)688-8180

Bradley, Jacquelyn, DO {1346627957} IntrMd<NJ-UMDNJ>
+ University Hospital
150 Bergen Street Newark, NJ 07103 (973)972-5672 Fax (973)972-0365

Bradley, Kathleen A., MD {1073694535} FamMed, Pedtrc, IntrMd(93,PA13)<NJ-VIRTMHBC>
+ Virtua Family Medicine
1605 Evesham Road/Suite 100 Voorhees, NJ 08043
(856)741-7100 Fax (856)424-2629

Bradshaw, Chanda M., MD {1962677971} Pedtrc, NnPnMd(NY20
+ CHOP Care Network at Princeton Medical Center
One Plainsboro Road Plainsboro, NJ 08536 (609)853-7000 Fax (609)497-4173

Bradway, William R., DO {1740224633} PulDis, SlpDis, IntrMd(77,IA75)<NJ-BURDTMLN>
+ Regional Heart & Lung Associates
207 Court House/S. Dennis Road Cape May Court House, NJ 08210 (609)465-2001 Fax (609)465-8440

Brady, Mary E., MD {1811093768} PhysMd(91,NJ05)<NJ-STCLR DOV, NJ-STCLRDEN>
+ St. Clare's Hospital-Dover
400 West Blackwell Street Dover, NJ 07801 (973)989-3000

Brady, Robert David, DO {1851335319} PhysMd, PainMd(94,NJ75)
+ New Jersey Spine and Sports Medicine PC
84 Orient Way Rutherford, NJ 07070 (201)964-0200 Fax (201)964-0220

Braff, Ricky A., MD {1083688956} IntrMd, Pedtrc(87,NY48)<NJ-HUNTRDN>
+ Hunterdon Pediatric Associates
1738 Route 31 North/Suite 201 Clinton, NJ 08809
(908)735-3960 Fax (908)735-3965

Braga, Gene J., MD {1336118835} Urolgy, IntrMd(83,MO07)<NJ-BURDTMLN, NJ-SHOREMEM>
+ Pagnani, Braga, & Kimmel Urologic Associates PA
229 Shore Road Somers Point, NJ 08244 (609)653-4343 Fax (609)653-2060
+ Pagnani, Braga, & Kimmel Urologic Associates PA
222 New Road/Building 700 Linwood, NJ 08221 (609)653-4343 Fax (609)601-9630
+ Pagnani, Braga, & Kimmel Urologic Associates PA
8 Court House South Dennis Rd Cape May Court House, NJ 08244 (609)465-4404

Braganza, Armando M., MD {1962565416} Psychy(76,PHIL)
+ Mt. Carmel Guild/Behavioral Health
285 Magnolia Avenue Jersey City, NJ 07304 (201)395-5400

Brahmbhatt, Gaurang Ravaji, MD {1225204266} FamMed(99,MNT01)
+ Riverside Medical Group
609 Washington Street Hoboken, NJ 07030 (201)706-8490 Fax (201)706-8491
+ Center for Family Health
122-132 Clinton Street Hoboken, NJ 07030 (201)706-8490 Fax (201)418-3148

Brahmbhatt, Ravikumar B., MD {1073816351} SrgTrm(97,INA21)<NJ-CHOSHUDC>
+ RR Surgical Associates
906 Oak Tree Road/Suite J South Plainfield, NJ 07080
(908)668-1400 Fax (908)222-8770
+ Hudson Surgeons
142 Palisade Avenue/Suite 108 Jersey City, NJ 07306

(908)668-1400   Fax (201)795-3550

Brahmbhatt, Sapna Sureshkumar, MD {1831163278} Otlryg, Otolgy(95,NJ05)<NJ-CENTRAST>
+ 222 Schanck Road/Suite 200
Freehold, NJ 07728 (732)683-2083

Brahms, Dana Lyn Satomi, MD {1588730667} IntrMd(01,NJ06)<NJ-HCKTSTWN, NJ-MORRISTN>
+ Physicians Health Alliance
28 Jackson Avenue Pompton Plains, NJ 07444 (973)835-2575 Fax (973)835-0531

Brahver, Danit Vera, MD {1952661514} FamMed(12,NJ02)
+ Planned Parenthood
69 East Newman Springs Road/PO Box 95 Shrewsbury, NJ 07702 (732)842-9300 Fax (732)842-9338

Braimbridge, Sandra P., MD {1538363833} IntrMd(95,NJ05)<NJ-SOMERSET>
+ RWJ University Hospital Somerset
110 Rehill Avenue Somerville, NJ 08876 (908)685-2200

Bram, Harris N., MD {1922056936} Anesth(88,AR01)<NJ-MONMOUTH, NJ-KIMBALL>
+ New Jersey Pain Care Specialists
1806 Highway 35/Suite 30 Oakhurst, NJ 07755 (732)720-0247 Fax (732)508-9100

Bramble, Charlene A., MD {1528048907} ObsGyn, IntrMd(83,NJ05)<NJ-VIRTBERL, NJ-VIRTVOOR>
+ Rowan SOM Department of Ob/Gyn
405 Hurffville-Cross Keys Road Sewell, NJ 08080
(856)589-1414 Fax (856)256-5772

Bramlette, James G.s., MD {1316070881} RadDia<NJ-HACKNSK>
+ Hackensack University Medical Center
30 Prospect Avenue Hackensack, NJ 07601 (551)996-2200 Fax (201)489-2812

Bramwell, Julia, MD {1740224773} Pedtrc(98,NJ06)<NJ-MOR RISTN, NJ-NWRKBETH>
+ Holistic Pediatrics
2200 Route 10 West/Suite 106 Parsippany, NJ 07054
(973)401-1818 Fax (973)401-1878
info@holisticpediatrics.net

Bramwit, Mark P., MD {1811979164} RadDia(93,NY47)<NJ-RWJUBRUN, NJ-STPETER>
+ University Radiology Group, P.C.
483 Cranbury Road East Brunswick, NJ 08816 (732)390-0030 Fax (732)390-5383
+ University Radiology Group, P.C.
10 Plum Street New Brunswick, NJ 08901 (732)390-0030 Fax (732)249-1208
+ University Radiology Group, P.C.
75 Veronica Avenue Somerset, NJ 08816 (732)246-0060 Fax (732)246-4188

Brana-Leon, Hazel A., MD {1750515227} ObsGyn(03,MEX14)<NJ-CHRIST>
+ WomenÆs Health Partners PC Teaneck
222 Cedar Lane/Suite 204 Teaneck, NJ 07666 (201)836-4025 Fax (201)836-4056

Brancato, Jaclyn, DO {1306195367} IntrMd(NJ75<NJ-JRSYCITY>
+ Summit Medical Group
6 Brighton Road/2 FL Clifton, NJ 07012 (973)777-7911 Fax (973)777-5403
+ Atlantic Medical Group
1395 Route 23/Suite 4 Butler, NJ 07405 (973)777-7911 Fax (973)838-1614

Brancato, Peter, Jr., MD {1760578892} PsyCAd, Psychy(75,PA01)<NJ-SJERSYHS, NJ-LOURDMED>
+ Center for Family Guidance, PC
765 East Route 70/Building A-101 Marlton, NJ 08053
(856)797-4800 Fax (856)810-0110

Brand-Abend, Lori M., MD {1184606329} RadDia, Radiol, IntrMd(87,NJ06)<NJ-STPETER, NJ-RWJUBRUN>
+ University Radiology Group, P.C.
48 Gilbert Street North Tinton Falls, NJ 07701 (732)530-5750 Fax (732)530-5848

Brandeisky, Thomas E., DO {1306816301} Otlryg, SrgFPl, SrgHdN(87,NJ75)<NJ-OCEANMC>
+ ENT & Facial Plastic Surgery Assocs
1608 Route 88/Suite 240 Brick, NJ 08724 (732)458-8575 Fax (732)206-0578

Brandi, Kristyn M., MD {1356630107} ObsGyn
+ University Physician Associates
140 Bergen Street/ACC Level C Newark, NJ 07103
(973)972-2700 Fax (973)972-2739

Brandon, Meredith, MD {1902172265} PsyCAd
+ St. Clare's Health Services
50 Morris Avenue Denville, NJ 07834 (973)625-7062

Brandsma, Erik, MD {1013243112} NnPnMd(04,NET03)
+ The Children's Regional Hospital at Cooper Univ Hosp
One Cooper Plaza/Drrnce 755 Camden, NJ 08103
(856)342-2000
+ Joseph M. Sanzari ChildrenÆs Hospital
30 Prospect Avenue Hackensack, NJ 07602 (856)342-2000 Fax (551)996-3051

Brandspiegel, Laura K., MD {1700830676} Pedtrc(95,PA02)<NJ-CHSMRCER, NJ-RWJUHAM>
+ Advocare Garden State Pediatrics
2133 Highway 33 Trenton, NJ 08690 (609)581-5100 Fax (609)581-5134
DrLauraB@netzero.net

Brandstaedter, Karen Hardy, MD {1730343468} Pedtrc(05,NY01)<NJ-OVERLOOK, NJ-STBARNMC>
+ Watchung Pediatrics
76 Stirling Road/Suite 201 Warren, NJ 07059 (908)755-5437 Fax (908)755-6905
+ Watchung Pediatrics
346 South Avenue/Suite 3 Fanwood, NJ 07023 (908)755-5437 Fax (908)889-0047
+ Watchung Pediatrics
225 Millburn Avenue/Suite 301 Millburn, NJ 07059
(973)376-7337 Fax (973)218-6647

Brandt, Frederick W., MD {1528008737} IntrMd, Rheuma(80,NY03)
+ Arthritis Center of New Jersey
600 Pavonia Avenue/5th Floor Jersey City, NJ 07306
(201)216-3050 Fax (201)499-0254

Brandt, Justin Samuel, MD {1184884140} MtFtMd, ObsGyn(08,PA02)<NJ-HACKNSK>
+ Hackensack University Medical Center
30 Prospect Avenue/OB/GYN Hackensack, NJ 07601
(551)996-2453 Fax (201)678-9189

Brandt, Suzanne Marie, MD {1508017427} PthACl
+ The Valley Hospital
223 North Van Dien Avenue Ridgewood, NJ 07450
(201)447-8242

Brandt-Park, Nicole, MD {1417419797} GenPrc
+ Sunset Road Medical Associates
911 Sunset Road Burlington, NJ 08016 (609)387-8787
Fax (609)386-8640

Brannan, Timothy S., MD {1619946431} Nrolgy(75,PA12)<NY-MTSINAI>
+ Liberty Medical Associates
377 Jersey Avenue/Suite 470 Jersey City, NJ 07302
(201)918-2239 Fax (201)918-2243

Branovan, Zhanna Emilia, MD {1881657328} IntrMd(96,NY46)<NJ-CHILTON>
+ Advanced Internal Medicine of NorthJersey
1680 Route 23 North/Suite 310 Wayne, NJ 07470
(973)835-6300 Fax (973)831-1460

Bransfield, Robert C., MD {1467449769} Psychy(72,DC01)<NJ-RIVERVW>
+ 225 Highway 35
Red Bank, NJ 07701 (732)741-3263 Fax (732)741-5308

Brar, Harleen, MD {1528177565} IntrMd, Rheuma(84,INA78)
+ Drs. Brar and Chatterjee
1031 McBride Avenue/Suite D-209 West Paterson, NJ 07424 (973)785-3455 Fax (973)785-4353
+ Drs. Brar and Chatterjee
542 East 29th Street Paterson, NJ 07504 (973)977-2250

Brar, Navdeep K., MD {1811254337} PulDis<NJ-DEBRAHLC>
+ Deborah Heart and Lung Center
200 Trenton Road Browns Mills, NJ 08015 (609)893-6611

Brar, Navtej Singh, DO {1255515292} CdvDis, IntrMd(04,AZ02)
+ St. Luke's Cardiology Associates
755 Memorial Parkway Phillipsburg, NJ 08865 (908)859-0514 Fax (908)859-0515

Brasile, Deanna Rose, DO {1457334047} ObsGyn, RprEnd(99,PA77)<NJ-COOPRUMC>
+ Cooper Institute for Reproductive Hormonal Disorders
17000 Commerce Parkway/Suite C Mount Laurel, NJ 08054
(856)751-5575 Fax (856)751-7289
+ Cooper Ob/Gyn
3 Cooper Plaza/Suite 300 Camden, NJ 08103 (856)751-5575 Fax (856)968-8575

Braslavsky, Gregory, MD {1255373726} Hemato, IntrMd, MedOnc(83,UKRA)<NJ-MONMOUTH, NJ-RIVERVW>
+ 127 Pavilion Avenue
Long Branch, NJ 07740 (732)222-4740 Fax (732)222-9345
gbrasl@hotmail.com

Brattelli, Gary Joseph, DO {1215973649} IntrMd(98,NJ75)<NJ-VIRTBERL, NJ-VIRTVOOR>
+ 532 Berlin Cross Keys Road
Sicklerville, NJ 08081 (856)728-8110 Fax (856)262-1936

Brauer, Howard E., MD {1164530838} Pedtrc(75,NJ05)<NJ-STPETER, NJ-RWJUBRUN>
+ Plaza Pediatrics
1950 State Highway 27 North/Suite HH North Brunswick, NJ 08902 (732)940-5511 Fax (732)940-0530

Brault, Peter V., MD {1306827258} Pedtrc(76,MA07)
+ Paterson Community Health Center
32 Clinton Street Paterson, NJ 07522 (973)790 6594 Fax (973)790-7703

Physicians by Name and Address

Braun, John E., DO {1891831244} IntrMd(83,IA75)<NJ-HOLY-NAME>
+ 550 Kinderamack Road
Oradell, NJ 07649 (201)967-7130 Fax (201)967-2270

Braun, Joshua Eugene, MD {1235350075} Psychy, PsyCAd(02,GA01)<NJ-MMHKEMBL>
+ Morristown Memorial Hospital/Mt. Kemble Division
95 Mount Kemble Avenue/Psych Morristown, NJ 07960 (973)971-4758

Brauner, Gary Jules, MD {1730149501} Dermat, SrgLsr(67,MA01)<NJ-ENGLWOOD, NY-MTSINAI>
+ Laser Medical Treatment Center of Greater New York
1625 Anderson Avenue Fort Lee, NJ 07024 (201)461-5522 Fax (201)461-2825
dermlaser@aol.com

Brauner, Rachel H., DO {1336414069}<NJ-HUNTRDN>
+ Hunterdon Medical Center
2100 Wescott Drive Flemington, NJ 08822 (908)415-5904
rhbrauner@gmail.com

Braunscheidel, Julie Ann, MD {1346211109} ObsGyn(95,IL02)
+ 2 Chesterfield Drive
Warren, NJ 07059

Braunstein, Edward A., MD {1003949322} Ophthl(76,MEX14)
+ PO Box 82
Manalapan, NJ 07726

Braunstein, Lior Z., MD {1548554769} IntrMd(11,MA01)<MA-MAEYEEAR>
+ Memorial Sloan Kettering Monmouth
480 Red Hill Road Middletown, NJ 07748 (201)775-7446
+ Memorial Sloan Kettering Bergen
225 Summit Avenue Montvale, NJ 07645 (201)775-7000

Braunstein, Robert Alan, MD {1891716262} Ophthl(72,IRE04)
+ 95 Madison Avenue
Morristown, NJ 07960 (973)540-1223

Braunstein, Scott N., MD {1578739199} IntrMd(90,NY46)<NJ-OVERLOOK>
+ 18 Thames Drive
Livingston, NJ 07039 Fax (973)758-1255

Braunstein, Steven W., MD {1821182494} Ophthl(82,MA07)
+ 7316 Kennedy Boulevard/PO Box 7266
North Bergen, NJ 07047 (201)869-3253 Fax (201)869-8235

Brauntuch, Glenn R., MD {1821012071} IntrMd, PulDis(78,NY01)<NJ-HOLYNAME>
+ Bergen Medical Alliance, P.A.
180 Engle Street Englewood, NJ 07631 (201)567-2050 Fax (201)568-8936

Braunwell, Arthur Henry, III, DO {1821094640} FamMed(88,PA77)<NJ-SOCEANCO>
+ Ocean County Family Care
901 Long Beach Boulevard Ship Bottom, NJ 08008 (609)361-2677 Fax (609)361-2469

Brautigan, Robert Anthony, MD {1932277118} Surgry(97,NJ05)
+ Amirata Surgical Group
5 Franklin Avenue/Suite 406 Belleville, NJ 07109 (973)759-4499
Brautiga@yahoo.com

Braver, Joel Keith, MD {1891791174} RadOnc(91,NJ06)<NJ-SOMERSET>
+ Steeplechase Cancer Center
30 Rehill Avenue/Suite 1100 Somerville, NJ 08876 (908)927-8777 Fax (908)927-8764

Braver, Vanita, MD {1811176415} PsyCAd, Psychy(91,NJ06)<NJ-MORRISTN>
+ Bonnie Brae Residential Treatment Center
3415 Valley Road/PO Box 825/Psych Liberty Corner, NJ 07938 (908)647-0800 Fax (908)647-5021

Braverman, Eric Randall, MD {1528186483} FamMed, IntrMd(83,NY19)<NY-CABRINI>
+ Total Health Nutrients
664 Route 518 Skillman, NJ 08558

Braverman, Gerald M., MD {1134166309} IntrMd(79,MEX03)<NJ-VIRTMARL>
+ 306 Posterity Place
Marlton, NJ 08053 (856)988-0114

Braverman, Isaac L., MD {1881619559} Pedtrc(95,ISR02)<NJ-COMMED, NJ-OCEANMC>
+ Pediatric Affiliates, PA
40 Bey Lea Road/Suite B203 Toms River, NJ 08753 (732)341-0720 Fax (732)244-6842
+ Pediatric Affiliates, PA
1616 Route 72 West/Suite 8 Manahawkin, NJ 08050 (732)341-0720 Fax (609)978-1229
+ Pediatric Affiliates, PA
400 Madison Avenue Lakewood, NJ 08753 (732)364-7770 Fax (732)364-9292

Braverman, Joel Morton, MD {1659488070} Anesth(94,NY09)<NY-PRSBWEIL>
+ New Jersey Anesthesia Associates, P.C.
252 Columbia Turnpike/PO Box 0037 Florham Park, NJ 07932 (973)660-9334 Fax (973)660-9779

Bravo, Holanda P., MD {1033268669} Pedtrc(94,ECU05)
+ Passaic Pediatrics II PA
913 Main Avenue Passaic, NJ 07055 (973)458-8000
+ Passaic Pediatrics II PC
93 Market Street Passaic, NJ 07055 (973)458-8000 Fax (973)458-8338

Bravoco, Michael C., MD {1699747311} ObsGyn(80,DOM02)<NJ-ACMCITY, NJ-SHOREMEM>
+ Somers Manor Obstetrics and Gynecology
599 Shore Road/Suite 101 Somers Point, NJ 08244 (609)926-8353 Fax (609)926-4579

Bravyak, James G., DO {1386642361} Anesth(83,PA77)<NJ-VIRTMARL>
+ West Jersey Anesthesia Associates
102-E Center Boulevard Marlton, NJ 08053 (856)988-6250 Fax (856)988-6270

Brawer, Arthur E., MD {1467550657} IntrMd, Rheuma(72,MA05)<NJ-BAYSHORE, NJ-RIVERVW>
+ 170 Morris Avenue
Long Branch, NJ 07740 (732)870-3133 Fax (732)222-0824

Brazaitis, Daiva, MD {1477555217} IntrMd(88,LITH)
+ Mercy Medical Group LLC
722 Sanford Avenue Newark, NJ 07106

Brazaitis, Edward, MD {1972614394} Psychy(79,LIT41)
+ 250 White Oak Ridge Road
Short Hills, NJ 07078

Brazeau, Chantal M., MD {1780796193} FamMed(83,ON09)<NJ-UMDNJ, NJ-RWJUBRUN>
+ New Jersey Family Practice Center (NJFPC)
90 Bergen Street/DOC 300/Lower Level Newark, NJ 07103 (973)972-2111 Fax (973)972-2754

Brazil, Deirdre A., MD {1386038792}
+ Hunterdon Medical Center
2100 Wescott Drive Flemington, NJ 08822 (908)788-6100
+ Delaware Valley Family Health Center
200 Frenchtown Road Milford, NJ 08848 (908)788-6100 Fax (908)995-2036

Brazzo, Brian Gerald, MD {1922083179} Ophthl(92,MA01)
+ Phillips Eye Center
619 River Drive Elmwood Park, NJ 07407 (201)796-2020 Fax (201)796-2833

Brecher, Linda S., DO {1346297215} Rheuma, IntrMd(87,IA75)
+ Atlantic Medical Imaging, LLC.
401 Bethel Road Somers Point, NJ 08244 (609)365-6200 Fax (609)365-6201

Bredin, Sherilyn A., MD {1689724932} ObsGyn(80,NJ06)<NJ-ACMCMAIN, NJ-SHOREMEM>
+ Ladies' Choice Ob-Gyn
314 Chris Gaupp Drive/Suite 101 Galloway, NJ 08205 (609)404-1400 Fax (609)404-1430

Breen, Gregory, MD {1538119961} PulCCr, IntrMd(94,PA07)
+ Penn Jersey Pulmonary Associates
52 West Red Bank Avenue/Suite 26 Woodbury, NJ 08096 (856)853-2025 Fax (856)845-8024
gbreen@pennjerseypulmonary.com

Breig, Jason Anthony, MD {1437545225} FamMed
+ Virtual Family Medicine - Mansfield
3242 Route 206/Building A Suite 2 Bordentown, NJ 08505 (609)298-4340 Fax (609)298-4370

Breit, Neal Gary, MD {1558419630} EnDbMt, IntrMd(97,NY45)<NJ-VALLEYHS, NY-MTSINAI>
+ Endocrinology & Diabetes Associates, LLC
333 Old Hook Road/Suite 103 Westwood, NJ 07675 (201)820-4646 Fax (201)820-4647

Breitbart, Gary B., MD {1073553400} SrgThr, SrgVas, Surgry(79,MEXI)
+ Garden State Surgical Associates
1511 Park Avenue South Plainfield, NJ 07080 (908)561-9500 Fax (908)561-7162

Breitbart, Seth Ilias, MD {1124266986} IntrMd(07,DMN01)<NJ-ENGLWOOD>
+ Englewood Hospital and Medical Center
350 Engle Street/Internal Med Englewood, NJ 07631 (201)894-3364 Fax (201)894-5693
+ The Valley Hospital
223 North Van Dien Avenue Ridgewood, NJ 07450 (201)447-8000

Brelvi, Zamir S., MD {1740213297} Gastrn, Hepato, IntrMd(91,NJ05)
+ UMDNJ Division of Gastroenterology & Hepatology
90 Bergen Street/DOC 2100/Hepatlgy Newark, NJ 07103 (973)972-2343 Fax (973)972-0752

Brener, Bruce J., MD {1053317636} OthrSp, SrgVas(66,MA01)<NJ-NWRKBETH, NJ-STBARNMC>
+ 200 South Orange Avenue
Livingston, NJ 07039 (973)322-7233 Fax (973)322-7499

Brenin-Goldfischer, Debra Sue, MD {1275583742} ObsGyn(93,NY46)<NJ-MORRISTN, NJ-STCLRDEN>
+ Women's Care Source
111 Madison Avenue/Suite 308 Morristown, NJ 07960 (973)285-0400 Fax (973)285-9848
+ Women's Care Source
16 Pocono Road/Suite 309 Denville, NJ 07834 (973)983-7695

Brennan, Alicia Ann, MD {1306853783} Pedtrc(94,MD07)<NJ-UN-VMCPRN, PA-CHILDHOS>
+ CHOP Newborn and Pediatric Care at UMCPP
One Plainsboro Road/6th Floor Plainsboro, NJ 08536 (609)853-7626 Fax (609)853-7630
+ University Medical Center of Princeton at Plainsboro
One Plainsboro Road Plainsboro, NJ 08536 (609)497-4076

Brennan, John A., MD {1508900069} EmrgMd, EmrgPedr(85,DC02)<NJ-NWRKBETH, NJ-STBARNMC>
+ Newark Beth Israel Medical Center
201 Lyons Avenue/EmergMed Newark, NJ 07112 (973)926-7000

Brennan, Laura Kaye, MD {1275579013} Pedtrc, PedEmg, IntrMd(01,PA12)<PA-CHILDHOS>
+ University Hospital-Cares Institute
42 East Laurel Road/Suite 1100 Stratford, NJ 08084 (856)566-7036 Fax (856)566-6108

Brennan, Mark D., MD {1326081357} AnesPain(90,PA02)
+ Lourdes Anesthesiology Associates
1600 Haddon Avenue Camden, NJ 08103 (856)757-3836

Brennan, William Frederick, DO {1306884515} FamMed(75,PA77)<NJ-UNDRWD>
+ Pitman Internal Medicine Associates
410 North Broadway/Suite 1 Pitman, NJ 08071 (856)589-3708 Fax (856)589-2662

Brenner, Dennis Jay, MD {1467487512} PedEnd, Pedtrc, IntrMd(97,NY08)<NJ-CHDNWBTH, NJ-NWRKBETH>
+ Children's Hospital of NJ Ped Cntr @ West Orange
375 Mount Pleasant Avenue/Suite 105 West Orange, NJ 07052 (973)322-6900 Fax (973)322-6999
+ Newark Beth Israel Medical Center
201 Lyons Avenue/Pedi Endo Newark, NJ 07112 (973)322-6900 Fax (973)705-3148

Brenner, Edward H., MD {1427138056} Ophthl(69,NC01)<NJ-CENTRAST, NJ-MONMOUTH>
+ Millennium Eye Care, LLC
500 West Main Street Freehold, NJ 07728 (732)462-8707 Fax (732)462-1296
+ Millennium Eye Care, LLC
Route 130 & Princeton Road Hightstown, NJ 08520 (732)462-8707 Fax (609)448-4197
+ Millennium Eye Care, LLC
515 Brick Boulevard/Suite G Brick, NJ 07728 (732)920-3800 Fax (732)920-5351

Brenner, Jeffrey Craig, MD {1558392217} FamMed(95,NJ06)
+ Camden Family Medicine PC
639 Cooper Street Camden, NJ 08102 (856)541-6800 Fax (856)541-1636

Brenner, Laura Ennis, MD {1235359019} Psychy(79,PA07)
+ 135 Country Road/Suite 6
Cresskill, NJ 07626 (201)871-7799 Fax (201)871-7799

Brenner, Robert W., MD {1639140148} FamMed(87,PA12)<NJ-OVERLOOK>
+ Westfield Family Practice
563 Westfield Avenue Westfield, NJ 07090 (908)232-5858 Fax (908)232-0439

Brenner-Gati, Leona, MD EnDbMt(79,MA01)
+ 71 Danville Drive
Princeton Junction, NJ 08550 (609)716-0089

Brennessel, Ryan William, DO {1639516701} EmrgMd<NJ-BAYSHORE>
+ Bayshore Community Hospital
727 North Beers Street Holmdel, NJ 07733 (732)739-5900

Brensilver, Jeffrey M., MD {1861452039} IntrMd, Nephro, OthrSp(70,NY01)<NJ-OVERLOOK>
+ Overlook Medical Center
99 Beauvoir Avenue/PO Box 210/Medicine Summit, NJ 07902 (908)522-2000

Brenza, Danielle, DO {1124047253} EmrgMd(98,NJ75)<NJ-UN-DRWD>
+ Inspira Health Network
509 North Broad Street/EmergencyMed Woodbury, NJ 08096 (856)845-0100

Bresalier, Howard J., DO {1114927159} Ophthl, GenPrc, Otlryg(92,IA75)
+ Advanced ENT - Washington Township
239 Hurffville Crosskeys Road Sewell, NJ 08080 (856)602-4000 Fax (856)629-3391
+ Advanced ENT - Voorhees
200 Bowman Drive/Suite D-285 Voorhees, NJ 08043 (856)602-4000 Fax (856)346-0757
+ Advanced ENT - Woodbury
620 North Broad Street Woodbury, NJ 08080 (856)602-4000 Fax (856)848-6029

Bresalier, Saul, DO {1518903244} Ophthl(64,IA75)<NJ-JFKMED, NJ-KMHCHRRY>
+ Eye Associates
251 South Lincoln Avenue   Vineland, NJ 08361   (856)691-8188   Fax (856)691-0421

Bresch, David, MD {1154419851} Psychy(97,NY08)
+ LifeCare Physicians, PC of Hamilton
1225 Whitehorse Mercerville Rd   Trenton, NJ 08619   (609)581-6087   Fax (609)581-9561

Brescia, Donald, MD {1265469480} FamMed(69,ITA01)<NJ-UN-VMCPRN>
+ 132 Route 31 North
Pennington, NJ 08534   (609)737-2714   Fax (609)737-1081

Brescia, Mark J., MD {1154537017} ObsGyn(85,MEXI)<NJ-HOBUNIMC>
+ Brescia-Migliaccio Ob/Gyn
609 Washington Street   Hoboken, NJ 07030   (201)659-7700   Fax (201)659-7701

Brescia, Michael Louis, MD {1033215819} CritCr, IntrMd, Pul-CCr(85,MEX34)
+ Drs. Maglaras and Brescia
236 East Westfield Avenue   Roselle Park, NJ 07204   (908)245-8222   Fax (908)245-6504

Breslauer, Lisa Marie, MD {1780779207} Dermat(96,NY01)<NJ-MORRISTN>
+ Laser & Skin Institute
417 Main Street   Chatham, NJ 07928   (973)635-5050   Fax (973)635-4567
+ Premier Health Associates-Administration
532 Lafayette Road/Suite 300   Sparta, NJ 07871   (973)635-5050   Fax (973)940-0399
+ Premier Health Associates
89 Sparta Avenue/Suite 100   Sparta, NJ 07928   (973)729-2121   Fax (973)729-3454

Breslow, Gary David, MD {1861461212} SrgPlstc(98,NY19)
+ The Breslow Center for Plastic Surgery
1 West Ridgewood Avenue/Suite 110   Paramus, NJ 07652   (201)444-9522   Fax (201)444-9277

Bressler, Jill Anne, MD {1306894217} Nrolgy, Acpntr(92,NY08)<NJ-HACKNSK>
+ Jill Ann Bressler MD, LLC
50 Hickory Street   Englewood Cliffs, NJ 07632   (201)568-4097

Bretan, Amy Faith, MD {1588696728} FamMed, IntrMd(03,NY46)
+ Flemington Medical Group, LLC
200 State Route 31 North/Suite 105   Flemington, NJ 08822   (908)782-5100   Fax (908)782-0290
ambrewh@att.net

Brett, Brian P., MD {1942386917} IntrMd, Pedtrc(94,NY06)<NJ-MORRISTN>
+ Medical Center at Budd Lake
125 US Highway 46   Budd Lake, NJ 07828   (973)691-9400   Fax (973)691-3283

Brewer, Arthur Martin, MD {1457360588} IntrMd(81,MO02)
+ Univ Correctional HealthCare-Colpitts
Whittessey Rd & Stuyvesant Ave   Trenton, NJ 08625   (609)292-9700

Brezel, Mitchell H., MD {1104939305} RadDia, Radiol, RadBdI(88,NY19)<NJ-ACMCMAIN, NJ-ACMCITY>
+ Atlantic Medical Imaging, LLC.
72 West Jimmie Leeds Road   Galloway, NJ 08205   (609)677-9729   Fax (609)653-8764
+ Atlantic Medical Imaging, LLC.
401 Bethel Road   Somers Point, NJ 08244   (609)677-9729
+ Atlantic Medical Imaging, LLC.
421 Route 9 North   Cape May Court House, NJ 08205   (609)463-9500   Fax (609)465-0918

Brezina, Eric Joseph, DO {1942360235} FamMed(01,NY75)<NJ-SOMERSET>
+ Comprehensive Family Medicine, PA
27 Mountain Boulevard/Suite 6   Warren, NJ 07059   (908)222-7777   Fax (908)222-9242
+ RWJ University Hospital Somerset
110 Rehill Avenue   Somerville, NJ 08876   (908)685-2200

Breznak, Cindy M., MD {1508904269} Ophthl(87,NJ06)<NJ-JFKMED>
+ 98 James Street/Suite 210
Edison, NJ 08820   (732)744-1800   Fax (732)744-1837

Brice, Marie F., MD {1497846869} FamMed, IntrMd(01,NET09)
+ Brice Medical Center, Inc.
300 Washington Avenue   Elizabeth, NJ 07202   (908)355-0664

Brickner, Gary R., MD {1699796607} ObsGyn(75,PA12)<NJ-CHSM-RCER, NJ-CHSFULD>
+ Brickner-Mantell Center for Womens' Health, LLC.
1-A Quakerbridge Plaza   Trenton, NJ 08619   (609)689-9991   Fax (609)689-9992
GBRICK2@comcast.net
+ Capital Health System/Mercer Campus
446 Bellevue Avenue/ObGyn   Trenton, NJ 08618   (609)394-4000

Bridge, Thomas Peter, MD {1134489487} Psychy(71,VA04)
+ Hoffman-La Roche Incorporated
340 Kingsland Street   Nutley, NJ 07110   (973)562-6580

Bridge-Jackson, Teresa A., MD {1366463986} EmrgMd, FamMed(78,NJ06)<NJ-BURDTMLN>
+ Cape Regional Medical Center
2 Stone Harbor Boulevard/EmergMed   Cape May Court House, NJ 08210   (609)463-2000   Fax (609)463-2946

Bridges, Kristen Leigh, MD {1649565748} Surgry
+ 714 Tenth Street
Secaucus, NJ 07094   (201)441-1450

Bridges, Yvette A., MD {1801805197} ObsGyn(82,NJ06)<NJ-STBARNMC>
+ St. Barnabas Medical Center
94 Old Short Hills Road   Livingston, NJ 07039   (973)322-5000

Bridges-White, Kimberly Gaye, MD {1770555948} ObsGyn(98,PA13)
+ Garden State Obstetrics and Gynecological Associates
2401 Evesham Road/Suite A   Voorhees, NJ 08043   (856)424-3323   Fax (856)424-4994

Brief, Andrew A., MD {1841206653} SrgOrt, SrgFAk(00,NY46)<NJ-HOLYNAME, NJ-ENGLWOOD>
+ Ridgewood Orthopedic Group, LLC
85 South Maple Avenue   Ridgewood, NJ 07450   (201)445-2830   Fax (201)445-7471

Brief, L. Paul, MD {1770585333} SrgOrt(64,NY09)
+ 162 Cortland Drive
Saddle River, NJ 07458   (845)359-1877
cyberdocs@aol.com

Brien, Michael J., MD {1003811043} PhysMd(80,DMN01)<NJ-STCLRDEN, NJ-STBARNMC>
+ 20 Valley Street
South Orange, NJ 07079   (973)762-2615

Briere, Misha H., DO {1396056941}
+ McGuire Air Force Base/Acute Health Care Clinic
3458 Neely Road   Trenton, NJ 08641   (609)754-9080   Fax (609)754-9015

Briggs, Jonathan Havens, MD {1700880069} RadOnc, Radiol(95,NJ06)<NJ-JRSYSHMC>
+ Jersey Shore University Medical Center
1945 Route 33/Radiology   Neptune, NJ 07753   (732)776-4404   Fax (732)776-4672
+ Shore Radiation Oncology, LLC
425 Jack Martin Boulevard   Brick, NJ 08724   (732)776-4404   Fax (732)836-4036

Briggs, Kari H., MD {1316012412} PthAcl(94,NJ06)<NJ-RWJUHAM>
+ Robert Wood Johnson University Hospital at Hamilton
1 Hamilton Health Place/Pathology   Hamilton, NJ 08690   (609)586-7900

Bright, Daniel J., MD {1952354169} Psychy, PsyGrt(88,NJ05)
+ 1051 West Sherman Avenue/Unit 3b
Vineland, NJ 08360

Bright, Nicole Jasmyn, DO {1578722856} Dermat(06,PA77)
+ Vause Dermatology Cosmetic Surgery Associates
545 Beckett Road/Suite 101   Logan Township, NJ 08085   (856)241-3311   Fax (856)241-3969
nbright@vausederm.com

Briglia, Francis A., MD {1699807446} PedCrC, Pedtrc(81,NJ06)<NJ-COOPRUMC>
+ Cooper University Medical Center/Camden
3 Cooper Plaza/Pedtrc/Suite 51   Camden, NJ 08103   (856)342-2546   Fax (856)963-2514
briglia-frank@chs

Briglia, William J., DO {1922291848} FamMed(88,PA77)<NJ-SJRSYELM, NJ-VIRTMHBC>
+ Bayside State Prison
4293 Route 47/Med Unit   Leesburg, NJ 08327   (856)785-9371

Brignola, Joseph John, MD {1508824897} IntrMd(01,NJ06)
+ The Internet Medical Group, P.C.
181 Franklin Avenue/Suite 204   Nutley, NJ 07110   (973)667-8117   Fax (973)667-6642

Briker, Alan J., MD {1942238654} IntrMd(71,NY46)<NJ-VALLEY>
+ Bergen Medical Associates
466 Old Hook Road/Suite 1   Emerson, NJ 07630   (201)967-8221   Fax (201)967-0340

Brill, Kristin Lynne, MD {1699706598} Surgry, SrgBst, SrgOnc(95,PA09)<NJ-COOPRUMC>
+ Cooper Surgical Associates
3 Cooper Plaza/Suite 411   Camden, NJ 08103   (856)342-2270   Fax (856)365-1180
+ Cooper University Medical Center/Camden
3 Cooper Plaza   Camden, NJ 08103   (856)342-2270   Fax (856)342-7606
+ 651 John F. Kennedy Way
Willingboro, NJ 08103   (856)342-3113

Brill, Susan R., MD {1487602033} AdolMd, Pedtrc(87,NY46)<NJ-NWRKBETH>
+ Adolescent Medicine of MMH
100 Madison Avenue   Morristown, NJ 07960   (973)971-4330
+ 11 Brookfall Road
Edison, NJ 08817   (732)819-8351

Brinkmann, Erika M., MD {1598822263} Surgry<NJ-HOLYNAME>
+ Holy Name Hospital
718 Teaneck Road/Breast Center   Teaneck, NJ 07666   (201)833-3000

Brinton, Karen J., MD {1962404434} Radiol(76,PA07)
+ Radiology Associates of Burlington County
1295 Route 38 West/PO Box 479   Hainesport, NJ 08036   (609)261-7017   Fax (609)261-4180

Briones, Renato J., MD {1194826099} Surgry(74,PHI01)<NJ-VIRTMHBC>
+ Virtua Medford Surgical Group
212 Creek Crossing Boulevard   Hainesport, NJ 08036   (609)267-1004   Fax (609)267-1044

Brisman, Daniel Aaron, MD {1790868081} PhysMd, IntrMd(94,MA07)<NJ-HOLYNAME>
+ Aspen Medical Associates, P.A.
1 DeGraw Square   Teaneck, NJ 07666   (201)928-0200   Fax (201)928-0820

Britt, Howard S., MD {1235358656} AdolMd, NnPnMd, Pedtrc(70,MA05)<NJ-NWRKBETH>
+ JRMC at George Washington Carver Elementary School
333 Clinton Place   Newark, NJ 07112   (973)679-7709   Fax (973)926-4510

Britton, Richard J., MD {1558392043} FamMed, EmrgMd(96,NJ05)
+ 651 Garwood Road
Moorestown, NJ 08057

Brizzio, Mariano Ezequiel, MD {1851468508} SrgThr(90,ARG01)<NJ-VALLEY>
+ Valley Columbia Heart Center
223 North Van Dien Avenue   Ridgewood, NJ 07450   (201)447-8377   Fax (201)447-8658

Brnouti, Fares, MD {1194957126}<NJ-STJOSHOS>
+ St. Peter's University Hospital
254 Easton Avenue   New Brunswick, NJ 08901   (732)745-8606
+ St Joseph's Medical Center Neonatology
703 Main Street   Paterson, NJ 07503   (973)754-2555

Broad, Daniel Gene, MD {1669562435} Anesth(90,PA09)<NJ-UN-VMCPRN>
+ University Medical Center of Princeton at Plainsboro
One Plainsboro Road/Anesthesiology   Plainsboro, NJ 08536   (609)497-4330

Brobyn, Tracy L., MD {1437230901} FamMed, IntrMd(94,NY06)
+ Drs. Chung & Shin
110 Marter Avenue/Suite 507   Moorestown, NJ 08057   (856)222-4766   Fax (856)222-1137

Brock, Donald J., MD {1659371334} CdvDis, IntrMd(65,NY01)<NJ-STBARNMC, NJ-OVERLOOK>
+ New Jersey Cardiology Associates
375 Mount Pleasant Avenue   West Orange, NJ 07052   (973)731-9442   Fax (973)731-8030

Brock, James Steven, MD {1477549954} Surgry, SrgVas(85,NY19)<NJ-RIVERVW>
+ Shrewsbury Surgical Associates
655 Shrewsbury Avenue/Suite 210   Shrewsbury, NJ 07702   (732)542-8118   Fax (732)747-4751

Brockman-Bitterman, Allyson Stacy, MD {1871535435} Dermat(00,NY08)
+ Millburn Laser Center
12 East Willow Street   Millburn, NJ 07041   (973)376-8500   Fax (973)376-1820

Broder, Arkady, MD {1336307529} Gastrn(07,NY46)<NJ-STPETER>
+ Saint Peter's Physician Associates
240 Easton Avenue/4th Floor   New Brunswick, NJ 08901   (732)565-5471   Fax (732)745-2163

Brodkey, Morris I., MD {1831179167} IntrMd(67,NE05)<NJ-OCEANMC>
+ Silverton Medical Center, PC
2446 Church Road/Suite 1A   Toms River, NJ 08753   (732)255-5915   Fax (732)255-5618

Brodkin, Joshua S., MD {1598763625} Radiol, RadDia(88,NJ05)<NJ-VIRTUAHS, NJ-VIRTMHBC>
+ South Jersey Radiology Associates, P.A.
901 Route 168/Suites 301-305   Turnersville, NJ 08012   (856)227-6600   Fax (856)227-8537
+ South Jersey Radiology Associates, P.A.
100 Carnie Boulevard/Suite B-5   Voorhees, NJ 08043   (856)227-6600   Fax (856)751-0535
+ South Jersey Radiology Associates, P.A.
315 Route 70 East/Suite B   Cherry Hill, NJ 08012   (856)428-4344   Fax (856)428-0356

Physicians by Name and Address

Brodkin, Lisa Faith, MD {1972561926} EnDbMt, IntrMd(94,ON05)<NJ-OVERLOOK>
+ Summit Medical Group
  34 Mountain Boulevard   Warren, NJ 07059   (908)561-8600   Fax (908)561-7265

Brodman, Richard R., MD {1831260702} IntrMd, Rheuma(73,NY08)<NJ-JFKMED>
+ 346 South Avenue/Suite 5
  Fanwood, NJ 07023   (908)889-4700   Fax (908)889-0867

Brodrick, Ian B., MD {1750336475} FamMed, IntrMd(85,NY20)<NJ-SOMERSET>
+ Rockaway Family Medicine Associates
  333 Mount Hope Avenue   Rockaway, NJ 07866   (973)895-6601   Fax (973)895-5324

Brodsky, Jonathan I., DO {1417633520} Anesth(91,NY75)
+ Red Bank Anesthesia, LLC
  1 Riverview Plaza   Red Bank, NJ 07701   (732)530-2255   Fax (732)450-2620

Brodsky, Michael C., MD {1487656997} RadDia(99,NC07)<NJ-VIRTMHBC>
+ Radiology Associates of Burlington County
  1295 Route 38 West/PO Box 479   Hainesport, NJ 08036   (609)261-7017   Fax (609)261-4180

Brodt, Zahava Nilly, MD {1841633369} Grtrcs
+ UH-RWJ General Internal Medicine
  125 Paterson Street/Suite 2300   New Brunswick, NJ 08901   (732)235-6968   Fax (732)235-7144

Brody, Joshua David, DO {1841220647} Radiol, RadNro, Rad-Dia(86,NJ75)<NJ-COOPRUMC>
+ Cooper University Hospital
  One Cooper Plaza/Radiology   Camden, NJ 08103   (856)342-2000   Fax (856)541-7219
+ Cooper University Medical Center/Camden
  3 Cooper Plaza/Radiology   Camden, NJ 08103   (856)342-2000
+ The Cooper Health System at Voorhees
  900 Centennial Boulevard/Suite E   Voorhees, NJ 08103   (856)325-6500

Brody, Robin Michelle, MD {1841239423} Otlryg, SrgHdN(94,NY03)<NJ-ENGLWOOD, NJ-HACKNSK>
+ ENT & Allergy Associates, LLP
  433 Hackensack Avenue/Suite 204   Hackensack, NJ 07601   (201)883-1062   Fax (201)883-9297

Brody, Zoltan, DO {1548221765} SrgC&R(79,PA77)
+ 1020 Galloping Hill Road
  Union, NJ 07083   (908)687-2062

Broizman, David T., MD {1952365645} ObsGyn, Gyneco(90,PA09)<NJ-HACKNSK, NJ-ENGLWOOD>
+ Tenafly Ob-Gyn Associates PA
  2 Dean Drive/2nd Floor   Tenafly, NJ 07670   (201)569-3300   Fax (201)569-7649

Brolin, Robert E., MD {1700923562} Surgry, Bariat(74,MI01)<NJ-UNVMCPRN>
+ New Jersey Bariatrics
  666 Plainsboro Road/Suite 640   Plainsboro, NJ 08536   (609)785-5870   Fax (609)785-5867

Brolis, Nils Viesturs, DO {1821385774} FamMed, IntrMd<NJ-VIRTBERL, NJ-VIRTMARL>
+ Partners in Primary Care
  19 West Main Street/Suite C   Maple Shade, NJ 08052   (856)779-7386   Fax (856)779-7563
+ Virtua Immediate Care Center
  239 Hurffville Crosskeys Road   Sewell, NJ 08080   (856)779-7386   Fax (856)341-8215

Bromberg, Assia, MD {1629047261} IntrMd, PulDis(74,RUSS)<NJ-VALLEY>
+ 19-20 Fair Lawn Avenue
  Fair Lawn, NJ 07410   (201)794-1963   Fax (201)794-2117
  assiabrombergmd@yahoo.com

Bromberg, David, MD {1376586412} Otlryg, OtgyFPlS(72,PA13)<NJ-UNDRWD, NJ-JFKMED>
+ 292 Hurffville-Grenloch Road/Suite 10
  Sewell, NJ 08080   (856)589-9200   Fax (856)589-1437
+ 600 Jessup Road
  Paulsboro, NJ 08066   (856)845-4931

Bromley, Steven Michael, MD {1962591586} Nrolgy(98,NJ06)<NJ-VIRTMARL, NJ-VIRTUAHS>
+ Virtua Nurosciences
  200 Bowman Drive/Suite E-385   Voorhees, NJ 08043   (856)247-7770   Fax (856)247-7766
+ Bromley Neurology, P.C.
  739 South White Horse Pike/Suite 1   Audubon, NJ 08106   (856)546-7770   Fax (856)546-2301

Bromley, William, II, DO {1205931797} FamMed(90,IA75)<NJ-VIRTVOOR, NJ-OURLADY>
+ 726 South White Horse Pike/Suite 2
  Audubon, NJ 08106   (856)546-6666   Fax (856)546-5345

Brondfeld, Raquel Lara, MD {1669639399} Pedtrc(05,NY03)<NJ-ENGLWOOD, NJ-HACKNSK>
+ Tenafly Pediatrics, PA
  1135 Broad Street/Suite 208   Clifton, NJ 07013   (973)471-8600   Fax (973)471-3068

+ Tenafly Pediatrics, PA
  32 Franklin Street   Tenafly, NJ 07670   (973)471-8600   Fax (201)569-6081

Bronikowski, John Anthony, DO {1932209483} IntrMd(64,IL76)<NJ-OVERLOOK>
+ NJ Heart/Linden Office
  520 North Wood Avenue   Linden, NJ 07036   (908)925-2100   Fax (908)587-0001
+ Union Medical Associates PA
  1308 Morris Avenue/Suite 101   Union, NJ 07083   (908)925-2100   Fax (908)687-8702

Bronshtein, Elena, MD {1205168309} ObsGyn<NJ-NWRKBETH>
+ Newark Beth Israel Medical Center
  201 Lyons Avenue   Newark, NJ 07112   (973)926-4882

Bronshteyn, Inessa, MD {1558785121}<NJ-ENGLWOOD>
+ Englewood Hospital and Medical Center
  350 Engle Street   Englewood, NJ 07631   (201)894-3000

Bronsnick, Tara A., MD {1447678313} Dermat
+ Summit Medical Group
  75 East Northfield Road   Livingston, NJ 07039   (973)436-1360   Fax (908)673-7336

Bronstein, Eric H., MD {1265401566} SrgThr, Surgry(87,NY48)<NJ-VALLEY>
+ The Valley Hospital
  223 North Van Dien Avenue/Surgery   Ridgewood, NJ 07450   (201)447-8000

Bronstein, Jagoda Ewa, MD {1205884574} Pedtrc(90,POL06)<NY-METHODST>
+ Willowbrook Pediatrics
  57 Willowbrook Boulevard/Suite 421   Wayne, NJ 07470   (973)754-4025   Fax (973)754-4044

Bronstein, Jeffrey Barry, MD {1528094463} Psychy(78,PA02)<NJ-COOPRUMC>
+ Cooper University Medical Center/Camden
  3 Cooper Plaza/Suite 310   Camden, NJ 08103   (856)342-2000

Bronstein, Regina, MD {1063408995} Pedtrc(83,RUS44)<NJ-MORRISTN>
+ Premier Health Associates
  89 Sparta Avenue/Suite 100   Sparta, NJ 07871   (973)729-2121   Fax (973)729-3454

Brooks, Ellen F., MD {1427195205} Psychy(78,PA02)<NJ-VIRTMHBC>
+ 1000 White Horse Road/Suite 704
  Voorhees, NJ 08043   (856)770-1555   Fax (856)770-9521

Brooks, Ira M., MD {1437172111} IntrMd(82,BELG)
+ 807 Kennedy Boulevard
  Bayonne, NJ 07002   (201)437-4073   Fax (201)437-1050

Brooks, Julius A., Jr., MD {1013905116} FamMed
+ Virtua Family Health Center
  1000 Atlantic Avenue   Camden, NJ 08104   (856)246-3542   Fax (856)246-3528

Brooks, Lee J., MD {1831108810} PedPul, Pedtrc, SlpDis(77,DC02)<PA-CHILDHOS>
+ CHOP Pediatric & Adolescent Specialty Care Center
  1012 Laurel Oak Road   Voorhees, NJ 08043   (856)435-1300   Fax (856)435-0091
+ CHOP Pediatric & Adolescent Specialty Care Center
  707 Alexander Road/Suite 205   Princeton, NJ 08540   (609)520-1717

Brooks, Monifa, MD {1386633105} PhysMd, OrtSpn(00,PA13)<NJ-KSLRWEST>
+ Kessler Institute for Rehabilitation West Orange
  1199 Pleasant Valley Way   West Orange, NJ 07052   (973)731-3600

Brooks, Nneka Offor, MD {1467614057} Ophthl(08,NY20)
+ Retina Associates of New Jersey, P.A.
  5 Franklin Avenue   Belleville, NJ 07109   (973)450-5100   Fax (973)450-9494
+ Retina Associates of New Jersey, P.A.
  1044 Route 23 North/Suite 207   Wayne, NJ 07470   (973)450-5100   Fax (973)633-3892

Brooks, Susan Sklower, MD {1023025764} ClnGnt, GntMCBch, Pedtrc(75,NY47)
+ Child Health Institute of New Jersey
  89 French Street/Suite 2300/2nd Floor   New Brunswick, NJ 08901   (732)235-9386   Fax (732)235-7088

Broslawski, Gregory E., DO {1578567350} IntrMd(89,NJ75)<NJ-HUNTRDN>
+ 6 Sand Hill Road/Suite 201
  Flemington, NJ 08822   (908)782-8019   Fax (908)782-7195

Bross, George, Jr., DO {1669493086} Pedtrc(87,PA77)<NJ-SHOREMEM>
+ Harborview KidsFirst
  505 Bay Avenue   Somers Point, NJ 08244   (609)927-4235   Fax (609)927-5590
+ Harborview KidsFirst Cape May
  1315 Route 9 South   Cape May Court House, NJ 08210   (609)927-4235   Fax (609)465-1539
+ Harborview Smithville
  48 South New York Road/Route 9   Smithville, NJ 08244   (609)748-2900   Fax (609)748-3067

Bross, Robert J., MD {1538142054} FamMed(84,NJ06)<NJ-VIRTMHBC>
+ Columbus Family Physicians
  23659 Columbus Road/Suite 4   Columbus, NJ 08022   (609)298-3304   Fax (609)298-7091

Brothers, Alexander Trexler, MD {1619318060}<NJ-STJOSHOS>
+ St. Joseph's Regional Medical Center
  703 Main Street   Paterson, NJ 07503   (973)754-2000

Brotman, Deborah L., MD {1275637530} IntrMd(83,NY09)
+ 3 Second Street/Suite 803
  Jersey City, NJ 07311   (201)416-3702

Brotman-O'Neill, Alissa Sue, DO {1649458540} SrgVas, Surgry(02,NJ75)<NJ-ENGLWOOD>
+ Diabetes and Endocrinology Associates
  3525 Quakerbridge Road/Suite 2000   Trenton, NJ 08619   (609)570-2071   Fax (609)689-2614
+ Englewood Hospital and Medical Center
  350 Engle Street   Englewood, NJ 07631   (201)894-3000

Brottman, Jeffrey S., MD {1699855239} Ophthl(88,NY47)<NJ-CENTRAST, NJ-MONMOUTH>
+ Millennium Eye Care, LLC
  500 West Main Street   Freehold, NJ 07728   (732)462-8707   Fax (732)462-1296

Brouder, Daniel J., MD {1659313963} Nephro, IntrMd(98,NY08)<NJ-JRSYSHMC, NJ-OCEANMC>
+ Ocean Renal Associates, P.A.
  210 Jack Martin Boulevard/Suite D-1   Brick, NJ 08724   (732)458-5854   Fax (732)458-8012
+ Ocean Renal Associates, P.A.
  508 Lakehurst Road/Suite 3 A   Toms River, NJ 08755   (732)458-5854   Fax (732)341-4993
+ Ocean Renal Associates, P.A.
  1145 Beacon Avenue/Suite B   Manahawkin, NJ 08724   (609)978-9940   Fax (609)978-9902

Broudy, Joseph Benjamin, MD {1689706434} RadV&I<NJ-OURLADY>
+ Our Lady of Lourdes Medical Center
  1600 Haddon Avenue   Camden, NJ 08103   (856)757-3500

Brouk, Alla, MD {1396933149} IntrMd(92,RUS14)
+ ED Medical Associates
  140 Grand Avenue   Englewood, NJ 07631   (201)569-9010   Fax (201)569-9063
  A_brouk@yahoo.com

Broussard, Crystal Naii Collins, MD {1114955846} IntrMd, Gastrn(92,OH06)<NJ-VALLEY>
+ Bergen Medical Associates
  466 Old Hook Road/Suite 1   Emerson, NJ 07630   (201)967-8221   Fax (201)967-0340
+ Bergen Medical Associates
  1 West Ridgewood Avenue/Suite 301   Paramus, NJ 07652   (201)967-8221   Fax (201)445-4296

Brower, Chelsea, MD {1548672249} FamMed
+ Erickson Health Medical Group
  1 Cedar Crest Village Drive   Pompton Plains, NJ 07444   (973)831-3540   Fax (973)831-3503

Brown, Alan Stuart, MD {1992898381} Psychy(87,PA02)
+ 163 Engle Street/Building 2
  Englewood, NJ 07631   (201)569-6768

Brown, Andrew Bennett, MD {1386800464} OncHem(03,PA02)
+ St. Barnabas Cancer Center
  94 Old Short Hills Road/Suite 1   Livingston, NJ 07039   (973)322-5650   Fax (973)422-1653

Brown, Andrew Carson, MD {1174595987} Ophthl(02,MA05)
+ Brown Eye Care Associates
  751 Teaneck Road   Teaneck, NJ 07666   (201)833-0006   Fax (201)833-9238

Brown, Anjeanette Tina, MD {1982872016} Surgry(98,MD01)<NJ-ACMCITY, NJ-SHOREMEM>
+ AtlantiCare Physician Group Joslin Diabetes Center
  2500 English Creek Avenue/Bldg 800   Egg Harbor Township, NJ 08234   (609)568-5606   Fax (609)568-5877

Brown, Anthony, DO {1780631150} IntrMd, Nephro(84,PA77)<NJ-WARREN>
+ Nephrology & Hypertension Associates of New Jersey
  201 Laurel Oak Road/Suite B   Voorhees, NJ 08043   (856)566-5478   Fax (856)566-9561

Brown, Arthur Samuel, MD {1598939878} SrgPlstc, Surgry(70,PA01)<NJ-COOPRUMC>
+ Cooper Surgical Associates
  3 Cooper Plaza/Suite 411   Camden, NJ 08103   (856)342-2270   Fax (856)365-1180
+ Cooper Surgical Associates
  110 Marter Avenue/Suite 402   Moorestown, NJ 08057   (856)342-2270   Fax (856)866-9846
+ The Cooper Health System at Voorhees
  900 Centennial Boulevard/Suite 403   Voorhees, NJ 08103   (856)325-6500

Brown, Barbara A., MD {1912926452} IntrMd(95,NJ06)
+ Princeton Lifestyle Medicine
  731 Alexander Road/Suite 200   Princeton, NJ 08540   (609)655-3800   Fax (609)655-5203

Brown, Christopher David, MD {1285650234} Ophthl(96,MA05)<NJ-HOLYNAME>
+ Brown Eye Care Associates
751 Teaneck Road   Teaneck, NJ 07666   (201)833-0006   Fax (201)833-9238

Brown, Christopher S., MD {1497732713} IntrMd(75,SPA05)<NJ-JRSYSHMC>
+ 1930 Highway 35/Suite 8
Wall Township, NJ 07719   (732)681-9363   Fax (732)681-0770

Brown, Colin Christopher, MD {1053371203} IntrMd, Gastrn(03,PA13)<MA-SSHREHOS>
+ Middlesex Monmouth Gastroenterology
222 Schanck Road/Suite 302   Freehold, NJ 07728   (732)577-1999   Fax (732)845-5356

Brown, David K., MD {1568468825} Allrgy, IntrMd(81,OH01)<NJ-STBARNMC>
+ Allergy Diagnostic & Treatment Center LLC
33 Overlook Road/Suite 307   Summit, NJ 07901   (908)522-9696   Fax (908)522-3070
billmgr@dkb-allergy.com

Brown, David P., DO {1255359477} PhysMd(85,PA77)<NJ-JFKJHNSN>
+ JFK Johnson Rehabilitation Institute
65 James Street/Phys Med&Rehab   Edison, NJ 08818   (732)321-7000   Fax (732)321-7330

Brown, Derrick M., MD {1942270848} IntrMd(93,GRNA)<NJ-BAYSHORE, NJ-RIVERVW>
+ Jersey Shore Medical Associates
734 North Beers Street/Suite U-4   Holmdel, NJ 07733   (732)264-8484   Fax (732)264-4324

Brown, Elliot M., MD {1285689315} CdvDis, IntrMd(88,NY09)<NJ-CHILTON, NJ-VALLEY>
+ Cardiology Center of North Jersey
1030 Clifton Avenue   Clifton, NJ 07013   (973)778-3777   Fax (973)778-3252
+ United Medical, P.C.
612 Rutherford Avenue   Lyndhurst, NJ 07071   (973)778-3777   Fax (201)460-1684

Brown, Gary Alan, DO {1891802302} Psychy(87,IA75)<NJ-CHSFULD, NJ-CHSMRCER>
+ Capital Health System/Fuld Campus
750 Brunswick Avenue/Psychiatry   Trenton, NJ 08638   (609)394-6085   Fax (609)815-7814

Brown, Gordon Andrew, DO {1124192489} Urolgy(98,NJ75)
+ Delaware Valley Urology LLC
570 Egg Harbor Road/Suite A-1   Sewell, NJ 08080   (856)582-9645   Fax (856)985-4583
+ New Jersey Urology LLC
2090 Springdale Road/Suite D   Cherry Hill, NJ 08003   (856)582-9645   Fax (856)985-9908
+ New Jersey Urology, LLC
2401 East Evesham Road/Suite F   Voorhees, NJ 08080   (856)673-1600   Fax (856)988-0636

Brown, Ingrid C., MD {1881629061} Pedtrc(82,NJ05)<NJ-STBARNMC>
+ 2801 Morris Avenue/Suite B
Union, NJ 07083   (908)688-8000   Fax (908)688-8039

Brown, James Harvey, MD {1689678039} RadDia, RadNro, Radiol(88,PA01)<NJ-CHOSHUDC>
+ University Radiology Group, P.C.
579A Cranbury Road   East Brunswick, NJ 08816   (732)390-0040   Fax (732)390-1856

Brown, Jeffrey G., MD {1992936942} PthAcl
+ Histopathology Services, LLC.
535 East Crescent Avenue   Ramsey, NJ 07446   (201)661-7280   Fax (201)661-7297

Brown, Jennifer A., DO {1538203054} Gastrn, IntrMd(98,MO78)<NJ-STMICHL>
+ St. Michael's Medical Center
268 MLK Jr. Boulevard   Newark, NJ 07102   (973)877-2580
+ Drs. Fedida and Brown
306 Martin Luther King Blvd/4th Floor   Newark, NJ 07102   (973)877-2580   Fax (973)877-2578

Brown, John M., MD {1063400323} PthAcl(77,CO02)<NJ-WARREN, PA-SCRDHRT>
+ Warren Hospital
185 Roseberry Street/Laboratory   Phillipsburg, NJ 08865   (908)859-6700   Fax (908)859-6849
mit69@rcn.com

Brown, John Muir, III, MD {1164424529} SrgThr, Surgry(86,NY20)<NJ-MORRISTN, NJ-JRSYSHMC>
+ Mid-Atlantic Surgical Associates
100 Madison Avenue   Morristown, NJ 07960   (973)971-7300   Fax (973)984-7019
john.brown@ahsys.org

Brown, Justin, MD {1740375310} Dermat(03,NJ05)
+ The Dermatology Group, P.C.
60 Pompton Avenue   Verona, NJ 07044   (973)571-2121   Fax (973)571-2126
+ The Dermatology Group, P.C.
347 Mount Pleasant Avenue/Suite 103   West Orange, NJ 07052   (973)571-2121   Fax (973)498-0535

Brown, Katherine E., MD {1851507628} Psychy(82,NJ05)
+ Raritan Bay Mental Health Center
570 Lee Street   Perth Amboy, NJ 08861   (732)442-1666   Fax (732)442-9512

Brown, Lemarra Rena, DO {1710120407} IntrMd
+ Atlantic Internal Medicine PA
310 Chris Gaupp Drive/Suite 102   Galloway, NJ 08205   (609)652-9933   Fax (609)652-9955

Brown, Lloyd Garth, MD {1114136645} SrgTpl
+ Rutgers- New Jersey Medical School
185 South Orange Avenue/MSB Rm G-594   Newark, NJ 07103   (973)972-4300

Brown, Melanie Antonietta, MD {1629202247} Surgry(03,GRN01)<NJ-STBARNMC>
+ St. Barnabas Medical Center
94 Old Short Hills Road/Surgery   Livingston, NJ 07039   (973)322-5000

Brown, Melinda Sheron, MD {1942456272} InfDis, IntrMd(01,JMA01)
+ 1 Carriage City Plaza/Apt 602
Rahway, NJ 07065   (347)585-1523
drmsbrown@yahoo.com

Brown, Michael James, MD {1639303969}<NJ-HACKNSK>
+ Hackensack University Medical Center
30 Prospect Avenue   Hackensack, NJ 07601   (201)996-2000

Brown, Michele Susan, MD {1932375276} RadV&I
+ Radiology Affiliates of Central New Jersey, P.A.
2501 Kuser Road   Hamilton, NJ 08691   (609)585-8800   Fax (609)585-1825

Brown, Miriam Renee, MD {1225035306} Ophthl(93,NY09)<NJ-VIRTMHBC>
+ South Jersey Eye Physicians PA
509 South Lenola Road/Suite 11   Moorestown, NJ 08057   (856)234-0222   Fax (856)727-9518
+ South Jersey Eye Physicians PA
25 Homestead Drive/Suite A   Columbus, NJ 08022   (856)234-0222   Fax (609)291-1972

Brown, Mitchell L., MD {1699883306} Grtrcs, IntrMd(87,DMN01)<NJ-BAYONNE, NJ-JRSYCITY>
+ 2 Joan Ree Terrace
Bayonne, NJ 07002   (201)339-2220   Fax (201)339-3667

Brown, Naomi Judith, MD {1184814949} Pedtrc, SprtMd(06,MA07)
+ CHOP Specialty Care Center at Virtua
200 Bowman Drive/2 FL/Suite D-260   Voorhees, NJ 08043   (267)425-5400
+ CHOP Care Network at Virtua Voorhees Hospital
100 Bowman Drive   Voorhees, NJ 08043   (267)425-5400   Fax (609)261-5842

Brown, Patricia J., MD {1144395617} IntrMd(81,NJ05)
+ Newark Community Health Centers Inc.
9 Coit Street   Irvington, NJ 07111   (973)399-6292

Brown, Patricia S., MD {1528262805} PsyCAd(99,PA02)
+ 155 County Road/Suite 18
Cresskill, NJ 07626   (201)541-8080   Fax (201)541-8084

Brown, Patti C., DO EmrgMd(85,NJ75)<NJ-VIRTMHBC>
+ SJ Emergency Physician, PA
175 Madison Avenue   Mount Holly, NJ 08060   (609)267-0700   Fax (609)261-5842

Brown, Rebecca Campau, MD {1164506721} PhysMd(03,NY08)
+ Physical Medicine & Rehabilitation Center
500 Grand Avenue/1st Floor   Englewood, NJ 07631   (201)567-2277   Fax (201)567-7506
+ Physical Medicine & Rehabilitation Center, PA
1530 Palisade Avenue   Fort Lee, NJ 07024   (201)567-2277   Fax (201)363-8873

Brown, Robert Henry, MD {1588617971} Ophthl(65,MA05)<NJ-HOLYNAME>
+ Brown Eye Care Associates
751 Teaneck Road   Teaneck, NJ 07666   (201)833-0006   Fax (201)833-9238
Brownkr@optonline.net

Brown, Robert Stephen, MD {1740206796} Ophthl(94,MA05)
+ Brown Eye Care Associates
751 Teaneck Road   Teaneck, NJ 07666   (201)833-0006   Fax (201)833-9238

Brown, Robert Theodore, MD {1962409037} AdolMd, Pedtrc(71,PA09)
+ The Cooper Hospital System-Univ Hospital
401 Haddon Avenue   Camden, NJ 08103   (856)342-2001   Fax (856)968-8206

Brown, Ryan P., MD {1396966750} Nephro, Pedtrc, IntrMd(00,LA01)
+ Medical Diagnostic Associates PA
215 North Avenue West   Westfield, NJ 07090   (908)232-4321
+ Medical Diagnostic Associates PA-Nephrology
1511 Park Avenue/3rd Floor   South Plainfield, NJ 07080   (908)232-4321   Fax (908)757-2470

Brown, Teresa V., DO {1194117127} IntrMd(PA77)
+ Summit Medical Group
890 New Mountain Avenue   New Providence, NJ 07974   (908)277-8601
+ Summit Medical Group
67 Walnut Avenue/Suite 202   Clark, NJ 07066   (908)277-8601   Fax (732)388-1330

Brown, William C., Jr., MD {1396713954} Ophthl(79,PA12)<NJ-CHSMRCER, NJ-CHSFULD>
+ 770 River Road
Trenton, NJ 08628   (609)771-1090   Fax (609)771-1045

Brown, William Howard, MD {1821012196} Gastrn, IntrMd(99,NY19)
+ Summit Medical Group-Berkeley Heights Campus
1 Diamond Hill Road   Berkeley Heights, NJ 07922   (908)277-8936   Fax (908)790-6576

Browne, Avery F., DO {1588777304} FamMSptM, IntrMd(03,NY75)<NJ-CHSFULD>
+ AFC Urgent Care South Plainfield
907 Oak Tree Avenue/Suite H   South Plainfield, NJ 07080   (908)222-3500

Browne, Mary Beth, MD {1285701094} NnPnMd, Pedtrc(88,NJ05)<NJ-MORRISTN, NJ-OVERLOOK>
+ Meridian Medical Group - Faculty Practice
61 Davis Avenue/Suite 1   Neptune, NJ 07753   (732)776-4524   Fax (732)776-4639

Browne, Patricia M., MD {1558372243} Pedtrc, Anesth(85,PA01)
+ CHOP Pediatric & Adolescent Specialty Care Center
1012 Laurel Oak Road   Voorhees, NJ 08043   (856)435-1300   Fax (856)435-0091

Browne, Satra Bianca, MD {1396067062}(06,NY46)
+ 5 Spruce Tree Lane
Randolph, NJ 07869   (973)953-2257

Brownstein, Gary M., MD {1235260035} SrgPlstc, Surgry(73,PA02)
+ 102 Browning Lane
Cherry Hill, NJ 08003   (856)424-5700   Fax (856)424-0333

Brozyna, David B., MD {1114042462} Psychy(85,POLA)
+ PO Box 1705
Rutherford, NJ 07070   (201)939-5500   Fax (201)939-1599

Bruce, Gullie E., IV, MD {1477562452} Anesth(93,NJ05)<NJ-OCEANMC>
+ Red Bank Anesthesia, LLC
1 Riverview Plaza   Red Bank, NJ 07701   (732)530-2255   Fax (732)450-2620

Brucia, Lauren A., MD {1922037506} Pedtrc(03,NJ05)<NJ-VALLEY, NJ-CHILTON>
+ PediatriCare Associates
20-20 Fair Lawn Avenue   Fair Lawn, NJ 07410   (201)791-4545   Fax (201)791-3765

Bruckler, Paula A., DO {1619336047} ObsGyn
+ Cooper Ob/Gyn
3 Cooper Plaza/Suite 220   Camden, NJ 08103   (856)342-2000

Bruder, Scott P., MD Ophthl(92,OH06)
+ Becton Dickinson & Company
1 Becton Drive/Suite 084   Franklin Lakes, NJ 07417   (201)847-6800

Brudie, Lorna Ann, DO {1942265517} ObsGyn(NY75
+ Atlantic Gynecologic Oncology
3349 State Route 138   Wall, NJ 07719   (732)280-5464   Fax (732)280-5443

Brug, Pamela, MD {1710950639} ObsGyn(89,NJ05)<NJ-RBAYPERT>
+ Raritan Bay Medical Center/Perth Amboy Division
530 New Brunswick Avenue/Ob/Gyn   Perth Amboy, NJ 08861   (732)442-3700

Bruk, George, MD {1417980095} Anesth(67,UKRA)<NJ-BAYSHORE>
+ Bayshore Community Hospital
727 North Beers Street/Anesthesiology   Holmdel, NJ 07733   (732)739-5900

Brumbaugh, Martha, MD {1649332974} FamMed(76,PA07)<NJ-COOPRUMC>
+ 436 Second Avenue
Haddon Heights, NJ 08035   (856)547-4734

Brumberg, Miles A., DO {1932144847} FamMed(76,PA77)
+ 601 Hurffville Crosskeys Road
Sewell, NJ 08080   (856)582-0470   Fax (856)256-0414
M.brumberg@comcast.net

Brundavanam, Hari Vs, MD {1073791950} Ophthl
+ 1450 Parkside Avenue/Suite 21
Ewing, NJ 08638   (732)751-4835

Bruneau, Eve Solange, DO {1093153728} Surgry
+ Rowan University-School of Osteopathic Medicine
1 Medical Center Drive   Stratford, NJ 08084   (856)566-7050

Bruneau, Lara A., MD {1669410445} Pedtrc, IntrMd(95,NJ05)<NJ-COOPRUMC>
+ Bruneau Family Care, P.C.
2963 Marne Highway   Mount Laurel, NJ 08054   (856)638-1990

Physicians by Name and Address

Bruner, David Glenn, MD {1679522999} Pedtrc(98,NJ06)<NJ-VIRTMHBC, NJ-VIRTUAHS>
+ Advocare Laurel Pediatrics
269 Fish Pond Road   Sewell, NJ 08080   (856)863-9999   Fax (856)863-9666

Bruner, Laurie Reid, MD {1508892829} Pedtrc(98,NJ06)<NJ-UNDRWD, NJ-VIRTUAHS>
+ Advocare Cornerstone Pediatrics
318 North Haddon Avenue/Suite A   Haddonfield, NJ 08033   (856)428-3746   Fax (856)310-0312

Bruner, Vanda, MD {1023066305} Pedtrc, AdolMd(82,YUGO)<NJ-MONMOUTH, NJ-RIVERVW>
+ 719 North Beers Street/Suite 1A
Holmdel, NJ 07733   (732)264-4646   Fax (732)264-4314

Brunetti, Jacqueline Carol, MD {1891722724} RadDia, Radiol, NuclMd(75,NY08)<NJ-HOLYNAME>
+ Holy Name Hospital
718 Teaneck Road/Radiology   Teaneck, NJ 07666   (201)833-7225   Fax (201)541-5919

Brunetti, Vito Anthony, MD {1336261056} OtgyFPIS, Otlryg, IntrMd(02,NY06)
+ ENT & Allergy Associates, LLP
1211 Hamburg Turnpike/Suite 205   Wayne, NJ 07470   (973)633-0808   Fax (973)633-8811

Brunetto, Jacqueline Marie Gerardi, MD {1689645806} Pedtrc, IntrMd(94,OH06)<NJ-MONMOUTH>
+ Monmouth Medical Center
300 Second Avenue/Pediatrics   Long Branch, NJ 07740   (732)923-6250   Fax (732)923-7255

Brunner, Eugenie, MD {1992732861} Otlryg, SrgFPI, OtgyFPIS(90,NJ06)<NJ-UNVMCPRN>
+ 256 Bunn Drive/Suite 4
Princeton, NJ 08540   (609)921-9497   Fax (609)921-7040
info@brunnermd.com

Brunner, Jaclyn Renee, MD {1619108347}
+ Cooper Univerisry Emergency Physicians
One Cooper Plaza   Camden, NJ 08103   (856)342-2627   Fax (856)968-8272

Brunnquell, Stephen B., MD {1740281310} IntrMd(89,NJ05)<NJ-ENGLWOOD>
+ The Park Medical Group
24 Elm Street   Harrington Park, NJ 07640   (201)784-0123   Fax (201)784-0065
+ The Park Medical Group
274 County Road/Suite A   Tenafly, NJ 07670   (201)784-0123   Fax (201)568-0483

Bruno, Basil, MD {1164509444} Pedtrc, IntrMd(89,NJ05)<NJ-HACKNSK>
+ Pedimedica, P.A.
18 Railroad Avenue/Suite 103   Rochelle Park, NJ 07662   (201)291-2323   Fax (201)291-2328

Bruno, Chantal Dominique, DO {1770946964} Pedtrc
+ University Medical Group Pediatrics
125 Paterson Street/MEB 3rd Fl   New Brunswick, NJ 08903   (732)235-7883   Fax (732)235-6609

Bruno, Christopher Ryan, MD {1255322079} Ophthl(98,PA14)<NJ-MEMSALEM>
+ Ophthalmic Associates
2835 South Delsea Drive   Vineland, NJ 08360   (856)696-0020   Fax (856)205-1721

Bruno, Robert, DO {1740220730} Nephro
+ Jersey Coast Nephrology & Hypertension Associates
1541 Route 88/Suite A   Brick, NJ 08724   (732)836-3200   Fax (732)836-3201

Bruno, Stephen F., MD {1891734406} EmrgMd, IntrMd(82,MNT01)<NJ-RIVERVW>
+ Riverview Medical Center
1 Riverview Plaza/EmergMed   Red Bank, NJ 07701   (732)741-2700   Fax (732)224-7498

Bruno, Victor P., MD {1073582276} Surgry(78,DC02)
+ Drs. Bruno and Hurwitz
104 North Euclid Avenue   Westfield, NJ 07090   (908)654-0888
+ Drs. Murphy & Williams, P.A.
33 Overlook Road/Suite 412   Summit, NJ 07901   (908)273-7274
+ Drs. Murphy & Williams, P.A.
867 St. Georges Avenue   Rahway, NJ 07090   (732)388-0990

Brunson, Rodney C., DO {1336247378} FamMed(91,NJ75)
+ 201 Tilton Road/Suite 12
Northfield, NJ 08225   (609)484-7000   Fax (609)484-1533

Brus, Christina R., MD {1265641120} Hemato, MedOnc, IntrMd(05,NY46)
+ MD Anderson Cancer Center at Cooper
2 Cooper Plaza   Camden, NJ 08103   (855)632-2667

Brusco, Louis, Jr., MD {1295779379} Anesth, CritCr, IntrMd(85,NY01)<NY-SLRLUKES>
+ Anesthesia Associates of Morristown
100 Madison Avenue   Morristown, NJ 07960   (973)971-1534
Louis.Brusco@gmail.com

Brustein, Fredric, MD {1881848125} PhysMd, IntrMd(73,NY09)
+ 3 Pilgrim Hollow Road
Asbury Park, NJ 07712   (732)493-4860   Fax (732)493-4860

Brutico, Anthony J., DO {1790728327} EmrgMd(01,PA78)<NJ-NWTNMEM>
+ Newton Medical Center
175 High Street/EmrgMed   Newton, NJ 07860   (973)383-2121

Brutus, Nadege A., DO {1154399392} NnPnMd<NJ-VIRTVOOR>
+ CHOP Care Network at Virtua Voorhees Hospital
100 Bowman Drive   Voorhees, NJ 08043   (856)325-3000   Fax (609)261-5842

Bruzzi-Ehrlich, Diane, MD {1912935875} IntrMd, FamMed(82,GRN01)
+ Medi Center of Edison
1813 Oak Tree Road   Edison, NJ 08820   (908)769-9494   Fax (908)755-3833

Bryan, Craigh Keith, MD {1588769178} IntrMd(98,NJ06)
+ Englewood Hospital and Medical Center
350 Engle Street/Medicine   Englewood, NJ 07631   (201)894-3364   Fax (201)894-5693

Bryan, Gregory Alan, MD {1376803650}<NJ-CHRIST>
+ Christ Hospital
176 Palisade Avenue   Jersey City, NJ 07306   (856)261-5165

Bryan, Margarette R.N., MD {1114019957} Hemato, IntrMd, MedOnc(79,JMAC)<NJ-UMDNJ>
+ University Hospital
150 Bergen Street/Hematology   Newark, NJ 07103   (973)972-6257   Fax (973)972-2384
bryanmr@umdnj.edu

Bryan, Sheila Curry, MD {1306895263} Pedtrc, IntrMd(88,FL03)<NJ-RWJUBRUN>
+ RWJ University Hospital New Brunswick
One Robert Wood Johnson Place   New Brunswick, NJ 08901   (732)937-8766   Fax (732)381-3144

Bryant, Dennie Antoinette, DO {1700174166}
+ 91 Kingsbridge Drive
Lumberton, NJ 08048

Bryant, Manmohan, MD {1639117583} FamMed(86,OH41)<NJ-HUNTRDN>
+ 6 Losey Road
Ringoes, NJ 08551   (908)237-2662   Fax (908)237-2663

Bryant, Tony Labree, Jr., MD {1548588072}
+ Rothman Institute
999 Route 73 North/3rd Fl   Marlton, NJ 08053   (856)821-6360   Fax (856)821-6359
bryantl@ortho.ufl.edu

Bryczkowski, Christopher J., MD {1992026348} EmrgMd(10,NJ06)
+ University Emergency Medicine
125 Paterson Street/MEB 104   New Brunswick, NJ 08901   (732)235-4296   Fax (732)235-7379
bryczkcj@rwjms.rutgers.edu

Bryczkowski, Sarah B., MD {1427375328}<NJ-UMDNJ>
+ University Hospital
150 Bergen Street   Newark, NJ 07103   (973)972-4300

Bryhn, Lisa Kristen, MD {1689648651} FamMed(95,NJ05)<NJ-HUNTRDN>
+ Delaware Valley Family Health Center
200 Frenchtown Road   Milford, NJ 08848   (908)995-2251   Fax (908)995-2036

Bryman, Paul N., DO {1609849819} Grtrcs(83,IA75)
+ 532 Old Marlton Pike
Marlton, NJ 08053   (732)367-4422

Brys, Agata K., MD {1447273487} Otlryg, SrgFPI, IntrMd(04,MA05)
+ ENT & Allergy Associates of Parsippany
900 Lanidex Plaza/Suite 300   Parsippany, NJ 07054   (973)394-1818   Fax (973)394-1810
+ ENT & Allergy Associates, LLP
3219 Route 46 East/Suite 203   Parsippany, NJ 07054   (973)394-1818   Fax (973)394-1810

Brzustowicz, Linda Marie, MD {1548632656} Psychy, IntrMd(87,NY01)
+ 40 Green Avenue
Madison, NJ 07940   (862)368-1153
brzustowicz@axon.rutgers.edu

Bshesh, Khaled Khalifa, MD {1083749998} Pedtrc, PedCrC(91,LIY02)<OH-CHLDAKRN>
+ Monmouth Medical Center
300 Second Avenue   Long Branch, NJ 07740   (732)923-7250   Fax (732)923-7255

Bucalo, Victor John, MD {1043258486} PhysMd(02,GRN01)<NJ-PALISADE, NJ-ENGLWOOD>
+ Physical Medicine & Rehabilitation Center
500 Grand Avenue/1st Floor   Englewood, NJ 07631   (201)567-2277   Fax (201)567-7506

Buccigrossi, Jennifer Leigh, MD {1598728131} Pedtrc, AdolMd(98,PA02)<NJ-VIRTUAHS, NJ-VIRTMHBC>
+ Advocare Medford Pediatric & Adolescent Medicine
520 Stokes Road   Medford, NJ 08055   (609)654-9112   Fax (609)654-7404

Bucek, John Ladislav, MD {1265432942} FamMed, OthrSp(93,NY47)<NJ-SOMERSET>
+ RWJ University Hospital Somerset
110 Rehill Avenue/FamMedResidency   Somerville, NJ 08876   (908)685-2900   Fax (908)685-2891
jbucek@somerset-healthcare.com
+ Somerset Family Practice
110 Rehill Avenue   Somerville, NJ 08876   (908)685-2900   Fax (908)685-2891

Buceta, Joseph, MD {1154392975} Psychy(78,URUG)<NJ-GRYSTPSY>
+ Greystone Park Psychiatric Hospital
59 Koch Avenue   Morris Plains, NJ 07950   (973)538-1800

Buch, David Leslie, MD {1467526756} PsyAdd, PsyGrt(77,TN05)
+ Univ Correctional HealthCare-Colpitts
Whittessey Rd & Stuyvesant Ave   Trenton, NJ 08625   (609)292-9700

Buch, Edward D., MD {1174575369} SrgVas, Surgry(81,NY08)<NJ-SOMERSET, NJ-STPETER>
+ Raritan Valley Surgical Associates PA
611 Courtyard Drive/Suite 600   Hillsborough, NJ 08844   (908)722-0030   Fax (908)722-8676

Buch, Raymond S., MD {1023016227} FamMed(79,NJ05)<NJ-WARREN>
+ St. Luke's Coventry Family Practice
755 Memorial Parkway/Suite 300   Phillipsburg, NJ 08865   (908)847-3300   Fax (866)281-6023

Buchalter, Maury, MD {1700842093} Pedtrc, InfDis, IntrMd(84,NY47)<NJ-ENGLWOOD, NJ-HACKNSK>
+ Tenafly Pediatrics, PA
1135 Broad Street/Suite 208   Clifton, NJ 07013   (973)471-8600   Fax (973)471-3068
+ Tenafly Pediatrics, PA
301 Bridge Plaza North   Fort Lee, NJ 07024   (973)471-8600   Fax (201)592-6350
+ The Valley Hospital
223 North Van Dien Avenue   Ridgewood, NJ 07013   (201)447-8000

Buchan, Shahindokh, MD {1235270471} Psychy(69,IRA01)
+ 718 Bernice Court
Toms River, NJ 08753   (732)244-2222

Buchanan, David J., DO {1639377120} CdvDis<NJ-DEBRAHLC>
+ Deborah Heart and Lung Center
200 Trenton Road   Browns Mills, NJ 08015   (609)893-6611   Fax (609)735-1856

Buchbinder, Howard J., MD {1952343998} Anesth(82,WI05)
+ 7 Rambling Drive
Scotch Plains, NJ 07076

Buchbinder, Marta Luisa H., MD {1134172893} Pedtrc(92,BRA44)
+ Hamilton Pediatric Associates
3 Hamilton Health Place/Suite A   Hamilton, NJ 08690   (609)581-4480   Fax (609)581-5222

Buchen, Daniel, MD {1922069467} Dermat, DerMOH(94,NY08)<NY-MTSINAI>
+ 730 Kennedy Boulevard
Bayonne, NJ 07002   (201)858-4300

Bucher, Joshua Thomas, MD {1700124765} EmrgMd
+ Robert Wood Johnson Emergency Medicine
One Robert Wood Johnson Place/MEB 104   New Brunswick, NJ 08901   (732)492-6158

Buchholz, Stacen, DO {1497168389}<NJ-SJHREGMC>
+ SJH Regional Medical Center
1505 West Sherman Avenue   Vineland, NJ 08360   (856)641-6023

Bucholtz, Harvey K., MD {1427020296} EnDbMt, IntrMd(68,NY15)<NJ-NWRKBETH, NJ-STBARNMC>
+ M.E.N.D., PA
2 Lincoln Highway/Suite 501   Edison, NJ 08820   (732)661-2020   Fax (732)661-2022

Buchwald, Eugene E., MD {1588724777} Nrolgy(69,DC03)<NJ-JFKMED, NJ-RWJURAH>
+ Edison Neurologic Associates
36 Progress Street/Suite B-3   Edison, NJ 08820   (908)757-6633   Fax (908)757-3912

Bucich, Joseph Marc, Jr., MD {1376594275} RadDia, Radiol, RadBdI(93,PA02)<NJ-WARREN>
+ Progressive Physician Associates, Inc.
185 Roseberry Street   Phillipsburg, NJ 08865   (610)868-1100   Fax (610)868-1111

Buck, Andrea S., DO {1447301700} Dermat(87,PA77)
+ 103 Old Marlton Pike/Suite 215
Medford, NJ 08055   (609)714-0202   Fax (609)714-0303

Buck, David Carmine, Jr., DO {1841507886}<NJ-DEBRAHLC>
+ Deborah Heart and Lung Center
200 Trenton Road   Browns Mills, NJ 08015   (609)893-6611

Physicians by Name and Address

Buck, Gary B., MD {1427054253} Anesth(93,NJ06)<NJ-LOURDMED>
+ Rancocas Anesthesiology, PA
  15000 Midlantic Drive/Suite 102   Mount Laurel, NJ 08054   (856)255-5479   Fax (856)393-8691
+ Rancocas Anesthesiology, PA
  700 Route 130 North/Suite 203   Cinnaminson, NJ 08077   (856)255-5479   Fax (856)829-3605
+ 34 Sheffield Drive
  Moorestown, NJ 08054

Buck, Melissa, MD {1235578840} Pedtrc
+ Goryeb Children's Hospital
  100 Madison Avenue   Morristown, NJ 07960   (973)971-7802

Buck, Murray D., DO {1841229309} FamMed(82,NJ75)<NJ-VIRTMHBC, NJ-KMHSTRAT>
+ Alliance for Better Care, PC/Mount Holly Division
  1613 Route 38   Lumberton, NJ 08048   (609)261-3716   Fax (609)261-5507
+ Alliance for Better Care, P.C.
  PO Box 1510   Medford, NJ 08055   (609)261-3716   Fax (609)953-8652

Buck, Warren G., MD {1720019532} CdvDis, IntrMd(73,ITAL)
+ Menlo Park Medical Group PA
  111 James Street   Edison, NJ 08820   (732)549-4066   Fax (732)549-2262

Buckley, Karen Marie, MD {1225094659} SrgPlstc, SrgRec(94,NY09)<NJ-COOPRUMC>
+ Cooper Surgical Associates
  3 Cooper Plaza/Suite 411   Camden, NJ 08103   (856)342-2270   Fax (856)365-1180

Buckley, Laura K., MD {1770745416} PulCCr, PulDis, IntrMd(05,NJ06)
+ Princeton Medicine
  5 Plainsboro Road/Suite 300   Plainsboro, NJ 08536   (609)853-7272   Fax (609)853-7271
+ Urology Group of Princeton PA
  281 Witherspoon Street/Suite 100   Princeton, NJ 08542   (609)853-7272   Fax (609)921-7020

Buckley, Michael K., MD {1891727350} SrgC&R, Surgry(79,IRE05)<NJ-STMRYPAS, NJ-STJOSHOS>
+ Surgery Associates of North Jersey, P.A.
  1100 Clifton Avenue   Clifton, NJ 07013   (973)778-0100   Fax (973)778-2029

Buckley, Patrick S., MD {1427315969} SprtMd
+ NJ Orthopedic Surgeons
  4810 Belmar Boulevard/1st Floor   Wall Township, NJ 07753   (732)938-6090

Buckley, Tinera Mcnair, MD {1720427669} PthAcl
+ St. Barnabas Medical Center
  94 Old Short Hills Road   Livingston, NJ 07039   (973)322-5760

Budak-Alpdogan, Tulin, MD {1942519004} OncHem, IntrMd(87)<NJ-COOPRUMC>
+ Cooper University Medical Center/Camden
  3 Cooper Plaza/Hema Oncology   Camden, NJ 08103   (856)356-4935

Budd, Daniel C., MD {1174588461} Surgry, IntrMd(69,NC07)<NJ-CHILTON, NJ-VALLEY>
+ General Surgeons of North Jersey
  707 Broadway   Paterson, NJ 07514   (973)742-3371   Fax (973)742-3168
+ General Surgeons of North Jersey
  535 Wanaque Avenue   Pompton Lakes, NJ 07442   (973)742-3371   Fax (973)742-3168
+ General Surgeons of North Jersey
  18-21 Fairlawn Avenue   Fair Lawn, NJ 07514   (201)796-9090   Fax (973)742-3168

Buddala, Sangeeta, MD {1659460509} IntrMd(97,INA83)
+ New Jersey Division of Developmental Disability
  Route 72 East   New Lisbon, NJ 08064   (609)726-1000   Fax (609)894-8430

Buddle, Patrick M., MD {1013904853} PhysMd(82,GRN01)<NJ-JRSYSHMC, NJ-OCEANMC>
+ Highway 71 & Crescent Place
  Sea Girt, NJ 08750   (732)974-8100

Budhwani, Anju, MD {1679795835} PulCCr, IntrMd(98,INA96)
+ NJ Heart/Elizabeth Office
  240 Williamson Street/Suite 402-406   Elizabeth, NJ 07202   (908)354-8900   Fax (908)354-0007
+ Global Tuberculosis Institute (GTBI)
  225 Warren Street/PO Box 1709   Newark, NJ 07101   (908)354-8900   Fax (973)972-3268
+ NJ MedCare
  1 Ethel Road/Suite 102 C   Edison, NJ 07202   (732)287-6663   Fax (732)287-6664

Budhwani, Navin, MD {1104990266} CdvDis, IntCrd, IntrMd(98,NJ05)<NY-MTSINAI, NJ-VALLEY>
+ Cardiac Associates of North Jersey
  43 Yawpo Avenue/Suite 2   Oakland, NJ 07436   (201)337-0066   Fax (201)337-7417

Budin, Joel A., MD {1821073180} Radiol, RadDia(69,NY01)<NJ-HACKNSK>
+ The Imaging Center
  30 South Newman Street   Hackensack, NJ 07601   (201)488-1188   Fax (201)488-5244
+ New Century Imaging at Oradell
  555 Kinderkamack Road   Oradell, NJ 07649   (201)488-1188   Fax (201)599-8333
+ Hackensack Radiology Group, P.A.
  30 Prospect Avenue   Hackensack, NJ 07601   (201)996-2200   Fax (201)336-8451

Budnick, Glenn R., MD {1497956940} Pedtrc(77,DC02)<NJ-ACMCITY>
+ Pediatric Associates of Atlantic County PA
  108 West Jimmie Leeds Road   Pomona, NJ 08240   (609)652-6872
+ Pediatric Associates of Atlantic County, P.A.
  9009 Ventnor Avenue   Margate, NJ 08402   (609)823-2773

Budnick, Lawrence D., MD {1801812136} OccpMd, PubHth, IntrMd(77,NY08)<NJ-UMDNJ>
+ The University Hospital
  65 Bergen Street   Newark, NJ 07107   (973)972-2900   Fax (973)972-2904

Budoff, Steven R., DO {1376517052} Psychy(89,NY75)<NJ-HUNTRDN>
+ CCVS Care LLC
  597 Springfield Avenue   Summit, NJ 07901   (908)654-7399

Buechel, Frederick F., MD {1770538894} SrgOrt(72,NJ05)
+ South Mountain Orthopaedic Associates, P.A.
  61 First Street   South Orange, NJ 07079   (973)762-8344   Fax (973)762-1626
+ The Joint Institute at Saint Barnabas Medical Center
  609 Morris Avenue   Springfield, NJ 07081   (973)762-8344   Fax (973)467-8647

Bueno, Hugo Felipe, MD {1881117877} IntrMd
+ Rutgers- New Jersey Medical School
  185 South Orange Avenue/MSB F508 B   Newark, NJ 07103   (973)972-6025   Fax (973)972-7429

Buerano, Thelma Mapa, MD {1487731543} IntrMd(79,PHI30)
+ 2142 Route 70
  Manchester, NJ 08759   (732)408-9585   Fax (732)408-9586

Bufalini, Bruno, MD {1740233956} Surgry(70,ITAL)<NJ-ENGLWOOD>
+ Dr. Bufalini and Associates
  200 Grand Avenue/Suite 203   Englewood, NJ 07631   (201)871-0303   Fax (201)871-4860

Bufalino, Kevin Thomas, MD {1518965748} RadDia, Radiol(90,PA13)<NJ-VIRTVOOR, NJ-VIRTUAHS>
+ South Jersey Radiology Associates, P.A.
  315 Route 70 East/Suite B   Cherry Hill, NJ 08034   (856)428-4344   Fax (856)428-0356
+ South Jersey Radiology Associates, P.A.
  1000 Lincoln Drive East   Marlton, NJ 08053   (856)428-4344   Fax (856)983-3226
+ South Jersey Radiology Associates, P.A.
  807 Haddon Avenue/Suite 5   Haddonfield, NJ 08034   (856)616-1130   Fax (856)616-1125

Bugay, Victor Valdes, MD {1568416352} IntrMd(97,PHI09)
+ Espineli Medical Associates PC
  1163 Route 37 West/Suite D-4   Toms River, NJ 08755   (732)341-9494   Fax (732)341-3416

Bui, Hoan K., MD {1780966788} SrgTrm, Surgry(GRN01)<NJ-STJOSHOS>
+ St. Joseph Medical Center Surgery
  703 Main Street   Paterson, NJ 07503   (973)754-2490   Fax (973)754-4332

Bui, Minh Ngoc, MD {1720037286} EmrgMd, IntrMd(87,PA13)<NJ-MEMSALEM>
+ Memorial Hospital of Salem County
  310 Woodstown Road/Emerg Med   Salem, NJ 08079   (856)339-6048   Fax (856)935-0962

Bui, Stephanie T., DO {1245461292}<NJ-DEBRAHLC>
+ Deborah Heart and Lung Center
  200 Trenton Road   Browns Mills, NJ 08015   (616)252-7200   stbui.do@gmail.com

Buinewicz, Anna Miller, MD {1700907110} FamMed(86,PA02)
+ Merck and Company Incorporated
  1 Merck Drive/PO Box 100   Whitehouse Station, NJ 08889   (908)423-1000   Fax (908)823-3142

Buirkle, James E., MD {1215041140} Pedtrc(85,NJ05)
+ Old Tappan Medical Group
  645 Westwood Avenue/2nd Floor   River Vale, NJ 07675   (201)666-1000   Fax (201)666-4108

Buisson, Valerie Fabiola, MD {1730409475} FamMed(DMN01)
+ Lutheran Senior Life at Jersey City
  377 Jersey Avenue/Suite 310   Jersey City, NJ 07302   (609)599-5433

Buker, Ibrahim S., MD {1295707636} Surgry(74,EGYP)<NJ-BAYSHORE, NJ-RBAYPERT>
+ One Bethany Road/Building 6/Suite 85
  Hazlet, NJ 07730

Bukhari, Sumera, MD {1467813279} IntrMd(PAK04)
+ St. Francis Medical Center
  601 Hamilton Avenue   Trenton, NJ 08629   (609)599-5000

Buksh, Wazim R., MD {1073893442}<NJ-MORRISTN>
+ Atlantic Medical Group
  One Health Plaza/Bldg. 125   East Hanover, NJ 07936   (862)778-7960   Fax (973)781-6505

Bulahan, Alvin, MD {1427347780} EmrgMd
+ 4 Rutgers Road
  Piscataway, NJ 08854

Bulan, Erwin Joseph, MD {1114953403} SrgPlstc(96,NY15)<NJ-MORRISTN, NJ-STBARNMC>
+ Bulan Plastic Surgery
  75 Main Street/Suite 105   Millburn, NJ 07041   (973)467-9744   Fax (973)467-7512
+ Bulan Plastic Surgery
  477 Route 10 East/Suite 204   Randolph, NJ 07869   (973)328-1357

Bulan, Jeanine Hermine, MD {1053357582} IntrMd(96,NY45)
+ Barnabas Medical Group
  560 Springfield Avenue/Suite 101   Westfield, NJ 07090   (908)233-8571   Fax (908)389-1411

Bulauitan, Constantine Spyridakis, MD {1477899359} Surgry(09,DMN01)
+ University Hospital-RWJ Medical School
  89 French Street/3/FL Suite 3265   New Brunswick, NJ 08901   (732)235-7766   Fax (732)235-2964

Bulei, Anita P., MD {1780844837} IntrMd(85,PA13)<NJ-COOPRUMC>
+ Cooper Physicians Washington Township
  1 Plaza Drive/Suite 103/Bunker Hill Pl   Sewell, NJ 08080   (856)270-4080   Fax (856)270-4085

Buli, Dolores M., MD {1497858468} Pedtrc(95,NJ05)<NJ-VALLEY, NJ-HACKNSK>
+ Garden State Pediatrics
  217 Old Hook Road/Suite 3C   Westwood, NJ 07675   (201)263-1477   Fax (201)263-0048

Bulik, Peter W., DO {1184987604}
+ Lourdes Cardiology Services
  1 Brace Road/Suite C   Cherry Hill, NJ 08034   (856)482-8900   Fax (856)482-7170
+ SOM - Department of Internal Medicine
  42 East Laurel Road/Suite 3100   Stratford, NJ 08084   (856)482-8900   Fax (856)566-6906

Bulkin, Yekaterina, MD {1912131152} RadDia, Radiol(02,NY47)
+ University Radiology Group, P.C.
  579A Cranbury Road   East Brunswick, NJ 08816   (732)390-0040   Fax (732)390-1856

Bullek, David D., MD {1417906439} SrgOrt(87,NJ06)<NJ-OVERLOOK>
+ Summit Medical Group
  574 Springfield Avenue   Westfield, NJ 07090   (908)232-7797   Fax (908)232-0540
  dbullek@smgnj.com

Bullinga, John Richard, MD {1699706994} IntrMd, ClcDEl, CdvDis(98,IA02)
+ Penn Medicine at Cherry Hill
  1400 East Route 70/Cardiology   Cherry Hill, NJ 08034

Bullock, Richard B., MD {1093704355} IntrMd, Grtrcs(81,NY47)<NJ-JFKMED>
+ Middlesex Medical Group
  225 May Street/Suite E   Edison, NJ 08837   (732)661-2020   Fax (732)661-2022

Bullock Palmer, Renee Patrice, MD {1972823334} CdvDis<NJ-DEBRAHLC>
+ Deborah Heart and Lung Center
  200 Trenton Road   Browns Mills, NJ 08015   (609)893-6611

Buna, Andrei, MD {1043309081} ObsGyn(78,ROM09)<NJ-MORRISTN, NJ-STCLRDEN>
+ Lifeline Medical Associates
  390 State Route 10/Suite 1   Randolph, NJ 07869   (973)328-1262   Fax (973)328-8576
  abuna@lma-llc.com

Bundens, David A., MD {1154321701} SrgOrt(78,PA13)<NJ-UNDRWD, NJ-KMHCHRRY>
+ 17 West Red Bank Avenue/Suite 104
  Woodbury, NJ 08096   (856)848-0665   Fax (856)384-1438

Buneviciute, Juste, MD {1578959748}
+ 248 Emmett Place
  Ridgewood, NJ 07450   (919)259-2626

Bunin, Sonalis, MD {1306007372} Nephro, IntrMd(06,NY0)<NY-SLOANKET, NY-PRSBCOLU>
+ Robert Wood Johnson Transplant Associates, P.A.
  10 Plum Street/7th Floor   New Brunswick, NJ 08901   (732)253-3699

Physicians by Name and Address

Bunn, Diane Marie, MD {1578986709} Pedtrc, IntrMd(SC01)
+ Princeton Nassau Pediatrics, P.A.
  25 South Route 31   Pennington, NJ 08534   (609)745-5300   Fax (609)745-5320
+ Princeton Nassau Pediatrics, P.A.
  196 Princeton-Hightstown Road   West Windsor, NJ 08550   (609)745-5300   Fax (609)799-2294

Bunnell, Eugene, MD {1770512089} CritCr, PulDis, IntrMd(86,PA02)<NJ-HACKNSK>
+ Hackensack University Medical Center
  30 Prospect Avenue/Critical Care   Hackensack, NJ 07601   (551)996-4838   Fax (551)996-3984

Buono, Amy C., MD {1881902799}
+ Buono Pediatrics & Wellness
  171 Millburn Avenue   Millburn, NJ 07041   (606)557-3085
+ PediatriCare Associates
  20-20 Fair Lawn Avenue   Fair Lawn, NJ 07410   (606)557-3085   Fax (201)791-3765
+ Morristown Medical Center
  100 Madison Avenue/4th floor   Morristown, NJ 07041   (973)971-7802

Buono, Lee M., MD {1134121981} SrgNro, IntrMd(PA02)
+ Capital Institute for Neurosciences
  2 Capital Way/Suite 456   Pennington, NJ 08534   (609)537-7300   Fax (609)537-7301

Buontempo, Angela J., DO {1861441461} ObsGyn, Gyneco(91,NY75)
+ Womens HealthCare of Union County
  950 West Chestnut Street/Suite 102   Union, NJ 07083   (908)688-8545   Fax (908)688-8447
+ Ambulatory Surgical Center of Union County
  950 West Chestnut Street/Suite 200   Union, NJ 07083   (908)688-8545   Fax (908)688-7424

Bupathi, Kavita Kishor, MD {1992732135} Pedtrc(91,INA16)
+ 2 Ethel Road/Suite 206C
  Edison, NJ 08817   (732)650-0350   Fax (732)650-0351
+ 1 Woodbridge Center/Suite 700
  Woodbridge, NJ 07095   (732)650-0350   Fax (732)320-0364

Burach, Ilene Heidi, MD {1184889925} RadDia
+ Coastal Imaging, LLC
  79 Route 37 West/Suite 103   Toms River, NJ 08755   (732)678-0087   Fax (732)276-2325

Burachinsky, Andrew E., DO {1093757429} CdvDis, IntrMd(77,PA77)<NJ-CLARMAAS, NJ-STBARNMC>
+ North Arlington Cardiology Associates
  62 Ridge Road   North Arlington, NJ 07031   (201)991-8565   Fax (201)991-2408

Burachinsky, Dennis Andrew, DO {1427376698} OtgyFPlS, Otlryg(07,PA77)<NJ-SOMERSET, NJ-RWJUBRUN>
+ ENT & Allergy Associates-Bridgewater
  245 US Highway 22/3rd Fl/Suite 300   Bridgewater, NJ 08807   (908)722-1022   Fax (908)722-2040

Burak, Edward, MD {1700995768} Radiol, RadDia(64,NY15)
+ South Mountain Imaging
  120 Millburn Avenue   Millburn, NJ 07041   (973)376-0900   Fax (973)376-0010

Burakgazi Dalkilic, Evren, MD {1164440483} Nrolgy
+ Cooper University Neurology
  1935 Route 70 East   Cherry Hill, NJ 08003   (856)342-2445   Fax (856)964-0504

Burbella, Ronald E., MD {1376523662} ObsGyn(74,NJ05)<NJ-CHSFULD, NJ-CHSMRCER>
+ 2500 US Highway 1/Suite 202
  Lawrenceville, NJ 08648   (609)530-9100   Fax (609)530-0743
  Burbellaron@cs.com

Burda, John F., MD {1922060268} RadV&I
+ Radiology Affiliates of Central New Jersey, P.A.
  2501 Kuser Road   Hamilton, NJ 08691   (609)585-8800   Fax (609)585-1825

Burden, Amanda R., MD {1245329861} Anesth(99,PA01)<NJ-COOPRUMC>
+ Cooper University Hospital
  One Cooper Plaza/Anesth   Camden, NJ 08103   (856)342-2000
+ Cooper Surgery Center
  900 Centennial Boulevard/Suite E   Voorhees, NJ 08043   (856)342-2000   Fax (856)325-6515

Burden, Yumie Nishida, DO {1467691709} FamMed
+ AFC Urgent Care West Orange
  464 Eagle Rock Avenue   West Orange, NJ 07052   (973)669-5900   Fax (973)669-5909

Burducea, Alexandru, DO {1558540807} Anesth, PainMd(03,NY75)
+ Newark Rehabilitation Center
  638 Mount Prospect Avenue   Newark, NJ 07104   (973)481-4040   Fax (973)481-1338

Burga, Ana Maria, MD {1285685909} Pthlgy, PthACl(96,IL11)<NJ-ENGLWOOD>
+ Englewood Hospital and Medical Center
  350 Engle Street   Englewood, NJ 07631   (201)894-3000
  Fax (201)871-2269

Burger, Max, MD {1386648004} FamMed(76,IREL)<NJ-VIRTUAHS>
+ 1805 Route 206/Suite 10
  Southampton, NJ 08088   (609)801-0300   Fax (609)801-0399
  maxburgermd@pol.net

Burgess, David B., MD {1215946215} PedDvl, Pedtrc(73,WI05)
+ CHOP Pediatric & Adolescent Specialty Care Center
  4009 Black Horse Pike   Mays Landing, NJ 08330   (609)677-7895   Fax (609)677-7835

Burghauser, Alan H., MD {1992806608} IntrMd, PulDis(79,NY08)<NJ-BAYONNE, NJ-STBARNMC>
+ Pulmonary and Critical Care Associates
  534 Avenue East   Bayonne, NJ 07002   (201)858-1021
  ahbmd@home.com
+ Pulmonary and Critical Care Associates
  2333 Morris Avenue/Suite B-15   Union, NJ 07083   (908)964-1964

Burgher, Sonia A., MD {1962431130} Pedtrc(76,NY03)
+ Drs. Burgher and Chikani
  2950 College Drive/Suite C   Vineland, NJ 08360   (856)692-6000   Fax (856)692-0609

Burghli, Rena F., DO {1255349957} IntrMd(03,IL76)<NJ-UMDNJ, NJ-HACKNSK>
+ Elan Laser MedSpa
  204 Summerhill Road/Suite C   East Brunswick, NJ 08816   (732)254-7601   Fax (732)254-7603
  info@elanlaser.com

Burgio, Michael T., MD {1811941339} IntrMd, EmrgMd(85,GRNA)<NJ-NWTNMEM>
+ Newton Medical Center
  175 High Street   Newton, NJ 07860   (973)383-2121

Burgos, Anthony, MD {1376702258} RadDia, Radiol, IntrMd(03,NJ06)
+ Radiology Affiliates of Central New Jersey, P.A.
  2501 Kuser Road   Hamilton, NJ 08691   (609)585-8800   Fax (609)585-1825
  aburgos@4rai.com

Burgos, Melissa, MD {1871753897} FamMed(05,NJ06)
+ Phillips Barber Family Health Center
  72 Alexander Avenue   Lambertville, NJ 08530   (609)397-3535   Fax (609)397-0301

Burhanna, Amy Scally, MD {1699725861} CdvDis, IntrMd(93,PA09)<NJ-BURDTMLN>
+ Cape Regional Physicians Associates-Cardiology
  217 North Main Street/Suite 205   Cape May Court House, NJ 08210   (609)463-5440   Fax (609)463-9888

Burke, Benita Mia, MD {1861684730} CdvDis, IntrMd(05,NJ03)
+ Valley Medical Group/Valley Heart Group
  1200 East Ridgewood Avenue   Ridgewood, NJ 07450   (201)670-3603   Fax (201)447-1957

Burke, Gary C., DO {1598744898} CdvDis, IntrMd(85,PA77)<NJ-OURLADY, NJ-VIRTUAHS>
+ Associated Cardiovascular Consultants-Lourdes
  1 Brace Road/Suite C & F   Cherry Hill, NJ 08034   (856)428-4100   Fax (856)428-5748

Burke, Gerald V., MD {1275611295} ObsGyn, RprEnd, IntrMd(79,PA09)<NJ-OURLADY, NJ-VIRTVOOR>
+ 1305 Kings Highway North/Suite 1
  Cherry Hill, NJ 08034   (856)429-2212   Fax (856)334-5896
  drburke@geraldburkemd.com

Burke, Hana Oswari, MD {1699764373} FamMed
+ Primary Care of Moorestown
  147 East 3rd Street/Suite 2   Moorestown, NJ 08057   (856)234-2500   Fax (856)234-3907
+ 10 Overlook Road/Apt 3 C
  Summit, NJ 07901

Burke, Margaret Linda, MD {1366531998} FamMed(91,PA02)<NJ-COOPRUMC>
+ Riverton Family Practice
  605 Main Street/Suite 104   Riverton, NJ 08077   (856)786-1717   Fax (856)786-2478

Burke, Meghan Deirdre, MD {1679740989} Pedtrc
+ Advocare Laurel Pediatrics
  269 Fish Pond Road   Sewell, NJ 08080   (856)863-9999   Fax (856)863-9666

Burke, Patricia A., MD {1952410680} Ophthl(86,NJ05)<NJ-HOLY-NAME>
+ One Sears Drive/4th Floor
  Paramus, NJ 07652   (201)599-0123   Fax (201)599-0934

Burke, Rachel Irene, MD {1417995614} EmrgMd(01,NJ06)<NJ-VIRTVOOR>
+ Virtua Voorhees
  100 Bowman Drive/EmrgMed   Voorhees, NJ 08043   (856)247-3000

Burke, Scott Walter, MD {1164488987} CdvDis, IntrMd(98,PA02)<NJ-BURDTMLN, NJ-SHOREMEM>
+ Mercer Bucks Cardiology
  3140 Princeton Pike/2nd Floor   Lawrenceville, NJ 08648   (609)895-1919   Fax (609)895-1200

Burkett, Eric Nelson, MD {1770550576} IntrMd, Grtrcs(71,PA09)<NJ-MONMOUTH>
+ Monmouth Medical Center
  300 Second Avenue   Long Branch, NJ 07740   (732)222-5200
+ Monmouth Medical Group, P.C.
  223 Monmouth Road   West Long Branch, NJ 07764   (732)222-5200   Fax (732)229-4562

Burkey, Brooke Alissa, MD {1649496340} SrgRec(01,PA01)
+ St. Christopher Care at Washington Township
  405 Hurffville-Cross Keys Road   Sewell, NJ 08080   (856)582-0644   Fax (856)582-0622

Burkey, Seth Micah, MD {1306031893} EmrgMd(06,PA13)<PA-STLKBTHL>
+ Coordinated Health
  222 Red Lane   Phillipsburg, NJ 08865   (610)861-8080   Fax (610)849-1013

Burn, Charlene H., MD {1568678555} Psychy(66,NJ05)
+ 49 Riverview Terrace
  Upper Saddle River, NJ 07458   (201)760-9709   Fax (201)760-9402

Burnett, Atuhani Seth, MD {1902125701}<NJ-UMDNJ>
+ University Hospital
  150 Bergen Street/Suite E-401   Newark, NJ 07103   (973)972-4300

Burns, Elizabeth Ann, DO {1255401402} PsyCAd, PsyFor(91,NJ75)
+ Ancora Psychiatric Hospital
  301 Spring Garden Road   Hammonton, NJ 08037   (609)561-1700   Fax (609)567-7252

Burns, Gerard Joseph, II, DO {1871783506} IntrMd
+ Advocare in-Patient Medicine
  100 Bowman Drive   Voorhees, NJ 08043   (856)247-3000

Burns, H. Patrick, MD {1538228432} IntrMd, Pedtrc(94,NJ05)
+ Morris County Primary Care
  2839 Route 10 East/Suite 101   Morris Plains, NJ 07950   (973)292-5600   Fax (973)292-6435

Burns, John J., MD {1962466284} CdvDis, IntCrd, IntrMd(75,PA09)<NJ-RWJUBRUN, NJ-STPETER>
+ Cardiology Associates of New Brunswick
  593 Cranbury Road/Suite 2   East Brunswick, NJ 08816   (732)390-3333   Fax (732)390-9244

Burns, Kenneth L., MD {1528155983} Psychy(84,NJ06)<NJ-RWJUBRUN>
+ UH-University Behavioral Hlth
  100 Metroplex Drive/Suite 200   Edison, NJ 08817   (732)235-8400   Fax (732)235-8395

Burns, Les A., MD {1528092608} ObsGyn(81,PA09)<NJ-CHILTON, NJ-STJOSHOS>
+ 1784 Hamburg Turnpike
  Wayne, NJ 07470   (973)831-9925   Fax (973)831-9926

Burns, Loren T., MD {1407952864} Dermat, SrgDer(67,IL11)<NJ-OURLADY>
+ Haddonfield Dermatology Associates
  24 West Kings Highway   Haddonfield, NJ 08033   (856)795-1341   Fax (856)795-5034

Burns, Paul Gerard, MD {1659348696} Surgry, SrgThr, CdvDis(89,NY01)<NJ-DEBRAHLC>
+ Deborah Heart and Lung Center
  200 Trenton Road/Surgery/Thorac   Browns Mills, NJ 08015   (973)971-7300   Fax (973)984-7019
+ Mid-Atlantic Surgical Associates
  100 Madison Avenue   Morristown, NJ 07960   (973)971-7300   Fax (973)984-7019

Burns, Richard Kent, MD {1093805855} SrgTrm, Surgry(85,CA14)
+ Cooper Surgical Associates
  3 Cooper Plaza/Suite 411   Camden, NJ 08103   (856)342-3340   Fax (856)365-1180

Burns, Talitha Mariana Hedley, DO {1578661856} Anesth(02,IA75)<NJ-OVERLOOK>
+ St. Joseph's Regional Medical Center Anesthesia
  703 Main Street   Paterson, NJ 07503   (973)754-2323   Fax (973)977-9455

Burroughs, Valentine J., MD {1689683369}(75,MI01)
+ 51 Dixon Drive
  Florham Park, NJ 07932   (973)520-8092
  vjbjrmd@aol.com

Burrows, Adria, MD {1841298932} Ophthl, PedOph(84,NY09)<NJ-STBARNMC>
+ Clifton Eye Care
  1016 Main Street   Clifton, NJ 07011   (973)546-5700   Fax (973)546-8898
+ Clifton Eye Care
  245 Engle Street   Englewood, NJ 07631   (973)546-5700   Fax (201)568-4233

Burrows, Andrew F., MD {1245385129} Ophthl(01,TX01)
+ 216 Engle Street/Suite 201
  Englewood, NJ 07631   (201)871-3415
+ Klein & Scannapiego MD PA
  230 West Jersey Street   Elizabeth, NJ 07202   (201)871-3415   Fax (908)352-4752

Physicians by Name and Address

Bursheh, Samar Samir, MD {1154573665}
+ Specialty Medconsultants LLC
6725 Ventnor Avenue/Suite C   Ventnor City, NJ 08406
(609)350-6780   Fax (609)350-6995

Burshtain, Ofer, MD {1376831297}<NJ-ENGLWOOD>
+ Englewood Hospital and Medical Center
350 Engle Street   Englewood, NJ 07631   (925)876-1227
boferb@gmail.com

Burshteyn, Mark, MD {1619118932} RadDia
+ Radiology Affiliates of Central New Jersey, P.A.
2501 Kuser Road   Hamilton, NJ 08691   (609)585-8800
Fax (609)585-1825

Burstein, Allan J., MD {1902087430} Psychy(68,TN07)
+ 505 Stillwells Corner Road
Freehold, NJ 07728   (732)462-5270   Fax (646)672-0446

Burstein, David Harris, MD {1164681524} Otlryg
+ Summit Medical Group-Berkeley Heights Campus
1 Diamond Hill Road   Berkeley Heights, NJ 07922
(908)273-4300   Fax (908)790-6576

Burstein, Mark Jeffrey, MD {1972788214} Otlryg
+ Premier ENT Associates
8 Quakerbridge Plaza   Hamilton, NJ 08619   (609)890-7800
Fax (609)890-6148

Burstin, Stuart J., MD {1528107588} InfDis, IntrMd(75,NY19)<NJ-RWJUBRUN, NJ-MORRISTN>
+ ID Associates PA/dba ID Care
8 Saddle Road   Cedar Knolls, NJ 07927   (973)993-5950
Fax (973)993-5953
+ ID Associates PA/dba ID Care
765 Route 10 East/Suite 201   Randolph, NJ 07869
(973)993-5950   Fax (973)361-8955

Burt, Clifton Daniel, MD {1588843163} PhyMPain(96,TN20)
+ Pain Managment Center of New Jersey
73 Main Street/Suite 36   Woodbridge, NJ 07095   (908)688-8880

Burt-Libo, Borislava, DO {1053532465} ObsGyn(03,NY75)
+ Healthy Woman Ob/Gyn
312 Professional View Drive   Freehold, NJ 07728
(732)431-1616   Fax (732)866-7962

Burtman, Elizabeth, MD {1679866255} Pedtrc
+ Pediatric Endocrinology
2 Dean Drive/Suite 2   Tenafly, NJ 07670   (201)871-4680
Fax (201)871-3815

Burton, Deniz Michelle, MD {1154538585} Pedtrc(92,TUR07)
+ 296 Clifton Avenue
Clifton, NJ 07011   (973)249-8211

Burton, Monica L., MD {1487684932} Pedtrc, IntrMd(85,VA07)<NJ-COOPRUMC>
+ CAMCare Health Corporation
817 Federal Street/Suite 100/Pedi   Camden, NJ 08103
(856)541-9811   Fax (856)541-4611

Burzon, Daniel Todd, MD {1134102015} Urolgy(91,NY06)<NJ-OCEANMC, NJ-JRSYSHMC>
+ Coastal Urology Associates
446 Jack Martin Boulevard   Brick, NJ 08724   (732)840-4300
Fax (732)840-4515
+ Coastal Urology Associates
444 Neptune Boulevard/Suite 3   Neptune, NJ 07753
(732)840-4300   Fax (732)988-8996
+ Coastal Urology Associates
814 River Avenue   Lakewood, NJ 08724   (732)370-2250
Fax (732)901-9119

Busbey, Shail, MD {1225168040} Dermat
+ 20 Park Place
Short Hills, NJ 07078   (973)218-1101   Fax (973)218-1101

Busch, Gregory Howard, DO {1598766131} FamMed(98,PA77)<NJ-VIRTMHBC>
+ Virtua Memorial
175 Madison Avenue/FamMed   Mount Holly, NJ 08060
(609)267-0700

Busch, Scott L., DO {1770507337} Otlryg, Otolgy, SrgPlstc(79,IA75)
+ Cherry Hill Center
1797 Springdale Road   Cherry Hill, NJ 08003   (856)424-0414   Fax (856)424-6335
slbusch@comcast.net

Bush, Nahndi, MD {1568504280} Ophthl(92,NJ05)<NJ-EAST-ORNG>
+ Healthcheck Medical and Eye Center
40 Union Avenue   Irvington, NJ 07111   (973)399-6270
Fax (973)374-3346
+ Health Excel PC
906 Oak Tree Road   South Plainfield, NJ 07080   (973)424-0776

Bushay, Stephen Lloyd, MD {1699867382} FamMed, IntrMd(97,PA02)
+ AtlantiCare Physician Group
1601 Tilton Road   Northfield, NJ 08225   (609)569-1900
Fax (609)569-1404

Busono, Stephanus Judi D., MD {1306888953} Nrolgy, OthrSp, IntrMd(93,NY46)
+ Princeton & Rutgers Neurology
77 Veronica Avenue/Suite 102   Somerset, NJ 08873
(732)246-1311   Fax (732)246-3089
+ Princeton Neuromuscular Center, PC
13 Clyde Road/Suite 103   Somerset, NJ 08873   (732)246-1311   Fax (732)649-3465

Bussard, Elizabeth S., MD {1497778757} Anesth(69,PA02)<NJ-HUNTRDN>
+ Hunterdon Medical Center
2100 Wescott Drive/Anesthesiology   Flemington, NJ 08822
(908)788-6181   Fax (908)788-6145

Bussey, Jonathan David, DO {1720296171} SrgNro, IntrMd(02,OK79)<NJ-COOPRUMC>
+ The Spine Institute of Southern New Jersey
512 Lippincott Drive   Marlton, NJ 08053   (856)797-9161
Fax (856)797-1288

Bussey, Paul George, MD {1356341424} FamMed(01,NET12)<NJ-MEMSALEM>
+ One Mill Street
Woodstown, NJ 08098   (856)769-1669

Bustamante, Irineo, Jr., MD {1154439420} EmrgMd(75,PHIL)<NJ-ACMCMAIN>
+ AtlantiCare Regional Med Ctr/Mainland
65 West Jimmie Leeds Road/EmergMed   Pomona, NJ 08240
(609)652-1000

Bustamante Dayanghirang, Alma, MD {1902135577} ObsGyn(96,PHI09)
+ SOMC Medical Group, P.C.
730 Lacey Road/Suite G-08   Forked River, NJ 08731
(609)693-2900   Fax (609)242-5437

Bustillo, Jose R., DO {1679972947} Pedtrc, IntrMd<NJ-NWRK-BETH, NJ-CHDNWBTH>
+ Newark Beth Israel Medical Center
201 Lyons Avenue/Internal Med   Newark, NJ 07112
(973)926-7472   Fax (973)926-5340

Butala, Rajesh M., MD {1619018512} PthAcl(79,INDI)<NJ-STMRY-PAS>
+ Bio-Reference Laboratory, Inc.
481 Edward H. Ross Drive   Elmwood Park, NJ 07407
(201)791-2600   Fax (201)791-1941

Butani, Rajen P., MD {1811920465} Urolgy(99,MA05)<NJ-OURLADY, NJ-VIRTVOOR>
+ New Jersey Urology, LLC
2401 East Evesham Road/Suite F   Voorhees, NJ 08043
(856)673-1600   Fax (856)988-0636
+ New Jersey Urology LLC
2090 Springdale Road/Suite D   Cherry Hill, NJ 08003
(856)673-1600   Fax (856)985-9908
+ Delaware Valley Urology LLC
570 Egg Harbor Road/Suite A-1   Sewell, NJ 08043
(856)582-9645   Fax (856)985-4583

Butani, Savita M., MD {1821086117} Nephro, IntrMd(98,NY19)
+ Haddon Renal Medical Specialists
401 Kings Highway South/Suite 5   Cherry Hill, NJ 08034
(856)428-8992   Fax (856)428-9614

Butch, Brian T., MD {1033657416}
+ 36 South Street
Manasquan, NJ 08736   (732)223-4673

Butensky, Arthur S., MD {1972570034} Pedtrc, AdolMd(80,NJ05)<NJ-MORRISTN, NJ-STBARNMC>
+ Pediatric Associates of West Essex PA
1129 Bloomfield Avenue/Suite 100   West Caldwell, NJ 07006   (973)575-8585   Fax (973)882-6914
+ Pediatric Associates of West Essex, PA
3155 Route 10/Suite 104   Denville, NJ 07834   (973)575-8585   Fax (973)361-1842

Butkiewicz, Elise Ann, MD {1023196979} FamMed(94,NJ05)<NJ-HOBUNIMC>
+ Overlook Family Medicine
33 Overlook Road/Suite 103   Summit, NJ 07901   (908)522-5700   Fax (908)273-8014

Butler, Barry K., MD {1770581449} IntrMd, FamMed(86,NJ05)<NJ-UNDRWD>
+ Drs. Bonett & Butler
50 Cooper Street   Woodbury, NJ 08096   (856)848-8081
Fax (856)848-1577

Butler, Charles J., MD {1073515045} Surgry(67,PA01)
+ Regional Surgical Associates
502 Centennial Boulevard/Suite 7   Voorhees, NJ 08043
(856)596-7440   Fax (856)596-6723

Butler, David George, MD {1316068448} ObsGyn(65,NY08)<NJ-HOLYNAME, NJ-ENGLWOOD>
+ Holy Name Physician Network
420 Grand Avenue/Suite 202   Englewood, NJ 07631
(201)871-4040   Fax (201)871-7326

Butler, Jill Kraft, MD {1295706158} IntrMd(92,NY48)<NJ-TRINI-WSC>
+ Trinitas Regional Medical Center-Williamson Street
225 Williamson Street/IntMed   Elizabeth, NJ 07207
(908)994-5000
JButler@trinitas.org

Butler, Mark S., MD {1063417905} SrgOrt, OrtTrm(84,NJ06)<NJ-STPETER, NJ-RWJUBRUN>
+ University Orthopaedic Associates, LLC.
Two Worlds Fair Drive   Somerset, NJ 08873   (732)979-2115
Fax (732)564-9032
+ University Orthopaedic Group
215 Easton Avenue   New Brunswick, NJ 08901   (732)979-2115   Fax (732)545-4011
+ University Orthopaedic Associates, LLC.
211 North Harrison Street   Princeton, NJ 08873   (609)683-7800   Fax (609)683-7875

Butt, Kambiz Reza, MD {1679758437} IntrMd(05,DMN01)
+ Cooper University Hospital
One Cooper Plaza   Camden, NJ 08103   (856)342-2000
+ 1 Westbrook Drive/Apt. 0202
Woolwich Township, NJ 08085

Butt, Saeed Ahmed, MD {1184684649} IntrMd(01,GRN01)<NJ-MEMSALEM>
+ Dorfner Family Medicine
811 Sunset Road/Suite 101   Burlington, NJ 08016
(609)387-9242   Fax (609)387-9408

Butt, Saima, MD {1205032364}
+ Somerset Family Practice
110 Rehill Avenue   Somerville, NJ 08876   (908)685-2900
Fax (908)685-2891
+ PO Box 5396
Somerset, NJ 08875   (765)714-5732

Butterman, Clifford Jay, MD {1104984749} Pedtrc(85,NY08)
+ Drs. Butterman & Goyco
228 60th Street   West New York, NJ 07093   (201)868-1120
Fax (201)868-5801
Cliff.butter@yahoo.com

Buttress, Sharon M., MD {1457380636} Pedtrc(80,NY48)
+ CAMCare Health Corporation
817 Federal Street   Camden, NJ 08103   (856)541-9811
Fax (856)541-4611

Butts, Christopher Alan, DO {1609137348} SrgTrm
+ RWJMG Acute Care Surgery
125 Paterson Street/Suite 6300   New Brunswick, NJ 08901
(315)404-2326   Fax (732)235-2964

Butzbach, Deborah Ann, MD {1871595348} RadOnc(97,PA09)
+ Radiology Associates of Burlington County
1295 Route 38 West/PO Box 479   Hainesport, NJ 08036
(609)261-7017   Fax (609)261-4180

Buwen, James P., DO {1679704761} Surgry
+ New Jersey Bariatric Center
193 Morris Avenue/2nd Floor   Springfield, NJ 07081
(908)481-1270   Fax (908)688-8861

Buxbaum, Eric Justin, DO {1427309210} SrgOrt<NJ-SJHREGMC>
+ SJH Regional Medical Center
1505 West Sherman Avenue/Box 93   Vineland, NJ 08360
(856)641-8661   Fax (856)575-4944

Buyer, David S., MD {1790759561} CdvDis, IntrMd(90,NY09)<NJ-NWTNMEM, NJ-MORRISTN>
+ Cardiology Associates of Sussex County LLP
222 High Street/Suite 205   Newton, NJ 07860   (973)579-2100   Fax (973)579-6638

Byahatti, Pramila, MD {1841212800} Anesth, PainMd(67,INA35)<NJ-SJRSYELM>
+ 1907 Park Avenue/Suite 103
South Plainfield, NJ 07080   (908)756-2080   Fax (908)668-0455

Byalik, Olga Viktoria, MD {1902994502} ObsGyn(97,CT02)<NJ-OVERLOOK>
+ Olga Byalik M.D. P. C.
90 Route 22 West   Springfield, NJ 07081   (973)467-0963
Fax (973)467-5385

Bye, Karen N., MD {1497700611} Pedtrc(79,PA13)<NJ-HACKNSK>
+ Hackensack University Medical Center
30 Prospect Avenue/Pediatrics   Hackensack, NJ 07601
(201)996-3186

Byers, Jason, MD {1033170394} Anesth(98,PA12)<NJ-OVER-LOOK>
+ Summit Anesthesia Associates, P.A.
33 Overlook Road/Suite 311   Summit, NJ 07901   (908)598-1500   Fax (908)598-0197
+ Overlook Medical Center
99 Beauvoir Avenue/PO Box 210   Summit, NJ 07902
(908)522-2000

Byk, Cheryl Jean, MD {1881756146} Radiol, RadDia(72,NJ05)
+ Hudson River Radiology
547 Summit Avenue   Jersey City, NJ 07306   (201)656-5050
Fax (201)656-0689

Byra, William M., MD {1851420251} IntrMd(78,NJ06)
+ 4 East High Street
Bound Brook, NJ 08805   (732)356-8100

Byrd, Lawrence H., MD {1619916756} IntrMd, Nephro(73,PA07)<NJ-STBARNMC, NJ-BAYONNE>
+ Hypertension & Renal Group, PA
930 Kennedy Boulevard   Bayonne, NJ 07002   (201)858-1509   Fax (201)858-2051

Physicians by Name and Address

Byrd, Raymond J., MD {1235127994} FamMed(74,NJ05)<NJ-HUNTRDN>
+ Hickory Run Family Practice Associates
  384 County Road 513   Califon, NJ 07830   (908)832-2125   Fax (908)832-6149

Byrd, Serena Ann, MD {1831450071} Otlryg
+ Summit Medical Group Florham Park Campus
  150 Park Avenue   Florham Park, NJ 07932   (908)977-9376

Byrne, Janet Marilyn, MD {1053425728} IntrMd(85,NJ05)<NJ-CENTRAST>
+ Patient first Urgent Care
  641 US Highway Route 130   Hamilton, NJ 08691   (609)568-9383   Fax (609)568-9384

Byrne, Kevin Joseph, MD {1205821675} RadDia(79,DC02)<NJ-MEMSALEM, PA-CHSTNHIL>
+ Memorial Hospital of Salem County
  310 Woodstown Road/Radiology   Salem, NJ 08079   (856)339-6054

Byrne, Richard George, MD {1093979353} EmrgMd, IntrMd(07,NJ06)
+ Cooper University Hospital
  One Cooper Plaza/Emerg Med   Camden, NJ 08103   (856)342-2351   Fax (856)968-8272

Byrne, William James, MD {1144329558} EnDbMt, IntrMd(86,CHI06)<NJ-VALYONS>
+ VA New Jersey Health Care System at Lyons
  151 Knollcroft Road   Lyons, NJ 07939   (908)647-0180

Byrnes, Curtis W., DO {1740228550} FamMed(96,PA77)
+ Allentown Family Medicine
  173 Walnford Road   Allentown, NJ 08501   (609)259-7400   Fax (609)259-4905

Byrnes, Michael John, DO {1245201102} FamMed
+ Walson Air Force Medical Facility
  5250 New Jersey Avenue   Fort Dix, NJ 08640

Byrom, Abbie R., MD {1508090267} Pedtrc<NJ-STPETER>
+ St. Peter's University Hospital
  254 Easton Avenue   New Brunswick, NJ 08901   (732)745-8600   Fax (732)745-2642
  Abbierommd@gmail.com

Caasi, Santiago J., Jr., MD {1194893354} Pedtrc(83,PHIL)
+ Edison Pediatric Associates PA
  7 Lincoln Highway/Suite 102   Edison, NJ 08820   (732)494-0866   Fax (732)494-1263

Cabahug, Wilfred Tan, MD {1659486462} Anesth(86,PHIL)<NJ-HUNTRDN>
+ Hunterdon Medical Center
  2100 Wescott Drive/Anesthesiology   Flemington, NJ 08822   (908)788-6100   Fax (908)237-9095

Cabaleiro, Renee J., MD {1407907256} Gastrn, IntrMd(86,MEXI)
+ 390 New York Avenue
  Newark, NJ 07105   (973)344-3518   Fax (973)344-1167

Cabales, Arthur L., MD {1407859705} IntrMd(84,PHIL)<NJ-CHRIST, NJ-BAYONNE>
+ Midland Medical Associates, LLC
  2726 Kennedy Boulevard   Jersey City, NJ 07306   (201)333-4115   Fax (201)333-6224
+ Hackensack Meridian Health-Oak Tree Primary Care
  904 Oak Tree Avenue/Suite M   South Plainfield, NJ 07080   (201)333-4115   Fax (732)283-0029

Cabales, Victor L., MD {1043317753} IntrMd(83,PHIL)<NJ-STMRY-PAS, NJ-HOBUNIMC>
+ Midland Medical Associates, LLC
  2726 Kennedy Boulevard   Jersey City, NJ 07306   (201)333-4115   Fax (201)333-6224

Caballes, Romeo A., Jr., MD {1891773610} IntrMd(97,GRN01)<NJ-HUNTRDN, NJ-SOMERSET>
+ Branchburg Internal Medicine
  9 Lamington Road   Somerville, NJ 08876   (908)203-0022   Fax (908)203-0122

Cabalu, Tyrone T., MD {1093841264} Pedtrc(64,PHI08)<NJ-CLARMAAS>
+ 108 Ridge Road/Suite 1
  North Arlington, NJ 07031   (201)998-5386   Fax (201)998-2973

Caban, Julio E., MD {1043286297} ObsGyn(70,SPA22)<NJ-NWRKBETH>
+ Newark Beth Israel Medical Center
  201 Lyons Avenue/Gyn   Newark, NJ 07112   (973)926-7000   Fax (973)705-8650

Caban, Michelle, MD {1184956286} ObsGyn, IntrMd(05,NY09)
+ Robert Wood Johnson Ob-Gyn Associates
  3270 State Route 27/Suite 2200   Kendall Park, NJ 08824   (732)422-8989   Fax (732)422-4526

Cabanas, Censon Lemuel Lizarondo, MD {1154760114}<NJ-MONMOUTH>
+ Monmouth Medical Center
  300 Second Avenue   Long Branch, NJ 07740   (862)367-6686

Cabanero, Camilo O., MD {1780649723} Anesth(69,PHIL)
+ Anesthesia Consultnts of NJ/Nova Pain
  285 Davidson Avenue/Suite 204   Somerset, NJ 08873   (732)271-1400   Fax (732)271-3543

Cabasso, Alan, MD {1710956438} Pedtrc, PedSpM(76,PHIL)<NJ-JRSYSHMC>
+ Jersey Shore University Medical Center
  1945 Route 33/Pedtrc   Neptune, NJ 07753   (732)776-4267   Fax (732)776-3161

Cabatu, Orsuville Guiang, MD {1447398508} PhysMd, NeuM-SptM(85,PHI09)
+ 4701 Broadway
  Union City, NJ 07087   (201)583-0551

Cabela, Gina Flores, MD {1225221278} FamMed(98,PHI09)
+ Valley Medical Group
  40 Washington Avenue   Dumont, NJ 07628   (201)387-7055   Fax (201)387-8605

Cabral, Carolina S., MD {1013183623}
+ 300 Winston Drive/Apt 2604
  Cliffside Park, NJ 07010   (201)240-4946

Cabral, Cesar A., Sr., MD {1639125610} IntrMd(69,DOM01)<NJ-CHRIST, NJ-HOBUNIMC>
+ 449 Avenue C
  Bayonne, NJ 07002   (201)823-2334   Fax (201)823-2344

Cabreros, Antonio T., MD {1396785176} PthAcl(79,PHI10)
+ 552 Andres Terrace
  Union, NJ 07083   (908)206-0571

Cacace, Cataldo P., MD {1740252907} Urolgy(79,MEXI)<NJ-HOBUNIMC>
+ 1815 Summit Avenue
  Union City, NJ 07087   (201)867-8555   Fax (201)601-0221

Caccavale, Robert J., MD {1386719318} SrgThr(81,NY06)<NJ-VALLEY>
+ New Jersey Thoracic Group
  35 Clyde Road/Suite 104   Somerset, NJ 08873   (732)247-3002   Fax (732)846-3819
+ New Jersey Thoracic Group
  901 West Main Street/MAB Suite 106   Freehold, NJ 07728   (732)247-3002

Cacciarelli, Andrea J., MD {1134231889} SrgPlstc(89,NY06)<NJ-CENTRAST, NJ-JRSYSHMC>
+ JFK Medical Center
  65 James Street   Edison, NJ 08820   (732)321-7668   Fax (732)767-2969

Cacciola, Thomas A., MD {1043273857} IntrMd, CdvDis, AltHol(83,PA02)<NJ-HACKNSK>
+ 403 Farview Avenue
  Paramus, NJ 07652   (201)261-8386   Fax (201)261-8827

Caceres, Maria Gabriela, MD {1730348129} Pedtrc<NJ-HACKNSK, NJ-HOLYNAME>
+ 7224 Bergenline Avenue
  North Bergen, NJ 07047   (201)869-4603   Fax (201)869-4605

Caces, Alan R., MD {1992064778} Anesth
+ Anesthesia Consultnts of NJ/Nova Pain
  285 Davidson Avenue/Suite 204   Somerset, NJ 08873   (732)271-1400   Fax (732)271-3543
+ Morris Anesthesia Group, PA
  3799 Route 46/Suite 211   Parsippany, NJ 07054   (732)271-1400   Fax (973)335-1448

Caces, Phyllis Adrienn Romero, MD {1962795864} EmrgMd(11,NY19)
+ Hackensack Medical Center Emergency Medicine
  30 Prospect Avenue/Main 3619   Hackensack, NJ 07601   (551)996-4230   Fax (201)968-1866
+ 1 Adrian Way
  River Edge, NJ 07661   (201)262-1867

Caci, Jerry A., MD {1912159856} Ophthl(92,NY08)
+ 30 Barclay Court
  Bordentown, NJ 08505   Fax (609)298-2622

Cackovic, Curt W., DO {1932107182} EmrgMd<NJ-SJHREGMC, NJ-SJRSYELM>
+ SJH Regional Medical Center
  1505 West Sherman Avenue/EmrgMed   Vineland, NJ 08360   (856)641-8000
+ SJH Elmer Hospital
  501 West Front Street/EmrgMed   Elmer, NJ 08318   (856)363-1000
+ SJH Bridgeton Health Center
  333 Irving Avenue/EmrgMed   Bridgeton, NJ 08360   (856)575-4500

Cadacio, Manolito G., MD {1447440680} IntrMd
+ Shore Physician Group
  401 Bethel Road   Somers Point, NJ 08244   (609)365-6200   Fax (609)365-6201

Cadet, Marc D., MD {1346268562} FamMed(77,HAI01)<NJ-GRYSTPSY, NJ-NWRKBETH>
+ Maplewood Family Medicine
  111 Dunnell Road/Suite 200   Maplewood, NJ 07040   (908)598-6690   Fax (973)762-0840

Cadoff, Evan M., MD {1659446763} Pthlgy, PthCln(81,NY48)<NJ-RWJUBRUN, NJ-CHLSMT>
+ UH- Robert Wood Johnson Med
  125 Paterson Street/MEB 212   New Brunswick, NJ 08901   (732)235-8120   Fax (732)235-4661

+ RWJ University Hospital New Brunswick
  One Robert Wood Johnson Place   New Brunswick, NJ 08901   (732)828-3000

Cadogan, Michael A., MD {1235149618} RadDia(75,JMA01)
+ RadPharm Inc.
  100 Overlook Center/3rd Floor   Princeton, NJ 08540   Fax (609)936-2602

Cadoo, Lisa K.A., MD {1538460498} IntrMd(PHI33)
+ United Medical, P.C.
  988 Broadway/Suite 201   Bayonne, NJ 07002   (201)339-6111   Fax (201)339-6333

Cafone, Michael D., DO {1588663728} Pedtrc(94,NJ75)<NJ-MEMSALEM>
+ Christiana Care Cardiology Consultants
  499 Beckett Road/Suite 202   Logan Township, NJ 08085   (856)769-3900   Fax (856)769-3903

Caga-Anan, Roberto Lagria, MD {1932192168} Psychy(87,PHI10)
+ New Bridge Services Inc.
  390 Main Road   Montville, NJ 07045   (973)316-9333   Fax (973)316-5790
+ New Bridge Services Inc.
  105 Hamburg Turnpike   Pompton Lakes, NJ 07442   (973)831-0613
+ New Bridge Services Inc.
  21 Evans Place   Pompton Plains, NJ 07045   (973)839-2520

Cagande, Consuelo Corazon, MD {1164520573} PsyCAd, Psychy(96,PHI10)<NJ-COOPRUMC>
+ The Cooper Hospital System-Univ Hospital
  401 Haddon Avenue/3rd Fl/Psych   Camden, NJ 08103   (856)342-2000

Cagen, Steven B., MD {1881635886} Anesth, CritCr, IntrMd(81,DC03)
+ 201 Belle Court
  Norwood, NJ 07648

Caggia, Josephine, DO {1023177409} FamMed, IntrMd(94,NJ75)
+ Roselle Park Medical Associates, LLC
  744 Galloping Hill Road   Roselle Park, NJ 07204   (908)241-0044   Fax (908)241-0526

Caguicla-Cruz, Natividad M., MD {1154324713} Anesth(74,PHI01)<NJ-STCLRDEN>
+ St. Clare's Hospital-Denville Campus
  25 Pocono Road/Anesthesiology   Denville, NJ 07834   (973)625-6000

Cahill, James W., MD {1124183694} PedOrt, SprtMd, SrgOrt(90,NY91)<NJ-HACKNSK>
+ Orthopedic Specialists NJ-Hackensack
  87 Summit Avenue   Hackensack, NJ 07601   (201)489-0022   Fax (201)489-6991
+ Orthopedic Specialists of NJ - Paramus
  277 Forest Avenue   Paramus, NJ 07652   (201)483-9228

Cahill, Kenneth Matthew, DO {1053336792} ObsGyn(92,NY75)
+ Ocean Gynecological & Obstetrical Associates PA
  475 Highway 70   Lakewood, NJ 08701   (732)364-8000   Fax (732)364-4601

Cahiwat, Ramona N., MD {1811901754} IntrMd
+ 310 Central Avenue/Suite 102
  East Orange, NJ 07018

Cai, Donghong, MD {1780880161} PthAcl<NJ-VAEASTOR>
+ VA New Jersey Health Care System-East Orange Campus
  385 Tremont Avenue/Pathology   East Orange, NJ 07018   (973)676-1000
  dcai2@hotmail.com

Cai, Kimberly, MD {1679967103} IntrMd
+ Hackensack Medical Center Internal Medicine
  385 Prospect Avenue   Hackensack, NJ 07601   (551)996-2000

Cai-Luo, Bonney Danhua, MD {1881641025} Pedtrc, IntrMd(84,CHNA)
+ 209 South Livingston Avenue/Suite 5
  Livingston, NJ 07039   (973)992-8189

Cailliau, Pamela Jean, MD {1336244292} ObsGyn, Gyneco(95,NJ05)<NJ-VAEASTOR>
+ VA New Jersey Health Care System-East Orange Campus
  385 Tremont Avenue/Ob/Gyn   East Orange, NJ 07018   (973)676-1000   Fax (973)395-7010

Cain, Courtney, MD {1710461314} PhysMd
+ Cross keys Physical Therapy
  151 Fries Mill Road/Suite 1   Turnersville, NJ 08012   (856)374-3707   Fax (856)374-3708

Cairns, Christine Dobrosky, MD {1578829859} Otlryg
+ Ear, Nose, & Throat Specialists of Morristown LLC
  95 Madison Avenue/Suite 105   Morristown, NJ 07960   (973)644-0808   Fax (973)644-9270

Cairoli, Maurice J., MD {1124051107} IntrMd, MedOnc, OncHem(84,NY09)<NJ-VIRTMHBC>
+ Virtua Memorial
  175 Madison Avenue/4th Fl   Mount Holly, NJ 08060   (609)702-1900   Fax (609)702-8455

Cairone, Stephen Scott, DO {1548260755} SrgOrt
+ Mercer-Bucks Orthopaedics, P.C.
  2501 Kuser Road   Hamilton, NJ 08691   (609)896-0444   Fax (609)587-4349

Physicians by Name and Address

Cajulis, Marivi Ora, MD {1174560536} PulDis(64,PHI01)<NJ-DEBRAHLC, NJ-SOCEANCO>
+ Deborah Heart and Lung Center
200 Trenton Road/Pulmonary Dis   Browns Mills, NJ 08015
(609)893-6611   Fax (609)893-1213

Cajulis, Michelle C., MD {1265425342} IntrMd(98,DC02)
+ Summit Medical Group-Berkeley Heights Campus
1 Diamond Hill Road/Suite C   Berkeley Heights, NJ 07922
(908)277-8991   Fax (908)790-6576

Calabrese, Carol E., MD {1972569671} Pedtrc(84,DC02)<NJ-NWT-NMEM>
+ Skylands Pediatrics
328-A Sparta Avenue   Sparta, NJ 07871   (973)729-2197   Fax (973)729-3653
+ Skylands Pediatrics
4 Oxbow Lane/Route 94   Franklin, NJ 07416   (973)729-2197   Fax (973)827-5093

Calabrese, David, MD {1437178217} IntrMd(79,MEX03)<NJ-RWJURAH, NJ-JFKMED>
+ Medical Diagnostic Associates
4 Progress Street/Suite B6   Edison, NJ 08820   (908)222-2806   Fax (908)222-2839

Calabrese, Karen Ann, DO {1154377687} FamMed(03,NJ75)
+ Center for Pediatrics and Adult Medicine
311 The Pavilions at Greentree   Marlton, NJ 08053
(856)985-8100   Fax (856)985-8374

Calabrese, Toni-Lynne, DO {1932240637} Psychy, PsyFor(92,NJ75)<NJ-ANNKLEIN>
+ Ann Klein Forensic Center
1609 Stuyvesant Avenue/PO Box 7717   West Trenton, NJ 08628   (609)633-0900

Calabro, John R., MD {1861471252} Anesth(75,NJ05)
+ Summit Anesthesia Associates, P.A.
33 Overlook Road/Suite 311   Summit, NJ 07901   (908)598-1500   Fax (908)598-0197

Calabro, Joseph John, DO {1972504413} EmrgMd(81,PA77)<NJ-STMICHL, NJ-RBAYPERT>
+ Pathlink, LLC
66 West Gilbert Street/Suite 100   Tinton Falls, NJ 07701
(732)212-0060   Fax (732)212-0061
+ St. Michael's Medical Center
268 MLK Jr. Boulevard/EmrgMed   Newark, NJ 07102
(973)877-5000
+ Raritan Bay Medical Center/Perth Amboy Division
530 New Brunswick Avenue/EmrgMed   Perth Amboy, NJ 07701   (732)442-3700

Calafiura, Peter C., MD {1578519211} Psychy(94,NJ02)
+ Genesis Counseling Center
566 Haddon Avenue   Collingswood, NJ 08108   (856)858-9314   Fax (856)858-5672

Calalang, Carolyn Clarice, MD {1437234648} Anesth(90,NY45)<NJ-UNVMCPRN>
+ Acute Rehab Unit / Med Ctr Princeton
One Plainsboro Road/2nd Floor   Plainsboro, NJ 08536
(609)853-7450   Fax (609)683-6899
+ University Medical Center of Princeton at Plainsboro
One Plainsboro Road/Anesthesiology   Plainsboro, NJ 08536
(609)497-4000

Calamari, Dawn E., DO {1124165501} IntrMd(95,NJ75)
+ Allied Medical Associates
510 Hamburg Turnpike   Wayne, NJ 07470   (973)942-6005
Fax (973)442-6009

Calata, Jed F., MD {1972828929}
+ Associated Colon & Rectal Surgeons PA
3900 Park Avenue/Suite 101   Edison, NJ 08820   (732)494-6640   Fax (732)549-8204

Calcara, Epifanio, MD {1790727337} IntrMd(82,NJ05)<NJ-OVERLOOK, NJ-MORRISTN>
+ Summit Medical Group
202 Elmer Street   Westfield, NJ 07090   (908)228-3675
Fax (908)654-1053
+ Summit Medical Group
552 Westfield Avenue   Westfield, NJ 07090   (908)228-3675
Fax (908)654-4044

Caldarella, Felice Antonino, MD {1093789158} EnDbMt, IntrMd(98,NY15)
+ Diabetes & Endocrine Associates of Hunterdon
9100 Westcott Drive/Suite 101   Flemington, NJ 08822
(908)237-6990   Fax (908)237-6995
+ Center for Endocrine Health
1738 Route 31 North/Suite 108   Clinton, NJ 08809
(908)237-6990   Fax (908)735-3981

Calder, Nicholas, MD {1477937217} IntrMd<NJ-COOPRUMC>
+ Cooper University Hospital
One Cooper Plaza   Camden, NJ 08103   (856)342-3150

Calderon, Dawn Michelle, DO {1336189976} CdvDis, IntrMd(90,NJ75)<NJ-DEBRAHLC>
+ 47 Bay Breeze Drive
Toms River, NJ 08753

Calderon, Dinorah, MD {1750467049} Pedtrc(00,PA13)<NJ-RBAYPERT>
+ Jewish Renaissance Medical Center
275 Hobart Street   Perth Amboy, NJ 08861   (732)376-9333
Fax (732)324-5765

Calderon, Mark J., MD {1902022270} FamMed(91,NJ06)
+ Associates in Cardiovascular Disease, LLC
29 South Street   New Providence, NJ 07974   (908)464-4200   Fax (908)464-1332
+ AmeriChoice of New Jersey, Inc.
2 Gateway Center/13th Floor   Newark, NJ 07102
(908)464-4200   Fax (973)645-1131

Calderon, Oscar R., MD {1659327286} EmrgMd(76,DOMI)<NJ-KIMBALL>
+ Kimball Medical Center
600 River Avenue/EmergMed   Lakewood, NJ 08701
(732)363-1900

Calderon, Rosa L., MD {1750497129} IntrMd(80,PER01)
+ Drs. Tello Valcarcel & Calderon
356 Totowa Avenue   Paterson, NJ 07502   (973)904-0100
Fax (973)595-8286

Calderone, Joseph, Jr., MD {1003841479} Ophthl, IntrMd(82,NJ05)<NJ-OVERLOOK, NJ-RWJURAH>
+ Cranford Ophthalmology
2 South Avenue East/Suite 1   Cranford, NJ 07016
(908)276-3030   Fax (908)276-3174
bettervisionnj@worldnet.att.net

Caldwell, Kathleen V., MD {1487690111} RadDia, Radiol, IntrMd(82,MEX03)
+ 40 Grover Lane
West Caldwell, NJ 07006   (973)980-9677

Caldwell, Shinelle, DO {1952705709} ObsGyn
+ St Joseph's Medical Center ObsGyn
1048 Main Street   Paterson, NJ 07503   (973)754-2000

Calello, Diane P., MD {1821018334} Pedtrc, PedEmg
+ 2 Martin Court
Martinsville, NJ 08836

Calem-Grunat, Jaclyn A., MD {1134116478} RadDia, Radiol(88,NY47)<NJ-VALLEY>
+ Radiology Associates of Ridgewood, P.A.
20 Franklin Turnpike   Waldwick, NJ 07463   (201)445-8822
Fax (201)447-5053
+ The Valley Hospital
223 North Van Dien Avenue/Radiology   Ridgewood, NJ 07450   (201)447-8210

Calenda, Brandon William, MD {1790074748} IntrMd(13,MA07)<NY-MTSINAI>
+ Cardiology Associates of North Jersey
242 West Parkway   Pompton Plains, NJ 07444   (973)831-7455   Fax (973)831-7585

Calero, Jose Manuel, MD {1700217353} FamMed(97,MI20)
+ 7100 Boulevard East
Guttenberg, NJ 07093

Calero-Bai, Rosario, MD {1851334361} Pedtrc(86,MNT01)<NJ-HACKNSK, NJ-VALLEY>
+ Riverside ENT Pediatric Group
324 Palisade Avenue/2nd Floor   Jersey City, NJ 07307
(201)386-1400   Fax (201)386-2343

Calesnick, Jay L., MD {1982654968} Ophthl(77,PA09)<NJ-MEM-SALEM>
+ 212 Lippincott Avenue
Riverton, NJ 08077   (856)786-2220
+ 261 Route 45
Salem, NJ 08079   (856)786-2220   Fax (856)935-8630

Calhoun, Sean Keith, DO {1598862617} Radiol, RadV&I, NeuMus(96,NJ75)<NJ-MORRISTN>
+ Memorial Radiology Associates
10 Lanidex Plaza West/Suite 125   Parsippany, NJ 07054
(973)503-5700   Fax (973)386-5701

Cali, Michael D., MD {1003856766} EmrgMd(79,NY01)<NJ-JFKMED>
+ JFK Medical Center
65 James Street/EmrgMed   Edison, NJ 08820   (732)321-7000

Califano, Antonio G., MD {1700955010} IntrMd(82,ITA01)<NJ-CLARMAAS, NJ-MTNSIDE>
+ 359 Centre Street
Nutley, NJ 07110   (973)667-3332   Fax (973)667-3332

Califano, Francesco, MD {1972597995} PulCCr, IntrMd, PulDis(94,ITA17)<NJ-ENGLWOOD>
+ Englewood Hospital and Medical Center
350 Engle Street   Englewood, NJ 07631   (201)894-3322
Fax (201)894-0585

Califano, Tiziana, MD {1861468431} IntrMd(96,ITA17)<NJ-MTNSIDE>
+ Hackensack UMC Mountainside
1 Bay Avenue/IntMed   Montclair, NJ 07042   (973)429-6000
Fax (973)429-6575

Calimlim, Grace T., MD {1922177336} Pedtrc(84,PHI01)
+ Pedi Health Medical Associates
720 Route 202-206 North/Suite 4   Bridgewater, NJ 08807
(908)722-5444   Fax (908)722-5071

Calise, Arthur G., DO {1184626509} FamMed, EmrgMd(92,FL75)<NJ-STMICHL>
+ Pathlink, LLC
66 West Gilbert Street/Suite 100   Tinton Falls, NJ 07701
(732)212-0060   Fax (732)212-0061

Callaghan, John Joseph, MD {1275842288}
+ New Jersey Orthopaedic Institute
504 Valley Road/Suite 200   Wayne, NJ 07470   (973)273-3439   Fax (973)694-2692

Callahan, James P., MD {1245236264} Radiol, RadDia(78,NY08)<NJ-RWJUHAM>
+ Quakerbridge Radiology Associates
8 Quakerbridge Plaza/Building 8   Mercerville, NJ 08619
(609)890-0033   Fax (609)689-6067
+ Quakerbridge Radiology MRI Center at Lawrenceville
21 Lawrenceville-Pennington Rd   Lawrenceville, NJ 08648
(609)890-0033   Fax (609)895-2647

Callahan, Kevin J., DO {1134125156} IntrMd, MedOnc, OncHem(87,ME75)<NJ-UNDRWD, NJ-VIRTUAHS>
+ Regional Cancer Care Associates, LLC
200 Bowman Drive/Suite E-125   Voorhees, NJ 08043
(856)424-3311   Fax (856)424-5634
+ The Center for Cancer & Hematologic Disease
609 North Broad Street/Suite 300   Woodbury, NJ 08096
(856)686-1002
+ The Center for Cancer & Hematologic Disease
856 South White Horse Pike/Suite 4   Hammonton, NJ 08043
(609)561-4444   Fax (609)561-2492

Callahan, Richard Allan, II, MD {1215378336} Psychy
+ Center for Family Guidance, PC
765 East Route 70/Building A-101   Marlton, NJ 08053
(856)797-4800   Fax (856)810-0110

Callahan, Troy Ezra, MD {1962444976} SrgPlstc(95,NY47)
+ Northern Jersey Plastic Surgery Center, LLC
140 Prospect Avenue/Suite 17   Hackensack, NJ 07601
(201)225-1811   Fax (201)616-7789

Callender, Gordon Erwin, MD {1215059399} SrgC&R(99,NY48)
+ Inspira Medical Group Surgical Associates
1206 West Sherman Avenue/Building 2   Vineland, NJ 08360
(856)696-9933   Fax (856)696-9939
+ Salartash Surgical Associates
301 Central Avenue/Suite D   Egg Harbor Township, NJ 08234   (856)696-9933   Fax (609)926-2020

Calligaro, Keith Don, MD {1326198946} SrgVas, Srgry(82,NJ02)
+ Pennsylvania Vascular Associates, PC
8 South Dennis Road   Cape May Court House, NJ 08210
(609)465-3939   Fax (609)465-4042

Calloway, Hollin Elizabeth, MD {1528325453} Otlryg
+ ENT and Allergy Associates (ENTA)
79 Hudson Street/Suite 303   Hoboken, NJ 07030
(201)792-1109   Fax (201)792-1145

Cally, Ronald G., MD {1720478837} Pedtrc(92,GRN01)<NJ-VALLEY>
+ Ronald G. Cally MD LLC
1250 East Ridgewood Avenue   Ridgewood, NJ 07450
(201)444-1133   Fax (201)444-4841

Caloustian, Marie-Louise, MD {1255421681} Anesth(90,PA09)<NJ-HACKNSK>
+ Hackensack Anesthesiology Associates
140 Prospect Avenue/Suite 8   Hackensack, NJ 07601
(201)488-0066   Fax (201)488-6769
+ Hackensack University MC-Anesthesia Dept
30 Prospect Avenue/Room 2703   Hackensack, NJ 07601
(201)488-0066   Fax (201)996-3962

Caltabiano, Claire L., MD {1457315665} Pedtrc(94,PA07)<NJ-OURLADY, NJ-VIRTUAHS>
+ Advocare Haddonfield Pediatric Association
220 North Haddon Avenue   Haddonfield, NJ 08033
(856)429-6719   Fax (856)429-6748

Calvert, Sara Marie, MD {1164689642} PsyCAd, Psychy(03,PA01)
+ Children's Aid and Family Services
240 Frisch Court   Paramus, NJ 07652   (201)226-0300   Fax (201)226-9262

Calvo, Ricardo A., MD {1356384705} CdvDis, IntrMd(77,PAN01)
+ 2 State Route 27/Suite 410
Edison, NJ 08820   (732)318-6858   Fax (732)318-6859

Calvosa, Michelle K., MD {1477684017} Psychy(96,NJ06)<NJ-UNIVBHC>
+ CPC Behavioral HealthCare
270 Highway 35   Red Bank, NJ 07701   (732)842-2000   Fax (732)224-0688
+ CPC Behavioral HealthCare
37 Court Street   Freehold, NJ 07728   (732)842-2000   Fax (732)780-5157

Calzada, Tania, MD {1356578041} IntrMd<NJ-CHSFULD>
+ Capital Health System/Fuld Campus
750 Brunswick Avenue   Trenton, NJ 08638   (609)394-6000
Fax (609)815-7814

Cam, Jenny G., MD {1134132889} EnDbMt, IntrMd(79,PHI01)<NJ-CHRIST, NJ-MEADWLND>
+ 10 Huron Avenue/Suite 1P
Jersey City, NJ 07306   (201)656-6003   Fax (201)656-4566

Physicians by Name and Address

Camacho, Brenda Y., MD {1821175134} Psychy(89,PA13)
+ New Point Behavioral Health Care
404 Tatum Street   Woodbury, NJ 08096   (856)845-8050   Fax (856)845-0688

Camacho, Jeanette M., MD {1952491730} Pthlgy, PthAcl(87,PA13)<NJ-COOPRUMC>
+ Cooper University Hospital
One Cooper Plaza/Pathology   Camden, NJ 08103   (856)342-2505

Camacho, Jose A., MD {1073612008} IntrMd(89,PA13)<NJ-UNDRWD>
+ Laskin Internal Medcine
400 Grove Road/PO Box 37   Thorofare, NJ 08086   (856)845-8010   Fax (856)845-9698

Camacho, Margarita T., MD {1164499620} SrgThr, Surgry, CdvDis(84,NY09)<NJ-NWRKBETH>
+ Newark Beth Israel Medical Center
201 Lyons Avenue/Suite G5   Newark, NJ 07112   (973)926-7000   Fax (973)923-4683

Camacho, Ricardo Miguel, MD {1124029228} IntrMd(99,NY46)<NJ-OVERLOOK, NJ-MORRISTN>
+ Summit Medical Group-Berkeley Heights Campus
1 Diamond Hill Road   Berkeley Heights, NJ 07922   (908)273-4300   Fax (908)277-8841

Camacho-Halili, Marie M., MD {1053578534} AlgyImmn, Pedtrc, IntrMd(06,NJ06)
+ ENT & Allergy Associates-Bridgewater
245 US Highway 22/3rd Fl/Suite 300   Bridgewater, NJ 08807   (908)722-1022   Fax (908)722-2040

Camacho-Pantoja, Jose A., MD {1801898804} Psychy(73,DOM04)
+ Medical Group Associates
190 North Evergreen Avenue/Suite 102   Woodbury, NJ 08096   (844)542-2273   Fax (856)845-9698

Camacho-Patterson, Evelyn Louise, MD {1063635332} EnDbMt, IntrMd(89,CUB06)<NJ-ENGLWOOD, NJ-HOLYNAME>
+ Comprehensive Endocrine Care Inc
Camacho-Patterson   North Bergen, NJ 07047   (201)868-0001   Fax (201)868-0999

Camal, Debra E., MD {1902833312} SrgBst, Surgry, IntrMd(88,NY08)<NJ-JRSYSHMC, NJ-RIVERVW>
+ Northern Monmouth County Medical Associates
656 Shrewsbury Avenue/Suite 300   Tinton Falls, NJ 07701   (732)531-5200   Fax (732)531-5836
dcamal@verizon.net

Cambareri, Gina M., MD {1952562019} PedUro(08,NY0)<NJ-NWRKBETH>
+ Children's Hospital of New Jersey
201 Lyons Avenue/Osborne Terrace/L5   Newark, NJ 07112   (973)926-7280

Cambria, Lina, MD {1144314824} Pedtrc, AdolMd(81,NJ05)<NJ-STPETER, NJ-RWJUBRUN>
+ Bethany Pediatrics PA
1 Bethany Road/Building 5/Suite 65   Hazlet, NJ 07730   (732)264-0700   Fax (732)264-1414

Cameron, James D., MD {1497794051} EmrgMd(77,ON06)<NJ-RIVERVW, NJ-JRSYSHMC>
+ Riverview Medical Center
1 Riverview Plaza/EmergMed   Red Bank, NJ 07701   (732)741-2700   Fax (732)224-7498

Camerota, Andrew Martin, MD {1568460459} Surgry, SrgLap(85,PA02)<NJ-STPETER>
+ 49 Veronica Avenue/Suite 104
Somerset, NJ 08873   (732)249-0977   Fax (732)249-1860
+ Cares Surgicenter, LLC.
240 Easton Avenue   New Brunswick, NJ 08901   (732)249-0977   Fax (732)296-8677

Camilo, Antonio Manuel, MD {1629047048} Pedtrc(89,DOM01)
+ Passaic Pediatrics PA
298 Passaic Street   Passaic, NJ 07055   (973)249-8100   Fax (973)249-8110
+ Passaic Pediatrics PA
200 Gregory Street/2nd Floor   Passaic, NJ 07055   (973)249-8100   Fax (973)249-8110

Camiolo, Mark A., DO {1932410172}
+ Newark Community Health Center, Inc.
741 Broadway   Newark, NJ 07104   (908)380-7912   Fax (973)676-1396
oloimac@hotmail.com

Camiolo, Melissa Rae, MD {1124339353} ObsGyn(10,KY02)<NJ-HUNTRDN>
+ Advanced Obstetrics & Gynecology, LLC
4 Walter E. Foran Boulevard/Suite 302   Flemington, NJ 08822   (908)806-0080   Fax (908)806-8570

Camiscoli, Deborah J., MD {1255304663} IntrMd(79,NJ05)<NJ-COMMED>
+ Coastal Health Care
1314 Hooper Avenue/Building B   Toms River, NJ 08753   (732)349-4994   Fax (732)341-1717

Camishion, Germaine Mary, MD {1477578011} Dermat(85,PA02)
+ Moorestown Dermatology Associates
702 East Main Street   Moorestown, NJ 08057   (856)235-6565   Fax (856)235-6566
germaine46@comcast.net

Cammarata, Lindsay, MD {1467784793} Anesth
+ Jersey Shore Anesthesiology Associates
1945 Route 33/PO Box 397   Neptune, NJ 07754   (732)775-5500

Cammarata, Sandra, MD {1215377338} PsyCAd, Psychy(83,ITA04)
+ The Center for Creative Lifestyles
66 Roseland Avenue   Caldwell, NJ 07006   (973)226-4773   Fax (973)226-4662
adeccl@att.net
+ 14 Smull Avenue
Caldwell, NJ 07006   (973)226-4773   Fax (973)401-2489

Campagnolo, Mary F., MD {1871576389} FamMed, Grtrcs(82,DC01)<NJ-VIRTMHBC>
+ Virtua Lumberton Family Physicians
1561 Route 38/Suite 6A/FamMed   Lumberton, NJ 08048   (609)267-2100   Fax (609)267-6921
mcampagnolo@virtua.org
+ Virtua Medical Group
401 Route 73/40 Lake Ctr Dr/Ste 201A   Marlton, NJ 08053   (609)267-2100   Fax (856)355-0346

Campagnuolo, Joann E., DO {1245200823} Anesth(93,NY75)<NJ-STPETER>
+ 91 Hunt Road
Freehold, NJ 07728

Campanella, Anthony J., Jr., MD {1982744413} IntrMd(79,MEX03)<NJ-HACKNSK, NJ-HOLYNAME>
+ Hackensack University Medical Center
30 Prospect Avenue/Internal Med   Hackensack, NJ 07601   (201)906-8407   Fax (201)556-0134
martialmd@hotmail.com
+ HackensackUMG Lodi
116 Terrace Avenue   Lodi, NJ 07644   (201)906-8407   Fax (973)473-4806

Campanella, Lisa Marie, MD {1720180623} EmrgMd(00,NY19)
+ Monmouth Medical Center
300 Second Avenue   Long Branch, NJ 07740   (732)222-5200

Campanile, Giovanni, MD {1013969377} CdvDis, IntCrd, IntrMd(83,ITA04)<NJ-MORRISTN, NJ-OVERLOOK>
+ Morristown Medical Center
100 Madison Avenue/Cardiology   Morristown, NJ 07962   (973)971-5000
+ Chambers Center
435 South Street/Suite 160   Morristown, NJ 07960   (973)971-6301

Campbell, Anthony E., MD {1114030962} Pedtrc, GenPrc(82,NJ05)
+ Woodbine Development Center/NJ Human Services
1175 Dehirsch Avenue   Woodbine, NJ 08270   (609)861-2164   Fax (609)861-2494

Campbell, Arthur Scott, MD {1023004389} IntrMd(86,NY09)<NJ-MORRISTN>
+ 2345 Lamington Road/Suite 105
Bedminster, NJ 07921   (908)234-0890   Fax (908)234-1432
Scampbell@aol.com

Campbell, Colin A., DO {1477518132} IntrMd(96,MO78)
+ Atco Medical Associates
289 White Horse Pike/Suite 101   Atco, NJ 08004   (856)767-2000   Fax (856)767-0073

Campbell, Damali M., MD {1467461772} ObsGyn(95,PA13)
+ New Margaret Hague Women's Health Institute
377 Jersey Avenue/Suite 220   Jersey City, NJ 07302   (201)795-9155   Fax (201)795-9157

Campbell, Jeffrey Wakeling, MD {1457442725} SrgNro, Pedtrc, IntrMd(91,PA02)<PA-TJHSP>
+ Nemours Dupont Pediatrics, Voorhees
443 Laurel Oak Road   Voorhees, NJ 08043   (856)309-8508   Fax (856)309-8556

Campbell, Joseph V., MD {1053351569} CdvDis, IntrMd(91,NJ05)<NJ-NWRKBETH>
+ Metropolitan Cardiovascular Center
1057 Sanford Avenue   Irvington, NJ 07111   (973)373-1875   Fax (973)373-9005
josephcampbellmd@verizon.net

Campbell, Neil Murdoch, DO {1154412542} ObsGyn(97,IL76)<NJ-SJHREGMC>
+ Women's Health at Hackettstown
108 Bilby Road/Suite 305   Hackettstown, NJ 07840   (908)813-8877   Fax (908)813-9984

Campeas, David, MD {1679616213} Ophthl(81,NY47)
+ 33 Overlook Road/Suite 106
Summit, NJ 07901   (908)522-0500
dcampeas@earthlink.net

Campeas, Sarah B., DO {1376962829}<NJ-MORRISTN>
+ Morristown Medical Center
100 Madison Avenue   Morristown, NJ 07962   (973)971-7926   Fax (973)290-7202

Campellone, Joseph V., Jr., MD {1902996796} Nrolgy(91,PA13)<NJ-COOPRUMC>
+ Cooper University Neurology
1935 Route 70 East   Cherry Hill, NJ 08003   (856)342-2445   Fax (856)964-0504

Campion, Thomas W., MD {1306883467} Surgry(80,NJ05)<NJ-HCKTSTWN>
+ Seber Road/Doctors Park/Suite 1A
Hackettstown, NJ 07840   (908)850-9548   Fax (908)813-3256
+ 195 Route 46 West/Atrium Prof Bldg
Mine Hill, NJ 07803   (973)366-5813

Campo, Anthony Guy, Jr., MD {1518034636} Dermat(71,PA09)<NJ-ACMCITY, NJ-SHOREMEM>
+ Dermatology of Somers Point
223 Shore Road   Somers Point, NJ 08244   (609)653-8040   Fax (609)653-1568

Campo, Richard Paul, MD {1609968676} Urolgy, SrgUro(89,NY47)<NJ-VALLEY, NJ-CHILTON>
+ 277 Forest Avenue/Suite 206
Paramus, NJ 07652   (201)489-8900   Fax (201)489-0877

Campo, Ruth A., MD {1538103965} EmrgMd(78,MEX55)<NJ-OVERLOOK>
+ Overlook Medical Center
99 Beauvoir Avenue/PO Box 210/EmrgMed   Summit, NJ 07902   (908)522-2000   Fax (908)522-0227

Campoalegre, Maria A., MD {1366609174} IntrMd
+ Cardio-Med Services
3196 Kennedy Boulevard/3rd Floor   Union City, NJ 07087   (201)974-0077   Fax (201)974-2232
+ Cardio-Med Services
635 Broadway   Paterson, NJ 07514   (973)742-6266

Campolattaro, Brian N., MD {1790794303} PedOph, Ophthl(90,NJ05)<NY-NYEYEINF, NY-MNTFMOSE>
+ Phillips Eye Center
619 River Drive   Elmwood Park, NJ 07407   (201)796-2020   Fax (201)796-2833

Campos, Danilo T., MD {1326014903} Psychy(69,PHI24)<NJ-MTNSIDE>
+ Hackensack UMC Mountainside
1 Bay Avenue/Psychiatry   Montclair, NJ 07042   (973)429-6000
danilo.campos@ahsys.org

Campos, Jose S., MD {1801057997} PhysMd, SprtMd(07,NJ05)
+ 2520 John F Kennedy Boulevard
Jersey City, NJ 07304   (201)942-4555   Fax (201)221-7577

Campos, Marite, MD {1366626509} PthAcl(99,IL11)
+ 85 Azalea Circle
Jackson, NJ 08527

Campos-Munoz, Magaly C., MD {1720113095} PsyCAd, Psychy(87,CHI08)
+ 824 Elizabeth Avenue
Elizabeth, NJ 07201   (908)352-0103   Fax (908)352-9134

Campton, Kristina Lee, MD {1902832777} Dermat(00,NY01)
+ Skin Laser & Surgery Specialists
20 Prospect Avenue/Suite 702   Hackensack, NJ 07601   (201)441-9890   Fax (201)441-9893

Can, Seyit A., MD {1205836319} Pthlgy, PthAcl, PthCyt(81,TURK)<NJ-ACMCITY, NJ-ACMCMAIN>
+ AtlantiCare Regional Medical Center/City Campus
1925 Pacific Avenue/Pathology   Atlantic City, NJ 08401   (609)441-2147   Fax (609)441-2107

Canabal, Vincent Paul, MD {1194912295} EmrgMd(06,NJ05)<NJ-JRSYCITY>
+ Jersey City Medical Center
355 Grand Street/EmrgMed   Jersey City, NJ 07304   (201)915-2000

Canals-Curtis, Elena, MD {1992712624}
+ Rancocas Anesthesiology, PA
700 Route 130 North/Suite 203   Cinnaminson, NJ 08077   (856)829-9345   Fax (856)829-3605

Canals-Ferrat, Pedro, MD {1811942709} Anesth(88,CUB06)
+ Bayonne Medical Center
29th Street at Avenue E   Bayonne, NJ 07002   (201)858-5000
+ Christ Hospital
176 Palisade Avenue   Jersey City, NJ 07306   (201)795-8200
+ Hoboken University Medical Center
308 Willow Avenue   Hoboken, NJ 07002   (201)418-1000

Canals-Navas, Carmen L., MD {1144277518} IntrMd, Nephro(88,PRO01)
+ Nephrology & Hypertension Associates of New Jersey
201 Laurel Oak Road/Suite B   Voorhees, NJ 08043   (856)566-5478   Fax (856)566-9561

Canario, Arthur T., MD {1568505832} SrgOrt(75,DC02)<NJ-NWRKBETH>
+ 206 Bergen Avenue
Kearny, NJ 07032   (201)998-9200   Fax (201)998-9201

Canavan, Brian F., DO {1760595516} IntrMd, OncHem(89,IA75)<NJ-RWJURAH>
+ Regional Cancer Care Specialists
34-36 Progress Street/Suite B-2   Edison, NJ 08820   (908)757-9696   Fax (908)757-9721

Cancel, Jaime, MD {1689778706} IntrMd, CritCr, IntHos(00,PRO03)<NJ-ATLANTHS, NJ-MORRISTN>
+ Pulmonary & Allergy Associates
1 Springfield Avenue/Suite 3-A   Summit, NJ 07901   (908)934-0555   Fax (908)934-0550
+ Pulmonary & Allergy Associates
8 Saddle Road/Suite 101   Cedar Knolls, NJ 07927   (908)934-0555   Fax (973)540-0472

Cancellieri, Francis Louis, MD {1285705053} Psychy, IntrMd(86,STM01)<NJ-RIVERVW, NJ-BAYSHORE>
+ Riverview Medical Center
1 Riverview Plaza/Behavioral Hlth   Red Bank, NJ 07701   (732)530-2478   Fax (732)224-3910
+ 279 Third Avenue/Suite 510
Long Branch, NJ 07740   (732)530-2478   Fax (732)870-8582

Candelore, Joseph Timothy, Jr., DO {1861742124} IntrMd(12,PA77)<NJ-SJERSYHS>
+ Internal Medicine Associates
201 Laurel Heights Drive/Suite 201   Bridgeton, NJ 08302   (856)455-4800   Fax (856)455-0650

Candido, Frank M., MD {1376646992} Gastrn, IntrMd(70,OH41)
+ 466 Old Hook Road
Emerson, NJ 07630   (201)265-4050   Fax (201)265-5183

Cane, Michael Elliot, MD {1689615213} SrgCdv, SrgCrC, Surgry(83,NY06)<NJ-DEBRAHLC>
+ Deborah Heart and Lung Center
200 Trenton Road/Surgery   Browns Mills, NJ 08015   (609)893-6611   Fax (609)893-1213
canem@deborah.org

Cangemi, Carla Primiani, MD {1154538759} Pedtrc, PedCrC(01,DMN01)
+ Children's Specialized Hospital
200 Somerset Street   New Brunswick, NJ 08901   (732)258-7065

Caniglia, James J., MD {1033117064} FamMed, GenPrc, EmrgMd(82,ITAL)<NJ-HOBUNIMC>
+ Hoboken University Medical Center
308 Willow Avenue   Hoboken, NJ 07030   (201)418-1000

Canillas, Elmo Maribao, MD {1073677555} AnesPain, Acpntr, IntrMd(85,PHI09)<NJ-MEADWLND, NY-DCTRSTAT>
+ Meadowlands Hospital Medical Center
55 Meadowlands Parkway/Anesthesia   Secaucus, NJ 07096   (201)819-2099

Canizales, Gloria M., DO {1295173185}<NJ-MORRISTN>
+ Morristown Medical Center
100 Madison Avenue/Box 157   Morristown, NJ 07962   (973)971-7065

Cann, Donald F., MD {1992785141} RadOnc(84,MA16)<NJ-STCLRDOV, NY-SLOANKET>
+ St. Clare's Hospital-Dover
400 West Blackwell Street   Dover, NJ 07801   (973)989-3000

Cannarozzi, Nicholas A., MD {1194810259} Rheuma, IntrMd(65,PA09)<NJ-MTNSIDE>
+ Drs. Weinberger & Cannarozzi
741 Northfield Avenue/Suite 210   West Orange, NJ 07052   (973)630-8950   Fax (973)669-9749
cannarozzimd@COMCAST.NET

Cannella, Michael, MD {1063512457} Psychy(91,NJ05)<NJ-STBARNMC>
+ Associates in Psychiatry
405 Northfield Avenue/Suite 204   West Orange, NJ 07052   (973)325-6120   Fax (973)325-6126

Cannon, Aileen Carol, MD {1841233434} Pedtrc, IntrMd(00,DMN01)<NJ-COMMED, NJ-KIMBALL>
+ Ocean Health Initiatives, Inc.
333 Haywood Road   Manahawkin, NJ 08050   (609)489-0110   Fax (609)489-0171

Cannon, Donald R., MD {1134145329} ObsGyn(02,DC03)<NJ-VIRTUAHS>
+ Ob-Gyn Care of Southern New Jersey
406 Gibbsboro Road East   Lindenwold, NJ 08021   (856)435-7007   Fax (856)435-7077

Canosa, Omar, MD {1841241494} PsyCAd(99,DOM15)<NJ-OVERLOOK>
+ 37 Kings Road/Suite 202
Summit, NJ 07902   (973)520-8848   Fax (973)200-8088

Canova, Amanda Derrick, MD {1164468161} ObsGyn(99,NJ05)<NJ-HCKTSTWN>
+ Obstetrics and Gynecology Associates
616 Willow Grove Street   Hackettstown, NJ 07840   (908)852-3443   Fax (908)852-0349

Canterino, Joseph C., MD {1760471122} ObsGyn, MtFtMd(91,NJ06)
+ Hackensack Meridian Maternal Fetal Medicine
19 Davis Avenue/Hope Tower 7th Floor   Neptune, NJ 07753   (732)776-4755   Fax (732)776-4754
+ Hackensack Meridian Medical Group Ob/Gyn, Neptune
1828 West Lake Avenue   Neptune, NJ 07753   (732)776-4755   Fax (732)776-4892
+ Southern Ocean County Medical Center
1140 Route 72 West   Manahawkin, NJ 07753   (732)776-4755   Fax (732)776-4754

Cantey, Mary Daisy, MD {1851422687} IntrMd, Pedtrc(98,NJ05)<NJ-UMDNJ>
+ University Hospital-Doctors Office Center
90 Bergen Street   Newark, NJ 07103   (973)972-6635   Fax (973)972-0956

Cantillo, Joaquin J., MD {1639183908} Anesth(84,PRO01)<NJ-CHSFULD, NJ-CHSMRCER>
+ Trenton Anesthesiology Associates, PA
One Capital Way/Second Floor   Pennington, NJ 08534   (609)396-4700   Fax (609)396-4900

Cantillon, Marc, MD {1427037803} Psychy, PsyGrt, PsyNro(87,SWE02)<NJ-MORRISTN>
+ Wellness Managements, Inc.
134 Walnut Street   Livingston, NJ 07039   (973)462-0496   Fax (973)486-8344
marcus219087@yahoo.com
+ Morristown Medical Center
100 Madison Avenue/Psych   Morristown, NJ 07962   (973)971-5000

Cantor, Susan J., MD {1275608408} IntrMd(82,NY19)<NJ-OVERLOOK>
+ Summit Medical Group
11 Cleveland Place   Springfield, NJ 07081   (973)378-8778   Fax (973)763-1748

Cantore, William Anthony, MD {1174587018} Ophthl<PA-PNSTHRSH>
+ Hackensack University Medical Group Emerson
452 Old Hook Road/2nd Floor   Emerson, NJ 07630   (201)666-3900   Fax (201)261-0505

Cantrell, Harry, MD {1972693760} Otlryg, IntrMd(82,PA14)<NJ-VIRTVOOR>
+ Advanced ENT - Voorhees
200 Bowman Drive/Suite D-285   Voorhees, NJ 08043   (856)602-4000   Fax (856)346-0757
+ Advanced ENT - Washington Township
239 Hurffville Crosskeys Road   Sewell, NJ 08080   (856)602-4000   Fax (856)629-3391
+ Advanced ENT - Haddonfield
130 North Haddon Avenue   Haddonfield, NJ 08043   (856)602-4000   Fax (856)429-1284

Canzoniero, Christian, MD {1144303439} Pedtrc(98,IL43)<NJ-NWTNMEM, NJ-MORRISTN>
+ Wellness Center Pediatrics LLC
21 Lafayette Road/Suite F   Sparta, NJ 07871   (973)726-4455   Fax (973)726-8445

Cao, Huyen Van, MD {1154364727} RadDia(89,VA07)<NJ-HOLYNAME, PA-EPHRATA>
+ Holy Name Hospital
718 Teaneck Road/Radiology   Teaneck, NJ 07666   (201)833-3000

Cao, Lan, MD {1639494677} IntrMd<NJ-HUNTRDN>
+ Hunterdon Medical Center
2100 Wescott Drive/Internal Med   Flemington, NJ 08822   (908)237-5486   Fax (908)237-5488

Capaci, Mary T., MD {1821001793} Pedtrc(88,TN06)
+ 171 Franklin Turnpike
Waldwick, NJ 07463   (201)689-0110   Fax (201)689-0114

Capalbo, Vincent J., MD {1134320013} Anesth(01,NET09)<NJ-STMICHL>
+ St. Michael's Medical Center
111 Central Avenue/Anesthesia   Newark, NJ 07102   (973)877-5034   Fax (973)877-5231
+ St. Joseph's Regional Medical Center Anesthesia
703 Main Street   Paterson, NJ 07503   (973)877-5034   Fax (973)977-9455

Capanescu, Cristina, MD {1316110422} IntrMd(02,PA02)
+ Cooper Digestive Health Institute
501 Fellowship Road/Suite 101   Mount Laurel, NJ 08054   (856)642-2133   Fax (856)642-2134

Capecci, Frank, MD {1184639940} SrgOrt(83,NJ05)
+ Morris County Orthopaedic Group
109 US Highway 46 East   Denville, NJ 07834   (973)625-1221   Fax (973)625-1594

Capecci, Louis J., MD {1922080381} RadDia, Radiol(76,PA13)<NJ-BURDTMLN>
+ Cape Regional Medical Center
2 Stone Harbor Boulevard/Radiology   Cape May Court House, NJ 08210   (609)463-2120
+ Cape Radiology
4011 Route 9 South/PO Box 244   Rio Grande, NJ 08242   (609)886-0100

Capella, Joseph Francis, MD {1518925130} SrgPlstc, Surgry(91,NY08)<NJ-HACKNSK, NJ-VALLEY>
+ Capella Plastic Surgery
545 Island Road/Suite 2-A   Ramsey, NJ 07446   (201)818-9199   Fax (201)818-0399

Capio, Christine Marie, MD {1063624823} Rheuma(91,PHI08)
+ 132 Perry Street
Trenton, NJ 08618   (609)394-8988   Fax (609)394-8842

Capio, Mario R., MD {1356383863} FamMed(95,NJ05)<NJ-CHILTON>
+ Pompton Plains Family Health Center
230 West Parkway/Suite 10   Pompton Plains, NJ 07444   (973)835-0800   Fax (973)616-2766

Capiola, David Raymond, MD {1316968647} Ortped, SprtMd(01,DC02)<NY-BETHKING, NY-METHODST>
+ Health East Medical Center
54 South Dean Street   Englewood, NJ 07631   (201)871-4000

Capiro, Rodney, MD {1174586333} ObsGyn, IntrMd(93,NY06)<NJ-STBARNAB>
+ Southern Jersey Family Medical Centers, Inc.
860 South White Horse Pike/Building A   Hammonton, NJ 08037   (609)567-0200   Fax (609)567-3492

Capitanelli, John R., MD {1538182688} CdvDis, IntrMd, IntCrd(82,MEXI)<NJ-VALLEY, NJ-COMMED>
+ Cardiology Associates LLC
999 McBride Avenue/Suite B-204   West Paterson, NJ 07424   (973)256-5667   Fax (973)256-7758
+ Cardiology Associates LLC
181 Franklin Avenue/Suite 301   Nutley, NJ 07110   (973)256-5667   Fax (973)667-0561

Capity, Domiciano V., MD {1124090360} IntrMd(68,PHIL)
+ 1907 Park Avenue/Suite 203
South Plainfield, NJ 07080   (908)561-3934   Fax (908)561-6881

Capko, Deborah M., MD {1447284450} Surgry, SrgOnc, SrgBst(89,NJ05)<NJ-HACKNSK, NJ-VALLEY>
+ Memorial Sloan-Kettering Cancer Center Basking Ridge
136 Mountain View Boulevard   Basking Ridge, NJ 07920   (908)542-3000   Fax (908)542-3220

Caplan, John L., MD {1386622769} CdvDis, IntrMd, ClCdEl(87,WIND)<NJ-RWJUHAM, NJ-STFRNMED>
+ Hamilton Cardiology Associates
2073 Klockner Road   Hamilton, NJ 08690   (609)584-1212   Fax (609)584-0103

Caplen, Stuart M., MD {1871529776} EmrgMd(76,MI07)<NJ-ENGLWOOD>
+ Englewood Hospital and Medical Center
350 Engle Street/EmrgMed   Englewood, NJ 07631   (201)984-3000   Fax (610)617-6280

Capo, Gerardo, MD {1225049505}<NJ-TRINIWSC>
+ Trinitas Regional Medical Center-Williamson Street
225 Williamson Street   Elizabeth, NJ 07207   (908)994-5000   Fax (908)994-8748

Capo, John Thomas, MD {1982781209} OrtSHand, SrgOrt, IntrMd(93,NJ06)<NY-NYUTISCH, NJ-HACKNSK>
+ NYU Langon Department of Orthopaedic Surgery
377 Jersey Avenue/Suite 280A   Jersey City, NJ 07302   (201)716-5851   Fax (201)309-2432

Capo', Aida P., MD {1235239369} CritCr(90,DOMI)<NJ-STMRYPAS>
+ Capo Medical Associates
700-79th Street   North Bergen, NJ 07047   (201)861-7900   Fax (201)861-5280

Capo', Maria Pilar, MD {1821199951} IntrMd, PulCCr, CritCr(83,DOM02)<NJ-HOLYNAME, NJ-PALISADE>
+ Capo Medical Associates
700-79th Street   North Bergen, NJ 07047   (201)861-7900   Fax (201)861-5280

Capone, Robert Anthony, MD {1528069663} CritCr, PulDis(78,NY01)<NJ-HCKTSTWN, NJ-ATLANTHS>
+ Pulmonary & Allergy Associates
8 Saddle Road/Suite 101   Cedar Knolls, NJ 07927   (973)267-9393   Fax (973)540-0472
+ Pulmonary & Allergy Associates
1 Springfield Avenue/Suite 3-A   Summit, NJ 07901   (973)267-9393   Fax (908)934-0556

Capotosta, Thomas J., Jr., MD {1518935436} SrgOrt(70,SPAI)<NJ-STFRNMED, NJ-RWJUHAM>
+ Mercer-Bucks Orthopaedics, P.C.
2501 Kuser Road   Hamilton, NJ 08691   (609)896-0444   Fax (609)587-4349

Capozzoli, Alexis Nicole, MD {1952743361} Pedtrc
+ Skylands Pediatrics
328-A Sparta Avenue   Sparta, NJ 07871   (973)729-2197   Fax (973)729-3653

Cappadona, Charles Richard, MD {1326054248} Surgry(95,NY19)<NJ-OCEANMC, NJ-COMMED>
+ 478 Brick Boulevard
Brick, NJ 08723   (732)701-4848   Fax (732)701-1244

Cappadona, James Louis, MD {1467517813} Rheuma(89,NJ05)<NJ-HACKNSK>
+ 75 Summit Avenue
Hackensack, NJ 07601   (201)968-9830   Fax (201)225-4702

93

Physicians by Name and Address

Cappadona, Joseph G., MD {1265441679} SrgOrt(95,NY19)<NJ-CHILTON>
+ SMG Orthopedic Surgery and Sports Medicine Center
2035 Hamburg Turnpike/Suite D   Wayne, NJ 07470   (973)616-0200   Fax (973)616-1792
+ SMG Orthopedic Surgery and Sports Medicine Center
61 Beaver Brook Road/Suite 201   Lincoln Park, NJ 07035   (973)616-0200   Fax (973)686-9294

Cappiello, Linda L., MD {1881853455} Dermat(86,NJ06)
+ 400 Grand Street
Hoboken, NJ 07030   (201)656-5257

Cappitelli, Jack V., MD {1851448492} IntrMd(94,NJ05)<NJ-VALLEY>
+ Summit Medical Group
31-00 Broadway   Fair Lawn, NJ 07410   (201)796-2255   Fax (201)796-7020

Caprio, Ralph E., MD {1174526636} Allrgy, Pedtrc(77,NY47)
+ Notchview Pediatrics, LLC.
1037 Route 46 East/Suite 201   Clifton, NJ 07013   (973)779-3911   Fax (973)471-2730

Capuano, Aaron Matthew, MD {1508064569} PlsSHNck, SrgPlstc, SrgPHand<NJ-MONMOUTH, NJ-CHILTON>
+ Northern Center for Plastic Surgery
700 East Palisade Avenue/1st Floor   Englewood Cliffs, NJ 07632   (201)820-5280   Fax (201)608-5156
+ 252 Broad Street
Red Bank, NJ 07701   (201)820-5280   Fax (201)608-5156

Caputo, Enza R., MD {1629041850} Pedtrc, IntrMd(89,ITAL)<NJ-OCEANMC, NJ-COMMED>
+ Brick Pediatric Group
1301 Route 70   Brick, NJ 08724   (732)892-8700   Fax (732)892-6689

Caputo, Francis John, MD {1790937175}
+ Cooper Perinatology Associates
3 Cooper Plaza/Suite 502   Camden, NJ 08103   (856)968-7433   Fax (856)968-8499

Caputo, Joseph L., MD {1972615896} Otlryg(79,MEX14)<NJ-VAEASTOR>
+ VA New Jersey Health Care System-East Orange Campus
385 Tremont Avenue/Otolaryngology   East Orange, NJ 07018   (973)676-1000

Caputo, Kevin P., MD {1255467106} Psychy(85,NY15)
+ 745 Lippincott Avenue
Moorestown, NJ 08057

Caraballo, Ricardo, MD {1275639783} ObsGyn(94,PA13)<NJ-COOPRUMC>
+ University Urogynecology Associates/Cooper Ob/Gyn
900 Centennial Boulevard/Suite L   Voorhees, NJ 08043   (856)325-6622   Fax (856)325-6522
+ Cooper Ob/Gyn
3 Cooper Plaza/Suite 300   Camden, NJ 08103   (856)325-6622   Fax (856)968-8575
+ Cooper Ob/Gyn
4 Plaza Drive/Suite 403/Bunker Hill Pl   Sewell, NJ 08043   (856)270-4020   Fax (856)270-4022

Carabelli, Robert A., MD {1467520692} PhysMd, PhyMPain(81,WIND)
+ Back Rehab Institute
1245 Whitehorse-Mercerville Rd   Hamilton, NJ 08619   (609)581-2400   Fax (609)581-2500

Carabin, Gari D., MD {1538121355} Ophthl, IntrMd(88,NY09)<NJ-HACKNSK>
+ 730 River Road/Suite 202
New Milford, NJ 07646   (201)692-1800   Fax (201)692-0403
Gcarabin@optonline.net

Caracitas, Alexandra Cristina, DO {1780642926} FamMed(00,NJ75)
+ Union County HealthCare Associates
300 South Avenue   Garwood, NJ 07027   (908)232-2273   Fax (908)232-1439
+ Union County HealthCare Associates
999 Raritan Road   Clark, NJ 07066   (908)232-2273   Fax (732)381-3733

Carafa, Ciro J., MD {1154485449} IntrMd, Rheuma(77,NY20)<NJ-HACKNSK>
+ 120 South Main Street
Lodi, NJ 07644   (973)473-7870   Fax (973)472-1455

Caravello, Andrew Benedetto, DO {1699973776} EmrgMd
+ 127 Oakdale Road
Cherry Hill, NJ 08034
+ Rowan University-School of Osteopathic Medicine
1 Medical Center Drive/Hse Staff   Stratford, NJ 08084   (856)566-7121

Caravello, Anthony Joseph, Jr., DO {1508813999} Radiol, RadDia(01,NY75)
+ University Radiology, PA
239 Route 22 East/Suite 302   Green Brook, NJ 08812   (732)968-4899   Fax (732)968-8096
+ University Radiology Group, P.C.
16 Mountain Boulevard   Warren, NJ 07059   (732)968-4899   Fax (908)769-9141
+ University Radiology Group, P.C.
3900 Park Avenue/Suite 107   Edison, NJ 08812   (732)548-6800   Fax (732)548-6290

Carayannopoulos, Leonidas Nicolas, MD {1043236367} PulDis(96,TX12)
+ Merck and Company Incorporated
126 East Lincoln Avenue/RY 34-A400   Rahway, NJ 07065   (732)574-4000

Carbonaro, Paul Anthony, MD {1841262185} Dermat(96,NJ05)
+ Advanced Dermatology, Laser & Cosmetic Center
2466 East Chestnut Avenue   Vineland, NJ 08361   (856)691-3442   Fax (856)691-6582

Carbone, Mary T., MD {1588617682} NnPnMd, Pedtrc(84,ITAL)<NJ-VALLEY>
+ Center for Pediatric Sleep Medicine
505 Goffle Road   Ridgewood, NJ 07450   (201)447-8152   Fax (201)447-8526

Carbonello, Justin Matthew, MD {1700179884}<NJ-HOBUNIMC>
+ Hoboken University Medical Center
308 Willow Avenue   Hoboken, NJ 07030   (973)975-7527

Carcia, Danielle, DO {1174962773} FamMed(13,PA77)
+ Capital Health Primary Care Columbus
23203 Columbus Road/Suite 1   Columbus, NJ 08022   (603)303-4450   Fax (603)303-4451

Cardamone, Kristen Elizabeth, DO {1487811055} PhysMd(04,NY75)
+ Sports and Spine Integrative Center
188 East Bergen Place/Suite 301   Red Bank, NJ 07701   (732)268-7250   Fax (732)268-7251
+ 35 Olcott Square/Fl. 1
Bernardsville, NJ 07924   (732)268-7250   Fax (844)321-1485

Cardiello, Gary P., MD {1114020690} IntrMd(82,ITAL)<NJ-CHRIST, NJ-BAYONNE>
+ Hudson Internal Medicine
744 Broadway   Bayonne, NJ 07002   (201)436-8888   Fax (201)436-6644

Cardiges, Nicholas Michael, MD {1831142124} RadOnc, Radiol(90,MD01)<PA-STLKBTHL>
+ Warren Hospital
185 Roseberry Street/Rad Onc   Phillipsburg, NJ 08865   (908)859-6700

Cardillo, Marina, MD {1902055569} Pthlgy, PthAna(85,ITA33)
+ Quest Diagnostics Inc.
1 Malcolm Avenue   Teterboro, NJ 07608   (201)393-5000   Fax (201)393-6127

Cardinale, Jan Foxman, MD {1578830592} EmrgMd(91,MD01)<NJ-JRSYSHMC>
+ Jersey Shore University Medical Center
1945 Route 33/EmergMed   Neptune, NJ 07753   (609)610-2847

Cardinale, Robert Michael, MD {1679500128} RadOnc(91,MD01)<NJ-CENTRAST, NJ-UNVMCPRN>
+ CentraState Medical Center
901 West Main Street/RadOncology   Freehold, NJ 07728   (732)431-2000
+ Princeton Radiation Oncology Center
9 Centre Drive/Suite 115   Jamesburg, NJ 08831   (732)431-2000   Fax (609)655-5725
+ Princeton Radiology Associates, P.A.
3674 Route 27   Kendall Park, NJ 07728   (732)821-5563   Fax (732)821-6675

Cardo, Amelia J., MD {1023044211} RadDia, Radiol(75,NJ05)
+ Atlantic Medical Imaging
455 Jack Martin Boulevard   Brick, NJ 08724   (732)223-9729   Fax (732)840-6459

Cardona, Shirley J., DO {1902104185} IntrMd<NJ-HOLYNAME>
+ Holy Name Hospital
718 Teaneck Road   Teaneck, NJ 07666   (201)833-3000   Fax (732)212-0713

Cardonick, Elyce Hope, MD {1831289529} ObsGyn, MtFtMd(91,PA07)<NJ-COOPRUMC, NJ-ACMCMAIN>
+ Cooper University Hospital
One Cooper Plaza/Ob/Gyn   Camden, NJ 08103   (856)342-2000
+ University Urogynecology Associates/Cooper Ob/Gyn
1230 Whitehorse Mercerville Rd/Suite B   Hamilton, NJ 08619   (609)581-5681

Cardoso, Gilbert Santos, DO {1477514818} Gastrn, IntrMd(95,MI12)<NJ-HUNTRDN>
+ Hunterdon Gastroenterology Associates, P.A.
1100 Wescott Drive/Suite 206-207   Flemington, NJ 08822   (908)483-4000   Fax (908)788-5090
+ Hunterdon Gastroenterology Associates, P.A.
135 West End Avenue/Suite 204   Somerville, NJ 08876   (908)483-4000   Fax (908)788-5090

Cardoso, Ronald J., MD {1891856456} Anesth(81,MEX62)<NJ-STBARNMC>
+ New Jersey Anesthesia Associates, P.C.
252 Columbia Turnpike/PO Box 0037   Florham Park, NJ 07932   (973)660-9334   Fax (973)660-9779

Cardullo, Alice Cecilia, MD {1801950480} Dermat, Pedtrc(82,NY47)<NJ-CHILTON>
+ 330 Ratzer Road
Wayne, NJ 07470   (973)696-4806   Fax (973)696-8980

Careaga, Eduardo, MD {1912166919} Surgry
+ Kennedy Health Alliance
900 Medical Center Drive/Suite 201   Sewell, NJ 08080   (856)218-2100   Fax (856)218-2101

Carela, Gendy, MD {1811255649} FamMed
+ Tatem Brown Family Practice
2225 East Evesham Road/Suite 101   Voorhees, NJ 08043   (856)325-3700   Fax (856)325-3704

Carey, Brittany Marie, DO {1962821132} Pedtrc
+ Pediatric Associates of Holmdel, PC
719 North Beers Street/Suite 1E   Holmdel, NJ 07733   (732)739-4414   Fax (732)739-9537

Carey, Christopher T., MD {1518069970} SrgOrt(94,PA02)
+ Orthopedic Reconstruction
600 Somerdale Road/Suite 113   Voorhees, NJ 08043   (856)795-1945   Fax (856)795-7472

Carfagno, Salvatore, Jr., DO {1851336671} ObsGyn(95,PA77)<NJ-ACMCITY, NJ-SHOREMEM>
+ 707 Whitehorse Pike/Suite D-4
Absecon, NJ 08201   (609)272-9596   Fax (609)272-0607

Cargan, Abba L., MD {1588727796} Pedtrc, NroChl, NrlgSpec(86,VA04)<NY-PRSBCOLU>
+ 1122 Route 22 West
Mountainside, NJ 07092   (908)233-5000   Fax (908)233-5523

Caride, Peter, MD {1689784381} IntrMd, Gastrn(90,NY09)<NJ-HOBUNIMC, NJ-HOLYNAME>
+ Drs. Caride and Sotiriadis
9226 Kennedy Boulevard/Suite A   North Bergen, NJ 07047   (201)869-9500   Fax (201)869-9501

Carideo, Ida M., MD {1578842977} IntrMd, Rheuma(88,DOMI)
+ Monmouth Total Health Care
285 Parker Road   Eatontown, NJ 07724   (732)229-3344   Fax (732)728-0870
+ Hazlet Family Care
3253 Route 35   Hazlet, NJ 07730   (732)229-3344   Fax (732)888-7649

Caringal, Cecilia G., MD {1639223498} Psychy(77,PHIL)<NJ-ANCPSYCH>
+ Ancora Psychiatric Hospital
301 Spring Garden Road   Hammonton, NJ 08037   (609)561-1700
Cecilia.caringal@dhs.state.nj.us

Carino, Samuel Comia, DO {1528069044} EmrgMd, OstMed(95,NY75)<NJ-CENTRAST>
+ CentraState Medical Center
901 West Main Street/Emergency Med   Freehold, NJ 07728   (732)431-2000

Carle, William J., MD {1366465924} EmrgMd(87,NJ05)
+ Hackettstown Regional Medical Center
651 Willow Grove Street   Hackettstown, NJ 07840   (908)850-6800   Fax (908)850-6896

Carlin, Elizabeth Berk, MD {1578582524} NnPnMd(90,MA05)<NJ-ENGLWOOD>
+ Englewood Hospital and Medical Center
350 Engle Street   Englewood, NJ 07631   (201)894-3000   Fax (201)569-5983

Carlin, Francis Scott, DO {1265578868} FamMed(88,PA77)
+ 2087 Route 9 Ste 9
Ocean View, NJ 08230   (609)486-5150   Fax (609)486-6798

Carlin, Teresa Mary, MD {1629026265} EmrgMd
+ Cape Urgent Care
900 Route 109   Cape May, NJ 08204   (609)884-4357   Fax (609)884-4377

Carlino, Anthony, MD {1649296310} IntrMd(00,NJ05)<NJ-STBARNMC>
+ St. Barnabas Medical Center
94 Old Short Hills Road   Livingston, NJ 07039   (973)322-5000
+ Barnabas Medical Group
560 Springfield Avenue/Suite 101   Westfield, NJ 07090   (973)322-5000   Fax (908)389-1411

Carlo, Jocelyn Ann, MD {1346235322} ObsGyn(01,MEX14)<NJ-JRSYSHMC>
+ Hackensack Meridian Medical Group Ob/Gyn, Wall
1924 Route 35/Suite 5   Wall, NJ 07719   (732)974-8404   Fax (732)974-8904
+ Monmouth County Associates
4788 US Highway 9   Howell, NJ 07731   (732)974-8404   Fax (732)905-1919

Carlo-Francisco, Kristen L., DO {1013244573} Psychy(09,NJ75)<NJ-UNIVBHC>
+ 281 Summerhill Road/Suite 103-B
East Brunswick, NJ 08816   (848)468-1307

Carlson, Joann Marie, MD {1932365400} Pedtrc, PedNph, IntrMd(08,DC01)
+ University Hospital-RWJ Medical School
89 French Street/Pediatrics   New Brunswick, NJ 08901   (732)235-7880   Fax (732)235-6620

Carlson, John A., MD {1710943121} ObsGyn, GynOnc(74,DC02)
+ Virtua Gynecologic Oncology Specialists
200 Bowman Drive/Suite E-315   Voorhees, NJ 08043   (856)247-7310   Fax (856)247-7309

Carlson, Roy Douglas, MD {1932142858} Otlryg, SrgHdN, IntrMd(79,CT01)<NJ-VIRTMHBC>
+ Advanced ENT - Mount Laurel
204 Ark Road/Building 1/Suite 102   Mount Laurel, NJ 08054   (856)602-4000   Fax (856)946-1747
+ Advanced ENT - Voorhees
200 Bowman Drive/Suite D-285   Voorhees, NJ 08043   (856)602-4000   Fax (856)346-0757

Carlson, Sandra Regina, MD {1033321302} IntrMd
+ Carlson Medical
385 South Maple Avenue/Suite 101   Glen Rock, NJ 07452   (201)345-1855

Carlucci, Michael Louis, MD {1194925750} IntrMd(07,NJ06)<NJ-RWJUBRUN>
+ Central Jersey Lung Center
333 Forsgate Drive/Suite 201   Jamesburg, NJ 08831   (732)521-3131   Fax (732)521-1116

Carman, Elise S., MD {1770552325} ObsGyn(92,NY47)<NJ-MORRISTN>
+ 127 Pine Street/Suite 5
Montclair, NJ 07042   Fax (973)655-9559

Carman, Roy L., MD {1760486476} Gastrn, IntrMd(72,DC02)<NJ-RIVERVW>
+ Parker Family Health Center
211 Shrewsbury Avenue   Red Bank, NJ 07701   (732)212-0777   Fax (732)212-9030

Carmickle, Lynne J., MD {1376877159} Nrolgy(81,NY46)
+ 2 The Crossing
North Caldwell, NJ 07006   (973)228-7933

Carneiro, Susete M., MD {1003170853}
+ 1759 Raleigh Court East/Apt 167b
Ocean, NJ 07712   (201)817-3485
swetecarneiro@gmail.com

Carness, Jason, MD {1184068223} Psychy
+ Immediate Care Psychiatric Center, LLC
22 Hill Road   Parsippany, NJ 07054   (973)335-9909   Fax (973)335-9910

Carneval, Patricia A., MD {1174643829} Psychy(87,PA12)<NJ-CARRIER>
+ 20 Nassau Street/Suite 318
Princeton, NJ 08542   (609)688-0066

Carnevale, Shawn A., DO {1184705113} EmrgMd(93,NJ75)<NJ-OURLADY>
+ Our Lady of Lourdes Medical Center
1600 Haddon Avenue/EmergMed   Camden, NJ 08103   (856)757-3500

Carney, Alexander S., MD {1154385466} Rheuma(66,NY20)<NJ-UNVMCPRN>
+ 8 Quakerbridge Plaza/Suite H
Mercerville, NJ 08619   (609)588-9044   Fax (609)588-0168

Carney, William P., MD {1982892188} SrgOrt(89,DC02)<NJ-VALLEY>
+ 127 Union Street
Ridgewood, NJ 07450   (201)444-4447   Fax (201)444-5155
+ Wayne Surgical Center, LLC.
1176 Hamburg Pike   Wayne, NJ 07470   (201)444-4447   Fax (973)709-1901

Carney-Gellella, Erin D., MD {1083882963} RadDia(03,NJ06)<NJ-STPETER, NJ-RWJUBRUN>
+ University Radiology Group, P.C.
483 Cranbury Road   East Brunswick, NJ 08816   (732)390-0030   Fax (732)390-5383
+ University Radiology Group, P.C.
579A Cranbury Road   East Brunswick, NJ 08816   (732)390-0030   Fax (732)390-1856

Carni, Abbe J., MD {1033293956} Anesth(79,NY46)
+ 1270 Fayette Street
Teaneck, NJ 07666   (201)837-8635

Carniol, Eric T., MD {1255698387} Otlryg, OtgyFPlS(12,MA05)
+ Carniol Plastic Surgery
33 Overlook Road/Suite 401   Summit, NJ 07901   (908)598-1400   Fax (908)273-1553

Carniol, Paul J., MD {1578591954} SrgFPl, Otlryg, SrgPlstc(76,PA01)
+ Carniol Plastic Surgery
33 Overlook Road/Suite 401   Summit, NJ 07901   (908)598-1400   Fax (908)273-1553
+ Short Hills Surgery Center
187 Millburn Avenue/Suite 101   Millburn, NJ 07041   (908)598-1400   Fax (973)671-0557

Carnow, David Robert, MD {1831434158} GPrvMd, OccpMd(79,IL01)
+ Pavonia Medical Associates
600 Pavonia Avenue/5th Floor   Jersey City, NJ 07306   (201)216-3050   Fax (201)499-0254

Caro, Marjorie, MD {1902811490} Psychy(95,DOM02)
+ AtlantiCare Behavioral Health/Cornerstone
6010 Black Horse Pike   Egg Harbor Township, NJ 08234   (609)646-5142   Fax (609)646-8715

Carolan, Owen J., MD {1134310667} FamMed
+ Shore Medical Group
1640 Highway 88/Suite 203   Brick, NJ 08724   (732)458-7777   Fax (732)458-6741

Carollo, Andrew, MD {1922189828} SrgOrt(71,MEXI)<NJ-TRINIJSC>
+ Suburban Orthopedic Medical Center
554 Bloomfield Avenue   Newark, NJ 07107   (973)483-2277   Fax (973)483-4577
doctors@rehabz.com

Carozza, Charles R., MD {1104982974} SrgOrt(70,NY03)<NJ-VALLEY>
+ 127 Union Street
Ridgewood, NJ 07450   (201)445-0880   Fax (201)445-7711

Carpenter, Bruce W., MD {1144256959} RadDia(82,NC05)<NJ-STBARNMC>
+ St. Barnabas Medical Center
94 Old Short Hills Road/Radiology   Livingston, NJ 07039   (973)322-5000

Carpenter, Duncan B., MD {1134295819} SrgNro, NeuMus(78,NY01)<NJ-VALLEY>
+ North Jersey Neurosurgical Associates PA
225 Dayton Street   Ridgewood, NJ 07450   (201)612-0020   Fax (201)612-0333

Carpenter, Todd Jared, MD {1770807794}<NJ-MORRISTN>
+ Morristown Medical Center
100 Madison Avenue   Morristown, NJ 07962   (212)241-7500
toddjcarpenter@gmail.com

Carpizo, Darren Richard, MD {1134377229} Surgry(97,IL11)<NY-SLOANKET, NJ-RWJUBRUN>
+ Rutgers Cancer Institute of New Jersey
195 Little Albany Street/PO Box 2681   New Brunswick, NJ 08903   (732)235-2465   Fax (732)235-6797

Carr, Alan D., DO {1184783375} Anesth, AnesPain(84,IA75)<NJ-JFKMED>
+ Neurology Associates & Ctr Pain
1030 North Kings Highway/Suite 200A   Cherry Hill, NJ 08034   (856)779-7774   Fax (609)567-8832
pain1@comcast.net
+ 1804 Berlin Road/Suite A
Cherry Hill, NJ 08003   (856)779-7774   Fax (856)489-3477
+ Professional Pain Management Associates
2007 North Black Horse Pike   Williamstown, NJ 08034   (856)740-4888   Fax (856)740-0558

Carracino, Robert L., MD {1093798571} IntrMd(91,SPAI)<NJ-RIVERVW>
+ Meridian Primary Care
55 North Gilbert Street/Suite 3201   Tinton Falls, NJ 07701   (732)450-0961   Fax (732)530-0213

Carrao, Vincent, MD {1417945767} SrgO&M, Surgry, IntrMd(97,NY01)<NY-MTSINAI>
+ Palisades Surgical Associates
1530 Palisade Avenue/Colony Building   Fort Lee, NJ 07024   (201)585-8282   Fax (201)585-0805
vcarrao@aol.com

Carrazzone, Peter Louis, MD {1962430371} FamMed(82,GRNA)<NJ-STJOSHOS, NJ-WAYNEGEN>
+ Wayne Primary Care
468 Parish Drive/Suite 1   Wayne, NJ 07470   (973)305-8300   Fax (973)305-8157
+ Vanguard Medical Group
535 High Mountain Road/Suite 111   North Haledon, NJ 07508   (973)305-8300   Fax (973)636-0913
+ North Jersey Family Medicine
19 Yawpo Avenue   Oakland, NJ 07470   (973)337-3412   Fax (201)337-3353

Carreno, Miguel Angel, MD {1295023489}<NJ-MORRISTN>
+ Morristown Medical Center
100 Madison Avenue   Morristown, NJ 07962   (973)971-5000

Carreno, Wilfredo, MD {1700803582} CdvDis, IntrMd(72,MEX14)<NJ-SHOREMEM, NJ-ACMCMAIN>
+ AtlantiCare Physicians
318 Chris Gaupp Drive/Suite 100   Galloway, NJ 08205   (609)404-9900   Fax (609)404-3653

Carrer, Alexandra, MD {1902047343} SrgOrt(06,NY08)<NJ-JRSYCITY>
+ Premier Orthopaedics and Sports Medicine, P.C.
111 Galway Place   Teaneck, NJ 07666   (201)833-9500   Fax (201)862-0095
+ Premier Orthopaedics and Sports Medicine, PC
663 Palisade Avenue/Suite 302   Cliffside Park, NJ 07010   (201)833-9500   Fax (201)943-7308
+ Premier Orthopaedics & Sports Medicine, PC.
1255 Bloomfield Street   Bloomfield, NJ 07666   (973)842-2100   Fax (973)338-0863

Carrieri, David A., DO {1831119643} FamMed(89,NY75)<NJ-SOMERSET>
+ MEDEMERGE
1005 North Washington Avenue   Green Brook, NJ 08812   (732)968-8900   Fax (732)968-4609

Carrigan, Robert Boyd, MD {1790725745} OrtSHand, SrgOrt(99,PA01)<PA-CHILDHOS>
+ CHOP Specialty Care Center at Virtua
200 Bowman Drive/2 FL/Suite D-260   Voorhees, NJ 08043   (267)425-5400

Carroccia, Eugene C., MD {1336279587} SrgPlstc(65,NJ05)<NJ-ACMCITY, NJ-SHOREMEM>
+ 8512 Ventnor Avenue
Margate, NJ 08402   (609)822-8200   Fax (609)822-8287
+ Volunteers in Medicine
423 North Route 9   Cape May Court House, NJ 08210   (609)822-8200   Fax (609)463-2830

Carroll, Gerard Gregori, MD {1982830097} EmrgMd(09,NH01)
+ Cooper University Hospital
One Cooper Plaza   Camden, NJ 08103   (856)968-7433   Fax (856)968-8499

Carroll, John F., MD {1396869210} Pedtrc, AdmMgt(70,NY08)
+ 108 Canal Walk Boulevard
Somerset, NJ 08873   (732)412-7324   Fax (732)412-7324

Carroll, Michael R., III, MD {1427053222} RadDia, Radiol, IntrMd(90,VA07)<NJ-JRSYSHMC>
+ University Radiology Group, P.C.
579A Cranbury Road   East Brunswick, NJ 08816   (732)390-0040   Fax (732)390-1856
+ Lacey Diagnostic Imaging LLC
833 Lacey Road/Suite 2   Forked River, NJ 08731   (732)390-0040   Fax (609)242-2402
+ University Radiology Group
900 West Main Street   Freehold, NJ 08816   (732)462-1900   Fax (732)462-1848

Carrozza, Anthony V., MD {1629269543}<NJ-OVERLOOK>
+ Overlook Medical Center
99 Beauvoir Avenue/PO Box 210   Summit, NJ 07902   (702)596-6326
antc78@aol.com

Carruth, Samuel G., Jr., MD {1841246675} Pedtrc(96,OH41)<NJ-STBARNMC, NJ-OVERLOOK>
+ 2 Cedar Street
Newark, NJ 07102   (973)733-7150   Fax (973)733-7154

Carruth Mehnert, Lauren Vales, MD {1477687200} FamMed(03,NJ06)<NJ-HUNTRDN>
+ Capital Health Primary Care - Mountainview
850 Bear Tavern Road/Suite 309   Ewing, NJ 08628   (609)656-8844   Fax (609)656-8845

Carson, Gregory B., MD {1063452720} Surgry, EmrgMd(84,PA13)<NJ-SOCEANCO>
+ Southern Ocean County Medical Center
1140 Route 72 West/Emerg Medicine   Manahawkin, NJ 08050   (609)597-6011   Fax (609)978-8948

Carson, Jeffrey L., MD {1174693873} IntrMd(77,PA09)
+ UH- Robert Wood Johnson Med
125 Paterson Street/CAB/IntrnlMdcn   New Brunswick, NJ 08901   (732)235-6968
+ 52 Ridgeview Drive
Belle Mead, NJ 08502   (908)874-0295

Carson, Milinda Ruth, MD {1275572034} ObsGyn, Obstet(92,NJ05)<NJ-HOLYNAME, NJ-HACKNSK>
+ Drs. Carson & Solomon
203 Passaic Avenue   Passaic, NJ 07055   (973)246-6999   Fax (973)685-7340

Carstens, Kathleen M., MD {1669736195}
+ 10 Berton Place
Nutley, NJ 07110   (201)317-4113

Carta, Maria C., MD {1043260250} Nrolgy(80,ITAL)<NJ-VIRTMARL, NJ-VIRTVOOR>
+ Integrative Neurological Care
663 South White Horse Pike   Hammonton, NJ 08037   (609)567-6042

Cartaxo, Kenneth W., MD {1083700702} FamMed, EmrgMd(80,MEX14)
+ 87 Chapel Hill Terrace
Kinnelon, NJ 07405

Carter, Alison F., MD {1710906482} IntrMd(85,NY08)<NJ-JRSYSHMC, NJ-CENTRAST>
+ Medical Associates of Marlboro PC
32 North Main Street   Marlboro, NJ 07746   (732)462-4100   Fax (732)462-3798

Carter, Brittany Nicole, MD {1265884605} IntrMd<NJ-ENGLWOOD>
+ Englewood Hospital and Medical Center
350 Engle Street   Englewood, NJ 07631   (201)894-3000

Physicians by Name and Address

Carter, Cheryl Ann, MD {1639188014} ObsGyn(98,NY08)
+ Metropolitan Family Health Network
935 Garfield Avenue Jersey City, NJ 07304 (201)478-5800 Fax (201)475-5814
+ New Margaret Hague Women's Health Institute
377 Jersey Avenue/Suite 220 Jersey City, NJ 07302 (201)478-5800 Fax (201)795-9157

Carter, Larry Ernest, DO {1164421491} EmrgMd(93,IA75)<NJ-RBAYPERT>
+ Raritan Bay Medical Center/Perth Amboy Division
530 New Brunswick Avenue/EmrgMed Perth Amboy, NJ 08861 (732)442-3700

Carter, Mitchel S., MD {1457341273} Surgry(79,IL42)
+ Summit Medical Group Florham Park Campus
150 Park Avenue/2nd FL Florham Park, NJ 07932 (973)404-9980

Carter, Susan Redfield, MD {1336191196} Ophthl(89,CT01)<NJ-UMDNJ, NJ-OVERLOOK>
+ The Eye Center
65 Mountain Boulevard Ext/Suite 105 Warren, NJ 07059 (732)356-6200 Fax (732)356-0228
+ The Eye Center
3900 Park Avenue/Suite 106 Edison, NJ 08820 (732)603-2101
+ The Eye Center
213 Stelton Road Piscataway, NJ 07059 (732)752-9090 Fax (732)752-9492

Cartnick, Gregory Alan, MD {1710082094} IntrMd(GRN01)
+ Neptune Pediatrics
1812 State Route 33 Neptune, NJ 07753 (732)988-3336 Fax (732)776-8668
+ Kristen A. Atienza, DO, FACOP
1812 Corlies Avenue Neptune, NJ 07753 (732)988-3336 Fax (732)776-8668

Cartwright, Charles N., MD {1497833735} Psychy, PsyCAd(88,SAF02)<NJ-UMDNJ>
+ University Psychiatric Associates
183 South Orange Avenue/E-F Levels Newark, NJ 07103 (973)972-2977 Fax (973)972-2979

Cartwright, Travante Mcnae, MD {1508111568} CdvDis<NJ-COOPRUMC>
+ Cooper University Hospital
One Cooper Plaza/Dorrance 261 Camden, NJ 08103 (856)342-2922

Carty, Robert W., MD {1689672800} FamMed(81,NJ06)
+ Capital Health Primary Care-Bordentown
1 Third Street Bordentown, NJ 08505 (609)298-2005 Fax (609)324-8267

Caruana, Lucia P., MD {1215975453} ObsGyn(89,NY47)<NJ-ENGLWOOD, NY-PRSBCOLU>
+ Metropolitan Pediatric Group
704 Palisade Avenue Teaneck, NJ 07666 (201)836-4301 Fax (201)836-5110
+ Metropolitan Pediatric Group
570 Piermont Road/17 Closter Commons Closter, NJ 07624 (201)836-4301 Fax (201)768-7316

Caruso, Donald A., MD {1891796801} IntrMd(69,ITAL)<NJ-COMMED>
+ Whiting Medical Associates
65 Lacey Road/Suite A Whiting, NJ 08759 (732)350-0404 Fax (732)350-2001

Caruso, Edward Francis, MD {1780658864} PsyGrt, Psychy, IntrMd(85,DMN01)
+ Coventry Cardiology Associates
960 Route 173 Bloomsbury, NJ 08804 (908)388-3500 Fax (908)388-3501

Caruso, Marco F., MD {1851476246} Anesth(01,NY46)
+ 65 Crine Lane
Morganville, NJ 07751 (732)915-2343
mcaruso1326@yahoo.com
+ Toms River Anesthesia Associates PC
409 Main Street/2nd Floor Toms River, NJ 08753 (732)915-2343 Fax (732)818-1567

Caruso, Meghan Murphy-Schmelze, DO {1821093436} Dermat, SrgDer(95,PA77)<NJ-MEMSALEM>
+ Drs. Schmelzer & Caruso
4 Bypass Road/Suite 104 Salem, NJ 08079 (856)983-4646 Fax (856)983-4760
+ Drs. Schmelzer & Caruso
427 Egg Harbor Road Sewell, NJ 08080 (856)589-2267

Caruso, Michael J., DO {1437124252} Ophthl(84,PA77)<NJ-BURDTMLN>
+ 207 Stone Harbor Boulevard
Cape May Court House, NJ 08210 (609)465-1616 Fax (609)465-3213
drcaruso@atlanticeye.net
+ Eye Max LASIK Center/Atlantic Eye Center
200 New Road Linwood, NJ 08221 (609)465-1616 Fax (609)653-2215
+ Cape Cataract Center
804 Route 9 South Cape May Court House, NJ 08210 (609)463-1525 Fax (609)463-1528

Caruso, Patrick A., MD {1588630784} Pedtrc(83,OH06)<NJ-HCKTSTWN, NJ-MORRISTN>
+ Plaza Family Care
657 Willow Grove Street/Suite 401 Hackettstown, NJ 07840 (908)850-7800 Fax (908)850-7801
+ Plaza Family Care
245 Main Street/Suite 300 & 302 Chester, NJ 07930 (908)850-7800 Fax (908)879-6738

Caruso, Robert Peter, MD {1588604557} Urolgy, SrgLap, OthrSp(98,NJ05)<NJ-MTNSIDE, NJ-CLARMAAS>
+ Essex Hudson Urology
256 Broad Street/Lap/RoboticSurg Bloomfield, NJ 07003 (973)743-4450 Fax (973)429-9076
+ Essex Hudson Urology
243 Chestnut Street Newark, NJ 07105 (973)743-4450 Fax (973)344-9188
+ Essex Hudson Urology
213 South Frank Rodgers Blvd Harrison, NJ 07003 (973)482-7070

Caruso, Steven A., MD {1104098995} SrgOrt
+ Trenton Orthopaedic Group
116 Washington Crossing Road Pennington, NJ 08534 (609)581-2200 Fax (609)581-1212

Caruthers, Samuel Grenville, MD {1225034887} Anesth, IntrMd(97,VA27)<NJ-VAEASTOR>
+ Interventional Pain Consultants
408 Main Street/Suite 101-D Boonton, NJ 07005 (862)222-4629 Fax (973)352-9519

Carvalho, Artur Meneses, MD {1821015546} IntrMd(97,GRN01)
+ 620 Essex Street/Suite 3
Harrison, NJ 07029 (973)535-5818 Fax (973)274-1959

Carvalho, Steven Evaristo, MD {1053608844} Anesth<NJ-TRINIWSC>
+ Trinitas Regional Medical Center-Williamson Street
225 Williamson Street/2 South Elizabeth, NJ 07207 (908)994-5390

Casagrande, Lisette Helene, MD {1912166877} IntrMd(07,NJ05)<NY-MTSINAI, NY-MTSINYHS>
+ Modern Nephrology & Transplant, LLC
767 Northfield Avenue West Orange, NJ 07052 (973)992-9022 Fax (973)992-9024

Casale, Alfred Stanley, MD {1598730384} SrgCdv, SrgThr(80,MD07)<PA-GSNGWYVL>
+ 15 Crescent Road
Madison, NJ 07940 (973)377-5996

Casale, Lisa M., MD {1982625984} IntrMd, PulDis, CritCr(88,PA13)<NJ-RWJBRUN, NJ-RWJURAH>
+ Pulmonary Internists, PA
2 Lincoln Highway/Suite 301 Edison, NJ 08820 (732)549-7380 Fax (732)548-8216
+ Pulmonary Internists, PA
3 Hospital Plaza/Suite 205 Old Bridge, NJ 08857 (732)360-2255

Casarona, Charles A., MD {1629164637} Pedtrc(84,DMN01)
+ 44 Pennington Ave.
Colonia, NJ 07067

Cascarina, Michael A., MD {1194732982} FamMed(91,PA07)<NJ-KIMBALL>
+ Our Family Practice
1899 State Highway 88 Brick, NJ 08723 (732)840-8177 Fax (732)840-2195

Cascarino, Raymond Patrick, DO {1326083544} EmrgMd, IntrMd(95,NJ75)<NJ-BURDTMLN>
+ Cape Regional Medical Center
2 Stone Harbor Boulevard/EmrgMed Cape May Court House, NJ 08210 (609)463-2000 Fax (609)463-2946

Case, John Gouyd, MD {1588756811} Psychy(80,NY06)<NJ-VIRTMHBC>
+ Virtua Memorial
175 Madison Avenue Mount Holly, NJ 08060 (609)267-0700
+ Center for Family Guidance
895 Beverly Rancocas Road Mount Holly, NJ 08060 (609)267-0700 Fax (856)797-4775

Case, Philip Lawrence, MD {1407906282} AlgyImmn, PedAlg, ImmAsm(80,VA07)<NJ-CENTRAST>
+ 3499 Route 9 North/Suite 2C-5
Freehold, NJ 07728 (732)577-1242 Fax (732)358-7250
+ 4251 Highway 9/Suite E
Freehold, NJ 07728 (732)577-1242 Fax (732)577-7019

Casella, Frank J., DO {1306888912} Nephro, IntrMd(86,MO79)<NJ-STMICHL>
+ Premier Health Associates
89 Sparta Avenue/Suite 100 Sparta, NJ 07871 (973)729-2121 Fax (973)729-3454

Casella, Joseph J., DO {1891781514} FamMed(81,MO79)<NJ-NWTNMEM>
+ Premier Health Associates-Administration
532 Lafayette Road/Suite 300 Sparta, NJ 07871 (973)940-0423 Fax (973)940-0399
+ Premier Health Associates
272 Route 206 North Andover, NJ 07821 (973)940-0423 Fax (973)729-3238
+ Premier Health Associates
89 Sparta Avenue/Suite 100 Sparta, NJ 07871 (973)729-2121 Fax (973)729-3454

Casey, Daniel T., MD {1366481962} FamMed
+ Partners in Primary Care
534 Lippincott Drive Marlton, NJ 08053 (856)985-7373 Fax (856)985-9611

Casey, Kathleen K., MD {1053398941} InfDis, IntrMd(82,NJ06)<NJ-JRSYSHMC, NJ-RIVERVW>
+ Jersey Shore University Medical Center
1945 Route 33 Neptune, NJ 07753 (732)776-4302

Casey, Meaghan M., MD {1700014008}<NJ-TRININPC>
+ Trinitas Regional Medical Center-New Point Campus
655 East Jersey Street Elizabeth, NJ 07206 (908)994-5000

Casey, Thomas James, MD {1972637585} PedNrD<NJ-HUNTRDN, PA-STCHRIS>
+ Hunterdon Medical Center
2100 Wescott Drive/Pedi Neuro Flemington, NJ 08822 (908)788-6650 Fax (908)788-2578

Cash, Stephen Laurence, MD {1508817669} SrgHnd, SrgOrt, OrtSHand(78,NY15)<NJ-MORRISTN>
+ Hand Surgery & Rehabilitation of North Jersey, P.C.
301 East Hanover Avenue Morristown, NJ 07960 (973)538-5200
+ Hand Surgery & Rehabilitation of North Jersey, PC
111 Madison Avenue/Suite 302 Morristown, NJ 07960 (973)538-5200

Casia, Jeffrey P., MD {1013066786} Pedtrc
+ 67 Central Avenue
Jersey City, NJ 07306 (201)798-6161 Fax (201)798-0432

Casiano Pagan, Hector Francisco, MD {1841630472}
+ Capital Institute for Neurosciences
2 Capital Way/Suite 456 Pennington, NJ 08534 (609)537-7300 Fax (609)537-7301

Casper, Ephraim S., MD {1174503320} IntrMd, MedOnc(74,IL01)<NY-SLOANKET>
+ Valley Mount Sinai Comprehensive Cancer Care
One Valley Health Plaza Paramus, NJ 07652 (201)634-5578 Fax (201)986-4702

Casper, Robert J., MD {1699832956} IntrMd(80,MEX55)<NJ-STPETER, NJ-RWJUBRUN>
+ RWJPE Dayton Medical Group
12 Stults Road/Suite 121 Dayton, NJ 08810 (732)329-4400 Fax (609)395-7519

Casser, Michael E., MD {1972667723} IntrMd(84,GRNA)<NJ-ENGLWOOD>
+ 200 Engle Street/Suite 26
Englewood, NJ 07631 (201)567-4444 Fax (201)567-2166

Cassetty, Christopher Todd, MD {1427002807} Dermat(00,OK01)<NJ-HUNTRDN>
+ Hunterdon Dermatology LLC
8 Main Street/Suite 20 Flemington, NJ 08822 (908)782-1647 Fax (908)782-7296

Cassidy, Thomas J., MD {1174612295} IntrMd(97,GRN01)<NJ-JFKMED>
+ Adult Medicine Specialists
3910 Park Avenue/Suite 8 Edison, NJ 08820 (732)767-3130 Fax (732)767-3134

Cassidy-Smith, Tara Nicole, MD {1124118815} EmrgMd, PedEmg(00,NJ06)<NJ-COOPRUMC>
+ Cooper University Hospital
One Cooper Plaza/EmrgMed Camden, NJ 08103 (856)342-2000

Cassilly, Ryan, MD {1235455924} SrgOrt
+ Garden State Orthopaedic Associates, P.A.
28-04 Broadway Fair Lawn, NJ 07410 (201)791-4434 Fax (201)791-9377

Cassir, Jorge F., MD {1356381636} RadOnc(68,COLO)<NJ-BURDTMLN, NJ-SHOREMEM>
+ Cape Regional Medical Center
2 Stone Harbor Boulevard/RadOnc Cape May Court House, NJ 08210 (609)463-2000

Cassotis, Maria, DO {1003112426} Anesth<NJ-COOPRUMC>
+ Cooper University Hospital
One Cooper Plaza Camden, NJ 08103 (856)342-2000

Cassotta, Joseph P., Jr., MD {1093870776} FamMed(79,MEX14)<NJ-HOLYNAME, NJ-ENGLWOOD>
+ 1600 Center Avenue
Fort Lee, NJ 07024 (201)585-7511 Fax (201)585-7079
+ Holy Name Hospital
718 Teaneck Road/Family Practice Teaneck, NJ 07666 (201)833-3000

Casta, Aurora Margarita, MD {1235169897} PsyCAd, Psychy(82,PRO01)
+ 8 Mount Vernon Avenue
Haddonfield, NJ 08033

Castaldi, Mark Whittaker, MD {1447275185} RadDia(99,NJ06)<NJ-HUNTRDN>
  + Hunterdon Medical Center
    2100 Wescott Drive/Radiology Flemington, NJ 08822 (908)788-6388 Fax (908)788-6442
  + Hunterdon Radiological Associate
    1 Dogwood Drive Clinton, NJ 08809 (908)788-6388 Fax (908)735-6532

Castaneda, Rachel Lim, MD {1619051646} EnDbMt, IntrMd(83,PHI01)<NJ-MORRISTN>
  + Summit Medical Group
    95 Madison Avenue Morristown, NJ 07960 (973)775-5115 Fax (973)285-7617

Castano, Albert Ruben, DO {1316912967} Pedtrc(86,PA77)<NJ-UNDRWD>
  + Inspira Health Network
    509 North Broad Street Woodbury, NJ 08096 (856)853-2001

Castel, Nikki, MD {1386007789} SrgPlstc
  + New Jersey Medical School Div Plastic & Hand Surgery
    140 Bergen Street/Suite E1620 Newark, NJ 07103 (973)972-5377 Fax (973)972-8268

Castellano, Charles Christopher, MD {1396845632} IntrMd(00,NY08)
  + Summit Medical Group
    140 Park Avenue/3rd Floor Florham Park, NJ 07932 (973)404-7880

Castellano, Lillian Checchio, MD {1609089283} IntrMd(93,NJ05)
  + 99 Jefferson Road/MS 125
    Parsippany, NJ 07054 (973)739-3518 Fax (973)739-3508

Castellano, Marissa D., MD {1952568818} Pedtrc, IntrMd(06,DC02)<NJ-UNVMCPRN>
  + University Medical Center of Princeton at Plainsboro
    One Plainsboro Road/6th Floor Plainsboro, NJ 08536 (609)853-7626 Fax (609)853-7630

Castellano, Nicolas Andre, MD {1215194337} IntrMd
  + 13 Wood View Drive
    Mount Laurel, NJ 08054 (856)206-9437

Castellino, Sharon Franklin, MD {1033346291} IntrMd(99,INA87)
  + Virtua Hospitalist Group Memorial
    175 Madison Avenue Mount Holly, NJ 08060 (609)914-6180 Fax (609)914-6182
  + 6111 Kaitlyn Court
    West Windsor, NJ 08550

Castello, Frank V., MD {1497720205} PedCrC, Pedtrc(82,PA12)<NJ-CHLSMT>
  + St. Barnabas Medical Center
    94 Old Short Hills Road Livingston, NJ 07039 (973)322-2770 Fax (973)322-5504

Castelluber, Gisele B V M, MD {1568500882} FamMed(88,BRA29)<NJ-CLARMAAS>
  + Ramesh C. Tandon MD PA
    477 Stuyvesant Avenue Lyndhurst, NJ 07071 (201)933-2333 Fax (201)933-3885

Castelo-Soccio, Leslie Ann, MD {1992865976} Dermat(05,NY20)
  + Warren S. Kurnick MD Dermatology Group PA
    215 Sunset Road/Suite 102 Willingboro, NJ 08046 (609)871-9500 Fax (609)871-7590

Castilla, William A., MD {1235283938} FamMed(66,COL02)
  + Drs. Sharma and Castilla
    293 Passaic Street Passaic, NJ 07055 (973)365-1377 Fax (973)365-1229

Castillo, Ana A., MD {1740216597} Pedtrc(86,PHI09)
  + Hunterdon Developmental Center
    40 Pittstown Road/PO Box 4003 Clinton, NJ 08809 (908)735-4031 Fax (908)730-1338

Castillo, Christine Capistran, DO {1831276294} FamMed(95,IA75)<NJ-JRSYSHMC>
  + Capital Health Primary Care-Hamilton
    1445 Whitehorse-Mercerville Rd Hamilton, NJ 08619 (609)587-6661 Fax (609)587-8503

Castillo, David Cinco, DO {1518142603} EmrgMd<NJ-MORRISTN>
  + Morristown Medical Center
    100 Madison Avenue/EmergMed Morristown, NJ 07962 (973)971-7926 Fax (973)290-7202

Castillo, Edwin F., MD {1598979155} Psychy(73,MEX62)
  + 95 Route 73 South
    Voorhees, NJ 08043 (856)768-1818 Fax (856)768-2058

Castillo, Elma D., MD {1467510859} Pedtrc, AdolMd(78,PHIL)<NJ-PALISADE>
  + Drs. Castillo and Castillo
    5801 Broadway West New York, NJ 07093 (201)869-4044 Fax (201)869-4105
  + Drs. Castillo and Castillo
    39 2nd Avenue Secaucus, NJ 07094 (201)617-1996

Castillo, Gregorio A. G., MD {1013095306} PsycAd, Psychy(91,PHIL)<NJ-UMDNJ, NJ-UNIVBHC>
  + UH-University Behavioral Hlth
    100 Metroplex Drive/Suite 200 Edison, NJ 08817 (732)235-8400 Fax (732)235-8395

Castillo, Hector L., MD {1528198124} IntrMd, Ophthl(80,MEXI)
  + Hector L. Castillo MD Associates
    1000 Madison Avenue Paterson, NJ 07501 (973)742-3937 Fax (973)742-4411

Castillo, Hilda A., MD {1689774598} Psychy(84,DOM02)
  + Hector L. Castillo MD Associates
    1000 Madison Avenue Paterson, NJ 07501 (973)742-3937

Castillo, Luciano, Jr., MD {1639173073} Radiol, NuclMd, RadDia(72,PHIL)<NJ-BAYONNE>
  + Bayonne Medical Center
    29th Street at Avenue E Bayonne, NJ 07002 (201)858-5000 Fax (201)243-4229

Castillo, Marianne Devilla, MD {1164718995} Pedtrc(11,NJ05)
  + Drs. Castillo and Castillo
    5801 Broadway West New York, NJ 07093 (201)869-4044

Castillo, Minerva R., MD {1538273727} NnPnMd, Pedtrc(74,PHI09)
  + On-Site Neonatal Partners
    1000 Haddonfield-Berlin Road/Suite 210 Voorhees, NJ 08043 (856)782-2212 Fax (856)782-2213

Castillo, Rodrigo I., MD {1821156480} Pedtrc, AdolMd(77,PHIL)
  + Drs. Castillo and Castillo
    39 2nd Avenue Secaucus, NJ 07094 (201)617-1996
  + Drs. Castillo and Castillo
    5801 Broadway West New York, NJ 07093 (201)869-4044

Castro, Christopher Paul, DO {1356422406} PhysMd, IntrMd(02,NY75)
  + The Orthopedic Institute of New Jersey
    108 Bilby Road/Suite 201 Hackettstown, NJ 07840 (908)684-3005 Fax (908)684-3301
  + The Orthopedic Institute of New Jersey
    254-B Mountain Avenue/Suite 201 Hackettstown, NJ 07840 (908)684-3005 Fax (908)684-3301
  + The Orthopedic Institute of New Jersey
    222 High Street/Suite 202 Newton, NJ 07840 (908)684-3005 Fax (908)684-3301

Castro, Dorothy, MD {1982848297} IntrMd<NJ-UMDNJ>
  + University Hospital
    150 Bergen Street/UH H-245 Newark, NJ 07103 (973)972-5672

Castro, Elsa Imelda, MD {1639146954} PedCrd(88,MEXI)<NJ-CENTRAST, NJ-JRSYSHMC>
  + Alpert Zales & Castro Pediatric Cardiology, PA
    1623 Route 88/Suite A/PO Box 1719 Brick, NJ 08723 (732)458-9666 Fax (732)458-0840 SusanJLesser@aol.com
  + Alpert Zales & Castro Pediatric Cardiology, PA
    2 Apple Farm Road/PO Box 4176 Middletown, NJ 07748 (732)458-9666 Fax (732)458-0840

Castro, Rodrigo Alejandro, DO {1477815538}
  + Overlook Family Medicine
    33 Overlook Road/Suite 103 Summit, NJ 07901 (908)522-5700 Fax (908)273-8014

Castro, Zoila Y., MD {1063616894} FamMed(86,MEXI)
  + Medi Center II
    2954 Kennedy Boulevard Jersey City, NJ 07306 (201)653-6666 Fax (201)653-4850

Castro-Chevere, Nancy Ann, MD {1144425851} FamMed
  + AtlantiCare Special Care Center
    1401 Atlantic Avenue/Suite 2500 Atlantic City, NJ 08401 (609)572-8800

Castro-Frenzel, Karla Jose, MD {1245228378} PedAne, Anesth(00,TX14)<NJ-HACKNSK>
  + Hackensack University Medical Center
    30 Prospect Avenue/Anesth Hackensack, NJ 07601 (201)996-2000

Casty, Frank Eugene, MD {1114915683} PulDis, CritCr, IntrMd(86,PA13)
  + 108th Medical Group Air National Guard
    3466 Neely Road Trenton, NJ 08641 (609)754-2635

Catalano, John B., MD {1659446607} SrgOrt, SrgTrm(88,PA02)<NJ-SJHREGMC, NJ-SJRSYELM>
  + Premier Orthopaedic Associates
    298 South Delsea Drive Vineland, NJ 08360 (856)690-1616 Fax (856)690-1089
  + Premier Orthopaedic Assocs of So NJ
    201 Tomlin Station Road/Suite C Mullica Hill, NJ 08062 (856)690-1616 Fax (856)223-9110
  + Premier Orthopaedic Assoc So NJ
    525 South State Street/Suite 2 Elmer, NJ 08360 (856)358-2559

Catalano, Mariano, MD {1245430909} Pedtrc
  + 18 Page Avenue
    Lyndhurst, NJ 07071 (201)925-7023

Cataldo, Ralph G., DO {1659567220} Anesth, PainMd(91,ME75)
  + 15-17 Black Horse Pike
    Haddon Heights, NJ 08035 (856)546-8800 Fax (856)547-7916
  + Pain Control Center of New Jersey
    561 Cranbury Road East Brunswick, NJ 08816 (856)546-8800 Fax (732)651-0375

Catalina, Gabriel Richard, DO {1336152206} IntrMd(96,PA77)<NJ-ACMCMAIN>
  + Shoreline Endocrine and Medical Associates PC
    707 White Horse Pike/Suite C1 Absecon, NJ 08201 (609)813-2200 Fax (609)813-2201
  + The Plastic Surgery Center
    2500 English Creek Avenue/Suite 605 Egg Harbor Township, NJ 08234 (609)813-2200 Fax (609)822-6611

Catanese, Anthony J., MD {1184682692} Urolgy, Onclgy, OthrSp(83,NY09)
  + Anthony J. Catanese MD
    315 East Main Street Somerville, NJ 08876 (908)722-6900 Fax (908)722-6699

Catanese, Vincent J., MD {1699755801} FamMed, Grtrcs(78,PA14)<NJ-JRSYSHMC, NJ-RIVERVW>
  + Jersey Shore Medical Associates
    734 North Beers Street/Suite U-4 Holmdel, NJ 07733 (732)264-8484 Fax (732)264-4324

Catania, Raymond, DO {1023094711} CdvDis, IntrMd(89,IA75)<NJ-MORRISTN>
  + Barone & Catania Cardiovascular
    786 Mountain Boulevard/Suite 200 Watchung, NJ 07069 (908)754-0975 Fax (908)754-0260 info@bccardio.com

Catanzaro, Donna, MD {1306838578} IntrMd(90,NJ05)
  + RWJPE Primary Care Raritan
    34 East Somerset Street Raritan, NJ 08869 (908)685-2532 Fax (908)685-2542

Capano, Anthony, DO {1598924987} EmrgMd<NJ-STJOSHOS>
  + St Joseph's Medical Center Emergency
    703 Main Street Paterson, NJ 07503 (973)754-2240 Fax (973)754-2249

Capano, Joseph A., MD {1942241435} CdvDis, IntrMd(76,NJ06)<NJ-NWRKBETH, NJ-JFKMED>
  + Health Med Associates, PC
    1080 Stelton Road/First FL Suite 202 Piscataway, NJ 08854 (732)985-2552 Fax (732)985-0552

Cataquet, David, MD {1346262029} EmrgMd, IntrMd(87,NY01)<NJ-HCKTSTWN>
  + Hackettstown Regional Medical Center
    651 Willow Grove Street/Emerg Med Hackettstown, NJ 07840 (877)714-1592 Fax (856)616-1919

Cathcart, Charles S., MD {1447273628} RadOnc(88,MA05)<NJ-UMDNJ>
  + Rutgers- New Jersey Medical School
    185 South Orange Avenue/CancerCtr Newark, NJ 07103 (973)972-4300

Cathcart, Kathleen Nell Sheber, MD {1508806050} IntrMd, OncHem(92,NJ05)<NJ-UMDNJ>
  + University Hospital
    150 Bergen Street/HemeOnc/D-Green Newark, NJ 07103 (973)972-4300

Cato-Varlack, Janice Antoinette, MD {1801965678} Pedtrc(95,NY20)<NJ-COMMED, NJ-OCEANMC>
  + Drs. Cato-Varlack & Sadik
    495 Iron Bridge Road/Suite 1 Freehold, NJ 07728 (732)577-0047
  + Pediatric Affiliates, PA
    1616 Route 72 West/Suite 8 Manahawkin, NJ 08050 (732)577-0047 Fax (609)978-1229
  + UMDNJ RWJ Neonatal-Perinatal
    125 Paterson Street/MEB 312 New Brunswick, NJ 07728 (732)235-7900 Fax (609)420-7255

Caucino, Julie A., DO {1366449142} AlgyImmn, IntrMd(87,MO79)<NJ-UNVMCPRN>
  + Princeton Allergy & Asthma Associates, P.A.
    24 Vreeland Drive Skillman, NJ 08558 (609)921-2202 Fax (609)924-1468
  + Princeton Allergy & Asthma Associates, P.A.
    1245 Whitehorse Mercerville Rd Hamilton, NJ 08619 (609)921-2202 Fax (609)924-1468
  + Princeton Allergy & Asthma Associates, P.A.
    666 Plainsboro Road/Building 100-B Plainsboro, NJ 08558 (609)799-8111 Fax (609)924-1468

Cauda, Joseph E., MD {1891771358} Surgry, SrgBst(80,MEXI)<NJ-BAYSHORE, NJ-RIVERVW>
  + Shrewsbury Surgical Associates
    655 Shrewsbury Avenue/Suite 210 Shrewsbury, NJ 07702 (732)542-8118 Fax (732)544-4090

Caudle, Jennifer Nicole, DO {1184821597} IntrMd
  + University Doctors
    570 Egg Harbor Road/Suite C-2 Sewell, NJ 08080 (856)589-1414 Fax (856)589-9487

Cauvin, Leslie R., DO {1669478483} IntrMd(95,NJ75)<NJ-COMMED, NJ-KIMBALL>
  + BC Medical Care
    1747 Hooper Avenue/Suite 8 Toms River, NJ 08753 (732)255-6777 Fax (732)255-6669

Cava, Thomas J., MD {1245203959} PhysMd(87,FL02)<NJ-MTN-SIDE>
  + PC Rehabilitation Medicine & Physical Therapy
    960 Pleasant Valley Way West Orange, NJ 07052 (973)243-1177 Fax (973)243-9077

Physicians by Name and Address

Cavaliere, Ava A., DO {1063596179} Pedtrc(99,NJ75)<NJ-ACMC-MAIN, NJ-ACMCITY>
+ Rainbow Pediatrics
2041 US Highway 9 Cape May Court House, NJ 08210 (609)624-9003 Fax (609)624-9002

Cavalieri, Thomas A., DO {1497735484} Grtrcs, IntrMd(76,IA75)<NJ-KMHSTRAT, NJ-KMHCHRRY>
+ New Jersey Institute for Successful Aging
42 East Laurel Road/Suite 1800 Stratford, NJ 08084 (856)566-6843 Fax (856)566-6781

Cavallaro, Barbara Ann, MD {1821058629} Gyneco(86,NY19)<NJ-HACKNSK>
+ Excelsior Women's Care
170 Prospect Avenue/Suite 4 Hackensack, NJ 07601 (201)488-2288 Fax (201)488-2298

Cavallaro, Joseph, III, DO {1568549335} FamMed(00,PA77)
+ Cavallaro Family Practice, P.C.
432 Ganttown Road/Suite 202 Sewell, NJ 08080 (856)344-7916 Fax (856)344-7920
cavvallarofamilypractice@yahoo.com

Cavalli, Nina Ann, MD {1164461810} Pedtrc(93,NJ05)<NY-NYACK-HOS>
+ Closter Medical Group
200 Closter Dock Road Closter, NJ 07624 (201)768-3900 Fax (201)768-3840

Cavallo, Danielle Janine, DO {1043383557} FamMed(01,NY75)
+ Comprehensive Family Medicine, PA
27 Mountain Boulevard/Suite 6 Warren, NJ 07059 (908)222-7777 Fax (908)220-9242

Cavan, Clodoveo N., MD {1750379806} GenPrc, Surgry(73,PHI10)
+ New Jersey Division of Developmental Disability
Route 72 East New Lisbon, NJ 08064 (609)726-1000 Fax (609)894-8430

Cavanagh, Yana, MD {1104189844} IntrMd
+ St Joseph's Medical Ctr Internal Med
703 Main Street Paterson, NJ 07503

Cavazos, Anthony Richard, MD {1104944263} FamMed, FamM-Grtc(88,MI01)
+ Erickson Health Medical Group
1 Cedar Crest Village Drive Pompton Plains, NJ 07444 (973)831-3540 Fax (973)831-3503

Cave, Marie, MD {1427109107} Pedtrc(75,HAI01)<NJ-JRSYCITY, NJ-HACKNSK>
+ Riverside Medical Group
714 Tenth Street/Suite 2 Secaucus, NJ 07094 (201)863-3346 Fax (201)865-0015

Caveng, Rocco F., Jr., DO {1780603381} FamMed(03,MO79)<NJ-KMHSTRAT, NJ-KMHTURNV>
+ Cooper University at Willingboro
218C Sunset Road Willingboro, NJ 08046 (609)877-0400 Fax (609)877-3542

Cavuto, John Nicholas, MD {1366483208} Pedtrc, AdolMd(89,PA07)
+ Westfield Pediatrics, P.A.
532 East Broad Street Westfield, NJ 07090 (908)232-3445 Fax (908)233-6184

Cavuto-Wilson, Carolyn Marie, DO {1295720035} FamMed, IntrMd(87,PA77)
+ Mobile Physician Group, PC
231 High Street/Suite 1 Mount Holly, NJ 08060 (609)534-5998 Fax (609)488-6023

Cawley, Christina M., DO {1063468866} SrgOrt
+ 42 East Laurel Road/UDP 1700
Stratford, NJ 08084 (856)566-7010 Fax (856)566-6956

Cayetano, Victoria F., MD {1194893347} Psychy(72,PHI01)<NJ-GRYSTPSY, NJ-HOBUNIMC>
+ Central Jersey Beharioral Health, LLC
216 North Avenue East Cranford, NJ 07016 (908)272-7500 Fax (908)272-7502
+ Greystone Park Psychiatric Hospital
59 Koch Avenue/Psych Morris Plains, NJ 07950 (973)538-1800

Cean, Daniela E., DO {1053622605} PedAne(05,NY75)
+ Anesthesia Consultnts of NJ/Nova Pain
285 Davidson Avenue/Suite 204 Somerset, NJ 08873 (732)271-1400 Fax (732)271-3543

Cece, John A., MD {1437198553} Otlryg, Otolgy(81,NJ06)<NJ-CHILTON, NJ-WAYNEGEN>
+ ENT & Allergy Associates, LLP
1211 Hamburg Turnpike/Suite 205 Wayne, NJ 07470 (973)633-0808 Fax (973)633-8811
+ Wayne Surgical Center, LLC.
1176 Hamburg Pike Wayne, NJ 07470 (973)633-0808 Fax (973)709-1901

Cecere, Antoinette M., MD {1831115633} IntrMd(85,GRN01)<NJ-STJOSHOS>
+ Cecere and Rubino Internal Medicine, LLC
1195 Clifton Avenue Clifton, NJ 07013 (973)471-4004 Fax (973)471-1180
+ Cecere and Rubino Internal Medicine, LLC
205 Browertown Road West Paterson, NJ 07424 (973)471-4004 Fax (973)471-1180

Ceci, Robert L., MD {1588863492} EmrgMd(73,PA09)<NJ-UNVM-CPRN>
+ Merrill-Lynch
101 Hudson Street/Suite 1/Medical Jersey City, NJ 07302 (973)733-2070
+ Bristol-Myers Squibb Company
One Squibb Drive New Brunswick, NJ 08903 (732)905-2640

Cedeno, Natalie Jeniece, MD {1669892410} IntrMd(14,NJ05)
+ Rutgers- New Jersey Medical School
185 South Orange Avenue Newark, NJ 07103 (973)972-6056

Cederbaum, Neil Kenneth, MD {1407855406} Pedtrc(99,NY47)
+ Mid Jersey Pediatrics
33 Brunswick Woods Drive East Brunswick, NJ 08816 (732)257-4330 Fax (732)257-1177
+ Mid Jersey Pediatrics
25 Kilmer Drive/Building 3/Suite 107 Morganville, NJ 07751 (732)257-4330 Fax (732)972-1677

Cefalu, Dimitri A., MD {1679505879} IntrMd, Grtrcs(84,ITA12)<NJ-JRSYSHMC>
+ Seabrook Village Medical Center
3000 Essex Road Tinton Falls, NJ 07753 (732)643-1200 Fax (732)643-2015

Cekleniak, Natalie A., MD {1790803773} ObsGyn(93,RI01)<NJ-ST-BARNMC, NJ-MONMOUTH>
+ The Institute for Reproductive Medicine and Science
94 Old Short Hills Road/Suite 403E Livingston, NJ 07039 (973)322-8286 Fax (973)322-2549
+ Inst of Repro Med and Science
609 Washington Street/2nd Floor Hoboken, NJ 07030 (973)322-8286 Fax (201)526-9319

Celebre, Louis J., MD {1871688440} Gastrn(84,ITAL)<NJ-MTN-SIDE>
+ 199 Broad Street/Suite 1-A
Bloomfield, NJ 07003 (973)680-5500 Fax (973)680-5561

Celestial, Rommel M., MD {1922159607} NnPnMd, Pedtrc(80,PHIL)<NJ-ACMCITY, NJ-ACMCMAIN>
+ AtlantiCare Regional Medical Center/City Campus
1925 Pacific Avenue/Neo-Peri Med Atlantic City, NJ 08401 (609)441-8087 Fax (609)441-8976
+ AtlantiCare/Dupont Children's Health Program
2500 English Creek Avenue Egg Harbor Township, NJ 08234 (609)441-8087 Fax (609)641-3652

Celestino, Cecilia Cruz, MD {1659307510} FamMed, Pedtrc(90,PHI32)
+ Hunterdon Developmental Center
40 Pittstown Road/PO Box 4003 Clinton, NJ 08809 (908)735-4031 Fax (908)730-1338

Celluzzi, Alex, DO {1770583536} Gastrn, IntrMd(84,IA75)
+ Advanced GI
2301 Evesham Road/Pav 800/Suite 110 Voorhees, NJ 08043 (856)772-1600 Fax (856)772-9031
+ Rancocas Anesthesiology, PA
151 Fries Mill Road/Suite 202 Turnersville, NJ 08012 (856)772-1600 Fax (856)228-7252

Celo, Jovenia S., MD {1497793996} IntrMd, PthACl, MedOnc(78,PHI02)<NJ-SOMERSET, NJ-JFKMED>
+ Somerset Hematology Oncology Associates, P.A.
30 Rehill Avenue/2nd Floor/Suite 2500 Somerville, NJ 08876 (908)927-8700 Fax (908)927-8706

Cencora, Barbara E., MD {1740248160} Gastrn, IntrMd(88,POLA)<NJ-CENTRAST>
+ Advanced Gastroenterology Associates LLC
475 County Road/Suite 201 Marlboro, NJ 07746 (732)370-2220 Fax (732)548-7408
+ Advanced Gastroenterology Associates LLC
403 Candlewood Commons/Building 4 Howell, NJ 07731 (732)370-2220 Fax (732)548-7408

Cennimo, David John, MD {1992722623} IntrMd, Pedtrc(01,NJ05)
+ 278 Longview Road
Union, NJ 07083 (908)964-0468

Cenon, Pearl L., MD {1811003619} Pedtrc(86,PHIL)<NJ-CHRIST, NJ-HOBUNIMC>
+ City Heights Pediatrics
511 22nd Street Union City, NJ 07087 (201)866-7740 Fax (201)223-1905
+ Christ Hospital
176 Palisade Avenue/Pediatrics Jersey City, NJ 07306 (201)795-8200
+ Hoboken University Medical Center
308 Willow Avenue/Pediatrics Hoboken, NJ 07087 (201)418-1000

Censullo, Michael Louis, MD {1770520835} RadDia, RadV&I(97,DC02)<NJ-STPETER, NJ-RWJUBRUN>
+ University Radiology Group, P.C.
483 Cranbury Road East Brunswick, NJ 08816 (732)390-0030 Fax (732)390-5383
+ University Radiology Group, P.C.
16 Mountain Boulevard Warren, NJ 07059 (732)390-0030 Fax (908)769-9141
+ University Radiology Group, P.C.
579A Cranbury Road East Brunswick, NJ 08816 (732)390-0040 Fax (732)390-1856

Centanni, Frank D., MD {1164563425} Psychy(74,MEX14)
+ Drs. Leung & Murphy
196 Speedwell Avenue Morristown, NJ 07960 (973)539-9580

Centanni, Marianne T., MD {1972549764} RadDia, Radiol(70,ITA01)
+ St. Joseph's Regional Medical Center
703 Main Street/Radiology Paterson, NJ 07503 (973)754-2000

Centanni, Monica Ann, MD {1942402664} IntrMd(02,DMN01)
+ Internal Medicine Consultants
765 State Route 10 East/Suite 201 Randolph, NJ 07869 (973)975-4830 Fax (973)271-1022

Centanni, Toni V., MD {1700832649} ObsGyn(82,DMN01)<NJ-CHILTON>
+ Physicians for Women
330 Ratzer Road/Suite 7 Wayne, NJ 07470 (973)694-2222 Fax (973)694-7664

Centeno, Galen Arcellana, MD {1255469938} IntrMd(86,PHIL)
+ Hackensack Meridian Health-Oak Tree Primary Care
904 Oak Tree Avenue/Suite M South Plainfield, NJ 07080 (732)283-0020 Fax (732)283-0029
+ JFK Medical Center
65 James Street Edison, NJ 08820 (732)283-0020 Fax (732)906-4927

Centeno-McNulla, Ligaya Victoria M., MD {1467479147} Allrgy, IntrMd, AlgyImmn(86,PHIL)
+ Adult & Pediatric Allergists of Central Jersey
1740 Oak Tree Road Edison, NJ 08820 (732)906-1717 Fax (732)906-1781
+ Adult & Pediatric Allergists of Central Jersey
3 Hospital Plaza/Suite 405 Old Bridge, NJ 08857 (732)906-1717 Fax (732)360-0033

Centurion, Santiago Alberto, MD {1710099585} Dermat, Pth-Drm(99,NJ05)
+ Dermatology Associates of Central NJ
3548 Route 9 Old Bridge, NJ 08857 (732)679-6300
+ Dermatology Associates of Central New Jersey
250 South Street Freehold, NJ 07728 (732)679-6300 Fax (732)679-9566

Ceppetelli, Lisa C., MD {1679679823} EmrgMd(94,PA02)<NJ-SOMERSET>
+ Emergency Medical Associates of NJ, P.A.
3 Century Drive Parsippany, NJ 07054 (973)740-0607 Fax (973)740-9895

Cerame, Barbara I., MD {1316918832} PedEnd, Pedtrc(85,MO34)<NJ-MORRISTN>
+ Morristown Medical Center
100 Madison Avenue/Box 53 Morristown, NJ 07962 (973)971-5000

Ceraulo, Philip, DO {1114180882} PhyMPain(04,NY75)
+ Freeman Spin & Pain Institute
102 James Street/Suite 101 Edison, NJ 08820 (732)906-9600 Fax (732)906-9300
+ Freeman Spin & Pain Institute
102 James Street/Suite 101 Edison, NJ 08820 (732)906-9600 Fax (908)272-7997

Cerbone, Joseph Eugene, MD {1235173709} Dermat(82,NY09)<NJ-JFKMED>
+ 1030 Saint Georges Avenue/Suite 306
Avenel, NJ 07001 (732)750-1331 Fax (732)750-3196

Cerceo, Elizabeth Ann, MD {1902969561} IntrMd(05,NJ06)<NJ-COOPRUMC>
+ Cooper University Hospital
One Cooper Plaza/Hospitalist Camden, NJ 08103 (856)342-2000

Cerda, Luis Mariano, MD {1780944702} SrgThr
+ St Joseph's Medical Thoracic Surgery
703 Main Street Paterson, NJ 07503 (973)754-2460 Fax (973)754-2462

Cerdena, Maria Corazon, MD {1457445637} Pedtrc(82,PHI08)
+ Kidz Doctor, LLC
11 Overlook Road/Suite 170 Summit, NJ 07901 (908)277-4480 Fax (908)277-4482

Cerefice, Mark L., MD {1417165416} Gastrn
+ Atlantic Coast Gastroenterology
1640 Route 88 West/Suite 202 Brick, NJ 08724 (732)458-8300 Fax (732)458-8529

Cerio, Dean Richard, MD {1407017767} SrgRec
+ East Coast Advanced Plastic Surgery
79 Hudson Street/Suite 700 Hoboken, NJ 07030 (201)449-1000 Fax (201)399-2433

Cerkvenik, Kathleen M., MD {1740249671} Pedtrc(81,ITA30)<NJ-VALLEY>
+ Bergen West Pediatric Center, PA
541 Cedar Hill Avenue Wyckoff, NJ 07481 (201)652-0300 Fax (201)444-6209

Cernadas, Maureen, MD {1427137066} ObsGyn(91,NJ05)<NJ-STPETER, NJ-RWJUBRUN>
+ Brunswick-Hills Ob/Gyn, PA
620 Cranbury Road/Suite LL90   East Brunswick, NJ 08816   (732)967-0033   Fax (732)613-4845
+ Brunswick-Hills Ob/Gyn, PA
751 Route 206/2nd Floor   Hillsborough, NJ 08844   (732)967-0033   Fax (908)725-2132

Cernea, Dana, MD {1699877084} GPrvMd, IntrMd(85,NY08)
+ 19-21 Fair Lawn Avenue/Suite 1E
Fair Lawn, NJ 07410   (201)475-9421   Fax (201)475-1555

Cerniglia, Salvatore Joseph, DO {1619076411} Anesth, PainMd, AnesPain(69,IA75)
+ South Jersey Pain Management
76 West Jimmie Leeds Road   Galloway, NJ 08205   (609)568-5567   Fax (609)568-5614

Cerone, Anthony J., Jr., DO {1558309773} GenPrc, Urolgy(79,PA77)
+ 745 Slate Court
Sewell, NJ 08080   (856)553-6553

Cerritelli, John A., MD {1437240553} FamMed, Gastrn, Surgry(87,ITAL)<NJ-CLARMAAS>
+ Medical first of NY & NJ
5 Franklin Avenue/Suite 501   Belleville, NJ 07109   (973)751-4477   Fax (973)751-4444
jcerrimd@sprintmail.com

Cerrone, Federico, MD {1184625220} CritCr, PulDis(86,DC02)<NY-VASSAR, NJ-MORRISTN>
+ Pulmonary & Allergy Associates
1 Springfield Avenue/Suite 3-A   Summit, NJ 07901   (908)934-0555   Fax (908)934-0556
F.Cerrone@mindspring.com
+ Pulmonary & Allergy Associates
8 Saddle Road/Suite 101   Cedar Knolls, NJ 07927   (908)934-0555   Fax (973)540-0472

Cervantes, Crisnoel, MD {1043211840} IntrMd(89,PHI08)<NJ-COMMED>
+ Whiting Medical Associates
65 Lacey Road/Suite A   Whiting, NJ 08759   (732)350-0404   Fax (732)350-2001

Cervantes, Luis A., MD {1215933353} SrgNro(76,MEX61)<NJ-VIRTMHBC>
+ 110 Marter Avenue/Suite 202
Moorestown, NJ 08057   (856)727-1000   Fax (856)727-9480

Cervenak-Panariello, Betty, MD {1134228679} Ophthl(78,NY09)
+ Palisade Eye Associates
203 Palisade Avenue   Jersey City, NJ 07306   (201)653-5722   Fax (201)792-9718

Cervi, Wendy Lee, DO {1336174416} ObsGyn(97,PA77)<NJ-CHS-FULD, NJ-CHSMRCER>
+ 321 North Warren Street
Trenton, NJ 08618   (609)278-5934

Cervone, Joseph Stephen, III, MD {1710991187} IntrMd, FamMed(82,MEXI)
+ Concierge Skin Care
200 South Orange Avenue/Suite 101   Livingston, NJ 07039   (973)325-8901   Fax (866)837-8133

Cervone, Maurizio, DO {1174653331} FamMed(88,IA75)
+ Drs. Cervone and Cervone
891 Tabor Road   Morris Plains, NJ 07950   (973)359-8859   Fax (973)359-8860

Cervone, Oswald, DO {1275661993} FamMed(88,IA75)
+ Drs. Cervone and Cervone
891 Tabor Road   Morris Plains, NJ 07950   (973)359-8859   Fax (973)359-8860

Cesarine, Joseph, MD {1821497520} EmrgMd
+ Cooper Univerisry Emergency Physicians
One Cooper Plaza   Camden, NJ 08103   (856)342-2627   Fax (856)968-8272

Cespedes, Lissette Maria, MD {1003238817}<NJ-RWJUBRUN>
+ RWJ University Hospital New Brunswick
One Robert Wood Johnson Place   New Brunswick, NJ 08901   (732)235-7742

Cespedes, Victoria Elena, MD {1578660163} EmrgMd(00,NY48)<NJ-JRSYCITY>
+ Jersey City Medical Center
355 Grand Street   Jersey City, NJ 07304   (201)915-2000

Cessario, Alison G., MD {1336275023} Pedtrc, AdolMd(87,ITA22)<NJ-OVERLOOK>
+ Maple Pediatric Associates LLC
47 Maple Street/Suite 107   Summit, NJ 07901   (908)273-5866   Fax (908)273-5811

Cetel, Marvin A., MD {1760642730} IntrMd(77,MA07)
+ 651 Route 73 North/Suite 406
Marlton, NJ 08053   (856)596-1872   Fax (856)596-9430

Cetta, Peter J., MD {1134183460} Ophthl(75,NJ05)<NJ-MORRISTN>
+ 10 West Hanover Avenue
Randolph, NJ 07869   (973)895-4600   Fax (973)895-4604

Cha, Andrew, DO {1568780500} SrgVas
+ University Medical Group/Vascular Surgery
One Robert Wood Johnson Place/MEB 541   New Brunswick, NJ 08901   (732)235-7816   Fax (732)235-8538

Cha, Doh Yoon, MD {1568605061} Urolgy(04,NJ06)
+ Urology Care Alliance
2 Hospital Plaza/Suite 110   Old Bridge, NJ 08857   (732)972-9000   Fax (732)972-0966
+ Urology Care Alliance
733 North Beers Street/Suite L-6   Holmdel, NJ 07733   (732)972-9000   Fax (732)739-8988
+ Urology Care Alliance
501 Iron Bridge Road   Freehold, NJ 08857   (732)780-7603   Fax (732)308-3323

Cha, Hak J., MD {1912934381} Anesth(72,KOR06)
+ Toms River Anesthesia Associates PC
409 Main Street/2nd Floor   Toms River, NJ 08753   (732)818-7575   Fax (732)818-1567

Cha, Jaeok, MD {1225175011} Psychy, PsyGrt, IntrMd(77,KOR05)
+ 45 Homestead Drive/Suite B
Columbus, NJ 08022   (609)291-1535   Fax (609)291-1235

Cha, Jisun, MD {1194950683} Dermat, PthDrm(01,KOR03)
+ Robert Wood Johnson Medical Group-Dermatology
1 World's Fair Drive/Suite 2400   Somerset, NJ 08873   (732)235-7993   Fax (732)235-7117

Cha, Min, MD {1124113535} EmrgMd(92,NJ06)<NJ-STPETER>
+ Brunswick Urgent Care
3185 State Route 27   Franklin Park, NJ 08823

Cha, Ri D., MD {1164502878} CdvDis, IntrMd, CritCr(77,KOR05)<NJ-DEBRAHLC>
+ Cooper Cardiology Associates
900 Centennial Boulevard   Voorhees, NJ 08043   (856)325-6700   Fax (856)325-6702
+ Cooper Cardiology Associates
1210 Brace Road/Suite 103   Cherry Hill, NJ 08034   (856)427-7254
+ University Cardiology
3 Cooper Plaza/Room 311   Camden, NJ 08043   (856)342-3000

Chaaban, Fadi Nemer, MD {1316947906} CdvDis, CarNuc, CarEle(90,LEB01)<NJ-CLARMAAS>
+ New Jersey Cardiology Associates
375 Mount Pleasant Avenue/Cardiology   West Orange, NJ 07052   (973)731-9442   Fax (973)731-8030
+ New Jersey Cardiology Associates
5 Franklin Avenue/Suite 502   Belleville, NJ 07109   (973)731-9442   Fax (973)450-8157

Chaaban, Janti, MD {1013169937} NroChl(01,MNT01)<NJ-STPETER>
+ St. Peter's University Hospital
254 Easton Avenue/PedNrolgy   New Brunswick, NJ 08901   (732)745-8600

Chaar, Mitchell Y., MD {1205021201} SrgTrm<NJ-JRSYCITY>
+ Jersey City Medical Center
355 Grand Street   Jersey City, NJ 07304   (201)915-2000

Chaaya, Adib H., MD {1124211925} IntrMd, Gastrn
+ Cooper Digestive Health Institute
501 Fellowship Road/Suite 101   Mount Laurel, NJ 08054   (856)642-2133   Fax (856)642-2134

Chabbott, David Robert, MD {1326330606} CdvDis
+ Heart & Vascular Associates of Northern Jersey
22-18 Broadway/Suite 201   Fair Lawn, NJ 07410   (201)475-5050   Fax (201)475-5522

Chacinski, Dariusz R., MD {1811088677} Psychy(81,POL03)<NJ-TRENTPSY>
+ Trenton Psychiatric Hospital
Sullivan Way/PO Box 7600/Psych   West Trenton, NJ 08628   (609)633-1500

Chacko-Varkey, Suneeta Esther, MD {1407035272} PsyCAd, Psychy(94,INA9A)<NJ-NWRKBETH>
+ Newark Beth Israel Medical Center
201 Lyons Avenue/Psychiatry   Newark, NJ 07112   (973)926-7000   Fax (973)705-9017

Chadehumbe, Madeline A., MD {1467577254} NrlgSpec
+ Ctr for Neurological/Neurodevelopment
250 Haddonfield-Berlin Road/Suite 105   Gibbsboro, NJ 08026   (856)346-0005   Fax (856)784-1799

Chadha, Inderpal S., MD {1689612335} Nephro, IntrMd(86,INDI)
+ Essex Medical and Nephrology
539 Bloomfield Avenue   Newark, NJ 07107   (973)566-9900   Fax (973)566-6692
Inderchad@aol.com

Chadha, Kanchi, MD {1245673797} ObsGyn<NJ-HACKNSK>
+ Hackensack University Medical Center
30 Prospect Avenue   Hackensack, NJ 07601   (551)996-2000

Chadha, Sonia, MD {1952341711} FamMed, IntrMd(01,WI05)
+ 1 Sears Drive/Suite 402
Paramus, NJ 07652   (201)483-9188   Fax (201)483-9189

Chae, Hung Y., MD {1760446322} Anesth, PthACl, IntrMd(76,KOR06)<NJ-RBAYPERT>
+ Raritan Bay Medical Center/Perth Amboy Division
530 New Brunswick Avenue/Suite 103   Perth Amboy, NJ 08861   (732)442-3700

Chae, Scott S., MD {1851409650} Gastrn, IntrMd(88,KORE)
+ Scott S. Chae M.D.
2 State Route 27/Suite 107   Edison, NJ 08820   (732)632-9777   Fax (732)632-8096

Chae, Sung Yeon, MD {1134280969} FamMed(96,NY06)
+ JFK Family Practice Group
65 James Street   Edison, NJ 08818   (732)321-7488   Fax (732)906-4927

Chae, Young Soo, MD {1124136031} Pedtrc(89,KORE)
+ 2 State Route 27/Suite 111
Edison, NJ 08820   (201)902-9094   Fax (201)902-9694

Chafos, John N., MD {1871673830} IntrMd, EmrgMd(88,MA07)<NJ-SOMERSET>
+ Family Care, P.A.
257 US Highway 22   Green Brook, NJ 08812   (732)968-7878   Fax (732)968-2187

Chagares, Stephen Arthur, MD {1619939758} Surgry, SrgBst(90,NJ06)<NJ-BAYSHORE, NJ-RIVERVW>
+ 1 Executive Drive/Suite 4
Tinton Falls, NJ 07701   (732)450-9700   Fax (732)450-1511

Chahal, Yashwant S., DO {1154513166}
+ Rowan University-School of Osteopathic Medicine
1 Medical Center Drive   Stratford, NJ 08084   (856)566-6835

Chahil, Neetu H., MD {1417118571} Gastrn, IntrMd<NJ-UMDNJ>
+ University Hospital
150 Bergen Street/Gastro   Newark, NJ 07103   (973)972-6000

Chai, Bob B., MD {1871898171} RadDia(06,NY08)
+ University Radiology Group, P.C.
483 Cranbury Road   East Brunswick, NJ 08816   (732)390-0030   Fax (732)390-5383
+ University Radiology Group, P.C.
16 Mountain Boulevard   Warren, NJ 07059   (732)390-0030   Fax (908)769-9141
+ University Radiology Group, P.C.
579A Cranbury Road   East Brunswick, NJ 08816   (732)390-0040   Fax (732)390-1856

Chai, George, MD {1942223458} Pedtrc(03,NY15)
+ Hand in Hand Pediatrics
725 River Road/Suite 201-A   Edgewater, NJ 07020   (201)840-8055   Fax (201)840-8099

Chai, Raymond, MD {1871948836} EmrgMd
+ 110 Arcadia Road/Apt I
Hackensack, NJ 07601   (347)308-3558

Chai, Yee Meen, MD {1306919915} CdvDis, IntCrd(92,DC01)
+ Cardio Intervent of Ctrl Jersey
465 Cranbury Road/Suite 201   East Brunswick, NJ 08816   (732)613-1988   Fax (732)651-7734

Chaikin, David Craig, MD {1750374823} Urolgy(92,NY46)<NJ-MORRISTN, NY-PRSBWEIL>
+ Morristown Urology Associates PC
261 James Street/Suite 1A   Morristown, NJ 07960   (973)539-1050   Fax (973)538-6111
chaikin@nac.net

Chaikin, Harry L., MD {1336139484} IntrMd, Grtrcs(78,PA02)<NJ-ACMCITY, NJ-ACMCMAIN>
+ Brigantine Medical Group
353 12th Street South/PO Box 129   Brigantine, NJ 08203   (609)266-7557   Fax (609)266-4450
+ Seashore Gardens Living Center
22 West Jimmie Leeds Road   Absecon, NJ 08205   (609)266-7557   Fax (609)404-4841

Chaise, Laurence S., MD {1881677664} RadDia, RadV&I(76,NC05)<NJ-RBAYOLDB, NJ-RBAYPERT>
+ University Radiology Group, P.C.
483 Cranbury Road   East Brunswick, NJ 08816   (732)390-0030   Fax (732)390-5383
+ University Radiology Group, P.C.
10 Plum Street   New Brunswick, NJ 08901   (732)390-0030   Fax (732)249-1208
+ University Radiology Group, P.C.
260 Amboy Avenue   Metuchen, NJ 08816   (732)548-2322   Fax (732)548-3392

Chait, Anita Irani, MD {1629143888} ObsGyn(96,FL02)
+ Women's Center For OB/GYN
21 East Park Place   Rutherford, NJ 07070   (201)438-7780

Chait Kessler, Dana Erica, MD {1750609558} Pedtrc
+ Denville Pediatrics Medical Associates PA
140 East Main Street   Denville, NJ 07834   (973)625-5090   Fax (973)625-8006

Chaitman, Edmund, MD {1659415198} Psychy(64,NY01)
+ 185 East Palisade Avenue/Apt A6a
Englewood, NJ 07631   (201)871-1121

Chak, Azfar Khalid, MD {1043475486} IntrMd(02,DMN01)
+ 75 Azalea Street
Paramus, NJ 07652

Physicians by Name and Address

Chaker, Antoine C., MD {1275559890} Otlryg, SrgHdN, SrgFPI(68,LEB01)<NJ-STBARNMC, NJ-COMMED>
+ 20 Hospital Drive/Suite 18
  Toms River, NJ 08755   (732)341-7400   Fax (732)341-7904
+ 70 Lacey Road/Irish Branch Mall
  Whiting, NJ 08759   (732)350-3330

Chakhtoura, Elie Youssef, MD {1376543868} CdvDis, IntCrd, Car-Nuc(91,LEB01)<NJ-STBARNMC, NJ-STMICHL>
+ New Jersey Cardiology Associates
  375 Mount Pleasant Avenue   West Orange, NJ 07052
  (973)731-9442   Fax (973)731-8030
+ Diagnostic & Clinical Cardiology
  111 Central Avenue/5th Floor   Newark, NJ 07102
  (973)731-9442   Fax (973)877-2567

Chakilam, Santhosh, MD {1184988628} IntrMd
+ first Care Medical Group
  50 Pompton Avenue   Verona, NJ 07044   (973)857-3400
  Fax (973)857-7034

Chakrabarti, Mukti, MD {1629156948} Psychy(74,INDI)<NJ-UMDNJ>
+ University Psychiatric Associates
  183 South Orange Avenue/E-F Levels   Newark, NJ 07103
  (973)972-5430   Fax (973)972-2979

Chakraborty, Anu, MD {1811943541} ObsGyn, Obstet(94,NJ05)<NJ-RIVERVW>
+ 224 Maple Avenue
  Red Bank, NJ 07701   (732)842-8400   Fax (973)852-1745
+ Womens Health Alliance of New Jersey, LLC
  142 State Highway 35/Suite 105   Eatontown, NJ 07724
  (732)842-8400   Fax (732)935-0731

Chakrapani, Soumya, MD {1902041999} IntrMd(01,INA28)
+ Shore Medical Specialists
  500 River Avenue/Suite 140   Lakewood, NJ 08701
  (732)363-7200   Fax (732)367-4461

Chakravarthi, Seshadri Shekar, MD {1316916166} Grtrcs(79,INA09)<NJ-HUNTRDN>
+ Hunterdon Medical Center
  2100 Wescott Drive/SeniorServices   Flemington, NJ 08822
  (908)788-6373   Fax (908)788-2525

Chakravarthy, Manu V., MD {1902847767} EnDbMt, IntrMd(01,TX14)<NJ-RWJUBRUN>
+ University Medical Group - General Internal Medicine
  125 Paterson Street/Suite 5100A   New Brunswick, NJ 08903
  (732)235-7219   Fax (732)235-7224
  manu_chakravarthy@merck.com

Chakravarti, Aloke, MD {1225459969} PulCCr, IntrMd(09,ANT02)<NY-BETHPETR>
+ VMG Respiratory Health & Pulmonary Medicine
  1200 East Ridgewood Avenue   Ridgewood, NJ 07450
  (201)689-7755   Fax (201)689-0521

Chakravarty, Arijit, MD {1386778199} Nephro(99,NJ05)
+ Our Lady Lourdes Transplant Ctr
  1601 Haddon Avenue   Camden, NJ 08103   (856)757-3840
  Fax (856)757-3519

Chakravarty, Mira, MD {1073719258} RadDia(74,INA7X)<NJ-JFKMED>
+ Edison Radiology Group, P.A.
  65 James Street   Edison, NJ 08820   (732)321-7917   Fax (732)737-2968

Chalabi, Dahlia, MD {1578797007} EmrgMd<NJ-JFKMED>
+ JFK Medical Center
  65 James Street/Emergency   Edison, NJ 08820   (732)321-7000

Chalal, Jeffrey, MD {1790707438} RadDia, Radiol(77,PA01)<NJ-CENTRAST>
+ CentraState Medical Center
  901 West Main Street/Radiology   Freehold, NJ 07728
  (732)462-4844
+ Freehold Radiology Group
  901 West Main Street   Freehold, NJ 07728   (732)462-4844

Chalal, Jo Ann, MD {1316944424} RadOnc(82,PA13)<NJ-STFRN-MED, NJ-RWJUHAM>
+ Radiology Affiliates of Central New Jersey, P.A.
  2501 Kuser Road   Hamilton, NJ 08691   (609)585-8800
  Fax (609)585-1825
+ Radiology Affiliates of Central New Jersey, P.A.
  3120 Princeton Pike   Lawrenceville, NJ 08648   (609)585-8800   Fax (609)219-0439
+ St. Francis Medical Center
  601 Hamilton Avenue/Radiation Onco   Trenton, NJ 08691
  (609)599-5179   Fax (609)599-6219

Chalasani, Krishna, MD {1427314202} EnDbMt
+ Hackensack Meridian Endocrinology
  2240 Route 33/Suite B   Neptune, NJ 07753   (732)897-3980
  Fax (732)897-3982

Chalasani, Sree Bhavani, MD {1285880039} OncHem, IntrMd(01,INA7C)
+ Memorial Sloan-Kettering Cancer Center Basking Ridge
  136 Mountain View Boulevard   Basking Ridge, NJ 07920
  (908)542-3300   Fax (908)542-3222

Chalemian, Bliss A., MD {1871718148} PsyCAd, Psychy(01,GRN01)
+ Excelsior II Psychiatric Services
  169 Ramapo Valley Road/Suite ML5   Oakland, NJ 07436
  (201)996-1120   Fax (201)996-0099

Chalemian, Robert J., MD {1144355322} Psychy, PsyFor, PainMd(72,NY46)
+ Excelsior II Psychiatric Services
  169 Ramapo Valley Road/Suite ML5   Oakland, NJ 07436
  (201)996-1120   Fax (201)996-0099

Chalfin, Matthew Bryan, MD {1285835074} Anesth(03,NJ05)<NJ-STJOSHOS, NJ-WAYNEGEN>
+ St. Joseph's Regional Medical Center Anesthesia
  703 Main Street   Paterson, NJ 07503   (973)754-2323   Fax (973)977-9455

Chalfin, Venus Helena, MD {1467617191} ObsGyn(03,NJ05)
+ Health East Medical Center
  54 South Dean Street   Englewood, NJ 07631   (201)871-4000   Fax (201)608-6938

Chalfoun, Charbel T., MD {1871775130} SrgPlstc
+ East Coast Advanced Plastic Surgery
  79 Hudson Street/Suite 700   Hoboken, NJ 07030
  (201)449-1000   Fax (201)399-2433

Chalikonda, Bhavani Prasad, MD {1790704955} Pedtrc, Ped-CrC(81,INA1L)<NJ-STPETER, NJ-MONMOUTH>
+ St. Peter's University Hospital
  254 Easton Avenue/Pediatrics   New Brunswick, NJ 08901
  (732)745-8600   Fax (732)745-0857

Challa, Sridevi, MD {1285981803}
+ 118 Victory Road/Unit 202
  Springfield, NJ 07081   (408)647-3603
  drsridevi.challa@gmail.com

Chalnick, David Lee, MD {1518918580} SrgOrt(92,NJ05)<NJ-MONMOUTH>
+ Shore Orthopaedic Group
  35 Gilbert Street South   Tinton Falls, NJ 07701   (732)530-1515   Fax (732)747-5433
+ Shore Orthopaedic Group
  1255 Route 70/Suite 11S   Lakewood, NJ 08701   (732)530-1515   Fax (732)942-2311

Chalom, Elizabeth Candell, MD {1154341147} PedRhm, Pedtrc(91,NY01)<NJ-STBARNMC, NJ-NWRKBETH>
+ Children's Hospital of NJ Ped Cntr @ West Orange
  375 Mount Pleasant Avenue/Suite 105   West Orange, NJ 07052   (973)322-6900   Fax (973)322-6999

Chalom, Rene, MD {1407816481} Pedtrc, PedCrC(89,NJ05)<NJ-VALLEY>
+ RWJ University Hospital New Brunswick
  One Robert Wood Johnson Place   New Brunswick, NJ 08901
  (732)235-7887   Fax (732)235-6609

Cham, Anita L., MD {1962416958} Dermat(64,PHIL)
+ 35 West Main Street/Suite 201
  Denville, NJ 07834   (973)627-9635   Fax (973)625-7484

Chambers, Bryan P., MD {1609866946} Anesth(87,NJ06)<NJ-SJHREGMC, NJ-SJRSYELM>
+ SJH Regional Medical Center
  1505 West Sherman Avenue/Anesthesia   Vineland, NJ 08360   (856)641-8000

Champey, Edward John, MD {1467458836} Anesth(99,NET09)
+ Generations Physical Medicine, LLC
  14 Cherry Tree Farm Road   Middletown, NJ 07748
  (732)671-3535
+ 1 Mount Prospect Avenue
  Verona, NJ 07044   (201)247-1747
+ Montclair Anesthesia Associates PC
  185 Fairfield Avenue/Suite 2A   West Caldwell, NJ 07748
  (973)226-1230   Fax (973)226-1232

Chan, Albert C., MD {1891800405} ObsGyn(83,PHIL)<NJ-JFKMED, NJ-STPETER>
+ 2301 Maple Avenue
  South Plainfield, NJ 07080   (908)754-9600   Fax (908)754-2043

Chan, Britton Miller, MD {1144455072} RadDia
+ Larchmont Medical Imaging
  210 Ark Road/Building 2   Mount Laurel, NJ 08054
  (856)778-8860   Fax (856)866-8102

Chan, Christina Yu-Yee, MD {1154625309} InfDis(89,TN06)<MA-MAGENHOS>
+ Merck and Company Incorporated
  1 Merck Drive/PO Box 100   Whitehouse Station, NJ 08889
  (908)423-6048

Chan, Diana, MD {1235399288} IntrMd
+ 35 Harkins Road
  Milltown, NJ 08850

Chan, Eric B.T., MD {1437202017} IntrMd(89,VT02)
+ 51 JFK Parkway
  Short Hills, NJ 07078   (973)417-8742

Chan, Florence Y., MD {1265497507} SrgVas, Surgry(76,NY01)<NJ-JRSYCITY>
+ Dr. Joven Dungo/NJ Impotence Ctr
  205 9th Street   Jersey City, NJ 07302   (201)653-1144   Fax (201)653-6104

Chan, Jennifer L., DO {1376870048}
+ Rowan University-School of Osteopathic Medicine
  1 Medical Center Drive   Stratford, NJ 08084   (856)566-6708

Chan, Jenny Sang, MD {1427217603} Anesth(04,NY08)<NJ-VALLEY>
+ The Valley Hospital
  223 North Van Dien Avenue/Anesth   Ridgewood, NJ 07450
  (201)447-8000
+ Bergen Anesthesia Group, P.C.
  500 West Main Street/Suite 16   Wyckoff, NJ 07481
  (201)447-8000   Fax (201)847-0059

Chan, Jose R., MD {1083684419} Anesth(72,PHI01)<NJ-NWRK-BETH>
+ Newark Beth Israel Medical Center
  201 Lyons Avenue/Anesthesiology   Newark, NJ 07112
  (973)926-7143   Fax (973)282-3285

Chan, Kar-Mei, MD {1629075783} Anesth(94,NY03)<NJ-STJOSHOS, NY-PRSBWEIL>
+ St. Joseph's Regional Medical Center Anesthesia
  703 Main Street   Paterson, NJ 07503   (973)754-2323   Fax (973)977-9455

Chan, Karen Rita Post, MD {1548240823} Anesth(93,DC02)<NJ-MORRISTN>
+ 90 Essex Road
  Summit, NJ 07901

Chan, Kim K., MD {1750383188} IntrMd, EmrgMd(72,PHI01)<NJ-MTNSIDE>
+ Teaneck Hospitalists, PA
  718 Teaneck Road   Teaneck, NJ 07666   (201)833-3000
  Fax (201)227-6207

Chan, Mei-Yung, MD {1760678205} EmrgMd(05,NJ05)<NJ-SOMERSET>
+ Emergency Medical Associates
  110 Rehill Avenue   Somerville, NJ 08876   (908)685-2920
  Fax (908)685-2968

Chan, Peter S., MD {1578549986} SrgOrt, SrgHnd(93,DC02)
+ Hand Surgery Specialists, L.L.C.
  1590 Route 206 North   Bedminster, NJ 07921   (908)470-4263   Fax (908)470-0001
  dr.pchan@yahoo.com

Chan, Phillip Pierre, MD IntrMd(00,CT01)
+ CytoSorbents Corporation
  7 Deer Park Drive/Suite K   Monmouth Junction, NJ 08852
  (732)329-8885   Fax (732)329-8650

Chan, Rolycito A., MD {1679541569} Anesth(73,PHIL)<NJ-ENGLWOOD>
+ Englewood Anesthesiology
  350 Engle Street   Englewood, NJ 07631   (201)894-3238
  Fax (201)894-0585

Chan, Russell K., DO {1801213640}<NJ-ENGLWOOD>
+ Morristown Medical Center
  100 Madison Avenue   Morristown, NJ 07962   (973)971-5000
+ Englewood Hospital and Medical Center
  350 Engle Street   Englewood, NJ 07631   (973)971-5000
  Fax (973)290-7202

Chan, Wai Ben, DO {1710291307} FamMed(10,NY75)<NJ-COOPRUMC>
+ Cooper Family Medicine
  110 Marter Avenue   Moorestown, NJ 08057   (856)608-8840   Fax (856)722-1898

Chan, Ying, MD {1174557979} MtFtMd, ObsGyn(91,NY48)<NJ-ENGLWOOD>
+ Englewood Hospital and Medical Center
  350 Engle Street/AntepartumTest   Englewood, NJ 07631
  (201)894-3669   Fax (201)541-3445

Chan-Ting, Rengena Eleanor, DO {1326149576} Grtrcs, In-trMd(00,NJ75)
+ Life at Lourdes
  2475 McClellan Avenue/Building C   Pennsauken, NJ 08109
  (856)675-3355   Fax (856)675-3686

Chanana, Manju, MD {1538318142} IntrMd
+ 10 Sunrise Drive
  Parsippany, NJ 07054   (973)240-7825   Fax (973)884-3388

Chandak, Ritu, MD {1033218531} Psychy(95,INDI)<NJ-JRSYCITY>
+ Jersey City Medical Center
  355 Grand Street/Psychiatry   Jersey City, NJ 07304
  (201)915-2000

Chandar, Ashwin, MD {1316320237}
+ RWJ Hospital Internal Medicine
  One Robert Wood Johnson Place/MEB 486   New Brunswick, NJ 08901   (732)235-7742   Fax (732)235-7427

Chandarana, Bhavini S., MD {1902826589} PhyMPain(98,DMN01)
+ 119-137 Clifford Street/Suite 106
  Newark, NJ 07105   (973)522-0008   Fax (973)522-0009

Chandarana, Shashikant A., MD {1568483824} Radiol(66,INA67)
+ 24 Nottingham Way
  Warren, NJ 07059

Chandela – Chanliecco

Chandela, Sweta, MD {1962655340} IntrMd(03)
+ 135 Heritage Road
Sewell, NJ 08080 (267)408-4687 Fax (267)408-4687

Chander, Harish, MD {1972595163} IntrMd(73,INDI)<NJ-KIMBALL, NJ-COMMED>
+ Shore Medical Specialists
500 River Avenue Lakewood, NJ 08701 (732)363-7200 Fax (732)367-4461
+ Shore Medical Specialists
9 Hospital Drive Toms River, NJ 08755 (732)363-7200 Fax (732)349-9697

Chander, Naresh, MD {1033284096} CritCr, IntrMd, PulDis(71,INDI)<NJ-HACKNSK>
+ 344 Prospect Avenue
Hackensack, NJ 07601 (201)342-4233 Fax (201)342-4840
Naresh.Chander@att.net

Chandiwala-Mody, Priti, DO {1225290463} RadDia
+ 29 East 29th Street
Bayonne, NJ 07002 (201)858-7341

Chandler, Khayriyyah Ebony Tahirah, DO {1104077130}
+ Virtua Family Medicine Center @Lumberton
1636 Route 38 & Eayrestown Rd. Lumberton, NJ 08048
(609)261-7035 Fax (609)914-8441

Chandra, Anurag, MD {1093716870} RadOnc(90,NY03)<NY-ALBANY>
+ 21st Century Oncology
220 Sunset Road/Suite 4 Willingboro, NJ 08046 (609)877-3064 Fax (609)877-2466

Chandra, Prasanta C., MD {1821043746} MtFtMd, ObsGyn(71,INA02)<NJ-VIRTVOOR, NJ-KMHSTRAT>
+ 468 Hurfville Crosskeys Road
Sewell, NJ 08080 (856)582-2111 Fax (856)582-9781

Chandra, Ram, MD {1598858854} Pedtrc, AdolMd, GPrvMd(88,INA35)<NJ-HACKNSK, NJ-HOLYNAME>
+ Inspira Health Network
509 North Broad Street/Hospitalist Woodbury, NJ 08096 (856)845-0100

Chandra, Shakuntala Nanjundaswamy, MD {1154386514} NnPnMd, Pedtrc(94,INA37)<NJ-STPETER>
+ St. Peter's University Hospital
254 Easton Avenue New Brunswick, NJ 08901 (732)745-8600 Fax (732)249-9572

Chandra, Sweta, MD {1770743163} IntrMd(00,INA70)
+ Hackensack Medical Center-Internal Medicine
30 Prospect Avenue/4 Main/Rm 4621 Hackensack, NJ 07601 (201)996-3664 Fax (551)996-0536

Chandran, Ankila Sharavati, DO {1093781114} FamMed, Psychy(01,CA23)
+ Center for Family Guidance, PC
765 East Route 70/Building A-101 Marlton, NJ 08053 (856)797-4800 Fax (856)810-0110

Chandran, Chandra B., MD {1164413266} IntrMd, Nephro(71,INDI)<NJ-CHILTON>
+ North Jersey Nephrology Associates PA
246 Hamburg Turnpike/Suite 207 Wayne, NJ 07470 (973)653-3366 Fax (973)653-3365

Chandrasekaran, Aparna, MD {1871544957} IntrMd(96,INA04)
+ Aparna Medical Associates
1527 Route 27/Suite 1600 Somerset, NJ 08873 (732)659-6650 Fax (732)659-6649

Chandrasekaran, Kulandaivelu, MD {1043327000} CdvDis, IntrMd(78,INA77)<NJ-VAEASTOR>
+ 1400 Rachel Terrace/Apt 16
Pine Brook, NJ 07058 (973)439-7273
KULCHANDRA@aol.com
+ VA New Jersey Health Care System-East Orange Campus
385 Tremont Avenue/MS111/Ste 9-165 East Orange, NJ 07018 (973)676-1000

Chandrasekhar, Sujana S. D., MD {1649363151} Otlryg, Neutgy(86,NY47)<NY-NYEYEINF, NY-LENOXHLL>
+ ENT & Allergy Associates, LLP
1211 Hamburg Turnpike/Suite 205 Wayne, NJ 07470 (973)633-0808 Fax (973)633-8811

Chandwani, Ashish, MD {1700053592} IntrMd, InfDis(98,INA6Z)<NJ-MORRISTN>
+ IPC The Hospitalist Company
220 Ridgedale Avenue/Suite C-2 Florham Park, NJ 07932 (973)538-5844 Fax (973)267-0181

Chaney, Arthur, Jr., MD {1346309119} FamMed(63,DC03)<NJ-HACKNSK>
+ 259 Berry Street
Hackensack, NJ 07601 (201)343-5035 Fax (201)996-1061

Chaney, Dewey A., MD {1689733610} FamMed(70,DC03)<NJ-HACKNSK>
+ Hackensack University Medical Center
20 Prospect Avenue/Suite 715 Hackensack, NJ 07601 (201)881-0721 Fax (201)881-0725

Chang, Basil Tzu Li, DO {1831175942}<NJ-RWJURAH>
+ Robert Wood Johnson University Hospital at Rahway
865 Stone Street Rahway, NJ 07065 (610)348-1917
btchang@att.net

Chang, Bernard P., MD {1922169093} ObsGyn(64,TAIW)<NJ-STJOSHOS, NJ-WAYNEGEN>
+ Comprehensive Women's Healthcare
220 Hamburg Turnpike/Suite 21 Wayne, NJ 07470 (973)790-8090 Fax (973)790-3198

Chang, Betty Chia-Wen, MD {1700923638} EmrgMd(99,DMN01)<NY-PRSBCOLU, NJ-HACKNSK>
+ Hackensack University Medical Center
30 Prospect Avenue/EmrgMed Hackensack, NJ 07601 (201)996-4614 Fax (201)996-4239

Chang, Bong M., MD {1720064827} RadOnc(72,KORE)<NJ-COMMED, NJ-SOCEANCO>
+ Community Medical Center
99 Route 37 West/Rad/Onco Toms River, NJ 08755 (732)240-8148
+ Southern Ocean County Medical Center
1140 Route 72 West Manahawkin, NJ 08050 (609)597-6011

Chang, Cindy Ching, MD {1396772349} AlgyImmn, IntrMd(97,NY48)<NJ-VALLEY, NJ-HACKNSK>
+ Forest HealthCare Associates, PC
277 Forest Avenue/Suite 200 Paramus, NJ 07652 (201)986-1881 Fax (201)986-1871
+ Allergy Associates of North Jersey
362 Union Boulevard Totowa, NJ 07512 (201)986-1881 Fax (973)790-1255

Chang, Connie Yachan, MD {1467879460} Anesth
+ 22 Hereford Drive
Princeton Junction, NJ 08550 (732)397-7725

Chang, David Tsuwei, MD {1487622718} Urolgy(94,NY01)<NJ-VALLEY>
+ Sovereign Medical Group
15-01 Broadway/Suite 1 Fair Lawn, NJ 07410 (201)791-4544 Fax (201)791-6585
+ Sovereign Medical Group, LLC.
205 Browertown Road/Suite 101 West Paterson, NJ 07424 (201)791-4544 Fax (973)890-9621
+ SurgiCare Surgical Associates, PA
630 East Palisade Avenue Englewood Cliffs, NJ 07410 (201)503-1503 Fax (201)503-1514

Chang, Eric, DO {1538321203} ObsGyn(02,IA75)<NJ-COOPRUMC>
+ The Cooper Hospital System-Univ Hospital
3 Cooper Plaza/Suite 215/Rm 221/ObGyn Camden, NJ 08103 (856)342-2439 Fax (856)365-1967

Chang, Eric I-Yun, MD {1831352871} Surgry(02,NJ06)<PA-FOXCAN>
+ The Plastic Surgery Ctr of NJ & Manhat
535 Sycamore Avenue Shrewsbury, NJ 07702 (732)741-0970 Fax (732)747-2606

Chang, Frances Yu-hsin, MD {1316996960} IntrMd, Grtrcs(99,NY48)<NJ-UNVMCPRN>
+ Princeton Medical Group, P.A.
419 North Harrison Street Princeton, NJ 08540 (609)924-9300 Fax (609)924-6552

Chang, Gene, MD {1174554851} CdvDis, IntCrd, IntrMd(91,MA07)<NJ-ACMCITY, NJ-SHOREMEM>
+ Penn Cardiac Care Shore Medical Center
1 East New York Avenue Somers Point, NJ 08244

Chang, Ho-Choong, MD {1679581458} Pedtrc(96,MD07)<NJ-SHOREMEM>
+ Tender Care Pediatrics
2322 New Road Northfield, NJ 08225 (609)641-0200

Chang, Hyun S., MD {1780619536} GenPrc(65,KOR04)
+ 500 South Burnt Mill Road
Voorhees, NJ 08043 (856)428-0386

Chang, James Kenneth, MD {1053501916} PhysMd, PainMd, IntrMd(06,NJ06)
+ Kenneth Sung Soo Chang MD PA
3144 Kennedy Boulevard Jersey City, NJ 07306 (201)792-9339 Fax (201)792-9818

Chang, Jimmy Chuming, MD {1629082300} Gastrn, IntrMd(92,IL06)<NJ-HCKTSTWN, NJ-MORRISTN>
+ Plaza Family Care
657 Willow Grove Street/Suite 401 Hackettstown, NJ 07840 (908)850-7800 Fax (908)850-7801
+ Plaza Family Care
245 Main Street/Suite 300 & 302 Chester, NJ 07930 (908)850-7800 Fax (908)879-6738

Chang, Joanne Meejin, MD {1336312271} ObsGyn<NJ-MONMOUTH>
+ Brielle Obstetrics & Gynecology, P.A.
117 County Line Road Lakewood, NJ 08701 (732)942-1900 Fax (732)942-1919

Chang, Kane L., MD {1871503920} SrgVas<NJ-DEBRAHLC>
+ Deborah Heart and Lung Center
200 Trenton Road Browns Mills, NJ 08015 (609)893-6611

Chang, Kenneth Sung Soo, MD {1053489997} ObsGyn, Gyneco(79,KOR13)<NJ-MEADWLND, NJ-CHRIST>
+ Kenneth Sung Soo Chang MD PA
3144 Kennedy Boulevard Jersey City, NJ 07306 (201)792-9339 Fax (201)792-9818

+ Kenneth Sung Soo Chang MD PA
605 Broad Avenue/Suite 201 Ridgefield, NJ 07657 (201)792-9339 Fax (201)941-9107

Chang, Leona, DO {1538539747} ObsGyn<NJ-COOPRUMC>
+ Cooper University Hospital
One Cooper Plaza Camden, NJ 08103 (856)342-2965

Chang, Luke, MD {1669563300} Psychy, PsyCAd(86,TAI05)<NJ-TRININPC>
+ Trinitas Regional Medical Center-New Point Campus
655 East Jersey Street/Psychiatry Elizabeth, NJ 07206 (908)994-5000

Chang, Michael Lin, MD {1366774697} EmrgMd(08,NY09)<RI-SJ-FATIMA>
+ Emergency Medical Associates of NJ, P.A.
3 Century Drive Parsippany, NJ 07054 (973)740-0607 Fax (973)740-9895

Chang, Michael Poyin, MD {1417978719} IntrMd, MedOnc, OncHem(87,PHI08)<NJ-HACKNSK, NJ-HOLYNAME>
+ 769 River Road
New Milford, NJ 07646 (201)261-0255 Fax (201)845-8485

Chang, Mimi A., MD {1992718530} PhysMd, PhyMPain(81,MYA04)
+ Integrated Paincare Center
27 Mountain Boulevard/Suite 7 Warren, NJ 07059 (908)822-2889
+ Integrated Paincare Center
1999 Route 27 Edison, NJ 08817 (732)287-9988
+ Integrated Paincare Center
252 Columbia Turnpike Florham Park, NJ 07059 (973)822-3338 Fax (973)822-8098

Chang, Ming Z., MD {1700985884} Radiol(74,TAIW)<NJ-HOBUNIMC>
+ Hoboken University Medical Center
308 Willow Avenue/Radiology Hoboken, NJ 07030 (201)418-1000
+ 343 Passaic Avenue/Suite C-1
Fairfield, NJ 07004 (201)418-1000 Fax (973)227-3475

Chang, Peiyun, DO {1558775825} FamMed
+ Care Station Medical Group
456 Prospect Avenue West Orange, NJ 07052 (973)731-6767 Fax (973)731-9881

Chang, Richard, MD {1790789618} Ortped, SrgOrt(94,NY19)
+ MidJersey Orthopaedics, P.A.
8100 Westcott Drive/Suite 101 Flemington, NJ 08822 (908)782-0600 Fax (908)782-7575

Chang, Richard Youngjae, DO {1548342488} CdvDis, IntrMd(00,MO78)
+ Cardiology Consultants
368 Lakehurst Road/Suite 301 Toms River, NJ 08755 (732)240-1048 Fax (732)240-3464
+ Cardiology Consultants of Toms River
401 Lacey Road/Suite D Whiting, NJ 08759 (732)240-1048 Fax (732)350-3350
+ Cardiology Consultants
63-C Lacey Road Whiting, NJ 08755 (732)350-3350 Fax (732)350-7054

Chang, Steven Yang-Liang, MD {1376515023} CritCr, PulDis, IntrMd(96,IL02)<NJ-UMDNJ>
+ University Hospital
150 Bergen Street/UH I-354 Newark, NJ 07103 (973)972-6111 Fax (973)972-6228

Chang, Victor Tsu-Shih, MD {1790795375} IntrMd, OncHem, PallCr(83,NY19)<NJ-VAEASTOR>
+ VA New Jersey Health Care System-East Orange Campus
385 Tremont Avenue/HemOnc East Orange, NJ 07018 (973)676-1000 Fax (973)395-7096
victor.chang@med.va.gov

Chang, Zhu Ping, MD {1255306775} IntrMd(01,CHN4A)<NJ-RWJUHAM>
+ Karaisz, Zhuping Chang
5 Schalks Crossing Road/Suite 228 Plainsboro, NJ 08536 (609)716-4800
+ Plainsboro Medical Associates
3 Market Street/Suite 422 Plainsboro, NJ 08536 (609)716-4800 Fax (609)275-5001

Changchien, Charlie J., MD {1265616908} Pedtrc(04,DMN01)<NJ-RIVERVW>
+ Millennium Pediatric Care, PA
1 Riverview Medical Center Red Bank, NJ 07701 (732)450-2801 Fax (732)450-2802

Chanin, Alan H., MD {1174517916} IntrMd(76,NY46)<NJ-MORRISTN>
+ Chester Medical Associates
385 Route 24/Suite 1-C Chester, NJ 07930 (908)879-6277 Fax (908)879-4464

Chanliecco, Ma Victoria C., MD {1518996776} IntrMd, EmrgMd(86,PHI09)<NJ-RWJUHAM>
+ Robert Wood Johnson University Hospital at Hamilton
1 Hamilton Health Place/EmrgMed Hamilton, NJ 08690 (609)586-7900 Fax (609)584-6428

Physicians by Name and Address

Channamsetty, Ramu, MD {1891908265} IntrMd(96,INA48)<PA-CROZER, NJ-MEMSALEM>
+ Memorial Hospital of Salem County
  310 Woodstown Road   Salem, NJ 08079   (856)935-1000
  Fax (856)935-9659

Channapragada, Srinivas, MD {1801944632} IntrMd, Gastrn(84,INDI)<NJ-JFKMED>
+ 904 Oak Tree Road/Suite C
  South Plainfield, NJ 07080   (908)754-1044   Fax (908)522-0849

Channell, Millicent King, DO {1043280159} FamMed, NeuMus(01,PA17)
+ University Pain Care Center
  42 East Laurel Road/Suite 1700   Stratford, NJ 08084
  (856)566-7010   Fax (856)566-6956

Chansky, Michael, MD {1245320944} EmrgMd, IntrMd(80,NY45)<NJ-COOPRUMC>
+ Cooper University Hospital
  One Cooper Plaza/EmergMed   Camden, NJ 08103
  (856)342-2351

Chao, Bo H., MD {1215144209} MedOnc, IntrMd(05,MN04)
+ 440 Route 22
  Bridgewater, NJ 08807   (908)203-6919

Chao, Chia Y., MD {1558460527} Pedtrc(83,GERM)<NJ-VIRTVOOR>
+ 539 Egg Harbor Road/Suite 3
  Sewell, NJ 08080   (856)582-8885   Fax (856)582-6556

Chao, Christina, MD {1588694657} ObsGyn(78,PA07)<NJ-VIRTMHBC>
+ Columbus Family Physicians
  23659 Columbus Road/Suite 4   Columbus, NJ 08022
  (609)261-0240   Fax (609)261-5181
+ Pinelands Obstetrics and Gynecology
  1617 Route 38   Mount Holly, NJ 08060   (609)261-0240
  Fax (609)261-8622
+ Penn Medicine Department of Ob/Gyn - Medford
  103 Old Marlton Pike/Suite 101   Medford, NJ 08022

Chapdelaine, Robert T., MD {1710080056} Anesth, AnesPain(02,MN04)
+ 390 North Broadway/Suite 500
  Pennsville, NJ 08070   (856)691-2211

Chapinski, Caren A., DO {1861887812} IntrMd
+ Drs. Eisenstat and Kershner
  1050 Galloping Hill Road/Suite 202   Union, NJ 07083
  (908)688-4845   Fax (908)687-2039

Chapman, Derek Q., MD {1972573244} ObsGyn(91,PA02)
+ Minoff Chapman Ob/Gyn
  110 Marter Avenue/Suite 504   Moorestown, NJ 08057
  (856)642-6580   Fax (856)273-8372

Chapman, John Robert, MD {1811971377} Urolgy(93,DC02)<NJ-OCEANMC, NJ-JRSYSHMC>
+ Coastal Urology Associates
  446 Jack Martin Boulevard   Brick, NJ 08724   (732)840-4300
  Fax (732)840-4515
+ Coastal Urology Associates
  444 Neptune Boulevard/Suite 3   Neptune, NJ 07753
  (732)840-4300   Fax (732)988-8996
+ Coastal Urology Associates
  814 River Avenue   Lakewood, NJ 08724   (732)370-2250
  Fax (732)901-9119

Chappell, Stephen E., MD {1578667911} EmrgMd(99,PA13)
+ 707 Rachel Drive
  Franklinville, NJ 08322

Chapple, Kyle Thomas, MD {1295961555} SrgNro(02,OH40)
+ Atlantic Neurosurgical Specialists
  310 Madison Avenue/Suite 300   Morristown, NJ 07960
  (973)285-7800   Fax (973)285-7839

Char, Daniel Jay, MD {1366518128} Surgry, SrgVas(95,NY48)<NJ-VALLEY>
+ NJ Endovascular Therapeutics
  1124 East Ridgewood Avenue/Suite 104   Ridgewood, NJ 07450   (201)444-5353

Charaipotra, Neelam, MD {1750476057} Pedtrc, AdolMd(71,INA23)<NJ-JFKMED, NJ-KMHSTRAT>
+ Woodbridge Pediatrics & Adolescent Care PC
  80 Lake Avenue   Colonia, NJ 07067   (732)396-4744   Fax (732)396-9604
  Wodbrgpeds@aol.com

Chardo, Francis, Jr., MD {1710979216} CdvDis, IntrMd(70,SC01)<NJ-LOURDMED>
+ Cooper University at Willingboro
  218C Sunset Road   Willingboro, NJ 08046   (609)877-0400
  Fax (609)877-3542
+ University Cardiology
  3 Cooper Plaza/Room 311   Camden, NJ 08103   (856)342-2034

Charen, Jeffrey H., MD {1891777942} SrgOrt(78,NY45)
+ Orthopedic Associates of Central Jersey
  205 May Street/Suite 202   Edison, NJ 08837   (908)757-1520   Fax (908)769-1388
+ Orthopedic Associates of Central Jersey PA
  3 Hospital Plaza/Suite 411   Old Bridge, NJ 08857

  (908)757-1520   Fax (732)360-0775

Chargualaf, Lisa Marie, MD {1255569661} Surgry<NJ-STBARNMC>
+ St. Barnabas Medical Center
  94 Old Short Hills Road/Surgery   Livingston, NJ 07039
  (973)322-5000

Charilaou, Paris, MD {1457734659}<NJ-STPETER>
+ St. Peter's University Hospital
  254 Easton Avenue   New Brunswick, NJ 08901   (203)550-7186

Charko, Gregory P., MD {1336189356} SrgOrt(82,NJ05)
+ Ortho Physicians & Surgeons
  975 Lehigh Avenue   Union, NJ 07083   (908)686-1488   Fax (908)687-7886
+ Ambulatory Surgical Center of Union County
  950 West Chestnut Street/Suite 200   Union, NJ 07083
  (908)686-1488   Fax (908)688-7424

Charles, Diane Isaacson, MD {1427314160} Pedtrc<NJ-HCKTSTWN>
+ Ocean Medical Center
  425 Jack Martin Boulevard   Brick, NJ 08723   (678)457-0765

Charles, Ellis B., MD {1013046341} Psychy(71,BRAZ)<NJ-EASTORNG>
+ 90 Washington Street
  East Orange, NJ 07019   (973)672-2555   Fax (973)672-2529
  EllisCharlesdoc@aol.com

Charles, James A., MD {1356457246} Nrolgy(78,NJ05)<NJ-CHRIST, NJ-BAYONNE>
+ 956 Kennedy Boulevard
  Bayonne, NJ 07002   (201)858-2457   Fax (201)858-1053
+ 8841 Kennedy Boulevard
  North Bergen, NJ 07047   (201)861-5674

Charles, Lydia N., MD {1598754509} AdolMd, Pedtrc, IntrMd(83,BUL03)<NJ-CHILTON>
+ New Jersey Pediatric & Adolescent Care, LLC.
  1680 Route 23/Suite 350   Wayne, NJ 07470   (973)521-9700   Fax (973)521-9707

Charles, Patrick, DO {1295138782} EmrgMd
+ Hackensack Medical Center Emergency Medicine
  30 Prospect Avenue/Main 3619   Hackensack, NJ 07601
  (551)996-2331   Fax (201)968-1866

Charney, Robert Howard, MD {1891736039} CdvDis, IntrMd(91,NY01)<NJ-NWRKBETH, NJ-STBARNMC>
+ The Heart Group, PA
  161 Millburn Avenue   Millburn, NJ 07041   (973)467-4220   Fax (973)467-9889
+ The Heart Group, PA
  654 Broadway   Bayonne, NJ 07002   (973)467-4220   Fax (201)243-9998

Charron, Mariane, MD {1982801684} CritCr, IntrMd(07,QU06)<CT-YALENHH>
+ Cooper University Hospital Critical Care
  One Cooper Plaza   Camden, NJ 08103   (856)342-2633
  Fax (856)968-8282
+ Inspira Health Network
  509 North Broad Street   Woodbury, NJ 08096   (856)845-0100
+ Frank & Edith Scarpa Regional Cancer
  1505 West Sherman Avenu/Suite B   Vineland, NJ 08103
  (856)641-8635   Fax (856)641-8636

Chartash, Elliot Keith, MD IntrMd, Rheuma(82,NY06)
+ 41 Summit Drive
  Basking Ridge, NJ 07920   (732)594-5901   Fax (732)594-2040
  chartash@optonline.net

Chasanov, William M., II, DO {1104028919} IntrMd(07,PA77)
+ EIP Clinic/Early Intervention Program (HIV/AIDS)
  3 Cooper Plaza/Suite 513   Camden, NJ 08103   (856)966-0735
+ 409 Haddon Avenue/Suite 259
  Camden, NJ 08103

Chase, Howard M., MD {1669429346} EmrgMd(78,CT01)<NJ-HACKNSK>
+ Hackensack University Medical Center
  30 Prospect Avenue/Emergency   Hackensack, NJ 07601
  (201)996-4614   Fax (201)968-1866

Chase, Mark D., MD {1699849711} SrgOrt(83,MA05)<NJ-MTNSIDE>
+ Montclair Orthopedic Group PA
  200 Highland Avenue   Glen Ridge, NJ 07028   (973)746-2200   Fax (973)429-2174
+ Active Orthopaedics & Sports Medicine
  440 Old Hook Road   Emerson, NJ 07630   (973)746-2200
  Fax (201)358-9777

Chase, Melissa Sussman, DO {1851355168} Pedtrc(00,PA77)<NJ-VIRTUAHS, NJ-COOPRUMC>
+ Advocare South Jersey Pediatrics Cherry Hill
  1949 Route 70 East/Suite 1 & 2   Cherry Hill, NJ 08003
  (856)424-6050   Fax (856)424-2943
+ Advocare South Jersey Pediatrics Collingswood
  204 White Horse Pike   Collingswood, NJ 08107   (856)424-

  6050   Fax (856)424-2943

Chase, Rachel Eisenbrock, DO {1003044884} EmrgMd<PA-DELCNTY>
+ Cooper University Hospital
  One Cooper Plaza   Camden, NJ 08103   (856)342-2000

Chase, Raymond Donald, DO {1174623896} Ophthl(85,PA77)<NJ-HCKTSTWN>
+ Hasting Sq Plaza/Schooley's Mt
  Hackettstown, NJ 07840   (908)850-4300

Chasen, David E., MD {1275599045} Pedtrc(94,PA02)<NJ-VIRTMARL>
+ Advocare The Farm Pediatrics
  975 Tuckerton Road/Suite 100   Marlton, NJ 08053
  (856)983-6190   Fax (856)983-3805
+ Advocare The Farm Pediatrics
  1001 Laurel Oak Boulevard/Suite B   Voorhees, NJ 08043
  (856)983-6190   Fax (856)782-7404

Chasin, Mitchell C., MD {1992746218} FamMed, SrgLap(85,NY15)<NJ-SOMERSET, NJ-OVERLOOK>
+ Refelctions Center for Skin & Body
  1924 Washington Valley Road   Martinsville, NJ 08836
  (732)356-1666
+ Reflections Center for Skin & Body
  299 East Northfield Road   Livingston, NJ 07039   (732)356-1666   Fax (973)740-0070

Chatelain, Martin P., MD {1538116611} IntrMd(92,NJ05)<NJ-HACKNSK>
+ Hackensack University Medical Center
  30 Prospect Avenue   Hackensack, NJ 07601   (201)996-3664   Fax (501)996-0536

Chatha, Anjum, MD {1205203452} IntrMd
+ 342 Mercer Loop
  Jersey City, NJ 07302   (201)687-8495

Chatha, Uzma Arshad, MD {1407174451} IntrMd(07,DMN01)<NJ-STBARNMC>
+ Drs. Chatha & Nasta
  90 Washington Street/Suite 311   East Orange, NJ 07017
  (973)676-7192   Fax (973)676-0525
  Uzmac80@gmail.com

Chatiwala, Jumana Safdar, MD {1215066980} IntrMd, OncHem(96,INA21)<NJ-STJOSHOS>
+ St. Joseph's Regional Medical Center
  703 Main Street/Hemat/Onc   Paterson, NJ 07503
  (973)754-2000

Chatlos, John Calvin, Jr., MD {1497752695} PsyCAd, PsyAdt, Addctn(78,MD01)<NJ-CENTRAST>
+ CentraState Medical Center
  901 West Main Street/Psychiatry   Freehold, NJ 07728
  (732)431-2000

Chatterjee, Abhijit, MD {1487692836} Grtrcs, IntrMd(87,INDI)<NJ-STPETER>
+ Abhijit Chatterjee MD PC
  312 Applegarth Road/Suite 207   Monroe Township, NJ 08831   (609)655-2700   Fax (609)655-2565

Chatterjee, Deelip, MD {1790894707} IntrMd, PulDis(84,INDI)
+ Drs. Brar and Chatterjee
  1031 McBride Avenue/Suite D-209   West Paterson, NJ 07424   (973)785-3455   Fax (973)785-4353
+ Drs. Brar and Chatterjee
  542 East 29th Street   Paterson, NJ 07504   (973)977-2250

Chatterjee, Monica, MD {1932138401} PthACl(94,INA69)
+ PLUS Diagnostics
  1200 River Avenue/Suite 10   Lakewood, NJ 08701
  (732)901-7575   Fax (732)901-1555

Chatterjee, Sonia, MD {1205132669} FamMed
+ Health Med Associates, PC
  1080 Stelton Road/First FL Suite 202   Piscataway, NJ 08854
  (732)985-2552   Fax (732)985-0552

Chattha, Savneet Kaur, MD {1629055181} IntrMd(00,VA04)
+ Montgomery Internal Medicine Group
  727 State Road   Princeton, NJ 08540   (609)921-6410   Fax (609)921-0406

Chaturvedi, Ratan B., MD {1962622720} IntrMd
+ 388 Pompton Avenue
  Cedar Grove, NJ 07009   (201)512-9494   Fax (973)239-4267

Chatyrka, George O., DO {1841226495} FamMed(74,PA77)<NJ-VIRTMHBC, NJ-KMHSTRAT>
+ Alliance for Better Care, PC/Mount Holly Division
  1613 Route 38   Lumberton, NJ 08048   (609)261-3716
  Fax (609)261-5507
+ Alliance for Better Care, P.C.
  PO Box 1510   Medford, NJ 08055   (609)261-3716   Fax (609)953-8652

Chau, Patricia Chang Wai, MD {1275852410} ObsGyn(NY48<NJ-JRSYCITY>
+ Jersey City Medical Center
  355 Grand Street/OB/GYN   Jersey City, NJ 07304
  (201)915-2466   Fax (201)915-2481

Chau, Wai Yip Y., MD {1467546325} Surgry(98,GRN01)
+ New Jersey Bariatrics
666 Plainsboro Road/Suite 640   Plainsboro, NJ 08536
(609)785-5870   Fax (609)785-5867
+ Princeton Health Medical & Surgical Associates
2 Centre Drive/Suite 200   Monroe, NJ 08831   (609)785-5870   Fax (609)860-5288

Chaubal, Abhijeet V., MD {1356456982} PthAClI(90,NJ05)<NJ-STPETER>
+ St. Peter's University Hospital
254 Easton Avenue   New Brunswick, NJ 08901   (732)745-8534   Fax (732)220-8595

Chaubey, Rakesh Kumar, MD {1386729341} Anesth(96,RUS76)<NJ-HOLYNAME>
+ Holy Name Hospital
718 Teaneck Road/Anesthesiology   Teaneck, NJ 07666
(201)833-3000   Fax (201)342-1259

Chaudhari, Anuja Parikh, DO {1477743920} IntrMd
+ 54 Corey Road
Flanders, NJ 07836

Chaudhari, Sameer Sadashiv, MD {1467680918} IntrMd<NJ-NWRKBETH>
+ Newark Beth Israel Medical Center
201 Lyons Avenue   Newark, NJ 07112   (973)926-7000

Chaudhari, Shilpa A., MD {1083952493}
+ 1507 Burroughs Mill Circle
Cherry Hill, NJ 08002   (718)877-7549
drshilpac@gmail.com
+ Infectious Disease Physicians PA
1001 Briggs Road/Suite 250   Mount Laurel, NJ 08054
(718)877-7549   Fax (856)866-9088

Chaudhari, Suvid, DO {1689871816} IntrMd<NJ-KMHSTRAT>
+ 54 Corey Road
Flanders, NJ 07836

Chaudhari, Umesh J., MD {1265761563} IntrMd(96,NJ06)<NJ-RWJUBRUN>
+ 14 Olsen Court
Kendall Park, NJ 08824

Chaudhary, Aliya Aslam, MD {1659655991}(02)
+ The Cooper Hospital System-Univ Hospital
401 Haddon Avenue/Suite 364   Camden, NJ 08103
(856)342-2001
+ Aliya Aslam Chaudhary
1132 Cooper Street   Deptford, NJ 08096   (856)342-2001
Fax (856)848-8038

Chaudhary, Jigisha S., MD {1114960705} Pedtrc(01,INA1D)
+ Drs. Gaurang R. Patel & Associates
1503 St Georges Avenue/Suite 205   Colonia, NJ 07067
(732)382-8111   Fax (732)381-0292

Chaudhary, Yasmeen Amjad, MD {1447261276} PhysMd(85,PAK12)<NJ-BAYONNE>
+ 398 Avenue East
Bayonne, NJ 07002   (201)455-2250   Fax (732)862-1201

Chaudhery, Shaukat A., MD {1821195363} CdvDis, IntrMd(68,PAKI)<NJ-RBAYOLDB, NJ-RBAYPERT>
+ Associates in Cardiology and Internal Medicine
530 Green Street   Iselin, NJ 08830   (732)283-0440   Fax (732)283-8943
+ Medical Associates of Marlboro
42 Throckmorton Lane/2nd flr   Old Bridge, NJ 08857
(732)283-0440   Fax (732)607-0552

Chaudhri, Eirum I., MD {1134461510} Gastrn, IntrMd(89,PA07)
+ 2 Stewart Court
Old Tappan, NJ 07675

Chaudhri, Imran I., MD {1790732998} EmrgMd(88,PAK01)<NJ-RWJUHAM>
+ Robert Wood Johnson University Hospital at Hamilton
1 Hamilton Health Place/EmergMed   Hamilton, NJ 08690
(609)586-7900   Fax (609)584-6428

Chaudhry, Ahmad N., MD {1881656635} Anesth(89,PAK20)<NJ-VALLEY>
+ The Valley Hospital
223 North Van Dien Avenue   Ridgewood, NJ 07450
(201)447-8000

Chaudhry, Ambareen Khan, MD {1295997872} Anesth<NJ-UNVMCPRN>
+ University Medical Center of Princeton at Plainsboro
One Plainsboro Road/Anesthesia   Plainsboro, NJ 08536
(609)853-7323   Fax (609)853-7324

Chaudhry, Anu, MD {1295709061} Nephro, IntrMd(94,INA82)<NJ-NWRKBETH, NJ-RWJUHAM>
+ 546 Saint Georges Avenue
Rahway, NJ 07065   (732)381-3642   Fax (732)396-4463

Chaudhry, Faiza N., MD {1356595805}
+ St. Lukes - Warren Hospital
Knj Hospitalist Group Llc   Phillipsburg, NJ 08865

Chaudhry, Faraz A., MD {1548401243} Anesth
+ Rutgers- New Jersey Medical School
185 South Orange Avenue/Anesth/LvlE   Newark, NJ 07103
(973)972-0470   Fax (973)972-0470

Chaudhry, Fatima N., MD {1598056079}
+ 12 Harvest Avenue
East Hanover, NJ 07936   (443)939-9212

Chaudhry, Humaira S., MD {1285895805} RadDia(05)<NJ-UMDNJ>
+ University Hospital
150 Bergen Street/C318   Newark, NJ 07103   (973)972-4300

Chaudhry, Iftikhar Manzoor, MD {1700874740} Ophthl, Glacma, Catrct(93,PA02)<PA-TMPHOSP>
+ IC Laser Eye Care
1725 Klockner Road   Hamilton, NJ 08619   (609)586-6700
Fax (609)586-8768

Chaudhry, Kunal, MD {1114138815} IntrMd<NJ-COOPRUMC>
+ Cooper University Hospital
One Cooper Plaza/4th Fl/Dorrance   Camden, NJ 08103
(856)342-2000

Chaudhry, Mohammad A., MD {1033119573} IntrMd(99,DOM18)<NJ-HOLYNAME>
+ Diligent Medical Care
3807 Bergenline Avenue   Union City, NJ 07087   (201)758-7250   Fax (201)758-7251

Chaudhry, Nadia Jahan, MD {1013115690} IntrMd(91,NJ05)<NJ-OURLADY>
+ Hope Medical Spa
12000 Lincoln Drive West/Suite 202   Marlton, NJ 08053
(856)988-8230
info@hopemedicalspa.com

Chaudhry, Nasser A., MD {1134108442} CdvDis, IntrMd(91,NJ05)<NJ-UNDRWD, NJ-VIRTUAHS>
+ Associated Cardiovascular Consultants-Lourdes
1 Brace Road/Suite C & F   Cherry Hill, NJ 08034   (856)428-4100   Fax (856)428-5748

Chaudhry, Shauhab, MD {1942599352} IntrMd<NJ-MTNSIDE>
+ Hackensack UMC Mountainside
1 Bay Avenue   Montclair, NJ 07042   (973)429-6000

Chaudhry, Sofia, MD {1700265543} IntrMd
+ Capital Health Hospitalist Group
750 Brunswick Avenue   Trenton, NJ 08638   (609)394-6031
Fax (609)394-6299

Chaudhry, Uzma, MD {1013320936}
+ IC Laser Eye Care
1725 Klockner Road   Hamilton, NJ 08619   (609)586-6700
Fax (609)586-8768

Chaudry, Ghazali Anwar, MD {1972619187} Surgry, SrgOnc(88,PAK10)
+ Somerset Surgical Associates
2 Lincoln Highway/Suite 402   Edison, NJ 08820   (732)744-0707   Fax (732)744-1717

Chaudry, Mansoora R., MD {1124097001} GenPrc, PthAClI(65,PAK08)<NJ-VALLEY>
+ Drs. Chaudry & Chaudry
41-04 Goldblatt Terrace   Fair Lawn, NJ 07410   (201)797-7129   Fax (201)703-6982

Chaudry, Sadia R., MD {1528079431} FamMed(91,DC03)<NJ-VALLEY, NJ-WAYNEGEN>
+ Drs. Chaudry & Chaudry
41-04 Goldblatt Terrace   Fair Lawn, NJ 07410   (201)797-7129   Fax (201)703-6982

Chaudry, Samia Riaz, DO {1366604605} FamMed, IntrMd(08,MO79)<NJ-STJOSHOS>
+ Drs. Chaudry & Chaudry
41-04 Goldblatt Terrace   Fair Lawn, NJ 07410   (201)797-7129   Fax (201)703-6982

Chauhan, Chetankumar K., MD {1801024559} IntrMd, IntHos(07)
+ Dr. Chetankumar Chauhan
171 Elmora Avenue   Elizabeth, NJ 07202   (908)388-1716
Fax (908)469-2821
+ Complete Care
1814 East Second Street   Scotch Plains, NJ 07076
(908)388-1716   Fax (908)322-8665

Chauhan, Dhaval B., MD {1528340130}
+ 125 Linden Avenue
Bloomfield, NJ 07003
dhavalchauhan86@gmail.com

Chauhan, Naresh, MD {1700039716} Rheuma
+ 359 Christopher Drive
Princeton, NJ 08540

Chauhan, Niravkumar M., MD {1538663869} Surgry
+ UMDNJ Surgery
185 South Orange Avenue/MSB I-508 B   Newark, NJ 07103
(973)972-5188   Fax (973)972-7429

Chauhan, Tusharsindhu Chhatrasinh, MD {1760447841} Gastrn, IntrMd(86,INA21)<NJ-OURLADY, NJ-VIRTVOOR>
+ Community Gastroenterology Center
1000 South Burnt Mill Road   Voorhees, NJ 08043
(856)795-5950   Fax (856)795-5951

Chaump, Michael, MD {1598963894}<NJ-MONMOUTH>
+ Monmouth Medical Center
300 Second Avenue   Long Branch, NJ 07740   (732)222-5200

Chaurasia, Preeti, MD {1801121850} IntrMd(98,INA74)<NJ-LOURDMED>
+ Lourdes Medical Center of Burlington County
218 Sunset Road/Suite A   Willingboro, NJ 08046   (609)835-3056   Fax (609)835-3061

Chava, Padma, MD {1508838186} IntrMd, Grtrcs(93,INA8Y)<NJ-HACKNSK>
+ New Jersey Physicians, LLC.
128 Union Avenue/Suite 2A   Rutherford, NJ 07070
(201)939-8834   Fax (201)939-7644

Chavarkar, Mrunalini R., MD {1003086398} NnPnMd, Pedtrc, IntrMd(93,INA69)<NJ-HUNTRDN>
+ Hunterdon Medical Center
2100 Wescott Drive/Pediatrics   Flemington, NJ 08822
(908)788-6695   Fax (908)788-6534

Chavez, Alberto M., MD {1255381802} NnPnMd, Pedtrc(72,PERU)<NJ-SOMERSET>
+ On-Site Neonatal Partners
1000 Haddonfield-Berlin Road/Suite 210   Voorhees, NJ 08043   (856)782-2212   Fax (856)782-2213

Chavez, Laura Monica, DO {1326136417} IntrMd, Grtrcs(98,NY75)<NJ-HACKNSK>
+ Holy Name Medical Partners Office
15 Anderson Street   Hackensack, NJ 07601   (201)487-3355
Fax (201)487-0960

Chavez, Martin R., MD {1356411375} ObsGyn, MtFtMd(96,NJ06)<NJ-RWJUBRUN>
+ University Medical Group/OBGYN
125 Paterson Street/2nd Floor   New Brunswick, NJ 08901
(732)235-6600   Fax (732)235-6627

Chavez, Rowland, MD {1356630172} IntrMd
+ 519 Broadway
Bayonne, NJ 07002   (908)273-4300

Chavez Santos, Maria, MD {1780061440} FamMed
+ Capital Health Primary Care-Hamilton
1445 Whitehorse-Mercerville Rd   Hamilton, NJ 08619
(609)587-6661   Fax (609)587-8503

Chavez-Cacho, Jose M., MD {1497854236} ObsGyn, UtlRQA, Gyneco(82,PER04)<NJ-STMRYPAS, NJ-MEADWLND>
+ Women & Children Primary Care of Passaic
61 Passaic Avenue   Passaic, NJ 07055   (973)473-5053
Fax (973)574-9430
J.m.chavez@verizon.net
+ Women's Primary Care
28-11 Kennedy Boulevard   North Bergen, NJ 07047
(201)319-1737

Chawla, Arun, MD {1568611630} Nephro
+ Advocare Nephrology of South Jersey
300 Sheppard Road   Voorhees, NJ 08043   (856)424-7390
Fax (856)424-7386
+ Advocare Sicklerville Internal Med
485 Williamstown Road   Sicklerville, NJ 08081   (856)424-7390   Fax (856)424-7386
+ Advocare Family Medicine Associates Williamstown
979 North Black Horse Pike   Williamstown, NJ 08043
(856)424-7390   Fax (856)424-7386

Chawla, Harbhajan Singh, MD {1801047253} NnPnMd, Pedtrc(64,MYA04)
+ 1605 Plymouth Rock Drive
Cherry Hill, NJ 08003

Chawla, Juhi, MD {1578502977} PsycAd(96,VA04)<NY-PRSB-COLU>
+ 300 Knickerbocker Road/Suite 3200
Cresskill, NJ 07626

Chawla, Neha Roshan, MD {1902056021} IntrMd
+ AtlantiCare Cancer Institute
2500 English Creek Avenue/Building 400   Egg Harbor Township, NJ 08234   (609)677-7777   Fax (757)686-0541

Chawla, Rajnish Paul Singh, MD {1932197456} IntrMd(99,INA03)<NJ-RWJUBRUN, NJ-CHSFULD>
+ Altus Medical Care
3840 Quakerbridge Road/Suite 206   Mercerville, NJ 08619
(609)890-4200   Fax (609)586-0399

Chawla, Rupinder, MD {1114194610} IntrMd(02,INA7Y)
+ Altus Medical Care
3840 Quakerbridge Road/Suite 206   Mercerville, NJ 08619
(609)890-4200   Fax (609)586-0399

Chazen, Diane R., MD {1336190560} IntrMd(82,NY09)<NJ-OVERLOOK>
+ 55 Morris Avenue/Suite 216
Springfield, NJ 07081   (973)379-8900   Fax (973)379-0580

Chazin, Norman S., MD {1710970553} Psychy, PsyFor(72,MA07)
+ 61A Central Square
Linwood, NJ 08221   (609)926-7001   Fax (609)926-7004

Cheatam, Consetta Mae, MD {1619989860} ObsGyn(96,NJ05)
+ 22 Sylvan Street/Suite 300
Rutherford, NJ 07070   (201)438-8860   Fax (201)438-1994

Chebotarev, Oleg, MD {1780647552} CdvDis<NJ-RWJUHAM>
+ Hamilton Cardiology Associates
2073 Klockner Road   Hamilton, NJ 08690   (609)584-1212
Fax (609)584-0103

Check, Jerome H., MD {1285617878} RprEnd, IntrMd(71,PA09)
+ Cooper Institute for Reproductive Hormonal Disorders
17000 Commerce Parkway/Suite C   Mount Laurel, NJ 08054
(856)751-5575   Fax (856)751-7289

Physicians by Name and Address

Checton, John B., MD {1962476416} CdvDis, CritCr, IntrMd(78,NJ05)<NJ-MONMOUTH, NJ-JRSYSHMC>
+ Monmouth Cardiology Associates, LLC
215 Brighton Avenue Long Branch, NJ 07740 (732)222-5143 Fax (732)222-4862
+ Monmouth Cardiology Associates, LLC
11 Meridian Road Eatontown, NJ 07724 (732)222-5143 Fax (732)663-0301
+ Monmouth Cardiology Associates, LLC
222 Schanck Road/Suite 104 Freehold, NJ 07740 (732)431-1332 Fax (732)431-1712

Chee, Michael Y., MD {1033387766} PedOto, Otlryg, IntrMd(PA14
+ RWJ University Hospital New Brunswick
One Robert Wood Johnson Place New Brunswick, NJ 08901 (732)235-5530 Fax (732)235-8882
michael.chee@rutgers.edu

Cheela, Santosh K., MD {1730169632} Gastrn, IntrMd(77,INA29)<NJ-JFKMED, NJ-RBAYPERT>
+ May Street Surgi Center
205 May Street/Suite 103 Edison, NJ 08837 (732)820-4566 Fax (732)661-9619
+ 200 Perrine Road/Suite 208
Old Bridge, NJ 08857 (732)820-4566 Fax (732)525-0275
+ 98 James Street/Suite 105
Edison, NJ 08837 (732)494-5400

Cheela, Shilpa, MD {1952714560}
+ 349 Mckinley Avenue
Edison, NJ 08820 (908)753-5262
shilpa.cheela@gmail.com

Cheema, Asad Mushtaq, MD {1639171457} IntrMd, CdvDis(97,PAK10)<NJ-STBARNMC, NJ-STMICHL>
+ Bart De Gregorio MD, LLC.
946 Bloomfield Avenue Glen Ridge, NJ 07028 (973)743-1121 Fax (973)743-2627

Cheema, Faiz Aslam, MD {1962602953} Psychy(97,PAK20)<NJ-BERGNMC>
+ New Bridge Medical Center
230 East Ridgewood Avenue Paramus, NJ 07652 (201)967-4000 Fax (201)967-4669
+ 1-14 Lyons Avenue
Fair Lawn, NJ 07410

Cheema, Humayun Mahmood, MD {1730227703} SrgOrt, IntrMd(63,PAKI)<NJ-STBARNMC>
+ St. Barnabas Medical Center
94 Old Short Hills Road/Suite 1172 Livingston, NJ 07039 (973)322-5195 Fax (973)322-2471

Cheeti, Kalpana, MD {1649352857} Grtrcs, IntrMd(96,INA83)
+ Summit Avenue Medical
5 Summit Avenue Hackensack, NJ 07601 (201)646-0001 Fax (201)646-9101

Chefitz, Dalya L., MD {1679650493} Pedtrc(90,NJ06)
+ UH- Robert Wood Johnson Med
125 Paterson Street/Pedi New Brunswick, NJ 08901 (732)828-3000

Chehade, Ghassan M., MD {1093717431} IntrMd(97,UKR05)
+ 236 East Westfield Avenue
Roselle Park, NJ 07204 (973)376-4216 Fax (973)771-3099
+ 221 Chestnut Street/Suite 101
Roselle, NJ 07203 (908)259-5775

Chekemian, Beth Ann, DO {1154567311} Anesth
+ Rancocas Anesthesiology, PA
15000 Midlantic Drive/Suite 102 Mount Laurel, NJ 08054 (856)255-5479 Fax (856)393-8691

Chekmareva, Marina A., MD {1598976573} PthACI(91,RUS37)<NJ-RWJUBRUN>
+ RWJ University Pathology
125 Paterson Street/MEB 212 New Brunswick, NJ 08901 (732)235-8121 Fax (732)235-8124

Chelemer, Scott Brain, MD {1063497329} IntrMd, PulDis(88,PA12)<NJ-VIRTMHBC>
+ Pulmonary and Sleep Physicians
204 Ark Road/Suite 206/Larchmont 1 Mount Laurel, NJ 08054 (856)778-4640 Fax (856)778-8862

Cheli, David J., MD {1043205685} FamMed(74,PA07)
+ 2640 Highway 70/Building 10
Manasquan, NJ 08736 (732)223-8200 Fax (732)223-3633

Chelliah, Padmini, MD {1710072350} Pedtrc(76,INDI)<NJ-HOLYNAME, NJ-STCLRDEN>
+ Holy Name Hospital
718 Teaneck Road Teaneck, NJ 07666 (201)833-3000

Chemaly, Philippe, Jr., DO {1346285434} PhysMd, PainMd, PhyMPain(94,NJ75)<NJ-WAYNEGEN, NJ-VALLEY>
+ Wayne Physical Med and Rehab Assocs
401 Hamburg Turnpike/Suite 105 Wayne, NJ 07470 (973)595-6066 Fax (973)595-1127
+ Wayne Physical Med and Rehab Assocs
730 Broad Street Clifton, NJ 07011 (973)595-6066 Fax (973)928-4340

Chen, Aileen Lim, MD {1194753350} OncHem, IntrMd(98,CA15)<NY-NYUTISCH>
+ Regional Cancer Care Associates, LLC
723 North Beers Street Holmdel, NJ 07733 (732)739-8644 Fax (732)739-4438

Chen, Anna, MD {1871690495} FamMed(93,PA02)<NJ-KMHSTRAT>
+ Wolfe-Simon Associates
511 Kings Highway North Cherry Hill, NJ 08034 (856)667-1654 Fax (856)482-8057

Chen, Arnold Yin-Ti, MD {1134299845} IntrMd(85,NY46)<NJ-RWJUBRUN>
+ Mathematica Policy Research, Inc.
PO Box 2393 Princeton, NJ 08543 (609)799-3535 Fax (609)799-0005
achen@mathematica-mpr.com
+ Eric B. Chandler Health Center
277 George Street New Brunswick, NJ 08901 (609)799-3535 Fax (732)235-6729

Chen, Bonnie L., MD {1750373486} IntrMd(83,CHN1C)
+ 243 Horseneck Road
Fairfield, NJ 07004
bonniechenmd@yahoo.com

Chen, Boqing, MD {1649291410} PhysMd, PainMd(83,CHN45)<NJ-STMICHL, NJ-JFKMED>
+ Center for Pain Management
102 Towne Centre Drive Hillsborough, NJ 08844 (908)359-3499
+ Center for Advanced Pain Management & Rehabilitation
249 Bridge Street/Building G Metuchen, NJ 08840 (908)359-3499 Fax (732)516-1015

Chen, Brian Youshane, DO {1053792366} IntrMd
+ SOM - Department of Internal Medicine
42 East Laurel Road/Suite 3100 Stratford, NJ 08084 (856)566-2753 Fax (856)566-6906

Chen, Catherine, MD {1073872073} IntrMd
+ UH-RWJ General Internal Medicine
125 Paterson Street/Suite 2300 New Brunswick, NJ 08901 (732)235-7122 Fax (732)235-7144
+ Patient first Urgent Care
641 US Highway Route 130 Hamilton, NJ 08691 (732)235-7122 Fax (609)568-9384

Chen, Chu-Kuang, MD {1013007707} Anesth, PainMd(83,TAIW)<NJ-UNVMCPRN>
+ University Medical Center of Princeton at Plainsboro
One Plainsboro Road/Anesthesiology Plainsboro, NJ 08536 (609)497-4330

Chen, Chunguang, MD {1093862138} CdvDis, IntrMd, OthrSp(81,GER21)<NJ-NWRKBETH>
+ Newark Beth Israel Medical Center
201 Lyons Avenue/CardioNonInvLab Newark, NJ 07112 (973)926-7475 Fax (973)923-4683

Chen, Cindy H., MD {1760506323} Anesth, IntrMd(06,IL42)<NJ-MORRISTN>
+ Morristown Medical Center
100 Madison Avenue/Anesthesia Morristown, NJ 07962 (201)388-5608

Chen, David, MD {1437120961} FamMed(02,PA02)
+ Family Medical Care of Clifton
1033 Clifton Avenue/Suite 209 Clifton, NJ 07013 (973)470-8377 Fax (973)470-8534

Chen, Deborah E., MD {1730190422} Pedtrc(83,TX12)
+ New Brunswick Pediatric Group, P.A.
1300 How Lane North Brunswick, NJ 08902 (732)247-1510 Fax (732)247-8885

Chen, Dehan, MD {1508806670} ObsGyn, RprEnd(95,NY46)<NY-NYUTISCH>
+ The Valley Hospital Fertility Center
140 East Ridgewood Avenue Paramus, NJ 07652 (212)263-7808 Fax (201)634-5503
+ Valley Hospital Fertility Center
One Valley Health Plaza Paramus, NJ 07652 (212)263-7808 Fax (201)634-5503

Chen, Dong, MD {1982607149} Anesth(81,CHN5D)<NJ-NWRKBETH>
+ Newark Beth Israel Medical Center
201 Lyons Avenue/Anesth Newark, NJ 07112 (973)926-7000

Chen, Donghui, MD {1578540597} Anesth(85,CHN42)<NJ-CHRIST>
+ Christ Hospital
176 Palisade Avenue/Anesth Jersey City, NJ 07306 (201)795-8200 Fax (201)943-8105

Chen, Edgar Y., MD {1871569616} Nrolgy(79,TAIW)<NJ-BAYSHORE, NJ-RIVERVW>
+ Greater Monmouth Neurology
130 Maple Avenue/Suite 1-A Red Bank, NJ 07701 (732)741-1378 Fax (732)741-1677
+ Greater Monmouth Neurology
733 North Beers Street Holmdel, NJ 07733 (732)741-1378

Chen, Elbert H., MD {1861553729} Dermat, SrgDer(99,NC07)
+ 12 Lorraine Drive
Pine Brook, NJ 07058

Chen, Emily Q., MD {1396947503} IntrMd, OncHem(93,CHN57)
+ Mercer County Hematology and Oncology PC
40 Fuld Street/Suite 404 Trenton, NJ 08638 (609)394-0660 Fax (609)394-1004
+ 8 Barley Court
Plainsboro, NJ 08536

Chen, Evan, MD {1265646707} Anesth
+ James Street Anesthesia
102 James Street/Suite 103 Edison, NJ 08820 (732)494-1444 Fax (732)494-7052

Chen, Fan, MD {1568634152} PthAna
+ 35 Homestead Road
Edison, NJ 08820

Chen, Franklin, MD {1245387554} SrgOrt, SrgHnd(90,MD07)<NJ-JFKMED>
+ Edison-Metuchen Orthopedic Group
10 Parsonage Road/5th Floor/Suite 500 Edison, NJ 08837 (732)494-6226 Fax (732)494-8762

Chen, Guo Ming, MD {1366583569} PedAne, IntrMd(86,CHNA)
+ St. Barnabas Medical Center
94 Old Short Hills Road/Anesthesia Livingston, NJ 07039 (973)322-5512 Fax (973)322-8165

Chen, Guo-Gang, MD {1710941943} Anesth(83,CHN63)<NJ-WARREN>
+ Morris Anesthesia Group, PA
3799 Route 46/Suite 211 Parsippany, NJ 07054 (973)335-1122 Fax (973)335-1448
+ Warren Hospital
185 Roseberry Street/Anesth Phillipsburg, NJ 08865 (908)859-6700

Chen, Hong, MD {1881669588} PsyCAd, Psychy(90,CHN40)<NJ-HUNTRDN>
+ Psychiatric Associates of Hunterdon
190 Route 31/Suite 100 Flemington, NJ 08822 (908)788-6654 Fax (908)788-6452

Chen, Ivan, MD {1467632364} PhyMPain, IntrMd
+ Algology Associates
905 Allwood Road/Suite 200 Clifton, NJ 07012 (973)815-0003 Fax (973)815-0030
info@mypainmd.com

Chen, James J., MD {1427092626} EnDbMt, IntrMd, NuclMd(80,TAI05)<NJ-OVERLOOK, NJ-ATLANTHS>
+ Overlook Medical Center
99 Beauvoir Avenue/PO Box 210 Summit, NJ 07902 (908)522-6995 Fax (908)522-5884

Chen, Janine Junying, MD {1649335621} ObsGyn, IntrMd(05,PA13)<NJ-VIRTVOOR, NJ-VIRTMHBC>
+ Virtua Maternal Fetal Medicine Center
100 Bowman Drive Voorhees, NJ 08043 (856)247-3328 Fax (856)247-3276
+ Virtua Memorial
175 Madison Avenue/OB/GYN Mount Holly, NJ 08060 (856)247-3328 Fax (609)914-7022
+ Virtua Maternal Fetal Medicine Center
239 Hurffville-Crosskeys Road Sewell, NJ 08043 (856)341-8300 Fax (856)341-8320

Chen, Jeffrey H., MD
+ Hunterdon Surgical Associates
1100 Wescott Drive/Suite 302 Flemington, NJ 08822 (908)788-6464 Fax (908)788-6459

Chen, Jennifer Yu-Chia, MD {1104124643} IntMSlpd
+ UMDNJ RWJ Sports Medicine
125 Paterson Street/Suite 6200 New Brunswick, NJ 08901 (732)235-7729

Chen, Jianping, MD {1962543173} Anesth(87,CHN4A)
+ New Jersey Anesthesia Associates, P.C.
30B Vreeland Road/Suite 200 Florham Park, NJ 07932 (973)660-9334 Fax (973)660-9779

Chen, Julie Eveline, MD {1073524542} IntrMd(97,GRN01)
+ 4 Conservancy Court
Franklin Park, NJ 08823

Chen, Karl Timothy, MD {1982600169} IntrMd(96,GRNA)<NJ-RWJUBRUN, NJ-STPETER>
+ Brunswick Medical Associates
620 Cranbury Road East East Brunswick, NJ 08816 (732)613-9335 Fax (732)613-9235

Chen, Kenneth H., DO {1902883010} ObsGyn(92,NJ75)<NJ-VIRTUAHS>
+ Rancocas Ob/Gyn Associates, LLC
200 Campbell Drive/Ste 101 Willingboro, NJ 08046 (609)877-8777 Fax (609)877-2497
chenkh@aol.com

Chen, Lee, MD {1174564991} EmrgMd(97,LA05)
+ Emergency Physician Associates, P.A.
307 South Evergreen Avenue/PO Box 298 Woodbury, NJ 08096 (856)848-3817 Fax (856)848-1431

Chen, Lucy L., MD {1366556615} Ophthl, IntrMd(85,MA05)<NJ-MORRISTN>
+ Pediatric Eye Physicians, PC
95 Madison Avenue/Suite 301 Morristown, NJ 07960 (973)540-8814 Fax (973)540-8556
+ Pediatric Eye Physicians, PC
70 Sparta Avenue/Suite 101 Sparta, NJ 07871 (973)540-8814 Fax (973)726-7005

Chen, Margaret G., MD {1770529430} Pedtrc, AdolMd(83,BRAZ)<NJ-OVERLOOK>
+ Westfield Pediatrics, P.A.
532 East Broad Street Westfield, NJ 07090 (908)232-3445 Fax (908)233-6184

Chen, Michael S., MD {1700101219} Psychy
+ Alexander Road Associates in Psychiatry & Psychology
707 Alexander Road/Bldg 2 Suite 202 Princeton, NJ 08540 (609)419-0400 Fax (609)419-9200

Chen, Michael T., MD {1790770642} IntrMd, CdvDis(72,TAI02)<NJ-RWJURAH, NJ-TRINIWSC>
+ Guarino & Chen PA
35-37 Progress Street/Suite B2 Edison, NJ 08820 (908)754-9292 Fax (908)754-3358

Chen, Natalie, DO {1265746697} Ophthl
+ Mid Atlantic Eye Center
70 East Front Street Red Bank, NJ 07701 (732)741-0858 Fax (732)219-0180

Chen, Pei-Jon, MD {1831223429} IntrMd(79,TAIW)
+ Bristol-Myers Squibb Co. - Occupational Health
Route 206 & Provinceline Road Princeton, NJ 08543 (609)252-4000 Fax (609)252-6383

Chen, Peter Jen-Chih, MD {1083646194} ObsGyn, IntrMd(96,PA09)<NJ-COOPRUMC>
+ Cooper University Medical Center/Camden
3 Cooper Plaza/Suite 502 Camden, NJ 08103 (856)356-4935
+ Cooper Faculty Ob/Gyn
1103 Kings Highway North/Suite 201 Cherry Hill, NJ 08034 (856)356-4935 Fax (856)321-0133
+ Cooper Ob/Gyn
4 Plaza Drive/Suite 403/Bunker Hill Pl Sewell, NJ 08103 (856)270-4020 Fax (856)270-4022

Chen, Roger L., MD {1528393204} FamMed, IntrMd(BWI01)<NJ-BAYSHORE, NJ-RIVERVW>
+ Meridian Primary Care
55 North Gilbert Street/Suite 3201 Tinton Falls, NJ 07701 (732)450-0961 Fax (732)530-0213

Chen, Roland Sangone, MD CmptMd, IntrMd(93,PA01)
+ 61 Maidenhead Road
Princeton, NJ 08540

Chen, Samuel Kuangzong, MD {1508891284} Urolgy, IntrMd(76,TAI05)<NJ-KMHSTRAT>
+ 760 Bound Brook Road/Suite B
Dunellen, NJ 08812 (732)321-1900

Chen, Serena Homei, MD {1598883571} RprEnd, Gyneco, Frt-Inf(88,NC07)<NJ-STBARNMC>
+ Inst of Repro Med and Science
609 Washington Street/2nd Floor Hoboken, NJ 07030 Fax (201)204-9319
+ The Institute for Reproductive Medicine and Science
94 Old Short Hills Road/Suite 403E Livingston, NJ 07039 Fax (973)322-8890

Chen, Shan, MD {1184940017} Nrolgy
+ JFK Neurosciences Institute
65 James Street/Second Floor Edison, NJ 08818 (732)632-1685 Fax (732)632-1669
+ University Hospital-RWJMS Neurology
125 Paterson Street/Suite 4100-6100 New Brunswick, NJ 08901 (732)632-1685 Fax (732)235-7041

Chen, Shwu-Miin Y., MD {1841282902} IntrMd, Nephro(75,TAI02)
+ Haddon Renal Medical Specialists
401 Kings Highway South/Suite 5 Cherry Hill, NJ 08034 (856)428-8992 Fax (856)428-9614

Chen, Sophia Wunchi, DO {1083846901} Pedtrc(03,IL76)<NJ-UMDNJ>
+ University Hospital
150 Bergen Street Newark, NJ 07103 (862)812-1930

Chen, Suann S., MD {1194959023} PhysMd<NJ-SHOREREH>
+ Shore Rehabilitation Institute
425 Jack Martin Boulevard Brick, NJ 08724 (732)836-4504 Fax (732)836-4532

Chen, Timothy, MD {1215935333} FamMed(00,PA13)
+ Virtual Family Medicine - Mansfield
3242 Route 206/Building A Suite 2 Bordentown, NJ 08505 (609)298-4340 Fax (609)298-4370

Chen, Timothy, MD {1578893947} RadDia
+ 99 Highway 37 West
Toms River, NJ 08755 (732)551-8151

Chen, Timothy H., MD {1336188549} RadOnc(89,DOM11)
+ Capital Health Radiation Oncology Department
One Capital Way Pennington, NJ 08534 (609)304-4244 Fax (609)303-4156

Chen, Tsuey-Ling, MD {1881604908} PthACl, Pthlgy(82,TAIW)<NJ-SOMERSET>
+ RWJ University Hospital Somerset
110 Rehill Avenue/Pathology Somerville, NJ 08876 (908)685-2938

Chen, Tzu-Shao, MD {1639361082} IntrMd
+ 9 Brownstone Way/Apt 414
Englewood, NJ 07631

Chen, Victoria Sheen, MD {1679982813} FamMSptM
+ Phillips Barber Family Health Center
72 Alexander Avenue Lambertville, NJ 08530 (609)397-3535 Fax (609)397-0301

Chen, Wei L., DO {1790018869} IntrMd
+ Rowan University-School of Osteopathic Medicine
1 Medical Center Drive Stratford, NJ 08084 (856)346-6000

Chen, Wen-Hong, MD {1043264856} Anesth(67,TAI04)
+ Englewood Anesthesiology
350 Engle Street Englewood, NJ 07631 (201)894-3238 Fax (201)871-0619

Chen, William Y., MD {1780784181} Gastrn, IntrMd(81,NY19)<NJ-STPETER, NJ-RWJUBRUN>
+ Associates in Digestive Disorders
561 Cranbury Road East Brunswick, NJ 08816 (732)238-4993 Fax (732)390-1751
+ Cares Surgicenter, LLC.
240 Easton Avenue New Brunswick, NJ 08901 (732)238-4993 Fax (732)296-8677

Chen, Xiaomei, MD {1982767828} IntrMd(89,CHN4A)<NJ-RWJUBRUN, NJ-UNVMCPRN>
+ 5 Schalks Crossing Road/Suite 228
Plainsboro, NJ 08536 (609)716-4800 Fax (609)716-4810

Chen, Yen Ping, MD {1962582791} PedGst, Pedtrc(83,BRA15)<NJ-RWJUBRUN>
+ Child Health Institute of New Jersey
89 French Street/Suite 2300 New Brunswick, NJ 08901 (732)235-6230 Fax (732)235-8766
chenyp@umdnj.edu

Chen, Yingying, MD {1710116199} IntrMd(02,CHN1S)
+ Virtua Voorhees
100 Bowman Drive/Internal Med Voorhees, NJ 08043 (856)762-1940

Chen, Yirong, MD {1588011597} Psychy
+ University Hospital-SOM Department of Psychiatry
2250 Chapel Avenue West/Suite 100 Cherry Hill, NJ 08002 (856)482-9000 Fax (856)482-1159

Chen, Zeng-Shan, MD {1174635502} Pedtrc(70,TAIW)
+ 1222 Route 46 West
Parsippany, NJ 07054 (973)299-0098 Fax (973)299-0916

Cheng, Adonis, DO {1639589666}<NJ-OVERLOOK>
+ Overlook Medical Center
99 Beauvoir Avenue/PO Box 210 Summit, NJ 07902 (908)522-2000

Cheng, Bonnie Kingman, MD {1053301010} IntrMd(98,NY06)
+ North Jersey Gastroenterology & Endoscopy Center
1825 State Route 23 South Wayne, NJ 07470 (973)633-1484 Fax (973)633-7980

Cheng, Chao T., MD {1841263183} CdvDis, IntrMd(69,TAI04)<NJ-SOMERSET>
+ Medicor Cardiology PA
225 Jackson Street Bridgewater, NJ 08807 (908)526-8668 Fax (908)231-6781
+ Medicor Cardiology PA
331 US Highway 206/Suite 1A Hillsborough, NJ 08844 (908)526-8668 Fax (908)431-0808

Cheng, Desmond H., DO {1073541744} FamMed(91,IA75)<NJ-OURLADY>
+ Kennedy Family Health Services
1 Somerdale Square Somerdale, NJ 08083 (856)309-7700 Fax (856)566-8944

Cheng, Eleanor Lillian, MD {1891914727} Ophthl(03,IL42)
+ The Rubino Ob/Gyn Group
101 Old Short Hills Road/Suite 101 West Orange, NJ 07052 (973)736-1313 Fax (973)731-8199

Cheng, Guo-Pao, MD {1598863649} Pedtrc(70,TAI05)<NJ-CLARMAAS>
+ 160 Bloomfield Avenue
Bloomfield, NJ 07003 (973)748-2220 Fax (973)748-2414

Cheng, Ho-Kan, MD {1881692374} PulCCr, IntrMd, PulDis(95,NJ05)<NJ-OURLADY, NJ-VIRTMARL>
+ Penn Jersey Pulmonary Associates
52 West Red Bank Avenue/Suite 26 Woodbury, NJ 08096 (856)853-2025 Fax (856)845-8024

Cheng, Jenfu, MD {1801862644} PhysMd, PedReh(99,NJ05)
+ 58 Roosevelt Boulevard
North Caldwell, NJ 07006

Cheng, Jennifer, DO {1699975037} EnDbMt
+ Hackensack Meridian Medical Group
19 Davis Avenue/5th-6th Floor Neptune, NJ 07753 (732)897-3980 Fax (732)897-3997
+ Meridian Medical Associates, P.C.
2240 State Route 33/2nd Floor Neptune, NJ 07753 (732)897-3980

Cheng, Peter F., MD {1417958505} EmrgMd, IntrMd(66,TAIW)<NJ-RBAYOLDB>
+ Raritan Bay Medical Center/Old Bridge Division
One Hospital Plaza/EmrgMed Old Bridge, NJ 08857 (732)360-1000
pficheng@verizon.net

Cheng, Ru-Fong J., MD {1881790384} ObsGyn(93,OH40)
+ University Medical Group/OBGYN
125 Paterson Street/2nd Floor New Brunswick, NJ 08901 (732)235-6600 Fax (732)235-6627

Cheng, Shiow-Jane L., MD {1114020526} CdvDis, IntrMd(72,TAIW)
+ Bridgewater Internal Medicine, PA
215 Union Avenue/Suite E Bridgewater, NJ 08807 (908)685-1818 Fax (908)685-8225

Cheng, Szu-Chi S., MD {1457343162} Anesth(86,TAI02)<NJ-CHILTON>
+ Chilton Medical Center
97 West Parkway/Anesthesiology Pompton Plains, NJ 07444 (973)831-5000

Cheng, Waina, MD {1922283126} OncHem, IntrMd(04,NY47)<NY-LINCOLN>
+ Sparta Health & Wellness
89 Sparta Avenu/Suite 207 Sparta, NJ 07871 (973)940-8780 Fax (973)726-9568

Cheng, Wunhuey, DO {1063651677} IntrMd
+ New Jersey Institute for Successful Aging
42 East Laurel Road/Suite 1800 Stratford, NJ 08084 (856)566-6843 Fax (856)566-6419

Cheng, Yihong Henry, MD {1629072046} IntrMd(01,NJ06)
+ Denville Associates of Internal Medicine
16 Pocono Road/Suite 317 Denville, NJ 07834 (973)627-2650 Fax (973)627-8383

Chenitz, Kara Beth, MD {1134306905} Nephro, IntrMd(07,NJ05)
+ St. Michael's Medical Center
111 Central Avenue/Bldg. B Level 4 Newark, NJ 07102 (973)624-4908 Fax (973)877-5595

Chenitz, William R., MD {1972531457} IntrMd, Nephro(65,NY46)<NJ-STMICHL>
+ St. Michael's Medical Center
268 MLK Jr. Boulevard Newark, NJ 07102 (973)624-4908

Chennapragada, Kausalya, MD {1003867607} IntrMd, IntHos(88,INA83)<NJ-VALLEY>
+ 1031 McBride Avenue/Suite D-208
Little Falls, NJ 07424 (973)812-1010
+ The Valley Hospital
223 North Van Dien Avenue Ridgewood, NJ 07450 (201)447-8000

Chennapragada, Ravi S., MD {1043211261} Pedtrc(91,INA48)<NJ-RWJUBRUN>
+ Pediatric and Adolescent Care
676 Route 202-206 North Bridgewater, NJ 08807 (908)927-1155 Fax (908)927-1133
+ 1667 Oak Tree Road
Edison, NJ 08820 (908)927-1155 Fax (908)927-1133

Cherciu, Doina M., MD {1043363179} FamMed(88,ROM01)
+ East Freehold Medical Associates
16 Thoreau Drive Freehold, NJ 07728 (732)761-0221 Fax (732)780-1886

Cherciu, Mugurel S., MD {1881747913} FamMed(88,ROMA)<NJ-KIMBALL, NJ-CENTRAST>
+ East Freehold Medical Associates
16 Thoreau Drive Freehold, NJ 07728 (732)761-0221 Fax (732)780-1886

Cherefko, Kathryn Baier, DO {1780022426} EmrgMd
+ Princeton Hospital
1 Plainsboro Road Plainsboro, NJ 08536 (609)853-7000

Cherian, Abraham, MD {1841491982} Anesth(INA9S)<NJ-UNDRWD>
+ Inspira Health Network
509 North Broad Street/Anesthesia Woodbury, NJ 08096 (856)845-0100

Cheriyan, Joshua M., MD {1780034827} PhysMd
+ 25 Grove Place
Whippany, NJ 07981 (973)884-2552

Chern, Joshua Saul, DO {1558689430}<NJ-COOPRUMC>
+ Cooper University Hospital
One Cooper Plaza/Suite B23 Camden, NJ 08103 (856)342-2383

Chern, Kenneth Y., MD {1821057886} SrgOrt(88,NY01)<NJ-JRSYSHMC, NJ-OCEANMC>
+ Seaview Orthopaedics
1200 Eagle Avenue Ocean, NJ 07712 (732)660-6200 Fax (732)660-6201
+ Seaview Orthopaedics
1640 Route 88 West Brick, NJ 08724 (732)660-6200 Fax (732)458-2743

Chern, Sy-Yeu Sue, MD {1790002343} Anesth
+ Anesthesia Associates
100 Madison Avenue Morristown, NJ 07960 (973)886-6784 Fax (973)631-8120

Chernack, William J., MD {1013941012} Allrgy, Pedtrc(70,NY09)<NY-PRSBCOLU, NJ-MORRISTN>
+ 28 Franklin Place
Morristown, NJ 07960 (973)538-7271 Fax (973)538-7491

Physicians by Name and Address

Chernock, Brad M., MD {1589967285}
+ Rutgers- New Jersey Medical School
  185 South Orange Avenue   Newark, NJ 07103   (908)447-7926

Chernoff, Brian Harris, MD {1013953660} IntrMd(92,PA09)<NJ-UNDRWD>
+ De Persia Medical Group
  17 West Red Bank Avenue/Suite 207   Woodbury, NJ 08096   (856)845-0664   Fax (856)845-7602

Chernyak, Anna, MD {1558437665} IntrMd, Addctn(78,BLAR)<NJ-OVERLOOK>
+ 2401 Morris Avenue/Suite 1
  Union, NJ 07083   (908)810-9330   Fax (908)810-9323
  annachdr@gmail.com

Chernyak, Arkadiy, MD {1780733147} Psychy(77,BLA46)
+ 2401 Morris Avenue/Suite 1
  Union, NJ 07083   (908)377-3273

Cherot, Elizabeth Kagel, MD {1629151733} ObsGyn(96,NY45)<NY-STRNGMEM, NJ-STPETER>
+ Brunswick-Hills Ob/Gyn, PA
  620 Cranbury Road/Suite LL90   East Brunswick, NJ 08816   (732)257-0081   Fax (732)613-4845
+ Brunswick-Hills Ob/Gyn, PA
  751 Route 206/2nd Floor   Hillsborough, NJ 08844   (732)257-0081   Fax (908)725-2132
+ Cares Surgicenter, LLC.
  240 Easton Avenue   New Brunswick, NJ 08816   (732)565-5400   Fax (732)296-8677

Cherry, Mohamad Ali, MD {1386690840} IntrMd<NJ-MORRISTN>
+ Morristown Medical Center
  100 Madison Avenue   Morristown, NJ 07962   (973)971-7960

Chertoff, Harvey R., MD {1689618845} Psychy, PsyFor, PsyAdd(66,NY46)<NJ-ENGLWOOD>
+ 205 Engle Street
  Englewood, NJ 07631   (201)567-4970

Cheruvu, Sunita, MD {1487850152} Pedtrc(04,NY15)<NJ-MORRISTN>
+ Morristown Medical Center
  100 Madison Avenue   Morristown, NJ 07962   (973)971-5000

Chervenak, Donald M., MD {1801863048} ObsGyn(80,MA05)<NJ-STBARNMC>
+ Florham Park Ob-Gyn
  15 James Street   Florham Park, NJ 07932   (973)822-3879   Fax (973)822-0850

Chery, Magdala, DO {1265852974} IntrMd
+ SOM - Department of Internal Medicine
  42 East Laurel Road/Suite 3100   Stratford, NJ 08084   (856)566-6845   Fax (856)566-6906

Chessler, Richard K., MD {1881632404} Gastrn, IntrMd(69,IL42)<NJ-HACKNSK, NJ-ENGLWOOD>
+ Advanced Gastroenterology of Bergen County
  140 Sylvan Avenue/Suite 101-A   Englewood Cliffs, NJ 07632   (201)945-6564   Fax (201)461-9038

Cheung, Deborah Jee Hae, MD {1255336004} IntrMd(97,DC01)<NJ-OVERLOOK, NJ-MORRISTN>
+ Summit Medical Group-Berkeley Heights Campus
  1 Diamond Hill Road   Berkeley Heights, NJ 07922   (908)273-4300   Fax (908)673-7391

Cheung, Sandy Wai Yi, DO {1740508969} NnPnMd<NJ-HACKNSK>
+ Hackensack University Medical Center
  30 Prospect Avenue   Hackensack, NJ 07601   (551)996-5308   Fax (201)996-9815

Chevinsky, Aaron H., MD {1598755316} SrgOnc, SrgCrC, SrgC&R(83,NY48)<NJ-MORRISTN>
+ Morristown Medical Center
  100 Madison Avenue/Suite C-4201   Morristown, NJ 07962   (973)971-7092   Fax (973)401-2481
+ Allied Surgical Group
  261 James Street/Suite 2-G   Morristown, NJ 07960   (973)971-7092   Fax (973)267-7295

Chew, Debra, MD {1366530982} InfDis, IntrMd(89,NY47)<NJ-UMDNJ>
+ University Physician Associates
  140 Bergen Street/ACC Level D   Newark, NJ 07103   (973)972-4071   Fax (973)972-3102

Chew, Jason M., DO {1891882254} FamMed(05,PA77)
+ Atlantic Care Physician Group
  201 West Avenue   Ocean City, NJ 08226   (609)391-7500   Fax (609)391-0963

Chew, Paul H., MD {1952698664} CdvDis, IntrMd(77,MD07)
+ Sanofi US-Sanofi-Aventis
  55 Corporate Drive   Bridgewater, NJ 08807

Chezian, Shanthi, MD {1114981735} Psychy, IntrMd(86,INA04)
+ Behavioral Medicine Associates, P.A.
  1550 Park Avenue/Suite 102   South Plainfield, NJ 07080   (908)561-6851   Fax (908)561-6863

Chhabra, Anjana R., MD {1780624718} IntrMd, Bariat(89,INA69)<NJ-HACKNSK>
+ Institute for Weight Management
  150 Overlook Avenue   Hackensack, NJ 07601   (201)487-8010   Fax (201)487-7010
  weightloss@mdslim.com

Chhabra, Mohina Singh, MD {1427261171} FamMed(96,GRN01)<NJ-HOBUNIMC>
+ 208 Russel Avenue/Apt 208
  Edgewater, NJ 07020

Chhabra, Rakesh S., MD {1962440677} Pedtrc, NnPnMd(82,INA69)<NJ-HACKNSK>
+ 30 Prospect Avenue
  Hackensack, NJ 07601   (201)996-5362   Fax (201)996-3232

Chhabra, Ravi, MD {1881893030} IntrMd<NJ-MEMSALEM>
+ Memorial Hospital of Salem County
  310 Woodstown Road   Salem, NJ 08079   (856)935-1000   Fax (856)935-9659

Chhada, Aditi, MD {1043415342} Gastrn
+ Hackensack Gastroenterology Associates
  130 Kinderkamack Road/Suite 301   River Edge, NJ 07661   (201)489-7772   Fax (201)489-2544

Chhatwal, Balwant K., MD {1235210808} ObsGyn(72,INDI)<NJ-KIMBALL, NJ-CENTRAST>
+ 705 Candlewood Commons
  Howell, NJ 07731   (732)367-7110   Fax (732)364-7054

Chheda, Monique Kamaria, MD {1588985188} Dermat
+ Moorestown Dermatology Associates
  110 Marter Avenue/Suite 102   Moorestown, NJ 08057   (856)235-6565

Chheda, Neha Das, MD {1295051696} Nephro
+ Bergen Hypertension & Renal Associates PA
  44 Godwin Avenue/Suite 301   Midland Park, NJ 07432   (201)447-0013   Fax (201)447-0438
  nmd630@gmail.com

Chheda, Samir Visanji, MD {1982831814} RadDia
+ Larchmont Medical Imaging
  210 Ark Road/Building 2   Mount Laurel, NJ 08054   (856)778-8860   Fax (856)866-8102

Chheda, Veena V., MD {1578622437} Psychy(73,INA67)<NJ-ANCPSYCH>
+ 33 Covington Lane
  Voorhees, NJ 08043

Chhibber, Geeta, MD {1851358360} MtFtMd, ObsGyn(74,INA79)<NJ-VIRTVOOR, NJ-VIRTMHBC>
+ Rowan SOM Department of Ob/Gyn
  405 Hurffville-Cross Keys Road   Sewell, NJ 08080   (856)589-1414   Fax (856)256-5772
+ The University Doctors - UMDNJ -SOM
  570 Egg Harbor Road/Suite C-2   Sewell, NJ 08080   (856)589-1414   Fax (856)589-6693

Chhipa, Irfan S., MD {1982962833} FamMSptM(10,GRN01)
+ Rothman Institute - Egg Harbor Township
  2500 English Creek Avenue/Bldg 1300   Egg Harbor Township, NJ 08234   (609)677-6060   Fax (609)677-6061

Chhokra, Renu, MD {1134201288} Anesth(91,INA72)<NJ-RWJUBRUN>
+ Robert Wood Johnson-UMDNJ Anesthesia Group
  125 Paterson Street/CAB 3100   New Brunswick, NJ 08901   (732)235-7827   Fax (732)418-8492
+ RWJ University Hospital New Brunswick
  One Robert Wood Johnson Place   New Brunswick, NJ 08901   (732)828-3000

Chi, Ching, MD {1780755058} Pedtrc(70,TAIW)<NJ-HCKTSTWN>
+ Ching-Hwa Chi MD PA
  3 State Route 57   Hackettstown, NJ 07840   (908)852-4404   Fax (908)979-0035

Chi, Jinhan, MD {1952383275} IntrMd(84,CHN4D)
+ The Heart Center of The Oranges
  310 Central Avenue/Suite 102   East Orange, NJ 07018   (973)395-1550   Fax (973)395-3711

Chi, Oak Z., MD {1275615320} Anesth(73,KOR11)<NJ-RWJUBRUN>
+ Robert Wood Johnson-UMDNJ Anesthesia Group
  125 Paterson Street/CAB 3100   New Brunswick, NJ 08901   (732)235-7827   Fax (732)235-6131

Chiang, Bessie, MD {1629160221} Ophthl(85,NY47)
+ 17 Sylvan Street/Suite 204
  Rutherford, NJ 07070   (201)507-1010   Fax (201)507-5900

Chiang, Chung, DO {1659507499} Pedtrc, IntrMd(06,NY75)<NJ-VIRTVOOR>
+ CHOP Care Network at Virtua Voorhees Hospital
  100 Bowman Drive   Voorhees, NJ 08043   (856)325-3000   Fax (609)261-5842

Chiang, Kou-Cheng, MD Anesth(78,JAPA)<NJ-ACMCMAIN>
+ 1450 Palisade Avenue
  Fort Lee, NJ 07024

Chiang, Peter Keh-dah, MD {1033281522} Ophthl(99,NJ05)<NJ-RIVERVW>
+ Eye Diagnostic Center
  3333 Fairmont Avenue   Asbury Park, NJ 07712   (732)988-4000   Fax (732)988-9502
+ Eye Diagnostic Center
  525 Route 70   Brick, NJ 08723   (732)988-4000   Fax (732)477-1444
+ Eye Diagnostic Center
  258 Broad Street   Red Bank, NJ 07712   (732)530-8500

Chiang, Robert Kent, MD {1306849526} Ophthl(99,CT01)<NJ-RWJUHAM>
+ Mercer Eye Associates, PA
  123 Franklin Corner Road/Suite 207   Lawrenceville, NJ 08648   (609)750-7300   Fax (609)896-7052

Chiang, Tom Shou, MD {1346345758} InfDis(00,DMN01)<NJ-VAEASTOR>
+ Infectious Disease Center of New Jersey
  22 Old Short Hills Road/Suite 106   Livingston, NJ 07039   (973)535-8355   Fax (973)535-8353
+ Infectious Disease Center of New Jersey
  653 Willow Grove Street/Suite 2700   Hackettstown, NJ 07840   (973)535-8355   Fax (973)535-8353

Chiang, Wendy M., MD {1083819916} OncHem, IntrMd(07,NJ05)
+ Hematology-Oncology Associates of Northern NJ
  100 Madison Avenue/PO Box 1089   Morristown, NJ 07962   (973)538-5210   Fax (973)644-9657

Chiappetta, Carl J., MD {1548258213} Psychy(73,NE06)
+ 1675 Whitehorse Mercerville Rd
  Trenton, NJ 08619   (609)890-1606

Chiappetta, Gino, MD {1124141858} SrgOrt(01,NJ06)<NJ-JRSYSHMC, NJ-RWJUBRUN>
+ University Orthopaedic Associates, LLC.
  Two Worlds Fair Drive   Somerset, NJ 08873   (732)979-2115   Fax (732)564-9032

Chiara, Bianca A., MD {1104031020} FamMed(04,NJ05)<NJ-BAYONNE, NJ-CHRIST>
+ Bayonne Medical Center
  29th Street at Avenue E/Fam Med   Bayonne, NJ 07002   (201)858-5000
+ Christ Hospital
  176 Palisade Avenue/Fam Med   Jersey City, NJ 07306   (201)795-8200
+ Hoboken University Medical Center
  308 Willow Avenue/Fam Med   Hoboken, NJ 07002   (201)418-1000

Chiaramida, Anthony J., MD {1477627750} CdvDis, IntrMd(78,CA06)
+ 280 Amboy Avenue
  Metuchen, NJ 08840   (732)902-6000   Fax (732)601-4757

Chiccarine, Anthony P., DO {1205897261} EmrgMd(96,PA77)<NJ-SHOREMEM>
+ Bayfront Emergency Physicians, P.A.
  1 East New York Avenue   Somers Point, NJ 08244   (609)653-3519   Fax (609)653-3247

Chiccone, Martha G., MD {1457512006} EmrgMd(77,MEX03)<NJ-COMMED>
+ Community Medical Center
  99 Route 37 West/EmergMed   Toms River, NJ 08755   (732)557-8000

Chichili, Eiswarya, MD {1376798074} IntrMd<NJ-WARREN>
+ KNJ Hospitalist Group, LLC.
  204 South Main Street   Manville, NJ 08835   (732)586-9035   Fax (908)213-6618

Chick, Charlene Elizabeth, DO {1386799245} FamMed, IntrMd(08,PA77)
+ University Hospital-University Family Medicine
  42 East Laurel Road/Suite 2100   Stratford, NJ 08084   (856)566-7020   Fax (856)566-6188

Chidambaram, Manjula S., MD {1447277132} Anesth(82,INDI)<NJ-RIVERVW>
+ Red Bank Anesthesia, LLC
  1 Riverview Plaza   Red Bank, NJ 07701   (732)530-2255   Fax (732)450-2620
+ Riverview Medical Center
  1 Riverview Plaza/Anesthesiology   Red Bank, NJ 07701   (732)741-2700

Chidyllo, Stephen A., MD {1578547311} SrgPlstc, SrgRec(87,PA09)<NJ-JRSYSHMC, NJ-RIVERVW>
+ Central Jersey Plastic Surgery
  107 Monmouth Road/Suite 106   West Long Branch, NJ 07764   (732)460-9566   Fax (732)460-9569
  Bodymakeover@optonline.net

Chieco, Michael Anthony, MD {1427027630} Pedtrc, EmrgMd(98,DMN01)<NY-LUTHERN>
+ Central Jersey Emergency Medicine Associates
  901 West Main Street   Freehold, NJ 07728   (732)942-2666   Fax (732)431-8267

Chien, Christina H., MD {1033556931} EmrgMd
+ Cooper Univerisry Emergency Physicians
  One Cooper Plaza   Camden, NJ 08103   (856)342-2000   Fax (856)968-8272

Chiesa, Drew Jonathan, DO {1689812505} Gastrn, IntrMd(08,PA77)
+ Kennedy Health Alliance Vascular Surgery
  333 Laurel Oak Road   Voorhees, NJ 08043   (844)542-2273   Fax (856)770-9194

Chiesa, Jennifer Elaine, DO {1154640050} FamMHPC
+ Samaritan HealthCare & Hospice
  5 Eves Drive/Suite 300   Marlton, NJ 08053   (856)896-1600   Fax (856)596-7881

Physicians by Name and Address

Chiesa, John C., DO {1649348582} Gastrn, IntrMd(73,PA77)<NJ-KMHSTRAT>
+ Kennedy Health Alliance
188 Fries Mill Road/Suite N-1   Turnersville, NJ 08012
(856)783-2241   Fax (856)783-2273
+ Kennedy Health Alliance Vascular Surgery
333 Laurel Oak Road   Voorhees, NJ 08043   (856)783-2241   Fax (856)770-9194

Chikani, Jignasa Ripal, MD {1447529045} Pedtrc
+ Drs. Burgher and Chikani
2950 College Drive/Suite C   Vineland, NJ 08360   (856)692-6000   Fax (856)692-0609

Chike-Obi, Toju O., MD {1356496129} Pedtrc(80,NIG03)<NJ-ST-BARNMC, NJ-NWRKBETH>
+ West Orange Pediatrics
81 Northfield Avenue/Suite 101   West Orange, NJ 07052
(973)324-5437   Fax (973)324-0356

Chikezie, Augustine O., MD {1669562393} PedEnd, Pedtrc(85,NIGE)<NJ-ACMCITY, NJ-ACMCMAIN>
+ South Jersey Pediatrics Endocrinology
6712 Washington Avenue/Suite 203   Egg Harbor Township, NJ 08234   (609)641-1155   Fax (609)641-1140

Chikezie, Pius U., MD {1609807379} IntrMd, InfDis(88,NIGE)<NJ-EASTORNG>
+ 6 Lahaway Creek Court
Millstone Township, NJ 08510   Fax (732)321-1150

Chilakapati, Manjula, MD {1568659779} Psychy(92,INA8Y)
+ 16 Bakley Terrace
West Orange, NJ 07052

Childs, Arthur L., DO {1871533620} IntrMd(86,NJ75)<NJ-BURDTMLN>
+ Dr. Arthur Childs Medical Home
307 Stone Harbor Boulevard/Suite 3   Cape May Court House, NJ 08210   (609)463-0555   Fax (609)463-0064
Drachilds@comcast.net

Childs, Julianne Wilkin, DO {1639166101} IntrMd, OncHem(86,MO78)<NJ-BURDTMLN, NJ-ACMCMAIN>
+ Hope Community Cancer Center LLC
210 South Shore Road/Suite 106-A   Marmora, NJ 08223
(609)390-7888   Fax (609)390-2614
HCCCChilds@aol.com

Childs, Kathryn Phyllis, MD {1023067741} Ophthl(91,NY08)
+ Ophthamology of Montclair, LLC
33 North Fullerton Avenue/Floor 1   Montclair, NJ 07042
(973)509-6039   Fax (973)509-6069
ophthamologyofmontclair@hotmail.com

Chillemi, Salvatore, MD {1285839431} IntHos
+ Rutgers- New Jersey Medical School
185 South Orange Avenue/I524   Newark, NJ 07103
(973)972-4300

Chilukuri, Neelima, MD {1619286226} IntrMd
+ 66 Berkshire Way
East Brunswick, NJ 08816

Chima, Kuljit Kaur, MD {1497794861} Dermat(96,NJ05)<NJ-CHILTON>
+ Corederm Dermatology and Cosmetic Center
246 Hamburg Turnpike/Suite 306   Wayne, NJ 07470
(973)956-0500   Fax (973)956-0522
+ K. Neena Chima MD LLC
508 Hamburg Turnpike/Suite 101   Wayne, NJ 07470
(973)956-0500   Fax (973)956-0522

Chimenti, James M., MD {1942203195} SrgNro(91,PA07)
+ Neurosurgical Associates of Central Jersey, P.A.
1200 Route 22 East/2nd Floor   Bridgewater, NJ 08807
(732)302-1720   Fax (732)302-1724
+ Raritan Valley Surgery Center
100 Franklin Square Drive/Suite 100   Somerset, NJ 08873
(732)302-1720   Fax (732)560-5999

Chin, Channing Yee, MD {1285870428} Surgry
+ New York Bariatric Group
1680 Route 23   Wayne, NJ 07470   (800)633-8446   Fax (516)625-2939

Chin, Christina W., MD {1225044654} Anesth, AnesPain(85,TAI04)
+ North Central New Jersey Periodonics
100 Town Center Drive   Warren, NJ 07059   (908)222-2777

Chin, Daisy Y., MD {1477501971} Pedtrc, PedEnd(92,NY08)<NJ-MORRISTN, NJ-OVERLOOK>
+ Morristown Medical Center
100 Madison Avenue/Pediatrics   Morristown, NJ 07962
(973)971-5000

Chin, Darren S., MD {1417934068} FamMed, IntrMd(96,NY03)<NJ-OVERLOOK>
+ Ohana Medical Spa
1765 East Second Street   Scotch Plains, NJ 07076
(908)322-2490   Fax (888)364-8160

Chin, Deanna G., MD {1275522609} RadDia(99,CT01)<NJ-STPETER, NJ-RWJUBRUN>
+ University Radiology Group, P.C.
579A Cranbury Road   East Brunswick, NJ 08816   (732)390-0040   Fax (732)390-1856
+ University Radiology Group, P.C.
10 Plum Street   New Brunswick, NJ 08901   (732)390-0040

Fax (732)249-1208

Chin, Kathleen L., MD {1811049430} Pedtrc(95,PA13)<NJ-ST-BARNMC, NJ-OVERLOOK>
+ The Pediatric Center
556 Central Avenue   New Providence, NJ 07974   (908)508-0400   Fax (908)508-0370

Chin, Meigra Myers, MD {1154512135} EmrgMd
+ University Emergency Medicine
125 Paterson Street/MEB 104   New Brunswick, NJ 08901
(732)235-8717   Fax (732)235-7379

Chin, Patrick K., MD {1396702783} Ophthl(89,NJ05)<NJ-VALLEY>
+ Westwood Ophthalmology Associates
300 Fairview Avenue/PO Box 698   Westwood, NJ 07675
(201)666-4014   Fax (201)664-4754
+ TLC New Jersey LASIK
475 Prospect Avenu   West Orange, NJ 07052

Chin, Stephanie Elaine, MD {1235344110} Pedtrc(06,NY06)
+ Alpert Zales & Castro Pediatric Cardiology, PA
1623 Route 88/Suite A/PO Box 1719   Brick, NJ 08723
(732)458-9666   Fax (732)458-0840

Chinai, Ronak N., MD {1235115312} IntrMd(00,DMN01)
+ Grove Medical Associates
129 Newark Avenue   Jersey City, NJ 07302   (201)451-8867
Fax (201)451-2819

Chinchankar, Rajeshree Prashant, MD {1003072034} ObsGyn
+ Hackensack University Medical Group Dumont
125 Washington Avenue   Dumont, NJ 07628   (201)374-2722   Fax (201)374-2723

Chinchilla, Miguel A., MD {1346217437} IntrMd, PulDis(64,MEXI)<NJ-RWJUBRUN, NJ-STPETER>
+ Drs. Hip Flores & Chinchilla
281 River Road   Piscataway, NJ 08854   (732)356-4665
Fax (732)356-4064
+ 4 East High Street
Bound Brook, NJ 08805   (732)356-8100

Chiniwala, Niyati Umesh, MD {1528219367} EnDbMt, IntrMd
+ Hackensack Meridian Endocrinology
2240 Route 33/Suite B   Neptune, NJ 07753   (732)897-3980
Fax (732)897-3982

Chinn, Bertram T., MD {1811968944} SrgC&R, Surgry(87,PA02)<NJ-JFKMED, NJ-SOMERSET>
+ Associated Colon & Rectal Surgeons PA
3900 Park Avenue/Suite 101   Edison, NJ 08820   (732)494-6640   Fax (732)549-8204

Chinn, Lawrence W., Sr., MD {1033379532} Anesth(04,NJ05)
+ Rutgers- New Jersey Medical School
185 South Orange Avenue/MSBE 547   Newark, NJ 07103
(973)230-2422

Chinn, Natasha R., MD {1609002419} ObsGyn
+ Brescia-Migliaccio Ob/Gyn
609 Washington Street   Hoboken, NJ 07030   (201)659-7700   Fax (201)659-7701
+ Hoboken University Medical Center
308 Willow Avenue   Hoboken, NJ 07030   (201)418-1000

Chinnici, Angelo A., MD {1417984659} IntrMd(82,ITAL)<NJ-JRSYSHMC, NJ-RIVERVW>
+ 601 Sunset Avenue
Asbury Park, NJ 07712   (732)775-7978   Fax (732)988-2545

Chinskey, Nicholas Daniel, MD {1174847941} Ophthl
+ Retina Associates of New Jersey, P.A.
525 Route 70 West/Suite B-14   Lakewood, NJ 08701
(732)363-2396   Fax (732)363-0403
+ Retina Associates of New Jersey, P.A.
2 Industrial Way West   Eatontown, NJ 07724   (732)363-2396   Fax (732)389-2788
+ Retina Associates of New Jersey, P.A.
530 Lakehurst Road/Suite 305   Toms River, NJ 08701
(732)797-3883   Fax (732)797-3886

Chinta, Bharath Kumar, MD {1033168422} RadDia(96,INA29)<PA-STVNCNT>
+ Coastal Imaging, LLC
79 Route 37 West/Suite 103   Toms River, NJ 08755
(732)678-0087   Fax (732)276-2325

Chinta, Viswanatha Reddy, MD {1326291089}<NJ-STFRNMED>
+ St. Francis Medical Center
601 Hamilton Avenue   Trenton, NJ 08629   (816)718-1059
drvisu3@gmail.com

Chintapalli, Nirmala K., MD {1497800619} Anesth(77,INDI)
+ 1 Richmond Street/Apt 4077
New Brunswick, NJ 08901   (732)514-1960   Fax (732)514-1960

Chinwalla, Farah, DO {1609038462} IntrMd
+ Americare Medical Associates, LLC
445 Whitehorse Avenue/Suite 202   Trenton, NJ 08610
(609)585-1122   Fax (609)585-0309

Chiodo, Damien F., MD {1548531502} Psychy
+ 48 Lehigh Street
Wharton, NJ 07885   (973)722-5439

Chiorazzi, Mary Lorraine, MD {1154412914} Psychy(70,DC02)
+ M. Lorraine Chiorazzi MD PA
163 Engle Street   Englewood, NJ 07631   (201)871-0646

Chirichella, Paul Sebastian, MD {1538553870}
+ North Jersey Brain and Surgical
680 Kinderkamack Road/Suite 300   Oradell, NJ 07649
(201)342-2550   Fax (201)342-7171

Chirico, Amy L., MD {1528326980}<NJ-HACKNSK>
+ Hackensack University Medical Center
30 Prospect Avenue   Hackensack, NJ 07601   (551)996-5455

Chiricolo, Antonio, MD {1295916997} Anesth
+ Robert Wood Johnson-UMDNJ Anesthesia Group
125 Paterson Street/CAB 3100   New Brunswick, NJ 08901
(732)235-7827   Fax (732)235-6131

Chiricolo, Heather Marie, MD {1184600595} PhysMd(00,MEX03)
+ Physical Medicine and Pain Center
34 Scotch Road   Trenton, NJ 08628   (609)883-0614   Fax (609)883-1606

Chirino, Maria E., MD {1114019163} IntrMd, EmrgMd(84,DOM02)<NJ-TRINIWSC, NJ-MEADWLND>
+ Trinitas Regional Medical Center-Williamson Street
225 Williamson Street/EmrgMed   Elizabeth, NJ 07207
(908)994-5000   Fax (908)994-5805

Chirla, Sujala, MD {1790946663} Gastrn, IntrMd(01,INA48)<NJ-JFKMED, NJ-RWJURAH>
+ Center for Digestive Diseases
695 Chestnut Street   Union, NJ 07083   (908)688-6565
Fax (908)688-3161

Chiromeras, Andrew, MD {1003201849} FamMed
+ Capital Health Primary Care-Hamilton
1445 Whitehorse-Mercerville Rd   Hamilton, NJ 08619
(609)587-6661   Fax (609)587-8503

Chism, Melissa A., MD {1861459596} Pedtrc(89,TX15)<NJ-VALLEY, NJ-CHILTON>
+ PediatriCare Associates
20-20 Fair Lawn Avenue   Fair Lawn, NJ 07410   (201)791-4545   Fax (201)791-3709
+ PediatriCare Associates
400 Franklin Turnpike   Mahwah, NJ 07430   (201)791-4545
Fax (201)529-1596
+ PediatriCare Associates
901 Route 23 South   Pompton Plains, NJ 07410   (973)831-4545   Fax (973)831-1527

Chitalia, Amit C., MD {1417280579}
+ 285 George Street/Unit 906
New Brunswick, NJ 08901   (603)598-6576
acc09@hotmail.com

Chithran, Payyanadan V., MD {1104804251} Anesth(69,INDI)
+ Englewood Anesthesiology
350 Engle Street   Englewood, NJ 07631   (201)894-3238
Fax (201)871-0619

Chitkara, Denesh Kumar, MD {1619996816} PedGst, IntrMd(96,OH40)
+ Celgene Global Health
86 Morris Avenue   Summit, NJ 07901   (732)673-9613
Fax (732)673-9001

Chitkara, Megha, MD {1356739338}<NJ-JRSYSHMC>
+ Jersey Shore University Medical Center
1945 Route 33   Neptune, NJ 07753   (732)775-5500

Chitnis, Subhanir Sunil, MD {1801152939} EmrgMd
+ University Hospital-New Jersey Medical School
30 Bergen Street/Bld 11/Rm1110   Newark, NJ 07107
(518)229-9083

Chityala, Haritha, MD {1306876305} Anesth(95,INA5B)<NJ-VIRTMARL>
+ Virtua Marlton Hospital
90 Brick Road/Anesthesiology   Marlton, NJ 08053
(856)355-6000

Chiu, Caroline, MD {1609865617} Pedtrc, AdolMd(95,NY09)<NJ-CHILTON>
+ New Jersey Pediatric & Adolescent Care, LLC.
1680 Route 23/Suite 350   Wayne, NJ 07470   (973)521-9700   Fax (973)521-9707

Chiu, Chi-Shin, MD {1437385424} AnesPain<NJ-NWRKBETH>
+ Newark Beth Israel Medical Center
201 Lyons Avenue   Newark, NJ 07112   (973)926-7655

Chiu, Kenny, MD {1518073782} IntrMd, Gastrn(99,NY47)<NJ-OCEANMC, NJ-SOCEANCO>
+ Coastal Gastroenterology Associates PA
525 Jack Martin Boulevard/Suite 301   Brick, NJ 08724
(732)840-0067   Fax (732)840-3169

Chiu, Nicholas, MD {1295736361} Anesth(95,NY08)<NJ-COMMED>
+ Red Bank Anesthesia, LLC
1 Riverview Plaza   Red Bank, NJ 07701   (732)530-2255
Fax (732)450-2620

Physicians by Name and Address

Chiu-Serodio, Lai-No, MD {1407839335} RadDia(92,NY19)<NJ-RWJUBRUN, NJ-RBAYOLDB>
+ University Radiology Group, P.C.
483 Cranbury Road   East Brunswick, NJ 08816   (732)390-0030   Fax (732)390-5383
+ University Radiology Group, P.C.
75 Veronica Avenue   Somerset, NJ 08873   (732)390-0030   Fax (732)246-4188
+ University Radiology Group, P.C.
260 Amboy Avenue   Metuchen, NJ 08816   (732)548-2322   Fax (732)548-3392

Chiumento, Marvin Joseph, MD {1497857635} Anesth, Dermat(84,BWI01)<NJ-CLARMAAS, NY-MTSINYHS>
+ 20 community Place/Suite 105
Morristown, NJ 07960   (973)538-4544   Fax (973)538-3703

Chiurco, Anthony A., MD {1578507620} SrgNro(67,PA02)<NJ-CHSFULD, NJ-CHSMRCER>
+ Neuro-Group, P.A.
3131 Princeton Pike   Lawrenceville, NJ 08648   (609)895-8898   Fax (609)895-8330
+ Neuro-Group PA at Hunterdon Medical Center
1100 Wescott Drive/Suite 301   Flemington, NJ 08822   (609)895-8898   Fax (609)788-6519

Chiusano, Emi A., MD {1205882438} FamMed, GenPrc(90,OH06)
+ MedExpress Urgent Care Woodbury
875 Mantua Pike   Woodbury, NJ 08096   (856)384-5949   Fax (856)384-5958

Chmara, Edward S., MD {1316258445} PthACl(99,NJ06)
+ 12 Crestmont Avenue
Ewing, NJ 08618

Chmarzewski, Barbara, MD {1194805655} PsyCAd, Psychy(97,NJ06)
+ St. Mary Community Mental Health Center
506 3rd Street   Hoboken, NJ 07030   (201)792-8200

Cho, Carleen K., MD {1205231982}
+ Cooper Surgical Associates
3 Cooper Plaza/Suite 411   Camden, NJ 08103   (949)466-8074   Fax (856)365-1180

Cho, Chang-Il, MD {1366470346} Pedtrc(67,KORE)
+ 1137 Park Avenue
Plainfield, NJ 07060   (908)756-2261   Fax (908)756-0513

Cho, Daniel P., MD {1598708679} Anesth, AnesPain(91,VA04)
+ Centennial Surgical Center LLC
502 Centennial Boulevard/Suite 1   Voorhees, NJ 08043   (856)874-0790

Cho, David Shen, MD {1801870365} RadOnc(98,VA04)<NJ-BURDTMLN>
+ Cape Regional Medical Center
2 Stone Harbor Boulevard/Rad Onc   Cape May Court House, NJ 08210   (609)463-2298   Fax (609)463-3071

Cho, Dong W., MD {1023190667} PhysMd(66,KORE)<NJ-EASTORNG, NJ-STCLRDEN>
+ 1001 Pleasant Valley Way
West Orange, NJ 07052   (973)325-7868   Fax (973)325-0211

Cho, Eun-Sook, MD {1780698803} PthAna, PthNro(65,KORE)<NJ-UMDNJ>
+ University Hospital
150 Bergen Street/Path   Newark, NJ 07103   (973)972-4145   Fax (973)972-5909

Cho, Grace C., MD {1396700282} Anesth(73,KOR03)<NJ-STPETER>
+ Anesthesia Consultnts of NJ/Nova Pain
285 Davidson Avenue/Suite 204   Somerset, NJ 08873   (732)271-1400   Fax (732)271-3543

Cho, Grace Shin, MD {1730990717} IntrMd, GenPrc(91,PA07)<NJ-OURLADY>
+ Cooper Physician Offices
900 Centennial Boulevard   Voorhees, NJ 08043   (856)325-6770   Fax (856)673-4300

Cho, Irene Soyoung, MD {1093910259} EnDbMt, IntrMd(03,NJ05)
+ Summit Medical Group
552 Westfield Avenue   Westfield, NJ 07090   (908)654-3377   Fax (908)654-4044
+ Rutgers- New Jersey Medical School
185 South Orange Avenue/MSB I-588   Newark, NJ 07103   (973)972-4300

Cho, Jason J., MD {1871589374} Pedtrc
+ McGuire Air Force Base/Acute Health Care Clinic
3458 Neely Road   Trenton, NJ 08641   (609)754-9201   Fax (609)754-9015

Cho, John S., MD {1417111600} PainMd, AnesPain(03,NJ06)<NJ-HOLYNAME>
+ Bethel Pain Management
385 Sylvan Avenue/Suite 23   Englewood Cliffs, NJ 07632   (201)871-4200   Fax (201)871-4211

Cho, Kun H., MD {1780619445} Surgry(63,KORE)<NJ-CHSFULD>
+ 40 Fuld Street/Suite 303
Trenton, NJ 08638   (609)393-3571   Fax (609)989-1153

Cho, Linda M., MD {1609884204} ObsGyn(02,NY09)<NJ-HACKNSK>
+ Bergen Ob-Gyn Associates, PA
130 Kinderkamack Road/Suite 300   River Edge, NJ 07661   (201)489-2727   Fax (201)489-5040
lindacho@gmail.com

Cho, Michael Ming-Huei, MD {1023101599} RprEnd, SrgGyn(93,PA12)<NJ-HACKNSK>
+ University Reproductive Associates, PC
214 Terrace Avenue/2nd Floor   Hasbrouck Heights, NJ 07604   (201)288-6330   Fax (201)288-6331
chomm@umdnj.edu

Cho, Seokkoon, MD {1740487628} Psychy(89,KOR11)<NJ-BERGNMC>
+ 121 Cedar Lane/Suite 3D
Teaneck, NJ 07666   (201)562-4736   Fax (201)580-4321

Cho, Soung Ick, MD {1801044557} IntrMd(04,PAR01)<NY-JACO-BIMC>
+ Heart & Vascular Associates of Northern Jersey
22-18 Broadway/Suite 201   Fair Lawn, NJ 07410   (201)475-5050   Fax (201)475-5522

Cho, Sung Hee, MD {1427220029} SrgO&M(10,GA05)
+ Riverside Oral Surgery
130 Kinderkamack Road/Suite 204   River Edge, NJ 07661   (201)487-6565
+ Riverside Oral Surgery
333 Old Hook Road/Suite 100   Westwood, NJ 07675   (201)664-2324

Chodha, Vicky, MD {1366884751} Psychy(11,NSK03)
+ Center for Family Guidance, PC
765 East Route 70/Building A-101   Marlton, NJ 08053   (856)797-4785   Fax (856)810-0110

Chodos, Wesley S., DO {1376970061} Gyneco, RprEnd(77,IA75)<NJ-VIRTVOOR, NJ-KMHCHRRY>
+ 16 Sunflower Circle
Lumberton, NJ 08048   (609)828-1131

Chodosh, Eliot Howard, MD {1235156969} Nrolgy(81,MEX03)<NJ-WAYNEGEN, NJ-CHILTON>
+ Neurologic Associates
220 Hamburg Turnpike/Suite 16   Wayne, NJ 07470   (973)942-4778   Fax (973)942-7020

Choe, Charles C., DO {1629081211} FamMed, GenPrc(03,AZ02)<NJ-HCKTSTWN>
+ Advocare Family Health at Mt. Olive
183 US Route 206/Suite 1   Flanders, NJ 07836   (973)347-3277   Fax (973)347-3141

Choe, Jin K., MD {1700893286} PthACl(70,KORE)<NJ-VAEASTOR, NJ-VANJHCS>
+ VA New Jersey Health Care System-East Orange Campus
385 Tremont Avenue   East Orange, NJ 07018   (973)676-1000   Fax (973)395-7126

Choe, Jisun Kim, MD {1649434366} IntrMd, IntHos(04,ARG01)<NJ-KMHSTRAT>
+ SOM - Department of Internal Medicine
42 East Laurel Road/Suite 3100   Stratford, NJ 08084   (856)566-6845   Fax (856)566-6906

Choe, Joseph Lee, MD {1912204777} Pedtrc
+ 45 West Columbia Avenue/Unit A
Palisades Park, NJ 07650   (201)450-7068

Choe, Jung Kyo, MD {1710963723} ObsGyn, RprEnd, FrtInf(71,KOR03)<NJ-COOPRUMC>
+ Cooper Institute for Reproductive Hormonal Disorders
17000 Commerce Parkway/Suite C   Mount Laurel, NJ 08054   (856)751-5575   Fax (856)751-7289

Choe, Philip Y., DO {1245512102}
+ Rowan University-School of Osteopathic Medicine
1 Medical Center Drive   Stratford, NJ 08084   (856)566-6708

Choe, Won Taek, MD {1790871416} Otlryg(00,CA11)<NJ-ENGLWOOD, NY-NYEYEINF>
+ ENT & Allergy Associates, LLP
433 Hackensack Avenue/Suite 204   Hackensack, NJ 07601   (201)883-1062   Fax (201)883-9297
wchoe@entandallergy.com

Choe, Wonsick, MD {1689070690}
+ Wayne Medical Care, PA
342 Hamburg Turnpike/Suite 101   Wayne, NJ 07470   (551)232-2532   Fax (973)942-5070
wonsick.choe@gmail.com

Choi, Bong H., MD {1083782783} Anesth(65,KOR07)<NJ-CLARMAAS>
+ Clara Maass Medical Center
1 Clara Maass Drive   Belleville, NJ 07109   (973)450-2000
+ Essex Ironbund Anesthesiologist LLC
155 Jefferson Street   Newark, NJ 07105   (973)450-2000   Fax (908)490-0067

Choi, Catherine Helen, MD {1467689018} Dermat(09,PA09)
+ Advanced Dermatology, P.C.
570 Egg Harbor Road/Suite C-1   Sewell, NJ 08080   (856)256-8899   Fax (856)256-8868

Choi, Chun W., MD {1952638132} SrgThr<NJ-RWJUBRUN>
+ RWJ University Hospital New Brunswick
One Robert Wood Johnson Place   New Brunswick, NJ 08901   (732)828-3000

Choi, Don W., MD {1548276769} IntrMd(70,KOR01)<NJ-JRSYSHMC>
+ 2100 Corlies Avenue/Suite 17
Neptune City, NJ 07753   (732)775-3187   Fax (732)775-6778

Choi, Edward Joung Myung, MD {1255362604} CdvDis, IntrMd(98,NC05)
+ Atlantic Cardiology LLC
444 Neptune Boulevard/Unit 2   Neptune, NJ 07753   (732)775-5300   Fax (732)988-9080
+ Atlantic Cardiology LLC
22 North Main Street   Marlboro, NJ 07746   (732)462-6666
+ Atlantic Cardiology, LLC
27 South Cooks Bridge Road/Suite 216   Jackson, NJ 07753   (848)217-3010

Choi, Hong Y., MD {1487677761} PthACl, PthCyt(68,KORE)<NJ-LOURDMED>
+ Lourdes Medical Center of Burlington County
218 Sunset Road   Willingboro, NJ 08046   (609)835-3065   Fax (609)835-3732
hychoi@aol.com

Choi, Hongsun, MD {1982665592} FamMed(84,GRN01)<NJ-VAEASTOR>
+ VA New Jersey Health Care System-East Orange Campus
385 Tremont Avenue   East Orange, NJ 07018   (973)676-1000

Choi, James, MD {1255321519} Urolgy(95,NY19)<NJ-OVERLOOK, NJ-MORRISTN>
+ Adult and Pediatric Urology of Hunterdon PA
5 Walter Foran Boulevard/Suite 4001   Flemington, NJ 08822   (908)751-5939   Fax (908)751-5938

Choi, Jay J., MD {1013925031} Anesth, PainMd(69,KORE)<NJ-EASTORNG>
+ 190 Midland Avenue
Saddle Brook, NJ 07663   (862)247-8080   Fax (862)247-8084

Choi, Jay Joonhyuk, MD {1821063199} ObsGyn, IntMBari(66,KORE)
+ United Medical, P.C.
612 Rutherford Avenue   Lyndhurst, NJ 07071   (201)460-0063   Fax (201)460-1684

Choi, Jea Keun, MD {1245329348} IntrMd(76,KORE)<NJ-CHRIST, NJ-JRSYCITY>
+ 550 Newark Avenue/Suite 301A
Jersey City, NJ 07306   (201)222-8288   Fax (201)222-8265

Choi, Jieun Susana, MD {1205881943} Anesth, PedAne(01,NY46)<NJ-SOMERSET, NJ-STPETER>
+ Anesthesia Consultnts of NJ/Nova Pain
285 Davidson Avenue/Suite 204   Somerset, NJ 08873   (732)271-1400   Fax (732)271-3543

Choi, Jong Eui, MD {1598787939} Anesth(75,KOR09)
+ Hackensack Anesthesiology Associates
140 Prospect Avenue/Suite 8   Hackensack, NJ 07601   (201)488-0066   Fax (201)488-6769

Choi, Jong I., MD {1568408904} FamMed(71,KORE)<NJ-BURDTMLN, NJ-SHOREMEM>
+ 6100 Landis Avenue/PO Box 143
Sea Isle City, NJ 08243   (609)263-1985   Fax (609)463-0654

Choi, Karmina, MD {1114223682} Surgry<NY-METHODST>
+ St. Joseph Medical Center Surgery
703 Main Street   Paterson, NJ 07503   (973)754-2490

Choi, Krissy, DO {1871864371}
+ Bergen Medical Associates
466 Old Hook Road/Suite 1   Emerson, NJ 07630   (201)967-8221   Fax (201)967-0340

Choi, Michael Namkyu, MD {1326350448} EmrgMd(06,IL01)<NJ-STPETER>
+ St. Peter's University Hospital
254 Easton Avenue/Emerg Med   New Brunswick, NJ 08901   (732)745-8600

Choi, Mingi, MD {1902802846} OthrSp, PainMd, PhysMd(87,NY47)<NJ-ENGLWOOD, NJ-SOMERSET>
+ Somerset Orthopedic Associates, PA
1081 Route 22 West   Bridgewater, NJ 08807   (908)722-0822   Fax (908)722-6318

Choi, Ok K., MD {1477668036} Pedtrc(74,KOR03)<NJ-MEADWLND, NJ-HACKNSK>
+ 1265 Paterson Plank Road/Suite 3E
Secaucus, NJ 07094   (201)330-1661

Choi, Patricia Hyunho, MD {1922078682} RadDia, Radiol(93,MD01)<NJ-STMRYPAS>
+ Diagnostic Radiology Associates of Northfield
772 Northfield Avenue   West Orange, NJ 07052   (973)325-0002   Fax (973)325-8140
+ Diagnostic Radiology Associates of Clifton
1339 Broad Street   Clifton, NJ 07013   (973)325-0002   Fax (973)778-4846
+ Diagnostic Radiology Associates of Cranford
25 South Union Avenue   Cranford, NJ 07052   (908)709-1323   Fax (908)709-1329

Choi, Sola, MD {1588644017} Dermat(01,MA01)
+ Princeton Medical Group, P.A.
419 North Harrison Street Princeton, NJ 08540 (609)924-9300 Fax (609)924-6552

Choi, Soon Chae, MD {1699778464} SrgOrt(66)<NJ-JFKMED>
+ Central Jersey Orthopaedic Specialists PA
1907 Park Avenue/Suite 102 South Plainfield, NJ 07080 (908)561-3400 Fax (908)769-5308

Choi, Stanley S., MD {1053337253} Surgry(67,KORE)
+ 34-36 Progess Street/Suite B-5
Edison, NJ 08820 (908)769-1020 Fax (908)668-1486

Choi, Sunny D., MD {1952360810} Anesth(80,VA01)<NJ-VALLEY>
+ The Valley Hospital
223 North Van Dien Avenue Ridgewood, NJ 07450 (201)447-8350
+ Bergen Anesthesia Group, P.C.
500 West Main Street/Suite 16 Wyckoff, NJ 07481 (201)447-8350 Fax (201)847-0059

Choi, Weekon, MD {1609806694} CritCr, PulDis, IntrMd(87,KOR14)
+ 17 Elm Avenue/3rd Floor
Hackensack, NJ 07601 (201)488-2210 Fax (201)488-2110
Wkchoimd@optonline.net

Choi, Yoonhee, MD {1669439543} Pedtrc(93,KOR05)<NJ-HACKNSK, NJ-ENGLWOOD>
+ Evergreen Pediatrics
1355 15th Street/Suite 190 Fort Lee, NJ 07024 (201)224-3344 Fax (201)224-4141

Choi, Yu-Jeong Alexis, MD {1942243035} IntrMd, Gastrn(99,NY01)<NJ-RIVERVW>
+ Red Bank Gastroenterology Associates PA
365 Broad Street/Suite 1-E Red Bank, NJ 07701 (732)842-4294 Fax (732)548-7408

Choi, Yun-Beom, MD {1194773192} Nrolgy(00,MA01)
+ Bergen Neurology Consultants
25 Rockwood Place/Suite 110 Englewood, NJ 07631 (201)894-5805 Fax (201)894-1956

Chokhavatia, Sita Shashikant, MD {1841219953} Gastrn, IntrMd(81,INA69)<NJ-UMDNJ, NJ-OVERLOOK>
+ RWJ Gastro & Hepatology
125 Paterson Street/CAB 5100B New Brunswick, NJ 08901 (732)235-7784 (732)235-7792
+ Gastrointestinal Associates PA
140 Chestnut Street/Suite 300 Ridgewood, NJ 07450 (732)235-7784 Fax (201)444-9471

Chokshi, Seema Patel, MD {1588893598} IntrMd(08,GRN01)
+ Premier Medicine & Wellness
231 Crosswicks Road/Suite 11 Bordentown, NJ 08505 (609)298-4750

Cholankeril, Mary G., MD {1588730212} IntrMd, OncHem(77,INA94)<NJ-TRINIWSC>
+ Drs. Reddy & Cholankeril
240 Williamson Street/Suite 205 Elizabeth, NJ 07202 (908)289-2070 Fax (908)289-4890
Marychol@yahoo.com

Cholankeril, Mathew V., MD {1588694780} CdvDis, IntrMd(79,INA97)
+ Cholankeril Medical Associates LLC
100 Grove Street Elizabeth, NJ 07202 (908)352-1738 Fax (908)820-0966
+ 1507 Saint Georges Avenue
Rahway, NJ 07065 (732)382-2177

Cholankeril, Matthew George, MD {1003204850} CdvDis
+ Cholankeril Medical Associates LLC
100 Grove Street Elizabeth, NJ 07202 (908)352-1738

Cholankeril, Michelle, MD {1801056155} OncHem<NJ-TRINI-WSC>
+ Trinitas Regional Medical Center-Williamson Street
225 Williamson Street Elizabeth, NJ 07207 (908)994-8771

Cholankeril, Thressiamma M., MD {1083644322} IntrMd(81,INA76)<NJ-TRINIWSC, NJ-RWJUBRUN>
+ Cholankeril Medical Associates LLC
100 Grove Street Elizabeth, NJ 07202 (908)352-1738 Fax (908)820-0966

Cholhan, Ruth C., MD {1447291653} IntrMd, Rheuma(86,GRN01)<NJ-ENGLWOOD>
+ 285 Engle Street
Englewood, NJ 07631 (201)871-0223 Fax (201)871-1117

Choma, Mtroslaw, MD {1689770042} ObsGyn, IntrMd(68,GER46)<NJ-OVERLOOK>
+ 2560 US Highway 22/Suite 226
Scotch Plains, NJ 07076 (908)316-8330 Fax (908)527-8550
+ 1156 Liberty Avenue/PO Box 248
Hillside, NJ 07205 (908)527-9555

Chomsky, Steven A., MD {1619016920} IntrMd(72,NJ05)
+ Comprehensive Care Center
297 16th Avenue Newark, NJ 07103 (973)485-3300 Fax (973)485-0226

Chon, Brian Hisuk, MD {1164459079} RadOnc(97,NJ06)<NJ-CENTRAST, NJ-HUNTRDN>
+ CentraState Medical Center
901 West Main Street/RadOncology Freehold, NJ 07728 (732)431-2000
+ Princeton Radiation Oncology Center
9 Centre Drive/Suite 115 Jamesburg, NJ 08831 (732)431-2000 Fax (609)655-5725

Chon, Jajin Thomas, MD {1346320553} EnDbMt(97,NY48)<NJ-MORRISTN>
+ Drs. Chon & Chon
435 South Street/Suite 230-A Morristown, NJ 07960 (973)971-6480 Fax (973)290-7435

Chong, Christopher K., MD {1851359962} ObsGyn(75,TAI02)<NJ-ACMCMAIN>
+ 76 West Jimmie Leeds Road/Suite 302
Galloway, NJ 08205 (609)652-3379 Fax (609)652-2078
chrischong@aol.com

Chong, Joseph K., MD {1366409476} ObsGyn(92,NY19)<NJ-HACKNSK>
+ 44 Sylvan Avenue/Suite 2-A
Englewood Cliffs, NJ 07632 (201)461-5770 Fax (201)461-5773

Chong, Penny Maria, MD {1710958665} Pedtrc(94,DC03)<NJ-OURLADY>
+ Lourdes Pediatric Associates
2475 McClellan Avenue/Building B201 Pennsauken, NJ 08109 (856)330-6300 Fax (856)330-6305

Chong, Raymond Ee-Mook, MD {1720239023} PsyCAd(03,NJ05)<NJ-UNIVBHC>
+ Central Jersey Beharioral Health, LLC
216 North Avenue East Cranford, NJ 07016 (908)272-7500 Fax (908)272-7502
+ Clifton Behavioral HealthCare
777 Bloomfield Avenue Clifton, NJ 07012 (973)594-0125

Choo, Nancy Hae-Jin, MD {1982791596} Ophthl(92,NY15)<NJ-WAYNEGEN>
+ Advanced Eye Care Center PA
220 Hamburg Turnpike/Suite 7 Wayne, NJ 07470 (973)790-1300 Fax (973)790-5310

Choo, Oliver Churl Jin, MD {1053540625}<NJ-STPETER>
+ St. Peter's University Hospital
254 Easton Avenue New Brunswick, NJ 08901 (732)745-8600

Choper, Joan Z., MD {1154327971} IntrMd(84,NY03)<NJ-KIMBALL, NJ-COMMED>
+ Blue Sky Medical, LLC
67 Lacey Road/Suite 5 Whiting, NJ 08759 (732)849-0707 Fax (732)849-0016

Choper, Niles E., MD {1083609069} ObsGyn, Gyneco(82,NY03)<NJ-OCEANMC, NJ-KIMBALL>
+ Women's Health Care & Aesthetics
1 Highway 70/Suite 6 Lakewood, NJ 08701 (732)364-1290 Fax (732)905-8649
drniles49@aol.com
+ Women's Health Care & Aesthetics
2290 West County Line Road Jackson, NJ 08527 (732)364-1290 Fax (732)905-8649
+ Women's Health Care & Aesthetics
1100 Route 70 West Whiting, NJ 08701 (732)364-1290 Fax (732)905-8649

Chopra, Anita, MD {1730169731} Grtrcs, IntrMd(73,INDI)<NJ-OURLADY, NJ-KMHSTRAT>
+ New Jersey Institute for Successful Aging
42 East Laurel Road/Suite 1800 Stratford, NJ 08084 (856)566-6843 Fax (856)566-6781

Chopra, Neeru Gera, MD {1619121498} BldBnk, PthAcl(87,INA72)
+ 4 North Longfellow Drive
Princeton Junction, NJ 08550

Chopra, Vinay, MD {1730329079} FamMed(08,DMN01)
+ 9 Dancer Lane
Freehold, NJ 07728

Chopra, Vinod Kumar, MD {1932427192} Surgry
+ Cooper Surgical Associates
3 Cooper Plaza/Suite 411 Camden, NJ 08103 (856)342-2000 Fax (856)365-1180

Chorney, Jeffrey R., MD {1619905775} OccpMd, OthrSp, Surgry(80,KS02)
+ 25 Manor House Drive
Cherry Hill, NJ 08003

Chorney, Stephanie Kim, MD (95,PA13)<NJ-UNVMCPRN>
+ University Medical Center of Princeton at Plainsboro
One Plainsboro Road Plainsboro, NJ 08536 (609)497-4000

Chottera, Shobha A., MD {1962579466} PsyCAd, Psychy, PsyAdd(82,INDI)<NJ-JRSYSHMC>
+ 3350 State Route 138/Suite 120
Wall, NJ 07719

Chou, Koulin L., MD {1588757165} Dermat(88,PA09)<NJ-VIRTVOOR>
+ Dermatology & Skin Care Center
2301 Evesham Road/Suite 103 Voorhees, NJ 08043 (856)772-6050 Fax (856)772-6404
koulin.chou@whallc.com

Chou, Lin W., MD {1083705560} IntrMd(84,CHNA)
+ Affiliates in Internal Medicine
311 Omni Drive Hillsborough, NJ 08844 (908)281-0632 Fax (908)281-9848
+ Affiliates in Internal Medicine
49 Route 202 Far Hills, NJ 07931 (908)281-0632 Fax (908)719-1091

Chou, Vivian K., MD {1780749945} ObsGyn, Gyneco(84,PA09)<NJ-OVERLOOK>
+ 340 Main Street
Madison, NJ 07940 (973)966-8590

Chouake, Benjamin S., MD {1891804654} EmrgMd, IntrMd(77,NY08)<NJ-HACKNSK, NJ-ENGLWOOD>
+ Emergimed
663 Palisade Avenue/Suite 101 Cliffside Park, NJ 07010 (201)945-6500 Fax (201)945-1157

Choubey, Sheela, MD {1023083441} ObsGyn(77,INA4X)<NJ-STPETER, NJ-RWJUBRUN>
+ Piscataway Somerset Ob/Gyn Group, LLP
31 Stelton Road/Suite 4 Piscataway, NJ 08854 (732)752-7755 Fax (732)752-7918
+ Piscataway Somerset Ob/Gyn Group, LLP
9 Clyde Road/Suite 101 Somerset, NJ 08873 (732)246-2280
+ Cares Surgicenter, LLC.
240 Easton Avenue New Brunswick, NJ 08854 (732)565-5400 Fax (732)296-8677

Choudhary, Anjali P., MD {1083703623} IntrMd(92,INA74)<NJ-JRSYCITY, NJ-CHRIST>
+ 550 Newark Avenue/Suite 406
Jersey City, NJ 07306 (201)216-9040 Fax (201)714-4828

Choudhary, Ratna, MD {1043253891} Anesth(91,INDI)
+ Morris Anesthesia Group, PA
3799 Route 46/Suite 211 Parsippany, NJ 07054 (973)335-1122 Fax (973)335-1448

Choudhry, Hammad S., MD {1346285079} Nephro, Grtrcs, IntrMd(00,GRN01)<NJ-BAYONNE>
+ 622 Broadway
Bayonne, NJ 07002 (201)436-2800 Fax (201)436-1353

Choudhry, Rafat S., MD {1467538835} IntrMd, FamMed(86,PAKI)<NJ-ACMCMAIN, NJ-SHOREMEM>
+ Regional Internal Medicine Associates
1004 South New Road Pleasantville, NJ 08232 (609)652-4141 Fax (609)652-9939

Choudhry-Akhter, Myra S., MD {1053666495}
+ Tatem Brown Family Practice
2225 East Evesham Road/Suite 101 Voorhees, NJ 08043 (856)795-4330 Fax (856)325-3704

Choudry, Abaid Ullah Anwar, MD {1235246588} IntrMd(98,NY08)
+ Parkside Medical Center
PO Box 4070 Jersey City, NJ 07304 (201)434-1111 Fax (201)432-0192
abaid@bigfoot.com

Choudry, Muhammad A., MD {1396828109} FamMed(01,DOM18)
+ 322 Sip Avenue
Jersey City, NJ 07306

Choudry, Omer F., MD {1922396647} Pedtrc
+ 322 Sip Avenue
Jersey City, NJ 07306

Choueiry, Rita, MD {1326271289}
+ 39 Allen Drive
Wayne, NJ 07470 (718)909-1187
rita-choueiry@hotmail.com

Choung, Edward W., MD {1073804027} Surgry(06,NJ05)
+ Northwest Surgical Associates
121 Center Grove Road Randolph, NJ 07869 (973)328-1414

Chovanes, John, DO {1124184577} Surgry
+ Cooper University Physician Trauma Center
One Cooper Plaza Camden, NJ 08103 (856)342-3014

Chow, Jessica C., MD {1992950232} FamMed(07,NJ75)
+ Health Consultants of New Jersey
516 Hamburg Turnpike/Suite 5 Wayne, NJ 07470 (973)925-7770 Fax (973)925-7772
+ Clifton Urgent and Primary Care
721 Clifton Avenue/Suite 2A Clifton, NJ 07013 (973)925-7770 Fax (973)779-7906

Chow, Matthew S.T., MD {1659367571} Anesth(89,NY01)<NJ-MORRISTN>
+ Morristown Medical Center
100 Madison Avenue/Anesthesiology Morristown, NJ 07962 (973)971-5000

Chow, Michael P., DO {1720286628}
+ Rowan University-School of Osteopathic Medicine
1 Medical Center Drive/Suite 162 Stratford, NJ 08084 (856)425-0796

Chow, Shih-Fen, MD {1861685588} IntrMd(91,NY01)<NJ-VIRTMHBC>
+ 2 Footes Lane
Morristown, NJ 07960 (973)656-1385 Fax (973)656-0856

Physicians by Name and Address

Chow, Shih-Han, MD {1245239466} Urolgy(92,NJ05)
+ Delaware Valley Urology LLC
63 Kresson Road/Suite 103 Cherry Hill, NJ 08034
(856)427-9004   Fax (856)267-2499

Chowdhrey, M. Salim, MD {1518092568} Psychy(68,PAK11)<NJ-STBARBHC, NJ-UNIVBHC>
+ St. Barnabas Behavioral Health Center
1691 US Highway 9/Attending Psych Toms River, NJ 08755
(800)300-0628
+ University Behavioral Health Care
671 Hoes Lane/PO Box 1392 Piscataway, NJ 08855
(732)235-5500

Chowdhrey, Mehar N., MD {1841326329} PhysMd(74,INDI)
+ 201 South Livingston Avenue/Suite 1B
Livingston, NJ 07039   (973)533-9370   Fax (973)533-9371

Chowdhry, Neil, MD {1881076610} IntrMd
+ Dr. Vinod K. Sinha, MD, PA
260 Hobart Street Perth Amboy, NJ 08861 (732)442-6464   Fax (732)442-6367

Chowdhury, Amina Kausar, MD {1760578785} PsyCAd(91,BAN03)
+ JFK Medical Center
65 James Street/BehavioralHlth Edison, NJ 08820
(732)321-7189

Chowdhury, Farhad Reza, DO {1063656882} OtgyFPlS(NJ75<NJ-RBAYOLDB>
+ ENT & Allergy Associates, LLP
3663 Route 9 North/Suite102 Old Bridge, NJ 08857
(732)679-7575   Fax (732)707-3850
+ ENT & Allergy Associates, LLP
485 Route 1 South/Bld B/Suite 350 Iselin, NJ 08830
(732)679-7575   Fax (732)549-7250

Chowdhury, Farys Reza, DO {1154556751} Anesth<NJ-JRSYSHMC>
+ 5 Ambrose Valley Lane
Piscataway, NJ 08854

Chowdhury, Khaza, MD {1831382340} IntHos
+ 7 White Hawk Way
Mays Landing, NJ 08330

Chowdhury, Shamima, MD {1154589026} IntrMd(97,BANG)
+ Heart & Vascular Medical Group
680 Broadway/Suite 116-A Paterson, NJ 07514   (973)684-3663   Fax (862)264-2386

Chowdhury, Shikha, MD {1225284607} IntrMd
+ After Hours Family Care
1001 Washington Boulevard Robbinsville, NJ 08691
(609)448-2401

Chowdhury, Zinnat A., MD {1528048527} IntrMd(87,BAN02)
+ New Jersey Institute for Successful Aging
42 East Laurel Road/Suite 1800 Stratford, NJ 08084
(856)566-6843   Fax (856)566-6781

Choy, Maria, MD {1093716268} Nrolgy, Elecmy, Acpntr(84,MA05)<NJ-BAYSHORE, NJ-CENTRAST>
+ Choy-Kwong, Maria
470 State Route 79/Suite 5 Morganville, NJ 07751
(732)591-5888   Fax (732)591-1133

Choy, Wanda Wai Ying, MD {1730187352} PulDis, IntrMd, CritCr(93,NY01)<NJ-VALLEY>
+ VMG Respiratory Health & Pulmonary Medicine
1200 East Ridgewood Avenue Ridgewood, NJ 07450
(201)689-7755   Fax (201)689-0521

Chrisanderson, Donna A., MD {1841251337} EnDbMt, IntrMd(88,GA01)<NJ-OVERLOOK>
+ 2040 Millburn Avenue/Suite 402
Maplewood, NJ 07040   (973)378-9070   Fax (973)378-8797

Chrisner, William Douglas, MD {1114154085}<NJ-VIRTMHBC>
+ Virtua Memorial
175 Madison Avenue Mount Holly, NJ 08060 (609)914-6000

Christensen, Brenda M., MD {1457327371} CdvDis, IntrMd(80,ITA01)
+ 466 Old Hook Road/Suite 12
Emerson, NJ 07630   (201)261-2228

Christian, Derick J., MD {1972594364} Surgry(98,NET09)<NJ-STPETER>
+ St. Peter's University Hospital
254 Easton Avenue New Brunswick, NJ 08901   (732)339-7633   Fax (732)745-8603

Christian, Sangita-Ann Justin, MD {1639276991} IntrMd, CritCr(98,NET09)<NJ-COOPRUMC>
+ Deborah Heart and Lung Center
200 Trenton Road Browns Mills, NJ 08015 (609)893-6611
Fax (609)735-0175

Christiana, William A., MD {1891884482} IntrMd(84,PA09)<NJ-CLARMAAS, NJ-MTNSIDE>
+ North Essex Medical Association
5 Franklin Avenue/Suite 609 Belleville, NJ 07109
(973)751-1410   Fax (973)751-9422

Christiano, Arthur A., MD {1578628764} PthACl, BldBnk, Pthlgy(67,DC02)<NJ-VALLEY>
+ The Valley Hospital
223 North Van Dien Avenue/Pathology Ridgewood, NJ 07450   (201)447-8242   Fax (201)447-8657

achrist@valleyhealth.com

Christiano, Arthur Patrick, MD {1780668483} Urolgy, IntrMd(94,NJ06)<NJ-RIVERVW, NJ-BAYSHORE>
+ Urology Associates, P.A.
595 Shrewsbury Avenue/Suite 103 Shrewsbury, NJ 07702
(732)741-5923   Fax (732)741-2759

Christiano, John M., MD {1477678126} IntrMd, OccpMd(79,PHI08)
+ Hoffman-La Roche Incorporated
340 Kingsland Street/Human Resources Nutley, NJ 07110
(973)235-3177   Fax (973)235-6228
john_m.christiano@roche.com

Christiano, Thomas R., MD {1487805800} Urolgy(06,NJ05)
+ New Jersey Center for Prostate Cancer & Urology
255 West Spring Valley Avenue Maywood, NJ 07607
(201)487-8866   Fax (201)487-2610
+ New Jersey Center for Prostate Cancer & Urology
200 South Orange Avenue/Suite 228 Livingston, NJ 07039
(201)487-8866   Fax (973)322-0135

Christiansen, David, MD {1811905318} EmrgMd(77,VA04)<NJ-HUNTRDN>
+ Pegasus Emergency Group
2100 Wescott Drive Flemington, NJ 08822 (908)788-6183
Fax (908)788-6516
dcedmd@juno.com

Christiansen, Keith Alan, MD {1679724694}
+ Sovereign Medical Group
15-01 Broadway/Suite 1 Fair Lawn, NJ 07410   (201)791-4544   Fax (201)791-6585

Christmas, Donald, MD {1841623170} IntrMd
+ St. Francis Medical Center
601 Hamilton Avenue Trenton, NJ 08629 (609)599-5000

Christodoulou, Evangelos, MD {1942232517} PsyCAd(94,NJ06)<NJ-SUMOAKSH>
+ St. Joseph's Regional Medical Center
703 Main Street/Psychiatry Paterson, NJ 07503   (973)754-3295

Christophe, Kathleen Mary, MD {1457390189} ObsGyn
+ CAMCare Health Corporation
817 Federal Street Camden, NJ 08103   (856)583-2415
Fax (856)541-3340

Christou, Alexander A., DO {1407992068} FamMed(04,PA77)<NJ-MORRISTN>
+ Summit Medical Group
95 Madison Avenue Morristown, NJ 07960   (973)267-1010   Fax (973)267-5521
+ Summit Medical Group
1 Anderson Hill Road/Suite 102 Bernardsville, NJ 07924
(973)267-1010   Fax (908)696-9943

Christoudias, George C., MD {1518043272} Surgry(69,GRE01)<NJ-HOLYNAME>
+ Surgical Oncology and Laparoscopy, P.A.
741 Teaneck/Suite B Teaneck, NJ 07666   (201)833-2888
Fax (201)833-1010

Christoudias, Moira Katherine, MD {1114139110} SrgBst(06,NJ05)
+ Robert and Audrey Luckow Pavilion
One Valley Health Plaza/Surgery Paramus, NJ 07652

Christoudias, Stavros George, MD {1679710875} Surgry
+ 95 Madison Avenue/Franklin/Surgery
Morristown, NJ 07960   (973)971-5684

Chrobok, Jan M., DO {1154544179} Psychy(66,PA77)
+ 930 Mt Kemble Avenue/1st Floor
Morristown, NJ 07960   (973)425-3434   Fax (973)425-8910
JANCHROBOK8@gmail.com

Chrucky, Roman, MD {1356384341} FamMed(70,SPA22)
+ North Jersey Developmental Center
169 Minisink Road/PO Box 169 Totowa, NJ 07512
(973)890-4542   Fax (973)890-4574

Chu, Alan, MD {1205178605}<NJ-HACKNSK>
+ Hackensack University Medical Center
30 Prospect Avenue Hackensack, NJ 07601   (551)996-3500

Chu, Alice, MD {1962513366} Rheuma, IntrMd(87,KOR05)
+ University Hospital Emergency Medicine
150 Bergen Street Newark, NJ 07103   (973)972-5128
Fax (973)972-6646
+ 889 Allwood Road
Clifton, NJ 07012   (973)972-5128   Fax (973)653-3028

Chu, Amy M., MD {1134127608} Anesth(93,NY48)<NJ-JFKMED, NJ-UMDNJ>
+ St. Joseph's Regional Medical Center Anesthesia
703 Main Street Paterson, NJ 07503   (973)754-2323   Fax (973)977-9455

Chu, Benny G., DO {1851483754} IntrMd(96,NY75)
+ Livingston Medical Associates, LLC.
449 Mount Pleasant Avenue/First Floor West Orange, NJ 07052   (973)535-8311   Fax (973)535-1210
+ Drs. Chu & Zauber
22 Old Short Hills Road/Suite 108 Livingston, NJ 07039
(973)535-8311   Fax (973)992-7648

Chu, Brian, MD {1154338556} Anesth, PainMd, FamMed(79,NY48)
+ Hand Surgery & Rehabilitation Center of New Jersey
5000 Sagemore Drive/Suite 103 Marlton, NJ 08053
(856)983-4263   Fax (856)983-9362

Chu, Chin-Chan, MD {1841514866} FamMed, IntrMd(06)
+ Patient first Urgent Care
630 Mantua Pike Woodbury, NJ 08096 (856)812-2220
Fax (856)812-2221

Chu, Ching-Huey, MD {1780725085} FamMed(94,PHI16)<NJ-WARREN>
+ St. Luke's Coventry Family Practice
755 Memorial Parkway/Suite 300 Phillipsburg, NJ 08865
(908)847-3300   Fax (866)281-6023

Chu, Daniel Yun, DO {1235222803} CritCr, IntrMd(86,NJ75)<NJ-HOBUNIMC>
+ Center for Family Health
122-132 Clinton Street Hoboken, NJ 07030   (201)418-3100   Fax (201)418-3148

Chu, David Shu-Chih, MD {1144260019} Ophthi, IntrMd(95,NY19)
+ St. Mary's Eye & Surgery Center
540 Bergen Boulevard Palisades Park, NJ 07650   (973)461-0021   Fax (201)242-9061
+ The Cornea & Laser Eye Institute
300 Frank W. Burr Boulevard Teaneck, NJ 07666
(973)461-0021   Fax (201)692-9646

Chu, Jae M., MD {1902992357} GenPrc(84,PHI14)
+ Woodbine Development Center/NJ Human Services
1175 Dehirsch Avenue Woodbine, NJ 08270   (609)861-2164   Fax (609)861-2494

Chu, Justin, DO {1275968570}<NJ-SJHREGMC>
+ SJH Regional Medical Center
1505 West Sherman Avenue Vineland, NJ 08360
(856)641-6023

Chu, Mary M., MD {1801025556} ObsGyn
+ Summit Medical Group
160 East Hanover Avenue/Suite 101 Cedar Knolls, NJ 07927
(973)605-5090   Fax (973)605-1705
+ 20 Second Street/Apt 202
Jersey City, NJ 07302

Chu, Regina Wong, MD {1659356558} RadDia, Radiol(93,NY03)<NJ-HACKNSK>
+ New Century Imaging at Oradell
555 Kinderkamack Road Oradell, NJ 07649   (201)599-1311
Fax (201)599-8333

Chu, Tony Nang-Tang, MD {1851370092} CdvDis, IntrMd, Int-Crd(87,TAI05)<NJ-JRSYSHMC, NJ-UNVMCPRN>
+ Shore Heart Group, P.A.
1820 State Route 33/Suite 4-B Neptune, NJ 07753
(732)776-8500   Fax (732)776-8946
+ Shore Heart Group, P.A.
9 Mule Road/Suite E-3 Toms River, NJ 08755   (732)776-8500   Fax (732)281-1105
+ Shore Heart Group, P.A.
35 Beaverson Boulevard/Suite 9-B Brick, NJ 07753
(732)262-4262   Fax (732)262-4317

Chu, Tsu M., MD {1518985548} ObsGyn(72,TAI04)<NJ-NWRKBETH>
+ 660 Springfield Avenue
Newark, NJ 07103   (973)375-2992   Fax (973)992-9204

Chu, Tun S., MD {1720048820} SrgVas, Surgry(74,TAIW)<NJ-COMMED>
+ ENT & Facial Plastic Surgery Assocs
1608 Route 88/Suite 240 Brick, NJ 08724   (732)458-8575
Fax (732)206-0578

Chu, Wei, MD {1073747739}(94,MD07)<NJ-RBAYPERT>
+ Jewish Renaissance Medical Center
275 Hobart Street Perth Amboy, NJ 08861   (732)376-9333
Fax (732)376-0139

Chu, Yie-Hsien, MD {1780644419} Pedtrc(98,PA02)<NJ-VALLEY>
+ Milestones Pediatric Group PA
11 East Oak Street Oakland, NJ 07436   (201)485-7557
Fax (201)485-7556

Chua, Jose, Jr., MD {1487651113} IntrMd(72,PHIL)<NJ-TRININPC, NJ-TRINIWSC>
+ Drs. Joshi & Chua
240 Williamson Street/Suite 203 Elizabeth, NJ 07202
(908)289-8060   Fax (908)289-8061

Chua, Lee Chadrick, MD {1942415716} IntrMd
+ 121 North Ohio Trail
Medford, NJ 08055

Chua Eoan, Pearl Davie, MD {1922068543} Pedtrc, AdolMd(91,NY48)
+ Summit Medical Group
75 East Northfield Road Livingston, NJ 07039   (973)436-1540   Fax (908)673-7336

Chuang, Connie T., MD {1275530313} IntrMd, GPrvMd(01,NY03)
+ EOHSI Clinical Center - UMDNJ
681 Frelinghuysen Road Piscataway, NJ 08855   (732)445-0123   Fax (732)445-0130

Physicians by Name and Address

Chuang, Ion S., MD {1821034448} EmrgMd(92,NJ06)<NJ-KMH-STRAT, NJ-KMHCHRRY>
+ Kennedy Memorial Hospital-University Medical Center
18 East Laurel Road/EmrgMed   Stratford, NJ 08084   (856)346-7985   Fax (856)346-6573
+ Kennedy Health System/Cherry Hill Campus
2201 Chapel Avenue West/EmrgMed   Cherry Hill, NJ 08002   (856)488-6500

Chuang, Linda I., MD {1518099175} Psychy, IntrMd(93,NY20)<NY-NYUTISCH>
+ Hudson Psychiatric Associates, LLC.
79 Hudson Street/Suite 203   Hoboken, NJ 07030   (201)222-8808   Fax (201)222-8803

Chuback, John A., MD {1124071261} Surgry, SrgThr(95,PA02)<NJ-MONMOUTH>
+ Cardiovascular Surgical Associates
350 Boulevard/Suite 130   Passaic, NJ 07055   (973)365-4567   Fax (973)916-5262
+ Cardiovascular Surgical Associates
11-01 Saddle River Road   Fair Lawn, NJ 07410   (973)365-4567   Fax (201)791-3538

Chubb, Paul Joseph, DO {1114121613} OrtSHand, IntrMd(05,PA77)
+ Advanced Orthopedics & Sports Medicine Institute
301 Professional View Drive   Freehold, NJ 07728   (732)720-2555   Fax (732)720-2556

Chudasama, Lalji S., MD {1174519250} CdvDis, IntrMd(68,UGA01)
+ Drs. Chudasama and Patel
1101 Raritan Road   Clark, NJ 07066   (732)381-3055   Fax (732)815-9330

Chudasama, Neelesh Lalji, MD {1740423805} IntrMd(09,NY01)
+ Drs. Chudasama and Patel
1101 Raritan Road   Clark, NJ 07066   (732)381-3055   Fax (732)815-9330

Chudner, Margarita, MD {1548544364} ObsGyn(08,PA09)<NJ-JFKMED>
+ 69 Brunswick Woods Drive
East Brunswick, NJ 08816   (732)927-1224   Fax (732)832-2946

Chudzik, Douglas W., MD {1477586931} IntrMd(72,MEX03)<NJ-BAYSHORE>
+ Drs. Chudzik and Chudzik
31 Village Court   Hazlet, NJ 07730   (732)264-1212   Fax (732)888-5452

Chudzik, Jeanmarie, DO {1679772495} IntrMd(05,NJ75)<NJ-MONMOUTH, NJ-BAYSHORE>
+ Drs. Chudzik and Chudzik
31 Village Court   Hazlet, NJ 07730   (732)264-1212   Fax (732)888-5452
+ Monmouth Medical Center
300 Second Avenue   Long Branch, NJ 07740   (732)222-5200

Chugh, Jagdish C., MD {1609980366} Pedtrc(80,INDI)<NJ-HCK-TSTWN, NJ-MORRISTN>
+ 182 Mountain Avenue
Hackettstown, NJ 07840   (908)852-8787   Fax (908)852-8187

Chugh, Rajinder P., MD {1316985724} IntrMd, EmrgMd(82,INA91)<NJ-VIRTBERL, NJ-VIRTVOOR>
+ Virtua Berlin
100 Townsend Avenue   Berlin, NJ 08009   (856)322-3000   Fax (856)322-3061

Chummar, Joseline, MD {1356761837} FamMed
+ Tatem Brown Family Practice
2225 East Evesham Road/Suite 101   Voorhees, NJ 08043   (856)325-3700   Fax (856)325-3705

Chun, Doreen Sze-Man, DO {1700836558} Pedtrc(94,PA77)<NJ-VIRTVOOR>
+ Cadoro Pediatrics, LLC
750 Route 73 South/Suite 307A   Marlton, NJ 08053   (856)983-9666   Fax (856)983-2662

Chun, Jay Y., MD {1548227663} SrgNro(98,NY01)<NJ-MORRISTN, NJ-ATLANTHS>
+ Atlantic Neurosurgical Specialists
310 Madison Avenue/Suite 300   Morristown, NJ 07960   (973)285-7800   Fax (973)285-7839
+ Short Hills Surgery Center
187 Millburn Avenue/Suite 101   Millburn, NJ 07041   (973)285-7800   Fax (973)671-0557

Chun, John Y., MD {1609858935} Anesth
+ Rancocas Anesthesiology Associates
700 US Highway 130 North/Suite 203   Cinnaminson, NJ 08077   (856)829-9345

Chun, Kye S., MD {1356371819} IntrMd(95,NJ03)
+ Prime Care Medical Group
55-59 Washington Avenue   Belleville, NJ 07109   (973)616-7117   Fax (973)616-7338

Chun, Shaun Joo Yup, MD EmrgMd(96,PA09)<NJ-UMDNJ>
+ University Hospital
150 Bergen Street/EmrgMed   Newark, NJ 07103   (973)972-4300

Chun, Thomas Young, MD {1407846827} Urolgy(91,DC01)<NJ-ENGLWOOD, NJ-HOLYNAME>
+ The Urology Center of Englewood, PA
663 Palisade Avenue/Suite 304   Cliffside Park, NJ 07010   (201)313-1933   Fax (201)313-9599
+ The Urology Center of Englewood, PA
300 Grand Avenue/Suite 102   Englewood, NJ 07631   (201)313-1933   Fax (201)816-1777

Chundru, Vasudha, MD {1184783490} Pedtrc, PedEmg(92,INDI)
+ RWJ University Pediatric Emergency Medicine
125 Paterson Street/MEB 342   New Brunswick, NJ 08903   (732)235-7893   Fax (732)235-9340
+ University Pediatric Associates PA
317 Cleveland Avenue   Highland Park, NJ 08904   (732)235-7893   Fax (732)249-7827

Chundury, Anupama, MD {1407199250}
+ Rutgers Cancer Institute of New Jersey
195 Little Albany Street/PO Box 2681   New Brunswick, NJ 08903   (732)235-8078   Fax (732)235-6797

Chung, Angela F., DO {1831520170} FamMed(13,NY75)
+ Blair Medical Associates PA
261 James Street/Suite 2A   Morristown, NJ 07960   (973)539-2468   Fax (973)539-7699

Chung, Dae S., MD {1376618892} Anesth(68,KOR01)<NJ-STBARNMC>
+ New Jersey Anesthesia Associates, P.C.
252 Columbia Turnpike/PO Box 0037   Florham Park, NJ 07932   (973)660-9334   Fax (973)660-9779

Chung, Daniel Hansam, MD {1578544078} Anesth(97,NY19)<NJ-MORRISTN>
+ Anesthesia Associates of Morristown
264 South Street/Suite 2A   Morristown, NJ 07960   (973)631-8119

Chung, Grace U., MD {1235111436} Dermat(85,NY15)
+ Center for Dermatology
17 West Red Bank Avenue/Suite 205   Woodbury, NJ 08096   (856)853-0900   Fax (856)853-5838

Chung, Haeyang, MD {1285670059} IntrMd, Pedtrc(81,KORE)<NJ-HOLYNAME>
+ 11 East Harwood Terrace
Palisades Park, NJ 07650   (201)313-1500   Fax (201)941-4157

Chung, Hei Jin, MD {1821077868} Surgry(89,BRA04)<NJ-WARREN>
+ 601 Coventry Drive
Phillipsburg, NJ 08865   (908)859-5676   Fax (908)859-2576

Chung, Inyoung, MD {1366595811} IntrMd, MedOnc, Hemato(71,KOR04)
+ 4 Progress Street/Suite A-7
Edison, NJ 08820   (908)755-7440   Fax (908)755-6999

Chung, Jacob H., MD {1245271717} Ophthl(02,NY19)
+ 621 Phillip Lane
Watchung, NJ 07069
+ Tenafly Eye Associates, PA
111 Dean Drive/Suite 2   Tenafly, NJ 07670   Fax (201)567-1354

Chung, Jae Won, MD {1629071840} Anesth(99,BLZ01)<NJ-STMRYPAS>
+ St. Mary's Hospital
350 Boulevard/Anesth   Passaic, NJ 07055   (973)365-4300

Chung, Jaehoon, MD {1205138500}
+ Drs. Di Vagno, Hasan & Chung
216 Route 17 North/Suite 201   Rochelle Park, NJ 07662   (201)753-1147   Fax (201)845-4040
jchung811@gmail.com

Chung, Jean Young, MD {1174737035} RadDia(01,PA01)<NJ-MORRISTN>
+ Memorial Radiology Associates
10 Lanidex Plaza West/Suite 125   Parsippany, NJ 07054   (973)503-5700   Fax (973)386-5701

Chung, Jeff, MD {1083684088} IntrMd, Rheuma(98,NY08)
+ Bergen Medical Associates
1 West Ridgewood Avenue/Suite 301   Paramus, NJ 07652   (201)445-1660   Fax (201)445-4296

Chung, John Wonkook, MD {1134224926} IntrMd(73,KOR06)<NJ-CHSFULD, NJ-STFRNMED>
+ 1450 Parkside Avenue/Suite 5
Trenton, NJ 08638   (609)882-2225   Fax (609)538-0177
johnwchung@comcast.net

Chung, Jooyeun, MD {1194932418} Surgry, IntrMd(02,PA01)<MA-BRIGWMN, MA-FAULKNR>
+ Capital Health Medical
2 Capital Way/Suite 356   Pennington, NJ 08534   (609)537-6000   Fax (609)537-6002

Chung, Kai B., MD {1437221306} GenPrc, PthAcl(70,KORE)
+ Vineland Developmental Center
1676 East Landis Avenue/PO Box 1513   Vineland, NJ 08362   (856)696-6000

Chung, Lynn S., MD {1902169832} FamMed
+ Patient first
2171 Route 70 West   Cherry Hill, NJ 08002   (856)406-0023   Fax (856)406-0024

Chung, Margaret U., MD {1578526489} IntrMd, InfDis(84,PHI08)<NJ-ACMCITY>
+ 20 Hospital Drive/Suite 9
Toms River, NJ 08755   (732)797-1979   Fax (732)797-1979

Chung, Myung K., MD {1609971803} FamMed, Acpntr, Pedtrc(81,WA04)
+ Drs. Chung & Shin
110 Marter Avenue/Suite 507   Moorestown, NJ 08057   (856)222-4766   Fax (856)222-1137

Chung, Nam Young, MD {1740586163} Pedtrc, IntrMd(89,KOR01)
+ Smart Care Pediatrics
158 Linwood plaza/Suite 326-328   Fort Lee, NJ 07024   (201)808-8610   Fax (201)875-5443
md@smartcarenj.com
+ Englewood Medical Associates Pediatrics
350 Engle Street   Englewood, NJ 07631   (201)808-8610   Fax (201)894-5649

Chung, Paul Kevin, MD {1669525093} OncHem, IntrMd, Onclgy(98,GRN01)<NJ-SOCEANCO>
+ Meridian Hematology & Oncology
1100 Route 72 West   Manahawkin, NJ 08050   (609)597-0547   Fax (609)597-8668

Chung, Soo K., MD {1952383416} Anesth(70,KOR06)
+ Campus Eye Group & Laser Center
1700 Whitehorse Hamilton Sq Rd   Hamilton Square, NJ 08690   (609)587-2020   Fax (609)588-9545

Chung, Sung K., MD {1477524742} Anesth, PainMd(70,KORE)
+ 212 Navajo Court
Morganville, NJ 07751

Chung, Uei K., MD {1487737193} ObsGyn(70,KOR05)
+ 975 Inman Avenue
Edison, NJ 08820   (908)561-0022   Fax (908)561-0054

Chung, Y. C. Emily, MD {1154391076} FamMed(98,NJ05)
+ Capital Health Primary Care
4056 Quakerbridge Road/Suite 101   Lawrenceville, NJ 08648   (609)528-9150   Fax (609)528-9151

Chung Loy, Harold E., MD {1811002728} Surgry, SrgVas(80,DC03)
+ All Care Family Medicine, LLC
3 Lincoln Highway/Suite 101   Edison, NJ 08820   (732)494-4500   Fax (732)494-2818

Church, Amy F., MD {1831191212} EmrgMd(94,MD01)<NJ-RWJUBRUN>
+ UH- Robert Wood Johnson Med
125 Paterson Street/MEB 388-C   New Brunswick, NJ 08901   (732)828-3000

Churgin, Warren K., MD {1447255583} IntrMd(80,MEX03)<NJ-MONMOUTH>
+ Eatontown Medical Associates
158 Wyckoff Road   Eatontown, NJ 07724   (732)544-9500   Fax (732)544-0132

Churlin, Donna M., MD {1164451340} Pedtrc, IntrMd(87,NJ05)
+ CAMCare Health Corporation
817 Federal Street/Suite 100   Camden, NJ 08103   (856)541-9811   Fax (856)541-4611

Churrango, Jose, MD {1386879914}
+ 46 Wedgewood Drive
Verona, NJ 07044   (862)686-8738

Chusid, Boris Gregory, MD {1518967769} Gastrn, IntrMd(95,RI01)<NY-LENOXHLL>
+ 700 High Woods Drive
Franklin Lakes, NJ 07417   (201)289-1121   Fax (201)560-1695

Chustek, Michael Aaron, MD {1609083393} Psychy<NJ-MORRISTN>
+ Morristown Medical Center
100 Madison Avenue   Morristown, NJ 07962   (973)971-5000

Chutke, Prashant Vithal, MD {1083782312} Pedtrc, EmrgMd(91,INA65)<NJ-STPETER>
+ EmCare
1945 Route 33   Neptune, NJ 07753   (732)776-4510   Fax (732)776-2329

Chuzhin, Yelena, MD {1881691707} Rheuma(86,RUSS)<NJ-STBARNMC>
+ The Osteoporosis and Metabolic Bone Disease Center
200 South Orange Avenue   Livingston, NJ 07039   (973)322-7302   Fax (973)322-7435

Chvala, Robert P., MD {1609458094} IntrMd, Nephro(76,NJ06)
+ Lyons & Chvala Nephrology Associates
730 North Broad Street/Suite 101   Woodbury, NJ 08096   (856)384-0147

Chyu, Darrick J., MD {1699901272} Anesth(PA13
+ Robert Wood Johnson-UMDNJ Anesthesia Group
125 Paterson Street/CAB 3100   New Brunswick, NJ 08901   (732)235-7827   Fax (732)235-6131

Ciambotti, Gary Francis, MD {1356327183} Gastrn, IntrMd(86,MNT01)<NJ-SOMERSET>
+ Digestive HealthCare Center
511 Courtyard Drive/Building 500   Hillsborough, NJ 08844   (908)218-9222   Fax (908)218-9818
gutman@po.com

Physicians by Name and Address

Ciatti, Sabatino, MD {1023002664} Dermat, SrgDer(92,NJ06)<NJ-OVERLOOK>
+ Advanced Dermatology, Laser, and MOHS Surgery Center
240 East Grove Street   Westfield, NJ 07090   (908)232-6446   Fax (908)232-6447
ciatti1@aol.com

Ciavarella, David Joseph, MD {1891810727} BldBnk, IntrMd, Pthlgy(77,CA14)<NY-NYUTISCH>
+ Johnson & Johnson Research & Develop
920 US Highway Route 202   Raritan, NJ 08869   (908)704-3819   Fax (908)218-4624
dciavare@odsos.jnj.com

Cicalese, Gerard R., MD {1871779579} ObsGyn(89,NJ05)<NJ-CLARMAAS>
+ 330 Washington Avenue
Belleville, NJ 07109   (973)751-4300   Fax (973)751-7577

Ciccone, Antonio, DO {1750413464} EmrgMd, FamMed, IntrMd(90,NJ75)<NJ-MORRISTN>
+ 727 Joralemon Street
Belleville, NJ 07109   (973)751-2060   Fax (973)751-2291
+ Silver Lake Medical
50 Newark Avenue/Suite 205   Belleville, NJ 07109   (973)751-2060   Fax (973)751-2291

Ciccone, Michael Paul, MD {1649294034} Urolgy(97,DC01)
+ Urology Consultants, PA
36 Newark Avenue/Suite 200   Belleville, NJ 07109   (973)759-6950   Fax (973)759-2006

Ciccone, Patrick N., MD {1477576643} Urolgy(67,DC02)
+ Urology Consultants, PA
36 Newark Avenue/Suite 200   Belleville, NJ 07109   (973)759-6950   Fax (973)759-2006

Ciceron, Andre, MD {1265526586} Urolgy, Onclgy(70,HAIT)<NJ-SHOREMEM>
+ Pavilion Ob/Gyn AtlantiCare
443 Shore Road/Suite 101   Somers Point, NJ 08244   (609)926-5838   Fax (609)926-5839

Ciceron, Asuncion V., MD {1588619258} ObsGyn(70,PHIL)<NJ-ACMCMAIN, NJ-SHOREMEM>
+ Pavilion Ob/Gyn AtlantiCare
443 Shore Road/Suite 101   Somers Point, NJ 08244   (609)677-7211   Fax (609)611-7210
mavcmd@msn.com

Ciciarelli, John G., II, MD {1629085691} IntrMd(81,MA07)<NJ-JRSYSHMC, NJ-MONMOUTH>
+ Ocean Park Medical Associates
1900 Highway 35/Suite 200   Oakhurst, NJ 07755   (732)663-0900   Fax (732)663-0901

Ciciola, Gerald F., MD {1003916297} ObsGyn(90,NJ05)<NJ-STBARNMC>
+ Partners for Women's Health PA
95 Northfield Avenue   West Orange, NJ 07052   (973)736-4505   Fax (973)376-9066

Cicogna, Cristina Emanuela, MD {1083681282} InfDis, IntrMd(86,SWIT)<NJ-HACKNSK>
+ Center for Infectious Diseases
20 Prospect Avenue/Suite 507   Hackensack, NJ 07601   (201)487-4088   Fax (201)489-8930

Cid, Georgina R., MD {1871672121} Psychy(76,PHIL)<NJ-JRSYSHMC>
+ 1222 Route 9
Howell, NJ 07731   (732)294-0165   Fax (732)294-0165

Cidambi, Indra Kumar, MD {1528097631} Psychy, PsyAdd(94,UZB03)<NY-BLVUENYU>
+ 43 Maple Avenue
Morristown, NJ 07960   (908)432-1929
Cidambi.Rumar@gmail.com

Ciechanowska, Malgorzata M., MD {1164514063} EnDbMt, IntrMd(81,POL03)
+ 142 Palisade Avenue/Suite 216
Jersey City, NJ 07306   (201)714-4668   Fax (201)714-9881

Ciechanowski, George J., MD {1407932650} IntrMd, PulDis(81,POL08)<NJ-CHRIST>
+ 408 Summit Avenue/First Floor
Jersey City, NJ 07306   (201)963-7000   Fax (201)963-8331

Ciencewicki, Michael, Jr., MD {1972670313} IntrMd(76,MEXI)<NJ-RBAYOLDB, NJ-RBAYPERT>
+ 51 Sandalwood Drive
Marlboro, NJ 07746   (732)577-0636   Fax (732)577-2877

Ciervo, Alfonso Clemente, MD {1457346918} Surgry(93,NY08)<NJ-BAYSHORE, NJ-RIVERVW>
+ 142 Highway 35/Suite 106
Eatontown, NJ 07724   (732)380-1222

Ciervo, Carman A., DO {1851371991} FamMed(88,PA77)<NJ-KMHCHRRY>
+ UMDNJ SOM Family Medicine
310 Creek Crossing Boulevard   Hainesport, NJ 08036   (609)702-7500   Fax (609)702-5928

Cifaldi, Ralph John, Jr., DO {1508965344} ObsGyn, IntrMd(92,NJ75)
+ Lozito Medical Associates
484 Lafayette Avenue   Hawthorne, NJ 07506   (973)423-4770   Fax (973)423-4816

Cifelli, Antonio, MD {1245228451} IntrMd(79,ITAL)<NJ-MORRISTN>
+ 116 Littleton Road
Morris Plains, NJ 07950   (973)829-0191   Fax (973)829-1562

Cifelli, John Riggio, MD {1295709566} SrgNro
+ 1054 Clifton Avenue
Clifton, NJ 07013

Cilursu, Ana Maria, MD {1275598104} IntrMd, Rheuma(82,BRA44)<NJ-ACMCITY, NJ-ACMCMAIN>
+ Shore Physician Group
401 Bethel Road   Somers Point, NJ 08244   (609)365-6200   Fax (609)365-6201
pal4life@comcast.net

Cimafranca, Daniel L., MD {1891877932} IntrMd, Grtrcs(78,PHI10)
+ Primary Care Medical Clinic
441 US Highway 130   East Windsor, NJ 08520   (609)336-7518   Fax (609)689-3888
danabell3@verizon.net

Ciminelli, Maria F., MD {1164447470} FamMed(96,NJ05)<NJ-RWJUBRUN, NJ-STPETER>
+ CentraState Family Medicine Residency Practice
1001 West Main Street/Suite B   Freehold, NJ 07728   (732)294-2540   Fax (732)294-9328
+ Family Medicine at Monument Square
317 George Street   New Brunswick, NJ 08901   (732)294-2540   Fax (732)246-7317

Ciminello, Frank Salvatore, MD {1699746875} SrgRec, SrgPlstc(00,NY09)<NJ-UMDNJ>
+ Vanguard Wellness Center
113 West Essex Street/Suite 204   Maywood, NJ 07607   (201)289-5551   Fax (201)843-2390
+ University Hospital-Doctors Office Center
90 Bergen Street/DOC 7200   Newark, NJ 07103   (201)289-5551   Fax (973)972-8268

Cimino, Robert, MD {1417992637} EmrgMd(02,NJ06)<NJ-BURDTMLN>
+ Cape Regional Medical Center
2 Stone Harbor Boulevard/EmrgMed   Cape May Court House, NJ 08210   (609)463-2000   Fax (609)463-2946

Cina, Anthony Joseph, MD {1114275641}<NJ-STBARNMC>
+ St. Barnabas Medical Center
94 Old Short Hills Road   Livingston, NJ 07039   (973)322-5000

Cinberg, James Z., MD {1801892732} Otlryg, Neutgy(70,NY01)
+ James Z. Cinberg MD PA
219 South Broad Street   Elizabeth, NJ 07202   (908)527-1717   Fax (908)527-1710

Cindrario, Dean P., MD {1063448207} Anesth, PainInvt(88,DC02)<NJ-JRSYSHMC>
+ Jersey Shore Anesthesiology Associates
1945 Route 33/PO Box 397   Neptune, NJ 07754   (732)922-3308   Fax (732)897-0263
+ Jersery Shore Anesthesiology
1945 Highway 33   Neptune, NJ 07753   (732)922-3308   Fax (732)897-0263

Cinotti, Donald J., MD {1255449153} Ophthl(76,MEXI)<NJ-CHRIST>
+ Hudson Eye Physicians & Surgeons, LLC
600 Pavonia Avenue/6th Floor   Jersey City, NJ 07306   (201)963-3937   Fax (201)963-8823
floor6@aol.com

Cioce, Anthony J., DO {1063466357} FamMed(93,MO79)<NJ-MORRISTN, NJ-SOMERSET>
+ Summit Medical Group
95 Madison Avenue   Morristown, NJ 07960   (973)285-7610

Cioce, Gerald, MD {1093817512} IntCrd, IntrMd(01,NJ02)
+ Cardiology Associates of Sussex County LLP
222 High Street/Suite 205   Newton, NJ 07860   (973)579-2100   Fax (973)579-6638

Cioce, Thomas G., DO {1386780310} FamMed
+ Summit Medical Group
95 Madison Avenue   Morristown, NJ 07960   (973)267-1010   Fax (973)267-5521
+ Summit Medical Group
1 Anderson Hill Road/Suite 102   Bernardsville, NJ 07924   (973)267-1010   Fax (908)696-9943

Ciocon, David Hermogenes, MD {1790878866} Dermat, DerMOH(02,NJ05)
+ Skin Laser & Surgery Specialists
105 Raider Boulevard/Suite 203   Hillsborough, NJ 08844   (201)441-9890   Fax (201)441-9893
+ Skin Laser & Surgery Specialists
20 Prospect Avenue/Suite 702   Hackensack, NJ 07601   (201)441-9890   Fax (201)441-9893

Cioffi, Francis J., MD {1396828208} ObsGyn(68,NJ05)<NJ-STPETER, NJ-JFKMED>
+ University Medical Group/OBGYN
125 Paterson Street/2nd Floor   New Brunswick, NJ 08901   (732)235-6600   Fax (732)235-6627

Ciolino, Charles P., MD {1841393121} Psychy(81,DC02)<NJ-OVERLOOK>
+ CCVS Care LLC
597 Springfield Avenue   Summit, NJ 07901   (908)654-7399
+ Summit Medical Group
654 Springfield Avenue   Berkeley Heights, NJ 07922   (908)654-7399   Fax (908)665-2794

Ciolino, Robert B., MD {1962577494} Anesth(83,NJ05)<NJ-STBARNMC>
+ New Jersey Anesthesia Associates, P.C.
252 Columbia Turnpike/PO Box 0037   Florham Park, NJ 07932   (973)660-9334   Fax (973)660-9779

Ciongoli, Bernard C., DO {1952535593} Anesth
+ Hackensack University MC-Anesthesia Dept
30 Prospect Avenue/Room 2703   Hackensack, NJ 07601   (201)996-2419   Fax (201)996-3962

Ciora, Cristian Dan, MD {1326067406} Psychy(96,ROM04)
+ 163 Engle Street/Suite 1A
Englewood, NJ 07631   (201)569-6100

Ciorlian, Cristina C., MD {1730160862} EnDbMt, IntrMd(91,ROM01)<NJ-JRSYSHMC>
+ 700 Highway 71
Sea Girt, NJ 08750   (732)282-1377   Fax (732)282-1377
+ Bergen Medical Associates
1 West Ridgewood Avenue/Suite 301   Paramus, NJ 07652   (732)282-1377   Fax (201)445-4296
+ Bergen Medical Associates
305 West Grand Avenue/Suite 200   Montvale, NJ 08750   (201)391-0071   Fax (201)391-1904

Cipriano, Joseph A., MD {1346295979} ObsGyn(92,NJ05)<NJ-RIVERVW>
+ Healthy Woman Ob/Gyn
312 Professional View Drive   Freehold, NJ 07728   (732)431-1616   Fax (732)866-7962

Cipriano, Rebecca J., MD {1396790135} ObsGyn, Obstet(94,IL42)<NJ-CENTRAST, NJ-JRSYSHMC>
+ Healthy Woman Ob/Gyn
312 Professional View Drive   Freehold, NJ 07728   (732)431-1616   Fax (732)866-7962

Cipriaso, Corazon Carrillo, MD {1851371801} PhysMd(93,PHI29)<NJ-JRSYSHMC>
+ 25 Mule Road/Suite B-1
Toms River, NJ 08755   (732)492-8241   Fax (732)521-7960

Cirangle, Lori Beth, MD IntrMd(85,NJ06)
+ PO Box 315
Berkeley Heights, NJ 07922   (973)635-0951

Cirella, Vincent N., MD {1073695136} Anesth(81,IL06)<NJ-RWJUBRUN>
+ Robert Wood Johnson-UMDNJ Anesthesia Group
125 Paterson Street/CAB 3100   New Brunswick, NJ 08901   (732)937-8841   Fax (732)418-8492
+ RWJ University Hospital New Brunswick
One Robert Wood Johnson Place   New Brunswick, NJ 08901   (732)828-3000

Cirello, Joseph Anthony, MD {1710144639} FamMed
+ Chatham Family Practice Associates
492 Main Street   Chatham, NJ 07928   (973)635-2432   Fax (973)635-6169

Cirello, Richard, MD {1770643215} FamMed, Grtrcs(75,MEXI)<NJ-MTNSIDE>
+ Town Medical Associates/Verona
271 Grove Avenue/Suite A   Verona, NJ 07044   (973)239-2600   Fax (973)239-0482

Cirelly, Francine Arlene, DO {1417094426} Nephro
+ 270 East Wheat Road/PO Box 618
Minotola, NJ 08341

Cirignano, Barbara M., MD {1053645739} FamMed
+ 31 Grant Avenue
Cliffside Park, NJ 07010

Cirullo, Pasquale Michael, MD {1912913682} Anesth, IntrMd(84,NY09)
+ Red Bank Anesthesia, LLC
1 Riverview Plaza   Red Bank, NJ 07701   (732)530-2255   Fax (732)450-2620

Cisnero, Maria Del Carmen, MD {1366617334} FamMed
+ P & C Medical Group LLC
605 South Broad Street/Unit B   Elizabeth, NJ 07202   (908)659-0075   Fax (908)469-4300

Citak, Kenneth A., MD {1578527941} Nrolgy(86,NY19)<NJ-VALLEY>
+ Neurology Group of Bergen County
1200 East Ridgewood Avenue   Ridgewood, NJ 07450   (201)444-0868   Fax (201)444-7363
kcitak@neurobergen.com

Citarelli, Louis J., MD {1063520484} IntrMd(82,MEX14)<NJ-CLARMAAS, NJ-MTNSIDE>
+ 181 Franklin Avenue/Suite 304
Nutley, NJ 07110   (973)667-3318   Fax (973)667-2134
+ New Jersey Plastic Surgery
29 Park Street   Montclair, NJ 07042   (973)667-3318   Fax (973)655-1228

Physicians by Name and Address

Citron, Andrew M., MD {1104859784} Anesth(90,MA07)<NJ-BAYSHORE>
+ Bayshore Community Hospital
727 North Beers Street/Anesthesiology Holmdel, NJ 07733 (732)739-5853

Citron, Barry S., MD {1942232301} IntrMd, SrgPlstc, Surgry(83,FL02)
+ 315 East Northfield Road/Suite 2 A
Livingston, NJ 07039 (973)535-5222 Fax (973)535-1450

Citron, Cheryl S., MD {1235168386} Dermat, IntrMd(84,FL02)
+ Summit Medical Group
315 East Northfield Road/Suite 1-E Livingston, NJ 07039 (973)535-3200 Fax (973)535-1450

Citta-Pietrolungo, Thelma Jean, DO {1912020322} PhysMd, PedReh(86,PA77)<NJ-VIRTVOOR>
+ New Life Rehab Medicine, P.C.
100 Springdale Road/Suite A-3,353 Cherry Hill, NJ 08003 (856)630-6000 Fax (856)795-9708
tjcitta@aol.com

Ciufalo, Marisa, MD {1598776056} Pedtrc(97,NH01)<NJ-MORRISTN>
+ Randolph Pediatrics
715 Route 10 East Randolph, NJ 07869 (973)328-9200 Fax (973)328-9144

Ciuffreda, Ronald V., MD {1831205871} IntrMd(75,ITAL)<NJ-MORRISTN>
+ Mendham Medical Group LLP
19 East Main Street/Suite 1 Mendham, NJ 07945 (973)543-6505 Fax (973)543-2967

Cizmar, Stephan, MD {1922014612} Anesth, PainMd(74,ITA22)<NJ-CLARMAAS>
+ Clara Maass Medical Center
1 Clara Maass Drive/Anesth Belleville, NJ 07109 (973)450-2000 Fax (908)653-9305

Clachko, Marc A., MD {1417919622} ObsGyn(71,MA05)<NJ-HACKNSK>
+ Bergen Ob-Gyn Associates, PA
130 Kinderkamack Road/Suite 300 River Edge, NJ 07661 (201)489-2727 Fax (201)489-5040

Clairvil, Jessie, DO {1538169909} Otlryg(98,OH75)
+ Kennedy Health Alliance - Swedesboro
545 Beckett Road/Suite 206 Swedesboro, NJ 08085 (856)339-0800 Fax (856)339-0884

Clancy, Joseph P., Jr., MD {1710914080} FamMed(81,SC04)
+ Vein Associates
382 West 9th Street Ship Bottom, NJ 08008 (609)361-7100 Fax (609)361-7105

Clancy, Kevin F., MD {1346245149} CdvDis, IntrMd(81,NJ06)
+ Cardiology Consultants
368 Lakehurst Road/Suite 301 Toms River, NJ 08755 (732)240-1048 Fax (732)240-3464
+ Cardiology Consultants
63-C Lacey Road Whiting, NJ 08759 (732)240-1048 Fax (732)350-7054
+ Cardiology Consultants of Toms River
401 Lacey Road/Suite D Whiting, NJ 08755 (732)350-3350 Fax (732)350-3350

Clancy, Lisa A., MD {1922173467} Anesth(87,NY09)<NJ-NWRKBETH>
+ New Jersey Anesthesia Associates, P.C.
252 Columbia Turnpike/PO Box 0037 Florham Park, NJ 07932 (973)660-9334 Fax (973)660-9779

Clanton, Chase P., MD {1477816429} Anesth
+ Morris Anesthesia Group, PA
3799 Route 46/Suite 211 Parsippany, NJ 07054 (973)335-1122 Fax (973)335-1448

Claps, Richard J., MD {1629008404} NuclMd, RadDia, RadNuc(68,NY09)
+ 15 Jason Lane
Morristown, NJ 07960

Clarin, Mitchell I., MD {1174597066} Pedtrc(88,NJ06)<NJ-HUNTRDN>
+ Hunterdon Pediatric Associates
8 Reading Road/Reading Ridge Flemington, NJ 08822 (908)788-6070 Fax (908)788-6005

Clark, Elizabeth C., MD {1558357996} FamMed, PubHth, GPrvMd(97,NC01)
+ Family Medicine at Monument Square
317 George Street New Brunswick, NJ 08901 (732)235-8993 Fax (732)246-7317

Clark, Kirpal, MD {1326468364}<NJ-NWRKBETH>
+ Newark Beth Israel Medical Center
201 Lyons Avenue Newark, NJ 07112 (973)926-6671 Fax (973)282-0562

Clark, Kristen S., MD {1447559455} Psychy(10,PA02)
+ Cedar Bridge Medical Associates
985 Cedarbridge Avenue Brick, NJ 08723 (732)477-5600 Fax (732)477-1899

Clark, Mary H., MD {1053355537} Pedtrc(76,NY01)<NJ-VALLEY>
+ Broadway Pediatric Associates
336 Center Avenue Westwood, NJ 07675 (201)664-7444 Fax (201)666-9476

Clark, Peter Joseph, DO {1164664967} Psychy<NJ-OVERLOOK>
+ Overlook Medical Center
99 Beauvoir Avenue/PO Box 210 Summit, NJ 07902 (908)522-4800 Fax (908)522-4888

Clark, Ruth L., MD {1740349968} Nrolgy(86,NJ05)<NJ-EASTORNG>
+ 310 Central Avenue/Suite 611
East Orange, NJ 07018 (973)678-5607 Fax (973)678-6319

Clark-Hamilton, Jill, MD {1861457020} Pedtrc, AdolMd(83,NY15)<NJ-MORRISTN>
+ Adolescent Medicine of MMH
100 Madison Avenue Morristown, NJ 07960 (973)971-4330
+ Morristown Medical Center
100 Madison Avenue Morristown, NJ 07962 (973)971-5000

Clark-Schoeb, James Scott, MD {1477523058} SrgSpn
+ New Jersey Spine Center
40 Main Street Chatham, NJ 07928 (973)635-0800 Fax (973)635-6254

Clarke, Dane Eric, MD {1710988050} EmrgMd(91,GA21)<NJ-RBAYPERT>
+ Raritan Bay Medical Center/Perth Amboy Division
530 New Brunswick Avenue Perth Amboy, NJ 08861 (732)442-3700

Clarke, Kevin O'Neil, MD {1598789265} Surgry, SrgOnc(98,CT02)<NJ-UMDNJ>
+ University Hospital-Doctors Office Center
90 Bergen Street/DOC 7100/OncSrg Newark, NJ 07103 (973)972-2400 Fax (973)972-2988

Clarke, Robert Anthony, MD {1114934007} IntrMd(00,DMN01)
+ 108 South Munn Avenue
East Orange, NJ 07018 (973)674-8100 Fax (973)674-8400

Clarkin, Kim Stephanie, MD {1235454042} RadDia
+ 47 Lynwood Road
Verona, NJ 07044 (973)650-7349
clarkiks@gmail.com

Clarkson, Philip Willie Bankole, MD {1073923835} IntrMd
+ Jersey Shore University Medical Center
1945 Route 33 Neptune, NJ 07753 (732)775-5500

Clayton, Elizabeth Noelle, DO {1932537529} ObsGyn
+ Community Health Care Inc
484 South Brewster Road Vineland, NJ 08360 (856)451-4700 Fax (856)696-2561

Clayton, Lisa M., DO {1487956728}<NJ-MORRISTN>
+ Morristown Medical Center
100 Madison Avenue Morristown, NJ 07962 (973)971-7926

Clayton, MaryAnn B., MD PthFor(81,NJ06)
+ Bergen County Medical Examiner's Office
351 East Ridgewood Avenue Paramus, NJ 07652 (201)634-2940 Fax (201)634-2950

Clear, Carolyn Elizabeth, DO {1205884681} Pedtrc(00,PA77)<NJ-UNDRWD, NJ-KMHSTRAT>
+ Advocare West Deptford Pediatrics
1050 Mantua Pike Wenonah, NJ 08090 (856)468-8330 Fax (856)468-9121
+ Advocare West Deptford Pediatrics
19 Village Center Drive Swedesboro, NJ 08085 (856)468-8330 Fax (856)879-2855
+ Advocare West Deptford Pediatrics
646 Kings Highway West Deptford, NJ 08090 (856)879-2887 Fax (856)879-2855

Cleary, Kelly, MD {1043449150} PedEmg(05,NY46)
+ PM Pediatrics
355 Route 22 Springfield, NJ 07081 (973)467-2767

Cleaves, Elle Sowa, MD {1538408646} GenPrc
+ McGuire Air Force Base/Acute Health Care Clinic
3458 Neely Road Trenton, NJ 08641 (609)754-9324 Fax (609)754-9015

Clement, Martinez Emmanuel, MD {1841235777} EmrgMd(86,MO34)<NJ-ENGLEWOOD>
+ Englewood Hospital and Medical Center
350 Engle Street/EmrgMed Englewood, NJ 07631 (201)984-3000 Fax (610)617-6280

Clemente, Jose D., MD {1932151917} GenPrc, Surgry(67,PHIL)
+ American Physician Services/Hudson HealthCare
679 Montgomery Street Jersey City, NJ 07306 (201)433-6500 Fax (201)433-8010

Clemente, Joseph, MD {1164425435} IntrMd, CritCr, CdvDis(83,MEX27)<NJ-BAYSHORE, NJ-RIVERVW>
+ Medical Health Center
1270 State Highway 35 Middletown, NJ 07748 (732)615-3900 Fax (732)615-0185

Clemente, Joseph Alfred, MD {1326129586} IntrMd(85,PA02)<NJ-JRSYSHMC>
+ Warren Primary Care
23 Mountain Boulevard Warren, NJ 07059 (908)598-7970 Fax (908)322-4989

Clemente, Maria F., MD {1932141108} Ophthl(89,NY47)<NJ-RIVERVW>
+ The Eye, Ear, Nose & Throat Institute

82 Bethany Road Hazlet, NJ 07730 (732)264-3937 Fax (732)264-1311

Clemente, Roderick J., MD {1053405654} SrgNro(78,ITA17)<NJ-MTNSIDE>
+ Neurological Care of New Jersey, P.A.
95 Gates Avenue Montclair, NJ 07042 (973)744-3166 Fax (973)744-3199

Clements, David, IV, MD {1932574118} Psychy
+ Cooper Psychiatric Associates
3 Cooper Plaza/Suite 307 Camden, NJ 08103 (856)342-2328 Fax (856)541-6137

Clements, David H., III, MD {1114995826} SrgOrt, SrgSpn(82,PA13)<NJ-COOPRUMC>
+ Cooper Bone and Joint Institute
401 South Kings Highway/Suite 3-A Cherry Hill, NJ 08003 (856)547-0201 Fax (856)547-0316

Cleri, Dennis J., MD {1487760070} InfDis, IntrMd(72,PA02)<NJ-STFRNMED, NJ-STJOSHOS>
+ St. Francis Medical Center
601 Hamilton Avenue Trenton, NJ 08629 (609)599-5000 Fax (609)599-6232

Clermont, Nadine Nattacha, MD {1598995375} IntrMd<NJ-VIRTMHBC>
+ Virtua Memorial
175 Madison Avenue Mount Holly, NJ 08060 (609)914-6180 Fax (609)914-6182

Clever, Marcia Sue, MD {1336261809} Psychy(81,NY20)
+ 25 Bridge Avenue/Suite 205
Red Bank, NJ 07701 (732)345-9100 Fax (732)345-9400

Clifford, Eileen M., MD {1730264052} IntrMd(77,NJ05)<NJ-STJOSHOS>
+ Medical Internists Associates PA
22-18 Broadway/Suite 104 Fair Lawn, NJ 07410 (201)797-4503 Fax (201)797-4270

Clifford, James R., MD {1881695336} CdvDis, IntrMd(82,BEL11)<NJ-HACKNSK, NJ-UMDNJ>
+ Rochelle Park Cardiac Center
186 Rochelle Avenue Rochelle Park, NJ 07662 (201)556-1225 Fax (201)556-1101
+ 255 West Spring Valley Avenue
Maywood, NJ 07607 (201)556-1225 Fax (201)996-0584

Clifford, Susan Michelle, MD {1518944768} IntrMd, Nephro(99,ISR02)<NJ-ENGLWOOD, NJ-HACKNSK>
+ Drs. Pattner, Grodstein, Fein & Davis
177 North Dean Street/Suite 207 Englewood, NJ 07631 (201)567-0446 Fax (201)567-8775

Cline, Douglas C., MD {1619934858} Allrgy, FamMed(86,PA13)
+ Broadway Family Practice
602 South Broadway Camden, NJ 08103 (856)964-4456 Fax (856)964-0670

Clinton, Cody, DO {1235425190} SrgOrt
+ 221 Victoria Street
Glassboro, NJ 08028 (856)536-1476

Clinton, Lawrence P., MD {1316003734} Psychy, PsyCAd, PsyFor(72,PA09)
+ 1138 East Chestnut Avenue
Vineland, NJ 08360 (609)696-2660 Fax (856)696-8548
lpclinton@mindspring.com

Closkey, Robert F., MD {1568498525} SrgOrt, SrgOARec(95,NJ06)<NJ-COMMED>
+ Ocean Orthopedic Associates, P.A.
530 Lakehurst Road/Suite 1 Toms River, NJ 08755 (732)349-8454 Fax (732)341-0259

Clott, Matthew Alan, MD {1801849096} SrgPlstc(97,PA09)
+ Somerset Cosmetic & Reconstructive Surgery
5 Mountain Boulevard/Suite 1 Warren, NJ 07059 (908)222-0070 Fax (908)222-8027

Clott, Shilpa Mahendra, MD {1083635940} ObsGyn(97,PA09)
+ Somerset Cosmetic & Reconstructive Surgery
5 Mountain Boulevard/Suite 1 Warren, NJ 07059 (908)222-0070 Fax (908)222-8027

Clouden, Tobechukwu A., MD {1669603387} Psychy
+ 852 Valley Street
Vauxhall, NJ 07088

Clouser, Katharine N., MD {1184990327}
+ Hackensack University Medical Center
30 Prospect Avenue Hackensack, NJ 07601 (201)996-2000

Cluley, Scott R., MD {1568434157} Surgry, SrgVas(85,NJ05)<NJ-JRSYSHMC, NJ-OCEANMC>
+ Jersey Coast Vascular Associates
425 Jack Martin Boulevard/Suite 2 Brick, NJ 08724 (732)202-1500 Fax (732)202-1058

Co, Anthony, MD {1780897447} Anesth
+ Hamilton Anesthesia Associates
2119 Highway 33/Suite B Trenton, NJ 08690 (609)581-5303 Fax (609)631-6839

Co, Demosthene E., MD {1942375498} Anesth(71,PHI10)<NJ-STBARNMC>
+ New Jersey Anesthesia Associates, P.C.
252 Columbia Turnpike/PO Box 0037 Florham Park, NJ 07932 (973)660-9334 Fax (973)660-9779

Physicians by Name and Address

Co, Dominador A., MD {1598753642} GenPrc, Surgry(76,PHI08)<NJ-VIRTMHBC>
+ New Jersey Division of Developmental Disability
  Route 72 East   New Lisbon, NJ 08064   (609)726-1000   Fax (609)894-8430
+ Virtua Memorial
  175 Madison Avenue   Mount Holly, NJ 08060   (609)267-0700

Co, Gerrie T., MD {1174617492} Psychy(79,PHI09)
+ 2 Jocama Boulevard/Suite A
  Old Bridge, NJ 08857   (732)591-1800   Fax (732)591-1881

Co, Jacqueline Ann B., MD {1548286842} Anesth(NJ02<NJ-OVERLOOK>
+ Summit Anesthesia Associates, P.A.
  33 Overlook Road/Suite 311   Summit, NJ 07901   (908)598-1500   Fax (908)598-0197

Co, John A., MD {1588620199} CdvDis, IntrMd(83,PHIL)<NJ-HACKNSK, NJ-VALLEY>
+ 140 Chestnut Street/Suite 202
  Ridgewood, NJ 07450   (201)445-0405   Fax (201)445-4282

Co, Margaret L., MD {1568494128} Allrgy, Pedtrc(84,PHI29)
+ 75 North Maple Avenue
  Ridgewood, NJ 07450   (201)652-7788   Fax (201)652-8644

Coant, Pierre N., MD {1669436945} Pedtrc(86,PA07)<NJ-COOPRUMC>
+ Gloucester County Pediatrics
  849 Cooper Street   Deptford, NJ 08096   (856)848-6346   Fax (856)848-5734

Coates, Robert G., MD {1740254994} FamMed(80,NY08)<NJ-HUNTRDN>
+ Hunterdon Medical Center
  2100 Wescott Drive   Flemington, NJ 08822   (908)788-6100

Coba, Miguel A., MD {1124223086} PhysMd, OrtSpn<NJ-KSLR-WEST>
+ 477 Rahway Avenue
  Woodbridge, NJ 07095   (732)527-0770   Fax (732)218-5872
+ Kessler Institute for Rehabilitation West Orange
  1199 Pleasant Valley Way   West Orange, NJ 07052   (973)731-3600

Cobb, William Stewart, MD {1972755254} SrgNro(06,NJ02)
+ Neurosurgeons of New Jersey
  1200 East Ridgewood Avenue   Ridgewood, NJ 07450   (201)824-6131

Coben, Robert M., MD {1891754891} Gastrn, IntrMd(85,PA13)<NJ-UNDRWD, NJ-SJRSYELM>
+ South Jersey Endoscopy Center
  26 East Red Bank Avenue   Woodbury, NJ 08096   (856)848-4464   Fax (856)848-8706

Cobert, Barton L., MD {1578739181} Gastrn, IntrMd, Rserch(74,NY19)
+ 31 Plymouth Road
  Westfield, NJ 07090   (908)654-1785

Cobert, Josiane C., MD {1982790432} PsyCAd, Psychy(76,FRA12)<NJ-TRININPC, NJ-TRINIWSC>
+ Trinitas Regional Medical Center-New Point Campus
  655 East Jersey Street/Psychiatry   Elizabeth, NJ 07206   (908)994-5000
+ Trinitas Regional Medical Center-Williamson Street
  225 Williamson Street/Psychiatry   Elizabeth, NJ 07207   (908)994-5000
+ Trinitas Regional Med Ctr-Jersey
  925 East Jersey Street/Psychiatry   Elizabeth, NJ 07206   (908)994-5000

Cobin, Rhoda Harriet, MD {1164588422} EnDbMt, IntrMd(69,PRO01)<NJ-HACKNSK, NJ-VALLEY>
+ Valley Medical Group-Endocrinology
  947 Linwood Avenue   Ridgewood, NJ 07450   (201)444-5963   Fax (201)444-4490
  rhcobin@gmail.com

Coblentz, Malcolm Guy, MD {1356301568} Surgry, SrgVas, IntrMd(71,ITA01)<NJ-STBARNMC>
+ 55 Morris Avenue/Suite 304
  Springfield, NJ 07081   (973)486-0108   Fax (973)762-5151

Coccaro, John A., MD {1841213121} EmrgMd, IntrMd(83,MEX34)<NJ-BAYONNE>
+ Bayonne Medical Center
  29th Street at Avenue E/EmrgMed   Bayonne, NJ 07002   (201)858-5000

Coccaro, John A., MD {1235280314} AnesPain(91,GRN01)<NJ-KIMBALL>
+ Precision Pain Managemant, LLC
  300 West Water Street/Suite A   Toms River, NJ 08753   (732)800-2760   Fax (732)505-5432
  drc@drcppm.com

Cocco, Frank A., MD {1982629622} ObsGyn, Gyneco(71,ITAL)<NJ-KIMBALL, NJ-COMMED>
+ Ocean Gynecological & Obstetrical Associates PA
  475 Highway 70   Lakewood, NJ 08701   (732)364-8000   Fax (732)364-4601
+ Ocean Gynecological & Obstetrical Associates PA
  2290 West County Line Road   Jackson, NJ 08527   (732)961-9205

Cochrane, Dennis G., MD {1922057132} EmrgMd, IntrMd(72,MN04)
+ Emergency Medical Associates of NJ, P.A.
  3 Century Drive   Parsippany, NJ 07054   (973)740-0607   Fax (973)740-9895
+ 241 Brook Valley Road
  Kinnelon, NJ 07405

Cocke, Thomas Preston, Jr., MD {1972508554} CdvDis, IntCrd(85,NY48)<NJ-HACKNSK, NJ-VALLEY>
+ Westwood Cardiology Associates PA
  333 Old Hook Road/Suite 200   Westwood, NJ 07675   (201)664-0201   Fax (201)666-7970
+ Westwood Cardiology Associates PA
  20 Prospect Avenue/Suite 810   Hackensack, NJ 07601   (201)664-0201   Fax (201)342-2422

Cocovinis, Barbara, MD {1285636563} PedCrd, Pedtrc, PedCrC(74,POLA)<NJ-STJOSHOS, NJ-HOBUNIMC>
+ St. Joseph's Children's Hospital
  703 Main Street/Critical Care   Paterson, NJ 07503   (973)754-2500   Fax (973)754-2567

Cocoziello, Alexander R., DO {1043384316} ObsGyn, IntrMd(70,MO78)<NJ-HACKNSK>
+ Coco OBGYN
  444 Market Street/Suite 2-B   Saddle Brook, NJ 07663   (201)794-8773   Fax (201)794-0335

Cocoziello, Ramin B., MD {1053344077} ObsGyn(91,NJ05)<NJ-HACKNSK, NJ-VALLEY>
+ 12-15 Broadway/Suite E
  Fair Lawn, NJ 07410   (201)794-0910   Fax (201)794-2164

Codel, Radu, MD {1821082827} CdvDis, IntrMd(77,ITAL)<NJ-ENGLWOOD, NJ-HOLYNAME>
+ 968 River Road
  Edgewater, NJ 07020   (201)969-0994   Fax (201)969-2453

Codella, Vincent Adrian, DO {1134111248} FamMed(01,NJ75)
+ Codella Family Practice
  1000 Galloping Hill Road/Suite 103   Union, NJ 07083   (908)688-1550   Fax (908)688-1552

Codispoti, Cindy A., DO {1366414427} CdvDis(00,CA22)
+ Cardiology Associates of Sussex County LLP
  222 High Street/Suite 205   Newton, NJ 07860   (973)579-2100   Fax (973)579-6638

Codjoe, Jessica R., MD {1659433084} FamMed
+ 52 Zaitz Farm Road
  West Windsor, NJ 08550

Codjoe, Paul Winfred, MD {1487790952} SrgOrt(01,NJ06)
+ Mercer-Bucks Orthopaedics PC
  3120 Princeton Pike   Lawrenceville, NJ 08648   (609)896-0444   Fax (609)896-1055
+ Mercer-Bucks Orthopaedics, P.C.
  2501 Kuser Road   Hamilton, NJ 08691   (609)896-0444   Fax (609)587-4349

Codoyannis, Aristides Basil, MD {1871565077} SrgCdv, SrgThr(71,GREE)<NJ-STMICHL>
+ 240 Williamson Street/Suite 403
  Elizabeth, NJ 07207   (973)553-5691   Fax (908)832-7034

Cody, Robert James, MD {1437227295} CdvDis
+ Merck and Company Incorporated
  1 Merck Drive/PO Box 100   Whitehouse Station, NJ 08889   (908)391-8284

Cody, William C., MD {1356390413} SrgC&R, Surgry(82,NY01)<NJ-VIRTUAHS, NJ-OURLADY>
+ Virtua Surgical Group, PA
  1935 Route 70 East   Cherry Hill, NJ 08003   (856)428-7700   Fax (856)424-9120

Coelho, Ryan, MD {1043703200} FamMed
+ Vanguard Medical Group, P.A.
  170 Changebridge Road/Suite C-3   Montville, NJ 07045   (973)559-3700   Fax (973)575-4885

Coelho-D'Costa, Vinette E., MD {1811919178} IntrMd, PulDis(91,INA6Y)
+ Advanced Pulmonary Assoc
  503 Raritan Avenue   Highland Park, NJ 08904   (908)333-6150   Fax (908)333-6154
+ RWJ University Hospital New Brunswick
  One Robert Wood Johnson Place   New Brunswick, NJ 08901   (732)828-3000

Coffey, Dennis Charles, MD {1578534210} Pedtrc, PedCrC(93,NJ06)<NJ-VALLEY, NY-CHLDCOPR>
+ The Valley Hospital
  223 North Van Dien Avenue/PICU   Ridgewood, NJ 07450   (201)447-8000
  coffde@valleyhealth.com

Coffin, Nina R., MD {1265527311} Gastrn(80,NJ06)<NJ-EASTORNG>
+ 185 Central Avenue
  East Orange, NJ 07018   (973)676-3918   Fax (973)676-5383

Cogan, Andrew M., DO {1346280591} FamMed(95,PA77)<NJ-VIRTVOOR, NJ-KMHTURNV>
+ Advocare Family Medicine Associates Williamstown
  979 North Black Horse Pike   Williamstown, NJ 08094   (856)629-5151   Fax (856)629-0281

+ Advocare Family Medicine Associates Mt. Laurel
  3115 Route 38/Suite 200B   Mount Laurel, NJ 08054   (856)629-5151   Fax (856)231-7543
+ Advocare Family Medicine Associates Vineland
  602 West Sherman Avenue/Suite B   Vineland, NJ 08094   (856)692-8484   Fax (856)896-3059

Cogliani, Ermes, MD {1588639348} ObsGyn(81,ITA17)<NJ-STPETER, NJ-RWJUBRUN>
+ Piscataway Somerset Ob/Gyn Group, LLP
  31 Stelton Road/Suite 4   Piscataway, NJ 08854   (732)752-7755   Fax (732)752-7918
+ Piscataway Somerset Ob/Gyn Group, LLP
  9 Clyde Road/Suite 101   Somerset, NJ 08873   (732)246-2280
+ Cares Surgicenter, LLC.
  240 Easton Avenue   New Brunswick, NJ 08854   (732)565-5400   Fax (732)296-8677

Cohen, Adam Jonathan, MD {1285873844} PsyCAd(03,NY06)
+ 261 James Street/Suite 3G
  Morristown, NJ 07960

Cohen, Alan, MD {1023070935} ObsGyn(82,DMN02)<NJ-MONMOUTH, NJ-RIVERVW>
+ 302 Candlewood Commons
  Howell, NJ 07731   (732)905-8111   Fax (732)886-9138
+ 279 Third Avenue/Suite 506
  Long Branch, NJ 07740   (732)222-8272

Cohen, Alan Polan, MD {1598836280} Dermat(85,TX12)
+ M.C. Medical Group
  1425 Pompton Avenue/Suite 1-1   Cedar Grove, NJ 07009   (973)785-8686   Fax (973)785-8680
+ Caldwell Center for Dermatology
  30 Westville Avenue   Caldwell, NJ 07006   (973)228-6866

Cohen, Alice J., MD {1528071164} IntrMd, OncHem(81,IL42)<NJ-NWRKBETH, NJ-STBARNMC>
+ Newark Beth Israel Medical Center
  201 Lyons Avenue/Hem/Onc   Newark, NJ 07112   (973)926-7230   Fax (973)926-9568

Cohen, Allan, MD {1205879152} Gastrn, IntrMd(79,NY08)
+ Gastroenterologists of Ocean County
  477 Lakehurst Road   Toms River, NJ 08755   (732)349-4422   Fax (732)349-5087

Cohen, Allan Bary, MD {1326137886} Gastrn, IntrMd(67,NY09)
+ Gastroenterology Associates
  1165 Park Avenue   Plainfield, NJ 07060   (908)754-2992   Fax (908)754-8366

Cohen, Aly G., MD {1346294188} IntrMd, Rheuma(99,PA09)<NJ-CENTRAST, NJ-RWJUHAM>
+ Arthritis & Osteoporosis Associates, P.A.
  4247 US Highway 9/Building 1   Freehold, NJ 07728   (732)780-7650   Fax (732)780-8817
+ Monroe Village Health Care Center
  1 David Brainerd Drive   Monroe Township, NJ 08831   (732)780-7650   Fax (732)521-6540

Cohen, Amir, MD {1841487220} Ophthl(03,NJ06)
+ 6 Troy Drive
  Livingston, NJ 07039

Cohen, Amy Marie Palmieri, MD {1336346709} Pedtrc(05,NJ05)
+ CHOP Care Network at Virtua Voorhees Hospital
  100 Bowman Drive   Voorhees, NJ 08043   (856)325-3000   Fax (609)261-5842

Cohen, Andrew Geoffrey, MD {1962431536} FamMed(03,PA14)
+ Virtua Family Medicine of Washington Township
  239 Hurffville Crosskeys Road   Sewell, NJ 08080   (856)341-8181   Fax (856)881-2071

Cohen, Andrew Nathan, DO {1508030610} EmrgMd(04,NY75)<NJ-NWRKBETH, NJ-STJOSHOS>
+ St Joseph's Medical Center Emergency
  703 Main Street   Paterson, NJ 07503   (973)754-2240   Fax (973)754-2249

Cohen, Avraham N., MD {1144269283} Ophthl(90,NY46)
+ Wills Eye Surgery Center in Cherry Hill
  408 Route 70 East   Cherry Hill, NJ 08034   (856)354-1600   Fax (856)429-7555

Cohen, Barbara Elisabeth, MD {1558304873} Pedtrc(76,PA07)<NJ-UMDNJ>
+ University Hospital-Cares Institute
  42 East Laurel Road/Suite 1100   Stratford, NJ 08084   (856)566-7036   Fax (856)566-6108

Cohen, Barry Alan, MD {1295839660} PedPul, Pedtrc, SlpDis(78,MD07)<NJ-STBARNMC, NJ-NWRKBETH>
+ St. Barnabas Medical Center
  94 Old Short Hills Road/Pedi Pulm   Livingston, NJ 07039   (973)322-9806   Fax (973)324-4908
+ Children's Hospital of NJ Ped Cntr @ West Orange
  375 Mount Pleasant Avenue/Suite 105   West Orange, NJ 07052   (973)322-9806   Fax (973)322-7310

Cohen, Barry Herbert, MD {1104856616} Nephro, IntrMd(65,PA09)<NJ-STFRNMED, NJ-CHSFULD>
+ Mercer Kidney Institute
  40 Fuld Street/Suite 401   Trenton, NJ 08638   (609)599-1004   Fax (609)599-3611

Physicians by Name and Address

Cohen, Barry Mark, MD {1275527707} CdvDis, IntrMd(80,QU06)
+ Associates in Cardiovascular Disease, LLC
211 Mountain Avenue   Springfield, NJ 07081   (973)467-0005   Fax (973)912-8989

Cohen, Benjamin, MD {1053301085} Dermat(88,ISR02)
+ Dermatology & Laser Center PA
279 Third Avenue/Suite 603   Long Branch, NJ 07740   (732)222-8323   Fax (732)870-9488
benjamin.cohen@dcneuro.net

Cohen, Brad J., MD {1871698951} ObsGyn, Gyneco(86,NJ05)<NJ-STPETER, NJ-RWJUBRUN>
+ 2477 Route 516/Suite 103
Old Bridge, NJ 08857   (732)679-6900   Fax (732)679-7900
+ Cares Surgicenter, LLC.
240 Easton Avenue   New Brunswick, NJ 08901   (732)679-6900   Fax (732)296-8677

Cohen, Dale L., MD {1417938770} Anesth, CritCr(87,PA13)<NJ-MORRISTN>
+ Morristown Medical Center
100 Madison Avenue   Morristown, NJ 07962   (973)971-5548   Fax (201)943-8733

Cohen, Dane Ryan, MD {1760825327} RadOnc
+ Kennedy Diagnostic & Treatment Center
900 Medical Center Drive/Suite 100   Sewell, NJ 08080   (856)582-3008

Cohen, Daniel Elliot, MD {1568494177} Psychy(71,NY01)<NJ-BERGNMC>
+ 60 West Ridgewood Avenue
Ridgewood, NJ 07450   (201)444-4588

Cohen, Daniel Jonathan, MD {1811993827} RadDia, RadV&I(83,TX12)<NJ-STFRNMED>
+ Radiology Affiliates of Central New Jersey, P.A.
2501 Kuser Road   Hamilton, NJ 08691   (609)585-8800   Fax (609)585-1825
+ Radiology Affiliates of Central New Jersey, P.A.
3120 Princeton Pike   Lawrenceville, NJ 08648   (609)585-8800   Fax (609)219-0439

Cohen, David Eliot, MD {1417950692} CdvDis, IntrMd, IntCrd(80,NY01)<NJ-VALLEY, NJ-STJOSHOS>
+ Circulatory Care of New Jersey
275 Forest Avenue/Suite 205   Paramus, NJ 07652   (201)265-5300   Fax (201)265-5350
info@cconj.com

Cohen, Douglas Jay, MD {1366427007} CritCr, PulDis(78,NY09)
+ Pulmonary and Sleep Physicians
204 Ark Road/Suite 206/Larchmont 1   Mount Laurel, NJ 08054   (856)778-4640   Fax (856)778-8862

Cohen, Ellen, MD {1598731754} IntrMd(80,NY20)<NJ-NWRKBETH>
+ Newark Beth Israel Medical Center
201 Lyons Avenue   Newark, NJ 07112   (973)926-7000
ecohen@sbhcs.com

Cohen, Eric R., DO {1356355044} Nrolgy, IntrMd(01,NY75)<NJ-OVERLOOK, NJ-MORRISTN>
+ Summit Medical Group-Berkeley Heights Campus
1 Diamond Hill Road/2nd Floor   Berkeley Heights, NJ 07922   (908)277-8639   Fax (908)790-6524

Cohen, Erik Gary, MD {1811921232} SrgHdN, Otlryg(96,NY46)<NY-SLOANKET, NJ-MORRISTN>
+ Morristown Medical Center
100 Madison Avenue/Cancer Center   Morristown, NJ 07962   (973)971-7355

Cohen, Hayley M., MD {1073607495} PsyCAd, Psychy(89,NY06)
+ 28 Millburn Avenue/Suite 3
Springfield, NJ 07081   (973)218-0777   Fax (973)921-1003

Cohen, Herman P., DO {1700966330} FamMed(93,PA77)<NJ-OURLADY, NJ-KMHCHRRY>
+ Advocare Cohen Family Medicine
5647 Westfield Avenue   Pennsauken, NJ 08110   (856)663-1470   Fax (856)665-2727
Hermcohen@aol.com

Cohen, Hillary Joy, MD {1104871912} EmrgMd(00,MI01)<NY-MAIMONMC>
+ Englewood Hospital Emergency
350 Engle Street   Englewood, NJ 07631   (201)894-3527

Cohen, Hillel D., MD {1124160320} Gastrn(01,NJ06)
+ 85 Raritan Avenue/Suite 120
Highland Park, NJ 08904

Cohen, Howard S., MD {1013913110} CdvDis, IntrMd(79,NY19)<NJ-JFKMED, NJ-SOMERSET>
+ Cardio Medical Group
98 James Street/Suite 313   Edison, NJ 08820   (732)635-1100   Fax (732)635-0918
+ Cardio Medical Group
5 Mountain Boulevard/Suite 2   Warren, NJ 07059   (732)635-1100   Fax (908)769-8182

Cohen, Howard Steven, DO {1306889514} FamMed, IntrMd(86,NJ75)<NJ-CENTRAST>
+ RWJPE Old Bridge Family Medicine
2107 Highway 516   Old Bridge, NJ 08857   (732)952-0626   Fax (732)463-6071

Cohen, Ian Thomas, MD {1073515524} PedSrg, Surgry(68,SAF01)<NJ-MONMOUTH>
+ Monmouth Medical Center
300 Second Avenue/Surgery   Long Branch, NJ 07740   (732)923-6091   Fax (732)923-6203

Cohen, Ilan, MD {1649374802} Ophthl, CrnExD, SrgRef(96,MA07)<NY-NYEYEINF, NY-MANHEYE>
+ World Class LASIK
28 Throckmorton Lane   Old Bridge, NJ 08857   (732)679-6100   Fax (732)673-6703
icohen@aol.com

Cohen, Jason D., MD {1417934449} SrgOrt, SrgSpn(94,NY46)<NJ-MONMOUTH, NJ-RIVERVW>
+ Professional Orthopaedic Associates
776 Shrewsbury Avenue/Suite 201   Tinton Falls, NJ 07724   (732)530-4949   Fax (732)530-3618
+ Professional Orthopaedic Associates
1430 Hooper Avenue/Suite 101   Toms River, NJ 08753   (732)530-4949   Fax (732)349-7722
+ Professional Orthopaedic Associates
303 West Main Street   Freehold, NJ 07724   (732)530-4949   Fax (732)577-0036

Cohen, Jason Leon, MD {1619199445} Psychy(99,NY08)
+ 8 School Road East
Marlboro, NJ 07746   (917)952-9422
gallocohen@aol.com

Cohen, Jason Ronald, MD {1578752572} PhyMSptM, Anesth, IntrMd(03,ISR02)<NJ-RWJUHAM>
+ Medical Associates of Central New Jersey
26 Throckmorton Lane/1st flr.   Old Bridge, NJ 08857   (732)952-5533   Fax (732)707-4732

Cohen, Jay A., MD {1588663231} Psychy(75,NJ06)<NJ-ANNKLEIN>
+ Ann Klein Forensic Center
1609 Stuyvesant Avenue/PO Box 7717   West Trenton, NJ 08628   (609)633-0900
jcohen@dhs.state.nj.us

Cohen, Joel S., MD {1053352385} Urolgy(72,MEX14)<NJ-MORRISTN, NJ-OVERLOOK>
+ 315 Lenox Avenue
Westfield, NJ 07090   (908)654-5577   Fax (908)654-4178
+ 384 Shunpike Road
Chatham, NJ 07928   (973)377-9500

Cohen, Jonathan, MD {1790709533} IntrMd, Gastrn(90,MA01)
+ Ocean County Internal Medicine Associates
1352 River Avenue   Lakewood, NJ 08701   (732)370-5100   Fax (732)901-9240

Cohen, Jonathan David, MD {1457890055} Psychy
+ 515 Cherry Hill Road
Princeton, NJ 08540   (609)658-0083

Cohen, Jonathan Ira, MD {1619077690} IntrMd, Grtrcs(81,NY47)
+ Ocean County Internal Medicine Associates
1352 River Avenue   Lakewood, NJ 08701   (732)370-5100   Fax (732)901-9240

Cohen, Kenneth Arthur, MD {1225089352} RadDia, Radiol(79,MEX03)<NJ-WARREN>
+ Progressive Physician Associates, Inc.
185 Roseberry Street   Phillipsburg, NJ 08865   (610)868-1100   Fax (610)868-1111

Cohen, Larry J., MD {1295731305} CdvDis, IntrMd(81,NJ05)<NJ-JFKMED, NJ-SOMERSET>
+ Cardio Medical Group
98 James Street/Suite 313   Edison, NJ 08820   (732)635-1100   Fax (732)635-0918
+ Cardio Medical Group
5 Mountain Boulevard/Suite 2   Warren, NJ 07059   (732)635-1100   Fax (908)769-8182

Cohen, Larry W., DO {1376544536} Surgry(74,PA77)<NJ-KMHCHRRY, NJ-KMHTURNV>
+ Advocare Associates in General Surgery
2201 Chapel Avenue West/Suite 100   Cherry Hill, NJ 08002   (856)665-2017   Fax (856)488-6769
+ Advocare Associates in General Surgery
570 Egg Harbor Road/Suite C-2   Sewell, NJ 08080   (856)665-2017   Fax (856)256-7789
+ Comprehensive Cancer & Hematology Specialists, P.C.
705 White Horse Road   Voorhees, NJ 08002   (856)435-1777   Fax (856)435-0696

Cohen, Liliana, MD {1225251408} IntrMd, CdvDis(02,PA09)
+ Summit Medical Group
140 Park Avenue/3rd Floor   Florham Park, NJ 07932   (973)404-9900   Fax (908)673-7108

Cohen, Marc, MD {1376510578} CdvDis, OthrSp(77,NY19)<NJ-NWRKBETH>
+ Newark Beth Israel Medical Center
201 Lyons Avenue/CardCathLab   Newark, NJ 07112   (973)926-7000   Fax (973)923-4683

Cohen, Marc Alan, MD {1124052295} SrgOrt(81,IL42)
+ Spine Institute
221 Madison Avenue   Morristown, NJ 07960   (973)538-4444   Fax (973)538-0420
+ Advanced Spine Surgery Center
855 Lehigh Avenue   Union, NJ 07083   (973)538-4444   Fax (908)557-9438

Cohen, Marc S., MD {1669436440} Ophthl(84,PA01)
+ 2301 Evesham Road/Suite 101
Voorhees, NJ 08043   (856)772-2552   Fax (856)772-1946

Cohen, Martin L., MD {1376513465} Pedtrc(67,NY15)
+ Morristown Pediatric Associates, LLC
261 James Street/Suite 1-G   Morristown, NJ 07960   (973)540-9393   Fax (973)540-1937

Cohen, Michael A., MD {1730479817}(11,PA0)
+ Rutgers NJ School of Medicine Neurology
90 Bergen Street/DOC 5200   Newark, NJ 07103   (973)972-2342   Fax (973)972-5059

Cohen, Michael B., MD {1598794588} Anesth(79,NJ05)<NJ-OCEANMC>
+ Morris Anesthesia Group, PA
3799 Route 46/Suite 211   Parsippany, NJ 07054   (973)335-1122   Fax (973)335-1448

Cohen, Michael B., MD {1396942231} IntrMd, IntCrd(04,FL02)<NJ-HOLYNAME>
+ Mulkay Cardiology Consultants, P.C.
493 Essex Street   Hackensack, NJ 07601   (201)996-9244   Fax (201)996-9243
+ Mulkay Cardiology Consultants, P.C.
529 39th Street   Union City, NJ 07087   (201)996-9244   Fax (201)601-0995

Cohen, Michael Scott, MD {1982875829} Urolgy(02,NY20)
+ Urology Care Alliance
2 Princess Road/Suite J   Lawrenceville, NJ 08648   (609)895-1991   Fax (609)895-6996

Cohen, Michele Marie-Liz, DO {1568661239} PedCrd(02,NY75)<NY-SCHNCHIL>
+ The Children's Hospital at Saint Peter's University
254 Easton Avenue/MOB 2nd Fl   New Brunswick, NJ 08901   (732)745-8538

Cohen, Morris, MD {1629099296} NnPnMd, Pedtrc(74,SAFR)<NJ-NWRKBETH>
+ Newark Beth Israel Medical Center
201 Lyons Avenue   Newark, NJ 07112   (973)926-7203   Fax (973)926-7203

Cohen, Neil M., MD {1689634438} Gastrn, IntrMd(84,PA13)<NJ-KMHCHRRY, NJ-VIRTMARL>
+ South Jersey Gastroenterology PA
406 Lippincott Drive/Suite E   Marlton, NJ 08053   (856)983-1900   Fax (856)983-5110
+ South Jersey Gastroenterology PA
807 Haddon Avenue/Suite 205   Haddonfield, NJ 08033   (856)983-1900   Fax (856)983-5110
+ South Jersey Gastroenterology PA
111 Vine Street   Hammonton, NJ 08053   (609)561-3080   Fax (856)983-5110

Cohen, Pamela E., MD {1811076755} PhysMd(83,PA13)<NY-NSUHMANH>
+ Westfield Center
1515 Lamberts Mill Road   Westfield, NJ 07090   (908)233-9700

Cohen, Penelope Jucowics, MD {1316029796} Dermat(86,NJ05)
+ 1527 Route 27/Suite 2800
Somerset, NJ 08873   (732)220-1222   Fax (732)220-2944

Cohen, Philip Jay, MD {1669566683} IntrMd, Dermat(85,NJ05)
+ 41 Ridge Road
Whitehouse Station, NJ 08889

Cohen, Rachael Anna, DO {1649447541} ObsGyn, RprEnd(04,PA77)
+ Cooper Institute for Reproductive Hormonal Disorders
17000 Commerce Parkway/Suite C   Mount Laurel, NJ 08054   (856)751-5575   Fax (856)751-7289
rachelariela.cohen@gmail.com

Cohen, Rachel Isabel Silliman, MD {1063711729} Pedtrc(11,MD01)
+ University Hospital-Cares Institute
42 East Laurel Road/Suite 1100   Stratford, NJ 08084   (856)566-7036   Fax (856)566-6108

Cohen, Randy Scott, MD {1871572354} Anesth
+ Hackensack Anesthesiology Associates
140 Prospect Avenue/Suite 8   Hackensack, NJ 07601   (201)488-0066   Fax (201)488-6769
+ Hackensack University MC-Anesthesia Dept
30 Prospect Avenue/Room 2703   Hackensack, NJ 07601   (201)488-0066   Fax (201)996-3962

Cohen, Ricky B., MD {1871559526} IntrMd(91,NY46)<NJ-VALLEY>
+ Prospect Medical Offices, LLC
301 Godwin Avenue   Midland Park, NJ 07432   (201)444-4526   Fax (201)301-1313

Cohen, Robert S., MD {1417535403} ObsGyn(65,NY09)
+ 140 Prospect Avenue/Suite 3
Hackensack, NJ 07601   (201)996-9449   Fax (201)342-0165

Physicians by Name and Address

Cohen, Ronald A., DO {1144273509} CdvDis(79,PA77)<NJ-KMHCHRRY, NJ-OURLADY>
+ Cardiovascular Associates of The Delaware Valley, PA
  1840 Frontage Road   Cherry Hill, NJ 08034   (856)795-2227   Fax (856)795-7436
+ Cardiovascular Associates
  210 West Atlantic Avenue   Haddon Heights, NJ 08035   (856)795-2227   Fax (856)547-5337
+ Cardiovascular Associates of The Delaware Valley, PA
  525 State Street/Suite 3   Elmer, NJ 08034   (856)358-2363   Fax (856)358-0725

Cohen, Ronald L., MD {1538271564} ObsGyn(70,NETH)<NJ-MONMOUTH>
+ Ocean Obstetric and Gynecologic Associates
  804 West Park Avenue/Building A   Ocean, NJ 07712   (732)695-2040   Fax (732)493-1640

Cohen, Sander M., MD {1649277351} Ophthl(83,MD07)<NJ-VIRTMHBC>
+ South Jersey Eye Physicians PA
  103 Old Marlton Pike/Suite 216   Medford, NJ 08055   (609)714-8761   Fax (609)714-8759
+ South Jersey Eye Physicians PA
  25 Homestead Drive/Suite A   Columbus, NJ 08022   (609)714-8761   Fax (609)291-1972
+ South Jersey Eye Physicians PA
  509 South Lenola Road/Suite 11   Moorestown, NJ 08055   (856)234-0222   Fax (856)727-9518

Cohen, Scott, DO {1497843288} Gastrn, IntrMd(93,NJ75)<NJ-COMMED>
+ Ocean Endosurgery Center
  129 Route 37 West   Toms River, NJ 08755   (732)606-4440   Fax (732)797-3963

Cohen, Scott Allan, MD {1528087319} Surgry(95,NY08)
+ Cohen Surgical Arts
  35 West Main Street/Suite 101   Denville, NJ 07834   (973)627-6006   Fax (973)627-4337

Cohen, Seth Aloe, MD {1134159684} Gastrn, IntrMd(86,NY01)
+ Center for Endocrine Health
  1121 route 22 west/Suite 205   Bridgewater, NJ 08807   (212)734-8874   Fax (212)249-5628

Cohen, Seth Daniel, MD {1548295306} IntrMd, Onclgy, Hemato(98,NY06)<NJ-MONMOUTH>
+ Monmouth Hematology Oncology Associates PA
  100 State Highway 36/Suite 1B   West Long Branch, NJ 07764   (732)222-1711   Fax (732)222-2060

Cohen, Shaul, MD {1013099175} Anesth(73,ISR01)<NJ-RWJUBRUN>
+ Robert Wood Johnson-UMDNJ Anesthesia Group
  125 Paterson Street/CAB 3100   New Brunswick, NJ 08901   (732)235-7827   Fax (732)235-6131

Cohen, Sherri Shubin, MD {1952324998} Pedtrc, PubHth, GPrvMd(99,PA13)<PA-CHILDHOS>
+ CHOP Specialty Care Center at Virtua
  200 Bowman Drive/2 FL/Suite D-260   Voorhees, NJ 08043   (267)425-5400
+ CHOP Pediatric & Adolescent Specialty Care Center
  1012 Laurel Oak Road   Voorhees, NJ 08043   (267)425-5400   Fax (856)435-0091

Cohen, Stephanie Gail, MD {1548271539} Pedtrc(02,NJ06)<NJ-RWJUBRUN, NJ-SOMERSET>
+ University Medical Group Pediatrics
  125 Paterson Street/MEB 3rd Fl   New Brunswick, NJ 08903   (732)235-7893   Fax (732)235-7345

Cohen, Stephanie Meryl, MD {1821031147} SrgPlstc(91,DC02)<NJ-HACKNSK>
+ Cohen/Winters Aesthetic & Reconstructive Surgery
  113 West Essex Street/Suite 202   Maywood, NJ 07607   (201)487-3400   Fax (201)487-2481
+ Aesthetic and Reconstructive Surgeons
  20 Prospect Avenue/Suite 501   Hackensack, NJ 07601   (201)487-3400

Cohen, Stephen Jonathan, MD {1417968355} PhysMd(02,NJ05)<NJ-COOPRUMC>
+ Cooper PM & R Assocs
  One Cooper Plaza/Suite 550   Camden, NJ 08103   (856)342-2040   Fax (856)968-8311
+ Cooper PM & R Assocs
  1101 North Kings Highway/Suite 100   Cherry Hill, NJ 08034   (856)342-2040   Fax (856)414-6121
+ Cooper PM & R Assocs
  3 Cooper Plaza/Suite 104   Camden, NJ 08103   (856)342-2040   Fax (856)968-8311

Cohen, Steven B., MD {1235133000} Ophthl(78,NY19)
+ Retina-Vitreous Consultants
  349 East Northfield Road/Suite 100   Livingston, NJ 07039   (973)716-0123   Fax (973)716-0441
+ Retina-Vitreous Consultants
  95 Madison Avenue/Suite A03   Morristown, NJ 07960   (973)716-0123   Fax (973)716-0441
+ Short Hills Surgery Center
  187 Millburn Avenue/Suite 101   Millburn, NJ 07039   (973)671-0555   Fax (973)671-0557

Cohen, Steven Craig, DO {1659301166} Nephro, IntrMd(96,PA77)<NJ-CHSMRCER>
+ Mercer Kidney Institute
  40 Fuld Street/Suite 401   Trenton, NJ 08638   (609)599-1004   Fax (609)599-3611

Cohen, Theodore, MD ObsGyn(74,NJ05)<NJ-STBARNMC>
+ Physicians for Women's HealthCare
  315 East Northfield Road/Suite 3-B   Livingston, NJ 07039   (973)422-1200   Fax (973)422-9169

Cohen, Todd S., DO {1780665265} CdvDis, IntrMd(89,PA77)<NJ-JRSYSHMC, NJ-OCEANMC>
+ Shore Cardiology Consultants, LLC
  1640 Route 88/Suite 201   Brick, NJ 08724   (732)840-1900   Fax (732)840-0355
+ Shore Cardiology Consultants, LLC
  3200 Sunset Avenue/Suite 208   Ocean, NJ 07712   (732)840-1900

Cohen, Zaza Isaac, MD {1245334721} PulDis, CritCr, IntrMd(97,VT02)<NJ-MTNSIDE>
+ Hackensack UMC Mountainside
  1 Bay Avenue/Pulm Disease   Montclair, NJ 07042   (973)429-6874   Fax (973)429-6575

Cohen-Schwartz, Dawn Sheri, MD {1083816227} RadDia(94,NY46)
+ Westfield Imaging Center
  118-122 Elm Street   Westfield, NJ 07090   (908)232-0610   Fax (908)232-7140

Cohler, Alan, MD {1407894322} RadThp, Radiol, RadOnc(70,PA01)<NJ-RWJUBRUN>
+ RWJ University Hospital New Brunswick
  One Robert Wood Johnson Place   New Brunswick, NJ 08901   (732)253-3939   Fax (732)253-3952
+ Rutgers Cancer Institute of New Jersey
  195 Little Albany Street/PO Box 2681   New Brunswick, NJ 08903   (732)253-3939   Fax (732)235-6797

Cohn, David B., MD {1740252261} CritCr, PulDis, IntrMd(86,PA02)<NJ-HUNTRDN>
+ Hunterdon Pediatric Associates
  6 Sand Hill Road/Suite 202   Flemington, NJ 08822   (908)237-4080   Fax (908)237-1749
+ Hunterdon Pediatric Associates
  8 Reading Road/Reading Ridge   Flemington, NJ 08822   (908)237-4080   Fax (908)788-6005
+ Hunterdon Pediatric Associates
  537 Route 22 East/3rd Floor   Whitehouse Station, NJ 08822   (908)823-1100   Fax (908)823-0433

Cohn, Joseph Theodore, MD {1831108935} FamMed(77,MA07)
+ 23 South First Avenue
  Highland Park, NJ 08904   (732)545-3434

Cohn, Steven M., MD {1649290453} CdvDis(82,MEX14)<NJ-SJRSYELM, NJ-SJHREGMC>
+ Cumberland Cardiology
  2848 South Delsea Drive/Suite 4-A   Vineland, NJ 08360
+ Cardiovascular Associates of The Delaware Valley, PA
  525 State Street/Suite 3   Elmer, NJ 08318   Fax (856)358-0725

Coia, Lawrence R., MD {1093791683} RadOnc(78,PA13)<NJ-COMMED>
+ Community Medical Center
  99 Route 37 West   Toms River, NJ 08755   (732)557-8000

Coifman, Robert E., MD {1477552024} Allrgy, ImmAsm, Imuno(64,WI05)<NJ-SJERSYHS, NJ-ACMCMAIN>
+ Allergy Asthma of South Jersey
  1122 North High Street   Millville, NJ 08332   (856)825-4100   Fax (856)825-1700
  rcoifman@aasj.com
+ Allergy Asthma of South Jersey
  5 East Jimmie Leeds Road   Galloway, NJ 08205   (609)652-1009

Coira, Diego L., MD {1750336038} Psychy(83,WIND)<NJ-HACKNSK>
+ Drs. Coira & Richards
  851 Franklin Lake Road/Suite 105   Franklin Lakes, NJ 07417   (201)904-2230   Fax (201)904-2232
+ Hackensack University Medical Center
  30 Prospect Avenue   Hackensack, NJ 07601   (201)904-2230   Fax (201)996-3602

Colaco, Rodolfo, MD {1912964537} Surgry(74,INDI)<NJ-TRINIWSC>
+ 431 Elmora Avenue
  Elizabeth, NJ 07208   (908)353-4177   Fax (908)353-7201

Colaneri, John A., MD {1326140088} GenPrc, FamMed(76,MEXI)
+ 310 Hoboken Road
  East Rutherford, NJ 07073   (201)939-4036

Colantoni, Matthew Steven, DO {1770840209} EmrgMd(12,NY75)
+ St Joseph's Medical Center Emergency
  703 Main Street   Paterson, NJ 07503   (973)754-2240   Fax (973)754-2249

Colao, Joseph A., Jr., DO {1154826774} OthrSp, PhysMd(92,NJ75)
+ University Hospital
  150 Bergen Street   Newark, NJ 07103   (973)972-4300

+ 86 North McClellan Avenue
  Manasquan, NJ 08736

Colarusso, Frank John Michael, DO {1558314047} PhysMd, PhyMSptM(96,PA77)
+ Mercer-Bucks Orthopaedics PC
  3120 Princeton Pike   Lawrenceville, NJ 08648   (609)896-0444   Fax (609)896-1055
+ Mercer-Bucks Orthopaedics, P.C.
  2501 Kuser Road   Hamilton, NJ 08691   (609)896-0444   Fax (609)587-4349

Colavita, Donato A., MD {1407811839} Surgry(80,DOMI)
+ 135 Bloomfield Avenue/Suite k
  Bloomfield, NJ 07003   (973)344-6897   Fax (973)344-3854

Colavita, Richard D., MD {1730144627} Anesth, PedAne, Acpntr(80,NC05)<NJ-SOMERSET, NJ-STPETER>
+ Anesthesia Consultnts of NJ/Nova Pain
  285 Davidson Avenue/Suite 204   Somerset, NJ 08873   (732)271-1400   Fax (732)271-3543

Colbert, Angelique L., DO {1801051875} FamMed(76,MI12)
+ 36 Lancaster Drive
  Westampton, NJ 08060   (609)265-9441   Fax (609)265-9628

Colcher, Amy, MD {1174554901} Nrolgy(89,PA02)<NJ-COOPRUMC>
+ Cooper University Neurology
  1935 Route 70 East   Cherry Hill, NJ 08003   (856)342-2445   Fax (856)964-0504

Cole, Brian Anthony, MD {1558315309} SrgOrt, SrgSpn(89,PA01)<NJ-ENGLWOD, NJ-HOLYNAME>
+ Englewood Orthopedic Associates
  401 South Van Brunt Street   Englewood, NJ 07631   (201)569-2770   Fax (201)569-1774

Cole, Bruno N., MD {1073532842} SrgThr, SrgVas, Surgry(78,PA01)
+ Princeton Primary and Urgent Care Center LLC
  707 Alexander Road/Suite 201   Princeton, NJ 08540   (809)919-0303   Fax (609)919-0008

Cole, Frederick, Jr., DO {1518076561} SrgHnd, SrgOrt, IntrMd(69,PA77)
+ 1 Secluded Lane
  Rio Grande, NJ 08242   (609)868-0710   Fax (609)886-8862

Cole, James R., MD {1114971595} SrgArt, SrgOrt, SrgSpn(65,NY01)<NY-SPCLSURG, NJ-ENGLWOD>
+ Englewood Orthopedic Associates
  401 South Van Brunt Street   Englewood, NJ 07631   (201)569-2770   Fax (201)569-1774

Cole, Janet M., MD {1669538153} FamMed(80,NY46)
+ Johnson & Johnson
  501 George Street   New Brunswick, NJ 08901   (908)218-3049
+ Johnson & Johnson
  1 Johnson & Johnson/EmpHlth Rm5G32   New Brunswick, NJ 08933   (908)218-3049   Fax (732)828-5493

Cole, Jeffrey Lewis, MD {1386646305} PhysMd, PhyMPain(77,MEX03)<NJ-KSLRWEST>
+ Kessler Institute for Rehabilitation West Orange
  1199 Pleasant Valley Way   West Orange, NJ 07052   (973)243-6999

Cole, Julie Barudin, MD {1962726588} RadDia, Radiol, IntrMd(86,NY01)
+ RadPharm Inc.
  100 Overlook Center/3rd Floor   Princeton, NJ 08540   (201)341-8376   Fax (609)936-2602

Cole, Peter D., MD {1376553057} PedHem, Pedtrc(93,NY20)<NJ-ENGLWOD, NJ-RWJUBRUN>
+ Englewood Hospital and Medical Center
  350 Engle Street/Pediatrics   Englewood, NJ 07631   (201)894-3000

Cole, Randolph Paul, MD {1073533022} IntrMd(73,NY08)<NJ-HOLYNAME>
+ Holy Name Hospital
  718 Teaneck Road/Intensive Care   Teaneck, NJ 07666   (201)833-3342   Fax (201)833-3098

Cole, Robert J., MD {1043482342} RadOnc, Radiol(79,NC05)<NJ-NWTNMEM, NJ-CHILTON>
+ Specialty Surgical Center
  380 Lafayette Road/Suite 110   Sparta, NJ 07871   (973)940-3166   Fax (973)940-3170

Colella, Robert Eugene, DO {1073574869} IntrMd(94,NY75)<NJ-STFRNMED>
+ St. Francis Medical Center
  601 Hamilton Avenue/Internal Med   Trenton, NJ 08629   (609)599-5000
+ Pathlink, LLC
  66 West Gilbert Street/Suite 100   Tinton Falls, NJ 07701   (609)599-5000   Fax (732)212-0061

Colella, Ryan Lawrence, MD {1265403737} ObsGyn(95,MA07)
+ Garden State Obstetrics and Gynecological Associates
  2401 Evesham Road/Suite A   Voorhees, NJ 08043   (856)424-3323   Fax (856)424-4994

Coleman, Ashley J., DO {1306009709} IntrMd(PA77<NJ-OURLADY>
  + Our Lady of Lourdes Medical Center
    1600 Haddon Avenue/Internal Med   Camden, NJ 08103   (856)757-3500
Coleman, Clenton Louis, MD {1730379025} Nephro, IntrMd(04,NJ05)<NJ-HOLYNAME>
  + Drs. Coleman & Adair
    222 Cedar Lane/Suite 111   Teaneck, NJ 07666   (201)836-7970   Fax (201)836-7973
  + Drs. Coleman & Adair
    211 60th Street   West New York, NJ 07093   (201)836-7970   Fax (201)868-7185
Coleman, Colleen Marie, MD {1215936836} Ophthl(00,MI07)
  + Soll Eye PC of New Jersey/Cooper Division
    3 Cooper Plaza/Suite 510   Camden, NJ 08103   (856)342-7200   Fax (856)342-6620
Coleman, Elliott H., MD {1487693990} CdvDis, IntrMd(65,PA13)
  + Penn Specialty Care of Burlington County
    200 Campbell Drive/Suite 115   Willingboro, NJ 08046   (609)871-7070   Fax (609)835-4510
Coleman, Jane L., MD {1730130550} Pedtrc, NnPnMd, AdolMd(78,PA09)<NJ-KMHSTRAT, NJ-KMHTURNV>
  + Kennedy Memorial Hospital-University Medical Center
    18 East Laurel Road/Pediatrics   Stratford, NJ 08084   (856)346-6000
Coleman, Reginald O., MD {1164596565} Pedtrc(75,NJ05)
  + 2728 Kennedy Boulevard
    Jersey City, NJ 07306   (201)433-7817   Fax (201)433-6044
Coleman, Scott L., MD {1275577074} IntrMd, FamMed(82,NJ05)
  + ImmediCenter/Clifton
    1355 Broad Street   Clifton, NJ 07013   (973)778-5566   Fax (973)778-2268
  + ImmediCenter/Totowa
    500 Union Boulevard   Totowa, NJ 07512   (973)778-5566   Fax (973)790-6070
Colen, Kari Lindsey, MD {1093972598} SrgPHand, SrgPlstc(02,NY19)<NY-NYEYEINF, NJ-HACKNSK>
  + Colen MD Plastic Surgery Center
    20 Prospect Avenue/Suite 902   Hackensack, NJ 07601   (201)996-5588   Fax (201)996-3518
Colen, Stephen R., MD {1154370245} SrgPlstc, Surgry, SrgBst(74,PA09)<NJ-HACKNSK, NY-NYUTISCH>
  + Colen MD Plastic Surgery Center
    20 Prospect Avenue/Suite 902   Hackensack, NJ 07601   (201)996-5588   Fax (201)996-3518
  + Hackensack University Medical Center
    20 Prospect Avenue/PlasticSurg   Hackensack, NJ 07601   (201)996-2000
Colenda, Maryann J., MD {1629006143} Pedtrc, PedAlg, Algy-Immn(71,NY09)<NJ-ENGLWOOD>
  + 810 Abbott Boulevard
    Fort Lee, NJ 07024   (201)224-2256
Coletta, Domenic, Jr., MD {1487681391} EmrgMd(82,PA09)<NJ-BURDTMLN>
  + Cape Regional Medical Center
    2 Stone Harbor Boulevard/EmergMed   Cape May Court House, NJ 08210   (609)463-2000   Fax (609)463-2946
Coletta, Umberto, MD {1437218641} PthACl, Pthlgy(80,NJ05)<NJ-OCEANMC>
  + Ocean Medical Center
    425 Jack Martin Boulevard/Pathology   Brick, NJ 08723   (732)840-2200
Coley, Marcelyn K., MD {1396906871}
  + Summit Medical Group-Berkeley Heights Campus
    1 Diamond Hill Road   Berkeley Heights, NJ 07922   (908)273-4300   Fax (973)921-9756
Colicchio, Alan Robert, MD {1477535375} Nrolgy, IntrMd(83,ITA17)<NJ-BAYSHORE, NJ-OCEANMC>
  + 99 Buena Vita Avenue
    Rumson, NJ 07760   (732)859-4214   Fax (732)842-7599   alancolicchio@yahoo.com
Colizza, Wayne A., MD {1568417137} OthrSp, SprtMd, SrgOrt(87,QU01)<NJ-MORRISTN>
  + Tri-County Orthopedics
    160 East Hanover Avenue   Morristown, NJ 07962   (973)538-2334   Fax (973)829-9174
  + Tri-County Orthopedics
    376 Lafayette Road/Suite 103   Sparta, NJ 07871   (973)538-2334   Fax (973)829-9174
  + Specialty Surgical Center
    380 Lafayette Road/Suite 110   Sparta, NJ 07962   (973)940-3166   Fax (973)940-3170
Collado, Anna A., DO {1215992011} ObsGyn(87,NJ75)<NJ-CHILTON, NJ-HACKNSK>
  + Women's Ob-Gyn PC
    150 Overlook Avenue/OFC 1   Hackensack, NJ 07601   (201)342-1191   Fax (201)342-1195   womobgyn@hotmail.com
Collado, Maria R., MD {1053340786} Pedtrc(93,PHI01)<NJ-OCEANMC>
  + Pediatric Care Physicians, LLC
    2211 Route 88/Suite 2-A   Brick, NJ 08724   (732)899-0008   Fax (732)899-0447
Collado, Marilyn Loh, MD {1952396053} ObsGyn(88,NY47)<NJ-RIVERVW>
  + Women Caring for Women
    43 North Gilbert Street/Suite 8   Tinton Falls, NJ 07701   (732)530-5550   Fax (732)345-8309
Collalto, Patrick Michael, MD {1649272998} SrgOrt, SrgSpn, NeuMSptM(80,NJ05)<NJ-HUNTRDN>
  + MidJersey Orthopaedics, P.A.
    8100 Westcott Drive/Suite 101   Flemington, NJ 08822   (908)782-0600   Fax (908)782-7575
Collazo, Edgar R., MD {1073596169} Pedtrc
  + Advocare Township Pediatrics
    123 Egg Harbor Road   Sewell, NJ 08080   (856)227-5437   Fax (856)227-5890
Collier, Jill A., MD {1740222702} Gastrn(90,NY47)
  + Gastroenterologists of Ocean County
    477 Lakehurst Road   Toms River, NJ 08755   (732)349-4422   Fax (732)349-5087   jcolliermd@comcast.net
Collin, Robert Daniel, MD {1700802790} IntrMd(81,MEX14)<NJ-CLARMAAS>
  + Essex Health Care
    23 Bran Ford Place   Newark, NJ 07107   (973)483-5551   Fax (973)484-0331
Collini, William R., MD {1922008036} Urolgy(66,PA02)<NJ-NWTNMEM, NJ-HCKTSTWN>
  + Drs. Mattes & Collini
    181 High Street   Newton, NJ 07860   (973)383-9898   Fax (973)383-9665
Collins, Beverly Ann, MD {1528063096}
  + University Health Plans, Inc.
    550 Broad Street/17th Floor   Newark, NJ 07102   (973)274-2102   Fax (973)623-3635   beverly.collins@wellcare.com
Collins, Caitlin, MD {1760965792} PhysMd<NJ-BERGNMC>
  + New Bridge Medical Center
    230 East Ridgewood Avenue   Paramus, NJ 07652   (908)222-6564
Collins, Christopher Michael, MD {1598083438} PedOrt
  + Seaview Orthopaedics
    1200 Eagle Avenue   Ocean, NJ 07712   (732)660-6200   Fax (732)988-4705
Collins, Gregory C., MD {1043229065} IntrMd(91,NJ06)<NJ-ACM-CITY>
  + Southern Jersey Family Medical Center
    1301 Atlantic Avenue   Atlantic City, NJ 08401   (609)572-0000   Fax (609)572-0039
  + Southern Jersey Family Medical Centers, Inc.
    860 South White Horse Pike/Building A   Hammonton, NJ 08037   (609)572-0000   Fax (609)567-3492
  + Southern Jersey Family Medical Centers Inc.
    932 South Main Street   Pleasantville, NJ 08401   (609)383-0880   Fax (609)383-0658
Collins, Harry, MD {1922078377} FamMed, Grtrcs, FamMAdlt(74,PA09)<NJ-JFKMED>
  + Mid Jersey Medical Associates
    1 Ethel Road/Suite 107b   Edison, NJ 08817   (732)287-2020   Fax (732)287-2071
Collins, Jared Andrew, DO {1891087979}<NJ-COOPRUMC>
  + Cooper University Hospital
    One Cooper Plaza   Camden, NJ 08103   (314)799-0974   drjc14@gmail.com
Collins, John Joseph, III, MD {1912976242} EmrgMd(02,MO34)<MA-NEMEDCEN>
  + University Emergency Medicine
    125 Paterson Street/MEB 104   New Brunswick, NJ 08901   (732)235-8717   Fax (732)235-7379
Collins, Joy Lynn, MD {1255428819} Surgry<PA-CHILDHOS>
  + CHOP Pediatric & Adolescent Specialty Care Center
    1012 Laurel Oak Road   Voorhees, NJ 08043   (856)435-1300   Fax (856)435-0091
  + CHOP Pediatric & Adolescent Specialty Care Center
    707 Alexander Road/Suite 205   Princeton, NJ 08540   (609)520-1717
Collins, Melinda Jean, DO {1407146400} Rheuma
  + Hackensack UMG
    150 Overlook Avenue   Hackensack, NJ 07601   (201)489-5999   Fax (201)489-1898
Collins, Neal, MD {1225578362} IntrMd
  + 19 North Hillside Avenue
    Chatham, NJ 07928   (973)665-1665
Collins, Patrice, MD {1407127400} Anesth(89,PA09)
  + 42 Christopher Drive
    Princeton, NJ 08540   (609)921-7472   Fax (609)228-4172
Collins, Philip, DO {1073945135} FamMed
  + Hammonton Family Medicine Center
    373 South White Horse Pike   Hammonton, NJ 08037   (609)704-0185   Fax (609)704-0195
Collins, Reid T., MD {1659637320} FamMed
  + Annandale Family Practice
    56 Payne Road/Suite 21   Lebanon, NJ 08833   (908)238-0100   Fax (908)238-0951
Collins, Robert S., MD {1710983507} Radiol, RadDia(78,NY09)<NJ-RWJUHAM>
  + Quakerbridge Radiology Associates
    8 Quakerbridge Plaza/Building 8   Mercerville, NJ 08619   (609)890-0033   Fax (609)689-6067
Collins, Ronald A., MD {1710995576} Pedtrc(68,MA07)<NJ-MORRISTN>
  + Pediatric Associates
    77 Union Street   Dover, NJ 07801   (973)366-5236   Fax (973)366-5236
Collopy, Edward M., MD {1134183007} PsyNro, Psychy(88,NY06)
  + 520 Speedwell Avenue/Suite 108
    Morris Plains, NJ 07950   (973)539-4466   Fax (973)984-9181
Collum, Robert G., MD {1912941899} IntrMd(92,NY01)<NJ-ENGLWOOD, NY-PRSBALLN>
  + Denville Associates of Internal Medicine
    16 Pocono Road/Suite 317   Denville, NJ 07834   (973)627-2650   Fax (973)627-8383
Collur, Surekha, MD {1750491015} Ophthl, IntrMd(86,INA5B)<NJ-BAYSHORE, NJ-RIVERVW>
  + Bayshore Ophthalmology, LLC.
    719 North Beers Street   Holmdel, NJ 07733   (732)264-6464   Fax (732)264-5114   surekha@pol.net
Colmer, Marc E., MD {1154376549} CdvDis, IntrMd, CarNuc(68,MA05)
  + Atlantic Cardiology LLC
    444 Neptune Boulevard/Unit 2   Neptune, NJ 07753   (732)775-5300   Fax (732)988-7364
  + Atlantic Cardiology LLC
    22 North Main Street   Marlboro, NJ 07746   (732)462-6666
  + Atlantic Cardiology LLC
    27 South Cooks Bridge Road/Suite 216   Jackson, NJ 07753   (848)217-3010
Colombo, Lynn N., MD {1871931204}
  + 812 Grand Street/Apt 504
    Hoboken, NJ 07030   (201)214-3408   lynn.castaldi@gmail.com
Colon, Deannon, MD {1093065542}
  + Eric B. Chandler Health Center
    277 George Street   New Brunswick, NJ 08901   (732)235-6700   Fax (732)235-6729
Colon, Francisco G., MD {1770574410} SrgPlstc, SrgRec(87,NY01)<NJ-MORRISTN, NJ-STBARNMC>
  + Peer Group Plastic Surgery Center
    124 Columbia Turnpike   Florham Park, NJ 07932   (973)822-3000   Fax (973)822-1726
Colon, German R., MD {1417389578} IntrMd<NJ-CLARMAAS>
  + Clara Maass Medical Center
    1 Clara Maass Drive   Belleville, NJ 07109   (973)450-2432
Colon, Jose F., MD {1154569044} IntrMd(78,NJ05)
  + Newark Rehabilitation Center
    638 Mount Prospect Avenue   Newark, NJ 07104   (973)481-4040   Fax (973)481-1338
  + Rehabilitation Medicine Associates, P.A.
    345 Main Street   West Orange, NJ 07052   (973)481-4040   Fax (973)325-8488
Colon, Vincent F., MD {1710011283} PsyCAd(89,NJ06)<NJ-MORRISTN>
  + 161 Washington Valley Road/Suite 206
    Warren, NJ 07059   (732)469-7717   Fax (732)469-7717
Colonna, Elizabeth Ann, MD {1831154269} ObsGyn(89,IL42)
  + Robert Wood Johnson Ob-Gyn Associates
    3270 State Route 27/Suite 2200   Kendall Park, NJ 08824   (732)422-8989   Fax (732)422-4526
Colopinto, Christopher F., DO {1659341923} FamMed(78,PA77)<NJ-KMHSTRAT>
  + 1168 Haddon Avenue
    Camden, NJ 08103   (856)365-3286   Fax (856)365-0293
  + Advocare Berlin Medical Associates
    175 Cross Keys Road/Suite 300A   Berlin, NJ 08009   (856)365-3286   Fax (856)767-6102
Colton, Marc D., MD {1427021732} Urolgy(89,PA07)<NJ-STCLRDEN, NJ-MORRISTN>
  + Morris Urology
    195 Route 46/Suite 100   Mine Hill, NJ 07803   (973)627-0060   Fax (973)627-6821
  + Morris Urology
    16 Pocono Road/Suite 205   Denville, NJ 07834   (973)627-0060   Fax (973)627-6821

Physicians by Name and Address

Colucciello, Michael, MD {1215934146} VitRet, Ophthl(86,NY15)<NJ-VIRTMHBC>
+ South Jersey Eye Physicians PA
509 South Lenola Road/Suite 11 Moorestown, NJ 08057 (856)234-0222 Fax (856)727-9518
michael@macula.us
+ South Jersey Eye Physicians PA
103 Old Marlton Pike/Suite 216 Medford, NJ 08055 (856)234-0222 Fax (609)714-8759
+ South Jersey Eye Physicians PA
25 Homestead Drive/Suite A Columbus, NJ 08057 (609)298-0888 Fax (609)291-1972

Colucio, Peter M., MD {1184625287} IntrMd(85,NJ06)<NJ-OVERLOOK, NJ-MORRISTN>
+ Summit Medical Group-Berkeley Heights Campus
1 Diamond Hill Road Berkeley Heights, NJ 07922 (908)273-4300 Fax (908)790-6524

Colyer-Aversa, Lori A., MD {1376582734} Pedtrc(89,NJ05)<NJ-MTNSIDE>
+ Bloomridge Pediatrics
206 Belleville Avenue/Suite 202 Bloomfield, NJ 07003 (973)748-9500 Fax (973)748-9492

Comandatore, Ann Marie, MD {1467454066} Pedtrc, AdolMd(90,NJ05)<NJ-STBARNMC, NJ-OVERLOOK>
+ Drs. Gruenwald & Comandatore
90 Millburn Avenue/Suite 101 Millburn, NJ 07041 (973)378-7990 Fax (973)378-7991

Comiskey, Walter M., DO {1457572802} IntrMd(71,PA77)
+ Dorfner Family Medicine
1 Mainbridge Lane Willingboro, NJ 08046 (609)877-0644 Fax (609)877-0370
+ Dorfner Family Medicine
811 Sunset Road/Suite 101 Burlington, NJ 08016 (609)877-0644 Fax (609)387-9408

Comizio, Renee Carol, MD {1982782124} SrgPlstc(00,NY09)
+ Surgical Practice of Rolando Rolandelli, MD
435 South Street/Suite 360 Morristown, NJ 07960 (973)775-9248 Fax (877)787-9098

Compagnone, Linda, MD {1720059371} IntrMd(85,PA07)<NJ-HUNTRDN>
+ Franklin Family Practice PA
29 Clyde Road/Suite 101 Somerset, NJ 08873 (732)873-0330 Fax (732)873-2077
+ Whitehouse Station Family Medicine
263 Main Street/PO Box 128 Whitehouse Station, NJ 08889 (732)873-0330 Fax (908)534-6634

Compito, Gerard Anthony, MD {1871527358} RadDia, RadNro(85,NY15)<NJ-UNVMCPRN>
+ Princeton Radiology Associates, P.A.
419 North Harrison Street Princeton, NJ 08540 (609)921-3345 Fax (609)683-8847
+ Princeton Radiology Associates, P.A.
9 Centre Drive Jamesburg, NJ 08831 (609)921-3345 Fax (609)655-4016
+ University Radiology Group, P.C.
375 Route 206/Suite 1 Hillsborough, NJ 08540 (908)874-7600 Fax (908)874-7052

Comsti, Eric A., MD {1598723827} IntrMd(90,PHIL)<NJ-JRSYSHMC, NJ-OCEANMC>
+ Physicians for Adults
681 Route 70 Lakehurst, NJ 08733 (732)657-8111 Fax (732)657-7828

Comsti, Maria Virginia, MD {1376501866} IntrMd(90,PHI09)<NJ-JRSYSHMC>
+ 3456 West Bangs Avenue
Neptune, NJ 07753 (732)922-1122 Fax (732)922-1957

Conaway, Herbert C., Jr., MD {1649387283} IntrMd(89,PA02)<NJ-STFRNMED>
+ St. Francis Medical Center
601 Hamilton Avenue/Internal Med Trenton, NJ 08629 (609)599-5050 Fax (609)599-4318

Concepcion, Cleo L., MD {1912942608} Anesth(68,PHIL)<NJ-CLARMAAS>
+ Clara Maass Medical Center
1 Clara Maass Drive Belleville, NJ 07109 (973)450-2000

Concepcion, Erika Kristina, MD {1477844660}
+ 4 Brittany Way
Kendall Park, NJ 08824 (732)513-4372
erika.concepcion@gmail.com

Concepcion, Kristin A., MD {1053524777} Pedtrc(97,GRN01)<NJ-HOLYNAME, NJ-ENGLWOOD>
+ 1C New Amwell Road
Hillsborough, NJ 08844 (908)874-5035 Fax (908)874-3288

Concha Leon, Alonso E., MD {1427149327} Pedtrc, IntrMd(00,PER02)<NJ-UNVMCPRN, NJ-SJHREGMC>
+ CHOP Care Network at Princeton Medical Center
One Plainsboro Road/Pediatrics Plainsboro, NJ 08536 (609)853-7000 Fax (609)497-4173
+ SJH Regional Medical Center
1505 West Sherman Avenue/Pediatrics Vineland, NJ 08360 (609)853-7000 Fax (856)641-7647
+ Nemours Dupont Pediatrics
1925 Pacific Avenue Atlantic City, NJ 08536 (609)345-4000 Fax (609)572-8523

Concodora, Charles William, MD {1942511373} PedUro
+ Urology for Children, LLC
200 Bowman Drive/Suite E-360 Voorhees, NJ 08043 (856)751-7880

Conde, Miguel A., MD {1093795270} Hemato, MedOnc, IntrMd(86,NY01)<NJ-STBARNMC>
+ St. Barnabas Medical Center
94 Old Short Hills Road Livingston, NJ 07039 (973)322-5525

Condemi, Giuseppe, MD {1083660781} OncHem, IntrMd, MedOnc(98,DMN01)<NJ-ENGLWOOD, NJ-HOLYNAME>
+ Regional Cancer Center at Holy Name Medical Center
718 Teaneck Road Teaneck, NJ 07666 (201)227-6008 Fax (201)227-6002

Condiotte, Shaw Brandon, MD {1134102387} Pedtrc(96,GRN01)<NJ-RIVERVW>
+ Navesink Pediatrics
55 North Gilbert Street/Suite 2101 Tinton Falls, NJ 07701 (732)842-6677 Fax (732)530-2946

Condo, Dominick, MD {1114019692} IntrMd(80,MEXI)<NJ-BAYONNE>
+ 622 Broadway Street
Bayonne, NJ 07002 (201)436-2800 Fax (201)436-1353

Condoluci, David V., DO {1245210459} InfDis(76,PA77)<NJ-KMHCHRRY, NJ-KMHSTRAT>
+ Garden State Infectious Diseases Associates, P.A.
709 Haddonfield Berlin Road Voorhees, NJ 08043 (856)566-3190 Fax (856)783-2193
+ Garden State Infectious Disease Associates
570 Egg Harbor Road/Suite B-5 Sewell, NJ 08080 (856)566-3190 Fax (856)566-1904

Condoluci, Mark, DO {1851603120} IntrMd
+ Rowan University-School of Osteopathic Medicine
1 Medical Center Drive/IntrMd Stratford, NJ 08084 (856)566-6708

Condren, Eileen, DO {1396009684} AdolMd
+ Pediatric Care Physicians, LLC
2211 Route 88/Suite 2-A Brick, NJ 08724 (732)899-0008 Fax (732)899-0447

Condren, Marc J., MD {1982757712} FamMed(84,NY06)
+ 7 Cedar Grove Lane/Suite 38
Somerset, NJ 08873 (732)469-2133 Fax (732)469-9777

Confino, Joel, MD {1710073069} Ophthl, Catrct(80,NY46)
+ Eye Care and Surgery Center
592 Springfield Avenue Westfield, NJ 07090 (908)789-8999 Fax (908)789-1379
jconfino@cox.com
+ Eye Care and Surgery Center
10 Mountain Boulevard Warren, NJ 07059 (908)789-8999 Fax (908)754-4803

Cong, Elaine Alice, MD {1710120944} EnDbMt(09,NY46)
+ Bergen Medical Alliance, P.A.
180 Engle Street Englewood, NJ 07631 (201)567-2050 Fax (201)567-5070

Coniaris, Harry J., MD {1992775563} IntrMd, Ophthl(86,NJ06)<NJ-BAYSHORE, NJ-RIVERVW>
+ 723 North Beers Street/Suite 1C
Holmdel, NJ 07733 (732)888-3688 Fax (732)888-3633

Conigliari, Matthew F., MD {1417958604} Nrolgy(94,NJ05)<NJ-MORRISTN>
+ Neuroscience Center of Northern New Jersey
310 Madison Avenue Morristown, NJ 07960 (973)285-1446 Fax (973)605-8854

Conkling, Robert F., MD {1174725477} FamMed
+ 2401 Algonkin Trail
Manasquan, NJ 08736 (202)320-8834 Fax (434)385-8616

Conley, Michael P., MD {1386632255} ObsGyn(88,NJ05)<NJ-MONMOUTH, NJ-RIVERVW>
+ Ob-Gyn Associates at Holmdel-Shrewsbury
704 North Beers Street Holmdel, NJ 07733 (732)739-2500 Fax (732)888-2778
+ Ob-Gyn Associates at Holmdel-Shrewsbury
39 Avenue of the Commons Shrewsbury, NJ 07702 (732)389-0003

Conliffe, Theodore David, Jr., MD {1285688747} PhyMPain(PA09<NJ-ATLANTHS>
+ Rothman Institute - Voorhees
443 Laurel Oak Road Voorhees, NJ 08043 (856)821-6360

Conn, Michael J., MD {1689755191} SrgPlstc, Surgry(86,DC02)<NJ-CHILTON, NJ-HOLYNAME>
+ 870 Palisade Avenue/Suite 206
Teaneck, NJ 07666 (201)836-9296 Fax (201)836-3571
+ 191 Hamburg Turnpike
Pompton Lakes, NJ 07442 (973)839-3900

Conn, Mitchell I., MD {1922067917} Gastrn, Hepato(80,NY19)<NJ-SJRSYELM, NJ-UNDRWD>
+ South Jersey Endoscopy Center
26 East Red Bank Avenue Woodbury, NJ 08096 (856)848-4464 Fax (856)848-8706

Connell, Rebecca Kathleen, MD {1467568139} CritCr, IntrMd, PulDis(88,GRN01)
+ VA New Jersey Health Care System-East Orange Campus
385 Tremont Avenue/Pulmonary East Orange, NJ 07018 (973)676-1000 Fax (973)395-7034

Connell, Thomas A., MD {1801974753} Psychy(87,PA07)<NJ-HAMPTBHC>
+ Hampton Behavioral Health Center
650 Rancocas Road Westampton, NJ 08060 (609)267-7000

Connelly, Brian, MD {1124103106} Anesth(89,NJ05)<NJ-VALLEY>
+ The Valley Hospital
223 North Van Dien Avenue/Anesth Ridgewood, NJ 07450 (201)847-9403
+ Bergen Anesthesia Group, P.C.
500 West Main Street/Suite 16 Wyckoff, NJ 07481 (201)847-9403 Fax (201)847-0059

Conner, Ellen Louise, MD {1609867100} ObsGyn, UroGyn, Gyneco(98,NY19)<NJ-JRSYSHMC>
+ Hackensack Meridian Urogynecolgy Medical Group
19 Davis Avenue/7th Floor Neptune, NJ 07753 (732)776-3797 Fax (732)776-3796
+ Jersey Shore University Medical Center
1945 Route 33 Neptune, NJ 07753 (732)775-5500

Conner, Patrick R., MD {1386880813} OccpMd(77,NC07)
+ BASF Corporation
100 Campus Drive Florham Park, NJ 07932 (973)895-8030 Fax (973)245-6947

Connolly, Adrian L., MD {1922001650} Dermat(75,NJ05)<NJ-STBARNMC>
+ 101 Old Short Hills Road/Suite 214
West Orange, NJ 07052 (973)731-9131 Fax (973)731-9201
Drconnolly@comcast.net

Connolly, Allison Carthan, MD {1760740757} IntrMd<NJ-MORRISTN>
+ Mendham Medical Group LLP
19 East Main Street/Suite 1 Mendham, NJ 07945 (973)543-6505 Fax (973)543-2967

Connolly, Coyle S., DO {1386601433} Dermat(92,PA77)<NJ-SHOREMEM>
+ Connolly Dermatology
2106 New Road/Suite D4 Linwood, NJ 08221 (609)926-8899 Fax (609)653-8713

Connolly, Karen Lynn, MD {1801116389} Dermat
+ 101 Old Short Hills Road/Suite 503
West Orange, NJ 07052 (973)731-9131

Connolly, Mark William, MD {1326010612} CdvDis, SrgThr(82,IL06)<NJ-STJOSHOS>
+ St. Joseph Medical Center Surgery
703 Main Street Paterson, NJ 07503 (973)754-2460 Fax (973)754-2462

Connolly, Melissa Jane, MD {1487758926} IntrMd, Pedtrc(95,NY48)
+ Pediatrics of Morris
16 Pocono Road/Suite 112 Denville, NJ 07834 (973)627-6010 Fax (973)625-9424

Connolly, Patrick Joseph, MD {1134113889} SrgNro(98,MD01)
+ Capital Institute for Neurosciences
2 Capital Way/Suite 456 Pennington, NJ 08534 (609)537-7300 Fax (609)537-7301

Connolly, Sandra M., MD {1023156825} EmrgMd, FamMed(89,NJ06)<NJ-CENTRAST>
+ CentraState Medical Center
901 West Main Street/HouseStaff Phys Freehold, NJ 07728 (732)431-2000

Connor, John Patrick, MD {1740267863} PedUro, Urolgy(83,IRE04)<NJ-MORRISTN, NY-PRSBCOLU>
+ Adult & Pediatric Urology Group PA
261 James Street/Suite 1-A Morristown, NJ 07960 (973)539-0333 Fax (973)539-8909
+ Morristown Medical Center
100 Madison Avenue Morristown, NJ 07962 (973)971-5000

Connor, Thomas M., MD {1194863407} PedCrd, Pedtrc(66,ITA01)<NJ-CHILTON, NJ-HACKNSK>
+ 101 Old Short Hills Road/Suite 104
West Orange, NJ 07052 (973)731-5550 Fax (973)243-0033
+ 4-14 Saddle River Road
Fair Lawn, NJ 07410 (201)794-1366

Connors, Anne, MD {1578500278} Anesth(98,IL42)<NJ-CENTRAST>
+ Liberty Anesthesia & Pain Management
901 West Main Street/2nd Floor Freehold, NJ 07728 (732)294-2876 Fax (732)294-2502
+ CentraState Medical Center
901 West Main Street/Anesthesiology Freehold, NJ 07728 (732)431-2000

Physicians by Name and Address

Connors, Barbara J., DO {1457525511} IntrMd, GPrvMd(81,NY75)
+ 658 North Saratoga Drive
Moorestown, NJ 08057

Connors, Daniel Bernard, MD {1821357435} Ophthl
+ Retinal & Ophthalmic Consultants, PC
1500 Tilton Road   Northfield, NJ 08225   (609)646-5200   Fax (609)646-9868

Connors, Diane, MD {1851333629} Radiol, RadDia, NuclMd(85,MI07)<NJ-OCEANMC>
+ Atlantic Medical Imaging
455 Jack Martin Boulevard   Brick, NJ 08724   (732)223-9729   Fax (732)840-6459

Connors, Robert Dedick, MD {1801030473} Nrolgy, ClNrPh(08,TN05)
+ Progressive Neurology
260 Old Hook Road/Suite 200   Westwood, NJ 07675   (201)546-8510   Fax (201)503-8142

Conover, Melissa, MD {1093109365} PhysMd
+ Linwood Care Center
201 New Road   Linwood, NJ 08221   (609)927-7837

Conrad, Michael James, MD {1871542134} Nephro, IntrMd(81,MA16)<NJ-VIRTMHBC, NJ-LOURDMED>
+ The Center for Kidney Care
1261 Route 38/Suite A   Hainesport, NJ 08036   (856)222-1975   Fax (856)222-0721

Conroy, Daniel, Jr., MD {1629098603} CdvDis, IntrMd(75,MEX14)<NJ-STMRYPAS>
+ Lyndhurst Medical Associates
358 Valley Brook Avenue   Lyndhurst, NJ 07071   (201)460-0142   Fax (201)460-1959
+ Lyndhurst Medical Associates
1033 Clifton Avenue   Clifton, NJ 07013   (201)460-0142   Fax (973)473-7085

Constable, Richard E., MD {1376572198} Surgry, SrgTrm(78,NY03)
+ 655 Amboy Avenue
Woodbridge, NJ 07095   (732)634-4440

Constad, William H., MD {1437267630} CrnExD, Ophthl(80,PA07)<NJ-JRSYCITY, NJ-CHRIST>
+ Hudson Eye Physicians & Surgeons, LLC
600 Pavonia Avenue/6th Floor   Jersey City, NJ 07306   (201)963-3937   Fax (201)963-8823
whconstad@hudsoneye.com

Constandis, Calin G., MD {1730297797} IntrMd(65,ROM06)
+ 867 Saint George Avenue
Rahway, NJ 07065   (732)381-0222

Constantino, Edwin M., MD {1083708309} Elecmy, PhysMd, OthrSp(83,PHIL)<NJ-CHRIST, NJ-HOBUNIMC>
+ 10 Huron Avenue/Suite 1L
Jersey City, NJ 07306   (201)656-0440   Fax (201)656-3444

Constantinopoulos, George S., MD {1588739742} SrgVas, Surgry(75,GRE01)<NJ-MONMOUTH>
+ 279 Third Avenue
Long Branch, NJ 07740   (732)229-8486

Conte, Daniel P., III, DO {1376616920} OstMed, NeuMus(86,NJ75)
+ Structure & Function
600 Midland Avenue   Garfield, NJ 07026   (973)253-1900   Fax (973)253-6323

Conte, Evan J., MD {1073883237}
+ Trenton Orthopaedic Group
1225 Whitehorse Mercerville Rd   Trenton, NJ 08619   (609)581-2200   Fax (609)581-1212
+ Trenton Orthopaedic Group
116 Washington Crossing Road   Pennington, NJ 08534   (609)581-2200   Fax (609)581-1212

Conte, Kenneth S., DO {1851436133} FamMed(66,MO78)
+ 600 Midland Avenue
Garfield, NJ 07026   (973)478-1212   Fax (973)478-5462
Lavinatconte@att.net

Conte, Louis J., DO {1952356651} Otlryg, SrgPlstc(90,IA75)
+ Associated Ear Nose & Throat Physicians
505 Chestnut Street   Roselle Park, NJ 07204   (908)241-0200   Fax (908)241-0445
+ Associated Ear Nose & Throat Physicians
778 Kennedy Boulevard   Bayonne, NJ 07002   (908)241-0200   Fax (201)829-1821

Conte, Patrick, Jr., MD {1235126772} NuclMd, Radiol(66,IL43)
+ Imaging Subspecialists of North Jersey LLC
703 Main Street   Paterson, NJ 07503   (973)754-2645

Conte, Salvatore A., MD {1174688493} IntrMd(91,WIND)<NJ-WAYNEGEN, NJ-STJOSHOS>
+ 1167 McBridge Avenue/Suite 1
West Paterson, NJ 07424   (973)790-8811   Fax (973)790-8817

Conte, Stephen John, DO {1750329900} Radiol(66,MO78)
+ Diagnostic Imaging Center and Group Practice
251 Rochelle Avenue   Rochelle Park, NJ 07662   (201)291-8800   Fax (201)291-0637

Conte, Theodore J., MD {1053366724} Nrolgy(98,NJ05)
+ 22 Madison Avenue/Suite 206
Paramus, NJ 07652   (201)291-8489   Fax (201)291-8487

Conti, John A., MD {1811973084} IntrMd, MedOnc, OncHem(86,NJ05)<NJ-CLARMAAS, NJ-STBARNMC>
+ Essex Hematology-Oncology Group, PA
36 Newark Avenue/Suite 304   Belleville, NJ 07109   (973)751-8880   Fax (973)751-8950
+ Essex Hematology-Oncology Group, PA
One Bay Avenue/Suite 2   Montclair, NJ 07042   (973)751-8880   Fax (973)744-8340

Conti, Joseph J., DO {1679552921} IntrMd(90,PA77)<NJ-KMHCHRRY, NJ-VIRTBERL>
+ Advocare Sicklerville Internal Medicine Associates
205 East Laurel Road/1 FL   Stratford, NJ 08084   (856)227-6575   Fax (856)374-9495

Contino, Krysta Marie, MD {1740695782} IntHos<NJ-COOPRUMC>
+ Cooper University Hospital
One Cooper Plaza   Camden, NJ 08103   (856)342-2000

Contractor, Daniel Gulammohammed, MD {1669495768} RadDia, RadV&I(88,INA67)<NJ-VAEASTOR>
+ 1815 Woodland Avenue
Edison, NJ 08820

Contractor, Sohail Gulammohamed, MD {1003871823} RadDia, IntrMd(92,INA67)<NY-NYUTISCH>
+ 15 Orchard Road
Watchung, NJ 07069
+ University Hospital-New Jersey Medical School
30 Bergen Street   Newark, NJ 07107   Fax (973)972-9355

Contreras, Diana Nancy, MD {1013088400} GynOnc, ObsGyn(91,NY01)<NY-LIJEWSH>
+ Morristown Medical Center
100 Madison Avenue   Morristown, NJ 07962   (973)971-5900   Fax (973)290-7257

Contreras, Jose A., MD {1558300145} PainMd, FamMed(99,GUA03)<NJ-HACKNSK>
+ Hackensack University Medical Center
20 Prospect Avenue/Ste 602/PainMed   Hackensack, NJ 07601   (201)996-2442   Fax (201)343-1045

Conyack, David G., DO {1558402768} Anesth(92,NY75)<NJ-STBARNMC>
+ New Jersey Anesthesia Associates, P.C.
252 Columbia Turnpike/PO Box 0037   Florham Park, NJ 07932   (973)660-9334   Fax (973)660-9779

Coohill, Lisa Marie, MD {1417958521} Nrolgy(91,NJ05)<NJ-OVERLOOK, NJ-MORRISTN>
+ Summit Medical Group-Berkeley Heights Campus
1 Diamond Hill Road   Berkeley Heights, NJ 07922   (908)273-4300   Fax (908)277-8767

Cook, Guillermo A., MD {1548267966} CdvDis, IntrMd(68,VENE)<NJ-MORRISTN>
+ Cardiology Consultants of North Morris, PA
356 US Highway 46/Suite B   Mountain Lakes, NJ 07046   (973)580-3400   Fax (973)586-1916

Cook, Jenny Lynn, DO {1255457552} FamMed(95,NY75)
+ North Wildwood Medical
1200 New Jersey Avenue   North Wildwood, NJ 08260   (609)522-3131   Fax (609)522-9024

Cook, Kristin M., MD {1093976466}
+ 26 Edison Drive
Summit, NJ 07901

Cook, Sean Michael, MD {1275584344} FamMed(00,NJ06)<NJ-SOMERSET>
+ Greenbrook Family Medicine
328 Greenbrook Road   Green Brook, NJ 08812   (732)356-0266   Fax (732)356-5022

Cook, Stuart D., MD {1720161375} Nrolgy(62,VT02)<NJ-UMDNJ, NJ-HACKNSK>
+ University Hospital
150 Bergen Street   Newark, NJ 07103   (201)456-5359   Fax (201)982-5059
+ Rutgers NJ School of Medicine Neurology
90 Bergen Street/DOC 5200   Newark, NJ 07103   (201)456-5359   Fax (973)972-5059

Cook, Wendy S., DO {1467422352} Pedtrc(87,IL76)<NJ-VIRTVOOR>
+ University Pediatrics
405 Hurffville Crosskeys Road   Sewell, NJ 08080   (856)582-0033   Fax (856)582-2305

Cook, Willard H., MD {1841874370} Grtrcs, IntrMd(72,PA09)
+ 59 Avenue at the Common
Shrewsbury, NJ 07702   (732)542-7010   Fax (732)542-0991

Cooke, Jacqueline P., MD {1275588550} IntrMd(82,MA07)
+ CAMCare Health Corporation
817 Federal Street/Suite 201   Camden, NJ 08103   (856)541-9811   Fax (856)541-4611
+ CAMCare Health Corporation
2610 Federal Street   Camden, NJ 08104   (856)635-0212

Cooke, John R., MD {1083895114} Psychy(96,NY01)
+ 516 Bloomfield Avenue/Suite 4
Montclair, NJ 07042   (973)509-1500   Fax (973)509-1919
drcookepatient@gmail.com

Cooke, Paul M., MD {1114952892} PhysMd(95,NJ05)<NY-SP-CLSURG>
+ Princeton Spine & Sports Physicians
389 Wall Street   Princeton, NJ 08540   (609)683-5500   Fax (609)683-0075

Cooley, Danielle Lynn, DO {1972701613} FamMed(07,NJ75)
+ The University Doctors
100 Century Parkway/Suite 140   Mount Laurel, NJ 08054   (856)380-2400   Fax (856)234-7870
+ University Pain Care Center
42 East Laurel Road/Suite 1700   Stratford, NJ 08084   (856)380-2400   Fax (856)566-6956
+ The University Doctors - UMDNJ -SOM
570 Egg Harbor Road/Suite C-2   Sewell, NJ 08054   (856)218-0300   Fax (856)589-5082

Cooley, Susan L., MD {1457321705} Ophthl(84,PA02)<NJ-WARREN, PA-EASTON>
+ Coventry Eye Associates, P.C.
10 Brass Castle Road   Washington, NJ 07882   (908)859-4268
+ Coventry Eye Associates, P.C.
800 Coventry Drive   Phillipsburg, NJ 08865   (908)859-4268   Fax (908)859-2042

Coons, Matthew S., MD {1548234099} SrgPlstc, SrgHnd(86,NY09)<NJ-CLARMAAS, NJ-STMICHL>
+ 2333 Morris Avenue/Suite C-216
Union, NJ 07083   (908)810-8550   Fax (908)810-8501
drcoons@verizon.net

Cooper, Alan Edward, MD {1720053341} SprtMd(PA0<NJ-STBARNMC>
+ St. Barnabas Medical Center
94 Old Short Hills Road/Surgery   Livingston, NJ 07039   (973)322-5195   Fax (973)322-2471

Cooper, David M., MD {1649272501} Otolgy, Otlryg, SrgHdN(85,NJ05)<NJ-OVERLOOK, NJ-MORRISTN>
+ Summit Medical Group-Berkeley Heights Campus
1 Diamond Hill Road   Berkeley Heights, NJ 07922   (908)277-8681   Fax (908)790-6524

Cooper, David Michael, MD {1619949716} PedPul, Pedtrc(88,VT02)<NJ-MORRISTN, NJ-CHILTON>
+ Pediatric Pulmonology
100 Madison Avenue   Morristown, NJ 07960   (973)971-4142   Fax (973)290-7360

Cooper, Dennis Lawrence, MD {1154319093} MedOnc, Onclgy, IntrMd(79,IL01)<CT-YALENHH>
+ Rutgers Health- RWJ Cancr Institute of New Jersey
335 George Street/Suite 370   New Brunswick, NJ 08901   (732)235-4161
+ Rutgers Cancer Institute of New Jersey
195 Little Albany Street/PO Box 2681   New Brunswick, NJ 08903   (732)235-4161   Fax (732)235-7355

Cooper, Eliyahu N., MD {1316258825} Anesth(10,NJ05)<NJ-CHILTON>
+ Chilton Medical Center
97 West Parkway/Anesthesia   Pompton Plains, NJ 07444   (973)831-5140

Cooper, Grant, MD {1528008869} PhysMd(03,NJ06)
+ Princeton Spine and Joint Center
601 Ewing Street/Suite A-2   Princeton, NJ 08540   (609)454-0760   Fax (609)454-0761

Cooper, Joel David, MD {1770529729} SrgThr, Surgry(MA01<PA-UPMCPHL>
+ Penn Medicine at Cherry Hill
409 Route 70 East/Surgery/Thorac   Cherry Hill, NJ 08034   (856)429-1519

Cooper, Kimberly Anne, DO {1780846915} CritCr, IntrMd<PA-UPMCMRCY>
+ Valley Diagnostic Medical Center
581 North Franklin Turnpike   Ramsey, NJ 07446   (201)327-0500   Fax (201)327-8612

Cooper, Lauren M., MD {1275629404} Dermat(84,NY19)
+ Affiliated Dermatology
Town Centre 66/Suite 301   Succasunna, NJ 07876   (973)267-0300   Fax (973)927-7512
+ Affiliated Dermatology
14 Church Street   Liberty Corner, NJ 07938   (973)267-0300   Fax (908)604-8544
+ Affiliated Dermatology
80 West End Avenue   Somerville, NJ 07876   (973)267-0300   Fax (908)429-8899

Cooper, Niti Dalal, DO {1881859080} AnesPain(04,NJ75)<NJ-COOPRUMC>
+ Rancocas Anesthesiology, PA
15000 Midlantic Drive/Suite 102   Mount Laurel, NJ 08054   (856)255-5479   Fax (856)393-8691

Cooper, Roger W., Jr., MD {1306807938} PedInf, Pedtrc(74,MEX14)<NJ-STMICHL>
+ 135 Bloomfield Avenue/Suite K
Bloomfield, NJ 07003   (973)748-8118

Physicians by Name and Address

Cooper, Sanford, MD {1326013202} IntrMd, Nephro(80,NY09)<NJ-CHRIST, NJ-NWRKBETH>
+ Nephrology Group
  111 Northfield Avenue/Suite 311   West Orange, NJ 07052   (973)325-2103   Fax (973)325-2254
+ Nephrology Group
  142 Palisade Avenue/Suite 202   Jersey City, NJ 07305   (201)963-1077

Cooperman, Alan Stewart, MD {1932214293} ObsGyn(68,ITA01)<NJ-OVERLOOK, NJ-STBARNMC>
+ Millburn Ob-Gyn Associates, P.A.
  233 Millburn Avenue   Millburn, NJ 07041   (973)467-9440   Fax (973)376-1680
+ Short Hills Surgery Center
  187 Millburn Avenue/Suite 101   Millburn, NJ 07041   (973)467-9440   Fax (973)671-0557

Cooperman, Harry Alan, MD {1932155702} Radiol, RadDia(81,PA07)<NJ-SHOREMEM, NJ-ACMCITY>
+ Shore Memorial Hospital
  1 East New York Avenue   Somers Point, NJ 08244   (609)653-3500
+ Atlantic Medical Imaging, LLC.
  3100 Hingston Avenue   Egg Harbor Township, NJ 08234   (609)653-3500   Fax (609)646-5469
+ Atlantic Medical Imaging, LLC.
  44 East Jimmie Leeds Road/Suite 101   Galloway, NJ 08244   (609)677-9729   Fax (609)652-6512

Cooperman, Ross D., MD {1407054109} SrgRec
+ 22 Old Short Hills Road/Suite 101
  Livingston, NJ 07039   (973)994-2021   Fax (973)994-7005

Cooperman, Todd J., MD {1053378935} PhysMd(93,NY48)<NJ-RHBHTNTN>
+ The Rehab Hosp of Tinton Falls
  2 Centre Plaza   Tinton Falls, NJ 07724   (732)460-5320

Cooperstein, Heidi B., DO {1104041722} PsyAdt, PsyCAd, Psychy(92,PA77)
+ 128 Borton Landing Road/Suite 2
  Moorestown, NJ 08057   (856)231-0590   Fax (856)231-1228

Cooray, Roshan, MD {1457778706} Pedtrc<NJ-CHDNWBTH>
+ Children's Hospital of New Jersey
  201 Lyons Avenue/Osborne Terrace   Newark, NJ 07112   (973)926-7471   Fax (973)926-6452

Copare, Fiore J., MD {1205869989} FamMed, IntrMd(82,MEXI)
+ Internal Medicine Associates
  201 Laurel Heights Drive/Suite 201   Bridgeton, NJ 08302   (856)455-4800   Fax (856)455-0650

Cope, Jennifer Anne, MD {1396706230} Pedtrc, Nrolgy, NroChl(95,NY08)<NJ-VALLEY>
+ Neurology Group of Bergen County
  1200 East Ridgewood Avenue   Ridgewood, NJ 07450   (201)444-0868   Fax (201)444-7363

Copeland, Lois J., MD {1255416970} IntrMd(68,NY20)<NJ-VALLEY, NJ-HOLYNAME>
+ 47 Central Avenue
  Hillsdale, NJ 07642   (201)664-1212   Fax (201)666-7433

Copeland, Marcia A., MD {1912926825} Anesth(92,PA14)
+ PO Box 4040
  Lindenwold, NJ 08021

Coplin, Bruce M., MD {1699755868} PhysMd(83,MEXI)<NJ-HLTHSRE, NJ-OCEANMC>
+ 7 Hospital Drive
  Toms River, NJ 08755   (732)505-5014   Fax (732)505-8770
+ HealthSouth Rehabilitation Hospital of New Jersey
  14 Hospital Drive   Toms River, NJ 08755   (732)505-5070

Coplin, Peter L., MD {1336239557} Anesth(79,MEXI)<NJ-UNVMCPRN>
+ University Medical Center of Princeton at Plainsboro
  One Plainsboro Road/Anesthesiology   Plainsboro, NJ 08536   (609)497-4330

Coppola, Danielle, MD {1033681432} IntrMd
+ 2 Cleveland Lane
  Princeton, NJ 08540   (609)876-0067

Coppola, Peter W., MD {1134116148} IntrMd(81,GRN01)<NJ-HACKNSK, NJ-HOLYNAME>
+ Wilton Internal Medicine
  751 Teaneck Road   Teaneck, NJ 07666   (201)837-3200   Fax (201)837-8993

Coppolecchia, Rosa, DO {1538318258} IntrMd, OccpMd(92,NJ75)
+ Bayer HealthCare
  100 Bayer Boulevard   Whippany, NJ 07981   (862)404-4984

Coppolino, Frank P., MD {1245379387} PulDis(85,MEX34)<NJ-CENTRAST>
+ Monmouth Ocean Pulmonary Medicine
  901 West Main Street/Suite 160   Freehold, NJ 07728   (732)577-0600   Fax (732)577-6332

Copur, Huseyin, MD {1982650545} ObsGyn(79,TURK)<NJ-HACKNSK, NJ-CLARMAAS>
+ first Choice Ob Gyn Group
  301 Beech Street/Unit 6   Hackensack, NJ 07601   (201)531-9006   Fax (201)531-9008

+ first Choice Ob Gyn Group
  1115 Clifton Avenue/Suite 104   Clifton, NJ 07013   (201)531-9006   Fax (201)525-1717
+ 14 Balmoral Lane
  Scotch Plains, NJ 07076   (201)216-1505

Coquia, Salvador F., MD {1417983594} CdvDis, IntrMd(64,PHIL)

Coraggio, Michael J., MD {1083688048} Pedtrc, SprtMd(84,NY09)<NJ-HUNTRDN>
+ Hunterdon Pediatric Associates
  1738 Route 31 North/Suite 201   Clinton, NJ 08809   (908)735-3960   Fax (908)735-3965

Corazon, Alexis J., MD {1770552614} IntrMd(89,DOM02)
+ Great Falls Medical Center
  354 Totowa Avenue/Apt 1   Paterson, NJ 07502   (973)389-1300   Fax (973)389-0138

Corazza, Douglas P., MD {1376520825} IntrMd(85,NJ06)<NJ-UNVMCPRN>
+ Montgomery Internal Medicine Group
  727 State Road   Princeton, NJ 08540   (609)921-6410   Fax (609)921-0406
+ Montgomery Internal Medicine Group
  719 Route 206 North/Suite 100   Hillsborough, NJ 08844   (609)921-6410   Fax (908)431-9407

Corbally, Brian Michael, DO {1619264637}<NJ-DEBRAHLC>
+ Deborah Heart and Lung Center
  200 Trenton Road   Browns Mills, NJ 08015   (609)893-1200

Corbett, Brian Joseph, DO {1649437690} IntrMd
+ 167 Lawnside Avenue
  Collingswood, NJ 08108

Corbett, Shonda Marcia, MD {1336140029} ObsGyn(99,NJ05)
+ Valley Medical Group
  70 Park Avenue   Park Ridge, NJ 07656   (201)476-0040   Fax (201)391-4837

Corbett, Siobhan Alden, MD {1093884835} Surgry(87,NJ06)<NJ-RWJUBRUN>
+ UMDNJ RWJ Surgery
  125 Paterson Street/CAB 4th FL 4100   New Brunswick, NJ 08901   (732)235-7920   Fax (732)235-7079
  corbetsi@umdnj.edu

Corbin, John C., DO {1790841484} Anesth(94,PA77)
+ Memorial Hospital of Salem County
  310 Woodstown Road/Anesthesia   Salem, NJ 08079   (856)339-6052   Fax (856)935-4757

Corbisiero, Raffaele, MD {1770523326} CdvDis, IntrMd, ClCdEl(87,NY09)<NJ-DEBRAHLC>
+ Deborah Heart and Lung Center
  200 Trenton Road   Browns Mills, NJ 08015   (609)893-6611   Fax (609)893-1213

Corbo, Emanuel, MD {1013000413} Pedtrc(85,GRN01)<NJ-OVERLOOK, NJ-TRININPC>
+ Park Pediatrics PA
  443 East Westfield Avenue   Roselle Park, NJ 07204   (908)245-2442   Fax (908)245-6258

Corcino, Ana J., MD {1184637415} Anesth(89,NJ45)
+ CHOP Pediatric & Adolescent Specialty Care Center
  1012 Laurel Oak Road   Voorhees, NJ 08043   (856)435-1300   Fax (856)435-0091
  corcino@email.chop.edu

Corcoran, Gavin R., MD InfDis, IntrMd(87,SAF01)
+ Schering-Plough Research Global Clinical Development
  2015 Galloping Hill Road   Kenilworth, NJ 07033   (908)298-4000

Corcoran, Gregory, MD {1023409323} EmrgMd
+ Robert Wood Johnson Emergency Medicine
  One Robert Wood Johnson Place/MEB 104   New Brunswick, NJ 08901   (732)235-8717

Corda, Peter D., DO {1861477192} Anesth(83,IL76)<NJ-ACMCITY, NJ-ACMCMAIN>
+ Professional Pain Management Associates
  2007 North Black Horse Pike   Williamstown, NJ 08094   (856)740-4888   Fax (856)740-0558

Cordal, Adriana, MD {1629166780} Psychy, IntrMd(85,URU02)<NJ-JRSYSHMC>
+ Jersey Shore University Medical Center - Psychiatry
  1200 Jumping Brook Road   Neptune, NJ 07753   (732)643-4356   Fax (732)643-4378
+ Jersey Shore Psychiatric Associates
  3535 Route 66/Building 5/Suite D   Neptune, NJ 07753   (732)643-4400

Cordell, Charles E., MD {1598767063} RadDia, Radiol(85,PA14)
+ Radiology Associates of Burlington County
  1295 Route 38 West/PO Box 479   Hainesport, NJ 08036   (609)261-7017   Fax (609)261-4180

Cordero, Hector Orlando, MD {1881629574} RadDia, Radiol(94,NJ05)<NJ-NWTNMEM>
+ Sparta Health and Wellness Center
  89 Sparta Avenue/Suite 120   Sparta, NJ 07871   (973)729-0002   Fax (973)729-1085
+ Image Care Centers
  222 High Street/Suite 101   Newton, NJ 07860   (973)729-0002   Fax (973)383-2774
+ Radiologic Associates of Northwest New Jersey

212 Route 94   Vernon, NJ 07871   (973)827-1961

Cordero, Orlando C., MD {1679780399} Radiol, RadDia(63,PHIL)<NJ-NWTNMEM>
+ Sparta Health and Wellness Center
  89 Sparta Avenue/Suite 120   Sparta, NJ 07871   (973)729-0002   Fax (973)729-1085
+ Image Care Centers
  222 High Street/Suite 101   Newton, NJ 07860   (973)729-0002   Fax (973)383-2774
+ Radiologic Associates of Northwest New Jersey
  212 Route 94   Vernon, NJ 07871   (973)827-1961

Cordero, Pedro E., MD {1295896231} SrgVas, Surgry(78,NY06)<NJ-NWRKBETH, NJ-TRINIWSC>
+ Center for Vascular Disorders
  236 East Westfield Avenue/Suite 4   Roselle Park, NJ 07204   (908)241-2401   Fax (908)241-2402

Cordoba, Isabelita Y., MD {1558375253} Gastrn, IntrMd(63,PHI08)<NJ-VAEASTOR>
+ VA New Jersey Health Care System-East Orange Campus
  385 Tremont Avenue   East Orange, NJ 07018   (973)676-1000   Fax (973)395-7076

Coren, Jennifer B., DO {1851496673} Pedtrc, IntrMd(03,PA77)
+ Cooper Peds/Children's Regional Ctr
  3 Cooper Plaza/Suite 200   Camden, NJ 08103   (856)342-2472   Fax (856)368-8297

Coren, Joshua Scott, DO {1750361820} FamMed, IntrMd(02,PA77)
+ The University Doctors
  100 Century Parkway/Suite 140   Mount Laurel, NJ 08054   (856)380-2400   Fax (856)234-7870
+ University Hospital-University Family Medicine
  42 East Laurel Road/Suite 2100   Stratford, NJ 08084   (856)380-2400   Fax (856)566-6188
+ The University Doctors - UMDNJ -SOM
  570 Egg Harbor Road/Suite C-2   Sewell, NJ 08054   (856)218-0300   Fax (856)589-5082

Corenthal Robins, Linda J., MD {1154579795} ObsGyn, RprEnd(83,NY19)
+ Montclair Homeopathy LLC
  50 Bentley Place   Upper Montclair, NJ 07043   (973)746-9888

Corey, Howard Erwin, MD {1710959036} PedNph, Pedtrc(83,NY08)<NJ-MORRISTN, NJ-OVERLOOK>
+ Morristown Medical Center
  100 Madison Avenue/POBox 24   Morristown, NJ 07962   (973)971-5000

Corey, Timothy J., MD {1235234949} Dermat(75,NY01)<NJ-VALLEY>
+ North Bergen Dermatologic Group, PA
  400 Route 17 South   Ridgewood, NJ 07450   (201)652-4536   Fax (201)652-4906
  klwtigger@aol.com
+ North Bergen Dermatologic Group, PA
  180 Ramapo Valley Road   Oakland, NJ 07436   (201)652-4536   Fax (201)337-7710

Corio, Frederick J., MD {1194750968} RadDia, Radiol(83,IL43)<NJ-NWTNMEM>
+ Sparta Health and Wellness Center
  89 Sparta Avenue/Suite 120   Sparta, NJ 07871   (973)729-0002   Fax (973)729-1085
+ Image Care Centers
  222 High Street/Suite 101   Newton, NJ 07860   (973)729-0002   Fax (973)383-2774
+ Radiologic Associates of Northwest New Jersey
  212 Route 94   Vernon, NJ 07871   (973)827-1961

Corley, David R., MD {1689612210} ObsGyn, EnDbMt, RprEnd(87,SC04)
+ Cooper Institute for Reproductive Hormonal Disorders
  17000 Commerce Parkway/Suite C   Mount Laurel, NJ 08054   (856)751-5575   Fax (856)751-7289

Cornejo, Juan Carlos, DO {1952568974} SprtMd, FamMed(05,MO79)
+ 113 White Horse Road West/Suite 7
  Voorhees, NJ 08043   (856)552-2208   Fax (856)283-3158

Cornel-Avendano, Beverly, MD {1255357349} IntrMd, Gastrn(82,PHI09)
+ Digestive Disease Specialists
  233 Middle Road/Suite 1   Hazlet, NJ 07730   (732)888-0411   Fax (732)888-3909
+ 875 Poole Avenue/#1
  Hazlet, NJ 07730   (732)888-0411   Fax (732)888-3909

Cornell, Russell John, MD {1285639088} CdvDis, IntrMd(75,NJ05)
+ Cardiology Consultants
  368 Lakehurst Road/Suite 301   Toms River, NJ 08755   (732)240-1048   Fax (732)240-3464
+ Cardiology Consultants
  63-C Lacey Road   Whiting, NJ 08759   (732)240-1048   Fax (732)350-7054
+ Cardiology Consultants of Toms River
  401 Lacey Road/Suite D   Whiting, NJ 08755   (732)350-3350   Fax (732)350-3350

Physicians by Name and Address

Cornett, Julia Kang, MD {1679884738} IntrMd, InfDis(05,NJ06)<NJ-UMDNJ>
+ Rutgers RWJ Allergy, Immunology and Infectious Group
125 Paterson Street   New Brunswick, NJ 08901   (732)235-7060

Cornett, Oriana Ellen, MD {1487977591} Nrolgy
+ Rutgers NJ School of Medicine Neurology
90 Bergen Street/DOC 5200   Newark, NJ 07103   (973)972-9274   Fax (973)972-5059

Coromilas, James, MD {1114004645} IntrMd, ClCdEl, CdvDis(75,QU01)<NJ-RWJUBRUN>
+ UH- Robert Wood Johnson Med
125 Paterson Street/# 5100   New Brunswick, NJ 08901   (732)235-6561   Fax (732)235-6530

Corona, Joseph T., MD {1720089840} Ortped, SrgOrt(71,QU01)<NJ-OVERLOOK, NJ-MORRISTN>
+ Summit Medical Group-Berkeley Heights Campus
1 Diamond Hill Road   Berkeley Heights, NJ 07922   (908)273-4300   Fax (908)790-6524

Coronato, Andrew, MD {1497747489} Gastrn, IntrMd(66,NY09)
+ Medical Diagnostic Associates PA
525 Central Avenue/Suite D   Westfield, NJ 07090   (908)232-5333   Fax (908)389-1930

Corpuz, Danielle M., MD {1023376647} Pedtrc
+ Touchpoint Pediatrics
17 Watchung Avenue   Chatham, NJ 07928   (973)665-0900   Fax (973)665-0901

Corradino, Christine M., MD {1699782821} SrgOrt(93,NJ05)<NJ-HACKNSK>
+ Premier Orthopaedics and Sports Medicine, PC
663 Palisade Avenue/Suite 302   Cliffside Park, NJ 07010   (201)943-9100   Fax (201)943-7308
+ Premier Orthopaedics and Sports Medicine, P.C.
3196 Kennedy Boulevard/Third Floor   Union City, NJ 07087   (201)943-9100   Fax (201)770-1010
+ Premier Orthopaedics and Sports Medicine, P.C.
111 Galway Place   Teaneck, NJ 07010   (201)833-9500   Fax (201)862-0095

Corrado, Anthony Charles, DO {1235338872} OtgyFPlS(02,NJ75)
+ Corrado Ctr Facial Plstic Cosmtic Srgy
1919 Greentree Road/Suite C   Cherry Hill, NJ 08003   (856)344-5906   Fax (856)229-7617
+ Cherry Hill Center
1797 Springdale Road   Cherry Hill, NJ 08003   (856)344-5906   Fax (856)424-6335
+ University Hospital -SOM University Doctors Surgeons
42 East Laurel Road/Suite 2500-2600   Stratford, NJ 08003   (856)344-5906   Fax (856)566-6873

Corrado, Peter M., DO {1972553436} FamMed(83,IA75)<NJ-BURDTMLN>
+ North Main Family Practice
108 North Main Street/Suite 3   Cape May Court House, NJ 08210   (609)463-9960   Fax (609)463-9980

Corrales, Michelle D., MD {1174736193} FamMed(01,PHI09)<NJ-ATLANTHS>
+ Reliance Medical Group, LLC
1325 Baltic Avenue   Atlantic City, NJ 08401   (609)441-0723   Fax (609)441-0953
+ Atlantic Care Physician Group
235 Shore Road/Suite C   Somers Point, NJ 08244   (609)441-0723   Fax (609)926-4177

Correa, Lilia M., MD {1316203110}
+ 1050 George Street/Apt 2l
New Brunswick, NJ 08901   (617)816-3321
liliacorreamd@gmail.com

Correa, Luis A., MD {1063771301} Pedtrc<NJ-NWRKBETH>
+ Newark Beth Israel Medical Center
201 Lyons Avenue   Newark, NJ 07112   (973)926-7000

Correa Orozco, Felipe A., MD {1659533370} IntrMd
+ IPC The Hospitalist Company
55 Madison Avenue/Suite 310   Morristown, NJ 07960   (973)993-9536   Fax (973)998-4237

Correia, Joaquim Jose Caldas, MD {1205945623} IntrMd, CdvDis, ClCdEl(86,NY19)<NJ-NWRKBETH>
+ Joaquim Jose Caldas Correia MD, LLC
243 Chestnut Street/Suite 2L   Newark, NJ 07105   (973)589-8668   Fax (973)589-7996

Corrigan, Frank John, MD {1164626834} SrgOrt, IntrMd(02,IRE03)
+ The Orthopedic Institute of New Jersey
108 Bilby Road/Suite 201   Hackettstown, NJ 07840   (908)684-3005   Fax (908)684-3301
+ The Orthopedic Institute of New Jersey
254-B Mountain Avenue/Suite 201   Hackettstown, NJ 07840   (908)684-3005   Fax (908)684-3301
+ The Orthopedic Institute of New Jersey
222 High Street/Suite 202   Newton, NJ 07840   (908)684-3005   Fax (908)684-3301

Corrigan, Lynn Ann, DO {1366526964} FamMed, IntrMd(96,NJ75)<NJ-WAYNEGEN, NJ-STJOSHOS>
+ Active Center for Health & Wellness
25 Prospect Avenue   Hackensack, NJ 07601   (201)487-4600   Fax (201)343-7410

Corrigan, Nicole Melissa, MD {1508182452} Nrolgy(NY47
+ St. Joseph's Regional Medical Center
703 Main Street/Neurology   Paterson, NJ 07503   (973)754-2463

Corrin, Courtney Wilczynski, DO {1619174315} EmrgMd
+ Kennedy Mem Hospital Emergency Medicine
18 East Laurel Road   Stratford, NJ 08084   (856)346-7985

Cors, William K., MD {1235134990} AdmMgt, Nrolgy(75,NJ05)<NJ-SOMERSET>
+ RWJ University Hospital Somerset
110 Rehill Avenue   Somerville, NJ 08876   (908)685-2200

Corsan, Gregory H., MD {1669403978} ObsGyn, RprEnd, Frt-Inf(83,NJ05)
+ Center for Advanced Reproductive Medicine/Fertility
4 Ethel Road/Suite 405A   Edison, NJ 08817   (732)339-9300   Fax (732)339-9400

Corso, Martin J., MD {1518067552} IntrMd(76,MEXI)<NJ-CHILTON>
+ 29 Station Road
Lincoln Park, NJ 07035   (609)628-8442   Fax (609)628-9516

Corso, Vincent Mark, MD {1609324300}
+ 37 Bruce Court
Cedar Grove, NJ 07009   (973)571-0053

Corson, Richard L., MD {1922089200} FamMed(83,NJ06)
+ 313 Courtyard Drive
Hillsborough, NJ 08844   (908)722-9962   Fax (908)722-9963
Drcorson@earthlink.net

Corson-Diaz, Cathy Lynn, MD {1609030089} OthrSp, FamMed(93,NJ05)<NJ-UNDRWD>
+ Creations Medical Spa
901 Route 168/Suite408   Blackwood, NJ 08012   (856)589-1151   Fax (856)589-1554

Cort, James T., MD {1851467294} IntrMd(80,DC03)<NJ-EASTORNG>
+ 98 South Munn Avenue
East Orange, NJ 07018   (973)673-2260   Fax (973)673-5110
Jamestcortmd@comcast.net

Cortazzo, Jessica A., MD {1679894224} Anesth<NJ-HACKNSK>
+ Hackensack University Medical Center
30 Prospect Avenue   Hackensack, NJ 07601   (201)488-0066   Fax (201)488-6769

Cortellino, Karen, MD {1205919396} Radiol(78,MEXI)
+ Wayne Urgent and Primary Care
246 Hamburg Turnpike/Suite 205   Wayne, NJ 07470   (973)389-1800   Fax (973)636-2734

Cortes, Andrew, MD {1588922678} RadV&I<NJ-HUNTRDN>
+ Hunterdon Medical Center
2100 Wescott Drive   Flemington, NJ 08822   (631)902-9033

Cortese, Bernard J., MD {1528039179} ObsGyn(80,MEXI)<NJ-VIRTBERL, NJ-VIRTVOOR>
+ Garden State Obstetrics and Gynecological Associates
2401 Evesham Road/Suite A   Voorhees, NJ 08043   (856)424-3323   Fax (856)424-4994

Cortese, Lisa Ann, MD {1629086061} Anesth(90,NY08)<NJ-STFRNMED>
+ St. Francis Medical Center
601 Hamilton Avenue/Anesthesiology   Trenton, NJ 08629   (609)599-5000   Fax (609)599-6312

Cortez, Jacqueline M., MD Psychy(81,PHIL)
+ American Institute for Counseling
1952 US Highway 22/Suite 102   Bound Brook, NJ 08805   (732)469-6444   Fax (732)469-6445

Cortina, Osvaldo, MD {1386630994} FamMed(86,DOM02)
+ Osvoldo Cortina MD PC
322-38th Street/Owner   Union City, NJ 07087   (201)865-9492   Fax (201)865-0306

Corvari, Steven Joseph, MD {1689793051} Psychy, PsyFor, IntrMd(03,GRN01)
+ AtlantiCare Behav Hlth/Hartford
13 North Hartford Avenue   Atlantic City, NJ 08401   (609)348-1161

Corzo, Jorge Francisco, MD {1497741367} PhysMd(98,NJ05)<NJ-RIVERVW>
+ Riverview Medical Center
1 Riverview Plaza/PhysRehab   Red Bank, NJ 07701   (732)741-2700   Fax (732)345-2034

Coscia, Sylvia, MD {1356417794} IntrMd(82,NJ05)<NJ-MTNSIDE>
+ 186 Long Hill Road
Little Falls, NJ 07424   (973)812-0979   Fax (973)812-0788

Cosentino, James P., DO {1821225715} IntrMd, PulDis(PA77
+ Shore Pulmonary PA
301 Bingham Avenue/Suite B   Ocean, NJ 07712   (732)775-9075   Fax (732)775-1212
+ Shore Pulmonary PA
2640 Highway 70/Building 6-A   Manasquan, NJ 08736   (732)775-9075   Fax (732)528-0887
+ Shore Pulmonary PA
1608 Route 88/Suite 117   Brick, NJ 07712   (732)575-1100

Cosentino, Mark O., MD {1447340385} Radiol, RadDia(86,NJ05)<NJ-MORRISTN>
+ Memorial Radiology Associates
10 Lanidex Plaza West/Suite 125   Parsippany, NJ 07054   (973)503-5700   Fax (973)386-5701
+ Morristown Medical Center
100 Madison Avenue/Radiology   Morristown, NJ 07962   (973)971-5370

Cosenza, Mario Anthony, DO {1588760102} EmrgMd(90,IA75)<NJ-MORRISTN>
+ Morristown Medical Center
100 Madison Avenue/PediEmrgMed   Morristown, NJ 07962   (973)971-5000

Cosimi, Katherine Rose, MD {1851870885} IntrMd<NJ-ACMC-MAIN>
+ AtlantiCare Regional Med Ctr/Mainland
65 West Jimmie Leeds Road   Pomona, NJ 08240   (609)748-7520
+ AtlantiCare Regional Medical Center/City Campus
1925 Pacific Avenue   Atlantic City, NJ 08401   (609)748-7520   Fax (609)441-8002

Cosmi, John Edward, MD {1558458950} IntrMd, IntCrd(97,NJ05)<NJ-MORRISTN>
+ Cardiology Associates of Morristown
95 Madison Avenue/Suite 10A   Morristown, NJ 07960   (973)889-9001   Fax (973)889-9051

Coss, Wanda I., MD {1326025404} Pedtrc(88,DOMI)<NJ-OURLADY>
+ Advocare Medford Pediatric & Adolescent Medicine
520 Stokes Road   Medford, NJ 08055   (609)654-9112   Fax (609)654-7404

Costa, Anthony Joseph, MD {1982677910} SrgOrt, SrgRec(00,NJ05)
+ Orthopaedic Sports Medicine
80 Oak Hill Road   Red Bank, NJ 07701   (732)741-2313   Fax (732)741-7154
+ Orthopaedic Sports Medicine & Rehabilitation Center
25 Kilmer Drive/Building 3/Suite 105   Morganville, NJ 07751   (732)741-2313   Fax (732)617-5959

Costa, Antoinette G., MD {1790791671} IntrMd, Grtrcs(82,NJ05)<NJ-VAEASTOR>
+ VA New Jersey Health Care System-East Orange Campus
385 Tremont Avenue   East Orange, NJ 07018   (973)676-1000   Fax (973)395-7010

Costa, Daria Ann, MD {1346418142}<NJ-STJOSHOS>
+ St. Joseph's Regional Medical Center Anesthesia
703 Main Street   Paterson, NJ 07503   (973)754-2323   Fax (973)754-2791

Costa, Gerald V., MD {1467690446} ObsGyn(85,MEX03)<NY-JACOBIMC>
+ 16 Sugarwood Way
Warren, NJ 07059   (908)607-0030

Costa, German H., MD {1639254634} Surgry(97,NJ05)<NJ-HOBUNIMC, NJ-PALISADE>
+ North Jersey Surgical Group PA
1 Marine View Plaza   Hoboken, NJ 07030   (201)795-9080   Fax (201)795-9434

Costa, Jose Carlos, MD {1043491830} Gastrn
+ 465 Cranbury Road
East Brunswick, NJ 08816   (732)390-1995   Fax (732)254-4610

Costa, Ralph F., MD {1740217652} FamMed(86,PA02)<NJ-VIRTVOOR>
+ Penn Medicine at Cherry Hill
409 Route 70 East   Cherry Hill, NJ 08034   (856)429-1519

Costa, Richard C., DO {1982693511} FamMed, IntrMd(85,IA75)<NJ-VIRTBERL, NJ-VIRTVOOR>
+ Advocare Berlin Medical Associates
339 North Route 73/Suite 1   Berlin, NJ 08009   (856)767-8228   Fax (856)753-7836
+ Advocare Berlin Medical Associates
175 Cross Keys Road/Suite 300A   Berlin, NJ 08009   (856)767-8228   Fax (856)767-6102

Costa, Ronald P., MD {1619006814} IntrMd(74,PA09)<NJ-RIVERVW>
+ 88 East Front Street
Red Bank, NJ 07701   (732)741-1256

Costabile, Jessica T., DO {1134236441} Anesth(02,NJ75)<NJ-ACM-CMAIN>
+ AtlantiCare Anesthesiology
65 West Jimmie Leeds Road   Pomona, NJ 08240   (609)748-7597
+ AtlantiCare Regional Med Ctr/Mainland
65 West Jimmie Leeds Road   Pomona, NJ 08240   (609)652-1000

Costabile, Joseph P., MD {1376592675} Surgry, SrgVas(86,NJ05)<NJ-VIRTUAHS, NJ-OURLADY>
+ Virtua Surgical Group, PA
1935 Route 70 East   Cherry Hill, NJ 08003   (856)428-7700   Fax(856)424-9120

Physicians by Name and Address

Costacurta, Gary A., MD {1679575856} CdvDis, IntrMd(84,PA09)<NJ-WARREN>
+ Drs. Costacurta & Nar
 96A Baltimore Street Phillipsburg, NJ 08865 (610)258-4337
 eastoncardiovascular@rcn.com

Costantini, Peter J., DO {1982704342} PulDis, IntrMd, CritCr(78,PA77)<NJ-SHOREMEM, NJ-ACMCMAIN>
+ Atlantic Pulmonary & Critical Care Associates, P.A.
 741 South Second Avenue/Suite A Galloway, NJ 08205
 (609)748-7300 Fax (609)748-7919
 pjc2@comcast.net

Costantini-Ferrando, Maria Fausta, MD {1861630451} RprEnd, ObsGyn
+ Reproductive Medicine Associates of New Jersey
 140 Allen Road Basking Ridge, NJ 07920 (908)604-7800
 Fax (973)290-8370
+ Reproductive Medicine Associates of New Jersey
 25 Rockwood Place Englewood, NJ 07631 (908)604-7800
 Fax (201)569-8143

Costanza, Carl, MD {1669400651} IntrMd(92,MA07)
+ Primary Care Physicians Inc.
 187 Chestnut Street Nutley, NJ 07110 (973)667-4402
 Fax (973)667-6974

Costanzo, Eric John, DO {1700977923} IntrMd, PulDis(01,NJ75)
+ Shore Pulmonary PA
 2640 Highway 70/Building 6-A Manasquan, NJ 08736
 (732)528-5900 Fax (732)528-0887
+ Shore Pulmonary PA
 301 Bingham Avenue/Suite B Ocean, NJ 07712 (732)528-5900 Fax (732)775-1212
+ Shore Pulmonary PA
 1608 Route 88/Suite 117 Brick, NJ 08736 (732)575-1100

Costanzo, William Edward, MD {1376531517} CdvDis, IntrMd(87,NY03)<NJ-CHSFULD, NJ-CHSMRCER>
+ Mercer Bucks Cardiology
 3140 Princeton Pike/2nd Floor Lawrenceville, NJ 08648
 (609)895-1919 Fax (609)895-1200

Costea-Misthos, Maria A., MD {1295872976} IntrMd(86,NY19)<NJ-MORRISTN>
+ Summit Medical Group
 1 Anderson Hill Road/Suite 102 Bernardsville, NJ 07924
 (908)696-0808 Fax (908)696-9943

Costeas, Constantinos A., MD {1255331849} ClCdEl, CdvDis, IntrMd(89,NY48)<NJ-STMICHL>
+ New Jersey Cardiology Associates
 375 Mount Pleasant Avenue West Orange, NJ 07052
 (973)731-9442 Fax (973)731-8030
+ Diagnostic & Clinical Cardiology
 111 Central Avenue/5th Floor Newark, NJ 07102
 (973)731-9442 Fax (973)877-2567
+ New Jersey Cardiology Associates
 201 Lyons Avenue/6th Floor Newark, NJ 07052 (973)926-7503 Fax (973)923-7267

Costello, Gregory Anthony, MD {1154411254} FamMed(94,PRO02)
+ Eastern Christian Children's Retreat
 700 Mountain Avenue Wyckoff, NJ 07481 (201)848-8005
 Fax (201)847-9619

Costello, Lauren E., MD {1326269440} EmrgMd, SprtMd, FamMed(85,NJ05)
+ McCosh Health Center
 Washington Road/McCosh Infirmary Princeton, NJ 08544
 (609)258-5357 Fax (609)258-1355

Costello, Robert, MD {1326454638} IntrMd
+ Drs. Morone and Costello
 220 Hamburg Turnpike Wayne, NJ 07470 (973)942-5230
 Fax (973)942-6652

Costin, Andrew, MD {1053475160} CdvDis, IntrMd(86,CT01)
+ Princeton Medical Group, P.A.
 419 North Harrison Street Princeton, NJ 08540 (609)924-9300 Fax (609)924-6552

Costomiris, Robert P., MD {1649382540} CdvDis(75,ITA01)
+ 331 Grand Street
 Hoboken, NJ 07030 (201)659-0942 Fax (201)659-1483

Cosulich, William F., MD {1427143312} Dermat(82,MO02)<NJ-JRSYSHMC>
+ Cosulich Dermatology
 3350 State Highway 138 Wall Township, NJ 07719
 (732)280-1200 Fax (732)280-1207
+ 1004 Commons Way/Building G
 Toms River, NJ 08755 (732)349-6868

Cote, Sean Arie, DO {1497963862}
+ 103 Louis Drive
 Montville, NJ 07045

Cotenoff, Melanie L., MD {1518940766} Pedtrc(87,GRN01)<NJ-RIVERVW>
+ Navesink Pediatrics
 55 North Gilbert Street/Suite 2101 Tinton Falls, NJ 07701
 (732)842-6677 Fax (732)530-2946

Cotler, Donald N., MD {1801853049} Pedtrc(83,IL43)<NJ-OVERLOOK, NJ-STBARNMC>
+ Buono Pediatrics & Wellness
 171 Millburn Avenue Millburn, NJ 07041 (606)557-3085

Cotler, Harold Mark, DO {1659355832} EmrgMd, FamMed(83,IA75)<NJ-JRSYSHMC>
+ Cotler Family Practice, LLC
 1937 State Highway 35/Suite 2 Wall, NJ 07719 (732)449-0914 Fax (732)449-5437

Cotler, Samantha, DO {1598142523} FamMed
+ Cotler Family Practice, LLC
 1937 State Highway 35/Suite 2 Wall, NJ 07719 (732)449-0914 Fax (732)449-5437

Cotov, Judith A., MD {1891763660} IntrMd(86,NJ05)<NJ-MONMOUTH>
+ Monmouth Family Center
 270 Broadway Long Branch, NJ 07740 (732)923-7100
 Fax (732)923-7104

Cotter, Ann C., MD {1932143807} PhysMd, OthrSp(90,NY06)<NJ-MMHKEMBL>
+ Morristown Memorial Hospital/Mt. Kemble Division
 95 Mount Kemble Avenue/MindBodyCtr Morristown, NJ 07960 (973)971-4575 Fax (973)267-3144

Cotto, Maritza, MD {1215034848} CdvDis, IntrMd(87,NY06)<NJ-COOPRUMC, NJ-DEBRAHLC>
+ Cooper University Hospital
 One Cooper Plaza Camden, NJ 08103 (856)342-2000
+ University Cardiology
 3 Cooper Plaza/Room 311 Camden, NJ 08103 (856)342-2034

Cotton, John M., MD {1871679100} Pedtrc(75,NY19)
+ The Pediatric Group PA
 66 Mount Lucas Road Princeton, NJ 08540 (609)924-4892
 Fax (609)921-9380
 cotton@pedgroup.com

Cottrill, Richard Z., Jr., MD {1124083811} Anesth(89,NY01)<NJ-STPETER, NJ-SOMERSET>
+ Anesthesia Consultnts of NJ/Nova Pain
 285 Davidson Avenue/Suite 204 Somerset, NJ 08873
 (732)271-1400 Fax (732)271-3543
+ Cares Surgicenter, LLC.
 240 Easton Avenue New Brunswick, NJ 08901 (732)271-1400 Fax (732)296-8677

Couch, Jonathan Darrell, DO {1689808107} SrgNro<NJ-STBARNMC>
+ St. Barnabas Medical Center
 94 Old Short Hills Road Livingston, NJ 07039 (973)322-5000

Coumbis, John J., MD {1992963060} OccpMd(85,ROM01)<NJ-STFRNMED>
+ St. Francis/Centers for Workers Health
 601 Hamilton Avenue/Suite 210 Hamilton, NJ 08629
 (609)890-7100

Coutermarsh, Andrew, DO {1740568716} FamMed
+ McGuire Air Force Base/Acute Health Care Clinic
 3458 Neely Road Trenton, NJ 08641 (609)754-9480 Fax (609)754-9015

Coutinho Haas, Sunita Patricia, MD {1770505828} Pedtrc(92,INA6Y)
+ CHOP Primary Care Mount Laurel
 3201 Marne Highway Mount Laurel, NJ 08054 (856)829-5545 Fax (856)829-9268

Covalesky, John, DO {1184845307} IntrMd, CdvDis, CarNuc(01,PA78)<NJ-JRSYSHMC, NJ-DEBRAHLC>
+ Garden State Heart Care, P.C.
 831 Tennent Road/Suite 1-F Englishtown, NJ 07726
 (732)851-4700 Fax (732)851-4703

Covelli, Joseph Michael, MD {1780622944} IntrMd, IntHos(96,NY08)<NJ-VALLEY>
+ The Valley Hospital
 223 North Van Dien Avenue Ridgewood, NJ 07450
 (201)447-8000

Covello, Lucy F., MD {1417058322} EnDbMt(84,DMN01)<NJ-CHILTON>
+ 1524 Route 23 North
 Butler, NJ 07405 (973)838-3112 Fax (973)838-3351

Coven, Roger A., MD {1518961143} ObsGyn(80,NJ05)<NJ-VALLEY>
+ Valley Center for Women's Health
 550 North Maple Avenue/Suite 102 Ridgewood, NJ 07450
 (201)444-4040 Fax (201)444-4473
+ Valley Center for Women's Health
 581 North Franklin Turnpike/2nd Floor Ramsey, NJ 07446
 (201)444-4040 Fax (201)236-5269

Coville, Frederick A., MD {1679728307} SrgPlstc(82,MEX03)
+ Drs. Sperling & Sperling
 162 South New York Road/Suite B-3 Galloway, NJ 08205
 (609)748-8200 Fax (609)748-9200

Covit, Andrew B., MD {1528058922} Hypten, IntrMd, Nephro(79,NY08)<NJ-RWJUBRUN, NJ-STPETER>
+ Nephrology Hypertension Associates of Central Jersey
 8 Old Bridge Turnpike/ManagingPartner South River, NJ 08882 (732)390-4888 Fax (732)390-0255
 acovit@nephrohibp.com
+ Nephrology Hypertension Associates of Central Jersey
 901 West Main Street/Suite 102 Freehold, NJ 07728
 (732)625-0707

Covone, Kenneth C., DO {1316138829} ObsGyn(03,ME75)
+ Kennedy Family Health Center
 445 Hurffville Crosskeys Road Sewell, NJ 08080 (856)218-2312

Cowan, Clayton Joseph, MD {1871599563} Anesth, AnesCrCr, IntrMd(91,PA02)<NJ-NWTNMEM>
+ Newton Medical Center
 175 High Street/Anesthesia Newton, NJ 07860 (973)383-2121

Cowan, James Rankin, Jr., MD {1063527026} Psychy, PsyFor(70,TN07)<NJ-EASTORNG>
+ The Cowan Wellness Center
 70 East Ridgewood Avenue Ridgewood, NJ 07450
 (201)670-4124 Fax (201)670-4120
+ East Orange General Hospital
 300 Central Avenue/Psych East Orange, NJ 07018
 (973)672-8400

Cowan, Robert Matthew, MD {1427098557} EmrgMd(02,PA12)<NJ-VIRTMHBC>
+ Virtua Memorial
 175 Madison Avenue/EmrgMed Mount Holly, NJ 08060
 (609)267-0700 Fax (609)914-6067

Cowell, Jennifer L., MD {1518374487} Anesth
+ Robert Wood Johnson-UMDNJ Anesthesia Group
 125 Paterson Street/CAB 3100 New Brunswick, NJ 08901
 (732)235-6153 Fax (732)235-6131

Cowen, Daniel S., MD {1659459980} Psychy, IntrMd(91,OH06)
+ UH- Robert Wood Johnson Med
 125 Paterson Street/Ste 2200/Psych New Brunswick, NJ 08901 (732)828-3000
+ Anxiety & Depression Treatment Center, LLC.
 2 Worlds Fair Drive/Suite 206 Somerset, NJ 08873
 (732)828-3000 Fax (732)805-9808

Cox, Courtney, DO {1356751317} EmrgMd
+ SJH Emergency Medicine
 1505 West Sherman Avenue Vineland, NJ 08360
 (856)641-8661 Fax (856)575-4944

Cox, Garrick Andrew, MD {1881613925} OrtTrm, SrgOrt, SprtMd(00,PA09)<NJ-STJOSHOS, NJ-WAYNEGEN>
+ North Jersey Orthopaedic Group
 246 Hamburg Turnpike/Suite 302 Wayne, NJ 07470
 (973)689-6266 Fax (973)689-6264

Cox, Gregory E., MD {1386607844} Ophthl(91,PA09)
+ 2 Hamilton Health Place/Building 2
 Hamilton, NJ 08690 (609)586-0849 Fax (609)586-7018

Cox, Mary Jude, MD {1144263500} Ophthl(97,VA01)
+ Eye Physicians PC
 1140 White Horse Road/Suite 1 Voorhees, NJ 08043
 (856)784-3366 Fax (856)784-4388

Cox, Trevor E., DO {1265842231} FamMed
+ Patient first
 606 Cross Keys Road Sicklerville, NJ 08081 (856)237-1016

Cox, Victoria Ryan, MD {1093087819} FamMed<NJ-HUNTRDN>
+ Hunterdon Medical Center
 2100 Wescott Drive Flemington, NJ 08822 (908)788-6160
+ Phillips Barber Family Health Center
 72 Alexander Avenue Lambertville, NJ 08530 (908)788-6160 Fax (609)397-0301

Coy, Deborah A., MD {1730261496} Pedtrc, AdolMd(88,GRNA)<NJ-MTNSIDE, NJ-STBARNMC>
+ 405 Northfield Avenue/Suite LL2
 West Orange, NJ 07052 (973)736-4442 Fax (973)736-8717

Coyle, Allison A., DO {1457615197} ObsGyn
+ Atlantic Coast Urology
 1944 Corlies Avenue/Suite 101/ObsGyn Neptune, NJ 07753
 (732)776-3790 Fax (732)776-4525

Coyle, Genoveva F., MD {1437228707} IntrMd(91,ROM01)
+ Med-Care of East Rutherford
 245 Park Avenue East Rutherford, NJ 07073 (201)939-7161 Fax (201)939-4053

Coyle, Michael P., Jr., MD {1285639120} SrgOrt, OrtSHand(68,NY01)<NJ-STPETER, NJ-RWJUBRUN>
+ University Orthopaedic Associates, LLC.
 Two Worlds Fair Drive Somerset, NJ 08873 (732)979-2115
 Fax (732)564-9032
+ University Orthopaedic Group
 215 Easton Avenue New Brunswick, NJ 08901 (732)979-2115 Fax (732)545-4011
+ University Orthopaedic Associates, LLC.
 211 North Harrison Street Princeton, NJ 08873 (609)683-7800 Fax (609)683-7875

Coyle, Raluca, MD {1417997701} Nephro(91,ROM01)<NJ-EASTORNG>
+ Kidney & Hypertension Associates
 733 Bloomfield Avenue Bloomfield, NJ 07003 (973)680-0400 Fax (973)680-0450

Coyne, Christine Ann, MD {1255451043} Pedtrc(94,TX04)<NJ-MORRISTN>
+ Basking Ridge Pediatric Association
150 North Finley Avenue   Basking Ridge, NJ 07920
(908)766-4660   Fax (908)204-9871

Coyne, Robert F., MD {1093746646} ClCdEl, CdvDis, IntrMd(90,TX12)<NJ-MORRISTN, NJ-OVERLOOK>
+ Electrophysiology Associates, PA
100 Madison Avenue/Suite 5   Morristown, NJ 07962
(973)971-4261   Fax (973)290-7253

Cozamanis, Steve G., DO {1770553042} IntrMd(PA77)
+ Atlantic Care Physician Group
201 West Avenue   Ocean City, NJ 08226   (609)391-7500
Fax (609)391-0963

Cozzarelli, James Francis, MD {1356315519} FamMed, SrgOrt(99,DC02)
+ Advanced Orthopedics & Sports Medicine Institute
301 Professional View Drive   Freehold, NJ 07728
(732)720-2555   Fax (732)720-2556

Cozzarelli-Franklin, Annette O., MD {1639230840} IntrMd(86,MEX03)<NJ-CLARMAAS>
+ Drs. Cozzarelli-Franklin and Franklin MD's
175 Franklin Avenue   Nutley, NJ 07110   (973)667-8535
Fax (973)667-8442

Cozzini, Nancy, MD {1265512321} Pedtrc(97,DMN01)<NJ-CLARMAAS>
+ Clara Maass Medical Center
1 Clara Maass Drive/Pediatrics   Belleville, NJ 07109
(973)450-2000

Cozzone, John T., MD {1639148802} SrgPlstc(78,ITA17)<NJ-HACKNSK, NJ-VALLEY>
+ 1 West Ridgewood Avenue/Suite 302
Paramus, NJ 07652   (201)689-1570   Fax (201)689-1559

Crabtree, Shawn M., MD {1831283910} FamMed, FamMAdlt(90,NJ05)<NJ-WAYNEGEN>
+ Wedgewood Primary Care
1055 Hamburg Turnpike/Suite 300   Wayne, NJ 07470
(973)904-1177   Fax (973)904-1166

Cracchiolo, Bernadette M., MD {1891721668} ObsGyn, GynOnc, PallCr(91,IL42)<NJ-UMDNJ>
+ University Hospital-Doctors Office Center
90 Bergen Street/Rm 4600   Newark, NJ 07103   (973)972-5554   Fax (973)972-4574
cracchiolo@umdnj.edu

Craciun, Liviu Ciprian, MD {1902022882} Nrolgy, ClNrPh(95,ROM02)
+ Summit Neurology Consulting, PC.
33 Overlook Road/Suite 401   Summit, NJ 07901   (908)273-9000   Fax (908)273-9022

Craft, Jeanne A., MD {1124093612} PedCrC, Pedtrc(89,PA02)<NJ-MORRISTN>
+ Morristown Medical Center
100 Madison Avenue   Morristown, NJ 07962   (973)971-7550   Fax (973)971-7364
jeanne.craft@ahsys.org

Craig, Gazelle A., MD {1730346826} Surgry
+ 70 South Munn Avenue/Suite 610
East Orange, NJ 07018   (214)727-8565

Craig, Krekamey Ropkui, MD {1376643437} Pedtrc(99,OH06)<NJ-MORRISTN, NJ-STCLRDEN>
+ Denville Pediatrics Medical Associates PA
140 East Main Street   Denville, NJ 07834   (973)625-5090
Fax (973)625-8006

Craig, Vicki L., MD {1538228705} Pedtrc, PedCrC(86,MEXI)<NJ-RWJUBRUN, NJ-JRSYSHMC>
+ RWJ University Hospital New Brunswick
One Robert Wood Johnson Place   New Brunswick, NJ 08901
(732)828-3000

Crain, Peter M., MD {1316132079} PsyNro, PsyFor(70,DC02)
+ Crain Medical Consultants PA
1 West Ridgewood Avenue/Suite 101   Paramus, NJ 07652
(201)444-9772   Fax (201)444-4220

Cramer, Kenneth E., MD {1306887005} EmrgMd(92,MD12)
+ Cape Urgent Care
900 Route 109   Cape May, NJ 08204   (609)884-4357   Fax (609)884-4377
+ Volunteers in Medicine
423 North Route 9   Cape May Court House, NJ 08210
(609)884-4357   Fax (609)463-2830

Crane, Charles J., MD {1710961917} Ophthl(88,NJ05)<NJ-ST-BARNMC>
+ Northern New Jersey Eye Institute
71 Second Street   South Orange, NJ 07079   (973)763-2203
Fax (973)762-9449
+ Northern New Jersey Eye Institute
616 Bloomfield Avenue   West Caldwell, NJ 07006
(973)763-2203   Fax (973)762-9449
+ Northern New Jersey Eye Institute
700 North Broad Street   Elizabeth, NJ 07079   (908)354-2138   Fax (908)354-9822

Crane, Stephen E., MD {1073613998} ObsGyn(86,NJ05)<NJ-ST-BARNMC>
+ Associates in Obstetrics Gynecology & Infertility
375 Mount Pleasant Avenue/Suite 202   West Orange, NJ 07052   (973)731-7707   Fax (973)669-0277

Cranley, Robert, MD {1336112242} RadDia(95,MA05)<NJ-KIMBALL>
+ Kimball Medical Center
600 River Avenue   Lakewood, NJ 08701   (732)363-1900
Fax (732)942-5658

Crasner, Joshua M., DO {1902898760} CdvDis, IntrMd(89,PA77)
+ South Jersey Heart Group
539 Egg Harbor Road/Suite 1   Sewell, NJ 08080   (856)589-0300   Fax (856)589-1753

Cravioto-Vaimakis, Stefanie Sara, MD {1396802633} Surgry, Bariat(96,NY19)<NJ-ENGLWOOD, NJ-HOLYNAME>
+ Englewood Laparoscopic and Bariatric Associates
309 Engle Street/Suite 1   Englewood, NJ 07631   (201)227-9444   Fax (201)227-8326
+ North Jersey Laparoscopic Associates
222 Cedar Lane/Room 201   Teaneck, NJ 07666   (201)227-9444   Fax (201)530-9300
+ North Jersey Laparoscopic Associates
6045 Kennedy Boulevard   North Bergen, NJ 07631
(201)453-2784   Fax (201)227-6282

Crawford, Carolyn S., MD {1518945369} NnPnMd(71,PA02)<NJ-OURLADY, NJ-BURDTMLN>
+ Our Lady of Lourdes Medical Center
1600 Haddon Avenue   Camden, NJ 08103   (856)757-3500

Crawford, Heather M., DO {1467789669} ObsGyn
+ 1114 South Park Avenue
Haddon Heights, NJ 08035

Crawford, Jeffrey R., DO {1275535064} CdvDis, IntrMd(83,PA77)
+ 37 East King's Highway
Audubon, NJ 08106   (856)573-9500   Fax (856)608-0501

Crawford, Steven G., MD {1841362746} IntrMd, IntrSptM(74,OH40)<NJ-JRSYSHMC, NJ-MONMOUTH>
+ Meridian Occupational Health
1430 Hooper Avenue/Suite 200-B   Toms River, NJ 08753
(732)557-0700

Crawford-Meadows, Robin A., MD {1881618130} ObsGyn, IntrMd(89,NJ06)
+ 1636 Route 38 Eayrestown Road
Lumberton, NJ 08048   (609)914-8450

Crawley, Joseph M., MD {1336182583} CritCr, IntrMd, PulDis(88,GRN01)<NJ-STMRYPAS>
+ JFK Medical Center
65 James Street   Edison, NJ 08820   (732)321-7605   Fax (732)744-5614

Crean, Christopher Arthur, MD {1588699409} EmrgMd(03,DC02)<NJ-RWJURAH, NJ-SOMERSET>
+ Emergency Medical Associates of NJ, P.A.
3 Century Drive   Parsippany, NJ 07054   (973)740-0607
Fax (973)740-9895

Creecy, Saundra K., MD {1760495493} Pedtrc(77,NC01)
+ CHOP Primary Care Mount Laurel
3201 Marne Highway   Mount Laurel, NJ 08054   (856)829-5545   Fax (856)829-9268

Creel, Marilyn U. Baruiz, MD {1932290137} IntrMd, InfDis(75,PHI10)
+ 758 Route 18 North/Suite 103A
East Brunswick, NJ 08816   (732)254-1911   Fax (732)679-1533

Cresanti-Daknis, Charles Brian, MD {1891753604} AnesPain, IntrMd(90,PA09)
+ Spine & Pain Centers
655 Shrewbury Avenue/Suite 202   Shrewsbury, NJ 07702
(732)345-1180   Fax (732)530-4476
+ Spine & Pain Centers
303 West Main Street/Lower Level   Freehold, NJ 07728
(732)345-1180   Fax (732)530-4476
+ Spine & Pain Centers
1430 Hooper Avenue/Suite 205   Toms River, NJ 07702
(732)473-9530   Fax (732)473-9574

Cricco, Carl F., Jr., MD {1114991510} Urolgy(75,DC01)<NJ-HOBUNIMC>
+ 315 Park Avenue
Hoboken, NJ 07030   (201)656-7688   Fax (201)656-1541

Cridge, Peter B., MD {1437236411} EmrgMd(94,PA09)<NJ-UNVMCPRN>
+ University Medical Center of Princeton at Plainsboro
One Plainsboro Road/Emergency   Plainsboro, NJ 08536
(609)497-4431   Fax (609)497-4988

Crighton, Kent Andrew, MD {1093764748} IntrMd, OccpMd(87,DMN01)
+ Prudential Employee Health Service
213 Washington Street   Newark, NJ 07102   (973)802-6380
Fax (973)802-2276

Crisan, Liviu C., MD {1730146051} IntrMd(78,ROMA)<NJ-COMMED>
+ 651 Lacey Road
Forked River, NJ 08731   (609)242-4322   Fax (609)242-4324

Crisanti, John, Jr., MD {1356379549} EmrgMd(76,PA13)<NJ-COMMED>
+ Community Medical Center
99 Route 37 West   Toms River, NJ 08755   (732)557-8056
Fax (732)557-8087
jcrisanti@barnabashealth.net

Criscitiello, Arnold A., MD {1245233634} SrgOrt(91,DC02)<NJ-VALLEY>
+ Ridgewood Orthopedic Group, LLC
85 South Maple Avenue   Ridgewood, NJ 07450   (201)445-2830   Fax (201)445-7471

Criscito, Mario A., MD {1063411957} CdvDis, IntrMd(67,ITAL)
+ Cardiology Center of New Jersey
50 Newark Avenue/Suite 204   Belleville, NJ 07109
(973)450-2158   Fax (973)450-2027

Crisman, Celina M., MD {1255699963}
+ 1180 Raymond Boulevard/Apt 25 E
Newark, NJ 07102   (617)201-4999

Crisp, Meredith Page, MD {1831300243} ObsGyn(00,KY12)<NJ-COOPRUMC, NJ-ACMCITY>
+ Cooper Gynecologic Oncology Associates
900 Centennial Boulevard/Suite F   Voorhees, NJ 08043
(856)325-6644   Fax (856)325-6643

Crist, Peter A., MD {1790139566} IntrMd, Psychy(77,CA14)
+ 62 Wagner Road
Stockton, NJ 08559

Cristini, John A., MD {1497854582} SrgOrt, SrgHnd(66,PA09)<NJ-ACMCMAIN, NJ-ACMCITY>
+ Atlantic Coast Orthopedics, LLC
401 New Road/Suite 200   Linwood, NJ 08221   (609)926-7400   Fax (609)926-9518

Cristoforo, Nancy Todd, MD {1215925136} CdvDis(98,PA13)
+ Raritan Bay Cardiology Group, P.A.
225 May Street/Suite F   Edison, NJ 08837   (732)738-8855
Fax (732)738-4141

Crivello, Keith Michael, MD {1902063167} SrgOrt(05,MA05)
+ Mercer-Bucks Orthopaedics, P.C.
2501 Kuser Road   Hamilton, NJ 08691   (609)896-0444
Fax (609)587-4349

Croce, Salvatore A., MD {1720192412} IntrMd, PulDis(80,DOM02)<NJ-KIMBALL, NJ-CENTRAST>
+ Monmouth Ocean Pulmonary Medicine
901 West Main Street/Suite 160   Freehold, NJ 07728
(732)577-0600   Fax (732)577-6332
+ Monmouth Ocean Pulmonary Medicine
886 River Avenue   Lakewood, NJ 08701   (732)577-0600
Fax (732)360-0336
+ Monmouth Ocean Pulmonary Medicine
312 Applegarth Road   Monroe Township, NJ 07728
(609)409-0029

Croff, William J., DO {1780656983} ObsGyn(72,PA77)<NJ-VIRTVOOR, NJ-JFKMED>
+ 188 Fries Mill Road/Suite B1
Blackwood, NJ 08012

Crompton, Thomas F., MD {1942255674} Anesth(68,VA01)<NJ-ACMCITY>
+ AtlantiCare Regional Medical Center/City Campus
1925 Pacific Avenue/Anesthesiology   Atlantic City, NJ 08401
(609)345-4000

Cronin, Leanne M., MD PthFor(03,NY47)
+ 10 Thomas Terrace
Wayne, NJ 07470

Cronin, Stephen R., MD {1720136153} IntrMd(82,PHI20)
+ 625 Broadway
Paterson, NJ 07514   (973)278-1100

Crooks, Michael H., MD {1760496350} IntrMd(88,NY46)
+ 474 Elkwood Terrace/Unit C
Englewood, NJ 07631

Crookshank, Aaron David, MD {1285875633} PulDis, PulCCr, IntrMd(03,PA13)<NJ-OURLADY, NJ-VIRTMARL>
+ Pulmonary & Sleep Associates of SJ, LLC.
107 Berlin Road   Cherry Hill, NJ 08034   (856)429-1800
Fax (856)429-1081
+ Pulmonary & Sleep Associates of SJ, LLC.
750 Route 73 South/Suite 401   Marlton, NJ 08053
(856)429-1800   Fax (856)375-2325
+ Pulmonary & Sleep Associates of SJ, LLC.
811 Sunset Road/Suite 201   Burlington, NJ 08034
(609)298-1776   Fax (609)531-2391

Cross, Gershwin A., MD {1306152400} Pedtrc, NnPnMd(93,BAR01)
+ 2 Garden Court
Lincoln Park, NJ 07035

Physicians by Name and Address

Crosta, Alan Michael, Jr., MD {1750362265} Anesth(90,NJ05)<NJ-MORRISTN>
  + Morristown Medical Center
    100 Madison Avenue/Anesthesiology   Morristown, NJ 07962   (973)971-5548   Fax (201)943-8733

Crowley, Elizabeth Ann, MD {1255374310} FamMed, IntrMd(97,PA02)<NJ-BURDTMLN>
  + Volunteers in Medicine
    423 North Route 9   Cape May Court House, NJ 08210   (609)463-2846   Fax (609)463-2830

Crowley, Elizabeth Ozimek, MD {1760733240} Psychy(95,NY09)
  + Drs. Hanna & Crowley
    545 Island Road/Suite 2B   Ramsey, NJ 07446   (201)995-1004   Fax (201)345-7121

Crowley, John G., MD SrgVas(65,IREL)<NJ-HUNTRDN>
  + UMDNJ RWJ Vascular Surgery Group
    125 Paterson Street/Suite 4100   New Brunswick, NJ 08901   (732)235-7816   Fax (732)235-8538
    crowlejg@umdnj.edu
  + Hunterdon Surgical Associates
    1100 Wescott Drive/Suite 302   Flemington, NJ 08822   (732)235-7816   Fax (908)788-6459

Crowley, Kathryn Ann, MD {1275506040} Pedtrc, NnPnMd(80,NY46)<NJ-MORRISTN, NJ-CHILTON>
  + MidAtlantic Neonatology Associates
    100 Madison Avenue   Morristown, NJ 07962   (973)971-5488   Fax (973)290-7175

Cruciani, Ricardo Alberto, MD {1881615268} PainMd, Nrolgy, IntrMd(79,ARG01)
  + Capital Institute for Neurosciences
    2 Capital Way/Suite 456   Pennington, NJ 08534   (609)537-7300   Fax (609)537-7301

Crudele, James E., MD {1073577920} FamMed, Grtrcs, OthrSp(85,MEX03)<NJ-VIRTVOOR, NJ-VIRTMARL>
  + James Crudele Family Medicine
    285 Church Street/Suite 1   Moorestown, NJ 08057   (856)235-6116   Fax (856)235-7329

Cruickshank, Royston Raleigh, MD {1548331622} Psychy(87,CHIL)<NJ-JRSYSHMC>
  + Jersey Shore University Medical Center
    1945 Route 33/2nd Floor   Neptune, NJ 07753   (732)775-5500

Crutchlow, William P., MD {1285069583} SrgOrt, IntrMd(67,PA02)
  + The Orthopedic Group, P.A.
    261 James Street/Suite 3-F   Morristown, NJ 07960   (973)538-0029   Fax (973)538-4957
  + The Orthopedic Group, P.A.
    50 Cherry Hill Road   Parsippany, NJ 07054   (973)538-0029   Fax (973)263-3243
  + 7 East 20th Street
    Barnegat Light, NJ 07960   (973)615-9398

Cruz, Avelino N., MD {1639118862} IntrMd, Nephro(72,PHIL)<NJ-SHOREMEM, NJ-ACMCMAIN>
  + 60 Tuckahoe Road
    Marmora, NJ 08223   (609)390-2632   Fax (609)390-9210
  + 1305 Route 50 South
    Mays Landing, NJ 08330   (609)390-2632   Fax (609)909-1402

Cruz, Bernardo V., MD {1215929153} Anesth(74,PHIL)<NJ-CHILTON>
  + Chilton Medical Center
    97 West Parkway/Anesthesiology   Pompton Plains, NJ 07444   (973)831-5000

Cruz, Catalina M., MD {1548323132} FamMed, IntMAdMd(66,PHIL)<NJ-TRININPC>
  + Trinitas Regional Medical Center-New Point Campus
    655 East Jersey Street   Elizabeth, NJ 07206   (908)994-5000

Cruz, Dionisio V., MD {1609833961} Nephro, IntrMd(72,PHI01)<NJ-JRSYSHMC, NJ-OCEANMC>
  + Shore Nephrology, P.A.
    2100 Corlies Avenue/Suite 15   Neptune, NJ 07753   (732)988-8228   Fax (732)774-1528
  + Shore Nephrology, P.A.
    35 Beaverson Boulevard   Brick, NJ 08723   (732)988-8228   Fax (732)451-0071
  + The Hernia Center
    495 Iron Bridge Road/Suite 3   Freehold, NJ 07753   (732)462-5995   Fax (732)845-1002

Cruz, Florencia Santos, MD {1083650808} Pedtrc, NnPnMd(88,PHI07)<NJ-KIMBALL, NJ-CENTRAST>
  + On-Site Neonatal Partners
    1000 Haddonfield-Berlin Road/Suite 210   Voorhees, NJ 08043   (856)782-2212   Fax (856)782-2213
    krdstfrei@aol.com

Cruz, Francisco Philomel Doming, MD {1184605339} EnDbMt(95,PHI02)
  + Drs. Ortiz, Villanueva and Cruz
    1163 Route 37 West/Suite A-1   Toms River, NJ 08755   (732)736-1000   Fax (732)736-8811
  + Drs. Ortiz, Villanueva and Cruz
    1255 Route 70/Suite 20-N   Lakewood, NJ 08701   (732)363-4770

Cruz, Gloria Maria, MD {1992760086} FamMed, ObsGyn(83,SPA03)<NJ-UNVMCPRN>
  + Princeton Occupational Medicine
    2271 Highway 33/Suite 109   Hamilton, NJ 08690   (609)584-0117   Fax (609)586-5103

Cruz, Joseph, DO {1417219239}
  + 32 Hanover Road
    Marlton, NJ 08053   (856)857-4261

Cruz, Mary Donna Mananghaya, MD {1922305952}
  + Cardiology Consultants
    246 Hamburg Turnpike/Suite 201   Wayne, NJ 07470   (973)942-1141   Fax (973)942-1250

Cruz, Wilfredo Tomas Correa, MD {1730116211} FamMed(98,PHI01)<NJ-JRSYCITY>
  + Horizon Health Center/Family Medicine
    412 Summit Avenue   Jersey City, NJ 07306   (201)963-5774   Fax (201)963-8274
  + Horizon Health Center
    714 Bergen Avenue   Jersey City, NJ 07306   (201)451-6300

Cruz Ithier, Mayra Alejandra, MD {1619263027} ObsGyn
  + University Medical Group/OBGYN
    125 Paterson Street/2nd Floor   New Brunswick, NJ 08901   (732)235-3362   Fax (732)235-6627

Cruz-Encarnacion, Merle C., MD {1043295579} CdvDis, IntrMd(76,PHI01)
  + 201 St. Pauls Avenue/Unit 1d
    Jersey City, NJ 07306

Cryan, Jeffrey M., MD {1831149566} Gastrn, IntrMd(79,MEX21)<NJ-OCEANMC>
  + 329 Commons Way
    Toms River, NJ 08755   (732)240-5656
  + 1673 Highway 88 West
    Brick, NJ 08724   (732)840-1222
  + 75 Lacey Road
    Whiting, NJ 08755   (732)350-7500

Crystal, Jessica S., MD {1285947945}
  + Robert Wood Johnson Surgery
    One Robert Wood Johnson Place/MEB 596   New Brunswick, NJ 08901   (732)235-7674

Cuadra, Salvador Alejandro, MD {1851310015} SrgVas, Surgry(97,NY48)<NJ-MTNSIDE>
  + The Cardiovascular Care Group
    433 Central Avenue   Westfield, NJ 07090   (908)654-5333   Fax (908)751-3730

Cubelli, Kenneth, MD {1346257581} SrgOrt(79,NY19)
  + Morris County Orthopaedic Group
    109 US Highway 46 East   Denville, NJ 07834   (973)625-1221   Fax (201)625-1594

Cubelli, Vincent, MD {1053353474} Urolgy(82,NY19)<NJ-STCLRDEN, NJ-STCLRDOV>
  + 16 Pocono Road/Suite 302
    Denville, NJ 07834   (973)627-3411   Fax (973)627-1095

Cuber, Shain A., MD {1992822126} SrgPlstc, SrgHnd(90,NY09)
  + Associates in Plastic Surgery
    1150 Amboy Avenue   Edison, NJ 08837   (732)548-3200   Fax (732)548-1919
  + Associates in Plastic Surgery
    203 Route 9 South/Marlboro   Englishtown, NJ 07726   (732)617-1800
  + Associates in Plastic Surgery
    5 Mountain Boulevard   Warren, NJ 08837   (908)222-8440

Cubero, John G., MD {1205856291} CdvDis, Gastrn(75,NJ05)
  + Lyndhurst Medical Associates
    358 Valley Brook Avenue   Lyndhurst, NJ 07071   (201)460-0142   Fax (201)460-1959

Cubina, Maria L., DO {1790765683} Anesth, PedAne(89,NY75)
  + New Jersey Ambulatory Anesthesia Consultants, LLC
    55 Schanck Road/Suite 8-A   Freehold, NJ 07728   (732)431-9544   Fax (732)431-9313

Cucci, Patricia, MD {1538135231} Ophthl(89,NJ05)<NJ-STMRYPAS, NY-MTSINYHS>
  + North Jersey Eye Associates PA
    1005 Clifton Avenue   Clifton, NJ 07013   (973)472-4114   Fax (973)472-0775
    cuccimd@aol.com

Cuccurullo, Sara J.M., MD {1982638904} PhysMd, IntrMd(87,NY08)<NJ-JFKJHNSN>
  + JFK Johnson Rehabilitation Institute
    65 James Street   Edison, NJ 08818   (732)321-7070   Fax (732)744-5846

Cucinella, Erica L., MD {1215343249}
  + 8b Sayre Court
    Madison, NJ 07940

Cucolo, Patricia Anne, MD {1598731879} Pedtrc(97,NY06)
  + Madison Pediatrics
    435 South Street/Suite 200   Morristown, NJ 07960   (973)822-0003   Fax (973)822-3349
    pcpedsid@att.net

Cuddihy, Kathleen Marie, MD {1699847285} Pedtrc(96,NJ05)<NJ-OVERLOOK, NJ-STBARNMC>
  + New Providence Pediatrics
    180 South Street/Suite 3   New Providence, NJ 07974   (908)771-9824   Fax (908)771-9674

Cuddihy, Laury A., MD {1740517457} SrgOrt, SrgSpn(04,NY46)<NY-MTSINAI, NY-MTSINYHS>
  + Institute for Spine & Scoliosis, P.A.
    3100 Princeton Pike/Building 1   Lawrenceville, NJ 08648   (609)912-1500   Fax (609)912-1600
    laury.cuddihy@gmail.com

Cuervo, Nieves, MD {1669657508} Psychy(85,CUB07)<NJ-STJOSHOS>
  + 810 Abbott Boulevard/Suite 204
    Fort Lee, NJ 07024
  + St. Joseph's Regional Medical Center
    703 Main Street/Psych   Paterson, NJ 07503   (973)754-2000

Cueto, Irene L., MD {1629001482} IntrMd(88,PHIL)<NJ-CHSMRCER>
  + Greater Mercer Pulmonary & Medical Assoc PC
    445 Whitehorse Avenue/Suite 103   Trenton, NJ 08610   (609)585-0300

Cueto, Victor, Jr., MD {1639439953} Pedtrc
  + Newark Community Health Center, Inc.
    741 Broadway   Newark, NJ 07104   (201)675-1900   Fax (973)676-1396

Cuffie, Cynthia A., MD {1366632721} EnDbMt, IntrMd(78,NJ05)
  + Schering Plough Research Institute
    2000 Galloping Hill Road   Kenilworth, NJ 07033   (908)740-4980   Fax (908)298-2834

Cugini, Donald A., MD {1225028640} Surgry, SrgBst(87,NJ06)<NJ-RIVERVW>
  + Navesink Surgical Associates MD, PA
    65 Mechanic Street/Suite 102   Red Bank, NJ 07701   (732)530-0151   Fax (732)741-3730

Culbert, Steven A., MD {1619904000} ObsGyn(95,MA07)<NJ-KIMBALL>
  + Women's Health Associates
    101 Prospect Street/Suite 202   Lakewood, NJ 08701   (732)942-4442   Fax (732)942-7024

Culin, Angelina Han, MD {1487613659} ObsGyn(01,NC05)<NJ-MORRISTN>
  + Morristown Obstetrics and Gynecology Associates
    101 Madison Avenue/Suite 405   Morristown, NJ 07960   (862)210-3217   Fax (973)267-7272

Cullen, Eugene A., MD {1487620407} FamMed, IntrMd(95,NJ05)<NJ-NWTNMEM>
  + Skylands Medical Group PA
    210 Route 94   Columbia, NJ 07832   (908)362-9285   Fax (908)362-7756

Cullen, Holly Doolittle, MD {1023048584} Gastrn, IntrMd(87,NJ05)<NJ-VALLEY>
  + Bergen Medical Associates
    466 Old Hook Road/Suite 1   Emerson, NJ 07630   (201)967-8221   Fax (201)967-0340
  + Bergen Medical Associates
    1 West Ridgewood Avenue/Suite 301   Paramus, NJ 07652   (201)967-8221   Fax (201)445-4296

Cullen, Kathryn Eva, DO {1437337219} IntrMd(04,NY75)<NJ-OVERLOOK>
  + Overlook Medical Center
    99 Beauvoir Avenue/PO Box 210   Summit, NJ 07902   (908)522-2000
    cullenK@emomedicalcare.com

Cullen, Michael E., MD {1013991181} Anesth(91,NJ05)<NJ-HACKNSK>
  + Hackensack University Medical Center
    30 Prospect Avenue/Anesthesiology   Hackensack, NJ 07601   (201)996-2419   Fax (201)488-6769
  + Hackensack University MC-Anesthesia Dept
    30 Prospect Avenue/Room 207   Hackensack, NJ 07601   (201)996-2419   Fax (201)996-3962

Culligan, Patrick John, MD {1497727721} ObsGyn, Gyneco(93,GA22)<NJ-MORRISTN, NJ-OVERLOOK>
  + Urogynecology & Reconstructive Pelvic Surgery
    435 South Street/Suite 370   Morristown, NJ 07960   (973)971-7267   Fax (973)290-7520
  + Urogynecology & Reconstructive Pelvic Surgery
    33 Overlook Road/Suite 409   Summit, NJ 07901   (908)522-7335
  + Morristown Medical Center
    100 Madison Avenue/Gynecology   Morristown, NJ 07960   (973)971-5000

Cultrara, Anthony, MD {1083619860} Otlryg(98,NJ05)
  + Advanced ENT - Haddonfield
    130 North Haddon Avenue   Haddonfield, NJ 08033   (856)602-4000   Fax (856)429-1284
  + Advanced ENT - Mount Laurel
    204 Ark Road/Building 1/Suite 102   Mount Laurel, NJ 08054   (856)602-4000   Fax (856)946-1747
  + Advanced ENT - Voorhees
    1307 White Horse Road   Voorhees, NJ 08033   (856)602-4000   Fax (856)346-0480

Culver, Kenneth Wayne, MD {1700036498} Pedtrc, Allrgy, IntrMd(81,IA02)
+ Novartis Pharmaceuticals Corporation
One Health Plaza East Hanover, NJ 07936 (862)778-3720 Fax (973)781-6504

Cumarasamy, Thayalan K., MD {1437292752} FamMed, SrgO&M(93,PA09)<NJ-VIRTVOOR, NJ-OURLADY>
+ Family Physicians at Burlington
1816 Route 151/Suite 102 Burlington, NJ 08016 (856)747-0870 Fax (856)747-0877

Cumbo, Edward J., DO {1891722047} GenPrc, FamMed(76,PA77)<NJ-WARREN>
+ Milford Medical Center
207 Strykers Road Phillipsburg, NJ 08865 (908)995-4125
+ Village Medical Center
207 Strykers Road Phillipsburg, NJ 08865 (908)995-4125 Fax (908)859-6697

Cummings, Allan H., MD {1043248487} RadDia, Radiol(82,PA02)
+ Tilton Dynamic Imaging
1226 Tilton Road Northfield, NJ 08225 (609)383-2400 Fax (609)383-2407
+ Ocean Upright MRI, LLC
864 Route 37 West/Suite 7B Toms River, NJ 08755 (609)383-2400 Fax (732)240-3795

Cummings, Dustin Randal, MD {1598021834} Surgry<NY-MTSI-NAI>
+ New Bridge Medical Center
230 East Ridgewood Avenue Paramus, NJ 07652 (201)967-4000

Cummings, Kenneth B., MD {1518133560} Surgry, Urolgy(65,IL06)
+ Pediatric Urology Associates PC
422 Morris Avenue Long Branch, NJ 07740 (732)613-9144 Fax (732)613-5121

Cummings-Becker, Stephanie Jane, MD {1548598063}
+ Summit Medical Group
890 New Mountain Avenue New Providence, NJ 07974 (908)277-8601
+ Summit Medical Group
34 Mountain Boulevard/Building B Warren, NJ 07059 (908)277-8601 Fax (908)769-8927

Cummins, Dean Robert, MD {1174549547} Ophthl(88,MA07)<NJ-HOLYNAME>
+ The New Jersey Eye Center
1 North Washington Avenue Bergenfield, NJ 07621 (201)384-7333 Fax (201)384-2564

Cummins, Tiffany Ann, MD {1174556914} Psychy(99,LA01)
+ Preferred Behavioral Health of New Jersey
700 Airport Road Lakewood, NJ 08701 (732)367-4700 Fax (732)364-2253

Cunanan, Joanne C., MD {1639152663} IntrMd(00,MEX03)
+ 542 Berlin Keys Road/Suite 3-247
Sicklerville, NJ 08081

Cunanan, Manuel Salas, MD {1144474636} PulDis, IntrMd
+ Shore Physicians Group
18 West New York Avenue Somers Point, NJ 08244 (609)926-1450 Fax (609)926-8419

Cunicella, Nicholas A., III, DO {1568514784} FamMed(80,MO78)
+ 2314 South Avenue
Scotch Plains, NJ 07076 (908)233-6660 Fax (908)654-7152

Cunningham, Bruce D., DO {1912031907} FamMed(70,PA77)<NJ-SJRSYELM>
+ 2630 East Chestnut Avenue
Vineland, NJ 08360 (856)691-1053 Fax (856)691-9561

Cunningham, Catherine M., MD {1578654901} ObsGyn, Gyneco(92,PA13)
+ Associates in OBGYN
522 East Broad Street Westfield, NJ 07090 (908)232-4449

Cunningham, Ellen Elizabeth, MD {1205902186} Dermat(95,IL43)<NJ-MTNSIDE>
+ M.C. Medical Group
1425 Pompton Avenue/Suite 1-1 Cedar Grove, NJ 07009 (973)785-8686 Fax (973)785-8680

Cunningham, Frank J., MD {1740358068} PedEmg, Pedtrc, EmrgMd(86,NY09)
+ JFK Medical Center
65 James Street Edison, NJ 08820 (732)321-6499 Fax (732)744-5614

Cunningham, Gregory J., MD {1063482396} PulDis, CritCr, IntrMd(87,GRNA)<NJ-JRSYSHMC>
+ Jersey Coast Pulmonary
700 Route 71 & Crescent Place Sea Girt, NJ 08750 (732)449-7171 Fax (732)449-7788

Cunningham, John David, MD {1992707863} SrgOnc, Surgry(85,WI05)<NJ-OVERLOOK, NJ-MORRISTN>
+ Summit Medical Group-Berkeley Heights Campus
1 Diamond Hill Road/Breast Care Ctr Berkeley Heights, NJ 07922 (908)277-8770 Fax (908)673-7171

Cunningham, Michael James, MD {1639365836} Psychy, IntrMd(03,GRN01)<NJ-STBARNMC>
+ Westfield Mental Health Specialists, LLC.
547 East Broad Street/2nd Floor Westfield, NJ 07090 (908)264-2454 Fax (908)603-8794
info@westfieldmentalhealth.com

Cunningham, Michael Joseph, MD {1033256243} SrgOrt, SrgHnd, SprtMd(85,NY19)<NJ-BAYSHORE, NJ-RIVERVW>
+ Immediate Care Medical Walk-in of Hazlet, P.A.
1376 State Highway 36 Hazlet, NJ 07730 (732)264-5500 Fax (732)264-5554

Cunningham, Robert D., MD {1306855861} Ophthl(80,DC03)<NJ-EASTORNG>
+ Central Parkway Eye Care Center
185 Central Avenue/Suite 509 East Orange, NJ 07018 (973)673-4620 Fax (973)673-3260

Cunningham, William J., MD {1346505518} Dermat(69,NY08)
+ 333 US Highway 46/Suite 203
Mountain Lakes, NJ 07046 (973)331-1620 Fax (973)331-1622

Cuomo, Thomas F., MD {1639107048} SrgOrt(71,ITAL)
+ The Joint Institute at Saint Barnabas Medical Center
609 Morris Avenue Springfield, NJ 07081 (973)379-1991 Fax (973)467-8647

Cuozzo, Gregory Joseph, MD {1013962166} IntrMd(96,NJ06)<NJ-COMMED>
+ 102 Commons Way/Building A
Toms River, NJ 08755 (732)349-4434 Fax (732)349-9290

Cuppari, Anthony L., MD {1063466902} Surgry(85,WIND)<NJ-MORRISTN, NJ-STBARNMC>
+ 222 Columbia Turnpike/Suite 177
Florham Park, NJ 07932 (973)966-8900 Fax (973)966-8910
+ 29 Columbia Turnpike/Suite 202
Florham Park, NJ 07932 (973)966-8900 Fax (973)966-8910
+ 85 South Jefferson Street
Orange, NJ 07932 (973)673-3522

Curato, Lauren Jennifer, DO {1235406778}
+ Emergency Medical Associates of NJ, P.A.
3 Century Drive Parsippany, NJ 07054 (877)692-4665 Fax (973)740-9895

Curato, Mark Anthony, DO {1366728693} EmrgMd
+ Emergency Medical Associates of NJ, P.A.
3 Century Drive Parsippany, NJ 07054 (973)740-0607 Fax (973)740-9895

Curatolo, Evan M., MD {1124367404} Ortped, PedOrt<NJ-MONMOUTH>
+ Atlantic Pediatric Orthopedics
1131 Broad Street/Suite 202 Shrewsbury, NJ 07702 (732)544-9000 Fax (732)544-9099

Curcio, Christine Marie, MD {1740440247} Anesth, PedAne(08,DMN01)<NY-STONYBRK>
+ Robert Wood Johnson-UMDNJ Anesthesia Group
125 Paterson Street/CAB 3100 New Brunswick, NJ 08901 (732)235-7827 Fax (732)235-6131

Curi, Michael A., MD {1033222161} SrgVas, Surgry, IntrMd(98,NJ05)<NJ-UMDNJ>
+ University Hospital-Doctors Office Center
90 Bergen Street/Suite 7200 Newark, NJ 07103 (973)972-9371 Fax (973)972-0092
+ Pediatric Clinic - UMDNJ
140 Bergen Street/E-Level Newark, NJ 07103 (973)972-9000
+ New Margaret Hague Women's Health Institute
377 Jersey Avenue/Suite 220 Jersey City, NJ 07103 (973)972-9371 Fax (201)795-9157

Curl, Kevin M., MD {1154611234} CdvDis<NJ-VIRTVOOR>
+ Virtua Cardiology Group
2309 East Evesham Road/Suites 201-202 Voorhees, NJ 08043 (856)325-5400 Fax (856)325-5416
+ Virtua Voorhees
100 Bowman Drive/1st Floor Voorhees, NJ 08043 (856)325-5400 Fax (856)247-2597

Curlik, Semena, MD {1003998568} Anesth(80,MEX03)<NJ-UNVMCPRN>
+ University Medical Center of Princeton at Plainsboro
One Plainsboro Road/Anesth Plainsboro, NJ 08536 (609)497-4000

Curnow, Hidalberto, DO {1174681688} IntrMd(87,NJ75)<NJ-ACMCMAIN, NJ-SHOREMEM>
+ Absecon Island Internal Medicine
6508 Ventnor Avenue/Suite F Ventnor City, NJ 08406 (609)822-3027 Fax (609)822-5195

Curran, Terrence, MD {1174845929} SrgCrC<NJ-MORRISTN>
+ Morristown Medical Center
100 Madison Avenue Morristown, NJ 07962 (732)828-3000

Curreri, Joseph P., DO {1609825623} IntrMd, PulDis(90,PA77)
+ Drs. Curreri and Curreri
124 Lexington Avenue Merchantville, NJ 08109 (856)663-1121 Fax (856)661-9818

Curreri, Peter Andrew, DO {1053397356} PulDis, IntrMd(97,PA77)
+ Drs. Curreri and Curreri
124 Lexington Avenue Merchantville, NJ 08109 (856)663-1121 Fax (856)661-9818

Curreri, Rosalie M., MD {1972895209} IntrMd(89,GRNA)<NY-CM-CSTVNY>
+ 25 Stonybrook Drive
North Caldwell, NJ 07006

Curry, Debra W., MD {1831164474} FamMed(87,NY15)<NJ-HUNTRDN>
+ Delaware Valley Family Health Center
200 Frenchtown Road Milford, NJ 08848 (908)995-2251 Fax (908)995-2036

Curtis, Bernadette M., MD {1407858970} RadDia, Radiol, IntrMd(90,PA13)<NJ-VIRTMHBC>
+ Radiology Associates of Burlington County
1295 Route 38 West/PO Box 479 Hainesport, NJ 08036 (609)261-7017 Fax (609)261-4180

Curtis, Paul A., MD {1609874551} RadDia, Radiol(79,PA09)<NJ-VIRTVOOR, NJ-VIRTMARL>
+ South Jersey Radiology Associates, P.A.
315 Route 70 East/Suite B Cherry Hill, NJ 08034 (856)428-4344 Fax (856)428-0356
+ South Jersey Radiology Associates, P.A.
901 Route 168/Suites 301-305 Turnersville, NJ 08012 (856)428-4344 Fax (856)227-8537
+ South Jersey Radiology Associates, P.A.
807 Haddon Avenue/Suite 5 Haddonfield, NJ 08034 (856)616-1130 Fax (856)616-1125

Curtis, Princena Maria, MD {1063678944} PedDrm(03,PHI02)
+ Robert Wood Johnson Dermatology
1 World's Fair Drive Somerset, NJ 08873 (732)235-7765 Fax (732)235-6568
+ The Dermatology Group, P.C.
347 Mount Pleasant Avenue/Suite 205 West Orange, NJ 07052 (732)235-7765 Fax (973)498-0512

Curtis, Scott Jeffrey, DO {1265852701}<NJ-MORRISTN>
+ Morristown Medical Center
100 Madison Avenue Morristown, NJ 07962 (973)971-5000

Curtiss, Steven Ian, MD {1144295486} Surgry(86,NY03)<NJ-RWJUBRUN, NJ-STPETER>
+ Highland Park Surgical Associates
31 River Road Highland Park, NJ 08904 (732)846-9500 Fax (732)846-3931
+ Highland Park Surgical Associates
B2 Brier Hill Court/Suite 3 East Brunswick, NJ 08816 (732)846-9500 Fax (732)238-9697
+ Cares Surgicenter, LLC.
240 Easton Avenue New Brunswick, NJ 08904 (732)565-5400 Fax (732)296-8677

Curwin, Jay Howard, MD {1396775391} CdvDis, ClCdEl, IntrMd(87,NY47)<NJ-MORRISTN, NJ-OVERLOOK>
+ Morristown Medical Center
100 Madison Avenue/Cardiology Morristown, NJ 07962 (973)971-4261 Fax (973)625-0349

Cusack, Carrie Ann Rishko, MD {1649238775} Dermat, PthDrm(99,PA02)
+ Dermatology Associates of South Jersey
715 Fellowship Road/Suite B Mount Laurel, NJ 08054 (856)206-0201 Fax (856)206-0209

Cusano, Paul, Jr., MD {1710924048} Psychy(72,NJ05)<NJ-STMRYPAS, NJ-BERGNMC>
+ 925 Clifton Avenue
Clifton, NJ 07013 (973)471-5256 Fax (973)471-5157

Cusumano, Robert J., MD {1457447195} Otlryg, Otolgy, IntrMd(82,NY19)<NJ-VALLEY>
+ ENT & Allergy Associates, LLP
690 Kinderkamack Road/Suite 101 Oradell, NJ 07649 (201)722-9850 Fax (201)722-9851

Cuthbert, Darren Patrick, MD {1326537036} EmrgMd
+ Robert Wood Johnson Emergency Medicine
One Robert Wood Johnson Place/MEB 104 New Brunswick, NJ 08901 (862)215-0870

Cuthbert, David, MD {1730594045} EmrgMd
+ Emergency Medical Associates of NJ, P.A.
3 Century Drive Parsippany, NJ 07054 (973)740-0607 Fax (973)740-9895

Cutler, David L., MD EnDbMt, IntrMd(82,SK01)
+ Schering Plough Research Institute
2000 Galloping Hill Road Kenilworth, NJ 07033 (908)740-2194 Fax (908)298-2834

Cutler, Jay M., MD {1700966249} IntrMd(73,MEXI)<NJ-CENTRAST>
+ 323 Route 9/Alex Plaza
Manalapan, NJ 07726 (732)728-7600

Cutler, Marna Alyse, DO {1558329961} FamMed(00,NJ75)
+ AtlantiCare Physician Group
802 Tilton Road/Suite 102 Northfield, NJ 08225 (609)569-1900

Physicians by Name and Address

Cutney, Carolyn A., MD {1740219310} Ophthl(99,PA02)
+ Carolyn Cutney MD, LLC.
  925 Route 73 North/Suite C   Marlton, NJ 08053   (856)983-2020   Fax (856)988-1087
+ Wills Eye Surgery Center in Cherry Hill
  408 Route 70 East   Cherry Hill, NJ 08034   (856)983-2020   Fax (856)429-7555

Cuttitta, Jerome D., MD {1083698443} Anesth(92,NJ06)<NJ-HACKNSK>
+ Hackensack University Medical Center
  30 Prospect Avenue/Anesthesiology   Hackensack, NJ 07601   (201)996-2000   Fax (201)488-6769
+ Hackensack University MC-Anesthesia Dept
  30 Prospect Avenue/Room 2703   Hackensack, NJ 07601   (201)996-2000   Fax (201)996-3962

Cuttler, Ira M., MD {1760462766} Grtrcs, IntrMd(82,NJ05)<NJ-KMHSTRAT>
+ University of Medicine & Dentistry of New Jersey-SOM
  42 East Laurel Road/Geriatrics   Stratford, NJ 08084   (856)566-6843
+ New Jersey Institute for Successful Aging
  42 East Laurel Road/Suite 1800   Stratford, NJ 08084   (856)566-6843   Fax (856)566-6781

Cuttler, Nirupa C., MD {1790097194} Ophthl
+ Clifton Eye Care
  1016 Main Street   Clifton, NJ 07011   (973)546-5700   Fax (973)546-8898

Cwik, Jason Charles, MD {1417900911} Anesth(88,PA02)<PA-PENNHOSP>
+ 404 East Oak Avenue
  Moorestown, NJ 08057

Cynn, Jhin J., MD {1124119284} FamMed(68,KORE)
+ Masonic Home of New Jersey
  902 Jacksonville Road   Burlington, NJ 08016   (609)239-3880   Fax (609)239-3808
+ Masonic Hospice Service
  902 Jacksonville Road   Burlington, NJ 08016   (609)589-4444

Cypel, David, MD {1396857389} Anesth(81,DOM03)
+ Rancocas Anesthesiology, PA
  700 Route 130 North/Suite 203   Cinnaminson, NJ 08077   (856)829-9345   Fax (856)829-3605

Cyriac, James Ignatius, MD {1265453559} Anesth(00,NY15)<NJ-TRINIWSC>
+ Trinitas Regional Medical Center-Williamson Street
  225 Williamson Street   Elizabeth, NJ 07207   (732)619-4856

Cyrulnik, Amanda Amy, MD {1417229683} Dermat
+ The Breslow Center for Plastic Surgery
  1 West Ridgewood Avenue/Suite 110   Paramus, NJ 07652   (201)444-9522   Fax (201)444-9277

Cyrus, Pamela A., MD {1972793073} Grtrcs, Nrolgy(89,WV02)
+ Bayer HealthCare
  100 Bayer Boulevard   Whippany, NJ 07981   (862)404-5727

Cytryn, Arthur S., MD {1447360961} IntrMd, InfDis, OrtSpn(77,NY09)<NJ-VAEASTOR, NY-BRNXVAMC>
+ VA New Jersey Health Care System-East Orange Campus
  385 Tremont Avenue/SpinalCordInjry   East Orange, NJ 07018   (973)676-1000

Cytryn, Richard A., MD {1841241379} CdvDis, IntrMd(79,NY47)<NJ-STPETER>
+ UH- Robert Wood Johnson Med
  125 Paterson Street/CAB 6100   New Brunswick, NJ 08901   (732)235-6561   Fax (732)235-8722

Czaja, Matthew T., MD {1225354491} IntrMd
+ UH-RWJ General Internal Medicine
  125 Paterson Street/Suite 2300   New Brunswick, NJ 08901   (732)235-7122   Fax (732)235-7441

Czaplicki-Margiotti, Marie A., MD {1528094927} SrgOrt(74,NJ05)
+ Sparta Health and Wellness Center
  89 Sparta Avenue/Suite 220   Sparta, NJ 07871   (973)940-8100   Fax (973)729-7235

Czar, Elizabeth Erin, DO {1417356189} Pedtrc
+ Cedar Bridge Pediatrics
  249 South Main Street/Suite 2   Barnegat, NJ 08005   (609)607-1010   Fax (609)607-9992

Czartorysky, Bohdan Nicholas, MD {1457640609} Psychy, PsyCAd(83,NY08)
+ Bridgeway Rehabilitation Services
  13 Fairfield Avenue   Little Falls, NJ 07424

Czenis, Ken, MD {1164816377} PhysMd
+ Bey Lea Village
  1351 Old Freehold Road   Toms River, NJ 08753   (732)240-0090   Fax (732)244-8551

Czernizer, Patricia L., MD {1235256223} Pedtrc(85,ARG03)<NJ-HACKNSK>
+ Carl J. Battista, MD, PC
  680 Kinderkamack Road/Suite 301   Oradell, NJ 07649   (201)634-1004   Fax (201)634-1028

Czyzewski, Ewa, MD {1467473173} IntrMd(92,POL06)<NJ-STMRYPAS, NJ-WAYNEGEN>
+ Drs. Czyzewski & Nowak
  515 North Wood Avenue/Suite 302   Linden, NJ 07036   (908)925-3300   Fax (908)925-4300

Czyzewski, Robert M., MD {1558304782} Nephro, IntrMd(92,POL06)
+ Edison Nephrology Consultants, LLC.
  34-36 Progress Street/Suite A-7   Edison, NJ 08820   (908)769-1440   Fax (908)769-0945
+ 2 State Route 27/Suite 410
  Edison, NJ 08820   (908)769-1440   Fax (732)318-6859

D'Aconti, John S., DO {1063460939} IntrMd(74,IL76)<NJ-MTN-SIDE, NJ-CLARMAAS>
+ Internet Medical Group, P.C.
  77 Newark Avenue/Suite 3 & 4   Belleville, NJ 07109   (973)528-2160   Fax (973)528-2165

D'Agostini, Robert J., MD {1407880115} SrgOrt(80,NJ05)<NJ-MORRISTN>
+ Tri-County Orthopedics
  197 Ridgedale Street/Suite 300   Cedar Knolls, NJ 07927   (973)538-2334   Fax (908)234-2022
+ Tri-County Orthopedics
  1590 Route 206 North   Bedminster, NJ 07921   (973)538-2334   Fax (908)234-2022

D'Agostino, Ralph S., MD {1790798437} FamMed, IntrMd(74,SPAI)
+ Primary Care Medical Group
  450 Bergen Street   Harrison, NJ 07029   (973)484-6900   Fax (973)484-0029

D'Aguillo, Anthony F., MD {1316969967} PthACl, PthCyt(72,NE06)<NJ-SOMERSET>
+ RWJ University Hospital Somerset
  110 Rehill Avenue/Pathology   Somerville, NJ 08876   (908)685-2935   Fax (908)704-3756

D'Alberti, Claudio F., MD {1174588545} Ophthl(75,MEX14)<NJ-HOBUNIMC>
+ 1126 Washington Street
  Hoboken, NJ 07030   (201)659-2020   Fax (201)659-8330   Dalberti@carroll.com

D'Alessandro, Angela Marie, MD {1619061652} PedReh, PhysMd(96,DC03)<NJ-VALLEY>
+ Kireker Center for Child Development
  505 Goffle Road/AttendPhysician   Ridgewood, NJ 07450   (201)447-8151   Fax (201)447-8526   dalean@valleyhealth.com

D'Alessandro, Daniel J., MD {1740237296} IntrMd, InfDis, IntHos(92,NY03)<NJ-HACKNSK>
+ Hackensack University Medical Center
  30 Prospect Avenue/4 Main/Rm4621   Hackensack, NJ 07601   (201)996-3664   Fax (201)996-0536

D'Alessio, Donna Giselda, MD {1760707392} PhysMd
+ Pain Medicine Physicians
  187 Millburn Avenue/Suite 103   Millburn, NJ 07041   (973)467-1466   Fax (973)467-1422

D'Amato, Anthony P., MD {1356457923} Ophthl(70,ITAL)<NJ-CLARMAAS, NJ-STCLRDOV>
+ Eye Surgeons of North Jersey, LLC
  199 Broad Street/Suite 2-B   Bloomfield, NJ 07003   (973)748-3300   Fax (973)748-3802
+ Eye Surgeons of North Jersey, LLC
  27 Baker Avenue   Dover, NJ 07801   (973)748-3300   Fax (973)328-1265

D'Amato, Pamela R., MD {1780872614} PainMd, Anesth(01,NET09)
+ University Spine Center
  504 Valley Road/Second Floor/Suite 203   Wayne, NJ 07470   (973)686-0700   Fax (973)686-0701

D'Amato, Thomas, MD {1912157116} Psychy(92,DMN01)<NY-CMCSTVSI>
+ 1810 Kennedy Boulevard
  Jersey City, NJ 07305

D'Ambola, Lesly A., DO {1285653097} IntrMd(94,NJ75)<NJ-STMICHL>
+ Athena Women's Institute for Pelvic Health
  151 Fries Mill Road/Suite 301   Turnersville, NJ 08012   (856)374-1881   Fax (856)302-1961
+ St. Luke's Catholic Medical Services
  511 State Street   Camden, NJ 08102   (856)374-1881   Fax (856)365-0539

D'Ambra-Cabry, Kimberly A., MD {1881619302} Dermat(91,PA13)
+ Moorestown Dermatology Associates
  702 East Main Street   Moorestown, NJ 08057   (856)235-6565   Fax (856)235-6566

D'Ambrosio, Anthony Louis, MD {1356463079} SrgNro(99,TN05)<NY-PRSBCOLU, NJ-STJOSHOS>
+ Neurosurgeons of New Jersey
  1200 East Ridgewood Avenue   Ridgewood, NJ 07450   (201)824-6131

D'Ambrosio, David Joseph, MD {1043485303} RadOnc, Radiol<NJ-SOCEANCO>
+ Southern Ocean County Medical Center
  1140 Route 72 West/Radiology   Manahawkin, NJ 08050   (609)978-2194   Fax (609)978-2843

D'Ambrosio, John C., DO {1740348853} IntrMd(03,MO78)<NJ-VIRTVOOR>
+ Virtua Voorhees
  100 Bowman Drive/IntMed   Voorhees, NJ 08043   (856)247-3000

D'Ambrosio, Robert Paul, DO {1497915391} FamMed(90,ME75)
+ 142 Saint Andrews Drive
  Egg Harbor Township, NJ 08234

D'Amelio, Louis F., MD {1447208897} Surgry, SrgCrC(83,PA02)<NJ-CHSFULD>
+ Capital Surgical Associates
  40 Fuld Street/Suite 303   Trenton, NJ 08638   (609)396-2600   Fax (609)396-3600
+ Capital Health System/Fuld Campus
  750 Brunswick Avenue/Surgery   Trenton, NJ 08638   (609)394-6000

D'Amico, James Charles, DO {1457353088} IntrMd(95,NJ75)<NJ-KMHSTRAT>
+ Medford Leas Health Center
  1 Medford Leas   Medford, NJ 08055   (609)654-3427   Fax (609)654-5519

D'Amico, Richard A., MD {1124074828} SrgPlstc(76,NY19)<NJ-ENGLWOOD, NJ-HOLYNAME>
+ 180 North Dean Street
  Englewood, NJ 07631   (201)567-9595   Fax (201)567-1813   RDamicops@aol.com

D'Amore, Katrina, DO {1215313812}<NJ-STJOSHOS>
+ St. Joseph's Regional Medical Center
  703 Main Street   Paterson, NJ 07503   (973)754-2918

D'Andrea, Christopher Ralph, MD {1609118298}<NJ-MTNSIDE>
+ Hackensack UMC Mountainside
  1 Bay Avenue   Montclair, NJ 07042   (973)429-6000

D'Andrea, Daniel Albert, MD {1992763866} Psychy(99,GRN01)<NJ-BAYSHORE>
+ Bayshore Community Hospital
  727 North Beers Street/Psychiatry   Holmdel, NJ 07733   (732)739-5660   Fax (732)739-5665   ddandrea@gmail.com

D'Andrea, John Louis, MD {1801213228} FamMed
+ Med-Care of East Rutherford
  245 Park Avenue   East Rutherford, NJ 07073   (201)939-7161

D'Angelo, Denis Gerard, MD {1326025842} RadDia, Radiol, RadMam(85,NY48)<NJ-BAYSHORE>
+ Bayshore Community Hospital
  727 North Beers Street/Diag Radiology   Holmdel, NJ 07733   (732)739-5900

D'Angelo, Michael Wayne, MD {1457493652} RadDia, RadV&I(01,VA04)<NJ-COMMED, NJ-SOCEANCO>
+ Community Medical Center
  99 Route 37 West   Toms River, NJ 08755   (732)557-8000

D'Angelo, Stephen Thomas, MD {1700813185} Anesth(89,MO78)<NY-STJOSHHC>
+ 480 Eagle Point Drive
  Toms River, NJ 08753   (732)240-2525

D'Angelo-Donovan, Desiree Diane, DO {1356517684} Surgry
+ GFH Surgical Associates
  718 Shore Road   Somers Point, NJ 08244   (609)927-8550   Fax (609)926-0273

D'Anton, Michael A., III, MD {1396784922} Otlryg, Otolgy, SrgHdN(84,PA09)<NJ-CHILTON, NJ-WAYNEGEN>
+ ENT & Allergy Associates, LLP
  1211 Hamburg Turnpike/Suite 205   Wayne, NJ 07470   (973)633-0808   Fax (973)633-8811
+ Wayne Surgical Center, LLC.
  1176 Hamburg Pike   Wayne, NJ 07470   (973)633-0808   Fax (973)709-1901

D'Aquino, Carol Madeleine, MD {1396816427} IntrMd(81,NY09)<NJ-VALLEY, NJ-HACKNSK>
+ Hackensack University Medical Group Emerson
  452 Old Hook Road/2nd Floor   Emerson, NJ 07630   (201)666-3900   Fax (201)261-0505

D'Auria, Daniel A., MD {1982704474} Gastrn, IntrMd(85,NJ06)
+ 485 Williamstown Road
  Sicklerville, NJ 08081   (856)237-8045   Fax (856)237-8042

D'Cruz, Cyril A., MD {1508822388} PthACl, PthCyt(66,INDI)<NJ-CHDNWBTH>
+ Children's Hospital of New Jersey
  201 Lyons Avenue/Osborne Terrace   Newark, NJ 07112   (973)926-4000   Fax (973)705-8301

D'Elia, Donna L., MD {1518039981} ObsGyn(85,MEXI)<NJ-VIRTVOOR>
+ Women's Group for OB/GYN
  2301 Evesham Road/Pav 800/Suite 122   Voorhees, NJ 08043   (856)770-8336   Fax (856)770-8238

D'Emic, Susan, DO {1043289606} Ophthl
+ Mid Atlantic Eye Center
  70 East Front Street   Red Bank, NJ 07701   (732)741-0858   Fax (732)219-0180

D'Guerra, Mignon Marie, MD {1841586062} FamMed(07,DMN01)
+ Southern Jersey Medical Center
651 High Street   Burlington City, NJ 08016   (609)386-0775   Fax (609)386-4372

D'Mello, Francisco C., MD {1023190972} Gastrn, IntrMd(71,INDI)<NJ-STPETER, NJ-RBAYOLDB>
+ 385 Route 18 South/Building K
East Brunswick, NJ 08816   (732)238-4343   Fax (732)238-6981
+ Cares Surgicenter, LLC.
240 Easton Avenue   New Brunswick, NJ 08901   (732)238-4343   Fax (732)296-8677

D'Mello, Maria W., MD {1154411478} Pedtrc(74,INA01)<NJ-STPETER>
+ 385 West Ferris Place/Highway 18 South
East Brunswick, NJ 08816   (908)238-4344

D'Mello, Sharon L., MD {1639375157} Pedtrc, PedGst(04,NJ05)<NJ-HACKNSK>
+ Joseph M. Sanzari Childrens' -Gastro
155 Polifly Road/Suite 102   Hackensack, NJ 07601   (551)996-8840   Fax (201)441-9949

D'Souza, Christabelle E., MD {1164589255} Psychy, PsyGrt(88,INA69)
+ 6 Kinglet Drive South
Cranbury, NJ 08512

D'Souza, Michael Gerard, MD {1225130206} Anesth, CritCr(81,INA69)<NJ-HOLYNAME>
+ Teaneck Anesthesia Group, P.A.
718 Teaneck Road   Teaneck, NJ 07666   (201)833-7149   Fax (201)833-6576

Da Costa, Theodore A., MD {1558395673} Gastrn, IntrMd(89,NJ05)
+ 85 South Jefferson Street
Orange, NJ 07050   (973)674-8866   Fax (973)672-9299

Da Torre, Steven D., MD {1083667380} CdvDis, ClCdEl, IntrMd(84,PA09)<NJ-OURLADY, NJ-KMHCHRRY>
+ Cardiovascular Associates
210 West Atlantic Avenue   Haddon Heights, NJ 08035   (856)546-3003   Fax (856)547-5337
+ Cardiovascular Associates of The Delaware Valley, PA
1840 Frontage Road   Cherry Hill, NJ 08034   (856)546-3003   Fax (856)795-7436
+ Cardiovascular Associates of The Delaware Valley, PA
525 State Street/Suite 3   Elmer, NJ 08035   (856)358-2363   Fax (856)358-0725

Dabaj, Dina, MD {1952551509} IntrMd(SYR02)
+ Valley Medical Group
44 Godwin Avenue/Suite 2   Midland Park, NJ 07432   (201)444-5992   Fax (201)444-9984

Dabrow, Jennifer, DO {1982085148} Psychy
+ University Hospital-SOM Department of Psychiatry
2250 Chapel Avenue West/Suite 100   Cherry Hill, NJ 08002   (856)482-9000   Fax (856)482-1159

Dabrowski, Peter A., MD {1447260229} IntrMd(97,DMN01)<NJ-HOLYNAME, NJ-MTNSIDE>
+ 115 Route 46 West/Suite A3
Mountain Lakes, NJ 07046   (973)335-3002   Fax (973)335-3118

Dabu, Joan K., MD {1891192696}
+ St. Michael's Medical Center
111 Central Avenue   Newark, NJ 07102   (973)877-5500

Dada-Ajulchukwu, Tokunbo T., MD {1144324559} AdolMd, Pedtrc(80,NIG03)<NJ-NWRKBETH, NJ-STBARNMC>
+ 50 Union Avenue/Suite 702
Irvington, NJ 07111   (973)373-7110   Fax (973)373-0476
tokidada@aol.com

Dadaian, Jon-Paul, MD {1629081013} Anesth(02,GRN01)
+ 434 Main Avenue
Wallington, NJ 07057   (973)365-5844

Dadaian, Susan, DO {1518254622} Anesth<NJ-CHRIST>
+ Christ Hospital
176 Palisade Avenue   Jersey City, NJ 07306   (201)795-8641

Dadhania, Jayantilal P., MD {1548298821} PedGst, Pedtrc(83,INA21)<NJ-CHSFULD, NJ-CHSMRCER>
+ 1303 State Route 27
Somerset, NJ 08873   (732)246-4727   Fax (732)246-0982

Dadhania, Ketki M., MD {1669465605} IntrMd(85,INDI)
+ 801 Route 73 North/Suite B
Marlton, NJ 08053   (856)596-3100   Fax (856)596-3133
ketki@greencardphysicals.com

Dadhania, Mahendrakumar P., MD {1356334353} Allrgy, IntrMd, AlgyImmn(85,INDI)<NJ-VIRTBERL, NJ-VIRTMARL>
+ Allergy & Asthma Consultants of NJ, P.A.
9004 Lincoln Drive West/Suite B   Marlton, NJ 08053   (856)596-3100   Fax (856)596-3133
drdadhania@allergyonweb.com
+ Allergy & Asthma Consultants of NJ, P.A.
110 South Dennisville Road   Cape May Court House, NJ 08210   (856)596-3100   Fax (856)596-3133

Dadhania, Manish Suresh, MD {1083711345} CdvDis, IntrMd(97,GRN01)<NJ-COOPRUMC>
+ University Cardiology
3 Cooper Plaza/Room 311   Camden, NJ 08103   (856)342-2034

Dadzie, Charles K., MD {1104882109} PedCrC, PedPul, Pedtrc(75,GHAN)<NJ-JRSYSHMC, NJ-RIVERVW>
+ Meridian Medical Group - Faculty Practice
61 Davis Avenue/Suite 1   Neptune, NJ 07753   (732)776-4268   Fax (732)776-4867
+ Jersey Shore University Medical Center
1945 Route 33/Pedtrc   Neptune, NJ 07753   (732)776-4268   Fax (732)776-3178

Dadzie, Daphne D., MD {1083945687} EnDbMt(NJ02)
+ Endocrinology Associates of Princeton, LLC
168 Franklin Corner Road   Lawrenceville, NJ 08648   (609)896-0075   Fax (609)896-0079

Dadzie, Kobena A., MD {1023332921}
+ Associated Renal & Hypertension Group, P.C.
7 Cedar Grove Lane/Suite 31   Somerset, NJ 08873   (732)873-1400   Fax (732)960-3444
+ The Valley Hospital
223 North Van Dien Avenue   Ridgewood, NJ 07450   (201)447-8000

Daftani, Kennedy Palwasha Fazli, MD {1043531726} FamMed
+ Mountainside Family Practice Associates
799 Bloomfield Avenue/Suite 201   Verona, NJ 07044   (973)746-7050   Fax (973)857-2831

Daftani, Mohammad Daoud Daoud, MD {1720316367} FamMed
+ Mountainside Family Practice Associates
799 Bloomfield Avenue/Suite 201   Verona, NJ 07044   (973)746-7050   Fax (973)857-2831

Daftari, Amita P., MD {1780677443} Anesth(71,INA15)
+ 19 Bennington Drive
Edison, NJ 08820   (732)388-0890   Fax (732)543-5941
amitaemail@yahoo.com

Daghistani, Lina, MD {1942262217} Pedtrc, IntrMd(83,SYR01)
+ 330 Jackson Mills Road
Freehold, NJ 07728

Daginawala, Naznin, MD {1811296080} RadDia
+ Hackensack Radiology Group, P.A.
30 Prospect Avenue   Hackensack, NJ 07601   (551)996-2200   Fax (201)336-8451

Dahal, Rama, MD {1407918550} IntrMd(91,INA12)
+ Barnegat Medical Associates, P.A.
41 Nautilus Drive   Manahawkin, NJ 08050   (609)978-0474   Fax (609)597-6186

Dahhan, Mohamed Zakaria, MD {1417279779} IntrMd(91,SYR02)
+ 871 McBride Avenue
Little Falls, NJ 07424   (973)569-4488   Fax (973)569-4743
+ Essex County Correctional Facility
354 Doremus Avenue   Newark, NJ 07105   (973)274-7500

Dahodwala, Nisrin Q., MD {1053378786} AdolMd, Pedtrc, IntrMd(83,INA53)
+ 290 North White Horse Pike
Hammonton, NJ 08037   (609)567-7882   Fax (609)567-3000

Dahrouj, Nabil I., MD {1720825331} Pedtrc(93,SYR01)<NJ-STJOSHOS>
+ St. Joseph's Regional Medical Center
703 Main Street   Paterson, NJ 07503   (973)754-2543
+ Drs. Serafino & Dahrouj
834 Avenue C   Bayonne, NJ 07002   (973)754-2543   Fax (201)339-4498

Daici, Silvia, MD {1598823643} Pedtrc(93,ROM01)<NJ-ENGLWOOD>
+ 401A South Van Brunt Street
Englewood, NJ 07631   (201)894-8829   Fax (201)894-8859

Daifotis, Anastasia Golfinos, MD EnDbMt(86,NY03)
+ 240 Watchung Fork
Westfield, NJ 07090

Daigle, Megan Elizabeth, MD {1457592420} RadDia
+ St. Barnabas Ambulatory Care Center
200 South Orange Avenue   Livingston, NJ 07039   (973)322-7000
mdaigle@barnabashealth.org

Dailey-Sterling, Felix G., MD {1194720540} CdvDis, IntrMd(90,NJ05)<NJ-STMICHL, NJ-HOBUNIMC>
+ St. Michael's Medical Center
268 MLK Jr. Boulevard   Newark, NJ 07102   (973)877-5770
+ Hudson Heart Associates
425 70th Street   Guttenberg, NJ 07093   (973)877-5770   Fax (201)854-2633

Daiter, Eric, MD {1184724957} ObsGyn, RprEnd(86,PA13)<NJ-RIVERVW, NJ-OCEANMC>
+ 34-36 Progress Street/Suite B4
Edison, NJ 08820   (908)226-0250   Fax (908)226-0830
+ 802 West Park Avenue/Suite 212
Ocean, NJ 07712   (732)695-9660

Dakake, Charles, Jr., MD {1316910474} Pedtrc(72,NJ05)<NJ-NWTNMEM, NJ-MORRISTN>
+ Advocare Sussex County Pediatrics Newton
39 Newton Sparta Road   Newton, NJ 07860   (973)383-9841   Fax (973)383-7989
+ Advocare Sussex County Pediatrics Montague
2B Myrtle Drive   Montague, NJ 07827   (973)383-9841   Fax (973)293-0138

Dakhel, Mahmoud, MD {1881644359} NuclMd, RadDia(90,SYR02)
+ New Jersey Institute of Radiology
630 Broad Street   Carlstadt, NJ 07072   (201)372-1020   Fax (201)372-1028

Dalal, Bhavna P., MD {1336123702} Anesth(70,INA20)<NJ-HACKNSK>
+ Hackensack University Medical Center
30 Prospect Avenue/Anesth   Hackensack, NJ 07601   (201)996-2000   Fax (201)488-6769
+ Hackensack University MC-Anesthesia Dept
30 Prospect Avenue/Room 2703   Hackensack, NJ 07601   (201)996-2000   Fax (201)996-3962

Dalal, Gita S., MD {1184649311} FamMed(69,INDI)
+ 49 Roxy Avenue
Edison, NJ 08820   (732)574-2796

Dalal, Kalpana S., MD {1235193954} Anesth(73,INA15)<NJ-RBAYPERT>
+ Raritan Bay Medical Center/Perth Amboy Division
530 New Brunswick Avenue/Anesth   Perth Amboy, NJ 08861   (732)442-3700

Dalal, Karambir S., MD {1881695757} IntrMd, Grtrcs(91,INA6Z)<NJ-CENTRAST, NJ-COMMED>
+ Ocean Medical Group PA Inc
63 Lacey Road/Suite F   Whiting, NJ 08759   (732)849-1075   Fax (732)849-1076

Dalal, Setu A., DO {1013180447} Surgry<NJ-STJOSHOS>
+ St. Joseph's Regional Medical Center
703 Main Street/Surgery   Paterson, NJ 07503   (973)754-2000

Dalal, Sima R., DO {1366421448} FamMed(00,NJ75)
+ Newark Department of Health
394 University Avenue/2nd Floor   Newark, NJ 07102   (973)877-6111   Fax (973)733-4328

Dalati, Nadia, MD Pedtrc(72,SYR01)
+ Novartis Pharmaceuticals Corporation
One Health Plaza   East Hanover, NJ 07936   (862)778-8081   Fax (973)781-6504

Dale, Elizabeth, MD {1811218332} Ophthl
+ Ophthalmic Partners of New Jersey
775 Route 70 East/Elmwood/Suite F 180   Marlton, NJ 08053   (856)596-1601   Fax (856)983-0396

Dalena, John Michael, MD {1215944582} Gastrn, IntrMd(85,NJ05)
+ Atlantic Gastroenterology Summit Medical Group
65 Ridgedale Avenue   Cedar Knolls, NJ 07927   (973)401-0500   Fax (973)401-9306

Dalgetty, Donna Earnice, MD {1891945390} Psychy, PsyCAd, IntrMd(96,NC01)
+ Northwest Essex Community HealthCare Network, Inc.
570 Belleville Avenue   Belleville, NJ 07109   (973)450-3100   Fax (973)450-1189
info@nechn.org

Dalkilic, Alican, MD {1700976198} Psychy(93,TUR07)
+ The Renfrew Center
15000 Midlantic Avenue   Mount Laurel, NJ 08054   (856)380-2768   Fax (856)778-0636

Dallapiazza, Michelle Lynn, MD {1871656215} InfDis, IntrMd(PA12)
+ University Physician Associates
140 Bergen Street/ACC Level D   Newark, NJ 07103   (973)972-5111   Fax (973)972-3102

Dallara Marsh, Alexis M., MD {1457642308}
+ Neurology Group of Bergen County
1200 East Ridgewood Avenue   Ridgewood, NJ 07450   (201)444-0868   Fax (201)444-7363
+ 383 Berkshire Road
Ridgewood, NJ 07450   (917)574-5525

Dallessio, Joseph J., MD {1629026919} PedCrC<NJ-STPETER>
+ St. Peter's University Hospital
254 Easton Avenue/PedCrCr   New Brunswick, NJ 08901   (732)745-8600

Dallhoff, Maureen Elizabeth, MD {1740533082} EmrgMd<NJ-RWJUBRUN>
+ RWJ University Hospital New Brunswick
One Robert Wood Johnson Place   New Brunswick, NJ 08901   (732)235-8122

Dalsey, Michael E., DO {1518997980} FamMed(71,PA77)<NJ-UNDRWD, NJ-KMHSTRAT>
+ Salem Medical Group
95 Woodstown Road/Suite B   Swedesboro, NJ 08085   (856)832-7359   Fax (856)832-4381

Dalsey, Nicholas R., DO {1306865431} EmrgMd, GenPrc(75,PA77)<NJ-UNDRWD>
+ Inspira Health Network
509 North Broad Street/EmergMed   Woodbury, NJ 08096   (856)845-0100

127

Physicians by Name and Address

Dalsey, Robert M., MD {1831139229} SrgHnd, SrgOrt, OrtS-Hand(82,PA13)
+ Orthopedic & Neurosurgical Specialists, LLC.
807 Haddon Avenue/Suite 1   Haddonfield, NJ 08033   (856)795-9222   Fax (856)795-0026

Dalsey, William Colwell, MD {1659315307} EmrgMd, IntrMd(81,PA07)<NJ-KIMBALL>
+ Kimball Medical Center
600 River Avenue/Emerg Med   Lakewood, NJ 08701   (732)363-1900

Dalton, John Boehmer, MD {1629041231} IntrMd(60,ON06)
+ Meridian Medical Group
552 Westwood Avenue   Long Branch, NJ 07740   (732)222-7800

Dalton, Laura J., DO {1750324943} ObsGyn(80,PA77)
+ Virtua Family Medicine Center @Lumberton
1636 Route 38 & Eayrestown Rd.   Lumberton, NJ 08048   (609)914-8440   Fax (609)914-8441

Dalton, Mark J K, MD {1710928536} EmrgMd(92,NJ05)
+ University Emergency Medicine
125 Paterson Street/MEB 104   New Brunswick, NJ 08901   (732)235-8717   Fax (732)235-7379

Daly, Eileen P., MD {1508969759} EmrgMd
+ 42 Goldfinch Lane
Neshanic Station, NJ 08853

Daly, John Christopher, MD {1801835905} IntrMd(97,NJ06)
+ St. Remi Behavioral Health
750 Route 73 South/Suite 106   Marlton, NJ 08053   (856)227-0306   Fax (856)396-9917
+ Seto Medical Providers
100 West Red Bank Avenue   West Deptford, NJ 08096   (856)227-0306   Fax (856)848-3011

Daly, M. Veronica, MD {1447219381} ObsGyn, Obstet(79,NC05)<NJ-MORRISTN>
+ Morristown Obstetrics and Gynecology Associates
101 Madison Avenue/Suite 405   Morristown, NJ 07960   (973)267-7272   Fax (973)455-0099
+ Morristown Obstetrics and Gynecology Associates
20 Commerce Boulevard/Unit C   Succasunna, NJ 07876   (973)267-7272   Fax (973)927-7408

Daly, Ronald A., MD {1124122866} SrgOrt(77,NJ05)<NJ-EASTORNG>
+ 96-98 Millburn Avenue/Suite 202
Millburn, NJ 07041   (973)378-9226   Fax (973)378-3969

Daly, Stephen J., DO {1063437523} CdvDis(76,IA75)<NJ-KMH-STRAT, NJ-KMHTURNV>
+ Southern New Jersey Cardiac Care Specialists
1020 Laurel Oak Road/Suite 102   Voorhees, NJ 08043   (856)435-8842   Fax (856)435-8665
+ Southern New Jersey Cardiac Care Specialists
151 Fries Mill Road/Suite 101   Turnersville, NJ 08012   (856)435-8842   Fax (856)374-3120

Dalzell, Frederick G., MD {1346536912} SrgOrt, SrgHnd, IntrMd(78,PA02)<NJ-ACMCMAIN, NJ-ACMCITY>
+ Shore Orthopedic University Associates
24 Macarthur Boulevard/First Floor   Somers Point, NJ 08244   (609)927-1991   Fax (609)927-4203

Dalzell, James G., MD {1417997719} RadOnc(88,NJ05)<NJ-ACMCMAIN, NJ-BURDTMLN>
+ AtlantiCare Regional Med Ctr/Mainland
65 West Jimmie Leeds Road/RadOnc   Pomona, NJ 08240   (609)652-3417   Fax (609)652-3538
+ Cape Regional Medical Center
2 Stone Harbor Boulevard/RadOnc   Cape May Court House, NJ 08210   (609)463-2000
+ Nazha Cancer Center
411 New Road   Northfield, NJ 08240   (609)383-6033   Fax (609)383-0064

Damani, Prabodhkum M., MD {1811931488} CdvDis, IntrMd(70,INDI)<NJ-CHSFULD>
+ Capital Cardiology Associates
40 Fuld Street/Suite 400   Trenton, NJ 08638   (609)396-1644   Fax (609)394-9526

Damani, Tanuja, MD {1235176272} Surgry(99,NY47)<NJ-STJOSHOS>
+ St. Joseph's Regional Medical Center
703 Main Street/Surgery   Paterson, NJ 07503   (973)754-2460
+ Wayne Cancer Center LLC
234 Hamburg Turnpike/Suite 202   Wayne, NJ 07470   (973)310-0309

Dambeck, Michael D., DO {1851562987} PhysMd(04,NY75)
+ Drs. Neuman & Dambeck
700 Highway 71/Suite 2   Sea Girt, NJ 08750   (732)974-8100   Fax (732)974-9125

Damerau, Keith R., MD {1558302349} IntrMd(95,NJ06)<NJ-VIRTVOOR, NJ-VIRTBERL>
+ Drs. Damerau, Todt & Dructor
1401 Marlton Pike East/Suite 26   Cherry Hill, NJ 08034   (856)479-9400   Fax (856)281-9913

Damico, Christopher R., DO {1386611218} FamMed(90,PA77)
+ Skylands Medical Group PA
150 Lakeside Boulevard   Landing, NJ 07850   (973)398-6300   Fax (973)398-6399

Damien, Miguel, MD {1821025925} ObsGyn, RprEnd(82,NH01)<NJ-CENTRAST, NJ-JRSYSHMC>
+ Damien Fertility Partners
655 Shrewsbury Avenue/Suite 300   Shrewsbury, NJ 07702   (732)758-6511   Fax (732)758-1048
+ Damien Fertility Partners
303 West Main Street/Lower Level   Freehold, NJ 07728   (732)758-6511   Fax (732)758-1048

Damle, Jagadish V., MD {1821106667} CdvDis, IntrMd(69,INDI)<NJ-HOBUNIMC>
+ 2 Marineview Plaza
Hoboken, NJ 07030   (201)420-1715   Fax (201)420-1179

Damle, Vasanti J., MD {1114035987} Hemato(73,INDI)<NJ-HOBUNIMC>
+ 2 Marine View Plaza
Hoboken, NJ 07030   (201)420-1715   Fax (201)420-1179

Damuth, Emily K., MD {1730347691} EmrgMd<NJ-COOPRUMC>
+ Cooper University Hospital
One Cooper Plaza   Camden, NJ 08103   (856)342-2000

Dancel, Concepcion A., MD {1558486092} Pedtrc, EmrgMd(68,PHIL)<NJ-RWJURAH, NJ-COMMED>
+ Robert Wood Johnson University Hospital at Rahway
865 Stone Street   Rahway, NJ 07065   (732)381-4200
+ Community Medical Center
99 Route 37 West   Toms River, NJ 08755   (732)557-8000

Dandavate, Varsha Mohan, MD {1710180039} InfDis<NJ-BERGNMC>
+ New Bridge Medical Center
230 East Ridgewood Avenue   Paramus, NJ 07652   (201)225-7130   Fax (201)967-4117

Dandu, Kartik Varma, MD {1841634771} Otlryg
+ Advanced ENT - Voorhees
200 Bowman Drive/Suite D-285   Voorhees, NJ 08043   (856)602-4000   Fax (856)946-1747

Dane, Alexander Ali, DO {1649619982} Dermat
+ Affiliated Dermatologists
182 South Street/Suite 1   Morristown, NJ 07960   (973)267-0300   Fax (973)984-2670

Dane, Steven H., MD {1245297100} Nrolgy, IntrMd(86,NY09)<NY-MTSINAI, NY-MTSINYHS>
+ Sall/Myers Medical Associates, PA
100 Hamilton Plaza/Suite 317/3rd Floor   Paterson, NJ 07505   (973)278-6254   Fax (973)279-5771
steven.dane@mountsinai.org

Daneshvar, Ali, MD {1962457366} Pthlgy, PthACli(71,IRAN)
+ Advanced Pathology Laboratory
1015 New Road   Northfield, NJ 08225   (609)646-7000

Daneshvar, Behdokht, MD {1093745473} IntrMd(91,IRA01)<NJ-ACMCITY, NJ-SHOREMEM>
+ 1015 New Road
Northfield, NJ 08225   (609)485-0300   Fax (609)485-0737

Dang, Jagdish G., MD {1629183678} Psychy, PsyGrt(64,INA23)<NJ-STJOSHOS>
+ 1031 McBride Avenue/Suite D-209
West Paterson, NJ 07424   (973)222-8387   Fax (973)227-8824

Dang, Saurabh, MD {1619267374} Anesth
+ Garden State Pain Control Center, P.A.
1117 Route 46 East/Suite 201   Clifton, NJ 07013   (973)777-5444   Fax (973)777-0304

Dangelo, Salvatore, MD {1245215664} Allrgy(70,ITA17)<NJ-VALLEY>
+ Center for Asthma & Allergy
611 79th Street   North Bergen, NJ 07047   (201)854-8119   Fax (201)854-4875
+ Center for Asthma & Allergy
18 North Third Avenue   Highland Park, NJ 08904   (201)854-8119   Fax (732)545-4087
+ Center for Asthma & Allergy
300 Hudson Street   Hoboken, NJ 07047   (201)792-5900   Fax (201)792-5320

Daniel, Beena Mary, MD {1386772515} FamMed, IntrMd(02,INA37)
+ Virtua Family Medicine
1605 Evesham Road/Suite 100   Voorhees, NJ 08043   (856)741-7100   Fax (856)424-2629

Daniel, Brian P., DO {1629196167} Anesth<NJ-OCEANMC>
+ Morris Anesthesia Group, PA
3799 Route 46/Suite 211   Parsippany, NJ 07054   (973)335-1122   Fax (973)335-1448

Daniel, Joseph N., DO {1801864392} SrgFAk
+ 204 Lippincott Avenue
Riverton, NJ 08077

Daniel, Joshua, MD {1841647823} Nrolgy
+ 58 West Aspen Way
Aberdeen, NJ 07747   (267)495-7955

Daniel, Robert J., MD {1962593723} Anesth(93,NJ06)
+ James Street Anesthesia
102 James Street/Suite 103   Edison, NJ 08820   (732)494-1444   Fax (732)494-7052

Daniels, Alicia L., MD {1831186733} RadDia(92,PA02)<NJ-COMMED>
+ Community Medical Center
99 Route 37 West/Radiology   Toms River, NJ 08755   (732)240-8150   Fax (732)557-2064
+ Coastal Imaging, LLC
79 Route 37 West/Suite 103   Toms River, NJ 08755   (732)240-8150   Fax (732)276-2325
+ Southern Ocean County Medical Center
1140 Route 72 West/Radiology   Manahawkin, NJ 08755   (609)978-8900   Fax (609)978-3415

Daniels, David Daizadeh, MD {1164520136} SrgPlstc, Surgry, SrgRec(95,NJ05)<NJ-OVERLOOK, NJ-STBARNMC>
+ 33 Overlook Road/Suite 302
Summit, NJ 07901   (908)598-8222   Fax (908)598-8222

Daniels, James W., III, MD {1750517728} Anesth(05,NY20)
+ Rancocas Anesthesiology, PA
700 Route 130 North/Suite 203   Cinnaminson, NJ 08077   (856)829-9345   Fax (856)829-3605

Daniels, Jeffrey B., MD {1538130471} SrgOrt(85,PA07)
+ South Jersey Orthopedic Associates PA
502 Centennial Boulevard/Suite 6   Voorhees, NJ 08043   (856)424-8866   Fax (856)424-2665
+ South Jersey Orthopedic Associates PA
901 Route 168/Suite 307   Turnersville, NJ 08012   (856)424-8866   Fax (856)228-1711

Daniels, Jeffrey S., MD {1659344307} CdvDis, CritCr, IntrMd(80,NY03)<NJ-JRSYSHMC, NJ-CENTRAST>
+ Monmouth Cardiology Associates, LLC
11 Meridian Road   Eatontown, NJ 07724   (732)663-0300   Fax (732)663-0301

Daniels, Lawrence B., MD {1669760856}
+ Advanced Neurosurgery Associates
201 Route 17 North/Suite 501   Rutherford, NJ 07070   (201)457-0044   Fax (201)457-0049

Daniels, Richard John, MD {1417905043} RadDia, RadV&I, Radiol(93,PA02)
+ Daniels Vein and Cosmetic Center
9500K Johnson Boulevard   Bordentown, NJ 08505   (609)316-4626
+ Michael W. Nagy MD FACS
2333 Highway 34   Manasquan, NJ 08736   (609)316-4626   Fax (732)282-1522
+ Bea Lea Ambulatory Surgical Center
54 Bey Lea Road/Suite 2   Toms River, NJ 08505   (609)316-4626

Daniels, Steven J., MD {1215901608} CdvDis, CritCr, IntrMd(77,IL42)<NJ-JRSYSHMC, NJ-CENTRAST>
+ Monmouth Cardiology Associates, LLC
11 Meridian Road   Eatontown, NJ 07724   (732)663-0300   Fax (732)663-0301
+ Monmouth Cardiology Associates, LLC
222 Schanck Road/Suite 104   Freehold, NJ 07728   (732)663-0300   Fax (732)431-1712

Danieu, Linda A., MD {1285614461} IntrMd, MedOnc, OncHem(79,TN05)<NJ-STBARNMC>
+ St. Barnabas Medical Center
94 Old Short Hills Road   Livingston, NJ 07039   (973)322-5000

Danish, Adnan F., MD {1265440903} RadOnc(01,NY46)
+ Shore Radiation Oncology, LLC
1 Riverview Plaza   Red Bank, NJ 07701   (732)530-2468   Fax (732)836-4036
+ Shore Radiation Oncology, LLC
425 Jack Martin Boulevard   Brick, NJ 08724   (732)530-2468   Fax (732)836-4036

Danish, Shabbar F., MD {1881757268} SrgNro(01,NJ06)<NJ-UMDNJ>
+ Rutgers - RWJMS
125 Paterson Street/Suite 2100   New Brunswick, NJ 08901   (732)235-7756   Fax (732)235-7095

Daniskas, Efthymios I., MD {1689668683} IntrMd, PulDis(77,NJ06)
+ Respiratory Disease Associates PA
200 Highland Avenue/Suite 100   Glen Ridge, NJ 07028   (973)746-7474   Fax (973)743-0265

Danko, Doris Julia, MD {1073791067} OccpMd, Ophthl, IntrMd(86,GER46)<NJ-CLARMAAS>
+ Clara Maass Medical Center
1 Clara Maass Drive/Ophthalmology   Belleville, NJ 07109   (973)450-2175   Fax (973)844-4779
dorisdanko@yahoo.com

Danks, John Michael, MD {1023308772} SrgVas
+ Vascular & Endovascular Associates of NJ
One West Ridgewood Avenue/Suite 106   Paramus, NJ 07652   (201)389-3700   Fax (201)389-6191

Dannemann, Brian R., MD IntrMd, InfDis(81,CO02)
+ 920 Route 202
Raritan, NJ 08869   (609)218-6142

Dannenbaum, Mark S., MD {1336147354} RadDia(86,NY47)<NJ-VIRTUAHS, NJ-VIRTMHBC>
  + **South Jersey Radiology Associates, P.A.**
    901 Route 168/Suites 301-305   Turnersville, NJ 08012   (856)227-6600   Fax (856)227-8537
  + **South Jersey Radiology Associates, P.A.**
    315 Route 70 East/Suite B   Cherry Hill, NJ 08034   (856)227-6600   Fax (856)428-0356
  + **South Jersey Radiology Associates, P.A.**
    807 Haddon Avenue/Suite 5   Haddonfield, NJ 08012   (856)616-1130   Fax (856)616-1125

Dannis, Seth Michael, MD {1710184064} SrgNro
  + **Neurological Care of New Jersey, P.A.**
    95 Gates Avenue   Montclair, NJ 07042   (973)744-3166   Fax (973)744-3199

Danoff, Madelyn S., MD {1558358093} Radiol, RadDia(91,PA01)<NJ-STJOSHOS>
  + **Imaging Subspecialists of North Jersey LLC**
    703 Main Street   Paterson, NJ 07503   (973)754-2645

Danowski, Kelli Mayo, DO {1508155300} Dermat
  + **Dr. Warmuth Skin Care Center**
    420 Front Street   Elmer, NJ 08318   (856)358-1500   Fax (856)358-1117

Dantas, Bruno Felipe, MD {1104909704} PthAna, PthCyt(04,MD01)
  + **Atlantic Pathologists, P.C.**
    1925 Pacific Avenue   Atlantic City, NJ 08401   (609)441-2147

Dantchenko, Victoria, MD {1811220924} FamMed(89,UKR08)
  + **15 Emily Road**
    Manalapan, NJ 07726

Dante, Karen L. Fung, MD {1285656124} Ophthl, IntrMd(85,PA01)<NJ-VIRTMARL>
  + **Eye Care Physicians & Surgeons of New Jersey**
    1701 Wynwood Drive   Cinnaminson, NJ 08077   (856)829-0600   Fax (856)829-2832
  + **Eye Care Physicians & Surgeons of New Jersey**
    2301 Evesham Road/Suite 501-502   Voorhees, NJ 08043   (856)829-0600   Fax (856)770-0840
  + **Eye Care Physicians & Surgeons of New Jersey**
    73 South Main Street   Medford, NJ 08077   (609)654-6140   Fax (609)953-2257

Dante, Stephen Joseph, MD {1669492625} SrgNro(83,CT02)<PA-PENNHOSP>
  + **Penn Medicine Egg Harbor**
    101 Atlantic City Airport/Bld 214   Egg Harbor Township, NJ 08234
  + **Penn Neurosurgery**
    409 Route 70 East   Cherry Hill, NJ 08034

Dantuluri, Hemamalini, MD {1235289307} IntrMd, IntHos(97,INA2Y)
  + **JFK Medical Center**
    65 James Street   Edison, NJ 08820   (908)315-3595   Fax (732)909-2070

Danzig, Jeffrey B., MD {1689653909} Gastrn, IntrMd(83,NY19)<NJ-VALLEY>
  + **Summit Medical Group**
    127 Union Street/Suite 108   Ridgewood, NJ 07450   (201)414-5477
  + **Bergen Medical Associates**
    466 Old Hook Road/Suite 1   Emerson, NJ 07630   (201)414-5477   Fax (201)967-0340

Danziger, Steven E., MD {1588187231}
  + **126 Montgomery Street/Apt C2**
    Highland Park, NJ 08904   (716)830-1414
  + **RWJ University Hospital New Brunswick**
    One Robert Wood Johnson Place   New Brunswick, NJ 08901   (732)828-3000

Daoko, Joseph, MD {1316100886} CdvDis, IntrMd(98,SYR02)<PA-WILLPORT>
  + **Emad Jacob, MD PC**
    714 Kearney Avenue   Kearny, NJ 07032   (201)772-5211   Fax (201)428-1627

Dapas, Frances, MD {1386880854} Pedtrc(78,NJ05)
  + **Novartis Pharmaceuticals Corporation**
    59 Route 10   East Hanover, NJ 07936   (908)277-5502
  + **Drs. Dapas and Traficante**
    2 Joanna Way   Chatham, NJ 07928   (908)277-5502   Fax (973)635-5826

Dapul, Gener M., MD {1316912629} NnPnMd, Pedtrc(69,PHI01)<NJ-CENTRAST, NJ-RWJUHAM>
  + **On-Site Neonatal Partners**
    1000 Haddonfield-Berlin Road/Suite 210   Voorhees, NJ 08043   (856)782-2212   Fax (856)782-2213

Dara, Michael R., MD {1356321780} IntrMd(81,ITAL)<NJ-CHILTON>
  + **Physicians Health Alliance**
    28 Jackson Avenue   Pompton Plains, NJ 07444   (973)835-2575   Fax (973)835-0531

Daramna, Yaser, MD {1902217300}<NJ-MORRISTN>
  + **Morristown Medical Center**
    100 Madison Avenue   Morristown, NJ 07962   (973)971-5000

Daras, Jason Glenn, DO {1386811164} Anesth
  + **Morris Anesthesia Group, PA**
    3799 Route 46/Suite 211   Parsippany, NJ 07054   (973)335-1122   Fax (973)335-1448

Darbouze, Jean R., MD {1639201510} IntrMd(75,HAI01)
  + **2630 John F. Kennedy Boulevard**
    Jersey City, NJ 07306   (201)432-0809   Fax (201)432-0074

Darcey, Jacqueline Marie, MD {1376515593} InsrMd, IntrMd(95,NY08)<NJ-MORRISTN>
  + **Family Health Center**
    200 South Street/Suite 4   Morristown, NJ 07960   (973)889-6800
  + **Morristown Medical Center**
    100 Madison Avenue   Morristown, NJ 07962   (973)971-5000

Dardanello, Marnie Cambria, MD {1679545529} Pedtrc(01,MD07)<PA-CHLHSPIT, NJ-OVERLOOK>
  + **Summit Medical Group-Berkeley Heights Campus**
    1 Diamond Hill Road   Berkeley Heights, NJ 07922   (908)273-4300   Fax (908)790-6576
  + **Summit Medical Group**
    560 Springfield Avenue   Westfield, NJ 07090   (908)228-3620

Dardashti, Omid A., MD {1639295686} IntrMd, CdvDis(01,NJ06)<NJ-VALLEY>
  + **Valley Medical Goup Cardioology Ridgewood**
    1124 East Ridgewood Avenue   Ridgewood, NJ 07450   (201)689-9400   Fax (201)689-9404

Darder, Michael C., MD {1254478624} FrtInf, ObsGyn, RprEnd(83,IL43)<NJ-STPETER, NJ-RWJUBRUN>
  + **Reproductive Medicine Associates of New Jersey**
    140 Allen Road   Basking Ridge, NJ 07920   (908)604-7800   Fax (973)290-8370
  + **Reproductive Medicine Associates of New Jersey**
    81 Veronica Avenue/Suite 101   Somerset, NJ 08873   (908)604-7800   Fax (732)220-1164

Dardik, Michael, MD {1386725059} PthACl(96,PA01)<NJ-STBARNMC>
  + **St. Barnabas Medical Center**
    94 Old Short Hills Road   Livingston, NJ 07039   (973)322-5000

Dardik, Raquel B., MD {1922064583} ObsGyn(96,PA01)<NJ-CHILTON, NJ-MORRISTN>
  + **Womens Health Care Associates of Sussex County**
    135 Newton Sparta Road/Suite 201   Newton, NJ 07860   (973)383-8555   Fax (973)383-8424

Darenkov, Ivan A., MD {1710172853} Pedtrc, PedGst(91,RUS15)<NJ-WAYNEGEN, NY-ARDNHILL>
  + **Erena Treskova and Co, LLC**
    510 Hamburg Turnpike/Suite 103   Wayne, NJ 07470   (845)341-0264   Fax (845)343-0962   ivan_darenkov@mail.ru

Dariani-Smith, Amanda Sarah, DO {1871970764}<NJ-SJHREGMC>
  + **SJH Regional Medical Center**
    1505 West Sherman Avenue   Vineland, NJ 08360   (856)641-8000

Darlington, Anne Marie, DO {1942514229}
  + **14 Ridgeview Court**
    Sewell, NJ 08080   (856)287-4102   adarlingdo@gmail.com

Darocha, Irene B., MD {1023040813} RadDia, IntrMd(86,PA07)
  + **Open Air MRI**
    430 Memorial Parkway/Suite 2   Phillipsburg, NJ 08865   (908)213-3600

Darocki, Mark, MD {1386062123} EmrgMd
  + **EmCare**
    425 Jack Martin Boulevard   Brick, NJ 08724   (732)840-3380   Fax (732)458-3745

Daroy, Christopher Felicano, MD {1386930378} FamMed(11,GRN01)
  + **Lourdes Medical Associates**
    200 Campbell Drive/Suite 102   Willingboro, NJ 08046   (609)877-4545   Fax (609)877-5129

Daruwala, Cherag A., MD {1003059676} Gastrn, IntrMd(03,PA09)
  + **Hunterdon Gastroenterology Associates, P.A.**
    1100 Wescott Drive/Suite 206-207   Flemington, NJ 08822   (908)483-4000   Fax (908)788-5090
  + **Hunterdon Gastroenterology Associates, P.A.**
    135 West End Avenue/Suite 204   Somerville, NJ 08876   (908)483-4000   Fax (908)788-5090

Darvin, Kenneth N., MD {1992786800} Ophthl, VitRet(90,NY08)<NJ-RWJUBRUN>
  + **Santamaria Eye Center**
    104 Market Street   Perth Amboy, NJ 08861   (732)826-5159   Fax (732)826-2107
  + **Santamaria Eye Center**
    100 Menlo Park Drive/Suite 408   Edison, NJ 08837   (732)826-5159   Fax (732)767-1871

Darvish, Arash, MD {1760860498} IntrMd
  + **6111 Bristol Station Court**
    Carteret, NJ 07008   (703)372-7274

Darvish, Cameron, DO {1275586711} ObsGyn(94,MO78)
  + **Drs. Darvish and Ephrem**
    401 Hamburg Turnpike/Suite 309   Wayne, NJ 07470   (973)942-1200

Das, Arvind K., MD {1770527756} CritCr, PulDis, SlpDis(82,INDI)<NJ-RWJUBRUN, NJ-STPETER>
  + **University Pulmonary & Sleep Medicine, LLC**
    81 Veronica Avenue/Suite 201   Somerset, NJ 08873   (732)246-1441   Fax (732)418-0676   Arvind_das@hotmail.com

Das, Dhirendra N., MD {1356440747} CdvDis, IntrMd(71,INDI)<NJ-CHILTON>
  + **342 Hamburg Turnpike/Suite 208**
    Wayne, NJ 07470   (973)790-5357   Fax (973)790-0007

Das, Dipali R., MD {1821387200} Psychy
  + **13 Lexington Road**
    Monmouth Junction, NJ 08852   (732)438-0965

Das, Kamala, MD {1821006065} ObsGyn(65,INDI)<NJ-MORRISTN>
  + **170 Changebridge Road/Suite B-6**
    Montville, NJ 07045   (973)227-8898   Fax (973)227-4633

Das, Kasturi, MD {1417970740} PthACl(89,INA6X)<NJ-UMDNJ>
  + **100 Columbus Drive/Apt 1121**
    Jersey City, NJ 07302

Das, Kiron M., MD {1033289756} Gastrn, IntrMd(65,INDI)<NJ-RWJUHAM>
  + **RWJ Gastro & Hepatology**
    125 Paterson Street/CAB 5100B   New Brunswick, NJ 08901   (732)235-7784   Fax (732)235-7792   daskm@umdnj.edu

Das, Mohan P., MD {1194769653} IntrMd(73,INDI)<NJ-MORRISTN, NJ-OVERLOOK>
  + **68 Ridgedale Avenue/PO Box 268**
    Florham Park, NJ 07932   (973)377-5459   Fax (973)377-0010

Das, Prabhat R., MD {1417983461} PulDis, IntrMd, CritCr(84,INA61)<NJ-KIMBALL, NJ-COMMED>
  + **495 Lakehurst Road**
    Toms River, NJ 08755   (732)473-0300   Fax (732)473-0700

Das, Saumya, MD {1922037472} IntrMd(91,INDI)<NJ-OCEANMC>
  + **1166 River Avenue**
    Lakewood, NJ 08701   (732)370-0576   Fax (732)736-6954

Das, Shyunti, MD {1861711269}
  + **331 Raymond Street**
    Hillsdale, NJ 07642

Das, Sudip S., MD {1659325074} Anesth
  + **Anesthesia Consultnts of NJ/Nova Pain**
    285 Davidson Avenue/Suite 204   Somerset, NJ 08873   (732)271-1400   Fax (732)271-3543

Das, Sumon Kumar, MD {1780831867} PedCrC, Pedtrc, IntrMd(02,ENG29)<NJ-CHDNWBTH, NJ-NWRKBETH>
  + **University Medical Group Pediatrics**
    125 Paterson Street/MEB 3rd Fl   New Brunswick, NJ 08903   (732)235-5709   Fax (732)235-6609
  + **Newark Beth Israel Medical Center**
    201 Lyons Avenue/Suite C5   Newark, NJ 07112   (732)235-5709   Fax (973)926-6452

Das, Urmi, MD {1235199449} Grtrcs, IntrMd(81,INDI)<NJ-HACKNSK, NJ-HOLYNAME>
  + **1 Sears Drive/2nd Floor**
    Paramus, NJ 07652   (201)634-8600   Fax (201)634-9011

Das, Vivek T., MD {1487684858} Anesth, PainMd, PainInvt(91,NJ06)<NJ-RWJUBRUN>
  + **Comprehensive Pain Management**
    501 Omni Drive   Hillsborough, NJ 08844   (908)704-8088   Fax (908)704-8820

Dasani, Bharatkumar M., MD {1073698049} Gastrn, IntrMd(79,INDI)<NJ-CHILTON>
  + **44 Route 23 North/Suite 7**
    Riverdale, NJ 07457   (973)248-1550   Fax (973)248-1560

Dasari, Rajasree V., MD {1811929045} IntrMd(93,INA7C)
  + **2 Maple Avenue**
    Metuchen, NJ 08840

Dash, Michael Roy, MD {1033164959} IntrMd(82,OR02)<NJ-CHSFULD, NJ-CHSMRCER>
  + **Internal Medicine Associates of Lawrence, PC**
    123 Franklin Corner Road/Suite 216   Lawrenceville, NJ 08648   (609)895-6800   Fax (609)895-6988

Dash, Sarat K., MD {1275680563} Surgry, SrgVas(67,INDI)<NJ-NWTNMEM>
  + **Northwest Jersey Surgical Associates, P.A.**
    71 Route 23 North/PO Box 59   Hamburg, NJ 07419   (973)827-2800   Fax (973)827-1495

Dash, Subasini, MD {1285693515} Nrolgy(92,INA25)
  + **Hackensack Neurology Group**
    211 Essex Street/Suite 202   Hackensack, NJ 07601   (201)488-1515   Fax (201)488-9471

Physicians by Name and Address

Dashefsky, Barry, MD {1003980467} Pedtrc, PedInf(73,MA07)<NJ-UMDNJ, NJ-STBARNMC>
+ University Hospital
150 Bergen Street/G102/PediInf   Newark, NJ 07103   (973)972-0382   Fax (973)972-0581
+ Rutgers- New Jersey Medical School
185 South Orange Avenue/MSB F570a   Newark, NJ 07103   (973)972-5066

Dashevsky, Nataliya, MD {1902857139} IntrMd(88,RUSS)<NJ-UNVMCPRN>
+ Medical Pediatrics Associates
256 Bunn Drive/Suite 3 A   Princeton, NJ 08540   Fax (609)683-7958

Dashow, Susan M., DO {1740277169} Anesth(87,IA75)
+ Hamilton Anesthesia and Pain Management
1 Hamilton Health Place   Hamilton, NJ 08690   (609)631-4200   Fax (609)631-6839

Dasika, Vijaya R., MD {1780625541} Nrolgy(68,INDI)
+ Bergen Neurology & Pain Management
600 Pavonia Avenue   Jersey City, NJ 07306   (201)420-1522

DaSilva, Annette Christina, DO {1326240284} PhysMd, PainMd(96,FL75)
+ 206 Bergen Avenue/Suite 203
Kearny, NJ 07032   (201)681-1800   Fax (888)485-0001

DaSilva, Robert Antonio, MD {1285791178} IntrMd, Pedtrc(96,NY47)
+ AstraHealth Urgent & Primary Care
95 Hudson Street   Hoboken, NJ 07030   (201)464-8888
+ AstraHealth Urgent & Primary Care
18 Lyons Mall   Basking Ridge, NJ 07920   (908)760-8888
+ AstraHealth Urgent & Primary Care
564 Broadway   Bayonne, NJ 07030   (201)464-8888

DaSilva, Shonola Samuel, MD {1548360498} PedCrC, Pedtrc(84,NIG13)
+ Cooper University Medical Center/Camden
3 Cooper Plaza   Camden, NJ 08103   (856)968-9575

Daskalakis, Nikki, MD {1376655878} Nephro, IntrMd(00,PA12)<NJ-RIVERVW, NJ-JRSYSHMC>
+ Sanofi US-Sanofi-Aventis
55 Corporate Drive/55c-315a   Bridgewater, NJ 08807   (908)981-5886   Fax (908)981-7708
nikki.daskalakis@sanofi.com

Dasmahapatra, Amita, MD   EnDbMt, IntrMd(74,INA30)
+ Medco Health Solutions, Inc.
100 Parsons Pond Drive   Franklin Lakes, NJ 07417   (201)269-3400   Fax (201)269-1109

Dasmahapatra, Kumar S., MD {1780644013} Surgry(74,INDI)<NJ-JFKMED, NJ-RBAYOLDB>
+ Comprehensive Surgical Associates
225 May Street/Suite A   Edison, NJ 08837   (732)346-5400   Fax (732)346-5404

Dasondi, Vivekkumar V., MD {1528129509} IntrMd(01,INA20)<NJ-SHOREMEM>
+ 72 West Jimmie Leeds Road/Suite 1600
Galloway, NJ 08205   (609)652-1115   Fax (609)652-1145

Dasti, Sofia J., MD {1548207954} FamMed, EmrgMd(96,DMN01)<NJ-RWJUHAM>
+ Robert Wood Johnson University Hospital at Hamilton
1 Hamilton Health Place/EmrgMed   Hamilton, NJ 08690   (609)586-7900   Fax (609)466-2772

Dasti, Umer R., MD {1497916845} SrgOrt(08,NJ05)
+ Ridgewood Orthopedic Group, LLC
85 South Maple Avenue   Ridgewood, NJ 07450   (201)445-2830   Fax (201)445-7471

Dastjerdi, Mohammad Hossein, MD {1831329291} Ophthl
+ University Ophthalmology Associates
90 Bergen Street/DOC 6100   Newark, NJ 07101   (973)972-2038   Fax (973)972-2068

Dateshidze, Konstantin, MD {1104873827} Anesth, CritCr(73,RUSS)<NJ-DEBRAHLC>
+ Deborah Heart and Lung Center
200 Trenton Road/Anesthesiology   Browns Mills, NJ 08015   (609)893-6611   Fax (609)893-1213
konstantin.dateshidze@demanddeborah.org

Datiashvili, Ramazi Otarovich, MD {1952466518} SrgPlstc, SrgRec(72,RUS81)<NJ-UMDNJ>
+ University Hospital-Doctors Office Center
90 Bergen Street   Newark, NJ 07103   (973)972-2500   Fax (973)972-2407

Datta, Samyadev, MD {1497778005} Anesth, AnesPain(79,INA09)<NJ-HOLYNAME>
+ Center for Pain Management
294 State Street/Suite 1   Hackensack, NJ 07601   (201)488-7246   Fax (201)488-2788

Datta-Bhutada, Subhashree, MD {1831192269} NnPnMd, Pedtrc(86,NIGE)<NJ-STJOSHOS>
+ St Joseph's Medical Center Neonatology
703 Main Street   Paterson, NJ 07503   (973)754-2555   Fax (973)754-2567

Datwani, Neeta D., MD {1700983061} IntrMd, CdvDis(91,INDI)
+ Cooper Physicians Washington Township
1 Plaza Drive/Suite 103/Bunker Hill Pl   Sewell, NJ 08080

(856)270-4080   Fax (856)270-4085
+ University Cardiology
3 Cooper Plaza/Room 311   Camden, NJ 08103   (856)342-2034

Daub, Denise M., MD {1437168432} IntrMd, GenPrc(84,NJ05)<NJ-CHRIST, NJ-HOBUNIMC>
+ 1808 Kennedy Boulevard
Union City, NJ 07087   (201)617-7771   Fax (201)617-0470

Daub, Horatio Guy, MD {1558345991} FamMed, Grtrcs, PubHth(81,MA07)<NJ-VIRTMHBC>
+ Virtua Family Medicine Center @Lumberton
1636 Route 38 & Eayrestown Rd.   Lumberton, NJ 08048   (609)914-8440   Fax (609)914-8441

Daud Ahmad, Sameera, MD {1073700381} EnDbMt, IntrMd(02,PAK11)
+ Hackensack University Medical Group Emerson
452 Old Hook Road/2nd Floor   Emerson, NJ 07630   (201)666-3900   Fax (201)261-0505

Daugherty, Dene Wesley, DO {1255564787}
+ 4508 Michael Lane
Voorhees, NJ 08043   (973)908-1779
dwdaugherty@gmail.com

Daugherty, Rhett L., MD {1679544365} Surgry, Urolgy(87,VT02)<NJ-VIRTMARL, NJ-VIRTMHBC>
+ New Jersey Urology
15000 Midlantic Drive/Suite 100   Mount Laurel, NJ 08054   (856)252-1000   Fax (856)985-4582
+ New Jersey Urology
911 Sunset Road   Willingboro, NJ 08046
+ New Jersey Urology
773 Route 70 East/Building H-120   Marlton, NJ 08054

Dauhajre, Teofilo A., MD {1245253442} SrgOrt(81,NY47)<NJ-CHRIST, NJ-MEADWLND>
+ 7000 Kennedy Boulevard East
Guttenberg, NJ 07093   (201)868-1200   Fax (201)868-0064

Dauito, Ralph, MD {1073562872} Radiol, RadDia(84,DC02)
+ Aims Diagnostics
434 New Jersey Avenue   Absecon, NJ 08201   (609)383-0500   Fax (609)383-0376
+ SJH Millville Imaging
1001 North High Street   Millville, NJ 08332   (609)383-0500   Fax (856)825-5576

Davanzo, Lawrence D., DO {1902834708} CritCr, IntrMd, PulDis(88,NJ75)<NJ-RWJUBRUN, NJ-SOMERSET>
+ Brunswick Pulmonary and Sleep Medicine
49 Veronica Avenue/Suite 105   Somerset, NJ 08873   (732)246-3066   Fax (732)246-3067
+ Brunswick Pulmonary and Sleep Medicine
10 Forrestal Road South/Suite 103   Princeton, NJ 08540   (732)246-3066   Fax (732)246-3067

Davanzo, Peter A., MD {1750497160} Anesth(84,GRN01)
+ 5 Syldeo Drive
Parsippany, NJ 07054

Davda, Niyati, MD {1659346419} ObsGyn(99,MEX14)<NJ-STPETER>
+ Davda Medical Group LLC
1100 Centennial Avenue/Suite 201   Piscataway, NJ 08854   (732)474-0909   Fax (732)474-0907

Dave, Akshay S., MD {1770563074} FamMed(86,INA2B)<NJ-UN-DRWD, NJ-OURLADY>
+ Akshay, Dave S.
321 East Broad Street   Gibbstown, NJ 08027   (856)423-2790   Fax (856)423-2798

Dave, Bijal A., MD {1770733321} FamMed, IntrMd(01,INA1P)<NY-CONEYISL>
+ Advanced Cardiology, LLC.
65 Ridgedale Avenue   Cedar Knolls, NJ 07927   (973)401-1100   Fax (973)401-1201

Dave, Chetna A., MD {1831179134} Nephro, IntrMd
+ New Jersey Institute for Successful Aging
42 East Laurel Road/Suite 1800   Stratford, NJ 08084   (856)566-6843   Fax (856)566-6781

Dave, Dhiren Sirish, MD {1023290533} Urolgy(03,TN05)
+ Somerset Urological Associates PA
72 West End Avenue   Somerville, NJ 08876   (908)927-0300   Fax (908)707-4988

Dave, Gazala, MD {1467745695}
+ Summit Medical Group-Berkeley Heights Campus
1 Diamond Hill Road   Berkeley Heights, NJ 07922   (908)273-4300   Fax (908)790-6576

Dave, Hemang U., MD {1891782371} Hemato, IntrMd, MedOnc(82,INA20)<NJ-SHOREMEM, NJ-BURDTMLN>
+ Hope Community Cancer Center LLC
210 South Shore Road/Suite 106-A   Marmora, NJ 08223   (609)390-7888   Fax (609)390-2614

Dave, Payal, MD {1689786501} IntrMd(01,VA09)
+ UH- Robert Wood Johnson Med
125 Paterson Street/MEB 486   New Brunswick, NJ 08901   (732)235-7742   Fax (732)235-7427

Dave, Sangeeta, MD {1154470839} ObsGyn(87,INDI)<NJ-JFKMED, NJ-SOMERSET>
+ 1 State Route 27/Suite 12

Edison, NJ 08820   (732)494-7025   Fax (732)875-0446
+ 201 Union Avenue/Building 2/Suite C
Bridgewater, NJ 08807   (732)494-7025   Fax (732)875-0446

Dave, Vinnidhy Hemang, DO {1437448115} PallCr, IntrMd(11,NY75)
+ Englewood Hospital and Medical Center
350 Engle Street   Englewood, NJ 07631   (201)894-3690   Fax (201)894-5264

Davenport, Leamon L., DO {1649230525} Pedtrc<NJ-ACMCITY>
+ AtlantiCare Regional Medical Center/City Campus
1925 Pacific Avenue   Atlantic City, NJ 08401   (609)345-4000

Daver, Nicole Rohinton, DO {1629205067} IntrMd(09,PA77)<NJ-OVERLOOK>
+ Institute for Rheumatic & Autoimmune Diseases
33 Overlook Road/MAC L01   Summit, NJ 07901   (908)598-7940   Fax (908)598-5447

David, Erica Nicola, MD {1780684167} PhysMd(00,NY47)
+ Associates in Rehabilitation Medicine
95 Mount Kemble Avenue   Morristown, NJ 07960   (973)267-2293   Fax (973)226-3144

David, Gwen Lynita, MD {1225138308} ObsGyn(89,NC01)
+ Partners for Women's Health PA
95 Northfield Avenue   West Orange, NJ 07052   (973)736-4505   Fax (973)376-9066

David, Henry Edward, DO {1649346776} SrgOrt(68,MO78)<NJ-VIRTVOOR>
+ David Orthopaedic Associates PA
3 Brendenwood Drive   Voorhees, NJ 08043   (856)751-0217   Fax (856)751-1967

David, Joseph, DO {1316235765}
+ 200 Mazdabrook Road
Parsippany, NJ 07054   (516)655-8640
jdavid9784@gmail.com

David, Kevin Andrew, MD {1336396357} OncHem
+ Rutgers Cancer Institute of New Jersey
195 Little Albany Street/PO Box 2681   New Brunswick, NJ 08903   (732)235-2465   Fax (732)235-6797

David, Lea H., MD {1134260821} Pedtrc(83,PHI07)<NJ-RIVERVW, NJ-MONMOUTH>
+ Miguelino and David Pediatrics
717 North Beers Street/Suite 1F   Holmdel, NJ 07733   (732)888-0777   Fax (732)888-0880

David, Steven, MD {1902896723} Gastrn, IntrMd(86,NY47)<NJ-CHILTON>
+ North Jersey Gastroenterology & Endoscopy Center
1825 State Route 23 South   Wayne, NJ 07470   (973)633-1484   Fax (973)633-7980

Davidoff, Ada, MD {1255758306} IntrMd
+ Drs. Davidoff and Davidoff
144 Speedwell Avenue   Morristown, NJ 07960   (973)267-7770   Fax (973)984-2933

Davidoff, Bernard M., MD {1649238106} IntrMd(73,NY01)
+ Drs. Davidoff and Davidoff
144 Speedwell Avenue   Morristown, NJ 07960   (973)267-7770   Fax (973)984-2933

Davidoff, Steven, MD {1841250685} Gastrn, IntrMd(74,VA04)<NJ-VIRTUAHS, NJ-KENEDYHS>
+ South Jersey Gastroenterology PA
406 Lippincott Drive/Suite E   Marlton, NJ 08053   (856)983-1900   Fax (856)983-5110
+ South Jersey Gastroenterology PA
807 Haddon Avenue/Suite 205   Haddonfield, NJ 08033   (856)983-1900   Fax (856)983-5110
+ South Jersey Gastroenterology PA
111 Vine Street   Hammonton, NJ 08053   (609)561-3080   Fax (856)983-5110

Davidov, Mark, MD {1154571164} Anesth, IntrMd(05,LAT03)
+ AtlantiCare Anesthesiology
65 West Jimmie Leeds Road   Pomona, NJ 08240   (609)748-7597

Davidov, Tomer, MD {1073560397} Surgry(00,MA05)
+ UMDNJ RWJ Surgery
125 Paterson Street/CAB 4th FL 4100   New Brunswick, NJ 08901   (732)235-7920   Fax (732)235-7079
davidoto@umdnj.edu

Davidson, Anne Stripling, MD {1356479026} PsyAdd, Psychy(82,VA01)
+ Princeton House Behavioral Health - Princeton
905 Herrontown Road   Princeton, NJ 08540   (609)497-3300   Fax (609)497-3370

Davidson, J. Thomas, MD {1700873817} SrgBst, SrgC&R, Surgry(66,NY20)
+ Princeton Gastrenterology
5 Plainsboro Road/Suite 260   Plainsboro, NJ 08536   (609)853-7204   Fax (609)853-6386

Davidson, Jean Marie, DO {1689866204} EnDbMt, IntrMd(03,NJ75)<NJ-VIRTVOOR>
+ Virtua Endocrinology
200 Bowman Drive   Voorhees, NJ 08043   (856)247-7220

Physicians by Name and Address

Davidson, Lawrence M., MD {1619970993} Ophthl(69,NY08)<NJ-STBARNMC, NJ-MTNSIDE>
 + 825 Bloomfield Avenue
  Verona, NJ 07044   (973)239-4000   Fax (973)239-5809
Davidson, Marson Tunde, MD {1699708412} Surgry, SrgOnc(99,DC01)<NJ-HACKNSK>
 + Drs. Karpeh & Davidson
  20 Prospect Avenue/Suite 406   Hackensack, NJ 07601
  (551)996-2959   Fax (551)996-2021
 + Hackensack University Medical Center
  30 Prospect Avenue/2 Conklin   Hackensack, NJ 07601
  (551)996-2959   Fax (201)336-8052
Davidson, Melissa, MD {1467410043} Pedtrc(87,NY09)<NJ-ENGLWOOD, NJ-HOLYNAME>
 + Drs. Baydar, Davidson & Tung
  370 Grand Avenue/Suite 203   Englewood, NJ 07631
  (201)568-3262   Fax (201)569-2634
Davidson, Stacy, MD {1043764061} PhysMd
 + 6 Elkin Drive
  Livingston, NJ 07039   (973)992-9622
Davidson, Stefanie Lynn, MD {1619067725} Ophthl<PA-CHILDHOS>
 + CHOP Pediatric & Adolescent Specialty Care Center
  1012 Laurel Oak Road   Voorhees, NJ 08043   (856)435-1300
  Fax (856)435-0091
Davine-Reicher, Joanne Erin, MD {1285996439} FamMed
 + Springfield Family Practice
  11 Overlook Road/Suite 140   Summit, NJ 07901   (908)277-0050   Fax (908)277-0201
Davis, Adriana, DO {1225373111} FamMed
 + Patient first Urgent Care
  630 Mantua Pike   Woodbury, NJ 08096   (856)812-2220
  Fax (856)812-2221
Davis, Alan L., MD {1033185327} PedCrC, Pedtrc(82,KY02)<NJ-MORRISTN, NJ-STBARNMC>
 + St. Barnabas Medical Center
  94 Old Short Hills Road/4th Fl/PICU   Livingston, NJ 07039
  (973)322-5000
Davis, Barbara, MD {1831395029} GenPrc(83,NJ05)
 + Newark Department of Health and Human Services
  110 William Street   Newark, NJ 07102   (973)733-5300
Davis, Bradley, DO {1790197101} FamMed<NJ-PALISADE>
 + Palisades Medical Center
  7600 River Road   North Bergen, NJ 07047   (201)854-5000
Davis, Brian Joseph, DO {1437199346} FamMed(00,PA77)
 + Cumberland Family Medicine Associates
  1203 North High Street/Suite A   Millville, NJ 08332
  (856)327-0182   Fax (856)327-7381
Davis, Bryan F., DO {1639425754} IntHos<NJ-KMHSTRAT>
 + Kennedy Memorial Hospital-University Medical Center
  18 East Laurel Road   Stratford, NJ 08084   (856)218-5634
  (856)218-5664
Davis, Cheryl Luise, MD {1194731083} NnPnMd, Pedtrc(78,VT02)<NJ-RWJUHAM, PA-RIDDLE>
 + On-Site Neonatal Partners
  1000 Haddonfield-Berlin Road/Suite 210   Voorhees, NJ
  08043   (856)782-2212   Fax (856)782-2213
Davis, Clifton Colby, MD {1518058973} Anesth(01,NET09)
 + New Jersey Anesthesia Associates PC
  25B Vreeland Road/Suite110/PO Box 0037   Florham Park,
  NJ 07932   (973)660-9334   Fax (973)660-9732
 + 35 Beachmont Terrace
  Caldwell, NJ 07006
Davis, Damien Ian, MD {1912181314} SrgOrt, OrtSHand(04,DC02)<NJ-ENGLWOOD, NJ-PALISADE>
 + Englewood Orthopedic Associates
  401 South Van Brunt Street   Englewood, NJ 07631
  (201)569-2770   Fax (201)569-1774
Davis, George C., MD {1295895993} PulDis, IntrMd, CritCr(73,PA09)
 + 279 Third Avenue/Suite 510
  Long Branch, NJ 07740   (732)870-0650   Fax (732)870-6950
Davis, George H., DO {1396725859} ObsGyn(78,TX78)<NJ-KMH-TURNV, NJ-JFKMED>
 + Kennedy Health Systems/Washington Township Campus
  435 Hurffville-Cross Keys Road   Turnersville, NJ 08012
  (856)582-2500
 + University Doctors-Ob Gyn
  42 East Laurel Road/Suite 3500   Stratford, NJ 08084
  (856)582-2500   Fax (856)566-6026
Davis, Glenn A., MD {1740275858} IntrMd(88,PA14)<NJ-MORRISTN>
 + Chester Medical Associates
  385 Route 24/Suite 1-C   Chester, NJ 07930   (908)879-6277
  Fax (908)879-4464
Davis, James Edward, MD {1811915408} IntrMd(01,PA13)
 + Horizon Blue Cross Blue Shield of N.J.
  250 Century Parkway/MT-03T   Mount Laurel, NJ 08054
  (856)638-3259
Davis, Jason Evan, MD {1285809475} SrgVas
 + 7912 River Road/Apt 611
  North Bergen, NJ 07047   (267)496-2964
  jdavis_is@hotmail.com
Davis, Kara Alison, MD {1184609117} PainMd, Anesth(93,TN07)
 + 289 White Horse Pike
  Atco, NJ 08004
Davis, Kenneth J., MD {1285650226} Pedtrc, IntrMd(62,NY46)<NJ-OVERLOOK, NJ-TRINIJSC>
 + Elizabeth Pediatric Group
  701 Newark Avenue/Suite 212   Elizabeth, NJ 07208
  (908)354-9500   Fax (908)354-9077
  Kjdmd@aol.com
Davis, Lawrence Jay, MD {1881675098} IntrMd(91,MD07)<NJ-ENGLWOOD>
 + Drs. Pattner, Grodstein, Fein & Davis
  177 North Dean Street/Suite 207   Englewood, NJ 07631
  (201)567-0446   Fax (201)567-8775
 + Drs. Pattner, Grodstein, Fein & Davis
  8100 Kennedy Boulevard   North Bergen, NJ 07047
  (201)868-5905
Davis, Lloyd A., MD {1851391064} FamMed, Grtrcs(75,DC02)
 + Somerset Family Practice
  110 Rehill Avenue   Somerville, NJ 08876   (908)685-2900
  Fax (908)685-2891
Davis, Maris R., MD {1841381076} EnDbMt, IntrMd(83,NY01)<NJ-MTNSIDE>
 + Montclair Endocrine Associates
  123 Highland Avenue/Suite 301   Glen Ridge, NJ 07028
  (973)744-3733   Fax (973)707-5821
Davis, Matthew B., MD {1548420193} EmrgMd<NJ-JRSYCITY>
 + Jersey City Medical Center
  355 Grand Street/Emerg Med   Jersey City, NJ 07304
  (201)915-2200
Davis, Matthew Jared, MD {1629238860} SlpDis
 + Neurology Specialists of Monmouth County
  107 Monmouth Road/Suite 110   West Long Branch, NJ
  07764   (732)935-1850   Fax (732)544-0494
Davis, Michael James, DO {1386639037} Anesth(94,NJ75)<NJ-UNDRWD>
 + Inspira Health Network
  509 North Broad Street/Anesthesiology   Woodbury, NJ
  08096   (856)845-0100   Fax (856)848-7023
Davis, Michele, DO {1164420352} FamMed, EmrgMd(01,IA75)<NJ-OVERLOOK, NJ-HOBUNIMC>
 + 614 Cranbury Road/Unit 81
  East Brunswick, NJ 08816   (908)360-5362
Davis, Nicole D., MD {1528082484} Gyneco, ObsGyn(88,CT01)<NJ-STPETER>
 + Brunswick-Hills Ob/Gyn, PA
  751 Route 206/2nd Floor   Hillsborough, NJ 08844
  (908)725-2510   Fax (908)725-2132
 + Brunswick-Hills Ob/Gyn, PA
  620 Cranbury Road/Suite LL90   East Brunswick, NJ 08816
  (908)725-2510   Fax (732)613-4845
Davis, Orrin, MD {1013908300} Otlryg(81,IL06)<NJ-HOLYNAME, NJ-VALLEY>
 + Northern Jersey Ear, Nose & Throat Associates, P.A.
  1 Degraw Avenue   Teaneck, NJ 07666   (201)837-2174
  Fax (201)836-7838
 + Northern Jersey Ear, Nose & Throat Associates, PA
  44 Godwin Avenue   Midland Park, NJ 07432   (201)837-2174   Fax (201)445-8679
Davis, Patrick Michael, MD {1649374000} EmrgMd(98,NY08)<NJ-CLARMAAS>
 + 22 Rose Lane
  Old Bridge, NJ 08857   (732)607-1196
 + Clara Maass Medical Center
  1 Clara Maass Drive   Belleville, NJ 07109   (973)450-2000
Davis, Paul K., MD {1255301552} SrgThr
 + LMA CardioThoracic Surgical Services
  1 Brace Road/Suite C   Cherry Hill, NJ 08034   (856)470-9029
  Fax (856)796-9391
Davis, Rachel B., MD {1740622422} Urolgy<NJ-RWJUBRUN>
 + RWJ University Hospital New Brunswick
  One Robert Wood Johnson Place   New Brunswick, NJ 08901
  (732)235-7775
 + 530 Village Road West
  Princeton Junction, NJ 08550   (609)275-5080
Davis, Robert A., DO {1720068851} FamMed(90,PA77)<NJ-VIRTBERL, NJ-VIRTMARL>
 + Integrated Family Medicine
  701 Cooper Road/Suite 16   Voorhees, NJ 08043   (856)783-5000   Fax (856)783-5041
Davis, Robert M., MD {1912970559} Psychy(99,PA14)
 + Catholic Charities-Delaware Mental Health Services
  25 Ikea Drive   Westampton, NJ 08060   (609)267-9339
Davis, Sampson M., MD {1346242310} EmrgMd(99,NJ06)<NJ-RBAYPERT>
 + Raritan Bay Medical Center/Perth Amboy Division
  530 New Brunswick Avenue/EmrgMed   Perth Amboy, NJ
  08861   (732)442-3700
Davis, Sanders W., MD {1730126350} PhyMPain(65,TX12)<NJ-MMHKEMBL>
 + Associates in Rehabilitation Medicine
  95 Mount Kemble Avenue   Morristown, NJ 07960
  (973)267-2293   Fax (973)226-3144
Davis, Steven L., DO {1811120918} SrgPlstc(87,PA77)
 + Center for Cosmetic Surgery
  1916 Marlton Pike East/Suite 1   Cherry Hill, NJ 08003
  (856)427-6900   Fax (856)427-0008
Davison, Beverly J., MD {1720029820} EmrgMd(93,NY15)<NJ-HACKNSK>
 + Hackensack Medical Center Emergency Medicine
  30 Prospect Avenue/Main 3619   Hackensack, NJ 07601
  (201)996-4614   Fax (201)342-7112
 + Hackensack University Medical Center
  30 Prospect Avenue/EmergMed   Hackensack, NJ 07601
  (201)996-4614   Fax (201)968-1866
Dawis, Maria Agnes Chaluangco, MD {1578565040} Pedtrc, Ped-Inf, IntrMd(92,PHI02)
 + Navesink Pediatrics
  55 North Gilbert Street/Suite 2101   Tinton Falls, NJ 07701
  (732)842-6677   Fax (732)530-2946
 + Meridian Medical Group - Faculty Practice
  61 Davis Avenue/Suite 1   Neptune, NJ 07753   (732)842-6677   Fax (732)776-4867
Dawlabani, Nassif E., MD {1184654261} Pedtrc(87,DOM10)<NJ-CHSFULD, NJ-CHSMRCER>
 + Drs. Dawlabani and Dawlabani
  908 West State Street   Trenton, NJ 08618   (609)503-5540
  Fax (609)503-5541
Dawlabani, Nickolas Elias, MD {1386820215} Pedtrc(04,DMN01)
 + Drs. Dawlabani and Dawlabani
  908 West State Street   Trenton, NJ 08618   (609)503-5540
  Fax (609)503-5541
Dawoud, Magy M., MD {1194770396} EmrgMd(97,NJ05)
 + 285 South Church Street/Suite 3
  Moorestown, NJ 08057
Dawson, Cleve R., MD {1316930605} IntrMd(70,PA13)
 + 72 Village Drive
  Basking Ridge, NJ 07920   (973)393-7756   Fax (908)718-5995
Dawson, George Anthony, MD {1629157482} RadOnc, RadThp(84,IA02)<NJ-WAYNEGEN, NJ-PALISADE>
 + Radiation Medicine
  785 Totowa Road   Totowa, NJ 07512   (973)904-0890   Fax
  (973)904-0695
Dawson, Martin S., MD {1609815836} CdvDis(93,PA09)
 + Owens Vergari Unwala Cardiology Associates PC
  17 West Red Bank Avenue/Suite 306   Woodbury, NJ 08096
  (856)845-6807   Fax (856)845-3760
Day, Brian Todd, MD {1164622270} ObsGyn
 + Totowa Ob/Gyn
  525 Union Boulevard   Totowa, NJ 07512   (973)790-1117
  Fax (973)790-1143
Day Salvatore, Debra-Lynn, MD {1851403539} ClnGnt, Pedtrc(86,OH06)<NJ-STPETER>
 + St. Peter's University Hospital
  254 Easton Avenue/ObsGyn/Peds   New Brunswick, NJ
  08901   (732)745-6659
Dayal, Rashmi P., MD {1609808708} Pedtrc(82,INA69)<NJ-COMMED, NJ-OCEANMC>
 + Pediatric Affiliates, PA
  3508 Route 9 South   Howell, NJ 07731   (732)905-9166
  Fax (732)905-9380
 + Pediatric Affiliates, PA
  40 Bey Lea Road/Suite B203   Toms River, NJ 08753
  (732)905-9166   Fax (732)244-6842
 + Pediatric Affiliates, PA
  400 Madison Avenue   Lakewood, NJ 07731   (732)364-7770
  Fax (732)364-9292
Dayal, Saraswati Devi, MD {1548208135} Surgry, SrgCrC(98,DC03)<NJ-HACKNSK>
 + Hackensack University Medical Center
  30 Prospect Avenue/Surgery/Trauma   Hackensack, NJ
  07601   (201)996-2000
 + Hackensack Surgical Critical Care Physicians
  5 Summit Avenue/Suite 105   Hackensack, NJ 07601
  (201)996-2000   Fax (201)883-1268
Dayan, Joseph Henry, MD {1962688978} SrgPlstc(02,VT02)
 + Memorial Sloan Kettering Bergen
  225 Summit Avenue   Montvale, NJ 07645   (212)639-8095
Dayner, Jeremy Joseph, MD {1922053222} EmrgMd(98,PA14)<NJ-CENTRAST>
 + CentraState Medical Center
  901 West Main Street/EmergMed   Freehold, NJ 07728
  (732)431-2000
Dayrit, Pedro Q., MD {1841343969} Gastrn, IntrMd(73,PHIL)<NJ-MEMSALEM>
 + 5 Pointers-Auburn Road
  Salem, NJ 08079   (856)935-8900   Fax (856)935-9399

Physicians by Name and Address

De Angelis, Thomas, MD {1336220193} ObsGyn, IntrMd(88,NY09)
+ Roseland Ob/Gyn Services
  27 Mountain Boulevard/Suite 6   Warren, NJ 07059
  (908)561-1102   Fax (908)561-1105

De Angelis, Vincent James, MD {1700968872} Anesth, IntrMd(87,NY09)<NJ-RWJUBRUN>
+ Robert Wood Johnson-UMDNJ Anesthesia Group
  125 Paterson Street/CAB 3100   New Brunswick, NJ 08901
  (732)937-8841   Fax (732)235-6131

De Angelo, Ann M., MD {1194839027} Pedtrc(92,NJ05)
+ Old Tappan Medical Group PA
  215 Old Tappan Road/Pediatrics   Old Tappan, NJ 07675
  (201)666-1001   (201)666-7610
+ Old Tappan Pediatrics
  136 North Washington Avenue   Bergenfield, NJ 07621
  (201)666-1001   Fax (201)385-4748

De Antonio, Joseph R., MD {1295745859} Gastrn, IntrMd(86,MO07)<NJ-CHSMRCER>
+ 3100 Princeton Pike
  Lawrenceville, NJ 08648   (609)882-2185   Fax (609)882-0347

De Antonio, Michele L., MD {1659304715} Pedtrc(81,PA12)<NJ-HOLYNAME, NJ-HACKNSK>
+ 160 Terrace Street
  Haworth, NJ 07641   (201)439-1200   Fax (201)439-1208

De Antonio, Sondra M., MD {1457368169} Nrolgy(86,NJ06)
+ Integrative Neurological Care
  663 South White Horse Pike   Hammonton, NJ 08037
  (609)567-6042   Fax (609)567-2722

De Biaso, Tracy A., MD {1831146802} FamMed(92,NJ06)
+ Family Practice Associates of Cumberland County, PC
  230 Laurel Heights Drive   Bridgeton, NJ 08302   (856)451-9595   Fax (609)451-1832

De Blasio, Thomas F., MD {1285790782} IntrMd, AltnMd(85,GRNA)<NJ-CENTRAST>
+ 200 Craig Road/1st Floor
  Manalapan, NJ 07726   (732)866-6600   Fax (732)866-6611

De Cotiis, Bruce A., MD {1750494613} Allrgy, IntrMd, Algy-Immn(75,NJ05)<NJ-JRSYSHMC, NJ-KIMBALL>
+ 1673 Highway 88 West
  Brick, NJ 08724   (732)458-2000   Fax (732)458-4523
+ Robert P. Rabinowitz, DO, PA
  462 Lakehurst Road   Toms River, NJ 08755   (732)458-2000   Fax (732)505-0862

De Cotiis, Dan A., MD {1285959650} RadV&I
+ Cooper University Hospital
  One Cooper Plaza   Camden, NJ 08103   (856)342-2000

De Crisce, Dean M., MD {1013923812} Psychy(99,CA06)<NJ-ANNKLEIN, NY-WOODHULL>
+ Ann Klein Forensic Center
  8 Production Way   Avenel, NJ 07001
+ Ann Klein Forensic Center
  1609 Stuyvesant Avenue/PO Box 7717   West Trenton, NJ 08628   (609)633-0900

De Cristofano, Robert E., MD {1881702165} Pedtrc(85,GRN01)<NJ-MORRISTN, NJ-STCLRDEN>
+ Pediatrics On Broadway
  10 Broadway   Denville, NJ 07834   (973)625-7734   Fax (973)625-4821

De Dan, Claudine Michele, MD {1124058367} FamMed(02,NJ05)
+ 34 Colson Lane/Suite B
  Mullica Hill, NJ 08062   (856)628-8120   Fax (856)628-8123

De Eugenio, Lewis, Jr., MD {1780664847} Grtrcs, IntrMd(76,NJ05)<NJ-SJRSYELM>
+ Pitman Internal Medicine Associates
  410 North Broadway/Suite 1   Pitman, NJ 08071   (856)589-3708   Fax (856)589-2662

De Falco, Robert Anthony, DO {1174554471} SrgOrt(98,ME75)<NJ-HCKTSTWN>
+ The Orthopedic Institute of New Jersey
  108 Bilby Road/Suite 201   Hackettstown, NJ 07840
  (908)684-3005   Fax (908)684-3301
+ The Orthopedic Institute of New Jersey
  380 Lafayette Road/Route 15   Sparta, NJ 07871   (908)684-3005   Fax (908)684-3301
+ The Orthopedic Institute of New Jersey
  66 Sunset Strip/Suite 400 Town Center   Succasunna, NJ 07840   (908)684-3005   Fax (908)684-3301

De Fazio, Ernest, MD {1477511707} IntrMd(75,ITA01)<NJ-MTN-SIDE>
+ 181 Franklin Avenue
  Nutley, NJ 07110   (973)667-6660   Fax (973)667-2134

De Feo, Daniel Scott, DO {1912147166} FamMed, EmrgMd(08,NY75)<NJ-STJOSHOS>
+ St Joseph's Medical Center Emergency
  703 Main Street   Paterson, NJ 07503   (973)754-2240   Fax (973)754-2249

De Flesco, Lindsay D., MD {1144352014} ObsGyn, IntrMd(03,PA14)<NJ-RBAYPERT>
+ Tri-County Ob-Gyn Associates, PA
  24 Stelton Road/Suite C   Piscataway, NJ 08854   (732)968-4444   Fax (732)968-1675

De Franco, Penny E., MD {1073625117} IntrMd, Nephro(85,DOM08)<NJ-CLARMAAS, NJ-MTNSIDE>
+ South Mountain Nephrology
  5 Franklin Avenue/Suite 401   Belleville, NJ 07109
  (973)450-8999

De Fronzo, Carl L., DO {1730415407} ObsGyn(88,NY75)
+ Drs. De Fronzo & De Fronzo
  216 Short Hills Avenue   Springfield, NJ 07081   (973)376-7838   Fax (973)912-4367

De Fronzo, Stephen D., MD {1922056548} InfDis, IntrMd(80,MEX03)
+ Drs. De Fronzo & De Fronzo
  216 Short Hills Avenue   Springfield, NJ 07081   (973)376-7838   Fax (973)912-4367

De Fusco, Carmine J., MD {1942270616} Allrgy, PedAlg, Algy-Immn(74,MEX03)<NJ-JRSYSHMC>
+ 224 Taylors Mills Road/Suite 106
  Manalapan, NJ 07726   (732)462-0666   Fax (732)462-0992

De Gennaro, Anthony, MD {1528137262} Otlryg, OtgyPSHN(83,OK01)<NJ-BAYSHORE, NJ-RIVERVW>
+ 370 Highway 35/Suite 100
  Red Bank, NJ 07701   (732)530-7799   Fax (732)530-9091

De Gennaro, Michael A., MD {1598713786} IntrMd(81,DMN01)
+ Bergenfield Internal Medicine
  161 North Washington Avenue/Suite A   Bergenfield, NJ 07621   (201)387-6900

De Gregorio, Bart, MD {1245205558} CdvDis, IntrMd(79,ITA03)<NJ-HACKNSK, NJ-STMICHL>
+ Bart De Gregorio MD, LLC.
  946 Bloomfield Avenue   Glen Ridge, NJ 07028   (973)743-1121   Fax (973)743-2627

De Gregorio, Joseph Anthony, MD {1023086691} CdvDis(91,NY15)<NJ-HACKNSK, NJ-MTNSIDE>
+ Bart De Gregorio MD, LLC.
  946 Bloomfield Avenue   Glen Ridge, NJ 07028   (973)743-1121   Fax (973)743-2627

De Guzman, Virginia H., MD {1144282450} FamMed(63,PHI01)<NJ-VALLEY, NJ-BERGNMC>
+ 688 Wyckoff Avenue
  Mahwah, NJ 07430   (201)891-3080   Fax (201)847-0995

De Jesus, Dino Nicol Enanoza, DO {1639298581} SrgOrt
+ Cooper University Medical Center/Camden
  3 Cooper Plaza/Suite 408   Camden, NJ 08103   (856)342-2000   Fax (856)541-2387

De Jesus, Joseph Ocampo, MD {1295946010} RadDia, Radiol(TN07<NJ-MEMSALEM>
+ Memorial Hospital of Salem County
  310 Woodstown Road/Radiology   Salem, NJ 08079
  (856)339-6054   Fax (856)935-4970

De Jesus, Luisito Garcia, MD {1801929286} IntrMd(86,PHI02)
+ UMDNJ Student Health Services
  249 University Avenue/Rm 104   Newark, NJ 07102
  (973)353-5231   Fax (973)353-1390

De Juliis, Aurora, MD {1881791903} IntrMd(80,ITA17)<NJ-MTN-SIDE>
+ 1018 Broad Street/Suite 1
  Bloomfield, NJ 07003   (973)338-6300   Fax (973)338-5347

De La Cruz, Angel Ramon, MD {1336444777} IntrMd<NJ-STJOSHOS>
+ A&S General Physician LLC
  1137 Main Avenue   Clifton, NJ 07011   (973)773-0303   Fax (973)773-0004

De La Cruz, Antonio A., MD {1467440776} Pedtrc, Allrgy, Algy-Immn(74,PHI08)<NJ-CLARMAAS>
+ 240 Williamson Street/Suite 503
  Elizabeth, NJ 07202   (908)469-4206   Fax (908)469-4207   tony@DLCruz.org
+ Allergy Consultants, PA
  197 Bloomfield Avenue   Verona, NJ 07044   (908)469-4206   Fax (973)857-0980
+ 559 Broad Street
  Newark, NJ 07202   (973)424-1300   Fax (973)424-1722

De La Cruz, Ernest Jose, MD {1821075334} IntrMd(94,NJ05)<NJ-UNVMCPRN>
+ Montgomery Internal Medicine Group
  727 State Road   Princeton, NJ 08540   (609)921-6410   Fax (609)921-0406

De La Cruz, Flavia Annette, MD {1538390950} IntrMd
+ 587 Westminster Avenue
  Elizabeth, NJ 07208   (908)351-6656   Fax (908)629-1634   FlaviaMD@direct.practicefusion.com
+ Dr. De La Cruz and Dhalla
  714 Tenth Street   Secaucus, NJ 07094   (908)351-6656   Fax (201)865-0015

De La Luz, Gustavo E., MD {1255333043} PulDis, IntrMd, CritCr(87,PRO01)<NJ-OCEANMC>
+ Shore Pulmonary PA
  2640 Highway 70/Building 6-A   Manasquan, NJ 08736   (732)528-5900   Fax (732)528-0887
+ Shore Pulmonary PA
  301 Bingham Avenue/Suite B   Ocean, NJ 07712   (732)528-5900   Fax (732)775-1212
+ Shore Pulmonary PA
  1608 Route 88/Suite 117   Brick, NJ 08736   (732)575-1100

De La Mota, Jessica Isabel, DO {1780898585} Anesth
+ 75 Orono Street
  Clifton, NJ 07013

De La Rosa, Benjamin Danny, MD {1467604843} InfDis
+ Institute for Clinical Research - Holy Name Hospital
  718 Teaneck Road   Teaneck, NJ 07666   (201)833-7274   Fax (201)833-7243
+ 302 Herman Street/Apt A
  Hackensack, NJ 07601

De La Rosa, Rita G., MD {1467532283} Pedtrc(69,PHI08)<NJ-JRSYCITY>
+ 779 Bergen Avenue
  Jersey City, NJ 07306   (201)433-0660   Fax (201)433-0444

De La Torre, Lily Shu, MD {1427012970} Psychy(75,DC02)<NJ-HCMEADPS>
+ 27 Valley Road
  Montclair, NJ 07042   (973)746-0795
+ Hudson County Meadowview Psychiatric Hospital
  595 County Avenue   Secaucus, NJ 07094   (201)369-5252

De La Torre, Pola, MD {1710084348} IntrMd, InfDis(94,DC02)<NJ-COOPRUMC>
+ The Cooper Hospital System-Univ Hospital
  401 Haddon Avenue/Room 268/Edu   Camden, NJ 08103   (856)342-2000

De Lara, Vilma A., MD {1023072980} ObsGyn(65,PHI08)<NJ-STM-RYPAS>
+ 178 Hamilton Avenue
  Passaic, NJ 07055   (973)777-1492   Fax (973)777-0873

De Laurentis, Joseph, MD {1932108156} RadDia(80,NJ05)<NJ-MEMSALEM>
+ Kennedy Health System/Cherry Hill Campus
  2201 Chapel Avenue West   Cherry Hill, NJ 08002
  (856)488-6500

De Laurentis, Mark, MD {1134127178} Radiol, RadNro, Rad-Dia(85,PA02)<NJ-VIRTMHBC, NJ-VIRTBERL>
+ South Jersey Radiology Associates, P.A.
  100 Carnie Boulevard/Suite B-5   Voorhees, NJ 08043
  (856)751-0123   Fax (856)751-0535
+ South Jersey Radiology Associates, P.A.
  315 Route 70 East/Suite B   Cherry Hill, NJ 08034   (856)751-0123   Fax (856)428-0356
+ The Women's Center at Voorhees
  100 Carnie Boulevard/Suite A-4   Voorhees, NJ 08043
  (856)751-5522   Fax (856)751-5650

De Leon, Essel Marie B., MD {1508090051} PthAcl<NJ-CLAR-MAAS>
+ Clara Maass Medical Center
  1 Clara Maass Drive/Pthlgy   Belleville, NJ 07109   (973)450-2480

De Leon, Michelle F., MD {1619261591}
+ 1050 George Street/Apt 19 I
  New Brunswick, NJ 08901   (856)308-4082   michellefdeleon@gmail.com

De Leonardis, John A., MD {1992851984} Pedtrc(84,DMN01)<NJ-UNDRWD>
+ Upper Deerfield Pediatrics
  1117 State Highway 77   Bridgeton, NJ 08302   (856)455-7337   Fax (856)455-0523
+ Mullica Hill Pediatrics
  8 High Street/Suite 1B   Mullica Hill, NJ 08062   (856)455-7337   Fax (856)223-1963

De Lillo, Anthony Rocco, MD {1356372536} Gastrn, IntrMd(94,NY20)<NJ-VALLEY>
+ Bergen Medical Associates
  1 West Ridgewood Avenue/Suite 301   Paramus, NJ 07652
  (201)445-1660   Fax (201)445-4296
+ Bergen Medical Associates
  466 Old Hook Road/Suite 1   Emerson, NJ 07630   (201)445-1660   Fax (201)967-0340

De Luca, Alfred A., Jr., MD {1265523021} InfDis(83,MEX14)<NJ-CENTRAST, NJ-MONMOUTH>
+ Central Jersey Infectious Diseases
  215 Gordons Corner Road/Suite 2J   Manalapan, NJ 07726
  (732)792-0741   Fax (732)792-0745   Adlmd216@aol.com

De Luca, Joseph Edward, MD {1942249552} EmrgMd, IntrMd(81,DOM06)<NJ-NWTNMEM>
+ Vernon Urgent Care Center
  212 Route 94/Suite 1A   Vernon, NJ 07462   (973)209-2260   Fax (973)209-1895

De Mais, John R., MD {1558320564} Anesth(79,MEX14)
+ Pain Medicine Physicians
  187 Millburn Avenue/Suite 103   Millburn, NJ 07041
  (973)467-1466   Fax (973)467-1422
+ 87 Horizon Terrace
  Hillsdale, NJ 07642

Physicians by Name and Address

De Marco, Angelo Albert, MD {1386681617} FamMed(80,MEX03)
+ Hoboken Family Practice
108 Washington Street   Hoboken, NJ 07030   (201)656-5688   Fax (201)656-8975

De Marco, Joseph A., Jr., MD {1639235476} SrgPlstc, SrgHnd(71,ITA01)<NJ-VALLEY, NJ-HACKNSK>
+ Joseph A. deMarco, M.D. P.C.
24 Godwin Avenue/2nd Floor   Midland Park, NJ 07432   (201)447-1160   Fax (201)447-9036
info@Josephdemarcomd.com

De Mare, Patrick J., DO {1245308402} FamMed, EmrgMd(74,MO78)<NJ-CHILTON>
+ 63 Beaverbrook Road/Suite 101
Lincoln Park, NJ 07035   (973)696-1087   Fax (973)686-1916

De Maria, Nicholas Anthony, MD {1942255286} IntrMd(80,MEXI)<NJ-VIRTBERL>
+ Winslow Primary Care Associates, PC
524 Williamstown Road/Suite A   Sicklerville, NJ 08081   (856)728-1181   Fax (856)728-1182

De Marsico, Richard, MD {1003983339} ObsGyn(74,DC02)<NJ-STBARNMC>
+ Essex Women's Health Care Center, P.A.
33 North Fullerton Avenue   Montclair, NJ 07042   (973)744-2226   Fax (973)509-0978

De Martino, Frank J., DO {1669415865} EmrgMd(90,NJ75)<NJ-KMHTURNV, NJ-KMHSTRAT>
+ Kennedy Health Systems/Washington Township Campus
435 Hurffville-Cross Keys Road   Turnersville, NJ 08012   (856)582-2816   Fax (856)582-2807
+ Kennedy Memorial Hospital-University Medical Center
18 East Laurel Road   Stratford, NJ 08084   (856)582-2816   Fax (856)346-6005

De Martino, Paul John, MD {1922104827} Gastrn, IntrMd(88,NJ06)<NJ-COMMED>
+ Ocean Endosurgery Center
129 Route 37 West   Toms River, NJ 08755   (732)606-4440   Fax (732)797-3963

De Masi, Christopher Louis, DO {1194759068} FamMed(01,NJ75)
+ Summit Medical Group
202 Elmer Street   Westfield, NJ 07090   (908)228-3675   Fax (908)664-1053
+ Summit Medical Group-Berkeley Heights Campus
1 Diamond Hill Road   Berkeley Heights, NJ 07922   (908)228-3675   Fax (908)232-1439

De Masi, Leon Gregory, MD {1518923796} PubHth
+ AmeriHealth HMO, Inc.
8000 Midlantic Drive/Suite 333   Mount Laurel, NJ 08054   (856)778-6376   Fax (856)778-6970

De Melo, Mauricio Garret, MD {1467825562} IntrMd
+ Riverside Pediatrics
714 Tenth Street   Secaucus, NJ 07094   (551)257-7038   Fax (201)552-2358

De Morat, Eugene John, MD {1255344818} SrgOrt(97,NJ06)<NJ-SHOREMEM>
+ Shore Orthopedic University Associates
24 Macarthur Boulevard/First Floor   Somers Point, NJ 08244   (609)927-1991   Fax (609)927-4203
+ Shore Orthopedic University Associates
18 East Jimmie Leeds Road   Galloway, NJ 08205   (609)927-1991   Fax (609)927-4203

De Noia, Anthony Philip, MD {1962409391} IntrMd(72,PA02)<NJ-JRSYSHMC, NJ-MONMOUTH>
+ Northern Monmouth County Medical Associates
1012 State Route 36   Atlantic Highlands, NJ 07716   (732)291-3865   Fax (732)291-3859

De Ocera, Zenaida Bascara, MD {1184660581} Anesth(67,PHI08)
+ 40 Oakland Road
Old Bridge, NJ 08857

De Paola, Anthony A., DO {1194711028} IntrMd(92,NJ75)
+ Premier Health Associates
202 Route 206 North/Suite A   Branchville, NJ 07826   (973)948-5577   Fax (973)729-6487
+ Premier Health Associates
5 Eisenhower Road   Columbia, NJ 07832   (908)362-5360
+ Premier Health Associates
89 Sparta Avenue/Suite 100   Sparta, NJ 07871   (973)729-2121   Fax (973)729-3454

De Persia, Rudolph T., Jr., MD {1134161813} Grtrcs, IntrMd(81,PA02)
+ De Persia Medical Group
17 West Red Bank Avenue/Suite 207   Woodbury, NJ 08096   (856)845-0664   Fax (856)845-7602

De Prince, Daniel, III, DO {1023080306} FamMed(93,PA77)
+ South Jersey Health & Wellness Center
1919 Greentree Road   Cherry Hill, NJ 08003   (856)761-8100   Fax (856)761-8107

De Priori, Elis Maria, MD {1598712861} Nephro, IntrMd(75,BRA50)<NJ-SJERSYHS>
+ Kidney & Hypertension Specialists PA
215 Laurel Heights Drive   Bridgeton, NJ 08302   (856)455-6002   Fax (856)455-6106
priorie@verizon.net

De Renzi, Paul D., MD {1164411773} CdvDis, IntrMd(86,CT01)<NJ-STCLRDEN>
+ Lakeland Cardiology Center, P.A.
415 Boulevard   Mountain Lakes, NJ 07046   (973)334-7700   Fax (973)402-5847

De Ritter, Lois M., MD {1629142245} Psychy, PsyCAd(82,NJ06)
+ 73 West End Avenue
Somerville, NJ 08876   (732)560-9770

De Rosa, Joseph, MD {1184671018} IntrMd(91,NJ06)
+ 505 East Broad Street
Westfield, NJ 07090   (908)232-0899   Fax (908)232-1728

De Rose, Marielaina S., MD {1346263779} IntrMd(95,PA02)<NJ-ENGLWOOD, NJ-HOLYNAME>
+ Englewood Hospital and Medical Center
350 Engle Street/Medicine   Englewood, NJ 07631   (201)894-3000

De Salvo, Eugene L., MD {1699757898} Urolgy(75,NJ05)
+ 515 Iron Bridge Road
Freehold, NJ 07728   (732)780-3434   Fax (732)780-9334

De Sanctis, Julia Tucker, MD {1083647887} RadV&I, Radiol, RadDia(91,MA01)<NJ-UNVMCPRN>
+ Princeton Radiology Associates, P.A.
419 North Harrison Street   Princeton, NJ 08540   (609)921-3345   Fax (609)683-8847
+ Princeton Radiology Associates, P.A.
9 Centre Drive   Jamesburg, NJ 08831   (609)921-3345   Fax (609)655-4016
+ Princeton Radiology Associates, P.A.
3674 Route 27   Kendall Park, NJ 08540   (732)821-5563   Fax (732)821-6675

De Santis, Fiorita G., DO {1922252519} Anesth, PainMd(93,NY75)
+ 6 Exeter Street
Morris Plains, NJ 07950   (973)402-1331

De Santis, Maryanne, MD {1174507594} Psychy, PsyFor(87,ITA27)
+ 50 Marion Street
Port Reading, NJ 07064   (732)541-5630

De Sarno, Carney Thomas, MD {1144296187} Surgry(93,PA09)<NJ-JRSYSHMC>
+ 1706 Corlies Avenue
Neptune, NJ 07753   (732)775-5005   Fax (732)775-0064

De Shaw, Max G., MD {1508808940} InfDis, IntrMd(88,MN04)<NJ-MORRISTN>
+ IPC The Hospitalist Company
220 Ridgedale Avenue/Suite C-2   Florham Park, NJ 07932   (973)538-5844   Fax (973)267-0181

De Silva, Malika Shani, MD {1992725857} FamMed, FamMAdM(01,GRN01)
+ Drs. Badin, De Silva, and Perera
1947 Kennedy Boulevard   Jersey City, NJ 07305   (201)433-4848   Fax (201)946-9292

De Sio, John Michael, MD {1578533329} Anesth, PainMd(87,MONT)<NJ-UNVMCPRN>
+ The De Sio Pain Institute, PA
452 Lakehurst Road   Toms River, NJ 08755   (732)349-9099   Fax (732)349-5485

De Stefano, Joseph L., MD {1083658728} Gyneco, SrgGyn(69,DC02)<NJ-ACMCITY, NJ-ACMCMAIN>
+ Absecon Island Centers for Women's Healthcare
4401 Ventnor Avenue   Atlantic City, NJ 08401   (609)345-2050   Fax (609)345-2052
+ Absecon Island Centers for Women's Healthcare
53 West White Horse Pike   Galloway, NJ 08205   (609)345-2050   Fax (609)652-2519

De Tata, Gerald C., MD {1902877079} FamMed, IntrMd(79,DC02)
+ AtlantiCare Family Medicine
120 South White Horse Pike   Hammonton, NJ 08037   (609)561-4211   Fax (609)561-0639

De Trespalacios, Jose A., DO {1073529764} Anesth(85,NJ75)<NJ-CLARMAAS>
+ Clara Maass Medical Center
1 Clara Maass Drive/Anesth   Belleville, NJ 07109   (973)450-2000

De Tulio, Anthony, MD {1205806064} IntrMd(85,MEX03)<NJ-JRSYSHMC, NJ-RIVERVW>
+ Jersey Shore Medical Associates
734 North Beers Street/Suite U-4   Holmdel, NJ 07733   (732)264-8484   Fax (732)264-4324

De Vastey, Gerard, MD {1235233347} IntrMd(87,NJ05)
+ 950 West Chestnut Street/Suite 101
Union, NJ 07083   (908)688-8630   Fax (908)688-1170

De Vera, Edmundo C., MD {1891752648} IntrMd(70,PHI01)<NJ-PALISADE>
+ NHCAC Health Center at North Bergen
1116 43rd Street   North Bergen, NJ 07047   (201)330-2632   Fax (201)330-2638
+ NHCAC Health Center at West New York
5301 Broadway   West New York, NJ 07093   (201)866-9320

Deacon, Nancy S., MD {1699746818} Pedtrc, IntrMd(91,NJ03)<NJ-JRSYSHMC>
+ Shore Touch Pediatrics LLC
600 Mule Road/Suie 10   Toms River, NJ 08757   (732)557-5555   Fax (732)557-9555

Deak, Steven T., MD {1548274111} SrgVas, Surgry(76,KY12)<NJ-STPETER, NJ-RWJUBRUN>
+ 37 Clyde Road/Suite 102
Somerset, NJ 08873   (732)873-0200   Fax (732)873-0255
deaksk@msn.com
+ Cares Surgicenter, LLC.
240 Easton Avenue   New Brunswick, NJ 08901   (732)873-0200   Fax (732)296-8677

Deal, Amanda E., DO {1750776126} FamMed
+ Woodstown Family Practice
125 East Avenue/Suite C   Woodstown, NJ 08098   (856)769-2800   Fax (856)769-4256

Deal, Edward R., DO {1558434654} Anesth(87,NJ75)<NJ-COOPRUMC>
+ Cooper University Hospital
One Cooper Plaza/Anesth   Camden, NJ 08103   (856)342-2000

Dealmeida, Patrick, DO {1851772008} IntrMd<NJ-CLARMAAS>
+ Clara Maass Medical Center
1 Clara Maass Drive   Belleville, NJ 07109   (973)251-1062

Dealwis, Jayakanthi, MD {1245285030} Psychy, PsyAdd(74,SRI01)<NJ-SUMOAKSH>
+ Summit Oaks Hospital
19 Prospect Street/Psych   Summit, NJ 07901   (330)758-4515   Fax (330)758-5121

Dealwis, Watutantrige T., MD {1396798120} Psychy, PsyCAd(73,SRI01)<NJ-VALLEY>
+ The Valley Hospital
223 North Van Dien Avenue/Psychiatry   Ridgewood, NJ 07450   (201)447-8000

Dean, Gregory Edwin, MD {1447226139} PedUro, Urolgy, IntrMd(88,NY01)<NJ-VIRTVOOR>
+ Urology for Children, LLC
120 Carnie Boulevard/Suite 2   Voorhees, NJ 08043   (856)751-7880
+ Urology for Children, LLC
239 Hurffville Crosskeys Road   Sewell, NJ 08080   (856)751-7880   Fax (856)751-9133
+ Urology for Children, LLC
1000 Atlantic Avenue   Camden, NJ 08043   (856)751-7880   Fax (856)751-9133

Dean-Davis, Ellen, MD {1679887103} PedOrt, SrgOrt(08,GRN01)
+ North Jersey Orthopaedic Group
246 Hamburg Turnpike/Suite 302   Wayne, NJ 07470   (865)405-3326   Fax (973)689-6264
ellendean.md@gmail.com

DeAngelis, Lawrence J., MD Anesth, IntrMd(71,NY06)
+ Summit Anesthesia Associates, P.A.
33 Overlook Road/Suite 311   Summit, NJ 07901   (908)598-1500   Fax (908)598-0197

Deangelis, Matthew Michael, DO {1548415706} Anesth
+ Cooper Anesthesia Associates
One Cooper Plaza/Suite 294-B   Camden, NJ 08103   (856)342-2000   Fax (856)968-8239

DeAngelo, Frank James, MD {1609973700}<NJ-ACMCITY>
+ AtlantiCare Regional Medical Center/City Campus
1925 Pacific Avenue   Atlantic City, NJ 08401   (215)301-5638
deang218@aol.com

DeAnnuntis, Liza Leluja, MD {1598919250} IntrMd(93,PA02)
+ 900 Route 168/Suite D1
Turnersville, NJ 08012   (856)227-0077

DeAntonio, Joseph Alexander, MD {1043477508} Anesth
+ 12 Adams Place
Freehold, NJ 07728   (908)692-5196
+ Red Bank Anesthesia, LLC
1 Riverview Plaza   Red Bank, NJ 07701   (908)692-5196   Fax (732)450-2620

Dearborn, Peyton Robert, MD {1346243219} Anesth(90,NJ05)<NJ-SHOREMEM>
+ Shore Memorial Hospital
1 East New York Avenue/Anesthesiology   Somers Point, NJ 08244   (609)653-3500

Deary, Michael J., MD {1144219130} ObsGyn
+ Osborn Family Health Center
1601 Haddon Road   Camden, NJ 08103   (856)757-3700   Fax (856)365-7972

DeAsis, Ma Lourdes, MD {1013912989} AlgyImmn(89,PHIL)<NY-NYACKHOS>
+ Allergy & Asthma Consultants
354 Old Hook Road   Westwood, NJ 07675   (201)666-8500   Fax (201)666-5241

Deb, Ashoke Kumar, MD {1124088760} IntrMd(80,BANG)<NJ-MEMSALEM>
+ Spotswood Medical Associates PA
498 Main Street   Spotswood, NJ 08884   (732)251-6900   Fax (732)251-5935
+ Cooper Primary Care
390 North Broadway/Suite 100   Pennsville, NJ 08070   (732)251-6900   Fax (856)678-7509

Physicians by Name and Address

Debbs, Robert H., DO {1295769396} MtFtMd, ObsGyn(89,PA77)<NJ-VIRTVOOR, NJ-ACMCITY>
+ Clin Health Care Assoc of NJ-Mat/Fetal
  2301 Evesham Road/Pav 800/Suite 221   Voorhees, NJ 08043
+ Clin Health Care Assoc of NJ-Mat/Fetal
  543 North Broad Street   Woodbury, NJ 08096

Debell, David Anthony, MD {1811938566} IntrMd(82,GRN01)
+ Summit Medical Group
  6 Brighton Road/2 FL   Clifton, NJ 07012   (973)777-7911   Fax (973)777-5403

DeBellis, Julia Angelina, MD {1417900150} OthrSp, Pedtrc(90,MA05)<NJ-HACKNSK>
+ Audrey Hepburn Children's House
  12 Second Street   Hackensack, NJ 07601   (201)996-2271   Fax (201)996-4926

DeBitetto, Nick P., DO {1083692933} IntrMd(88,NY75)<NJ-NWTNMEM>
+ Premier Health Associates
  123 Newton Sparta Road   Newton, NJ 07860   (973)579-6300   Fax (973)579-1524

DeBlasi, Richard A., MD {1538353255} Psychy(71,NJ05)<NJ-JRSYSHMC>
+ Monmouth County Department of Correction
  1 Waterworks Road/Psychiatry   Freehold, NJ 07728   (732)431-7860

Deblasio, Joseph, MD {1669544003} IntrMd(83,GRNA)<NJ-RWJUHAM, NJ-STFRNMED>
+ Hamilton Medical Group
  2275 State Route 33/Suite 301   Hamilton Square, NJ 08690   (609)586-6006

Deblasio, Joseph, Jr., MD {1871896864} IntrMd
+ 2275 Route 33/Suite 301
  Hamilton Square, NJ 08690   (609)586-7833

DeBruin, William J., MD {1457353757} Pedtrc, PedCrC(84,NJ05)<NJ-HOBUNIMC, NJ-STJOSHOS>
+ St. Joseph's Children's Hospital
  703 Main Street/PICU   Paterson, NJ 07503   (973)754-2560
  Debruinw@sjhmc.org

DeCastro, Amante N., MD {1649331620} ObsGyn(65,PHI01)<NJ-MEMSALEM, NJ-UNDRWD>
+ Amante N. DeCastro MD PC
  4 Bypass Road/Suite 202   Salem, NJ 08079   (856)935-7200   Fax (856)935-9655
+ Amante N. DeCastro MD PC
  218 Laurel Heights Drive   Bridgeton, NJ 08302   (856)455-7283

Decker, Ashley, MD {1972861102} SrgDer
+ Cooper Center for Dermatologic Surgery
  10000 Sagemore Drive/Suite 10103   Marlton, NJ 08053   (856)356-4924   Fax (856)356-4793

Decker, Edmund J., DO {1851308779} FamMed(85,NJ75)<NJ-VIRTBERL, NJ-VIRTVOOR>
+ 3820 Church Road
  Mount Laurel, NJ 08054   (856)727-4774   Fax (856)727-4715

Decker, Edward Bruce, MD {1942243829} Ophthl(90,NY15)
+ Marano Eye Care Center
  200 South Orange Avenue/Suite 209   Livingston, NJ 07039   (973)322-0102   Fax (973)322-0102

Decker, Eugene Michael, DO {1619975687} FamMed(87,NJ75)<NJ-WARREN>
+ St. Luke's Coventry Family Practice
  755 Memorial Parkway/Suite 300   Phillipsburg, NJ 08865   (908)847-3300   Fax (866)281-6023

Decker, Jerome Elliot, MD {1366449449} OthrSp, SrgHnd, SrgOrt(84,DC02)<NJ-HUNTRDN>
+ MidJersey Orthopaedics, P.A.
  8100 Westcott Drive/Suite 101   Flemington, NJ 08822   (908)782-0600   Fax (908)782-7575
+ Hunterdon Orthopaedic Institute, P.A.
  80 West End Avenue   Somerville, NJ 08876   (908)182-0600

Decker, Raymond, Jr., MD {1801880695} SrgHnd(84,DC02)<NJ-JRSYSHMC, NJ-BAYSHORE>
+ Central Jersey Hand Surgery
  2 Industrial Way West   Eatontown, NJ 07724   (732)542-4477   Fax (732)935-0355
+ Central Jersey Hand Surgery
  535 Iron Bridge Road   Freehold, NJ 07728   (732)542-4477   Fax (732)431-4770
+ Central Jersey Hand Surgery
  780 Route 37 West/Suite 140   Toms River, NJ 07724   (732)286-9000   Fax (732)240-0036

Decker, Robert James, V, DO {1326470139}
+ University Hospital-University Family Medicine
  42 East Laurel Road/Suite 2100   Stratford, NJ 08084   (856)566-4677   Fax (856)566-6188

Decorso, Joseph A., MD {1023176682} IntrMd(83,DMN01)<NJ-STBARNMC, NJ-MTNSIDE>
+ 20 Montreal Court
  Toms River, NJ 08757   (973)699-1830   Fax (973)575-5307

DeCosimo, Diana R., MD {1962437731} CdvDis, Grtrcs, IntrMd(74,MA05)<NJ-UMDNJ, NJ-HACKNSK>
+ University Hospital-Doctors Office Center
  90 Bergen Street/DOC 4400   Newark, NJ 07103   (973)972-1880   Fax (973)972-1879

DeCosmo, Michael J., DO {1376519645} Dermat(71,IA75)<NJ-KMHCHRRY>
+ Kennedy Health System/Cherry Hill Campus
  2201 Chapel Avenue West/Dermatology   Cherry Hill, NJ 08002   (856)662-7883   Fax (856)662-5838

Decter, Edward M., MD {1033215298} SrgOrt(75,NE06)
+ Tri-County Orthopedics
  197 Ridgedale Street/Suite 300   Cedar Knolls, NJ 07927   (973)538-2334   Fax (973)829-9174
  emdecter@gmail.com

Decter, Julian A., MD {1295810141} MedOnc, Hemato, IntrMd(66,NY19)<NY-PRSBWEIL, NJ-STBARNMC>
+ 200 South Orange Avenue
  Livingston, NJ 07039   (212)517-5900   Fax (212)744-0029
  jdecter@yahoo.com

DeDona, Anna, DO {1194721902} IntrMd(93,MO78)<NJ-COMMED, NJ-KIMBALL>
+ Ocean County Family Care
  2125 Route 88 East   Brick, NJ 08724   (732)892-4548   Fax (732)892-0961
+ Ocean County Family Care
  400 New Hampshire Avenue   Lakewood, NJ 08701   (732)892-4548   Fax (732)901-0744

Dedousis, John, Jr., MD {1164515706} IntrMd(85,WIND)<NJ-BAYONNE>
+ Carepoint Health Medical Group
  1166 Kennedy Boulevard   Bayonne, NJ 07002   (201)339-1133   Fax (201)339-1073
+ Carepoint Health
  10 Exchange Place   Jersey City, NJ 07302   (201)339-1133

Deehan, Michael A., MD {1306857461} SrgOrt(88,NJ05)<NJ-HCKTSTWN, NJ-MORRISTN>
+ Skylands Orthopaedics PC
  57 US Highway 46/Suite 107   Hackettstown, NJ 07840   (908)813-9700   Fax (908)813-2861
+ Skylands Orthopaedics PC
  1 Robertson Drive/Suite 11   Bedminster, NJ 07921   (908)813-9700   Fax (908)813-2861
+ Emmaus Surgical Center
  57 US Highway 46/Suite 104   Hackettstown, NJ 07840   (908)813-9600   Fax (908)813-9611

Deen, Malik F., MD {1881769909} PthCln, PthAna, PthCyt(73,SRI01)<NJ-RWJUBRUN, NJ-BAYSHORE>
+ UH- Robert Wood Johnson Med
  125 Paterson Street/MEB 222   New Brunswick, NJ 08901   (732)235-8120   Fax (732)235-8124
+ RWJ University Hospital New Brunswick
  One Robert Wood Johnson Place   New Brunswick, NJ 08901   (732)828-3000

Deen, Shereelah, MD {1649287756} IntrMd(78,SRI01)<NJ-NWRKBETH>
+ 372 Valley Road
  West Orange, NJ 07052   (973)324-1190   Fax (973)736-8355
  Sdeenmd@comcast.net

Deendyal, Yoganand, MD {1023120615} EmrgMd, IntrMd(84,ROM07)<NJ-CHSFULD>
+ Capital Health System/Fuld Campus
  750 Brunswick Avenue/Emergency   Trenton, NJ 08638   (609)394-6000

Deery, Kimberly Jeanne, DO {1992081392} Pedtrc
+ Dr. G. Lee Lerch and Associates
  63 North Lakeview Drive/Suite 202   Gibbsboro, NJ 08026   (856)435-6000   Fax (856)782-1667

Defalco, Lisa May, DO {1659478691} ObsGyn(98,ME75)<NJ-HCKTSTWN>
+ All About Women Gyn Associates
  653 Willow Grove Street/Suite 2200   Hackettstown, NJ 07840   (908)852-7770   Fax (908)852-7755

DeFelice, Magee Lindinger, MD {1194854851} Pedtrc(06,PA02)<NJ-VIRTVOOR, NJ-VIRTMHBC>
+ Children's Health Associates II LLC
  101 Carnie Boulevard   Voorhees, NJ 08043   (856)782-3300   Fax (856)504-8029
+ Virtua Memorial
  175 Madison Avenue   Mount Holly, NJ 08060   (609)267-0700

Defilippis, Nicholas A., MD {1518962257} IntrMd(85,NJ05)<NJ-OVERLOOK>
+ Union Internal Medicine Group
  2027 Morris Avenue   Union, NJ 07083   (908)688-2480   Fax (908)688-7518

DeFranco, Paul David, DO {1952453839} IntrMd(00,MO78)<NJ-WAYNEGEN, NJ-VALLEY>
+ Allied Medical Associates
  510 Hamburg Turnpike   Wayne, NJ 07470   (973)942-6005   Fax (973)442-6009

Defrank, Joseph Miguel, MD {1801095864} IntrMd(00,DOM01)
+ 336-338 Ridge Street
  Newark, NJ 07104   (973)230-7522
  josephmiguel2@hotmail.com

DeFusco, Kenneth T., MD {1790779148} IntrMd, PulDis(68,ITA01)<NJ-STBARNMC>
+ 2 West Northfield Road/Suite 206
  Livingston, NJ 07039   (973)994-1544

Degaeta, Linda R., MD {1053562942} RadDia(80,PA02)
+ 20 Sheephill Drive
  Gladstone, NJ 07934   (908)234-0125   Fax (732)469-9180

Degapudi, Bhargavi, MD {1033384706} Nephro, IntrMd(02,INA83)<NJ-ACMCITY>
+ AtlantiCare Regional Medical Center/City Campus
  1925 Pacific Avenue/Nephrology   Atlantic City, NJ 08401   (609)441-8146   Fax (609)441-8002

Degen, Michael Conrad, MD {1174962757} Urolgy, IntrMd(05)
+ Drs. Fagelman, Degen & Fagelman
  360 Essex Street/Suite 403   Hackensack, NJ 07601   (551)996-8090   Fax (551)996-8221

DeGennaro, Marianne E., DO {1124113691} Pedtrc(87,MO78)<NY-STATNRTH, NY-STATNSTH>
+ Degennaro Pediatrics Associates
  370 State Route 35/Suite 200   Red Bank, NJ 07701   (732)534-5437   Fax (732)219-5437

Deger, Randolph Bruce, MD {1598754400} ObsGyn, IntrMd(86,NY47)
+ Virtua Gynecologic Oncology Specialists
  200 Bowman Drive/Suite E-315   Voorhees, NJ 08043   (856)247-7310   Fax (856)325-4309

DeGoma, Rolando L., MD {1194724195} CdvDis, IntrMd(72,PHI01)<NJ-CHSMRCER>
+ NJ Preventive Cardiology/Cholesterol
  416 Bellevue Avenue/Suite 303   Trenton, NJ 08618   (609)396-6363   Fax (609)695-7747

Degraaff, Doreen E., MD {1629142401} ObsGyn(88,NJ05)
+ Associates in Obstetrics Gynecology & Infertility
  375 Mount Pleasant Avenue/Suite 202   West Orange, NJ 07052   (973)731-7707   Fax (973)669-0277

Degrande, Gary C., MD {1275609380} ObsGyn(78,MEX03)<NJ-MTNSIDE>
+ Essex Women's Health Care Center, P.A.
  33 North Fullerton Avenue   Montclair, NJ 07042   (973)744-2226   Fax (973)509-0978

Degregorio, Scott David, MD {1588869655} RadDia, IntrMd(06,CT01)
+ Radiology Associates of Ridgewood, P.A.
  20 Franklin Turnpike   Waldwick, NJ 07463   (201)445-4822   Fax (201)447-5053

DeGroote, Richard J., MD {1104875947} Pedtrc(73,DC02)<NJ-MONMOUTH, NJ-JRSYSHMC>
+ Ocean Pediatric Group
  1 Industrial Way West/Suite 1-C   Eatontown, NJ 07724   (732)542-6451   Fax (732)542-1654
+ Ocean Pediatric Group
  2640 Route 70/Suite 1-B   Manasquan, NJ 08736   (732)542-6451   Fax (732)223-5792
+ Monmouth Family Center
  270 Broadway   Long Branch, NJ 07724   (732)923-7100   Fax (732)923-7104

DeGuzman, Richelle T., MD {1588641609} Anesth(72,PHI01)<NJ-CHRIST>
+ Christ Hospital
  176 Palisade Avenue/Anesthesiology   Jersey City, NJ 07306   (201)795-8310   Fax (201)943-8105

DeGuzman, Ronaldo Cruz, DO {1659478212} FamMed(94,NY75)<NJ-VIRTUAHS, NY-MTSINYHS>
+ Meetinghouse Family Physicians
  330 East Greentree Road   Marlton, NJ 08053   (856)596-9050   Fax (856)596-0320

Dehnert, Michele Chun, MD {1851533358} PedDvl
+ Center for Children with Special Needs
  953 Garfield Avenue   Jersey City, NJ 07304   (201)915-2059   Fax (201)915-2551

Deignan, Dianna T., MD {1841219359} FamMed, IntrMd(03,NJ06)
+ Cape Regional Physicians Associates
  211 North Main Street/Suite 203   Cape May Court House, NJ 08210   (609)536-8272   Fax (609)536-8273

Deingeniis-Depasquale, Antoinette M., DO {1922192517} FamMed(93,NY75)<NJ-STJOSHOS, NJ-WAYNEGEN>
+ Wayne Primary Care
  468 Parish Drive/Suite 1   Wayne, NJ 07470   (973)305-8300   Fax (973)305-8157

Deitch, Christopher William, MD {1528154903} Gastrn, IntrMd(93,PA09)
+ Cooper Digestive Health Institute
  501 Fellowship Road/Suite 101   Mount Laurel, NJ 08054   (856)642-2133   Fax (856)642-2134

Deitch, Edwin A., MD {1841218088} SrgCrC, Surgry(73,MD01)<NJ-UMDNJ>
+ University Hospital-Doctors Office Center
90 Bergen Street/DOC 7100   Newark, NJ 07103   (973)972-2400   Fax (973)972-2988

Deitz, Justina May, DO {1699922880} IntrMd, EnDbMt<NJ-ENGLWOOD, NJ-HOLYNAME>
+ Summit Medical Group
19-21 Fair Lawn Avenue   Fair Lawn, NJ 07410   (201)414-5095   Fax (201)414-5390
+ Bergen Medical Associates
466 Old Hook Road/Suite 1   Emerson, NJ 07630   (201)414-5095   Fax (201)967-0340
+ Bergen Medical Alliance, P.A.
180 Engle Street   Englewood, NJ 07410   (201)567-2050   Fax (201)568-8936

Deitz, Ruth Ellen Thisbe, MD {1114942836} FamMed(94,NY20)
+ Summit Medical Group-Berkeley Heights Campus
1 Diamond Hill Road   Berkeley Heights, NJ 07922   (908)277-8878   Fax (908)790-6576

Dejene, Brook A., MD {1013918416} SrgThr, Surgry(83,ETHI)<NJ-JRSYSHMC, NJ-MORRISTN>
+ Mid-Atlantic Surgical Associates
1944 Route 33/Suite 201   Neptune, NJ 07753   (732)776-4622   Fax (732)776-3765
+ Mid-Atlantic Surgical Associates
100 Madison Avenue   Morristown, NJ 07960   (732)776-4622   Fax (973)984-7019

Dejesus, Jennifer, MD {1710206818}(09,MNT01)
+ Riverside Medical Group
6045 Kennedy Boulevard/Suite A   North Bergen, NJ 07047   (201)861-4443   Fax (201)861-0941

Deka, Bharati, MD {1154520534} InfDis, IntrMd(90,INA18)
+ Drs. Deka and Ata
2090 State Route 27/Suite 101   North Brunswick, NJ 08902   (732)979-0035   Fax (908)829-4408

Dekermenjian, Rony, MD {1972766657} NrlgMusM
+ JFK Neurosciences Institute
65 James Street/Second Floor   Edison, NJ 08818   (732)321-7010   Fax (732)632-1669

Dekko, Samar, MD {1669766861} IntrMd<NJ-MORRISTN>
+ Morristown Medical Center
100 Madison Avenue   Morristown, NJ 07962   (973)971-5000   Fax (973)290-8325

Del Alcazar, Carlos O., MD {1255365912} IntrMd(82,NY01)<NJ-RWJUBRUN, NJ-RBAYOLDB>
+ Associates in Internal Medicine HealthCare Inc
1810 Englishtown Road   Old Bridge, NJ 08857   (732)416-6900   Fax (732)416-4823

Del Casale, Thomas Ernest, DO {1386683266} FamMed(86,NY75)
+ ImmediCenter/Clifton
1355 Broad Street   Clifton, NJ 07013   (973)778-5566   Fax (973)778-2268
+ ImmediCenter/Totowa
500 Union Boulevard   Totowa, NJ 07512   (973)778-5566   Fax (973)790-6070
+ ImmediCenter/Bloomfield
557 Broad Street   Bloomfield, NJ 07013   (973)680-8300   Fax (973)743-5601

Del Castillo, Luisa Rita, MD {1376549196} Pedtrc(82,DOM01)
+ Pediatric Health, P.A.
69 West Main Street   Freehold, NJ 07728   (732)409-3633   Fax (732)409-7133

Del Castillo, Ma Dolores, MD {1952741209} IntrMd<NJ-JRSYCITY>
+ Jersey City Medical Center
355 Grand Street   Jersey City, NJ 07304   (201)915-2000

Del Giorno, Joseph John, MD {1003871203} Pedtrc, IntrMd(98,PA02)<NJ-VIRTVOOR, NJ-VIRTUAHS>
+ Advocare DelGiorno Pediatrics
535 South Black Horse Pike   Blackwood, NJ 08012   (856)228-1061   Fax (856)228-1907
+ Advocare DelGiorno Pediatrics
412 Ewan Road   Mullica Hill, NJ 08062   (856)228-1061   Fax (856)343-3919

Del Giudice, Gina C., MD {1447292321} IntrMd, Rheuma(86,NY47)<NY-SPCLSURG, NJ-RWJUBRUN>
+ Rheumatology Center of Princeton
123 Franklin Corner Road/Suite 106   Lawrenceville, NJ 08648   (609)896-2505   Fax (609)896-2530

Del Monaco, Magaly Patricia, DO {1861567067} Dermat(92,PA77)<NJ-KMHSTRAT>
+ Academy Dermatology and Cosmetic Center
110 Marter Avenue/Suite 306   Moorestown, NJ 08057   (856)642-6450   Fax (856)642-6451

Del Moro, Ellen C., MD {1538137567} Pedtrc(00,PA09)<NJ-VIRTMHBC, NJ-VIRTUAHS>
+ Advocare Laurel Pediatrics
269 Fish Pond Road   Sewell, NJ 08080   (856)863-9999   Fax (856)863-9666

Del Negro, Ralph G., DO {1033297155} Ophthl(86,NJ75)<NJ-JRSYSHMC, NJ-RIVERVW>
+ Jersey Shore Eye Associates
1809 Corlies Avenue/Suite 1   Neptune City, NJ 07753   (732)774-5566   Fax (732)988-7574

Del Re, Sallustio, MD {1306802988} PulDis, CritCr, IntrMd(89,ITA22)<NJ-ACMCMAIN, NJ-SHOREMEM>
+ Shore Physicians Group
18 West New York Avenue   Somers Point, NJ 08244   (609)926-1450   Fax (609)926-8419
+ Atlantic Pulmonary & Critical Care Associates, P.A.
741 South Second Avenue/Suite A   Galloway, NJ 08205   (609)926-1450   Fax (609)748-7919

Del Rosario, Elizabeth C., MD {1316012578} ObsGyn, IntrMd(78,PHI30)
+ Hackensack University Medical Group Westwood
250 Old Hook Road   Westwood, NJ 07675   (201)781-1750   Fax (201)781-1753

Del Rosario, Michael Patrick, MD {1427158831} Surgry, SrgC&R(97,NY08)
+ 76 West Jimmie Leeds Road
Absecon, NJ 08205   (609)652-3655

Del Rosario Torres, Leonida, MD {1649356817} ObsGyn(63,PHI07)
+ Union Fertility Center
2166 Morris Avenue   Union, NJ 07083   (908)686-3933   Fax (908)686-3549

Del Rosario-Garcia, Mariza, MD {1245205491} Psychy(76,PHI01)<NJ-TRININPC, NJ-TRINIJSC>
+ Trinitas Regional Medical Center-New Point Campus
655 East Jersey Street   Elizabeth, NJ 07206   (908)994-5000

Del Valle, Francisco I., MD {1235126616} PhysMd, PainMd(86,PHI02)<NJ-BAYSHORE, NJ-CENTRAST>
+ HealthCare Pain and Rehabilitation
3 Hospital Plaza/Suite 309   Old Bridge, NJ 08857   (732)607-9000   Fax (732)607-7706

Del Valle, Heather Marie, DO {1164721908} IntrMd(10,NJ75)<NJ-MORRISTN>
+ Anesthesia Associates of Morristown
100 Madison Avenue   Morristown, NJ 07960   (973)971-5000

Del Valle, Jacqueline P., MD {1679560908} AnesPain, IntrMd(85,PHIL)
+ HealthCare Pain and Rehabilitation
3 Hospital Plaza/Suite 309   Old Bridge, NJ 08857   (732)607-9000   Fax (732)383-6026

Del Valle, Mario James, DO {1972698421} FamMed<PA-NZRTH>
+ 55 Corporate Drive/Mail Stop 55c-100a
Bridgewater, NJ 08807   (908)981-6925

Del Vento, Robert A., MD {1659438158} IntrMd(75,MEX03)<NJ-STBARNMC>
+ 81 Northfield Avenue
West Orange, NJ 07052   (973)736-1000   Fax (973)736-2166

Dela Cruz, Danna, MD {1689602369} IntrMd(95,PHI07)<NJ-COMMED>
+ Whiting Medical Associates
65 Lacey Road/Suite A   Whiting, NJ 08759   (732)350-0404   Fax (732)350-2001

Dela Cruz, Leo A., MD {1770662140} Psychy, PsyGrt, PssoMd(86,PHIL)<NJ-CHRIST, NJ-HOBUNIMC>
+ 142 Palisade Avenue/Suite 105
Jersey City, NJ 07306   (201)233-2447   Fax (201)792-8851
+ 395 Grand Street
Jersey City, NJ 07302   (201)233-2447   Fax (201)369-6301

Dela Gente, Robert Saladaga, DO {1891886230} FamMed(02,CA22)<NJ-STJOSHOS, NJ-WAYNEGEN>
+ North Jersey Family Medicine
19 Yawpo Avenue   Oakland, NJ 07436   (201)337-3412   Fax (201)337-3353

Dela Rosa, Aurora P., MD {1639149149} PhyMPain, Acpntr(73,PHI01)<NJ-RWJUHAM>
+ 1245 Whitehorse-Mercerville Rd
Hamilton, NJ 08619   (609)581-2700   Fax (609)581-2725

Dela Torre, Andrew Nelson, MD {1184659823} Surgry, SrgTpl(89,MD07)<NJ-STJOSHOS>
+ St. Joseph Medical Center Surgery
703 Main Street/Room A2404   Paterson, NJ 07503   (973)754-2315   Fax (973)754-3528

DeLaCalzada Jeanlouie, Mae Faye, DO {1275853897} EmrgMd
+ 60 Northfield Avenue
West Orange, NJ 07052

deLacy, Lee M., MD {1174576359} Gastrn(81,PA09)
+ Gastroenterology Consultants of South Jersey
693 Main Street/Suite 2   Lumberton, NJ 08048   (609)265-1700   Fax (609)265-9005
+ Burlington County Endoscopy Center
140 Mount Holly Bypass/Unit 5   Lumberton, NJ 08048   (609)267-1555

DeLago, Cynthia W., MD {1972573947} Pedtrc(86,PA02)<PA-ENSTEIN>
+ University Hospital-Cares Institute
42 East Laurel Road/Suite 1100   Stratford, NJ 08084   (856)566-7036   Fax (856)566-6108

Delaleu, Harold, MD {1073760039} Anesth<NJ-CHILTON>
+ Chilton Medical Center
97 West Parkway/Anesth   Pompton Plains, NJ 07444   (973)831-5000

Delaney, Beverly Renay, MD {1356376214} Psychy(85,NJ05)<NJ-UMDNJ, NJ-VAEASTOR>
+ VA New Jersey Health Care System-East Orange Campus
385 Tremont Avenue   East Orange, NJ 07018   (973)676-1000
+ University Psychiatric Associates
183 South Orange Avenue/E-F Levels   Newark, NJ 07103   (973)676-1000   Fax (973)972-2979

Delasotta, Fernando J., MD {1710051305} SrgNro(74,CHIL)<NJ-ACMCITY, NJ-SHOREMEM>
+ 598 New Road/PO Box 385
Linwood, NJ 08221   (609)927-1000   Fax (609)653-6852

Delavaux, Laurent, MD {1356684583} PhysMd<NJ-JFKJHNSN>
+ JFK Johnson Rehabilitation Institute
65 James Street   Edison, NJ 08818   (732)321-7070   Fax (732)321-7330

Delaverdac, Claude L., DO {1851438675} CdvDis, IntrMd(70,IL76)<NJ-ACMCMAIN>
+ Atlantic Internal Medicine PA
310 Chris Gaupp Drive/Suite 102   Galloway, NJ 08205   (609)652-9933   Fax (609)652-9955
+ AtlantiCare Regional Med Ctr/Mainland
65 West Jimmie Leeds Road   Pomona, NJ 08240   (609)652-1000

Delcurla, Gina M., DO {1275694358} FamMed(91,NJ75)
+ CentraState Family Medicine Residency Practice
1001 West Main Street/Suite B   Freehold, NJ 07728   (732)294-2540   Fax (732)294-9328

DeLeon, Edgardo S., MD {1316995392} Anesth(76,PHIL)<NJ-SJRSYELM>
+ SJH Elmer Hospital
501 West Front Street/Anesth   Elmer, NJ 08318   (856)363-1000

Deleon, Miguel L., MD {1104875400} SrgC&R, Surgry(75,PHIL)<NJ-VIRTUAHS, NJ-OURLADY>
+ Virtua Surgical Group, PA
1935 Route 70 East   Cherry Hill, NJ 08003   (856)428-7700   Fax (856)424-9120

DeLeon, Zorayda Olaya, MD {1023081338} IntrMd(86,PHI15)
+ Jae Medical Clinic
311 Palisade Avenue   Jersey City, NJ 07307   (201)963-5500   Fax (201)963-5563

Delev, Nikolay G., MD {1720277387}
+ 1712 Sun Valley
Florham Park, NJ 07932

Delfico, Anthony John, MD {1275535379} SrgOrt(92,NJ05)<NJ-VALLEY>
+ Ridgewood Orthopedic Group, LLC
85 South Maple Avenue   Ridgewood, NJ 07450   (201)445-2830   Fax (201)445-7471

Delgado, Jorge L., MD {1730227141} IntrMd, Gastrn(70,PER01)
+ 114 Elmora Avenue
Elizabeth, NJ 07202   (908)355-6122   Fax (908)355-9097
Delgadojorgeluismd@yahoo.com

Delgado, Mercedes, MD {1083646277} NnPnMd, Pedtrc(94,NJ06)<NJ-ENGLWOOD>
+ Englewood Hospital and Medical Center
350 Engle Street/Neo-Peri Med   Englewood, NJ 07631   (201)894-3000   Fax (201)569-5983

Delgado, Wilson Eduardo, MD {1275844516} Pedtrc
+ Riverside Pediatric Group
4201 New York Avenue   Union City, NJ 07087   (201)601-9515   Fax (201)601-9516

Delgaizo, Anthony, MD {1639192800} Urolgy(64,DC02)<NJ-CLARMAAS>
+ Urology Consultants, PA
36 Newark Avenue/Suite 200   Belleville, NJ 07109   (973)759-6950   Fax (973)759-2006

DelGiorno, Charles J., MD {1548455314} EnDbMt, IntrMd(06,PA02)
+ Advocare DelGiorno Endocrinology
239 Hurffville Crosskeys Road   Sewell, NJ 08080   (856)728-3636   Fax (856)728-3633

Delgiorno, John Michael, MD {1104970359} Pedtrc
+ Advocare DelGiorno Pediatrics
535 South Black Horse Pike   Blackwood, NJ 08012   (856)228-1061   Fax (856)228-1907

Delgra, Alexander B., MD {1154313526} IntrMd(80,PHI13)
+ Dr. Delgra Internal Medicine PC
5 Ravine Avenue   Nutley, NJ 07110   (973)429-0178   Fax (973)429-0297
drdelgra@aol.com

Delice, Anael Destin, Jr., DO {1851734669} FamMed
+ Health Med Associates, PC
24 South Carolina Avenue   Atlantic City, NJ 08401   (856)832-7145   Fax (609)345-2885

Physicians by Name and Address

Delio, Constance Mary, MD {1033284393} FamMed, IntrMd(98,NY48)
+ Medical Diagnostic Associates, P.A.
1801 East Second Street/Suite 1 Scotch Plains, NJ 07076 (908)322-7786 Fax (908)322-0191

Delis, Aristidis G., MD {1730373390} Anesth(04,IRE05)
+ Morris Anesthesia Group, PA
3799 Route 46/Suite 211 Parsippany, NJ 07054 (973)335-1122 Fax (973)335-1448

Delisa, Joel A., MD {1528147220} PhysMd(68,WA04)<NJ-UMDNJ>
+ University Hospital-Doctors Office Center
90 Bergen Street/DOC 3100 Newark, NJ 07103 (973)972-2802 Fax (973)972-2825

Delisfort, Guy J., MD {1407803539} Pedtrc(64,HAI01)<NJ-NWRK-BETH>
+ 815 South 12th Street
Newark, NJ 07108 (973)375-4479 Fax (973)375-3699

Delisi, Michael David, MD {1275575110} FamMed, Grtrcs(80,MEX14)<NJ-STJOSHOS>
+ St. Joseph's Family Medicine @ Clifton
1135 Broad Street/Suite 201 Clifton, NJ 07013 (973)754-4100 Fax (973)472-9062
+ St. Joseph's Regional Medical Center
703 Main Street/FamMed Paterson, NJ 07503 (973)754-2000

Deliwala, Tejas Pramodrai, MD {1881647188} ClNrPh(92,INA87)
+ Community Medical Center Department of Cardiology
20 Hospital Drive/Suite 1 Toms River, NJ 08755 (732)240-9222 Fax (732)240-5757

Deliz, Yasmin D., DO {1093040321} Pedtrc
+ Harborview KidsFirst Cape May
1315 Route 9 South Cape May Court House, NJ 08210 (609)465-6100 Fax (609)465-1539

Dell'Aquila, Paul V., MD {1275594707} IntrMd, Grtrcs(86,MEX14)<NJ-STBARNMC, NJ-CLARMAAS>
+ 339 Passaic Avenue
Nutley, NJ 07110 (973)542-2880 Fax (973)542-2881

Della Bella, Peter, MD {1235329103} PsyCAd(88,NY06)
+ 210 Bellevue Avenue/2 nd Floor
Montclair, NJ 07043

Della Croce, David R., DO PthACl, Pthlgy(72,MO78)
+ 311 Red Lion Road
Southampton, NJ 08088

Della Peruta, Joseph, MD {1912915497} Radiol, RadDia(93,NY47)<NJ-OURLADY, NJ-LOURDMED>
+ Lourdes Imaging Associates, PA
1600 Haddon Avenue Camden, NJ 08103 (856)635-2654 Fax (856)668-8436
+ Lourdes Imaging Associates, PA
218-A Sunset Road Willingboro, NJ 08046 (856)635-2654 Fax (609)835-3190

Della Torre, Kara E., MD {1649491978} Ophthl
+ 620 North Broad Street
Woodbury, NJ 08096 (856)853-5554 Fax (856)853-5650

Dellacroce, Joseph Michael, MD {1780677567} Surgry, SrgVas, IntrMd(84,PA02)<NJ-CHSMRCER>
+ Doctors Dellacroce and Lee
2 Capital Way/Suite 390 Pennington, NJ 08534 (609)818-0040 Fax (609)818-0049

Dellapi, Andrew Thomas, MD {1619935160} EmrgMd(94,NJ05)<NJ-CHILTON>
+ Chilton Medical Center
97 West Parkway/EmrgMed Pompton Plains, NJ 07444 (973)831-5000 Fax (973)831-5443
+ The Doctor's Office New Jersey Urgent Care
85 Godwin Avenue Midland Park, NJ 07432 (973)831-5000 Fax (201)857-8406

Dellavalle, Lindsay Joy, DO {1154529220} FamMed
+ Pleasant Run Family Physicians
925 US Highway 202 Neshanic Station, NJ 08853 (908)788-9468 Fax (908)788-5720

Dellinger, Richard Phillip, MD {1336246453} CritCr, IntrMd(75,SC01)<NJ-COOPRUMC>
+ Cooper University Hospital
One Cooper Plaza/Critical Care Camden, NJ 08103 (856)342-2000

Dello Russo, Jeffrey, MD {1912011826} Ophthl(98,NY09)
+ The New Jersey Eye Center
1 North Washington Avenue Bergenfield, NJ 07621 (201)384-7333 Fax (201)384-2564

Dellorso, John, MD {1013952332} IntrMd, OccpMd, OthrSp(83,ITAL)<NJ-NWRKBETH>
+ Newark International Airport
Newark Airport/Medical Offices/Bld 339 Newark, NJ 07102 (973)643-8383 Fax (973)643-4744

DelMaestro, Steven R., MD {1851442206} IntrMd(81,MEXI)
+ RWJPE Franklin Internal Medicine
454 Elizabeth Avenue/Suite 210 Somerset, NJ 08873 (908)685-2526 Fax (908)685-2527

Delmonico, Gerard J., MD {1184683690} FamMed(85,WIND)<NJ-WARREN>
+ Village Medical Center
207 Strykers Road Phillipsburg, NJ 08865 (908)859-6568 Fax (908)859-6697

Delong, Donald H., II, MD {1841261609} Anesth(67,NY19)<NJ-NWTNMEM>
+ Newton Medical Center
175 High Street/Anesthesiology Newton, NJ 07860 (973)579-8525 Fax (973)383-9475
dhdiiwj@EMBARQMAIL.com
+ 355 Ridge Road
Newton, NJ 07860 (973)579-8525 Fax (973)383-6341

DeLorenzo, Arthur J., MD {1093754277} Pedtrc(80,MEX03)<NJ-STBARNMC>
+ 616 Bloomfield Avenue/Suite 1A
West Caldwell, NJ 07006 (973)226-4439 Fax (973)226-4452
drcarea2z@verizon.net

DeLorio, Nicola Anne, DO Otlryg, Rhinol(93,NJ75)<NJ-BURDTMLN, NJ-SHOREMEM>
+ Drs. Matlick, DeLorio, and Mucci
307 Stone Harbor Boulevard/Suite 3 Cape May Court House, NJ 08210 (609)465-4667 Fax (609)465-9387
+ Court House Surgery Center
106 Courthouse South Dennis Rd Cape May, NJ 08204 (609)465-4667 Fax (609)465-8771

Delphin, Ellise S., MD {1437181997} Anesth, Pedtrc(75,NY01)<NJ-UMDNJ>
+ University Hospital
150 Bergen Street/Anesth Newark, NJ 07103 (973)972-5006 Fax (973)972-4172

Delsardo, Anthony C., MD {1154308203} IntrMd(74,MEX14)<NJ-NWTNMEM>
+ Premier Health Associates
123 Newton Sparta Road Newton, NJ 07860 (973)579-6300 Fax (973)579-1524

Delston, Damon D., MD {1720297963} Psychy(79,BEL07)
+ 665 Newark Avenue
Jersey City, NJ 07306 (201)963-9331 Fax (212)581-9860
damondelston@hotmail.com

Deltieure, Michele H., MD {1821241779} OccpMd, IntrMd(84,DMN01)
+ E. I. Dupont
250 Cheesequake Road Parlin, NJ 08859 (732)613-2140
MDsquared@att.net

DeLuca, Alison Kay, MD {1457507022} Psychy(04,PA12)<NJ-UNIVBHC>
+ University Behavioral Health Care
671 Hoes Lane/PO Box 1392/Psych Piscataway, NJ 08855 (732)235-5500

DeLuca, Debra J., MD {1669423463} Nrolgy, SlpDis(80,OH41)<NJ-CHSMRCER, NJ-CHSFULD>
+ Mercer Neurology
2 Princess Road/Suite 2F Lawrenceville, NJ 08648 (609)895-9000 Fax (609)895-1006
+ Snoring and Sleep Apnea Center Mercer County
1401 Whitehorse Mercerville Rd Hamilton, NJ 08619 (609)895-9000 Fax (609)584-5144

DeLuca, Francis N., MD {1669449344} SrgOrt(71,PA09)
+ Orthopedic Surgical Associates
33 Overlook Road/Suite 201 Summit, NJ 07901 (908)522-4555 Fax (908)522-1128

DeLuca, Joseph A., MD {1205916509} Ophthl(85,NJ06)<NJ-CLARMAAS>
+ 20 Park Avenue/Suite 1A
Lyndhurst, NJ 07071 (201)896-0096 Fax (201)896-0062
+ Eye Institute of Essex, PA
5 Franklin Avenue/Suite 209 Belleville, NJ 07109 (201)896-0096 Fax (973)450-1464

Deluca, Matthew J., MD {1982680302} Nrolgy(79,MEXI)<NJ-CLARMAAS, NJ-MTNSIDE>
+ 36 Newark Avenue/Suite 326
Belleville, NJ 07109 (973)450-0444 Fax (973)566-0303
+ 1600 Saint Georges Avenue/Suite 116
Rahway, NJ 07065 (973)450-0444 Fax (732)396-1588

DeLuca, Peter Francis, MD {1013954262} SrgOrt(86,DC02)<NJ-VIRTUAHS, NJ-ATLANTHS>
+ Rothman Institute - Voorhees
443 Laurel Oak Road Voorhees, NJ 08043 (856)821-6360
+ Rothman Institute-The Performance Lab
2005 Route 7 East Cherry Hill, NJ 08003 Fax (856)874-1188

Deluca, Samantha, DO {1871525188} ObsGyn(99,PA77)<NJ-VIRTMHBC>
+ Pinelands Obstetrics and Gynecology
1617 Route 38 Mount Holly, NJ 08060 (609)261-0240 Fax (609)261-8622

DeLucia, Carolyn Ann, MD {1346288685} Gyneco(88,NY09)
+ 349 Rt 206 and Doctors Way/Bld. B
Hillsborough, NJ 08844

DeLue, Erik Nathaniel, MD {1134166937} IntHos(97,OH43)<NJ-VIRTMHBC>
+ Virtua Hospitalist Group Memorial
175 Madison Avenue Mount Holly, NJ 08060 (609)267-0700 Fax (856)355-0346

Deluty, Sheldon H., MD {1871595314} Anesth(81,NY01)<NY-BLVUENYU, NY-NYUTISCH>
+ PO Box 5513
Englewood, NJ 07631 (917)279-3383 Fax (201)569-8878
mdshd@earthlink.net

Deluzio, Antonio John, DO {1992701585} PthACl(97,MO78)
+ 10 Longview Drive
Bordentown, NJ 08505

Delvadia, Dipak R., DO {1386624773} ObsGyn(90,IL76)<NJ-JFKMED, NJ-KENEDYHS>
+ Drexel University Physicians
400 East Church Street Blackwood, NJ 08012 (856)228-8066

Delvalle, Yissell, MD {1750585709} Psychy
+ Santana, Yissell
235 Vernon Avenue Paterson, NJ 07503

Delvecchio, Joanna Catherine, MD {1700144094} EmrgMd<NJ-COOPRUMC>
+ Cooper University Hospital
One Cooper Plaza/EmergMed Camden, NJ 08103 (856)342-2006

Delvers, Dilek Sunay, MD {1881620631} FamMed(87,MNT01)
+ Hunterdon Developmental Center
40 Pittstown Road/PO Box 4003/Ext 1070 Clinton, NJ 08809 (908)735-4031 Fax (908)730-1338
Dilek.delvers@dhs.nj.us

Demangone, Dawn Adele, MD {1194761114} EmrgMd(93,PA02)
+ 143 Renaissanre Drive
Cherry Hill, NJ 08003

Demario, Irena Lisa, DO {1538502075}<NJ-STBARNMC>
+ St. Barnabas Medical Center
94 Old Short Hills Road Livingston, NJ 07039 (973)322-5000

Demartin, Robert, MD {1043260870} IntrMd(86,COLO)<NJ-OCEANMC, NJ-JRSYSHMC>
+ 1330 Laurel Avenue/Suite 201
Sea Girt, NJ 08750 (732)449-6681

Demauro, Linda Dell, MD RadDia(78,MEXI)
+ 888 Hilltop Terrace
Franklin Lakes, NJ 07417

Dembner, Alan G., MD {1487681649} RadDia(73,MA07)<NJ-STBARNMC>
+ St. Barnabas Medical Center
94 Old Short Hills Road/DiagRad Livingston, NJ 07039 (973)322-5804
ADEMBNER@sbhcs.com
+ St. Barnabas Ambulatory Care Center
200 South Orange Avenue/DiagRad Livingston, NJ 07039 (973)322-7700

Demchuk, Beverly Jean, MD {1932922554} IntrMd, IntCrd, Cd-vDis(86,BC01)
+ American Heart Center PC
1900 Corlies Avenue State Rout Neptune, NJ 07753 (732)663-1123 Fax (732)663-1179

Dementyeva, Yuliya, MD {1811192255} Psychy, PssoMd, Psy-Grt(94,BLA02)<NJ-STJOSHOS>
+ St. Joseph's Regional Medical Center
703 Main Street/Psych Paterson, NJ 07503 (973)754-3298

DeMercurio, Robert Edward, DO {1992833396} Psychy(94,MI12)
+ Hampton Behavioral Health Center
650 Rancocas Road Westampton, NJ 08060 (609)267-7000

Demeritt, John S., III, MD {1275518532} Radiol, RadNro(86,NY45)<NJ-HACKNSK>
+ The Imaging Center
30 South Newman Street Hackensack, NJ 07601 (201)996-2200 Fax (201)489-2812
+ New Century Imaging at Oradell
555 Kinderkamack Road Oradell, NJ 07649 (201)996-2200 Fax (201)599-8333
+ Hackensack Radiology Group, P.A.
30 Prospect Avenue Hackensack, NJ 07601 (201)996-2200 Fax (201)336-8451

Demesmin, Didier, MD {1336170216} PainInvt, Anesth, PainMd(00,NJ06)<NJ-STPETER, NJ-RWJUBRUN>
+ University Pain Medicine Center
33 Clyde Road/Suite 105 & 106 Somerset, NJ 08873 (732)875-3033 Fax (732)873-6869
+ University Pain Medicine Center
111 Union Valley Road/Suite 202 Monroe, NJ 08831 (732)875-3033 Fax (732)873-6869
+ Raritan Valley Surgery Center
100 Franklin Square Drive/Suite 100 Somerset, NJ 08873 (732)828-1003 Fax (732)560-5999

Demetriades, Haralambos, MD {1730148719} SrgOrt, SrgSpn(93,NY47)<NJ-OCEANMC, NJ-JRSYSHMC>
+ Seaview Orthopaedics
1200 Eagle Avenue   Ocean, NJ 07712   (732)660-6200   Fax (732)660-6201
+ Seaview Orthopaedics
1640 Route 88 West   Brick, NJ 08724   (732)660-6200   Fax (732)458-2743
+ Seaview Orthopaedics
222 Schanck Road/3rd Floor   Freehold, NJ 07712   (732)462-1700   Fax (732)303-8314

Demidowich, George, MD {1679594923} CdvDis, IntrMd(75,NY09)
+ Cardiovascular Consultants of New Jersey
340 East Northfield Road   Livingston, NJ 07039   (973)994-0880   Fax (973)994-9408

DeMilio, Lawrence T., MD {1588783237} Psychy, PsyCAd, Nrolgy(76,NY09)
+ 10 Fairmount Avenue/Suite 2
Chatham, NJ 07928

Demoll, Ashleigh, DO {1598184806}<NJ-SJHREGMC>
+ SJH Regional Medical Center
1505 West Sherman Avenue   Vineland, NJ 08360   (240)409-4208

Demos, James P., MD {1457353872} IntrMd(83,DMN01)<NJ-RWJUBRUN, NJ-STPETER>
+ Old Bridge Primary Care
300 Perrine Road/Suite 324   Old Bridge, NJ 08857   (732)753-9890   Fax (732)753-9893

DeMoss, Jeanne Lorraine, DO {1245263144} IntrMd(90,NJ75)
+ Cardiology Associates of New Brunswick
593 Cranbury Road/Suite 2   East Brunswick, NJ 08816   (732)390-3333   Fax (732)390-9244

DeMuro, Paul G., Jr., DO {1992883235} FamMed(79,MO79)<NJ-STMRYPAS>
+ 338 Chestnut Street
Passaic, NJ 07055   (973)471-9494   Fax (973)778-4649

Demyen, Michael Frank, MD {1568611465} IntrMd, Gastrn(00,NJ06)
+ UMDNJ Division of Gastroenterology & Hepatology
90 Bergen Street/DOC 2100   Newark, NJ 07103   (973)972-2343   Fax (973)972-0752
+ 904 Jefferson Street/Unit 3 G, Suite 2
Hoboken, NJ 07030   (973)989-0800

Denbo, Nancy J., MD {1750545752} PsyCAd, Psychy(NY09)
+ 412 Kings Croft
Cherry Hill, NJ 08034   (856)482-8493

Denbow, Frank Alstein, MD {1063641975} IntrMd(81,IRE01)
+ Executive Health Group, Inc.
44 Whippany Road   Morristown, NJ 07960   (973)540-0177   Fax (973)984-9351

Dendrinos, George Aristidis, MD {1982776118} FamMed(95,DMN01)<NJ-SJERSYHS>
+ Excelcare Alliance, LLC
2020 East Chestnut Avenue   Vineland, NJ 08361   (856)563-1600   Fax (856)563-1212

Denehy, Ann Smith, MD   Radiol(92,CT01)
+ Montclair Radiology
20 High Street   Nutley, NJ 07110   (973)284-1881   Fax (973)284-0269

Denehy, Thad R., MD {1912904756} GynOnc, SrgGyn, ObsGyn(84,NC05)<NJ-STBARNMC, NJ-MORRISTN>
+ Gynecologic Cancer and Pelvic Surgery, LLC
101 Old Short Hills Road/Suite 400   West Orange, NJ 07052   (973)243-9300   Fax (973)325-8254

Denenberg, Howard W., MD {1992841548} Anesth(86,MA05)<NJ-RWJUBRUN>
+ Robert Wood Johnson-UMDNJ Anesthesia Group
125 Paterson Street/CAB 3100   New Brunswick, NJ 08901   (732)235-7827   Fax (732)235-6131
+ Robert Wood Johnson-UMDNJ Anesthesia Group
1140 Route 72 West   Manahawkin, NJ 08050   (609)978-8900

DeNeve, Albert A., MD {1558453498} OncHem, IntrMd(83,KORE)<NJ-VALLEY>
+ 143 East Ridgewood Avenue/Suite 539
Ridgewood, NJ 07451   (201)251-9030   Fax (201)251-9032
+ 1 Demercurio Drive/Suite 3
Allendale, NJ 07401   (201)251-9030   Fax (201)251-9032

Deng, Yingzi, MD {1346689403} IntrMd<NJ-STPETER>
+ Cooper Primary Care
390 North Broadway/Suite 100   Pennsville, NJ 08070   (856)678-6411   Fax (856)678-7509

Dengrove, Robert S., MD {1780722421} PsyFor, Psychy(74,NJ05)
+ 541 North Edgemere Drive
Allenhurst, NJ 07711   (732)531-8100   Fax (732)531-8133

Denick, Kimberly Keane, MD {1124082508} Pedtrc, IntrMd(93,PA13)<NJ-VIRTUAHS, NJ-COOPRUMC>
+ Advocare The Farm Pediatrics
975 Tuckerton Road/Suite 100   Marlton, NJ 08053   (856)983-6190   Fax (856)983-3805

+ Advocare The Farm Pediatrics
1001 Laurel Oak Boulevard/Suite B   Voorhees, NJ 08043   (856)983-6190   Fax (856)782-7404

DeNicola, Nancy Ann, DO {1568450690} Pedtrc
+ Childrens Health Center
2139 State Route 35   Holmdel, NJ 07733   (732)264-6070   Fax (732)264-6076

Deniro, Lauren Victoria, MD {1518255181}(10,DC02)<NY-MNTF-MOSE>
+ Bergen Neurology Consultants
25 Rockwood Place/Suite 110   Englewood, NJ 07631   (201)894-5805   Fax (201)894-1956

Denis, Frantz, MD {1457518615} ObsGyn(89,NY09)
+ American Women's Services - Voorhees
1 Alpha Avenue/Suite 27   Voorhees, NJ 08043   (856)427-6245   Fax (856)427-6952

Denis, Joanna M., MD {1528129475} IntrMd(90,POL02)<NJ-BAYSHORE, NJ-MORRISTN>
+ 1145 Bordentown Avenue/Suite 4
Parlin, NJ 08859   (732)553-1901
+ 415 Parsippany Road
Parsippany, NJ 07054   (732)553-1901   Fax (973)560-9166

DeNittis, Albert Stephen, MD {1134129349} RadOnc(95,NJ05)
+ 5 St. James Gate
Medford, NJ 08055

Denker, Michael, MD {1164417580} IntrMd(82,ROM01)<NJ-HACKNSK, NJ-HOLYNAME>
+ Wilton Internal Medicine
751 Teaneck Road   Teaneck, NJ 07666   (201)837-3200   Fax (201)837-8993

Denley, Ryan Christopher, DO {1386038560}<NJ-MORRISTN>
+ Morristown Medical Center
100 Madison Avenue   Morristown, NJ 07962   (973)971-5000

Denner, Michael J., MD {1528154077} Nrolgy(79,NJ05)
+ Woodbury Neurology Associates
17 West Red Bank Avenue/Suite 204   Woodbury, NJ 08096   (856)853-1133   Fax (856)845-5405

Dennis, Charles A., MD {1669436127} CdvDis, IntCrd, IntrMd(79,AZ01)<NJ-DEBRAHLC>
+ The Cardiology Group, P.A.
401 Young Avenue/Suite 275   Moorestown, NJ 08057   (856)291-8855   Fax (856)291-8844   cdennis51@comcast.net
+ The Cardiology Group, P.A.
128 State Highway Route 70/Suite 1-B   Medford, NJ 08055   (856)291-8855   Fax (609)444-5521

Dennis, Elaine Debra, MD {1356368971} EmrgMd(97,NY47)
+ Family Walk-in LLC
4013 Route 9 North/suite 1-N   Howell, NJ 07731   (732)905-5255   Fax (732)905-5266

Dennis, Philip S., MD {1942391313} FamMed(01,GRN01)
+ 17 Casino Drive
Farmingdale, NJ 07727   Fax (732)256-4281

Dennis, Robert I., MD {1437220159} SrgOrt(71,PA13)<NJ-JRSYSHMC>
+ Robert I. Dennis MD PA
2040 Sixth Avenue/Suite 1/Door B   Neptune, NJ 07753   (732)775-5189   Fax (732)775-3065

Dennison, Alan D., MD {1033216163} FamMed(77,PA09)
+ Cooper Family Medicine
110 Marter Avenue   Moorestown, NJ 08057   (856)608-8840   Fax (856)722-1898
+ Cooper Family Medicine
1001-F Lincoln Drive West   Marlton, NJ 08053   (856)608-8840   Fax (856)810-1879

Denniston, Robert B., MD {1740215144} IntrMd(72,SC01)
+ 120 Madison Avenue
Mount Holly, NJ 08060   (609)261-1144   Fax (609)267-4399
+ One Sheffield Drive/Suite 101
Columbus, NJ 08022   (609)949-9092

Denny, Ashleigh, MD {1376801134} ObsGyn
+ Cherry Hill Ob/Gyn
150 Century Parkway/Suite A   Mount Laurel, NJ 08054   (856)778-4700   Fax (856)222-0482

Denny, Donald, Jr., MD {1184657975} RadDia, RadV&I(78,PA09)<NJ-UNVMCPRN>
+ Princeton Radiology Associates, P.A.
253 Witherspoon Street   Princeton, NJ 08540   (609)497-4310   Fax (609)497-4989   ddennyjr@nerc.com
+ Princeton Radiology Associates, P.A.
419 North Harrison Street   Princeton, NJ 08540   (609)497-4310   Fax (609)683-8847
+ Princeton Radiology Associates, P.A.
9 Centre Drive   Jamesburg, NJ 08540   (609)655-1448   Fax (609)655-4016

Denny, John T., MD {1982786067} Anesth, CritCr, OthrSp(88,WI05)<NJ-RWJUBRUN>
+ Robert Wood Johnson-UMDNJ Anesthesia Group
125 Paterson Street/CAB 3100   New Brunswick, NJ 08901   (732)937-8841   Fax (732)235-6131

Denoble, Peter Hart, MD {1285947689} OrtSHand(05,MA16)
+ Advanced Orthopedics & Hand Surgery Institute
504 Valley Road/Suite 201   Wayne, NJ 07470   (973)942-1315   Fax (973)942-8724

DeNoble, Shaghayegh Moghaddam, MD {1770726564} ObsGyn(05,MA16)<NJ-CHILTON>
+ Advanced Gynecology and Laparoscopy of North Jersey
20 Wilsey Square/Suite C   Ridgewood, NJ 07450   (201)957-7220   Fax (201)977-6747   info@advancedgynnj.com

Denson, H. Mark, MD {1184789562} CdvDis, IntrMd(83,PA14)<NJ-HACKNSK>
+ Cardiac Medical Associates PA
920 Main Street   Hackensack, NJ 07601   (201)342-7733   Fax (201)342-7998

Dent, Dean A., MD {1265413785} Anesth(78,DC01)
+ 3 Bell Aire Court
Denville, NJ 07834

Denysenko, Lex, MD {1871737759} Psychy, IntrMd<NJ-KMHCHRRY, NJ-KMHTURNV>
+ University Hospital-SOM Department of Psychiatry
2250 Chapel Avenue West/Suite 100   Cherry Hill, NJ 08002   (856)482-9000   Fax (856)482-1159

Deora-Bhens, Sonia, DO {1235134297} FamMAdlt, FamMed(97,NJ75)<NJ-JFKMED>
+ Garden State Physicians P.C.
21 Jefferson Plaza   Princeton, NJ 08540   (732)274-1274   Fax (732)355-0321
+ Garden State Physicians P.C.
1002 Amboy Avenue   Edison, NJ 08837   (732)274-1274   Fax (732)355-0321
+ Garden State Physicians P.C.
10 Jefferson Plaza/Suite 100   Princeton, NJ 08540   (732)274-1274   Fax (732)355-0321

DePace, Nicholas L., MD {1467496687} CdvDis(78,NY47)
+ 438 Ganttown Road/Suite B8-B9
Sewell, NJ 08080   (856)589-6034   Fax (856)589-6036

DePalma, John Anthony, DO {1407054471} Nephro, IntrMd(06,PA77)
+ Ocean Renal Associates, P.A.
1617 Route 88 West/Suite 101   Brick, NJ 08724   (732)458-5854   Fax (732)458-8012

DePaola, Frederick A., MD {1538156815} SrgOrt(83,WIND)<NJ-JRSYSHMC>
+ 2444 Route 34 North
Manasquan, NJ 08736   (732)528-4407   Fax (732)528-4525

DePasquale, Joseph R., MD {1194796953} Gastrn, IntrMd(83,ITA07)<NJ-MTNSIDE>
+ North Jersey Gastroenterology Associates PA
741 Northfield Avenue/Suite 101   West Orange, NJ 07052   (973)736-1991   Fax (973)736-9377
+ North Jersey Gastroenterology Associates PA
5 Franklin Avenue/Suite 109   Belleville, NJ 07109   (973)736-1991   Fax (973)759-7243

DePass, Lorraine Francis, MD {1194738203} FamMed(95,DC03)<NJ-CHSFULD>
+ Family Care of Somerset, LLC.
80 North Gaston Avenue   Somerville, NJ 08876   (908)218-1121   Fax (908)253-9031
+ Complete Care
1814 East Second Street   Scotch Plains, NJ 07076   (908)218-1121   Fax (908)322-8665

DePerio, Alicia G., MD {1578535035} Pedtrc(80,PHI01)
+ 4679 US Highway 9
Howell, NJ 07731   (732)905-9505   Fax (732)905-2448

DePerio, Elizabeth P., MD {1033138540} IntrMd(87,PHI09)<NJ-JRSYSHMC, NJ-KIMBALL>
+ 4677 US Highway 9
Howell, NJ 07731   (732)901-4080

Depersia, Lori Angela, MD {1295727352} RadDia, Radiol(81,PA02)
+ Radiology Associates of New Jersey
2201 Chapel Avenue West/Suite 106   Cherry Hill, NJ 08002   (856)488-6844   Fax (856)488-6507

Dephillips, Donna M., MD {1386657971} PhysMd, PhyMPain(93,NY09)
+ 7 Westminster Place
Old Tappan, NJ 07675   (201)666-5564

DePietro, Joseph Anthony, MD {1770798092} FamMed, GPrvMd(76,MEX03)
+ 86 Radcliffe Drive
Lincroft, NJ 07738

Deramo, David Michael, MD {1063562445} SprtMd, SrgOrt(01,NJ05)<NJ-OVERLOOK>
+ Englewood Knee & Sports Medicine
370 Grand Avenue/Suite 100   Englewood, NJ 07631   (201)567-5700   Fax (201)567-8049

Physicians by Name and Address

DeRemigio, David Michael, DO {1316921489} Anesth(90,NJ75)<NJ-HACKNSK>
+ Hackensack University Medical Center
30 Prospect Avenue/Anesth   Hackensack, NJ 07601   (201)996-2000
+ Hackensack University MC-Anesthesia Dept
30 Prospect Avenue/Room 2703   Hackensack, NJ 07601   (201)996-2000   Fax (201)996-3962

DeRespinis, Patrick A., MD {1144282997} Ophthl, PedOph(80,MEXI)<NY-CMCSTVSI, NY-STATNRTH>
+ University Hospital-Doctors Office Center
90 Bergen Street/Ophthl/6th Floo   Newark, NJ 07103   (973)972-2065
+ Pediatric Eye Care of Monmouth, LLC
33 Village Court   Hazlet, NJ 07730   (973)972-2065   Fax (732)217-3504

DeRisio, Vincent James, II, DO {1427538701} PthAcl(82,NY75)
+ University Hospital-Cares Institute
42 East Laurel Road/Suite 1100   Stratford, NJ 08084   (856)566-7036   Fax (856)566-6108

Derivaux, Christopher Charles, MD {1790733004} SrgCTh, Surgry, SrgCrC(93,NJ02)<NJ-OURLADY, NJ-VIRTUAHS>
+ Virtua Surgical Group, PA
1935 Route 70 East   Cherry Hill, NJ 08003   (856)428-7700   Fax (856)424-9120

Derman, Arnold, MD {1275515504} RadDia(63,NY15)<NJ-RBAYPERT, NJ-RBAYOLDB>
+ University Radiology Group, P.C.
483 Cranbury Road   East Brunswick, NJ 08816   (732)390-0030   Fax (732)390-5383
+ University Radiology Group, P.C.
3 Hospital Plaza/Suite LL-4   Old Bridge, NJ 08857   (732)390-0030   Fax (732)360-2828
+ University Radiology Group, P.C.
579A Cranbury Road   East Brunswick, NJ 08816   (732)390-0040   Fax (732)390-1856

Derman, Seth G., MD {1093715161} RprEnd, FrtInf, ObsGyn(88,PA12)<NJ-UNVMCPRN, NJ-CHSMRCER>
+ Princeton IVF
2 Princess Road/Suite C   Lawrenceville, NJ 08648   (609)896-4984   Fax (609)896-3266
fertilmd@aol.com
+ Delaware Valley Ob/Gyn & Infertility Group, PC
300B Princeton Hightstown Road   East Windsor, NJ 08520   (609)896-4984   Fax (609)443-4506

Dermendjian, Mariette, MD {1194745968} NnPnMd, Pedtrc(84,LEB03)<NJ-CHDNWBTH, NJ-UMDNJ>
+ Children's Hospital of New Jersey
201 Lyons Avenue/Osborne Terrace   Newark, NJ 07112   (973)926-7203

Dermer, Alicia R., MD {1316058852} FamMed(77,ON01)
+ CentraState Family Medicine Residency Practice
1001 West Main Street/Suite B   Freehold, NJ 07728   (732)294-2540   Fax (732)294-9328

DeRosa, William T., DO {1902894991} OncHem(80,MO79)<NJ-MORRISTN>
+ Summit Medical Group Florham Park Campus
150 Park Avenue/3rd FL   Florham Park, NJ 07932   (973)538-5210

Derr, Lisa M., DO {1124218540} Surgry(NJ75}
+ LMA Surgical Associates
120 White Horse Pike/Suite 103   Haddon Heights, NJ 08035   (856)546-3900   Fax (856)546-3908

Dershem, Jonel M., MD {1003988403} ObsGyn(91,PA02)<NJ-VIRTVOOR>
+ Women's Group for OB/GYN
2301 Evesham Road/Pav 800/Suite 122   Voorhees, NJ 08043   (856)770-9300   Fax (856)770-9518

Desai, Aaditya A., DO {1053517268} EmrgMd(03,IL76)<NJ-RIVERVW>
+ Riverview Medical Center
1 Riverview Plaza/EmrgMed   Red Bank, NJ 07701   (732)530-2204
+ St Joseph's Medical Center Emergency
703 Main Street   Paterson, NJ 07503   (732)530-2204   Fax (973)754-2249

Desai, Aashish P., MD {1992016125} FamMed, IntrMd
+ New Jersey Doctors Urgent Care
620 Route 23 North   Pompton Plains, NJ 07444   (973)530-4362
adesai76@gmail.com

Desai, Ajay Kishor, DO {1295962462} PedEmg<PA-STCHRIS, PA-CHILDHOS>
+ CHOP Care Network at Virtua Voorhees Hospital
100 Bowman Drive   Voorhees, NJ 08043   (856)325-3000   Fax (609)261-5842

Desai, Akhilesh S., MD {1043287402} RadDia(70,INA21)
+ Advanced Open MRI and Diagnostic Imaging
751 Highway 37 West   Toms River, NJ 08755   (732)240-7756   Fax (732)240-7761

Desai, Amee B., MD {1063570299} IntrMd
+ 850 West Bay Avenue
Barnegat, NJ 08005

Desai, Amita Jayantilal, MD {1780685362} IntrMd, InfDis(83,NY09)<NJ-HOLYNAME>
+ Holy Name Hospital
718 Teaneck Road   Teaneck, NJ 07666   (201)833-3000

Desai, Amita S., MD {1477600971} Psychy, IntrMd(81,INA65)<NJ-ANCPSYCH>
+ Ancora Psychiatric Hospital
301 Spring Garden Road   Hammonton, NJ 08037   (609)561-1700

Desai, Anagha Kishor, MD {1023306495} ObsGyn
+ Southern Jersey Family Medical Centers Inc.
932 South Main Street   Pleasantville, NJ 08232   (609)383-0880   Fax (609)383-0658

Desai, Anil G., MD {1639177504} NuclMd, Radiol, RadV&I(72,INA21)
+ South Jersey Radiology Associates, P.A.
Severan Profess Mews/Suite 105   Sewell, NJ 08080   (856)848-4998   Fax (856)589-6142
+ South Jersey Radiology Associates, P.A.
748 Kings Highway   West Deptford, NJ 08096   (856)848-4998   Fax (856)853-7362
+ South Jersey Radiology Associates, P.A.
807 Haddon Avenue/Suite 5   Haddonfield, NJ 08080   (856)616-1130   Fax (856)616-1125

Desai, Anjali Ashok, MD {1225137797} IntrMd(01,NY08)
+ Cooper Physicians Office
196 Grove Avenue/Suite C   Thorofare, NJ 08086   (856)848-7577   Fax (856)848-6554

Desai, Ankur Akhilesh, MD {1568545846} PsyCAd, Psychy(01,MA07)<NJ-CENTRAST>
+ CentraState Medical Center
901 West Main Street/Bldg/A Suite367   Freehold, NJ 07728   (732)637-6323   Fax (732)845-5407

Desai, Aruna A., MD {1518985795} Acpntr, Anesth, PainMd(65,INA65)
+ Advanced Pain Control Ctr, PC
300 Winston Drive/Apt 1621   Cliffside Park, NJ 07010

Desai, Avani Mahesh, MD {1669817433} IntrMd(NJ06<NY-MTSI-NAI, NY-MTSINYHS>
+ UH-RWJ General Internal Medicine
125 Paterson Street/Suite 2300   New Brunswick, NJ 08901   (732)235-7112   Fax (732)235-7144

Desai, Bankimchandra D., MD {1780618868} GenPrc, IntrMd(79,INA53)<NJ-BAYONNE>
+ Bayonne Medical Center
29th Street at Avenue E   Bayonne, NJ 07002   (201)858-5000

Desai, Bharat V., MD {1992701189} IntrMd(70,INA21)<NJ-RWJUHAM, NJ-STLAWRN>
+ Drs. Desai & Yanamadula
123 Franklin Corner Road/Suite 104   Lawrenceville, NJ 08648   (609)512-1690   Fax (609)512-1674

Desai, Bhumika, MD {1306105820} Pedtrc(11,GRN01)
+ Hand in Hand Pediatrics
725 River Road/Suite 201-A   Edgewater, NJ 07020   (201)840-8055   Fax (201)840-8099

Desai, Bijal, MD {1104963230} IntrMd, Nephro(97,DMN01)<NJ-OVERLOOK>
+ Kidney & Hypertension Center of Central Jersey
23 Clyde Road/Suite 101   Somerset, NJ 08873   (732)873-9500   Fax (732)873-0261

Desai, Chaitanya M., MD {1780707398} EmrgMd
+ 6 Pheasant Run
Green Brook, NJ 08812

Desai, Darshana A., MD {1760546758} ObsGyn, Gyneco(73,INA69)
+ Drs. Desai and Patel
2177 Oak Tree Road/Suite 205   Edison, NJ 08820   (732)549-3700   Fax (732)549-3203

Desai, Deep G., DO {1265798078}
+ 11 Avenue at Port Imperial/Apt 834
West New York, NJ 07093   (973)405-0343
deepdesai227@gmail.com

Desai, Dilip Navnitlal, MD {1144213794} IntrMd(90,IN20)
+ 20 Hospital Drive/Suite 19
Toms River, NJ 08755   (732)341-8044   Fax (732)341-8055

Desai, Foram R., MD {1174722011} IntrMd, IntHos(04,GRN01)<NY-SLRLUKES>
+ Excelcare
375 South Washington Avenue   Bergenfield, NJ 07621   (201)384-0036   Fax (201)384-7304

Desai, Gautam J., MD {1245242510} IntrMd(91,INA71)<NJ-JRSYSHMC>
+ RWJBH Primary Care Eatontown
145 Wyckoff Road/Suite 301   Eatontown, NJ 07724   (732)220-0180   Fax (732)935-1590
+ 842 Broadway
West Long Branch, NJ 07764   (732)222-0180   Fax (732)222-3990

Desai, Gautamkumar T., MD {1639116742} IntrMd, PulDis, SlpDis(70,INA21)<NJ-HCKTSTWN, NJ-STCLRDOV>
+ 447 Route 10/Suite 2
Randolph, NJ 07869   (973)361-4555   Fax (973)361-6360
+ 653 Willow Grove Street/Suite 2700
Hackettstown, NJ 07840   (973)361-4555   Fax (908)852-7404

Desai, Gopal Rao, MD {1104870450} RadOnc(79,INA9D)<NJ-STPETER, NJ-RWJUBRUN>
+ St. Peter's University Hospital
254 Easton Avenue/RadOnc   New Brunswick, NJ 08901   (732)745-8590   Fax (732)390-1856

Desai, Harit, DO {1548472905} IntrMd
+ Capital Health-Heart Care Specialists
2 Capital Way/Suite 385   Pennington, NJ 08534   (609)303-4838   Fax (609)303-4835

Desai, Hemlata K., MD {1578643193} PthAcl(72,INDI)
+ New Jersey Division of Developmental Disability
Route 72 East/HealthServPCP   New Lisbon, NJ 08064   (609)726-1000   Fax (609)894-8430

Desai, Jagdip, MD {1194761593} Anesth, PainInvt(01,NJ06)
+ Metropolitan Pain Consultants
1640 Schlosser Street/Suite C-3   Fort Lee, NJ 07024   (201)729-0001   Fax (201)729-0006
+ Metropolitan Pain Consultants
464 Valley Brook Avenue   Lyndhurst, NJ 07071   (201)729-0001   Fax (201)729-0006
+ Metropolitan Pain Consultants
1340 State Highway 34/Suite A   Aberdeen, NJ 07024   (201)729-0001   Fax (201)729-0006

Desai, Jigar, DO {1518353705} EmrgMd
+ University Hospital Emergency Medicine
150 Bergen Street   Newark, NJ 07103   (732)331-3506   Fax (973)972-6646

Desai, Jignesh, MD {1265857114} IntrMd
+ 600 Pavonia Avenue/8th Floor
Jersey City, NJ 07306   (201)216-3060   Fax (201)499-0253

Desai, Kiritkumar T., MD {1538166004} Ophthl(69,INDI)<NJ-CHSMRCER, NJ-CHSFULD>
+ Monique Eye Center, Inc.
2095 Klockner Road   Hamilton Square, NJ 08690   (609)890-7621   Fax (609)890-6950
KathyMagner@aol.com

Desai, Mahesh R., MD {1366541690} Gastrn, IntrMd(69,INDI)<NJ-STBARNMC, NJ-NWRKBETH>
+ 120 Millburn Avenue/Suite M2
Millburn, NJ 07041   (973)763-7716   Fax (973)763-4646

Desai, Maheshwari M., MD {1356482053} RadOnc(70,INDI)<NJ-NWRKBETH>
+ 61 Spenser Drive
Short Hills, NJ 07078

Desai, Maya G., MD {1508891342} PsyCAd, Psychy(70,INDI)
+ 447 Route 10/Suite 2
Randolph, NJ 07869   (973)361-4555

Desai, Meghna M., MD {1629384821}
+ 636 Doris Place
Ridgewood, NJ 07450

Desai, Navtika R., DO {1053376954} EnDbMt(01,NJ75)
+ 105 Raider Boulevard/Suite 200
Hillsborough, NJ 08844   (908)829-4244   Fax (908)382-3280

Desai, Neel, MD {1083952436} IntrMd(NJ05
+ UH-RWJ General Internal Medicine
125 Paterson Street/Suite 2300   New Brunswick, NJ 08901   (732)235-7112   Fax (732)235-7144

Desai, Nicky, MD {1710248166} IntHos
+ Summit Medical Group-Berkeley Heights Campus
1 Diamond Hill Road   Berkeley Heights, NJ 07922   (908)273-4300   Fax (908)790-6576

Desai, Priya Vasudev, MD {1750414157} Ophthl
+ Matossian Eye Associates
2 Capital Way/Suite 326   Pennington, NJ 08534   (609)882-8833   Fax (609)882-0077
+ Matossian Eye Associates
1445 Whitehorse-Mercerville Rd   Hamilton, NJ 08619   (609)882-8833   Fax (609)890-0774

Desai, Rajendra R., MD {1144338641} IntrMd, CdvDis(81,INDI)<NJ-EASTORNG>
+ New Jersey Cardiovascular Care Center
116 Millburn Avenue/Suite 214   Millburn, NJ 07041   (973)218-6000   Fax (973)679-8636

Desai, Rashmikant Sumantlal, MD {1437186814} CdvDis, IntrMd(71,INDI)<NJ-SOCEANCO>
+ Womens Health & Wellness
2500 English Creek Avenue   Egg Harbor Township, NJ 08234   (609)677-7776   Fax (609)677-7509

Desai, Renuka C., MD {1245324862} Pedtrc(70,INA69)
+ Advocare Township Pediatrics
123 Egg Harbor Road   Sewell, NJ 08080   (856)227-5437   Fax (856)227-5890

Desai, Ronak G., DO {1629181987} Anesth
+ Cooper Anesthesia Associates
One Cooper Plaza/Suite 294-B Camden, NJ 08103
(856)342-2425   Fax (856)968-8239

Desai, Ruchit B., MD {1770901472} IntrMd<NJ-NWRKBETH>
+ Newark Beth Israel Medical Center
201 Lyons Avenue Newark, NJ 07112 (732)995-3941

Desai, Sagar R., MD {1386649861} IntrMd(93,INA21)<NJ-JFKMED, NJ-SOMERSET>
+ Edison Emergi Med
98 James Street/Suite 313 Edison, NJ 08820 (732)635-1600 Fax (732)635-1402

Desai, Sameer P., MD {1487776373} OncHem
+ Drs. Fein, Porcelli & Richards
75 Veronica Avenue/Suite 201 Somerset, NJ 08873
(732)246-4882   Fax (732)249-5633
+ Regional Cancer Care Associates
111 Union Valley Road/Suite 205 Monroe, NJ 08831
(732)246-4882   Fax (609)395-7955

Desai, Samit Sharad, MD {1730103789} InfDis, IntrMd(01,NJ06)<NJ-HACKNSK>
+ Center for Infectious Diseases
20 Prospect Avenue/Suite 507 Hackensack, NJ 07601
(201)487-4088   Fax (201)489-8930

Desai, Shailendra A., MD {1073553152} RadDia, Radiol(75,INDI)<NJ-LOURDMED>
+ Center for Diagnostic Imaging
1450 East Chestnut Avenue Vineland, NJ 08360 (856)794-8664   Fax (856)794-2671

Desai, Shalin P., MD {1689841017} CdvDis
+ Cardiovascular Associates of Teaneck
954 Teaneck Road Teaneck, NJ 07666 (201)833-2300
Fax (201)833-7600

Desai, Sunit Bipinchandra, MD {1861496457} IntrMd(97,INDI)
+ 809 Highway 36/Suite 101
Union Beach, NJ 07735 (732)856-5299   Fax (732)856-5222

Desai, Suruchi Bankim, MD {1932456951}<NJ-UNVMCPRN>
+ University Medical Center of Princeton at Plainsboro
One Plainsboro Road Plainsboro, NJ 08536 (732)740-5019
desai.suruchi@gmail.com

Desai, Ved, DO {1871869511} OncHem
+ Advanced Care Hematology & Oncology Associates
385 Morris Avenue/Suite 100 Springfield, NJ 07081
(973)379-2111   Fax (973)379-2807

Desai, Veena C., MD {1548594211} FamMed
+ Bergen Medical Associates
466 Old Hook Road/Suite 1 Emerson, NJ 07630 (201)967-8221   Fax (201)967-0340

Desai, Vidhi Parikh, MD {1437497880} OncHem, IntrMd(10,NY09)<NJ-RWJUBRUN>
+ UH-RWJ General Internal Medicine
125 Paterson Street/Suite 2300 New Brunswick, NJ 08901
(732)235-7112   Fax (732)235-7144
+ RWJ University Hospital New Brunswick
One Robert Wood Johnson Place New Brunswick, NJ 08901
(732)235-7115

Desai, Vijaya S., MD {1841218468} Pedtrc(71,INDI)<NJ-CHRIST, NJ-HOBUNIMC>
+ 121 Saint Paul's Avenue
Jersey City, NJ 07306 (201)792-4286   Fax (201)659-1004

Desai, Vinay M., MD {1972532331} IntrMd, EmrgMd(90,INA09)<NY-CMCSTVSI>
+ JFK Medical Center
65 James Street Edison, NJ 08820 (732)321-7605

Desai, Viren, MD {1568401636} IntrMd, PulDis(86,INDI)<NJ-CLARMAAS>
+ Dr. Desai and Associates
221 Kearny Avenue Kearny, NJ 07032 (201)997-0808
Fax (201)997-0013
+ 639 Ridge Road
Lyndhurst, NJ 07071 (201)997-0808   Fax (201)460-3850

Desai, Vishal, MD {1063774776} RadDia<NJ-KMHCHRRY>
+ Kennedy Health System/Cherry Hill Campus
2201 Chapel Avenue West Cherry Hill, NJ 08002
(856)488-6500   Fax (856)488-6507

Desani, Jatin Karsandas, MD {1689868440} OncHem
+ Meridian Hematology & Oncology
1100 Route 72 West Manahawkin, NJ 08050 (609)597-0547   Fax (609)597-8668

DeSanti, Michelina, DO {1487766416} ObsGyn(89,NJ75)<NJ-HCKTSTWN>
+ Woman to Woman Ob/Gyn Associates
576 State Route 94 Columbia, NJ 07832 (908)496-9400
Fax (908)496-9414
+ Woman to Woman Ob/Gyn Associates
46 Main Street Sparta, NJ 07871 (973)726-7300

DeSantis Mastrangelo, Rosemarie, MD {1336112606} IntrMd, Rheuma(96,NY08)
+ Coastal HealthCare
44 Nautilus Drive/Suite 2A Manahawkin, NJ 08050
(609)597-4178   Fax (609)597-4387

Desantos, Victoria Christina, MD {1891061065}(10,WI06)<NJ-ST-BARNMC>
+ Women first Health Center
520 Pleasant Valley Way West Orange, NJ 07052
(973)669-5711   Fax (973)669-5722

Deshaw, Barbara Blank, MD {1528205630} Nutrtn(95,NY46)
+ 3 Edwards Place
Short Hills, NJ 07078 (973)376-9664

Deshields, Manley S., MD {1245345743} IntrMd, Addctn(80,PA13)
+ Kennedy Clinic
300 Woodbury-Turnersville Road Blackwood, NJ 08012
(856)227-5254
+ Camden County Health Services Center
20 N Woodbury-Turnersville Rd Blackwood, NJ 08012
(856)227-5254   Fax (856)374-6436

Deshmukh, Kalpana S., MD {1780682575} Radiol, RadDia(72,INA11)<NJ-VIRTMHBC, NJ-VIRTBERL>
+ The Women's Center at Voorhees
100 Carnie Boulevard/Suite A-4 Voorhees, NJ 08043
(856)751-5522   Fax (856)751-5650
+ South Jersey Radiology Associates, P.A.
315 Route 70 East/Suite B Cherry Hill, NJ 08034 (856)751-5522   Fax (856)428-0356
+ South Jersey Radiology Associates, P.A.
1000 Lincoln Drive East Marlton, NJ 08043 (856)983-1818
Fax (856)983-3226

Deshmukh, Poornima Vasudeo, MD {1609821776} Anesth(94,INDI)<NJ-CENTRAST>
+ CentraState Medical Center
901 West Main Street/Anesthesiology Freehold, NJ 07728
(732)431-2000

Deshmukh, Pratibha S., MD {1508802349} Pedtrc, AdolMd(74,INA4X)<NJ-CHILTON, NJ-HACKNSK>
+ DP Pediatrics
142 Totowa Road/Suite 8 Totowa, NJ 07512 (973)904-1000   Fax (973)904-1480

Deshpande, Jyoti M., MD {1982625448} Pthlgy, PthAcl(85,INA4X)
+ 16 Pine Valley Road
Livingston, NJ 07039 (973)325-5098

Deshpande, Kalyani Kumari, MD {1932299922} PsyCAd, Psychy(92,INA48)<NJ-UNIVBHC>
+ University Behavioral Health Care
671 Hoes Lane/PO Box 1392 Piscataway, NJ 08855
(732)235-5500
+ University Behavioral Health Care
4326 Route 1 North Monmouth Junction, NJ 08852
(732)235-5500   Fax (732)235-5799

Deshpande, Mohan S., MD {1134101934} CdvDis, IntrMd(65,INDI)
+ 806 Kearny Avenue
Kearny, NJ 07032 (201)997-8806

Deshpande, Neha A., MD {1073992129}
+ Princeton Medical Group, P.A.
419 North Harrison Street Princeton, NJ 08540 (609)924-9300   Fax (609)924-6552

Deshpande, Nikhil, MD {1003869041} Gastrn(93,INA74)
+ Jersey Shore Gastroenterology
408 Bethel Road/Suite E Somers Point, NJ 08244
(609)926-3330   Fax (609)926-8578

Deshpande, Sanjay V., MD {1417187303} Pedtrc, IntrMd(85,INA67)
+ 285 Durham Avenue/Suite 2
South Plainfield, NJ 07080 (732)756-7500

Desiderio, Abelardo C., MD {1487768610} PthAcl(66,PHIL)<NJ-HCKTSTWN>
+ Hackettstown Regional Medical Center
651 Willow Grove Street/Pathology Hackettstown, NJ
07840 (908)852-5100

Desiderio, Carl M., DO {1992748495} EmrgMd(76,PA77)
+ 69 East Cartwright Drive
Princeton Junction, NJ 08550

Desiderio, Michael Carl, DO {1720388143}<NJ-MORRISTN>
+ Morristown Medical Center
100 Madison Avenue Morristown, NJ 07962 (973)682-2136

DeSilva, Derrick, Jr., MD {1467541755} IntrMd(82,DOM02)
+ 629 Amboy Avenue
Edison, NJ 08837 (732)738-8801   Fax (732)738-8802

DeSilverio, Robert Vincent, Jr., MD {1972591147} SrgDer
+ Atlantic Dermatology & Laser Center
1401 New Road Linwood, NJ 08221 (609)927-5885   Fax (609)927-5565

Desimone, Alexandra, MD {1306228143} FamMed
+ Virtua Family Medicine of Washington Township
239 Hurffville Crosskeys Road Sewell, NJ 08080 (856)341-8181   Fax (856)341-8180

Desimone, Dennis Charles, DO {1255599130} ObsGyn<NJ-OURLADY>
+ Osborn Family Health Center
1601 Haddon Road Camden, NJ 08103 (856)757-3700

Fax (856)365-7972
+ Our Lady of Lourdes Medical Center
1600 Haddon Avenue/OB/GYN Camden, NJ 08103
(856)757-3500

DeSimone, Luca, MD {1104897388} IntrMd, Nephro, Hypten(92,ITA33)<NJ-JFKMED, NJ-RBAYOLDB>
+ 4 Progress Street/Suite B-4
Edison, NJ 08820 (908)834-8030   Fax (908)834-8033

DeSimone, Robert Anthony, MD {1932102589} Anesth(90,NJ05)<NJ-STCLRDEN, NJ-STCLRBOO>
+ Morris Anesthesia Group, PA
3799 Route 46/Suite 211 Parsippany, NJ 07054 (973)335-1122   Fax (973)335-1448

DeSipio, Joshua Peter, MD {1063628360} Gastrn
+ The Cooper Hospital System-Univ Hospital
3 Cooper Plaza/Suite 215 Camden, NJ 08103 (856)342-2439   Fax (856)342-7832

DeSouza, Sylvie D., MD {1477590875} EmrgMd(89,NY08)<NJ-HACKNSK>
+ Hackensack Medical Center Emergency Medicine
30 Prospect Avenue/Main 3619 Hackensack, NJ 07601
(201)996-4614   Fax (201)996-4239
sylviedesouza@gmail.com

DeSouza, Trevor G., MD {1972699205} NroChl, Pedtrc, Nrolgy(77,KENY)<NJ-NWTNMEM>
+ Advocare Pediatric Neurology Associates
25 Lindsley Drive/Suite 205 Morristown, NJ 07960
(973)993-8777   Fax (973)993-8577

Desouza-Sanders, Kelly R., MD {1912929860} ObsGyn, IntrMd(89,PA14)<NJ-VIRTMHBC>
+ Penn Medicine at Cherry Hill
409 Route 70 East Cherry Hill, NJ 08034 (856)795-0587

Desplat, Philippe, DO {1033166798} FamMed(81,NJ75)<NJ-VALLEY>
+ Valley Medical Group
40 Washington Avenue Dumont, NJ 07628 (201)387-7055
Fax (201)387-8605

DesRochers, Laurence R., MD {1861437295} EmrgMd(93,NJ05)<NJ-COMMED>
+ Community Medical Center
99 Route 37 West/EmrgMed Toms River, NJ 08755
(732)557-8080
LDesRochers@sbhcs.com
+ Jersey Emergency Medicine Specialists
99 Highway 37 West Toms River, NJ 08755 (732)557-8080

Dessalines, Normy, MD {1740607316} IntrMd<NJ-STFRNMED>
+ St. Francis Medical Center
601 Hamilton Avenue/Rm B-158 Trenton, NJ 08629
(609)599-5061   Fax (609)599-6232

Dessio, Whitney Charnell, MD {1679862049} GPrvMd, PubHth, IntrMd(06,NY48)
+ 30 Landau Road
Basking Ridge, NJ 07920 (631)398-6591

DeStefano, Michael William, MD {1326369943} RadDia(10,CT01)<NY-MTSINAI, NY-MTSINYHS>
+ Cooper University Hospital
One Cooper Plaza Camden, NJ 08103 (856)342-2000

DeStefano, Peter M., MD CdvDis, IntrMd(87,PRO01)<NJ-STFRNMED, NJ-RWJUHAM>
+ 669 Chambers Street
Trenton, NJ 08611 (609)695-2676   Fax (609)895-9581
petermd@alumni.princeton.edu

DeStefano, Sabrina Gloria, DO {1336161496}<NJ-OVERLOOK>
+ Overlook Medical Center
99 Beauvoir Avenue/PO Box 210 Summit, NJ 07902
(908)522-0000
sabrinagd@aol.com

Desueza, Juan A., MD {1871683821} IntrMd(86,DOM02)
+ Centro Medico Iberoamericano
416 Park Avenue Paterson, NJ 07501 (973)684-8138
Fax (973)684-0032
+ Centro-Ibero-Americano
406 Mountain Avenue Franklin Lakes, NJ 07417 (973)684-8138

DeTorres, Wayne Raymond, MD {1811039357} Urolgy(88,MA07)<NJ-VALLEY>
+ Urology Group PA
4 Godwin Avenue Midland Park, NJ 07432 (201)444-7070
Fax (201)444-7228

Detrizio Carotenuto, Isabel, MD {1376622159} Pedtrc(82,DOM02)
+ 24 Heritage Drive
East Hanover, NJ 07936 (973)884-3155   Fax (973)884-3523

Dettmer, Matthew Robert, MD {1972814309} CritCr
+ Cooper University Hospital Critical Care
One Cooper Plaza Camden, NJ 08103 (843)819-7660
Fax (856)968-8282
dettmerm@wusm.wustl.edu

Physicians by Name and Address

DeTullio, John P., MD {1184738940} CritCr, IntrMd, PulDis(81,ITA17)<NJ-KIMBALL, NJ-CENTRAST>
+ Monmouth Ocean Pulmonary Medicine
  901 West Main Street/Suite 160 Freehold, NJ 07728 (732)577-0600 Fax (732)577-6332
+ Monmouth Ocean Pulmonary Medicine
  886 River Avenue Lakewood, NJ 08701 (732)577-0600 Fax (732)360-0336
+ Monmouth Ocean Pulmonary Medicine
  312 Applegarth Road Monroe Township, NJ 07728 (609)409-0029

Deutsch, Alan D., DO {1528040011} Nrolgy(87,NJ75)<NJ-JRSYSHMC, NJ-OCEANMC>
+ Monmouth Ocean Neurology
  1944 State Route 33/Suite 206 Neptune, NJ 07753 (732)774-8282 Fax (732)774-4407
+ Monmouth Ocean Neurology
  190 Jack Martin Boulevard/Building B-3 Brick, NJ 08724 (732)774-8282 Fax (732)785-0116

Deutsch, Jason Alexander, MD {1285665141} EmrgMd, IntrMd(99,MA16)<NJ-HACKNSK>
+ Hackensack Medical Center Emergency Medicine
  30 Prospect Avenue/Main 3619 Hackensack, NJ 07601 (201)996-4614 Fax (201)968-1866

Deutsch, Jonathan S., MD {1053746057} Anesth(88,ISRA)
+ 5 Brush Hill Road
  Kinnelon, NJ 07405

Deutsch, Lawrence Steven, MD {1588636534} SrgOrt, SrgSpn, IntrMd(82,NY15)<NJ-COOPRUMC>
+ Coastal Spine
  4000 Church Road Mount Laurel, NJ 08054 (856)222-4733 Fax (856)222-0049

Deutsch, Michael, MD {1356668602} SrgC&R
+ Associated Colon & Rectal Surgeons PA
  3900 Park Avenue/Suite 101 Edison, NJ 08820 (732)494-6640 Fax (732)549-8204

Deutsch, Paul Jan, MD {1225262355} EnDbMt(82,NY46)<NY-PRSBWEIL>
+ 50 Maybury Hill Road
  Princeton, NJ 08540 (609)688-9547 Fax (908)304-7572

Deutsch, Robert Jay, MD {1588674824} Pedtrc, PedEmg(03,DC01)<NJ-STBARNMC, NJ-JRSYCITY>
+ Emergency Medical Associates of NJ, P.A.
  3 Century Drive Parsippany, NJ 07054 (973)740-0607 Fax (973)740-9895

Deutsch, Stuart, MD {1285620799} Pedtrc(81)<NY-MAIMONMC>
+ Drs. Indich and Deutsch
  619 West County Line Road Lakewood, NJ 08701 (732)730-9111 Fax (732)730-9154

Dev, Rajesh K., MD {1255447975} EnDbMt(01,WA04)
+ Summit Medical Group
  552 Westfield Avenue Westfield, NJ 07090 (908)654-3377 Fax (908)654-4044
+ Thyroid & Diabetes Ctr
  240 Easton Avenue/4th Floor New Brunswick, NJ 08901 (908)654-3377 Fax (732)249-0969
+ Saint Peter's Physician Associates
  294 Applegarth Road Monroe Township, NJ 07090 (609)409-1363 Fax (609)409-9493

Devadan, Phillip Sunil, MD {1740335892} Pedtrc, EmrgPedr(97,GRN01)<NJ-CHILTON>
+ Chilton Medical Center
  97 West Parkway/Pediatrics Pompton Plains, NJ 07444 (973)831-5120 Fax (973)831-5342

Devalla, Meena, MD {1497765358} ObsGyn(88,INA83)<NJ-STMICHL, NJ-STMRYPAS>
+ Special Care Ob-Gyn
  14 Franklin Street/2nd Floor Belleville, NJ 07109 (973)759-4802 Fax (973)759-4805
+ Special Care Ob-Gyn
  465 Mount Prospect Avenue Newark, NJ 07102 (973)482-6070
+ Special Care Ob-Gyn
  905 Allwood Road/Sute 103 Clifton, NJ 07109 (973)340-9400 Fax (973)340-1518

Devarajan, Anandan, MD {1619932837} IntrMd(77,INDI)
+ 230 West End Avenue
  Green Brook, NJ 08812 (908)251-5114 Fax (201)437-2419
  Adevarajan@somerset-healthcare.com

Dever, Lisa Lynn, MD {1619901014} InfDis, IntrMd(86,TX02)<NJ-VAEASTOR>
+ University Physician Associates
  140 Bergen Street/ACC Level D Newark, NJ 07103 (973)972-4071 Fax (973)972-3102

Dever, Matthew Patrick, MD {1639104706} Pedtrc(94,NY15)<NJ-OCEANMC, NJ-COMMED>
+ Pediatric Affiliates, PA
  40 Bey Lea Road/Suite B203 Toms River, NJ 08753 (732)341-0720 Fax (732)244-6842
+ Pediatric Affiliates, PA
  218 Jack Martin Boulevard/Building E-1 Brick, NJ 08724 (732)341-0720 Fax (732)458-9329
+ Pediatric Affiliates, PA
  1616 Route 72 West/Suite 8 Manahawkin, NJ 08753 (609)597-6200 Fax (609)978-1229

Devereux, Corinne K., MD {1710172127} RadOnc, Radiol, RadThp(71,PA07)<NJ-CLARMAAS>
+ Clara Maass Medical Center
  1 Clara Maass Drive Belleville, NJ 07109 (201)450-2270 Fax (201)751-2943

Devereux, Linda, MD {1720187206} MedOnc, Hemato, IntrMd(74,PA02)<NJ-COOPRUMC>
+ The Cooper Hospital System-Univ Hospital
  3 Cooper Plaza/Suite 215/Hematology Camden, NJ 08103 (856)342-2439 Fax (856)338-9211

Devers, Paul Dix, MD {1376514968} FamMed(97,VA07)
+ Virtual Family Medicine - Mansfield
  3242 Route 206/Building A Suite 2 Bordentown, NJ 08505 (609)298-4340 Fax (609)298-4370

DeVincenzo, Raven, MD {1104844117} RadDia, Radiol(98,NY48)<NY-STATNRTH>
+ Red Bank Radiologists, P.A.
  200 White Road/Suite 115 Little Silver, NJ 07739 (732)741-9595 Fax (732)741-0985
+ Coastal Imaging, LLC
  79 Route 37 West/Suite 103 Toms River, NJ 08755 (732)741-9595 Fax (732)276-2325

deVinck, Oana, DO {1306103593} PedDvl, Pedtrc(06,NJ75)
+ 242 Warren Avenue
  Fort Lee, NJ 07024

Devine, Mary Ann, MD {1508885153} CritCr, IntrMd, SrgCrC(90,DC02)<NJ-RWJUHAM>
+ Capital Health Stroke and Cerebrovascular Center
  1401 Whitehorse Mercerville Rd Hamilton, NJ 08619 (609)588-5081 Fax (609)588-5086

Devinsky, Orrin, MD {1679581623} Nrolgy(82,MA01)
+ St. Barnabas Institute of Neurology & Neurosurgery
  200 South Orange Avenue/Suite 101 Livingston, NJ 07039 (973)322-6600 Fax (973)322-6631

Devita, Jack Joseph, MD {1586624340} Gastrn, IntrMd(95,NY09)<NJ-VIRTUAHS, NJ-KENEDYHS>
+ South Jersey Gastroenterology PA
  406 Lippincott Drive/Suite E Marlton, NJ 08053 (856)983-1900 Fax (856)983-5110
+ South Jersey Gastroenterology PA
  807 Haddon Avenue/Suite 205 Haddonfield, NJ 08033 (856)983-1900 Fax (856)983-5110
+ South Jersey Gastroenterology PA
  111 Vine Street Hammonton, NJ 08053 (609)561-3080 Fax (856)983-5110

DeVita, Michael G., DO {1790766277} IntrMd, CarNuc, IntCrd(95,NY75)<NJ-OCEANMC, NJ-JRSYSHMC>
+ Shore Cardiology Consultants, LLC
  1640 Route 88/Suite 201 Brick, NJ 08724 (732)840-1900 Fax (732)840-0355
+ Shore Cardiology Consultants, LLC
  3200 Sunset Avenue/Suite 208 Ocean, NJ 07712 (732)840-1900

Devito, Fiore J., MD {1679599609} Gastrn(81,MEXI)
+ 733 Bloomfield Avenue
  Bloomfield, NJ 07003 (973)743-6447 Fax (973)743-6918

Devito, Marc J., MD {1295920262} IntrMd, Pedtrc
+ Deborah C. Rose Family Chiropractic Center
  180 White Road/Suite 205 Little Silver, NJ 07739 (732)530-7229 Fax (732)842-4119

Devli, Aynur A., MD {1144262403} Pedtrc, InfDis, EmrgMd(84,AUST)<NJ-CHILTON>
+ JFK Medical Center
  65 James Street Edison, NJ 08820 (732)321-7601 Fax (732)744-5614
+ 504 Hamburg Turnpike/Suite 206
  Wayne, NJ 07470

Dewil, Frederic, MD {1790711810} CritCr, IntrMd, PulDis(86,NY48)<NJ-SOCEANCO>
+ Medical Associates of Ocean County, P.A.
  1301 Route 72 West/Suite 300 Manahawkin, NJ 08050 (609)597-6513 Fax (609)597-4593
  fdewil@maochealth.com

Deworsop, Richard, MD {1629011598} Psychy, PsyGrt, PsyFor(81,INA94)<NJ-COMMED, NJ-KIMBALL>
+ ADAPT
  1163 Route 37 West/Suite 1 Toms River, NJ 08755 (732)244-4807 Fax (732)244-3667

Dewyke, Kathleen Michelle, MD {1588151898} Psychy
+ Veterans Affairs Department Outpatient Clinic
  654 East Jersey Street Elizabeth, NJ 07206 (908)994-7233 Fax (908)994-0131

Dey, Chaitali, MD {1841238334} IntrMd, Nephro(84,INA7B)<NJ-COOPRUMC>
+ 54 Manor House Drive
  Cherry Hill, NJ 08003 (856)489-0662
+ The Cooper Hospital System-Univ Hospital
  3 Cooper Plaza/Suite 215 Camden, NJ 08103 (856)342-2439

DeYoung, Chad M., MD {1225063456} RadOnc<NJ-VALLEY>
+ Valley Radiation Oncology Associates
  One Valley Health Plaza Paramus, NJ 07652 (201)634-5403

Dhadwal, Ajay Kapoor, MD {1629206032} SrgVas, Surgry, IntrMd(95,ENG25)<NJ-UMDNJ>
+ University Hospital
  150 Bergen Street/UH F102 Newark, NJ 07103 (973)972-6295
  ajay.dhadwal@rutgers.edu

Dhadwal, Neetu, MD {1962842492} Nrolgy, ClNrPh(08,VA07)
+ Bergen Medical Associates
  466 Old Hook Road/Suite 1 Emerson, NJ 07630 (201)967-8221 Fax (201)967-0340

Dhaibar, Yeshuschandra R., MD {1831259282} Psychy, PsyCAd(79,INA70)<NJ-MTNSIDE>
+ 622 Eagle Rock Avenue
  West Orange, NJ 07052 (973)699-1100

Dhakhwa, Raj B., MD {1891839239} PulDis, IntrMd(70,ISRA)
+ 200 Perrine Road/Suite 230
  Old Bridge, NJ 08857 (732)727-0060
  Rbdhakhwa@comcast.net

Dhaliwal, Harleen, MD {1942654470} IntHos
+ AtlantiCare Hospitalist Program
  1925 Pacific Avenue/8th Floor Atlantic City, NJ 08401 (609)441-8990

Dhalla, Sameer, MD {1417121898} Gastrn
+ Dr. De La Cruz and Dhalla
  714 Tenth Street Secaucus, NJ 07094 (201)865-2050 Fax (201)865-0015

Dhamotharan, Shakira N., MD {1699102848} FamMed
+ St. Joseph's Family Medicine @ Clifton
  1135 Broad Street/Suite 201 Clifton, NJ 07013 (973)754-4100 Fax (973)472-9062

Dhanani, Harsha Narendra, MD {1346359122} RadDia, Radiol(74,INDI)<NY-CONEYISL>
+ Emergimed
  663 Palisade Avenue/Suite 101 Cliffside Park, NJ 07010 (201)945-6500 Fax (201)945-1157

Dhanaraj, Dinesh, MD {1093982654} SrgOrt(TX13<NY-JTORTHO>
+ Princeton Bone & Joint
  5 Plainsboro Road/Suite 100 Plainsboro, NJ 08536 (609)750-1600 Fax (609)750-1611

Dhar, Gargi, MD {1639365729} FamMed
+ Visiting Nurse Association of Central Jersey
  1301 Main Street Asbury Park, NJ 07712 (732)774-6333 Fax (732)774-0313
+ 406 Green Hollow Drive
  Iselin, NJ 08830 (732)602-2441

Dhar, Rajat K., MD {1023073277} IntrMd, Rheuma(88,GRN01)<NJ-COMMED>
+ 442D Commons Way
  Toms River, NJ 08755 (732)505-3510 Fax (732)505-5308

Dhar, Seema, MD {1912056045} Pedtrc
+ 237 Ferry Street
  Newark, NJ 07105 (973)344-7614 Fax (973)466-1535

Dhar, Vasudha, MD {1659574770} IntrMd, Gastrn(96,INA67)<NJ-CENTRAST, NJ-UNVMCPRN>
+ 300 B Princeton-Hightstown Rd
  East Windsor, NJ 08520 (609)918-1222 Fax (609)918-1235

Dhar, Veena, MD {1841248796} AdolMd, Pedtrc(75,INA36)<NJ-STBARNMC>
+ 237 Ferry Street
  Newark, NJ 07105 (973)344-7614 Fax (973)466-1535
  V.dhasm.d@aol.com

Dharia, Amishi, DO {1538457338} PhysMd(11,NY75)
+ National Health Rehabilitation
  103 River Road/Suite 101 Edgewater, NJ 07020 (201)654-6397 Fax (201)917-3603

Dhawan, Aman, MD {1861558280} SrgOrt
+ University Orthopaedic Associates, LLC.
  4810 Belmar Boulevard/Suite 102 Wall, NJ 07753 (732)938-6090 Fax (732)938-5720

Dhawan, Denise Marie, MD {1053481390} Pedtrc, AdolMd
+ Wee Care Pediatrics
  831 Tennent Road/Suite A Manalapan, NJ 07726 (732)536-6222 Fax (732)536-9272

Dhawlikar, Sripad H., MD {1659327898} SrgOrt, SrgSpn, PedOrt(85,INDI)<NJ-COMMED>
+ Ocean Orthopedic Associates, P.A.
  530 Lakehurst Road/Suite 1 Toms River, NJ 08755 (732)349-8454 Fax (732)341-0259
+ Community Medical Center
  99 Route 37 West Toms River, NJ 08755 (732)557-8000
+ Physician Surgery Center
  1 Plaza Drive Toms River, NJ 08755 (732)818-0059

Physicians by Name and Address

Dhawlikar, Sunita Sripad, MD {1053540419} Anesth(85,INDI)<NJ-BAYSHORE>
+ Bayshore Community Hospital
727 North Beers Street/Anesthesiology Holmdel, NJ 07733 (732)739-5900

Dhebaria, Tina, DO {1124361878} PedEmg
+ Jersey Shore Medical Pediatric Emergency
1945 Route 33 Neptune, NJ 07753 (732)776-4220

Dheer, Sachin, MD {1427160449} RadDia
+ Radiology Associates of New Jersey
2201 Chapel Avenue West/Suite 106 Cherry Hill, NJ 08002 (856)488-6844 Fax (856)488-6507
+ 12 Forrest Hills Drive
Voorhees, NJ 08043 (856)210-6408

Dhib Jalbut, Suhayl S., MD {1518032093} Nrolgy(80,LEB03)<NJ-RWJUBRUN>
+ UH- Robert Wood Johnson Med
125 Paterson Street/CAB 6200 New Brunswick, NJ 08901 (732)235-7733 Fax (732)235-7041
+ RW Johnson University Medical Group Neurology
97 Paterson Street New Brunswick, NJ 08901 (732)235-7733 Fax (732)235-8115
+ Rutgers NJ School of Medicine Neurology
90 Bergen Street/DOC 5200 Newark, NJ 08901 (973)972-5209 Fax (973)972-5059

Dhillon, Navdeep, MD {1356509095} Nephro, IntrMd(00,INA4E)<NJ-STBARNMC>
+ St. Barnabas Medical Center Renal Transplant Center
94 Old Short Hills Road Livingston, NJ 07039 (973)322-5065 Fax (973)322-8930

Dhillon, Ravinder S., MD {1629290556} IntrMd, Gastrn(02,IL06)
+ Mercer Gastroenterology
2 Capital Way/Suite 487 Pennington, NJ 08534 (609)818-1900 Fax (609)818-1908

Dhillon, Satvinder K., MD {1437296548} IntrMd(73,INA67)<NJ-CHSMRCER>
+ Mercer Regional Medical Associates, LLC
2 Capital Way/Suite 315 Pennington, NJ 08534 (609)730-0010 Fax (609)730-3939

Dhillon, Shamina, MD {1992779300} Gastrn, IntrMd(98,NJ05)<NJ-MONMOUTH, NJ-JRSYSHMC>
+ Shore Gastroenterology Associates, P.C.
1907 Highway 35/Suite 1 Oakhurst, NJ 07755 (732)517-0060 Fax (732)548-7408
+ Shore Gastroenterology Associates, P.C.
1907 Highway 35/Suite 1 Oakhurst, NJ 07755 (732)517-0060 Fax (732)548-7408
+ Shore Gastroenterology Associates, P.C.
233 Middle Road Hazlet, NJ 07755 (732)361-2476

Dhillon, Sudeep S., MD {1780904094} EnDbMt, IntrMd
+ Mercer Regional Medical Associates, LLC
2 Capital Way/Suite 315 Pennington, NJ 08534 (732)668-2000 Fax (609)730-3939

Dhillon, Swapna K., MD {1508135823}
+ Capital Health System/Fuld Campus
750 Brunswick Avenue/Psychiatry Trenton, NJ 08638 (609)394-6085 Fax (609)394-6205
+ Princeton Center for Eating Disorders
One Plainsboro Road Plainsboro, NJ 08536 (609)853-7575

Dhillon, Yadwinder Singh, MD {1245528637}<NJ-MORRISTN>
+ Morristown Medical Center
100 Madison Avenue Morristown, NJ 07962 (973)971-5000

Dhillon-Acosta, Raminder Kaur, DO {1790749984} Radiol, RadBdI(97,IA75)
+ Shore Imaging
1166 River Avenue/Suite 102 Lakewood, NJ 08701 (732)364-9565 Fax (732)364-1908

Dhillon-Athwal, Narinder Kaur, MD {1629249321} FamMed(05,DMN01)
+ Advance Hospital Care @ Somerset Medical Center
110 Rehill Avenue Somerville, NJ 08876 (908)429-5833 Fax (908)203-5970

Dhindsa, Sumeet, MD {1972750776} Grtrcs, IntrMd(01,INA9Y)
+ 1028 New Durham Road
Edison, NJ 08817 (848)229-2484
docsumeetj@yahoo.com

Dhingra, Monica, MD {1235211608} PsyGrt, Psychy(95,INA72)<NJ-BERGNMC>
+ New Bridge Medical Center
230 East Ridgewood Avenue Paramus, NJ 07652 (201)967-4000 Fax (201)967-4205

Dhir, Nisha Solanki, MD {1760470579} Surgry(93,PA01)
+ Princeton Surgical Associates, P.A.
5 Plainsboro Road/Suite 400 Plainsboro, NJ 08536 (609)936-9100 Fax (609)936-9700
NDhir@princeton-surgical.com

Dhirmalani, Rajesh A., DO {1073522819} IntrMd, Gastrn(99,IA75)<NJ-OVERLOOK, NJ-RWJURAH>
+ Advanced Gastroenterology Group
1308 Morris Avenue Union, NJ 07083 (908)851-2770 Fax (908)851-7706

Dhorajia, Seema P., DO {1891985214} Surgry
+ Advanced Laparoscopic Associates
81 Route 4 West/Suite 401/35 Plaza Paramus, NJ 07652 (201)646-1121 Fax (201)646-1110

Dhorajia, Shruti P., DO {1073751848} IntrMd
+ 14 Asnius Road
Closter, NJ 07624

Dhru, Sahil H., DO {1912065921} Anesth, IntrMd(02,NY75)<NJ-VIRTVOOR>
+ Virtua Hospitalist Group Memorial
175 Madison Avenue Mount Holly, NJ 08060 (609)914-6180 Fax (609)914-6182
+ Union County HealthCare Associates
689 Inman Avenue Colonia, NJ 07067 (609)914-6180 Fax (732)381-0070

Dhupar, Shanti, MD {1346242815} Pedtrc, AdolMd(69,INA8Z)<NJ-HACKNSK>
+ Pediatric Medical Office
501 North Avenue Wood Ridge, NJ 07075 (201)460-9362 Fax (201)460-0258

Di Biase, John J., MD {1336117332} SrgOrt(79,NY01)<NJ-STFRN-MED, NJ-RWJUHAM>
+ Trenton Orthopaedic Group
1225 Whitehorse Mercerville Rd Trenton, NJ 08619 (609)581-2200 Fax (609)581-1212
+ Trenton Orthopaedic Group
116 Washington Crossing Road Pennington, NJ 08534 (609)581-2200 Fax (609)581-1212
+ Trenton Orthopaedic Group, PA
1 Sheffield Drive/Suite 202A Columbus, NJ 08619 (609)581-2200 Fax (609)581-1212

Di Bruno, Donna, DO {1851371983} IntrMd(02,PA77)
+ SOM - Department of Internal Medicine
42 East Laurel Road/Suite 3100 Stratford, NJ 08084 (856)566-6845 Fax (856)566-6906

Di Cicco Bloom, Emanuel M., MD {1578658720} NroChl(77,NY20)
+ Child Health Institute of New Jersey
89 French Street/Suite 2300 New Brunswick, NJ 08901 (732)235-7875 Fax (732)235-6620

Di Cindio, William D., DO {1982715967} EmrgMd(93,NJ75)<NJ-SJHREGMC, NJ-SJERSYHS>
+ SJH Regional Medical Center
1505 West Sherman Avenue/EmrgMed Vineland, NJ 08360 (856)641-8000

Di Fazio, Louis Thomas, Jr., MD {1376510032} Surgry, SrgCrC(90,PA12)<NJ-MORRISTN, NJ-JRSYSHMC>
+ Surgical Practice of Rolando Rolandelli, MD
435 South Street/Suite 360 Morristown, NJ 07960 (973)971-7200 Fax (973)290-7521

Di Filippo, John A., MD {1558353565} CdvDis, IntrMd(77,ITAL)
+ Summit Medical Group Cardiology
62 South Fullerton Avenue Montclair, NJ 07042 (973)746-8585 Fax (973)746-0088

Di Fiore, Richard, MD {1902000995} SrgVas(01,GRN01)
+ LMA Surgical Associates
120 White Horse Pike/Suite 103 Haddon Heights, NJ 08035 (856)546-3900 Fax (856)546-3908

Di Giacomo, Eric D., MD {1467431312} IntrMd(77,MEX22)
+ 205 Ridgedale Avenue
Florham Park, NJ 07932 (973)377-1884

Di Gioia, Julia Marie, MD {1902964448} Surgry, SrgBst, SrgRec(79,ITA17)
+ Hall-DiGioia Center for Breast Care
33 Overlook Road/Suite 205 Summit, NJ 07901 (908)522-3200 Fax (908)522-1222

Di Giorgio, Christopher B., MD {1548575137} CdvDis, IntrMd(08,NY48)
+ Bart De Gregorio MD, LLC.
946 Bloomfield Avenue Glen Ridge, NJ 07028 (973)743-1121 Fax (973)743-2627

Di Guglielmo, Nicola, MD {1063488484} IntrMd(84,SPAI)<NJ-JRSYSHMC>
+ 1900 Route 35/Suite 300
Oakhurst, NJ 07755 (732)531-5509 Fax (732)531-5164

Di Joseph, Benjamin D., Jr., DO {1841375565} ObsGyn(94,FL75)<NJ-UNDRWD>
+ Westwood Womens Health Center
600 Jessup Road West Deptford, NJ 08066 (856)845-4061 Fax (856)812-2880
+ Westwood Womens Center
155 Bridgeton Pike/Suite B Mullica Hill, NJ 08062 (856)845-4061 Fax (856)812-2880

Di Lisi, Joseph P., DO {1396824256} FamMed(77,PA77)<NJ-UNDRWD>
+ Di Lisi Family Medicine LLC
110 North Woodbury Road Pitman, NJ 08071 (856)589-1212 Fax (856)589-6635

Di Marcangelo, Mark T., DO {1336149319} Radiol, RadDia, NuclMd(82,PA77)<NJ-KMHCHRRY>
+ Radiology Associates of New Jersey
2201 Chapel Avenue West/Suite 106 Cherry Hill, NJ 08002 (856)488-6844 Fax (856)488-6507

Di Marcangelo, Michael C., Jr., DO {1881673275} FamMed(85,PA77)
+ Partners in Primary Care
19 West Main Street Maple Shade, NJ 08052 (856)779-7386 Fax (856)779-7563

Di Marco, Eugene M., DO {1780601369} Ophthl(84,PA77)<NJ-ACMCITY>
+ Brigantine Eye Care Center
4274 Harbour Beach Boulevard Brigantine, NJ 08203 (609)266-8000 Fax (609)266-9555

Di Mari, Connie Lee, MD {1891841920} Ophthl(80,NY48)
+ 334 Kinderkamack Road
Oradell, NJ 07649 (201)265-4122

Di Marino, Michael C., MD {1619936515} IntrMd, Gastrn(98,PA09)
+ South Jersey Endoscopy Center
26 East Red Bank Avenue Woodbury, NJ 08096 (856)848-4464 Fax (856)848-8706

Di Medio, Lisa C., DO {1013028844} IntrMd(92,PA77)
+ Jefferson Health Primary & Specialty Care
1A Regulus Drive Turnersville, NJ 08012 (844)542-2273

Di Paolo, Jeffrey C., MD {1295829588} Radiol, RadNro(87,PA02)<NJ-OCEANMC>
+ Open MRI of Wall
1975 Route 34 Wall, NJ 07719 (732)974-8060
+ Coastal Imaging, LLC
79 Route 37 West/Suite 103 Toms River, NJ 08755 (732)974-8060 Fax (732)276-2325
+ Ocean Medical Center
425 Jack Martin Boulevard Brick, NJ 07719 (732)836-4040 Fax (732)836-4047

Di Paolo, Patrick J., MD {1245341171} OncHem, IntrMd(83,ITA17)<NJ-MTNSIDE>
+ 781 Bloomfield Avenue/Suite 1
Montclair, NJ 07042 (973)744-7979 Fax (973)744-8120
+ Medical first of NY & NJ
5 Franklin Avenue/Suite 501 Belleville, NJ 07109 (973)744-7979 Fax (973)751-4444

Di Paolo, Peter F., MD {1437219045} SrgOrt(82,NJ05)
+ 1225 McBride Avenue/Unit 111
Little Falls, NJ 07424 (973)239-1699 Fax (973)239-1692

Di Paolo, Raymond Paul, MD {1275598799} Pedtrc(75,MEX14)<NJ-NWTNMEM>
+ Skylands Pediatrics
328-A Sparta Avenue Sparta, NJ 07871 (973)729-2197 Fax (973)729-3653
+ Skylands Pediatrics
4 Oxbow Lane/Route 94 Franklin, NJ 07416 (973)729-2197 Fax (973)827-5093

Di Pasquale, Anthony J., DO {1215975446} EmrgMd(77,PA77)<NJ-VIRTVOOR>
+ Emergency Physician Associates, P.A.
307 South Evergreen Avenue/PO Box 298 Woodbury, NJ 08096 (856)848-3817 Fax (856)848-1431

Di Pasquale, Laurene, MD {1164499430} IntrMd, PulDis, SlpDis(82,DOM02)<NJ-ENGLWOOD>
+ 55 Orchard Street
Hillsdale, NJ 07642 (201)664-8663 Fax (201)664-8705

Di Piero, Alfred M., DO {1396857629} IntrMd(66,IA75)<NJ-UNDRWD, NJ-KMHSTRAT>
+ 400 Medical Center Drive/Suite E
Sewell, NJ 08080 (856)582-5678 Fax (856)582-8868

Di Ruggiero, Roger P., MD {1457301699} IntrMd(81,ITA22)<NJ-MORRISTN>
+ Omni-Med
131 Columbia Turnpike/Suite 3 Florham Park, NJ 07932 (973)377-8776 Fax (973)822-2393

Di Saverio, Joseph, MD {1740331495} Surgry(75,PA02)<NJ-VALLEY>
+ 140 Chestnut Street/Suite 301
Ridgewood, NJ 07450 (201)447-2777 Fax (201)445-3835

Di Stefano, Valeria M., MD {1457614679} ObsGyn
+ University Medical Group/OBGYN
125 Paterson Street/2nd Floor New Brunswick, NJ 08901 (732)235-6632 Fax (732)235-6627

Di Trolio, Joseph V., MD {1295767804} Urolgy(79,NJ05)
+ 556 Eagle Rock Avenue/Suite 204
Roseland, NJ 07068 (973)228-2771 Fax (973)228-7477

Di Turi, Richard Michael, MD {1093781106} Psychy, PsyCAd(95,NY15)<NJ-MMHKEMBL, NJ-MORRISTN>
+ Morristown Memorial Hospital/Mt. Kemble Division
95 Mount Kemble Avenue/Psych Morristown, NJ 07960 (973)971-4758

Di Turi, Suzanne V., MD {1598877789} Pedtrc, AdolMd(95,NY15)<NJ-MORRISTN>
+ Pediatrics On Broadway
10 Broadway Denville, NJ 07834 (973)625-7734 Fax (973)625-4821

Physicians by Name and Address

Di Vagno, Leonardo Joseph, MD {1851392435} CdvDis, IntrMd(89,ITA17)<NJ-HACKNSK>
+ Drs. Di Vagno, Hasan & Chung
  216 Route 17 North/Suite 201 Rochelle Park, NJ 07662 (201)845-3535   Fax (201)845-4040

Di Verniero, Richard Charles, Jr., MD {1609941657} SrgOrt(97,NJ05)<NJ-SJHREGMC, NJ-SJRSYELM>
+ Premier Orthopaedic Associates
  298 South Delsea Drive Vineland, NJ 08360 (856)690-1616   Fax (856)690-1089
  rcdmd@excite.com
+ Premier Orthopaedic Assocs of So NJ
  201 Tomlin Station Road/Suite C Mullica Hill, NJ 08062 (856)690-1616   Fax (856)223-9110
+ Premier Orthopaedic Assoc So NJ
  525 South State Street/Suite 2 Elmer, NJ 08360 (856)358-2559

Diab, Khaled D., MD {1750729679}<NJ-UNVMCPRN>
+ University Medical Center of Princeton at Plainsboro
  One Plainsboro Road Plainsboro, NJ 08536 (305)600-1176
  kdiabmd@gmail.com

Diah, Paulett, MD {1396799573} Pedtrc(97,NY20)
+ Audrey Hepburn Children's House
  12 Second Street Hackensack, NJ 07601 (201)996-2271   Fax (201)996-4926

Diakolios, Constantine E., MD {1366584724} IntrMd, Addctn(87,GREE)
+ 404 Dogwood Court
  Leonia, NJ 07605

Diamantopoulos, Vasilios T., MD {1184718371} EmrgMd(90,NJ05)
+ 1018 Boynton Avenue
  Westfield, NJ 07090 (908)518-1593   Fax (973)989-3092

Diamond, Elan Shlomo, MD {1659530608} IntrMd(08,NY20)<NJ-HOLYNAME>
+ Regional Cancer Center at Holy Name Medical Center
  718 Teaneck Road/Internal Med Teaneck, NJ 07666 (201)227-6008   Fax (201)227-6002

Diamond, Gigi R., MD {1295757359} InfDis, IntrMd(82,SPAI)<NJ-STBARNMC>
+ Livingston Subspecialty Group, P.A.
  349 East Northfield Road/Suite 200 Livingston, NJ 07039 (973)597-0900   Fax (973)597-0910
+ St. Barnabas Medical Center
  94 Old Short Hills Road/ID Livingston, NJ 07039 (973)322-5000

Diamond, Mark S., MD {1073514113} Nrolgy(77,PA02)
+ Neuroscience Center of Northern New Jersey
  310 Madison Avenue Morristown, NJ 07960 (973)285-1446   Fax (973)605-8854

Diamond, Martin, MD {1184694846} PedReh, PhysMd, Elecmy(75,PA12)<NJ-CHLSMT, NJ-CHLSOCEN>
+ Children's Specialized Hospital
  150 New Providence Road Mountainside, NJ 07092 (908)233-3720
  mdiamond@childrens-specialized.org
+ Children's Specialized Hospital-Ocean
  94 Stevens Road Toms River, NJ 08755 (732)914-1100
+ 116 South Euclid Avenue
  Westfield, NJ 07092 (908)233-4801   Fax (908)233-1364

Diamond, Paul M., MD {1518920461} IntrMd(77,MA07)<NJ-HOLYNAME, NJ-ENGLWOOD>
+ Bergenfield Medical
  205 North Washington Avenue Bergenfield, NJ 07621 (201)384-9255   Fax (201)384-2758

Diamond, Shari E., DO {1912926254} UrgtCr, IntrMd(85,IA75)<NJ-CHSFULD>
+ Professional HealthCare Services of Lawrenceville
  2500 US Highway 1 Lawrenceville, NJ 08648 (609)771-6660   Fax (609)530-0966

Diamond, Steven H., MD {1679582764} PedHem, Pedtrc(74,PA01)<NJ-HACKNSK, NJ-CHILTON>
+ Tomorrow's Children's Inst/HUMC
  30 Prospect Avenue/WFAN - PC 116 Hackensack, NJ 07601 (201)996-5437   Fax (201)487-7340
  sdiamond@humed.com

Diamond, Stuart M., MD {1174589709} Urolgy, IntrMd(92,NY03)<NJ-MEMSALEM>
+ Center for Advanced Urology Associates, PA
  330 Salem Woodstown Road/Suite 8 Salem, NJ 08079 (856)339-4466   Fax (856)339-6580
+ Center for Advanced Urology Associates, PA
  811 Sunset Road Burlington, NJ 08016 (856)339-4466   Fax (856)339-6580

Diana, Joseph N., MD {1649370131} IntrMd(77,ITA01)
+ 15 Liddy Place
  West Caldwell, NJ 07006

Diano, Rowen Gumapas, MD {1992862585} IntrMd, Grtrcs(83,PHIL)<NJ-MTNSIDE>
+ 48 North Fullerton Avenue
  Montclair, NJ 07042 (973)744-3371

Diao, Carolina Efren, MD {1275602344} Psychy(71,PHI09)<NJ-TRENTPSY>
+ 3131 Princeton Pike/Suite 109
  Lawrenceville, NJ 08648 (609)633-1500

Diar Bakerli, Hala, MD {1952532236} IntrMd
+ 716 Broad Street/Suite 2 D
  Clifton, NJ 07013 (973)435-6070   Fax (973)435-6090

Diarbakerli, Fares, MD {1508011602} ObsGyn
+ SA HealthCare Management, LLC
  145 Route 46 West/Suite 304 Wayne, NJ 07470 (973)826-8290   Fax (866)760-4555
+ NJ Best OBGYN
  716 Broad Street/Suite 6 A Clifton, NJ 07013 (973)826-8290   Fax (973)574-1008

Dias, Alan Steven, MD {1609821685} EmrgMd(95,FL02)<NJ-VIRTMHBC>
+ Virtua Memorial
  175 Madison Avenue/EmergMed Mount Holly, NJ 08060 (609)267-0700   Fax (609)914-6067

Dias, Magna M., MD {1609886381} Pedtrc(96,MD07)<NJ-SHOREMEM>
+ Nemours Dupont Pediatrics
  1925 Pacific Avenue Atlantic City, NJ 08401 (609)345-4000   Fax (609)572-8523

Dias Martin, Karen A., MD {1407914542} ObsGyn(84,OH41)
+ 200 Highland Avenue/Suite 230
  Glen Ridge, NJ 07028 (973)743-8585   Fax (973)743-1549

Diaz, Agustin, MD {1174582720} IntrMd(87,DOM14)<NJ-MEADWLND, NJ-PALISADE>
+ East Hudson Primary Care, PC
  435 57th Street West New York, NJ 07093 (201)863-2620   Fax (201)863-4804

Diaz, Elizabeth Ann, MD {1619189123} PedAne, Anesth, Rserch(81,NY19)
+ Forest Research Institute
  201 Strykers Road/Suite 19-249 Phillipsburg, NJ 08865 (908)399-6626

Diaz, Francis L., MD {1932314382} RadDia(03,PA02)<NJ-STCLRDEN>
+ Northwest Radiology Associates, P.A.
  400 West Blackwell Street Dover, NJ 07801 (973)625-6648   Fax (973)983-5206
+ St. Clare's Hospital-Denville Campus
  25 Pocono Road Denville, NJ 07834 (973)625-6000

Diaz, Francisco J., MD {1972509958} FamMed(89,DOMI)<NJ-STMRYPAS, NJ-CHRIST>
+ Bayonne Family Practice
  391 Kennedy Boulevard Bayonne, NJ 07002 (201)858-4110   Fax (201)858-2240

Diaz, Jose F., MD {1467528299} Urolgy(68,COL04)
+ Genito Urinary Associates
  20 Magnolia Avenue/Suite D Bridgeton, NJ 08302 (856)455-5770   Fax (856)453-8458
+ Genito Urinary Associates
  125 State Street/Suite 4 Elmer, NJ 08318 (856)358-2330

Diaz, Julio C., MD {1881682300} Pedtrc(88,MEX03)<NJ-OVERLOOK, NJ-MORRISTN>
+ Summit Medical Group
  85 Woodland Road Short Hills, NJ 07078 (973)376-0080   Fax (973)921-0669
+ Summit Medical Group-Berkeley Heights Campus
  1 Diamond Hill Road Berkeley Heights, NJ 07922 (973)376-0080   Fax (908)790-6576

Diaz, Julio E., MD {1831192129} IntrMd(90,NJ06)<NJ-JFKMED, NJ-MEADWLND>
+ Care Station Medical Group
  328 West St. Georges Avenue Linden, NJ 07036 (908)925-2273   Fax (908)925-2235
+ Care Station Medical Group
  456 Prospect Avenue West Orange, NJ 07052 (908)925-2273   Fax (973)731-9881

Diaz, Laura M., MD {1720593288} Pedtrc
+ Children's Specialized Hospital
  200 Somerset Street New Brunswick, NJ 08901 (973)768-1646

Diaz, Lissa, DO {1487066924} EmrgMd<NJ-KMHSTRAT>
+ Kennedy Memorial Hospital-University Medical Center
  18 East Laurel Road Stratford, NJ 08084 (856)346-7985

Diaz, Lloyd P., MD {1265634489} Anesth(03,OH44)<NJ-HACKNSK>
+ Hackensack University MC-Anesthesia Dept
  30 Prospect Avenue/Room 2703 Hackensack, NJ 07601 (201)996-2419   Fax (201)996-3962
+ Hackensack University Medical Center
  30 Prospect Avenue/Anesth Hackensack, NJ 07601 (201)996-2000

Diaz, Roberto R., MD {1912918400} IntrMd, CdvDis(70,PHIL)
+ 4 Bypass Road/Suite 203
  Salem, NJ 08079 (856)339-4444   Fax (856)339-9437

Diaz, Yanirys, MD {1831431493} Obstet
+ Cooper University Hospital
  One Cooper Plaza Camden, NJ 08103 (856)342-2000

+ Mercer Ob/Gyn Associates at Mercer
  446 Bellevue Avenue Trenton, NJ 08618 (856)342-2000   Fax (609)394-4070

Diaz Gonzalez, Rodolfo, MD {1851360663} Otlryg(81,PRO02)
+ Ear Nose & Throat Specialist
  1206 West Sherman Avenue/Suite B2 Vineland, NJ 08360 (856)696-5510   Fax (856)696-5590

Diaz Jimenez, Jose Eduardo, MD {1396906178} OthrSp, UrgtCr, IntrMd(94,NJ05)
+ Creations Medical Spa
  901 Route 168/Suite408 Blackwood, NJ 08012 (856)589-1151   Fax (856)589-1554

Diaz-Hernandez, Jose Juan, MD {1346592417} Radiol(06,PRO02)<NY-MTSINAI, NY-MTSINYHS>
+ Newark Beth Israel Medical Center
  201 Lyons Avenue Newark, NJ 07112 (973)926-7038

Diaz-Johnson, Nereida, MD {1013939917} IntrMd(82,NY47)
+ Union Medical Group LLC
  2401 Morris Avenue/Suite 101 Union, NJ 07083 (908)688-5000   Fax (908)688-5220

Dib, Haitham R., MD {1225124613} CdvDis, IntrMd, CritCr(86,SYR01)<NJ-ACMCMAIN, NJ-ACMCITY>
+ Shore Memorial Hospital
  1 East New York Avenue/Cardiology Somers Point, NJ 08244 (609)365-3100   Fax (609)652-0150
+ Atlantic Cardiology in Ventor
  6725 Atlantic Avenue/2nd Floor Ventnor, NJ 08406 (609)822-2006
+ Atlantic Cardiology in Galloway
  436 Chris Gaupp Drive/Suite 204 Galloway, NJ 08244 (609)652-0100   Fax (609)652-7616

Dib, Joe Elias, MD {1700820933} EmrgMd, IntrMd(94,NY08)<NJ-CLARMAAS, NJ-CHRIST>
+ Clara Maass Medical Center
  1 Clara Maass Drive/EmergMed Belleville, NJ 07109 (973)450-2000

Dibadj, Khosro, MD {1831264399} Anesth(96,IRA01)
+ New Jersey Anesthesia Associates, P.C.
  252 Columbia Turnpike/PO Box 0037 Florham Park, NJ 07932 (973)660-9334   Fax (973)660-9779

Dibba, Prameela, MD {1730434598}
+ Tatem Brown Family Practice
  2225 East Evesham Road/Suite 101 Voorhees, NJ 08043 (856)795-4330   Fax (856)325-3704

DiBella, Louis J., Jr., MD {1437304250} Urolgy(72,NJ05)<NJ-MEADWLND, NJ-HACKNSK>
+ New Jersey Urology Associates, PA
  110 Meadowlands Parkway Secaucus, NJ 07094 (201)867-1297   Fax (201)867-4165
+ Meadowlands Hospital Medical Center
  55 Meadowlands Parkway Secaucus, NJ 07096 (201)392-3100

Dibenedetto, Robert J., MD {1861592586} ObsGyn(73,NJ05)<NJ-STBARNMC>
+ 23 Crestfield Road
  Boonton, NJ 07005 (973)216-6049

DiBernardo, Barry E., MD {1164599262} SrgPlstc, SrgBst(84,NY20)
+ New Jersey Plastic Surgery
  29 Park Street Montclair, NJ 07042 (973)509-2000   Fax (973)655-1228

Dibona, Anthony D., Jr., DO {1194785717} FamMed(81,IA75)<NJ-SJRSYELM, NJ-KENEDYHS>
+ Wedgewood Family Practice Associates PA
  302 Hurffville Cross-Keys Road Sewell, NJ 08080 (856)589-4610   Fax (609)589-1624

DiCarlo, Frederick J., MD PthAcl(83,GRN01)<NJ-HACKNSK>
+ Bergen County Medical Examiner's Office
  351 East Ridgewood Avenue Paramus, NJ 07652 (201)634-2940   Fax (201)634-2950
+ 123 Knollwood Drive
  Watchung, NJ 07069

DiCarlo, Jilma Patricia, MD {1467513119} Pedtrc(79,PAN01)<NJ-STPETER, NJ-JFKMED>
+ 285 Durham Avenue/Suite 2B
  South Plainfield, NJ 07080 (908)756-7500   Fax (908)756-8025
  Jpdicarlo@yahoo.com

Dicenzo-Flynn, Carla F., MD {1114942075} IntrMd(89,BRA11)<NJ-MORRISTN, NJ-OVERLOOK>
+ 146 Columbia Turnpike/Suite 308
  Florham Park, NJ 07932 (973)410-0452   Fax (973)410-0057

DiChiara, Frank P., DO {1053382291} GenPrc, FamMed(76,PA77)<NJ-OCEANMC>
+ Drs. DiChiara and Lozowski
  2446 Church Road/Suite 10 Toms River, NJ 08753 (732)255-3636   Fax (732)864-0176

Dichter, Eric Kyle, DO {1033557772} EmrgMd
+ Rowan University-School of Osteopathic Medicine
  1 Medical Center Drive Stratford, NJ 08084 (856)566-7050

Dick, Adam M., MD {1770597551} Pedtrc(86,NY09)<NJ-HCK-TSTWN, NJ-MORRISTN>
+ Plaza Family Care
657 Willow Grove Street/Suite 401   Hackettstown, NJ 07840   (908)850-7400   Fax (908)850-7801
+ Plaza Family Care
245 Main Street/Suite 300 & 302   Chester, NJ 07930   (908)850-7800   Fax (908)879-6738

Dick, Charles, MD {1639263882} Psychy
+ 1057 Shunpike Road
Cape May, NJ 08204

Dick, Donna Rosalind, MD {1134344781} Pedtrc(94,MA05)<NJ-STCLRDEN>
+ Franklin Pediatrics, PA
91 South Jefferson Road/Suite 200   Whippany, NJ 07981   (973)538-6116   Fax (973)538-3712

Dick, Leon S., MD {1811036130} SrgVas, Surgry(72,JMAC)<NJ-EASTORNG>
+ 2232 Millburn Avenue
Maplewood, NJ 07040   (973)763-8087   Fax (973)763-6482

Dick, Susan E., MD {1669442935} FamMed, Grtrcs(79,PA01)<NJ-JRSYSHMC>
+ 230 Neptune Boulevard/Suite 202
Neptune, NJ 07753   (732)774-4040   Fax (732)774-2143

Dicker, Adam P., MD {1558383984} RadOnc
+ 418 Silver Hill Road
Cherry Hill, NJ 08002

Dicker, Paul M., MD {1528145059} ObsGyn(92,NY19)<NJ-VALLEY, NJ-HACKNSK>
+ The Center for Women's Health
270 Old Hook Road/2nd Floor   Westwood, NJ 07675   (201)358-0505   Fax (201)358-1515

Dicker, Richard Irving, MD {1154436863} Pedtrc(78,MEX03)
+ Pediatrics On Broadway
10 Broadway   Denville, NJ 07834   (973)625-7734   Fax (973)625-4821

Dickerson, David B., MD {1033317219} SrgOrt(03,LA06)<NJ-MONMOUTH, NJ-COMMED>
+ Performance Orthopaedics & Sports Medicine
9 Hospital Drive   Toms River, NJ 08755   (732)691-4898   Fax (732)608-8950
info@performanceorthonj.com
+ Performance Orthopaedics & Sports Medicine
1131 Broad Street/Suite 201/Building B   Shrewsbury, NJ 07702   (732)691-4898   Fax (732)608-8950

Dickes, Richard A., MD {1013005180} Psychy(67,NY46)
+ 310 Madison Avenue/Suite 220
Morristown, NJ 07960   (973)267-1238   Fax (973)540-8849

Dickson, David Gordon, MD {1063482545} CdvDis, IntrMd, Int-Crd(85,NY01)<NJ-MORRISTN>
+ Morristown Cardiology Associates, P.A.
435 South Street/Suite 100   Morristown, NJ 07960   (973)267-3944   Fax (973)889-1107

Dickson, Robert W., III, MD {1851314017} IntrMd(88,TX13)
+ Shiloh Medical Group
351 Main Street/PO Box 110   Shiloh, NJ 08353   (856)455-1464   Fax (856)453-8401

Dickson, Scott Vincent, DO {1043235328} EmrgMd(99,NJ75)<NJ-VIRTMHBC>
+ Virtua Memorial
175 Madison Avenue/EmrgMed   Mount Holly, NJ 08060   (609)267-0700   Fax (609)914-6067

Dickstein, Richard A., MD {1376595108} CdvDis(70,KY02)<NJ-SJRSYELM, NJ-OURLADY>
+ Cardiovascular Associates of The Delaware Valley, PA
1840 Frontage Road   Cherry Hill, NJ 08034   (856)795-2227   Fax (856)795-7436
+ Cardiovascular Associates
210 West Atlantic Avenue   Haddon Heights, NJ 08035   (856)795-2227   Fax (856)547-5337
+ Cardiovascular Associates of The Delaware Valley, PA
525 State Street/Suite 3   Elmer, NJ 08034   (856)358-2363   Fax (856)358-0725

Dicola, May Bersalona, MD {1215000708} FamMed(01,NJ06)
+ Comprehensive Family Medicine, PA
27 Mountain Boulevard/Suite 6   Warren, NJ 07059   (908)222-7777   Fax (908)222-9242

Didie, William J., MD {1609815463} Radiol, RadDia(00,NY15)<NJ-COMMED>
+ Community Medical Center
99 Route 37 West/Radiol   Toms River, NJ 08755   (732)557-8000   Fax (732)505-0325

Diefenbacher, Jaclyn, MD {1386203487}<NJ-CHSFULD>
+ Capital Health System/Fuld Campus
750 Brunswick Avenue   Trenton, NJ 08638   (609)394-6000

Diehl, William L., MD {1629068457} SrgOnc, Surgry(81,MEXI)
+ Summit Medical Group Orthopedics and Sports Medicine
140 Park Avenue/2nd Floor   Florham Park, NJ 07932   (973)404-9980   Fax (973)267-7295
+ Allied Surgical Group
261 James Street/Suite 2-G   Morristown, NJ 07960

(973)404-9980   Fax (973)267-7295

Diener, Melissa Ann, MD {1316106347} IntrMd<PA-TMPHOSP>
+ Atlantic Gastroenterology Associates, P.A.
3205 Fire Road/Suite 4   Egg Harbor Township, NJ 08234   (609)407-1220   Fax (609)407-0220

Dienna, Erik, MD {1003109893} Pedtrc
+ St. Barnabas Cancer Center
94 Old Short Hills Road/Suite 1   Livingston, NJ 07039   (973)322-5650

Dierkes, Thomas F., DO {1336142041} Pedtrc(94,MO78)<NJ-BUR-DTMLN, NJ-SHOREMEM>
+ Rainbow Pediatrics
2041 US Highway 9   Cape May Court House, NJ 08210   (609)624-9003   Fax (609)624-9002
+ Volunteers in Medicine
423 North Route 9   Cape May Court House, NJ 08210   (609)624-9003   Fax (609)463-2830

Dierlam, Paul T., MD {1487679551} Anesth(84,GRNA)<NJ-HCK-TSTWN>
+ Hackettstown Regional Medical Center
651 Willow Grove Street   Hackettstown, NJ 07840   (908)852-5100

Dietzek, Charles L., DO {1639283344} SrgVas, Surgry(83,NY75)<NJ-KMHSTRAT>
+ Center for Vascular Surgery
1000 White Horse Road/Suite 703   Voorhees, NJ 08043   (856)346-1500   Fax (856)309-9774
+ University Hospital -SOM University Doctors Surgeons
42 East Laurel Road/Suite 2500-2600   Stratford, NJ 08084   (856)346-1500   Fax (856)566-6873

Dieudonne, Arry, MD {1649349333} Pedtrc, PedInf(82,HAI01)<NJ-UMDNJ>
+ University Hospital
150 Bergen Street/G102 /Pedi   Newark, NJ 07103   (973)972-0380   Fax (973)972-6443

Difabio, Kelly Ann, DO {1265870091} EmrgMd
+ 1825 Route 35
Wall Township, NJ 07719   (732)280-2600

Difazio, Matthew C., MD {1649203191} RadDia(92,MI01)<NJ-UN-VMCPRN>
+ Princeton Radiology Associates, P.A.
419 North Harrison Street   Princeton, NJ 08540   (609)921-3345   Fax (609)683-8847
+ Princeton Radiology Associates, P.A.
9 Centre Drive   Jamesburg, NJ 08831   (609)921-3345   Fax (609)655-4016
+ Princeton Radiology Associates, P.A.
3674 Route 27   Kendall Park, NJ 08540   (732)821-5563   Fax (732)821-6675

Difelice, Gregory Scott, MD {1639148208} SrgOrt, SprtMd(94,NJ05)<NY-PRSBWEIL>
+ HSS Paramus Outpatient Center
140 East Ridgewood Avenue/Suite 175-S   Paramus, NJ 07652   (201)796-2255   Fax (201)796-3711

DiFerdinando, George Thomas, Jr., MD {1669746327} PubHth(78,NC01)
+ New Jersey Department of Health and Senior Services
50 East State/PO Box 360   Trenton, NJ 08625   (609)292-9354   Fax (609)292-6523
gdiferdinando@doh.state.nj.us

DiGaetano, Andrea F., MD {1548231624} ObsGyn(77,PA07)<NJ-VIRTMHBC, NJ-VIRTVOOR>
+ Womens Health Associates PA
2301 East Evesham Road/Suite 602   Voorhees, NJ 08043   (856)772-2066   Fax (856)772-9159

Digby, Thomas E., MD {1386600294} Pedtrc(66,MD07)<NJ-NWT-NMEM, NJ-MORRISTN>
+ Advocare Sussex County Pediatrics Newton
39 Newton Sparta Road   Newton, NJ 07860   (973)383-9841   Fax (973)383-7989
+ Advocare Sussex County Pediatrics Montague
2B Myrtle Drive   Montague, NJ 07827   (973)383-9841   Fax (973)293-0138

Digenio, Andres German, MD {1568748499} GPrvMd(81,URU01)
+ 265 North Garden Court
Egg Harbor City, NJ 08215

Digenio, Ines Elena, MD {1215113477} FamMed
+ 1401 Atlantic Avenue
Atlantic City, NJ 08401

DiGiacomo, Dennis A., MD {1649218421} IntrMd(78,MEX14)<NJ-OVERLOOK, NJ-STMICHL>
+ Vailsburg Medical Associates PA
1072 South Orange Avenue   Newark, NJ 07106   (973)623-5309   Fax (973)399-8562
+ Vailsburg Medical Associates PA
2801 Morris Avenue   Union, NJ 07083   (908)851-2500

Digiacomo, Jody Christopher, MD {1063449551} SrgTrm, SrgCrC(86,PA13)<NJ-CENTRAST>
+ CentraState Medical Center
901 West Main Street/Emergency   Freehold, NJ 07728   (732)431-2000

Digiacomo, Michael B., MD {1821389958} Anesth
+ Englewood Anesthesiology
350 Engle Street   Englewood, NJ 07631   (201)894-3238   Fax (201)894-0585

DiGiacomo, William A., MD {1184672172} IntrMd(74,MEX03)<NJ-OVERLOOK, NJ-STMICHL>
+ 25 Coniston Road
Short Hills, NJ 07078

DiGiacomo, William S., MD {1982652970} Gastrn(01,NET09)<NJ-STMICHL, NJ-CLARMAAS>
+ William Scott DiGiacomo LLC
2801 Morris Drive   Union, NJ 07083   (908)857-2500   Fax (908)851-0708
+ William Scott DiGiacomo LLC
1072 South Orange Avenue   Newark, NJ 07106   (973)623-5309

Digioia, John J., Jr., MD {1154359255} IntrMd(85,ITAL)<NJ-HOBUNIMC>
+ Drs. DiGioia & Singh
1971 Kennedy Boulevard   Jersey City, NJ 07305   (201)432-5222   Fax (201)333-2503

DiGiovanni, Leonard G., DO {1013903228} FamMed(63,MO79)<NJ-ENGLWOOD>
+ The Park Medical Group
220 Livingston Street/Suite 202   Northvale, NJ 07647   (201)768-9090   Fax (201)768-9009
lendee@webtv.net

Digiovanni, Marianne, DO {1831169184} ObsGyn(85,NJ75)
+ Obstetrics & Gynecology Associates
239 Hurffville Crosskeys Road   Sewell, NJ 08080   (856)262-8300   Fax (856)262-1635

Digiovanni, Vincent Mathew, DO {1154361277} Surgry(00,PA77)
+ AtlantiCare Physician Group Joslin Diabetes Center
2500 English Creek Avenue/Bldg 800   Egg Harbor Township, NJ 08234   (609)407-2277   Fax (609)272-6306

Dignam, Ritchell Rodriguez, MD {1467432476} IntrMd, Grtrcs(88,PHI08)
+ New Jersey Institute for Successful Aging
42 East Laurel Road/Suite 1800   Stratford, NJ 08084   (856)566-6843   Fax (856)566-6781
+ University of Medicine & Dentistry of New Jersey-SOM
42 East Laurel Road   Stratford, NJ 08084   (856)566-6843

DiGregorio, Kenneth J., MD {1598726382} Gastrn, IntrMd(86,VA04)
+ Hunterdon Gastroenterology Associates, P.A.
1100 Wescott Drive/Suite 206-207   Flemington, NJ 08822   (908)483-4000   Fax (908)788-5090
+ Hunterdon Gastroenterology Associates, P.A.
135 West End Avenue/Suite 204   Somerville, NJ 08876   (908)483-4000   Fax (908)788-5090

Diiorio, Emil John, MD {1922005826} SrgOrt
+ Coordinated Health
222 Red Lane   Phillipsburg, NJ 08865   (610)861-8080   Fax (610)849-1013
jlaychock@coordinatedhealth.com

Dikengil, Asim G., MD {1295838845} Radiol, RadDia(82,NJ06)
+ A.G. Dikengil MD PA
736 Page Avenue   Lyndhurst, NJ 07071   (201)729-1234   Fax (201)729-1233

Dikengil, Yahya Mete, MD {1073687273} PulDis, CritCr, SlpDis(89,NJ05)<NJ-MTNSIDE>
+ 388 Pompton Avenue/Suite 8
Cedar Grove, NJ 07009   (973)433-0665   Fax (973)433-0668
+ Hackensack UMC Mountainside
1 Bay Avenue/Sleep Ctr   Montclair, NJ 07042   (973)433-0665   Fax (973)433-0668

Diko, Sindi, DO {1154812071}<NJ-STJOSHOS>
+ St. Joseph's Regional Medical Center
703 Main Street   Paterson, NJ 07503   (973)754-2000

Dilallo, Denis, MD {1710980131} Pedtrc, NnPnMd(82,NJ05)<NJ-STJOSHOS>
+ St. Joseph's Children's Hospital
703 Main Street   Paterson, NJ 07503   (973)754-2555   Fax (973)754-2567

Dileonardo, Francesca, MD {1770520645} EmrgMd(87,PA13)<NJ-KMHSTRAT>
+ 2250 Chapel Avenue West
Cherry Hill, NJ 08002   (610)892-3999

Dilks, Robert H., MD {1871565671} ObsGyn(74,MO34)<NJ-UN-DRWD, NJ-VIRTBERL>
+ 188 Fries Mill Road/Suite B1
Turnersville, NJ 08012

Dill, Barbara A., MD {1962458851} ObsGyn(91,VT02)<NJ-EN-GLWOOD>
+ 440 Curry Avenue/Suite C
Englewood, NJ 07631   (201)894-0525   Fax (201)894-8666
drdillobgyn@verizon.net
+ JFK Medical Center
65 James Street   Edison, NJ 08820   (201)894-0525   Fax (732)906-4961

Physicians by Name and Address

Dillaway, Winthrop Chalmers, III, MD {1194943191} FamMed, IntrMd(75,MEX03)
+ New Jersey Universal HealthCare Coalition
11 Willard Place   Morristown, NJ 07960   (862)268-0986

Dillner, Jill Sue, DO {1386969830}
+ 15 Fletcher Drive
Morganville, NJ 07751   (732)754-9551

Dillon, John J., MD {1033409412} EmrgMd<NJ-COOPRUMC>
+ Cooper University Hospital
One Cooper Plaza/EmergMed   Camden, NJ 08103
(856)342-2351

Dillon, Richard Lansing, MD {1306806237} RadDia, Radiol(93,PA02)<NJ-OCEANMC>
+ Ocean Medical Center
425 Jack Martin Boulevard/Radiology   Brick, NJ 08723
(732)840-2200

DiLorenzo, William Richard, DO {1013199538} IntrMd, CdvDis(02,NY75)<NY-NSUHMANH>
+ Shore Cardiac Institute
367 Lakehurst Road   Toms River, NJ 08755   (732)473-0158
Fax (732)473-0033

Dimaculangan, Nelo De Gala, MD {1164492971} Pedtrc(89,PHIL)<NJ-CHSMRCER>
+ Old Bergen Pediatrics PC
4 Highland Avenue   Jersey City, NJ 07306   (201)434-3997
Fax (201)434-3304
+ Capital Health System/Mercer Campus
446 Bellevue Avenue/Pedi   Trenton, NJ 08618   (609)394-4000

Dimaio, Andrea Lynne, DO {1225553217} Psychy<NJ-COOPRUMC>
+ Cooper University Hospital
One Cooper Plaza/Suite 307   Camden, NJ 08103   (856)342-2328

DiMaio, Robert D., DO {1932149226} FamMed(85,PA77)<NJ-OURLADY, NJ-KMHCHRRY>
+ Cherry Hill Primary and Specialty Care
457 Haddonfield Road/Suite 110   Cherry Hill, NJ 08002
(844)542-2273   Fax (856)406-4570
+ Family Care Associates
6705 Park Avenue   Pennsauken, NJ 08109   (844)542-2273
Fax (856)663-3038

Dimapilis, Ann B., DO {1245229913} FamMed(88,NJ75)<NJ-VIRTVOOR>
+ Tatem Brown Family Practice
2225 East Evesham Road/Suite 101   Voorhees, NJ 08043
(856)795-4330   Fax (856)325-3704

DiMarco, Jack Peter, MD {1841234341} PhysMd, IntrMd(79,MO02)<NJ-OURLADY>
+ Associated Physiatrists of Southern New Jersey
1600 Haddon Avenue/Room R-122   Camden, NJ 08103
(856)757-3878   Fax (856)757-3760
+ Associated Physiatrists of Southern New Jersey
501 West Front Street   Elmer, NJ 08318   (856)757-3878
Fax (856)757-3760

DiMarino, Anthony J., Jr., MD {1780643775} Gastrn, IntrMd(68,PA09)<NJ-UNDRWD, NJ-SJRSYELM>
+ South Jersey Endoscopy Center
26 East Red Bank Avenue   Woodbury, NJ 08096   (856)848-4464   Fax (856)848-8706

Dimino, Michael L., MD {1386662872} ObsGyn, IntrMd(90,DC01)<NJ-CENTRAST>
+ Women's Physicians & Surgeons
501 Iron Bridge Road/Suite 10   Freehold, NJ 07728
(732)431-2999   Fax (732)431-2993
+ Women's Physicians & Surgeons
510 Bridge Plaza Drive   Englishtown, NJ 07726   (732)431-2999   Fax (732)536-4570
+ Women's Physicians & Surgeons
245A Main Street   Matawan, NJ 07728   (732)566-9466
Fax (732)566-0343

Dimitrova, Dessislava Iv, MD {1548465552} IntrMd(95,BUL02)<NJ-CAPITLHS>
+ 11 South Mill Road
Princeton Junction, NJ 08550   (609)750-8547
ddimitrova@aol.com

Dimitry, Edward, Jr., MD {1275534323} CritCr, PulDis(88,PA09)<NJ-MORRISTN, NJ-OVERLOOK>
+ Pulmonary & Allergy Associates
8 Saddle Road/Suite 101   Cedar Knolls, NJ 07927
(973)267-9393   Fax (973)540-0472
edward.dimitry@pulmonaryandallergyassociates.com
+ Pulmonary & Allergy Associates
1 Springfield Avenue/Suite 3-A   Summit, NJ 07901
(973)267-9393   Fax (908)934-0556

Dimov, Nikolay D., MD {1033588041} PthAcl
+ 103 River Road/Apt A6
Nutley, NJ 07110

Ding, Yifeng, MD {1255422960} Anesth(86,CHN1I)
+ James Street Anesthesia
102 James Street/Suite 103   Edison, NJ 08820   (732)494-1444   Fax (732)494-7052

Ding, You-Guang, MD {1346292786} NuclMd, CarNuc(84,CHN1J)
+ 44 Sylvan Avenue/Suite 1-E
Englewood Cliffs, NJ 07632   Fax (201)632-7000

Dinh, Cung T., MD {1538186994} Anesth(03,VA07)
+ Hamilton Anesthesia Associates
2119 Highway 33/Suite B   Trenton, NJ 08690   (609)581-5303   Fax (609)631-6839

Dinh, Megan, MD {1306943410} Pedtrc(03,VA07)<NJ-UNVM-CPRN>
+ Princeton Nassau Pediatrics, P.A.
196 Princeton-Hightstown Road   West Windsor, NJ 08550
(609)799-5335   Fax (609)799-2294
+ Princeton Nassau Pediatrics, P.A.
301 North Harrison Street   Princeton, NJ 08540   (609)799-5335   Fax (609)924-3577

Dinh, Tuan A., MD {1588674386} ObsGyn, MtFtMd, FamMed(86,TX02)<NJ-COOPRUMC>
+ Cooper University Hospital
One Cooper Plaza   Camden, NJ 08103   (856)342-2000

Dinks-Brown, Shantay M., DO {1013112390} FamMed(05,TX78)
+ CAMCare Health Corporation
817 Federal Street   Camden, NJ 08103   (856)541-8217
Fax (856)541-4611

Dinneen, Henry Scott, DO {1417247784}<NJ-VAEASTOR>
+ VA New Jersey Health Care System-East Orange Campus
385 Tremont Avenue   East Orange, NJ 07018   (973)908-1474
hsdinneen@gmail.com

Dinovitser, Jay Daniel, DO {1649583808} IntrMd(09,NY75)
+ Dover Woods Health Care Center
1001 State Route 70   Toms River, NJ 08755   (732)370-4600

Dinowitz, Seth, MD {1336186667} EmrgMd(96,NY48)<NJ-SOCEANCO>
+ Southern Ocean County Medical Center
1140 Route 72 West/EmrgMed   Manahawkin, NJ 08050
(609)597-6011

Dinsmore, Steven Thomas, DO {1396705976} Nrolgy, IntrMd(82,PA77)<NJ-KMHSTRAT>
+ The Neurological Management Group
55 East Cuthbert Boulevard   Haddon Township, NJ 08108

Dinu, Catalina, MD {1730184110} ObsGyn(96)<NJ-STJOSHOS>
+ 1187 Main Avenue/Suite 1-A
Clifton, NJ 07011   (862)247-8440

Dinu, Veronica Carmen, MD {1699968743} PthAcl, PthDrm(89,ROM05)
+ Inform Diagnostics
825 Rahway Avenue   Union, NJ 07083   (732)901-7575
Fax (732)901-1555

Dionne-McCracken, Laura, MD {1659507945} Pedtrc(93,NJ05)
+ Pedi Health Medical Associates
720 Route 202-206 North/Suite 4   Bridgewater, NJ 08807
(908)722-5444   Fax (908)722-5071
+ Advocare Sinatra & Peng Pediatrics
169 Minebrook Road   Bernardsville, NJ 07924   (908)722-5444   Fax (908)766-5065

Diorio, Dominic A., MD {1275588196} EmrgMd, IntrMd, EmrgEMed(65,NJ15)<NJ-SJHREGMC>
+ SJH Regional Medical Center
1505 West Sherman Avenue   Vineland, NJ 08360
(856)641-8000
whitebeard39@aol.com

Diorio, Joseph J., MD {1891711826} EmrgMd(00,DMN01)<NJ-VALLEY>
+ The Valley Hospital
223 North Van Dien Avenue/Emerg Med   Ridgewood, NJ 07450   (201)447-8000

DiPaola, Douglas Joseph, MD {1699003145} SrgThr, Surgry, SrgCTh(82,DC02)<NJ-OURLADY, NJ-VIRTUAHS>
+ 5 Fullerton Road
Moorestown, NJ 08057   (856)866-5529   Fax (856)866-9268

DiPaola, Rocco J., MD {1285692053} Nrolgy(91,NJ05)<NJ-COMMED, NJ-OCEANMC>
+ Shore Neurology, P.A.
633 Route 37 West   Toms River, NJ 08755   (732)240-4787
Fax (732)240-3114
+ Shore Neurology, PA
1613 Route 88/Suite 3   Brick, NJ 08724   (732)240-4787
Fax (732)785-2599

DiPaolo, Ann, DO {1285604041} FamMed(01,NY75)
+ Toms River Family Medical Center PA
1028 Hooper Avenue   Toms River, NJ 08753   (732)349-8866   Fax (732)349-7842
+ Lacey Medical Group
411 US Highway 9/Suite 2   Lanoka Harbor, NJ 08734
(732)349-8866   Fax (609)971-0834

Dipasquale, Albert M., MD {1740284595} Dermat(81,CT02)<NJ-VIRTBERL, NJ-VIRTMARL>
+ 813 East Gate Drive/Suite B
Mount Laurel, NJ 08054   (856)222-9119   Fax (856)222-9907
adipasquale104@comcast.net

DiPisa, Leonard R., MD {1730176611} CdvDis, IntrMd(78,MEXI)
+ Toms River Cardiology Associates, LLP.
780 Route 37 West/Suite 310   Toms River, NJ 08755
(732)240-0599   Fax (732)240-3039

Dippl, Julia M., MD {1356377949} IntrMd(89,PA13)<NJ-STFRN-MED>
+ JFK Medical Center
65 James Street   Edison, NJ 08820   (732)321-7601   Fax (732)744-5614

Dippo, Grace E., MD {1689089641} Anesth
+ Cooper Anesthesia Associates
One Cooper Plaza/Suite 294-B   Camden, NJ 08103
(856)342-2425   Fax (856)968-8239

DiProspero, Elizabeth J., MD {1649579152} IntrMd
+ Warren Primary Care
23 Mountain Boulevard   Warren, NJ 07059   (908)598-7970
Fax (908)322-4989

DiRenzo, Joseph P., Jr., DO FamMed(94,PA77)
+ Partners in Primary Care
239 Hurffville Crosskeys Road   Sewell, NJ 08080   (856)881-1940
+ Drs. Gilliss and DiRenzo
27 East Chestnut Avenue   Merchantville, NJ 08109
(856)881-1940   Fax (856)662-7404

DiRico, Julie, MD {1417905001} IntrMd(78,MEX03)
+ Womens HealthCare of Union County
950 West Chestnut Street/Suite 102   Union, NJ 07083
(908)688-8545   Fax (908)688-8447

DiSabatino, Daniel, DO {1295120699} ObsGyn(PA77
+ West Essex Ob/Gyn Associates
200 South Orange Avenue/Suite 290   Livingston, NJ 07039
(973)740-1330   Fax (973)740-8998

Disabella, Vincent N., DO {1487632170} EmrgSptM, IntrMd(92,PA77)
+ Premier Orthopaedic Associates
298 South Delsea Drive   Vineland, NJ 08360   (856)690-1616   Fax (856)690-1089

Disandro, Daniel G., MD {1609804160} EmrgMd, IntrMd(93,PA13)<NJ-COOPRUMC>
+ Cooper University Medical Center/Camden
3 Cooper Plaza/Suite 500   Camden, NJ 08103   (856)356-4935
+ Cooper University Hospital
One Cooper Plaza/Emerg Med   Camden, NJ 08103
(856)342-2627

DiSandro, Theresa Maria, DO {1750544391} Gastrn, IntrMd(03,PA77>
+ Lourdes Medical Associates
500 Grove Street/Suite 100   Haddon Heights, NJ 08035
(856)796-9200   Fax (856)310-5603
+ LMA Gastroenterology Associates
63 Kresson Road/Suite 104   Cherry Hill, NJ 08034
(856)796-9200   Fax (856)424-3113

DiSanto, Vinson Michael, DO {1932300134} GenPrc, FamMAdlt(86,PA77)
+ 107 Monmouth Road/Suite 104
West Long Branch, NJ 07764   (732)542-2638   Fax (732)542-2620

Discepola, Patrick Joseph, MD {1669746368} Anesth<NJ-UMDNJ>
+ University Hospital
150 Bergen Street   Newark, NJ 07103   (973)972-0470

Discepola, Paul, MD {1427315340} EmrgMd<NJ-JRSYSHMC>
+ Jersey Shore University Medical Center
1945 Route 33/EmergMed   Neptune, NJ 07753   (732)776-4203

Disciglio, Michael J., MD {1922075373} Grtrcs, IntrMd(84,WIND)<NJ-MONMOUTH>
+ Barnabas Health Medical Group
1300 Highway 35 South/Suites 101-103   Ocean, NJ 07712
(732)531-6400   Fax (732)517-0223

Dise, Craig A., MD {1710921879} PthAcl, Pthlgy(75,PA01)<NJ-MORRISTN, NJ-OVERLOOK>
+ Morristown Medical Center
100 Madison Avenue/Path   Morristown, NJ 07962
(973)971-5600   Fax (973)290-7370
+ Overlook Medical Center
99 Beauvoir Avenue/PO Box 210   Summit, NJ 07902
(908)522-2000

Dishler, Elyse Lyn, MD {1700058385} FamMed(97,PA13)
+ 3002 Lincoln Drive West/Suite E
Marlton, NJ 08053   (856)701-8979   Fax (856)810-7662

Dismukes, Jennifer Bright, DO {1396818076} PsyCAd
+ 88 Orchard Road/Suite 2-6
Skillman, NJ 08558   (609)228-6896   Fax (940)293-8585

Dispenziere, Benjamin R., MD {1780734962} ObsGyn(78,NJ05)<NJ-VALLEY>
+ 43 Yawpo Avenue/Suite 4
Oakland, NJ 07436   (201)337-7201   Fax (201)337-9621

DiStefano, Kelly Frances, MD {1679511000} Anesth(01,NET09)
+ 20 Longeran Lane
West Orange, NJ 07052

Distefano, Kenneth Louis, MD {1619146677} FamMed
+ 1 Mount Prospect Avenue
Verona, NJ 07044 (973)239-7777 Fax (973)239-7082

Distefano, Michael C., MD {1407883887} SrgOrt(77,NY46)<NJ-HACKNSK, NJ-VALLEY>
+ Dr. Distefano and Associates
140 Route 17 North/Suite 225 Paramus, NJ 07652
(201)261-5501 Fax (201)261-3350

Ditkoff, Jonathan W., MD {1386600823} Ophthl(89,NY15)<NJ-MTNSIDE>
+ The Eye Care Ctr of New Jersey
108 Broughton Avenue Bloomfield, NJ 07003 (973)743-1331 Fax (973)743-6577

Ditmar, Mark F., MD {1629168356} Pedtrc(83,MA01)<NJ-ACMC-MAIN, NJ-ACMCITY>
+ AtlantiCare/Dupont Children's Health Program
2500 English Creek Avenue Egg Harbor Township, NJ 08234
(609)641-3700 Fax (609)641-3652

Dittrich, Richard J., DO {1528030327} ObsGyn, IntrMd(73,IA75)<NJ-VIRTVOOR>
+ 1000 White Horse Road/Suite 612
Voorhees, NJ 08043 (856)435-9090 Fax (856)435-8753

Ditullio, Anthony Joseph, MD {1942347323} AdmMgt, AeroMd, IntrMd(73,PA09)
+ 21 Andrew Drive
Lawrenceville, NJ 08648

Dituro, Joseph William, MD {1194871459} IntrMd(78,MEXI)
+ 242 Paterson Avenue
East Rutherford, NJ 07073 (201)460-0302 Fax (201)460-0348

Ditusa, Diane Michele, DO {1225283278} ObsGyn<NJ-JRSYSHMC, NJ-OCEANMC>
+ Brielle Obstetrics & Gynecology, P.A.
2671 Highway 70/Wall Township Manasquan, NJ 08736
(732)528-6999 Fax (732)528-3397
+ Brielle Obstetrics & Gynecology, P.A.
117 County Line Road Lakewood, NJ 08701 (732)528-6999 Fax (732)942-1919
+ Jersey Shore University Medical Center
1945 Route 33/OB/GYN Neptune, NJ 08736 (732)776-3790

Diventi, Christina G., MD {1922112291} ObsGyn(02,NJ06)
+ Princeton Medical Group, P.A.
419 North Harrison Street Princeton, NJ 08540 (609)924-9300 Fax (609)924-6552

Divilov, Vadim, MD {1841678422} IntHos
+ Cooper University Hospital Hospitalists
One Cooper Plaza/Suite 222/Drrnce Camden, NJ 08103
(856)342-2000

Divino, Eumena M., MD {1225076235} ObsGyn(64,PHI01)<NJ-RBAYOLDB, NJ-RBAYPERT>
+ Bay Obstetrics & Gynecology
740 US Highway 1 North Iselin, NJ 08830 (732)362-3840
Fax (732)362-3850
+ Bay Obstetrics & Gynecology
2 Hospital Plaza/Suite 314 Old Bridge, NJ 08857
(732)362-3840 Fax (732)360-4081

Diwan, Nauman Abdul, MD {1609802057} IntrMd(89,PAKI)<NJ-CHSMRCER>
+ Medical Associates at Hamilton PC
1235 Whitehorse Mercerville Rd Hamilton, NJ 08619
(609)581-9000 Fax (609)585-7228
+ 1760 White Horse Hamilton Road/Suite 4
Hamilton, NJ 08690 (609)581-9000 Fax (609)890-8410

Diwan, Ravi, MD {1376792382} CdvDis, IntrMd, IntCrd(06,IRE04)
+ Shore Heart Group, P.A.
1820 State Route 33/Suite 4-B Neptune, NJ 07753
(732)776-8500 Fax (732)776-8946
+ Shore Heart Group, P.A.
555 Iron Bridge Road/Suite 15 Freehold, NJ 07728
(732)776-8500 Fax (732)333-1366
+ Shore Heart Group, P.A.
115 East Bay Avenue Manahawkin, NJ 07753 (609)971-3300 Fax (609)597-4656

Dixit, Seema P., DO {1144476417} Nrolgy
+ Princeton & Rutgers Neurology
77 Veronica Avenue/Suite 102 Somerset, NJ 08873
(732)246-1311 Fax (732)246-3089
+ Saint PeterÆs Physician Associates
240 Easton Avenue/4th Floor New Brunswick, NJ 08901
(732)937-6008
+ Princeton & Rutgers Neurology
9 Centre Drive/Suite 130 Monroe Township, NJ 08873
(609)395-7615 Fax (609)395-1885

Dixon, George C., MD {1548341464} IntrMd(80,NJ06)<NJ-JFKMED, NJ-MEADWLND>
+ ImmediCenter/Clifton
1355 Broad Street Clifton, NJ 07013 (973)778-5566 Fax (973)778-2268
+ Care Station Medical Group
456 Prospect Avenue West Orange, NJ 07052 (973)778-5566 Fax (973)731-9881

Dixon, Keith Raymond, MD {1982606810} IntrMd, SlpDis(00,NJ05)<CT-GAYLORD>
+ Riverside Medical Group
1 Maywood Avenue Maywood, NJ 07607 (201)249-6394
Fax (201)880-8117

Dixon, Melissa Kaye, MD {1891745790} Dermat(00,MA01)<NJ-COMMED, NJ-KIMBALL>
+ Schweiger Dermatology
368 Lakehurst Road/Suite 201 Toms River, NJ 08755
(732)244-4700 Fax (732)731-6134
kenneth899@msn.com

Dixon, Rosina B., MD {1134353907} IntrMd(68,NY01)
+ 43 Old Wood Road
Bernardsville, NJ 07924 (908)766-3558 Fax (908)766-7561

Dixon Dahms, Victoria Ann, MD {1619030541} Pedtrc(02,NY47)<NJ-VALLEY, NJ-HACKNSK>
+ North Jersey Pediatrics
17-10 Fair Lawn Avenue Fair Lawn, NJ 07410 (201)794-8585 Fax (201)703-9889

Diziki, Donna C., DO {1902850167} FamMed(86,NJ75)<NJ-SOMERSET>
+ US Healthworks
16 Ethel Road Edison, NJ 08817 (732)248-0088 Fax (732)248-4408

Dizon, Alita L., MD {1003926932} Gastrn, IntrMd(82,PHI01)<NJ-JRSYCITY>
+ Drs. Barber and Dizon
377 Jersey Avenue/Suite 460 Jersey City, NJ 07302
(201)332-4110 Fax (201)332-4122

Djebiyan, Eli S., MD {1841215969} IntrMd(86,BUL03)<NJ-ENGLWOOD, NJ-HOLYNAME>
+ ED Medical Associates
140 Grand Avenue Englewood, NJ 07631 (201)569-9010
Fax (201)569-9063

Dlugi, Alexander M., MD {1891799532} RprEnd, ObsGyn(77,PA01)<NJ-MONMOUTH>
+ OptumHealth
8 Barberry Row/Infertility Chester, NJ 07930 (908)879-0112

Dmytrienko, Igor, MD {1881730026} IntrMd(83,UKR25)<NJ-VALLEY>
+ 51 Chestnut Street
Ridgewood, NJ 07450 (201)670-9215

Do, Minh-Tu, MD {1023433794} PedEmg
+ RWJ University Pediatric Emergency Medicine
125 Paterson Street/MEB 342 New Brunswick, NJ 08903
(732)235-7893 Fax (732)235-9340

Dobesh, David P., MD {1083838890} ClCdEl, CdvDis(00,IL11)<NJ-STBARNMC, NJ-STMICHL>
+ New Jersey Cardiology Associates
375 Mount Pleasant Avenue West Orange, NJ 07052
(973)731-9442 Fax (973)731-8030
+ New Jersey Cardiology Associates
201 Lyons Avenue/6th Floor Newark, NJ 07112 (973)731-9442 Fax (973)923-7267

Dobken, Jeffrey Hall, MD {1457460966} Allrgy, Pedtrc(73,NY09)<NJ-RIVERVW>
+ 200 White Road/Suite 204
Little Silver, NJ 07739 (732)842-8818 Fax (732)842-9788
jdobken@monmouth.com

Dobrescu, Andrei Mihnea, MD {1093949224} IntrMd(98,ROM01)
+ Somerset Hematology Oncology Associates, P.A.
30 Rehill Avenue/2nd Floor/Suite 2500 Somerville, NJ 08876 (908)927-8700 Fax (908)927-8706

Dobrescu, Delia J., MD {1790910966} ClCdEl, IntrMd(98,ROM01)
+ Medical Health Center
1270 State Highway 35 Middletown, NJ 07748 (732)615-3900 Fax (732)615-0865

Dobro, Jeffrey Steven, MD {1790778405} IntrMd, Rheuma(81,PA07)
+ Physicians Health Alliance
28 Jackson Avenue Pompton Plains, NJ 07444 (973)835-2575 Fax (973)835-0531

Dobrosky, Joseph D., MD {1831146323} EmrgMd(86,MEX14)
+ Emergency Physician Associates, P.A.
307 South Evergreen Avenue/PO Box 298 Woodbury, NJ 08096 (856)848-3817 Fax (856)848-1431

Dobrow, Michael Craig, DO {1952508087} FamMed(04,NY75)
+ Silver Lake Medical, P.C.
1084 Main Avenue Clifton, NJ 07011 (973)751-2060
Fax (973)751-3334

Dobruskin, Yelizaveta, MD {1578647939} SrgEnd, Surgry, IntrMd(00,NY09)<NJ-CENTRAST>
+ Endo-Surgical Associates
901 West Main Street/Suite 104 Freehold, NJ 07728
(732)761-1740 Fax (732)761-8320

Dobrzynski, Carol A., MD {1255407367} Psychy, PsyCAd(94,NJ05)
+ C. A. Dobrzynski MD PC
2240 Church Road Toms River, NJ 08753 (732)864-2240 Fax (732)864-2240

MJDeMOLA@hotmail.com

Dockery, Keith Forrest, MD {1972512754} RadDia, Radiol, NuclMd(04,NY45)
+ Radiology Associates of Ridgewood, P.A.
20 Franklin Turnpike Waldwick, NJ 07463 (201)445-8822
Fax (201)447-5053

Doctoroff, Alexander, DO {1881648970} Dermat, SrgDer(98,NJ75)<NJ-STBARNMC>
+ Dermatology Associates-Warren
122 Mount Bethel Road Warren, NJ 07059 (908)756-7999
Fax (908)756-8017
+ Dermatology Associates-Livingston
201 South Livingston Avenue/Suite 1F Livingston, NJ 07039
(908)756-7999 Fax (973)994-1052

Doctoroff, Ella, DO {1790941433} FamMed(03,NY75)
+ 252 County Road
Belle Mead, NJ 08502

Dodaro, John P., MD {1407817562} Otlryg, IntrMd(89,NY47)<NY-LICOLLGE>
+ ENT & Allergy Associates, LLP
3663 Route 9 North/Suite102 Old Bridge, NJ 08857
(732)679-7575 Fax (732)707-3850
jdodaro@entandallergy.com

Dodge, Sarah Ann, MD {1235143504} Radiol(05,NY45)
+ Summit Medical Group-Berkeley Heights Campus
1 Diamond Hill Road Berkeley Heights, NJ 07922
(908)277-8673 Fax (908)790-6576

Doerr, Alphonsus L., MD {1295780096} GenPrc, SrgPlstc(89,IL42)
+ Clifton Center for Plastic Surgery
914 Clifton Avenue Clifton, NJ 07013 (973)458-1788

Doerr, John J., MD {1194808717} Radiol(80,MEXI)
+ Allwood Imaging
914 Clifton Avenue Clifton, NJ 07013 (973)777-5022
Fax (973)594-4769

Dogra, Vijay K., MD {1568464311} IntrMd, EmrgMd(84,INDI)<NJ-RBAYPERT>
+ Raritan Bay Medical Center/Perth Amboy Division
530 New Brunswick Avenue Perth Amboy, NJ 08861
(732)324-5095

Doherty, Leo Francis, MD {1144498718} ObsGyn, RprEnd, IntrMd(06,MA16)
+ Reproductive Medicine Associates of New Jersey
140 Allen Road Basking Ridge, NJ 07920 (908)604-7800
Fax (973)290-8370

Doidge, Robert W., DO {1326113416} SrgOrt(86,PA77)
+ Englewood Knee & Sports Medicine
370 Grand Avenue/Suite 100 Englewood, NJ 07631
(201)567-5700 Fax (201)567-8049

Doiranlis, Zenaida P., MD {1346308087} IntrMd, Grtrcs(63,PHI01)<NJ-HOLYNAME>
+ 985 River Road
New Milford, NJ 07646 (201)261-5856 Fax (201)265-1774

Doka, Najah I., MD {1598929416} InfDis
+ ID Associates PA/dba ID Care
765 Route 10 East/Suite 201 Randolph, NJ 07869
(973)989-0068 Fax (973)361-8955
+ ID Associates PA/dba ID Care
8 Saddle Road Cedar Knolls, NJ 07927 (973)989-0068
Fax (973)993-5953

Dokko, John Hoon, DO {1003804550} IntrMd, Nephro(97,NY75)<NJ-OVERLOOK, NJ-MORRISTN>
+ Summit Medical Group-Berkeley Heights Campus
1 Diamond Hill Road Berkeley Heights, NJ 07922
(908)273-4300 Fax (908)277-8808
+ Summit Medical Group
95 Madison Avenue Morristown, NJ 07960 (908)273-4300 Fax (973)267-5521

Doktor, Katherine Leigh, MD {1386909752} IntHos
+ Cooper University Medical Center/Camden
3 Cooper Plaza/Suite 502 Camden, NJ 08103 (856)968-7433 Fax (856)968-8499

Dolan, Eileen A., MD {1851556773} PedDvl(05,GRN01)
+ Institute for Child Development
30 Prospect Avenue Hackensack, NJ 07601 (201)996-4559

Dolgin, James S., MD {1679655864} ObsGyn, RprEnd(77,TN05)<NJ-VALLEY>
+ Valley Medical Group Ob/Gyn in Fairlawn
5-22 Saddle River Road Fair Lawn, NJ 07410 (201)796-2025 Fax (201)796-0587

Dolitsky, Shelley Nicole, MD {1851880652} ObsGyn
+ University Medical Group/OBGYN
125 Paterson Street/2nd Floor New Brunswick, NJ 08901
(732)235-6200 Fax (732)235-6627

Dolorico, Valentin N., MD {1841400736} Anesth(67,PHIL)<NJ-CHILTON>
+ Chilton Medical Center
97 West Parkway/Anesthesiology Pompton Plains, NJ 07444 (973)831-5000

Physicians by Name and Address

Domanski, John D., MD {1073593083} Grtrcs, FamMed(75,PA01)
+ Gericare Associates LLC
1405 Chews Landing Road/Suite 4 Laurel Springs, NJ 08021
(856)228-1118   Fax (856)228-9928

Domanski, Joseph E., MD {1326011909} IntrMd(74,MEXI)<NJ-UNVMCPRN, NJ-OCEANMC>
+ 2911 Highway 88/Suite 1
Point Pleasant Beach, NJ 08742   (732)295-2337

Dombchewsky, Orest A., MD {1376706416}<NJ-ACMCMAIN>
+ AtlantiCare Regional Med Ctr/Mainland
65 West Jimmie Leeds Road Pomona, NJ 08240   (610)574-7339

Dombo, Kudzai Rebecca, MD {1326010505} ObsGyn(01,NJ06)<NJ-CHILTON>
+ Associates in Women's Healthcare
1900 Union Valley Road Hewitt, NJ 07421   (973)831-1800
Fax (973)831-8820

Dombrowski, Henry Timothy, DO {1417937582} IntrMd(81,PA77)<NJ-VIRTMARL, NJ-VIRTVOOR>
+ University of Medicine & Dentistry of New Jersey-SOM
42 East Laurel Road/3100 Stratford, NJ 08084   (856)566-6845

Dombrowski, Mark A., MD {1043263916} FamMed, IntrMd(85,ITAL)<NJ-STJOSHOS, NJ-VALLEY>
+ Hackensack University Medical Group Emerson
452 Old Hook Road/2nd Floor Emerson, NJ 07630
(201)666-3900   Fax (201)261-0505

Domingo, Connie Dela Pena, MD {1902896889} PhysMd, Pedtrc, PedReh(94,NJ05)
+ Weisman Children's Rehabilitation Hospital
92 Brick Road/3rd Floor Marlton, NJ 08053   (856)489-4520   Fax (856)983-1065
CDomingo@weismanchildrens.com

Domingo, Joselito B., MD {1609936806} Psychy(83,PHI01)<NJ-GRYSTPSY>
+ Greystone Park Psychiatric Hospital
59 Koch Avenue Morris Plains, NJ 07950   (973)538-1800

Dominguez, Jonathan Manuel, MD {1376923755} FamMed
+ Dr Jerry L. Jurado and Assoc
2401 Palisade Avenue Union City, NJ 07087   (201)867-5791   Fax (201)223-1905

Dominguez Mustafa, Rolando, MD {1508145251} IntrMd<NJ-MORRISTN>
+ Morristown Medical Center
100 Madison Avenue Morristown, NJ 07962   (973)971-5912

Dominik, Jeremy A., MD {1679778823} Anesth
+ Summit Anesthesia Associates, P.A.
33 Overlook Road/Suite 311 Summit, NJ 07901   (908)598-1500   Fax (908)598-0197

Domnitz, Steven W., MD {1427096254} ObsGyn(86,DC01)<NJ-CHILTON>
+ Associates in Women's Healthcare
1777 Hamburg Turnpike/Suite 202 Wayne, NJ 07470
(973)831-1800   Fax (973)831-8820
+ Associates in Women's Healthcare
1900 Union Valley Road Hewitt, NJ 07421   (973)831-1800
Fax (973)831-8820
+ Associates in Women's Healthcare
329 Main Road/Suite 101 Montville, NJ 07470   (973)831-1800   Fax (973)831-8820

Domovich, Ora, MD {1427444256} FamMed
+ Morristown Medical Center Family Medicine
435 South Street/Suite 220-A Morristown, NJ 07960
(973)971-4222   Fax (973)290-7050

Dona, Samuel Torres, Jr., MD {1982043857} PhyMSptM
+ Tri-County Orthopedics
197 Ridgedale Street/Suite 300 Cedar Knolls, NJ 07927
(973)538-2334   Fax (973)829-9174

Donaire, Michael Jeremie, MD {1952740185} Surgry, SrgLap, Bariat(08,ENG29)
+ Advanced Surgical & Bariatrics of NJ, PA
49 Veronica Avenue/Suite 202 Somerset, NJ 08873
(732)640-5316   Fax (800)689-2361
m_donaire@hotmail.com

Donald, Gordon D., III, MD {1912936162} SrgSpn, SrgOrt(87,VT02)<NJ-RIVERVW>
+ Jersey Shore CardioThoracic & Vascular Surgery
234 Industrial Way West/Suite A-103 Eatontown, NJ 07724
(848)208-2055   Fax (848)208-2078

Donaldson, James Kenneth, DO {1871522763} EmrgMd(96,PA77)<NJ-ACMCITY>
+ AtlantiCare Regional Medical Center/City Campus
1925 Pacific Avenue/Emerg Med Atlantic City, NJ 08401
(609)572-8300   Fax (609)572-8305
+ 443 Shore Road/Suite 103
Somers Point, NJ 08244   (609)569-7077

Donat-Flowers, Rhoda J., DO {1841458874} FamMed
+ 298 Applegarth Road
Monroe, NJ 08831   (609)409-0600

Donato, Michele Lyne, MD {1346202439} IntrMd, MedOnc(92,QU01)<NJ-HACKNSK>
+ John Theurer Cancer Center - HUMC
92 Second Street Hackensack, NJ 07601   (201)336-8297
Fax (551)996-0575

Donde, Dilip M., MD {1669563367} IntrMd(71,INA67)<NJ-CENTRAST>
+ 555 Iron Bridge Road
Freehold, NJ 07728   (732)294-9373   Fax (732)333-1366

Donde, Mrunalini D., MD {1952399446} Pedtrc(69,INDI)<NJ-JRSYSHMC>
+ Allergy & Pediatric Associates of Jersey Shore
222 Schanck Road/Suite 105 Freehold, NJ 07728
(732)431-3373   Fax (732)303-0172
+ Allergy & Pediatric Associates of Jersey Shore
500 West Kennedy Boulevard Lakewood, NJ 08701
(732)431-3373   Fax (732)905-8773

Dondero, Stephanie K., DO {1578978656}
+ 37 Hillside Avenur
Riverdale, NJ 07457

Donepudi, Saila B., MD {1609893627} Psychy(91,INDI)<NJ-VAEASTOR>
+ VA New Jersey Health Care System-East Orange Campus
385 Tremont Avenue/Psych East Orange, NJ 07018
(973)676-1000

Donepudi, Srilalitha, MD {1417048208} Grtrcs, IntrMd(91,INA3D)<NJ-ANCPSYCH>
+ Ancora Psychiatric Hospital
301 Spring Garden Road/Geriatrics Hammonton, NJ 08037
(609)561-1700

Donetz, Pamela Suzanne, MD {1780753079} FamMed, GenPrc(94,NJ05)<NJ-HUNTRDN>
+ Branchburg Medical Group
3322 Route 22 West/Bldg. 6, Suite 601 Branchburg, NJ 08876   (908)800-7330   Fax (732)463-6050

Dong, Feiyan, MD {1619264611} Pedtrc(99,CHN59)
+ Pediatric Professional Associates PA
330 Ratzer Road/Suite 20 Wayne, NJ 07470   (973)835-5556   Fax (973)628-7942

Dong, Karen, MD {1255629424}
+ 360 Hadden Avenue
Collingswood, NJ 08108
karenkedong@gmail.com

Doniguian, Ann-Elizabeth E., MD {1699758052} BldBnk, PthACl(89,NY01)<NJ-STJOSHOS>
+ St Joseph's Medical Center Pathology
703 Main Street Paterson, NJ 07503   (973)754-3516   Fax (973)754-3649

Donikyan, Mardik Martin, DO {1245337054} GenPrc, EmrgMd(90,MO79)
+ 250 Old Hook Road
Westwood, NJ 07675   (201)358-3646

Donkina, Luiza, MD {1174625263} IntrMd, Pedtrc(81,UKRA)<NJ-HACKNSK>
+ 40-06 Morlot Avenue
Fair Lawn, NJ 07410   (201)797-5836   Fax (201)797-5836

Donkor, Lawrence Tawiah, MD {1760492524} IntrMd(97,NJ06)
+ Apogee Medical Group of New Jersey
425 Jack Martin Boulevard Brick, NJ 08724   (732)836-4817
Fax (732)836-4818

Donlon, Margaret, MD {1003053976} PhysMd
+ Orthopaedic Sports Medicine
80 Oak Hill Road Red Bank, NJ 07701   (732)741-2313
Fax (732)936-8445

Donnabella, Vincent, MD {1710988860} CritCr, IntrMd, PulDis(87,NJ05)<NJ-OVERLOOK, NJ-MORRISTN>
+ Pulmonary & Allergy Associates
1 Springfield Avenue/Suite 3-A Summit, NJ 07901
(908)934-0555   Fax (908)934-0556
V.Donnabella@tampabay.rr.com
+ Pulmonary & Allergy Associates
8 Saddle Road/Suite 101 Cedar Knolls, NJ 07927
(908)934-0555   Fax (973)540-0472

Donnellan, Joseph Anthony, MD {1649366089} Psychy(86,NJ05)<NJ-SOMERSET>
+ 422 Courtyard Drive/Route 206
Hillsborough, NJ 08844   (908)725-5595   Fax (908)725-3314
+ RWJ University Hospital Somerset
110 Rehill Avenue/Psych Somerville, NJ 08876   (908)685-2200

Donnelly, Brian, MD {1538157094} RadDia(71,PA02)<NJ-OVERLOOK>
+ Overlook Medical Center
99 Beauvoir Avenue/PO Box 210 Summit, NJ 07902
(908)522-2065   Fax (908)273-1920
+ Westfield Imaging Center
118-122 Elm Street Westfield, NJ 07090   (908)522-2065
Fax (908)232-7140

Donnelly, Christine M., MD {1104898394} PedCrd, Pedtrc(78,NY01)<NJ-MORRISTN, NY-CHLDCOPR>
+ Morristown Medical Center
100 Madison Avenue/PediCardio Morristown, NJ 07962
(973)971-5996   Fax (973)290-7979

Donnelly, Michael G., MD {1255310330} IntrMd, Grtrcs(87,PA07)<NJ-MORRISTN>
+ 4 Glenbrook Drive
Mendham, NJ 07945   (973)543-7966

Donnon, Henry P., MD {1831119171} FamMed, GenPrc(67,PA02)
+ 4 Twin Hill Drive
Willingboro, NJ 08046   (609)877-5088   Fax (609)877-2177
+ 701 East Main Street
Moorestown, NJ 08057   (856)235-3610

Donofrio, Scott D., MD {1538182423} Psychy
+ 100 Straube Center Boulevard/Box H-1
Pennington, NJ 08534   (609)737-7797   Fax (609)737-7499

Donohue, Robert, III, MD {1659385144} Ophthl(85,NJ05)
+ 1262 Whitehorse Hamilton Road
Trenton, NJ 08690   (609)585-9595   Fax (609)585-9444
rdonohue@cox.com

Donovan, Colleen Mary, MD {1639371016} EmrgMd
+ University Emergency Medicine
125 Paterson Street/MEB 104 New Brunswick, NJ 08901
(732)235-8717   Fax (732)235-7379

Dooley, Christina Yick, MD {1508984147} Pedtrc(02,NJ05)<NJ-MEADWLND>
+ Meadowlands Hospital Medical Center
55 Meadowlands Parkway/Pediatrics Secaucus, NJ 07096
(201)392-3100
cdyick@gmail.com

Dooley, James R., MD {1023030228} Anesth(71,PA02)<NJ-RIVERVW>
+ Red Bank Anesthesia, LLC
1 Riverview Plaza Red Bank, NJ 07701   (732)530-2255
Fax (732)450-2620
+ Riverview Medical Center
1 Riverview Plaza/Anesthesiology Red Bank, NJ 07701
(732)741-2700
+ 718 Boston Boulevard
Sea Girt, NJ 07701   (732)974-2115

Doolin, Edward John, MD {1154419471} PedSrg, SrgCrC, Surgry(79,IL06)<PA-CHILDHOS>
+ CHOP Pediatric & Adolescent Specialty Care Center
1012 Laurel Oak Road Voorhees, NJ 08043   (856)435-1300
Fax (856)435-0091
+ CHOP Pediatric & Adolescent Specialty Care Center
4009 Black Horse Pike Mays Landing, NJ 08330   (856)435-1300   Fax (609)677-7835

Dorai, Bhuvaneswari, MD {1396837969} PthACl(82,INDI)<NJ-STMICHL, NY-NYACKHOS>
+ St. Michael's Medical Center
268 MLK Jr. Boulevard/Pathology Newark, NJ 07102
(973)877-5200   Fax (973)877-2712

Dorazio, John L., MD {1205832904} CdvDis(82,NY08)<NJ-STPETER, NJ-RWJUBRUN>
+ RWJPE/New Brunswick Cardiology Group, P.A.
75 Veronica Road/Suite 101 Somerset, NJ 08873
(732)247-7444   Fax (732)247-5119
+ RWJPE New Brunswick Cardiology Group, P.A.
111 Union Valley Road/Suite 201 Monroe Township, NJ 08831   (732)247-7444   Fax (609)409-6882
+ RWJPE New Brunswick Cardiology Group, P.A.
15H Briar Hill Court East Brunswick, NJ 08873   (732)613-9313

Dorcely, Brenda, MD {1104182062} EnDbMt<NY-VAHARBOR>
+ 573 Broughton Avenue/Apt 4B
Bloomfield, NJ 07003   (973)303-3722

Dorflinger, Ernest Edward, Jr., MD {1750555892} Nrolgy, IntrMd(80,NJ05)
+ 10 Schindler Court
Chatham, NJ 07928   (973)701-1732

Dorfman, Aaron Todd, MD {1003006214} PedCrd, Pedtrc(04,PA01)<PA-CHILDHOS>
+ CHOP Pediatric & Adolescent Specialty Care Center
1012 Laurel Oak Road/Cardiology Voorhees, NJ 08043
(856)783-0287   Fax (856)435-0091
+ CHOP Specialty Care Center at Virtua
200 Bowman Drive/2 FL/Suite D-260 Voorhees, NJ 08043
(267)425-5400

Dorfman, Joseph Charles, MD {1780664722} Pedtrc(99,NJ05)
+ David J. Strader MD, PHD
799 Bloomfield Avenue/Suite 304 Verona, NJ 07044
(973)618-9990   Fax (973)618-9991
+ Princeton Nassau Pediatrics, P.A.
301 North Harrison Street Princeton, NJ 08540   (973)618-9990   Fax (609)921-3410

Dorfman, Neil H., MD {1902855463} Ophthl(82,NY45)<NJ-KENEDYHS, NJ-VIRTUAHS>
+ 20 East Taunton Road/Bldg 2
Berlin, NJ 08009   (856)753-9090   Fax (856)753-9001

Dorfner, Scott M., DO {1699783985} IntrMd(88,PA77)
+ Dorfner Family Medicine
811 Sunset Road/Suite 101 Burlington, NJ 08016 (609)387-9242 Fax (609)387-9408
+ Dorfner Family Medicine
950 A Chester Avenue/Suite 10 Delran, NJ 08075 (609)387-9242 Fax (856)764-8335

Doria, Cataldo, MD {1255357877} SrgTpl
+ Capital Health Medical
2 Capital Way/Suite 356 Pennington, NJ 08534 (609)537-6000 Fax (609)537-6002

Doria, Marie E., MD {1518118231} Psychy(69,PA07)
+ 408 South White Horse Pike
Audubon, NJ 08106 (856)858-1843
+ Southern State Correctional Facility
4295 Route 47 Delmont, NJ 08314 (856)785-1300

Dorio, Nicole Marie, DO {1356549661} Psychy, PsyFor(07,PA77)
+ New Jersey State Prison
Third and Federal Streets Trenton, NJ 08625 (609)292-9700

Dorkhom, Stephan Joseph, DO {1578872776} OncHem
+ Wayne Cancer Center LLC
234 Hamburg Turnpike/Suite 202 Wayne, NJ 07470 (973)310-0309
sdorkhom@nyit.edu

Dorn, Eric A., MD {1457529299} PedEmg, Pedtrc, EmrgMd(05,PA02)<NJ-VIRTMARL>
+ CHOP Care Network at Virtua Voorhees Hospital
100 Bowman Drive Voorhees, NJ 08043 (856)325-3000 Fax (609)261-5842
+ Advocare Township Pediatrics
123 Egg Harbor Road Sewell, NJ 08080 (856)325-3000 Fax (856)227-5890

Dorneo, Aurora B., MD {1427025956} Pedtrc(89,PHI09)<NJ-CHS-FULD, NJ-CHSMRCER>
+ Pediatrics by Night
1230 Whitehorse Mercerville Ro Hamilton, NJ 08619 (609)581-1700 Fax (609)581-8472

Dornfeld, David B., DO {1346210820} UndsMd, OstMed, GPrvMd(84,ME75)<NJ-RIVERVW>
+ Family Wellness Center
1680 State Route 35 Middletown, NJ 07748 (732)671-3730 Fax (732)706-1078
DrDave@osteodocs.net

Doroudi, Shideh, MD {1427452465} FamMed(96,IRAN)<NJ-WAY-NEGEN>
+ St. Joseph's Family Medicine @ Clifton
1135 Broad Street/Suite 201 Clifton, NJ 07013 (973)754-4100 Fax (973)472-9062

Dorr, Jeffrey, MD {1013279595} RadDia(12,FL03)
+ University Radiology Group, P.C.
579A Cranbury Road East Brunswick, NJ 08816 (732)390-0040 Fax (732)390-1856

Dorri, Mohammad Hossein, MD {1366754293} PhysMd, Surgry(00,IRA08)
+ Premier Orthopaedics and Sports Medicine, P.C.
111 Galway Place Teaneck, NJ 07666 (201)833-9500 Fax (201)862-0095

Dorsey, Philip J., Jr., MD {1215179452} Urolgy
+ Delaware Valley Urology
1138 East Chestnut Avnue/Suite 8-B Vineland, NJ 08360 (856)213-4035 Fax (856)213-4036

Dorsky, Seth Michael, MD {1245597426} Psychy
+ 40 Main Street/Suite 7
Chatham, NJ 07928 (973)635-4244 Fax (973)635-4246

Dorsky, Steven G., MD {1124090337} SrgOrt(80,RI01)<NJ-MOR-RISTN, NJ-STBARNMC>
+ New Jersey Spine Center
40 Main Street Chatham, NJ 07928 (973)635-0800 Fax (973)635-6254
+ New Jersey Spine Center
1222 Kennedy Boulevard Bayonne, NJ 07002 (973)635-0800 Fax (973)635-6254
+ New Jersey Spine Center
25 East Willow Street Millburn, NJ 07928 (973)379-1114 Fax (973)635-6254

Dort, Christian, MD {1255503793} FamMed
+ 64-66 Grumman Avenue
Newark, NJ 07112
+ Clark Surgical Care
100 Commerce Place Clark, NJ 07066 (732)499-0606

Dos Santos, Stephanie, MD {1093740458} Pedtrc(96,PAR01)<NJ-HACKNSK>
+ 17D River Road
Nutley, NJ 07110
+ Advanced Pediatrics
5 Summit Avenue/Suite 203 Hackensack, NJ 07601 Fax (201)343-4668

Doshi, Anish, MD {1346568797}
+ Rancocas Anesthesiology, PA
15000 Midlantic Drive/Suite 102 Mount Laurel, NJ 08054 (201)873-6223 Fax (856)393-8691

doshiai@gmail.com

Doshi, Arvind K., MD {1457302259} IntrMd(80,INA21)<NJ-JFKMED>
+ 906 Oak Tree Road/Suite K
South Plainfield, NJ 07080 (908)822-2277 Fax (908)822-1121
+ 5 Stenworth Road
Kendall Park, NJ 08824 (908)822-2277 Fax (732)297-2039

Doshi, Deepa, MD {1992989156} Pedtrc, IntrMd
+ Princeton Nassau Pediatrics, P.A.
312 Applegarth Road/Suite 104 Monroe Township, NJ 08831 (609)409-5600 Fax (609)409-5610
deepa0579@gmail.com
+ Princeton Nassau Pediatrics, P.A.
196 Princeton-Hightstown Road West Windsor, NJ 08550 (609)409-5600 Fax (609)799-2294

Doshi, Dhvani, MD {1700152626} IntHos
+ University Hospital
150 Bergen Street/Rm H245 Newark, NJ 07103 (973)972-5672

Doshi, Ila H., MD {1265537773} IntrMd(71,INA69)<NJ-VIRT-MARL>
+ 717 South Black Horse Pike
Blackwood, NJ 08012 (856)227-2020 Fax (856)227-2646
+ Virtua Marlton Hospital
90 Brick Road Marlton, NJ 08053 (856)355-6000

Doshi, Manish, MD {1336302314} InfDis, IntrMd<PA-TMPHOSP>
+ ID Associates PA/dba ID Care
105 Raider Boulevard/Suite 101 Hillsborough, NJ 08844 (908)281-0221 Fax (908)281-0940
+ ID Associates PA/dba ID Care
81 Veronica Avenue/Suite 203 Somerset, NJ 08873 (908)281-0221 Fax (732)729-0924

Doshi, Mona, MD {1598064537} CritCr, PulDis(91,INDI)<NJ-RBAYPERT>
+ Raritan Bay Medical Center/Perth Amboy Division
530 New Brunswick Avenue Perth Amboy, NJ 08861 (732)442-3700

Doshi, Nilesh M., MD {1518929272} RadV&I, Radiol, RadDia(92,OH44)<NJ-KMHSTRAT, NJ-COOPRUMC>
+ South Jersey Radiology Associates, P.A.
100 Carnie Boulevard/Suite B-5 Voorhees, NJ 08043 (856)751-0123 Fax (856)751-0535
+ South Jersey Radiology Associates, P.A.
315 Route 70 East/Suite B Cherry Hill, NJ 08034 (856)751-0123 Fax (856)428-0356
+ South Jersey Radiology Associates, P.A.
901 Route 168/Suites 301-305 Turnersville, NJ 08043 (856)227-6600 Fax (856)227-8537

Doshi, Pankaj Ajay, MD {1821029745} IntrMd, InfDis(96,INA9B)<NJ-BAYSHORE, NJ-CENTRAST>
+ Central Jersey Bariatrics
668 North Beers Street/Suite 103 Holmdel, NJ 07733 (732)739-9090 Fax (732)739-9094
+ Central Jersey Bariatrics
901 West Main Street/MAB Suite 103 Freehold, NJ 07728 (732)739-9090 Fax (732)761-8320

Doshi, Pankaj Manilal, MD {1366487746} Pedtrc(80,INA20)<NJ-SOMERSET, NJ-COMMED>
+ RWJ University Hospital Somerset
110 Rehill Avenue Somerville, NJ 08876 (908)685-2200

Doshi, Prakash J., MD {1790733491} GenPrc, IntrMd(84,INA65)<NJ-CLARMAAS, NJ-WESTHDSN>
+ Premier Care Associates of West Hudson
206 Bergen Avenue/Suite 201 Kearny, NJ 07032 (201)998-7474
+ 213 River Road
East Hanover, NJ 07936 (201)998-7474 Fax (201)998-6550

Doshi, Samir Kirankumar, MD {1427006691} Pedtrc(96,PA02)<NJ-VIRTMHBC>
+ Virtua Memorial
175 Madison Avenue/Pediatrics Mount Holly, NJ 08060 (609)914-6610 Fax (609)261-5842
+ Virtua Voorhees
100 Bowman Drive Voorhees, NJ 08043 (856)247-3000

Doshi, Sangita K., MD {1376505057} FamMed(99,PA02)
+ Cooper Family Medicine
504 White Horse Pike Haddon Heights, NJ 08035 (856)546-7990 Fax (856)546-6686

Doshi, Vatsal Suryakant, MD {1831394899} Ophthl(03,MA01)<NJ-STBARNMC, NY-NYEYEINF>
+ Vitreous Retina Macula Specialists of NJ
225 Millburn Avenue/Suite 206 Millburn, NJ 07041 (973)467-2020 Fax (973)467-2030
+ Vitreous Retina Macula Specialists of NJ
1543 Route 27/Suite 12 Somerset, NJ 08873 (973)467-2020 Fax (732)253-5259

Dosik, Jonathan Scott, MD {1396704755} Dermat(96,NY19)<NJ-VALLEY>
+ Dermatology Associates
348 South Maple Avenue Glen Rock, NJ 07452 (201)652-6060 Fax (201)652-1882

Doskow, Jeffrey B., MD {1164489670} CdvDis, IntrMd(85,NY15)
+ Suburban Heart Group, P.A.
1000 Galloping Hill Road/Suite 107 Union, NJ 07083 (908)964-7333 Fax (908)687-7855

Doss, Anthony, MD {1750775987} PhysMd
+ 75 Bourbon Street
Wayne, NJ 07470 (973)641-3820

Doss, Emile F., MD {1699790931} CdvDis, IntrMd(81,EGYP)<NJ-CHILTON>
+ 510 Hamburg Turnpike/Suite 107
Wayne, NJ 07470 (973)942-7377 Fax (973)942-7030

Doss, George S., MD {1104917814} Anesth(89,EGY03)
+ Montclair Anesthesia Associates PC
185 Fairfield Avenue/Suite 2A West Caldwell, NJ 07006 (973)226-1230 Fax (973)226-1232

Doss, Michael Nader, MD {1316940521} IntrMd, Anesth, PainMd(84,EGY04)
+ Wayne Surgical Center, LLC.
1176 Hamburg Pike Wayne, NJ 07470 (973)709-1900 Fax (973)709-1901
+ The AIPM Group
1037 Route 46 East/Suite G-5 Clifton, NJ 07013 (973)709-1900 Fax (973)928-5359

Doss, Nermine N., MD {1063509958} Pedtrc(88,EGY04)<NJ-HACKNSK, NJ-HOLYNAME>
+ Riverside Medical Group
714 Tenth Street/Suite 2 Secaucus, NJ 07094 (201)863-3346 Fax (201)865-0015

Doss, Peter S., MD {1609869098} RadDia(97,TX14)<NJ-TRINIWSC, NJ-BAYSHORE>
+ Red Bank Radiologists, P.A.
200 White Road/Suite 115 Little Silver, NJ 07739 (732)741-9595 Fax (732)741-0985
+ Coastal Imaging, LLC
79 Route 37 West/Suite 103 Toms River, NJ 08755 (732)741-9595 Fax (732)276-2325
+ Doctors Radiology Center - MRI of Woodbridge
1500 St. George Avenue/Peach Plaza Avenel, NJ 07739 (732)574-1414 Fax (732)574-0845

Dostal, Courtney Lynne, DO {1063618619} PulDis, IntrMd<PA-LHVLYMHL>
+ Pulmonary & Sleep Associates of SJ, LLC.
107 Berlin Road Cherry Hill, NJ 08034 (856)429-1800 Fax (856)429-1081
+ Pulmonary & Sleep Associates of SJ, LLC.
750 Route 73 South/Suite 401 Marlton, NJ 08053 (856)429-1800 Fax (856)375-2325

Dosunmu, Ronke Y., MD {1619903069} Pedtrc(87,NIGE)<NJ-STBARNMC, NJ-NWRKBETH>
+ Foundation Pediatrics
344 South Harrison Street East Orange, NJ 07018 (973)674-8373 Fax (973)552-2805

Dotto, Myles E., MD {1346215761} ObsGyn, Gyneco(76,NJ05)<NJ-VALLEY>
+ Ob-Gyn Associates of Bergen County, PA
680 Kinderkamack Road/Suite 204 Oradell, NJ 07649 (201)391-5443 Fax (201)391-8019

Doubek, Marnie Lynn, MD {1720070980} FamMed(97,NY08)
+ Springfield Family Practice
11 Overlook Road/Suite 140 Summit, NJ 07901 (908)277-0050 Fax (908)277-0201

Doubrava, Suzanne M., MD {1104076058} Psychy
+ University Medical Group
125 Paterson Street/Suite 5100 New Brunswick, NJ 08901 (732)235-7993 Fax (732)235-7117

Douedi, Hani R., MD {1922073949} CdvDis, IntrMd(82,EGYP)
+ Dover Cardiology Center
PO Box 1729 Toms River, NJ 08754 (732)557-4777 Fax (732)557-4887

Douge, Simone Alicia, MD {1093133746} FamMHPC
+ 700 Route 46 East/Suite 450
Fairfield, NJ 07004 (973)559-3701 Fax (973)559-8650

Dougherty, Barbara D., DO {1780608083} Anesth(76,PA77)<NJ-KMHSTRAT, NJ-KENEDYHS>
+ Kennedy Surgical Center
540 Egg Harbor Road Sewell, NJ 08080 (856)218-4900

Dougherty, Joseph F., MD {1114060647} FamMed(80,PA13)
+ 12 Harlow Circle
Medford, NJ 08055

Dougherty, Renee Maria, DO {1609260835} IntrMd
+ Meridian Primary Care
55 North Gilbert Street/Suite 3201 Tinton Falls, NJ 07701 (732)450-0961 Fax (732)530-0213

Douglas, Barbara L., MD {1417925124} PhysMd(94,PA07)
+ University Pain Care Center
42 East Laurel Road/Suite 1700 Stratford, NJ 08084 (856)566-7010 Fax (856)566-6956

Physicians by Name and Address

Douglas, Elaine, MD {1841371853} FamMed(86,CO02)<NJ-MTNSIDE>
+ 160 Lincoln Street
Montclair, NJ 07042   (973)744-0528

Douglas, Nataki Celeste, MD {1376702407} RprEnd, ObsGyn(02,CT01)<NY-PRSBCOLU>
+ University Physician Associates
140 Bergen Street/ACC Level C   Newark, NJ 07103   (973)972-2700   Fax (973)972-2739

Douglass-Bright, April M., MD {1447357405} Pedtrc(91,CT02)<NJ-COOPRUMC>
+ Cooper Peds/Children's Regional Ctr
3 Cooper Plaza/Suite 200/Pediatrics   Camden, NJ 08103   (856)342-2472   Fax (856)368-8297

Doujaiji, Bassam Mouhin, MD CritCr, IntrMd, PulDis(87,GRN01)
+ 192 Berger Street
Somerset, NJ 08873

Doujaiji, Hala Badaoui, MD
+ 192 Berger Street
Somerset, NJ 08873

Doumas, Christopher, MD {1235295239} OrtSHand(01)
+ University Orthopaedic Associates, LLC.
4810 Belmar Boulevard/Suite 102   Wall, NJ 07753   (732)938-6090   Fax (732)938-5680
+ University Orthopaedic Associates, LLC.
211 North Harrison Street   Princeton, NJ 08540   (732)938-6090   Fax (609)683-7875
+ University Orthopaedic Associates, LLC.
Two Worlds Fair Drive   Somerset, NJ 07753   (732)979-2115   Fax (732)564-9032

Doumas, Stacy James, MD {1447343678} PsyCAd, Psychy
+ 19 Forest Avenue
Rumson, NJ 07760

Dounis, Harry James, DO {1124286083} Nephro, IntrMd(05,NY75)<NJ-JRSYSHMC, NJ-OCEANMC>
+ Shore Nephrology, P.A.
35 Beaverson Boulevard   Brick, NJ 08723   (732)451-0063   Fax (732)451-0071
+ Shore Nephrology, P.A.
2100 Corlies Avenue/Suite 15   Neptune, NJ 07753   (732)451-0063   Fax (732)774-1528
+ Shore Nephrology, PA
27 South Cookbridge Road/Suite 211   Jackson, NJ 08723   (732)987-5990   Fax (732)987-5994

Douvris, John S., MD {1871517060} Pedtrc(91,DMN01)<NJ-OVERLOOK, NJ-MORRISTN>
+ Hunterdon Pediatric Associates
6 Sand Hill Road/Suite 202   Flemington, NJ 08822   (908)782-6700   Fax (908)788-5861

Douyon, Erwin, MD {1649420464} SrgTrm, SrgCrC(99,DC02)<NJ-STJOSHOS, NJ-WAYNEGEN>
+ Drs. Douyon & Bernstein
220 Hamburg Turnpike/Suite 11   Wayne, NJ 07470   (973)942-4941   Fax (973)942-4259

Douyon, Philippe Gerard, MD {1306169487} Nrolgy(07,NY19)<NY-JTORTHO>
+ Northeast Regional Epilepsy Group
20 Prospect Avenue/Suite 800   Hackensack, NJ 07601   (201)343-6676   Fax (201)343-6689

Dover, Marcia Anne, MD {1356452312} Nrolgy(98,CT01)<NJ-HCKTSTWN, NJ-NWTNMEM>
+ Neuro-Specialists of Morris-Sussex, PA
369 West Blackwell Street   Dover, NJ 07801   (973)361-7606   Fax (973)361-8942
+ Neuro-Specialists of Morris-Sussex, PA
350 Sparta Avenue   Sparta, NJ 07871   (973)361-7606   Fax (973)579-9618
+ Neuro-Specialists of Morris-Sussex, PA
254 Mountain Avenue   Hackettstown, NJ 07801   (908)850-5505   Fax (908)813-8848

Dovlatyan, Raida, MD {1700874898} PhysMd(74,ARM27)<NJ-KSLRSADB>
+ Kessler Institute for Rehabilitation
300 Market Street   Saddle Brook, NJ 07663   (201)587-8500

Dovnarsky, Michael K., MD {1891729372} CdvDis, IntrMd(81,PA09)
+ Cumberland Medical Associates
1206 West Sherman Avenue   Vineland, NJ 08360   (856)691-8444   Fax (856)691-8325

Dow, William A., MD {1669462636} FamMed(68,WV01)
+ 455 Broad Street
Beverly, NJ 08010   (609)387-0110   Fax (609)387-1304

Dowd, Heather Lynn, DO {1225237480} IntrMd(06,PA77)
+ 217 White Horse Pike
Haddon Heights, NJ 08035   (856)672-1115

Dowd, Mary Katherine, MD {1235104340} CdvDis, IntrMd(79,MA16)<NJ-ACMCITY, NJ-SHOREMEM>
+ Shore Memorial Hospital
1 East New York Avenue/MOB 2nd Floor   Somers Point, NJ 08244   (609)365-3100   Fax (609)365-3165
+ Penn Medicine Somers Point
155 Brighton Avenue/Second Floor   Somers Point, NJ 08244   (609)365-3100   Fax (609)365-3165

Dowd, Timothy Joseph, MD {1598762171} Anesth, Pedtrc(82,NY20)<NY-VASSAR>
+ Summit Anesthesia Associates, P.A.
33 Overlook Road/Suite 311   Summit, NJ 07901   (908)598-1500   Fax (908)598-0197

Dower, Samuel M., MD {1942260690} EnDbMt, IntrMd(81,NY19)<NJ-STBARNMC>
+ The Joslin Center for Diabetes
200 South Orange Avenue/2nd Floor   Livingston, NJ 07039   (973)322-7200   Fax (973)322-7250

Dowling, Peter E., MD {1952373144} ObsGyn(80,DC02)<NY-NATHNLIT>
+ Rutgers NJ School of Medicine Neurology
90 Bergen Street/DOC 5200   Newark, NJ 07103   (973)972-5209   Fax (973)972-5059
dowlinpc@njms.rutgers.edu

Dowling, Ryan Martin, MD {1790916138} SrgOrt(07,PA13)<NJ-STJOSHOS, NJ-WAYNEGEN>
+ North Jersey Orthopaedic Group
246 Hamburg Turnpike/Suite 302   Wayne, NJ 07470   (973)689-6266   Fax (973)689-6264

Dowling, William J., Jr., MD {1629048855} SrgOrt(71,NJ05)<NJ-MORRISTN>
+ Atlantic Orthopedic Institute
111 Madison Avenue/Suite 400   Morristown, NJ 07960   (973)984-0404   Fax (973)984-2516

Downey, Laura L., MD {1215932553} Otlryg(89,NY19)
+ Associates in Otolaryngology
741 Northfield Avenue/Suite 104   West Orange, NJ 07052   (973)243-0600   Fax (973)736-9607
+ Short Hills Surgery Center
187 Millburn Avenue/Suite 101   Millburn, NJ 07041   (973)243-0600   Fax (973)671-0557

Downey, Margaret Kelly, MD {1265589600} PedDvl, Pedtrc(81,IL42)
+ 110 Hazel Court
Norwood, NJ 07648   (201)767-8696

Downie, Jeanine Bernice, MD {1811959232} Dermat(92,NY08)<NJ-MTNSIDE, NJ-OVERLOOK>
+ Image Dermatology
51 Park Street   Montclair, NJ 07042   (973)509-6900   Fax (973)509-6939

Downs, Elvira Foglia, MD {1275661845} PsyCAd, Psychy(75,NY20)
+ Children's Specialized Hospital
3575 Quakerbridge Road   Hamilton, NJ 08619   (609)631-2800

Downs, William R., Jr., DO {1801833132} EmrgMd(95,NY75)<NJ-MONMOUTH>
+ Monmouth Medical Center
300 Second Avenue/EmergMed   Long Branch, NJ 07740   (732)222-5200

Doyle, Stephanie L., MD {1679747729} FamMed(93,NJ05)
+ 118 West Cottage Avenue
Haddonfield, NJ 08033

Doyle, Werner K., MD {1164534301} SrgNro, Eplpsy(82,NY01)<NY-NYUTISCH, NY-BLVUENYU>
+ St. Barnabas Institute of Neurology & Neurosurgery
200 South Orange Avenue/Suite 101   Livingston, NJ 07039   (973)322-7580   Fax (973)322-7505

Drabik, Thomas Edward, DO {1619967064} Nephro, IntrMd(94,NY75)<NJ-CENTRAST, NJ-RWJUBRUN>
+ Nephrology Hypertension Associates of Central Jersey
8 Old Bridge Turnpike   South River, NJ 08882   (732)390-4888   Fax (732)390-0255
+ Nephrology Hypertension Associates of Central Jersey
901 West Main Street/Suite 102   Freehold, NJ 07728   (732)625-0707

Drachman, Brian Michael, MD {1801827597} CdvDis, IntrMd(89,PA01)<NJ-VIRTVOOR, NJ-VIRTMARL>
+ Penn Medicine at Cherry Hill
1400 East Route 70/Cardiology   Cherry Hill, NJ 08034
+ Penn Medicine at Cherry Hill
409 Route 70 East   Cherry Hill, NJ 08034   (856)429-1519

Drachtman, Richard A., MD {1609958248} PedHem, Pedtrc(84,IL42)<NJ-CHSFULD, NJ-CHSMRCER>
+ Rutgers Cancer Institute of New Jersey
195 Little Albany Street/PO Box 2681   New Brunswick, NJ 08903   (732)235-5437   Fax (732)235-8234
drachtri@umdnj.edu
+ 416 Bellevue Avenue/Suite 103
Trenton, NJ 08618   (732)235-5437   Fax (732)235-8234

Dracxler Meaker, Roberta, MD {1588009971} Psychy
+ 222 Columbia Turnpike
Florham Park, NJ 07932   (973)261-9075   Fax (973)593-2063

Dragalin, Daniel J., MD {1124116363} Pedtrc(75,DC02)
+ 14 Prospect Street
Mendham, NJ 07945   (973)543-6867   Fax (440)447-3195

Draganescu, Mirela, MD {1932135696} IntrMd, Grtrcs(97,ROM01)
+ Haddonfield Internal Medicine
216 Haddon Avenue   Haddon Township, NJ 08108   (856)854-6600   Fax (856)854-6700

Dragert, Robert Joseph, DO {1558522821} Psychy(04,PA77)<NJ-CARRIER>
+ Carrier Clinic
252 Route 601   Belle Mead, NJ 08502   (908)281-1000

Drago, Lisa Anne Marie, DO {1467640458} EmrgPedr(00,PA78)
+ The Children's Regional Hospital at Cooper Univ Hosp
One Cooper Plaza   Camden, NJ 08103   (856)342-2351

Dragomir, Dan, MD {1427071091} IntrMd(97,ROM01)<NJ-COOPRUMC>
+ Cooper University Hospital
One Cooper Plaza/Internal Med   Camden, NJ 08103   (856)342-3150   Fax (856)968-8573

Dragon, Glenn M., MD {1275528366} Anesth(90,PA13)<NJ-UNDRWD>
+ Inspira Health Network
509 North Broad Street/Anesthesiology   Woodbury, NJ 08096   (856)845-0100

Dragon, Greg R., MD {1861467128} Anesth, PainMd(86,PA02)<NJ-BURDTMLN>
+ Cape Regional Medical Center
2 Stone Harbor Boulevard   Cape May Court House, NJ 08210   (609)463-2458   Fax (609)463-2757

Dragone, Daniel Claudio, MD {1306828827} Anesth(99,NJ05)<NJ-HACKNSK>
+ Hackensack Anesthesiology Associates
140 Prospect Avenue/Suite 8   Hackensack, NJ 07601   (201)488-0066   Fax (201)488-6769
+ Hackensack University MC-Anesthesia Dept
30 Prospect Avenue/Room 2703   Hackensack, NJ 07601   (201)488-0066   Fax (201)996-3962

Dragone, Sergio D., MD {1639140355} Anesth(88,MEXI)<NJ-HACKNSK>
+ Hackensack Anesthesiology Associates
140 Prospect Avenue/Suite 8   Hackensack, NJ 07601   (201)488-0066   Fax (201)488-6769
+ Hackensack University MC-Anesthesia Dept
30 Prospect Avenue/Room 2703   Hackensack, NJ 07601   (201)488-0066   Fax (201)996-3962
+ Hackensack University Medical Center
30 Prospect Avenue/Anesthesiology   Hackensack, NJ 07601   (201)996-2000

Dragos, Simona E., MD {1326344011}
+ 2041 North Route 9
Cape May Court House, NJ 08210

Dragun, Anthony E., MD {1710068036} RadOnc
+ Two Cooper Plaza/Suite C 1030
Camden, NJ 08103   (856)735-6119   Fax (856)735-6467

Dragun, Elena, MD {1467413583} IntrMd(89,BLA01)
+ Elizabeth Medical Associates
469 Morris Avenue/1st Floor   Elizabeth, NJ 07208   (908)351-3535   Fax (908)351-0161

Draikiwicz, Steven M., MD {1902228703}<NJ-RWJUBRUN>
+ RWJ University Hospital New Brunswick
One Robert Wood Johnson Place   New Brunswick, NJ 08901   (732)235-7742

Drake, Andrew F., DO {1033251442} FamMed(74,PA77)<NJ-BURDTMLN>
+ Cape Regional Physicians Associates
3806 Bayshore Road/Suite 101   North Cape May, NJ 08204   (609)898-7447   Fax (609)898-1912

Drake, William, III, MD {1861489890} Otlryg(89,NJ05)
+ Westfield Ear Nose & Throat Surgical Associates
213 Summit Road/Suite 1   Mountainside, NJ 07092   (908)233-5500   Fax (908)233-5776

Drakh, Alexander, DO {1104192897} PhysMd<NJ-HLTHSRE>
+ HealthSouth Rehabilitation Hospital of New Jersey
14 Hospital Drive   Toms River, NJ 08755   (732)279-7656

Dralle, James G., MD {1992795918} SrgThr, SrgCdv, Surgry(82,NY19)<NJ-ACMCMAIN>
+ Cardiac Surgery Group PC
65 Jimmie Leeds Road   Pomona, NJ 08240   (609)748-7089   Fax (609)652-3460
+ AtlantiCare Regional Med Ctr/Mainland
65 West Jimmie Leeds Road   Pomona, NJ 08240   (609)652-1000

Drascher, Gary A., MD {1871536474} Surgry, SrgVas, VasDis(81,NY47)<NJ-SOMERSET, NJ-RWJUBRUN>
+ Surgical Associates of Central NJ
30 Rehill Avenue/Suite 3300   Somerville, NJ 08876   (908)927-8994   Fax (908)927-8995

Draucikas, Lisa A., DO {1003243981} FamMed(11,NY75)
+ Valley Medical Group
140 Franklin Turnpike/Suite 6-A   Waldwick, NJ 07463   (201)447-3603   Fax (201)447-5184

Dravid, Anjana, MD {1881782605} Pedtrc(96,INA9B)<NJ-JFKMED>
+ 1630 Stelton Road/Suite 205
Piscataway, NJ 08854   (732)626-5635   Fax (732)626-5636

Dreier, Marc Max, MD {1902856222} EmrgMd(89,NJ06)<NJ-VAL-LEY>
+ The Valley Hospital
223 North Van Dien Avenue/Emergency   Ridgewood, NJ 07450   (201)447-8300   Fax (201)443-8174

Dreizen, Neil G., MD {1831149293} Ophthl(80,MA05)
+ Erickson, Dreizen & Lee Eye Center
1206 Route 72 West   Manahawkin, NJ 08050   (609)597-8087   Fax (609)597-7192
+ Erickson, Dreizen & Lee Eye Center
730 West Lacey Road/Suite G-07   Forked River, NJ 08731   (609)971-8822

Dresdner, Michael T., MD {1962567172} ObsGyn, IntrMd(92,NY19)
+ South Orange Ob/Gyn & Infertility Group
106 Valley Street   South Orange, NJ 07079   (973)763-4334

Dressner, Ivan R., MD {1699802736} Nrolgy(64,NY46)<NJ-ST-BARNMC>
+ Essex Neurological Associates PA
50 Union Avenue/Suite 406   Irvington, NJ 07111   (973)994-3322

Dressner, Roy M., DO {1124040910} SrgC&R, Surgry(91,NY75)<NJ-MONMOUTH, NJ-RIVERVW>
+ Specialty Surgical Associates
10 Industrial Way East/Suite 104   Eatontown, NJ 07724   (732)389-1331   Fax (732)542-8587

Drews, Michael Robert, MD {1568496453} RprEnd, ObsGyn(86,NY20)
+ Reproductive Medicine Associates of New Jersey
140 Allen Road   Basking Ridge, NJ 07920   (908)604-7800   Fax (973)290-8370
+ Reproductive Medicine Associates of New Jersey
111 Madison Avenue/Suite 100   Morristown, NJ 07962   (908)604-7800   Fax (973)290-8370
+ Reproductive Medicine Associates of New Jersey
475 Prospect Avenue/Suite 101   West Orange, NJ 07920   (973)325-2229   Fax (973)290-8370

Drexler, Christopher W., DO {1699798413} Pedtrc(95,NJ75)<NJ-SHOREMEM>
+ Harborview KidsFirst
505 Bay Avenue   Somers Point, NJ 08244   (609)927-4235   Fax (609)927-5590
+ Harborview KidsFirst Cape May
1315 Route 9 South   Cape May Court House, NJ 08210   (609)927-4235   Fax (609)465-1539
+ Harborview Smithville
48 South New York Road/Route 9   Smithville, NJ 08244   (609)748-2900   Fax (609)748-3067

Drey, Iris Antonella, MD {1689680209} SrgOrt(92,DC01)
+ The Orthopedic Group, P.A.
261 James Street/Suite 3-F   Morristown, NJ 07960   (973)538-0029   Fax (973)538-4957
+ The Orthopedic Group, P.A.
50 Cherry Hill Road   Parsippany, NJ 07054   (973)538-0029   Fax (973)263-3243
+ Premier Orthopaedics and Sports Medicine, PC
663 Palisade Avenue/Suite 302   Cliffside Park, NJ 07960   (201)943-9100   Fax (201)943-7308

Dreyfuss, Patricia O., MD {1841201936} ObsGyn(79,NJ05)<NJ-MORRISTN, NJ-STBARNMC>
+ 115 US Highway 46/Building D/Suite 27
Mountain Lakes, NJ 07046   (973)334-3345   Fax (973)263-3142

Drezner, Dean Andrew, MD {1760589725} Otlryg, IntrMd(84,PA13)<NJ-VIRTMHBC>
+ Princeton Eye and Ear
5 Plainsboro Road/Suite 510   Plainsboro, NJ 08536   (609)403-8840   Fax (609)403-8852

Dreznin, Howard N., MD {1255338224} Anesth, IntrMd(83,DOM02)<NJ-STJOSHOS>
+ St. Joseph's Regional Medical Center
703 Main Street/Anesthesia   Paterson, NJ 07503   (973)754-2790   Fax (973)754-2791

Drillings, Gary J., MD {1033208491} SrgOrt(85,NY15)<NJ-CHILTON>
+ 1777 Hamburg Turnpike/Suite 305
Wayne, NJ 07470   (973)831-6666   Fax (973)831-8661

Drimmer, Marc A., MD {1215082367} SrgPlstc(74,BELG)<NJ-UNVMCPRN>
+ 842 State Road
Princeton, NJ 08540   (609)924-1026   Fax (609)924-8249

Driscoll, Eric Joseph, DO {1730192691} IntrMd(96,PA77)<NJ-ACMCMAIN>
+ Shoreline Endocrine and Medical Associates PC
707 White Horse Pike/Suite C1   Absecon, NJ 08201   (609)813-2200   Fax (609)813-2201
+ The Plastic Surgery Center
2500 English Creek Avenue/Suite 605   Egg Harbor Township, NJ 08234   (609)813-2200   Fax (609)813-2201

Driscoll, Lorraine Eva, MD {1104847979} ObsGyn(81,NY09)<NJ-HACKNSK, NJ-HOLYNAME>
+ 9 Ridge Road
Rutherford, NJ 07070   (201)933-3203   Fax (201)933-7901

Driscoll, Michael Joseph, DO {1497946792} IntrMd(02,NJ75)
+ Pulmonary & Sleep Associates of SJ, LLC.
107 Berlin Road   Cherry Hill, NJ 08034   (856)429-1800   Fax (856)429-1081
+ Pulmonary & Sleep Associates of SJ, LLC.
750 Route 73 South/Suite 401   Marlton, NJ 08053   (856)429-1800   Fax (856)375-2325
+ Pulmonary & Sleep Associates of SJ, LLC.
811 Sunset Road/Suite 201   Burlington, NJ 08034   (609)298-1776   Fax (609)531-2391

Drivas, Antonios, MD {1083787485} EmrgMd, IntrMd(01,NJ05)<NJ-OVERLOOK>
+ Summit Medical Group-Berkeley Heights Campus
1 Diamond Hill Road   Berkeley Heights, NJ 07922   (908)273-4300   Fax (908)790-6576
tonydrivas@yahoo.com
+ Summit Medical Group
574 Springfield Avenue   Westfield, NJ 07090   (908)273-4300   Fax (908)232-0540

Driver, Paul J., MD {1477550002} Ophthl(90,PA13)<NJ-COOPRUMC>
+ Soll Eye PC of New Jersey/Cooper Division
3 Cooper Plaza/Suite 510   Camden, NJ 08103   (856)342-7200   Fax (856)342-6620

Droney, Timothy J., III, MD {1902832892} Anesth(83,GRN01)<NJ-ACMCITY>
+ AtlantiCare Regional Medical Center/City Campus
1925 Pacific Avenue/Anesthesiology   Atlantic City, NJ 08401   (609)345-4000

Drossner, Robbie Beth, MD {1659324440} Dermat(82,PA01)<NJ-OVERLOOK>
+ 2350 South Avenue
Scotch Plains, NJ 07076   (908)232-6668   Fax (908)232-0691

Drout, David I., MD {1366449787} CdvDis, IntrMd(73,NJ05)<NJ-RIVERVW>
+ Riverview Medical Associates, PA
4 Hartford Drive/Suite 1   Tinton Falls, NJ 07701   (732)741-3600   Fax (732)741-3603

Druce, Howard M., MD {1871658476} AlgyImmn, IntrMd(77,ENGL)<NJ-UMDNJ>
+ Ear, Nose & Throat Care, P.C.
242 East Main Street   Somerville, NJ 08876   (908)704-9696   Fax (908)704-0097

Druck, Mark, MD {1124109178} IntrMd, OncHem(77,NY08)<NJ-HOLYNAME>
+ Combine Hematology Oncology
210 Palisade Avenue   Jersey City, NJ 07306   (201)963-2213   Fax (201)963-7070

Drucker, David Wayne, MD {1730179854} CdvDis, IntCrd, IntrMd(90,MO02)
+ Mercer Bucks Cardiology
3140 Princeton Pike/2nd Floor   Lawrenceville, NJ 08648   (609)895-1919   Fax (609)895-1200

Druckman, Scott Jonathan, DO {1871582304} FamMed, IntrMd(94,NJ75)<NJ-VIRTBERL, NJ-VIRTMARL>
+ Jackson Family Medicine
27 South Cooks Bridge Road/Suite 2-1   Jackson, NJ 08527   (732)367-0166   Fax (732)367-7220

Dructor, Lisa Ann, DO {1245296169} IntrMd(96,PA77)
+ Drs. Damerau, Todt & Dructor
1401 Marlton Pike East/Suite 26   Cherry Hill, NJ 08034   (856)479-9400   Fax (856)281-9913

Drudy, Elena R., MD {1700835121} Ophthl(02,NY19)<NJ-SOCEANCO>
+ Erickson, Dreizen & Lee Eye Center
1206 Route 72 West   Manahawkin, NJ 08050   (609)597-8087   Fax (609)597-7192
+ Erickson, Dreizen & Lee Eye Center
730 West Lacey Road/Suite G-07   Forked River, NJ 08731   (609)971-8822

Drzala, Mark R., MD {1538261250} SrgOrt, SrgSpn(91,NJ05)<NJ-MTNSIDE, NJ-STBARNMC>
+ 33 North Fullerton Avenue
Montclair, NJ 07042   (973)233-9600   Fax (973)783-0144
msdrzala@aol.com

Du, Bing, MD {1912904434} Anesth(82,CHNA)<NJ-MONMOUTH>
+ Monmouth Medical Center
300 Second Avenue/Anesth   Long Branch, NJ 07740   (732)222-5200

Du, Doantrang Thi, MD {1699782474} IntrMd(95,NY47)<NJ-MONMOUTH>
+ Monmouth Medical Center
300 Second Avenue/InternalMed   Long Branch, NJ 07740   (732)222-5200
+ Monmouth Family Center
270 Broadway   Long Branch, NJ 07740   (732)222-5200   Fax (732)923-7104
+ Monmouth Medical Group, P.C.
279 Third Avenue/Suite 604   Long Branch, NJ 07740   (732)222-4474   Fax (732)222-4472

Dubbaka-Rajaram, Arunasree, MD {1558515213} Pedtrc(97,INA1I)<NJ-NWRKBETH, NJ-CHDNWBTH>
+ Drs. Gaurang R. Patel & Associates
1503 St Georges Avenue/Suite 205   Colonia, NJ 07067   (732)382-8111   Fax (732)381-0292

Dube, Bianca, MD {1740535152} FamMed
+ New Jersey Family Practice Center (NJFPC)
90 Bergen Street/DOC 300/Lower Level   Newark, NJ 07103   (973)972-2112   Fax (973)972-2754

Dube, Neerja, MD {1174697312} Surgry(69,INA7Y)
+ 13 Bretton Way
Mount Laurel, NJ 08054

Dube, Veena, MD {1558452011} Psychy(79,INDI)
+ Raritan Bay Mental Health Center
570 Lee Street   Perth Amboy, NJ 08861   (732)442-1666   Fax (732)376-6768

Dubin, David M., MD {1205881703} RadOnc(86,NY46)<NJ-ENGLWOOD>
+ Englewood Hospital and Medical Center
350 Engle Street/RadOnc   Englewood, NJ 07631   (201)894-3125   Fax (201)541-2463

Dubin, Reva, MD {1508812371} EmrgMd(81,WIND)<NJ-ACMCITY, NJ-ACMCMAIN>
+ AtlantiCare Regional Medical Center/City Campus
1925 Pacific Avenue/EmergMed   Atlantic City, NJ 08401   (609)345-4000
+ AtlantiCare Regional Med Ctr/Mainland
65 West Jimmie Leeds Road   Pomona, NJ 08240   (609)652-1000

Dubois, Yves Georges, MD {1043300833} Psychy, PsyGrt(83,HAI01)<NJ-TRENTPSY>
+ Y. Georges Dubois, MD
5603 Westfield Avenue   Pennsauken, NJ 08110   (856)665-1045   Fax (609)665-1046
ygdub@aol.com
+ Trenton Psychiatric Hospital
Sullivan Way/PO Box 7600   West Trenton, NJ 08628   (609)633-1500
+ River Primary Care
2809 River Road   Camden, NJ 08110   (856)966-8088   Fax (856)966-8088

Dubov, Glenn A., MD {1407846884} IntrMd, Nephro(83,IL42)<NJ-CENTRAST>
+ Nephrology Hypertension Associates of Central Jersey
8 Old Bridge Turnpike   South River, NJ 08882   (732)390-4888   Fax (732)390-0255
+ Nephrology Hypertension Associates of Central Jersey
901 West Main Street/Suite 102   Freehold, NJ 07728   (732)625-0707

Dubowitch, Stuart G., DO {1003861758} SrgOrt(82,PA77)<NJ-KMHCHRRY>
+ Regional Orthopedic, P.A.
2201 West Chapel Avenue/PO Box 8566   Cherry Hill, NJ 08002   (856)663-7080   Fax (856)663-4945
+ Regional Orthopedic, P.A.
163 Hurffville Crosskeys Road   Turnersville, NJ 08012   (856)663-7080   Fax (856)875-1368

Duca, Maria Diane, MD {1790754059} CdvDis, IntrMd(91,PA02)
+ The Cardiology Group, P.A.
401 Young Avenue/Suite 275   Moorestown, NJ 08057   (856)291-8855   Fax (856)291-8844
+ The Cardiology Group, P.A.
128 State Highway Route 70/Suite 1-B   Medford, NJ 08055   (856)291-8855   Fax (609)444-5521
+ The Cardiology Group, P.A.
1 Sheffield Drive/Suite 102   Columbus, NJ 08057   (856)291-8855

Ducey, Stephen Alexander, MD {1265462733} SrgOrt, IntrMd(93,NC05)<NJ-CLARMAAS>
+ Femino-Ducey Orthopaedic Group
45 Franklin Avenue   Nutley, NJ 07110   (973)751-0111   Fax (973)235-0110

Duch, Michael R., MD {1962408856} SrgOrt(90,PA13)<NJ-CHSMRCER, NJ-STFRNMED>
+ Trenton Orthopaedic Group
1225 Whitehorse Mercerville Rd   Trenton, NJ 08619   (609)581-2200   Fax (609)581-1212
+ Trenton Orthopaedic Group
116 Washington Crossing Road   Pennington, NJ 08534   (609)581-2200   Fax (609)581-1212

Duch, Peter M., MD {1730108150} CdvDis, IntrMd(86,MONT)
+ Molk Cardiology
4 Ethel Road/Suite 406-A   Edison, NJ 08817   (732)287-2888   Fax (732)287-1176
+ Monk Cardiology
167 Main Street/Suite 1 B   Metuchen, NJ 08840   (732)287-2888   Fax (732)662-9848

Ducheine, Yvan D., MD {1578638136} Surgry, SrgLap, SrgLsr(90,NJ05)<NJ-NWRKBETH>
+ Drs. Ducheine and Joseph
310 Central Avenue/Suite 203   East Orange, NJ 07018

Physicians by Name and Address

Duchin, Sybil E., MD {1528048758} ObsGyn(77,CT01)<NJ-VALLEY>
+ 483 Old Post Road
Wyckoff, NJ 07481

Duck, Evander, Jr., MD {1679673636} PhysMd(92,OH43)<NJ-CENTRAST>
+ Strategic Rehabilitation Services
PO Box 190   Tennent, NJ 07763   (732)780-8477
strategicrehab@yahoo.com

Duckles, Benjamin Jeffrey, MD {1073679767} PainInvt, PainMd, IntrMd(PA01<PA-PENNHOSP>
+ Reconstructive Orthopedics, P.A.
401 Young Avenue/Suite 245   Moorestown, NJ 08057
(609)267-9400   Fax (609)267-9457

Dudda Subramanya, Raghunandan, MD {1114243516} CdvDis, IntrMd(00,INA96)
+ Virtua Cardiology Group
2309 East Evesham Road/Suites 201-202   Voorhees, NJ 08043   (856)325-5400   Fax (856)325-5416

Dudick, Catherine A., MD {1912971607} SrgCrC, SrgTrm, Surgry(91,PA07)<NJ-ACMCITY>
+ AtlantiCare Regional Medical Center/City Campus
1925 Pacific Avenue/Trauma   Atlantic City, NJ 08401
(609)441-8023   Fax (609)441-8178

Dudick, Stephen T., MD {1508890526} SrgPlstc, SrgRec(75,MEXI)<NJ-MONMOUTH, NJ-JRSYSHMC>
+ 252 Broad Street
Red Bank, NJ 07701   (732)741-1303   Fax (732)741-7613
+ 76 West Jimmie Leeds Road/Suite 103
Galloway, NJ 08205   (732)741-1303   Fax (732)741-7613
+ 180 White Road/Suite 102
Little Silver, NJ 07701   (732)741-1303   Fax (732)741-7613

Dudiy, Yuriy, MD {1134416001} SrgThr<NJ-HACKNSK>
+ Hackensack University Medical Center
30 Prospect Avenue   Hackensack, NJ 07601   (519)963-8805   Fax (551)996-4833

Dudley, Larissa Sophia, MD {1003251422} EmrgMd
+ Newark Beth Israel Medical Center Emergency Medicine
201 Lyons Avenue/Suite D11   Newark, NJ 07112   (973)926-6671

Dudnick, Michael, DO {1699710343} EmrgMd(76,PA77)<NJ-BURDTMLN, NJ-SHOREMEM>
+ Cape Regional Medical Center
2 Stone Harbor Boulevard/EmergMed   Cape May Court House, NJ 08210   (609)463-2000

Duffoo, Frantz Michel, MD {1669544953} IntrMd, Nephro(79,TN07)<NY-WYCKOFF>
+ St. Peter's University Hospital
254 Easton Avenue   New Brunswick, NJ 08901   (732)745-8600

Duffy, Joseph M., MD {1033117171} FamMed, EmrgMd(87,DMN01)
+ 220 Hamburg Turnpike/Suite 14
Wayne, NJ 07470   (973)696-4440   Fax (973)942-0202

Duffy, Kevin James, Jr., MD {1790907673} CdvDis, IntrMd(00,PA01)<PA-UPMCPHL, PA-JEANES>
+ Penn Cardiology @ Cherry Hill
1400 Route 70 East   Cherry Hill, NJ 08034   (856)216-0300

Dufreney, Margaret S. Durante, MD {1922310705} ObsGyn(06,PA14)
+ Women's Health Specialists of CentraState
479 County Road 520/Suite 202A   Marlboro, NJ 07746
(732)837-1130

Dugan, John Donald, Jr., MD {1699717553} Ophthl(90,MD07)
+ Eye Physicians PC
1140 White Horse Road/Suite 1   Voorhees, NJ 08043
(856)784-3366   Fax (856)784-4388

Dugar, Vikash, MD {1154541175} AnesPain<NJ-CHILTON>
+ Chilton Medical Center
97 West Parkway   Pompton Plains, NJ 07444   (973)831-5000

Duhaney, Michael Owen, MD {1144201831} Radiol, RadDia(89,MD01)<NJ-WAYNEGEN>
+ Point View Radiology Associates
246 Hamburg Turnpike/Suite 101   Wayne, NJ 07470
(973)904-0404   Fax (973)904-0423
+ St. Joseph's Wayne Hospital
224 Hamburg Turnpike   Wayne, NJ 07470   (973)942-6900

Duhl, Jozsef S., MD {1043393317} Gastrn, IntrMd(82,ROMA)<NJ-RWJUBRUN, NJ-STPETER>
+ 1030 St. Georges Avenue/Suite 103A
Avenel, NJ 07001   (732)596-0155   Fax (732)596-0158
+ Medigest Associates P.A.
21 Clyde Road/Suite 102   Somerset, NJ 08873   (732)873-0033

Duke, Stephanie D., MD {1982756961} ObsGyn, IntrMd(83,NY05)
+ Brunswick-Hills Ob/Gyn, PA
620 Cranbury Road/Suite LL90   East Brunswick, NJ 08816
(732)257-0081   Fax (732)613-4845
+ Brunswick-Hills Ob/Gyn, PA
751 Route 206/2nd Floor   Hillsborough, NJ 08844

(732)257-0081   Fax (908)725-2132

Dukshtein, Mark, MD {1275944340} IntrMd<NJ-NWRKBETH>
+ Newark Beth Israel Medical Center
201 Lyons Avenue   Newark, NJ 07112   (973)926-8431

Dukuly, Zwannah D., MD {1710958392} PthACl, Pthlgy, PthCyt(83,LIBE)<NJ-RIVERVW, NJ-JRSYSHMC>
+ Riverview Medical Center
1 Riverview Plaza/Pathology   Red Bank, NJ 07701
(732)741-2700   Fax (732)345-2045
+ Jersey Shore University Medical Center
1945 Route 33/Pathology   Neptune, NJ 07753   (732)775-5500

Dultz, Rachel Paula, MD {1386631489} Surgry(91,NY08)<NJ-UNVMCPRN>
+ 300 B Princeton-Hightstown Rd
East Windsor, NJ 08520   (609)688-2729   Fax (609)688-2709
rrpd2000@aol.com

Dumapit, Gerardo D., MD {1619929627} Grtrcs, IntrMd(86,PHIL]<NJ-JFKMED>
+ Dr. Dumapit and Associates
906 Oak Tree Road/Suite C   South Plainfield, NJ 07080
(908)822-1213   Fax (908)822-1088

Dumay, Serge, MD {1760409411} IntrMd, PulDis(81,PRO03)<NJ-HACKNSK>
+ Paramus Pulmonary Clinic
211 Howland Avenue   Paramus, NJ 07652   (201)587-1321

Dumbroff, Steven A., MD {1396844023} Anesth(89,NJ05)
+ 4 Pittsfield Court
Livingston, NJ 07039   (973)992-9482

Dumitru, Dan Lucian, MD {1073639530} Nrolgy(95,ROM01)
+ 1810 John F. Kennedy Boulevard
Jersey City, NJ 07305   (201)710-0948

Dunaway, David Ryan, MD {1902030265} RadDia<NJ-STBARNMC>
+ St. Barnabas Medical Center
94 Old Short Hills Road   Livingston, NJ 07039   (973)322-8945

Duncan, Beth R., MD {1124143482} Surgry
+ Cooper Surgical Associates
3 Cooper Plaza/Suite 411   Camden, NJ 08103   (856)342-3275   Fax (856)968-8468

Duncan, David Brian, MD {1053364430} Nrolgy, IntrMd(88,IN20)<NJ-HOLYNAME>
+ MS Center at Holy Name Hospital
718 Teaneck Road   Teaneck, NJ 07666   (201)837-0727
Fax (201)837-8504

Duncan, Eva, MD {1194763540} Pedtrc, NnPnMd(80,ISR01)<NJ-HACKNSK>
+ Hackensack University Medical Center
30 Prospect Avenue/NeoPeri/Pedi   Hackensack, NJ 07601
(201)996-2000   Fax (201)996-3232

Duncan, Kathyann Sylvia, MD {1215049630} FamMed(93,NJ05)<NJ-UMDNJ>
+ University Hospital
150 Bergen Street/FamMed   Newark, NJ 07103   (973)972-4300

Duncan, Samuel T., MD {1063419810} IntrMd, Ophthl(86,NJ05)
+ 378 Marion Street
Union, NJ 07083

Dundeva Baleva, Pavlinka Vanyova, MD {1932358074} IntrMd, Rheuma(95,BUL02)
+ Ewing Rheumatology
1901 North Olden Avenue Ext/Suite 13-A   Ewing, NJ 08618
(609)883-1171   Fax (609)883-7777

Dundon, John M., MD {1831325166} SrgOARec
+ The Orthopedic Institute of New Jersey
108 Bilby Road/Suite 201   Hackettstown, NJ 07840
(908)684-3005   Fax (908)684-3301
+ The Orthopedic Institute of New Jersey
254-B Mountain Avenue/Suite 201   Hackettstown, NJ 07840
(908)684-3005   Fax (908)684-3301
+ The Orthopedic Institute of New Jersey
222 High Street/Suite 202   Newton, NJ 07840   (908)684-3005   Fax (908)684-3301

Dungo, Joven P., MD {1386726230} IntrMd, CdvDis(81,PHIL)<NJ-JRSYCITY, NJ-STMRYPAS>
+ Dr. Joven Dungo/NJ Impotence Ctr
205 9th Street   Jersey City, NJ 07302   (201)653-1144   Fax (201)653-6104
Jovendungo@yahoo.com
+ Westside Medical Associates
562 West Side Avenue   Jersey City, NJ 07304   (201)653-1144   Fax (201)434-6715

Dunham, Brian Philip, MD {1336275197} PedOto, Otlryg(98,CA11)<PA-CHILDHOS>
+ CHOP Pediatric & Adolescent Specialty Care Center
4009 Black Horse Pike   Mays Landing, NJ 08330   (609)677-7895   Fax (609)677-7835
+ CHOP Pediatric & Adolescent Specialty Care Center
707 Alexander Road/Suite 205   Princeton, NJ 08540

(609)520-1717

Dunham, Gerald, MD {1528173788} Ophthl, IntrMd(81,NJ06)<NJ-HUNTRDN>
+ Princeton Flemington Eye Institute
1100 Wescott Drive/Suite 305   Flemington, NJ 08822
(908)237-7037

Dunham, Rozy D., MD {1164576872} CdvDis, IntrMd(99,PA02)<NJ-OURLADY, NJ-VIRTUAHS>
+ Associated Cardiovascular Consultants-Lourdes
1 Brace Road/Suite C & F   Cherry Hill, NJ 08034   (856)428-4100   Fax (856)428-5748

Dunn, Anna Maria L., MD {1306865019} PhysMd(92,NY08)<NJ-JFKJHNSN, NJ-RWJUBRUN>
+ JFK Johnson Rehabilitation Institute
65 James Street   Edison, NJ 08818   (732)321-7070   Fax (732)744-5833

Dunn, Beverly A., MD {1568578847} IntrMd(82,NJ05)<NJ-VALLEY>
+ Drs. Belov & Dunn
61 Crescent Avenue   Waldwick, NJ 07463   (201)445-0033
Fax (201)857-0453

Dunn, Davonnie Marie, MD {1144302530} FamMed(98,NJ05)
+ Columbus Family Physicians
23659 Columbus Road/Suite 4   Columbus, NJ 08022
(609)298-3304   Fax (609)298-7091

Dunn, Eric Scott, MD {1144380452} Ophthl(93,PA02)<NJ-ACMCITY, NJ-SHOREMEM>
+ Drs. Dunn & Smith
4 East Jimmie Leeds Road/Suites 1-2   Galloway, NJ 08205
(609)652-6100
+ Drs. Dunn & Smith
4807 Atlantic Avenue   Ventnor, NJ 08406   (609)823-8488

Dunn, Ernest Charles, Jr., MD {1003840430} FamMed(98,PA02)<NJ-SHOREMEM>
+ 133 Folger Court
Ocean City, NJ 08226   (609)432-6442   Fax (609)432-6442

Dunn, Jonathan C., MD {1124090881} EnDbMt, IntrMd(83,TN05)
+ M.E.N.D., PA
2 Lincoln Highway/Suite 501   Edison, NJ 08820   (732)549-7470   Fax (732)494-8596

Dunn, Kevin B., MD {1891950366} PhysMd
+ New Jersey Sports Medicine
197 Ridgedale Avenue/Suite 210   Cedar Knolls, NJ 07927
(973)998-8301   Fax (973)998-8302

Dunn, Michael Joseph, MD {1700856184} IntrMd, FamMed(81,MNT01)<NJ-ACMCMAIN, NJ-ACMCITY>
+ Medical One
4248 Harbour Beach Boulevard   Brigantine, NJ 08203
(609)266-0400   Fax (866)912-0605

Dunn, Sarah Ruth, MD {1548404759} EmrgMd<NJ-RIVERVW>
+ Riverview Medical Center
1 Riverview Plaza   Red Bank, NJ 07701   (732)741-2700

Dunn, Timothy John, MD {1669523445} Nrolgy(95,GRN01)<NJ-LOURDMED, NJ-VIRTMARL>
+ The Neurological Center
231 Van Sciver Parkway   Willingboro, NJ 08046   (609)871-7500   Fax (609)877-5555

Dunzik, Scott Dennis, MD {1023100203} Psychy(92,PA13)
+ 29 Lee Avenue
Haddonfield, NJ 08033

Dupre, Callum Michael, DO {1942438999} SlpDis, IntrMd(09,NY75)
+ Snoring and Sleep Apnea Center Mercer County
1401 Whitehorse Mercerville Rd   Hamilton, NJ 08619
(609)584-5150   Fax (609)584-5144

Dupree, David Joseph, MD {1386843126} Surgry(NET09)<NJ-MONMOUTH>
+ 776 Shrewsbury Avenue/Suite 405
Tinton Falls, NJ 07724   (732)450-1200   Fax (732)450-1220
+ Monmouth Medical Center
300 Second Avenue/Surgery   Long Branch, NJ 07740
(732)923-6769

Dupree, William Brion, MD {1336189943} PthCyt, Pthlgy(76,VT02)
+ Bio-Reference Laboratory, Inc.
481 Edward H. Ross Drive   Elmwood Park, NJ 07407
(201)791-2600   Fax (201)791-1941
+ PLUS Diagnostics
1200 River Avenue/Suite 10   Lakewood, NJ 08701
(201)791-2600   Fax (732)901-1555

Duprey, Kevin M., DO {1417278789} FamMSptM(10,PA77)
+ 1 Brace Road/Suite H
Cherry Hill, NJ 08034   (856)470-9230   Fax (856)357-2011

Durante, Michael F., MD {1730369430} IntrMd(84,NY03)<NJ-OVERLOOK, NJ-STBARNMC>
+ 460 Franklin Avenue/Suite 1
Nutley, NJ 07110   (973)667-8640   Fax (973)667-0401

Durback, Mark Andrew, MD {1689615601} Rheuma
+ 228 Roseberry Street
Phillipsburg, NJ 08865

Durelli, Gloria S., MD {1427015130} Pedtrc(80,PA07)<NJ-ACMC-MAIN, NJ-ACMCITY>
 + Pediatric Associates of Atlantic County, P.A.
   9009 Ventnor Avenue Margate, NJ 08402 (609)823-2773
 + Genesis Pediatrics Assocociates LLC
   297 Westwood Drive/Suite 101 Woodbury, NJ 08096
   (856)848-2332

Durham, Booth H., MD {1740392075} Dermat(75,PA13)<NJ-UNDRWD>
 + South Jersey Dermatology Associates
   900 Route 168/Suite F6 Turnersville, NJ 08012 (856)227-7488 Fax (856)228-3476

Durnan, Rosemary, MD {1811998750} Anesth(89,NJ05)
 + 1706 Route 35 South
   Seaside Heights, NJ 08751

Durojaye, Abike Ogunrenike, MD {1154459568} RadDia
 + The Connie Dwyer Breast Center
   111 Central Avenue Newark, NJ 07102 (973)877-5189
   Fax (973)877-5205

Durrani, Mohamed Sohail, MD {1396804910} IntrMd(70,PAK18)<NJ-WARREN>
 + 218 S First Street
   Phillipsburg, NJ 08865 (908)454-5080 Fax (908)454-4105

Durrani, Muhammad I., MD {1295783371} Radiol, Anesth(92,PAK10)<NJ-SJHREGMC>
 + SJH Regional Medical Center
   1505 West Sherman Avenue Vineland, NJ 08360 (856)641-8000 Fax (856)641-7671

Durrani-Tariq, Siama H., DO {1417196320}<NJ-MORRISTN>
 + Emergency Medical Associates of NJ, P.A.
   3 Century Drive Parsippany, NJ 07054 (973)740-0607 Fax (973)740-9895

Duryee, John Jourdan, MD {1992797427} FamMed(02,VA01)
 + Medical Care Associates
   137 Mountain Avenue Hackettstown, NJ 07840 (908)852-1887 Fax (908)852-0614

Dutka, Michael Vincent, MD {1255547717} Radiol, RadDia(02,CT01)
 + Radiology Affiliates of Central New Jersey, P.A.
   2501 Kuser Road Hamilton, NJ 08691 (609)585-8800 Fax (609)585-1825

Dutkowsky, Charles J., DO {1477573798} PhysMd, FamMed(83,PA77)
 + Physical Medicine & Rehabilitation Center
   500 Grand Avenue/1st Floor Englewood, NJ 07631 (201)567-2277 Fax (201)567-7506

Dutta, Kamal K., MD {1952433062} ObsGyn(71,INDI)<NJ-HACKNSK, NJ-STMRYPAS>
 + 426 Passaic Avenue/Suite 2
   Lodi, NJ 07644 (973)777-9889

Duvvuri, Krishna, MD {1073574745} CdvDis, IntrMd(86,JMAC)<NJ-CHILTON>
 + Care Point Health
   637 Route 23 South Pompton Plains, NJ 07444 (973)248-8403 Fax (973)839-6015

Duvvuri, Uma, MD {1891765573} IntrMd(96,TN07)<NJ-CHILTON>
 + Firstmed Family HealthCare LLC
   637 Route 23 South Pompton Plains, NJ 07444 (973)859-7277 Fax (862)666-9215

Duzyj-Buniak, Christina Maria, MD {1982888111}
 + UH- Robert Wood Johnson Med
   125 Paterson Street/Rm 2124 New Brunswick, NJ 08901 (732)235-6632 Fax (732)235-7349
   christina.duzyj@rutgers.edu

Dvir, David, MD {1972558633} Anesth(75,GA01)
 + Associated Surgeons of Northern New Jersey
   25 Rockwood Place Englewood, NJ 07631 (201)567-3999 Fax (201)567-9288

Dvorin, Donald J., MD {1316095664} AlgyImmn, Pedtrc(78,PHI08)<NJ-VIRTMHBC>
 + Allergic Disease Associates, PC - Mount Laurel
   210 Ark Road & Route 38/Suite 109 Mount Laurel, NJ 08054 (856)235-8282 Fax (856)235-2154
 + Allergic Disease Associates, PC - Woodbury
   608 North Broad Street/Suite 310 Woodbury, NJ 08096 (856)235-8282 Fax (856)251-0966

Dvorzhinskiy, Olga, MD {1386667764} PthACl, PthAna(84,RUS06)<NJ-RWJUBRUN>
 + RWJ University Hospital New Brunswick
   One Robert Wood Johnson Place New Brunswick, NJ 08901 (732)828-3000

Dvoskin, Dmitriy, MD {1518224583} PhyMPain(12,GRN01)
 + Bogdan Pain Management Services
   112 Professional View Drive/Bld 100 Freehold, NJ 07728 (732)577-9126 Fax (732)577-9127
 + Bogdan Pain Management
   200 Perrine Road/Suite 224 Old Bridge, NJ 08857 (732)577-9126 Fax (732)553-1215

Dweck, Isaac Jay, MD {1881785343} FamMed, IntrMd(88,MEXI)<NJ-JRSYSHMC>
 + Oakhurst Medical Group LLC
   40 Monmouth Road Oakhurst, NJ 07755 (732)222-3243

Fax (732)222-3019

Dwivedi, Shaunak A., DO {1144488321} Nephro, IntrMd(06,NY75)
 + Hypertension & Nephrology Specialists, LLC
   2 Research Way/Suite 301 Monroe, NJ 08831 (732)521-0800 Fax (732)521-0833
 + Hypertension & Nephrology Specialists, LLC
   49 Veronica Avenue/Suite 104 Somerset, NJ 08873 (732)521-0800 Fax (732)521-0833
 + Hypertension & Nephrology Specialists, LLC
   601 Ewing Street/Suite C-7 Princeton, NJ 08831 (732)521-0800 Fax (732)521-0833

Dwivedi, Sukrut A., DO {1003082660} InfDis, IntrMd(03,NY75)
 + Infectious Disease Care
   1912 State Route 35/Suite 101 Oakhurst, NJ 07755 (732)222-4762 Fax (732)222-4764

Dworkin, Gerald E., DO {1578673208}
 + Pain and Spine Treatment Center
   811 Sunset Road Burlington, NJ 08016 (610)237-4612
   ged@painfix.com

Dworkin, Jack H., MD {1619063963} CdvDis, IntrMd(81,NY19)<NJ-CENTRAST>
 + 225 Gordons Corner Road/Suite 1-B
   Manalapan, NJ 07726

Dwosh, Jack, MD {1033180724} PedUro, Urolgy(80,NY01)
 + New Jersey Urology
   15000 Midlantic Drive/Suite 100 Mount Laurel, NJ 08054 (856)252-1000 Fax (856)985-4582
 + New Jersey Urology
   773 Route 70 East/Building H-120 Marlton, NJ 08053

Dwyer, James P., DO {1164469383} IntrMd, Rheuma(75,PA77)<NJ-VIRTUAHS>
 + 401 Route 73 North/Suite 401
   Marlton, NJ 08053
 + Arthritis, Rheumatic & Back Disease Associates
   2309 East Evesham Road/Suite 101 Voorhees, NJ 08043 Fax (856)424-4716

Dwyer, James W., MD {1629072541} SrgOrt(82,NJ05)<NJ-HACKNSK, NJ-HCKTSTWN>
 + The Orthopedic Health Center
   720 Monroe Street/Suite C209 Hoboken, NJ 07030 (201)286-3622

Dwyer, Joseph Michael, MD {1285899203} SrgOrt, SprtMd(08,PA13)
 + Reconstructive Orthopedics, P.A.
   401 Young Avenue/Suite 245 Moorestown, NJ 08057 (609)267-9400 Fax (609)267-9457

Dwyer, Kevin Thomas, DO {1063774859}<NJ-VIRTVOOR>
 + Rowan University-School of Osteopathic Medicine
   1 Medical Center Drive Stratford, NJ 08084 (856)566-7050
 + Virtua Voorhees
   100 Bowman Drive Voorhees, NJ 08043 (856)247-3000

Dwyer, Thomas A., MD {1972678027} SprtMd, SrgOrt(90,NY15)<NJ-SJHREGMC, NJ-SJRSYELM>
 + Premier Orthopaedic Associates
   298 South Delsea Drive Vineland, NJ 08360 (856)690-1616 Fax (856)690-1089
 + Premier Orthopaedic Assocs of So NJ
   201 Tomlin Station Road/Suite C Mullica Hill, NJ 08062 (856)690-1616 Fax (856)223-9110

Dyakina, Nika, DO {1699971937} Psychy, IntrMd(04)
 + 36 Franklin Turnpike
   Waldwick, NJ 07463 (201)250-1579 Fax (201)283-9094

Dyal, Cherise Malinda, MD {1699874487} SrgOrt(89,CT01)<NJ-CHILTON, NY-MNTFMOSE>
 + Advanced Orthopaedic Associates
   1777 Hamburg Turnpike/Suite 301 Wayne, NJ 07470 (973)839-5700 Fax (973)616-4343

Dyce, Michael Constantine, MD {1881645331} EmrgMd(96,MA01)<NJ-JRSYSHMC>
 + Jersey Shore University Medical Center
   1945 Route 33/EmergMed Neptune, NJ 07753 (732)775-5500

Dyckman, Steven Ira, MD {1396864385} PsyCAd, PsyAdt, Psychy(97,DC01)<NJ-MONMOUTH>
 + D-4 Brier Hill Court
   East Brunswick, NJ 08816 (732)238-7711 Fax (732)238-1977
 + 137 Pavilion Avenue
   Long Branch, NJ 07740 (732)238-7711
 + Monmouth Medical Center
   300 Second Avenue Long Branch, NJ 08816 (732)222-5200

Dye, Autumn J., DO {1225323801} Pedtrc
 + Cooper University Medical Center/Camden
   3 Cooper Plaza Camden, NJ 08103 (856)342-2000

Dyme, Joshua L., MD {1215973730} PedCrd(00,NY45)
 + The Pediatric Center for Heart Disease
   155 Polifly Road/Suite 106 Hackensack, NJ 07601 (201)487-7617 Fax (201)342-5341

Dyme, Rachel Sarah, MD {1265497150} Pedtrc(01,MI01)<NJ-ENGLWOOD, NJ-HACKNSK>
 + Hackensack Univ Medical Center Pediatric Emerg Room
   30 Prospect Avenue Hackensack, NJ 07601 (201)996-5430 Fax (201)996-3676

Dynof, Francis R., MD {1386602829} EmrgMd, GenPrc(77,DC01)<NJ-CHILTON, NJ-RIVERVW>
 + Chilton Medical Center
   97 West Parkway/EmergMed Pompton Plains, NJ 07444 (973)831-5000 Fax (973)444-3604

Dzhalturova, Nadire, DO {1124467444} EnDbMt<NJ-BERGNMC>
 + New Bridge Medical Center
   230 East Ridgewood Avenue Paramus, NJ 07652 (201)225-7130 Fax (201)967-4117

Dziadosz, Margaret, MD {1922232388} ObsGyn
 + St. Barnabas Medical ObsGyn
   94 Old Short Hills Road/Suite 402 Livingston, NJ 07039 (973)322-5287 Fax (973)322-2309

Dziarmaga, Ewa R., MD {1144278904} Pedtrc(86,POL06)<NJ-VALLEY>
 + Ridgewood Pediatrics LLC
   265 Ackerman Avenue/Suite 204 Ridgewood, NJ 07450 (201)444-3309 Fax (201)444-3349

Dziezanowski, Margaret Ann, MD {1659560308} IntrMd(80,NY19)
 + VMG-Internal Medicine Midland Park
   44 Goodwin Street/Suite 201 Midland Park, NJ 07432 (201)891-5044 Fax (201)891-1119

Eagan, Michael Patrick, MD {1003965237} EmrgMd(94,NY09)<NJ-MONMOUTH>
 + Emergency Medical Offices
   651 West Mount Pleasant Avenue Livingston, NJ 07039 (973)740-9396 Fax (973)251-1165
 + Monmouth Medical Center
   300 Second Avenue Long Branch, NJ 07740 (732)923-8882

Eagle, Robert Selig, MD {1922012335} Gastrn, IntrMd(79,BELG)
 + 405 Northfield Avenue/Suite LL3
   West Orange, NJ 07052 (973)731-9855 Fax (973)731-9855

Eagle, Steven B., MD {1609012806} Pedtrc(07,NJ05)<NJ-UMDNJ>
 + 705 Suffern Road
   Teaneck, NJ 07666 (201)357-2169

Eakin, David Eugene, DO {1518076579} SrgOrt(95,NJ75)
 + LMA Professional Orthopaedics
   2103 Burlington Mount Burlington Township, NJ 08016 (609)747-9200 Fax (609)747-1408

Eang, Rosanna, DO {1366857997} FamMed
 + 1238 Chews Landing Road
   Laurel Springs, NJ 08021 (856)545-9560 Fax (856)497-5214

Eapen, Elizabeth, MD {1407855216} PthAna, PthCyt, PthACl(94,INA76)<NJ-VALLEY>
 + The Valley Hospital
   223 North Van Dien Avenue/Path Ridgewood, NJ 07450 (201)447-8000

Eapen, Prema Mary, MD {1972510097} FamMed(96,OH44)
 + Our Family Practice
   1899 State Highway 88 Brick, NJ 08723 (732)840-8177 Fax (732)840-2195

Eapen, Santhosh, MD {1962464503} PedEnd, Pedtrc(89,NIGE)<NJ-JRSYSHMC>
 + Meridian Medical Group - Faculty Practice
   61 Davis Avenue/Suite 1 Neptune, NJ 07753 (732)776-4860 Fax (732)776-4867
 + Jersey Shore University Medical Center
   1945 Route 33/Pediatrics Neptune, NJ 07753 (732)776-4860

Eardley, Anna Mary, MD {1043210461} RadDia, Radiol(98,NY47)
 + University Radiology Group, P.C.
   483 Cranbury Road East Brunswick, NJ 08816 (732)390-0030 Fax (732)390-5383
 + University Radiology Group, P.C.
   579A Cranbury Road East Brunswick, NJ 08816 (732)390-0030 Fax (732)390-1856

Earl, Lawrence N., MD {1376625723} GenPrc, OccpMd(82,WI06)
 + Concentra Urgent Care at Parsippany
   190 Baldwin Road Parsippany, NJ 07054 (973)882-0444 Fax (973)882-3217
   laryearl@aol.com

Early, Ellen Marie, MD {1912995960} Hemato, Onclgy, OncHem(91,DC02)<NY-SLOANKET, NJ-MORRISTN>
 + Hematology-Oncology Associates of Northern NJ
   100 Madison Avenue/PO Box 1089 Morristown, NJ 07962 (973)538-5210 Fax (973)644-9657

Easaw, Saramma John, MD {1265424253} IntrMd, Hemato, Onclgy(85,INDI)<NJ-VALLEY>
 + Northern Valley Medical Associates
   221 Old Hook Road Westwood, NJ 07675 (201)666-4949 Fax (201)666-6920

Physicians by Name and Address

Easterling, Torian J., MD {1578881090} FamMed
+ New Jersey Family Practice Center (NJFPC)
  90 Bergen Street/DOC 300/Lower Level Newark, NJ 07103
  (973)972-2111 Fax (973)972-2754

Eastern, Joseph S., MD {1447395991} Dermat(77,CA02)
+ 36 Newark Avenue/Suite 214
  Belleville, NJ 07109 (973)751-1200 Fax (973)450-9395
  joseph.eastern@verizon.net

Eastman, Ralph M., MD {1700883683} RadOnc, Radiol, RadThp(73,WI06)<NJ-VIRTVOOR, NJ-TRINIWSC>
+ The Center for Cancer & Hematologic Disease
  750 Route 73 South/Suite 401/Radiology Marlton, NJ 08053 (856)797-1507 Fax (856)797-1597
+ Regional Cancer Care Associates, LLC
  200 Bowman Drive/Suite E-125 Voorhees, NJ 08043
  (856)797-1507 Fax (856)424-5634

Eastwick, Gary, MD {1801206776} RadOnc
+ MD Anderson Cancer Center at Cooper
  2 Cooper Plaza Camden, NJ 08103 (856)735-6119

Eatman, Florence B., MD {1942252374} Grtrcs, IntrMd(81,NJ05)
+ 20 Valley Street/Suite 320
  South Orange, NJ 07079 (973)761-6203 Fax (973)761-4347
  featmanmd@aol.com

Eaton, Edward E., MD {1699726422} Anesth(02,NY46)
+ 401 Ridge Road
  Newton, NJ 07860
+ Synergy Anesthesia
  2740 State Route 10/Suite 104 Morris Plains, NJ 07950
  Fax (973)695-1324

Ebani, Jack E., MD {1962563932} Urolgy(79,NY08)<NJ-JRSYSHMC, NJ-OCEANMC>
+ 1820 Corlies Avenue
  Neptune, NJ 07753 (732)774-4551 Fax (732)774-8933

Ebeid, Hasan Samir, MD {1861606394} Pedtrc(05,GRN01)<NJ-STJOSHOS, NJ-STCLRDEN>
+ St. Joseph's Regional Medical Center
  703 Main Street/Pediatrics Paterson, NJ 07503 (973)754-2000

Ebel, Keren Zahav, MD {1386685006} Pedtrc, GenPrc(01,NY47)
+ Somerset Pediatric Group PA
  2345 Lamington Road/Suite 101 Bedminster, NJ 07921
  (908)470-1124 Fax (908)470-2845
+ Somerset Pediatric Group PA
  155 Union Avenue Bridgewater, NJ 08807 (908)470-1124
  Fax (908)203-8825

Eberly, Andrea Cecilia, MD EmrgMd(90,CA14)
+ 1 Innisbrook Road
  Skillman, NJ 08558

Ebersole, John S., MD {1568513547} Psychy, Nrolgy
+ Northeast Regional Epilepsy Group
  20 Prospect Avenue/Suite 800 Hackensack, NJ 07601
  (201)343-6676 Fax (201)343-6689

Ebert, Ellen C., MD {1477635522} Gastrn, Hepato, IntrMd(77,NY20)<NJ-RWJUBRUN>
+ Hypertension & Nephrology Specialists, LLC
  49 Veronica Avenue/Suite 104 Somerset, NJ 08873
  (732)873-1600 Fax (732)873-1606
+ Kavita Bupathi, LLC
  2 Ethel Road/Suite 206C Edison, NJ 08817 (732)873-1600
  Fax (732)650-0351

Ebert, Gary A., MD {1750487161} ObsGyn(93,NJ06)<NJ-RWJUBRUN, NJ-STPETER>
+ University Medical Group
  125 Paterson Street/Suite 5100 New Brunswick, NJ 08901
  (732)235-7627 Fax (732)235-7349
+ University Medical Group/OBGYN
  125 Paterson Street/2nd Floor New Brunswick, NJ 08901
  (732)235-7627 Fax (732)235-6627

Ebert, Karl H., MD {1831156421} Urolgy(78,GA01)<NJ-UNDRWD, NJ-VIRTVOOR>
+ Delaware Valley Urology LLC
  17 West Red Bank Avenue/Suite 303 Woodbury, NJ 08096
  (856)853-0955 Fax (856)985-4583
+ New Jersey Urology LLC
  2090 Springdale Road/Suite D Cherry Hill, NJ 08003
  (856)853-0955 Fax (856)985-9908
+ New Jersey Urology, LLC
  2401 East Evesham Road/Suite F Voorhees, NJ 08096
  (856)673-1600 Fax (856)988-0636

Eboli, Dominick Joseph, MD {1649228065} Surgry(95,NJ06)<NJ-CHSFULD, NJ-CHSMRCER>
+ Capital Surgical Associates
  40 Fuld Street/Suite 303 Trenton, NJ 08638 (609)396-2600 Fax (609)396-3600
  deboli@chsnj.org
+ Capital Health Primary Care
  832 Brunswick Avenue Trenton, NJ 08638 (609)396-2500
  Fax (609)815-7401

Eccles, Shannon, DO {1386179083} Pedtrc
+ 20 David Court
  Perrineville, NJ 08535 (732)792-1171

Echeverri, Samuel David, MD {1174874481} Surgry
+ Strafford Surgical Specialists, P.A.
  1100 Route 72 West/Suite 303 Manahawkin, NJ 08050
  (609)978-3325 Fax (609)978-3123
+ Monmouth Surgical Specialists
  727 North Beers Street Holmdel, NJ 07733 (609)978-3325
  Fax (732)290-7067

Echols, Karolynn T., MD {1992716419} Gyneco(96,PA13)<NJ-COOPRUMC>
+ University Urogynecology Associates
  6012 Piazza at Main Street Voorhees, NJ 08043 (856)325-6622 Fax (856)325-6522
+ Cooper University Hospital
  One Cooper Plaza Camden, NJ 08103 (856)342-2000

Eck, Alieta R., MD {1720093107} IntrMd(80,MO34)
+ Eck, Apelian & Mathews
  1056 Stelton Road Piscataway, NJ 08854 (732)463-0303
  Fax (732)463-2289

Eck, John M., MD {1639186158} FamMed(80,MO34)
+ Eck, Apelian & Mathews
  1056 Stelton Road Piscataway, NJ 08854 (732)463-0303
  Fax (732)873-8099

Eck, Philip Ofosu, MD {1003251349} Anesth
+ Hackensack University MC-Anesthesia Dept
  30 Prospect Avenue/Room 2703 Hackensack, NJ 07601
  (551)996-2419 Fax (551)996-3962

Eckardt, Gerald William, MD {1013189737} Nrolgy
+ Global Neuroscience Institute
  750 Brunswick Avenue Trenton, NJ 08638 (414)405-0398
  geckardt@mcw.edu

Ecker, Teresa, MD {1902803604} RadDia, Radiol, IntrMd(86,NJ05)<NJ-STFRNMED, NJ-RWJUHAM>
+ University Radiology Group, P.C.
  579A Cranbury Road East Brunswick, NJ 08816 (732)390-0040 Fax (732)390-1856

Eckert, Jessica, DO {1164841391} Pedtrc
+ Madison Pediatrics
  435 South Street/Suite 200 Morristown, NJ 07960
  (973)971-4222 Fax (973)822-3349

Eckman, Ari S., MD {1386859585} EnDbMt
+ 1199 Pershing Circle
  Teaneck, NJ 07666

Eckstein, Devin Brazill, DO {1942628912} Pedtrc<NJ-MORRISTN>
+ Morristown Medical Center
  100 Madison Avenue Morristown, NJ 07962 (973)971-5000

Edara, Srinivasa R., MD {1629268218} IntrMd, CritCr(92,INA62)<NJ-VALLEY>
+ The Valley Hospital
  223 North Van Dien Avenue Ridgewood, NJ 07450
  (201)447-8288 Fax (201)251-3599

Eddey, Gary E., MD {1942273388} Pedtrc(83,NY20)<NJ-MATHENY>
+ The Matheny School and Hospital
  Main Street/PO Box 339 Peapack, NJ 07977 (908)234-0011

Edelman, Bruce Allen, MD {1639276009} Otlryg, PedOto(84,NY19)
+ ENT & Allergy Associates
  B-3 Cornwall Drive East Brunswick, NJ 08816 (732)238-0300 Fax (732)238-4066
+ ENT & Allergy Associates
  1543 Route 27/Suite 21 Somerset, NJ 08873 (732)238-0300 Fax (732)873-6853

Edelman, Carrie Allysia, MD {1821061110} IntrMd, Rheuma(96,NY08)<NJ-OCEANMC>
+ Shore Medical Group
  1640 Highway 88/Suite 203 Brick, NJ 08724 (732)458-7777 Fax (732)263-9470
+ 2640 Route 70/Suite 11
  Manasquan, NJ 08736 (732)458-7777 Fax (732)458-6741

Edelman, Douglas Jay, MD {1437283280} Psychy, PsycAd, Pedtrc(92,PA14)<NJ-STFRNMED, NJ-SJERSYHS>
+ Center for Family Guidance, PC
  765 East Route 70/Building A-101 Marlton, NJ 08053
  (856)797-4800 Fax (856)810-0110
+ St. Francis Medical Center
  601 Hamilton Avenue/Psychiatry Trenton, NJ 08629
  (609)599-5000

Edelman, Robert Benedict, Jr., MD {1700858545} Anesth(83,PHIL)
+ Kimball Medical Center
  600 River Avenue Lakewood, NJ 08701 (732)797-3890
  Fax (732)797-3893

Eden, Avrim Reuben, MD {1831145226} Otlryg, Otolgy(68,SAF02)<NJ-OVERLOOK, NJ-MORRISTN>
+ Summit Medical Group-Berkeley Heights Campus
  1 Diamond Hill Road Berkeley Heights, NJ 07922
  (908)273-4300 Fax (908)277-8662

Eder, Scott E., MD {1083614150} ObsGyn(82,BEL04)<NJ-CHSFULD, NJ-UNVMCPRN>
+ Delaware Valley Ob/Gyn & Infertility Group, PC
  300B Princeton Hightstown Road East Windsor, NJ 08520
  (609)336-3266 Fax (609)443-4506

Edison, Barry Jay, DO {1447283510} Ophthl(96,NY75)<NJ-JRSYSHMC, NJ-RIVERVW>
+ Barry Edison Ophthalmology
  10 Industrial Way/Suite 2 Eatontown, NJ 07724 (732)542-0300 Fax (732)935-0533
  info@drbarryedison.com
+ Barry Edison Ophthalmology
  100 Drum Point Road Brick, NJ 08723 (732)542-0300
  Fax (732)477-7170

Edlin, Dale E., MD {1740250117} CdvDis, IntrMd(79,OH41)<NJ-RIVERVW, NJ-BAYSHORE>
+ Shore Heart Group, PA
  179 Avenue at the Commons/Suite 102 Shrewsbury, NJ 07702 (732)542-7655 Fax (732)542-7600
+ Shore Heart Group, P.A.
  1820 State Route 33/Suite 4-B Neptune, NJ 07753
  (732)542-7655 Fax (732)776-8946
+ Shore Heart Group, P.A.
  555 Iron Bridge Road/Suite 15 Freehold, NJ 07702
  (732)308-0774 Fax (732)333-1366

Edman, Joel B., MD {1316015613} Pedtrc(78,NY46)<NJ-RIVERVW>
+ Middletown Pediatrics
  529 Highway 35 Red Bank, NJ 07701 (732)741-9800 Fax (732)758-6367

Edmonston, Tina B., MD {1679581284} PthyMGen
+ 57 Linden Avenue
  Haddonfield, NJ 08033

Edobor-Osula, Osamuede, MD {1689996142} SrgOrt, PedOrt, IntrMd(07,NY20)<NJ-UMDNJ>
+ University Hospital-Doctors Office Center
  90 Bergen Street/Suite 7300 Newark, NJ 07103 (973)972-0244 Fax (973)972-1080

Edoga, John K., MD {1962759126} SrgVas, Surgry(71,NY01)
+ John K. Edoga MD LLC
  177 Madison Avenue/Suite 7 Morristown, NJ 07960
  (973)656-0777 Fax (973)656-0717

Edokwe, Obunike O.J., MD {1306848080} FamMed(81,ROM06)
+ Pathlink, LLC
  66 West Gilbert Street/Suite 100 Tinton Falls, NJ 07701
  (732)212-0060 Fax (732)212-0061

Edrich, Dina Rachel, MD {1891074746} FamMed
+ CentraState Family Medicine Residency Practice
  1001 West Main Street/Suite B Freehold, NJ 07728
  (732)294-2540 Fax (732)409-2621

Edula, Raja Gopal Reddy, MD {1568454064} Hepato, IntrMd(97,INA5B)
+ Rutgers- New Jersey Medical School
  185 South Orange Avenue/MSB H-538 Newark, NJ 07103
  (973)972-5252 Fax (973)972-3144

Edwards, Barbara Ruth, MD {1699790972} IntrMd(88,PA01)
+ Princeton Medicine
  5 Plainsboro Road/Suite 300 Plainsboro, NJ 08536
  (609)853-7272 Fax (609)853-7271

Edwards, Daniel James, DO {1326081134} EmrgMd(97,FL75)<NJ-MORRISTN, NJ-WAYNEGEN>
+ Morristown Medical Center
  100 Madison Avenue/EmrgMed Morristown, NJ 07962
  (973)971-5000
+ St. Joseph's Wayne Hospital
  224 Hamburg Turnpike/EmrgMed Wayne, NJ 07470
  (973)942-6900
+ Hackensack UMC Mountainside
  1 Bay Avenue/EmrgMed Montclair, NJ 07962 (973)429-6000

Edwards, Jennifer L., MD {1033275300} PsycAd, Psychy(91,NY09)<NJ-RIVERVW>
+ 661 Shrewsbury Avenue/Suite 1
  Shrewsbury, NJ 07702 (732)450-2900 Fax (732)345-3401

Edwards, Jillian, DO {1104110964} Nrolgy(09,PA78)<NJ-BURDTMLN>
+ Cape Regional Physicians Associates
  11 Village Drive Cape May Court House, NJ 08210
  (609)465-2273 Fax (609)463-0235

Edwards, Kathryn Payne, MD {1326197039} Pedtrc
+ Becker ENT
  One Union Street/Suite 203 Robbinsville, NJ 08691
  (609)436-5740 Fax (609)436-5741

Edwards, Linda J., MD {1114073269} ObsGyn(83,PA07)<NJ-VIRTVOOR>
+ Alliance Ob/Gyn Consultants
  5045 Route 130 South/Suite 1 Delran, NJ 08075
  (856)764-7660 Fax (856)764-5723

Physicians by Name and Address

Edwards, Michael J., MD {1689644213} RadDia, RadV&I(82,NY19)<NJ-STMRYPAS>
+ Diagnostic Radiology Associates of Northfield
  772 Northfield Avenue   West Orange, NJ 07052   (973)325-0002   Fax (973)325-8140
+ Diagnostic Radiology Associates of Clifton
  1339 Broad Street   Clifton, NJ 07013   (973)325-0002   Fax (973)778-4846
+ Diagnostic Radiology Associates of Cranford
  25 South Union Avenue   Cranford, NJ 07052   (908)709-1323   Fax (908)709-1329

Edwards, Teresa Michelle, MD {1265768709} Radiol, RadDia(09,OH06)
+ University Radiology Group, P.C.
  579A Cranbury Road   East Brunswick, NJ 08816   (732)390-0040   Fax (732)390-1856

Effron, Charles Richard, MD {1558499350} Nrolgy(83,RI01)
+ 365 West Passaic Street
  Rochelle Park, NJ 07662   (201)489-8006
  ceffronmd@nyc.rr.com

Effron-Gurland, Frances R., MD {1710064720} PsyCAd, Psychy(89,NY08)
+ 216 Engle Street/Suite 202
  Englewood, NJ 07631   (201)568-4066   Fax (201)568-5595

Efremova, Irina Vladimirovna, MD {1316020035} Psychy, PsyGrt(89,RUS80)<NJ-UNIVBHC>
+ Rutgers Health Services
  17 Senior Street   New Brunswick, NJ 08901

Efros, Barry J., MD {1093879579} IntrMd, Rheuma(74,NJ05)<NJ-MORRISTN>
+ 95 Madison Avenue
  Morristown, NJ 07960   (973)540-8744   Fax (973)540-1614

Eftychiadis, Angela S., MD {1982840898} PthAcl, Pthlgy(73,GRE01)
+ Quest Diagnostics Inc.
  1 Malcolm Avenue   Teterboro, NJ 07608   (201)393-5000   Fax (201)393-6127

Egan, Daniel J., MD {1962493585} EmrgMd, IntrMd(02,NY47)<NJ-VALLEY>
+ The Valley Hospital
  223 North Van Dien Avenue/Emerg Med   Ridgewood, NJ 07450   (201)447-8000

Egan, Elizabeth Anne, MD {1174685416} Gastrn, IntrMd(00)
+ Advanced GI
  2301 Evesham Road/Pav 800/Suite 110   Voorhees, NJ 08043   (856)772-1600   Fax (856)772-9031

Egan, Kevin J., MD {1669567368} SrgOrt(81,MEXI)
+ 200 South Orange Avenue/Suite 230
  Livingston, NJ 07039   (973)322-7223
+ The Joint Institute at Saint Barnabas Medical Center
  609 Morris Avenue   Springfield, NJ 07081   (973)322-7223   Fax (973)467-8647

Egan, Sean Christopher, MD {1164588711} Urolgy(93,NJ05)<NJ-CLARMAAS>
+ 443 Northfield Avenue/Suite 301
  West Orange, NJ 07052   Fax (973)718-4611

Egazarian, Marc M., MD {1306976097} Surgry(95,NY09)<NJ-HOLYNAME>
+ 477 Bergen Boulevard
  Ridgefield, NJ 07657   (201)941-6999   Fax (201)945-6476

Eggerding, Caroline, MD {1285645689} Pedtrc, OthrSp, PedNrD(77,MO07)
+ Bancroft NeuroHealth
  425 Kings Highway East/PO Box 20   Haddonfield, NJ 08033   (856)429-0010   Fax (856)429-1613

Eggert, Bryan George, MD {1538459995} RadOnc
+ Garden State Radiation Oncology
  512 Lakehurst Road   Toms River, NJ 08755   (732)240-0053   Fax (732)240-9360
+ Manchester Surgery Center
  1100 Route 70   Whiting, NJ 08759   (732)240-0053   Fax (732)849-1511

Egodage, Tanya, MD {1477825891} SrgTrm<NJ-COOPRUMC>
+ Cooper University Hospital
  One Cooper Plaza   Camden, NJ 08103   (856)342-2000
+ Cooper University Physician Trauma Center
  One Cooper Plaza   Camden, NJ 08103   (856)342-3014

Eguino Conde, Damaris Alejandra, MD {1376708263} Pedtrc(91,CUB08)
+ Santa Clara Pediatrics
  7524 Kennedy Boulevard   North Bergen, NJ 07047   (201)751-4746   Fax (201)751-4747
  stclarapd@aol.com

Ehrenreich, Michael, MD {1124249644} Dermat
+ Soma Skin and Laser LLC
  90 Millburn Avenue/Suite 206   Millburn, NJ 07041   (973)763-7546   Fax (973)288-2188

Ehrlich, Harold B., MD {1114921582} IntrMd(82,GRNA)
+ AFC Urgent Care Bound Brook
  601 West Union Avenue/Suite 1   Bound Brook, NJ 08805   (732)469-3627   Fax (732)667-3708

Ehrlich, Jerry S., MD {1346297611} Pedtrc(63,NETH)
+ 1999 East Marlton Pike
  Cherry Hill, NJ 08003   (856)424-2485   Fax (856)424-3885

Ehrlich, Paul, MD {1629287560} ObsGyn, Gyneco(87,NY19)
+ 9 Beaumont Terrace
  West Orange, NJ 07052

Ehrlichman, Richard S., MD {1083956429} EmrgMd
+ SJH Emergency Medicine
  1505 West Sherman Avenue   Vineland, NJ 08360   (856)641-8000   Fax (888)395-8975

Eichel, Richard L., MD {1104817576} Gastrn, IntrMd(78,PA09)<NJ-BAYSHORE, NJ-RIVERVW>
+ 180 White Road/Suite 104
  Little Silver, NJ 07739   (732)530-3228   Fax (732)224-0144

Eicher, Peggy Smith, MD {1184666885} Pedtrc(81,GA05)<NJ-STJOSHOS>
+ St. Joseph's Children's Hospital
  703 Main Street/FeedingCtr   Paterson, NJ 07503   (973)754-2500

Eichler, Joel D., MD {1326033598} Ophthl(88,DC01)<NJ-CLARMAAS, NJ-STBARNMC>
+ Eye Institute of Essex, PA
  5 Franklin Avenue/Suite 209   Belleville, NJ 07109   (973)751-6060   Fax (973)450-1464
+ Eye Institute of Essex, PA
  5 Franklin Avenue/Suite 209   Belleville, NJ 07109   (973)751-6060   Fax (973)450-1464
+ Roxbury Eye Center, PC
  66 Sunset Strip/Suite 107   Succasunna, NJ 07109   (973)584-4451   Fax (973)584-2099

Eichman, Gerard T., MD {1699774950} CdvDis, IntrMd(88,DMN01)<NJ-HOLYNAME, NJ-HACKNSK>
+ Cardiovascular Associates of Teaneck
  954 Teaneck Road   Teaneck, NJ 07666   (201)833-2300   Fax (201)833-7600

Eichman, Margaret J., MD {1558335455} FamMed(89,PA02)<NJ-HUNTRDN>
+ Phillips Barber Family Health Center
  72 Alexander Avenue   Lambertville, NJ 08530   (609)397-3535   Fax (609)397-0301

Eichner, Craig N., MD {1477541571} IntrMd(80,NJ05)<NJ-KSLR-SADB>
+ Kessler Institute for Rehabilitation
  300 Market Street   Saddle Brook, NJ 07663   (201)368-6052   Fax (201)368-6184

Eid, Hala Milad, MD {1760583801} IntrMd, Rheuma(91,LEB01)
+ Cooper Rheumatology
  900 Centennial Boulevard/Suite 203   Voorhees, NJ 08043   (856)968-7019   Fax (856)482-5621

Eid, Joseph E., MD {1710057385} Hemato, Onclgy, IntrMd(93,LEB03)<NJ-RWJUBRUN>
+ Hematology Clinic
  125 Paterson Street/Room 5230   New Brunswick, NJ 08901   (732)235-7223
+ RWJ University Hospital New Brunswick
  One Robert Wood Johnson Place   New Brunswick, NJ 08901   (732)828-3000

Eid, Mahmoud Mohamed, MD {1508968561} IntrMd, EmrgMd(90,EGY09)<NJ-STJOSHOS>
+ St Joseph's Medical Center Emergency
  703 Main Street   Paterson, NJ 07503   (973)754-2222   Fax (973)754-2249

Eid, Sebastian R., MD {1811151699} Surgry
+ Advanced Laparoscopic Associates
  81 Route 4 West/Suite 401/35 Plaza   Paramus, NJ 07652   (201)646-1121   Fax (201)646-1110
+ 747 Edgewater Avenue
  Ridgefield, NJ 07657

Eida, Emily Kott, MD {1457585440} Pedtrc(09,NJ03)
+ Franklin Pediatrics, PA
  91 South Jefferson Road/Suite 200   Whippany, NJ 07981   (973)538-6116   Fax (973)538-3712

Eigen, Karen Lori, MD {1417987553} Pedtrc(93,NY46)<NJ-HACKNSK>
+ Hackensack University Medical Center
  30 Prospect Avenue/Pediatrics   Hackensack, NJ 07601   (201)996-2000

Eilenberg, Eli, MD {1376639799} Pedtrc(76,NY09)
+ 150 James Street/Suite 204
  Lakewood, NJ 08701   (732)363-4003   Fax (732)363-4447

Eilers, Robert Paul, MD {1205207339} Psychy(76,PA02)
+ 222 South Warren Street
  Trenton, NJ 08625   (609)777-0686

Eilers, Steven Edwin, MD {1306250790} Dermat
+ Skin Laser & Surgery Specialists
  20 Prospect Avenue/Suite 702   Hackensack, NJ 07601   (201)299-4521   Fax (201)441-9893

Einbinder, Lynne C., MD {1780687129} IntrMd, CdvDis(97,MD07)
+ Monmouth Heart Specialists
  274 Highway 35   Eatontown, NJ 07724   (732)440-7336   Fax (732)440-9404

+ Samir S. Jain MD PC
  599 Route 37 West/Suite 5   Toms River, NJ 08755   (732)440-7336   Fax (732)608-9744

Eingorn, David S., MD {1821094723} SrgOrt(79,PA13)<NJ-CHS-FULD, NJ-CHSMRCER>
+ Mercer-Bucks Orthopaedics PC
  3120 Princeton Pike   Lawrenceville, NJ 08648   (609)896-0444   Fax (609)896-1055
+ Mercer-Bucks Orthopaedics, P.C.
  2501 Kuser Road   Hamilton, NJ 08691   (609)896-0444   Fax (609)587-4349

Einhorn, Robert, MD {1265414999} RadDia(72,NY06)<NJ-RBAYPERT, NJ-RBAYOLDB>
+ University Radiology Group, P.C.
  260 Amboy Avenue   Metuchen, NJ 08840   (732)548-2322   Fax (732)548-3392
+ University Radiology Group, P.C.
  483 Cranbury Road   East Brunswick, NJ 08816   (732)548-2322   Fax (732)390-5383
+ University Radiology Group, P.C.
  579A Cranbury Road   East Brunswick, NJ 08840   (732)390-0040   Fax (732)390-1856

Einreinhofer, Stephen V., DO {1396848982} CritCr, PulDis, SlpDis(90,MO78)<NJ-SOMERSET, NJ-RWJUBRUN>
+ 491 Amwell Road/Suite 200
  Hillsborough, NJ 08844   (908)829-3788   Fax (908)829-3789

Einstein, Mark H., MD {1356421812} GynOnc, ObsGyn, Gyneco(95,FL02)
+ University Reproductive Association
  185 South Orange Avenue/MSB E-506   Newark, NJ 07103   (973)972-5266   Fax (973)972-4574

Eiras, Maria E., MD {1285640037} IntrMd(79,SPA22)<NJ-JRSYSHMC>
+ 702 Brewers Bridge Road
  Jackson, NJ 08527   (732)905-9630   Fax (732)905-0837

Eis, Amanda, MD {1104061753} EmrgMd<NJ-UMDNJ>
+ University Hospital
  150 Bergen Street/M-219   Newark, NJ 07103   (973)972-5128

Eisele, Joseph Carl, DO {1376818450} Anesth<NJ-CLARMAAS>
+ Clara Maass Medical Center
  1 Clara Maass Drive   Belleville, NJ 07109   (973)450-2000

Eisen, David Jeffrey, MD {1104899434}
+ Histopathology Services, LLC.
  535 East Crescent Avenue   Ramsey, NJ 07446   (301)693-5317   Fax (201)661-7297

Eisen, Deborah Ida, MD {1265428874} CritCr, IntrMd, PulDis(90,PA02)
+ 530 Lakehurst Road/Suite 306
  Toms River, NJ 08755   (732)818-9400   Fax (732)818-0210

Eisen, Morris M., DO {1558326579} SrgCdv, SrgThr(79,IA75)<NJ-KMHCHRRY>
+ 2301 East Evesham Road/Suite 406
  Voorhees, NJ 08043   (856)667-1970   Fax (856)667-0409

Eisenberg, Joshua Aaron, MD {1689602229} SrgVas, Surgry(99,PA02)<PA-TJCNTR>
+ Capital Health Medical
  2 Capital Way/Suite 356   Pennington, NJ 08534   (609)537-6000   Fax (609)537-6002

Eisenberg, Lee D., MD {1649219320} Otolgy, PedOto, Otlryg(71,NY08)<NJ-ENGLWOOD, NJ-HACKNSK>
+ ENT & Allergy Associates, LLP
  433 Hackensack Avenue/Suite 204   Hackensack, NJ 07601   (201)883-1062   Fax (201)883-9297
  Leisenberg@entandallergy.com

Eisenberg, Richard R., MD {1225148307} Dermat, IntrMd(82,NY20)<NJ-OVERLOOK>
+ 40 Stirling Road/Suite 203
  Watchung, NJ 07069   (908)753-4144   Fax (908)753-3743

Eisenberg, Ronald Lee, DO {1124042205} FamMed(64,PA77)
+ Advocare Berlin Medical Associates
  175 Cross Keys Road/Suite 300A   Berlin, NJ 08009   (856)767-0077   Fax (856)767-6102

Eisenberg, Scott R., DO {1891778353} CdvDis, IntrMd(89,PA77)<NJ-JRSYSHMC, NJ-OCEANMC>
+ Change of Heart Cardiology
  2130 Highway 35/Building C Suite 321   Sea Girt, NJ 08750   (732)974-6700   Fax (732)974-6707

Eisenberg, Sheldon B., MD {1144225723} CdvDis, CritCr, IntrMd(76,NY20)<NJ-HACKNSK, NJ-VALLEY>
+ Westwood Cardiology Associates PA
  333 Old Hook Road/Suite 200   Westwood, NJ 07675   (201)664-0201   Fax (201)666-7970
  wca@cybernet.net
+ Westwood Cardiology Associates PA
  20 Prospect Avenue/Suite 810   Hackensack, NJ 07601   (201)664-0201   Fax (201)342-2422

Eisenberg, Stuart Richard, MD {1912087552} Psychy, IntrMd(70,NY19)
+ 10 Shawnee Drive/Suite 7A
  Watchung, NJ 07069   (973)753-0916   Fax (908)753-4616

Physicians by Name and Address

Eisenbrock, Howard J., DO {1447568839} SrgNro(09,PA77)<MA-NEBAPTST>
+ Meridian Medical Group Specialties/Nuerosurgery
  65 Mechanic Street/Suite 105   Red Bank, NJ 07701   (732)268-7130   Fax (732)268-7131

Eisengart, Charles Andrew, MD {1063465342} SrgC&R, Surgry(95,MA07)
+ Drs. Hardy and Eisengart
  3131 Princeton Pike   Lawrenceville, NJ 08648   (609)896-1700   Fax (609)896-1087

Eisenstat, Carol M., MD {1669761037} Anesth
+ Morris Anesthesia Group, PA
  3799 Route 46/Suite 211   Parsippany, NJ 07054   (973)335-1122   Fax (973)335-1448

Eisenstat, Steven Alan, DO {1134104516} FamMed, FamM-Grtc(84,OH75)<NJ-OVERLOOK>
+ Drs. Eisenstat and Kershner
  1050 Galloping Hill Road/Suite 202   Union, NJ 07083   (908)688-4845   Fax (908)687-2039

Eisenstat, Theodore Ellis, MD {1619948536} SrgC&R, Surgry, IntrMd(68,NY09)<NJ-RWJUBRUN>
+ UMDNJ RWJ Surgery
  125 Paterson Street/CAB 4th FL 4100   New Brunswick, NJ 08901   (732)235-7920   Fax (732)235-7079

Eisenstein, Robert Mark, MD {1598796112} EmrgMd(92,IL42)<NJ-VIRTVOOR>
+ University Emergency Medicine
  125 Paterson Street/MEB 104   New Brunswick, NJ 08901   (732)235-8717   Fax (732)235-7379

Ejimofor, Ebikaboere, MD {1033538616} FamMed<NJ-RIVERVW>
+ Riverview Medical Center
  1 Riverview Plaza   Red Bank, NJ 07701   (732)741-2700

Ekbote, Radha N., MD {1518261486}
+ 69 Tammy Place
  Iselin, NJ 08830

Ekekwe, Ikemefula E., MD {1952505570} SlpDis
+ St. Peter's University Hospital
  254 Easton Avenue   New Brunswick, NJ 08901   (732)745-8564   Fax (732)745-9156

Ekulide, Emmanuel N., MD {1386803989} ObsGyn(67,NIG01)
+ Suburban Clinic
  43 Progress Street   Union, NJ 07083   (908)687-7188   Fax (908)687-0294

Ekulide, Ifeyinwa Ndidi, MD {1740444603} Anesth<NJ-STMRYPAS>
+ St. Mary's Hospital
  350 Boulevard/Anesthesia   Passaic, NJ 07055   (973)365-4300   Fax (845)357-5777

El Abidin, Mohammad NazirZ., MD {1205823192} Radiol, RadDia(72,SYR01)<NJ-COMMED>
+ Community Medical Center
  99 Route 37 West/Radiology   Toms River, NJ 08755   (732)557-8000

El Amir, Mazhar E., MD {1972527950} IntrMd, PulDis(81,EGYP)<NJ-CHRIST>
+ Drs. Elamir & El Amir
  192 Harrison Avenue   Jersey City, NJ 07304   (201)333-5363   Fax (201)333-4710

El Amir, Medhat Elsayed, MD {1770568461} IntrMd(78,EGY03)<NJ-BAYONNE, NJ-CHRIST>
+ Immediate Care, PC
  1856 Kennedy Boulevard   Jersey City, NJ 07305   (201)333-7606   Fax (201)333-8789
+ Immediate Care, PC
  6815 Bergenline Avenue   Guttenberg, NJ 07093   (201)453-2025
+ Immediate Care, PC
  621 Kennedy Boulevard   North Bergen, NJ 07305   (201)325-9500   Fax (201)325-0385

El Attar, Ayman Fatehy, MD {1881752665} FamMed, Dermat, Surgry(87,EGY05)
+ Derma Laser Centers
  2239 Whitehorse Mercerville Ro/Suite B   Mercerville, NJ 08619   (609)631-8558   Fax (609)631-8118

El Badawi, Khaled Iqbal, MD {1124244637} SrgC&R, Surgry(02,GRN01)
+ Virtua Surgical Group, PA
  1935 Route 70 East   Cherry Hill, NJ 08003   (856)428-7700   Fax (856)424-9120

El Banna, Mahmoud, MD {1194036483} IntrMd(NET09)
+ Regional Internal Medicine
  59 Veronica Avenue/Suite 201   Somerset, NJ 08873   (732)828-0200   Fax (732)828-0300

El Deeb, Mokhtar M., MD {1780917989} ObsGyn(06)<NJ-STJOSHOS>
+ St. Joseph's Regional Medical Center
  703 Main Street/OB/GYN   Paterson, NJ 07503   (973)754-2700   Fax (973)754-2725
+ St. Joseph's DePaul Center ObsGyn
  11 Getty Avenue   Paterson, NJ 07503   (973)754-4200

El Gazzar, Yaser S., MD {1033416995}
+ Sovereign Oncology, LLC.
  631 Grand Street   Jersey City, NJ 07304   (201)942-3999   Fax (201)942-3998

El Habr, Abdallah H., MD {1689767915} PulDis, IntrMd(91,LEB01)
+ Hamilton Pulmonary & Critical Care Associates
  3606 Nottingham Way   Hamilton, NJ 08690   (609)587-9140

El Kadi, Hisham S., MD {1184698466} IntrMd, Rheuma(81,EGY05)<NJ-CENTRAST, NJ-CLARMAAS>
+ Arthritis & Osteoporosis Associates, P.A.
  4247 US Highway 9/Building 1   Freehold, NJ 07728   (732)780-7650   Fax (908)780-8817
+ Arthritis and Osteoporosis Associates
  5 Franklin Avenue/Suite 403   Belleville, NJ 07109   (973)844-0049
+ Arthritis and Osteoporosis Associates
  9 Mule Road/Suite A-2   Toms River, NJ 07728   (732)341-1166   Fax (732)341-0018

El Khashab, Mostafa A. F., MD {1689790669} SrgNro(82,EGY03)<NJ-HACKNSK, NJ-NWRKBETH>
+ Advanced Neurosurgery Associates
  201 Route 17 North/Suite 501   Rutherford, NJ 07070   (201)457-0044   Fax (201)457-0049

El Mansoury, Hassan M., MD {1407076862} Surgry(73,EGY05)
+ JFK Medical Center
  65 James Street   Edison, NJ 08820   (732)321-7668

El Mouelhi, Mohamed H., MD {1003902545} IntrMd(74,EGY03)
+ 53 Quail Run
  Randolph, NJ 07869

El Rehim, Mohsen Sayed Abd, MD {1972655355} Psychy, PsyGrt(79,EGY04)<NJ-CENTRAST>
+ 615 Newman Springs Road
  Lincroft, NJ 07738   (732)842-1122   Fax (732)842-1191

El Sioufi, Sherene M., DO {1205940657} IntrMd, CritCr, PulCCr(00,NJ75)
+ 20-24 Branford Place/Suite 605
  Newark, NJ 07102

El Zein, Lama, MD {1003058074} FamMed, PallCr(07,LEB03)<NY-PRSBWEIL>
+ Summit Medical Group-Berkeley Heights Campus
  1 Diamond Hill Road   Berkeley Heights, NJ 07922   (908)273-4300   Fax (908)790-6576
+ Summit Medical Group
  315 East Northfield Road/Suite 1-E   Livingston, NJ 07039   (908)273-4300   Fax (973)535-1450

El-Atat, Fadi Ahmed, MD {1386776797} CdvDis, IntCrd, IntrMd(99,LEB03)
+ FACV Consultants PC
  127 Pine Street/Suite 1   Montclair, NJ 07042   (973)744-4075   Fax (973)744-2179
+ FACV Consultants PC
  1945 Morris Avenue/Suite 8   Union, NJ 07083   (973)744-4075   Fax (908)686-2637

El-Halabi, Waseem, MD {1770857419} EmrgMd
+ 231 South Park Drive/Apt E3
  Woodbridge, NJ 07095   (732)666-7622

El-Harazy, Essam, MD {1801977533} IntrMd(83,EGY05)
+ New Jersey Division of Developmental Disability
  Route 72 East   New Lisbon, NJ 08064   (609)726-1000   Fax (609)894-8430

El-Kholy, Nahed M., MD {1518939800} Psychy(77,EGY12)<NJ-NWTNMEM>
+ Atlantic Behavioral Health at Newton Medical Center
  175 High Street   Newton, NJ 07860   (973)381-1533   Fax (973)579-8430

Elagami, Mohamed Mohamed Baheild, MD {1417440439} IntrMd<NJ-STJOSHOS>
+ St. Joseph's Regional Medical Center
  703 Main Street   Paterson, NJ 07503   (973)754-2000

Elahi, Abdul Wadood, MD {1689654691} Grtrcs, IntrMd
+ New Jersey Institute for Successful Aging
  42 East Laurel Road/Suite 1800   Stratford, NJ 08084   (856)566-6843   Fax (856)566-6781

Elamir, Mohammed, MD {1811371420} IntrMd
+ Drs. Elamir & El Amir
  192 Harrison Avenue   Jersey City, NJ 07304   (201)333-5363   Fax (201)333-4710

Elango, Adhithaselvi Kandasamy, MD {1376620609} IntrMd(97,INDI)<NJ-STBARNMC>
+ St. Barnabas Medical Center
  94 Old Short Hills Road   Livingston, NJ 07039   (973)322-5000

Elango, Sitalakshmi, MD {1821095340} Anesth, PedAne(78,INDI)<NJ-MONMOUTH>
+ Monmouth Medical Center
  300 Second Avenue/Anesthesiology   Long Branch, NJ 07740   (732)222-5200

Elbasty, Azza A., MD {1588732614} Pedtrc(75,EGYP)<NJ-RIVERVW, NJ-BAYSHORE>
+ 100 Commons Way/Suite 130
  Holmdel, NJ 07733   (732)615-0700   Fax (732)615-9152

Elbaum, Philip, MD {1235484031} IntrMd<NJ-COOPRUMC>
+ Cooper University Hospital
  One Cooper Plaza   Camden, NJ 08103   (856)342-2000

Elber, Daniel A., DO {1174538938} FamMed, IntrMd(62,PA77)<NJ-JFKMED, NJ-RWJURAH>
+ Preventive HealthCare Associates
  102 James Street/Suite 202   Edison, NJ 08820   (732)548-5541   Fax (732)548-2610

Elber, Lee Bennett, DO {1104831973} OccpMd, IntrMd, PubHth(96,PA77)<NJ-JFKMED, NJ-MORRISTN>
+ Preventive HealthCare Associates
  102 James Street/Suite 202   Edison, NJ 08820   (732)548-5541   Fax (732)548-2610

Elden, Lisa Melinda, MD {1609966720} Otlryg(88,QU01)<PA-CHILDHOS>
+ CHOP Pediatric & Adolescent Specialty Care Center
  1012 Laurel Oak Road   Voorhees, NJ 08043   (856)435-1300   Fax (856)435-0091

Elder, Demian, MD {1811910623} IntrMd(99,PA02)
+ Horizon NJ Health
  210 Silvia Street   West Trenton, NJ 08628   (609)538-0700

Elder, James P., Jr., MD {1366441016} RadDia(88,NJ05)<NJ-VIRTUAHS, NJ-VIRTMHBC>
+ South Jersey Radiology Associates, P.A.
  100 Carnie Boulevard/Suite B-5   Voorhees, NJ 08043   (856)751-0123   Fax (856)751-0535
+ The Women's Center at Voorhees
  100 Carnie Boulevard/Suite A-4   Voorhees, NJ 08043   (856)751-0123   Fax (856)751-5650
+ South Jersey Radiology Associates, P.A.
  901 Route 168/Suites 301-305   Turnersville, NJ 08043   (856)227-6600   Fax (856)227-8537

Elder, Sandra Depadova, MD {1538122668} Dermat(88,NJ05)
+ Aesthetic Dermatology, LLC.
  771 East Route 70/Suite D-150   Marlton, NJ 08053   (856)596-3393   Fax (856)596-3394

Eldrich, Samuel Reich, MD {1457713554} EmrgMd
+ Cooper Univerisry Emergency Physicians
  One Cooper Plaza   Camden, NJ 08103   (856)342-2000   Fax (856)968-8272

Eleff, Michael, MD {1598857591} MedOnc, IntrMd, AdmMgt(79,OH06)<NJ-RWJUBRUN>
+ Rutgers Cancer Institute of New Jersey
  195 Little Albany Street/PO Box 2681   New Brunswick, NJ 08903   (732)235-2465   Fax (732)235-6797   meleff@juno.com
+ The Cancer Institute of New Jersey at Hamilton
  5 Hamilton Health Place/Suite 120   Hamilton, NJ 08690   (732)235-2465   Fax (609)631-6888

Elenewski, John Francis, MD {1710059803} Anesth(78,MEX14)<NJ-CHSMRCER, NJ-CHSFULD>
+ 407 Saint Andrews Place
  Manalapan, NJ 07726   (609)947-3970   Fax (609)947-3970

Elepano, Richard G., DO {1427176718} Pedtrc(03,MO79)<NJ-STCLRDEN>
+ Totowa Pediatric Group, P.A.
  290 Union Boulevard/Suite 2   Totowa, NJ 07512   (973)595-0600   Fax (973)595-0206
+ St. Clare's Hospital-Denville Campus
  25 Pocono Road   Denville, NJ 07834   (973)625-6000

Eletto, Vincent Joseph, MD {1558300327} EmrgMd(82,MEX34)<NJ-STMRYPAS, NY-MAIMONMC>
+ St. Mary's Hospital
  350 Boulevard   Passaic, NJ 07055   (973)365-4489   Fax (973)916-2032

Elfanagely, Sarah Hedy, MD {1427345313} Pedtrc
+ Totowa Pediatric Group, P.A.
  290 Union Boulevard/Suite 2   Totowa, NJ 07512   (973)595-0600   Fax (973)595-0206

Elfant, Adam B., MD {1508930298} Gastrn, IntrMd(89,NJ06)<NJ-COOPRUMC>
+ Cooper Digestive Health Institute
  501 Fellowship Road/Suite 101   Mount Laurel, NJ 08054   (856)642-2133   Fax (856)642-2134

Elfayoumi, Islam Moustafa, MD {1063450591} IntrMd<NJ-HOLYNAME>
+ Holy Name Hospital
  718 Teaneck Road   Teaneck, NJ 07666   (201)833-3000   polymathmedical@gmail.com

Elfenbein, Cherie, MD {1902019797} Psychy(83,NY08)
+ Montclair Counseling Center
  183 Inwood Avenue   Upper Montclair, NJ 07043   (973)783-6977   Fax (973)509-6597

Elfenbein, Emanuel, MD {1881808756} PsyCAd, Psychy(73,PA09)<NJ-STBARNMC>
+ 204 Eagle Rock Avenue
  Roseland, NJ 07068   (973)228-8943

Elga, Shana Stein, MD {1528235991} Psychy(05,CA14)<NJ-UNIVBHC>
+ University Behavioral Health Care
  671 Hoes Lane/PO Box 1392   Piscataway, NJ 08855   (732)235-5500

Elgawli, Philip Raef, DO {1124058102} FamMed(03,NJ75)
+ **Elmer Family Practice, P.C.**
330 West Front Street/P.O. Box 577   Elmer, NJ 08318
(856)358-0770   Fax (856)358-0108

Elgenaidi, Hisham, MD {1073573663} Hepato, IntrMd<NJ-VIRTMHBC>
+ **Southern New Jersey Center for Liver Disease**
63 Kresson Road/Suite 105   Cherry Hill, NJ 08034
(856)796-9340   Fax (856)547-0390
+ **Virtua Memorial**
175 Madison Avenue/Hepatlgy   Mount Holly, NJ 08060
(609)267-0700

Elgenaidi, Mona E., MD {1336274927} Pedtrc(82,EGYP)<NJ-ACMCITY>
+ **Mainland Pediatric Association**
741 South Second Avenue/Suite B   Galloway, NJ 08205
(609)748-8500   Fax (609)748-6700

Elhagaly, Hatem, MD {1063491496} Pedtrc
+ **1135 Main Avenue**
Clifton, NJ 07011

Elhelw, Ramy, MD {1649794587} AnesAddM
+ **50 Bergen Street**
Newark, NJ 07103   (862)232-3613   Fax (908)276-3666

Elhussein, Khalid Ali, MD {1992898134} EmrgMd(99,NY08)<NJ-UMDNJ>
+ **St Joseph's Medical Center Emergency**
703 Main Street   Paterson, NJ 07503   (973)754-2240   Fax (973)754-2249

Elia, Anna, MD {1811183866} Anesth
+ **103 Forest Road**
Moorestown, NJ 08057

Elias, Ahdi I., MD {1700808219} IntrMd, EmrgMd, Surgry(78,EGYP)<NJ-MORRISTN, NJ-NWRKBETH>
+ **Elias Medical Associates**
2839 Route 10 East/Suite 202   Morris Plains, NJ 07950
(973)292-9248   Fax (973)944-1228

Elias, Charles, MD {1710378690} Dermat<NJ-PALISADE>
+ **Palisades Medical Center**
7600 River Road/GME   North Bergen, NJ 07047   (862)223-9234

Elias, Maurice, MD {1073536256} Pedtrc(86,SYRI)<NJ-STJOSHOS>
+ **Totowa Pediatric Group, P.A.**
290 Union Boulevard/Suite 2   Totowa, NJ 07512   (973)595-0600   Fax (973)595-0206
+ **Totowa Pediatric Group, P.A.**
400 West Blackwell Street   Dover, NJ 07801   (973)595-0600   Fax (973)989-3651

Elias, Nivin, MD {1770507949} FamMed
+ **3 Rubino Road**
West Caldwell, NJ 07006

Elias, Salwa E.G., MD {1568482073} AlgyImmn, PedAlg, Pedtrc(78,EGY04)<NJ-MORRISTN, NJ-NWRKBETH>
+ **Elias Medical Associates**
2839 Route 10 East/Suite 202   Morris Plains, NJ 07950
(973)292-9248   Fax (973)944-1228

Elias, Sameh S., MD {1417092172} IntrMd(85,EGYP)<NJ-JRSYCITY, NJ-CHRIST>
+ **1610 Summit Avenue**
Union City, NJ 07087   (201)863-5696   Fax (201)863-5612

Eligulashvili, Victoria, MD {1427219310} EmrgMd<NJ-SJHREGMC>
+ **SJH Regional Medical Center**
1505 West Sherman Avenue   Vineland, NJ 08360
(856)641-8000

Elisha, Daniel, MD {1619918695} EmrgMd, FamMed(79,ISR02)<NJ-VIRTMHBC>
+ **Virtua Memorial**
175 Madison Avenue   Mount Holly, NJ 08060   (609)267-0700   Fax (609)914-6067

Elisha, Neely S., DO {1508293978}<NJ-SJHREGMC>
+ **SJH Regional Medical Center**
1505 West Sherman Avenue   Vineland, NJ 08360
(856)641-8000

Elitsur, Noeet, MD {1275793507} NnPnMd, Pedtrc, IntrMd(08,WV02)<NJ-SJHREGMC>
+ **SJH Regional Medical Center**
1505 West Sherman Avenue/Neonatology   Vineland, NJ 08360   (856)641-8160   Fax (856)641-7650

Eljarrah, Fouad, MD {1831185008} Psychy(83,SYRI)
+ **Catholic Community Services**
1160 Raymond Boulevard   Newark, NJ 07102   (973)596-4190

Elkassir, Amina, MD {1518909290} Pedtrc, AdolMd(74,EGY04)<NJ-HOLYNAME>
+ **487 Edsall Boulevard**
Fort Lee, NJ 07024   (201)224-4300   Fax (201)224-4397

Elkhalili, Walid, MD {1205186756}<NJ-STJOSHOS>
+ **St. Joseph's Regional Medical Center**
703 Main Street   Paterson, NJ 07503   (973)754-2000

Elkholy, Neveen A., DO {1346245560} FamMed(01,NJ75)
+ **Express Medical Group**
1042 Main Street   Paterson, NJ 07503   (973)510-2444

Elkholy, Wael Talaat, MD {1437240298} Acpntr, PainMd, Anesth(86,EGY03)
+ **New Jersey Pain Spine & Sports Associates**
2050 Route 27/Suite 105   North Brunswick, NJ 08902
(732)565-3777   Fax (732)746-0223
+ **New Jersey Pain Spine & Sports Associates**
601 Ewing Street/Suite C-3   Princeton, NJ 08540   (732)565-3777   Fax (732)746-0223
+ **New Jersey Pain Spine & Sports Associates**
1255 Whitehorse Mercerville Rd   Hamilton, NJ 08902
(609)688-6866   Fax (732)746-0223

Elkin, Avigayil H., MD {1720044233} Pedtrc(01,NY46)<NJ-ENGLWOOD, NJ-HACKNSK>
+ **Tenafly Pediatrics, PA**
32 Franklin Street   Tenafly, NJ 07670   (201)569-2400   Fax (201)569-6081

Elkind, Barry M., MD {1790726990} CdvDis, IntrMd(76,NJ05)
+ **Associates in Cardiovascular Care, P.A.**
1061 Avenue C   Bayonne, NJ 07002   (201)858-0800   Fax (201)858-3367
+ **Associates in Cardiovascular Care, P.A.**
33 Overlook Road/Suite 205   Summit, NJ 07901   (201)858-0800   Fax (201)858-3367
+ **Carepoint Health Bayonne Med Center**
29 East 29th Street   Bayonne, NJ 07002   (201)858-5000

Elkins, Michele, MD {1073736005} IntrMd, Grtrcs(78,FRA08)<NJ-STBARNMC>
+ **Community Health Center at Vauxhall**
3 Farrington Street   Vauxhall, NJ 07088   (908)598-7950   Fax (908)686-1163
+ **Atlantic Surgical Oncology**
99 Beauvoir Street   Summit, NJ 07901   (908)598-7950   Fax (908)598-2392

Elkwood, Andrew I., MD {1396714804} SrgPlstc, Surgry(88,NY03)<NJ-JRSYSHMC, NJ-BAYSHORE>
+ **The Plastic Surgery Ctr of NJ & Manhat**
535 Sycamore Avenue   Shrewsbury, NJ 07702   (732)741-0970   Fax (732)747-2606

Ellabbad, Essam-Eldin Moussa A., MD {1679510143} PsyAdd, Psychy(80,EGY04)
+ **Center for Family Guidance, PC**
765 East Route 70/Building A-101   Marlton, NJ 08053
(856)797-4800   Fax (856)810-0110

Ellern, Michelle Lynn, DO {1740412477} IntrMd
+ **Rowan University-School of Osteopathic Medicine**
1 Medical Center Drive   Stratford, NJ 08084   (856)566-6708

Ellinghaus, Eric J., MD {1275539496} Gastrn, IntrMd(73,DC02)<NJ-HACKNSK>
+ **Hackensack Digestive Diseases Associates, P.A.**
52 First Street   Hackensack, NJ 07601   (201)488-3003   Fax (201)488-6911
+ **Holy Name Medical Partners Office**
15 Anderson Street   Hackensack, NJ 07601   (201)488-3003   Fax (201)487-0960

Elliott, Andrew J., MD {1649356486} SrgOrt(91,MA01)<NJ-ENGLWOOD, NY-SPCLSURG>
+ **HSS Paramus Outpatient Center**
140 East Ridgewood Avenue/Suite 175-S   Paramus, NJ 07652   (201)796-2255   Fax (201)796-3711

Elliott, Nancy L., MD {1508811282} SrgBst, SrgOnc, Surgry(81,NY47)<NJ-STBARNMC, NJ-MTNSIDE>
+ **Montclair Breast Center**
37 North Fullerton Avenue   Montclair, NJ 07042   (973)509-1818   Fax (973)509-0532
+ **Glen Ridge Surgicenter**
230 Sherman Avenue   Glen Ridge, NJ 07028   (973)509-1818   Fax (973)680-4211

Ellis, Daniel Thomas, MD {1134162522} EmrgMd(01,PA02)<NJ-KMHSTRAT>
+ **Kennedy Memorial Hospital-University Medical Center**
18 East Laurel Road/EmrgMed   Stratford, NJ 08084
(856)346-7816   Fax (856)346-6385

Ellis, George David, MD {1487729141} Psychy(89,NJ05)
+ **New Point Behavioral Health Care - Outpost Division**
1070 Main Street   Sewell, NJ 08080   (856)256-3320
+ **New Point Behavioral Health Care**
404 Tatum Street/Ext 113   Woodbury, NJ 08096   (856)256-3320   Fax (856)845-0688

Ellis, Michael Joseph, DO {1972986693} IntrMd
+ **St. Michael's Medical Center**
111 Central Avenue   Newark, NJ 07102   (973)877-5487

Ellis, Stephen J., MD {1801831854} Nephro, IntrMd(71,DC02)<NJ-COMMED, NJ-OCEANMC>
+ **Ocean Renal Associates, P.A.**
210 Jack Martin Boulevard/Suite D-1   Brick, NJ 08724
(732)458-5854   Fax (732)458-8012
+ **Ocean Renal Associates, P.A.**
508 Lakehurst Road/Suite 3 A   Toms River, NJ 08755
(732)458-5854   Fax (732)341-4993
+ **Ocean Renal Associates, P.A.**
1145 Beacon Avenue/Suite B   Manahawkin, NJ 08724

(609)978-9940   Fax (609)978-9902

Ellis, Steven P., MD {1225031453} Ophthl(82,NY19)<NJ-RWJUHAM>
+ **Mercer Eye Associates, PA**
123 Franklin Corner Road/Suite 207   Lawrenceville, NJ 08648   (609)750-7300   Fax (609)896-7052

Ellison, Christian Eric, MD {1306838305} FamMed(95,NJ05)
+ **Medical Diagnostic Associates PA**
525 Central Avenue/Suite D   Westfield, NJ 07090
(908)232-5333   Fax (908)389-1922

Elliston, Jason Taiwo Jos, MD {1669520375} Allrgy(99,NM01)<NJ-UMDNJ>
+ **Metropolitan Family Health Network**
935 Garfield Avenue   Jersey City, NJ 07304   (201)478-5800   Fax (201)475-5814

Ellman, Barry R., MD {1578661351} Surgry(70,PA01)<NJ-JFKMED>
+ **98 James Street/Suite 100**
Edison, NJ 08820   (732)906-8501   Fax (732)906-8502

Ellner, Jerrold Jay, MD {1174736797} InfDis, IntrMd(70,MD07)<MA-BOSTMC>
+ **University Physician Associates**
140 Bergen Street/ACC Level D   Newark, NJ 07103
(973)972-4071   Fax (973)972-3102

Elman, Igor, MD {1548221559} Psychy, PsyAdd(91,ISR05)<MA-MAGENHOS>
+ **The Cooper Hospital System-Univ Hospital**
401 Haddon Avenue   Camden, NJ 08103   (856)342-2000
+ **Cooper Psychiatric Associates**
3 Cooper Plaza/Suite 307   Camden, NJ 08103   (856)342-2000   Fax (856)541-6137

Elmann, Elie Marco, MD {1225138290} SrgCdv, SrgThr, OthrSp(87,NY09)<NJ-HACKNSK, NJ-HOLYNAME>
+ **Hackensack University Medical Center**
20 Prospect Avenue/Cardio Surgery   Hackensack, NJ 07601
(201)996-2261   Fax (201)343-0609
elmannCTS@aol.com
+ **Cardiac Surgery Group, P.A.**
20 Prospect Avenue/Suite 900   Hackensack, NJ 07601
(201)996-2261   Fax (201)343-0609

Elmore, Erin Maureen, MD {1780711382} Psychy, Nrolgy, IntrMd(97,NY46)<NJ-STBARNMC>
+ **Essex Neurological Associates, P.A.**
81 Northfield Avenue/Suite 301   West Orange, NJ 07052
(973)373-8000   Fax (973)373-5265

Elmoursi, Sedeek, MD {1982049441} Nrolgy
+ **University Hospital-Doctors Office Center**
90 Bergen Street/Suite 8100   Newark, NJ 07103   (973)972-2550   Fax (973)972-5059

Elnahal, Mohamed H., MD {1912949199} CdvDis, IntrMd(81,EGYP)<NJ-ACMCITY, NJ-ACMCMAIN>
+ **Womens Health & Wellness**
2500 English Creek Avenue   Egg Harbor Township, NJ 08234
(609)677-7776   Fax (609)677-7509

Elnahar, Yaser, MD {1831409531} IntrMd(07,GRN01)
+ **Hunterdon Cardiovascular Associates**
1100 Wescott Drive/Suite G-3   Flemington, NJ 08822
(908)788-6471   Fax (908)788-6460

Eloy, Jean Anderson, MD {1295997500} Otlryg, Rhinol(02,NJ05)<NJ-UMDNJ>
+ **University Hospital-Doctors Office Center**
90 Bergen Street/Suite 8100   Newark, NJ 07103   (973)972-2500   Fax (973)972-3767

Eloy, Jean D., MD {1538328851} Anesth(04,NJ05)<NJ-UMDNJ>
+ **Rutgers- New Jersey Medical School**
185 South Orange Avenue/Anesth   Newark, NJ 07103
(973)972-4300

Elrabie, Nazmi A., MD {1124046917} Surgry, SrgVas(69,EGY05)<NJ-WAYNEGEN, NJ-STJOSHOS>
+ **1020 Main Street**
Paterson, NJ 07503   (973)648-1103   Fax (973)684-2332
+ **Wayne Surgical Center, LLC.**
1176 Hamburg Pike   Wayne, NJ 07470   (973)648-1103   Fax (973)709-1901

ElRafei, Mohamed A., MD {1114955895} Psychy(81,EGY04)<NJ-CHILTON>
+ **Wayne Behavioral Services**
401 Hamburg Turnpike/Suite 303   Wayne, NJ 07470
(973)790-9222   Fax (973)790-0671

Elreda, Lauren, MD {1952479073} OncHem, IntrMd(03,DMN01)<NJ-NWRKBETH>
+ **Newark Beth Israel Medical Center**
201 Lyons Avenue/HemaOnc   Newark, NJ 07112
(973)926-7000
Lelreda@sbhcs.com

ElSahwi, Karim Samir, MD {1508909995} ObsGyn(94,EGY05)<NJ-JRSYSHMC>
+ **Meridian Obstetrics amd Gynecology Associates PC**
19 Davis Avenue/Fl 1   Neptune, NJ 07753   (732)897-7944   Fax (732)922-8264

Physicians by Name and Address

Elsakka, Maha Fathy, MD {1679501779} Anesth, PainInvt(86,EGY03)<NJ-JRSYSHMC>
+ Jersey Shore University Medical Center
1945 Route 33/Anesthesiology   Neptune, NJ 07753   (732)775-5500   Fax (732)897-0263
+ Jersery Shore Anesthesiology
1945 Highway 33   Neptune, NJ 07753   (732)775-5500   Fax (732)897-0263

Elsamman, Wael A., MD {1831419126} IntrMd
+ Ocean County Family Care
9 Mule Road   Toms River, NJ 08755   (732)818-0004   Fax (732)818-7775

Elsamra, Sammy E., MD {1992907034} Urolgy(07,NJ05)<NJ-RWJUBRUN>
+ RWJ University Hospital Urology
125 Paterson Street/CAB 4100   New Brunswick, NJ 08901   (732)235-7775   Fax (732)235-6042
+ Rutgers Cancer Institute of NJ at Univ Hospital
205 South Orange Avenue/B Level   Newark, NJ 07101   (973)972-5108

Elsawaf, Mohamed Ashraf, MD {1447419718} PulDis, IntrMd
+ Shore Pulmonary PA
301 Bingham Avenue/Suite B   Ocean, NJ 07712   (732)775-9075   Fax (732)775-1212
+ Shore Pulmonary PA
2640 Highway 70/Building 6-A   Manasquan, NJ 08736   (732)775-9075   Fax (732)528-0887
+ Shore Pulmonary PA
1608 Route 88/Suite 117   Brick, NJ 07712   (732)575-1100

Elsawy, Osama Ahmed, DO {1962732115} Surgry(06,NJ75)
+ St. Joseph Medical Center Surgery
703 Main Street   Paterson, NJ 07503   (973)754-2490

Elsayed, Ali Elsayed Mohamme, MD {1871702977} IntrMd<NJ-MTNSIDE>
+ Hackensack UMC Mountainside
1 Bay Avenue   Montclair, NJ 07042   (973)429-6000

Elsayed, Yusri Ali, MD {1043460538} IntrMd, MedOnc(90,SUD02)
+ Johnson & Johnson Research & Develop
920 US Highway Route 202   Raritan, NJ 08869   (908)704-4000

Elshinawy, Ashgan A., DO {1417907528} IntrMd, PulDis(99,NJ75)<NJ-STPETER>
+ St. Peter's University Hospital
254 Easton Avenue   New Brunswick, NJ 08901   (732)745-8600   Fax (732)745-9156

Elshoreya, Hazem Mohamed, MD {1801094099} ObsGyn(95,EGY05)
+ Cooper Ob/Gyn
3 Cooper Plaza/Suite 300   Camden, NJ 08103   (856)342-2186   Fax (856)968-8575

Elson, Abe, MD {1689778136} CdvDis, IntrMd(80,ITA17)<NJ-VALLEY>
+ 1 West Ridgewood Avenue/Suite 210
Paramus, NJ 07652   (201)652-0402

Eltaki, Madiha Ahmed, MD {1588628283} GenPrc(71,EGY05)<NJ-ESSEXCO>
+ Essex County Hospital Center
204 Grove Avenue   Cedar Grove, NJ 07009   (973)571-2800   Fax (973)571-2899

Eltawansy, Sherif Mahmoud, MD {1518308949}<NJ-MONMOUTH>
+ Monmouth Medical Center
300 Second Avenue   Long Branch, NJ 07740   (732)923-5000

Eltemsah, Nagi I., MD {1568535367} Pedtrc(84,EGY09)<NJ-JRSYCITY>
+ Pediatrics A1-LLC
2775 John F. Kennedy   Jersey City, NJ 07306   (201)222-7899   Fax (201)222-7801

Eltom, Alaeldin Abdalla, MD {1033373386} IntrMd<NJ-TRINIWSC>
+ Trinitas Regional Medical Center-Williamson Street
225 Williamson Street   Elizabeth, NJ 07207   (908)994-5000

Elvey, Sharon Marie, MD {1851360101} Pedtrc, IntrMd(78,PA07)<PA-TJHSP>
+ Pediatric and Adolescent Medicine Group
400 East Church Street   Blackwood, NJ 08012   (856)374-8446

Elvove, Robert M., MD {1710033972} Psychy(66,IL02)<NJ-VALLEY>
+ 1250 East Ridgewood Avenue
Ridgewood, NJ 07450   (201)447-4765   Fax (201)447-4698

Elyash, Igor Gary, DO {1952630444} Surgry<NJ-UNVMCPRN>
+ Morristown Surgical Associates
344 South Street   Morristown, NJ 07960   (973)267-2838   Fax (973)267-7909

Emami, Arash, MD {1558302935} SrgSpn, SrgOrt(94,IL02)
+ University Spine Center
504 Valley Road/Second Floor/Suite 203   Wayne, NJ 07470   (973)686-0700   Fax (973)686-0701

Emanuel, Anthony, MD {1528088473} Pedtrc(79,NJ05)<NJ-CENTRAST, NJ-JRSYSHMC>
+ Pediatric Health, P.A.
470 Stillwells Corner Road   Freehold, NJ 07728   (732)780-3333   Fax (732)780-6968
+ Pediatric Health, PA
4537 Route 9 North   Howell, NJ 07731   (732)780-3333   Fax (732)367-6524
+ Pediatric Health, PA
23 Kilmer Drive/Building 1 Suite B   Morganville, NJ 07728   (732)972-0900   Fax (732)972-2892

Emanuele, William Anthony, DO {1144658337} SprtMd
+ 1280 Almonesson Road
Deptford, NJ 08096   (856)537-7060   Fax (856)805-9370

Embrescia, Mary Megan, MD {1659556934} PsyCAd(CA06)
+ Center for Family Guidance, PC
765 East Route 70/Building A-101   Marlton, NJ 08053   (856)983-3900   Fax (856)810-0110

Emelle, Emmanuel M., MD {1558343756} Pedtrc(83,NIGE)<NJ-NWRKBETH, NJ-STMICHL>
+ 40 Union Avenue/Suite 306
Irvington, NJ 07111   (973)374-3544   Fax (973)374-3554
mdemelle@yahoo.com

Emenari, Chibuzo U., MD {1659692887} FamMed
+ 200 Strykers Road
Phillipsburg, NJ 08865   (484)526-4000

Emery, Robert C., MD {1386745693} CdvDis, IntrMd(65,SWIT)<NJ-WARREN, MA-STLUKES>
+ Warren Hospital
185 Roseberry Street/Cardiology   Phillipsburg, NJ 08865   (908)859-6700
+ Premier Heart Specialists
200 Coventry Drive   Phillipsburg, NJ 08865   (908)213-1030

Emiliani, Vincent J., MD {1487634457} Gastrn(82,MEXI)<NJ-STCLRDEN, NJ-MORRISTN>
+ Morris County Gastroenterology Associates
16 Pocono Road/Suite 201   Denville, NJ 07834   (973)627-4430   Fax (973)586-2336

Emma, Sheri Lynn, MD {1699889469} Dermat(00,NJ05)
+ 2130 Highway 35/Suite A-113
Sea Girt, NJ 08750

Emmolo, Joana S., MD {1073825543} RadOnc, Radiol, IntrMd(05,NJ05)
+ Radiation Oncology at Overlook Medical Center
33 Overlook Road/MAC 1 Suite L-05   Summit, NJ 07901   (908)522-2871   Fax (908)522-5628

Emmons, Alyson, DO {1891733010} IntrMd<NJ-VIRTVOOR>
+ Virtua Voorhees
100 Bowman Drive   Voorhees, NJ 08043   (856)247-3000   Fax (856)504-8029

Empaynado, Edwin Abogado, MD {1326071713} Surgry(99,NJ06)
+ Colon & Rectal Surgical Associates of South Jersey
502 Centennial Boulevard/Suite 5   Voorhees, NJ 08043   (856)429-8030   Fax (856)428-2718

Empedrad, Albert Barcelona, MD {1699899914} EnDbMt(91,PHI02)
+ 2139 Route 33/Suite 2
Hamilton, NJ 08690   (609)915-8781

Empedrad, Raquel B., MD {1902896988} AlgyImmn, IntrMd(91,PHI18)<NJ-VIRTUAHS, NJ-SOCEANCO>
+ Allergic Disease Associates, PC - Forked River
1044 Lacey Road/suite 9   Forked River, NJ 08731   (609)693-5317   Fax (609)693-0351
+ Allergic Disease Associates, PC - Mount Laurel
210 Ark Road & Route 38/Suite 109   Mount Laurel, NJ 08054   (609)693-5317   Fax (856)235-2154

Emy, Margaret Yoko, MD {1699750877} Radiol, RadDia(91,NY01)<NJ-HACKNSK>
+ New Century Imaging at Oradell
555 Kinderkamack Road   Oradell, NJ 07649   (201)599-1311   Fax (201)599-8333

Enabosi, Ellis, MD {1669866158} GenPrc
+ 460 North Maple Avenue
East Orange, NJ 07017   (973)280-9600

Encarnacion, Cirilo, MD {1578788048} Surgry, OccpMed(76,PHIL)<NJ-JFKMED>
+ JFK Medical Center
65 James Street/OccupHlth   Edison, NJ 08820   (732)321-7610   Fax (732)906-4928

Endaya-Aguila, Thelma, MD {1841223534} Pedtrc(73,PHIL)<NJ-HOBUNIMC>
+ 550 Newark Avenue/Suite 305
Jersey City, NJ 07306   (201)963-2320   Fax (201)222-2099

Ende, Leigh S., MD {1578535860} SrgHnd, SrgOrt(78,LA01)<NJ-STCLRDEN, NJ-STCLRDOV>
+ Leigh Ende MD LLC
121 Center Grove Road   Randolph, NJ 07869   (973)366-5565   Fax (973)361-2308
handsurg715@optonline.net
+ Leigh Ende MD, LLC
380 Lafayette Road/Suite 204   Sparta, NJ 07871   (973)366-5565

Ende, Mark, DO {1518006584} IntrMd(83,PA77)<NJ-COMMED>
+ 1228 Route 37 West/Suite 6
Toms River, NJ 08755   (732)244-2700   Fax (732)244-7666
+ Meridian Primary Care
138 Route 9 South   Forked River, NJ 08731   (732)244-2700   Fax (609)488-1613

Ende, Theodore, DO {1093722480} IntrMd, Grtrcs(73,PA77)<NJ-COMMED, NJ-HLTHSRE>
+ Forked River Medical Specialties
422 West Lacey Road   Forked River, NJ 08731   (609)693-1992   Fax (609)971-3199

Enescu, Cristian C., MD {1518920925} Nrolgy(83,ROM01)
+ Ultimed HealthCare PC
50 Franklin Lane   Manalapan, NJ 07726   (732)972-1267   Fax (732)972-1026

Eng, Jeffrey M., MD {1174828065} Pedtrc
+ Watchung Pediatrics
76 Stirling Road/Suite 201   Warren, NJ 07059   (908)755-5437   Fax (908)755-6905

Eng, Kenneth, DO {1134193865} FamMed(96,NY75)<NJ-CENTRAST, NJ-COMMED>
+ 800 West Main Street
Freehold, NJ 07728   (732)409-2822

Eng, Leonard K., MD {1205055928} Psychy, PsyCAd(83,NJ05)
+ 385 Main Street/PO Box 343
Metuchen, NJ 08840   (732)494-5858   Fax (732)494-7060
+ Raritan Bay Mental Health Center
570 Lee Street   Perth Amboy, NJ 08861   (732)494-5858   Fax (732)442-9512

Eng, Margaret Hom, MD {1386693448} InfDis, IntrMd(80,NY46)<NJ-MONMOUTH>
+ Monmouth Family Center
270 Broadway   Long Branch, NJ 07740   (732)923-7100   Fax (732)923-7104

Eng, Robert H., MD {1043234529} InfDis, IntrMd, Grtrcs(75,NY46)<NJ-VAEASTOR>
+ VA New Jersey Health Care System-East Orange Campus
385 Tremont Avenue   East Orange, NJ 07018   (973)676-1000

Eng, Tiffany, MD {1801174636} EmrgMd<NJ-COMMED>
+ Community Medical Center
99 Route 37 West   Toms River, NJ 08755   (732)557-8000

Engel, Barbara M., MD {1295725745} Pedtrc(71,NY08)<NJ-RIVERVW>
+ Bayshore Pediatric Association
717 North Beers Street/Suite 1C   Holmdel, NJ 07733   (732)888-0010   Fax (732)888-0012
barbara@bayshore.pcc.com

Engel, Jennifer Duck, MD {1609808567} Pedtrc(00,MONT)<NJ-RIVERVW, NJ-JRSYSHMC>
+ Bayshore Pediatric Association
717 North Beers Street/Suite 1C   Holmdel, NJ 07733   (732)888-0010   Fax (732)888-0012

Engel, John Mark, MD {1104806553} PedOph, Ophthl(86,IL43)<NJ-RWJUBRUN, NJ-STPETER>
+ University Children's Eye Center, P.C.
4 Cornwall Court   East Brunswick, NJ 08816   (732)613-9191   Fax (732)613-1139
+ University Children's Eye Center, P.C.
678 Route 202-206 North/Bld 5   Bridgewater, NJ 08807   (732)613-9191   Fax (908)203-9010

Engel, Margaret A., MD {1245394436} IntrMd, Nephro(83,NY09)
+ 327 Avenue C
Bayonne, NJ 07002   (201)437-8500

Engel, Mark L., MD {1487648457} Ophthl, PedOph(71,NY08)<NJ-BAYSHORE, NJ-RIVERVW>
+ University Children's Eye Center, P.C.
4 Cornwall Court   East Brunswick, NJ 08816   (732)613-9191   Fax (732)613-1139
+ University Children's Eye Center, P.C.
678 Route 202-206 North/Bld 5   Bridgewater, NJ 08807   (732)613-9191   Fax (908)203-9010
+ Ophthalmic Physicians of Monmouth PA
733 North Beers Street/Suite U-4   Holmdel, NJ 08816   (732)739-0707   Fax (732)739-6722

Engel, Samuel Henry, MD {1083820518} Otlryg, PedOto(02,NJ06)<NJ-JRSYSHMC>
+ Coastal Ear Nose and Throat LLC
3700 Route 33/Suite 101   Neptune, NJ 07753   (732)280-7855   Fax (732)280-7815
+ Coastal Ear Nose and Throat LLC
1301 Route 72/Suite 340   Manahawkin, NJ 08050   (732)280-7855   Fax (732)280-7815

Engelbach, Ludmila, MD {1336174945} PthACl, Pthlgy(73,CZE07)<NJ-COMMED, NJ-KIMBALL>
+ PLUS Diagnostics
1200 River Avenue/Suite 10   Lakewood, NJ 08701   (732)901-7575   Fax (732)901-1555

Engell, Christian August, MD {1831374305} InfDis, IntrMd(02,DEN04)<NJ-NWRKBETH>
+ Newark Beth Israel Medical Center
201 Lyons Avenue/Inf Disease   Newark, NJ 07112   (973)926-5212   Fax (973)926-8182

Engelman, James E., DO {1528002110} PhysMd(93,CA22)<NJ-CENTRAST>
+ CentraState Medical Center
901 West Main Street/PhysRehab   Freehold, NJ 07728   (732)431-5024   Fax (732)431-2561

Engle, Edward A., MD {1134327869} SrgNro(75,PA02)
+ 10 Cambridge Court
Randolph, NJ 07869

Engle, Edward Issac, DO {1417021627} Otlryg, SrgHdN(94,NY75)
+ NJ Regional Ear, Nose & Throat Center LLC
1145 Beacon Avenue   Manahawkin, NJ 08050   (609)597-7110   Fax (609)597-7113
Eengl@comcast.net
+ NJ Regional Ear, Nose & Throat Center LLC
300 Water Street   Toms River, NJ 08753   (609)597-7110   Fax (609)597-7113

Engler, Mitchell S., MD {1326061755} IntrMd, PulDis, SlpDis(78,MA05)<NJ-ENGLWOOD, NJ-HOLYNAME>
+ Bergen Medical Alliance, P.A.
180 Engle Street   Englewood, NJ 07631   (201)568-8010   Fax (201)568-8936

Englert, Christopher A., MD {1134240138} ObsGyn(85,OH41)<NJ-HOLYNAME>
+ Holy Name Physician Network
420 Grand Avenue/Suite 202   Englewood, NJ 07631   (201)871-4040   Fax (201)871-7326

Enis, Sean, MD {1417104399} GenPrc<NJ-MORRISTN>
+ Morristown Medical Center
100 Madison Avenue   Morristown, NJ 07962   (973)971-5000

Enjamuri, Devendra, MD {1861745135} IntrMd<NJ-STPETER>
+ Newark Beth Israel Medical Center
201 Lyons Avenue   Newark, NJ 07112   (973)926-7000

Enlow, Tracey S., MD {1780884858} Anesth(03,NJ06)
+ Robert Wood Johnson-UMDNJ Anesthesia Group
125 Paterson Street/CAB 3100   New Brunswick, NJ 08901   (732)235-7827   Fax (732)235-6131
traceysenlow@aol.com

Enriquez, Alfred Vasquez, MD {1912249145} FamMed
+ Tatem Brown Family Practice
2225 East Evesham Road/Suite 101   Voorhees, NJ 08043   (856)325-3700   Fax (856)325-3704

Enriquez, Carla, MD {1548385578} BhvrMd, PedDvl, Pedtrc(71,MA05)
+ 1138 East Chestnut Avenue
Vineland, NJ 08360   (856)691-8426   Fax (856)696-7053

Enriquez, Eduardo F., MD {1063573616} IntrMd(84,MEXI)<NJ-VIRTUAHS>
+ Enriquez Medical Center
3 Brendenwood Drive   Voorhees, NJ 08043   (856)874-0202   Fax (856)874-0220

Enriquez, Joseph E., MD {1801909247} Anesth(84,NY09)<NJ-CHS-FULD, NJ-CHSMRCER>
+ Trenton Anesthesiology Associates, PA
One Capital Way/Second Floor   Pennington, NJ 08534   (609)396-4700   Fax (609)396-4900

Enriquez, Melissa J., MD {1447469473} EmrgMd(04,NJ05)<NJ-HOBUNIMC>
+ Hoboken University Medical Center
308 Willow Avenue/EmrgMed   Hoboken, NJ 07030   (201)418-1900

Enriquez, Miriam Lynn, MD {1467517565} PthAClt(PA01<NJ-COOPRUMC>
+ Cooper University Medical Center/Camden
3 Cooper Plaza/Suite 502   Camden, NJ 08103   (856)342-2506   Fax (856)968-8806

Enriquez, Santiago, Jr., MD {1790722429} EnDbMt, EmrgMd, NuclMd(67,PHIL)
+ Drs. Delaney, Merlin & Pourmasiha
66 West Gilbert Street/2nd Floor   Tinton Falls, NJ 07701   (732)212-0051   Fax (732)212-0713

Enriquez-Leff, Liza Jeanne, MD {1770724528} Anesth(04,DMN01)<NJ-MEADWLND>
+ St. Joseph's Regional Medical Center Anesthesia
703 Main Street   Paterson, NJ 07503   (973)754-2323   Fax (973)977-9455

Entmacher, Michael S., MD {1053346304} IntrMd, MedOnc, OncHem(79,NC07)<NJ-VIRTMHBC>
+ Virtua Memorial
175 Madison Avenue/4th Floor   Mount Holly, NJ 08060   (609)267-0700   Fax (609)702-8455

Entmacher, Susan D., MD {1558369629} EnDbMt, IntrMd(79,PA07)
+ Endocrine Associates of Southern Jersey
703 East Main Street/Suite 5   Moorestown, NJ 08057   (856)727-0900   Fax (856)231-8428

Entrada, Julian, Jr., MD {1104823921} Anesth(69,PHIL)
+ 51 Leonard Terrace
Roseland, NJ 07068

Enukashvili, Rafael R., MD {1073554838} Grtrcs, IntrMd(89,RUSS)<NJ-BAYSHORE, NJ-HOBUNIMC>
+ 3310 Route 9
Old Bridge, NJ 08857   (732)617-2988   Fax (732)970-8703

Enyeribe, Chioma J., MD {1700192275} FamMed, IntrMd, IntHos(98,NIG02)<NJ-COOPRUMC>
+ Cooper University Hospital
One Cooper Plaza/Hospitalist   Camden, NJ 08103   (856)342-3150   Fax (856)968-8418

Epelboim Feldman, Joyce, MD {1033323779} IntrMd(93,VEN04)
+ Penn Medicine at Cherry Hill
409 Route 70 East/Sleep Center   Cherry Hill, NJ 08034   (856)429-1519

Ephrat, Moshe, MD {1447357025} IntrMd(87,NY46)<NJ-HACKNSK>
+ 101 Prospect Avenue
Hackensack, NJ 07601   (201)342-6550   Fax (201)342-8549

Ephrat, Roni, MD {1528143591} Anesth(91,NJ05)<NJ-HOLY-NAME>
+ Holy Name Hospital
718 Teaneck Road/Anesthesiology   Teaneck, NJ 07666   (201)833-3000   Fax (201)342-1259

Ephrem, Yasmina Marie Therese, MD {1336180793} ObsGyn(94,NY09)
+ Drs. Darvish and Ephrem
401 Hamburg Turnpike/Suite 309   Wayne, NJ 07470   (973)942-1200

Ephros, Hillel, MD {1346254752} SrgO&M(92,GRN01)
+ St. Joseph's Regional Medical Center
703 Main Street/Dentistry   Paterson, NJ 07503   (973)754-2050

Eppanapally, Shanti Sree, MD {1306872635} PainMd, Anesth(90,INA83)<NJ-STMRYPAS>
+ St. Mary's Hospital
350 Boulevard   Passaic, NJ 07055   (973)365-4300   Fax (973)779-7385
+ Pain Centers of America
1060 Clifton Avenue   Clifton, NJ 07013   (973)365-4300   Fax (608)571-1035

Epperlein, Jennifer I., DO {1205084357} PhysMd
+ 282 Woodland Avenue
Summit, NJ 07901   (908)277-2172

Eppinger, Barry A., DO {1336233956} Nephro, IntrMd(87,NY75)<NJ-MORRISTN>
+ Kidney Care
131 Madison Avenue/Suite 3   Morristown, NJ 07960   (973)631-6223   Fax (973)631-6225
+ Nephrology Hypertension Assocs
2 Franklin Place   Morristown, NJ 07960   (973)631-6223   Fax (973)267-3270

Epstein, Britany Faith, MD {1689018251} EnDbMt
+ 8501 Fulton Avenue
Margate City, NJ 08402   (609)287-6462   Fax (609)601-1981

Epstein, David Israel, MD {1801864699} Anesth(90,CT02)
+ 500 Grand Avenue
Englewood, NJ 07631

Epstein, David Michael, MD {1609034560} SrgOrt, SrgFAk(05,NY48)<NY-JTORTHO>
+ Tri-County Orthopedics
160 East Hanover Avenue   Morristown, NJ 07962   (973)538-2334   Fax (973)829-9174

Epstein, Debra M., MD {1821060005} ObsGyn(88,IL06)<NJ-VIRTMHBC>
+ Epstein Gynocology Associates Maple Shade
1000 South Linola Road   Maple Shade, NJ 08052   (856)234-4436   Fax (856)234-4469
+ Epstein Gynocology Associates Turnersville
151 Fries Mill Road/Suite 403   Turnersville, NJ 08012   (856)234-4436   Fax (856)234-4469

Epstein, Jeffrey E., MD {1689755860} Grtrcs, IntrMd(85,NJ06)<NJ-VIRTMHBC>
+ Epstein Internal Medicine
2906 Route 130 North   Delran, NJ 08075   (856)764-4115   Fax (856)764-4116
JeffreyEpsteinMD@gmail.com
+ AmeriHealth HMO, Inc.
8000 Midlantic Drive/Suite 333   Mount Laurel, NJ 08054   (856)778-6500

Epstein, John Arthur, MD {1851304612} Ophthl(00,MD07)
+ The Princeton Eye Group
419 North Harrison Street/Suite 104   Princeton, NJ 08540   (609)921-9437   Fax (609)921-0277
+ The Princeton Eye Group
1600 Perrinville Road   Monroe Township, NJ 08831   (609)921-9437   Fax (609)655-3685
+ The Princeton Eye Group
900 Eastern Avenue/Suite 50   Somerset, NJ 08540   (732)565-9550   Fax (732)565-0946

Epstein, Matthew D., MD {1922000793} PulCCr, IntrMd, SlpDis(90,QU01)<NJ-MORRISTN>
+ Pulmonary & Allergy Associates
8 Saddle Road/Suite 101   Cedar Knolls, NJ 07927   (973)267-9393   Fax (973)540-0472
+ Pulmonary & Allergy Associates
1 Springfield Avenue/Suite 3-A   Summit, NJ 07901   (973)267-9393   Fax (908)934-0556

Epstein, Nina, MD {1245317676} Pedtrc(97,NY46)
+ Metropolitan Pediatric Group
704 Palisade Avenue   Teaneck, NJ 07666   (201)836-4301   Fax (201)836-5110
+ Metropolitan Pediatric Group
570 Piermont Road/17 Closter Commons   Closter, NJ 07624   (201)836-4301   Fax (201)768-7316

Epstein, Richard William, MD {1700882081} RadDia(96,CT01)
+ University Radiology, PA
239 Route 22 East/Suite 302   Green Brook, NJ 08812   (732)968-4899   Fax (732)968-8096
+ University Radiology Group, P.C.
3900 Park Avenue/Suite 107   Edison, NJ 08820   (732)968-4899   Fax (732)548-6290
+ University Radiology Group, P.C.
16 Mountain Boulevard   Warren, NJ 08812   (908)769-7200   Fax (908)769-9141

Epstein, Robert E., MD {1356323083} RadDia(90,NC07)<NJ-RWJUBRUN, NJ-STPETER>
+ University Radiology Group, P.C.
483 Cranbury Road   East Brunswick, NJ 08816   (732)390-0030   Fax (732)390-5383
+ University Radiology Group, P.C.
105 Raider Boulevard/Suite 101   Hillsborough, NJ 08844   (732)390-0030   Fax (908)359-9273
+ University Radiology Group, P.C.
579A Cranbury Road   East Brunswick, NJ 08816   (732)390-0040   Fax (732)390-1856

Epstein, Samuel E., DO {1609872555} SrgOrt(84,PA77)<NJ-SOCEANCO>
+ Stafford Orthopedics PA
1168 Beacon Avenue   Manahawkin, NJ 08050   (609)597-6092   Fax (609)597-7458

Epstein, Steven Brian, MD {1356349641} RadV&I, RadDia(82,NY08)<NY-STBARNAB>
+ Vascular Epicenter
7000 Boulevard East   Guttenberg, NJ 07093   (201)861-9900   Fax (201)861-9977

Eraiba, Ayman E., MD {1467589085} IntrMd(84,EGY05)<NJ-CHILTON>
+ Eraiba & Eraiba Internal Medicine
510 Hamburg Turnpike/Suite 208   Wayne, NJ 07470   (973)904-3480   Fax (973)904-3485

Eraiba, Magda A., MD {1841327384} IntrMd(83,EGYP)<NJ-CHILTON>
+ Eraiba & Eraiba Internal Medicine
510 Hamburg Turnpike/Suite 208   Wayne, NJ 07470   (973)904-3480   Fax (973)904-3485

Eraky, Waheed K., MD {1649271761} Anesth(81,EGY05)<NJ-MONMOUTH>
+ Monmouth Medical Center
300 Second Avenue/Anesthesiology   Long Branch, NJ 07740   (732)222-5200

Erb, Erica, MD {1801943303} FamMed(01,NJ06)<NJ-SOMERSET>
+ RWJPE Towne Centre Family Care
302 Towne Centre Drive   Hillsborough, NJ 08844   (908)359-8613   Fax (908)874-8509

Erbicella, John Michael, MD {1992722649} Surgry(88,PA14)<NJ-UNDRWD>
+ Woodbury Surgical Associates
127 North Broad Street   Woodbury, NJ 08096   (856)845-0500   Fax (856)384-8757

Erguder, Iris, MD {1508095159} FamMed, IntrMd(01,DOM18)
+ Holy Name Physician Network
175 Bergen Boulevard   Fairview, NJ 07022   (201)945-1400   Fax (201)945-4441

Ergun-Longmire, Berrin, MD {1306898812} PedEnd, Pedtrc(89,TUR01)<NY-MTSINYHS>
+ RUW Pediatric Endocrinology
89 French Street/Room 1363   New Brunswick, NJ 08901   (732)235-9378   Fax (732)235-5002

Erianne, John A., MD {1750486221} Dermat(68,NJ05)
+ 3285 Kennedy Boulevard
Jersey City, NJ 07307   (201)656-5263   Fax (201)656-3931
J.Erianne@verizon.net

Erickson, Alan R., MD {1538119169} Ophthl(79,PA02)<NJ-SOCEANCO>
+ Erickson, Dreizen & Lee Eye Center
1206 Route 72 West   Manahawkin, NJ 08050   (609)597-8087   Fax (609)597-7192
+ Erickson, Dreizen & Lee Eye Center
730 West Lacey Road/Suite G-07   Forked River, NJ 08731   (609)971-8822

Physicians by Name and Address

Erickson, John A., MD {1528346962} SrgOrt<NJ-RWJUBRUN>
+ RWJ University Hospital New Brunswick
One Robert Wood Johnson Place   New Brunswick, NJ 08901   (609)457-3145

Ericsson, Dawn Marie, MD {1639229628} ObsGyn(01,NY48)
+ Union & Cranford Ob/Gyn & Infertility Group
1323 Stuyvesant Avenue   Union, NJ 07083   (908)686-4334   Fax (908)686-1744
+ Union & Cranford Ob/Gyn & Infertility Group
118 South Avenue East   Cranford, NJ 07016   (908)276-7333
+ Union & Cranford Ob/Gyn & Infertility Group
349 Valley Street   South Orange, NJ 07083   (973)763-4334

Erlebacher, Jay A., MD {1285737080} CdvDis, CarNuc, IntrMd(75,NY15)<NJ-ENGLWOOD, NJ-HACKNSK>
+ Englewood Cardiology Consultants
177 North Dean Street/Suite 100   Englewood, NJ 07631   (201)569-4901   Fax (201)569-6111

Erler, Brian S., MD {1366414294} PthACl, PthCyt, Pthlgy(89,NY08)<NJ-JRSYSHMC, NJ-RIVERVW>
+ Jersey Shore University Medical Center
1945 Route 33/Pathology   Neptune, NJ 07753   (732)776-4148   Fax (732)776-4146
+ Riverview Medical Center
1 Riverview Plaza/Pathology   Red Bank, NJ 07701   (732)741-2700

Erlikhman, Alla, MD {1871827501} EmrgMd, Pedtrc
+ University Pediatric Associates PA
317 Cleveland Avenue   Highland Park, NJ 08904   (732)249-8999   Fax (732)249-7827
+ University Pediatric Associates
D-1 Brier Hill Court   East Brunswick, NJ 08816   (732)238-3310
+ Advocare Sinatra & Peng Pediatrics
169 Minebrook Road   Bernardsville, NJ 08904   (908)766-0034   Fax (908)766-4387

Erondu, Ngozi Emmanuel, MD {1003065780} EnDbMt(79,NIG03)
+ Johnson & Johnson Research & Develop
920 US Highway Route 202   Raritan, NJ 08869   (908)816-1233   Fax (908)927-7977
ngerondu@aol.com

Errickson, Carla V., MD {1255730537} Dermat(92,NJ05)
+ 198 Changewater Road
Changewater, NJ 07831   (908)391-2548

Errico, Carmine P., MD {1144278771} ObsGyn(64,DC02)<NJ-STPETER, NJ-SOMERSET>
+ Somerset Ob-Gyn Associates
215 Union Avenue/Suite A   Bridgewater, NJ 08807   (908)722-2900   Fax (908)722-1856
+ Somerset Ob-Gyn Associates
1 New Amwell Road   Hillsborough, NJ 08844   (908)874-5900

Errion, Christine, MD {1780078816} PhysMd
+ Bey Lea Village
1351 Old Freehold Road   Toms River, NJ 08753   (732)240-0090   Fax (732)244-8551

Erskine, Jennifer Grantham, MD {1477796811} IntrMd, IntHos(98,PA09)
+ Shore Hospitalists Associates
100 Medical Center Way   Somers Point, NJ 08244   (609)653-3500   Fax (609)926-4799

Esber, Natacha, MD {1568626836} IntrMd(04,LEB01)
+ Regional Cancer Center Associates
250 Old Red Hook Road/Suite 301   Westwood, NJ 07675   (201)383-1035   Fax (201)383-4824

Escaldi, Steven V., DO {1720004625} PhysMd(93,NY75)<NJ-JFKJHNSN, NJ-RWJUBRUN>
+ JFK Johnson Rehabilitation Institute
65 James Street   Edison, NJ 08818   (732)321-7070   Fax (732)321-7330

Escandon, Pedro J., MD {1215917737} IntCrd, CdvDis, IntrMd(88,NJ05)<NJ-JRSYSHMC, NJ-OCEANMC>
+ Coastal Cardiovascular Consultants, PA
459 Jack Martin Boulevard/Suite 4   Brick, NJ 08724   (732)458-6200   Fax (732)458-9464
+ Coastal Cardiovascular Consultants, PA
1930 Highway 35/Suite 3   Wall, NJ 07719   (732)458-6200   Fax (732)974-6209

Escandon, Sandra L., MD {1114985942} Nrolgy(90,PA09)<NJ-COMMED, NJ-OCEANMC>
+ Shore Neurology, PA
1613 Route 88/Suite 3   Brick, NJ 08724   (732)785-3335   Fax (732)785-2599
+ Shore Neurology, P.A.
633 Route 37 West   Toms River, NJ 08755   (732)785-3335   Fax (732)240-3114

Escano, Jude Thaddeus, DO {1831180561}
+ 165 Parlin Lane
Watchung, NJ 07069   (908)757-2149
jescano10@yahoo.com

Escareal, Myrna S., MD {1962466086} NnPnMd, Pedtrc(71,PHI01)<NJ-ACMCITY, NJ-ACMCMAIN>
+ AtlantiCare Regional Medical Center/City Campus
1925 Pacific Avenue/Neonatology   Atlantic City, NJ 08401   (609)441-8087
+ AtlantiCare/Dupont Children's Health Program
2500 English Creek Avenue   Egg Harbor Township, NJ 08234   (609)441-8087   Fax (609)641-3652

Esche, Clemens, MD {1790826394} Dermat(GER55)
+ Cosulich Dermatology
3350 State Highway 138   Wall Township, NJ 07719   (732)280-1200   Fax (732)280-1207

Eschinger, Amy Folio, MD {1396713418} InfDis, IntrMd(97,DC02)<NJ-RIVERVW, NJ-JRSYSHMC>
+ Meridian Medical Associates-Infectious Disease
1 Riverview Plaza/Suite 2 West   Red Bank, NJ 07701   (732)530-2421

Eschinger, Eric Jon, MD {1720184625} Gastrn, IntrMd(97,DC02)
+ Ocean Endosurgery Center
129 Route 37 West   Toms River, NJ 08755   (732)606-4440   Fax (732)797-3963

Escobar, Javier I., MD {1306926035} Psychy(67,COLO)
+ UH- Robert Wood Johnson Med
125 Paterson Street/CAB/Rm 7038   New Brunswick, NJ 08901   (732)235-6383   Fax (732)235-6663

Escobar, Juan Nicolas, MD {1780079145} ObsGyn
+ Palisades Women's Group
7650 River Road/Suite 230   North Bergen, NJ 07047   (201)868-6755   Fax (201)868-8442

Escobar-Barboza, Vanessa, MD {1558580936} EnDbMt, IntrMd(02,COL14)
+ Liberty Medical Associates
377 Jersey Avenue/Suite 470   Jersey City, NJ 07302   (201)309-2380   Fax (201)918-2243

Esfahanizadeh, Abdolreza, MD {1659507275} NroChl, ClNrPh(89,IRA06)<NJ-RWJUBRUN>
+ Child Health Institute of New Jersey
89 French Street/Suite 2300   New Brunswick, NJ 08901   (732)235-7875   Fax (732)235-6620

Esformes, Ira, MD {1104914084} SrgOrt, IntrMd(77,NY03)
+ Active Orthopaedics & Sports Medicine
440 Old Hook Road   Emerson, NJ 07630   (201)358-0707   Fax (201)358-9777

Eshkar, Noam Simon, MD {1811977440} RadDia, Radiol(91,NY08)<NJ-JFKMED>
+ JFK Medical Center
65 James Street/Radiology   Edison, NJ 08820   (732)321-7917   Fax (732)767-2968

Esiely, Mohamed A., MD {1083942635} ObsGyn
+ 82 Van Houten Place
Belleville, NJ 07109   (201)647-6794

Eskin, Barnet, MD {1457377699} EmrgMd(83,NJ05)<NJ-MORRISTN>
+ Morristown Medical Center
100 Madison Avenue/EmrgMed   Morristown, NJ 07962   (973)971-8919   Fax (973)290-7202
phdmd@prodigy.net

Eskin, Evamaria Ursula, MD {1275617730} OccpMd, GPrvMd(82,PA13)<NJ-VIRTVOOR, NJ-VIRTMHBC>
+ Virtua at Work
2309 Evesham Road/Suite 104   Voorhees, NJ 08043   (856)325-5310
+ Virtua at Work
895 Rancocas Road/Suite 1   Westampton, NJ 08060   (856)325-5310   Fax (609)914-8626

Eskinazi, Daniel, MD {1154768000} Anesth
+ Hackensack University MC-Anesthesia Dept
30 Prospect Avenue/Room 2703   Hackensack, NJ 07601   (551)996-2419   Fax (201)996-3962

Eskow, Eugene S., MD {1831213743} FamMed(88,NJ05)
+ 4 Walter E. Foran Boulevard/Suite 103
Flemington, NJ 08822   (908)782-7625   Fax (908)284-2582

Eskow, Raymond P., MD {1548207202} FamMed(91,NJ05)<NJ-CHILTON, NJ-VALLEY>
+ Valley Medical Group
44 Godwin Avenue/Suite 2   Midland Park, NJ 07432   (201)444-5992   Fax (201)444-9984

Esmail, Ali Raza, MD {1134673502} OtgyFPIS
+ 1 Spring Street/Suite 2304
New Brunswick, NJ 08901   (609)906-3551

Espana, Madesa A., MD {1205874781} Pedtrc, EmrgMd(89,PHI30)<NJ-STJOSHOS>
+ St Joseph's Medical Pedicatic EmerMed
703 Main Street   Paterson, NJ 07503   (973)754-4901

Espina, Luis Alberto, MD {1396184784} FamMed(13,NJ05)
+ Barnabas Health Medical Group
339 Passaic Avenue   Nutley, NJ 07110   (973)542-2880   Fax (973)542-2881

Espinal-Mariotte, Jose D., MD {1952384042} Pthlgy, PthAna(78,MEX62)<NJ-WAYNEGEN>
+ St. Joseph's Wayne Hospital
224 Hamburg Turnpike/Pathology   Wayne, NJ 07470   (973)956-3589   Fax (973)389-4019
jespinal@sjwh.org
+ Ideal Labs, LLC
307 Hamburg Turnpike/Suite 201   Wayne, NJ 07474   (973)720-5733

Espinar Ho, Maria Elena, MD {1306253083} FamMed
+ CentraState Family Medicine Residency Practice
1001 West Main Street/Suite B   Freehold, NJ 07728   (732)294-4570   Fax (732)431-8267

Espineli, Dino O., MD {1992807382} IntrMd(00,PHI08)<NJ-COMMED>
+ Espineli Medical Associates PC
1163 Route 37 West/Suite D-4   Toms River, NJ 08755   (732)341-9494   Fax (732)341-3416

Espineli, Rosalinda O., MD {1982706370} IntrMd(69,PHI08)
+ Espineli Medical Associates PC
1163 Route 37 West/Suite D-4   Toms River, NJ 08755   (732)341-9494   Fax (732)341-3416

Espinosa, James A., MD {1235165259} EmrgMd, FamMed(80,PA09)<NJ-KMHSTRAT>
+ Emergency Physician Associates, P.A.
307 South Evergreen Avenue/PO Box 298   Woodbury, NJ 08096   (856)848-3817   Fax (856)848-1431
+ Kennedy Memorial Hospital-University Medical Center
18 East Laurel Road/EmrgMed   Stratford, NJ 08084   (856)346-6000

Espinoza, Andrey, MD {1255384897} IntrMd, CdvDis, IntCrd(97,NET09)<NJ-MORRISTN>
+ 1465 State Route 31 South/Suite 1
Annandale, NJ 08801   (908)237-9092   Fax (908)237-9095

Espinoza, Lisa C., MD {1053534628} FamMed(04,PA09)
+ 287 South Main Street
Lambertville, NJ 08530

Espiritu-Fuller, Maria Concepcion, MD {1215956982} PedInf(88,PHIL)<NJ-NWRKBETH>
+ Newark Beth Israel Medical Center
201 Lyons Avenue   Newark, NJ 07112   (973)926-8094   Fax (973)926-4203

Esposito, Amanda Santoro, MD {1922492917} EmrgMd
+ Morristown Medical Center Emergency Medicine
100 Madison Avenue   Morristown, NJ 07960   (973)971-5000

Esposito, Michael P., MD {1154390458} Urolgy(94,NJ05)<NJ-HACKNSK, NJ-HOLYNAME>
+ New Jersey Center for Prostate Cancer & Urology
255 West Spring Valley Avenue   Maywood, NJ 07607   (201)487-8866   Fax (201)487-2602

Esquerre, Rene B., MD {1033150172} Pedtrc(79,NJ06)<NJ-CLAR-MAAS>
+ North End Family Health Center
644 Mount Prospect Avenue   Newark, NJ 07104   (973)483-4702   Fax (973)483-0955
+ Springfield Pediatrics
190 Meisel Avenue   Springfield, NJ 07081   (973)483-4702   Fax (973)467-7836

Esquieres, Raymond Edel, MD {1932180924} PhysMd(99,NJ05)
+ Brielle Orthopedics PA
457 Jack Martin Boulevard   Brick, NJ 08724   (732)840-7500   Fax (732)840-2088
+ Brielle Orthopedics PA
823 Lacey Road   Forked River, NJ 08731   (732)840-7500   Fax (732)840-2088
+ Brielle Orthopedics PA
1301 Route 72 West   Manahawkin, NJ 08724   (609)971-7616   Fax (609)971-7639

Essa, Noorjehan, MD {1417083072} Surgry(63,MYAN)<NJ-CHS-FULD, NJ-CHSMRCER>
+ 40 Fuld Street/Suite 309
Trenton, NJ 08638   (609)396-3209   Fax (609)777-5419

Essandoh, Louisa Efua, MD {1902059025} ObsGyn
+ Fleisch OBGYN Group
3 Lincoln Boulevard/Suite 315   Edison, NJ 08820   (732)738-7600   Fax (732)635-9810

Esses, Steven J., MD {1154600427} RadDia<NJ-MORRISTN>
+ Morristown Medical Center
100 Madison Avenue   Morristown, NJ 07962   (973)971-5000

Estacio, Joseph M., DO {1841257565} RadDia(93,IL76)
+ Coordinated Health
222 Red Lane   Phillipsburg, NJ 08865   (610)861-8080   Fax (610)849-1013
+ 19 Old Schoolhouse Road
Asbury, NJ 08802   (856)401-8740

Estavillo, Aileen Casambre, MD {1558413617} IntrMd(98,PHI09)
+ 3084 Route 27/Suite 1
Kendall Park, NJ 08824

Estella, Faustino F., Jr., MD {1023119757} Surgry, SrgVas, SrgThr(73,PHIL)<NJ-MEMSALEM>
+ Memorial Hospital of Salem County
310 Woodstown Road/Surgery   Salem, NJ 08079   (856)935-1000

Estephan, Amir E., MD {1457673246} EmrgMd
 + Christ Hospital
  176 Palisade Avenue   Jersey City, NJ 07306   (201)795-8200
  Fax (201)795-8280
Esterova, Elizaveta, MD {1275535858} Pedtrc(81,RUS15)
 + 2206 Route 130
  North Brunswick, NJ 08902   (732)422-1420   Fax (732)422-1439
Estevez, Gerardo V., MD {1659379865} FamMed, Grtrcs, ErgMd(87,PHI09)<NJ-JFKMED>
 + 1931 OakTree Road/Suite 201
  Edison, NJ 08820   (732)452-0680   Fax (732)452-9137
  gbestevez@comcast.net
Estilo, Genevieve Kristina, MD {1558560482} Nephro, IntrMd(00,NY47)
 + Nephrological Associates, P.A.
  83 Hanover Road/Suite 290   Florham Park, NJ 07932   (973)736-2212   Fax (973)736-2989
  genevieve.estilo@mssm.edu
Estin, David, MD {1598726283} SrgNro(91,NY19)<NJ-RIVERVW, NJ-JRSYSHMC>
 + Neurosurgeons of New Jersey
  121 Highway 36 West/Suite 330   West Long Branch, NJ 07764   (732)963-4631   Fax (732)870-6342
 + Neurosurgeons of New Jersey
  530 Lakehurst Road/Suite 308   Toms River, NJ 08755   (732)443-1372
Estok, Jason E., MD {1841496098}
 + Tenafly Psychiatric Associates
  111 Dean Drive   Tenafly, NJ 07670
Estrada, Aristides M., MD {1114970068} Grtrcs, IntrMd(71,DOMI)
 + Internal Medicine of Morris County LLC
  195 Route 46 West/Suite 102   Mine Hill, NJ 07803   (973)366-6060   Fax (973)366-1423
Estrada, Christian, MD {1598019937} Anesth
 + Rutgers- New Jersey Medical School
  185 South Orange Avenue/MSB E-547   Newark, NJ 07103   (908)425-6378   Fax (973)972-3835
Estrada, Elsie C., MD {1851368849} AdolMd, Pedtrc(77,PHI01)<NJ-OVERLOOK, NJ-STBARNMC>
 + Chatham Pediatrics
  12 Parrot Mill Road   Chatham, NJ 07928   (973)635-4511   Fax (973)701-1520
Estrellas, Bernabe A., MD {1952471435} IntrMd(79,PHI01)<NJ-RWJURAH>
 + New Jersey Veterans Memorial Home - Menlo Park
  132 Evergreen Road/PO Box 3013   Edison, NJ 08818   (732)452-4100
Eswar, Anastasia Maria, MD {1043515471} Nrolgy
 + Monmouth Ocean Neurology
  1944 State Route 33/Suite 206   Neptune, NJ 07753   (732)774-8282   Fax (732)774-4407
Eswarapu, Srinivasa, MD {1346215225} IntrMd(83,INA5B)<NJ-CLARMAAS, NJ-STBARHCS>
 + Sai Medical Center
  252 Washington Avenue   Belleville, NJ 07109   (973)450-9600   Fax (973)450-4054
 + Clara Maass Continuing Care Center
  1 Clara Maass Drive   Belleville, NJ 07109   (973)450-2900
Etheridge, Barbara Anne, MD {1184792814} FamMed(95,PA02)<NJ-RWJUBRUN, NJ-STPETER>
 + Etheridge Family Medicine LLC
  81 Veronica Avenue/Suite 202   Somerset, NJ 08873   (732)246-0057   Fax (732)745-7070
Ettinger, Leigh Mark, MD {1194765859} Pedtrc, PedNph(98,MA07)<NJ-HACKNSK, NY-MNTFMOSE>
 + Hackensack University Medical Center
  30 Prospect Avenue   Hackensack, NJ 07601   (201)336-8228   Fax (201)996-5397
Etzi, Susan, MD {1003081423} PubHth, GPrvMd, OccpMd(88,PA02)
 + 2200 North Central Road/Apt 9D
  Fort Lee, NJ 07024
Eufemia, Joann M., MD {1326033275} IntrMd(81,DOM03)
 + 105 Atsion Road/Suite A
  Medford, NJ 08055   (609)953-1700   Fax (609)953-1208
Evageliou, Nicholas Fontaine, MD {1659401149} Pedtrc<PA-CHESTRCT, PA-CHILDHOS>
 + CHOP Pediatric & Adolescent Specialty Care Center
  1012 Laurel Oak Road   Voorhees, NJ 08043   (856)435-1300   Fax (856)435-0091
Evangelisto, Amy Marie, MD {1023119195} Rheuma, IntrMd(97,PA13)<NJ-COOPRUMC>
 + Arthritis, Rheumatic & Back Disease Associates
  2309 East Evesham Road/Suite 101   Voorhees, NJ 08043   (856)424-5005   Fax (856)424-4716
 + Cooper Physicians
  1103 North Kings Highway/Suite 203   Cherry Hill, NJ 08034   (856)424-5005   Fax (856)321-0206
 + Cooper Rheumatology
  900 Centennial Boulevard/Suite 203   Voorhees, NJ 08043

  (856)968-7019   Fax (856)482-5621
Evans, Barbara J. Marcelo, MD {1518050129} Pedtrc, OthrSp, PedNrD(68,PA07)<NJ-COOPRUMC>
 + 36 Knickerbocker Drive
  Belle Mead, NJ 08502   (609)915-4318   Fax (908)874-3397
 + Cooper University Medical Center/Camden
  3 Cooper Plaza/ChldDevelCtr   Camden, NJ 08103   (609)915-4318   Fax (856)968-8581
Evans, Carrie Marie, DO {1386884419} IntrMd, IntHos(05,PA77)<NJ-VIRTMHBC, NJ-VIRTMARL>
 + Virtua Hospitalist Group Marlton
  90 Brick Road   Marlton, NJ 08053   (609)914-6180   Fax (609)914-6182
Evans, Charles, III, MD {1669432472} Pedtrc(97,NJ06)<NJ-WARREN>
 + New Beginnings Pediatrics
  755 Memorial Parkway/Suite 115   Phillipsburg, NJ 08865   (908)454-3737   Fax (908)454-0402
Evans, Ed Nelvyn Lezette, MD {1043231574} Grtrcs(78,NJ05)
 + 385 Prospect Avenue
  Hackensack, NJ 07601   (201)342-4536   Fax (201)342-7962
Evans, Hugh E., MD {1356415525} Pedtrc(58,NY08)<NJ-UMDNJ>
 + University Hospital-Doctors Office Center
  90 Bergen Street/DOC 4300/Pedi   Newark, NJ 07103   (973)972-2100   Fax (973)972-2102
 + University Pediatric Group
  90 Bergen Street/DOC 4300   Newark, NJ 07103   (973)972-2100
Evans, Matthew, DO {1083876940} CdvDis<NJ-DEBRAHLC>
 + Deborah Heart and Lung Center
  200 Trenton Road   Browns Mills, NJ 08015   (609)893-6611   Fax (609)735-0175
Evans, Nathaniel Rutherford, II, MD {1659437549} EmrgMd, OccpMd, IntrMd(73,MD07)
 + Burlington Medical Center
  640 Beverly Rancocas Road   Willingboro, NJ 08046   (609)835-9555   Fax (609)835-2313
Evans, Rachael Blackburn, MD {1922056167} FamMed(01,NY19)
 + 70 North Main Street
  Pennington, NJ 08534
Evans Murage, Julene Opalene, MD {1356356919} ObsGyn(93,NY06)<NJ-CHSMRCER, NJ-RWJUHAM>
 + Drs. Lendor and Evans Murage
  1301 Whitehorse Mercerville Rd   Hamilton, NJ 08619   (609)585-9901   Fax (609)585-9919
Evdokimow, David Z., MD {1508930678} SrgPlstc, SrgRec, SrgHnd(84,BUL04)<NJ-OVERLOOK, NJ-MORRISTN>
 + 96 South Finley Avenue
  Basking Ridge, NJ 07920   (908)859-5676
Evens, Andrew M., DO {1265468110} OncHem, Hemato, IntrMd(96,IL76)<MA-NEMEDCEN>
 + Rutgers Cancer Institute of New Jersey
  195 Little Albany Street/PO Box 2681   New Brunswick, NJ 08903   (732)235-5459   Fax (732)235-6797
Evering, Daniel, Jr., DO {1174937395} FamMSptM
 + Reconstructive Orthopedics
  994 West Sherman Avenue   Vineland, NJ 08360   (609)267-9400   Fax (609)267-9457
Ewald, Edward A., MD {1730268749} IntrMd, Rheuma(81,NY19)<NJ-VALLEY>
 + 127 Union Street
  Ridgewood, NJ 07450   (201)447-0660   Fax (201)447-2830
Ewing, Clinton Alexander, MD {1639112337} Pthlgy, PthCyt, PthAClf(97,NC05)<NJ-JFKMED>
 + JFK Medical Center
  65 James Street/Path   Edison, NJ 08820   (732)321-7000   Fax (732)321-7008
Ewing, Douglas R., MD {1245397017} Surgry, SrgLap(97,NY01)<NJ-HACKNSK>
 + Advanced Laparoscopic Associates
  81 Route 4 West/Suite 401/35 Plaza   Paramus, NJ 07652   (201)646-1121   Fax (201)646-1110
 + Paramus Surgical Center
  30 West Century Road/Suite 300   Paramus, NJ 07652   (201)986-9000
Ewing, Jacqueline L., DO {1740269018} FamMed(91,PA77)<NJ-VIRTBERL, NJ-VIRTVOOR>
 + Partners in Primary Care
  239 Hurffville Crosskeys Road   Sewell, NJ 08080   (856)881-1940
Eyerkuss, Emily Abra, DO {1699214759} Pedtrc<NJ-JRSYSHMC>
 + Jersey Shore University Medical Center
  1945 Route 33   Neptune, NJ 07753   (732)775-5500
Eyerman, Luke Edmund, MD {1225021405} FamMed(01,DMN01)
 + 175 Bergen Boulevard
  Fairview, NJ 07022   (201)943-2900   Fax (201)943-2903
Eytan, Shira B., MD {1215252580} IntrMd
 + Rutgers- New Jersey Medical School
  185 South Orange Avenue   Newark, NJ 07103   (973)972-5307

Physicians by Name and Address

Eyzner, Igor, DO {1396164554}<NJ-UMDNJ>
 + University Hospital
  150 Bergen Street/Uh H-245   Newark, NJ 07103   (973)972-5672   Fax (973)972-0365
Ezati, Omid, MD {1518120658} Radiol
 + Radiology Affiliates of Central New Jersey, P.A.
  2501 Kuser Road   Hamilton, NJ 08691   (609)585-8800   Fax (609)585-1825
Eze, Schakia Yolanda, DO {1679702567}<NJ-STJOSHOS>
 + St. Joseph's Regional Medical Center
  703 Main Street   Paterson, NJ 07503   (973)754-2918
Ezeadichie, Chioma A., DO {1023267465} PhyMPain
 + ASAP - Advanced Spine and Pain
  2 Eighth Street   Hammonton, NJ 08037   (609)567-8832
Ezeala, Ugochi Gucci, MD {1154663664}
 + MedExpress Urgent Care
  135 Bloomfield Avenue   Bloomfield, NJ 07003   (973)748-7459
Ezeanya, Ebere Nneka, MD {1053547919} FamMed
 + NJ South Coast Medical Center
  415 Chris Gaupp/Suite D   Galloway, NJ 08205
  njsouthcoast@njscmc.com
Ezekowitz, Raymond Alan B., MD {1174509335} Pedtrc, PedHem(77,SAF02)
 + Merck and Company Incorporated
  1 Merck Drive/PO Box 100   Whitehouse Station, NJ 08889   (908)423-1000
Ezema, James N., MD {1003818881} IntrMd(86,NIG03)
 + 27 Nashaway Drive
  Ringoes, NJ 08551
Ezer, Mayer Roy, MD {1417925538} IntrMd(98,MA01)<NJ-JRSYSHMC>
 + Hackensack Meridian Medical Group
  195 Route 9 South/Suite 106   Manalapan, NJ 07726   (732)536-7144   Fax (732)536-7520
Ezon, Frederick C., MD {1538142187} Otlryg, SrgFPl(75,TX13)<NJ-JRSYSHMC, NJ-MONMOUTH>
 + 1025 Highway 35
  Ocean, NJ 07712   (732)531-8200   Fax (732)531-8201
  fredezonmd@msn.com
 + 921 East Countyline Road
  Lakewood, NJ 08701
Ezon, Isaac C., MD {1801057781} Ophthl
 + 133 Van Nostrand Avenue
  Englewood, NJ 07631   (732)241-6666
  ice202@gmail.com
Ezrokhi, Marina B., MD {1235172545} PedAne, Anesth(96,RUS15)
 + St. Joseph's Regional Medical Center Anesthesia
  703 Main Street   Paterson, NJ 07503   (973)754-2323   Fax (973)977-9455
Faber, Mark P., MD {1134237019} PsyCAd, Psychy(88,DMN01)
 + 594 Valley Road
  Upper Montclair, NJ 07043   (973)746-6711
Fabia, Candida M., MD {1255319224} NnPnMd, Pedtrc(67,PHIL)<NJ-OURLADY>
 + Our Lady of Lourdes Medical Center
  1600 Haddon Avenue/Neonatology   Camden, NJ 08103   (856)757-3826
Fabila, Jocelyn E., MD {1437184504} Psychy(79,PHIL)<NJ-TRENTPSY>
 + Ocean Mental Health Services, Inc.
  160 Atlantic City Boulevard   Bayville, NJ 08721   (732)349-5550   Fax (732)349-0841
 + Trenton Psychiatric Hospital
  Sullivan Way/PO Box 7600   West Trenton, NJ 08628   (609)633-1500
Fabius, Daniel, MD {1073884680} IntrMd<NJ-COOPRUMC>
 + Cooper Perinatology Associates
  3 Cooper Plaza/Suite 502   Camden, NJ 08103   (856)968-7433   Fax (856)968-8499
Fabricant, Christopher James, MD {1275502072} ObsGyn, Gyneco(94,DC02)<NJ-JRSYSHMC, NJ-OCEANMC>
 + Hackensack Meridian Urogynecolgy Medical Group
  19 Davis Avenue/7th Floor   Neptune, NJ 07753   (732)776-3797   Fax (732)776-3796
 + Jersey Shore University Medical Center
  1945 Route 33/Ob/Gyn   Neptune, NJ 07753   (732)775-5500
 + Meridian Obstetrics amd Gynecology Associates PC
  19 Davis Avenue/Fl 1   Neptune, NJ 07753   (732)897-7944   Fax (732)922-8264
Fabrizio, Lawrence, DO {1215937891} CdvDis, IntrMd(88,WV75)<NJ-STBARNMC, NJ-MORRISTN>
 + Essex Cardiology Group PC
  10 James Street/Suite 130   Florham Park, NJ 07932   (973)736-9557   Fax (973)736-9757
Facciolo, Jack, DO {1558330076} SrgOrt, Ortped(80,PA77)<NJ-BURDTMLN>
 + 1 Secluded Lane
  Rio Grande, NJ 08242   (609)886-0837

Physicians by Name and Address

Faccone, Jacqueline M., DO {1659594455} Anesth(92,IA75)<NJ-OVERLOOK>
+ Overlook Medical Center
  99 Beauvoir Avenue/PO Box 210   Summit, NJ 07902   (908)522-2000

Faccone, John A., DO {1447259122} SrgOrt(94,IA75)<NJ-BAYONNE, NJ-OVERLOOK>
+ Summit Medical Group
  574 Springfield Avenue   Westfield, NJ 07090   (908)389-6294   Fax (908)232-0540
+ Summit Medical Group
  34 Mountain Boulevard/Building B   Warren, NJ 07059   (908)389-6294   Fax (908)769-8927

Facey, Maxine Elizabeth, MD {1407920564} IntrMd(96,DC03)<NJ-STMICHL>
+ Paterson Community Health Center
  32 Clinton Street   Paterson, NJ 07522   (973)790-6594   Fax (973)790-7703

Faches, Allison L., MD {1336397785} FamMed(93,IA02)<NJ-JFKMED>
+ Mid Jersey Medical Associates
  1 Ethel Road/Suite 107b   Edison, NJ 08817   (732)452-0057   Fax (732)287-2071

Factor, Steven Daniel, MD {1730472408}
+ 700 US Highway 46/Suite 420
  Fairfield, NJ 07004   (973)882-3456   Fax (973)882-3450

Fadden, Kathleen Selvaggi, MD {1871561266} PedDvl, Pedtrc(83,PA07)<NJ-MORRISTN, NJ-OVERLOOK>
+ Morristown Medical Center
  100 Madison Avenue/ChildDev/Box100   Morristown, NJ 07962   (973)971-5227
  kathleen.fadden@ahsys.org

Faden, Justin B., DO {1972758142} Psychy
+ University Hospital-SOM Department of Psychiatry
  2250 Chapel Avenue West/Suite 100   Cherry Hill, NJ 08002   (856)482-9000   Fax (856)482-1159

Faderl, Stefan H., MD {1689770844} MedOnc
+ John Theurer Cancer Center - HUMC
  92 Second Street   Hackensack, NJ 07601   (551)996-3925   Fax (551)996-0574

Fadil, Tina Marie, MD {1932101516} IntrMd(86,IL43)
+ The Park Medical Group
  24 Elm Street   Harrington Park, NJ 07640   (201)784-0123   Fax (201)784-0065

Fadugba, Olawale Akindiran, MD {1457391674} Anesth(92,NIG05)<NJ-ACMCMAIN, NJ-ACMCITY>
+ AtlantiCare Regional Med Ctr/Mainland
  65 West Jimmie Leeds Road   Pomona, NJ 08240   (609)652-1000
+ AtlantiCare Regional Medical Center/City Campus
  1925 Pacific Avenue/PainManagement   Atlantic City, NJ 08401   (609)345-4000

Faelnar, Luis B., MD {1992752034} Anesth(68,PHIL)<NJ-BAYSHORE>
+ Bayshore Community Hospital
  727 North Beers Street   Holmdel, NJ 07733   (732)739-5900

Fagan, Elizabeth Owens, MD {1295707156} FamMed, IntrMd(01,PA02)
+ 12 Bank Street/Suite 201
  Summit, NJ 07901   (908)376-6550

Fagan, Linda Nadine, MD {1861864654} ObsGyn(92,DC02)
+ 24 Independence Drive
  Basking Ridge, NJ 07920

Fagel, Jonathan Val C., DO {1639507510} FamMed
+ Patients first
  705 Haddonfield Berlin Road   Voorhees, NJ 08043   (856)679-0537

Fagel, Valentin L., MD {1053411058} RadDia, Radiol(73,PHIL)
+ The Osteoporosis Center at Pennsville Radiology
  248 South Broadway   Pennsville, NJ 08070   (856)678-8118   Fax (856)678-8130

Fagelman, Elliot, MD {1184668808} Urolgy(95,NY15)
+ Drs. Fagelman, Degen & Fagelman
  360 Essex Street/Suite 403   Hackensack, NJ 07601   (551)996-8090   Fax (845)354-5966

Fagelman, Mark, MD {1497798896} Urolgy(67,MI07)<NY-NYACKHOS>
+ Drs. Fagelman, Degen & Fagelman
  360 Essex Street/Suite 403   Hackensack, NJ 07601   (551)996-8090   Fax (845)354-5966

Fahey, Ann Leilani, MD {1386737997} SrgPlstc, Surgry(88,NY20)<NJ-COOPRUMC>
+ Cooper Orthopaedics
  2 Plaza Drive/Suite 202   Sewell, NJ 08080   (856)270-4150   Fax (856)270-4012
+ Cooper Surgical Associates
  3 Cooper Plaza/Suite 411   Camden, NJ 08103   (856)270-4150   Fax (856)365-1180

Fahim, Farheen, MD {1730257502} Psychy, PsyCAd(89,PAK11)<NJ-TRINIJSC>
+ Livingston HealthCare, LLC
  107 East Mount Pleasant Avenue/Suite 1   Livingston, NJ 07039   (973)535-3999   Fax (973)535-3222

Fahimi, Nader, MD {1346326956} SrgOrt, SprtMd(98,DC02)
+ Elite Orthopedics & Sports Medicine, P.A.
  342 Hamburg Turnpike/Suite 209   Wayne, NJ 07470   (973)956-8100   Fax (973)956-8104
+ Elite Orthopedics & Sports Medicine, P.A.
  44 Route 23 North/Suite 3   Riverdale, NJ 07457   (973)513-9646
+ Elite Orthopedics & Sports Medicine, P.A.
  1035 Route 46 East/Suite G-2   Clifton, NJ 07470   (973)513-9646

Fahmy, Hannan Adel, DO FamMed(89,NY75)
+ Concentra Medical Centers
  30 Seaview Drive/Suite 2   Secaucus, NJ 07094   (201)319-1611   Fax (201)319-1233
+ Care Station
  90 Route 22 West   Springfield, NJ 07081   (973)467-2273

Fahmy, Nader M., MD {1780627794} Anesth(98,EGY03)<NJ-CENTRAST>
+ Liberty Anesthesia & Pain Management
  901 West Main Street/2nd Floor   Freehold, NJ 07728   (732)294-2876   Fax (732)294-2502
+ CentraState Medical Center
  901 West Main Street/Anesth   Freehold, NJ 07728   (732)431-2000

Fahmy, Nevine Karam, MD {1801099684} Psychy, PsyCAd(90,EGY04)
+ 251 Bridge Street
  Metuchen, NJ 08840   (732)754-4354   Fax (732)744-1344

Fahmy, Samir Awadalla, MD {1831183599} IntrMd, PulDis, CritCr(82,EGY05)
+ Drs. Fahmy and Fahmy
  58 Wildwood Terrace   Watchung, NJ 07069   Fax (908)822-2234

Fahmy, Sandra Patricia, DO {1144317439} OthrSp(03,PA77)
+ Bay Family Medicine
  26 Throckmorton Lane   Old Bridge, NJ 08857   (732)360-0287   Fax (732)360-1279

Fahrenbruch, Gretchen B., MD {1396954145} Surgry, SrgTrm, EmrgMd(87,NC08)<NJ-CHSFULD, NJ-UMDNJ>
+ Capital Health System/Fuld Campus
  750 Brunswick Avenue/AdjunctSrgStaff   Trenton, NJ 08638   (609)394-6000
  cobaltwam@comcast.net
+ University Hospital
  150 Bergen Street/Clinical/Surg   Newark, NJ 07103   (973)972-4300

Faiena, Izak, MD {1447562418} Urolgy<NJ-RWJUBRUN>
+ RWJ University Hospital New Brunswick
  One Robert Wood Johnson Place   New Brunswick, NJ 08901   (732)235-7718

Faigenbaum, Steven J., MD {1235226978} Ophthl(70,NY06)
+ Paul Phillips Eye & Surgery Center
  1 Monroe Street   Bridgewater, NJ 08807   (908)526-4588   Fax (908)231-6718

Failey, Colin Leander, MD {1992957922} Surgry, SrgRec(04,NY03)
+ Peer Group Plastic Surgery Center
  124 Columbia Turnpike   Florham Park, NJ 07932   (973)822-3000   Fax (973)822-1726

Fain, Richard A., MD {1962576918} ObsGyn(73,MEXI)
+ West Essex Ob/Gyn Associates
  200 South Orange Avenue/Suite 290   Livingston, NJ 07039   (973)740-1330   Fax (973)740-8998

Fair-Covely, Rose Mary, DO {1245324334} EnDbMt, IntrMd(91,PA77)
+ Martin K. Belsky, D.O., P.C.
  100 Brick Road/Suite 108   Marlton, NJ 08053   (856)810-7337   Fax (856)810-7917
+ Martin K. Belsky DO PC
  608 North Broad Street/Suite 201   Woodbury, NJ 08096   (856)384-9239

Fairbanks, Janet A., MD {1053567602} Psychy(81,NY47)
+ 28 Prospect Avenue
  Haworth, NJ 07641   (201)384-2242   Fax (201)385-9864

Faisal, Khaja Tajuddin, MD {1366562902} Psychy, PsyCAd, IntrMd(95,INA75)<NJ-BERGNMC>
+ Princeton House Behavioral Health
  300 Clocktower Drive/Suite 101   Hamilton, NJ 08690   (609)683-3283   Fax (609)683-3291

Faisal, Siddiq A., MD {1780797423} FamMed(97,PAK12)
+ 12 Petunia Drive/Apt 1H
  North Brunswick, NJ 08902

Faistl, Kenneth W., MD {1154395622} FamMed, Grtrcs(75,NJ05)<NJ-CENTRAST>
+ Family Practice of CentraState
  901 West Main Street/Suite 106   Freehold, NJ 07728   (732)462-0100   Fax (732)462-0348
+ Family Practice of CentraState
  281 Route 34/Suite 813   Colts Neck, NJ 07722   (732)462-0100   Fax (732)431-3707
+ Family Practice of CentraState
  319 Route 130 North   East Windsor, NJ 07728   (609)426-1555   Fax (609)447-8070

Faiz, Arifa, MD {1164452975}<NJ-HOLYNAME>
+ Holy Name Hospital
  718 Teaneck Road   Teaneck, NJ 07666   (201)833-3000

Faizan, Anila, MD {1184937930} IntrMd<NJ-OVERLOOK, NJ-STBARNMC>
+ St. Barnabas Medical Center
  94 Old Short Hills Road   Livingston, NJ 07039   (973)322-5000

Fajardo, Gil Valdez, MD {1336226463} FamMed(81,PHIL)<NJ-HOBUNIMC>
+ Bergenline Family Medicine LLC
  333 60th Street   West New York, NJ 07093   (201)453-8777   Fax (201)453-8804

Fakayode, Abisoye Victoria, MD {1225415227} IntrMd
+ Southern Jersey Family Medical Centers, Inc.
  860 South White Horse Pike/Building A   Hammonton, NJ 08037   (609)567-0200   Fax (609)567-1951

Fakharzadeh, Frederick F., MD {1497790067} SrgHnd, SrgOrt, OrtSHand(80,NY01)<NJ-HACKNSK, NJ-VALLEY>
+ Drs. Rosenstein & Fakharzadeh
  22 Madison Avenue/Suite 3-1   Paramus, NJ 07652   (201)587-7767   Fax (201)587-8090

Fakhry, Michael, MD {1649531039} Anesth<NY-NYUTISCH>
+ 30 Shawn Court
  North Brunswick, NJ 08902   (732)422-4107
  fakhrymi@gmail.com

Faktor, Mitchell J., DO {1013209626} Otlryg(87,NJ75)
+ 2528 River Road
  Manasquan, NJ 08736   (732)223-7444

Fakulujo, Adeshola D., MD {1528297678} Surgry, IntrMd(NIG01)
+ Advocare Associates in General Surgery
  2201 Chapel Avenue West/Suite 100   Cherry Hill, NJ 08002   (856)665-2017   Fax (856)488-6769
+ Advocare Associates in General Surgery
  570 Egg Harbor Road/Suite C-2   Sewell, NJ 08080   (856)665-2017   Fax (856)256-7789
+ Kennedy Health System/Cherry Hill Campus
  2201 Chapel Avenue West   Cherry Hill, NJ 08002   (856)488-6500

Falciani, Amerigo, DO {1093765414} Radiol(92,NJ75)<NJ-ACMCITY, NJ-SHOREMEM>
+ Atlantic Medical Imaging, LLC.
  72 West Jimmie Leeds Road   Galloway, NJ 08205   (609)677-9729   Fax (609)653-8764
+ Atlantic Medical Imaging, LLC.
  401 Bethel Road   Somers Point, NJ 08244   (609)677-9729
+ Atlantic Medical Imaging, LLC.
  421 Route 9 North   Cape May Court House, NJ 08205   (609)463-9500   Fax (609)465-0918

Falco, David J., MD {1639106016} IntrMd(79,PA09)<NJ-MONMOUTH>
+ 280 Norwood Avenue
  West Long Branch, NJ 07764   (732)222-4653   Fax (732)222-2524

Falco, Sharon Anne, MD {1154531283} Psychy(96,PA09)
+ 39 Avenue at The Common/Suite 106
  Shrewsbury, NJ 07702   (732)345-1999

Falcon, Christopher Ryan, DO {1851582332}
+ Rowan University-School of Osteopathic Medicine
  1 Medical Center Drive   Stratford, NJ 08084   (856)566-6835

Falcon, Lisa Fern, MD {1427097526} RadDia(82,WIND)
+ 26 Polktown Road
  Hampton, NJ 08827   (908)638-5357

Falcone, Michael, MD {1689787129} PhysMd(87,DMN01)<NJ-ACMCITY, NJ-ATLANTHS>
+ Rothman Institute - Egg Harbor Township
  2500 English Creek Avenue/Bldg 1300   Egg Harbor Township, NJ 08234   (609)677-7002   Fax (609)677-7000

Falconiero, Robert Paul, DO {1376500967} SrgOrt, SprtMd(84,PA77)
+ South Jersey Sports Medicine Center
  556 Egg Harbor Road/Suite A   Sewell, NJ 08080   (856)589-0650   Fax (856)589-2720
+ South Jersey Sports Medicine Center
  1004 Haddonfield Road   Cherry Hill, NJ 08002   (856)589-0650   Fax (856)662-7727

Faleck, Herbert J., DO {1285069948} Pedtrc(80,MO78)
+ 19 Lakeview Drive
  West Orange, NJ 07052   (973)669-3547

Falescky, Allan Jeffrey, MD {1427161777} IntrMd(82,NY08)<NY-BROOKDAL>
+ SOM - Department of Internal Medicine
  42 East Laurel Road/Suite 3100   Stratford, NJ 08084   (856)566-6853   Fax (856)566-6342
+ Kennedy Health System/Cherry Hill Campus
  2201 Chapel Avenue West/Internal Med   Cherry Hill, NJ 08002   (856)488-6500

Physicians by Name and Address

Falivena, Richard Peter, DO {1154578227} Surgry<NJ-BURDTMLN>
+ Cape Regional Medical Center
2 Stone Harbor Boulevard   Cape May Court House, NJ 08210   (609)463-2000   Fax (609)463-2318

Falk, Michael Alexander, MD {1316905425} Pedtrc(94,VA04)<NJ-VIRTVOOR, NJ-VIRTUAHS>
+ Advocare Atrium Pediatrics
301 Old Marlton Pike West/Suite 1   Marlton, NJ 08053   (856)988-9101   Fax (856)988-7712
+ Advocare Atrium Pediatrics Cedar Brook
41 South Route 73/Building 1/Suite 101   Hammonton, NJ 08037   (856)988-9101   Fax (609)567-4904

Falk, Theodore, MD {1912967464} Pedtrc, PedAlg, AlgyImmn(77,BELG)<NJ-ENGLWOOD, NJ-HOLYNAME>
+ Teaneck Allergy & Immunology Associates
63 Grand Avenue   River Edge, NJ 07661   (201)487-2900   Fax (201)487-1022

Fallek, Steve R., MD {1548238280} SrgPlstc, Surgry, SrgRec(91,NY47)<NJ-ENGLWOOD, NY-LENOXHLL>
+ 300 Sylvan Avenue/Suite 301
Englewood Cliffs, NJ 07632   (201)541-4181   Fax (201)541-1990
info@fallekplasticsurgery.com

Fallick, Mark Lawrence, MD {1245297837} Urolgy(91,MA07)<NJ-VIRTVOOR, NJ-VIRTBERL>
+ New Jersey Urology LLC
2090 Springdale Road/Suite D   Cherry Hill, NJ 08003   (856)751-9010   Fax (856)985-9908
+ New Jersey Urology
731 Bay Avenue   Somers Point, NJ 08244   Fax (609)653-9411
+ New Jersey Urology, LLC
2401 East Evesham Road/Suite F   Voorhees, NJ 08003   (856)673-1600   Fax (856)988-0636

Fallil, Zianka Huzailyn, MD {1376861948} Nrolgy, Eplpsy(07,NY15)
+ Northeast Regional Epilepsy Group
20 Prospect Avenue/Suite 800   Hackensack, NJ 07601   (201)343-6676   Fax (201)343-6689

Fallon, Jill C., MD {1043345242} OccpMd, IntrMd(73,NJ05)<NJ-MORRISTN>
+ Prudential Financial
290 West Mount Pleasant Avenue   Livingston, NJ 07039   (973)992-6363

Fallon, Joseph, Jr., MD {1760429369} EnDbMt, IntrMd(79,IL42)
+ 603 North Broad Street/Suite 200
Woodbury, NJ 08096   (856)853-1111   Fax (856)853-1288
+ SOM - Department of Internal Medicine
42 East Laurel Road/Suite 3100   Stratford, NJ 08084   (856)853-1111   Fax (856)566-6906
+ 2301 East Evesham Road/Suite 210
Voorhees, NJ 08096   (856)772-1700   Fax (856)772-5949

Fallon, Kimberly L., MD {1477674737} ObsGyn(97,NY47)
+ Valley Medical Group
70 Park Avenue   Park Ridge, NJ 07656   (201)476-0040   Fax (201)391-7733

Falls, Ingrid T., MD {1235204975} Psychy(86,NJ06)<NJ-SOMERSET>
+ RWJ University Hospital Somerset
110 Rehill Avenue/PsychEmrgScrnng   Somerville, NJ 08876   (908)526-4100   Fax (908)218-0466
+ 2 Worlds Fair Drive/Suite 111
Somerset, NJ 08873   (908)526-4100   Fax (732)563-2930

Faloba, Kathryn, MD {1689094443}<NJ-JRSYSHMC>
+ Jersey Shore University Medical Center
1945 Route 33   Neptune, NJ 07753   (732)776-4945

Faloon, Michael J., MD {1043420136} SrgOrt(NY20)
+ University Spine Center
504 Valley Road/Second Floor/Suite 203   Wayne, NJ 07470   (973)686-0700   Fax (973)686-0701

Faltas, Ashraf Kamal, MD {1275635070} IntrMd(93,EGY03)<NJ-MEADWLND>
+ Meadowlands Hospital Medical Center
55 Meadowlands Parkway   Secaucus, NJ 07096   (201)392-3100

Faltas-Fouad, Suzan L., MD {1609960921} FamMed(80,EGY05)<NJ-STMRYPAS>
+ The Valley Hospital
223 North Van Dien Avenue/Hospitalist   Ridgewood, NJ 07450   (201)447-8618

Faludi, Christopher, MD {1497121743} IntrMd<NJ-JRSYCITY>
+ Jersey City Medical Center
355 Grand Street   Jersey City, NJ 07304   (201)915-2431

Falzon, Andrea, MD {1487819736} PthACl, PthFor, IntrMd(86,MLT01)
+ Middlesex County-Medical Examiner
1490 Livingston Avenue/Suite 800   North Brunswick, NJ 08902   (732)745-3190   Fax (732)745-3491
falzonandrew@hotmail.com

Falzon, Andrew L., MD {1689186579} PthFor, PthACl(86,MLT01)
+ Office of The Regional Medical Examiner State of NJ
325 Norfolk Street   Newark, NJ 07103   (973)648-7220   Fax (973)648-3692
+ Middlesex County-Medical Examiner
1490 Livingston Avenue/Suite 800   North Brunswick, NJ 08902   (973)648-7220   Fax (732)745-3491

Fam, Alfred M., MD {1295013225} Anesth<NJ-HACKNSK>
+ Hackensack University Medical Center
30 Prospect Avenue   Hackensack, NJ 07601   (201)996-2419   Fax (201)996-3962

Fam, Mina, MD {1659661338} Urolgy
+ Coastal Urology Associates
446 Jack Martin Boulevard   Brick, NJ 08724   (732)840-4300   Fax (732)840-4515

Fan, Foun-Chung, MD {1255466017} Anesth(72,TAIW)<NJ-STBARNMC>
+ St. Barnabas Medical Center
94 Old Short Hills Road/PO Box 39   Livingston, NJ 07039   (973)322-5000
+ New Jersey Anesthesia Associates, P.C.
252 Columbia Turnpike/PO Box 0037   Florham Park, NJ 07932   (973)322-5000   Fax (973)660-9779

Fan, Liqi, MD {1083910830} EmrgMd<NJ-TRINIWSC>
+ Trinitas Regional Medical Center-Williamson Street
225 Williamson Street/EmergMed   Elizabeth, NJ 07207   (860)869-7642
liqi.fan@gmail.com

Fan, Lu, MD {1548687742} IntrMd<NJ-COOPRUMC>
+ Cooper University Hospital
One Cooper Plaza   Camden, NJ 08103   (856)356-4924   Fax (856)356-4793

Fan, Pang-Dian, MD {1184878837} MedOnc(01,NY01)
+ 149 Alexandria Way
Basking Ridge, NJ 07920

Fan, Sarah Y., MD {1821035411} IntrMd, CdvDis, CarNuc(03,PA01)<NJ-NWRKBETH, NJ-STMICHL>
+ New Jersey Cardiology Associates
653 Willow Grove Street/Suite 1000   Hackettstown, NJ 07840   (908)852-9020   Fax (908)852-5056
+ New Jersey Cardiology Associates
375 Mount Pleasant Avenue   West Orange, NJ 07052   (908)852-9020   Fax (973)731-8030

Fan, Schuber C., MD {1245205376} Nrolgy(69,TAIW)<NJ-BAYSHORE, NJ-RIVERVW>
+ Greater Monmouth Neurology
130 Maple Avenue/Suite 1-A   Red Bank, NJ 07701   (732)741-1378   Fax (732)741-1677
jack@scfanmd.com
+ Greater Monmouth Neurology
733 North Beers Street   Holmdel, NJ 07733   (732)741-1378

Fan, Wen Lin, MD {1437122611} RadDia, RadV&I(98,TX13)<PA-HHNMANN>
+ South Jersey Radiology Associates, P.A.
100 Carnie Boulevard/Suite B-5   Voorhees, NJ 08043   (856)751-0123   Fax (856)751-0535
+ South Jersey Radiology Associates, P.A.
6650 Browning Road/Suite M14   Pennsauken, NJ 08109   (856)751-0123   Fax (856)661-0686

Fan, Wen-Ling Lee, MD {1427115708} PhysMd(74,TAI05)
+ Preakness Hospital
305 Oldham Road   Wayne, NJ 07470   (973)904-6126   Fax (973)904-9843

Fand, Benjamin, MD {1134232291} Urolgy(79,NJ06)
+ Premier Urology Group, LLC
10 Parsonage Road/Suite 118   Edison, NJ 08837   (732)494-9400   Fax (732)548-3931
+ Premier Urology Group, LLC
2 Hospital Plaza/Suite 430   Old Bridge, NJ 08857   (732)494-9400   Fax (732)679-2077
+ Premier Urology Group, LLC
570 South Avenue East/Building A   Cranford, NJ 08837   (908)603-4200   Fax (908)497-1633

Fanelle, Joseph W., MD {1578563334} RadOnc, RadThp(87,PA09)
+ South Jersey Radiation Oncology P.C.
PO Box 866   Millville, NJ 08332   (856)293-2910

Fanelli, Allison Sagan, DO {1326006636} Pedtrc(00,NJ75)<NJ-VIRTVOOR, NJ-VIRTUAHS>
+ Advocare Atrium Pediatrics
301 Old Marlton Pike West/Suite 1   Marlton, NJ 08053   (856)988-9101   Fax (856)988-7712
+ Advocare Atrium Pediatrics Cedar Brook
41 South Route 73/Building 1/Suite 101   Hammonton, NJ 08037   (856)988-9101   Fax (609)567-4904

Fang, Bruno S., MD {1982692851} OncHem, IntrMd(91,BRA04)<NJ-RWJUBRUN, NJ-STPETER>
+ Regional Cancer Care Associates - Central Jersey Div
454 Elizabeth Avenue/Suite 240   Somerset, NJ 08873   (732)390-7750   Fax (732)390-7725
+ Central Jersey Oncology Center, P.A.
Brier Hill Court/Building J-2   East Brunswick, NJ 08816   (732)390-7750   Fax (732)390-7725
+ Central Jersey Oncology Center, P.A.
205 Easton Avenue   New Brunswick, NJ 08873   (732)828-9570   Fax (732)828-7638

Fang, Margaret Wu, MD {1740386788} PsyGrt, Psychy(98,NJ06)<NJ-MONMOUTH>
+ Monmouth Medical Center
300 Second Avenue/Psych   Long Branch, NJ 07740   (732)923-6912

Fanning, Christine M., MD {1881015659} IntHos
+ Princeton Medicine
5 Plainsboro Road/Suite 300   Plainsboro, NJ 08536   (609)853-7230   Fax (609)853-7271

Fanous, Michelle, DO {1558598292}<NJ-OCEANMC>
+ Ocean Medical Center
425 Jack Martin Boulevard   Brick, NJ 08723   (732)840-3380

Fanous, Venis F., MD {1871594432} IntrMd(76,EGY04)
+ 59 Brunswick Woods Drive
East Brunswick, NJ 08816   (732)238-3883   Fax (732)238-4826

Fanouse, John A., DO {1205193422} Anesth
+ Morris Anesthesia Group, PA
3799 Route 46/Suite 211   Parsippany, NJ 07054   (973)335-1122   Fax (973)335-1448

Fantasia, Michele Elaine, MD {1447226261} Pedtrc, PedReh(94,NJ05)<NJ-CHLSOCEN, NJ-CHLSMT>
+ Children's Specialized Hospital
200 Somerset Street   New Brunswick, NJ 08901   (732)258-7000   Fax (908)301-5456
+ Children's Specialized Hospital-Ocean
94 Stevens Road   Toms River, NJ 08755   (732)914-1100

Fantazzio, Michele Adrienne, MD {1326036245} Surgry, SrgTrm, SrgVas(96,PA02)<NJ-VIRTUAHS>
+ Kennedy Health Alliance
900 Medical Center Drive/Suite 201   Sewell, NJ 08080   (856)218-2100   Fax (856)218-2101
+ Breast Specialty Care Group
1605 East Evesham Road/Suite 2-B   Voorhees, NJ 08043   (856)218-2100   Fax (856)424-8007

Fantini, Domenica Alexandra, DO {1548609464}<NJ-MORRISTN>
+ Morristown Medical Center
100 Madison Avenue   Morristown, NJ 07962   (908)418-2831

Farag, Amanda S., MD {1548421910} OrtSpn, IntrMd(CT02<NJ-VAEASTOR>
+ VA New Jersey Health Care System-East Orange Campus
385 Tremont Avenue   East Orange, NJ 07018   (973)676-1000
amanda.farag@va.gov

Farag, Magdy M., MD {1346302411} Pedtrc, NnPnMd(77,EGY04)<NJ-HACKNSK, NJ-HOLYNAME>
+ Riverside Medical Group
714 Tenth Street/Suite 2   Secaucus, NJ 07094   (201)863-3346   Fax (201)865-0015

Farag, Marianne, DO {1306167721}
+ 245 Prospect Avenue/Apt 4c
Hackensack, NJ 07601

Faragalla, Emad T., MD {1457515322} Anesth<NJ-MEADWLND>
+ Meadowlands Hospital Medical Center
55 Meadowlands Parkway   Secaucus, NJ 07096   (201)392-3100

Farajallah, Awny Sb, MD {1831327337} IntrMd, InfDis(91,EGY03)<NJ-COOPRUMC>
+ Cooper University Hospital
One Cooper Plaza   Camden, NJ 08103   (856)342-2000

Faraz, Haroon Ahmed, MD {1629250535} IntCrd, IntrMd(01,PAK11)
+ Cross Country Cardiology
103 River Road/2nd Floor   Edgewater, NJ 07020   (201)941-8100   Fax (201)941-2899
haroonafaraz@gmail.com

Farber, Charles M., MD {1144218215} IntrMd, MedOnc, Hemato(86,NY19)<NJ-MORRISTN>
+ Hematology-Oncology Associates of Northern NJ
100 Madison Avenue/PO Box 1089   Morristown, NJ 07962   (973)538-5210   Fax (973)644-9657

Farber, Liora Judith, MD {1912261009}
+ Palisades Medical Center
705B Anderson Avenue   Cliffside Park, NJ 07010   (201)861-1851   Fax (201)861-1853
+ 613 Martense Avenue
Teaneck, NJ 07666   (401)456-2179

Farber, Michael A., MD {1154301679} Gastrn, IntrMd(81,MEX14)<NJ-SJRSYELM, NJ-UNDRWD>
+ Pitman Internal Medicine Associates
410 North Broadway/Suite 1   Pitman, NJ 08071   (856)589-3708   Fax (856)589-2662

Farber, Michael Seth, MD {1538107867} IntrMd(95,GRNA)<NJ-HACKNSK>
+ Executive Health
20 Prospect Avenue/Suite 100   Hackensack, NJ 07601   (201)996-3166   Fax (201)968-0537

Physicians by Name and Address

Farbowitz, Michael Aron, MD {1740276393}
Ophthl(94,NY19)<NJ-OVERLOOK, NJ-STBARNMC>
+ Short Hills Ophthalmology Group
551 Millburn Avenue   Short Hills, NJ 07078   (973)379-2544   Fax (973)379-1317

Fardman, Emiliya, MD {1497826630} Psychy, PsyCAd(90,KAZ02)<NJ-MONMOUTH>
+ Monmouth Medical Center
300 Second Avenue/Psychiatry   Long Branch, NJ 07740   (732)222-5200

Fares, Louis G., II, MD {1417903998} SrgVas, Surgry(78,PHI01)<NJ-RWJUHAM, NJ-STFRNMED>
+ Louis B. Fares II MD FACS LLC
116 Washington Crossing Road/Suite 1   Pennington, NJ 08534   (609)737-2223   Fax (609)737-2350

Farghani, Saima Obaid, MD {1982922183} EnDbMt<NJ-RWJUBRUN>
+ Mid-Atlantic Endocrinology & Diabetes Associates
555 Iron Bridge Road/Suite 18   Freehold, NJ 07728   (732)409-6233   Fax (732)409-6414

Farhangfar, Reza, MD {1184709297} IntrMd, PulDis(86,GRNA)<NJ-CHILTON>
+ Drs. Singh & Farhangfar
401 Hamburg Turnpike/Suite 109   Wayne, NJ 07470   (973)595-7456   Fax (973)904-9119

Farhat, Salman, MD {1356780274} IntrMd<NJ-MORRISTN>
+ Morristown Medical Center
100 Madison Avenue   Morristown, NJ 07962   (973)971-5000

Farhath, Sabeena, MD {1023142676} PedGst(91,INA8Y)<NJ-COOPRUMC>
+ Cooper University Hospital
One Cooper Plaza/Pediatrics   Camden, NJ 08103   (856)342-2000

Farion, George Z., MD {1558420364} IntrMd(76,OH40)<NJ-CLARMAAS>
+ 87 Franklin Avenue
Nutley, NJ 07110   (973)542-0800   Fax (973)542-0133

Farjo, Sara, DO {1851648695}
+ Family Medicine at Monument Square
317 George Street   New Brunswick, NJ 08901   (732)235-8993   Fax (732)246-7317

Farkas, Andrew, MD {1699982165} Obstet(04,NJ06)
+ Eric B. Chandler Health Center
277 George Street   New Brunswick, NJ 08901   (732)235-6700   Fax (732)235-6729

Farkas, Attila Istvan, MD {1639114614} IntrMd(99,NY08)<NJ-MORRISTN>
+ Internal Medicine Consultants
765 State Route 10 East/Suite 201   Randolph, NJ 07869   (973)975-4830   Fax (732)271-1022

Farkas, Edward L., MD {1154313955} Psychy, PsyGrt(79,ITAL)<NJ-HOLYNAME>
+ 175 Cedar Lane/Suite A
Teaneck, NJ 07666   (201)692-8354   Fax (201)692-0234   elfmd2@aol.com

Farkas, Jeffrey, MD {1942315163} RadDia, RadNro, IntrMd(91,NY08)<NY-LUTHERN>
+ Interventional Neuro Associates, LLC
777 Terrace Avenue/Suite 401   Hasbrouck Heights, NJ 07604   (201)387-1957   Fax (201)351-0656

Farkas, John J., MD {1205924248} Gastrn, IntrMd(83,DMN01)
+ Gastroenterology Associates of New Jersey
842 Clifton Avenue   Clifton, NJ 07013   (973)777-5717   Fax (201)632-4815

Farkas, Jordan Phillip, MD {1548434665} SrgPlstc
+ 570 Sylvan Avenue/Suite 202
Englewood Cliffs, NJ 07632   (201)587-4961

Farkas, Klara, MD {1891722468} Anesth(88,HUN02)
+ Toms River Anesthesia Associates PC
409 Main Street/2nd Floor   Toms River, NJ 08753   (732)818-7575   Fax (732)818-1567
+ Community Medical Center
99 Route 37 West   Toms River, NJ 08755   (732)818-7575

Farley-Loftus, Rachel L., MD {1285845941} Dermat, PedDrm, IntrMd(06,NY01)<NY-NYUTISCH>
+ M.C. Medical Group
1425 Pompton Avenue/Suite 1-1   Cedar Grove, NJ 07009   (973)785-8686   Fax (973)785-8680   richard.farley@mssm.edu

Farmer, Alka Rajesh, MD {1821207143} IntrMd(02,INA20)<NJ-COOPRUMC>
+ Cooper University Hospital
One Cooper Plaza/Hospitalist   Camden, NJ 08103   (856)342-3150   Fax (856)968-8418

Farnacio, Yvonne, MD {1528331022}
+ JFK Medical Center
65 James Street   Edison, NJ 08820   (732)321-7610

Farnath, Denise Anne, MD {1134225907} Ophthl(85,NJ06)
+ Burlington County Eye Physicians
225 Sunset Road   Willingboro, NJ 08046   (609)877-2800   Fax (609)877-1813

Farner, Michael Charles, MD {1467415729} RadDia, RadV&I(96,CA02)
+ South Jersey Radiology Associates, P.A.
100 Carnie Boulevard/Suite B-5   Voorhees, NJ 08043   (856)751-0123   Fax (856)751-0535
+ South Jersey Radiology Associates, P.A.
6650 Browning Road/Suite M14   Pennsauken, NJ 08109   (856)751-0123   Fax (856)661-0686
+ South Jersey Radiology Associates, P.A.
315 Route 70 East/Suite B   Cherry Hill, NJ 08043   (856)428-4344   Fax (856)428-0356

Farnese, Jeffrey Jason, MD {1730269994} IntrMd(97,GRNA)<NJ-MTNSIDE>
+ Drs. Farnese and Farnese
109 Newark Pompton Turnpike   Little Falls, NJ 07424   (973)890-0330   Fax (973)890-0705

Farnese, Joseph T., MD {1922188184} IntrMd(84,GRN01)
+ Drs. Farnese and Farnese
109 Newark Pompton Turnpike   Little Falls, NJ 07424   (973)890-0330   Fax (973)890-0705

Farnsworth, Marie N., MD {1023061157} EmrgMd<NJ-ACMCITY, NJ-ACMCMAIN>
+ AtlantiCare Regional Medical Center/City Campus
1925 Pacific Avenue/EmergMed   Atlantic City, NJ 08401   (609)345-4000

Faro, Revital D., MD {1275892812} ObsGyn, MtFtMd
+ University Medical Group/OBGYN
125 Paterson Street/2nd Floor   New Brunswick, NJ 08901   (732)235-6632   Fax (732)235-6627
+ St. Peter's Family Health
123 How Lane   New Brunswick, NJ 08901   (732)235-6632   Fax (732)729-0869

Farooki, Adil, MD {1073718235} IntrMd
+ 35 Evergreen Place
Demarest, NJ 07627   (201)467-5303

Farooki, Alima Bibi, MD {1275748717} Psychy, PsyCAd, OthrSp(78,INA5B)
+ 127 Union Street/Suite 106
Ridgewood, NJ 07450   (201)444-6140   Fax (201)444-6148

Farooki, Zahid A., MD {1578505988} IntrMd(70,PAK01)
+ Hackensack University Medical Group Closter
1 Ruckman Road   Closter, NJ 07624   (201)385-6161   Fax (201)385-1671

Farooqi, Ahmad, MD {1396754776} IntrMd, PallCr, Grtrcs(88,PAK20)<NJ-JRSYCITY>
+ 377 Jersey Avenue/Suite 310
Jersey City, NJ 07302   (201)499-3900   Fax (201)706-2092   Ahmad.Farooq@va.gov

Farooq, Omer, MD {1952333262}
+ Apogee Physicians
201 Lyons Avenue   Newark, NJ 07112   (973)926-2164   Fax (214)764-6683

Farooq, Sadaf, MD {1598964090} Pedtrc(99,PAK01)
+ 93 Fountayne Lane
Lawrenceville, NJ 08648

Farooq, Tahir, MD {1376759100} InfDis
+ Infectious Disease Consultants
1245 Whitehorse-Mercerville Rd   Mercerville, NJ 08619   (609)581-2000   Fax (609)581-5450

Farooq, Taliya, MD {1215339221} PthAcl<NJ-RIVERVW>
+ Riverview Medical Center
1 Riverview Plaza   Red Bank, NJ 07701   (732)741-2700

Farooqui, Ozer A., MD {1285054650} IntrMd<NJ-UMDNJ>
+ University Hospital
150 Bergen Street/Suite H245   Newark, NJ 07103   (973)972-4672   Fax (973)972-0365

Farooqui, Shahid Waseem, MD {1205804127} IntrMd(83,EGYP)<NJ-RIVERVW>
+ 20 White Road/Suite B
Shrewsbury, NJ 07702   (732)747-4723   Fax (732)747-5998

Farooqui, Syeda Saleha, MD {1538233358} IntrMd, Grtrcs(79,INA39)
+ Drs. Hossain, Hossain, and Farooqui
26-01 Broadway/Suite 105   Fair Lawn, NJ 07410   (201)703-3664

Farooqui, Zaheerulla A., MD {1578544599} IntrMd, FamMed(71,INDI)<NJ-BURDTMLN>
+ 3018 Bayshore Road
North Cape May, NJ 08204   (609)886-5637   Fax (609)886-0713

Farrales, Caroline P., MD {1255445128} PsyGrt, Psychy(83,PHI01)<NJ-MORRISTN>
+ Morristown Medical Center
100 Madison Avenue/Psych   Morristown, NJ 07962   (973)971-5000

Farrar, Robert, MD {1245288273} Anesth, CritCr, IntrMd(81,ITA16)
+ Summit Anesthesia Associates, P.A.
33 Overlook Road/Suite 311   Summit, NJ 07901   (908)598-1500   Fax (908)598-0197

Farrell, Charles W., MD {1790891802} Anesth(91,PA09)<NJ-COMMED>
+ Red Bank Anesthesia, LLC
1 Riverview Plaza   Red Bank, NJ 07701   (732)530-2255   Fax (732)450-2620

Farrell, Christopher James, MD {1922134394} SrgNro(02,PA13)
+ 443 Laurel Oak Road/Suite 230
Voorhees, NJ 08043   (215)503-7008

Farrell, Joseph E., DO {1821043456} SrgOrt, SprtMd(78,PA77)<NJ-VIRTMHBC, NJ-VANJHCS>
+ Reconstructive Orthopedics, P.A.
243 Route 130/Suite 100   Bordentown, NJ 08505   (609)267-9400   Fax (609)267-9457
+ Reconstructive Orthopedics, P.A.
131 Route 70 West/Suite 100   Medford, NJ 08055   (609)267-9400   Fax (609)267-9457

Farrell, Lynda A., MD {1346338340} IntrMd(78,NJ05)<NJ-CHILTON>
+ 9 Post Road/Suite M-7
Oakland, NJ 07436   (201)337-9498   Fax (201)337-9031

Farrell, Michael Louis, DO {1326003914} Surgry(94,NJ75)<NJ-CHILTON>
+ 547 Union Boulevard
Totowa, NJ 07512   (973)790-9301   Fax (973)790-9390   louie6838@aol.com

Farrell, Paul R., MD {1679534176} Pedtrc(74,DC02)<NJ-JRSYSHMC, NJ-MONMOUTH>
+ Ocean Pediatric Group
1 Industrial Way West/Suite 1-C   Eatontown, NJ 07724   (732)542-6451   Fax (732)542-1654
+ Ocean Pediatric Group
2640 Route 70/Suite 1-B   Manasquan, NJ 08736   (732)542-6451   Fax (732)223-5792

Farrer, William E., MD {1114997012} InfDis, IntrMd(75,MA01)<NJ-TRINIWSC>
+ Trinitas Regional Medical Center-Williamson Street
225 Williamson Street   Elizabeth, NJ 07207   (908)994-5010   Fax (908)351-7930   wfarrer@trinitas.org
+ Union County Infectious Disease Group
240 Williamson Street/Suite 502   Elizabeth, NJ 07207   (908)994-5010   Fax (908)994-5308

Farrow, Syrita Shantell, DO {1942596564}<NJ-VIRTVOOR>
+ Virtua Voorhees
100 Bowman Drive   Voorhees, NJ 08043   (856)247-3060   syrita_farrow@teamhealth.com

Farrugia, Peter Michael, MD {1003142530} IntrMd(04,NY48)
+ Barnabas Health Medical Group
1270 Highway 35 South/Suite 1   Middletown, NJ 07748   (732)615-3900   Fax (732)671-0395
+ Barnabas Health Medical Group
166 Morris Avenue/2nd Floor   Long Branch, NJ 07740   (732)615-3900   Fax (732)263-5029
+ Monmouth Heart Specialists
274 Highway 35   Eatontown, NJ 07748   (732)440-7336   Fax (732)440-9404

Farry, John Patrick, MD {1174517635} CdvDis, CarNuc, IntrMd(71,DC02)<NJ-OVERLOOK, NJ-MMHKEMBL>
+ Associates in Cardiovascular Disease, LLC
571 Central Avenue/Suite 115   New Providence, NJ 07974   (908)464-4200   Fax (908)464-1332

Farzad, Ahmad, MD {1578591533} Otlryg(66,IRAN)
+ 2480 Pennington Road/Suite 105
Pennington, NJ 08534   (609)737-7555   Fax (609)737-7032

Fasano, Armand P., MD {1467487736} Ophthl(95,CA06)<NJ-PALISADE, NJ-HACKNSK>
+ 229 60th Street
West New York, NJ 07093   (201)869-0707   Fax (201)861-8878

Faschan, Steven Michael, DO {1922374081} FamMed(12,NY76)
+ MedExpress Urgent Care Watchung
1569 US Highway 22   Watchung, NJ 07069   (908)322-2631   Fax (908)322-2679

Fascitelli, David A., MD {1962451880} EmrgMd, IntrMd(72,NY06)<NJ-VALLEY, NJ-CHILTON>
+ The Valley Hospital
223 North Van Dien Avenue/EmergMed   Ridgewood, NJ 07450   (201)447-8300   Fax (201)447-8174

Fass, Barry D., MD {1740396308} PhysMd, IntrMd(82,DC03)
+ Hamilton HealthCare Center
3840 Quakerbridge Road/Suite 100   Hamilton, NJ 08619   (609)890-2222   Fax (609)890-0715

Fastag Guttman, Eduardo, MD {1699150177} Pedtrc
+ St Joseph's Medical Center Pediatrics
703 Main Street   Paterson, NJ 07503   (973)754-2543

Fatima, Uzma, MD {1831357656}<NJ-STJOSHOS>
+ St. Joseph's Regional Medical Center
703 Main Street   Paterson, NJ 07503   (973)754-2000

Faugno, Gerard L., MD {1710073408} FamMed(81,DOM02)
+ 160 Ridge Road
Lyndhurst, NJ 07071   (201)933-1480   Fax (201)933-5937

Physicians by Name and Address

Faulkner, Adriana Danielle, MD {1942511688} RadDia
 + Hackensack Radiology Group, P.A.
  30 Prospect Avenue Hackensack, NJ 07601 (551)996-2200 Fax (201)489-2812

Faust, Michael G., MD {1962406595} ObsGyn, IntrMd(83,PA12)<NJ-VALLEY>
 + Valley Center for Women's Health
  581 North Franklin Turnpike/2nd Floor Ramsey, NJ 07446 (201)236-2100 Fax (201)236-5269
 + Valley Center for Women's Health
  One Godwin Avenue Midland Park, NJ 07432 (201)444-4040

Faustino, Alan Herbert, MD {1669482568} IntrMd, GenPrc(95,VA07)
 + 28 West Gilmar Circle
  Margate City, NJ 08402

Favata, Elissa A., MD {1619039971} IntrMd, OccpMd(80,VA01)
 + Enviromental & Occupational Health Associates
  1401 Route 70 East/Suite 14 Cherry Hill, NJ 08034 (856)216-1100 Fax (856)216-0484

Favetta, John R., MD {1497861090} Ophthl(75,NJ05)
 + 70 Ridge Road
  North Arlington, NJ 07031 (201)997-2332 Fax (201)997-6845
  Johnfavetta@comcast.net

Fayemi, Alfred O., MD {1649345794} PthACl, FamMed(70,ISRA)<NJ-HOBUNIMC>
 + Hoboken University Medical Center
  308 Willow Avenue/Pathology Hoboken, NJ 07030 (201)418-1000 Fax (201)418-1983

Fayngersh, Alla, MD {1801816103} IntrMd(01,NY45)<NJ-ENGLWOOD>
 + Englewood Hospital and Medical Center
  350 Engle Street/Medicine Englewood, NJ 07631 (201)894-3000

Fayngersh, David, MD {1124082532} Pedtrc(86,RUS35)<NJ-CLARMAAS>
 + NHCAC Health Center at West New York
  5301 Broadway West New York, NJ 07093 (201)866-9320 Fax (201)867-9183
  Dfayn@wsu.com
 + NHCAC Health Center at North Bergen
  1116 43rd Street North Bergen, NJ 07047 (201)866-9320 Fax (201)330-2638

Fayyaz, Imran, MD {1952385692} IntrMd, Gastrn(87,PAK01)<NJ-RWJUBRUN>
 + RWJ University Hospital New Brunswick
  One Robert Wood Johnson Place New Brunswick, NJ 08901 (732)828-3000

Fayyaz, Tooba, DO {1679716740}
 + Cape Regional Physicians Associates
  11 Village Drive Cape May Court House, NJ 08210 (609)465-2273 Fax (609)463-0235

Fazal, Zoheb, MD {1538578489}
 + 2601 Larchmont Place
  Mount Laurel, NJ 08054 (732)543-4569
  zohebfazal@gmail.com

Fazekas, Jessica Eden, DO {1609938281} RadDia, RadBdI(01,NJ75)<NJ-KMHCHRRY>
 + Kennedy Health System/Cherry Hill Campus
  2201 Chapel Avenue West/Radiology Cherry Hill, NJ 08002 (856)661-5473 Fax (856)488-6507

Fazio, Ignazio, Jr., MD {1972500528} IntrMd, Nephro(89,NY15)
 + Suburban Nephrology Group
  1031 McBride Avenue/Suite D-210 Little Falls, NJ 07424 (973)389-1119
 + Suburban Nephrology Group
  342 Hamburg Turnpike/Suite 201 Wayne, NJ 07470 (973)389-1119 Fax (973)389-1145

Febbraro, Terri, MD {1396975520} GynOnc, ObsGyn(09,NY46)
 + Summit Medical Group Florham Park Campus
  150 Park Avenue Florham Park, NJ 07932 (908)273-4300

Febin, John, MD {1619385606}
 + St. Peter's University Hospital
  254 Easton Avenue New Brunswick, NJ 08901 (732)745-8600

Fechisin, Joel Patrick, MD {1366641029} SrgOrt<NJ-MONMOUTH>
 + Monmouth Medical Center
  300 Second Avenue Long Branch, NJ 07740 (732)222-5200

Fechner, Adam Jeffrey, MD {1982845426} ObsGyn(05,NJ05)
 + University Reproductive Associates, PC
  214 Terrace Avenue/2nd Floor Hasbrouck Heights, NJ 07604 (201)288-6330 Fax (201)288-6331
 + Rutgers- New Jersey Medical School
  185 South Orange Avenue Newark, NJ 07103 (973)972-4300

Fechtner, Robert D., MD {1871527259} Ophthl, Glacma(82,MI01)<NJ-UMDNJ>
 + University Ophthalmology Associates
  90 Bergen Street/DOC 6100 Newark, NJ 07101 (973)982-2065 Fax (973)972-1244

Fede, Jean M., DO {1598820730} PthAna(00,NJ75)<NJ-UNVM-CPRN>
 + University Medical Center of Princeton at Plainsboro
  One Plainsboro Road Plainsboro, NJ 08536 (609)497-4000

Fede, Robert Michael, MD {1407948243} IntrMd(86,NJ05)<NJ-UMDNJ>
 + University Hospital
  150 Bergen Street/Critical Care Newark, NJ 07103 (973)972-6111
 + University Hospital-New Jersey Medical School
  30 Bergen Street Newark, NJ 07107 (973)972-4511

Fedele, Dara, MD {1316101439} RadDia<NY-STATNRTH>
 + Riverview Medical Center
  1 Riverview Plaza Red Bank, NJ 07701 (732)530-2305 Fax (732)224-8410

Feder, Craig A., MD {1952494106} Anesth, PainInvt(83,NY08)
 + Anesthesia Pain Treatment Center
  1666 Hamilton Avenue/Suite 2 Hamilton, NJ 08629 (609)584-9080 Fax (609)584-0139

Feder, Marc T., MD {1255662284} Urolgy
 + Genito-Urinary Surgeons of New Jersey
  579-A Cranbury Road/Suite 104 East Brunswick, NJ 08816 (732)390-8700 Fax (732)390-8555
 + Genito-Urinary Surgeons of New Jersey
  211 Courtyard Drive Hillsborough, NJ 08844 (732)390-8700 Fax (908)685-7594

Federbush, Joel S., MD {1417000332} Psychy, PsyFor(86,NY08)
 + 16 Arcadian Way
  Paramus, NJ 07652 (201)845-9800 Fax (201)845-8663

Federici, Peter J., MD {1265464473} Urolgy(74,NH01)
 + 2815 East Chestnut Avenue
  Vineland, NJ 08360 (856)691-3273 Fax (856)691-4649

Federico, Cheryl L., MD {1689647810} NnPnMd, Pedtrc(93,PA01)<NJ-MORRISTN>
 + MidAtlantic Neonatology Associates
  100 Madison Avenue Morristown, NJ 07962 (973)971-5488 Fax (973)290-7175

Fedida, Andre Armand, MD {1891839312} IntrMd, Gastrn(86,GRN01)
 + Drs. Fedida and Brown
  306 Martin Luther King Blvd/4th Floor Newark, NJ 07102 (973)877-2580 Fax (973)877-2578
 + Harrison Endo Surgical Center
  620 Essex Street/Suite 3 Harrison, NJ 07029 (973)877-2580 Fax (973)474-1030

Fedorcik, Gregory Gerard, MD {1164499786} SrgHnd, OrtSHand(00,GRN01)<NJ-COMMED, NJ-MONMOUTH>
 + Central Jersey Hand Surgery
  2 Industrial Way West Eatontown, NJ 07724 (732)542-4477 Fax (732)935-0355
 + Central Jersey Hand Surgery
  535 Iron Bridge Road Freehold, NJ 07728 (732)542-4477 Fax (732)431-4770
 + Central Jersey Hand Surgery
  780 Route 37 West/Suite 140 Toms River, NJ 07724 (732)286-9000 Fax (732)240-0036

Fedorciw, Boris Jaroslaw, MD {1538178306} PthACl, PthCyt(87,NY15)<NJ-STPETER>
 + St. Peter's University Hospital
  254 Easton Avenue/Pathology New Brunswick, NJ 08901 (732)745-8534 Fax (732)220-8595

Feehan, Brian Patrick, DO {1457513319} IntrMd(05,PA77)<NJ-DEBRAHLC>
 + Empire Medical Associates
  5 Franklin Avenue/Suite 302 Belleville, NJ 07109 (973)759-1221 Fax (973)759-1997
 + Empire Medical Associates
  264 Boyden Avenue Maplewood, NJ 07040 (973)759-1221 Fax (973)761-7617
 + Empire Medical Associates
  382 West Passaic Avenue Bloomfield, NJ 07109 (973)338-1900

Feeney, Charlee Wallis, DO {1427138882} Radiol, RadDia(00,MO79)<NJ-OCEANMC>
 + Ocean Medical Center
  425 Jack Martin Boulevard/Radiology Brick, NJ 08723 (732)840-2200 Fax (732)974-8820
 + Coastal Imaging, LLC
  79 Route 37 West/Suite 103 Toms River, NJ 08755 (732)840-2200 Fax (732)276-2325

Fegan, Robert James, MD {1841291580} Ophthl(97,NY46)<NJ-MONMOUTH>
 + Atlantic Eye Physicians
  279 Third Avenue/Suite 204 Long Branch, NJ 07740 (732)222-7373 Fax (732)571-9212

Fehder, Carl G., MD {1497769244} Anesth(77,CA11)<NJ-MEMSALEM>
 + Memorial Hospital of Salem County
  310 Woodstown Road/Anesthesiology Salem, NJ 08079 (856)935-1000

Fehmian, Carol Janice, MD {1114963923} PthACl(91,NJ05)<NJ-HACKNSK>
 + Hackensack University Medical Center
  30 Prospect Avenue/Pathology Hackensack, NJ 07601 (201)996-2000

Fehrle, Wilfrid Martin, MD {1700926094} PthACl, Hemato, Pthlgy(92,PA09)
 + Bio-Reference Laboratory, Inc.
  481 Edward H. Ross Drive Elmwood Park, NJ 07407 (201)791-2600 Fax (201)791-1941

Feibusch, Evan Lawrence, MD {1831172261} PsyFor(93,NJ06)<NJ-ANNKLEIN, NJ-TRENTPSY>
 + Trenton Psychiatric Hospital
  Sullivan Way/PO Box 7600/Psychiatric West Trenton, NJ 08628 (609)633-1500
 + Ann Klein Forensic Center
  1609 Stuyvesant Avenue/PO Box 7717 West Trenton, NJ 08628 (609)633-0900

Feigelis, Robin Y., MD {1023087533} CdvDis, IntrMd(83,NY08)<NJ-VALLEY>
 + 74 Pascack Road/Suite 10
  Park Ridge, NJ 07656 (201)573-9266 Fax (201)573-8082

Feigelman, Theodor, MD {1447222641} IntrMd(76,MI07)<NJ-MORRISTN, NJ-OVERLOOK>
 + Morristown Medical Center
  100 Madison Avenue/IntMed Morristown, NJ 07962 (973)971-4095 Fax (973)290-7172
  Ted.Feigelman@atlantichealth.org
 + Overlook Hospital-Dvpmt Disabilities
  1000 Galloping Hill Road Union, NJ 07083 (973)971-4095 Fax (908)686-8374

Feigenbaum, Howard, MD {1982700340} Surgry(71,NY19)<NJ-CHILTON>
 + 227 Hamburg Turnpike
  Pompton Lakes, NJ 07442 (973)839-7999 Fax (973)839-5878

Feigenblum, David Yehuda, MD {1356357420} CdvDis, ClCdEl, IntrMd(97,NY19)<NJ-ENGLWOOD>
 + North Jersey Electrophysiology Associates
  350 Engle Street Englewood, NJ 07631 (201)894-3533 Fax (201)541-2188
 + North Jersey Electrophysiology Associates
  20 Prospect Avenue/Suite 615 Hackensack, NJ 07601 (201)894-3533 Fax (201)518-8739

Feigin, Gerald A., MD {1548444532} PthFor, PthACl(81,NC05)<NJ-UNDRWD>
 + Gloucester County - Medical Examiner
  254 County House Road Clarksboro, NJ 08020 (856)384-6910 Fax (856)384-6915

Feigin, Joel Stanley, MD {1356466296} FamMed(76,NY15)
 + 8 West View Drive
  Flemington, NJ 08822 (908)788-0909

Feigin, Leslie C., MD {1447336250} Grtrcs, IntrMd(73,NJ05)<NJ-STCLRDEN>
 + Feigin & Las
  56 Diamond Springs Road Denville, NJ 07834 (973)625-1000 Fax (973)625-9122
  doc@beagleweb.com

Feigl, Frances Marie, MD {1518960202} PsyCAd(94,PA02)
 + Youth Consultation Service
  20 East Evergreen Avenue Somerdale, NJ 08083

Feiler, Michael Augustus, MD {1114057866} Anesth, FamMed(79,NY48)<NJ-VALLEY>
 + The Valley Hospital
  223 North Van Dien Avenue Ridgewood, NJ 07450 (201)447-8350

Fein, David A., MD {1780721704} IntrMd(83,NY19)<NJ-MORRISTN>
 + The Princeton Longevity Center
  136 Main Street Princeton, NJ 08540 (609)430-0752 Fax (609)430-8470

Fein, Deborah Allen, MD {1295768901} RadDia(89,LA01)<NJ-UNVMCPRN>
 + Princeton Radiology Associates, P.A.
  419 North Harrison Street Princeton, NJ 08540 (609)921-3345 Fax (609)683-8847
 + Princeton Radiology Associates, P.A.
  9 Centre Drive Jamesburg, NJ 08831 (609)921-3345 Fax (609)655-4016
 + Princeton Radiology Associates, P.A.
  3674 Route 27 Kendall Park, NJ 08540 (732)821-5563 Fax (732)821-6675

Fein, Deborah Anne, MD {1013998210} Nephro, IntrMd(80,MA07)<NJ-ENGLWOOD, NJ-PALISADE>
 + Drs. Pattner, Grodstein, Fein & Davis
  8100 Kennedy Boulevard North Bergen, NJ 07047 (201)868-5905
 + Drs. Pattner, Grodstein, Fein & Davis
  177 North Dean Street/Suite 207 Englewood, NJ 07631 (201)868-5905 Fax (201)567-8775

Physicians by Name and Address

Fein, Douglas Allen, MD {1851317739} RadOnc(89,NC05)<NJ-UN-VMCPRN, NJ-HUNTRDN>
+ University Medical Center of Princeton at Plainsboro
One Plainsboro Road   Plainsboro, NJ 08536   (609)497-4000
+ Princeton Radiation Oncology Center
9 Centre Drive/Suite 115   Jamesburg, NJ 08831   (609)497-4000   Fax (609)655-5725

Fein, Edward Dennis, MD {1629070305} PulDis, CritCr, IntrMd(89,NY47)<NJ-STPETER, NJ-RWJUBRUN>
+ Central Jersey Lung Center
333 Forsgate Drive/Suite 201   Jamesburg, NJ 08831   (732)521-3131   Fax (732)521-1116

Fein, Eric N., MD {1104987502} Anesth(79,SWI05)<NJ-STBARNMC, NJ-NWRKBETH>
+ New Jersey Anesthesia Associates, P.C.
252 Columbia Turnpike/PO Box 0037   Florham Park, NJ 07932   (973)660-9334   Fax (973)660-9779

Fein, Lesley A., MD {1568535664} IntrMd, Rheuma
+ 1099 Bloomfield Avenue
West Caldwell, NJ 07006   (973)575-0338   Fax (973)575-9340

Fein, Robert P., MD {1801887286} Hemato, IntrMd, MedOnc(79,NY19)<NJ-STPETER, NJ-RWJUHAM>
+ Drs. Fein, Porcelli & Richards
75 Veronica Avenue/Suite 201   Somerset, NJ 08873   (732)246-4882   Fax (732)249-5633
+ Regional Cancer Care Associates
111 Union Valley Road/Suite 205   Monroe, NJ 08831   (732)246-4882   Fax (609)395-7955

Feinberg, Craig Harlan, MD {1548258007} IntrMd(99,NY06)<NJ-OVERLOOK, NJ-MORRISTN>
+ Summit Medical Group-Berkeley Heights Campus
1 Diamond Hill Road/1st Fl Suite B   Berkeley Heights, NJ 07922   (908)277-8625   Fax (908)277-8841

Feinberg, Gary L., MD {1417940230} Surgry, SrgVas(82,PA02)<NJ-SHOREMEM, NJ-ACMCMAIN>
+ GFH Surgical Associates
718 Shore Road   Somers Point, NJ 08244   (609)927-8550   Fax (609)926-0273

Feinberg, Joseph H., MD {1497783211} Elecmy, PhysMd, SprtMd(83,NY03)<NY-SPCLSURG, NJ-KSLRWEST>
+ Kessler Institute for Rehabilitation West Orange
1199 Pleasant Valley Way/Sports Med   West Orange, NJ 07052   (973)243-6907   Fax (973)243-6861

Feiner, Laurel A., MD {1972556454} Ophthl, OthrSp, OphNeu(81,NY09)<NJ-COMMED>
+ 40 Bey Lea Road/Suite B103
Toms River, NJ 08753   (732)349-1012   Fax (732)349-1082

Feiner, Leonard, MD {1841208014} Ophthl, IntrMd(00,PA01)<NJ-CLARMAAS, NJ-ENGLWOOD>
+ Retina Associates of New Jersey, P.A.
628 Cedar Lane   Teaneck, NJ 07666   (201)837-7300   Fax (201)836-6426
+ Retina Associates of New Jersey, P.A.
200 South Broad Street/Unit B   Ridgewood, NJ 07450   (201)837-7300   Fax (201)445-0262

Feiner, Shoshana N., MD {1508049867} IntrMd
+ Summit Medical Group
31-00 Broadway   Fair Lawn, NJ 07410   (201)796-2255   Fax (201)796-7020

Feinerman, Larry Robert, MD {1962419572} Anesth(80,MEX14)<NJ-KMHCHRRY>
+ Rancocas Anesthesiology Associates
700 US Highway 130 North/Suite 203   Cinnaminson, NJ 08077   (856)829-9345

Feingold, Aaron J., MD {1811947328} CdvDis, IntrMd(76,IL42)
+ Raritan Bay Cardiology Group, P.A.
225 May Street/Suite F   Edison, NJ 08837   (732)738-8855   Fax (732)738-4141
+ Raritan Bay Cardiology Group, P.A.
3 Hospital Plaza/Suite 305   Old Bridge, NJ 08857   (732)738-8855   Fax (732)738-4141
+ Raritan Bay Cardiology Group, P.A.
337 Applegarth Road   Monroe Township, NJ 08837   (609)655-8860   Fax (732)738-4141

Feingold, Anat Rachel, MD {1609969146} Pedtrc, PedInf(83,MO02)<NJ-COOPRUMC>
+ Cooper Peds/Children's Regional Ctr
3 Cooper Plaza/Suite 200/Rm 202   Camden, NJ 08103   (856)342-2617   Fax (856)968-8414   feingold-anat@cooperhealth.edu
+ The Cooper Hospital System-Univ Hospital
401 Haddon Avenue   Camden, NJ 08103   (856)342-2617

Feingold, David Yitzchak, MD {1669571584} Pedtrc(87,ISRA)<NJ-NWRKBETH, NY-BLVUENYU>
+ St Joseph's Medical Center Emergency
703 Main Street   Paterson, NJ 07503   (973)754-2240   Fax (973)754-2249

Feingold, Gail J., MD {1386655199} AdolMd, IntrMd(77,DC01)<NJ-MORRISTN>
+ 70 Brooklawn Drive
Morris Plains, NJ 07950   (973)984-8085   Fax (973)984-0061

Feingold, Jay Marshall, MD {1639512841} Pedtrc
+ Daiichi Sankyo, Inc.
Two Hilton Court   Parsippany, NJ 07054   (973)944-2955   Fax (973)944-2680

Feingold, Katherine Linda, MD {1447476155} Psychy, PsyCAd(00,NJ06)
+ Bartky HealthCare Center, LLC
513 West Mount Pleasant Avenue   Livingston, NJ 07039   (973)533-1195   Fax (973)533-1305

Feingold, Marc Benjamin, MD {1306805015} FamMed, IntrMd(99,NY03)
+ 420 Bridge Plaza Drive
Manalapan, NJ 07726   (732)536-8008   Fax (732)536-8849

Feinstein, David E., DO {1477568707} Rheuma, IntrMd(00,NJ75)<NJ-COOPRUMC>
+ Cooper Rheumatology
900 Centennial Boulevard/Suite 203   Voorhees, NJ 08043   (856)968-7019   Fax (856)482-5621

Feinstein, Richard S., MD {1952383689} RadDia(77,MD07)<NJ-STPETER, NJ-RWJUBRUN>
+ University Radiology Group, P.C.
483 Cranbury Road   East Brunswick, NJ 08816   (732)390-0030   Fax (732)390-5383
+ University Radiology Group, P.C.
10 Plum Street   New Brunswick, NJ 08901   (732)390-0030   Fax (732)249-1208

Feintisch, Adam, MD {1962729863} SrgRec
+ Vanguard Wellness Center
113 West Essex Street/Suite 204   Maywood, NJ 07607   (201)289-5551   Fax (201)843-2390

Feit, David L., MD {1962409045} Gastrn, IntrMd(81,NY01)<NJ-HACKNSK>
+ Hackensack Digestive Diseases Associates, P.A.
52 First Street   Hackensack, NJ 07601   (201)488-3003   Fax (201)488-6911

Feit, Russell, MD {1942613989} PainInvt
+ North American Spine & Pain
310 Central Avenue   East Orange, NJ 07018   (908)425-6574

Feitell, Leonard A., MD {1396745949} CdvDis, IntrMd(76,NY09)<NJ-HCKTSTWN, NJ-STBARNMC>
+ Advanced Cardiology, LLC.
65 Ridgedale Avenue   Cedar Knolls, NJ 07927   (973)401-1100   Fax (973)401-1201

Feld, Ross J., DO {1376749630} EmrgMd
+ 165 Tavistock
Cherry Hill, NJ 08034   (609)206-8877

Feld, Steven M., MD {1538158613} MtFtMd, ObsGyn(76,MA07)<NJ-COOPRUMC, NJ-JRSYSHMC>
+ Cooper University Hospital
One Cooper Plaza/Dorrance/Rm 623   Camden, NJ 08103   (856)342-2000   Fax (856)342-7023
+ The Cooper Hospital System-Univ Hospital
3 Cooper Plaza/Suite 215   Camden, NJ 08103   (856)342-2439

Feldan, Paul E., MD {1063517860} IntrMd, Grtrcs(85,NJ06)
+ Besen-Goldstein Medical Associates PC
1000 Birchfield Drive/Suite 1004   Mount Laurel, NJ 08054   (856)866-1557   Fax (856)231-7955

Felderman, Howard E., MD {1033394366}<NJ-MORRISTN>
+ Morristown Medical Center
100 Madison Avenue   Morristown, NJ 07962   (973)971-5000

Feldman, Alan J., MD {1114961851} ObsGyn(72,PA13)<NJ-ACMCITY, NJ-ACMCMAIN>
+ 53 West Whitehorse Pike
Galloway, NJ 08205   (609)652-7045

Feldman, Alexander, MD {1023381662} NnPnMd
+ Rutgers- New Jersey Medical School
185 South Orange Avenue   Newark, NJ 07103   (973)972-5000

Feldman, Arthur E., MD {1518991934} Urolgy(72,PA13)
+ Somerset Urological Associates PA
72 West End Avenue   Somerville, NJ 08876   (908)927-0300   Fax (908)707-4988

Feldman, Brad Hal, MD {1750554507} Ophthl, IntrMd(NY45)
+ Philadelphia Eye Associates
1113 Hospital Drive/Suite 302   Willingboro, NJ 08046   (609)871-1112

Feldman, David C., MD {1588948392} EmrgMd<NJ-MORRISTN>
+ Morristown Medical Center
100 Madison Avenue/Box 8   Morristown, NJ 07962   (973)971-7926

Feldman, David J., MD {1619990371} SrgOrt, NeuMSptM(72,MA05)<NJ-STCLRDEN, NJ-STCLRDOV>
+ 16 Pocono Road/Suite 100
Denville, NJ 07834   (973)625-5700   Fax (973)625-3381

Feldman, David Nathan, MD {1982667317} SrgOrt(85,NY08)<NJ-ENGLWOOD, NJ-HOLYNAME>
+ Advanced Pain Care
2040 Millburn Avenue   Maplewood, NJ 07040   (908)242-3688   Fax (908)242-3902
+ Active Joints Orthopedics
25 Rockwood Place/Suite 425   Englewood, NJ 07631   (908)242-3688   Fax (201)567-4039

Feldman, Elad, MD {1275686412} Ophthl(03,NY48)<NY-NYEYEINF, NJ-RWJUHAM>
+ Mercer Eye Associates, PA
123 Franklin Corner Road/Suite 207   Lawrenceville, NJ 08648   (609)750-7300   Fax (609)896-7052

Feldman, Jeffrey N., MD {1124081336} VasDis, Nephro, IntrMd(76,PA09)<NJ-OVERLOOK>
+ Union-Plainfield Medical Associates, PA
440 Chestnut Street   Union, NJ 07083   (908)686-9330   Fax (732)686-5614   jfeldmanmd@upmed.com

Feldman, Jenna Aviv, DO {1689136012} SrgOrt
+ SJH Medical Center Orthopedic Surgery
1505 West Sherman Avenue   Vineland, NJ 08360   (856)641-8000

Feldman, Kira, MD {1629071014} Pedtrc(92,BLA02)<NJ-JRSYSHMC, NJ-ATLANCHS>
+ Cedar Bridge Pediatrics
249 South Main Street/Suite 2   Barnegat, NJ 08005   (609)607-1010   Fax (609)607-9992

Feldman, Liliya A., MD {1689714768} PthACl, PthHem(87,UKR14)
+ 26 Chris Court
Fair Lawn, NJ 07410

Feldman, Marc D., MD {1548350242} Otlryg, SrgHnd, SrgPlstc(82,NY15)<NJ-ACMCMAIN, NJ-SHOREMEM>
+ Feldman-Rayfield Cosmetic Surgery, PA
222 New Road/Suite 6   Linwood, NJ 08221   (609)601-1000   Fax (609)601-1010

Feldman, Nathaniel Seth, MD {1558331132} IntrMd, Nephro(83,NY08)<NJ-NWTNMEM>
+ Newton Medical Center
175 High Street/Hospitalist   Newton, NJ 07860   (973)383-2121

Feldman, Russett P., MD {1801942107} Psychy(76,NY46)
+ 16 Holly Drive
Short Hills, NJ 07078   (973)376-7774

Feldman, Ruth S., MD {1750459426} RadDia, Radiol(74,NJ05)
+ Women's Mammography Center
121 State Route 31/Suite 500   Flemington, NJ 08822   (908)782-4700

Feldman, Tamara Lee, MD {1588699755} Pedtrc, PedGst(00,NY15)<NJ-OVERLOOK, NJ-MORRISTN>
+ Overlook Medical Center
99 Beauvoir Avenue/PO Box 210/Pedi GI   Summit, NJ 07902   (908)522-8714
+ Morristown Medical Center
100 Madison Avenue/Pedi GI   Morristown, NJ 07962   (973)971-5676

Feldman, Tatyana A., MD {1578528089} Hemato, IntrMd, MedOnc(92,BLA02)<NY-JTORTHO>
+ John Theurer Cancer Center - HUMC
92 Second Street   Hackensack, NJ 07601   (201)996-3033   Fax (551)996-0573

Feldman-Winter, Lori, MD {1588757025} Pedtrc(86,NY46)<NJ-COOPRUMC>
+ Cooper Peds/Children's Regional Ctr
3 Cooper Plaza/Suite 200   Camden, NJ 08103   (856)342-2472   Fax (856)368-8297
+ The Cooper Hospital System-Univ Hospital
401 Haddon Avenue/Rm 366   Camden, NJ 08103   (856)342-2000

Feldstein, Neil Arthur, MD {1588608186} SrgNro, IntrMd(84,NY19)
+ Neurosurgeons of New Jersey
1200 East Ridgewood Avenue   Ridgewood, NJ 07450   (201)824-6131

Felegi, William B., DO {1760408918} EmrgMd(89,ME75)<NJ-MORRISTN>
+ Morristown Medical Center
100 Madison Avenue/EmrgMed   Morristown, NJ 07962   (973)971-7973   Fax (973)290-7202   william.felegi@ahsys.org
+ Travel MD
95 Madison Avenue/Suite 106   Morristown, NJ 07962   (973)971-7291

Feliberti, Jason Paul, MD {1811215692}
+ 700 Cranbury Cross Road/Apt B
North Brunswick, NJ 08902   (646)360-5611   jfeliberti@gmail.com

Felibrico, Oliver G., MD {1649249715} IntrMd(82,PHIL)<NJ-JRSYSHMC>
+ Jersey Shore University Medical Center
1945 Route 33/Medicine   Neptune, NJ 07753   (732)776-4420   Fax (732)776-3795
+ Hackensack Meridian Medical Group
19 Davis Avenue/5th-6th Floor   Neptune, NJ 07753   (732)776-4420   Fax (732)897-3997

Physicians by Name and Address

Feliciano, Edward, MD {1265587802} SrgOrt(99,NY20)
+ The Orthopedic Health Center
720 Monroe Street/Suite C209 Hoboken, NJ 07030
(201)286-3622

Feliciano, Migdalia, MD {1841533684}
+ Apogee Physicians
201 Lyons Avenue Newark, NJ 07112 (973)926-2164
Fax (214)764-6683

Felig, David M., MD {1780681866} Gastrn, IntrMd(88,IL06)<NJ-HACKNSK>
+ Hackensack Digestive Diseases Associates, P.A.
52 First Street Hackensack, NJ 07601 (201)488-3003
Fax (201)488-6911

Feliksik Watorek, Elzbieta Barbara, MD {1992822936} Pedtrc(79,POL17)<NJ-STPETER>
+ 1145 Bordentown Avenue/Suite 4
Parlin, NJ 08859 (732)553-1901 Fax (732)553-1903

Felipe, Ronald Anthony, MD {1306968805} IntrMd(97,PHI32)<NJ-CHSFULD, NJ-CHSMRCER>
+ Pathlink, LLC
66 West Gilbert Street/Suite 100 Tinton Falls, NJ 07701
(732)212-0060 Fax (732)212-0061

Fellenbaum, Paul, MD {1922063031} Anesth(80,WI06)<NJ-SOMERSET, NJ-STPETER>
+ Anesthesia Consultnts of NJ/Nova Pain
285 Davidson Avenue/Suite 204 Somerset, NJ 08873
(732)271-1400 Fax (732)271-3543

Feller, Matthew F., MD {1659323970} IntrMd(80,NY01)<NJ-HOLY-NAME, NJ-ENGLWOOD>
+ 1475 Bergen Boulevard/Suite 16
Fort Lee, NJ 07024 (201)461-4852 Fax (201)461-6018

Fellman, Damon M., MD {1982671830} Nrolgy(70,OH41)<NJ-HACKNSK, NJ-HOLYNAME>
+ Hackensack Neurology Group
211 Essex Street/Suite 202 Hackensack, NJ 07601
(201)488-1515 Fax (201)488-9471

Fellman, Katherine, MD {1528387396} EmrgMd
+ Capital Emergency Physicians & Associates
One Capital Way Pennington, NJ 08534 (800)637-2374

Fellmeth, Wayne G., MD {1891769857} Pedtrc(81,DC02)<NJ-HUNTRDN>
+ Hunterdon Pediatric Associates
6 Sand Hill Road/Suite 202 Flemington, NJ 08822
(908)782-6700 Fax (908)788-5661

Fellows, Wayne, DO {1265869952} FamMed
+ Patient first Urgent Care
630 Mantua Pike Woodbury, NJ 08096 (856)812-2220
Fax (856)812-2221

Felman, Rina Lita, MD {1447447750} RadDia(95,MA07)<NJ-HOLY-NAME>
+ Holy Name Hospital
718 Teaneck Road/Radiology Teaneck, NJ 07666
(201)833-3000

Felsen, Alan K., MD {1619979317} IntrMd(74,NY47)<NJ-HACKNSK, NJ-HOLYNAME>
+ 344 Prospect Street
Hackensack, NJ 07601 (201)342-2771 Fax (201)342-8377

Felsenstein, Bruce W., MD {1821048273} EmrgMd, Pedtrc, IntrMd(83,NY08)<NJ-VALLEY>
+ The Valley Hospital
223 North Van Dien Avenue/EmrgMed Ridgewood, NJ 07450 (201)447-8300 Fax (201)447-8174

Felsenstein, Roberta G., MD {1245453646} ObsGyn(98,PA07)
+ Advocare Premier Ob/Gyn of South Jersey
903 Sheppard Road Voorhees, NJ 08043 (856)772-2300
Fax (856)772-2301

Felser, James M., MD {1821335043} IntrMd, InfDis(79,CA14)
+ Novartis Pharmaceuticals Corporation
59 Route 10 East Hanover, NJ 07936 (973)503-7500

Felton, Stephen M., MD {1083627806} Ophthl(76,NJ06)
+ The Princeton Eye Group
419 North Harrison Street/Suite 104 Princeton, NJ 08540
(609)921-9437 Fax (609)921-0277
+ The Princeton Eye Group
1600 Perrinville Road Monroe Township, NJ 08831
(609)921-9437 Fax (609)655-3685
+ The Princeton Eye Group
900 Eastern Avenue/Suite 50 Somerset, NJ 08540
(732)565-9550 Fax (732)565-0946

Feltz, John P., MD {1619928934} ObsGyn(80,NJ06)<NJ-MORRISTN, NJ-STCLRDEN>
+ Women's Care Source
111 Madison Avenue/Suite 308 Morristown, NJ 07960
(973)285-0400 Fax (973)285-9848

Felzenberg, Emily R., DO {1063684702} IntrMd(05,NY75)
+ JFK Medical Center
65 James Street/Hospitalists Edison, NJ 08820 (732)321-7000

Felzenberg, Jeffrey D., MD {1083719165} IntrMd(78,MEX03)<NJ-MONMOUTH>
+ 23 White Street
Shrewsbury, NJ 07702 (732)747-1555 Fax (732)741-8262

Femino, Frank Placido, MD {1487683645} SrgOrt, SrgOARec, IntrMd(90,NJ05)<NJ-CLARMAAS>
+ Femino-Ducey Orthopaedic Group
45 Franklin Avenue Nutley, NJ 07110 (973)751-0111
Fax (973)235-0110

Fendley, Ann Ehrke, MD {1346305851} IntrMd(71,OR02)
+ Open Air MRI
430 Memorial Parkway/Suite 2 Phillipsburg, NJ 08865
(908)213-3600 Fax (908)213-3601

Fendrick, Jeffrey Scott, MD {1093739385} Pedtrc(88,PA02)<PA-CHOPHIL, PA-CHESTRCT>
+ Primary Care at Gibbsboro
13 South Lakeview Drive Gibbsboro, NJ 08026 (856)783-2802 Fax (856)783-2806

Feng, Bo, MD {1669672994} PthAna, PthHem<NJ-STBARNMC>
+ St. Barnabas Medical Center
94 Old Short Hills Road/PathLabMed Livingston, NJ 07039
(973)322-2772 Fax (973)322-8917

Feng, David H., MD {1659465896} RadV&I, Radiol(96,PA09)<NJ-OCEANMC>
+ Center for Vein Restoration
1015 New Road/Suite D Northfield, NJ 08225 (844)897-6159 Fax (609)677-6032
+ Center for Vein Restoration
456 Chestnut Street/Suite 301 Lakewood, NJ 08701
(844)897-6159 Fax (732)987-6715
+ 200 Tilton Road/Unit G-5
Northfield, NJ 08225 Fax (609)484-0894

Feng, Jing Jing, MD {1003177676} Ophthl
+ 680 Broadway/Suite 114
Paterson, NJ 07514 (973)742-4747

Feng, Shufang, MD {1285686667} IntrMd(83,CHNA)<NJ-BAYSHORE, NJ-RIVERVW>
+ The Doctor's Office
1070 Highway 34/Suite C Matawan, NJ 07747 (732)290-0300 Fax (732)290-9661

Fenichel, Stefan, MD {1750685848} Dermat, FamMed(76,IREL)<NJ-ACMCITY, NJ-ACMCMAIN>
+ Community Health Care Inc
53 South Laurel Street Bridgeton, NJ 08302 (856)451-4700 Fax (856)453-8495

Fenkart, Douglas R., MD {1205895224} Pedtrc(91,NJ05)<NJ-VALLEY>
+ Bergen West Pediatric Center, PA
541 Cedar Hill Avenue Wyckoff, NJ 07481 (201)652-0300
Fax (201)444-6209

Fenkel, Jonathan M., MD {1811031222} Gastrn
+ 17 West Red Bank Avenue/Suite 302
Woodbury, NJ 08096

Fennell, Vernard Sharif, MD {1801152244} SrgNro
+ Capital Institute for Neurosciences
2 Capital Way/Suite 456 Pennington, NJ 08534 (609)537-7300 Fax (609)537-7301

Fennelly, Bryan William, MD {1669588406} PsyCAd, Psychy(89,NJ05)<NJ-MORRISTN>
+ 8 Shunpike Road
Madison, NJ 07940 (973)660-0084 Fax (973)966-0332

Fenster, Gerald F., MD {1568441970} Otlryg, OtgyFPIS(65,NY09)
+ ENT & Allergy Associates-Bridgewater
245 US Highway 22/3rd Fl/Suite 300 Bridgewater, NJ 08807
(908)722-1022 Fax (908)722-5122

Fenster, William R., MD {1841482635} Pedtrc<NJ-COMMED, NJ-OCEANMC>
+ 1201 River Road/Unit 10
Lakewood, NJ 08701 (732)775-0222 Fax (732)775-0224

Fenyar, Bonnie Ann M., MD {1669504478} PsyFor, Psychy, IntrMd(87,ANT01)
+ AtlantiCare Regional Med Ctr/Mainland
65 West Jimmie Leeds Road/Psychiatry Pomona, NJ 08240
(609)652-1000

Feoli, Enrique Alfredo, MD {1629097852} Nrolgy(93,ARG02)
+ Northeast Regional Epilepsy Group
20 Prospect Avenue/Suite 800 Hackensack, NJ 07601
(201)343-6676 Fax (201)343-6689

Ferber, Andres, MD {1841213048} OncHem, IntrMd(URU01)
+ The Cooper Health System at Voorhees
900 Centennial Boulevard Voorhees, NJ 08043 (856)673-4215 Fax (856)673-4286

Ferdinand, Brett D., MD {1588701213} RadDia(01,NY19)
+ 4 Brighton Road/Suite 200
Clifton, NJ 07012 (973)284-0020 Fax (973)284-6310

Ferdinand, Michel-Ange, MD {1770686289} GenPrc, FamMed(74,HAI01)<NJ-EASTORNG, NJ-TRININPC>
+ La Familia Medical Care
115 Jefferson Avenue Elizabeth, NJ 07201 (908)351-6663
Fax (908)351-1760
+ 60 Evergreen Place/Suite 307
East Orange, NJ 07018 (973)675-0097

Ferdinand, Pascale, MD {1487067856} FamMed
+ La Familia Medical Care
115 Jefferson Avenue Elizabeth, NJ 07201 (908)447-7221
Fax (908)351-6663

Ferencz, Gerald J., MD {1275583379} Nrolgy, SlpDis, VasNeu(80,PA07)<NJ-COMMED, NJ-OCEANMC>
+ Shore Neurology, P.A.
633 Route 37 West Toms River, NJ 08755 (732)240-4787
Fax (732)240-3114
+ Shore Neurology, PA
1613 Route 88/Suite 3 Brick, NJ 08724 (732)240-4787
Fax (732)785-2599

Ferenz, Clint C., MD {1104805647} SrgOrt, OrtSHand(82,NY08)<NJ-JRSYSHMC>
+ Orthopaedic Institute of Central Jersey
2315A Highway 34/Suite D Manasquan, NJ 08736
(732)974-0404 Fax (732)974-2653
+ Orthopaedic Institute of Central Jersey
226 Highway 37 West/Suite 203 Toms River, NJ 08755
(732)974-0404 Fax (732)240-5329
+ Orthopaedic Institute of Central Jersey
365 Broad Street Red Bank, NJ 08736 (732)933-4300
Fax (732)933-1444

Feret, Eve Anne, MD {1356338875} GenPrc(80,MEX14)
+ 4121-B New York Avenue
Union City, NJ 07087 (201)319-9722 Fax (201)319-1707

Ferges, Mitchell L., MD {1407853310} Gastrn, IntrMd(75,NJ06)<NJ-STPETER, NJ-RWJUBRUN>
+ Digestive Disease Center of New Jersey, LLC
33 Clyde Road/Suite 102 Somerset, NJ 08873 (732)873-9200 Fax (732)873-1699
+ Digestive Disease Center of New Jersey, LLC
810 Ryders Lane East Brunswick, NJ 08816 (732)873-9200
Fax (732)257-0229
+ Cares Surgicenter, LLC.
240 Easton Avenue New Brunswick, NJ 08873 (732)565-5400 Fax (732)296-8677

Ferges, William James, MD {1982909040} Gastrn, IntrMd
+ Digestive Disease Center of New Jersey, LLC
33 Clyde Road/Suite 102 Somerset, NJ 08873 (732)873-9200 Fax (732)873-1699

Ferlise, Kathleen M., MD {1174742712} CdvDis, SrgThr, Surgry(79,ITAL)<NJ-DEBRAHLC>
+ Deborah Heart and Lung Center
200 Trenton Road Browns Mills, NJ 08015 (609)893-6611
Fax (609)735-0175

Ferlise, Victor J., MD {1528088861} Urolgy(01,NJ06)<NJ-COMMED>
+ Urologic Health Center of New Jersey
67 Route 37 West/Building 2/Suite 1 Toms River, NJ 08755
(732)914-1300 Fax (732)914-0849
+ Urologic Health Center of New Jersey
63C Lacey Road Whiting, NJ 08759 (732)914-1300 Fax (732)350-7054
+ Urologic Health Center of New Jersey
949 Lacey Road Forked River, NJ 08755 (609)242-6930
Fax (609)242-6932

Fermaglich, Matis A., MD {1386603785} Urolgy(64,BEL07)<NJ-HOLYNAME>
+ Urology Specialty Care, P.A.
630 East Palisade Avenue Englewood Cliffs, NJ 07632
(201)837-0606 Fax (201)837-1319

Fermin, Carlos Miguel, MD {1043534506} IntrMd, IntHos(05,DOM02)<NJ-JRSYCITY>
+ Jersey City Medical Center
355 Grand Street/Medicine Jersey City, NJ 07304
(201)915-2160 Fax (201)915-2219

Fernandes, Gregory M., MD {1417012337} Pthlgy, PthACl, PthCyt(73,INA67)<NJ-STMRYPAS>
+ St. Mary's Hospital
350 Boulevard/Pathology Passaic, NJ 07055 (973)365-4300

Fernandes, Jaxon James, MD {1073675740} IntrMd<NJ-CLARMAAS>
+ Clara Maass Medical Center
1 Clara Maass Drive Belleville, NJ 07109 (973)450-2000

Fernandes, John, MD {1073589883} CdvDis, Pedtrc, PedCrd(82,QU01)<NJ-MTNSIDE, NJ-NWRKBETH>
+ 349 East Northfield Avenue/Suite 201
Livingston, NJ 07039 (973)533-1031 Fax (973)533-1033

Fernandes, Margaret C., MD {1982682696} NnPnMd, Pedtrc(74,INDI)<NJ-OURLADY>
+ Our Lady of Lourdes Medical Center
1600 Haddon Avenue/Neonatology Camden, NJ 08103
(856)757-3826
fernandesm@lourdesnet.org

Fernandes, Michael Alexandre, MD {1861656076} EmrgMd
+ Cooper Univerisry Emergency Physicians
One Cooper Plaza Camden, NJ 08103 (856)342-2000
Fax (856)968-8272

Fernandes, Rinet Philomena, MD {1104036680} Pedtrc(96,INA94)<NJ-STJOSHOS>
+ St. Joseph's Pediatrics DePaul Center
11 Getty Avenue/2nd Floor Paterson, NJ 07503 (973)754-2727

Physicians by Name and Address

Fernandez, Afranio L., MD {1720086465} Anesth(63,COLO)<NJ-STJOSHOS>
+ St. Joseph's Regional Medical Center Anesthesia
 703 Main Street   Paterson, NJ 07503   (973)754-2323   Fax (973)977-9455

Fernandez, Ann Marie, DO {1356572507}
+ Rowan University-School of Osteopathic Medicine
 1 Medical Center Drive   Stratford, NJ 08084   (856)566-6708

Fernandez, Carlos O., MD {1720074362} MtFtMd, NnPnMd, ObsGyn(89,MA07)<NJ-JRSYSHMC, NJ-RIVERVW>
+ 1416 Hooper Avenue/Suite 1
 Toms River, NJ 08753

Fernandez, Christine Alison, MD {1053340513} EmrgMd(02,NJ05)<NJ-HACKNSK>
+ Hackensack University Medical Center
 30 Prospect Avenue/EmrgMed   Hackensack, NJ 07601   (201)996-2300   Fax (201)968-1866

Fernandez, Claudio Miguel, DO {1891081881} EmrgMd
+ Rowan University-School of Osteopathic Medicine
 1 Medical Center Drive   Stratford, NJ 08084   (856)566-6708

Fernandez, Eduardo E., MD {1174589493} OncHem(89,NJ06)<NJ-VIRTMHBC, NJ-LOURDMED>
+ Lourdes Medical Associates Hematology Oncology
 101 Burrs Road/Suite C   Westampton, NJ 08060   (609)702-7550   Fax (609)702-1277
+ Lourdes Medical Associates Hematology Oncology
 1 Brace Road/Suite B   Cherry Hill, NJ 08034   (609)702-7550   Fax (609)702-1277

Fernandez, Edwin Paras, MD {1891860524} IntrMd(83,PHI01)<NJ-ANCPSYCH>
+ Ancora Psychiatric Hospital
 301 Spring Garden Road/Internal Med   Hammonton, NJ 08037   (609)561-1700

Fernandez, Fredy A., MD {1932329570} Pedtrc(76,BOL01)<NJ-JRSYCITY>
+ Metropolitan Family Health Network
 935 Garfield Avenue   Jersey City, NJ 07304   (201)478-5800   Fax (201)478-5856

Fernandez, Gregory Scott, MD {1194927863} Psychy
+ Princetown House Behavioral Health
 615 Hope Road/1B, 2nd flr.   Eatontown, NJ 07724   (848)208-2600   Fax (848)208-2601
+ Princeton House Behavioral Health - Princeton
 905 Herrontown Road   Princeton, NJ 08540   (848)208-2600   Fax (609)497-3370

Fernandez, Jacinto J., MD {1578567103} ObsGyn, IntrMd(67,GRNA)<NJ-HOLYNAME>
+ 222 Cedar Lane/Suite 207
 Teaneck, NJ 07666   (201)833-7087   Fax (201)833-7123

Fernandez, Jacqueline A., MD {1982628335} IntrMd(91,PA09)<NJ-OVERLOOK>
+ 2027 Morris Avenue
 Union, NJ 07083   (908)810-9147   Fax (908)688-7518

Fernandez, Manuel A., MD {1487619144} Anesth(71,PHIL)<NJ-RBAYPERT>
+ Raritan Bay Medical Center/Perth Amboy Division
 530 New Brunswick Avenue   Perth Amboy, NJ 08861   (732)442-3700

Fernandez, Maria Elmina, MD {1891047957} Nrolgy, IntrMd(91,PHI09)
+ Salem Inernal Medicine
 316 Merion Avenue   Carneys Point, NJ 08069   (856)299-0345   Fax (856)299-9438

Fernandez, Marlyn A., MD {1124253752} EnDbMt, IntrMd(06,DOM11)<NJ-HACKNSK>
+ Forest HealthCare Associates, PC
 277 Forest Avenue/Suite 200   Paramus, NJ 07652   (201)986-1881   Fax (201)986-1871
+ Hackensack UMG
 150 Overlook Avenue   Hackensack, NJ 07601   (201)986-1881   Fax (201)489-1898

Fernandez, Osbert, MD {1740252477} ObsGyn, Gyneco(97,GRN01)<NJ-HOBUNIMC>
+ Horizon Health Center
 714 Bergen Avenue   Jersey City, NJ 07306   (201)451-6300

Fernandez, Ricardo J., MD {1114080215} Psychy, PsyCAd, Psyphm(79,NJ06)
+ Princeton Family Care Associates, LLC
 12 Roszel Road/Suite A-103   Princeton, NJ 08540   (609)419-0123   Fax (609)419-0126

Fernandez, Richard E., MD {1376530113} RadDia, RadNro(79,NY19)<NJ-SOCEANCO, NJ-COMMED>
+ Southern Ocean County Medical Center
 1140 Route 72 West   Manahawkin, NJ 08050   (609)597-6011
+ Ocean Medical Imaging Center
 21 Stockton Drive   Toms River, NJ 08754   (609)597-6011   Fax (732)505-0325
+ Community Medical Center
 99 Route 37 West   Toms River, NJ 08050   (732)557-8000

Fernandez, Ronald Leonardo, MD {1942373345} EmrgMd(01,NJ05)<NJ-JFKMED>
+ JFK Medical Center
 65 James Street/Emergency   Edison, NJ 08820   (732)321-7000

Fernandez, Sofia Ramona, MD {1174678114} FamMed(99,GRN01)<NJ-STCLRDEN>
+ Washington Family Medicine PC
 191 US Highway 206   Flanders, NJ 07836   (973)584-0045   Fax (973)584-0094

Fernandez, Yocasta Mabel, MD {1316909674} Pedtrc(89,DOM11)<NJ-STJOSHOS, NJ-STMRYPAS>
+ Kind Care Pediatrics
 289 Monroe Street/2nd Floor   Passaic, NJ 07055   (973)574-8688

Fernandez Ginorio, Enoc Jose, MD {1205102464}<NJ-UMDNJ>
+ University Hospital
 150 Bergen Street   Newark, NJ 07103   (973)972-5672   Fax (973)972-0365

Fernandez Ledon, Ramon A., MD {1083621460} Gastrn, IntrMd(82,SPA22)<NY-MTSINYHS>
+ Advanced Gastroenterology Group
 1308 Morris Avenue   Union, NJ 07083   (908)851-2770   Fax (908)851-7706

Fernandez Santiago, Angela, DO {1942664511} FamMed
+ Center for Adult Medicine & Preventive Care
 293 Passaic Street   Passaic, NJ 07055   (973)859-9165   Fax (973)773-0336

Fernandez-Cos, Henry, MD {1881698157} ObsGyn(79,SPA06)<NJ-HOBUNIMC, NJ-CHRIST>
+ Women's Health Partners, PC
 419 66th Street   West New York, NJ 07093   (201)861-9229   Fax (201)861-9272
+ WomenÆs Health Partners, Cliffside Park
 574 Anderson Avenue   Cliffside Park, NJ 07010   (201)861-9229   Fax (201)943-4839

Fernandez-Moure, Joseph L., MD {1174693006} Pedtrc(80,SPA06)<NJ-STBARNMC>
+ Elmora Pediatrics
 425 Westfield Avenue   Elizabeth, NJ 07208   (908)351-7584   Fax (908)351-0914

Fernandez-Obregon, Adolfo C., MD {1316944051} Dermat, SrgDer, DerImm(78,NY09)<NJ-HOBUNIMC, NJ-CHRIST>
+ Hudson Dermatology & Skin Cancer Center
 10 Church Towers   Hoboken, NJ 07030   (201)795-3376   Fax (201)795-5515

Fernandez-Piparo, May Anne Malinis, MD {1275768798} Anesth
+ Summit Anesthesia Associates, P.A.
 33 Overlook Road/Suite 311   Summit, NJ 07901   (908)598-1500   Fax (908)598-0197

Fernando, Chandani D., MD {1679513501} InfDis, IntrMd(90,DMN01)<NJ-UNVMCPRN>
+ Princeton Primary and Urgent Care Center LLC
 707 Alexander Road/Suite 201   Princeton, NJ 08540   (609)919-0009   Fax (609)919-0008

Fernando, Rosario P., MD {1437153897} Anesth(69,PHI09)<NJ-EASTORNG>
+ 4 Clarken Drive
 West Orange, NJ 07052

Fernando-Flores, Avelina M., MD {1104899582} IntrMd(70,PHIL)
+ Comprehensive Medical Associates
 411 Route 9/Suite 6   Lanoka Harbor, NJ 08734   (609)971-1711   Fax (609)971-3390

Fernbach, Barry R., MD {1427076736} Hemato, IntrMd, MedOnc(71,MA01)<NJ-VALLEY>
+ Valley Medical Group-Hematology/Oncology
 One Valley Health Plaza   Paramus, NJ 07652   (201)634-5353   Fax (201)986-4702

Fernicola, Charles P., MD {1063472694} Urolgy(82,NJ05)<NJ-OCEANMC>
+ 1145 Beacon Avenue
 Manahawkin, NJ 08050   (609)597-1991   Fax (609)597-8198
+ 730 Lacey Road
 Forked River, NJ 08731   (609)971-3213

Fernicola, Joseph Robert, MD {1063467314} IntrMd(95,NY47)<NJ-VALLEY>
+ Valley Medical Group
 470 North Franklin Turnpike   Ramsey, NJ 07446   (201)327-8765   Fax (201)327-8496

Fernicola, Richard G., MD {1487723615} PhysMd(92,NJ05)<NJ-JRSYSHMC, NJ-OCEANMC>
+ PO Box 334
 Allenhurst, NJ 07711   (732)660-0202
+ 1451 Route 88 West/Suite 5
 Brick, NJ 08723   (732)785-9552

Ferra, Michael John, MD {1427391457} RadDia
+ One Nancy Road
 Marlboro, NJ 07746   (908)907-0038

Ferrante, Christopher R., MD {1013904416} SrgOrt(96,NJ05)<NJ-WARREN>
+ Orthopedic Associates of Greater Lehigh Valley
 755 Memorial Parkway/Suite 101   Phillipsburg, NJ 08865   (908)859-5585   Fax (908)859-3990
+ Coordinated Health
 222 Red Lane   Phillipsburg, NJ 08865   (908)859-5585   Fax (610)849-1013

Ferrante, Daniel P., MD {1316998859} ObsGyn(87,NJ06)
+ Women's Care Source
 111 Madison Avenue/Suite 308   Morristown, NJ 07960   (973)285-0400   Fax (973)285-9848

Ferrante, Francis L., MD {1134204779} IntrMd, Pedtrc(77,NJ05)<NJ-STJOSHOS>
+ West Paterson Family Medical Center
 1031 McBride Avenue/Suite D109   West Paterson, NJ 07424   (973)785-4020   Fax (973)785-3186
+ West Paterson Family Medical Center
 154 Union Avenue   Paterson, NJ 07502   (973)942-3618

Ferrante, Jeanne Min-Li, MD {1659302941} FamMed(87,PA02)<NJ-RWJUBRUN, NJ-UMDNJ>
+ University Hospital-New Jersey Medical School
 30 Bergen Street/ADMC 1205   Newark, NJ 07107   (973)972-0037

Ferrante, Maurice Andrew, MD {1437154192} IntrMd(87,PA02)<NJ-OVERLOOK>
+ Summit Medical Group
 34 Mountain Boulevard   Warren, NJ 07059   (908)561-8600   Fax (908)561-7265

Ferrante, Robyn, MD {1669416665} Pedtrc(96,NJ06)
+ Somerset Pediatric Group PA
 155 Union Avenue   Bridgewater, NJ 08807   (908)725-1802   Fax (908)203-8825

Ferrari, Albert N., MD {1346280138} Anesth(77,IL06)<NJ-VIRTMHBC>
+ Burlington Anesthesia Associates
 120 Madison Ave/Suite E/PO Box 174   Mount Holly, NJ 08060   (609)261-1660   Fax (609)261-1779

Ferrari, Anna C., MD {1316948268} IntrMd, MedOnc, OncHem(74,URUG)
+ Rutgers Cancer Institute of New Jersey
 195 Little Albany Street/PO Box 2681   New Brunswick, NJ 08903   (732)235-2465   Fax (732)235-6797

Ferrari, Arthur J., MD {1932196482} Otlryg(75,DC02)<NJ-SJERSYHS>
+ 112 South East Avenue
 Vineland, NJ 08360   (856)692-5516   Fax (856)692-3799

Ferraris, Ambra, MD {1255578399} PulDis, IntrMd(00,DOM11)<NJ-MORRISTN>
+ JFK Medical Center
 65 James Street/Med/Pulm   Edison, NJ 08820   (732)321-7660

Ferraro, Donna J., MD {1760414882} PhysMd, IntrMd(88,MEX03)<NJ-HOLYNAME>
+ 31 Pine Lake Terrace
 River Vale, NJ 07675   (201)316-5325   Fax (201)505-1767
 ddjrf3@gmail.com

Ferraro, Frank James, Jr., MD {1891764478} SrgPlstc, Surgry, IntrMd(88,NJ05)<NJ-VALLEY, NJ-CLARMAAS>
+ Plastic Surgery Specialists of New Jersey
 2 Sears Drive/Suite 103   Paramus, NJ 07652   (201)664-8000
 frankferraro@email.com

Ferraro, Lisa, MD {1659302925} IntrMd(84,DMN01)<NJ-STJOSHOS>
+ Ferraro Medical Associates
 414 Broadway   Paterson, NJ 07501   (973)742-1761   Fax (973)742-2033
 Ferraro@attglobal.net

Ferraz, Ricardo J. P., MD {1275505844} Pedtrc(78,POR02)<NJ-STBARNMC>
+ 374 Chestnut Street/Suite A
 Newark, NJ 07105   (973)690-5995   Fax (973)589-2405
 RICJFERRAZ-PRF@yahoo.com

Ferrazzo-Weller, Marissa G., DO {1780943001} IntrMd(09,NY75)<NY-NYACKHOS>
+ Summit Medical Group
 6 Brighton Road/2 FL   Clifton, NJ 07012   (973)777-7911   Fax (973)777-5403

Ferreira, Gabriela Simoes, MD {1972673549} IntrMd(92,NH01)<NJ-RWJUBRUN>
+ UH- Robert Wood Johnson Med
 125 Paterson Street/IntMed   New Brunswick, NJ 08901   (732)235-7145
 ferreiga@umdnj.edu

Ferrer, Angel Salvador, MD {1497724819} Pedtrc(00,RI01)<NJ-STJOSHOS>
+ Passaic Pediatrics PA
 298 Passaic Street   Passaic, NJ 07055   (973)249-8100   Fax (973)249-8110
+ Passaic Pediatrics PA
 200 Gregory Street/2nd Floor   Passaic, NJ 07055   (973)249-8100   Fax (973)249-8110

Physicians by Name and Address

Ferrer, Gerrard F. A., DO {1689719353} PthNro, Nrolgy(95,NY75)
+ Hudson Neurosciences, PC
605 Broadway Bayonne, NJ 07002 (201)339-6531 Fax (201)339-6536
+ Hudson Neurosciences PC
142 Palisade Avenue/Suite 205 Jersey City, NJ 07306 (201)339-6531 Fax (201)216-9211

Ferrer, Steven Michael, MD {1346590924} PhyMPain, IntrMd(08,NJ05)
+ Progressive Spine & Sports Medicine
48 South Franklin Turnpike/Suite 101 Ramsey, NJ 07446 (201)962-9199 Fax (201)962-9198
info@progressivespineandsports.com

Ferrer, Waldo L., MD {1881772978} IntrMd
+ Valley Health Medical Group
780 Cedar Lane Teaneck, NJ 07666 (201)836-7664 Fax (201)836-5710

Ferreras, Jessie A.M., MD {1548205404} FamMed(82,PHI01)<NJ-VALLEY>
+ Valley Medical Group
140 Franklin Turnpike/Suite 6-A Waldwick, NJ 07463 (201)447-3603 Fax (201)447-5184
FERRJE@valleyhealth.com

Ferretti, James Christian, DO {1821395955} RadDia(06,PA78)<NY-NASSAUMC>
+ Atlantic Medical Imaging, LLC.
72 West Jimmie Leeds Road Galloway, NJ 08205 (732)433-1087 Fax (609)653-8764

Ferrier, Austin Seymour, DO {1477604270} IntrMd, CdvDis(97,NJ75)
+ Morris Heart Associates PA
400 Valley Road/Suite 102 Mount Arlington, NJ 07856 (973)770-7899 Fax (973)770-7840

Ferro, Joseph James, MD {1679692008} IntrMd(85,NJ05)<NJ-RWJUBRUN>
+ Johnson & Johnson
1 Johnson & Johnson/EmpHlth Rm5G32 New Brunswick, NJ 08933 (732)524-3000 Fax (732)828-5493

Ferrone, George J., MD {1023093101} RadDia(95,NY15)<NJ-HACKNSK>
+ Hackensack University Medical Center
30 Prospect Avenue/Radiology Hackensack, NJ 07601 (201)996-2000 Fax (201)489-2812
+ Hackensack Radiology Group, P.A.
30 Prospect Avenue Hackensack, NJ 07601 (201)996-2000 Fax (201)336-8451

Ferroni, Bryan R., DO {1508836339} IntrMd, CritCr, PulCCr(94,PA77)
+ Carlos A. Obregon, D.O., P.C.
100A Kings Way West Sewell, NJ 08080 (856)218-8080 Fax (856)218-8070

Fersel, Jordan S., MD {1881685519} Anesth, PainMd(84,NY47)<NJ-TRININPC>
+ Center for Pain Relief
138 West 8th Street/Suite 5 Bayonne, NJ 07002 (201)243-9140
info@njcenterforpainrelief.com

Ferstandig, Russell A., MD {1780779702} Psychy(75,NJ05)
+ 2446 Church Road
Toms River, NJ 08753

Fertakos, Roy J., MD {1356448773} RadDia, Radiol, IntrMd(89,NJ06)<NJ-STBARNMC>
+ Imaging Consultants of Essex
94 Old Short Hills Road Livingston, NJ 07039 (973)322-5800 Fax (973)322-5536

Fertels, Scott H., DO {1871544718} CdvDis, IntrMd(92,NJ75)<NJ-OURLADY, NJ-KMHTURNV>
+ Cardiovascular Associates of The Delaware Valley, PA
1840 Frontage Road Cherry Hill, NJ 08034 (856)795-2227 Fax (856)795-7436
+ Cardiovascular Associates
210 West Atlantic Avenue Haddon Heights, NJ 08035 (856)795-2227 Fax (856)547-5337
+ Cardiovascular Associates of The Delaware Valley, PA
570 Egg Harbor Road/Suite B-1 Sewell, NJ 08034 (856)582-2000 Fax (856)582-2061

Fertig, Brian J., MD {1528119146} EnDbMt, IntrMd(88,GRN01)<NJ-JFKMED, NJ-RWJURAH>
+ Diabetes & Osteoporosis Center
20 Wills Way Piscataway, NJ 08854 (732)562-0027 Fax (732)562-0041

Fesnak, Susan Gail, DO {1043436371} FamMed(83,PA77)
+ 2 Riverside Drive/1 Port/Suite 401
Camden, NJ 08103 (856)614-2870 Fax (856)614-2575

Fessler, Sue Atherton, MD {1174512636} IntrMd, CritCr, PulDis(95,MA07)<NJ-ATLANTHS, NJ-MORRISTN>
+ Pulmonary & Allergy Associates
1 Springfield Avenue/Suite 3-A Summit, NJ 07901 (908)934-0555 Fax (908)934-0556
+ Pulmonary & Allergy Associates
8 Saddle Road/Suite 101 Cedar Knolls, NJ 07927

(908)934-0555 Fax (973)540-0472

Festa, Alfredo Gerardo, MD {1013131861} Otlryg(63,ARG01)<NJ-HOBUNIMC>
+ 4508 Kennedy Boulevard
Union City, NJ 07087 (201)864-3168 Fax (201)864-4488
+ 451 Clifton Avenue
Clifton, NJ 07011 (973)340-8787

Festa, Anthony Nmi, MD {1154455947} SprtMd, SrgOrt(02,NJ06)<NJ-STJOSHOS, NJ-WAYNEGEN>
+ New Jersey Orthopaedic Institute
504 Valley Road/Suite 200 Wayne, NJ 07470 (973)694-2690 Fax (973)694-2762
anthonyfestamd@gmail.com

Festa, Christopher James, MD {1366430266} PedCrC, Pedtrc(89,PA07)<NJ-VIRTVOOR>
+ Virtua Voorhees
100 Bowman Drive Voorhees, NJ 08043 (856)782-3300 Fax (267)425-9331

Festa, Eugene Daniel, MD {1629395629} IntrMd
+ Complete Medical & Skin Caree, LLC
245 Diamond Bridge Avenue Hawthorne, NJ 07506 (973)427-0600 Fax (973)427-0604
+ The Valley Hospital
223 North Van Dien Avenue Ridgewood, NJ 07450 (201)447-8000

Festa, Michelle G., MD {1679662712} FamMed(90,PA07)
+ Cooper Family Medicine
1001-F Lincoln Drive West Marlton, NJ 08053 (856)810-1800 Fax (856)810-1879

Festa, Steven, MD {1467433813} RadV&I, RadDia(94,NJ05)<NJ-STLAWRN, NJ-STJOSHOS>
+ Point View Radiology Associates
246 Hamburg Turnpike/Suite 101 Wayne, NJ 07470 (973)904-0404 Fax (973)904-0423

Feteiha, Muhammad S., MD {1447241567} SrgAbd, SrgLap, SrgVas(95,MA07)<NJ-TRINIWSC, NJ-OVERLOOK>
+ Advanced Surgical Associates LLC
155 Morris Avenue/2nd Floor Springfield, NJ 07081 (973)232-2300 Fax (973)232-2301
+ Ambulatory Surgical Center of Union County
950 West Chestnut Street/Suite 200 Union, NJ 07083 (973)232-2300 Fax (908)688-7424

Feuer, Elizabeth Janet, MD {1053461467} Psychy(79,CT01)
+ 29 State Highway No 34
Colts Neck, NJ 07722 (732)780-9119

Feuer Razin, Zippora, DO {1639227796} Psychy(02,NY75)
+ Palisades General Hospital Mental Health Center
7101 Kennedy Boulevard North Bergen, NJ 07047 (201)854-0500

Feurdean, Mirela Cristina, MD {1629040423} IntrMd(95,ROM02)
+ Community Health Center at Vauxhall
3 Farrington Street Vauxhall, NJ 07088 (908)598-7950 Fax (908)686-1163

Fialkoff, Cheryl N., MD {1376636852} Dermat, IntrMd(86,NY46)
+ Affiliated Dermatologists
182 South Street/Suite 1 Morristown, NJ 07960 (973)267-0300 Fax (973)695-1480
+ Affiliated Dermatology
Town Centre 66/Suite 301 Succasunna, NJ 07876 (973)267-0300 Fax (973)927-7512
+ Affiliated Dermatology
14 Church Street Liberty Corner, NJ 07960 (973)267-0300 Fax (908)604-8544

Fianko, Felix Akwasi-Owusu, MD {1982645750} Anesth(02,NY45)
+ Jersery Shore Anesthesiology
1945 Highway 33 Neptune, NJ 07753 (732)897-0200 Fax (732)897-0263

Fibison, Diana, MD {1932479706}
+ Somerset Family Practice
110 Rehill Avenue Somerville, NJ 08876 (908)685-2900 Fax (908)704-3764

Fiderer, Stefanie C., DO {1720259856} Pedtrc(88,NJ75)<NJ-VIRTMHBC, NJ-VIRTUAHS>
+ Advocare Laurel Pediatrics
269 Fish Pond Road Sewell, NJ 08080 (856)863-9999 Fax (856)863-9666

Fiedler, Joel Mark, MD {1346259363} AlgyImmn, Pedtrc(81,NY06)
+ CHOP Pediatric & Adolescent Specialty Care Center
1012 Laurel Oak Road Voorhees, NJ 08043 (856)435-0086 Fax (856)435-0091

Fiel, Stanley Bruce, MD {1497727697} IntrMd, PulDis(73,PA07)<NJ-MORRISTN, NJ-OVERLOOK>
+ Morristown Medical Center
100 Madison Avenue Morristown, NJ 07962 (973)971-5000

Fiel Cagande, Venerande, MD {1851390991} Anesth(63,PHIL)<NJ-MEMSALEM>
+ Memorial Hospital of Salem County
310 Woodstown Road/Anesthesiology Salem, NJ 08079 (856)935-1000 Fax (856)935-0962

Field, Charles K., MD {1720037039} SrgVas, Surgry(86,NJ02)<NJ-VIRTUAHS, NJ-OURLADY>
+ Virtua Surgical Group, PA
1935 Route 70 East Cherry Hill, NJ 08003 (856)428-7700 Fax (856)424-9120

Field, Shawn Michael, MD {1417913021} FamMed, IntrMd(97,NJ06)<NJ-BAYSHORE, NJ-RIVERVW>
+ 628 Beers Street
Hazlet, NJ 07730 (732)888-4100 Fax (732)888-0430
+ 226 Middle Road/Suite 1
Hazlet, NJ 07730 (732)888-4100

Fielding, Dennis P., MD {1619917929} Grtrcs, IntrMd(84,GRNA)<NJ-STCLRSUS>
+ Drs. Fielding and Geisen
17 Route 23 North Hamburg, NJ 07419 (973)827-7800 Fax (973)209-7855
dennispfielding@tellurian.net

Fieldman, Robert J., MD {1992700223} Otlryg(81,LA01)<NJ-STBARNMC>
+ Associates in Otolaryngology
741 Northfield Avenue/Suite 104 West Orange, NJ 07052 (973)243-0600 Fax (973)731-9208
+ Short Hills Surgery Center
187 Millburn Avenue/Suite 101/Surgery Millburn, NJ 07041 (973)243-0600 Fax (973)671-0557
+ St. Barnabas Medical Center
94 Old Short Hills Road Livingston, NJ 07052 (973)322-5000

Fields, Ryan G., DO {1427092386} Anesth(02,PA77)
+ Jersery Shore Anesthesiology
1945 Highway 33 Neptune, NJ 07753 (732)897-0200 Fax (732)897-0263

Fields, Scott G., MD {1609825033} IntrMd
+ 90 Mount Kemble Avenue/Unit 11
Morristown, NJ 07960

Fields, Sheila M., MD {1649270240} IntrMd(68,NY08)<NJ-VALLEY>
+ Northern Valley Medical Associates
221 Old Hook Road Westwood, NJ 07675 (201)666-4949 Fax (201)666-6920

Fiesseler, Frederick William, DO {1033177415} EmrgMd(97,PA78)<NJ-MORRISTN>
+ Morristown Medical Center
100 Madison Avenue/EmrgMed Morristown, NJ 07962 (800)290-5309 Fax (803)434-4354

Fiest, Thomas C., DO {1265533772} Gastrn, IntrMd(85,PA77)<NJ-MONMOUTH, NJ-JRSYSHMC>
+ Monmouth Gastroenterology
142 Route 35 Eatontown, NJ 07724 (732)389-5004 Fax (732)389-1850
+ Monmouth Gastroenterology
142 State Route 35 South/Suite 103 Eatontown, NJ 07724 (732)389-5004 Fax (732)389-1850

Fife, Kelly D., MD {1356343743} RadOnc(77,IL43)<NJ-VIRTMHBC>
+ Virtua Memorial
175 Madison Avenue Mount Holly, NJ 08060 (609)261-7074 Fax (609)265-9303

Figarola, Carlos J., MD {1306999768} Psychy(81,WIND)<NJ-CENTRAST>
+ 501 Iron Bridge Road/Suite 8
Freehold, NJ 07728 (732)431-4277

Figliola, Robin A., DO {1841290343} FamMed(97,NJ75)
+ Virtua Family Health Center
1000 Atlantic Avenue Camden, NJ 08104 (856)246-3542 Fax (856)246-3528

Figueredo, Nicole Dionesia, MD {1609038702} Surgry(01,DOM18)
+ Virtua Breast Specialty Care
200 Bowman Drive/Suite E-300 Voorhees, NJ 08043 (856)247-7515 Fax (856)247-7525
+ Drs Figueredo and Kimbaris
239 Hurffville CrossKeys Road Sewell, NJ 08080 (856)247-7515 Fax (856)247-7525

Figueroa, Astrid Giselle, DO {1003127861}
+ 1311 Stonybrook Drive
Deptford, NJ 08096 (856)534-8269
astridgfigueroa@gmail.com

Figueroa, Delia, MD {1801815675} EmrgMd(79,NY46)
+ Emergency Medical Associates of NJ, P.A.
3 Century Drive Parsippany, NJ 07054 (973)740-0607 Fax (973)740-9895

Figueroa, Marciano Tiu, Jr., MD {1689623936} FamMed, Grtrcs, IntrMd(85,PHI16)<NJ-HOBUNIMC, NJ-CLARMAAS>
+ Divine Grace Medical Service Inc
260 Washington Avenue Nutley, NJ 07110 (973)235-1772 Fax (973)235-1774
+ Valley Medical Group of Montvale
85 Chestnut Ridge Road/Suite 111 Montvale, NJ 07645 (973)235-1772 Fax (201)930-0705

Figueroa, Nilka, MD {1497083091} IntrMd
+ St Joseph's Medical Ctr Internal Med
703 Main Street Paterson, NJ 07503 (973)754-3424

Physicians by Name and Address

Figueroa, Pablo T., MD {1992702997} Anesth(89,PHIL)<NJ-TRINI-WSC>
+ St. Joseph's Regional Medical Center Anesthesia
703 Main Street   Paterson, NJ 07503   (973)754-2323   Fax (973)977-9455

Figueroa, Wanda E., MD {1194811463} InfDis, IntrMd(94,NJ05)
+ Newark Department of Health and Human Services
110 William Street   Newark, NJ 07102   (973)733-5300
figueroaw@ci.newark.nj.us

Figurasin, Rick Ornum, DO {1053705566}
+ 240 East Clinton Avenue
Bergenfield, NJ 07621   (201)951-1223

Filardo, Josephine, MD {1174602858} ObsGyn(86,PA07)<NJ-OCEANMC>
+ Brielle Obstetrics & Gynecology, P.A.
2671 Highway 70/Wall Township   Manasquan, NJ 08736   (732)528-6999   Fax (732)528-3397
+ Brielle Obstetrics & Gynecology, P.A.
117 County Line Road   Lakewood, NJ 08701   (732)528-6999   Fax (732)942-1919

Filart, Michael Valencia, DO {1629283312} EmrgMd
+ 1 Bennington Drive
Medford, NJ 08055

Filer, Joshua Michael, DO {1790118933} IntrMd<NJ-KMHSTRAT>
+ Kennedy Memorial Hospital-University Medical Center
18 East Laurel Road   Stratford, NJ 08084   (856)513-4124

Filion, Dean Thomas, DO {1679513188} PhysMd(91,PA77)<NJ-STBARNMC>
+ New Jersey Spine and Sports Medicine PC
84 Orient Way   Rutherford, NJ 07070   (201)964-0200   Fax (201)964-0220
+ New Jersey Spine and Sports Medicine PC
137 Main Road/Suite 200   Montville, NJ 07045   (201)964-0200   Fax (201)964-0220

Filion, Jacqueline D. Weil, DO {1184704934} FamMed(91,PA77)<NJ-STCLRDEN>
+ Montville Primary Care Physicians
137 Main Road   Montville, NJ 07045   (973)402-0025   Fax (973)402-0508

Filippis, Philip J., II, MD {1003851288} InfDis, IntrMd(88,DMN01)<NJ-CHILTON>
+ Saint JWH Infectious Diseases
220 Hamburg Turnpike/Suite 2   Wayne, NJ 07470   (973)389-9975   Fax (973)389-9976

Filippone, Lisa M., MD {1275563702} EmrgMd<NJ-COOPRUMC>
+ Cooper University Hospital
One Cooper Plaza/EmergMd   Camden, NJ 08103   (856)342-2000

Filippone, Mark A., MD {1710063797} PhysMd(74,DC02)<NJ-CHRIST, NJ-HOBUNIMC>
+ 15 Morrissee Avenue
Wallington, NJ 07057   (201)528-7851   Fax (201)528-7853

Filler, Sharon Lee, MD {1801837687} Pedtrc, GenPrc(98,NJ06)
+ Somerset Pediatric Group PA
65 Mountain Boulevard Ext/Suite 205   Warren, NJ 07059   (732)560-9080   Fax (732)560-8085
+ Somerset Pediatric Group PA
1-C New Amwell Road   Hillsborough, NJ 08844   (732)560-9080   Fax (908)874-3288

Finamore, Christina Lucy, MD {1245437052} Dermat<NY-VAHAR-BOR>
+ Advanced Dermatology, Laser, and MOHS Surgery Center
240 East Grove Street   Westfield, NJ 07090   (908)232-6446   Fax (908)232-6447

Finan, Cathleen M., DO {1063456911} FamMed(94,NJ75)<NJ-OURLADY, NJ-VIRTBERL>
+ Finan Family Medicine, P.C.
36 Kresson Road/Suite B   Cherry Hill, NJ 08034   (856)616-2444   Fax (856)616-2376

Finan-Duffy, Colleen M., DO {1013954429} FamMed, OstMed(94,NJ75)<NJ-KMHCHRRY, NJ-OURLADY>
+ Finan Family Medicine, P.C.
36 Kresson Road/Suite B   Cherry Hill, NJ 08034   (856)616-2444   Fax (856)616-2376

Finch, Daniel Garrett, MD {1861709347} Psychy(08,NJ06)<NJ-HACKNSK>
+ Hackensack University Medical Center
30 Prospect Avenue/4 Main RM 4620   Hackensack, NJ 07601   (551)996-4793   Fax (551)996-3620

Finch, Mark T., MD {1336116995} CdvDis, IntrMd(84,NY20)<NJ-VIRTMHBC>
+ The Cardiology Group, P.A.
401 Young Avenue/Suite 275   Moorestown, NJ 08057   (856)291-8855   Fax (856)291-8844
+ The Cardiology Group, P.A.
128 State Highway Route 70/Suite 1-B   Medford, NJ 08055   (856)291-8855   Fax (609)444-5521
+ The Cardiology Group, P.A.
1 Sheffield Drive/Suite 102   Columbus, NJ 08022   (856)291-8855

Finch, Vlada E., MD {1821380262}
+ MedExpress Urgent Care Watchung
1569 US Highway 22   Watchung, NJ 07069   (908)322-2631   Fax (908)322-2679
vlada15@yahoo.com

Finder, Susan M., DO {1770558918} FamMed(87,MO78)
+ 2462 Graiffs Way
Vineland, NJ 08361   (856)692-6663   Fax (856)692-5726

Findley, Thomas Wagner, Jr., MD {1841210614} PhysMd, IntrMd(77,DC02)
+ 3 Royal Avenue/Suite 4
Livingston, NJ 07039   Fax (973)302-8463

Findura, Michael James, DO {1922072420} IntrMd(01,PA77)<NJ-JRSYSHMC>
+ 1930 Highway 35 North/Suite 10
Wall, NJ 07719   (732)974-7007   Fax (732)974-7131

Fine, Howard Frederick, MD {1295810059} Ophthl(01,MA01)
+ Retina Associates of New Jersey, P.A.
10 Plum Street/Suite 600   New Brunswick, NJ 08901   (732)220-1600   Fax (732)220-1603
+ Retina Associates of New Jersey, P.A.
2 Industrial Way West   Eatontown, NJ 07724   (732)220-1600   Fax (732)389-2788

Fine, Jeffrey Scott, MD {1811963960} PedEmg, Pedtrc, Txclgy(83,DC01)<NY-BLVUENYU>
+ Hackensack Univ Medical Center Pediatric Emerg Room
30 Prospect Avenue   Hackensack, NJ 07601   (201)996-5430   Fax (201)996-3676

Fine, Manette K., DO {1194769034} FamMed, FamMGrtc(84,MO78)
+ 2027 Queen Anne Road
Cherry Hill, NJ 08003   (856)428-8101   Fax (856)428-7801
+ New Jersey Institute for Successful Aging
42 East Laurel Road/Suite 1800   Stratford, NJ 08084   (856)428-8101   Fax (856)566-6781

Fine, Paul L., MD {1164517918} Nephro, IntrMd(79,CT01)<NJ-MORRISTN, NJ-STCLRDEN>
+ Nephrology Hypertension Assocs
2 Franklin Place   Morristown, NJ 07960   (973)267-7673   Fax (973)267-3270

Fine, Shari R., DO {1124099288} FamMed(85,NY75)<NJ-CHRIST>
+ 25 Wildwood Drive
Short Hills, NJ 07078

Finegan, James, Jr., MD {1750332532} Ophthl(85,VA01)<NJ-WARREN>
+ 236 Roseberry Street
Phillipsburg, NJ 08865   (908)859-4311   Fax (908)859-4499

Finelli, Peter K., DO {1427067156} FamMed, IntrMd(66,MO79)
+ 67 Broadway
Elmwood Park, NJ 07407   (201)796-4444   Fax (201)796-4034

Fineman, Mitchell S., MD {1013965276} Ophthl, IntrMd(93,GA05)<PA-TJHSP>
+ Mid Atlantic Retina - Wills Eye Retina Surgeons
501 Cooper Landing Road   Cherry Hill, NJ 08002   (856)667-2246   Fax (856)755-1223

Fineman, Sanford, MD {1851362768} SrgNro(76,PA13)<NJ-OVERLOOK, NJ-TRINIJSC>
+ 617 Viscaya Court
Somerset, NJ 08873   (908)487-7176   Fax (732)302-0434

Fineman, William, MD {1962688564} PulDis, IntrMd
+ Horizon Blue Cross Blue Shield of N.J.
250 Century Parkway/MT-03T   Mount Laurel, NJ 08054   (856)638-3259

Finfer, Michael D., MD {1932142684} PthACl, PthCyt(86,PA09)<NJ-JFKMED>
+ JFK Medical Center
65 James Street/Pathology   Edison, NJ 08820   (732)321-7680   Fax (732)321-7008

Fingerman, Jarad Scott, DO {1376529966} SrgUro, Urolgy(96,PA77)<NJ-CHSFULD, NJ-CHSMRCER>
+ Urology Care Alliance
2 Princess Road/Suite J   Lawrenceville, NJ 08648   (609)895-1991   Fax (609)895-6996

Fink, Andrew Nathen, MD {1366483380} IntrMd(96,NY46)<NJ-HACKNSK>
+ 160 Overlook Avenue/Suite 1-A
Hackensack, NJ 07601   (201)488-3131   Fax (201)488-0430

Fink, Glenn D., MD {1205870300} EmrgMd, FamMed(76,MI01)<NJ-STBARNMC, NJ-SOMERSET>
+ St. Barnabas Medical Center
94 Old Short Hills Road   Livingston, NJ 07039   (973)322-5000
+ Emergency Medical Associates
110 Rehill Avenue   Somerville, NJ 08876   (973)322-5000   Fax (908)685-2968

Finkel, Arkady, MD {1558548599} RadNro, RadDia(98,PA14)<NJ-COMMED, NJ-SOCEANCO>
+ Community Medical Center
99 Route 37 West/NeuroRad   Toms River, NJ 08755   (732)557-8000

+ Coastal Imaging, LLC
79 Route 37 West/Suite 103   Toms River, NJ 08755   (732)557-8000   Fax (732)276-2325

Finkel, Diana Gurevich, DO {1780704205} InfDis, IntrMd(97,MO78)
+ University Physician Associates
140 Bergen Street/ACC Level D   Newark, NJ 07103   (973)972-5111   Fax (973)972-3102
+ Crossroads Medical Group
975 Clifton Avenue   Clifton, NJ 07013   (973)972-5111   Fax (973)778-7559

Finkel, Martin A., DO {1033189006} Pedtrc(74,MI12)
+ University Hospital-Cares Institute
42 East Laurel Road/Suite 1100   Stratford, NJ 08084   (856)566-7036   Fax (856)566-6108

Finkel, Richard I., MD {1124079520} CritCr, IntrMd, PulDis(86,NY47)<NJ-MORRISTN>
+ Associates in Pulmonary Medicine, PA
16 Pocono Road/Suite 217   Denville, NJ 07834   (973)625-5651
+ Associates in Pulmonary Medicine, PA
765 State Highway 10 East   Randolph, NJ 07869   (973)625-5651   Fax (973)366-6385

Finkelstein, David Hal, MD {1518034628} Dermat(97,PA02)
+ Alta Dermatology & Skin Care Center LLC
7014 Cooper Road/Suite 13   Voorhees, NJ 08043   (856)344-2849   Fax (856)344-2938
info@altaskincenter.com

Finkelstein, Mario, MD {1962478255} Psychy(79,ARG01)<NJ-UMDNJ>
+ University Psychiatric Associates
183 South Orange Avenue/E-F Levels   Newark, NJ 07103   (973)972-2977   Fax (973)972-2979
+ 135 Newcomb Road
Tenafly, NJ 07670   (201)871-7067

Finkelstein, Norman M., MD {1639367014} SrgVas, Surgry(65,NY01)<NJ-STPETER, NJ-RWJUBRUN>
+ 31 River Road
Highland Park, NJ 08904   (732)545-0212   Fax (732)545-2223

Finkelstein, Warren, MD {1376543223} Gastrn, IntrMd(72,VA04)
+ Gastroenterology Group of NJ, PA
123 Highland Avenue/Suite 103   Glen Ridge, NJ 07028   (973)429-8800   Fax (973)748-7076

Finkenstadt, Eric V., MD {1851340061} PulDis(78,PA09)
+ Inspira Medical Group Pulmonary Associates
17 West Red Bank Avenue/Suite 104   Woodbury, NJ 08096   (856)853-2025   Fax (856)845-8024

Finkielstein, Vadim Aaron, MD {1336188481} Nephro, IntrMd(98,MD07)
+ Princeton Hypertension-Nephrology
88 Princeton Hightstown Road/Suite 203   Princeton Junction, NJ 08550   (609)750-7330   Fax (609)750-7336

Finley, Stephanie Elena, DO {1811283757} ObsGyn
+ Kennedy Family Health Services
1 Somerdale Square   Somerdale, NJ 08083   (856)309-7700   Fax (856)566-8944

Finn, Roman E., MD {1144330580} IntrMd, Nutrtn, PainMd(81,MOL02)
+ Advanced Medical Care Center
22 Madison Avenue/Suite 1   Paramus, NJ 07652   (201)291-0401   Fax (201)291-5670

Finn Wedmid, Myra Elizabeth, MD {1881858736} RadDia, Radiol, IntrMd(NY19)
+ University Radiology, PA
239 Route 22 East/Suite 302   Green Brook, NJ 08812   (732)968-4899   Fax (732)968-8096
+ University Radiology Group, P.C.
16 Mountain Boulevard   Warren, NJ 07059   (732)968-4899   Fax (908)769-9141

Finnegan, Matthew J., MD {1003845223} Surgry, WundCr, SrgGst(88,PA09)<NJ-UNDRWD, NJ-COOPRUMC>
+ LMA Surgical Associates
120 White Horse Pike/Suite 103   Haddon Heights, NJ 08035   (856)546-3900   Fax (856)546-3908

Finnesey, Kevin Sean, MD {1952371791} SrgSpn
+ Premier Orthopaedics and Sports Medicine, PC
663 Palisade Avenue/Suite 302   Cliffside Park, NJ 07010   (201)943-9100   Fax (201)943-7308

Finston, Peggy Anne, MD {1376664201} Psychy
+ 200 Dee Court
Lakewood, NJ 08701   (928)713-6577

Fiore, Edward D., MD {1043300817} FamMed(66,ITAL)<NJ-COMMED>
+ Edward D. Fiore MD PA
20 Hospital Drive/Suite 12 A   Toms River, NJ 08755   (732)349-2067   Fax (732)341-9164

Fiore, Elizabeth Jill, DO {1386676427} Pedtrc(00,PA77)<NJ-COMMED, NJ-OCEANMC>
+ Pediatric Affiliates, PA
40 Bey Lea Road/Suite B203   Toms River, NJ 08753
(732)341-0720   Fax (732)244-6842
+ Pediatric Affiliates, PA
1616 Route 72 West/Suite 8   Manahawkin, NJ 08050
(732)341-0720   Fax (609)978-1229

Fiore, Philip M., MD {1306826581} Ophthl(84,NJ05)
+ 213 Chestnut Street
Nutley, NJ 07110   (973)667-2020

Fiore, Rosemary P., MD {1093819674} MedOnc, Hemato(88,NJ05)
+ Monmouth Hematology Oncology Associates PA
100 State Highway 36/Suite 1B   West Long Branch, NJ 07764   (732)222-1711   Fax (732)222-2060

Fiore, Vicki M., MD {1508883406} Psychy(82,CA14)<NJ-VALLEY>
+ 75 Grand Avenue
Englewood, NJ 07631   (201)569-9059

Fiorentino, Diego M., DO {1265449326} IntrMd(86,MO78)<NJ-SHOREMEM, NJ-ACMCMAIN>
+ Diego M. Fiorentino DO FACP
200 South New Road/Suite 1   Absecon, NJ 08201
(609)641-2062   Fax (609)641-4633

Fiorentino, Grace, DO {1780792051} FamMed, IntrMd(97,NJ75)<NJ-ACMCITY, NJ-ACMCMAIN>
+ Shore Physicians Group
2605 Shore Road   Northfield, NJ 08225   (609)365-5300
Fax (609)365-5301
+ Diego M. Fiorentino DO FACP
200 South New Road/Suite 1   Absecon, NJ 08201
(609)365-5300   Fax (609)641-4633

Fiorillo, Marc Anthony, MD {1477712636} Gastrn
+ Advanced Gastroenterology of Bergen County
140 Sylvan Avenue/Suite 101-A   Englewood Cliffs, NJ 07632
(201)945-6564   Fax (201)461-9038

Fiorillo, Michael A., MD {1275520991} SrgPlstc(91,IL42)<NJ-HOLYNAME>
+ Rockland Plastic Surgery
390 Old Hook Road   Westwood, NJ 07675   (201)358-0478
Fax (201)634-3613
info@rpsinternet.com

Fioriti, Gina Marie, DO {1558394536} IntrMd(97,IA75)<NJ-MMHKEMBL, NJ-VAEASTOR>
+ Morristown Memorial Hospital/Mt. Kemble Division
95 Mount Kemble Avenue   Morristown, NJ 07960
(973)971-4758   Fax (973)267-3144
+ VA New Jersey Health Care System-East Orange Campus
385 Tremont Avenue   East Orange, NJ 07018   (973)676-1000

Firdu, Tikikil, MD {1235478033} ObsGyn, GenPrc
+ Lawrence Ob/Gyn Associates
123 Franklin Corner Road/Suite 214   Lawrenceville, NJ 08648   (609)896-1400   Fax (609)896-3986

Firestone, Debra A., MD {1083664585} Ophthl(96,NY46)<NJ-OVERLOOK>
+ The Eye Center
65 Mountain Boulevard Ext/Suite 105   Warren, NJ 07059
(732)356-6200   Fax (732)356-0228
+ The Eye Center
213 Stelton Road   Piscataway, NJ 08854   (732)356-6200
Fax (732)752-9492
+ The Eye Center
3900 Park Avenue/Suite 106   Edison, NJ 07059   (732)603-2101

Firoozi, Babak, MD {1891734828} IntrMd, Gastrn(95,NJ05)<NJ-HACKNSK, NJ-VALLEY>
+ 275-277 Forest Ave/Suite 200
Paramus, NJ 07652   (201)986-1881

Firoozi, Tahmoures, MD {1659326486} Urolgy, IntrMd(64,IRAN)<NJ-CHILTON>
+ The Stone Center of New Jersey, LLC.
376 Hamburg Turnpike   Wayne, NJ 07470   (973)595-8554
Fax (973)790-4804
firoozi@optonline.net

Firoz, Bahar F., MD {1932249943} Dermat, IntrMd(04,CT01)
+ Robert Wood Johnson Medical Group-Dermatology
1 World's Fair Drive/Suite 2400   Somerset, NJ 08873
(732)235-7993   Fax (732)235-7117
+ 47 Orient Way
Rutherford, NJ 07070   (732)235-7993   Fax (201)460-8084

Fisch, Amy Heather, DO {1235202094} Anesth(01,PA77)<NJ-HOLYNAME>
+ 300 Avalon Drive/Suite 3274
Wood Ridge, NJ 07075   (201)669-7640   Fax (887)598-9776

Fisch, Arthur P., MD {1184622193} CdvDis, IntrMd, CarNuc(69,MA05)<NJ-MORRISTN>
+ Morristown Cardiology Associates, P.A.
435 South Street/Suite 100   Morristown, NJ 07960
(973)267-3944   Fax (973)455-0399

Fisch, Shirley B.D., MD {1972579621} NrlgSpec(NY46<NJ-ST-BARNMC, NJ-MONMOUTH>
+ Monmouth Medical Center
300 Second Avenue/Pediatrics   Long Branch, NJ 07740
(732)923-7790   Fax (732)923-7722
+ Monmouth Medical Group, P.C.
255 Third Avenue/SH 001   Long Branch, NJ 07740
(732)923-7790

Fisch, Tobe M., MD {1689608283} IntrMd(90,NY20)<NJ-UNVM-CPRN>
+ Princeton Health Medical & Surgical Associates
2 Centre Drive/Suite 200   Monroe, NJ 08831   (609)395-2470   Fax (609)860-5288
+ Princeton Medicine
5 Plainsboro Road/Suite 300   Plainsboro, NJ 08536
(609)395-2470   Fax (609)853-7271

Fischer, Beverly Ruth, MD {1700961307} Nrolgy, Pedtrc, NrlgSpec(70,DC03)<NJ-JRSYCITY>
+ 4 Chiplou Lane
Scotch Plains, NJ 07076   (908)561-3620

Fischer, Emily Frances, MD {1659631331} Pedtrc
+ North Jersey Pediatrics
17-10 Fair Lawn Avenue   Fair Lawn, NJ 07410   (201)794-8585   Fax (201)703-9889

Fischer, Evan S., MD {1992714182} SrgOrt, SrgHnd(92,CT01)<NJ-MTNSIDE, NJ-STBARNMC>
+ Summit Medical Group
103 Park Street/Suite 1-G   Montclair, NJ 07042   (973)744-7900   Fax (973)744-7995
+ Short Hills Surgery Center
187 Millburn Avenue/Suite 101   Millburn, NJ 07041
(973)744-7900   Fax (973)671-0557

Fischer, Joel M., MD {1619997749} Urolgy(85,NY09)<NJ-SOMERSET>
+ Somerset Urological Associates PA
72 West End Avenue   Somerville, NJ 08876   (908)927-0300
Fax (908)707-4988

Fischer, John F., MD {1245276310} Pedtrc, GenPrc(88,SC01)<NJ-SOMERSET, NJ-RWJUBRUN>
+ Somerset Pediatric Group PA
2345 Lamington Road/Suite 101   Bedminster, NJ 07921
(908)470-1124   Fax (908)253-6559
+ Somerset Pediatric Group PA
1390 Route 22 West/Suite 106   Lebanon, NJ 08833
(908)470-1124   Fax (908)236-7557

Fischer, Lauren Jane, MD {1366657181} Surgry(02,NJ05)
+ Matawan Medical Associates
213 Main Street   Matawan, NJ 07747   (732)566-2363
Fax (732)566-0502

Fischer, Mitchell Steven, DO {1487640157} EmrgMd(89,NY75)<NY-LDYMRCY>
+ St Joseph's Medical Center Emergency
703 Main Street   Paterson, NJ 07503   (973)754-2240   Fax (973)754-2249

Fischer, Richard L., MD {1386739480} MtFtMd, ObsGyn(83,PA01)<NJ-COOPRUMC>
+ Cooper University Hospital
One Cooper Plaza/Drrnc/Rm 628   Camden, NJ 08103
(856)342-2491   Fax (856)342-7023
Fischer-richard@cooperhealth.edu

Fischer, Robert S., MD {1174695001} SrgPlstc, SrgCsm, SrgLsr(63,IL42)<NJ-WAYNEGEN, NJ-HOLYNAME>
+ The Aesthetic Plastic Surgery & Laser Center
19-21 Fair Lawn Avenue/Suite 2-B   Fair Lawn, NJ 07410
(201)796-4100   Fax (201)796-4102

Fischer, Stuart J., MD {1790832616} SrgOrt(75,NY01)<NJ-OVERLOOK>
+ Summit Orthopaedics & Sports Medicine
33 Overlook Road/Suite 301   Summit, NJ 07901   (908)277-1122   Fax (908)277-0140

Fischer, Zvi, MD {1437108339} Gastrn(78,NY47)<NJ-VALLEY>
+ Gastrointestinal Associates PA
140 Chestnut Street/Suite 300   Ridgewood, NJ 07450
(201)444-2600   Fax (201)444-9471

Fischetti-Galvin, Jessica, DO {1700177854} ObsGyn
+ Sunrise Obstetrics & Gynecology
831 Tennent Road   Manalapan, NJ 07726   (732)972-4200
Fax (732)333-4643
+ Sunrise Obstetrics & Gynecology
921 East County Line Road   Lakewood, NJ 08701
(732)987-5950

Fischkoff, James Daniel, MD {1972895373} IntrMd
+ Arthritis and Osteporosis Associates
4247 Route 9 North Building/Unit 1   Freehold, NJ 07728

Fischler, David Ross, MD {1275622540} IntrMd, PulCCr, PulDis(98,NY46)<NJ-STPETER, NJ-RWJUBRUN>
+ Pulmonary & Intensive Care Specialists of NJ
593 Cranbury Road   East Brunswick, NJ 08816   (732)613-8880   Fax (732)613-0077

Fisgus, John R., MD {1902840846} Anesth(82,NY06)<NJ-ACMC-MAIN>
+ AtlantiCare Anesthesiology
65 West Jimmie Leeds Road   Pomona, NJ 08240   (609)748-7597

Fish, Frank H., MD {1265409817} CdvDis, IntrMd(70,NJ05)<NJ-DEBRAHLC>
+ Deborah Heart and Lung Center
200 Trenton Road   Browns Mills, NJ 08015   (609)893-6611
Fax (609)735-1856

Fish, Gabrielle A., DO {1891862090} FamMAdlt, FamMed, IntrMd(91,CA22)
+ Brookmead Medical Associates, P.C.
432 Columbia Boulevard   Cherry Hill, NJ 08002   (856)427-4001   Fax (856)427-4003

Fish, Heidi, MD {1730343427} PthAcl, PthCyt(93,RI01)<NJ-HOLYNAME, NJ-TRINIJSC>
+ Holy Name Hospital
718 Teaneck Road/Pathology   Teaneck, NJ 07666
(201)833-3000   Fax (201)661-7297
+ Trinitas Regional Medical Center-Williamson Street
225 Williamson Street/Path   Elizabeth, NJ 07207
(201)833-3000   Fax (908)994-5573

Fish, Michelle Leigh Karam, DO {1851539613} Pedtrc
+ Cooper University Hospital Pediatrics/Endocrinology
3 Cooper Plaza/Suite 200   Camden, NJ 08103   (856)342-2001   Fax (856)963-2499

Fishbein, Richard J., MD {1841355419} CdvDis, CritCr(81,NJ05)<NJ-HOBUNIMC>
+ Hoboken University Medical Center
308 Willow Avenue/Cardiology   Hoboken, NJ 07030
(201)418-1240   Fax (201)418-1245

Fishbein, Susan, MD {1205945086} Gastrn, IntrMd(82,NY08)<NY-BETHPETR, NY-SLRLUKES>
+ Emergimed
663 Palisade Avenue/Suite 101   Cliffside Park, NJ 07010
(201)945-6500   Fax (201)945-1157

Fishbein, Vitaly A., MD {1467410381} Gastrn, IntrMd(80,UKR25)<NJ-STBARNMC>
+ 401 Pleasant Valley Way
West Orange, NJ 07052   (973)736-1112   Fax (973)736-5590
+ 3300 Broadway/Suite 204
Fair Lawn, NJ 07410   (201)797-3003

Fishberg, Robert Daniel, MD {1871587345} CdvDis(81,NY15)<NJ-MORRISTN>
+ Associates in Cardiovascular Disease, LLC
211 Mountain Avenue   Springfield, NJ 07081   (973)467-0005   Fax (973)912-8989

Fisher, Adrian Alex, MD {1912925157} SrgTpl, Surgry(86,MA01)<NJ-UMDNJ>
+ Liver Transplant & Hepatobiliary Diseases/UMDNJ
140 Bergen Street/ACC Bldg   Newark, NJ 07101   (973)972-7218
+ University Hospital-Doctors Office Center
90 Bergen Street/7100   Newark, NJ 07103   (973)972-7218
Fax (973)972-2988

Fisher, Bruce D., MD {1861401135} InfDis, IntrMd(70,MO02)<NJ-STPETER>
+ Qualcare, Inc.
30 Knightsbridge Road   Piscataway, NJ 08854   (732)562-7802   Fax (732)562-1023

Fisher, Deneishia Shramaine, MD {1891878914} ObsGyn(00,VA01)<NJ-STPETER>
+ Brunswick-Hills Ob/Gyn, PA
620 Cranbury Road/Suite LL90   East Brunswick, NJ 08816
(732)967-0033   Fax (732)613-4845
+ Brunswick-Hills Ob/Gyn, PA
751 Route 206/2nd Floor   Hillsborough, NJ 08844
(732)967-0033   Fax (908)725-2132

Fisher, Emery, IV, DO {1558434548} Anesth(94,IA75)<NJ-NWRKBETH, NJ-UMDNJ>
+ New Jersey Anesthesia Associates, P.C.
252 Columbia Turnpike/PO Box 0037   Florham Park, NJ 07932   (973)660-9334   Fax (973)660-9779

Fisher, Frederick S., MD {1639171663} SrgVas, Surgry(88,NY47)
+ Regional Surgical Associates
502 Centennial Boulevard/Suite 7   Voorhees, NJ 08043
(856)596-7440   Fax (856)751-3320

Fisher, Howard J., MD {1710955240} Pedtrc(78,MEX14)<NJ-HOLYNAME, NJ-HACKNSK>
+ 960 Teaneck Road
Teaneck, NJ 07666   (201)837-2121   Fax (201)837-0679
Howardjfishermd@aol.com

Fisher, John F., MD {1073583720} IntrMd(79,DC02)
+ 16 East Main Street
Sussex, NJ 07461   (973)875-3646   Fax (973)875-2021

Fisher, Joie, DO {1124293329} Pedtrc, NnPnMd(00,IA75)<NJ-NWRKBETH>
+ Newark Beth Israel Medical Center
201 Lyons Avenue/Neontlgy   Newark, NJ 07112   (973)926-7000

Physicians by Name and Address

Fisher, Margaret Catharine, MD {1932165701} Pedtrc, PedInf(75,CA14)<NJ-MONMOUTH>
+ Monmouth Medical Center
300 Second Avenue/Pediatrics   Long Branch, NJ 07740   (732)222-5200

Fisher, Margaret Elizabeth, MD {1407813611} Anesth(75,CA06)
+ Ambulatory Anesthesia Care, PC
1450 Route 22 West   Mountainside, NJ 07092   (908)233-2020   Fax (908)233-9322

Fisher, Mark, MD {1609961937} IntrMd, Rheuma(73,PA09)
+ Arthritis & Rheumatology Physicians
713 Station Avenue   Haddon Heights, NJ 08035   (856)547-8004   Fax (856)547-8377

Fisher, Matthew Adam, MD {1730271727} Pedtrc(95,NJ06)
+ Pediatric Associates, LLC.
1318 South Main Street   Vineland, NJ 08360   (856)691-8585   Fax (856)691-8489

Fisher, Scott Robert, MD {1437306107} Anesth(07,PA09)<NJ-MONMOUTH>
+ Monmouth Medical Center
300 Second Avenue   Long Branch, NJ 07740   (732)923-6980

Fisher-Swartz, Lucinda, MD {1750364261} FamMed(99,PA02)
+ Tatem Brown Family Practice
2225 East Evesham Road/Suite 101   Voorhees, NJ 08043   (856)795-4330   Fax (856)325-3704

Fishkin, Igor V., MD {1225108673} RadDia, Ultsnd(82,RUS21)
+ 364 Mauro Road
Englewood Cliffs, NJ 07632

Fishkin, Joseph D., MD {1407953540} Ophthl(98,IL42)<NJ-HOLYNAME, NY-MANHEYE>
+ 85 Kinderkamack Road/Suite 201
Emerson, NJ 07630   (201)383-9140   Fax (201)262-7800

Fishkind, Perry Neal, MD {1306950233} Pedtrc(93,NY15)<NJ-VALLEY, NJ-ENGLWOOD>
+ Old Tappan Medical Group PA
215 Old Tappan Road   Old Tappan, NJ 07675   (201)666-1001   Fax (201)666-4108
info@otpediatrics.com
+ Old Tappan Pediatrics
136 North Washington Avenue   Bergenfield, NJ 07621   (201)666-1001   Fax (201)385-4748

Fishman, Claire Margaret, DO {1396771408}
+ 2 Kathleen Drive
Jackson, NJ 08527   (732)979-4116

Fishman, Jordan E., MD {1366606147}<NJ-UMDNJ>
+ University Hospital
150 Bergen Street/Suite E-401   Newark, NJ 07103   (201)417-3249

Fishman, Miriam, MD {1396845269} Dermat, SrgDer(78,NY19)<NJ-ENGLWOOD>
+ Fishman & Fishman
216 Engle Street   Englewood, NJ 07631   (201)569-5678   Fax (201)569-6225
miriam.fishman@ehmc.com

Fishman, S. Jose, MD Dermat(67,PER04)<NJ-CHRIST>
+ Academic Dermatology & Dermatologic Surgery Group
703 Kearny Avenue   Kearny, NJ 07032   (201)998-4699
+ Fishman & Fishman
216 Engle Street   Englewood, NJ 07631   (201)998-4699   Fax (201)569-6225

Fisicaro, Tamara Marie, MD {1700094075} FamMed, IntrMd(05,PA02)
+ Advocare DelGiorno Pediatrics
527 South Black Horse Pike   Blackwood, NJ 08012   (856)302-5322   Fax (856)245-7719

Fisk, Marc Saslow, DO {1669472213} CdvDis, IntrMd(92,NY75)<NJ-NWTNMEM, NJ-STBARNMC>
+ New Jersey Cardiology Associates
375 Mount Pleasant Avenue   West Orange, NJ 07052   (973)731-9442   Fax (973)731-8030
+ New Jersey Cardiology Associates
5 Franklin Avenue/Suite 502   Belleville, NJ 07109   (973)731-9442   Fax (973)450-8157

Fiske, Joshua Michael, MD {1508853458} Urolgy(99,NY19)<NJ-CLARMAAS, NJ-TRINIWSC>
+ Premier Urology Group, LLC
275 Orchard Street   Westfield, NJ 07090   (908)654-5100   Fax (908)789-8755
+ Premier Urology Group, LLC
659 Kearny Avenue   Kearny, NJ 07032   (908)654-5100   Fax (201)789-8755
+ Premier Urology Group, LLC
776 East Third Avenue   Roselle Park, NJ 07090   (908)241-5268   Fax (908)241-8755

Fiske, Steven C., MD {1093754236} Gastrn, IntrMd(74,NY19)<NJ-STBARNMC, NJ-CLARMAAS>
+ Premier Urology Group, LLC
1500 Pleasant Valley Road   West Orange, NJ 07052   (973)325-5775   Fax (973)325-5770

Fitz, Rachel Myra, DO {1306265673} Anesth
+ New Jersey Anesthesia Associates, P.C.
30B Vreeland Road/Suite 200   Florham Park, NJ 07932   (973)660-9334   Fax (973)660-9779

Fitzgerald, Denis B., MD {1265427223} MedOnc, Hemato, IntrMd(78,NY08)<NJ-RIVERVW>
+ Regional Cancer Care Associates, LLC
180 White Road   Little Silver, NJ 07739   (732)530-8666   Fax (732)530-4139
+ Riverview Medical Center
1 Riverview Plaza   Red Bank, NJ 07701   (732)741-2700

Fitzgerald, Timothy E., MD {1225019599} Anesth(86,NJ05)<NJ-MORRISTN>
+ Morristown Medical Center
100 Madison Avenue   Morristown, NJ 07962   (973)971-5548   Fax (973)943-8733

Fitzhenry, Laurence N., IV, MD {1275745655} Anesth(03,PA02)
+ Premier Orthopaedic Associates
298 South Delsea Drive   Vineland, NJ 08360   (856)690-1616   Fax (856)690-1089

Fitzhugh, Valerie A., MD {1508025164} PthACl<NJ-UMDNJ>
+ University Hospital
150 Bergen Street/Suite E156   Newark, NJ 07103   (973)972-4300

Fitzpatrick, Brendan Thomas, MD {1043294754} Pthlgy, PthACl, PthCyt(79,IRE06)<NJ-OURLADY, NJ-BAYONNE>
+ Our Lady of Lourdes Medical Center
1600 Haddon Avenue/Path   Camden, NJ 08103   (856)757-3500

Fitzpatrick, Hendrieka Ann, MD {1821124959} FamMed(81,DC01)<OH-FHNRTHSD>
+ 435 South Street/Suite 160
Morristown, NJ 07960   (973)971-8552

Fitzpatrick, John E., MD {1699740753} Nrolgy(86,NY08)<NJ-JRSYSHMC, NJ-OCEANMC>
+ Jersey Shore Neurology Associates PA
1900 Corlies Avenue/Third Floor   Neptune, NJ 07753   (732)775-2400   Fax (732)775-5673
+ Jersey Shore Neurology Associates PA
222 Jack Martin Boulevard   Brick, NJ 08723   (732)840-4666

Fitzpatrick, Maurice, MD {1225011703} RadNro, RadDia(81,DC02)<NJ-STPETER, NJ-RWJUBRUN>
+ University Radiology Group, P.C.
483 Cranbury Road   East Brunswick, NJ 08816   (732)390-0030   Fax (732)390-5383
+ University Radiology Group, P.C.
10 Plum Street   New Brunswick, NJ 08901   (732)390-0030   Fax (732)249-1208
+ University Radiology Group, P.C.
579A Cranbury Road   East Brunswick, NJ 08816   (732)390-0040   Fax (732)390-1856

Fitzsimmons, Adriana Marie, MD {1285606921} Psychy(98,NJ06)<NJ-RIVERVW, NJ-OCEANMC>
+ Jersey Shore Psychiatric Associates
3535 Route 66/Building 5/Suite D   Neptune, NJ 07753   (732)643-4350   Fax (732)643-4398

Fitzsimmons, John Michael, MD {1932166527} ObsGyn, MtFtMd<NJ-VIRTBERL, NJ-VIRTMARL>
+ Virtua Maternal Fetal Medicine Center
100 Bowman Drive   Voorhees, NJ 08043   (856)247-3328   Fax (856)247-3276

Fix, Cecilia Crane, MD {1679991806} IntrMd
+ EIP Clinic/Early Intervention Program (HIV/AIDS)
3 Cooper Plaza/Suite 513   Camden, NJ 08103   (856)963-3715

Fix, Daniel Jonas, MD {1750672119} PthAna<NJ-HACKNSK>
+ Hackensack University Medical Center
30 Prospect Avenue   Hackensack, NJ 07601   (551)996-4808

Flaherty, Stephanie, DO {1720414584}
+ CompleteCare Adult & Specialty Medical Professionals
1038 East Chestnut Avenue/Suite 110   Vineland, NJ 08360   (856)498-2083

Flannery, Ashley Laura, DO {1215255013} EmrgMd<NJ-MORRISTN>
+ St Joseph's Medical Center Emergency
703 Main Street   Paterson, NJ 07503   (973)754-2240   Fax (973)754-2249

Flannery, Todd W., MD {1033253679} RadOnc(03,MD01)
+ Princeton Radiology Associates, P.A.
3674 Route 27   Kendall Park, NJ 08824   (732)821-5563   Fax (732)821-6675
+ Westfield Pediatrics, P.A.
532 East Broad Street   Westfield, NJ 07090   (908)232-3445   Fax (908)233-6184

Flanzman, Richard M., MD {1083702021} RadDia(90,NJ05)<NY-BETHPETR>
+ Medical Park Imaging
330 Ratzer Road/Suite 6-A   Wayne, NJ 07470   (973)696-5770   Fax (973)633-1204

Flanzman, Susan Amy, MD {1609870245} IntrMd(87,NY47)<NJ-VALLEY>
+ Bergen Medical Associates
466 Old Hook Road/Suite 1   Emerson, NJ 07630   (201)967-8221   Fax (201)967-0340
+ Valley Center for Women's Health
581 North Franklin Turnpike/2nd Floor   Ramsey, NJ 07446   (201)967-8221   Fax (201)236-5269
+ Valley Center for Women's Health
One Godwin Avenue   Midland Park, NJ 07630   (201)444-4040

Flashburg, Michael H., MD {1093712515} Anesth(79,NY08)<NJ-MONMOUTH>
+ Monmouth Medical Center
300 Second Avenue/Anesth   Long Branch, NJ 07740   (732)222-5200

Flaxman, Alexander, MD {1497870133} AnesCrCr, EmrgMd, CritCr(03,NJ05)
+ Chronic Pain Management of New Jersey
1930 Route 70 East/Suite N-70   Cherry Hill, NJ 08003   (856)581-9157   Fax (856)581-9159
info@ChronicPainNJ.com

Flaxman, Daena Meredith, MD {1710195961} IntrMd(04,NY08)<NJ-KMHTURNV>
+ Kennedy Health Systems/Washington Township Campus
435 Hurffville-Cross Keys Road   Turnersville, NJ 08012   (856)218-5634   Fax (856)218-5664

Fleisch, Charles M., DO {1679686224} ObsGyn(70,IA75)<NJ-JFKMED>
+ Fleisch OBGYN Group
3 Lincoln Boulevard/Suite 315   Edison, NJ 08820   (732)635-9800   Fax (732)635-9810
+ Preventive HealthCare Associates
102 James Street/Suite 202   Edison, NJ 08820   (732)635-9800   Fax (732)548-2610

Fleischer, Gilbert E., MD {1104915354} Pedtrc(90,GHA01)<NJ-MONMOUTH, NJ-RBAYOLDB>
+ first Step Pediatrics
206 Laurel Heights Drive   Bridgeton, NJ 08302   (856)459-2270   Fax (856)459-9674
+ Elmer Pediatrics
525 State Street/Suite 1/PO Box 603   Elmer, NJ 08318   (856)459-2270   Fax (856)358-1141

Fleischer, Jessica Beth, MD {1851464978} IntrMd, EnDbMt(97,NY48)
+ Englewood Orthopedic Associates
401 South Van Brunt Street   Englewood, NJ 07631   (201)569-2770   Fax (201)569-1774

Fleischer, Joseph S., MD {1386670206} IntrMd(97,NY48)<NJ-VALLEY>
+ Bergen Medical Associates
466 Old Hook Road/Suite 1   Emerson, NJ 07630   (201)967-8221   Fax (201)967-0340
+ Bergen Medical Associates
1 West Ridgewood Avenue/Suite 301   Paramus, NJ 07652   (201)967-8221   Fax (201)445-4296

Fleischer, Michael S., MD {1588621973} Ophthl(95,NJ06)
+ Westwood Ophthalmology Associates
300 Fairview Avenue/PO Box 698   Westwood, NJ 07675   (201)666-4014   Fax (201)664-4754

Fleischhacker, Wayne, DO {1386637270} Anesth, AnesPain(90,NY75)
+ Union Anesthesia & Pain Management
695 Chestnut Street   Union, NJ 07083   (908)851-7161   Fax (908)851-7536

Fleischman, Keith A., DO {1073674487} Anesth(84,ME75)
+ 34 Little Wolf Road
Summit, NJ 07901   (908)918-1291

Fleischman, William, MD {1316264468} EmrgMd(10,NY06)<CT-YALENHH, CT-HOSPSTRA>
+ Hackensack University Medical Center
30 Prospect Avenue   Hackensack, NJ 07601   (201)996-2000

Fleischner, Charles Alan, MD {1023262037} EmrgMd(06,NJ05)
+ University Hospital-New Jersey Medical School
30 Bergen Street/ADMC 1110   Newark, NJ 07107   (973)972-4511

Fleischner, Nathaniel P., MD {1083880926} IntrMd
+ 56 Duke Drive
Paramus, NJ 07652

Fleisher, Michael H., MD {1972595593} PedUro, Urolgy(77,NY08)<NJ-STPETER, NJ-MONMOUTH>
+ Pediatric Urology Associates PC
557 Cranbury Road/Suite 4   East Brunswick, NJ 08816   (732)613-9144   Fax (732)613-5121
+ Pediatric Urology Associates PC
422 Morris Avenue   Long Branch, NJ 07740   (732)613-9144   Fax (732)613-5121

Fleming, Gregory John, MD {1255372165} Otlryg, Otolgy(82,MA16)
+ Summit Medical Group
140 Park Avenue/3rd Floor/ENT   Florham Park, NJ 07932   (973)404-9970

Physicians by Name and Address

Fleming, Jacqueline, MD {1558457614} Pedtrc(88,NJ06)
+ Eric B. Chandler Health Center
277 George Street   New Brunswick, NJ 08901   (732)235-6700   Fax (732)235-6713
+ UH- RWJ Medical School
One Robert Wood Johnson Place/Pedi   New Brunswick, NJ 08903   (732)235-5600

Fleming, Richard E., Jr., MD {1649290917} SrgOrt(72,NY01)<NJ-VANJHCS>
+ Princeton Orthopaedic Associates, P.A.
325 Princeton Avenue   Princeton, NJ 08540   (609)924-8131   Fax (609)924-8532
+ Princeton Orthopaedic Associates, P.A.
11 Centre Drive   Jamesburg, NJ 08831   (609)655-4848

Fleming, Talya K., MD {1679712327} PhysMd, IntrMd(NJ02<NJ-JFKMED>
+ JFK Medical Center
65 James Street/Phys Rehab   Edison, NJ 08820   (732)321-7070   Fax (732)321-7330

Flescher, Sylvia Evelyn, MD {1033393111} Psychy, Psynls(75,NY09)
+ 76 West Ridgewood Avenue
Ridgewood, NJ 07450   (201)445-0322   Fax (201)447-8799

Fleser, Cecilia, MD {1932370913} Psychy(93,ROM06)
+ 47 Conover Avenue
Nutley, NJ 07110

Fless, Kristin Gail, MD {1043305493} CritCr, PulDis, IntrMd(95,NJ05)
+ University Hospital-New Jersey Medical School
30 Bergen Street/Room 1205   Newark, NJ 07107   (973)972-4511

Fletcher, Daniel J., MD {1558339564} SrgHnd, SrgOrt, OrtS-Hand(90,NY15)<NJ-STFRNMED, NJ-RWJUHAM>
+ Trenton Orthopaedic Group
1225 Whitehorse Mercerville Rd   Trenton, NJ 08619   (609)581-2200   Fax (609)581-1212
+ Trenton Orthopaedic Group
116 Washington Crossing Road   Pennington, NJ 08534   (609)581-2200   Fax (609)581-1212

Fletcher, H. Stephen, MD   SrgVas, Srgry(67,DC01)<NJ-STBARNMC>
+ St. Barnabas Medical Center
94 Old Short Hills Road/Suite 1172   Livingston, NJ 07039   (201)404-8148   Fax (973)322-2471

Fleurantin, Jean J., MD {1376739888} GenPrc, EmrgMd(73,HAIT)<NJ-MEMSALEM>
+ Memorial Hospital of Salem County
310 Woodstown Road/EmergMed   Salem, NJ 08079   (856)935-1000

Flick, Jeffrey L., DO {1174526875} Pedtrc(87,MO78)<NJ-SHOREMEM, NJ-BURDTMLN>
+ Rainbow Pediatrics
2041 US Highway 9   Cape May Court House, NJ 08210   (609)624-9003   Fax (609)624-9002

Flint, Laurence E., MD {1700098076} Pedtrc
+ 66 Annin Road
West Caldwell, NJ 07006   (973)228-6487

Flood, Mark J., MD {1376729046} Psychy(87,TX15)<NJ-HACKNSK>
+ Psychiatric Associates
218 State Route 17 North/Suite 13   Rochelle Park, NJ 07662   (201)488-6543

Flood, Stephen James, MD {1427130186} SrgOrt
+ Sall/Myers Medical Associates, PA
100 Hamilton Plaza/Suite 317/3rd Floor   Paterson, NJ 07505   (973)279-2323   Fax (973)279-7551

Florczyk, Margaret, MD {1013927755} IntrMd(75,POLA)<NJ-BAYSHORE>
+ M & M Florczyk, Inc.
3 Parlin Drive/Suite G   Parlin, NJ 08859   (732)651-7005   Fax (732)651-7707

Florczyk, Miroslaw, MD {1780694364} IntrMd, OncHem(75,POLA)<NJ-RWJUBRUN, NJ-RBAYPERT>
+ M & M Florczyk, Inc.
3 Parlin Drive/Suite G   Parlin, NJ 08859   (732)651-7005

Florence, Isaiah Meyer, MD {1114906377} Anesth, PainMd, Anes-Pain(89,NY08)<NJ-ENGLWOOD>
+ IFPAIN Associates, PLLC
222 Cedar Lane/Suite 210   Teaneck, NJ 07666   (201)287-1100   Fax (201)586-0409

Florentino, Hector Leandro, MD {1154363661} IntrMd, OncHem(75,DOM01)<NJ-HOBUNIMC>
+ 316 Monastery Place
Union City, NJ 07087   (201)867-3535   Fax (201)867-2433

Flores, Alejandro Alberto, MD {1578737300} Pedtrc(08,MD01)
+ Drs. Flores and Flores
819 Main Street   Hackensack, NJ 07601   (201)489-3678   Fax (201)489-7618

Flores, Belen P., MD {1386664332} Pedtrc(71,PHIL)<NJ-CHSMRCER, NJ-STFRNMED>
+ Pediatrics by Night
1230 Whitehorse Mercerville Ro   Hamilton, NJ 08619   (609)581-1700   Fax (609)581-8472

Flores, Charles Edward, MD {1962659953} Pedtrc(04,NJ05)
+ Endurance Sports Medicine LLC
1230 Whitehorse Mercerville Rd   Hamilton, NJ 08619   (609)581-1700   Fax (609)581-9957
+ Pediatrics by Night
1230 Whitehorse Mercerville Ro   Hamilton, NJ 08619   (609)581-1700   Fax (609)581-8472

Flores, David, MD {1710943154} Grtrcs, IntrMd, PulDis(82,MEXI)<NJ-JRSYCITY>
+ Liberty Medical Associates
377 Jersey Avenue/Suite 470   Jersey City, NJ 07302   (201)918-2239   Fax (201)918-2243
dfloresmd@aol.com

Flores, Eduardo G., MD {1497710974} ObsGyn(72,PHIL)<NJ-CHSMRCER, NJ-RWJUHAM>
+ 1230 Whitehorse-Mercerville Rd
Trenton, NJ 08619   (609)581-9950   Fax (609)581-9957

Flores, Jose C., DO {1205808300} FamMed(88,NJ75)<NJ-MTNSIDE>
+ Montclair Family Practice
230 Sherman Avenue/Suite A   Glen Ridge, NJ 07028   (973)743-2321   Fax (973)259-0600

Flores, Lisa, MD {1720496755} FamMed, IntMBari(03,INA3Y)
+ Pediatrics by Night
1230 Whitehorse Mercerville Ro   Hamilton, NJ 08619   (609)581-1700   Fax (609)581-9957

Flores, Marc E., DO {1740202779} FamMed(95,NJ75)<NJ-VIRTMARL>
+ Virtua Marlton Hospital
90 Brick Road   Marlton, NJ 08053   (856)355-6000   Fax (856)355-6061

Flores, Maria S., MD {1851399604} FamMed, Acpntr(82,NJ05)<NJ-JFKMED, NJ-RBAYPERT>
+ 616 Grove Avenue
Edison, NJ 08820   (732)548-6303   Fax (732)548-9822
msfloresmd@optonline.net

Flores, Ramon L., MD {1043279227} NnPnMd, Pedtrc(80,ELSA)<NJ-HACKNSK, NJ-HOLYNAME>
+ Drs. Flores and Flores
819 Main Street   Hackensack, NJ 07601   (201)489-3678   Fax (201)489-7618

Flores Penilla, Jose G., MD {1013151695}<NJ-MORRISTN>
+ Morristown Medical Center
100 Madison Avenue   Morristown, NJ 07962   (973)971-6279

Florino, Guy Michael, MD {1235110560} IntrMd(84,MEX48)
+ 1160 Kennedy Boulevard/51st Street
Bayonne, NJ 07002   (201)823-0303   Fax (201)436-6180

Florio, Francesco, DO {1558479667} RadDia, RadV&I, RadBdI(91,NJ75)<NJ-SHOREMEM>
+ Coastal Imaging, LLC
79 Route 37 West/Suite 103   Toms River, NJ 08755   (732)678-0087   Fax (732)276-2325
+ Shore Memorial Hospital
1 East New York Avenue/Radiology   Somers Point, NJ 08244   (609)653-3500

Florou, Vaia, MD {1205190568} IntrMd
+ St. Peter's University Hospital
254 Easton Avenue   New Brunswick, NJ 08901   (732)745-8600

Flowers, Raphael G., DO {1083622500} IntrMd(00,PA77)<NJ-VALLEY>
+ The Valley Hospital
223 North Van Dien Avenue/IntMed   Ridgewood, NJ 07450   (201)447-8000

Flowers, Rashonda R., MD {1679721831} PhysMd(04,NJ06)
+ Integrated Physiatry Services
45 South Park Place/Suite 259   Morristown, NJ 07960   (908)490-0036   Fax (908)490-0067

Flowers, Robert M., DO {1407143951}
+ Overlook Family Medicine
33 Overlook Road/Suite 103   Summit, NJ 07901   (908)522-5700   Fax (908)273-8014

Flowers, Sakhshat William Knox, III, MD {1225064769} ObsGyn, FamMed(75,DC02)
+ 2 Plymouth Place
Maplewood, NJ 07040   (973)378-8322

Flowers, Shari Carla, MD {1902067937} Rheuma
+ Summit Medical Group-Berkeley Heights Campus
1 Diamond Hill Road   Berkeley Heights, NJ 07922   (908)273-4300   Fax (908)790-6576

Floyd, Darryl Bracey, MD {1689676421} IntrMd(94,PA12)<NJ-LOURDMED>
+ Cooper University Internal Medicine Group
651 John F. Kennedy Way   Willingboro, NJ 08046   (609)835-2838   Fax (690)589-3897
floyd-daryl@cooperhealth.edu

Flyer, Richard H., MD {1104892546} Pedtrc(76,MA01)<NJ-STBARNMC>
+ Park Avenue Pediatrics
36 Park Avenue   Verona, NJ 07044   (973)239-7001   Fax (973)239-8867

Flynn, Anthony M., MD {1912115254} CdvDis
+ Atlantic Cardiology in Galloway
436 Chris Gaupp Drive/Suite 204   Galloway, NJ 08205   (609)652-0100   Fax (609)652-7616
+ Atlantic Cardiology in Ventor
6725 Atlantic Avenue/2nd Floor   Ventnor, NJ 08406   (609)822-2006

Flynn, Daniel E., MD {1881699684} RadDia, Radiol, IntrMd(87,MD01)<NJ-JRSYSHMC>
+ University Radiology Group, P.C.
579A Cranbury Road   East Brunswick, NJ 08816   (732)390-0040   Fax (732)390-1856
+ University Radiology Group
2100 Route 33/Neptune City Med Bld   Neptune, NJ 07753   (732)390-0040   Fax (732)502-0368

Flynn, Jamie, DO {1013391911} FamMed
+ Capital Health Primary Care-Bordentown
1 Third Street   Bordentown, NJ 08505   (609)298-2005   Fax (609)324-8267
+ Capital Health Primary Care Columbus
23203 Columbus Road/Suite 1   Columbus, NJ 08022   (609)298-2005   Fax (603)303-4451

Flynn, Patrick Joseph, DO {1518055243} IntrMd, Grtrcs(72,PA77)<NJ-SJRSYELM, NJ-KMHTURNV>
+ 340 Front Street/Suite 102
Elmer, NJ 08318   (856)358-3747   Fax (856)358-8907

Flynn, Sean A., MD {1154576049} Pedtrc, IntrMd(05,NC08)
+ Step by Step Pediatrics, P.C.
299 Glenwood Avenue/2nd Floor Suite 6   Bloomfield, NJ 07003   (973)743-5639   Fax (973)743-5840

Flynn-Abdalla, Jane, DO {1295820322} FamMed
+ Capital Health Primary Care - Mountainview
850 Bear Tavern Road/Suite 309   Ewing, NJ 08628   (609)656-8844   Fax (609)656-8845

Foca, Francis J., MD {1871516344} PhysMd, OthrSp(66,ITA01)<NJ-OVERLOOK>
+ 507 Westfield Avenue
Westfield, NJ 07090   (908)233-4475   Fax (973)635-2707

Focazio, William John, MD {1205817277} Gastrn, IntrMd(81,GRN01)<NJ-CHILTON>
+ 2 South Main Street
Lodi, NJ 07644   (973)777-3130
+ Endosurgical Center
999 Clifton Avenue   Clifton, NJ 07012   Fax (973)777-6738

Focella, Salvatore, MD {1013901511} IntrMd(90,ITA22)<NJ-HACKNSK, NJ-VALLEY>
+ 1 West Ridgewood Avenue/Suite 203
Paramus, NJ 07652   (201)652-8800   Fax (201)444-8560

Fockler, Raechel Ann, DO {1780934042} ObsGyn
+ Luciano Jose Bispo, MD, LLC
2950 College Drive/Suite 2F   Vineland, NJ 08360   (856)205-0606   Fax (856)205-0044

Foda, Randa Baher, MD {1881629178} FamMed(92,EGY04)
+ Foda Family Practice LLC
2000 Academy Drive/Suite 600   Mount Laurel, NJ 08054   (856)985-9100   Fax (856)985-9106
rfodamd@aol.com

Foddai, Paul A., MD {1457443103} SrgOrt(75,SC04)
+ 142 Palisade Avenue
Jersey City, NJ 07306   (201)795-0904   Fax (201)795-3450

Fodero, Joseph Peter, MD {1073541314} SrgPlstc(93,CT01)<NJ-MORRISTN>
+ 239 West Northfield Road
Livingston, NJ 07039   (973)992-4460   Fax (973)992-2466

Fofah, Onajovwe O., MD {1720187883} Pedtrc(84,NICA)<NJ-UMDNJ>
+ Joseph M. Sanzari ChildrenÆs Hospital
30 Prospect Avenue   Hackensack, NJ 07602   (551)996-8340   Fax (551)996-3051
+ University Hospital
150 Bergen Street/NICU   Newark, NJ 07103   (551)996-8340   Fax (973)972-7711

Fog, Denise Susan, DO {1548268733} RadDia(98,NJ75)
+ South Jersey Radiology Associates, P.A.
748 Kings Highway   West Deptford, NJ 08096   (856)848-4998   Fax (856)853-7362
+ South Jersey Radiology Associates, P.A.
Severan Profess Mews/Suite 105   Sewell, NJ 08080   (856)848-4998   Fax (856)589-6142
+ South Jersey Radiology Associates, P.A.
807 Haddon Avenue/Suite 5   Haddonfield, NJ 08096   (856)616-1130   Fax (856)616-1125

Fog, Edward Roland, DO {1699707232} FamMed, EmrgMd(98,NJ75)<NJ-ACMCITY, NJ-ACMCMAIN>
+ AtlantiCare Regional Medical Center/City Campus
1925 Pacific Avenue/EmergMed   Atlantic City, NJ 08401   (609)345-4000
+ AtlantiCare Regional Med Ctr/Mainland
65 West Jimmie Leeds Road   Pomona, NJ 08240   (609)652-1000

Physicians by Name and Address

Fogari, Robert A., MD {1952499006} IntrMd, Rheuma(69,ITAL)
+ 3053 Kennedy Boulevard
Jersey City, NJ 07306 (201)795-2999 Fax (201)795-5211

Foglio, Elsie Jazmin, DO {1801183926} PedGst<NJ-NWRKBETH>
+ Newark Beth Israel Medical Center
201 Lyons Avenue/Bld L-5 Newark, NJ 07112 (973)926-7280 Fax (926)705-3146

Fojas, Felicia Regina, MD {1881936482} Pedtrc<NJ-CHDNWBTH>
+ Children's Hospital of New Jersey
201 Lyons Avenue/Osborne Terrace Newark, NJ 07112 (973)926-7040

Fojas, Ma. Conchitina Manas, MD {1043594344} EnDbMt
+ Endocrinology Consultants P.C.
229 Engle Street Englewood, NJ 07631 (201)567-5385 Fax (201)567-5385

Foley, James, MD {1689709297} FamMed(89,NY03)
+ St. Peter's University Hospital
254 Easton Avenue New Brunswick, NJ 08901 (732)565-5432 Fax (732)981-0388
+ 149 North Mountain Avenue
Montclair, NJ 07042 (732)565-5432 Fax (973)746-7234

Folk, David, MD {1417215971} OtgyFPlS<NJ-STJOSHOS>
+ St. Joseph's Regional Medical Center
703 Main Street Paterson, NJ 07503 (973)754-2460

Folkman, Michelle Gabrielle, MD {1457386575} PhysMd(89,PA02)
+ 701 White Horse Road
Voorhees, NJ 08043

Follo, Joseph Michael, MD {1003874397} IntrMd(99,NJ05)<NJ-MTNSIDE>
+ 616 Bloomfield Avenue/Suite 3D
West Caldwell, NJ 07006 (973)227-2272 Fax (973)227-2279

Fomin, Svetlana, MD {1326219924} EnDbMt, IntrMd(97,UZB44)<NJ-OCEANMC>
+ Shore Endocrinology Associates, LLC
2200 River Road/Suite A Point Pleasant Boro, NJ 08742 (732)892-7300 Fax (732)892-7301

Fomitchev, Oleg V., MD {1427025105} FamMed<NJ-STMRYPAS>
+ St. Mary's Hospital
350 Boulevard Passaic, NJ 07055 (973)365-4300

Fondacaro, Paul Francis, MD {1770597643} Surgry(81,NY19)
+ 242 Haven Road
Franklin Lakes, NJ 07417

Fong, Dean Kimton, MD {1326164724} EmrgMd, Acpntr(05,NY08)<NJ-STBARNAB>
+ EMedical Urgent Care
2 Kings Highway Middletown, NJ 07748 (732)957-0707 Fax (732)957-9852

Fong, Donald Patrick, MD {1386690683} PsyCAd, Psychy(91,TX15)
+ 100 Straube Center Boulevard/H-1
Pennington, NJ 08534 (609)737-7797 Fax (609)737-7499

Fong DeLeon, Elizabeth Y., MD {1922098813} NnPnMd(75,PHIL)<NJ-VIRTVOOR, NJ-VIRTMHBC>
+ Virtua Voorhees
100 Bowman Drive/Section Chief Voorhees, NJ 08043 (215)529-3191 Fax (215)829-7123
+ Virtua Memorial
175 Madison Avenue/Neontlgy Mount Holly, NJ 08060 (609)261-7053
+ Continuum Health Alliance
1020 Laurel Oak Road/Suite 201 Voorhees, NJ 08043 (856)782-3300 Fax (856)504-8029

Fontana, Leo John, MD {1194722637} RadNro, RadDia(91,VA07)<NJ-RWJURAH>
+ Doctors Radiology Center - MRI of Woodbridge
1500 St. George Avenue/Peach Plaza Avenel, NJ 07001 (732)574-1414 Fax (732)574-0845
+ Coastal Imaging, LLC
79 Route 37 West/Suite 103 Toms River, NJ 08755 (732)574-1414 Fax (732)276-2325
+ Red Bank Radiologists, P.A.
200 White Road/Suite 115 Little Silver, NJ 07001 (732)741-9595 Fax (732)741-0985

Fontana, Victor, DO {1003922113} SrgPlstc(01,NJ15)
+ Fontana Plastic Surgery
879 Poole Avenue Hazlet, NJ 07730 (732)888-8388 Fax (732)888-5595

Fontanazza, Paul, MD {1225041965} IntrMd(75,NJ05)<NJ-CLARMAAS, NJ-WESTHDSN>
+ Primary Care Medical Group
450 Bergen Street Harrison, NJ 07029 (973)484-6900 Fax (973)484-0029

Fontanetta, John Anthony, MD {1457380701} EmrgMd, IntrMd, PulDis(83,NY20)<NJ-CLARMAAS>
+ Clara Maass Medical Center
1 Clara Maass Drive/EmrgMed Belleville, NJ 07109 (973)450-2046

Fontanilla, Hiral P., MD {1093905184} RadOnc(07,NJ05)<PA-ENSTEIN>
+ Princeton Radiology Associates, P.A.
3674 Route 27 Kendall Park, NJ 08824 (732)821-5563 Fax (732)821-6675
+ Princeton Radiology Associates, P.A.
9 Centre Drive Jamesburg, NJ 08831 (732)821-5563 Fax (609)655-4016

Fooks, Tanya, MD {1104141589}
+ 1080 Cambridge Road
Teaneck, NJ 07666 (718)360-3323
talbukh@gmail.com

Foon, Kenneth Alan, MD {1942271945} Hemato(72,MI07)<OH-UNIVCINC>
+ Celgene Global Health
86 Morris Avenue Summit, NJ 07901 (732)673-9613 Fax (732)673-9001

Foos, Gregg Robert, MD {1710964770} SrgOrt, SprtMd(90,NY15)<NJ-MONMOUTH, NJ-RIVERVW>
+ Professional Orthopaedic Associates
776 Shrewsbury Avenue/Suite 201 Tinton Falls, NJ 07724 (732)530-4949 Fax (732)530-3618
+ Professional Orthopaedic Associates
1430 Hooper Avenue/Suite 101 Toms River, NJ 08753 (732)530-4949 Fax (732)349-7722
+ Professional Orthopaedic Associates
303 West Main Street Freehold, NJ 07724 (732)530-4949 Fax (732)577-0036

Foote, Holly Christine, DO {1558706564} Surgry(12,NY76)
+ 326 Edgewater Towne Center
Edgewater, NJ 07020

Foran, Daniel J., DO {1649248402} Pedtrc, AdolMd(81,NJ75)<NJ-VIRTMHBC, NJ-SOCEANCO>
+ Advocare Medford Pediatric & Adolescent Medicine
520 Stokes Road Medford, NJ 08055 (609)654-9112 Fax (609)654-7404

Forbes, Darlene Henderson, MD {1619909504} Pedtrc(97,NY15)<NJ-JRSYSHMC, NJ-OCEANMC>
+ Jewish Renaissance Medical Center
275 Hobart Street Perth Amboy, NJ 08861 (732)376-9333 Fax (732)376-0139

Forbes, Jennifer Rebecca Hughes, MD {1376787994} Pedtrc
+ Franklin Pediatrics, PA
91 South Jefferson Road/Suite 200 Whippany, NJ 07981 (973)538-6116 Fax (973)538-3712

Forbes, Trevor G., MD {1225109390} Psychy(84,NY46)<NY-JACOBIMC, NY-NRTHCBRX>
+ 1010 Park Avenue
Plainfield, NJ 07060 (908)822-9099 Fax (908)822-0449

Forcina, Salvatore John, MD {1124124425} SrgVas, Surgry(68,ARG03)<NJ-HOLYNAME>
+ 810 Main Street
Hackensack, NJ 07601 (201)488-2666 Fax (201)488-1655

Ford, Lisa M., MD {1659445013} Nrolgy, NroChl, NrlgSpec(80,PA13)<NJ-UMDNJ, NJ-NWRKBETH>
+ University Hospital
150 Bergen Street/Bldg-h506 Newark, NJ 07103 (973)972-4300

Ford, Robert R., MD {1093731879} RadDia, Radiol(83,NJ06)
+ Princeton Radiology Associates, P.A.
419 North Harrison Street Princeton, NJ 08540 (609)921-3345 Fax (609)683-8847
+ Princeton Radiology Associates, P.A.
9 Centre Drive Jamesburg, NJ 08831 (609)921-3345 Fax (609)655-4016
+ University Radiology Group, P.C.
375 Route 206/Suite 1 Hillsborough, NJ 08540 (908)874-7600 Fax (908)874-7052

Ford, Stephen D., MD {1447290408} IntrMd(84,TN07)
+ Union County HealthCare Associates
999 Raritan Road Clark, NJ 07066 (732)381-3740 Fax (732)381-3733
+ 1503 Saint Georges Avenue/Suite 201
Colonia, NJ 07067 (732)381-3740 Fax (732)382-5201

Forde, Frank, MD {1902291800} EmrgMd
+ University Hospital-New Jersey Medical School
30 Bergen Street/Room 1110 Newark, NJ 07107 (973)972-9261

Forde Baker, Jenice Michelle Letici, MD {1851565501} EmrgMd(04,NY20)<NJ-OURLADY>
+ Our Lady of Lourdes Medical Center
1600 Haddon Avenue/EmrgMed Camden, NJ 08103 (856)757-3500

Foreman, Michael J., MD {1801844188} Pedtrc(81,PA09)<NJ-VIRTMHBC>
+ Advocare Delran Pediatrics
5045 Route 130 South/Suite F Delran, NJ 08075 (856)461-1717 Fax (856)461-1143

Forester, Gary P., MD {1154352698} Gastrn, IntrMd(75,PA01)<NJ-UNVMCPRN>
+ Princeton Health Medical & Surgical Associates
2 Centre Drive/Suite 200 Monroe, NJ 08831 (609)395-2470 Fax (609)860-5288
+ Princeton Medicine
5 Plainsboro Road/Suite 300 Plainsboro, NJ 08536 (609)395-2470 Fax (609)853-7271

Forman, Eric Jason, MD {1053521500} RprEnd
+ Reproductive Medicine Associates of New Jersey
111 Madison Avenue/Suite 100 Morristown, NJ 07962 (973)971-4600 Fax (973)290-8370

Forman, Glenn M., MD {1457376642} PhysMd(88,DC02)
+ Orthopaedic Sports Medicine
80 Oak Hill Road Red Bank, NJ 07701 (732)741-2313 Fax (732)741-7154

Forman, Jeffrey S., MD {1427056050} Ophthl(85,NY47)<NJ-VIRTUAHS>
+ 1233 Haddonfield Berlin Road/Unit 5
Voorhees, NJ 08043 (856)767-7800 Fax (856)767-7833

Forman, Lawrence S., DO {1437175544} FamMed(68,IA75)
+ Springside Road Medical Associates
2428 Route 38/Suite 306 Cherry Hill, NJ 08002 (856)348-8444 Fax (856)348-8446

Forman, Mark H., MD {1235190190} SrgThr, Surgry(76,LA01)<NJ-STBARNMC, NJ-CLARMAAS>
+ Forman-Hertz, MD LLC
1500 Pleasant Valley Way/Suite 302 West Orange, NJ 07052 (973)324-0988 Fax (973)324-1064

Forman-Chou, Alexandra Catherine, MD {1730231200} Psychy(99,PA12)
+ Integrated Behavioral Care, P.A.
35 Beechwood Road/Suite 3-A & 3-B Summit, NJ 07901 (908)598-2400 Fax (908)598-2408

Fornari, Marcella, DO {1427310192} SrgBst(12,WV75)<NJ-MORRISTN>
+ Atlantic Breast Associates
100 Madison Avenue/3rd Floor Morristown, NJ 07962 (973)971-4166 Fax (973)290-7152

Forosisky, Garett John, MD {1750642393}
+ 473 Salter Court
Glassboro, NJ 08028 (856)889-8831
garett.forosisky@drexelmed.edu

Foroush, Pejman, MD {1528233202} Anesth(03,GRN01)<NJ-BAYSHORE>
+ Bayshore Community Hospital
727 North Beers Street Holmdel, NJ 07733 (732)739-5900
+ 30 Cape May Drive
Marlboro, NJ 07746

Foroutan, Janelle, MD {1215222534} MtFtMd<NY-SLRRSVLT>
+ St. Peter's Family Health
123 How Lane New Brunswick, NJ 08901 (732)745-8600 Fax (732)729-0869

Forouzan-Gandashmin, Iraj, MD {1376500942} MtFtMd, ObsGyn(76,IRA09)<NJ-CHSMRCER, PA-HLYRDMER>
+ Capital Health System/Mercer Campus
446 Bellevue Avenue/Mat-Fetal/3rd F Trenton, NJ 08618 (609)394-4000

Forouzesh, Avisheh, MD {1346273778} InfDis, IntrMd(01,NY15)<NJ-HOBUNIMC>
+ Carepoint Health Medical Group
331 Grand Street/Ground Floor Hoboken, NJ 07030 (201)238-2888 Fax (201)656-5989

Forrest, Robert, MD {1104890953} Anesth(90,NY15)<NJ-HCKTSTWN, CT-ALLIANCE>
+ Montclair Anesthesia Associates PC
185 Fairfield Avenue/Suite 2A West Caldwell, NJ 07006 (973)226-1230 Fax (973)226-1232

Forrester, Catherine A., MD {1568413201} IntrMd(79,NJ05)<NJ-COMMED>
+ Ocean Adult Medical Group LLC
147 Route 37 West/Suite 1 Toms River, NJ 08755

Forrester, Dara Lynn, MD {1851563662} ObsGyn(01,GRN01)
+ 115 North Road
Berkeley Heights, NJ 07922

Forrester, Glenn Joseph, MD {1043475643} Surgry, Bariat(01,GRN01)<NJ-OVERLOOK, NJ-TRINIWSC>
+ New Jersey Bariatric Center
193 Morris Avenue/2nd Floor Springfield, NJ 07081 (908)481-1270 Fax (908)688-8861
gforrester@njbcenter.com

Forsberg, Martin M., MD {1790881944} Psychy, PsyGrt
+ New Jersey Institute for Successful Aging
42 East Laurel Road/Suite 1800 Stratford, NJ 08084 (856)566-6843 Fax (856)566-6781

Forster, Brian, MD {1407396328}<NJ-JRSYSHMC>
+ Jersey Shore University Medical Center
1945 Route 33 Neptune, NJ 07753 (732)776-4263

Forster, Judith Karen, MD {1598828931} ObsGyn(93,NJ05)<NJ-STPETER>
+ Womens Health first
114 Stanhope Street Princeton, NJ 08540 (609)683-7979 Fax (609)683-1972

Physicians by Name and Address

Forster, Susan A., MD {1518026913} ObsGyn(84,NJ06)<NJ-RWJUBRUN, NJ-STPETER>
+ Womens Health first
  114 Stanhope Street   Princeton, NJ 08540   (609)683-7979   Fax (609)683-1972
+ Cares Surgicenter, LLC.
  240 Easton Avenue   New Brunswick, NJ 08901   (609)683-7979   Fax (732)296-8677

Fort, Prem, MD {1639345580} NnPnMd
+ 3307 Autumn Drive
  Tinton Falls, NJ 07753

Forte, Francis A., MD {1063467645} OncHem, IntrMd(64,NY46)<NJ-ENGLWOOD, NJ-HOLYNAME>
+ Forte Schleider & Attas MD PA
  350 Engle Street/Berrie Building/1 FL   Englewood, NJ 07631   (201)568-5250   Fax (201)568-5358

Forti, Viviana Claure, MD {1225438963} Pedtrc
+ 6 Apache Trail
  Rockaway, NJ 07866   (973)925-3425

Fortin, Robert Glenn, MD {1932178217} Pedtrc, AdolMd(89,PA01)<NJ-RWJUBRUN, NJ-STPETER>
+ Tiefenbrunn & Fortin Pediatrics, PA
  503 Cranbury Road   East Brunswick, NJ 08816   (732)390-8400   Fax (732)390-8970

Fortino, Gregg L., MD {1245232995} CdvDis, IntrMd(87,NJ06)<NJ-COOPRUMC, NJ-VIRTMARL>
+ Cardiovascular Associates
  210 West Atlantic Avenue   Haddon Heights, NJ 08035   (856)546-3003   Fax (856)547-5337
+ Cardiovascular Associates of The Delaware Valley, PA
  1840 Frontage Road   Cherry Hill, NJ 08034   (856)546-3003   Fax (856)795-7436
+ Cardiovascular Associates of The Delaware Valley, PA
  525 State Street/Suite 3   Elmer, NJ 08035   (856)358-2363   Fax (856)358-0725

Fortunato, Diane L., MD {1053313718} IntrMd(81,GRN01)
+ 509 Roseville Avenue/PO Box 7129
  Newark, NJ 07107   (973)482-0339

Fortunato Sieglen, Linda Marie, MD {1922188051} Anesth(83,NJ06)<NJ-UNVMCPRN>
+ University Medical Center of Princeton at Plainsboro
  One Plainsboro Road/Anesthesiology   Plainsboro, NJ 08536   (609)497-4000

Forward, John B., MD {1477507192} IntrMd, AltHol(81,MEX03)<NJ-STCLRBOO>
+ Internal Medicine of Morris County LLC
  195 Route 46 West/Suite 102   Mine Hill, NJ 07803   (973)366-8884   Fax (973)366-1423

Foschetti, Felix P., Jr., DO {1790799492} FamMed(70,PA77)<NJ-WARREN>
+ Warren County Family Practice
  23 West Church Street   Washington, NJ 07882   (908)689-7171

Foss, Roberta, DO {1316154438} FamMed, IntrMd(92,PA77)
+ 124 Kings Highway West
  Haddonfield, NJ 08033   (856)216-9001   Fax (856)616-9837

Fossati, Jeffrey Joseph, MD {1093875015} PhysMd, OthrSp(91,NJ05)
+ Northern New Jersey Pain & Rehabilitation Center
  37 West Century Road/Suite 111   Paramus, NJ 07652   (201)262-2244   Fax (201)262-2246

Fost, Arthur F., MD {1881682185} Allrgy, Pedtrc, AlgyImmn(63,PA02)<NJ-NWTNMEM, NJ-CLARMAAS>
+ Allergy Consultants, PA
  197 Bloomfield Avenue   Verona, NJ 07044   (973)857-0330   Fax (973)857-0980
  affost@pol.net
+ Allergy Consultants, PA
  5 Franklin Avenue   Belleville, NJ 07109   (973)857-0330   Fax (973)759-0403
+ Allergy Consultants, PA
  89 Sparta Avenue/Suite 230   Sparta, NJ 07044   (973)726-8850   Fax (973)726-8924

Fost, David A., MD {1356339410} Allrgy, AlgyImmn(92,PA02)<NJ-NWTNMEM, NJ-CLARMAAS>
+ Allergy Consultants, PA
  197 Bloomfield Avenue   Verona, NJ 07044   (973)857-0330   Fax (973)857-0980
+ Allergy Consultants, PA
  89 Sparta Avenue/Suite 230   Sparta, NJ 07871   (973)857-0330   Fax (973)726-8924
+ Allergy Consultants, PA
  5 Franklin Avenue   Belleville, NJ 07044   (973)759-2029   Fax (973)759-0403

Foster, Jonathan A., MD {1093909483} RadDia(93,NY01)<NJ-ENGLWOOD>
+ Englewood Radiologic Group PA
  350 Engle Street   Englewood, NJ 07631   (201)894-3000   Fax (201)894-5244

Foster, Ronald D., MD {1760484273} IntrMd(83,PA09)<NJ-RWJUBRUN, NJ-STPETER>
+ 7 Centre Drive/Suite 13
  Monroe Township, NJ 08831   (609)655-7752   Fax (609)655-8065

Foster, Sarah Jeanmarie, MD {1811212715} RadNro
+ Hackensack Radiology Group, P.A.
  30 Prospect Avenue   Hackensack, NJ 07601   (551)996-2200   Fax (201)489-2812

Foster, Wayne Paul, MD {1316052699} Otlryg, SrgFPl(88,PA13)
+ ENT of NJ/Foster Facial PlasticSurgery
  500 Lakehurst Road   Toms River, NJ 08755   (732)914-1461   Fax (732)914-8974
+ ENT of NJ/Foster Facial PlasticSurgery
  2041 Highway 35   Wall, NJ 07719   (732)449-2099

Foti, Frederick D., Jr., MD {1972528495} Dermat, PthAna(91,LA05)
+ Dermatology Associates
  303 Chester Avenue   Moorestown, NJ 08057   (856)235-1178   Fax (856)722-9244
  fratfo3@comcast.net
+ Moorestown Dermatology Associates
  702 East Main Street   Moorestown, NJ 08057   (856)235-1178   Fax (856)235-6566

Fourcand, Farah Yolanda, MD {1013302421} Nrolgy
+ JFK Neurosciences Institute
  65 James Street/Second Floor   Edison, NJ 08818   (732)321-7010   Fax (732)632-1669

Fowlie, Thomas, Jr., MD {1770528168} EmrgMd(92,NJ06)<NJ-COMMED>
+ Community Medical Center
  99 Route 37 West/Emerg Medicine   Toms River, NJ 08755   (732)240-8080

Fowls, Brianna, MD {1801146378} FamMed
+ Your Doctors Care, PA
  71 Route 206 South   Hillsborough, NJ 08844   (908)685-1887   Fax (908)707-0816
+ 161 West Cliff Street/Apt 2
  Somerville, NJ 08876   (201)787-9696

Fox, Alissa B., MD {1780688697} Dermat(80,NY19)<NJ-SOMERSET, NJ-HUNTRDN>
+ Fox Skin & Allergy Associates
  3461 Route 22   Branchburg, NJ 08876   (908)725-4777   Fax (908)725-7439
  alissa.fox@foxskinandallergy.mymedfusion.com

Fox, Daniel E., MD {1538131560} SrgOrt(83,NJ05)<NJ-COMMED>
+ Center for Orthopedics & Sports Medicine
  111 West Water Street/PO Box 5016   Toms River, NJ 08754   (732)505-8844   Fax (732)505-4485

Fox, David B., MD {1427098631} IntrMd, PhysMd(86,WIND)
+ Center for Physical Medicine and Rehabilitation
  30 North Main Street   Marlboro, NJ 07746   (732)761-0500
+ Center for Physical Medicine and Rehabilitation
  776 Shrewsbury Avenue/Suite 203   Tinton Falls, NJ 07724   (732)761-0500   Fax (732)219-6526

Fox, Ellen H., MD {1285775775} Pthlgy, PthAna, PthACl(82,CHNA)<NJ-CHSMRCER, NJ-CHSFULD>
+ Capital Health System/Hopewell
  One Capital Way/Pathology   Pennington, NJ 08534   (609)303-4019

Fox, Howard D., DO {1811956576} ObsGyn(71,MO79)<NJ-JFKMED, NJ-RWJURAH>
+ The Rubino Ob/Gyn Group
  101 Old Short Hills Road/Suite 101   West Orange, NJ 07052   (732)396-1881   Fax (732)396-3262

Fox, James A., MD {1144224056} AlgyImmn, PedAlg(77,CT01)<NJ-SOMERSET, NJ-HUNTRDN>
+ Fox Skin & Allergy Associates
  3461 Route 22   Branchburg, NJ 08876   (908)725-4777   Fax (908)725-7439
+ Fox Skin & Allergy Associates
  1100 Wescott Drive/Suite 303   Flemington, NJ 08822   (908)725-4777   Fax (908)788-6668

Fox, Jerry C., MD {1043374523} Anesth(75,NY01)<NJ-STBARNMC>
+ St. Barnabas Medical Center
  94 Old Short Hills Road/Anesthesia   Livingston, NJ 07039   (973)322-5512

Fox, Jonathan L., MD {1538208301} SrgHnd, SrgOrt, IntrMd(74,PA01)<NJ-ACMCITY, NJ-ACMCMAIN>
+ Fox Orthopedic Center
  1601 Tilton Road   Northfield, NJ 08225   (609)407-1600   Fax (609)641-6776

Fox, Justin Michael, MD {1629269600} IntrMd, CdvDis, IntCrd(04,NY19)<NJ-RWJUHAM>
+ Hamilton Cardiology Associates
  2073 Klockner Road   Hamilton, NJ 08690   (609)584-1212   Fax (609)584-0103

Fox, Katherine, MD {1063672905} IntMHPC<NJ-HUNTRDN>
+ Hunterdon Medical Center
  2100 Wescott Drive   Flemington, NJ 08822   (908)237-7018   Fax (908)788-6361

Fox, Martin Lee, MD {1831264225} Ophthl, CrnExD, SrgRef(76,PA09)<NY-NYEYEINF>
+ Cornea & Refractive Surgery Practice of New Jersey
  61 North Maple Avenue   Ridgewood, NJ 07450   (201)493-1885
+ Cornea & Refractive Surgery Practice of New Jersey
  91 Millburn Avenue   Millburn, NJ 07041   (973)218-9050

Fox, Melissa D., MD {1326266776} Pthlgy<NJ-RWJUBRUN>
+ RWJ University Hospital New Brunswick
  One Robert Wood Johnson Place   New Brunswick, NJ 08901   (304)654-1491
  mfoxis@gmail.com

Fox, Michael L., MD {1316007040} FamMAdlt
+ 550 Bay Avenue/Harbour Cove 503
  Somers Point, NJ 08244

Fox, Michelle Candice, MD {1790717619} ObsGyn(97,MD07)
+ 60 Fairhill Drive
  Westfield, NJ 07090   (732)594-2312

Fox, Nicole M., MD {1023147816} Surgry<NJ-COOPRUMC>
+ Cooper University Hospital
  One Cooper Plaza   Camden, NJ 08103   (856)342-2000
+ Cooper University Physician Trauma Center
  One Cooper Plaza   Camden, NJ 08103   (856)342-3014

Fox, Richard David, MD {1578531133} Dermat(67,PA02)<NJ-CHRIST>
+ Academic Dermatology & Dermatologic Surgery Group
  3202 Kennedy Boulevard   Jersey City, NJ 07307   (201)792-4500   Fax (201)792-5983
+ Academic Dermatology & Dermatologic Surgery Group
  703 Kearny Avenue   Kearny, NJ 07032   (201)998-4699

Fox, Ross J., MD {1689698128} SrgHnd, SrgOrt, OrtSHand(94,NY45)
+ North Jersey Hand Surgery
  385 Morris Avenue/Third Floor   Springfield, NJ 07081   (973)664-9899   Fax (973)664-1875
+ North Jersey Hand Surgery
  75 Bloomfield Avenue/Suite 102   Denville, NJ 07834   (973)664-9899   Fax (973)664-1875

Fox, Steven N., MD {1114998218} CdvDis, IntrMd(81,NY19)<NJ-VIRTMARL, NJ-OURLADY>
+ Associated Cardiovascular Consultants-Lourdes
  1 Brace Road/Suite C & F   Cherry Hill, NJ 08034   (856)428-4100   Fax (856)428-5748
+ Associated Cardiovascular Consultants, P.A.
  730 North Broad Street/Suite 200   Woodbury, NJ 08096   (856)428-4100   Fax (856)251-2344

Fox, Stuart W., MD {1063413102} Nrolgy, IntrMd(75,NY20)<NJ-MORRISTN>
+ Neuroscience Center of Northern New Jersey
  310 Madison Avenue   Morristown, NJ 07960   (973)285-1446   Fax (973)605-8854

Fox-Mellul, Jodi V., MD {1053616631} EnDbMt, IntrMd(02,ISR05)<NJ-UNDRWD>
+ Inspira Medical Group Endocrinolgy Mullica Hill
  34 Colson Lane   Mullica Hill, NJ 08062   (856)223-0965   Fax (856)223-1357

Foxman, Brett T., MD {1376518738} Ophthl(82,MA05)<NJ-SHOREMEM, NJ-ACMCMAIN>
+ Retinal & Ophthalmic Consultants, PC
  1500 Tilton Road   Northfield, NJ 08225   (609)646-5200   Fax (609)646-9868
+ Retinal & Ophthalmic Consultants, PC
  2466 East Chestnut Avenue   Vineland, NJ 08360   (609)646-5200   Fax (856)507-0040
+ Retinal & Ophthalmic Consultants, PC
  211 South Main Street/Suite 102   Cape May Court House, NJ 08225   (609)463-4610   Fax (609)463-4616

Foxman, Scott G., MD {1447224175} Ophthl(79,MA05)<NJ-ACMCITY, NJ-ACMCMAIN>
+ Retinal & Ophthalmic Consultants, PC
  1500 Tilton Road   Northfield, NJ 08225   (609)646-5200   Fax (609)646-9868
+ Retinal & Ophthalmic Consultants, PC
  2466 East Chestnut Avenue   Vineland, NJ 08360   (609)646-5200   Fax (856)507-0040
+ Retinal & Ophthalmic Consultants, PC
  211 South Main Street/Suite 102   Cape May Court House, NJ 08225   (609)463-4610   Fax (609)463-4616

Foye, Patrick M., MD {1013942853} PhysMd, Elecmy, PainInvt(92,NJ05)<NJ-UMDNJ>
+ University Hospital-Doctors Office Center
  90 Bergen Street/PhysMed/DOC3100   Newark, NJ 07103   (973)972-2802   Fax (973)972-2825

Fradkin, Yuli, MD {1255589461}
+ 63 Claremont Avenue
  Montclair, NJ 07042   (646)685-9836
  julikfradkin@gmail.com

Fradlis, Alina, MD {1619210366} Anesth<NJ-HOLYNAME>
+ Holy Name Hospital
  718 Teaneck Road   Teaneck, NJ 07666   (201)833-3000

Physicians by Name and Address

Fragoso, Jose, MD {1164497624} Pedtrc, AdolMd(81,DOMI)<NJ-HOBUNIMC>
+ 4808 Bergenline Avenue/5th Floor
Union City, NJ 07087 (201)865-3444 Fax (201)865-0038

Fraimow, Henry S., MD {1821183963} InfDis, IntrMd(82,PA01)<NJ-COOPRUMC>
+ EIP Clinic/Early Intervention Program (HIV/AIDS)
3 Cooper Plaza/Suite 513 Camden, NJ 08103 (856)963-3715 Fax (856)635-1052

Franasiak, Jason Michael, MD {1871727016}
+ 140 Allen Ridge
Basking Ridge, NJ 07920

France, Jeffrey W., DO {1942280219} NnPnMd, Pedtrc, LeglMd(82,NJ75)<NJ-JRSYSHMC, NJ-RIVERVW>
+ 59 Avenue at the Common/Suite 103
Shrewsbury, NJ 07702 (732)935-3500

France, Matthew P., MD {1467450387} SrgArt, SprtMd, SrgOrt(86,NJ05)<NJ-MORRISTN>
+ Arthroscopic Surgery & Sports Medicine Center
1 Robertson Drive/Suite 11 Bedminster, NJ 07921 (908)234-9800 Fax (908)234-2070
+ Arthroscopic Surgery & Sports Medicine Center
101 Madison Avenue/Suite 401 Morristown, NJ 07960 (908)234-9800 Fax (908)234-2070

Franceschini, Chloe Nicole, MD {1023351558} ObsGyn(PRO03)
+ University Consultants in Ob-Gyn & Womens Health
33 Overlook Road/Mac 405 Summit, NJ 07902 (908)522-3688 Fax (908)522-3687

Francis, Amanda Rachael, DO {1679833727} ObsGyn
+ University Medical Group/OBGYN
125 Paterson Street/2nd Floor New Brunswick, NJ 08901 (732)235-7755 Fax (732)235-6627

Francis, Bruce H., MD {1285890343} EnDbMt, IntrMd(79,ITA01)
+ Novartis Pharmaceuticals Corporation
One Health Plaza East Hanover, NJ 07936 (973)432-2743 Fax (973)781-6504

Francis, Charles Kenneth, MD {1801837356} IntrMd, CdvDis(65,PA02)
+ University Cardiology Group
125 Paterson Street/Suite 5200 New Brunswick, NJ 08901 (732)235-6561 Fax (732)235-6530

Francis, Guy Anthony, MD {1376554378} FamMed(96,NJ05)<NJ-UMDNJ, NJ-HOBUNIMC>
+ 2130 Millburn avenue/Suite C5
Maplewood, NJ 07040 (973)763-2555 Fax (973)763-2558
+ St. Mary Center for Family Health
122-132 Clinton Street Hoboken, NJ 07030 (973)763-2555 Fax (201)418-3140

Francis, Kathleen D., MD {1578669164} PhysMd(89,NJ05)<NJ-STBARNMC>
+ Lymphedema Physician Services, P.C.
200 South Orange Avenue/Suite 111 Livingston, NJ 07039 (973)322-7366 Fax (973)322-7450

Francis, Thomas Paul, DO {1497894091} IntrMd, Pedtrc, FamMed(92,PA77)
+ 38 Ridge Road
North Arlington, NJ 07031 (201)998-6100 Fax (201)998-6232
Tfrancis2280@yahoo.com

Francisco, Rowena Rebano, MD {1518045954} Psychy, IntrMd(80,PHI09)
+ Center for Family Guidance, PC
765 East Route 70/Building A-101 Marlton, NJ 08053 (856)797-4800 Fax (856)810-0110

Franckle, William C., IV, MD {1770785685} Surgry, SrgPlstc(96,NJ06)
+ 23 Staffordshire Road
Cherry Hill, NJ 08003 (732)545-4520

Franco, Charles D., MD {1942393012} SrgVas, Surgry(82,NJ05)<NJ-RWJUBRUN>
+ 2 Research Way/Suite 307
Monroe Township, NJ 08831 (609)409-4500 Fax (609)409-9050
+ RWJ University Hospital New Brunswick
One Robert Wood Johnson Place New Brunswick, NJ 08901 (732)828-3000

Franco, Hugo C., MD {1629022769} Psychy, PsyAdd(78,BRA04)<NJ-CARRIER>
+ 111 Broad Street
Eatontown, NJ 07724 (732)915-0461 Fax (732)389-3533

Franco, Maria M., MD {1861548166} Pedtrc(82,PHI02)<NJ-JRSYCITY>
+ Metropolitan Family Health Network
935 Garfield Avenue Jersey City, NJ 07304 (201)478-5800 Fax (201)478-5823

Francois, Emmanuel J., MD {1457383382} Pedtrc(82,FRA40)<NJ-NWRKBETH, NJ-STBARNMC>
+ Washington Pediatrics Center
41 Washington Avenue Irvington, NJ 07111 (973)373-3199 Fax (973)373-0480

Francois, Jean-Marie L., MD {1821152125} IntrMd(77,HAI01)<NJ-GRYSTPSY>
+ Greystone Park Psychiatric Hospital
59 Koch Avenue/IntMed Morris Plains, NJ 07950 (973)538-1800

Francois, Vincent, MD {1386696755} IntrMd(68,MEXI)<NJ-BAYONNE>
+ American Physician Services/Hudson HealthCare
679 Montgomery Street Jersey City, NJ 07306 (201)433-6500 Fax (201)433-8010
+ Immediate Care, PC
621 Kennedy Boulevard North Bergen, NJ 07047 (201)433-6500 Fax (201)325-0385

Francolla, Karen Ann, MD {1609890433} PedGst, Pedtrc, IntrMd(02,NY15)
+ Joseph M. Sanzari Childrens' -Gastro
155 Polifly Road/Suite 102 Hackensack, NJ 07601 (551)996-8840 Fax (201)441-9949

Francos, George Charles, MD {1457374530} IntrMd, Nephro(78,PA02)
+ 285 Merion Avenue
Haddonfield, NJ 08033

Franger, Margaret Mary, MD {1164470753} Nephro, IntrMd(99,PA02)<NJ-VIRTMHBC, NJ-LOURDMED>
+ The Center for Kidney Care
1261 Route 38/Suite A Hainesport, NJ 08036 (856)222-1975 Fax (856)222-0721

Franjul Diaz, Rafael Eduardo, MD {1972866291}
+ 127 Old Short Hills Road/Apt 176
West Orange, NJ 07052 (516)376-2558
Franjul@gmail.com

Frank, Daniel B., MD {1457593709} EmrgMd(09,NY48)
+ Hackensack Medical Center Emergency Medicine
30 Prospect Avenue/Main 3619 Hackensack, NJ 07601 (551)996-2000 Fax (201)968-1866

Frank, David J., MD {1174633648} Nrolgy(88,PA09)<NJ-JRSYSHMC, NJ-CENTRAST>
+ Central Jersey Neurology Associates
501 Iron Bridge Road/Suite 2 Freehold, NJ 07728 (732)462-7030 Fax (732)308-3562

Frank, Elliot, MD {1205805009} InfDis, IntrMd(78,CT01)<NJ-JRSYSHMC>
+ Hackensack Meridian Medical Group
19 Davis Avenue/5th-6th Floor Neptune, NJ 07753 (732)897-3995 Fax (732)897-3997
+ Jersey Shore University Medical Center
1945 Route 33/Medicine Neptune, NJ 07753 (732)897-3995 Fax (732)776-3795

Frank, Howard, MD {1043356348} Anesth(71,PA09)
+ 22 Hidden Lake Circle
Barnegat, NJ 08005

Frank, Marcella M., DO {1083611255} PulDis, IntrMd(78,PA77)<NJ-CHSFULD>
+ Capital Health System/Fuld Campus
750 Brunswick Avenue/InternalMed Trenton, NJ 08638 (609)278-6990 Fax (609)278-6982
+ Snoring and Sleep Apnea Center Mercer County
1401 Whitehorse Mercerville Rd Hamilton, NJ 08619 (609)278-6990 Fax (609)584-5144

Frank, Martin J., MD {1821016155} OncHem, IntrMd(82,DC01)<NJ-CHILTON, NJ-VALLEY>
+ Chilton Medical Center
97 West Parkway/Hemat/Oncology Pompton Plains, NJ 07444 (973)831-5000
+ The Valley Hospital
223 North Van Dien Avenue Ridgewood, NJ 07450 (201)447-8000

Frank, Oleg, MD {1457469090} IntrMd(96,DMN01)
+ 40 Ferry Street/Rear
Newark, NJ 07105 (973)344-4470 Fax (973)344-4476
Olegfrank@optionline.com

Frank, Ronald Gary, MD {1760426829} Urolgy, Surgry(85,NY09)
+ Lincoln P. Miller, MD, LLC
1500 Pleasant Valley Way/Suite 201 West Orange, NJ 07052 (973)966-6400 Fax (973)731-5690

Frank-Gerszberg, Robin G., MD {1104813658} PedRad, RadDia(87,NY46)<NJ-STJOSHOS>
+ Imaging Subspecialists of North Jersey LLC
703 Main Street Paterson, NJ 07503 (973)754-2645

Frank-Shrensel, Bettie, MD {1114995750} Pedtrc(84,NJ05)<NJ-MORRISTN, NJ-STBARNMC>
+ Pediatric Associates of West Essex PA
1129 Bloomfield Avenue/Suite 100 West Caldwell, NJ 07006 (973)575-8585 Fax (973)882-6914

Frankel, David Zelig, MD {1689862799} FamMed, FamMSptM, IntrMd(02,PA02)
+ Frankel Sports Medicine
8512 Ventnor Avenue Margate City, NJ 08402 (609)225-9625 Fax (609)541-2727

Frankel, Kathryn A., MD {1023407616}<NJ-MORRISTN>
+ Morristown Medical Center
100 Madison Avenue Morristown, NJ 07962 (973)971-7926

Frankel, Renee Ellen, MD {1790852739} InfDis, IntrMd(89,NJ05)
+ IPC The Hospitalist Company
220 Ridgedale Avenue/Suite C-2 Florham Park, NJ 07932 (973)538-5844 Fax (973)267-0181

Frankel, Robert, MD {1205880978} EmrgMd(02,GRN01)
+ 200 Atlantic Avenue/Suite E
Manasquan, NJ 08736 (866)821-7655

Frankel, Susan L., DO {1760522163} Grtrcs, IntrMd(89,MO78)<NY-MTSINAI, NJ-HACKNSK>
+ New Jersey Institute for Successful Aging
42 East Laurel Road/Suite 1800 Stratford, NJ 08084 (856)566-6843 Fax (856)566-6781
+ Hackensack University Medical Center
30 Prospect Avenue Hackensack, NJ 07601 (201)996-2000

Frankel, Trina N., MD {1407847932} IntrMd(68,NY46)<NJ-STBARNMC>
+ Millburn Primary Care LLC
120 Millburn Avenue/Suite 206 Millburn, NJ 07041 (973)467-9282 Fax (973)467-0340

Frankel, Victor R., MD {1356303648} SrgOrt, SprtMd(81,NJ05)<NJ-BURDTMLN, NJ-ACMCITY>
+ Pace Orthopedics & Sports Medicine
547 New Road Somers Point, NJ 08244 (609)927-9200 Fax (609)927-1616
+ Fox Orthopedic Center
1601 Tilton Road Northfield, NJ 08225 (609)927-9200 Fax (609)641-6776

Frankel, Zev Binyamin, MD {1477758670} IntrMd, CdvDis(02,MA01)
+ Valley Medical Group/Valley Heart Group
1200 East Ridgewood Avenue Ridgewood, NJ 07450 (201)670-8660 Fax (201)447-1957

Frankel-Tiger, Robyn F., MD {1669588380} Radiol, RadBdl(91,PA07)<NJ-VIRTUAHS, NJ-VIRTMHBC>
+ Atlantic Medical Imaging, LLC.
72 West Jimmie Leeds Road Galloway, NJ 08205 (609)677-9729 Fax (609)653-8764
+ Atlantic Medical Imaging, LLC.
401 Bethel Road Somers Point, NJ 08244 (609)677-9729
+ Atlantic Medical Imaging, LLC.
421 Route 9 North Cape May Court House, NJ 08205 (609)463-9500 Fax (609)465-0918

Franklin, Barry I., MD {1821023672} RadDia, Radiol(75,OH41)<NJ-NWTNMEM>
+ Sparta Health and Wellness Center
89 Sparta Avenue/Suite 120 Sparta, NJ 07871 (973)729-0002 Fax (973)729-1085
+ Image Care Centers
222 High Street/Suite 101 Newton, NJ 07860 (973)729-0002 Fax (973)383-2774
+ Radiologic Associates of Northwest New Jersey
212 Route 94 Vernon, NJ 07871 (973)827-1961

Franklin, James D., MD {1801957014} IntrMd(86,MEX03)<NJ-CLARMAAS, NJ-MTNSIDE>
+ Drs. Cozzarelli-Franklin and Franklin MD's
175 Franklin Avenue Nutley, NJ 07110 (973)667-8535 Fax (973)667-8442

Franks, Lori Genevieve Pihl, MD {1932391612} IntHos<NJ-VIRTVOOR>
+ Virtua Voorhees
100 Bowman Drive Voorhees, NJ 08043 (225)636-0254 lori.franks1@gmail.com

Franks, Ralph Robert, Jr., DO {1386739449} FamMed, SprtMd(99,NJ75)<NJ-COOPRUMC>
+ Cooper University Medical Center/Camden
3 Cooper Plaza/Ste411/SportMed Camden, NJ 08103 (856)342-2000
franks-robert@cooperhealth.edu
+ Cooper Bone and Joint Institute
900 Centennial Boulevard Voorhees, NJ 08043 (856)342-2000 Fax (856)325-6678

Frantz, Mildred Marie, MD {1497816995} FamMed(02,NJ06)<NJ-MONMOUTH>
+ HealthCare for Life
1 Industrial Way W/Bldg. B Eatontown, NJ 07724 (732)935-0500
+ HealthCare for Life LLC
212 Monmouth Road Oakhurst, NJ 07755 (732)935-0500 Fax (732)531-9901

Franz, Stacey, DO {1306018668} PhysMd(04,PA77)
+ Northeast Spine & Sports Medicine
1104 Arnold Avenue Point Pleasant Beach, NJ 08742 (732)714-0070 Fax (732)714-0188
+ Northeast Spine and Sports Medicine
728 Bennetts Mills Road Jackson, NJ 08527 (732)714-0070 Fax (732)415-1403

Franzblau, Natali R., MD {1598847071} ObsGyn(89,NY46)
  + Cooper Ob/Gyn
    4 Plaza Drive/Suite 403/Bunker Hill Pl   Sewell, NJ 08080
    (856)270-4020   Fax (856)270-4022
  + Cooper Ob/Gyn
    3 Cooper Plaza/Suite 300   Camden, NJ 08103   (856)270-4020   Fax (856)968-8575
  + Cooper Faculty Ob/Gyn
    1103 Kings Highway North/Suite 201   Cherry Hill, NJ 08080
    (856)321-1800   Fax (856)321-0133
Franzen Saad, Jillian Leigh, MD {1871814269}
  + Drs. Saad and Saad
    139 Sequoia Drive   Berlin, NJ 08009   (856)767-2783
    jillianfranzen@gmail.com
Franzese, John, MD {1053390104} Gastrn, IntrMd(88,GRNA)<NJ-OVERLOOK, NJ-STBARNMC>
  + John N. Franzese MD
    396 Main Street   Chatham, NJ 07928   (973)701-8277   Fax (973)701-9546
Franzl, Wojciech, MD {1508033242} Anesth(06,NY08)
  + Teaneck Anesthesia Group, P.A.
    718 Teaneck Road   Teaneck, NJ 07666   (201)833-7149
    Fax (201)833-6576
Franzoni, David Fred, MD {1447291646} Urolgy(95,DC02)<NJ-MTNSIDE>
  + Essex Hudson Urology
    256 Broad Street   Bloomfield, NJ 07003   (973)743-4450
    Fax (973)429-9076
  + Essex Hudson Urology
    243 Chestnut Street   Newark, NJ 07105   (973)743-4450
    Fax (973)344-9188
  + Essex Hudson Urology
    213 South Frank Rodgers Blvd   Harrison, NJ 07003
    (973)482-7070
Frascella, Rosemary C., MD {1750495057} IntrMd(80,NJ06)<NJ-STFRNMED>
  + Premier Medicine & Wellness
    231 Crosswicks Road/Suite 11   Bordentown, NJ 08505
    (609)298-4750
  + St. Francis Medical Center
    601 Hamilton Avenue/Internal Med   Trenton, NJ 08629
    (609)599-5171
Frasco, Franklin J., MD {1316908676} SrgVas, Surgry(83,MA07)<NJ-JRSYSHMC, NJ-OCEANMC>
  + 2051 State Highway 35
    Belmar, NJ 07719   (732)449-7776   Fax (732)974-1039
Fraser, Iain Peter, MD {1306827563} PedInf, ClnPhm(87,SAF02)
  + Merck and Company Incorporated
    126 East Lincoln Avenue/RY 34-A500   Rahway, NJ 07065
    (732)594-3931
Fraser, Keith E., MD {1881621266} SrgHnd(82,PA01)<NJ-NWRKBETH, NJ-STMICHL>
  + PO Box 6
    Verona, NJ 07044
Fraser, Margaret Cameron, MD {1659443943} Psychy, PsyFor(88,NY46)
  + 65 North Maple Street
    Ridgewood, NJ 07450   (201)444-6844
Fratello, Joseph J., MD {1851334429} IntrMd, Allrgy(83,GRN01)<NJ-HOLYNAME>
  + Holy Name Hospital
    718 Teaneck Road/InternalMed   Teaneck, NJ 07666
    (201)833-3000
Fratello, Laura F., MD {1174885420} InfDis, IntrMd(84,MEX34)
  + 385 Summit Avenue
    Leonia, NJ 07605   (201)302-9431   Fax (201)302-9431
Frates, Angela Dawn, MD {1144423765} Gastrn
  + The Gastroenterology Group, PA
    103 Old Marlton Pike/Suite 102   Medford, NJ 08055
    (609)953-3440   Fax (609)996-4002
  + The Gastroenterology Group, PA
    15000 Midlantic Drive/Suite 110   Mount Laurel, NJ 08054
    (609)953-3440   Fax (856)996-4002
Frattarola, John D., MD {1609836592} ObsGyn(78,PHI08)<NJ-HOLYNAME, NJ-HACKNSK>
  + Women's Health Care Group
    870 Palisade Avenue/Suite 301   Teaneck, NJ 07666
    (201)907-0770   Fax (201)907-0229
Frattarola, Michael A., MD {1184674160} ObsGyn, Gyneco(73,NJ05)<NJ-OURLADY>
  + Our Lady of Lourdes Medical Center
    1600 Haddon Avenue/OB/GYN   Camden, NJ 08103
    (856)757-3700   Fax (856)365-7972
Fratzola, Christine Hunter, MD {1033291703} Anesth, IntrMd(85,DC03)<NJ-RWJUBRUN>
  + RWJ University Hospital New Brunswick
    One Robert Wood Johnson Place   New Brunswick, NJ 08901
    (732)937-8841
Frauwirth, Howard David, MD {1992789697} Gastrn, IntrMd(00,NJ05)
  + VMG-Internal Medicine Midland Park
    44 Goodwin Street/Suite 201   Midland Park, NJ 07432

(201)891-5044   Fax (201)891-1119
Frazer, Keith Evan, DO {1730161258} Anesth(01,FL75)<NJ-HACKNSK>
  + Hackensack University Medical Center
    30 Prospect Avenue/Anesthesiology   Hackensack, NJ 07601
    (201)996-2000   Fax (201)488-6769
Frazier, Daveed Damon, MD {1518048446} SrgSpn, SrgOrt(90,MA01)<NY-SLRLUKES, NY-LENOXHLL>
  + New York City Spine
    261 James Street/Suite 2-G   Morristown, NJ 07960
    (973)998-9651   Fax (212)265-0739
  + Advanced Spine Surgery Center
    855 Lehigh Avenue   Union, NJ 07083   (973)998-9651   Fax (908)557-9438
Frazier, Hawwa Sharif, DO {1881889277} FamMed(07,NJ75)<NJ-STPETER>
  + 1145 Bordentown Avenue/Suite 1
    Parlin, NJ 08859   (732)638-4688   Fax (732)416-6085
  + 1 Bethany Road/Suite 97
    Hazlet, NJ 07730   (732)638-4688   Fax (732)416-6085
Freas, Glenn Curtis, MD {1730111451} EmrgMd, IntrMd(81,PA02)<NJ-VIRTMHBC>
  + Virtua Memorial
    175 Madison Avenue/Emerg Med   Mount Holly, NJ 08060
    (609)261-7045   Fax (609)261-5842
Fred, Matthew Ross, MD {1831235860} IntrMd(03,NY20)<NJ-VIRTMHBC>
  + Virtua Memorial
    175 Madison Avenue   Mount Holly, NJ 08060   (609)267-0700
Freda, John Jeffrey, MD {1952498040} Anesth(88,PA13)<NJ-UMDNJ, NY-PRSBWEIL>
  + Rutgers- New Jersey Medical School
    185 South Orange Avenue   Newark, NJ 07103   (973)972-4300
  + University Hospital
    150 Bergen Street   Newark, NJ 07103   (973)972-4300
    Fax (973)972-1587
Fredericks, Duane A., MD {1184618886} Surgry, Bariat(96,PA13)
  + North Jersey Laparoscopic Associates
    222 Cedar Lane/Room 201   Teaneck, NJ 07666   (201)530-1900   Fax (201)530-9300
  + North Jersey Laparoscopic Associates
    6045 Kennedy Boulevard   North Bergen, NJ 07047
    (201)530-1900   Fax (201)227-6282
Frederickson, Anne M., MD {1629259288}<NJ-NWRKBETH>
  + Newark Beth Israel Medical Center
    201 Lyons Avenue   Newark, NJ 07112   (973)926-3393
    anne.frederickson@gmail.com
Frederikse, Melissa Ellison, MD {1710910294} Psychy(91,NY46)<NJ-UMDNJ>
  + University Psychiatric Associates
    183 South Orange Avenue/E-F Levels   Newark, NJ 07103
    (973)972-2977   Fax (973)972-2979
Freed, Brian, DO {1073951554} PhyMPain
  + Summit Medical Group-Berkeley Heights Campus
    1 Diamond Hill Road   Berkeley Heights, NJ 07922
    (908)277-8897   Fax (908)277-8901
Freedenfeld, Stuart H., MD {1164498333} FamMed(75,NJ05)<NJ-HUNTRDN>
  + Stockton Family Practice
    56 South Main Street/Stockton Center   Stockton, NJ 08559
    (609)397-8585   Fax (609)397-9335
Freedman, Amy L., MD {1134626310} IntrMd(84,PA01)
  + Janssen Pharmaceutical/Drug Safety and Surveillance
    1125 Trenton Harbourton Road   Titusville, NJ 08560
    (609)730-2000
Freedman, Andrew R., MD {1598766743} CritCr, IntrMd, PulDis(79,NJ05)
  + Raritan Bay Cardiology
    7 Centre Dtrive/Suite 13   Monroe Township, NJ 08831
    (609)655-8860   Fax (609)655-8065
Freedman, Gary Mitchel, MD {1073534830} RadOnc<PA-FOXCAN>
  + Penn Medicine at Cherry Hill
    409 Route 70 East   Cherry Hill, NJ 08034   (856)429-1519
Freedman, Jennifer Emi Chan, MD {1457545576} EmrgMd(06,NY19)<NJ-UNVMCPRN>
  + University Medical Center of Princeton at Plainsboro
    One Plainsboro Road/Emerg Med   Plainsboro, NJ 08536
    (609)853-7700
Freedman, Joshua R., MD {1265721674} Dermat
  + 1700 Whitehorse-Hamilton Squar
    Hamilton Square, NJ 08690   (215)840-1311
    jrfreedman@gmail.com
Freeland, Erik Christopher, DO {1912147745} SrgOrt(08,PA77)<NJ-COOPRUMC>
  + Cooper University Medical Center/Camden
    3 Cooper Plaza/Suite 502   Camden, NJ 08103   (856)356-4935
  + Underwood-Memorial Hospital Family Health Center
    1120 North Delsea Drive/2nd Floor   Glassboro, NJ 08028

(856)356-4935   Fax (856)582-0163
  + Cooper Bone and Joint Institute
    401 South Kings Highway/Suite 3-A   Cherry Hill, NJ 08103
    (856)547-0201   Fax (856)547-0316
Freeman, Amy Ilyse, MD {1467448514} Dermat(99,NY47)
  + Millburn Laser Center
    12 East Willow Street   Millburn, NJ 07041   (973)376-8500
    Fax (973)376-1820
Freeman, Barry C., MD {1760577761} Hemato, IntrMd, MedOnc(70,NY15)
  + 505 East Broad Street
    Westfield, NJ 07090   (908)233-0259   Fax (908)232-9553
Freeman, Benjamin B., MD {1912206434}
  + Regional Cancer Care Associates
    100 Madison Avenue   Morristown, NJ 07960   (973)538-5210   Fax (973)539-2664
Freeman, Darren Keith, DO {1326184896} PhysMd(00,CA22)<NJ-BAYSHORE>
  + Freeman Integrated Spine & Pain, P.C.
    3499 Route 9 North/Suite 2B   Freehold, NJ 07728
    (973)893-7246   Fax (732)970-4012
Freeman, Eliot, MD {1598740458} RadDia(65,PA13)<NJ-STPETER, NJ-RWJUBRUN>
  + University Radiology Group, P.C.
    483 Cranbury Road   East Brunswick, NJ 08816   (732)390-0030   Fax (732)390-5383
  + University Radiology Group, P.C.
    10 Plum Street   New Brunswick, NJ 08901   (732)390-0030
    Fax (732)249-1208
Freeman, Eric D., DO {1184720930} PainInvt, PhyMPain, NrlgPain(96,NY75)<NJ-RWJURAH>
  + Freeman Spin & Pain Institute
    102 James Street/Suite 101   Edison, NJ 08820   (732)906-9600   Fax (732)906-9300
Freeman, Hank Jason, MD {1124050331} RadV&I, RadDia(99,PA13)<NJ-JFKMED>
  + Edison Radiology Group, P.A.
    65 James Street   Edison, NJ 08820   (732)321-7917   Fax (732)737-2968
Freeman, Neil J., MD {1114963857} RadDia, RadV&I(85,NY01)<NJ-STCLRDOV, NJ-STCLRDEN>
  + St. Clare's Hospital-Dover
    400 West Blackwell Street/Radiology   Dover, NJ 07801
    (973)537-3806   Fax (973)989-3194
  + St. Clare's Hospital-Denville Campus
    25 Pocono Road/Radiology   Denville, NJ 07834   (973)625-6650
Freeman, Ted Lawrence, DO {1881762029} PhysMd, PainMd(93,NY75)<NJ-CENTRAST, NJ-OCEANMC>
  + Freeman Spine & Disc Center
    186 Jack Martin Boulevard   Brick, NJ 08724   (732)785-1600
    Fax (732)785-1642
    ginaangel40@yahoo.com
Freer, Christopher F., DO {1952399420} EmrgMd(95,NJ75)<NJ-STBARNMC>
  + Emergency Medical Associates of NJ, P.A.
    3 Century Drive   Parsippany, NJ 07054   (973)740-0607
    Fax (973)740-9895
Freeze, Brian, MD {1679990840} EmrgMd
  + Cooper Univerisry Emergency Physicians
    One Cooper Plaza   Camden, NJ 08103   (856)342-2930
    Fax (856)968-8272
Freiberg, Evan, MD {1386887636} Radiol, RadDia(09,NY48)<NY-STONYBRK>
  + University Radiology Group, P.C.
    483 Cranbury Road   East Brunswick, NJ 08816   (732)390-0030   Fax (732)390-1856
  + University Radiology Group, P.C.
    579A Cranbury Road   East Brunswick, NJ 08816   (732)390-0030   Fax (732)390-1856
Freiberg, Scott Tyler, MD {1669851515}<NJ-HOBUNIMC>
  + Hoboken University Medical Center
    308 Willow Avenue   Hoboken, NJ 07030   (201)418-3127
Freid, Robert S., MD {1659474104} IntrMd(83,NJ06)<NJ-MORRISTN>
  + 205 Ridgedale Avenue
    Florham Park, NJ 07932   (973)377-0164   Fax (973)377-0063
  + Alliance Center for Weight Management
    95 Mount Kemble Avenue   Morristown, NJ 07960
    (973)971-4555
Freid, Russell Marc, MD {1033195391} Urolgy(92,PA09)<NJ-CHSFULD, NJ-CHSMRCER>
  + Urology Care Alliance
    2 Princess Road/Suite J   Lawrenceville, NJ 08648
    (609)895-1991   Fax (609)895-6996
Freifeld, Stephen F., MD {1881685352} Otlryg(65,NY09)
  + 454 Morris Avenue
    Springfield, NJ 07081   (973)277-3875   Fax (973)564-5251
    sfreifeld@sf-md.com

Physicians by Name and Address

Freiheiter, John Scott, MD {1073688438} IntrMd, Pedtrc(90,NJ06)<NJ-MORRISTN>
+ 16 Old Brookside Road/Suite 2
Randolph, NJ 07869   (973)895-8884   Fax (973)895-2530

Freilich, Benjamin Douglas, MD {1831298488} Ophthl(89,NY08)
+ Freilich Eye Associates
15 Engle Street/Suite 106   Englewood, NJ 07631
(201)871-9595   Fax (201)871-2323
benfmd@gmail.com

Freilich, David Eric, MD {1295783611} Ophthl(97,NY45)
+ Freilich Eye Associates
15 Engle Street/Suite 106   Englewood, NJ 07631
(201)871-9595   Fax (201)871-2323

Freilich, David I., MD {1043307440} CdvDis, IntCrd(83,NY01)
+ Cardiology Associates of Morristown
95 Madison Avenue/Suite 10A   Morristown, NJ 07960
(973)889-9001   Fax (973)889-9051

Freilich, Jonathan Michael, MD {1366404402} Ophthl, IntrMd(91,NY47)<NJ-STBARNMC, NJ-OVERLOOK>
+ Associates in Eye Care
155 Morris Avenue/Suite 302   Springfield, NJ 07081
(973)232-6900   Fax (973)232-6911

Freire, Jorge Efrain, MD {1902847411} RadOnc(72,ECU01)
+ CyberKnife Center at Capital Health
446 Bellevue Avenue   Trenton, NJ 08618   (609)394-4244   Fax (609)394-4156

Freis, Peter C., MD {1578622767} Pedtrc, FamMed, AdolMd(70,DC01)<NJ-RWJUBRUN, NJ-STPETER>
+ Robert Wood Johnson University Hospital
443 Middlesex Avenue   Metuchen, NJ 08840   (732)548-5991   Fax (732)548-8370

Freiss, Rebecca, MD {1487098588}
+ Drs. Bogusz & Weiss
44 State Route 23 North/Suite 6   Riverdale, NJ 07457
(973)248-9199   Fax (973)248-9299

Freitag, Warren Barry, MD {1336129980} RadDia(85,NY08)<NJ-STJOSHOS>
+ Imaging Subspecialists of North Jersey LLC
703 Main Street   Paterson, NJ 07503   (973)754-2645

Fremed, Daniel, MD {1548536436}
+ The Cardiovascular Care Group
649 Morris Avenue   Springfield, NJ 07081   (973)759-9000

Fremed, Eric L., MD {1992700843} Nrolgy(83,NY15)<NJ-HOLYNAME>
+ Drs. Rabin, Fremed, Prince, P.C.
700 Palisade Avenue   Englewood Cliffs, NJ 07632
(201)568-3412   Fax (201)568-8249

French, Eugene C., MD {1215927843} IntrMd, InfDis(88,WIND)<NJ-HACKNSK>
+ ID CareGuard
255 West Spring Valley Ave/Suite 200   Maywood, NJ 07607
(201)343-2778   Fax (201)343-1990

Frenia, Douglas Scott, MD {1902969769} PulDis, SlpDis
+ St. Peter's University Hospital
254 Easton Avenue   New Brunswick, NJ 08901   (732)745-8564   Fax (732)745-9156

Frenkel, Daniel, MD {1144427832} ClCdEl, IntrMd(06,NY19)
+ Medicor Cardiology PA
225 Jackson Street   Bridgewater, NJ 08807   (908)526-8668   Fax (908)231-6781

Fresca, Diane Elizabeth, MD {1104084649} EnDbMt, IntrMd(01,NJ06)
+ Endocrinology Associates of Princeton, LLC
168 Franklin Corner Road   Lawrenceville, NJ 08648
(609)896-0075   Fax (609)896-0079

Fresco, Silvia, MD {1497805832} Surgry(92,NJ05)<NJ-BAYSHORE, NJ-SOCEANCO>
+ Strafford Surgical Specialists, P.A.
1100 Route 72 West/Suite 303   Manahawkin, NJ 08050
(609)978-3325   Fax (609)978-3123
+ Monmouth Surgical Specialists
727 North Beers Street   Holmdel, NJ 07733   (609)978-3325   Fax (732)290-7067

Fretta, Joseph, MD {1538113626} IntrMd(77,MEXI)<NJ-STBARNMC, NJ-NWRKBETH>
+ New Jersey Vein and Cosmetic Surgery Center
741 Northfield Avenue/Suite 105   West Orange, NJ 07052
(973)243-2200   Fax (973)243-1409
+ Total Vein Care
480 Shrewsbury Plaza   Shrewsbury, NJ 07702   (973)243-2200

Freund, William Roy, DO {1831192541} Pedtrc(98,MO78)<NJ-SHOREMEM>
+ Rainbow Pediatrics
2041 US Highway 9   Cape May Court House, NJ 08210
(609)624-9003   Fax (609)624-9002

Freundlich, Nancy Lynn, MD {1992716021} IntrMd(86,NJ05)<NJ-STBARNMC, NJ-NWRKBETH>
+ Associates in Internal Medicine & Nephrology
225 Millburn Avenue/Suite 104-B   Millburn, NJ 07041
(973)218-9330   Fax (973)218-9351

Freundlich, Richard E., MD {1265443238} Nephro, IntrMd(82,GRN01)<NJ-NWRKBETH, NJ-STBARNMC>
+ Associates in Internal Medicine & Nephrology
225 Millburn Avenue/Suite 104-B   Millburn, NJ 07041
(973)218-9330   Fax (973)218-9351

Frey, Howard L., MD {1932241361} Urolgy(77,MD07)<NJ-VALLEY>
+ Urology Group PA
4 Godwin Avenue   Midland Park, NJ 07432   (201)444-7070   Fax (201)444-7228

Frey, Patricia E., DO {1538426796} Psychy<NJ-SUMOAKSH>
+ Summit Oaks Hospital
19 Prospect Street   Summit, NJ 07901   (908)277-9722

Frey, Steven, MD {1396943619} SrgOrt(03,DC02)
+ Advanced Orthopaedic Centers
414 Tatum Street   Woodbury, NJ 08096   (856)848-3880   Fax (856)848-4895

Freyman, Boris, DO {1184676934} IntrMd, FamMed(98,NY75)<NJ-HCKTSTWN, NJ-NWTNMEM>
+ North Warren Medical Associates PC
Route 517/Building B   Hackettstown, NJ 07840   (908)852-0107   Fax (908)850-9160
+ North Warren Medical Associates
155 State Highway 94   Blairstown, NJ 07825   (908)852-0107   Fax (908)362-6984

Frias, Carlos, MD {1235132440} Anesth(80,PER01)
+ Advanced Interventional Pain Management
1176 Hamburg Turnpike   Wayne, NJ 07470   (973)365-4747   Fax (973)365-4596

Frick, Glen Steven, MD {1699760629} Pedtrc(98,NY08)
+ 1804 Champlain Drive
Voorhees, NJ 08043

Fridman, Esther D., MD PsyCAd, Psychy(83,FL02)
+ 185 East Palisade Avenue/Apt A-6
Englewood, NJ 07631   (201)816-0002

Fridman, Morton Zvi, MD {1679799316} PsyCAd, Psychy(84,NY47)
+ 185 East Palisade Avenue/Apt A-6
Englewood, NJ 07631   (201)816-0002

Fried, Arno H., MD {1063452514} SrgNro, PedSrg, IntrMd(80,TN07)<NJ-HACKNSK, NJ-STPETER>
+ Advanced Neurosurgery Associates
201 Route 17 North/Suite 501   Rutherford, NJ 07070
(201)457-0044   Fax (201)457-0049

Fried, Harry A., MD {1609810126} Gastrn, IntrMd(86,NY06)<NJ-ENGLWOOD>
+ 333 Old Hook Riad/Suite 101
Westwood, NJ 07675   (201)594-0535   Fax (201)594-0538

Fried, Kenneth S., MD {1225085152} SrgVas, Surgry(78,NY19)<NJ-ENGLWOOD, NJ-HOLYNAME>
+ 180 North Dean Street
Englewood, NJ 07631   (201)568-8666   Fax (201)568-2941
Eliasfried1@aol.com

Fried, Martin D., MD {1578557344} Pedtrc, PedGst, Nutrtn(85,NY15)<NJ-JRSYSHMC, NJ-RIVERVW>
+ Healthy Days, LLC
3200 Sunset Avenue/Suite 100   Ocean, NJ 07712
(732)682-3425   Fax (732)455-3309
martinfried@optonline.net

Fried, Ruthellen, MD {1093876450} Pedtrc(76,NY09)<NJ-ENGLWOOD>
+ 180 North Dean Street
Englewood, NJ 07631   (201)568-1120   Fax (201)568-2941

Fried, Sharon Z., MD {1740236975} Dermat, IntrMd(80,NY19)<NJ-ENGLWOOD>
+ 180 North Dean Street
Englewood, NJ 07631   (201)569-9800   Fax (201)568-2941

Fried, Steven H., MD {1629146733} SrgOrt, IntrMd(75,NJ06)
+ Brunswick Orthopaedic Associates, P.C.
303 George Street/Suite 105   New Brunswick, NJ 08901
(732)846-6100   Fax (732)846-6113
+ Brunswick Orthopaedic Associates, P.C.
252 Bridge Street/Building G   Metuchen, NJ 08840
(732)321-9700

Friedberg, Andrea, MD {1922004456} Ophthl(83,GA05)
+ Friedberg Eye Associates
661 North Broad Street   Woodbury, NJ 08096   (856)845-7968   Fax (856)845-8544
drandrea@comcast.net

Friedberg, Eric Brian, MD {1932218625} RadDia, RadV&I, Radiol(93,PA09)
+ Montclair Radiology
20 High Street   Nutley, NJ 07110   (973)284-1881   Fax (973)284-0269

Friedberg, Howard L., MD {1164427696} Ophthl(81,GA05)
+ Friedberg Eye Associates
661 North Broad Street   Woodbury, NJ 08096   (856)845-7968   Fax (856)845-8544

Friedberg, Mark A., MD {1114999356} Ophthl, VitRet(86,PA01)<NJ-RIVERVW>
+ Mid Atlantic Eye Center
70 East Front Street   Red Bank, NJ 07701   (732)741-0858   Fax (732)219-0180
+ Edison Eye Group
7 State Route 27/Suite 101   Edison, NJ 08820   (732)741-0858   Fax (732)549-5869
+ Altima Eye Associates
100 Morris Avenue   Springfield, NJ 07081   (973)379-5200   Fax (973)376-3157

Friedel, Mark Erik, MD {1972708139} Otlryg, IntrMd(07,PA02)
+ Advanced ENT - Washington Township
239 Hurffville Crosskeys Road   Sewell, NJ 08080   (856)602-4000   Fax (856)629-3391
+ Advanced ENT - Voorhees
200 Bowman Drive/Suite D-285   Voorhees, NJ 08043   (856)602-4000   Fax (856)667-3020
+ Advanced ENT - Haddonfield
11A Laurel Road East   Stratford, NJ 08080   (856)602-4000   Fax (856)346-0757

Friedel, Steven P., MD {1124018270} SrgOrt(89,MD12)<NJ-RIVERVW>
+ Orthopaedic Sports Medicine
80 Oak Hill Road   Red Bank, NJ 07701   (732)741-2313   Fax (732)741-7154

Friedel, Walter E., MD {1124013602} Gyneco(69,IL42)<NJ-STCLRDEN, NJ-MORRISTN>
+ Drs. Friedel & Lam
1259 US Highway 46 East/Suite 314   Parsippany, NJ 07054
(973)316-9800   Fax (973)316-9805
+ 70 Sparta Avenue
Sparta, NJ 07871   (973)316-9800   Fax (973)729-5667

Friedenberg, Barry, MD {1023030640} Radiol, RadDia(68,DC02)<NJ-CENTRAST>
+ Freehold Radiology Group
901 West Main Street   Freehold, NJ 07728   (732)462-4844
+ CentraState Medical Center
901 West Main Street/Radiology   Freehold, NJ 07728
(732)294-2946

Friedenberg, Jeffrey Scott, MD {1427070069} RadDia(98,NJ05)<NJ-CENTRAST>
+ Freehold Radiology Group
901 West Main Street   Freehold, NJ 07728   (732)462-4844

Friedenthal, Roy B., MD {1609814870} SrgOrt(73,NY09)
+ Central Physicians and Surgeons
820 South White Horse Pike   Hammonton, NJ 08037
(609)561-8787   Fax (609)567-9546

Friedhoff, Stephen G., MD {1679535306} FamMed(91,NJ05)<NJ-VIRTMHBC>
+ Cooper Family Medicine
1001-F Lincoln Drive West   Marlton, NJ 08053   (856)810-1800   Fax (856)810-1879

Friedland, Howard M., DO {1275586422} EmrgMd(96,MO78)<NJ-NWRKBETH>
+ St Joseph's Medical Center Emergency
703 Main Street   Paterson, NJ 07503   (973)754-2240   Fax (973)754-2249

Friedland, Richard James, MD {1437157583} IntrMd(84,NY08)<NJ-STFRNMED>
+ 4 Princess Road/Suite 210
Lawrenceville, NJ 08648   (609)895-0100   Fax (609)895-6966

Friedlander, Beverly, MD {1467563338} SrgPlstc, Surgry(80,NY08)<NJ-OVERLOOK, NJ-STBARNMC>
+ 636 Morris Turnpike
Short Hills, NJ 07078   (973)912-9120   Fax (973)912-8070

Friedlander, Devin S., MD {1487695623} Nrolgy(89,NJ06)
+ Princeton & Rutgers Neurology
9 Centre Drive/Suite 130   Monroe Township, NJ 08831
(609)395-7615   Fax (609)395-1885
+ Princeton & Rutgers Neurology
77 Veronica Avenue/Suite 102   Somerset, NJ 08873
(609)395-7615   Fax (732)246-3089

Friedlander, Jeffrey Dean, MD {1356323885} Anesth(90,PA09)<NJ-HACKNSK>
+ Hackensack University Medical Center
30 Prospect Avenue/Anesthesiology   Hackensack, NJ 07601
(201)996-2000   Fax (201)488-6769
+ Hackensack University MC-Anesthesia Dept
30 Prospect Avenue/Room 2703   Hackensack, NJ 07601
(201)996-2000   Fax (201)996-3962

Friedlander, Joseph Raymond, MD {1033106117} IntrMd, EnDbMt(82,PHI08)<NJ-HACKNSK, NJ-HOLYNAME>
+ 200 The Plaza
Teaneck, NJ 07666   (201)833-8840   Fax (201)833-8886
DocJoe13@ipinet.com

Friedlander, Marvin E., MD {1073513545} SrgNro(82,NY08)
+ The Back Institute
700 Rahway Avenue/Suite A-14   Union, NJ 07083
(908)688-1999   Fax (908)688-8180

Physicians by Name and Address

Friedler-Eisenberg, Susan F., DO {1205885431} Pedtrc(90,PA77)<NJ-VIRTUAHS, NJ-VIRTMARL>
  + **Advocare Greentree Pediatrics**
    127 Church Road/Suite 800   Marlton, NJ 08053   (856)988-7899   Fax (856)988-9499
  + **Advocare Laurel Pediatrics**
    269 Fish Pond Road   Sewell, NJ 08080   (856)988-7899   Fax (856)863-9666
Friedlin, Forrest Jeffrey, DO {1427014455} FamMed(87,PA77)
  + 147 Grandview Avenue
    Pitman, NJ 08071
Friedman, Alan L., MD {1215955166} ObsGyn, Gyneco(82,IL02)<NJ-UNVMCPRN>
  + **Princeton Ob/Gyn**
    5 Plainsboro Road/Suite 500   Plainsboro, NJ 08536   (609)936-0700   Fax (609)936-0750
Friedman, Alan Mark, MD {1104959527} IntrMd, PhysMd(93,NY46)
  + **Physical Medicine & Rehabilitation Center**
    500 Grand Avenue/1st Floor   Englewood, NJ 07631   (201)567-2277   Fax (201)567-7506
Friedman, Alan Stanley, MD {1982617312} Radiol, RadBdI, IntrMd(72,PA02)<NJ-ACMCMAIN, NJ-ACMCITY>
  + **Atlantic Medical Imaging, LLC.**
    72 West Jimmie Leeds Road   Galloway, NJ 08205   (609)677-9729   Fax (609)653-8764
  + **Atlantic Medical Imaging, LLC.**
    401 Bethel Road   Somers Point, NJ 08244   (609)677-9729
  + **Atlantic Medical Imaging, LLC.**
    421 Route 9 North   Cape May Court House, NJ 08205   (609)463-9500   Fax (609)465-0918
Friedman, Amir Mordechai, MD {1417907361} ObsGyn, IntrMd(95,NY47)
  + 390 North Broadway/Suite 500
    Pennsville, NJ 08070   (856)514-3992
Friedman, Arielle Jordana Cohen, MD {1972762482} PedAne, Anesth(08,MA01)<NJ-ENGLEWOOD>
  + **Englewood Hospital and Medical Center**
    350 Engle Street/Anesthesia   Englewood, NJ 07631   (201)894-3322
Friedman, Barton J., MD {1710941562} Pedtrc(66,PA02)<NJ-OURLADY, NJ-VIRTUAHS>
  + **Advocare Haddonfield Pediatric Association**
    220 North Haddon Avenue   Haddonfield, NJ 08033   (856)429-6719   Fax (856)429-6748
Friedman, Bernard, MD {1932190048} IntrMd, PulDis(76,NY47)
  + 100 Winston Drive
    Cliffside Park, NJ 07010
Friedman, Bruce I., MD {1457480113} PedCrC, Pedtrc(79,NY09)<NJ-HACKNSK>
  + **Hackensack University Medical Center**
    30 Prospect Avenue/Pediatrics/PICU   Hackensack, NJ 07601   (201)996-5303   Fax (201)996-4277
Friedman, Bruce Phillip, MD {1154544518} Psychy, PsyCAd(98,AZ01)
  + 209 Cooper Avenue/Suite 8
    Montclair, NJ 07043   (973)509-8400   Fax (973)337-5097
Friedman, Daniel Marc, DO {1457513533} EmrgMd<NJ-CENTRAST>
  + **CentraState Medical Center**
    901 West Main Street   Freehold, NJ 07728   (732)431-2000
Friedman, David Lewis, MD {1922199678} PedSrg, Pedtrc(71,NY08)<NJ-VALLEY, NJ-HACKNSK>
  + **Pediatric Surgery**
    30 West Century Road/Suite 235   Paramus, NJ 07652   (201)996-0010   Fax (201)225-9430
  + **Paramus Surgical Center**
    30 West Century Road/Suite 300   Paramus, NJ 07652   (201)986-9000
Friedman, Debbie, MD {1003004656} Pedtrc<NJ-CHDNWBTH>
  + **Children's Hospital of New Jersey**
    201 Lyons Avenue/Osborne Terrace   Newark, NJ 07112   (973)926-3500
Friedman, Dena Seifer, MD {1194873380} Psychy(82,IL02)
  + **BeginWithin**
    272 Broad Street   Red Bank, NJ 07701   (732)747-3663
Friedman, Ella, MD {1255459475} Psychy(79,RUSS)
  + **Raritan Valley Psychiatric Care, PC**
    105 East Union Avenue/Suite 1   Bound Brook, NJ 08805   (732)469-7899
    friedman1@usa.net
Friedman, Eric Stephen, MD {1538132337} Ophthl, VitRet(89,RI01)<NJ-RWJUBRUN, NJ-KIMBALL>
  + **Retina Associates of New Jersey, P.A.**
    10 Plum Street/Suite 600   New Brunswick, NJ 08901   (732)220-1600   Fax (732)220-1603
  + **Retina Associates of New Jersey, P.A.**
    140 Franklin Corner Road   Lawrenceville, NJ 08648   (732)220-1600   Fax (609)895-0853
  + **Retina Associates of New Jersey, P.A.**
    1200 Route 22 East   Bridgewater, NJ 08901   (908)218-4303   Fax (908)218-4307

Friedman, Gary S., MD {1952393431} Nephro, IntrMd(87,NJ05)
  + 11 Glenbrook Court
    Lawrenceville, NJ 08648
Friedman, Gina Y., DO {1518106616} Anesth
  + 1265 15th Street/Apt 17J
    Fort Lee, NJ 07024
Friedman, Glenn T., MD {1053384305} CdvDis(81,MEX03)<NJ-MORRISTN, NJ-SOMERSET>
  + **Medicor Cardiology PA**
    225 Jackson Street   Bridgewater, NJ 08807   (908)526-8668   Fax (908)231-6781
  + **Medicor Cardiology PA**
    331 US Highway 206/Suite 1A   Hillsborough, NJ 08844   (908)526-8668   Fax (908)431-0808
Friedman, Harvey Y., MD {1982663191} ObsGyn(81,NY19)<NJ-HACKNSK, NJ-ENGLEWOOD>
  + **Comprehensive Women's Care**
    401A South Van Brunt Street/Suite 405   Englewood, NJ 07631   (201)871-4346   Fax (201)871-5953
Friedman, Howard Michael, MD {1669496634} Pedtrc, Allrgy, AdolMd(84,NY08)<NJ-ENGLEWOOD, NJ-HOLYNAME>
  + **Washington Avenue Pediatrics**
    95 North Washington Avenue   Bergenfield, NJ 07621   (201)384-0300   Fax (201)384-9518
Friedman, Inga, MD {1376635417} IntrMd(83,RUSS)<NJ-RBAYOLDB, NJ-RBAYPERT>
  + 6 Cornwall Court/Suite E
    East Brunswick, NJ 08816   (732)257-0003   Fax (732)651-8023
Friedman, James Keith, MD {1760573471} Anesth, IntrMd(82,NY09)
  + **Red Bank Anesthesia, LLC**
    1 Riverview Plaza   Red Bank, NJ 07701   (732)530-2255   Fax (732)450-2620
Friedman, Jared Evan, MD {1174815799}
  + 5 Taylor Lake Court
    Manalapan, NJ 07726   (732)823-8226
Friedman, Jay Lawrence, MD {1669447587} PsyGrt, Psychy(92,ISR02)<NY-PRSBWEST, NJ-ENGLEWOOD>
  + **Tenafly Psychiatric Associates, LLC**
    111 Dean Drive   Tenafly, NJ 07670   (201)568-8288   Fax (201)568-8105
Friedman, Jeffrey R., DO {1477532802} IntrMd(89,IA75)<NJ-VIRTBERL, NJ-VIRTVOOR>
  + **Advocare Sicklerville Internal Medicine Associates**
    205 East Laurel Road/1 FL   Stratford, NJ 08084   (856)227-6575   Fax (856)374-9495
  + 1 Chadwick Court
    Voorhees, NJ 08043
Friedman, Jerrold Aaron, MD {1841249497} PhysMd, Acpntr(95,NY15)<NJ-COOPRUMC>
  + **Voorhees Center**
    3001 Evesham Road   Voorhees, NJ 08043   (856)751-1600   Fax (856)751-1548
Friedman, Lawrence, MD {1972571990} Urolgy(89,NJ06)<NJ-HCKTSTWN>
  + **Garden State Urology**
    282 US Highway 46   Denville, NJ 07834   (973)895-6636   Fax (973)895-5327
  + **Associates in Pediatric & Adult Urology**
    20 Commerce Boulevard/Suite D   Succasunna, NJ 07876   (973)895-6636   Fax (973)927-6831
  + **Associates in Pediatric & Adult Urology**
    653 Willow Grove Street   Hackettstown, NJ 07834   (908)684-4670
Friedman, Louis Alexander, DO {1124099197} IntrMd(92,PA77)<NJ-RBAYOLDB, NJ-JFKMED>
  + **Woodbridge Internal Medicine Associates**
    1000 Route 9 North/Suite 302   Woodbridge, NJ 07095   (732)634-0036   Fax (732)634-9182
Friedman, Michael J., DO {1104897586} Psychy, Nrolgy(94,FL75)<NJ-KMHTURNV, NJ-LOURDEHS>
  + **University Hospital-SOM Department of Psychiatry**
    2250 Chapel Avenue West/Suite 100   Cherry Hill, NJ 08002   (856)482-9000   Fax (856)482-1159
Friedman, Paul Dean, DO {1780605253} Radiol, RadDia(96,FL75)<NJ-MORRISTN>
  + **Memorial Radiology Associates**
    10 Lanidex Plaza West/Suite 125   Parsippany, NJ 07054   (973)503-5700   Fax (973)386-5701
  + **Morristown Medical Center**
    100 Madison Avenue/Breast Ctr   Morristown, NJ 07962   (973)971-5000
Friedman, Paul Martin, MD {1386646040} CritCr, IntrMd, PulDis(77,NY08)<NJ-JRSYSHMC, NJ-OCEANMC>
  + **Shore Pulmonary PA**
    2640 Highway 70/Building 6-A   Manasquan, NJ 08736   (732)528-5900   Fax (732)528-0887
  + **Shore Pulmonary PA**
    301 Bingham Avenue/Suite B   Ocean, NJ 07712   (732)528-5900   Fax (732)775-1212
  + **Shore Pulmonary PA**

  1608 Route 88/Suite 117   Brick, NJ 08736   (732)575-1100
Friedman, Robert A., MD {1750361127} RadDia(88,OH06)
  + **Edison Imaging Associates at JFK**
    60 James Street   Edison, NJ 08820   (732)321-7540   Fax (732)318-3883
  + **JFK Medical Center**
    65 James Street   Edison, NJ 08820   (732)321-7540   Fax (732)767-2968
Friedman, Robert Lawrence, MD {1790772499} SrgOrt, Ortped, SprtMd(88,CA14)<NJ-WARREN>
  + **Coordinated Health**
    222 Red Lane   Phillipsburg, NJ 08865   (610)861-8080   Fax (610)849-1013
Friedman, Samara, MD {1821298688} PedOrt, SrgOrt(01,NY48)
  + **Advocare The Orthopedic Center**
    218 Ridgedale Avenue/Suite 104   Cedar Knolls, NJ 07927   (973)538-7700   Fax (973)538-9478
Friedman, Samuel, MD {1366836611} FamMed
  + **Advocare Family Health at Mt. Olive**
    183 US Route 206/Suite 1   Flanders, NJ 07836   (973)347-3277   Fax (973)347-3141
Friedman, Samuel H., MD {1356363352} IntrMd, CdvDis(79,NY08)<NJ-HACKNSK>
  + 211 Essex Street/Suite 304
    Hackensack, NJ 07601   (201)487-2924   Fax (201)487-2853
Friedman, Samuel L., DO {1558579631} FamMed, GenPrc(63,MO79)<NJ-VIRTBERL, NJ-VIRTVOOR>
  + **Patient first**
    4000 Route 130/Bldg. C   Delran, NJ 08075   (856)705-0685   Fax (856)705-0686
Friedman, Susan R., MD {1902803422} Anesth(80,NY47)<NJ-MONMOUTH>
  + **Monmouth Medical Center**
    300 Second Avenue/Anesth   Long Branch, NJ 07740   (732)222-5200
Friedman, Terry David, MD {1760419659} CdvDis, IntrMd(77,NY08)<NJ-VIRTVOOR, NJ-VIRTMARL>
  + **Penn Medicine at Cherry Hill**
    1400 East Route 70/Cardiology   Cherry Hill, NJ 08034
Friedman-Cohen, Heather Naomi, MD {1376649707} EmrgMd, EmrgPedr, Pedtrc(02,GRN01)<NY-PRSBWEIL, NJ-HACKNSK>
  + **Hackensack University Medical Center**
    30 Prospect Avenue   Hackensack, NJ 07601   (201)996-2000
Friedrich, Ivan A., MD {1306890165} Gastrn, IntrMd(76,NY03)<NJ-ENGLEWOOD, NJ-HOLYNAME>
  + **Englewood Endoscopic Assocociates**
    420 Grand Avenue/Suite 101/Partner   Englewood, NJ 07631   (201)569-7044   Fax (201)569-1999
Friehling, Jane Susan, DO {1336109164} Gastrn, IntrMd(78,MO79)<NJ-KMHCHRRY, NJ-VIRTUAHS>
  + **South Jersey Gastroenterology PA**
    406 Lippincott Drive/Suite E   Marlton, NJ 08053   (856)983-1900   Fax (856)983-5110
  + **South Jersey Gastroenterology PA**
    111 Vine Street   Hammonton, NJ 08037   (856)983-1900   Fax (856)983-5110
  + **South Jersey Gastroenterology PA**
    807 Haddon Avenue/Suite 205   Haddonfield, NJ 08053   (856)428-2112   Fax (856)983-5110
Friel, David M., MD {1821161290} Psychy(87,PA07)
  + 704 A Shiloh Pike
    Bridgeton, NJ 08302   (856)451-5511   Fax (856)451-3589
Frieman, Amy Porter, MD {1255359907} PallCr, IntrMd(00,MO46)<NJ-OCEANMC, NJ-BAYSHORE>
  + 1355 Campus Parkway/Suite 103
    Neptune, NJ 07753   (732)202-8076   Fax (732)922-6026
Frieman, Brett Justin, DO {1669467536} Ophthl(00,MO78)
  + **Frieman Ophthalmology**
    75 West Front Street   Red Bank, NJ 07701   (732)741-4242
Frieman, Lawrence, MD {1609861913} Ophthl(72,NJ05)<NJ-RIVERVW, NJ-BAYSHORE>
  + **Frieman Ophthalmology**
    75 West Front Street   Red Bank, NJ 07701   (732)741-4242
    lfrieman@earthlink.net
Friend, Adam Seth, MD {1235109927} Ophthl(93,NY46)<NJ-VALLEY>
  + **Eye Care Associates of New Jersey, PA**
    One Broadway/Suite 404   Elmwood Park, NJ 07407   (201)797-5100   Fax (201)797-4160
Frier, Steven F., MD {1386734739} IntrMd, Nephro(63,NY09)<NJ-ENGLWOOD>
  + **Primary Care NJ**
    370 Grand Avenue/Suite 102   Englewood, NJ 07631   (201)567-3370   Fax (201)816-1265

Physicians by Name and Address

Frinjari, Hassan, MD {1811127764} ObsGyn<NJ-RHBHSPSJ>
+ Community Health Care Inc
  484 South Brewster Road   Vineland, NJ 08360   (856)451-4700   Fax (856)863-5732
+ Community Health Care, Inc.
  1200 North High Street   Millville, NJ 08332   (856)451-4700   Fax (856)327-4208
+ Community Health Care, Inc.
  70 Cohansey Street   Bridgeton, NJ 08360   (856)451-4700   Fax (856)451-0029

Frisch, Katalin Andrea, MD {1578739983} IntrMd, EnDbMt(04,NJ06)<NJ-ENGLWOOD, NJ-HOLYNAME>
+ Bergen Medical Alliance, P.A.
  180 Engle Street   Englewood, NJ 07631   (201)567-2050   Fax (201)567-5070

Frisoli, Anthony, MD {1851385751} FamMed(83,NJ06)<NJ-SOMERSET>
+ Martinsville Family Practice
  1973 Washington Valley Road   Martinsville, NJ 08836   (732)560-9225   Fax (732)560-8095
  anthonyfrisoli@mfpnj.allscriptsdirect.net

Frisoli, Gaetano, MD {1780772020} MtFtMd(70,ITAL)
+ 33 Overlook Road/Suite 110
  Summit, NJ 07901   (908)598-1020

Frisoni, Lorenza, MD {1013246099} IntrMd
+ Advocare DelGiorno Pediatrics
  527 South Black Horse Pike   Blackwood, NJ 08012   (856)302-5322   Fax (856)245-7719

Fritz, Gerard D., MD {1326084088} Pedtrc, GenPrc(89,NJ05)<NJ-SOMERSET, NJ-STPETER>
+ Somerset Pediatric Group PA
  65 Mountain Boulevard Ext/Suite 205   Warren, NJ 07059   (732)560-9080   Fax (732)560-8085
+ Somerset Pediatric Group PA
  155 Union Avenue   Bridgewater, NJ 08807   (732)560-9080   Fax (908)203-8825
+ Somerset Pediatric Group PA
  2345 Lamington Road/Suite 101   Bedminster, NJ 07059   (908)470-1124   Fax (908)470-2845

Fritz, John A., DO {1316032394} FamMed(95,NJ75)<NJ-JRSYCITY>
+ 709 Newark Avenue
  Jersey City, NJ 07306   (201)239-9200   Fax (201)239-7788
  Jfdoc@att.net

Fritz, John Patrick, DO {1083700868} FamMed, IntrMd(93,IL76)<NJ-WARREN>
+ 500 Greenwich Street
  Belvidere, NJ 07823   (908)475-9990   Fax (908)475-9993

Fritz, Melinda D., MD {1922184688} PedHem<NJ-MORRISTN>
+ Morristown Medical Center
  100 Madison Avenue/Box 70   Morristown, NJ 07962   (973)971-5000

Froehlich, Allison Ann, MD {1962619189} EnDbMt, IntrMd(03,NJ05)<NJ-VALLEY>
+ Endocrine Associates
  30 West Century Drive/Suite 255   Paramus, NJ 07652   (201)444-4363   Fax (201)444-4590

Frohman, Larry P., MD {1760588180} Ophtl, OphNeu(80,PA01)
+ University Hospital-Doctors Office Center
  90 Bergen Street/Ophtha/Ste 6100   Newark, NJ 07103   (973)972-2065   Fax (973)972-2068
  lpf2584@aol.com
+ Institute of Ophthalmology & Visual Science
  556 Eagle Rock Avenue/Suite 206   Roseland, NJ 07068   (973)972-2065   Fax (973)972-2389

From, Stuart B., MD {1831142736} Allrgy, IntrMd, PedAlg(87,NY09)<NJ-ENGLWOOD, NJ-HOLYNAME>
+ Englewood Allergy Associates
  309 Engle Street   Englewood, NJ 07631   (201)568-1480   Fax (201)568-1326

Fromer, Debra Lynn, MD {1801839642} Urolgy(98,MA07)<NJ-HACKNSK>
+ HUMC Faculty Practice
  360 Essex Street/Suite 403   Hackensack, NJ 07601   (201)336-8090   Fax (201)336-8221

Frometa, Ayme Veronica, MD {1669600995} Psychy
+ NBIMC Psychiatry
  201 Lyons Avenue   Newark, NJ 07112   (973)926-3693   Fax (973)926-2862

Fromowitz, Frank B., MD {1578675278} PthAna(73,PA02)
+ PLUS Diagnostics
  1200 River Avenue/Suite 10   Lakewood, NJ 08701   (732)901-7575   Fax (732)901-1555

Froncek, Michael Jude, MD {1386687713} Rheuma, Immuno(94,NY45)<NJ-UNVMCPRN, NJ-RWJUHAM>
+ Rheumatology Center of Princeton
  123 Franklin Corner Road/Suite 106   Lawrenceville, NJ 08648   (609)896-2505   Fax (609)896-2530

Frost, James H., MD {1235120981} SrgVas, Surgry(82,MEX03)<NJ-TRINIWSC, NJ-OVERLOOK>
+ AtlantiCare Cancer Institute
  2500 English Creek Avenue/Building 400   Egg Harbor Township, NJ 08234   (609)677-7700   Fax (609)677-7701

Fruchter, Joseph S., MD {1427082304} Pedtrc(73,NY09)<NJ-HACKNSK, NJ-VALLEY>
+ Haclensack Bergen Pediatrics
  385 Prospect Avenue/Suite 210   Hackensack, NJ 07601   (551)996-9160   Fax (551)996-9165

Fruchtman, Deborah S., MD {1154520047} Ophthl(80,NJ05)<NJ-STBARNMC>
+ 11 Rappleye Court
  West Orange, NJ 07052

Frys, Kelly Ann, DO {1588923833} ObsGyn
+ All Women's Healthcare
  1100 Wescott Drive/Suite 105   Flemington, NJ 08822   (908)788-6469   Fax (908)788-6483

Fucanan, Vilma D., MD {1518059013} Psychy<NJ-TRENTPSY>
+ Trenton Psychiatric Hospital
  Sullivan Way/PO Box 7600   West Trenton, NJ 08628   (609)633-1500

Fuchs, Eliyahu Elliot, MD {1952339509} IntrMd, Gastrn(86,ON01)<NJ-MORRISTN>
+ Medical Institute of New Jersey
  11 Saddle Road   Cedar Knolls, NJ 07927   (973)267-2122   Fax (973)267-3478

Fuchs, Susan, MD {1902980915} Psychy
+ 396 Whitehorse Avenue
  Trenton, NJ 08610   (609)585-4200

Fuhrman, Joel H., MD {1386765287} FamMed(88,PA01)<NJ-HUNTRDN>
+ The Center for Nutritional Medicine
  4 Walter E. Foran Boulevard/Suite 409   Flemington, NJ 08822   (908)237-0200   Fax (908)237-0210

Fuhrman, Michael Alexander, MD {1720077746} IntrMd, Gastrn(97,NJ05)
+ Associates in Digestive Disease
  25 Morris Avenue   Springfield, NJ 07081   (973)467-1313   Fax (973)467-3133

Fuhrman, Mitchell J., MD {1619969474} CdvDis, IntrMd(77,NJ05)<NJ-OURLADY, NJ-VIRTUAHS>
+ Associated Cardiovascular Consultants-Lourdes
  1 Brace Road/Suite C & F   Cherry Hill, NJ 08034   (856)428-4100   Fax (856)428-5748
+ South Jersey Heart Group
  539 Egg Harbor Road/Suite 1   Sewell, NJ 08080   (856)428-4100   Fax (856)589-1753

Fuhrman, Robert A., MD {1518962919} EnDbMt, IntrMd(66,IL42)<NJ-OVERLOOK, NJ-CHLSMT>
+ Summit Medical Group
  552 Westfield Avenue/Endocrinology   Westfield, NJ 07090   (908)654-3377   Fax (908)654-4044
+ Summit Medical Group
  67 Walnut Avenue/Suite 202   Clark, NJ 07066   (908)654-3377   Fax (732)388-1330

Fujita, Kenji Peter, MD {1154461655} IntrMd, SrgCdv(00,MA01)<NJ-CLARMAAS>
+ UH-RWJ General Internal Medicine
  125 Paterson Street/Suite 2300   New Brunswick, NJ 08901   (732)235-7122   Fax (732)235-7144

Fuksina, Natasha, MD {1053398065} IntrMd(97,NY03)
+ Astra MD PC
  550 Bloomfield Avenue   Newark, NJ 07107   (973)483-1500   Fax (973)483-4577

Fule, Vilma G., MD {1104907740} SrgPlstc(74,PHIL)
+ 2730 Kennedy Boulevard
  Jersey City, NJ 07306   (201)435-1660   Fax (201)435-8409

Fullenkamp, Mark P., MD {1528089414} Anesth(02,NE06)<NJ-RWJUBRUN>
+ RWJ University Hospital New Brunswick
  One Robert Wood Johnson Place   New Brunswick, NJ 08901   (732)937-8841   Fax (732)418-8492

Fuller, David Alden, MD {1548359979} SrgOrt, SrgHnd(91,PA01)
+ Cooper Surgical Associates
  3 Cooper Plaza/Suite 411   Camden, NJ 08103   (856)342-2270   Fax (856)365-1180

Fulop, Eugene, MD {1558489716} IntrMd, GPrvMd(79,ROMA)<NJ-HACKNSK>
+ Drs. Fulop and Fulop
  653 Maywood Avenue   Maywood, NJ 07607   (201)845-9053

Fulop, Luminita, MD {1720037609} IntrMd(81,ROMA)<NJ-HACKNSK>
+ Drs. Fulop and Fulop
  653 Maywood Avenue   Maywood, NJ 07607   (201)845-9053

Fuloria, Mamta, MD {1063496149} Pedtrc, NnPnMd(92,INA05)
+ 100 Pollard Road
  Mountain Lakes, NJ 07046

Fumento, Robert S., MD {1740254002} EmrgMd
+ Lourdes Medical Center of Burlington County
  218 Sunset Road/Suite A   Willingboro, NJ 08046   (609)835-5240

Fumia, Fred Daniel, MD {1639149099} ObsGyn
+ Hackensack Meridian Urogynecolgy Medical Group
  19 Davis Avenue/7th Floor   Neptune, NJ 07753   (732)776-3797   Fax (732)776-3796
+ Jersey Shore Medical Center Obs/Gyn
  1945 Route 33   Neptune, NJ 07753   (732)776-3797   Fax (732)776-4525
+ Meridian Obstetrics amd Gynecology Associates PC
  19 Davis Avenue/Fl 1   Neptune, NJ 07753   (732)897-7944   Fax (732)922-8264

Funches, Antonio, MD {1659630895} FamMed
+ 3840 Quakerbridge Road/Suite 110
  Hamilton, NJ 08619   (609)528-2144   Fax (609)584-1023

Funches, Judith Melton, MD {1932171824} ObsGyn, IntrMd(87,NJ05)<NJ-CHSFULD, NJ-CHSMRCER>
+ Lawrence Ob/Gyn Associates
  123 Franklin Corner Road/Suite 214   Lawrenceville, NJ 08648   (609)896-1400   Fax (609)896-3986

Fune, Jose M.C., MD {1043289184} InfDis, IntrMd(83,PHIL)<NJ-JRSYSHMC, NJ-RIVERVW>
+ Jersey Shore University Medical Center
  1945 Route 33/InfectiousDis   Neptune, NJ 07753   (732)776-4302   Fax (732)776-4619
+ Riverview Medical Center
  1 Riverview Plaza   Red Bank, NJ 07701   (732)741-2700
+ Hackensack Meridian Medical Group
  19 Davis Avenue/5th-6th Floor   Neptune, NJ 07753   (732)897-3990   Fax (732)897-3997

Fung, Kent C., MD {1730347212} FamMed, IntrMd(07,GRN01)
+ Cedar Bridge Medical Associates
  985 Cedarbridge Avenue   Brick, NJ 08723   (732)477-5600   Fax (732)477-1899

Fung, Phoenix C., MD {1619214285} IntrMd(10,NY09)<NJ-UMDNJ>
+ University Hospital
  150 Bergen Street/Internal Med   Newark, NJ 07103   (973)972-5672   Fax (973)972-0365

Funicello, Alex Vincent, MD {1992906432} Surgry(97,GRN01)<NY-LUTHERN>
+ Dr. Barry L. Cohen
  695 US Highway 46/Suite 400-A   Fairfield, NJ 07004   (973)826-8080   Fax (866)309-3354

Funiciello, Marco, DO {1750607321} PhysMd
+ Princeton Spine and Joint Center
  601 Ewing Street/Suite A-2   Princeton, NJ 08540   (609)454-0760   Fax (609)454-0761

Funkhouser, Martha E., MD {1235195157} Dermat, IntrMd(89,MN04)<NJ-UNVMCPRN>
+ Princeton Dermatology Associates
  208 Bunn Drive/Suite 1-E   Princeton, NJ 08540   (609)683-4999   Fax (609)683-0298
  jeannieeronj@yahoo.com
+ Princeton Dermatology Associates
  5 Centre Street/Suite 1-A   Monroe Township, NJ 08831   (609)683-4999   Fax (609)655-2390

Furer, Steven K., MD {1366481343} CarNuc, IntrMd(NY08<NJ-OVERLOOK, NJ-STBARHCS>
+ Associates in Cardiovascular Disease, LLC
  211 Mountain Avenue   Springfield, NJ 07081   (973)467-0005   Fax (973)912-8989
+ Associates in Cardiovascular Disease, LLC
  571 Central Avenue/Suite 115   New Providence, NJ 07974   (973)467-0005   Fax (908)464-1332

Furey, Sandy Anselm, III, MD {1336350099} OthrSp, Rserch, AdmMgt(84,OH06)
+ The Medical Center Warner Lambert Co.
  201 Tabor Road   Morris Plains, NJ 07950   (908)277-7056   Fax (908)540-3828

Furey, William J., DO {1790822427} FamMed(88,PA77)<NJ-VIRTVOOR>
+ Kennedy Care Center
  705 White Horse Road/Suite D-101-2   Voorhees, NJ 08043   (856)783-0695   Fax (856)783-8083

Furiato, Anthony John, DO {1780948935}
+ 133 Aberdeen Road/Unit 10
  Aberdeen, NJ 07747   (732)245-2500

Furka, Natalie C., DO {1588808869}
+ 3438 Riverside Boulevard
  Secaucus, NJ 07094

Furlan, Louis E., MD {1588613665} Ophtl, PedOph(92,PA02)<NY-NYEYEINF>
+ Eye Care and Surgery Center
  592 Springfield Avenue   Westfield, NJ 07090   (908)789-8999   Fax (908)789-1379

Furman, Boris, DO {1164695011} Nrolgy(04,NY75)<NJ-CENTRAST>
+ 6 Maple Knoll Lane
  Manalapan, NJ 07726   Fax (732)851-5566

Furman, Jasmin W., MD {1942254503} Pedtrc, PedDvl(78,ASTL)<NJ-HACKNSK>
+ Hackensack University Medical Center
  30 Prospect Avenue/Pediatrics   Hackensack, NJ 07601   (201)996-2000

Furman, Lesley P., MD {1265466684} ObsGyn(74,PA12)<NJ-COMMED>
  + Woman to Woman Obstetrics & Gynecology
    615 Main Street   Toms River, NJ 08753   (732)797-1510   Fax (732)797-2377
Furst, Alan David, MD {1164459962} FamMed, IntrMd, LeglMd(76,NJ05)
  + first Urgent Medical Care
    3175 Route 10 East/Suite 500   Denville, NJ 07834   (973)537-1400   Fax (973)366-1648
Fury, Mary Anne, DO {1568555290} Pedtrc(03,NJ75)<NJ-MONMOUTH>
  + Meridian Medical Group
    2130 Route 35/Suite B216   Sea Girt, NJ 08750   (732)974-0228   Fax (732)263-7938
Fusco, Joseph M., MD {1194751099} Radiol, RadDia(87,NY46)<NJ-CLARMAAS>
  + Essex Imaging Associates
    5 Franklin Avenue/Suite 510   Belleville, NJ 07109   (973)751-2011   Fax (973)751-4456
Fuseini, Nurain M., MD {1932493764} ObsGyn<NJ-OURLADY>
  + Lourdes Medical Associates
    1601 Haddon Avenue   Camden, NJ 08103   (856)757-3700   Fax (856)385-7972
Fusilli, Louis D., MD {1790702678} CdvDis, IntrMd(81,ITAL)<NJ-VALLEY, NJ-STJOSHOS>
  + Cardiology Associates LLC
    181 Franklin Avenue/Suite 301   Nutley, NJ 07110   (973)667-5511   Fax (973)667-0561
  + Cardiology Associates LLC
    999 McBride Avenue/Suite B-204   West Paterson, NJ 07424   (973)667-5511   Fax (973)256-7758
Fusman, Benjamin, MD {1376540351} IntCrd, CdvDis(88,PA02)<NJ-STCLRDEN, NJ-MORRISTN>
  + Cardiology Consultants of North Morris, PA
    356 US Highway 46/Suite B   Mountain Lakes, NJ 07046   (973)586-3400   Fax (973)586-1916
Fussa, Mark J., DO {1942407374} IntrMd, InfDis
  + Garden State Infectious Diseases Associates, P.A.
    709 Haddonfield Berlin Road   Voorhees, NJ 08043   (856)566-3190   Fax (856)783-2193
  + Garden State Infectious Disease Associates
    570 Egg Harbor Road/Suite B-5   Sewell, NJ 08080   (856)566-3190   Fax (856)566-1904
Futterman, Noah D., DO {1184007858} EmrgMd
  + Clara Maass Medical Center
    1 Clara Maass Drive   Belleville, NJ 07109   (516)510-5291
Fyfe-Kirschner, Billie Shawn, MD {1003981127} Pthlgy, PthAna(87,FL02)<NJ-RWJUBRUN>
  + RWJ University Pathology
    125 Paterson Street/MEB 212   New Brunswick, NJ 08901   Fax (732)418-8445
Fyffe, Ullanda P., MD {1932481546} FamMed
  + Clifton Urgent and Primary Care
    721 Clifton Avenue/Suite 2A   Clifton, NJ 07013   (973)777-7727   Fax (973)779-7906
  + Wayne Urgent and Primary Care
    246 Hamburg Turnpike/Suite 205   Wayne, NJ 07470   (973)777-7727   Fax (973)636-2734
Gaafer-Ahmed, Hany M., MD {1518990381} ObsGyn(90,EGY04)<NJ-HACKNSK>
  + Hackensack University Medical Center
    30 Prospect Avenue/Suite 711   Hackensack, NJ 07601   (201)996-2000
Gabay, Jacqueline Estelle, MD {1245310531} Ophthl(95,NY46)
  + Hudson Eye Specialists
    2201 Bergen Line Avenue/3rd Floor   Union City, NJ 07087   (201)601-2020
  + Phillips Eye Center
    619 River Drive   Elmwood Park, NJ 07407   (201)601-2020   Fax (201)796-2833
Gabel, Molly Mary, MD {1518900117} RadOnc(88,MA16)<NJ-RWJUBRUN>
  + Summit Medical Group-Berkeley Heights Campus
    1 Diamond Hill Road   Berkeley Heights, NJ 07922   (908)588-3651   Fax (908)673-7336
  + Rutgers Cancer Institute of New Jersey
    195 Little Albany Street/PO Box 2681   New Brunswick, NJ 08903   (908)588-3651   Fax (732)235-6797
Gabel, Robert L., MD {1164419206} IntrMd, Rheuma, Addctn(77,BELG)<NJ-BAYSHORE, NJ-MONMOUTH>
  + 27 Pinckney Road/Building 2/Suite 35
    Red Bank, NJ 07701   (732)936-1900   Fax (732)936-9119   rgabel48@aol.com
Gabelman, Mark Scott, MD {1750371290} CdvDis, CritCr, IntrMd(80,NY47)<NJ-ENGLWOOD, NJ-HACKNSK>
  + Northern New Jersey Cardiology Associates PA
    7704 Marine Road   North Bergen, NJ 07047   (201)869-1313   Fax (201)854-7945
  + Northern New Jersey Cardiology Associates PA
    200 Grand Avenue   Englewood, NJ 07631   (201)869-1313   Fax (201)854-7945
Gabisan, Glenn Gacula, MD {1346227428} SrgOrt, SrgFAk, OrtSpn(97,NJ05)<NJ-RIVERVW, NJ-MONMOUTH>
  + Professional Orthopaedic Associates
    1430 Hooper Avenue/Suite 101   Toms River, NJ 08753   (732)341-6777   Fax (732)349-7722
  + Professional Orthopaedic Associates
    776 Shrewsbury Avenue/Suite 201   Tinton Falls, NJ 07724   (732)341-6777   Fax (732)530-3618
  + Professional Orthopaedic Associates
    303 West Main Street   Freehold, NJ 08753   (732)530-4949   Fax (732)577-0036
Gable, Brian Philip, MD {1336244672} IntrMd(03,NJ06)
  + 216 Buckingham Avenue
    Somerset, NJ 08873
Gable-Selmon, Chana H., MD {1447294368} EmrgMd(97,NY20)<NJ-HACKNSK>
  + Hackensack Medical Center Emergency Medicine
    30 Prospect Avenue/Main 3619   Hackensack, NJ 07601   (201)996-4614   Fax (201)996-4239
  + Englewood Hospital and Medical Center
    350 Engle Street   Englewood, NJ 07631   (201)894-3000
Gabler, Scott Joseph, MD {1972652840} IntrMd(05,LA01)
  + Associated Cardiovascular Consultants, P.A.
    1105 Laurel Oak Road/Suite 165   Voorhees, NJ 08043   (856)424-3600   Fax (856)424-7154
Gabre, Kennedy Ogbazion, MD {1730149139} Surgry(00,MD01)<NJ-MORRISTN, NJ-STCLRDEN>
  + Summit Medical Group Orthopedics and Sports Medicine
    140 Park Avenue/2nd Floor   Florham Park, NJ 07932   (973)404-9980   Fax (973)267-7295
  + Allied Surgical Group
    261 James Street/Suite 2-G   Morristown, NJ 07960   (973)404-9980   Fax (973)267-7295
Gabrial, Irene Gamalnoub, MD {1710074158} PsyGrt(93,EGY03)
  + Rutgers Hurtado Health Center
    11 Bishop Place   New Brunswick, NJ 08901   (732)932-7402   Fax (732)932-1223
Gabriel, Ahab M., MD {1285729319} IntrMd, Grtrcs(95,EGY05)
  + East Brunswick Medical Associates PA
    63 West Prospect Avenue   East Brunswick, NJ 08816   (732)651-7122
Gabriel, Andre C., MD {1043630833}
  + Internal Medicine Associates
    201 Laurel Heights Drive/Suite 201   Bridgeton, NJ 08302   (856)455-4800   Fax (856)451-0650
Gabriel, Chantal Delise, MD {1366584195} EmrgMd(98,KY02)
  + 9 Nottingham Court
    Ringwood, NJ 07456
Gabriel, Courtney Ann, MD {1144385451} IntrMd
  + Penn Medicine at Cherry Hill
    409 Route 70 East   Cherry Hill, NJ 08034   (856)429-1519
Gabriel, John, MD {1265524110} Pedtrc, PedEmg(97,DMN01)
  + 6 Cornwall Court/Suite A
    East Brunswick, NJ 08816   (732)698-0082   Fax (732)698-0679
Gabriel, Laurice Helen, MD {1104089226} FamMed
  + 4 Pollis Drive
    East Hanover, NJ 07936
Gabriel, Nathaniel F., MD {1104217488} InfDis(10,PA09)<NJ-COOPRUMC>
  + Cooper University Medical Center/Camden
    3 Cooper Plaza/Suite 215   Camden, NJ 08103   (856)342-2000
Gabriel, Timothy Cayco, MD {1992710875} IntrMd(88,PHI01)
  + Alberto Medical Associates PA
    25 Mule Road/Unit A-3   Toms River, NJ 08755   (732)240-0404   Fax (732)244-3555
Gabriele, Elizabeth Ann, MD {1659403319} Pedtrc, IntrMd(06,PA02)<NJ-VIRTVOOR, NJ-VIRTMHBC>
  + CHOP Care Network at Virtua Voorhees Hospital
    100 Bowman Drive/Pediatrics   Voorhees, NJ 08043   (856)325-3000   Fax (609)261-5842
Gabros, David E., MD {1144268426} IntrMd(80,EGY16)<NJ-ACMCMAIN, NJ-ACMCITY>
  + Lighthouse Medical Care LLC
    217 34th Street   Brigantine, NJ 08203   (609)264-7252   Fax (609)264-8657
Gabucan, Maximo B., Jr., MD {1801833264} Surgry(72,PHI10)<NJ-RBAYPFRT>
  + Raritan Bay Medical Center/Perth Amboy Division
    530 New Brunswick Avenue/Surgery   Perth Amboy, NJ 08861   (732)442-3700   Fax (732)324-4811
Gabuzda, George Mark, MD {1033103957} SrgHnd(87,PA02)<NJ-JRSYSHMC, NJ-BAYSHORE>
  + Central Jersey Hand Surgery
    2 Industrial Way West   Eatontown, NJ 07724   (732)542-4477   Fax (732)935-0355
  + Central Jersey Hand Surgery
    535 Iron Bridge Road   Freehold, NJ 07728   (732)542-4477   Fax (732)431-4770
  + Central Jersey Hand Surgery

780 Route 37 West/Suite 140   Toms River, NJ 07724   (732)286-9000   Fax (732)240-0036
Gachette, Emmanuel Amilcar, MD {1306874979} FamMed(00,MEX34)
  + Careplus Medical Associates
    473 Main Street   Paterson, NJ 07501   (973)707-8243
Gad, Gamal Eldin, MD {1578695714} Psychy(74,EGYP)<NJ-STJOSHOS>
  + Gamal E Gad MD PC
    541 East 29th Street   Paterson, NJ 07504   (973)523-6830   Fax (973)523-3145   Eila5@aol.com
Gada, Alaine E., MD {1871794339}
  + 1200 Geiger Lane
    Bridgewater, NJ 08807   (201)836-0897   Fax (201)836-8042   mcgarrygada@gmail.com
Gadalla, Hisham Hussein, MD {1689666257} Pedtrc(83,EGY03)<NJ-STJOSHOS>
  + Fayrouz Pediatrics
    1300 Main Avenue/Suite 2-C   Clifton, NJ 07011   (973)928-3388   Fax (973)404-8525
Gadarla, Mamatha R., MD {1124167879} IntrMd(99,INA5B)<NJ-CHILTON>
  + Chilton Medical Center
    97 West Parkway   Pompton Plains, NJ 07444   (973)831-5000
Gadgil, Nandini S., MD {1871559088} Pedtrc(69,INDI)<NJ-STJOSHOS>
  + St. Joseph's Family Health Center
    21 Market Street   Paterson, NJ 07501   (973)754-4200   Fax (973)754-4259
Gadhvi, Pragnesh Harish, MD {1306865571} IntCrd, IntrMd, CdvDis(97,MNT01)
  + Newark International Airport
    Newark Airport/Medical Offices   Newark, NJ 07102   (973)596-1200
Gadin, Erlita Pagaduan, MD {1689799702}
  + CHOP Specialty Care Center at Virtua
    200 Bowman Drive/2 FL/Suite D-260   Voorhees, NJ 08043   (856)719-9926
Gadiraju, Silpa, MD {1003105750} EnDbMt, IntrMd
  + Summit Medical Group
    95 Madison Avenue   Morristown, NJ 07960   (973)775-5115   Fax (973)267-5521
Gadomski, Stephen P., MD {1376549832} Otlryg, PedOto(81,PA02)<NJ-VIRTVOOR, NJ-VIRTMARL>
  + Advanced ENT - Haddonfield
    130 North Haddon Avenue   Haddonfield, NJ 08033   (856)602-4000   Fax (856)429-1284
  + Advanced ENT - Mount Laurel
    204 Ark Road/Building 1/Suite 102   Mount Laurel, NJ 08054   (856)602-4000   Fax (856)946-1747
  + Advanced ENT - Voorhees
    1307 White Horse Road   Voorhees, NJ 08033   (856)602-4000   Fax (856)346-0480
Gaela, Joan Fontelera, MD FamMed(84,PHIL)
  + 11 Magnolia Lane
    Mount Arlington, NJ 07856
Gaffin, Neil, MD {1649259045} IntrMd, InfDis, MRImag(93,PA09)<NJ-VALLEY>
  + Ridgewood Infectious Disease Associates
    947 Linwood Avenue/Suite 2E   Ridgewood, NJ 07450   (201)447-6468   Fax (201)447-3189
Gaffney, John L., DO {1710985387} FamMed(88,PA77)<NJ-ACMC-ITY, NJ-SHOREMEM>
  + The Medical Center of Margate
    9501 Ventnor Avenue   Margate, NJ 08402   (609)823-6161   Fax (856)823-3413
Gaffney, Joseph W., MD {1437125952} PedCrd, Pedtrc(81,NY09)<NJ-RWJUBRUN>
  + Rutgers Pediatric Cardiology
    125 Paterson Street/CAB 6100   New Brunswick, NJ 08901   (732)235-7905   Fax (732)235-8259
  + RWJ University Hospital New Brunswick
    One Robert Wood Johnson Place   New Brunswick, NJ 08901   (732)828-3000
Gagliano, Salvatore M., MD {1104915297} ObsGyn(74,NJ05)
  + 258 Passaic Avenue
    Passaic, NJ 07055   (973)471-8887   Fax (973)471-9162
Gagliardi, Anthony J., MD {1265582746} IntrMd, PulDis(81,NJ05)<NY-CMCSTVNY>
  + 25 Stonybrook Drive
    North Caldwell, NJ 07006
Gagliardi, Carol L., MD {1184633570} FrtInf, ObsGyn, RprEnd(80,PA14)<NJ-JRSYCITY, NJ-MEADWLND>
  + New Margaret Hague Women's Health Institute
    377 Jersey Avenue/Suite 220   Jersey City, NJ 07302   (201)795-9155   Fax (201)795-9157
Gaioni, Kathleen A., MD {1831352665} IntrMd(82,NJ05)
  + Rutgers Hurtado Health Center
    11 Bishop Place   New Brunswick, NJ 08901   (732)932-7402   Fax (732)932-1223

Physicians by Name and Address

Gaito, Andrea D., MD {1487781787} IntrMd, Rheuma(86,GRNA)<NJ-MORRISTN>
 + 211 South Finley Avenue
  Basking Ridge, NJ 07920 (908)766-0339

Gaitour, Larisa, MD {1760715288}(94,MOL02)
 + Aspen Medical Associates, P.A.
  1 DeGraw Square Teaneck, NJ 07666 (201)928-0807
  Fax (201)928-0820
  lgaitour@gmail.com

Gajarawala, Jatin M., MD {1538103213} NuclMd, Radiol, RadDia(68,INDI)
 + Toms River X-Ray
  154 Highway 37 West Toms River, NJ 08753 (732)244-0777 Fax (732)244-0428
 + University Imaging
  246 Hamburg Turnpike/Suite 101 Wayne, NJ 07470 (732)244-0777 Fax (973)790-7397

Gajarawala, Raksha J., MD {1730295502} Pedtrc, FamMed(72,INDI)<NJ-NWRKBETH, NJ-UMDNJ>
 + 1096 Broad Street
  Newark, NJ 07114 (973)242-0191 Fax (973)242-0593

Gajdos, Robert M., MD {1649347964} IntrMd(85,GRNA)<NJ-STMRYPAS, NJ-MTNSIDE>
 + 1005 Clifton Avenue
  Clifton, NJ 07013 (973)777-2005 Fax (973)777-7758

Gajera, Bhavinkumar, MD {1205063005} Psychy(06,INA15)
 + Hudson Psychiatric Associates, LLC.
  79 Hudson Street/Suite 203 Hoboken, NJ 07030 (201)222-8808 Fax (201)222-8803

Gajera, Sangeeta Jadav, MD Pedtrc(97,NJ06)
 + New Brunswick Pediatric Group, P.A.
  1300 How Lane North Brunswick, NJ 08902 (732)247-1510 Fax (732)247-8885

Gajewski, Jan Peter, MD {1437114097} Anesth(90,NJ05)<NJ-STPETER>
 + Anesthesia Consultnts of NJ/Nova Pain
  285 Davidson Avenue/Suite 204 Somerset, NJ 08873 (732)271-1400 Fax (732)271-3543
 + Cares Surgicenter, LLC.
  240 Easton Avenue New Brunswick, NJ 08901 (732)271-1400 Fax (732)296-8677

Gajewski, Michael M., DO {1326351271} Anesth(09,NY75)
 + Rutgers- New Jersey Medical School
  185 South Orange Avenue/ESB E-538 Newark, NJ 07103 (973)972-2518

Gajian, Garen Edward, MD {1417928789} AnesPain(85,UKR05)
 + 251 Powers Street
  New Brunswick, NJ 08901 (732)745-2989

Gajraj Singh Sachan, Reena Sachan, MD {1649431263}
 + Cooper University Hospital
  One Cooper Plaza Camden, NJ 08103 (856)342-2000

Gajula, Ramarao Sundara, MD {1801843297} Pedtrc, EmrgMd, AdolMd(79,INA11)<NJ-CENTRAST>
 + CentraState Medical Center
  901 West Main Street/Pediatrics Freehold, NJ 07728 (732)431-2000

Gak, Alexander V., MD {1396724555} Anesth, IntrMd(97,NY48)
 + Englewood Anesthesiology
  350 Engle Street Englewood, NJ 07631 (201)894-3238 Fax (201)894-0585

Gal, Stephen, MD {1073544326} Anesth, Pedtrc(82,VA07)<NJ-VALLEY>
 + The Valley Hospital
  223 North Van Dien Avenue Ridgewood, NJ 07450 (201)447-8350

Gala, Indira H., MD {1881757292} PthACl(74,INDI)<NJ-UNDRWD>
 + Inspira Health Network
  509 North Broad Street Woodbury, NJ 08096 (856)845-0100

Gala, Ketan M., MD {1932381035} CdvDis
 + Mercer Bucks Cardiology
  One Union Street/Suite 101 Robbinsville, NJ 08691 (609)890-6677 Fax (609)890-7292

Gala, Payal K., MD {1215221437} PedEmg<PA-CHILDHOS>
 + Virtua Voorhees
  100 Bowman Drive Voorhees, NJ 08043 (856)247-3000

Galabi, Michael, MD {1205129533} IntrMd(11,PA0)
 + Penn Medicine at Cherry Hill
  409 Route 70 East/2nd Floor Cherry Hill, NJ 08034 (856)429-0589

Galaktionova, Dina, DO {1316364144}
 + 37-19 Stelton Terrace
  Fair Lawn, NJ 07410 (917)373-3412

Galandauer, Isaac, MD {1356543276} Gastrn, IntrMd(02,NY09)<NJ-MORRISTN>
 + Summit Medical Group
  140 Park Avenue/3rd Floor Florham Park, NJ 07932 (908)273-4300

Galbraith, Michael, MD {1093912867} RadDia(01,NJ06)
 + 6 Monica Drive
  Edison, NJ 08820 (732)687-8208

Galdi, Balazs, MD {1316108806} SprtMd, SrgOrt(08,NY46)
 + 8200 Boulevard/Suite 7-K
  North Bergen, NJ 07047 (201)923-0921

Galdieri, Louis C., MD {1124024146} Urolgy(79,MEXI)
 + New Jersey Urology, LLC
  741 Northfield Avenue/Suite 206 West Orange, NJ 07052 (973)325-6100 Fax (973)325-1616
 + New Jersey Urology, LLC
  375 Mounain Pleasant Ave/Suite 250 West Orange, NJ 07052 (973)325-6100 Fax (973)323-1311
 + New Jersey Urology, LLC
  1515 Broad Street/Suite B-130 Bloomfield, NJ 07052 (973)873-7000 Fax (973)873-7035

Galea, Marina, MD {1649242793} Psychy(87,ROM01)<NJ-TRIN-INPC>
 + 2143 Morris Avenue/Suite 106
  Union, NJ 07083 (908)687-6344

Galeano, Narmer E., MD {1528003985} Pedtrc, PedGst, Nutrtn(75,COL01)<NJ-STJOSHCS>
 + St. Joseph's Pediatrics DePaul Center
  11 Getty Avenue/2nd Floor Paterson, NJ 07503 (973)754-2727

Galeos, Warren L., MD {1275502114} Otlryg, Otolgy(80,NJ05)<NJ-NWTNMEM>
 + Skylands Medical Group PA
  135 Newton Sparta Road/Suite 101 Newton, NJ 07860 (973)383-9966 Fax (973)383-7772

Galetto, David W., MD {1871574962} InfDis, IntrMd(81,NJ05)<NJ-SJERSYHS, NJ-SJHREGMC>
 + Cumberland Internal Medicine
  1450 East Chestnut Avenue Vineland, NJ 08361 (856)794-8700 Fax (856)794-2752

Galezniak, John, DO {1730560988} FamMed
 + Advocare Gigliotti Family Medicine
  181 West White Horse Pike/Suite 100 Berlin, NJ 08009 (856)767-3234 Fax (856)767-3518

Gali, Lavanya, MD {1730347915} IntrMd, SlpDis(01,INA2Y)
 + 20 Forest Center South
  Monmouth Junction, NJ 08852 (908)420-6755

Galimidi Hodara, Salomon, MD {1750415626} Pedtrc(78,URUG)<NJ-NWRKBETH, NJ-CHDNWBTH>
 + 29 Elmora Avenue
  Elizabeth, NJ 07202 (908)289-2239 Fax (908)659-1001

Galitzin, Joseph C., MD {1356402127} SrgHnd
 + Premier Orthopaedics and Sports Medicine, P.C.
  111 Galway Place Teaneck, NJ 07666 (201)833-9500 Fax (201)862-0095

Galkin, Vadim, MD {1003819293} Anesth(86,UZB44)
 + Advanced Interventional Pain Management
  1176 Hamburg Turnpike Wayne, NJ 07470 (973)365-4747 Fax (973)365-4596

Galkowski, Dariusz Bohdan, MD {1285893834} GntMMPty(90,POL06)
 + RWJ University Pathology
  125 Paterson Street/MEB 212 New Brunswick, NJ 08901 (732)235-8801 Fax (732)418-8445

Galla, Jan David, MD {1376716274} SrgCdv, SrgThr, Surgry(81,TX04)<NY-MTSINAI, NJ-ENGLWOOD>
 + Englewood Hospital and Medical Center
  350 Engle Street/Suite 5200 Englewood, NJ 07631 (201)894-3636 Fax (201)541-2188
 + Englewood Cardiac Surgery Associates
  350 Engle Street Englewood, NJ 07631 (201)894-3636
 + Heart and Vascular Institute at EHMC
  350 Engle Street/Suite 1000 Englewood, NJ 07631 (201)894-3636

Gallagher, Christopher John, MD {1669409587} RadOnc(88,NJ05)<NJ-CHSMRCER>
 + Capital Health System/Mercer Campus
  446 Bellevue Avenue/RadOnc Trenton, NJ 08618 (609)394-4244

Gallagher, Cornelius T., MD {1194727982} CritCr, IntrMd, PulDis(86,NJ05)<NJ-JRSYSHMC, NJ-OCEANMC>
 + Shore Pulmonary PA
  2640 Highway 70/Building 6-A Manasquan, NJ 08736 (732)528-5900 Fax (732)528-0887
 + Shore Pulmonary PA
  301 Bingham Avenue/Suite B Ocean, NJ 07712 (732)528-5900 Fax (732)775-1212
 + Shore Pulmonary PA
  1608 Route 88/Suite 117 Brick, NJ 08736 (732)575-1100

Gallagher, Edward J., MD {1881637965} PhysMd(78,WV02)<NJ-OURLADY, NJ-UNDRWD>
 + 636 Kings Highway/Suite B
  Woodbury, NJ 08096 (856)848-1688 Fax (856)848-6886
 + Inspira Health Network
  509 North Broad Street/Phys Med&Rehab Woodbury, NJ 08096 (856)853-2081
 + Associated Physiatrists of Southern New Jersey
  1600 Haddon Avenue/Room R-122 Camden, NJ 08096 (856)757-3878 Fax (856)757-3760

Gallagher, Joseph L., III, DO {1841229457} FamMed
 + Kennedy Family Health Services
  1 Somerdale Square Somerdale, NJ 08083 (856)309-7700 Fax (856)566-8944

Gallagher, Michael J., MD {1598760431} IntrMd, RadThp, MedOnc(73,OH06)
 + Sparta Cancer Center
  89 Sparta Avenue/Suite 130 Sparta, NJ 07871 (973)729-7001

Gallagher, Peter K., MD {1174517841} Psychy, PsyFor(80,IL11)<NJ-ANNKLEIN>
 + Ann Klein Forensic Center
  1609 Stuyvesant Avenue/PO Box 7717 West Trenton, NJ 08628 (609)633-0900

Gallagher, Thomas Jude, DO {1972542280} RadDia(99,NJ75)
 + South Jersey Radiology Associates, P.A.
  901 Route 168/Suites 301-305 Turnersville, NJ 08012 (856)227-6600 Fax (856)227-8537
 + South Jersey Radiology Associates, P.A.
  100 Carnie Boulevard/Suite B-5 Voorhees, NJ 08043 (856)227-6600 Fax (856)751-0535
 + South Jersey Radiology Associates, P.A.
  6650 Browning Road/Suite M14 Pennsauken, NJ 08012 (856)665-3330 Fax (856)661-0686

Gallagher, William Joseph, MD {1295170082}<NJ-HOBUNIMC>
 + Hoboken University Medical Center
  308 Willow Avenue Hoboken, NJ 07030 (732)567-5284

Gallardo, Mario L., MD {1285635201} IntrMd(87,PHIL)<NJ-COMMED>
 + Whiting Medical Associates
  65 Lacey Road/Suite A Whiting, NJ 08759 (732)350-0404 Fax (732)350-2001

Gallardo, Mary Rose Ramos, MD {1255412391} Pedtrc, AdolMd(88,PHI02)<NJ-OCEANMC>
 + 1608 Route 88/Suite 104 C
  Brick, NJ 08724 (732)785-9080 Fax (732)785-9084

Galldin, Lars Michael, MD {1063640902} Anesth, IntrMd(09,GRN01)
 + St. Joseph's Regional Medical Center Anesthesia
  703 Main Street Paterson, NJ 07503 (973)754-2323 Fax (973)977-9455

Gallegos, Analysa, MD {1003219155}<NJ-HACKNSK>
 + Hackensack University Medical Center
  30 Prospect Avenue Hackensack, NJ 07601 (551)996-2331

Galler, Leonard, MD {1013909530} Surgry, SrgVas(77,NY47)<NJ-SHOREMEM, NJ-ACMCMAIN>
 + GFH Surgical Associates
  718 Shore Road Somers Point, NJ 08244 (609)927-8550 Fax (609)926-0273
  lap1818@aol.com

Gallerstein, Peter E., MD {1902957749} CdvDis, IntrMd(74,MD07)<NJ-MORRISTN>
 + Honeywell Inc.
  115 Tabor Road Morris Plains, NJ 07950 (973)455-3306 Fax (973)455-4416

Gallick, Gregory S., MD {1538138656} SrgOrt(80,NJ06)<NJ-STBARNMC, NJ-OVERLOOK>
 + 2780 Morris Avenue/Suite 2-C
  Union, NJ 07083 (908)686-6665 Fax (908)686-5245

Gallina, David J., MD {1760492946} Psychy(67,NJ05)
 + 541 Cedar Hill Avenue
  Wyckoff, NJ 07481 (201)447-0500 Fax (201)447-5233

Gallina, Gregory J., MD {1356437198} SrgC&R, Surgry(92,DC01)<NJ-HACKNSK, NJ-HOLYNAME>
 + Colon and Rectal Specialists PA
  255 West Spring Valley Avenue Maywood, NJ 07607 (201)525-1031 Fax (201)880-4560

Gallina, Jessica Blair, MD {1245330885} SrgOrt, SrgFAk(98,NY47)<NY-SLRRSVLT, NY-SLRLUKES>
 + Srino Bharam MD PC
  541 Cedar Hill Avenue Wyckoff, NJ 07481 (201)904-2121 Fax (201)904-2125

Gallinson, David Herschel, DO {1124020052} IntrMd, OncHem(98,NJ75)<NJ-MORRISTN>
 + Carol G. Simon Cancer Center
  100 Madison Avenue/Suite 4101 Morristown, NJ 07962 (973)538-5210 Fax (973)644-9657

Gallo, Leza N., MD {1083709208} PthACl, PthCyt, PthAna(80,DC03)
 + Quest Diagnostics Inc.
  1 Malcolm Avenue Teterboro, NJ 07608 (201)393-5035 Fax (201)393-6127

Gallo, Richard James, MD {1144306317} CdvDis, IntrMd(86,GRNA)<NJ-HOLYNAME>
 + Bergen Internal Medicine, LLC
  6 Horizon Road Fort Lee, NJ 07024 (201)886-8989 Fax (201)886-8990

Gallo, Robert James, MD {1750385225} ObsGyn, IntrMd(77,ITA17)<NJ-HACKNSK>
+ 125 Prospect Avenue
Hackensack, NJ 07601 (201)342-6633 Fax (201)342-3570
drgallo@mac.com
+ Bergen Ob-Gyn Associates, PA
130 Kinderkamack Road/Suite 300 River Edge, NJ 07661
(201)342-6633 Fax (201)489-5040

Gallo, Vincent, MD {1568699403} RadV&I
+ Advanced Interventional Radiology Services, LLP
718 Teaneck Road Teaneck, NJ 07666 (973)219-5530
Fax (201)643-3077

Galloway, Joseph, MD {1821449604} Surgry
+ 140 Bergen Street/Suite D1610
Newark, NJ 07103

Gallucci, John Gerard, MD {1245295153} PedSrg, Surgry(90,NJ05)<NJ-STPETER>
+ St. Peter's University Hospital
254 Easton Avenue/PediSurgery New Brunswick, NJ 08901
(732)745-8600 Fax (732)249-5284
+ Cares Surgicenter, LLC.
240 Easton Avenue New Brunswick, NJ 08901 (732)745-8600 Fax (732)296-8677

Galope, Roel Pangilinan, DO {1629021779} Radiol(98,CA22)
+ Diagnostic Imaging Center and Group Practice
251 Rochelle Avenue Rochelle Park, NJ 07662 (201)291-8800 Fax (201)291-1619

Galowitz, Stacey, DO {1972825719} Pedtrc, AllmCLIm(09,NJ75)
+ ENT & Allergy Associates
1543 Route 27/Suite 21 Somerset, NJ 08873 (732)873-6863 Fax (732)873-6853

Galperina, Klara, DO {1447539143} Pedtrc
+ 7 Doral Drive
Marlboro, NJ 07746

Galski, Thomas M., DO {1811966187} CdvDis, IntrMd(95,NJ75)
+ The Cardiology Group, P.A.
401 Young Avenue/Suite 275 Moorestown, NJ 08057
(856)291-8855 Fax (856)291-8844
+ The Cardiology Group, P.A.
128 State Highway Route 70/Suite 1-B Medford, NJ 08055
(856)291-8855 Fax (609)444-5521
+ Avnet Memec
7000 Atrium Way/Suite 6 Mount Laurel, NJ 08057
(856)291-6818 Fax (856)291-6819

Galumyan, Yelena V., MD {1356587828} IntrMd<NJ-ENGLWOOD>
+ Englewood Hospital and Medical Center
350 Engle Street Englewood, NJ 07631 (201)894-3364
Fax (201)894-5693

Galvin, Sharon A., MD {1962461400} Dermat(85,NY19)<NJ-VALLEY>
+ Dermatology Associates
348 South Maple Avenue Glen Rock, NJ 07452 (201)652-6060 Fax (201)652-1882

Gamallo, Ma. Bernardita Ricafort, MD {1952544272} Pedtrc<OH-CHLDHOSP>
+ Goryeb Children's Hospital
100 Madison Avenue Morristown, NJ 07960 (973)971-5232

Gamao, Eddie M., MD {1770500423} IntrMd(65,PHI26)
+ 1032 Stelton Road
Piscataway, NJ 08854 (732)981-9336 Fax (732)981-9339

Gambale, Joseph Gerard, DO {1851599120} IntrMd(NJ75<NJ-KMHTURNV>
+ Kennedy Health Systems/Washington Township Campus
435 Hurffville-Cross Keys Road Turnersville, NJ 08012
(856)218-5634 Fax (856)218-5664

Gambescia, Richard Alan, MD {1427031343} IntrMd, Gastrn(71,PA09)
+ Philadelphia Gastroenterology Group, P.C.
570 Egg Harbor Road/Suite A-2 Sewell, NJ 08080
(856)218-1410 Fax (856)218-0193

Gambhir, Priyanka, MD {1518124528} FamMed(04,GCY01)
+ Nu U MedSpa
32 Washington Street/Suite 2-A Tenafly, NJ 07670
(201)696-1880 Fax (801)618-4476
+ Nu U MedSpa
1346 Clifton Avenue Clifton, NJ 07012 (201)696-1880

Gamble, James D., MD {1154310829} Grtrcs, IntrMd(82,MO34)<NJ-VIRTVOOR>
+ Tatem Brown Family Practice
2225 East Evesham Road/Suite 101 Voorhees, NJ 08043
(856)795-4330 Fax (856)325-3704

Gamboa, Elmer Salvador, MD {1205973666} Pthlgy, PthACl(85,PHI01)<NJ-STPETER>
+ St. Peter's University Hospital
254 Easton Avenue/Diagnostics New Brunswick, NJ 08901
(732)745-8600

Gamburg, David, MD {1134120298} AnesPain, IntrMd(93,ISR02)<NY-BENEDCTN, NY-KINGSTON>
+ Pain Management Associates
255 East Main Street Ramsey, NJ 07446 (201)326-4777
Fax (201)391-1196

Gamburg, Eugene Samuel, MD {1043293624} ObsGyn(00,KY12)<NJ-UNVMCPRN>
+ Delaware Valley Ob/Gyn & Infertility Group, PC
300B Princeton Hightstown Road East Windsor, NJ 08520
(609)336-3266 Fax (609)443-4506
+ Delaware Valley Ob/Gyn & Infertility Group, PC
2 Princess Road/Suite C Lawrenceville, NJ 08648
(609)336-3266 Fax (609)896-3266

Gami, Nishith Madhusudan, MD {1295786440} IntrMd(89,INA20)
+ Vital Medical Care, LLC.
212 West Route 38/Suite 540 Moorestown, NJ 08057
(856)396-0260 Fax (856)787-0262

Gamss, Jonathan, MD {1598922874} IntrMd, EmrgMd(04,NY46)<NJ-CLARMAAS>
+ Clara Maass Medical Center
1 Clara Maass Drive/EmrgMed Belleville, NJ 07109
(973)450-2010 Fax (973)450-0383

Gamss, Rebecca, MD {1598053746} RadDia
+ Hackensack Radiology Group, P.A.
30 Prospect Avenue Hackensack, NJ 07601 (201)996-2200 Fax (201)489-2812

Gan, Richard A., MD {1063588481} Nrolgy, IntrMd(83,OK01)
+ Edison Neurologic Associates
36 Progress Street/Suite B-3 Edison, NJ 08820 (908)757-6633 Fax (908)757-3912

Gan, Yuebo, MD {1972769768}
+ 88 Running Deer Trail
Elmer, NJ 08318 (215)485-7054
ganyuebo@yahoo.com

Ganapathy, Jayalakshmi, MD {1942292479} Pedtrc, IntrMd(64,INDI)<NJ-HACKNSK>
+ 8 Hedden Terrace
North Arlington, NJ 07031 (201)991-6363 Fax (201)991-6330

Ganatra, Nikita, MD {1104236298} EmrgMd<NJ-RBAYPERT>
+ Raritan Bay Medical Center/Perth Amboy Division
530 New Brunswick Avenue Perth Amboy, NJ 08861
(732)324-5104

Ganchi, Amir, MD {1467527424} PedSrg, Surgry(64,IRA01)<NJ-WAYNEGEN, NJ-CHILTON>
+ Ganchi Plastic Surgery
246 Hamburg Turnpike/Suite 307 Wayne, NJ 07470
(973)942-6600 Fax (973)595-5964
Ganchi@aol.com

Ganchi, Parham Amir, MD {1972570240} SrgPlstc, IntrMd(94,NC07)<NJ-HACKNSK, NJ-UMDNJ>
+ Ganchi Plastic Surgery
246 Hamburg Turnpike/Suite 307 Wayne, NJ 07470
(973)942-6600 Fax (973)595-5964

Ganchi, Pedramine, MD {1619918463} SrgPlstc, Surgry(92,NY46)<NJ-VALLEY>
+ Village Plastic Surgery
75 Oak Street Ridgewood, NJ 07450 (201)444-6646 Fax (201)444-6642
info@drpedyganchi.com
+ Paramus Surgical Center
30 West Century Road/Suite 300 Paramus, NJ 07652
(201)986-9000
+ Wayne Surgical Center, LLC.
1176 Hamburg Pike Wayne, NJ 07450 (973)709-1900
Fax (973)709-1901

Gandehok, Jasneet K., MD {1922307248} IntrMd<NJ-UMDNJ>
+ University Hospital
150 Bergen Street/Room I-248 Newark, NJ 07103
(973)972-6056 Fax (973)972-3129

Gandhi, Achyut Natvarial, MD {1740288521} EmrgMd, IntrMd(79,INDI)
+ Allied Medical Associates
510 Hamburg Turnpike Wayne, NJ 07470 (973)653-9485
Fax (973)442-6009

Gandhi, Alpana D., MD {1003871484} Pedtrc(70,INA9B)<NJ-STCLRDEN, NJ-MORRISTN>
+ 170 Changebridge Road/Suite B-6
Montville, NJ 07045 (973)882-4994
dinesh111@optonline.net

Gandhi, Champaklal K., MD {1568408573} IntrMd, Nephro(68,INDI)<NJ-STBARNMC>
+ 707 South Orange Avenue
South Orange, NJ 07079 (973)762-4720 Fax (973)762-3731

Gandhi, Chirag D., MD {1316068927} SrgNro<NJ-RWJUBRUN>
+ Center for Neurological Surgery UMDNJ
90 Bergen Street/DOC 8100 Newark, NJ 07103 (973)972-2323 Fax (973)972-2333

Gandhi, Devang Amrat, MD {1225038755} CdvDis, CarNuc(92,NJ05)<NJ-STBARNMC, NJ-CLARMAAS>
+ New Jersey Cardiology Associates
375 Mount Pleasant Avenue West Orange, NJ 07052
(973)731-9442 Fax (973)731-8030

Gandhi, Dhiren K., MD {1295792919} FamMed(00,DMN01)<NJ-COMMED, NJ-SOCEANCO>
+ 240 Mathistown Road
Little Egg Harbor, NJ 08087 (609)294-4232 Fax (732)505-5495
Dgandhi1412@yahoo.com

Gandhi, Jinesh Mulraj, MD {1043217342} IntrMd(92,INA69)
+ 59 Roseberry Street
Phillipsburg, NJ 08865 (908)454-8600 Fax (908)454-3524
+ Coordinated Health
222 Red Lane Phillipsburg, NJ 08865 (908)454-8600 Fax (610)849-1013

Gandhi, Kirit V., MD {1629180344} IntrMd(78,INDI)<NJ-JRSYCITY, NJ-CHRIST>
+ Drs. Gandhi and Roy
3665 Kennedy Boulevard Jersey City, NJ 07306 (201)963-1155 Fax (201)963-7957

Gandhi, Nabila Asif, MD {1669452553} IntrMd(92,INDI)<NJ-JFKMED, NJ-RBAYOLDB>
+ North Edison Family Practice Group
35-37 Progress Street/Suite A-3 Edison, NJ 08820
(908)755-9797 Fax (908)668-4848

Gandhi, Neel Jitendra, MD {1033385877} IntrMd(06,TN06)
+ Mercer Bucks Hematology Oncology
2 Capital Way/Suite 220 Pennington, NJ 08534 (609)303-0747 Fax (609)303-0771

Gandhi, Nisha R., MD {1891744355} IntrMd, CritCr(98,DMN01)<NJ-ENGLWOOD>
+ Englewood Hospital and Medical Center
350 Engle Street/Crtcl Care Med Englewood, NJ 07631
(201)894-3000 Fax (201)871-0619

Gandhi, Rajinder P., MD {1184716953} PedSrg, Gastrn, Surgry(66,MYA02)<NJ-VALLEY, NJ-ENGLWOOD>
+ Pediatric Surgery
30 West Century Road/Suite 235 Paramus, NJ 07652
(201)996-0010 Fax (201)225-9430
+ Paramus Surgical Center
30 West Century Road/Suite 300 Paramus, NJ 07652
(201)986-9000

Gandhi, Senthamara, MD {1033385257} IntrMd(67,INA04)<NJ-CLARMAAS>
+ Clara Maass Medical Center
1 Clara Maass Drive Belleville, NJ 07109 (973)450-2000

Gandhi, Shefali, DO {1952634750} Nrolgy, IntrMd(05,NY75)<NJ-BAYSHORE, NJ-JRSYSHMC>
+ 670 North Beers Street
Holmdel, NJ 07733 (732)788-6537 Fax (732)254-1558

Gandhi, Shveta V., DO {1023402534} IntrMd
+ 23 Chestnut Oak Drive
Cape May Court House, NJ 08210

Gandhi, Snehal V., MD {1760509533} IntrMd(04,NJ06)<NJ-COOPRUMC>
+ Cooper University Hospital
One Cooper Plaza/Ste 222/Dorrnce Camden, NJ 08103
(856)342-2000

Gandhi, Sulakshana, MD {1669819744} IntrMd
+ 707 South Orange Avenue
South Orange, NJ 07079 (973)761-6111

Gandhi, Thimma S., MD {1487771325} EnDbMt(72,INA47)<NJ-HOBUNIMC>
+ 122 Clinton Street/3rd Floor
Hoboken, NJ 07030 (201)861-2918 Fax (201)861-2859
+ Endocrine Associates
30 West Century Drive/Suite 255 Paramus, NJ 07652
(201)861-2918 Fax (201)444-6590

Gandhi, Veena S., MD {1144250200} Gyneco(66,INDI)<NJ-VIRTVOOR, NJ-VIRTBERL>
+ 314 South Burnt Mill Road
Voorhees, NJ 08043 (856)428-2522 Fax (856)428-8022
+ 925B Black Horse Pike
Williamstown, NJ 08094 (856)428-2522 Fax (856)629-7801

Gandhi, Vijaykumar K., MD {1619930617} Hemato, IntrMd, MedOnc(81,INA21)<NJ-BURDTMLN, NJ-SHOREMEM>
+ 301 Stone Harbor Boulevard/Unit C
Cape May Court House, NJ 08210 (609)465-3995 Fax (609)465-4913
Vkg1@verizon.net

Gandhi, Zindadil Manoj, MD {1215196043} Psychy, PsyCAd, IntrMd(03,INA21)<NJ-UNIVBHC>
+ University Behavioral Health Care
4326 Route 1 North Monmouth Junction, NJ 08852
(732)235-5790 Fax (732)235-5799

Gandolfi, Brad Michael, MD {1003131053} Surgry, SrgRec(08,LA05)<NY-BETHPETR>
+ Robert Zubowski MD Ctr Cosmetic/Recon
1 Sears Drive Paramus, NJ 07652 (201)261-7550 Fax (201)261-7515

Gandotra, Puneet, MD {1780728105} IntCrd(05,MD01)
+ Cardiology Associates of Morristown
95 Madison Avenue/Suite 10A Morristown, NJ 07960
(973)889-9001 Fax (973)889-9051

Physicians by Name and Address

Gandrabura, Tatiana, MD {1861602740} IntrMd
+ Endocrine Associates of Southern Jersey
703 East Main Street/Suite 5   Moorestown, NJ 08057
(856)727-0900   Fax (856)231-8428

Ganek, Ellen Beth, MD {1750379228} Pedtrc(99,NJ03)<NJ-OVERLOOK, NJ-MORRISTN>
+ Advocare Sinatra & Peng Pediatrics
169 Minebrook Road   Bernardsville, NJ 07924   (908)766-0034   Fax (908)766-5065

Ganek, Martin E., MD {1639146798} Pedtrc(71,DC02)<NJ-MORRISTN, NJ-STBARNMC>
+ Pediatric Associates of West Essex, PA
3155 Route 10/Suite 104   Denville, NJ 07834   (973)361-4900   Fax (973)361-1842

Ganepola, Ganepola Araccige Padmaj, MD {1487680260} Surgry, SrgOnc(67,JAP01)<NJ-VALLEY>
+ 400 Franklin Turnpike/Suite 110
Mahwah, NJ 07430   (201)236-0400   Fax (201)236-8463

Ganesan, Azhagasund, MD {1285722736} IntrMd, OncHem(67,INDI)
+ 534 Clifton Avenue
Clifton, NJ 07011   (973)365-1330   Fax (973)365-2410

Ganesan, Balamurugan, MD {1760692263} FamMed, IntrMd(02,INA04)<NJ-BURDTMLN, NJ-SHOREMEM>
+ Shore Memorial Hospital
1 East New York Avenue/Fam Med   Somers Point, NJ 08244
(609)653-3500   Fax (609)926-4311
+ Cape Regional Medical Center
2 Stone Harbor Boulevard/FamMed   Cape May Court House, NJ 08210   (609)463-2000
+ Shore Hospitalists Associates
100 Medical Center Way   Somers Point, NJ 08244
(609)653-3500   Fax (609)926-4799

Ganesan, Shridar, MD {1619916566} OncHem, Onclgy, MedOnc(93,CT01)<NJ-RWJUBRUN>
+ Rutgers Cancer Institute of New Jersey
195 Little Albany Street/PO Box 2681   New Brunswick, NJ 08903   (732)235-2465   Fax (732)235-6797

Ganescu, Daniela Florentina, MD {1669572228} Psychy(90,ROM01)<NJ-CAPITLHS, NJ-CHSFULD>
+ Capital Health System/Fuld Campus
750 Brunswick Avenue/Psychiatry   Trenton, NJ 08638
(609)394-6085   Fax (609)394-6205

Ganesh, Manickam, MD {1962419838} Grtrcs, IntrMd, Nephro(69,SRIL)<NJ-STBARNMC>
+ Drs. Ganesh and Theivanayagam
24 Park Avenue   West Orange, NJ 07052   (973)669-8181
Fax (973)669-1687

Ganesh, Vijaya L., MD {1346275096} ObsGyn, MtFtMd(67,INDI)<NJ-UMDNJ, NJ-CLARMAAS>
+ University Physician Associates
140 Bergen Street/ACC Level C   Newark, NJ 07103
(973)972-2700   Fax (973)972-2739
+ University Hospital
150 Bergen Street   Newark, NJ 07103   (973)982-2700

Ganeshamurthy, Agrahara, MD {1508966052} IntrMd(71,INA28)
+ 13 Colasurdo Court
Edison, NJ 08820

Gang, Maureen A., MD {1912990680} EmrgMd, EmrgEMed(78,NY19)<NY-NYUTISCH>
+ University Hospital Emergency Medicine
150 Bergen Street   Newark, NJ 07103   (973)972-5128
Fax (973)972-6646

Gangat, Mariam A., MD {1396060315} PedEnd(06,GRN01)
+ RUW Pediatric Endocrinology
89 French Street/Room 1363   New Brunswick, NJ 08901
(732)235-9378   Fax (732)235-5002

Gangavalli, Ravi Venkata, MD {1104027390} Anesth(02,INA5B)<NJ-SOMERSET>
+ Anesthesia Consultnts of NJ/Nova Pain
285 Davidson Avenue/Suite 204   Somerset, NJ 08873
(732)271-1400   Fax (732)271-3543
+ RWJ University Hospital Somerset
110 Rehill Avenue/Anesth   Somerville, NJ 08876   (908)685-2200

Gangemi, Edwin Michael, MD {1962433524} PhysMd(86,MEXI)
+ Jersey Rehab, P.A.
15 Newark Avenue/Suite 1   Belleville, NJ 07109   (973)844-9220   Fax (973)844-9221
+ Jersey Rehab, P.A.
77 Newark Avenue   Belleville, NJ 07109   (973)844-9220
Fax (973)751-0498
+ Jersey Rehab, PA
409 39th Street   Union City, NJ 07109   (201)319-1539

Gangemi, Frederick D., MD {1356446108} PhysMd(80,MEX14)
+ Empire Medical Associates
5 Franklin Avenue/Suite 302   Belleville, NJ 07109
(973)751-8454   Fax (973)751-0071
fdgmdoffice@aol.com

Ganguly, Kingsuk, MD {1336584762} Anesth, PhyMSptM
+ Cooper Anesthesia Associates
One Cooper Plaza/Suite 294-B   Camden, NJ 08103
(856)342-2425   Fax (856)968-8239

Ganguly, Panchali, MD {1407805914} IntrMd(87,INA7X)
+ MedExpress Urgent Care Hamilton Square
811 Route 33   Hamilton, NJ 08619   (609)216-0927   Fax (609)587-8570
docpg19@gmail.com

Ganguly, Tarun, DO {1144259912} EmrgMd(95,NY75)
+ Browns Mills Family Practice
212 Trenton Road/Second Floor   Browns Mills, NJ 08015
(609)893-3599   Fax (609)893-8806

Ganime, Peter David, MD {1174609580} Psychy, PsyCAd, PsyFor(66,LA01)<NJ-JRSYSHMC>
+ Jersey Shore University Medical Center
1945 Route 33/Psychiatry   Neptune, NJ 07753   (732)775-5500
pdganime@aol.com

Ganitsch, Christine A., MD {1619935871} ObsGyn(79,NJ05)<NJ-MORRISTN>
+ 33 Main Street
Chatham, NJ 07928   (908)745-8110
Cganit01@gmail.com

Ganley, Theodore John, MD {1023107117} SrgOrt, SprtMd(90,PA09)<PA-CHILDHOS>
+ CHOP Specialty Care Center at Virtua
200 Bowman Drive/2 FL/Suite D-260   Voorhees, NJ 08043
(267)425-5400

Gannamani, Vedavyas, MD {1881028884}<NJ-STPETER>
+ St. Peter's University Hospital
254 Easton Avenue   New Brunswick, NJ 08901   (732)745-8600   Fax (732)745-2980

Ganne, Sudha, MD {1376747618} IntrMd(99,INA28)<NJ-MONMOUTH>
+ Monmouth Medical Center
300 Second Avenue/Suite 005   Long Branch, NJ 07740
(732)728-0628

Gannon, Michael A., MD {1225441215}(10,DMN01)
+ Martinsville Family Practice
1973 Washington Valley Road   Martinsville, NJ 08836
(732)560-9225   Fax (732)560-8095
michaelgannon@mfpnj.allscriptsdirect.net

Gannu, Rajyalakshmi M., MD {1770600769} IntrMd
+ St. Clare's Hospital-Dover
400 West Blackwell Street   Dover, NJ 07801   (973)989-3000

Ganon, Michael R., DO {1992758007} FamMed, EmrgMd(82,NY75)<NJ-NWTNMEM>
+ Premier Health Associates
89 Sparta Avenue/Suite 100   Sparta, NJ 07871   (973)729-2121   Fax (973)729-3454

Ganopolsky, Elizabeth, MD {1518181791} Anesth(78,UKR25)<NJ-STFRNMED>
+ St. Francis Medical Center
601 Hamilton Avenue/Anesthesiology   Trenton, NJ 08629
(609)599-5000

Gans, Bruce Merrill, MD {1437147816} PhysMd(73,PA01)<NJ-KSLRWEST>
+ Kessler Institute for Rehabilitation West Orange
1199 Pleasant Valley Way   West Orange, NJ 07052
(973)324-3658   Fax (973)324-3656
BGANS@Kessler-Rehab.com

Ganti, Kennedy U., MD {1235322165} FamMed, IntrMd(02,INA3D)
+ Cooper University Internal Medicine Group
651 John F. Kennedy Way   Willingboro, NJ 08046
(609)835-2838   Fax (609)589-3841

Ganti, Subrahmanyam, MD {1407920606} Pedtrc(79,INA62)<NJ-JFKMED, NJ-STPETER>
+ 906 Oak Tree Road/Suite E
South Plainfield, NJ 07080   (908)822-1181   Fax (908)822-1480
gantimd@yahoo.com

Ganti, Suryaprakash, MD {1740340355} Anesth, Pedtrc(81,INA62)<NJ-NWRKBETH>
+ New Jersey Anesthesia Associates, P.C.
252 Columbia Turnpike/PO Box 0037   Florham Park, NJ 07932   (973)660-9334   Fax (973)660-9779

Gantner, Mark, MD {1750324588} Anesth(99,NJ05)<NJ-OCEANMC>
+ Ocean Medical Center
425 Jack Martin Boulevard/Anesth   Brick, NJ 08723
(732)840-2200

Gantt, Robyn K., MD {1821009309} FamMed(94,NJ05)<NJ-UMDNJ, NJ-STMRYPAS>
+ University Family Practice Center at Vailsburg
1040-1044 South Orange Avenue   Newark, NJ 07106
(973)972-1510   Fax (973)972-1518
+ University Hospital
150 Bergen Street/Family Medicine   Newark, NJ 07103
(973)972-1510   Fax (973)972-1518

Gantz, Kenneth B., MD {1972544161} CdvDis, IntrMd(76,NY20)
+ The Heart Group, PA
161 Millburn Avenue   Millburn, NJ 07041   (973)467-4220
Fax (973)467-9889
+ The Heart Group, PA
654 Broadway   Bayonne, NJ 07002   (973)467-4220   Fax (201)243-9998

Ganzon-Zampino, Gilda E., MD {1245313527} IntrMd(89,PHIL)
+ Absecon Medical Associates LLC
408 Chris Gaupp Drive/Suite 100   Galloway, NJ 08205
(609)748-5015   Fax (609)748-0303

Gao, Hong-Guang, MD {1205982162} PthACl, PthCyt(82,CHN9D)<NJ-KENEDYHS>
+ Kennedy Health System/Cherry Hill Campus
2201 Chapel Avenue West/Pathology   Cherry Hill, NJ 08002
(856)488-6560   Fax (856)488-6848
+ University Hospital -SOM Department of Pathology
42 East Laurel Road/Suite 3700   Stratford, NJ 08084
(856)488-6560   Fax (856)566-6176

Gao, Michael Yuan, MD {1477592228} ObsGyn(00,NJ06)
+ 49 Veronica Avenue/Suite 201
Somerset, NJ 08873   (732)246-0495   Fax (732)246-0503

Gapinski, Magdalena Maria, MD {1316445778} Pedtrc
+ Jersey Shore University Medical Center
1945 Route 33   Neptune, NJ 07753   (732)775-5500

Garabedian, Hamlet Charmahali, MD {1316081623} SrgO&M(03,CA14)<NJ-RIVERVW>
+ Middletown Oral/Maxillofacial Surgery
21 New Monmouth Road   Middletown, NJ 07748
(732)671-5822

Garabedian, J. Andre, DO {1609038298} CdvDis<NJ-DEBRAHLC>
+ Deborah Heart and Lung Center
200 Trenton Road   Browns Mills, NJ 08015   (609)893-6611

Garakani Nejad, Houshang, MD {1255382966} Psychy, IntrMd(65,IRA01)
+ Vantage Health System
93 West Palisade Avenue   Englewood, NJ 07631   (201)567-0500   Fax (201)567-9335
hgarakani@hotmail.com

Garay, Kenneth F., MD {1518055730} Otlryg, SrgHdN(78,PA13)<NJ-JRSYCITY>
+ 377 Jersey Avenue/Suite 220
Jersey City, NJ 07302   (201)224-4155   Fax (201)224-4580
+ Jersey City Medical Center
355 Grand Street/Otolaryngology   Jersey City, NJ 07304
(201)915-2832

Garay, Luis Alberto, MD {1821080490} Pedtrc(74,PER01)
+ Washington Park Medical Associates
559 Broad Street   Newark, NJ 07102   (973)622-3890   Fax (973)622-6443

Garbaccio, Charles G., MD {1801857388} SrgPlstc, Surgry(68,DC02)<NJ-HACKNSK, NJ-HOLYNAME>
+ Charles G. Garbaccio MD PA
2 Dean Drive   Tenafly, NJ 07670   (201)567-1380   Fax (201)567-9106

Garbarini Carty, Elyse, MD {1992703177} FamMed(82,NY09)<NJ-RWJUHAM>
+ Capital Health Primary Care-Bordentown
1 Third Street   Bordentown, NJ 08505   (609)298-2005
Fax (609)324-8267

Garbarino, Charles L., MD {1952326522} Pedtrc(78,NY09)<NJ-MTNSIDE>
+ Deborah A Coy, MD, LLC
405 Northfield Avenue/Suite LL2   West Orange, NJ 07052
(973)736-4442   Fax (973)736-8717

Garber, Brett A., DO {1477594117} GenPrc, SrgRec(92,IA75)
+ Prestige Institute for Plastic Surgery
1605 East Evesham Road/Suite 201   Voorhees, NJ 08043
(856)304-1114   Fax (267)454-7196

Garber, Todd Ryan, MD {1558467357} Nrolgy, ClNrPh(99,VA01)<NJ-WARREN>
+ Riverfront Neurology
755 Memorial Parkway   Phillipsburg, NJ 08865   (908)387-8811   Fax (908)387-6772

Garberina, Matthew J., MD {1659367100} SrgOrt, SrgOARec(97,PA13)<NJ-OVERLOOK, NJ-MORRISTN>
+ Summit Medical Group-Berkeley Heights Campus
1 Diamond Hill Road   Berkeley Heights, NJ 07922
(908)273-4300   Fax (908)790-6576

Garberman, Scott F., MD {1871564880} SrgHnd, Surgry(86,PA09)<NJ-VIRTMHBC>
+ Burlington County Hand Surgical Associates, PA
1338 Route 38   Hainesport, NJ 08036   (609)261-2662
Fax (609)261-6980

Garbowit, David L., MD {1548525578} EnDbMt, IntrMd(83,NY01)
+ The Joslin Center for Diabetes
200 South Orange Avenue/2nd Floor   Livingston, NJ 07039
(973)322-7200   Fax (973)322-7250

Garcia, Calixto G., DO {1154313724} IntrMd, EmrgMd(91,IA75)<NJ-STMICHL>
+ 22 Langon Hollow Road
Bridgewater, NJ 08807

Physicians by Name and Address

Garcia, Carmen Josefina, MD {1639105331} Dermat(77,NY01)
+ Center for Dermatology & Skin Surgery, LLC
1 West Ridgewood Avenue/Suite 103   Paramus, NJ 07652   (201)857-4200   Fax (201)857-4199

Garcia, Christopher M., MD {1619103306} Radiol(09,NJ05)
+ Hoboken University Medical Center
308 Willow Avenue   Hoboken, NJ 07030   (201)418-1000
+ Carepoint Health Bayonne Med Center
29 East 29th Street   Bayonne, NJ 07002   (201)858-5000

Garcia, Dianelys, MD {1407103500} PsyCAd<NJ-STJOSHOS>
+ St. Joseph Medical Center Mental Health Clinic
56 Hamilton Street   Paterson, NJ 07505   (973)754-4771

Garcia, Gerald Matthew, MD {1902177819} Anesth
+ St. Joseph's Regional Medical Center Anesthesia
703 Main Street   Paterson, NJ 07503   (973)754-2323   Fax (973)754-3131

Garcia, Guillermo A., MD {1629024526} EmrgMd(69,COLO)<NJ-RWJUBRUN>
+ RWJ University Hospital New Brunswick
One Robert Wood Johnson Place   New Brunswick, NJ 08901   (732)937-8550

Garcia, Jason P., MD {1114989829} SrgOrt(01,NJ05)
+ 741 Northfield Avenue/Suite 200
West Orange, NJ 07052   (973)736-9980   Fax (973)736-9981

Garcia, Joaquin B., MD {1669436861} FamMed(89,NJ06)
+ Whippany Family Practice
53 Whippany Road   Whippany, NJ 07981   (973)887-7776   Fax (973)884-1727

Garcia, Joseph, MD {1053306357} Surgry(77,NY09)<NJ-CHILTON>
+ 502 Hamburg Turnpike/Suite 105
Wayne, NJ 07470   (973)790-7655   Fax (973)942-8818
+ Wayne Surgical Center, LLC.
1176 Hamburg Pike   Wayne, NJ 07470   (973)790-7655   Fax (973)709-1901

Garcia, Julia Griggs, MD {1164402889} OccpMd
+ University Hospital-School of Public Health
170 Frelinghuysen Road   Piscataway, NJ 08854   (732)445-0123   Fax (732)445-3644

Garcia, Maria E., MD {1336536697} Psychy(90,CUB08)
+ University Behavioral Health Care
303 George Street/Suite 200   New Brunswick, NJ 08901   (732)235-6800   Fax (732)235-6187

Garcia, Maria Teresa, MD {1629070354} FamMed(95,NJ05)
+ PrimeCare Medical Group
561 Middlesex Avenue   Metuchen, NJ 08840   (732)549-9363   Fax (732)603-0397
+ Family Connections Inc
395 South Center Street   Orange, NJ 07050   (732)549-9363   Fax (973)673-5782

Garcia, Michael J., DO {1326353913} EmrgMd(10,NJ75)
+ 344 South Jackson Street
Woodbury, NJ 08096   (856)491-5066

Garcia, Nicole DeVincenzo, MD {1124293865} Pedtrc
+ Summit Medical Group
560 Springfield Avenue   Westfield, NJ 07090   (908)228-3620
+ Summit Medical Group-Berkeley Heights Campus
1 Diamond Hill Road   Berkeley Heights, NJ 07922   (908)228-3620   Fax (908)790-6576

Garcia, Raudel, MD {1629362520} FamMed(94,CUB06)
+ Center for Family Health
122 Clinton Street   Hoboken, NJ 07030   (201)418-3100

Garcia, Raul Angel, DO {1083100895} IntrMd<NJ-TRININPC>
+ Trinitas Regional Medical Center-New Point Campus
655 East Jersey Street   Elizabeth, NJ 07206   (908)994-5030

Garcia, Steven Jesus, MD {1073668679} FamMed(89,DOMI)<NJ-HOBUNIMC>
+ Center for Family Health
122-132 Clinton Street   Hoboken, NJ 07030   (201)418-3100   Fax (201)418-3148

Garcia Marotta, Ylonka, MD {1215190178} FamMed(03,BLZ02)
+ ImmediCenter/Bloomfield
557 Broad Street   Bloomfield, NJ 07003   (973)680-8300   Fax (973)743-5601
+ Mountainside Medical Group
1129 Bloomfield Avenue/Suite 220   West Caldwell, NJ 07006   (973)680-8300   Fax (973)244-9062

Garcia Rodriguez, Magdelyn, MD {1720322274} Pedtrc
+ St. Joseph's Children's Hospital
703 Main Street   Paterson, NJ 07503   (973)754-2575   Fax (973)754-2546

Garcia-Lat, Zenda, MD {1629311857} PthAcl(72,PHI02)
+ Paramus Plastic Surgery, Skin Care & Laser Center
17 Arcadian Avenue/Suite 103   Paramus, NJ 07652   (201)843-0700

Garcia-Perez, Felix A., MD {1841266145} SrgCrC, Surgry, SrgTrm(82,DOMI)<NJ-JRSYSHMC>
+ Meridian Trauma Associates
530 Prospect Avenue/Suite 2-A   Little Silver, NJ 07739   (201)240-6853   Fax (201)530-5516

Gardella, Dean, MD {1174667034} RadDia
+ Hackensack Radiology Group, P.A.
30 Prospect Avenue   Hackensack, NJ 07601   (551)996-2200   Fax (201)336-8451

Garden, Marc David, MD {1447252333} Ophthl(80,PA12)
+ Philadelphia Eye Associates
1113 Hospital Drive/Suite 302   Willingboro, NJ 08046   (609)871-1112

Garden, Richard J., MD {1689642985} Urolgy(87,NY47)<NJ-HACKNSK>
+ 555 Kinderkamack Road/Suite 2
Oradell, NJ 07649   (201)834-1890   Fax (201)834-1898
+ Northern Valley ENT
354 Old Hook Road/Suite 204   Westwood, NJ 07675   (201)834-1890   Fax (201)358-6686

Gardilla, Kalyani Ila, MD {1831196278} IntrMd(95,INA38)<NJ-RIVERVW>
+ Riverview Medical Associates, PA
4 Hartford Drive/Suite 1   Tinton Falls, NJ 07701   (732)741-3600   Fax (732)741-3603

Gardin, Julius Markus, MD {1245226794} IntrMd, CdvDis(72,MI01)<NJ-HACKNSK>
+ Hackensack University Medical Center
30 Prospect Avenue/IntMed   Hackensack, NJ 07601   (201)996-3500   Fax (201)996-3298
JGardin@humed.com

Gardine, Robert L., MD {1659372167} SrgC&R, Surgry(80,NY01)<NJ-VIRTVOOR>
+ Colon & Rectal Surgical Associates of South Jersey
502 Centennial Boulevard/Suite 5   Voorhees, NJ 08043   (856)429-8030   Fax (856)428-2718

Gardner, Allan Lee, MD {1144272667} SrgNro(65,VT02)<NJ-STCLRDEN, NJ-MORRISTN>
+ PO Box 1253
Morristown, NJ 07962   (973)267-4355   Fax (973)538-1042

Gardner, Beth C., MD {1457334369} Gastrn, IntrMd(83,PA09)
+ Philadelphia Gastroenterology Group, P.C.
570 Egg Harbor Road/Suite A-2   Sewell, NJ 08080   (856)218-1410   Fax (856)218-0193

Gardner, James Nicholas, MD {1386676088} SrgHnd, SrgPlstc, IntrMd(87,NJ06)<NJ-UMDNJ, NY-STBARNAB>
+ Summit Plastic Surgery, P.C.
33 Overlook Road/Suite 310   Summit, NJ 07901   (908)918-1969   Fax (908)918-1995
info@JamesGardnerMD.com

Gardner, Kimberly Ruth, MD {1023247061}<NJ-MORRISTN>
+ Morristown Medical Center
100 Madison Avenue   Morristown, NJ 07962   (973)971-5684

Gardy, Mark Alan, MD   EmrgMd(93,IL42)<NJ-HACKNSK>
+ 518 Dorchester Drive
River Vale, NJ 07675
+ Emergency Medical Associates of NJ, P.A.
3 Century Drive   Parsippany, NJ 07054   Fax (973)740-9895

Garfinkel, David A., MD {1760476899} ObsGyn(88,NY47)<NJ-MORRISTN>
+ One to One Female Care, P.A.
111 Madison Avenue/Suite 305   Morristown, NJ 07960   (973)683-1400   Fax (973)683-0700
DGarfinkel@1to1femalecare.com
+ One to One Female Care, PA
2345 Lamington Road   Bedminster, NJ 07921   (973)683-1400   Fax (908)719-2004

Garfinkel, Matthew J., MD {1497802649} SrgOrt(86,NY20)<NJ-JFKMED>
+ Edison-Metuchen Orthopedic Group
10 Parsonage Road/5th Floor/Suite 500   Edison, NJ 08837   (732)494-6226   Fax (908)494-8762

Garg, Anil, MD {1912922956} IntrMd, IntMAdMd(75,INDI)<NJ-HCKTSTWN, NJ-WARREN>
+ 173 East Washington Avenue/Box 338
Washington, NJ 07882   (908)689-0547   Fax (908)689-0649

Garg, Anju, MD   IntrMd(95,PA07)
+ 53 Crestmont Road
Bedminster, NJ 07921

Garg, Deepika, MD {1679879373} IntrMd, IntHos(06,INA92)
+ IPC The Hospitalist Company
55 Madison Avenue/Suite 310   Morristown, NJ 07960   (973)993-9536   Fax (973)998-4237

Garg, Delyse, MD {1811340813} IntrMd<NJ-TRINIWSC>
+ Trinitas Regional Medical Center-Williamson Street
225 Williamson Street   Elizabeth, NJ 07207   (908)994-5000

Garg, Geetanjali Davuluri, MD {1477574531} Ophthl(99,NY45)
+ Advanced Eye Care Center PA
220 Hamburg Turnpike/Suite 7   Wayne, NJ 07470   (973)790-1300   Fax (973)790-5310

Garg, Lorraine Freed, MD {1568669497} AdolMd, Pedtrc(93,CA02)
+ New Jersey Department of Health and Senior Services
50 East State/PO Box 360   Trenton, NJ 08625   (609)777-0686   Fax (609)292-6523

Garg, Neha, MD {1134360902} Nephro
+ 24 Beacon Way/Unit 803
Jersey City, NJ 07304

Garg, Rakesh K., MD {1841270741} CritCr, IntrMd, PulDis(73,INA1F)<NJ-NWTNMEM, NJ-HCKTSTWN>
+ Pulmonary Medical Associates, L.L.P
222 High Street/Suite 102   Newton, NJ 07860   (973)579-5090   Fax (973)579-2994

Garg, Sangeeta, MD {1801874284} CdvDis, IntCrd, IntrMd(93,INA92)<NJ-RWJUHAM, NJ-STFRNMED>
+ 555 Iron Bridge Road/Suite 15
Freehold, NJ 07728   (732)294-9373   Fax (732)333-1366

Garg, Shyamala, MD {1780834101} IntrMd(96)
+ 115 Emily Place
Parsippany, NJ 07054

Garg, Siddharth Rajesh, MD {1972997229} IntrMd
+ Jersey Shore University Medical Center
1945 Route 33   Neptune, NJ 07753   (732)775-5500

Garg, Sunir Jain, MD {1427056134} Ophthl(98,MI01)
+ Mid Atlantic Retina - Wills Eye Retina Surgeons
501 Cooper Landing Road   Cherry Hill, NJ 08002   (856)667-2246   Fax (856)667-2238

Garg, Vipin, MD {1881662062} PulDis, SlpDis, CritCr(94,INA92)<NJ-TRINIWSC>
+ 240 Williamson Street/Suite 300
Elizabeth, NJ 07202   (908)994-8880   Fax (908)994-8882
Vipin.Garg@comcast.net

Gargani, Stephanie, MD {1386812188} Anesth
+ St. Joseph's Regional Medical Center Anesthesia
703 Main Street   Paterson, NJ 07503   (973)754-2323   Fax (973)977-9455

Gargano, Francesco, MD {1831359421} SrgPlstc(97,ITA17)
+ St Joseph's Medical Center Plastic Surgery
703 Main Street   Paterson, NJ 07503   (973)754-2413

Gargano, Joseph A., DO {1518054899} FamMed(84,IA75)
+ Montville Primary Care Physicians
137 Main Road   Montville, NJ 07045   (973)402-0025   Fax (973)402-0508

Garger, Alexander, MD {1376730325} RadNro
+ 115 River Road
Edgewater, NJ 07020   (201)840-1980

Garger, Yana Basis, MD {1366604704} EnDbMt, IntrMd(07,NY09)
+ Drs. Anchipolovsky and Garger
77 Prospect Avenue/Suite 1 K   Hackensack, NJ 07601   (201)820-3596   Fax (201)322-2170

Gargiulo, Andrew Michael, MD {1699805705} RadDia, IntrMd(06,PA14)
+ Larchmont Medical Imaging
204-210 Ark Road/LMC 1-2   Mount Laurel, NJ 08054   (609)914-7017   Fax (856)866-8102

Gargiulo, Katherine Anne, MD {1700044047} Pedtrc
+ Advocare Kressville Pediatrics Cherry Hill
710 Kresson Road   Cherry Hill, NJ 08003   (856)795-3320   Fax (856)795-1213

Gargiulo, Richard F., MD {1780628750} Anesth(83,NJ06)
+ Burlington Anesthesia Associates
120 Madison Ave/Suite E/PO Box 174   Mount Holly, NJ 08060   (609)261-1660   Fax (609)261-1779

Garibaldi, Pia M., MD {1538214028} EmrgMd, IntrMd(85,OH40)<NJ-UNVMCPRN>
+ University Medical Center of Princeton at Plainsboro
One Plainsboro Road/EmergMed   Plainsboro, NJ 08536   (609)497-4000

Garibaldi, Thomas A., MD {1629071279} Anesth(83,MEX14)<NJ-STCLRDEN>
+ Morris Anesthesia Group, PA
3799 Route 46/Suite 211   Parsippany, NJ 07054   (973)335-1122   Fax (973)335-1448

Garipalli, Lakshmi, MD {1184736696} Anesth(74,INA39)
+ 1201 Morris Avenue
Union, NJ 07083   (908)688-3727   Fax (908)688-3036

Garla, Sudha, MD {1659330629} IntrMd(90,NJ06)<NJ-RWJUBRUN, NJ-JRSYSHMC>
+ Atlantic Medical Associates
1200 Eagle Avenue/Suite 101   Ocean, NJ 07712   (732)660-6200   Fax (732)660-6201
+ Atlantic Medical Associates
1640 Route 88 West   Brick, NJ 08724   (732)660-6200   Fax (732)458-2743

Garmkhorani, Abolghassem, MD {1851332704} IntrMd(80,IRAN)<NJ-MONMOUTH>
+ Walk-in Center of Freehold
3333 Route 9 North/Chadwick Square   Freehold, NJ 07728   (732)683-1975   Fax (732)683-1978

Garner, Eve Marybeth, MD {1750511796} RadDia, IntrMd(07,NY08)
+ University Radiology Group, P.C.
483 Cranbury Road   East Brunswick, NJ 08816   (732)390-0030   Fax (732)390-5383

Physicians by Name and Address

Garnet, Daniel, MD {1538428453} RadDia
+ Princeton Radiology Associates, P.A.
3674 Route 27/B   Kendall Park, NJ 08824   (732)821-5563
Fax (732)821-6675

Garnier, Katharine M., MD {1114934932} FamMed(88,NJ06)<NJ-VIRTBERL, NJ-VIRTMARL>
+ University Hospital-University Family Medicine
42 East Laurel Road/Suite 2100   Stratford, NJ 08084
(856)566-7020   Fax (856)566-6188

Garrett, Kenneth M., MD {1467491944} ObsGyn(75,NY19)<NJ-CHILTON>
+ Physicians for Women
330 Ratzer Road/Suite 7   Wayne, NJ 07470   (973)694-2222
Fax (973)694-7664
+ Wayne Surgical Center, LLC.
1176 Hamburg Pike   Wayne, NJ 07470   (973)694-2222
Fax (973)709-1901

Garrett, Parisa Mousavi, MD {1891850756} Pedtrc(02,PA02)<NJ-VIRTUAHS, NJ-COOPRUMC>
+ AtlantiCare/Dupont Children's Health Program
2500 English Creek Avenue   Egg Harbor Township, NJ 08234
(609)641-3700   Fax (609)641-3652
+ Advocare Haddon Pediatric Group
119 White Horse Pike   Haddon Heights, NJ 08035
(609)641-3700   Fax (856)547-4573

Garrett, Paul R., MD {1164523312} RadDia, Radiol(81,PA02)<NJ-BURDTMLN>
+ Cape Regional Medical Center
2 Stone Harbor Boulevard/Radiology   Cape May Court House, NJ 08210   (609)463-2000
pgarrett@caperegional.com

Garrett, Rebecca Ann, MD {1790756922} PhysMd, PainMd(73,CA14)<NJ-OVERLOOK>
+ Overlook Medical Center
99 Beauvoir Avenue/PO Box 210   Summit, NJ 07902
(908)522-5338   Fax (908)522-2734

Garrido, Eddy O., MD {1194712430} SrgNro(PA02<NJ-KENEDYHS>
+ 445 Hurffville Crosskeys Road
Sewell, NJ 08080   (856)256-7591   Fax (856)256-7585

Garrisi, Margaret Graf, MD {1780702761} ObsGyn, RprEnd(79,NY06)<NJ-STBARNMC>
+ Inst of Repro Med and Science
609 Washington Street/2nd Floor   Hoboken, NJ 07030   Fax (201)204-9319
+ The Institute for Reproductive Medicine and Science
94 Old Short Hills Road/Suite 403E   Livingston, NJ 07039
Fax (973)322-8890

Garrison, Jordan Milton, MD {1780756999} Surgry, IntrMd(82,NJ05)<NJ-STCLRDOV>
+ St. Clare's Hospital-Dover
400 West Blackwell Street/Surgery   Dover, NJ 07801
(973)437-8021

Garstang, Susan Veronica, MD {1235119686} PhysMd(94,MO02)<NJ-VAEASTOR, NJ-UMDNJ>
+ VA New Jersey Health Care System-East Orange Campus
385 Tremont Avenue   East Orange, NJ 07018   (973)676-1000

Garten, Alan J., MD {1932137569} RadDia, RadV&I(86,MA07)<NJ-STBARNMC>
+ St. Barnabas Medical Center
94 Old Short Hills Road   Livingston, NJ 07039   (973)322-5800

Gartland, John, Jr., MD {1417045030} FamMed(87,MEXI)<NJ-UNDRWD>
+ 636 Kings Highway/Suite B
Woodbury, NJ 08096   (856)845-3443   Fax (856)845-4544

Gartner, Joseph J., MD {1861455644} ObsGyn, Gynecol(71,NY47)<NJ-VALLEY>
+ Bergen-Passaic Women's Health
258 Godwin Avenue   Wyckoff, NJ 07481   (201)891-3336
Fax (201)891-5535

Gartner, Michael C., DO {1780619171} SrgPlstc(93,NJ75)<NJ-VALLEY, NJ-MONMOUTH>
+ 3 Winslow Place
Paramus, NJ 07652   (201)546-1890   Fax (201)546-1893
+ TriState Surgery Center
3 Winslow Place   Paramus, NJ 07652   (201)546-1890

Garuba, Mariam I., MD {1275748261}
+ 300 Grand Street/Apt 204
Hoboken, NJ 07030   (973)738-2272
mischni33@gmail.com

Garvey, Karen Marie, MD {1932300399} OccpMd, GPrvMd(88,DC03)
+ Novartis Pharmaceuticals Corporation
One Health Plaza   East Hanover, NJ 07936   (862)778-8081
Fax (973)781-6504
Karen.Garvey@Novartis.com
+ Cornerstone Medical and Wellness LLC
235 Millburn Avenue/Suite 101   Millburn, NJ 07041
(862)778-8081   Fax (973)467-3102

Gasalberti, Richard Anthony, MD {1043324759} PhysMd, PhyM-Pain(84,DMN01)<NY-METHODST>
+ Bloomfield Rehabilitation Group
50 Park Place/Lobby Level   Newark, NJ 07102   (973)642-2277

Gasalberti, Robert P., MD {1346247780} Anesth, IntrMd(86,MEXI)<NY-STATNRTH>
+ Wound Healing & Hyperbaric Medicine
240 Williamson Street/Suite 104   Elizabeth, NJ 07202
(908)994-5480   Fax (908)994-8802

Gashi, Sheremet, MD {1114093564} IntrMd(86)<NJ-CLARMAAS, NJ-MTNSIDE>
+ 11 Ridge Road
North Arlington, NJ 07031   (201)998-1800   Fax (201)998-1891

Gaskel, Virginia M., DO {1295833825} FamMed(92,NJ75)<NJ-CHSMRCER>
+ Corporate Health Center
832 Brunswick Avenue   Trenton, NJ 08638   (609)695-7471
Fax (609)815-7814

Gaspard, Henry Claude, MD {1881646172} Surgry, IntrMd(77,HAIT)>
+ 17 Dahlia Road
Somerset, NJ 08873   (732)937-8374
+ American Physician Services/Hudson HealthCare
679 Montgomery Street   Jersey City, NJ 07306   (732)937-8374   Fax (201)433-8010

Gastell, Gilberto F., MD {1942200472} IntrMd(81,DOM02)<NJ-PALISADE, NJ-MEADWLND>
+ Excelcare Medical Associates
408 37th Street   Union City, NJ 07087   (201)864-4477
Fax (201)864-9727
Gastellmd@aol.com

Gatchalian, Luningning C., MD {1801863675} FamMed(85,PHI32)<NJ-HACKNSK>
+ Center for Occupational Medicine
360 Essex Street/Suite 203   Hackensack, NJ 07601
(201)336-8686   Fax (201)342-3546
+ Montville Primary Care Physicians
137 Main Road   Montville, NJ 07045   (201)336-8686   Fax (973)402-0508

Gatla, Nandita, MD {1306166632} Rheuma
+ Riverside Pediatrics
714 Tenth Street   Secaucus, NJ 07094   (551)257-7038
Fax (201)552-2358

Gatoulis, Maria K., MD {1215239124} Pedtrc(DC01
+ Summit Medical Group
1 Diamond Hill Road/Bensley Pav/2 FL   Berkeley, NJ 07922
(908)277-8700   Fax (908)288-7993
+ Summit Medical Group
890 New Mountain Avenue   New Providence, NJ 07974
(908)277-8601
+ Wellness Center Pediatrics LLC
21 Lafayette Road/Suite F   Sparta, NJ 07922   (973)726-4455   Fax (973)726-8445

Gatt, Charles J., Jr., MD {1861497257} SprtMd, SrgOrt(89,NJ06)<NJ-RWJUBRUN, NJ-STPETER>
+ University Orthopaedic Associates, LLC.
Two Worlds Fair Drive   Somerset, NJ 08873   (732)979-2115
Fax (732)564-9032
+ University Orthopaedic Group
215 Easton Avenue   New Brunswick, NJ 08901   (732)979-2115   Fax (732)545-4011
+ University Orthopaedic Associates, LLC.
211 North Harrison Street   Princeton, NJ 08873   (609)683-7800   Fax (609)683-7875

Gatti, Eugene A., MD {1144200601} Allrgy, Pedtrc(82,DC02)<NJ-VIRTUAHS, NJ-OURLADY>
+ Advocare Allergy & Asthma
54 East Main Street   Marlton, NJ 08053   (856)988-0570
Fax (856)988-0303
+ Advocare Allergy & Asthma
239 Hurffville Crosskeys Road   Sewell, NJ 08080   (856)988-0570   Fax (856)988-0303
+ Advocare Allergy & Asthma
409 Kings Highway South   Cherry Hill, NJ 08053   (856)988-0570   Fax (856)988-0303

Gatti, John E., MD {1942336060} SrgPlstc, Surgry(78,DC02)<NJ-VIRTMARL, NJ-OURLADY>
+ 409 Kings Highway South
Cherry Hill, NJ 08034   (856)354-6100   Fax (856)354-3288
Jgattimd@aol.com

Gatto, Charles Anthony, MD {1619068616} SrgOrt(92,NY03)<NJ-MORRISTN>
+ Tri-County Orthopedics
160 East Hanover Avenue   Morristown, NJ 07962
(973)538-2334   Fax (973)829-9174
+ Tri-County Orthopedics
197 Ridgedale Street/Suite 300   Cedar Knolls, NJ 07927
(973)538-2334   Fax (973)829-9174

Gauchan, Dron, MD {1487805784}
+ 18 Washington Drive/Apt H
Little Falls, NJ 07424

Gaudino, Silvana, MD {1467520239} ObsGyn, IntrMd(83,NY15)
+ 127 Pine Street/Suite 10 & 11
Montclair, NJ 07042   (973)707-2122   Fax (973)655-9559

Gaukler, Carolyn J., MD {1194715516} IntrMd(84,PA13)<NJ-CHSMRCER, NJ-RWJUHAM>
+ 1230 Parkway Avenue/Suite 203
Trenton, NJ 08628   (609)844-0084   Fax (609)844-0085
CGauklerMD@aol.com
+ Capital Health Primary Care
1230 Parkway Avenue/Suite 203   Ewing, NJ 08628
(609)844-0084   Fax (609)883-2564

Gault, Janice Ann, MD {1780673137} Ophthl(91,NC07)<PA-WILLSEYE>
+ Eye Physicians PC
1140 White Horse Road/Suite 1   Voorhees, NJ 08043
(856)784-3366   Fax (856)784-4388
+ Eye Physicians of Southern New Jersey
401 South Kings Highway   Cherry Hill, NJ 08034   (856)795-4040

Gaur, Sunanda, MD {1467511311} PedInf, Pedtrc(77,INDI)<NJ-RWJUBRUN, NJ-JRSYSHMC>
+ RWJ University Pediatric Infectious Disease
125 Paterson Street/MEB 322   New Brunswick, NJ 08901
(732)235-7894   Fax (732)235-7419

Gavai, Medha A., MD {1104849181} Pedtrc, AdolMd(87,INA00)<NJ-RWJUBRUN>
+ University Pediatric Associates PA
317 Cleveland Avenue   Highland Park, NJ 08904   (732)249-8999   Fax (732)249-7827

Gavi, Shai, DO {1396761292} IntrMd, IntHos(98,FL75)<NJ-MORRISTN>
+ Morristown Medical Center
100 Madison Avenue/Internal Med   Morristown, NJ 07962
(973)971-7135   Fax (973)290-8349

Gavini, Jaya L., MD {1871687392} PsyCAd(78,INA11)<NJ-TRININPC>
+ Trinitas Regional Medical Center-New Point Campus
655 East Jersey Street/Chld&AdolPsy   Elizabeth, NJ 07206
(908)994-5000

Gaviola, Durga C., MD {1750341491} Pedtrc(78,PHI08)<NJ-JFKMED, NJ-STPETER>
+ 1550 Park Avenue
South Plainfield, NJ 07080   (908)757-4222   Fax (908)757-1538

Gaviola, Gerry F., MD {1881761054} Psychy(83,PHI08)<NJ-GRYSTPSY>
+ Greystone Park Psychiatric Hospital
59 Koch Avenue/ClinicalPsych   Morris Plains, NJ 07950
(973)538-1800

Gavrilovic, Igor T., MD {1518938554} Nrolgy(99,DMN01)<NY-SLOANKET>
+ Memorial Sloan-Kettering Cancer Center Basking Ridge
136 Mountain View Boulevard   Basking Ridge, NJ 07920
(908)542-3000   Fax (908)542-3220

Gayam, Vani, MD {1366442659} Pedtrc(95,INA5B)<NJ-JFKMED>
+ JFK Medical Center
65 James Street   Edison, NJ 08820   (732)321-7000   Fax (732)744-5873

Gayed, Noha, MD {1386148989} IntrMd<NJ-HACKNSK>
+ Hackensack University Medical Center
30 Prospect Avenue   Hackensack, NJ 07601   (551)996-2000

Gayeski, David R., MD {1053516005} Anesth
+ AtlantiCare Anesthesiology
65 West Jimmie Leeds Road   Pomona, NJ 08240   (609)748-7597

Gayle, Catherine, MD {1528039146} GenPrc, OthrSp, Psychy(80,PA01)
+ Rowan Medical Department of Psychiatry
42 Laurel Road East/Suite 3610   Stratford, NJ 08084
(856)482-9000   Fax (856)482-1159

Gayle-Barton, Delores C., MD {1508886664} IntrMd(76,NJ05)<NJ-NWRKBETH, NJ-EASTORNG>
+ Gayle, Delores C.
742 Clinton Avenue   Newark, NJ 07108   (973)374-2550
Fax (973)374-2081

Gayner, Robert S., MD Nephro(86,NY47)<NJ-WARREN>
+ Warren Hospital
185 Roseberry Street/Nephrology   Phillipsburg, NJ 08865
(908)859-6700

Gaynor, James William, MD {1346338746} SrgThr, Surgry(82,SC01)<PA-CHOPHIL, PA-CHILDHOS>
+ CHOP Pediatric & Adolescent Specialty Care Center
1012 Laurel Oak Road   Voorhees, NJ 08043   (856)435-1300
Fax (856)435-0091

Gazi, Mukaram A., MD {1679527188} Urolgy, SrgLap, OthrSp(95,FL02)<NJ-STBARNMC, NJ-RWJUHAM>
+ University Urology Associates of New Jersey
1374 Whitehorse Hamilton Sq/Suite 101 Hamilton, NJ 08690 (609)581-5900 Fax (609)581-5901
+ 2364 Route 9 South/Unit B-2
Howell, NJ 07731 (732)928-5300

Gazurian, Raina, MD {1619135530} FamMed(PA09
+ Cornerstone Family Practice
9100 Wescott Drive/Suite 103 Flemington, NJ 08822 (908)237-6910 Fax (908)237-6919
+ AtlantiCare Physician Group
712 East Bay Avenue/Suite 19 Manahawkin, NJ 08050 (908)237-6910 Fax (609)597-0746

Gazzillo, Frank L., MD {1376643973} Nrolgy(72,NJ05)<NJ-WAYNE-GEN, NJ-CHILTON>
+ Neurologic Associates
220 Hamburg Turnpike/Suite 16 Wayne, NJ 07470 (973)942-4778 Fax (973)942-7020

Gbadamosi, Sikiru Aderoju, MD {1326074618} IntrMd, EmrgMd(82,NIG01)
+ 2177 Oak Tree Road/Suite 206
Edison, NJ 08820 (732)755-4000 Fax (732)755-4006

Gbeve-Hill, Dorcas, MD {1609331735} PsyNro
+ 43 Rockingham Way
Manchester, NJ 08759 (848)221-9295

Ge, Shuping, MD {1811077167} Pedtrc, PedCrd(86,CHN1J)<PA-STCHRIS>
+ St. Christopher Care at Washington Township
405 Hurffville-Cross Keys Road Sewell, NJ 08080 (856)582-0644 Fax (856)582-0622

Gealt, David Benjamin, DO {1386733673} FamMed, SprtMd, FamMSptM(01,NJ75)
+ Cooper Bone and Joint Institute
900 Centennial Boulevard Voorhees, NJ 08043 (856)673-4914 Fax (856)325-6678
+ Cooper Bone and Joint Institute
401 South Kings Highway/Suite 3-A Cherry Hill, NJ 08003 (856)673-4914 Fax (856)547-0316

Gebre Medhin, Hanna, MD {1598944415} AdolMd, Pedtrc(99,DMN01)
+ Pediatrician in Jamesburg
10A West Railroad Avenue Jamesburg, NJ 08831 (732)561-7810 Fax (732)631-0742
Hannage@verizon.net

Gecha, Steven R., MD {1710906698} SrgOrt, SprtMd(80,NJ06)<NJ-UNVMCPRN, NJ-VANJHCS>
+ Princeton Orthopaedic Associates, P.A.
325 Princeton Avenue Princeton, NJ 08540 (609)924-8131 Fax (609)924-8532
+ Princeton Orthopaedic Associates, P.A.
11 Centre Drive Jamesburg, NJ 08831 (609)655-4848
+ Princeton Orthopaedic Associates, P.A.
340 Scotch Road Ewing, NJ 08540 (609)924-8131 Fax (609)924-8532

Geck, Wilma Santiago, MD {1124010798} EmrgMd(91,PHI09)<NJ-MTNSIDE, NJ-RBAYPERT>
+ Hackensack UMC Mountainside
1 Bay Avenue/EmrgMed Montclair, NJ 07042 (973)429-6000
+ Raritan Bay Medical Center/Perth Amboy Division
530 New Brunswick Avenue/EmrgMed Perth Amboy, NJ 08861 (732)442-3700

Gecys, Gintare T., DO {1982684056} FamMed(86,PA77)
+ South Jersey Medical Associates, PA
1504 Blackwood Clementon Road Blackwood, NJ 08012 (856)228-0144 Fax (856)232-0320

Gedroic, Kristine Lynn, MD {1760699474} FamMed
+ 465 South Street/Suite 101
Morristown, NJ 07960 (973)993-4445 Fax (973)993-4942

Geelan, Caroline C., DO {1184873523} PsyCAd, Psychy(06,NJ75)
+ 89 East Clinton Avenue
Tenafly, NJ 07670

Gefen, Ron, MD {1427282524} RadDia, Radiol, IntrMd(04,PA02)<NJ-COOPRUMC>
+ Cooper University Hospital
One Cooper Plaza/Radiology Camden, NJ 08103 (856)342-2380 Fax (856)365-0472

Geffner, Michael Howard, MD {1619199551} PedNrD, Pedtrc(94,NY03)
+ Merck and Company Incorporated
1 Merck Drive/PO Box 100/WS3D-90 Whitehouse Station, NJ 08889 (908)423-3426 Fax (908)259-2535

Geffner, Rami E., MD {1366491110} Dermat, PthDrm(79,NJ05)<NJ-COMMED, NJ-KIMBALL>
+ Schweiger Dermatology
712 East Bay Avenue/Suite 19 Manahawkin, NJ 08050 (609)597-5850 Fax (609)597-9667
+ Accredited Dermatology
525 Route 70 West/Suite A1 Lakewood, NJ 08701 (609)597-5850 Fax (732)370-1526
+ Schweiger Dermatology

67 Lacey Road Whiting, NJ 08050 (732)849-4410 Fax (732)849-4421

Geffner, Stuart R., MD {1649213422} Surgry(88,NJ05)
+ 94 Old Short Hills Road/Suite 1
Livingston, NJ 07039 (973)597-9005 Fax (973)322-9807

Gefter, Igor, MD {1528013547} Psychy(83,RUS59)<NJ-WAYNE-GEN>
+ Ramapo Ridge Psychiatric Hospital
301 Sicomac Avenue Wyckoff, NJ 07481 (201)848-5500

Gehring, David J., MD {1740288091} IntrMd, FamMed(85,GRN01)<NJ-UNDRWD>
+ 223 South Evergreen Avenue
Woodbury, NJ 08096 (856)384-0400 Fax (856)453-8495

Gehringer, Travis James, MD {1982973046} RadDia
+ Larchmont Medical Imaging
204-210 Ark Road/LMC 1-2 Mount Laurel, NJ 08054 (609)914-7017 Fax (856)866-8102

Gehrmann, Robin Michael, MD {1871675512} SrgOrt(95,PA09)<NJ-UMDNJ>
+ North Jersey Orthopaedic Group
799 Bloomfield Avenue/Suite 111 Verona, NJ 07044 (973)689-6266 Fax (973)689-6264
+ North Jersey Orthopaedic Group
33 Bleeker Street Millburn, NJ 07041 (973)689-6266 Fax (973)564-8928
+ North Jersey Orthopaedic Group
246 Hamburg Turnpike/Suite 302 Wayne, NJ 07044 (973)689-6266 Fax (973)689-6264

Geisen, Amy Grace, MD {1538101282} IntrMd(02,DMN01)<NJ-ATLANTHS, NJ-NWTNMEM>
+ Drs. Fielding and Geisen
17 Route 23 North Hamburg, NJ 07419 (973)827-7800 Fax (973)209-7855
+ Internal Medicine of Vernon
212 State Route 94/Suite 1-C Vernon, NJ 07462 (973)827-7800 Fax (973)823-8811

Geisler, Alan K., DO {1831129659} CdvDis(80,PA77)<NJ-KMH-STRAT, NJ-KMHTURNV>
+ Southern New Jersey Cardiac Care Specialists
1020 Laurel Oak Road/Suite 102 Voorhees, NJ 08043 (856)435-8842 Fax (856)435-8665
+ Southern New Jersey Cardiac Care Specialists
151 Fries Mill Road/Suite 101 Turnersville, NJ 08012 (856)435-8842 Fax (856)374-3120

Gejerman, Glen, MD {1972565182} Radiol, RadOnc(90,NJ05)<NJ-HACKNSK>
+ John Theurer Cancer Center - HUMC
92 Second Street Hackensack, NJ 07601 (201)996-2210 Fax (551)996-0730
+ Hackensack University Medical Center
30 Prospect Avenue/Radiology Hackensack, NJ 07601 (201)996-2210 Fax (201)996-2965

Gekowski, Kathleen M., MD {1942295761} InfDis, IntrMd(76,PA09)<NJ-CHSMRCER, NJ-RWJUHAM>
+ 1450 Parkside Avenue/Suite 4
Ewing, NJ 08638 (609)882-3500 Fax (609)882-3501

Gelber, Lawrence J., MD {1346202009} RadDia(73,MO34)
+ Tri County MRI & Diagnostic Radiology
97 Main Street Chatham, NJ 07928 (973)635-2000 Fax (973)635-1749
+ Tri County Open MRI
188 Route 10 West East Hanover, NJ 07936 (973)635-2000 Fax (973)884-8893

Gelernt, Mark D., MD {1972556207} CdvDis(86,NY01)<NJ-OURLADY, NJ-SJRSYELM>
+ Cardiovascular Associates of The Delaware Valley, PA
1840 Frontage Road Cherry Hill, NJ 08034 (856)795-2227 Fax (856)795-7436
+ Cardiovascular Associates of The Delaware Valley, PA
525 State Street/Suite 3 Elmer, NJ 08318 (856)795-2227 Fax (856)358-0725
+ Cardiovascular Associates of The Delaware Valley, PA
570 Egg Harbor Road/Suite B-1 Sewell, NJ 08034 (856)582-2000 Fax (856)582-2061

Gelfand, Robert Matthew, MD {1407855612} IntrMd, Hemato, MedOnc(90,NY08)<NY-PRSBWEIL>
+ Hudson Hematology Oncologny
377 Jersey Avenue/Suite 160 Jersey City, NJ 07302 (201)333-8248 Fax (201)333-8469

Geliebter, Ari, MD {1316210990} IntrMd<NY-JACOBIMC>
+ 211 Essex Street/Suite 304
Hackensack, NJ 07601 (201)903-0070 Fax (201)322-0287

Gellella, Erik Leonard, MD {1952563520} RadDia
+ Radiology Affiliates of Central New Jersey, P.A.
2501 Kuser Road Hamilton, NJ 08691 (609)585-8800 Fax (609)585-1825

Geller, Arthur J., MD {1629073127} IntrMd, Gastrn(85,NY01)<NJ-BAYSHORE, NJ-CENTRAST>
+ Middlesex Monmouth Gastroenterology
222 Schanck Road/Suite 302 Freehold, NJ 07728 (732)577-1999 Fax (732)845-5356

Geller, Bradley David, MD {1780607580} Ophthl(98,NY45)<NJ-VALLEY, NJ-HACKNSK>
+ 466 Old Hook Road/Suite 24E
Emerson, NJ 07630 (201)265-7515 Fax (201)265-8626
+ 19-21 Fair Lawn Avenue/Suite 1-E
Fair Lawn, NJ 07410 (201)265-7515 Fax (201)265-8626

Geller, Debora Klein, MD {1083659064} AlgyImmn(99,NY45)<NJ-HACKNSK, NJ-CHILTON>
+ ENT & Allergy Associates, LLP
433 Hackensack Avenue/Suite 204 Hackensack, NJ 07601 (201)883-1062 Fax (201)883-9297

Geller, Eric Bernard, MD {1780788992} Nrolgy, Eplpsy(89,RI01)<NJ-STBARNMC>
+ St. Barnabas Institute of Neurology & Neurosurgery
200 South Orange Avenue/Suite 101 Livingston, NJ 07039 (973)322-7580 Fax (973)322-7505
egeller@sbhcs.com

Geller, Felix A., MD {1902073216} Psychy, IntrMd(08,STM01)<NJ-COMMED, NJ-KIMBALL>
+ Stress Care Clinic of New Jersey, LLC
4122 Route 516/Suite C & D Matawan, NJ 07747 (732)679-4500 Fax (732)679-4549
+ Community Medical Center
99 Route 37 West Toms River, NJ 08755 (732)679-4500 Fax (732)557-4015
+ Specialty Hospital at Monmouth
300 Second Avenue/Greenwall 6 Long Branch, NJ 07747 (732)923-6912

Geller, Ian B., DO {1679667273} Psychy(77,IA75)
+ New Jersey Division of Developmental Disability
Route 72 East New Lisbon, NJ 08064 (609)726-1000 Fax (609)894-8430

Geller, Jay D., MD {1548261266} Dermat, PthDrm(86,NH01)<NJ-HCKTSTWN, NJ-SOMERSET>
+ 310 Route 24 East/PO Box 399
Chester, NJ 07930 (908)879-8800 Fax (908)879-2955

Geller, Judy Irene, MD {1568509305} IntrMd(91,NY47)<NJ-EN-GLWOOD>
+ Englewood Hospital and Medical Center
350 Engle Street/InternalMed Englewood, NJ 07631 (201)894-3510 Fax (201)894-0857

Geller, Matthew Al, MD {1346317013} Psychy(72,UZB44)<NJ-MONMOUTH>
+ Monmouth Medical Center
300 Second Avenue/Psychiatry Long Branch, NJ 07740 (732)222-5200

Geller, Robert J., DO {1518932979} EmrgMd(71,IL76)<NJ-STFRN-MED>
+ St. Francis Medical Center
601 Hamilton Avenue/EmrgMed Trenton, NJ 08629 (609)599-5000

Geller, Toby A., MD {1255490488} FamMed(75,NJ06)
+ East Brunswick Family Practice Associates
123 Dunhams Corner Road East Brunswick, NJ 08816 (732)254-3300 Fax (732)651-0822

Gellerstein, Alan Stuart, MD {1588695712} FamMed(96,VA04)
+ Medical Institute of New Jersey
11 Saddle Road Cedar Knolls, NJ 07927 (973)267-2122 Fax (973)267-3478

Gellis, Dana B., MD {1477500577} IntrMd(98,NY08)<NJ-HACKNSK>
+ 6 Village Square East
Clifton, NJ 07011 (973)253-9566 Fax (973)253-8835

Gellman, Alexander C., MD {1295798775} Urolgy(69,PA02)<NJ-MORRISTN>
+ North Jersey Center for Urological Care PA
16 Pocono Road/Suite 114 Denville, NJ 07834 (973)586-3056 Fax (973)625-0116
doc943@aol.com
+ Specialty Surgical Center
380 Lafayette Road/Suite 110 Sparta, NJ 07871 (973)586-3056 Fax (973)940-3170

Gellman, Elliott, MD {1831136795} ObsGyn(72,SC01)
+ 177 North Dean Street/Suite 203
Englewood, NJ 07631 (201)747-9412 Fax (201)801-9012

Gellman, Marc D., MD {1366495194} Anesth(80,PA13)<NJ-UN-DRWD>
+ 82 Blue Heron Way
Gibbsboro, NJ 08026 (856)435-4233 Fax (856)435-4233

Gellrick, Judith C., MD {1093799124} IntrMd, Nephro(68,DC02)<NJ-HACKNSK>
+ 77 Prospect Avenue
Hackensack, NJ 07601 (201)342-5555 Fax (201)343-3389

Gelman, Beth Paula, MD {1295838530} Pedtrc, AdolMd(91,NY46)<NJ-MORRISTN, NJ-HCKTSTWN>
+ College Plaza Pediatrics
765 State Route 10 East/Suite 203 Randolph, NJ 07869 (973)659-9991 Fax (973)659-9632
+ 22 Tammy Hill Trail
Randolph, NJ 07869

Physicians by Name and Address

Gelman, Scott Franklin, MD {1316980006} Gastrn, IntrMd(91,NY46)<NJ-MORRISTN>
+ 477 Route 10 East
  Randolph, NJ 07869   (973)361-4343   Fax (973)361-4355
+ 111 Madison Avenue/Suite 305
  Morristown, NJ 07960   (973)361-4343   Fax (973)252-0052

Geltzeiler, Jules M., MD {1083693394} Urolgy(79,PA09)<NJ-JRSYSHMC, NJ-RIVERVW>
+ New Jersey Urologic Institute
  10 Industrial Way East   Eatontown, NJ 07724   (732)963-9091   Fax (732)963-9092

Genau, Young J., MD {1215948344}
+ 66 Mill Park Lane
  Marlton, NJ 08053   (856)296-0458
  youngg9@comcast.net

Genco, John Joseph, DO {1255523585} Pedtrc, GenPrc(88,NY75)
+ 16 West River Road
  Rumson, NJ 07760   (732)842-9889   Fax (732)741-8209

Genco, Thomas Albert, MD {1497714398} Pedtrc(94,NJ06)
+ 395 Ridge Road/Suite 6
  Dayton, NJ 08810   (732)274-2727   Fax (732)274-1662

Gendel, Vyacheslav, MD {1992954283} RadV&I, RadDia
+ University Radiology Group, P.C.
  579A Cranbury Road   East Brunswick, NJ 08816   (732)390-0040   Fax (732)390-1856
+ University Radiology Group, P.C.
  483 Cranbury Road   East Brunswick, NJ 08816   (732)390-0040   Fax (732)390-5383

Gendler, Leah S., MD {1306836127} SrgBst, Surgry, SrgOnc(99,NY46)<NJ-MORRISTN>
+ Atlantic Breast Associates
  100 Madison Avenue/3rd Floor   Morristown, NJ 07962   (973)971-4166   Fax (973)290-7152

Gendy, Hany Moris, MD {1861411134} IntrMd(92,EGY05)
+ Franklin Medical Center
  514 Route 33 West/Suite 6   Millstone Township, NJ 08535   (732)851-7007   Fax (732)786-0012

Generelli, Patricia Ann, MD {1255301826} ObsGyn(95,NJ06)
+ Coastal Monmouth Obstetrics & Gynecology
  521 Newman Springs Road/Suite 12   Lincroft, NJ 07738   (732)747-0022   Fax (732)747-0086

Geneslaw, Charles H., MD {1619940814} Pedtrc(82,NJ06)<NJ-COMMED, NJ-OCEANMC>
+ Coastal Health Care
  1314 Hooper Avenue/Building B   Toms River, NJ 08753   (732)349-4994   Fax (732)341-1717

Geng, Qingdi, MD {1821237520} IntrMd(93,CHN57)
+ Henry J. Austin Health Center
  321 North Warren Street   Trenton, NJ 08618   (609)278-4900   Fax (609)695-3532

Gengel, Natalie, MD {1437690914} AdolMd
+ Mid Jersey Pediatrics
  33 Brunswick Woods Drive   East Brunswick, NJ 08816   (732)257-4330   Fax (732)257-1177

Genin, Ilya D., MD {1205814696} CdvDis, IntrMd(75,UKRA)<NJ-RWJUHAM>
+ Hamilton Cardiology Associates
  2073 Klockner Road   Hamilton, NJ 08690   (609)584-1212   Fax (609)584-0103

Genkin, Igor, MD {1700802972} IntrMd(90,RUS05)<NY-STBARNAB>
+ 220 Hamburg Tpke/Suite 20
  Wayne, NJ 07470   (973)200-8955

Gennace, Ronald E., MD {1497836241} SrgOrt(76,NJ05)<NJ-WESTHDSN>
+ 32 Belleville Turnpike
  North Arlington, NJ 07031   (201)997-8777

Gennaro, Anthony J., MD {1790859494} IntrMd(75,MEX14)<NJ-HACKNSK>
+ 413 Boulevard
  Hasbrouck Heights, NJ 07604   (201)288-6335   Fax (201)393-0890

Gennaro, Paul, MD {1942268412} Nrolgy(79,NJ05)<NJ-MONMOUTH, NJ-RIVERVW>
+ Neurology Specialists of Monmouth County
  107 Monmouth Road/Suite 110   West Long Branch, NJ 07764   (732)935-1850   Fax (732)544-0494

Genova-Goldstein, Jeanne, MD Pedtrc(86,NY08)
+ West Park Pediatrics
  219 Taylors Mills Road   Manalapan, NJ 07726   (732)577-0088   Fax (732)577-9643
+ West Park Pediatrics
  804 West Park Avenue   Ocean, NJ 07712   (732)577-0088   Fax (732)493-0903

Genovese, Cynthia Marie, MD {1902034242} FamMed(01,ITA01)
+ Monmouth Medical Group, P.C.
  1 Route 70   Lakewood, NJ 08701   (848)222-4690   Fax (848)222-4688
+ Dorfner Family Medicine
  639 Stokes Road/Suite 102   Medford, NJ 08055   (848)222-4690   Fax (609)714-9288
+ Dorfner Family Medicine

811 Sunset Road/Suite 101   Burlington, NJ 08701   (609)387-9242   Fax (609)387-9408

Gentile, David R., MD {1023095007} SrgOrt, SprtMd(92,NJ05)<NJ-MONMOUTH, NJ-RIVERVW>
+ Professional Orthopaedic Associates
  776 Shrewsbury Avenue/Suite 201   Tinton Falls, NJ 07724   (732)530-4949   Fax (732)530-3618
+ Professional Orthopaedic Associates
  1430 Hooper Avenue/Suite 101   Toms River, NJ 08753   (732)530-4949   Fax (732)349-7722
+ Professional Orthopaedic Associates
  303 West Main Street   Freehold, NJ 07724   (732)530-4949   Fax (732)577-0036

Gentile, James, DO {1376507814} Anesth, NeuMSptM(88,PA77)
+ Suburban Endoscopy
  799 Bloomfield Avenue/Suite 101   Verona, NJ 07044   (973)571-1600
+ North Fullerton Surgery Center
  37 North Fullerton Avenue   Montclair, NJ 07042   (973)571-1600   Fax (973)233-0144
+ Columbia Anesthesia Associates
  37 West Century Road/Suite 101   Paramus, NJ 07044   (201)634-9000   Fax (201)634-9014

Gentile, Michael P., MD {1649386020} PsyCAd, PsyFor, Psychy(90,NY08)
+ 145 Prospect Street
  Ridgewood, NJ 07450   (201)444-0528   Fax (201)444-0634

Gentile, Michael R., MD {1982675773} IntrMd(85,GRN01)
+ 655 Franklin Avenue
  Nutley, NJ 07110   (973)542-1122   Fax (973)661-1300
  grenadamd@ipninet.com

Gentile, Victor G., MD {1821060187} Otlryg, OtgyFPIS(91,NJ05)<NJ-HCKTSTWN>
+ Ear, Nose, & Throat Medical Associates
  108 Bilby Road/Suite 301   Hackettstown, NJ 07840   (908)979-0662   Fax (908)979-0713
+ Specialty Surgical Center
  380 Lafayette Road/Suite 110   Sparta, NJ 07871   (908)979-0662   Fax (973)940-3170

Gentlesk, Michael J., MD {1083899645} Allrgy, ImmAsm, Immuno(64,DC02)
+ 2301 East Evesham Road/Suite 607
  Voorhees, NJ 08043   (856)651-9393   Fax (856)651-9222

George, Bettina, MD {1861854739}
+ Mountainside Family Practice Associates
  799 Bloomfield Avenue/Suite 201   Verona, NJ 07044   (973)746-7050   Fax (973)857-2831

George, Bibbin Philip, MD {1780971028}
+ Complete Care Family Medicine
  75 West Red Bank Avenue   Woodbury, NJ 08096   (856)853-2055   Fax (856)848-2879

George, Brian Philip, MD {1992953434} SrgOrt<PA-STLKBTHL>
+ Reconstructive Orthopedics, P.A.
  200 Bowman Drive/Suite E-100   Voorhees, NJ 08043   (609)267-9400   Fax (609)267-9457

George, Cyriac, DO {1629239884} Pedtrc(05,PA77)<NJ-VIRTVOOR, NJ-COOPRUMC>
+ Advocare DelGiorno Pediatrics
  535 South Black Horse Pike   Blackwood, NJ 08012   (856)228-1061   Fax (856)228-1907

George, Geny Ann, MD {1073870697}
+ 199 Engle Street
  Englewood, NJ 07631   (201)567-8008   Fax (201)567-3003

George, Gina, DO {1952539181} Anesth<NJ-RWJUBRUN>
+ Robert Wood Johnson-UMDNJ Anesthesia Group
  125 Paterson Street/CAB 3100   New Brunswick, NJ 08901   (732)235-7827   Fax (732)235-6131

George, James E., MD {1215956347} EmrgMd, LeglMd(70,KY02)
+ Emergency Physician Associates, P.A.
  307 South Evergreen Avenue/PO Box 298   Woodbury, NJ 08096   (856)848-3817   Fax (856)848-1431

George, Jason C., MD {1861759490} CritCr
+ VA New Jersey Health Pulmonary & Critical Care
  385 Tremont Avenue   East Orange, NJ 07018   (973)676-1000   Fax (973)395-7034

George, Louis C., MD {1669452215} Radiol, RadDia(83,NJ05)<NJ-JFKMED>
+ Edison Radiology Group, P.A.
  65 James Street   Edison, NJ 08820   (732)321-7917   Fax (732)737-2968
+ JFK Medical Center
  65 James Street   Edison, NJ 08820   (732)321-7000

George, Malini Susan, MD {1962766352} FamMed
+ Riverside Medical Group
  714 Tenth Street/Suite 2   Secaucus, NJ 07094   (860)368-7018   Fax (201)865-0015
  mg8270@gmail.com

George, Mridula A., MD {1285997569}
+ 111 Delmonica Avenue
  Somerset, NJ 08873   (848)228-1544

George, Philip M., MD {1851472070} IntrMd(96,INDI)
+ Cooper University at Willingboro
  218C Sunset Road   Willingboro, NJ 08046   (609)877-0400   Fax (609)877-3542

George, Preethi Sara, MD {1922107440} FamMed(98,INA5Y)<NJ-STCLRDEN, NJ-HOLYNAME>
+ 765 Teaneck Road/Suite 1R
  Teaneck, NJ 07666   (201)837-2500   Fax (201)837-2511

George, Renu, MD {1144753021} IntrMd
+ University Medical Group - General Internal Medicine
  125 Paterson Street/Suite 5100A   New Brunswick, NJ 08903   (732)235-6968   Fax (732)235-8935

George, Roshini, DO {1700866951} OncHem, IntrMd(94,NJ75)
+ Summit Medical Group Florham Park Campus
  150 Park Avenue   Florham Park, NJ 07932   (973)538-5210   Fax (973)644-9657
+ Hematology-Oncology Associates of Northern NJ
  3219 US Highway 46/Suite 108   Parsippany, NJ 07054   (973)538-5210   Fax (973)316-5990

George, Tony, MD {1215916606} PedAne, Anesth(00,NET12)
+ Summit Anesthesia Associates, P.A.
  33 Overlook Road/Suite 311   Summit, NJ 07901   (908)598-1500   Fax (908)598-0197

George, Tony Kuttikattu, DO {1891006359} PhysMd(10,WV75)
+ University Pain Medicine Center
  33 Clyde Road/Suite 105 & 106   Somerset, NJ 08873   (732)873-6868   Fax (732)873-6869

George-Varghese, Blessit, DO {1225343874} EmrgMd<NJ-STJOSHOS>
+ St. Joseph's Regional Medical Center
  703 Main Street   Paterson, NJ 07503   (973)754-2000

George-Vickers, Jonelle, DO {1700226693} FamMed
+ Carepoint Health Bayonne Med Center
  29 East 29th Street   Bayonne, NJ 07002   (201)858-5000

Georgekutty, Jason, DO {1053750299} PhysMd<NJ-KSLRWELK>
+ Kessler Institute for Rehab
  201 Pleasant Hill Road   Chester, NJ 07930   (973)252-6300

Georgelos, Panagiotis, MD {1528027406} Pedtrc
+ Advocare South Jersey Pediatrics Collingswood
  204 White Horse Pike   Collingswood, NJ 08107   (856)424-6050   Fax (856)424-2943
+ Advocare South Jersey Pediatrics Cherry Hill
  1949 Route 70 East/Suite 1 & 2   Cherry Hill, NJ 08003   (856)424-6050   Fax (856)424-2943

Georges, Peter T., MD {1861699944} OncHem, IntrMd<MA-UMMBELM>
+ South Jersey Health Care Center
  Two Cooper Plaza/Suite 3200   Camden, NJ 08103   (856)735-6260   Fax (856)342-6662

Georges, Renee N., MD {1356409130} Surgry(88,DC03)
+ PO Box 816
  Lakewood, NJ 08701   (732)886-9966   Fax (732)886-9943

Georgescu, Anca D., MD {1407157506} InfDis
+ Summit Medical Group
  315 East Northfield Road/Suite 1-E   Livingston, NJ 07039   (973)436-4170   Fax (973)436-4169

Georgeson, Steven E., MD {1487627741} CdvDis(86,NY09)<NJ-MORRISTN, NJ-SOMERSET>
+ Medicor Cardiology PA
  225 Jackson Street   Bridgewater, NJ 08807   (908)526-8668   Fax (908)231-6781
+ Medicor Cardiology PA
  331 US Highway 206/Suite 1A   Hillsborough, NJ 08844   (908)526-8668   Fax (908)431-0808

Georgsson, Maria Anna, MD {1700804101} Gastrn, IntrMd(90,NY01)<NJ-HUNTRDN>
+ Hunterdon Gastroenterology Associates, P.A.
  1100 Wescott Drive/Suite 206-207   Flemington, NJ 08822   (908)483-4000   Fax (908)788-5090
+ Hunterdon Gastroenterology Associates, P.A.
  135 West End Avenue/Suite 204   Somerville, NJ 08876   (908)483-4000   Fax (908)788-5090

Georgy, John, MD {1972921948} PhyMPain
+ 1116 Giordano Avenue
  Parlin, NJ 08859   (908)705-4467

Georgy, Mary Sarah, MD {1326228982} IntrMd, AlgyImmn(04,NJ06)<PA-NZRTH, NJ-COMMED>
+ Bruce A. De Cotiis, MD, PA
  1673 Highway 88 West   Brick, NJ 08724   (732)458-2000   Fax (732)458-4523
+ Robert P. Rabinowitz, DO, PA
  462 Lakehurst Road   Toms River, NJ 08755   (732)458-2000   Fax (732)505-0862

Geraci, Brian Anthony, MD {1487661096} IntrMd(89,PA13)<NJ-ACMCMAIN>
+ Shore Physician Group
  401 Bethel Road   Somers Point, NJ 08244   (609)365-6200   Fax (609)365-6201
  bgeraci@shorephysiansgroup.com

Gerardi, Michael J., MD {1194763425} EmrgMd, IntrMd, PedEmg(85,DC02)<NJ-MORRISTN>
+ Morristown Medical Center
100 Madison Avenue/Pedi Emerg Med   Morristown, NJ 07962   (973)971-8919   Fax (973)290-7202
michael.gerardi@ahsys.org

Gerardis, Judi R., MD {1528028313} ObsGyn(93,DC01)<NJ-HACKNSK>
+ Obstetrics and Gynecology PA
20 Prospect Avenue/Suite 607   Hackensack, NJ 07601   (201)487-3464   Fax (201)487-0232

Gerber, Austin J., DO {1801943220} FamMed, Grtrcs(78,PA77)<NJ-ACMCITY>
+ 850 North Main Street
Pleasantville, NJ 08232   (609)641-1118   Fax (609)383-9370

Gerber, David R., DO {1861580219} CritCr, IntrMd(82,NY75)<NJ-COOPRUMC>
+ Cooper University Hospital
One Cooper Plaza   Camden, NJ 08103   (856)342-2400

Gerber, Marina, MD {1003063082} PthAna(71,RUSS)
+ Quest Diagnostics Inc.
1 Malcolm Avenue   Teterboro, NJ 07608   (201)393-5357   Fax (201)462-4712

Gerber, Steven Lewis, MD {1558378034} IntrMd(84,PA13)<NJ-VIRTVOOR>
+ 1025 West Marlton Pike
Cherry Hill, NJ 08002   (856)429-6858   Fax (856)429-0916

Gerber, Susan Marie, MD {1568627545} IntrMd(08,PA02)
+ Cooper Endocrinology Associates
1210 Brace Road/Suite 107   Cherry Hill, NJ 08034   (856)795-3597   Fax (856)795-7590

Gerewitz, Fredric B., MD {1396724035} CdvDis, IntrMd(84,NY08)<NJ-VIRTVOOR, NJ-OURLADY>
+ Associated Cardiovascular Consultants, P.A.
1105 Laurel Oak Road/Suite 165   Voorhees, NJ 08043   (856)424-3600   Fax (856)424-7154
+ Associated Cardiovascular Consultants-Lourdes
1 Brace Road/Suite C & F   Cherry Hill, NJ 08034   (856)424-3600   Fax (856)428-5748

Gerges, Christine Nabil, DO {1023034006} IntrMd(02,FL75)<NJ-STCLRDEN, NJ-STCLRDOV>
+ St. Clare's Hospital-Denville Campus
25 Pocono Road/VitalMedForces   Denville, NJ 07834   (973)625-6000   Fax (973)989-3106
+ Internal Medicine Consultants
765 State Route 10 East/Suite 201   Randolph, NJ 07869   (973)625-6000   Fax (732)271-1022

Gerges, Jocelyn, MD {1821416538} IntrMd<NJ-UMDNJ>
+ University Hospital
150 Bergen Street/Suite H245   Newark, NJ 07103   (973)972-5672

Gerges, Maged Moussa, MD {1194738708} Anesth(87,EGY04)<NJ-CLARMAAS>
+ Clara Maass Medical Center
1 Clara Maass Drive/Anesthesiology   Belleville, NJ 07109   (973)450-2000

Gerges, Theresa, DO {1700203965}
+ Summit Anesthesia Associates, P.A.
33 Overlook Road/Suite 311   Summit, NJ 07901   (908)598-1500   Fax (908)598-0197

Gerhard, Harvey, MD {1982797551} IntrMd, PulDis(74,CT01)
+ 416 Mount Airy Road
Basking Ridge, NJ 07920   (732)776-6605   Fax (908)766-0439

Gerhardstein, Brian Lee, MD {1790982064} Nrolgy(03,MI07)
+ University Hospital-RWJMS Neurology
125 Paterson Street/Suite 4100-6100   New Brunswick, NJ 08901   (732)235-7733   Fax (732)235-7041
+ Rutgers NJ School of Medicine Neurology
90 Bergen Street/DOC 5200   Newark, NJ 07103   (732)235-7733   Fax (973)972-5059

Gerhardt, Amy Ilene Katz, MD {1245419928} ObsGyn(06,NY19)
+ Valley Center for Women's Health
550 North Maple Avenue/Suite 102   Ridgewood, NJ 07450   (201)444-4040   Fax (201)444-4473

Gerhardt, William J., MD {1831207950} Radiol, RadDia(84,PA09)<NJ-ACMCITY, NJ-SHOREMEM>
+ Atlantic Medical Imaging, LLC.
72 West Jimmie Leeds Road   Galloway, NJ 08205   (609)677-9729   Fax (609)653-8764
+ Atlantic Medical Imaging, LLC.
401 Bethel Road   Somers Point, NJ 08244   (609)677-9729
+ Atlantic Medical Imaging, LLC.
421 Route 9 North   Cape May Court House, NJ 08205   (609)463-9500   Fax (609)465-0918

Geria, Michael J., DO {1497706089} ObsGyn, IntrMd(90,IL76)<NJ-SJERSYHS>
+ Community Health Care, Inc.
1200 North High Street   Millville, NJ 08332   (856)451-4700   Fax (856)825-8167

Geria, Rajesh Navin, MD {1700864410} EmrgMd(00,POL18)<NJ-RWJUBRUN>
+ University Emergency Medicine
125 Paterson Street/MEB 104   New Brunswick, NJ 08901   (732)235-6071   Fax (732)235-7379
+ RWJ University Hospital New Brunswick
One Robert Wood Johnson Place   New Brunswick, NJ 08901   (732)235-6071   Fax (732)235-7379

Germaine, Pauline, DO {1700077625} RadDia
+ 1036 Heartwood Drive
Cherry Hill, NJ 08003

German, Yelena, MD {1952344632} CdvDis, IntrMd(79,RUS59)
+ 805 Cooper Road/Suite 1
Voorhees, NJ 08043   (856)489-3200   Fax (856)489-3254

Germiller, John Andrew, MD {1104916121} Otlryg(97,MI01)<PA-CHILDHOS>
+ CHOP Pediatric & Adolescent Specialty Care Center
1012 Laurel Oak Road   Voorhees, NJ 08043   (856)435-1300   Fax (856)435-0091

Germinario, Carla Ann, MD {1356362180} IntrMd(00,HUN01)<NJ-HOLYNAME>
+ Holy Name Medical Partners Office
15 Anderson Street   Hackensack, NJ 07601   (201)487-3355   Fax (201)487-0960

Germond, Christopher John, DO {1952560526} Anesth(08,PA78)<NJ-STJOSHOS>
+ St. Joseph's Regional Medical Center
703 Main Street/Anesthiology   Paterson, NJ 07503   (973)754-2323

Gershenbaum, Eric Andrew, MD {1548227309} Ophthl(00,NJ06)
+ Freehold Ophthalmology, LLC
509 Stillwells Corner Road/Suite E-5   Freehold, NJ 07728   (732)431-9333   Fax (732)431-3312
+ Freehold Ophthalmology, LLC
20 Hospital Drive   Toms River, NJ 08755   (732)431-9333   Fax (732)505-4322
+ Freehold Ophthalmology, LLC
202 Jack Martin Boulevard   Brick, NJ 07728   (732)458-5700   Fax (732)458-0693

Gershenbaum, Mark R., DO {1982665782} FamMed(84,PA77)<NJ-CENTRAST, NJ-JRSYSHMC>
+ CentraState Medical Center
901 West Main Street   Freehold, NJ 07728   (732)431-2000   Fax (732)431-8267

Gershman, Larisa Khaimovna, MD {1447223201} IntrMd(80,UZB44)<NJ-CHILTON>
+ 191 Hamburg Turnpike/Suite 2-B
Pompton Lakes, NJ 07442   (973)248-9446   Fax (973)248-9445

Gershteyn, Eduard, MD {1932171766} Anesth(72,UKRA)
+ Ocean Anesthesia Group PA
1200 Hooper Avenue   Toms River, NJ 08753   (732)797-3890   Fax (732)942-5603

Gershuny, Kevin Michael, DO {1023341047}
+ 30 Mountain Avenue/Unit 8
Paterson, NJ 07501

Gerson, Ronald L., MD {1235179813} SrgOrt(78,PA09)
+ Central Physicians and Surgeons
820 South White Horse Pike   Hammonton, NJ 08037   (609)561-8787   Fax (609)567-9546

Gerstein, Gary, MD {1689662769} Hemato, IntrMd, OncHem(73,PA02)<NJ-MORRISTN>
+ Hematology-Oncology Associates of Northern NJ
100 Madison Avenue/PO Box 1089   Morristown, NJ 07962   (973)538-5210   Fax (973)644-9657

Gerstel, Alan Victor, MD {1417915737} EmrgMd(98,MD07)<NJ-VALLEY>
+ The Valley Hospital
223 North Van Dien Avenue/EmrgMed   Ridgewood, NJ 07450   (201)447-8000

Gersten, Michael, MD {1699872218} Gastrn, IntrMd(78,MEXI)<NJ-CHSFULD, NJ-CHSMRCER>
+ 2097 Klockner Road/Building 5
Hamilton, NJ 08690   (609)588-0888   Fax (609)588-0159

Gerstman, Brett A., MD {1760687636} PainMd
+ New Jersey Spine Center
40 Main Street   Chatham, NJ 07928   (732)616-5713   Fax (973)635-6254

Gerstmann, Michael Adam, MD {1073510947} FamMed(93,NM01)
+ Yaffa-Rose Integrated Health Care Center-Newark
183 South Orange Avenue/BHSB B1455   Newark, NJ 07103   (973)972-6479   Fax (973)972-8626
gerstmma@umdnj.edu
+ New Jersey Family Practice Center (NJFPC)
90 Bergen Street/DOC 300/Lower Level   Newark, NJ 07103   (973)972-6479   Fax (973)972-2754
+ Westfield Family Practice
563 Westfield Avenue   Westfield, NJ 07103   (908)232-5858   Fax (908)232-0439

Gerszberg, Ted M., MD {1225075237} Ophthl(86,NY46)<NJ-CHILTON>
+ 150 River Road/Suite C-2
Montville, NJ 07045   (973)402-9200   Fax (973)402-7788

Gertz, Shira J., MD {1740237759} Pedtrc, PedCrC(01,GRN01)<NJ-NWRKBETH, NJ-HACKNSK>
+ Hackensack University Medical Center
30 Prospect Avenue   Hackensack, NJ 07601   (201)996-2403

Gertzman, Jerrold Scott, MD {1194799106} FamMed(97,MA05)<NJ-HUNTRDN>
+ Hunterdon Family Medicine
190 State Highway 31/Suite 500   Flemington, NJ 08822   (908)788-6161   Fax (908)788-6522

Gertzman-Dafilou, Sharon D., DO {1487821054} FamMed(91,ME75)
+ Pleasant Run Family Physicians
925 US Highway 202   Neshanic Station, NJ 08853   (908)788-9468   Fax (908)788-5720
+ Priority Medical Care/Family Health Center
350 Grove Street   Bridgewater, NJ 08807   (908)788-9468   Fax (908)722-6031

Gerula, Christine Marie, MD {1619908878} IntrMd, CdvDis(96,NJ05)<NJ-UMDNJ>
+ University Hospital-Doctors Office Center
90 Bergen Street/DOC 3500/Cardio   Newark, NJ 07103   (973)972-2573   Fax (973)972-4695

Gervasoni, James Edmund, Jr., MD {1396807145} Surgry, SrgOnc(93,NJ06)<NJ-STPETER>
+ 562 Easton Avenue
Somerset, NJ 08873   (732)339-7770   Fax (732)745-8603

Gerwin, Kenneth S., MD {1326155417} Otlryg(63,IA02)
+ 4 Kissel Lane
Morristown, NJ 07960   (973)267-6891

Gery, Brian F., MD {1114084423} IntrMd(93,RI01)<NJ-SHOREMEM>
+ Coastal Physicians and Surgeons
110 Harbor Lane/Suite A   Somers Point, NJ 08244   (609)653-0850   Fax (609)927-3934

Gesell, Mark William, MD {1083654990} SrgOrt(01,IL43)
+ Professional Orthopaedic Associates
776 Shrewsbury Avenue/Suite 201   Tinton Falls, NJ 07724   (732)530-4949   Fax (732)530-3618
+ Professional Orthopaedic Associates
1430 Hooper Avenue/Suite 101   Toms River, NJ 08753   (732)530-4949   Fax (732)349-7722
+ Professional Orthopaedic Associates
303 West Main Street   Freehold, NJ 07724   (732)530-4949   Fax (732)577-0036

Gesner, Lyle Robert, MD {1023055654} RadDia, RadNro, Radiol(90,NY09)<NY-MNTFMOSE, NJ-STBARNMC>
+ St. Barnabas Medical Center
94 Old Short Hills Road/Radiology   Livingston, NJ 07039   (973)322-5000

Gesser, Gail A., DO {1922053289} Pedtrc(83,NY75)<NJ-HACKNSK>
+ Hackensack Univ Medical Center Pediatric Emerg Room
30 Prospect Avenue   Hackensack, NJ 07601   (201)996-5430   Fax (201)996-3676
+ Hackensack University Medical Center
30 Prospect Avenue   Hackensack, NJ 07601   (201)996-5454

Gessman, Lawrence J., MD {1730277195} CdvDis, ClCdEl, IntrMd(74,PA01)<NJ-DEBRAHLC>
+ University Cardiology
3 Cooper Plaza/Room 311   Camden, NJ 08103   (856)342-2034   Fax (856)342-6608
+ Cooper Cardiology Associates
900 Centennial Boulevard   Voorhees, NJ 08043   (856)342-2034   Fax (856)325-6702
+ Cooper Cardiology Associates
1210 Brace Road/Suite 103   Cherry Hill, NJ 08103   (856)427-7254

Gesumaria, Robert Cosmo, DO {1437560828} EmrgMd
+ Kennedy Mem Hospital Emergency Medicine
18 East Laurel Road   Stratford, NJ 08084   (908)510-1945

Getson, Philip, DO {1083749501} FamMed(75,PA77)
+ 100 Brick Road/Suite 206
Marlton, NJ 08053   (856)983-7246   Fax (856)983-0908

Gettings, Matthew James, DO {1962693432} FamMed(NJ75<NJ-LOURDMED>
+ Lourdes Medical Associates/Triboro Family Physicians
1104 Route 130/Suite K   Cinnaminson, NJ 08077   (856)786-8010   Fax (856)786-0529

Physicians by Name and Address

Gettys, Jacqueline Brown, MD {1508806951} IntrMd, Grtrcs(84,NH01)<NJ-CHSMRCER>
+ Capital Health Primary Care
  1230 Parkway Avenue/Suite 203 Ewing, NJ 08628 (609)883-5454 Fax (609)883-2564
+ West Trenton Medical Associates
  1230 Parkway Avenue/Suite 203 Trenton, NJ 08638 (609)883-5454 Fax (609)883-2565

Geuder, James W., MD {1619022068} SrgVas, Surgry(81,WI06)<NJ-HACKNSK, NJ-VALLEY>
+ Wound Healing & Hyperbaric Medicine
  240 Williamson Street/Suite 104 Elizabeth, NJ 07202 (908)994-5480 Fax (908)994-8802

Gewirtz, George P., MD {1477516615} EnDbMt, IntrMd(65,MA01)
+ The Joslin Center for Diabetes
  200 South Orange Avenue/2nd Floor Livingston, NJ 07039 (973)322-7200 Fax (973)322-7250

Gewirtz, Jonathan D., MD {1639155542} ObsGyn(81,NY06)
+ Community Health Care Inc
  484 South Brewster Road Vineland, NJ 08360 (856)696-0300 Fax (856)696-2561
+ Women's Medical Center
  3980 Black Horse Pike Mays Landing, NJ 08330 (856)696-0300 Fax (609)625-2610

Gewirtz, Matthew B., MD {1417909771} Ophthl(02,NJ05)<NJ-OVERLOOK>
+ The Eye Center
  65 Mountain Boulevard Ext/Suite 105 Warren, NJ 07059 (732)356-6200 Fax (732)356-0228
+ The Eye Center
  213 Stelton Road Piscataway, NJ 08854 (732)356-6200 Fax (732)752-9492
+ The Eye Center
  3900 Park Avenue/Suite 106 Edison, NJ 07059 (732)603-2101

Gewolb, Eric B., MD {1326094871} Psychy(74,LA01)<NJ-BAYONNE>
+ 830 Kennedy Boulevard
  Bayonne, NJ 07002 (201)339-0200 Fax (201)339-0201 EBGMDPA@gmail.com
+ Bayonne Medical Center
  29th Street at Avenue E/Psychiatry Bayonne, NJ 07002 (201)858-5000

Ghaben, Kamel Mostafa, MD {1396951158} NnPnMd, Pedtrc(01,PAK20)
+ On-Site Neonatal Partners
  1000 Haddonfield-Berlin Road/Suite 210 Voorhees, NJ 08043 (856)782-2212 Fax (856)782-2213

Ghabious, Emad Faiek, MD {1265429666} Anesth(92,EGY04)<NJ-RWJUHAM, NJ-RWJUBRUN>
+ Robert Wood Johnson University Hospital at Hamilton
  1 Hamilton Health Place/Anesth Hamilton, NJ 08690 (609)586-7900

Ghabour, Rose Ann Sameh, MD {1770994386} FamMed
+ AFC Urgent Care
  2100 88th Street/Bldg G1A North Bergen, NJ 07047 (201)588-1300 Fax (201)588-1300

Ghabras, Magda S., DO {1841407749} IntrMd(05,NY75)<NJ-RWJUBRUN, NJ-JFKMED>
+ Matawan Medical Associates
  213 Main Street Matawan, NJ 07747 (732)566-2363 Fax (732)566-0502
+ Matawan Medical Center
  158 Main Street/Suite 101 Matawan, NJ 07747 (732)566-2363 Fax (732)970-6163

Ghacibeh, Georges A., MD {1851331680} Nrolgy, ClNrPh, IntrMd(97,LEB04)<NJ-HACKNSK, NJ-MORRISTN>
+ Progressive Neurology
  260 Old Hook Road/Suite 200 Westwood, NJ 07675 (201)546-8510 Fax (201)503-8142

Ghadiali, Farida Hashim, MD {1518055482} Psychy(71,INA72)<NJ-TRENTPSY>
+ Trenton Psychiatric Hospital
  Sullivan Way/PO Box 7600 West Trenton, NJ 08628 (609)633-1500 Fax (609)777-4095

Ghaffar, Sadia, MD {1154582500} Psychy(94,PAK11)
+ 1 Waters Edge Drive
  Delran, NJ 08075 (856)495-8927

Ghafoor, Sadia, DO {1275722951} Rheuma(04,NJ75)
+ Midstate Rheumatology Center
  900 West Main Street Freehold, NJ 07728 (732)431-4335 Fax (732)818-3320
+ Midstate Rheumatology Center
  508 Lakehurst Road/Suite 1 A Toms River, NJ 08755 (732)431-4335 Fax (732)431-4771

Ghali, Anwar Y., MD {1093787145} Psychy, AdmMgt(66,EGY03)<NJ-TRINIPC>
+ Trinitas Regional Medical Center-New Point Campus
  655 East Jersey Street/Physiatry Elizabeth, NJ 07206 (908)994-5000 aghali@trinitas.org

+ Central Jersey Behariaral Health, LLC
  216 North Avenue East Cranford, NJ 07016 (908)994-5000 Fax (908)272-7502

Ghali, Wael, MD {1467518118}<NJ-MONMOUTH>
+ Monmouth Medical Center
  300 Second Avenue Long Branch, NJ 07740 (480)543-7004 Fax (480)393-2989 wael.ghali@apogeephysicians.com

Ghaly, Alan George, DO {1245463520}
+ Rowan University-School of Osteopathic Medicine
  1 Medical Center Drive Stratford, NJ 08084 (856)566-6708 Fax (856)566-6222

Ghaly, Aziz S., MD {1669538997} SrgCTh
+ RWJ University Hospital New Brunswick
  One Robert Wood Johnson Place New Brunswick, NJ 08901 (732)235-7806 Fax (732)235-8727

Ghaly, Maged Antoine, MD {1154327880} Pedtrc(94,EGY05)<NJ-JRSYCITY>
+ 840 Bergen Avenue/Floor 1
  Jersey City, NJ 07306 (201)333-5934 Fax (201)333-5353 Jalmghaly@yahoo.com

Ghaly, Nader Naguib, MD {1396777967} CdvDis, ClCdEl, IntrMd(81,EGY04)<NJ-ACMCMAIN, NJ-COOPRUMC>
+ Atlantic Heart Rhythm Center
  415 Chris Gaupp Drive/Suite C Galloway, NJ 08205 (609)748-7580 Fax (609)748-7574
+ AtlantiCare Regional Med Ctr/Mainland
  65 West Jimmie Leeds Road Pomona, NJ 08240 (609)652-1000

Ghanbari, Cecilia W., MD {1801962212} GenPrc, IntrMd(80,POLA)<NJ-RUNNELLS>
+ Runnells Specialized Hospital of Union County
  40 Watchung Way Berkeley Heights, NJ 07922 (908)771-5700

Ghanekar, Geeta R., MD {1295837078} ObsGyn(69,INDI)<NJ-JFKMED, NJ-RBAYOLDB>
+ 515 Route 27
  Iselin, NJ 08830 (732)283-3850 Fax (732)283-3854

Ghanem, Osama K., MD {1689679565} IntrMd(84,EGYP)
+ Howell Medical Care, PA
  8 Scenic Way Monroe Township, NJ 08831 (732)414-9825

Ghanem, Roland, MD {1952405482} Allrgy, FamMed(67,SYR01)<NJ-STJOSHOS>
+ Allergy Associates of North Jersey
  362 Union Boulevard Totowa, NJ 07512 (973)790-6707 Fax (973)790-1255 rghanem@att.com

Ghani, Muhammad Rehan, MD {1699861443} PsyGrt, Psychy(90,PAK11)<NJ-UNIVBHC>
+ 288 Leonard Place
  Paramus, NJ 07652

Ghanny, Bryan Abdul, MD {1639442619}<NJ-UMDNJ>
+ University Hospital
  150 Bergen Street Newark, NJ 07103 (973)229-4288

Ghanta, Suma Bala, MD {1609818756} FamMed, GenPrc(98,GRN01)<NJ-STCLRDEN, NJ-HCKTSTWN>
+ Advocare Family Health at Mt. Olive
  183 US Route 206/Suite 1 Flanders, NJ 07836 (973)347-3277 Fax (973)347-3141

Gharibo, Mecide M., MD {1700968245} MedOnc<NJ-RWJUBRUN>
+ Rutgers Cancer Institute of New Jersey
  195 Little Albany Street/PO Box 2681 New Brunswick, NJ 08903 (732)235-2465 Fax (732)235-6797

Ghassemi, Rex, MD {1942388921} CdvDis, IntrMd(88,NJ06)<NJ-CHILTON>
+ Cardiology Consultants
  246 Hamburg Turnpike/Suite 201 Wayne, NJ 07470 (973)942-1141 Fax (973)942-7071

Ghattas, Maged L., MD {1770574626} Anesth, IntrMd(92,EGY04)<NJ-CENTRAST>
+ Complete Care Pain and Palliative Center
  901 West Main Street/Suite 203 Freehold, NJ 07728 (732)336-1806 Fax (732)333-8178

Ghaul, Mark R., MD {1053354191} Anesth, AnesPain(89,PA14)<NJ-OURLADY>
+ Our Lady of Lourdes Medical Center
  1600 Haddon Avenue Camden, NJ 08103 (856)757-3836

Ghavam, Sarvin, MD {1972637569} Pedtrc, NnPnMd(MD01
+ CHOP Care Network at Virtua Voorhees Hospital
  100 Bowman Drive Voorhees, NJ 08043 (856)325-3000 Fax (609)261-5842

Ghavami, Roozbeh Mofid, MD {1730541103} IntrMd
+ Capital Health Hospitalist Group
  750 Brunswick Avenue Trenton, NJ 08638 (609)394-6031 Fax (609)394-6299

Ghavami-Maibodi, Seyed Zia, MD {1033154570} Pedtrc, PedEnd(67,IRA07)<NY-MNTFMOSE, NY-MNTFWEIL>
+ Comprehensive Pediatric Care
  119 Propect Street Ridgewood, NJ 07450 (551)220-3378 Fax (201)445-9515

Ghavimi, Shima, MD {1811316458} IntrMd
+ Rutgers- New Jersey Medical School
  185 South Orange Avenue Newark, NJ 07103 (202)480-3808

Ghayad, Zeina Rita, DO {1649461930} InfDis, IntrMd(07,PA78)
+ Garden State Infectious Diseases Associates, P.A.
  709 Haddonfield Berlin Road Voorhees, NJ 08043 (856)566-3190 Fax (856)783-2193

Ghayal, Mahesh, MD {1841217635} CdvDis, IntrMd(80,ENG22)<NJ-ACMCMAIN, NJ-SHOREMEM>
+ AtlantiCare Physicians
  318 Chris Gaupp Drive/Suite 100 Galloway, NJ 08205 (609)404-9900 Fax (609)404-3653

Ghayal, Payal Patel, MD {1477878130} Pedtrc(05,INA3D)<NJ-HACKNSK, NJ-HOLYNAME>
+ Riverside Medical Group
  714 Tenth Street/Suite 2 Secaucus, NJ 07094 (201)863-3346 Fax (201)865-0015
+ Riverside Medical Group
  10 First Street Hackensack, NJ 07601 (201)863-3346 Fax (201)968-5349

Ghazarian, Zeron, MD {1063785756}<NJ-STJOSHOS>
+ St. Joseph's Regional Medical Center
  703 Main Street Paterson, NJ 07503 (973)754-2431

Ghazi, Elizabeth Rose, MD {1669732467} Dermat
+ Cooper University Medical Center/Camden
  3 Cooper Plaza Camden, NJ 08103 (908)528-1251

Ghazi, John, MD {1548288905} RadDia, RadNuc(86,NJ05)
+ Princeton Radiology Associates, P.A.
  419 North Harrison Street Princeton, NJ 08540 (609)921-3345 Fax (609)683-8847
+ Princeton Radiology Associates, P.A.
  9 Centre Drive Jamesburg, NJ 08831 (609)921-3345 Fax (609)655-4016
+ University Radiology Group, P.C.
  375 Route 206/Suite 1 Hillsborough, NJ 08540 (908)874-7600 Fax (908)874-7052

Ghazi, Mohammad, MD {1831265826} ObsGyn, Gyneco, PsyAdt(64,IRA01)<NJ-GRYSTPSY>
+ Greystone Park Psychiatric Hospital
  59 Koch Avenue/Ob/Gyn Morris Plains, NJ 07950 (973)538-1800

Ghelani, Sujal, DO {1700213055}<NJ-SJHREGMC>
+ SJH Regional Medical Center
  1505 West Sherman Avenue Vineland, NJ 08360 (856)641-8000

Ghetia, Ditina, MD {1750698171} IntrMd
+ AtlantiCare Hospitalist Program
  1925 Pacific Avenue/8th Floor Atlantic City, NJ 08401 (609)345-4000

Ghetiya, Vinodrai V., MD {1568410249} IntrMd(79,INA71)<NJ-COMMED>
+ 1749 Hooper Avenue/Suite 203
  Toms River, NJ 08753 (732)864-7030 Fax (732)864-7032

Ghisletta, Leslie C., MD {1851537705} Surgry
+ RWJMG Acute Care Surgery
  125 Paterson Street/Suite 6300 New Brunswick, NJ 08901 (732)235-7766 Fax (732)235-2964

Ghobadi, Fereydoon, MD {1912952607} SrgHnd, SrgOrt(64,IRA24)
+ Advanced Orthopedics & Hand Surgery Institute
  504 Valley Road/Suite 201 Wayne, NJ 07470 (973)942-1315 Fax (973)942-8724

Ghobadi, Ramin, MD {1811944200} SrgHnd, SrgOrt, OrtS-Hand(94,NY48)<NJ-STJOSHOS>
+ Advanced Orthopedics & Hand Surgery Institute
  504 Valley Road/Suite 201 Wayne, NJ 07470 (973)942-1315 Fax (973)942-8724
+ Wayne Surgical Center, LLC.
  1176 Hamburg Pike Wayne, NJ 07470 (973)942-1315 Fax (973)709-1901

Ghobraiel, Raafat Tawfek, MD {1053490359} IntrMd(78,EGY07)<NJ-BAYONNE, NJ-JFKMED>
+ Dr. Ghobraiel Internal Medicine & Weight Loss Mgmt.
  79 Brunswick Woods Drive East Brunswick, NJ 08816 (732)254-7778 Fax (732)254-1443
+ Bayonne Medical Center
  29th Street at Avenue E Bayonne, NJ 07002 (201)858-5000
+ Dr. Ghobraiel Internal Medicine & Weight Loss Mgmt.
  834 Avenue C Bayonne, NJ 08816 (201)471-7750 Fax (201)471-7749

Ghobrial, John M., MD {1508868290} Ophthl, CrnExD(97,NJ05)
+ The Eye Professionals, P.A.
  1205 North High Street Millville, NJ 08332 (856)825-8700 Fax (856)825-8640

Ghobrial, Mark Nashaat, DO {1730442443} SrgOrt
+ Union County Orthopaedic Group
  210 West St. Georges Avenue/PO Box 330 Linden, NJ 07036 (908)486-1111 Fax (908)583-1876

Ghobrial, Peter Morcos Ibrah, MD {1407176621} IntrMd, IntHos(03,EGY03)<NJ-VIRTMHBC>
+ Virtua Hospitalist Group Memorial
175 Madison Avenue/1 FL   Mount Holly, NJ 08060   (609)914-6180   Fax (609)914-6182

Ghodsi, Mohammad, MD {1982645990} Surgry, SrgThr(74,IRA09)<NJ-HACKNSK>
+ Hackensack University Medical Center
30 Prospect Avenue/Surgery   Hackensack, NJ 07601   (201)996-2000

Ghosh, Arpita, MD {1093975864} Anesth(95,INA02)<NJ-ST-BARNMC>
+ Morris Anesthesia Group, PA
3799 Route 46/Suite 211   Parsippany, NJ 07054   (973)335-1122   Fax (973)335-1448

Ghosh, Propa, MD {1659601102} Urolgy
+ Hunterdon Urological Associates
121 Highway 31/Suite 1200   Flemington, NJ 08822   (908)782-0019   Fax (908)782-0630
+ Hunterdon Somerset Medical Office Building
1121 Route 22/Suite 202   Bridgewater, NJ 08807   (908)782-0019

Ghotb, Sara, MD {1124312277} IntrMd<MA-NSSALEM>
+ Monmouth Medical Center
300 Second Avenue   Long Branch, NJ 07740   (732)929-6056   Fax (732)923-6052

Ghotra, Navjot, MD {1558652099}
+ Carepoint Health
10 Exchange Place   Jersey City, NJ 07302   (917)753-2279

Ghuman, Damanjit K., MD {1649366832} IntrMd, MedOnc, OncHem(03,DMN01)
+ Hudson Hematology Oncologny
377 Jersey Avenue/Suite 160   Jersey City, NJ 07302   (201)333-8248   Fax (201)333-8469

Ghusson, Mahmoud Saleh, MD {1336127380} CdvDis, IntrMd(81,EGY04)<NJ-RWJUHAM>
+ Hamilton Cardiology Associates
2073 Klockner Road   Hamilton, NJ 08690   (609)584-1212   Fax (609)584-0103

Ghusson, Soheir F., MD {1588634703} CdvDis, InfDis, IntrMd(81,EGY04)<NJ-RWJUHAM>
+ Hamilton Infectious Disease Associates
2073 Klockner Road   Hamilton, NJ 08690   (609)584-7771   Fax (609)584-5520
+ Hamilton Cardiology Associates
2073 Klockner Road   Hamilton, NJ 08690   (609)584-7771   Fax (609)584-0103

Giacchi, Renato John, MD {1841224847} Otlryg, SrgHdN(93,NY19)<NJ-MORRISTN>
+ Ear, Nose, & Throat Specialists of Morristown LLC
95 Madison Avenue/Suite 105   Morristown, NJ 07960   (973)644-0808   Fax (973)644-9270

Giacobbe, Dean Thomas, MD {1639165939} Anesth, AnesCrCr, IntrMd(95,NH01)
+ Anesthesia Consultnts of NJ/Nova Pain
285 Davidson Avenue/Suite 204   Somerset, NJ 08873   (732)271-1400   Fax (732)271-3543

Giacobbo, Kenneth V., DO {1689618639} IntrMd(90,MO78)
+ Care-at-Home Connections
282 Chester Avenue   Moorestown, NJ 08057   (856)222-3292   Fax (856)222-3293

Giacona, Caryn Marie, MD {1982686010} FamMed(94,NJ05)<NJ-BAYSHORE, NJ-RIVERVW>
+ Family Practice of Middletown
18 Leonardville Road   Middletown, NJ 07748   (732)671-0860   Fax (732)671-6467

Gialanella, Craig David, MD {1467596502} IntrMd(96,ITA17)
+ 50 Newark Avenue/Suite 307
Belleville, NJ 07109   (973)751-0020   Fax (973)751-4454

Gialanella, Francis J., MD {1265448237} IntrMd, FamMed(95,PA02)
+ Primary Medical Care
85 South Jefferson Street   Orange, NJ 07050   (973)673-3522   Fax (973)673-0018
+ Primary Medical Care
76 Prospect Street   Newark, NJ 07105   (973)673-3522   Fax (973)344-1811

Gialanella, Robert J., MD {1144224858} Gastrn, IntrMd(93,GRNA)<NJ-OCEANMC>
+ Red Bank Gastroenterology Associates PA
365 Broad Street/Suite 1-E   Red Bank, NJ 07701   (732)842-4294   Fax (732)548-7408

Giampapa, Vincent C., MD {1801961446} SrgPlstc(78,NY47)<NJ-HACKNSK>
+ Plastic Surgery Center Internationale
89 Valley Road   Montclair, NJ 07042   (973)746-3535   Fax (973)746-4385

Giamporcaro, Steven J., MD {1255356994} GenPrc, FamMed(81,MEXI)
+ Center City Family Practice
2512 Atlantic Avenue   Atlantic City, NJ 08401   (609)347-7333   Fax (609)347-1632

Gianatiempo, Carmine, MD {1558310748} IntrMd, CritCr, EmrgUHyM(86,ITA22)<NJ-ENGLWOOD, NY-BRNXVAMC>
+ Englewood Hospital and Medical Center
350 Engle Street/ICU/CritCare   Englewood, NJ 07631   (201)894-3000   Fax (201)871-0619
carmine.gianatiempo@ehmc.com

Gianchandani, Deepa A., MD Radiol(67)
+ 2 Morning Glory Circle
Mullica Hill, NJ 08062

Giangola, Joseph, MD {1922174457} IntrMd, EnDbMt(78,ITAL)<NJ-HACKNSK>
+ Forest HealthCare Associates, PC
277 Forest Avenue/Suite 200   Paramus, NJ 07652   (201)986-1881   Fax (201)986-1871
+ Hackensack University Medical Center
30 Prospect Avenue/DiabetesTeam   Hackensack, NJ 07601   (201)996-3500

Giangrante, Matthew E., MD {1427200245} FamMed
+ Phillips Barber Family Health Center
72 Alexander Avenue   Lambertville, NJ 08530   (609)397-3535   Fax (609)397-0301

Giangrasso, Thomas A., MD {1609810449} Rheuma, Allrgy(75,PA07)<NJ-STCLRDEN>
+ Allergy & Arthritis Associates PA
66 Sunset Strip/Suite 207   Succasunna, NJ 07876   (973)584-1391   Fax (973)584-7017
+ Allergy & Arthritis Associates PA
600 Mount Pleasant Avenue/Suite C   Dover, NJ 07801   (973)584-1391   Fax (973)989-5046

Gianis, John Thomas, Jr., MD {1467492678} Urolgy(81,MEX03)
+ Drs. Gianis and Gianis
475 Springfield Avenue   Summit, NJ 07901   (908)273-8854   Fax (908)273-4585

Gianis, Thomas J., MD {1376587501} Urolgy(78,OH41)<NJ-OVER-LOOK>
+ Drs. Gianis and Gianis
475 Springfield Avenue   Summit, NJ 07901   (908)273-8854   Fax (908)273-4585

Giannakopoulos, Georgios, DO {1093776759} IntrMd, InfDis(93,ME75)<NJ-BAYSHORE, NJ-CENTRAST>
+ 717 North Beers Street/Suite 2E
Holmdel, NJ 07733   (732)888-7381

Giannattasio, Theresa, DO {1558620690}
+ Essex-Morris Pediatric Group P.A.
203 Hillside Avenue   Livingston, NJ 07039   (973)992-5588   Fax (973)992-1005
+ Pediatric & Adolescent Center
1911 Route 46/PO Box 100   Ledgewood, NJ 07852   (973)992-5588   Fax (973)347-7320

Giannone, Dean Francis, MD {1013907245} IntrMd(96,NY08)<NY-STATNRTH>
+ 10 Cambridge Road
Freehold, NJ 07728   (848)444-9096

Giannuzzi, Rosanne Frances, MD {1861477309} Anesth(93,NJ05)<NJ-HCKTSTWN, NJ-MTNSIDE>
+ Montclair Anesthesia Associates PC
185 Fairfield Avenue/Suite 2A   West Caldwell, NJ 07006   (973)226-1230   Fax (973)226-1232

Giardina, Jennifer, DO {1427221738} FamMed(88,PA77)
+ Toms River Primary Care LLC
3 Plaza Drive/Suite 6   Toms River, NJ 08757   (732)914-0070   Fax (732)914-0071

Giardina-Beckett, Marieanne, MD {1679634414} Dermat(86,NY09)<NJ-BAYONNE>
+ 71 Union Avenue/Suite 108
Rutherford, NJ 07070   (201)804-8900   Fax (201)804-8901
mark.ciavattone@state.mn.us

Giardino, John Domenic, Jr., MD {1790709624} Pedtrc(00,PA09)
+ Moorestown Pediatrics
212 West Route 38/Suite 400   Moorestown, NJ 08057   (856)235-0264   Fax (856)235-4635

Giardino, V. J., MD GenPrc(66,ITA01)<NJ-STMRYPAS>
+ 109 Marsellus Place
Garfield, NJ 07026   (973)340-0283

Giarraputo, Leonard J., MD {1174745657} Psychy, Psyphm, Psythp(91,NJ06)
+ 189 Lakeview Drive South/Suite 102
Gibbsboro, NJ 08026   (856)784-7744   Fax (856)784-7530

Giasi, William George, Jr., MD {1821297680} Pedtrc, IntrMd(03,DC01)<NJ-UNVMCPRN>
+ Princeton Nassau Pediatrics, P.A.
301 North Harrison Street   Princeton, NJ 08540   (609)924-5510   Fax (609)924-3577
+ Princeton Nassau Pediatrics, P.A.
312 Applegarth Road/Suite 104   Monroe Township, NJ 08831   (609)924-5510   Fax (609)409-5610
+ Princeton Nassau Pediatrics, P.A.
196 Princeton-Hightstown Road   West Windsor, NJ 08540   (609)799-5335   Fax (609)799-2294

Gibbens, Douglas T., MD {1447247382} Radiol, RadDia, RadV&I(89,CA06)<NJ-COMMED>
+ Community Medical Center
99 Route 37 West   Toms River, NJ 08755   (732)557-8000   Fax (732)577-2064

Gibbons, James Vernon, Jr., MD {1528098076} FamMed(00,NJ05)<NJ-MORRISTN>
+ Medical Institute of New Jersey
11 Saddle Road   Cedar Knolls, NJ 07927   (973)267-2122   Fax (973)267-3478

Gibbon, Darlene Grace, MD {1972687010} ObsGyn, GynOnc(89,NY08)<NJ-RWJUBRUN>
+ Summit Medical Group Florham Park Campus
150 Park Avenue/Gyn-Oncology   Florham Park, NJ 07932   (973)404-9700
+ Summit Medical Group
315 East Northfield Road/Suite 1-E   Livingston, NJ 07039   (973)404-9700   Fax (973)535-1450

Gibbons, Alice B., MD {1649268012} ObsGyn(84,NY19)<NJ-OVERLOOK, NJ-MORRISTN>
+ Summit Medical Group
890 New Mountain Avenue   New Providence, NJ 07974   (908)277-8601
+ Summit Medical Group-Berkeley Heights Campus
1 Diamond Hill Road/3rd Fl   Berkeley Heights, NJ 07922   (908)277-8601   Fax (908)790-6524

Gibiezaite, Sandra, MD {1255651873} EnDbMt<NJ-STJOSHOS>
+ 57 Willowbrook Boulevard/Suite 303
Wayne, NJ 07470   (973)754-4060
+ St. Joseph's Regional Medical Center
703 Main Street/Medicine   Paterson, NJ 07503   (973)754-4060   Fax (973)754-3376

Gibilisco, Raffaele A., MD {1124134002} Gastrn, IntrMd(85,ITAL)<NJ-HOBUNIMC, NJ-MEADWLND>
+ 435 59th Street/1st Floor
West New York, NJ 07093   (201)295-1456   Fax (201)295-0266

Gibreal, Mohammed, MD {1710242086} CdvDis
+ Hamilton Cardiology Associates
2073 Klockner Road   Hamilton, NJ 08690   (609)584-1212   Fax (609)584-0103

Gibson, Jeffrey T., MD {1851323141} ObsGyn(80,PA13)<NJ-UNDRWD>
+ Premier Women's Health of South Jersey
603 North Broad Street/Suite 300   Woodbury, NJ 08096   (856)223-8930   Fax (856)223-8948
+ Premier Women's Health of South Jersey
340 West Front Street/Suite 201   Elmer, NJ 08318   (856)223-8930   Fax (856)223-8948
+ Premier Women's Health of South Jersey
100 Lexington Road/Bldg 1   Swedesboro, NJ 08096   (856)223-8930   Fax (856)223-8948

Gibson, Lisa Kay, MD {1225294796} FamMed
+ 201 Route 34/Bldg C-3
Colts Neck, NJ 07722   (732)866-2690   Fax (732)866-1165

Gibson-Gill, Carol M., MD {1811098437} InfDis, IntrMd(88,NJ05)<NJ-VAEASTOR>
+ VA New Jersey Health Care System-East Orange Campus
385 Tremont Avenue/Suite 6B   East Orange, NJ 07018   (973)676-1000

Gidding, Samuel S., MD {1124110903} PedCrd, Pedtrc(78,NJ06)<NJ-ACMCMAIN, NJ-ACMCITY>
+ Nemours Dupont Pediatrics, Voorhees
443 Laurel Oak Road   Voorhees, NJ 08043   (856)309-8508   Fax (856)309-8556
+ AtlantiCare/Dupont Children's Health Program
2500 English Creek Avenue   Egg Harbor Township, NJ 08234   (856)309-8508   Fax (609)641-3652

Gidea, Claudia Gabriela, MD {1356374748} CdvDis<NJ-NWRKBETH>
+ Newark Beth Israel Medical Center
201 Lyons Avenue/L4   Newark, NJ 07112   (973)926-7205   Fax (973)923-8993

Gidwaney, Neelam Gail, MD {1538320551}
+ 125 Patterson Street/5th Floor
New Brunswick, NJ 08901   (914)263-2046
neelam.gidwaney@gmail.com

Gieger, Andrew, MD {1205281730} GenPrc
+ McGuire Air Force Base/Acute Health Care Clinic
3458 Neely Road   Trenton, NJ 08641   (609)754-9080   Fax (609)754-9015

Gifford, Deana Marie, MD {1629395595}<NJ-VIRTVOOR>
+ Virtua Voorhees
100 Bowman Drive   Voorhees, NJ 08043   (856)247-3921

Gigante, Paul R., MD {1609026145} SrgNro
+ Neurosurgeons of New Jersey
200 South Orange Avenue/Suite 116   Livingston, NJ 07039   (973)718-9919

Giglio, Michael, MD {1891808259} Otlryg(76,ITAL)<NJ-VALLEY>
+ 623 Lafayette Avenue
Hawthorne, NJ 07506   (973)423-3833   Fax (973)423-4335

Physicians by Name and Address

Gigliotti, David T., DO {1518920552} FamMed(94,PA77)<NJ-KMHCHRRY>
+ Advocare Gigliotti Family Medicine
  181 West White Horse Pike/Suite 100 Berlin, NJ 08009 (856)767-0069 Fax (856)767-2531
  dgigliotti@challc.net

Gigliuto, Christine M., MD {1952374266} IntrMd(87,GRN01)<NJ-SOCEANCO>
+ Coastal Health Care
  1314 Hooper Avenue/Building B Toms River, NJ 08753 (732)349-4994 Fax (732)341-1717

Gigos-Costeas, Sophia, MD {1013977651} Pedtrc, AdolMd, IntrMd(93,NY48)
+ Avenue Pediatrics, LLC
  1140 Bloomfield Avenue/Suite 213 West Caldwell, NJ 07006 (973)228-6302 Fax (973)228-6305

Gil, Constante, MD {1063479335} IntrMd(81,DOMI)<NJ-UNVM-CPRN, NJ-RBAYOLDB>
+ 408 New Brunswick Ave
  Fords, NJ 08863 (732)826-1609 Fax (732)826-0075

Gilad, Ronit, MD {1770743429} SrgNro(03,NY19)<NJ-OVERLOOK, NJ-STBARNMC>
+ IGEA Brain & Spine
  1057 Commerce Avenue Union, NJ 07083 (908)688-8800 Fax (908)688-2377
  rgilad@ucneurosurgery.com

Gilani, Asim Haider, MD {1598756173} IntrMd, FamMed(00,POL12)<NJ-OCEANMC>
+ Total Patient Care
  2401 Route 35 Manasquan, NJ 08736 (732)292-9222 Fax (732)292-9633
+ Total Patient Care LLC
  459 Jack Martin Boulevard Brick, NJ 08724 (732)292-9222 Fax (732)785-1222

Gilbert, Steven L., MD {1174523302} Radiol, RadDia(91,PA13)
+ South Jersey Radiology Associates, P.A.
  748 Kings Highway West Deptford, NJ 08096 (856)848-4998 Fax (856)853-7362
+ South Jersey Radiology Associates, P.A.
  Severan Profess Mews/Suite 105 Sewell, NJ 08080 (856)848-4998 Fax (856)589-6142
+ SJRA South Jersey Radiology Associates, P.A.
  113 East Laurel Road Stratford, NJ 08096 (856)566-2552

Gilbert, Tricia Todisco, MD {1720177090} PulCCr, CritCr, SlpDis(97,NJ06)
+ Pulmonary & Intensive Care Specialists of NJ
  593 Cranbury Road East Brunswick, NJ 08816 (732)613-8880 Fax (732)613-0077

Gildengers, Jaime N., MD {1699761924} Surgry(65,ARG01)
+ 313 60th Street
  West New York, NJ 07093 (201)854-0406 Fax (201)854-8437

Gilder, Mark E., MD {1356316525} SrgC&R(87,NY08)<NJ-OVER-LOOK>
+ Associates in Colon and Rectal Diseases
  231 Millburn Avenue Millburn, NJ 07041 (973)467-2277 Fax (973)467-4037

Gildiner, Lennard R., MD {1457322596} ObsGyn(86,PA09)<NJ-VIRTBERL, NJ-VIRTVOOR>
+ Ob-Gyn Care of Southern New Jersey
  406 Gibbsboro Road East Lindenwold, NJ 08021 (856)435-7007 Fax (856)435-7077

Giles, Robert A., MD {1093759649} EmrgMd(95,MI07)<NJ-CLARMAAS>
+ Clara Maass Medical Center
  1 Clara Maass Drive/EmergMed Belleville, NJ 07109 (973)450-2000

Giles, Thomas William, DO {1366470767} EmrgMd(97,MO78)<NJ-COMMED>
+ Community Medical Center
  99 Route 37 West/EmergMed Toms River, NJ 08755 (732)557-8000

Gilhooly, Patricia Eileen, MD {1073627949} Urolgy(76,NY01)<NJ-VAEASTOR, NJ-UMDNJ>
+ VA New Jersey Health Care System-East Orange Campus
  385 Tremont Avenue/Urology(112) East Orange, NJ 07018 (973)676-1000 Fax (973)395-7197
  patricia.gilhooly@mcd.va.gov
+ New Jersey Urology, LLC
  700 North Broad Street/Suite 302 Elizabeth, NJ 07208 (973)676-1000 Fax (908)289-0716

Giliberti, Francesca Marie, MD {1790001279}
+ Giliberti Eye & Laser Center PC
  415 Totowa Road Totowa, NJ 07512 (973)595-0011 Fax (973)595-5155

Giliberti, Orazio L., MD {1407896475} Ophthl(82,GRN01)<NJ-CLARMAAS, NJ-UMDNJ>
+ Giliberti Eye & Laser Center PC
  415 Totowa Road Totowa, NJ 07512 (973)595-0011 Fax (973)595-5155

Giliberti, Rocco A., DO {1013970086} IntrMd, Grtrcs(82,PA77)<NJ-OCEANMC>
+ 2911 Route 88/Suite B-3
  Point Pleasant Beach, NJ 08742 (732)892-9920 Fax (732)295-6625

Giliberti, William S., MD {1801802459} SrgOrt, IntrMd(74,ITAL)<NJ-HCKTSTWN>
+ The Orthopedic Institute of New Jersey
  108 Bilby Road/Suite 201 Hackettstown, NJ 07840 (908)684-3005 Fax (908)684-3301
+ The Orthopedic Institute of New Jersey
  254-B Mountain Avenue/Suite 201 Hackettstown, NJ 07840 (908)684-3005 Fax (908)684-3301
+ The Orthopedic Institute of New Jersey
  222 High Street/Suite 202 Newton, NJ 07840 (908)684-3005 Fax (908)684-3301

Gilkey, Edward A., MD {1982152138} FamMed(83,NY08)<NJ-VIRTMHBC, NJ-WARREN>
+ Warren Hospital
  185 Roseberry Street Phillipsburg, NJ 08865 (908)859-6700

Gill, Jasrai Singh, MD {1538336904} CdvDis, IntCrd(06,NY03)
+ Shore Heart Group, P.A.
  1820 State Route 33/Suite 4-B Neptune, NJ 07753 (732)776-8500 Fax (732)776-8946
+ Shore Heart Group, P.A.
  9 Mule Road/Suite E-3 Toms River, NJ 08755 (732)776-8500 Fax (732)281-1105
+ Shore Heart Group, P.A.
  555 Iron Bridge Road/Suite 15 Freehold, NJ 07753 (732)308-0774 Fax (732)333-1366

Gill, Melissa, MD {1467602581} PthDrm, PthAna(01,RI01)
+ Quest Diagnostics Inc.
  1 Malcolm Avenue Teterboro, NJ 07608 (201)393-5000 Fax (201)393-6127

Gill, Ramneet Kaur, MD {1598928103} Pedtrc(05,GRN01)
+ Pediatric Pulmonology
  100 Madison Avenue Morristown, NJ 07960 (973)971-4142 Fax (973)290-7360

Gill, Rupinder K., MD {1649484791} PedGst(04,WV02)<NJ-STPETER>
+ St. Peter's University Hospital
  254 Easton Avenue/Gastro New Brunswick, NJ 08901 (732)745-8600 Fax (732)937-9428

Gillam, Linda Dawn, MD {1457359382} CdvDis, IntrMd(76,ON05)<NY-PRSBCOLU>
+ Electrophysiology Associates, PA
  100 Madison Avenue/Suite 5 Morristown, NJ 07962 (973)971-5899 Fax (973)290-7253

Gillard, Bonita Dee, MD {1760446918} Pedtrc(95,NJ06)<NJ-OVERLOOK>
+ Watchung Pediatrics
  346 South Avenue/Suite 3 Fanwood, NJ 07023 (908)889-8687 Fax (908)889-0047
+ Watchung Pediatrics
  76 Stirling Road/Suite 201 Warren, NJ 07059 (908)889-8687 Fax (908)755-6905
+ Watchung Pediatrics
  225 Millburn Avenue/Suite 301 Millburn, NJ 07023 (973)376-7337 Fax (973)218-6647

Gillespie, Christine, MD {1902956998} Otlryg
+ Ocean Otolaryngology Associates
  54 Bey Lea Road/Suite 3 Toms River, NJ 08753 (732)281-0100 Fax (732)281-0400

Gillespie, Kevin A., MD {1831139559} EmrgMd, FamMed(80,MEX14)<NJ-JFKMED>
+ JFK Medical Center
  65 James Street/EmergMed Edison, NJ 08820 (732)321-7605 Fax (732)744-5614

Gillick, John, MD {1821499344} SrgNro
+ Center for Neurological Surgery UMDNJ
  90 Bergen Street/DOC 8100 Newark, NJ 07103 (973)972-2323 Fax (973)972-2333

Gillin, James Scott, MD {1639167000} Gastrn, IntrMd(79,NJ05)<NJ-OVERLOOK, NJ-MORRISTN>
+ Summit Medical Group-Berkeley Heights Campus
  1 Diamond Hill Road Berkeley Heights, NJ 07922 (908)673-7140 Fax (908)790-6576

Gillio, Alfred Peter, III, MD {1588602270} PedHem, Pedtrc(81,VA04)<NJ-HACKNSK>
+ Hackensack University Medical Center
  30 Prospect Avenue/Pedtrcs Hackensack, NJ 07601 (201)996-5600 Fax (201)996-5336
+ Tomorrow's Children's Inst/HUMC
  30 Prospect Avenue/WFAN - PC 116 Hackensack, NJ 07601 (201)996-5437

Gillis, Christopher Charles, MD {1669891180} SrgNro
+ Neurosurgical Associates of NJ
  121 Highway 36 West/Suite 330 West Long Branch, NJ 07764 (732)222-8866 Fax (732)870-6432

Gillis Funderburk, Sheri Anita, MD {1922078195} EnDbMt(01,NJ06)
+ Capital Endocrinology
  2 Capital Way/Suite 290 Pennington, NJ 08534 (609)303-4300 Fax (609)303-4301

Gillis-Harry, Deinso Abayomi, MD (82,NIGE)
+ 87 Knickerbocker Road
  Englewood, NJ 07631

Gilliss, Adam C., DO {1982741328} FamMed(92,PA77)<NJ-OURLADY>
+ Drs. Gilliss and DiRenzo
  27 East Chestnut Avenue Merchantville, NJ 08109 (856)662-0424 Fax (856)662-7404
+ University Hospital-University Family Medicine
  42 East Laurel Road/Suite 2100 Stratford, NJ 08084 (856)662-0424 Fax (856)566-6188

Gilliss, Matthew J., DO {1629107941} FamMed
+ Drs. Gilliss and DiRenzo
  27 East Chestnut Avenue Merchantville, NJ 08109 (856)662-0424 Fax (856)662-7404

Gillon, Steven D., DO {1285668376} Gastrn, IntrMd(86,FL75)<NJ-ENGLWOOD, NJ-HOLYNAME>
+ 401 South Van Brunt Street/Suite 400
  Englewood, NJ 07631 (201)569-0555 Fax (201)569-3111

Gillum, Diane, MD {1174511091} Surgry(81,PA02)
+ Kennedy Health Alliance
  900 Medical Center Drive/Suite 201 Sewell, NJ 08080 (856)218-2100 Fax (856)218-2101
+ Breast Specialty Care Group
  1605 East Evesham Road/Suite 2-B Voorhees, NJ 08043 (856)218-2100 Fax (856)424-8007

Gilly, Frank J., Jr., MD {1891785291} FamMed, Grtrcs(77,MD07)<NJ-WARREN>
+ Warren Hills Family Health Center
  315 Route 31 South Washington, NJ 07882 (908)689-0777 Fax (908)835-3037

Gilman, Arthur Michael, MD {1710045901} SrgNro(86,VA07)<NJ-NWRKBETH>
+ SBMC-Institute for Neurosurgery
  94 Old Short Hills Road Livingston, NJ 07039 (973)322-6732

Gilman, Elizabeth Ann, MD {1316963853} EmrgMd(99,NY03)<NJ-MONMOUTH>
+ Monmouth Medical Center
  300 Second Avenue Long Branch, NJ 07740 (732)222-5200

Gilman, Howard E., MD {1669492229} Psychy, PsyFor, PsyGrt(78,WI06)
+ 1172 East Ridgewood Avenue
  Ridgewood, NJ 07450 (201)612-6050 Fax (201)612-0422

Gilmandyar, Dzhamala, MD {1609016815} ObsGyn
+ University Medical Group/OBGYN
  125 Paterson Street/2nd Floor New Brunswick, NJ 08901 (732)235-6632 Fax (732)235-7349

Gilmartin, Andrew Philip, MD {1205119807} IntrMd(08,GRN01)
+ Vanguard Medical Group, P.A.
  170 Changebridge Road/Suite C-3 Montville, NJ 07045 (973)575-5540 Fax (973)575-4885

Gilmour, Kevin P., DO {1275540106} IntrMd, PulDis(86,NY75)
+ South Jersey Chest Diseases
  107 Vine Street Hammonton, NJ 08037 (609)561-7666 Fax (609)561-8347

Gilo, Belen Frias, MD {1871515775} Pedtrc(73,PHIL)
+ 492 Ferry Street
  Newark, NJ 07105 (973)344-3444 Fax (973)344-3444

Gilo, Elmer S., MD {1598764912} FamMed(73,PHI09)
+ Denville Family Practice
  16 Pocono Road/Suite 307 Denville, NJ 07834 (973)625-3515 Fax (973)627-2842

Gilsenan, Michele T., DO {1821066283} FamMed, SprtMd, FamMSptM(88,ME75)<NJ-OVERLOOK>
+ Summit Medical Group
  67 Walnut Avenue/Suite 202 Clark, NJ 07066 (732)388-7300 Fax (732)388-1330
+ Sports Extra
  67 Walnut Avenue/Suite 202B Clark, NJ 07066 (732)388-7300 Fax (732)388-1330

Gilson, Cynthia T., MD {1811947047} Dermat(83,NY08)
+ Drs. Gilson, Orsini & Miller
  223 Monmouth Road West Long Branch, NJ 07764 (732)870-2992 Fax (732)870-2533

Gilson, Noah R., MD {1821054230} Nrolgy(82,IL43)<NJ-MONMOUTH, NJ-RIVERVW>
+ Neurology Specialists of Monmouth County
  107 Monmouth Road/Suite 110 West Long Branch, NJ 07764 (732)935-1850 Fax (732)544-0494

Gimovsky, Martin Larry, MD {1497721823} ObsGyn, MtFtMd(76,NY19)<NJ-NWRKBETH>
+ Newark Beth Israel Medical Center
  201 Lyons Avenue/ViceChair/ObGyn Newark, NJ 07112 (973)926-4787 Fax (973)923-7497
  mgimovsky@SBHCS.com

Physicians by Name and Address

Ginalis, Ernest M., MD {1629151048} Surgry(85,GRE03)<NJ-MONMOUTH>
  + 279 Third Avenue/Suite 407
    Long Branch, NJ 07740 (732)229-8486 Fax (732)229-1576

Ginart, Gaspar L., MD {1891741765} Pedtrc, AdolMd(88,DOM02)<NJ-STJOSHOS>
  + Paterson Community Health Center
    227 Broadway Paterson, NJ 07501 (973)278-2600 Fax (973)278-5837

Gingerelli, Frank, MD {1285704387} Radiol, RadOnc(67,NE06)
  + 250 Old Hook Road
    Westwood, NJ 07675 (201)358-3666 Fax (201)358-1140

Gingold, Alan R., DO {1578670253} Gastrn, IntrMd(00,NY75)<NJ-SOMERSET>
  + Digestive HealthCare Center
    511 Courtyard Drive/Building 500 Hillsborough, NJ 08844 (908)218-9222 Fax (908)218-9818

Ginn-Scott, Elizabeth J., MD {1326252941} Psychy, PsyNro(04,ISR05)
  + CPC Behavioral HealthCare
    270 Highway 35 Red Bank, NJ 07701 (732)842-2000 Fax (732)224-0688
  + CPC Behavioral HealthCare
    37 Court Street Freehold, NJ 07728 (732)842-2000 Fax (732)780-5157

Ginsberg, Claudia Lisa, MD {1366533309} IntrMd, SprtMd(99,NY20)<NJ-MORRISTN>
  + Tri-County Orthopedics
    160 East Hanover Avenue Morristown, NJ 07962 (973)538-2334 Fax (973)829-9174

Ginsberg, Ferris, DO {1326111378} Radiol, RadDia(81,NJ75)
  + Central Jersey Radiologists
    2128 State Route 35 Oakhurst, NJ 07755 (732)493-8444 Fax (732)493-4185

Ginsberg, Fredric L., MD {1528156981} CdvDis, IntrMd(77,PA02)<NJ-COOPRUMC>
  + Cooper University Hospital
    One Cooper Plaza/Cardiology Camden, NJ 08103 (856)342-2000
  + University Cardiology
    3 Cooper Plaza/Room 311 Camden, NJ 08103 (856)342-2034

Ginsberg, Hal N., MD {1194815068} RadDia(83,DOM03)<NJ-MORRISTN>
  + Morris Imaging Associates
    66 Maple Avenue/Suite 2 Morristown, NJ 07960 (973)267-1274 Fax (973)267-2912
  + Morristown Medical Center
    100 Madison Avenue/Radiology Morristown, NJ 07962 (973)971-5000
  + Memorial Radiology Associates
    10 Lanidex Plaza West/Suite 125 Parsippany, NJ 07960 (973)503-5700 Fax (973)386-5701

Ginsberg, Janet A., MD {1447667449} Pedtrc
  + 321 Forest Avenue
    Lyndhurst, NJ 07071 (201)745-2512

Ginsberg, Sanford Ginsberg, MD {1750601068} Anesth
  + Anesthesia Consultnts of NJ/Nova Pain
    285 Davidson Avenue/Suite 204 Somerset, NJ 08873 (732)271-1400 Fax (732)271-3543

Ginsberg, Steven H., MD {1205918059} Anesth, CdvDis(85,MEX03)<NJ-RWJUBRUN>
  + Robert Wood Johnson-UMDNJ Anesthesia Group
    125 Paterson Street/CAB 3100 New Brunswick, NJ 08901 (732)235-7827 Fax (732)235-6131

Ginsberg, Terrie Beth, DO {1750361663} Grtrcs
  + New Jersey Institute for Successful Aging
    42 East Laurel Road/Suite 1800 Stratford, NJ 08084 (856)566-6843 Fax (856)566-6781

Ginsburg, Deborah J., MD {1750397642} FamMed(92,CA14)<NJ-CHSFULD, NJ-CHSMRCER>
  + Capital Health Family Health Center
    433 Bellevue Avenue/4th Floor Trenton, NJ 08618 (609)815-7296 Fax (609)815-7178
  + Capital Health Primary Care
    4056 Quakerbridge Road/Suite 101 Lawrenceville, NJ 08648 (609)815-7296 Fax (609)528-9151

Ginsburg, Jeffrey B., MD {1043204332} Otlryg, PedOto(92,NY09)<NJ-CHILTON, NY-NYEYEINF>
  + ENT and Facial Plastic Surgeons
    51 Route 23 South/2nd Floor Riverdale, NJ 07457 (973)831-1220 Fax (973)831-0029
    JMGINS@optonline.net
  + Wayne Surgical Center, LLC.
    1176 Hamburg Pike Wayne, NJ 07470 (973)831-1220 Fax (973)709-1901

Ginty, Catherine, MD {1912265331}<NJ-COOPRUMC>
  + Cooper University Hospital
    One Cooper Plaza/EmergMed Camden, NJ 08103 (856)342-2627

Ginwala, Khatoon T., MD {1235169202} ObsGyn(68,INDI)<NJ-VIRTMHBC>
  + Alliance Ob/Gyn Consultants
    5045 Route 130 South/Suite 1 Delran, NJ 08075 (856)764-7660 Fax (856)764-5723

Giobbe, Raphael C., MD {1710075775} RadDia, Radiol(68,ITAL)
  + 5 Dellmead Drive
    Livingston, NJ 07039

Gioia, Kevin Thomas, MD {1053578831}
  + Coastal Urology Associates
    446 Jack Martin Boulevard Brick, NJ 08724 (732)840-4300 Fax (732)840-4515

Gioia, Mario, MD {1285098830}<NJ-MORRISTN>
  + Morristown Medical Center
    100 Madison Avenue Morristown, NJ 07962 (973)971-5000

Giordano, Carl P., MD {1497710511} SrgOrt, SrgSpn, NeuM-SptM(86,NJ05)<NJ-MORRISTN, NJ-OVERLOOK>
  + Atlantic Spine Specialists
    131 Madison Avenue Morristown, NJ 07960 (973)971-3500 Fax (973)683-0016

Giordano, Samuel Nicholas, MD {1780892968} IntrMd
  + 1805 Roberts Way
    Voorhees, NJ 08043 (732)674-1081

Giordano Farmer, Jill Marie, DO {1851548671} Nrolgy
  + Drexel Neurosciences Institute
    3100 Princeton Pike Lawrenceville, NJ 08648 (215)762-6915 Fax (215)762-6914
  + Drexel Neurosciences Institute
    601 Route 73 North Marlton, NJ 08053 (215)762-6915 Fax (215)762-6914

Giorgi, Marilyn V., MD {1457466559} Pedtrc, NnPnMd(00,DC03)
  + 15 Snowden Road
    East Brunswick, NJ 08816

Giorgio, Anthony Richard, MD {1740446442} Anesth, IntrMd, PainMd(73,PA13)<NJ-UNDRWD, NJ-MEMSALEM>
  + Inspira Health Network
    509 North Broad Street/Anesth Woodbury, NJ 08096 (856)845-0100

Giorlando, Mary Elizabeth, MD {1306887724} FamMed(87,MEX03)<NJ-VALLEY>
  + Prospect Medical Offices, LLC
    301 Godwin Avenue Midland Park, NJ 07432 (201)444-4526 Fax (201)301-1313

Giove, Gian-Carlo, MD {1700194966} IntrMd(05,PER11)<NJ-MORRISTN>
  + Morristown Medical Center
    100 Madison Avenue/Suite 5 Morristown, NJ 07962 (973)971-7496

Giovine, Anthony P., MD {1780632281} ObsGyn(86,NJ05)<NJ-MONMOUTH, NJ-RIVERVW>
  + A Woman's Place
    34 Sycamore Avenue Little Silver, NJ 07739 (732)747-9310 Fax (732)747-9320
  + A Woman's Place - Lakewood
    820 East County Line Road/Suite A Lakewood, NJ 08701 (732)747-9310 Fax (732)364-7271
  + A Woman's Place - Colts Neck
    310 Route 34/Suite 1 Colts Neck, NJ 07739 (732)845-0606 Fax (732)845-3606

Gips, Sanford J., MD {1366493942} CdvDis, IntCrd(89,MD07)<NJ-COOPRUMC, NJ-VIRTMARL>
  + Cardiovascular Associates
    210 West Atlantic Avenue Haddon Heights, NJ 08035 (856)546-3003 Fax (856)547-5337
  + Cardiovascular Associates of The Delaware Valley, PA
    1840 Frontage Road Cherry Hill, NJ 08034 (856)546-3003 Fax (856)795-7436
  + Cardiovascular Associates of The Delaware Valley, PA
    525 State Street/Suite 3 Elmer, NJ 08035 (856)358-2363 Fax (856)358-0725

Giraldo, Juan Pablo, MD {1114958626} Anesth, PainMd(85,COLO)<NJ-BERGNMC>
  + New Bridge Medical Center
    230 East Ridgewood Avenue Paramus, NJ 07652 (201)967-4000

Girardy, James Douglas, MD {1497756936} PhysMd, IntrMd(96,NY03)<NJ-SOMERSET>
  + Robalino-Sanghavi, Michelle Marie
    120 Eagle Rock Avenue/Suite 154 East Hanover, NJ 07936 (201)447-4772
  + Rehabilitation Specialists of New Jersey
    505 Goffle Road/Suite 3 Ridgewood, NJ 07450 (201)447-4772 Fax (201)447-4277

Girgis, Ihab, MD {1134109895} ClCdEl, CdvDis, IntrMd(88,NY48)<NJ-JRSYSHMC, NJ-COMMED>
  + Shore Heart Group, P.A.
    1820 State Route 33/Suite 4-B Neptune, NJ 07753 (732)776-8500 Fax (732)776-8946
  + Shore Heart Group, P.A.
    35 Beaverson Boulevard/Suite 9-B Brick, NJ 08723 (732)776-8500 Fax (732)262-4317
  + Shore Heart Group, P.A.
    9 Mule Road/Suite E-3 Toms River, NJ 07753 (732)281-1101 Fax (732)281-1105

Girgis, Linda Mae, MD {1295721108} FamMed(94,GRN01)
  + Girgis Family Medicine
    171 Main Street/Suite 4 South River, NJ 08882 (732)254-9494 Fax (732)254-9903

Girgis, Magdy S., MD {1497729867} Anesth(80,EGY04)<NJ-BAYSHORE, NJ-EASTORNG>
  + Bayshore Community Hospital
    727 North Beers Street/Anesth Holmdel, NJ 07733 (732)739-5900

Girgis, Moris Beachay, MD {1699761502} FamMed(84,EGY05)
  + Girgis Family Medicine
    171 Main Street/Suite 4 South River, NJ 08882 (732)254-9494 Fax (732)254-9903

Girgis, Raymond Michael, MD {1851464234} Ophthl, IntrMd(91,ON02)<NJ-KENEDYHS, NJ-VIRTUAHS>
  + Center for Eye Care
    123 Egg Harbor Road/Suite 300 Sewell, NJ 08080 (856)290-4548 Fax (856)290-4552

Girgis, Wahid S., MD {1073518205} RadDia, Radiol(96,NJ05)<NJ-JRSYSHMC>
  + University Radiology Group, P.C.
    579A Cranbury Road East Brunswick, NJ 08816 (732)390-0040 Fax (732)390-1856
  + University Radiology Group
    2100 Route 33/Neptune City Med Bld Neptune, NJ 07753 (732)390-0040 Fax (732)502-0368
  + University Radiology Group
    900 West Main Street Freehold, NJ 08816 (732)462-1900 Fax (732)462-1848

Giri, Janaki, MD {1215959879} IntrMd, OncHem(66,INDI)<NJ-RBAYOLDB, NJ-BAYSHORE>
  + 200 Perrine Road/Suite 210
    Old Bridge, NJ 08857 (732)525-0028 Fax (732)525-2460

Giri, Kartik S., MD {1104878768} CdvDis, IntCrd, IntrMd(97,PA02)<NJ-COOPRUMC, NJ-OURLADY>
  + Cardiovascular Associates
    210 West Atlantic Avenue Haddon Heights, NJ 08035 (856)546-3003 Fax (856)547-5337
  + Cardiovascular Associates of The Delaware Valley, PA
    1840 Frontage Road Cherry Hill, NJ 08034 (856)546-3003 Fax (856)795-7436
  + Cardiovascular Associates of The Delaware Valley, PA
    525 State Street/Suite 3 Elmer, NJ 08035 (856)358-2363 Fax (856)358-0725

Giri, Suresh C., MD {1245313931} Otlryg, OtgyPSHN(75,INDI)<NJ-KIMBALL, NJ-COMMED>
  + 101 Prospect Street/Suite 117
    Lakewood, NJ 08701 (732)364-7776 Fax (732)905-9407

Girnar, Digvijaysi, MD {1215919741} Anesth(63,INDI)<NJ-HACKNSK>
  + Hackensack University Medical Center
    30 Prospect Avenue Hackensack, NJ 07601 (201)996-2000 Fax (201)488-6769
  + Hackensack University MC-Anesthesia Dept
    30 Prospect Avenue/Room 2703 Hackensack, NJ 07601 (201)996-2000 Fax (201)996-3962

Giron, Miguel, MD {1912927930} EmrgMd(95,NY08)<NJ-CENTRAST>
  + CentraState Medical Center
    901 West Main Street/EmergMed Freehold, NJ 07728 (732)431-2000

Giron-Jimenez, Sandra, MD {1568430189} ObsGyn(97,NY15)
  + Ob-Gyn Associates of North Jersey
    7400 Bergenline Avenue North Bergen, NJ 07047 (201)869-5488 Fax (201)869-6944

Girone, Joseph Francis, MD {1366692253} Nephro, IntrMd(83,NJ05)
  + CompleteCare Adult & Specialty Medical Professionals
    1038 East Chestnut Avenue/Suite 110 Vineland, NJ 08360 (856)451-4700

Gironta, Michael Gerard, DO {1013985928} IntrMd, VasDis(91,NY75)<NJ-STCLRDEN, NJ-MORRISTN>
  + Eastern Vascular Associates
    16 Pocono Road/Suite 313 Denville, NJ 07834 (973)625-0112 Fax (973)625-0721

Giroski, Laura J., DO {1891739561} EmrgMd(88,PA77)<NJ-SOMERSET>
  + Emergency Medical Associates of NJ, P.A.
    3 Century Drive Parsippany, NJ 07054 (973)740-0607 Fax (973)740-9895

Girshovich, Irina, MD {1043287212} IntrMd(72,LAT03)<NJ-CHRIST>
  + Dr. Girshovich Medical Care
    810 Abbott Boulevard/Suite 20 Fort Lee, NJ 07024 (201)886-9699 Fax (201)886-9015

Physicians by Name and Address

Girz, Barbara A., DO {1487685780} MtFtMd(82,OH75)<NJ-STCLR-DEN>
+ St. Clare's Hospital-Denville Campus
  25 Pocono Road Denville, NJ 07834 (973)625-6000 Fax (973)983-2107

Gistrak, Michael Andrew, MD {1396793972} PthAcl, Pthlgy(90,NY20)<NJ-RWJURAH>
+ Robert Wood Johnson University Hospital at Rahway
  865 Stone Street/Path Rahway, NJ 07065 (732)381-4200 Fax (732)499-6122

Gitler, Steven F., DO {1669559266} FamMed(90,PA77)<NJ-SJRSYELM>
+ Drs. Gitler and Kleeman
  2961 Yorkship Square Camden, NJ 08104 (856)541-5588

Gittell, Amy, DO {1164592648} Pedtrc(81,NY75)
+ Mercer Pediatrics Associates
  3131 Princeton Pike Lawrenceville, NJ 08648 (609)896-2922 Fax (609)896-2502

Gittens-Williams, Lisa Nadine, MD {1043243504} ObsGyn, MtFtMd(87,PA13)<NJ-UMDNJ>
+ University Physician Associates
  140 Bergen Street/ACC Level C Newark, NJ 07103 (973)972-2700 Fax (973)972-2739

Gitterman, Benjamin Eric, MD {1447349162} IntrMd(94,PA13)<NJ-UNVMCPRN>
+ Princeton Medical Group, P.A.
  419 North Harrison Street Princeton, NJ 08540 (609)924-9300 Fax (609)924-6552
+ Princeton Medical Group PA
  2 Research Way/Bldg 2/Suite 302 Monroe Township, NJ 08831 (609)924-9300 Fax (609)655-7466

Gittleman, Neal D., MD {1255379772} Pedtrc(84,MA05)<NJ-KIMBALL>
+ Dr. Gittleman & Associates
  450 East Kennedy Boulevard Lakewood, NJ 08701 (732)901-0050 Fax (732)370-2386

Giudice, James C., DO {1053381244} PulDis, IntrMd(68,PA77)
+ SOM - Department of Internal Medicine
  42 East Laurel Road/Suite 3100 Stratford, NJ 08084 (856)566-6859 Fax (856)566-6906

Giuffrida, Angela Ylenia, MD {1457562548} SrgHnd, SrgOrt(03,NJ05)<NJ-HACKNSK, NJ-VALLEY>
+ Active Orthopaedics & Sports Medicine
  25 Prospect Avenue Hackensack, NJ 07601 (201)343-2277 Fax (201)343-7410
+ Active Orthopaedics & Sports Medicine
  440 Old Hook Road Emerson, NJ 07630 (201)343-2277 Fax (201)358-9777

Giuglianotti, Daniel Scott, DO {1154682979} FamMed
+ Kennedy Care Center
  705 White Horse Road/Suite D-101-2 Voorhees, NJ 08043 (856)783-0695 Fax (856)783-8083

Giuliano, Michael A., MD {1295850063} PsycAd, Psychy(70,WI06)
+ 261 James Street/Suite 3-G
  Morristown, NJ 07960 (973)540-9492 Fax (973)540-0716

Giuliano, Michael Gerard, DO {1376546325} FamMed, Grtrcs, FamMGrtc(81,PA77)<NH-MONADNK>
+ 622 Franklin Avenue
  Nutley, NJ 07110 (973)661-1900 Fax (973)661-3658

Giunta, Michael Anthony, MD {1558651737} IntrMd
+ The Advanced Pulmonary Diagnostic Center
  100 Medical Center Way Somers Point, NJ 08244 (609)653-3500 Fax (609)653-3586

Giuseffi, Vincent J., III, MD {1760433973} Ophthl, IntrMd(89,LA01)<NJ-OVERLOOK>
+ The Eye Center
  65 Mountain Boulevard Ext/Suite 105 Warren, NJ 07059 (732)356-6200 Fax (732)356-0228
+ The Eye Center
  213 Stelton Road Piscataway, NJ 08854 (732)356-6200 Fax (732)752-9492
+ The Eye Center
  3900 Park Avenue/Suite 106 Edison, NJ 07059 (732)603-2101

Giyanani, Sunita M., MD {1972535060} ObsGyn(64,INA67)<NJ-SJHREGMC>
+ Drs. Babalola and Giyanani
  1601 North 2nd Street/Suite C1 Millville, NJ 08332 (856)691-3145 Fax (856)691-0625
+ Community Health Care Inc
  484 South Brewster Road Vineland, NJ 08360 (856)691-3145 Fax (856)696-2561
+ Community Health Care, Inc.
  70 Cohansey Street Bridgeton, NJ 08332 (856)451-4700 Fax (856)451-0029

Gjenvick, Timothy C., MD {1003905498} IntrMd, Grtrcs(76,WI06)<NJ-UNVMCPRN>
+ Princeton Medical Group PA
  2 Research Way/Bldg 2/Suite 302 Monroe Township, NJ 08831 (609)655-8800 Fax (609)655-7466
+ Princeton Medical Group, P.A.
  419 North Harrison Street Princeton, NJ 08540 (609)655-8800 Fax (609)924-6552

Gjoni, Indira, MD {1992094726}
+ Mountainside Family Practice Associates
  799 Bloomfield Avenue/Suite 201 Verona, NJ 07044 (973)746-7050 Fax (973)857-2831

Gladstone, Clifford D., MD {1548266265} CdvDis(89,NY19)<NJ-STPETER, NJ-RWJUBRUN>
+ RWJPE/New Brunswick Cardiology Group, P.A.
  75 Veronica Road/Suite 101 Somerset, NJ 08873 (732)247-7444 Fax (732)247-5119
+ RWJPE New Brunswick Cardiology Group, P.A.
  111 Union Valley Road/Suite 201 Monroe Township, NJ 08831 (732)247-7444 Fax (609)409-6882
+ RWJPE New Brunswick Cardiology Group, P.A.
  15H Briar Hill Court East Brunswick, NJ 08873 (732)613-9313

Glantz, Eric J., DO {1821385568}
+ Rowan University-School of Osteopathic Medicine
  1 Medical Center Drive Stratford, NJ 08084 (856)566-6707

Glaser, Ariella N., MD {1477650067} EmrgMd(02,NY47)<NJ-ENGLWOOD>
+ Englewood Hospital and Medical Center
  350 Engle Street/EmrgMed Englewood, NJ 07631 (201)894-3000

Glaser, Aylon Y., MD {1598938433} Otlryg(03,NY46)
+ ENT and Allergy Associates (ENTA)
  79 Hudson Street/Suite 303 Hoboken, NJ 07030 (201)792-1109 Fax (201)792-1145

Glaser-Schanzer, Felice, MD {1205163706} Pedtrc(93,NY46)
+ University Pediatric Associates PA
  317 Cleveland Avenue Highland Park, NJ 08904 (732)249-8999 Fax (732)249-7827

Glasgold, Mark J., MD {1487729034} Otlryg, SrgFPl, SrgRec(88,PA02)
+ Glasgold Group for Plastic Surgery
  31 River Road Highland Park, NJ 08904 (732)846-6540 Fax (732)846-8231

Glasgold, Robert Alexander, MD {1558436113} SrgFPl(97,NJ06)
+ Glasgold Group for Plastic Surgery
  31 River Road Highland Park, NJ 08904 (732)846-6540 Fax (732)846-8231

Glashofer, Marc David, MD {1851340418} Dermat, DerMOH, SrgDer(01,DC01)
+ The Dermatology Group, P.C.
  347 Mount Pleasant Avenue/Suite 103 West Orange, NJ 07052 (973)571-2121 Fax (973)498-0569
  mglashofer@thedermatologygroup.com

Glashow, Marisa Brittany, DO {1609216811} EmrgMd<NJ-JRSYSHMC>
+ Jersey Shore University Medical Center
  1945 Route 33 Neptune, NJ 07753 (732)775-5500

Glasnapp, Angela Jack, MD {1497076012} Surgry
+ New Jersey Bariatric Center
  193 Morris Avenue/2nd Floor Springfield, NJ 07081 (908)481-1270 Fax (908)688-8861

Glasofer, Adam K., MD {1376679563} Pedtrc, IntrMd(05,PA02)<NJ-VIRTVOOR, NJ-VIRTBERL>
+ Virtua Perinatology Associates
  101 Carnie Boulevard/Antenatal Unit Voorhees, NJ 08043 (856)325-3328
+ Virtua Voorhees
  100 Bowman Drive/Pediatrics Voorhees, NJ 08043 (856)325-3328 Fax (856)247-3922
+ Virtua Memorial
  175 Madison Avenue/Pediatrics Mount Holly, NJ 08043 (609)914-7051 Fax (609)265-7931

Glasofer, Eric David, MD {1033176136} Allrgy, Pedtrc(78,PA02)<NJ-OURLADY, NJ-VIRTVOOR>
+ Lourdes Pediatric Associates
  2475 McClellan Avenue/Building B201 Pennsauken, NJ 08109 (856)330-6300 Fax (856)330-6305

Glasofer, Sidney, MD {1699932343} CdvDis, IntrMd, CarNuc(03,NJ05)<NJ-OVERLOOK, NJ-MMHKEMBL>
+ Associates in Cardiovascular Disease, LLC
  571 Central Avenue/Suite 101 New Providence, NJ 07974 (908)464-4200 Fax (908)464-1332
+ Associates in Cardiovascular Disease
  2253 South Avenue Scotch Plains, NJ 07076 (908)654-3300

Glass, Andrew S., MD {1679622500} SrgNro(86,NY47)<NJ-ACMCITY, NJ-SHOREMEM>
+ Coastal Physicians and Surgeons
  110 Harbor Lane/Suite A Somers Point, NJ 08244 (609)653-9110 Fax (609)653-4105

Glass, Charles Adam, MD {1467748632} Ophthl
+ Garden State Community Medical Center
  100 Brick Road/Suite 115 Marlton, NJ 08053 (856)983-1400 Fax (856)983-1681

Glass, Gary M., MD {1831241371} Psychy, PsyFor(74,MEX14)
+ 3137 Fire Road/Suite A
  Egg Harbor Township, NJ 08234 (609)646-3272 Fax (609)646-3129

Glass, Gina Gill, MD {1518940394} FamMed(94,LA01)<NJ-UNDRWD>
+ Complete Care Family Medicine
  75 West Red Bank Avenue Woodbury, NJ 08096 (856)853-2055 Fax (856)848-2879

Glass, James M., MD {1790841666} IntrMd(94,LA01)
+ Virtua Medford Medical Center
  128 Route 70 Medford, NJ 08055 (609)953-7111 Fax (609)953-1544

Glass, Joel Bennett, MD {1861537219} Psychy(68,PA01)<NJ-VIRT-MARL, NJ-COOPRUMC>
+ 8004-E Lincoln Drive West
  Marlton, NJ 08053 (856)983-3830 Fax (856)983-3837
  drjpsych68@aol.com

Glass, Nina Elizabeth, MD {1346483815} SrgTrm
+ Rutgers- New Jersey Medical School
  185 South Orange Avenue/MSB G-526 Newark, NJ 07103 (973)972-6293 Fax (973)972-6803

Glass, Phillip, MD {1467590992} ObsGyn(71,PA02)<NJ-VIRTMHBC>
+ 514 Knight Place
  Cherry Hill, NJ 08003 (856)427-0097 Fax (856)427-0047

Glass, Robert M., MD {1316039027} Ophthl, PthACl(64,CA02)<NJ-STPETER>
+ Brunswick Eye Associates
  317 Cleveland Avenue Highland Park, NJ 08904 (732)828-5190 Fax (732)828-0677

Glass, Steven J., MD {1659599918} Psychy(76,PA02)<NJ-UNDRWD>
+ 93 Remsterville Road
  Elmer, NJ 08318 (856)358-8419

Glassberg, Robert M., MD {1982717187} Radiol, RadNro, RadBdI(87,VT02)<NJ-ACMCITY, NJ-ACMCMAIN>
+ Atlantic Medical Imaging, LLC.
  72 West Jimmie Leeds Road Galloway, NJ 08205 (609)677-9729 Fax (609)653-8764
+ Atlantic Medical Imaging, LLC.
  401 Bethel Road Somers Point, NJ 08244 (609)677-9729
+ Atlantic Medical Imaging, LLC.
  421 Route 9 North Cape May Court House, NJ 08205 (609)463-9500 Fax (609)465-0918

Glassburn, John Robertson, MD {1669404984} RadOnc(66,PA09)
+ Kennedy Diagnostic & Treatment Center
  900 Medical Center Drive/Suite 100 Sewell, NJ 08080 (856)582-3008

Glasser, Barry D., MD {1487689162} IntrMd, PainMd(81,WIND)<NJ-ACMCITY, NJ-ACMCMAIN>
+ Medical One
  4248 Harbour Beach Boulevard Brigantine, NJ 08203 (609)266-0400 Fax (866)912-0605

Glasser, Laurie, MD {1679552103} PhysMd(92,GA05)<NJ-JRSYSHMC>
+ Orthopaedic Institute of Central Jersey
  2315A Highway 34/Suite D Manasquan, NJ 08736 (732)974-0404 Fax (732)974-2653
+ Orthopaedic Institute of Central Jersey
  226 Highway 37 West/Suite 203 Toms River, NJ 08755 (732)974-0404 Fax (732)240-5329
+ Orthopaedic Institute of Central Jersey
  365 Broad Street Red Bank, NJ 08736 (732)933-4300 Fax (732)933-1444

Glassman, Adam M., MD {1710046800} IntrMd, PulDis, SlpDis(87,GRN01)<NJ-HOLYNAME, NJ-ENGLWOOD>
+ S. L. Silverstein MD LLC
  180 North Dean Street Englewood, NJ 07631 (201)871-8366 Fax (201)871-8356

Glassman, Ronald M., MD {1316930936} Ophthl(83,MI01)<NJ-ENGLWOOD>
+ Glassman Eye Associates
  185 Cedar Lane Teaneck, NJ 07666 (201)836-0888 Fax (201)836-6662

Glassner, Norman, MD {1972526887} SrgOrt(68,NY19)<NJ-HUNTRDN>
+ Pulmonary & Sleep Associates of Hunterdon County
  1100 Wescott Drive/Suite G-2 Flemington, NJ 08822 (908)788-6457 Fax (908)806-2529

Glassner, Philip Justin, MD {1013174689} SrgOrt(04,NJ05)
+ MidJersey Orthopaedics, P.A.
  8100 Wescott Drive/Suite 101 Flemington, NJ 08822 (908)782-0600 Fax (908)782-7575

Glastein, Cary D., MD {1154371557} SrgOrt(79,NY09)<NJ-MONMOUTH, NJ-RIVERVW>
+ Shore Orthopaedic Group
  35 Gilbert Street South Tinton Falls, NJ 07701 (732)530-1515 Fax (732)747-5433
+ Shore Orthopaedic Group
  1255 Route 70/Suite 11S Lakewood, NJ 08701 (732)530-1515 Fax (732)942-2311
+ Shore Orthopaedic Group
  1322 Route 72 West Manahawkin, NJ 07701 (609)597-1377 Fax (609)597-0204

Physicians by Name and Address

Glatman, Marina, MD {1033420955} Ophthl
+ Jersey Shore Eye Associates
1809 Corlies Avenue/Suite 1   Neptune City, NJ 07753
(732)774-5566   Fax (732)988-7574

Glatt, Brian Steven, MD {1184691875} SrgPlstc(98,PA01)<NJ-ST-BARHCS, NJ-MTNSIDE>
+ Dr. Brian Steven Glatt and Associates
310 Madison Avenue/Suite 100   Morristown, NJ 07960
(973)889-9300   Fax (973)889-9400

Glatt, Herbert L., MD {1730259623} Ophthl(79,MEXI)<NJ-EASTORNG>
+ 1025 Broad Street
Bloomfield, NJ 07003   (973)338-1001   Fax (973)338-1221

Glatter, Frederic G., MD {1679551832} FamMed(84,PA14)
+ 27 South Fifth Avenue
Highland Park, NJ 08904   (732)819-9696

Glatthorn, Haley, MD {1578052338} ObsGyn
+ University Medical Group/OBGYN
125 Paterson Street/2nd Floor   New Brunswick, NJ 08901
(732)235-6375   Fax (732)235-6627

Glaubiger, Carol, MD {1912953068} IntrMd, Acpntr(86,MI20)<NH-MONADNK>
+ Hackensack University Medical Group Emerson
452 Old Hook Road/2nd Floor   Emerson, NJ 07630
(201)666-3900   Fax (201)261-0505

Glazer, Joyce H., MD {1104915552} IntrMd(80,PA01)<NJ-UNVM-CPRN>
+ Princeton Medical Group, P.A.
419 North Harrison Street   Princeton, NJ 08540   (609)924-9300   Fax (609)924-6552
+ Princeton Medical Group PA
2 Research Way/Bldg 2/Suite 302   Monroe Township, NJ 08831   (609)924-9300   Fax (609)655-7466

Glazer, Robert Dean, MD {1619114600} IntrMd(80,NJ06)
+ 109 Wyckoff Avenue
Piscataway, NJ 08854   Fax (732)563-4194

Glazier, Kenneth David, MD {1245296243} IntrMd, Gastrn(95,IL06)<NJ-CENTRAST>
+ Gastroenterologists of Ocean County
477 Lakehurst Road   Toms River, NJ 08755   (732)349-4422   Fax (732)349-5087

Glazier, Kim Steinberg, MD {1598795528} PedHem, Pedtrc(95,IL43)<NJ-JRSYSHMC>
+ Northern Ocean County Medical Associates
10 Neptune Boulevard/Suite 201   Neptune, NJ 07753
(732)455-8559   Fax (732)774-1394

Gleason, Abigail Hott, MD {1720045750} ObsGyn(93,NY47)
+ Ob & Gyn Group of E Brunswick
172 Summerhill Road/Suite 1   East Brunswick, NJ 08816
(732)254-1500   Fax (732)254-1436
+ Cares Surgicenter, LLC.
240 Easton Avenue   New Brunswick, NJ 08901   (732)254-1500   Fax (732)296-8677

Gleason, Catherine Elizabeth, MD {1700849759} Surgry, SrgBst(82,MS01)<NJ-HUNTRDN>
+ Hunterdon Breast Surgery
121 State Route 31/Suite 1000   Flemington, NJ 08822
(908)968-3162   Fax (908)968-3181
Cegcatherine@aol.com

Gleeson, Tara Elizabeth, DO {1558302620} EmrgMd(91,PA77)<NJ-VIRTVOOR>
+ Virtua Voorhees
100 Bowman Drive/EmergMed   Voorhees, NJ 08043
(856)247-3000

Gleimer, Barry S., DO {1306891627} SrgOrt(79,MO79)<NJ-KMHCHRRY, NJ-KMHSTRAT>
+ Regional Orthopedic, P.A.
2201 West Chapel Avenue/PO Box 8566   Cherry Hill, NJ 08002   (856)663-7080   Fax (856)663-4945
+ Regional Orthopedic, P.A.
163 Hurffville Crosskeys Road   Turnersville, NJ 08012
(856)663-7080   Fax (856)875-1368

Gleimer, Emily R., DO {1174844484} ObsGyn<NJ-COOPRUMC>
+ Virtua Gynecologic Oncology Specialists
200 Bowman Drive/Suite E-315   Voorhees, NJ 08043
(856)247-7310   Fax (856)247-7309
+ Cooper Perinatology Associates
3 Cooper Plaza/Suite 502   Camden, NJ 08103   (856)247-7310   Fax (856)968-8499

Gleimer, Evan Michael, DO {1184985095} EmrgMd<NJ-OVERLOOK>
+ Overlook Medical Center
99 Beauvoir Avenue/PO Box 210   Summit, NJ 07902
(908)522-2000

Gleimer, Jeffrey Robert, DO {1548469232} SrgOrt(05,NJ75)<NJ-KMHCHRRY>
+ Regional Orthopedic, P.A.
2201 West Chapel Avenue/PO Box 8566   Cherry Hill, NJ 08002   (856)663-7080   Fax (856)663-4945
+ Regional Orthopedic, P.A.
163 Hurffville Crosskeys Road   Turnersville, NJ 08012

(856)663-7080   Fax (856)875-1368

Glenn, April, MD {1902242126} EmrgMd
+ 307 South Evergreen Avenue
Woodbury, NJ 08096   (813)245-0135

Glenn, Danette, MD {1720028921} IntrMd
+ Cooper Physicians Washington Township
1 Plaza Drive/Suite 103/Bunker Hill Pl   Sewell, NJ 08080
(856)270-4080   Fax (856)270-4085

Glenn, William B., DO {1629150024} FamMed, Grtrcs, SprtMd(80,PA77)<NJ-SOCEANCO>
+ Family Medicine Center
279 Mathistown Road   Little Egg Harbor, NJ 08087
(609)296-1101
+ Family Medicine Center
1301 Route 72 West/Suite 240   Manahawkin, NJ 08050
(609)296-1101   Fax (609)597-6833

Glessner, Robyn, DO {1831547637} EmrgMd<NJ-OVERLOOK>
+ Overlook Medical Center
99 Beauvoir Avenue/PO Box 210   Summit, NJ 07902
(908)522-2000

Glezen-Schneider, Priscilla Ann, MD {1093707812} FamMed(95,NY15)
+ Millburn Family Practice
425 Essex Street   Millburn, NJ 07041   (973)379-3051   Fax (973)379-8828

Glick, Craig S., MD {1356454540} Radiol, RadBdI(86,NY45)<NJ-ACMCITY, NJ-ACMCMAIN>
+ Atlantic Medical Imaging, LLC.
72 West Jimmie Leeds Road   Galloway, NJ 08205
(609)677-9729   Fax (609)653-8764
+ Atlantic Medical Imaging, LLC.
401 Bethel Road   Somers Point, NJ 08244   (609)677-9729
+ Atlantic Medical Imaging, LLC.
421 Route 9 North   Cape May Court House, NJ 08205
(609)463-9500   Fax (609)465-0918

Glick, Ronald S., MD {1588623169} SrgOrt(68,MD01)<NJ-CHSFULD, NJ-CHSMRCER>
+ Lawrence Orthopaedics
4065 Quakerbridge Road   Princeton Junction, NJ 08550
(609)394-3804   Fax (609)989-1501

Glick, Sarah Rachel, MD {1316137037} Pedtrc
+ St Barnabas Medical Center Pediatrics
94 Old Short Hills Road   Livingston, NJ 07039   (973)322-5690   Fax (973)322-5504
sglick@barnabashealth.org

Glickman, Alexander B., MD {1801847629} Otlryg(91,PA09)
+ 331 Grand Street/Suite 1
Hoboken, NJ 07030   (201)420-6300

Glickman, Amy Borg, MD {1710045323} Psychy, PsyCAd(89,PA09)
+ Bancroft NeuroHealth
425 Kings Highway East   Haddonfield, NJ 08033   (856)429-0010

Glickman, Lee M., MD {1295702884} CdvDis, IntrMd(86,NY08)<NJ-CHSMRCER, NJ-CHSFULD>
+ Capital Health Medical Center Hopewell
Two Capital Way/Suite 380/Cardiology   Pennington, NJ 08534   (609)303-4838   Fax (609)303-4835
+ Capital Health-Heart Care Specialists
1445 Whitehorse-Mercerville Rd   Hamilton, NJ 08619
(609)303-4838   Fax (609)303-4835

Glickman, Leonard, MD {1730355272} Urolgy(08,NY19)
+ HUMC Faculty Practice
360 Essex Street/Suite 403   Hackensack, NJ 07601
(201)336-8090   Fax (201)336-8221

Glicksman, Caroline A., MD {1467429027} SrgPlstc(85,NY08)<NJ-JRSYSHMC, NJ-OCEANMC>
+ 2164 Route 35
Sea Girt, NJ 08750   (732)974-2424   Fax (732)974-0134

Gliebus, Gediminas Peter, MD {1174789044} Nrolgy
+ Drexel Neurosciences Institute
601 Route 73 North   Marlton, NJ 08053   (215)762-6915
Fax (215)762-6914

Gliksman, Felicia Joyce, MD {1003041716} NrlgSpec(04)<NJ-HACKNSK>
+ Hackensack University Medical Center
30 Prospect Avenue/Imus Room 338   Hackensack, NJ 07601
(201)996-3200   Fax (201)968-0163

Gliksman, Michele Isaacs, MD {1851374326} ObsGyn, IntrMd(90,NY47)<NJ-VALLEY, NJ-HACKNSK>
+ Hackensack University Medical Group Emerson
452 Old Hook Road/2nd Floor   Emerson, NJ 07630
(201)666-3900   Fax (201)261-0505

Gloria, Stephen B., DO {1407825920} FamMed(82,PA77)
+ Skylands Medical Group PA
5678 Berkshire Valley Road   Oak Ridge, NJ 07438
(973)697-0200   Fax (973)697-6844

Gloth, Jonathan Michael, MD {1932361110} Ophthl(05,NJ06)<NY-ALBANY>
+ Ocean County Retina, P.C.
780 Route 37 West/Suite 200   Toms River, NJ 08755
(732)797-1855   Fax (732)797-1856

Glotzer, Taya Valerie, MD {1376510792} CdvDis, ClCdEl(87,NY19)<NJ-HACKNSK>
+ Electrophysiology Associates
20 Prospect Avenue/Suite 701   Hackensack, NJ 07601
(201)996-2997   Fax (201)996-2571

Glowacki, Carol Ann, MD {1346236536} ObsGyn(92,IA02)
+ 6012 Pazza At Main Street
Voorhees, NJ 08043

Gluck, Ian J., MD {1053391458} ObsGyn(79,NY09)<NJ-MORRISTN>
+ Obstetrical & Gynecological Associates of Morris
59 Franklin Street   Morristown, NJ 07960   (973)538-1515
Fax (973)538-5542

Gluck, Karen, MD {1124286794} NnPnMd
+ MidAtlantic Neonatology Associates
100 Madison Avenue   Morristown, NJ 07962   (973)971-5488   Fax (973)290-7175

Gluckman, William Alan, DO {1336225424} EmrgMd(95,NY75)<NJ-UMDNJ>
+ University Hospital
150 Bergen Street/Emerg Medicine   Newark, NJ 07103
(973)972-5076   Fax (973)972-6646
gluckmwa@umdnj.edu

Glushakow, Allen S., MD {1720062243} IntrMd, SrgOrt(67,MD01)<NJ-EASTORNG>
+ The Joint Institute at Saint Barnabas Medical Center
609 Morris Avenue   Springfield, NJ 07081   (973)379-1991
Fax (973)467-8647

Glynn, Nicole Lasasso, MD {1235134479} RadDia, Radiol, IntrMd(98,NJ06)
+ University Radiology Group, P.C.
579A Cranbury Road   East Brunswick, NJ 08816   (732)390-0040   Fax (732)390-1856
+ University Radiology Group
2100 Route 33/Neptune City Med Bld   Neptune, NJ 07753
(732)390-0040   Fax (732)502-0368
+ University Radiology Group
900 West Main Street   Freehold, NJ 08816   (732)462-1900
Fax (732)462-1848

Gmyrek, Glenn A., MD {1740249143} Urolgy(96,NY01)<NJ-WAYNEGEN, NJ-VALLEY>
+ 246 Hamburg Tpke/Suite 308
Wayne, NJ 07470   (973)956-1555   Fax (973)956-9875
+ SurgiCare Surgical Associates of Wayne, LLC
246 Hamburg Turnpike   Wayne, NJ 07470   (973)790-0954

Gnoy, Alexander Roman, MD {1336137827} Otlryg(94,NJ06)<NY-MTSINAI, NJ-OVERLOOK>
+ Summit Medical Group-Berkeley Heights Campus
1 Diamond Hill Road   Berkeley Heights, NJ 07922
(908)273-4300   Fax (908)277-8662

Go, Ernesto B., MD {1265489207} Radiol, RadDia, IntrMd(67,PHI01)
+ Center for Diagnostic Imaging
1450 East Chestnut Avenue   Vineland, NJ 08360   (856)794-8664   Fax (856)794-2671

Go, Jane O., MD {1861506958} Pedtrc(73,PHI10)<NJ-OCEANMC, NJ-JRSYSHMC>
+ Pediatric Medical Group
2640 US Highway 70/Suite 2-A   Manasquan, NJ 08736
(732)223-1440

Go, Richard Au Yeung, MD {1649283102} InfDis
+ 214 Pomponio Avenue
South Plainfield, NJ 07080

Goa, Cristobal Javier, MD {1528201993} IntrMd(09,NY19)
+ Physician Specialists of New Jersey
1 Sears Drive/Suite 306   Paramus, NJ 07652   (201)830-2287   Fax (201)830-2286

Gochfeld, Linda G., MD {1972650448} Psychy(65,NY46)
+ 40 Witherspoon Street
Princeton, NJ 08542   (609)921-1370   Fax (609)406-0307
gochfeli@aol.com
+ Serv Behavioral Health System
20 Scotch Road   Ewing, NJ 08628   (609)921-1370   Fax (609)406-0307

Gochfeld, Michael, MD {1083768360} IntrMd, OccpMd, GPrvMd(65,NY46)
+ University Hospital-School of Public Health
170 Frelinghuysen Road/EOHSI Rm 200   Piscataway, NJ 08854   (732)445-0123   Fax (732)445-0130

Godek, Christopher P., MD {1558300889} SrgPlstc(94,MA05)<NJ-CENTRAST, NJ-OCEANMC>
+ Personal Enhancement Center
1430 Hooper Avenue/Suite 204   Toms River, NJ 08753
(732)281-1988   Fax (732)281-1977

Godfrey, John Trevor, DO {1770704850} IntrMd(01,MO78)<NJ-DEBRAHLC>
+ Deborah Heart and Lung Center
200 Trenton Road/Internal Med   Browns Mills, NJ 08015
(609)893-6611

Physicians by Name and Address

Godfrey, Loren, MD {1780645911} RadOnc(95,NY08)<NJ-HACKNSK>
+ John Theurer Cancer Center - HUMC
  92 Second Street   Hackensack, NJ 07601   (201)996-2210   Fax (551)996-0730

Godin, Willis Eugene, DO {1508944570} CdvDis, IntrMd(00,PA77)
+ South Jersey Heart Group
  3001 Chapel Avenue/Suite 101   Cherry Hill, NJ 08002   (856)482-8900   Fax (856)482-7170

Godin-Ostro, Evelyn R., MD {1457503039} IntrMd(81,SWI04)
+ 23 West Shore Drive
  Pennington, NJ 08534

Godkar, Darshan, MD {1952515264} CdvDis, IntrMd
+ Advanced Cardiology, LLC.
  65 Ridgedale Avenue   Cedar Knolls, NJ 07927   (973)401-1100   Fax (973)401-1201
+ Advanced Cardiology, LLC.
  117 Seber Road/Suite 1-B   Hackettstown, NJ 07840   (973)401-1100   Fax (908)979-1493

Godleski, Thomas D., DO {1235168709} FamMed(98,NJ75)<NJ-VIRTMHBC, NJ-KMHSTRAT>
+ Alliance for Better Care, P.C.
  PO Box 1510   Medford, NJ 08055   (609)953-4099   Fax (609)953-8652
+ Alliance for Better Care, PC/Mount Holly Division
  1613 Route 38   Lumberton, NJ 08048   (609)953-4099   Fax (609)261-5507

Godlewska-Janusz, Elzbieta, MD {1326235441} Pedtrc(96,POL02)
+ Kang Lee and Lee Allergy/Pediatrics
  2177 Oak Tree Road/Suite 207   Edison, NJ 08820   (732)549-7007

Godorecci, Michele, MD {1255402079} ObsGyn(94,PA09)
+ Advocare Heights Primary Care
  318 White Horse Pike   Haddon Heights, NJ 08035   (856)547-6000   Fax (856)546-3189
+ Ob-Gyn Specialists
  157 Route 73   Voorhees, NJ 08043   (856)547-6000   Fax (856)874-9555

Godwin Karolak, Allison M., DO {1700818275} FamMed(02,NJ75)
+ Makowski Medical Associates
  44 Dune Terrace   Seaside Heights, NJ 08751   (732)528-5626

Godyn, Janusz J., MD {1174698203} PthACl, Hemato, Immuno(70,POLA)<NJ-RWJUHAM, NJ-KMHSTRAT>
+ Kennedy Health System/Cherry Hill Campus
  2201 Chapel Avenue West/Hematology   Cherry Hill, NJ 08002   (856)488-6560   Fax (856)566-6176

Goel, Kriti, MD {1063689040}
+ 58 Spruce Street
  Princeton Junction, NJ 08550

Goel, Narender, MD {1710131537} Nephro
+ Drs. Ahmed, Haddad & Batwara
  26 Greenville Avenue   Jersey City, NJ 07305   (201)333-8222   Fax (201)333-0095

Goel, Rajiv, MD {1366500332} NnPnMd, Pedtrc(75,INA05)<NY-METROHOS>
+ CHOP Newborn and Pediatric Care at UMCPP
  One Plainsboro Road/6th Floor   Plainsboro, NJ 08536   (609)853-7626   Fax (609)853-7630
+ Somerset Medical Center Neonatology
  110 Rehill Avenue   Somerville, NJ 08876   (908)685-2473

Goel, Ravi Desh, MD {1376576108} Ophthl(97,NJ02)<NJ-VIRTU-AHS>
+ Regional Eye Associates
  741 Route 70 West   Cherry Hill, NJ 08002   (856)795-8787   Fax (856)795-8688
  rea741@aol.com
+ Regional Eye Associates
  200 White Horse Pike   Haddon Heights, NJ 08035   (856)547-0200
+ Regional Eye Associates
  8 North White Horse Pike/Suite 106   Hammonton, NJ 08002   (856)795-8787

Goel, Surendra P., MD {1912958521} Surgry, WundCr(63,INDI)
+ 159 Mountain Avenue
  Hawthorne, NJ 07506   (973)557-6731
  goelusa@hotmail.com

Goett, Rebecca R., MD {1588985337} EmrgMd<RI-RIHOSPTL, RI-MIRIAM>
+ 185 South Orange Avenue
  Newark, NJ 07103   (973)972-9151

Gof, Sonia M., MD {1386732600} ObsGyn(81,TN07)<NJ-WAYNE-GEN, NJ-STJOSHOS>
+ Wayne Obstetrics & Gynecology
  510 Hamburg Turnpike/Suite 202   Wayne, NJ 07470   (973)942-3500   Fax (973)942-3881
+ Wayne Surgical Center, LLC.
  1176 Hamburg Pike   Wayne, NJ 07470   (973)942-3500   Fax (973)709-1901

Gogineni, Rama Rao, MD {1295823656} Psychy, IntrMd(73,INA1I)
+ Cooper Psychiatric Associates
  3 Cooper Plaza/Suite 307   Camden, NJ 08103   (856)342-2328   Fax (856)541-6137

Goglia, Kara Defilippis, MD {1427282987}
+ Advanced Obstetrics & Gynecology, LLC
  4 Walter E. Foran Boulevard/Suite 302   Flemington, NJ 08822   (908)806-0080   Fax (908)806-3478

Goh, Jean Sian Li, MD {1124138920} Pedtrc(97,IL06)
+ North Brunswick Pediatrics
  1598 US Highway 130   North Brunswick, NJ 08902   (732)297-0603   Fax (732)297-2866

Gohel, Rekha M., MD {1679653992} Grtrcs, IntrMd(95,INA2B)<NJ-CENTRAST>
+ Elite Medical Care, LLC
  318 Professional View Drive   Freehold, NJ 07728   (732)409-6440   Fax (732)409-6466

Gohil, Kartik Narendra, MD {1649432097} Surgry
+ Ballem Surgical
  230 Sherman Avenue/Suite C   Glen Ridge, NJ 07028   (973)744-8585   Fax (973)748-5990

Gohsler, Steven P., MD {1184643983} EmrgMd(86,PA02)<NJ-MORRISTN>
+ Morristown Medical Center
  100 Madison Avenue/EmrgMed   Morristown, NJ 07962   (973)971-5000

Goil, Sunita, MD {1578651535} NnPnMd(84,INA36)<NJ-MTN-SIDE>
+ Morristown Medical Center
  100 Madison Avenue/Simon A   Morristown, NJ 07962   (973)971-5000
+ Hackensack UMC Mountainside
  1 Bay Avenue   Montclair, NJ 07042   (973)429-6932

Gojaniuk, Jeffrey David, DO {1770879703} EmrgMd(04,PA77)<NJ-RWJUHAM, NJ-KMHSTRAT>
+ Robert Wood Johnson University Hospital at Hamilton
  1 Hamilton Health Place/EmrgMed   Hamilton, NJ 08690   (609)586-7900
+ Kennedy Memorial Hospital-University Medical Center
  18 East Laurel Road/EmrgMed   Stratford, NJ 08084   (856)346-6000

Gokcen, Eric C., MD {1821094764} SrgOrt(88,PA02)<NJ-CHSM-RCER>
+ Mercer-Bucks Orthopaedics PC
  3120 Princeton Pike   Lawrenceville, NJ 08648   (609)896-0444   Fax (609)896-1055

Gokhale, Kedar Arvind, MD {1437134061} IntrMd(91,GA05)<NJ-VALLEY>
+ Bergen Medical Associates
  466 Old Hook Road/Suite 1   Emerson, NJ 07630   (201)967-8221   Fax (201)967-0340
+ Bergen Gastroenterology PC
  236 Grand Avenue   Park Ridge, NJ 07656   (201)967-8221   Fax (201)390-1904

Gokli, Khyati, MD {1790792893} AdolMd, IntrMd(87,NY15)
+ McCosh Health Center
  Washington Road/McCosh Infirmary   Princeton, NJ 08544   (609)258-5357   Fax (609)258-1355

Golbe, Lawrence I., MD {1215002795} Nrolgy, OthrSp(78,NY19)<NJ-RWJUBRUN>
+ UH- Robert Wood Johnson Med
  125 Paterson Street/Room 6214/Neuro   New Brunswick, NJ 08901   (732)235-7729   Fax (732)235-7041
+ RW Johnson University Medical Group Neurology
  97 Paterson Street   New Brunswick, NJ 08901   (732)235-7729   Fax (732)235-7041

Golbert, Thomas Melvin, MD {1538144951} Allrgy(62,CO02)<NJ-RWJUHAM, NJ-CENTRAST>
+ Center for Asthma & Allergy
  18 North Third Avenue   Highland Park, NJ 08904   (732)545-0094   Fax (732)545-4087
+ Center for Asthma & Allergy
  300 Hudson Street   Hoboken, NJ 07030   (732)545-0094   Fax (201)792-5320
+ Center for Asthma & Allergy
  90 Milburn Avenue/Suite 200   Maplewood, NJ 08904   (973)763-5787   Fax (973)763-8568

Gold, David A., MD {1891704292} SrgOrt(89,NY20)<NJ-CHILTON>
+ SMG Orthopedic Surgery and Sports Medicine Center
  2035 Hamburg Turnpike/Suite D   Wayne, NJ 07470   (973)616-0200   Fax (973)616-1792
+ SMG Orthopedic Surgery and Sports Medicine Center
  61 Beaver Brook Road/Suite 201   Lincoln Park, NJ 07035   (973)616-0200   Fax (973)686-9294

Gold, Edward J., MD {1831168194} OncHem, IntrMd(77,MI07)<NJ-VALLEY>
+ Hackensack University Medical Group Emerson
  452 Old Hook Road/2nd Floor   Emerson, NJ 07630   (201)666-3900   Fax (201)261-0505

Gold, Jared Z., MD {1962455063} Gastrn, IntrMd(00,ISR02)<NJ-CENTRAST>
+ Advanced Gastroenterology Associates LLC
  475 County Road/Suite 201   Marlboro, NJ 07746   (732)370-2220   Fax (732)548-7408
+ Advanced Gastroenterology Associates LLC
  403 Candlewood Commons/Building 4   Howell, NJ 07731   (732)370-2220   Fax (732)548-7408

Gold, Jeffrey L., MD {1083647165} IntrMd(77,MEX03)<NJ-STJOSHOS>
+ Wayne Primary Care
  468 Parish Drive/Suite 1   Wayne, NJ 07470   (973)305-8300   Fax (973)305-8157

Gold, Jeffrey M., DO {1104884659} IntrMd, CdvDis(88,NY75)
+ Suburban Heart Group, P.A.
  1000 Galloping Hill Road/Suite 107   Union, NJ 07083   (908)964-7333   Fax (908)687-7855

Gold, Jessica Frances, DO {1760546733} IntrMd(03,NY75)
+ Pathlink, LLC
  66 West Gilbert Street/Suite 100   Tinton Falls, NJ 07701   (732)212-0060   Fax (732)212-0061

Gold, Jonathan Allan, MD {1841219797} Dermat(82,QU01)
+ Dermatology Center of North Jersey
  1033 Clifton Avenue   Clifton, NJ 07013   (973)777-6444   Fax (973)777-5277

Gold, Marcia D., MD {1710921804} IntrMd(85,NY08)
+ Family Practice of Middletown
  18 Leonardville Road   Middletown, NJ 07748   (732)671-0860   Fax (732)671-6467

Gold, Michael J., MD {1215151162} RadDia(05,NY08)
+ Radiology Affiliates of Central New Jersey, P.A.
  2501 Kuser Road   Hamilton, NJ 08691   (609)585-8800   Fax (609)585-1825

Gold, Nina A., MD {1326091562} Pedtrc, PedEmg(91,ISR02)<NJ-STJOSHOS, NJ-HACKNSK>
+ Hackensack University Medical Center
  30 Prospect Avenue   Hackensack, NJ 07601   (201)996-5430

Gold, Ruth Leah, MD {1740241074} Allrgy, Pedtrc(89,NY20)<NJ-CHILTON, NJ-VALLEY>
+ Allergy and Asthma Specialists
  51 State Route 23   Riverdale, NJ 07457   (973)831-5799   Fax (973)831-7422
+ Allergy and Asthma Specialists
  82 East Allendale Road/Suite 7-B   Saddle River, NJ 07458   (973)831-5799   Fax (201)236-0138

Gold, Steven M., MD {1164461877} Otlryg, SrgHdN(93,NY09)<NJ-ENGLWOOD, NJ-HACKNSK>
+ ENT & Allergy Associates, LLP
  433 Hackensack Avenue/Suite 204   Hackensack, NJ 07601   (201)883-1062   Fax (201)883-9297
  steven.gold@direct.entandallergy.nextgen

Goldberg, Alexander, MD {1952371734} FamMed(89,RUSS)<NJ-CENTRAST, NJ-JRSYSHMC>
+ Taylors Mills Family Medical, PC
  224 Taylors Mills Road/Suite 112   Manalapan, NJ 07726   (732)577-1066   Fax (732)577-0049

Goldberg, Alvin Hugh, MD {1396759270} EmrgMd(76,NJ05)
+ Doctors' Office Walk-in Urgent Care
  110 East Ridgewood Avenue   Paramus, NJ 07652   (201)265-9500   Fax (201)265-1355
+ Manalapan Urgent Care
  120 Craig Road   Manalapan, NJ 07726   (201)265-9500   Fax (732)414-2995

Goldberg, Daniel B., MD {1861493488} Ophthl(74,NY08)<NJ-MONMOUTH>
+ Atlantic Eye Physicians
  279 Third Avenue/Suite 204   Long Branch, NJ 07740   (732)222-7373   Fax (732)571-9212
+ Atlantic Eye Physicians
  180 White Road/Suite 202   Little Silver, NJ 07739   (732)222-7373   Fax (732)219-9557

Goldberg, David Felheimer, MD {1255727954} EmrgMd
+ SJ Emergency Physician, PA
  175 Madison Avenue   Mount Holly, NJ 08060   (609)914-6000   Fax (609)261-5842

Goldberg, David Israel, MD {1669413324} Pedtrc, PedInf(81,MD12)<NJ-STJOSHOS, NJ-VALLEY>
+ St. Joseph's Pediatrics DePaul Center
  11 Getty Avenue/2nd Floor   Paterson, NJ 07503   (973)754-3729

Goldberg, David Jay, MD {1528001583} Dermat, SrgDer, Sr-gLsr(80,CT01)<NJ-HACKNSK, NY-MTSINYHS>
+ Skin Laser & Surgery Specialists
  20 Prospect Avenue/Suite 702   Hackensack, NJ 07601   (201)441-9890   Fax (201)441-9893
+ Skin Laser & Surgery Specialists
  105 Raider Boulevard/Suite 203   Hillsborough, NJ 08844   (201)441-9890   Fax (201)441-9893

Goldberg, Grigory, MD {1033142112} SrgSpn, SrgOrt, IntrMd(00,NY08)
+ Advanced Orthopedics & Sports Medicine Institute
  301 Professional View Drive   Freehold, NJ 07728   (732)720-2555   Fax (732)720-2556

Physicians by Name and Address

Goldberg, Irwin L., DO {1821002452} IntrMd(73,IA75)<NJ-COMMED>
+ 600 Mule Road/Unit 9
Toms River, NJ 08757 (732)914-8118 Fax (732)914-8887
Lgoldberg.do@stuffz.net

Goldberg, Jack, MD {1548372022} OncHem, IntrMd(73,NY15)<PA-PNPRSBYT>
+ Penn Medicine at Cherry Hill
409 Route 70 East/Hema Oncology Cherry Hill, NJ 08034 (856)429-1519
goldberj10@gmail.com

Goldberg, Jory J., MD {1407841638} IntrMd, PulDis(76,MEXI)<NJ-UNVMCPRN>
+ 18 Centre Drive/Suite 103
Monroe Township, NJ 08831 (609)655-1700 Fax (609)655-4455

Goldberg, Judah Lev, MD {1669629218} EmrgMd<NJ-CHILTON>
+ Chilton Medical Center
97 West Parkway Pompton Plains, NJ 07444 (973)831-5447

Goldberg, Leah, MD {1649768144} ObsGyn
+ University Medical Group/OBGYN
125 Paterson Street/2nd Floor New Brunswick, NJ 08901 (908)963-1642 Fax (732)235-6627

Goldberg, Lon E., DO {1972574713} EmrgMd(84,PA77)
+ Access Medical Associates
3322 Route 22 West/Building 1 Branchburg, NJ 08876 (908)704-0100 Fax (908)704-0090

Goldberg, Marc A., MD {1376599563} IntrMd, Rheuma(69,VA04)
+ Summit Medical Group
6 Brighton Road/2 FL Clifton, NJ 07012 (973)777-7911 Fax (973)777-5403

Goldberg, Marc B., MD Anesth(79,PA02)<NJ-LOURDMED>
+ Rancocas Anesthesiology, PA
700 Route 130 North/Suite 203 Cinnaminson, NJ 08077 (856)829-9345 Fax (856)829-3605

Goldberg, Mark C., MD {1114914389} CdvDis, IntrMd(86,NJ05)
+ Consultants in Cardiology
741 Northfield Avenue/Suite 205 West Orange, NJ 07052 (973)467-1544 Fax (973)467-9586

Goldberg, Michael E., MD {1083710677} Anesth, PainMd(82,PA02)<NJ-COOPRUMC>
+ Cooper University Medical Center/Camden
3 Cooper Plaza/Suite 314 Camden, NJ 08103 (856)963-6770
+ The Cooper Health System at Voorhees
900 Centennial Boulevard/Suite E Voorhees, NJ 08043 (856)325-6365

Goldberg, Michael I., MD {1528117926} GynOnc, Gyneco(70,ITAL)<NJ-STPETER, NJ-RWJUBRUN>
+ Saint Peter's Physician Associates
78 Easton Avenue New Brunswick, NJ 08901 (732)828-3300 Fax (732)937-5739

Goldberg, Michael Scott, MD {1184622151} Gastrn(88,NY48)
+ Gastroenterology Consultants PA
205 May Street/Suite 201 Edison, NJ 08837 (732)661-9225 Fax (732)661-9259

Goldberg, Paul E., MD {1316943574} IntrMd(75,PA02)<NJ-CHSM-RCER>
+ Princeton Pike Internal Medicine
3100 Princeton Pike/Bldg 3/ 3rd Fl Lawrenceville, NJ 08648 (609)896-1793 Fax (609)896-1847

Goldberg, Rina Freida, MD {1306954730} ClNrPh, Pedtrc, Nrolgy(92,NY46)
+ St. Barnabas Institute of Neurology & Neurosurgery
200 South Orange Avenue/Suite 101 Livingston, NJ 07039 (973)322-7580 Fax (973)322-6631

Goldberg, Robert M., MD {1215054168} MedOnc, Hemato, OncHem(75,NY15)<NJ-SHOREMEM, NJ-ACMCITY>
+ 727 Shore Road
Somers Point, NJ 08244 (609)927-3772 Fax (609)926-3543

Goldberg, Ryan J., MD {1427104041} IntrMd<NJ-STBARNMC>
+ St. Barnabas Medical Center
94 Old Short Hills Road Livingston, NJ 07039 (973)322-8892

Goldberg, Shira, MD {1710181607} Grtrcs, IntrMd(NY47<NJ-MONMOUTH>
+ Monmouth Medical Center
300 Second Avenue/Suite 005 Long Branch, NJ 07740 (732)923-7550 Fax (732)923-7553

Goldberg, Steven C., MD {1487688537} ObsGyn(83,IL02)<NJ-STPETER, NJ-SOMERSET>
+ Bay Obstetrics & Gynecology
740 US Highway 1 North Iselin, NJ 08830 (732)362-3840 Fax (732)362-3850
+ 2045 Route 355
South Amboy, NJ 08879

Goldberg, Stuart Lee, MD {1215996376} Hemato, MedOnc, IntrMd(86,PA14)<NJ-HACKNSK>
+ John Theurer Cancer Center - HUMC
92 Second Street Hackensack, NJ 07601 (201)996-3925

Fax (201)996-0582
+ Regional Cancer Care Center
7650 River Road/2nd Floor North Bergen, NJ 07047 (212)464-0008

Goldberg, William P., MD {1215191994} CdvDis, Grtrcs, IntrMd(80,NJ05)<NJ-JFKMED>
+ Metuchen Cardiology Associates
579 Main Street Metuchen, NJ 08840 (732)906-2332 Fax (732)906-9433

Goldberg, Yana Pavel, MD {1336368646} RadOnc, Radiol(04,PA09)<NJ-MORRISTN>
+ Radiation Oncology Associates of North Jersey, P.A.
100 Madison Avenue Morristown, NJ 07962 (973)971-5329 Fax (973)290-7393

Goldberger, Gerardo V., DO {1306810726} SrgOrt, SrgSpn, IntrMd(91,IA75)<NJ-CENTRAST>
+ Advanced Orthopedics & Sports Medicine Institute
301 Professional View Drive Freehold, NJ 07728 (732)720-2555 Fax (732)720-2556

Goldberger, Michael Irwin, MD {1316034002} SrgOrt(92,PA02)<NJ-MORRISTN>
+ Tri-County Orthopedics
160 East Hanover Avenue Morristown, NJ 07962 (973)538-2334 Fax (973)829-9174

Goldblatt, Kenneth H., MD {1720019052} IntrMd, PulDis(72,NY09)<NJ-UNVMCPRN>
+ Princeton Medicine
5 Plainsboro Road/Suite 300 Plainsboro, NJ 08536 (609)853-7272 Fax (609)853-7271

Goldbloom, David Lee, MD {1487810081} PsyAdd(04,NY46)
+ 450 Hamburg Turnpike/Suite 2-F
Wayne, NJ 07470 (973)617-6352 Fax (617)677-5012

Golden, Daniel Martin, DO {1154332294} FamMed
+ Atlantic Off Shore Medical Associates
5401 Harding Highway/Suite 5 Mays Landing, NJ 08330 (609)909-0200 Fax (609)909-0267

Golden, Lee Scott, MD CdvDis(93,NY19)
+ 728 Shoshone Trail
Franklin Lakes, NJ 07417

Golden, Richard F., DO {1356381388} FamMed(84,IA75)<NJ-KMHCHRRY, NJ-VIRTVOOR>
+ Advocare Family Medicine Associates Mt. Laurel
3115 Route 38/Suite 200B Mount Laurel, NJ 08054 (856)231-9666 Fax (856)231-7543
+ Advocare Family Medicine Associates Vineland
602 West Sherman Avenue/Suite B Vineland, NJ 08360 (856)231-9666 Fax (856)896-3059
+ Advocare Family Medicine Associates Williamstown
979 North Black Horse Pike Williamstown, NJ 08094 (856)629-5151 Fax (856)629-0281

Golden, Richard Frederick, MD {1083666879} InfDis, IntrMd(88,MNT01)<NJ-VIRTMHBC, NJ-OURLADY>
+ Infectious Disease Physicians PA
1001 Briggs Road/Suite 250 Mount Laurel, NJ 08054 (856)866-7466 Fax (856)866-9088

Golden-Tevald, Jean M., DO {1184608853} FamMed(87,PA77)<NJ-HUNTRDN>
+ MorningStar Family Health Center
416 Mechlin Corner Road Pittstown, NJ 08867 (908)735-9344 Fax (908)735-7136
info@morningstarfhc.com
+ Hunterdon Medical Center
2100 Wescott Drive/FamMed Flemington, NJ 08822 (908)788-6100

Goldenberg, Bruce S., MD {1538168745} SrgCdv, SrgCth, SrgThr(76,IL06)<NJ-MTNSIDE, NJ-STCLRDEN>
+ 30 Chatham Road/Suite 377
Short Hills, NJ 07078 (973)467-5550 Fax (973)467-9511
bgoldenbergmd@att.net
+ Hackensack UMC Mountainside
1 Bay Avenue Montclair, NJ 07042 (973)429-6000
+ St. Clare's Hospital-Denville Campus
25 Pocono Road Denville, NJ 07078 (973)625-6000

Goldenberg, David A., MD {1194814624} Gastrn, IntrMd(74,NY09)
+ Gastroenterology Associates
1165 Park Avenue Plainfield, NJ 07060 (908)754-2992 Fax (908)754-8366

Goldenberg, Elie Adam, MD {1063432680} Surgry, SrgVas(99,PRO02)<NH-DRTMTHMC>
+ Mercer Surgical Group
2063 Klockner Road/Suite 1 Hamilton, NJ 08690 (609)631-1001 Fax (609)588-5970

Goldenberg, Gennifer E., MD {1922017102} EmrgMd(01,FL02)<NJ-VIRTMHBC>
+ Virtua Memorial
175 Madison Avenue/EmrgMed Mount Holly, NJ 08060 (609)267-0700

Goldenberg, Samuel F., MD {1619977642} Urolgy(85,LA01)
+ New Jersey Urology, LLC
2401 East Evesham Road/Suite F Voorhees, NJ 08043 (856)673-1600 Fax (856)988-0636

Goldenberg-Sandau, Anna, DO {1679884431} Surgry
+ Cooper University Hospital
One Cooper Plaza Camden, NJ 08103 (856)342-2000
+ Cooper University Physician Trauma Center
One Cooper Plaza Camden, NJ 08103 (856)342-3014

Goldenring, Debra Semel, MD {1558322651} AdolMd, Pedtrc, IntrMd(91,NJ05)<NJ-STBARNMC>
+ Summit Medical Group
75 East Northfield Road Livingston, NJ 07039 (973)436-1540 Fax (908)673-7336

Goldfaden, Isabel, MD {1154416550} Dermat, IntrMd(90,MI01)
+ Summit Medical Group-Berkeley Heights Campus
1 Diamond Hill Road Berkeley Heights, NJ 07922 (908)273-4300 Fax (908)646-6816

Goldfarb, Adam S., MD {1275534174} IntrMd(92,NJ05)<NJ-HACKNSK>
+ Summit Avenue Medical
5 Summit Avenue Hackensack, NJ 07601 (201)646-0001 Fax (201)646-9101

Goldfarb, David Steven, MD {1629018908} IntrMd, Nephro(81,CT01)<NY-VAHARBOR>
+ Pulmonary & Sleep Associates of SJ, LLC.
750 Route 73 South/Suite 401 Marlton, NJ 08053 (856)375-1288 Fax (856)375-2325

Goldfarb, Helene, MD {1619089364} RadDia, Radiol(78,NY09)<NJ-UMDNJ>
+ University Hospital-Doctors Office Center
90 Bergen Street/DOC 1700 & 1500 Newark, NJ 07103 (973)972-2300 Fax (973)972-2307

Goldfarb, Irvin D., MD {1972530707} CdvDis, IntrMd(73,NJ05)<NJ-STMICHL>
+ St. Michael's Medical Center
268 MLK Jr. Boulevard Newark, NJ 07102 (201)624-0805 Fax (201)854-2844
+ 306 Martin Luther King Blvd
Newark, NJ 07102 (201)624-0805 Fax (973)824-2844

Goldfarb, Mark S., MD {1093801920} Ophthl(70,NY19)<NJ-HACKNSK, NJ-HOLYNAME>
+ Advanced Eye Care
130 Kinderkamack Road/Suite 205 River Edge, NJ 07661 (201)488-2020 Fax (201)488-1582
m-goldfarb@mail.holyname.org

Goldfarb, Michael, MD {1720062227} Gastrn, IntrMd(78,DC02)
+ 2130 Millburn Avenue/Suite C-6
Maplewood, NJ 07040 (973)762-8200 Fax (973)762-8203

Goldfarb, Michael A., MD {1497724702} Surgry(67,NY19)
+ 279 Third Avenue/Suite 103/Surgery
Long Branch, NJ 07740 (732)870-6060 Fax (732)571-4114
mgoldfarb@sbhcs.com

Goldfarb, Olga, MD {1952407546} Pedtrc, NroChl, IntrMd(75,RUSS)
+ Capital Institute for Neurosciences
2 Capital Way/Suite 456 Pennington, NJ 08534 (609)537-7300 Fax (609)537-7301

Goldfarb, Sidney J., MD {1093776916} Urolgy(75,NY46)<NJ-UNVMCPRN, NJ-RWJUBRUN>
+ 419 North Harrison Street/Suite 206
Princeton, NJ 08540 (609)921-3008 Fax (609)921-7533

Goldfarb, Stephen A., MD {1497769970} EmrgMd(72,MEXI)<NJ-HCKTSTWN>
+ Hackettstown Regional Medical Center
651 Willow Grove Street/EmergMed Hackettstown, NJ 07840 (908)852-5100 Fax (856)616-1919

Goldfeder, Alan W., MD {1841256757} Ophthl(74,NY20)
+ Eye Clinic PA
155 Jefferson Street Newark, NJ 07105 (973)622-2020 Fax (973)817-8666
+ Eye Clinic PA
2333 Morris Avenue/Suite D111 Union, NJ 07083 (973)622-2020 Fax (908)810-9046

Goldfine, Stephen P., MD {1578608162} FamMed, IntrMd(87,PA13)<NJ-VIRTMHBC>
+ Samaritan HealthCare & Hospice
5 Eves Drive/Suite 300 Marlton, NJ 08053 (856)896-1600 Fax (856)552-3268
+ Primary Care of Moorestown
147 East 3rd Street/Suite 2 Moorestown, NJ 08057 (856)896-1600 Fax (856)234-3907

Goldfine, Yvette Bernice, MD {1508949900} Psychy(75,NJ05)
+ Richard Hall Community Mental Health Center
500 North Bridge Street Bridgewater, NJ 08807 (908)725-2800

Goldfischer, Michael J., MD {1336178862} Pthlgy, PthAcl(91,NY46)<NJ-HACKNSK>
+ Hackensack University Medical Center
30 Prospect Avenue/Pathology Hackensack, NJ 07601 (201)996-4893 Fax (201)996-2156

Physicians by Name and Address

Goldfischer, Mindy A., MD {1144285057} Radiol, RadDia(77,NY19)<NJ-ENGLWOOD>
+ Englewood Radiologic Group PA
350 Engle Street   Englewood, NJ 07631   (201)894-3000   Fax (201)894-5244
+ Advanced Medical Imaging of North Jersey
452 Old Hook Road/Suite 301   Emerson, NJ 07630   (201)894-3000   Fax (201)262-2330
+ Englewood Hospital and Medical Center
350 Engle Street/Radiology   Englewood, NJ 07631   (201)894-3400   Fax (201)894-5244

Goldhill, Vicki B., MD {1558304618} EmrgMd(91,NY20)<NJ-HACKNSK>
+ Hackensack University Medical Center
30 Prospect Avenue/Emrg/Trauma   Hackensack, NJ 07601   (201)996-2000   Fax (201)968-1866

Goldin, Michael R., MD {1558353102} Psychy(69,PA02)
+ Drs. Nelson and Goldin
541 Clubhouse Court/Unit 3   Union, NJ 07083
+ 601 Jefferson Road/Suite 107
Parsippany, NJ 07054   Fax (973)956-9549

Goldin, Nancy Jean, MD {1073680351} Psychy(93,NY47)<NJ-UNVMCPRN>
+ 4446 Route 27
Kingston, NJ 08528   Fax (609)688-1256

Golding, Richard C., MD {1306842539} Gastrn, IntrMd(75,PA13)<NJ-HACKNSK, NJ-HOLYNAME>
+ Hackensack Digestive Diseases Associates, P.A.
52 First Street   Hackensack, NJ 07601   (201)488-3003   Fax (201)488-6911

Golding-Granado, Lisa Michelle, MD {1538163928} IntrMd(97,NY20)<NJ-BAYSHORE>
+ Immediate Care Medical Walk-in of Hazlet, P.A.
1376 State Highway 36   Hazlet, NJ 07730   (732)264-5500   Fax (732)264-5554

Goldis, Michael E., DO {1982603247} FamMed, Grtrcs, IntrMd(88,IA75)<NJ-JFKMED, NJ-VIRTVOOR>
+ Abigail House for Nursing and Rehabilitation LLC
1105-1115 Linden Street   Camden, NJ 08101   (856)365-8500   Fax (856)365-8027
+ Innova Health & Rehabilitation - Deptford
1511 Clements-Bridge Road   Deptford, NJ 08096   (856)365-8500   Fax (856)567-8997

Goldlust, Robert W., MD {1629021126} Urolgy(78,ON01)<NJ-LOURDMED, NJ-VIRTMHBC>
+ New Jersey Urology
243 Route 130/Suite 100   Bordentown, NJ 08505   Fax (856)252-1100
+ New Jersey Urology
15000 Midlantic Drive/Suite 100   Mount Laurel, NJ 08054   Fax (856)985-4582
+ New Jersey Urology
911 Sunset Road   Willingboro, NJ 08505

Goldlust, Samuel Aaron, MD {1225221922} Nrolgy(05,OH40)<NJ-HACKNSK>
+ John Theurer Cancer Center - HUMC
92 Second Street/NeuroOnc   Hackensack, NJ 07601   (201)996-5266   Fax (201)996-9246

Goldman, Alice Ruth, MD {1609971472} Radiol, RadDia, RadBdI(88,NY19)<NJ-UMDNJ>
+ University Hospital-Doctors Office Center
90 Bergen Street/DOC 1700 & 1500   Newark, NJ 07103   (973)972-2300   Fax (973)972-2307

Goldman, Clifford D., MD {1275656803} Psychy(84,NY19)
+ Moreines & Goldman PC
577 Westfield Avenue   Westfield, NJ 07090   (908)232-6566   Fax (908)232-6628

Goldman, Daniel Marc, MD {1417950767} IntrMd(94,PA12)
+ 205 East Laurel Road/2nd Floor
Stratford, NJ 08084   (856)783-1987   Fax (856)783-1403

Goldman, Faith Renee, MD {1861487894} ObsGyn(01,NY46)<NJ-ENGLWOOD>
+ Englewood Hospital and Medical Center
350 Engle Street/Brst Svc   Englewood, NJ 07631   (201)894-3893   Fax (201)894-3764

Goldman, Frieda Shepsel, MD {1841270329} FamMed(88,ESTO)
+ Middlebrook Family Practice
101 East Union Avenue   Bound Brook, NJ 08805   (732)560-0490   Fax (732)560-3681

Goldman, Gerald A., MD {1578650826} Urolgy(72,MEXI)
+ 66 West 35th Street
Bayonne, NJ 07002

Goldman, Howard Warren, MD {1497851927} SrgNro(73,NY09)<NJ-COOPRUMC>
+ The Cooper Hospital System-Univ Hospital
3 Cooper Plaza/Suite 215/Surgery   Camden, NJ 08103   (856)342-2439   Fax (856)968-8222
+ Cooper Surgical Associates
3 Cooper Plaza/Suite 411   Camden, NJ 08103   (856)342-2439   Fax (856)365-1180

Goldman, Iosif, DO {1477615466} FamMed(99,NY75)
+ Global Pediatrics
7 Auer Court   East Brunswick, NJ 08816   (732)432-7777   Fax (732)432-9030

Goldman, Jane Cleary, MD {1538274477} MtFtMd, ObsGyn, IntrMd(97,NY01)<NJ-VALLEY>
+ Maternal Fetal Medicine Associates
140 East Ridgewood Avenue/Suite 390S   Paramus, NJ 07652   (201)291-6321   Fax (201)291-6318

Goldman, Jeffrey Philip, MD {1114004009} Radiol, RadDia(90,CA11)<NJ-STPETER, NJ-RWJUBRUN>
+ University Radiology Group, P.C.
483 Cranbury Road   East Brunswick, NJ 08816   (732)390-0030   Fax (732)390-5383
+ University Radiology Group, P.C.
16 Mountain Boulevard   Warren, NJ 07059   (732)390-0030   Fax (908)769-9141
+ University Radiology Group, P.C.
579A Cranbury Road   East Brunswick, NJ 08816   (732)390-0040   Fax (732)390-1856

Goldman, Kara J., MD {1457666539} ObsGyn
+ Summit Medical Group
34 Mountain Boulevard/Building B   Warren, NJ 07059   (908)769-0100   Fax (908)769-8927
+ Summit Medical Group
574 Springfield Avenue   Westfield, NJ 07090   (908)769-0100   Fax (908)232-0540

Goldman, Kenneth A., MD {1821085937} SrgVas, Surgry(88,NY19)
+ Princeton Surgical Associates, P.A.
5 Plainsboro Road/Suite 400   Plainsboro, NJ 08536   (609)936-9100   Fax (609)936-9700   KGoldman@princeton-surgical.com

Goldman, Marvin, MD {1821183336} Pedtrc, AdoIMd(68,NY04)<NJ-STPETER, NJ-RWJUBRUN>
+ Mid Jersey Pediatrics
33 Brunswick Woods Drive   East Brunswick, NJ 08816   (732)257-4330   Fax (732)257-1177
+ Mid Jersey Pediatrics
25 Kilmer Drive/Building 3/Suite 107   Morganville, NJ 07751   (732)257-4330   Fax (732)972-1677

Goldman, Michael H., MD {1376517094} EnDbMt, IntrMd(73,NY09)<NJ-ENGLWOOD>
+ Michael Goldman MD PA
600 East Palisade Avenue   Englewood Cliffs, NJ 07632   (201)568-1108   Fax (201)568-9249

Goldman, Noah Adam, MD {1790786416} ObsGyn, GynOnc(96,NJ05)<NJ-VALLEY>
+ University Physician Associates
140 Bergen Street/ACC Level C   Newark, NJ 07103   (973)972-2714   Fax (973)972-5214
+ VMG Gynecology Oncology Associates
One Valley Health Plaza   Paramus, NJ 07652   (973)972-2714   Fax (201)986-4701

Goldman, Raimonda, DO {1639482581}
+ Regional Cancer Center at Holy Name Medical Center
718 Teaneck Road   Teaneck, NJ 07666   (201)227-6008   Fax (201)227-6002

Goldman, Robert T., MD {1396831129} SrgOrt, SprtMd, IntrMd(89,MD07)<NJ-MORRISTN>
+ Tri-County Orthopedics
197 Ridgedale Street/Suite 300   Cedar Knolls, NJ 07927   (973)538-2334   Fax (973)829-9174
+ Tri-County Orthopedics
160 East Hanover Avenue   Morristown, NJ 07962   (973)538-2334   Fax (973)829-9174

Goldman, Stuart J., MD {1841258233} Pedtrc(79,MEX03)<NJ-ACMCITY, NJ-ACMCMAIN>
+ Hamilton Pediatrics
5401 Harding Highway/Suite 6   Mays Landing, NJ 08330   (609)625-8585   Fax (609)625-3415

Goldman-Gorelov, Victoria, MD {1932155074} IntrMd(87,GEO02)<NJ-HUNTRDN>
+ Summit Medical Group-Berkeley Heights Campus
1 Diamond Hill Road   Berkeley Heights, NJ 07922   (908)273-4300   Fax (908)790-6576

Goldofsky, Sheldon E., MD {1902802374} Anesth, PainMd(81,PA07)<NJ-BAYSHORE, NJ-RIVERVW>
+ 450 Shrewsbury Place/Suite 292
Shrewsbury, NJ 07702   (201)342-1205   neuros@attglobal.net

Goldrich, Michael Seth, MD {1487748844} Otlryg, Lryngo, SrgHdN(89,DC01)<NJ-RWJUBRUN>
+ University Otolaryngology Associates
181 Somerset Street   New Brunswick, NJ 08901   (732)247-2401   Fax (732)247-6920

Goldschmidt, Howard Z., MD {1619940038} CdvDis, IntrMd(83,NY01)<NJ-HACKNSK, NJ-VALLEY>
+ Valley Medical Group/Valley Heart Group
1200 East Ridgewood Avenue   Ridgewood, NJ 07450   (201)670-8660   Fax (201)447-1957

Goldschmidt, Marc Eliot, MD {1932109493} CdvDis, IntrMd(94,NY46)<NJ-MORRISTN>
+ Gagnon Cardiovasular Institute
100 Madison Avenue/Level C   Morristown, NJ 07962   (973)971-7184   Fax (973)290-8349

Goldschmiedt, Judah, MD {1396065421} RadDia
+ University Hospital Emergency Medicine
150 Bergen Street/Level C   Newark, NJ 07103   (973)972-5128   Fax (973)972-6646

Goldshlack, Jack S., DO {1316991458} IntrMd, PulDis(73,IA75)<NJ-MORRISTN>
+ Associates in Pulmonary Medicine, PA
16 Pocono Road/Suite 217   Denville, NJ 07834   (973)625-5651

Goldsmith, Daniel French, MD {1265574016} IntrMd(95,NY20)<NJ-CHSFULD, NJ-CHSMRCER>
+ Capital Health System/Fuld Campus
750 Brunswick Avenue/InternalMed   Trenton, NJ 08638   (609)394-6000   Fax (609)394-6028

Goldsmith, Joel W., MD {1124005020} Urolgy(68,NY08)
+ UH- Robert Wood Johnson Med
125 Paterson Street/MEB 588C   New Brunswick, NJ 08901   (732)235-8853   Fax (732)235-8018

Goldsmith, Joyce, MD {1174868038} GenPrc(76,SPAI)
+ 205 Henfield Avenue
Cherry Hill, NJ 08003   (856)266-1201

Goldsmith, Steven Matthew, MD {1821087222} CdvDis, IntrMd(77,MEXI)<NJ-CHSFULD, NJ-CHSMRCER>
+ Mercer Bucks Cardiology
3140 Princeton Pike/2nd Floor   Lawrenceville, NJ 08648   (609)895-1919   Fax (609)895-1200

Goldson, Howard J., MD {1013021674} SrgVas, Surgry, WundCr(71,NY08)
+ Wound Care Institute of Central NJ
103 Omni Drive   Hillsborough, NJ 08844   (908)874-5630   Fax (908)359-6813

Goldstein, Adam S., DO {1497757462} Surgry(98,NY75)
+ Woodbury Primary and Specialty Care
159 South Broad Street   Woodbury, NJ 08096   (844)542-2273   Fax (856)384-0218
+ Advocare Associates in General Surgery
2201 Chapel Avenue West/Suite 100   Cherry Hill, NJ 08002   (844)542-2273   Fax (856)488-6769
+ Advocare Associates in General Surgery
570 Egg Harbor Road/Suite C-2   Sewell, NJ 08096   (856)256-7777   Fax (856)256-7789

Goldstein, Alan F., MD {1144219155} IntrMd, EmrgMd, FamMed(71,MO34)
+ Clark Urgent Care
100 Commerce Place   Clark, NJ 07066   (732)499-0606   Fax (732)499-8128

Goldstein, Andrea E., MD {1467653055} Gastrn
+ Hunterdon Gastroenterology Associates, P.A.
1100 Wescott Drive/Suite 206-207   Flemington, NJ 08822   (908)483-4000   Fax (908)788-5090
+ Hunterdon Gastroenterology Associates, P.A.
135 West End Avenue/Suite 204   Somerville, NJ 08876   (908)483-4000   Fax (908)788-5090

Goldstein, Arthur Meyer, MD {1316032287} Ophthl(63,PA01)
+ Drs. Kresloff and Young
900 Haddon Avenue/Suite 102   Collingswood, NJ 08108   (856)854-4242   Fax (856)854-3585

Goldstein, Asher C., MD {1790725661} PhysMd, PainMd(00,NY08)
+ 354 Old Hook Road/Suite 207
Westwood, NJ 07675   (201)645-4336   Fax (201)917-1452

Goldstein, Carl S., MD {1861497315} Hypten, IntrMd, Nephro(78,MO02)<NJ-OVERLOOK, NJ-RWJURAH>
+ Medical Diagnostic Associates PA
215 North Avenue West   Westfield, NJ 07090   (908)232-4321   Fax (908)232-7788
+ Medical Diagnostic Associates PA
525 Central Avenue/Suite D   Westfield, NJ 07090   (908)232-4321   Fax (908)389-1922

Goldstein, Charles, MD {1295737708} RadDia(74,NY19)<NJ-VIRTMHBC>
+ Radiology Associates of Burlington County
1295 Route 38 West/PO Box 479   Hainesport, NJ 08036   (609)261-7017   Fax (609)261-4180
+ Larchmont Medical Imaging
204-210 Ark Road/LMC 1-2   Mount Laurel, NJ 08054   (609)261-7017   Fax (856)866-8102
+ Larchmont Medical Imaging
219 Sunset Road   Willingboro, NJ 08036   (609)835-6540   Fax (609)835-6544

Goldstein, Craig Russell, DO {1700973203} IntrMd, Nephro(02,NY75)<NJ-NWRKBETH, NJ-CHRIST>
+ Nephrology Group
111 Northfield Avenue/Suite 311   West Orange, NJ 07052   (973)325-2103   Fax (973)325-2254
+ Nephrology Group
142 Palisade Avenue/Suite 202   Jersey City, NJ 07305   (201)963-1077

Physicians by Name and Address

Goldstein, David D., MD {1063453348} Gastrn, IntrMd(81,NY09)<NH-MONADNK>
+ Hackensack University Medical Group Emerson
452 Old Hook Road/2nd Floor   Emerson, NJ 07630
(201)666-3900   Fax (201)261-0505

Goldstein, David S., MD {1730103797} PulDis, IntrMd, CritCr(80,NY46)
+ Pulmonary Internists, PA
2 Lincoln Highway/Suite 301   Edison, NJ 08820   (732)549-7380   Fax (732)548-8216
+ Pulmonary Internists, PA
3 Hospital Plaza/Suite 205   Old Bridge, NJ 08857
(732)360-2255

Goldstein, David Wayne, DO {1831119544} Radiol, RadV&I, RadDia(89,MO78)<NJ-KMHSTRAT>
+ Kennedy Memorial Hospital-University Medical Center
18 East Laurel Road/Radiology   Stratford, NJ 08084
(856)346-6000

Goldstein, Debra R., MD {1619966850} Gastrn, IntrMd(87,MN04)<NJ-STBARNMC>
+ Summit Medical Group
75 East Northfield Road   Livingston, NJ 07039   (973)436-1540   Fax (908)673-7336

Goldstein, Elisabeth Rachel, MD {1245596741} Anesth<NJ-STBARNMC>
+ St. Barnabas Medical Center
94 Old Short Hills Road   Livingston, NJ 07039   (973)322-5000   Fax (855)851-4405

Goldstein, Gary N., MD {1265593255} IntrMd, SrgOrt, SrgPlstc(76,PA01)
+ 600 Somerdale Road/Suite 215
Voorhees, NJ 08043   (856)795-8884   Fax (856)795-7870

Goldstein, Harold A., MD {1225228315} NuclMd(74,SC01)
+ 147 Shady Lane
Randolph, NJ 07869   (973)895-5351

Goldstein, Ira Morris, MD {1427088590} SrgNro(97,IL02)<NJ-UMDNJ, NJ-JRSYCITY>
+ Center for Neurological Surgery UMDNJ
90 Bergen Street/DOC 8100   Newark, NJ 07103   (973)972-2323   Fax (973)972-2333

Goldstein, Jack, MD {1114929858} Gastrn, IntrMd(77,PA09)<NJ-LOURDMED>
+ Cooper University at Willingboro
218C Sunset Road   Willingboro, NJ 08046   (609)877-0400   Fax (609)877-3542

Goldstein, Jay R., MD {1194198739} GenPrc
+ 96 Tulip Lane
Freehold, NJ 07728   (732)859-3193

Goldstein, Joel M., MD {1396724704} SrgOrt, SrgSpn(83,IL42)<NJ-JRSYSHMC>
+ Orthopaedic Institute of Central Jersey
2315A Highway 34/Suite D   Manasquan, NJ 08736   (732)974-0404   Fax (732)974-2653
+ Orthopaedic Institute of Central Jersey
226 Highway 37 West/Suite 203   Toms River, NJ 08755   (732)974-0404   Fax (732)240-5329
+ Orthopaedic Institute of Central Jersey
365 Broad Street   Red Bank, NJ 08736   (732)933-4300   Fax (732)933-1444

Goldstein, Jonathan Edward, MD {1679532287} CdvDis, IntrMd, IntCrd(73,NJ05)<NJ-STMICHL>
+ St. Michael's Medical Center
268 MLK Jr. Boulevard/Medicine   Newark, NJ 07102   (973)877-5000

Goldstein, Joshua D., MD {1205094372} Anesth
+ New Jersey Anesthesia Associates PC
25B Vreeland Road/Suite110/PO Box 0037   Florham Park, NJ 07932   (973)660-9334   Fax (973)660-9732

Goldstein, Keith Ty, MD {1275506453} CritCr, PulDis, IntrMd(83,NY06)<NJ-HUNTRDN>
+ Hunterdon Pediatric Associates
6 Sand Hill Road/Suite 202   Flemington, NJ 08822   (908)237-4080   Fax (908)237-1749
+ Hunterdon Pediatric Associates
8 Reading Road/Reading Ridge   Flemington, NJ 08822   (908)237-4080   Fax (908)788-6005
+ Hunterdon Pediatric Associates
537 Route 22 East/3rd Floor   Whitehouse Station, NJ 08822   (908)823-1100   Fax (908)823-0433

Goldstein, Kenneth Brian, MD {1659473239} IntrMd, Grtrcs(86,PA13)
+ Besen-Goldstein Medical Associates PC
1000 Birchfield Drive/Suite 1004   Mount Laurel, NJ 08054   (856)866-1557   Fax (856)231-7955

Goldstein, Lauren T., MD {1730257551} Psychy(89,NY08)
+ 495 Iron Bridge Road/Suite 11
Freehold, NJ 07728   (732)683-1283   Fax (732)683-1619

Goldstein, Marc, DO {1770569568} FamMed(75,PA77)<NJ-HOBUNIMC>
+ Palisades Medical Center
8100 Kennedy Boulevard   North Bergen, NJ 07047   (201)866-6770   Fax (201)866-6771

Goldstein, Marc F., MD {1093863334} AlgyImmn, IntrMd, Diagns(79,PA01)<NJ-VIRTMHBC, NJ-LOURDMED>
+ Allergic Disease Associates, PC - Mount Laurel
210 Ark Road & Route 38/Suite 109   Mount Laurel, NJ 08054   (856)235-8282   Fax (856)235-2154

Goldstein, Marcy A., MD {1942209028} Dermat(90,NY46)<NY-MNTFMOSE, NJ-VALLEY>
+ 21st Century Dermatology LLC
1 West Ridgewood Avenue/Suite 305   Paramus, NJ 07652   (201)445-8786   Fax (201)445-8811
joshlochala@yahoo.com

Goldstein, Martin M., MD {1831162189} Urolgy, IntrMd(94,NJ06)<NJ-HACKNSK, NJ-VALLEY>
+ New Jersey Center for Prostate Cancer & Urology
255 West Spring Valley Avenue   Maywood, NJ 07607   (201)342-6600   Fax (201)342-4222

Goldstein, Michael Bruce, MD {1669469581} Gastrn, IntrMd(78,NY46)
+ South Jersey Gastrointestinal
2301 Evesham Road/Suite 110   Voorhees, NJ 08043   (856)772-1600   Fax (856)772-9031

Goldstein, Monte Jay, MD {1770590432} Anesth(86,NY08)
+ Jandee Anesthesiology
500 North Franklin Turnpike/Suite 206   Ramsey, NJ 07446   (201)962-7282   Fax (201)962-7283

Goldstein, Richard Alan, MD {1285625897} IntrMd(94,NY46)<NJ-JFKMED, NJ-RBAYOLDB>
+ The Doctor's Office
1 Woodbridge Center/Suite 900   Woodbridge, NJ 07095   (732)965-1050   Fax (732)791-2153
+ The Doctor's Office
3897 Route 516/Suite 2-C   Old Bridge, NJ 08857   (732)965-1050   Fax (732)394-6436

Goldstein, Richard M., MD {1386678613} Pedtrc, Nephro(64,FL02)<NJ-VIRTMHBC, NJ-SOCEANCO>
+ Pediatric Affiliates, PA
40 Bey Lea Road/Suite B203   Toms River, NJ 08753   (732)341-0720   Fax (732)244-6842
+ Pediatric Affiliates, PA
1616 Route 72 West/Suite 8   Manahawkin, NJ 08050   (732)341-0720   Fax (609)978-1229

Goldstein, Robert Glen, MD {1194807891} Psychy(89,NY47)<NY-LICOLLGE>
+ 1 Springfield Avenue
Summit, NJ 07901   (908)277-6065

Goldstein, Sheldon, MD {1467453662} Anesth, IntrMd(83,PA09)<NY-FRANKLIN, NJ-RWJUBRUN>
+ UH-New Jersey Med Sch Anesthesia
185 Bergen Street/MSB E538   Newark, NJ 07101   (973)972-5007
+ University Hospital
150 Bergen Street/Anesthesia   Newark, NJ 07103   (973)972-4300

Goldstein, Sodi H., DO {1598726366} EmrgMd(00,PA77)<NJ-LOURDMED>
+ Emergency Physician Associates, P.A.
307 South Evergreen Avenue/PO Box 298   Woodbury, NJ 08096   (856)848-3817   Fax (856)848-1431

Goldstein, Steven A., MD {1790772432} ObsGyn(85,NY08)<NJ-CENTRAST>
+ Back, Seigel & Goldstein, MD, PA
501 Iron Bridge Road   Freehold, NJ 07728   (732)431-1807   Fax (732)409-2777
+ Back, Seigel & Goldstein, MD PA
4200 Route 9 South   Howell, NJ 07731   (732)431-1807   Fax (732)409-2777

Goldstein, Steven Charles, MD {1780740860} Gastrn, IntrMd(83,NY46)<NY-SLRRSVLT, NJ-MEADWLND>
+ East Hudson Medical Group
3196 Kennedy Boulevard/Suite 2   Union City, NJ 07087   (201)325-9393   Fax (201)325-0696

Goldwaser, Alberto Mario, MD {1083766000} PsyFor, Psychy, Psynls(76,PER04)
+ Forensic Psychiatric Associates
239 Washington Street/Suite 409   Jersey City, NJ 07302   (201)314-8637   Fax (201)435-3400
AGoldwaserMD@nyumc.org

Goldwaser, Elan Luria, DO {1215378369} FamMed
+ SOM - Department of Internal Medicine
42 East Laurel Road/Suite 3100   Stratford, NJ 08084   (856)566-6477   Fax (856)566-6906

Goldweit, Richard S., MD {1053414854} CdvDis, IntrMd(82,NY20)<NJ-ENGLWOOD>
+ Heart and Vascular Institute at EHMC
350 Engle Street/Suite 1000   Englewood, NJ 07631   (201)894-3636
+ Englewood Cardiology Consultants
177 North Dean Street/Suite 100   Englewood, NJ 07631   (201)894-3636   Fax (201)569-6111

Goldzweig, Peter Allan, DO {1194774828} Anesth(93,NY75)<NJ-ENGLWOOD>
+ Englewood Hospital and Medical Center
350 Engle Street/Anesth   Englewood, NJ 07631   (201)894-3000   Fax (201)871-0619

Golestaneh, Fazlollah, MD {1780785311} Radiol, RadDia(66,IRA01)
+ SJH Millville Imaging
1001 North High Street   Millville, NJ 08332   (856)825-0005   Fax (856)825-5576

Goli, Sridhar Reddy, MD {1851528103} PedGst, Pedtrc<NJ-MEADWLND>
+ Meadowlands Physicians
6017 Bergenline Avenue   West New York, NJ 07093   (201)766-9668   Fax (201)766-9677
+ Meadowlands Physicians
913 Main Street   Passaic, NJ 07055   (201)766-9668   Fax (973)778-0809

Golin, Alexander Mark, MD {1750328639} Psychy(97,NJ06)<NJ-BERGNMC>
+ 217 First Street/Suite te 2C
Ho Ho Kus, NJ 07423   (201)670-5750   Fax (201)670-5752

Golin, Gratsiana, MD {1174557300} Psychy(65,LAT02)<NJ-RAMAPO>
+ Christian Health Care Heritage Manor Nursing Home
301 Sicomac Avenue/Psych   Wyckoff, NJ 07481   (201)848-5200   Fax (201)848-9758
ggolin@chccnj.org

Golin, Thomas, MD {1831252642} ObsGyn(83,NY20)<NJ-VALLEY>
+ 1 West Ridgewood Avenue/Suite 209
Paramus, NJ 07652   (201)444-5744   Fax (201)444-8990

Gollance, Stephen Andrew, MD {1215996517} Ophthl(99,ISR02)
+ Eye Associates of Wayne PA
968 Hamburg Turnpike   Wayne, NJ 07470   (973)696-0300   Fax (973)696-0465

Gollapudi, Devi P., MD {1841248036} IntrMd(85,INA39)<NJ-HCKTSTWN, NJ-NWTNMEM>
+ 47 Route 46
Hackettstown, NJ 07840   (908)852-8750   Fax (908)852-8820

Gollapudi, Praveen Choudary, MD {1740482231} Anesth, IntrMd(99,NY19)<NJ-VIRTMHBC>
+ Virtua Memorial
175 Madison Avenue   Mount Holly, NJ 08060   (609)267-0700

Gollotto, Kathryn T., DO {1730302274} PhysMd(05,PA77)<NJ-VIRTUAHS, NJ-KENEDYHS>
+ Orthopedic Reconstruction
600 Somerdale Road/Suite 113   Voorhees, NJ 08043   (856)795-1945   Fax (856)795-7472

Gollotto, Michael R., DO {1437368834} Anesth<NJ-OURLADY>
+ Our Lady of Lourdes Medical Center
1600 Haddon Avenue   Camden, NJ 08103   (856)757-3500

Golloub, Cory A., MD {1508867235} IntrMd, Pedtrc(86,MEXI)<NJ-CHILTON>
+ Primary Care Associates of NJ, P.A.
329 Main Road/Suite 101   Montville, NJ 07045   (973)334-9404   Fax (973)334-7615

Gollup, Andrew M., MD {1538123799} IntrMd(77,MEX14)<NJ-RIVERVW, NJ-BAYSHORE>
+ 145 Route 34
Matawan, NJ 07747   (732)525-0400

Gologorsky, Yakov, MD {1548429038} SrgNro, SrgSpn(07,PA12)<NY-MTSINAI>
+ Metropolitan Neurosurgery Associates, PA
309 Engle Street/Suite 6   Englewood, NJ 07631   (201)569-7737   Fax (201)569-1494

Golombek, Steven J., MD {1760449565} IntrMd, Rheuma(81,MD07)<NJ-HCKTSTWN>
+ Allergy & Arthritis Associates PA
600 Mount Pleasant Avenue/Suite C   Dover, NJ 07801   (973)989-0500   Fax (973)989-5046
+ Allergy & Arthritis Associates PA
66 Sunset Strip/Suite 207   Succasunna, NJ 07876   (973)989-0500   Fax (973)584-7017

Golsaz, Cyrus Michael, MD {1295017762} RadDia
+ Coastal Imaging, LLC
79 Route 37 West/Suite 103   Toms River, NJ 08755   (732)678-0087   Fax (732)276-2325

Golub, Larisa, MD {1710956586} FamMed, FamMGrtc(00,UKR16)<NJ-HUNTRDN>
+ Hunterdon Medical Center
2100 Wescott Drive/SeniorServices   Flemington, NJ 08822   (908)788-6100

Physicians by Name and Address

Golub, Michael L., MD {1336177369} Pedtrc(97,NY08)<NJ-COMMED, NJ-OCEANMC>
+ Pediatric Affiliates, PA
40 Bey Lea Road/Suite B203   Toms River, NJ 08753   (732)341-0720   Fax (732)244-6842
+ Pediatric Affiliates, PA
1616 Route 72 West/Suite 8   Manahawkin, NJ 08050   (732)341-0720   Fax (609)978-1229
+ Pediatric Affiliates, PA
400 Madison Avenue   Lakewood, NJ 08753   (732)364-7770   Fax (732)364-9292

Golubchik, Anneta V., MD {1861511610} IntrMd(95,RUS05)
+ Prudent MD
5 Dundee Avenue   Iselin, NJ 08830   (732)404-0044   Fax (732)218-3933
+ Infectious Disease Center of New Jersey
22 Old Short Hills Road/Suite 106   Livingston, NJ 07039   (732)404-0044   Fax (973)535-8353
+ Infectious Disease Center of New Jersey
653 Willow Grove Street/Suite 2700   Hackettstown, NJ 08030   (973)535-8355   Fax (973)535-8353

Gombas, George Frank, MD {1134142219} PhysMd, IntrMd(90,NJ05)<NJ-HOLYNAME>
+ 42 Chuckanutt Drive
Oakland, NJ 07436   (201)337-3638

Gomberg, Jacqueline S., MD {1285675389} Radiol, RadDia, IntrMd(82,PA07)<NJ-SJHREGMC>
+ SJH Regional Medical Center
1505 West Sherman Avenue/Radiology   Vineland, NJ 08360   (856)641-8000

Gomberg, Richard M., DO {1497747257} CdvDis, IntrMd(78,PA77)<NJ-OURLADY, NJ-KMHSTRAT>
+ Associated Cardiovascular Consultants-Lourdes
1 Brace Road/Suite C & F   Cherry Hill, NJ 08034   (856)428-4100   Fax (856)428-5748

Gomes, Ana P., DO {1750348900} FamMed(94,ME75)<NJ-WARREN>
+ Kaleidoscope Medical Associates
410 Coventry Drive   Phillipsburg, NJ 08865   (908)454-9902   Fax (908)454-9905
+ Warren Hospital
185 Roseberry Street   Phillipsburg, NJ 08865   (908)859-6700

Gomes, Eric Arvind, MD {1205831807} IntrMd(95,CT01)<NJ-CHSMRCER>
+ Princeton Pike Internal Medicine
3100 Princeton Pike/Bldg 3/ 3rd Fl   Lawrenceville, NJ 08648   (609)896-1793   Fax (609)896-1847

Gomez, Andrew Thomas, MD {1841619418} FamMed
+ Reconstructive Orthopedics, P.A.
131 Route 70 West/Suite 100   Medford, NJ 08055   (609)267-9400   Fax (609)267-9457

Gomez, Arturo A., MD {1679595912} Psychy(76,SPAI)<NJ-ACMCITY>
+ AtlantiCare Behav Hlth/Hartford
13 North Hartford Avenue   Atlantic City, NJ 08401   (609)348-1161

Gomez, Johnson Lim, MD {1649534918} IntrMd<NJ-MONMOUTH>
+ Monmouth Medical Center
300 Second Avenue   Long Branch, NJ 07740   (732)923-6537   Fax (732)923-6536

Gomez, Jose F., MD {1801893326} Anesth(86,COL22)<NJ-MONMOUTH>
+ Monmouth Medical Center
300 Second Avenue/Anesth   Long Branch, NJ 07740   (732)222-5200

Gomez, Rene S., MD {1255316766} Nrolgy(76,PERU)<NJ-UNVM-CPRN, NJ-CHSFULD>
+ Lawrenceville Neurology Center, PA
3131 Princeton Pike   Lawrenceville, NJ 08648   (609)896-1701   Fax (609)896-3735

Gomez, Syeda Rabia, DO {1255693867} ObsGyn
+ Virtua Obstetrics & Gynocology
401 Young Avenue   Moorestown, NJ 08057   (856)291-8865   Fax (856)291-8880

Gomez, William, MD {1649248634} SrgOrt(82,NY01)<NJ-STFRNMED, NJ-RWJUHAM>
+ Trenton Orthopaedic Group
1225 Whitehorse Mercerville Rd   Trenton, NJ 08619   (609)581-2200   Fax (609)581-1212
+ Trenton Orthopaedic Group
116 Washington Crossing Road   Pennington, NJ 08534   (609)581-2200   Fax (609)581-1212
+ Trenton Orthopaedic Group, PA
1 Sheffield Drive/Suite 202A   Columbus, NJ 08619   (609)581-2200   Fax (609)581-1212

Gomez Gonzalez, Vivian Katherine, MD {1730476995}
+ 1 New York Avenue
Somers Point, NJ 08244   (609)814-9550

Gomez Leonardelli, Dominic Theodore, MD {1992966493}
+ South Jersey Hand Center
1888 Marlton Pike East/Suite E-F-G   Cherry Hill, NJ 08003   (856)489-5630   Fax (856)489-5631

Gomez-Vasquez, Ricardo Antonio, MD {1801053715} FamMed
+ Wayne Medical Care, PA
342 Hamburg Turnpike/Suite 101   Wayne, NJ 07470   (973)942-4140   Fax (973)942-5070

Gong, Bing, MD {1306238100} IntrMd<NJ-HACKNSK>
+ Hackensack University Medical Center
30 Prospect Avenue   Hackensack, NJ 07601   (201)658-3148

Gong, Jeffrey, DO {1780771626} Grtrcs, IntrMd(77,MO79)<NJ-ACMCITY, NJ-ACMCMAIN>
+ 101 South New York Road
Galloway, NJ 08205   (609)652-2730   Fax (609)652-7463
+ Seashore Gardens Living Center
22 West Jimmie Leeds Road   Absecon, NJ 08205   (609)652-2730   Fax (609)404-4841

Gong, Ping, MD {1356584650} PthACl
+ Riverview Medical Center
1 Riverview Plaza/Pathology   Red Bank, NJ 07701   (732)530-2347   Fax (732)345-2045
+ Bayshore Community Hospital
727 North Beers Street/Pathology   Holmdel, NJ 07733   (732)530-2347   Fax (732)888-5243
+ Jersey Shore University Medical Center
1945 Route 33/Pathology   Neptune, NJ 07701   (732)776-4148   Fax (732)776-4146

Gongireddy, Srinivas Vamshidharan Re, MD {1316106305} IntrMd(99,INA9D)<NJ-JRSYCITY>
+ Jersey City Medical Center
355 Grand Street/Medicine   Jersey City, NJ 07304   (201)915-2000

Gonnella, Eleanor A., MD {1255432688} IntrMd(82,DOMI)
+ Sall/Myers Medical Associates, PA
100 Hamilton Plaza/Suite 317/3rd Floor   Paterson, NJ 07505   (973)279-2323   Fax (201)939-0562
egonnella@hotmail.com

Gonsorcik, Victoria K., DO {1487876637} PthACl<NJ-SOMERSET>
+ RWJ University Hospital Somerset
110 Rehill Avenue   Somerville, NJ 08876   (908)685-2935

Gonter, Neil Jeffrey, MD {1760465579} IntrMd, Rheuma(98,NY15)<NJ-HACKNSK, NJ-HOLYNAME>
+ Rheumatology Associates of North Jersey, PA
1415 Queen Anne Road   Teaneck, NJ 07666   (201)837-7788   Fax (201)837-2077
+ Rheumatology Associates of North Jersey, PA
420 Grand Avenue   Englewood, NJ 07631   (201)837-7788   Fax (201)837-2077
+ Rheumatology Associates of North Jersey, PA
8305A Bergenline Avenue   North Bergen, NJ 07666   (201)837-7788   Fax (201)837-2077

Gonzaga, Zenaida Palma, MD {1013072800} Pedtrc(63,PHIL)<NJ-NWRKBETH>
+ 50 Union Avenue/Suite 604
Irvington, NJ 07111   (973)374-2283   Fax (973)374-2936

Gonzales, Antero B., MD {1245322866} IntrMd(82,PHI15)<NJ-CENTRAST, NJ-COMMED>
+ I.M. Care Medical Group
246 South Street   Freehold, NJ 07728   (732)462-8388   Fax (732)462-8521
imbrick@aol.com
+ I.M. Care Medical Group
35 Beaverson Boulevard/Suite 2B   Brick, NJ 08723   (732)462-8388   Fax (732)970-5387

Gonzales, Antonio M., MD {1801980313} PedOph(68,PHIL)
+ 52 Ryerson Place
Closter, NJ 07624   (201)768-8453

Gonzales, Emelito T., MD {1497709091} RadOnc(69,PHIL)<NY-ARDNHILL>
+ 7 Eckerson Avenue
Closter, NJ 07624

Gonzales, Marjorie M., MD {1952341232} IntrMd(88,SPAI)
+ 650 Route 33
Hamilton Square, NJ 08690   (609)588-0158   Fax (609)588-5791

Gonzales, Santos O., MD {1538198148} EmrgMd, IntrMd(77,PHI01)<NJ-RWJUHAM>
+ Robert Wood Johnson University Hospital at Hamilton
1 Hamilton Health Place   Hamilton, NJ 08690   (609)586-7900   Fax (609)584-6428

Gonzales, Sharon Frances, MD {1720034135} RadDia, Radiol, OthrSp(95,NJ06)<NY-BETHPETR>
+ 110 South Grove Street
East Orange, NJ 07018   (973)677-1027

Gonzalez, Abel Ernesto, MD {1568711448} IntrMd
+ Hackensack Medical Center-Internal Medicine
30 Prospect Avenue/4 Main/Rm 4621   Hackensack, NJ 07601   (201)996-3664   Fax (551)996-0536

Gonzalez, David, Jr., MD {1992772594} ObsGyn, MtFtMd(90,PA13)<NJ-MONMOUTH>
+ Monmouth Medical Group, P.C.
73 South Bath Avenue   Long Branch, NJ 07740   (732)870-3600   Fax (732)870-0119
+ Monmouth Family Center
270 Broadway   Long Branch, NJ 07740   (732)870-3600   Fax (732)923-7104

Gonzalez, Felicia Ellen, DO {1598850935} IntrMd(93,WV75)
+ 1205 Green View Way
Toms River, NJ 08753   (609)314-8132   Fax (732)240-0644

Gonzalez, Francisco D., MD {1518954882} FamMed(89,DOM02)
+ 420 38th Street
Union City, NJ 07087   (201)325-9009   Fax (201)325-0113
+ Hoboken University Medical Center
308 Willow Avenue   Hoboken, NJ 07030   (201)418-1000

Gonzalez, Isabel V., MD {1497779680} Pedtrc(02,NJ05)
+ Newark Department of Health and Human Services
110 William Street/Rm 110/Pedi   Newark, NJ 07102   (973)733-5300   Fax (973)733-7617

Gonzalez, Jaime Abel, MD {1730113143} Anesth(84,DOM02)
+ 4 Glengorra Court
Mahwah, NJ 07430

Gonzalez, Joanne, MD {1235515081}
+ University Hospital-SOM Department of Psychiatry
2250 Chapel Avenue West/Suite 100   Cherry Hill, NJ 08002   (856)482-9000   Fax (856)482-1159

Gonzalez, Joselyn, MD {1063491629} IntrMd(90,DMN01)<NJ-MORRISTN>
+ 100 Madison Avenue
Morristown, NJ 07960   (973)971-4192   Fax (973)290-7148

Gonzalez, Juan A., Jr., MD {1568556520} Surgry(80,WIND)<NJ-HOBUNIMC>
+ North Jersey Surgical Group PA
1 Marine View Plaza   Hoboken, NJ 07030   (201)795-9080   Fax (201)795-9434
+ North Jersey Surgical Group PA
6040 Kennedy Boulevard East/Suite L-7   West New York, NJ 07093   (201)795-9080   Fax (201)861-5560

Gonzalez, Lenis Marisa, MD {1316145329} Dermat
+ 109 Eisenhower Drive
Cresskill, NJ 07626   (201)741-0614

Gonzalez, Lily W., MD {1780698167} ObsGyn(66,PHIL)<NJ-HOBUNIMC>
+ 359 Grove Street
Jersey City, NJ 07302   (201)432-8717   Fax (201)946-0360
Lilyg130@aol.com

Gonzalez, Marcia M., MD {1780790568} IntrMd(81,WIND)
+ Palisades Medical Center
8100 Kennedy Boulevard   North Bergen, NJ 07047   (201)866-6770   Fax (201)866-6771
+ 6115 Granton Avenue/Apt.17 F
North Bergen, NJ 07047

Gonzalez, Mario Segundo, MD {1952414476} PthACl(76,SPA06)<NJ-STMICHL>
+ St. Michael's Medical Center
268 MLK Jr. Boulevard/Path   Newark, NJ 07102   (973)877-5000

Gonzalez, Orlando V., MD {1871742700} FamMed
+ Mountainside Family Practice Associates
799 Bloomfield Avenue/Suite 201   Verona, NJ 07044   (973)746-7050   Fax (973)857-2831

Gonzalez, Patria Ramona, MD {1730111402} IntrMd(87,DOM01)
+ 1059 Soldier Hill Road
Oradell, NJ 07649   (201)262-8890

Gonzalez, Peter G., MD {1790878148} PhyMSptM
+ Orthopaedic Institute of Central Jersey
2315A Highway 34/Suite D   Manasquan, NJ 08736   (732)974-0404   Fax (732)974-2653

Gonzalez, Priscila N., MD {1508816679} PhysMd(96,PRO02)<NJ-SOMERSET>
+ Water's Edge Healthcare and Rehabilitation Center
512 Union Street   Trenton, NJ 08611   (609)393-8622   Fax (609)393-5409

Gonzalez, Raimundo, MD {1184719478} Pthlgy, PthACI(74,TX13)<NJ-MORRISTN>
+ 56 Tremont Drive
East Hanover, NJ 07936

Gonzalez, Ronald H., MD {1639277528} PhysMd(83,PRO03)<NJ-CAPITLHS>
+ Capital Institute for Neurosciences
2 Capital Way/Suite 456   Pennington, NJ 08534   (609)537-7300   Fax (609)537-7301

Gonzalez, Rosa M., MD {1033153143} ObsGyn(75,SPA06)<NJ-ENGLWOOD>
+ 7800 Palisades Avenue
North Bergen, NJ 07047   (201)861-3346   Fax (201)861-6435
docgonzd@c.net

Gonzalez Abella, Beatriz C., MD {1316974819}
+ 150 Providence Road
Mountainside, NJ 07092   (908)233-3720   Fax (908)301-5456

Gonzalez Acuna, Jose M., MD {1174758767} FamMed(85,PA13)
+ 116 Weldon Way
Pennington, NJ 08534   (609)213-5901

Gonzalez Braile, Dinah A., MD {1326040767} ObsGyn, IntrMd(90,PA07)<NJ-RWJUHAM, NJ-CHSMRCER>
+ Robert Wood Johnson Ob/Gyn Group
1 Hamilton Health Place   Hamilton, NJ 08690   (609)631-6899   Fax (609)631-6898

Gonzalez Ibarra, Fernando P., MD {1841615317}
+ 355 Jersey Avenue
Jersey City, NJ 07302   (201)915-2000

Gonzalez Monserrate, Evelyn, MD {1619905163} NroChl
+ Cooper Peds/Children's Regional Ctr
3 Cooper Plaza/Suite 200   Camden, NJ 08103   (856)342-2001   Fax (856)963-2499

Gonzalez Pantaleon, Adalberto D., MD {1306916531} EnDbMt, IntrMd
+ Endocrinology Associates
740 Marne Highway/Suite 206   Moorestown, NJ 08057   (856)234-0645   Fax (856)234-0498

Gonzalez Rivera, Tania Celeste, MD {1528260932} Rheuma
+ Penn Medicine at Cherry Hill
409 Route 70 East   Cherry Hill, NJ 08034   (856)429-1519

Gonzalez Rivera, Veronica, MD {1578722740} Pedtrc
+ Community Health Care, Inc.
3700 New Jersey Avenue   Wildwood, NJ 08260   (856)451-4700   Fax (856)794-7183

Gonzalez-Gomez, Luis A., MD {1225199698} CdvDis(81,DOMI)
+ 319 60th Street
West New York, NJ 07093   (201)868-6626   Fax (201)868-2966

Gonzalez-Mejia, Johanna Jacqueline, MD {1669565396} Pedtrc(89,DOM01)
+ Meija Pediatrics, LLC.
433 North Broad Street   Elizabeth, NJ 07208   (908)436-1002   Fax (908)436-1109

Gonzalez-Valle, Marijesmar, MD {1154649424} IntrMd<NJ-UMDNJ>
+ University Hospital
150 Bergen Street   Newark, NJ 07103   (973)972-5672

Gooberman, Bruce D., MD {1568424448} IntrMd, PsyAdd, Pedtrc(82,MEX29)<NJ-VIRTUAHS, NJ-COOPRUMC>
+ Advocare Merchantville Pediatrics
1600 Chapel Avenue/Suite 100   Cherry Hill, NJ 08002   Fax (856)665-3938

Gooberman, Lance L., MD {1194998682} Addctn(78,MEX29)
+ NaltrexZone, LLC.
1 South Centre Street/Suite 201   Merchantville, NJ 08109   (856)663-4447   Fax (856)488-6380

Goodchild, Caroline Gagel, MD {1104116409} ObsGyn
+ Garden State Obstetrics and Gynecological Associates
2401 Evesham Road/Suite A   Voorhees, NJ 08043   (856)424-3323   Fax (856)424-4994

Goode, Dale Norman, MD {1891737722} EmrgMd, IntrMd(77,PA02)
+ Patient first Urgent Care
630 Mantua Pike   Woodbury, NJ 08096   (856)812-2220   Fax (856)812-2221
+ Patient first Urgent Care
641 US Highway Route 130   Hamilton, NJ 08691   (856)812-2220   Fax (609)568-9384

Goodell, Lauri A., MD {1508931635} Pthlgy, PthACl, PthHem(91,NJ06)<NJ-RWJUBRUN>
+ RWJ University Pathology
125 Paterson Street/MEB 212   New Brunswick, NJ 08901   (732)937-8595   Fax (732)418-8445
+ RWJ University Hospital New Brunswick
One Robert Wood Johnson Place   New Brunswick, NJ 08901   (732)828-3000

Goodgold, Abraham, MD {1184791980} IntrMd(73,NY19)
+ Elizabeth Medical Group
310 West Jersey Avenue   Elizabeth, NJ 07202   (908)351-2222   Fax (908)351-1977

Gooding, Susane Lavern, MD {1902028897} GPrvMd, IntrMd(00,NJ06)
+ Capital Health Primary Care - Mountainview
850 Bear Tavern Road/Suite 309   Ewing, NJ 08628   (609)656-8844   Fax (609)656-8845

Goodman, Aimee R., DO {1235232513} Pedtrc, IntrMd(03,PA78)<NJ-UNVMCPRN>
+ East Windsor Pediatric Group
300B Princeton Hightstown/Suite 201   Hightstown, NJ 08520   (609)448-7300   Fax (609)448-8022

Goodman, Alan Jay, MD {1447255351} Allrgy, IntrMd, Algy-Immn(82,NY15)<NJ-STBARNMC>
+ Allergy, Asthma & Immunology PA
209 South Livingston Avenue   Livingston, NJ 07039   (973)992-4171   Fax (973)992-6325   Ajgoodman@att.net
+ Allergy, Asthma & Immunology PA
381 Chestnut Street   Union, NJ 07083   (973)992-4171   Fax (908)688-4416

Goodman, Arlene Michelle, MD {1629274865} PedSpM, IntrMd(04,NC05)
+ Sports Medicine Institute

562 Easton Avenue   New Brunswick, NJ 08901   (732)565-5455   Fax (732)565-5454

Goodman, Daniel J., MD {1922075639} CdvDis(70,NY08)<NJ-HACKNSK>
+ Cardiovascular Consultants of North Jersey
777 Terrace Avenue   Hasbrouck Heights, NJ 07604   (201)288-4252   Fax (201)288-7172

Goodman, Elizabeth Anne, MD {1740449743} Pedtrc(07,CT02)
+ RWJ University Medical Group/Somerset Pediatrics
1 Worlds Fair Drive/Suite 1   Somerset, NJ 08873   (732)743-5437   Fax (732)564-0212
+ RWJ University Hospital New Brunswick
One Robert Wood Johnson Place   New Brunswick, NJ 08901   (732)828-3000

Goodman, Elliot S., DO {1538214812} EmrgMd(03,PA78)<NJ-JRSYSHMC>
+ EmCare
1945 Route 33   Neptune, NJ 07753   (732)776-4510   Fax (732)776-2329

Goodman, Jeffrey W., MD {1316977416} IntrMd, Nephro(00,MA16)
+ Nephrological Associates, P.A.
83 Hanover Road/Suite 290   Florham Park, NJ 07932   (973)736-2212   Fax (973)736-2989
+ South Mountain Nephrology
5 Franklin Avenue/Suite 401   Belleville, NJ 07109   (973)450-8999
+ Fresenius Kidney Care Dialysis Center
114 Valley Road   Montclair, NJ 07932   (973)744-2059   Fax (973)744-2078

Goodman, Jonathan L., DO {1639100530} Radiol, RadDia(80,IA75)
+ Medical Institute of New Jersey
11 Saddle Road   Cedar Knolls, NJ 07927   (973)267-2122   Fax (973)267-3478

Goodman, Karen Natalie, MD {1700821402} Pedtrc(02,NY46)<NY-NYUTISCH>
+ Hackensack Univ Medical Center Pediatric Emerg Room
30 Prospect Avenue   Hackensack, NJ 07601   (201)996-5430   Fax (201)996-3676

Goodman, Robert Leon, MD {1649217779} RadThp, Radiol, MedOnc(66,NY01)<NJ-STBARNMC>
+ St. Barnabas Medical Center
94 Old Short Hills Road/Rad Onc   Livingston, NJ 07039   (973)322-5000

Goodnight, James W., MD {1144313131} Otlryg, SrgFPl(88,MA07)<NJ-WAYNEGEN>
+ Optimum Vitality
535 High Mountain Road/Suite 110   North Haledon, NJ 07508   (973)427-2711   Fax (973)427-2770   goodnig@aol.com

Goodstein, Carolyn E., MD {1932104254} Allrgy, IntrMd, Algy-Immn(64,NY08)<NJ-ENGLWOOD, NJ-HACKNSK>
+ 180 North Dean Street
Englewood, NJ 07631   (201)871-4755   Fax (201)871-8389

Goodwin, James E., MD {1699765099} FamMed(77,PA13)<NJ-WARREN>
+ Warren Hills Family Health Center
315 Route 31 South   Washington, NJ 07882   (908)689-0777   Fax (908)835-3037

Goodworth, Gregory J., MD {1528017803} RadDia
+ South Jersey Radiology Associates, P.A.
315 Route 70 East/Suite B   Cherry Hill, NJ 08034   (856)428-4344   Fax (856)428-0356
+ South Jersey Radiology Associates, P.A.
100 Carnie Boulevard/Suite B-5   Voorhees, NJ 08043   (856)428-4344   Fax (856)751-0535
+ South Jersey Radiology Associates, P.A.
6650 Browning Road/Suite M14   Pennsauken, NJ 08034   (856)665-3330   Fax (856)661-0686

Gooriah, Vinobha, MD {1912985565} Psychy(80,INA04)<NJ-CHS-FULD, NJ-ANNKLEIN>
+ Capital Health System/Fuld Campus
750 Brunswick Avenue/Physiatry   Trenton, NJ 08638   (609)394-6205   Fax (609)943-5769   vin.gooriah@dhs.state.nj.us
+ Ann Klein Forensic Center
1609 Stuyvesant Avenue/PO Box 7717   West Trenton, NJ 08628   (609)394-6205   Fax (609)633-1384
+ Medical Evaluations
268 Academy Street   Hightstown, NJ 08638   (732)940-7669   Fax (732)348-3660

Gopal, Indumathi, MD {1275607897} IntrMd(75,INA47)<NJ-CENTRAST>
+ 555 Iron Bridge Road/Suite 17
Freehold, NJ 07728   (732)294-9922

Gopal, Krishnan T., MD {1255411716} Hemato, IntrMd, MedOnc(72,INDI)<NJ-BAYSHORE, NJ-CENTRAST>
+ Monmouth-Middlesex Hematology/Oncology
326 Professional View Drive   Freehold, NJ 07728   (732)431-8400   Fax (732)431-0114

+ Regional Cancer Care Associates, LLC
723 North Beers Street   Holmdel, NJ 07733   (732)431-8400   Fax (732)739-4438

Gopal, Lekha Hareshbhai, MD {1689624173} Ophthl(91,INDI)
+ Ophthalmology & Neuro-Ophthalmology Associates
25-15 Fair Lawn Avenue   Fair Lawn, NJ 07410   (201)791-7773   Fax (201)791-7355
+ Ophthalmology & Neuro-Ophthalmology Associates
218 Ridgedale Avenue/Suite 100   Cedar Knolls, NJ 07927   (973)326-6805

Gopal, Manish, MD {1205981230} ObsGyn, UroGyn, IntrMd(00,PA09)
+ Urogynecology Associates of Central NJ, P.C.
49 Veronica Avenue/Suite 207   Somerset, NJ 08873   Fax (732)640-5320
+ Urogynecology Associates of Central NJ, P.C.
111 Union Valley Road/Suite 22   Monroe, NJ 08831   Fax (732)640-5320

Gopal, Richa, MD {1235266867} IntrMd(00,INA08)<NJ-RWJUBRUN, NJ-CENTRAST>
+ Family Practice of CentraState
312 Applegarth Road/Suite 107   Monroe, NJ 08831   (609)395-2939   Fax (609)395-4179

Gopal, Srihari, MD {1811934946} FamMed(95,NJ06)
+ Emergency Physician Associates, P.A.
307 South Evergreen Avenue/PO Box 298   Woodbury, NJ 08096   (856)848-3817   Fax (856)848-1431

Gopalam, Mrunalini, MD {1184814808} FamMed(02,INA5B)
+ 115 Berkley Avenue
Belle Mead, NJ 08502
+ 871 Allwood Road/Suite 2
Clifton, NJ 07012   Fax (862)249-4903
+ Advocare Aygen Pediatrics and Adult Care
530 East Main Street   Chester, NJ 08502   (908)879-4300   Fax (908)879-8956

Gopin, Joan M., MD {1073555686} FamMed, Grtrcs(83,NJ06)
+ Medical Institute of New Jersey
11 Saddle Road   Cedar Knolls, NJ 07927   (973)267-2122   Fax (973)267-3478

Gopinathan, Kastooril, MD {1689668139} CdvDis, IntrMd(64,INDI)
+ Union County Cardiology Associates, P.A.
1317 Morris Avenue   Union, NJ 07083   (908)964-9370   Fax (908)964-9308

Gor, Hetal Bankim, MD {1003911280} ObsGyn(94,INA65)<NJ-CLARMAAS>
+ Womens Own OBGYN LLC
180 Grand Avenue   Englewood, NJ 07631   (201)541-6868   Fax (201)541-6869

Gor, Jyotsna H., MD {1366544157} ObsGyn(70,INA21)<NJ-MEAD-WLND, NJ-HOBUNIMC>
+ 2787 Kennedy Boulevard
Jersey City, NJ 07306   (201)656-1836   Fax (201)963-8118   ranne@bellatlantic.com

Gor, Pradip D., MD {1326026899} Surgry(66,INDI)<NJ-CHRIST, NJ-HOBUNIMC>
+ 149 Palisade Avenue
Jersey City, NJ 07306   (201)792-5151   Fax (201)792-5159

Gor, Priya P., MD {1710915269} IntrMd, MedOnc, OncHem(00,NJ06)<NJ-VIRTVOOR, NJ-COOPRUMC>
+ Regional Cancer Care Associates, LLC
200 Bowman Drive/Suite E-125   Voorhees, NJ 08043   (856)424-3311   Fax (856)424-5634

Gor, Ronak, DO {1558657924} Urolgy
+ Cooper Surgical Care at Voorhees
6015 Main Street/Suite G   Voorhees, NJ 08043   (856)325-6565   Fax (856)325-6555

Gora, Jill Suzanne, MD {1356372080} FamMed(96,NJ05)<PA-SMRST>
+ Summit Medical Group
465 Union Avenue/Suite B   Bridgewater, NJ 08807   (908)864-4820   Fax (908)864-4819

Goradia, Rita U., MD {1174626774} FamMed(92,INDI)<NJ-JFKMED>
+ Harshen Family Practice
1003 St. Georges Avenue   Rahway, NJ 07065   (732)388-3006   Fax (732)388-9878

Goraya, Sukhjender, MD {1710931498} IntrMd, NeuMSptM(91,INA5Z)
+ Carteret Medical Center
606 Roosevelt Avenue   Carteret, NJ 07008   (732)541-6521   Fax (732)541-0060

Gorcey, Steven A., MD {1679512941} Gastrn, IntrMd(86,ISR02)<NJ-MONMOUTH, NJ-JRSYSHMC>
+ Monmouth Gastroenterology
142 Route 35   Eatontown, NJ 07724   (732)389-5004   Fax (732)389-1850
+ Monmouth Gastroenterology
142 State Route 35 South/Suite 103   Eatontown, NJ 07724

Physicians by Name and Address

Gordin, Mark, MD {1588693642} Psychy(87,DMN02)<NJ-VAN-JHCS, NJ-VAEASTOR>
+ VA New Jersey Health Care System-East Orange Campus
385 Tremont Avenue/Psych   East Orange, NJ 07018
(973)676-1000

Gordin, Stephen Joshua, MD {1821328527} IntrMd
+ Horizon Blue Cross Blue Shield of N.J.
250 Century Parkway/MT-03T   Mount Laurel, NJ 08054
(856)638-3259

Gordina, Alla, MD {1982766978} Pedtrc(83,RUSS)<NJ-STPETER, NJ-RWJUBRUN>
+ Global Pediatrics
7 Auer Court   East Brunswick, NJ 08816   (732)432-7777
Fax (732)432-9030

Gordon, Anne M., MD {1669564753} Pedtrc(03,PA01)<NJ-VIRTU-AHS, NJ-VIRTMARL>
+ Cooper Pediatrics
110 Marter Avenue/Bldg. 500, Suite 505   Moorestown, NJ 08057   (856)536-1400   Fax (856)536-1402
+ Advocare Marlton Pediatrics
525 Route 73 South   Marlton, NJ 08053   (856)536-1400
Fax (856)596-9110
+ Advocare Hammonton Pediatrics
856 South Whitehorse Pike   Hammonton, NJ 08057
(609)704-8848   Fax (609)704-8849

Gordon, Clifford Avery, MD {1720089816} Gastrn, IntrMd(68,PA02)<NJ-CHILTON>
+ 13 Donald Court
Wayne, NJ 07470   (862)220-4000   Fax (201)815-2000

Gordon, Emily, MD {1760762710} IntrMd
+ 140 Bergen Street/Suite 1779
Newark, NJ 07103   (973)972-9523

Gordon, Eric Michael, MD {1336312727} SrgOARec(02,NY20)
+ MidJersey Orthopaedics, P.A.
8100 Westcott Drive/Suite 101   Flemington, NJ 08822
(908)782-0600   Fax (908)782-7575

Gordon, F. Kennedy, MD {1548354897} SprtMd, IntrMd, Acp-ntr(87,NJ05)
+ Gordon Elite Sports Medicine
2500 Morris Avenue/Suite 200   Union, NJ 07083
(908)688-8630   Fax (908)688-0869
gordonelite@hotmail.com

Gordon, Jeffrey, MD {1649287251} Anesth(88,NY01)
+ Rancocas Anesthesiology, PA
700 Route 130 North/Suite 203   Cinnaminson, NJ 08077
(856)829-9345   Fax (856)829-3605

Gordon, Karen Ann, MD {1770555856} Dermat(92,NY19)<NJ-STBARNMC, NJ-VALLEY>
+ The Dermatology Group, P.C.
30 West Century Road/Suite 320   Paramus, NJ 07652
(973)571-2121   Fax (201)986-0702

Gordon, Leslie Ellen, MD {1104038231} Ophthl
+ 57 Herrick Avenue
Teaneck, NJ 07666

Gordon, Marc William, MD {1134448509} EmrgMd<NJ-NWRK-BETH>
+ Newark Beth Israel Medical Center
201 Lyons Avenue   Newark, NJ 07112   (973)926-7000

Gordon, Marilyn L., MD {1174562896} IntrMd(92,PA13)<NJ-COOPRUMC>
+ Cooper University Medical Center/Camden
3 Cooper Plaza/Room 220   Camden, NJ 08103   (856)342-2000

Gordon, Michael H., MD SrgOrt(73,IL42)<NJ-OCEANMC>
+ 3350 State Highway 138 West
Wall, NJ 07719   (732)681-2552

Gordon, Michael Stuart, MD {1013904333} Anesth(89,PA13)
+ Hamilton Anesthesia and Pain Management
1 Hamilton Health Place   Hamilton, NJ 08690   (609)631-6824   Fax (609)631-6839

Gordon, Nancy Deborah, MD {1679621734} AlgyImmn, IntrMd(95,PA13)<NJ-VIRTMHBC, NJ-VIRTUAHS>
+ Allergic Disease Associates, PC - Mount Laurel
210 Ark Road & Route 38/Suite 109   Mount Laurel, NJ 08054   (856)235-8282   Fax (856)235-2154

Gordon, Richard Dennis, MD {1295755254} Rheuma, IntrMd(75,PA02)
+ 2121 Klockner Road
Hamilton, NJ 08690   (609)587-9898   Fax (609)584-1774

Gordon, Richard L., DO {1407859259} Hemato, IntrMd, OncHem(68,PA77)<NJ-KMHCHRRY, NJ-KENEDYHS>
+ Comprehensive Cancer & Hematology Specialists, P.C.
705 White Horse Road   Voorhees, NJ 08043   (856)435-1777   Fax (856)435-0696
+ Comprehensive Cancer & Hematology Specialists, P.C.
17 West Red Bank Avenue/Suite 202   Woodbury, NJ 08096
(856)435-1777   Fax (856)848-0958
+ Comprehensive Cancer & Hematology Specialists, P.C.
900 Medical Center Drive/Suite 200   Sewell, NJ 08043
(856)582-0550   Fax (856)582-7640

Gordon, Robert, DO {1013945799} IntrMd, PulDis(75,PA77)<NJ-KMHTURNV>
+ SOM - Department of Internal Medicine
42 East Laurel Road/Suite 3100   Stratford, NJ 08084
(856)566-6859   Fax (856)566-6952
+ University Doctors Family Practice
100 Centruy Parkway/Suite 140   Mount Laurel, NJ 08054
(856)566-6859   Fax (856)566-6952

Gordon, Robert P., MD {1053349191} Anesth(82,DMN01)<NY-WESTCHMC>
+ Jandee Anesthesiology
500 North Franklin Turnpike/Suite 206   Ramsey, NJ 07446
(201)962-7282   Fax (201)962-7283

Gordon, Stephen J., MD {1801829734} Ophthl(77,NY09)<NJ-RWJUBRUN>
+ Ophthalmology Surgical Associates
317 Cleveland Avenue/2nd Floor   Highland Park, NJ 08904
(732)545-0362   Fax (732)545-7499
+ Ophthalmology Surgical Associates
579a Cranbury Road/Suite 101   East Brunswick, NJ 08816
(732)254-0097

Gordon, Stuart Leon, MD {1154361103} SrgOrt(81,PA02)
+ Cooper Bone and Joint Institute
401 South Kings Highway/Suite 3-A   Cherry Hill, NJ 08003
(856)547-0201   Fax (856)547-0316
+ Cooper Bone and Joint Institute
900 Centennial Boulevard   Voorhees, NJ 08043   (856)547-0201   Fax (856)325-6678

Gordon, Susan Master, MD {1003034034} Ophthl(04,PA02)
+ Eye Physicians PC
1140 White Horse Road/Suite 1   Voorhees, NJ 08043
(856)784-3366   Fax (856)784-4388

Gorechlad, John W., MD {1881788065} Surgry(05,NJ05)<NY-LINCOLN>
+ Meridian Trauma Associates PC
1945 State Route 33   Neptune, NJ 07754   (732)776-4949

Gorelik, Dmitry David, MD {1942375654} IntrMd(01,ISR02)
+ 197 Wyckoff Avenue
Wyckoff, NJ 07481   (646)331-9154

Gorelli, Lucy Ann, MD {1700276532} GenPrc
+ Walson Air Force Medical Facility
5250 New Jersey Avenue   Fort Dix, NJ 08640
+ Fort Dix Military Entrance Processing Station
5645 Texas Avenue   Fort Dix, NJ 08640   (609)562-6050

Gorgo, Jessica, DO {1861657397} Psychy<NJ-HACKNSK>
+ Vantage Health System
2 Park Avenue   Dumont, NJ 07628   (201)385-4400   Fax (201)385-9689
jlh2980@aol.com

Gorgy, Raafat A., DO {1700137734}<NJ-SJHREGMC>
+ SJH Regional Medical Center
1505 West Sherman Avenue   Vineland, NJ 08360
(856)641-7675   Fax (856)705-4944

Gorin, Risa Jill, DO {1770524274} Dermat(00,NJ75)
+ Dermatology & Skin Cancer Center
55 North Gilbert Street   Tinton Falls, NJ 07701   (732)747-5500   Fax (732)747-1212

Gorlitsky, Helen, MD {1164458683} ObsGyn(99,PA13)<NJ-VIRTMHBC>
+ Virtua Phoenix OBGYN
120 Madison Avenue/Suite B   Mount Holly, NJ 08060
(609)444-5500   Fax (609)444-5501
+ Virtua Phoenix OBGYN
3242 Route 206   Bordentown, NJ 08505   (609)444-5500
Fax (609)444-5606
+ Virtua Obstetrics & Gynocology
401 Young Avenue   Moorestown, NJ 08060   (856)291-8865
Fax (856)291-8867

Gorloff, Victor, MD {1194794396} PulDis, IntrMd, CritCr(92,NJ06)<NJ-HACKNSK, NJ-HOLYNAME>
+ Holy Name Pulmonary Associates PC
200 Grand Avenue/Suite 102   Englewood, NJ 07631
(201)871-3636   Fax (201)871-2286
vgorloff@njlung.com

Gorman, Eugene S., MD {1548238447} Anesth(84,NY46)
+ Ambulatory Surgery Center Association Inc.
556 Eagle Rock Avenue   Roseland, NJ 07068   (973)618-2200   Fax (973)403-8945

Gorman, James G., Jr., DO {1720002967} Ophthl(93,NJ75)<NJ-KMHSTRAT>
+ 102 West Whitehorse Road/Suite 103
Voorhees, NJ 08043   (856)309-5800   Fax (856)309-8600

Gorman, Robert T., MD {1265592786} FamMed(82,NJ05)<NJ-MTNSIDE>
+ Town Medical Associates/Verona
271 Grove Avenue/Suite A   Verona, NJ 07044   (973)239-2600   Fax (973)239-0482

Gorman, Saul David, MD {1982676045} Psychy(73,VA04)<NJ-TRININPC>
+ Trinitas Regional Medical Center-New Point Campus
655 East Jersey Street/Psychiatry   Elizabeth, NJ 07206
(908)994-5000

Gormley, Jillian, DO {1063830297} Pedtrc
+ Cooper Peds/Children's Regional Ctr
3 Cooper Plaza/Suite 200   Camden, NJ 08103   (856)356-4924   Fax (856)368-8297

Gormus, Margarita, MD {1366642340}
+ St. Clare's Health Services
50 Morris Avenue/Psychiatry M.D.   Denville, NJ 07834
(973)625-7051   Fax (973)625-7128
ritagormus@gmail.com

Gorney, Marilyn A., DO GPrvMd(93,NJ75)
+ 50 East State Street/6th Floor
Trenton, NJ 08625

Gornish, Aron L., MD {1902871437} Surgry(86,NY09)<NJ-JRSYSHMC, NJ-OCEANMC>
+ Atlantic Surgical Group, PA
255 Monmouth Road   Oakhurst, NJ 07755   (732)531-5445
Fax (732)531-1776
+ Atlantic Surgical Group, PA
459 Jack Martin Boulevard/Suite 7   Brick, NJ 08724
(732)531-5445   Fax (732)836-1592

Gorodokin, Gary I., MD {1619996774} Gastrn, IntrMd(89,NY08)<NJ-VALLEY>
+ Gastroenterology Consultants of North Jersey, PC
24-07 A Broadway   Fair Lawn, NJ 07410   (201)791-7760
Fax (201)791-7746
gorodokin@earthlink.net

Gorski, Robert Mitchell, MD {1922202399} EmrgMd(04,MI20)<NJ-MTNSIDE>
+ Hackensack UMC Mountainside
1 Bay Avenue/Emergency   Montclair, NJ 07042   (973)429-6000

Gorsky, Mila, MD {1679695928} IntrMd
+ Memorial Sloan-Kettering Cancer Center Basking Ridge
136 Mountain View Boulevard/Medicine   Basking Ridge, NJ 07920   (908)542-3000   Fax (908)542-3220

Gosalia, Tanmay Pradip, DO {1184064347} IntrMd<NJ-PALISADE>
+ Palisades Medical Center
7600 River Road   North Bergen, NJ 07047   (201)854-5000

Gosin, Jeffrey Stuart, MD {1386752012} SrgVas, Surgry, IntrMd(89,PA02)
+ Shore Vascular & Vein Center
442 Bethel Road   Somers Point, NJ 08244   (609)927-8346

Goss, Deborah Anne Marie, MD {1790765949} PulDis, IntrMd(97,NE06)<NJ-HACKNSK>
+ Hackensack Sleep & Pulmonary Center
170 Prospect Avenue/Suite 20   Hackensack, NJ 07601
(201)996-0232   Fax (201)996-0095

Goss, Graydon G., MD {1306937529} PsycAd, Psychy(77,NH01)
+ 79 Oak Hill Road
Red Bank, NJ 07701   (732)530-1181   Fax (732)530-1182
GRAYDON@GGOSS.com

Gosselin, Edward M., MD {1821015330} EmrgMd(90,MA05)<NJ-CHILTON>
+ Chilton Medical Center
97 West Parkway/EmrgMed   Pompton Plains, NJ 07444
(973)831-5000   Fax (201)444-3604

Goswami, Amit, MD {1972605137} AnesPain(99,INA69)
+ Plastic Surgery Specialists of New Jersey
2 Sears Drive/Suite 103   Paramus, NJ 07652   (201)664-8000

Gotesman, Alexander, MD {1003002072} Urolgy(99,NY48)
+ University Urology Associates of New Jersey
1374 Whitehorse Hamilton Sq/Suite 101   Hamilton, NJ 08690   (609)586-1319   Fax (609)581-5901

Gotfried, Fern, MD {1649282419} Pedtrc, AdolMd(80,NJ06)<NJ-MORRISTN>
+ Franklin Pediatrics, PA
91 South Jefferson Road/Suite 200   Whippany, NJ 07981
(973)538-6116   Fax (973)538-3712

Goth, Melanie Michele, MD {1447346838} Pedtrc(98,NC01)<NY-STANTHNY>
+ Herbert Kania Pediatric Center
1900 Union Valley Road   Hewitt, NJ 07421   (973)728-4480
Fax (973)728-4375

Gottdiener, Alexandra H., MD {1710907019} IntrMd(97,IL11)<NJ-ENGLWOOD>
+ Englewood Hospital and Medical Center
350 Engle Street/Medicine   Englewood, NJ 07631
(201)894-3000

Gottesman, Brian Tod, MD {1306874615} ObsGyn(95,NY08)<NJ-SOCEANCO>
+ SOMC Medical Group, PC
1100 Route 72 West/Suite 305   Manahawkin, NJ 08050
(609)978-9841   Fax (609)978-9843

Gottfried, Maureen, DO {1972652832} Elecmy, Nrolgy(92,PA77)<NJ-ACMCITY, NJ-ACMCMAIN>
+ Coastal Physicians and Surgeons
110 Harbor Lane/Suite A   Somers Point, NJ 08244
(609)653-9110   Fax (609)653-4105

Gottfried, Michael S., MD {1417905985} IntrMd(70,IL11)<NJ-CHSMRCER>
+ Pathlink, LLC
66 West Gilbert Street/Suite 100   Tinton Falls, NJ 07701   (732)212-0060   Fax (732)212-0061

Gottlieb, Joel M., MD {1174529705} Ophthl(79,NY03)<NJ-STCLR-DOV>
+ Roxbury Eye Center, PC
66 Sunset Strip/Suite 107   Succasunna, NJ 07876   (973)584-4451   Fax (973)584-2099
joelg@roxburyeyecenter.com
+ Mountain Lakes Eye Center
19 Pocono Road/Suite 212   Denville, NJ 07834   (973)584-4451   Fax (973)584-2099

Gottlieb, Ricki L., MD {1437836039} Pedtrc(88,MEX03)<NJ-HCKTSTWN>
+ College Plaza Pediatrics
765 State Route 10 East/Suite 203   Randolph, NJ 07869   (973)659-9991   Fax (973)659-9632

Gottlieb, Stanley, MD {1982752200} Psychy(65,IL42)
+ 575 Cranbury Road
East Brunswick, NJ 08816   (732)238-0035

Goudsward, Sean M., DO {1114972999} FamMed(88,IA75)<NJ-VIRTBERL>
+ Cedar Brook Family Practice
187 South Route 73/Building B   Hammonton, NJ 08037   (609)567-2101   Fax (609)704-9351

Goulart, Hamilton C., MD {1104992890} SrgNro, SrgSpn(75,BRAZ)<NJ-VALLEY>
+ North Jersey Neurosurgical Associates PA
225 Dayton Street   Ridgewood, NJ 07450   (201)612-0020   Fax (201)612-0333

Gould, Carolyn L., MD {1649294703} Pedtrc(75,MD07)<NJ-VIRTMHBC, NJ-LOURDMED>
+ Kids first
2006 Salem Road   Burlington, NJ 08016   (609)877-1500   Fax (609)877-4262

Gould, Jack R., DO {1235241258} ObsGyn(89,NJ75)<NJ-MONMOUTH, NJ-RIVERVW>
+ Ocean Obstetric and Gynecologic Associates
804 West Park Avenue/Building A   Ocean, NJ 07712   (732)695-2040   Fax (732)493-1640

Gould, Joshua Mark, DO {1043238876} Ophthl, IntrMd(02,NY75)
+ The Eye Care Ctr of New Jersey
108 Broughton Avenue   Bloomfield, NJ 07003   (973)743-1331   Fax (973)743-6577

Gould, Lawrence, MD {1548206337} Radiol(66,BEL04)<NJ-HOBUNIMC>
+ Hoboken University Medical Center
308 Willow Avenue/Radiology   Hoboken, NJ 07030   (201)418-1000   Fax (201)418-1822

Gould, Michael Alan, MD {1902825847} EmrgMd(94,PA07)<NJ-SOMERSET>
+ Emergency Medical Associates of NJ, P.A.
3 Century Drive   Parsippany, NJ 07054   (973)740-0607   Fax (973)740-9895

Gould, Peter L., MD {1801944921} FamMed, IntrMd(92,NJ06)
+ Cina Medical Associates
50 Newark Avenue/Suite 308   Belleville, NJ 07109   (973)450-1155   Fax (973)751-5741

Goulet, Nicole, MD {1336434257} SrgCrC
+ Rutgers- New Jersey Medical School
185 South Orange Avenue/MSB G-514   Newark, NJ 07103   (973)972-6439

Goulko, Olga, MD {1710094578} Dermat, FamMed(79,RUS06)
+ 2125 Center Avenue/Suite 200
Fort Lee, NJ 07024   (201)461-5655   Fax (201)461-1181
friendship_dusti@yahoo.com

Goulston, Michael Keith, MD {1992957203} SrgO&M
+ Oral & Maxillofacial Surgery Middlesex
213 Durham Avenue   South Plainfield, NJ 07080   (908)222-0040   Fax (908)222-0041

Gourishankar, Ruplanaik, MD {1629138235} Anesth(70,INA3Y)
+ 15 Brayton Road
Livingston, NJ 07039   (973)533-5512

Gourkanti, Bharathi, MD {1720188402} Anesth(79,INA39)<NJ-COOPRUMC>
+ Cooper University Hospital
One Cooper Plaza   Camden, NJ 08103   (856)342-2000

Gourkanti, Rao S., MD {1881630028} IntrMd(83,INDI)<NJ-RIVERVW, NJ-BAYSHORE>
+ PG Medical Associates
31 Seven Bridges Road   Little Silver, NJ 07739   (732)741-4668   Fax (732)219-1681
+ PG Medical Associates
25 First Avenue/Suite 104   Atlantic Highlands, NJ 07716   (732)741-4668   Fax (732)219-1681

Govan, Satyen Manilal, DO {1639195910} IntrMd(01,NJ75)<NJ-VIRTVOOR, NJ-VIRTMHBC>
+ Virtua Hospitalist Group Memorial
175 Madison Avenue/1 FL   Mount Holly, NJ 08060   (609)914-6180   Fax (609)914-6182

+ Virtua Voorhees
100 Bowman Drive/Hospitalist   Voorhees, NJ 08043   (856)247-3000

Gove, Ronald C., MD {1033170030} IntrMd(73,PA13)<NJ-SHOREMEM>
+ 222 New Road/Suite 304/Central Park E
Linwood, NJ 08221   (609)927-9790   Fax (609)646-9663

Goveas, Roveena Noeline, MD {1487895363} Nephro<NJ-JFKJHNSN>
+ Hackensack UMC Mountainside
1 Bay Avenue   Montclair, NJ 07042   (973)429-6000

Govil, Sushama, MD {1386615284} PthACl, Pthlgy, PthHem(64,INA72)<NJ-JRSYSHMC, NJ-RIVERVW>
+ Jersey Shore University Medical Center
1945 Route 33/Pathology   Neptune, NJ 07753   (732)776-4143   Fax (732)776-4146

Govindani, Niketa Vinod, MD {1619943446} ObsGyn(01,DMN01)
+ Excelsior Women's Care
170 Prospect Avenue/Suite 4   Hackensack, NJ 07601   (201)488-2288   Fax (201)488-2298

Gowali, Neha M., MD {1538592084} RadDia(12,GRN01)
+ Summit Radiological Associates, PA
1811 Springfield Avenue   New Providence, NJ 07974   (908)522-9111

Gowda, Mamatha Ramesh, MD {1881630671} RadDia(93,INDI)<NJ-HOBUNIMC>
+ Hoboken University Medical Center
308 Willow Avenue/Radiology   Hoboken, NJ 07030   (201)418-1000   Fax (201)418-1822

Gowda, Nidagalle, MD {1851346399} PsyCAd, Pedtrc(90,INA68)
+ University Behavioral Health Care
303 George Street/Suite 200   New Brunswick, NJ 08901   (732)235-6863   Fax (732)235-6187
+ University Behavioral Health Care
671 Hoes Lane/PO Box 1392   Piscataway, NJ 08855   (732)235-5500

Gowda, Sharada Hiranya, MD {1063452555} EmrgMd, Pedtrc, IntrMd(99,INA68)<NJ-VIRTVOOR>
+ CHOP Care Network at Virtua Voorhees Hospital
100 Bowman Drive/MEB 396   Voorhees, NJ 08043   (732)235-5699   Fax (609)261-5842
+ RWJ University Hospital New Brunswick
One Robert Wood Johnson Place   New Brunswick, NJ 08901   (732)235-5699   Fax (732)235-5668

Gowda, Srisai, MD {1801995352} Psychy, PssoMd(91,INA9Z)<NJ-SHOREMEM, NJ-ACMCITY>
+ Srisai Gowda MD LLC
408 Bethel Road/Suite D201   Somers Point, NJ 08244   (609)927-1030   Fax (609)927-9985

Gowda, Subhashini Anande, MD {1225058423} ClCdEl, CdvDis(95,INA28)<NJ-STPETER, NJ-RWJUBRUN>
+ RWJPE/New Brunswick Cardiology Group, P.A.
75 Veronica Road/Suite 101   Somerset, NJ 08873   (732)247-7444   Fax (732)247-5119
+ RWJPE New Brunswick Cardiology Group, P.A.
111 Union Valley Road/Suite 201   Monroe Township, NJ 08831   (732)247-7444   Fax (609)409-6882
+ RWJPE New Brunswick Cardiology Group, P.A.
15H Briar Hill Court   East Brunswick, NJ 08873   (732)613-9313

Goy, Andre Henri, MD {1215992912} IntrMd, OncHem, MedOnc(88,FRA22)<NJ-HACKNSK>
+ John Theurer Cancer Center - HUMC
92 Second Street   Hackensack, NJ 07601   (201)996-3033   Fax (551)996-0573

Goyal, Ajai K., MD {1578594446} Pedtrc(66,INDI)<NJ-CHILTON, NJ-VALLEY>
+ 130 Skyline Drive
Ringwood, NJ 07456   (973)962-6165   Fax (973)962-4409

Goyal, Ajay, MD {1922196815} Surgry(96,NY08)<NJ-OVERLOOK>
+ New Jersey Bariatric Center
193 Morris Avenue/2nd Floor   Springfield, NJ 07081   (908)481-1270   Fax (908)688-8861
agoyal@njbariatriccenter.com

Goyal, Alok, MD {1003848805} Gastrn, IntrMd(84,NY01)<NJ-JFKJHNSN, NJ-JFKMED>
+ South Plainfield Primary Care
2509 Park Avenue/Suite 1A   South Plainfield, NJ 07080   (908)668-8290   Fax (908)561-4914

Goyal, Janak R., MD {1417903477} IntrMd, Rheuma(74,INDI)<NJ-RBAYPERT, NJ-RBAYOLDB>
+ 528 Amboy Avenue
Perth Amboy, NJ 08861

Goyal, Madhu A., MD {1538102413} MtFtMd, NnPnMd, Pedtrc(85,INDI)<NJ-NWRKBETH>
+ South Plainfield Primary Care
2509 Park Avenue/Suite 1A   South Plainfield, NJ 07080   (908)668-8290   Fax (908)561-4914

Goyal, Madhu B., MD {1467457226} IntrMd, Grtrcs(72,INA72)<NJ-JFKMED>
+ Goyal & Natarajan MDs LLC
904 Oak Tree Road/Suite M   South Plainfield, NJ 07080   (908)757-1414   Fax (908)757-3317
mbgoyal@gmail.com

Goyal, Neil Kamal, MD {1275559718} IntrMd, IntCrd, CdvDis(99,NY01)
+ Summit Medical Group
6 Brighton Road/2 FL   Clifton, NJ 07012   (973)777-7911   Fax (973)777-5403

Goyal, Seema Agrawal, MD {1609043082} Rheuma
+ Princeton Medical Group, P.A.
419 North Harrison Street   Princeton, NJ 08540   (312)497-1212   Fax (609)924-6552
+ Princeton Medical Group, P.A.
3 Liberty Street   Plainsboro, NJ 08536   (609)924-9300
+ Princeton Medical Group PA
2 Research Way/Bldg 2/Suite 302   Monroe Township, NJ 08540   (609)655-8800   Fax (609)655-7466

Goyal, Sharad, MD {1447416417} RadOnc(02,VA01)<NJ-RWJUBRUN>
+ Rutgers Cancer Institute of New Jersey
195 Little Albany Street/PO Box 2681   New Brunswick, NJ 08903   (732)235-6777   Fax (732)235-6797

Goyal, Shefali, MD {1669662334} ObsGyn<NJ-UNVMCPRN>
+ Delaware Valley Ob/Gyn & Infertility Group, PC
2 Princess Road/Suite C   Lawrenceville, NJ 08648   (609)896-0777   Fax (609)896-3266

Goyal, Vinod K., MD {1902971971} Pedtrc, BhvrMd, PedDvl(72,INDI)<NJ-CHDNWBTH, NJ-NWRKBETH>
+ St. Barnabas Ambulatory Care Center
200 South Orange Avenue   Livingston, NJ 07039   (973)322-7600   Fax (973)322-7685
+ Children's Hospital of New Jersey
201 Lyons Avenue/Osborne Terrace   Newark, NJ 07112   (973)926-4000

Goycer, Emelina A., MD {1396766101} Pedtrc(72,PHI09)<NJ-HOLYNAME>
+ 140 Henley Avenue/PO Box 3
New Milford, NJ 07646   (201)262-9229   Fax (201)262-9288

Goyco, Luis A., MD {1558333724} Pedtrc(75,NY08)<NJ-HOLYNAME, NJ-HACKNSK>
+ Drs. Butterman & Goyco
228 60th Street   West New York, NJ 07093   (201)868-1120   Fax (201)868-5801

Goydos, James S., MD {1346324217} SrgOnc, Surgry(88,NJ06)<NJ-RWJUBRUN>
+ Rutgers Cancer Institute of New Jersey
195 Little Albany Street/PO Box 2681   New Brunswick, NJ 08903   (732)235-6777   Fax (732)235-8098
goydosjs@umdnj.edu

Goykhman, Stanislav, MD {1740488402} EnDbMt, IntrMd(97,RUS05)<NJ-BAYONNE, NJ-MEADWLND>
+ United Medical, P.C.
988 Broadway/Suite 201   Bayonne, NJ 07002   (201)339-6111   Fax (201)339-6333
+ United Medical, P.C.
612 Rutherford Avenue   Lyndhurst, NJ 07071   (201)339-6111   Fax (201)460-1684
+ United Medical, P.C.
533 Lexington Avenue   Clifton, NJ 07002   (973)546-6844   Fax (973)546-7707

Gozo, Ave O., MD {1306812037} Pedtrc(75,PHIL)<NJ-CHLSOCEN, NJ-NWRKBETH>
+ CSH Pediatric Practice of Union
150 New Providence Road   Mountainside, NJ 07092   (908)353-8998   Fax (908)527-6766
+ Children's Specialized Hospital-Ocean
94 Stevens Road   Toms River, NJ 08755   (732)914-1100

Gozzo, Yvette Marie, MD {1952351066} IntrMd, CritCr, PulDis(99,NJ06)<NJ-STPETER>
+ St. Peter's University Hospital
254 Easton Avenue/PulmDisease   New Brunswick, NJ 08901   (732)745-8564   Fax (735)745-9156

Grabell, Daniel, MD {1851764336} GenPrc<NJ-RWJUBRUN>
+ RWJ University Hospital New Brunswick
One Robert Wood Johnson Place   New Brunswick, NJ 08901   (732)235-8377

Graber, Cheryl L., MD {1760615983} Psychy<NJ-JRSYSHMC>
+ Jersey Shore University Medical Center
1945 Route 33   Neptune, NJ 07753   (732)775-5500

Graber, David J., MD {1952345126} IntrMd, Grtrcs, Gastrn(75,NY19)
+ Summit Medical Group
6 Brighton Road/2 FL   Clifton, NJ 07012   (973)777-7911   Fax (973)777-5403

Grabiak, Thomas A., MD {1710988852} Surgry, IntrMd(80,PA02)
+ Regional Surgical Associates
502 Centennial Boulevard/Suite 7   Voorhees, NJ 08043   (856)596-7440   Fax (856)751-3320

Physicians by Name and Address

Grabowski, Wayne M., MD {1588774046} Ophthl(77,NY03)
+ Outlook Eyecare
  5 Centre Drive/1B   Monroe Township, NJ 08831   (609)409-2777   Fax (609)409-2718
+ Outlook Eyecare
  100 Canal Pointe Boulevard/Suite 100   Princeton, NJ 08540   (609)409-2777   Fax (609)279-0150
+ Wills Surgery Center of Central New Jersey
  107 North Center Drive   North Brunswick, NJ 08831   (732)297-8001   Fax (732)297-8007

Grabowy, Thaddeus John, MD {1679570006} Gastrn, IntrMd(86,NJ05)<NJ-RIVERVW>
+ Riverview Medical Associates, PA
  4 Hartford Drive/Suite 1   Tinton Falls, NJ 07701   (732)741-3600   Fax (732)741-6079

Grabski, Karsten, MD {1518944677} NuclMd(97,GER55)<NJ-COOPRUMC>
+ Cooper University Hospital
  One Cooper Plaza/Nuclear Med   Camden, NJ 08103   (856)342-2000   Fax (856)365-0472

Grace, Rashy, MD {1912175603} Anesth
+ Liberty Anesthesia & Pain Management
  901 West Main Street/2nd Floor   Freehold, NJ 07728   (732)641-0744   Fax (732)294-2502

Grachev, Sergey, MD {1487629614} Surgry(80,UKR13)<NJ-COMMED, NJ-ACMCMAIN>
+ Southern Ocean County Surgical Associates, LLC
  44 Nautilus Drive/Suite 2b   Manahawkin, NJ 08050   (609)597-9477   Fax (609)489-0226
  serggrachev@hotmail.com
+ Community Medical Center
  99 Route 37 West/Surgery   Toms River, NJ 08755   (732)557-8000
+ AtlantiCare Regional Med Ctr/Mainland
  65 West Jimmie Leeds Road/Surgery   Pomona, NJ 08050   (609)652-1000

Gracia, Anne Marie G., MD {1447328018} Grtrcs, IntrMd(78,MEXI)<NJ-STBARNMC, NJ-MTNSIDE>
+ 59 Main Street/Suite 204
  West Orange, NJ 07052   (973)243-0220   Fax (973)243-2441

Gracias, Vicente H., MD {1841227774} SrgCrC, Surgry(91,UT01)
+ UMDNJ RWJ Surgery
  125 Paterson Street/CAB 4th FL 4100   New Brunswick, NJ 08901   (732)235-7920   Fax (732)235-7079

Gradinger, Lynne S., MD {1285614198} IntrMd(73,MA05)
+ University of Medicine & Dentistry of New Jersey-SOM
  42 East Laurel Road/Suite 3200   Stratford, NJ 08084   (856)566-6843   Fax (856)566-6781

Graebe, Kerry, MD {1053742262} ObsGyn(10,DMN01)<NJ-MORRISTN>
+ Morristown Medical Center
  100 Madison Avenue/OB/GYN   Morristown, NJ 07962   (973)971-9550

Graebe, Robert A., MD {1427174028} ObsGyn, RprEnd(77,MEXI)<NJ-RIVERVW>
+ Monmouth Medical Center
  300 Second Avenue/Ob/Gyn   Long Branch, NJ 07740   (732)222-5200

Graebe, Robert S., MD {1447672373}<NJ-STPETER>
+ St. Peter's University Hospital
  254 Easton Avenue   New Brunswick, NJ 08901   (732)745-8600

Graessle, William R., MD {1700986486} Pedtrc(91,NJ05)<NJ-COOPRUMC>
+ Cooper Peds/Children's Regional Ctr
  3 Cooper Plaza/Suite 200   Camden, NJ 08103   (856)342-2001   Fax (856)368-8297
+ Cooper Peds/Children's Regional Ctr
  6400 Main Street Complex   Voorhees, NJ 08043   (856)342-2000

Graf, Jennifer A., DO {1841239696} ObsGyn(01,NJ75)
+ Contemporary Women's Care
  338 Belleville Turnpike   Kearny, NJ 07032   (201)991-3838   Fax (201)998-4643

Graf, Kenneth W., Jr., MD {1477528321}(98,PA0)
+ 3 Kendles Run Road
  Moorestown, NJ 08057   (828)545-8295   Fax (856)968-8661
  pdrkwg@gmail.com

Graff, Michael A., MD {1649243684} NnPnMd, Pedtrc(76,ITAL)<NJ-JRSYSHMC, NJ-CENTRAST>
+ Meridian Medical Group - Faculty Practice
  61 Davis Avenue/Suite 1   Neptune, NJ 07753   (732)776-4860   Fax (732)776-4867
+ Meridian Medical Group - Faculty Practice
  61 Davis Avenue/Suite 1   Neptune, NJ 07753   (732)776-4860   Fax (732)776-4639

Graffino, Donatella B., MD {1952302192} AlgyImmn, Pedtrc(81,ITA22)<NJ-MORRISTN, NJ-OVERLOOK>
+ Pulmonary & Allergy Associates
  8 Saddle Road/Suite 101   Cedar Knolls, NJ 07927   (973)267-9393   Fax (973)540-0472
+ Pulmonary & Allergy Associates
  1 Springfield Avenue/Suite 3-A   Summit, NJ 07901   (973)267-9393   Fax (908)934-0556

Grafilo, Antonio C., MD {1104927920} Surgry(71,PHIL)<NJ-ACMCITY, NJ-ACMCMAIN>
+ 252 West Father Keis Drive/Box 710
  Pomona, NJ 08240   (609)965-4858   Fax (609)965-4859

Graham, April Danielle, DO {1144588674} Pedtrc
+ Southern Jersey Medical Center
  651 High Street   Burlington City, NJ 08016   (609)386-0775   Fax (609)386-4372

Graham, Daniel, DO {1083008460}
+ Integrated Medical Alliance/IMA Medical Care Center
  30 Shrewsbury Plaza   Shrewsbury, NJ 07702   (732)542-0002   Fax (732)542-2992

Graham, Deena Mary-Atieh, MD {1790716926} IntrMd, Hemato, MedOnc(00,MA05)<NY-SLOANKET, NJ-STCLRDEN>
+ John Theurer Cancer Center - HUMC
  92 Second Street/MedOnc   Hackensack, NJ 07601   (201)996-5811   Fax (201)996-9246
+ Regional Cancer Care Center
  7650 River Road/2nd Floor   North Bergen, NJ 07047   (212)464-0008

Graham, Dennis C., DO {1700855384} Nrolgy(73,PA77)<NJ-MEM-SALEM>
+ 385 South Golfwood Avenue
  Carneys Point, NJ 08069   (856)299-7400   Fax (856)249-0498

Graham, Patricia Ann, MD {1124114079} PhysMd, IntrMd(92,PA02)<NJ-UNVMCPRN, NJ-RWJUHAM>
+ 106 Straube Center Boulevard/Suite 118
  Pennington, NJ 08534   (609)303-0120   Fax (609)303-0151

Graham, Peter E., MD {1841385226} IntrMd, MedOnc(73,NY08)
+ 19 Old Pascak Road
  Woodcliff Lake, NJ 07677

Grana, Generosa, MD {1588773824} IntrMd, OncHem(85,IL06)<NJ-COOPRUMC>
+ The Cooper Hospital System-Univ Hospital
  3 Cooper Plaza/Suite 215   Camden, NJ 08103   (856)342-2439
  grana-generosa@cooperhealth.edu

Granas, Andrew Daniel, MD {1083607162} FamMed(01,NJ02)
+ Valley Medical Group
  140 Franklin Turnpike/Suite 6-A   Waldwick, NJ 07463   (201)447-3603   Fax (201)447-5184

Granatir, Charles E., MD {1740388545} SrgOrt(79,PA09)<NJ-WESTHDSN, NJ-STBARNMC>
+ 586 Kearny Avenue
  Kearny, NJ 07032   (201)997-7667   Fax (201)997-3324

Granato, Anthony Alexander, MD {1508838202} IntrMd, PulDis(96,NY20)<NJ-HUNTRDN>
+ Pulmonary & Sleep Associates of Hunterdon County
  1100 Wescott Drive/Suite G-2   Flemington, NJ 08822   (908)237-1560   Fax (908)806-2529

Grand, Elliot S., MD {1184704744} Glacma, Ophthl(85,NY08)<NJ-CENTRAST, NJ-MONMOUTH>
+ Millennium Eye Care, LLC
  500 West Main Street   Freehold, NJ 07728   (732)462-8707   Fax (732)462-1296
+ Millennium Eye Care, LLC
  Route 130 & Princeton Road   Hightstown, NJ 08520   (732)462-8707   Fax (609)448-4197
+ Millennium Eye Care, LLC
  515 Brick Boulevard/Suite G   Brick, NJ 07728   (732)920-3800   Fax (732)920-5351

Grande, Nancy J., MD {1205042876} IntrMd(87,NY20)
+ Novartis Pharmaceuticals Corporation
  One Health Plaza   East Hanover, NJ 07936   (862)778-8081   Fax (973)781-6504

Granderson, Lisa Irene, MD {1508892324} ObsGyn(89,NY46)<NJ-CHSMRCER>
+ Capital Health Family Health Center
  433 Bellevue Avenue/4th Floor   Trenton, NJ 08618   (609)394-4111   Fax (609)394-4070
+ Capital Health System/Mercer Campus
  446 Bellevue Avenue/Obs & Gynecolog   Trenton, NJ 08618   (609)394-4111   Fax (609)815-7814

Grandhi, Miral Sadaria, MD {1134275803} Surgry
+ Rutgers Cancer Institute of New Jersey
  195 Little Albany Street/PO Box 2681   New Brunswick, NJ 08903   (732)253-3939   Fax (732)235-6797

Grandhi, Sreeram, MD {1871822056} CdvDis, IntrMd(04,NJ03)
+ 500 Summit Avenue
  Union City, NJ 07087   (732)804-7087

Granet, Kenneth M., MD {1164569257} IntrMd(84,NY08)<NJ-MONMOUTH>
+ 166 Morris Avenue
  Long Branch, NJ 07740   (732)229-2020   Fax (732)229-2255

Granet, Roger B., MD {1366536914} Psychy(74,NJ05)<NY-PRSB-WEIL, NJ-MORRISTN>
+ The Center for Psychiatry & Psycho-Oncology
  261 James Street/Unit 2-E L   Morristown, NJ 07960   (973)540-9490   Fax (973)292-4905

Granick, Mark Stephen, MD {1235239328} Otlryg, SrgPlstc, PlsSHNck(77,MA01)
+ New Jersey Medical School Div Plastic & Hand Surgery
  140 Bergen Street/Suite E1620   Newark, NJ 07103   (973)972-8092   Fax (973)972-8268
+ Rutgers- New Jersey Medical School
  185 South Orange Avenue   Newark, NJ 07103   (973)972-4300

Granito, Joseph Louis, MD {1083663769} EmrgMd, IntrMd(PA01<PA-UPMCPHL>
+ Patient first Urgent Care
  630 Mantua Pike   Woodbury, NJ 08096   (856)812-2220   Fax (856)812-2221

Grann, Alison, MD {1992751853} RadOnc(91,DC01)<NJ-ST-BARNMC>
+ St. Barnabas Medical Center
  94 Old Short Hills Road/RadOnc   Livingston, NJ 07039   (973)322-5000

Granowitz, Gail F., MD {1487619003} Anesth(90,NY01)<NJ-SOM-ERSET>
+ RWJ University Hospital Somerset
  110 Rehill Avenue/Anesthesiology   Somerville, NJ 08876   (908)685-2200

Grant, Geordie P., MD {1861544280} Anesth(78,NJ05)<NJ-UMDNJ>
+ University Hospital
  150 Bergen Street/Level E/Anesth   Newark, NJ 07103   (973)972-5787   Fax (973)972-4172

Grant, Gwendolyn Hunter, DO {1285077800} ObsGyn
+ Lawrence Ob/Gyn Associates
  123 Franklin Corner Road/Suite 214   Lawrenceville, NJ 08648   (609)896-1400   Fax (609)896-3986

Grant, Maurice R., MD {1770782153} PthAna
+ 1 Richmond Street/Apt 3014
  New Brunswick, NJ 08901

Grant, Susan J., MD {1528143237} PsyCAd, Psychy(94,NH01)
+ CPC Behavioral HealthCare
  270 Highway 35   Red Bank, NJ 07701   (732)842-2000   Fax (732)224-0688

Grasso, Antonio Michael, MD {1497930408}
+ 1 Richmond Street/Apt 4065
  New Brunswick, NJ 08901

Grasso, Armand J., MD {1578678876} ObsGyn(79,MEX03)
+ Comprehensive Women's Healthcare
  44 Ridge Road   North Arlington, NJ 07031   (201)991-2880   Fax (201)991-0027

Grasso, Mario Lucio, MD {1972664522} Anesth(05,PA01)
+ Morris Anesthesia Group, PA
  3799 Route 46/Suite 211   Parsippany, NJ 07054   (973)335-1122   Fax (973)335-1448

Grasso, Michael A., MD {1821063785} IntrMd, Nephro(70,MD01)<NJ-NWRKBETH, NJ-STBARNMC>
+ Nephrology Group
  111 Northfield Avenue/Suite 311   West Orange, NJ 07052   (973)325-2103   Fax (973)325-2254

Grasso, Santo Vincent, DO {1487788758} GenPrc(91,IA75)
+ 1 Orient Way/Unit 203
  Rutherford, NJ 07070

Gratz, Irwin, DO {1518687297} Anesth, IntrMd(PA77<NJ-COOPRUMC>
+ Cooper Anesthesia Associates
  One Cooper Plaza/Suite 294-B/Residency   Camden, NJ 08103   (856)342-2425   Fax (856)968-8239

Graule, Melissa J., MD {1104876242} RadDia, RadV&I(92,NJ06)<NJ-ACMCITY, NJ-SHOREMEM>
+ Atlantic Medical Imaging, LLC.
  72 West Jimmie Leeds Road   Galloway, NJ 08205   (609)677-9729   Fax (609)653-8764
+ Atlantic Medical Imaging, LLC.
  401 Bethel Road   Somers Point, NJ 08244   (609)677-9729
+ Atlantic Medical Imaging, LLC.
  421 Route 9 North   Cape May Court House, NJ 08205   (609)463-9500   Fax (609)465-0918

Graves, Holly Lynn, MD {1427256080} Surgry
+ Woodbury Primary and Specialty Care
  159 South Broad Street   Woodbury, NJ 08096   (844)542-2273   Fax (856)384-0218
+ Kennedy Vascular Surgery
  1001 Laurel Oak Road/Suite D1   Voorhees, NJ 08043   (844)542-2273   Fax (856)783-0264

Graves, Linda M., MD {1528066610} GenPrc, PhysMd(94,NJ05)
+ 705 Broadway
  Paterson, NJ 07503   (973)278-0707   Fax (973)278-0709

Gray, Edward Harlan, DO {1588843015} CritCr, IntrMd(99,NY75)<NJ-COOPRUMC>
+ Cooper University Hospital
One Cooper Plaza/Critical Care   Camden, NJ 08103   (973)600-7447

Gray, John Michael, MD {1871532010} SrgOrt, SprtMd, SrgArt(88,NY15)<NJ-VIRTMHBC, NJ-VANJHCS>
+ Reconstructive Orthopedics, P.A.
243 Route 130/Suite 100   Bordentown, NJ 08505   (609)267-9400   Fax (609)267-9457
+ Reconstructive Orthopedics, P.A.
401 Young Avenue/Suite 245   Moorestown, NJ 08057   (609)267-9400   Fax (609)267-9457
+ Reconstructive Orthopedics, P.A.
131 Route 70 West/Suite 100   Medford, NJ 08505   (609)267-9400   Fax (609)267-9457

Gray, Sonja B., MD {1043304108} Psychy(88,NY20)<NJ-SUMOAKSH>
+ Summit Oaks Hospital
19 Prospect Street   Summit, NJ 07901   (908)522-7000

Gray, Terence Bay, MD {1518917129} Anesth<NY-BRKLNDWN>
+ Rancocas Anesthesiology, PA
700 Route 130 North/Suite 203   Cinnaminson, NJ 08077   (856)829-9345   Fax (856)829-3605

Grayer, Nicole C., MD {1902052749} Anesth
+ Robert Wood Johnson-UMDNJ Anesthesia Group
125 Paterson Street/CAB 3100   New Brunswick, NJ 08901   (732)235-7827   Fax (732)235-6131

Grayson, Douglas Keane, MD {1689674129} Ophthl(89,RI01)<NY-BETHPETR, NY-MANHEYE>
+ Omni Eye Services
485 Route 1 South/Building A   Iselin, NJ 08830   (732)750-0400   Fax (732)602-0749
+ Omni Eye Services
218 State Route 17 North   Rochelle Park, NJ 07662   (732)750-0400   Fax (201)368-0254
+ Omni Eye Services
2200 Route 10 West/Suite 102   Parsippany, NJ 08830   (973)538-7400   Fax (973)538-3007

Grayson, Janine Denise, MD {1215036397} EmrgMd(01,DC03)<NJ-UMDNJ>
+ 724 Firethorn Drive
Union, NJ 07083

Grayson, Jeremy Seth, MD {1912089772} Anesth, PedAne(99,PA02)<NJ-RWJUBRUN>
+ Robert Wood Johnson-UMDNJ Anesthesia Group
125 Paterson Street/CAB 3100   New Brunswick, NJ 08901   (732)235-7827   Fax (732)235-6131
+ Robert Wood Johnson-UMDNJ Anesthesia Group
1140 Route 72 West   Manahawkin, NJ 08050   (609)978-8900

Grayson, Leila S., MD {1790818102} Surgry, SrgCsm(87,NY06)<NJ-CENTRAST, NJ-RIVERVW>
+ 3350 State Route 138
Wall, NJ 07719   (732)681-0001   Fax (732)681-9112

Grayson, Stephanie Anne, MD {1164613477} NnPnMd, Pedtrc, IntrMd(06,PA13)<NJ-ACMCMAIN>
+ AtlantiCare - Neonatology Department
65 West Jimmie Leeds Road   Pomona, NJ 08240   (609)404-3817   Fax (609)404-3818
stephanie.grayson@atlanticare.org

Graziani, Virginia, MD {1467557629} PhysMd(86,PA02)<NJ-ACMCITY, NJ-ACMCMAIN>
+ Lowe-Greenwood-Zerbo Spinal Associates
1999 New Road/Suite B   Linwood, NJ 08221   (609)601-6363   Fax (609)601-6364

Graziano, Andrew A., MD {1154748994}
+ 208 River Place
Butler, NJ 07405   (973)998-0190
graziaaa@gmail.com

Graziano, Linda M., MD {1609830934} AlgyImmn, IntrMd(83,PA09)<NJ-COOPRUMC, NJ-VIRTVOOR>
+ South Jersey Allergy & Asthma
108 Kings Highway South   Cherry Hill, NJ 08034   (856)428-5120   Fax (856)428-0264

Graziano, Robert J., MD {1184730947} RadDia, RadBdI(87,PA13)<NJ-ACMCITY, NJ-SHOREMEM>
+ Atlantic Medical Imaging, LLC.
72 West Jimmie Leeds Road   Galloway, NJ 08205   (609)677-9729   Fax (609)653-8764
+ Atlantic Medical Imaging, LLC.
401 Bethel Road   Somers Point, NJ 08244   (609)677-9729
+ Atlantic Medical Imaging, LLC.
421 Route 9 North   Cape May Court House, NJ 08205   (609)463-9500   Fax (609)465-0918

Graziano, Vincent Angelo, MD {1578554796} IntrMd, Nephro(75,DC02)
+ North Jersey Nephrology Associates PA
246 Hamburg Turnpike/Suite 207   Wayne, NJ 07470   (973)653-3366   Fax (973)653-3365

Graziano, Vincent Anthony, MD {1003002809} RadDia(04,NJ06)
+ 416 Old Mill Lane
Wyckoff, NJ 07481

Graziano-Wilcox, Donna, DO {1437159027} FamMed(85,PA77)
+ Delran Family Practice
8008 Route 130/Suite 120   Delran, NJ 08075   (856)764-7997   Fax (856)764-1840

Greaney, Kathleen Margaret, MD {1952367898} Pedtrc(01,NJ06)
+ Maple Avenue Pediatrics
23-00 Route 208   Fair Lawn, NJ 07410   (201)797-1900   Fax (201)797-4457

Greatrex, Kathleen Mae V., MD {1801819123} RadDia, Radiol(90,PA13)<NJ-OURLADY>
+ Our Lady of Lourdes Medical Center
1600 Haddon Avenue/Radiology   Camden, NJ 08103   (856)757-3500

Greaves, Keiron W., MD {1447257969} Anesth(89,NJ06)<NJ-MONMOUTH>
+ Monmouth Medical Center
300 Second Avenue/Anesthesiology   Long Branch, NJ 07740   (732)222-5200

Greaves, Mark Leslie, MD {1518139914} IntrMd, Gastrn(02,OH06)<NJ-SLOANKET>
+ Digestive HealthCare Center
511 Courtyard Drive/Building 500   Hillsborough, NJ 08844   (908)218-9222   Fax (908)218-9818

Grebenau, Mark David, MD {1912154881} Immuno(78,NY19)
+ Novartis Pharmaceuticals Corporation
One Health Plaza/MedInfoCommun   East Hanover, NJ 07936   (862)778-8081   Fax (973)781-6504

Grech, Dennis George, MD {1144314022} Anesth(01,STM01)<NJ-HACKNSK>
+ Hackensack University Medical Center
30 Prospect Avenue   Hackensack, NJ 07601   (201)488-0066   Fax (201)488-6769

Greco, Dante, MD {1083649032} SrgPlstc, SrgPHand(65,QU01)<NJ-HACKNSK, NJ-VALLEY>
+ 970 Clifton Avenue
Clifton, NJ 07013   (973)779-0681   Fax (973)916-1853

Greco, Gregory A., DO {1083764187} Surgry, SrgPlstc(93,NJ75)<NJ-RIVERVW, NJ-JRSYSHMC>
+ Monmouth Plastic Surgery
264 Broad Street   Red Bank, NJ 07701   (732)842-3737   Fax (732)842-3110

Greco, John, Jr., MD {1770686867} Ophthl(88,DC01)<NJ-RIVERVW, NJ-MONMOUTH>
+ 130 Maple Avenue/Building 4/Suite 4-B
Red Bank, NJ 07701   (732)741-7997   Fax (732)741-8741

Greco, Richard Yackshaw, DO {1992039085} Surgry(07,PA78)
+ Strafford Surgical Specialists, P.A.
1100 Route 72 West/Suite 300   Manahawkin, NJ 08050   (609)978-3325   Fax (609)978-3123
+ Monmouth Surgical Specialists
727 North Beers Street   Holmdel, NJ 07733   (609)978-3325   Fax (732)290-7067

Greco, Sandra Jeanne, MD {1346204153} UroGyn, ObsGyn(91,NY09)<NJ-MONMOUTH>
+ 279 Third Avenue/Suite 307
Long Branch, NJ 07740   (732)571-0972   Fax (732)571-0748
+ 1 Route 70 West
Lakewood, NJ 08701   (732)901-0271
+ Monmouth Medical Center
300 Second Avenue/Ob/Gyn   Long Branch, NJ 07740   (732)222-5200

Gredell, Elizabeth S., DO {1851566525} FamMed(98,MO78)
+ 7 First Street
Fair Haven, NJ 07704
+ Hazlet Family Care
3253 Route 35   Hazlet, NJ 07730   Fax (732)888-7649

Greeley, Drew Peter, MD {1518968932} SrgThr, Surgry(92,NJ05)<NJ-MORRISTN, NJ-JRSYSHMC>
+ Mid-Atlantic Surgical Associates
100 Madison Avenue   Morristown, NJ 07960   (973)971-7300   Fax (973)984-7019

Green, Adam Godfrey, MD {1871882258} CritCr
+ Cooper University Hospital Critical Care
One Cooper Plaza   Camden, NJ 08103   (856)342-2000   Fax (856)968-8282

Green, Amy, MD {1972662526} Psychy(64,QU01)<NJ-MTNSIDE>
+ 326 Park Street
Upper Montclair, NJ 07043   (973)783-4669   Fax (973)783-6288

Green, Anthony J., MD {1972677003} Psychy(94,NJ05)
+ CPC Behavioral HealthCare
1088 Highway 34   Aberdeen, NJ 07747   (732)290-1700   Fax (732)290-0040

Green, Aron M., MD {1891726238} SrgOrt(01,NJ05)
+ 130 Van Orden Avenue
Leonia, NJ 07605

Green, Ashlee, MD {1518455112} ObsGyn<NJ-RWJUBRUN>
+ RWJ University Hospital New Brunswick
One Robert Wood Johnson Place   New Brunswick, NJ 08901   (732)828-3000

Green, Camille P J, MD {1811293921}<NJ-COOPRUMC>
+ Cooper University Hospital
One Cooper Plaza   Camden, NJ 08103   (856)342-2000
green-camille@cooperhealth.edu

Green, Donald H., MD {1760573125} Ophthl(72,NY19)
+ 1135 Clifton Avenue/Suite 105
Clifton, NJ 07013   (973)773-9882   Fax (973)773-9884
+ Associated Eye Physicians, P.A.
1033 Clifton Avenue/Suite 107   Clifton, NJ 07013   (973)773-9882   Fax (973)472-4832

Green, Douglas S., MD {1790753523} PulDis, IntrMd(82,PHI08)<NJ-KSLRWEST>
+ Kessler Institute for Rehabilitation West Orange
1199 Pleasant Valley Way   West Orange, NJ 07052   (973)731-3600   Fax (973)243-6861

Green, Jason D., MD {1851376271} SrgC&R, Surgry, IntrMd(87,VT02)
+ Premier Health Associates
532 Lafayette Road/Suite 100   Sparta, NJ 07871   (973)383-3730   Fax (973)383-2285

Green, Jeffrey H., MD {1558499137} Psychy(82,IL02)
+ Cedar Glen Professional Association
170 Cold Soil Road   Princeton, NJ 08540   (609)896-1122   Fax (609)896-2688

Green, Jeremy Charles, MD {1629090055} RadDia(99,NY19)<NJ-NWRKBETH>
+ Newark Diagnostic Radiologists, PA
201 Lyons Avenue   Newark, NJ 07112   (973)926-7466
+ Newark Beth Israel Medical Center
201 Lyons Avenue/Radiology   Newark, NJ 07112   (973)926-7466

Green, Jon David, MD {1245283563} Gastrn, IntrMd(74,NJ05)
+ Diagnostic & Clinical Cardiology
449 Mount Pleasant Avenue/2nd Floor   West Orange, NJ 07052   (973)731-7868   Fax (973)731-7907

Green, Justin Jacob, MD {1104894872} Dermat(98,NJ06)
+ Heymann, Manders & Green LLC
100 Brick Road/Suite 306   Marlton, NJ 08053   (856)596-0111   Fax (856)596-7194
+ The Cooper Hospital System-Univ Hospital
3 Cooper Plaza/Suite 215   Camden, NJ 08103   (856)342-2439

Green, Kirsten M., DO {1093942807}
+ Rowan University-School of Osteopathic Medicine
1 Medical Center Drive   Stratford, NJ 08084   (856)566-6708

Green, Minda A., MD {1245493022} ObsGyn
+ 601 Angielee Avenue
Williamstown, NJ 08094

Green, Patricia, MD {1578950390} Pedtrc
+ CAMCare Health Corporation
817 Federal Street   Camden, NJ 08103   (856)583-2400   Fax (856)541-4611

Green, Robert S., MD {1275500886} NnPnMd, Pedtrc, IntrMd(74,MD07)<NY-MTSINAI, NJ-ENGLWOOD>
+ Englewood Hospital and Medical Center
350 Engle Street/Pediatrics   Englewood, NJ 07631   (201)894-3000

Green, Stuart N., MD {1841263647} Ophthl, VitRet(74,NY47)<NJ-RWJUBRUN, NJ-KIMBALL>
+ Retina Associates of New Jersey, P.A.
10 Plum Street/Suite 600   New Brunswick, NJ 08901   (732)220-1600   Fax (732)220-1603
+ Retina Associates of New Jersey, P.A.
98 James Street/Suite 209   Edison, NJ 08820   (732)220-1600   Fax (732)906-1883
+ Retina Associates of New Jersey, P.A.
2 Industrial Way West   Eatontown, NJ 08901   (732)389-2333   Fax (732)389-2788

Green, Suzanne E., MD {1730205105} Surgry, SrgC&R(91,NJ05)<NJ-JFKMED>
+ JFK Medical Center
65 James Street   Edison, NJ 08820   (732)321-7000

Green, Tamar Buchsbaum, MD {1457460271} IntrMd, ErgMd(90,NC07)
+ Ocean County Internal Medicine Associates
1352 River Avenue   Lakewood, NJ 08701   (732)370-5100   Fax (732)901-9240

Green, William M., MD {1114943909} RadDia, Radiol(67,NY46)<NJ-UNVMCPRN>
+ University Medical Center of Princeton at Plainsboro
One Plainsboro Road   Plainsboro, NJ 08536   (609)497-4000
+ Princeton Radiology Associates, P.A.
419 North Harrison Street   Princeton, NJ 08540   (609)497-4000   Fax (609)683-8847
+ Princeton Radiology Associates, P.A.
9 Centre Drive   Jamesburg, NJ 08536   (609)655-1448   Fax (609)655-4016

Greenawald, Lawrence Edward, MD {1063726925} Surgry
+ LMA Surgical Associates
120 White Horse Pike/Suite 103   Haddon Heights, NJ 08035   (856)546-3900   Fax (856)546-3908

Physicians by Name and Address

Greenbaum, Barbara H., MD {1386653335} PedHem, Pedtrc(77,NY15)<NJ-VIRTVOOR>
+ CHOP Pediatric & Adolescent Specialty Care Center
1012 Laurel Oak Road/Hematology/Onc Voorhees, NJ 08043 (856)435-7502 Fax (856)627-2183

Greenbaum, David F., MD {1851392955} SrgThr, Surgry(80,PA01)
+ Rancocas Valley Surgical Associates PA
1000 Salem Road/Suite A Willingboro, NJ 08046 (609)877-1737 Fax (609)877-1589

Greenbaum, Roy L., MD {1255338463} RadDia(81,SC01)<NJ-STFRNMED>
+ Radiology Affiliates of Central New Jersey, P.A.
2501 Kuser Road Hamilton, NJ 08691 (609)585-8800 Fax (609)585-1825
+ St. Francis Medical Center
601 Hamilton Avenue/Radiology Trenton, NJ 08629 (609)599-5000

Greenberg, Aaron Joseph, MD {1609127869} SrgOrt
+ Kayal Orthopaedic Center, P.C.
784 Franklin Avenue/Suite 250 Franklin Lakes, NJ 07417 (844)777-0910 Fax (201)560-0712

Greenberg, Alan, MD {1326092180} Grtrcs, IntrMd, NuclMd(77,PA12)<NJ-COOPRUMC>
+ Cooper University Hospital
One Cooper Plaza/Internal Med Camden, NJ 08103 (856)342-3150 Fax (856)968-8573

Greenberg, Andrew Seth, MD {1548286339} RadOnc(87,NJ05)<NJ-HUNTRDN, NJ-UNVMCPRN>
+ Princeton Radiation Oncology Center
9 Centre Drive/Suite 115 Jamesburg, NJ 08831 (609)655-5755 Fax (609)655-5725
+ Hunterdon Medical Center
2100 Wescott Drive/RadOncology Flemington, NJ 08822 (908)788-6100
+ University Medical Center of Princeton at Plainsboro
One Plainsboro Road Plainsboro, NJ 08831 (609)497-4000

Greenberg, Anthony, MD {1487641239} FamMed(89,NJ06)<NJ-NWTNMEM>
+ 576 State Route 94/Suite 3
Columbia, NJ 07832 (908)496-8014 Fax (908)496-8016

Greenberg, Bram, MD {1124285788} Pedtrc(81,PA09)
+ 555 Hope Chapel Road
Lakewood, NJ 08701

Greenberg, Caroline M., MD {1104808310} RadDia(89,PA02)<NJ-STPETER, NJ-RWJUBRUN>
+ University Radiology Group, P.C.
483 Cranbury Road East Brunswick, NJ 08816 (732)390-0030 Fax (732)390-5383
+ University Radiology Group, P.C.
10 Plum Street New Brunswick, NJ 08901 (732)390-0030 Fax (732)249-1208
+ University Radiology Group, P.C.
16 Mountain Boulevard Warren, NJ 08816 (908)769-7200 Fax (908)769-9141

Greenberg, Carrie Lynn, MD {1386623668} Anesth(88,NY06)<NJ-OVERLOOK>
+ Summit Anesthesia Associates, P.A.
33 Overlook Road/Suite 311 Summit, NJ 07901 (908)598-1500 Fax (908)598-0197
+ Overlook Medical Center
99 Beauvoir Avenue/PO Box 210 Summit, NJ 07902 (908)522-2000

Greenberg, David Benjamin, MD {1053413500} OncHem, IntrMd(01,NY08)
+ Atlantic Hematology Oncology Associates, L.L.C.
1707 Atlantic Avenue Manasquan, NJ 08736 (732)528-0760 Fax (732)528-0764

Greenberg, E. Jeffrey, MD {1710929989} Nrolgy(98,PA07)
+ Princeton & Rutgers Neurology
77 Veronica Avenue/Suite 102 Somerset, NJ 08873 (732)246-1311 Fax (732)246-3089
+ Princeton & Rutgers Neurology
9 Centre Drive/Suite 130 Monroe Township, NJ 08831 (732)246-1311 Fax (609)395-1885

Greenberg, Eric N., MD {1205975901} Anesth(85,IL42)
+ 717 Ocean Avenue/Unit 205
Long Branch, NJ 07740

Greenberg, Heather Ellyn, MD {1407121684}
+ Summit Medical Group
95 Madison Avenue Morristown, NJ 07960 (973)267-1010 Fax (973)775-5115

Greenberg, Jeffrey David, MD {1982783981} Rheuma, IntrMd(98,QU01)<NJ-OVERLOOK>
+ 33 Overlook Road/Suite L-01
Summit, NJ 07901 (905)598-7940 Fax (908)598-7940

Greenberg, John P., MD {1164452439} Nrolgy(63,NJ05)<NJ-SOMERSET>
+ 8 Loch Arbour Court
Waretown, NJ 08758

Greenberg, Karen Julie, DO {1912041575} EmrgMd<NJ-VIRTMARL>
+ Virtua Marlton Hospital
90 Brick Road Marlton, NJ 08053 (856)355-6000

Greenberg, Leslie M., MD {1952480337} Anesth, Otolgy(77,MA01)<NJ-UNVMCPRN>
+ University Medical Center of Princeton at Plainsboro
One Plainsboro Road/Anesthesiology Plainsboro, NJ 08536 (609)497-4330

Greenberg, Leslie Robin, MD {1871735118} Pedtrc, IntrMd(MA07
+ Princeton Nassau Pediatrics, P.A.
301 North Harrison Street Princeton, NJ 08540 (609)924-5510 Fax (609)924-3577
+ Princeton Nassau Pediatrics, P.A.
312 Applegarth Road/Suite 104 Monroe Township, NJ 08831 (609)924-5510 Fax (609)409-5610
+ Princeton Nassau Pediatrics, P.A.
196 Princeton-Hightstown Road West Windsor, NJ 08540 (609)799-5335 Fax (609)799-2294

Greenberg, Martin J., MD {1760474308} PulDis, IntrMd(83,DMN01)<NJ-STBARNMC>
+ 124 East Mount Pleasant Avenue
Livingston, NJ 07039 (973)994-4130 Fax (973)994-2977

Greenberg, Richard H., MD {1902803349} IntrMd, OncHem(90,PA01)<NJ-VIRTBERL, NJ-VIRTMARL>
+ Regional Cancer Care Associates, LLC
200 Bowman Drive/Suite E-125 Voorhees, NJ 08043 (856)424-3311 Fax (856)424-5634
+ The Center for Cancer & Hematologic Disease
856 South White Horse Pike/Suite 4 Hammonton, NJ 08037 (856)424-3311 Fax (609)561-2492

Greenberg, Robert M., MD {1912079070} Psychy, PsyGrt(78,NY47)<NJ-HOBUNIMC>
+ Hoboken University Medical Center
308 Willow Avenue/GeriatricPsych Hoboken, NJ 07030 (201)418-1000

Greenberg, Rosalie, MD {1821164278} Psychy, PsyCAd(76,NY01)<NJ-OVERLOOK>
+ Medical Arts Psychotherapy Associates, P.A.
33 Overlook Road/Suite 406 Summit, NJ 07901 (908)598-0200 Fax (908)598-0924

Greenberg, Scott Ross, MD {1972653384} FamMed(96,PA07)
+ Magaziner Medical Center
1907 Greentree Road Cherry Hill, NJ 08003 (856)424-8222 Fax (856)424-2599

Greenberg, Susan Nancy, MD {1477533172} IntrMd, OncHem, Onclgy(78,PA07)<NJ-JRSYSHMC, NJ-MONMOUTH>
+ Adult Medical Oncology-Hematology LLC
39 Sycamore Avenue Little Silver, NJ 07739 (732)576-8610 Fax (732)576-8827

Greenberg, William M., MD {1316047889} Psychy(78,NY46)
+ Forest Research Institute, Inc
Plaza V/28th Floor Jersey City, NJ 07311 (201)427-8000 william.greenberg@frx.com
+ 65 North Maple Avenue
Ridgewood, NJ 07450

Greenblatt, Adrienne Masin, MD {1215097886} RadDia, Radiol, RadBdI(79,NY15)
+ University Radiology Group, P.C.
579A Cranbury Road East Brunswick, NJ 08816 (732)390-0040 Fax (732)390-1856

Greenblatt, David R., MD {1063465490} RadOnc, RadThp(80,NY15)<NJ-VALLEY>
+ The Valley Hospital
223 North Van Dien Avenue/Radiology Ridgewood, NJ 07450 (201)447-8000

Greenblatt, Naomi H., MD {1083815591} Psychy
+ 60 Grand Avenue
Englewood, NJ 07631 (201)830-5325

Greenblatt, Robert, MD {1104171198} EmrgMd(08,ISR06)<NY-KINGSTON, RI-SJFATIMA>
+ Emergency Medical Associates of NJ, P.A.
3 Century Drive Parsippany, NJ 07054 (973)740-0607 Fax (973)740-9895

Greenblatt, Robert I., MD {1861580433} Gastrn, IntrMd(79,CA06)
+ 2333 Morris Avenue/Suite B-6
Union, NJ 07083 (908)964-1144 Fax (908)964-7646
+ 623 North Wood Avenue
Linden, NJ 07036 (908)964-1144 Fax (908)486-3568

Greenblum, Robert, MD {1073575551} SrgOrt(83,NY01)<NJ-VALLEY>
+ Orthopedic Associates
15-01 Broadway/Suite 20 Fair Lawn, NJ 07410 (201)794-6008 Fax (201)794-6190

Greene, Arthur J., MD {1508834359} RadDia, Radiol(81,MO34)
+ Excalibur HealthCare
1000 South Lenola Road Moorestown, NJ 08057 (856)231-4300 info@excaliburmed.com
+ Excalibur HealthCare
710 Dominion Drive Moorestown, NJ 08057 (856)231-4300

Greene, Bruce H., DO {1770683153} PsyCAd, Psychy(85,NJ75)<NJ-STBARNMC>
+ Associates in Psychiatry
405 Northfield Avenue/Suite 204 West Orange, NJ 07052 (973)325-6120 Fax (973)325-6126

Greene, Damon Alan, MD {1619262763}
+ Shore Orthopedic University Associates
24 Macarthur Boulevard/First Floor Somers Point, NJ 08244 (609)927-1991 Fax (609)927-4203

Greene, Glenn Joel, MD {1932397742} GPrvMd, OccpMd(96,PA01)
+ University Hospital-School of Public Health
170 Frelinghuysen Road Piscataway, NJ 08854 (732)445-0123 Fax (732)445-3644

Greene, Jennifer Yvonne, MD {1689730269} ObsGyn(84,DC03)<NJ-STJOSHOS, NJ-STBARNMC>
+ 57 Willowbrook Road/Suite 203
Wayne, NJ 07470 (973)754-4000 Fax (973)754-4003
+ St. Joseph's Regional Medical Center
703 Main Street/Teen OB Paterson, NJ 07503 (973)754-2000

Greene, Samuel James, MD {1053722850} RadDia
+ Princeton Radiology Associates, P.A.
3674 Route 27 Kendall Park, NJ 08824 (732)325-7721 Fax (732)821-6675

Greene, Tobi B., MD {1861501009} Surgry
+ Institute for Breast Care
20 Prospect Avenue/Suite 513 Hackensack, NJ 07601 (201)996-2222

Greene, Tricia Danielle, MD {1801090576} Urolgy
+ Adult and Pediatric Urology Center, P.A.
1033 Clifton Avenue Clifton, NJ 07013 (973)473-5700 Fax (973)473-3367

Greene, Wayne L., MD {1881705879} Nrolgy(73,PA09)<NJ-NWT-NMEM, NJ-HCKTSTWN>
+ Neuro-Specialists of Morris-Sussex, PA
350 Sparta Avenue Sparta, NJ 07871 (973)579-1089 Fax (973)579-9618
+ Neuro-Specialists of Morris-Sussex, PA
369 West Blackwell Street Dover, NJ 07801 (973)579-1089 Fax (973)361-8942
+ Neuro-Specialists of Morris-Sussex, PA
254 Mountain Avenue Hackettstown, NJ 07871 (908)850-5505 Fax (908)813-8848

Greenfeld, Alan L., MD {1437385531} Anesth(76,NY15)<NJ-WARREN>
+ Warren Hills Family Health Center
315 Route 31 South Washington, NJ 07882 (908)689-0777 Fax (908)835-3037
+ Warren County - Warren Haven Nursing Home
350 Oxford Road Oxford, NJ 07863 (908)689-0777 Fax (908)475-7722

Greenfield, Brett Steven, DO {1134159601} EmrgMd(97,NJ75)<NJ-VIRTVOOR, NJ-ACMCITY>
+ Emergency Physician Associates, P.A.
307 South Evergreen Avenue/PO Box 298 Woodbury, NJ 08096 (856)848-3817 Fax (856)848-1431
+ Virtua Voorhees
100 Bowman Drive/EmrgMed Voorhees, NJ 08043 (856)247-3000

Greenfield, Daniel P., MD {1558582650} Addctn, Psychy, PubHth(75,NC01)<NY-MNTFMOSE>
+ 62 Old Short Hills Road
Short Hills, NJ 07078 (973)376-0026 Fax (973)376-1196 dpgreenfieldmdpsychiatry@msn.com

Greenfield, Donald A., MD {1477545481} Ophthl(68,PA13)<NJ-NWRKBETH, NJ-STBARNMC>
+ Hudson Eye Physicians & Surgeons, LLC
288 Millburn Avenue Millburn, NJ 07041 (973)912-9100 Fax (973)912-0800 dagmd@home.com
+ Newark Beth Israel Medical Center
201 Lyons Avenue Newark, NJ 07112 (973)926-7000

Greenfield, Efrem L., MD {1730274796} Pedtrc(85,NY08)<NJ-HACKNSK>
+ 185 Cedar Lane
Teaneck, NJ 07666 (201)836-5858 Elgreenfieldmd@yahoo.com
+ 16 Pocono Road/Suite 111
Denville, NJ 07834 (201)836-5858 Fax (973)625-8465

Greenhill, Philip A., MD {1295787711} PedCrd, Pedtrc(71,NY08)
+ 151 State Route 10 East/Suite 106
Succasunna, NJ 07876 (973)584-0400 Fax (973)584-6090

Greenhut, William H., DO {1205098563} EmrgMd<NY-NYACK-HOS>
+ Emergency Medical Associates of NJ, P.A.
3 Century Drive Parsippany, NJ 07054 (973)740-0607 Fax (973)740-9895

Greenleaf, Betsy Alice, DO {1700893948} Gyneco(98,NJ75)
+ New Jersey Urologic Institute
10 Industrial Way East   Eatontown, NJ 07724   (732)963-9091   Fax (732)963-9092

Greenleaf, Robert Martin, MD {1225289903} SrgOrt, IntrMd(05,PA09)<NJ-VIRTMHBC, NJ-VIRTUAHS>
+ Reconstructive Orthopedics, P.A.
401 Young Avenue/Suite 245   Moorestown, NJ 08057   (609)267-9400   Fax (609)267-9457

Greenman, James L., MD {1811989635} InfDis(82,NY46)<NJ-OVERLOOK>
+ Medical Diagnostic Associates PA
525 Central Avenue/Suite D   Westfield, NJ 07090   (908)232-5333   Fax (908)389-1933

Greenman, Rachelle A., MD {1598865271} EmrgMd, IntrMd(85,NJ05)<NJ-COOPRUMC>
+ Cooper University Hospital
One Cooper Plaza/EmergMed   Camden, NJ 08103   (856)342-2000

Greenseid, Keri Lee, MD {1235219791} RprEnd(01,NY08)
+ The Valley Hospital Fertility Center
140 East Ridgewood Avenue   Paramus, NJ 07652   (201)963-7640   Fax (201)204-9319
+ Inst of Repro Med and Science
609 Washington Street/2nd Floor   Hoboken, NJ 07030   (201)963-7640   Fax (201)204-9319
+ The Institute for Reproductive Medicine and Science
94 Old Short Hills Road/Suite 403E   Livingston, NJ 07652   (973)322-8286   Fax (973)322-8890

Greenspan, Joshua N., MD {1215978861} Gastrn, IntrMd(81,NY47)<NJ-VALLEY>
+ 1 Sears Drive/Suite 3
Paramus, NJ 07652   (201)265-0001   Fax (201)265-0061

Greenstein, Elizabeth Louise, MD {1427085612} RadDia, Rad-Nuc(96,PA01)<NJ-HOLYNAME>
+ Holy Name Hospital
718 Teaneck Road/Radiology   Teaneck, NJ 07666   (201)833-3000

Greenstein, Gary David, MD {1235111493} ObsGyn, IntrMd(94,ISR02)
+ Women's Health Associates
101 Prospect Street/Suite 202   Lakewood, NJ 08701   (732)942-4442

Greenstein, Steven, MD {1255627501} Ophthl
+ University Ophthalmology Associates
90 Bergen Street/DOC 6100   Newark, NJ 07101   (973)972-2020

Greenstein, Steven E., MD {1619046380} IntrMd(73,NY09)
+ The Cornea & Laser Eye Institute
300 Frank W. Burr Boulevard   Teaneck, NJ 07666   (201)883-0505   Fax (201)692-9646

Greenstein, Yonatan Yosef, MD {1902123458} IntrMd
+ University Hospital
150 Bergen Street   Newark, NJ 07103   (973)972-6111   Fax (888)950-7753

Greenwald, Bob, MD {1144275207} RadDia, IntrMd(74,NY09)<NY-ARDNHILL, MA-ARDHILL>
+ Hackensack University Medical Center
30 Prospect Avenue/Radiology   Hackensack, NJ 07601   (551)996-2194   Fax (201)489-2812

Greenwald, Brian David, MD {1518935089} PhysMd, IntrMd(95,NY48)<NJ-JFKMED>
+ JFK Medical Center
65 James Street/Phys Rehab   Edison, NJ 08820   (732)321-7070   Fax (732)321-7330
+ Rehabilitation Specialists
18-01 Pollitt Drive/Suite 1-A   Fair Lawn, NJ 07410   (732)321-7070   Fax (201)478-4202

Greenwood, Beth M., MD {1578798617} FamMed
+ Advocare Heights Primary Care
318 White Horse Pike   Haddon Heights, NJ 08035   (856)547-6000   Fax (856)546-3189

Greer, Jeannete G., MD {1932106127} Radiol(89,MA05)
+ University Radiology Group, P.C.
579A Cranbury Road   East Brunswick, NJ 08816   (732)390-0040   Fax (732)390-1856
+ University Radiology Group, P.C.
16 Mountain Boulevard   Warren, NJ 07059   (732)390-0040   Fax (908)769-9141
+ University Radiology Group, P.C.
3900 Park Avenue/Suite 107   Edison, NJ 08816   (732)548-6800   Fax (732)548-6290

Gregg, John A., DO {1013118660} FamMed, Grtrcs(03,FL75)<NJ-VALLEY, NJ-WAYNEGEN>
+ Allied Medical Associates
510 Hamburg Turnpike   Wayne, NJ 07470   (973)942-4455   Fax (973)442-6009
+ The Doctor's Office New Jersey Urgent Care
85 Godwin Avenue   Midland Park, NJ 07432   (973)942-6005   Fax (201)857-8406

Gregory, John Joseph, Jr., MD {1457307340} PedHem, Pedtrc(92,NJ06)<NJ-OVERLOOK>
+ The Valerie Fund Children's Center
33 Overlook Road/Suite 211   Summit, NJ 07901   (908)522-2353   Fax (908)522-0440
+ The Valerie Fund Children's Ctr/Goryeb
100 Madison Avenue/Simon 2/Suite 70   Morristown, NJ 07962   (908)522-2353   Fax (973)401-2410

Gregory, Naomi D., DO {1780902775}
+ Becker Nose & Sinus Center, LLC.
570 Egg Harbor Road   Sewell, NJ 08080   (856)589-6673   Fax (856)589-3443
ngregory@beckerentcenter.com
+ Becker ENT
2 Princess Road/Suite East   Lawrenceville, NJ 08648   (856)589-6673   Fax (610)303-5164

Greifinger, David J., MD {1043213499} SrgOrt(73,MD01)<NJ-CLARMAAS>
+ Essex Orthopedic Group
36 Newark Avenue/Suite 220   Belleville, NJ 07109   (973)759-8284   Fax (973)751-4156
esexortho@aol.com

Greisberg, Justin Kenneth, MD {1326063371} SrgOrt, SrgFAk(95,NY46)<NY-PRSBCOLU>
+ Columbia Grand Orthopaedics
500 Grand Avenue/Suite 101   Englewood, NJ 07631   (201)569-0440   Fax (201)569-4949

Greiss, Christine, DO {1043537947}
+ 23 Lee Court
Jersey City, NJ 07305   Fax (201)437-7117

Grelecki, Stephen, MD {1508838665} Psychy(87,NY19)<NJ-TRININPC>
+ Trinitas Regional Medical Center-New Point Campus
655 East Jersey Street/Psychiatry   Elizabeth, NJ 07206   (908)994-5000

Grella, William F., MD {1568497824} IntrMd(97,GRNA)<NJ-WAYNEGEN>
+ St. Joseph's Wayne Hospital
224 Hamburg Turnpike/Suite 4023   Wayne, NJ 07470   (973)956-3357   Fax (973)389-4050

Greller, Michael Jon, MD {1194799346} SrgOrt, SrgOARec, IntrMd(94,NY46)<NJ-CENTRAST>
+ Advanced Orthopedics & Sports Medicine Institute
301 Professional View Drive   Freehold, NJ 07728   (732)720-2555   Fax (732)720-2556
mgbones@optonline.net

Grenis, Michael Steven, MD {1669546834} SrgHnd, SrgOrt, IntrMd(84,NY09)
+ Princeton Orthopaedic Associates, P.A.
325 Princeton Avenue   Princeton, NJ 08540   (609)924-8131   Fax (609)924-8532

Gresham, Keith A., MD {1063599215} ObsGyn(82,WIND)<NJ-ENGLWOOD>
+ Ob-Gyn Associates of Englewood
177 North Dean Street/Suite 208   Englewood, NJ 07631   (201)569-0200   Fax (201)569-8287

Gressianu, Monica Terezia, MD {1811956840} CdvDis(86,ROMA)<NJ-STBARNMC>
+ Cardiac Care of North Jersey
340 East Northfield Road/Suite 2C   Livingston, NJ 07039   (973)994-0069   Fax (973)994-0567

Gressock, Joseph Neal, MD {1376654129} ObsGyn(02,OH40)
+ Horizon Health Center
714 Bergen Avenue   Jersey City, NJ 07306   (201)451-6300

Grewal, Amrit K., MD {1154382331} Nrolgy
+ Neurology Group of Bergen County
1200 East Ridgewood Avenue   Ridgewood, NJ 07450   (201)444-0868   Fax (201)444-7363

Grewal, Harpreet Singh, MD {1114215126} Anesth, Surgry(85,INA79)
+ Newark Beth Israel Pulmonary Critical Care
201 Lyons Avenue/L4   Newark, NJ 07112   (201)655-5712

Grewal, Harsh, MD {1740278779} PedSrg, Surgry(84,INA30)<NJ-COOPRUMC>
+ Cooper Peds/Children's Regional Ctr
6400 Main Street Complex   Voorhees, NJ 08043   (856)342-3113
+ Cooper University Medical Center/Camden
3 Cooper Plaza/Ste 403/PediSrg   Camden, NJ 08103   (856)342-3113   Fax (856)541-2634
+ Cooper Surgical Associates
3 Cooper Plaza/Suite 411/PediSurgery   Camden, NJ 08043   (856)342-3412   Fax (856)365-1180

Grewal, Jasbir, MD {1881731560} RadDia(69,INDI)
+ 28 Wildwood Avenue
West Orange, NJ 07052

Grewal, Kamaldeep K., MD {1306226931}<NJ-ACMCITY>
+ AtlantiCare Regional Medical Center/City Campus
1925 Pacific Avenue   Atlantic City, NJ 08401   (818)267-6632
kkgrewal@gmail.com

Grewal, Perminder Singh, MD {1053381715} CdvDis, IntrMd(80,INA78)<NY-NYACKHOS, NY-GOODSAM>
+ Bergen Heart Center
85 Chestnut Ridge Road/Suite 111   Montvale, NJ 07645   (201)444-9913   Fax (201)444-6158

Grewal, Raji Paul, MD {1407856792} Nrolgy, NeuMus(82,AB01)
+ LifeCare Physicians, PC of Hamilton
1225 Whitehorse Mercerville Rd   Trenton, NJ 08619   (609)581-6060   Fax (609)581-9561

Grewal, Roopinder K., MD {1740327527} Ophthl(90,IL06)<NJ-RWJUBRUN, NJ-STPETER>
+ Somerset Ophthalmology Associates
49 Veronica Avenue/Suite 204   Somerset, NJ 08873   (732)565-1500   Fax (732)565-1501

Grey, Glenn Allen, MD {1558368472} Anesth, IntrMd(93,NY46)<NJ-STJOSHOS>
+ St. Joseph's Regional Medical Center Anesthesia
703 Main Street   Paterson, NJ 07503   (973)754-2323   Fax (973)754-2791

Gribbin, Christopher E., MD {1295718989} RadV&I, Radiol(84,NY20)<NJ-STPETER, NJ-RWJUBRUN>
+ University Radiology Group, P.C.
483 Cranbury Road   East Brunswick, NJ 08816   (732)390-0030   Fax (732)390-5383
+ University Radiology Group, P.C.
579A Cranbury Road   East Brunswick, NJ 08816   (732)390-0030   Fax (732)390-1856
+ University Radiology Group, P.C.
579A Cranbury Road   East Brunswick, NJ 08816   (732)390-0040   Fax (732)390-1856

Gribbin, Dorota M., MD {1003951112} PhysMd(84,POLA)<NJ-RWJUHAM, NY-PRSBCOLU>
+ Comprehensive Pain & Rehabilitation Center
2333 Whitehorse-Mercerville Rd/Suite A   Hamilton, NJ 08619   (609)588-0540   Fax (609)588-0197

Gribbon, John J., MD {1639224728} IntrMd(77,NJ05)<NJ-MTNSIDE>
+ Internal Medicine of Essex
62 S Fullerton Avenue   Montclair, NJ 07042   (973)744-3382   Fax (973)509-3205

Gribin, Bradley Jay, MD {1205868304} Pedtrc, IntrMd(95,NJ06)<NJ-COMMED, NJ-OCEANMC>
+ East Windsor Pediatric Group
300B Princeton Hightstown/Suite 201   Hightstown, NJ 08520   (609)448-7300   Fax (609)448-8022

Griech-McCleery, Cynthia, MD {1952401630} Gastrn, IntrMd(91,NJ05)<NJ-COOPRUMC, NJ-MEMSALEM>
+ Cooper University Medical Center/Camden
3 Cooper Plaza/Rm 220   Camden, NJ 08103   (856)342-2000   Fax (856)342-7832

Grieco, Rachael D., MD {1376773671} Pedtrc<NJ-RWJUBRUN>
+ UH- Robert Wood Johnson Med
125 Paterson Street/MEB 344   New Brunswick, NJ 08901   (732)235-7893   Fax (732)235-7077

Griesback, Russell, DO {1598745085} IntrMd, PulDis(67,PA77)<NJ-KMHCHRRY, NJ-KENEDYHS>
+ SOM - Department of Internal Medicine
42 East Laurel Road/Suite 3100   Stratford, NJ 08084   (856)566-6859   Fax (856)566-6906

Grife, Robert M., MD {1306042130} FamMed, IntrMd(04,DMN01)<NJ-UNDRWD>
+ 6601 Ventnor Avenue/Suite 12
Ventnor, NJ 08406   (609)350-6680   Fax (609)823-9505
+ Atlantic Care Physician Group
201 West Avenue   Ocean City, NJ 08226   (609)350-6680   Fax (609)391-0963
+ Comprehensive Wellness
501 Tilton Road   Egg Harbor City, NJ 08406   (609)823-9300   Fax (609)823-9505

Griffel, Louis H., MD {1902976582} Gastrn, Hepato, IntrMd(90,PA09)<NJ-RWJUBRUN>
+ RWJ Gastro & Hepatology
125 Paterson Street/CAB 5100B   New Brunswick, NJ 08901   (732)235-7784   Fax (732)235-7792
griffelh@umdnj.edu

Griffin, Amanda, MD {1518386135} FamMed
+ Burlington Family Medical Center
666 Madison Avenue   Burlington, NJ 08016   (609)386-0023   Fax (609)386-4648

Griffin, Francis L., MD {1770675308} IntrMd(74,MA01)
+ JFK Medical Center - Muhlenberg Campus
Park Avenue & Randolph Road   Plainfield, NJ 07061   (908)668-2000   Fax (908)668-3149

Griffin, John P., MD {1770571986} IntrMd(84,MEX03)<NJ-HACKNSK, NJ-STBARNMC>
+ IPC The Hospitalist Company
55 Madison Avenue/Suite 310   Morristown, NJ 07960   (973)993-9536   Fax (973)998-4237

Griffin, Mark, MD {1669998167} PhysMd
+ 500 Lippincott Drive
Marlton, NJ 08053   (856)334-4100   Fax (856)334-4015

Physicians by Name and Address

Griffith, Heidi E., MD {1558649020}
+ 2438 Atlantic Avenue/Apt 206
Atlantic City, NJ 08401

Griffith, Negin Noorchashm, MD {1588778096} SrgPlstc(00,PA12)<NJ-RIVERVW>
+ Avicenna Plastic Surgery
721 North Beers Street/Suite 2B   Holmdel, NJ 07733   (732)335-0335   Fax (732)335-0338

Griffith, Rebecca Anne, MD {1215909320} IntrMd(95,MA16)<NJ-MORRISTN>
+ Family Health Center
200 South Street/Suite 4   Morristown, NJ 07960   (973)889-6800

Griffith, Rebecca N., MD {1356532832} Anesth(03,NJ02)<NJ-UNVMCPRN>
+ University Medical Center of Princeton at Plainsboro
One Plainsboro Road/Anesthesia   Plainsboro, NJ 08536   (609)853-6500

Griffiths, Shernett Olivine, MD {1245495423} Rheuma(08,OH06)
+ Bergen Medical Alliance, P.A.
180 Engle Street   Englewood, NJ 07631   (201)567-2050   Fax (201)568-8936

Grigaux, Claire Nathalie, MD {1992883557} IntrMd(98,NY15)
+ Overlook Hospital-Dvpmt Disabilities
1000 Galloping Hill Road   Union, NJ 07083   (908)598-6655   Fax (908)686-8374

Griggs, Abeer S., DO {1861669137} IntrMd(04,NY75)<NJ-JRSYSHMC>
+ 444 Neptune Boulevard/Suite 13
Neptune, NJ 07753   (732)455-8090   Fax (732)455-8091

Griggs, Allen R., DO {1912935669} IntrMd(73,IA75)<NJ-VALLEY, NJ-HOLYNAME>
+ Bergen Medical Associates
466 Old Hook Road/Suite 1   Emerson, NJ 07630   (201)967-8221   Fax (201)967-0340
+ Valley Health Medical Group
15 Essex Road/Fifth Floor   Paramus, NJ 07652   (201)967-8221   Fax (201)291-6129

Grigorescu, Catalina Anca, MD {1376657205} PhysMd(87,ROM01)
+ Spine & Sports Rehabilitation Center LLC
205 Robin Road/Suite 118   Paramus, NJ 07652   (201)225-1522   Fax (201)342-1259

Grigorescu, Traian Andrei, MD {1205927787} Anesth(88,ROM01)<NJ-JRSYCITY>
+ 270 Bluff Road
Fort Lee, NJ 07024

Grigoriu, Adriana, MD {1841237534} InfDis, IntrMd(79,ROMA)<NJ-JRSYCITY>
+ Liberty Medical Associates
377 Jersey Avenue/Suite 470   Jersey City, NJ 07302   (201)918-2239   Fax (201)918-2243
+ Jersey City Medical Center
355 Grand Street   Jersey City, NJ 07304   (201)915-2000

Grigoryan, Galina, MD {1619923067} IntrMd(96,NY08)<NJ-HACKNSK>
+ Hackensack University Medical Center
30 Prospect Avenue   Hackensack, NJ 07601   (201)996-2000

Griinke, Sheila Lynn, DO {1477572584} Psychy(97,MO79)
+ 2500 English Creek Avenue/Bldg E
Egg Harbor Township, NJ 08234   (609)272-0909

Grill, Lawrence J., MD {1063543844} CdvDis, IntrMd(78,OK01)
+ 1166 River Avenue
Lakewood, NJ 08701   (732)367-8272   Fax (732)367-3693

Grim, Keith Case, MD {1992766760} EmrgMd(01,PA02)<NJ-VIRTVOOR>
+ Virtua Voorhees
100 Bowman Drive   Voorhees, NJ 08043   (856)247-3000

Grimaldi, Matthew Porter, MD {1851590863} Anesth(07,PA13)
+ Morris Anesthesia Group, PA
3799 Route 46/Suite 211   Parsippany, NJ 07054   (973)335-1122   Fax (973)335-1448

Grimes, Julia P., DO {1336219914} IntrMd(94,NJ75)
+ UH-RWJ General Internal Medicine
125 Paterson Street/Suite 2300   New Brunswick, NJ 08901   (732)235-6968   Fax (732)235-7144

Grimes, Kathryn Leigh, MD {1962793935}<NJ-COOPRUMC>
+ Cooper University Hospital
One Cooper Plaza/EmrgMed   Camden, NJ 08103   (856)342-2351   Fax (856)968-8272

Grimes, Sara, MD {1891081782} ObsGyn(11,HI01)<NJ-HUNTRDN>
+ All Women's Healthcare
1100 Wescott Drive/Suite 105   Flemington, NJ 08822   (908)788-6469   Fax (908)788-6483

Grimmett, Brian L., MD {1629053434} Grtrcs, IntrMd, Rheuma(70,NJ05)<NJ-VIRTUAHS, NJ-VIRTMHBC>
+ Arthritis, Rheumatic & Back Disease Associates
2309 East Evesham Road/Suite 101   Voorhees, NJ 08043   (856)424-5005   Fax (856)424-4716

Grinberg, Diana, MD {1679769111} EmrgMd
+ 12-55 Lyle Terrace
Fair Lawn, NJ 07410

Grinberg, Sagy, MD {1093177503}<NJ-NWRKBETH>
+ Newark Beth Israel Medical Center
201 Lyons Avenue   Newark, NJ 07112   (973)926-7000

Grinblat, Inessa, MD {1962473884} IntrMd(91,RUS15)
+ 87 Brunswick Woods Drive
East Brunswick, NJ 08816   (732)254-0081   Fax (732)254-2851
+ 345 Route 9 South
Manalapan, NJ 07726

Grinchenko, Tatyana, DO {1770627713} IntrMd, Rheuma(02,NY75)
+ 506 Hamburg Turnpike/Suite 201
Wayne, NJ 07470   (201)282-8356

Grinman, Lev, MD {1457511743} NeuMus<NY-NSUHMANH>
+ 37 West Century Road/Suite 107
Paramus, NJ 07652   (201)967-1111

Gritsman, Andrey, MD {1134277601} Pthlgy(72,RUSS)<NJ-VALLEY>
+ The Valley Hospital
223 North Van Dien Avenue/Pathology   Ridgewood, NJ 07450   (201)447-8000   Fax (201)447-8657

Gritsus, Vadim, MD {1336170182} Surgry(92,RUS01)<NJ-CHILTON>
+ 7 Industrial Road/Suite 203
Pequannock, NJ 07440   Fax (973)696-9055

Grizzanti, Joseph N., DO {1932107554} PulDis, IntrMd, Allrgy(76,PA77)<NJ-VALLEY>
+ Sovereign Medical Goup
85 Harristown Road/Soite 101   Glen Rock, NJ 07452   (973)790-4111   Fax (973)790-4330

Grob, Alexandra, DO {1588927354} Dermat
+ Affiliated Dermatologists
182 South Street/Suite 1   Morristown, NJ 07960   (973)936-1802   Fax (973)695-1480

Grob, Patricio, DO {1316912884} SrgOrt, OrtTrm, SrgSpn(96,PA77)
+ Atlantic Orthopedic Associates
91 South Jefferson Road/Suite 201   Whippany, NJ 07981   (973)599-9779   Fax (973)599-1179

Grobstein, Naomi S., MD {1427121631} FamMed(80,NJ05)<NJ-MTNSIDE, NJ-CLARMAAS>
+ Summit Medical Group
48-50 Fairfield Street   Montclair, NJ 07042   (973)744-8511   Fax (973)744-6356
Ngrobstein@gmail.com

Grochmal, Stephen A., MD {1124153028} Gyneco, ObsGyn(77,MEXI)
+ The Childbirth & Women's Wellness Center
29 The Crescent   Montclair, NJ 07042   (201)696-6945
+ Care Station Medical Group
328 St. Georges Avenue   Linden, NJ 07036   (201)696-6945   Fax (908)925-2841

Grochowalska, Ewa Malgorzata, MD {1659572311} Pedtrc, PedEmg(80,POL03)
+ SAMRA Pediatrics
300 Perrine Road/Suite 331   Old Bridge, NJ 08857   (732)727-8800   Fax (732)727-0955
+ SAMRA Pediatrics
733 North Beers Street/Suite L-5   Holmdel, NJ 07733   (732)727-8800   Fax (732)727-0955

Grochowalski, Tomasz K., MD {1265495980} IntrMd(81,POLA)<NJ-RBAYPERT>
+ Gregory Shypula MD PA
2045 Route 35 South/Suite 202   South Amboy, NJ 08879   (732)721-5511   Fax (732)721-2007
+ Raritan Bay Medical Center/Perth Amboy
535 New Brunswick Avenue   Perth Amboy, NJ 08861   (732)324-5231

Grodberg, Michele, MD {1225047038} Dermat(87,NY19)<NJ-ENGLWOOD>
+ 106 Grand Avenue/Suite 330
Englewood, NJ 07631   (201)567-8884   Fax (201)567-5799
michele.grodberg@ehmc.com

Grodman, Marc D., MD {1487704797} IntrMd(77,NY01)
+ Bio-Reference Laboratory, Inc.
481 Edward H. Ross Drive/Suite B   Elmwood Park, NJ 07407   (201)791-2600   Fax (201)791-1941

Grodstein, Gerald P., MD {1245211440} IntrMd, Nephro(74,NY08)<NJ-ENGLWOOD, NJ-PALISADE>
+ Drs. Pattner, Grodstein, Fein & Davis
177 North Dean Street/Suite 207   Englewood, NJ 07631   (201)567-0446   Fax (201)567-8775
+ Drs. Pattner, Grodstein, Fein & Davis
8100 Kennedy Boulevard   North Bergen, NJ 07047   (201)868-5905

Groff, Walter L., MD {1437116423} SrgC&R(70,NY03)<NJ-OVERLOOK>
+ Atlantic Colon & Rectal
33 Overlook Road/Suite 412   Summit, NJ 07901   (908)598-0220   Fax (908)598-0415
+ Atlantic Colon & Rectal
8 Mountain Boulevard   Warren, NJ 07059   (908)769-9111
+ Gastrosurgical Center of NJ
7132 Spruce Street   Mountainside, NJ 07901   (908)317-0071   Fax (908)317-0081

Grogan, Rita J., MD {1730395229} Psychy(88,NY06)
+ 1250 East Ridgewood Avenue/Suite B
Ridgewood, NJ 07450   (201)445-0506   Fax (201)612-8960

Groh, William Carl, MD {1063444362} CdvDis, IntrMd, IntCrd(76,PA01)<NJ-COOPRUMC, NJ-ACMCITY>
+ Penn Medicine at Cherry Hill
1400 East Route 70/Cardiology   Cherry Hill, NJ 08034

Groisberg, Roman, MD {1235404450} MedOnc
+ Rutgers Cancer Institute of New Jersey
195 Little Albany Street/PO Box 2681   New Brunswick, NJ 08903   (732)235-2465   Fax (732)235-6797

Groisser, Daniel S., MD {1376514745} Dermat(86,NY20)<NJ-STBARNMC, NJ-MTNSIDE>
+ The Dermatology Group, P.C.
347 Mount Pleasant Avenue/Suite 103   West Orange, NJ 07052   (973)571-2121   Fax (973)498-0535
+ The Dermatology Group, P.C.
310 Madison Avenue/Suite 206   Morristown, NJ 07960   (973)571-2121   Fax (973)539-1180

Groman, David I., MD {1790717890} EmrgMd
+ 4 Meadowbrook Road
Short Hills, NJ 07078

Gronczewski, Craig Anthony, MD {1992841621} EmrgMd(98,NJ06)<NJ-UNVMCPRN>
+ University Medical Center of Princeton at Plainsboro
One Plainsboro Road/EmrgMed   Plainsboro, NJ 08536   (609)497-4000

Gronowitz, Steven D., MD {1093772030} Gastrn, IntrMd(90,NY06)
+ Gastroenterology Associates of New Jersey
1011 Clifton Avenue   Clifton, NJ 07013   (973)471-8200   Fax (973)471-3032
+ United Medical, P.C.
988 Broadway/Suite 201   Bayonne, NJ 07002   (973)471-8200   Fax (201)339-6333
+ United Medical, P.C.
612 Rutherford Avenue   Lyndhurst, NJ 07013   (201)460-0063   Fax (201)460-1684

Gronsky, Rudolph Edward, DO {1841249059} EmrgMd, IntrMd(86,MO78)<NJ-OCEANMC, NJ-JRSYSHMC>
+ Ocean County Family Care
2125 Route 88 East   Brick, NJ 08724   (732)892-4548   Fax (732)892-0961
+ Ocean County Family Care
9 Mule Road   Toms River, NJ 08755   (732)892-4548   Fax (732)818-7775
+ Ocean County Family Care
27 South Cooks Bridge Road   Jackson, NJ 08724   (732)364-3881   Fax (732)364-4625

Grookett, Thomas Wister, MD {1033356027} IntrMd, PulCCr(03,VA04)
+ Pulmonary & Sleep Associates of SJ, LLC.
750 Route 73 South/Suite 401   Marlton, NJ 08053   (856)375-1288   Fax (856)375-2325
+ Pulmonary & Sleep Associates of SJ, LLC.
107 Berlin Road   Cherry Hill, NJ 08034   (856)375-1288   Fax (856)429-1081

Grosh, Taras, MD {1255691564} Anesth
+ Penn Medicine Cherry Hill
1865 Route 70 East/Suite 220   Cherry Hill, NJ 08003   (856)429-1519   Fax (856)427-2933

Grosiak, David Matthew, DO {1942447073}
+ Team Health East
307 South Evergeen Avenue/Suite 201   Woodbury, NJ 08096   (856)686-4300   Fax (856)848-8536

Gross, Arthur H., MD {1134217292} ObsGyn, IntrMd(92,RI01)<NJ-ENGLWOOD, NJ-HACKNSK>
+ Englewood Women's Health
25 Rockwood Place/Suite 305   Englewood, NJ 07631   (201)894-0003   Fax (201)894-0006

Gross, Carey E., MD {1902028863} Psychy, PsyCAd(87,GRNA)
+ 260 Engle Street
Tenafly, NJ 07670   (201)567-6000

Gross, David D., MD {1538130398} IntrMd(87,GRNA)<NJ-VIRTMHBC, NJ-LOURDMED>
+ Moorestown Internal Medicine PC
147 East Third Street/Suite One   Moorestown, NJ 08057   (856)234-7754   Fax (856)234-2290

Gross, David E., MD {1467447011} SrgOrt(86,NY47)
+ Union Middlesex Orthopedic
2333 Morris Avenue/Suite A15 Union, NJ 07083
(908)686-5444 Fax (908)686-3599
+ Union Middlesex Orthopedic
329 Amboy Avenue Woodbridge, NJ 07095 (732)636-9788
+ Short Hills Surgery Center
187 Millburn Avenue/Suite 101 Millburn, NJ 07083
(973)671-0555 Fax (973)671-0557

Gross, Eric L., MD {1215937602} Surgry, SrgOnc(88,NY47)<NJ-HCKTSTWN>
+ 657 Willow Grove Street/Suite 302
Hackettstown, NJ 07840 (908)852-7482 Fax (908)852-1167

Gross, Gary L., MD {1336143247} Allrgy, Pedtrc, AlgyImmn(81,NY19)<NJ-JRSYSMC, NJ-MONMOUTH>
+ Allergy Partners of New Jersey PC
802 West Park Avenue/Suite 213 Ocean, NJ 07712
(732)695-2555 Fax (732)695-2552
+ Allergy Partners of New Jersey PC
8 Tindall Road Middletown, NJ 07748 (732)695-2555
Fax (732)671-0144

Gross, Harvey R., MD {1407897689} FamMed, Grtrcs, FamM-Grtc(70,MA05)<NJ-ENGLWOOD, NJ-HOLYNAME>
+ Primary Care NJ
370 Grand Avenue/Suite 102 Englewood, NJ 07631
(201)567-3370 Fax (201)816-1265

Gross, Howard J., MD {1104821610} Ophthl(71,DC01)<NJ-ACMCITY, NJ-ACMCMAIN>
+ Horizon Eye Care
9701 Ventnor Avenue Margate City, NJ 08402 (609)822-4242 Fax (609)822-3211
drgross@horizoneyecare.com
+ Horizon Eye Care
4 Village Drive Cape May Court House, NJ 08210
(609)465-7100
+ Horizon Eye Care
655 Route 72 Manahawkin, NJ 08402 (609)597-0666

Gross, Jeffrey K., MD {1053343327} ObsGyn(82,NY19)<NJ-UNVMCPRN>
+ Princeton Ob/Gyn
5 Plainsboro Road/Suite 500 Plainsboro, NJ 08536
(609)936-0700 Fax (609)936-0750
+ University Medical Center of Princeton at Plainsboro
One Plainsboro Road Plainsboro, NJ 08536 (609)497-4000

Gross, Joshua David, MD {1255362570} RadMam, Radiol, RadPhy(80,NY46)
+ HNMC The Breast Center
718 Teaneck Road/Radiology Teaneck, NJ 07666
(201)833-7100 Fax (201)833-7248

Gross, Michael L., MD {1386701654} Rheuma, IntrMd(95,ISR02)<NJ-VALLEY>
+ Physician Specialists of New Jersey
1 Sears Drive/Suite 306 Paramus, NJ 07652 (201)703-5500 Fax (201)830-2286

Gross, Michael Lee, MD {1396712337} SrgOrt, SprtMd(83,NY19)<NJ-HACKNSK, NJ-VALLEY>
+ Active Orthopaedics & Sports Medicine
440 Old Hook Road Emerson, NJ 07630 (201)358-0707
Fax (201)358-9777
+ Active Orthopaedics & Sports Medicine
25 Prospect Avenue Hackensack, NJ 07601 (201)358-0707 Fax (201)343-7410
+ Active Center for Health & Wellness
25 Prospect Avenue Hackensack, NJ 07630 (201)487-4600 Fax (201)343-7410

Gross, Peter A., MD {1891763769} InfDis(64,CT01)<NJ-HACKNSK>
+ Hackensack University Medical Center
30 Prospect Avenue/InternalMed Hackensack, NJ 07601
(201)996-2000
pgross@humed.com

Gross, Renee, MD {1164488557} ObsGyn(81,MEXI)<NJ-STPETER, NJ-RWJUBRUN>
+ Ob & Gyn Group of E Brunswick
172 Summerhill Road/Suite 1 East Brunswick, NJ 08816
(732)254-1500 Fax (732)254-1878
+ Obstetrical & Gynecological Grou
319 Route 9 South/Alexander Plaza Manalapan, NJ 07726
(732)780-6970
+ Cares Surgicenter, LLC.
240 Easton Avenue New Brunswick, NJ 08816 (732)565-5400 Fax (732)296-8677

Gross, Robert M., MD {1629114327} Anesth(93,NY09)
+ Holy Name Hospital
718 Teaneck Road/Anesthesia Teaneck, NJ 07666
(201)833-3000

Gross, Russell A., MD {1255305686} IntrMd(77,NJ05)<NJ-CENTRAST>
+ Medical Health Center
1270 State Highway 35 Middletown, NJ 07748 (732)615-3900 Fax (732)615-0865

+ Barnabas Health Medical Group
1029 Sycamore Avenue Tinton Falls, NJ 07753 (732)615-3900 Fax (732)544-1479

Gross, Steven C., MD {1437155470} RadDia, Radiol(72,MI01)<NJ-SOMERSET>
+ University Radiology, PA
239 Route 22 East/Suite 302 Green Brook, NJ 08812
(732)968-4899 Fax (732)968-8096
+ University Radiology Group, P.C.
3900 Park Avenue/Suite 107 Edison, NJ 08820 (732)968-4899 Fax (732)548-6290

Gross, Tiberiu A., MD {1366478844} IntrMd(83,ROMA)<NJ-OCEANMC>
+ 450 University Court
Brick, NJ 08723 (732)279-9400

Grossi, Eugene Andrew, MD {1205821949} SrgCTh, Surgry, SrgThr(81,NY01)<NJ-ACMCMAIN, NY-BLVUENYU>
+ AtlantiCare Regional Med Ctr/Mainland
65 West Jimmie Leeds Road Pomona, NJ 08240 (609)652-1000

Grossi, Maureen A., MD {1205942661} Pedtrc(03,NY06)<NJ-ENGLWOOD, NJ-HACKNSK>
+ Tenafly Pediatrics, PA
74 Pascack Road Park Ridge, NJ 07656 (201)326-7120
Fax (201)326-7130
+ Tenafly Pediatrics, PA
26 Park Place Paramus, NJ 07652 (201)326-7120 Fax (201)261-8413

Grossman, Abigail Michael, MD {1083894182} Pedtrc(96,NY20)
+ 815 Frederick Court
Wyckoff, NJ 07481

Grossman, Andrew Brian, MD {1013127422} PedGst, Pedtrc(02,NJ06)<PA-CHILDHOS>
+ CHOP Pediatric & Adolescent Specialty Care Center
4009 Black Horse Pike/Pedi GI Mays Landing, NJ 08330
(609)677-7895 Fax (609)677-7835
+ CHOP Pediatric & Adolescent Specialty Care Center
1012 Laurel Oak Road Voorhees, NJ 08043 (609)677-7895
Fax (856)435-0091

Grossman, Andrew G., MD {1528026853} EmrgMd(80,NY09)<NJ-CHILTON>
+ Chilton Medical Center
97 West Parkway/EmergMed Pompton Plains, NJ 07444
(973)831-5000 Fax (201)444-3604

Grossman, Bernard, MD {1487668265} IntrMd, OncHem(74,PA13)<NJ-CHSMRCER>
+ Mercer Bucks Hematology Oncology
2 Capital Way/Suite 220 Pennington, NJ 08534 (609)303-0747 Fax (609)303-0771

Grossman, Bruce Jay, MD {1720057409} PedCrC, Pedtrc(96,NJ05)<NJ-JRSYSHMC>
+ RWJ University Pediatric Critical Care
125 Paterson Street/MEB 343 New Brunswick, NJ 08901
(732)235-7887 Fax (732)235-6609

Grossman, David R., MD {1407822380} IntrMd, Ophthl(82,NJ06)
+ Ocean Eye Institute
601 Route 37 West Toms River, NJ 08755 (732)244-4400
Fax (732)505-2171

Grossman, Davida S., MD {1649270372} Anesth(94,CA11)<NJ-VIRTMARL>
+ West Jersey Anesthesia Associates
102-E Center Boulevard Marlton, NJ 08053 (856)988-6250 Fax (856)988-6270

Grossman, Elliot A., MD {1194755710} NroChl, Nrolgy(80,TN07)<NJ-MORRISTN>
+ 205 Ridgedale Avenue
Florham Park, NJ 07932 (973)966-6333 Fax (973)301-0435
pdneuro@aol.com
+ 2780 Morris Avenue/Suite 1C
Union, NJ 07083

Grossman, Eric Brian, MD {1659342202} ObsGyn(98,PA02)
+ Advocare Premier Ob/Gyn of South Jersey
903 Sheppard Road Voorhees, NJ 08043 (856)772-2300
Fax (856)772-2301

Grossman, Harry D., MD {1043309487} Ophthl(93,PA02)<NJ-COOPRUMC>
+ Garden State Community Medical Center
100 Brick Road/Suite 115 Marlton, NJ 08053 (856)983-1400 Fax (856)983-1681
+ The Cooper Health System at Voorhees
900 Centennial Boulevard Voorhees, NJ 08043 (856)325-6500

Grossman, Israel Robert, MD {1255311445} OncHem, IntrMd(93,CT01)<NJ-STBARNMC>
+ St. Barnabas Cancer Center
94 Old Short Hills Road Livingston, NJ 07039 (973)322-5200 Fax (973)322-5666
+ St. Barnabas Cancer Center
94 Old Short Hills Road/Suite 1 Livingston, NJ 07039
(973)322-5650

Grossman, Kenneth A., MD {1427012533} Dermat, IntrMd, SrgDer(77,NY08)<NJ-RIVERVW>
+ 180 White Road/Suite 103
Little Silver, NJ 07739 (732)842-5222 Fax (732)741-6285

Grossman, Leonard, MD {1457388563} ObsGyn(75,PA02)<NJ-VIRTMHBC>
+ Virtua Phoenix OBGYN
120 Madison Avenue/Suite B Mount Holly, NJ 08060
(609)444-5500 Fax (609)444-5501
+ Phoenix Ob-Gyn Associates
1 Sheffield Drive/Suite 101 Columbus, NJ 08022
(609)444-5500 Fax (609)291-5603
+ Phoenix Ob-Gyn Associates
110 Marter Avenue/Suite 505 Moorestown, NJ 08060
(856)235-4840 Fax (856)235-3795

Grossman, Leonard A., MD {1578600136} FamMed, Rheuma(75,NY46)
+ Princeton Medical Group PA
2 Research Way/Bldg 2/Suite 302 Monroe Township, NJ 08831 (609)655-8800 Fax (609)655-7466
+ Princeton Medical Group, P.A.
3 Liberty Street Plainsboro, NJ 08536 (609)924-9300

Grossman, Leonard J., MD {1174563761} Pedtrc, PedAlg(69,DC01)<NJ-STCLRDEN>
+ Pediatric & Adolescent Center
1911 Route 46/PO Box 100 Ledgewood, NJ 07852
(973)347-8500 Fax (973)347-7320
LJGMD@msn.com

Grossman, Matthew Aaron, MD {1063618908} Gastrn, IntrMd(04,NJ06)
+ Gastroenterology Associates of New Jersey
1124 East Ridgewood Avenue/Suite 203 Ridgewood, NJ 07450 (201)882-1080 Fax (201)857-8646
+ Gastroenterology Associates of New Jersey
205 Browertown Road/Suite 204 Little Falls, NJ 07424
(201)882-1080 Fax (973)812-5235

Grossman, Perry, MD {1881082774} PhysMd(80,MEX03)
+ Maplewood Holistic Center
137 Parker Avenue Maplewood, NJ 07040 (973)763-0032

Grossman, Rachel M., MD {1548225477} Dermat(84,NC07)
+ University Medical Group
125 Paterson Street/Suite 5100/CAB New Brunswick, NJ 08901 (732)235-7993 Fax (732)235-7117
+ Princeton Dermatology Associates
208 Bunn Drive/Suite 1-E Princeton, NJ 08540 (732)235-7993 Fax (609)683-0298
+ Johnson & Johnson
199 Grandview Road Skillman, NJ 08901 (908)874-1000

Grossman, Robert B., MD {1801847942} SrgOrt(72,MD01)<NJ-CENTRAST, NJ-RIVERVW>
+ Shore Orthopaedic Group
35 Gilbert Street South Tinton Falls, NJ 07701 (732)530-1515 Fax (732)747-5433
+ Shore Orthopaedic Group
1255 Route 70/Suite 11S Lakewood, NJ 08701 (732)530-1515 Fax (732)942-2311

Grossman, Sandra Lynn, MD {1205151115} Pedtrc<NJ-COOPRUMC>
+ Cooper University Hospital
One Cooper Plaza Camden, NJ 08103 (856)342-2351
Fax (856)968-8272

Grossman, Steven H., MD {1710901491} CdvDis, IntrMd, CarNuc(79,ITA01)<NJ-VALLEY>
+ Heart & Vascular Associates of Northern Jersey
22-18 Broadway/Suite 201 Fair Lawn, NJ 07410 (201)475-5050 Fax (201)475-5522

Grosso, Dominick A., DO {1568486249} IntrMd, FamMAdlt(83,PA77)<NJ-RIVERVW>
+ 5 Globe Court
Red Bank, NJ 07701 (732)219-0110 Fax (732)212-8818

Grosso, Joseph X., MD {1619989456} PsycAd, Psychy(65,PA02)
+ 1 Deerfield Drive
Woodcliff Lake, NJ 07677 (201)391-4141 Fax (201)391-4141
jxgmd@aol.com

Grosso-Rivas, Suejane, MD {1770563413} Radiol, RadDia(85,MA01)
+ Westfield Imaging Center
118-122 Elm Street Westfield, NJ 07090 (908)232-0610
Fax (908)232-7140

Grosu, Victor George, MD {1376789487}
+ Princeton House Behavioral Health - Princeton
905 Herrontown Road Princeton, NJ 08540 (609)497-3300 Fax (609)497-3370

Grote, Walter R., DO {1811983745} IntrMd(79,MO78)<NJ-NWTNMEM>
+ Premier Health Associates
5 Eisenhower Road Columbia, NJ 07832 (908)362-5360
Fax (973)729-0291

Physicians by Name and Address

Grotkowski, Carolyn E., MD {1275746331} PthACl, PthCyt(76,OH41)
+ Quest Diagnostics Inc.
907 Pleasant Valley Avenue   Mount Laurel, NJ 08054
(856)222-0675   Fax (856)222-0946

Ground, Christen Denise, DO {1689021842} FamMed
+ Patient first Urgent Care
630 Mantua Pike   Woodbury, NJ 08096   (856)812-2220
Fax (856)812-2221

Grove, Michele Sak, MD {1528054608} ObsGyn(95,NJ05)<NJ-HUNTRDN>
+ Affiliates in Obstetrics & Gynecology, P.A.
111 Route 31/Suite 121 2nd FL Bldg B   Flemington, NJ 08822   (908)782-2825   Fax (908)782-0196
+ All Women's Healthcare
1100 Wescott Drive/Suite 105   Flemington, NJ 08822
(908)782-2825   Fax (908)788-6483

Grover, Anjali, MD {1881891109} EnDbMt, IntrMd
+ Montclair Endocrine Associates
123 Highland Avenue/Suite 301   Glen Ridge, NJ 07028
(973)744-3733   Fax (973)707-5821

Grover, Arvind K., MD {1306986914} IntrMd(82,DOM03)<NJ-STBARNMC>
+ 8 Fords Road
Randolph, NJ 07869   (973)366-6232   Fax (973)763-0505
+ 2168 Millburn Avenue
Maplewood, NJ 07040   (973)366-6232   Fax (973)763-0505

Grover, Kunal, MD {1346445574} IntrMd, Gastrn(03,GRN01)<NJ-OVERLOOK, NJ-RWJURAH>
+ Advanced Gastroenterology Group
1308 Morris Avenue   Union, NJ 07083   (908)851-2770
Fax (908)851-7706

Grover, Manisha B., MD {1336311927} IntrMd(97,INA57)
+ IPC The Hospitalist Company
55 Madison Avenue/Suite 310   Morristown, NJ 07960
(973)993-9536   Fax (973)998-4237

Grover, Meenu, MD {1518115336} EmrgEMed
+ 21 Surrey Lane
Mahwah, NJ 07430

Grover, Pamela, MD {1649450990} IntrMd(04,NY03)
+ 8 Fords Road
Randolph, NJ 07869

Grover, Surender M., MD {1437370004} SrgOrt, PedOrt(66,INDI)<NJ-BAYSHORE>
+ 1632 Oak Tree Road
Edison, NJ 08820   (732)548-2600

Groves, Danielle Breitman, MD {1679580823} PhysMd(00,NY09)
+ Premier Orthopaedics and Sports Medicine, PC
663 Palisade Avenue/Suite 302   Cliffside Park, NJ 07010
(201)943-9100   Fax (201)943-7308
+ Premier Orthopaedics and Sports Medicine, P.C.
111 Galway Place   Teaneck, NJ 07666   (201)943-9100
Fax (201)862-0095

Groves, Gerald A., MD {1942285887} Psychy(69,JMA01)
+ Family Guidance Center of Warren County
492 State Route 57 West   Washington, NJ 07882
(908)852-0333   Fax (908)852-8370
+ 178 Tamarack Circle
Skillman, NJ 08558   (609)924-5757
+ The Mentor Network of New Jersey
2000 Crawford Place/Suite 700   Mount Laurel, NJ 07882
(856)533-4100

Grubb, Charles R., DO {1780644831} GenPrc, FamMed(76,PA77)<NJ-WARREN>
+ 39 Roseberry Street
Phillipsburg, NJ 08865   (908)454-8787   Fax (908)454-1192

Grubb, William R., MD {1699857458} Anesth, PainMd(85,DC01)<NJ-RWJUBRUN>
+ New Jersey Pain Institute
125 Paterson Street/CAB 6100   New Brunswick, NJ 08901
(732)235-6444
+ Robert Wood Johnson-UMDNJ Anesthesia Group
125 Paterson Street/CAB 3100   New Brunswick, NJ 08901
(732)235-6444   Fax (732)235-6131

Gruber, Amy D., MD {1578588851} FamMed(88,NJ06)<NJ-OVERLOOK>
+ Chatham Family Practice Associates
492 Main Street   Chatham, NJ 07928   (973)635-2432   Fax (973)635-6169

Gruber, Gabriel G., MD {1073514105} Dermat(72,MA01)<NJ-OVERLOOK, NJ-MORRISTN>
+ Summit Medical Group-Berkeley Heights Campus
1 Diamond Hill Road   Berkeley Heights, NJ 07922
(908)273-4300   Fax (908)277-8629

Gruber, Melvin S., MD {1912019332} Dermat(64,KS02)<NJ-UN-DRWD>
+ South Jersey Dermatology Associates
900 Route 168/Suite F6   Turnersville, NJ 08012   (856)227-7488   Fax (856)228-3476
+ South Jersey Dermatology Associates
52 West Red Bank Avenue   Woodbury, NJ 08096

(856)227-7488   Fax (856)845-3719

Gruber, Todd A., MD {1467568451} IntrMd(90,NY08)
+ 25 Empress Court
Freehold, NJ 07728

Gruczynski, Tomasz A., MD {1497707087} Pedtrc(85,POLA)<NJ-STJOSHOS, NJ-RIVERVW>
+ North Wayne Pediatrics
508 Hamburg Turnpike/Suite 106   Wayne, NJ 07470
(973)942-7800   Fax (973)942-9680

Gruen, Amy Beth, DO {1316054588} Anesth(02,NJ75)<NJ-VIRT-MARL>
+ Virtua Marlton Hospital
90 Brick Road   Marlton, NJ 08053   (856)355-6000

Gruenwald, Laurence D., MD {1508868191} Pedtrc(75,NJ05)<NJ-STBARNMC, NJ-OVERLOOK>
+ Drs. Gruenwald & Comandatore
90 Millburn Avenue/Suite 101   Millburn, NJ 07041
(973)378-7990   Fax (973)378-7991

Grujic, Dejan, MD {1972791705}
+ Capital Health System/Hopewell
One Capital Way   Pennington, NJ 08534   (215)955-2570

Grujic, Slobodan, MD {1487650149} Anesth(75,BOS01)<NJ-CHSMRCER, NJ-CHSFULD>
+ Trenton Anesthesiology Associates, PA
One Capital Way/Second Floor   Pennington, NJ 08534
(609)396-4700   Fax (609)396-4900

Grullon Okumus, Ariolis Carmelina, MD {1801024856} Pedtrc(12,DOM09)
+ Fayrouz Pediatrics
1300 Main Avenue/Suite 2-C   Clifton, NJ 07011   (973)340-6666   Fax (973)404-8525

Grundy, Kia Calhoun, MD {1992819338} Pedtrc, IntrMd(97,NJ05)<NJ-STBARNMC>
+ Trinity Pediatrics
430 Morris Avenue/1st Floor   Elizabeth, NJ 07208
(908)353-5437   Fax (908)353-0727
+ 2130 Millburn Avenue/Suite C-7
Maplewood, NJ 07040   (908)353-5437   Fax (973)843-7154

Grunstein, Erno, MD {1437227048} Anesth(76,HUN01)<NY-CABRINI>
+ 20 Brodil Court
Closter, NJ 07624   (201)750-9865

Grutzmacher, June Edith, MD {1932199361} Ophthl(82,PA13)<NJ-HUNTRDN>
+ 173 North Union Street
Lambertville, NJ 08530   (609)397-0007   Fax (609)397-0696
+ 4 Walter E. Foran Boulevard/Suite 103
Flemington, NJ 08822   (908)782-8541

Grygotis, Anthony E., MD {1568486231} PthCln(90,NJ05)<NJ-UMDNJ>
+ University Hospital
150 Bergen Street/Pathology   Newark, NJ 07103
(973)972-4520   Fax (973)972-5909

Grygotis, Laura Anne, MD {1609859610} RadDia, Radiol(93,NJ06)<NJ-RBAYOLDB>
+ University Radiology Group, P.C.
483 Cranbury Road   East Brunswick, NJ 08816   (732)390-0030   Fax (732)390-5383
+ University Radiology Group, P.C.
260 Amboy Avenue   Metuchen, NJ 08840   (732)390-0030   Fax (732)548-3392
+ University Radiology Group, P.C.
579A Cranbury Road   East Brunswick, NJ 08816   (732)390-0040   Fax (732)390-1856

Grzybowski, Jacek, MD {1225038508} Pedtrc(92,POL02)<NJ-TRINIWSC>
+ 812 North Wood Avenue/Suite 201
Linden, NJ 07036   (908)587-9611   Fax (908)587-9622

Gu, Lingping, MD {1134133481} IntrMd(88,CHN4A)<NJ-STPETER, NJ-RWJURAH>
+ Patient first Medical Care, LLC
3084 State Route 27/Suite 9   Kendall Park, NJ 08824
(732)297-4321   Fax (732)297-2202

Gu, Ping, MD {1336383637} Hemato, MedOnc, IntrMd(85,CHN91)
+ Memorial Sloan Kettering Bergen
225 Summit Avenue   Montvale, NJ 07645   (201)775-7183   Fax (201)691-6661

Gualberti, Joann, MD {1669482220} IntrMd(97,NY08)<NY-STAT-NRTH>
+ Orchard Medical Group
9 Professional Circle/Suite 101   Colts Neck, NJ 07722
(732)431-1520   Fax (732)431-1567

Gualberti-Girgis, Lisa, MD {1134139710} IntrMd(95,NY08)<NY-STATNRTH, NY-STATNSTH>
+ Orchard Medical Group
9 Professional Circle/Suite 101   Colts Neck, NJ 07722
(732)431-1520   Fax (732)431-1567

Gualtieri, Louis Robert, DO {1265540397} Radiol(84,NJ75)<NJ-ACMCITY, NJ-SHOREMEM>
+ Atlantic Medical Imaging, LLC.

3100 Hingston Avenue   Egg Harbor Township, NJ 08234
(609)677-9729   Fax (609)646-5469
+ Atlantic Medical Imaging, LLC.
401 Bethel Road   Somers Point, NJ 08244   (609)677-9729
+ Atlantic Medical Imaging, LLC.
72 West Jimmie Leeds Road   Galloway, NJ 08234
(609)677-9729   Fax (609)653-8764

Gualtieri, Sara Liliana, MD {1902839509} IntrMd(94,ECU03)
+ 1 Wexford Lane
Linwood, NJ 08221   (609)927-6989

Guanci, Nicole Alexis, MD {1225356165} Psychy(10,NJ05)
+ 421 East Passaic Avenue
Bloomfield, NJ 07003   (973)985-8628
+ Advanced Psychiatric Associates
211 Essex Street/Suite 204   Hackensack, NJ 07601
(973)985-8628   Fax (201)487-1241

Guariglia, Anthony R., MD {1093971236} Pedtrc<NJ-SOCEANCO>
+ Southern Ocean County Medical Center
1140 Route 72 West   Manahawkin, NJ 08050   (609)597-6011

Guariglia, George Angelo, DO {1730276437} FamMed(96,NJ75)<NJ-CHILTON>
+ Highlander Family Medicine
1900 Union Valley Road/Suite 303   Hewitt, NJ 07421
(973)076-8535   Fax (973)706-8536
+ Chilton Medical Center
97 West Parkway/Fam Med   Pompton Plains, NJ 07444
(973)831-5000

Guarini, Vincent, MD {1811935216} Anesth(86,PA01)<NJ-DEBRAHLC>
+ Deborah Heart and Lung Center
200 Trenton Road/Anesthesiology   Browns Mills, NJ 08015
(609)893-6611   Fax (609)893-1213
Shelly_berkowitz@cooley-dickinson.org

Guarino, Joseph J., Jr., MD {1558479436} CdvDis, IntrMd(80,ARG07)<NJ-COMMED, NJ-OCEANMC>
+ Brick Cardiovascular Specialists/Toms River
147 Route 37 West   Toms River, NJ 08753   (732)240-3700
Fax (732)929-9179
+ Brick Cardiovascular Specialists/Brick Office
525 Jack Martin Boulevard/3rd Floor   Brick, NJ 08724
(732)240-3700   Fax (732)206-1563

Guarino, Joseph M., DO {1689681421} FamMed(90,PA77)<NJ-CHSFULD>
+ 1345 Kuser Road/Suite 4
Hamilton, NJ 08619   (609)581-1878   Fax (609)581-2632

Guarino, Lawrence A., MD {1508909037} Surgry(00,BWI01)
+ 376 Hamburg Tpke/Suite 1-A
Wayne, NJ 07470   (866)696-1118

Guarino, Ralph V., MD {1134140767} IntrMd(80,DOM21)
+ Drs. Guarino & O'Brien
160 Highway 37 West   Toms River, NJ 08755   (732)286-0440   Fax (732)286-2885

Guarrera, James Vincent, MD {1417998782} Surgry(98,NY47)
+ New Jersey Medical School Div Plastic & Hand Surgery
140 Bergen Street/Suite E1620   Newark, NJ 07103
(973)972-8092   Fax (973)972-8268

Guba, Russell F., Jr., MD {1932288628} Ophthl(81,NY46)
+ 220 Knickerbocker Road
Cresskill, NJ 07626   (201)568-2020   Fax (201)568-4213

Gubbi, Renukamba Nagaraju, MD {1255363719} Grtrcs, IntrMd<NJ-UMDNJ>
+ 12 Bernart Court
Hillsborough, NJ 08844   (732)356-3103

Gubbi, Smitha Ayodhyarama, MD {1275620650} FamMed, Grtrcs(98,INDI)
+ Bridgewater Internal Medicine, PA
215 Union Avenue/Suite E   Bridgewater, NJ 08807
(908)685-1818   Fax (908)685-8225

Gubenko, Yuriy Aronovich, MD {1295882231} Anesth, CarAne(85,UKR04)<NJ-UMDNJ>
+ University Hospital
150 Bergen Street/Level E/Anesth   Newark, NJ 07103
(973)972-5254   Fax (973)972-4172

Guda, Sivakoti Nagireddy, MD {1013043520} IntrMd
+ 2117 Klockner Road
Trenton, NJ 08690

Gudapati, Raghu, MD {1629087622} IntrMd(79,INA48)
+ NJ VA/James J Howard Outpatient Clinic
970 Route 70 West/IntMed   Brick, NJ 08724   (732)206-8900   Fax (732)836-6001

Gudapati, Ramakrishna, MD {1275589202} Psychy(00,DMN01)<NJ-UMDNJ>
+ University Psychiatric Associates
183 South Orange Avenue/E-F Levels   Newark, NJ 07103
(973)972-2977   Fax (973)972-2979

Gude, Prabhavat Venkata, MD {1205952173} PsyCAd, Psychy(69,INA48)<NJ-NWRKBETH>
+ Newark Beth Israel Medical Center
201 Lyons Avenue/Psychiatry   Newark, NJ 07112
(973)926-7026   Fax (973)926-2862

Physicians by Name and Address

Gudimella, Lakshmi, MD {1619068475} Anesth(92,INA48)<NJ-JFKMED>
+ JFK Medical Center
65 James Street/Anesthesiology   Edison, NJ 08820   (732)321-7000

Gudin, Jeffrey Alan, MD {1831133420} AnesPain, Addctn, IntrMd(92,NY03)<NJ-ENGLWOOD>
+ Ctr for Pain Management/Englwood Hosp
350 Engle Street   Englewood, NJ 07631   (201)894-3595   Fax (201)894-9046
pain2dr@yahoo.com

Gudis, Steven M., MD {1396719845} IntrMd, Nephro(77,NY47)
+ Randolph Medical & Renal Associates
121 Center Grove Road/Suite 13-14   Randolph, NJ 07869   (973)361-3737   Fax (973)361-9884

Gudofsky, Gina Lynn, MD {1992753099} EmrgMd(99,NY15)<NJ-OVERLOOK>
+ Overlook Medical Center
99 Beauvoir Avenue/PO Box 210/EmergMed   Summit, NJ 07902   (908)522-2000

Gudz, Alexandr, MD {1346280336} Gyneco, ObsGyn(88,UKRA)
+ 749 Irvington Avenue
Maplewood, NJ 07040   (973)762-6033   Fax (973)762-6088

Gudz, Ludmila, MD {1386747806} IntrMd(77,UKR25)<NJ-STBARNMC>
+ 2333 Morris Avenue/Suite B-115
Union, NJ 07083   (908)624-0090   Fax (908)624-0091
+ 749 Irvington Drive
Maplewood, NJ 07040   (908)624-0090   Fax (973)762-6088

Gue, Jean B., MD {1831434257} IntrMd, IntHos(09,NY09)
+ Cooper University Hospital
One Cooper Plaza/Hospitalist   Camden, NJ 08103   (856)342-3150

Guena, Luisa, MD {1972710366} Anesth, Surgry, IntrMd(79,NY09)<NJ-SOLARIHS>
+ JFK Medical Center
65 James Street   Edison, NJ 08820   (732)321-7668   Fax (732)767-2969

Guenin, Alla Mikhaylovna, MD {1275802324}<NJ-CHILTON>
+ Chilton Medical Center
97 West Parkway   Pompton Plains, NJ 07444   (763)843-0129

Guercio-Hauer, Catherine A., MD {1083670079} FamMed, IntrMd(87,GRN01)
+ Morristown Medical Center Family Medicine
435 South Street/Suite 220-A   Morristown, NJ 07960   (973)971-4222   Fax (973)290-7050

Guerin, Bonni Lee, MD {1922090802} OncHem, IntrMd(88,NY48)<NJ-OVERLOOK>
+ Medical Diagnostic Associates, P.A.
99 Beauvoir Avenue   Summit, NJ 07901   (908)608-0078   Fax (908)608-1504
+ Atlantic Surgical Oncology
99 Beauvoir Street   Summit, NJ 07901   (908)608-0078   Fax (908)598-2392

Guernica, Adele Marie, DO {1073547048} AlgyImmn
+ Allergy & Asthma Consultants of NJ, P.A.
9004 Lincoln Drive West/Suite B   Marlton, NJ 08053   (856)596-3100   Fax (856)596-3133
+ Allergy & Asthma Consultants of NJ, P.A.
110 South Dennisville Road   Cape May Court House, NJ 08210   (856)596-3100   Fax (856)596-3133

Guerra, Julio C., MD {1154432276} AdolMd, Pedtrc(87,MEXI)<NJ-OVERLOOK, NJ-STBARNMC>
+ College Plaza Pediatrics
765 State Route 10 East/Suite 203   Randolph, NJ 07869   (973)659-9991   Fax (973)659-9632
+ College Plaza Pediatrics
653 Willow Grove Street/Suite 2300   Hackettstown, NJ 07840   (973)659-9991   Fax (908)852-1900

Guerra-Deluna, Myrna T., MD {1508803990} ObsGyn(76,PHIL)<NJ-JFKMED>
+ 904 Oak Tree Road/Suite B
South Plainfield, NJ 07080   (908)757-8400

Guerrera, Angela Dixon, MD {1962734913} EmrgMd<NJ-COOPRUMC>
+ Cooper University Hospital
One Cooper Plaza   Camden, NJ 08103   (856)342-2000

Guerrero, Isabel C., MD {1568456580} InfDis, IntrMd(72,PHI02)<NJ-COMMED>
+ 25 Mule Road/Suite B-1
Toms River, NJ 08755   (732)286-2565   Fax (732)286-7669

Guerrero Miranda, Cesar Yvan, MD {1508028960}<NJ-NWRKBETH>
+ Newark Beth Israel Medical Center
201 Lyons Avenue   Newark, NJ 07112   (973)926-7000

Guerzon, Pearl Tolentino, MD {1851599765} FamMed(02,PHI22)<MA-DEACGLOV>
+ 4 Brighton Road/Suite 208
Clifton, NJ 07012   (973)321-9884   Fax (978)645-6871

Guevarra, Andres T., MD {1427009588} Pedtrc(78,PHIL)<NJ-VIRTMHBC>
+ Moorestown Pediatrics
212 West Route 38/Suite 400   Moorestown, NJ 08057   (856)235-0264   Fax (856)235-4635

Guevarra, Jesusita H., MD {1003867177} Pedtrc(78,PHIL)
+ Moorestown Pediatrics
212 West Route 38/Suite 400   Moorestown, NJ 08057   (856)235-0264   Fax (856)235-4635

Guevarra, Keith Poscablo, DO {1699925263} IntrMd
+ 4 Lackawanna Place
Passaic, NJ 07055

Guggenheim, Douglas Eric, MD {1790974889}
+ Regional Cancer Care Associates, LLC
200 Bowman Drive/Suite E-125   Voorhees, NJ 08043   (609)468-7888   Fax (856)424-5634
dguggenheim@regionalcancercare.org

Guglielmi, Gwen E., MD {1851317036} RadDia, Radiol(83,PA14)
+ Princeton Radiology Associates, P.A.
419 North Harrison Street   Princeton, NJ 08540   (609)921-3345   Fax (609)683-8847
+ Princeton Radiology Associates, P.A.
9 Centre Drive   Jamesburg, NJ 08831   (609)921-3345   Fax (609)655-4016
+ University Radiology Group, P.C.
375 Route 206/Suite 1   Hillsborough, NJ 08540   (908)874-7600   Fax (908)874-7052

Gugliotta, Joseph L., MD {1619949575} InfDis, IntrMd(74,NY46)<NJ-HUNTRDN>
+ Hunterdon Infection Disease
1100 Wescott Drive/Suite 306   Flemington, NJ 08822   (908)788-6474   Fax (908)788-6616
+ Hunterdon Medical Center
2100 Wescott Drive   Flemington, NJ 08822   (908)788-6474   Fax (908)788-6616

Gugnani, Manish K., MD {1558327221} PulDis, IntrMd, CritCr(93,NIG02)
+ Mercer Bucks Pulmonary
416 Bellevue Avenue/Suite 405   Trenton, NJ 08618   (609)394-2900   Fax (609)394-2916
+ Snoring and Sleep Apnea Center Mercer County
1401 Whitehorse Mercerville Rd   Hamilton, NJ 08619   (609)394-2900   Fax (609)584-5144

Guha, Koel, MD {1073760930} Pedtrc<NJ-UNVMCPRN>
+ CHOP Care Network at Princeton Medical Center
One Plainsboro Road   Plainsboro, NJ 08536   (609)853-7000   Fax (609)497-4173

Guha, Surya, MD {1548553951}
+ 3 Wedgewood Drive
West Orange, NJ 07052   (917)572-6630

Guibor, Pierre, MD {1093922569} EmrgMd, UndsMd(66,IL11)<NJ-MEADWLND>
+ 1018 Harmon Cove Towers
Secaucus, NJ 07094   (201)392-3438   Fax (201)271-3688
drpierre@aol.com

Guida, Vincent C., DO {1285677427} IntrMd(93,NY75)<NJ-COMMED>
+ Stafford Medical, P.A.
1364 Route 72 West/Suite 5   Manahawkin, NJ 08050   (609)597-3416   Fax (609)597-9608

Guido, Stephanie, DO {1992140313} FamMed
+ Virtua Family Medicine
128 Route 70   Medford, NJ 08055   (609)953-7105

Guiliano, Philip M., MD {1609843762} FamMed(74,NY15)<NJ-VIRTMHBC>
+ Columbus Family Physicians
23659 Columbus Road/Suite 4   Columbus, NJ 08022   (609)298-7333   Fax (609)298-7091

Guillaume, Stephanie Ann, MD {1891936589} Anesth(06,NY48)<NJ-ENGLWOOD>
+ Englewood Anesthesiology
350 Engle Street   Englewood, NJ 07631   (201)894-3238   Fax (201)894-0585

Guillen, Gregorio J., MD {1538252226} Grtrcs, IntrMd(82,DOM11)
+ 400 State Street/Suite 2
Perth Amboy, NJ 08861   (732)442-6020   Fax (732)442-1995

Guillen, Steven E., MD {1710911029} EmrgMd<NJ-HUNTRDN>
+ Hunterdon Medical Center
2100 Wescott Drive   Flemington, NJ 08822   (908)788-6100

Guillermety, Esperanza E., MD {1720184104} PhysMd(81,PRO01)<NJ-UNVMCPRN>
+ 9 Brookdale Drive
Lawrenceville, NJ 08648

Guinto, Danilo M., MD {1598702094} Pedtrc(76,PHIL)<NJ-CLARMAAS>
+ Forest Hill Family Health Associates, P.A.
465 Mount Prospect Avenue/Pediatrics   Newark, NJ 07104   (973)483-3640   Fax (973)483-4895

Guinto, Wilson Desquitado, MD {1619497708}
+ 144 Chilton Street
Elizabeth, NJ 07202   (908)956-5850

Guirguis, George, DO {1407087711} MtFtMd, ObsGyn(09,PA78)
+ Hackensack Univ. Maternal Fetal Med
20 Prospect Avenue/Suite 601   Hackensack, NJ 07601   (201)996-2765   Fax (201)487-8516
+ Hackensack University Medical Center
30 Prospect Avenue/Suite 2W-73   Hackensack, NJ 07601   (551)996-2453

Guirguis, Nagy Nimr, MD {1346294873} IntrMd(76,EGYP)<NJ-BAYSHORE>
+ Guirguis Medical Care LLC
301 Church Street   Aberdeen, NJ 07747   (732)566-0595   Fax (732)566-0597

Guirguis, Soad George, MD {1326212531} Psychy(71,EGYP)
+ Neighborhood Health Center Plainfield
1700-58 Myrtle Avenue   Plainfield, NJ 07060   (908)753-6401   Fax (908)226-6743

Guirguis, Sonia S., MD {1215968136} Allrgy, Pedtrc(81,EGY04)
+ 172 Summerhill Road/Suite 2
East Brunswick, NJ 08816   (732)613-6161   Fax (732)613-9090
sguirguis1000@gmail.com

Guittari, Nicholas S., MD {1841354537} IntrMd, Grtrcs(86,NJ05)
+ 946 Avenue C
Bayonne, NJ 07002   (201)436-3900   Fax (973)746-8508

Gujar, Priti S., MD {1356382600} Grtrcs, IntrMd, FamMGrtc(94,INA65)<NJ-HUNTRDN>
+ Hunterdon Medical Center
2100 Wescott Drive   Flemington, NJ 08822   (908)788-6575   Fax (908)237-5439

Gujja, Rajitha Reddy, MD {1558362202} IntrMd(97,INA5B)<NJ-MTNSIDE>
+ Rajitha Gujja MD LLC
239 Claremont Avenue/Suite A/223250   Montclair, NJ 07042   (973)338-4900   Fax (973)338-4420

Gujjula, Prashanthi, MD {1134407547} FamMed
+ Atlantic Medical Care Primary Care
3322 Route 22/Suite 1204   Branchburg, NJ 08876   (908)378-7227   Fax (908)252-0127

Gujral, Manmeet Kaur, MD {1891090353}
+ 302 Summit Avenue/First Floor
Jersey City, NJ 07306

Gul, Sheba, MD {1528120110} Pedtrc(90,PAK11)
+ Highland Park Pediatrics
85 Raritan Avenue   Highland Park, NJ 08904   (732)246-0202   Fax (732)246-8334

Gulab, Nazli E., MD {1598736118} Psychy(78,PAK08)<NJ-OURLADY, NJ-KMHCHRRY>
+ University Hospital-SOM Department of Psychiatry
2250 Chapel Avenue West/Suite 100   Cherry Hill, NJ 08002   (856)482-9000   Fax (856)482-1159

Gulati, Rita, MD {1467489906} RprEnd, ObsGyn, FrtInf(91,NY03)
+ Reproductive Medicine Associates of New Jersey
475 Prospect Avenue/Suite 101   West Orange, NJ 07052   (973)325-2229   Fax (973)290-8370
+ Reproductive Medicine Associates of New Jersey
140 Allen Road   Basking Ridge, NJ 07920   (973)325-2229   Fax (973)290-8370

Gulati, Sunita, MD {1861677791} Pedtrc
+ 66 Avenue K
Monroe Township, NJ 08831   (732)656-1962

Gulevski, Vasko Kole, MD {1528011517} Nrolgy
+ Central Jersey Neurology Associates
501 Iron Bridge Road/Suite 2   Freehold, NJ 07728   (732)462-7030   Fax (732)308-3562

Guliano, Jaclyn M., MD {1225445737} FamMed(NET12)
+ Family Practice of CentraState
479 Newman Springs Rd/Suite A-101   Marlboro, NJ 07746   (732)780-1601

Gulli, Maria T., MD {1174674238} Pedtrc(81,ITA08)<NJ-MONMOUTH>
+ 1 Channel Drive/Unit 1213
Monmouth Beach, NJ 07750   (732)229-4933

Gulli, Vito M., MD {1255491023} Hemato, PthACl, PthAna(81,ITA08)<NJ-BAYSHORE>
+ RWJ University Pathology
125 Paterson Street/MEB 212   New Brunswick, NJ 08901   (732)235-8120   Fax (732)235-8120

Gultom, Yanto Meiyer, MD {1851444228} IntrMd(98,GRN01)<NJ-VIRTMHBC, NJ-KMHSTRAT>
+ Hillsborough Internal Medicine
403 Towne Centre Drive   Hillsborough, NJ 08844   (908)428-4840   Fax (908)382-3288
+ Alliance for Better Care, P.C.
PO Box 1510   Medford, NJ 08055   (908)428-4840   Fax (609)953-8652

Guma, Michael, DO {1376655407} IntrMd, Rheuma(89,MO79)<NJ-BAYONNE, NJ-WESTHDSN>
+ 312 Belleville Turnpike/Suite 3-A
North Arlington, NJ 07031   (201)998-2800   Fax (201)998-0800

Physicians by Name and Address

Gumaste, Sandhya V., MD {1811943418} IntrMd(86,INDI)<NJ-ENGLWOOD, NJ-HOLYNAME>
+ 185 Cedar Lane/Suite 8
Teaneck, NJ 07666 (201)836-6441 Fax (201)836-6448

Gumbs, Andrew Alexander, MD {1487849725} SrgOnc, Surgry(98,CT01)<NJ-OVERLOOK>
+ Summit Medical Group-Berkeley Heights Campus
1 Diamond Hill Road Berkeley Heights, NJ 07922 (908)277-8950 Fax (908)790-6576

Gumidyala, Lalitha V., MD {1831160027} IntrMd(94,INA5B)<NJ-NWRKBETH>
+ Corporate Health Center
832 Brunswick Avenue Trenton, NJ 08638 (609)695-7471

Gumidyala, Padmasree, MD {1699075127} Pedtrc
+ ABC Pediatrics, LLC.
974 Inman Avenue/Suite 1-A Edison, NJ 08820 (908)412-8866 Fax (908)412-9363

Gumina, John D., MD {1831169515} FamMed(74,NJ05)<NJ-JRSYSHMC>
+ Howell Jackson Medical Center
4764 Route 9 South Howell, NJ 07731 (732)370-3563
+ Wall Family Medical
500 Candlewood Commons Howell, NJ 07731 (732)370-3563 Fax (732)364-7713

Gummadi, Vedam, MD InfDis(88,INDI)
+ 138 Country Club Drive
Moorestown, NJ 08057

Gumnic, Blair Rachel, DO {1043657059} ObsGyn
+ Hackensack Meridian Medical Group Ob/Gyn, Wall
1924 Route 35/Suite 5 Wall, NJ 07719 (732)974-8404 Fax (732)974-8904

Gumnit, Robert Y., MD {1902803471} Anesth(75,PA02)<NJ-VIRTMHBC>
+ Burlington Anesthesia Associates
120 Madison Ave/Suite E/PO Box 174 Mount Holly, NJ 08060 (609)261-1660 Fax (609)261-1779
+ Virtua Memorial
175 Madison Avenue Mount Holly, NJ 08060 (609)267-0700

Gunadasa, Susanthi N., MD {1639331861} IntrMd(05,SRI08)<NJ-HACKNSK>
+ Hackensack University Medical Center
30 Prospect Avenue/Internal Med Hackensack, NJ 07601 (201)996-2000

Gunawan, Rita R., MD {1720021827} Pedtrc(78,GER54)<NJ-STPETER, NJ-RWJUBRUN>
+ 3 Clyde Road/Suite 102
Somerset, NJ 08873 (732)545-6464

Gundapuneni, Satish Babu, MD {1982018826} IntrMd<NJ-PALISADE>
+ Palisades Medical Center
7600 River Road North Bergen, NJ 07047 (201)854-5000

Gungor, Semih, MD {1033104534} Anesth, IntrMd(90,TUR04)
+ HSS Paramus Outpatient Center
140 East Ridgewood Avenue/Suite 175-S Paramus, NJ 07652 (201)796-2255 Fax (201)796-3711

Gunja, Sakina Zahir, MD {1639257934} Psychy(79,INA1Y)<NJ-UNIVBHC>
+ University Behavioral Health Care
671 Hoes Lane/PO Box 1392 Piscataway, NJ 08855 (732)235-5500
+ University Behavioral Health Care
303 George Street/Suite 200 New Brunswick, NJ 08901 (732)235-5500 Fax (732)235-6187

Gunn, Angela Lijoi, MD {1780641514} Pedtrc(85,DC02)
+ Notchview Pediatrics, LLC.
1037 Route 46 East/Suite 201 Clifton, NJ 07013 (973)779-3911 Fax (973)471-2730
+ St. Joseph's Pediatrics DePaul Center
11 Getty Avenue/2nd Floor Paterson, NJ 07503 (973)754-4690

Gunn Russell, Ian Neil, MD {1801858576} FamMed, GenPrc(77,SCO02)<NJ-MORRISTN>
+ 71 Hanover Road
Florham Park, NJ 07932 (973)712-3517 Fax (973)712-3520

Gunvantlal, Desai A., MD {1730137308} Anesth(76,INA69)
+ Anesthesia Consultnts of NJ/Nova Pain
285 Davidson Avenue/Suite 204 Somerset, NJ 08873 (732)271-1400 Fax (732)271-3543

Gunzburg, Allison B., MD {1235132804} Ophthl
+ Northern New Jersey Eye Institute
71 Second Street South Orange, NJ 07079 (973)763-2203 Fax (973)762-9449

Guo, H. Jennifer, MD {1154595692} IntrMd(86,CHN19)<NJ-STJOSHOS, NJ-VALLEY>
+ CGF Medical Center PA
1254 Route 27 North Brunswick, NJ 08902 (732)640-2777 Fax (732)317-8148

Guo, Jianhua, MD {1457356925} Anesth(82,CHN42)<NJ-SOCEANCO>
+ Robert Wood Johnson-UMDNJ Anesthesia Group
1140 Route 72 West Manahawkin, NJ 08050 (609)978-8900

Guo, Jin Ping, MD {1205852464} IntrMd(85,CHN8A)<NJ-LOURDMED>
+ Lourdes Medical Center of Burlington County
218 Sunset Road Willingboro, NJ 08046 (609)835-2900

Guo, Shuang, MD {1821385386}
+ University Physician Associates of New Jersey
125 Paterson Street/CAB 5200 New Brunswick, NJ 08901 (732)235-7226 Fax (732)235-7115

Guo, Suqin, MD {1740394667} Ophthl(95,CHNA)
+ University Hospital-Doctors Office Center
90 Bergen Street/Ophth/DOC 6th F Newark, NJ 07103 (973)972-2500 Fax (973)972-2068

Guo, Xiaotao, MD {1437239670} Anesth(82,CHNA)<NJ-UNVM-CPRN>
+ University Medical Center of Princeton at Plainsboro
One Plainsboro Road/Anesthesiology Plainsboro, NJ 08536 (609)497-4000

Guo, Yijun, MD {1215924170} PthACl(88,CHN57)
+ PLUS Diagnostics
1200 River Avenue/Suite 10 Lakewood, NJ 08701 (732)901-7575 Fax (732)901-1555

Gupta, Abhinai K., MD {1699784298} IntrMd, IntHos(01,INA30)<ME-EASTMAIN>
+ Lyons & Chvala Nephrology Associates
730 North Broad Street/Suite 101 Woodbury, NJ 08096 (856)384-0238 Fax (856)384-4788

Gupta, Adarsh Kumar, DO {1003896523} FamMed(00,NJ75)
+ University Hospital-University Family Medicine
42 East Laurel Road/Suite 2100 Stratford, NJ 08084 (856)566-7020 Fax (856)566-6188

Gupta, Ajay K., MD {1215974225} CdvDis, IntrMd(80,INA92)<NJ-STJOSHOS, NJ-MTNSIDE>
+ 401 Hamburg Turnpike/Suite 109
Wayne, NJ 07470 (973)595-5345 Fax (973)595-5069
+ 50 Mount Prospect Avenue/Suite 101
Clifton, NJ 07013 (973)595-5345 Fax (973)595-5069

Gupta, Amit, MD {1740274612} Surgry
+ Union County HealthCare Associates
300 South Avenue Garwood, NJ 07027 (908)232-2273 Fax (908)232-1439
+ Union County HealthCare Associates
999 Raritan Road Clark, NJ 07066 (908)232-2273 Fax (732)381-3733

Gupta, Amit Kumar, MD {1245423573} EmrgMd, Txclgy(04,GRN01)<NY-STATNRTH>
+ Hackensack University Medical Center
30 Prospect Avenue Hackensack, NJ 07601 (201)996-2000
agupta1@hotmail.com

Gupta, Angela, MD {1497912315} IntrMd(99,NJ05)
+ Rutgers Hurtado Health Center
11 Bishop Place New Brunswick, NJ 08901 (732)932-7402 Fax (732)932-1223

Gupta, Anil Kumar, MD {1932184728} CdvDis, IntrMd(85,INA57)<NJ-COMMED, NJ-KIMBALL>
+ 780 Route 37 West/Suite 220
Toms River, NJ 08755 (732)286-4801

Gupta, Anita, DO {1376746834} Anesth, PainMd(03,NJ75)
+ Drexel College of Medicine
312 North Berlin Road/Medical Lindenwold, NJ 08021
+ Atrium Spine and Pain
3100 Quakerbridge Road Mercerville, NJ 08619 (732)654-2772

Gupta, Anupama, MD {1679513105} PthCyt, PthACl, Pthlgy(98,INA72)<NJ-CHILTON>
+ Hackensack University Medical Center
30 Prospect Avenue/Cytopathology Hackensack, NJ 07601 (201)996-2000
+ 826 Sunset Avenue
Haworth, NJ 07641

Gupta, Archana, MD {1609894898} Pedtrc, NnPnMd(95,INA23)
+ 826 Sunset Avenue
Haworth, NJ 07641

Gupta, Asha, MD {1609804038} Nrolgy(70,INA43)<NJ-VIRTVOOR>
+ Echelon Medical Center
600 Somerdale Road Voorhees, NJ 08043 (856)429-8445 Fax (856)429-1962

Gupta, Ashmit, MD {1245220151} Otlryg(97,DC01)<NJ-VIRTVOOR, NJ-VIRTMARL>
+ Advanced Mount Laurel
204 Ark Road/Building 1/Suite 102 Mount Laurel, NJ 08054 (856)602-4000 Fax (856)946-1747
+ Advanced ENT - Washington Township
239 Hurffville Crosskeys Road Sewell, NJ 08080 (856)602-4000 Fax (856)629-3391
+ Advanced ENT - Voorhees
200 Bowman Drive/Suite D-285 Voorhees, NJ 08054 (856)602-4000 Fax (856)346-0757

Gupta, Ashok, MD {1205846904} Gastrn, IntrMd(73,INDI)<NJ-CHILTON>
+ Gastroenterology Associates of New Jersey
842 Clifton Avenue/Suite 6 Clifton, NJ 07013 (973)470-0101 Fax (973)470-3024
+ Gastroenterology Associates of New Jersey
332 Lafayette Avenue Hawthorne, NJ 07506 (973)470-0101 Fax (973)777-3024

Gupta, Atul Kumar, MD {1912976093} RadDia(81,NY15)<NY-VIAROCHS>
+ Coastal Imaging, LLC
79 Route 37 West/Suite 103 Toms River, NJ 08755 (732)678-0087 Fax (732)276-2325

Gupta, Avinash Chandra, MD {1265531487} CdvDis, IntrMd(80,INA3C)<NJ-KIMBALL>
+ Avinash Gupta MD PC
637 River Avenue Lakewood, NJ 08701 (732)886-9101 Fax (732)886-9523

Gupta, Bhavna, MD {1801074455} MedOnc, IntrMd(97,INA1P)
+ Jersey HemOnc LLC
9238 Kennedy Blvd North Bergen, NJ 07047 (201)751-4004

Gupta, Charu, MD {1457506792}
+ Concentra Medical Centers
30 Seaview Drive/Suite 2 Secaucus, NJ 07094 (201)272-8900 Fax (201)319-1233

Gupta, Chiraag U., MD {1083868673} EmrgMd
+ University Emergency Medicine
125 Paterson Street/MEB 104 New Brunswick, NJ 08901 (732)235-8717 Fax (732)235-7379

Gupta, Dev R., MD {1720055502} Elecen, Nrolgy, SrgNro(63,INDI)<NJ-HACKNSK, NJ-HOLYNAME>
+ Hackensack Neurology Group
211 Essex Street/Suite 202 Hackensack, NJ 07601 (201)488-1515 Fax (201)488-9471

Gupta, Divya, MD {1477559763} Nrolgy, ClNrPh, SlpDis(94,INA23)<NJ-JFKMED>
+ JFK Neurosciences Institute
65 James Street/Second Floor Edison, NJ 08818 (732)321-7950 Fax (732)632-1584

Gupta, Gaurav, MD {1285898312} SrgNro, Surgry(98,INA28)<NJ-UMDNJ>
+ Rutgers - RWJMS
125 Paterson Street/Suite 2100 New Brunswick, NJ 08901 (732)235-7756 Fax (732)235-7095

Gupta, Juhee, MD {1053318063} Hemato, IntrMd, Onclgy(79,INA39)<NJ-JFKMED, NJ-RWJURAH>
+ Juhee Gupta MD PC
35-37 Progress Street/Suite A-1 Edison, NJ 08820 (908)226-1500 Fax (908)755-3200
+ Linden Medical Associates MD PC
540 South Wood Avenue Linden, NJ 07036 (908)226-1500 Fax (908)862-5810

Gupta, Kanika, MD {1821475898} IntHos<NJ-SJHREGMC>
+ SJH Regional Medical Center
1505 West Sherman Avenue Vineland, NJ 08360 (856)845-1000

Gupta, Kavita, DO {1699745828} PhysMd, PainMd(98,NJ75)
+ Kennedy Care Center
705 White Horse Road/Suite D-101-2 Voorhees, NJ 08043 (856)783-0695 Fax (856)783-8083
+ Institute for Pain Relief
120 Carnie Boulevard/Suite 4 Voorhees, NJ 08043 (856)783-0695 Fax (856)751-6660

Gupta, Kavita, MD {1073833554} IntrMd
+ Center for Healthy Senior Living
360 Essex Street/Suite 401 Hackensack, NJ 07601 (551)996-1140 Fax (551)996-0543

Gupta, Kunal, MD {1023256567} Gastrn
+ Middlesex Monmouth Gastroenterology
222 Schanck Road/Suite 302 Freehold, NJ 07728 (732)577-1999 Fax (732)845-5356

Gupta, Mala Rani, MD {1407973001} PsyCAd, Psychy, PsyFor(87,INA6Z)
+ CENTRA Comprehensive Psychotherapy
5000 Sagemore Drive/Suite 205 Marlton, NJ 08053 (856)983-3866 Fax (856)985-8148

Gupta, Mamta Bansal, MD {1255528618} Pedtrc(99,INA07)
+ Piscataway Pediatrics
47 Wills Way Piscataway, NJ 08854 (908)834-8534 Fax (908)922-4880
piscatawaypeds@gmail.com

Gupta, Manjari, MD {1710275672} ObsGyn
+ Ob & Gyn Group of E Brunswick
172 Summerhill Road/Suite 1 East Brunswick, NJ 08816 (732)254-1500 Fax (732)254-1436

Gupta, Manju, MD {1790717528} IntrMd(77,INA6Z)<NJ-WAYNEGEN, NJ-CHILTON>
+ 332 Lafayette Avenue
Hawthorne, NJ 07506 (973)423-0145 Fax (973)423-0667

Gupta, Meera, MD {1750351433} PedInf, Pedtrc, AdolMed(77,INDI)
+ Morristown Pediatric Associates, LLC
261 James Street/Suite 1-G   Morristown, NJ 07960   (973)540-9393   Fax (973)540-1937

Gupta, Mini, MD {1528117389} FamMed(96,OH44)
+ Haddonfield Internal Medicine
216 Haddon Avenue   Haddon Township, NJ 08108   (856)854-6600   Fax (856)854-6610

Gupta, Monika, MD {1134270846} Pedtrc<NJ-COOPRUMC>
+ Cooper University Hospital
One Cooper Plaza   Camden, NJ 08103   (856)342-2000   Fax (856)968-9598

Gupta, Namita J., MD {1255591905} PthACl
+ Riverview Medical Center
1 Riverview Plaza   Red Bank, NJ 07701   (732)530-2347   Fax (732)345-2045

Gupta, Narendra K., MD {1386750255} IntrMd(86,MEXI)<NJ-BAYSHORE, NJ-JRSYSHMC>
+ Marlboro Medical Center
203 Route 9 South   Englishtown, NJ 07726   (732)617-8800   Fax (732)617-8808

Gupta, Neena, MD {1598784308} EmrgMd(91,PA07)<NJ-STBARNMC>
+ St. Barnabas Medical Center
94 Old Short Hills Road   Livingston, NJ 07039   (973)322-5000
+ St. Barnabas Cancer Center
94 Old Short Hills Road/Suite 1   Livingston, NJ 07039   (973)322-5650

Gupta, Neeti, MD {1538226980} AlgyImmn, IntrMd(01,NJ06)
+ Mercer Allergy & Asthma Center
300A Princeton Hightstown Road   East Windsor, NJ 08520   (609)371-6222   Fax (609)371-6282
mercerallergy@gmail.com

Gupta, Neha, MD {1962798033} Psychy(10,BLZ02)
+ Juhee Gupta MD PC
35-37 Progress Street/Suite A-1   Edison, NJ 08820   (908)226-1500   Fax (908)755-3200

Gupta, Pooja, MD {1801281845}<NY-MNTFMOSE>
+ St. Joseph's HealthCare System
703 Main Street/Administration   Paterson, NJ 07503   (973)754-2000

Gupta, Pradip, MD {1861686305} Nrolgy, Psychy(71,INDI)<NJ-VAEASTOR>
+ VA New Jersey Health Care System-East Orange Campus
385 Tremont Avenue   East Orange, NJ 07018   (973)676-1000
+ Essex Diagnostic Group
280 South Harrison Street   East Orange, NJ 07018   (973)678-8839

Gupta, Punit Kumar, MD {1336118975} InfDis, IntrMd(99,NJ05)
+ 285 Lexington Avenue
Passaic, NJ 07055   (973)779-5879   Fax (973)239-4267

Gupta, Punita, MD {1073709457} Grtrcs(02,INA96)<MA-NEMEDCEN>
+ St. Joseph's Pediatrics DePaul Center
11 Getty Avenue/2nd Floor   Paterson, NJ 07503   (973)754-2727

Gupta, Rachna, MD {1134132475} InfDis
+ ID Associates PA/dba ID Care
765 Route 10 East/Suite 201   Randolph, NJ 07869   (973)989-0068   Fax (973)361-8955
+ ID Associates PA/dba ID Care
8 Saddle Road   Cedar Knolls, NJ 07927   (973)989-0068   Fax (973)993-5953

Gupta, Rajan, MD {1922014422} Surgry, SrgTrm, SrgCrC(91,MA05)<NH-DRTMTHMC>
+ RWJMG Acute Care Surgery
125 Paterson Street/Suite 6300   New Brunswick, NJ 08901   (732)235-4959   Fax (732)235-2964

Gupta, Rajan S., MD {1114997962} PhysMd, PainMd, IntrMd(96,INA20)
+ Gupta Institute for Integrative Medicine
951 Berlin Road   Cherry Hill, NJ 08034   (856)482-7246   Fax (856)482-7245
+ Gupta Institute for Integrative Medicine
2301 Evesham Road/Suite 305   Voorhees, NJ 08043   (856)482-7246   Fax (856)482-7245
+ Gupta Institute for Integrative Medicine
860 Route 168/Suite 104   Turnersville, NJ 08034   (856)482-7246   Fax (856)482-7245

Gupta, Rajendra Prasad, MD {1124035886} Gastrn, IntrMd(70,INA32)<NJ-CHSMRCER, NJ-CHSFULD>
+ Hopewell Valley Medical Group, PA
1871 Pennington Road   Trenton, NJ 08618   (609)882-5317   Fax (609)538-8031
RGUPTAMD@hotmail.com
+ Delaware Valley Cardiovascular
1401 Whitehorse Mercerville Rd   Hamilton, NJ 08619   (609)882-5317   Fax (609)752-3036

Gupta, Rakesh Chander, MD {1639197783} Anesth, PainMd, AnesPain(80,INDI)<NJ-VIRTMHBC, NJ-VIRTVOOR>
+ Advanced Pain Consultants, P.A.
120 Madison Avenue/Suite D   Mount Holly, NJ 08060   (609)267-1707

Gupta, Rakesh Vardhan, MD {1972554020} IntCrd, CdvDis, IntrMd(99,NY48)
+ Drs. Gupta and Patel
20 Hospital Drive/Suite 12B   Toms River, NJ 08755   (732)240-7777   Fax (732)240-7710

Gupta, Raksha R., MD {1295816270} Pedtrc(76,INA92)<NJ-HACKNSK>
+ 952 Main Street
Hackensack, NJ 07602   (201)488-2200   Fax (201)488-0211

Gupta, Ramesh C., MD {1205813391} Gastrn, IntrMd(70,INA32)<NJ-STJOSHOS, NJ-CHILTON>
+ 15-01 Broadway/Suite 28
Fair Lawn, NJ 07410   (201)794-8900   Fax (201)794-9424
Ramesh.Gupta@Verizon.net

Gupta, Ravi, MD {1437532819} IntrMd<NJ-COOPRUMC>
+ Cooper University Hospital
One Cooper Plaza   Camden, NJ 08103   (856)342-2000

Gupta, Rohit Kumar, MD {1245646330}<NJ-STJOSHOS>
+ St. Joseph's Regional Medical Center
703 Main Street   Paterson, NJ 07503   (973)754-2000

Gupta, Sanchita, MD {1932302924} IntrMd(04,INA70)
+ Bergen Medical Associates
190 Dayton Street   Ridgewood, NJ 07450   (201)670-7800   Fax (201)670-7720

Gupta, Shabnam, MD {1427097039} Nephro, IntrMd(91,INA83)<NJ-STBARNMC, NJ-BAYONNE>
+ United Medical, P.C.
988 Broadway/Suite 201   Bayonne, NJ 07002   (201)339-6111   Fax (201)339-6333
+ Hypertension & Renal Group, P.A.
22 Old Short Hills Road/Suite 212   Livingston, NJ 07039   (201)339-6111   Fax (973)994-7085
+ Hypertension & Renal Group, P.A.
930 Kennedy Boulevard   Bayonne, NJ 07002   (201)858-1509   Fax (201)858-2051

Gupta, Shalini, MD {1912294042} ObsGyn(03,INA05)<NJ-HACKNSK>
+ Hackensack University Medical Center
30 Prospect Avenue/4E-90/ObGyn   Hackensack, NJ 07601   (201)996-2755

Gupta, Simhadri M., MD {1760483895} Nrolgy(79,INA13)
+ 2 Lincoln Highway/Suite 302
Edison, NJ 08820

Gupta, Suraj P., MD {1770518425} IntrMd(64,INDI)
+ 3 Plaza Drive/Suite 4
Toms River, NJ 08757   (732)240-1555   Fax (732)240-5007

Gupta, Suresh Kumar, MD {1558383331} PthACl, Pthlgy(74,INA82)<NJ-EASTORNG>
+ East Orange General Hospital
300 Central Avenue/Pathology   East Orange, NJ 07018   (973)672-8400   Fax (973)266-2932

Gupta, Swati, MD {1386035772} IntrMd
+ Avenel Iselin Medical Group
400 Gill Lane   Iselin, NJ 08830   (732)404-1580   Fax (732)404-1594

Gupta, Vijay, MD {1508068693} Anesth(04,INA30)<NJ-HOLYNAME>
+ Teaneck Anesthesia Group, P.A.
718 Teaneck Road   Teaneck, NJ 07666   (201)833-7149   Fax (201)833-6576

Gupta, Vikram, MD {1750538609} FamMed, GenPrc(01)
+ 246 Clifton Avenue/Suite 4
Clifton, NJ 07011   (973)330-6765   Fax (973)939-8489
+ West Paterson Family Medical Center
154 Union Avenue   Paterson, NJ 07502   (973)942-3618

Gupta, Vinod K., MD {1356350888} FamMed, Pedtrc, AdolMed(83,INA82)<NJ-CHSMRCER, NJ-CHSFULD>
+ Hopewell Valley Medical Group, PA
1871 Pennington Road   Trenton, NJ 08618   (609)882-5317   Fax (609)538-8031

Gupta, Vinod K., MD {1558472241} FamMed(71,INA7P)<NJ-RBAYOLDB>
+ Freehold Insta-Care Medical Center
3681 Route 9 North   Freehold, NJ 07728   (732)863-7100   Fax (732)863-7001

Gupta, Vipan Kumar, MD {1871588988} IntrMd, GenPrc(83,INA07)<NJ-HOLYNAME>
+ Holy Name Hospital
718 Teaneck Road/PracticeMngmnt   Teaneck, NJ 07666   (201)833-3000   Fax (201)881-6295

Gupta, Vipin K., MD {1851351035} Nrolgy(78,INDI)<NJ-SJERSYHS>
+ 2848 South Delsea Drive/Suite 2B
Vineland, NJ 08360   (856)691-7474   Fax (856)691-0372

Gupte, Chaitali Rajan, MD {1437301231}
+ Pulmonary & Allergy Associates
1 Springfield Avenue/Suite 3-A   Summit, NJ 07901

(908)934-0555   Fax (908)934-0556
chaitaligupte@yahoo.com

Gupte, Meenal A., MD {1770612962} Pedtrc(92,INA69)
+ Med 4 Kids Pediatrics
322 Shore Road   Somers Point, NJ 08244   (609)927-1353

Gura, Russell Saul, MD {1962400119} IntrMd(95,NY08)<NJ-ENGLWOOD, NJ-HOLYNAME>
+ Leonia Medical Associates, P.A.
25 Rockwood Place/Suite 120   Englewood, NJ 07631   (201)568-3335   Fax (201)568-2450

Gurak, Randall B., MD {1770659799} PsyCAd, Psychy, PsyFor(86,PA09)
+ One Mall Drive/Suite 920
Cherry Hill, NJ 08002   (856)482-2777

Gurando, Kate, DO {1467734707}
+ 3 Aberdeen Road
Chatham, NJ 07928   (917)449-4975
kategurando@gmail.com

Gurbuxani, Geeta, MD {1912171356}
+ 314 Oak Street/Unit b
Ridgewood, NJ 07450   (917)655-5862
geeta.gurbuxani@gmail.com

Gurell, Daniel Steven, MD {1336164029} RadDia, Radiol, RadBdI(99,NY46)<NJ-MTNSIDE, NY-STATNRTH>
+ Hackensack UMC Mountainside
1 Bay Avenue/Radiology   Montclair, NJ 07042   (973)429-6000

Gurey, Lowell Evan, MD {1558519918} Otlryg(06,NJ03)
+ Summit Medical Group-Berkeley Heights Campus
1 Diamond Hill Road/Otolaryngology   Berkeley Heights, NJ 07922   (908)273-4300   Fax (908)790-6576

Gurey Wasserstein, Allison P., MD {1740302249} Pedtrc(00,NJ06)
+ Summit Medical Group
85 Woodland Road   Short Hills, NJ 07078   (973)379-2488   Fax (973)921-0669

Gurkan, Sevgi, MD {1093976656} Pedtrc, PedNph(01,TUR04)
+ Child Health Institute of New Jersey
89 French Street/Suite 2300   New Brunswick, NJ 08901   (732)235-6230   Fax (732)235-8766

Gurland, Ira Alan, MD {1730159476} IntrMd, InfDis(95,PA12)
+ Highland Park Medical Associates
579A Cranbury Road/Suite 102   East Brunswick, NJ 08816   (732)613-0711   Fax (732)613-5783

Gurland, Jake, MD {1174028435} IntrMd<NJ-OVERLOOK>
+ Overlook Medical Center
99 Beauvoir Avenue/PO Box 210   Summit, NJ 07902   (908)522-2000

Gurland, Keith G., MD {1013098805} Ophthl(77,MEXI)<NJ-HOBUNIMC>
+ 521 Broadway
Bayonne, NJ 07002   (201)339-1266   Fax (201)339-0069

Gurland, Mark A., MD {1023127537} SrgHnd, SrgMcr, SrgOrt(79,NY19)<NJ-ENGLWOOD, NJ-HACKNSK>
+ 216 Engle Street
Englewood, NJ 07631   (201)568-4066   Fax (201)568-5595
+ 235 Prospect Avenue
Hackensack, NJ 07601   (201)489-0099

Gurnaney, Harshad Govindram, MD {1841304326} Anesth(97,INA69)<PA-CHOPHIL, PA-CHILDHOS>
+ CHOP Pediatric & Adolescent Specialty Care Center
1012 Laurel Oak Road/Anesth   Voorhees, NJ 08043   (856)435-1300   Fax (856)435-0091

Guron, Gunwant K., MD {1417926429} IntrMd(85,INDI)<NJ-STMICHL>
+ St. Michael's Medical Center
268 MLK Jr. Boulevard   Newark, NJ 07102   (973)877-5340

Gurrieri, John E., MD {1528137122} FamMed(84,SPA04)<NJ-VIRTMARL>
+ 301 Morris Drive
Cherry Hill, NJ 08003   (856)354-2232   Fax (856)354-9319

Gursky, Elliot J., MD {1578655890} PsyCAd, Psychy(71,WI05)
+ 92 Nassau Street
Princeton, NJ 08542   (609)924-6294   Fax (609)924-6352

Gurtovy, Mark, MD {1053332072} Psychy(74,UKRA)
+ Drs. Shapnik & Gurtovy
2150 Center Avenue/Suite 1-B   Fort Lee, NJ 07024   (201)461-2444   Fax (201)461-7148

Gurubhagavatula, Sarada, MD {1942390869} OncHem, IntrMd(98,MD07)
+ Summit Medical Group Florham Park Campus
150 Park Avenue   Florham Park, NJ 07932   (908)273-4300
+ Hematology-Oncology Associates of Northern NJ
100 Madison Avenue/PO Box 1089   Morristown, NJ 07962   (908)273-4300   Fax (973)644-9657
+ Hematology-Oncology Associates of Northern NJ
3219 US Highway 46/Suite 108   Parsippany, NJ 07932   (973)316-5900   Fax (973)316-5990

Gururajarao, Lakshmi, MD {1275540379} Pedtrc(69,INDI)
+ Beth Prime Care
166 Lyons Avenue/Ground Floor   Newark, NJ 07112   (973)926-3535   Fax (973)926-6187

Physicians by Name and Address

Guruswamy, Parvathi, MD {1477612737} Pedtrc, IntrMd(DMN01)
+ Milestones Pediatric Group PA
11 East Oak Street   Oakland, NJ 07436   (201)485-7557   Fax (201)485-7556

Gurwin, Eric B., MD {1275535312} Ophthl(80,NY09)<NJ-OVERLOOK, NJ-MORRISTN>
+ Summit Medical Group-Berkeley Heights Campus
1 Diamond Hill Road   Berkeley Heights, NJ 07922   (908)273-4300   Fax (908)790-6524

Gushue, George F., Jr., DO {1093761678} PulDis, IntrMd(76,IA75)<NJ-CHSMRCER>
+ Allergy and Pulmonary Associates
1542 Kuser Road/Suite B-7   Trenton, NJ 08619   (609)581-1400   Fax (609)585-5234

Guss, Howard N., DO {1831162403} Gastrn, IntrMd(90,NY75)<NJ-JRSYSHMC, NJ-MONMOUTH>
+ Dr. Howard N. Guss & Dr. Gagan D. Beri
3200 Sunset Avenue/Suite 208   Ocean, NJ 07712   (732)775-9000   Fax (732)775-6660

Guss, Stephen B., MD {1386642395} CdvDis, IntrMd(68,MA01)<NJ-MORRISTN>
+ Morristown Cardiology Associates, P.A.
435 South Street/Suite 100   Morristown, NJ 07960   (973)267-3944   Fax (973)455-0399

Gussak, Hiie M., MD {1689641292} Nephro, IntrMd(84,EST01)<NJ-HACKNSK, NJ-HOLYNAME>
+ Nephrology Associates PA
870 Palisade Avenue/Suite 202   Teaneck, NJ 07666   (201)836-0897   Fax (201)836-8042

Gussman, Debra, MD {1770559858} ObsGyn, IntrMd(82,PA01)<NJ-JRSYSHMC>
+ Hackensack Meridian Urogynecolgy Medical Group
19 Davis Avenue/7th Floor   Neptune, NJ 07753   (732)776-3797   Fax (732)776-3796
+ Jersey Shore UMC - Urogynecology
1944 Route 33/Suite 101B   Neptune, NJ 07754   (732)776-3797   Fax (732)776-3796

Guterman, Carl B., MD {1881603959} Ophthl, PedOph(86,NY47)<NJ-HACKNSK, NJ-HOLYNAME>
+ Pediatric Eye Associates of Northern New Jersey
385 Prospect Avenue   Hackensack, NJ 07601   (201)342-5544   Fax (201)342-8488

Guterman, Jonathan Glenn, MD {1720285349} VasNeu(06,GRN01)<NJ-ACMCITY>
+ AtlantiCare Regional Medical Center/City Campus
1925 Pacific Avenue   Atlantic City, NJ 08401   (609)407-2277

Gutfreund, Devra A., MD {1528298742} PedEmg(07,ISR02)<NJ-NWRKBETH>
+ St Joseph's Medical Center Emergency
703 Main Street   Paterson, NJ 07503   (973)754-2240   Fax (973)754-2249

Gutierrez, Alejandra Isabel, MD {1689003998}
+ 10 Landing Lane/Apt 6G
New Brunswick, NJ 08901   (617)963-4863

Gutierrez, Alvaro M., MD {1174615769} Psychy(74,NICA)<NJ-STMRYPAS>
+ 223 Bloomfield Street
Hoboken, NJ 07030   (201)222-1370   Fax (201)217-8189
+ 520 Westfield Avenue/Suite 204
Elizabeth, NJ 07201   (908)353-0270

Gutierrez, Christine V., MD {1487975306} ObsGyn(07,NJ05)
+ Ob-Gyn Associates of North Jersey
7400 Bergenline Avenue   North Bergen, NJ 07047   (201)869-5488   Fax (201)869-6944

Gutierrez, Juan Alberto, MD {1790750404} Pedtrc, PedCrC(88,CHI02)<NJ-MORRISTN>
+ Morristown Medical Center
100 Madison Avenue/Pedi Crtcl Care   Morristown, NJ 07962   (973)971-7550

Gutierrez, Martin Eduardo, MD {1558562793} IntrMd, MedOnc, Hemato(91,COL05)
+ John Theurer Cancer Center - HUMC
92 Second Street   Hackensack, NJ 07601   (201)996-5863   Fax (551)996-0580
+ Regional Cancer Care Center
7650 River Road/2nd Floor   North Bergen, NJ 07047   (212)464-0008

Gutierrez, Pedro M., MD {1093880239} SrgOrt, Surgry(79,SPA09)
+ 464 North Avenue
Elizabeth, NJ 07208   (908)351-0790   Fax (908)355-5966

Gutierrez Mena, Maria, MD {1154318111} Pedtrc(71,SPA12)<NJ-MEADWLND, NJ-ENGLWOOD>
+ 418 57th Street
West New York, NJ 07093   (201)868-5391   Fax (201)453-1054

Gutin, Faina M., MD {1578666707} AlgyImmn, PedAlg, IntrMd(84,RUS01)<NJ-COOPRUMC>
+ Center for Asthma & Allergy
18 North Third Avenue   Highland Park, NJ 08904   (732)545-0094   Fax (732)545-4087

+ Center for Asthma & Allergy
300 Hudson Street   Hoboken, NJ 07030   (732)545-0094   Fax (201)792-5320
+ Center for Asthma & Allergy
90 Milburn Avenue/Suite 200   Maplewood, NJ 08904   (973)763-5787   Fax (973)763-8568

Gutkin, Michael, MD {1033152244} IntrMd, Nephro(62,PA01)<NJ-STBARNMC>
+ Drs. Gutkin & Peos
349 East Northfield Road/Suite 210   Livingston, NJ 07039   (973)597-1107   Fax (973)597-1407

Gutkin, Michael Scott, MD {1083695258} PhysMd, IntrMd(97,GRN01)<NJ-HCKTSTWN>
+ The Orthopedic Institute of New Jersey
108 Bilby Road/Suite 201   Hackettstown, NJ 07840   (908)684-3005   Fax (908)684-3301
+ The Orthopedic Institute of New Jersey
380 Lafayette Road/Route 15   Sparta, NJ 07871   (908)684-3005   Fax (908)684-3301
+ The Orthopedic Institute of New Jersey
254-B Mountain Avenue/Suite 201   Hackettstown, NJ 07840   (908)684-3005   Fax (908)684-3301

Gutman, Gabriella, MD {1902005721} PhysMd, IntrMd(GRN01)
+ Reconstructive Orthopedics, P.A.
401 Young Avenue/Suite 245   Moorestown, NJ 08057   (609)267-9400   Fax (609)267-9457

Gutman, Julius A., MD {1174525976} CdvDis, IntrMd(72,MA07)
+ Summit Medical Group Cardiology
62 South Fullerton Avenue   Montclair, NJ 07042   (973)746-8585   Fax (973)746-0088
+ Essex Heart Group LLC
1310 Broad Street   Bloomfield, NJ 07003   (973)746-8585   Fax (973)338-1140

Gutowski, Christina, MD {1902196272} SrgOrt
+ Cooper University Medical Center/Camden
3 Cooper Plaza   Camden, NJ 08103   (856)361-1754

Gutowski, Ted, MD {1669476073} CdvDis, IntrMd, IntCrd(83,NY01)<NJ-CENTRAST>
+ Heart Specialists/Central Jersey
901 West Main Street/Suite 205   Freehold, NJ 07728   (732)866-8000   Fax (732)463-6082
+ Heart Specialists/Central Jersey
901 West Main Street/Suite 205   Freehold, NJ 07728   (732)866-8000   Fax (732)463-6082

Gutowski, Walter Thomas, III, MD {1205855061} SrgOrt, OrtHKn, Ortped(80,NY20)<NJ-UNVMCPRN, NJ-VANJHCS>
+ Princeton Orthopaedic Associates, P.A.
325 Princeton Avenue   Princeton, NJ 08540   (609)924-8131   Fax (609)924-8532
+ Princeton Orthopaedic Associates, P.A.
11 Centre Drive   Jamesburg, NJ 08831   (609)655-4848

Gutterman, Lily Z., MD {1689752925} Psychy(84,CHN57)<NJ-UNIVBHC>
+ University Behavioral Health Care
671 Hoes Lane/PO Box 1392   Piscataway, NJ 08855   (732)235-5500

Gutwein, Marina Ayzenberg, MD {1831170414} RadDia(00,NY46)<NJ-ENGLWOOD>
+ Englewood Radiologic Group PA
350 Engle Street   Englewood, NJ 07631   (201)894-3000   Fax (201)894-5244
+ Englewood Hospital and Medical Center
350 Engle Street   Englewood, NJ 07631   (201)894-3000
+ Advanced Medical Imaging of North Jersey
452 Old Hook Road/Suite 301   Emerson, NJ 07631   (201)262-0001   Fax (201)262-2330

Guy, Stephen Reed, MD {1417934977} SrgTpl, Surgry, SrgVas(85,MA05)
+ Our Lady Lourdes Transplant Ctr
1601 Haddon Avenue   Camden, NJ 08103   (856)757-3840

Guy Rodriguez, Eva Porter, MD {1770742827} RadDia
+ Hackensack Radiology Group, P.A.
30 Prospect Avenue   Hackensack, NJ 07601   (201)996-2200   Fax (201)336-8451

Guyotte, Jason Arnold, MD {1306024427}
+ 89 Washington Street/Apt A
Morristown, NJ 07960   (478)918-3592
jguyotte@gmail.com

Guyton, Margaret Louise, MD {1750381802} FamMed, OthrSp(95,NJ06)<NJ-SOMERSET>
+ Somerset Family Practice
110 Rehill Avenue   Somerville, NJ 08876   (908)685-2900   Fax (908)685-2891

Guzas, Ronald P., DO {1437240363} EmrgMd<NJ-STCLRDEN>
+ St. Clare's Hospital-Denville Campus
25 Pocono Road   Denville, NJ 07834   (973)625-6511

Guzewicz, Richard Michael, MD {1437122181} SrgPlstc, Surgry(83,NJRSYSHMC, NJ-OCEANMC)
+ 2399 Highway 34/Unit A/Suite A 2
Manasquan, NJ 08736   (732)223-5665   Fax (732)528-1983

Guzik, David J., DO {1881687986} FamMed(91,NJ75)
+ Union County HealthCare Associates

689 Inman Avenue   Colonia, NJ 07067   (732)381-4575   Fax (732)381-0070

Guzik, Ryan, DO {1639531064}<NJ-NWTNMEM>
+ Newton Medical Center
175 High Street   Newton, NJ 07860   (973)383-2121

Gwertzman, Alan R., MD {1619052693} Anesth(89,NJ05)<NJ-HOLYNAME>
+ Teaneck Anesthesia Group, P.A.
718 Teaneck Road   Teaneck, NJ 07666   (201)833-7149   Fax (201)833-6576

Gwertzman, Rachel, DO {1740696996} Pedtrc
+ Chemed Family Health Center
1771 Madison Avenue   Lakewood, NJ 08701   (732)364-2144   Fax (732)364-3559

Gwozdz, Paul William, MD {1396786000} FamMed(97,NJ06)
+ Paul William Gwozdz MD LLC
710 Easton Avenue/Suite 1A   Somerset, NJ 08873   (732)545-4100   Fax (732)545-4102

Gyi, Jennifer, DO {1902060619} PainMd, PhysMd(08,NY75)
+ Center for Neurological Surgery UMDNJ
90 Bergen Street/DOC 8100   Newark, NJ 07103   (973)972-4836   Fax (973)972-2333

Ha, Victor Vinh, MD {1437385085} SrgTrm
+ Liberty Surgical Associates
355 Grand Street   Jersey City, NJ 07302   (201)915-2450   Fax (201)915-2192

Haacker, David S., MD {1902879000} IntrMd(85,NJ05)<NJ-MTNSIDE>
+ Abbas Shehadeh Cardiology & Internal Medicine
443 Northfield Avenue/Suite 301   West Orange, NJ 07052   (973)731-0203   Fax (973)731-0017

Haag, Jerry L., MD {1699717165} FamMed(72,IL42)<NJ-SJRSYELM>
+ 350 West Front Street
Elmer, NJ 08318   (856)358-8113   Fax (856)358-1305

Haas, Kent Steven, MD {1528089018} SrgVas, Surgry, IntrMd(93,NY19)<NJ-UNDRWD>
+ Woodbury Surgical Associates
127 North Broad Street   Woodbury, NJ 08096   (856)845-0500   Fax (856)384-8757

Habba, Saad F., MD {1649476076} Gastrn(78,IREL)
+ 12 Bank Street/Suite 102
Summit, NJ 07901   (908)273-3434   Fax (908)273-3210

Haber, Daran W., MD {1205858404} Anesth, PainMd(86,PRO03)<NJ-RIVERVW>
+ Red Bank Anesthesia, LLC
1 Riverview Plaza   Red Bank, NJ 07701   (732)530-2255   Fax (732)450-2620
+ Riverview Medical Center
1 Riverview Plaza/Anesthesiology   Red Bank, NJ 07701   (732)741-2700

Haber, Monte Arthur, MD {1669567202} PhysMd, SprtMd, PainMd(91,ISR02)
+ North Jersey Spine Group
1680 State Route 23/Suite 250   Wayne, NJ 07470   (973)633-1132
+ North Jersey Spine Group
1 West Ridgewood Avenue/Suite 207   Paramus, NJ 07652   (973)633-1122

Haber-Kuo, Sheryl Ann, MD {1376507806} IntrMd(93,PA09)<NJ-CHSMRCER>
+ 2312 Whitehorse Mercer Rd/Suite 105
Mercerville, NJ 08619   (609)586-9566   Fax (609)586-9055

Haberman, Fredric, DO {1912901695} Dermat, SrgDer(67,MO78)<NJ-HOLYNAME, NY-MNTFMOSE>
+ Haberman Dermatology Institute
50 Market Street   Saddle Brook, NJ 07663   (201)368-0011   Fax (201)368-2380
drfhaberman@gmail.com
+ Haberman Dermatology Institute
75 North Maple Avenue   Ridgewood, NJ 07450   (201)368-0011   Fax (201)445-3662

Haberman, James E., MD {1023019171} Ophthl(83,NY09)
+ Excel Eye Care and Laser Surgery Center
2401 Morris Avenue   Union, NJ 07083   (908)688-4000   Fax (908)688-1717

Habib, Fatimah, MD {1497135123} Anesth
+ Cooper Anesthesia Associates
One Cooper Plaza/Suite 294-B   Camden, NJ 08103   (856)342-2425   Fax (856)968-8239

Habib, Habib, MD {1831471093}<NJ-STJOSHOS>
+ St. Joseph's Regional Medical Center
703 Main Street   Paterson, NJ 07503   (973)745-2000

Habib, Michael George, MD {1376678276} IntrMd, CdvDis(79,EGY04)<NY-STATNRTH>
+ Drs. Abdelmalek and Habib
E5 Brier Hill Court   East Brunswick, NJ 08816   (732)698-1331   Fax (732)698-1379

Habib, Mirette G., MD {1700121365} IntrMd
+ St. Michael's Medical Center
111 Central Avenue   Newark, NJ 07102   (732)266-5161

Habib, Misha, MD {1477866549} IntrMd
+ Pathlink, LLC
  66 West Gilbert Street/Suite 100   Tinton Falls, NJ 07701
  (732)212-0060   Fax (732)212-0061

Habib, Nader Nagy, MD {1598977753}
+ 626 Lukas Boulevard
  Morganville, NJ 07751   (203)535-9060
  nhabib1@yahoo.com

Habib, Tehmina, MD {1487068409} IntrMd
+ Capital Health System/Hopewell
  One Capital Way   Pennington, NJ 08534   (734)620-0514

Habib, Thomas G., MD {1184822389} Pedtrc
+ Pediatrix Medical Group
  255 Third Avenue   Long Branch, NJ 07740   (732)222-7006

Habiel, Miriam, MD {1285991737} Glacma
+ University Ophthalmology Associates
  90 Bergen Street/DOC 6100   Newark, NJ 07101   (973)972-2020

Habida, Ladislav, MD {1508947037} Anesth, PainMd, Anes-Pain(82,CZE07)
+ North Jersey Pain Management Center
  39 Newton-Sparta Road   Newton, NJ 07860   (973)383-0173   Fax (201)567-1432
+ Clifton Surgery Center
  1117 Route 46 East/Suite 303   Clifton, NJ 07013   (973)779-7210

Habj Bik, Ynal, MD {1952353427}
+ 503 Lafayette Avenue/2nd Fl
  Hawthorne, NJ 07506   (580)229-0079
  ynalbik@hotmail.com

Hackett, Gladston Randall, MD {1801182845} EmrgMd<NJ-RWJUBRUN>
+ RWJ University Hospital New Brunswick
  One Robert Wood Johnson Place   New Brunswick, NJ 08901
  (732)235-3381   Fax (732)235-3384

Hackett, Thomas Everett, DO {1619069424} GynOnc, ObsGyn(83,NJ75)<NJ-MONMOUTH, NJ-OCEANMC>
+ Atlantic Gynecologic Oncology
  3349 State Route 138   Wall, NJ 07719   (732)280-5464
  Fax (732)280-5443

Hackford, Robert R., MD {1790786689} PedDvl(72,NY20)
+ 211 South Main Street
  Cape May Court House, NJ 08210   (609)463-1577

Hadaya, Ola, MD {1861981664} ObsGyn
+ University Medical Group/OBGYN
  125 Paterson Street/2nd Floor   New Brunswick, NJ 08901
  (732)235-6375   Fax (732)235-6627

Hadaya, Ziad, MD {1841312055} IntrMd(80,SYR01)<NJ-RWJUHAM, NJ-CHSFULD>
+ Hamilton Medical Center
  994 Whitehorse Avenue   Hamilton, NJ 08610   (609)585-4100

Haddad, Ahmad J., MD {1982686457} FamMed(82,ITAL)<NJ-RIVERVW>
+ Chapel Hill Family Medicine
  100 Village Court/Suite 302   Hazlet, NJ 07730   (732)758-0048   Fax (732)758-0052

Haddad, Bassam M., MD {1790784510} Nephro, IntrMd(72,SYR01)<NJ-BAYONNE, NJ-CHRIST>
+ Drs. Ahmed, Haddad & Batwara
  26 Greenville Avenue   Jersey City, NJ 07305   (201)333-8222   Fax (201)333-0095
+ Bayonne Medical Center
  29th Street at Avenue E/Nephrology   Bayonne, NJ 07002
  (201)858-5000
+ Christ Hospital
  176 Palisade Avenue/Nephrology   Jersey City, NJ 07305
  (201)795-8200

Haddad, Charles George, MD {1750329538} ObsGyn(93,SYR01)<NJ-STJOSHOS, NJ-STMRYPAS>
+ Clifton Ob/Gyn
  1033 Route 46 East/Suite 102   Clifton, NJ 07013   (973)779-7979   Fax (973)779-7970

Haddad, Danny B., MD {1235351297} Nephro, IntrMd(07,PA02)<NJ-BAYONNE, NJ-CHRIST>
+ Drs. Ahmed, Haddad & Batwara
  26 Greenville Avenue   Jersey City, NJ 07305   (201)333-8222   Fax (201)333-0095
+ Bayonne Medical Center
  29th Street at Avenue E/Nephrology   Bayonne, NJ 07002
  (201)858-5000
+ Christ Hospital
  176 Palisade Avenue/Nephrology   Jersey City, NJ 07305
  (201)795-8200

Haddad, Ghada, MD {1689632440} EnDbMt, IntrMd(87,LEBA)<NJ-COOPRUMC>
+ Cooper Endocrinology Associates
  1210 Brace Road/Suite 107   Cherry Hill, NJ 08034
  (856)795-3597   Fax (856)795-7590
+ Cooper University Medical Center/Camden
  3 Cooper Plaza   Camden, NJ 08103   (856)342-2439
+ The Cooper Hospital System-Univ Hospital
  3 Cooper Plaza/Suite 215   Camden, NJ 08034   (856)342-2439

Haddad, Joanne T., MD {1285844175} IntrMd, EmrgMd(82,MEX14)
+ 8 Clarissa Drive
  Middletown, NJ 07748   (732)706-0495   Fax (732)706-5115

Haddad, Richard Hani, MD {1750382800} IntrMd(99,MNT01)
+ Allegra Arthritis Associates
  282 Broad Street   Red Bank, NJ 07701   (732)842-3600
  Fax (732)842-3665

Haddad, Sohail G., MD {1417143678} IntrMd, InfDis(94,SYR01)
+ Hunterdon Infection Disease
  1100 Wescott Drive/Suite 306   Flemington, NJ 08822
  (908)788-6474   Fax (908)788-6616

Haddad, Stephanie I., MD {1275875437} EmrgMd
+ 10 Julia Way
  Dayton, NJ 08810   (732)735-8475

Hade, Jason R., MD {1497929509} Ophthl(04,NJ05)
+ Hade Eye Care, LLC
  1 Indian Road/Suite 9   Denville, NJ 07834   (973)586-2188
  Fax (973)586-2218

Hadeed, Jodi Louisa, MD {1649711433}
+ 743 Passaic Avenue/Apt 128
  Clifton, NJ 07012   (347)421-1033

Haders, Allison Lula, MD {1255595583} EmrgMd(05,NJ06)<NJ-TRINIWSC>
+ Trinitas Regional Medical Center-Williamson Street
  225 Williamson Street/EmrgMed   Elizabeth, NJ 07207
  (908)994-5000   Fax (919)425-0478

Hadi, Ahmed Suhail, MD {1831490614} Dermat(10,NY19)
+ Westwood Dermatology
  390 Old Hook Road   Westwood, NJ 07675   (201)666-9550
  Fax (201)666-1251
+ Dr. Ahmed S. Hadi
  85 Harristown Road/Suite 101   Glen Rock, NJ 07452
  (201)666-9550   Fax (201)621-0854
+ Sovereign Medical Group
  85 Harristown Road/Suite 104   Glen Rock, NJ 07675
  (201)855-8300   Fax (201)857-2541

Hadjistavrinos, Kriss, MD {1205059672} ObsGyn(67,GREE)
+ Metropolitan Medical Associates
  40 Engle Street   Englewood, NJ 07631   (201)567-0522
  Fax (201)567-5955

Haenel, Louis C., III, DO {1871549436} IntrMd, EnDbMt(70,PA77)<NJ-KMHSTRAT, NJ-KMHCHRRY>
+ Stratford - Endocrinology
  25 East Laurel Road   Stratford, NJ 08084   Fax (856)783-8537
+ Haenel-Haenel
  25 East Laurel Road   Stratford, NJ 08084   (856)783-2244
+ Kennedy Health Alliance Vascular Surgery
  333 Laurel Oak Road   Voorhees, NJ 08084   (844)542-2273
  Fax (856)783-8537

Hafez, Nagwa I., MD {1487853875} IntrMd, Grtrcs
+ 246 Hamburg Turnpike/Suite 208
  Wayne, NJ 07470   (973)790-3433   Fax (973)790-0433

Haffty, Bruce George, MD {1033108782} RadOnc, RadThp(84,CT01)<NJ-RWJUBRUN>
+ Rutgers Cancer Institute of New Jersey
  195 Little Albany Street/PO Box 2681   New Brunswick, NJ 08903   (732)235-2465   Fax (732)235-6797

Hafiz, Mohammad A., MD {1306896964} Pthlgy, PthACl(71,INDI)<NJ-COMMED>
+ Community Medical Center
  99 Route 37 West   Toms River, NJ 08755   (732)557-8000

Haflin, Mary Ann, MD {1982652731} FamMed(71,PA07)<NJ-BURDTMLN>
+ North Wildwood Medical
  1200 New Jersey Avenue   North Wildwood, NJ 08260
  (609)522-3131   Fax (609)522-9024

Hagans, Iris, MD {1669888129} IntrMd
+ Cooper University Medical Center/Camden
  3 Cooper Plaza   Camden, NJ 08103   (856)342-2000

Hage, Charles W., MD {1053593954} ObsGyn(85,RI01)<NJ-JRSYSHMC>
+ 250 Monmouth Road
  Oakhurst, NJ 07755   (732)517-8887

Hageboutros, Alexandre, MD {1598874042} OncHem, MedOnc, IntrMd(87,LEBA)<NJ-COOPRUMC>
+ Cooper University Medical Center/Camden
  3 Cooper Plaza/Suite 211   Camden, NJ 08103   (856)342-2000
+ The Cooper Health System at Voorhees
  900 Centennial Boulevard/Suite M   Voorhees, NJ 08043
  (856)325-6750
+ 1000 Salem Road/Suite C
  Willingboro, NJ 08103

Hager, George W., III, MD {1730181660} Surgry(72,PA02)
+ Regional Surgical Associates
  502 Centennial Boulevard/Suite 7   Voorhees, NJ 08043
  (856)596-7440   Fax (856)751-3320

Hager, Jeffrey C., DO {1992706030} SrgVas, Surgry(87,PA77)<NJ-DEBRAHLC>
+ Surgical Specialists of New Jersey
  37 Nautilus Drive   Manahawkin, NJ 08050   (609)978-0778
  Fax (609)978-1377

Hages, Harry A., MD {1477667301} Pedtrc(66,PA12)
+ Old Tappan Medical Group PA
  215 Old Tappan Road   Old Tappan, NJ 07675   (201)666-1000   Fax (201)666-4108
+ Old Tappan Pediatrics
  136 North Washington Avenue   Bergenfield, NJ 07621
  (201)666-1000   Fax (201)385-4748

Haggerty, Mary A., MD {1770551988} Grtrcs, IntrMd(79,NJ05)<NJ-NWRKBETH, NJ-UMDNJ>
+ University Hospital
  150 Bergen Street/H-245   Newark, NJ 07103   (973)972-4300

Haghdoost, Mohammad, MD {1710291570} GenPrc<NJ-STBARNMC>
+ St. Barnabas Medical Center
  94 Old Short Hills Road   Livingston, NJ 07039   (973)322-5000

Haghighi, Kayvon, MD {1306912720} SrgO&M, Surgry(99,NJ05)<NJ-JRSYSHMC>
+ 276 Broad Street
  Red Bank, NJ 07701   (732)530-1110

Haghour Vwich, Marina, MD {1063612059}
+ 29 Bow Fell Court
  Wayne, NJ 07470

Haghverdi, Mojdeh, MD {1730815612} IntrMd(91,GRNA)
+ Physicians Health Alliance
  1777 Hamburg Turnpike/Suite 205   Wayne, NJ 07470
  (973)248-1440   Fax (973)248-1448

Hagino, Owen Rinzo, MD {1225262793} PsyCAd, Psychy, Pedtrc(88,HI01)
+ Sanofi US-Sanofi-Aventis
  55 Corporate Drive   Bridgewater, NJ 08807

Hagler, Rhonda A., MD {1487666202} IntrMd(85,NJ05)<NJ-STMRYPAS>
+ Park Avenue Medical Associates
  30 Park Avenue/Suite 202   Lyndhurst, NJ 07071   (201)438-5900   Fax (201)438-5980

Hagopian, Ellen Joyce, MD {1982628327} Surgry, IntrMd(92,PA02)<NJ-JRSYSHMC>
+ New Jersey HPB Surgery, LLC.
  142 Route 35/Suite 105   Eatontown, NJ 07724   (732)380-9200   Fax (732)380-9202
  ellenhagopian@aol.com
+ Jersey Shore University Medical Center
  1945 Route 33/Surgery   Neptune, NJ 07753   (732)380-9200   Fax (732)776-3763

Hagopian, Vahe H., MD {1982665683} Anesth(87,DMN01)
+ North Jersey Pain Management Center
  39 Newton-Sparta Road   Newton, NJ 07860   (973)383-0173   Fax (201)567-1432

Hahn, Edward, Jr., MD {1356669162} SrgRec
+ Vanguard Wellness Center
  113 West Essex Street/Suite 204   Maywood, NJ 07607
  (201)289-5551   Fax (201)843-2390

Hahn, John C., MD {1538272091} Gastrn, IntrMd(85,NJ05)<NJ-BAYONNE>
+ 534 Avenue E/Suite 1-C
  Bayonne, NJ 07002   (201)823-0450   Fax (201)823-3311
+ Hudson Pain Management Center
  183 Avenue B   Bayonne, NJ 07002   (201)823-0450   Fax
  (201)339-7250

Hahn, Paul, MD {1043360704} Ophthl(06,PA01)
+ Retina Associates of New Jersey, P.A.
  628 Cedar Lane   Teaneck, NJ 07666   (201)837-7300   Fax
  (201)836-6426
+ Retina Associates of New Jersey, P.A.
  182 South Street/Suite 5   Morristown, NJ 07960   Fax
  (973)605-5807
+ Retina Associates of New Jersey, P.A.
  1044 Route 23 North/Suite 207   Wayne, NJ 07666
  (973)633-9898   Fax (973)633-3892

Hahn, Robert Douglas, MD {1881786523} Ophthl(69,NY08)<NY-METHODST>
+ 10 Bridge Street/Box 518
  Milford, NJ 08848   (908)995-9555   Fax (908)995-4500

Hahn, Robert Francis, DO {1811941115} PhysMd(02,NJ75)<NJ-KMHTURNV, NJ-KMHSTRAT>
+ Bacharach Institute for Rehabilitation
  61 West Jimmie Leeds Road   Pomona, NJ 08240   (609)748-5380   Fax (609)652-8749

Hai, Nabila, MD {1902120066} Radiol(10,DC01)
+ Radiology Associates of Ridgewood, P.A.
  20 Franklin Turnpike   Waldwick, NJ 07463   (201)445-8822
  Fax (201)447-5053

213

Physicians by Name and Address

Haider, Nadeem Z., MD {1508801390} Nephro, IntrMd(95,GRN01)<NJ-OCEANMC, NJ-COMMED>
+ Ocean Renal Associates, P.A.
210 Jack Martin Boulevard/Suite D-1   Brick, NJ 08724   (732)458-5854   Fax (732)458-8012
+ Ocean Renal Associates, P.A.
508 Lakehurst Road/Suite 3 A   Toms River, NJ 08755   (732)458-5854   Fax (732)341-4993
+ Ocean Renal Associates, P.A.
1301 Route 72 West/Suite 206   Manahawkin, NJ 08724   (609)978-9940   Fax (609)978-9902

Haig, Joseph Michael, MD {1063677029} EmrgMd<NJ-TRINIWSC>
+ Trinitas Regional Medical Center-Williamson Street
225 Williamson Street/EmergMed   Elizabeth, NJ 07207   (908)994-5000   Fax (908)351-7930

Haig, Lauren Grace, MD {1124277421} Anesth
+ Hamilton Anesthesia Associates
2119 Highway 33/Suite B   Trenton, NJ 08690   (609)581-5303   Fax (609)631-6839

Haik, Bruce Joseph, MD {1023018520} CdvDis, IntCrd(82,GRN01)<NJ-STBARNMC, NJ-CLARMAAS>
+ New Jersey Cardiology Associates
375 Mount Pleasant Avenue   West Orange, NJ 07052   (973)731-9442   Fax (973)731-8050

Haim, Alain, MD {1245207646} RadDia, Radiol(71,BOL01)<NJ-VAEASTOR>
+ Advanced Open MRI and Diagnostic Imaging
751 Highway 37 West   Toms River, NJ 08755   (732)240-7756   Fax (732)240-7761
+ Roseland Medical Imaging
107 Cedar Grove Lane/Suite 108   Somerset, NJ 08873   (732)560-7172

Haim, Sara Rose, MD {1508010885} Psychy, NroChl(04,ISR05)
+ 2 Driftway
Dunellen, NJ 08812

Haimowitz, Ira L., DO {1538191697} Pedtrc(85,NY75)<NJ-COMMED, NJ-OCEANMC>
+ Pediatric Affiliates, PA
40 Bey Lea Road/Suite B203   Toms River, NJ 08753   (732)341-0720   Fax (732)244-6842
+ Pediatric Affiliates, PA
1616 Route 72 West/Suite 8   Manahawkin, NJ 08050   (732)341-0720   Fax (609)978-1229
+ Pediatric Affiliates, PA
218 Jack Martin Boulevard/Building E-1   Brick, NJ 08753   (732)458-0010   Fax (732)458-9329

Hain, Joshua Meir, MD {1578709317} Psychy
+ 526 Rutland Avenue
Teaneck, NJ 07666

Hainer, Meg M., MD {1942389028} ObsGyn<NJ-VALLEY>
+ Bergen-Passaic Women's Health
258 Godwin Avenue   Wyckoff, NJ 07481   (201)891-3336   Fax (201)891-5535
+ Bergen-Passaic Women's Health
2024 Macopin Road/Suite D   West Milford, NJ 07480   (201)891-3336   Fax (973)728-7707

Haines, Elizabeth Jane, DO {1073783486} PedEmg, EmrgMd(05,NY75)<NJ-MTNSIDE>
+ Hackensack UMC Mountainside
1 Bay Avenue/EmrgMed   Montclair, NJ 07042   (973)429-6200   Fax (973)680-7847
ejhaines@gmail.com

Haines, Kathleen Ann, MD {1912952417} PedRhm, AlgyImmn, Pedtrc(75,NY46)<NJ-HACKNSK, NY-JTORTHO>
+ Hackensack University Medical Center
30 Prospect Avenue/WFAN/RM PC360   Hackensack, NJ 07601   (551)996-5306   Fax (201)996-9815

Hait, William N., MD {1982788832} IntrMd, MedOnc(78,PA07)
+ Rutgers Cancer Institute of New Jersey
195 Little Albany Street/PO Box 2681   New Brunswick, NJ 08903   (732)235-2465   Fax (732)235-6797

Haj-Ibrahim, Mouna, MD {1205873643} Pedtrc(88,SYR01)<NJ-STJOSHOS>
+ St. Joseph's Regional Medical Center
703 Main Street/Ped/Xavier 701   Paterson, NJ 07503   (973)754-2000

Hajal, Hussam, MD {1558450775} IntrMd, Nephro(81,SYR02)<NJ-MEADWLND, NJ-HOBUNIMC>
+ Hudson Essex Nephrology
510 31st Street   Union City, NJ 07087   (201)866-3322   Fax (201)866-2289

Hajee, Feryal, MD {1841438447} Allrgy
+ 617 79th Street
North Bergen, NJ 07047   (201)854-8119   Fax (201)854-4875

Hajee, Mohammedyusuf Ebrahimadham, MD {1316085566} Ophthl
+ Ocean County Retina, P.C.
780 Route 37 West/Suite 200   Toms River, NJ 08755   (732)797-1855   Fax (732)797-1856

Hajela, Amitabh, MD {1548329840} Nephro, IntrMd(99,GRN01)<NJ-MORRISTN>
+ Infectious Disease Center of New Jersey
653 Willow Grove Street/Suite 2700   Hackettstown, NJ 07840   (973)535-8355   Fax (973)535-8353

Hajela, Durgesh, MD {1619957867} RadOnc, RadThp(68,INDI)<NJ-STCLRDEN>
+ St. Clare's Cancer Center
23 Pocono Road   Denville, NJ 07834   (973)983-7300   Fax (973)983-7301

Hajela, Shailendra, MD {1093786212} PhysMd(87,INA23)
+ Jersey Rehab, P.A.
15 Newark Avenue/Suite 1   Belleville, NJ 07109   (973)844-9220   Fax (973)844-9221

Hajjar, Bassam, MD {1316024946} IntrMd(90,SYR01)
+ Carepoint Gastroenterology Center
1300 Main Avenue/Suite 1-B   Clifton, NJ 07011   (973)595-6444   Fax (973)782-4819

Hajjar, John H., MD {1104894435} Urolgy(81,DC02)<NJ-HACKNSK, NJ-VALLEY>
+ SurgiCare Surgical Associates, P.A.
15-01 Broadway/Suites 1 & 3   Fair Lawn, NJ 07410   (201)791-4544   Fax (201)791-6585
+ Sovereign Medical Group
15-01 Broadway/Suite 1   Fair Lawn, NJ 07410   (201)791-4544   Fax (201)791-6585
+ Sovereign Medical Group, LLC.
205 Browertown Road/Suite 101   West Paterson, NJ 07410   (973)890-9168   Fax (973)890-9621

Hakim, James, MD {1881856631} EmrgMd(08,NY48)
+ Trinitas Regional Medical Center-Williamson Street
225 Williamson Street/Emerg Med   Elizabeth, NJ 07207   (607)592-3335

Hakim, James J., MD {1457411019} IntrMd(86,NJ06)<NJ-OVERLOOK>
+ New Providence Internal Medical Associates
571 Central Avenue/Suite 112   New Providence, NJ 07974   (908)464-7300   Fax (908)464-7350

Hakimi, Daniel, DO {1033160890} ObsGyn, SrgLap(98,NY75)<NJ-HACKNSK, NJ-HOLYNAME>
+ Ob/Gyn and Infertility Services of Northern NJ
721 Clifton Avenue/Suite 1A   Clifton, NJ 07013   (973)471-0707   Fax (973)471-2112

Hakimzadeh, Parisa, DO {1104826718} Nephro, IntrMd(98,NJ75)
+ Associated Renal & Hypertension Group, P.C.
7 Cedar Grove Lane/Suite 31   Somerset, NJ 08873   (732)873-1400   Fax (732)960-3444

Hal-Ibrahim, Ahmad, MD   IntrMd(87,SYR01)<NY-MARGRTVL, NJ-VIRTMHBC>
+ Florence Medical, PC
691 Delaware Avenue/PO Box 301   Roebling, NJ 08554   (609)499-8100

Halas, Francis P., Jr., MD {1326110446} Pedtrc, FamMAdM(75,IL43)<NJ-MONMOUTH>
+ Doctors Halas & Lutz
2130 Highway 35/Suite 214   Sea Girt, NJ 08750   (732)974-0228   Fax (732)974-7458

Haldar, Pranab K., MD {1437253549} Grtrcs, IntrMd(90,GRNA)<NJ-JFKMED>
+ Adult Treatment Center
512 New Brunswick Avenue   Fords, NJ 08863   (732)738-5401   Fax (732)738-5409
haldarp@exite.com

Hale, James Joseph, MD {1528079654} SrgOrt, SrgSpn(98,NY19)<NJ-HOLYNAME>
+ Eastern Orthopedic Associates
222 Cedar Lane/Suite 120   Teaneck, NJ 07666   (201)836-5332   Fax (201)836-4002

Hale, Paula M., MD {1598901647} PedEnd, Pedtrc(81,WI06)
+ Novo Nordisk Inc.
100 College Road West   Princeton, NJ 08540   (609)987-5925   Fax (609)921-8082

Haleem, Burhan, DO {1467740811} Anesth
+ Rancocas Anesthesiology, PA
15000 Midlantic Drive/Suite 102   Mount Laurel, NJ 08054   (718)352-2959   Fax (856)393-8691
burhan.haleem@gmail.com

Halejian, Barry A., MD {1528152832} OccpMd(82,ITAL)
+ Occupational Medical Associates
17-15 Maple Avenue/Suite 100   Fair Lawn, NJ 07410   (201)794-8055   Fax (201)794-8086
halejian@hotmail.com

Halevy, Jonathan D., MD   Anesth(84,ISR02)<NJ-LOURDMED>
+ Rancocas Anesthesiology, PA
700 Route 130 North/Suite 203   Cinnaminson, NJ 08077   (856)829-9345   Fax (856)829-3605

Haliasos, Helen C., MD {1679591358} Dermat(01,NY06)
+ Memorial Sloan-Kettering Cancer Center Basking Ridge
136 Mountain View Boulevard   Basking Ridge, NJ 07920   (908)542-3000   Fax (908)542-3220
+ Dermatology Associates-Warren
122 Mount Bethel Road   Warren, NJ 07059   (908)542-3000   Fax (908)756-8017

Halibey, Bohdan E., MD {1841277803} MedOnc(77,MEX14)<NJ-NWTNMEM>
+ Premier Health Associates
89 Sparta Avenue/Suite 130   Sparta, NJ 07871   (973)726-0005   Fax (973)726-4668

Halickman, Isaac J., MD {1437323250} IntrMd, CdvDis(02,QU01)
+ 5 Isaac Lane
Cherry Hill, NJ 08002
+ Cooper Cardiology Associates
900 Centennial Boulevard   Voorhees, NJ 08043   Fax (856)325-6702

Haliczer, Abraham T., MD {1982672978} AnesPain(83,NJ06)<NJ-HACKNSK, NJ-MEADWLND>
+ Interventional Pain Management
75 Orient Way/Suite 302   Rutherford, NJ 07070   (201)372-0401   Fax (201)372-0402

Halifman, Dorina, MD {1134390792} Pedtrc(94,LAT03)
+ Glen Rock Pediatrics
385 South Maple Avenue/Suite107A   Glen Rock, NJ 07452   (201)857-3111   Fax (201)857-3110
glenrockpediatrics@gmail.com

Halioua, Solomon, MD {1093864563} AnesPain, IntrMd(95,ISR02)
+ 255 East Main Street
Ramsey, NJ 07446   (201)845-6555   Fax (201)845-5599

Halko, George J., DO {1932178928} Rheuma, IntrMd(85,PA77)<NJ-SHOREMEM>
+ 408 Bethel Road/Unit C-1
Somers Point, NJ 08244   (609)601-1080   Fax (609)601-1077

Hall, Alvin J., MD {1154537140} PthAcl, PthDrm(88,LIB01)
+ Laboratory Corporation of America
69 First Avenue   Raritan, NJ 08869

Hall, Andrew Robert, MD {1336470640} PhyMPain
+ Englewood Orthopedic Associates
401 South Van Brunt Street/3rd Floor   Englewood, NJ 07631   (201)569-2770   Fax (201)808-6786

Hall, Bianca Elena, DO {1104488188} ObsGyn
+ Cooper University Hospital OBGYN
3 Cooper Plaza/Suite 221   Camden, NJ 08103   (856)342-2000   Fax (856)365-1967

Hall, Dahlia Annmarie, MD {1538158928} Pedtrc(97,MA07)<NJ-RIVERVW, NJ-MONMOUTH>
+ Monmouth Family Center
270 Broadway   Long Branch, NJ 07740   (732)923-7100   Fax (732)923-7104
+ Personal Care Pediatrics, LLC
241B Millburn Avenue   Millburn, NJ 07041   (732)923-7100   Fax (973)376-7610

Hall, Dennis B., MD {1104908862} Anesth, PainMd(81,VA04)<NJ-RWJUBRUN>
+ Robert Wood Johnson-UMDNJ Anesthesia Group
125 Paterson Street/CAB 3100   New Brunswick, NJ 08901   (732)235-7827   Fax (732)418-8492

Hall, Jason O., MD {1356313878} CdvDis(85,NJ06)<NJ-MORRISTN, NJ-SOMERSET>
+ Medicor Cardiology PA
225 Jackson Street   Bridgewater, NJ 08807   (908)526-8668   Fax (908)231-6781
+ Medicor Cardiology PA
331 US Highway 206/Suite 1A   Hillsborough, NJ 08844   (908)526-8668   Fax (908)431-0808

Hall, Jeffrey, MD {1285923573} Psychy
+ 101 Eisenhower Parkway/Suite 300
Roseland, NJ 07068   (973)795-1260   Fax (973)795-1259

Hall, Kendria, MD {1174835839} Pedtrc
+ RWJ University Hospital Somerset
110 Rehill Avenue/Pedtrc   Somerville, NJ 08876   (908)203-6247

Hall, Kevin Arthur, MD {1467708271} GenPrc
+ Haskell Towne Medical LLC
1141 Ringwood Avenue/Suite 7   Haskell, NJ 07420   (201)259-0289   Fax (973)215-2052

Hall, Lanniece F., MD {1326091992} ObsGyn(02,PA14)<NJ-UNVM-CPRN>
+ Delaware Valley Ob/Gyn & Infertility Group, PC
2 Princess Road/Suite C   Lawrenceville, NJ 08648   (609)896-0777   Fax (609)896-3266

Hall, Matthew Scott, MD {1356509319} Urolgy(08,NJ05)
+ Skylands Urology Group
  89 Sparta Avenue/Suite 200   Sparta, NJ 07871   (973)726-7220   Fax (973)726-7230
+ New Jersey Urology, LLC
  700 North Broad Street/Suite 302   Elizabeth, NJ 07208   (973)726-7220   Fax (908)289-0716

Hall, Patrick J., MD {1194725143} Otlryg, Otolgy(86,NJ05)
+ Advanced ENT - Cherry Hill
  1910 Route 70 East/Suite 3   Cherry Hill, NJ 08003   (856)602-4000   Fax (856)424-4695
+ Advanced ENT - Woodbury
  620 North Broad Street   Woodbury, NJ 08096   (856)602-4000   Fax (856)848-6029
+ Advanced ENT - Washington Township
  239 Hurffville Crosskeys Road   Sewell, NJ 08003   (856)602-4000   Fax (856)629-3391

Hall, Philip Isaac, DO {1790166197} EmrgMd
+ Kennedy Hlth Syst/Cherry Hill Emergency
  2201 Chapel Avenue West   Cherry Hill, NJ 08002   (856)488-6816

Hall, Stephen C., MD {1639237241} SrgPlstc, SrgRec(80,ITAL)<NJ-HOBUNIMC, NJ-CHRIST>
+ Hall-DiGioia Center for Breast Care
  33 Overlook Road/Suite 205   Summit, NJ 07901   (908)522-3200   Fax (908)522-1222

Hallenbeck, John P., DO {1033152277} EmrgMd(96,ME75)<NJ-HACKNSK>
+ Hackensack Medical Center Emergency Medicine
  30 Prospect Avenue/Main 3619   Hackensack, NJ 07601   (201)996-4614   Fax (201)968-1866

Haller, Kate, MD {1962474213} PsyNro, IntrMd(78,MA07)<NJ-MORRISTN, NJ-OVERLOOK>
+ Hackensack UMC Mountainside
  1 Bay Avenue/DDC-3N   Montclair, NJ 07042   (973)429-6272   Fax (973)680-7806
+ Developmental Disability Center
  350 Boulevard/4th Floor/Reid Building   Passaic, NJ 07055   (973)429-6272   Fax (973)916-5272
+ Overlook Hospital-Dvpmt Disabilities
  1000 Galloping Hill Road   Union, NJ 07042   (973)971-5595   Fax (908)686-8374

Hallit, Janice A., DO {1720199730} FamMed(87,MO78)
+ Center for Family Health, LLC.
  431 Route 22 East/Suite 79   Whitehouse Station, NJ 08889   (908)534-5559   Fax (888)256-4023

Hallit, Rabih Riad, MD {1114217296} IntrMd
+ St. Michael's Medical Center
  111 Central Avenue/MedEdu   Newark, NJ 07102   (973)877-5000

Halper-Erkkila, Ruby A., MD {1699722330} FamMed(85,PA13)
+ 48 Robbins Road
  Somerville, NJ 08876   (908)526-8300   Fax (908)685-1925

Halperin, John Jacob, MD {1124010079} Nrolgy, ClNrPh, IntrMd(75,MA01)<NJ-OVERLOOK, NY-NSUHMANH>
+ Overlook Medical Center
  99 Beauvoir Avenue/PO Box 210   Summit, NJ 07902   (908)522-2829
  John.Halperin@atlantichealth.org

Halperin, William Edward, MD {1467706119} PubHth, GenPrc(73,MA01)<NJ-UMDNJ>
+ Preventive Medicine & Community Health
  185 South Orange Avenue/MSB F-506   Newark, NJ 07101   (973)972-4422   Fax (973)972-7625
+ University Hospital
  150 Bergen Street/PrevMed   Newark, NJ 07103   (973)972-4300

Halpern, Analisa Vincent, MD {1619029527} Dermat
+ Heymann, Manders & Green LLC
  100 Brick Road/Suite 306   Marlton, NJ 08053   (856)596-0111   Fax (856)596-7194
  analisa_halpern@yahoo.com

Halpern, Steven L., MD {1396791117} PedHem, Pedtrc, IntrMd(76,IL42)<NJ-MORRISTN>
+ Morristown Medical Center
  100 Madison Avenue/Pedi Hem Onc   Morristown, NJ 07962   (973)971-6720   Fax (973)971-6720

Halvorsen, Julie Beth, DO {1356395594} Pedtrc(99,PA77)<NJ-CHSMRCER, NJ-RWJUHAM>
+ Delaware Valley Pediatric Associates PA
  132 Franklin Corner Road   Lawrenceville, NJ 08648   (609)896-4141   Fax (609)896-3940

Ham, Antoinette Lucy, MD {1245343821} ObsGyn(01,NJ06)
+ Robert Wood Johnson Ob-Gyn Associates
  3270 State Route 27/Suite 2200   Kendall Park, NJ 08824   (732)422-8989   Fax (732)422-4526
+ Robert Wood Johnson Ob-Gyn Associates
  50 Franklin Lane/Suite 203   Manalapan, NJ 07726   (732)422-8989   Fax (732)536-7118
+ Robert Wood Johnson Ob-Gyn Associates
  525 Route 70/Suite B-11   Lakewood, NJ 08824   (732)905-6466   Fax (732)905-6467

Hamada, Aboulnasr H., MD {1710905773}
+ 27 Morning Glory Circle
  Mullica Hill, NJ 08062

Hamada, Murray S., MD {1821107608} IntrMd, EmrgMd, CdvDis(80,SPAI)<NJ-HOLYNAME>
+ Emergimed
  663 Palisade Avenue/Suite 101   Cliffside Park, NJ 07010   (201)945-6500   Fax (201)945-1157

Hamal, Rekha, MD {1225227176} FamMed(83,INDI)<NJ-MORRISTN>
+ NHCAC Health Center at West New York
  5301 Broadway   West New York, NJ 07093   (201)866-9320   Fax (201)330-3803

Hamaoui, Manuela Belda, MD {1457798829} IntrMd
+ Medical Center Partners
  108 Bilby Road/Suite 104   Hackettstown, NJ 07840   (908)441-1352

Hamaty, Edward G., Jr., DO {1932122819} PulDis, IntrMd(82,MO79)<NJ-OURLADY, NJ-KMHCHRRY>
+ Exel-Med Inc.
  100 Springdale Road/Suite A3   Cherry Hill, NJ 08003   (856)651-1400   Fax (856)651-1401

Hamaty, John N., DO {1306838164} CdvDis, IntrMd(88,PA77)
+ Associated Cardiovascular Consultants-Lourdes
  1 Brace Road/Suite C & F   Cherry Hill, NJ 08034   (856)428-4100   Fax (856)428-5748
+ South Jersey Heart Group
  400 Creek Crossing Boulevard/Suite 404   Hainesport, NJ 08036   (856)428-4100   Fax (609)261-5072

Hamawy, Adam Hisham, MD {1205015617} SrgPlstc, Surgry, IntrMd(96,NJ05)<CT-GRENWCH>
+ Princeton Plastic Surgeons PC
  106 Stanhope Street   Princeton, NJ 08540   (609)301-0760   Fax (888)415-3270
  plasticsurgeon@live.com
+ Princeton Plastic Surgeons PC
  155 Willowbrook Boulevard/Suite 340   Wayne, NJ 07470   (973)380-0690

Hamed, Kamal Abdel-Jabbar, MD {1679747844} IntrMd, InfDis(85,LEB03)
+ Novartis Pharmaceuticals Corporation
  One Health Plaza/InfDis   East Hanover, NJ 07936   (862)778-8081   Fax (973)781-6504

Hameed, Fauzia, MD {1750479705} IntrMd(92,PAKI)
+ Raritan Valley Medical Care, LLC.
  616 Amboy Avenue   Woodbridge, NJ 07095   (732)636-1010   Fax (732)636-1018

Hameed, Nida, MD {1881866218} InfDis<NJ-MONMOUTH>
+ Monmouth Medical Center
  300 Second Avenue   Long Branch, NJ 07740   (732)222-5200

Hameed, Samar, MD {1861640518} IntrMd, Grtrcs(06,PAK11)<NJ-STPETER>
+ Internal Medicine Faculty Practice
  101 Old Short Hills Road/Suite 106   West Orange, NJ 07052   (973)322-6256   Fax (973)322-6241

Hameer, Muneer, MD {1376943183} EmrgMd
+ Jersey City Medical Center Emergency
  355 Grand Street   Jersey City, NJ 07302   (201)915-2218   Fax (201)915-2157

Hamel, Marianne, MD {1447468616} PthACI, PthFor(04,PA02)
+ 1 Convention Boulevard/Suite 2 #361
  Atlantic City, NJ 08401   (609)225-4865

Hamer, Orlee, DO {1922390574} PhysMd
+ Physical Medicine & Rehabilitation Center
  500 Grand Avenue/1st Floor   Englewood, NJ 07631   (917)439-9499   Fax (201)567-7506

Hametz, Irwin, MD {1992720999} Dermat(73,NY09)<NJ-CENTRAST>
+ Drs. Hametz & Picascia
  77-55 Schanck Road/Suite B-3   Freehold, NJ 07728   (732)462-9800
  hpderm@optonline.net

Hamilton, Audrey May, MD {1073593224} MedOnc, Hemato(83,MA01)
+ Memorial Sloan-Kettering Cancer Center Basking Ridge
  136 Mountain View Boulevard   Basking Ridge, NJ 07920   (908)542-3300   Fax (908)542-3222

Hamilton, Cliff Scott, MD {1487991105}<NJ-OVERLOOK>
+ Summit Medical Group
  465 Union Avenue/Suite B   Bridgewater, NJ 08807   (908)219-6767   Fax (908)864-4819

Hamilton, Kathryn Diane, MD {1447224688} FamMed(99,PA12)<NJ-HUNTRDN>
+ Hunterdon Family Medicine
  250 Route 28/Suite 100   Bridgewater, NJ 08807   (908)237-4135   Fax (908)237-4136

Hamilton, Monique S., MD {1366909356} IntrMd(05,PA13)<NY-STBARNAB>
+ Leonia Medical Associates, P.A.
  25 Rockwood Place/Suite 120   Englewood, NJ 07631   (201)568-3335   Fax (201)568-2450

Hamilton, Sylvester Sutton, IV, MD {1265415798} FamMed(97,PA12)<NJ-UNDRWD>
+ Complete Care Family Medicine
  75 West Red Bank Avenue   Woodbury, NJ 08096   (856)853-2055   Fax (856)848-2879

Hamilton, Tammy Joan, MD {1720148349} ObsGyn(95,DC02)<NJ-STBARNMC>
+ Associates in Obstetrics Gynecology & Infertility
  375 Mount Pleasant Avenue/Suite 202   West Orange, NJ 07052   (973)731-7707   Fax (973)669-0277

Hamilton, Thanuja Kumari, MD {1073774691} IntrMd(06,GRN01)
+ Pulmonary and Sleep Physicians
  204 Ark Road/Suite 206/Larchmont 1   Mount Laurel, NJ 08054   (856)778-4640   Fax (856)778-8862

Hamirani, Kamran Ismail, MD {1033291711} CdvDis, IntrMd, IntCrd(90,PAK04)
+ Cardiovascular Associates of NJ, P.A.
  377 Jersey Avenue/Suite 410   Jersey City, NJ 07302   (201)200-0318   Fax (201)200-0319
+ Cardiovascular Associates of NJ P.A.
  1931 Oak Tree Road/Suite 202   Edison, NJ 08820   (201)200-0318   Fax (732)372-7634
+ Rochelle Park Cardiac Center
  186 Rochelle Avenue   Rochelle Park, NJ 07302   (201)556-1225   Fax (201)556-1101

Hammer, Ashley Morgan, MD {1043506603} ObsGyn<NJ-LOURDMED, NJ-VIRTMHBC>
+ Advocare Burlington County Obstetrics & Gynecology
  1000 Salem Road/Suite B   Willingboro, NJ 08046   (609)871-2060   Fax (609)871-5478
+ Advocare Burlington County Obstetrics & Gynecology
  45b Homestead Drive/Homestead Plaza   Columbus, NJ 08022   (609)871-2060   Fax (609)871-3535

Hammer, Stacey R., MD {1588756662} Pedtrc(03,LA01)<NJ-VIRTMARL, NJ-VIRTUAHS>
+ Advocare Marlton Pediatrics
  525 Route 73 South   Marlton, NJ 08053   (856)596-3434   Fax (856)596-9110
+ Advocare Township Pediatrics
  123 Egg Harbor Road   Sewell, NJ 08080   (856)596-3434   Fax (856)227-5890

Hammerman, Louis, MD {1194724310} IntrMd(78,PA02)
+ 360 Hawkins Place
  Boonton, NJ 07005   (973)334-3006   Fax (973)402-9778

Hammerschlag, Warren A., MD {1104981679} SrgOrt(82,PA07)<NJ-ENGLWOOD, NJ-HACKNSK>
+ Orthopedic Specialists NJ-Hackensack
  87 Summit Avenue   Hackensack, NJ 07601   (201)489-0022   Fax (201)489-6991
+ Orthopedic Specialists of NJ - Paramus
  277 Forest Avenue   Paramus, NJ 07652   (201)483-9228

Hammod, Riyadh Shakir, MD {1568556512} IntrMd, Gastrn(79,IRQ02)
+ 1051 West Sherman Avenue/Suite 1C
  Vineland, NJ 08360   (856)692-9900   Fax (856)692-9911

Hammond, Betty L., MD {1952345753} FamMed(81,NC01)<NJ-STPETER, NJ-RWJUBRUN>
+ RWJ University Hospital New Brunswick
  One Robert Wood Johnson Place   New Brunswick, NJ 08901   (732)235-7657   Fax (732)235-8084
+ Robert Wood Johnson Monroe
  16 Centre Drive   Monroe, NJ 08831   (609)655-5178
+ Bay Family Medicine
  26 Throckmorton Lane   Old Bridge, NJ 08901   (732)360-0287   Fax (732)360-1279

Hammond, Carla Chambers, MD {1407889355} Psychy, PsyAdd, PsyCAd(93,TX12)
+ 43 Lakeside Drive North
  Piscataway, NJ 08854   (732)754-9049

Hammond, Deborah Ellen, MD {1891784310} IntrMd(77,OK01)
+ Healthfirst
  668 Alanon Road   Ridgewood, NJ 07450   (201)251-9655
+ Healthfirst
  1 Washington Square/VP   Newark, NJ 07105

Hammond, Jeffrey S., MD {1114096815} SrgCrC, Surgry, IntrMd(75,FL02)<NJ-RWJUBRUN>
+ 15 Mendham Road
  Gladstone, NJ 07934   (908)208-8236

Hammond, Kelly C., MD {1770572786} ObsGyn(91,RI01)<NJ-RIVERVW>
+ Drs. Karoly, Kaskiw, Hammond & Jacoby
  180 White Road/Suite 209   Little Silver, NJ 07739   (732)842-0673   Fax (732)842-7352
+ Drs. Karoly, Kaskiw, Hammond & Jacoby
  1 Bethany Road/Building 2/Suite 31   Hazlet, NJ 07730

Hammonds, Charles Dewey, MD {1831283290} Anesth(03,NC08)
+ Hackensack University MC-Anesthesia Dept
  30 Prospect Avenue/Room 2703   Hackensack, NJ 07601   (201)996-2419   Fax (201)996-3962

Physicians by Name and Address

Hammoud, Marwan Fahim, MD {1851390470} FamMed
+ MEDEMERGE
  1005 North Washington Avenue   Green Brook, NJ 08812
  (732)968-8900   Fax (732)968-5607
+ Med-Care of East Rutherford
  245 Park Avenue   East Rutherford, NJ 07073   (201)939-7161

Hampel, Howard, MD {1700825635} IntrMd, Gastrn(99,PA12)
+ Red Bank Gastroenterology Associates PA
  365 Broad Street/Suite 1-E   Red Bank, NJ 07701   (732)842-4294   Fax (732)548-7408

Hampton, Stephen, MD {1578827929} PhysMd<NJ-KSLRWEST>
+ Kessler Institute for Rehabilitation West Orange
  1199 Pleasant Valley Way   West Orange, NJ 07052
  (973)731-3600

Hamsa, Gangaswamaiah, MD {1700829496} IntrMd(97,INA68)<NJ-JRSYCITY>
+ 1555 Ruth Road/Suite 6
  North Brunswick, NJ 08902   (732)821-9200   Fax (732)821-9202

Hamza, Hisham M., MD {1154439610} Pedtrc(87,EGY05)
+ Bayshore Pediatrics LLC
  558 Commons Way   Toms River, NJ 08755   (732)736-0110
  Fax (732)736-0990
  Hmmd99@yahoo.com

Hamzeh Langroudi, Mehrdad, MD {1164413084} Anesth, IntrMd(93,BEL07)
+ SJH Regional Medical Center
  1505 West Sherman Avenue/Anesthesia   Vineland, NJ 08360   (856)641-8000

Han, Chang H., MD {1750574158} SrgO&M(05,NY01)<NJ-HACKNSK, NY-PRSBCOLU>
+ Bergen Oral & Maxillofacial Surgery
  920 Main Street   Hackensack, NJ 07601   (201)343-8297
  Fax (201)343-2535

Han, Dennis, MD {1881956050}
+ Summit Medical Group
  140 Park Avenue/3rd Floor   Florham Park, NJ 07932
  (973)404-9700

Han, Gene, MD {1275699001} RadDia(99,NY19)<NJ-HACKNSK>
+ Hackensack University Medical Center
  30 Prospect Avenue/Radiology   Hackensack, NJ 07601
  (201)996-2000   Fax (201)489-2812
+ Hackensack Radiology Group, P.A.
  30 Prospect Avenue   Hackensack, NJ 07601   (201)996-2000   Fax (201)336-8451

Han, Ji Soo, MD {1649436205} ObsGyn(88,KOR03)
+ Best Choice-Gyn
  2 State Route 27/Suite 311A   Edison, NJ 08820   (732)603-2122   Fax (732)603-3566
  info@bestchoiceobgyn.com

Han, Kwang Hoon, MD {1740201615} Rheuma
+ Cooper Physician Offices
  900 Centennial Boulevard   Voorhees, NJ 08043   (856)325-6770   Fax (856)673-4510

Han, Lu, MD {1619922127} PhysMd(83,CHN11)<NJ-RBAYPERT>
+ Jersey Rehabilitation Medical Clinic, P.C.
  620 Cranbury Road/Suite 118   East Brunswick, NJ 08816
  (732)390-8866   Fax (732)390-6550
  rehabmedicalclinic@yahoo.com
+ Raritan Bay Medical Center/Perth Amboy Division
  530 New Brunswick Avenue   Perth Amboy, NJ 08861
  (732)390-8866   Fax (732)324-3121

Han, Min, MD {1386707701} IntrMd(69,TAI05)
+ 249 State Route 94/Suite 3
  Vernon, NJ 07462   (973)827-3150   Fax (973)827-5845

Han, Min Woo, MD {1053341578} PthAcl(75,KOR04)<NJ-HACKNSK>
+ Hackensack University Medical Center
  30 Prospect Avenue/Pathology   Hackensack, NJ 07601
  (201)996-2000

Han, Paul S., MD {1174590558} PulDis, SlpDis, IntrMd(98,NJ06)<NJ-HOLYNAME, NJ-ENGLWOOD>
+ Holy Name Pulmonary Associates PC
  200 Grand Avenue/Suite 102   Englewood, NJ 07631
  (201)871-3636   Fax (201)871-2286

Han, Stella Insook, MD {1619957610} Ophthl(91,NY19)<NJ-STPETER, NJ-RWJUBRUN>
+ University Children's Eye Center, P.C.
  4 Cornwall Court   East Brunswick, NJ 08816   (732)613-9191   Fax (732)613-1139
+ University Children's Eye Center, P.C.
  678 Route 202-206 North/Bld 3   Bridgewater, NJ 08807
  (732)613-9191   Fax (908)203-9010

Hanan, Scott H., MD {1487649372} Surgry, SrgOnc(90,NJ06)
+ Summit Medical Group
  6 Brighton Road/2 FL   Clifton, NJ 07012   (973)436-1530
  Fax (973)777-5403
+ Summit Medical Group
  75 East Northfield Road   Livingston, NJ 07039   (973)436-1530   Fax (908)673-7336

Hanauske Abel, Hartmut Martin, MD {1972716058} Pedtrc(77,GER15)
+ Rutgers- New Jersey Medical School
  185 South Orange Avenue/MSB E-506   Newark, NJ 07103
  (973)972-4300

Hanchuk, Hilary T., MD {1760447197} Psychy, Nrolgy, PsyGrt(86,PA14)
+ 764 Easton Avenue/Suite 6
  Somerset, NJ 08873   (908)781-6242   Fax (908)782-6242
  Hthanchuk@aol.com

Hancock, Joseph Patrick, MD {1073788964} Anesth(04,TX13)<NJ-UNVMCPRN>
+ Princeton Anesthesia Services PC
  253 Witherspoon Street   Princeton, NJ 08540   (609)497-4000   Fax (609)497-4331
+ University Medical Center of Princeton at Plainsboro
  One Plainsboro Road/Anesth   Plainsboro, NJ 08536
  (609)497-4000

Hancq, Nicole Elizabeth, MD {1942400205} FamMed
+ Bruneau Family Care, P.C.
  2963 Marne Highway   Mount Laurel, NJ 08054   (856)638-1990

Hand, Steven Casey, MD {1831536440}
+ 1422 Greene Lane
  Cherry Hill, NJ 08003   (404)849-4571
  steve.hand15@gmail.com

Handa Nayyar, Seema, DO {1144295445} Anesth
+ May Street Surgi Center
  205 May Street/Suite 103   Edison, NJ 08837   (732)826-4177   Fax (732)607-1160

Handel, David B., MD {1518970953} RadDia, Radiol, RadBdl(80,PA09)<NJ-ACMCITY, NJ-SHOREMEM>
+ Atlantic Medical Imaging, LLC.
  72 West Jimmie Leeds Road   Galloway, NJ 08205
  (609)677-9729   Fax (609)653-8764
+ Atlantic Medical Imaging, LLC.
  401 Bethel Road   Somers Point, NJ 08244   (609)677-9729
+ Atlantic Medical Imaging, LLC.
  421 Route 9 North   Cape May Court House, NJ 08205
  (609)463-9500   Fax (609)465-0918

Handelsman, Cory, MD {1437458924} IntrMd(11,GA01)<NY-MTSINAI, NY-MTSINYHS>
+ RWJ Gastro & Hepatology
  125 Paterson Street/CAB 5100B   New Brunswick, NJ 08901
  (732)235-6512   Fax (732)235-7792

Handler, Eric Todd, DO {1700820446} EmrgMd(01,FL75)<NJ-STBARNMC>
+ St. Barnabas Medical Center
  94 Old Short Hills Road   Livingston, NJ 07039   (973)322-5000

Handler, Heidi L., MD {1578737987} FamMed(04,PA02)<NJ-VIRTMHBC>
+ Lourdes Medical Associates
  500 Grove Street/Suite 100   Haddon Heights, NJ 08035
  (856)796-9200   Fax (856)310-5603

Handler, Marc Z., MD {1376854836}
+ Rutgers- New Jersey Medical School
  185 South Orange Avenue   Newark, NJ 07103   (973)972-6255

Handler, Robert W., MD {1720038235} Pedtrc(75,NJ05)<NJ-MORRISTN, NJ-STCLRSUS>
+ Parsippany Pediatrics
  1140 Parisppany Boulevard/Suite 102   Parsippany, NJ 07054
  (973)263-0066   Fax (973)263-3160

Handler, Steven Douglas, MD {1790872323} PedOto, Otlryg(72,CA14)<PA-CHILDHOS>
+ CHOP Pediatric & Adolescent Specialty Care Center
  1012 Laurel Oak Road   Voorhees, NJ 08043   (856)435-1300
  Fax (856)435-0091

Handlin, David S., MD {1003821363} Anesth(80,NY01)<NJ-BAYSHORE>
+ Bayshore Community Hospital
  727 North Beers Street/Anesthesiology   Holmdel, NJ 07733
  (732)739-5853

Hands, Robert A., Jr., MD {1306160056} Pedtrc(68,NY20)<NY-PRSBCOLU, NJ-VALLEY>
+ 331 East Saddle River Road
  Upper Saddle River, NJ 07458   (201)327-9080   Fax (201)327-2678

Hanes, Douglas James, MD {1225138910} IntrMd(00,PA13)<NJ-COOPRUMC>
+ Cooper University Medical Center/Camden
  3 Cooper Plaza   Camden, NJ 08103   (856)342-2000

Haney, James Joseph, III, MD {1952300139} RadDia, Radiol, Rad-Nuc(76,PA13)<NJ-MEMSALEM>
+ Kennedy Health System/Cherry Hill Campus
  2201 Chapel Avenue West   Cherry Hill, NJ 08002
  (856)661-5454   Fax (856)488-6507

Hanfling, Marcus, DO {1922015007} CdvDis, IntrMd(81,NY75)<NJ-BAYSHORE, NJ-RIVERVW>
+ Shore Heart Group, P.A.
  555 Iron Bridge Road/Suite 15   Freehold, NJ 07728

  (732)308-0774   Fax (732)333-1366
+ Shore Heart Group, P.A.
  115 East Bay Avenue   Manahawkin, NJ 08050   (732)308-0774   Fax (609)597-4656
+ Shore Heart Group, P.A.
  35 Beaverson Boulevard/Suite 9-B   Brick, NJ 07728
  (732)262-4262   Fax (732)262-4317

Hanft, Simon J., MD {1679732960}
+ Robert Wood Johnson Neurosurgery
  125 Patterson Street/Suite 2100   New Brunswick, NJ 08901
  (732)235-7756

Hanhan, Stephanie B., MD {1629286315} PedRad, RadDia(03,NJ02)
+ University Radiology Group, P.C.
  483 Cranbury Road   East Brunswick, NJ 08816   (732)390-0030   Fax (732)390-5383
+ University Radiology Group, P.C.
  579A Cranbury Road   East Brunswick, NJ 08816   (732)390-0030   Fax (732)390-1856

Hanhan, Ziad George, MD {1841306149} Surgry(99,NET09)<NJ-JRSYCITY>
+ Carepoint Medical-Surgery
  142 Palisades Avenue/Suite 213   Jersey City, NJ 07306
  (201)217-1200

Hanif, Ghalia, MD {1952556326} IntrMd
+ 300 Etra Road
  East Windsor, NJ 08520   (609)426-6815   Fax (609)426-6871

Hanif, Muhammad Shahzad, MD {1487792503} IntrMd
+ 502 West Side Avenue
  Jersey City, NJ 07304

Hankin, William H., MD {1356354898} Psychy(83,PA13)<NJ-BUR-DTMLN>
+ 303 Court House/S. Dennis Road
  Cape May Court House, NJ 08210   (609)465-4424   Fax (609)465-4864
  wh@whhmd.com

Hanley, Daniel Lee Wilburn, MD {1407268600} FamMed
+ 5 Allen Lane
  Lawrence Township, NJ 08648   (833)742-6276   Fax (609)435-1356

Hanley, Debra A., MD {1659300069} Hemato, IntrMd, MedOnc(80,MEXI)
+ Wayne Hematology-Oncology Associates PA
  468 Parish Drive/Suite 4   Wayne, NJ 07470   (973)694-5005
  Fax (973)694-5990

Hanley, Maryellen L., MD {1255446183} MtFtMd, ObsGyn(91,NJ06)<NJ-MORRISTN, NJ-CHILTON>
+ Atlantic Maternal Fetal Medicine
  435 South Street/Suite 380   Morristown, NJ 07960
  (973)971-7080   Fax (973)290-8312
+ Maternal Fetal Medicine of Practice Associates
  11 Overlook Road/Suite LL 102   Summit, NJ 07901
  (973)971-7080   Fax (908)522-5557

Hanley, Thomas T., MD {1235166133} FamMed(86,PA09)<NJ-VIRTVOOR>
+ Penn Medicine at Cherry Hill
  409 Route 70 East   Cherry Hill, NJ 08034   (856)429-1519

Hanlon, Catherine A., MD {1346283496} EmrgMd, IntrMd(83,PA09)<NJ-CHSFULD, NJ-CHSMRCER>
+ Monmouth Medical Center
  300 Second Avenue   Long Branch, NJ 07740   (732)222-5200

Hanna, Aghnatious A Ha Awadalla, MD {1366954091} Ophthl
+ 316 Prospect Avenue
  Hackensack, NJ 07601   (201)923-0454   Fax (973)827-6636
  AGHIHANNA@GMAIL.COM

Hanna, Amir, MD {1376881920} Anesth<NJ-VIRTMHBC>
+ 1 Bennington Drive
  Medford, NJ 08055

Hanna, Amir Atallaha, MD {1750391041} NroChl, Nrolgy(78,EGY05)<NJ-CHRIST, NJ-HOBUNIMC>
+ 253 Academy Street/Second Floor
  Jersey City, NJ 07306   (201)876-5550   Fax (201)876-8995
+ 579 Bergen Boulevard
  Ridgefield, NJ 07657

Hanna, Bishoy F., MD {1538507389} IntrMd
+ 73 Winding Wood Drive/Apt 4A
  Sayreville, NJ 08872   (908)202-9198

Hanna, Dalia N., MD {1053402479} FamMed(02,DMN01)<NJ-MERIDNHS>
+ Matawan Medical Associates
  213 Main Street   Matawan, NJ 07747   (732)566-2363
  Fax (732)566-0502

Hanna, Dina W., MD {1386759447} Pedtrc(95,NJ05)<NJ-STPETER, NJ-RWJUBRUN>
+ Plaza Pediatrics
  1950 State Highway 27 North/Suite HH   North Brunswick, NJ 08902   (732)940-5511   Fax (732)940-0530
  drdhanna@yahoo.com

Physicians by Name and Address

Hanna, Ekram Labeb, MD {1730273772} IntrMd(86,EGY07)
+ Internal Medicine Associates
201 Laurel Heights Drive/Suite 201   Bridgeton, NJ 08302   (856)455-4800   Fax (856)455-0650

Hanna, Emad Zareef Ayoub, MD {1679911572} Pedtrc(02,EGYP)<NY-CMCSTVSI>
+ Raritan Bay Medical Center/Perth Amboy Division
530 New Brunswick Avenue   Perth Amboy, NJ 08861   (732)442-3700
ehanna@rbmc.org

Hanna, Gamal Kamel, MD {1467444968} Surgry, EmrgMd(72,EGY03)<NJ-STMRYPAS>
+ St. Mary's Hospital
350 Boulevard/Surgery   Passaic, NJ 07055   (973)365-4300

Hanna, Gamil Sabet Fawzy, MD {1104849231} IntrMd, OncHem(88,EGY04)
+ Penn Medicine at Cherry Hill
409 Route 70 East   Cherry Hill, NJ 08034   (856)429-1519   Fax (856)427-0250

Hanna, George J., MD {1801928304} InfDis
+ 1805 Stuart Road West
Princeton, NJ 08540   (609)897-5055

Hanna, George M., MD {1902033723} Anesth(08,PA01)<MA-BRIGWMN>
+ Chilton Medical Center
97 West Parkway   Pompton Plains, NJ 07444   (973)831-5000

Hanna, Hossam H., MD {1124002605} IntrMd, IntHos(83,EGY04)<NY-CGHSEELG>
+ The Valley Hospital
223 North Van Dien Avenue   Ridgewood, NJ 07450   (201)447-8000

Hanna, John M., MD {1922396266} VasNeu
+ NE Regional Epilepsy/Atlantic Neuro
99 Beauvoir Avenue/5th Fl   Summit, NJ 07902   (908)522-5545

Hanna, John Patrick, DO {1699086058} Otlryg(06,NY75)
+ Hunterdon Otolaryngology Associates
6 Sand Hill Road/Suite 302   Flemington, NJ 08822   (908)788-9131   Fax (908)788-0945

Hanna, Joseph S., MD {1326126590} SrgCrC, Surgry(06,IL02)
+ RWJMG Acute Care Surgery
125 Paterson Street/Suite 6300   New Brunswick, NJ 08901   (732)235-7766   Fax (732)235-2964

Hanna, Madouna Gamal, DO {1740546266}
+ New Bridge Medical Center
230 East Ridgewood Avenue   Paramus, NJ 07652   (201)967-4000
+ MidJersey Orthopaedics, P.A.
8100 Westcott Drive/Suite 101   Flemington, NJ 08822   (201)967-4000   Fax (908)782-7575
+ 353 Weart Avenue
Lyndhurst, NJ 07652   (201)889-7519

Hanna, Mamdouh Soliman, MD {1073517462} Anesth, Pain-Invt(87,EGY05)<NJ-BAYONNE, NJ-STFRNMED>
+ Bayonne Medical Center
29th Street at Avenue E   Bayonne, NJ 07002   (201)858-5000
+ Hudson Pain Management Center
183 Avenue B   Bayonne, NJ 07002   (201)858-5000   Fax (201)339-7250

Hanna, Manar H., MD {1588625859} IntrMd(88,SYR03)
+ Drs. Hanna and Recho
117 State Route 35   Eatontown, NJ 07724   (732)542-4411   Fax (732)542-1070

Hanna, Michael, MD {1679823645} IntrMd
+ St Joseph's Medical Ctr Internal Med
703 Main Street   Paterson, NJ 07503   (973)754-2450

Hanna, Mohab, MD {1629129093} PsyCAd(97,NJ05)
+ Drs. Hanna & Crowley
545 Island Road/Suite 2B   Ramsey, NJ 07446   (201)995-1004   Fax (201)345-7121

Hanna, Moneer K., MD {1215968540} Urolgy, PedUro(63,EGY03)<NY-PRSBWEIL, NY-SCHNCHIL>
+ 101 Old Short Hills Road/Suite 203
West Orange, NJ 07052   (973)325-7188   Fax (973)325-7409
mkhanna@mkhanna.com

Hanna, Niveen, MD {1780668889} Surgry, IntrMd(96,NJ05)
+ Advanced Surgical Associates of New Jersey
40 Fuld Street/Suite 403   Trenton, NJ 08638   (609)396-2600   Fax (609)396-3600
+ Capital Health Primary Care
832 Brunswick Avenue   Trenton, NJ 08638   (609)396-2600   Fax (609)815-7401

Hanna, Philip Andre, MD {1306846647} Nrolgy(93,IL06)<NJ-JFKMED>
+ JFK Neurosciences Institute
65 James Street/Second Floor/Balance   Edison, NJ 08818   (732)321-7010   Fax (732)632-1669
+ JFK Medical Center
65 James Street/NroSci   Edison, NJ 08820   (732)321-7010

Fax (732)632-1584

Hanna, Ruba, MD {1629071188} Pedtrc(94,SYR03)<NJ-STJOSHOS>
+ Notchview Pediatrics, LLC.
1037 Route 46 East/Suite 201   Clifton, NJ 07013   (973)779-3911   Fax (973)471-2730

Hanna, Sherine Farag, MD {1003886417} Anesth(92,IL01)
+ Robert Wood Johnson-UMDNJ Anesthesia Group
1140 Route 72 West   Manahawkin, NJ 08050   (609)978-8900

Hanna, Sherry Kamal, MD {1770750655} FamMed(04,EGY04)
+ 3102 Saxony Drive
Mount Laurel, NJ 08054

Hannallah, Benyamin A., MD {1831126945} CdvDis, IntCrd, IntrMd(81,EGY16)<NJ-CHRIST, NJ-STJOSHOS>
+ 142 Palisade Avenue/Suite 216
Jersey City, NJ 07306   (201)714-4900   Fax (201)459-9040
bhannallah@pol.net

Hannallah, Youssef A., MD {1760424378} IntrMd, Pedtrc(83,EGYP)<NJ-EASTORNG>
+ 142 Palisade Avenue
Jersey City, NJ 07306   (201)714-4900

Hannani, Afshin K., MD {1154353290} Nephro, IntrMd(87,TUR04)<NJ-CHSFULD>
+ Mercer Renal Associates PA
1345 Kuser Road/Suite 2   Hamilton, NJ 08619   (609)585-1344   Fax (609)585-1355

Hannema, Erica L., DO {1780012609} FamMed(11,ME75)
+ Hunterdon Family Medicine
1100 Wescott Drive/Suite 101   Flemington, NJ 08822   (908)788-6535   Fax (908)788-6536

Hannoush, Peter Yousef, MD {1184760811} EnDbMt, IntrMd(92,NJ06)<NJ-HACKNSK>
+ 380 Sutton Avenue
Hackensack, NJ 07601   (201)488-8766   Fax (201)488-8646

Hanono, Joseph A., MD {1356575971} RadDia
+ Our Lady of Lourdes Medical Center
1600 Haddon Avenue   Camden, NJ 08103   (718)757-2552

Hanrahan, Maureen A., MD {1184635930} FamMed(85,IL43)
+ Matula Medical, P.C.
435 Liberty Lane   Marlton, NJ 08053   (856)985-3406   Fax (856)988-8835

Hansalia, Riple Jayamtilal, MD {1669511721} IntrMd
+ Shore Heart Group, P.A.
35 Beaverson Boulevard/Suite 9-B   Brick, NJ 08723   (732)262-4262   Fax (732)262-4317
+ Shore Heart Group, P.A.
1820 State Route 33/Suite 4-B   Neptune, NJ 07753   (732)262-4262   Fax (732)776-8946
+ Shore Heart Group, P.A.
555 Iron Bridge Road/Suite 15   Freehold, NJ 08723   (732)308-0774   Fax (732)333-1366

Hansch, Lalitha Therese Waldron, MD {1568462505} FamMed(99,OH45)<NJ-SOMERSET, NJ-STPETER>
+ Somerset Family Practice
110 Rehill Avenue   Somerville, NJ 08876   (908)685-2900   Fax (908)685-2891

Hansen, David Wayne, MD {1851367056} Anesth(00,GRN01)
+ 183 West Oakland Avenue
Oakland, NJ 07436   (201)953-3840   Fax (201)337-7056

Hansen, Eric Andrew, DO {1508956533} InfDis, IntrMd(96,NY75)<NJ-BURDTMLN, NJ-SHOREMEM>
+ Cape May Infectious Disease, LLC
8 South Dennisville Road   Cape May Court House, NJ 08210   (609)465-0678   Fax (609)465-9958

Hansen, Eric S., DO {1306823364} IntrMd(94,NJ75)<NJ-NWTN-MEM>
+ Premier Health Associates
212 State Route 94/Suite 1-D   Vernon, NJ 07462   (973)209-2162   Fax (973)209-2665
+ Premier Health Associates
123 Newton Sparta Road   Newton, NJ 07860   (973)209-2162   Fax (973)579-1524

Hansen, Luke, MD {1063861664} Psychy
+ Rowan Medical Psychiatry
100 Century Parkway/Suite 350   Mount Laurel, NJ 08054   (856)482-9000

Hanson, Anna Jang, MD {1679639496} ObsGyn(NC08
+ Premier Women's Health of South Jersey
603 North Broad Street/Suite 300   Woodbury, NJ 08096   (856)223-8930   Fax (856)223-8948
+ Premier Women's Health of South Jersey
340 West Front Street/Suite 201   Elmer, NJ 08318   (856)223-8930   Fax (856)223-8948
+ Premier Women's Health of South Jersey
34 Colson Lane   Mullica Hill, NJ 08096   (856)223-1385

Hanson, Claudia A., MD IntrMd(83,DMN01)
+ 15 Lewis Drive
Maplewood, NJ 07040

Hanusey, Robert William, MD {1316505894} Anesth
+ Trenton Anesthesiology Associates, PA
One Capital Way/Second Floor   Pennington, NJ 08534

(800)637-2374   Fax (609)396-4900

Hao, Irene, MD {1598807521} IntrMd<NJ-UMDNJ>
+ University Hospital
150 Bergen Street/Lvl 354   Newark, NJ 07103   (973)972-6111   Fax (973)972-6228

Hao, Tong Karen, MD {1023085263} IntrMd(91,CHN57)
+ 402 New Castle Court
Morganville, NJ 07751

Hapner, Byron S., DO {1548290695} ObsGyn, IntrMd(90,NY75)<NJ-UNDRWD>
+ Premier Women's Health of South Jersey
603 North Broad Street/Suite 300   Woodbury, NJ 08096   (856)223-8930   Fax (856)223-8948
+ Premier Women's Health of South Jersey
340 West Front Street/Suite 201/West   Elmer, NJ 08318   (856)223-8930   Fax (856)223-8948
+ Premier Women's Health of South Jersey
34 Colson Lane   Mullica Hill, NJ 08096   (856)223-1385

Haq, Imran Ul, MD {1770537326} Surgry(85,PAK02)<NJ-SJHREGMC, NJ-SJRSYELM>
+ Iqbal & Khan Surgical Associates, P.A.
10 Magnolia Avenue/Suite E   Bridgeton, NJ 08302   (856)455-2399   Fax (856)451-7791

Haq, Mehnaz A., MD {1881648541} IntrMd(89,PAKI)
+ 2648 State Route 7
North Brunswick, NJ 08902   (732)951-8585   Fax (732)951-9112
Mehnazhaqmd@hotmail.com

Haque, A. F. M. Z., MD {1649309170} Psychy, PsyCAd(90,BAN05)
+ CPC Behavioral HealthCare
1 Highpoint Center Way   Morganville, NJ 07751   (732)591-1750   Fax (732)591-2516
+ Princeton Develeopmental and Psychiatric Center
24 Jefferson Plaza   Princeton, NJ 08540   (732)647-6000

Haque, Anwar Mohammed, MD {1689833402} IntrMd, PulDis, PulCCr(05,GRN01)<NJ-COOPRUMC>
+ Cooper University at Willingboro
218C Sunset Road   Willingboro, NJ 08046   (609)877-0400   Fax (609)877-1682

Haque, Maahir Ul, MD {1871883181} Surgry
+ Robert Wood Johnson University Hospital
51 French Street/MEB-234B/MEB 422A   New Brunswick, NJ 08903   (732)235-7869

Haque, Nadeem U., MD {1538121926} IntrMd(87,PAKI)<NJ-BAYONNE, NJ-JRSYCITY>
+ 630 Broadway/Suite 2R
Bayonne, NJ 07002   (201)823-4400

Haque, Salma, MD {1528107315} IntrMd(72,PAK08)<NJ-COMMED>
+ Coastal Health Care
1314 Hooper Avenue/Building B   Toms River, NJ 08753   (732)349-4994   Fax (732)341-1717

Haque, Shahid N., MD {1811080310} SrgVas, Surgry(70,PAKI)<NJ-OCEANMC>
+ 218 Commonsway/Building B
Toms River, NJ 08755   (732)244-4448   Fax (732)244-4818

Haramis, Harry Theodore, MD {1386861177} SrgPlstc, SrgRec, Surgry(87,NJ05)
+ New Jersey Plastic Surgery
29 Park Street   Montclair, NJ 07042   (973)509-2000   Fax (973)655-1228

Haran, Pahirathi E., MD {1366528531} PedNrD(75,INDI)<NJ-STCLRDEN>
+ Child Development Medicine
76 Broadway/Suite 200 B   Denville, NJ 07834   (973)627-3366   Fax (973)539-5537

Harangozo, Andrea M., MD {1982793253} CritCr, IntrMd, PulDis(84,NY19)
+ Pulmonary & Intensive Care Specialists of NJ
593 Cranbury Road   East Brunswick, NJ 08816   (732)613-8880   Fax (732)613-0077

Haratz, Alan B., MD {1336155688} IntrMd, Nephro(79,PA09)<NJ-RIVERVW, NJ-MONMOUTH>
+ Hypertension & Nephrology Association, PA
6 Industrial Way West/Suite B   Eatontown, NJ 07724   (732)460-1200   Fax (732)460-1211
+ Atlantic Artificial Kidney Center
6 Industrial Way West/Suite B   Eatontown, NJ 07724   (732)460-1414

Harawi, Sami J., MD {1902842719} Pthlgy, PthACl(74,LEB03)<NJ-HACKNSK>
+ Institute for Breast Care
20 Prospect Avenue/Suite 513   Hackensack, NJ 07601   (201)996-2222
+ Hackensack University Medical Center
30 Prospect Avenue/Pathology   Hackensack, NJ 07601   (201)996-4817

Harb, George E., MD IntrMd(83,LEB03)
+ 148 Park Street
Montclair, NJ 07042

Physicians by Name and Address

Harback, Edward R., MD {1720075070} CdvDis, IntrMd(86,NJ05)<NJ-MORRISTN>
+ Consultants in Cardiology
741 Northfield Avenue/Suite 205   West Orange, NJ 07052   (973)467-1544   Fax (973)467-9586

Harbison, Margaret S., MD {1245357235} Psychy(92,PA07)
+ CENTRA Comprehensive Psychotherapy
5000 Sagemore Drive/Suite 205   Marlton, NJ 08053   (856)983-3866   Fax (856)985-8148

Harbist, Noel Rebecca, MD Pedtrc(83,PA12)
+ Kids first
2006 Salem Road   Burlington, NJ 08016   (609)877-1500   Fax (609)877-4262

Hardeski, David Paul, MD {1497940290} SrgOrt, SrgTrm
+ Mercer-Bucks Orthopaedics, P.C.
2501 Kuser Road/3rd Fl   Hamilton, NJ 08691   (609)896-0444   Fax (609)587-4349
+ Mercer-Bucks Orthopaedics PC
3120 Princeton Pike   Lawrenceville, NJ 08648   (609)896-0444   Fax (609)896-1055

Harding, John Arthur, MD {1487652392} RadDia(81,WI06)<NJ-VIRTUAHS, NJ-VIRTMHBC>
+ South Jersey Radiology Associates, P.A.
901 Route 168/Suites 301-305   Turnersville, NJ 08012   (856)227-6600   Fax (856)227-8537
+ South Jersey Radiology Associates, P.A.
807 Haddon Avenue/Suite 5   Haddonfield, NJ 08033   (856)227-6600   Fax (856)616-1125
+ South Jersey Radiology Associates, P.A.
315 Route 70 East/Suite B   Cherry Hill, NJ 08012   (856)428-4344   Fax (856)428-0356

Harding, Mark, MD {1386011666} FamMed
+ 214 State Highway 36
West Long Branch, NJ 07764   (732)222-8000   Fax (732)963-2246

Hardy, Caitlin Judith, MD {1962692806} RadNuc<NJ-COOPRUMC>
+ Cooper University Hospital
One Cooper Plaza   Camden, NJ 08103   (856)342-2390

Hardy, Howard, III, MD {1821041054} SrgC&R(80,NY01)<NJ-STFRNMED, NJ-CHSFULD>
+ Drs. Hardy and Eisengart
3131 Princeton Pike   Lawrenceville, NJ 08648   (609)896-1700   Fax (609)896-1087

Hardy, Samuel Solomon, MD {1851714141}<NJ-COOPRUMC>
+ Cooper University Hospital
One Cooper Plaza   Camden, NJ 08103   (856)342-2000

Hargrave, Douglas M., DO {1497700355} FamMed(95,PA77)
+ Buena Family Practice
1315 Harding Highway/Box 310   Richland, NJ 08350   (856)697-0300   Fax (856)697-8944

Harhay, Joseph S., MD {1508972183} SrgOrt, SprtMd(77,DC01)<NJ-ACMCITY, NJ-ACMCMAIN>
+ 611 New Road
Northfield, NJ 08225   (609)645-1500   Fax (609)484-9122   jharhay@asoaortho.com

Hariharan, Subramanian, MD {1497755847} IntrMd, OncNeu, Nrolgy(88,INDI)<NJ-JFKMED>
+ JFK Medical Center
65 James Street/Neuroscience   Edison, NJ 08820   (732)321-7010   Fax (732)632-1584
+ JFK Neurosciences Institute
65 James Street/Second Floor   Edison, NJ 08818   (732)321-7010   Fax (732)632-1669

Harish, Ziv, MD {1821041831} Allrgy, Pedtrc(84,ISR05)<NJ-ENGLWOOD, NJ-HACKNSK>
+ 200 Engle Street/Suite 18
Englewood, NJ 07631   (201)871-7475   Fax (201)871-6091   allergy@covad.net
+ Englewood Hospital and Medical Center
350 Engle Street/Allergy & Immun   Englewood, NJ 07631   (201)894-3000

Harjani, Vashdeo Daulat, MD {1528105640} IntrMd(92,INDI)
+ Berkeley Internal Medicine
391 Springfield Avenue/Suite 1B   Berkeley Heights, NJ 07922   (908)665-1177   Fax (908)665-8420

Harkaway, Karen S., MD {1093817280} Dermat, IntrMd(69,PA01)
+ 8001 US Highway 130 South
Delran, NJ 08075   (856)461-1400   Fax (856)461-2366

Harkins, Michael J., MD {1497726764} CdvDis, IntCrd, IntrMd(69,PA13)<NJ-OURLADY, NJ-COOPRUMC>
+ Associated Cardiovascular Consultants-Lourdes
1 Brace Road/Suite C & F   Cherry Hill, NJ 08034   (856)428-4100   Fax (856)428-5748
+ Associated Cardiovascular Consultants, P.A.
1105 Laurel Oak Road/Suite 165   Voorhees, NJ 08043   (856)428-4100   Fax (856)424-7154

Harlow, Paul J., MD {1659349272} PedHem, Pedtrc(74,NY08)<NJ-HACKNSK, NJ-VALLEY>
+ Pediatric Specialties PA
90 Prospect Avenue/Suite 1-A   Hackensack, NJ 07601   (201)342-4001   Fax (201)342-9569

+ Pediatric Specialties PA
50 South Franklin Turnpike   Ramsey, NJ 07446   (201)342-4001   Fax (201)934-2947
+ Tomorrow's Children's Inst/HUMC
30 Prospect Avenue/WFAN - PC 116   Hackensack, NJ 07601   (201)996-5437

Harmady, Debra, MD {1053383455} Pedtrc(98,PA09)
+ Venture Pediatrics
1275 State Route 35/Unit 6   Middletown, NJ 07748   (732)957-9200   Fax (732)957-9203

Harman, John A., MD {1386692135} PulDis, IntrMd(69,PA01)<NJ-CHSMRCER>
+ Capital Health Primary Care - Mountainview
850 Bear Tavern Road/Suite 309   Ewing, NJ 08628   (609)656-8844   Fax (609)656-8845

Harman, Robert Ashworth, MD {1376914382} Psychy, IntrMd(80,CA14)
+ 67 Burnt Hill Road
Skillman, NJ 08558   (609)466-3598

Harmon, Keith Andrew, MD {1396776910} Urolgy(92,MA01)
+ Somerset Urological Associates PA
72 West End Avenue   Somerville, NJ 08876   (908)927-0300   Fax (908)707-4988

Harnly, Heather Withington, MD {1548331952} SrgOrt, PedOrt(00,PA01)
+ Pediatric Orthopedic Associates, P.A.
585 Cranbury Road/Suite A   East Brunswick, NJ 08816   (732)390-1160   Fax (732)390-8449
+ Pediatric Orthopedic Associates, P.A.
3700 State Route 33   Neptune, NJ 07753   (732)390-1160   Fax (732)897-4205

Haroldson, Kathryn, MD {1831544493} IntrMd
+ Cooper University Hospital Hospitalists
One Cooper Plaza/Suite 222/Drrnce   Camden, NJ 08103   (856)342-3150

Haroun, Sandra, MD {1528455664} EmrgMd
+ Ocean Medical Center Emergency
425 Jack Martin Boulevard   Brick, NJ 08724   (716)859-1993

Harowitz, Robert J., MD {1417942772} Anesth(89,NY09)<NJ-UNDRWD>
+ Inspira Health Network
509 North Broad Street/Anesth   Woodbury, NJ 08096   (856)845-0100   Fax (856)848-7023

Haroz, Rachel, MD {1093815789} EmrgMd<NJ-COOPRUMC>
+ Cooper University Hospital
One Cooper Plaza/Emerg Med   Camden, NJ 08103   (856)342-2351   Fax (856)968-8272

Harper, Andrea A., MD {1700853892} Ophthl, Glacma(93,GA21)<NJ-WESTHDSN, NJ-CLARMAAS>
+ 39 Seeley Avenue
Kearny, NJ 07032   (201)998-1717   Fax (201)998-1793   aharpermd@aol.com

Harper, Harry D., MD {1811958481} OncHem, IntrMd(77,TX04)<NJ-HACKNSK, NJ-HOLYNAME>
+ John Theurer Cancer Center - HUMC
92 Second Street   Hackensack, NJ 07601   (201)996-5900   Fax (201)996-9246

Harper, Leannah L., MD {1598708448} Pedtrc(83,PA13)
+ 80 South Main Road/Suite 103
Vineland, NJ 08360   (856)690-0050   Fax (856)690-9499

Harrell, Angela Duley, MD {1871541623} Pedtrc(97,PA09)<NJ-VIRTMHBC>
+ Advocare Delran Pediatrics
5045 Route 130 South/Suite F   Delran, NJ 08075   (856)461-1717   Fax (856)461-1143

Harrell, Russell L., MD {1619912920} ObsGyn(83,MEXI)<NJ-COMMED>
+ North Dover Ob-Gyn Associates
222 Oak Avenue/3rd Floor/Suite 301   Toms River, NJ 08753   (732)914-1919   Fax (732)914-0725
+ North Dover Ob-Gyn Associates
442 Lacey Road   Forked River, NJ 08731   (732)914-1919   Fax (609)971-9712
+ North Dover Ob-Gyn Associates
214 Jack Martin Boulevard/Building D-3   Brick, NJ 08753   (732)840-3900   Fax (732)840-9270

Harrer, Michael F., MD {1194829762} SrgOrt(93,PA02)
+ Orthopedic Reconstruction
600 Somerdale Road/Suite 113   Voorhees, NJ 08043   (856)795-1945   Fax (856)795-7472

Harrigan, John T., MD {1902801053} RadDia, Radiol, IntrMd(89,NJ06)<NJ-JRSYSHMC>
+ University Radiology Group, P.C.
579A Cranbury Road   East Brunswick, NJ 08816   (732)390-0040   Fax (732)390-1856
+ University Radiology Group
2100 Route 33/Neptune City Med Bld   Neptune, NJ 07753   (732)390-0040   Fax (732)502-0368
+ University Radiology Group
900 West Main Street   Freehold, NJ 08816   (732)462-1900   Fax (732)462-1848

Harrigan, Michael Richard, MD {1104207687} Psychy<NJ-BERGNMC>
+ New Bridge Medical Center
230 East Ridgewood Avenue/Psychy   Paramus, NJ 07652   (201)967-4132

Harris, Brenda D., MD {1427024975} PedNrD(75,NY20)<NJ-CHLSMT>
+ CSH Pediatric Practice of Union
150 New Providence Road   Mountainside, NJ 07092   (908)353-8998   Fax (908)527-6766

Harris, Brian E., MD {1013977453} EmrgMd, IntrMd(82,TN07)
+ Worknet Occupational Medicine
510 Heron Drive/Suite 108   Bridgeport, NJ 08014   (856)467-8550   Fax (856)467-3361

Harris, Colin B., MD {1194979435} SrgSpn<NY-STJOSHHC>
+ University Hospital
150 Bergen Street   Newark, NJ 07103   (973)972-5929   Fax (973)972-3897

Harris, Elliott Michael, MD {1639279326} PedEmg, EmrgPedr(87,NY19)<NJ-COOPRUMC>
+ Cooper University Hospital
One Cooper Plaza/PedEmrgMd   Camden, NJ 08103   (856)342-2000

Harris, Esther R., MD {1740243187} Pedtrc(92,PA07)<NJ-VIRTVOOR, NJ-COOPRUMC>
+ Advocare Merchantville Pediatrics
1600 Chapel Avenue/Suite 100   Cherry Hill, NJ 08002   Fax (856)665-3938

Harris, Jazmine A., MD {1881693844} Pedtrc(99,PA01)
+ Community Health Care Inc
53 South Laurel Street/Second Floor   Bridgeton, NJ 08302   (856)451-4700   Fax (856)453-8495

Harris, Kenneth Barton, MD {1861492027} IntrMd, CdvDis(95,NY15)<NJ-JRSYSHMC>
+ Atlantic Cardiology LLC
444 Neptune Boulevard/Unit 2   Neptune, NJ 07753   (732)775-5300   Fax (732)988-9080
+ Atlantic Cardiology LLC
22 North Main Street   Marlboro, NJ 07746   (732)462-6666
+ Atlantic Cardiology, LLC
27 South Cooks Bridge Road/Suite 216   Jackson, NJ 07753   (848)217-3010

Harris, Michael, MD {1346247954} Ophthl(70,NY15)<NJ-ST-BARNMC>
+ 315 East Northfield Road/Suite 2 B
Livingston, NJ 07039   (973)994-0010   Fax (973)994-2342

Harris, Michael B., MD {1699744037} PedHem, Pedtrc, IntrMd(69,NY46)<NJ-HACKNSK>
+ Tomorrow's Children's Inst/HUMC
30 Prospect Avenue/WFAN - PC 116   Hackensack, NJ 07601   (201)996-5437   mbharris@humed.com
+ Rutgers- New Jersey Medical School
185 South Orange Avenue/Pediatrics   Newark, NJ 07103   (973)972-4300

Harris, Michael J., MD {1912915125} Ophthl, VitRet, IntrMd(80,MD07)<NJ-ENGLWOOD, NJ-HACKNSK>
+ Retina Associates of New Jersey, P.A.
200 South Broad Street/Unit B   Ridgewood, NJ 07450   (201)445-6622   Fax (201)445-0262
+ Retina Associates of New Jersey, P.A.
1044 Route 23 North/Suite 207   Wayne, NJ 07470   (201)445-6622   Fax (973)633-3892
+ Retina Associates of New Jersey, P.A.
628 Cedar Lane   Teaneck, NJ 07450   (201)837-7300   Fax (201)836-6426

Harris, Michael T., MD {1699741066} SrgC&R, Surgry(88,NY01)<NJ-ENGLWOOD, NY-MTSINAI>
+ Englewood Hospital and Medical Center
350 Engle Street/2 NW/Surgery   Englewood, NJ 07631   (201)608-2800   Fax (201)608-2478   michael.harris@ehmchealth.org

Harris, Robert M., MD {1225066533} IntrMd, UtlRQA(74,NY19)<NJ-HOLYNAME, NJ-HACKNSK>
+ 185 Cedar Lane/Suite U4
Teaneck, NJ 07666   (201)928-1930   Fax (201)928-1217

Harris, Ronald K., MD {1003894023} Surgry, SrgOnc(71,NY20)<NJ-NWTNMEM>
+ Medical & Surgical Specialty Group
135 Newton Sparta Road/Suite 201   Newton, NJ 07860   (973)383-6244   Fax (973)383-0573

Harris, Timothy Wayne, DO {1447364294} FamMed(96,ME75)<NJ-MEMSALEM>
+ Southern Jersey Family Medical
238 East Broadway   Salem, NJ 08079   (856)935-7711   Fax (856)935-2193

Harris, Tracey Dionne, MD {1467429746} PhysMd(94,NJ05)<NJ-OURLADY, NJ-COOPRUMC>
+ 230 North Maple Avenue/Suite B-1
Marlton, NJ 08053   (856)334-2000   Fax (866)528-3728

Physicians by Name and Address

Harris, William G., MD {1023024718} GenPrc, FamMed(65,NC05)
+ 79 South Main Street/PO Box 368
Mullica Hill, NJ 08062 (856)478-2160 Fax (856)417-3005
wgharrisjr@comcast.net

Harris, William Matthew, MD {1437549482} Surgry<NJ-OURLADY>
+ Our Lady of Lourdes Medical Center
1600 Haddon Avenue Camden, NJ 08103 (856)757-3500

Harrison, Andrew, MD {1457303166} SprtMd, SrgOrt, IntrMd(88,PA01)<NJ-COMMED, NJ-KIMBALL>
+ Ultimed HealthCare PC
50 Franklin Lane Manalapan, NJ 07726 (732)972-1267
Fax (732)972-1026

Harrison, David E., DO {1689653313} Psychy(90,PA77)<NJ-BURDTMLN>
+ 211 South Main Street/Suite 302-A
Cape May Court House, NJ 08210 (609)465-4442

Harrison, Lawrence Evan, MD {1386733186} SrgHdN, Surgry, SrgOnc(88,PA13)<NJ-UMDNJ>
+ Atlantic Surgical Oncology
100 Madison Avenue Morristown, NJ 07960 (973)971-7111 Fax (973)397-2901

Harrison, Stephen Jay, DO {1043362080} EmrgMd(85,IA75)<NJ-UNVMCPRN>
+ University Medical Center of Princeton at Plainsboro
One Plainsboro Road/Emerg Medicine Plainsboro, NJ 08536 (609)497-4432

Harrop, Elyse Horn, MD {1164472023} Dermat(95,PA02)
+ Dermatology and Laser Center
622 Stokes Road/Suite A Medford, NJ 08055 (609)953-0908 Fax (609)953-5978

Harrop, James Shields, MD {1215957337} SrgNro(95,PA02)
+ Jefferson HealthCare - Voorhees
443 Laurel Oak Road Voorhees, NJ 08043

Hart, Daniel, MD {1548330061} InfDis, IntrMd(00,NJ05)<NJ-MORRISTN>
+ Summit Medical Group Florham Park Campus
150 Park Avenue Florham Park, NJ 07932 (908)273-4300
+ Summit Medical Group
315 East Northfield Road/Suite 1-E Livingston, NJ 07039
(908)273-4300 Fax (973)515-1450

Hart, Karen Manheimer, MD {1679539332} IntrMd(97,MO02)<NJ-VALLEYHS>
+ Prospect Medical Offices, LLC
301 Godwin Avenue Midland Park, NJ 07432 (201)444-4526 Fax (201)301-1313

Hartanowicz, Stanley J., MD {1851421325} Urolgy, GenPrc(74,MEX14)
+ Toms River Wellness Center
10 Kettle Creek Road Toms River, NJ 08753 (732)255-8880 Fax (732)255-8885

Hartanto, Victor H., MD {1376679639} Urolgy(96,WI06)<NJ-VALLEY>
+ Urology Group PA
4 Godwin Avenue Midland Park, NJ 07432 (201)444-7070
Fax (201)444-7228

Hartford, Jeffrey D., MD {1043238439} Gastrn(85,PA07)<NJ-HUNTRDN>
+ Huntendon Gastroenterology
1100 Wescott Drive/Suite 201 Flemington, NJ 08822
(908)788-4022 Fax (908)788-4066
+ Advanced Gastroenterology & Nutrition
1100 Wescott Drive/Suite 304 Flemington, NJ 08822
(908)788-4022 Fax (908)788-4066
+ Advanced Gastroenterology & Nutrition
1738 Route 31 North/Suite 108 Clinton, NJ 08822
(908)788-4022 Fax (908)788-4066

Hartigan, Thomas P., MD {1588782262} Pedtrc, NnPnMd(93,GRNA)<NJ-HUNTRDN>
+ Hunterdon Medical Center
2100 Wescott Drive/Peds/Neonatal Flemington, NJ 08822
(908)788-6100

Hartman, Eric J., MD {1265424337} Ophthl(91,NY08)<NJ-VIRTU-AHS>
+ The Eye Center at Lumberton-Mt. Holly
200 Madison Avenue Mount Holly, NJ 08060 (609)265-9363 Fax (609)265-9424
hollyeye02@aol.com

Hartman, Rachael Dalya, MD {1568636314} Dermat(07,NY01)<NY-VAHARBOR>
+ Dr. Deborah Ruth Spey
101 Old Short Hills Road/Suite 410 West Orange, NJ 07052
(973)731-9600 Fax (973)731-1635

Hartmann, Anthony William, MD {1578582425} EmrgMd(84,NY15)<NJ-SOMERSET>
+ Emergency Medical Associates of NJ, P.A.
3 Century Drive Parsippany, NJ 07054 (973)740-0607
Fax (973)740-9895
+ Emergency Medical Associates
110 Rehill Avenue Somerville, NJ 08876 (973)740-0607
Fax (908)685-2968

Hartmann, Rupert C., II, DO {1003817313} FamMed(73,PA77)
+ 943 Cinnaminson Avenue
Palmyra, NJ 08065 (856)829-4007 Fax (856)786-7729

Hartwell, Richard Conrad, MD {1669581534} SrgNro(82,IL42)
+ Coastal Neurosurgery
9 Hospital Drive Toms River, NJ 08755 (732)341-1881
Fax (732)505-4453

Hartzband, Mark A., MD {1386639722} SrgOrt(94,QU01)<NJ-HACKNSK>
+ Hartzband Center for Hip & Knee Replacement
10 Forest Avenue Paramus, NJ 07652 (201)291-4040
Fax (201)291-0440

Harutyunyan, Anna, MD {1467610014} IntrMd(97,ARM27)<NY-LINCOLN>
+ Physicians Practice at New Bridge Med Ctr
230 East Ridgewood Avenue Paramus, NJ 07652
(201)225-4700 Fax (201)225-4702

Harvey, Alexis, MD {1578559050} RadOnc(85,PA09)<NJ-VIRTVOOR, NJ-LOURDMED>
+ 21st Century Oncology
130 Carnie Boulevard Voorhees, NJ 08043 (856)424-0003
Fax (856)424-0055
+ 21st Century Oncology
17 West Red Bank Avenue Woodbury, NJ 08096
(856)424-0003 Fax (856)848-5855
+ 21st Century Oncology
220 Sunset Road/Suite 4 Willingboro, NJ 08043 (609)877-3064 Fax (609)877-2466

Harvey, Arthur James, MD {1962425843} RadOnc(83,PA07)
+ Urology Care Alliance
3311 Brunswick Pike Lawrenceville, NJ 08648 (609)895-1991 Fax (609)895-6996

Harvey, Danielle Nicole, MD {1437305612} Pedtrc
+ Princeton Nassau Pediatrics, P.A.
301 North Harrison Street Princeton, NJ 08540 (609)924-5510 Fax (609)924-3577

Harvey, Karanja, MD {1952346991} Pedtrc, GenPrc, IntrMd(96,CT01)
+ Princeton Nassau Pediatrics, P.A.
301 North Harrison Street Princeton, NJ 08540 (609)924-5510 Fax (609)924-3577

Harvey, Robert Todd, MD {1104828615} RadDia(95,PA01)
+ Radiology Associates of Burlington County
1295 Route 38 West/PO Box 479 Hainesport, NJ 08036
(609)261-7017 Fax (609)261-4180

Harvey, Samantha K., MD {1043472004} Anesth
+ Bergen Anesthesia Group, P.C.
500 West Main Street/Suite 16 Wyckoff, NJ 07481
(201)847-9320 Fax (201)847-0059

Harwani, Nita R., MD {1073706347} FamMed
+ Summit Medical Group
140 Park Avenue/3rd Floor Florham Park, NJ 07932
(908)273-4300

Harwitz, David Marc, MD {1760541098} Psychy, PsyCAd(96,PA09)<NJ-SJERSYHS, NJ-LOURDMED>
+ Center for Family Guidance, PC
765 East Route 70/Building A-101 Marlton, NJ 08053
(856)797-4800 Fax (856)810-0110

Harwood, David A., MD {1144025079} SrgOrt, SrgOARec(84,NJ06)<NJ-STPETER, NJ-RWJUBRUN>
+ University Orthopaedic Associates, LLC.
Two Worlds Fair Drive Somerset, NJ 08873 (732)979-2115
Fax (732)564-9032
+ University Orthopaedic Group
215 Easton Avenue New Brunswick, NJ 08901 (732)979-2115 Fax (732)545-4011
+ University Orthopaedic Associates, LLC.
211 North Harrison Street Princeton, NJ 08873 (609)683-7800 Fax (609)683-7875

Harwood, Katerina K., MD {1861563249} Pedtrc, PedEnd(98,CZE02)<NJ-STJOSHOS, NJ-HOBUNIMC>
+ St. Joseph's Regional Medical Center
11 Getty Avenue/Peds Endocrine Paterson, NJ 07503
(973)754-2541 Fax (973)754-2548
+ Pediatric Sub Specialty Outpatient Center
186 Rochelle Avenue Rochelle Park, NJ 07662 (973)754-2541 Fax (201)843-6546

Hasaj, Mario Jorge, MD {1043263809} Psychy, PsyGrt(90,ARG01)
+ Palisades Behavioral Care
221 Palisade Avenue Jersey City, NJ 07306 (201)656-3116
Fax (201)656-9044
+ St Joseph's Medical Center Psychiatry
703 Main Street Paterson, NJ 07503 (973)754-2841

Hasan, Bassam I., MD {1346246097} IntrMd, InfDis(81,JOR01)<NJ-KIMBALL>
+ Ocean County Family Care
2125 Route 88 East Brick, NJ 08724 (732)892-4548 Fax (732)892-0961

Hasan, Izhar U., MD {1003919572} FamMed(95,PAK11)
+ Complete Care
1814 East Second Street Scotch Plains, NJ 07076
(908)322-6611 Fax (908)322-8665

+ Primary Care Physicians Inc.
155 Park Avenue/Suite 206 Lyndhurst, NJ 07071
(201)939-1007

Hasan, Omar S., MD {1669602975} IntrMd(01,BAN02)<NJ-NWRKBETH>
+ Drs. Di Vagno, Hasan & Chung
216 Route 17 North/Suite 201 Rochelle Park, NJ 07662
(201)845-3535 Fax (201)845-4040

Hasan, Saba Ali, MD {1700988334} IntrMd(86,PAKI)<NJ-CHSFULD>
+ Capital Health System/Fuld Campus
750 Brunswick Avenue/Medicine Trenton, NJ 08638
(609)394-6000

Hasan, Sanjida, MD {1427189679} GenPrc(66,INA29)
+ 16 Manor Drive
Wayne, NJ 07470

Hasan, Syeda I., MD {1447370259} PsyCAd, PsyGrt, Psychy(82,DOM03)<NJ-OVERLOOK, NJ-STBARNMC>
+ 28 Beechwood Road/Suite 4
Summit, NJ 07901 (908)608-1414 Fax (908)608-9441

Hasan, Uzma Naveen, MD {1679729792} PedInf
+ 18 Ocean Street/2nd Floor
Millburn, NJ 07041

Hasbun, Rafael D., MD {1477533545} IntrMd(82,DOM01)<NJ-VIRTVOOR, NJ-VIRTMARL>
+ Associates in Family HealthCare, P.C.
73 North Maple Avenue/Suite B Marlton, NJ 08053
(844)542-2273 Fax (856)569-4043

Hasbun, William Miguel, MD {1295762466} Grtrcs, IntrMd, FamMGrtc(77,DOMI)<NJ-VIRTVOOR>
+ TLC HealthCare
2070 Springdale Road/Suite 100 Cherry Hill, NJ 08003
(856)985-0590 Fax (856)985-2866
+ 414 Hadon Avenue
Collingswood, NJ 08108 (856)985-0590 Fax (856)854-1687

Hasham, Mohamed H., MD {1982985594} IntrMd
+ Raritan Bay Infectious Disease Consultants
3 Hospital Plaza/Suite 208 Old Bridge, NJ 08857
(732)360-2700 Fax (732)360-2703

Hashem, Bassam Emile, MD {1003900242} CritCr, IntrMd(84,FRA04)<NJ-VAEASTOR>
+ VA New Jersey Health Care System-East Orange Campus
385 Tremont Avenue/IntMed East Orange, NJ 07018
(973)676-1000

Hashem, Jenifer, MD {1861550857}<NY-MAIMONMC>
+ Drs. Sheikh & Weber
201 Route 17 North Rutherford, NJ 07070 (201)549-8860
Fax (201)549-8861

Hashemi, Zaher Mohammad Said, MD {1356345755} Anesth(90,HUN03)<NJ-BAYONNE>
+ Bayonne Medical Center
29th Street at Avenue E/Anesth Bayonne, NJ 07002
(201)858-5000
+ Montclair Anesthesia Associates PC
185 Fairfield Avenue/Suite 2A West Caldwell, NJ 07006
(201)858-5000 Fax (973)226-1232

Hasher-Mascoveto, Wendy M., DO {1295774198} Anesth, AnesPain(91,PA77)<NJ-OURLADY>
+ Our Lady of Lourdes Medical Center
1600 Haddon Avenue/Anesthesiology Camden, NJ 08103
(856)757-3500

Hashim, Anjum, MD {1245410885} Pedtrc(87,PAK01)<NJ-NWRKBETH>
+ Newark Beth Israel Medical Center
201 Lyons Avenue/Pediatrics Newark, NJ 07112 (973)926-7000 Fax (973)923-2978

Hashish, Hisham A., MD {1285718817} PthACl
+ Woodbine Development Center/NJ Human Services
1175 Dehirsch Avenue Woodbine, NJ 08270 (609)861-2164 Fax (609)861-2494

Hashmi, M. Arif, MD {1497743975} Gastrn, IntrMd(76,PAK11)<NJ-VIRTBERL, NJ-VIRTVOOR>
+ Allied Gastrointestinal Associates
502 Centennial Boulevard/Suite 3 Voorhees, NJ 08043
(856)751-2300 Fax (856)751-2333

Haskel, Steven A., MD {1639163561} ObsGyn(84,PA12)<NJ-MORRISTN, NJ-STCLRDEN>
+ 3699 Route 46 East
Parsippany, NJ 07054 (973)335-4466 Fax (973)335-8723

Haskins, Danielle, MD {1144232893} Nrolgy, ClNrPh(04,OH41)
+ Drs. Mehta & Haskins
101 Old Short Hills Road/Suite 401 West Orange, NJ 07052
(973)322-6500 Fax (973)322-6418

Hasni, Syed Shayan Ahmed, MD {1740259746} IntrMd, AdolMd, IntHos(96,PAK11)<NJ-ACMCITY>
+ AtlantiCare Regional Medical Center/City Campus
1925 Pacific Avenue/8th Floor Atlantic City, NJ 08401
(609)441-8146 Fax (609)441-8002

Physicians by Name and Address

Hassab, Joseph E., MD {1235438813}<NJ-VIRTMHBC>
+ Virtua Memorial
  175 Madison Avenue   Mount Holly, NJ 08060   (609)261-4076

Hassan, Ahmad Mohamed, MD {1427391598} PsyCAd
+ Princeton House Behavioral Health - Princeton
  905 Herrontown Road   Princeton, NJ 08540   (800)242-2550   Fax (609)497-3370

Hassan, Farida, MD {1962677583} IntrMd(02,PAK11)
+ 19 North County Line Road
  Jackson, NJ 08527

Hassan, Hardawan Ahmed, MD {1861855991} IntHos
+ Capital Health Hospitalist Group
  750 Brunswick Avenue   Trenton, NJ 08638   (609)394-6031   Fax (609)394-6299

Hassan, Khaled A., MD {1437197837} FamMed, ObsGyn(84,EGY03)<NJ-WAYNEGEN>
+ St. Joseph's Family Health Center
  21 Market Street   Paterson, NJ 07501   (973)754-4200   Fax (973)754-4201
  khassanmd@aol.com
+ St. Joseph's Wayne Hospital
  224 Hamburg Turnpike   Wayne, NJ 07470   (973)942-6900
+ St. Joseph's DePaul Center ObsGyn
  11 Getty Avenue   Paterson, NJ 07501   (973)754-4200

Hassan, Sheref E., MD {1003112244} SrgOrt, SprtMd(07,NY46)<NY-MTSINAI, NY-MTSINYHS>
+ Landa Spine Center
  300 Perrine Road/Suite 333   Old Bridge, NJ 08857   (732)289-9335   Fax (732)289-9336

Hassan, Sherif A., MD {1528279320} Otlryg(02,MO34)
+ The Family Center for Otolaryngology
  47 Orient Way/Lower Level   Rutherford, NJ 07070   (201)935-5508   Fax (201)465-6088
+ The Family Center for Otolaryngology
  1265 Paterson Plank Road   Secaucus, NJ 07094   (201)935-5508   Fax (201)465-6088
+ The Family Center for Otolaryngology
  6 Brighton Road/Suite 104   Clifton, NJ 07070   (973)470-0282   Fax (201)465-6088

Hassan, Syed R., MD {1891922589} IntrMd
+ JFK Medical Center
  65 James Street   Edison, NJ 08820   (732)321-7000

Hassanien, Gammal A., DO {1528262961} IntrMd(04,NY75)
+ 91 Main Street/1st Floor
  Paterson, NJ 07505   (973)523-4000

Hassanin, Ahmed, MD {1851635981} IntrMd<NJ-MORRISTN>
+ Morristown Medical Center
  100 Madison Avenue/Medicine   Morristown, NJ 07962   (973)971-5912

Hassman, David R., DO {1922001841} FamMed(91,PA77)
+ Advocare Berlin Medical Associates
  175 Cross Keys Road/Suite 300A   Berlin, NJ 08009   (856)767-0077   Fax (856)767-6102

Hassman, Howard A., DO {1891915427} IntrMd, FamMed(83,PA77)
+ CRI Worldwide LLC
  1113 Hospital Drive   Willingboro, NJ 08046

Hassman, Joseph M., DO {1831193671} FamMed(65,PA77)<NJ-VIRTVOOR, NJ-VIRTMARL>
+ Advocare Berlin Medical Associates
  175 Cross Keys Road/Suite 300A   Berlin, NJ 08009   (856)767-0077   Fax (856)767-6102
+ Advocare Berlin Medical Associates
  339 Route 73/Suite 1   Berlin, NJ 08009   (856)767-0077   Fax (856)753-7836

Hassman, Michael A., DO {1922002765} FamMed(94,PA77)<NJ-VIRTUAHS, NJ-KENEDYHS>
+ Advocare Berlin Medical Associates
  175 Cross Keys Road/Suite 300A   Berlin, NJ 08009   (856)767-0077   Fax (856)767-6102

Hasson, Marie Elena, MD {1033152707} Psychy, IntrMd(95,PA02)<NJ-ACMCMAIN, NJ-ANCPSYCH>
+ ARMC Faculty Practice Psychiatry
  65 West Jimmie Leeds Road   Pomona, NJ 08240   (609)652-3551   Fax (609)404-7686

Hassoun, Patrice, MD {1841220175} PthAna, PthACl(75,LEBA)<NJ-HACKNSK>
+ Institute for Breast Care
  20 Prospect Avenue/Suite 513   Hackensack, NJ 07601   (201)996-2222

Hastings, Shirin Elizabeth, MD {1245472208} IntrMd(09)
+ UH- Robert Wood Johnson Med
  125 Paterson Street/Rm 2322   New Brunswick, NJ 08901   (732)235-7122   Fax (732)235-7144

Hatchard, John R. E., MD {1669435657} ObsGyn(77,NJ05)<NJ-NWRKBETH, NJ-STJOSHOS>
+ Newark Beth Israel Medical Center
  201 Lyons Avenue/WomensHlthClnc   Newark, NJ 07112   (973)926-7000   Fax (973)923-7497

Hatefi, Homayoon, MD {1285695015} Gastrn, IntrMd(70,IRA01)<NJ-VALLEY>
+ Bergen Medical Associates
  1 West Ridgewood Avenue/Suite 301   Paramus, NJ 07652   (201)445-1660   Fax (201)445-4296
+ 145 Prospect Street
  Ridgewood, NJ 07450   (201)445-1660   Fax (201)445-4209

Hathaway, Elaine G., MD {1588756209} Ophthl(77,IN20)<NJ-STPETER, NJ-UNVMCPRN>
+ Brunswick Eye Associates
  317 Cleveland Avenue   Highland Park, NJ 08904   (732)828-5190   Fax (732)828-0677
+ Ophthalmology Associates
  800 Bunn Drive/Suite 301   Princeton, NJ 08540   (609)924-3700

Hathout, Lara, MD {1588005904} RadOnc
+ Rutgers Cancer Institute of New Jersey
  195 Little Albany Street/PO Box 2681   New Brunswick, NJ 08903   (732)235-2465   Fax (732)235-6797

Hattab, Raed Abdulla, MD {1497701718} PhysMd(93,PAK12)
+ 18 Mulberry Court
  Paramus, NJ 07652

Hatzantonis, John Emanuel, MD {1467551374} IntrMd(89,GRN01)
+ Internal Medicine Associates
  201 Laurel Heights Drive/Suite 201   Bridgeton, NJ 08302   (856)455-4800   Fax (856)455-0650

Hauck, Lisanne Constance, MD {1013076975} Pedtrc, PedCrC(90,PA09)<NJ-RWJUBRUN>
+ RWJ University Hospital New Brunswick
  One Robert Wood Johnson Place   New Brunswick, NJ 08901   (732)828-3000

Hauck, Robert Martin, MD {1437121035} Radiol, RadDia(76,MEX03)<NJ-SJHREGMC>
+ SJH Regional Medical Center
  1505 West Sherman Avenue/Radiology   Vineland, NJ 08360   (856)641-8000

Haupt, Helen M., MD {1548295504} PthAna(81,MD07)<NJ-COOPRUMC>
+ Cooper University Hospital
  One Cooper Plaza   Camden, NJ 08103   (856)342-2506   Fax (856)968-8312

Hauptman, Jonathan B., MD {1457527558} EnDbMt, IntrMd, Rserch(78,NY47)
+ Hoffman-La Roche Incorporated
  340 Kingsland Street   Nutley, NJ 07110   (973)235-5000

Hausdorff, Mark Alan, MD {1093876310} Anesth, PedAne(85,NY47)<NJ-CHDNWBTH, NJ-NWRKBETH>
+ New Jersey Anesthesia Associates PC
  25B Vreeland Road/Suite110/PO Box 0037   Florham Park, NJ 07932   (973)660-9334   Fax (973)660-9732

Hauser, Adam Dankner, MD {1427471972} Psychy, PsyCAd(99,PA01)
+ 1930 Marlton Pike East/Suite D-25
  Cherry Hill, NJ 08003

Hauter, Moneef S., MD {1720220635} FamMed
+ 512 Bloomfield Avenue/Apt 9F
  Caldwell, NJ 07006

Haverty, Thomas Patrick, MD {1922241546} Nephro, IntrMd(80,CA18)
+ Johnson & Johnson Pharmaceuticals Research
  700 US Highway Route 202/PO Box 300   Raritan, NJ 08869   (908)704-5180

Havriliak, Damian John, MD {1720046857} SrgHnd, SrgPlstc, Surgry(87,NY06)<NJ-ENGLWOOD, NY-GOODSAM>
+ 106 Grand Avenue
  Englewood, NJ 07631   (201)227-8500

Hawes, Ruppert Augustus, MD {1982655320} FamMed(91,OH40)<NJ-CHSFULD, NJ-CHSMRCER>
+ Capital Health Family Health Center
  433 Bellevue Avenue/4th Floor   Trenton, NJ 08618   (609)815-2671   Fax (609)815-2672
+ Capital Health Primary Care
  4056 Quakerbridge Road/Suite 101   Lawrenceville, NJ 08648   (609)815-2671   Fax (609)528-9151

Hawkins, Nancy S., MD {1225084973} EmrgMd(85,PA14)<NJ-ACMCITY, NJ-ACMCMAIN>
+ AtlantiCare Regional Medical Center/City Campus
  1925 Pacific Avenue/EmrgMed   Atlantic City, NJ 08401   (609)345-4000

Hawkins, Yolanda C., MD {1598926008}
+ Concentra Medical Centers
  30 Seaview Drive/Suite 2   Secaucus, NJ 07094   (201)223-8530   Fax (201)319-1233

Hawruk, Elizabeth A., MD {1720107741} IntrMd, Rheuma(82,POL02)<NJ-CHILTON>
+ North Jersey Center for Arthritis and Osteoporosis
  45 Carey Avenue/Suite 250   Butler, NJ 07405   (973)283-2700   Fax (973)283-2707

Hawrylo, Richard R., MD {1477529717} SrgPlstc, Surgry(72,NC05)<NJ-MORRISTN, NJ-STBARNMC>
+ Peer Group Plastic Surgery Center

124 Columbia Turnpike   Florham Park, NJ 07932   (973)822-3000   Fax (973)822-1726

Hawthorne, Keith Allen, MD {1265432918} CdvDis, IntCrd, IntrMd(84,CHI06)<NJ-STBARNMC, NJ-NWRKBETH>
+ New Jersey Cardiology Associates
  375 Mount Pleasant Avenue   West Orange, NJ 07052   (973)731-9442   Fax (973)731-8030

Hawthorne-Nardini, Christa, MD {1720472921} PhysMd
+ Bey Lea Village
  1351 Old Freehold Road   Toms River, NJ 08753   (732)240-0090   Fax (732)244-8551

Hayashi, Fumitaka, MD {1255656344}
+ 45 Fox Hedge Road
  Saddle River, NJ 07458   (862)222-0295
  fumitaka.hayashi@gmail.com

Hayes, Ciana Tyiesh, MD {1689836264} Pedtrc
+ Advocare Delran Pediatrics
  5045 Route 130 South/Suite F   Delran, NJ 08075   (856)461-1717   Fax (856)461-1143

Hayes, Lisa Erin, MD {1972907164}<NJ-STBARNMC>
+ St. Barnabas Medical Center
  94 Old Short Hills Road   Livingston, NJ 07039   (973)322-5000   Fax (973)533-4492

Hayes, William P., MD {1881716801} PsyCAd, Psychy, IntrMd(81,NY08)
+ Alexander Road Associates in Psychiatry & Psychology
  707 Alexander Road/Bldg 2 Suite 202   Princeton, NJ 08540   (609)419-0400   Fax (609)419-9200

Hayes Rosen, Caroline Diane, MD {1942368550} NroChl, Pedtrc(98,NY08)
+ Rutgers NJ School of Medicine Neurology
  90 Bergen Street/DOC 5200   Newark, NJ 07103   (973)972-5209   Fax (973)972-5059
  hayesrca@njms.rutgers.edu
+ Pediatric Clinic - UMDNJ
  140 Bergen Street/PediNeuro/G Lvl   Newark, NJ 07103   (973)972-9000

Hayet, Bill, MD {1679548127} Grtrcs, IntrMd(81,NJ05)<NJ-MONMOUTH, NJ-JRSYSHMC>
+ Ocean Park Medical Associates
  1900 Highway 35/Suite 200   Oakhurst, NJ 07755   (732)663-0900   Fax (732)663-0901

Hayet, Rose F., MD {1134204332} ObsGyn(80,NJ05)<NJ-MONMOUTH>
+ Ocean Park Ob Gyn
  1900 Highway 35/Suite 100   Oakhurst, NJ 07755   (732)663-0030   Fax (732)663-0882

Haymond, Jean R., MD {1578504403} Pedtrc, AdolMd(81,IA02)<NJ-OVERLOOK, NJ-STBARNMC>
+ Westfield Pediatrics, P.A.
  532 East Broad Street   Westfield, NJ 07090   (908)232-3445   Fax (908)233-6184

Hayne, Charles W., DO {1194816207} FamMed(78,PA77)<NJ-CENTRAST>
+ Medical Associates of Freehold
  27 Wildhedge Lane   Holmdel, NJ 07733

Haynes, Paul Thomas, II, MD {1669796868} SrgOrt(03,NJ03)
+ Seaview Orthopaedics
  1200 Eagle Avenue   Ocean, NJ 07712   (732)660-6200   Fax (732)660-6201

Hayter, William Aaron, MD {1972028009}
+ North Hudson Community Action Corporation
  197 South Van Brunt Street   Englewood, NJ 07631   (201)537-4442   Fax (201)568-1876

Hayward, Denise H., MD {1881669950} IntrMd(96,NJ06)
+ Fair Haven Internal Medicine
  569 River Road/Suite 1   Fair Haven, NJ 07704   (732)530-0100   Fax (732)530-5895

Hazelton, Joshua Paul, DO {1881915684} SrgTrm, Surgry
+ Cooper Surgical Associates
  3 Cooper Plaza/Suite 411   Camden, NJ 08103   (856)342-2241   Fax (856)365-1180
+ Cooper University Physician Trauma Center
  One Cooper Plaza   Camden, NJ 08103   (856)342-3014

Hazen, Jill, DO {1376624254} SrgPlstc(85,OK79)
+ 311 Commons Way
  Princeton, NJ 08540   (609)921-7747   Fax (609)921-7748

Hazley, Donald J., MD {1588631295} IntrMd(87,BWI01)<NJ-MONMOUTH>
+ Horizon NJ Health
  210 Silvia Street   West Trenton, NJ 08628   (609)718-9350

Hazra, Anup K., MD {1285709311} PthACl(75,INA7X)<NJ-SOCEANCO, NJ-RWJUHAM>
+ UH-Robert Wood Jhnsn Med Sch
  97 Paterson Street/Pathology   New Brunswick, NJ 08901   (609)584-6569   Fax (609)584-6439
  hazraan@umdnj.edu

Hazzah, Marwa Mohamed, MD {1891956876} IntrMd(98,EGY03)
+ United Medical, P.C.
  612 Rutherford Avenue   Lyndhurst, NJ 07071   (201)460-0063   Fax (201)460-1684

He, Ming, MD {1497911531} Nrolgy, OphNeu(89,CHN40)<NJ-JFKMED>
+ JFK Medical Center
65 James Street   Edison, NJ 08820   (732)321-7010   Fax (732)744-5873

He, Ningning, MD {1164699955} Anesth(07,AR01)
+ Advanced Pain Care
2040 Millburn Avenue   Maplewood, NJ 07040   (908)242-3688   Fax (908)242-3902
+ Advanced Pain Care
65 Springfield Avenue/Suite 1   Springfield, NJ 07081   (908)242-3688
+ Advanced Pain Care
2177 Oak Tree Road/Suite 209   Edison, NJ 07040   (732)979-2288

He, Wenlei, MD {1912201930} PthAcl(93,CHN1J)<NJ-HACKNSK>
+ Hackensack University Medical Center
30 Prospect Avenue   Hackensack, NJ 07601   (201)996-2322   Fax (201)996-2156

He, Xiaoli, MD {1255349767} Anesth(83,CHN07)<NJ-RWJUBRUN>
+ RWJ University Hospital New Brunswick
One Robert Wood Johnson Place   New Brunswick, NJ 08901   (732)828-3000

Heacock, James K., MD {1992778153} IntrMd(75,MEXI)<NJ-OCEANMC>
+ Shore Medical Group
1640 Highway 88/Suite 203   Brick, NJ 08724   (732)458-7777   Fax (732)263-9470

Head, William Bryan, Jr., MD {1417013160} Nrolgy(70,CA06)
+ 2333 Morris Avenue/Suite B-17
Union, NJ 07083   (908)353-7111   Fax (908)688-6194

Headley, Adrienne J., MD {1811157936} FamMed(91,NY08)
+ UH- RWJ Medical School
One Robert Wood Johnson Place   New Brunswick, NJ 08903   (732)235-7665

Headley, David F., MD {1649295239} Grtrcs, IntrMd(74,DC02)<NJ-VIRTMHBC>
+ 737 Main Street/Suite 4
Mount Holly, NJ 08060   (609)267-7370   Fax (609)261-6715

Headly, Anna, MD {1629178314} IntrMd(MI01<NJ-COOPRUMC>
+ The Cooper Hospital System-Univ Hospital
3 Cooper Plaza/Suite 215   Camden, NJ 08103   (856)342-2439

Healy, Christine B., DO {1457443954} FamMed(03,ME75)
+ Leonia Medical Associates, P.A.
25 Rockwood Place/Suite 120   Englewood, NJ 07631   (201)568-3335   Fax (201)568-2450

Heard, Delano R., DO {1114086642} Psychy(71,MO78)
+ Nease Associates
111 Chestnut Street/Suite 104   Cherry Hill, NJ 08002   (856)779-0111   Fax (856)779-0936

Heary, Robert F., MD {1659407542} SrgNro, SrgSpn(86,PA12)
+ University Hospital-Doctors Office Center
90 Bergen Street/8th Fl/Ste 8100   Newark, NJ 07103   (973)972-2334   Fax (973)972-2333
heary@umdnj.edu

Heath, Cathryn Batutis, MD {1598842288} FamMed(83,PA09)<NJ-RWJUBRUN, NJ-STPETER>
+ Family Medicine at Monument Square
317 George Street   New Brunswick, NJ 08901   (732)235-8993   Fax (732)246-7317

Heath, John Michael, MD {1487731170} FamMed, Grtrcs(83,PA09)<NJ-RWJUBRUN, NJ-STPETER>
+ UH- RWJ Medical School
One Robert Wood Johnson Place   New Brunswick, NJ 08903   (732)235-7669
+ Family Medicine at Monument Square
317 George Street   New Brunswick, NJ 08903   (732)235-7669   Fax (732)246-7317
+ Center for Healthy Aging
18 Centre Drive/Suite 104   Monroe Township, NJ 08903   (609)655-5178   Fax (609)655-5284

Heaton, Caryl Joan, DO {1063500767} FamMed(80,MI12)
+ University Hospital-University Family Medicine
42 East Laurel Road/Suite 2100   Stratford, NJ 08084   (856)566-7020   Fax (856)566-6188

Hebbalu, Praphulla, MD {1174549331} IntrMd(93,INA28)
+ 63 South Main Street
Cranbury, NJ 08512

Hebbe, Karl Albert, Jr., DO {1063486132} PulDis, IntrMd(97,PA77)<NJ-TRINIJSC, NJ-TRINIWSC>
+ JFK Critical Care
65 James Street   Edison, NJ 08818   (732)321-7680   Fax (732)906-4946
+ Drs. Sarraf and Hebbe
1907 Park Avenue   South Plainfield, NJ 07080   (732)321-7680   Fax (908)561-3917

Hebela, Nader M., MD {1255340410} SrgOrt<PA-UPMCPHL>
+ Brielle Orthopedics PA
457 Jack Martin Boulevard   Brick, NJ 08724   (732)840-7500   Fax (732)840-2088

+ Brielle Orthopedics PA
823 Lacey Road   Forked River, NJ 08731   (732)840-7500   Fax (732)840-2088
+ Brielle Orthopedics PA
1301 Route 72 West   Manahawkin, NJ 08724   (609)971-7616   Fax (609)971-7639

Heching, Moshe, MD {1295078863}
+ 6 Martin Avenue
Clifton, NJ 07012   (973)246-3573

Hecht, Stacey Markowitz, MD {1578579587} Pedtrc(89,NJ06)<NJ-VALLEY>
+ Hecht and Segal MDs
171 Franklin Turnpike/Suite 110   Waldwick, NJ 07463   (201)612-5100   Fax (201)612-4499

Heck, Gary X., DO {1316984180} GenPrc, FamMed(77,PA77)
+ Drs. Heck & Schiavone
222 Gibbsboro Road   Clementon, NJ 08021   (856)784-4999   Fax (856)784-0258
+ Drs. Heck & Schiavone
416 Haddon Avenue   Collingswood, NJ 08108   (856)858-1240

Hector, Christina, DO {1366679169} FamMed, FamMSptM, IntrMd
+ Princeton Sports & Family Medicine
3131 Princeton Pike   Lawrenceville, NJ 08648   (609)896-9190   Fax (609)896-3555

Hedaya, Edward L., MD {1891883997} Ophthl(81,NY09)
+ Invision, Inc.
One Route 70   Lakewood, NJ 08701   (732)905-5600

Hede, Madan M., MD {1053369769} Pedtrc(02,NJ06)<NJ-RWJUBRUN, NJ-STPETER>
+ Somerset Pediatric Group PA
1-C New Amwell Road   Hillsborough, NJ 08844   (908)874-5035   Fax (908)874-3288
+ Somerset Pediatric Group PA
155 Union Avenue   Bridgewater, NJ 08807   (908)874-5035   Fax (908)203-8825

Hedlund, Edward L., MD {1386668622} IntrMd(73,NY20)<NJ-HOLYNAME>
+ 268 Kinderkamack Road
River Edge, NJ 07661   (201)343-4332   Fax (201)343-3991

Heether, Joseph J., MD {1962510842} Surgry, SrgThr(89,NJ06)<NJ-CHSFULD, NJ-CHSMRCER>
+ Capital Health System/Fuld Campus
750 Brunswick Avenue/Cardio Disease   Trenton, NJ 08638   (609)394-6266   Fax (609)815-7814

Hefferan, James J., MD {1508807710} CdvDis, IntrMd(86,NJ05)
+ Associates in Cardiovascular Care, P.A.
1061 Avenue C   Bayonne, NJ 07002   (201)858-0800   Fax (201)858-3367
+ Associates in Cardiovascular Care, P.A.
33 Overlook Road/Suite 205   Summit, NJ 07901   (201)858-0800   Fax (201)858-3367

Heffernan, Kathleen Anne, MD {1891797957} ObsGyn, IntrMd(81,NY09)<NJ-OVERLOOK>
+ Summit Medical Group
34 Mountain Boulevard/Building B   Warren, NJ 07059   (908)769-0100   Fax (908)769-8927

Heffner, Catherine D'aprix, DO {1922075696} Psychy, Nrolgy(00,NJ75)<NJ-MMHKEMBL, NJ-UMDNJ>
+ University Psychiatric Associates
183 South Orange Avenue/E-F Levels   Newark, NJ 07103   (973)972-2977   Fax (973)972-2979
+ Morristown Memorial Hospital/Mt. Kemble Division
95 Mount Kemble Avenue/Psych   Morristown, NJ 07960   (973)971-4758

Hefler, Stephen Edward, MD {1215028196} Pedtrc(68,NY01)<NJ-UNVMCPRN, NJ-RWJUHAM>
+ Princeton Windsor Pediatrics
88 Princeton Hightstown Road/Suite 103   Princeton Junction, NJ 08550   (609)799-4700   Fax (609)799-4545

Hegedus Bispo, Sandra, MD {1194803296} Pedtrc, IntrMd(95,GRNA)<NJ-STJOSHOS, NJ-STCLRSUS>
+ Pediatric Associates, LLC.
1318 South Main Street   Vineland, NJ 08360   (856)691-8585   Fax (856)691-8489

Hegyi, Thomas, MD {1386710754} NnPnMd, Pedtrc(72,NY46)<NJ-RWJUBRUN, NJ-STPETER>
+ UMDNJ RWJ Neonatal-Perinatal
125 Paterson Street/MEB 312   New Brunswick, NJ 08901   (732)235-7354   Fax (732)235-6609

Heidary, Noushin, MD {1487850871} Dermat(05,NY19)
+ Dermatology & Laser Center of Northern New Jersey
347 Mount Pleasant Avenue/Suite 205   West Orange, NJ 07052   (973)740-0101   Fax (973)740-0103

Heideman, Alan J., MD {1114971827} RadDia(87,NY46)<NJ-NWRKBETH>
+ Millburn Medical Imaging
2130 Millburn Avenue/Suite A-8   Maplewood, NJ 07040   (973)912-0404   Fax (973)912-0444

+ Newark Diagnostic Radiologists, PA
201 Lyons Avenue   Newark, NJ 07112   (973)926-7466
+ Millburn Medical Imaging
210 West St. Georges Avenue   Linden, NJ 07040   (908)587-0035   Fax (908)587-0037

Heifler, Gregory Dean, MD {1902998685} FamMed(94,NJ05)
+ 103 Park Street
Montclair, NJ 07042   (973)783-4117   Fax (973)783-5236

Heilbroner, Peter Louis, MD {1861453011} Pedtrc, NroChl, Nrolgy(93,NJ06)
+ Neurology Group of Bergen County
1200 East Ridgewood Avenue   Ridgewood, NJ 07450   (201)444-0868   Fax (201)444-7363

Heim, John A., MD {1538117825} SrgThr, Surgry(85,NJ05)<NJ-OURLADY, NJ-VIRTUAHS>
+ 645 Garwood Road
Moorestown, NJ 08057

Heimann, James A., MD {1528099900} RadDia, RadV&I, IntrMd(82,NY45)<NJ-CLARMAAS>
+ Essex Imaging Associates
5 Franklin Avenue/Suite 510   Belleville, NJ 07109   (973)751-2011   Fax (973)751-4456
DocH301454@aol.com
+ Essex Imaging Associates
1 Clara Maass Drive   Belleville, NJ 07109   (973)751-2011   Fax (973)751-4456
+ Essex Imaging Associates
32 Newark Avenue/Suite 100   Belleville, NJ 07109   (973)844-4170   Fax (973)844-4192

Heimmel, Mark Robert, MD {1942427125} Ophthl(05,NJ06)
+ Freehold Ophthalmology, LLC
20 Hospital Drive   Toms River, NJ 08755   (732)349-7167   Fax (732)505-4322
+ Freehold Ophthalmology, LLC
509 Stillwells Corner Road/Suite E-5   Freehold, NJ 07728   (732)349-7167   Fax (732)431-3312
+ Freehold Ophthalmology, LLC
202 Jack Martin Boulevard   Brick, NJ 08755   (732)458-5700   Fax (732)458-0693

Heinrich, Art, MD {1386665701} IntrMd, OccpMd, OthrSp(80,ROMA)<NJ-RWJUBRUN>
+ Compli-Med
6 Hawthorne Drive   Somerset, NJ 08873   (732)545-2200   Fax (732)545-2693

Heintz, Kathleen M., DO {1437259124} CdvDis, IntrMd(92,PA77)<NJ-COOPRUMC, NJ-MEMSALEM>
+ University Cardiology
3 Cooper Plaza/Room 311   Camden, NJ 08103   (856)342-2034   Fax (856)342-6608
+ Cooper Cardiology Associates
900 Centennial Boulevard   Voorhees, NJ 08043   (856)342-2034   Fax (856)325-6702
+ Cooper Cardiology Associates
1210 Brace Road/Suite 103   Cherry Hill, NJ 08103   (856)427-7254

Heinz, Kristann Wilmore, MD {1720285752} FamMed
+ Stockton Family Practice
56 South Main Street/Stockton Center   Stockton, NJ 08559   (609)397-8585   Fax (609)397-9335

Heisler, Samantha, DO {1366989907} Pedtrc
+ Jersey Shore Medical Pediatrics
1945 Route 33   Neptune, NJ 07753   (732)776-4333

Heist, Jon S., DO {1760501373} FamMed(91,PA77)
+ 361 North Main Street
Glassboro, NJ 08028   (856)881-8618   Fax (856)881-5368

Heist, Kenneth C., DO {1730269481} Ophthl, FamMed(87,PA77)<NJ-KMHTURNV>
+ South Jersey Laser Vision
101A Kingsway West   Sewell, NJ 08080   (856)582-9507   Fax (856)582-4472

Heit, Peter, MD {1912952763} Gastrn, IntrMd(84,MA05)
+ Ridgedale Surgery Center
16 Pocono Road/Suite 310   Denville, NJ 07834   (973)627-7570

Heitzer, Frederic M., MD {1750499034} IntrMd(82,NJ05)<NJ-CENTRAST>
+ 55 Schanck Road/Suite A-12
Freehold, NJ 07728   (732)577-5525   Fax (732)577-0045

Heitzman, Christopher James, DO {1487682605} FamMed(00,NJ75)<NJ-STCLRDEN>
+ Rockaway Family Medicine Associates
333 Mount Hope Avenue   Rockaway, NJ 07866   (973)895-6601   Fax (973)895-5324

Hekiert, Adrianna Maria, MD {1073679916} Otlryg(04,NY03)<NJ-SOMERSET>
+ ENT & Allergy Associates-Bridgewater
245 US Highway 22/3rd Fl/Suite 300   Bridgewater, NJ 08807   (908)722-1022   Fax (908)722-2040
+ Raritan Valley Surgery Center
100 Franklin Square Drive/Suite 100   Somerset, NJ 08873   (908)722-1022   Fax (732)560-5999

Physicians by Name and Address

Helbig, Thomas E., MD {1962457028} SrgOrt(81,NJ05)
  + South Mountain Orthopaedic Associates, P.A.
    61 First Street   South Orange, NJ 07079   (973)762-8344   Fax (973)762-1626
  + The Joint Institute at Saint Barnabas Medical Center
    609 Morris Avenue   Springfield, NJ 07081   (973)762-8344   Fax (973)467-8647

Helbraun, Mark E., MD {1376690032} SrgC&R, Surgry(72,MI07)<NJ-HACKNSK, NJ-HOLYNAME>
  + The Center for Advanced Neurosurgery
    20 Prospect Avenue/Suite 811   Hackensack, NJ 07601   (201)781-5964   Fax (201)881-0700
  + Hackensack University Medical Center
    20 Prospect Avenue/Colon&Rect Srg   Hackensack, NJ 07601   (201)781-5964   Fax (201)525-1667

Held, Sharon L., DO {1609897180} Pedtrc(87,PA77)
  + Harborview KidsFirst
    505 Bay Avenue   Somers Point, NJ 08244   (609)927-4235   Fax (609)927-5590
  + Harborview KidsFirst Cape May
    1315 Route 9 South   Cape May Court House, NJ 08210   (609)927-4235   Fax (609)465-1539
  + Harborview Smithville
    48 South New York Road/Route 9   Smithville, NJ 08244   (609)748-2900   Fax (609)748-3067

Heldman, Jay P., MD {1821087982} Dermat(77,NY01)<NJ-VAL-LEY>
  + 23-00 Route 208 South
    Fair Lawn, NJ 07410   (201)797-7770   Fax (201)797-1660   jcsm10@msn.com

Helfer, Elizabeth L., MD {1891775979} EnDbMt, IntrMd(83,MA05)<NJ-VIRTVOOR, NJ-KMHTURNV>
  + SOM - Department of Internal Medicine
    42 East Laurel Road/Suite 3100   Stratford, NJ 08084   (856)566-6845   Fax (856)566-6906
  + University Doctors
    2301 East Evesham Road/Suite 202   Voorhees, NJ 08043   (856)566-6845   Fax (856)770-1732

Helfman, Alan S., MD {1982610879} Urolgy(82,MEXI)<NJ-NWRK-BETH, NJ-STBARNMC>
  + Essex Urology Associates/UGNJ
    225 Millburn Avenue/Suite 304   Millburn, NJ 07041   (973)218-9400   Fax (973)218-9420
  + New Jersey Urology, LLC
    700 North Broad Street/Suite 302   Elizabeth, NJ 07208   (973)218-9400   Fax (908)289-0716

Heller, Allen H., MD {1417381823} IntrMd, Nrolgy(73,MD07)
  + Bayer HealthCare Corporation
    PO Box 1000   Montville, NJ 07045

Heller, Debra S., MD {1528196615} ObsGyn, PthAna(77,NY09)<NJ-UMDNJ, NJ-HACKNSK>
  + University Hospital
    150 Bergen Street/Pathology   Newark, NJ 07103   (973)972-0751   Fax (973)972-5909

Heller, Diane Beth, MD {1437268109} EmrgMd(99,NY20)
  + 34 Glen Oaks Avenue
    Summit, NJ 07901

Heller, Elliot M., MD {1770688723} Otlryg, SrgPlstc, SrgRec(83,NY08)
  + Associates in Plastic Surgery
    1150 Amboy Avenue   Edison, NJ 08837   (732)548-3200   Fax (732)548-1919

Heller, James Norman, MD {1972546083} SrgCdv, SrgThr, Surgry(76,MA07)<NJ-BAYONNE, NJ-JFKMED>
  + 98 James Street/Suite 100
    Edison, NJ 08820   (732)635-9300   Fax (973)921-9644

Heller, Michelle, DO {1710156799} Pedtrc
  + Advocare West Morris Pediatrics
    151 Route 10/Suite 105   Succasunna, NJ 07876   (973)584-0002   Fax (973)584-7107

Heller, Mitchell J., MD {1275504052} EmrgMd(93,NJ06)<NY-BRKLNDWN>
  + Emergency Medical Associates of NJ, P.A.
    3 Century Drive   Parsippany, NJ 07054   (973)740-0607   Fax (973)740-9895

Heller, Paul B., MD {1508838863} GynOnc, ObsGyn(68,NY09)<NJ-MORRISTN, NJ-OVERLOOK>
  + Carol G. Simon Cancer Center
    100 Madison Avenue/Suite 4101   Morristown, NJ 07962   (973)971-6100

Heller, Philip Arthur, MD {1528190840} Psychy(84,PA13)
  + Cedar Glen Professional Association
    170 Cold Soil Road   Princeton, NJ 08540   (609)896-1122   Fax (609)896-2688

Hellman, Laura J., MD Dermat(86,NY48)
  + 73 Fox Hedge Road
    Saddle River, NJ 07458

Hellmann, Mira C., MD {1730372079} GynOnc, ObsGyn(00,NY08)<NJ-RWJUBRUN>
  + Rutgers Cancer Institute of New Jersey
    195 Little Albany Street/PO Box 2681   New Brunswick, NJ 08903   (732)235-2465   Fax (732)235-6797

Helmer, Diana Lynn, MD {1154547685} IntrMd(82,NJ06)<NJ-COOPRUMC>
  + Cooper University Medical Center/Camden
    3 Cooper Plaza   Camden, NJ 08103   (856)342-2000
  + Volunteers in Medicine
    423 North Route 9   Cape May Court House, NJ 08210   (856)342-2000   Fax (609)463-2830

Helmrich, Robert Florian, MD {1780654269} Pedtrc, IntrMd(98,NJ06)
  + Princeton Nassau Pediatrics, P.A.
    301 North Harrison Street   Princeton, NJ 08540   (609)924-5510   Fax (609)924-3577
  + Princeton Nassau Pediatrics, P.A.
    25 South Route 31   Pennington, NJ 08534   (609)924-5510   Fax (609)745-5320

Helmy, Nayel Ahmed, MD {1356592265}<NJ-MORRISTN>
  + Morristown Medical Center
    100 Madison Avenue/Suite 20   Morristown, NJ 07962   (973)971-5000

Hemrajani, Payal, MD {1528155595} Pedtrc, IntrMd(NJ15
  + Princeton Nassau Pediatrics, P.A.
    312 Applegarth Road/Suite 104   Monroe Township, NJ 08831   (609)409-5600   Fax (609)409-5610

Hemsley, Michael, MD {1851407720} IntrMd
  + Drs. Sunderam and Sunderam
    310 Central Avenue/Suite 102   East Orange, NJ 07018   (973)266-9111   Fax (973)266-1227

Hendershott, Karen Jean, MD {1336310168} Surgry
  + Cooper Surgical Associates
    3 Cooper Plaza/Suite 411   Camden, NJ 08103   (856)342-2270   Fax (856)365-1180

Henderson, Craig E., DO {1902870967} ObsGyn, OstMed(93,NY75)<NJ-MONMOUTH, NJ-RIVERVW>
  + Ocean Obstetric and Gynecologic Associates
    804 West Park Avenue/Building A   Ocean, NJ 07712   (732)695-2040   Fax (732)493-1640
  + Ocean Obstetric and Gynecologic Associates
    2164 Route 35   Sea Girt, NJ 08750   (732)695-2040   Fax (732)493-1640
  + Ocean Obstetric and Gynecologic Associates
    3469 Route 9 North   Howell, NJ 07712   (732)695-2040   Fax (732)493-1640

Henderson, Thomas J., MD {1720095664} FamMed(85,GRN01)<NJ-HCKTSTWN>
  + JFK Family Practice Group
    65 James Street   Edison, NJ 08818   (732)321-7601   Fax (732)744-5614

Henderson Chen, Jessica L., MD {1417994021} EmrgMd(99,NY20)<NJ-HACKNSK>
  + Hackensack Medical Center Emergency Medicine
    30 Prospect Avenue/Main 3619   Hackensack, NJ 07601   (201)996-4614   Fax (201)968-1866
  + DoctorsÆ Office Walk-in Urgent Care
    110 East Ridgewood Avenue   Paramus, NJ 07652   (201)996-4614   Fax (201)265-1355
  + Hackensack University Medical Center
    30 Prospect Avenue/EmrgMed   Hackensack, NJ 07601   (201)996-2000

Hendi, Jennifer Michelle, MD {1053576132} RadDia
  + 70 Valley View Terrace
    Montvale, NJ 07645

Henick, David H., MD {1447366901} Otlryg, SrgHdN(87,NY06)<NJ-ENGLWOOD, NJ-HOLYNAME>
  + 301 Bridge Plaza North
    Fort Lee, NJ 07024   (201)592-8200   Fax (201)592-7786   dhenick@nj.rr.com

Hennawy, Randa Philip, MD {1669451704} BldBnk, Pthlgy(87,EGY03)
  + 535 Coles Mill Road
    Haddonfield, NJ 08033

Henner, Benjamin Joseph, MD {1477880615} GenPrc(99,NY08)
  + 304 Verona Avenue
    Elizabeth, NJ 07208

Henner, Rochelle, MD {1447273420} Pedtrc, AdolMd(82,OH06)<NJ-RWJUBRUN, NJ-STPETER>
  + University Pediatric Associates
    D-1 Brier Hill Court   East Brunswick, NJ 08816   (732)238-3310
  + University Pediatric Associates PA
    317 Cleveland Avenue   Highland Park, NJ 08904   (732)238-3310   Fax (732)249-7827

Hennessey, Adam S., DO {1689818197} EmrgMd<NJ-OURLADY>
  + Our Lady of Lourdes Medical Center
    1600 Haddon Avenue/Emerg Med   Camden, NJ 08103   (856)757-3803

Henning, Jeffrey Scott, DO {1538181045} Dermat, IntrMd(00,CA22)
  + Princeton Dermatology Associates
    307 Omni Drive   Hillsborough, NJ 08844   (908)281-6633   Fax (908)281-6690
  + Princeton Dermatology Associates
    208 Bunn Drive/Suite 1-E   Princeton, NJ 08540   (908)281-6633   Fax (609)683-0298

Henningson, Carl Thomas, Jr., MD {1609858463} IntrMd, OncHem(96,CT01)
  + Atlantic Hematology Oncology Associates, L.L.C.
    1707 Atlantic Avenue   Manasquan, NJ 08736   (732)528-0760   Fax (732)528-0764

Henningson, Karen Jeanne, DO {1609959881} Psychy, PsyCAd(00,MO78)
  + Catholic Community Services
    1160 Raymond Boulevard   Newark, NJ 07102   (973)596-4190

Henriquez, Karina A., MD {1326201484} IntrMd<NJ-STBARNMC>
  + St. Barnabas Medical Center
    94 Old Short Hills Road   Livingston, NJ 07039   (973)322-5000

Henry, Audrey W., MD {1073684031}
  + Capital Health System/Hopewell
    One Capital Way   Pennington, NJ 08534   (609)394-4000
  + Princeton House Behavioral Health - Princeton
    905 Herrontown Road   Princeton, NJ 08540   (609)394-4000   Fax (609)497-3370

Henry, Camille Angela Nicole, MD {1093865115} IntrMd, Pedtrc(06,PA01)
  + Cooper Family Medicine
    1865 Harrison Avenue/Suite 1300   Camden, NJ 08103   (856)963-0126   Fax (856)365-0279

Henry, Elizabeth Robinson, MD {1386769859} Pedtrc(94,PA01)
  + New Brunswick Pediatric Group, P.A.
    1300 How Lane   North Brunswick, NJ 08902   (732)247-1510   Fax (732)247-8885

Henry, James R., MD {1841368958} CdvDis(78,MN04)
  + Medical Associates of Ocean County, P.A.
    1301 Route 72 West/Suite 300   Manahawkin, NJ 08050   (609)597-6513   Fax (609)597-4593

Henry, Ricki M., MD {1205075470} Surgry(77,NJ05)<NJ-JFKMED>
  + JFK Medical Center
    65 James Street   Edison, NJ 08820   (732)321-7000

Henry, Sharon M., MD {1164767109} Surgry, IntrMd(76,NY19)<NY-SUNYBRKL>
  + 3551 Lawrenceville Road
    Princeton, NJ 08540   (609)252-4153

Henry-Dindial, Nicole A., MD {1629174669} FamMed(94,NY48)<NJ-OVERLOOK>
  + Paramount MedGrou -Westfield FamPract
    592 Springfield Avenue   Westfield, NJ 07090   (908)301-0888   Fax (908)301-0883
  + Westfield Family Practice
    563 Westfield Avenue   Westfield, NJ 07090   (908)301-0888   Fax (908)232-0439

Henseler, Roy A., MD {1942379300} Surgry, SrgHdN(69,NJ05)<NJ-MORRISTN, NJ-OVERLOOK>
  + 21 Perry Street
    Morristown, NJ 07960   (973)267-2715   Fax (973)326-6768

Hensle, Terry W., MD {1932253309} PedUro, Surgry, IntrMd(68,NY20)
  + Castle Connolly Medical, LTD.
    699 Teaneck Road/Suite 103   Teaneck, NJ 07666   (201)645-3362   Fax (201)692-1363

Henson, Bernard, MD {1952331746} Surgry(79,MEXI)<NJ-CHILTON>
  + 220 Hamburg Turnpike/Suite 18A
    Wayne, NJ 07470   (973)904-1704   Fax (973)595-8741

Henson, Clarissa F., MD {1568411908} RadOnc(00,NJ06)<NJ-COOPRUMC>
  + Cooper University Hospital
    One Cooper Plaza   Camden, NJ 08103   (856)342-2300   Fax (856)968-8361

Hepburn, Valerie J., MD {1770670481} EmrgMd(83,DC02)<NJ-CHRIST>
  + Christ Hospital
    176 Palisade Avenue/EmrgMed   Jersey City, NJ 07306   (201)795-8200

Herbert, Lisa R., MD {1518070424} FamMed(92,NY15)
  + AstraHealth Urgent & Primary Care
    1100 Centennial Avenue/Suite 104   Piscataway, NJ 08854   (732)981-1111   Fax (732)981-1113
  + AstraHealth Urgent & Primary Care
    95 Hudson Street   Hoboken, NJ 07030   (201)464-8888
  + AstraHealth Urgent & Primary Care
    18 Lyons Mall   Basking Ridge, NJ 08854   (908)760-8888

Herbst, Allison B., MD {1689675068} EnDbMt(92,MA05)
  + Endocrine Associates of Southern Jersey
    703 East Main Street/Suite 5   Moorestown, NJ 08057   (856)727-0900   Fax (856)231-8428

Herbstman, Charles A., MD {1184659344} Radiol, RadDia(75,NY47)
  + Radiology Center of Fair Lawn
    0-100 28th Street   Fair Lawn, NJ 07410   (201)475-1300   Fax (201)475-1709

Herbstman, Robert A., MD {1972557627} SrgPlstc(82,NY45)<NJ-RWJUHAM, NJ-STPETER>
+ Contemporary Plastic Surgery LLC
579A Cranbury Road/Suite 202   East Brunswick, NJ 08816   (732)254-1919   Fax (732)254-0703
drherbstman@cosmeticsurgerynj.com
+ Courts of Red Bank
130 Maple Avenue   Red Bank, NJ 07701   (732)530-6450

Herera, Daniel Joe, MD {1164424958} PhysMd(99,GRN01)
+ The Park Medical Group
24 Elm Street   Harrington Park, NJ 07640   (201)784-0123   Fax (201)784-0065

Heresniak, Victor A., DO {1336194596} EmrgMd, IntrMd(86,NJ75)
+ PO Box 189
Swedesboro, NJ 08085

Herlich, Michael B., MD {1891748109} CdvDis, IntrMd(82,PA09)<NJ-COOPRUMC, NJ-VIRTMARL>
+ Cardiovascular Associates
210 West Atlantic Avenue   Haddon Heights, NJ 08035   (856)546-3003   Fax (856)547-5337
+ Cardiovascular Associates of The Delaware Valley, PA
1840 Frontage Road   Cherry Hill, NJ 08034   (856)546-3003   Fax (856)795-7436
+ Cardiovascular Associates of The Delaware Valley, PA
525 State Street/Suite 3   Elmer, NJ 08035   (856)358-2363   Fax (856)358-0725

Herman, Barry Eugene, MD {1700865607} Gastrn, IntrMd(85,PA09)<NJ-WARREN, PA-WARRNGEN>
+ Twin Rivers Gastroenterology Center
755 Memorial Parkway/Suite 202A   Phillipsburg, NJ 08865   (908)859-5400

Herman, Brad Morris, MD {1760484729} CdvDis, IntrMd, FamMAdlt(84,NY09)<NJ-VALLEY>
+ Medical Multispecialty Associates PA
11-26 Saddle River Road   Fair Lawn, NJ 07410   (201)796-9200   Fax (201)796-7606

Herman, David J., MD {1326014390} InfDis, IntrMd(85,MO03)<NJ-RWJUBRUN, NJ-STPETER>
+ ID Associates PA/dba ID Care
105 Raider Boulevard/Suite 101   Hillsborough, NJ 08844   (908)281-0221   Fax (908)281-0940
+ ID Associates PA/dba ID Care
81 Veronica Avenue/Suite 203   Somerset, NJ 08873   (908)281-0221   Fax (732)729-0924
+ ID Associates PA/dba ID Care
10 Forrestal Road South/Suite 203   Princeton, NJ 08844   (609)759-2750   Fax (609)919-9700

Herman, Eric W., MD {1073605291} Dermat(76,NY47)
+ 411 60th Street
West New York, NJ 07093   (201)867-8550   Fax (201)861-2223

Herman, Glenn O., MD {1790727857} MtFtMd, ObsGyn(71,NY09)<NJ-VIRTMHBC, NJ-VIRTVOOR>
+ Virtua Maternal Fetal Medicine Center
100 Bowman Drive   Voorhees, NJ 08043   (856)247-3328   Fax (856)247-3276
+ Memorial Maternal Fetal Medicine Center
175 Madison Avenue   Mount Holly, NJ 08060   (609)265-7914
+ Barnabas Health Medical Group
166 Morris Avenue/2nd Floor   Long Branch, NJ 08043   (732)263-5024   Fax (732)263-5029

Herman, Gregory E., MD {1760465603} FamMed(88,PA02)<NJ-UNDRWD>
+ Family Health Center of Mullica Hill
155 Bridgeton Pike/Suite A   Mullica Hill, NJ 08062   (856)223-0500   Fax (856)223-1098
fhcmh@snip.net

Herman, Jeffrey P., MD {1659338234} Pedtrc(73,NY06)<NJ-STPETER, NJ-RWJUBRUN>
+ 100 Perrine Road
Old Bridge, NJ 08857   (732)679-5100   Fax (732)679-0452

Herman, Kenneth L., DO {1356382550} IntrMd, EmrgMd(86,MO78)
+ Emergency Physician Associates, P.A.
307 South Evergreen Avenue/PO Box 298   Woodbury, NJ 08096   (856)848-3817   Fax (856)848-1431
kenneth.herman@umhospital.org
+ JFK Medical Center
65 James Street   Edison, NJ 08820   (856)848-3817   Fax (732)744-5614

Herman, Kenneth Louis, DO {1013998756} Dermat, PthDrm, FamMed(84,MO78)<NJ-UNDRWD>
+ Center for Dermatology
17 West Red Bank Avenue/Suite 205   Woodbury, NJ 08096   (856)853-0900   Fax (856)853-5838
kenneth.herman@umhospital.org

Herman, Kevin, MD {1619107703} RadDia<NJ-HOLYNAME, NJ-CHRIST>
+ Advanced Interventional Radiology Services, LLP
718 Teaneck Road   Teaneck, NJ 07666   (201)227-6210   Fax (201)643-3077
kherman@airsllp.com
+ Holy Name Hospital
718 Teaneck Road/Radiology   Teaneck, NJ 07666   (201)227-6210   Fax (201)643-3077

Herman, Marc Arthur, MD {1104881374} Radiol, RadDia(88,PA07)<NJ-ENGLWOOD>
+ Englewood Hospital and Medical Center
350 Engle Street/Radiology   Englewood, NJ 07631   (201)894-3000   Fax (201)894-5244
+ Englewood Radiologic Group PA
350 Engle Street   Englewood, NJ 07631   (201)894-3000   Fax (201)894-5244
+ Advanced Medical Imaging of North Jersey
452 Old Hook Road/Suite 301   Emerson, NJ 07631   (201)262-0001   Fax (201)262-2330

Herman, Martin N., MD {1902862345} Nrolgy, IntrMd(64,IL06)<NJ-JFKMED>
+ JFK Medical Center
65 James Street/Neurology   Edison, NJ 08820   (732)321-7010   Fax (732)744-5873

Herman, Perry Mitchell, MD {1447200878} PhysMd(95,NJ06)<NJ-UNVMCPRN>
+ 18 Centre Drive/Suite 207
Monroe Township, NJ 08831   (609)655-1500   Fax (609)655-4900
+ 3131 Princeton Pike/Building 1/Suite B
Lawrenceville, NJ 08648   (609)655-1500   Fax (609)655-4900

Herman, Samantha Paige, MD {1417199050}
+ 411 60th Street
West New York, NJ 07093   (201)867-8550   Fax (201)861-2223

Herman, Steven Douglas, MD {1255390787} SrgCdv, SrgThr(69,MD07)<NY-MTSINYHS, NJ-RBAYPERT>
+ 268 MLK Jr. Boulevard
Newark, NJ 07102   (973)877-4500

Hermann, Allan J., MD {1649311259} Psychy(65,LA01)<NJ-OVERLOOK, NJ-TRINIJSC>
+ 159 Millburn Avenue
Millburn, NJ 07041   (973)376-4306   Fax (908)889-5201

Hermann, Daniel Eric, MD {1902845746} Pedtrc(99,GRN01)<NJ-MORRISTN, NJ-OVERLOOK>
+ Summit Medical Group-Berkeley Heights Campus
1 Diamond Hill Road   Berkeley Heights, NJ 07922   (908)273-4300   Fax (908)228-3621
+ Summit Medical Group
560 Springfield Avenue   Westfield, NJ 07090   (908)228-3620

Hermann, Todd G., MD {1235138678} Anesth(94,TX04)<NJ-VIRTMARL>
+ West Jersey Anesthesia Associates
102-E Center Boulevard   Marlton, NJ 08053   (856)988-6250   Fax (856)988-6270

Hermosilla, Elias P., Jr., MD {1790887412} Surgry(66,PHI01)<NJ-SOMERSET>
+ 95 Hidden Lake Drive
North Brunswick, NJ 08902

Hernandez, Allyn, MD {1659391274} RadDia(93,PRO03)
+ 9 Honeyman Road
Basking Ridge, NJ 07920
+ University Radiology Group, P.C.
16 Mountain Boulevard   Warren, NJ 07059   Fax (908)769-9141
+ University Radiology Group, P.C.
579A Cranbury Road   East Brunswick, NJ 07920   (732)390-0040   Fax (732)390-1856

Hernandez, Alyssa Kate, MD {1285071043} FamMed
+ Medical Diagnostic Associates, P.A.
1801 East Second Street/Suite 1   Scotch Plains, NJ 07076   (908)322-7786   Fax (908)322-0191

Hernandez, Jacqueline, DO {1477780021} Pedtrc
+ Passaic Pediatrics II PA
913 Main Avenue   Passaic, NJ 07055   (973)458-8000

Hernandez, Marcia Lynn, DO {1902177074} ObsGyn
+ Women's Care Center
3 Cooper Plaza/Suite 301   Camden, NJ 08103   (856)342-2959   Fax (856)968-8575

Hernandez, Michael Dennis, MD {1700830098} IntrMd(99,NJ05)<NJ-HOLYNAME>
+ Bergen Internal Medicine, LLC
6 Horizon Road   Fort Lee, NJ 07024   (201)886-8989   Fax (201)886-8990

Hernandez, Monica M., MD {1235171166} EmrgMd(95,NY08)<NJ-HACKNSK>
+ Hackensack University Medical Center
30 Prospect Avenue/EmergMed   Hackensack, NJ 07601   (201)996-2000   Fax (201)968-1866

Hernandez, Osnel, MD {1447635081} IntrMd
+ St. Michael's Medical Center
111 Central Avenue   Newark, NJ 07102   (973)877-5000

Hernandez, Robert Nicholas, MD {1043552409}
+ Center for Neurological Surgery UMDNJ
90 Bergen Street/DOC 8100   Newark, NJ 07103   (973)972-2326   Fax (973)972-2333

Hernandez, Victor F., MD {1518904036} Psychy, PsyCAd(80,COL06)<NJ-JRSYCITY>
+ Liberty Behavioral Health
395 Grand Avenue   Jersey City, NJ 07302   (201)915-2278
+ Hudson Medical & Mental Health Integrated Service
301 60th Street   West New York, NJ 07093   (201)295-3033

Hernandez, Victor Hugo, MD {1417282971} SrgOARec
+ Rothman Institute - Egg Harbor Township
2500 English Creek Avenue/Bldg 1300   Egg Harbor Township, NJ 08234   (609)677-7002   Fax (609)677-7000

Hernandez, Yanill, MD {1801101472}
+ Invision, Inc.
One Route 70   Lakewood, NJ 08701   (848)222-4690
yanillh@hotmail.com

Hernandez, Zachary Kris, DO {1245677004} EmrgMd<NJ-OVERLOOK>
+ Overlook Medical Center
99 Beauvoir Avenue/PO Box 210   Summit, NJ 07902   (908)522-2000

Hernandez Colon, Agdel Jose, MD {1326195009} Psychy(04,PRO01)<NY-BROOKDAL>
+ Jersey Shore University Medical Center
1945 Route 33   Neptune, NJ 07753   (732)643-4363   Fax (732)643-4376

Hernandez Comesanas, Gricel, MD Pedtrc(83,MEX03)
+ PO Box 451
East Hanover, NJ 07936   (973)344-6190

Hernandez Eguez, Carolina De Lourdes, MD {1598064693} ObsGyn, IntrMd(05,ECU08)<NJ-HACKNSK>
+ Hackensack University Medical Group Westwood
250 Old Hook Road   Westwood, NJ 07675   (201)781-1750   Fax (201)781-1753

Hernando, Franklin P., MD {1053481879} Surgry(65,PHIL)<NJ-BAYSHORE, NJ-RIVERVW>
+ 55 Village Court
Hazlet, NJ 07730   (732)264-7171   Fax (732)264-5388

Hernando, Michael T., MD {1902017296} Surgry, SrgBst, SrgLap(01,MEX03)<NJ-MORRISTN, NJ-STCLRDEN>
+ Morristown Surgical Associates
435 South Street/Suite 230-B   Morristown, NJ 07960   (973)267-2838   Fax (973)267-7909
+ Morristown Surgical Associates
183 High Street/Suite 1500   Newton, NJ 07860   (973)267-2838   Fax (973)267-7909
+ Morristown Surgical Associates
344 South Street   Morristown, NJ 07960   (973)267-2838   Fax (973)267-7909

Hernberg, Scott Alan, DO {1538164009} Anesth, OthrSp(80,IA75)
+ TomorrowÆs Wellness Center
1601 Tilton Road/Suite 4   Northfield, NJ 08225   (609)407-1119   Fax (609)407-1138
twc4u@comcast.net

Heron, Joseph, MD {1629639976} EmrgEMed
+ Kennedy Mem Hospital Emergency Medicine
18 East Laurel Road   Stratford, NJ 08084   (856)346-7985

Herrera, Alejandro J., MD {1558512855} IntrMd<NJ-STPETER>
+ Saint PeterÆs Physician Associate
59 Veronica Avenue/Suite 203   Somerset, NJ 08873   (732)937-6008
+ St. Peter's Family Health
123 How Lane   New Brunswick, NJ 08901   (732)937-6008   Fax (732)729-0869

Herrera, Iris Del Carmen, MD {1457446643} IntrMd(88,DOM14)
+ 90 Bergen Street/DOC 4400
Newark, NJ 07103   (973)972-1438   Fax (973)972-6651

Herrera, Jennifer Emma, MD {1801183793} IntrMd<NJ-STJOSHOS>
+ St. Joseph's Regional Medical Center
703 Main Street   Paterson, NJ 07503   (973)754-2000

Herrera, Juan Carlos, MD {1194832766} FamMed(87,ECU01)<NJ-STMRYPAS>
+ 1034 Salem Road
Union, NJ 07083   (908)258-0045   Fax (908)258-0802
+ United Medical, P.C.
533 Lexington Avenue   Clifton, NJ 07011   (908)258-0045   Fax (973)546-7707

Herrera, Saturnino Domingo, MD {1245324581} IntrMd(78,PHI01)<NJ-HOBUNIMC>
+ Hoboken University Medical Center
308 Willow Avenue/House Physician   Hoboken, NJ 07030   (201)418-2840

Herrera-Figueira, Diego Alberto, MD {1376746362} SrgOrt
+ Advanced Orthopaedics & Sports Medicine Center, PC
1907 Oak Tree Road/Suite 201   Edison, NJ 08820   (732)548-7332   Fax (732)548-7350
dr.diegoherrera@gmail.com

Physicians by Name and Address

Herrera-Garcia, Guadalupe, DO {1497073704} NnPnMd
+ UMDNJ RWJ Maternal Fetal Medicine
  125 Paterson Street/Suite 4200   New Brunswick, NJ 08901   (732)235-6632   Fax (732)235-7349
  gh268@rutgers.edu

Herreros, Claudia, MD {1558851915} ObsGyn
+ University Medical Group/OBGYN
  125 Paterson Street/2nd Floor   New Brunswick, NJ 08901   (732)235-6700   Fax (732)235-6627

Herridge, Peter Lamont, MD {1972833655} Psychy(80,NY47)<NJ-OVERLOOK>
+ Johnson & Johnson
  1 Johnson & Johnson/EmpHlth Rm5G32   New Brunswick, NJ 08933   (732)524-3000   Fax (732)828-5493

Herrigel, Dana J., MD {1760799449} IntrMd
+ RWJ University Hospital New Brunswick
  One Robert Wood Johnson Place   New Brunswick, NJ 08901   (732)235-7742   Fax (732)235-7427

Herrighty, Marianne K., MD {1992740385} ObsGyn, IntrMd(95,NJ05)
+ Contemporary Women's Care
  338 Belleville Turnpike   Kearny, NJ 07032   (201)991-3838   Fax (201)998-4643

Herriman, Daniel Lee, MD {1144256629} IntrMd, EmrgMd(86,OH44)<NJ-KMHCHRRY, NJ-KMHSTRAT>
+ 201 Burrs Road
  Westampton, NJ 08060   (609)652-4858

Herring, Gary S., MD {1669576187} FamMed(89,NJ06)
+ Bergen Medical Associates, PC
  1 Sears Drive/Third Floor   Paramus, NJ 07652   (201)261-5220   Fax (201)261-5223
  doctorgh@aol.com
+ Bergen Medical Associates, PC
  10 East 22nd Street   Bayonne, NJ 07002   (201)339-8889

Herrington, James William, MD {1629061437} Surgry, SrgVas(98,NJ05)<NJ-SHOREMEM>
+ GFH Surgical Associates
  718 Shore Road   Somers Point, NJ 08244   (609)927-8550   Fax (609)926-0273

Herron, Garland Ella, MD {1497808752} ObsGyn(00,MEX14)
+ Meridian Medical Group
  514 Bangs Avenue   Asbury Park, NJ 07712   (732)774-0200   Fax (732)774-1019

Herschmann, Yehuda, MD {1659614089}
+ Center for Neurological Surgery UMDNJ
  90 Bergen Street/DOC 8100   Newark, NJ 07103   (973)972-2326   Fax (973)972-2329

Herscu, Joseph I., MD {1598964686} IntrMd(82,ROMA)<NJ-BAYONNE>
+ Bayonne Medical Center
  29th Street at Avenue E   Bayonne, NJ 07002   (201)858-5000

Hersh, Craig M., MD   FamMed, IntrMd(87,NY08)<NJ-HOLYNAME, NJ-ENGLWOOD>
+ Holy Name Hospital
  718 Teaneck Road/Fam Med   Teaneck, NJ 07666   (201)833-3000
  hersh1@optonline.net

Hersh, Joshua Neil, MD {1457679987} Nrolgy(05,NY08)<NY-MNTFMOSE>
+ Princeton & Rutgers Neurology
  77 Veronica Avenue/Suite 102   Somerset, NJ 08873   (732)246-1311   Fax (732)246-3089
+ Princeton & Rutgers Neurology
  9 Centre Drive/Suite 130   Monroe Township, NJ 08831   (732)246-1311   Fax (609)395-1885

Hersh, Judith Ellen, MD {1922152909} ObsGyn, Gyneco(90,NJ06)<NJ-SOMERSET>
+ Central Jersey Women's Health Associates, PC
  1 Robertson Drive/Suite 25   Bedminster, NJ 07921   (908)532-0788   Fax (908)532-0787
+ Pedi Health Medical Associates
  720 Route 202-206 North/Suite 4   Bridgewater, NJ 08807   (908)532-0788   Fax (908)722-5071

Hersh, Peter S., MD {1366564346} Ophthl(82,MD07)<NJ-UMDNJ>
+ The Cornea & Laser Eye Institute
  300 Frank W. Burr Boulevard   Teaneck, NJ 07666   (201)883-0505   Fax (201)692-9646
  phersh@vision-institute.com
+ Rutgers- New Jersey Medical School
  185 South Orange Avenue/Ophthalmology   Newark, NJ 07103   (973)972-4300

Hershkopf, Richard Jay, MD {1881647063} Pedtrc, PedEnd(74,NY06)<NJ-ENGLWOOD, NY-PRSBCOLU>
+ Pediatric Endocrinology
  214 Engle Street/Suite G-2   Englewood, NJ 07631   (201)871-4680   Fax (201)871-3815

Hershenbaum, Esther, MD {1538278312} Dermat(82,NY08)<NJ-HOLYNAME>
+ Emergimed
  663 Palisade Avenue/Suite 101   Cliffside Park, NJ 07010   (201)945-6500   Fax (201)945-1157
  esther.hershenbaum@emedmag.com

Hershkin, Paige B., DO {1902957723} Ophthl(96,NY75)<NJ-HOBUNIMC>
+ Associated Eye Physicians & Surgeons of NJ, P.A.
  724 Jersey Avenue   Jersey City, NJ 07302   (201)795-0808   Fax (201)795-9797
+ Associated Eye Physicians & Surgeons of NJ, P.A.
  1050 Galloping Hill Road/Suite 104   Union, NJ 07083   (201)795-0808   Fax (908)964-5434

Hershkowitz, Robert P., MD {1003822966} IntrMd(71,PA09)
+ 153 Pavilion Avenue
  Long Branch, NJ 07740   (732)229-3833   Fax (732)229-4080

Hershman, Ilene M., MD {1255300059} Pedtrc, AdolMd(80,DOMI)<NJ-STCLRDEN>
+ 181 Route 46 West
  Mine Hill, NJ 07803   (973)361-1172   Fax (973)361-2415
  nunruch@aol.com

Hershman, Jerald B., MD {1699783019} IntrMd, GenPrc(80,DOMI)<NJ-VALLEY>
+ 1 Demercurio Drive
  Allendale, NJ 07401   (201)327-1800   Fax (201)327-7747

Hersi, Kenadeed, MD {1750792883} EmrgMd
+ University Hospital-New Jersey Medical School
  30 Bergen Street/Room 1110   Newark, NJ 07107   (434)466-1316

Herskovic, Thomas M., MD {1811009483} RadOnc, RadThp(69,MD01)<NJ-STJOSHOS, NJ-CHILTON>
+ St. Joseph's Regional Medical Center
  703 Main Street/Radiation Onco   Paterson, NJ 07503   (973)754-2675   Fax (973)625-0349
  Therskovic@aol.com

Hertz, Marcie B., MD {1164477857} SrgBst, Surgry, IntrMd(84,NY46)<NJ-MTNSIDE>
+ Montclair Breast Center
  37 North Fullerton Avenue   Montclair, NJ 07042   (973)509-1818   Fax (973)509-0532
+ Glen Ridge Surgicenter
  230 Sherman Avenue   Glen Ridge, NJ 07028   (973)509-1818   Fax (973)680-4211

Hertz, Steven M., MD {1326009283} SrgVas, Surgry(87,NY46)<NJ-STBARNMC>
+ Forman-Hertz, MD LLC
  1500 Pleasant Valley Way/Suite 302   West Orange, NJ 07052   (973)324-0988   Fax (973)324-1064

Herzberg, Steven Michael, MD {1093714487} Dermat(69,CT01)<NJ-TRINIWSC>
+ 236 East Westfield Avenue
  Roselle Park, NJ 07204   (908)241-8277   Fax (908)241-8277
  sherzberg@verizon.net

Hesquijarosa, Alexander, MD {1457573586} IntrMd(07,NJ05)<NJ-HOLYNAME>
+ Excelcare Medical Associates
  408 37th Street   Union City, NJ 07087   (201)864-4477   Fax (201)864-9727
+ Holy Name Hospital
  718 Teaneck Road   Teaneck, NJ 07666   (201)864-4477   Fax (201)379-5759

Hess, Jocelyn S., MD {1619062692} Ophthl(90,NY08)<NJ-HCK-TSTWN>
+ Eye Care Northwest
  350 Sparta Avenue   Sparta, NJ 07871   (973)729-5757   Fax (973)729-8322

Hessami, Sam H., MD {1831167162} ObsGyn, Gyneco(93,NY09)<NJ-HACKNSK>
+ Sovereign Medical Group
  15-01 Broadway/Suite 1   Fair Lawn, NJ 07410   (201)791-4544   Fax (201)791-6585
+ SurgiCare Surgical Associates, PA
  630 East Palisade Avenue   Englewood Cliffs, NJ 07632   (201)791-4544   Fax (201)503-1514
+ SurgiCare Surgical Associates, P.A.
  15-01 Broadway/Suites 1 & 3   Fair Lawn, NJ 07410   (201)703-8487   Fax (201)791-6585

Hesselink, Laura, DO {1194141465}
+ GenPsych
  5 Regent Street/Suite 518   Livingston, NJ 07039   (973)994-1011   Fax (973)994-1220

Hessert, Eva Marie, MD {1659353191} Anesth(98,NY15)<NJ-HACKNSK>
+ Hackensack University Medical Center
  30 Prospect Avenue/Anesthesiology   Hackensack, NJ 07601   (201)996-2000   Fax (201)488-6769

Hessler, Sarah Catherine, MD {1891927372} ObsGyn, RprEnd(07,NJ05)
+ The Institute for Reproductive Medicine and Science
  94 Old Short Hills Road/Suite 403E   Livingston, NJ 07039   (973)322-8286   Fax (973)322-8890

Hetling, Kristina, MD {1871550582} Pedtrc(02,NY19)<NJ-VALLEY, NJ-CHILTON>
+ PediatriCare Associates
  20-20 Fair Lawn Avenue   Fair Lawn, NJ 07410   (201)791-4545   Fax (201)791-3765
+ PediatriCare Associates
  400 Franklin Turnpike   Mahwah, NJ 07430   (201)791-4545   Fax (201)529-1596
+ PediatriCare Associates
  901 Route 23 South   Pompton Plains, NJ 07410   (973)831-4545   Fax (973)831-1527

Hetzler, Peter T., MD {1730143751} SrgPlstc, Surgry(81,MI01)<NJ-RIVERVW>
+ 200 White Road/Suite 211
  Little Silver, NJ 07739   (732)219-0447   Fax (732)219-6563

Heverling, Harry Euston, DO {1649443466}<NJ-VIRTMARL>
+ Virtua Marlton Hospital
  90 Brick Road   Marlton, NJ 08053   (856)355-6000

Hevert, Robert A., DO {1073699294} FamMed(66,MO79)<NJ-RWJURAH, NJ-OVERLOOK>
+ 1240 Summit Avenue
  Westfield, NJ 07090   (908)233-6330   Fax (908)233-5636

Hewens, Jeremy C., MD {1306810379} FamMed(76,OH06)<NJ-HUNTRDN>
+ Delaware Valley Family Health Center
  200 Frenchtown Road   Milford, NJ 08848   (908)995-2251   Fax (908)995-2036

Hewitt, James L., MD {1629155544} Psychy(74,GA01)
+ 442 Warwick Road North
  Lawnside, NJ 08045   (856)547-1166   Fax (856)547-5228

Hewitt, Kevin Joseph, MD {1447294046} EmrgMd(89,NY08)<NJ-HACKNSK>
+ Hackensack University Medical Center
  30 Prospect Avenue/EmrgMed   Hackensack, NJ 07601   (201)996-2000   Fax (201)968-1866

Hewlett, Guy Stewart, MD {1437217759} ObsGyn, IntrMd(PA02)<NJ-COOPRUMC>
+ Cooper Ob/Gyn
  3 Cooper Plaza/Suite 300   Camden, NJ 08103   (856)342-2186   Fax (856)968-8575

Heyman, David Mark, DO {1386639854} Anesth, PainMd(85,PA77)
+ Regional Orthopedic, P.A.
  2201 West Chapel Avenue/PO Box 8566   Cherry Hill, NJ 08002   (856)663-7080   Fax (856)663-4945

Heymann, Warren R., MD {1144297318} Dermat, PthDrm(79,NY46)<NJ-COOPRUMC>
+ Heymann, Manders & Green LLC
  100 Brick Road/Suite 306   Marlton, NJ 08053   (856)596-0111   Fax (856)596-7194
  Heymanwr@umdnj.edu
+ The Cooper Hospital System-Univ Hospital
  3 Cooper Plaza/Suite 215   Camden, NJ 08103   (856)342-2439

Heyrich, George Patrick, MD {1316938707} CdvDis, IntCrd, IntrMd(89,DC02)<NJ-BURDTMLN, NJ-SHOREMEM>
+ Mercer Bucks Cardiology
  3140 Princeton Pike/2nd Floor   Lawrenceville, NJ 08648   (609)895-1919   Fax (609)895-1200

Heyt, Gregory John, MD {1861496572} Gastrn, IntrMd(96,NJ05)<NJ-RIVERVW>
+ Red Bank Gastroenterology Associates PA
  365 Broad Street/Suite 1-E   Red Bank, NJ 07701   (732)842-4294   Fax (732)548-7408

Hiatt, I. Mark, MD {1003870163} NnPnMd, Pedtrc(72,NY20)<NJ-STPETER, NJ-JRSYSHMC>
+ St. Peter's University Hospital
  254 Easton Avenue/Neo-Natal Med   New Brunswick, NJ 08901   (732)745-8523   Fax (732)249-9572

Hickey, John Selano, Jr., MD {1033133129} Pedtrc(79,PA13)
+ Kids first
  2006 Salem Road   Burlington, NJ 08016   (609)877-1500   Fax (609)877-4262

Hickey, Joseph J., MD {1639197239} IntrMd(85,PA02)<NJ-VIRTMHBC, NJ-VIRTUAHS>
+ Advocare Medford Station Internal Medicine
  69 North Main Street   Medford, NJ 08055   (609)953-9000   Fax (609)953-9696

Hickman, Renee Booker, MD {1619917788} FamMed
+ Capital Health Primary Care-Bordentown
  1 Third Street   Bordentown, NJ 08505   (609)298-2005   Fax (609)324-8267
+ Capital Health Primary Care Columbus
  23203 Columbus Road/Suite 1   Columbus, NJ 08022   (609)298-2005   Fax (603)303-4451

Hicks, Kristina Elizabeth, MD {1437314606} PhysMd(04,NJ05)
+ North Atlantic Rehab Medicine
  799 Bloomfield Avenue/Suite 303   Verona, NJ 07044   (973)857-7800   Fax (973)857-7822

Hicks, Michael James, MD {1245232198} EmrgMd
+ Patient first
  4000 Route 130/Bldg. C   Delran, NJ 08075   (856)705-0685   Fax (856)705-0686

Physicians by Name and Address

Hicks, Patricia Margaret, MD {1164488284} Allrgy(73,PA14)<NJ-VALLEY, PA-CHILDHOS>
+ Summit Medical Group
574 Springfield Avenue Westfield, NJ 07090 (908)389-6366 Fax (908)232-0540
+ Summit Medical Group-Berkeley Heights Campus
1 Diamond Hill Road Berkeley Heights, NJ 07922 (908)389-6366 Fax (908)790-6576

Hidalgo, Andrea, MD {1427101302} Nrolgy(91,NY20)<NJ-UMDNJ>
+ University Hospital
150 Bergen Street Newark, NJ 07103 (973)972-2550
+ Rutgers NJ School of Medicine Neurology
90 Bergen Street/DOC 5200 Newark, NJ 07103 (973)972-2550 Fax (973)972-5059

Hidalgo, Marla, MD {1164866547} Psychy
+ Summit Medical Group
890 New Mountain Avenue New Providence, NJ 07974 (908)277-8601
+ Summit Medical Group-Berkeley Heights Campus
1 Diamond Hill Road Berkeley Heights, NJ 07922 (908)277-8601 Fax (908)790-6576

Hiemenz, Matthew Charles, MD {1306075379} PthyMGen
+ 104 East 39th Street
Paterson, NJ 07514 (267)648-3057
matthew.hiemenz@gmail.com

Hierholzer, Paul D., DO {1467415851} IntrMd(90,PA77)<NJ-BURDTMLN, NJ-SHOREMEM>
+ 2778 Dune Drive
Avalon, NJ 08202 (609)967-4070 Fax (609)967-4115
+ Point Medical
750 Shore Road Somers Point, NJ 08244 (609)967-4070 (609)653-2247

Higginbotham, Monique Renee, MD {1225006208} Pedtrc(90,OH41)
+ University Hospital-Cares Institute
42 East Laurel Road/Suite 1100 Stratford, NJ 08084 (856)566-7036 Fax (856)566-6108

Higgins, Alexander J., MD {1720077001} FamMed(69,PA13)<NJ-VIRTVOOR, NJ-VIRTUAHS>
+ Advocare Heights Primary Care
318 White Horse Pike Haddon Heights, NJ 08035 (856)547-6000 Fax (856)546-3189

Higgins, Annlouise Maria, MD {1114960317} Anesth(90,GRN01)
+ Paramus Surgical Center
30 West Century Road/Suite 300 Paramus, NJ 07652 (201)986-9000
+ Ambulatory Surgical Center of Union County
950 West Chestnut Street/Suite 200 Union, NJ 07083 (201)986-9000 Fax (908)688-7424

Higgins, James Martin, MD {1225067218} Anesth(88,NJ05)<NJ-OCEANMC>
+ Ocean Medical Center
425 Jack Martin Boulevard Brick, NJ 08723 (732)840-2200

Higgins, Lisa Marie, MD {1386794576} Ophthl(94,NJ05)
+ The Eye Centre
10 Elizabeth Street/Suite 2 River Edge, NJ 07661 (201)488-4412 Fax (201)488-6524

Higgins, Nancy C., MD {1164522652} CritCr, IntrMd, PulDis(86,NJ06)<NJ-ACMCITY, NJ-ACMCMAIN>
+ Atlantic Pulmonary & Critical Care Associates, P.A.
741 South Second Avenue/Suite A Galloway, NJ 08205 (609)748-7300 Fax (609)748-7919

Higgins, Patrick M., MD {1285642470} Ophthl, VitRet(93,NJ05)<NJ-VALLEY>
+ Retina Associates of New Jersey, P.A.
628 Cedar Lane Teaneck, NJ 07666 (201)837-7300 Fax (201)836-6426
+ Retina Center of New Jersey
1086 Teaneck Road/Suite 2a Teaneck, NJ 07666 (201)837-7300 Fax (201)871-4830

High, David A., MD {1972554400} Dermat(81,PA02)<NJ-VIRTMHBC>
+ Dermatology and Laser Center
622 Stokes Road/Suite A Medford, NJ 08055 (609)953-0908 Fax (609)953-5978
kotttonmouf24_7@yahoo.com

Highbloom, Richard Yale, MD {1417984311} SrgThr, IntrMd(PA13<NJ-COOPRUMC>
+ Cooper University Medical Center/Camden
3 Cooper Plaza/Suite 403 Camden, NJ 08103 (856)342-2141 Fax (856)968-7082
Richard_highbloom@chs.net
+ Cooper University Medical Center/Camden
3 Cooper Plaza/Suite 104 Camden, NJ 08103 (856)342-2141 Fax (856)968-7082

Highstein, Charles I., MD {1750478145} Otlryg(79,MD01)
+ Advanced Otolaryngology Associates
557 Cranbury Road/Suite 3 East Brunswick, NJ 08816 (732)613-0600 Fax (732)613-0508

Hijazi, Rana, MD {1538379953} PedNph, Pedtrc, IntrMd(01,GRN01)
+ Children of Joy Pediatrics
134 Summit Avenue Hackensack, NJ 07601 (201)525-0077 Fax (201)525-0072

Hilal-Campo, Diane M., MD {1538151147} Ophthl(91,NY01)<NJ-VALLEY, NJ-CHILTON>
+ 43 Yawpo Avenue/Suite 1
Oakland, NJ 07436 (201)337-9300 Fax (201)405-0558

Hildebrant, Laura Nadine, DO {1043212970} IntrMd(96,NY75)
+ Montgomery Internal Medicine Group
719 Route 206 North/Suite 100 Hillsborough, NJ 08844 (908)904-0920 Fax (908)431-9407
+ Montgomery Internal Medicine Group
727 State Road Princeton, NJ 08540 (908)904-0920 Fax (609)921-0406

Hilderbrand, Rene Francis, DO {1861716292} FamMed, IntrMd(07,NY75)
+ Jersey Rehab, P.A.
15 Newark Avenue/Suite 1 Belleville, NJ 07109 (973)844-9220 Fax (973)844-9221

Hiley, Paul C., MD {1336145176} Gastrn, IntrMd(64,MD01)<NJ-KIMBALL, NJ-COMMED>
+ Ocean County Family Care
2125 Route 88 East Brick, NJ 08724 (732)892-4548 Fax (732)892-0961
+ Ocean County Family Care
400 New Hampshire Avenue Lakewood, NJ 08701 (732)892-4548 Fax (732)901-0744

Hilkert, Robert Joseph, MD {1427355569} CdvDis, IntrMd(85,OH43)<NJ-RWJUBRUN, NJ-STPETER>
+ UH- Robert Wood Johnson Med
125 Paterson Street/Room 2302B New Brunswick, NJ 08901 (732)235-7786 Fax (732)235-8371
hilkert@umdnj.edu

Hill, Eileen G., MD {1245342740} FamMed(80,PA01)
+ Rutgers Hurtado Health Center
11 Bishop Place New Brunswick, NJ 08901 (732)932-7402 Fax (732)932-1223

Hill, Everett Huntington, MD {1770557464} Psychy(82,RI01)<NJ-HUNTRDN>
+ Psychiatric Associates of Hunterdon
190 Route 31/Suite 100 Flemington, NJ 08822 (908)788-6654 Fax (908)788-6452

Hill, Robert B., MD {1700800802} Surgry(74,TX12)<NJ-OURLADY, NJ-COOPRUMC>
+ 80 Tanner Street/PO Box 2028
Haddonfield, NJ 08033 (856)795-1952 Fax (856)429-0335

Hill, Ryan Davidson, DO {1093150880} EmrgMd<NJ-JFKMED>
+ JFK Medical Center
65 James Street Edison, NJ 08820 (732)321-7000

Hill-Hugh, Naomi Lynette, MD {1801851647} Pedtrc(96,DC03)<NJ-COOPRUMC, NJ-VIRTUAHS>
+ Advocare Kressville Pediatrics Sicklerville
431 Sicklerville Road Sicklerville, NJ 08081 (856)875-7444 Fax (856)875-4042
+ Advocare Kressville Pediatrics Cherry Hill
710 Kresson Road Cherry Hill, NJ 08003 (856)875-7444 Fax (856)795-1213

Hillen, Machteld E., MD {1255362463} Nrolgy(95,OTHR)<NJ-UMDNJ>
+ University Hospital
150 Bergen Street/Neurology Newark, NJ 07103 (973)972-4300
+ Rutgers NJ School of Medicine Neurology
90 Bergen Street/DOC 5200 Newark, NJ 07103 (973)972-4300 Fax (973)972-5059

Hilsenrath, Robin Elaine, MD {1659367118} ObsGyn, RprEnd(87,BWI01)
+ Delaware Valley Ob/Gyn & Infertility Group, PC
2 Princess Road/Suite C Lawrenceville, NJ 08648 (609)896-0777 Fax (609)896-3266

Hilty, Amy, MD {1730468489}<NJ-UNIVBHC>
+ University Behavioral Health Care
671 Hoes Lane/PO Box 1392 Piscataway, NJ 08855 (732)235-4433

Hinchliffe, Susan, MD {1356388235} EmrgMd(88,NJ05)<NJ-KMHCHRRY>
+ Kennedy Health System/Cherry Hill Campus
2201 Chapel Avenue West/EmrgMed Cherry Hill, NJ 08002 (856)488-6500 Fax (856)488-6511

Hindin, Lee Eban, MD {1194804153} Psychy, PsyAdd, IntrMd(77,NJ05)
+ 22 Old Short Hills Road/Suite 217
Livingston, NJ 07039 (973)535-0627 Fax (973)535-0628

Hinds, Audrey M., MD {1861461337} IntrMd, Nephro(69,DC03)<NJ-NWRKBETH, NJ-EASTORNG>
+ 310 Central Avenue
East Orange, NJ 07018 (973)678-1631 Fax (973)678-6361

Hinds, Jonathan Anthony, MD {1134564222}<NJ-JRSYSHMC>
+ Jersey Shore University Medical Center
1945 Route 33 Neptune, NJ 07753 (732)776-5000

Hinds, Peter R., MD {1245436518} Urolgy(05,NY08)
+ 140 Bergen Street/ACC Urology
Newark, NJ 07101

Hines, Patrick J., MD {1073614939} Radiol, RadDia(87,NY09)<NJ-CHILTON>
+ Fair Lawn Diagnostic Imaging
19-04 Fair Lawn Avenue Fair Lawn, NJ 07410 (201)794-3132 Fax (201)794-6291

Hinfey, Patrick Blaine, MD {1588616460} EmrgMd(97,NJ05)<NJ-NWRKBETH>
+ Newark Beth Israel Medical Center
201 Lyons Avenue/EmrgMed Newark, NJ 07112 (973)926-7000 Fax (610)617-6280

Hingrajia, Rashmin M., MD {1225260490} AdolMd(03,INA20)
+ JFK Medical Center
65 James Street/EmergMed Edison, NJ 08820 (732)321-7605

Hinkle, Mary Katrina, MD {1447240106} IntrMd<NJ-ACMCITY>
+ AtlantiCare Regional Medical Center/City Campus
1925 Pacific Avenue Atlantic City, NJ 08401 (585)922-4003

Hinrichs, Clay Robert, MD {1295756062} RadDia(98,GRN01)<NJ-UMDNJ>
+ University Hospital
150 Bergen Street/Rm C-320 Newark, NJ 07103 (973)972-4300

Hip-Flores, Julio, MD {1033103528} IntrMd(76,NJ06)<NJ-SOMERSET, NJ-STPETER>
+ Drs. Hip Flores & Chinchilla
281 River Road Piscataway, NJ 08854 (732)356-4665 Fax (732)356-4064

Hira, Ajay, MD {1952660060} RadDia
+ University Radiology Group, P.C.
579A Cranbury Road East Brunswick, NJ 08816 (732)390-0040 Fax (732)390-1856
+ University Radiology Group, P.C.
16 Mountain Boulevard Warren, NJ 07059 (732)390-0040 Fax (908)769-9141

Hiramoto, Harlan E., MD {1528061975} SrgOrt, IntrMd(80,AL06)
+ Hiramoto Orthopaedics & Sports Medicine, P.A.
465 Union Avenue/Suite A Bridgewater, NJ 08807 (908)429-7600 Fax (908)429-7960

Hirawat, Samit, MD {1619102878} MedOnc, IntrMd(94,INA9B)
+ 5 Buxton Road
Chatham, NJ 07928

Hiremath, Vijay, MD {1255328704} Radiol, RadDia, RadV&I(70,INA2A)<NJ-STJOSHOS>
+ Imaging Subspecialists of North Jersey LLC
703 Main Street Paterson, NJ 07503 (973)754-2645

Hirsch, Andrew C., MD {1275588972} AlgyImmn, Pedtrc, Allrgy(88,PA13)<NJ-RIVERVW, NJ-MONMOUTH>
+ Allergy & Asthma Associates
258 Broad Street Red Bank, NJ 07701 (732)741-8900 Fax (732)741-8911
sneezedoctor@msn.com
+ Allergy & Asthma Associates
219 Taylors Mills Road Manalapan, NJ 07726 (732)741-8900 Fax (732)741-8911

Hirsch, Daniel Shawn, MD {1427033513} NnPnMd, Pedtrc(89,PA13)<NJ-SOMERSET>
+ RWJ University Hospital Somerset
110 Rehill Avenue Somerville, NJ 08876 (908)685-2200

Hirsch, David Jay, MD {1588657423} ObsGyn(77,IL42)<NJ-MORRISTN>
+ Lifeline Medical Associates, LLC
50 Cherry Hill Road/Suite 303 Parsippany, NJ 07054 (973)335-8500 Fax (973)335-8429

Hirsch, Gregory D., MD {1831114362} ObsGyn(93,NY48)<NJ-SOMERSET>
+ 203 Omni Drive
Hillsborough, NJ 08844 (908)904-4966 Fax (908)904-4968

Hirsch, Harvey Alan, MD {1972620516} Pedtrc(79,MEXI)<NJ-CENTRAST>
+ Chemed Family Health Center
1771 Madison Avenue Lakewood, NJ 08701 (732)364-2144 Fax (732)364-3559

Hirsch, Howard J., MD {1699863720} MRIimag, Radiol, RadDia(84,NY08)<NJ-CHRIST>
+ Magnetic Resonance Imaging
142 Palisade Avenue Jersey City, NJ 07306 (201)795-0700 Fax (201)795-0874
+ Christ Hospital
176 Palisade Avenue/Radiology Jersey City, NJ 07306 (201)795-8200

Hirsch, Laurence J., MD {1558467068} EnDbMt(78,MA01)
+ Becton Dickinson & Company
1 Becton Drive/Suite 084/Diabetes Care Franklin Lakes, NJ 07417 (201)847-6800 Fax (201)848-0457

Physicians by Name and Address

Hirsch, Martin A., MD {1881694214} Radiol, RadDia(80,NY20)
+ Hirsch & Ratakonda MD, PA
290 Madison Avenue/Suite 4   Morristown, NJ 07960
(973)538-8181   Fax (973)538-6565

Hirschfeld, James M., MD {1023022407} Ophthl(96,NY19)<NJ-STCLRDOV>
+ Silverstein Eye Group
408 Main Street   Chester, NJ 07930   (908)879-7297   Fax (908)879-4798
+ Lakeland Ophthalmology
3799 Route 46 East/Suite 300   Parsippany, NJ 07054
(908)879-7297   Fax (973)331-9777

Hirschfeld, Laura Ann, MD {1376577445} Ophthl(96,NY19)<NJ-NWTNMEM, NJ-STCLRDOV>
+ Eye Physicians of Sussex County
183 High Street/Suite 2200   Newton, NJ 07860   (973)383-6345   Fax (973)383-0032
+ Lakeland Ophthalmology
3799 Route 46 East/Suite 300   Parsippany, NJ 07054
(973)383-6345   Fax (973)331-9777

Hirsh, Alina Z., MD {1609008333} RadOnc(05,NY48)
+ New Jersey Urology LLC
2090 Springdale Road/Suite D   Cherry Hill, NJ 08003
(856)751-9010   Fax (856)985-1600

Hirsh, Andrew L., MD {1912182189} Urolgy, Surgry(05,NY48)
+ Jersey Urology Group
403 Bethel Road   Somers Point, NJ 08244   (609)927-8746   Fax (609)601-1406

Hirsh, Ellen J., MD {1992771976} InfDis, IntrMd(88,NJ06)<NJ-UNVMCPRN, NJ-HCKTSTWN>
+ ID Associates PA/dba ID Care
105 Raider Boulevard/Suite 101   Hillsborough, NJ 08844
(908)281-0221   Fax (908)281-0940
+ ID Associates PA/dba ID Care
81 Veronica Avenue/Suite 203   Somerset, NJ 08873
(908)281-0221   Fax (732)729-0924

Hirsh, Jennifer L., MD {1587744742} Anesth(89,CT01)<NJ-UNVMCPRN>
+ University Medical Center of Princeton at Plainsboro
One Plainsboro Road/Anesth   Plainsboro, NJ 08536
(609)497-4329

Hirsh, Robert Alan, MD {1518067206} Anesth, PainMd, Anes-Pain(84,NY46)<NJ-COOPRUMC>
+ Cooper University Hospital
One Cooper Plaza   Camden, NJ 08103   (856)342-2425

Hirsh, Ron, MD {1710925094} Psychy(83,ITAL)<NJ-STJOSHOS>
+ St. Joseph's Regional Medical Center
703 Main Street/Pschtry/X6500   Paterson, NJ 07503
(973)754-2000   Fax (973)754-2839

Hirshfield, Kim Marie, MD {1841374790} IntrMd, OncHem, MedOnc(99,NJ06)<NJ-RWJUBRUN>
+ Rutgers Cancer Institute of New Jersey
195 Little Albany Street/PO Box 2681   New Brunswick, NJ 08903   (732)235-6028   Fax (732)235-5331

Hirth, Thomas G., MD {1538120514} Anesth(02,NJ05)<NJ-HACKNSK>
+ Hackensack University Medical Center
30 Prospect Avenue/Anesth   Hackensack, NJ 07601
(201)996-2000   Fax (201)488-6769
+ Hackensack University MC-Anesthesia Dept
30 Prospect Avenue/Room 2703   Hackensack, NJ 07601
(201)996-2000   Fax (201)996-3962

Hmoud, Talat Yousef, MD {1295727758} IntrMd, EmrgMd(80,JOR01)
+ 34 Bluffs Court
Hamburg, NJ 07419

Ho, Allen C., MD {1922056712} Ophthl, VitRet(88,NY01)
+ Mid Atlantic Retina - Wills Eye Retina Surgeons
501 Cooper Landing Road   Cherry Hill, NJ 08002   (856)667-2246   Fax (856)667-2238
Acho@att.net
+ Mid Atlantic Retina - Wills Eye Retina Surgeons
1417 Cantillon Boulevard   Mays Landing, NJ 08330
(856)667-2246   Fax (609)625-0788

Ho, Bryan Tao, MD {1417960238} Otlryg(89,NY47)<NJ-ENGLWOOD>
+ Englewood Ear Nose & Throat, P.C.
216 Engle Street/Suite 101   Englewood, NJ 07631
(201)816-9800   Fax (201)567-1569

Ho, Christopher, MD {1578563797}
+ Pathlink, LLC
66 West Gilbert Street/Suite 100   Tinton Falls, NJ 07701
(212)732-0060   Fax (212)732-0061

Ho, Diana, MD {1730677527} Obstet
+ University Medical Group/OBGYN
125 Paterson Street/2nd Floor   New Brunswick, NJ 08901
(732)235-6735   Fax (732)235-6627

Ho, Eddie Kasing, MD {1104864925} IntrMd(95,NY08)<NJ-HOLYNAME>
+ Primary Care NJ
370 Grand Avenue/Suite 102   Englewood, NJ 07631
(201)567-3370   Fax (201)816-1365

Ho, Henry C., MD {1841412624} Gastrn, IntrMd(06,NJ02)
+ Cooper Digestive Health Institute
501 Fellowship Road/Suite 101   Mount Laurel, NJ 08054
(856)642-2133   Fax (856)380-7712

Ho, John, MD {1518963933} FamMed(91,NY09)
+ 16 Pocono Road/Suite 110
Denville, NJ 07834   (973)586-3700   Fax (973)586-8666

Ho, Leo E., MD {1700057817} Pedtrc
+ Children's Health Associates II LLC
101 Carnie Boulevard   Voorhees, NJ 08043   (856)782-3300   Fax (856)504-8029

Ho, Linden D., MD {1881754794} Allrgy, Pedtrc, AlgyImmn(76,CA14)<NJ-CENTRAST, NJ-BAYSHORE>
+ The Allergy & Asthma Group
717 North Beers Street/Suite 2 A   Holmdel, NJ 07733
(732)739-0660   Fax (732)739-1406
+ The Allergy & Asthma Group
100 Craig Road/Suite 204   Manalapan, NJ 07726
(732)739-0660   Fax (732)683-1070
+ The Allergy & Asthma Group
368 Lakehurst Road/Suite 304   Toms River, NJ 07733
(732)349-6856   Fax (732)349-0117

Ho, Maggie May, DO {1073516613} Anesth(92,NY75)<NJ-STCLR-DEN>
+ St. Clare's Hospital-Denville Campus
25 Pocono Road/Anest/ViceChair   Denville, NJ 07834
(973)625-6000
+ Morris Anesthesia Group, PA
3799 Route 46/Suite 211   Parsippany, NJ 07054   (973)625-6000   Fax (973)335-1448

Ho, Victor T., MD {1356424659} SrgNro(76,NY15)<NJ-NWRK-BETH>
+ Newark Beth Israel Medical Center
201 Lyons Avenue/Surgry/L3   Newark, NJ 07112   (973)926-7000

Ho, Vincent Yih, MD {1720390891} Ophthl
+ Retina Associates of New Jersey, P.A.
3196 Kennedy Boulevard   Union City, NJ 07087   (201)867-2999   Fax (201)867-4440
+ Retina Associates of New Jersey, P.A.
2952 Vauxhall Road   Vauxhall, NJ 07088   (201)867-2999   Fax (908)349-8134
+ Retina Associates of New Jersey, P.A.
5 Franklin Avenue   Belleville, NJ 07087   (973)450-5100   Fax (973)450-9494

Hoang, Loan Kim, MD {1720405798} EmrgMd
+ Emergency Physician Associates, P.A.
307 South Evergreen Avenue/PO Box 298   Woodbury, NJ 08096   (856)848-3817   Fax (856)848-1431

Hoang, Michelle Phi, MD {1174967426}
+ Warren Primary Care
23 Mountain Boulevard   Warren, NJ 07059   (908)598-7970   Fax (908)322-4989

Hobayan, Edgar R., MD {1023072469} Surgry(71,PHIL)<NJ-RWJURAH, NJ-JFKMED>
+ 1907 Park Avenue
South Plainfield, NJ 07080   (908)561-7739   Fax (908)757-3671

Hobson, Lendbergh, Jr., DO {1437177284}<NJ-NWRKBETH>
+ Newark Beth Israel Medical Center
201 Lyons Avenue   Newark, NJ 07112   (973)926-7000

Hocbo, Aileen Aileen, MD {1912130105} IntrMd, IntHos(04,PHI01)<NJ-ACMCITY>
+ AtlantiCare Hospitalist Program
1925 Pacific Avenue/8th Floor   Atlantic City, NJ 08401
(609)441-8146   Fax (609)441-8002

Hochberg, Michael Lawrence, MD {1932279114} EmrgMd(00,NJ06)<NJ-STPETER>
+ St. Peter's University Hospital
254 Easton Avenue   New Brunswick, NJ 08901   (732)745-8600

Hochman, Lisa G., MD {1992799134} Dermat(87,NJ05)<NJ-OVERLOOK>
+ Advanced Dermatology, Laser, and MOHS Surgery Center
240 East Grove Street   Westfield, NJ 07090   (908)232-6446   Fax (908)232-6447
+ Morristown Dermatology
290 Madison Avenue/Bldg 5   Morristown, NJ 07960
(973)538-7171

Hochman, Steven Mark, MD {1538175633} EmrgMd, EmrgEMed(01,NJ05)<NJ-STJOSHOS>
+ St Joseph's Medical Center Emergency
703 Main Street   Paterson, NJ 07503   (973)754-2240   Fax (973)754-2249

Hochstadt, Bruce A., MD {1174022347} InsrMd(85,MA05)
+ 2 Tower Center Boulevard/Suite 1101g
East Brunswick, NJ 08816   (646)668-4507

Hochstein, Martin A., MD {1255406427} EnDbMt, IntrMd(69,KY02)<NJ-VALLEY, NJ-HACKNSK>
+ Bergen Medical Associates
466 Old Hook Road/Suite 1   Emerson, NJ 07630   (201)967-8221   Fax (201)967-0340

+ 1 Sears Drive
Paramus, NJ 07652   (201)967-8221   Fax (201)986-0608

Hock, Doreen L., MD {1235169061} FrtInf, ObsGyn, RprEnd(91,NJ06)<NJ-STPETER>
+ Reproductive Medicine Associates of New Jersey
25 Rockwood Place   Englewood, NJ 07631   (201)569-7773   Fax (201)569-8143
+ Reproductive Medicine Associates of New Jersey
475 Prospect Avenue/Suite 101   West Orange, NJ 07052
(201)569-7773   Fax (973)290-8370
+ Reproductive Medicine Associates of New Jersey
111 Madison Avenue/Suite 100   Morristown, NJ 07631
(973)971-4600   Fax (973)290-8370

Hodach-Avalos, Meredith J., MD {1144407412}
+ Princeton Medicine
5 Plainsboro Road/Suite 300   Plainsboro, NJ 08536
(609)240-1153   Fax (609)853-7271
mhavalos@gmail.com

Hodes, Steven E., MD {1578561759} Gastrn, IntrMd(74,NY46)
+ Gastroenterology Consultants PA
205 May Street/Suite 201   Edison, NJ 08837   (732)661-9225   Fax (732)661-9259

Hodges, David M., MD {1881734168} CdvDis, IntrMd(84,NY19)<NJ-HOLYNAME, NJ-ENGLWOOD>
+ Englewood Health Care Associates
200 Grand Avenue   Englewood, NJ 07631   (201)816-9266   Fax (201)816-9242

Hodgson, Elizabeth Susan, MD {1821017914} Pedtrc(78,CT01)<NJ-RWJUBRUN, NJ-STPETER>
+ St. Peter's Dorothy B. Hersh Child Protection Center
123 How Lane   New Brunswick, NJ 08901   (732)448-1000

Hodosh, Richard M., MD {1861580755} SrgNro(72,OH41)
+ Atlantic Brain & Spine, LLC
99 Beauvoir Avenue   Summit, NJ 07902   (908)522-4979   Fax (908)522-5377

Hoebich, Karen A., MD {1407903594} ObsGyn(83,DOM03)<NJ-SOMERSET, NJ-JFKMED>
+ 1139 Raritan Road/Suite 204
Clark, NJ 07066   (732)669-0999   Fax (732)669-0994

Hoelzel, Donald W., MD {1194797456} Pedtrc(89,NJ06)<NJ-MORRISTN>
+ Family Health Center
200 South Street/Suite 4   Morristown, NJ 07960   (973)889-6800

Hoelzer, Dennis James, MD {1922192749} PedSrg(72,NY45)<NJ-COOPRUMC>
+ Cooper Surgical Associates
3 Cooper Plaza/Suite 411   Camden, NJ 08103   (856)342-2270   Fax (856)365-1180
+ Cooper Orthopaedics
2 Plaza Drive/Suite 202   Sewell, NJ 08080   (856)342-2270   Fax (856)270-4012

Hoenig, Sandra R., MD {1043473309} FamMed
+ 170 Changebridge Road
Montville, NJ 07045   (973)575-5540   Fax (973)575-4885

Hoette, Petra, MD {1841283298} FamMed(00,GER07)<NJ-HUNTRDN>
+ Hunterdon Family Medicine
1100 Wescott Drive/Suite 101   Flemington, NJ 08822
(908)788-6535   Fax (908)788-6536

Hoey, Courtney Leigh, MD {1992904072}
+ Summit Radiological Associates, PA
1811 Springfield Avenue   New Providence, NJ 07974
(908)522-9111

Hoey, Kathleen Marie, MD {1619193240} FamMed(88,MNT01)
+ 125 Route 46
Budd Lake, NJ 07828

Hoey, Stephen E., DO {1548359607} IntrMd(81,NJ75)
+ South Woods State Prison/NJ Dept of Corrections
215 South Burlington Road   Bridgeton, NJ 08302
(856)459-7000

Hoffler, Charles E., II, MD {1043496896} SrgOrt
+ Rothman Institute
999 Route 73 North/3rd Fl   Marlton, NJ 08053   (856)821-6360   Fax (856)821-6359

Hoffman, Barry M., DO {1194743641} FamMed(69,PA77)<NJ-VIRTVOOR>
+ University Hospital-University Family Medicine
42 East Laurel Road/Suite 2100   Stratford, NJ 08084
(856)566-7020   Fax (856)566-6188

Hoffman, Christian T., III, MD {1427097674} ObsGyn(91,NJ06)<NJ-KIMBALL>
+ Women's Health Associates
101 Prospect Street/Suite 202   Lakewood, NJ 08701
(732)942-4442
+ Kimball Medical Center
600 River Avenue   Lakewood, NJ 08701   (732)363-1900

Hoffman, David Sandor, MD {1013972322} Ophthl(83,PA07)<NJ-OVERLOOK>
+ 803 Springfield Avenue
Summit, NJ 07901   (908)273-9500   Fax (908)273-4626

Hoffman, Esther Sima, DO {1730558354} IntrMd
+ Hackensack University Medical Group Dumont
125 Washington Avenue   Dumont, NJ 07628   (201)374-2722   Fax (201)374-2723

Hoffman, Jenna Whylings, MD {1942627575}<NJ-COOPRUMC>
+ Virtua Voorhees
100 Bowman Drive   Voorhees, NJ 08043   (856)247-3000

Hoffman, Joseph Henry, MD {1619103629} CritCr, IntrMd, PulDis(83,CT02)
+ 273 Vitmar Place
Park Ridge, NJ 07656

Hoffman, Mark Andrew, MD {1639174048} IntrMd(83,DMN01)<NJ-BAYONNE, NJ-STMRYPAS>
+ United Medical, P.C.
988 Broadway/Suite 201   Bayonne, NJ 07002   (201)339-6111   Fax (201)339-6333
+ South Hudson Medical Associates, PA
19 East 27th Street   Bayonne, NJ 07002   (201)339-6111   Fax (201)339-0506

Hoffman, Michael J., MD {1447215165} Surgry, SrgVas(80,MD01)
+ Northwest Surgical Associates
121 Center Grove Road   Randolph, NJ 07869   (973)328-1414   Fax (973)361-1085

Hoffman, Russell R., MD {1356476063} ObsGyn(87,MEX03)<NJ-OVERLOOK>
+ 576 Springfield Avenue
Summit, NJ 07901   (908)273-3335   Fax (908)273-4648

Hoffman-Wadhwa, Nancy I., MD {1689732216} IntrMd(82,GRN01)
+ 215 East Camden Avenue/Suite H-13
Moorestown, NJ 08057

Hofgaertner, Wolfgang Theodor, MD PthCln(92,GER05)
+ 89 Brooklake Road/Suite A
Florham Park, NJ 07932

Hofmann, William Andrew, III, DO {1376549642} IntMAdMd, IntrMd(84,PA77)
+ Cape Regional Physicians Associates
336 96th Street/Suite 1   Stone Harbor, NJ 08247   (609)967-0070   Fax (609)967-0077

Hogan, Elizabeth Anne, MD {1073598561} Psychy(93,NJ06)<NJ-ANNKLEIN>
+ Ann Klein Forensic Center
1609 Stuyvesant Avenue/PO Box 7717   West Trenton, NJ 08628   (609)633-0900

Hogan, James R., MD {1093079121} PedRad
+ University Radiology Group, P.C.
579A Cranbury Road   East Brunswick, NJ 08816   (732)390-0040   Fax (732)390-1856

Hogan, Jonathan James, MD {1366644791}
+ Penn Medicine at Woodbury Heights
1006 Mantua Pike   Woodbury Heights, NJ 08097   (215)662-2638   Fax (856)845-0535
jonathan.hogan2@uphs.upenn.edu

Hogan, Kimberly Ann, MD {1588854459} FamMed(94,WI06)
+ Family Medicine Center
1301 Route 72 West/Suite 240   Manahawkin, NJ 08050   (609)597-7394   Fax (609)597-6833

Hogan, Robert P., DO {1396708632} Hemato, IntrMd, MedOnc(86,NJ75)<NJ-STPETER, NJ-RWJUBRUN>
+ 1239 Parkway Ave./Suite 203
Ewing, NJ 08628   (609)833-5454   Fax (609)882-2565

Hogshire, Lauren Christine, MD {1083871479} IntrMd(07,NY01)
+ University Medical Group - General Internal Medicine
125 Paterson Street/Suite 5100A   New Brunswick, NJ 08903   (732)235-6968   Fax (732)235-8935

Hogue, Donna J., DO {1215939061} PulDis, PulCCr, IntrMd(91,PA77)
+ The Cooper Health System at Voorhees
900 Centennial Boulevard   Voorhees, NJ 08043   (856)325-6789   Fax (856)325-6545

Hohl, Rosario DeFatima M., MD {1144321472} IntrMd(88,MEX14)<NJ-CHSFULD, NJ-CHSMRCER>
+ Drs. Stillwell & Hohl
1423 Pennington Road   Trenton, NJ 08618   (609)882-8080   Fax (609)882-8433

Hohmuth, Benjamin Adam, MD {1508822081} IntHos, IntrMd(99,NJ05)<NJ-ENGLWOOD>
+ Englewood Hospital and Medical Center
350 Engle Street/Hospitalist   Englewood, NJ 07631   (201)894-3000

Holaday, William J., MD {1851392112} SrgVas, Surgry(79,OH06)
+ Rancocas Valley Surgical Associates PA
1000 Salem Road/Suite A   Willingboro, NJ 08046   (609)877-1737   Fax (609)877-1589

Holahan, Joseph A., MD {1871534230} Pedtrc, PedNrD(70,NJ05)<NJ-STJOSHOS>
+ St. Joseph's Children's Hospital
703 Main Street/Dvlpmntl Pdtrcs   Paterson, NJ 07503   (973)754-2510

Holahan, Nancy C., MD {1518908441} Pedtrc, OthrSp, PedNrD(70,NJ05)<NJ-STJOSHOS, NJ-HOBUNIMC>
+ St. Joseph's Children's Hospital
703 Main Street/Dvlpmntl Pdtrcs   Paterson, NJ 07503   (973)754-2510

Holbrook, David Vining, MD {1609943885} Psychy, PsyCAd(97,NY46)
+ 1109a Highway 31 South
Lebanon, NJ 08833   (908)730-5900   Fax (908)730-5900

Holcomb, Brenda E., DO {1982030474} Grtrcs, IntrMd(88,NJ75)<NJ-STBARNMC>
+ 82 Roland Road
New Providence, NJ 07974

Holdbrook, Thomas, MD {1568663326} PthACli(07,PA02)<NJ-COOPRUMC>
+ Cooper University Hospital
One Cooper Plaza/Pathology   Camden, NJ 08103   (856)356-4935

Holdcraft, Suzanne, MD {1578503405} FamMed(83,PA02)<NJ-HUNTRDN>
+ Hopewell Family Practice & Sports Medicine
84 Route 31 North/Suite 103   Pennington, NJ 08534   (609)730-1771   Fax (609)730-1274

Holden, Douglas Scott, MD {1861469694} SrgOrt(95,NY01)<NJ-HACKNSK, NJ-VALLEY>
+ Garden State Orthopaedic Associates, P.A.
400 Franklin Turnpike/Suite 112   Mahwah, NJ 07430   (201)825-2266   Fax (201)825-9727
+ Garden State Orthopaedic Associates, P.A.
33-41 Newark Street   Hoboken, NJ 07030   (201)825-2266   Fax (201)876-5305
+ Garden State Orthopaedic Associates, P.A.
28-04 Broadway   Fair Lawn, NJ 07430   (201)791-4434   Fax (201)791-9377

Holden, Emily C., MD {1962796193} ObsGyn
+ Damien Fertility Partners
655 Shrewsbury Avenue/Suite 300   Shrewsbury, NJ 07702   (732)758-6511   Fax (732)758-1048
+ Rutgers- New Jersey Medical School
185 South Orange Avenue/Ob/Gyn   Newark, NJ 07103   (201)704-6849

Holder, Dawn Paulette, MD {1134296288} FamMed(03,NJ05)
+ Mountainside Family Practice Associates
799 Bloomfield Avenue/Suite 201   Verona, NJ 07044   (973)746-7050   Fax (973)857-2831

Holder, Kevin D., MD {1063543254} IntrMd(83,NJ05)
+ 5 Stanley Road
South Orange, NJ 07079   (973)762-6077   Fax (973)762-4331

Holder, Sarah Schell, DO {1316142177} FamMed<NJ-ACMCITY>
+ AtlantiCare Regional Medical Center/City Campus
1925 Pacific Avenue   Atlantic City, NJ 08401   (609)441-8146   Fax (609)441-8002

Holder, William B., MD {1316168602} GenPrc, IntrMd, FamMAdlt(81,NJ06)
+ Cntr for Preventive Medicine
285 North Beverwyck Road   Parsippany, NJ 07054

Hole, Robert L., MD {1982795241} SrgOrt(88,NJ05)
+ Passaic County Orthopaedic Associates LLC
1011 Clifton Avenue/Suite 6   Clifton, NJ 07013   (973)458-0772   Fax (973)458-0864

Holgado, Cesar B., MD {1811930027} ObsGyn(82,PHIL)<NJ-TRINIWSC>
+ 102 James Street/Suite 203
Edison, NJ 08820   (732)548-8897   Fax (732)548-8898

Holgado, Marco Patrick Guinto, DO {1053329524} FamMed(97,NJ75)<NJ-NWTNMEM, NJ-STCLRDEN>
+ Skylands Medical Group PA
406 Route 23/Suite 1   Franklin, NJ 07416   (973)827-2120   Fax (973)827-9445

Holgado, Maynard R., MD {1679526396} IntrMd(91,NJ06)<NJ-VIRTVOOR, NJ-KMHSTRAT>
+ Advocare Sicklerville Internal Med
485 Williamstown Road   Sicklerville, NJ 08081   (856)237-8100   Fax (856)237-8042

Holguin, Leonardo Fabio, MD {1154632701} IntrMd
+ Hospital Medicine Associates
157 Broad Street/Suite 317   Red Bank, NJ 07701   (732)530-2960   Fax (732)530-7446

Holland, David Andersson, MD {1790782522} Anesth(98,ISR02)<NJ-STJOSHOS, NJ-WAYNEGEN>
+ St. Joseph's Regional Medical Center
703 Main Street/Anesthesiology   Paterson, NJ 07503   (973)754-2000

Holland, Elbridge T., Jr., MD {1225089261} FamMed, Grtrcs(75,IL02)<NJ-OVERLOOK>
+ Chatham Family Practice Associates
492 Main Street   Chatham, NJ 07928   (973)635-2432   Fax (973)635-6169

Holland, Soemiwati Weidris, MD {1740549864} EnDbMt<PA-DVNPRVD>
+ Hackensack Meridian Medical Group
19 Davis Avenue/5th-6th Floor   Neptune, NJ 07753   (732)897-3990   Fax (732)897-3997

Hollander, Adrienne R., MD {1417994633} IntrMd, Rheuma(96,PA13)
+ Arthritis, Rheumatic & Back Disease Associates
2309 East Evesham Road/Suite 101   Voorhees, NJ 08043   (856)424-5005   Fax (856)424-4716

Hollander, Annette J., MD Psychy(66,NY01)
+ 282 Sunset Avenue
Englewood, NJ 07631   (201)871-0560

Hollander, Jason Michael, MD {1093890303} IntrMd, Pedtrc(99,NJ05)<NY-ARDNHILL, MA-ARDHILL>
+ Endocrinology Associates of Princeton, LLC
168 Franklin Corner Road   Lawrenceville, NJ 08648   (609)896-0075   Fax (609)896-0079
+ Endocrinology Associates of Princeton, LLC
256 Bunn Drive/Suite D   Princeton, NJ 08540   (609)896-0075   Fax (609)924-4423
+ Endocrinology Associates of Princeton, LLC
579A Cranberry Road/Suite 101   East Brunswick, NJ 08648   (732)579-6444   Fax (609)896-0079

Hollander, Philip, DO {1831128370} FamMed(68,IA75)<NJ-VIRTMHBC, NJ-VIRTBERL>
+ Virtua Family Medicine
103 Old Marlton Pike/Suite 103   Medford, NJ 08055   (609)953-7105   Fax (609)953-0042
+ Alliance for Better Care, P.C.
PO Box 1510   Medford, NJ 08055   (609)953-7105   Fax (609)953-8652

Hollander, Scott Craig, DO {1609030758} RadV&I, Radiol, RadDia(03,NY75)
+ Vascular Access Centers
4622 Black Horse Pike/Suite 102   Mays Landing, NJ 08330   (609)829-3285

Hollander, Steven Barry, MD FamMed(91,NJ05)
+ Celgene Global Health
86 Morris Avenue   Summit, NJ 07901   (732)673-9613   Fax (732)673-9001

Hollenberg, Steven M., MD {1811979130} CdvDis, CritCr, IntrMd(84,GA05)<NJ-COOPRUMC>
+ Cooper Cardiology Associates
1210 Brace Road/Suite 103   Cherry Hill, NJ 08034   (856)938-2052   Fax (856)429-1561
+ University Cardiology
3 Cooper Plaza/Room 311   Camden, NJ 08103   (856)342-2034
+ Cooper Cardiology Associates
900 Centennial Boulevard   Voorhees, NJ 08034   (856)325-6700   Fax (856)325-6702

Holler, Marianne Marie, DO {1336195676} IntrMd, PallCr(03,NJ75)<NJ-LOURDMED>
+ Visiting Physician Services
23 Main Street/Suite D1   Holmdel, NJ 07733   (732)571-1000

Hollingsworth, Jessie, MD {1326606070} ObsGyn
+ UMDNJ OBGYN
125 Paterson Street/Suite 4200   New Brunswick, NJ 08901   (732)235-6375   Fax (732)235-6650

Hollywood, Jacqueline, MD {1770589608} CdvDis(96,NY47)<NJ-ENGLWOOD, NJ-HOLYNAME>
+ Advanced Cardiology Institute
2200 Fletcher Avenue/Suite 1   Fort Lee, NJ 07024   (201)461-6200   Fax (201)461-7204

Holman, Michael Jeffrey, MD {1275596629} Surgry(79,CA15)<NJ-UMDNJ>
+ UH- RWJ Medical School
One Robert Wood Johnson Place   New Brunswick, NJ 08903   (732)235-5600

Holmes, Raymond Joseph, MD {1699771220} SrgVas(97,GRN01)<NJ-MTNSIDE, NJ-CLARMAAS>
+ The Cardiovascular Care Group
1401 Broad Street/Suite 1   Clifton, NJ 07013   (973)759-9000   Fax (973)751-3730
+ The Cardiovascular Care Group
433 Central Avenue   Westfield, NJ 07090   (973)759-9000   Fax (908)490-1698

Holmes-Bricker, Mary E., DO Pedtrc(91,PA77)<NJ-VIRTMARL>
+ Advocare The Farm Pediatrics
975 Tuckerton Road/Suite 100   Marlton, NJ 08053   (856)983-6190   Fax (856)983-3805
+ Advocare The Farm Pediatrics
1001 Laurel Oak Boulevard/Suite B   Voorhees, NJ 08043   (856)983-6190   Fax (856)782-7404

Holowinsky, Mary I., MD InfDis, IntrMd(84,NJ06)<NJ-STPETER>
+ 162 Wilshire Drive
Belle Mead, NJ 08502

Holt, Elaine Marie, MD {1447363254} IntrMd(95,NY46)<NJ-VALLEY>
+ 352 Godwin Avenue
Ridgewood, NJ 07450   (201)493-9311   Fax (201)493-9314

Holt, Stephen, MD Gastrn, IntrMd, Nutrtn(72,ENGL)
+ 47 Center Avenue
Little Falls, NJ 07424

Physicians by Name and Address

Holton, James Jeffrey, MD {1740215938} IntrMd(85,NJ06)<NJ-VIRTMHBC, NJ-VIRTUAHS>
+ Advocare Medford Station Internal Medicine
69 North Main Street   Medford, NJ 08055   (609)953-9000
Fax (609)953-9696

Holtsclaw, John David, MD {1235309915} IntrMd, Pedtrc(94,TN06)
+ Camden Treatment Associates
424 Market Street   Camden, NJ 08102   (856)338-1811
Fax (856)338-1754

Holtzberg, Nathan, MD {1295714715} PainMd, Anesth, Anes-Pain(91,NY08)<NJ-RIVERVW>
+ Orthopaedic Institute of Central Jersey
226 Highway 37 West/Suite 203   Toms River, NJ 08755
(732)240-6060   Fax (732)240-5329
+ Orthopaedic Institute of Central Jersey
365 Broad Street   Red Bank, NJ 07701   (732)240-6060
Fax (732)933-1444
+ Orthopaedic Institute of Central Jersey
2315A Highway 34/Suite D   Manasquan, NJ 08755
(732)974-0404   Fax (732)449-4271

Holtzin, Robert M., DO {1073602082} FamMed(80,PA77)<NJ-ACMCMAIN, NJ-ACMCITY>
+ 802 Tilton Road/Suite 103
Northfield, NJ 08225   (609)277-7382   Fax (609)569-1404

Holtzman, Gayle S., MD Hemato, IntrMd, MedOnc(81,NY19)
+ The Cancer Institute of New Jersey at Hamilton
5 Hamilton Health Place/Suite 120   Hamilton, NJ 08690
(609)631-6960   Fax (609)631-6888

Holubka, Jacquelin Pickford, MD {1174577373} IntrMd(86,MI20)<NJ-STBARNMC>
+ Mayor Group
53 School House Lane   Morristown, NJ 07960   (973)867-6565   Fax (973)998-4237
+ St. Barnabas Medical Center
94 Old Short Hills Road/IntMed   Livingston, NJ 07039
(973)322-5000

Holwell, Michael, DO {1609800754} FamMed(03,PA77)
+ Collingwood Family Practice
600 Atlantic Avenue   Collingswood, NJ 08108   (856)854-1050   Fax (856)854-2453

Holwitt, Dana M., MD {1043435548} SrgOnc, Surgry, IntrMd(00,VA04)<NJ-STCLRDEN>
+ St. Clare's Hospital-Denville Campus
25 Pocono Road/Surgery   Denville, NJ 07834   (973)537-5600   Fax (973)625-6293

Holwitt, Kenneth N., MD {1225083751} SrgThr, SrgVas, Surgry(68,WV01)
+ Monmouth Surgical Specialists
123 Highland Avenue/Suite 202   Glen Ridge, NJ 07028
(973)429-7600   Fax (973)429-7602

Holyk, Brian William, DO {1013201946}
+ 117 Winstead Drive
Westampton, NJ 08060   (215)603-3583
bwholyk@gmail.com

Holz, Matthew Andrew, DO {1568897999}(13,ME75)<NJ-SJHREGMC>
+ SJH Regional Medical Center
1505 West Sherman Avenue   Vineland, NJ 08360
(856)641-7675   Fax (856)575-4944

Holzberg, Adam S., DO {1952495798} ObsGyn, UroGyn(95,NY75)<NJ-COOPRUMC, NJ-RWJUHAM>
+ University Urogynecology Associates/Cooper Ob/Gyn
900 Centennial Boulevard/Suite L   Voorhees, NJ 08043
(856)325-6622   Fax (856)325-6522
holzberg-adam@cooperhealth.edu
+ University Urogynecology Associates/Cooper Ob/Gyn
1230 Whitehorse Mercerville Rd/Suite B   Hamilton, NJ 08619   (609)581-5681

Holzberg, Norman, MD {1689679904} Otlryg(85,IL42)<NJ-STBARNMC, NJ-NWRKBETH>
+ Associates in Otolaryngology
741 Northfield Avenue/Suite 104   West Orange, NJ 07052
(973)243-0600   Fax (973)736-9607
+ Short Hills Surgery Center
187 Millburn Avenue/Suite 101   Millburn, NJ 07041
(973)243-0600   Fax (973)671-0557

Holzinger, Karl Anthony, MD {1245206226} Ophthl(83,NY19)<NJ-VIRTUAHS>
+ Eye Associates
251 South Lincoln Avenue   Vineland, NJ 08361   (856)691-8188   Fax (856)691-0421
+ Eye Associates
1401 Route 70 East   Cherry Hill, NJ 08034   (856)691-8188
Fax (856)428-6359
+ Eye Associates
141 Black Horse Pike/Suite 7   Blackwood, NJ 08012
(856)227-6262   Fax (856)227-8830

Holzman, Kevin Jay, MD {1790907657} SrgC&R, IntrMd(04,GRN01)<NJ-STBARNMC, NJ-NWRKBETH>
+ Summit Medical Group
75 East Northfield Road   Livingston, NJ 07039   (973)436-1530   Fax (908)673-7336
+ Summit Medical Group
6 Brighton Road/2 FL   Clifton, NJ 07012   (973)436-1530
Fax (973)777-5403

Hom, William L., MD {1487783338} Psychy(76,MA07)
+ 33 State Road/Suite A2
Princeton, NJ 08540   (609)924-5997   Fax (609)924-0135

Homayouni, Homayoun, MD {1083686174} InfDis, IntrMd(71,IRA15)<NJ-ACMCITY, NJ-ACMCMAIN>
+ 334 West Oakcrest Avenue
Northfield, NJ 08225   (609)485-0808   Fax (609)485-0737

Homb, Kris, MD {1366767006} PhysMd
+ University Hospital-Doctors Office Center
90 Bergen Street/Suite 3100   Newark, NJ 07103   (973)972-2802

Homer, Stuart M., MD {1760488373} IntrMd, Nephro(77,MA07)
+ Stuart Homer and Associates, PA
1030 Saint Georges Avenue/Suite 201   Avenel, NJ 07001
(732)602-0244   Fax (732)602-2577

Hon, Beverly J., MD {1619315934} PhysMd<NJ-JFKJHNSN>
+ JFK Johnson Rehabilitation Institute
65 James Street   Edison, NJ 08818   (732)321-7070   Fax (732)321-7330

Hon, David C., MD {1013054725} Surgry
+ AtlantiCare Urgent Care Center
2500 English Creek Avenue   Egg Harbor Township, NJ 08234
(609)407-2273

Hong, Alice, DO {1891180956} FamMed(15,PA78)
+ Morristown Medical Center
100 Madison Avenue   Morristown, NJ 07962   (973)971-5000

Hong, John S., MD {1871573063} IntrMd(98,VA01)<NJ-BURDTMLN>
+ Cape Regional Physicians Associates
11 Village Drive   Cape May Court House, NJ 08210
(609)465-2273   Fax (609)463-0236

Hong, Joseph Johnson, MD {1548231228} Dermat(93,PA02)
+ Atlantic Dermatology & Laser Center
1401 New Road   Linwood, NJ 08221   (609)927-5885   Fax (609)927-5565

Hong, Kathleen H., MD {1255583829} ObsGyn
+ Reproductive Medicine Associates of New Jersey
140 Allen Road   Basking Ridge, NJ 07920   (908)604-7800
Fax (973)290-8370

Hong, Matthew H., MD {1841299534} FamMed(91,DC02)
+ Cape Regional Physicians Associates
3806 Bayshore Road/Suite 101   North Cape May, NJ 08204
(609)898-7447   Fax (609)898-1912

Hong, Rick, MD {1851379473} EmrgMd(01,PA01)<NJ-COOPRUMC>
+ Cooper University Hospital
One Cooper Plaza/EmergMed   Camden, NJ 08103
(856)342-2000

Hong, Rolando Y., MD {1720072242} PsyCAd, NrlgAddM(78,PHI02)<NJ-MTCARMEL>
+ Central Jersey Beharioral Health, LLC
216 North Avenue East   Cranford, NJ 07016   (908)272-7500   Fax (908)272-7502

Hong, William Y. C., MD {1225077456} CdvDis, CarNuc, IntrMd(79,NY46)<NJ-SOCEANCO>
+ Stafford Medical, P.A.
1364 Route 72 West/Suite 5   Manahawkin, NJ 08050
(609)597-3416   Fax (609)597-9608

Hong, Young Ki, MD {1952543548} Surgry
+ MD Anderson Cancer Center at Cooper
2 Cooper Plaza   Camden, NJ 08103   (856)342-3113

Honickman, Steven P., MD {1790781094} RadDia(76,NC05)<NJ-SOMERSET>
+ University Radiology, PA
239 Route 22 East/Suite 302   Green Brook, NJ 08812
(732)968-4899   Fax (732)968-8096
+ University Radiology Group, P.C.
3900 Park Avenue/Suite 107   Edison, NJ 08820   (732)968-4899   Fax (732)548-6290

Hood, Ian C., MD {1801344825} PthFor, Pthlgy, PthACl(77,NEW02)
+ Burlington County Medical Examiner
4 Academy Drive   Westampton, NJ 08060   (609)702-7030

Hooda, Anjali, MD {1346468709} IntrMd(98,INA06)<NJ-MORRISTN, NJ-OVERLOOK>
+ Storch Nutritional Medical Assoc
147 Columbia Turnpike/Suite 308   Florham Park, NJ 07932

Hooper, William, Jr., MD {1336173442} IntrMd(74,PA13)<NJ-SHOREMEM>
+ Shore Physicians Group
52 East New York Avenue   Somers Point, NJ 08244
(609)365-6202   Fax (609)653-1925

Hooshangi, Nossratollah, MD {1598846990} Nrolgy, SrgNro(66,IRA01)<NJ-JFKMED>
+ JFK Medical Center
65 James Street   Edison, NJ 08820   (732)321-7000   Fax (732)632-1584
+ 98 James Street/Suite 309
Edison, NJ 08820   (732)321-7000   Fax (732)549-9251

Hope, Lisa Dawn, MD {1669415410} IntrMd(02,NJ05)
+ Prospect Medical Offices, LLC
301 Godwin Avenue   Midland Park, NJ 07432   (201)444-4526   Fax (201)301-1313

Hopkins, Leigh Hastings, MD {1679512883} SrgOrt, IntrMd(89,MD07)
+ Endocrinology Associates
1 Brace Road/Suite B   Cherry Hill, NJ 08034   (856)234-0645
Fax (856)234-0498
+ Leigh H. Hopkins MD, P.C.
Route 70 and Brace Road   Cherry Hill, NJ 08002   (856)234-0645   Fax (877)277-2897

Hopkins, Lisa Anne, MD {1144347675} Surgry
+ Somerset Medical Associates
1553 Highway 27/Suite 3100   Somerset, NJ 08873
(732)846-3300   Fax (732)846-3323
+ St. Peter's Family Health
123 How Lane   New Brunswick, NJ 08901   (732)846-3300
Fax (732)729-0869

Hopkins, Rebecca Jane, MD {1740228634} Psychy(01,PA14)
+ Integrated Behavioral Care
35 Beachwood Road/Suite 3A   Summit, NJ 07901
rebecca.hopkins@mssm.edu

Hoppe, James Robert, MD {1174587661} FamMed(98,NJ06)
+ Family Practice & Gynecology
273 Durham Avenue   South Plainfield, NJ 07080   (908)561-9900   Fax (908)561-6650

Hoppenfeld, Brad M., MD {1396773776} RadV&I, RadDia(94,PA09)<NJ-KMHCHRRY, NJ-KMHSTRAT>
+ Capital Health System/Fuld Campus
750 Brunswick Avenue   Trenton, NJ 08638   (609)815-7532

Horak, Ivan D., MD IntrMd, MedOnc(75,CZE03)
+ Symphogen Inc
50 Division Street/Suite 503   Somerville, NJ 08876
(908)378-9630

Horan, Corinne E., DO {1952643884} EmrgMd<NJ-SJHREGMC>
+ SJH Regional Medical Center
1505 West Sherman Avenue   Vineland, NJ 08360
(856)881-9150
choran02@gmail.com

Horana, Lasanta S., MD {1861548158} EmrgMd<NJ-RWJUHAM>
+ Robert Wood Johnson University Hospital at Hamilton
1 Hamilton Health Place/EmergMed   Hamilton, NJ 08690
(609)586-7900

Horenstein, Marcelo G., MD {1508837253} PthACl, DrmtPthy(90,ARG06)
+ The Dermatology Group, P.C.
60 Pompton Avenue   Verona, NJ 07044   (973)571-2121
Fax (973)571-2126
+ The Dermatology Group, P.C.
44 Route 23 North/Suite 213   Riverdale, NJ 07457
(973)571-2121   Fax (973)839-5751
+ The Dermatology Group, P.C.
30 West Century Road/Suite 320   Paramus, NJ 07044
(973)571-2121   Fax (201)986-0702

Horiuchi, Jonathan K., MD {1659338077} CdvDis(85,HI01)<NJ-HUNTRDN>
+ Hunterdon Cardiovascular Associates
1100 Wescott Drive/Suite G-3   Flemington, NJ 08822
(908)788-6471   Fax (908)788-6460
+ Hunterdon Cardiovascular Associates
1738 Route 31/Suite 210   Clinton, NJ 08809   (908)788-6471   Fax (908)823-9211

Horkheimer, Ian Christin, MD {1316924772}
+ Regional Cancer Care Associates, LLC
180 White Road   Little Silver, NJ 07739   (732)530-8666
Fax (732)530-4139

Hormilla, Amador N., MD {1710984521} IntrMd(81,DOM02)<NJ-COMMED>
+ 508 Lakehurst Road/Suite 3 B
Toms River, NJ 08755   (732)505-0500
Hormilla@comcast.net

Horn, Abraham S., DO {1053371815} Gastrn, IntrMd(81,NJ75)<NJ-OURLADY, NJ-VIRTUAHS>
+ South Jersey Gastroenterology PA
406 Lippincott Drive/Suite E   Marlton, NJ 08053   (856)983-1900   Fax (856)983-5110
+ South Jersey Gastroenterology PA
807 Haddon Avenue/Suite 205   Haddonfield, NJ 08033
(856)983-1900   Fax (856)983-5110
+ South Jersey Gastroenterology PA
111 Vine Street   Hammonton, NJ 08053   (609)561-3080
Fax (856)983-5110

Horn, Bernard David, MD {1639251085} SrgOrt, PedOrt(86,OH43)<PA-CHILDHOS>
+ CHOP Pediatric & Adolescent Specialty Care Center
1012 Laurel Oak Road   Voorhees, NJ 08043   (856)435-1300   Fax (856)435-0091
+ CHOP Specialty Care Center at Virtua
200 Bowman Drive/2 FL/Suite D-260   Voorhees, NJ 08043   (267)425-5400

Horn, Christopher Michael, DO {1821095605} FamMed<NJ-MORRISTN>
+ Skylands Medical Group PA
66 East Main Street   Rockaway, NJ 07866   (973)627-4499   Fax (973)627-5083

Horn, Eva M., MD {1922042266} RadDia, Radiol, IntrMd(78,NY19)<NJ-HOLYNAME, NJ-NWRKBETH>
+ Holy Name Hospital
718 Teaneck Road/Radiology   Teaneck, NJ 07666   (201)833-7023   Fax (201)541-5919

Horn, Robert John, DO {1104137785} EmrgMd
+ Rowan University-School of Osteopathic Medicine
1 Medical Center Drive   Stratford, NJ 08084   (856)566-6708

Horn, Russell J., MD {1720061849} Anesth(83,NY19)<NJ-HACKNSK>
+ Hackensack University MC-Anesthesia Dept
30 Prospect Avenue/Room 2703   Hackensack, NJ 07601   (201)996-2419   Fax (201)996-3962
+ Hackensack University Medical Center
30 Prospect Avenue/Anesth   Hackensack, NJ 07601   (201)996-2419   Fax (201)488-6769

Horne, Howard Krutzel, MD {1356395883} ObsGyn(00,IL06)
+ Phillipsburg Ob/Gyn Associates
700 Coventry Drive   Phillipsburg, NJ 08865   (908)454-4666

Horner, Neil B., MD {1083694731} RadDia, RadNro, RadNuc(83,NJ06)
+ Westfield Imaging Center
118-122 Elm Street   Westfield, NJ 07090   (908)232-0610   Fax (908)232-7140
+ Summit Radiology Associates
99 Beauvoir Avenue   Summit, NJ 07901   (908)522-2066

Hornstein, Joshua Scott, MD {1366405813} SrgOrt(96,NJ06)<NJ-RWJUHAM, NJ-STFRNMED>
+ Trenton Orthopaedic Group
1225 Whitehorse Mercerville Rd   Trenton, NJ 08619   (609)581-2200   Fax (609)581-1212
+ Trenton Orthopaedic Group
116 Washington Crossing Road   Pennington, NJ 08534   (609)581-2200   Fax (609)581-1212

Horowitz, Alyssa G., MD {1013943901} ObsGyn(91,NY19)
+ Premier Ob/Gyn HealthCare LLC
971 Route 202   Branchburg, NJ 08876   (908)429-0044   Fax (908)429-0048

Horowitz, Carolyn J., MD {1275512600} RadOnc(81,NJ06)
+ Kennedy Diagnostic & Treatment Center
900 Medical Center Drive/Suite 100   Sewell, NJ 08080   (856)582-3008   Fax (856)582-3009   C.horowitz@kennedyhealth.org

Horowitz, Deborah L., MD {1447227202} Pedtrc, IntrMd(96,NJ06)<NJ-CHILTON>
+ Advocare Pediatric Arts
1403 Route 23 South   Butler, NJ 07405   (973)283-2200   Fax (973)283-0406
+ Advocare Pediatric Arts
1777 Hamburg Turnpike/Suite 103   Wayne, NJ 07470   (973)283-2200   Fax (973)283-0406

Horowitz, Elisabeth W., MD {1952310930} EnDbMt, IntrMd(85,PA09)<NJ-VIRTMARL, NJ-VIRTVOOR>
+ Regional Pulmonary Associates PA
2301 East Evesham Road/Suite 402   Voorhees, NJ 08043   (856)528-2583   Fax (856)528-2585

Horowitz, Ira David, MD {1780682278} CritCr, IntrMd, PulDis(85,PA09)<NJ-OURLADY, NJ-VIRTBERL>
+ Pulmonary & Sleep Associates of SJ, LLC.
107 Berlin Road   Cherry Hill, NJ 08034   (856)429-1800   Fax (856)429-1081
+ Pulmonary & Sleep Associates of SJ, LLC.
750 Route 73 South/Suite 401   Marlton, NJ 08053   (856)429-1800   Fax (856)375-2325
+ Pulmonary & Sleep Associates of SJ, LLC.
811 Sunset Road/Suite 201   Burlington, NJ 08034   (609)298-1776   Fax (609)531-2391

Horowitz, Jay B., MD {1255421673} Otlryg, Otolgy(87,CT01)
+ Advanced Otolaryngology Associates
557 Cranbury Road/Suite 3   East Brunswick, NJ 08816   (732)613-0600   Fax (732)613-0508
+ ENT & Allergy Associates, LLP
3663 Route 9 North/Suite102   Old Bridge, NJ 08857   (732)613-0600   Fax (732)707-3850

Horowitz, Jeffrey Scot, MD {1558469437} Pedtrc(81,NY47)<NY-STANTHNY>
+ Herbert Kania Pediatric Center
1900 Union Valley Road   Hewitt, NJ 07421   (973)728-4480   Fax (973)728-4375

Horowitz, Jerry A., DO {1225065311} FamMed(88,FL75)
+ 618 North Shore Road
Marmora, NJ 08223   (609)390-0693   Fax (609)390-1147

Horowitz, Mark Lawrence, MD {1477649853} Pedtrc(77,NY09)<NY-STANTHNY>
+ Herbert Kania Pediatric Center
1900 Union Valley Road   Hewitt, NJ 07421   (973)728-4480   Fax (973)728-4375

Horowitz, Meggan Elise, DO {1396972030} Pedtrc, IntrMd<NJ-ATLANTHS>
+ Morristown Medical Center Family Medicine
435 South Street/Suite 220-A   Morristown, NJ 07960   (973)971-4222   Fax (973)290-7050

Horowitz, Michael S., MD {1275647174} CdvDis, IntrMd(69,DC01)<NJ-MTNSIDE, NJ-STBARNMC>
+ North Jersey Cardiovascular Consultants
329 Belleville Avenue   Bloomfield, NJ 07003   (973)748-3800   Fax (973)748-3540

Horowitz, Mitchell Loyd, MD {1316922883} IntrMd, PulDis, CritCr(86,MEX34)<NY-STATNRTH, NY-STATNSTH>
+ 21 Ottowa Road North
Morganville, NJ 07751   (732)915-0217   Fax (732)970-4445
+ 762 Highway 18 North
East Brunswick, NJ 08816   (732)915-0217   Fax (732)970-4445

Horowitz, Philip, MD {1801893516} Ophthl(65,MD07)<NJ-VIRTMHBC, NJ-LOURDMED>
+ South Jersey Eye Physicians PA
509 South Lenola Road/Suite 11   Moorestown, NJ 08057   (856)234-0222   Fax (856)727-9518
+ South Jersey Eye Physicians PA
103 Old Marlton Pike/Suite 216   Medford, NJ 08055   (856)234-0222   Fax (609)714-8759
+ South Jersey Eye Physicians PA
25 Homestead Drive/Suite A   Columbus, NJ 08057   (609)298-0888   Fax (609)291-1972

Horowitz, Stephen M., MD {1386676054} SrgOrt(83,NY09)
+ 750 Route 73 South/Suite 207
Marlton, NJ 08053   (856)988-1966   Fax (856)988-1965

Horten, James, MD {1760405138} Pedtrc(87,PA13)
+ Kids first
2006 Salem Road   Burlington, NJ 08016   (609)877-1500   Fax (609)877-4262

Horton, Daniel B., MD {1528224193} Pedtrc
+ Child Health Institute of New Jersey
89 French Street/Suite 2300   New Brunswick, NJ 08901   (732)235-4980   Fax (732)235-5002

Horvath, Katalin, MD {1609884303} IntrMd(89,HUN03)
+ Hackensack Meridian Health-Oak Tree Primary Care
904 Oak Tree Avenue/Suite M   South Plainfield, NJ 07080   (732)283-0020   Fax (732)283-0029
+ Health Med Associates, PC
1080 Stelton Road/First FL Suite 202   Piscataway, NJ 08854   (732)283-0020   Fax (732)985-0552

Horvath, Kedron Nicole, MD {1346450723} FamMed
+ Cooper Family Medicine
1001-F Lincoln Drive West   Marlton, NJ 08053   (856)810-1800   Fax (856)810-1879

Horvath Matthews, Jessica Erin, MD {1740357953} FamMed(03,PA02)<NJ-COOPRUMC>
+ Cooper Family Medicine
141 South Black Horse Pike/Suite 1   Blackwood, NJ 08012   (856)232-6471   Fax (856)232-7028

Horvick, David, MD {1205897808} RadOnc, Radiol(82,PA02)
+ 21st Century Oncology
220 Sunset Road/Suite 4   Willingboro, NJ 08046   (609)877-3064   Fax (609)877-2466

Horvitz, Steven P., DO {1689784894} FamMed(91,PA77)<NJ-KMHCHRRY, NJ-VIRTVOOR>
+ 128 Borton Landing Road/Suite 2
Moorestown, NJ 08057   (856)231-0590   Fax (856)231-1228

Horwitz, Jerome M., DO {1740272509} CdvDis, IntrMd(73,PA77)
+ South Jersey Heart Group
3001 Chapel Avenue/Suite 101   Cherry Hill, NJ 08002   (856)482-8900   Fax (856)482-7170
+ Associated Cardiovascular Consultants-Lourdes
1 Brace Road/Suite C & F   Cherry Hill, NJ 08034   (856)482-8900   Fax (856)428-5748

Horwitz, Michael J., DO {1386842987} CdvDis, CarNuc, IntrMd(05,NJ75)
+ South Jersey Heart Group
1113 Hospital Drive/Suite 202   Willingboro, NJ 08046   (609)835-3550   Fax (609)835-3557

Horwitz, Morris, MD {1235394057} IntrMd, LeglMd(81,GRN01)
+ 175 Cedar Lane
Teaneck, NJ 07666   (201)692-1300   Fax (201)692-0081

Horwitz, Steven Mankowitz, MD {1972899425} Pedtrc(08,GRN01)
+ 791 John Street
Teaneck, NJ 07666   (201)357-0103

+ RWJ University Hospital New Brunswick
One Robert Wood Johnson Place   New Brunswick, NJ 08901   (732)235-7887

Hosadurga, Supriya S., MD {1437211109} IntrMd(02,INA28)
+ IPC The Hospitalist Company
55 Madison Avenue/Suite 310   Morristown, NJ 07960   (973)993-9536   Fax (973)998-4237

Hosay, John J., Jr., MD {1255432886} Urolgy(77,MEX14)<NJ-CHRIST, NJ-MEADWLND>
+ 2555 Kennedy Boulevard
Jersey City, NJ 07304   (201)433-9666   Fax (201)432-9647

Hoskin, Jane F., MD {1194738195} IntrMd(81,DC02)<NJ-STMRY-PAS>
+ Park Avenue Medical Associates
30 Park Avenue/Suite 202   Lyndhurst, NJ 07071   (201)438-5900   Fax (201)438-5980

Hosler, Matthew Robert, MD {1346462637} Ophthl
+ Associated Eye Physicians & Surgeons of NJ, P.A.
1530 Saint Georges Avenue   Rahway, NJ 07065   (732)382-9000   Fax (732)382-7455

Hosmer, Stephan E., DO {1750327375} ObsGyn(78,MI12)<NJ-VIRTVOOR, NJ-KENEDYHS>
+ 1000 White Horse Road/Suite 502
Voorhees, NJ 08043   (856)627-9898   Fax (856)627-7647

Hossain, Akhtar, MD {1295836633} PsyCAd, Psychy(89,RUS76)
+ 153 North Auten Avenue
Somerville, NJ 08876   (908)231-7700   Fax (908)231-6144   ahossain@fgcwc.org
+ Somerset Medical Center Psychiatry
110 Rehill Avenue   Somerville, NJ 08876   (908)685-2200

Hossain, Asghar S.M., MD {1295824381} Psychy(78,BANG)<NJ-BERGNMC, NJ-HOLYNAME>
+ Drs. Hossain, Hossain, and Farooqui
26-01 Broadway/Suite 105   Fair Lawn, NJ 07410   (201)703-3664   Fax (201)652-7233

Hossain, Feroza K., MD {1801847397} IntrMd(83,BANG)<NJ-UNVMCPRN>
+ Medical Pediatrics Associates
256 Bunn Drive/Suite 3 A   Princeton, NJ 08540   Fax (609)683-7958

Hossain, Mohammad Amir, MD {1639559438} IntrMd<NJ-JRSYSHMC>
+ Hackensack Meridian Medical Group
19 Davis Avenue/5th-6th Floor   Neptune, NJ 07753   (732)775-5500   Fax (732)897-3997
+ Jersey Shore University Medical Center
1945 Route 33   Neptune, NJ 07753   (732)775-5500

Hossain, Nazma A., MD {1518997360} IntrMd(78,BANG)<NJ-HOLYNAME>
+ Drs. Hossain, Hossain, and Farooqui
26-01 Broadway/Suite 105   Fair Lawn, NJ 07410   (201)703-3664   Fax (201)652-7233

Hossain, Shahreen Rafa, MD {1184970139} Grtrcs<NJ-STJOSHOS>
+ St. Joseph's Regional Medical Center
703 Main Street   Paterson, NJ 07503   (973)754-2000

Hossain, Shawn Isteak, DO {1457511776} Psychy
+ Advocare Berlin Medical Associates
175 Cross Keys Road/Suite 300A   Berlin, NJ 08009   (856)753-7335   Fax (856)767-6102

Hostetler, Caecilia E., MD {1578621413} FamMed(94,NY19)<NJ-MTNSIDE>
+ Summit Medical Group
48-50 Fairfield Street   Montclair, NJ 07042   (973)744-8511   Fax (973)744-6356

Hotchkin, Karen Lynn, MD {1215996731} IntrMd(94,PA02)<NJ-WARREN>
+ Village Medical Center
207 Strykers Road   Phillipsburg, NJ 08865   (908)859-6568   Fax (908)859-6697

Hou, Cindy Meng, DO {1902096530} InfDis
+ Garden State Infectious Diseases Associates, P.A.
709 Haddonfield Berlin Road   Voorhees, NJ 08043   (856)566-3190   Fax (856)783-2193
+ Garden State Infectious Disease Associates
570 Egg Harbor Road/Suite B-5   Sewell, NJ 08080   (856)566-3190   Fax (856)566-1904

Hou, Hui Ying, MD {1184911687} ObsGyn(11,PA14)
+ Jersey Womens Care Center
435 Central Avenue   Jersey City, NJ 07307   (201)217-5600

Hou, Lisa Jenny, DO {1891904967} Otlryg(96,NJ75)
+ Medical Command - National Guard
Academy Way/Building 64   Sea Girt, NJ 08750   (732)974-5910

Hou, Shunli, MD {1356401806} Pedtrc(84,CHN40)<NJ-CHD-NWBTH, NJ-NWRKBETH>
+ 56 Union Avenue/Suite 3
Somerville, NJ 08876   (908)723-0796   Fax (732)377-8568

Hou, Stephanie W., MD {1598089823} RadDia
+ Hackensack Radiology Group, P.A.
30 Prospect Avenue   Hackensack, NJ 07601   (201)996-2200   Fax (201)489-2812

Physicians by Name and Address

Houck, Karen Leigh, MD {1154393205} ObsGyn, GynOnc(94,NY06)<NJ-MORRISTN, NJ-OVERLOOK>
+ Rutgers- New Jersey Medical School
185 South Orange Avenue/MSB E510   Newark, NJ 07103   (973)972-5554   Fax (973)972-4574

Houck, Meghan Mcfee, DO {1235545401} Pedtrc
+ Mainland Pediatric Association
741 South Second Avenue/Suite B   Galloway, NJ 08205   (609)748-8500   Fax (609)748-6700
+ 114 Franklin Street/Apt Sh2
Morristown, NJ 07960   (609)828-2410

Houlihan, Christopher M., MD {1114983590} NnPnMd, ObsGyn, MtFtMd(89,NJ05)<NJ-STJOSHCS, NJ-STPETER>
+ Perinatal Services of Northern New Jersey
57 Willowbrook Road/3rd Floor   Wayne, NJ 07470   (973)754-3800   Fax (973)244-0476
+ St. Peter's University Hospital
254 Easton Avenue/Suite1-H   New Brunswick, NJ 08901   (732)745-8600

Houlis, Nicholas J., DO {1508023466} Surgry
+ 31 Stone Hame Drive
Brick, NJ 08724

Houng, Abraham Pohan, MD {1649226135} Surgry, SrgTrm, SrgCrC(01,NJ05)<NJ-STBARNMC>
+ Burn Surgeons of Saint Barnabas
94 Old Short Hills Road   Livingston, NJ 07039   (973)322-5924   Fax (973)322-5447
+ St. Barnabas Medical Center
94 Old Short Hills Road/Surgery   Livingston, NJ 07039   (973)322-5000

Houng, Mindy S., MD {1992704993} IntrMd, Pedtrc(00,NJ05)<NJ-CLARMAAS>
+ Clara Maass Medical Center
1 Clara Maass Drive   Belleville, NJ 07109   (973)450-2000

Housam, Ryan Ann, MD {1336345313} Pedtrc
+ Somerset Pediatric Group PA
3322 Route 22/Suite 1002   Branchburg, NJ 08876   (908)725-5530   Fax (908)253-6559

Housri, Ibrahim, MD {1033222369} Hemato, IntrMd(72,SYR01)<NJ-MORRISTN, NJ-STBARNMC>
+ 321 Old Bergen Road
Jersey City, NJ 07305   (973)887-3883

Houston, Patrick J., MD {1376637124} Otlryg, SrgHdN(65,NY06)<NJ-VIRTMARL, NJ-COOPRUMC>
+ 1509 Sagemore Drive
Marlton, NJ 08053   (856)596-9442

Houston, Sean David, MD {1598769259} Otlryg(92,DC02)<NJ-JRSYSHMC>
+ Coastal Ear Nose and Throat LLC
3700 Route 33/Suite 101   Neptune, NJ 07753   (732)280-7855   Fax (732)280-7815
+ Coastal Ear Nose and Throat LLC
1301 Route 72/Suite 340   Manahawkin, NJ 08050   (732)280-7855   Fax (732)280-7815

Howard, Brandon Trevor, MD {1720267081} IntrMd(02,GRN01)
+ 192 Prospect Avenue/Grnd Fl
Hackensack, NJ 07601   (201)336-0095   Fax (201)820-0817

Howard, L. Deanna, MD {1326066812} ObsGyn, IntrMd(92,NJ05)<NJ-NWRKBETH>
+ Women & Wellness, LLC
349 East Northfield Road/Suite 212   Livingston, NJ 07039   (973)758-9311   Fax (973)758-1430

Howard, Michael Lawrence, MD {1174595508} Urolgy(91,PA12)<NJ-JRSYSHMC, NJ-OCEANMC>
+ Drs. Rotolo, Howard, and Leitner
2401 Highway 35   Manasquan, NJ 08736   (732)223-7877   Fax (732)223-7151
+ Drs. Rotolo and Howard
525 Jack Martin Boulevard/Suite 102   Brick, NJ 08724   (732)206-9830

Howard, Peter Carson, MD {1952357543} Urolgy(00,PA02)<NJ-COMMED>
+ Urologic Health Center of New Jersey
67 Route 37 West/Building 2/Suite 1   Toms River, NJ 08755   (732)914-1300   Fax (732)914-0849
+ Urologic Health Center of New Jersey
63C Lacey Road   Whiting, NJ 08759   (732)914-1300   Fax (732)350-7054
+ Urologic Health Center of New Jersey
949 Lacey Road   Forked River, NJ 08755   (609)242-6930   Fax (609)242-6932

Howard, Tanya Dayell, MD {1669628673} EmrgMd(05,NJ06)<NJ-CHSFULD, NJ-CHSMRCER>
+ Capital Health System/Fuld Campus
750 Brunswick Avenue/EmrgMed   Trenton, NJ 08638   (609)394-6000

Howard, Thomas R., Jr., MD {1639243348} FamMed(71,OK01)<NJ-MEMSALEM>
+ Cooper Primare Care
567 Salem Quinton Road/Suite C   Salem, NJ 08079   (856)696-4932

Howard, Timothy S., MD {1992723266} RadDia(95,VT02)<NJ-UN-VMCPRN>
+ Princeton Radiology Associates, P.A.
253 Witherspoon Street   Princeton, NJ 08540   (609)497-4310   Fax (609)497-4989
+ Princeton Radiology Associates, P.A.
419 North Harrison Street   Princeton, NJ 08540   (609)497-4310   Fax (609)683-8847
+ Princeton Radiology Associates, P.A.
9 Centre Drive   Jamesburg, NJ 08540   (609)655-1448   Fax (609)655-4016

Howarth, David F., MD {1750466439} FamMed(83,GRNA)
+ UH- Robert Wood Johnson Med
125 Paterson Street/MEB 268   New Brunswick, NJ 08901   (732)235-6969   Fax (732)246-8084
+ Family Medicine at Monument Square
317 George Street/1st Fl   New Brunswick, NJ 08901   (732)235-6969   Fax (732)246-7317
+ Center for Healthy Aging
18 Centre Drive/Suite 104   Monroe Township, NJ 08901   (609)655-5178   Fax (609)655-5284

Howe, Joseph H., MD {1043309750} IntrMd(75,MEXI)<NJ-OURLADY>
+ 512 East Browning Road
Bellmawr, NJ 08031   (856)931-2311   Fax (856)931-3688

Howe, Matthew R., MD {1154462240} Pedtrc(03,NJ05)
+ East Windsor Pediatric Group
300B Princeton Hightstown/Suite 201   Hightstown, NJ 08520   (609)448-7300   Fax (609)448-8022

Howe, Michele Margaret, DO {1679534093} FamMed, GenPrc(81,MO79)<NJ-ENGLWOOD, NJ-VALLEY>
+ Valley Health Medical Group
72 Hamburg Turnpike   Riverdale, NJ 07457   (973)835-7290   Fax (973)835-0696

Howe, Thomas Arthur, MD {1962794412} IntrMd(73,PA13)
+ Aetna, Inc.
55 Lane Road   Fairfield, NJ 07004   (973)575-5600

Howell, Emily Ruth, DO {1114328390} ObsGyn
+ Hackensack Hospital Obs/Gyn
30 Prospect Avenue/4E-90   Hackensack, NJ 07601   (551)996-2000

Howell, Melanie Ann, DO {1295022606}
+ 530 Gregory Avenue/Unit C202
Weehawken, NJ 07086   (973)896-8013
dr.mhowell@gmail.com

Howhannesian, Andranik, MD {1174591762} Urolgy, IntrMd(90,MA05)<NJ-HACKNSK, NJ-VALLEY>
+ Sovereign Medical Group
15-01 Broadway/Suite 1   Fair Lawn, NJ 07410   (201)791-4544   Fax (201)791-6585
drhowh@aol.com

Hoye, Vincent Joseph, III, MD {1508910803} Ophthl(93,NH01)<NJ-STBARNMC, NJ-MORRISTN>
+ Hoye Eye Care
385 Route 24/Suite 2-C   Chester, NJ 07930   (908)879-9555   Fax (908)879-9545

Hozack, William James, MD {1497709075} SrgOrt(81,QU01)<NJ-ATLANTHS>
+ Rothman Institute - Voorhees
443 Laurel Oak Road   Voorhees, NJ 08043   (856)821-6360

Hozayen, Ossama, MD {1922162122} Nephro, IntrMd(88,EGY05)<NJ-BAYSHORE>
+ Drs. Awad and Hozayen
1 Bethany Road/Building 6   Hazlet, NJ 07730   (732)264-5005   Fax (732)264-1843

Hrabarchuk, Eugene S., MD {1396704938} FamMed, GenPrc(81,DOM02)<NJ-NWTNMEM>
+ 165 State Highway 23
Franklin, NJ 07416   (973)827-5255   Fax (973)827-0026

Hraniotis, Nicole J., MD {1265751531} Psychy<NJ-UNIVBHC>
+ University Behavioral Health Care
671 Hoes Lane/PO Box 1392   Piscataway, NJ 08855   (732)235-5500

Hric, Jerome Joseph, MD {1437164290} NnPnMd, Pedtrc(81,PA09)
+ On-Site Neonatal Partners
1000 Haddonfield-Berlin Road/Suite 210   Voorhees, NJ 08043   (856)782-2212   Fax (856)782-2213

Hrishikesan, Geetha, MD {1326117599} FamMed(89,INA76)<NJ-MTNSIDE>
+ Summit Medical Group
48-50 Fairfield Street   Montclair, NJ 07042   (973)744-8511   Fax (973)744-6356

Hriso, Emmanuel, MD {1942217328} Psychy, PsyAdd, PsyGrt(82,DOM02)<NJ-CHRIST, NJ-JFKMED>
+ 54 Main Street
Woodbridge, NJ 07095   (732)855-1199   Fax (732)855-1138
+ 654 Avenue C
Bayonne, NJ 07002   (732)855-1199   Fax (201)436-1601
+ Christ Hospital
176 Palisade Avenue/Psych&Behavrl   Jersey City, NJ 07095   (201)795-8375

Hriso, Paul, MD {1295754158} Psychy(88,FRA13)
+ 54 Main Street
Woodbridge, NJ 07095   (732)855-1199

Hrymoc, Zofia, MD {1891728481} EnDbMt, IntrMd(75,POL03)<NJ-STPETER, NJ-RWJUBRUN>
+ Endocrinology Associates of New Jersey
9 Auer Court/Suite A   East Brunswick, NJ 08816   (732)390-6666   Fax (732)390-7711

Hsieh, Allen, MD {1912992769} CdvDis, CarNuc, IntrMd(91,MD07)<NJ-MORRISTN>
+ Morristown Cardiology Associates, P.A.
435 South Street/Suite 100   Morristown, NJ 07960   (973)267-3944   Fax (973)455-0399

Hsieh, Ching C., MD {1497758031} Anesth(67,TAI06)<NJ-STCLRDEN>
+ 5 Harbeson Court
Montville, NJ 07045

Hsieh, Jennifer, MD {1629357835} Gastrn, IntrMd(09,NY46)
+ Gastrointestinal Associates PA
140 Chestnut Street/Suite 300   Ridgewood, NJ 07450   (212)444-2600   Fax (201)444-9471

Hsieh, Kuang-Yiao, MD {1114968260} Urolgy(96,NY08)
+ Essex Hudson Urology
256 Broad Street   Bloomfield, NJ 07003   (973)743-4450   Fax (973)429-9076
+ Essex Hudson Urology
243 Chestnut Street   Newark, NJ 07105   (973)743-4450   Fax (973)344-9188

Hsu, Chia-En, MD {1104872894} RadDia, Radiol, RadBdl(95,PA07)
+ 10 Smoke Tree Close
Piscataway, NJ 08854

Hsu, Christopher Tzu-Yao, MD {1467589903} NnPnMd
+ On-Site Neonatal Partners
1000 Haddonfield-Berlin Road/Suite 210   Voorhees, NJ 08043   (856)782-2212   Fax (856)782-2213

Hsu, George Chiahung, MD {1780892901} Anesth(04,VA01)<PA-TJCNTR, PA-TJHSP>
+ Cooper Anesthesia Associates
One Cooper Plaza/Suite 294-B   Camden, NJ 08103   (856)356-4924   Fax (856)968-8239

Hsu, Jason, MD {1548218787} Ophthl(01,PA01)<PA-WILLSEYE>
+ Mid Atlantic Retina - Wills Eye Retina Surgeons
501 Cooper Landing Road   Cherry Hill, NJ 08002   (856)667-2246   Fax (856)667-2238
+ Mid Atlantic Retina - Wills Eye Retina Surgeons
1417 Cantillon Boulevard   Mays Landing, NJ 08330   (856)667-2246   Fax (609)625-0788

Hsu, Kevin Kaiwen, MD {1477740751} PhyMPain
+ Northeast Spine and Sports Medicine
728 Bennetts Mills Road   Jackson, NJ 08527   (732)415-1401   Fax (732)415-1403
+ Northeast Spine & Sports Medicine
1104 Arnold Avenue   Point Pleasant Beach, NJ 08742   (732)415-1401   Fax (732)714-0188
+ Northeast Spine & Sports Medicine
367 Lakehurst Road   Toms River, NJ 08527   (732)653-1000

Hsu, Madeleine F., MD {1508826249} Anesth(88,DC01)<NJ-OVERLOOK>
+ Overlook Medical Center
99 Beauvoir Avenue/PO Box 210   Summit, NJ 07902   (908)522-2000

Hsu, Pochien Gregory, MD {1407945314} ObsGyn(93,NY47)<NJ-STPETER>
+ 22 Bridge Street
Metuchen, NJ 08840   (732)906-8689   Fax (732)906-8689
+ Cares Surgicenter, LLC.
240 Easton Avenue   New Brunswick, NJ 08901   (732)906-8689   Fax (732)296-8677

Hsu, Stanley Cho Hsien, MD {1992939235} IntrMd, Gastrn(03,PA09)
+ Princeton Medical Group, P.A.
419 North Harrison Street   Princeton, NJ 08540   (609)924-9300   Fax (609)924-6552

Hsu, Vivien M., MD {1992875421} IntrMd, Rheuma(83,NJ05)
+ University Physician Associates of New Jersey
125 Paterson Street/CAB 5200   New Brunswick, NJ 08901   (732)235-7217   Fax (732)235-7217

Hsueh, Linda, MD {1902895253} Ophthl(81,MA05)<NJ-OVERLOOK, NJ-MORRISTN>
+ Summit Medical Group-Berkeley Heights Campus
1 Diamond Hill Road   Berkeley Heights, NJ 07922   (908)273-4300   Fax (908)790-6524

Hsueh, Wayne Daniel, MD {1407113921}
+ Center for Neurological Surgery UMDNJ
90 Bergen Street/DOC 8100   Newark, NJ 07103   (973)972-4588   Fax (973)972-2333

Hu, Andre Min-Teh, MD {1194762971} PainMd, PhysMd(99,NJ06)<NJ-VIRTMHBC, NJ-VIRTUAHS>
+ Synergy Joint and Spine
525 Route 73 South/Suite 302   Marlton, NJ 08053
(856)267-5319   Fax (856)267-5483

Hu, Judy Y., MD {1205897840} Dermat, IntrMd(VA07)
+ Advanced Dermatology, P.C.
33 Overlook Road/MAC 1/Suite 405   Summit, NJ 07901
+ Advanced Dermatology, P.C.
1200 East Ridgewood Avenue   Ridgewood, NJ 07450   Fax (201)493-1009

Hu, Long-Gue, MD {1154330520} ObsGyn(80,TAIW)<NJ-JRSYCITY, NJ-MEADWLND>
+ New Margaret Hague Women's Health Institute
377 Jersey Avenue/Suite 220   Jersey City, NJ 07302
(201)714-2538   Fax (201)795-9157

Hu, Xin Tian, MD {1720081599} Anesth(84,CHN9D)<NJ-SHORE-MEM>
+ Shore Memorial Hospital
1 East New York Avenue/Anesthesiology   Somers Point, NJ 08244   (609)653-3500

Hu, Yiqun, MD {1972529592} Psychy, Nrolgy(91,CHN11)
+ 19 Andover Way
Hamilton, NJ 08610

Hu, Yuan, MD {1497716757} Anesth(99,NY47)
+ Summit Anesthesia Associates, P.A.
33 Overlook Road/Suite 311   Summit, NJ 07901   (908)598-1500   Fax (908)598-0197

Hu, Yuange, MD {1649290180} Psychy, IntrMd(90,CHN07)<NJ-UNIVBHC>
+ Advanced Eyecare & Vision Gallery
105 Omni Drive   Hillsborough, NJ 08844   (732)693-1317   Fax (732)521-3098
eyecare-nj@comcast.net

Hua, Xingjia, MD {1689763971} Grtrcs, IntrMd(87,CHN4A)<NJ-UNVMCPRN>
+ Princeton Medical Group, P.A.
419 North Harrison Street   Princeton, NJ 08540   (609)924-9300   Fax (609)924-6552

Hua, Zhongxue, MD {1376601120} PthAna, PthFor, PthNro(89,CHN19)<NY-JACOBIMC>
+ Office of The Regional Medical Examiner State of NJ
325 Norfolk Street   Newark, NJ 07103   (973)648-3914   Fax (973)648-3692
zxhua@hotmail.com

Huan, Victoria Y., MD {1740431972} Psychy
+ St. Peter's University Hospital
254 Easton Avenue   New Brunswick, NJ 08901   (732)745-8600

Huang, Bei Barbara, MD {1780740605} Psychy(86,CHN2C)<NJ-RUNNELLS, NJ-UNIVBHC>
+ Runnells Specialized Hospital of Union County
40 Watchung Way   Berkeley Heights, NJ 07922   (732)603-8809

Huang, Chen Ya, MD {1801901202} FamMed(65,TAIW)<NJ-STCLR-DOV>
+ 270 Route 206/Bartley Square
Flanders, NJ 07836   (973)584-0233   Fax (973)584-0037

Huang, Chien-Yao, MD {1922154319} Anesth<NJ-HACKNSK>
+ Hackensack University Medical Center
30 Prospect Avenue/Anesth   Hackensack, NJ 07601   (201)996-2000   Fax (201)488-6769
+ Hackensack University MC-Anesthesia Dept
30 Prospect Avenue/Room 2703   Hackensack, NJ 07601   (201)996-2000   Fax (201)996-3962

Huang, Diana, MD {1467686162} ObsGyn
+ The Rubino Ob/Gyn Group
101 Old Short Hills Road/Suite 101   West Orange, NJ 07052   (973)736-1100   Fax (973)736-1834

Huang, Doris Amy, MD {1659684694} Pedtrc
+ Rutherford Pediatrics
338 Union Avenue/Suite 2   Rutherford, NJ 07070   (201)842-0501   Fax (201)842-9190

Huang, Eric A., MD {1477594133} PedEnd(00,NJ06)<NJ-OVERLOOK, NJ-MORRISTN>
+ Overlook Medical Center
99 Beauvoir Avenue/PO Box 210/PediEndo   Summit, NJ 07902   (908)522-2000

Huang, Eric Y., MD {1306000229} Dermat(PA02)
+ Summit Medical Group Florham Park Campus
150 Park Avenue   Florham Park, NJ 07932   (908)273-4300

Huang, Eric Yuchueh, MD {1952320962} Dermat(02,PA01)<NY-NYUTISCH>
+ Summit Medical Group Florham Park Campus
150 Park Avenue   Florham Park, NJ 07932   (973)775-5156
+ Summit Medical Group
34 Mountain Boulevard/Building B   Warren, NJ 07059   (973)775-5156   Fax (908)769-8927

Huang, Grace, MD {1467876268} Pedtrc<NJ-NWRKBETH>
+ Newark Beth Israel Medical Center
201 Lyons Avenue   Newark, NJ 07112   (973)926-7471   Fax (973)926-6452

Huang, Guojie, MD Anesth(82,CHN21)
+ Summit Anesthesia Associates, P.A.
33 Overlook Road/Suite 311   Summit, NJ 07901   (908)598-1500   Fax (908)598-0197

Huang, Hoi Pan, MD {1376770354} RadDia(09,NY0)
+ Our Lady of Lourdes Medical Center
1600 Haddon Avenue/Radiol   Camden, NJ 08103   (856)757-3500

Huang, Ih-Ping, MD {1295759041} Surgry(99,MA05)<NJ-STCLR-DOV>
+ Northwest Surgical Associates
121 Center Grove Road   Randolph, NJ 07869   (973)328-1414

Huang, Jianzhong, MD {1023373818} Surgry
+ Mid-Atlantic Surgical Associates
100 Madison Avenue/Box 88   Morristown, NJ 07960   (646)305-0028   Fax (973)984-7019

Huang, Joe T., MD {1083858872} Surgry<NJ-UMDNJ>
+ University Hospital
150 Bergen Street   Newark, NJ 07103   (973)972-6295

Huang, John Jan, MD {1689613747} Otlryg, SrgFPl(94,PA02)<NJ-VALLEY, NJ-HACKNSK>
+ ENT & Allergy Associates, LLP
690 Kinderkamack Road/Suite 101   Oradell, NJ 07649   (201)722-9850   Fax (201)722-9851
jhuang@entandallergy.com

Huang, Jun C., MD {1700838166} Ophthl, IntrMd(83,CHN21)<NJ-ACMCITY>
+ Horizon Eye Care
2401 Bay Avenue   Ocean City, NJ 08226   (609)399-6300   Fax (609)399-6284
+ Horizon Eye Care
4 Village Drive   Cape May Court House, NJ 08210   (609)465-7100
+ Horizon Eye Care
3003 English Creek Avenue   Egg Harbor Township, NJ 08226   (609)569-8168

Huang, Kevin, MD {1205014420} Surgry(02,PA13)
+ Atlantic Shore Surgical Associates
478 Brick Boulevard   Brick, NJ 08723   (732)701-1244   Fax (732)701-1244

Huang, Kuei-Huang, MD {1609942952} IntrMd(83,NJ05)<NJ-STBARNMC, NJ-MTNSIDE>
+ 912 Pompton Avenue/Suite B-1
Cedar Grove, NJ 07009

Huang, Michael Shu Hsien, DO {1659566628} CdvDis, IntCrd, CarEch(NJ75<NJ-RWJUBRUN, NJ-SOMERSET>
+ 24/7 Heart and Vascular
3084 State Route 27/Suite 5   Kendall Park, NJ 08824   Fax (800)336-7779
+ 24/7 Heart and Vascular
312 Applegarth Road/Suite 207   Monroe, NJ 08831   Fax (800)336-7779
+ 24/7 Heart and Vascular
503 Omni Drive   Hillsborough, NJ 08824   Fax (800)336-7779

Huang, Michelle, MD {1790084473} ObsGyn(10,NJ05)
+ Brunswick-Hills Ob/Gyn, PA
620 Cranbury Road/Suite LL90   East Brunswick, NJ 08816   (732)257-0081   Fax (732)613-4845

Huang, Ming Y., MD {1891897583} FamMed(69,CHN48)<NJ-SOMERSET>
+ 183 West High Street
Somerville, NJ 08876   (908)725-0732   Fax (908)253-0251

Huang, Patty P., MD {1760693287} Pedtrc, PedDvl<PA-CHILDHOS>
+ CHOP Pediatric & Adolescent Specialty Care Center
4009 Black Horse Pike   Mays Landing, NJ 08330   (609)677-7895   Fax (609)677-7835

Huang, Renee, MD {1700041902} SrgC&R
+ St. Barnabas Colon & Rectal Srgy
200 South Orange Avenue/Suite 232   Livingston, NJ 07039   (973)322-0250

Huang, Robert D., MD {1740200096} Otlryg(84,NJ06)<NJ-JFKMED, NJ-RWJURAH>
+ Associates in ENT/Allergy
470 North Avenue   Elizabeth, NJ 07208   (908)352-6700   Fax (908)352-6734
+ Ear Nose & Throat Group of Central NJ
2124 Oak Tree Road/2nd floor   Edison, NJ 08820   (908)352-6700   Fax (732)205-9648

Huang, Shyuan, MD {1699797894} Anesth(81,MEXI)<NJ-RIVERVW>
+ Riverview Medical Center
1 Riverview Plaza/Anesthesiology   Red Bank, NJ 07701   (732)741-2700

Huang, Tammy, MD {1922036896} RadDia, Radiol, IntrMd(90,NY20)<NY-SLOANKET>
+ St. Barnabas Medical Center
94 Old Short Hills Road/Radiology   Livingston, NJ 07039   (973)322-5000

+ Memorial Sloan-Kettering Cancer Center Basking Ridge
136 Mountain View Boulevard   Basking Ridge, NJ 07920   (973)322-5000   Fax (908)542-3220

Huang, Tony T., MD {1639146475} ObsGyn(87,NY47)<NJ-HACKNSK>
+ 40 West Palisade Avenue/Suite 208
Englewood, NJ 07631   (201)568-6588   Fax (201)568-6488

Huang, Wendy, MD {1932272853} AltHol, Acpntr(79,TAIW)<NJ-RIVERVW>
+ 9 Professional Circle/Suite 212
Colts Neck, NJ 07722   (732)780-1155
ask@holisticwendy.com

Hubbard, Sean Tomar, DO {1598779670} Nrolgy(96,FL75)
+ The Neurological Management Group
55 East Cuthbert Boulevard   Haddon Township, NJ 08108

Hubbi, Basil, MD {1316116270} Radiol, RadBdI(03,NJ05)<NJ-UMDNJ>
+ University Hospital
150 Bergen Street/Room C-318   Newark, NJ 07103   (973)972-4300

Hubbs, James E., DO {1922078906} FamMed, IntrMd(92,NJ75)<NJ-UNDRWD, NJ-KMHCHRRY>
+ Maternity & Women's Health
187 East Avenue   Woodstown, NJ 08098   (856)628-0909   Fax (856)624-4496

Huber, Elaine E., MD {1225052624} ObsGyn(83,NY06)<NJ-SOMERSET>
+ Women's Care
903 US Highway 202/Suite 2-A   Raritan, NJ 08869   (908)231-6836   Fax (908)231-6680

Huber, Michael D., DO {1518916162} Anesth(99,NY75)<NJ-ENGLWOOD>
+ Englewood Anesthesiology
350 Engle Street   Englewood, NJ 07631   (201)894-3238   Fax (201)894-0585

Huberman, Daniel Tzvi, MD {1629231279} IntrMd(05,NJ06)<NJ-RWJUBRUN>
+ Sharon E. Selinger MD PA
1 Springfield Avenue/Suite 1A   Summit, NJ 07901   (908)273-8300   Fax (908)273-8807

Hubert, Julio Alejandro, MD {1386770493} IntrMd(80,MEXI)
+ 20 Ferry Street
Newark, NJ 07105   (973)589-5841   Fax (973)589-8446

Hubert, Steven Lee, MD {1770586430} Dermat(93,NY20)<NJ-UNVMCPRN>
+ Lawrenceville Dermatology Associates PC
74 Franklin Corner Road   Lawrenceville, NJ 08648   (609)896-3232   Fax (609)896-3233
hubs@att.net

Hubschmann, Andrea Gibbons, MD {1952643355} ObsGyn
+ Summit Medical Group
34 Mountain Boulevard/Building B   Warren, NJ 07059   (908)769-0100   Fax (908)769-8927
+ Summit Medical Group-Berkeley Heights Campus
1 Diamond Hill Road   Berkeley Heights, NJ 07922   (908)769-0100   Fax (908)608-2376
+ Summit Medical Group
574 Springfield Avenue   Westfield, NJ 07059   (908)389-6391   Fax (908)232-0540

Hubschmann, Otakar R., MD {1528126711} SrgNro(67,CZEC)
+ SBMC-Institute for Neurosurgery
94 Old Short Hills Road   Livingston, NJ 07039   (973)322-6732

Hubsher, Merritt S., MD {1275752404} PsyCAd, Psychy(80,NY08)
+ ADHD, Mood & Behavior Center of New Jersey
210 Malapardis Road   Cedar Knolls, NJ 07927   (973)605-5000   Fax (973)898-9305

Huch, Shane M., DO {1023396769}<NH-DRTMTHMC>
+ Red Bank Anesthesia, LLC
1 Riverview Plaza   Red Bank, NJ 07701   (732)530-2255   Fax (732)450-2620

Huda, Rafeul, MD {1982798294} IntrMd(73,PAK01)<NJ-TRINIWSC>
+ 240 Williamson Street/Suite 506
Elizabeth, NJ 07207   (908)352-4579   Fax (908)352-3540
+ Trinitas Regional Medical Center-Williamson Street
225 Williamson Street/Medicine   Elizabeth, NJ 07207   (908)994-5000

Hudacko, Rachel Mary, MD {1407173941} PthACl(06,NJ06)
+ 4 O'Brien Court
Bayonne, NJ 07002

Hudgins, Joan Leonard, MD {1154430924} PulDis, CritCr(85,DC03)<NJ-NWRKBETH, NJ-STBARNMC>
+ 400 Osborne Terrace at Lyons
Newark, NJ 07112   (973)926-8205   Fax (973)923-5741
+ 90 Washington Street
East Orange, NJ 07017   (973)674-6400

Hudock, Jude A., MD {1710040563} PthCyt, Pthlgy, PthACl(88,PA02)<NJ-UNDRWD>
+ Inspira Health Network
509 North Broad Street/Pathology   Woodbury, NJ 08096   (856)845-0100

Physicians by Name and Address

Hudome, Susan M., MD {1578574877} Pedtrc, NnPnMd(88,PA14)<NJ-MONMOUTH>
+ Pediatrix Medical Group
 255 Third Avenue Long Branch, NJ 07740 (732)222-7006

Hudrick, Robert Eugene, DO {1972583060} GenPrc, FamMed, IntrMd(88,PA77)<NJ-KMHSTRAT, NJ-KMHCHRRY>
+ University Hospital-University Family Medicine
 42 East Laurel Road/Suite 2100 Stratford, NJ 08084 (856)566-7020 Fax (856)566-6188
+ University Doctors Family Practice
 100 Centruy Parkway/Suite 140 Mount Laurel, NJ 08054 (856)566-7020 Fax (856)667-9054
+ The University Doctors - UMDNJ -SOM
 570 Egg Harbor Road/Suite C-2 Sewell, NJ 08084 (856)218-0300 Fax (856)589-5082

Hudson, Claudia Scalorbi, MD {1477524544} FamThp, FamMed(96,ITA01)
+ Whitehouse Station Family Medicine
 263 Main Street/PO Box 128 Whitehouse Station, NJ 08889 (908)534-2249 Fax (908)534-6634

Huege, Steven Fredrick, MD {1598716367} PsyGrt, Psychy, IntrMd(02,TX12)<NJ-HAMPTBHC, PA-UPMCPHL>
+ Hampton Behavioral Health Center
 650 Rancocas Road/Psych Westampton, NJ 08060 (609)267-7000

Huegel, Claudia Marie, MD {1770553455} FamMed(01,DMN01)
+ Integrated Medicine Alliance, P.A.
 30 Shrewsbury Plaza Shrewsbury, NJ 07702 (732)460-9840 Fax (732)460-9848

Hufnal-Miller, Carrie Ann, MD {1861509564} Pedtrc<PA-CHILDHOS>
+ Princeton HealthCare System
 253 Witherspoon Street Princeton, NJ 08540
+ CHOP Newborn and Pediatric Care at UMCPP
 One Plainsboro Road/6th Floor Plainsboro, NJ 08536 Fax (609)853-7630

Hug, Eugene Boris, MD {1114964855} RadOnc, IntrMd, Radiol(86,GER16)<NH-DRTMTHMC>
+ Princeton Radiology Associates, P.A.
 3674 Route 27 Kendall Park, NJ 08824 (732)821-5563 Fax (732)821-6675

Hug, Vickie Beth, MD {1235116781} IntrMd(94,NJ05)
+ Montgomery Internal Medicine Group
 727 State Road Princeton, NJ 08540 (609)921-6410 Fax (609)921-0406

Huggins, Iris A., MD {1235396227} ObsGyn(79,DC03)
+ 101 Church Street
 Teaneck, NJ 07666

Huggins, Juanita Kimberly, DO {1376585950} ObsGyn(92,PA77)<NJ-ACMCMAIN, NJ-ACMCITY>
+ Obstetrics & Gynecology Associates
 239 Hurffville Crosskeys Road Sewell, NJ 08080 (856)262-8300 Fax (856)262-1635

Hugh-Goffe, Judith Colleen, MD {1346232964} Pedtrc(88,NY08)
+ Pathlink, LLC
 66 West Gilbert Street/Suite 100 Tinton Falls, NJ 07701 (732)212-0060 Fax (732)212-0061

Hughes, Alexander Philip, MD {1043488281} SrgSpn(03,TN05)
+ HSS Paramus Outpatient Center
 140 East Ridgewood Avenue/Suite 175-S Paramus, NJ 07652 (201)796-2255 Fax (201)796-3711

Hughes, Ann M., MD {1649292236} Radiol, RadDia(80,NY03)<NJ-CENTRAST>
+ Freehold Radiology Group
 901 West Main Street Freehold, NJ 07728 (732)462-4844
+ CentraState Medical Center
 901 West Main Street/Radiology Freehold, NJ 07728 (732)294-2946

Hughes, Charles R., MD {1902807282} SrgC&R, Surgry(90,PA14)
+ Surgical Specialists of New Jersey
 668 Main Street/Suite 4 Lumberton, NJ 08048 (609)267-7050 Fax (609)267-7065

Hughes, Eric Anton, MD {1700984952} InfDis(99,CT01)
+ Bristol-Myers Squibb Co. - Occupational Health
 Route 206 & Provinceline Road Princeton, NJ 08543 (609)252-4000
 eric.hughes@aya.yale.edu

Hughes, Janey Ballin, DO {1326098930} FamMed(95,NY75)
+ Capital Health Primary Care-Bordentown
 1 Third Street Bordentown, NJ 08505 (609)298-2005 Fax (609)324-8267

Hughes, Kristin Lynne, MD {1366882862} EmrgMd(09,GRN01)<NJ-CHSFULD>
+ Capital Health System/Fuld Campus
 750 Brunswick Avenue/Emerg Med Trenton, NJ 08638 (609)394-6000

Hughes, Lesley Ann, MD {1508818808} RadOnc(98,PA09)<NJ-COOPRUMC>
+ Cooper University Hospital
 One Cooper Plaza/B-122 Keleman Camden, NJ 08103 (856)342-2300 Fax (856)365-8504

Hughes, Naomi Teutel, MD {1255372819} Pedtrc<NJ-VIRTVOOR>
+ Virtua Voorhees
 100 Bowman Drive Voorhees, NJ 08043 (443)722-2370

Hughes, Patricia L., MD {1851486765} ObsGyn, RprEnd(80,NY03)<NJ-HACKNSK>
+ 140 Prospect Avenue/Suite 10
 Hackensack, NJ 07601 (201)342-3428 Fax (201)342-3904

Hughes, Susan M., MD {1528060365} SrgFPl, OthrSp, Ophthl(75,DC01)<NJ-VIRTUAHS, NJ-VIRTMARL>
+ Hughes Center for Aesthetic Medicine
 1765 S Springdale Road/Suite B-2 Cherry Hill, NJ 08003 (856)751-4554 Fax (856)751-6888
 drhughes@drnewyou.com

Hughes, Wray, DO {1669761128} Anesth
+ Cooper Anesthesia Associates
 One Cooper Plaza/Suite 294-B Camden, NJ 08103 (856)342-2425 Fax (856)968-8239

Hugo, Manuel C., MD {1760568836} Pedtrc(69,PHIL)<NJ-HOBUNIMC>
+ Palisades Pediatrics
 2009 Palisade Avenue Union City, NJ 07087 (201)865-6750 Fax (201)601-1336

Huh, Chan Woo, MD {1417937178} Anesth(73,KOR07)<NJ-BAYSHORE>
+ Red Bank Anesthesia, LLC
 1 Riverview Plaza Red Bank, NJ 07701 (732)530-2255 Fax (732)450-2620

Huhn-Werner, Maryann, MD {1194787606} Gyneco, ObsGyn(83,DOM03)
+ 854 Mountain Avenue
 Mountainside, NJ 07092 (908)317-9922 Fax (908)317-9544

Hui, Dao, MD {1285730283} FamMed(99,PA13)<NJ-UNVMCPRN>
+ Menla HealthCare, LLC
 411 Executive Drive Princeton, NJ 08540 (609)688-1608 Fax (609)688-1648
 menlahealthcare@yahoo.com

Hui, Kenny Pingchi, MD {1588637540} Gastrn, IntrMd(93,NY19)<NJ-JRSYSHMC, NJ-OCEANMC>
+ Atlantic Coast Gastroenterology
 1944 Corlies Avenue/Suite 205 Neptune, NJ 07753 (732)776-9300 Fax (732)776-8059
+ Atlantic Coast Gastroenterology
 1640 Route 88 West/Suite 202 Brick, NJ 08724 (732)776-9300 Fax (732)458-8529

Hui, Thomas P., MD {1629236989} IntrMd, Nephro(79,NY19)<NJ-RWJUBRUN>
+ Horizon NJ Health
 210 Silvia Street West Trenton, NJ 08628 (609)538-0700 Fax (609)538-1510

Hui, Ying-Kei, MD {1982866430} IntrMd(05,CHN1P)<NJ-UNVMCPRN>
+ Penn Medicine Princeton Medicine Phys
 5 Plainsboro Road/Suite 350 Plainsboro, NJ 08536 (609)853-6049 Fax (609)853-7271

Huish, Stephen H., DO {1235214339} PainMd, PhysMd, SprtMd(91,MO78)<NJ-MEADWLND>
+ Boulevard Medical
 801 Kennedy Boulevard Bayonne, NJ 07002 (201)437-0250

Huk, Matthew David, MD {1184911356} SrgC&R
+ Surgical Practice of Rolando Rolandelli, MD
 435 South Street/Suite 360 Morristown, NJ 07960 (973)971-7200 Fax (973)290-7521

Hulbert, David S., MD {1609864370} ObsGyn(87,PA14)<NJ-LOURDMED, NJ-VIRTMHBC>
+ Advocare Burlington County Obstetrics & Gynecology
 1000 Salem Road/Suite B Willingboro, NJ 08046 (609)871-2060 Fax (609)871-3535
+ Burlington County Ob-Gyn
 8008 Route 130 N/Suite 320 Delran, NJ 08075 (856)871-2060 Fax (856)764-0103
+ Burlington County Ob-Gyn
 210 Ark Road/Suite 216 Mount Laurel, NJ 08046 (856)778-2060 Fax (856)778-8182

Hullinger, Heidi, MD {1942461033} SrgSpn
+ 33 Overlook Road/Suite 305
 Summit, NJ 07901 (908)376-1532 Fax (908)634-9555

Hulse, Andrea Doria, DO {1679532220} FamMed(00,MO79)
+ Columbus Family Physicians
 23659 Columbus Road/Suite 4 Columbus, NJ 08022 (609)298-3304 Fax (609)298-7091

Huma, Sabahath, MD {1144674847} IntHos
+ AtlantiCare Hospitalist Program
 1925 Pacific Avenue/8th Floor Atlantic City, NJ 08401 (609)576-9089

Hume, Edward Samuel, MD {1225197502} Psychy(75,MO02)
+ Center for Family Guidance, PC
 765 East Route 70/Building A-101 Marlton, NJ 08053 (856)797-4800 Fax (856)810-0110

Hume, Eric Lynn, MD {1871688192} SrgOrt, IntrMd(78,NY15)<PA-UPMCPHL>
+ Penn Medicine at Cherry Hill
 409 Route 70 East/Surgery/Ortho Cherry Hill, NJ 08034 (856)429-1519

Humera, Rafath Khatoon, MD {1376871202} IntrMd(98,INA83)
+ Park Medical Center
 535 Getty Avenue/Suite 3 Clifton, NJ 07011 (973)782-4905 Fax (973)782-4893
 contact@parkmedicalnj.com

Hummel, Andrew E., DO {1457334005} Anesth(86,PA77)<NJ-HACKNSK>
+ Hackensack Anesthesiology Associates
 140 Prospect Avenue/Suite 8 Hackensack, NJ 07601 (201)488-0066 Fax (201)488-6769
+ Hackensack University MC-Anesthesia Dept
 30 Prospect Avenue/Room 2703 Hackensack, NJ 07601 (201)488-0066 Fax (201)996-3962
+ Hackensack University Medical Center
 30 Prospect Avenue/Anesthesiology Hackensack, NJ 07601 (201)996-2000

Hummel, Jennifer E., DO {1134327026} ObsGyn(05,NJ75)<NJ-KMHTURNV>
+ Rowan SOM Department of Ob/Gyn
 405 Hurffville-Cross Keys Road Sewell, NJ 08080 (856)589-1414 Fax (856)256-5772

Hummel, Joseph C., DO {1275565616} EmrgMd, FamMed(70,PA77)<NJ-VIRTVOOR>
+ Virtua Camden
 1000 Atlantic Avenue/EmrgServices Camden, NJ 08104 (856)246-3000 Fax (856)246-3061
+ Emergency Physician Associates, P.A.
 307 South Evergreen Avenue/PO Box 298 Woodbury, NJ 08096 (856)246-3000 Fax (856)848-1431

Hummel, Mark J., MD {1598787673} Pedtrc(85,PA02)<NJ-VIRTVOOR>
+ Virtua Voorhees
 100 Bowman Drive Voorhees, NJ 08043 (856)325-3563
 mhummel@wjhs.org

Humoee, Nidal Michel, MD {1326186396} Pedtrc, NnPnMd(93,SYR01)<NJ-HUNTRDN>
+ Hunterdon Medical Center
 2100 Wescott Drive/NeoPeri/Pedi Flemington, NJ 08822 (908)788-6100

Humphrey, Frederick James, II, DO {1841439163} PsyCAd(66,PA77)<NJ-KMHTURNV, NJ-KMHSTRAT>
+ Kennedy Memorial Hospital-University Medical Center
 18 East Laurel Road Stratford, NJ 08084 (856)346-6000

Humphreys, Erika, MD {1922054931} Pedtrc(87,CZE15)<NJ-COMMED>
+ Drs. Lee and Humphreys
 1479 Route 539/Suite 1 A Little Egg Harbor, NJ 08087 (609)296-1900 Fax (609)296-1906

Hundle, Rameet Kaur, MD {1427477785} FamMed
+ MedExpress Urgent Care Hazlet
 2880 Highway 35 Hazlet, NJ 07730 (732)888-1238 Fax (732)888-1230

Hundle, Sukhwinder K., MD {1306811773} IntrMd, Grtrcs(78,INA13)<NJ-JRSYSHMC, NJ-MONMOUTH>
+ 721 North Beers Street/Suite 1-A
 Holmdel, NJ 07733 (732)739-3555

Hung, Deborah Liu, MD {1770531055} Pedtrc(95,PA12)
+ Advocare West Deptford Pediatrics
 1050 Mantua Pike Wenonah, NJ 08090 (856)468-8330 Fax (856)468-9121
+ Advocare West Deptford Pediatrics
 19 Village Center Drive Swedesboro, NJ 08085 (856)468-8330 Fax (856)879-2855
+ Advocare West Deptford Pediatrics
 646 Kings Highway West Deptford, NJ 08090 (856)879-2887 Fax (856)879-2855

Hung, Oliver Li-Ping, MD {1356390173} EmrgMd, UndsMd(92,MA05)<NJ-MORRISTN>
+ Morristown Medical Center
 100 Madison Avenue/EmrgMed Morristown, NJ 07962 (800)290-5309 Fax (803)434-4354

Hung, Yvonne, MD {1538233804} Pedtrc(98,NJ05)<NJ-MTNSIDE, NJ-STBARNMC>
+ Montclair Pediatrics
 73 Park Street Montclair, NJ 07042 Fax (973)746-6772

Hunninghake, Leroy H., MD {1144263773} Rheuma, OrtOst, IntrMd(83,KS02)<NJ-UNVMCPRN, NJ-CHSFULD>
+ Princeton Rheumatology & Osteoporosis Center
 281 Witherspoon Street/Suite 200 Princeton, NJ 08540 (609)921-3331 Fax (609)252-0722
+ Princeton Rheumatology & Osteoporosis Center
 11 Centre Drive Jamesburg, NJ 08831 (609)921-3331

Hunt, Charles D., MD SrgNro(77,OH40)
+ 1031 Garden Street
 Hoboken, NJ 07030
 huntneurosurgery@mac.com

Hunt, Judith A., MD {1366470320} Pedtrc(78,PA13)<NJ-SJHREGMC>
+ Vineland Children's Residential Treatment Center
2000 Maple Avenue   Vineland, NJ 08360
Hunt, Mary Elizabeth, MD {1497799563} ObsGyn(98,NY19)<NJ-SUMOAKSH>
+ Lifeline Medical Associates
530 Morris Avenue   Springfield, NJ 07081   (973)379-7477   Fax (973)379-9094
Hunt, Rameck R., MD {1932130267} IntrMd(99,NJ06)<NJ-RWJUBRUN>
+ Princeton Medicine
5 Plainsboro Road/Suite 300   Plainsboro, NJ 08536   (609)853-7272   Fax (609)853-7271
Hunt, Stephen A., MD {1457440711} SrgOrt, SprtMd(00,NY19)<NJ-MORRISTN>
+ Tri-County Orthopedics
197 Ridgedale Street/Suite 300   Cedar Knolls, NJ 07927   (908)234-2022   Fax (973)829-9174
+ Tri-County Orthopedics
1590 Route 206 North   Bedminster, NJ 07921   (908)234-2022   Fax (908)234-2022
Hunter, James Blaine, MD {1194766360} Surgry, SrgThr(86,DC03)<NJ-HACKNSK>
+ Hackensack University Medical Center
30 Prospect Avenue/Surgery   Hackensack, NJ 07601   (201)996-2000
Hunter, Kevin Edward, MD {1831248780} Nrolgy(92,PA12)<NJ-ACMCMAIN>
+ AtlantiCare Physician Group Joslin Diabetes Center
2500 English Creek Avenue/Bldg 800   Egg Harbor Township, NJ 08234   (609)407-2277   Fax (609)677-7280
Hunter, Robert L., MD {1871688101} ObsGyn(96,MI07)<NJ-COOPRUMC>
+ Cooper Faculty Ob/Gyn
1103 Kings Highway North/Suite 201   Cherry Hill, NJ 08034   (856)321-1800   Fax (856)321-0133
+ Cooper Ob/Gyn
4 Plaza Drive/Suite 403/Bunker Hill Pl   Sewell, NJ 08080   (856)321-1800   Fax (856)270-4022
+ Women's Care Center
3 Cooper Plaza/Suite 301   Camden, NJ 08034   (856)342-2959   Fax (856)968-8575
Hupart, Preston Arthur, DO {1487610796} CdvDis, IntrMd(87,NY75)
+ Total Cardiology Care
120 Franklin Street   Jersey City, NJ 07307   (201)216-9791   Fax (201)216-1362
+ Total Cardiology Care
2035 Hamburg Pike/Suite L   Wayne, NJ 07470   (201)216-9791   Fax (973)248-3455
+ Total Cardiology Care
150 Warren Street   Jersey City, NJ 07307   (201)216-9791   Fax (201)216-1362
Huppert, Leon J., MD {1407815947} Ophthl(74,NY19)
+ Cataract & Laser Institute, P.A.
101 Prospect Street/Suite 102   Lakewood, NJ 08701   (732)367-0699   Fax (732)367-0937
Huq, Irfan-Ul, MD {1225080229} Gastrn, IntrMd(69,BAN02)<NJ-CHSFULD, NJ-RWJUHAM>
+ Capital Medical Associates
1235 Whitehorse Mercerville Rd   Trenton, NJ 08619   (609)587-3003   Fax (609)587-4512
+ Capital Medical Associates
132 Delaware Avenue   Florence, NJ 08518   (609)587-3003   Fax (609)499-9384
Hurckes, Lisa Carabelli, MD {1518901503} IntrMd(93,NJ03)<NJ-OVERLOOK>
+ Community Health Center at Vauxhall
3 Farrington Street   Vauxhall, NJ 07088   (908)598-7950   Fax (908)686-1163
DrHurckes@aol.com
Hurley, Kathleen Lenore, MD {1508200270} Anesth<NJ-STBARNMC>
+ St. Barnabas Medical Center
94 Old Short Hills Road   Livingston, NJ 07039   (973)322-5512
Hurley, Margaret L., DO {1659392413} FamMed(88,NJ75)<NJ-UNDRWD, NJ-SJRSYELM>
+ 303 North Main Street
Woodstown, NJ 08098   (856)769-7737   Fax (856)769-8291
Huron, Randye F., MD {1689612822} PedDvl(83,NY08)<NJ-HACKNSK>
+ Hackensack University Medical Center
30 Prospect Avenue/DevlpmntlPeds   Hackensack, NJ 07601   (201)996-2000
Hurst, Wendy Robin, MD {1215025440} FrtInf, ObsGyn(86,MA07)<NJ-ENGLWOOD, NJ-HACKNSK>
+ Englewood Ob/Gyn Associates
370 Grand Avenue   Englewood, NJ 07631   (201)894-9599   Fax (201)894-9192

Hurwitz, James Bennett, MD {1023087236} SrgCrC, Surgry(84,IL02)<NJ-STBARNMC, NJ-OVERLOOK>
+ Drs. Bruno and Hurwitz
104 North Euclid Avenue   Westfield, NJ 07090   (908)654-0888
+ Drs. Murphy & Williams, P.A.
33 Overlook Road/Suite 412   Summit, NJ 07901   (908)273-7274
+ Drs. Murphy & Williams, P.A.
867 St. Georges Avenue   Rahway, NJ 07090   (732)388-0990
Husain, Abbas M., MD {1164449641} FamMed(72,INA87)<NJ-OURLADY>
+ Drs Husain and Shen
5 West Chestnut Avenue   Merchantville, NJ 08109   (856)665-9424
Husain, Abid, MD {1275658577} PhysMd(82,PAK04)
+ Cardiac Care
1314 Park Avenue/Suite 9   Plainfield, NJ 07060   (908)222-8970   Fax (908)222-8762
Husain, Aftab, MD {1235131616} Urolgy(76,INA54)<NJ-RBAY-OLDB, NJ-RBAYPERT>
+ Avenel Iselin Medical Group
400 Gill Lane   Iselin, NJ 08830   (732)404-1580   Fax (732)404-1594
+ 663 Bruce Avenue
Perth Amboy, NJ 08861   (732)404-1580   Fax (732)826-6576
Husain, Ali, DO {1790073419} FamMed
+ 663 Brace Avenue
Perth Amboy, NJ 08861   (732)826-0059
Husain, Mansoor Ul-Haque, MD {1497723548} Anesth(86,AB01)
+ 16 Autumn Drive
Moorestown, NJ 08057
Husain, Qasim M., MD {1982835849} SrgSpn, SrgOrt(NJ05<NY-MTSINAI>
+ Orthopaedic Sports Medicine
80 Oak Hill Road   Red Bank, NJ 07701   (732)741-2313   Fax (732)741-7154
+ Coastal Ear Nose and Throat LLC
1301 Route 72/Suite 340   Manahawkin, NJ 08050   (732)741-2313   Fax (732)280-7815
Husain, Sajidah I., MD {1225204852} Pedtrc(80,PAKI)
+ 24 Even Drive
Morganville, NJ 07751   (609)562-6748
Husain, Saleem, MD {1134197346} CdvDis, IntrMd(90,NJ06)<NJ-JFKMED, NJ-RWJURAH>
+ Cardiac Care
1314 Park Avenue/Suite 9   Plainfield, NJ 07060   (908)222-8970   Fax (908)222-8762
Husain, Sara, MD {1912285701} IntrMd
+ Shore Nephrology, P.A.
2100 Corlies Avenue/Suite 15   Neptune, NJ 07753   (732)988-8228   Fax (732)774-1528
Husain, Syed Asif, DO {1326054008} InfDis, IntrMd(06,NY75)
+ Infectious Disease Consultants
1245 Whitehorse-Mercerville Rd   Mercerville, NJ 08619   (609)581-2000   Fax (609)581-5450
Husain, Syeda Amna, MD {1629463468} Pedtrc
+ 479 County Road 520/Suite A201
Marlboro, NJ 07746   (732)786-3484
Husain, Zaheer, MD {1144429697} IntrMd(99,INA1K)<NJ-VIRTMHBC>
+ Virtua Memorial
175 Madison Avenue/Hospitalist   Mount Holly, NJ 08060   (609)914-6180   Fax (609)914-6182
Husain, Zain, MD {1225325848} Dermat
+ 479 County Road 520/Suite A201
Marlboro, NJ 07746   (732)702-1212   Fax (732)702-1214
Husar, Walter G., MD {1619974466} Nrolgy(88,NJ05)<NJ-STCLR-DEN>
+ Rutgers- New Jersey Medical School
185 South Orange Avenue/Neuroscience   Newark, NJ 07103   (973)972-5208
husar@umdnj.edu
+ Rutgers NJ School of Medicine Neurology
90 Bergen Street/DOC 1201   Newark, NJ 07103   (973)972-5208   Fax (973)972-5059
Huskowski, Piotr, MD {1710932959} IntrMd, Gastrn(82,POLA)<NJ-STMRYPAS>
+ 1005 Clifton Avenue/Suite 1
Clifton, NJ 07013   (973)778-7882   Fax (973)778-3827
Husnain, Zia F., MD {1225418783}<NJ-HOBUNIMC>
+ Hoboken University Medical Center
308 Willow Avenue   Hoboken, NJ 07030   (201)418-3127
Hussain, Aazim Syed, MD {1134167596} Pedtrc(99,NJ06)<NJ-RWJUBRUN>
+ Hillsborough Pediatrics
390 Amwell Road/Suite 106   Hillsborough, NJ 08844   (908)431-3100   Fax (908)431-3101
Hussain, Adnan, MD {1215297429} IntrMd
+ Pulmonary & Allergy Associates
8 Saddle Road/Suite 101   Cedar Knolls, NJ 07927

(908)934-0555   Fax (973)540-0472
Hussain, Aijaz, MD {1851364301} FamMGrtc, IntrMd(95,INA32)<NJ-STPETER>
+ Saint Peter's Physician Associates
294 Applegarth Road   Monroe Township, NJ 08831   (609)409-1363
Hussain, Arif, MD {1053402784} IntrMd(99,PAK18)<PA-UPMCBDFD, NJ-ACMCITY>
+ AtlantiCare Regional Medical Center/City Campus
1925 Pacific Avenue/Internal Med   Atlantic City, NJ 08401   (609)441-8146   Fax (609)441-8002
Hussain, Arif Syed, MD {1548554249} IntrMd(08,NSK03)<NJ-STFRNMED>
+ LMA LifeCare Physicians
1001 Washington Road   Robbinsville, NJ 08691   (609)944-4500
+ St. Francis Medical Center
601 Hamilton Avenue/IntMed   Trenton, NJ 08629   (609)599-5061
Hussain, Asad R., MD {1376858043}
+ 364 Spotswood Englishtown Road
Monroe Township, NJ 08831   (210)567-7000
Hussain, Asher Ferjad, MD {1780921288} Nephro(NJ02<NJ-JRSYSHMC>
+ Mercer Kidney Institute
40 Fuld Street/Suite 401   Trenton, NJ 08638   (609)599-1004   Fax (609)599-3611
asherh@gmail.com
Hussain, Asim, MD {1871910455} IntHos<NJ-RWJURAH>
+ Robert Wood Johnson University Hospital at Rahway
865 Stone Street   Rahway, NJ 07065   (732)381-4200
Hussain, Asiya, MD {1679984843} IntrMd<NJ-ACMCITY>
+ AtlantiCare Regional Medical Center/City Campus
1925 Pacific Avenue/Medicine   Atlantic City, NJ 08401   (609)345-4000
Hussain, Kashif, MD {1710399365} Pedtrc<NJ-CHDNWBTH>
+ Children's Hospital of New Jersey
201 Lyons Avenue/Osborne Terrace   Newark, NJ 07112   (973)926-7040
Hussain, Mahboob, MD {1336231828} Anesth(75,INA16)
+ Endo Surgi Center at Union
11 Hanson Court   Princeton, NJ 08540   (732)355-1569
mahboobhuss@gmail.com
Hussain, Mohammed Jawaad, MD {1932337144} Pedtrc
+ Cooper Peds/Children's Regional Ctr
3 Cooper Plaza/Suite 200   Camden, NJ 08103   (856)342-2472   Fax (856)368-8297
Hussain, Muhammad N., DO {1992719652} FamMed, EnDbMt(95,IA75)<NJ-CHSFULD, NJ-CHSMRCER>
+ Muhammad N. Hussain MD PHD
512 Hamilton Avenue   Trenton, NJ 08609   (609)395-5787   Fax (609)394-3777
Hussain, Najeeb Ullah, MD {1376626093} PsyGrt, Psychy(90,PAK11)<NJ-UNIVBHC>
+ University Behavioral HealthCare
183 South Orange Avenue   Newark, NJ 07103   (973)972-5479
Hussain, Rubaba, MD {1194913681} FamMed<NJ-HACKNSK>
+ Hackensack University Medical Center
30 Prospect Avenue   Hackensack, NJ 07601   (201)996-2000
Hussain, Sabiha, MD {1881764314} IntrMd, PulDis, CritCr(95,NJ05)
+ UH- Robert Wood Johnson Med
125 Paterson Street/MEB 568/PmCrtc   New Brunswick, NJ 08901   (732)828-3000
Hussain, Sajjad, MD {1780672188} IntrMd, EnDbMt(88,PAK01)<NJ-SOCEANCO>
+ Southern Ocean County Medical Center
1140 Route 72 West   Manahawkin, NJ 08050   (609)597-6011
Hussain, Saleha, MD {1093804965} FamMed(79,INA16)<NJ-CHSFULD, NJ-CHSMRCER>
+ 100 Federal City Road/Suite C103
Lawrenceville, NJ 08648   (609)883-1700
Hussain, Sarah, MD {1801134119} FamMed
+ Associates in Ophthalmology
22 Old Short Hills Road/Suite 102   Livingston, NJ 07039   (973)992-5200   Fax (973)535-5741
Hussain, Shahzad, MD {1982795191} IntrMd, Allrgy, Rheuma(90,PAK12)
+ 101 Prospect Street
Lakewood, NJ 08701   (732)370-7711   Fax (732)370-6519
Shahzadhussainmd@yahoo.com
Hussain, Suhaila S., MD {1225055775} Pedtrc(78,IRQ01)<NJ-CHSFULD, NJ-CHSMRCER>
+ 512 Hamilton Avenue
Trenton, NJ 08609   (609)394-5787   Fax (609)394-3777
Hussain, Syed, MD {1194279786} RadDia
+ Monmouth Medical Imaging
300 Second Avenue   Long Branch, NJ 07740   (732)923-6806   Fax (732)923-6006

Physicians by Name and Address

Hussain, Syed Faiyaz, MD {1013017284} IntrMd, EnDbMt(77,PAKI11)
+ 208 Bridge Street
Metuchen, NJ 08840   (732)603-2001   Fax (732)906-8540

Hussain, Zaheda M., MD {1487853727} Pedtrc(70,PAKI)<NJ-HACKNSK, NJ-HOLYNAME>
+ Riverside Medical Group
714 Tenth Street/Suite 2   Secaucus, NJ 07094   (201)863-3346   Fax (201)865-0015

Hussain, Zahid, MD {1992733232} FamMed(02,DMN01)<NJ-CHSFULD, NJ-CHSMRCER>
+ Summit Medical Arts
9225 John F Kennedy Boulevard   North Bergen, NJ 07047   (201)453-2800

Hussain-Rizvi, Ambrin, MD {1831227875} Pedtrc, PedEmg(00,DMN01)<NY-JACOBIMC>
+ St Joseph's Medical Center Emergency
703 Main Street   Paterson, NJ 07503   (973)754-2240   Fax (973)754-2249

Hussaini, Azmatullah Syed, MD {1366725335}
+ Virtua Voorhees
100 Bowman Drive   Voorhees, NJ 08043   (856)247-2594   Fax (856)247-2597

Hussaini, Syed Azharullah, MD {1518929728} IntrMd, Grtrcs(91,INA2Y)<NJ-NWRKBETH>
+ Newark Beth Israel Medical Center
201 Lyons Avenue/GeriatricMed   Newark, NJ 07112   (973)926-8491

Hussein, Ahmed Hamdy, MD {1104294685} IntrMd<NJ-MORRISTN>
+ Morristown Medical Center
100 Madison Avenue   Morristown, NJ 07962   (973)971-5000

Hussein, Hussein A., MD {1154654648}<NJ-CHSFULD>
+ Capital Health System/Fuld Campus
750 Brunswick Avenue   Trenton, NJ 08638   (609)394-6031   Fax (609)394-6031

Husserl, Toby B., MD {1548249063} SrgOrt, SprtMd(79,PA09)<NJ-JRSYSHMC, NJ-OCEANMC>
+ Orthopaedic Institute of Central Jersey
2315A Highway 34/Suite D   Manasquan, NJ 08736   (732)974-0404   Fax (732)449-4271
+ Orthopaedic Institute of Central Jersey
226 Highway 37 West/Suite 203   Toms River, NJ 08755   (732)974-0404   Fax (732)240-5329
+ Orthopaedic Institute of Central Jersey
365 Broad Street   Red Bank, NJ 08736   (732)933-4300   Fax (732)933-1444

Huston, Donald, Jr., DO {1316973563} IntrMd, PulDis(80,IA75)
+ Cumberland Medical Associates
1206 West Sherman Avenue   Vineland, NJ 08360   (856)691-8444   Fax (856)691-8325

Huston, Whitney Leigh, DO {1790072411}
+ Rowan University-School of Osteopathic Medicine
1 Medical Center Drive   Stratford, NJ 08084   (856)566-6748   Fax (856)566-6222

Hutcheson, Jonathan Justin, DO {1144500554} FamMed
+ AtlantiCare Family Medicine
210 South Shore Road/Suite 201   Marmora, NJ 08223   (609)407-2273   Fax (609)390-2753

Hutchinson-Colas, Juana A., MD {1689780587} ObsGyn(90,NY08)
+ UMDNJ OBGYN
125 Paterson Street/Suite 4200   New Brunswick, NJ 08901   (732)235-6600   Fax (732)235-6550
+ New Margaret Hague Women's Health Institute
377 Jersey Avenue/Suite 220   Jersey City, NJ 07302   (732)235-6600   Fax (201)795-9157

Hutchison, Melissa M., MD {1285664615} FamMed(91,IL01)
+ AtlantiCare Family Medicine
210 South Shore Road/Suite 201   Marmora, NJ 08223   (609)407-2273   Fax (609)390-2753

Hutt, Douglas A., MD {1457440729} PulDis, CritCr, IntrMd(82,NY01)
+ Pulmonary & Intensive Care Specialists of NJ
593 Cranbury Road   East Brunswick, NJ 08816   (732)613-8880   Fax (732)613-0077

Hutter, Andrew M., MD {1710087747} SrgOrt(83,DC03)<NJ-STBARNMC>
+ Center for Orthopaedics
1500 Pleasant Valley Way/Suite 101   West Orange, NJ 07052   (973)669-5600   Fax (973)669-0269
+ Short Hills Surgery Center
187 Millburn Avenue/Suite 101   Millburn, NJ 07041   (973)669-5600   Fax (973)671-0557

Huttner, Ruby P., MD {1053586146} ObsGyn, IntrMd(76,NY45)<NJ-HUNTRDN>
+ Affiliates in Obstetrics & Gynecology, P.A.
111 Route 31/Suite 121 2nd FL Bldg B   Flemington, NJ 08822   (908)782-2825   Fax (908)782-0196
+ Affiliates in Obstetrics & Gynecology, P.A.
99 Grayrock Road/Second Floor   Clinton, NJ 08809

(908)782-2825   Fax (908)730-8504
+ Affiliates in Obstetrics & Gynecology, P.A.
431 Highway 22 East   Whitehouse, NJ 08822   (908)823-1600   Fax (908)823-1640

Hutton-Cassie, Donna Pauline, MD {1639101272} Pedtrc(96,DC03)
+ NHCAC Health Center at West New York
5301 Broadway   West New York, NJ 07093   (201)866-9320   Fax (201)867-9183

Hux, Charles Howard, MD {1609861616} MtFtMd, ObsGyn(81,OH06)<NJ-JRSYSHMC, NJ-MONMOUTH>
+ 2130 Highway 35/Suite A123
Sea Girt, NJ 08750   (732)449-9900
+ Shore Perinatal Associates
475 Route 70/Suite 201   Lakewood, NJ 08701   (732)449-9900   Fax (732)449-4407

Huynh, Nha T., DO {1376709758} IntrMd<NJ-DEBRAHLC>
+ Deborah Heart and Lung Center
200 Trenton Road   Browns Mills, NJ 08015   (609)893-1200

Huzar, Diana, DO {1336310788} Pedtrc<NJ-MORRISTN, NJ-STCLRDEN>
+ Advocare Vernon Pediatrics
249 Route 94   Vernon, NJ 07462   (973)827-4550   Fax (973)827-5845

Hwang, Cheng-Hong, DO {1063509362} IntrMd, PulDis, CritCr(78,IA75)<NJ-RWJURAH>
+ 1457 Raritan Road
Clark, NJ 07066   (908)272-2270   Fax (908)272-0558
Cheng-Hong.Hwang@yahoo.com

Hwang, Eric Jesse, DO {1922312289} EmrgMd<NJ-STJOSHOS>
+ St Joseph's Medical Center Emergency
703 Main Street   Paterson, NJ 07503   (973)754-2240   Fax (973)754-2249

Hwang, Evelyn R., DO {1558375311} IntrMd, Nephro(78,IA75)<NJ-VALYONS>
+ VA New Jersey Health Care System at Lyons
151 Knollcroft Road   Lyons, NJ 07939   (908)647-0180   Fax (908)604-5219

Hwang, John M., MD {1457349177} IntrMd(94,NY08)
+ The Park Medical Group
220 Livingston Street/Suite 202   Northvale, NJ 07647   (201)768-9090   Fax (201)768-9009
+ The Park Medical Group
274 County Road/Suite A   Tenafly, NJ 07670   (201)768-9090   Fax (201)568-0483

Hwang, Ki S., MD {1205846680} SrgOrt(99,NJ05)
+ New Jersey Orthopaedic Institute
504 Valley Road/Suite 200   Wayne, NJ 07470   (973)694-2690   Fax (973)686-0701

Hwee, Lillian, DO {1750325312} IntrMd(88,PA77)
+ CAMCare Health Corporation
2610 Federal Street   Camden, NJ 08104   (856)635-0203   Fax (856)225-0753

Hyans, Peter, MD {1528060605} SrgPlstc, Surgry, SrgHnd(86,NJ06)<NJ-OVERLOOK, NJ-STBARNMC>
+ Summit Medical Group-Berkeley Heights Campus
1 Diamond Hill Road   Berkeley Heights, NJ 07922   (908)273-4300   Fax (908)790-6524

Hyatt, Adam Extein, MD {1497080105} SrgOrt<NJ-RWJUBRUN>
+ RWJ University Hospital New Brunswick
One Robert Wood Johnson Place   New Brunswick, NJ 08901   (732)828-3000

Hyatt, Alexander Charles, MD {1578503595} Pedtrc, PedInf(75,NY47)<NJ-ENGLWOOD>
+ Englewood Hospital and Medical Center
350 Engle Street/Pedi Clinic   Englewood, NJ 07631   (201)894-3245   Fax (201)894-3759
hyatta@aol.com
+ Englewood Medical Associates Pediatrics
350 Engle Street   Englewood, NJ 07631   (201)894-3245   Fax (201)894-5649

Hyatt, Gayon Marie, MD {1538401781} FamMed
+ 1310 Broad Street
Bloomfield, NJ 07003   (973)338-0935   Fax (973)338-1097

Hyder, Carl Franklin, MD {1245371129} Ophthl(84,PA07)
+ Eye Care Physicians & Surgeons of New Jersey
73 South Main Street   Medford, NJ 08055   (609)654-6140   Fax (609)953-2257
+ Eye Care Physicians & Surgeons of New Jersey
2301 Evesham Road/Suite 501-502   Voorhees, NJ 08043   (609)654-6140   Fax (856)770-0840
+ Eye Care Physicians & Surgeons of New Jersey
1701 Wynwood Drive   Cinnaminson, NJ 08055   (856)829-0600   Fax (856)829-2832

Hyett, Marvin R., MD {1538271275} Gyneco, ObsGyn(63,PA02)<NJ-ACMCITY, NJ-ACMCMAIN>
+ 2021 New Road/Suite 10
Linwood, NJ 08221   (609)653-1444   Fax (609)926-2308

Hyman, Daniel J., DO {1346335023} IntrMd(90,PA77)<NJ-COOPRUMC>
+ 14 South Broadway
Gloucester City, NJ 08030   (856)465-0518   Fax (856)456-

4359
+ South Jersey Health Care Center
Two Cooper Plaza   Camden, NJ 08103   (856)465-0518   Fax (856)342-6662
+ Cooper University Hospital
One Cooper Plaza   Camden, NJ 08030   (856)342-3150

Hyman, Francine, MD {1346655495} ObsGyn<NJ-OURLADY>
+ Our Lady of Lourdes Medical Center
1600 Haddon Avenue/L&D   Camden, NJ 08103   (856)757-3786   Fax (856)365-7865

Hyman, Kristin Lepore, MD {1871799270}
+ Continuum Health Alliance LLC
402 Lippincott Drive   Marlton, NJ 08053

Hyman, Martin C., MD {1700836087} ObsGyn(76,MEX03)<NJ-OVERLOOK>
+ Womens HealthCare of Union County
950 West Chestnut Street/Suite 102   Union, NJ 07083   (908)688-8545   Fax (908)688-8447

Hyman, Richard Louis, MD {1770572422} CdvDis, IntrMd(89,PA13)<NJ-CHSFULD, NJ-CHSMRCER>
+ Mercer Bucks Cardiology
3140 Princeton Pike/2nd Floor   Lawrenceville, NJ 08648   (609)895-1919   Fax (609)895-1200
+ Penn Cardiac Care Mercer Bucks
2 Capitol Way/Suite 487A   Pennington, NJ 08534

Hynes, Peter James, MD {1497953210} CdvDis<NJ-JRSYSHMC, NJ-CENTRAST>
+ Change of Heart Cardiology
2130 Highway 35/Building C Suite 321   Sea Girt, NJ 08750   (732)974-6700   Fax (732)974-6707

Hyon, Joseph K., DO {1245281773} IntrMd, NeuMus(91,MO78)<NJ-VALLEY>
+ 555 Kinderkamack Road/Suite D
Oradell, NJ 07649   (201)265-1133   Fax (201)265-1135
+ Valley Medical Group
70 Park Avenue   Park Ridge, NJ 07656   (201)265-1133   Fax (201)391-7733

Hypolite, Renee E., DO {1053647222}
+ Capital Health Family Health Center
433 Bellevue Avenue/4th Floor   Trenton, NJ 08618   (609)394-4111   Fax (609)815-7178
+ 9 Thornhill Drive
Lumberton, NJ 08048   (856)764-7660

Hyppolite, Alex, MD {1881868511} Pedtrc(04,NY08)<NJ-HACKNSK>
+ Hackensack Univ Medical Center Pediatric Emerg Room
30 Prospect Avenue   Hackensack, NJ 07601   (201)996-5430   Fax (201)996-3676

Hyppolite, David, MD {1508856394} IntrMd, FamMed(85,BELG)<NJ-RIVERVW, NJ-BAYSHORE>
+ 66 C Bridge Avenue
Red Bank, NJ 07701   (732)747-6600

Hyun, Aerin M., MD {1992970065} Psychy(07,IL11)
+ 82 North Summit Street/Suite B
Tenafly, NJ 07670

Hyun, Chul Soo, MD {1467540401} Gastrn, IntrMd(86,FL02)
+ 35 Van Nostrand Avenue
Englewood, NJ 07631   (201)568-6222

Hyun, Youngsoon, MD {1215026554} IntrMd(80,NC01)
+ Princeton Medical Group, P.A.
419 North Harrison Street   Princeton, NJ 08540   (609)924-9300   Fax (609)924-6552
+ Princeton Medical Group PA
2 Research Way/Bldg 2/Suite 302   Monroe Township, NJ 08831   (609)924-9300   Fax (609)655-7466

Iacobas, Ionela, MD {1265743108} PedHem<NJ-STPETER>
+ St. Peter's University Hospital
254 Easton Avenue   New Brunswick, NJ 08901   (732)745-6674   Fax (732)418-9708

Iacobucci, Audrey J., MD {1154589869} Pedtrc(05,PA02)<NJ-VIRTUAHS, NJ-VIRTVOOR>
+ Advocare DelGiorno Pediatrics
527 South Black Horse Pike   Blackwood, NJ 08012   (856)302-5322   Fax (856)245-7719
+ Advocare DelGiorno Pediatrics
412 Ewan Road   Mullica Hill, NJ 08062   (856)302-5322   Fax (856)343-3919

Iammatteo, Matthew D., MD {1346203593} ObsGyn(85,WIND)<NJ-MORRISTN>
+ 111 Madison Avenue/Suite 311/3rd Floor
Morristown, NJ 07960   (973)971-9950   Fax (973)971-9958

Ianacone, Mary R., DO {1386966257} IntrMd(84,PA77)<NJ-VIRTMHBC, NJ-VIRTBERL>
+ Alliance for Better Care, P.C.
PO Box 1510   Medford, NJ 08055   (609)953-4099   Fax (609)953-8652

Iannaccone, Ferdinand, DO {1851658397} AnesPain
+ Comprehensive Pain Center
90 Bergen Street/DOC 3400   Newark, NJ 07103   (973)972-2085   Fax (973)972-2130

Physicians by Name and Address

Iannacone, Richard F., DO {1295795458} Anesth(89,NJ75)<NJ-VALLEY>
+ The Valley Hospital
223 North Van Dien Avenue   Ridgewood, NJ 07450   (201)447-8350

Iannacone, Ronald J., DO {1558346825} Otlryg, SrgFPl, OtgyF-PlS(89,NJ75)<NJ-JRSYSHMC, NJ-OCEANMC>
+ Ear Nose and Throat Associates
2640 Highway 70/Building 6B   Manasquan, NJ 08736   (732)223-8686   Fax (732)223-6572
+ Ear Nose and Throat Associates
1 Plaza Drive/Plaza II/Unit 10   Toms River, NJ 08757   (732)557-4480

Iannetta, Frank, MD {1881621217} FamMed(87,NJ05)
+ Vanguard Medical Group, P.A.
170 Changebridge Road/Suite C-3   Montville, NJ 07045   (973)575-5540   Fax (973)575-4885

Iannotta, Patricia N., MD {1942255633} Dermat(89,PA02)<NJ-RWJUBRUN>
+ 6 Auer Court/Suite E
East Brunswick, NJ 08816   (732)651-0009   Fax (732)651-0015
pni6@verizon.net

Iavicoli, Michelle A., MD {1306931092} ObsGyn(91,DC02)
+ Cooper Ob/Gyn
4 Plaza Drive/Suite 403/Bunker Hill Pl   Sewell, NJ 08080   (856)270-4020   Fax (856)270-4022
+ Cooper Faculty Ob/Gyn
1103 Kings Highway North/Suite 201   Cherry Hill, NJ 08034   (856)270-4020   Fax (856)321-0133

Ibale, Florence E., MD {1255386876} Pedtrc, PedEmg(89,UGA01)<NJ-CENTRAST>
+ CentraState Medical Center
901 West Main Street/Emergency   Freehold, NJ 07728   (732)431-2000

Ibanez, Delfin George C., MD {1144292210} Psychy(77,PHI08)
+ CPC Behavioral HealthCare
37 Court Street   Freehold, NJ 07728   (732)780-7387   Fax (732)780-5257

Ibarbia, Jose D., MD {1881857902} PhysMd<NJ-STMRYPAS>
+ Summit Medical Group
6 Brighton Road/2 FL   Clifton, NJ 07012   (973)777-7911   Fax (973)473-5958
+ New Jersey Physicians, LLC.
128 Union Avenue/Suite 2A   Rutherford, NJ 07070   (973)777-7911   Fax (201)939-7644

Ibay, Annamarie D., MD {1003805763} FamMed(01,PA13)
+ Virtua Family Medicine Center @Lumberton
1636 Route 38 & Eayrestown Rd.   Lumberton, NJ 08048   (609)914-8440   Fax (609)914-8441

Ibay, Maria Lourdes D., MD {1871709972} Pedtrc(04,PA09)<NJ-VIRTUAHS, NJ-KENEDYHS>
+ Advocare Kressville Pediatrics Cherry Hill
710 Kresson Road   Cherry Hill, NJ 08003   (856)795-3320   Fax (856)795-1213
+ Advocare Kressville Pediatrics Sicklerville
431 Sicklerville Road   Sicklerville, NJ 08081   (856)795-3320   Fax (856)875-4042

Ibeabuchi, Adaeze Nneka, MD {1811219918} Nephro
+ Physicians Practice at New Bridge Med Ctr
230 East Ridgewood Avenue   Paramus, NJ 07652   (201)225-4700   Fax (201)225-4702

Ibch, Khadija Hakiya, MD {1588892079} Psychy(09,NY48)<NJ-TRININPC>
+ Trinitas Regional Medical Center-New Point Campus
655 East Jersey Street/Psychiatry   Elizabeth, NJ 07206   (908)994-7166

Ibeku, Chukwuemeka A., MD {1023059722} FamMed(92,NIG02)<NJ-NWRKBETH, NJ-STJOSHOS>
+ North Jersey Developmental Center
169 Minisink Road/PO Box 169   Totowa, NJ 07512   (973)256-1700   Fax (973)256-3468

Ibekwe, Ola, MD {1386029080} IntHos<NJ-COOPRUMC>
+ Cooper University Hospital
One Cooper Plaza   Camden, NJ 08103   (856)342-2000

Ibikunle, Olumuyiwa Adedotun, MD {1013112069} IntrMd(92,NIG01)<NJ-OVERLOOK>
+ Overlook Medical Center
99 Beauvoir Avenue/PO Box 210   Summit, NJ 07902   (908)522-2000

Ibragimov, Araz, DO {1689838159} AnesCrCr, Anesth, IntrMd(03,NY75)<NY-KINGSCO>
+ Newton Medical Center
175 High Street/Anesthesia   Newton, NJ 07860   (973)383-2121

Ibrahim, Adel, MD {1093709529} IntrMd(77,EGYP)<NJ-BAYSHORE, NJ-RIVERVW>
+ Metropolitan Asthma & Allergy
551 Newman Springs Road/Unit 1   Lincroft, NJ 07738   (732)530-9200   Fax (732)530-8820

Ibrahim, Ayman M., DO {1508025834} Nrolgy, IntrMd(07,NY75)
+ Neurology Consultants of North Jersey PA
92 Summit Avenue/2nd Floor   Hackensack, NJ 07601   (201)630-0012   Fax (201)630-0014

Ibrahim, Candace, MD {1548720055} Psychy
+ UMCPP Outpatient Rehabilitation
1315 Whitehorse Mercerville Ro   Hamilton, NJ 08619   (609)581-5910

Ibrahim, Christine M., MD {1114158987} FamMed, IntrMd(09,DMN01)
+ Integrated Medicine Alliance, PA.
363 Highway 36   Port Monmouth, NJ 07758   (732)471-0400   Fax (732)471-7949

Ibrahim, Ehab Fawzy, MD {1942395108} IntrMd(95,EGY05)<NJ-HACKNSK>
+ Neurology Consultants of North Jersey PA
92 Summit Avenue/2nd Floor   Hackensack, NJ 07601   (201)630-0012   Fax (201)630-0014

Ibrahim, Gehan M., MD {1538405147} ObsGyn<NY-FLUSHNG>
+ Women's Physician
35 Journal Square/Suite 822   Jersey City, NJ 07306   (201)222-2682   Fax (201)222-2692

Ibrahim, Ghassan Jerjous, MD {1740456136} PthAcl<NJ-COMMED>
+ Community Medical Center
99 Route 37 West   Toms River, NJ 08755   (732)557-8141

Ibrahim, Ibrahim M., MD {1467465724} SrgLap, Surgry, Bariat(66,NY19)<NJ-ENGLWOOD, NJ-HOLYNAME>
+ Bergen Laparoscopy & Bariatric, LLC
97 Engle Street   Englewood, NJ 07631   (201)227-5533   Fax (201)227-5537
imibrahim@gmail.com

Ibrahim, Jennifer, MD {1932163342} GnetMd, ClnGnt(95,NJ05)<NJ-NWRKBETH, NJ-ENGLWOOD>
+ Genetics Associates of New Jersey, P.C.
154 Vista Terrace   Pompton Lakes, NJ 07442   (973)831-6020   Fax (973)831-6001
+ Newark Beth Israel Medical Center
201 Lyons Avenue/MedicalGenetics   Newark, NJ 07112   (973)926-7000
+ Genetics Associates of New Jersey, P.C.
405 Northfield Avenue   West Orange, NJ 07442   (973)831-6020

Ibrahim, Joseph Georgy Amin Aze, MD {1225068281} PainMd(93,EGY05)<NJ-STCLRDEN, NJ-STCLRDOV>
+ New Jersey Spine & Pain Institute, LLC
19 East 27th Street   Bayonne, NJ 07002   (201)436-0033   Fax (201)436-0079

Ibrahim, Maher, MD {1053301309} Anesth, PainMd(89,EGY05)
+ Interventional Pain Management Associates
1374 Whitehorse-Hamilton Sq Rd   Hamilton, NJ 08690   (609)838-2900   Fax (609)838-2901

Ibrahim, Mariane, MD {1669748695}
+ Deborah A Coy, MD, LLC
405 Northfield Avenue/Suite LL2   West Orange, NJ 07052   (201)552-2256   Fax (973)736-8717

Ibrahim, Mary I., MD {1801983127} IntrMd(72,EGYP)<NJ-CHRIST, NJ-JRSYCITY>
+ 130 Bentley Avenue
Jersey City, NJ 07304   (201)434-9110   Fax (201)918-5118

Ibrahim, Mohammad S., MD {1265494645} EnDbMt, IntrMd, InfDis(89,SYR01)<NJ-CHILTON>
+ Amana Medical Group
871 McBride Avenue   West Paterson, NJ 07424   (973)569-4488   Fax (973)565-4743

Ibrahim, Mohammad Younis, MD {1649641226} IntrMd<NJ-STFRNMED>
+ St. Francis Medical Center
601 Hamilton Avenue/Rm B-158   Trenton, NJ 08629   (609)599-5061

Ibrahim, Samih A., MD {1407848237} ObsGyn(93,PA09)
+ Princeton Health Medical & Surgical Associates
2 Centre Drive/Suite 200   Monroe, NJ 08831   (609)395-2470   Fax (609)860-5288
+ Robert Wood Johnson Ob/Gyn Group
1 Hamilton Health Place   Hamilton, NJ 08690   (609)395-2470   Fax (609)631-6898

Ibrahim, Zuhaib, MD {1780840173} SrgPlstc
+ The Plastic Surgery Ctr of NJ & Manhat
535 Sycamore Avenue   Shrewsbury, NJ 07702   (717)608-2250   Fax (732)747-2606

Icasiano, Evelyn J., MD {1619189164} Ophthl(03,IL42)
+ 500 Central Avenue/Suite 220
Union City, NJ 07087

Idank, David M., DO {1831256098} PhysMd(90,ME75)<NJ-JFKMED>
+ Edison-Metuchen Orthopedic Group
10 Parsonage Road/5th Floor/Suite 500   Edison, NJ 08837   (732)494-6226   Fax (732)494-8762

Ie, Darmakusuma, MD {1881690956} Ophthl(88,LA01)<NJ-CHSM-RCER>
+ Delaware Valley Retina Associates
4 Princess Road/Suite 101   Lawrenceville, NJ 08648   (609)896-1414   Fax (609)896-2982
delawarevalleyretina@worldnet.att.net
+ Delaware Valley Retina Associates
121 Highway 31 North/Suite 700   Flemington, NJ 08822   (908)806-6191

Ierardi-Curto, Lynne A., MD {1942590484} GnetMd, GntMCBCh, Pedtrc(86,MA01)
+ LabCorp
151 Fries Mills Road/Suites 205-206   Turnersville, NJ 08012   (609)510-9157   Fax (856)401-1304

Ietta, Michael Angelo, MD {1356319735} Anesth(85,NY48)<NJ-VALLEY>
+ The Valley Hospital
223 North Van Dien Avenue   Ridgewood, NJ 07450   (201)447-8000

Ifabiyi, Lubunmi, MD {1497796445} FamMed
+ MedExpress Urgent Care East Brunswick
418 State Route 18   East Brunswick, NJ 08816   (732)613-6168   Fax (732)613-6178

Iftekhar, Ruksana, MD {1760577464} Psychy(78,INDI)<NJ-COOPRUMC, NJ-HAMPTBHC>
+ Cooper Psychiatric Associates
3 Cooper Plaza/Suite 307   Camden, NJ 08103   (856)342-2328   Fax (856)541-6137

Igbanugo, Anselm, MD {1780658187} IntrMd(84,NIG01)<NJ-COMMED, NJ-OCEANMC>
+ 508 Lakehurst Road/Suite 2 A
Toms River, NJ 08755   (732)281-3100   Fax (732)281-3311

Igbokwe, Jennifer, MD {1124043930} FamMed, IntrMd(00,DC01)
+ Summit Medical Group
6 Brighton Road/2 FL   Clifton, NJ 07012   (973)777-7911   Fax (973)777-5403

Ighama-Amegor, Ibilola, MD {1659453173} Pedtrc(86,NIGE)<NJ-NWRKBETH>
+ Quality Care Pediatrics
88 Chancellor Avenue   Newark, NJ 07112   (973)926-4400   Fax (973)926-4660
ibilolai@selema.net
+ Alberta-Bey Community Health Center
300 Chancellor Avenue   Newark, NJ 07112   (973)926-4400   Fax (973)926-6281

Iglesias, Hector R., MD {1447324389} Pedtrc(84,DOM01)<NJ-RIVERVW>
+ Tinton Falls Pediatrics
776 Shrewsbury Avenue   Tinton Falls, NJ 07724   (732)758-1223   Fax (732)758-0866

Iglesias, Jose Ignacio, DO {1467498402} Nephro, CritCr, IntrMd(93,NJ75)<NJ-COMMED, NJ-KIMBALL>
+ Ocean Renal Associates, P.A.
210 Jack Martin Boulevard/Suite D-1   Brick, NJ 08724   (732)458-5854   Fax (732)458-8012
+ Ocean Renal Associates, P.A.
1301 Route 72 West/Suite 206   Manahawkin, NJ 08050   (732)458-5854   Fax (609)978-9902
+ Ocean Renal Associates, P.A.
508 Lakehurst Road/Suite 3 A   Toms River, NJ 08724   (732)341-4600   Fax (732)341-4993

Ignacio, Cristina Usi, MD {1053503532}
+ Family Practice of CentraState-Jackson
161 Bartley Road   Jackson, NJ 08527   (732)363-6140   Fax (732)363-6196

Ignatius, Nandini, MD {1235462128} OncHem, IntrMd(00,INA68)
+ Rutgers Cancer Institute of NJ at Univ Hospital
205 South Orange Avenue/B Level   Newark, NJ 07101   (973)972-6257   Fax (973)972-2384

Ijaz, Muhammad Shabbir, MD {1306298377} EmrgMd<NJ-STFRN-MED>
+ St. Francis Medical Center
601 Hamilton Avenue   Trenton, NJ 08629   (609)599-5061   Fax (609)599-6232

Ijehsedeh, Anthony, MD {1689194094}
+ Rudolph C. Willis, Inc.
12 Krotik Place   Irvington, NJ 07111   (973)373-3000

Ikegami, Hirohisa, MD {1982851887} SrgThr
+ UMDNJ RWJ CardioThoracic Surgery
125 Paterson Street/Suite 4100/P1528   New Brunswick, NJ 08901   (732)235-7800   Fax (732)235-8727

Ikelheimer, Douglas Mark, MD {1508979519} Psychy(97,NY48)
+ InSight LLC
765 East Route 70/Bldg A   Marlton, NJ 08053   (856)983-3900   Fax (856)810-0110

Ilangovan, Kani Mozhi, MD {1932322419} Psychy, PsyCAd(03,IL11)<NJ-STFRNMED>
+ 20 Nassau Street/Suite 309
Princeton, NJ 08542

Ilardi, Jeffrey Michael, MD {1639193618} Psychy(00,NJ05)<NJ-STCLRBOO>
+ St. Clare's Hospital-Boonton
130 Powerville Road/Psych   Boonton, NJ 07005   (973)316-1800   Fax (973)316-1839

Physicians by Name and Address

Ilaria, Philip V., MD {1235105081} Nrolgy(85,MEXI)<NJ-BAYSHORE, NJ-RIVERVW>
+ Greater Monmouth Neurology
130 Maple Avenue/Suite 1-A   Red Bank, NJ 07701   (732)741-1378   Fax (732)741-1677
+ Greater Monmouth Neurology
733 North Beers Street   Holmdel, NJ 07733   (732)741-1378

Ilaria, Shawen Maryrose, MD {1386051860} PsyCAd<NJ-UNIVBHC>
+ University Behavioral Health Care
671 Hoes Lane/PO Box 1392   Piscataway, NJ 08855   (732)235-4433

Ilario, Marius John-Marc, MD {1720024995} PthACl, Pthlgy(97,GRN01)
+ Histopathology Services, LLC.
535 East Crescent Avenue   Ramsey, NJ 07446   (201)661-7280   Fax (201)661-7297

Iledan, Liesl P., MD {1659416360} EmrgPedr
+ 374 Hopedale Drive SE
Bayville, NJ 08721

Iliadis, Elias, MD {1326133034} IntrMd, CdvDis, IntCrd(92,NJ06)<NJ-ACMCITY>
+ Cooper Cardiology Associates
900 Centennial Boulevard   Voorhees, NJ 08043   (856)325-6700   Fax (856)325-6702
+ Cooper Cardiology Associates
1210 Brace Road/Suite 103   Cherry Hill, NJ 08034   (856)427-7254
+ University Cardiology
3 Cooper Plaza/Room 311   Camden, NJ 08043   (856)342-2034

Ilic Bogojevic, Zvezdana, MD {1104159896}
+ 7 Wilmer Street/Apt G
Madison, NJ 07940   (973)845-2855
zvezdana@aol.com

Ilievski, Petar Mihajlo, MD {1093788465}
+ 215 Nuthatch Court
Three Bridges, NJ 08887   (917)647-2738
petaril@pvtnetworks.net

Ilkhanizadeh, Ladan, MD {1023315918} IntrMd<NY-METHODST>
+ Cedar Bridge Medical Associates
985 Cedarbridge Avenue   Brick, NJ 08723   (732)477-5600   Fax (732)477-1899

Ilogu, Noel O., MD {1518063551} IntrMd, Addctn(85,NIG07)<NJ-RWJUBRUN, NJ-STPETER>
+ University Medical & Treatment Center
33 Clyde Road/Suite 105   Somerset, NJ 08873   (732)247-9001   Fax (732)247-9002
office@umtcenter.com

Ilonzo, Chiamaka, MD {1750729406} ObsGyn
+ Drs. Wong and Ilonzo
20 Prospect Avenue   Hackensack, NJ 07601   (551)996-2000

Ilowite, Peter G., DO {1699792382} Dermat, SrgDer(90,NY75)<NJ-HOLYNAME>
+ Skin & Allergy Center
275 Market Street   Saddle Brook, NJ 07663   (201)843-7177   Fax (201)556-0970
drpeterilowite@gmail.com

Ilowite, Robert K., DO {1003887704} Dermat(92,PA77)<NJ-HUNTRDN>
+ The Dermatology Center
505 Omni Drive   Hillsborough, NJ 08844   (908)359-6685   Fax (908)359-0649

Ilustre, Joanne Marie, DO {1750545661}
+ 128 Cuffys Lane
Cherry Hill, NJ 08003   (856)428-4289
joanne.ilustre@gmail.com

Ilut, Irina Claudia, MD {1962916833} Surgry<NJ-JFKMED>
+ JFK Medical Center
65 James Street   Edison, NJ 08820   (732)321-7668

Im, Chae K., MD {1457372443} PhysMd(89,NY06)<NJ-VAEASTOR>
+ VA New Jersey Health Care System-East Orange Campus
385 Tremont Avenue   East Orange, NJ 07018   (973)676-1000

Im-Imamura, Lauren H., DO {1003262783} FamMed<NJ-OVERLOOK>
+ Overlook Medical Center
99 Beauvoir Avenue/PO Box 210   Summit, NJ 07902   (908)522-2000

Imaizumi, Sonia O., MD {1376638080} Pedtrc, NnPnMd(71,BRA04)<NJ-COOPRUMC>
+ The Children's Regional Hospital at Cooper Univ Hosp
One Cooper Plaza   Camden, NJ 08103   (856)342-2000
+ Cooper Peds/Children's Regional Ctr
3 Cooper Plaza/Suite 200   Camden, NJ 08103   (856)342-2000   Fax (856)368-8297

Imbesi, John J., MD {1487654349} Gastrn, IntrMd(99,NY15)<NJ-HACKNSK, NJ-MTNSIDE>
+ Summit Medical Group
75 East Northfield Road   Livingston, NJ 07039   (973)436-1400   Fax (908)673-7336
+ Gastroenterology Group of NJ, PA
123 Highland Avenue/Suite 103   Glen Ridge, NJ 07028   (973)436-1400   Fax (973)748-7076

Imbesi, Joseph Thomas, DO {1457330755} EmrgMd, FamMed, OccpMd(69,IL76)<NJ-JRSYSHMC>
+ 100 Commons Way
Holmdel, NJ 07733   (732)450-2930   Fax (732)450-2931

Imbornone, Peter J., MD {1568531432} IntrMd, IntMAdMd(80,ITA15)<NJ-HACKNSK>
+ Rochelle Park Medical Center PA
96 Park Way   Rochelle Park, NJ 07662   (201)291-1010   Fax (201)587-0313

Imbriano, Michael A., DO {1740485267} Nephro
+ Nephrology Consultants of New Jersey
19 Holly Street   Cranford, NJ 07016   (908)276-4711   Fax (908)276-6490

Imegwu, Obi J., MD {1043261001} SrgVas, Surgry(92,PA02)<NJ-SOMERSET>
+ Breast Cancer Prevention Institute
30 Rehill Avenue/Suite 3400   Somerville, NJ 08876   (908)725-2400   Fax (908)927-8990

Imm, James T., MD {1942567201}
+ 2516 Leslie Street
Union, NJ 07083   (908)687-8049
immjames@gmail.com

Immerman, Sara Beth, MD {1922204429} Otlryg(07,NY19)<NY-NYUTISCH>
+ Ear, Nose, & Throat Specialists of Morristown LLC
95 Madison Avenue/Suite 105   Morristown, NJ 07960   (973)644-0808   Fax (973)644-9270

Impeduglia, Theresa Maria, MD {1336189786} SrgVas, Surgry, IntrMd(92,NY48)<NJ-ENGLWOOD>
+ Bergen Thoracic & Vascular Associates
350 Engle Street/2 East   Englewood, NJ 07631   (201)569-1101   Fax (201)569-1108
+ North Jersey Surgical Specialists
83 Summit Avenue   Hackensack, NJ 07601   (201)569-1101   Fax (201)646-0600

Implicito, Dante A., MD {1578586632} SrgOrt, SrgSpn(90,NJ05)<NJ-HACKNSK, NJ-VALLEY>
+ New Jersey Spinal Medicine & Surgery
266 Harristown Road/Suite 100   Glen Rock, NJ 07452   (201)251-7725   Fax (201)251-2599

Imran, Uzma, MD {1164697041} FamMed(PAK12)
+ 16 Saint Andrews Lane
Annandale, NJ 08801

Imsirovic-Starcevic, Dubravka, MD {1801846829} CdvDis, IntrMd(86,CRO01)<NJ-HUNTRDN>
+ Hunterdon Cardiovascular Associates
1100 Wescott Drive/Suite G-3   Flemington, NJ 08822   (908)788-6471   Fax (908)788-6460
+ Hunterdon Cardiovascular Associates
1738 Route 31/Suite 210   Clinton, NJ 08809   (908)788-6471   Fax (908)823-9211

Incandela, Nicholas J., MD {1336176767} Anesth(89,MEX03)<NY-WESTCHMC>
+ AtlantiCare Anesthesiology
65 West Jimmie Leeds Road   Pomona, NJ 08240   (609)748-7597   Fax (609)748-7586

Incorvati, Jason A., MD {1467687392} OncHem, IntrMd(PA13
+ Sparta Health & Wellness
89 Sparta Avenu/Suite 207   Sparta, NJ 07871   (973)940-8780   Fax (973)726-9568

Incremona, Brian R., MD {1992752810} SprtMd, IntrMd(88,WIND)<NJ-STPETER, NJ-RIVERVW>
+ East-West Medical Care of NJ
560 Main Street/Suite 1-E   Loch Arbour, NJ 07711   (732)517-8914   Fax (732)531-4049
admin@east-westmedicalcareofnj.com

Indich, Norman, MD {1427005602} Pedtrc(84,OH06)<NJ-KIMBALL, NJ-JRSYSHMC>
+ Drs. Indich and Deutsch
619 West County Line Road   Lakewood, NJ 08701   (732)730-9111   Fax (732)730-9154

Indruk, William L., MD {1205825254} EmrgMd(74,DC02)
+ Emergency Medical Associates of NJ, P.A.
3 Century Drive   Parsippany, NJ 07054   (973)740-0607   Fax (973)740-9895

Infantino, Dorian, MD {1780121723} Pedtrc
+ Robert Wood Johnson University Hospital
51 French Street/MEB-234B/Pthlgy   New Brunswick, NJ 08903   (215)590-1220

Infantino, Salvatore, MD {1477557759} CdvDis, IntrMd, FamMAdlt(71,ITAL)<NJ-VALLEY>
+ Medical Multispecialty Associates PA
11-26 Saddle River Road   Fair Lawn, NJ 07410   (201)796-9200   Fax (201)796-7606

Infantino, Edward, MD {1184650111} IntrMd(73,MEXI)<NJ-ACMCITY, NJ-ACMCMAIN>
+ Ocean Internal Medicine Associates
4301 Ventnor Avenue   Atlantic City, NJ 08401   (609)344-3787
+ Ocean Internal Medicine Associates
634 Shore Road   Somers Point, NJ 08244   (609)653-0808

Infantolino, John A., MD {1215902325} IntrMd, NeuMus(83,MEXI)<NJ-JRSYSHMC, NJ-OCEANMC>
+ 5 Princeton Avenue
Brick, NJ 08724   (732)840-0010   Fax (732)840-9770

Infantolino, Philip L., MD {1790759983} CdvDis, IntrMd(68,NJ05)<NJ-OCEANMC>
+ 2640 Highway 70/Building 11
Manasquan, NJ 08736   (732)528-8500   Fax (732)528-6710
+ Ocean Heart Group
1530 Route 88/Suite A   Brick, NJ 08724   (732)528-8500   Fax (732)840-0611

Ing, Richard Daniel, MD {1003817339} Surgry(90,OH41)
+ Rancocas Valley Surgical Associates PA
1000 Salem Road/Suite A   Willingboro, NJ 08046   (609)877-1737   Fax (609)877-1589

Ingala, Erin Einbinder, MD {1659506202} Nrolgy<PA-UPMCPHL>
+ Penn Medicine at Cherry Hill
409 Route 70 East   Cherry Hill, NJ 08034   (856)427-4336
erin.ingala@uphs.upenn.edu

Ingato, Steven P., MD {1497851836} IntrMd(85,TN20)<NJ-SHOREMEM, NJ-COMMED>
+ Frank C. Alario MD Inc
355 Route 9/Suite 2   Bayville, NJ 08721   (732)269-0001   Fax (732)269-9636
+ Frank C. Alario MD Inc
1220 Route 70 West   Whiting, NJ 08759   (732)350-3784

Ingber, Michael S., MD {1861606329} Urolgy, IntrMd(02,MI07)
+ The Center For Specialized Women's Health
3155 State Route 10/Suite 100   Denville, NJ 07834   (973)537-5557   Fax (973)537-5547
+ The Center For Specialized Women's Health
16 Eden Lane   Whippany, NJ 07981   (973)537-5557   Fax (973)947-9056
+ The Center For Specialized Women's Health
16 Pocono Road/Suite 103   Denville, NJ 07834   (973)947-9066   Fax (973)947-9056

Ingenito, Anthony C., MD {1710940127} RadOnc(91,NJ05)<NJ-HACKNSK>
+ John Theurer Cancer Center - HUMC
92 Second Street   Hackensack, NJ 07601   (201)996-2210   Fax (551)996-0730
+ Hackensack University Medical Center
30 Prospect Avenue/Radiology   Hackensack, NJ 07601   (201)996-2210   Fax (201)996-2965

Ingis, David Alan, MD {1083637722} Gastrn, IntrMd(68,NY19)
+ Penn Medicine at Cherry Hill
409 Route 70 East/GI   Cherry Hill, NJ 08034   (856)429-1519

Ingram, Karen M., MD {1811910607} Pedtrc(78,NJ05)<NJ-STPETER, NJ-RWJUBRUN>
+ Rutgers Hurtado Health Center
11 Bishop Place   New Brunswick, NJ 08901   (732)932-7402   Fax (732)932-1223

Ingram, Mark Anthony, MD {1710040621} Surgry, Gastrn(90,JMA01)<NY-LINCOLN>
+ St. Joseph Medical Center Surgery
703 Main Street   Paterson, NJ 07503   (973)754-2480

Ingrassia-Squiers, Keri Lynn, DO {1467465203} IntrMd(99,NJ75)<NJ-HCKTSTWN, NJ-MORRISTN>
+ Hackettstown Medical Group
Hastings Sq Plaza/Building 5   Hackettstown, NJ 07840   (908)979-0050   Fax (908)979-0044

Inguaggiato, Anthony J., MD {1336219948} CdvDis, IntrMd(86,ITAL)<NJ-HOBUNIMC, NJ-HACKNSK>
+ 4302 Palisade Avenue
Union City, NJ 07087   (201)863-5673   Fax (201)863-1372

Inkeles, David M., MD {1194759613} Ophthl(72,NY46)<NJ-NWTNMEM>
+ Eye Physicians of Sussex County
183 High Street/Suite 2200   Newton, NJ 07860   (973)383-6345   Fax (973)383-0032

Innella, Robin R., DO {1578562245} SrgOrt(82,PA77)<NJ-OVERLOOK, NJ-BAYONNE>
+ Associated Orthopaedics
1000 Galloping Hill Road,/Suite 202   Union, NJ 07083   (908)964-6600   Fax (908)364-1025
+ Associated Orthopaedics
654 Broadway   Bayonne, NJ 07002   (908)964-6600   Fax (201)436-8110

Innerfield, Caitlin, MD {1548492127}
+ Rancocas Anesthesiology, PA
151 Fries Mill Road/Suite 202   Turnersville, NJ 08012   (856)228-7246   Fax (856)228-7252
cailin.innterfield@gmail.com

Inouye, Masayuki, MD {1861480295} Otlryg(96,NY48)
+ Bergen Ear Nose & Throat Associates PA
20 Prospect Avenue/Suite 909   Hackensack, NJ 07601   (201)489-6520   Fax (201)489-6530

Inoyama, Katherine S., MD {1902032188} Nrolgy
+ Northeast Regional Epilepsy Group
20 Prospect Avenue/Suite 800 Hackensack, NJ 07601
(201)343-6676   Fax (201)343-6689

Intili, John J., MD {1831243682} Pedtrc(89,ITAL)
+ 715 Fischer Boulevard
Toms River, NJ 08753 (732)929-4566

Introcaso, Lucian J., MD {1386795680} OccpMd, IntrMd(81,MEXI)
+ Worknet Occupational Medicine
9370 Route 130 North/Suite 200 Pennsauken, NJ 08110
(856)662-0660   Fax (856)662-0798

Inverno, Anthony J., MD {1942390331} Ophthl, IntrMd(68,ITAL)<NJ-RWJURAH, NJ-JFKMED>
+ Anthony J Inverno & Associates
95 Westfield Avenue   Clark, NJ 07066   (732)381-5555
Fax (732)381-5055

Inwood, Richard J., MD {1881619112} NnPnMd, Pedtrc(72,CT01)<NJ-NWRKBETH>
+ Newark Beth Israel Medical Center
201 Lyons Avenue Newark, NJ 07112   (973)926-7203
Fax (973)926-2332
rinwood@bethi.com

Inzerillo, Angela Mary, MD {1346300852} EnDbMt, IntrMd(93,NY46)
+ Princeton Endocrinology Associates, LLC
10 Forrestal Road South/Suite 106   Princeton, NJ 08540
(609)921-1511   Fax (609)921-3316
amei16@aol.com
+ Princeton Endocrinology Associates, LLC
1315 Whitehorse Mercerville Rd   Hamilton, NJ 08610
(609)921-1511   Fax (609)921-3316

Iofel, Elizaveta, MD {1124198288} Pedtrc, PedGst(90,LAT02)
+ University Hospital-RWJ Medical School
89 French Street/Rm 2208/Pedi New Brunswick, NJ 08901
(732)828-3000   Fax (732)235-6620

Ioffe, Inna S., MD {1285774901} Pedtrc(64,BLAR)
+ 204 Eagle Rock Avenue/Suite 1
Roseland, NJ 07068 (973)226-5212   Fax (973)226-5447

Ioffe, Julia, MD {1043471808} PhysMd
+ 1187 Main Avenue/Suite 1D
Clifton, NJ 07011

Ioffe, Michail, MD {1316008642} Anesth(80,RUSS)<NJ-STBARNMC>
+ St. Barnabas Medical Center
94 Old Short Hills Road   Livingston, NJ 07039   (973)322-5000

Ioffreda, Richard E., MD {1780752964} Urolgy(87,PA02)<NJ-STPETER, NJ-UMDNJ>
+ P. F. Ioffreda, MD, PA
1250 Marigold Street North Brunswick, NJ 08902
(732)545-8259   Fax (732)247-5574

Iofin, Alexander, MD {1053565630} PsyCAd, Psychy, Psyphm(80,AZE01)<NJ-TRININPC, NJ-HAGEDORN>
+ Advance Psychiatric Care PA
444 Neptune Boulevard/Suite 17   Neptune, NJ 07753
(732)528-3232   Fax (732)528-5495
advpsychcopc@yahoo.com

Iofin, Ilya, MD {1639337108} SrgOrt(03,MO02)<NY-MTSINAI>
+ University Orthopaedic Center, PA
433 Hackensack Avenue/Second Floor   Hackensack, NJ 07601   (201)343-1717   Fax (201)343-3217

Iones, Anna, MD {1558597336} Nrolgy, ClNrpPh(09,GRN01)
+ Advocare Comprehensive Neurology of New Jersey
95 Madison Avenue/Suite 103 Morristown, NJ 07960
(973)455-7444   Fax (973)455-7447

Iorio, Louis Michael, MD {1831184522} SrgPlstc, Surgry(92,OH44)<NJ-MONMOUTH, NJ-JRSYSHMC>
+ Iorio Plastic Surgery & CosMedical Center
780 Route 34   Colts Neck, NJ 07722   (732)780-9191 Fax (732)780-0961
+ Iorio Plastic Surgery & CosMedical Center
1140 Burnt Tavern Road/Unit 1-D   Brick, NJ 08724
(732)780-9191   Fax (732)458-7435

Iorio, Richard, MD {1922139070} IntrMd, PulDis(72,ITAL)
+ 1130 Route 202 South/Building A
Raritan, NJ 08869   (908)526-1216   Fax (908)526-8351

Ippolito, Tobi, MD {1659401636} IntrMd(96,NJ05)
+ Summit Medical Group
75 East Northfield Road Livingston, NJ 07039   (973)436-1460   Fax (908)673-7336

Iqbal, Javid, MD {1710941414} IntHos, IntrMd(92,DOM16)<NJ-ACMCITY>
+ AtlantiCare Hospitalist Program
1925 Pacific Avenue/8th Floor   Atlantic City, NJ 08401
(609)441-8146   Fax (609)441-8002

Iqbal, Mohammad Javed, MD {1205913423} Psychy(63,PAK11)
+ 299 Forest Avenue/Suite C
Paramus, NJ 07652   (201)599-2926

Iqbal, Nauveed, MD {1104851492} Surgry, SrgVas, Bariat(72,PAK01)<NJ-SJERSYHS, NJ-MEMSALEM>
+ Iqbal & Khan Surgical Associates, P.A.
10 Magnolia Avenue/Suite E   Bridgeton, NJ 08302

(856)455-2399   Fax (856)451-7791
+ Inspira Medical Group Surgical Associates
1206 West Sherman Avenue/Building 2   Vineland, NJ 08360
(856)455-2399   Fax (856)696-9939
+ Iqball & Khan Surgical Associates, P. A.
900 Route 168/Suite G   Blackwood, NJ 08302 (856)369-6887   Fax (856)696-9939

Iqbal, Sheeraz, MD {1336151901} Pedtrc(02,GRN01)<NJ-VALLEY>
+ 735 Linwood Avenue
Ridgewood, NJ 07450   (201)670-1231   Fax (201)612-0922
info@DoctorIqbal.com

Iqbal, Wasie Jawed, MD {1407275274} Pedtrc
+ 435 Huffville Crosskeys Road
Turnersville, NJ 08012   (856)661-5199

Iqbal-Hussain, Farida, MD {1710037593} Psychy(82,PAK01)
+ 13 Walnut Street
Livingston, NJ 07039

Iraj Shaari, Gita M., MD {1134147192} ObsGyn(93,NY47)
+ The Doctors Shaari
413 60th Street   West New York, NJ 07093   (201)867-5557
Fax (201)867-5566

Irakam, Anitha, MD {1003849571} NnPnMd, Pedtrc(92,INA2X)<NJ-NWRKBETH>
+ Newark Beth Israel Medical Center
201 Lyons Avenue/Suite C 10   Newark, NJ 07112
(973)926-7203   Fax (973)926-2332

Irakam, Surya Prakash, MD {1114971397} IntrMd, Gastrn(91,INA40)
+ Gastromed HealthCare, PA
25 Monroe Street   Bridgewater, NJ 08807   (908)231-1999
Fax (908)231-1612
+ Gastromed HealthCare PA
203 Towne Centre Drive   Hillsborough, NJ 08844
(908)359-1639

Irani, Bakhtaver A., MD {1679648828} ObsGyn(68,INDI)<NJ-HACKNSK>
+ Women's Center For OB/GYN
21 East Park Place   Rutherford, NJ 07070   (201)438-7780
+ 101 Prospect Avenue
Hackensack, NJ 07601   (201)996-0070

Irby, Dahlia Jean, MD {1649228248} Nrolgy(97,PA09)<NJ-KENEDYHS>
+ Kennedy Health Alliance- Neurology
151 Fries Mill Road/Suite 102   Turnersville, NJ 08012
(844)542-2273   Fax (856)269-4258
dahlia5@comcast.net

Irving, Carol, MD {1457340788} EmrgMd(90,NJ06)<NJ-MORRISTN>
+ Atlantic Medical Group
One Health Plaza/Bldg. 125   East Hanover, NJ 07936
(862)778-7960   Fax (973)781-6505
+ Morristown Medical Center
100 Madison Avenue/EmrgMed   Morristown, NJ 07962
(973)971-5000

Irving, Henry C., III, MD {1427118223} SrgOrt(72,TN07)<NJ-CHRIST, NJ-JRSYCITY>
+ Drs. Tolentino & Irving MD PA
600 Pavonia Avenue/7th Floor   Jersey City, NJ 07306
(201)216-9300   Fax (201)216-0091

Irving, Robert John, MD {1033354907} FamMed(83,MEX03)
+ 2 Wharfside Drive
Monmouth Beach, NJ 07750

Irvis, Kenneth M., MD {1306864202} ObsGyn(77,PA12)<NJ-ACMCMAIN>
+ Southern Jersey Family Medical Center
1301 Atlantic Avenue   Atlantic City, NJ 08401   (609)572-0000   Fax (609)572-0039
+ Southern Jersey Family Medical Centers, Inc.
860 South White Horse Pike/Building A   Hammonton, NJ 08037   (609)572-0000   Fax (609)567-3492
+ Southern Jersey Family Medical Centers Inc.
932 South Main Street   Pleasantville, NJ 08401   (609)383-0880   Fax (609)383-0658

Irwin, Eytan A., MD {1801897319} SrgC&R, Surgry(84,NJ06)<NJ-VIRTVOOR>
+ Colon & Rectal Surgical Associates of South Jersey
502 Centennial Boulevard/Suite 5   Voorhees, NJ 08043
(856)429-8030   Fax (856)428-2718

Irwin-Obregon, Virginia, DO {1578565180} Nephro, OstMed, IntrMd(93,NJ75)<NJ-KENEDYHS>
+ Center for Kidney Disease & Hypertension
129 Johnson Road/Suite 4   Turnersville, NJ 08012
(856)374-4440   Fax (856)374-4445
+ Center for Kidney Disease & Hypertension
100 Brick Road/Suite 216   Marlton, NJ 08053   (856)374-4440   Fax (856)374-4445

Isaac, Fikry W., MD {1649394123} IntrMd(80,EGY04)
+ 501 George Street/Johnson Hall 120
New Brunswick, NJ 08901   (732)524-3404

Isaac, Irene V., MD {1750405239} PthAcl, PthCyt(81,EGY04)
+ 2 Crystal Glenn Court
Flemington, NJ 08822

Isaac, Roman, MD {1881913622} SrgOrt, SrgHnd(08,NY09)
+ Hudson Pro Orthopaedics and Sports Medicine
1320 Adams Street/Unit D-E   Hoboken, NJ 07030
(201)241-2044   Fax (646)681-2599

Isaac, Vina H., MD {1669547071} ObsGyn(77,DC03)<NJ-MORRISTN>
+ Lifeline Medical Associates
290 Madison Avenue/Suite 2   Morristown, NJ 07960
(973)267-8266   Fax (973)267-2103
vhisaacmd@aol.com

Isaacson, Brian Eric, MD {1740340694} Psychy, PsyCAd
+ AtlantiCare Hospitalist Program
1925 Pacific Avenue/8th Floor   Atlantic City, NJ 08401
(609)345-4000

Isang, Emmanuel Emmanuel, MD {1215347174} IntrMd<NJ-JRSYSHMC>
+ Jersey Shore University Medical Center
1945 Route 33   Neptune, NJ 07753   (732)775-5500

Isani, Sara, MD {1992973275} GynOnc
+ Rutgers Cancer Institute of New Jersey
195 Little Albany Street/PO Box 2681   New Brunswick, NJ 08903   (732)235-2465   Fax (732)235-6797

Isayeva, Eleonora, DO {1851315998} Pedtrc(98,NY75)<NJ-STPETER, NJ-RWJUBRUN>
+ Taylors Mills Family Medical, PC
224 Taylors Mills Road/Suite 112   Manalapan, NJ 07726
(732)577-1066   Fax (732)577-0049

Isbitan, Ahmad Abbad, MD {1477805919}
+ St. Michael's Medical Center
111 Central Avenue   Newark, NJ 07102   (973)877-5000

Isecke, Dorothy Ann, MD {1811935521} PsyCAd, Psychy(99,NJ05)<NJ-UMDNJ>
+ University Psychiatric Associates
183 South Orange Avenue/E-F Levels   Newark, NJ 07103
(973)972-2977   Fax (973)972-2979

Isedeh, Cynthia O., DO {1093059404} Pedtrc
+ Irvington Community Health Center
1148-1150 Springfield Avenue   Irvington, NJ 07111
(973)399-6292   Fax (973)372-4534

Ishikawa, Yoshihiro, MD {1356426324} CdvDis(84,JAP88)<NJ-UMDNJ>
+ Rutgers- New Jersey Medical School
185 South Orange Avenue   Newark, NJ 07103   (973)972-4300

Isidro, Jose R., Jr., MD {1558337972} Anesth(67,PHI01)<NJ-HOBUNIMC>
+ 2 Lincoln Highway/Suite 109
Edison, NJ 08820   (732)318-6869   Fax (732)494-9112
+ Hoboken University Medical Center
308 Willow Avenue/Anesth   Hoboken, NJ 07030   (732)318-6869   Fax (201)943-8105

Iskandarani, Nimer M., MD {1457498768} Psychy(69,SYRI)
+ 255 State Route 3
Secaucus, NJ 07094   (201)348-3118   Fax (201)348-5592

Iskander, Andrew J., MD {1982919775} Anesth
+ 178 Starmond Avenue
Clifton, NJ 07013
+ St. Barnabas Medical Center
94 Old Short Hills Road   Livingston, NJ 07039   Fax (973)660-9732

Iskaros, Basem F., MD {1659521524} PthAcl, PthCyt(79,EGY04)
+ Quest Diagnostics Inc.
1 Malcolm Avenue   Teterboro, NJ 07608   (201)393-5000
Fax (201)393-6127

Islam, Javedul M., MD {1457491599} FamMed(95,PAK01)
+ PromptMD Urgent Care Center
309 First Street   Hoboken, NJ 07030   (201)222-8411   Fax (201)222-8711
+ PromptMD Urgent Care Center
1122 Washington Street   Hoboken, NJ 07030   (201)706-8411

Islam, Mohammed Areful, MD {1114938461} IntrMd(88,BAN01)<NJ-RBAYPERT>
+ Raritan Bay Medical Center/Perth Amboy Division
530 New Brunswick Avenue/IntMed   Perth Amboy, NJ 08861   (732)324-5080   Fax (732)324-4669
+ Jewish Renaissance Medical Center
275 Hobart Street   Perth Amboy, NJ 08861   (732)324-5080
Fax (732)376-7402

Islam, Mohammed Nazrul, MD {1558472977} Psychy, PsyCAd(89,BAN03)<NJ-UNVMCPRN>
+ Princeton House Behavioral Health - Cherry Hill
375 North Kings Highway   Cherry Hill, NJ 08034   (856)779-8455   Fax (856)779-2988

Physicians by Name and Address

Islinger, Richard Barnard, MD {1043223605} SrgOrt, SrgTrm(91,NY01)
+ Shore Orthopedic University Associates
24 Macarthur Boulevard/First Floor   Somers Point, NJ 08244   (609)927-1991   Fax (609)927-4203
+ Shore Orthopedic University Associates
18 East Jimmie Leeds Road   Galloway, NJ 08205   (609)927-1991   Fax (609)927-4203

Ismail, Elham Mohamed, MD {1225057276} IntrMd(90,EGY05)
+ Community Health Care, Inc.
70 Cohansey Street   Bridgeton, NJ 08302   (856)451-4700   Fax (856)863-5732

Ismail, Medhat E., MD {1982665600} PulDis, IntrMd, SlpDis(80,EGY04)<NJ-CHILTON>
+ 246 Hamburg Turnpike/Suite 208
Wayne, NJ 07470   (973)790-3433   Fax (973)790-0433

Ismail, Mona S. A., MD {1053355834} PsyCAd, Psychy(96,EGY03)
+ American Institute for Counseling
1952 US Highway 22/Suite 102   Bound Brook, NJ 08805   (732)469-6444   Fax (732)469-6445

Ismail, Mourad Mohamed Farrag, MD {1386686269} IntrMd, PulDis(97,EGY05)<NJ-STJOSHOS>
+ St. Joseph's Regional Medical Center
703 Main Street/Medicine   Paterson, NJ 07503   (973)754-3970

Isnar, Noyemi, MD {1780758607} FamMed(72,TUR01)
+ 296 Garfield Street
Haworth, NJ 07641   (201)384-3733   Fax (201)384-8251

Isola, Anthony John, MD {1528220027} PedGst(06,NJ03)
+ Cooper Perinatology Associates
3 Cooper Plaza/Suite 502   Camden, NJ 08103   (856)968-7433   Fax (856)968-8499

Isola, Venkatarao, MD {1114944568} Pedtrc(85,INA62)<NJ-CHSMRCER>
+ Bellevue Pediatrics
416 Bellevue Avenue/Suite 207   Trenton, NJ 08648   (609)989-9801   Fax (609)989-9896

Israel, Alan M., MD {1710987730} Hemato, IntrMd, MedOnc(79,NY19)<NJ-VALLEY>
+ Northern Valley Medical Associates
221 Old Hook Road   Westwood, NJ 07675   (201)666-4949   Fax (201)666-6920
amis2@att.net

Israel, Arthur R., MD {1740273788} Urolgy(78,NY20)<NJ-MORRISTN>
+ Morristown Urology Associates PC
261 James Street/Suite 1A   Morristown, NJ 07960   (973)539-1050   Fax (973)538-6111

Israel, Jessica Leigh, MD {1629017843} IntrMd(95,NY47)<NJ-MONMOUTH, NY-MTSINAI>
+ Monmouth Medical Center
300 Second Avenue   Long Branch, NJ 07740   (732)222-5200

Israelite, Craig L., MD {1154359610} SrgOrt, IntrMd(87,PA09)<PA-UPMCPHL>
+ Penn Medicine at Cherry Hill
409 Route 70 East/Surgery/Ortho   Cherry Hill, NJ 08034   (856)429-1519

Isralowitz, David L., MD {1417929092} IntrMd, Grtrcs(75,NJ05)<NJ-HACKNSK>
+ New Jersey Physicians, LLC.
128 Union Avenue/Suite 2A   Rutherford, NJ 07070   (201)939-8834   Fax (201)939-7644

Issa, Amir Karam, MD {1386110799} IntrMd
+ St. Michael's Medical Center
111 Central Avenue   Newark, NJ 07102   (973)877-5000

Issa, Ebrahim S., MD {1578524864} CdvDis(82,INDI)<NJ-HOLYNAME, NJ-HACKNSK>
+ North Jersey Heart
800 Grange Road   Teaneck, NJ 07666   (201)907-0995   Fax (201)907-0996
+ North Jersey Heart
155 Cedar Lane   Teaneck, NJ 07666   (201)907-0995

Isserow, Jonathan Arnold, MD {1255337127} RadDia(91,SAF02)
+ University Radiology, PA
239 Route 22 East/Suite 302   Green Brook, NJ 08812   (732)968-4899   Fax (732)968-8096
+ University Radiology Group, P.C.
16 Mountain Boulevard   Warren, NJ 07059   (732)968-4899   Fax (908)769-9141
+ University Radiology Group, P.C.
579A Cranbury Road   East Brunswick, NJ 08812   (732)390-0040   Fax (732)390-1856

Istafanous, Rafik Monir, MD {1184713059} Psychy, PsyAdd(89,EGY05)<NJ-TRININPC, NJ-UMDNJ>
+ 125 Academy Street
Belleville, NJ 07109

Istvan, David Joseph, MD {1467473892} EmrgMd(96,PA01)<NJ-BAYONNE>
+ Bayonne Medical Center
29th Street at Avenue E/EmergMed   Bayonne, NJ 07002   (201)858-5000

Isukapalli, Padmaja, MD {1275543027} IntrMd(94,INA69)
+ Inman Medical Associates
1024 Park Avenue/Suite 6A   Plainfield, NJ 07060   (908)222-8400   Fax (908)222-8402
+ Inman Medical Associates
805 Inman Avenue   Colonia, NJ 07067   (908)222-8400   Fax (908)222-8402
+ Inman Medical Associates
322 State Street   Perth Amboy, NJ 07060   (732)751-4200

Ital, Rosa, MD {1831178235} IntrMd(80,IRA01)<NJ-JRSYSHMC>
+ Brick Town Medical
34 Lanes Mill Road   Brick, NJ 08724   (732)458-0300   Fax (732)458-8449

Itani, Mazen S., MD {1770555930} SrgVas, Surgry, RadV&I(96,LEB03)
+ 653 Willow Grove Street/Suite 1200
Hackettstown, NJ 07840   (908)684-0004

Itskovich, Alexander, MD {1427283712} Surgry
+ Comprehensive Surgical Associates
225 May Street/Suite A   Edison, NJ 08837   (732)346-5400   Fax (732)346-5404

Ittoop, Paul T., MD {1104900844} IntrMd, PulDis(74,INDI)
+ 2001 Palisade Avenue
Union City, NJ 07087   (201)863-4547   Fax (201)316-0459

Iturbides, Victor D., MD {1366545170} IntrMd(83,DOMI)<NJ-UNVMCPRN, NJ-CHSFULD>
+ We Care MD PC
2 Capital Way/Suite 359   Pennington, NJ 08534   (609)303-0590   Fax (609)303-0592

Itzeva, Youlia I., MD {1730356627} IntrMd<NJ-CHSFULD>
+ Capital Health System/Fuld Campus
750 Brunswick Avenue   Trenton, NJ 08638   (609)815-7887   Fax (609)394-6776

Itzkovich, Chad Jason, MD {1063478014} Anesth, IntrMd(02,NY47)
+ Synergy Anesthesia
2740 State Route 10/Suite 104   Morris Plains, NJ 07950   (973)200-8224   Fax (973)695-1324
+ Synergy Anestesia
2312 Gates Court   Morris Plains, NJ 07950   (973)200-8224   Fax (973)695-1324

Iucci, Gene, DO {1053674390} IntrMd
+ Rowan University-School of Osteopathic Medicine
1 Medical Center Drive   Stratford, NJ 08084   (856)346-6000

Iucci, Lisa Diane, DO {1275975161} Surgry
+ University Hospital -SOM University Doctors Surgeons
42 East Laurel Road/Suite 2500-2600   Stratford, NJ 08084   (856)566-6875   Fax (856)566-6873

Iula, Frank J., Jr., MD {1952309940} Anesth(90,DC02)<NJ-VIRTBERL, NJ-VIRTMARL>
+ West Jersey Anesthesia Associates
102-E Center Boulevard   Marlton, NJ 08053   (856)988-6250   Fax (856)988-6270

Iuliano, Frank David, MD {1679540850} Anesth, IntrMd(83,MEX34)<NJ-HOLYNAME>
+ Westwood Anesthesia Associates
250 Old Hook Road/2nd Floor   Westwood, NJ 07675   (201)358-3190   Fax (201)358-6622
+ Bergen Anesthesia Associates
718 Teaneck Road   Teaneck, NJ 07666   (201)358-3190   Fax (201)833-6576

Iuzzolino, Anthony, MD {1528153996} CdvDis, IntrMd(82,MEXI)
+ 33 Overlook Road/Suite 303
Summit, NJ 07901   (908)522-1000   Fax (908)522-9521

Ivan, Joseph R., MD {1770559221} ObsGyn(89,NJ05)<NJ-NWRKBETH>
+ Martinsville Women's Health
16 Mount Bethel Road/Suite 261   Warren, NJ 07059   (908)331-3470   Fax (732)271-9477

Ivanov, Alexander, MD {1790825222} Psychy(80,LAT02)
+ Drs. Rasin and Ivanov
2143 Morris Avenue/Suite 3   Union, NJ 07083   (908)686-4145

Ivanov, Alexander, MD {1770583163} CdvDis, ClCdEl(83,RUS01)
+ RWJPE Cardiology Associates of Somerset County, P.A.
487 Union Avenue/Suite A   Bridgewater, NJ 08807   (908)722-6410   Fax (908)722-4638

Ivanov, Ilya, DO {1487848149} Psychy(05,NJ75)
+ University Hospital-SOM Department of Psychiatry
2250 Chapel Avenue West/Suite 100   Cherry Hill, NJ 08002   (856)482-9000   Fax (856)482-1159

Ivanovic, Sasa, MD {1881072106}<NJ-STBARNMC>
+ St. Barnabas Medical Center
94 Old Short Hills Road   Livingston, NJ 07039   (973)322-5000

Ivchenko, Ludmila, MD {1720070345} IntrMd(76,UKR18)<NJ-RBAYOLDB>
+ Raritan Bay Medical Center/Old Bridge Division
One Hospital Plaza/IntMed   Old Bridge, NJ 08857   (732)360-1000

Ivelja-Hill, Danijela, MD {1831351865} Psychy<NJ-UNIVBHC>
+ University Behavioral Health Care
671 Hoes Lane/PO Box 1392   Piscataway, NJ 08855   (732)235-6114

Iversen, Robin J., MD {1306595135} IntrMd(85,TX14)<NJ-VALLEY, NJ-BERGNMC>
+ Valley Institute for Pain
One Valley Health Plaza/3 FL   Paramus, NJ 07652   (201)634-5555   Fax (201)634-5454
+ The Valley Hospital
223 North Van Dien Avenue   Ridgewood, NJ 07450   (201)447-8000

Ives, Elizabeth Payne, MD {1265635056} RadDia(11,MD01)
+ Cooper University Hospital
One Cooper Plaza   Camden, NJ 08103   (856)342-2000
+ Radiology Affiliates of Central New Jersey, P.A.
2501 Kuser Road   Hamilton, NJ 08691   (856)342-2000   Fax (609)585-1825

Ivker, Robert Alan, DO {1922133057} RadOnc, Radiol(91,IA75)<NJ-NWRKBETH, NJ-COMMED>
+ Prostate Cancer Center of New Jersey
375 Mount Pleasant Avenue/Suite 251   West Orange, NJ 07052   (973)323-1300   Fax (973)323-1319
+ Newark Beth Israel Medical Center
201 Lyons Avenue/RadiationOnc E2   Newark, NJ 07112   (973)926-7000
+ New Jersey Urology, LLC
700 North Broad Street/Suite 302   Elizabeth, NJ 07052   (908)289-3666   Fax (908)289-0716

Iwamoto, Marian, MD {1215101910} IntrMd(95,GA05)
+ Merck and Company Incorporated
126 East Lincoln Avenue   Rahway, NJ 07065   (732)594-4947   Fax (908)823-3620

Iwata, Isao, MD {1295921773} IntrMd(94,JAP50)<MA-CARNEY>
+ UH-RWJ General Internal Medicine
125 Paterson Street/Suite 2300   New Brunswick, NJ 08901   (732)235-7122   Fax (732)235-7144

Iwelumo, Ifeoma N., MD {1205897865} Pedtrc(83,NIG03)<NJ-STMRYPAS>
+ Lakeview Medical Center
266 Lakeview Avenue   Clifton, NJ 07011   (973)340-1222
driwelumo@aol.com

Iwu, Adaeze Anneliese, MD {1639437437}
+ 704 Cranbury Circle
East Brunswick, NJ 08816   (973)420-4146
iwuanne@gmail.com

Iyanoye, Abimbola Olamide, MD {1093961732} Pedtrc
+ 1702 Van Wickle Drive
Franklin Park, NJ 08823

Iyanoye, Adeyemi, MD {1124287479} IntCrd, IntrMd(02,MD07)
+ Cardiology Consultants
368 Lakehurst Road/Suite 301   Toms River, NJ 08755   (732)240-1048   Fax (732)240-3464
+ Cardiology Consultants of Toms River
401 Lacey Road/Suite D   Whiting, NJ 08759   (732)240-1048   Fax (732)350-3350
+ Cardiology Consultants
63-C Lacey Road   Whiting, NJ 08755   (732)350-3350   Fax (732)350-7054

Iyengar, Arjun D., MD {1053603340} OncHem, IntrMd(11)
+ Comprehensive Cancer Care LLC
27 East 29th Street   Bayonne, NJ 07002   (201)858-1211   Fax (201)858-4171

Iyengar, Devarajan Parthasarthy, MD {1689620700} IntrMd, MedOnc, OncHem(77,INA21)
+ Comprehensive Cancer Care LLC
27 East 29th Street   Bayonne, NJ 07002   (201)858-1211   Fax (201)858-4171

Iyer, Asha Muthuraman, MD {1831410299} SrgNro
+ JFK Neurosciences Institute
65 James Street/Second Floor   Edison, NJ 08818   (732)321-7010   Fax (732)744-5873

Iyer, Deepa Balasubramanian, MD {1174755144} CdvDis, IntrMd(96,INA69)
+ 10 Plum Street/7th Street
New Brunswick, NJ 08901   (732)253-3699   Fax (732)253-3467

Iyer, Malini, MD {1023014230} Surgry, SrgOnc, SrgBst(87,INA30)<NJ-UNDRWD>
+ Lourdes Medical Associates Hematology Oncology
1 Brace Road/Suite B   Cherry Hill, NJ 08034   (609)702-7550   Fax (609)702-1277
+ CancerCare of Southern New Jersey
51 Haddonfield Road/Suite 145   Cherry Hill, NJ 08002   (609)702-7550   Fax (856)488-8050

Iyer, Neel Subramanian, DO {1689235418} ObsGyn
+ Cooper University Hospital Obstetrics & Gynecology
One Cooper Plaza   Camden, NJ 08103   (856)342-2000

Iyer, Rajesh V., MD {1558317149} RadOnc(96,PA13)<NJ-COMMED>
+ Community Medical Center
99 Route 37 West   Toms River, NJ 08755   (732)557-8000

Iyer, Sekhar Gopalan, MD {1679576045}<NJ-STBARNMC>
+ St. Barnabas Medical Center
94 Old Short Hills Road/Rm 4225   Livingston, NJ 07039
(973)322-5777

Izakov, Natalya B., DO {1861837965} EmrgMd
+ 105 Roseland Avenue/Unit 1104
Caldwell, NJ 07006   (973)287-6485

Izanec, James L., MD {1235356148} Gastrn(01,NY20)
+ Allied Gastroenterology Associates
217 White Horse Pike   Haddon Heights, NJ 08035
(856)547-1212   Fax (856)547-6117

Izeogu, Chinweike, MD {1598789141} Anesth(01,AL02)<NJ-HACKNSK>
+ Montclair Anesthesia Associates PC
185 Fairfield Avenue/Suite 2A   West Caldwell, NJ 07006
(973)226-1230   Fax (973)226-1232

Izgur, Vitaly, MD {1164664421} RadDia<NJ-MEADWLND>
+ Meadowlands Hospital Medical Center
55 Meadowlands Parkway   Secaucus, NJ 07096   (201)392-3100

Jaaj, Hedoneia C., MD {1326158197} IntrMd(71,BRAZ)<NJ-CHILTON>
+ 34 Main Street/Suite A
Bloomingdale, NJ 07403   (973)838-0714

Jabbour, Salma K., MD {1184707234} RadOnc(01,MD01)<NJ-RWJUBRUN>
+ Rutgers Cancer Institute of New Jersey
195 Little Albany Street/PO Box 2681   New Brunswick, NJ 08903   (732)235-2465   Fax (732)235-6797
+ UH- Robert Wood Johnson Med
125 Paterson Street/RadOnc G2N45   New Brunswick, NJ 08901   (732)828-3000

Jaber Iqbal, Reem, DO {1326231879} IntrMd, OstMed(05,NY75)
+ 735 Linwood Avenue
Ridgewood, NJ 07450   (201)670-1231   Fax (201)612-0922

Jablons, Mitchell L., MD {1164483418} Anesth(77,MO34)
+ Summit Anesthesia Associates, P.A.
33 Overlook Road/Suite 311   Summit, NJ 07901   (908)598-1500   Fax (908)598-0197

Jabush, Jondavid H., MD {1649486705} Surgry(01,NJ05)
+ 108 Bilby Road/Suite 303
Hackettstown, NJ 07840   (908)850-9548   Fax (908)813-3256
+ Hackensack University Medical Center
20 Prospect Avenue   Hackensack, NJ 07601   (201)996-2000

Jachens, Adrian William, MD {1063673408} Ophthl
+ Ridgewood Ophthalmology PC
1200 East Ridgewood Avenue   Ridgewood, NJ 07450
(201)612-4400   Fax (201)612-9446

Jacir, Nabil N., MD {1841262995} PedSrg(73,LEBA)<NJ-OVERLOOK>
+ Overlook Medical Center
99 Beauvoir Avenue/PO Box 210   Summit, NJ 07902
(973)522-3523   Fax (973)522-3525

Jackman, Earl Francis, DO {1881639011} ObsGyn(81,MO78)<NJ-COMMED, NJ-MONMOUTH>
+ North Dover Ob-Gyn Associates
222 Oak Avenue/3rd Floor/Suite 301   Toms River, NJ 08753
(732)914-1919   Fax (732)341-3303
+ North Dover Ob-Gyn Associates
442 Lacey Road   Forked River, NJ 08731   (732)914-1919
Fax (609)971-9712
+ North Dover Ob-Gyn Associates
214 Jack Martin Boulevard/Building D-3   Brick, NJ 08753
(732)840-3900   Fax (732)840-9270

Jacknin, Mark A., DO {1033179338} IntrMd(02,NY75)
+ ImmediCenter/Clifton
1355 Broad Street   Clifton, NJ 07013   (973)778-5566   Fax
(973)778-2268

Jacks, Maryann, MD {1548322977} FamMed(91,NJ05)<NJ-JFKMED>
+ PO Box 4162
Middletown, NJ 07748   (732)391-5269

Jackson, Douglas T., MD {1962472407} Anesth, AnesCrCr(83,PA13)<NJ-UMDNJ>
+ University Hospital
150 Bergen Street/Anesthesiology   Newark, NJ 07103
(973)972-4300

Jackson, Eric Marc, MD {1235131251} IntrMd(78,NY47)<NJ-CLARMAAS, NJ-WESTHDSN>
+ 16-18 Ridge Road
North Arlington, NJ 07031   (201)997-1010   Fax (201)997-7436

Jackson, Kurt T., MD {1619161858} Ophthl
+ NJ Retina
1255 Broad Street/Suite 104   Bloomfield, NJ 07003
(973)707-5632   Fax (973)707-7349

Jackson, Michael B., MD {1073600896} Psychy, PsyFor, Psyphm(01,NJ06)
+ 80 River Street/Suite 302
Hoboken, NJ 07030   (201)244-7799

mbjacksonMD@hotmail.com

Jackson, Olga E., MD {1396947792} ObsGyn(07,MA05)
+ Pinelands Obstetrics and Gynecology
1617 Route 38   Mount Holly, NJ 08060   (609)261-0240
Fax (609)261-8622
+ Penn Medicine Department of Ob/Gyn - Medford
103 Old Marlton Pike/Suite 101   Medford, NJ 08055

Jackson, Sharon, MD {1992152987} ObsGyn
+ West Long Branch Obstetrics & Gynecology
1019 Broadway   West Long Branch, NJ 07764   (732)229-6797   Fax (732)229-6893

Jackson, Thomas Edward, MD {1245330950} IntrMd(81,MEX03)
+ 47 Maple Street/Suite 205
Summit, NJ 07901   (908)522-9400   Fax (908)522-3226

Jackson, Unjeria C., MD {1477608677} MtFtMd, ObsGyn(81,MA05)<NJ-MORRISTN>
+ 5 Wooded Acres Lane
Morristown, NJ 07960   (973)829-1711

Jacob, David E., MD {1063466381} CdvDis, IntrMd(85,MEX34)<NJ-STPETER>
+ St. Peter's University Hospital
254 Easton Avenue   New Brunswick, NJ 08901   (732)745-8600   Fax (732)729-1990

Jacob, Emad, MD {1669622015} IntrMd(93,POL10)<NJ-STMICHL>
+ 714 Kearney Avenue
Kearny, NJ 07032   (201)772-5211   Fax (201)428-1627

Jacob, Jeena, MD {1285898684} EmrgMd
+ University Hospital Emergency Medicine
150 Bergen Street   Newark, NJ 07103   (973)972-5128
Fax (973)972-6646

Jacob, Leena Rachel, DO {1851655765}
+ Samaritan HealthCare & Hospice
5 Eves Drive/Suite 300   Marlton, NJ 08053   (610)772-1161
Fax (856)596-7881
leenarachelphilip@gmail.com

Jacob, Mariamma, MD {1477539567} FamMed(75,INDI)<NJ-HACKNSK>
+ Hackensack University Medical Center
30 Prospect Avenue/Pediatrics   Hackensack, NJ 07601
(201)996-2000

Jacob, Seby Mathewkutty, MD {1730340621} IntrMd(08,NY08)
+ Princeton Wound Care Center
3626 Route 1 North   Princeton, NJ 08540   (609)945-3611
Fax (609)945-3688

Jacob, Sharon Leigh, MD {1649461708} EmrgMd<NJ-JRSYSHMC>
+ EmCare
1945 Route 33   Neptune, NJ 07753   (732)776-4510   Fax
(732)776-2329

Jacob, Sneha Elizabeth, MD {1265569602} IntrMd
+ Eric B. Chandler Health Center
277 George Street   New Brunswick, NJ 08901   (732)235-6700   Fax (732)235-6729

Jacob, Tess, MD {1679838163} EnDbMt
+ Summit Medical Group
75 East Northfield Road   Livingston, NJ 07039   (973)436-1450   Fax (908)964-5718
+ Summit Medical Group-Berkeley Heights Campus
1 Diamond Hill Road   Berkeley Heights, NJ 07922
(973)436-1450   Fax (203)384-4294

Jacobowitz, Esther, MD {1881884583} Psychy, PsyCAd(86,MA05)
+ 265 Cedar Lane/Suite 2
Teaneck, NJ 07666   (201)329-4314

Jacobs, Abbie D., MD {1811042575} FamMed(86,NY47)<NJ-STMRYPAS, NJ-HOBUNIMC>
+ Center for Family Health
122-132 Clinton Street   Hoboken, NJ 07030   (201)418-3100   Fax (201)418-3148

Jacobs, David Jay, MD {1205846342} PhysMd(79,MEX14)<NJ-OVERLOOK, NJ-STBARNMC>
+ 2780 Morris Avenue
Union, NJ 07083   (908)769-0137
+ 5 Mountain Boulevard
Warren, NJ 07059   (908)769-0137

Jacobs, David S A, MD {1952701468} IntrMd(96,NJ06)
+ 46 Timberhill Drive
Franklin Park, NJ 08823

Jacobs, Emily J., MD {1669715959}{PA02
+ Miller Ophthalmology Associates, LLC
101 Old Short Hills Road/Suite 430   West Orange, NJ 07052
(973)325-3300   Fax (973)325-3320

Jacobs, Glenn Paul, MD {1417952219} CdvDis, IntrMd(75,NJ05)<NJ-COMMED>
+ Cardiology Consultants
368 Lakehurst Road/Suite 301   Toms River, NJ 08755
(732)240-1048   Fax (732)240-3464
+ Cardiology Consultants
63-C Lacey Road   Whiting, NJ 08759   (732)240-1048   Fax
(732)350-7054
+ Cardiology Consultants of Toms River
401 Lacey Road/Suite D   Whiting, NJ 08755   (732)350-3350   Fax (732)350-3350

Physicians by Name and Address

Jacobs, Ian Neal, MD {1720178742} PedOto, Otlryg(86,NY47)<PA-CHILDHOS>
+ CHOP Pediatric & Adolescent Specialty Care Center
1012 Laurel Oak Road   Voorhees, NJ 08043   (856)435-1300
Fax (856)435-0091
+ CHOP Pediatric & Adolescent Specialty Care Center
707 Alexander Road/Suite 205   Princeton, NJ 08540
(609)520-1717

Jacobs, Ivan H., MD {1871689109} Ophthl, Glacma, Catrct(73,PA02)
+ Eye Care and Surgery Center
10 Mountain Boulevard   Warren, NJ 07059   (908)754-4800
Fax (908)754-4803
ijacobs@newjerseyvision.com
+ Eye Care and Surgery Center
592 Springfield Avenue   Westfield, NJ 07090   (908)754-4800   Fax (908)789-1379
+ Eye Care and Surgery Center
517 Route 1 South/Suite 1100   Iselin, NJ 07059   (732)636-7355   Fax (732)636-7497

Jacobs, Jeffry Lance, DO {1134169279} SrgPlstc, SrgPHand(90,NJ75)<NJ-ENGLWOOD, NJ-HOLYNAME>
+ Jeffrey Lance Jacobs, DO
680 Kinderkamack Road/Suite 205   Oradell, NJ 07649
(201)969-9900   Fax (201)969-9925
+ Personal Image PC
PO Box 98   Hillsdale, NJ 07642

Jacobs, Lyssa Sorkin, MD {1245499870} PhysMd, IntrMd(07,NY46)
+ Pain Management Associates
255 East Main Street   Ramsey, NJ 07446   (201)326-4777
Fax (201)391-1196

Jacobs, Miriam, MD {1205264694} Ophthl, IntrMd(83,NY47)
+ Anthony J Inverno & Associates
95 Westfield Avenue   Clark, NJ 07066   (732)381-5555
Fax (732)381-5055

Jacobs, Sharon G., MD {1902046531} ClnPhm, Pedtrc, Rserch(75,BELG)
+ Daiichi Sankyo Research Institute
399 Thornhall Street/Suite 7   Edison, NJ 08837   (732)590-5000

Jacobs, Stefanie S., MD {1144288507} RadDia, RadNuc(87,GRN01)<NJ-ENGLWOOD>
+ Englewood Hospital and Medical Center
350 Engle Street/Radiology   Englewood, NJ 07631
(201)894-3000   Fax (201)541-2193

Jacobs, Stephen H., MD {1740370204} IntrMd(64,DC02)<NJ-BERGNMC>
+ New Bridge Medical Center
230 East Ridgewood Avenue   Paramus, NJ 07652
(201)967-4000   Fax (201)967-7924

Jacobson, Louis Robert, MD {1376625145} Pedtrc(88,MD01)
+ Sparta Pediatrics, LLC
106 Main Street   Sparta, NJ 07871   (973)729-7400   Fax
(973)729-2201

Jacobson, Marina, MD {1831145473} ObsGyn, AdolMd(01,PA13)<NJ-ENGLWOOD>
+ Complete Women's Healthcare
200 Engle Street/Suite 14   Englewood, NJ 07631
(201)735-5700   Fax (201)735-5750
info@drmarinajacobson.com

Jacobson, Mark, DO {1659394484} Pedtrc(74,IA75)<PA-CHOPHIL>
+ Harborview KidsFirst
505 Bay Avenue   Somers Point, NJ 08244   (609)927-4235
Fax (609)927-5590
+ Harborview KidsFirst Cape May
1315 Route 9 South   Cape May Court House, NJ 08210
(609)927-4235   Fax (609)465-1539
+ Harborview Smithville
48 South New York Road/Route 9   Smithville, NJ 08244
(609)748-2900   Fax (609)748-3067

Jacobson, Martin Alexander, MD {1316173446} Anesth
+ Morris Anesthesia Group, PA
3799 Route 46/Suite 211   Parsippany, NJ 07054   (973)335-1122   Fax (973)335-1448

Jacobson, Nina Stella, MD {1154619500} ObsGyn, IntrMd(09,ISR02)<NY-MTSINAI, NY-MTSINYHS>
+ Hackensack Meridian Urogynecology Medical Group
19 Davis Avenue/7th Floor   Neptune, NJ 07753   (732)776-3797   Fax (732)776-3796
+ Jersey Shore University Medical Center
1945 Route 33   Neptune, NJ 07753   (732)775-5500

Jacobson, Sayre K., MD {1447302864} CdvDis, IntrMd(64,PA01)
+ Marven Wallen & S. Kenneth Jacobson MD PA
1985 Springfield Avenue   Maplewood, NJ 07040   (973)763-5010   Fax (973)761-6980

Jacoby, Dana R., MD {1356311609} ObsGyn(93,PA09)<NJ-RIVERVW, NJ-MONMOUTH>
+ 766 Shrewsbury Avenue
Tinton Falls, NJ 07724   (732)530-4545   Fax (732)530-5741

Physicians by Name and Address

Jacoby, Douglas Scott, MD {1477580371} CarNuc, CdvDis, IntrMd(99,MA01)
+ Penn Medicine at Cherry Hill
  1400 East Route 70/Cardiology   Cherry Hill, NJ 08034

Jacoby, Jacob Herman, MD {1174648232} Psychy, Addctn, NrlgAddM(80,NY06)<NJ-BAYONNE, NJ-STBARNMC>
+ 654 Avenue C/Suite 201
  Bayonne, NJ 07002   (201)339-0323   Fax (201)339-0349
  JHJacoby@hotmail.com
+ Bayonne Medical Center
  29th Street at Avenue E/Psych   Bayonne, NJ 07002
  (201)858-5000
+ 127 East Mt. Pleasant Avenue
  Livingston, NJ 07002   (201)339-0323   Fax (201)339-0349

Jacoby, James Howard, MD {1174522072} Radiol, RadPhy, IntrMd(68,PA02)<NJ-COOPRUMC>
+ Cooper University Hospital
  One Cooper Plaza/Radiology   Camden, NJ 08103
  (856)342-2383
+ Heights Imaging Center
  17 White Horse Pike   Haddon Heights, NJ 08035   (856)342-2383   Fax (856)546-0666

Jacoby, Michelle P., MD {1841289857} ObsGyn(93,PA09)<NJ-RIVERVW>
+ Drs. Karoly, Kaskiw, Hammond & Jacoby
  180 White Road/Suite 209   Little Silver, NJ 07739
  (732)842-0673   Fax (732)842-7352
+ Drs. Karoly, Kaskiw, Hammond & Jacoby
  1 Bethany Road/Building 2/Suite 31   Hazlet, NJ 07730

Jacoby, Richard, MD {1811428493} Dermat
+ 8 Collins Mill Court
  Moorestown, NJ 08057   (609)458-6304

Jacoby, Sari H., MD {1740430529} IntrMd(04,NY46)<NJ-NWRK-BETH>
+ Newark Beth Israel Medical Center
  201 Lyons Avenue/IntMed   Newark, NJ 07112   (973)926-7231
+ 590 Ogden Avenue
  Teaneck, NJ 07666

Jacoby, Sidney Mark, MD {1750415527} SrgOrt
+ South Jersey Hand Center
  1888 Marlton Pike East/Suite E-F-G   Cherry Hill, NJ 08003
  (856)489-5630   Fax (856)489-5631

Jacoby, Steven Clifford, MD {1619977667} IntrMd, CritCr, PulDis(99,CT01)<NJ-VALLEY>
+ Respiratory Health & Critical Care Associates
  1114 Goffle Road/Suite 103   Hawthorne, NJ 07506
  (973)790-4111   Fax (973)790-4330
+ VMG Respiratory Health & Pulmonary Medicine
  1200 East Ridgewood Avenue   Ridgewood, NJ 07450
  (973)790-4111   Fax (201)689-0521

Jacome-Bohorquez, Gloria C., MD {1225186075} PedEmg, Pedtrc, EmrgMd(85,ECU01)<NJ-MONMOUTH, NJ-STBARNMC>
+ Monmouth Medical Center
  300 Second Avenue   Long Branch, NJ 07740   (732)923-7300   Fax (732)923-8882

Jacowitz, Joel D., MD {1922009760} CdvDis, IntrMd, IntCrd(77,NY08)<NY-ARDNHILL, NJ-VALLEY>
+ Hackensack University Medical Group Emerson
  452 Old Hook Road/2nd Floor   Emerson, NJ 07630
  (201)666-3900   Fax (201)261-0505

Jacque, Celeste A., MD {1194765206} PsyCAd, Psychy(78,NY48)
+ 201 South Livingston Avenue/Suite 1-A
  Livingston, NJ 07039   (973)994-1500   Fax (973)994-1606

Jacques, Walter J., MD {1619932860} Pedtrc, AdolMd(89,NJ06)<NJ-RWJUHAM, NJ-CHSMRCER>
+ Hamilton Pediatric Associates
  3 Hamilton Health Place/Suite A   Hamilton, NJ 08690
  (609)581-4480   Fax (609)581-5222

Jacquette, Germaine Marie, MD {1528090099} IntrMd, InfDis(79,NY19)
+ Global Tuberculosis Institute (GTBI)
  225 Warren Street/PO Box 1709   Newark, NJ 07101
  (973)972-3270   Fax (973)972-3268
  jacquegm@umdnj.edu

Jadav, Jitendra K., MD {1578535316} Anesth(82,INDI)<NJ-KIMBALL>
+ Ocean Anesthesia Group PA
  1200 Hooper Avenue   Toms River, NJ 08753   (732)797-3890   Fax (732)942-5603

Jadeja, Kiranben J., MD {1669595310} Psychy, PssoMd(92,INA53)
+ NBIMC Psychiatry
  201 Lyons Avenue   Newark, NJ 07112   (973)926-7026
  Fax (973)926-2862

Jadeja, Poiyniba Dilip, MD {1962426171} FamMed(94,DMN01)
+ 20 Millennium Drive
  Columbus, NJ 08022

Jadeja, Priya Hari, MD {1912296427}
+ Summit Medical Group
  75 East Northfield Road   Livingston, NJ 07039   (973)436-1530   Fax (973)422-0414

Jadhav, Ashwin R., MD {1457675159} ObsGyn, MtFtMd<NY-NYUTISCH>
+ UMDNJ RWJ Maternal Fetal Medicine
  125 Paterson Street/Suite 4200   New Brunswick, NJ 08901
  (732)235-6632   Fax (732)235-7349

Jadhav, Latha, MD {1396075636} Pedtrc
+ Drs. Ballem and Jadhav
  715 Broadway   Paterson, NJ 07514   (973)279-2294   Fax (973)279-7341
  Drjadhav@yahoo.com

Jadhav, Pallavi Dinkar, MD {1356531768} FamMed
+ 1 Weaver Drive
  Marlton, NJ 08053

Jadhav, Surekha Ashwin, MD {1164899704} Pedtrc
+ Central Jersey Pediatrics PC
  1553 Ruth Road/Suite 1   North Brunswick, NJ 08902
  (732)418-1700   Fax (732)249-9599

Jadico, Suzanne K., MD {1376744342} Ophthl(06,PA01)
+ The Princeton Eye Group
  419 North Harrison Street/Suite 104   Princeton, NJ 08540
  (609)921-9437   Fax (609)921-0277
+ The Princeton Eye Group
  1600 Perrinville Road   Monroe Township, NJ 08831
  (609)921-9437   Fax (609)655-3685
+ The Princeton Eye Group
  900 Eastern Avenue/Suite 50   Somerset, NJ 08540
  (732)565-9550   Fax (732)565-0946

Jadidi, Shirin, MD {1386070340} Allrgy, Pedtrc(83,IA02)<NJ-WARREN>
+ 12 McVickers Lane
  Mendham, NJ 07945

Jadun, Wamiq, MD {1144336777} Pedtrc(87,PAK06)<NJ-HACKNSK, NJ-HOLYNAME>
+ Riverside Medical Group
  710 Tenth Street   Secaucus, NJ 07094   (201)865-2050
  Fax (201)865-0015

Jaeckle, Kurt Alfred, MD {1205825650} MedOnc
+ Medical Diagnostic Associates, P.A.
  99 Beauvoir Avenue   Summit, NJ 07901   (973)971-4179
  Fax (973)971-7905

Jafari, Mortaza, MD {1053498097} IntrMd(76,IRA08)
+ Jafari Medical Associates
  176 Bloomfield Avenue   Newark, NJ 07104   (973)484-7702
  Fax (973)484-8954

Jaferi, Barkat A., MD {1932148137} IntrMd(76,PAK01)<NJ-RWJUHAM>
+ 2067 Klockner Road
  Trenton, NJ 08690   (609)584-6221   Fax (609)584-6224

Jaffari, Syed Moosa Raza, MD {1063526168} Otlryg(70,INA5B)<NJ-KIMBALL>
+ 814 River Road
  Lakewood, NJ 08701   (732)367-7707   Fax (732)367-7860

Jaffe, Brian C., MD {1346401023} IntrMd
+ Virtua Pulmonology - Marlton
  141 Route 70/Suite B   Marlton, NJ 08053   (856)596-9057
  Fax (856)596-0837

Jaffe, Jane K., DO {1144485152} IntrMd(07,PA77)
+ South Jersey Gastroenterology PA
  406 Lippincott Drive/Suite E   Marlton, NJ 08053   (856)983-1900   Fax (856)983-1914

Jaffe, Joel D., MD {1659366318} Otlryg(75,PA13)<NJ-STFRNMED, NJ-RWJUHAM>
+ Premier ENT Associates
  8 Quakerbridge Plaza   Hamilton, NJ 08619   (609)890-7800
  Fax (609)890-6148

Jaffe, Leonard, MD {1467514083} SrgOrt(78,IL42)
+ Specialty Orthopedics, LLC
  609 Morris Avenue   Springfield, NJ 07081   (973)467-9500
  Fax (973)467-2364

Jaffe, Robert M., MD {1164428033} NuclMd, Radiol(78,MA07)
+ University Radiology Group, P.C.
  3900 Park Avenue/Suite 107   Edison, NJ 08820   (732)548-6800   Fax (732)548-6290
+ University Radiology Group, P.C.
  16 Mountain Boulevard   Warren, NJ 07059   (732)548-6800
  Fax (908)769-9141
+ University Radiology Group, P.C.
  579A Cranbury Road   East Brunswick, NJ 08820   (732)390-0040   Fax (732)390-1856

Jaffe, Seth L., DO SrgOrt(87,NJ75)
+ 17 Academy Street
  Newark, NJ 07102

Jaffery, Fatema, MD {1003877663} Pedtrc(80,PAK23)<NJ-CHD-NWBTH, NJ-NWRKBETH>
+ Children's Hospital of New Jersey
  201 Lyons Avenue/Osborne Terrace   Newark, NJ 07112
  (973)926-7282
+ Prime Pediatrics
  50 Union Avenue/Suite 704   Irvington, NJ 07111
  (973)373-9600

Jaffery, Fizza Aftab, MD {1730467374}
+ 366 Lincoln Avenue
  Cherry Hill, NJ 08002

Jaffry, Syed Ali Hasan, MD {1487615050} IntrMd, InfDis(91,INA2Y)<NJ-PALISADE, NJ-TRININPC>
+ Central Jersey Health Care Associates
  240 Williamson Street/Suite 305   Elizabeth, NJ 07201
  (908)354-5353   Fax (908)351-6911

Jafri, Abida Y., MD {1093845729} PhysMd(78,PAK04)
+ 2 State Route 27/Suite 405
  Edison, NJ 08820   (732)318-6623   Fax (732)318-6623

Jafri, Iqbal H., MD {1811913692} PhysMd, PainMd, OthrSp(78,PAKI)<NJ-JFKJHNSN, NJ-JFKMED>
+ JFK Johnson Rehabilitation Institute
  65 James Street   Edison, NJ 08818   (732)321-7070   Fax (732)321-7330

Jafri, Jaffar M., MD {1477562007} IntrMd
+ 6 Sasha Court
  Matawan, NJ 07747

Jafri, Rana B., MD {1912938747} IntrMd(83,PAKI)<NJ-BAYSHORE>
+ Medical Associates of Marlboro
  42 Throckmorton Lane/2nd flr   Old Bridge, NJ 08857
  (732)607-1111   Fax (732)607-0552
+ Associates in Cardiology and Internal Medicine
  790 Amboy Avenue   Perth Amboy, NJ 08861   (732)607-1111   Fax (732)324-8095

Jafri, Syed S., MD {1235198169} Nrolgy(84,PAK11)<NJ-CHRIST, NJ-PALISADE>
+ 1031 McBride Avenue/Suite C-203
  West Paterson, NJ 07424   (973)890-0710
+ 8534 Kennedy Boulevard
  North Bergen, NJ 07047   (201)854-2774

Jafry, Behjath, MD {1043402456} IntrMd(04,NJ06)<NJ-COOPRUMC>
+ Cooper Physicians
  1210 Brace Road/Suite 102   Cherry Hill, NJ 08034
  (856)428-6616   Fax (856)428-4823

Jafry, Yasmeen, MD {1235277054} FamMed
+ Integrated Medical Alliance/IMA Medical Care Center
  30 Shrewsbury Plaza   Shrewsbury, NJ 07702   (732)542-0002   Fax (732)542-2992

Jagadeesh, Jyothi, MD {1053512269} Grtrcs, IntrMd(02,INA7C)<NJ-VIRTMHBC>
+ Virtua Memorial
  175 Madison Avenue   Mount Holly, NJ 08060   (609)914-6180   Fax (609)914-6182

Jagamony, Sandhya, MD {1801047220} IntrMd
+ 83 Alderberry Court
  Edison, NJ 08820

Jaggi, Mona, MD {1912004508} EmrgMd(95,NJ05)<NJ-JRSYCITY>
+ Jersey City Medical Center
  355 Grand Street/EmrgMed   Jersey City, NJ 07304
  (201)915-2000

Jagpal, Karandeep, DO {1457632572} GenPrc
+ Rowan University-School of Osteopathic Medicine
  1 Medical Center Drive   Stratford, NJ 08084   (856)566-6708

Jagpal, Sugeet K., MD {1326215179} CritCr
+ 46 Treetops Circle
  Princeton, NJ 08540   (732)422-7708

Jahn, Anthony Frederick, MD {1073546743} Otlryg, Otolgy(74,ON01)<NY-SLRLUKES>
+ Englewood Ear Nose & Throat, P.C.
  216 Engle Street/Suite 101   Englewood, NJ 07631
  (201)816-9800   Fax (201)567-1569

Jahn, Eric G., MD {1265542633} IntrMd(88,NJ06)<NJ-RWJUBRUN>
+ Eric B. Chandler Health Center
  277 George Street   New Brunswick, NJ 08901   (732)235-6700   Fax (732)235-6726

Jain, Ami J., MD {1124124649} Pedtrc(98,MA07)<NJ-STPETER>
+ Pedi Health Medical Associates
  720 Route 202-206 North/Suite 4   Bridgewater, NJ 08807
  (908)722-5444   Fax (908)722-5071

Jain, Archna, MD {1235107301} Pedtrc(81,INDI)
+ Vineland Pediatrics
  1138 East Chestnut Avenue   Vineland, NJ 08360   (856)692-1108   Fax (609)692-2077

Jain, Asha, MD {1891754982} Pedtrc, AdolMd(76,INA72)<NJ-BAYSHORE, NJ-RIVERVW>
+ 35 Village Court
  Hazlet, NJ 07730   (732)739-8866   Fax (732)739-5652

Jain, Chandru U., MD {1427053024} RadDia, Radiol, IntrMd(83,INA67)<NJ-OCEANMC>
+ Ocean Medical Center
  425 Jack Martin Boulevard/Radiology   Brick, NJ 08723
  (732)836-4046   Fax (732)836-4047
+ Coastal Imaging, LLC
  79 Route 37 West/Suite 103   Toms River, NJ 08755
  (732)836-4046   Fax (732)276-2325

Physicians by Name and Address

Jain, Deepak K., MD {1356368823} IntrMd(98,GRN01)
+ Central Jersey Internal Medicine
  75 Veronica Avenue/Suite 204   Somerset, NJ 08873
  (732)828-0002   Fax (732)828-0153
+ Central Jersey Internal Medicine
  111 Union Valley Road/Suite 203   Monroe, NJ 08831
  (732)828-0002   Fax (609)655-2253

Jain, Deepika, MD {1750551875} IntrMd
+ Drs. Ahmed, Haddad & Batwara
  26 Greenville Avenue   Jersey City, NJ 07305   (201)333-8222   Fax (201)333-0095

Jain, Doney B., MD {1720484777} Pedtrc(09,GRN01)
+ V 1 Brothers, Inc.
  751 Bergen Avenue   Jersey City, NJ 07306   (201)946-1200
  Fax (201)946-1201

Jain, Keshani, MD {1376557546} Nephro(00,NJ05)<NJ-OCEANMC, NJ-JRSYSHMC>
+ Jersey Coast Nephrology & Hypertension Associates
  1541 Route 88/Suite A   Brick, NJ 08724   (732)836-3200
  Fax (732)836-3201

Jain, Madhu, MD {1033211255} IntrMd, PhysMd(91,NJ05)<NJ-STLAWRN, NJ-RWJUHAM>
+ St. Lawrence Rehabilitation Center
  2381 Lawrenceville Road   Lawrenceville, NJ 08648
  (609)896-9500   Fax (609)896-4107
  Mjain@slnc.org

Jain, Manoj Prakash, MD {1972717676} FamMed(03,DMN01)
+ Cape Hospitalist Associates, P.A.
  2 Stone Harbor Boulevard   Cape May Court House, NJ 08210   (609)463-2058   Fax (732)212-0713

Jain, Monica, MD {1588615157} RadDia(01,NJ05)
+ 69 Lawrence Drive
  Short Hills, NJ 07078

Jain, Navjot, DO {1609284397}
+ Cooper University Hospital
  One Cooper Plaza   Camden, NJ 08103   (856)342-2000

Jain, Rajesh K., MD {1588644405} SrgOrt(00,NY15)<NJ-VIRTMHBC, NJ-VIRTUAHS>
+ Reconstructive Orthopedics, P.A.
  243 Route 130/Suite 100   Bordentown, NJ 08505
  (609)267-9400   Fax (609)267-9457
+ Reconstructive Orthopedics, P.A.
  131 Route 70 West/Suite 100   Medford, NJ 08055
  (609)267-9400   Fax (609)267-9457

Jain, Ratnam, MD {1679583546} ObsGyn(85,INA9Y)<NJ-CLARMAAS, NJ-STMRYPAS>
+ Special Care Ob-Gyn
  14 Franklin Street/2nd Floor   Belleville, NJ 07109
  (973)759-4802   Fax (973)759-4805
+ Special Care Ob-Gyn
  905 Allwood Road/Sute 103   Clifton, NJ 07011   (973)759-4802   Fax (973)340-1518

Jain, Rishabh Kumar, MD {1679887822} IntrMd<NJ-MONMOUTH>
+ Monmouth Medical Center
  300 Second Avenue   Long Branch, NJ 07740   (732)923-6537   Fax (732)923-6536

Jain, Samir S., MD {1851312656} CdvDis, CarNuc, IntrMd(96,INA26)<NJ-COMMED, NJ-SOCEANCO>
+ Samir S. Jain MD PC
  599 Route 37 West/Suite 5   Toms River, NJ 08755
  (732)608-9737   Fax (732)608-9744

Jain, Sandesh, MD {1831236967} Nephro, IntrMd(00,GRN01)<NJ-RWJUBRUN, NJ-STPETER>
+ Kidney & Hypertension Center of Central Jersey
  23 Clyde Road/Suite 101   Somerset, NJ 08873   (732)873-9500   Fax (732)873-0261

Jain, Sanjay K., MD {1063345780} EmrgMd, FamMed(76,INA69)<NJ-NWTNMEM, NJ-HCKTSTWN>
+ North Warren Medical Associates PC
  Route 517/Building B   Hackettstown, NJ 07840   (908)852-0107   Fax (908)850-9160
  Drsanjayjain@hotmail.com
+ North Warren Medical Associates
  155 State Highway 94   Blairstown, NJ 07825   (908)852-0107   Fax (908)362-6984

Jain, Sanjeevani, MD {1902887235} Psychy(81,INDI)<NJ-NWTNMEM, NJ-HCKTSTWN>
+ Route 517/Building B
  Hackettstown, NJ 07840   (908)852-4084
+ Highland Psychiatric Associates
  89 Sparta Avenue/Suite 240   Sparta, NJ 07871   (908)852-4084   Fax (973)729-7641

Jain, Sapna, MD {1568415990} IntrMd(84,INA5A)
+ Neighborhood Health Center Plainfield
  1700-58 Myrtle Avenue   Plainfield, NJ 07060   (908)753-6401   Fax (908)226-6743
+ Inman Medical Associates
  805 Inman Avenue   Colonia, NJ 07067   (908)753-6401
  Fax (908)222-8402
+ Inman Medical Associates
  322 State Street   Perth Amboy, NJ 08861   (732)751-4200

Jain, Sejal, MD {1073900445} FamMed
+ Drs. Kharazi and Jain
  7 Vose Avenue   South Orange, NJ 07079   (973)630-8989
  Fax (973)761-1694

Jain, Sneh, MD {1912971730} IntrMd(70,INA72)<NJ-VIRTBERL, NJ-VIRTVOOR>
+ 900 Route 168/Suite A-6
  Blackwood, NJ 08012   (856)232-6500   Fax (856)232-0022

Jain, Subhash, MD {1770559882} PainMd, Anesth(70,INA9B)
+ 79 East Madison Avenue
  Dumont, NJ 07628   (201)501-0079   Fax (201)501-8380
  admin@nycpain.com

Jain, Suman Singhal, MD {1114027109} Pedtrc(82,INA54)<NJ-COMMED>
+ Lakewood Pediatric Associates
  101 Prospect Street/Suite 112   Lakewood, NJ 08701
  (732)363-1424   Fax (732)370-0714
+ Lakewood Pediatric Associates
  US Highway 9 North   Lanoka Harbor, NJ 08734   (732)363-1424   Fax (609)693-3548
+ Lakewood Pediatric Associates
  500 Route 9/3B   Lanoka Harbor, NJ 08701   (609)693-8131

Jain, Vikalp, MD {1073747705} SrgVas
+ Jersey Coast Vascular Associates
  425 Jack Martin Boulevard/Suite 2   Brick, NJ 08724
  (732)202-1500

Jain, Vishal K., MD {1710185467} IntrMd
+ Coastal Gastroenterology Associates PA
  525 Jack Martin Boulevard/Suite 301   Brick, NJ 08724
  (732)840-0067   Fax (732)840-3169

Jain Bhalodia, Sapna, DO {1508892845} FamMed(97,NJ75)<NJ-VIRTMHBC, NJ-KMHSTRAT>
+ Alliance for Better Care, PC/Mount Holly Division
  1613 Route 38   Lumberton, NJ 08048   (609)261-3716
  Fax (609)261-5507
+ Alliance for Better Care, P.C.
  PO Box 1510   Medford, NJ 08055   (609)261-3716   Fax (609)953-8652

Jain Lakhani, Neelu, MD {1568407302} RadNro, MRIImag, RadDia(92,NY46)<NJ-OCEANMC>
+ Atlantic Medical Imaging
  455 Jack Martin Boulevard   Brick, NJ 08724   (732)223-9729
  Fax (732)840-6459

Jaiswal, Paresh, MD {1376510891} Pedtrc(00,NF01)<NJ-VIRTVOOR, NJ-VIRTMHBC>
+ CHOP Care Network at Virtua
  101 Carnie Boulevard   Voorhees, NJ 08043   (856)325-3831
  Fax (856)325-3750

Jaiyebo, Omotola Olubunmi, MD {1912077421} IntrMd(89,NIG01)
+ PO Box 90
  Paramus, NJ 07653

Jaiyeola, Patti Jo, MD {1699041343} Pedtrc
+ Nemours Dupont Pediatrics
  2950 College Drive/Suite 2b   Vineland, NJ 08360
  (856)309-8508   Fax (856)309-2714

Jaker, Michael A., MD {1609968445} EmrgMd, IntrMd(72,MA07)<NJ-UMDNJ>
+ University Hospital
  150 Bergen Street/EmrgMed   Newark, NJ 07103   (973)972-7846   Fax (973)972-2384

Jalali, Shailen, MD {1427021351} PainInvt, Anesth(85,PA02)<PA-LNKNAU>
+ South Jersey Spine and Pain Physicians, LLC
  310 Egg Harbor Road/Suite B-3   Sewell, NJ 08080
  (856)589-4500   Fax (856)589-5380

Jalan, Suman L., MD {1982661971} Psychy(71,INA7B)<NJ-STCLRBOO>
+ St. Clare's Hospital-Boonton
  130 Powerville Road/Psychiatry   Boonton, NJ 07005
  (973)316-1800
  Slbpj17@aol.com

Jalandoon, Cynthia Tabligan, MD {1780617415} Psychy(87,PHI31)<NJ-RAMAPO>
+ Christian Health Care Counseling Center
  301 Sicomac Avenue/AttendingPhys   Wyckoff, NJ 07481
  (201)848-5809   Fax (201)848-5547

Jaleel, Syed, MD {1386034007} IntHos
+ AtlantiCare Hospitalist Program
  1925 Pacific Avenue/8th Floor   Atlantic City, NJ 08401
  (609)345-4000

Jalil, Kiran, MD {1639132400} Pedtrc(89,PAK11)
+ Bound Brook Pediatrics
  27 West Union Avenue   Bound Brook, NJ 08805   (732)356-3737   Fax (732)356-6934
+ 20 Pinecone Avenue
  Bridgewater, NJ 08807   (732)356-3737   Fax (908)725-5025

Jalil, Sheema, MD {1336399963} Pedtrc(97,PAK01)<NJ-STFRNMED>
+ St. Francis Medical Center
  601 Hamilton Avenue/Medicine   Trenton, NJ 08629
  (609)599-5000

Jallad, Maisa Z., MD {1861789752}
+ 45 Kennedy Drive
  Lodi, NJ 07644

Jamal, Sameer Mustafa, MD {1245455799} IntrMd(05,VA04)<NJ-HACKNSK>
+ Electrophysiology Associates
  20 Prospect Avenue/Suite 701   Hackensack, NJ 07601
  (201)996-2997   Fax (201)996-2571

Jamdar, Niteen Subhash, MD {1407846173} IntrMd, Grtrcs(00,GRN01)<NJ-HCKTSTWN, NJ-STCLRDEN>
+ Drs. Lewis & Jamdar
  346 South Avenue   Fanwood, NJ 07023   (908)889-4700
  Fax (908)889-0867

James, David Joel, MD {1205093846} IntrMd<NY-SLOANKET>
+ Advanced Cardiology, LLC.
  65 Ridgedale Avenue   Cedar Knolls, NJ 07927   (973)401-1100   Fax (973)401-1201
+ Advanced Cardiology, LLC.
  117 Seber Road/Suite 1-B   Hackettstown, NJ 07840
  (973)401-1100   Fax (908)979-1493

James, Kevin V., MD {1700811353} Surgry, SrgVas(89,PA01)<NJ-NWTNMEM>
+ Advanced Vascular Associates, PC
  131 Madison Avenue/2nd Floor   Morristown, NJ 07960
  (973)755-9206   Fax (973)540-9717

James, Todd C., MD {1306989223} Grtrcs
+ Drs. James and Kovaleva
  125 Chubb Avenue/Suite 100-S   Lyndhurst, NJ 07071
  (201)559-7600

Jamieson, Janine, DO {1770610818} SrgOrt, NeuMSptM(85,NJ75)<NJ-JFKMED>
+ Edison Orthopedic Institute
  3 Progress Street/Suite 106   Edison, NJ 08820   (908)834-8343   Fax (908)834-8347

Jamil, Erum, MD {1124124706} Pedtrc(94,PAK08)
+ Holly City Pediatrics
  10 East Main Street/Suite A   Millville, NJ 08332   (856)825-5932   Fax (856)825-4819

Jamil, Zafar, MD {1932276755} SrgVas, Surgry(71,PAKI)
+ General Vascular Surgical Associates
  306 Martin Luther King Blvd   Newark, NJ 07102   (973)877-5059   Fax (973)877-2954

Jampol, Francis Michael, MD {1871551812} Allrgy, Otlryg, OtgyFPIS(78,MEXI)<NJ-HCKTSTWN>
+ ENT & Allergy Associates of Parsippany
  900 Lanidex Plaza/Suite 300   Parsippany, NJ 07054
  (973)394-1818   Fax (973)394-1810
+ ENT & Allergy Associates, LLP
  3219 Route 46 East/Suite 203   Parsippany, NJ 07054
  (973)394-1818   Fax (973)394-1810

Jan, Louis C. W., MD {1831152966} IntrMd, Nephro(95,PA02)<NJ-ENGLWOOD, NJ-HACKNSK>
+ Drs. Abramovici, Jan & Zelkowitz
  140 Grand Avenue/Suite B   Englewood, NJ 07631
  (201)567-5787   Fax (201)567-7652
  louisjan@mac.com

Jan, Naveed A., MD {1285743542} Hemato, IntrMd, OncHem(90,PAK11)<NJ-MORRISTN>
+ Oncology & Hematology Specialists, PA
  23 Pocono Road/Suite 100   Denville, NJ 07834   (973)316-1701   Fax (973)316-1708
+ Oncology & Hematology Specialists, PA
  100 Madison Avenue/Suite C3402   Morristown, NJ 07960
  (973)316-1701   Fax (973)267-2550

Jan, Thomas, MD {1093071466} Anesth
+ Robert Wood Johnson-UMDNJ Anesthesia Group
  125 Paterson Street/CAB 3100   New Brunswick, NJ 08901
  (347)770-0003   Fax (732)235-6131

Jana, Kumar P., MD {1649249459} IntrMd(77,INA04)<NJ-VIRTMHBC>
+ Cardio Medical Group
  98 James Street/Suite 313   Edison, NJ 08820   (732)635-1100   Fax (732)635-0918
+ Cardio Medical Group
  5 Mountain Boulevard/Suite 2   Warren, NJ 07059
  (732)635-1100   Fax (908)769-8182

Janakiraman, Arun, MD {1891116729}
+ Cooper University Internal Medicine Group
  651 John F. Kennedy Way   Willingboro, NJ 08046
  (609)835-2838   Fax (609)877-5421

Janardhan, Yellagonda V., MD {1912900556} Anesth(70,INA37)<NJ-STCLRDEN>
+ Morris Anesthesia Group, PA
  3799 Route 46/Suite 211   Parsippany, NJ 07054   (973)335-1122   Fax (973)335-1448

Janeczek, Susan, DO {1235209982} ObsGyn, MtFtMd, IntrMd(95,NJ75)
+ Rowan SOM Department of Ob/Gyn
  405 Hurffville-Cross Keys Road   Sewell, NJ 08080
  (856)589-1414   Fax (856)256-5772

Physicians by Name and Address

Janes, Laura C., DO {1952494940} FamMed(96,MO78)<NJ-SHOREMEM>
+ Point Medical
750 Shore Road   Somers Point, NJ 08244   (609)653-2101   Fax (609)653-2247

Janes, Susan F., DO {1205847514} EmrgMd, Psychy(92,MO79)<NJ-COMMED>
+ Community Medical Center
99 Route 37 West/EmrgMd   Toms River, NJ 08755   (732)557-8000

Jang, Thomas Lee, MD {1699927566} Urolgy, Surgry, IntrMd(00,IL06)
+ Rutgers Cancer Institute of New Jersey
195 Little Albany Street/PO Box 2681   New Brunswick, NJ 08903   (732)235-2043   Fax (732)235-6596

Jani, Beena Harendra, MD {1255499109} FamMed(00,NJ05)
+ Summit Medical Group
85 Woodland Road   Short Hills, NJ 07078   (973)379-4496   Fax (973)921-0669

Jani, Chandrashekhar C., MD {1750422499} EmrgMd, OccpMd(67,INA65)
+ PromptMD Urgent Care Center
309 First Street   Hoboken, NJ 07030   (201)222-8411   Fax (201)222-8711

Jani, Samir Ranjit, MD {1184912826} AnesPain
+ Manchester Surgery Center
1100 Route 70   Whiting, NJ 08759   (732)716-8116   Fax (732)849-1511
+ Prima Pain Relief
300-A Princeton Highstown Road   East Windsor, NJ 08520   (732)716-8116   Fax (609)371-9109

Janik, Nancy E., MD {1548249949} FamMed
+ Partners in Primary Care
19 West Main Street   Maple Shade, NJ 08052   (856)779-7386   Fax (856)779-7563

Janjua, Tanveer Ahmed, MD {1285623132} Otlryg, SrgFPl, OtgyFPlS(91,PAK14)
+ 2345 Lamington Road/Suite 108
Bedminster, NJ 07921   (908)470-2600   Fax (908)470-1660

Jankowski, Marcin Andrew, DO {1538489687} Surgry
+ 60 Upland Way
Haddonfield, NJ 08033   (610)447-6238

Janniger, Camila K., MD {1659499010} Dermat(84,POL03)
+ 42 Locust Avenue
Wallington, NJ 07057   (973)472-5044   Fax (973)472-4235
camila.janniger@mental-health-centers.healthguru.c

Jannone, Joel P., MD {1811911225} IntrMd(78,IL43)<NY-CMNTYMEM>
+ 801 Lacey Road
Forked River, NJ 08731   (609)242-0040   Fax (609)242-1019

Janoff, Larry Stewart, DO {1245200864} Nrolgy(73,IA75)<NJ-KMHCHRRY, NJ-KMHSTRAT>
+ LMA Neurology Consultants
63 Kresson Road/Suite 101   Cherry Hill, NJ 08034   (856)218-1770   Fax (856)795-3625
+ LMA Neurology Consultants
570 Egg Harbor Road/Suite B-3   Sewell, NJ 08080   (856)218-1770   Fax (856)795-3625

Janora, Deanna Marie, MD {1427064823} PhysMd(91,PA13)<NJ-KMHSTRAT>
+ University Pain Care Center
42 East Laurel Road/Suite 1700   Stratford, NJ 08084   (856)566-7010   Fax (856)566-6956

Janosky, Maxwell, MD {1972739308} OncHem, IntrMd(07,CA12)<NJ-ENGLWOOD>
+ Forte Schleider & Attas MD PA
350 Engle Street/Berrie Building/1 FL   Englewood, NJ 07631   (201)568-5250   Fax (201)568-5358

Janow, Ginger Lee, MD {1609109818}<NJ-HACKNSK>
+ Hackensack University Medical Center
30 Prospect Avenue   Hackensack, NJ 07601   (551)996-5306

Janowski, Kenneth J., DO {1629017017} IntrMd(92,NJ75)<NJ-HCKTSTWN>
+ Hackettstown Regional Medical Center
651 Willow Grove Street   Hackettstown, NJ 07840   (908)852-5100   kjanowsk@hch.org
+ Hackettstown Medical Group
Hastings Sq Plaza/Building 5   Hackettstown, NJ 07840   (908)852-5100   Fax (908)979-0044

Jansons, Uldis J., MD {1255312054} IntrMd(74,NE05)<NJ-HCKTSTWN>
+ 115 Church Street
Hackettstown, NJ 07840   (908)850-0150   Fax (908)850-9061

Janvier, Yvette Marie, MD {1952377509} Pedtrc, OthrSp, PedDvl(84,POL03)<NJ-CHLSOCEN, NJ-CENTRAST>
+ Children's Specialized Hospital-Ocean
94 Stevens Road   Toms River, NJ 08755   (732)914-1100
+ CentraState Medical Center
901 West Main Street/Pediatrics   Freehold, NJ 07728   (732)431-2000

Japa-Camilo, Judelka, MD {1659418978} Pedtrc(89,DOM01)
+ Passaic Pediatrics PA
298 Passaic Street   Passaic, NJ 07055   (973)249-8100   Fax (973)249-8110
+ Passaic Pediatrics PA
200 Gregory Street/2nd Floor   Passaic, NJ 07055   (973)249-8100   Fax (973)249-8110

Jaques, James Phillip, DO {1558351767} FamMed(86,MO79)<NJ-WARREN>
+ Warren Hills Family Health Center
315 Route 31 South   Washington, NJ 07882   (908)689-0777   Fax (908)835-3037   d2502787@aol.com

Jarahian, George, Jr., MD {1154394310} IntrMd(78,MEXI)<NJ-OCEANMC>
+ Shore Medical Center
1640 Highway 88/Suite 203   Brick, NJ 08724   (732)458-7777   Fax (732)263-9470

Jaramillo, Luis Fernando, MD {1952361784} FamMed(86,COL03)
+ Hudson Medical & Mental Health Integrated Service
301 60th Street   West New York, NJ 07093   (201)295-3033

Jaramillo, Marina A., MD {1548235195} PthACl(88,CHI02)<NJ-MORRISTN>
+ Morristown Medical Center
100 Madison Avenue/Path   Morristown, NJ 07962   (973)971-5000

Jardim, Carla Mia, MD {1184698169} FamMed(88,NJ05)<NJ-HUNTRDN>
+ Delaware Valley Family Health Center
200 Frenchtown Road   Milford, NJ 08848   (908)995-2251   Fax (908)995-2036

Jardosh, Kunal Rashmin, MD {1588906879} Anesth
+ Hackensack University MC-Anesthesia Dept
30 Prospect Avenue/Room 2703   Hackensack, NJ 07601   (551)996-2000   Fax (201)996-3962

Jarecki, Jennifer A., DO {1639266638} EmrgMd(95,NJ75)<NJ-COOPRUMC>
+ Cooper University Hospital
One Cooper Plaza/EmergMed   Camden, NJ 08103   (856)342-2000

Jarillo, Maria Roca Cami, MD {1679968028} PhysMd
+ Linwood Care Center
201 New Road   Linwood, NJ 08221   (609)927-6131

Jariwala, Nilesh R., MD {1073572848} Pedtrc(82,INDI)<NJ-STJOSHOS, NJ-CHILTON>
+ Preakness Pediatrics Associates
150 Hinchman Avenue/Suite 4   Wayne, NJ 07470   (973)595-6996   Fax (973)595-6706

Jariwala, Punit Rajnikant, MD {1386060507} IntrMd
+ West Park Medical, LLC.
100 Highway 36/Suite 2-K   West Long Branch, NJ 07764   (732)531-6600   Fax (732)660-6606

Jarmain, Scott Joseph, MD {1225017460} PhysMd(97,MNT01)
+ Coastal Spine
4000 Church Road   Mount Laurel, NJ 08054   (856)222-4444   Fax (856)222-0049

Jarmon, Nicholas Albert, MD {1265696389} SrgOrt
+ Orthopaedic Institute of Central Jersey
2315A Highway 34/Suite D   Manasquan, NJ 08736   (732)974-0404   Fax (732)449-4271
+ Orthopaedic Institute of Central Jersey
1100 Route 72 West/Suite 203   Manahawkin, NJ 08050   (732)974-0404   Fax (609)489-4085

Jaroslow, Amy E., MD {1568557064} Pedtrc(82,PA07)<NJ-RWJUBRUN, NJ-STPETER>
+ Mid Jersey Pediatrics
33 Brunswick Woods Drive   East Brunswick, NJ 08816   (732)257-4330   Fax (732)257-1177
+ Mid Jersey Pediatrics
25 Kilmer Drive/Building 3/Suite 107   Morganville, NJ 07751   (732)257-4330   Fax (732)972-1677

Jarrett, Vincent A., DO {1447200407} RadDia(94,PA77)<NJ-COOPRUMC>
+ Cooper University Hospital
One Cooper Plaza/Radiology   Camden, NJ 08103   (856)342-2000

Jarvis, Lori J., MD {1366525198} FamMed(93,CT02)
+ Mosaic Health
136 Franklin Corner Road   Lawrenceville, NJ 08648   (609)482-3701   Fax (609)482-3702

Jasani, Anita, MD {1912012519} FamMed(95,INA9B)<NJ-JFKMED>
+ PrimeCare Medical Group
561 Middlesex Avenue   Metuchen, NJ 08840   (732)549-9363   Fax (732)603-0397

Jasani, Sona, MD {1437412186} ObsGyn
+ University Medical Group/OBGYN
125 Paterson Street/2nd Floor   New Brunswick, NJ 08901   (732)235-6623   Fax (732)235-7349

Jasey, Neil N., Jr., MD {1659538551} PhysMd(03,NJ05)
+ 45 Marquette Road
Montclair, NJ 07043

Jaskolski, Joseph A., MD {1295723807} FamMed(95,WI05)<NJ-HUNTRDN>
+ Hickory Run Family Practice Associates
384 County Road 513   Califon, NJ 07830   (908)832-2125   Fax (908)832-6149

Jasmin, Diane, DO {1922441377}
+ 300 Avalon Drive/Apt 3261
Wood Ridge, NJ 07075   (732)470-3506   emerald203@msn.com

Jasper, Gabriele P., MD {1669543443} Anesth, AnesPain(87,ITA01)<NJ-COMMED>
+ Center for Pain Control
74 Brick Boulevard/Building 3   Brick, NJ 08723   (732)262-0700   Fax (732)262-0400
+ Center for Pain Control
440 South Main Street   Milltown, NJ 08850   (732)967-0050

Jasper, Josephine V., MD {1962571752} EnDbMt, IntrMd(85,ITA01)
+ 829 Allwood Road
Clifton, NJ 07012   (973)777-0900   Fax (973)777-4463

Jasper, Theodore F., MD {1528171972} Psychy(89,ITA01)<NJ-HACKNSK>
+ 1010 Clifton Avenue
Clifton, NJ 07013   (973)472-8550   Fax (973)472-8580

Jass, Daniel K., MD {1184715542} FamMed, GPrvMd(83,NJ05)<NJ-CHSFULD, NJ-UNVMCPRN>
+ 1330 Parkway Avenue/Suite 5
Ewing, NJ 08628   (609)538-1212

Jassal, Peter, MD {1548495252} Anesth(06,DMN01)<NJ-SJHREGMC>
+ SJH-Pinnacle Mid-Atlantice Anesthesia Associates
1505 West Sherman Avenue/Box 51   Vineland, NJ 08360   (856)641-8000   Fax (856)641-7668
+ SJH Regional Medical Center
1505 West Sherman Avenue/Anesthesia   Vineland, NJ 08360   (856)641-8000

Jasutkar, Ashwini, MD {1245472836} Pedtrc
+ Hunterdon Pediatric Associates
6 Sand Hill Road/Suite 202   Flemington, NJ 08822   (908)782-6700   Fax (908)788-5861

Jathavedam, Ashwin, MD {1609862747} IntrMd, InfDis(02,NY19)
+ Leonia Medical Associates, P.A.
25 Rockwood Place/Suite 120   Englewood, NJ 07631   (201)568-3335   Fax (201)568-2450

Javaiya, Hemangkumar, MD {1952604464} IntrMd
+ Lisa A. Rink Family Medicine, LLC.
217 White Horse Pike   Haddon Heights, NJ 08035   (856)672-1115   Fax (856)672-9111

Javed, Arshad, MD {1932202868} SlpDis, PulDis, IntrMd(67,PAK10)<NJ-CHILTON, NJ-HACKNSK>
+ Pulmonary Associates of Morris County, P.A.
282 Route 46/PO Box 911   Denville, NJ 07834   (973)625-0888   Fax (973)625-3142

Javed, Mohammad Tariq, MD {1699750158} SrgCdv, IntrMd(85,PAK15)<NJ-NWRKBETH>
+ Cardiovascular Associates of NJ P.A.
1931 Oak Tree Road/Suite 202   Edison, NJ 08820   (732)373-7633   Fax (732)372-7634
+ Cardiovascular Associates of NJ, P.A.
377 Jersey Avenue/Suite 410   Jersey City, NJ 07302   (732)373-7633   Fax (201)200-0319

Javed, Omair, MD {1043578974} CdvDis
+ The Cooper Hospital System-Univ Hospital
401 Haddon Avenue/Room 369   Camden, NJ 08103   (856)757-7848

Javia, Subhashchandra Jethalal, MD {1730148321} Psychy(78,INDI)<NJ-WARREN, PA-EASTON>
+ Subhash Javia, MD PC
300 Coventry Drive   Phillipsburg, NJ 08865   (908)454-7726   Fax (908)213-0560

Javidian, Parisa, MD {1366503377} Pthlgy, PthACl(89,DC01)<NJ-RWJUBRUN>
+ RWJ University Hospital New Brunswick
One Robert Wood Johnson Place   New Brunswick, NJ 08901   (732)828-3000

Jawaharani, Shobha, MD {1376583773} Pedtrc(93,INA65)<NJ-JFKMED, NJ-HACKNSK>
+ Riverside Medical Group
714 Tenth Street/Suite 2   Secaucus, NJ 07094   (201)863-3346   Fax (201)865-0015

Jawaid, Nosheen, DO {1912311408} IntrMd
+ SOM - Department of Internal Medicine
42 East Laurel Road/Suite 3100   Stratford, NJ 08084   (856)566-2753   Fax (856)566-6906

Jawed, Aram Elahi, MD {1356654206} SrgLap, SrgBrtc<NJ-JFKMED>
+ JFK for Life
  98 James Street/Suite 212   Edison, NJ 08820   (732)343-7484
+ Advanced Laparoscopic Surgeons of Morris
  83 Hanover Road/Suite 190   Florham Park, NJ 07932   (732)343-7484   Fax (973)410-9703

Jawetz, Harold I., MD {1972543585} IntrMd, PulDis(71,NY46)
+ Summit Medical Group
  6 Brighton Road/2 FL   Clifton, NJ 07012   (973)777-7911   Fax (973)777-5403

Jawetz, Robert Evan, MD {1326004847} Pedtrc(99,NY01)<NJ-ENGLWOOD, NJ-HACKNSK>
+ Tenafly Pediatrics, PA
  1135 Broad Street/Suite 208   Clifton, NJ 07013   (973)471-8600   Fax (973)471-3068
+ Tenafly Pediatrics, PA
  32 Franklin Street   Tenafly, NJ 07670   (973)471-8600   Fax (201)569-6081

Jawetz, Seth Gerald, MD {1104010131} CdvDis, CarEch, CarNuc(03,NY01)<NJ-HACKNSK, NJ-STJOSHOS>
+ Summit Medical Group
  6 Brighton Road/2 FL   Clifton, NJ 07012   (973)473-2597   Fax (973)473-5958

Jawetz, Sheryl Andrea, MD {1265497267} Pedtrc, IntrMd(99,NY01)<NJ-ENGLWOOD, NJ-HACKNSK>
+ Tenafly Pediatrics, PA
  32 Franklin Street   Tenafly, NJ 07670   (201)569-2400   Fax (201)569-6081

Jaworski, Alison, MD {1861810152} EmrgMd
+ Cooper Univerisry Emergency Physicians
  One Cooper Plaza   Camden, NJ 08103   (856)342-3278   Fax (856)968-8272

Jaworski, Joseph Mark, MD {1366761298} PthAcl
+ RWJ University Hospital New Brunswick
  One Robert Wood Johnson Place   New Brunswick, NJ 08901   (732)235-7816

Jayakumar, Lalithapriya, MD {1891020640} Surgry
+ UMDNJ RWJ Surgery
  125 Paterson Street/CAB 4th FL 4100   New Brunswick, NJ 08901   (732)235-7674   Fax (732)235-7079

Jayakumaran, Jenani Sarah, MD {1790289775} ObsGyn<NJ-RWJUBRUN>
+ RWJ University Hospital New Brunswick
  One Robert Wood Johnson Place   New Brunswick, NJ 08901   (732)828-3000

Jayanathan, Chelvakumaran R., MD {1588692701} IntrMd, EmrgMd(83,SRIL)<NJ-COMMED>
+ Community Medical Center
  99 Route 37 West/EmergMed   Toms River, NJ 08755   (732)557-8000

Jayanathan, Subendrini G., MD {1356565634} IntrMd, OccpMd(83,SRI01)
+ New Jersey Transit Medical Department
  180 Boyden Avenue   Maplewood, NJ 07040   (973)378-6300

Jayaraj, Kasthuri E., MD {1275578619} PulDis, IntrMd(72,INA2X)<NJ-JFKMED>
+ Neighborhood Health Center Plainfield
  1700-58 Myrtle Avenue   Plainfield, NJ 07060   (908)753-6401   Fax (908)226-6743

Jayasinghe, Swarnathilaka, MD {1437176237} CdvDis, IntrMd(75,SRI02)<NJ-SHOREMEM, NJ-ACMCMAIN>
+ AtlantiCare Physicians
  318 Chris Gaupp Drive/Suite 100   Galloway, NJ 08205   (609)404-9900   Fax (609)404-3653

Jean, Nagaeda, MD {1568755866} ObsGyn(07,DMN01)<NH-MONADNK>
+ Hackensack University Medical Group Montvale
  305 West Grand Avenue   Montvale, NJ 07645   (201)746-9150   Fax (201)746-9151
+ Hackensack University Medical Group Westwood
  250 Old Hook Road   Westwood, NJ 07675   (201)746-9150   Fax (201)781-1753

Jean Philippe, Carolyne, MD {1912134404} EmrgMd<NJ-JFKMED>
+ JFK Medical Center
  65 James Street/EmrgMed   Edison, NJ 08820   (732)321-7601

Jeanlouie, Odler R., MD {1881655686} Nephro(84,HAIT)<NJ-EASTORNG>
+ 60 Northfield Avenue
  West Orange, NJ 07052   (973)731-1919   Fax (973)731-0408

Jeanty, Moise, MD {1851883573} PhysMd
+ 1430 West Sherman Avenue
  Vineland, NJ 08360   (856)641-7875

Jedlinski, Barbara, MD {1679525224} Pedtrc(85,POLA)<NJ-VALLEY>
+ The Valley Hospital
  223 North Van Dien Avenue/Pediatrics   Ridgewood, NJ 07450   (201)447-8000   Fax (201)447-8491

Jedlinski, Tadeusz, MD {1033151469} Pedtrc, AdolMd(81,POL10)<NJ-CHILTON>
+ 50 Mount Prospect Avenue/Suite 202
  Clifton, NJ 07013   (973)458-0407   Fax (973)458-0889
  Jedlinskimd@hotmail.com

Jedlinski, Zbigniew J., MD {1538209283} Pedtrc(74,POLA)<NJ-CHRIST, NJ-HACKNSK>
+ Riverside Medical Group
  714 Tenth Street/Suite 2   Secaucus, NJ 07094   (201)863-3346   Fax (201)865-0015

Jedynak, Andrzej R., MD {1891959466} RadDia(04,NJ05)<NJ-UMDNJ>
+ University Hospital
  150 Bergen Street/Radiology   Newark, NJ 07103   (973)972-4300

Jee, Jimmy Hoon, MD {1396807905} Ophthl(97,NJ05)
+ 401A South Van Brunt Street/Suite 200
  Englewood, NJ 07631   (201)541-6806   Fax (201)541-6807

Jeereddy, Bhavani, MD {1689833485} IntrMd<NJ-OVERLOOK>
+ 391 Springfield Avenue
  Berkeley Heights, NJ 07922
+ Overlook Medical Center
  99 Beauvoir Avenue/PO Box 210   Summit, NJ 07902   (908)522-2000

Jeffries, Emily L., MD {1093704934} IntrMd(91,NY08)<NJ-OVERLOOK>
+ Summit Internal Medicine, LLC
  33 Overlook Road/Suite LO6   Summit, NJ 07901   (908)522-0050   Fax (908)522-6575

Jeganathan, Narayanan, MD {1558452946} CdvDis, IntrMd(73,SRI01)
+ Brunswick Cardiology Associates
  1140 Somerset Street   New Brunswick, NJ 08901   (732)246-4699   Fax (732)246-4889

Jehangir, Waqas, MD {1659752541} IntrMd
+ 61 Evergreen Avenue
  Blackwood, NJ 08012   (267)844-7119

Jenci, Joseph D., MD {1508821448} ObsGyn(73,MD01)<NJ-STPETER>
+ St. Peter's University Hospital
  254 Easton Avenue/ObGyn/4th Floor   New Brunswick, NJ 08901   (732)745-8600   Fax (732)828-8929
+ Cares Surgicenter, LLC.
  240 Easton Avenue   New Brunswick, NJ 08901   (732)745-8600   Fax (732)296-8677

Jendrek, Paul, MD {1356328082} PhysMd(84,NJ05)
+ Physical Medicine & Rehabilitation Center
  500 Grand Avenue/1st Floor   Englewood, NJ 07631   (201)567-2277   Fax (201)567-7506
+ Regent Care Center
  50 Polifly Road   Hackensack, NJ 07601   (201)567-2277   Fax (201)487-3835

Jeney, Heather A., MD {1982867800} Pedtrc, Acpntr(05,NJ05)<NJ-MORRISTN, NJ-JFKMED>
+ Whole Child Center
  690 Kinderkamack Road/Suite 102   Oradell, NJ 07649   (201)634-1600   Fax (201)634-1606

Jenkins, Angela Virginia, MD {1508919549} SrgOrt
+ 300 Creek Crossing Boulevard/Suite 307
  Hainesport, NJ 08036   (609)267-2333   Fax (609)267-2533

Jenkins, David W., MD {1609817170} FamMed, FamMAdlt(66,PA02)
+ 22 Crestmont Avenue
  Trenton, NJ 08618   (609)882-6610   Fax (609)882-3470

Jenkins, Lauren Anne, MD {1467764464} ObsGyn
+ Cherry Hill Ob/Gyn
  150 Century Parkway/Suite A   Mount Laurel, NJ 08054   (856)778-4700   Fax (856)778-1572
+ Cherry Hill Ob/Gyn
  777 South White Horse Pike/Suite A-1   Hammonton, NJ 08037   (856)778-4700   Fax (609)561-6309

Jenkins, Lisa Michelle, MD {1265468243} Pedtrc(96,DC03)
+ NHCAC Health Center at Jersey City
  324 Palisade Avenue   Jersey City, NJ 07306   (201)459-8888   Fax (201)459-8872

Jenkins, Paul B., MD {1831154129} Anesth(86,NJ06)<NJ-STPETER>
+ Anesthesia Consultnts of NJ/Nova Pain
  285 Davidson Avenue/Suite 204   Somerset, NJ 08873   (732)271-1400   Fax (732)271-3543
+ Cares Surgicenter, LLC.
  240 Easton Avenue   New Brunswick, NJ 08901   (732)271-1400   Fax (732)296-8677

Jenkins, Reginald Alexander, MD {1306869409} ObsGyn(74,NJ05)<NJ-EASTORNG>
+ Reginald Alexander Jenkins MD PA
  393 Bloomfield Avenue   Montclair, NJ 07042   (973)746-8181   Fax (973)746-0955

Jennings, Anthony S., MD {1962490243} EnDbMt, IntrMd(70,GA05)
+ 27 Covered Bridge Road   Cherry Hill, NJ 08034   (856)428-6728   Fax (856)429-1926

Jennings, Gloria Ann, MD {1770506602} Pedtrc, AdolMd(84,MI01)<NY-HELNHAYS, NJ-UNVMCPRN>
+ University Pediatric Associates
  D-1 Brier Hill Court   East Brunswick, NJ 08816   (732)238-3310

Jennis, Andrew A., MD {1720049398} IntrMd, OncHem(85,NY01)<NJ-HACKNSK, NJ-HOLYNAME>
+ John Theurer Cancer Center - HUMC
  92 Second Street   Hackensack, NJ 07601   (201)996-5863   Fax (551)996-0580

Jennison, Elizabeth A., MD {1922217272} OccpMd
+ Honeywell Inc.
  115 Tabor Road   Morris Plains, NJ 07950   (973)455-3306   Fax (973)455-4416

Jensen, Edwin A., DO {1306025549} GenPrc(70,PA77)
+ 1736 Lark Lane
  Cherry Hill, NJ 08003   (856)428-1506

Jensen, Michael Edward, MD {1902048978} Surgry
+ 224 Florence Road
  Harrington Park, NJ 07640   (917)930-0413   Fax (201)621-0115

Jensen, Sharone Lynn, MD {1710994744} EmrgMd(00,VT02)<NJ-OURLADY>
+ Our Lady of Lourdes Medical Center
  1600 Haddon Avenue/EmergMed   Camden, NJ 08103   (856)757-3500   Fax (856)365-7773

Jergens, Paul B., MD {1437152675} Ophthl, IntrMd(76,OH43)<NJ-RIVERVW>
+ Del Negro and Senft Eye Associates, PC
  152 Broad Street   Red Bank, NJ 07701   (732)747-7725   Fax (732)741-7930

Jermyn, Richard T., DO {1992775050} PhysMd(92,PA77)
+ Burlington Medical Center
  640 Beverly Rancocas Road   Willingboro, NJ 08046   (609)835-9555   Fax (609)835-2313
+ University Pain Care Center
  42 East Laurel Road/Suite 1700   Stratford, NJ 08084   (609)835-9555   Fax (856)566-6956

Jeshion, Wendy Cheryl, MD {1851338644} PedGst, Pedtrc(92,NY47)<NJ-HACKNSK>
+ Joseph M. Sanzari Childrens' -Gastro
  155 Polifly Road/Suite 102   Hackensack, NJ 07601   (551)996-8840   Fax (201)441-9949

Jessel, Nele, MD {1982648135} Pedtrc(00,GER15)<NJ-MORRISTN, NJ-OVERLOOK>
+ Bridgewater-Raritan Pediatrics
  475 North Bridge Street/Suite 204   Bridgewater, NJ 08807   (908)526-2100   Fax (908)526-2155

Jethva, Purvi Jitendra, MD {1083669295} NnPnMd, Pedtrc, IntrMd(01,DMN01)
+ On-Site Neonatal Partners
  1000 Haddonfield-Berlin Road/Suite 210   Voorhees, NJ 08043   (856)782-2212   Fax (756)782-2266

Jethwa, Kusum A., MD {1578679544} Pedtrc(67,INA2B)<NJ-TRINIJSC, NJ-STBARNMC>
+ 117 Westfield Avenue
  Elizabeth, NJ 07208   (908)354-1400   Fax (908)354-1400
  Kusumjethwa@hotmail.com

Jethwa, Pinakin R., MD {1427253665} SrgNro(07,NJ05)
+ Center for Neurological Surgery UMDNJ
  90 Bergen Street/DOC 8100   Newark, NJ 07103   (973)972-2323   Fax (973)972-2333

Jethwa, Samir C., DO {1871736108} RadV&I
+ Ocean Medical Center
  425 Jack Martin Boulevard   Brick, NJ 08723   (732)836-4046   Fax (732)836-4047
+ Coastal Imaging, LLC
  79 Route 37 West/Suite 103   Toms River, NJ 08755   (732)836-4046   Fax (732)276-2325

Jetty, Siva Teja, MD {1073977278} IntrMd<NJ-JRSYCITY>
+ Jersey City Medical Center
  355 Grand Street   Jersey City, NJ 07304   (201)915-2431

Jewel, Kenneth L., MD {1386753077} RadDia(68,NY06)
+ Montclair Radiology
  116 Park Street   Montclair, NJ 07042   (973)746-2525   Fax (973)746-5802
+ Montclair Radiology
  1140 Bloomfield Avenue   West Caldwell, NJ 07006   (973)746-2525   Fax (973)439-6885
+ Montclair Radiology
  20 High Street   Nutley, NJ 07042   (973)284-1881   Fax (973)284-0269

Jeyakumar, Anusuya, MD {1447453329} IntrMd, Grtrcs(86,SRI03)
+ Calhoun Medical Center
  1330 Rev S Howard Woodson/Junior Way   Trenton, NJ 08638   (609)396-4222   Fax (609)396-4378

Jeyarajasingam, Aravindan V., MD {1871848663}
+ 357 New Castle Lane
  Swedesboro, NJ 08085   (267)258-3403

Physicians by Name and Address

Jez, Mieczyslaw Z., MD {1689758864} Pedtrc(67,POLA)<NJ-NWRKBETH>
+ 25 West Henry Street
Linden, NJ 07036   (908)925-6290   Fax (908)925-8433

Jhaveri, Bharat J., MD {1356341473} GenPrc, PthACl, PthCyt(71,INDI)<NJ-ACMCITY, NJ-ACMCMAIN>
+ 544 New Jersey Avenue
Absecon, NJ 08201   (609)484-7009   Fax (609)484-7571
bjjhaveri@pol.net

Jhaveri, Lajwanti R., MD {1922078799} Anesth(64,INDI)<NJ-NWRKBETH>
+ Newark Beth Israel Medical Center
201 Lyons Avenue/Anesthesiology   Newark, NJ 07112
(973)926-7000   Fax (201)943-8105

Jhaveri, Mukesh J., MD {1275526709} Nrolgy, Psychy(74,INDI)<NJ-STCLRSUS>
+ 71 Route 23 North/PO Box 87
Hamburg, NJ 07419   (973)209-1110

Jhaveri, Sujata Ketan, MD {1710932918} RadDia(93,INA20)
+ Millburn Medical Imaging
2130 Millburn Avenue/Suite A-8   Maplewood, NJ 07040
(973)912-0404   Fax (973)912-0444
+ Coastal Imaging, LLC
79 Route 37 West/Suite 103   Toms River, NJ 08755
(973)912-0404   Fax (732)276-2325

Jhawer, Minaxi P., MD {1487760930} MedOnc, IntrMd(98,INA5Y)<NJ-ENGLWOOD>
+ Forte Schleider & Attas MD PA
350 Engle Street/Berrie Building/1 FL   Englewood, NJ 07631
(201)568-5250   Fax (201)568-5358

Jhee, Yoon-Bok, MD {1366493058} ObsGyn(67,KORE)
+ Englewood Ob Gyn Women's Group
286 Engle Street   Englewood, NJ 07631   (201)569-6190
Fax (201)569-6940

Ji, Yong, MD {1518963875} IntrMd, OncHem(84,CHN93)<NJ-OURLADY>
+ Regional Cancer Care Associates, LLC
200 Bowman Drive/Suite E-125   Voorhees, NJ 08043
(856)424-3311   Fax (856)424-5634
+ The Center for Cancer & Hematologic Disease
609 North Broad Street/Suite 300   Woodbury, NJ 08096
(856)686-1002
+ The Center for Cancer & Hematologic Disease
856 South White Horse Pike/Suite 4   Hammonton, NJ 08043
(609)561-4444   Fax (609)561-2492

Jiang, Heng, MD {1689674327} Anesth(83,CHN57)<NJ-VIRTBERL, NJ-VIRTMARL>
+ West Jersey Anesthesia Associates
102-E Center Boulevard   Marlton, NJ 08053   (856)988-6250   Fax (856)988-6270

Jiang, Li, MD {1841448974} Pedtrc(85,CHN38)
+ Hills Pediatrics
613 Courtyard Drive   Hillsborough, NJ 08844   (908)240-8285

Jiang, Rongjie, MD {1851527733} Anesth(94,CHN57)<NJ-NWTN-MEM>
+ Newton Medical Center
175 High Street/Anesthesia   Newton, NJ 07860   (973)383-2121

Jiang, Tony T., MD {1205169885} PthACl(84,ITAL)
+ Integrated Paincare Center
27 Mountain Boulevard/Suite 7   Warren, NJ 07059
(908)822-2889
+ Integrated Paincare Center
252 Columbia Turnpike   Florham Park, NJ 07932   (908)822-2889   Fax (973)822-8098
+ Integrated Paincare Center
1999 Route 27   Edison, NJ 07059   (732)287-9988

Jiang, Yihao, MD {1649539248} Anesth
+ 401 Avalon Drive/Unit 4212
Wood Ridge, NJ 07075   (405)414-5286

Jih, Ting-Yu Yu, MD {1588951867}
+ RWJ University Hospital New Brunswick
One Robert Wood Johnson Place   New Brunswick, NJ 08901
(732)357-7158
+ 35 East Elizabeth Avenue/Apt C3
Linden, NJ 07036

Jilani, Mohammad Imran, MD {1962482331} RadNro, Radiol(95,NJ05)<NJ-JFKMED>
+ JFK Medical Center
65 James Street   Edison, NJ 08820   (732)321-7917   Fax (732)767-2968

Jilani, Usman Khan, MD {1053774844} IntrMd
+ Ocean Health Initiatives, Inc.
101 Second Street   Lakewood, NJ 08701   (732)363-6655
Fax (732)363-6236

Jimenez, Arnaldo M., MD {1669533113} IntrMd, Gastrn(91,PRO02)<NJ-TRININPC>
+ 240 Williamson Street/Suite 303
Elizabeth, NJ 07207   (908)282-0500   Fax (908)282-1482

+ 616 Grove Avenue
Edison, NJ 08820   (908)282-0500   Fax (908)282-1482
+ 2401 Morris Avenue
Union, NJ 07207   (908)282-0500   Fax (908)282-1482

Jimenez, Arturo De La Caridad, MD {1164532909} IntrMd(87,CUB06)
+ 86 New Brunswick Avenue
Perth Amboy, NJ 08861   (732)826-1881   Fax (732)826-1108

Jimenez, Jennifer E., MD {1073789905} PedGst
+ Meridian Medical Group - Faculty Practice
61 Davis Avenue/Suite 1   Neptune, NJ 07753   (732)776-4860   Fax (732)776-4867

Jimenez, Joseph C., MD {1437310448} PhysMd(04,NJ06)
+ 816 Meacham Avenue
Linden, NJ 07036

Jimenez, Manuel, MD {1548427420} PedDvl
+ University Hospital-RWJ Medical School
89 French Street/RM 1349   New Brunswick, NJ 08901
(732)235-6188

Jimenez, Martin Zaratan, MD {1043225923} IntrMd(91,PHI01)
+ Alberto Medical Associates PA
25 Mule Road/Unit A-3   Toms River, NJ 08755   (732)240-0404   Fax (732)244-3555

Jimenez-Silva, Jeanette, MD {1982798914} IntrMd(87,MA07)
+ Internal Medicine Associates
201 Laurel Heights Drive/Suite 201   Bridgeton, NJ 08302
(856)455-4800   Fax (856)455-0650

Jimma, Lulu A., MD {1669428793} FamMed(91,ETH01)<NJ-RBAYPERT>
+ Capital Health Primary Care-Bordentown
1 Third Street   Bordentown, NJ 08505   (609)298-2005
Fax (609)324-8267
+ Jewish Renaissance Medical Center
275 Hobart Street   Perth Amboy, NJ 08861   (609)298-2005
Fax (732)376-0139

Jin, Jie, MD {1225006117} Anesth(82,CHN69)<NJ-HOLYNAME>
+ Westwood Anesthesia Associates
250 Old Hook Road/2nd Floor   Westwood, NJ 07675
(201)358-3190   Fax (201)358-6622
+ Bergen Anesthesia Associates
718 Teaneck Road   Teaneck, NJ 07666   (201)358-3190
Fax (201)833-6576

Jin, Li, MD {1922121102} PthCln(82,CHN39)
+ Newark Department of Health and Human Services
110 William Street   Newark, NJ 07102   (973)733-5300

Jindal, Jagdish R., MD {1780698068} IntrMd(64,INA1H)
+ 166 Main Street/Suite 1A
Lincoln Park, NJ 07035   (973)694-6260   Fax (973)694-2359

Jines, N. Patricia, MD {1487876306}
+ St Barnabas Medical Center Pediatrics
94 Old Short Hills Road   Livingston, NJ 07039   (973)322-5690   Fax (973)322-5504
+ 528 Greene Lane
Cherry Hill, NJ 08003   (310)415-3567

Jinivizian, Hasmig Barkeve, MD {1336304096} EmrgMd<NJ-MORRISTN>
+ Morristown Medical Center
100 Madison Avenue/Box 8   Morristown, NJ 07962
(973)971-5000

Jitan, Raed Abdalla, MD {1033167986} IntrMd, CdvDis(81,JOR01)
+ 15 McCampbell Road
Holmdel, NJ 07733   (732)946-0995   Fax (732)946-0995

Jiu, Wun-Ye, MD {1104025170} IntrMd(97,NY47)<NY-CMC-STVNY>
+ Am/PM Walk in Urgent Care Center
19 South Washington Avenue   Bergenfield, NJ 07621
(201)387-0177   Fax (201)387-0114

Jivani, Rasik M., MD {1265476576} IntrMd(80,INA2B)
+ 611 Route 539
Cream Ridge, NJ 08514   (609)758-3200

Jiwani, Ameena Javed, DO {1902259393} FamMed
+ University Hospital-University Family Medicine
42 East Laurel Road/Suite 2100   Stratford, NJ 08084
(856)566-6477   Fax (856)566-6188

Jmeian, Ashraf, MD {1023443074} IntrMd<NJ-STJOSHOS>
+ St. Joseph's Regional Medical Center
703 Main Street   Paterson, NJ 07503   (973)754-2000

Jo, Young I., MD {1255498804} IntrMd, PulDis(74,KOR04)<NJ-STMRYPAS>
+ 930 Clifton Avenue
Clifton, NJ 07013   (973)778-2665   Fax (973)778-9753

Jobanputra, Aesha M., MD {1770872004}
+ 125 paterson street/Suite 568
New Brunswick, NJ 08901   (732)235-7840
aeshaj@gmail.com

Jobbagy, Zsolt, MD {1588717474} PthACl(89,HUN08)<NJ-NWRKBETH>
+ Newark Beth Israel Medical Center
201 Lyons Avenue/Path   Newark, NJ 07112   (973)926-8556
Fax (973)705-8301

Jobes, David Richard, MD {1174550065} Anesth(67,PA07)<PA-CHILDHOS>
+ CHOP Pediatric & Adolescent Specialty Care Center
1012 Laurel Oak Road/Anesth   Voorhees, NJ 08043
(856)435-1300   Fax (856)435-0091

Jodorkovsky, Roberto Alex, MD {1457391880} Pedtrc, PedNph(74,CHI06)<NJ-STJOSHOS, NY-BRKLNDWN>
+ St. Joseph's Regional Medical Center
11 Getty Avenue/Pedi Nephro   Paterson, NJ 07503
(973)754-2570
+ St. Joseph's Children's Hospital
703 Main Street/Pedi Nephro   Paterson, NJ 07503
(973)754-2570   Fax (973)754-2628

Joffe, Avrum L., MD {1962656579} SrgOrt(07,NJ05)<NY-SLR-LUKES>
+ North Jersey Pediatric Orthopedics PA
140 Chestnut Street/Suite 201   Ridgewood, NJ 07450
(201)612-9988   Fax (201)445-9050

Joffe, Ian I., MD {1891766622} CdvDis(87,SAF02)<NJ-ACMC-MAIN, NJ-OURLADY>
+ Associated Cardiovascular Consultants, P.A.
1105 Laurel Oak Road/Suite 165   Voorhees, NJ 08043
(856)424-3600   Fax (856)424-7154
+ Associated Cardiovascular Consultants-Lourdes
1 Brace Road/Suite C & F   Cherry Hill, NJ 08034   (856)424-3600   Fax (856)428-5748

Joffe, Libby, MD {1831199645} IntrMd(90,UKR01)
+ Advanced Internal Medicine of NorthJersey
1680 Route 23 North/Suite 310   Wayne, NJ 07470
(973)831-9222   Fax (973)831-1460

Johal, Gurvindra Singh, DO {1871551721} EmrgMd(94,NJ75)
+ Medi Center of Edison
1813 Oak Tree Road   Edison, NJ 08820   (908)769-9494
Fax (908)755-3833

John, Asha, MD {1356679823} IntrMd(03,INA98)<NJ-VALLEY>
+ Prospect Medical Offices, LLC
301 Godwin Avenue   Midland Park, NJ 07432   (201)444-4526   Fax (201)301-1313

John, Eirene George, MD {1639514169} FamMed
+ Radburn Medical Associates
20-20 Fair Lawn Avenue/Suite 104   Fair Lawn, NJ 07410
(201)703-0202   Fax (201)703-1231

John, Elizabeth Sheena, MD {1346794815}
+ 34 Kanouse Lane
Montville, NJ 07045   (973)592-6116

John, Jeanie Elizabeth, MD {1972759199} Pedtrc(05,NJ05)<NJ-HACKNSK, NJ-HOLYNAME>
+ Riverside Medical Group
714 Tenth Street/Suite 2   Secaucus, NJ 07094   (201)863-3346   Fax (201)865-0015
+ Riverside Pediatric Group
1425 Bloomfield Street   Hoboken, NJ 07030   (201)863-3346   Fax (201)876-3218
+ Riverside Pediatric Group
609 Washington Street/Ground Floor   Hoboken, NJ 07094
(201)706-8488   Fax (201)706-8489

John, Miriam, MD {1669425369} EmrgMd(01,NY09)<NJ-NWRK-BETH>
+ Newark Beth Israel Medical Center
201 Lyons Avenue/EmrgMed   Newark, NJ 07112   (973)926-7000   Fax (610)617-6280

John, Sheena J., DO {1275794794} EmrgMd(04,NY75)<NJ-NWRK-BETH>
+ Newark Beth Israel Medical Center
201 Lyons Avenue/Ste D11/EmrgMed   Newark, NJ 07112
(973)926-7000

John, Sheryl Mary, MD {1992963409} Pedtrc, AdolMd
+ University Pediatric Associates PA
317 Cleveland Avenue   Highland Park, NJ 08904   (732)249-8999   Fax (732)249-7827

John, Sunitha Sara, MD {1114971777} IntrMd
+ 3 Gatheringhill Court
Morris Plains, NJ 07950

John, Thomas, Jr., MD {1619248457} IntHos(05,POLA)
+ Hospital Medicine Associates
157 Broad Street/Suite 317   Red Bank, NJ 07701
(732)530-2960   Fax (732)530-7446

John, Thomas Karoor, MD {1104021427} SrgOrt
+ Active Orthopaedics & Sports Medicine
25 Prospect Avenue   Hackensack, NJ 07601   (201)358-0707   Fax (201)343-7410
+ Active Orthopaedics & Sports Medicine
440 Old Hook Road   Emerson, NJ 07630   (201)358-0707
Fax (201)358-9777

Johnsen, Peter Edward, MD {1336361450} Pedtrc, AdolMd(72,NY08)
+ Princeton University
307 Nassau Hall/HealthServices   Princeton, NJ 08544
(609)258-3000
johnsenp@princeton.edu

Physicians by Name and Address

Johnson, Andrew, DO {1386610319} PainInvt, AnesPain(98,NJ75)<NJ-MONMOUTH>
+ Monmouth Medical Center
300 Second Avenue/Anesthesia   Long Branch, NJ 07740
(732)222-5200   Fax (732)923-6977

Johnson, Christina Nicole, MD {1336568419} IntrMd<NJ-OVERLOOK>
+ Overlook Medical Center
99 Beauvoir Avenue/PO Box 210   Summit, NJ 07902
(908)522-2000

Johnson, Christopher D., MD {1841277993} SrgHnd, SrgOrt(83,NJ06)<NJ-JRSYSHMC, NJ-RIVERVW>
+ Professional Orthopaedic Associates
776 Shrewsbury Avenue/Suite 201   Tinton Falls, NJ 07724
(732)530-4949   Fax (732)530-3618
+ Professional Orthopaedic Associates
1430 Hooper Avenue/Suite 101   Toms River, NJ 08753
(732)530-4949   Fax (732)349-7722
+ Professional Orthopaedic Associates
303 West Main Street   Freehold, NJ 07724   (732)530-4949
Fax (732)577-0036

Johnson, Curtis, Jr., MD {1780771030} Pedtrc(79,NJ05)<NJ-STBARNMC>
+ 280 South Harrison Street/Suite 403
East Orange, NJ 07018   (973)678-5698   Fax (973)678-3420

Johnson, David L., MD {1114928652} SrgThr, Surgry(83,MD07)<NJ-MORRISTN, NJ-JRSYSHMC>
+ Mid-Atlantic Surgical Associates
1944 Route 33/Suite 201   Neptune, NJ 07753   (732)776-4622   Fax (732)776-3765
+ Mid-Atlantic Surgical Associates
100 Madison Avenue   Morristown, NJ 07960   (732)776-4622   Fax (732)984-7019

Johnson, Deborah Anne, MD {1851481477} FamMed(00,NJ05)<NJ-SOMERSET>
+ New Jersey Division of Developmental Disability
Route 72 East   New Lisbon, NJ 08064   (609)726-1000   Fax (609)894-8430

Johnson, Deborah J., MD {1194880021} Pedtrc(83,NJ05)<NJ-UMDNJ, NJ-NWRKBETH>
+ University Hospital
150 Bergen Street/ChildrnsHlthCtr   Newark, NJ 07103
(973)972-0543

Johnson, Edward S., MD {1184699290} InfDis, IntrMd(75,ITA01)
+ Drs. Johnson and Beggs
5 Franklin Avenue/Suite 103   Belleville, NJ 07109
(973)751-3399

Johnson, Elizabeth, MD {1982043725}<NJ-HOBUNIMC>
+ Hoboken University Medical Center
308 Willow Avenue   Hoboken, NJ 07030   (201)418-1000

Johnson, Erin Margaret, MD {1093039034}<NJ-MORRISTN>
+ Morristown Medical Center
100 Madison Avenue/PICU 89   Morristown, NJ 07962
(973)971-5324

Johnson, George A., MD {1326145590} Urolgy(77,NJ05)<NJ-EASTORNG, NJ-STBARNMC>
+ Urology Group of NJ
258-264 Central Avenue   Orange, NJ 07050   (973)677-1144
Fax (973)677-9145

Johnson, Judith Ann, MD {1962571620} Anesth(89,NJ06)<NJ-MONMOUTH>
+ Monmouth Medical Center
300 Second Avenue/Anesth   Long Branch, NJ 07740
(732)222-5200

Johnson, Karen Teresa, DO {1508278052} Pedtrc
+ The Cooper Hospital System-Univ Hospital
401 Haddon Avenue   Camden, NJ 08103   (856)757-7904
Fax (856)968-9598

Johnson, Keith Patrick, MD {1487616967} SrgOrt(97,VA01)<MA-BEVNHS>
+ Oasis Medical and Wellness
85 Harristown Road/Suite 103   Glen Rock, NJ 07452   Fax (844)366-8900

Johnson, Mark Raymond, MD {1578670931} IntrMd, Nephro(03,NY19)<NJ-MORRISTN>
+ Morristown Medical Center
100 Madison Avenue/Medicine   Morristown, NJ 07962
(973)971-7165   Fax (973)290-7521

Johnson, Natalie A., MD {1114032059} IntrMd(87,NY06)
+ Drs. Alves & Johnson
470 Prospect Avenue/Suite 200   West Orange, NJ 07052
(973)243-0290   Fax (973)243-1863

Johnson, Paul B., MD {1992062855}
+ Soll Eye PC of New Jersey/Cooper Division
3 Cooper Plaza/Suite 510   Camden, NJ 08103   (856)342-7200   Fax (856)342-6622
johnson.paul.b@gmail.com

Johnson, Robert Lee, MD {1134149230} AdolMd, Pedtrc(72,NJ05)<NJ-UMDNJ, NJ-RWJUBRUN>
+ University Hospital-New Jersey Medical School
30 Bergen Street/ADMC 12 1205   Newark, NJ 07107
(973)972-0037

Johnson, Ryan P., MD {1417007071}
+ Cooper Center for Dermatologic Surgery
10000 Sagemore Drive/Suite 10103   Marlton, NJ 08053
(856)596-3040   Fax (856)596-5651
ryan.p.johnson50.mil@mail.mil

Johnson, Sharon, MD {1750412573} ObsGyn(76,NJ05)<NJ-NWRKBETH>
+ Newark Community Health Center Inc.
982 Broad Street   Newark, NJ 07102   (973)353-0699
+ Newark Community Health Centers Inc.
9 Coit Street   Irvington, NJ 07111   (973)399-6292
+ Irvington Community Health Center
1148-1150 Springfield Avenue   Irvington, NJ 07102
(973)399-6292   Fax (973)372-4534

Johnson, Steven A., DO {1710965702} IntrMd, EmrgMd(97,PA77)<PA-LHVLYCED>
+ Capital Health Medical
2 Capital Way/Suite 356   Pennington, NJ 08534   (609)537-6000   Fax (609)537-6002

Johnson, Steven A., MD {1881665560} Surgry
+ Capital Health Medical
2 Capital Way/Suite 356   Pennington, NJ 08534   (609)537-6000   Fax (609)537-6002

Johnson, Swati, DO {1033435011} Pedtrc(04,NY75)
+ On-Site Neonatal Partners
1000 Haddonfield-Berlin Road/Suite 210   Voorhees, NJ 08043   (856)782-2212   Fax (856)782-2213

Johnson, Terry D., MD {1982663183} NnPnMd, Pedtrc(86,DC01)<NJ-HACKNSK>
+ 30 Prospect Avenue
Hackensack, NJ 07601   (201)996-5305

Johnson, Timothy David, MD {1104129204} IntrMd, EmrgMd(05,NJ03)<NY-LIJEWSH, RI-SJFATIMA>
+ Clara Maass Medical Center
1 Clara Maass Drive   Belleville, NJ 07109   (973)450-2100
Fax (973)450-0383

Johnson, William Gessner, MD {1477628956} Nrolgy, GnetMd(67,NY01)<NJ-UNIVBHC, NJ-RWJUBRUN>
+ University Medical Group/UMDNJ
125 Paterson Street/Suite 2200   New Brunswick, NJ 08901
(732)235-7647   Fax (732)235-7677

Johnson-Sena, Leonie J., MD {1245454842} Psychy, PsyCAd, IntrMd(91,NY20)
+ 2 Highland Avenue
Jersey City, NJ 07306   (201)332-0016   Fax (877)246-9995

Johnson-Villanueva, Norma J., MD {1154335602} EmrgMd(96,PA02)<NJ-HUNTRDN>
+ Hunterdon Medical Center
2100 Wescott Drive   Flemington, NJ 08822   (908)788-6100
Fax (856)616-1919

Johnston, Christopher K., MD {1790760775} FamMed(81,NJ05)
+ Integrated Medicine Alliance, P.A.
30 Shrewsbury Avenue   Shrewsbury, NJ 07702   (732)460-9840   Fax (732)460-9848
+ Integrated Medicine Alliance, PA.
363 Highway 36   Port Monmouth, NJ 07758   (732)460-9840   Fax (732)471-7949

Johnston, William E., MD {1467486142} IntrMd(81,NJ06)
+ 10 Plum Tree Drive
Sewell, NJ 08080

Joki, Jaclyn Beth, MD {1386949576} PhysMd
+ JFK Medical Center
65 James Street   Edison, NJ 08820   (732)321-7070

Jokic, Dragana, MD {1700081163} EnDbMt, IntrMd(00,BOS02)<NJ-RBAYPERT>
+ Raritan Bay Medical Center/Perth Amboy Division
530 New Brunswick Avenue/Endo Diab Mt   Perth Amboy, NJ 08861   (732)442-3700

Jokubaitis, Leonard Anthony, MD {1295164507} IntrMd(81,NJ06)
+ 1125 Trenton Harbourton Road
Titusville, NJ 08560   (609)730-3475   Fax (609)730-2104

Jolitz, Whitney, DO {1407269053} Gyneco
+ University Hospital -SOM University Doctors Surgeons
42 East Laurel Road/Suite 2500-2600   Stratford, NJ 08084
(856)566-2700   Fax (856)566-6873

Jolley, Michael N., MD {1326067232} SrgOrt(73,NJ05)<NJ-UNVMCPRN>
+ Princeton Orthopaedic Associates, P.A.
11 Centre Drive   Jamesburg, NJ 08831   (609)655-4848
+ Princeton Orthopaedic Associates, P.A.
325 Princeton Avenue   Princeton, NJ 08540   (609)655-4848   Fax (609)924-8532

Joneja, Upasana, MD {1902245608} PthAcl
+ Cooper University Hospital Pathology
One Cooper Plaza   Camden, NJ 08103   (800)826-6737

Jones, Angela Marie, MD {1770536047} Anesth(93,IL43)
+ PO Box 874
Elmer, NJ 08318

Jones, Angela Renee, MD {1558357640} ObsGyn(01,OH01)<NJ-COMMED>
+ Woman to Woman Obstetrics & Gynecology
615 Main Street   Toms River, NJ 08753   (732)797-1510

Fax (732)797-2370

Jones, Caitlin Maria, MD {1275686057} EmrgMd(99,NY0)<NJ-CHRIST>
+ Christ Hospital
176 Palisade Avenue   Jersey City, NJ 07306   (201)912-5291
caitlin.jones@carepointhealth.org

Jones, Christopher Warren, MD {1851552426} EmrgMd, IntrMd(08,MI01)<NJ-COOPRUMC>
+ Cooper University Hospital
One Cooper Plaza/Suite 152   Camden, NJ 08103   (856)342-2627   Fax (856)968-8272

Jones, Clifford W., DO {1952435349} Psychy(85,NJ75)<NJ-SJRSYELM, NJ-SJERSYHS>
+ PO Box 2162
Medford, NJ 08055

Jones, Debra Y., MD {1376661306} IntrMd(77,NJ05)
+ 1235 Whitehorse-Mercerville Rd
Hamilton, NJ 08619   (609)581-5124   Fax (609)581-5129

Jones, Eva R., MD {1528168598} ObsGyn(80,MEXI)<NJ-CHSMRCER>
+ Women's Health Choice
2420 Nottingham Way   Mercerville, NJ 08619   (609)586-4474   Fax (609)586-8195

Jones, Frank A., Jr., MD {1790747152} Psychy(72,OH06)
+ 2186 Route 27/Suite 2A
North Brunswick, NJ 08902   (732)422-0800   Fax (732)422-2485
fajonesmd@yahoo.com

Jones, Graham P., MD {1699707364} FamMed, IntrMd(60,PA12)
+ Medford Family Practice
152 Himmelein Road/Suite 100   Medford, NJ 08055
(609)654-7117   Fax (609)654-8555

Jones, Howard D., MD {1326012378} FamMed(69,PA09)<NJ-HUNTRDN>
+ Delaware Valley Family Health Center
200 Frenchtown Road   Milford, NJ 08848   (908)995-2251
Fax (908)995-2036

Jones, Howard Harris, MD {1598914152} ObsGyn(07,GRN01)<NJ-VALLEY>
+ VMG Gynecology Oncology Associates
One Valley Health Plaza   Paramus, NJ 07652   (201)634-5401   Fax (201)986-4701
haljones@gmail.com

Jones, James Brian, MD {1184646614} EmrgMd(94,PA01)
+ 32 Graham Avenue
Metuchen, NJ 08840

Jones, Jane W., MD {1790853851} Psychy(77,NY20)
+ 137 Summit Avenue
Summit, NJ 07901   (908)277-1552

Jones, Kathryn M., MD {1730148545} ObsGyn(96,PA02)<NJ-MORRISTN>
+ Morristown Obstetrics and Gynecology Associates
101 Madison Avenue/Suite 405   Morristown, NJ 07960
(973)267-7272   Fax (973)455-0099

Jones, Kevin Errol, MD {1851365217} Anesth(00,IL06)<NJ-STMRYPAS>
+ St. Mary's Hospital
350 Boulevard/Anesthesia   Passaic, NJ 07055   (973)669-1743   Fax (845)357-5777

Jones, Kimberley L., MD {1841403730} EmrgMd(04,PA02)<NJ-SOCEANCO>
+ Southern Ocean County Medical Center
1140 Route 72 West/EmrgMed   Manahawkin, NJ 08050
(609)597-6011

Jones, Krister J., MD {1952621229} PthAna
+ Capital Emergency Physicians & Associates
One Capital Way   Pennington, NJ 08534   (609)303-4019
Fax (609)537-6251

Jones, Lori Elizabeth, MD {1891990016}
+ 1115 Willow Avenue/Apt 407
Hoboken, NJ 07030

Jones, Marvin M., MD {1689620361} EmrgMd(85,DC03)<NJ-CENTRAST>
+ CentraState Medical Center
901 West Main Street/EmergMed   Freehold, NJ 07728
(732)294-2667

Jones, Michael R., MD {1720002991} Anesth(70,DC01)<NJ-KMHSTRAT>
+ Kennedy Memorial Hospital-University Medical Center
18 East Laurel Road   Stratford, NJ 08084   (856)346-6000

Jones, Rhys E., MD {1457394538} FamMed, IntrMd(95,NJ05)
+ Valley Health Medical Group
780 Cedar Lane   Teaneck, NJ 07666   (201)836-7664   Fax (201)836-5710

Jones, Tamika Lillian, MD {1861560336} Pedtrc, IntrMd(99,PA09)
+ Advocare Woodbury Pediatrics
1050 Mantua Pike/Suite 200   Wenonah, NJ 08090
(856)853-0848   Fax (856)853-1889

Jones Burton, Charlotte Michelle, MD {1205870052} IntrMd, Nephro(99,MD01)
+ 50 Valley Wood Drive
Somerset, NJ 08873

245

Physicians by Name and Address

Jones-Dillon, Shelley A., MD {1174576870}
EmrgMd(01,NY08)<NJ-NWRKBETH>
+ Newark Beth Israel Medical Center
201 Lyons Avenue/EmrgMed   Newark, NJ 07112   (973)926-7000   Fax (610)617-6280

Jones-Hicks, Linda N., DO {1750339453} Pedtrc, AdolMd(79,IA75)<NJ-VIRTUAHS>
+ Genesis Pediatrics Assocoiates LLC
297 Westwood Drive/Suite 101   Woodbury, NJ 08096   (856)848-2332   Fax (856)848-5955

Jones-Mudd, Kimberly M., DO {1093000549} FamMed(11,NJ75)
+ AtlantiCare Family Medicine
219 North White Horse Pike/Suite 101   Hammonton, NJ 08037   (609)561-4211   Fax (609)561-0639

Jongco, Robert D., MD {1477848919}
+ 11 Bridle Court
Somerset, NJ 08873   (862)250-0936
rjongco@gmail.com

Jonna, Harsha R., MD {1063648871} Radiol
+ University Radiology Group, P.C.
579A Cranbury Road   East Brunswick, NJ 08816   (908)698-2254   Fax (732)390-1856
harshajonna@gmail.com

Jonna, Siva Prasad, MD {1245259332} Pedtrc, PedCrC(81,INDI)<NJ-STPETER, NJ-CENTRAST>
+ St. Peter's University Hospital
254 Easton Avenue/Pediatrics   New Brunswick, NJ 08901   (732)565-5434   Fax (732)745-0857

Jonna, Vaidehi, MD {1770502882} Pedtrc(81,INA4D)<NJ-RWJUHAM, NJ-STPETER>
+ 110 New Brunswick Avenue
Perth Amboy, NJ 08861   (732)826-5500

Jonna, Venkata Karthik, MD {1396905667} SrgOARec
+ 222 Easton Avenue/Suite D2
New Brunswick, NJ 08901   (732)339-7779   Fax (732)745-8029

Jonnalagadda, Balathripura S., MD {1922111558} Pedtrc(75,INDI)<NJ-CENTRAST, NJ-RWJUBRUN>
+ CentraState Family Medicine Residency Practice
1001 West Main Street/Suite B   Freehold, NJ 07728   (732)294-2540   Fax (732)294-9328
+ CentraState Medical Center
901 West Main Street/Family Practice   Freehold, NJ 07728   (732)294-2540

Jonnalagadda, Padmavathi, MD {1144228891} IntrMd(96,INA7C)<NJ-BAYONNE, NJ-CHRIST>
+ Padmavathi Jonnalagadda MD PA
3438 JF Kennedy Boulevard   Jersey City, NJ 07307   (201)420-0366   Fax (201)420-6422

Jonnalagadda, Vasudeva Rao, MD {1669470308} IntrMd, Nephro(89,INDI)<NJ-CHRIST, NJ-BAYONNE>
+ Padmavathi Jonnalagadda MD PA
3438 JF Kennedy Boulevard   Jersey City, NJ 07307   (201)420-0366   Fax (201)420-6422

Joo, Eui-Don, MD {1952421612} Psychy(64,KOR04)<NY-SOUTH-PSY>
+ 6305 Westover Way
Somerset, NJ 08873   (908)472-4999
euidonjoo@gmail.com

Joo, Richard H., MD {1851351282} IntrMd(01,KOR05)
+ Joo Medical Center
388 Broad Street   Leonia, NJ 07605   (201)292-1567   Fax (201)585-0692

Jordan, Daniel Robert, MD {1043307051} IntrMd(97,NJ06)<NJ-COOPRUMC>
+ Dorfner Family Medicine
811 Sunset Road/Suite 101   Burlington, NJ 08016   (609)387-9242   Fax (609)387-1948

Jordan, Jo-Ann, MD {1558358358} Pedtrc(99,NJ06)<NJ-RIVERVW>
+ Monmouth Pediatric Group, P.A.
272 Broad Street   Red Bank, NJ 07701   (732)741-0456   Fax (732)219-9477
+ Monmouth Pediatric Group, P.A.
3350 Highway 138   Wall, NJ 07719   (732)741-0456   Fax (732)681-6939

Jordan, Karen T., MD {1760691257} Psychy, Bariat(83,MI07)
+ The K Jordan Associates LLC
1000 White Horse Road/Suite 902   Voorhees, NJ 08043   (856)309-1363   Fax (856)309-1369

Jordan, Lawrence Joseph, III, MD {1588651608} Surgry(83,NY20)<NJ-UNVMCPRN>
+ Princeton Surgical Associates, P.A.
5 Plainsboro Road/Suite 400   Plainsboro, NJ 08536   (609)936-9100   Fax (609)936-9700
LJordan@princeton-surgical.com

Jordan, Nicole, MD {1013304989} IntrMd<NJ-PALISADE>
+ Palisades Medical Center
7600 River Road   North Bergen, NJ 07047   (201)854-5005

Jordan-Scalia, Lisa Judith, DO {1659388858} FamMed(97,NY75)
+ Raritan Family Health Care
901 US Highway 202   Raritan, NJ 08869   (908)253-6640

Fax (908)253-6908

Jordanovski, Daniel, MD {1053739318} IntrMd<NJ-OVERLOOK>
+ Overlook Medical Center
99 Beauvoir Avenue/PO Box 210   Summit, NJ 07902   (908)522-2000

Jorgensen, Otto B., MD {1578578332} FamMed(85,NJ06)<NJ-STPETER>
+ Immedi-Care Urgent Family HealthCare Center
2300 State Route 27   North Brunswick, NJ 08902   (732)940-7770   Fax (732)422-0202

Jose, Jaison, DO {1871752600} Pedtrc
+ Princeton Family Care
100 Federal City Road/Suite A   Lawrenceville, NJ 08648   (609)620-1380   Fax (609)771-8991

Joseffer, Seth S., MD {1851445910} SrgNro
+ Princeton Brain & Spine Care LLC
731 Alexander Road/Suite 200   Princeton, NJ 08540   (609)921-9001   Fax (609)921-9055
+ Princeton Brain & Spine Care LLC
190 Route 31N/Suite 300B   Flemington, NJ 08822   (609)921-9001   Fax (908)806-6625

Joseph, Albert M. Duverglas, MD {1518051499} IntrMd(78,MEXI)
+ Heart & Vascular Medical Group
680 Broadway/Suite 116-A   Paterson, NJ 07514   (973)684-3663   Fax (862)264-2386

Joseph, Anita, MD {1780698282} Pedtrc(72,INA68)<NJ-STPETER>
+ 2010 Park Avenue
South Plainfield, NJ 07080   (908)753-6660

Joseph, Charles A., MD {1285675090} FamMed(76,NJ06)<NJ-MORRISTN>
+ Morris Family Medicine Associates, PA
340 Speedwell Avenue/PO Box 190   Morris Plains, NJ 07950   (973)267-9899   Fax (973)538-3522

Joseph, Eddy M., MD {1952465163} ObsGyn(78,MEX03)
+ 44 Elmora Avenue
Elizabeth, NJ 07202   (908)353-1171   Fax (908)353-4660
eddyjosephmd@aol.com

Joseph, Eric M., MD {1558462556} Otlryg, OtgyFPIS(92,NY08)
+ 1500 Pleasant Valley Way/Suite 206
West Orange, NJ 07052   (973)325-1155   Fax (973)325-8668

Joseph, Frederique Mirlene, MD {1710089917} Pedtrc, GenPrc(80,MEX03)<NJ-MEADWLND, NJ-MTNSIDE>
+ Lyons Medical Center LLC
669 Elizabeth Avenue/Owner/Partner   Newark, NJ 07112   (973)923-6452   Fax (973)923-1979

Joseph, Gipsa Ann, MD {1013335041} IntrMd<NJ-UMDNJ>
+ University Hospital
150 Bergen Street/Suite H245   Newark, NJ 07103   (973)972-5672

Joseph, Jain, MD {1265745111} SrgRec
+ Summit Medical Group-Berkeley Heights Campus
1 Diamond Hill Road   Berkeley Heights, NJ 07922   (908)277-8759   Fax (908)790-6576

Joseph, John K., MD {1003131038} PthAcl
+ Histopathology Services, LLC.
535 East Crescent Avenue   Ramsey, NJ 07446   (201)661-7280   Fax (201)661-7297

Joseph, Joslyn, DO {1861886137} EmrgMd
+ Newark Beth Israel Medical Center Emergency Medicine
201 Lyons Avenue   Newark, NJ 07112   (973)926-7240

Joseph, Judith Fiona, MD {1841487014} Psychy, Psyphm, IntrMd(07,NY01)<NJ-HOBUNIMC>
+ Hoboken University Medical Center
308 Willow Avenue/Psychiatry   Hoboken, NJ 07030   (201)418-1892   Fax (201)418-1800

Joseph, Junie Lorna, MD {1215302112} FamMed
+ Hunterdon Family Medicine
1100 Wescott Drive/Suite 101   Flemington, NJ 08822   (908)788-6535   Fax (908)788-6536

Joseph, Lisa V., MD {1417085937} IntrMd(94,MO34)<NJ-STCLR-DEN>
+ 179 Cahill Cross Road/Suite 210
West Milford, NJ 07480   (973)728-6935
Lisa.joseph@bshsi.org
+ Summit Medical Group
477 Route 10 East/Suite 204   Randolph, NJ 07869   (862)260-3020

Joseph, Merab, MD {1053421032} IntrMd, EnDbMt(92,GEO02)
+ North Jersey Diabetes and Endocrinology
596 Anderson Avenue/Suite 208   Cliffside Park, NJ 07010   (201)467-5775   Fax (201)949-5779
+ North Jersey Diabetes and Endocrinology
24-07 A Broadway   Fair Lawn, NJ 07410   (201)941-5757

Joseph, Monalisa, MD {1578849345} Nephro, IntrMd(05)
+ Suburban Nephrology Group
342 Hamburg Turnpike/Suite 201   Wayne, NJ 07470   (973)389-1119   Fax (973)389-1145

Joseph, P. Dilip, MD {1891709697} IntrMd(71,INA37)
+ 2010 Park Avenue
South Plainfield, NJ 07080   (908)753-2110

Joseph, Richard S., MD {1467452805}(62,NY46)
+ UniMed Center LLC
190 Route 18/Suite 202   East Brunswick, NJ 08816   (516)286-4467   Fax (732)828-1010
drjogger@gmail.com

Joseph, Romane, MD {1801197447} Surgry
+ Drs. Ducheine and Joseph
310 Central Avenue/Suite 203   East Orange, NJ 07018   (973)674-4042   Fax (973)674-5070
Josephsurgery@gmail.com

Joseph, Rosy E., MD {1497774350} Nephro, IntrMd(90,NY01)<NJ-HACKNSK>
+ BSD Nephrology & Hypertension
360 Essex Street/Suite 304   Hackensack, NJ 07601   (201)646-0110   Fax (201)646-0219

Josephberg, Robert G., MD {1588601793} Ophthl, VitRet, OthrSp(76,NY03)<NY-WESTCHMC, NY-STJOSHHC>
+ 710 Tennent Road
Englishtown, NJ 07726   (732)972-0800   Fax (732)972-7742
rj2526@aol.com

Josephs, Joshua, MD {1609263102} IntHos
+ Hackensack Univ Medical Center Hospitalists
30 Prospect Avenue   Hackensack, NJ 07601   (551)996-4466

Josephson, Tina M., MD {1164493086} IntrMd(88,PA09)<NJ-VIRTVOOR, NJ-VIRTMARL>
+ Cherry Hill Family Care & Internal Medicine
101 Barclay Pavilion West   Cherry Hill, NJ 08034   (856)429-4179   Fax (856)429-3794

Josephson, Youssef, DO {1598928608} PhyMPain, IntrMd(05,NJ75)<NJ-KMHCHRRY, NJ-KMHTURNV>
+ The Pain Management Center at Hamilton
2271 Highway 33/Suite 103   Hamilton, NJ 08690   (609)890-4080   Fax (609)890-4090

Joshi, Anuja, MD {1881004588} FamMed<NJ-HOBUNIMC>
+ Hoboken University Medical Center
308 Willow Avenue   Hoboken, NJ 07030   (201)418-1000

Joshi, Archana N., MD {1578725255} IntrMd(97,INA1P)
+ Dr. Archana Joshi LLC
1856 Oak Tree Road   Edison, NJ 08820   (732)910-1134   Fax (732)906-7820

Joshi, Hetal Chaitanyaprasad, MD {1790729879} EmrgEMed(95)<NJ-STFRNMED>
+ St. Francis Medical Center
601 Hamilton Avenue/Emergency   Trenton, NJ 08629   (609)599-5000
+ JFK Medical Center
65 James Street/Emergency   Edison, NJ 08820   (732)321-7000

Joshi, Jyotika D., MD {1447221205} ObsGyn, Gyneco, IntrMd(70,INDI)<NJ-CENTRAST, NJ-JRSYSHMC>
+ Hackensack Meridian Medical Group Ob/Gyn, Freehold
3499 Route 9 North/Suite 2B   Freehold, NJ 07728   (732)577-1199   Fax (732)577-8922

Joshi, Kiran M., MD {1215001698} ObsGyn(70,INA69)
+ Garden State Women's Center
301 Beech Street   Hackensack, NJ 07601   (201)880-7641   Fax (201)546-1621

Joshi, Kumud Gada, MD {1760674360} Psychy
+ 137 Westley Road
Old Bridge, NJ 08857   (732)696-2779

Joshi, Meeta Yatinkumar, MD {1518974815} PainMd, Anesth(87,INA15)<NJ-VAEASTOR>
+ VA New Jersey Health Care System-East Orange Campus
385 Tremont Avenue/Anesth   East Orange, NJ 07018   (973)676-1000

Joshi, Meherwan Burzor, MD {1598938391} CdvDis, IntrMd(01,INA1N)
+ Drs. Joshi & Chua
240 Williamson Street/Suite 203   Elizabeth, NJ 07202   (732)491-9597   Fax (973)261-5142

Joshi, Namita V., MD {1982875696} FamMed, IntrMd(05,DMN01)
+ Morristown Medical Center Family Medicine
435 South Street/Suite 220-A   Morristown, NJ 07960   (973)971-4222   Fax (973)290-7050

Joshi, Nandita, MD {1619991866} IntrMd(96,INA5B)<NJ-ENGLEWOOD, NJ-HOLYNAME>
+ Bergen Medical Alliance, P.A.
180 Engle Street   Englewood, NJ 07631   (201)567-2050   Fax (201)568-8936

Joshi, Puja, MD {1811248164}
+ 802 Evergreen Forest Boulevard
Avenel, NJ 07001   (215)375-4477
puja.aggarwal@nyumc.org

Joshi, Rachna B., MD {1477849800}
+ Shore Hospitalists Associates
100 Medical Center Way   Somers Point, NJ 08244   (609)653-3500   Fax (609)926-4799
+ Shore Memorial Hospital
1 East New York Avenue   Somers Point, NJ 08244   (609)653-3500

Physicians by Name and Address

Joshi, Raksha, MD {1174517619} ObsGyn(80,INDI)<NJ-MON-MOUTH>
+ Monmouth Medical Center
300 Second Avenue/Ob-Gyn Long Branch, NJ 07740 (732)222-5200
+ Monmouth Family Center
270 Broadway Long Branch, NJ 07740 (732)222-5200 Fax (732)923-7104

Joshi, Samir V., MD {1528036787} EmrgPedr, Pedtrc
+ JFK Medical Center
65 James Street Edison, NJ 08820 (732)321-7605 Fax (732)744-5614

Joshi, Tapankumar, MD {1710150115} PhysMd
+ Advanced Medical Care Center
901 Route 73 North/Suite C Marlton, NJ 08053 (856)581-9711 Fax (856)581-9712
+ Gupta Institute for Integrative Medicine
951 Berlin Road Cherry Hill, NJ 08034 (856)581-9711 Fax (856)482-7245

Josias, Fernande, MD {1477813848}
+ 242 East 5th Avenue
Roselle, NJ 07203 (973)943-3474
sweetnande@gmail.com

Josyula, Leela S., MD {1730293903} Pedtrc, NnPnMd(75,INA62)<NJ-RWJUBRUN, NJ-CENTRAST>
+ On-Site Neonatal Partners
1000 Haddonfield-Berlin Road/Suite 210 Voorhees, NJ 08043 (856)782-2212 Fax (856)782-2213

Jotwani, Madhu M, MD {1700040482} Anesth<NJ-STMRYPAS>
+ St. Mary's Hospital
350 Boulevard Passaic, NJ 07055 (973)365-4300 Fax (973)779-7385

Jourdan, Cassie, MD {1407261787} PedEmg
+ Morristown Medical Center Emergency Medicine
100 Madison Avenue Morristown, NJ 07960 (973)971-5000

Jow, William W., MD {1164424057} Urolgy(86,NY19)<NJ-RWJUBRUN, NJ-BAYSHORE>
+ Center for Urology at Holmdel
723 North Beers Street/Ste 1F Holmdel, NJ 07733 (732)888-0809 Fax (732)888-5559

Joy, Ansu Varughese, MD {1629278536} EnDbMt(DMN01)
+ Endocrinology Associates of Princeton, LLC
256 Bunn Drive/Suite D Princeton, NJ 08540 (609)924-4433 Fax (609)924-4423
+ Endocrinology Associates of Princeton, LLC
168 Franklin Corner Road Lawrenceville, NJ 08648 (609)924-4433 Fax (609)896-0079

Joyce, Katherine Ellen, MD {1255779401}
+ Virtua Nurosciences
200 Bowman Drive/Suite E-385 Voorhees, NJ 08043 (856)247-7720 Fax (856)247-7766

Joyce, Michael Walter, MD {1780644005} PulDis, IntrMd(91,NY08)
+ Coastal Pulmonary PA
20 Hospital Drive/Suite 5 Toms River, NJ 08755 (732)341-2411 Fax (732)341-2447

Joynes, Robert Joseph, MD {1942267240} IntrMd(72,PA09)
+ 4 Hibiscus Drive
Marlton, NJ 08053 (856)577-6963 Fax (856)854-6700

Ju, Albert Changwon, MD {1609010917} Anesth
+ New Jersey Anesthesia Associates, P.C.
30B Vreeland Road/Suite 200 Florham Park, NJ 07932 (973)660-9334 Fax (973)660-9779
drokosny@hnmanagement.com

Ju, Tashil Kim, MD {1730314972} PedAne, Anesth(06,IL11)<NY-PRSBCOLU>
+ Bergen Anesthesia Group, P.C.
500 West Main Street/Suite 16 Wyckoff, NJ 07481 (201)847-9320 Fax (201)847-0059

Ju, William D., MD {1982852661} Dermat(82,PA01)
+ 100 Corporate Court
South Plainfield, NJ 07080 (908)222-7000

Juarez, Veronica Jean, MD {1871988527}<NJ-NWRKBETH>
+ Newark Beth Israel Medical Center
201 Lyons Avenue Newark, NJ 07112 (973)926-7000

Juco, Henry P., MD {1154350007} EmrgMd(67,PHI01)<NJ-NWTN-MEM>
+ Newton Medical Center
175 High Street/EmrgMed Newton, NJ 07860 (973)383-2121

Juco, Jonathan W., MD {1871798595} PthHem, PthAcl
+ Merck and Company Incorporated
126 East Lincoln Avenue Rahway, NJ 07065 (551)427-9564
jwjuco@yahoo.com

Juco, Judy M., MD {1326113465} PthAcl, Pthlgy, FamMed(69,PHIL)<NJ-BERGNMC>
+ Institute of Preventive Medicine
95 East Main Street/Suite 106 Denville, NJ 07834 (973)586-4111 Fax (973)586-8466

Judge, Thomas Aloysius, MD {1407945462} Gastrn, IntrMd(87,PA13)<NJ-COOPRUMC>
+ Cooper Digestive Health Institute
501 Fellowship Road/Suite 101 Mount Laurel, NJ 08054 (856)642-2133 Fax (856)642-2134
+ The Cooper Hospital System-Univ Hospital
3 Cooper Plaza/Suite 215 Camden, NJ 08103 (856)642-2133 Fax (856)642-2134

Juele, Nicholas J., DO {1710929427} GenPrc, FamMed(79,PA77)<NJ-VIRTMARL>
+ 205 Tuckerton Road
Medford, NJ 08055 (856)983-4560 Fax (856)983-4264

Juengst-Mitchell, Jannine, DO {1902847254} Radiol, RadBdi(88,NY75)<NJ-ENGLWOOD>
+ Englewood Radiologic Group PA
350 Engle Street Englewood, NJ 07631 (201)894-3000 Fax (201)894-5244

Juha, Ramez, MD {1265738223} Surgry, IntrMd(00,SYR02)
+ Princeton Surgical Associates, P.A.
5 Plainsboro Road/Suite 400 Plainsboro, NJ 08536 (609)936-9100 Fax (609)936-9700

Juliano, Julieann S., MD {1174570774} FamMed(84,NY46)
+ South Branch Family Practice
48 Robbins Road Somerville, NJ 08876 (908)685-8080 Fax (908)685-1925

Juliano, Nickolas Daniel, MD {1114192101} IntCrd, CdvDis, IntrMd(00,NY01)
+ Summit Medical Group-Berkeley Heights Campus
1 Diamond Hill Road Berkeley Heights, NJ 07922 (908)277-8700 Fax (908)277-8993

Julie, Edward, MD {1497701163} CdvDis, IntrMd(80,NY46)<NJ-CHILTON, NJ-VALLEY>
+ Cardiology Center of North Jersey
1030 Clifton Avenue Clifton, NJ 07013 (973)778-3777 Fax (973)778-3252
+ Cardiology Center of North Jersey
61 Beaver Brook Road/Suite 202 Lincoln Park, NJ 07035 (973)778-3777

Julius, Barry D., MD {1508886763} RadDia, NuclMd(98,NY46)
+ 171 Westcott Road
Princeton, NJ 08540

Jumao-As, Joseph Maben Aparece, MD {1346331667} EmrgMd
+ Advocare in-Patient Medicine
100 Bowman Drive Voorhees, NJ 08043 (856)247-3000

Juneau, Jeffrey Evan, MD {1851681167} IntrMd
+ UH-RWJ General Internal Medicine
125 Paterson Street/Suite 2300 New Brunswick, NJ 08901 (732)235-7122 Fax (732)235-7144

Juneja, Tony, MD {1871519215} Psychy, NrlgSpec, PsyAdt(01,GRN01)
+ 1215 Route 70/Suite 1001
Lakewood, NJ 08701 (732)942-5056

Jung, Herbert Michael, DO {1568418101} FamMed(85,NJ75)
+ Advocare Advanced Primary Care
111 Vine Street Hammonton, NJ 08037 (609)561-2518 Fax (609)567-0934

Junior, John L., MD {1043484181} Anesth, IntrMd(80,POLA)
+ 658 North Saratoga Drive
Moorestown, NJ 08057

Junker, Elizabeth Elsa, MD {1518983808} EmrgMed<NJ-MORRISTN>
+ Morristown Medical Center
100 Madison Avenue/EmrgMed Morristown, NJ 07962 (973)971-5000

Jurado, Jerry L., MD {1720004021} FamMed(86,PHIL)<NJ-STFRN-MED, NJ-STMRYPAS>
+ Dr Jerry L. Jurado and Assoc
2401 Palisade Avenue Union City, NJ 07087 (201)867-5791 Fax (201)223-1905
+ 768 Westside Avenue
Jersey City, NJ 07306 (201)867-5791 Fax (201)435-2351

Jurasinski, Craig M., MD {1225038995} Pthlgy, PthCln(90,PA07)<NJ-BURDTMLN>
+ Cape Regional Medical Center
2 Stone Harbor Boulevard/Pathology Cape May Court House, NJ 08210 (609)463-2000

Jurema, Marcus W., MD {1184654824} ObsGyn, RprEnd, IntrMd(96,CA11)<NJ-HUNTRDN, NJ-STPETER>
+ Reproductive Medicine Associates of New Jersey
140 Allen Road Basking Ridge, NJ 07920 (908)604-7800 Fax (973)290-8370

Jurewicz, Stephen S., MD {1679570089} IntrMd, Grtrcs(77,PA09)<NJ-RIVERVW>
+ Riverview Medical Associates, PA
4 Hartford Drive/Suite 1 Tinton Falls, NJ 07701 (732)741-3600 Fax (732)741-6079
+ Chapin Hill at Red Bank
100 Chapin Avenue Red Bank, NJ 07701 (732)741-3600 Fax (732)842-8269

Juusela, Alexander Lawrence, MD {1184036352} ObsGyn<NJ-NWRKBETH>
+ Newark Beth Israel Medical Center
201 Lyons Avenue Newark, NJ 07112 (973)926-4882 Fax (973)923-7497

Jyonouchi, Harumi, MD {1225177090} Pedtrc, AlgyImmn, Ped-Alg(76,JAP88)<NJ-UMDNJ>
+ St. Peter's Family Health
123 How Lane New Brunswick, NJ 08901 (732)745-8600 Fax (732)729-0869
+ University Hospital-Doctors Office Center
90 Bergen Street/Doc 4600 Newark, NJ 07103 (732)745-8600 Fax (973)972-5895

Jyung, Robert Wha, MD {1093283138} Otolgy, Otlryg(89,MI01)
+ University Physician Associates
140 Bergen Street/ACC Level E Newark, NJ 07103 (973)972-4966 Fax (973)972-3923

Kaari, Jacqueline Marie, DO {1457321127} Pedtrc(98,NJ75)<NJ-KMHTURNV, NJ-KMHCHRRY>
+ The University Doctors - UMDNJ -SOM
570 Egg Harbor Road/Suite C-2 Sewell, NJ 08080 (856)218-0300 Fax (856)589-5082
+ University Pediatrics
405 Hurffville Crosskeys Road Sewell, NJ 08080 (856)218-0300 Fax (856)582-2305

Kabadi, Rajesh Mahesh, MD {1316155088} IntHos, IntrMd(06,IL42)<NJ-COOPRUMC>
+ Cooper University Hospital
One Cooper Plaza/3rd Floor Camden, NJ 08103 (856)342-2000 Fax (856)968-7420

Kabakibi, Riad A., MD {1609896406} FrtInf, ObsGyn, SrgMcr(70,EGYP)<NJ-MEADWLND, NJ-STJOSHOS>
+ 255 Route 3 East/Suite 206A
Secaucus, NJ 07094 (201)867-6677 Fax (201)520-0316

Kabaria, Sunit P., MD {1134266240} Nephro(97,DMN01)<NJ-OVERLOOK>
+ Overlook Medical Center
99 Beauvoir Avenue/PO Box 210 Summit, NJ 07902 (908)522-2000

Kabarwal, Navneesh Kaur, MD {1568645646} Pedtrc, AdolMd(04,NY15)
+ Advocare Vernon Pediatrics
249 Route 94 Vernon, NJ 07462 (973)827-4550 Fax (973)827-5845

Kabba, Chidinma Dawn, MD {1659647873} EmrgMd
+ University Hospital-New Jersey Medical School
30 Bergen Street/Bld 11/Rm 1110 Newark, NJ 07107 (973)972-9200 Fax (973)972-9268

Kabel, Stephen E., DO {1134129125} IntrMd(88,IA75)<NJ-LOUR-DMED, NJ-VIRTUAHS>
+ Delran Medical Practice
26 Haines Mill Road Delran, NJ 08075 (856)461-6200 Fax (856)461-4013

Kabel-Kotler, Caroline, DO {1932157419} Pedtrc(95,NJ75)<NJ-VIRTUAHS, NJ-VIRTMARL>
+ Advocare Laurel Pediatrics
269 Fish Pond Road Sewell, NJ 08080 (856)863-9999 Fax (856)863-9666
+ Advocare Greentree Pediatrics
127 Church Road/Suite 800 Marlton, NJ 08053 (856)863-9999 Fax (856)988-9499
+ Advocare South Jersey Pediatrics Collingswood
204 White Horse Pike Collingswood, NJ 08080 (856)424-6050 Fax (856)424-2943

Kabis, Suzanne M., MD {1386665628} Nephro, IntrMd(79,NJ06)<NJ-RWJUBRUN, NJ-STPETER>
+ The Renal Group of Central NJ, P.A.
1350 Hamilton Street Somerset, NJ 08873 (732)246-2626 Fax (732)249-5480
+ Somerset Dialysis DAVITA
240 Churchill Avenue Somerset, NJ 08873 (732)937-5000

Kabnick, Lowell Stuart, MD {1477533925} SrgVas, Surgry(76,DC01)<NJ-MORRISTN, NY-NYUTISCH>
+ 95 Madison Avenue/Suite 415
Morristown, NJ 07960 (973)538-2000

Kachadourian, Anise A., MD {1750349395} IntrMd, OncHem(95,GRN01)<NJ-OVERLOOK>
+ 2333 Morris Avenue/Suite A121
Union, NJ 07083 (908)442-7920 Fax (908)258-0350

Kachirayan, Vasanthi, MD {1578697090} IntrMd, Grtrcs(91,INA04)
+ 68 Alder Lane
Basking Ridge, NJ 07920

Kachroo, Arun, MD {1609840602} Nrolgy(94,NJ05)
+ Neurology Associaates of South Jersey
693 Main Street/Building D Lumberton, NJ 08048 (609)261-7600 Fax (609)265-8205
+ Advocare Neurology of South Jersey
200-B Route 73 North/Suite 2 Voorhees, NJ 08043 (609)261-7600 Fax (856)335-0406

Kachroo, Puja, MD {1881899714}<NJ-UMDNJ>
+ University Hospital
150 Bergen Street/E 401 Newark, NJ 07103 (973)972-4300

Physicians by Name and Address

Kaczaj, Olga, MD {1518055755} IntrMd(93,UKR25)
+ Millville Medical Center
1700 North Tenth Street Millville, NJ 08332 (856)327-6446

Kaddaha, Raja'A Mohammed, MD {1578584736} CdvDis, IntrMd, ClCdEl(93,LEB03)
+ Cardiology Associates LLC
999 McBride Avenue/Suite B-204 West Paterson, NJ 07424 (973)256-5667 Fax (973)256-7758

Kaddissi, Georges Ibrahim, MD {1821040478} CdvDis(96,LEB01)<NJ-COOPRUMC, NJ-OURLADY>
+ Cardiovascular Associates
210 West Atlantic Avenue Haddon Heights, NJ 08035 (856)546-3003 Fax (856)547-5337
+ Cardiovascular Associates of The Delaware Valley, PA
1840 Frontage Road Cherry Hill, NJ 08034 (856)546-3003 Fax (856)795-7436
+ Cardiovascular Associates of The Delaware Valley, PA
525 State Street/Suite 3 Elmer, NJ 08035 (856)358-2363 Fax (856)358-0725

Kaden, Ian H., MD {1871560474} Ophthl(87,MD07)<NJ-MORRISTN>
+ Morris Ophthalmology Consultants
121 Center Grove Road Randolph, NJ 07869 (973)328-6622 Fax (973)328-4495

Kader, Richard A., DO {1003983594} FamMed(88,NJ75)<NJ-SHOREMEM>
+ Virtua Primary Care
1201 New Road/Suite 150a Linwood, NJ 08221 (609)788-3338
+ Atlantic Shore Family Practice PA
1423 Tilton Road/Suite 3 Northfield, NJ 08225 (609)788-3338 Fax (609)272-8306
+ Virtua Primary Care
401 Young Avenue/Suite 260 Moorestown, NJ 08221 (856)291-8920 Fax (856)291-8922

Kadimcherla, Praveen, MD {1700182946} SrgOrt(08,NY06)
+ Atlantic Spine Center
475 Prospect Avenue/Suite 110 West Orange, NJ 07052 (973)419-0200 Fax (973)419-0223

Kadivar, Khadijeh, MD {1881833853} Radiol, RadNro
+ University Radiology Group, P.C.
579A Cranbury Road East Brunswick, NJ 08816 (732)390-0040 Fax (732)390-1856

Kadiyam, Sandhya, MD {1093034308} IntrMd<NY-LUTHERN>
+ Monmouth Medical Center
300 Second Avenue Long Branch, NJ 07740 (732)222-5200

Kadosh, Yisrael, MD {1417917907} CdvDis, IntrMd
+ Ocean Cardiology
1166 River Avenue/Suite 204 Lakewood, NJ 08701 (732)905-4142 Fax (732)905-4160

Kadri, Iftekhar S., MD {1093711947} CdvDis, IntrMd(78,INDI)<NJ-NWRKBETH, NJ-EASTORNG>
+ 372 Valley Road
West Orange, NJ 07052 (973)736-2600 Fax (973)736-8355

Kadrmas-Iannuzzi, Tanya Lynn, DO {1205806957} Pedtrc(99,NJ75)
+ University Doctors Pavilion
42 East Laurel Road/Suite 2545 Stratford, NJ 08084 (856)566-7040 Fax (856)566-6826

Kaelin Wooton, Kathleen M., MD {1275893950} IntrMd
+ 223 Woodward Avenue
Rutherford, NJ 07070 (201)964-1806

Kaftal, Sergiusz I., MD {1740204361} FamMed, Grtrcs(78,POLA)<NJ-MORRISTN, NJ-SOMERSET>
+ Serge I. Kaftal, MD, PA
10 Anderson Hill Road Bernardsville, NJ 07924 (908)766-1223 Fax (908)766-0765
SKAFTAL@comcast.net

Kaga, Mira Kamal, MD {1760707327} IntrMd
+ 4255 US Highway 9/Suite 5B
Freehold, NJ 07728 (732)719-2001
info@drmirakaga.com

Kagan, Eduard, MD {1679511257} RadOnc, Radiol(99,MI20)<NJ-RWJUBRUN>
+ New Jersey Urology, LLC
1515 Broad Street/Suite B-130 Bloomfield, NJ 07003 (973)873-7000 Fax (973)873-7035

Kagan, Mikhail, MD {1871936237} Anesth
+ Summit Anesthesia Associates, P.A.
33 Overlook Road/Suite 311 Summit, NJ 07901 (718)309-5855 Fax (908)598-0197

Kagan, Peter Evan, MD {1932281219} SrgVas, Surgry(97,GRN01)<NJ-HACKNSK>
+ North Jersey Surgical Specialists
83 Summit Avenue Hackensack, NJ 07601 (201)646-0010 Fax (201)646-0600

Kaganovskaya, Margarita, MD {1932188190} Anesth(99,GRN01)<NJ-ENGLWOOD>
+ Englewood Hospital and Medical Center
350 Engle Street/Anesth Englewood, NJ 07631 (201)894-3000 Fax (201)871-0619

Kahanovitz, Neil, MD {1124123864} Ortped, SrgOrt(75,MD01)
+ Hahemann Orthopedics and Sports Medicine
13000 Route 73 South Marlton, NJ 08053 (856)396-0940 Fax (856)396-0127
+ Short Hills Surgery Center
187 Millburn Avenue/Suite 101 Millburn, NJ 07041 (856)396-0940 Fax (973)671-0557

Kahf, Ahmad N., MD {1922069517} IntrMd, CdvDis(72,SYRI)<NJ-STJOSHOS>
+ Medical Group of North Jersey
401 Haledon Avenue/2nd Floor Haledon, NJ 07508 (973)942-3767 Fax (973)942-1027

Kahf, Amr, MD {1326257668} IntrMd
+ Medical Group of North Jersey
401 Haledon Avenue/2nd Floor Haledon, NJ 07508 (973)942-3767 Fax (973)942-1027

Kahlam, Sarwan S., MD {1710958137} Gastrn, IntrMd(82,SCOT)<NJ-NWTNMEM, NJ-HCKTSTWN>
+ 37 US Highway 46
Hackettstown, NJ 07840 (908)852-8588 Fax (908)852-8588
+ 183 High Street
Newton, NJ 07860 (973)579-1775

Kahlon, Tejinderpaul Singh, MD {1164703534} FamMed
+ ImmediCenter/Clifton
1355 Broad Street Clifton, NJ 07013 (973)778-5566 Fax (973)778-4044

Kahn, Alissa Rachel, MD {1598924011} PedHem, Pedtrc, IntrMd(06,NY47)<NJ-STJOSHOS>
+ St. Joseph's Regional Medical Center
703 Main Street/Pedi Hem Onc Paterson, NJ 07503 (973)754-3230

Kahn, Daniel Efraim, MD {1962442525} Pedtrc(97,NY47)<NJ-MORRISTN, NJ-STCLRDEN>
+ Parsippany Pediatrics
1140 Parsippany Boulevard/Suite 102 Parsippany, NJ 07054 (973)263-0066 Fax (973)263-3160

Kahn, Frederick E., MD {1316160039} Psychy, PssoMd(76,MI07)
+ Forest Psychiatric Associates
6 Forest Avenue Paramus, NJ 07652 (201)587-0414 Fax (201)655-7851

Kahn, Jason Peter, DO {1538572425} FamMed
+ 161 Bellevue Avenue/2nd Floor
Montclair, NJ 07043 (201)280-2755

Kahn, Laura H., MD IntrMd, PubHth(89,NY47)
+ 14 Journeys End Lane
Princeton, NJ 08540

Kahn, Marc L., MD {1609955756} SrgOrt(82,PA09)<NJ-VIRTVOOR, NJ-KENEDYHS>
+ Garden State Orthopedics & Sports Medicine
455 Route 70 West Cherry Hill, NJ 08002 (609)616-2999 Fax (856)616-1437

Kahn, Mark Elliot, MD {1285632281} SrgVas, Surgry(74,NY03)<NJ-ENGLWOOD, NJ-HOLYNAME>
+ Englewood Surgical Associates
375 Engle Street/Ground Floor Englewood, NJ 07631 (201)894-0400 Fax (201)894-1022

Kahn, Milton, MD {1750477006} Ophthl(87,MA05)<NJ-OVERLOOK>
+ Eye Care and Surgery Center
10 Mountain Boulevard Warren, NJ 07059 (908)754-4800 Fax (908)754-4803
+ Eye Care and Surgery Center
592 Springfield Avenue Westfield, NJ 07090 (908)754-4800 Fax (908)789-1379
+ Eye Care and Surgery Center
517 Route 1 South/Suite 1100 Iselin, NJ 07059 (732)636-7355 Fax (732)636-7497

Kahn, Randolph, DO {1235122144} Anesth(90,NY75)<NJ-RWJUBRUN>
+ Union Anesthesia & Pain Management
695 Chestnut Street Union, NJ 07083 (908)851-7161 Fax (908)851-7536

Kahn, Steven H., DO {1164461356} SrgOrt(94,MI12)<NJ-KMHCHRRY, NJ-KMHSTRAT>
+ Regional Orthopedic, P.A.
2201 West Chapel Avenue/PO Box 8566 Cherry Hill, NJ 08002 (856)663-7080 Fax (856)663-4945
+ Regional Orthopedic, P.A.
163 Hurffville Crosskeys Road Turnersville, NJ 08012 (856)663-7080 Fax (856)875-1368

Kahn, Walter J., MD {1669452660} Ophthl(59,IL02)<NJ-BAYSHORE, NJ-RIVERVW>
+ Mid Atlantic Eye Center
70 East Front Street Red Bank, NJ 07701 (732)741-0858 Fax (732)219-0180

Kahng, He-Yeun, MD {1811168321} PhysMd, IntrMd(74,KOR01)<NJ-BAYSHORE, NJ-RIVERVW>
+ 335 Dorn Drive
Shrewsbury, NJ 07702 (732)493-0065

Kahyaoglu, Aret Y., MD {1811023682} IntrMd, Pedtrc(85,TUR01)
+ 165 Summit Avenue
Hackensack, NJ 07601 (201)488-5892 Fax (201)488-5892

Kaiafas, Costas Andreas, MD {1528057866} EmrgMd(96,PA09)<NJ-MORRISTN, NJ-MTNSIDE>
+ Morristown Medical Center
100 Madison Avenue/EmrgMed Morristown, NJ 07962 (973)971-5000
+ Hackensack UMC Mountainside
1 Bay Avenue/EmrgMed Montclair, NJ 07042 (973)429-6000
+ Emergency Medical Associates
110 Rehill Avenue Somerville, NJ 07962 (908)685-2920 Fax (908)685-2968

Kaicker, Shipra, MD {1194770574} PedHem, Pedtrc(92,INA72)<NY-MAIMONMC, NY-NYPRESHS>
+ St Joseph's Medical Center Pediatrics
703 Main Street Paterson, NJ 07503 (973)754-2544

Kaid, Khalil Ahmed, MD {1285651109} IntrMd(03,DMN01)
+ Drs. Kaid & Tanwir
2168 Millburn Avenue/Suite 204 Maplewood, NJ 07040 (973)762-3353 Fax (973)762-3370
+ Avenel Iselin Medical Group
400 Gill Lane Iselin, NJ 08830 (973)762-3353 Fax (732)404-1594

Kaiden, Jeffrey S., MD {1871559005} Ophthl(73,FL03)<NJ-VALLEY>
+ Westwood Ophthalmology Associates
300 Fairview Avenue/PO Box 698 Westwood, NJ 07675 (201)666-4014 Fax (201)664-4754

Kaighn, Karen Chicalo, MD {1386674406} Pedtrc(96,NJ05)<NJ-VIRTMHBC>
+ Advocare Pedi Phys of Burlington Co
693 Main Street/PO Box 367 Lumberton, NJ 08048 (609)261-4058 Fax (609)261-8381
+ Advocare Pedi Phys of Burlington Co
204 Ark Road/Suite 209 Mount Laurel, NJ 08054 (609)261-4058 Fax (856)234-9402

Kailas, Michael G., MD {1013001478} Nrolgy(80,ITA01)<NJ-HOLYNAME>
+ 699 Teaneck Road/Suite 2
Teaneck, NJ 07666 (201)287-0300 Fax (201)287-1550
+ Holy Name Hospital
718 Teaneck Road Teaneck, NJ 07666 (201)833-3000

Kaim, Oleg, MD {1730133141} IntrMd(84,LATV)<NJ-ENGLWOOD>
+ Oleg Kaim MD PC
214 Engle Street/Suite 11 Englewood, NJ 07631 (201)567-4488 Fax (201)567-4771

Kainth, Inderjit S., MD {1194763029} IntrMd(94,INA92)<NJ-MONMOUTH>
+ Brunswick Internal Medical Group
17 Bridge Street Metuchen, NJ 08840 (732)321-1600 Fax (732)321-1699

Kairam, Hemant, MD {1629062633} Pedtrc, IntrMd(97,NET09)<NJ-OVERLOOK>
+ Summit Pediatric Associates
33 Overlook Road/Suite 101 Summit, NJ 07901 (908)273-1112 Fax (908)273-1146
+ Florham Park Pediatrics
195 Columbia Turnpike/Suite 105 Florham Park, NJ 07932 (908)273-1112 Fax (973)845-2883

Kairam, Neeraja, MD {1487691135} Pedtrc, EmrgMd(97,NET09)<NJ-OVERLOOK>
+ Morristown Medical Center
100 Madison Avenue/Box 8 Morristown, NJ 07962 (973)971-5000
+ Emergency Medical Offices
651 West Mount Pleasant Avenue Livingston, NJ 07039 (973)971-5000 Fax (973)251-1165

Kairys, Steven W., MD {1316927734} Pedtrc, AdolMd(75,PA13)<NJ-JRSYSHMC, NJ-RWJUBRUN>
+ UH- Robert Wood Johnson Med
125 Paterson Street/Pediatrics New Brunswick, NJ 08901 (732)828-3000
+ Jersey Shore University Medical Center
1945 Route 33/Pediatrics Neptune, NJ 07753 (732)775-5500

Kaiser, Anthony J., MD {1376668558} SrgOrt(69,NJ05)<NJ-MTNSIDE>
+ 2333 Morris Avenue/Suite C-9
Union, NJ 07083 (908)687-0810 Fax (908)964-6090

Kaiser, Bruce A., MD Pedtrc, PedNph(72,PA13)<NJ-VIRTMHBC, NJ-ACMCITY>
+ AtlantiCare/Dupont Children's Health Program
2500 English Creek Avenue Egg Harbor Township, NJ 08234 (609)641-3700 Fax (609)641-3652

Kaiser, Michael Guenther, MD {1598818817} Nrolgy, SrgNro, IntrMd(94,CT01)<NY-NYPRESHS, NY-PRSBCOLU>
+ Neurosurgeons of New Jersey
1200 East Ridgewood Avenue Ridgewood, NJ 07450 (201)824-6131

Kaiser, Paul K., MD {1689658460} Nrolgy(88,PA02)<NJ-UNVM-CPRN, NJ-CHSFULD>
+ Lawrenceville Neurology Center, PA
3131 Princeton Pike   Lawrenceville, NJ 08648   (609)896-1701   Fax (609)896-3735

Kaiser, Richard Scott, MD {1124076930} Ophthl, IntrMd(95,NY19)
+ Mid Atlantic Retina - Wills Eye Retina Surgeons
501 Cooper Landing Road   Cherry Hill, NJ 08002   (856)667-2246   Fax (856)667-2238
+ Mid Atlantic Retina - Wills Eye Retina Surgeons
1417 Cantillon Boulevard   Mays Landing, NJ 08330   (856)667-2246   Fax (609)625-0788

Kaiser, Susan, MD {1417988809} Surgry, SrgTrm, SrgBst(81,NY46)<NJ-JRSYCITY>
+ Jersey City Medical Center
355 Grand Street/Surgery/3 East   Jersey City, NJ 07304   (201)915-2000
+ Liberty Medical Associates
377 Jersey Avenue/Suite 470   Jersey City, NJ 07302   (201)915-2000   Fax (201)918-2243

Kaiser-Smith, Joanne, DO {1750361838} IntrMd(84,NJ75)<NJ-VIRTVOOR>
+ University of Medicine & Dentistry of New Jersey-SOM
42 East Laurel Road/3100/IntMed   Stratford, NJ 08084   (856)566-6845   Fax (856)566-6906

Kaji, Anand, MD {1962798173}
+ 57 Avenue East
Lodi, NJ 07644   (973)246-4084

Kakarla, Madhavi, MD {1598952632} FamMed(99,KS02)
+ Hopewell Family Practice & Sports Medicine
84 Route 31 North/Suite 103   Pennington, NJ 08534   (609)730-1771   Fax (609)730-1274

Kaki, Sujatha, MD {1407825375}
+ 724, Cedar Court
New Brunswick, NJ 08901   (813)436-9266
kakisujatha@yahoo.com

Kaki, Sushma R., MD {1427260850} Pedtrc(99,INA4D)<NJ-STPETER>
+ Drs. Politis and Kaki
3526 Kennedy Boulevard   Jersey City, NJ 07307   (201)653-5933   Fax (201)653-3930

Kakkar, Pankaj, MD {1912278615} Nrolgy
+ Progressive Neurology
260 Old Hook Road/Suite 200   Westwood, NJ 07675   (201)546-8510   Fax (201)503-8142

Kakkilaya, Harish, MD {1902064140} Surgry, Bariat
+ LMA Surgical Associates
120 White Horse Pike/Suite 103   Haddon Heights, NJ 08035   (856)546-3900   Fax (856)546-3908
+ Salem Medical Group
66 East Avenue   Woodstown, NJ 08098   (856)546-3900   Fax (856)624-4329

Kakkilaya, Harshila, MD {1326231242} Pedtrc(92,INA4X)
+ Advocare, LLC.
402 Lippincott Drive   Marlton, NJ 08053   (856)504-8028   Fax (856)504-8029

Kaladas, Jeffrey J., MD {1295758258} FamMed, IntrMd, OccpMd(92,NJ06)<NJ-RWJUHAM>
+ RWJPE UrgentMed
141 Main Street   South Bound Brook, NJ 08880   (732)560-1234   Fax (732)560-1883
urgentmedpc@pol.com

Kalambakas, Stacey Anastasia, MD {1285606335} PedHem(96,MNT01)<NJ-MORRISTN, NJ-OVERLOOK>
+ The Valerie Fund Children's Ctr/Goryeb
100 Madison Avenue/Simon 2/Box 70   Morristown, NJ 07962   (973)971-5161

Kalariya, Rupal S., MD {1114152808} Anesth
+ 120 Madison Avenue/Suite East
Mount Holly, NJ 08060   (609)267-0700

Kalatoudis, Haris Angelo, MD {1144587502}(11,NSK03)
+ St. Joseph's Wayne Hospital
224 Hamburg Turnpike   Wayne, NJ 07470   (973)942-6900

Kalawadia, Jay Vinodrai, MD {1417186156} SrgOrt
+ Advanced Orthopaedic Centers
414 Tatum Street   Woodbury, NJ 08096   (856)848-3880   Fax (856)848-4895

Kalaydjian, Garine, MD {1184657660} IntrMd(98,DMN01)<NJ-STCLRDEN>
+ St. Clare's Hospital-Denville Campus
25 Pocono Road   Denville, NJ 07834   (973)625-6000   Fax (973)989-3106

Kalayjian, Tro, DO {1558660720} IntrMd(11,NY76)
+ 328 Bridge Plaza North/Suite 1-H
Fort Lee, NJ 07024

Kaldany, Herbert A., DO {1962636498} Psychy(92,NY75)
+ 1930 East Marlton Pike/Suite M-69
Cherry Hill, NJ 08003

Kale, Meera V., MD {1043338254} Pedtrc(96,INDI)
+ Pediatrix Medical Group
255 Third Avenue   Long Branch, NJ 07740   (732)222-7006

Kalevich, Serge F., MD {1538151329} IntrMd(74,NJ05)<NJ-CHILTON>
+ West Milford Medical Center
1485 Union Valley Road   West Milford, NJ 07480   (973)728-1880   Fax (973)728-1559

Kalia, Amita, MD {1376619353} IntrMd, OncHem(94,INA07)<NJ-VALLEY>
+ RS Hematology Oncology
1124 East Ridgewood Avenue   Ridgewood, NJ 07450   (201)652-8585   Fax (201)612-1439

Kalia, Jessica Leigh, DO {1588875306} Pedtrc, NnPnMd(02,IA75)<NJ-NWRKBETH>
+ Newark Beth Israel Medical Center
201 Lyons Avenue   Newark, NJ 07112   (973)926-7000

Kalika, Sanna, MD {1396700795} IntrMd(00,DMN01)<NJ-STBARNMC>
+ Doctors MediCenter
835 Roosevelt Avenue/Plaza 12/Suite 4A   Carteret, NJ 07008   (732)969-2240   Fax (732)969-2152
+ Healthpoint Medical Group of Keyport LLC
39 West Front Street   Keyport, NJ 07735   (732)969-2240   Fax (732)264-4291

Kalika, Valery, MD {1891844429} NuclMd, RadDia(65,RUS06)
+ Imaging Subspecialists of North Jersey LLC
703 Main Street   Paterson, NJ 07503   (973)754-2645

Kalina, Michael, DO {1861574329} SrgCrC, Surgry<NJ-CHSFULD>
+ Capital Health Medical
2 Capital Way/Suite 356   Pennington, NJ 08534   (609)537-6000   Fax (609)537-6002

Kalinine, Viatcheslav, MD {1184765307} Anesth(88,RUS66)<NJ-STBARNMC>
+ St. Barnabas Medical Center
94 Old Short Hills Road   Livingston, NJ 07039   (973)322-5000

Kalischer, Alan L., MD {1598727299} CdvDis, IntrMd(77,NY09)<NJ-OVERLOOK, NJ-JFKMED>
+ Fanwood Westfield Cardiology
313 South Avenue   Fanwood, NJ 07023   (908)889-1900   Fax (908)889-0800
mhansen284@gmail.com
+ Fanwood Westfield Cardiology
134 South Euclid Avenue   Westfield, NJ 07090   (908)301-0441

Kalish, Joanne B., DO {1790724292} IntrMd(88,NY75)
+ 863 State Road
Princeton, NJ 08540   (609)924-5440   Fax (609)921-3438

Kalisher, Lester, MD {1558306969} Radiol, RadDia(66,MI07)<NJ-STBARNMC>
+ St. Barnabas Medical Center
94 Old Short Hills Road   Livingston, NJ 07039   (973)533-5822

Kalishman, Raffaella Linda, MD {1255610507} InfDis, IntrMd(09,GRN01)
+ 1 Degraw Avenue/Suite B
Teaneck, NJ 07666   (201)855-8480   Fax (201)836-7838
+ 85 Harristown Road/Suite 104
Glen Rock, NJ 07452   (201)855-8480

Kaliyadan, George, MD {1679960959} Pedtrc
+ University Medical Group Pediatrics
125 Paterson Street/MEB 3rd Fl   New Brunswick, NJ 08903   (732)235-7883   Fax (732)235-7345

Kallich, Marsha M., MD {1053381624} InfDis, IntrMd(80,NY08)
+ Highland Park Medical Associates
579A Cranbury Road/Suite 102   East Brunswick, NJ 08816   (732)613-0711   Fax (732)613-5783

Kallina, Lauren A., MD {1023017357} Ophthl, OthrSp(92,DC02)<NY-NYEYEINF>
+ NJ Retina
1255 Broad Street/Suite 104   Bloomfield, NJ 07003   (973)707-5632   Fax (973)707-7349

Kallini, Ronnie N., MD {1417389339} IntrMd<NJ-MORRISTN>
+ Morristown Medical Center
100 Madison Avenue   Morristown, NJ 07962   (862)881-9874

Kalliny, Mohsen Ayad, MD {1629009568} Anesth(76,EGY04)<NJ-JRSYSHMC>
+ Jersey Shore University Medical Center
1945 Route 33/Anesthesiology   Neptune, NJ 07753   (732)775-5500   Fax (732)897-0263
+ Jersery Shore Anesthesiology
1945 Highway 33   Neptune, NJ 07753   (732)775-5500   Fax (732)897-0263

Kalmar, Edward T., MD {1356399000} IntrMd(73,NJ05)<NJ-CLARMAAS, NJ-MTNSIDE>
+ The Internet Medical Group, P.C.
181 Franklin Avenue/Suite 204   Nutley, NJ 07110   (973)667-8117   Fax (973)667-6642

Kalnins, Linda Y., MD {1003825514} Ophthl(87,DC02)
+ 12 Knollwood Trail West
Mendham, NJ 07945   (973)539-1900   Fax (973)539-1901

Kalola, Vijay K., MD {1649373978} IntrMd(91,INA20)<NJ-OURLADY, NJ-KMHSTRAT>
+ PO Box 40
Somerdale, NJ 08083   (856)309-1866   Fax (856)309-1868

Kalra, Amit, MD {1467673467} CdvDis(01,MD01)<NJ-RWJUBRUN, NJ-STPETER>
+ Cardiology Associates of New Brunswick
593 Cranbury Road/Suite 2   East Brunswick, NJ 08816   (732)390-3333   Fax (732)390-9244

Kalra, Krishan G., MD {1871537472} CdvDis, IntrMd(86,INDI)<NJ-CHSFULD>
+ Capital Cardiology Associates
40 Fuld Street/Suite 400   Trenton, NJ 08638   (609)396-1644   Fax (609)394-9526

Kalra, Rakhi, MD {1922178466} IntrMd(96,NY15)
+ UH- Robert Wood Johnson Med
125 Paterson Street/Suite 2300   New Brunswick, NJ 08901   (732)828-3000

Kalra, Ritesh, MD {1043436348} IntrMd(02,POLA)
+ 196 Paterson Avenue/1st Floor
East Rutherford, NJ 07073   (201)460-8060   Fax (201)460-8070

Kalra, Tamanna H., MD {1588851398} Nephro, IntrMd(02,NJ05)
+ Brunswick Nephrology and Hypertension, LLC.
18 Centre Drive/Suite 201   Monroe, NJ 08831   (609)655-1100   Fax (732)289-6239

Kalsi, Kamaljeet Singh, DO {1649430950}<NJ-STJOSHOS>
+ Urgent Care
282 East Route 4   Paramus, NJ 07652   (551)222-0800
+ St. Joseph's Regional Medical Center
703 Main Street/EmergMed   Paterson, NJ 07503   (973)754-2000

Kaltman, Leah B., MD {1972505550} IntrMd(90,NY09)<NJ-OVERLOOK, NJ-STBARNMC>
+ West Orange Primary Care
449 Mount Pleasant Street   West Orange, NJ 07052   (973)736-2290   Fax (973)736-0105

Kalu, Eke N., MD {1659503837} IntrMd
+ 2806 Burroughs Mill Circle
Cherry Hill, NJ 08002

Kalu, Ogori N., MD {1992942676} Surgry(04,NY09)<NJ-MORRISTN, NJ-MTNSIDE>
+ Summit Breast Care/The Connie Dwyer Breast Center
111 Central Avenue   Newark, NJ 07102   (973)877-2770   Fax (973)877-5205
+ St. Michael's Medical Center
268 MLK Jr. Boulevard   Newark, NJ 07102   (973)877-5000

Kaluhiokalani, Leiloni Heather, DO {1891923884} EmrgMd
+ SJH Emergency Medicine
1505 West Sherman Avenue   Vineland, NJ 08360   (856)881-9150   Fax (888)395-8975

Kaluski, Edo, MD {1245321249} CdvDis, IntrMd(84,ISRA)
+ 36 West Mcclellan Avenue
Livingston, NJ 07039

Kalyanaraman, Meena, MD {1821174558} Pedtrc, PedCrC(91,INA2X)<NJ-NWRKBETH>
+ Newark Beth Israel Medical Center
201 Lyons Avenue/PediCriticlCare   Newark, NJ 07112   (973)926-7000   Fax (973)926-6452

Kalyoussef, Evelyne, MD {1053516765} Otlryg<NJ-UMDNJ>
+ Rutgers NJ School of Medicine Neurology
90 Bergen Street/DOC 5200   Newark, NJ 07103   (973)972-4588   Fax (973)972-5059

Kalyoussef, Sabah, DO {1598089195} EmrgPedr<NY-CHMONTEF>
+ St. Peter's University Hospital
254 Easton Avenue   New Brunswick, NJ 08901   (732)339-7041

Kamakshi, Savithri, MD {1801958640} Psychy(70,INA47)<NJ-GRYSTPSY>
+ 127 Patriots Road
Morris Plains, NJ 07950

Kamal, Roohi, MD {1326090135} ObsGyn(80,PAKI)<NJ-CLARMAAS, NJ-HCKTSTWN>
+ Summit OBGYN LLC
331 Summit Avenue   Hackensack, NJ 07601   (201)457-2300   Fax (201)457-1715

Kamal-Mostafavi, Noreen, MD {1073748018} ObsGyn(06,GRN01)
+ Clifton Ob/Gyn
1033 Route 46 East/Suite 102   Clifton, NJ 07013   (973)779-7979   Fax (973)779-7970

Kamalakar, Peri, MD {1598780371} PedHem, Pedtrc(67,INA62)<NJ-MONMOUTH, NJ-NWRKBETH>
+ Valerie Fund Childrens Center
201 Lyons Avenue   Newark, NJ 07112   (973)926-7161   Fax (973)282-0395
pkamalakar@barnabashealth.org
+ The Valerie Fund Children's Center
95 Old Short Hills Road   Livingston, NJ 07039   (973)926-7161   Fax (973)322-2856
+ Monmouth Medical Center
300 Second Avenue   Long Branch, NJ 07112   (732)222-5200

Physicians by Name and Address

Kamalu, Okebugwu, MD {1053720847} IntHos<NJ-COOPRUMC>
+ Cooper University Hospital
One Cooper Plaza Camden, NJ 08103 (856)342-2000

Kamat, Sanjay Dattatraya, DO {1205886421} Ophthl(98,MO78)
+ Campus Eye Group & Laser Center
1700 Whitehorse Hamilton Sq Rd Hamilton Square, NJ 08690 (609)587-2020 Fax (609)588-9545

Kamath, Ashwin S., MD {1891950010} Surgry(06,INA1D)
+ Atlantic Shore Surgical Associates
478 Brick Boulevard Brick, NJ 08723 (514)803-1741 Fax (732)701-1244
k.ashwin.kamath@gmail.com

Kamath, Chandrakal Y., MD {1134149545} Surgry(68,INA69)<NJ-STPETER>
+ C. Y. Kamath M.D.
26 Kingston Terrace Princeton, NJ 08540 (609)921-6992 Fax (609)921-2847
+ C. Y. Kamath M.D.
1520 Route 130 North/Suite 202 North Brunswick, NJ 08902 (732)821-1616
+ Cares Surgicenter, LLC.
240 Easton Avenue New Brunswick, NJ 08540 (732)565-5400 Fax (732)296-8677

Kamath, Sudha P., MD {1720002900} IntrMd, Rheuma(81,INDI)<NJ-STPETER, NJ-UNVMCPRN>
+ Spectrum Medical Associates
3250 State Route 27/Suite 103 Kendall Park, NJ 08824 (732)398-9100 Fax (732)398-9101

Kamath, Vijay, MD {1467616995} SrgVas, Surgry(06,INA68)
+ Deborah Heart and Lung Center
200 Trenton Road/Surgery/Vascul Browns Mills, NJ 08015 (609)893-6611
+ 25 Mule Road/Suite B5
Toms River, NJ 08753 (609)893-6611 Fax (732)557-5016
+ 1322 Route 72 West/Suite 1
Manahawkin, NJ 08015 (609)597-4479 Fax (609)597-8382

Kambam, Shravan R., MD {1124055272} RadOnc(00,TN06)<NJ-VALLEY>
+ The Valley Hospital
223 North Van Dien Avenue/Radiology Ridgewood, NJ 07450 (201)447-8000

Kambolis, Joanne Peter, MD {1184642126} Pedtrc(98,HUN02)<NJ-HOLYNAME>
+ Holy Name Hospital
718 Teaneck Road/EmrgMed Teaneck, NJ 07666 (201)833-3210 Fax (201)833-7095

Kamdar, Mehul R., MD {1275786089} SrgPlstc
+ 53 Whitewood Drive
Morris Plains, NJ 07950 (917)656-1977 Fax (973)577-6049

Kamel, Emad R., MD {1083676746} PulDis, CritCr, IntrMd(94,EGY05)<NJ-OCEANMC, NJ-COMMED>
+ Ocean Pulmonary Associates PA
457 Jack Martin Boulevard/Suite 4 Brick, NJ 08724 (732)840-4200 Fax (732)840-6444
+ Ocean Pulmonary Associates PA
3 Plaza Drive/Suite 2 Toms River, NJ 08757 (732)840-4200 Fax (732)505-9296
+ Ocean Pulmonary Associates PA
70 Lacey Road/Irish Branch Mall Whiting, NJ 08724 (732)350-4777

Kamerling, Joseph M., MD {1972591634} Ophthl(89,PA02)<NJ-OURLADY, NJ-VIRTBERL>
+ 423 Clements Bridge Road
Barrington, NJ 08007 (856)547-0804 Fax (856)547-2780
+ Wills Eye Surgery Center in Cherry Hill
408 Route 70 East Cherry Hill, NJ 08034 (856)547-0804 Fax (856)429-7555

Kamieniecki, Robert Edward, MD {1093935835} RadDia(01,NJ06)
+ 9 Debby Lane
Warren, NJ 07059

Kamin, Marc, MD {1760625263} Nrolgy(75,NY08)
+ 22-10 Route 208 South
Fair Lawn, NJ 07410

Kamin, Stephen S., MD {1538182704} Nrolgy(84,MA01)<NJ-UMDNJ>
+ University Hospital-Doctors Office Center
90 Bergen Street/Ste 8100 Newark, NJ 07103 (973)972-2550 Fax (973)972-2559
kaminst@umdnj.edu
+ Rutgers NJ School of Medicine Neurology
90 Bergen Street/DOC 5200 Newark, NJ 07103 (973)972-2550 Fax (973)972-5059

Kaminek, Alexandra, DO {1922584853}
+ Atlantic Eye Physicians
279 Third Avenue/Suite 204 Long Branch, NJ 07740 (732)222-7373 Fax (732)222-7372

Kaminetsky, Eric Jay, DO {1093969164} FamMed
+ first Urgent Medical Care
3175 Route 10 East/Suite 500 Denville, NJ 07834 (973)891-1213 Fax (973)891-1216

Kaminski, Donna Marie, DO {1033489802}
+ Somerset Family Practice
110 Rehill Avenue Somerville, NJ 08876 (908)685-2900 Fax (908)704-3764

Kaminski, Mitchell Anthony, MD {1013060466} FamMed, IntrMd(79,MI01)
+ AtlantiCare Family Medicine
120 South White Horse Pike Hammonton, NJ 08037 (609)561-4211 Fax (609)561-0639

Kaminsky, Lillian M., MD {1174563969} ObsGyn
+ University Medical Group/OBGYN
125 Paterson Street/2nd Floor New Brunswick, NJ 08901 (732)235-6600 Fax (732)235-6627

Kaminskyj, Megan Elizabeth, MD {1982991618} ObsGyn
+ St. Joseph's Regional Medical Center
703 Main Street Paterson, NJ 07503 (973)617-7401

Kamm, Ronald L., MD {1851439103} Psychy(68,PA09)
+ 257 Monmouth Road/Suite A5
Oakhurst, NJ 07755 (732)517-0595 Fax (732)517-8585

Kammiel, Rita R., MD {1427142736} Psychy(76,EGYP)<NJ-ACMC-MAIN, NJ-ACMCITY>
+ 707 White Horse Pike/Suite A-3
Absecon, NJ 08201 (609)383-3330 Fax (609)383-3301

Kamoun, Layla, MD {1922087774} Ophthl, IntrMd(93,PA01)
+ Garden State Community Medical Center
100 Brick Road/Suite 115 Marlton, NJ 08053 (856)983-1400 Fax (856)983-1681

Kampf, Richard S., MD {1366614315} IntrMd(75,NY20)
+ 16 Seminole Avenue
Oakland, NJ 07436

Kampf, Robyn A., MD {1285665919} Pedtrc(94,NY47)<NJ-ENGLEWOOD>
+ Englewood Hospital and Medical Center
350 Engle Street/PedsClinic Englewood, NJ 07631 (201)894-3000 Fax (201)569-5983

Kamplain, Trey Lee, MD {1053305680} RadDia(98,AL02)<PA-CHSTNHL, NJ-MEMSALEM>
+ Memorial Hospital of Salem County
310 Woodstown Road/Diag Radiology Salem, NJ 08079 (856)935-1000

Kamra, Roopama, MD {1083996003} IntrMd(97,BLA02)
+ Dorfner Family Medicine
811 Sunset Road/Suite 101 Burlington, NJ 08016 (609)387-9242 Fax (609)387-9408

Kanamori, Hiromi, MD {1427141829} EmrgMd, GenPrc(79,NY19)<NJ-MONMOUTH>
+ Monmouth Medical Center
300 Second Avenue/EmergMed Long Branch, NJ 07740 (732)222-5200

Kanarek, Ninette Marciano, MD {1295876514} Pedtrc(96,NY46)<NJ-VALLEY, NJ-HACKNSK>
+ Teaneck Pediatric Associates PA
197 Cedar Lane Teaneck, NJ 07666 (201)836-7171 Fax (201)928-4227

Kanarek, Samantha Leigh, DO {1912174012} PhysMd, IntrMd(NY75
+ Brielle Orthopedics PA
457 Jack Martin Boulevard Brick, NJ 08724 (732)840-7500 Fax (732)840-2088

Kanarek, Steven Edward, MD {1851429518} CdvDis, IntrMd(96,NY46)<NJ-HACKNSK>
+ Cardiac Medical Associates PA
920 Main Street Hackensack, NJ 07601 (201)342-7733 Fax (201)342-7998

Kancherla, Sandarsh Raj, MD {1568641058} Gastrn, IntrMd(06,NJ05)
+ Englewood Endoscopic Assocociates
420 Grand Avenue/Suite 101 Englewood, NJ 07631 (201)569-7044 Fax (201)569-1999

Kanchwala, Suhail Khuzema, MD {1174689038} SrgPlstc
+ Virtua Primary Care
401 Young Avenue/Suite 260 Moorestown, NJ 08057 (856)291-8920 Fax (856)291-8922

Kandasamy, Rajaram, MD {1134269954} IntrMd, Nephro(89,SRI03)<NJ-CHSMRCER>
+ 5 Rushton Court
Princeton, NJ 08550

Kandathil, Mathew K., MD {1346232097} Gastrn, IntrMd(74,INA67)<NJ-KIMBALL, NJ-COMMED>
+ Shore Medical Specialists
500 River Avenue Lakewood, NJ 08701 (732)363-7200 Fax (732)367-4461
+ Shore Medical Specialists
9 Hospital Drive Toms River, NJ 08755 (732)363-7200 Fax (732)349-9697

Kandinov, Fanya, MD {1811943277} IntrMd(72,UZB44)<NJ-HACKNSK>
+ 540A Glen Avenue
Palisades Park, NJ 07650 (201)328-2888

Kandra, Arun M., MD {1376703132} Anesth(98,INA7C)<NJ-RWJUBRUN>
+ Robert Wood Johnson-UMDNJ Anesthesia Group

125 Paterson Street/CAB 3100 New Brunswick, NJ 08901 (732)235-7827 Fax (732)235-6131

Kandula, Praveena, MD {1114123239} RadDia
+ University Radiology Group, P.C.
483 Cranbury Road East Brunswick, NJ 08816 (732)390-0030 Fax (732)390-1856

Kandula, Sridevi, MD {1194942805} FamMed<NJ-JFKMED>
+ JFK Family Practice Group
65 James Street Edison, NJ 08818 (732)321-7487 Fax (732)906-4927

Kandula, Swetha, MD {1861604795} Dermat(03,INA97)
+ M.C. Medical Group
1425 Pompton Avenue/Suite 1-1 Cedar Grove, NJ 07009 (217)801-3989 Fax (973)785-8680
+ Advanced Laser & Skin Cancer Center
870 Palisade Avcenue/Suite 302 Teaneck, NJ 07666 (217)801-3989 Fax (201)836-4716

Kane, Edwin P., MD {1720012545} Surgry(78,ITA17)<NJ-STMRY-PAS, NJ-STJOSHOS>
+ Surgery Associates of North Jersey, P.A.
1100 Clifton Avenue Clifton, NJ 07013 (973)778-0100 Fax (973)778-2029

Kane, Frank L., MD {1154390540} FamMed(82,NJ05)<NJ-STCLR-SUS, NJ-NWTNMEM>
+ MDVIP Office at DrakeÆs Pond Professional Building
33 Newton-Sparta Road/Suite 2 Newton, NJ 07860 (973)383-5844 Fax (973)383-8692
+ Skylands Medical Group PA
33 Newton-Sparta Road/Suite 1 Newton, NJ 07860 (973)383-5844 Fax (973)383-0448

Kane, Haresh Shaba, MD {1134290224} IntrMd
+ Princeton Wound Care Center
3626 Route 1 North Princeton, NJ 08540 (609)945-3611 Fax (609)945-3688

Kane, Michelle Christine, DO {1740204551} FamMed
+ Partners in Primary Care
239 Hurffville Crosskeys Road Sewell, NJ 08080 (856)341-8181 Fax (856)341-8180

Kane, Patrick, MD {1730576117} Psychy
+ 1945 State Route 33
Neptune City, NJ 07753 (732)775-5000

Kane, Patrick Martin, MD {1396907838} Ortped, SrgOrt(08,NJ06)
+ South Jersey Hand Center
1888 Marlton Pike East/Suite E-F-G Cherry Hill, NJ 08003 (856)489-5630 Fax (856)489-5631

Kane, Seth O., MD {1679614358} SrgOrt(73,NY19)<NJ-HACKNSK, NJ-BERGNMC>
+ 550 Kindermack Road/Suite 204
Oradell, NJ 07649 (201)261-7980 Fax (201)261-8050
SethKaneMD@aol.com

Kanellakos, James George, MD {1750499455} SrgOrt(96,NS01)<NY-LDYLORDS, NY-UHSBINGH>
+ The Orthopedic Group, P.A.
261 James Street/Suite 3-F Morristown, NJ 07960 (973)538-0029 Fax (973)538-0029

Kanengiser, Bruce Evan, MD {1801956271} Ophthl(78,NY19)<NY-NYUTISCH>
+ Clinical Research Laboratories, Inc.
371 Hoes Lane Piscataway, NJ 08854 (732)981-1444 Fax (732)562-1586

Kanengiser, Steven Jay, MD {1316032998} PedPul, Pedtrc(84,CA02)<NJ-VALLEY>
+ Kireker Center for Child Development
505 Goffle Road/PediPulm Ridgewood, NJ 07450 (201)447-8026 Fax (201)251-3333
kanest@valleyhealth.com

Kanetkar, Madhavi Jayat, MD {1205833944} Anesth(92,INA4X)<NJ-STJOSHOS>
+ St. Joseph's Regional Medical Center Anesthesia
703 Main Street Paterson, NJ 07503 (973)754-2323 Fax (973)977-9455

Kang, Ashley Eunhye, MD {1891141958}<NJ-HACKNSK>
+ Hackensack University Medical Center
30 Prospect Avenue Hackensack, NJ 07601 (551)996-7548

Kang, Chang H., MD {1831109917} AnesPain, IntrMd(71,JAPA)
+ 1101 Palisade Avenue
Fort Lee, NJ 07024 (201)224-8477 Fax (201)224-8479

Kang, David H., MD {1659318285} IntrMd(79,KOR11)<NJ-RWJU-RAH>
+ 1457 Raritan Road/Suite 203
Clark, NJ 07066 (908)709-4114 Fax (908)709-8011

Kang, Katherine E. Lee, MD {1356374631} ObsGyn(98,NY46)
+ Gene Medical Group
464 Hudson Terrace/Suite 203 Englewood Cliffs, NJ 07632 (201)567-7725 Fax (201)567-5255

Kang, Mohleen, MD {1184967713} IntrMd
+ University Hospital Medicine
150 Bergen Street/Room I-248 Newark, NJ 07103 (973)972-6056 Fax (973)972-3129

Kang, Richard, MD {1407874100} AnesPain, PainInvt, IntrMd(00,MNT01)<NJ-CHRIST>
+ Metropolitan Pain Consultants
  1640 Schlosser Street/Suite C-3 Fort Lee, NJ 07024 (201)729-0001 Fax (201)729-0006
+ Metropolitan Pain Consultants
  464 Valley Brook Avenue Lyndhurst, NJ 07071 (201)729-0001 Fax (201)729-0006
+ Metropolitan Pain Consultants
  1340 State Highway 34/Suite A Aberdeen, NJ 07024 (201)729-0001 Fax (201)729-0006

Kang, Richard T., MD {1730340118} Anesth, PainMd(03,NY08)
+ The AIPM Group
  1037 Route 46 East/Suite G-5 Clifton, NJ 07013 (973)928-5363 Fax (973)928-5359

Kang, Soonmo Peter, MD {1306009279} OncHem
+ Merck and Company Incorporated
  126 East Lincoln Avenue/PO Box 2000 Rahway, NJ 07065 (732)574-4000

Kang, Yong, MD {1609932433} PthACl(84,CHN4A)<NJ-MONMOUTH>
+ Laboratory Medicine Associates, PA
  300 Second Avenue/Dept of Pathology Long Branch, NJ 07740 (732)923-7380 Fax (732)923-7355

Kang-Lee, Elica J., MD Pedtrc(84,VA04)
+ Kang Lee and Lee Allergy/Pediatrics
  2177 Oak Tree Road/Suite 207 Edison, NJ 08820 (732)549-7007

Kania, Nirmala R., MD {1831118009} IntrMd, Onclgy, OncHem(78,INA53)<NJ-STBARNMC, NJ-EASTORNG>
+ Orange Medical Group
  310 Central Avenue/Suite 106 East Orange, NJ 07018 (973)674-4542 Fax (973)674-3901

Kanikicharla, Uma, MD {1487840039} Pedtrc(95,INA1L)
+ Internet Medical Group, P.C.
  66 Somme Street Newark, NJ 07105 (973)589-7337 Fax (973)589-1905

Kanj, Hassan A., MD {1598815987} IntrMd, EnDbMt(82,LEB03)<NJ-JFKMED, NJ-SOMERSET>
+ Diabetes & Osteoporosis Center
  20 Wills Way Piscataway, NJ 08854 (732)562-0027 Fax (732)562-0041

Kankanala, Sucharitha, MD {1356580054}
+ Endocrine Associates of Southern Jersey
  703 East Main Street/Suite 5 Moorestown, NJ 08057 (856)727-0900 Fax (856)231-2428

Kann, Brian Robert, MD {1689763179} SrgC&R, Surgry(97,PA09)<NJ-COOPRUMC>
+ Cooper Surgical Associates
  3 Cooper Plaza/Suite 411 Camden, NJ 08103 (856)342-2270 Fax (856)365-1180

Kanna, Sowjanya, MD {1851624787}
+ Rutgers- New Jersey Medical School
  185 South Orange Avenue/Room H-538 Newark, NJ 07103 (973)972-5252
  drsowjanyakanna@gmail.com

Kannankeril, Mary C., MD {1629115126} Psychy(76,INDI)
+ 170 Changebridge Road/Building B-34
  Montville, NJ 07045 (973)276-0041

Kanner Liebman, Rachel Brooke, DO {1780858118} FamMed
+ Kaleidoscope Medical Associates
  410 Coventry Drive Phillipsburg, NJ 08865 (908)454-9902 Fax (908)454-9905

Kannisto, Cheryl Lynne, MD Surgry(94,KY02)
+ 18 Oak Park Drive
  Morristown, NJ 07960

Kanoff, Jack M., DO {1902813843} PulDis(82,PA77)
+ South Jersey Chest Diseases
  107 Vine Street Hammonton, NJ 08037 (609)561-7666 Fax (609)561-8347

Kanoff, Martin E., DO {1285664854} ObsGyn(81,PA77)<NJ-KENEDYHS, NJ-KMHTURNV>
+ Harmony HealthCare for Women, LLC
  139 Ganttown Road/PO Box 1109 Turnersville, NJ 08012 (856)232-0050 Fax (856)232-0251

Kanouka, Indira Jouma, MD {1023193356} IntrMd(92,SYR02)<NJ-KIMBALL, NJ-MONMOUTH>
+ Medical Associates of Marlboro PC
  32 North Main Street Marlboro, NJ 07746 (732)462-4100 Fax (732)462-3798
+ Kimball Medical Center
  600 River Avenue/Internal Med Lakewood, NJ 08701 (732)598-3308
+ Specialty Hospital at Monmouth
  300 Second Avenue/Greenwall 6 Long Branch, NJ 07746 (732)923-5037 Fax (732)923-6580

Kanowitz, Seth J., MD {1649375759} Otlryg, PedOto, PlsSH-Nck(01,FL04)<NJ-MORRISTN>
+ 95 Madison Avenue/Suite 105
  Morristown, NJ 07960 (973)644-0808 Fax (973)644-9270

Kansagra, Ashwin Maganlal, MD {1508984519} Surgry, OccpMd(88,SCO05)
+ Concentra Medical Centers
  595 Division Street Elizabeth, NJ 07201 (908)289-5646 Fax (908)351-1099

Kansagra, Chunilal H., MD {1538146030} Psychy(73,INDI)<NJ-JRSYSHMC, NJ-CENTRAST>
+ 1540 State Route 138/Suite 208
  Wall, NJ 07719 (732)449-0290 Fax (732)614-4343
+ Jersey Shore University Medical Center
  1945 Route 33/Psychiatry Neptune, NJ 07753 (732)776-4339
+ CentraState Medical Center
  901 West Main Street/Psych Freehold, NJ 07719 (732)431-2000

Kansagra, Ketan Vallabh, MD {1609839331} Pedtrc, NnPnMd(97,PA02)<NJ-HUNTRDN>
+ Newark Beth Israel Medical Center
  201 Lyons Avenue/Suite C 9 Newark, NJ 07112 (973)926-7203 Fax (973)926-2332

Kansagra, Nilesh V., MD {1437286002} EmrgMd(04,NJ05)<NJ-WAYNEGEN>
+ St. Joseph's Wayne Hospital
  224 Hamburg Turnpike/Emergency Wayne, NJ 07470 (973)740-0607 Fax (973)740-8595
+ Emergency Medical Associates of NJ, P.A.
  3 Century Drive Parsippany, NJ 07054 (973)740-0607 Fax (973)740-9895

Kanter, Alan I., MD {1184678328} Pedtrc(70,NY46)<NJ-ENGLEWOOD, NY-PRSBCOLU>
+ Metropolitan Pediatric Group
  704 Palisade Avenue Teaneck, NJ 07666 (201)836-4301 Fax (201)836-5110
+ Metropolitan Pediatric Group
  570 Piermont Road/17 Closter Commons Closter, NJ 07624 (201)836-4301 Fax (201)768-7316

Kanter, Eric D., MD {1558365411} Ophthl, VitRet(89,NY46)<NJ-STBARNMC, NJ-MORRISTN>
+ Retina-Vitreous Consultants
  349 East Northfield Road/Suite 100 Livingston, NJ 07039 (973)716-0123 Fax (973)716-0441
  Kanter@rvc-nj.com
+ Retina-Vitreous Consultants
  95 Madison Avenue/Suite A03 Morristown, NJ 07960 (973)716-0123 Fax (973)716-0441
+ Short Hills Surgery Center
  187 Millburn Avenue/Suite 101 Millburn, NJ 07039 (973)671-0555 Fax (973)671-0557

Kanter, Lawrence E., MD {1710067970} Anesth(89,PA01)
+ 381 Christopher Drive
  Princeton, NJ 08540

Kantha, Brinda Sri, DO {1851452007} PhysMd, PainInvt, SprtMd(00,PA77)
+ 575 Route 28
  Raritan, NJ 08869 (908)252-9900 Fax (908)252-9901

Kantha Bhatnagar, Rajashree, MD {1417991381} FamMed(91,INA75)<NJ-VALLEY>
+ Valley Health Medical Group
  15 Essex Road/Fifth Floor Paramus, NJ 07652 (201)291-6120 Fax (201)291-6129

Kanthala, Trishla Reddy, DO {1124361944} PhysMd
+ AP Diagnostic Imaging
  1692 Oak Tree Road/Suite 1 Edison, NJ 08820 (732)692-0542

Kanthan, Rajeswari, MD {1124074091} Pedtrc, IntrMd(79,INDI)
+ Williamstown Pediatrics
  925-A South Black Horse Pike Williamstown, NJ 08094 (856)629-9000 Fax (856)629-6440

Kanthan, Sudha, MD {1922027010} GenPrc, Pedtrc(73,INA97)<NJ-COMMED, NJ-OCEANMC>
+ Pediatric Affiliates, PA
  40 Bey Lea Road/Suite B203 Toms River, NJ 08753 (732)341-0720 Fax (732)244-6842
+ Pediatric Affiliates, PA
  400 Madison Avenue Lakewood, NJ 08701 (732)341-0720 Fax (732)364-9292
+ Pediatric Affiliates, PA
  3508 Route 9 South Howell, NJ 08753 (732)905-9166 Fax (732)905-9380

Kantor, Ruth B., MD {1235265620} Psychy(86,NJ05)<NJ-STBARNMC>
+ Ruth B. Kantor MD PA
  212 Short Hills Avenue Springfield, NJ 07081 (973)467-3267 Fax (973)564-9070
  rbkantor@comcast.net

Kantor, Thomas E., MD {1962579490} Gastrn, IntrMd(76,NY09)<NJ-WARREN>
+ 100 Coventry Drive/Red School Lane
  Phillipsburg, NJ 08865 (908)454-9728

Kanuga, Dharmishtha Jayesh, MD {1982858361} Pthlgy, PthACl, Hemato(70,INA20)
+ Quest Diagnostics Inc.
  1 Malcolm Avenue Teterboro, NJ 07608 (201)393-5000 Fax (201)393-6127

Kanuga, Jayesh G., MD {1689607871} Allrgy, Pedtrc, AlgyImmn(74,INA20)<NJ-JFKMED, NJ-RWJURAH>
+ Adult & Pediatric Allergists of Central Jersey
  1740 Oak Tree Road Edison, NJ 08820 (732)906-1717 Fax (732)906-1781
+ Adult & Pediatric Allergists of Central Jersey
  3 Hospital Plaza/Suite 405 Old Bridge, NJ 08857 (732)906-1717 Fax (732)360-0033

Kanumury, Sunita, MD {1205806924} Allrgy, Pedtrc(86,INDI)<NJ-HCKTSTWN, NJ-MORRISTN>
+ Asthma & Allergy Care, P.C.
  183 Adams Street Newark, NJ 07105 (973)589-8888
+ Asthma & Allergy Care, P.C.
  496 East Main Street/Suite 1 Denville, NJ 07834 (973)589-8888 Fax (973)627-0443
+ Asthma & Allergy Care, P.C.
  402 Chestnut Street Union, NJ 07105 (908)206-0606

Kanuri, Kavitha, MD {1053382341} PhysMd(89,INA8Y)<NJ-SOMERSET, NJ-UNVMCPRN>
+ New Jersey Rehab & Electrodiagnostics, PA
  201 Union Avenue/Suite 1A Bridgewater, NJ 08807 (908)429-7799 Fax (908)595-6331
+ New Jersey Rehab & Electrodiagnostics, PA
  71 Route 206 Hillsborough, NJ 08844 (908)203-0202

Kanwal, Sunil, MD {1780940205}
+ University Hospital Medicine
  150 Bergen Street/Room I-248 Newark, NJ 07103 (973)972-6056 Fax (973)972-3129

Kanzaria, Mitul, MD {1639499023} CdvDis
+ AtlantiCare Physicians
  318 Chris Gaupp Drive/Suite 100 Galloway, NJ 08205 (609)404-9900 Fax (609)404-3653

Kao, Sen-Pin, MD {1366418782} Anesth(68,CHNA)<NJ-HOBUNIMC>
+ Hoboken University Medical Center
  308 Willow Avenue/Anesthesiology Hoboken, NJ 07030 (201)418-1000 Fax (201)943-8105

Kapadia, Bhupendra A., MD {1316992118} FamMed, Surgry(69,INDI)<NJ-CHRIST, NJ-EASTORNG>
+ American Physician Services/Hudson HealthCare
  679 Montgomery Street Jersey City, NJ 07306 (201)433-6500 Fax (201)433-8010

Kapadia, Cyrus Baji, MD {1538140066} Anesth(80,INDI)
+ 7 Jacob Arnold Road
  Morristown, NJ 07960

Kapadia, Milan R., MD {1255483012} Pedtrc(79,INDI)<NJ-CHSFULD, NJ-CHSMRCER>
+ Quakerbridge Pediatrics
  3564 Quakerbridge Road Hamilton, NJ 08619 (609)631-9006 Fax (609)631-9008
  quakerbridgepediatrics@yahoo.com

Kapadia, Rina, MD {1679567184} IntrMd(01,GRN01)<NJ-STCLRDEN>
+ St. Clare's Hospital-Denville Campus
  25 Pocono Road Denville, NJ 07834 (973)625-6000

Kapadia, Ruby Rabiya-Sheikh, DO {1134544307}<NJ-CHRIST>
+ Christ Hospital
  176 Palisade Avenue Jersey City, NJ 07306 (201)795-8201

Kapchits, Elmira, MD {1609808807} IntrMd(75,RUS31)<NJ-RBAYOLDB>
+ Comprehensive Rehabilitation
  69 Brunswick Woods Drive East Brunswick, NJ 08816 (732)238-0080 Fax (732)238-0070

Kapila, Bina, MD {1003063595} Pedtrc(64,INDI)
+ 145 Copper Tree Court
  Edison, NJ 08820

Kapila, Rajendra, MD {1669554036} InfDis, IntrMd(64,INDI)<NJ-UMDNJ>
+ University Hospital-Doctors Office Center
  90 Bergen Street/DOC 4500 Newark, NJ 07103 (973)972-2500 Fax (973)972-2510

Kapitanyan, Raffi S., MD {1245269083} EmrgMd, EmrgEMed(02,NY08)
+ UH- RWJ Medical School
  One Robert Wood Johnson Place New Brunswick, NJ 08903 (732)235-5600

Kaplan, Adam Chaim, MD {1013330018} IntrMd(10,DMN01)<NJ-MERIDNHS>
+ Hackensack Meridian Medical Group
  19 Davis Avenue/5th-6th Floor Neptune, NJ 07753 (732)897-3990 Fax (732)897-3997

Physicians by Name and Address

Kaplan, Barnard A., MD {1558305581} Ophthl(74,PA01)<NJ-VIRTVOOR>
+ Eye Associates
  1401 Route 70 East   Cherry Hill, NJ 08034   (856)428-5797   Fax (856)428-6359
+ Eye Associates
  650 South White Horse Pike   Hammonton, NJ 08037   (856)428-5797   Fax (609)567-3705
+ Eye Associates
  141 Black Horse Pike/Suite 7   Blackwood, NJ 08034   (856)227-6262   Fax (856)227-8830

Kaplan, Bruce Zachary, MD {1982639795} Anesth, AnesPain(78,NY45)<NJ-ACMCITY>
+ AtlantiCare Anesthesiology
  65 West Jimmie Leeds Road   Pomona, NJ 08240   (609)748-7597

Kaplan, Carol Ellen, MD {1801835137} Radiol, RadMam(88,NJ05)
+ Cooper University Medical Center/Camden
  3 Cooper Plaza   Camden, NJ 08103   (856)342-3300

Kaplan, Eliot F., MD {1972527174} Psychy, IntrMd(80,PA02)<NJ-UNDRWD, NJ-ACMCMAIN>
+ ARMC Faculty Practice Psychiatry
  65 West Jimmie Leeds Road   Pomona, NJ 08240   (609)652-3551   Fax (609)404-7686

Kaplan, Ellen B., MD {1730126772} PedPul, AlgyImmn, Pedtrc(83,NY15)<NJ-HACKNSK>
+ Hackensack University Medical Center
  30 Prospect Avenue/Pedtrcs   Hackensack, NJ 07601   (201)996-5207   Fax (201)996-4969

Kaplan, Emily A., MD {1801181979} EmrgMd(11,NJ06)<MA-BIDMCEST>
+ St. Barnabas Medical Center
  94 Old Short Hills Road   Livingston, NJ 07039   (973)322-5000

Kaplan, Gabriel, MD {1639228190} PsyCAd, Psychy(80,ARG01)<NJ-HOBUNIMC>
+ 535 Morris Avenue/Suite 108
  Springfield, NJ 07081   (973)659-6060
+ B. Silver, MD & G. Kaplan, MD, PA
  535 Morris Avenue   Springfield, NJ 07081   (973)659-6060   Fax (973)376-0802

Kaplan, Gary Peter, MD {1962596015} EmrgMd, IntrMd(89,PA09)
+ Hackensack Meridian Urgent Care-Freehold
  315 West Main Street   Freehold, NJ 07728   (732)414-6850   Fax (732)414-6851
+ AFC Urgent Care Hamilton
  2222 Route 33   Hamilton, NJ 08690   (609)890-4100

Kaplan, Gordon Marc, MD {1871799080} SrgPlstc, SrgRec(99,NY03)<NJ-HACKNSK, NJ-VALLEYHS>
+ The Kaplan Center for Plastic Surgery
  1033 River Road/Unit 1   Edgewater, NJ 07020   (201)786-1977   Fax (201)731-5247
  gordonkaplanmd@gmail.com

Kaplan, Joshua Michael, MD {1407881287} IntrMd, Nephro(95,NY20)<NJ-UMDNJ>
+ University Physician Associates
  140 Bergen Street/ACC Level F   Newark, NJ 07103   (973)972-8087   Fax (973)972-6651

Kaplan, Kenneth A., MD {1376629147} Otlryg(91,NY46)<NJ-STPETER, NJ-RWJUHAM>
+ Advanced Otolaryngology Associates
  557 Cranbury Road/Suite 3   East Brunswick, NJ 08816   (732)613-0600   Fax (732)613-0508
+ ENT & Allergy Associates, LLP
  3663 Route 9 North/Suite102   Old Bridge, NJ 08857   (732)613-0600   Fax (732)707-3850

Kaplan, Leonard F., MD {1194788067} Pedtrc(84,GRN01)<NJ-VIRTVOOR, NJ-COOPRUMC>
+ Advocare Merchantville Pediatrics
  1600 Chapel Avenue/Suite 100   Cherry Hill, NJ 08002   Fax (856)665-3938

Kaplan, Murray C., MD {1346288537} IntrMd(67,NY06)<NJ-RWJUBRUN>
+ Brier Hill Court/Unit E-6B
  East Brunswick, NJ 08816   (732)238-2010   Fax (732)238-2973

Kaplan, Regina Mpakarakes, MD {1609887165} ObsGyn, IntrMd(89,NY08)<NJ-STBARNMC>
+ Center for Women's Care, P.C.
  340 Main Street/Suite 207   Madison, NJ 07940   (973)301-0081   Fax (973)301-0098

Kaplan, Richard D., MD {1073553137} Psychy(76,NY47)<NJ-ENGLWOOD>
+ Englewood Hospital and Medical Center
  350 Engle Street/Psych   Englewood, NJ 07631   (201)894-3000
  Rkaplan1@nshs.edu

Kaplan, Sarah, MD {1376665406} IntrMd, CdvDis(01,NY09)
+ Cardiovascular Associates of North Jersey
  25 Rockwood Place/Suite 440   Englewood, NJ 07631   (201)568-3690   Fax (201)568-3667

+ Cardiovascular Associates of North Jersey
  1555 Center Avenue   Fort Lee, NJ 07024   (201)568-3690   Fax (201)568-3667

Kaplan, Sheldon B., MD {1437185493} RadDia, RadNro(83,NY03)
+ Atlantic Medical Imaging
  455 Jack Martin Boulevard   Brick, NJ 08724   (732)223-9729   Fax (732)840-6459

Kaplan, Stacy M., DO {1164585659} SrgPlstc, Surgry, SrgRec(92,PA77)<NJ-UNVMCPRN, NY-NYEYEINF>
+ Godiva Plastic & Reconstructive Surgery, P.C.
  601 Ewing Street/Suite B-17   Princeton, NJ 08540   (609)688-8800   Fax (609)688-8801
  skaplando@aol.com

Kaplan, Steven Mark, MD {1942578323} RadDia
+ Bioclinica
  100 Princeton Overlook   Princeton, NJ 08540   (609)936-2600

Kaplan-Sagal, Lauren Ellen, MD {1457463671} Psychy(88,NY46)
+ 332 Springfield Avenue
  Summit, NJ 07901   (908)522-1166   Fax (908)522-1186
+ Summit Medical Group
  654 Springfield Avenue   Berkeley Heights, NJ 07922   (908)522-1166   Fax (908)665-2794

Kaplin, Aviva Wallace, DO {1346676988} Surgry<NJ-SJHREGMC>
+ SJH Regional Medical Center
  1505 West Sherman Avenue/GME   Vineland, NJ 08360   (856)641-8000

Kaplitz, Neil H., MD {1467407445} ObsGyn(90,NJ05)<NJ-ACMC-ITY>
+ Pavilion Ob/Gyn AtlantiCare
  443 Shore Road/Suite 101   Somers Point, NJ 08244   (609)677-7211   Fax (609)611-7210

Kaplounova, Irina, MD {1548487432} Gastrn, IntrMd(96,RUS15)<NJ-ENGLWOOD, NJ-HOLYNAME>
+ Englewood Endoscopic Assocociates
  420 Grand Avenue/Suite 101   Englewood, NJ 07631   (201)569-7044   Fax (201)569-1999

Kaplun, Olga, MD {1871913863} IntrMd
+ The Cooper Hospital System-Univ Hospital
  401 Haddon Avenue   Camden, NJ 08103   (856)757-7767   Fax (856)757-7803

Kapoian, Toros, MD {1083630628} Nephro, IntrMd(90,NY47)<NJ-RWJUBRUN, NJ-STPETER>
+ Robert Wood Johnson Dialysis Center
  117 North Center Drive   North Brunswick, NJ 08902   (732)677-5629   Fax (732)422-0473
  kapoiato@umdnj.edu
+ UMDNJ RWJ Nephrology
  125 Paterson Street/Suite 5100-B   New Brunswick, NJ 08901   (732)677-5629   Fax (732)235-6524

Kapoor, Amee Patel, DO {1760426894} Pedtrc(02,NY75)
+ Monmouth Family Center
  270 Broadway   Long Branch, NJ 07740   (732)923-7100   Fax (732)923-7104

Kapoor, Anil, MD {1437259751} IntrMd, Rheuma(66,INDI)<NJ-CHILTON>
+ 1680 Route 23 North/Suite 160
  Wayne, NJ 07470   (973)633-8830   Fax (973)633-8840

Kapoor, Anuj, MD {1871885509} IntrMd, IntHos
+ Allied Medical Associates
  510 Hamburg Turnpike   Wayne, NJ 07470   (973)653-9485   Fax (973)442-6009
+ St. Joseph's Wayne Hospital
  224 Hamburg Turnpike/Hospitalist   Wayne, NJ 07470   (973)956-3357

Kapoor, Ashika Patil, MD {1003841503} Psychy
+ 200 Starboard Way
  Mount Laurel, NJ 08054

Kapoor, Ashima, MD {1750811030} IntrMd
+ St Joseph's Medical Ctr Internal Med
  703 Main Street   Paterson, NJ 07503   (973)754-2000

Kapoor, Ashish, MD {1164733739} Nrolgy
+ Carepoint Health Medical Group
  631 Broadway/3rd Floor   Bayonne, NJ 07002   (732)763-2269   Fax (201)243-0377
+ 85 Maple Court
  Highland Park, NJ 08904   (646)420-0122
  karnika.kapoor@gmail.com

Kapoor, Kusum, MD {1114989738} Pedtrc, IntrMd(72,INA8A)<NJ-STPETER, NJ-RWJUBRUN>
+ Somerhills Pediatrics
  1553 Route 27/Suite 1800   Somerset, NJ 08873   (732)828-4850   Fax (732)828-4290
+ Somerhills Pediatrics
  450 Amwell Road/Suite M   Belle Mead, NJ 08502   (908)359-3338

Kapoor, Mahim, MD {1841452513} CdvDis, IntrMd
+ Monmouth Cardiology Associates, LLC
  11 Meridian Road   Eatontown, NJ 07724   (732)663-0300   Fax (732)663-0301

+ Monmouth Cardiology Associates, LLC
  222 Schanck Road/Suite 104   Freehold, NJ 07728   (732)663-0300   Fax (732)431-1712

Kapoor, Radhika, DO {1447493184} IntrMd(09,NY75)
+ Bergen Medical Alliance, P.A.
  180 Engle Street   Englewood, NJ 07631   (201)567-2050   Fax (201)568-8936

Kapoor, Rajat, DO {1881867232} Nephro, IntrMd(02,NY75)
+ Jersey Coast Nephrology & Hypertension Associates
  1541 Route 88/Suite A   Brick, NJ 08724   (732)836-3200   Fax (732)836-3201
+ Jersey Coast Nephrology & Hypertension Associates
  1008 Commons Way/Suite Q   Toms River, NJ 08755   (732)836-3200   Fax (732)818-0730

Kapoor, Saurabh, MD {1235376864} CdvDis
+ Hackensack Heart Failure Program
  20 Prospect Avenue   Hackensack, NJ 07601   (201)996-4849   Fax (201)996-5703

Kapoor, Tarun Kumar, MD {1538197900} IntrMd(00,NJ06)<NJ-VIRTMHBC>
+ Virtua Memorial
  175 Madison Avenue   Mount Holly, NJ 08060   (609)914-6180   Fax (609)614-6182

Kapoor, Vidhi, MD {1518257476}
+ 29 Point Of Woood Drive
  North Brunswick, NJ 08902   (732)777-1480
  vidhi.kapoor@gmail.com

Kapoor, Vinod, MD {1053457986} Nrolgy(80,INA3C)
+ Carepoint Health Medical Group
  631 Broadway/3rd Floor   Bayonne, NJ 07002   (201)243-0700   Fax (201)243-0377

Kappy, Kenneth Allen, MD {1295063410} MtFtMd, ObsGyn, IntrMd(74,NJ05)<NJ-NWRKBETH>
+ 9 Harrison Way
  Mount Arlington, NJ 07856   (973)601-7562

Kaptain, George J., MD {1306813621} SrgNro(93,VA01)
+ North Jersey Brain and Surgical
  680 Kinderkamack Road/Suite 300   Oradell, NJ 07649   (201)342-2550   Fax (201)342-7171

Kaptain, Stamatina, MD {1124001110} PthAcl, PthHem(93,MA01)<NJ-WAYNEGEN, NJ-CHILTON>
+ St. Joseph's Wayne Hospital
  224 Hamburg Turnpike/Pathology   Wayne, NJ 07470   (973)942-6900   Fax (973)389-4019
+ Chilton Medical Center
  97 West Parkway/Pathology   Pompton Plains, NJ 07444   (973)831-5000

Kapur, Sakshi, MD {1538509716} IntrMd
+ Berkeley Internal Medicine
  391 Springfield Avenue/Suite 1B   Berkeley Heights, NJ 07922   (908)665-1177   Fax (908)665-8420

Kapusuz, Tolga, MD {1316919004} Anesth, PainMd(92,TUR04)<NY-SLOANKET>
+ RejuV Aesthetic Gynecology
  285 Durham Avenue/Suite 1A, Bldg. 6   South Plainfield, NJ 07080   (732)338-0228   Fax (908)941-5963

Karabach, Maxim, MD {1144381005} IntrMd(84,RUSS)
+ 2101 Lake Road/Suite 1
  Whiting, NJ 08759   (732)716-1700   Fax (732)716-0500

Karabulut, Nigahus, MD {1396881280} InfDis, IntrMd(81,TUR01)<NJ-CHSFULD, NJ-CHSMRCER>
+ Pennington Medical Group
  820 Bear Tavern Road/Suite 106   Ewing, NJ 08628   (609)882-5400   Fax (609)882-5224

Karagiannis, Paul, MD {1558603704} EmrgMd
+ Cooper Univerisry Emergency Physicians
  One Cooper Plaza/Suite 152   Camden, NJ 08103   (856)342-2627   Fax (856)968-8272

Karakashian, Gary V., MD {1649227174} Dermat(84,NY03)<NJ-OCEANMC>
+ Affordable Cosmetic Surgery Center
  107 Monmouth Road/Suite 108   West Long Branch, NJ 07764   (732)544-9200   Fax (732)449-3272
+ Affordable Cosmetic Surgery Ctr
  2100 Highway 35   Sea Girt, NJ 08750   (732)449-9200

Karam, Christopher S., MD {1477866986} PhysMd(10,GRN01)
+ Performance Spine & Sports Medicine
  9500 K Johnson Boulevard/Suite 1   Bordentown, NJ 08505   (609)817-0050   Fax (609)588-8602

Karam, Edmund Thomas, MD {1932211646} IntrMd, CdvDis, CICdEI(02,DC02)<NJ-BAYSHORE, NJ-JRSYSHMC>
+ Shore Heart Group, P.A.
  35 Beaverson Boulevard/Suite 9-B   Brick, NJ 08723   (732)262-4262   Fax (732)262-4317
+ Shore Heart Group, P.A.
  1820 State Route 33/Suite 4-B   Neptune, NJ 07753   (732)262-4262   Fax (732)776-8946
+ Shore Heart Group, P.A.
  555 Iron Bridge Road/Suite 15   Freehold, NJ 08723   (732)308-0774   Fax (732)333-1366

Karam, Sara R., MD {1386850774} CdvDis, ClCdEl, IntrMd(01,VA01)<NJ-JRSYSHMC>
+ American Heart Center PC
1900 Corlies Avenue State Rout   Neptune, NJ 07753   (732)663-1123   Fax (732)663-1179

Karanam, Deepthi, MD {1093906109}
+ North Jersey Nephrology Associates PA
246 Hamburg Turnpike/Suite 207   Wayne, NJ 07470   (973)653-3366   Fax (973)653-3365

Karanam, Ravindra N., MD {1922075506} SrgCdv, SrgThr, Surgry(72,INDI)<NJ-NWRKBETH>
+ Newark Beth Israel Medical Center
201 Lyons Avenue   Newark, NJ 07112   (973)926-7747   Fax (201)923-7552

Karandikar, Shaila Y., MD {1700960465} Anesth(66,INDI)
+ Wills Surgery Center of Central New Jersey
107 North Center Drive   North Brunswick, NJ 08902   (732)297-8001   Fax (732)297-8007

Karanikolas, Steven, MD {1134202286} ObsGyn(80,GRE03)<NJ-STPETER, NJ-RWJUBRUN>
+ Brunswick-Hills Ob/Gyn, PA
751 Route 206/2nd Floor   Hillsborough, NJ 08844   (908)725-2510   Fax (908)725-2132
+ Brunswick-Hills Ob/Gyn, PA
620 Cranbury Road/Suite LL90   East Brunswick, NJ 08816   (908)725-2510   Fax (732)613-4845

Karanjgaokar, Seema Jeevan, MD {1841521598} Nephro, IntrMd(04,INA69)<NY-LINCOLN, NJ-NWRKBETH>
+ Newark Beth Israel Medical Center
201 Lyons Avenue/Nephrology   Newark, NJ 07112   (973)926-7000

Karantza-Wadsworth, Vassiliki, MD {1710928189} OncHem(01,NJ06)<NJ-RWJUBRUN>
+ Rutgers Cancer Institute of New Jersey
195 Little Albany Street/PO Box 2681   New Brunswick, NJ 08903   (732)235-2465   Fax (732)235-6797

Karanzalis, Demetrius, DO {1972803864} Anesth
+ West Jersey Anesthesia Assoc PA
102 Centre Boulevard/Suite East   Marlton, NJ 08053   (856)988-6260   Fax (856)988-6270

Karatas, Meltem, MD {1467427963} Pedtrc, NnPnMd, IntrMd(83,TUR01)
+ Meridian Medical Group - Faculty Practice
61 Davis Avenue/Suite 1   Neptune, NJ 07753   (732)776-4860   Fax (732)776-4867

Karatepe, Murat, MD {1043256134} CdvDis, IntrMd(89,TUR16)<NJ-JRSYSHMC>
+ 25 Mule Road/Suite B-2
Toms River, NJ 08755   (732)505-9005   Fax (732)505-9919

Karatoprak, Ohan, MD {1588757058} FamMed, Grtrcs(77,TURK)<NJ-HACKNSK, NJ-HOLYNAME>
+ 420 Deerwood Road
Fort Lee, NJ 07024   (201)886-8877   Fax (201)886-9335

Karcnik, Margaret A., DO {1194881730} PhysMd(88,NY75)
+ 18 Redneck Avenue
Little Ferry, NJ 07643   (201)641-3115   Fax (201)641-3116

Karetzky, Monroe Stuart, MD {1821060880} PulDis, SlpDis, Grtrcs(63,NY20)
+ 200 Engle Street
Englewood, NJ 07631   (201)569-0404   Fax (201)569-0422
mkaretzkymd@aol.com

Karger, Louise D., MD {1245202522} IntrMd(86,PA01)<NJ-MORRISTN>
+ 137 Hillcrest Avenue
Morristown, NJ 07960   (973)656-9888   Fax (973)656-9777

Kargman, Jeffrey M., MD {1942280409} Psychy, PsyGrt, PsyFor(81,NY48)<NJ-OCEANMC, NJ-JRSYSHMC>
+ 2130 Highway 35/Building A Suite 124
Sea Girt, NJ 08750   (732)974-3500   Fax (732)974-3501
jeffreykargmanmd@msn.com

Kargman, Kevin Jerome, DO {1407810302} Pedtrc, IntrMd(95,MO78)
+ Washington Pediatrics
400 Medical Drive   Sewell, NJ 08080   (856)589-0011   Fax (856)589-5015

Kargul, George John, MD {1538376421}<NJ-VIRTVOOR>
+ Virtua Voorhees
100 Bowman Drive   Voorhees, NJ 08043   (248)259-5765

Kargutkar, Smita Nandkumar, MD {1043482631} EnDbMt<NJ-MONMOUTH>
+ 225 Highway 35 North/Suite 102b
Red Bank, NJ 07701   (732)413-8000   Fax (732)400-6745
+ Monmouth Medical Center
300 Second Avenue/Suite 005   Long Branch, NJ 07740   (732)413-8000   Fax (732)923-7553
+ Barnabas Health Medical Group
1029 Sycamore Avenue   Tinton Falls, NJ 07701   (732)544-1048   Fax (732)544-1479

Karia, Roopal M., MD {1467452722} Nrolgy, NroChl, NrlgSpec(95,FL04)<NJ-JRSYSHMC>
+ Jersey Shore Child Evaluation Center
81-04 Davis Avenue   Neptune, NJ 07753   (732)776-4178

Fax (732)776-4946

Karim, Anjum Hasan, MD {1639328685} InfDis, IntrMd
+ Summit Medical Group-Berkeley Heights Campus
1 Diamond Hill Road/Inf Disease   Berkeley Heights, NJ 07922   (973)738-2285   Fax (908)790-6576

Karim, Karim Issa, MD {1417917717} IntrMd(87,SYR02)<NJ-SELSPNNJ>
+ Select Specialty Hospital-Northeast New Jersey
96 Parkway/Internal Med   Rochelle Park, NJ 07662   (201)845-0099
+ Sovereign Medical Group
15-01 Broadway/Suite 1   Fair Lawn, NJ 07410   (201)845-0099   Fax (201)791-6585
+ Urology Specialty Care, P.A.
555 Kindermack Road/Suite D   Oradell, NJ 07662   (201)834-1890   Fax (201)834-1898

Karim, Minhaz, MD {1831154426} IntrMd
+ Lourdes Medical Associates
200 Campbell Drive/Suite 102   Willingboro, NJ 08046   (609)877-4545   Fax (609)877-5129

Karim, Mona, MD {1255386371} RadOnc, Radiol, IntrMd(99,NY46)<NJ-MORRISTN>
+ Radiation Oncology Associates of North Jersey, P.A.
100 Madison Avenue   Morristown, NJ 07962   (973)971-6233   Fax (973)290-7393
mona.el-gabry@atlantichealth.org
+ Morristown Medical Center
100 Madison Avenue/Rad Onc   Morristown, NJ 07962   (973)971-6233   Fax (973)290-7393

Karim, Nuzhat, MD {1215070289} ObsGyn, Gyneco(71,PAK08)<NJ-STPETER, NJ-RWJUBRUN>
+ 3084 State Highway 27
Kendall Park, NJ 08824   (732)821-5100   Fax (732)940-1873
+ 317 Cleveland Avenue
Highland Park, NJ 08904   (732)545-8181

Karimi, Michael M., MD {1801979762} Pedtrc, FamMed(61,IRA01)<NY-BRNXLFUL>
+ 50 Kinderkamack Road
Woodcliff Lake, NJ 07677   (201)391-6700   Fax (201)391-4784

Karimi, Reza J., MD {1891950788} SrgNro(05,NJ05)<NJ-VALLEY>
+ North Jersey Brain and Surgical
680 Kinderkamack Road/Suite 300   Oradell, NJ 07649   (201)342-2550   Fax (201)342-7171

Karl, Justin Adam, MD {1134366958} CdvDis, IntrMd(06,NJ06)
+ Mercer Bucks Cardiology
3140 Princeton Pike/2nd Floor   Lawrenceville, NJ 08648   (609)895-1919   Fax (609)895-1200

Karlekar, Kripalaxmi R., MD {1598920571} CdvDis, IntrMd(70,INDI)
+ 559 Winnie Avenue
Oradell, NJ 07649

Karlin, Gary S., MD {1457334575} Urolgy(84,IL42)<NJ-CHSMRCER>
+ Urology Care Alliance
2 Princess Road/Suite J   Lawrenceville, NJ 08648   (609)895-1991   Fax (609)895-6996

Karlson, Karen B., MD RadDia, Radiol(75,NY01)<NJ-STBARNMC>
+ St. Barnabas Medical Center
94 Old Short Hills Road/Radiology   Livingston, NJ 07039   (973)322-5000

Karluk, Diane, MD PthFor(91,MN04)
+ Middlesex County-Medical Examiner
1490 Livingston Avenue/Suite 800   North Brunswick, NJ 08902   (732)745-3190   Fax (732)745-3491

Karmaker, Shekhar Chandra, MD {1134190408} Anesth(88,BAN05)
+ Institute of Ophthalmology & Visual Science
556 Eagle Rock Avenue/Suite 206   Roseland, NJ 07068   (973)228-2771   Fax (973)228-7477

Karmazin, Polina, MD {1861471161} FamMed(76,ROMA)<NJ-VIRTBERL, NJ-VIRTVOOR>
+ Integrated Family Medicine
701 Cooper Road/Suite 16   Voorhees, NJ 08043   (856)783-5000   Fax (856)783-5041

Karmel, Bruce A., MD {1568468510} Ophthl(80,NY08)<NJ-CENTRAST>
+ 710 Tennent Road
Englishtown, NJ 07726   (732)536-7600   Fax (732)972-7742

Karmel, Mitchell I., MD {1992700058} RadDia, Radiol(83,NY06)<NJ-OCEANMC>
+ Ocean Medical Center
425 Jack Martin Boulevard/Radiology   Brick, NJ 08723   (732)840-2200

Karmilovich, Beth Ann, DO {1598853228} Pedtrc, IntrMd(98,NJ75)<NJ-COOPRUMC>
+ Cooper Perinatology Associates
3 Cooper Plaza/Suite 502   Camden, NJ 08103   (856)356-4935   Fax (856)968-8499
+ Cooper University Hospital Pediatrics/Endocrinology
3 Cooper Plaza/Suite 200   Camden, NJ 08103   (856)356-

4935   Fax (856)968-8597
+ Cooper Peds/Children's Regional Ctr
6400 Main Street Complex   Voorhees, NJ 08103   (856)751-9339   Fax (856)751-8940

Karnaugh, Ronald Daniel, MD {1194965905} PhysMd, PainMd
+ JFK Neurosciences Institute
65 James Street/Second Floor   Edison, NJ 08818   (732)321-7010   Fax (732)632-1584

Karolak, Mark, DO {1063482651} Otlryg, OtgyFPlS(04,NJ75)
+ Refelctions Center for Skin & Body
1924 Washington Valley Road   Martinsville, NJ 08836   (732)356-1666

Karolchyk, Mary A., DO Nrolgy(88,MI12)
+ 103 Skyline Drive
Morristown, NJ 07960

Karoly, Michael D., MD {1902895923} ObsGyn(79,NJ06)<NJ-RIVERVW>
+ Drs. Karoly, Kaskiw, Hammond & Jacoby
180 White Road/Suite 209   Little Silver, NJ 07739   (732)842-0673   Fax (732)842-7352
+ Drs. Karoly, Kaskiw, Hammond & Jacoby
1 Bethany Road/Building 2/Suite 31   Hazlet, NJ 07730

Karou, Fadi, MD {1780870444}
+ 716 Broad Street/Suite 2 D
Clifton, NJ 07013   (423)262-7151
fadi.karoy@gmail.com

Karounos, Marianna, DO {1831536336} EmrgMd(07,NY75)<NY-PRSBWEIL>
+ St Joseph's Medical Center Emergency
703 Main Street   Paterson, NJ 07503   (973)754-2240   Fax (973)754-2249

Karp, Eric A., MD {1811972607} RadOnc(86,NY47)
+ Rahway Regional Cancer Center
892 Trussler Place   Rahway, NJ 07065   (732)382-5550   Fax (732)382-2407

Karp, George I., MD {1518955491} OncHem(76,NY01)
+ Regional Cancer Care Associates - Central Jersey Div
454 Elizabeth Avenue/Suite 240   Somerset, NJ 08873   (732)390-7750   Fax (732)390-7725

Karp, Hillel J., MD {1902851421} RadDia, Ultsnd, NuclMd(75,NY46)<NJ-CHRIST>
+ Christ Hospital
176 Palisade Avenue/Radiology   Jersey City, NJ 07306   (201)795-8250   Fax (201)795-8629
+ Radiology Professional Association
142 Palisade Avenue   Jersey City, NJ 07306   (201)795-8250   Fax (201)795-0874

Karp, Howard M., DO {1619986841} IntrMd, Nephro(69,MO79)<NJ-SHOREMEM, NJ-BURDTMLN>
+ Shore Physicians Group
2605 Shore Road   Northfield, NJ 08225   (609)365-5300   Fax (609)365-5301

Karpeh, Martin Sieh, Jr., MD {1962421339} SrgOnc, Surgry, IntrMd(83,PA14)<NJ-MTNSIDE>
+ Drs. Karpeh & Davidson
20 Prospect Avenue/Suite 406   Hackensack, NJ 07601   (551)996-2959   Fax (551)996-2021

Karpf, Gary A., MD {1679691679} Psychy(80,PA09)
+ Cedar Glen Professional Association
170 Cold Soil Road   Princeton, NJ 08540   (609)896-1122   Fax (609)896-2688

Karpf, Robin R., MD {1417070400} Psychy(81,AL02)
+ Lawrenceville School Infirmary
2500 Main Street/PO Box 6011   Lawrenceville, NJ 08648   (609)896-0400   Fax (609)895-2056

Karpinos, Robert D., MD {1972587046} Anesth, CritCr(91,ISR02)<NJ-HACKNSK>
+ Hackensack University MC-Anesthesia Dept
30 Prospect Avenue/Room 2703   Hackensack, NJ 07601   (201)996-2419   Fax (201)996-3962
+ Hackensack University Medical Center
30 Prospect Avenue/Anesth   Hackensack, NJ 07601   (201)996-2419   Fax (201)488-6769

Karpinski-Failla, Susan Ellen, DO {1801860838} FamMed(98,ME75)<NJ-WARREN>
+ Riverfield Family Health Center
1738 State Route 31 North   Clinton, NJ 08809   (908)735-4645   Fax (908)735-7361

Karpman, Jesse, MD {1801997515} PulDis, IntrMd, CritCr(86,GRN01)
+ Pulmonary and Critical Care Associates
2333 Morris Avenue/Suite B-15   Union, NJ 07083   (908)964-1964   Fax (908)964-6286
+ Pulmonary and Critical Care Associates
534 Avenue East   Bayonne, NJ 07002   (201)858-1021

Karpova, Natalia M., MD {1174850564} Pedtrc
+ 31 Alan Avenue
Glen Rock, NJ 07452

Physicians by Name and Address

Karroum, Kamil Hanna, MD {1831286517} Pedtrc(79,SYRI)<NJ-OCEANMC>
+ Family Health Center/Community Medical Center
  301 Lakehurst Road Toms River, NJ 08755 (732)557-3380 Fax (732)557-3390
+ ABC Pediatric Associates PA
  131 Drum Point Road Brick, NJ 08723 (732)477-8988

Karry Mohanrao, Shailender K., MD {1093745077} IntrMd(00,INA83)
+ 2115 Millburn Avenue/Suite L-2
  Maplewood, NJ 07040 (973)275-1322 Fax (973)900-8917

Kartika, Gunawan, MD {1225030604} Pthlgy, PthAcl, PthCyt(80,BEL03)<NJ-JRSYCITY, NJ-MEADWLND>
+ PLUS Diagnostics
  1200 River Avenue/Suite 10 Lakewood, NJ 08701 (732)901-7575 Fax (732)901-1555
+ Jersey City Medical Center
  355 Grand Street/Path Jersey City, NJ 07304 (201)915-2000

Karu, Moiz S., MD {1902871999} IntrMd, Gastrn(74,INA67)
+ 760 Bound Brook Road
  Dunellen, NJ 08812 (732)968-2811 Fax (732)968-7769

Karunanithi, Subhathra, MD {1992855258} FamMed
+ 9-10 5th Street
  Fair Lawn, NJ 07410

Karwowska, Helena, MD {1023173382} NnPnMd, Pedtrc(79,POL14)<NJ-COMMED>
+ Meridian Medical Group - Faculty Practice
  61 Davis Avenue/Suite 1 Neptune, NJ 07753 (732)776-4860 Fax (732)776-4867
+ Meridian Medical Group - Faculty Practice
  61 Davis Avenue/Suite 1 Neptune, NJ 07753 (732)776-4860 Fax (732)776-4639
+ Community Medical Center
  99 Route 37 West/Peds/Neonatlgy Toms River, NJ 07753 (732)557-8000

Kasama, Richard K., MD {1912095647} Nephro, IntrMd(85,PA09)<NJ-COOPRUMC>
+ The Cooper Hospital System-Univ Hospital
  401 Haddon Avenue Camden, NJ 08103 (856)342-2000

Kasarda, Frances E., MD {1801895693} Anesth(83,PA13)
+ West Jersey Anesthesia Associates
  102-E Center Boulevard Marlton, NJ 08053 (856)988-6250 Fax (856)988-6270

Kasaryan, Hrach Ike, DO {1023296936} IntrMd
+ Bergen Cardiology Associates
  400 Frank W. Burr Boulevard Teaneck, NJ 07666 (201)928-2300 Fax (201)692-3263
+ 36 Byrne Place
  Bergenfield, NJ 07621 (201)637-8002

Kasatkin, Alexander E., MD {1144270323} CdvDis, IntrMd(96,RUS80)<NJ-OVERLOOK>
+ 28-02 Fairlawn Avenue
  Fair Lawn, NJ 07410 (201)475-2225 Fax (201)475-2221
  Anna_kasatkin@yahoo.com

Kasdaglis, Tania Luna, MD {1366644601} MtFtMd, ObsGyn<NJ-STBARNMC>
+ St. Barnabas Medical Center
  94 Old Short Hills Road Livingston, NJ 07039 (973)322-5287 Fax (973)322-2309

Kashani, John S., DO {1700931680} EmrgMTx(00,NY75)<NJ-STMICHL>
+ St Joseph's Medical Center Emergency
  703 Main Street Paterson, NJ 07503 (973)754-2240 Fax (973)754-2249
+ New Jersey Poison Center
  65 Bergen Street/4th Floor Newark, NJ 07107 (973)754-2240 Fax (973)972-2679

Kashani, Massoud, MD {1003867722} Pthlgy, PthAcl, PthAcl(67,IRAN)<NJ-ENGLWOOD>
+ Englewood Hospital and Medical Center
  350 Engle Street/Pathology Englewood, NJ 07631 (201)894-3424 Fax (201)871-2269

Kashanian, Franciska K., MD {1154524866} Rserch, IntrMd(76,PA13)
+ Bayer HealthCare Corporation
  PO Box 1000/Pharmaceuticals Montville, NJ 07045 Fax (973)857-8168
  Fran.Kashanian@bayer.com

Kashif, Shumaila, MD {1578839775}
+ 27 Yellowstone Drive
  Old Bridge, NJ 08857 (908)965-1916
  shumkash@gmail.com

Kashif, Soofia, MD {1659641983} IntHos, IntrMd(01,PAK11)<NJ-ACMCITY>
+ Kennedy Hospitalist Office
  2201 Chapel Avenue West Cherry Hill, NJ 08002 (856)513-4124 Fax (856)302-5932
+ AtlantiCare Hospitalist Program
  1925 Pacific Avenue/8th Floor Atlantic City, NJ 08401 (856)513-4124 Fax (609)441-8002

Kashkin, Jay Michael, MD {1235128497} Allrgy, Immuno, PedAlg(83,DOMI)<NJ-HACKNSK, NJ-VALLEY>
+ 23-00 Route 208 South/1st Floor
  Fair Lawn, NJ 07410 (201)794-7400 Fax (201)475-9669

Kashlan, Bassam T., MD {1093817637} Surgry(72,SYRI)<NJ-JRSYSHMC, NJ-OCEANMC>
+ Kashlan & Schreiber
  1540 Highway 138/Suite 201 Wall, NJ 07719 (732)280-0020 Fax (732)681-0261

Kashlan, Fawaz T., MD {1205040425} NnPnMd, Pedtrc(90,SYR01)<NJ-STPETER, NJ-RWJUBRUN>
+ 5 Springhouse Road
  Ocean, NJ 07712

Kashnikow, Constantine, MD {1811956881} CdvDis, IntrMd(80,DOMI)<NJ-STBARNMC>
+ Cardiac Care of North Jersey
  340 East Northfield Road/Suite 2C Livingston, NJ 07039 (973)994-0069 Fax (973)994-0567

Kashoqa, Amer H., MD {1972615078} Psychy(82,ROMA)<NJ-CHILTON>
+ 506 HamburgTurnpike/Suite 203
  Wayne, NJ 07470 (973)633-1996 Fax (973)633-8078

Kashyap, Arun Kumar, MD {1114290996} Pedtrc(DMN01)<NJ-RWJUBRUN, NJ-SOMERSET>
+ RWJ University Hospital New Brunswick
  One Robert Wood Johnson Place New Brunswick, NJ 08901 (932)235-5709 Fax (732)235-6609

Kashyap, Meeta Parashar, MD {1760578025} ObsGyn(94,NY15)
+ AFC Urgent Care South Plainfield
  907 Oak Tree Avenue/Suite H South Plainfield, NJ 07080 (732)491-1790

Kashyap, Rupa R., MD {1699831461} IntrMd(97,INA08)<NJ-KIMBALL>
+ Kimball Medical Center
  600 River Avenue Lakewood, NJ 08701 (732)363-1900
+ 2 Dorset Court
  Princeton, NJ 08540

Kasibhotla, Sumabala, MD {1700910288} IntrMd(94,INA9D)
+ 59 East Cartwright Drive
  West Windsor, NJ 08550

Kasica, Patricia R., DO {1417013905} Anesth, IntrMd(91,NJ75)
+ Kasica Pain Management
  76 West Jimmie Leeds Road/Suite 501 Galloway, NJ 08205 (609)748-0505 Fax (609)748-0515

Kasim, Nader Q., MD {1538241955} SprtMd, SrgOrt(91,PA01)<NJ-JFKMED>
+ Advanced Orthopaedics & Sports Medicine Center, PC
  1907 Oak Tree Road/Suite 201 Edison, NJ 08820 (732)548-7332 Fax (732)548-7350

Kasimis, Basil S., MD {1720001183} Hemato, IntrMd, MedOnc(70,GRE01)<NJ-VAEASTOR, NJ-UMDNJ>
+ VA New Jersey Health Care System-East Orange Campus
  385 Tremont Avenue/Chief/Hemat/Onc East Orange, NJ 07018 (973)395-7809 Fax (973)395-7096
  basil.kasimis@med.va.gov
+ University Hospital-Doctors Office Center
  90 Bergen Street/MSB I 506 Newark, NJ 07103 (973)972-5257

Kaskiw, Eugene H., MD {1518956531} ObsGyn(84,PA09)<NJ-RIVERVW>
+ Drs. Karoly, Kaskiw, Hammond & Jacoby
  180 White Road/Suite 209 Little Silver, NJ 07739 (732)842-0673 Fax (732)842-7352
+ Drs. Karoly, Kaskiw, Hammond & Jacoby
  1 Bethany Road/Building 2/Suite 31 Hazlet, NJ 07730

Kasmin, Franklin Ethan, MD {1336178581} Gastrn, IntrMd(87,NY45)
+ Center for Endocrine Health
  1121 route 22 west/Suite 205 Bridgewater, NJ 08807 (212)734-8874 Fax (212)249-5628

Kasowitz, Andrea Ruth, DO {1659661643}
+ Mountainside Family Practice Associates
  799 Bloomfield Avenue/Suite 201 Verona, NJ 07044 (973)746-7050 Fax (973)857-2831

Kaspareck, Joseph, Jr., MD {1285615989} Ophthl(80,NJ06)
+ Central Jersey Eye Associates
  56 Union Avenue Somerville, NJ 08876 (908)725-6225 Fax (908)218-0802

Kasper, Andrew, MD {1013007459} CdvDis, IntrMd(77,NJ05)<NJ-VALLEY>
+ Saddle River Medical Group
  82 East Allendale Road/Suite 3-A Saddle River, NJ 07458 (201)825-3933 Fax (201)236-1460

Kasper, John F., DO {1205842473} IntrMd(93,NJ75)
+ 6725 Ventnor Avenue/Suite A
  Ventnor, NJ 08406 (609)487-0100 Fax (609)487-1144

Kasper, Joseph E., MD {1437247558} IntrMd(93,NJ05)<NJ-VALLEY>
+ Saddle River Medical Group
  82 East Allendale Road/Suite 3-A Saddle River, NJ 07458 (201)236-2000 Fax (201)236-1460

Kasper, Laura Carol, DO {1710098702} EmrgMd(95,NJ75)<NJ-SJHREGMC>
+ SJH Regional Medical Center
  1505 West Sherman Avenue/EmrgMed Vineland, NJ 08360 (856)641-8000

Kasper, Lydia Marie, DO {1134420565}
+ Emergency Medical Associates of NJ, P.A.
  3 Century Drive Parsippany, NJ 07054 (973)740-0607 Fax (973)740-9895

Kasper, Mark T., MD {1336189026} SrgOrt(81,PA13)<NJ-COMMED, NJ-HLTHSRE>
+ Ocean Orthopedic Associates, P.A.
  530 Lakehurst Road/Suite 1 Toms River, NJ 08755 (732)349-8454 Fax (732)341-0259

Kasper, Michael E., MD {1124280250} CdvDis
+ Saddle River Medical Group
  82 East Allendale Road/Suite 3-A Saddle River, NJ 07458 (201)825-3933 Fax (201)236-1460

Kass, Jonathan Eliot, MD {1700974441} IntrMd, PulDis, SlpDis(79,OH41)<NJ-COOPRUMC>
+ Cooper University Medical Center/Camden
  3 Cooper Plaza/Pulm/Crit Care Camden, NJ 08103 (856)342-2478 Fax (856)541-3968

Kassem, Jawad Nadim, MD {1417110438} EmrgMd(06,GRN01)<NJ-MORRISTN>
+ Morristown Medical Center
  100 Madison Avenue/Emerg Med Morristown, NJ 07962 (973)971-5000 Fax (973)251-1109
+ Robert Wood Johnson University Hospital at Rahway
  865 Stone Street/Emerg Med Rahway, NJ 07065 (732)499-6100

Kassenoff, Lisa Adrian, DO {1912960436} FamMed, IntrMd(02,PA77)<NJ-OCEANMC>
+ 138 South Main Street
  Forked River, NJ 08731 (609)756-0000 Fax (609)488-1613
+ Meridian Primary Care
  138 Route 9 South Forked River, NJ 08731 (609)756-0000 Fax (609)488-1613

Kassim, Andrea Tinuola, MD {1689802647} Dermat, IntrMd(08,DC03)
+ The Dermatology Group, P.C.
  60 Pompton Avenue Verona, NJ 07044 (973)571-2121 Fax (973)571-2126

Kassir, Ramtin Ronald, MD {1477591048} Otlryg, SrgFPl(91,TX02)<NJ-STJOSHOS, NY-LENOXHLL>
+ Mona Lisa Cosmetic Surgery Center
  1176 Hamburg Turnpike/Suite 2 Wayne, NJ 07470 (973)692-9300
  drkassir@drkassir.com
+ Ridgewood ENT and Dermatology
  81 North Maple Avenue Ridgewood, NJ 07450 (973)692-9300 Fax (201)857-2371

Kassis, Kamal F., MD {1831292010} Surgry, SrgVas(73,SYRI)<NJ-ACMCITY, NJ-ACMCMAIN>
+ Kamal F. Kassis MD, PC
  415 South Chris Gaupp Drive/Suite E Galloway, NJ 08205 (609)652-5577 Fax (609)652-1977

Kassoff, David B., MD {1619091014} Psychy(74,NY15)
+ 223 Highway 18/Suite 102
  East Brunswick, NJ 08816 (732)246-1969 Fax (732)843-3705

Kassouf, Michael J., MD {1609812528} SrgVas, Surgry(70,LEB01)<NJ-BAYSHORE>
+ 1145 Bordentown Road/Suite 10
  Parlin, NJ 08859 (732)553-0101
  doc@veinmedic.com

Kassutto, Zach, MD {1598715690} EmrgMd, EmrgPedr
+ Emergency Medical Associates of NJ, P.A.
  3 Century Drive Parsippany, NJ 07054 (973)740-0607 Fax (973)740-9895

Kastenberg, Charles A., DO {1063441400} FamMed(74,PA77)<NJ-VIRTMHBC, NJ-KMHSTRAT>
+ Alliance for Better Care, PC/Mount Holly Division
  1613 Route 38 Lumberton, NJ 08048 (609)261-3716 Fax (609)261-5507
+ Alliance for Better Care, P.C.
  PO Box 1510 Medford, NJ 08055 (609)261-3716 Fax (609)953-8652

Kastner, Theodore A., MD {1942226154} Pedtrc, PedDvl, PedNrD(81,CT02)<NJ-MTNSIDE, NJ-RWJUHAM>
+ Developmental Disabilities Health Alliance
  1285 Broad Street Bloomfield, NJ 07003 (973)338-4200

Kastuar, Satya P., MD {1861402562} Gastrn, IntrMd(79,INA7B)
+ 2480 State Highway 27
  North Brunswick, NJ 08902 (732)821-0011 Fax (732)821-2998

Kasturi, Sanjay Srinivas, MD {1285832600} Urolgy(07,IL06)
+ Delaware Valley Urology
  1138 East Chestnut Anvue/Suite 8-B Vineland, NJ 08360 (856)213-4037 Fax (856)267-2499

Kasuni, William Tatsuo, MD {1649342627} IntrMd(96,NY46)<NJ-ENGLWOOD, NJ-HACKNSK>
+ Riverside Kenshin Center
401 Hackensack Avenue/5th Floor   Hackensack, NJ 07601   (201)678-1900

Kasuri, Jasbir K., MD {1841234473} IntrMd, Nephro(78,INDI)<NJ-JFKMED>
+ 340 Route 1 North
Edison, NJ 08817   (732)777-1010   Fax (732)777-1266
JasbirKasuri@yahoo.com

Kaszubski, Priscilla D., DO {1174561781} PhysMd, PedReh(90,NY75)<NJ-STJOSHOS>
+ St. Joseph's Regional Medical Center
703 Main Street/Rehab Med   Paterson, NJ 07503   (973)754-2946

Kat, Yousef A., MD {1801818711} Psychy, PsyGrt(84,RUS78)<NJ-CHILTON>
+ 99 Warbler Drive
Wayne, NJ 07470   (973)720-6655   Fax (973)720-6644

Katava, Gordana L., DO {1285944652} PthAcl<NY-MTSINAI, NY-MTSINYHS>
+ Morristown Pathology Associates
100 The American Road/Suite 118   Morris Plains, NJ 07950   (973)867-7298

Katdare, Umesh Vasudeo, MD {1447255898} CdvDis, IntCrd(97,DMN01)<NJ-NWRKBETH>
+ Hudson Heart Associates
425 70th Street   Guttenberg, NJ 07093   (201)854-0055   Fax (201)854-2633

Katebian, Manoucher E., MD {1356378202} CdvDis, IntrMd(68,IRA01)<NJ-HACKNSK>
+ 274 Summit Avenue
Hackensack, NJ 07601   (201)342-3800   Fax (201)343-7320

Katechis, Dennis, DO {1033129978} CdvDis, CarNuc, CarEch(97,NY75)<NJ-ENGLWOOD>
+ Englewood Cardiology Consultants
177 North Dean Street/Suite 100   Englewood, NJ 07631   (201)816-2508   Fax (201)569-6111
+ Englewood Cardiology Consultants
220 Livingston Street   Northvale, NJ 07647   (201)569-4901

Kater, Mitchell Jay, MD {1083625842} Anesth(81,PA14)
+ Gastroenterology Associates
2275 Whitehorse-Mercerville Rd   Trenton, NJ 08619   (609)890-0200   Fax (609)890-8335

Kath, Heaton, MD {1295184463}<NJ-COOPRUMC>
+ Cooper University Hospital
One Cooper Plaza   Camden, NJ 08103   (856)342-2000

Kathrotia, Mitesh Gordhan, MD {1154612430} FamMed, IntrMd(POL06)
+ Family Practice of CentraState
901 West Main Street/Suite 106   Freehold, NJ 07728   (732)462-0100   Fax (732)462-0348
+ Family Practice of CentraState
281 Route 34/Suite 813   Colts Neck, NJ 07722   (732)462-0100   Fax (732)431-3707
+ Family Practice of CentraState
319 Route 130 North   East Windsor, NJ 07728   (609)426-1555   Fax (609)447-8070

Kathuria, Kanik, MD {1609118140} IntHos<NJ-NWRKBETH>
+ Newark Beth Israel Medical Center
201 Lyons Avenue   Newark, NJ 07112   (973)926-7425   Fax (973)926-6130

Kathuria, Richa, MD {1477582260} EmrgMd(00,NJ05)<NJ-OCEANMC>
+ Ocean Medical Center
425 Jack Martin Boulevard/EmergMed   Brick, NJ 08723   (732)840-2200

Katikaneni, Swapna, MD {1134526189} IntrMd
+ Riverside Medical Group
714 Tenth Street/Suite 2   Secaucus, NJ 07094   (201)865-2050   Fax (201)865-0015

Katona, John J., MD {1841201811} SrgOrt(70,DC01)<NJ-HACKNSK, NJ-HOLYNAME>
+ Eastern Orthopedic Associates
222 Cedar Lane/Suite 120   Teaneck, NJ 07666   (201)836-5332   Fax (201)836-4002

Katowitz, William Rocamora, MD {1851484745} Ophthl<PA-VAPHIL>
+ CHOP Pediatric & Adolescent Specialty Care Center
1012 Laurel Oak Road   Voorhees, NJ 08043   (856)435-1300   Fax (856)435-0091

Katpally, Ram Reddy, MD {1316285372}
+ St. Michael's Medical Center
111 Central Avenue   Newark, NJ 07102   (973)877-5487

Katragadda, Rama Sastrulu, MD {1518981083} Anesth(71,INA11)
+ Montclair Anesthesia Associates PC
185 Fairfield Avenue/Suite 2A   West Caldwell, NJ 07006   (973)226-1230   Fax (973)226-1232
+ 230 Sherman Avenue
Glen Ridge, NJ 07028

Katsetos, Suzanne A., MD {1477642631} EmrgMd
+ University Hospital-New Jersey Medical School
30 Bergen Street/Rm 1110   Newark, NJ 07107   (973)972-9261

Katseva, Alla, MD {1871547950} IntrMd, Grtrcs, FamMed(81,UKR01)<NJ-STPETER, NJ-RWJUBRUN>
+ Dr. Alla Katseva and Associates
561 Cranbury Road   East Brunswick, NJ 08816   (732)238-8200   Fax (732)651-6500

Katsman, Tatyana, DO {1447259841} FamMed, OstMed(00,NY75)
+ Steinbaum & Levine Associates
789 Avenue C   Bayonne, NJ 07002   (201)339-2620   Fax (201)339-2785

Katsnelson, Marcella, DO {1942663158}<NJ-HACKNSK>
+ Hackensack University Medical Center
30 Prospect Avenue   Hackensack, NJ 07601   (551)996-1548

Katsoulis-Emnace, Maria G., MD {1699748848} Pedtrc(95,PA02)<NJ-OCEANMC>
+ Coastal HealthCare
525 Jack Martin Boulevard/Suite 102   Brick, NJ 08724   (732)458-5300   Fax (732)458-6356

Katt, Brian Matthew, MD {1386625382} SrgOrt(99,NY15)
+ Brielle Orthopedics PA
457 Jack Martin Boulevard   Brick, NJ 08724   (732)840-7500   Fax (732)840-2088
+ Brielle Orthopedics PA
823 Lacey Road   Forked River, NJ 08731   (732)840-7500   Fax (732)840-2088
+ Brielle Orthopedics PA
1301 Route 72 West   Manahawkin, NJ 08724   (609)971-7616   Fax (609)971-7639

Katta, Madhavi R., MD {1356490056} FamMed(97,INA7C)
+ Newark Community Health Center, Inc.
444 William Street   East Orange, NJ 07017   (973)675-1900   Fax (973)675-5418

Katta, Pratyusha Reddy, MD {1699013045} IntHos(07,INA5B)<NJ-SJHREGMC>
+ SJH Regional Medical Center
1505 West Sherman Avenue/Hospitalist   Vineland, NJ 08360   (856)641-8000   Fax (856)641-7650

Katturupalli, Madhavi, MD {1538450457} Pedtrc
+ Allergy & Pediatric Associates of Jersey Shore
222 Schanck Road/Suite 105   Freehold, NJ 07728   (732)431-3373   Fax (732)303-0172

Katz, Adriana, MD {1952355356} EnDbMt, IntrMd(86,WIND)<NJ-HACKNSK>
+ 211 Essex Street/Suite 203
Hackensack, NJ 07601   (201)488-8882   Fax (201)883-0404

Katz, Alvin, MD {1700948650} Otlryg(63,NY08)<NY-LENOXHLL, NY-MANHEYE>
+ 200 Grand Avenue/Suite 204
Englewood, NJ 07631   (201)816-0600   Fax (201)816-0900

Katz, Amos, MD {1952411340} Nrolgy(79,NY09)<NJ-CENTRAST>
+ Central Jersey Neurology Associates
501 Iron Bridge Road/Suite 2   Freehold, NJ 07728   (732)462-7030   Fax (732)308-3562

Katz, Andrea M., MD {1124011903} Pedtrc(88,NY09)<NJ-OVERLOOK, NJ-STBARNMC>
+ Watchung Pediatrics
76 Stirling Road/Suite 201   Warren, NJ 07059   (908)755-5437   Fax (908)755-6905
+ Watchung Pediatrics
346 South Avenue/Suite 3   Fanwood, NJ 07023   (908)755-5437   Fax (908)889-0047
+ Watchung Pediatrics
225 Millburn Avenue/Suite 301   Millburn, NJ 07059   (973)376-7337   Fax (973)218-6647

Katz, Anna Beth, MD {1346401429} SrgOnc
+ 20 Livingston Avenue/Unit 1105
New Brunswick, NJ 08901

Katz, Arthur M., MD {1790866895} Dermat(69,ITA01)
+ Dermatology Affiliates
2954 Kennedy Boulevard/2nd Floor   Jersey City, NJ 07306   (201)653-5555   Fax (201)963-9202

Katz, Avery S., MD {1083600662} Nrolgy, Eplpsy, VasNeu(92,NY08)<NJ-STJOSHOS>
+ Neurology Group of North Jersey PA
905 Allwood Road/Suite 105   Clifton, NJ 07012   (973)471-3680   Fax (973)471-6360

Katz, Barry Harmon, MD {1942206818} Radiol, RadNro(82,NY45)
+ University Radiology, PA
239 Route 22 East/Suite 302   Green Brook, NJ 08812   (732)968-4899   Fax (732)968-8096
+ University Radiology Group, P.C.
16 Mountain Boulevard   Warren, NJ 07059   (732)968-4899   Fax (908)769-9141
+ University Radiology Group, P.C.
579A Cranbury Road   East Brunswick, NJ 08812   (732)390-0040   Fax (732)390-1856

Katz, Brian Charles, MD {1538261136} IntrMd, Gastrn(97,NY20)<NJ-STPETER>
+ 85 Raritan Avenue/Suite 125
Highland Park, NJ 08904   (732)246-1028   Fax (732)246-1045
+ Cares Surgicenter, LLC.
240 Easton Avenue   New Brunswick, NJ 08901   (732)246-1028   Fax (732)296-8677

Katz, Doron Zvi, MD {1053351106} IntrMd(01,NY46)<NY-MTSINAI, NJ-HACKNSK>
+ Access Medical Associates PC
177 North Dean Street/Suite 203   Englewood, NJ 07631   (201)503-0833   Fax (201)503-0844
doron@onlysimchas.com

Katz, Harry, MD {1508857814} Otlryg(77,NY19)<NJ-VALLEY, NJ-HOLYNAME>
+ Sovereign Northern Jersey ENT
85 Harristown Road/Suite 105   Glen Rock, NJ 07452   (201)455-2900   Fax (201)703-0390
+ Northern Jersey Ear, Nose & Throat Associates, P.A.
1 Degraw Avenue   Teaneck, NJ 07666   (201)455-2900   Fax (201)836-7838

Katz, Herbert I., MD {1801995790} Urolgy(74,PA13)<NJ-BAYONNE>
+ Specialists in Urology, P.A.
534 Avenue E   Bayonne, NJ 07002   (201)823-1303   Fax (201)823-0944
+ Short Hills Surgery Center
187 Millburn Avenue/Suite 101   Millburn, NJ 07041   (201)823-1303   Fax (973)671-0557

Katz, Howard A., DO {1962443135} IntrMd(93,NY75)<NJ-BAYSHORE, NJ-CENTRAST>
+ 9 Professional Circle/Suite 210
Colts Neck, NJ 07722   (732)761-8170   Fax (732)761-8175

Katz, James M., MD {1568486785} Dermat(73,NY09)<NJ-VALLEY>
+ 15-01 Broadway/Suite 38
Fair Lawn, NJ 07410   (201)797-4009

Katz, Jeffrey I., MD {1831195320} Urolgy, IntrMd(70,ITA01)<NJ-STBARNMC>
+ Physicians for Women's HealthCare
315 East Northfield Road/Suite 3-B   Livingston, NJ 07039   (973)436-1070   Fax (973)422-9169
JKatz0785@Hotmail.com
+ Summit Medical Group
315 East Northfield Road/Suite 1-E   Livingston, NJ 07039   (973)436-1070   Fax (973)535-1450

Katz, Jodie H., MD {1114960259} FamMed(86,ISR01)<NJ-VALLEY>
+ Valley Medical Group-Center for Integrative Medicine
1200 East Ridgewood Ave/Suite 308   Ridgewood, NJ 07450   (201)389-0075

Katz, John W., Jr., MD {1548377443} Anesth, CritCr, AnesCrCr(75,NJ05)<NJ-UMDNJ>
+ University Hospital
150 Bergen Street/Anesthesiology   Newark, NJ 07103   (973)972-4300

Katz, Kristina, MD {1689081945} Gastrn
+ Center for Digestive Health
5 Plainsboro Road/Suite 450   Plainsboro, NJ 08536   (609)853-6390

Katz, Lawrence, MD {1508815903} IntrMd(75,PA09)<NJ-MONMOUTH>
+ 812 Poole Avenue
Hazlet, NJ 07730   (732)888-0600   Fax (732)264-8194

Katz, Manuel David, MD {1376541359} IntrMd(97,NY46)<NJ-ENGLWOOD, NJ-HOLYNAME>
+ Leonia Medical Associates, P.A.
25 Rockwood Place/Suite 120   Englewood, NJ 07631   (201)568-3335   Fax (201)568-2450

Katz, Melvin I., MD {1407878242} Pedtrc(70,NY19)<NJ-STPETER, NJ-RWJUBRUN>
+ North Brunswick Pediatrics
1598 US Highway 130   North Brunswick, NJ 08902   (732)297-0603   Fax (732)297-2866

Katz, Michael Dennis, MD {1922160068} NroChl, PedNrD, Pedtrc(84,GRN01)
+ 77 Prospect Avenue/Suite 1 K
Hackensack, NJ 07601   (201)525-4777   Fax (201)524-7705

Katz, Michael Geoffrey, MD {1831382506} ClCdEl, CdvDis, IntrMd(07,NY45)<NJ-MORRISTN>
+ Morristown Medical Center
100 Madison Avenue/Box 5   Morristown, NJ 07962   (973)971-4261   Fax (973)290-7253

Katz, Michael Jonathan, MD {1124124805} Otlryg(97,MA05)<NJ-HACKNSK>
+ The Family Center for Otolaryngology
47 Orient Way/Lower Level   Rutherford, NJ 07070   (201)935-5508   Fax (201)465-6088
+ The Family Center for Otolaryngology
1265 Paterson Plank Road   Secaucus, NJ 07094   (201)935-5508   Fax (201)465-6088
+ The Family Center for Otolaryngology
6 Brighton Road/Suite 104   Clifton, NJ 07070   (973)470-0282   Fax (201)465-6088

Physicians by Name and Address

Katz, Randi J., DO {1871540328} OncHem(01,NY75)
+ Regional Cancer Care Associates, LLC
4632 US Highway 9   Howell, NJ 07731   (732)367-1535
Fax (732)367-9514

Katz, Robert Samuel, MD {1164575759} Pthlgy, PthACl, Hemato(75,NY46)<NJ-MORRISTN>
+ 11 Van Beuren Road
Morristown, NJ 07960

Katz, Stanley Norman, MD {1790846095} Dermat(74,NJ05)
+ 523 Westwood Avenue
Long Branch, NJ 07740   (732)842-2790   Fax (732)842-2790
snk0529@aol.com

Katz, Steven A., MD {1477555993} Urolgy(69,NY06)<NJ-ENGLWOOD, NJ-HOLYNAME>
+ The Urology Center of Englewood, PA
300 Grand Avenue/Suite 102   Englewood, NJ 07631
(201)816-1900   Fax (201)816-1777
+ The Urology Center of Englewood, PA
663 Palisade Avenue/Suite 304   Cliffside Park, NJ 07010
(201)816-1900   Fax (201)313-9599

Katz, Terri F., MD {1588764005} Grtrcs, IntrMd(86,DC01)<NJ-ENGLWOOD, NJ-HOLYNAME>
+ 655 Pomander Walk
Teaneck, NJ 07666   (201)836-2990   Fax (201)836-2994
+ 15 Anderson Street
Hackensack, NJ 07601   (201)836-2990   Fax (201)487-0960

Katzenbach, George Francis, III, MD {1225085400} Pedtrc(98,PA01)<NJ-KMHTURNV, NJ-KMHSTRAT>
+ Kennedy Health Systems/Washington Township Campus
435 Hurffville-Cross Keys Road   Turnersville, NJ 08012
(856)582-2816   Fax (856)582-2807
+ Kennedy Memorial Hospital-University Medical Center
18 East Laurel Road/Pediatrics   Stratford, NJ 08084
(856)582-2816   Fax (856)346-6005

Katzman, Jay David, MD {1043284227} IntrMd, Gastrn(91,NY19)<NJ-CHILTON>
+ 1777 Hamburg Turnpike/Suite 203
Wayne, NJ 07470   (973)633-9933   Fax (973)839-1681

Kaufer, Melanie Erin, MD {1750663209}
+ Rutgers- New Jersey Medical School
185 South Orange Avenue   Newark, NJ 07103   (973)972-5266

Kaufer, Michael Jason, MD {1922419167} EmrgMd<NJ-OCEANMC>
+ Ocean Medical Center
425 Jack Martin Boulevard   Brick, NJ 08723   (732)840-2200

Kaufer, Seth Woodrow, DO {1225292105} Gastrn, IntrMd(08,PA77)
+ Philadelphia Gastroenterology Group, P.C.
570 Egg Harbor Road/Suite A-2   Sewell, NJ 08080
(856)218-1410   Fax (856)218-0193

Kauffman, Patricia Joan, MD {1376975813} PthAna, PthFor(93,PA13)
+ 502 Carnegie Center/Suite 300
Princeton, NJ 08540   (609)250-6936

Kaufman, Andrew Greg, MD {1437201332} Anesth, PallCr, PainInvt(88,VA01)<NJ-UMDNJ>
+ Comprehensive Pain Center
90 Bergen Street/DOC 3400   Newark, NJ 07103   (973)972-2085   Fax (973)972-2130

Kaufman, Barry P., MD {1154499085} Gastrn, IntrMd(71,NY46)<NJ-ACMCITY, NJ-ACMCMAIN>
+ Atlantic Gastroenterology Associates, P.A.
3205 Fire Road/Suite 4   Egg Harbor Township, NJ 08234
(609)407-1220   Fax (609)407-0220
+ Atlantic Gastroenterology Associates, P.A.
72 West Jimmie Leeds Road/Suite 2600   Galloway, NJ 08205
(609)407-1220   Fax (609)407-0220

Kaufman, Bradley S., MD {1730509706} CdvDis, IntrMd(82,MA16)<NJ-VALLEY>
+ Hackensack University Medical Group Emerson
452 Old Hook Road/2nd Floor   Emerson, NJ 07630
(201)666-3900   Fax (201)261-0505

Kaufman, David H., MD {1659352292} InfDis, IntrMd(74,NY19)<NJ-MEMSALEM>
+ Cumberland Internal Medicine
1450 East Chestnut Avenue   Vineland, NJ 08361   (856)794-8700   Fax (856)794-2752

Kaufman, Deborah Louise, DO {1285602375} ObsGyn(94,TX17)<NJ-VALLEY>
+ Bergen-Passaic Women's Health
2024 Macopin Road/Suite D   West Milford, NJ 07480
(973)728-7787   Fax (973)728-7707

Kaufman, Gregory Joel, MD {1164522363} ObsGyn(92,MD07)<NY-SOUTHNAS, NY-NSUHMANH>
+ Partners for Women's Health PA
95 Northfield Avenue   West Orange, NJ 07052   (973)736-4505   Fax (973)376-9066

Kaufman, Harvey Willard, MD {1104130954} PthACl, PthChm(82,MA05)
+ Quest Diagnostics Inc.
1 Malcolm Avenue   Teterboro, NJ 07608   (201)393-6383
Fax (201)393-6127

Kaufman, Irving H., MD {1942341458} FamMed, Grtrcs(83,ITAL)<NJ-RWJUBRUN, NJ-STPETER>
+ Be Well Family Practice
1303 State Route 27   Somerset, NJ 08873   (732)249-1500
Fax (732)249-8749

Kaufman, Jarrod Peter, MD {1154364073} SrgVas, Surgry, IntrMd(97,ISR02)<NJ-CENTRAST, NJ-KIMBALL>
+ Premier Surgical
525 Route 70 East Brick Office   Brick, NJ 08723   (732)262-1600   Fax (732)262-1606
jarrodkaufman@gmail.com

Kaufman, Jodi D., MD {1265403935} IntrMd(87,PA07)<NJ-VIRTMHBC, NJ-LOURDMED>
+ Moorestown Internal Medicine PC
147 East Third Street/Suite One   Moorestown, NJ 08057
(856)235-1870   Fax (856)234-2290

Kaufman, Keith, MD {1801240015} EnDbMt
+ Merck and Company Incorporated
126 East Lincoln Avenue/RY 34-A248   Rahway, NJ 07065
(732)594-5821

Kaufman, Kenneth R., MD {1831277169} Psychy(74,MO02)<NJ-UNIVBHC>
+ University Behavioral Health Care
671 Hoes Lane/PO Box 1392/Psych   Piscataway, NJ 08855
(732)235-5500

Kaufman, Larry J., MD {1558304568} ObsGyn(84,PA07)<NJ-ACMCITY, NJ-ACMCMAIN>
+ 2500 English Creek Avenue/Suite 604
Egg Harbor Township, NJ 08234   (609)485-0885   Fax (609)485-0882

Kaufman, Lee D., MD {1528020591} IntrMd, Rheuma(77,ITA17)<NJ-STBARNMC>
+ Center for Rheumatic & Autoimmune Diseases
200 South Orange Avenue/Suite 107   Livingston, NJ 07039
(973)322-7400   Fax (973)322-7420

Kaufman, Margit I., MD {1700157286} AnesCrCr
+ 545 West Englewood Avenue
Teaneck, NJ 07666   (201)833-8545

Kaufman, Matthew Roy, MD {1134188378} SrgPlstc, OtgyPSHN(98,NY15)
+ The Plastic Surgery Ctr of NJ & Manhat
535 Sycamore Avenue   Shrewsbury, NJ 07702   (732)741-0970   Fax (732)747-2606

Kaufman, Michael S., MD {1922000439} NuclMed(93,PA12)
+ Radiology Associates of Burlington County
1295 Route 38 West/PO Box 479   Hainesport, NJ 08036
(609)261-7017   Fax (609)261-4180

Kaufman, Nathan, MD {1275537144} RadOnc, Radiol(85,MI07)<NJ-OCEANMC, NJ-JRSYSHMC>
+ Shore Radiation Oncology, LLC
425 Jack Martin Boulevard   Brick, NJ 08724   (732)836-4109
Fax (732)836-4036
+ Ocean Medical Center
425 Jack Martin Boulevard/RadOnc   Brick, NJ 08723
(732)836-4109   Fax (732)836-4036
+ Riverview Medical Center
1 Riverview Plaza/Cyberknife   Red Bank, NJ 08724
(732)530-2468

Kaufman, Steven Todd, MD {1144279639} EnDbMt(95,PA13)
+ Cooper Endocrinology Associates
1210 Brace Road/Suite 107   Cherry Hill, NJ 08034
(856)795-3597   Fax (856)795-7590

Kaufman, Stuart, MD {1871572487} PedCrd, Pedtrc(80,PA07)<NY-CHLDCOPR, NJ-MORRISTN>
+ Morristown Medical Center
100 Madison Avenue/PediCardio   Morristown, NJ 07962
(973)971-5996   Fax (973)290-7979
stuart.kaufman@ahsys.org

Kaufman, Susan I., DO {1275504193} ObsGyn(81,PA77)<NJ-COOPRUMC, NJ-VIRTUAHS>
+ Center for Specialized Gynecology
1930 State Highway 70 East   Cherry Hill, NJ 08003
(856)424-8091   Fax (856)424-0704

Kaufman, William N., DO {1710976519} ObsGyn(73,IA75)<NJ-MONMOUTH>
+ Shore Area Ob-Gyn
200 White Road/Suite 105   Little Silver, NJ 07739
(732)741-3331   Fax (732)741-5119
+ Shore Area Ob-Gyn
302 Candlewood Commons   Howell, NJ 07731   (732)741-3331   Fax (732)886-9138

Kaufmann, Gregory A., MD {1659391647} RadDia, Radiol, RadNro(86,NJ06)
+ Princeton Radiology Associates, P.A.
419 North Harrison Street   Princeton, NJ 08540   (609)921-3345   Fax (609)683-8847
+ Princeton Radiology Associates, P.A.
9 Centre Drive   Jamesburg, NJ 08831   (609)921-3345   Fax (609)655-4016
+ University Radiology Group, P.C.
375 Route 206/Suite 1   Hillsborough, NJ 08540   (908)874-7600   Fax (908)874-7052

Kaufmann, Roderick, Jr., MD {1740245539} Dermat(81,NJ05)
+ Princeton Dermatology Associates
5 Centre Street/Suite 1-A   Monroe Township, NJ 08831
(609)655-4544   Fax (609)655-2390
+ Princeton Dermatology Associates
208 Bunn Drive/Suite 1-E   Princeton, NJ 08540   (609)655-4544   Fax (609)683-0298

Kauh, John S., MD {1972610731} CdvDis(97,PA02)
+ Rutgers Cancer Institute of New Jersey
195 Little Albany Street/PO Box 2681   New Brunswick, NJ 08903   (732)235-2465   Fax (732)235-7355

Kaul, Rachna, MD {1073776340} FamMed
+ 468 Cambridge Road
Ridgewood, NJ 07450

Kaul, Reena Sonya, MD {1821089715} Pedtrc(02,CA06)<NJ-VALLEY, NJ-CHILTON>
+ PediatriCare Associates
20-20 Fair Lawn Avenue   Fair Lawn, NJ 07410   (201)791-4545   Fax (201)791-3765

Kaul, Sameer, MD {1699006445} IntrMd
+ Cardiology Center of New Jersey
50 Newark Avenue/Suite 204   Belleville, NJ 07109
(973)450-2158   Fax (973)450-2027

Kaul, Sanjeev Kumar, MD {1144267683} Surgry, SrgTrm, SrgCrC(90,INA23)<NJ-HACKNSK>
+ Hackensack University Medical Center
30 Prospect Avenue/St. John G834   Hackensack, NJ 07601
(201)996-2000
skaulmd@yahoo.com
+ Hackensack Surgical Critical Care Physicians
5 Summit Avenue/Suite 105   Hackensack, NJ 07601
(201)996-2000   Fax (201)883-1268

Kaul, Shailja, MD {1780841270} EnDbMt
+ Endocrinology Associates
1 Brace Road/Suite B   Cherry Hill, NJ 08034   (856)234-0645
Fax (856)234-0498

Kaul, Sushma Dhar, MD {1447285069} PedEnd, Pedtrc(75,INA72)<NJ-ENGLWOOD, NJ-HACKNSK>
+ Edgewater Pediatrics
115 River Road/Suite 1003   Edgewater, NJ 07020
(201)945-9453   Fax (201)945-9484

Kaulback, Kurt W., MD {1902852957} CdvDis, IntrMd, IntCrd(88,PA09)
+ Owens Vergari Unwala Cardiology Associates PC
17 West Red Bank Avenue/Suite 306   Woodbury, NJ 08096
(856)845-6807   Fax (856)845-3760

Kaune, Maureen, MD {1265459101} PsyCAd, Psychy, PsyAdd(87,MNT01)<NJ-VALYONS>
+ VA New Jersey Health Care System at Lyons
151 Knollcroft Road/Psychiatry   Lyons, NJ 07939   (908)647-0180   Fax (908)604-5251

Kaunzinger, Christian M., MD {1912976010} IntrMd(93,NJ05)<NJ-JRSYSHMC>
+ Hackensack Meridian Medical Group
19 Davis Avenue/5th-6th Floor   Neptune, NJ 07753
(732)897-3990   Fax (732)897-3997

Kaur, Amrita, DO {1568660439} InfDis, IntrMd(03,NJ75)
+ Atlantic Heart Rhythm Center
415 Chris Gaupp Drive/Suite C   Galloway, NJ 08205
(609)568-0599   Fax (609)748-7574

Kaur, Birinder Jeet, MD {1992706733} IntrMd(87,INA72)<MA-ARDHILL>
+ 1200 East Ridgewood Avenue
Ridgewood, NJ 07450   (201)670-7557   Fax (201)670-5757

Kaur, Dvinder, MD {1285605238} IntrMd(95,NJ05)<NJ-STPETER, NJ-RWJUBRUN>
+ Brunswick Internal Medical Group
17 Bridge Street   Metuchen, NJ 08840   (732)321-1600
Fax (732)321-1699

Kaur, Harleen, MD {1922267012} FamMed(01,INA5Z)<NJ-RBAYOLDB, NJ-RBAYPERT>
+ Ansonya Family Care
238 Ernston Road   Parlin, NJ 08859   (732)727-5110   Fax (732)316-2323
staff@ansonya.com

Kaur, Harmanjot, MD {1699909564} Anesth(09,DMN01)<NJ-SJHREGMC>
+ SJH Regional Medical Center
1505 West Sherman Avenue/Box #51   Vineland, NJ 08360
(856)641-7859   Fax (856)641-7671

Kaur, Harneet, MD {1700019742} Nephro<NY-WESTCHMC>
+ Shore Nephrology, PA
27 South Cookbridge Road/Suite 211   Jackson, NJ 08527
(732)987-5990   Fax (732)987-5994
+ Shore Nephrology, P.A.
2100 Corlies Avenue/Suite 15   Neptune, NJ 07753
(732)987-5990   Fax (732)774-1528
+ Shore Nephrology, P.A.
1000 West Main Street/Suite 3   Freehold, NJ 08527
(732)303-9390   Fax (732)414-1591

Kaur, Harpreet, MD {1609923432} Pedtrc(97,INA21)<NY-FLUSHNG>
+ The Children's Hospital at Saint Peter's University
254 Easton Avenue/Pediatrics   New Brunswick, NJ 08901   (732)745-8566

Kaur, Harsohena, MD {1538258454} Pedtrc<NJ-STPETER>
+ St. Peter's University Hospital
254 Easton Avenue   New Brunswick, NJ 08901   (732)745-8600

Kaur, Jasneet, MD {1609208925} FamMed, IntrMd(11,NJ05)
+ Summit Medical Group
31-00 Broadway   Fair Lawn, NJ 07410   (201)796-2255   Fax (201)796-7020
+ Summit Medical Group Internal Medicine
127 Union Street/Suite 101   Ridgewood, NJ 07450   (201)796-2255   Fax (201)444-2399

Kaur, Jaspreet, DO {1235416140} EmrgMd<NJ-CHSFULD>
+ Capital Health System/Fuld Campus
750 Brunswick Avenue   Trenton, NJ 08638   (609)815-7091   Fax (609)815-7886

Kaur, Jasrup, MD {1154635423}
+ 788 Shrewsbury Avenue/Suite 103
Tinton Falls, NJ 07724   (732)450-0961   Fax (732)530-0213

Kaur, Narinder, MD {1508072224} FamMed
+ 666 Plainsboro Road/Suite 1020
Plainsboro, NJ 08536

Kaur, Navjot, MD {1871156810}
+ Capital Health Hospitalist Group
750 Brunswick Avenue   Trenton, NJ 08638   (609)394-6031   Fax (609)394-6299
+ Capital Health Primary Care - Mountainview
850 Bear Tavern Road/Suite 309   Ewing, NJ 08628   (609)394-6031   Fax (609)656-8845

Kaur, Navneet, MD {1861427635} IntrMd(98,INA82)
+ 27 Carter Avenue
Marlton, NJ 08053

Kaur, Ranbir, DO {1689810186} Pedtrc, IntrMd(NJ75)
+ JFK Neurosciences Institute
65 James Street/Second Floor   Edison, NJ 08818   (732)321-7010   Fax (732)906-4906

Kaur, Sundip, MD {1134380314} IntrMd(DMN01)<NJ-OCEANMC>
+ Cedar Bridge Medical Associates
985 Cedarbridge Avenue   Brick, NJ 08723   (732)477-5600   Fax (732)477-1899

Kaus, Sharon M., DO {1003083312} Pedtrc(05,NJ75)<NJ-VIRTUAHS, NJ-COOPRUMC>
+ Advocare Greentree Pediatrics
127 Church Road/Suite 800   Marlton, NJ 08053   (856)988-7899   Fax (856)988-9499

Kaushal, Neil, MD {1275943110} PedOrt
+ UMDNJ Orthopaedics
205 South Orange Avenue/Suite C1200   Newark, NJ 07103   (973)972-2150   Fax (973)972-2155

Kaushik, Raj Ramanuj, MD {1164464608} SrgThr, Surgry(78,INA65)<NJ-MTNSIDE>
+ Cardiovascular Surgical Associates
350 Boulevard/Suite 130   Passaic, NJ 07055   (973)365-4567   Fax (973)916-5262

Kaushik, Sridhar, MD {1174586739} NnPnMd, Pedtrc, IntrMd(85,INA30)<NJ-RWJUBRUN>
+ RWJ University Hospital New Brunswick
One Robert Wood Johnson Place   New Brunswick, NJ 08901   (732)235-7887
+ On-Site Neonatal Partners
1000 Haddonfield-Berlin Road/Suite 210   Voorhees, NJ 08043   (732)235-7887   Fax (856)782-2213

Kavaler, Robert, MD {1932148913} IntrMd(92,NY08)<NJ-HACKNSK, NJ-VALLEY>
+ Forest HealthCare Associates, PC
277 Forest Avenue/Suite 200   Paramus, NJ 07652   (201)986-1881   Fax (201)986-1871

Kavanagh, Mark Lawrence, MD {1558514380} SrgOrt(03,VA07)<NJ-CHILTON>
+ SMG Orthopedic Surgery and Sports Medicine Center
61 Beaver Brook Road/Suite 201   Lincoln Park, NJ 07035   (973)686-9292   Fax (973)686-9294
+ Summit Medical Group
6 Brighton Road/2 FL   Clifton, NJ 07012   (973)686-9292   Fax (973)777-5403
+ Summit Medical Group
34 Mountain Boulevard/Building B   Warren, NJ 07035   (908)769-0100   Fax (908)769-8927

Kavathia, Sanjay G., MD {1124078142} IntrMd(94,INA2B)<NJ-HCKTSTWN, NJ-STCLRDEN>
+ PriMed Medical Care PC
616 Willow Grove Street/Suite 1-A   Hackettstown, NJ 07840   (908)852-8484   Fax (908)852-4197   SKAVATHIA@yahoo.com

Kaveney, Amanda Davis, MD {1508154162}
+ Rutgers Cancer Institute of New Jersey
195 Little Albany Street/PO Box 2681   New Brunswick, NJ 08903   (732)235-2465   Fax (732)235-6797

Kavi, Tapan, MD {1780008748}
+ Cooper University Medical Center/Camden
3 Cooper Plaza/Suite 320   Camden, NJ 08103   (856)342-2000

Kavuru, Sudha, MD {1689765190} OncHem, IntrMd(94,INA5B)<NJ-KIMBALL, NJ-JRSYSHMC>
+ Shore Hematology Oncology
40 Bey Lea Road/Suite C-202   Toms River, NJ 08753   (732)240-0068   Fax (732)240-1574

Kawalec, Maksymilian Antoni, MD {1659323673}
+ 115 White Owl Trail
Mullica Hill, NJ 08062

Kawata, Michitaka, MD {1417186859} SrgC&R
+ Cooper Surgical Associates
3 Cooper Plaza/Suite 411   Camden, NJ 08103   (856)342-2270   Fax (856)365-1180

Kaweblum, Jaime, DO {1164534798} Pedtrc(01,NJ75)<NJ-JRSYSHMC>
+ Chemed Family Health Center
1771 Madison Avenue   Lakewood, NJ 08701   (732)364-2144   Fax (732)364-3559
+ EmCare
1945 Route 33   Neptune, NJ 07753   (732)364-2144   Fax (732)776-2329

Kaweblum, Moises, MD {1790785921} PhysMd, PainMd, PhyM-SptM(84,MEX61)<NJ-KIMBALL>
+ Center for Advanced Pain Management & Clinical Ortho
500 River Avenue/Suite 255   Lakewood, NJ 08701   (732)905-4446   Fax (732)961-7233

Kawecki, Jerzy Stanislaw, MD {1619045531} FamMed(72,POL03)
+ 4 Garwood Court South
Garfield, NJ 07026   (973)340-9790   Fax (973)772-3911

Kay, Andrea C., MD {1609185602} Hemato, IntrMd, MedOnc(84,PA07)
+ Novartis Pharmaceuticals Corporation
180 Park Avenue/OncClnclResrch   Florham Park, NJ 07932   (862)778-8152   Fax (973)781-6598

Kay, Elizabeth E., DO {1942434139} EmrgMd<NJ-NWRKBETH>
+ Englewood Hospital and Medical Center
350 Engle Street   Englewood, NJ 07631   (201)894-3450
+ Newark Beth Israel Medical Center
201 Lyons Avenue   Newark, NJ 07112   (973)926-6671

Kay, Scott Lawrence, MD {1689736589} Otlryg, Otolgy, SrgFPl(86,PA01)
+ Princeton Otolaryngology Associates, PA
7 Schalks Crossing Road/Suite 324   Plainsboro, NJ 08536   (609)897-0203   Fax (609)897-0213

Kayal, Robert Albert, MD {1053365676} SrgOrt(94,NJ05)<NJ-VALLEY, NJ-HACKNSK>
+ Kayal Orthopaedic Center, PC
385 South Maple Avenue/Suite 206   Ridgewood, NJ 07450   (201)447-3880   Fax (201)447-9326   rkayalmd@kayalortho.com
+ Kayal Orthopaedic Center, P.C.
784 Franklin Avenue/Suite 250   Franklin Lakes, NJ 07417   (201)447-3880   Fax (201)560-0712

Kayal, Thomas Joseph, MD {1316081268} SrgC&R, Surgry(82,MEX14)
+ Advanced Surgical Health Associates
901 West Main Street/MAB Suite 101   Freehold, NJ 07728   (732)308-4202   Fax (732)308-4212

Kayal, William Jesse, MD {1104080860} FamMed
+ Delaware Valley Family Health Center
200 Frenchtown Road   Milford, NJ 08848   (908)995-2251   Fax (908)995-2036

Kayastha, Shital, DO {1053734632} FamMed
+ Medical Associates of Marlboro PC
32 North Main Street   Marlboro, NJ 07746   (732)462-4100   Fax (732)462-3798

Kaye, Alissa Ellen, MD {1700951589} ObsGyn(00,PA02)
+ Drs. Kaye and Kaye
31 South Union Avenue   Cranford, NJ 07016   (908)272-8676   Fax (908)272-7052

Kaye, Gary L., MD {1124190293} ObsGyn(74,IL42)<NJ-OVERLOOK>
+ Drs. Kaye and Kaye
31 South Union Avenue   Cranford, NJ 07016   (908)272-8676   Fax (908)272-7052

Kaye, Rachel, MD {1861783615} Otlryg
+ Center for Neurological Surgery UMDNJ
90 Bergen Street/DOC 8100   Newark, NJ 07103   (973)972-2548   Fax (973)972-2333

Kaye, Shana Malka, MD {1235167594} Pedtrc(03,NY09)
+ Washington Avenue Pediatrics
95 North Washington Avenue   Bergenfield, NJ 07621   (201)384-0300   Fax (201)384-9518

Kaye, Susan T., MD {1760404115} FamMed, IntrMd(79,NY19)<NJ-OVERLOOK>
+ Overlook Family Medicine
33 Overlook Road/Suite 103   Summit, NJ 07901   (908)522-5700   Fax (908)273-8014

Kayiaros, Stephen, MD {1669699542} SrgOrt(05,NJ06)<NY-SP-CLSURG>
+ University Orthopaedic Associates, LLC.
Two Worlds Fair Drive   Somerset, NJ 08873   (732)979-2115   Fax (732)564-9032
+ University Orthopaedic Associates, LLC.
4810 Belmar Boulevard/Suite 102   Wall, NJ 07753   (732)979-2115   Fax (732)938-5680
+ University Orthopaedic Associates, LLC.
211 North Harrison Street   Princeton, NJ 08873   (609)683-7800   Fax (609)683-7875

Kaylen, Thomas G., MD {1538131727} IntrMd(94,NJ06)
+ 904 Oak Tree Road/Suite F
South Plainfield, NJ 07080   (908)755-7688   Fax (908)755-2960

Kaynan, Ayal Menashe, MD {1023095122} Urolgy(94,NC07)
+ Adult & Pediatric Urology Group PA
261 James Street/Suite 1-A   Morristown, NJ 07960   (973)539-0333   Fax (973)539-8909

Kaynan, Riva Lori, MD {1245368554} PhysMd, IntrMd(95,NY46)
+ Care Station Medical Group
456 Prospect Avenue   West Orange, NJ 07052   (973)731-6767   Fax (973)731-9881
+ Care Station Medical Group
328 West St. Georges Avenue   Linden, NJ 07036   (973)731-6767   Fax (908)925-2842

Kayser, Robert Granville, Jr., MD {1346260999} CdvDis
+ Change of Heart Cardiology
2130 Highway 35/Building C Suite 321   Sea Girt, NJ 08750   (732)974-6700   Fax (732)974-6707

Kayserman, Larisa, MD {1417926361} Ophthl(89,NY08)<NJ-VALLEY, NY-NYEYEINF>
+ Retina Consultants PA
1200 East Ridgewood Avenue/Suite 207   Ridgewood, NJ 07450   (201)612-9600   Fax (201)612-0428
+ Retina Consultants PA
39 South Fullerton Avenue   Montclair, NJ 07042   (973)783-7830
+ Vitreo-Retinal Associates of NJ
119 Prospect Street   Ridgewood, NJ 07450   (201)444-3878

Kazahaya, Ken, MD {1891885810} Otlryg, PedOto(93,PA01)<PA-CHILDHOS>
+ CHOP Pediatric & Adolescent Specialty Care Center
1012 Laurel Oak Road   Voorhees, NJ 08043   (856)435-1300   Fax (856)435-0091
+ CHOP Pediatric & Adolescent Specialty Care Center
4009 Black Horse Pike   Mays Landing, NJ 08330   (856)435-1300   Fax (609)677-7835

Kazam, Bonnie B., MD {1083609804} Dermat(73,NY08)<NJ-MORRISTN>
+ 2 Washington Place
Morristown, NJ 07960   (973)267-8585   Fax (973)267-6265

Kazam, Ezra S., MD {1891713384} Ophthl(73,NY08)<NJ-MORRISTN>
+ 2 Washington Place
Morristown, NJ 07960   (973)267-8755   Fax (973)267-8755

Kazemi, Ahmad, MD {1588640874} FamMed(66,IRA01)<NJ-CLARMAAS>
+ 562 Boulevard
Kenilworth, NJ 07033   (973)375-2900   Fax (908)272-3231

Kazemian, Pedram, MD {1891078358}<NJ-DEBRAHLC>
+ Deborah Heart and Lung Center
200 Trenton Road   Browns Mills, NJ 08015   (609)893-6611

Kazenoff, Steven, MD {1841371507} Dermat, IntrMd(79,PA02)<NJ-UNVMCPRN>
+ Princeton Medical Group, P.A.
419 North Harrison Street   Princeton, NJ 08540   (609)924-9300   Fax (609)924-6552
+ Princeton Medical Group PA
2 Research Way/Bldg 2/Suite 302   Monroe Township, NJ 08831   (609)924-9300   Fax (609)655-7466

Kazi, Abdul Haseeb, MD {1902837503} Psychy(90,PAK11)<NJ-TRENTPSY>
+ Trenton Psychiatric Hospital
Sullivan Way/PO Box 7600/Psych   West Trenton, NJ 08628   (609)633-1500

Kazi, Moazzem, MD {1053577874}<NJ-COOPRUMC>
+ Cooper University Hospital
One Cooper Plaza   Camden, NJ 08103   (856)342-2000

Kazim, Debra Ann, MD {1770564205} Anesth(92,NY01)<NJ-MORRISTN>
+ Morristown Medical Center
100 Madison Avenue   Morristown, NJ 07962   (973)971-5000   Fax (201)943-8733

Kazmi, Aasim, MD {1770612111} Surgry
+ Meridian Surgical Associates
2101 Route 34 South   Wall, NJ 07719   (732)974-0003   Fax (732)974-0366

Physicians by Name and Address

Kazmi, Ahsan Mahmood, MD {1013212570} IntrMd(88,PAK01)<NJ-STBARNMC>
+ St. Barnabas Medical Center
  94 Old Short Hills Road/Hospitalist   Livingston, NJ 07039   (973)867-6565

Kazmi, Faaiza K., MD {1710942883} RadDia
+ 1051 West Sherman Avenue
  Vineland, NJ 08360   (856)692-1198   Fax (856)692-1449

Kazmi, Najam U., MD {1417066010} SrgNro(65,PAKI)<NJ-MEM-SALEM>
+ PO Box 178
  Vineland, NJ 08362   (856)692-4244   Fax (856)794-1254

Kazmi, Syed Iftikhar Ahmed, MD {1699922856} IntrMd(87,PAK13)<NJ-CHRIST>
+ Christ Hospital
  176 Palisade Avenue   Jersey City, NJ 07306   (201)560-6840   Fax (732)212-0713

Kazmouz, Hasna M., MD {1548374747} FamMed(89,SYR01)<NJ-STJOSHOS>
+ Kazmouz Medical Center
  7 Lee Place   Paterson, NJ 07505   (973)742-1824   Fax (973)742-1818
+ NHCAC Health Center at Passaic
  110 Main Avenue   Passaic, NJ 07055   (973)742-1824   Fax (973)777-3910

Keagle, Jessica Marie, MD {1225362957}<NJ-HOBUNIMC>
+ Hoboken University Medical Center
  308 Willow Avenue   Hoboken, NJ 07030   (201)418-2840

Kean Chong, Maria R., MD {1174586788} ObsGyn(92,NJ05)<NJ-HACKNSK>
+ Mria R. Kean Chong MD PA
  20 Prospect Avenue/Suite 810   Hackensack, NJ 07601   (201)880-4949   Fax (201)880-4950

Keating, William G., DO {1770670101} FamMed(86,IA75)<NJ-MORRISTN>
+ Montville Primary Care Physicians
  137 Main Road   Montville, NJ 07045   (973)402-0025   Fax (973)402-0508
+ The Doctor's Office New Jersey Urgent Care
  85 Godwin Avenue   Midland Park, NJ 07432   (973)402-0025   Fax (201)857-8406

Keddis, Robert N., MD {1932333648}<NY-NYUTISCH>
+ Deborah Heart and Lung Center
  200 Trenton Road   Browns Mills, NJ 08015   (609)893-6611

Kedersha, Thomas A., MD {1609957976} SrgVas, Surgry(78,MEX03)
+ Route 37 West/Bld E/552 Cmmns Way
  Toms River, NJ 08755

Kedzierska, Ksymena, MD {1326045295} Pedtrc(95,POL02)<NJ-LIBTYHCS>
+ 4 Doctors Park/Suite C
  Hackettstown, NJ 07840   (908)852-8096   Fax (908)852-5012
  canlas@verizon.net

Kedziora, Halina M., MD {1871573782} Grtrcs, IntrMd(78,POLA)<NJ-VIRTMHBC>
+ New Jersey Institute for Successful Aging
  42 East Laurel Road/Suite 1800   Stratford, NJ 08084   (856)566-6843   Fax (856)566-6781
+ University of Medicine & Dentistry of New Jersey-SOM
  42 East Laurel Road/#3200   Stratford, NJ 08084   (856)566-6825

Keedy, Jennifer, MD {1447265897} RadDia
+ Monmouth Medical Imaging
  300 Second Avenue   Long Branch, NJ 07740   (732)923-7700   Fax (732)923-7710

Keefer, Keith J., MD {1770688038} FamMed(81,PA09)
+ Route 72 East
  New Lisbon, NJ 08064

Keegan, Brian Robert, MD {1053516351} Dermat, IntrMd(06,NY19)
+ Windsor Dermatology
  59 One Mile Road Extension/Suite G   East Windsor, NJ 08520   (609)619-3433   Fax (609)426-0530
  brkeegan@gmail.com

Keegan, Debbra Ames, MD {1689737173} ObsGyn(00,NY19)
+ The Institute for Reproductive Medicine and Science
  94 Old Short Hills Road/Suite 403E   Livingston, NJ 07039   (973)322-8286   Fax (973)322-8890

Keegan, Leo Martin, Jr., MD {1114934783} SrgPlstc(86,NY47)<NJ-ENGLWOOD>
+ 370 Grand Avenue
  Englewood, NJ 07631   (201)567-7020

Keelan, Michael E., MD {1316026933} ObsGyn(90,NJ06)<NJ-OCEANMC>
+ Brielle Obstetrics & Gynecology, P.A.
  2671 Highway 70/Wall Township   Manasquan, NJ 08736   (732)528-6999   Fax (732)528-3397
+ Brielle Obstetrics & Gynecology, P.A.
  117 County Line Road   Lakewood, NJ 08701   (732)528-6999   Fax (732)942-1919

Keeler, Louis L., III, MD {1366409955} Urolgy(86,PA02)<NJ-VIRTVOOR, NJ-VIRTBERL>
+ New Jersey Urology LLC
  2090 Springdale Road/Suite D   Cherry Hill, NJ 08003   (856)751-9010   Fax (856)985-9908
+ New Jersey Urology, LLC
  2401 East Evesham Road/Suite F   Voorhees, NJ 08043   (856)751-9010   Fax (856)988-0636

Keeler, Sean Michael, MD {1205997277}<NJ-STBARNMC>
+ St. Barnabas Medical Center
  94 Old Short Hills Road   Livingston, NJ 07039   (973)322-5287   Fax (973)322-2309
  sean.keeler@gmail.com

Keenaghan, Michael Andrew, MD {1396074456} PedCrC, Pedtrc(06,GRN01)<NJ-MORRISTN>
+ Morristown Medical Center
  100 Madison Avenue/Pedi Crtcl Care   Morristown, NJ 07962   (973)971-7550

Keenan, Christopher Joseph, DO {1497778237} Pedtrc(82,PA77)
+ Harborview KidsFirst
  505 Bay Avenue   Somers Point, NJ 08244   (609)927-4235   Fax (609)927-5590
+ Harborview Smithville
  48 South New York Road/Route 9   Smithville, NJ 08205   (609)927-4235   Fax (609)748-3067
+ Harborview KidsFirst Cape May
  1315 Route 9 South   Cape May Court House, NJ 08244   (609)465-6100   Fax (609)465-1539

Keene, Nilda M., MD {1881030575} Psychy(76,PRO01)
+ 414 Stokess Road/Suite 204
  Medford, NJ 08055   (609)654-4990   Fax (609)654-4992

Keflemariam, Yodit J., MD {1801989777} ObsGyn(94)<NJ-JFKMED>
+ JFK Medical Center
  65 James Street/Ob/Gyn   Edison, NJ 08820   (732)839-9341   Fax (732)906-4961

Kehar, Mira, MD {1124341433} Anesth<NJ-HACKNSK>
+ Hackensack University Medical Center
  30 Prospect Avenue   Hackensack, NJ 07601   (201)488-0066

Keiman, Isidore Michael, MD {1174532022} Psychy(87,PRO02)
+ Clifton Psychiatric Services
  469 Clifton Avenue   Clifton, NJ 07011   (973)253-0266   Fax (973)253-0399

Keiner, Lisa R., DO {1497865497} FamMed, IntrMd(95,PA77)<NJ-ACMCITY, NJ-ACMCMAIN>
+ AtlantiCare Special Care Center
  1401 Atlantic Avenue/Suite 2500   Atlantic City, NJ 08401   (609)572-8800

Keir, Donald R., MD {1114969748} EmrgMd(95,NJ06)<NJ-VIRTMHBC>
+ Virtua Memorial
  175 Madison Avenue   Mount Holly, NJ 08060   (609)267-0700   Fax (609)914-6067

Keise, Lydia Nicole, MD {1346562857} Psychy(06,NJ06)
+ Insyte Psychiatric LLC
  33 Plymouth Street/Suite 108   Montclair, NJ 07042   (973)744-6440
  drkeise@insytecenter.com
+ GenPsych
  5 Regent Street/Suite 518   Livingston, NJ 07039   (973)744-6440   Fax (973)994-1220

Keiser, Oren S., MD {1548203383} ObsGyn(01,NY46)
+ West Essex Ob/Gyn Associates
  200 South Orange Avenue/Suite 290   Livingston, NJ 07039   (973)740-1330   Fax (973)740-8998

Keklak, C. Stephen, MD {1164440053} RadDia(75,NJ05)<NJ-CENTRAST>
+ Freehold Radiology Group
  901 West Main Street   Freehold, NJ 07728   (732)462-4844
+ CentraState Medical Center
  901 West Main Street/Radiology   Freehold, NJ 07728   (732)294-2946

Kelemen, Ina J., MD {1871533646} IntrMd, Pedtrc(90,NY48)<NJ-JRSYSHMC, NJ-KIMBALL>
+ Farmingdale Medical Associates
  21 Main Street   Farmingdale, NJ 07727   (732)938-7002   Fax (732)751-9492

Kella, Venkata Krishnam Naidu, MD {1164699195} SrgGst, Bariat(93,INA48)<NJ-UNVMCPRN>
+ University Medical Center of Princeton at Plainsboro
  One Plainsboro Road   Plainsboro, NJ 08536   (609)497-4000

Kelleher, Maureen Michelle, MD {1710910930} IntrMd, FamMed(78,MA01)
+ ImmediCenter/Clifton
  1355 Broad Street   Clifton, NJ 07013   (973)778-5566   Fax (973)778-4044

Keller, Barnes D., MD {1255375135} CdvDis(63,PA01)<NJ-RWJUBRUN, NJ-STPETER>
+ Cardiology Associates of New Brunswick
  593 Cranbury Road/Suite 2   East Brunswick, NJ 08816   (732)390-3333   Fax (732)390-9244

Keller, Betty Sue, MD {1972836781} Rheuma(86,GRN01)<NJ-CHILTON>
+ Optimal Wellness Center
  172 Franklin Avenue/Suite 4-A   Ridgewood, NJ 07450   (201)485-7930   Fax (201)485-7931
  info@optimalwellnessctr.com

Keller, Brett A., DO {1306104419}
+ St. Luke's Orthopedics
  755 Memorial Parkway/Suite 201   Phillipsburg, NJ 08865   (908)847-8884

Keller, Irwin A., MD {1457334237} RadDia, RadNro, Radiol(80,NY09)<NJ-STPETER, NJ-RWJUBRUN>
+ University Radiology Group, P.C.
  483 Cranbury Road   East Brunswick, NJ 08816   (732)390-0030   Fax (732)390-5383
+ University Radiology Group, P.C.
  579A Cranbury Road   East Brunswick, NJ 08816   (732)390-0030   Fax (732)390-1856

Keller, Julie Michelle, MD {1619134285} OrtTrm, SrgOrt(04,NY01)<NJ-STJOSHOS>
+ Restoration Orthopaedics
  113 West Essex Street/Suite 201   Maywood, NJ 07607   (201)226-0145   Fax (201)226-0147

Keller, Malvin S., MD {1013967520} CdvDis, IntrMd(75,MEXI)
+ Raritan Bay Cardiology Group, P.A.
  225 May Street/Suite F   Edison, NJ 08837   (732)738-8855   Fax (732)738-4141

Keller, Maureen Reilly, DO {1154406932} FamMed(98,PA77)
+ Epstein Internal Medicine
  2906 Route 130 North   Delran, NJ 08075   (856)764-4115   Fax (856)764-4116

Keller, Seth Martin, MD {1366557043} Nrolgy(89,DC01)
+ Neurology Associaetes of South Jersey
  693 Main Street/Building D   Lumberton, NJ 08048   (609)261-7600   Fax (609)265-8205
+ Advocare Neurology of South Jersey
  200-B Route 73 North/Suite 2   Voorhees, NJ 08043   (609)261-7600   Fax (856)335-0406

Kellerman, Joshua David, MD {1598906000} RadDia
+ Radiology Associates of Burlington County
  1295 Route 38 West/PO Box 479   Hainesport, NJ 08036   (609)261-7017   Fax (609)261-4180
+ Coastal Imaging, LLC
  79 Route 37 West/Suite 103   Toms River, NJ 08755   (609)261-7017   Fax (732)276-2325

Kellum, Sandra, MD {1669881397} Pedtrc
+ 24 Yantecaw Avenue
  Bloomfield, NJ 07003   (201)275-8742

Kelly, Brendan S., DO {1629222781} IntrMd, IntHos<NJ-ACMC-ITY>
+ AtlantiCare Hospitalist Program
  1925 Pacific Avenue/8th Floor   Atlantic City, NJ 08401   (609)441-8146   Fax (609)441-8002

Kelly, Dennis Hughes, III, MD {1417947748} IntCrd, CdvDis(95,NJ05)<NJ-ENGLWOOD, NJ-PALISADE>
+ Drs. Kelly & Stein
  One Marine Road/Suite 100   North Bergen, NJ 07047   (201)869-1313   Fax (201)854-7945
  nnjca@optonline.net

Kelly, Francis J., MD {1457453847} Surgry, IntrMd(76,ITA17)<NJ-COMMED>
+ Atlantic Shore Surgical Associates
  478 Brick Boulevard   Brick, NJ 08723   (732)701-4848   Fax (732)701-1244
+ Atlantic Shore Surgical Associates
  67 Riverwood/Building 2   Toms River, NJ 08755   (732)701-4848   Fax (732)557-3518

Kelly, Hortensia, DO {1114181443} FamMed(01,NY75)
+ 68 James Street/1st Floor
  Newark, NJ 07102

Kelly, John D., MD SrgOrt(84,OH41)
+ Temple University Orthopaedics & Sports Medicine
  One Greentree Center/Suite 104   Marlton, NJ 08053   (856)596-0906

Kelly, John V., Jr., MD {1265540686} IntrMd(85,DMN01)<NJ-CLARMAAS, NJ-MTNSIDE>
+ Empire Medical Associates
  382 West Passaic Avenue   Bloomfield, NJ 07003   (973)338-1900
+ Empire Medical Associates
  5 Franklin Avenue/Suite 302   Belleville, NJ 07109   (973)338-1900   Fax (973)759-1997
+ Empire Medical Associates
  264 Boyden Avenue   Maplewood, NJ 07003   (973)761-5200   Fax (973)761-7617

Kelly, Kathleen M., MD SrgCrC, Surgry(81,NY19)<NJ-MORRISTN>
+ 19 Junard Drive
  Morristown, NJ 07960

Kelly, Michael, DO {1265583884} IntrSptM(00,NY75)<NJ-STBARNMC, NJ-MTNSIDE>
+ Procare Medical Associates LLC
124 E Mount Pleasant Avenue   Livingston, NJ 07039
(973)535-8300   Fax (973)535-6334

Kelly, Michael E., DO {1730330861} Surgry<NH-CAPITHS>
+ Advanced Surgical Associates of New Jersey
40 Fuld Street/Suite 403   Trenton, NJ 08638   (856)261-3242   Fax (609)537-6002
+ Capital Surgical Associates
40 Fuld Street/Suite 303   Trenton, NJ 08638   (856)261-3242   Fax (609)396-3600
+ Capital Health Primary Care
832 Brunswick Avenue   Trenton, NJ 08638   (609)815-7400   Fax (609)815-7401

Kelly, Michael John, MD {1144389602} Pedtrc, PedCrC(92,NY08)<NJ-PRSBWEIL>
+ 125 Paterson Street/MEB 308A
New Brunswick, NJ 08901   (732)235-7671   Fax (732)235-9340

Kelly, Michelle, MD {1679698450} Pedtrc, NnPnMd(01,MA05)<NJ-VIRTVOOR>
+ Virtua Voorhees
100 Bowman Drive/Pediatrics   Voorhees, NJ 08043   (856)247-3000   Fax (856)504-8029
+ CHOP Specialty Care Center at Virtua
200 Bowman Drive/2 FL/Suite D-260   Voorhees, NJ 08043   (267)425-5400
+ CHOP Virtua Mount Holly
175 Madison Avenue   Mount Holly, NJ 08043   (609)267-0700

Kelly, Peter Hamilton, MD {1205080850} EmrgMd, IntrMd, OccpMd(77,NY03)<NY-ALBANY, NY-STPETERS>
+ Access Health Systems
622 Georges Road   North Brunswick, NJ 08902   (732)951-8000

Kelly, Peter J., MD {1649271883} Ophthl(76,DC02)<MA-WING-MEM>
+ Cooper Family Medicine
110 Marter Avenue   Moorestown, NJ 08057   (856)608-8840   Fax (856)722-1898

Kelly, Robert B., DO {1922202738} ObsGyn(86,NJ75)
+ 508 Lakehurst Road/Suite 3 B
Toms River, NJ 08755

Kelman, Adam Scott, MD {1912065442} EnDbMt, IntrMd(93,IL01)<NJ-VALLEY, NJ-STJOSHOS>
+ Valley Medical Group-Endocrinology
947 Linwood Avenue   Ridgewood, NJ 07450   (201)444-5552   Fax (201)444-4490
drkelman@optonline.net

Kelsey, Alan G., MD {1295735231} FamMed(79,NJ06)<NJ-HUNTRDN>
+ Whitehouse Station Family Medicine
263 Main Street/PO Box 128   Whitehouse Station, NJ 08889   (908)534-2249   Fax (908)534-6634

Kelter, Richard J., MD {1154394286} Grtrcs, IntrMd(74,FRAN)<NJ-CENTRAST>
+ 368 Union Hill Road
Manalapan, NJ 07726   (732)536-5302   Fax (732)972-8638

Kemeny, Alexa C., MD {1619979200} Pedtrc(98,MA01)<NJ-OVERLOOK, NJ-MORRISTN>
+ Summit Medical Group-Berkeley Heights Campus
1 Diamond Hill Road   Berkeley Heights, NJ 07922   (908)273-4300   Fax (908)277-8706

Kemmann, Ekkehard, MD ObsGyn, RprEnd(67,GER25)<NJ-RWJUBRUN, NJ-STPETER>
+ RWJ University Hospital New Brunswick
One Robert Wood Johnson Place   New Brunswick, NJ 08901   (732)828-3000

Kempf, Jeffrey Scott, MD {1851373864} NuclMd, RadDia(84,NJ06)<NJ-STPETER, NJ-RWJUBRUN>
+ University Radiology Group, P.C.
483 Cranbury Road   East Brunswick, NJ 08816   (732)390-0040   Fax (732)390-1856
+ University Radiology Group, P.C.
105 Raider Boulevard/Suite 101   Hillsborough, NJ 08844   (732)390-0040   Fax (908)359-9273
+ University Radiology Group, P.C.
10 Plum Street   New Brunswick, NJ 08816   (732)249-4410   Fax (732)249-1208

Kemps, Anton P., MD {1497843148} IntrMd(73,PA02)<NJ-VIRTVOOR>
+ Cooper Physician Offices
1210 Brace Road/Suite 102   Cherry Hill, NJ 08034   Fax (856)428-4823

Kendall, Roxanne E., MD {1134133234} Pedtrc(79,CT01)<NJ-RWJUBRUN, NJ-UNVMCPRN>
+ RWJ University Hospital New Brunswick
One Robert Wood Johnson Place   New Brunswick, NJ 08901   (732)828-3000

Kendzierski, Renee Marie, DO {1952399883} RadDia(99,PA77)
+ South Jersey Radiology Associates, P.A.
100 Carnie Boulevard/Suite B-5   Voorhees, NJ 08043   (856)751-0123   Fax (856)751-0535
+ South Jersey Radiology Associates, P.A.
6650 Browning Road/Suite M14   Pennsauken, NJ 08109   (856)751-0123   Fax (856)661-0686
+ South Jersey Radiology Associates, P.A.
315 Route 70 East/Suite B   Cherry Hill, NJ 08043   (856)428-4344   Fax (856)428-0356

Keni, Sanjay P., MD {1720273378} Otlryg(03,IL06)<NJ-RWJUBRUN>
+ University Otolaryngology
31 River Road   Highland Park, NJ 08904   (732)846-6540   Fax (732)846-8231

Kenigsberg, David R., MD {1396856696} EmrgMd, FamMed(79,CA02)<NJ-CLARMAAS, NJ-CHRIST>
+ Christ Hospital
176 Palisade Avenue   Jersey City, NJ 07306   (201)795-8200

Kennard, William Francis, MD {1174548112} SrgOrt(73,PA01)<NJ-SOCEANCO, NJ-COMMED>
+ JB Orthopaedics PA
1173 Beacon Avenue   Manahawkin, NJ 08050   (609)597-1556   Fax (609)597-0911
+ JB Orthopaedics PA
9 Mule Road/Suite E-13   Toms River, NJ 08755   (732)244-4600

Kennedy, Cheryl A., MD {1457418618} Psychy(87,WEST)<NJ-UMDNJ>
+ University Hospital-Doctors Office Center
90 Bergen Street/Fl 5, Rm 5300   Newark, NJ 07103   (973)972-2977
kennedy@umdnj.edu

Kennedy, Daniel F., DO {1881658250} IntrMd(97,IA75)<NJ-JRSYSHMC>
+ Jersey Shore University Medical Center
1945 Route 33   Neptune, NJ 07753   (732)775-5500
+ Meridian Medical Associates, P.C.
1945 Route 33   Neptune, NJ 07753   (732)775-5500   Fax (732)776-3795

Kennedy, Eugene Cullen, MD {1639151632} RadDia(88,IRE04)
+ University Radiology Group, P.C.
483 Cranbury Road   East Brunswick, NJ 08816   (732)390-0030   Fax (732)390-5383
+ Trinitas Regional Medical Center-Williamson Street
225 Williamson Street   Elizabeth, NJ 07207   (908)994-5000
+ 4 Sylvan Terrace
Summit, NJ 08816

Kennedy, Harvey Ronald, MD {1902034937} PthAna, Adm-Mgt(79,FL04)
+ Quest Diagnostics Inc.
1 Malcolm Avenue   Teterboro, NJ 07608   (201)393-5559   Fax (201)393-5446
kennedyr@questdiagnostics.com

Kennedy, Kevin J., MD {1639111735} EmrgMd(79,MO07)<NJ-OVERLOOK, NJ-MORRISTN>
+ Summit Medical Group-Berkeley Heights Campus
1 Diamond Hill Road   Berkeley Heights, NJ 07922   (908)273-4300   Fax (908)277-8779

Kennedy, Paul, MD {1194763904} PsyCAd, Psychy(72,WI06)<NJ-STCLRBOO, NJ-MTNSIDE>
+ 117 Watchung Avenue/2nd Floor
Montclair, NJ 07043   (973)783-2984   Fax (973)783-5074

Kennedy, Timothy John, MD {1235394255} SrgOnc, Gastrn(99,DC02)
+ Rutgers Cancer Institute of New Jersey
195 Little Albany Street/PO Box 2681   New Brunswick, NJ 08903   (732)235-6572   Fax (732)235-6797

Kennedy-Little, Dawn Marie, DO {1316994601} PulCCr, SlpDis, IntrMd(94,PA77)<NJ-COOPRUMC, NJ-SOCEANCO>
+ Cooper University Hospital
One Cooper Plaza   Camden, NJ 08103   (856)342-2000

Kenner, George R., Jr., MD {1073529244} Otlryg(78,PA02)
+ Pinnacle ENT Alliance of NJ
2835 South Delsea Drive/Suite D   Vineland, NJ 08360   (856)839-2313   Fax (856)839-2318

Kennett, Shar, MD {1225027568} EmrgMd(90,NJ05)<NJ-STMRYPAS>
+ St. Mary's Hospital
350 Boulevard/Emerg Med   Passaic, NJ 07055   (973)365-4501   Fax (973)365-4641
+ Emergency Medical Associates of NJ, P.A.
3 Century Drive   Parsippany, NJ 07054   (973)365-4501   Fax (973)740-9895

Kenney, Adam, MD {1083956114} EmrgMd<NJ-UMDNJ>
+ University Hospital
150 Bergen Street   Newark, NJ 07103   (973)972-5128   Fax (973)972-6646

Kenney, Ellen N., MD {1366456055} OncHem, IntrMd(88,NY03)<NJ-CHSMRCER>
+ Bellevue Hematology-Oncology
2997 Princeton Pike   Lawrenceville, NJ 08648

Kenney, Meredith Ann, DO {1104056282} FamMed
+ Advocare Grove Family Medical Associates
132 Grove Street/Suite A   Haddonfield, NJ 08033   (856)354-2211   Fax (856)354-6181

Kennish, Lauren M., MD {1508690998} Rheuma
+ Summit Medical Group-Berkeley Heights Campus
1 Diamond Hill Road   Berkeley Heights, NJ 07922   (908)273-4300   Fax (908)790-6576

Kenny, David Anthony, DO {1942476700} RadDia(03,PA77)
+ Atlantic Medical Imaging, LLC.
72 West Jimmie Leeds Road   Galloway, NJ 08205   (609)677-9729   Fax (609)652-6270

Kenny, John J., DO {1891877288} FamMed, Grtrcs, IntrMd(77,PA77)<NJ-SOCEANCO>
+ Family Medicine Center
1301 Route 72 West/Suite 240   Manahawkin, NJ 08050   (609)597-7394   Fax (609)597-6833
+ Family Medicine Center
279 Mathistown Road   Little Egg Harbor, NJ 08087   (609)296-1101

Kenny, Raymond P., MD {1982604831} Gastrn, IntrMd(81,NY48)<NJ-MTNSIDE, NJ-STBARNMC>
+ Gastroenterology Group of NJ, PA
123 Highland Avenue/Suite 103   Glen Ridge, NJ 07028   (973)429-8800   Fax (973)746-0344

Keno, Deborah, MD {1255702536} GenPrc
+ 18 Emerson Street
East Orange, NJ 07018   (973)789-8300

Kent, Justine Marie, MD {1902878077} Psychy(91,NY19)<NJ-MMHKEMBL>
+ Morristown Memorial Hospital/Mt. Kemble Division
95 Mount Kemble Avenue/Psych/6th Fl   Morristown, NJ 07960   (973)971-4758

Kent, Maria Candice, MD {1992781298} FamMed(00,NJ05)<NJ-UNDRWD>
+ Family Health Center of Mullica Hill
155 Bridgeton Pike/Suite A   Mullica Hill, NJ 08062   (856)223-0500   Fax (856)223-1098
+ Family Health Center of Paulsboro
One West Broad Street   Paulsboro, NJ 08066   (856)223-0500   Fax (856)423-4444

Kenton, Alicia Nicole, MD {1821358565} PedSpM
+ Rutgers Hurtado Health Center
11 Bishop Place   New Brunswick, NJ 08901   (848)932-7402   Fax (732)932-1223

Kenwood, Alan L., MD {1669498945} EmrgMd(71,MO34)<NJ-MORRISTN>
+ Morristown Medical Center
100 Madison Avenue   Morristown, NJ 07962   (973)971-5000

Kepecs, Gilbert, MD {1093710014} Rheuma, IntrMd(86,NY46)<NJ-HACKNSK, NJ-HOLYNAME>
+ Hackensack Rheumatology LLC
385 Prospect Avenue/2nd Floor   Hackensack, NJ 07601   (201)498-9060   Fax (201)498-1988

Kepler, Christopher Keppel, MD {1114184389} SrgOrt, IntrMd(05,NY01)
+ South Jersey Physicians Associates
327 Haddon Avenue   Westmont, NJ 08108   (856)869-0009   Fax (856)869-0008

Kepler, Karen Lynn, DO {1982625232} PhysMd, OrtSpn(99,NJ75)<NJ-UMDNJ>
+ University Hospital
150 Bergen Street/PhysRehab   Newark, NJ 07103   (973)972-7954

Kerensky, Kirk M., MD {1811968134} PedEnd, Pedtrc(78,PA01)<NJ-JRSYSHMC>
+ West Park Pediatrics
804 West Park Avenue   Ocean, NJ 07712   (732)531-0010   Fax (732)493-0903
+ West Park Pediatrics
219 Taylors Mills Road   Manalapan, NJ 07726   (732)531-0010   Fax (732)577-9643
+ West Park Pediatrics
921 East County Line Road/Suite B   Lakewood, NJ 07711   (732)370-8500   Fax (732)370-5550

Kerlegrand, Pascale, MD {1144344094} FamMed(92,NY06)
+ Step by Step Pediatrics, P.C.
299 Glenwood Avenue/2nd Floor Suite 6   Bloomfield, NJ 07003   (973)743-5639   Fax (973)743-5840

Kerley, Sara Shelton, MD {1932388642} FamMed
+ 3131 Route 38
Mount Laurel, NJ 08054   (856)866-8700   Fax (856)866-1302

Kern, Allen J., MD {1770584823} Urolgy(78,NJ06)<NJ-HUNTRDN>
+ Hunterdon Urological Associates
121 Highway 31/Suite 1200   Flemington, NJ 08822   (908)782-0019   Fax (908)782-0630

Kern, Carrie Catherine, DO {1659327401} FamMed, IntrMd(03,NJ75)
+ AtlantiCare Physician Group
2500 English Creek Avenue   Egg Harbor Township, NJ 08234   (609)909-0200   Fax (609)909-0267

Physicians by Name and Address

Kern, Hilary Beth, MD {1033282934} PhysMd(89,NY03)
+ 185 Grand Avenue
  Englewood, NJ 07631

Kern, John Matthew, DO {1588930879} IntrMd
+ University Hospital Medicine
  150 Bergen Street/Room I-248   Newark, NJ 07103
  (973)972-6056   Fax (973)972-3129

Kerner, Michael B., MD {1982693990} Gastrn, IntrMd(71,NC05)<NJ-OVERLOOK>
+ Associates in Digestive Disease
  25 Morris Avenue   Springfield, NJ 07081   (973)467-1313
  Fax (973)467-3133
  MBKerner@gmail.com
+ Gastrosurgical Center of NJ
  7132 Spruce Street   Mountainside, NJ 07092   (973)467-1313   Fax (908)317-0081

Kerner, Michael B., DO {1144248154} Anesth(95,PA77)
+ 12 Furlong Drive
  Cherry Hill, NJ 08003   (856)795-0543   Fax (856)795-0544

Kerner, Sheldon P., DO {1376631028} Radiol, RadBdI(68,PA77)<NJ-COOPRUMC>
+ Cooper University Hospital
  One Cooper Plaza/Radiology   Camden, NJ 08103
  (856)342-2000

Kerness, Wayne Jared, MD {1922281997} SrgOrt(71,ITA01)
+ 128 Somerset Road
  Norwood, NJ 07648   (201)767-9450
  arthrodoc@aol.com

Kernis, Elyse Beth, DO {1538275458} FamMed
+ Drs. Vitola & Kernis
  900 Route 168/Suite C3   Turnersville, NJ 08012   (856)374-0430   Fax (856)374-0048

Kernis, Steven J., MD {1336103845} CdvDis, IntCrd, CarNuc(97,MI07)<NJ-VALLEY, NY-GOODSAM>
+ Associated Cardiovascular Consultants-Lourdes
  1 Brace Road/Suite C & F   Cherry Hill, NJ 08034   (856)428-4100   Fax (856)428-5748

Kernitsky, Roman G., MD {1407936966} Ophthl(66,NY19)<NJ-CENTRAST, NJ-MONMOUTH>
+ Millennium Eye Care, LLC
  500 West Main Street   Freehold, NJ 07728   (732)462-8707   Fax (732)462-1296
+ Millennium Eye Care, LLC
  Route 130 & Princeton Road   Hightstown, NJ 08520
  (732)462-8707   Fax (609)448-4197
+ Millennium Eye Care, LLC
  515 Brick Boulevard/Suite G   Brick, NJ 07728   (732)920-3800   Fax (732)920-5351

Kernizan, Daphney, MD {1518493352} Pedtrc
+ 901 Montague Avenue
  Iselin, NJ 08830   (347)885-9918

Kernizan, Eddy, MD Surgry(76,HAIT)
+ 3 East Dogwood Court
  Westampton, NJ 08060

Kernodle, Judith M., MD {1043373400} Psychy(73,TN06)
+ 37 King Street
  Englewood, NJ 07631   (201)652-6099
+ 75 Oak Street
  Ridgewood, NJ 07450   (201)652-6099

Kerns, John F., MD {1083796403} Urolgy(75,DC02)<NJ-HOLY-NAME>
+ Urologic Specialties PA
  177 North Dean Street/Suite 305   Englewood, NJ 07631
  (201)569-7777   Fax (201)569-6861
+ Urologic Specialties PA
  6045 Kennedy Boulevard   North Bergen, NJ 07047
  (201)569-7777   Fax (201)569-6861

Kerr, Brian S., MD {1669441952} PulDis, IntrMd(83,NY09)<NJ-OCEANMC, NJ-COMMED>
+ Ocean Pulmonary Associates PA
  457 Jack Martin Boulevard/Suite 4   Brick, NJ 08724
  (732)840-4200   Fax (732)840-6444
+ Ocean Pulmonary Associates PA
  3 Plaza Drive/Suite 2   Toms River, NJ 08757   (732)840-4200   Fax (732)505-9296
+ Ocean Pulmonary Associates PA
  70 Lacey Road/Irish Branch Mall   Whiting, NJ 08724
  (732)350-4777

Kerr, Eric S., MD {1457445538} Urolgy(92,NY08)<NJ-CHRIST>
+ Specialists in Urology, P.A.
  534 Avenue E   Bayonne, NJ 07002   (201)823-1303   Fax (201)823-0944
+ Short Hills Surgery Center
  187 Millburn Avenue/Suite 101   Millburn, NJ 07041
  (201)823-1303   Fax (973)671-0557

Kerr, Kathy Rosen, MD {1396707741} Pedtrc, IntrMd(84,PA06)<NJ-MORRISTN>
+ 26 Madison Avenue/Suite 1
  Morristown, NJ 07960   (973)455-1234   Fax (973)455-1561

Kerr, Ruthann Warnell, MD {1376665307} IntrMd(87,PA01)
+ 126 East Lincoln Avenue/RY 59-10
  Rahway, NJ 07065   (732)594-7663   Fax (732)594-3548

Kerrigan, Margot I., MD {1730361676} Pedtrc
+ 71 North Maple Avenue
  Basking Ridge, NJ 07920   (908)447-1054
+ Touchpoint Pediatrics
  17 Watchung Avenue   Chatham, NJ 07928   (908)447-1054
  Fax (973)665-0901

Kershner, Gary Brian, DO {1518937234} IntrMd, FamMed(00,NJ75)<NJ-RIVERVW>
+ Drs. Eisenstat and Kershner
  1050 Galloping Hill Road/Suite 202   Union, NJ 07083
  (908)688-4845   Fax (908)687-2039

Kertesz, Jennifer L., MD {1063688034} RadDia
+ 5 Valley View Drive
  Mendham, NJ 07945

Kerven, Elliot Sean, MD {1144207192} Anesth(99,NET09)<NJ-MTNSIDE>
+ Hackensack UMC Mountainside
  1 Bay Avenue/Anesthesia   Montclair, NJ 07042   (973)429-6219   Fax (845)357-5777

Kerwin, Lauren Michelle, MD {1669797304} RadDia
+ 21 Ford Hill Road
  Whippany, NJ 07981   (818)640-1864

Kesarwala, Hemant, MD {1831243708} Allrgy, PedInf, Pedtrc(71,INA87)<NJ-STPETER, NJ-RWJUBRUN>
+ Central NJ Allergy Asthma Associates
  3084 State Route 27/Suite 6   Kendall Park, NJ 08824
  (732)821-0595   Fax (732)821-1174

Kesavan, Dhanalakshmi, MD {1881873982} Pedtrc
+ 100 Westgate Drive
  Edison, NJ 08820

Keselman, Ira G., MD {1821076472} Urolgy(89,MA05)<NJ-CENTRAST, NJ-MONMOUTH>
+ New Jersey Urologic Institute
  10 Industrial Way East   Eatontown, NJ 07724   (732)963-9091   Fax (732)963-9092
+ CentraState Medical Center
  901 West Main Street/Surgical Center   Freehold, NJ 07728
  (732)431-2000

Keshav, Gayithri R., MD {1588767875} Nephro, IntrMd(82,INDI)<NJ-MTNSIDE>
+ 140 Belmont Avenue/Suite 103
  Belleville, NJ 07109   (973)751-7870

Keshav, Roger, MD {1942525316} Nephro, IntrMd<NJ-UMDNJ>
+ Drs. Keshav & Shivashankar
  140 Belmont Avenue/Suite 102   Belleville, NJ 07109
  (973)751-7870   Fax (973)751-7875

Keshishian, Paul, DO {1437207610} FamMed(79,PA77)<NJ-HACKNSK>
+ Redi-Med
  186 Rochelle Avenue/Suite 2-A   Rochelle Park, NJ 07662
  (201)368-3384   Fax (201)587-0300

Kessel, Allan David, MD {1326070376} ObsGyn(98,MI07)
+ The Rubino Ob/Gyn Group
  101 Old Short Hills Road/Suite 101   West Orange, NJ 07052
  (973)736-1100   Fax (973)736-1834

Kessel, Daniel S., MD {1063449700} Dermat(83,PA13)<NJ-RWJUHAM, NJ-STFRNMED>
+ Drs. Kessel & Mercer
  1700 White Horse Hamilton Road   Hamilton Square, NJ 08690   (609)890-2600   Fax (609)890-0265

Kesselhaut, Marc D., MD {1649242181} IntrMd(86,GRN01)<NJ-STJOSHOS, NJ-VALLEY>
+ Valley Medical Group
  43 Yawpo Avenue/Suite 3   Oakland, NJ 07436   (201)337-9600

Kesselheim, Howard I., DO {1003812231} OncHem, IntrMd(74,MO78)<NJ-VIRTMARL, NJ-OURLADY>
+ MD Anderson Cancer Center at Cooper
  2 Cooper Plaza   Camden, NJ 08103   (855)632-2667
+ Regional Cancer Care Associates, LLC
  200 Bowman Drive/Suite E-125   Voorhees, NJ 08043
  (855)632-2667   Fax (856)424-5634
+ The Center for Cancer & Hematologic Disease
  856 South White Horse Pike/Suite 4   Hammonton, NJ 08103
  (609)561-4444   Fax (609)561-2492

Kesselman, Gayle, MD {1447331046} Psychy(75,MI07)
+ Northern State Prison Corrections Department
  168 Frontpage Road   Newark, NJ 07106   (973)465-0068
+ Clifton Behavioral HealthCare
  777 Bloomfield Avenue   Clifton, NJ 07012   (973)594-0125

Kessler, Alex, DO {1487600839} Nephro, IntrMd<NJ-ACMCITY>
+ AtlantiCare Regional Medical Center/City Campus
  1925 Pacific Avenue/8th Floor   Atlantic City, NJ 08401
  (609)441-8146   Fax (609)441-8002

Kessler, Barry M., MD {1902882855} Pedtrc(77,IL06)<NJ-ACMC-MAIN>
+ Kids Care Pediatrics
  6529 Blackhorse Pike   Egg Harbor Township, NJ 08234
  (609)645-8500   Fax (609)272-8886

Kessler, Howard, MD {1881707693} Radiol, NuclMd, RadDia(69,BEL06)<NJ-STMRYPAS>
+ Union Imaging Associates PA
  445 Chestnut Street   Union, NJ 07083   (908)687-6054
  Fax (908)688-1131
+ Open MRI of Morristown PA
  95 Madison Avenue   Morristown, NJ 07960   (908)687-6054   Fax (973)539-7677

Kessler, Jason Adam, MD {1255598850} InfDis, IntrMd(00,NY08)<NJ-MORRISTN>
+ Internal Medicine Faculty Associates
  435 South Street/Suite 210   Morristown, NJ 07960
  (973)971-7165   Fax (973)290-7675

Kessler, Martin, MD {1164446472} FamMed(81,PA07)<NJ-UNDRWD, NJ-KMHCHRRY>
+ Delaware Valley Primary Care & Occupational Medicine
  1458 West Landis Avenue/Suite 2   Vineland, NJ 08360
  (856)696-0669   Fax (856)696-1424
  dvpc@gmail.com

Kessler, Michael A., MD {1952305393} RadDia, IntrMd(72,DC01)
+ Diagnostic Radiology Associates of Northfield
  772 Northfield Avenue   West Orange, NJ 07052   (973)325-0002   Fax (973)325-8140
+ Diagnostic Radiology Associates of Clifton
  1339 Broad Street   Clifton, NJ 07013   (973)325-0002   Fax (973)778-4846
+ Diagnostic Radiology Associates of Cranford
  25 South Union Avenue   Cranford, NJ 07052   (908)709-1323   Fax (908)709-1329

Kessler, William W., MD {1083710842} MedOnc(75,NY46)<NJ-TRINIWSC>
+ Trinitas Regional Medical Center-Williamson Street
  225 Williamson Street   Elizabeth, NJ 07207   (908)994-5349
  Fax (908)994-5633

Kessous, Deborah Lynne, MD {1588860100} Pedtrc(98,GRN01)<NJ-OCEANMC, NJ-COMMED>
+ New Brunswick Pediatric Group, P.A.
  1300 How Lane   North Brunswick, NJ 08902   (732)247-1510   Fax (732)247-8885

Keswani, Ashok Kumar, MD {1740237551} ObsGyn(91,IL42)<NJ-KMHSTRAT, NJ-UNDRWD>
+ 992 Mantua Pike/Suite 104
  Woodbury Heights, NJ 08097   (856)845-5645   Fax (856)845-1666

Keswani, Deepak Pessu, MD {1235339755} IntrMd
+ 7400 River Road/Apt 204
  North Bergen, NJ 07047

Keswani, Rohit, MD {1952358673} PhysMd(96,NJ05)<NJ-STBARNMC, NJ-HOBUNIMC>
+ North Atlantic Rehab Medicine
  799 Bloomfield Avenue/Suite 303   Verona, NJ 07044
  (973)857-7800   Fax (973)857-7822

Ketelaar, Pieter J., MD {1659350189} ObsGyn, Gyneco(70,NJ05)<NJ-OCEANMC>
+ Pineland Associates PA
  1608 Route 88/Suite 208   Brick, NJ 08724   (732)458-7878
  Fax (732)840-6378

Kett, Attila G., MD {1821053372} Anesth(90,HUN02)<NJ-STPETER
+ Anesthesia Consultnts of NJ/Nova Pain
  285 Davidson Avenue/Suite 204   Somerset, NJ 08873
  (732)271-1400   Fax (732)271-3543

Kewalramani, Kavita Rajiv, MD {1952528432} IntrMd(90,INA65)
+ K Primary Care & Medical Nutrition Center
  571 Central Avenue/Suite 104   New Providence, NJ 07974
  (908)206-4676   Fax (908)206-4707
+ State of New Jersey Medicaid Office
  153 Halsey Street/Floor 4   Newark, NJ 07102   (908)206-4676   Fax (973)631-6448

Keys, Roger C., MD {1750349759} SrgVas, Surgry(68,SCOT)<NJ-HACKNSK>
+ Bergen Surgical Specialists
  20 Prospect Avenue/Suite 707   Hackensack, NJ 07601
  (201)343-0040   Fax (201)343-2733

Keyser, Bruce J., MD {1558334359} Ophthl, VitRet(86,PA02)<NJ-RWJUBRUN, NJ-KIMBALL>
+ Retina Associates of New Jersey, P.A.
  10 Plum Street/Suite 600   New Brunswick, NJ 08901
  (732)220-1600   Fax (732)220-1603
+ Retina Associates of New Jersey, P.A.
  530 Lakehurst Road/Suite 305   Toms River, NJ 08753
  (732)220-1600   Fax (732)797-3886
+ Retina Associates of New Jersey, P.A.
  525 Route 70 West/Suite B-14   Lakewood, NJ 08901
  (732)363-2396   Fax (732)363-0403

Keyser, Joseph W., MD {1801945977} Psychy, PsyFor(75,NJ05)
+ 382 Springfield Avenue/Suite 412
  Summit, NJ 07901   (908)277-2655

Khaddash, Ibrahim Saleh, MD {1477840247}<NJ-STJOSHOS>
+ St. Joseph's Regional Medical Center
  703 Main Street   Paterson, NJ 07503   (973)754-2000

Khaddash, Saleh I., MD {1174551824} EnDbMt, IntrMd(80,JOR01)<NJ-STJOSHOS>
+ 40 Union Avenue
  Clifton, NJ 07011   (973)546-3355   Fax (973)546-8501

Physicians by Name and Address

Khademi, Allen Mansour, MD {1427070077} PhysMd(92,DC02)<NJ-SHOREREH>
+ Summit Medical Group-Berkeley Heights Campus
1 Diamond Hill Road   Berkeley Heights, NJ 07922   (908)277-8897   Fax (908)277-8901

Khadka Kunwar, Erina, MD {1043568488} IntrMd
+ Birch Tree Medical Associates
718 Teaneck Road   Teaneck, NJ 07666   (201)833-7274

Khadke, Neelam, MD {1528222882}
+ 64 Middlesex Avenue
Edison, NJ 08820   (347)989-7481
neelam@gmail.com

Khakoo, Rafiya Shabbir, MD {1770558843} Nrolgy(82,INDI)<NJ-BAYSHORE, NJ-RIVERVW>
+ 721 North Beers Street/Suite 2-G
Holmdel, NJ 07733   (732)264-5051

Khaleel, Abdul R., MD {1487650073} SrgOrt(63,INA68)<NJ-SOCEANCO, NJ-VIRTMHBC>
+ 1020 D Long Beach Boulevard
Beach Haven, NJ 08008

Khalid, Aysha, MD {1952522732} OncHem, IntrMd(01,DMN01)
+ Somerset Hematology Oncology Associates, P.A.
30 Rehill Avenue/2nd Floor/Suite 2500   Somerville, NJ 08876   (908)927-8700   Fax (908)927-8706
+ Regional Cancer Care Specialists
34-36 Progress Street/Suite B-2   Edison, NJ 08820   (908)927-8700   Fax (908)757-9721

Khalid, Khaula, DO {1164698445} IntrMd, CdvDis(04,NY75)
+ 892 Avenue C
Bayonne, NJ 07002

Khalid, Samira, DO {1467795476} ObsGyn
+ Lifeline Medical Associates, LLC
900 Lanidex Plaza/Suite 220   Parsippany, NJ 07054   (973)831-2777   Fax (973)831-2780

Khalighi, Koroush, MD {1356345193} IntrMd, CdvDis(86,CHI06)<NJ-WARREN>
+ Easton Cardiovascular Associates
123 Roseberry Street   Phillipsburg, NJ 08865   (908)213-3100

Khalil, Chaza H., MD {1982974739}
+ Hackensack University Medical Faculty Practice
25 East Salem Street   Hackensack, NJ 07601   (201)464-7844   Fax (551)996-4432

Khalil, Christina, DO {1689943821} FamMed
+ Raritan Family Health Care
901 US Highway 202   Raritan, NJ 08869   (908)253-6640   Fax (908)253-6908

Khalil, Erum, MD {1598174583} Pedtrc<NJ-MONMOUTH>
+ Monmouth Medical Center
300 Second Avenue   Long Branch, NJ 07740   (732)923-7251

Khalil, Hossam M., MD {1295733970} IntrMd(90,EGYP)<NJ-BAYSHORE>
+ Meleis Medical Associates
233 Middle Road/Suite 2   Hazlet, NJ 07730   (732)335-0900   Fax (732)335-8080

Khalil, Marwa A., MD {1790126183} NnPnMd(03,EGY05)
+ RWJ University Hospital New Brunswick
One Robert Wood Johnson Place   New Brunswick, NJ 08901   (732)235-5709

Khalil, Monica B., MD {1740234491} Ophthl(01,NY08)<NJ-OVERLOOK, NJ-MORRISTN>
+ Summit Medical Group-Berkeley Heights Campus
1 Diamond Hill Road   Berkeley Heights, NJ 07922   (908)273-4300   Fax (908)277-8694

Khalil, Rahab M., MD {1053487363} ObsGyn(94,EGY03)<NJ-MONMOUTH>
+ Monmouth Family Center
270 Broadway   Long Branch, NJ 07740   (732)923-7100   Fax (732)923-7104

Khalil, Samir Walid, MD {1396087987} FamMed
+ Tatem Brown Family Practice
2225 East Evesham Road/Suite 101   Voorhees, NJ 08043   (856)325-3700   Fax (856)325-3704

Khalil, Sara Adel, MD {1740519834} IntrMd
+ SJH Regional Medical Center
1505 West Sherman Avenue   Vineland, NJ 08360   (856)641-8000

Khalil, Steve, MD {1568738268} Nephro
+ RWJ University Hospital New Brunswick
One Robert Wood Johnson Place   New Brunswick, NJ 08901   (732)828-3000

Khalil, Suzan Y., MD {1265534820} IntrMd(72,EGYP)
+ Green Brook Regional Center
275 Green Brook Road   Green Brook, NJ 08812   (732)968-6000   Fax (732)968-8125
sukhalil@dhs.state.nj.us

Khalil, Venus T., MD {1073559860} FamMed, ObsGyn(69,EGYP)<NJ-STPETER, NJ-RBAYOLDB>
+ 3 Brunswick Woods Drive
East Brunswick, NJ 08816   (732)432-9923   Fax (732)432-0030

Khalil, Yasmine Ossama, DO {1376777102}
+ 325 Lafayette Street
Linden, NJ 07036

Khalina, Svetlana Petrovna, MD {1003041062} IntrMd
+ 22 Rector Street
Millburn, NJ 07041   (973)258-1941

Khamis, Khamis Gerious, DO {1942473269} FamMed, EmrgMd(04,NY75)<NJ-TRINIWSC, NJ-JFKMED>
+ Trinitas Regional Medical Center-Williamson Street
225 Williamson Street/Emergency   Elizabeth, NJ 07207   (908)994-5422
+ JFK Medical Center
65 James Street/Emergency   Edison, NJ 08820   (732)321-7000

Khan, Abrar Maqsood, MD {1043471667} IntrMd(94,INA44)
+ Atlantic Medical Associates, P.A.
499 Emston Road/Suite B6   Parlin, NJ 08859   (732)707-4676   Fax (732)372-0211

Khan, Adnan Iqbal, MD {1770537797} PsyCAd, Psychy(94,PAK20)<NJ-BERGNMC>
+ New Bridge Medical Center
230 East Ridgewood Avenue   Paramus, NJ 07652   (201)967-4000

Khan, Afshan R., DO {1578802591} FamMed
+ Summit Medical Group
48-50 Fairfield Street   Montclair, NJ 07042   (973)744-8511   Fax (973)744-6356

Khan, Aftab A., MD {1558316299} SrgVas, Surgry(67,PAK11)<NJ-MEMSALEM, NJ-SJHREGMC>
+ Iqbal & Khan Surgical Associates, P.A.
10 Magnolia Avenue/Suite E   Bridgeton, NJ 08302   (856)455-2399   Fax (856)451-7791
+ Inspira Medical Group Surgical Associates
1206 West Sherman Avenue/Building 2   Vineland, NJ 08360   (856)455-2399   Fax (856)696-9939

Khan, Akbar Ali, MD {1831155639} IntrMd(96,NET09)<NH-ANDROSGN>
+ Southern Ocean County Medical Center
1140 Route 72 West   Manahawkin, NJ 08050   (609)597-6011

Khan, Aliya W., MD {1366473654} IntrMd(96,PAK11)<NJ-UNVM-CPRN>
+ Princeton Family Care
100 Federal City Road/Suite A   Lawrenceville, NJ 08648   (609)620-1380   Fax (609)771-8991
+ Community Health Care, Inc.
319 Landis Avenue/Suites A & B   Vineland, NJ 08360   (609)620-1380   Fax (856)696-0344
+ Cooper University Internal Medicine Group
651 John F. Kennedy Way   Willingboro, NJ 08648   (609)835-2838   Fax (609)877-5421

Khan, Amber Manzoor, MD {1508958471} IntrMd, Gastrn(90,PHI02)
+ 1500 Mountain Top Road
Bridgewater, NJ 08807   (908)522-1313   Fax (908)522-1302

Khan, Amjad A., MD {1649272022} PthACl, Pthlgy, IntrMd(79,PAKI)<NJ-JRSYCITY>
+ QDx Pathology Services
46 Jackson Drive   Cranford, NJ 07016   Fax (908)272-1478

Khan, Aneela, MD {1972732543} Psychy
+ 823 Richard Road
Cherry Hill, NJ 08034   (856)482-1064

Khan, Anwar Ahmad, MD {1629168919} IntrMd(89,PAK13)
+ 66 York Street/Suite 101
Jersey City, NJ 07302   (201)626-7201   Fax (201)526-7202

Khan, Asim Haleem, MD {1174780100} Anesth<NJ-OURLADY>
+ Our Lady of Lourdes Medical Center
1600 Haddon Avenue   Camden, NJ 08103   (856)757-3500   Fax (856)755-0098

Khan, Atif Jalees, MD {1255545653} RadOnc(99,PAK14)<NJ-RWJUBRUN>
+ Rutgers Cancer Institute of New Jersey
195 Little Albany Street/PO Box 2681   New Brunswick, NJ 08903   (732)235-2465   Fax (732)235-6797

Khan, Basma, MD {1194875260} IntrMd, IntHos(96,PAK15)
+ JFK Medical Center
65 James Street   Edison, NJ 08820   (908)325-3595   Fax (732)909-2070
+ JFK Medical Center - Muhlenberg Campus
Park Avenue & Randolph Road   Plainfield, NJ 07061   (908)325-3595   Fax (908)668-3149

Khan, Dewan S., MD {1306914825} IntrMd(85,BAN08)<NJ-BAYSHORE, NJ-RBAYPERT>
+ 146 New Brunswick Avenue
Perth Amboy, NJ 08861   (732)697-1919   Fax (732)954-0789

Khan, Fahad, MD {1336303890} Gastrn, IntrMd(08,NY0)
+ Hackensack Digestive Diseases
52 First Street   Hackensack, NJ 07601   (201)488-3003   Fax (201)488-6911

Khan, Farah Asim, MD {1639325442} Psychy, PsyCAd, NrlgAddM<NJ-MORRISTN, NJ-CARRIER>
+ Behavioral Health Solution
85 Raritan Avenue   Highland Park, NJ 08904   (908)867-8766
dr.khan.@behavioralhealthsolution.com
+ AAMH - All Access Mental Health
819 Alexander Road   Princeton, NJ 08540   (908)867-8766   Fax (609)452-0627
+ NuView Academy
1 Park Avenue   Piscataway, NJ 08904   (732)878-0070

Khan, Farhana Haleem, MD {1033392642} ObsGyn(03,GRN01)
+ OB/GYN Women's Wellness, P.C.
1040 Clifton Avenue   Clifton, NJ 07013   (973)272-3136   Fax (973)547-9144

Khan, Fariha, MD {1770878423}
+ Hampton Behavioral Health Center
650 Rancocas Road   Westampton, NJ 08060   (609)267-7000   Fax (609)518-2190
+ 1173 Kaye Court
Burlington, NJ 08016   (609)949-3319

Khan, Ferdaus A., MD {1700838752} IntrMd(83,BAN04)
+ 5 Brian Court
Piscataway, NJ 08854

Khan, Ferhana, MD {1740371053} Pedtrc(73,INDI)<NJ-STJOSHOS>
+ Paterson Community Health Center
227 Broadway   Paterson, NJ 07501   (973)278-2600   Fax (973)278-5837

Khan, Habib, MD {1437393063} SrgVas
+ Meridian Surgical Associates
3700 Route 33/Suite C   Neptune, NJ 07753   (732)212-6598   Fax (732)922-2026

Khan, Ibraheem, MD {1396137683} Anesth
+ Robert Wood Johnson-UMDNJ Anesthesia Group
125 Paterson Street/CAB 3100   New Brunswick, NJ 08901   (732)235-6153   Fax (732)235-6131

Khan, Imran Ahmad, MD {1184826526} IntHos(00,PAK22)
+ SOM - Department of Internal Medicine
42 East Laurel Road/Suite 3100   Stratford, NJ 08084   (856)566-6845   Fax (856)566-6906

Khan, Imran Ahmad, MD {1003981499} IntrMd(00,PAK12)
+ University Physician Associates of New Jersey
125 Paterson Street/CAB 5200   New Brunswick, NJ 08901   (732)235-6531   Fax (732)235-7115

Khan, Imteyaz Ahmad, MD {1871751875} NnPnMd, Pedtrc, IntrMd(03,INA54)<NJ-STPETER>
+ St. Peter's University Hospital
254 Easton Avenue   New Brunswick, NJ 08901   (732)745-8600
+ St. Peter's University Hospital
254 Easton Avenue/Pediatrics   New Brunswick, NJ 08901   (732)565-1555

Khan, Inamul, MD {1265726939}
+ Carepoint Health
10 Exchange Place/16th Floor   Jersey City, NJ 07302   (201)884-5289
inamkhanmd@gmail.com

Khan, Irfana B., MD {1750660924} IntHos, IntrMd(03,PAK26)<NJ-BAYONNE>
+ Bayonne Medical Center
29th Street at Avenue E   Bayonne, NJ 07002   (201)858-5000   Fax (201)858-5080

Khan, Khuram Adnan, DO {1982865671} Anesth
+ 921 Azalea Drive
North Brunswick, NJ 08902

Khan, Majid K., MD {1568557346} CdvDis, IntrMd(71,GER07)
+ first Health
10 Parsonage Road/Suite 102   Edison, NJ 08837   (732)662-4680   Fax (732)662-3354

Khan, Malik Adnan Ullah, MD {1295905370} IntrMd(01,PAK15)
+ 21 Orta Court
Sayreville, NJ 08872

Khan, Mansoor Ali, MD {1114067667} EmrgMd(01,NY48)<NJ-WAYNEGEN>
+ St. Joseph's Wayne Hospital
224 Hamburg Turnpike   Wayne, NJ 07470   (973)740-0607
+ Emergency Medical Associates of NJ, P.A.
3 Century Drive   Parsippany, NJ 07054   (973)740-0607   Fax (973)740-9895

Khan, Maryam Ijaz, MD {1780893826}
+ Corrado Ctr Facial Plstic Cosmtic Srgy
1919 Greentree Road/Suite C   Cherry Hill, NJ 08003   (856)344-5906   Fax (856)229-7617
+ The Cooper Hospital System-Univ Hospital
3 Cooper Plaza/Suite 215   Camden, NJ 08103   (856)342-2439
+ Cooper Endocrinology Associates
1210 Brace Road/Suite 107   Cherry Hill, NJ 08003   (832)651-8436   Fax (856)795-7590

Physicians by Name and Address

Khan, Mateen Abdul Rahman, MD {1558387480} EmrgMd(04,PA13)
+ RWJ Hamilton/Emergency Services
1 Hamilton Health Place   Hamilton, NJ 08690   (609)586-7900

Khan, Mehtab A., MD {1154414431} Psychy(01,INA2Y)
+ 113 East Centre Street/Apt 2105
Nutley, NJ 07110   (765)935-0629
mehtabkhan@yahoo.com

Khan, Mohammad F., MD {1982880316} IntrMd(00,PAK21)<NJ-CHSFULD>
+ Capital Health System/Fuld Campus
750 Brunswick Avenue   Trenton, NJ 08638   (609)394-6000

Khan, Mohammed Faraz, MD {1487894820} SrgNro
+ North Jersey Brain and Surgical
680 Kinderkamack Road/Suite 300   Oradell, NJ 07649
(201)342-2550   Fax (201)342-7171

Khan, Mohammed Nasir, MD {1932214095} FamMed, IntrMd(87,DOM01)
+ My Family Practice Associates
37 South Main Street   Manville, NJ 08835   (908)722-9333
Fax (908)722-9990

Khan, Mubashar H., MD {1497175707} CdvDis<NJ-COOPRUMC>
+ Cooper University Hospital
One Cooper Plaza/Drrance/3rd Fl   Camden, NJ 08103
(856)342-2624

Khan, Muhammad Anees, MD {1295762516} PulDis, IntrMd(66,PAKI)<NJ-STJOSHOS>
+ St. Joseph's Regional Medical Center
703 Main Street/Pulmonary   Paterson, NJ 07503
(973)754-2450   Fax (973)754-2469

Khan, Muhammad B.H., MD {1225045990} Anesth(81,PAKI)<NJ-CLARMAAS>
+ Clara Maass Medical Center
1 Clara Maass Drive/Anesthesiology   Belleville, NJ 07109
(973)450-2000

Khan, Muhammad Khurram, MD {1528253408} CritCr
+ Hunterdon Pulmonary & Critical Care Associates
6 Sand Hill Road/Suite 202   Flemington, NJ 08822
(908)237-1148   Fax (908)237-1749

Khan, Mujahid A., MD {1548376205} Psychy, PssoMd(83,EGY03)<PA-STLKBTHL>
+ Capital Health System/Fuld Campus
750 Brunswick Avenue   Trenton, NJ 08638   (609)394-6000

Khan, Munaza Anwar, MD {1619117926} Psychy(03,PAK18)
+ University Hospital-SOM Department of Psychiatry
2250 Chapel Avenue West/Suite 100   Cherry Hill, NJ 08002
(856)482-9000   Fax (856)482-1159

Khan, Musaid A., MD {1134263460} Nrolgy, Psychy(92,PAK11)
+ 142 Palisade Avenue/Suite 111
Jersey City, NJ 07306   (201)918-2568   Fax (201)360-0453
+ New Jersey Medical Group
464 Hudson Terrace/Suite 201   Englewood Cliffs, NJ 07632
(201)918-2568   Fax (201)503-0848

Khan, Naheed A., MD {1144326034} PhysMd, SrgOrt, PhyM-Pain(66,PAKI)<NJ-ACMCITY, NJ-ACMCMAIN>
+ PO Box 712
Absecon, NJ 08201   (609)641-6666   Fax (609)641-4674

Khan, Nazia, MD {1700196581} IntrMd(04,INA23)<NJ-STJOSHOS>
+ St. Joseph's Regional Medical Center
703 Main Street/Internal Med   Paterson, NJ 07503
(732)890-1138

Khan, Noroze Jalil, MD {1972580835} InfDis, IntrMd(74,PAKI)<NJ-CHRIST>
+ 20 Lincoln Street
Jersey City, NJ 07307   (201)963-3570   Fax (201)526-0461
rosemedical20@yahoo.com

Khan, Rafay Tariq, MD {1194258012} IntrMd
+ 11 Hop Brook Lane
Holmdel, NJ 07733   (848)391-3245

Khan, Rizwana, MD {1154558419} IntrMd(98,PAK22)
+ Westside Medical Associates
562 West Side Avenue   Jersey City, NJ 07304   (201)434-7800   Fax (201)434-6715

Khan, Sabeen, MD {1589979181} IntrMd(01)
+ Union County HealthCare Associates
400 Westfield Avenue   Elizabeth, NJ 07208   (908)620-3800   Fax (908)620-3243

Khan, Sadaf Ahmad, MD {1073522033} Pedtrc, PedCrd(98,MD01)
+ CHOP Pediatric & Adolescent Specialty Care Center
1012 Laurel Oak Road   Voorhees, NJ 08043   (856)435-1300   Fax (856)435-0091

Khan, Saima, MD {1881890416} IntrMd(00,PAK18)<NJ-STPETER>
+ Diabetes & Endocrine Associates of Hunterdon
9100 Westcott Drive/Suite 101   Flemington, NJ 08822
(908)237-6990   Fax (908)237-6995

Khan, Samina K., MD {1992764906} IntrMd(87,PAK20)<NJ-STMICHL>
+ 327 Valley Road
West Orange, NJ 07052   (973)736-0909   Fax (973)736-8355

+ St. Michael's Medical Center
268 MLK Jr. Boulevard/Internal Med   Newark, NJ 07102
(973)877-5000

Khan, Saqiba, MD {1336192509} Pedtrc, PedEmg(87,PAK15)<NJ-HACKNSK>
+ Hackensack University Medical Center
30 Prospect Avenue   Hackensack, NJ 07601   (551)996-5061   Fax (551)996-3676
+ St Joseph's Medical Center Emergency
703 Main Street   Paterson, NJ 07503   (551)996-5061   Fax (973)754-2249

Khan, Sarah, MD {1093794448} IntrMd, EnDbMt(94,ENG22)
+ 245 Baldwin Road/Suite 107
Parsippany, NJ 07054   (973)402-1477   Fax (973)402-1488

Khan, Sarosh, MD {1366799199} IntrMd<NJ-HCKTSTWN>
+ Hackettstown Regional Medical Center
651 Willow Grove Street   Hackettstown, NJ 07840
(908)441-1161

Khan, Shameen, DO {1386975324} InfDis
+ Center for Asthma & Allergy
18 North Third Avenue   Highland Park, NJ 08904
(732)545-0094   Fax (732)545-4087
+ Center for Asthma & Allergy
300 Hudson Street   Hoboken, NJ 07030   (732)545-0094
Fax (201)792-5320
+ Center for Asthma & Allergy
90 Milbum Avenue/Suite 200   Maplewood, NJ 08904
(973)763-5787   Fax (973)763-8568

Khan, Sohaila, MD {1669541264} Pedtrc(88,PAK20)<NJ-RBAY-OLDB, NJ-STPETER>
+ 11 Burlew Place
Parlin, NJ 08859   (732)316-5444   Fax (732)316-0330

Khan, Sophia S., MD {1417186842} FamMed
+ The University Doctors
100 Century Parkway/Suite 140   Mount Laurel, NJ 08054
(856)380-2400   Fax (856)234-7870
+ Cooper Family Medicine
1001-F Lincoln Drive West   Marlton, NJ 08053   (856)380-2400   Fax (856)810-1879

Khan, Sunniya, MD {1992065593} PainMd
+ Hackensack Medical Center Pain & Palliative
20 Prospect Avenue/Suite 602   Hackensack, NJ 07601
(551)996-2442

Khan, Taj G., DO {1851480917} Ophthl, IntrMd(96,NY75)<NJ-HOBUNIMC, NJ-STBARNMC>
+ Associated Eye Physicians & Surgeons of NJ, P.A.
1530 Saint Georges Avenue   Rahway, NJ 07065   (732)382-9000   Fax (732)382-7455
+ Associated Eye Physicians & Surgeons of NJ, P.A.
724 Jersey Avenue   Jersey City, NJ 07302   (732)382-9000
Fax (201)795-9797
+ Associated Eye Physicians & Surgeons of NJ, P.A.
1050 Galloping Hill Road/Suite 104   Union, NJ 07065
(908)964-7878   Fax (908)964-5434

Khan, Talha Ehsan, MD {1356573646} CritCr<NJ-STPETER>
+ St. Peter's University Hospital
254 Easton Avenue/Cares/4th Fl   New Brunswick, NJ 08901
(716)374-1271

Khan, Umer, MD {1548657034}<NJ-RWJUHAM>
+ Robert Wood Johnson University Hospital at Hamilton
1 Hamilton Health Place   Hamilton, NJ 08690   (509)586-7900

Khan, Ummais N., MD {1649543380} PhysMd<NJ-KSLRWEST>
+ Integrated Physiatry Services
45 South Park Place/Suite 259   Morristown, NJ 07960
(908)490-0036   Fax (908)490-0067

Khan, Wajahat Hussain, MD {1932426905} PulDis, IntrMd(06,NET12)
+ Respiratory & Sleep Specialists, LLC.
3546 State Route 27   Kendall Park, NJ 08824   (732)737-7801   Fax (877)632-3456

Khan, Yusra, MD {1184987927} IntHos<NJ-SJHREGMC>
+ SJH Regional Medical Center
1505 West Sherman Avenue   Vineland, NJ 08360
(856)845-0100   Fax (302)651-4945

Khan, Yusuf Mujtaba, MD {1962442655} IntrMd, PulDis(81,BWI01)<NJ-CHSMRCER>
+ Snoring and Sleep Apnea Center Mercer County
1401 Whitehorse Mercerville Rd   Hamilton, NJ 08619
(609)584-5150   Fax (609)584-5144

Khan, Zeeshan, MD {1922449206} FamMGrtc
+ CentraState Family Medicine Residency Practice
1001 West Main Street/Suite B   Freehold, NJ 07728
(732)294-2540   Fax (732)409-2621

Khan-Jaffery, Kaniz F., MD {1629143979} IntrMd(89,PAK11)
+ Premier HealthCare
1129 North New Road/Suite C   Absecon, NJ 08201
(609)377-8516   Fax (609)377-8607

Khandelwal, Anil, MD {1669630356} FamMed(97,INA9B)
+ Visiting Nurse Association of Central Jersey
1301 Main Street   Asbury Park, NJ 07712   (732)774-6333
Fax (732)219-6625
+ 1 Faith Avenue
Edison, NJ 08820

Khandelwal, Meena, MD {1841377942} ObsGyn, IntrMd, MtFtMd(86,INA72)<NJ-COOPRUMC>
+ Cooper University Hospital
One Cooper Plaza/Rm 623/Dorrance   Camden, NJ 08103
(856)342-2000

Khandelwal, Priyank, MD {1225347727} Nrolgy
+ Center for Neurological Surgery UMDNJ
90 Bergen Street/DOC 8100   Newark, NJ 07103   (973)972-2323   Fax (973)972-2333

Khani, Ghassan, MD {1124190616} Surgry(71,SYR01)<NJ-MEADWLND, NJ-CHRIST>
+ 255 Route 3 East/Suite 202
Secaucus, NJ 07094   (201)866-3266   Fax (201)866-0887

Khanijow, Vikresh, MD {1962768531} Gastrn, IntrMd
+ Gastroenterology Consultants of South Jersey
693 Main Street/Suite 2   Lumberton, NJ 08048   (609)265-1700   Fax (609)265-9005

Khanna, Anirudh, MD {1104909712} IntrMd, CdvDis(93,INA69)<NJ-HCKTSTWN>
+ Medical Care Associates
137 Mountain Avenue   Hackettstown, NJ 07840   (908)852-1887   Fax (908)852-0614
+ Medical Care Associates
262 Route 10 West   Succasunna, NJ 07876   (908)852-1887
Fax (973)252-1422

Khanna, Anisha, DO {1912110826} Pedtrc(04,MO78)
+ 401 Ridgewood Avenue
Glen Ridge, NJ 07028   (973)748-6470   Fax (973)748-1834

Khanna, Ashish, MD {1770833188} Surgry
+ Kessler Institute for Rehabilitation West Orange
1199 Pleasant Valley Way   West Orange, NJ 07052
(973)731-3600

Khanna, Bindu Chiranjit, MD {1427004472} PsyCAd, Psychy(91,INA65)<NJ-HACKNSK>
+ 90 Arverne Road
West Orange, NJ 07052

Khanna, Kamlesh, MD {1487782579} Pedtrc(70,INA56)<NJ-CLARMAAS, NJ-MTNSIDE>
+ 401 Ridgewood Avenue
Glen Ridge, NJ 07028   (973)748-6470   Fax (973)748-1834

Khanna, Malini M., MD {1306087200} PhysMd, Anesth(07,DC01)<PA-UPMCPHL>
+ Reconstructive Orthopedics, P.A.
570 Egg Harbor Road/Suite C-4   Sewell, NJ 08080
(609)267-9400   Fax (609)267-9457

Khanna, Pawandeep S., MD {1578774618} RadDia, Radiol, IntrMd(00,INA9F)
+ Shore Imaging
1166 River Avenue/Suite 102   Lakewood, NJ 08701
(732)364-9565   Fax (732)364-1908

Khanna, Pravien K., MD {1497932149} CdvDis, IntrMd(06,NY01)<NY-PRSBWEIL>
+ RWJPE/New Brunswick Cardiology Group, P.A.
75 Veronica Road/Suite 101   Somerset, NJ 08873
(732)247-7444   Fax (732)247-5119
+ RWJPE New Brunswick Cardiology Group, P.A.
15H Briar Hill Court   East Brunswick, NJ 08816   (732)613-9313
+ RWJPE New Brunswick Cardiology Group, P.A.
111 Union Valley Road/Suite 201   Monroe Township, NJ 08873   (609)409-6856   Fax (609)409-6882

Khanna, Priya, DO {1295940161} Nephro(03,MO78)
+ 401 Ridgewood Avenue
Glen Ridge, NJ 07028   (973)930-9344   Fax (973)748-1834
Khannanephrology@yahoo.com

Khanna, Roohi, DO {1285900928} FamMed(12,VA75)<MA-LAWR-GEN>
+ Summit Medical Group
383 Ridgedale Avenue/Suite 8   East Hanover, NJ 07936
(973)887-0200   Fax (973)887-4965
+ Summit Medical Group
6 Brighton Road/2 FL   Clifton, NJ 07012   (973)887-0200
Fax (973)777-5403

Khanna, Santosh B., MD {1326189812} Pedtrc(63,INA72)
+ Drs Khanna & Kukla MDs
817 Inman Avenue   Edison, NJ 08820   (732)381-8600   Fax (732)381-8690

Khanna, Sunil K., MD {1063404242} IntrMd, CdvDis(93,NY03)<NJ-JFKMED, NJ-RWJBURN>
+ 579 Main Street
Metuchen, NJ 08840   (732)906-2332   Fax (732)806-9433

Khanna, Veena W., MD {1881795417} FamMed(66,INDI)<NJ-TRENTPSY>
+ Trenton Psychiatric Hospital
Sullivan Way/PO Box 7600/FamMed   West Trenton, NJ 08628   (609)633-1500

Physicians by Name and Address

Khanna, Vikas, MD {1851331904} EmrgMd(01,GRN01)<NJ-JFKMED>
+ JFK Medical Center
65 James Street/EmrgMed Edison, NJ 08820 (732)321-7000 Fax (732)744-5614

Kharaz, Marina, MD {1194790899} Psychy(82,RUSS)
+ Preferred Behavioral Health of New Jersey
725 Airport Road Lakewood, NJ 08701 (732)367-4700 Fax (732)364-2253
+ Preferred Behavioral Health of New Jersey
700 Airport Road Lakewood, NJ 08701 (732)367-4700 Fax (732)364-2253

Kharazi, Fariba, DO {1326428152} FamMed
+ Drs. Kharazi and Jain
7 Vose Avenue South Orange, NJ 07079 (973)630-8989 Fax (908)277-0201

Khare, Madhurani, MD {1508950684} PsyCAd, Psychy(91,INDI)
+ Princeton House Behavioral Health - Princeton
905 Herrontown Road Princeton, NJ 08540 (609)497-3300 Fax (609)497-3370

Kharitonova, Anna A., DO {1619032539} Psychy(96,NY75)
+ 776 East Third Avenue
Roselle, NJ 07203 (718)238-2285 Fax (718)322-7412

Kharkover, Mark Y., MD {1902849847} Pedtrc(81,RUSS)
+ Advocare Scotch Plains Pediatrics
1608 East 2nd Street Scotch Plains, NJ 07076 (908)322-6000 Fax (908)322-7770
drkharkover1@yahoo.com

Kharod, Amit S., MD {1003804964} Surgry, SrgBst(96,PA13)
+ Advanced Surgical Health Associates
901 West Main Street/MAB Suite 101 Freehold, NJ 07728 (732)308-4202 Fax (732)308-4212

Kharod, Sudhakar J., MD {1518937580} Pedtrc(69,INDI)<NJ-JRSYSHMC>
+ 507 Fourth Avenue
Asbury Park, NJ 07712 (732)774-5600

Khasak, Dmitry, MD {1649258286} Dermat(92,NY19)<NY-MTSINYHS, NY-NRTHGEN>
+ Better Skin Dermatology, LLC
100 Town Square/Suite 409 Jersey City, NJ 07310 (201)626-4040 Fax (201)626-4041
ebetterskin@yahoo.com
+ 844 Avenue C
Bayonne, NJ 07002 (201)626-4040 Fax (201)339-6688

Khatib, Amira, MD {1861584773} Pedtrc(72,SYR01)<NJ-CLARMAAS>
+ Clara Maass Medical Center
1 Clara Maass Drive Belleville, NJ 07109 (973)450-2000

Khatib, Samara, MD {1366754152} IntrMd(10,ANT02)<NJ-STJOSHOS>
+ St. Joseph's Regional Medical Center
703 Main Street/Medicine Paterson, NJ 07503 (973)754-2549

Khatiwala, Colleen Pravin, MD {1679724553} Anesth<NJ-SHOREMEM>
+ Shore Memorial Hospital
1 East New York Avenue Somers Point, NJ 08244 (609)653-3500

Khatiwala, Jayesh Ramesh, MD {1881665628} CdvDis, IntrMd(96,NJ05)<NJ-VIRTUAHS, NJ-OURLADY>
+ Associated Cardiovascular Consultants-Lourdes
1 Brace Road/Suite C & F Cherry Hill, NJ 08034 (856)428-4100 Fax (856)428-5748

Khatiwala, Manisha P., MD {1003924259} EmrgMd(97,NJ05)<NJ-ACMCITY, NJ-ACMCMAIN>
+ AtlantiCare Regional Medical Center/City Campus
1925 Pacific Avenue Atlantic City, NJ 08401 (609)345-4000
+ AtlantiCare Regional Med Ctr/Mainland
65 West Jimmie Leeds Road Pomona, NJ 08240 (609)652-1000

Khattar, Vimi, MD {1053484709} PhysMd, IntrMd(94,NJ05)
+ Integrated Physiatry Services
45 South Park Place/Suite 259 Morristown, NJ 07960 (908)490-0036 Fax (908)490-0067

Khavarian, Javad, MD {1851462212} SrgOrt(63,IRAN)<NJ-BAYSHORE>
+ 733 North Beers Street
Holmdel, NJ 07733 (732)739-3130 Fax (732)739-1783

Khaw, Kenneth, MD {1336119601} CdvDis, IntCrd, IntrMd(88,NY09)<NJ-OURLADY, NJ-VIRTUAHS>
+ Associated Cardiovascular Consultants-Lourdes
1 Brace Road/Suite C & F Cherry Hill, NJ 08034 (856)428-4100 Fax (856)428-5748

Khawaja, Aftab A., MD {1730157587} SrgVas, Surgry(66,PAKI)<NJ-CHRIST>
+ Hudson Surgeons
142 Palisade Avenue/Suite 108 Jersey City, NJ 07306 (201)795-0101 Fax (201)795-3550

Khawaja, Asia B., MD {1619084696} PthAcl, Pthlgy(66,PAK01)<NJ-CHRIST>
+ Christ Hospital
176 Palisade Avenue/Path/Lab Med Jersey City, NJ 07306 (201)795-8339 Fax (201)795-8118
asiakhawaja@christhospital.org

Khawaja, Hasan Sajjad, MD {1215099379} Anesth, IntrMd(02,DMN01)<PA-MRCYFTZG, PA-MRCYPHIL>
+ Deborah Heart and Lung Center
200 Trenton Road/Anesthesia Browns Mills, NJ 08015 (770)643-5619

Khawja, Yasmin, MD {1407116452} IntrMd(12,NY46)<NY-MTSINAI>
+ Cooper University Internal Medicine Group
651 John F. Kennedy Way Willingboro, NJ 08046 (609)835-2838 Fax (609)877-5421

Khazai, Kamran, MD {1578667119} ObsGyn(86,DOM10)
+ Preferred Women HealthCare LLC
240 Williamson Street/Suite 405 Elizabeth, NJ 07202 (908)353-5551 Fax (908)353-5052
+ Neighborhood Health Center Plainfield
1700-58 Myrtle Avenue Plainfield, NJ 07060 (908)353-5551 Fax (908)226-6743

Khebzou, Zaki, MD {1750334710} EmrgMd(78,FRAN)<NJ-ACMCITY, NJ-ACMCMAIN>
+ AtlantiCare Regional Medical Center/City Campus
1925 Pacific Avenue/EmergMed Atlantic City, NJ 08401 (609)345-4000

Khedekar, Surekha D., MD {1396745980} RadDia(78,INA67)<NJ-EASTORNG>
+ 3 Murphy Court
West Orange, NJ 07052 (973)325-2968

Kheder, Abdul-Hady M., MD {1487631909} IntrMd(88,EGY05)<NJ-STFRNMED, NJ-RWJUHAM>
+ Americare Medical Associates, LLC
445 Whitehorse Avenue/Suite 202 Trenton, NJ 08610 (609)585-1122 Fax (609)585-0309

Khedkar, Meera, MD {1306973870} AlgyImmn, IntrMd(99,PA09)<NJ-JFKMED, NJ-RWJUBRUN>
+ Summit Medical Group-Berkeley Heights Campus
1 Diamond Hill Road Berkeley Heights, NJ 07922 (908)273-4300 Fax (908)790-6576
+ Asthma, Sinus & Allergy Centers
19 Holly Street Cranford, NJ 07016 (908)273-4300 Fax (908)276-7434

Khedkar, Mona S., MD {1013023423} Radiol(72,INDI)
+ Magnetic Resonance of New Jersey
410 Centre Street Nutley, NJ 07110 (973)661-0006 Fax (973)661-4473

Khelemsky, Serge, DO {1528405420} Nrolgy
+ University Hospital-RWJMS Neurology
125 Paterson Street/Suite 4100-6100 New Brunswick, NJ 08901 (732)235-7757 Fax (732)235-7041

Khelil, Jennifer Lynn, DO {1740323443} IntrMd(95,NJ75)
+ Pulmonary and Sleep Physicians
204 Ark Road/Suite 206/Larchmont 1 Mount Laurel, NJ 08054 (856)778-4640 Fax (856)778-8862

Khella, Hani Joseph, MD {1518394840} FamMed(89,NY03)
+ 9901 Seapoint Boulevard
Wildwood Crest, NJ 08260

Kheny, Mira, MD {1083653521} FamMed(76,INA68)<NJ-VIRTBERL, NJ-VIRTVOOR>
+ 6650 Browning Road/Room M21
Pennsauken, NJ 08109 (856)910-8100 Fax (856)910-8101

Kher, Neeta Yogesh, MD {1922115351} Psychy, IntrMd(89,INA65)<NJ-CHSFULD>
+ Capital Health System/Fuld Campus
750 Brunswick Avenue/Psychy Trenton, NJ 08638 (609)815-7829 Fax (609)815-7814

Khera, Gurbir Singh, MD {1871667204} Psychy(81,MEX29)
+ 1 Main Street/Suite 308
Eatontown, NJ 07724 (732)530-2900
+ PO Box 148
Manalapan, NJ 07726 (732)530-2900

Khesin, Yevgeniy I., MD {1821098500} Nrolgy(95,RUS15)
+ Neurological Arts Associated, LLC.
183 High Street/Suite 1200 Newton, NJ 07860 (973)300-0579 Fax (973)300-5535

Khetani, Manish P., MD {1447430244} Psychy, Anesth(96,INA5Y)
+ James Street Anesthesia
102 James Street/Suite 103 Edison, NJ 08820 (732)494-1444 Fax (732)494-7052

Kheterpal, Neil M., DO {1609891415} Gastrn, IntrMd(03,NY75)<NJ-HACKNSK>
+ Hackensack University Medical Center
20 Prospect Avenue/Suite 715 Hackensack, NJ 07601 (201)881-0721 Fax (201)881-0725

Khety, Shabnam N., MD {1104063734}
+ 289 Mckinley Avenue
Edison, NJ 08820 (732)668-4292

Kheyfets, Irina, MD {1407813355} IntrMd(79,RUSS)<NJ-STJOSHOS>
+ St. Joseph's Family Health Center
21 Market Street Paterson, NJ 07501 (973)754-4222 Fax (973)754-4201

Khianey, Reena, MD {1215195268} Rheuma, AlgyImmn, IntrMd(07,VA04)
+ University Hospital-Doctors Office Center
90 Bergen Street/Suite 4500 Newark, NJ 07103 (973)972-2500

Khimani, Karim J., MD {1962460196} IntrMd, Grtrcs(82,DMN01)
+ 240 Williamson Street/Suite 306
Elizabeth, NJ 07202 (908)352-5071 Fax (908)352-0538
+ Overlook Medical Center
99 Beauvoir Avenue/PO Box 210 Summit, NJ 07902 (908)352-5071 Fax (908)352-0538

Khinda, Navjot, MD {1932454998} Psychy
+ 221 Park Avenue
Rutherford, NJ 07070 (201)293-0976

Khine, Mary L., MD {1891762571} ObsGyn(92,PA02)<NJ-MORRISTN, NJ-OVERLOOK>
+ Atlantic Maternal Fetal Medicine
435 South Street/Suite 380 Morristown, NJ 07960 (973)971-7080 Fax (973)290-8312
+ Maternal Fetal Medicine of Practice Associates
11 Overlook Road/Suite LL 102 Summit, NJ 07901 (973)971-7080 Fax (908)522-5557

Khokhar, Rizwana T., MD {1508828567} Pedtrc(83,PAK01)<NJ-STBARNMC>
+ Park Avenue Pediatrics
36 Park Avenue Verona, NJ 07044 (973)239-7001 Fax (973)239-8867

Khokher, Sairah M., MD {1376798454}
+ 19 Kyle Way
Trenton, NJ 08628

Kholdarov, Boris, MD {1578000519} OccpMd
+ EOHSI
170 Frelinghuysen Road/Room 212 Piscataway, NJ 08854 (848)445-6071

Khona, Nithyashuba B., MD PhysMd(73,INA67)
+ South Jersey Health Care Center
Two Cooper Plaza Camden, NJ 08103 (856)342-7600 Fax (856)342-6662

Khong, Darmadi S., MD {1902957657} IntrMd(95,GER25)<NY-LICOLLGE>
+ 73 Linden Street
Millburn, NJ 07041

Khoo, Patrick S., MD {1689686743} IntrMd(81,MYAN)<NY-BRNXVAMC, NJ-HOLYNAME>
+ Holy Name Hospital
718 Teaneck Road Teaneck, NJ 07666 (201)833-3000

Khoo, Robert Eng Hong, MD {1659315760} SrgC&R<PA-GSNGER>
+ Surgical Specialists of New Jersey
1364 Route 72 West/Suite 5 Manahawkin, NJ 08050 (609)978-0778 Fax (609)978-1377
+ Robert Eng Hong Khoo MD
44 Nautilus Drive/Suite 201 Manahawkin, NJ 08050 (609)978-0778 Fax (609)978-3190

Khorenian, Sylvie D., MD {1275625246} Dermat(91,NJ05)<NJ-ENGLWOOD, NY-MTSINAI>
+ 630 East Palisade Avenue
Englewood Cliffs, NJ 07632 (201)503-0302 Fax (201)503-0309
sdkhorenian@aol.com

Khorrami, Cyrus, MD {1902079262} RadDia(03,PA13)<NJ-COOPRUMC>
+ Cooper University Hospital
One Cooper Plaza Camden, NJ 08103 (856)342-2000

Khorrami, Parviz, MD {1598709271} Radiol, RadDia(68,IRAN)
+ Toms River X-Ray
154 Highway 37 West Toms River, NJ 08753 (732)244-0777 Fax (732)244-0428

Khorsandi, Shayan, MD {1083159305}
+ Alliance Ob/Gyn Consultants
5045 Route 130 South/Suite 1 Delran, NJ 08075 (856)764-7660 Fax (856)764-5723

Khoshnu, Esha, MD {1689775942} Nrolgy, Psychy(93,CT01)
+ 1140 Bloomfield Avenue/Suite 202
West Caldwell, NJ 07006 (973)575-1107 Fax (732)563-0035

Khosla, Jayasree, MD {1962821140} ObsGyn
+ Penn Medicine at Cherry Hill
409 Route 70 East Cherry Hill, NJ 08034 (856)427-4336

Khosla, Meenakshi, MD {1154685386} Pedtrc<NJ-STPETER>
+ St. Peter's University Hospital
254 Easton Avenue New Brunswick, NJ 08901 (732)745-8600

Khosla, Savita, MD {1265424238} ObsGyn, Gyneco(76,INDI)<NJ-VALLEY, NJ-HACKNSK>
+ Physicians for Womens Health
1124 East Ridgewood Avenue/Suite 105 Ridgewood, NJ 07450 (201)489-2255 Fax (201)447-1231
+ Physicians for Womens Health
58 Summit Avenue Hackensack, NJ 07601 (201)489-2255 Fax (201)489-4799

Physicians by Name and Address

Khosravi, Abtin Hajiloo, MD {1356583033} Surgry
+ Surgical Associates
  90 Prospect Avenue/Room 1D   Hackensack, NJ 07601   (201)343-3433   Fax (201)343-0420

Khot, Ashish Abhay, MD {1871822619} OncHem
+ Advanced Care Hematology & Oncology Associates
  385 Morris Avenue/Suite 100   Springfield, NJ 07081   (973)379-2111   Fax (973)379-2807

Khoudary, Maryann Lisa, MD {1578686424} ObsGyn, IntrMd(97,NJ06)<NJ-OVERLOOK>
+ Overlook Medical Center
  99 Beauvoir Avenue/PO Box 210/OB/GYN   Summit, NJ 07902   (908)522-2000

Khouri, Albert S., MD {1093915837} Ophthl
+ University Ophthalmology Associates
  90 Bergen Street/DOC 6100   Newark, NJ 07101   (973)972-2065   Fax (973)972-1746

Khouri, Philippe J., MD {1689768830} PsyGrt, Psychy(72,LEBA)<NJ-UNVMCPRN>
+ Princeton House Behavioral Health - Princeton
  905 Herrontown Road/Psychiatry   Princeton, NJ 08540   (609)497-3300   Fax (609)497-3370

Khoury, Aldo D., MD {1154356830} NnPnMd, ObsGyn(78,SYRI)<NJ-STJOSHOS>
+ Perinatal Services of Northern New Jersey
  57 Willowbrook Road/3rd Floor   Wayne, NJ 07470   (973)754-3800   Fax (973)244-0476
+ St. Joseph's Regional Medical Center
  703 Main Street   Paterson, NJ 07503   (973)754-2710

Khoury, Hani A., MD {1558440925} SrgC&R, Surgry(73,SYR01)<NJ-STJOSHOS, NJ-WAYNEGEN>
+ 502 Hamburg Turnpike/Suite 107
  Wayne, NJ 07470   (973)942-6611   Fax (973)942-5906
+ 1815 Kennedy Boulevard
  Jersey City, NJ 07305   (201)432-0110

Khrizman, Polina, MD {1861673089} IntrMd
+ The Cooper Hospital System-Univ Hospital
  3 Cooper Plaza/Suite 215   Camden, NJ 08103   (856)342-2312

Khuddus, Munawara S., MD {1528037272} Pedtrc(69,INDI)<NJ-BAYSHORE, NJ-RIVERVW>
+ 51 Village Court
  Hazlet, NJ 07730   (732)739-1908   Fax (732)739-1565
+ SAMRA Pediatrics
  300 Perrine Road/Suite 331   Old Bridge, NJ 08857   (732)739-1908   Fax (732)727-0955

Khullar, Ritu, MD {1912167701}
+ 2619 Forest Haven Boulevard
  Edison, NJ 08817   (609)457-5941

Khulusi, Nami, MD {1841361771} IntrMd(89,SYRI)
+ 615 Hope Road/Building 2A
  Eatontown, NJ 07724   (848)456-4485   Fax (848)456-4492

Khurana, Pavan, MD {1992932636} Radiol, RadDia(06,NY08)
+ University Radiology, PA
  239 Route 22 East/Suite 302   Green Brook, NJ 08812   (732)968-5160   Fax (973)716-9250
+ University Radiology Group, P.C.
  579A Cranbury Road   East Brunswick, NJ 08816   (732)968-5160   Fax (732)390-1856
+ University Radiology Group, P.C.
  16 Mountain Boulevard   Warren, NJ 08812   (908)769-7200   Fax (908)769-9141

Khutorskoy, Tamara, MD {1548502891} EnDbMt
+ UMDNJ Otolaryonology
  185 South Orange Avenue/MSB I-590   Newark, NJ 07103   (973)972-6170   Fax (973)972-5185

Khwaja, Tahir Nisar, MD {1881804938} PsyCAd
+ Princeton House Behavioral Health - North Brunswick
  1460 Livingston Avenue   North Brunswick, NJ 08902   (732)435-0202   Fax (732)435-0222

Kiamzon, Harald James, MD {1447358858} Anesth
+ Anesthesia Consultnts of NJ/Nova Pain
  285 Davidson Avenue/Suite 204   Somerset, NJ 08873   (732)271-1400   Fax (732)271-3543

Kianfar, Hormoz, MD {1306008727} IntrMd<NY-NYHQUEEN>
+ Ocean Heart Group
  1530 Route 88/Suite A   Brick, NJ 08724   (732)840-0600   Fax (732)840-0611

Kibilska Borowski, Jolanta M., MD {1356434591} IntrMd(82,POLA)
+ Drs. Borowski & Kibilska-Borowski
  812 North Wood Avenue/Suite 101   Linden, NJ 07036   (908)486-3366

Kiblawi, Fuad Moh'D, MD {1710065107} Pedtrc, PedCrd(93,JOR01)<NJ-STJOSHOS, NJ-CHILTON>
+ Pediatric Cardiology Associates
  1 Broadway/Suite 203   Elmwood Park, NJ 07407   (973)569-6250   Fax (973)569-6270

Kibrea, S. M. Golam, MD {1306012182} InfDis, IntrMd(98,BAN02)
+ 170 Prospect Avenue/Suite 6
  Hackensack, NJ 07601   (201)621-5820   Fax (201)621-5820

+ Capital Health System/Fuld Campus
  750 Brunswick Avenue   Trenton, NJ 08638   (609)394-6000

Kicenuik, Michael T., MD {1487652988} ObsGyn, Gyneco(76,NJ05)<NJ-STPETER, NJ-RWJUBRUN>
+ St. Peter's Family Health
  123 How Lane   New Brunswick, NJ 08901   (732)745-8600   Fax (732)729-0869
+ University of Urogynecology of New Jersey
  254 Easton Avenue/3 FL/Cares Blg   New Brunswick, NJ 08901   (732)745-8600   Fax (732)249-6140

Kidangan, Julie Thomas, DO {1437470119} FamMed, IntrMd(10,IL76)<NJ-MTNSIDE>
+ Montclair Endocrine Associates
  123 Highland Avenue/Suite 301   Glen Ridge, NJ 07028   (973)744-3733   Fax (973)707-5821
+ Hackensack UMC Mountainside
  1 Bay Avenue/Suite 5   Montclair, NJ 07042   (973)259-3417

Kiehlmeier, Scott Louis, MD {1750479424} Pedtrc(81,PA09)
+ Cooper Peds/Children's Regional Ctr
  6400 Main Street Complex   Voorhees, NJ 08043   (856)342-2000

Kiel, Samuel Yol, MD {1245382100} Anesth(87,NJ05)<NJ-RWJUBRUN>
+ Robert Wood Johnson-UMDNJ Anesthesia Group
  125 Paterson Street/CAB 3100   New Brunswick, NJ 08901   (732)937-8841   Fax (732)235-6131

Kielar, Francis, MD {1104945138} FamMed(82,POLA)<NJ-CHILTON>
+ 45 Carey Avenue
  Butler, NJ 07405   (973)283-9300   Fax (973)283-9311

Kierce, Roger P., MD {1740216605} ObsGyn(86,NJ05)<NJ-STJOSHOS>
+ Willowbrook Ob/Gyn
  57 Willowbrook Boulevard/Suite 301   Wayne, NJ 07470   (973)754-4075   Fax (973)754-4097

Kierson, Malca Ester, DO {1497911648} PthAcl
+ UH- RWJ Medical School
  One Robert Wood Johnson Place/MEB 212   New Brunswick, NJ 08903   (732)235-8121

Kihiczak, George, MD {1376696997} Dermat(70,NJ05)
+ 116 Millburn Avenue/Suite 111
  Millburn, NJ 07041   (973)467-5499

Kiken, David Adam, MD {1801004114} Dermat(03,NY19)<NY-ST-BARNAB>
+ Dermatology & Skin Surgery Center
  220 Ridgedale Avenue/2nd Floor Suite 4   Florham Park, NJ 07932   (973)301-9500   Fax (973)301-0435

Kikta, Kevin J., DO {1376648915} EmrgMd(96,OK79)<NJ-STPETER>
+ 12 Crowel Road
  Hillsborough, NJ 08844   (908)369-0827
  kevinkikta@comcast.net

Kilgannon, Jennifer Hope, MD {1609964386} EmrgMd(00,NJ06)<NJ-COOPRUMC>
+ Cooper University Hospital
  One Cooper Plaza/EmergMed   Camden, NJ 08103   (856)342-2000

Kilinsky, Vladimir, MD {1942218623} ObsGyn(81,MA05)<NJ-HOLYNAME, NJ-HACKNSK>
+ Ob-Gyn Associates of Englewood
  177 North Dean Street/Suite 208   Englewood, NJ 07631   (201)569-0200   Fax (201)569-8287

Kilkenny-Trainor, Kerryann A., MD {1265461925} IntrMd(91,NJ06)<NJ-MORRISTN>
+ IPC The Hospitalist Company
  220 Ridgedale Avenue/Suite C-2   Florham Park, NJ 07932   (973)538-5844   Fax (973)267-0181
+ Poblete Medical Practice PC
  1033 US Highway 46   Clifton, NJ 07013   (973)253-7800

Killeen, Thomas Joseph, III, MD {1902126121} Pedtrc
+ Advocare, LLC.
  402 Lippincott Drive   Marlton, NJ 08053   (856)782-3300   Fax (856)504-8029
+ Advocare Haddonfield Pediatric Assoc
  220 Haddon Avenue   Haddonfield, NJ 08033

Killilea, Edward M., MD {1982654406} IntrMd(72,DC02)
+ 111 Grand Place
  Kearny, NJ 07032   (201)998-2142   Fax (201)997-7650

Kim, Amy, MD {1780773143} Psychy<PA-CHILDHOS>
+ CHOP Pediatric & Adolescent Specialty Care Center
  1012 Laurel Oak Road   Voorhees, NJ 08043   (856)435-1300   Fax (856)435-0091

Kim, Andrew Edward, MD {1053349449} RadDia, NuclMd(96,NY09)<NJ-CHSFULD>
+ Capital Health System/Fuld Campus
  750 Brunswick Avenue/Radiology   Trenton, NJ 08638   (609)815-7565   Fax (609)815-7545

Kim, Andrew Hanyoung, MD {1306823778} Anesth, PedAne(01,NY01)
+ Princeton Anesthesia Services PC
  253 Witherspoon Street   Princeton, NJ 08540   (609)497-4000   Fax (609)497-4331

Kim, Andrew Young, MD {1134539976} IntrMd<NJ-RWJUHAM>
+ Robert Wood Johnson University Hospital at Hamilton
  1 Hamilton Health Place   Hamilton, NJ 08690   (609)586-7900

Kim, Anthony Junghoi, MD {1790048254}
+ Neurology Consultants of North Jersey PA
  92 Summit Avenue/2nd Floor   Hackensack, NJ 07601   (201)342-0066   Fax (201)630-0014

Kim, Brian Hangil, MD {1053568873} OncHem, IntrMd<NJ-HOLYNAME>
+ Forte Schleider & Attas MD PA
  350 Engle Street/Berrie Building/1 FL   Englewood, NJ 07631   (201)568-5250   Fax (201)568-5358
+ Holy Name Hospital
  718 Teaneck Road/CancerCtr   Teaneck, NJ 07666   (201)568-5250   Fax (201)227-6002

Kim, Catherine Sun Joo, MD {1871700781} RadOnc(02,PA02)<NJ-VIRTMHBC, NJ-VIRTBERL>
+ Virtua Memorial
  175 Madison Avenue/Rad Onc   Mount Holly, NJ 08060   (609)261-7074   Fax (609)265-9303
+ Virtua Fox Chase Cancer Center
  200 Bowman Drive/Suite D-190   Voorhees, NJ 08043   (609)261-7074   Fax (856)217-7331

Kim, Chang N., MD {1063516458} Psychy(69,KOR04)<NJ-STMRY-PAS>
+ 1200 Route 46 West
  Clifton, NJ 07013   (973)773-9228   Fax (973)773-3029

Kim, Chee Gap, MD {1093723314} PhysMd(79,KORE)<NJ-ENGLWOOD, NJ-HACKNSK>
+ 535 Grand Avenue/2nd Floor
  Englewood, NJ 07631   (201)541-1111   Fax (201)541-0777

Kim, Chong M., MD {1295750701} Urolgy
+ Atlantic Coast Urology
  525 Jack Martin Boulevard/Suite 304   Brick, NJ 08723   (732)840-6606   Fax (732)840-6601
  drcmkim@gmail.com

Kim, Chong S., MD {1265478036} Otlryg, SrgHdN, OtgyFPlS(95,NY15)<NJ-RIVERVW>
+ Holmdel Medical Group, Inc
  100 Commons Way/Suite 701   Holmdel, NJ 07733   (732)796-0182
+ Holmdel Medical Group, Inc
  200 Perrine Road/Suite 207   Old Bridge, NJ 08857   (732)796-0182   Fax (732)796-0186

Kim, Christian C. K., MD {1457580177} IntrMd(06,GRN01)<NJ-STPETER>
+ Endocrinology Associates of New Jersey
  9 Auer Court/Suite A   East Brunswick, NJ 08816   (732)390-6666   Fax (732)390-7711
  vizcoz@yahoo.com

Kim, Christopher C., MD {1164430468} PhysMd(87,KOR01)<NJ-RBAYPERT, NJ-JFKMED>
+ Christopher Kim Rehab Inc
  34-36 Progress Street/Suite A-7   Edison, NJ 08820   (732)669-0077   Fax (732)669-0076

Kim, Christopher E., MD {1962757690} RadV&I
+ Atlantic Medical Imaging, LLC.
  44 East Jimmie Leeds Road/Suite 101   Galloway, NJ 08205   (609)677-9729   Fax (609)652-6512

Kim, Claudia, MD {1023205135} Pedtrc(05,ARG01)<NJ-STJOSHOS>
+ St. Joseph's Pediatrics DePaul Center
  11 Getty Avenue/2nd Floor   Paterson, NJ 07503   (973)754-2727

Kim, Dae U., MD {1225110034} PthACl, Pthlgy(65,KOR04)<NJ-STBARNMC>
+ St. Barnabas Medical Center
  94 Old Short Hills Road   Livingston, NJ 07039   (973)322-5000

Kim, Daniel Y., MD {1477500866} Ophthl(92,NY19)
+ St. Mary's Eye & Surgery Center
  540 Bergen Boulevard   Palisades Park, NJ 07650   (201)461-3970   Fax (201)242-9061
  dkim@dicare.com

Kim, Daryl Kyung, MD {1730175431} IntrMd, Pedtrc(96,GA01)<NJ-NWTNMEM, NJ-MORRISTN>
+ Premier Health Associates
  89 Sparta Avenue/Suite 100   Sparta, NJ 07871   (973)729-2121   Fax (973)729-3454
+ Premier Health Associates
  5 Eisenhower Road   Columbia, NJ 07832   (908)362-5360

Kim, David Howard, MD {1245356971} PhysMd(92,NJ05)
+ 704 East Main street/Suite A
  Moorestown, NJ 08057   (856)608-1130   Fax (856)608-7630
  DKACNMD@aol.com

Kim, David Yhoshin, MD {1972763530} Ophthl, IntrMd(07,NY01)
+ Retina Associates of New Jersey, P.A.
200 South Broad Street/Unit B   Ridgewood, NJ 07450
(201)445-6622   Fax (201)445-0262
+ Retina Associates of New Jersey, P.A.
628 Cedar Lane   Teaneck, NJ 07666   (201)445-6622   Fax (201)836-1757
+ Retina Associates of New Jersey, P.A.
3196 Kennedy Boulevard   Union City, NJ 07450   (201)867-2999   Fax (201)867-4440

Kim, Dong Hyun, MD {1588829352} IntrMd(04,KOR05)
+ 44 Sylvan Avenue/Suite 2D
Englewood Cliffs, NJ 07632   (201)961-2808

Kim, Duk Hee, MD {1578574414} IntrMd(97,NY48)<NJ-ACMCITY>
+ Absecon Medical Associates LLC
408 Chris Gaupp Drive/Suite 100   Galloway, NJ 08205
(609)748-5015   Fax (609)748-0303

Kim, Eugene J., MD {1174963672} ObsGyn(09,PA09)
+ Robert Wood Johnson Ob-Gyn Associates
3270 State Route 27/Suite 2200   Kendall Park, NJ 08824
(732)422-8989   Fax (732)422-4526
+ Robert Wood Johnson Ob-Gyn Associates
50 Franklin Lane/Suite 203   Manalapan, NJ 07726
(732)422-8989   Fax (732)536-7118
+ Robert Wood Johnson Ob-Gyn Associates
525 Route 70/Suite B-11   Lakewood, NJ 08824   (732)905-6466   Fax (732)905-6467

Kim, Eun-Joo Song, MD {1760448161} Pedtrc, IntrMd(94,CA18)<NJ-ENGLWOOD, NJ-HACKNSK>
+ Tenafly Pediatrics, PA
301 Bridge Plaza North   Fort Lee, NJ 07024   (201)592-8787   Fax (201)592-6350

Kim, Eunja, MD {1770679409} Pedtrc(91,NY08)<NJ-HACKNSK>
+ Pedimedica PA
810 Abbott Boulevard/Suite 101   Fort Lee, NJ 07024
(201)224-3200   Fax (201)224-4045
+ Pedimedica PA
500 Piermont Road/Suite 102   Closter, NJ 07624   (201)224-3200   Fax (201)784-3321

Kim, Eunjung, MD {1689923427}<NJ-ENGLWOOD>
+ Englewood Hospital and Medical Center
350 Engle Street   Englewood, NJ 07631   (201)894-3000

Kim, Hannah Seonghyun, MD {1811239114}
+ 155 Polifly Road
Hackensack, NJ 07601   (201)441-9980

Kim, Harold J., MD {1659331221} IntrMd, CdvDis, CarNuc(98,NY15)
+ Summit Medical Group Cardiology
62 South Fullerton Avenue   Montclair, NJ 07042   (973)746-8585   Fax (973)746-0088
+ Summit Medical Group
75 East Northfield Road   Livingston, NJ 07039   (973)746-8585   Fax (908)673-7336

Kim, Hazel Hae-sook, MD {1215970967} PthAcl, PthHem(77,KOR06)<NJ-JFKMED>
+ JFK Medical Center
65 James Street   Edison, NJ 08820   (732)321-7680   Fax (732)321-7008
HAZELHKIM@gmail.com

Kim, Hee Jin, MD {1306155395}
+ 800 Park Avenue/Apt 1902
Fort Lee, NJ 07024   (213)999-9503
heejin.m.kim@gmail.com

Kim, Hei Y., MD {1558308569} Pedtrc(70,KOR01)<NJ-RWJUBRUN, NJ-STPETER>
+ Drs. Kim & Kim
61 Brunswick Woods Drive   East Brunswick, NJ 08816
(732)257-8777

Kim, Hong Suk, MD {1942384128} IntrMd, EmrgMd(93,NJ05)
+ 494 Knickerbocker Road
Tenafly, NJ 07670

Kim, Hoon, MD {1073597787} Pthlgy, PthAcl(71,KOR04)<NJ-OURLADY>
+ Our Lady of Lourdes Medical Center
1600 Haddon Avenue   Camden, NJ 08103   (856)757-3567

Kim, Hyon S., MD {1326003302} Anesth(92,NJ06)<NJ-STPETER>
+ Anesthesia Consultnts of NJ/Nova Pain
285 Davidson Avenue/Suite 204   Somerset, NJ 08873
(732)271-1400   Fax (732)271-3543
+ Cares Surgicenter, LLC.
240 Easton Avenue   New Brunswick, NJ 08901   (732)271-1400   Fax (732)296-8677

Kim, Hyung G., MD {1609813781} CdvDis, IntrMd(70,KOR01)<NJ-STPETER, NJ-RWJUBRUN>
+ Drs. Kim & Kim
61 Brunswick Woods Drive   East Brunswick, NJ 08816
(732)257-8777   Fax (732)613-6171

Kim, Isaac Yi, MD {1235217985} Urolgy<NJ-RWJUBRUN>
+ Rutgers Cancer Institute of New Jersey
195 Little Albany Street/PO Box 2681   New Brunswick, NJ 08903   (732)235-2043   Fax (732)235-6596

Kim, Jeffrey S., MD {1073648994} IntrMd, CritCr, PulDis(00,PA02)
+ Pulmonary & Medical Associates of Pasack Valley
466 Old Hook Road/Suite 26   Emerson, NJ 07630
(201)261-0821   Fax (201)261-0823

Kim, Jenny Hyunjung, MD {1619024510} PulDis, CritCr, IntrMd(97,NY08)<NJ-VAEASTOR>
+ VA New Jersey Health Care System-East Orange Campus
385 Tremont Avenue/7/FL Suite 135   East Orange, NJ 07018
(973)676-1000   Fax (973)395-7034
+ Summit Medical Group
75 East Northfield Road   Livingston, NJ 07039   (973)676-1000   Fax (973)436-1404

Kim, Jeongwon, MD {1831199199} InfDis, IntrMd(97,NET09)
+ 1608 Lemoine Avenue/Suite 206
Fort Lee, NJ 07024   (917)301-5821

Kim, Jiwon, MD {1548427545} CdvDis, CarNuc, CarEle(07,NY46)<NJ-JRSYSHMC>
+ Monmouth Cardiology Associates, LLC
11 Meridian Road   Eatontown, NJ 07724   (732)663-0300
Fax (732)663-0301
+ Monmouth Cardiology Associates, LLC.
2102 Corlies Avenue/State Highway 33   Neptune, NJ 07753
(732)663-0300   Fax (732)774-9148

Kim, Joh W., MD {1932292109} Pedtrc(65,KORE)
+ 10 Magnolia Avenue/Suite B1
Bridgeton, NJ 08302   (856)451-4140   Fax (856)451-3657

Kim, John, MD {1659359263} Grtrcs, IntrMd(89,KOR17)<NJ-HACKNSK, NJ-BERGNMC>
+ Bethel Pain Management
158 Linwood Plaza/Suite 324-325   Fort Lee, NJ 07024
(201)871-4200   Fax (201)849-5097

Kim, John Sung, MD {1831152867} Ophthl(77,NY19)<NJ-ENGLWOOD>
+ 2500 Lemoine Avenue
Fort Lee, NJ 07024   (201)461-8110   Fax (201)461-3614

Kim, John Yohan, MD {1467442384} AlgyImmn, IntrMd(03,IL42)
+ Cornerstone Asthma and Allergy Associates
103 Old Marlton Pike/Suite 211   Medford, NJ 08055
(609)953-7500   Fax (609)953-9085

Kim, Jong Hyun, MD {1871736256} PhysMd, GenPrc(66,KOR14)
+ Pain & Rehab Center, P.C.
158 Linwood Plaza/Suite 208-2010   Fort Lee, NJ 07024
(201)252-4014

Kim, Joseph, MD {1689640625} IntrMd, InfDis(99,NJ06)<NJ-RWJUBRUN, NJ-SOMERSET>
+ ID Associates PA/dba ID Care
765 Route 10 East/Suite 201   Randolph, NJ 07869
(973)989-0068   Fax (973)361-8955
+ ID Associates PA/dba ID Care
8 Saddle Road   Cedar Knolls, NJ 07927   (973)989-0068
Fax (973)993-5953

Kim, Joseph J., MD {1073774246} RadBdI, RadDia, Radiol(03,NJ06)
+ Radiology Affiliates of Central New Jersey, P.A.
2501 Kuser Road   Hamilton, NJ 08691   (609)585-8800
Fax (609)585-1825

Kim, Joseph Jongbum, MD {1356667158} SrgOnc
+ Summit Medical Group Florham Park Campus
150 Park Avenue   Florham Park, NJ 07932   (973)404-9980
Fax (855)307-9476

Kim, Juen, MD {1578862413} AlgyImmn, Pedtrc(96,MI01)
+ Allergic Disease Associates, PC - Mount Laurel
210 Ark Road & Route 38/Suite 109   Mount Laurel, NJ 08054   (856)235-8282   Fax (856)235-2154
+ Allergic Disease Associates, PC - Forked River
1044 Lacey Road/suite 9   Forked River, NJ 08731
(856)235-8282   Fax (609)693-0351

Kim, Julia G., MD {1205254620} ObsGyn
+ Reproductive Medicine Associates of New Jersey
140 Allen Road   Basking Ridge, NJ 07920   (973)971-4600
Fax (973)290-8370

Kim, Julia J., MD {1457515785} FamMGrtc
+ Overlook Family Medicine
33 Overlook Road/Suite 103   Summit, NJ 07901   (908)522-5700   Fax (908)273-8014

Kim, Justin, MD {1063904134}
+ 7 Broad Avenue/Suite 206
Palisades Park, NJ 07650   (201)313-0131

Kim, Kathlyn M., MD {1730174715} ObsGyn(90,NY47)<NJ-VALLEY>
+ Valley Center for Women's Health
550 North Maple Avenue/Suite 102   Ridgewood, NJ 07450
(201)444-4040   Fax (201)444-4473
+ Valley Center for Women's Health
581 North Franklin Turnpike/2nd Floor   Ramsey, NJ 07446
(201)444-4040   Fax (201)236-5269

Kim, Kun, MD {1083691091} Anesth(63,KOR14)
+ 18 Woodland Avenue
North Caldwell, NJ 07006   (973)744-7119

Kim, Kyur Gsook Cho, MD {1205916251} FamMed(81,KORE)
+ Cooper Family Medicine
3156 River Road   Camden, NJ 08105   (856)963-0126

Kim, Maria Batraki, DO {1679831739} Pedtrc
+ North Brunswick Pediatrics
1598 US Highway 130   North Brunswick, NJ 08902
(732)297-0603   Fax (732)297-2866

Kim, Miah, MD {1720053838} FamMed(92,NJ03)<NJ-CENTRAST>
+ 55-77 Schanck Road/Suite A-20
Freehold, NJ 07728   (732)683-0010   Fax (732)409-6997

Kim, Michelle Joosun, MD {1689896722} Urolgy(01,NJ05)<NJ-HACKNSK>
+ HUMC Faculty Practice
360 Essex Street/Suite 403   Hackensack, NJ 07601
(201)336-8090   Fax (201)336-8221

Kim, Mina Jung, MD {1568704054} Anesth
+ Summit Medical Group
140 Park Avenue/3rd Floor   Florham Park, NJ 07932
(973)404-9700   Fax (908)673-7336

Kim, Minbae, MD {1588647614} Pthlgy, PthAcl(81,KORE)<NJ-STJOSHOS>
+ St. Joseph's Regional Medical Center
703 Main Street/Pathology   Paterson, NJ 07503   (973)754-2000   Fax (973)754-3649

Kim, Mirye, MD {1982694626} NnPnMd, Pedtrc(96,KOR04)<NJ-VIRTMHBC, NJ-VIRTVOOR>
+ Virtua Voorhees
100 Bowman Drive/Pediatrics   Voorhees, NJ 08043
(856)247-3244
+ Virtua Memorial
175 Madison Avenue/Pediatrics   Mount Holly, NJ 08060
(856)247-3244   Fax (856)247-3504

Kim, Nami, DO {1366633612} IntrMd<NJ-COOPRUMC>
+ Cooper University Medical Center/Camden
3 Cooper Plaza/Suite 215   Camden, NJ 08103   (856)342-2000   Fax (856)966-0735

Kim, Okja, MD {1760435101} PhysMd(70,KOR03)<NJ-JFKJHNSN, NJ-STPETER>
+ Metuchen Electrodiagnostics
239 Bridge Street/Building H   Metuchen, NJ 08840
(732)635-1577   Fax (732)635-1576

Kim, Regina Siobhan, MD {1447492038} Pedtrc<PA-CHILDHOS>
+ CHOP Newborn and Pediatric Care at UMCPP
One Plainsboro Road/6th Floor   Plainsboro, NJ 08536
(609)853-7626   Fax (609)853-7630

Kim, Richard Young Jin, MD {1407833932} SrgPlstc, SrgOrt(99,NY47)<NJ-HACKNSK>
+ Hackensack University MedCtr-Plastic & Ortho Surgery
360 Essex Street/Suite 303   Hackensack, NJ 07601
(201)996-5439   Fax (201)996-4743
rkim@humed.com

Kim, Rose, MD {1437175916} InfDis, IntrMd(99,NY19)<NJ-COOPRUMC>
+ EIP Clinic/Early Intervention Program (HIV/AIDS)
3 Cooper Plaza/Suite 513   Camden, NJ 08103   (856)963-3715   Fax (856)635-1052
+ Cooper University Hospital
One Cooper Plaza/E&R Rm259   Camden, NJ 08103
(856)342-2000

Kim, Ruby E., MD {1972762730} PhysMd(05,NJ06)
+ Premier Spine & Sports Medicine
1555 Center Avenue/2nd Floor   Fort Lee, NJ 07024
(201)242-1600   Fax (201)299-2555

Kim, Ryul, DO {1407864895} PhysMd, IntrMd(02,IA75)
+ Chestnut Hill Convalescent Center
360 Chestnut Street   Passaic, NJ 07055   (973)777-7800
Fax (973)778-9013

Kim, Sam, MD {1740226950} Dermat(98,PA01)<NJ-OVERLOOK, NJ-MORRISTN>
+ Summit Medical Group-Berkeley Heights Campus
1 Diamond Hill Road   Berkeley Heights, NJ 07922
(908)273-4300   Fax (908)790-6576

Kim, Sam Kwang, MD {1558307579} Pedtrc(67,KOR05)<NJ-WARREN>
+ 228 Roseberry Street/Suite 3
Phillipsburg, NJ 08865   (908)454-4545   Fax (908)454-3227

Kim, Sang K., MD {1487765509} Anesth(70,KORE)<NJ-COMMED>
+ Community Medical Center
99 Route 37 West/Anesthesiology   Toms River, NJ 08755
(732)557-8000

Kim, Sarang, MD {1538231873} IntrMd(98,IL02)
+ University Medical Group
125 Paterson Street/Suite 5100   New Brunswick, NJ 08901
(732)235-7993   Fax (732)235-7117

Kim, Seyun, MD {1508197591}
+ St. Michael's Medical Center
111 Central Avenue   Newark, NJ 07102   (916)812-1062
seyunk24@gmail.com

Kim, Sion, DO {1861920787} GenPrc
+ McGuire Air Force Base/Acute Health Care Clinic
3458 Neely Road   Trenton, NJ 08641   (609)754-9080   Fax (609)754-9015

Physicians by Name and Address

Kim, Sonia, MD {1558525840} ObsGyn(06,DMN01)<NJ-HACKNSK>
+ Hackensack University Medical Group Dumont
  125 Washington Avenue   Dumont, NJ 07628   (201)374-2722   Fax (201)374-2723
+ Hackensack University Medical Group Westwood
  250 Old Hook Road   Westwood, NJ 07675   (201)374-2722   Fax (201)781-1753

Kim, Soon K., MD {1942217617} Pedtrc(75,KOR03)<NJ-STBARNMC, NJ-TRINIWSC>
+ 230 West Jersey Street/Suite 102
  Elizabeth, NJ 07202   (908)352-8383

Kim, Stanley S., MD {1306850433} IntrMd, Nephro(89,KOR01)
+ Edison Nephrology Consultants, LLC.
  34-36 Progress Street/Suite A-7   Edison, NJ 08820   (908)769-1440   Fax (908)769-0945
+ Avenel Iselin Medical Group
  400 Gill Lane   Iselin, NJ 08830   (908)769-1440   Fax (732)404-1594

Kim, Steve Sang-Yoon, MD {1548213796} CdvDis, IntCrd(98,OH06)<NJ-ENGLWOOD, NJ-HOLYNAME>
+ Advanced Cardiology Institute
  2200 Fletcher Avenue/Suite 1   Fort Lee, NJ 07024   (201)461-6200   Fax (201)461-7204

Kim, Steve Yun, MD {1225105414} Otlryg, SrgFPl, IntrMd(92,NY15)
+ 2185 Lemoine Avenue/Suite 1-P
  Fort Lee, NJ 07024   (201)569-9130   Fax (201)569-9131

Kim, Steven Namgi, MD {1356574099} IntrMd(96,NY08)
+ AFC Urgent Care South Plainfield
  907 Oak Tree Avenue/Suite H   South Plainfield, NJ 07080   (908)222-3500

Kim, Sue Hyun, MD {1194932350} RadDia(02,NY19)<NJ-STPETER, NJ-RWJUBRUN>
+ University Radiology Group, P.C.
  483 Cranbury Road   East Brunswick, NJ 08816   (732)390-0030   Fax (732)390-5383
+ University Radiology Group, P.C.
  10 Plum Street   New Brunswick, NJ 08901   (732)390-0030   Fax (732)249-1208
+ University Radiology Group, P.C.
  260 Amboy Avenue   Metuchen, NJ 08816   (732)548-2322   Fax (732)548-3392

Kim, Sung N., MD {1164591152} RadOnc(01,CT01)
+ Rutgers Cancer Institute of New Jersey
  195 Little Albany Street/PO Box 2681   New Brunswick, NJ 08903   (732)235-2465   Fax (732)235-6797

Kim, Sung Hyun, MD {1447665369} IntrMd<NJ-ENGLWOOD>
+ Englewood Hospital and Medical Center
  350 Engle Street   Englewood, NJ 07631   (201)894-3000

Kim, Sunmee Louise, MD {1285713917} Pedtrc(00,NY15)<NJ-ENGLWOOD, NJ-HACKNSK>
+ Tenafly Pediatrics, PA
  26 Park Place   Paramus, NJ 07652   (201)262-1140   Fax (201)261-8413
+ Tenafly Pediatrics, PA
  32 Franklin Street   Tenafly, NJ 07670   (201)262-1140   Fax (201)569-6081

Kim, Tae Won Benjamin, MD {1780846246} SrgOrt(08,NY46)<NJ-COOPRUMC>
+ Cooper Perinatology Associates
  3 Cooper Plaza/Suite 502   Camden, NJ 08103   (856)356-4935   Fax (856)968-8499
+ Cooper University Medical Center/Camden
  3 Cooper Plaza/Suite 400   Camden, NJ 08103   (856)356-4935   Fax (856)361-1761

Kim, Urian, MD {1851487292} Pedtrc(99,NY15)
+ Valley Pediatric Associates, P.A.
  201 East Franklin Turnpike   Ho Ho Kus, NJ 07423   (201)652-1888   Fax (201)652-6485

Kim, William J., MD {1962444943} Radiol(99,NJ06)<NJ-HACKNSK>
+ Hackensack Radiology Group, P.A.
  30 Prospect Avenue   Hackensack, NJ 07601   (201)996-2200   Fax (201)336-8451
+ Hackensack University Medical Center
  30 Prospect Avenue/Radiology   Hackensack, NJ 07601   (201)996-2200   Fax (201)489-2812

Kim, Wun Jung, MD {1982690525}<NJ-UNIVBHC>
+ University Behavioral Health Care
  671 Hoes Lane/PO Box 1392   Piscataway, NJ 08855   (724)235-2804   Fax (724)235-3923

Kim, Yon Sook, MD {1205983558} ObsGyn, IntrMd
+ Cooper Ob/Gyn
  3 Cooper Plaza/Suite 300   Camden, NJ 08103   (856)342-2186   Fax (856)968-8575
+ Ripa Center for Women's Health & Wellness
  6100 Main Street   Voorhees, NJ 08043   (856)342-2186   Fax (856)325-6677

Kim, Yongjung, MD {1548429806} SrgOrt(85,KOR04)
+ Columbia Grand Orthopaedics
  500 Grand Avenue/Suite 101   Englewood, NJ 07631   (201)569-0440   Fax (201)569-4949

Kim, Yoonjoo, MD {1598841942} FamMed(88,KORE)<NJ-PALISADE>
+ Hanmi Medical Associates
  232 Broad Avenue/Suite 208   Palisades Park, NJ 07650   (201)346-0999   Fax (201)346-0118

Kim, Yooree, MD {1235557679}<NJ-CHSFULD>
+ Capital Health System/Fuld Campus
  750 Brunswick Avenue   Trenton, NJ 08638   (609)394-6000

Kim, Young-Min, MD {1881771160} EmrgMd(97,PA09)<NJ-HACKNSK>
+ Hackensack University Medical Center
  30 Prospect Avenue/EmrgMed   Hackensack, NJ 07601   (201)996-3285

Kim, Yumi, MD {1659383669} MedOnc, Hemato(95,NY09)
+ Aly Internal Medicine/Hematology Oncology
  883 Poole Avenue/Suite 4   Hazlet, NJ 07730   (732)203-9500   Fax (732)203-0851

Kim, Yung H., MD {1093856668} PthAcl, Pthlgy(63,KOR01)<NJ-CHSMRCER>
+ Capital Health System/Mercer Campus
  446 Bellevue Avenue/Pathology   Trenton, NJ 08618   (609)394-4014   Fax (609)394-4685

Kimbaris, James Nicholas, MD {1124310370} Gastrn
+ Drs Figueredo and Kimbaris
  239 Hurffville CrossKeys Road   Sewell, NJ 08080   (856)237-8045   Fax (856)237-8047

Kimel, Alexandru F., MD {1992940860} IntrMd, Rheuma(03,NY09)
+ Rheumatology Associates of North Jersey, PA
  1415 Queen Anne Road   Teaneck, NJ 07666   (201)837-7788   Fax (201)837-2077
+ Rheumatology Associates of North Jersey, PA
  420 Grand Avenue   Englewood, NJ 07631   (201)837-7788   Fax (201)837-2077
+ Rheumatology Associates of North Jersey, PA
  8305A Bergenline Avenue   North Bergen, NJ 07666   (201)837-7788   Fax (201)837-2077

Kimel, Ana Josephine, MD {1982884045} Pedtrc(03,IRE02)<NY-LICOLLGE>
+ Children of Joy Pediatrics
  134 Summit Avenue   Hackensack, NJ 07601   (201)525-0077   Fax (201)525-0072

Kimler, Christine Marie, DO {1346328770} FamMed(96,NJ75)
+ University Hospital-University Family Medicine
  42 East Laurel Road/Suite 2100   Stratford, NJ 08084   (856)566-7020   Fax (856)566-6188
+ Inspira Medical Group
  660 Woodbury Glassboro Road/Suite 26   Sewell, NJ 08080   (856)566-7020   Fax (856)464-1855

Kimler, Stephen C., MD {1902961543} Pthlgy(70,NY08)<NJ-MTNSIDE>
+ Hackensack UMC Mountainside
  1 Bay Avenue/Path   Montclair, NJ 07042   (973)429-6164   Fax (973)429-6992

Kimmel, Barry S., MD {1326017559} Urolgy, IntrMd(88,FL02)<NJ-ACMCITY, NJ-SHOREMEM>
+ Pagnani, Braga, & Kimmel Urologic Associates PA
  229 Shore Road   Somers Point, NJ 08244   (609)653-4343   Fax (609)653-2060
+ Pagnani, Braga, & Kimmel Urologic Associates PA
  222 New Road/Building 700   Linwood, NJ 08221   (609)653-4343   Fax (609)601-9630
+ Pagnani, Braga, & Kimmel Urologic Associates PA
  8 Court House South Dennis Rd   Cape May Court House, NJ 08244   (609)465-4404

Kimmel, Craig S., MD {1255307591} FamMSptM, SprtMd(87,PA09)<NJ-LOURDEHS>
+ Endocrinology Associates
  1 Brace Road/Suite B   Cherry Hill, NJ 08034   (856)234-0645   Fax (856)234-0498

Kimura, Yukiko, MD {1417900135} PedRhm(82,NY46)<NJ-HACKNSK>
+ Hackensack University Medical Center
  30 Prospect Avenue/WFAN Bldg/3rd F   Hackensack, NJ 07601   (201)996-5306   Fax (201)996-9815

Kincaid, Leah Celia, MD {1710401203} Dermat
+ Alliance Dermatology Associates
  3311 Brunswick Pike   Lawrenceville, NJ 08648   (609)799-1600   Fax (609)799-1677

Kincel, David Nathaniel, DO {1972789162} EmrgMd<PA-ARHTRRDL>
+ Virtua Marlton Hospital
  90 Brick Road   Marlton, NJ 08053   (856)355-6000

Kinchelow-Schmidt, Tosca E., MD {1316027105} InfDis, IntrMd(76,NJ05)<NJ-EASTORNG>
+ 471 East Saddle River Road
  Ridgewood, NJ 07450   (201)925-2400   Fax (201)612-1104

Kinder, Michael L., DO {1780025080}
+ 159 Chancellor Drive
  Deptford, NJ 08096   (973)464-1080
  drmkinder@gmail.com

Kindermann, Wilfred Reed, MD {1285604918} Ophthl(75,NY45)<NJ-VIRTMARL, NJ-COOPRUMC>
+ W. Reed Kindermann, M.D. and Associates
  3001 Chapel Avenue West/Suite 200   Cherry Hill, NJ 08002   (856)667-3937   Fax (856)667-0661

Kindsfather, Scott K., MD {1659385615} Hemato, MedOnc, IntrMd(89,NJ06)<NJ-CHSFULD, NJ-CHSMRCER>
+ Mercer Bucks Hematology Oncology
  2 Capital Way/Suite 220   Pennington, NJ 08534   (609)303-0747   Fax (609)303-0771

Kindzierski, John A., MD {1396811485} ObsGyn(76,NJ05)<NJ-STBARNMC>
+ Physicians for Women's HealthCare
  315 East Northfield Road/Suite 3-B   Livingston, NJ 07039   (973)422-1200   Fax (973)422-9169

Kindzierski, Michael A., DO {1770656597} FamMed(94,PA77)<NJ-RWJURAH>
+ 76 Carteret Avenue
  Carteret, NJ 07008   (732)541-9060   Fax (732)541-9220

King, Alexander B., MD {1073830717}<NJ-STBARNMC>
+ St. Barnabas Medical Center
  94 Old Short Hills Road   Livingston, NJ 07039   (732)768-9593

King, Alina, MD {1053837864} PhysMd
+ 123 Egg Harbor Road/Suite 305
  Sewell, NJ 08080   (856)481-3513   Fax (856)228-2105

King, Andrew P., MD {1164515953} ObsGyn(81,DOMI)<NJ-COMMED>
+ Drs. O'Donnell and King
  1163 Route 37 West/Suite A-2   Toms River, NJ 08755   (732)349-2424   Fax (732)349-8130

King, Anne H., DO {1952565475} RadBdl
+ South Jersey Radiology Associates, P.A.
  100 Carnie Boulevard/Suite B-5   Voorhees, NJ 08043   (856)751-0123   Fax (856)751-0535
+ South Jersey Radiology Associates, P.A.
  6650 Browning Road/Suite M14   Pennsauken, NJ 08109   (856)751-0123   Fax (856)661-0686
+ South Jersey Radiology Associates, P.A.
  315 Route 70 East/Suite B   Cherry Hill, NJ 08043   (856)428-4344   Fax (856)428-0356

King, Cecile Carol-Ann, MD {1114361748} IntHos<NJ-COOPRUMC>
+ Cooper University Hospital
  One Cooper Plaza   Camden, NJ 08103   (856)356-4924

King, John Wayne, DO {1730129800} SrgOrt(90,NY75)<NJ-TRININPC>
+ Ortho Physicians & Surgeons
  975 Lehigh Avenue   Union, NJ 07083   (908)686-1488   Fax (908)687-7886

King, Kevin J., MD {1073578381} Pedtrc(94,PA13)<NJ-OURLADY, NJ-VIRTUAHS>
+ Advocare Haddonfield Pediatric Association
  220 North Haddon Avenue   Haddonfield, NJ 08033   (856)429-6719   Fax (856)429-6748

King, Krista H., MD {1053372136} IntrMd(98,OH41)<NJ-VIRTUAHS>
+ Advocare Heights Primary Care
  318 White Horse Pike   Haddon Heights, NJ 08035   (856)547-6000   Fax (856)546-3189

King, Lorraine C., MD {1922181262} ObsGyn(71,PA07)
+ PO Box 188
  Stone Harbor, NJ 08247   (609)368-7618

King, Richard A., MD {1386687853} Pedtrc(78,DC02)<NJ-VIRTMHBC>
+ Advocare Pedi Phys of Burlington Co
  693 Main Street/PO Box 367   Lumberton, NJ 08048   (609)261-4058   Fax (609)261-8381
+ Advocare Pedi Phys of Burlington Co
  204 Ark Road/Suite 209   Mount Laurel, NJ 08054   (609)261-4058   Fax (856)234-9402

Kingsbery, Mina Yassaee, MD {1760719967} Dermat(09,PA01)
+ Dermatology Associates of Morris PA
  199 Baldwin Road   Parsippany, NJ 07054   (973)335-2560   Fax (973)335-9421

Kingsly, Jill H., MD {1992732937} RadDia(89,NY46)
+ Tri County MRI & Diagnostic Radiology
  97 Main Street   Chatham, NJ 07928   (973)635-2000   Fax (973)635-1749
+ Diagnostic Radiology Associates of Northfield
  772 Northfield Avenue   West Orange, NJ 07052   (973)635-2000   Fax (973)325-8140
+ Diagnostic Radiology Associates of Clifton
  1339 Broad Street   Clifton, NJ 07928   (973)778-9600   Fax (973)778-4846

Kinoshita, Ken, MD {1801059258} FamMed(02,JAP34)
+ Warren Hills Family Health Center
  315 Route 31 South   Washington, NJ 07882   (908)689-0777   Fax (908)835-3037

Physicians by Name and Address

Kinsler, Kristin J., DO {1538570833} ObsGyn
+ Brunswick-Hills Ob/Gyn, PA
620 Cranbury Road/Suite LL90   East Brunswick, NJ 08816   (610)657-5003   Fax (732)613-4845
kristinkinsler@hotmail.com

Kintiroglou, Constantinos, MD {1205966124} AdolMd, NnPnMd, Pedtrc(69,GREE)
+ Kintiroglou Pediatrics
1500 Pleasant Valley Way/Suite 301   West Orange, NJ 07052   (973)243-0002   Fax (973)243-1227

Kintiroglou, John, MD {1528198645} Pedtrc(97,NJ06)
+ Kintiroglou Pediatrics
1500 Pleasant Valley Way/Suite 301   West Orange, NJ 07052   (973)243-0002   Fax (973)243-1227

Kintiroglou, Marietta, MD {1598846263} PthACl, PthCyt(69,GRE01)<NJ-STBARNMC>
+ St. Barnabas Medical Center
94 Old Short Hills Road   Livingston, NJ 07039   (973)322-5000

Kintzel, Timothy J., MD {1578509618} EmrgMd(98,PA09)<NJ-ENGLWOOD, NY-JACOBIMC>
+ Englewood Hospital and Medical Center
350 Engle Street   Englewood, NJ 07631   (201)984-3000   Fax (610)617-6280

Kinyon, Jeffrey James, DO {1326268871} EmrgMd, IntrMd(02,IA75)
+ St Joseph's Medical Center Emergency
703 Main Street   Paterson, NJ 07503   (973)754-2240   Fax (973)754-2249

Kipel, George, MD {1548216690} PedCrd, Pedtrc(85,MEXI)<NJ-HACKNSK>
+ The Pediatric Center for Heart Disease
155 Polifly Road/Suite 106   Hackensack, NJ 07601   (201)487-7617   Fax (201)342-5341

Kipen, Howard M., MD {1871605006} IntrMd, OccpMd, GPrvMd(79,CA02)<NJ-RWJUBRUN>
+ EOHSI Clinical Center - UMDNJ
681 Frelinghuysen Road   Piscataway, NJ 08855   (732)445-0123   Fax (732)445-0131

Kipnis, Ilana Ariel, DO {1164680799} Anesth(04,NY75)
+ 88 Brownstone Way/Suite 112
Englewood, NJ 07631

Kipnis, Seth Michael, MD {1871559096} Surgry(00,NY15)<NJ-VIRTUAHS>
+ 1706 Corlies Avenue/Suite 5
Neptune, NJ 07753

Kirby, John A., MD {1164502126} IntrMd(90,PA01)<NJ-COOPRUMC, NJ-VIRTVOOR>
+ Cooper Physicians
1210 Brace Road/Suite 102   Cherry Hill, NJ 08034   (856)428-6616   Fax (856)428-4823

Kirchhoff, Michael Anthony, MD {1578643532} EmrgMd(97,NJ06)<NJ-COOPRUMC>
+ Cooper University Hospital
One Cooper Plaza/EmergMed   Camden, NJ 08103   (856)342-2000

Kirchner, Brian K., MD {1205846862} IntrMd(87,NJ05)<NJ-ACMCITY, NJ-ACMCMAIN>
+ Absecon Medical Associates LLC
408 Chris Gaupp Drive/Suite 100   Galloway, NJ 08205   (609)748-5015   Fax (609)748-0303

Kirk, Michael John, Jr., DO {1023339124} GenPrc, IntrMd(09,FL75)<NJ-SOCEANCO>
+ Southern Ocean County Medical Center
1140 Route 72 West/Internal Med   Manahawkin, NJ 08050   (609)978-3331   Fax (609)978-3113

Kirkham, Jay G., Jr., DO {1225319130} CritCr
+ Rowan University-School of Osteopathic Medicine
1 Medical Center Drive   Stratford, NJ 08084   (856)566-6096

Kirkpatrick, Christopher Thomas, MD {1508908088} RadDia
+ Radiology Affiliates Imaging
3625 Quakerbridge Road   Hamilton, NJ 08619

Kirkpatrick-Reese, Gina Brazylle, DO {1407101611}
+ HUMC Faculty Practice
360 Essex Street/Suite 403   Hackensack, NJ 07601   (201)336-8090   Fax (201)336-8221

Kirmani, Jawad F., MD {1871527721} Nrolgy, VasNeu(95,PAK14)<NJ-UMDNJ>
+ JFK Neurosciences Institute
65 James Street/Second Floor   Edison, NJ 08818   (732)321-7010   Fax (732)632-1584

Kirn, Thomas Joseph, Jr., MD {1457418444} PthClLab, Pthlgy<NJ-RWJUBRUN>
+ RWJ University Hospital New Brunswick
One Robert Wood Johnson Place   New Brunswick, NJ 08901   (732)235-5338

Kirsch, Victoria Susan, DO {1902986821} PhysMd(97,NY75)<NJ-KSLRWEST>
+ Kessler Institute for Rehabilitation West Orange
1199 Pleasant Valley Way   West Orange, NJ 07052   (973)731-3600

Kirschenbaum, Abram Eugene, MD {1205861168} SrgHnd, SrgOrt, OrtSHand(88,NY19)<NJ-MORRISTN, NJ-OVERLOOK>
+ North Jersey Hand Surgery
385 Morris Avenue/Third Floor   Springfield, NJ 07081   (973)664-9899   Fax (973)664-1875
+ North Jersey Hand Surgery
75 Bloomfield Avenue/Suite 102   Denville, NJ 07834   (973)664-9899   Fax (973)664-1875

Kirschenbaum, David, MD {1639274061} SrgHnd, SrgOrt, OrtTrm(86,NJ06)<NJ-CENTRAST>
+ Affiliated Orthopaedic Specialists
2186 Route 27/Suite 1A   North Brunswick, NJ 08902   (732)422-1222   Fax (732)422-3636
+ Affiliated Orthopaedic Specialists
50 Franklin Lane/Suite 102   Manalapan, NJ 07726   (732)617-9500

Kirshblum, Steven C., MD {1033107347} PhysMd, SrgSpn(86,IL42)<NJ-KSLRWEST>
+ Kessler Institute for Rehabilitation West Orange
1199 Pleasant Valley Way   West Orange, NJ 07052   (973)731-3600
+ Rutgers-Department of Physical Med
183 South Orange Ave/Suite F-1555   Newark, NJ 07101   (973)972-3606

Kirshenbaum, Alexander, MD {1447306345} Urolgy, PedUro(01,NJ06)
+ Central Jersey Urology Associates LLC
23 Kilmer Drive/Suite C/Building 1   Morganville, NJ 07751   (732)972-9000   Fax (732)972-0966
+ Urology Care Alliance
501 Iron Bridge Road/Suite 5   Freehold, NJ 07728   (732)972-9000   Fax (732)308-3323
+ Urology Care Alliance
2 Hospital Plaza/Suite 110   Old Bridge, NJ 07751   (732)972-9000   Fax (732)972-0966

Kirshner, Eli David, MD {1376627737} OncHem, IntrMd(87,NJ06)<NJ-VALLEY>
+ 400 Old Hook Road/Suite 1-6
Westwood, NJ 07675   (201)664-3900   Fax (201)664-7800
+ Valley Medical Group-Hematology/Oncology
One Valley Health Plaza   Paramus, NJ 07652   (201)664-3900   Fax (201)986-4702

Kirshner, Steven B., MD {1518906767} SrgOrt, SrgSpn(83,PA09)<NJ-VIRTMHBC, NJ-VANJHCS>
+ The Spine Institute of Southern New Jersey
512 Lippincott Drive   Marlton, NJ 08053   (856)797-9161   Fax (856)797-3637

Kirstein, Laurie Jill, MD {1285677922} Surgry, SrgBst(01,NY08)<NY-SLOANKET>
+ Memorial Sloan Kettering Monmouth
480 Red Hill Road/Breast Srvcs   Middletown, NJ 07748   (848)225-6000

Kirszrot, James, MD {1447234117} Ophthl(01,NY46)
+ Westwood Ophthalmology Associates
300 Fairview Avenue/PO Box 698   Westwood, NJ 07675   (201)666-4014   Fax (201)664-4754
+ Eye Care Associates of New Jersey, PA
One Broadway/Suite 404   Elmwood Park, NJ 07407   (201)666-4014   Fax (201)797-4160
+ Eye Associates of Wayne PA
968 Hamburg Turnpike   Wayne, NJ 07675   (973)696-0300   Fax (973)696-0465

Kirwin, Michael S., MD {1548286164} ObsGyn, IntrMd(91,NY08)<NJ-CENTRAST>
+ Women's Physicians & Surgeons
501 Iron Bridge Road/Suite 10   Freehold, NJ 07728   (732)431-2999   Fax (732)431-2993
+ Women's Physicians & Surgeons
510 Bridge Plaza Drive   Englishtown, NJ 07726   (732)431-2999   Fax (732)536-4570
+ Women's Physicians & Surgeons
245A Main Street   Matawan, NJ 07747   (732)566-9466   Fax (732)566-0343

Kirzner, Howard L., MD {1124188792} RadDia, Radiol, RadBdI(83,NY08)
+ Teaneck Radiology Center, LLC.
699 Teaneck Road   Teaneck, NJ 07666   (201)836-2500   Fax (201)836-0083

Kisch, Agnes M., MD {1326197021} Psychy(75,FRA19)<NJ-GRYSTPSY, NJ-BERGNMC>
+ Greystone Park Psychiatric Hospital
59 Koch Avenue   Morris Plains, NJ 07950   (973)538-1800

Kiselev, Marianna L., MD {1366510927} Psychy(90,UZB44)<NJ-MONMOUTH>
+ Monmouth Medical Center
300 Second Avenue/Psych   Long Branch, NJ 07740   (732)222-5200

Kishen, Anita, MD {1407989395} Pedtrc(96,INA75)<NJ-JFKMED>
+ 795 Inman Avenue
Colonia, NJ 07067   (732)396-0700   Fax (732)396-0701

+ 120 West 7th Street/Suite 203
Plainfield, NJ 07060   (908)757-8687

Kiss, Geza Kalmar, MD {1699857367} Anesth(95,NJ05)<NJ-RWJUBRUN>
+ Robert Wood Johnson-UMDNJ Anesthesia Group
125 Paterson Street/CAB 3100   New Brunswick, NJ 08901   (732)235-7827   Fax (732)235-6131

Kissin, Anna, MD {1336254762} IntrMd, EnDbMt(96,ISR02)<NJ-MORRISTN>
+ Drs. Siegel and Kissin
10 James Street/Suite 140   Florham Park, NJ 07932   (973)665-8100   Fax (973)665-8097

Kissin, Yair David, MD {1619182276} SrgOrt(02,ISR02)<NJ-BURDTMLN>
+ Hackensack University MedCtr-Plastic & Ortho Surgery
360 Essex Street/Suite 303   Hackensack, NJ 07601   (551)996-8867   Fax (551)996-8873

Kisza, Piotr Slawomir, MD {1013960079} Radiol, RadV&I(90,POL08)<NJ-UMDNJ, NJ-VAEASTOR>
+ University Hospital
150 Bergen Street/Suite 318   Newark, NJ 07103   (973)972-4300

Kithinji, Kagendo M., MD {1992983977} ObsGyn<NY-MTSINYHS>
+ Tenafly Ob-Gyn Associates PA
2 Dean Drive/2nd Floor   Tenafly, NJ 07670   (201)569-3300   Fax (201)569-7649

Kitts, Lori M., MD {1891781043} FamMed(00,MI07)
+ Integrated Family Medicine
701 Cooper Road/Suite 16   Voorhees, NJ 08043   (856)783-5000   Fax (856)783-5041

Kitzis, Hugo D., MD {1902874506} ObsGyn(67,ARG01)<NJ-HACKNSK>
+ Ob-Gyn Associates of North Jersey
7400 Bergenline Avenue   North Bergen, NJ 07047   (201)869-5488   Fax (201)869-6944

Kizina, Christopher Allen, MD {1164674024} AnesPain(04,PA13)
+ The AIPM Group
1037 Route 46 East/Suite G-5   Clifton, NJ 07013   (973)928-5363   Fax (973)928-5359

Kjellberg, Sten I., MD {1285665034} Surgry(91,NY09)<NJ-WARREN>
+ 224 Roseberry Street/Suite 8
Phillipsburg, NJ 08865   (908)859-5222   Fax (908)859-3261
+ Coordinated Health
222 Red Lane   Phillipsburg, NJ 08865   (908)859-5222   Fax (610)849-1013

Klachko, Daria A., MD {1255449724} ObsGyn(93,NJ05)
+ Summit Medical Group
75 East Northfield Road   Livingston, NJ 07039   (973)436-1410   Fax (973)325-5677
dklachko@smgnj.com

Klafter, George, MD {1114929635} Urolgy, PedUro(74,NY09)<NJ-ENGLWOOD, NJ-HOLYNAME>
+ The Urology Center of Englewood, PA
663 Palisade Avenue/Suite 304   Cliffside Park, NJ 07010   (201)313-1933   Fax (201)313-9599
+ The Urology Center of Englewood, PA
300 Grand Avenue/Suite 102   Englewood, NJ 07631   (201)313-1933   Fax (201)816-1777

Klansky, Megan A., DO {1023304789}
+ Rowan University-School of Osteopathic Medicine
1 Medical Center Drive   Stratford, NJ 08084   (856)566-6708   Fax (856)566-6222

Klapholz, Marc, MD {1063447829} CdvDis, IntrMd(86,NY46)<NJ-UMDNJ>
+ University Hospital-Doctors Office Center
90 Bergen Street/DOC 3500/Cardio   Newark, NJ 07103   (973)972-2573   Fax (973)972-4695

Klapper, Daniel A., MD {1538106703} Ophthl, SrgLsr, Glacma(84,NY46)<NY-MANHEYE, NY-NYEYEINF>
+ 185 Cedar Lane/Suite U-3
Teaneck, NJ 07666   (201)530-0555
drdaniel@lasereyemd.com

Klausman, Kenneth Barry, MD {1306803549} IntrMd, OccpMd(81,DMN01)
+ 508 Gatewood Road
Cherry Hill, NJ 08003

Klausner, Anna Jill, MD {1710252804} Anesth
+ Princeton Anesthesia Services PC
One Plainsboro Road   Plainsboro, NJ 08536   (609)497-4000

Klausner, Mark A., MD {1346412012} IntrMd(77,MA01)
+ 2332 Town Court North
Lawrence, NJ 08648

Klauss, Gunnar, MD {1962685305} Anesth<NJ-HACKNSK>
+ Hackensack University Medical Center
30 Prospect Avenue/Anesth   Hackensack, NJ 07601   (201)996-2419   Fax (201)996-3962

Klazmer, Jay, DO {1356341556} Nrolgy, VasNeu(00,PA77)<NJ-KENEDYHS>
+ Associates in Family HealthCare, P.C.
73 North Maple Avenue/Suite B   Marlton, NJ 08053   (844)542-2273   Fax (856)569-4043

267

Physicians by Name and Address

Klebacher, Ronald John, DO {1508894759} IntrMd, EmrgMd(01,MO78)<NJ-COMMED>
+ Community Medical Center
  99 Route 37 West/EmrgMed   Toms River, NJ 08755   (732)557-8000

Klebanov, Vladimir, MD {1033227525} Psychy, NrlgAddM(72,UZB44)<NY-MAIMONMC>
+ 2101 Route 516/Suite B
  Old Bridge, NJ 08857   (732)607-7700   Fax (732)607-3770

Klebba, Kevin Edmund, MD {1386729697} Anesth(95,FL02)<NJ-STBARNMC>
+ St. Barnabas Medical Center
  94 Old Short Hills Road   Livingston, NJ 07039   (973)322-5000

Klecz, Robert J., MD {1104814318} PhysMd(90,POL03)<NJ-KSLR-WEST, NJ-KSLRSADB>
+ Kessler Institute for Rehabilitation West Orange
  1199 Pleasant Valley Way   West Orange, NJ 07052   (201)368-6054
  Michael.sheehy@reliantmedicalgroup.org
+ Associates in Rehabilitation Medicine
  95 Mount Kemble Avenue   Morristown, NJ 07960   (201)368-6054   Fax (973)226-3144

Kleeman, Jeffrey A., DO {1598777310} FamMed(87,IA75)<NJ-VIRTBERL, NJ-VIRTVOOR>
+ Drs. Gitler and Kleeman
  2961 Yorkship Square   Camden, NJ 08104   (856)541-5588   Fax (856)338-9223

Klees, Julia E., MD {1669644779} IntrMd, OccpMd(94,PA09)
+ BASF Corporation
  100 Campus Drive   Florham Park, NJ 07932   (973)243-6000   Fax (973)245-6947

Kleiber, Maria A., MD {1285672048} EnDbMt, InfDis, IntrMd(70,URUG)<NJ-ACMCITY, NJ-ACMCMAIN>
+ 2106 New Road/Suite C-3
  Linwood, NJ 08221   (609)653-2966   Fax (609)653-8900
+ Seashore Gardens Living Center
  22 West Jimmie Leeds Road   Absecon, NJ 08205   (609)653-2966   Fax (609)404-4841

Klein, Alan C., MD {1710069471} IntrMd(80,MEXI)<NJ-JRSYSHMC>
+ Shore Primary Care
  1944 Corlies Avenue/Suite 103   Neptune, NJ 07753   (732)774-2336   Fax (732)774-2337

Klein, Bradley Marc, MD {1619314705} Pedtrc
+ Neurology Group of Bergen County
  1200 East Ridgewood Avenue   Ridgewood, NJ 07450   (201)444-0868   Fax (201)447-0581

Klein, Bruce M., MD {1275640302} Pedtrc(77,NY08)<NJ-VIRT-MARL, NJ-VIRTBERL>
+ Southern Jersey Family Medical Centers, Inc.
  860 South White Horse Pike/Building A   Hammonton, NJ 08037   (609)567-0200   Fax (609)567-3492

Klein, Edward M., MD {1679549398} ObsGyn, IntrMd(78,PA13)<NJ-OURLADY, NJ-VIRTVOOR>
+ Ob-Gyn Care of Southern New Jersey
  406 Gibbsboro Road East   Lindenwold, NJ 08021   (856)435-7007   Fax (856)435-7077

Klein, Eileen C., MD {1336141928} Nephro, IntrMd(86,NY19)<NJ-OVERLOOK>
+ Summit Medical Group
  75 East Northfield Road   Livingston, NJ 07039   (973)436-1400   Fax (908)673-7336
+ Summit Medical Group-Berkeley Heights Campus
  1 Diamond Hill Road/4th flr   Berkeley Heights, NJ 07922   (973)436-1400   Fax (908)673-7391
+ Somerset Hematology Oncology Associates, P.A.
  30 Rehill Avenue/2nd Floor/Suite 2500   Somerville, NJ 07039   (908)927-8700   Fax (908)927-8706

Klein, Gregg Roger, MD {1528053642} SrgOrt(97,PA02)
+ Hartzband Center for Hip & Knee Replacement
  10 Forest Avenue   Paramus, NJ 07652   (201)291-4040   Fax (201)291-0440

Klein, Harvey A., MD {1164595534} SrgOrt, PainMd, AltHol(80,MA07)
+ The Klein Center for Integrative Med
  1029 Teaneck Road/Suite 3-D   Teaneck, NJ 07666   (201)357-8747

Klein, Ira A., MD {1629073945} Anesth(91,NY15)<NJ-BAYONNE, NY-STFRNCIS>
+ Bayonne Medical Center
  29th Street at Avenue E   Bayonne, NJ 07002   (201)858-5000

Klein, Irving J., DO {1659378321} FamMed(64,PA77)<NJ-KMH-STRAT, NJ-UNDRWD>
+ 165 Princeton Avenue
  West Deptford, NJ 08096   (856)456-0400   Fax (856)456-3011

Klein, James Joseph, Jr., MD {1407814007} SrgCTh, Srgry, SrgThr(90,NY48)<NJ-ENGLWOOD>
+ Englewood Cardiac Surgery Associates
  350 Engle Street   Englewood, NJ 07631   (201)894-3636
  Fax (201)541-2188
+ Englewood Hospital and Medical Center
  350 Engle Street   Englewood, NJ 07631   (201)894-3000
+ Heart and Vascular Institute at EHMC
  350 Engle Street/Suite 1000   Englewood, NJ 07631   (201)894-3636

Klein, Kathryn Suzanne, MD {1598961484} Ophthl
+ Pediatric Eye Physicians, PC
  95 Madison Avenue/Suite 301   Morristown, NJ 07960   (646)784-4679   Fax (973)540-8556
  kathysklein@gmail.com

Klein, Kenneth Michael, MD {1912920240} PthAClf(67,BELG)<NJ-UMDNJ>
+ University Hospital
  150 Bergen Street/Path   Newark, NJ 07103   (973)972-4716   Fax (973)972-5724
  kklein@umdnj.edu
+ Rutgers- New Jersey Medical School
  185 South Orange Avenue/Path/Lab Med   Newark, NJ 07103   (973)972-4716   Fax (973)972-5724

Klein, Kenneth Stuart, MD {1427115906} SrgOrt(66,PA13)<NJ-RWJUBRUN, NJ-STPETER>
+ Mid Atlantic Orthopedic Associates LLP
  557 Cranbury Road/Suite 10   East Brunswick, NJ 08816   (732)238-8800   Fax (732)238-8246

Klein, Laura Ann, MD {1043383672} Srgry, SrgBst(98,ISR02)<NJ-VALLEY>
+ Daniel and Gloria Blumenthal Cancer Center
  One Valley Health Plaza   Paramus, NJ 07652   (201)634-5557

Klein, Laura B., MD {1073643706} RadBdI
+ Hunterdon Radiology
  PO Box 5388   Clinton, NJ 08809

Klein, Martin Edward, MD {1235209560} FamMed(00,NJ05)<NJ-HUNTRDN>
+ Hunterdon Family Medicine
  250 Route 28/Suite 100   Bridgewater, NJ 08807   (908)237-4135   Fax (908)237-4136

Klein, Matthew Seth, MD {1265434005} Anesth, IntrMd(86,IL06)<NJ-MONMOUTH>
+ Monmouth Medical Center
  300 Second Avenue/Anesthesia   Long Branch, NJ 07740   (732)222-5200   Fax (732)923-6977

Klein, Patricia G., MD {1720048648} Nrolgy(76,NJ05)<NJ-HOLY-NAME>
+ David D. Van Slooten MD, PA
  99 Kinderamack Road/Suite 307   Westwood, NJ 07675   (201)261-6222   Fax (201)261-4411

Klein, Patti S., MD {1538244397} Anesth(82,DC01)<NJ-HOLY-NAME>
+ Bergen Anesthesia Associates
  718 Teaneck Road   Teaneck, NJ 07666   (201)833-7149   Fax (201)342-1259
+ Holy Name Hospital
  718 Teaneck Road/Anesthesiology   Teaneck, NJ 07666   (201)833-3000

Klein, Philip S., MD {1952393522} Nephro, IntrMd(82,NY46)<NJ-OVERLOOK, NJ-RWJURAH>
+ Medical Diagnostic Associates PA
  215 North Avenue West   Westfield, NJ 07090   (908)232-4321   Fax (908)232-7788
+ Medical Diagnostic Associates PA-Nephrology
  1511 Park Avenue/3rd Floor   South Plainfield, NJ 07080   (908)232-4321   Fax (908)757-2427

Klein, Rachel S., MD {1871813709} IntrMd(10,PA01)
+ Dermatology and Laser Center
  622 Stokes Road/Suite A   Medford, NJ 08055   (609)953-0908   Fax (609)953-5978

Klein, Randy S., MD {1265549042} FamMed(83,NY03)<NJ-HUNTRDN>
+ The Doctor Is in
  149 Highway 31   Flemington, NJ 08822   (908)782-7700   Fax (908)782-3644
+ The Doctor Is in
  59 Old Highway 22   Clinton, NJ 08809   (908)782-7700   Fax (908)730-8185
+ The Doctor Is in
  6701 Bergenline Avenue   West New York, NJ 08822   (201)758-9100

Klein, Richard Ashley, MD {1992833651} SrgOrt(02,PA13)
+ Mid Atlantic Orthopedic Associates LLP
  557 Cranbury Road/Suite 10   East Brunswick, NJ 08816   (732)238-8800   Fax (732)238-8246

Klein, Richard M., MD {1407864663} Ophthl, VitRet, IntrMd(70,MD07)<NJ-HACKNSK, NJ-ENGLWOOD>
+ Retina Associates of New Jersey, P.A.
  628 Cedar Lane   Teaneck, NJ 07666   (201)837-7300   Fax (201)836-6426
+ Retina Associates of New Jersey, P.A.
  1044 Route 23 North/Suite 207   Wayne, NJ 07470   (201)837-7300   Fax (973)633-3892
+ Retina Associates of New Jersey, P.A.
  3196 Kennedy Boulevard   Union City, NJ 07666   (201)867-2999   Fax (201)867-4440

Klein, Robert Michael, MD {1235196452} Allrgy, Pedtrc(76,NY09)<NJ-STMRYPAS, NY-PRSBCOLU>
+ Allergy & Asthma Medical Associates
  1005 Clifton Avenue/Suite 1   Clifton, NJ 07013   (973)773-7400   Fax (973)779-5224
  amjb@verizon.net

Klein, Roger Scott, MD {1295756708} Gastrn, Hepato, IntrMd(91,NY19)
+ Summit Medical Group-Berkeley Heights Campus
  1 Diamond Hill Road   Berkeley Heights, NJ 07922   (908)273-4300   Fax (908)673-7140
  rkleinmd@gmail.com

Klein, Sanford L., MD {1154493732} Anesth(71,NY03)<NJ-RWJUBRUN>
+ UH- Robert Wood Johnson Med
  125 Paterson Street/Anesthesiology   New Brunswick, NJ 08901   (732)235-7827
+ Robert Wood Johnson-UMDNJ Anesthesia Group
  125 Paterson Street/CAB 3100   New Brunswick, NJ 08901   (732)235-7827   Fax (732)235-6131

Klein, Shawn Richard, MD {1982690574} Ophthl(99,NJ06)<NJ-UMDNJ>
+ Klein & Scannapiego MD PA
  230 West Jersey Street   Elizabeth, NJ 07202   (908)289-1166   Fax (908)352-4752
+ Paterson Eye Associates
  100 Main Street   Paterson, NJ 07505   (908)289-1166   Fax (973)278-7207

Klein, Steven, DO {1972676716} FamMed, OccpMd(84,IA75)<NJ-KMHCHRRY, NJ-OURLADY>
+ 104 South Broadway/PO Box 389
  Gloucester City, NJ 08030   (856)456-3888   Fax (856)456-6444

Klein, Walter A., MD {1821099078} Gastrn, IntrMd(87,NY20)<NJ-ENGLWOOD>
+ The Park Medical Group
  274 County Road/Suite A   Tenafly, NJ 07670   (201)568-0493   Fax (201)568-0483

Klein, Warren M., MD {1114912342} Ophthl(72,NJ05)<NJ-TRIN-INPC, NJ-UMDNJ>
+ Klein & Scannapiego MD PA
  230 West Jersey Street   Elizabeth, NJ 07202   (908)289-1166   Fax (908)352-4752
+ Paterson Eye Associates
  100 Main Street   Paterson, NJ 07505   (908)289-1166   Fax (973)278-7207

Kleinbart, Fredric Alan, MD {1396714747} SrgOrt(86,PA01)
+ Mercer-Bucks Orthopaedics, P.C.
  2501 Kuser Road   Hamilton, NJ 08691   (609)896-0444   Fax (609)587-4349

Kleiner, Alexander, MD {1174774251} Anesth(05,DMN01)<NJ-STCLRDEN>
+ St. Clare's Hospital-Denville Campus
  25 Pocono Road/Anesthesia   Denville, NJ 07834   (973)335-1122

Kleinfeld, David I., MD {1881605491} InfDis, IntrMd(80,NJ05)<NJ-OCEANMC>
+ 1200 Riverview Drive
  Brielle, NJ 08730   (732)292-0355   Fax (732)292-0357

Kleinman, David S., MD {1639123755} EnDbMt, IntrMd(78,ASTL)<NJ-KIMBALL, NJ-OCEANMC>
+ 40 Bey Lea Road/Suite B-103
  Toms River, NJ 08753   (732)341-9965   Fax (732)341-9588

Kleinman, Michael Ari, DO {1740394949} IntrMd(99,PA77)<NJ-VIRTMHBC, NJ-KMHSTRAT>
+ Alliance for Better Care, PC/Madison Avenue Division
  103 Madison Avenue   Mount Holly, NJ 08060   (609)267-7456   Fax (609)261-8670

Kleinmann, Richard, MD {1679817777} PsycCAd(98,NJ05)
+ PO Box 4516
  Highland Park, NJ 08904   (732)452-0990

Klele, Christo Selim, MD {1992708184} Anesth(89,NJ05)
+ Wayne Surgical Center, LLC.
  1176 Hamburg Pike   Wayne, NJ 07470   (973)709-1900   Fax (973)709-1901

Klele, Michael A, MD {1861512030} FamMed, IntrMd(05,SEN02)
+ Family Care, P.A.
  257 US Highway 22   Green Brook, NJ 08812   (732)968-7878   Fax (732)968-2187

Klempner, William L., MD {1730255423} SrgNro(69,VA04)<NJ-VALLEY>
+ North Jersey Neurosurgical Associates PA
  225 Dayton Street   Ridgewood, NJ 07450   (201)612-0020   Fax (201)612-0333

Klenoff, Paul H., MD {1649244930} Dermat(66,NY46)<NJ-JRSYSHMC>
+ 804 West Park Avenue
  Ocean, NJ 07712   (732)493-3337   Fax (732)493-4463
  dameekz@verizon.net

Kleshchelskaya, Valeria, MD {1417907171} IntrMd(92,UKR18)<NJ-JFKMED>
 + Edison Emergi Med
  98 James Street/Suite 313   Edison, NJ 08820   (732)635-1100   Fax (732)635-0918

Kleyn, Michael, MD {1275761207} CritCr, IntrMd
 + 6 Highpoint Drive
  Mountainside, NJ 07092   (718)207-3140

Klier, Steven W., MD {1184652638} CdvDis, IntrMd(82,NY08)
 + Penn Specialty Care of Burlington County
  200 Campbell Drive/Suite 115   Willingboro, NJ 08046   (609)871-7070   Fax (609)835-4510

Klifto, Eugene J., DO {1689609083} RadDia(80,PA77)<NJ-OURLADY>
 + Our Lady of Lourdes Medical Center
  1600 Haddon Avenue/Radiology   Camden, NJ 08103   (856)757-3500

Klimczak, Amber, MD {1790165405} RprEnd
 + Reproductive Medicine Associates of New Jersey
  140 Allen Road   Basking Ridge, NJ 07920   (973)871-2238   Fax (973)290-8370

Klimowicz-Mallon, Elizabeth, MD {1235579129} ObsGyn
 + Physicians for Womens Health
  1124 East Ridgewood Avenue/Suite 105   Ridgewood, NJ 07450   (201)489-2255   Fax (201)489-4799
 + 470 North Franklin Turnpike
  Ramsey, NJ 07446   (201)327-8765

Kline, Bradley H., DO {1134161987} FamMed, OccpMd, SprtMd(81,PA77)<NJ-UNVMCPRN, NJ-RWJUHAM>
 + Brunswick Princeton Industrial Medical Center
  4105 US Highway 1/Suite 1   Monmouth Junction, NJ 08852   (732)329-8585   Fax (732)329-5668
  DrKline@Workers-Comp.Org

Kline, David M., DO {1568653558} Pedtrc(04,NJ75)<NJ-COOPRUMC>
 + Cooper Peds/Children's Regional Ctr
  3 Cooper Plaza/Suite 200   Camden, NJ 08103   (856)342-2472   Fax (856)368-8297

Kline, Gary Michael, MD {1497825830} Surgry, SrgCTh, SrgThr(86,MI07)<NY-WINTHROP, NY-NSUHMANH>
 + Summit Surgical Institute
  332 Summit Avenue   Hackensack, NJ 07601   (201)488-6445   Fax (201)488-6441

Kline, Jason Andrew, MD {1912115296} Nephro(02,PA02)
 + The Cooper Hospital System-Univ Hospital
  3 Cooper Plaza/Suite 215   Camden, NJ 08103   (856)342-2439   Fax (856)757-7778

Kline, John A., MD {1255306049} SrgOrt, SprtMd(70,PA02)<NJ-RWJURAH, NJ-TRINIJSC>
 + Union County Orthopaedic Group
  210 West St. Georges Avenue/PO Box 330   Linden, NJ 07036   (908)486-1111   Fax (908)583-1034

Kline, Philip E., MD {1942347281} ObsGyn(80,MEX14)<NJ-JFKMED, NJ-RWJURAH>
 + Ob & Gyn Group of Central NJ
  1500 St. Georges Avenue/Suite F   Avenel, NJ 07001   (732)669-9600   Fax (732)669-9800
  pekmd@aol.com

Kline, Roxana Gabriela, MD {1215037981} SrgVas, Surgry(91,MI07)<NJ-HACKNSK, NJ-VALLEY>
 + Summit Surgical Institute
  332 Summit Avenue   Hackensack, NJ 07601   (201)488-6445   Fax (201)488-6441

Kline-Kim, Johanna F., MD {1952562381} FamMed(07,PA09)
 + Penn Medicine at Woodbury Heights
  1006 Mantua Pike   Woodbury Heights, NJ 08097   (856)845-8600   Fax (856)845-0535

Kling, Maureen C., MD {1336140649} Surgry(86,PA07)<NJ-VIRTMHBC>
 + Virtua Athena Breast Care Center
  110 Marter Avenue/Suite 508   Moorestown, NJ 08057   (856)581-8500   Fax (856)581-8503

Klingenstein, Gregory Gillman, MD {1952517963} SrgOrt(05,NY47)
 + Reconstructive Orthopedics, P.A.
  200 Bowman Drive/Suite E-100   Voorhees, NJ 08043   (609)267-9400   Fax (609)267-9457

Klinger, Frederick Boyd, III, DO {1871888354} InfDis
 + Infectious Disease Physicians PA
  1001 Briggs Road/Suite 250   Mount Laurel, NJ 08054   (856)866-7466   Fax (856)866-9088

Klingmeyer, Dorothy Marie, DO {1487996062} FamMed
 + Morristown Medical Center Family Medicine
  435 South Street/Suite 220-A   Morristown, NJ 07960   (973)971-4222   Fax (973)290-7050

Klingsberg, Gary P., DO {1801833413} FamMed(81,NY75)<NJ-HOLYNAME>
 + Center for Nutrition and Preventive Medicine
  66 North Van Brunt Street   Englewood, NJ 07631   (201)503-0007   Fax (201)503-0008

Klitzman, Donna Leslie, MD {1295824563} CritCr, IntrMd, PulDis(87,MA05)
 + Pulmonary & Intensive Care Specialists of NJ
  593 Cranbury Road   East Brunswick, NJ 08816   (732)613-8880   Fax (732)613-0077

Klodnicki, Walter E., MD {1437120078} CdvDis, IntrMd(82,NJ05)<NJ-OURLADY, NJ-COOPRUMC>
 + Associated Cardiovascular Consultants-Lourdes
  1 Brace Road/Suite C & F   Cherry Hill, NJ 08034   (856)428-4100   Fax (856)428-1517

Kloepping, Carolyn H., MD {1477978294}
 + UMDNJ Anesthesiology-Pain Medicine
  185 South Orange Avenue   Newark, NJ 07103   (973)972-5007   Fax (973)972-0582

Kloos, Thomas H., MD {1295833556} IntrMd(79,KY02)<NJ-OVERLOOK>
 + Warren Primary Care
  23 Mountain Boulevard   Warren, NJ 07059   (908)598-7970   Fax (908)322-4989

Klos, Andrzej E., MD {1104932144} Pedtrc(77,POLA)<NJ-HOBUNIMC, NJ-STBARNMC>
 + Hoboken East
  5 Marine View Plaza   Hoboken, NJ 07030   (201)479-5206   Fax (201)963-3924
 + Hoboken University Medical Center
  308 Willow Avenue   Hoboken, NJ 07030   (201)418-1000

Kloser, Patricia C., MD {1801988787} InfDis, IntrMd, HivAid(83,DMN01)<NJ-UMDNJ>
 + University Hospital-Doctors Office Center
  90 Bergen Street/DOC 4500   Newark, NJ 07103   (973)972-2500   Fax (973)972-2510

Klots, Larisa, DO {1053361550} FamMed(97,NY75)<NJ-STPETER, NY-BRNXLFUL>
 + B-3 Brier Hill Court
  East Brunswick, NJ 08816   (732)254-1405   Fax (732)254-2247

Kloupar, Dagmar S., MD {1497739312} Psychy(75,CZE07)<NJ-NWTNMEM>
 + Highland Psychiatric Associates
  89 Sparta Avenue/Suite 240   Sparta, NJ 07871   (973)729-2991   Fax (973)729-7641

Klug, Ronald David, MD {1376537340} Ophthl, VitRet(80,NY19)<NJ-BAYSHORE, NJ-RIVERVW>
 + Ophthalmic Physicians of Monmouth PA
  733 North Beers Street/Suite U-4   Holmdel, NJ 07733   (732)739-0707   Fax (732)739-6722

Klughaupt, Stanley, MD {1912933656} IntrMd(72,NY06)<NJ-CLARMAAS>
 + 50 Newark Avenue/Suite 306
  Belleville, NJ 07109   (973)450-0220   Fax (973)450-0162

Klukowicz, Alan J., MD {1912959685} IntrMd, PulDis(80,MEXI)<NJ-MTNSIDE>
 + Better Breathing Center
  62 South Fullerton Avenue   Montclair, NJ 07042   (973)744-9125   Fax (973)744-7281

Klyashtorny, Alexander, MD {1417996836} Anesth, PainMd, AnesPain(91,PA02)<NJ-STMRYPAS>
 + Jersey Anesthesia & Pain Management Consultants, LLC
  940 Amboy Avenue/Suite 104A   Edison, NJ 08837   (732)738-3963   Fax (732)738-3965
 + Paramus Surgical Center
  30 West Century Road/Suite 300   Paramus, NJ 07652   (732)738-3963   Fax (201)634-9014

Klyde, David Philip, MD {1447204946} RadDia, RadV&I(93,NY46)
 + Renex Dialysis Clinic
  110 South Grove Street   East Orange, NJ 07018   (973)414-6100   Fax (973)414-6109

Knackmuhs, Gary Glenn, MD {1649259037} InfDis, IntrMd(76,NY09)<NJ-VALLEY>
 + Ridgewood Infectious Disease Associates
  947 Linwood Avenue/Suite 2E   Ridgewood, NJ 07450   (201)447-6468   Fax (201)447-3189
 + The Valley Hospital
  223 North Van Dien Avenue/Inf Disease   Ridgewood, NJ 07450   (201)447-8000

Knafel, Natalya, MD {1720487648} Psychy
 + Tenafly Psychiatric Associates, LLC
  2 Dean Drive/1st Floor S   Tenafly, NJ 07670   (201)568-8288

Knapp, Stefanie, MD {1376651257} Ophthl(02,TN05)
 + Eyecare MD of New Jersey
  261 James Street/Suite 2-D & 3EL   Morristown, NJ 07960   (973)984-3937   Fax (973)984-0059

Knappertz, Volker Armin, MD {1831355981} Nrolgy(90,GER22)
 + 22 Three Gables Road
  Morristown, NJ 07960   Fax (973)695-1462

Knause, Rita Vinod, MD {1649218173} ObsGyn(98,GRN01)
 + Holy Name Ob-Gyn Associates
  49 Woodmere Lane   Tenafly, NJ 07670   (201)960-0920   Fax (201)866-9067

Knee, C. Michael, MD {1225123961} Rheuma, PedRhm(72,NY46)<NJ-STJOSHOS>
 + 44 Godwin Avenue
  Midland Park, NJ 07432   (201)444-5004   Fax (201)670-0356
  cmknee7@aol.com
 + St. Joseph's Regional Medical Center
  703 Main Street/Rheumatology   Paterson, NJ 07503   (201)444-5004   Fax (973)754-2724

Knee, Robert, MD {1669454666} RadOnc, RadThp, Radiol(78,NY08)
 + Radiation Oncology at Overlook Medical Center
  33 Overlook Road/MAC 1 Suite L-05   Summit, NJ 07901   (908)522-2871   Fax (908)522-5628
 + JFK Medical Center
  65 James Street   Edison, NJ 08820   (908)522-2871   Fax (732)906-4914

Kneisser, George, MD {1982600433} Ophthl(78,LEB01)
 + Middletown Eye Care
  565 Highway 35   Red Bank, NJ 07701   (732)747-4443   Fax (732)747-4439
  drgeorge@aol.com

Knep, Stanley J., MD {1518952803} Nrolgy(65,SAF01)<NJ-STJOSHOS>
 + Neurology Group of North Jersey PA
  905 Allwood Road/Suite 105   Clifton, NJ 07012   (973)471-3680   Fax (973)471-6360

Knepa, Valdone Elena, MD {1134224637} Anesth(89,LIT02)
 + 25b Vreeland Road/Suite 110
  Florham Park, NJ 07932

Knestaut, Angela Gaudiano, DO {1881642569} Pedtrc(92,PA77)
 + Advocare West Deptford Pediatrics
  1050 Mantua Pike   Wenonah, NJ 08090   (856)468-8330   Fax (856)468-9121
 + Advocare West Deptford Pediatrics
  19 Village Center Drive   Swedesboro, NJ 08085   (856)468-8330   Fax (856)879-2855
 + Advocare West Deptford Pediatrics
  646 Kings Highway   West Deptford, NJ 08090   (856)879-2887   Fax (856)879-2855

Knezevic, Dusan Svetozar, MD {1023062866} CdvDis, IntrMd(94,SER03)
 + Montclair Cardiology Group PA
  123 Highland Avenue/Suite 302   Glen Ridge, NJ 07028   (973)748-9555   Fax (973)748-2003

Knifong, Genoveva, MD {1508856279} Pedtrc(01,MI01)<NJ-VIRTVOOR>
 + Virtua Voorhees
  100 Bowman Drive/Pediatrics   Voorhees, NJ 08043   (856)247-3000   Fax (856)325-3157

Knight, Jennifer Mary, MD {1548422603} Psychy, IntrMd(04,PA07)
 + Salerno Medical Associates, LLP
  613 Park Avenue   East Orange, NJ 07017   (973)672-8573   Fax (973)676-4099

Knight, Michael Robert, MD {1487852570} CdvDis, SrgCrC, Surgry(07,GRN01)<NJ-MERIDNHS, NJ-JRSYSHMC>
 + Jersey Shore University Medical Center
  1945 Route 33/Surgery/Trauma   Neptune, NJ 07753   (732)776-4747   Fax (732)776-4843

Knight, Phillip Thomas, DO {1639557598} Pedtrc
 + Progressive Pediatrics
  3196 Kennedy Boulevard   Union City, NJ 07087   (201)319-9800   Fax (201)319-9849

Knightly, John J., MD {1912964008} SrgNro(85,NJ05)<NJ-ATLANTHS, NJ-OVERLOOK>
 + Atlantic Neurosurgical Specialists
  310 Madison Avenue/Suite 300   Morristown, NJ 07960   (973)285-7800   Fax (973)285-7839

Knights, Jayci Elenor, MD {1184704140} ObsGyn(97,NJ06)
 + Cooper University Hospital OBGYN
  3 Cooper Plaza/Suite 221   Camden, NJ 08103   (856)325-6600   Fax (856)968-8575
 + University Urogynecology Associates/Cooper Ob/Gyn
  900 Centennial Boulevard/Suite L   Voorhees, NJ 08043   (856)325-6600   Fax (856)325-6522
 + Cooper Ob/Gyn
  3 Cooper Plaza/Suite 300   Camden, NJ 08103   (856)342-2186   Fax (856)968-8575

Knihnicky, Alexander, DO {1295141448}<NJ-CHRIST>
 + Christ Hospital
  176 Palisade Avenue   Jersey City, NJ 07306   (201)795-8201

Knod, George Albert, DO {1700825783} PhysMd(83,PA77)<NJ-OURLADY, NJ-VIRTMHBC>
 + Associated Physiatrists of Southern New Jersey
  435 Hurffville-Cross Keys Road   Turnersville, NJ 08012   (856)757-3878   Fax (856)757-3760
 + Associated Physiatrists of Southern New Jersey
  175 Madison Avenue/Cardiology   Mount Holly, NJ 08060   (856)757-3878   Fax (856)757-3760

Knoflicek, Lisa E., MD {1720184807} Pedtrc, IntrMd(03,TN05)
 + CAMCare Health Corporation
  817 Federal Street/Pediatrics   Camden, NJ 08103   (856)541-9811   Fax (856)225-1678

Physicians by Name and Address

Knoll, Abraham, MD {1932143633} Urolgy(99,NY08)<NJ-CHILTON, NJ-VALLEY>
+ Associates in Urology, PA
1777 Hamburg Turnpike/Suite 304   Wayne, NJ 07470   (973)616-8400   Fax (973)616-8485
aiunjpa@aol.com

Knoll, Frank J., III, MD {1609938018} Anesth
+ West Jersey Anesthesia Associates
102E Centre Boulevard   Marlton, NJ 08053   (856)988-6260   Fax (856)988-6270

Knops, Karen M., MD {1609843382} IntrMd(01,CA14)<NJ-MORRISTN>
+ Morristown Medical Center
100 Madison Avenue/Medicine   Morristown, NJ 07962   (973)971-5000

Knowles, Kelly Petrison, MD {1003895798} Pedtrc(90,NY45)<NJ-OVERLOOK>
+ Millburn Pediatrics PA
159 Millburn Avenue   Millburn, NJ 07041   (973)912-0155   Fax (973)912-8714

Knowles, William O., MD {1386683134} Allrgy, IntrMd(77,PA09)
+ CAMCare Health Corporation
2610 Federal Street   Camden, NJ 08104   (856)635-0212

Ko, Albert Edward, MD {1396892758} SrgPlstc(92,PA09)
+ Northern New Jersey Plastic Surgery
95 Madison Avenue/Suite 305   Morristown, NJ 07960   (973)270-0283

Ko, Haeng S., MD {1134230774} Psychy(67,KOR14)
+ New Point Behavioral Health Care
404 Tatum Street   Woodbury, NJ 08096   (856)845-8050   Fax (856)845-0688

Ko, James H., MD {1972773935} ClNrPh, Nrolgy(02,PA02)
+ 177 North Dean Street/Suite 201
Englewood, NJ 07631   (201)347-4012

Ko, Pan Sok, MD {1083851687} IntrMd(04,GRN01)
+ PSK Infectious Disease
400 Sylvan Avenue/Suite 108   Englewood Cliffs, NJ 07632   (201)408-5314   Fax (201)408-4431
+ 260 Old Hook Road/Suite 300
Westwood, NJ 07675   (201)408-5314   Fax (201)408-4431

Ko, So Hun, MD {1336171461} NnPnMd, Pedtrc(69,KORE)<NJ-STBARNMC>
+ St. Barnabas Medical Center
94 Old Short Hills Road/Pediatrics   Livingston, NJ 07039   (973)322-5000   Fax (973)322-8833

Koblenzer, Caroline S., MD {1588621320} Dermat(63,ENGL)
+ Dermatology Associates
303 Chester Avenue   Moorestown, NJ 08057   (856)235-1178   Fax (856)722-9244

Kobylarz, Fred A., MD {1023710749} FamMed(88,MEXI)
+ Center for Healthy Aging
18 Centre Drive/Suite 104   Monroe Township, NJ 08831   (609)655-5178   Fax (609)655-5284
kobylafr@umdnj.edu

Kocaj, Stephen Mark, MD {1275568446} SrgOrt(00,NJ05)
+ Summit Medical Group Orthopedics and Sports Medicine
140 Park Avenue/2nd Floor   Florham Park, NJ 07932   (973)404-9800   Fax (973)267-1737

Koch, Donna Marie, DO {1083652853} FamMed(97,NJ75)
+ Comprehensive Family Care LLC
297 Passaic Street/Suite 2   Garfield, NJ 07026   (973)777-2293   Fax (973)777-9117
+ Midtown Primary Care LLC
550 Newark Avenue/Suite 308   Jersey City, NJ 07306   (973)777-2293   Fax (201)656-2390

Koch, Marjan Leoni, MD {1164608816} OncHem
+ The Cooper Hospital System-Univ Hospital
3 Cooper Plaza/Suite 215/Hematology   Camden, NJ 08103   (856)963-3573   Fax (856)338-9211

Koch, Peter Benjamin, MD {1720172505} EmrgMd(98,NJ06)<NJ-JRSYCITY>
+ Jersey City Medical Center
355 Grand Street/EmrgMed   Jersey City, NJ 07304   (201)915-2000

Koch, Robert K., MD {1477691293} ObsGyn(88,NJ05)<NJ-STBARNMC>
+ Dr. Anthony Quartell and Associates
316 Eisenhower Parkway/Suite 202   Livingston, NJ 07039   (973)716-9600   Fax (973)716-9650

Kocher, Jeffrey, MD {1053319202} InfDis, IntrMd(80,NY20)<NJ-ENGLWOOD, NJ-HOLYNAME>
+ Leonia Medical Associates, P.A.
25 Rockwood Place/Suite 120   Englewood, NJ 07631   (201)568-3335   Fax (201)568-2450

Kocher, William D., MD {1942218599} PthAcl, Hemato(81,PA02)<NJ-COOPRUMC>
+ Cooper University Hospital
One Cooper Plaza/Path   Camden, NJ 08103   (856)342-2506   Fax (856)968-8312

Kochhar, Seema, MD {1861545519} PsyCAd
+ Jersey Shore Psychiatric Associates
3535 Route 66/Building 5/Suite D   Neptune, NJ 07753

(732)643-4350   Fax (732)643-4398

Kochlatyi, Sergei G., MD {1104877836} IntrMd(93,RUSS)
+ 110 Fifth Street
Cresskill, NJ 07626

Kocia, Orjeta, MD {1194020164} IntHos<NJ-HOBUNIMC>
+ Hoboken University Medical Center
308 Willow Avenue   Hoboken, NJ 07030   (201)418-1000

Kocinski, Michael Stephen, I, DO {1295798262} FamMed(97,PA77)<NJ-COOPRUMC>
+ Cooper Physicians
1210 Brace Road/Suite 102   Cherry Hill, NJ 08034   (856)428-6616   Fax (856)428-4823

Kociuba, Marcin K., DO {1285859488} EmrgMd(03,MI12)<NJ-VAEASTOR>
+ VA New Jersey Health Care System-East Orange Campus
385 Tremont Avenue   East Orange, NJ 07018   (973)676-1000

Kocsis, Cynthia A., MD {1780659219} Surgy(81,OH43)<NJ-CENTRAST, NJ-MONMOUTH>
+ Kocsis Surgical Services
1451 Route 34/Suite 304   Wall, NJ 07719   (732)577-8338   Fax (732)972-6095

Kocun, Christopher C., MD {1134358088} ObsGyn(96,NJ05)
+ 845 Adelaide Avenue
Woodbridge, NJ 07095

Kodali, Padmaja, MD {1790747764} Nephro, IntrMd(92,INA5B)<NJ-EASTORNG>
+ 2040 Millburn Avenue/Suite 306
Maplewood, NJ 07040   (973)763-1100   Fax (973)763-1122

Kodavali, Lavanya A., MD {1477598068} IntrMd(96,INA48)<NJ-NWTNMEM>
+ 71 Holly Oak Drive
Voorhees, NJ 08043
+ Newton Medical Center
175 High Street   Newton, NJ 07860   (973)383-2121

Kodery, Chitra, DO {1538422993}
+ New Bridge Medical Center
230 East Ridgewood Avenue   Paramus, NJ 07652   (201)967-4000
+ 199 Nebula Road
Piscataway, NJ 08854   (848)248-0633

Kodiyalam, Uthra K., MD {1770545501} IntrMd(92,INDI)<NJ-STBARNMC>
+ 55 Morris Avenue/Suite 300
Springfield, NJ 07081   (973)379-9601   Fax (973)467-6779

Koduah, Doris Afreh, MD {1275592735} IntrMd(91,GHA02)<NJ-NWRKBETH>
+ Hackensack Medical Center-Internal Medicine
30 Prospect Avenue/4 Main/Rm 4621   Hackensack, NJ 07601   (201)996-3664   Fax (551)996-0536

Koduri, Beaula V., MD {1972505311} OncHem, IntrMd(93<NJ-RBAYOLDB>
+ Hematology Oncology Consultants, LLC.
2110 Oak Tree Road   Edison, NJ 08820   (732)483-4501   Fax (732)483-4502

Koduri, Hemanth Kumar, MD {1801065198} PhysMd(98,NSK01)
+ Aspen Medical Associates, P.A.
1 DeGraw Square   Teaneck, NJ 07666   (201)928-0200   Fax (201)928-0820

Koduru, Sobha R., MD {1114232428} IntrMd<NJ-UMDNJ>
+ University Hospital
150 Bergen Street   Newark, NJ 07103   (973)972-5672   Fax (973)972-0365

Koenig, Andrew Stuart, DO IntrMd, Rheuma(96,NJ75)<NJ-LOURDMED>
+ Penn Specialty Care of Burlington County
200 Campbell Drive/Suite 115   Willingboro, NJ 08046   (609)871-7070   Fax (609)835-4510

Koenig, Christopher, MD {1831127323} OthrSp, Pthlgy, PthACl(87,NJ06)<NJ-HACKNSK>
+ Hackensack University Medical Center
30 Prospect Avenue/Pathology   Hackensack, NJ 07601   (201)996-4808   Fax (201)996-2156
ckoenig@humed.com

Koenig, Michele L., MD {1144494964} Psychy(81,FRA33)
+ 30 Constitution Hill West
Princeton, NJ 08540

Koenigsberg, Alan M., MD {1407828312} Pedtrc(82,NY08)<NJ-MORRISTN, NJ-STCLRDEN>
+ Parsippany Pediatrics
1140 Parisppany Boulevard/Suite 102   Parsippany, NJ 07054   (973)263-0066   Fax (973)263-3160

Koenigsberg, Martin Allen, DO {1770534000} FamMed, IntrMd(76,IA75)
+ Martin Allen Koenigsberg DO, P.A.
235 Main Street/Suite 101   Hackensack, NJ 07601   (201)773-6600   Fax (201)773-6602
Koenigsberg88@yahoo.com

Koenigsberg, Tova Chava, MD {1164515300} RadDia, Radiol(93,NY46)
+ The Imaging Center
30 South Newman Street   Hackensack, NJ 07601   (201)488-1188   Fax (201)488-5244
+ New Century Imaging at Oradell
555 Kinderkamack Road   Oradell, NJ 07649   (201)488-1188   Fax (201)599-8333

Koerner, David M., DO {1477528529} FamMed(96,PA77)
+ Voorhees Family Practice
102 West White Horse Road/Suite 102   Voorhees, NJ 08043   (856)783-6200   Fax (856)783-8434

Koerner, Steven, DO {1558434308} Gastrn(89,MO78)<NJ-SOCEANCO>
+ Medical Associates of Ocean County, P.A.
1301 Route 72 West/Suite 300   Manahawkin, NJ 08050   (609)597-6513   Fax (609)597-4593

Koerner, Theodore G., DO {1245225366} GenPrc, FamMed(75,PA77)
+ 4911 Route 42/PO Box 1107
Turnersville, NJ 08012   (856)227-7048

Kofman, Igor, MD {1780845180} Surgry
+ North Jersey Surgical Group PA
3196 Kennedy Boulevard/2nd Floor   Union City, NJ 07087   (201)795-9080   Fax (201)795-9434

Kogan, Irina, MD {1679730477} Nrolgy(02,DMN01)
+ Medico-Legal Evaluations, PA
50 Franklin Lane/Suite 201   Manalapan, NJ 07726   (732)972-4771   Fax (732)972-8610

Kogan, Robert, MD {1114003936} Gastrn, IntrMd(81,NY09)
+ 700 North Broad Street
Elizabeth, NJ 07208   (908)354-1045

Koganti, Monika, MD {1669523981} IntrMd, PulCCr(97,INA29)<NJ-UNVMCPRN, NJ-VIRTMHBC>
+ Respiratory & Sleep Specialists, LLC.
3546 State Route 27   Kendall Park, NJ 08824   (732)737-7801   Fax (877)632-3456
+ Princeton Medicine
5 Plainsboro Road/Suite 300   Plainsboro, NJ 08536   (732)737-7801   Fax (609)853-7271
+ Princeton Plainsboro Hospitalists
253 Witherspoon Street/Suite J1   Princeton, NJ 08824   Fax (609)497-4020

Koh, Elsie, MD {1679548234} RadV&I, RadDia, IntrMd(96,MA07)
+ Verona Veins @ Access Care Physicians of NJ
1225 McBride Avenue/Suite 116   Little Falls, NJ 07424   (973)837-1018   Fax (973)837-1329
veronaveins@aac-llc.com
+ American Access Care, LLC.
2401 Morris Avenue/Suite West 112   Union, NJ 07083   (973)837-1018   Fax (908)686-0014

Kohan, Feraydoon, MD {1831134311} IntrMd, CdvDis(92,NY08)
+ 550 Newark Avenue/Suite 301-A
Jersey City, NJ 07306   (201)222-9900   Fax (201)222-9929

Kohlberg, William I., MD {1063523892} Urolgy, SrgUro(75,PA12)<NJ-CENTRAST>
+ Urology Care Alliance
501 Iron Bridge Road   Freehold, NJ 07728   (732)780-7603   Fax (732)308-3323
wkohlberg@yahoo.com
+ Urology Care Alliance
2 Hospital Plaza/Suite 110   Old Bridge, NJ 08857   (732)780-7603   Fax (732)972-0966
+ Urology Care Alliance
733 North Beers Street/Suite L-6   Holmdel, NJ 07728   (732)739-2200   Fax (732)739-8988

Kohler, Frank R., DO {1659314953} FamMed(63,PA77)
+ Center for Family Health/Doctors & Midwives
105 Manheim Avenue/Suite 1   Bridgeton, NJ 08302   (856)455-2700   Fax (856)455-7051

Kohler, John Patrick, MD {1861508954} Surgry, Acpntr, PainMd
+ 151 Fries Mill Road/Suite 506
Turnersville, NJ 08012   (856)232-8161

Kohlhapp, Caroline R., DO {1245599984}
+ Virtual Family Medicine - Mansfield
3242 Route 206/Building A Suite 2   Bordentown, NJ 08505   (507)261-2639   Fax (609)298-4370
caroline.kohlhapp@gmail.com

Kohli, Jatinder, MD {1518224567} Nephro<NJ-NWRKBETH>
+ Newark Beth Israel Medical Center
201 Lyons Avenue   Newark, NJ 07112   (973)926-7000

Kohli, Manpreet K., MD {1205097581} SrgOnc
+ 1501 Ocean Avenue/Suite 1309
Asbury Park, NJ 07712

Kohlitz, Patrick, MD {1962720482} IntHos<NY-UPSTSYRA>
+ Inspira Health Network
509 North Broad Street   Woodbury, NJ 08096   (856)845-0100

Kohn, Gary Lawrence, MD {1710954409} PedPul, PedCrC, Pedtrc(94,IL42)<NJ-MORRISTN, NJ-OVERLOOK>
  + Pulmonary & Allergy Associates
    8 Saddle Road/Suite 101   Cedar Knolls, NJ 07927
    (973)267-9393   Fax (973)540-0472
  + Pulmonary & Allergy Associates
    1 Springfield Avenue/Suite 3-A   Summit, NJ 07901
    (973)267-9393   Fax (908)934-0556

Kohn, Jocelyn Cramer, MD {1083682181} Pedtrc(96,IL06)<NJ-MORRISTN>
  + Basking Ridge Pediatric Association
    150 North Finley Avenue   Basking Ridge, NJ 07920
    (908)766-4660   Fax (908)204-9871

Kohut, Adrian, MD {1629578257} ObsGyn
  + UMDNJ OBGYN
    125 Paterson Street/Suite 4200   New Brunswick, NJ 08901
    (609)922-0729   Fax (732)235-6650

Kokkola-Korpela, Marjut Hellen, MD {1316387376} InfDis, IntrMd(94,FIN05)
  + Infectious Disease Center of New Jersey
    22 Old Short Hills Road/Suite 106   Livingston, NJ 07039
    (973)535-8355   Fax (973)535-8353

Kolaczynski, Jerzy Wiktor, MD {1376615625} EnDbMt
  + UH- Robert Wood Johnson Med
    125 Paterson Street/CAB/Suite 510   New Brunswick, NJ 08901   (732)828-3000

Kolakowski, Stephen, Jr., MD {1003971102} Surgry
  + Vascular Access Centers
    10 Industrial Way East   Eatontown, NJ 07724   (732)380-0730   Fax (732)380-0735

Kolander, Scott A., MD {1942242748} IntrMd, Grtrcs(82,PA09)<NJ-CHSMRCER>
  + Capital Health Primary Care - Mountainview
    850 Bear Tavern Road/Suite 309   Ewing, NJ 08628
    (609)656-8844   Fax (609)656-8845
  + West Trenton Medical Associates
    1230 Parkway Avenue/Suite 203   Trenton, NJ 08638
    (609)656-8844   Fax (609)883-2565

Kolansky, Glenn, MD {1740351683} Dermat(89,NY08)<NJ-RIVERVW>
  + 4 Hartford Drive
    Tinton Falls, NJ 07701   (732)933-8500   Fax (732)933-4177

Kolarov, Sanja, MD {1215106778} IntrMd(97,YUG13)<NJ-MORRISTN>
  + Morristown Medical Center
    100 Madison Avenue   Morristown, NJ 07962   (973)971-5000
    sanjakolarov@yahoo.com
  + Internal Medicine Consultants
    765 State Route 10 East/Suite 201   Randolph, NJ 07869
    (973)971-5000   Fax (732)271-1022

Kolasa, Christopher, MD {1073680062} IntrMd, Nephro(83,POL09)<NJ-RWJUBRUN, NJ-STPETER>
  + 6 Auer Court/Suite C
    East Brunswick, NJ 08816   (732)254-4200   Fax (732)254-4256

Kolber, Ronald B., MD {1962484410} RadDia(71,NY09)<NJ-RBAYOLDB, NJ-STPETER>
  + University Radiology Group, P.C.
    260 Amboy Avenue   Metuchen, NJ 08840   (732)548-2322
    Fax (732)548-3392
  + University Radiology Group, P.C.
    483 Cranbury Road   East Brunswick, NJ 08816   (732)548-2322   Fax (732)390-5383

Kole, Alison S., MD {1770704116} IntrMd, SlpDis(MA07
  + Summit Medical Group
    1 Diamond Hill Road/Bensley Pav/2 FL   Berkeley, NJ 07922
    (908)277-8674   Fax (908)288-7993
  + Summit Medical Group
    140 Park Avenue/3rd Floor   Florham Park, NJ 07932
    (973)404-9930

Kole, Thomas Pedicino, MD {1598064545} RadOnc, Radiol<NY-WINTHROP>
  + Valley Radiation Oncology Associates
    One Valley Health Plaza   Paramus, NJ 07652   (201)634-5403

Kolesk, Stephen J., MD {1972570802} FamMed, Grtrcs(78,CT02)
  + Virtua Family Medicine Center @Lumberton
    1636 Route 38 & Eayrestown Rd.   Lumberton, NJ 08048
    (609)914-8440   Fax (609)914-8441

Koliopoulos, John S., DO {1053353516} GenPrc, EmrgMd(92,IA75)<NJ-OVERLOOK>
  + Overlook Medical Center
    99 Beauvoir Avenue/PO Box 210/EmrgMed   Summit, NJ 07902   (908)522-2000   Fax (908)522-0227

Kolipakam, Vani S., MD {1871524264} Psychy, PsyCAd(91,INA48)<NJ-BAYSHORE>
  + Ocean Mental Health Services, Inc.
    160 Atlantic City Boulevard   Bayville, NJ 08721   (732)349-1977   Fax (732)349-5553

Koliver, Maria Gabriela Riera, MD {1043276827} IntrMd(89,BRA06)<NJ-MTNSIDE>
  + NJ Heart/Newark Office
    635 Market Street   Newark, NJ 07105   (973)344-5454
    Fax (973)344-5488

Kolla, Sairamachandra Rao, MD {1174503205} PhysMd(97,INA75)<NY-STJOHNSS>
  + 2757 Kennedy Boulevard/First Floor
    Jersey City, NJ 07306   (201)333-8004   Fax (201)333-8425

Kollar, John C., DO {1841227352} Surgry(87,NJ75)<NJ-VALLEY>
  + Saddle Brook Medical Center
    449 Market Street/Suite B   Saddle Brook, NJ 07663
    (201)712-7900   Fax (201)712-7902

Kolli, Sireesha K., MD {1194929372} Psychy<PA-WPSYCH>
  + 25 Birch Drive
    Freehold, NJ 07728

Kolli, Sudha Rani, MD {1174623508} IntrMd, Grtrcs(91,INDI)<NJ-SOMERSET, NJ-STPETER>
  + RWJPE Sudha Kolli
    262 Livingston Avenue   New Brunswick, NJ 08901
    (732)249-2044   Fax (732)790-2626

Kollimuttathuillam, Sudarsan, MD {1902324528} IntrMd
  + St. Michael's Medical Center
    111 Central Avenue   Newark, NJ 07102   (973)877-5000

Kollmeier, Brett R., MD {1295722601} Anesth(00,DMN01)<NJ-CHSFULD, NJ-CHSMRCER>
  + Trenton Anesthesiology Associates, PA
    One Capital Way/Second Floor   Pennington, NJ 08534
    (609)396-4700   Fax (609)396-4900

Kollmer, W. Lance, MD SrgFPI(77,MN08)
  + 38 Hampshire Drive
    Mendham, NJ 07945

Kolman-Taddeo, Diana, MD {1982866646} IntrMd
  + Capital Health Primary Care - Mountainview
    850 Bear Tavern Road/Suite 309   Ewing, NJ 08628
    (609)815-7390   Fax (609)815-7391

Kolnik, John P., DO {1902894496} Gastrn, IntrMd(92,PA77)<NJ-OURLADY, NJ-VIRTUAHS>
  + Allied Gastroenterology Associates
    217 White Horse Pike   Haddon Heights, NJ 08035
    (856)547-1212   Fax (856)547-6117

Kolon, Thomas Francis, MD {1558445957} Surgry, Urolgy(89,DC02)<PA-CHILDHOS>
  + CHOP Pediatric & Adolescent Specialty Care Center
    707 Alexander Road/Suite 205   Princeton, NJ 08540
    (609)520-1717
  + CHOP Pediatric & Adolescent Specialty Care Center
    4009 Black Horse Pike   Mays Landing, NJ 08330   (609)520-1717   Fax (609)677-7835

Kolpan, Brett Heath, MD {1598739757} FamMed(98,NJ06)
  + Charlestown Medical Associates
    140 Boulevard   Washington, NJ 07882   (908)689-3200
    Fax (908)689-8295

Kolsky, Neil H., MD {1164424032} Pedtrc(66,NJ15)<NJ-HOLYNAME, NJ-HACKNSK>
  + Pedimedica PA
    870 Palisade Avenue/Suite 201   Teaneck, NJ 07666
    (201)692-1661   Fax (201)692-9219

Komansky, Henry J., DO {1508049578} PulDis, CritCr, IntrMd(73,PA77)<NJ-BURDTMLN>
  + 17 Court House South Dennis Ro
    Cape May Court House, NJ 08210   (609)465-7662   Fax (609)465-9365

Komati, Naga Malleswari, MD {1902014525} Nephro, IntrMd(00,INA48)<NJ-STBARNMC, NJ-CLARMAAS>
  + 767 Northfield Avenue
    West Orange, NJ 07052   (973)419-0417   Fax (862)766-5904
  + St. Barnabas Medical Center
    94 Old Short Hills Road/Nephrology   Livingston, NJ 07039
    (973)322-5000
  + Modern Nephrology & Transplant, LLC
    767 Northfield Avenue   West Orange, NJ 07052   (973)992-9022   Fax (973)992-9024

Komboz, Rita Fares, MD {1275508541} IntrMd, Rheuma(91,LEBA)<NJ-CLARMAAS>
  + Arthritis & Osteoporosis Associates, P.A.
    4247 US Highway 9/Building 1   Freehold, NJ 07728
    (732)780-7650   Fax (732)780-8817
  + Arthritis and Osteoporosis Associates
    5 Franklin Avenue/Suite 403   Belleville, NJ 07109
    (973)844-0049

Komer, Claudia A., DO {1922005669} Anesth, CritCr, IntrMd(84,NY75)<NJ-STMICHL>
  + St. Michael's Medical Center
    111 Central Avenue   Newark, NJ 07102   (973)877-5034
    Fax (973)877-5231

Kominos, Vivian A., MD {1780688192} CdvDis, IntrMd(84,MO34)<NJ-CENTRAST>
  + Heart Specialists/Central Jersey
    901 West Main Street/Suite 205   Freehold, NJ 07728
    (732)866-0800   Fax (732)463-6082

Kommireddi, Sowmini, MD {1518064260} Pedtrc(96,INA47)<NJ-RIVERVW>
  + Millennium Pediatric Care, PA
    1 Riverview Medical Center   Red Bank, NJ 07701
    (732)450-2801   Fax (732)450-2802

Komorowski, Thomas W., MD {1154382224} CdvDis, IntrMd, IntCrd(93,POL03)<NJ-OCEANMC, NJ-JRSYSHMC>
  + Ocean Heart Group
    1530 Route 88/Suite A   Brick, NJ 08724   (732)840-0600
    Fax (732)840-0611
  + Cardiology Associates of Ocean County PA
    495 Jack Martin Boulevard/Suite 2   Brick, NJ 08724
    (732)840-0600   Fax (732)458-0874

Komotar, Ana M., MD {1114976230} Nrolgy(69,URUG)
  + 10 Huron Avenue/Suite 1P
    Jersey City, NJ 07306   (201)963-8203   Fax (201)963-9155

Konakondla, Krishna, MD {1457761223} FamMSptM
  + Performance Spine & Sports Medicine
    9500 K Johnson Boulevard/Suite 1   Bordentown, NJ 08505
    (609)817-0050   Fax (609)588-8602

Konchak, Peter Stephen, DO {1669452025} MtFtMd, ObsGyn(80,IA75)<NJ-KMHSTRAT, NJ-JFKMED>
  + University Doctors-Ob Gyn
    42 East Laurel Road/Suite 3500   Stratford, NJ 08084
    (856)566-7090   Fax (856)566-6026
  + Kennedy Memorial Hospital-University Medical Center
    18 East Laurel Road/Perinatology   Stratford, NJ 08084
    (856)566-7090   Fax (856)346-6003

Konda, Kalpana Reddy, MD {1770646267} Pedtrc(72,INDI)<NJ-RBAYPERT>
  + Raritan Bay Medical Center/Perth Amboy Division
    530 New Brunswick Avenue   Perth Amboy, NJ 08861
    (732)442-3700   Fax (732)324-3320

Kondamudi, Noah Praveen Kaur, MD {1114958451} Pedtrc, PedEmg(80,INA5B)<NY-BRKLNDWN, NJ-UMDNJ>
  + University Hospital
    150 Bergen Street/PediEmrgMed   Newark, NJ 07103
    (973)972-4300

Kondapaneni, Srikant, MD {1447273867} PulDis, IntrMd, CritCr(99,MI07)<NJ-ENGLWOOD, NJ-HOLYNAME>
  + Bergen Medical Alliance, P.A.
    180 Engle Street   Englewood, NJ 07631   (201)567-2050
    Fax (201)568-8936
    srikant.kondapaneni@bergenmedical.com
  + Englewood Hospital and Medical Center
    350 Engle Street   Englewood, NJ 07631   (201)894-3000
  + Holy Name Hospital
    718 Teaneck Road   Teaneck, NJ 07631   (201)833-3000

Kondoleon, Mary Therese, MD {1083643597} ObsGyn(93,NJ05)<NJ-HACKNSK>
  + Hackensack University Medical Center
    30 Prospect Avenue/OB/GYN   Hackensack, NJ 07601
    (201)996-2000

Kondrashin, Sofia, MD {1750460754} PsyCAd(89,RUS06)
  + 103 River Road
    Edgewater, NJ 07020   (201)945-6633

Koneru, Baburao, MD {1588694558} Surgry, SrgTpl(72,INDI)<NJ-UMDNJ>
  + Liver Transplant & Hepatobiliary Diseases/UMDNJ
    140 Bergen Street/ACC Bldg   Newark, NJ 07101   (973)972-7218

Koneru, Jayanth, MD {1962736801} IntrMd
  + 46 Mollet Pitcher Drive
    Manalapan, NJ 07726

Kong, Henry Woongjae, MD {1629057971} IntrMd(95,NJ06)
  + 730 Jamaica Boulevard
    Toms River, NJ 08757   (732)341-4400   Fax (732)341-4450

Kong, Ji Yong, MD {1235450693} Pedtrc
  + Princeton Nassau Pediatrics, P.A.
    301 North Harrison Street   Princeton, NJ 08540   (609)924-5510   Fax (609)924-3577

Kong, Yekyung, MD {1134117419} PhysMd(90,NY09)<NJ-KSLRWEST>
  + Kessler Institute for Rehabilitation West Orange
    1199 Pleasant Valley Way   West Orange, NJ 07052
    (973)731-3600

Kong, Young D., MD {1770672412} IntrMd(70,KOR01)<NJ-JRSYSHMC>
  + 97 Central Avenue
    Ocean Grove, NJ 07756   (732)774-4418

Koniaris, Lauren Solanko, MD {1568424570} PulDis, CritCr(94,MA01)<NJ-HACKNSK>
  + University Respiratory Medicine, P.A.
    75 Summit Avenue   Hackensack, NJ 07601   (201)487-4595

Koniaris, Soula G., MD {1942380779} Pedtrc, PedGst(88,TN06)
  + UH- RWJ Medical School
    One Robert Wood Johnson Place   New Brunswick, NJ 08903
    (732)235-7885   Fax (732)235-7077

Physicians by Name and Address

Koniges, Frank C., MD {1417037482} SrgBst, Surgry(81,TX12)<NJ-COOPRUMC>
+ Cooper Surgical Associates
3 Cooper Plaza/Suite 411   Camden, NJ 08103   (856)342-2270   Fax (856)365-1180
+ Cooper Surgical Associates
110 Marter Avenue/Suite 402   Moorestown, NJ 08057   (856)342-2270   Fax (856)866-9846

Konigsberg, David, DO {1114178142} FamMed
+ Ocean County Family Care
2125 Route 88 East   Brick, NJ 08724   (732)892-4548   Fax (732)892-0961

Konigsberg, David Eric, MD {1578614723} SrgOrt, PedOrt(94,NJ06)<NJ-HACKNSK, NJ-VALLEY>
+ Konigsberg Pediatric Orthopaedics, P.A.
600 Godwin Avenue/Suite 4   Midland Park, NJ 07432   (201)445-9000   Fax (201)445-7400

Koniuta, Robert L., MD {1346225448} Anesth(85,TX13)<NJ-HOLY-NAME>
+ Holy Name Hospital
718 Teaneck Road/PedAne   Teaneck, NJ 07666   (201)833-3000   Fax (201)831-9856

Konkesa, Anuradha R., MD {1013908268} IntrMd(98,INA39)
+ New Bridge Medical Center
230 East Ridgewood Avenue   Paramus, NJ 07652   (201)967-4000
+ North Jersey Health PA
502 Hamburg Turnpike/Suite 108   Wayne, NJ 07470   (201)967-4000   Fax (973)942-7443
+ Rutgers- New Jersey Medical School
185 South Orange Avenue   Newark, NJ 07652   (973)772-4100

Konlian, Donna Marie, MD {1144308115} CdvDis, IntrMd(89,PA02)<NJ-CHILTON>
+ Cardiology Consultants
246 Hamburg Turnpike/Suite 201   Wayne, NJ 07470   (973)942-1141   Fax (973)942-1250
+ Clifton Urgent and Primary Care
721 Clifton Avenue/Suite 2A   Clifton, NJ 07013   (973)942-1141   Fax (973)779-7906

Konnick, Patrina A., MD {1942239843} Pedtrc(82,DOMI)<NJ-CHS-FULD, NJ-CHSMRCER>
+ Medical Pediatrics Associates
256 Bunn Drive/Suite 3 A   Princeton, NJ 08540   Fax (609)683-7958

Koo, Bon Chang Andy, MD {1396960043} IntrMd, Gastrn(00,NY19)<NY-BLVUENYU>
+ Bergen Medical Associates
466 Old Hook Road/Suite 1   Emerson, NJ 07630   (201)967-8221   Fax (201)967-0340

Koo, Charles H., MD {1396782595} CdvDis, ClCdEl, IntrMd(95,NY48)<NJ-OURLADY, NJ-CENTRAST>
+ Monmouth Cardiology Associates, LLC
11 Meridian Road   Eatontown, NJ 07724   (732)663-0300   Fax (732)663-0301
+ Monmouth Cardiology Associates, LLC
222 Schanck Road/Suite 104   Freehold, NJ 07728   (732)663-0300   Fax (732)431-1712

Koo, Harry P., MD {1114005568} Surgry
+ HUMC Faculty Practice
360 Essex Street/Suite 403   Hackensack, NJ 07601   (201)336-8090   Fax (201)336-8222

Koo, Jennifer S., MD {1730331059} RadDia
+ 20 Franklin Turnpike
Waldwick, NJ 07463

Koorie, Elizabeth L., MD {1619137767} FamMed(05,NJ06)<NJ-HUNTRDN>
+ Phillips Barber Family Health Center
72 Alexander Avenue   Lambertville, NJ 08530   (609)397-3535   Fax (609)397-0301

Koota, David H., MD {1548367006} Surgry(91,NY45)
+ Genito-Urinary Surgeons of New Jersey
211 Courtyard Drive   Hillsborough, NJ 08844   (908)685-0080   Fax (908)685-7594
+ Genito-Urinary Surgeons of New Jersey
579-A Cranbury Road/Suite 109   East Brunswick, NJ 08816   (908)685-0080   Fax (732)390-8555

Kopacz, Kenneth J., MD {1205944709} SrgOrt, SrgSpn(88,PA01)<NJ-STBARNMC, NJ-CLARMAAS>
+ Spine Care and Rehabilitation
200 South Orange Ave./Suite 180   Livingston, NJ 07039   (973)226-2725   Fax (973)226-3270
+ Spine Care and Rehabilitation
36 Newark Avenue/Suite 220   Belleville, NJ 07109   (973)226-2725   Fax (973)226-3270
+ St. Barnabas Ambulatory Care Center
200 South Orange Avenue   Livingston, NJ 07039   (973)226-2725   Fax (973)226-3270

Kopacz, Magdaline S., MD {1558543876} Pedtrc(99,POL02)<NJ-HACKNSK>
+ Hackensack Univ Medical Center Pediatric Emerg Room
30 Prospect Avenue   Hackensack, NJ 07601   (201)996-5430   Fax (201)996-3676
+ Hackensack University Medical Center
30 Prospect Avenue/PedsEmergency   Hackensack, NJ 07601   (201)996-5430   Fax (201)996-5435

Kopec, Anna V., MD {1477644599} Dermat, OthrSp(75,NJ05)
+ 730 Kennedy Boulevard
Bayonne, NJ 07002   (201)858-4300   Fax (201)339-0708   jeter4ever_101@yahoo.com

Kopelan, Adam Michael, MD {1679573307} Surgry(96,NY19)<NJ-NWRKBETH, NJ-STBARNMC>
+ Millburn Surgical Associates
225 Millburn Avenue/Suite 104-B   Millburn, NJ 07041   (973)379-5888   Fax (973)912-9757

Kopelan, Leah Michelle, MD {1417915422} IntrMd, IntHos(97,IL11)<NJ-NWRKBETH>
+ IPC The Hospitalist Company
55 Madison Avenue/Suite 310   Morristown, NJ 07960   (973)993-9536   Fax (973)998-4237

Kopelman, Joel E., MD {1427053537} Ophthl, SrgPlstc(77,NJ05)<NJ-VALLEY, NJ-HACKNSK>
+ 1200 East Ridgewood Avenue
Ridgewood, NJ 07450   (201)444-4499   Fax (201)612-8114

Kopelman, Rima G., MD {1023074754} Rheuma, IntrMd(77,NY01)<NJ-VALLEY>
+ Prospect Medical Offices, LLC
301 Godwin Avenue   Midland Park, NJ 07432   (201)444-4526   Fax (201)301-1313

Kopeloff, Iris H., MD {1518934058} Dermat, IntrMd(89,NY47)<NJ-VALLEY, NY-NYUTISCH>
+ The Dorothy B. Kraft Center
15 Essex Road   Paramus, NJ 07652   (201)291-6000   kopeir@valleyhealth.com
+ Daniel and Gloria Blumenthal Cancer Center
One Valley Health Plaza   Paramus, NJ 07652   (201)634-5339
+ The Valley Hospital
223 North Van Dien Avenue   Ridgewood, NJ 07652   (201)447-8000

Koplik, Andrew D., MD {1346462165} Anesth(05,NJ06)
+ Synergy Anesthesia
485 Speedwell Avenue/PO Box 305   Morris Plains, NJ 07950   (973)200-8224   Fax (973)695-1324   koplikan@yahoo.com

Kopolovich, Harry, MD {1144351156} EmrgMd(06,NY08)<NY-JA-COBIMC>
+ Emergency Medical Associates of NJ, P.A.
3 Century Drive   Parsippany, NJ 07054   (973)740-0607   Fax (973)740-9895

Kopp, Lizabeth A., MD {1205804358} ObsGyn(86,VA01)<NJ-HACKNSK>
+ Obstetrics and Gynecology PA
20 Prospect Avenue/Suite 607   Hackensack, NJ 07601   (201)487-3464   Fax (201)487-0232

Kopp Mulberg, F. Elyse, DO {1699077909} FamMed(89,NY75)
+ Family and Community Medicine
1050 North Kings Highway/Suite 105   Cherry Hill, NJ 08034   (856)321-0303
+ Cooper Family Medicine
3 Cooper Plaza/Suite 502   Cherry Hill, NJ 08003   (856)963-0126

Koppel, Alexander Joshua, MD {1649446006} CdvDis<PA-TJC-NTR>
+ Mercer Bucks Cardiology
3140 Princeton Pike/2nd Floor   Lawrenceville, NJ 08648   (609)895-1919   Fax (609)895-1200

Koppel, Todd Sloan, MD {1932109170} Anesth, PainMd, Anes-Pain(92,NY20)<NY-NYACKHOS>
+ Garden State Pain Control Center, P.A.
1117 Route 46 East/Suite 201   Clifton, NJ 07013   (973)777-5444   Fax (973)777-0304

Kor, Danuta C., MD {1518965599} Anesth(82,POL08)<NJ-VIRT-MARL>
+ Rancocas Anesthesiology, PA
700 Route 130 North/Suite 203   Cinnaminson, NJ 08077   (856)829-9345   Fax (856)829-3605

Koranyi, Peter, MD {1255312708} Anesth(95,NY01)<NJ-MOR-RISTN>
+ Morristown Medical Center
100 Madison Avenue/Anesthesiology   Morristown, NJ 07962   (973)971-5548   Fax (201)943-8733

Korban, Anna, MD {1003158718} Anesth
+ Rutgers- New Jersey Medical School
185 South Orange Avenue/MSB F-611   Newark, NJ 07103   (973)972-5007   Fax (973)972-0582

Kordula, Charles E., MD {1578999116} Surgry(76,FRA04)
+ 9 Elm Place
Woodcliff Lake, NJ 07677

Korenblit, Pearl, MD {1043248131} IntrMd, GPrvMd, PubHth(79,ON01)<NJ-HACKNSK, NJ-STMRYPAS>
+ 1011 Clifton Avenue/First Floor
Clifton, NJ 07013   (973)928-5490   Fax (973)928-5493

Korenfeld, Alexander, MD {1063428803} IntrMd(77,RUSS)<NJ-MEADWLND>
+ Renaissance General Medicine
596 Anderson Avenue/Suite 302   Cliffside Park, NJ 07010   (201)943-2700   Fax (201)943-2646

Korenfeld, Yelena, MD {1720094576} IntrMd(77,RUSS)
+ Renaissance General Medicine
596 Anderson Avenue/Suite 302   Cliffside Park, NJ 07010   (201)943-2700   Fax (201)943-2646

Koretzky, Jeffrey Robert, MD {1942271283} IntrMd(93,NJ05)<NJ-KIMBALL>
+ Community Health Associates
4618 Route 9 South   Howell, NJ 07731   (732)364-5533   Fax (732)367-1325

Korkis, Anna Maria, MD {1912014887} Gastrn, IntrMd(86,VA04)<NJ-VALLEY>
+ 206 Dayton Street
Ridgewood, NJ 07450   (201)444-0009   Fax (201)444-2181
+ 200 South Broad Street
Ridgewood, NJ 07450

Korkmazsky, Yelena N., MD {1306801733} Pedtrc(84,RUS11)<NJ-STBARNMC, NJ-OVERLOOK>
+ Springfield Pediatrics
190 Meisel Avenue   Springfield, NJ 07081   (973)467-1009   Fax (973)467-7836
+ Springfield Pediatrics
939 Park Avenue   Plainfield, NJ 07060   (973)467-1009   Fax (908)226-5481

Korman, Andrew Stephen, MD {1780833343} Gastrn(08,ISR02)
+ St. Peter's University Hospital
254 Easton Avenue   New Brunswick, NJ 08901   (732)565-5471

Korman, Linda Z., MD {1437290079} IntrMd, Bariat, GPrvMd(82,NY08)<NJ-RWJUBRUN>
+ RWJ University Hospital New Brunswick
One Robert Wood Johnson Place   New Brunswick, NJ 08901   (732)828-3000

Korn, Barry Allen, DO {1790714293} PainMd, FamMed(91,PA77)<NJ-KMHSTRAT>
+ Neurology Associates & Ctr Pain
1030 North Kings Highway/Suite 200A   Cherry Hill, NJ 08034   (856)779-7774   Fax (856)779-7787

Korn, Elizabeth Amy, MD {1588869952} Pedtrc, PedEnd(85,PA01)<NJ-STPETER, NJ-UMDNJ>
+ St. Peter's University Hospital
254 Easton Avenue/MOB 3rd FL   New Brunswick, NJ 08901   (732)745-8574   Fax (732)514-1956   kornel@umdnj.edu
+ University Hospital- Department of Pediatrics
90 Bergen Street/DOC 5100   Newark, NJ 07101   (732)745-8574   Fax (732)514-7356

Kornberg, Steven Edward, MD {1427089069} CdvDis, IntrMd(80,NJ05)<NJ-SHOREMEM>
+ Shore Memorial Hospital
1 East New York Avenue/Cardiology   Somers Point, NJ 08244   (609)653-3500
+ Penn Medicine Somers Point
155 Brighton Avenue/Second Floor   Somers Point, NJ 08244   (609)653-3500   Fax (609)926-8096

Kornfeld, Howard Neil, MD {1770539181} Pedtrc(95,BWI01)<NJ-OVERLOOK, NJ-MORRISTN>
+ Summit Medical Group-Berkeley Heights Campus
1 Diamond Hill Road   Berkeley Heights, NJ 07922   (908)273-4300   Fax (908)277-8706

Kornicki, Janusz S., MD {1013914035} IntrMd(81,POL03)
+ 67 Walnut Avenue/Suite 402
Clark, NJ 07066   (908)276-6644   Fax (908)276-3862

Kornitzer, Jeffrey Michael, MD {1932499266}
+ University Behavioral HealthCare
183 South Orange Avenue/Room F-603   Newark, NJ 07103   (973)972-6015   Fax (973)972-1019
+ Rutgers NJ School of Medicine Neurology
90 Bergen Street/DOC 5200   Newark, NJ 07103   (973)972-6015   Fax (973)972-5059

Kornmehl, Carol, MD {1164467924} RadOnc(84,NY08)<NJ-TRINI-JSC>
+ Cancer Treatment Center
2090 Springdale Road/Suite B   Cherry Hill, NJ 08003   (856)751-9010   Fax (856)985-9908

Kornweiss, Steven Alexander, MD {1205179058} EmrgEMed<NJ-SJHREGMC>
+ SJH Regional Medical Center
1505 West Sherman Avenue   Vineland, NJ 08360   (856)686-4319

Korsakoff, Kristopher Paul, MD {1174589246} Gastrn, IntrMd(99,NJ05)<NY-BONSECRS>
+ 521 State Route 515/suite 304
Vernon, NJ 07462   (973)864-6029   Fax (973)864-1010

Korshunova, Valeria S., MD {1407904253} PsyCAd, Psychy(81,RUSS)<NJ-HACKNSK>
+ Psychiatric Associates
218 State Route 17 North/Suite 13 Rochelle Park, NJ 07662 (201)488-6543

Korst, Robert J., MD {1821185901} SrgThr, Surgry, IntrMd(89,CT02)<NJ-VALLEY>
+ VPS Thoracic Surgery
One Valley Health Plaza Paramus, NJ 07652 (201)634-5722 Fax (201)986-4704

Kortebein, Patrick, MD {1568552131} PhysMd
+ Novartis Pharmaceuticals Corporation
One Health Plaza East Hanover, NJ 07936 (862)778-9800 Fax (973)781-6504

Korya, Dani, MD {1235426347} Nrolgy, VasNeu, IntrMd(10,GRN01)
+ Carepoint Health Neurology
142 Palisade Avenue/Suite 200 Jersey City, NJ 07306 (201)795-8596 Fax (201)418-7067
+ Christ Hospital
176 Palisade Avenue Jersey City, NJ 07306 (201)795-8200

Korzeniowski, Philip A., MD {1720050776} ObsGyn(91,CA14)<NJ-ACMCMAIN, NJ-ACMCITY>
+ Somers Manor Obstetrics and Gynecology
599 Shore Road/Suite 101 Somers Point, NJ 08244 (609)926-8353 Fax (609)926-4579

Kos, Cynthia A., DO {1952716805}<NJ-DEBRAHLC>
+ Deborah Heart and Lung Center
200 Trenton Road Browns Mills, NJ 08015 (609)893-6611 Fax (609)893-6038

Kos, Luke Bronislaw, MD {1134350028} Anesth
+ 24 Nobhill/Unit K
Roseland, NJ 07068 (978)944-6310

Kosarin, Kristi, DO {1114384328} IntrMd
+ Jersey Shore University Medical Center
1945 Route 33 Neptune, NJ 07753 (732)775-5500

Kosc, Gary J., MD {1932105236} Gastrn(80,MEXI)
+ Gastroenterology Associates of New Jersey
205 Browertown Road/Suite 201 Little Falls, NJ 07424 (973)812-8120 Fax (973)812-8144

Koscica, Karen Lynn, DO {1437184389} ObsGyn, MtFtMd(95,NY75)<NJ-RWJUBRUN>
+ Hackensack Meridian Maternal Fetal Medicine
19 Davis Avenue/Hope Tower 7th Floor Neptune, NJ 07753 (732)776-4755 Fax (732)776-4754
+ Newark Beth Israel Medical Center
201 Lyons Avenue Newark, NJ 07112 (732)776-4755 Fax (973)923-7497

Koshenkov, Vadim P., MD {1376785360} SrgOnc
+ Rutgers Cancer Institute of New Jersey
195 Little Albany Street/PO Box 2681 New Brunswick, NJ 08903 (732)235-2465 Fax (732)235-6797

Koshibe, Gen, MD {1609004787} Anesth<NJ-HOLYNAME>
+ Holy Name Hospital
718 Teaneck Road Teaneck, NJ 07666 (201)833-3000

Koshy, Ranie, MD {1558392720} BldBnk(70,INDI)<NJ-UMDNJ>
+ University Hospital
150 Bergen Street/C101 Newark, NJ 07103 (973)972-4300 Fax (973)972-5909

Kosiborod, Roman, DO {1831192079} Anesth(98,NY75)<NJ-COMMED>
+ Bergen Ambulatory Surgery Center
190 Midland Avenue/Anesth Saddle Brook, NJ 07663 (973)405-6888

Kosinski, Mark S., MD {1184661597} Allrgy, PedAlg, IntrMd(72,POL08)<NJ-STJOSHOS>
+ St. Joseph's Regional Medical Center
703 Main Street/Allergy/Immun Paterson, NJ 07503 (973)754-2000
+ 81 Two Bridges Road/Building 2
Fairfield, NJ 07004 (973)754-2000 Fax (973)569-6380

Kosinski, Robert M., MD {1780655068} IntrMd, PulDis, SlpDis(87,OH43)<NJ-MONMOUTH, NJ-JRSYSHMC>
+ Monmouth Pulmonary Consultants
30 Corbett Way Eatontown, NJ 07724 (732)380-0020 Fax (732)380-1990
+ Monmouth Medical Center
300 Second Avenue/SleepDsrdrsCtr Long Branch, NJ 07740 (732)222-5200

Koskinen, Jason Alexander, DO {1801970215} FamMed, IntrMd(FL75
+ Cape Regional Urgent Care
11 Court House South Dennis RD Cape May Court House, NJ 08210 (609)465-6364 Fax (609)465-1696

Koskinen, Kjersti, MD {1790774685} FamMed
+ Coast Guard Health Services
1 Munroe Avenue Cape May, NJ 08204 (609)898-6567

Koslowe, Oren Lewis, MD {1023142395} Pedtrc(02,NY46)<NY-PRSBWEIL, NJ-MORRISTN>
+ Morristown Medical Center
100 Madison Avenue Morristown, NJ 07962 (973)971-5000

Kosmetatos, Elizabeth, MD {1386725281} Pedtrc
+ Mainland Pediatric Association
741 South Second Avenue/Suite B Galloway, NJ 08205 (609)748-8500 Fax (609)748-6700

Kososky, Charles S., MD {1245254531} Nrolgy(75,NJ05)
+ 1100 Wescott Drive
Flemington, NJ 08822 (908)788-6452

Kosoy, Edward, MD {1871561571} FamMed(00,DMN01)<NJ-MTNSIDE>
+ Denville Medical & Sports Rehabilitation Center
161 East Main Street Denville, NJ 07834 (973)627-7888 Fax (973)627-7040

Koss, Debra Elvira, MD {1114044997} Psychy, PsyCAd(89,VA01)
+ 46 Main Street/Suite 201
Sparta, NJ 07871 (973)726-4137 Fax (973)726-4138

Koss, James C., MD {1669474052} Radiol(76,NJ05)<NJ-VIRTMHBC>
+ Radiology Associates of Burlington County
1295 Route 38 West/PO Box 479 Hainesport, NJ 08036 (609)261-7017 Fax (609)261-4180

Koss, Stephen Dennis, MD {1265482897} SrgOrt, IntrMd(89,VA01)<NJ-NWTNMEM>
+ The Orthopedic Institute of New Jersey
108 Bilby Road/Suite 201 Hackettstown, NJ 07840 (908)684-3005 Fax (908)684-3301
+ The Orthopedic Institute of New Jersey
254-B Mountain Avenue/Suite 201 Hackettstown, NJ 07840 (908)684-3005 Fax (908)684-3301
+ The Orthopedic Institute of New Jersey
222 High Street/Suite 202 Newton, NJ 07840 (908)684-3005 Fax (908)684-3301

Kossev, Viliana D., MD {1881661510} IntrMd(89,BUL03)
+ Sea Girt Medical Associates
235 Route 71 Manasquan, NJ 08736 (732)223-4300 Fax (732)223-5273

Kossow, Lynne Becker, MD {1659390193} IntrMd(88,PA01)
+ Princeton Lifestyle Medicine
731 Alexander Road/Suite 200 Princeton, NJ 08540 (609)655-3800 Fax (609)655-5203

Kostis, William J., MD {1922203439} IntrMd(07,NJ06)<MA-MAGENHOS>
+ University Physician Associates of New Jersey
125 Paterson Street/CAB 5200 New Brunswick, NJ 08901 (732)235-6561 Fax (732)235-7115

Kostoulakos, Paul M., DO {1982817326} ClNrPh, Nrolgy(02,ME75)<NJ-JRSYSHMC, NJ-OCEANMC>
+ Monmouth Ocean Neurology
1944 State Route 33/Suite 206 Neptune, NJ 07753 (732)774-8282 Fax (732)774-4407
+ Monmouth Ocean Neurology
190 Jack Martin Boulevard/Building B-3 Brick, NJ 08724 (732)774-8282 Fax (732)774-6216
+ Hackensack Meridian Medical Group
53 Nautilus Drive/Suite 201 Manahawkin, NJ 07753 (609)978-8870 Fax (609)978-8903

Kostroma, Boris Vladimirovich, MD {1760550537} PainMd, Anesth(92,RUS06)<NJ-EASTORNG>
+ Essex Ironbund Anesthesiologist LLC
155 Jefferson Street Newark, NJ 07105 (908)490-0036 Fax (908)490-0067

Kota, Karthik, MD {1982022505}
+ UH-RWJ General Internal Medicine
125 Paterson Street/Suite 2300 New Brunswick, NJ 08901 (732)235-7122 Fax (732)235-7144

Kotb, Mohy Eldin A., MD {1871739748} PedCrd, Pedtrc, IntrMd(96,EGY03)
+ Saint Peter's Physician Associates
33-41 Newark Street/Suite 4c Hoboken, NJ 07030 (201)533-0222 Fax (201)533-0223

Kotch, Hannah Rapaport, MD {1780826016} RadDia, Radiol(09,NY46)
+ Imaging Consultants of Essex
94 Old Short Hills Road Livingston, NJ 07039 (973)322-5804 Fax (973)322-5536
+ St. Barnabas Ambulatory Care Center
200 South Orange Avenue/Radiology Livingston, NJ 07039 (973)322-5804

Kotch, Michael J., MD {1194881607} Ophthl(76,MEX14)
+ 1905 North Wood Avenue
Linden, NJ 07036 (908)925-2020 Fax (908)925-3373

Kotecha, Nisha Suresh, MD {1073873956} PulDis
+ Pulmonary & Allergy Associates
1 Springfield Avenue/Suite 3-A Summit, NJ 07901 (908)934-0555 Fax (908)934-0556

Kothapally, Jaya Reddy, MD {1790894954}
+ Cooper University at Willingboro
218C Sunset Road Willingboro, NJ 08046 (609)877-0400 Fax (609)877-3542

Kothari, Anil G., MD {1831181692} CdvDis, IntrMd, IntCrd(72,INDI)<NJ-OURLADY>
+ Associated Cardiovascular Consultants-Lourdes
1 Brace Road/Suite C & F Cherry Hill, NJ 08034 (856)428-4100 Fax (856)428-5748
+ Our Lady of Lourdes Medical Center
1600 Haddon Avenue/Cardiology Camden, NJ 08103 (856)428-4100 Fax (856)580-6350

Kothari, Gautam Himanshu, DO {1821251968} PhysMd, IntrMd(04,NY75)<PA-NZRTH, PA-ARHBUCKS>
+ Mercer-Bucks Orthopaedics PC
3120 Princeton Pike Lawrenceville, NJ 08648 (609)896-0444 Fax (609)896-1055
+ Mercer-Bucks Orthopaedics, P.C.
2501 Kuser Road Hamilton, NJ 08691 (609)896-0444 Fax (609)587-4349

Kothari, Harish B., MD {1003878943} Allrgy(70,INA20)<NJ-JFKMED>
+ 906 Oak Tree Road/Suite N
South Plainfield, NJ 07080 (908)412-6588 Fax (908)412-6558

Kothari, Jay, MD {1700142924} Anesth
+ Anesthesia Associates of Morristown
100 Madison Avenue Morristown, NJ 07960 (973)971-5000

Kothari, Kaumudi H., MD {1215028923} Anesth(71,INA15)
+ 9 Sherman Boulevard
Edison, NJ 08820

Kothari, Kinnari A., MD {1659439644} Psychy(84,INDI)
+ 1 Britton Place/Suite 6
Voorhees, NJ 08043 (856)772-0700 Fax (856)864-0310

Kothari, Megha Mukesh, MD {1215170816} IntrMd(GRN01)
+ 484 Liberty Avenue
Jersey City, NJ 07307 (201)966-9335

Kothari, Nayan K., MD {1881648244} Grtrcs, IntrMd, Rheuma(61,INA68)<NJ-STPETER, NJ-RWJUBRUN>
+ St. Peter's Family Health
123 How Lane New Brunswick, NJ 08901 (732)745-8600 Fax (732)729-0869
+ Saint PeterÆs Physician Associate
59 Veronica Avenue/Suite 203 Somerset, NJ 08873 (732)745-8600 Fax (732)745-1339

Kothari, Neha A., MD {1457370330} RadDia(93,NJ05)<NJ-STBARNMC>
+ St. Barnabas Medical Center
94 Old Short Hills Road Livingston, NJ 07039 (973)322-5000

Kothari, Neil, MD {1639100233} IntrMd(00,NJ05)<NJ-UMDNJ>
+ University Hospital
150 Bergen Street/H-251/IntMed Newark, NJ 07103 (973)972-5672 Fax (973)972-0365

Kothari, Nita H., MD {1598728552} Pedtrc(76,INA65)<NJ-VIRTVOOR, NJ-COOPRUMC>
+ Advocare Merchantville Pediatrics
1600 Chapel Avenue/Suite 100 Cherry Hill, NJ 08002 Fax (856)665-3938

Kothari, Rajesh Suryakant, DO {1659363174} EmrgMd(97,NY75)
+ 27 Bolton Boulevard
Berkeley Heights, NJ 07922

Kothari, Raksha Anil, MD {1992785083} IntrMd(76,INA15)
+ Our Lady of Lourdes Medical Center
1600 Haddon Avenue Camden, NJ 08103 (856)757-3500

Kothari, Sona A., DO {1013148683} IntHos, IntrMd
+ Rowan University-School of Osteopathic Medicine
1 Medical Center Drive Stratford, NJ 08084 (856)566-6096

Kothavale, Avinash Annash, MD {1285672584} CdvDis, IntrMd, CarEch(99,OH06)<NJ-OVERLOOK, NJ-MORRISTN>
+ Summit Medical Group-Berkeley Heights Campus
1 Diamond Hill Road Berkeley Heights, NJ 07922 (908)273-4300 Fax (908)673-7108

Kotla, Revathi, MD {1063506434} Nephro(91,INA5B)<NJ-STBARNMC>
+ 349 Northfield Avenue/Suite 107
Livingston, NJ 07039 (973)758-1650

Kotler, Amy Maxine, MD {1356384234} Pedtrc(97,PA02)<NJ-MORRISTN, NJ-STCLRDOV>
+ A to Z Pediatrics
369 West Blackwell Street Dover, NJ 07801 (973)328-8300 Fax (973)328-8315
doctor@atozpeds.org

Kotler, Lisa A., MD {1700902079} Psychy, PsyCAd(93,CT01)
+ Care PLUS NJ, Inc. - Mid-Bergen Center
610 Valley Health Plaza Paramus, NJ 07652 (201)265-8200 Fax (201)265-0366
lisak@careplusnj.org

Kotler, Mitchell N., MD {1427057785} Urolgy(84,DC01)<NJ-UNDRWD, NJ-OURLADY>
+ Delaware Valley Urology LLC
17 West Red Bank Avenue/Suite 303 Woodbury, NJ 08096 (856)853-0955 Fax (856)985-4583

Physicians by Name and Address

Kotler, Stuart M., MD {1992787626} Radiol, RadDia(66,CT01)<NJ-STPETER, NJ-RBAYPERT>
+ University Radiology Group, P.C.
483 Cranbury Road   East Brunswick, NJ 08816   (732)390-0030   Fax (732)390-5383
+ University Radiology Group, P.C.
260 Amboy Avenue   Metuchen, NJ 08840   (732)390-0030   Fax (732)548-3392

Kotlov, Mikhail, MD {1891840872} IntrMd, Nephro(03,NY46)<NJ-VALLEY, NJ-HACKNSK>
+ Bergen Hypertension & Renal Associates PA
44 Godwin Avenue/Suite 301   Midland Park, NJ 07432   (201)447-0013   Fax (201)447-0438

Kotlyar, Boleslav, MD {1386986669}
+ Vitreous Retina Macula Specialists NJ
306 Main Street/Suite 2   Millburn, NJ 07041   (973)467-2020

Kottahachchi, Wijepala, MD {1275644064} Pedtrc(69,SRIL)<NJ-RBAYOLDB, NJ-RBAYPERT>
+ 468 Amboy Avenue
Perth Amboy, NJ 08861   (732)442-1820   Fax (732)442-2918

Kottler, William F., MD {1275642373} PedPul, Pedtrc(87,DMN01)<NJ-STBARNMC>
+ Children's Asthma and Breathing Center
48 Essex Street   Millburn, NJ 07041   (973)218-0900   Fax (973)218-0909

Kotturi, Shiva Kumar, MD {1013168251} Pedtrc, IntrMd(78,INDI)
+ Northern New Jersey Pain & Rehabilitation Center
37 West Century Road/Suite 111   Paramus, NJ 07652   (201)262-2244   Fax (201)262-2246

Kotturi, Vijendra B., MD {1669679700} IntHos
+ 1900 Frontage Road/Unit 705
Cherry Hill, NJ 08034

Kotwal, Anoop Pramod, MD {1912297896}
+ 142 Tower Boulevard
Piscataway, NJ 08854   (215)720-6081

Kotys, Ola, DO {1861728727} Anesth(03,NY75)
+ 701 Newcomb Road
Ridgewood, NJ 07450

Kou, Jen Lih, MD {1386731354} IntrMd, Grtrcs(94,NJ05)<NJ-ANCPSYCH>
+ Ancora Psychiatric Hospital
301 Spring Garden Road   Hammonton, NJ 08037   (609)561-1700   Fax (609)561-2509

Kou, Victoria Wei-Li, MD {1972541621} EmrgMd(97,DC01)
+ Cardiology Associates of North Jersey
242 West Parkway   Pompton Plains, NJ 07444   (973)831-7455   Fax (973)831-7585

Koul, Mrinal, MD {1114067527} ObsGyn(99,GRN01)
+ 341 Walnut Street
Newark, NJ 07105   (973)589-8800   Fax (908)490-0067

Koulogiannis, Konstantinos Peter, MD {1407042203} IntrMd, CdvDis(04,NJ05)
+ Gagnon Cardiovasular Institute
100 Madison Avenue/Level C   Morristown, NJ 07962   (973)971-5597   Fax (973)290-7145

Kountz, David S., MD {1679645931} IntrMd(85,NY06)<NJ-RWJUBRUN, NJ-STPETER>
+ University Medical Group
125 Paterson Street/Suite 5100   New Brunswick, NJ 08901   (732)235-6968   Fax (732)235-7117
kountzds@umdnj.edu

Koury, Kenneth Louis, MD {1376855643}
+ 625 Washington Street
Hoboken, NJ 07030   (201)788-4929

Koutcher, Gary Lewis, MD {1477622884} EmrgMd(78,NY48)<NJ-STCLRSUS>
+ St. Clare's Hospital-Sussex
20 Walnut Street/EmrgMed   Sussex, NJ 07461   (973)702-2600

Kouvaras, John Nikolaos, DO {1437194081} Anesth(02,ME75)<NJ-NWTNMEM>
+ Newton Medical Center
175 High Street/Anesth   Newton, NJ 07860   (973)383-2121

Kouveliotes, Peter J., MD {1144242686} RadDia(95,PA09)<NJ-CENTRAST>
+ CentraState Medical Center
901 West Main Street/Radiology   Freehold, NJ 07728   (732)431-2000
+ Freehold Radiology Group
901 West Main Street   Freehold, NJ 07728   (732)462-4844

Kouyoumdji, Paul R., MD {1124027172} Pedtrc(91,LEB01)<NJ-MEMSALEM>
+ Salem Medical Group
4 Bypass Road/Suite 101   Salem, NJ 08079   (856)935-3582   Fax (856)935-4382

Kovacs, Daniel Douglas, MD {1649590217}
+ 41 Anderson Hill Road
Bernardsville, NJ 07924   (973)723-0309
ddkovacs@gmail.com

Kovacs, Gabor, MD {1003955113} SrgVas, Surgry(87,BEL06)<NJ-CENTRAST>
+ Central Jersey Surgical Associates
495 Iron Bridge Road/Suite 3   Freehold, NJ 07728   (732)845-0222   Fax (732)845-1002

Kovacs, James E., DO {1447335039} RadDia, FamMed, RadBdI(85,MO78)<NJ-COOPRUMC>
+ Cooper University Hospital
One Cooper Plaza   Camden, NJ 08103   (856)342-2000
+ The Cooper Health System at Voorhees
900 Centennial Boulevard/Suite E   Voorhees, NJ 08043   (856)325-6500

Kovacs, Jeffrey Peter, DO {1578569265} SrgOrt, SprtMd, IntrMd(84,ME75)
+ Reconstructive Orthopedics, P.A.
570 Egg Harbor Road/Suite C-4   Sewell, NJ 08080   (609)267-9400   Fax (609)267-9457

Kovacs, Lauren R., MD {1598062259}
+ Partners for Women's Health PA
95 Northfield Avenue   West Orange, NJ 07052   (973)736-4505   Fax (973)376-9066

Kovacs, Tiberiu, MD {1780684506} CdvDis, IntrMd, CarNuc(75,ROMA)<NJ-JFKMED, NJ-RWJUBRUN>
+ RWJPE Heart Specialists of Edison
4 Ethel Road/Suite 406-B   Edison, NJ 08817   (732)287-6622   Fax (732)287-2233

Kovaleva, Alexandra, MD {1487063855} Grtrcs
+ Drs. James and Kovaleva
125 Chubb Avenue/Suite 100-S   Lyndhurst, NJ 07071   (201)559-7600   Fax (201)559-7601

Kovalsky, David Joseph, DO {1164782694} IntrMd<NJ-KMH-TURNV>
+ Kennedy Health Systems/Washington Township Campus
435 Hurffville-Cross Keys Road   Turnersville, NJ 08012   (856)218-5634   Fax (856)218-5664

Kovatis, Paul Evan, MD {1669475083} SrgOrt, SrgFak(89,NJ05)<NJ-HACKNSK>
+ Orthopedic Spine and Sports Medicine Center
2 Forest Avenue   Paramus, NJ 07652   (201)587-1111   Fax (201)587-8192

Koven, Marshall B., MD {1538196308} Radiol, RadDia(86,NY15)<NJ-OCEANMC>
+ Atlantic Medical Imaging
455 Jack Martin Boulevard   Brick, NJ 08724   (732)223-9729   Fax (732)840-6459

Kovtun, Marina, MD {1801804034} IntrMd(91,UKR10)<NJ-VA-LYONS>
+ VA New Jersey Health Care System at Lyons
151 Knollcroft Road/IntMed   Lyons, NJ 07939   (908)647-0180   Fax (908)607-6367

Kowal, Noel, MD {1528493574}
+ University Hospital Pathology
150 Bergen Street   Newark, NJ 07103   (973)972-5722

Kowal, Timothy S., MD {1760626048} IntrMd
+ 321 Summit Avenue
Hackensack, NJ 07601   (201)343-2437   Fax (201)343-3917

Kowalczyk, Matthew A., MD {1972548931} Pedtrc, AdolMd(88,NJ06)
+ Westfield Pediatrics, P.A.
532 East Broad Street   Westfield, NJ 07090   (908)232-3445   Fax (908)233-6184

Kowalec, Joan K., MD {1497703474} IntrMd, Rheuma(74,NJ05)<NJ-NWRKBETH>
+ Newark Beth Israel Medical Center
201 Lyons Avenue   Newark, NJ 07112   (973)926-7000

Kowalenko, Karen F., DO {1043288582} FamMed(89,NJ75)
+ 808 Raritan Road
Clark, NJ 07066   (732)381-2100

Kowalenko, Thomas Alex, DO {1538136429} FamMed(96,PA77)
+ 808 Raritan Road
Clark, NJ 07066   (732)381-2100   Fax (732)382-3576

Kowalik, Sharon, MD {1639230915} PsycAd, Psychy(89,NJ05)
+ CPC Behavioral HealthCare
270 Highway 35   Red Bank, NJ 07701   (732)842-2000   Fax (732)224-0688

Kowalski, Albert A., MD {1992978514} IntrMd, OccpMd(79,MEXI)
+ Prudential Financial
290 West Mount Pleasant Avenue   Livingston, NJ 07039   (973)992-6363

Koward, Donna Marie, MD {1386622256} Pedtrc(96,NJ05)<NJ-STBARNMC, NJ-OVERLOOK>
+ Watchung Pediatrics
346 South Avenue/Suite 3   Fanwood, NJ 07023   (908)889-8687   Fax (908)889-0047
+ Watchung Pediatrics
76 Stirling Road/Suite 201   Warren, NJ 07059   (908)889-8687   Fax (908)755-6905
+ Watchung Pediatrics
225 Millburn Avenue/Suite 301   Millburn, NJ 07023   (973)376-7337   Fax (973)218-6647

Kowzun, Maria Ji, MD {1619138765} Surgry
+ 195 Little Albany Street
New Brunswick, NJ 08901   (732)235-8524   Fax (732)235-8099

Kozak, Margaret Zsuzsa, DO {1891781720} FamMed(96,ME75)<NJ-NWTNMEM>
+ Premier Health Associates
225 Route 23 South   Hamburg, NJ 07419   (973)209-1550   Fax (973)729-6487
+ Premier Health Associates
89 Sparta Avenue/Suite 100   Sparta, NJ 07871   (973)209-1550   Fax (973)729-3454

Kozakowski, Edward, Jr., MD {1902852064} IntrMd(75,PA13)<NJ-ACMCMAIN, NJ-ACMCITY>
+ Seashore Medical Associates
48 Ansley Boulevard   Pleasantville, NJ 08232   (609)641-1077   Fax (609)641-1023

Kozakowski, Stanley M., MD {1255305231} FamMed, Grtrcs(81,NY09)<NJ-HUNTRDN>
+ Delaware Valley Family Health Center
200 Frenchtown Road   Milford, NJ 08848   (908)995-2251   Fax (908)995-2036

Kozanitis Mentakis, Irene D., MD NroChl(72,GRE01)
+ Total Care Pediatrics in Jersey City
550 Newark Avenue/Suite 200   Jersey City, NJ 07306   (201)714-7902   Fax (201)795-4999

Kozel, Joseph M., MD {1346376464} IntrMd, PulDis(73,MEXI)<NJ-HOBUNIMC>
+ 331 Grand Street/Suite 1
Hoboken, NJ 07030   (201)656-3519   Fax (201)656-5989

Kozich, Jeanine Masington, MD {1649437385} Pedtrc(07,NJ06)
+ Summit Medical Group
574 Springfield Avenue   Westfield, NJ 07090   (908)673-7227   Fax (908)232-0540
+ Summit Medical Group
75 East Northfield Road   Livingston, NJ 07039   (908)673-7227   Fax (908)673-7336
+ Summit Medical Group
1 Diamond Hill Road/Bensley Pav/2 FL   Berkeley, NJ 07090   (908)227-8601   Fax (908)288-7993

Kozielski, Joseph A., MD {1013080090} SrgOrt(71,PA02)<NJ-OURLADY, NJ-VIRTUAHS>
+ Professional Orthopedic Assocs of South Jersey PA
17 White Horse Pike/Suite 1   Haddon Heights, NJ 08035   (856)547-2323   Fax (856)547-7932

Koziol, Joseph M., MD {1942378070} SrgNro(83,NJ06)<NJ-STBARNMC>
+ St. BarnabasMedCtr-Int Neurosurgery
101 Old Short Hills Road/Suite 409   West Orange, NJ 07052   (973)322-6732   Fax (973)322-6545

Kozlov, Zinovy, MD {1679505002} GenPrc(68,RUSS)
+ 1044 East Hazelwood Avenue
Rahway, NJ 07065   (732)381-3636   Fax (732)381-5977

Kozlowski, Jeffrey P., MD {1558352369} IntrMd, Nephro(78,NY19)<NJ-VALLEY, NJ-HACKNSK>
+ Bergen Hypertension & Renal Associates PA
44 Godwin Avenue/Suite 301   Midland Park, NJ 07432   (201)447-0013   Fax (201)447-0438
+ Bergen Hypertension & Renal Associates PA
20 Prospect Avenue/Suite 709   Hackensack, NJ 07601   (201)447-0013   Fax (201)678-1072

Krachman, Amy Nicole, DO {1669645800} FamMed(00,PA77)
+ Style Family Medicine
502 Hillside Terrace   Pennsauken, NJ 08110   (856)663-7874   Fax (856)633-5158

Krachman, Donald A., DO {1265507214} FamMed, IntrMd(73,PA77)<NJ-VIRTBERL, NJ-VIRTVOOR>
+ Dermalogic Laser Center
777 South White Horse Pike/Suite D1   Hammonton, NJ 08037   (609)561-0033   Fax (609)561-2748

Krachman, Joel E., DO {1467529792} Gastrn(85,MO79)<NJ-ACMCITY, NJ-ACMCMAIN>
+ Jersey Shore Gastroenterology
408 Bethel Road/Suite E   Somers Point, NJ 08244   (609)926-3330   Fax (609)926-8578

Krachman, Michael S., MD {1649347345} Gastrn, IntrMd(87,CA15)<NJ-ACMCMAIN, NJ-BURDTMLN>
+ Jersey Shore Gastroenterology
408 Bethel Road/Suite E   Somers Point, NJ 08244   (609)926-3330   Fax (609)926-8578
+ Jersey Shore Gastroenterology
108 North Main Street   Cape May Court House, NJ 08210   (609)465-0060

Krachman, Samuel Lee, DO {1093703043} PulDis, IntrMd, SlpDis(84,MO79)<NJ-CENTRAST>
+ CentraState Medical Center
901 West Main Street/Sleep Center   Freehold, NJ 07728   (732)303-5070

Kraft, Jeffrey Joseph, MD {1427348721}
+ John Theurer Cancer Center - HUMC
20 Prospect Avenue/Suite 703   Hackensack, NJ 07601   (551)996-4424

Kraidin, Jonathan L., MD {1902988694} Anesth(91,PA07)<NJ-RWJUBRUN>
+ RWJ University Hospital New Brunswick
One Robert Wood Johnson Place   New Brunswick, NJ 08901   (732)828-3000

Krain, Samuel, MD {1831254333} RadDia<NJ-MEMSALEM>
+ Memorial Hospital of Salem County
310 Woodstown Road/Radiology   Salem, NJ 08079   (856)935-1000

Krajewski, Jennifer Anne, MD {1174698096} PedHem, Pedtrc(03,IL42)<NY-CHLDCOPR, NY-PRSBCOLU>
+ Hackensack University Medical Center
30 Prospect Avenue/Wfan Bldg 137   Hackensack, NJ 07601   (201)996-5600   Fax (201)996-5336
+ St Joseph's Medical Center Emergency
703 Main Street   Paterson, NJ 07503   (201)996-5600   Fax (973)754-2249

Krakauer, Randall Sheldon, MD {1588811012} IntrMd, Rheuma(72,NY03)
+ Arthritis & Osteoporosis Associates, P.A.
4247 US Highway 9/Building 1   Freehold, NJ 07728   (732)780-7650   Fax (732)780-8817

Krakowski, Andrew Charles, MD {1962651679} Dermat
+ 200 Tilton Road/Suite 5
Northfield, NJ 08225   (484)240-6598   Fax (484)585-1594

Kral, Felix E., MD {1306985114} PsyAdt, PsyGrt, Psychy(91,NJ05)<NJ-MORRISTN>
+ 17 Hanover Road/Suite 300
Florham Park, NJ 07932   (973)660-4900   Fax (973)660-0494

Kral, Michael George, MD {1306825716} Anesth(90,NE06)
+ Summit Anesthesia Associates, P.A.
33 Overlook Road/Suite 311   Summit, NJ 07901   (908)598-1500   Fax (908)598-0197

Kramberg, Robert David, MD {1154499549} PhysMd(81,MEXI)
+ Newark Rehabilitation Center
638 Mount Prospect Avenue   Newark, NJ 07104   (973)481-4040   Fax (973)481-1338
+ Rehabilitation Medicine Center of NJ, P.A.
1350 Route 23 North   Wayne, NJ 07470   (973)481-4040   Fax (973)709-9207

Kramer, Alan D., MD {1316918956} CdvDis, IntrMd(82,MA05)<NJ-ACMCMAIN, NJ-OURLADY>
+ Associated Cardiovascular Consultants, P.A.
1105 Laurel Oak Road/Suite 165   Voorhees, NJ 08043   (856)424-3600   Fax (856)424-7154
+ Associated Cardiovascular Consultants-Lourdes
1 Brace Road/Suite C & F   Cherry Hill, NJ 08034   (856)424-3600   Fax (856)428-5748

Kramer, David C., MD {1053394833} Anesth, IntrMd(84,NY46)<NJ-MONMOUTH>
+ Monmouth Medical Center
300 Second Avenue/Anesthesia   Long Branch, NJ 07740   (732)923-3980   Fax (732)923-6977

Kramer, David H., MD {1205835949} RadDia, Radiol(92,PA13)<NJ-VIRTUAHS, NJ-VIRTMHBC>
+ South Jersey Radiology Associates, P.A.
100 Carnie Boulevard/Suite B-5   Voorhees, NJ 08043   (856)751-0123   Fax (856)751-0535
+ The Women's Center at Voorhees
100 Carnie Boulevard/Suite A-4   Voorhees, NJ 08043   (856)751-0123   Fax (856)751-5650
+ South Jersey Radiology Associates, P.A.
315 Route 70 East/Suite B   Cherry Hill, NJ 08043   (856)428-4344   Fax (856)428-0356

Kramer, Isaac, MD {1104829712} IntrMd(84,GEO02)
+ 349 East Northfield Road/Suite 101
Livingston, NJ 07039   (973)716-0300   Fax (973)716-0005

Kramer, Neil, MD {1306808746} Rheuma, IntrMd(74,PA01)<NJ-OVERLOOK>
+ Institute for Rheumatic & Autoimmune Diseases
33 Overlook Road/MAC L01   Summit, NJ 07901   (908)598-7940   Fax (908)598-5447

Kramer, Neil Robert, MD {1073512869} RadDia, Radiol(80,PA13)<NJ-VIRTUAHS, NJ-VIRTMHBC>
+ South Jersey Radiology Associates, P.A.
315 Route 70 East/Suite B   Cherry Hill, NJ 08043   (856)428-4344   Fax (856)428-0356
+ South Jersey Radiology Associates, P.A.
901 Route 168/Suites 301-305   Turnersville, NJ 08012   (856)428-4344   Fax (856)227-8537
+ South Jersey Radiology Associates, P.A.
807 Haddon Avenue/Suite 5   Haddonfield, NJ 08033   (856)616-1130   Fax (856)616-1125

Kramer, Noel Melitta, DO {1801864095} RadOnc(99,PA77)<NJ-COOPRUMC>
+ Cooper University Hospital
One Cooper Plaza   Camden, NJ 08103   (856)342-2000

Kramer, Phillip D., MD {1053311233} Nrolgy, Neutgy(89,CT02)
+ JFK Neurosciences Institute
65 James Street/Second Floor   Edison, NJ 08818   (732)321-7010   Fax (732)632-1584

Kramer, Rachel Laurie, MD {1003814260} ObsGyn(94,NY47)
+ Virtua Phoenix OBGYN
3242 Route 206   Bordentown, NJ 08505   (609)444-5505   Fax (609)444-5606
+ Virtua Obstetrics & Gynocology
401 Young Avenue   Moorestown, NJ 08057   (609)444-5505   Fax (856)291-8880

Kramer, Radu, MD {1326036898} IntrMd, Nephro(82,ROM01)<NJ-VALLEY, NJ-HACKNSK>
+ 800 Kinderkamack Road/Suite 205N
Oradell, NJ 07649   (201)967-0800   Fax (201)942-0492
+ Integrative Medicine Associates PC
1 Sears Drive/3rd Floor   Paramus, NJ 07652   (201)967-0800   Fax (201)967-0811

Kramer, Sarah R., MD {1881758365} Pedtrc(02,PA02)<NJ-STBARNMC, NJ-OVERLOOK>
+ Watchung Pediatrics
76 Stirling Road/Suite 201   Warren, NJ 07059   (908)755-5437   Fax (908)755-6905
+ Watchung Pediatrics
346 South Avenue/Suite 3   Fanwood, NJ 07023   (908)755-5437   Fax (908)889-0047
+ Watchung Pediatrics
225 Millburn Avenue/Suite 301   Millburn, NJ 07059   (973)376-7337   Fax (973)218-6647

Kramer, Sherri Lynn, MD {1720246226} IntrMd(90,PA02)<NJ-KMHTURNV>
+ Kennedy Health Systems/Washington Township Campus
435 Hurffville-Cross Keys Road   Turnersville, NJ 08012   (856)582-2500

Kramer, Theodore Ian, MD {1730334988} IntrMd(83,MD01)
+ 73 Whitney Road
Short Hills, NJ 07078

Kramer, Violet Elizabeth, MD {1033314745} CritCr, IntrMd, PulDis(04,IN20)
+ Monmouth Pulmonary Consultants
30 Corbett Way   Eatontown, NJ 07724   (732)380-0020   Fax (732)380-1990

Kranias, Hristos K., MD {1689951980} ObsGyn
+ Metropolitan Family Health Network
935 Garfield Avenue   Jersey City, NJ 07304   (201)478-5850   Fax (201)475-5814

Kranzler, Harvey N., MD {1134244023} PsyCAd, Psychy(73,NY46)
+ 265 Cedar Lane/2nd Floor
Teaneck, NJ 07666   (201)907-0185   Fax (201)907-0185

Krasikov, Tatiana, MD {1205982949} CdvDis, IntrMd(98,MA01)<NY-PRSBWEIL>
+ Advanced Cardiology Institute
2200 Fletcher Avenue/Suite 1   Fort Lee, NJ 07024   (201)461-6200   Fax (201)461-7204

Krathen, Jonathan, DO {1598023996} IntrMd<NJ-STFRNMED>
+ St. Francis Medical Center
601 Hamilton Avenue   Trenton, NJ 08629   (609)599-5000

Kraus, Jennifer Lynn, MD {1558314906} InfDis, IntrMd(92,GA05)<NJ-VIRTMHBC>
+ Infectious Disease Physicians PA
1001 Briggs Road/Suite 250   Mount Laurel, NJ 08054   (856)866-7466   Fax (856)866-9088

Kraus, Warren M., MD {1902808991} Otlryg, OtgyFPIS(88,NY47)<NJ-SOMERSET>
+ 35-37 Progress Street/Suite B1
Edison, NJ 08820   (908)412-9599   Fax (908)753-6226
+ RWJ University Hospital Somerset
110 Rehill Avenue/Otolaryngology   Somerville, NJ 08876   (908)685-2200

Krause, Tyrone J., MD {1477525574} CdvDis, SrgThr(85,NY09)<NJ-RWJUBRUN>
+ RWJ University Hospital New Brunswick
One Robert Wood Johnson Place   New Brunswick, NJ 08901   (732)235-7810

Krauser, Paula S., MD {1841234028} FamMed, Grtrcs, PallCr(78,NJ06)<NJ-RWJUBRUN, NJ-RBAYOLDB>
+ Center for Healthy Aging
18 Centre Drive/Suite 104   Monroe Township, NJ 08831   (609)655-5178   Fax (609)655-5284
+ Bay Family Medicine
26 Throckmorton Lane   Old Bridge, NJ 08857   (609)655-5178   Fax (732)360-1279

Krauss, Elliot A., MD {1194753616} Pthlgy, PthACl, PthChm(77,MO02)<NJ-UNVMCPRN, NJ-RWJUBRUN>
+ University Medical Center of Princeton at Plainsboro
One Plainsboro Road/Pathology   Plainsboro, NJ 08536   (609)497-4351   Fax (609)497-4982

Krauss, Joel Martin, MD {1629120472} Pedtrc, IntrMd, IntHos(92,NY47)
+ CHOP Care Network at Princeton Medical Center
One Plainsboro Road/Hospitalist   Plainsboro, NJ 08536   (609)853-7000   Fax (215)590-2180

Kraut, Bruce H., MD {1205836509}
+ Lawrenceville School Infirmary
2500 Main Street/PO Box 6011   Lawrenceville, NJ 08648   (609)896-0391

Kraut, Evelyn S., MD {1669464657} Allrgy, Pedtrc(78,NY09)<NJ-HACKNSK>
+ Pedimedica, P.A.
18 Railroad Avenue/Suite 103   Rochelle Park, NJ 07662   (201)291-2323   Fax (201)291-2328

Kraut, Lawrence, MD {1245267079} SrgOrt(78,NY09)
+ Orthopedic Sports Medicine
1136 Clifton Avenue   Clifton, NJ 07013   (973)777-1677   Fax (973)773-1553

Krauthamer, Matthew J., DO {1619109121} EmrgMd(06,ME75)<NJ-CHILTON>
+ Chilton Medical Center
97 West Parkway/EmrgMed   Pompton Plains, NJ 07444   (973)831-5000

Kravets, Felix G., MD {1841226008} RadDia, RadNro(00,NY48)<NJ-COMMED>
+ Community Medical Center
99 Route 37 West/Radiology   Toms River, NJ 08755   (732)557-8000

Kravitz, Elaine K., MD {1659351757} Allrgy(79,NY47)<NJ-VIRTMHBC, NJ-VIRTBERL>
+ Allergy & Asthma Associates
525 Route 73 South/Suite 106   Marlton, NJ 08053   (856)596-5585   Fax (856)596-3178
+ Allergy & Asthma Associates
127 Ark Road/Suite 1   Mount Laurel, NJ 08054   (856)596-5585   Fax (856)727-9595

Kravitz, John Jay, MD {1588612105} Gastrn, IntrMd(72,PA13)
+ The Gastroenterology Group, PA
103 Old Marlton Pike/Suite 102   Medford, NJ 08055   (609)953-3440   Fax (609)996-4002
+ The Gastroenterology Group, PA
15000 Midlantic Drive/Suite 110   Mount Laurel, NJ 08054   (609)953-3440   Fax (856)996-4002

Kravitz, Stuart A., MD {1235119330} Allrgy, ImmAsm(76,PA13)<NJ-VIRTMHBC, NJ-VIRTVOOR>
+ Allergy & Asthma Associates
127 Ark Road/Suite 1   Mount Laurel, NJ 08054   (856)778-4222   Fax (856)727-9595
+ Allergy & Asthma Associates
525 Route 73 South/Suite 106   Marlton, NJ 08053   (856)778-4222   Fax (856)596-3178

Krawet, Steven Howard, MD {1467554956} Gastrn(89,NJ06)<NJ-RWJUBRUN, NJ-STPETER>
+ 557 Cranbury Road/Suite 1
East Brunswick, NJ 08816   (732)390-5534   Fax (732)390-6141
+ Cares Surgicenter, LLC.
240 Easton Avenue   New Brunswick, NJ 08901   (732)390-5534   Fax (732)296-8677

Krawitz, Mark J., MD {1659323194} Ophthl(80,PA02)<NJ-OVERLOOK>
+ The Eye Center
65 Mountain Boulevard Ext/Suite 105   Warren, NJ 07059   (732)356-6200   Fax (732)356-0228
+ The Eye Center
213 Stelton Road   Piscataway, NJ 08854   (732)356-6200   Fax (732)752-9492
+ The Eye Center
3900 Park Avenue/Suite 106   Edison, NJ 07059   (732)603-2101

Krawitz, Steven, MD {1285959056} Gastrn
+ UMDNJ Division of Gastroenterology & Hepatology
90 Bergen Street/DOC 2100   Newark, NJ 07103   (973)972-5252   Fax (973)972-0752

Kraynock, John, MD {1215024906} Pedtrc, EmrgMd(87,MEXI)<NJ-OCEANMC>
+ ABC Pediatric Associates PA
131 Drum Point Road   Brick, NJ 08723   (732)477-8988
+ Family Health Center/Community Medical Center
301 Lakehurst Road   Toms River, NJ 08755   (732)477-8988   Fax (732)557-3390

Krblich, Diana, MD {1811212939} FamMed
+ MedExpress Urgent Care Springfield
200 US Highway 22 West   Springfield, NJ 07081   (973)376-4341   Fax (973)376-4342

Kreibich, Thomas Alfred, MD {1700089166} Nrolgy
+ New Jersey Neurological Specialists
20 Prospect Avenue/Suite 800   Hackensack, NJ 07601   (201)518-7290   Fax (201)604-6428

Kreidy, Mazen Pierre, MD {1972741635} CritCr
+ Cooper University Hospital Critical Care
One Cooper Plaza   Camden, NJ 08103   (856)448-3051   Fax (856)968-8282

Krel, Regina, MD {1053068257} Nrolgy(11,ANT02)
+ Multiple Sclerosis Center
300 Essex Street/Suite 203   Hackensack, NJ 07601   (551)996-8100   Fax (551)996-4140

Krell, Mark J., MD {1558456822} CdvDis, IntrMd(79,NY19)
+ Summit Cardiology, LLC
One Springfield Avenue/Suite 2-A   Summit, NJ 07901   (908)273-1999   Fax (908)273-1332

Physicians by Name and Address

Krell, Todd P., MD {1043204985} SrgOrt(82,NY09)<NJ-OVERLOOK, NJ-MTNSIDE>
+ Westfield Orthopedic Group
541 East Broad Street   Westfield, NJ 07090   (908)232-3879   Fax (908)232-5789

Kresloff, Michael Scott, MD {1164514857} Ophthl(96,NJ05)<NJ-VANJHCS>
+ Drs. Kresloff and Young
900 Haddon Avenue/Suite 102   Collingswood, NJ 08108   (856)854-4242   Fax (856)854-3585

Kresloff, Richard S., MD {1770674236} Ophthl(70,PA01)<NJ-VAN-JHCS>
+ Drs. Kresloff and Young
900 Haddon Avenue/Suite 102   Collingswood, NJ 08108   (856)854-4242   Fax (856)854-3585
+ Wills Eye Surgery Center in Cherry Hill
408 Route 70 East   Cherry Hill, NJ 08034   (856)854-4242   Fax (856)429-7555

Kretov, Aleksey, MD {1811184211} IntrMd, Grtrcs(96,UKR13)<NJ-JRSYSHMC, NJ-RIVERVW>
+ Dr. Kretov and Associates
230 Neptune Boulevard   Neptune, NJ 07753   (732)414-2005   Fax (732)414-2006

Krever, Kristine Wang, MD {1366533721} FamMed(00,VA07)
+ Tatem Brown Family Practice
2225 East Evesham Road/Suite 101   Voorhees, NJ 08043   (856)795-4330   Fax (856)325-3704
+ Rowan University Student Health Center
201 Mullica Hill Road   Glassboro, NJ 08028   (856)795-4330   Fax (856)256-4427

Kricko, Michael J., DO {1215029905} IntrMd(93,IA75)<NJ-MTN-SIDE, NJ-CLARMAAS>
+ first Care Medical Group
750 Valley Brook Avenue   Lyndhurst, NJ 07071   (201)896-0900   Fax (201)896-2726

Krieg, Eileen M., MD {1639174485} RadDia, Radiol, IntrMd(76,NY08)<NJ-JRSYSHMC>
+ University Radiology Group, P.C.
579A Cranbury Road   East Brunswick, NJ 08816   (732)390-0040   Fax (732)390-1856
+ Lacey Diagnostic Imaging LLC
833 Lacey Road/Suite 2   Forked River, NJ 08731   (732)390-0040   Fax (609)242-2402
+ University Radiology Group
2100 Route 33/Neptune City Med Bld   Neptune, NJ 08816   (732)988-1234   Fax (732)502-0368

Krieg, Karen Sue, DO {1700859113} ObsGyn, IntrMd(97,NJ75)<NJ-STPETER>
+ Rowan SOM Department of Ob/Gyn
405 Hurffville-Cross Keys Road   Sewell, NJ 08080   (856)589-1414   Fax (856)256-5772
+ Women's Physicians & Surgeons
501 Iron Bridge Road/Suite 10   Freehold, NJ 07728   (856)589-1414   Fax (732)431-2993
+ Women's Physicians & Surgeons
510 Bridge Plaza Drive   Englishtown, NJ 08080   (732)536-5552   Fax (732)536-4570

Kriegel, Marni Ruth, MD {1760640403} Pedtrc<NJ-HACKNSK>
+ Hackensack Univ Medical Center Pediatric Emerg Room
30 Prospect Avenue   Hackensack, NJ 07601   (201)996-5430   Fax (201)996-3676
+ Hackensack University Medical Center
30 Prospect Avenue   Hackensack, NJ 07601   (201)996-2000

Krieger, Alan P., MD {1740385772} Urolgy(84,MEXI)
+ New Jersey Urology, LLC
700 North Broad Street/Suite 302   Elizabeth, NJ 07208   (908)289-3666   Fax (908)289-0716
+ New Jersey Urology, LLC
1600 George Avenue/Suite 202   Rahway, NJ 07065   (908)289-3666   Fax (732)499-0432

Krieger, Richard E., MD {1184648347} InfDis, IntrMd(78,NJ05)<NJ-CHILTON, NJ-WAYNEGEN>
+ ID Associates PA/dba ID Care
765 Route 10 East/Suite 201   Randolph, NJ 07869   (973)989-0068   Fax (973)361-8955
+ ID Associates PA/dba ID Care
8 Saddle Road   Cedar Knolls, NJ 07927   (973)989-0068   Fax (973)993-5953
+ ID Associates PA/dba ID Care
2035 Hamburg Turnpike/Suite F   Wayne, NJ 07869   (973)513-9475   Fax (973)513-9478

Kriegman, Audrey Gail, MD {1669645560} GenPrc, OthrSp(76,NJ05)
+ 131 Barchester Way
Westfield, NJ 07090   (973)781-6549

Krigsman, Suzanne Karimi, MD {1669402798} FamMed(99,PA09)
+ Valley Medical Group
140 Franklin Turnpike/Suite 6-A   Waldwick, NJ 07463   (201)447-3603   Fax (201)447-5184

Krikhely, Abraham, MD {1861698870} Surgry, SrgBrtc(07,NY19)<NY-PRSBCOLU>
+ 140 Route 17 North/Suite 102
Paramus, NJ 07652   (212)305-9506   Fax (212)345-1996

Krinsky, Glenn Andrew, MD {1356338180} RadDia, Radiol(88,NY19)<NJ-VALLEY>
+ Radiology Associates of Ridgewood, P.A.
20 Franklin Turnpike   Waldwick, NJ 07463   (201)445-8822   Fax (201)447-5053

Kriplani, Anuja, MD {1831484419} MedOnc
+ Memorial Sloan Kettering Bergen
225 Summit Avenue   Montvale, NJ 07645   (201)775-7443

Kripsak, John P., DO {1275576910} FamMed, FamMSptM(87,MO79)<NJ-SOMERSET>
+ RWJPE Bridgewater Medical Group
766 Route 202-206/Suite 1   Bridgewater, NJ 08807   (908)722-0808   Fax (908)722-7645

Krisa, Paul C., MD {1588608525} IntrMd(80,MEX03)<NJ-STJOSHOS, NJ-STMRYPAS>
+ Broad Street Medical Associates
1135 Broad Street/Suite 205   Clifton, NJ 07013   (973)471-8850   Fax (973)471-5232
+ Broad Street Medical Associates
201 Route 17/Floor 11   Rutherford, NJ 07070   (973)471-8850   Fax (973)471-5232

Krisch, Evan B., MD {1588621189} Urolgy(83,PA02)<NJ-COOPRUMC, NJ-VIRTBERL>
+ Cooper University Urology
3 Cooper Plaza/Suite 411   Camden, NJ 08103   (856)963-3577
+ New Jersey Urology, LLC
2401 East Evesham Road/Suite F   Voorhees, NJ 08043   (856)963-3577   Fax (856)988-0636
+ Center for Urologic Care PA
485 Williamstown-New Freedom R   Sicklerville, NJ 08103   (856)237-8035   Fax (856)237-8039

Krish, Nagesh B., MD {1710918115} Nrolgy(82,INDI)<NJ-CHRIST, NJ-MEADWLND>
+ Nagesh B. Krish MD, PA
727 10th Street   Union City, NJ 07087   (201)864-5252   Fax (201)864-9555

Krishan, Mona, DO {1992182802}
+ Radiology Affiliates Imaging
3625 Quakerbridge Road   Hamilton, NJ 08619   (609)890-8844

Krishna, Sunanda, MD {1245205145} IntrMd(94,INAZ6)<NJ-CENTRAST>
+ 3 Plaza Drive/Suite 14
Toms River, NJ 08753   (732)240-0303   Fax (732)240-2430

Krishnaiah, Muralidhar, MD {1427071729} PsyGrt(82,INA37)
+ 39 Keswick Circle
Monroe Township, NJ 08831

Krishnamoorthy, Ambalavaner, MD {1679634968} MtFtMd, ObsGyn(74,SRIL)
+ High Risk Pregnancy Center of New Jersey PC
1 Auer Court/Suites A & B   East Brunswick, NJ 08816   (732)390-1020   Fax (732)390-8035
+ High Risk Pregnancy Center of New Jersey PC
908 Oak Tree Road/Suite M & N   South Plainfield, NJ 07080   (732)390-1020   Fax (908)753-2473

Krishnamoorthy, Sripriya, MD {1083824999}
+ 200 Hospital Plaza/Suite 104
Paterson, NJ 07503

Krishnamsetty, Nanditha, MD {1174582746} PsyCAd(96,INA83)
+ Bay Family Medicine
26 Throckmorton Lane   Old Bridge, NJ 08857   (732)360-0287   Fax (732)360-1279
+ 14 Venezia Drive
Monroe, NJ 08831

Krishnan, Lalitha B., MD {1538152293} IntrMd(80,INA2X)
+ 11 Golden Valley Drive
North Brunswick, NJ 08902

Krishnan, Lalitha G., MD {1669555793} EnDbMt, IntrMd(77,INDI)<NJ-CENTRAST>
+ Drs. Krishnan and Krishnan
14 Hospital Drive   Toms River, NJ 08755   (732)502-5292   Fax (732)818-4810

Krishnan, Mahadevan Gopa, MD {1699849620} Surgry, SrgVas(76,INDI)
+ Drs. Krishnan and Krishnan
14 Hospital Drive   Toms River, NJ 08755   (732)502-5292   Fax (732)818-4810

Krishtul, Eduard, MD {1396717021} Anesth(96,DOM10)<NJ-KIMBALL>
+ Bey Lea Anesthesia Associates
54 Bey Lea Road/Bldg. 2   Toms River, NJ 08753   (732)281-1020

Krisiloff, Edward B., MD {1548359151} SrgOrt(84,NJ06)
+ Raritan Valley Surgery Center
100 Franklin Square Drive/Suite 100   Somerset, NJ 08873   (732)560-1000   Fax (732)560-5999

Kriso, Stephen A., MD {1922004654} IntrMd(66,DC02)<NJ-STMRYPAS>
+ 44 Union Boulevard/PO Box 3338
Wallington, NJ 07057   (973)779-3030   Fax (973)779-0225
Skrisomd@dessk.net

Kristan, Ronald W., MD {1114928843} Ophthl(80,NY19)<NJ-JRSYSHMC, NJ-MONMOUTH>
+ Atlantic Eye Physicians
279 Third Avenue/Suite 204   Long Branch, NJ 07740   (732)222-7373   Fax (732)571-9212
+ Atlantic Eye Physicians
180 White Road/Suite 202   Little Silver, NJ 07739   (732)222-7373   Fax (732)219-9557
+ Atlantic Eye Physicians
100 Commons Way/Suite 230   Holmdel, NJ 07740   (732)671-4060

Krisza, Mary L., MD {1710969241} IntrMd(80,PA09)<NJ-RIVERVW>
+ 61 Spruce Drive
Fair Haven, NJ 07704   (908)902-5593
mlkrisza@verizon.net

Kritharis-Agrusa, Athena, MD {1598907982} OncHem, IntrMd
+ Rutgers Cancer Institute of New Jersey
195 Little Albany Street/PO Box 2681   New Brunswick, NJ 08903   (732)235-2465   Fax (732)235-7355

Kritzberg, William S., MD {1780725010} IntrMd(91,ISR02)<NJ-STBARNMC>
+ 100 Northfield Road
West Orange, NJ 07052   (973)243-1400   Fax (973)243-1415

Krivoshik, Mark P., MD {1669409306} EmrgMd, IntrMd(86,PA01)<NJ-COMMED, NJ-SOCEANCO>
+ 16 Yeger Drive
Allentown, NJ 08501   (609)259-1439
docmark758@aol.com
+ Community Medical Center
99 Route 37 West/EmergMed   Toms River, NJ 08755   (732)557-8283
+ Southern Ocean County Medical Center
1140 Route 72 West/EmrgMed   Manahawkin, NJ 08501   (609)597-6011

Krohn, David Isaac, MD {1689643298} IntrMd(74,NY47)
+ Chemed Family Health Center
1771 Madison Avenue   Lakewood, NJ 08701   (732)364-2144   Fax (732)364-3559

Krohn, Douglas R., MD {1891734471} FamMed(81,MEXI)
+ Piscataway Dunellen Family Practice
24 Stelton Road/Suite A   Piscataway, NJ 08854   (732)424-0440   Fax (732)424-0443

Krohn, Natan Nata, MD {1306005962} Gastrn<NY-MTSINAI, NY-MTSINYHS>
+ Gastroenterology Associates of New Jersey
1011 Clifton Avenue   Clifton, NJ 07013   (973)471-8200   Fax (973)471-3032
+ Gastroenterology Associates of New Jersey
20 Prospect Avenue/Suite 813   Hackensack, NJ 07601   (973)471-8200
+ Gastroenterology Associates of New Jersey
71 Union Avenue/Suite 210   Rutherford, NJ 07013   (201)896-0400   Fax (201)896-0863

Krok, Elion J., MD {1538468491} IntrMd(83,SAF02)
+ IMMC Health
737 Northfield Avenue   West Orange, NJ 07052   (973)544-8901   Fax (973)544-8991

Krol, Anna, MD {1679522908} Pedtrc(00,DMN01)<NJ-VIRTMHBC, NJ-VIRTUAHS>
+ Cooper University Hospital Pediatrics/Endocrinology
3 Cooper Plaza/Suite 200   Camden, NJ 08103   (856)968-8898
+ Advocare Laurel Pediatrics
269 Fish Pond Road   Sewell, NJ 08080   (856)968-8898   Fax (856)863-9666

Krol, David Matthew, MD {1710963863} Pedtrc, IntrMd(96,CT01)
+ 148 Bertrand Drive
Princeton, NJ 08540   (609)627-7567
+ Robert Wood Johnson Foundation
PO Box 2316   Princeton, NJ 08540   (609)627-7567   Fax (609)452-1865

Krol, Kristine, MD {1275528465} Allrgy, AlgyImmn(81,NY08)<NY-STATNSTH, NJ-SOMERSET>
+ Allercare
177 West High Street   Somerville, NJ 08876   (908)725-8666   Fax (908)725-2223

Krol, Roman, MD {1477500569} IntrMd(00,DMN01)
+ 310 Woodstown Road/4th Floor
Salem, NJ 08079   (856)935-0276   Fax (856)935-1638

Krol, Ryszard B., MD {1750463741} CdvDis, IntrMd, ClCdEl(73,POL02)<NJ-NWRKBETH>
+ 164 Brighton Road
Clifton, NJ 07012   (973)778-3111   Fax (973)778-0403

Kroll, Mark S., MD {1174598619} IntrMd, MedOnc, Hemato(72,PA01)<NJ-BAYSHORE, NJ-CENTRAST>
+ 501 Ironbridge Road/Suite 15
Freehold, NJ 07728 (732)780-0100 Fax (732)780-8452

Kroll, Spencer Daniel, MD {1891738498} IntrMd(95,DC01)<NJ-RBAYOLDB, NJ-CENTRAST>
+ The Kroll Medical Group
25 Kilmer Drive/Building 3/Suite 215 Morganville, NJ 07751 (732)591-8840 Fax (732)591-2822

Krommes, Janet Filemyr, MD {1659398675} Rheuma, IntrMd(89,PA13)
+ Arthritis, Rheumatic & Back Disease Associates
2309 East Evesham Road/Suite 101 Voorhees, NJ 08043 (856)424-5005 Fax (856)424-4716

Kron, Stanley M., MD {1770566564} RadDia(68,NY08)<NJ-STPETER, NJ-RWJUBRUN>
+ University Radiology Group, P.C.
483 Cranbury Road East Brunswick, NJ 08816 (732)390-0030 Fax (732)390-5383
+ University Radiology Group, P.C.
10 Plum Street New Brunswick, NJ 08901 (732)390-0030 Fax (732)249-1208

Kronengold, Charles J., MD {1679648596} Ophthl(73,NJ05)<NJ-STBARNMC>
+ The Laser Care Center of Livingston
22 Old Short Hills Road Livingston, NJ 07039 (973)992-5005 Fax (973)992-5024
CKRONENGOLD@pol.net

Kronhaus, Kenneth E., MD {1104918242} FamMed(02,DMN01)
+ 10 Sandy Point Drive
Brick, NJ 08723 (908)208-7417
+ Jersey Coast Family Medicine
495 Jack Martin Boulevard/Suite 5 Brick, NJ 08724 (908)208-7417 Fax (732)458-8020

Kroning, David R., MD {1922058346} Pedtrc, PedEmg(86,BWI01)<NJ-VALLEY>
+ The Valley Hospital
223 North Van Dien Avenue Ridgewood, NJ 07450 (201)447-8000

Kronish, Anne L., MD {1467491381} FamMed, GenPrc(83,MEX03)<NJ-VALLEY>
+ Valley Health Medical Group
780 Cedar Lane Teaneck, NJ 07666 (201)836-7664 Fax (201)836-5710

Kroon, David Fleming, MD {1104854991} Otlryg(98,NJ06)<NJ-HUNTRDN>
+ Hunterdon Otolaryngology Associates
6 Sand Hill Road/Suite 302 Flemington, NJ 08822 (908)788-9131 Fax (908)788-0945

Kroon, Jody Lynn, MD {1619941671} Pedtrc(98,NJ06)<NJ-HUNTRDN>
+ Hunterdon Pediatric Associates
1738 Route 31 North/Suite 201 Clinton, NJ 08809 (908)735-3960 Fax (908)735-3965

Kroop, Howard S., MD {1427027614} Gastrn, IntrMd(72,NC01)
+ South Jersey Endoscopy Center
26 East Red Bank Avenue Woodbury, NJ 08096 (856)848-4464 Fax (856)848-8706

Kropa, Jill, MD {1558628776} FamMed
+ Family Medicine at Monument Square
317 George Street New Brunswick, NJ 08901 (732)235-8993 Fax (732)246-7317

Kropf, Laura Dawn, DO {1841259363} FamMed(01,NJ75)
+ Village Medical Center
207 Strykers Road Phillipsburg, NJ 08865 (908)859-6568 Fax (908)859-6697
+ Warren Hospital
185 Roseberry Street Phillipsburg, NJ 08865 (484)526-3319

Krotenberg, Robert, MD {1366547424} PhysMd(74,ITAL)<NJ-KSLRSADB, NJ-KSLRWELK>
+ Kessler Institute for Rehabilitation
300 Market Street Saddle Brook, NJ 07663 (201)587-8500
+ Kessler Institute for Rehab
201 Pleasant Hill Road Chester, NJ 07930 (973)584-7500
+ Kessler Institute for Rehabilitation West Orange
1199 Pleasant Valley Way West Orange, NJ 07663 (973)243-6961

Kroth, Patricia Haeusler, DO {1306817150} FamMed(96,PA77)<NJ-WARREN>
+ Delaware Valley Family Health Center
200 Frenchtown Road Milford, NJ 08848 (908)995-2251 Fax (908)995-2036

Krottapalli, Harini, MD {1285631929} Anesth(93,INA84)<NJ-STJOSHOS>
+ St. Joseph's Regional Medical Center Anesthesia
703 Main Street Paterson, NJ 07503 (973)754-2323 Fax (973)977-9455

Krueger, Kelly A., MD {1861663528}
+ Atlantic Gastroenterology Summit Medical Group
65 Ridgedale Avenue Cedar Knolls, NJ 07927 (973)401-0500 Fax (973)401-9306

Krueger, Paul M., DO {1861646234} ObsGyn, IntrMd(75,NJ75)
+ 25 Chestnut Street/Suite 203
Haddonfield, NJ 08033 (856)428-7211
krueger@umdnj.edu

Kruger, Eric N., MD {1487634952} FamMed(77,PA02)<NJ-VIRTBERL, NJ-VIRTVOOR>
+ Inspira Medical Group
660 Woodbury Glassboro Road/Suite 26 Sewell, NJ 08080 (856)415-6868 Fax (856)464-1855

Kruger, Hillary Anne, MD {1073521571} PedDvl, Pedtrc(90,NY19)
+ CHOP Pediatric & Adolescent Specialty Care Center
4009 Black Horse Pike Mays Landing, NJ 08330 (609)677-7895 Fax (609)677-7835
+ CHOP Pediatric & Adolescent Specialty Care Center
1012 Laurel Oak Road Voorhees, NJ 08043 (609)677-7895 Fax (856)435-0091

Krugman, Richard S., MD {1821037193}<NJ-KMHCHRRY>
+ Kennedy Health System/Cherry Hill Campus
2201 Chapel Avenue West Cherry Hill, NJ 08002 (856)488-6500

Krugman, Robert L., MD {1659356749} Radiol, RadDia(66,PA01)<NJ-HACKNSK>
+ New Century Imaging at Oradell
555 Kinderkamack Road Oradell, NJ 07649 (201)599-1311 Fax (201)599-8333
+ The Imaging Center
30 South Newman Street Hackensack, NJ 07601 (201)599-1311 Fax (201)488-5244
+ Hackensack Radiology Group, P.A.
30 Prospect Avenue Hackensack, NJ 07649 (201)996-2200 Fax (201)336-8451

Krul, Geddy J., MD {1215936604} Pedtrc(80,MEXI)<NJ-STBARNMC, NJ-NWRKBETH>
+ Union Pediatric Associate PA
381 Chestnut Street Union, NJ 07083 (908)688-8007 Fax (908)688-3884

Krulish, Sean P., DO {1861821738}
+ 3 Cooper Plaza/Suite 520
Camden, NJ 08103 (856)342-2298

Krumerman, Martin Saul, MD {1972641371} PthAClI(65,NY19)
+ Ocean County Medical Lab
525 Route 70 Brick, NJ 08723 (732)920-1772 Fax (732)920-6171
KRmsmart@optonline.net

Krupinski, Donna J., MD {1528032588} Pedtrc(89,TX12)<NJ-HUNTRDN>
+ Hunterdon Pediatric Associates
8 Reading Road/Reading Ridge Flemington, NJ 08822 (908)788-6070 Fax (908)788-6005

Krupnick, Matthew E., MD {1629005566} Gastrn(90,PA02)<NJ-HCKTSTWN>
+ Gastroenterology Associates of North Jersey
369 West Blackwell Street Dover, NJ 07801 (973)361-7660 Fax (973)361-0455
+ Gastroenterology Associates of North Jersey
16 Pocono Road/Suite 210 Denville, NJ 07834 (973)361-7660 Fax (973)627-7610

Krupp, Edward Todd, DO {1760583868} IntrMd(99,NJ75)<NJ-MTNSIDE>
+ Crescent Internal Medicine Group
98 Park Street Montclair, NJ 07042 (973)783-0800 Fax (973)744-1274

Kruse, Christopher Bryant, MD {1083636898} Dermat, DerMOH(96,NY19)<NJ-MTNSIDE>
+ Dermatology & Skin Cancer Center
55 North Gilbert Street Tinton Falls, NJ 07701 (732)747-5500 Fax (877)843-7654
+ Dr. Deborah Ruth Spey
101 Old Short Hills Road/Suite 410 West Orange, NJ 07052 (732)747-5500 Fax (973)731-1635

Kruse, Lakota K., MD GPrvMd, Pedtrc(90,PA01)
+ New Jersey Department of Health and Senior Services
50 East State/PO Box 360 Trenton, NJ 08625 (609)292-4043 Fax (609)292-9599
lkruse@doh.state.nj.us

Kruse, Laurel Anita Farnham, MD {1871515973} Pedtrc(86,NJ06)<NJ-CAPITLHS, PA-CHILDHOS>
+ Capital Emergency Physicians & Associates
One Capital Way Pennington, NJ 08534 (609)394-6063 Fax (609)278-5420

Krutak-Krol, Halina M., MD {1619063922} IntrMd, Nephro(73,POL02)
+ 164 Brighton Road
Clifton, NJ 07012 (973)777-9950 Fax (973)778-2763

Krutchik, Allan N., MD {1619938289} IntrMd, MedOnc, OncHem(73,IL42)<NJ-CHILTON, NJ-HACKNSK>
+ Northern New Jersey Cancer Center
795 Franklin Avenue Franklin Lakes, NJ 07417 (201)848-8791 Fax (201)848-9604

Kruvant-Gornish, Nancy J., MD {1669441465} InfDis, IntrMd(87,GRNA)<NJ-JRSYSHMC, NJ-RIVERVW>
+ Hackensack Meridian Medical Group

19 Davis Avenue/5th-6th Floor Neptune, NJ 07753 (732)897-3990 Fax (732)897-3997
+ Jersey Shore University Medical Center
1945 Route 33 Neptune, NJ 07753 (732)775-5500

Krynska, Elzbieta B., MD {1619970852} Anesth(82,POL17)
+ Advanced Interventional Pain Management
1176 Hamburg Turnpike Wayne, NJ 07470 (973)365-4747 Fax (973)365-4596

Krynyckyi, Borys Roman, MD {1003892613} NuclMd(91,IL42)
+ Personal Care Molecular
1514 State Route 138/PCMI Wall, NJ 07719 (732)681-2700 Fax (732)681-2701

Krystofiak, Jason Anthony, MD {1679991145} FamMSptM
+ RWJBH Primary Care Eatontown
145 Wyckoff Road/Suite 301 Eatontown, NJ 07724 (848)208-5250 Fax (732)935-1590

Krzanowski, Tracey J., MD {1154306637} Anesth, PedAne(00,GRN01)<NJ-STCLRDEN>
+ St. Clare's Hospital-Denville Campus
25 Pocono Road/Anesthesiology Denville, NJ 07834 (973)625-6000
+ Malo Clinic Center for Ambulatory Surgery
210 Route 17 North/12th Fl Rutherford, NJ 07070

Krzemieniecki, Thomas Gerald, DO {1609015627} Anesth
+ 75 Broadway/Unit 107
Somers Point, NJ 08244

Ksiazek, Stephen Jude, MD {1851346738} CdvDis, IntrMd(91,PA01)<NJ-WARREN>
+ Coordinated Health
222 Red Lane Phillipsburg, NJ 08865 (610)861-8080 Fax (610)849-1013

Ku, James Chien, MD {1366408247} Anesth(01,NJ05)<NJ-STPETER>
+ Anesthesia Consultnts of NJ/Nova Pain
285 Davidson Avenue/Suite 204 Somerset, NJ 08873 (732)271-1400 Fax (732)271-3543
+ Cares Surgicenter, LLC.
240 Easton Avenue New Brunswick, NJ 08901 (732)271-1400 Fax (732)296-8677
+ St. Peter's University Hospital
254 Easton Avenue/Anesth New Brunswick, NJ 08873 (732)745-8600

Ku, Min Jung, MD {1740281955} AlgyImmn, IntrMd(99,PA14)
+ Allergy & Asthma Care, P.C.
213 North Haddon Avenue Haddonfield, NJ 08033 (856)795-5600 Fax (856)795-6644
+ Allergy & Asthma Care, P.C.
2301 East Evesham Road/Suite 207 Voorhees, NJ 08043 (856)795-5600 Fax (856)795-6644

Kubeck, Justin P., MD {1063613339} SrgOrt, SrgSpn(02,PA02)
+ Ocean Orthopedic Associates, P.A.
530 Lakehurst Road/Suite 1 Toms River, NJ 08755 (732)349-8454 Fax (732)341-0259

Kubicek, Gregory John, MD {1558427153} RadOnc, RadThp(04,MN07)<NJ-COOPRUMC>
+ CUH Cancer & Radiation Oncology Institute
715 Fellowship Road Mount Laurel, NJ 08054 (856)638-1180 Fax (856)638-1188
+ Cooper University Hospital
One Cooper Plaza/Rad Onc Camden, NJ 08103 (856)342-2300

Kubichek, Marilyn Ann, MD {1750449286} NroChl, Pedtrc, NrlgSpec(88,DMN01)
+ St. Barnabas Ambulatory Care Center
200 South Orange Avenue Livingston, NJ 07039 (973)322-7600 Fax (973)322-7685
+ 256 Columbia Turnpike/Suite 109
Florham Park, NJ 07932 (973)322-7600 Fax (973)377-7821

Kuchar, Sarah Driscoll, MD {1376851709} IntrMd<PA-WILLSEYE>
+ The Princeton Eye Group
419 North Harrison Street/Suite 104 Princeton, NJ 08540 (609)921-9437 Fax (609)921-0277
+ The Princeton Eye Group
900 Eastern Avenue/Suite 50 Somerset, NJ 08873 (609)921-9437 Fax (732)565-0946

Kucharski, Jarrod Michael, MD {1225360217} Pedtrc(PA0<NJ-STCLRDEN>
+ Riverside Pediatric Group
609 Washington Street/Ground Floor Hoboken, NJ 07030 (201)706-8488 Fax (201)706-8489

Kuchera, James Joseph, MD {1356454813} ObsGyn, IntrMd(76,NY01)<NJ-MORRISTN>
+ Summit Medical Group
160 East Hanover Avenue/Suite 101 Cedar Knolls, NJ 07927 (973)605-5090 Fax (973)605-1705

Kuchera, Michael W., MD {1215041348} ObsGyn(87,NJ05)<NJ-MORRISTN>
+ Summit Medical Group
160 East Hanover Avenue/Suite 101 Cedar Knolls, NJ 07927 (973)605-5090 Fax (973)605-1705

Physicians by Name and Address

Kuchipudi, Solomon Sudhakar, MD {1073544284} IntrMd(97,INA7C)
+ Prompt Medical Care
  636 Easton Avenue   Somerset, NJ 08873   (732)220-8811   Fax (732)220-1300
+ Solomon Kuchipudi MD LLC
  1814 East 2nd Street   Scotch Plains, NJ 07076   (908)322-6611

Kuchler, Joseph A., MD {1538117189} SrgCdv, SrgThr, Surgry(74,PA02)<NJ-OURLADY, NJ-VIRTUAHS>
+ Virtua Surgical Group, PA
  1935 Route 70 East   Cherry Hill, NJ 08003   (856)428-7700   Fax (856)424-9120

Kucuk, Erhan, MD {1528069416} IntrMd(81,TURK)<NJ-WAYNE-GEN>
+ Wayne Primary Care, P.A.
  508 Hamburg Turnpike/Suite 102   Wayne, NJ 07470   (973)595-0096   Fax (973)595-6414
+ St. Joseph's Wayne Hospital
  224 Hamburg Turnpike   Wayne, NJ 07470   (973)942-6900

Kudakachira, Shaismy, DO {1205248192} IntrMd
+ Capital Health Primary Care - Mountainview
  850 Bear Tavern Road/Suite 309   Ewing, NJ 08628   (609)656-8844   Fax (609)656-8845

Kudipudi, Ramanasri V., MD {1447325311} IntrMd, InfDis(95,INA11)<NJ-CENTRAST>
+ CentraState Medical Center
  901 West Main Street/Ste 260/CN 5050   Freehold, NJ 07728   (732)685-9243   Fax (732)631-9924

Kudryk, Alexander B., MD {1912938671} IntrMd, Addctn, Alc-Sub(85,MEXI)<NJ-OVERLOOK>
+ Clark Urgent Care
  100 Commerce Place   Clark, NJ 07066   (732)499-0606

Kuehn, Adam, MD {1972608313} PthAcl, Pthlgy(00,NJ05)
+ Urology Care Alliance
  3311 Brunswick Pike   Lawrenceville, NJ 08648   (609)895-1991   Fax (609)895-6996

Kufelnicka, Anna M., MD {1376847517} InfDis
+ Hackensack Meridian Medical Group
  19 Davis Avenue/5th-6th Floor   Neptune, NJ 07753   (732)897-3990   Fax (732)897-3997
+ 81 Pleasant Run Road
  Flemington, NJ 08822

Kuflik, Avery S., MD {1952415705} Dermat(93,IL42)<NJ-COMMED, NJ-KIMBALL>
+ Kuflik Dermatology
  453 Lakehurst Road   Toms River, NJ 08755   (732)341-0515   Fax (732)505-6006
+ Kuflik Dermatology
  150 East Kennedy Boulevard   Lakewood, NJ 08701   (732)341-0515   Fax (732)364-6006
+ Kuflik Dermatology
  63D Lacey Road   Whiting, NJ 08755   (732)849-9444   Fax (732)849-9456

Kuflik, Emanuel G., MD {1467566208} Dermat(63)<NJ-COMMED, NJ-KIMBALL>
+ Kuflik Dermatology
  453 Lakehurst Road   Toms River, NJ 08755   (732)341-0515   Fax (732)505-6006
+ Kuflik Dermatology
  150 East Kennedy Boulevard   Lakewood, NJ 08701   (732)341-0515   Fax (732)364-6006
+ Kuflik Dermatology
  63D Lacey Road   Whiting, NJ 08755   (732)849-9444   Fax (732)849-9456

Kuflik, Julianne Helen, MD {1295849065} Dermat, IntrMd(98,IL42)
+ Kuflik Dermatology
  150 East Kennedy Boulevard   Lakewood, NJ 08701   (732)364-0515   Fax (732)364-6006
+ Kuflik Dermatology
  453 Lakehurst Road   Toms River, NJ 08755   (732)364-0515   Fax (732)505-6006
+ Kuflik Dermatology
  63D Lacey Road   Whiting, NJ 08701   (732)849-9444   Fax (732)849-9456

Kugay, Natalya P., MD {1134326655} ObsGyn(73,UKR18)<NJ-MONMOUTH>
+ Monmouth Medical Center
  300 Second Avenue/OB/GYN   Long Branch, NJ 07740   (732)923-6795

Kugler, Edward F., MD {1326093204} ObsGyn(86,MEXI)<NJ-STJOSHOS>
+ Clifton Ob/Gyn Associates
  716 Broad Street/First Floor   Clifton, NJ 07013   (973)754-4141   Fax (973)754-4161

Kuhfahl, Keith Joseph, DO {1609087733} EmrgMd<NJ-VIRTMHBC>
+ Virtua Memorial
  175 Madison Avenue/EmergMed   Mount Holly, NJ 08060   (609)267-0700

Kuhlmann, Sarah Elizabeth, MD {1538430707} EmrgMd<NJ-STBARNMC>
+ St. Barnabas Medical Center
  94 Old Short Hills Road   Livingston, NJ 07039   (973)322-5000

Kuhn, Theresa Marie, MD {1255727707} ObsGyn
+ University Reproductive Association
  185 South Orange Avenue/MSB E-506   Newark, NJ 07103   (973)972-5266   Fax (973)972-4574

Kukafka, Sheldon Jay, MD {1982600607} CdvDis(92,NY08)<NJ-STPETER, NJ-RWJUBRUN>
+ RWJPE/New Brunswick Cardiology Group, P.A.
  75 Veronica Road/Suite 101   Somerset, NJ 08873   (732)247-7444   Fax (732)247-5119
+ RWJPE New Brunswick Cardiology Group, P.A.
  111 Union Valley Road/Suite 201   Monroe Township, NJ 08831   (732)247-7444   Fax (609)409-6882
+ RWJPE New Brunswick Cardiology Group, P.A.
  15H Briar Hill Court   East Brunswick, NJ 08873   (732)613-9313

Kukla, Leon F., MD {1871506576} PedInf, Pedtrc(66,NJ05)
+ Drs Khanna & Kukla MDs
  817 Inman Avenue   Edison, NJ 08820   (732)381-8600   Fax (732)381-8690
+ 1503 St. Georges Avenue
  Colonia, NJ 07067   (732)381-2273

Kukreja, Meenakshi, MD {1740318559} GenPrc, PhysMd, FamMed(73,INDI)
+ 35-37 Progress Street/Suite B5
  Edison, NJ 08820   (908)755-0550

Kulak, David, MD {1114208725} Gyneco
+ Rutgers- New Jersey Medical School
  185 South Orange Avenue/E-561   Newark, NJ 07103   (973)972-5136

Kulczycki, Alexander, MD {1992932248} IntrMd
+ Ocean County Family Care
  27 South Cooks Bridge Road   Jackson, NJ 08527   (732)364-3881   Fax (732)364-4625
+ Ocean County Family Care
  9 Mule Road   Toms River, NJ 08755   (732)364-3881   Fax (732)818-7775
+ Ocean County Family Care
  2125 Route 88 East   Brick, NJ 08527   (732)892-4548   Fax (732)892-0961

Kulessa-Dussias, Renata, DO {1972582336} PhysMd, FamMed, IntrMd(95,NJ75)
+ The Wholeistic You, LLC.
  335 East Main Street   Somerville, NJ 08876   (908)864-4200   Fax (908)864-4201

Kulesza, Elizabeth Ann, MD {1043236466} IntrMd, Nephro(79,MEX03)
+ 7 Stem Brook Road
  Montvale, NJ 07645   (201)476-0196

Kulesza-Galvez, Theodora, MD {1013323450} FamMed
+ MedExpress Urgent Care Lodi
  184 Essex Street   Lodi, NJ 07644   (201)843-3207   Fax (201)843-3215

Kulik, Alfred D., MD {1518043165} Ophthl, IntrMd(87,NJ06)<NJ-ENGLWOOD>
+ 1 Bridge Plaza North/2nd Floor
  Fort Lee, NJ 07024   (201)346-3937   Fax (201)944-0099   askdrkulik@kulikmd.com

Kulikova-Schupak, Romana, MD {1245263441} NrlgSpec(92,CZE01)
+ 114 Essex Street/3rd Floor
  Rochelle Park, NJ 07662   (201)845-0055   meds@njneurology.com

Kulin, John C., DO {1720024482} EmrgMd(91,MO79)<NJ-SOCEANCO>
+ Southern Ocean County Medical Center
  1140 Route 72 West/EmergMed   Manahawkin, NJ 08050   (609)597-6011

Kulischenko, Alexander W., MD {1447204565} IntrMd(81,DOM15)<NJ-RWJUBRUN, NJ-STPETER>
+ Drs. Kulischenko & Kulischenko
  495 Ryders Lane   East Brunswick, NJ 08816   (732)613-9155   Fax (732)651-0804

Kulischenko, Idelma, MD {1679527790} IntrMd(81,DOM15)
+ Drs. Kulischenko & Kulischenko
  495 Ryders Lane   East Brunswick, NJ 08816   (732)613-9155   Fax (732)651-0804

Kulkarni, Anand U., MD {1063418655} CdvDis, IntrMd(81,INDI)<NJ-STPETER, NJ-RWJUBRUN>
+ RWJPE/New Brunswick Cardiology Group, P.A.
  75 Veronica Road/Suite 101   Somerset, NJ 08873   (732)247-7444   Fax (732)247-5119
+ RWJPE New Brunswick Cardiology Group, P.A.
  111 Union Valley Road/Suite 201   Monroe Township, NJ 08831   (732)247-7444   Fax (609)409-6882
+ RWJPE New Brunswick Cardiology Group, P.A.
  15H Briar Hill Court   East Brunswick, NJ 08873   (732)613-9313

Kulkarni, Jyothi, MD {1689608168} IntrMd, IntHos(94,INA35)<NJ-VALLEY>
+ The Valley Hospital
  223 North Van Dien Avenue/IntMed   Ridgewood, NJ 07450   (201)447-8000

Kulkarni, Kedar, MD {1588620686} RadNro, RadDia(89,INA67)
+ Radiology Affiliates of Central New Jersey, P.A.
  2501 Kuser Road   Hamilton, NJ 08691   (609)585-8800   Fax (609)585-1825

Kulkarni, Miriam L., MD {1871758359} EmrgMd(04,NJ06)<NJ-UMDNJ>
+ University Hospital
  150 Bergen Street/EmrgMed/M-12   Newark, NJ 07103   (973)972-4300

Kulkarni, Mohan H., MD {1891856878} Anesth(67,INA69)<NJ-STBARNMC>
+ St. Barnabas Medical Center
  94 Old Short Hills Road   Livingston, NJ 07039   (973)322-5000

Kulkarni, Nandini N., MD {1598929218} Surgry
+ AtlantiCare Physician Group
  1601 Tilton Road/Suite 4   Northfield, NJ 08225   (609)568-5606   Fax (609)303-2482
+ Court House Surgery Center
  106 Courthouse South Dennis Rd   Cape May, NJ 08204   (609)568-5606   Fax (609)463-3224

Kulkarni, Prashant P., MD {1215124979} Anesth
+ Red Bank Anesthesia, LLC
  1 Riverview Plaza   Red Bank, NJ 07701   (732)530-2255   Fax (732)450-2620

Kulkarni, Pratibha A., MD {1306867478} IntrMd(77,INDI)<NJ-STBARNMC>
+ 297 Walnut Street
  Livingston, NJ 07039   (973)373-4023
+ 320 Union Avenue
  Irvington, NJ 07111   (973)373-4023

Kulkarni, Rachana A., MD {1912971185} CdvDis, IntrMd(89,INDI)<NJ-MORRISTN, NJ-SOMERSET>
+ Medicor Cardiology PA
  225 Jackson Street   Bridgewater, NJ 08807   (908)526-8668   Fax (908)231-6781
+ Medicor Cardiology PA
  331 US Highway 206/Suite 1A   Hillsborough, NJ 08844   (908)526-8668   Fax (908)431-0808

Kulkarni, Renuka Sanjay, MD {1316169428}<NJ-STBARNMC>
+ St. Barnabas Medical Center
  94 Old Short Hills Road   Livingston, NJ 07039   (973)322-5000

Kulkarni, Sumedha V., MD {1538126537} Anesth(66,INDI)
+ Englewood Anesthesiology
  350 Engle Street   Englewood, NJ 07631   (201)894-3238   Fax (201)894-0585
+ Hackensack University MC-Anesthesia Dept
  30 Prospect Avenue/Room 2703   Hackensack, NJ 07601   (201)894-3238   Fax (201)996-3962

Kulkarni, Vijaykumar A., MD {1184681173} Surgry(66,INDI)<NJ-HOBUNIMC>
+ North Jersey Surgical Group PA
  6040 Kennedy Boulevard East/Suite L-7   West New York, NJ 07093   (201)861-0720   Fax (201)861-5560

Kull, Elizabeth J., MD {1912391046} PhysMd
+ Linwood Care Center
  201 New Road   Linwood, NJ 08221   (609)927-6131

Kullmann, Valerie L., MD {1932179447} Pedtrc, IntrMd(89,NJ06)<NJ-UNVMCPRN>
+ Princeton Nassau Pediatrics, P.A.
  196 Princeton-Hightstown Road   West Windsor, NJ 08550   (609)799-5335   Fax (609)799-2294
+ Princeton Nassau Pediatrics, P.A.
  312 Applegarth Road/Suite 104   Monroe Township, NJ 08831   (609)799-5335   Fax (609)409-5610

Kulper, Bernard J., MD {1063499218} Hemato, Onclgy, OncHem(79,MEXI)
+ Gregory Shypula MD PA
  1030 St. Georges Avenue/Suite 307   Avenel, NJ 07001   (732)750-1200   Fax (732)602-4044
+ Gregory Shypula MD PA
  2045 Route 35 South/Suite 202   South Amboy, NJ 08879   (732)750-1200   Fax (732)602-4044

Kulwatdanaporn, Somchai, MD {1225255243} ObsGyn, Gyneco(71,THA04)
+ 645 Broadway
  Paterson, NJ 07514   (973)742-2077   Fax (973)881-0439

Kumar, Ajay, MD {1871545111} PhysMd(91,INA30)
+ 10 Sunrise Drive
  Parsippany, NJ 07054

Physicians by Name and Address

Kumar, Akshat, MD {1962767764} IntrMd
+ St. Peter's Family Health
   123 How Lane   New Brunswick, NJ 08901   (732)745-8600   Fax (732)729-0869
+ St. Peter's University Hospital
   254 Easton Avenue   New Brunswick, NJ 08901   (408)800-8443

Kumar, Anand, MD {1932289915} IntrMd, InfDis, CritCr(86,ON02)<NJ-COOPRUMC>
+ Cooper University Hospital
   One Cooper Plaza/Dorrance 372A   Camden, NJ 08103   (856)342-3084   Fax (856)968-7420   anand.kumar@cooperhealth.org

Kumar, Anand K., MD {1912964875} IntrMd(71,INA04)
+ St. Joseph's Family Health Center
   21 Market Street   Paterson, NJ 07501   (973)754-4200   Fax (973)754-4201

Kumar, Anita Kiran, MD {1518133313} Pedtrc(91,INA68)
+ Child Health Associates
   666 Plainsboro Road/Suite 1300   Plainsboro, NJ 08536   (609)750-1521   Fax (609)750-1523

Kumar, Anshul, MD {1558674226} IntrMd(01,INA14)
+ Cumberland Nephrology Associates, PA
   1318 South Main Road   Vineland, NJ 08360   (856)205-9900   Fax (856)205-0041

Kumar, Arun S., MD {1114077211} Otlryg(95,INA77)<NJ-CENTRAST>
+ Freehold ENT Associates, PA
   222 Schanck Road   Freehold, NJ 07728   (732)431-1666   Fax (732)431-1665

Kumar, Arvind, MD {1356357479} IntrMd, MedOnc, OncHem(84,DOM02)
+ Oncology & Hematology Associates
   2177 Oak Tree Road/Suite 104   Edison, NJ 08820   (908)755-1165   Fax (908)755-2093

Kumar, Ashok, MD {1962438036} CdvDis, IntrMd(71,INA07)<NJ-RWJUBRUN, NJ-STPETER>
+ Drs. Kumar and Kumar
   75 Brunswick Woods Drive/Building L   East Brunswick, NJ 08816   (732)254-1450   Fax (732)613-8525
+ RWJ University Hospital New Brunswick
   One Robert Wood Johnson Place   New Brunswick, NJ 08901   (732)828-3000

Kumar, Awani, MD {1497720635} PulDis, IntrMd, CritCr(87,INA3C)<NJ-KIMBALL, NJ-COMMED>
+ 780 Route 37 West/Suite 110
   Toms River, NJ 08755   Awanikumar2000@yahoo.com

Kumar, Chitra, MD {1083663496} IntrMd, OncHem(76,INDI)<NJ-PALISADE, NJ-CHRIST>
+ 5311 Boulevard E
   West New York, NJ 07093   (201)864-7172   Fax (201)864-5599

Kumar, Geeta L., DO {1992706311} Pedtrc(97,NJ75)<NJ-HACKNSK, NJ-HOLYNAME>
+ Bridge Pediatrics
   2175 Lemoine Avenue/Suite 502   Fort Lee, NJ 07024   (201)585-7337   Fax (201)585-7333

Kumar, Geetha, MD {1326010349} PsyCAd, Psychy(75,INA68)<NJ-KMHTURNV, NJ-KMHSTRAT>
+ 42 East Laurel Road/Suite 3610
   Stratford, NJ 08084

Kumar, Harini C., MD {1821380940} FamMed(08,NJ06)
+ Center for Family Health
   122-132 Clinton Street   Hoboken, NJ 07030   (201)418-3131   Fax (201)418-3148

Kumar, Kusum Lata, MD {1871516443} IntrMd
+ 27 Palmer Circle
   Perrineville, NJ 08535   (732)446-0583

Kumar, Mark Hemanth, MD {1114929395} Surgry, SrgVas(96,VA01)<NJ-OVERLOOK, NJ-STBARNMC>
+ The Cardiovascular Care Group
   433 Central Avenue   Westfield, NJ 07090   (908)490-1699   Fax (908)490-1698
+ The Cardiovascular Care Group
   1401 Broad Street/Suite 1   Clifton, NJ 07013   (908)490-1699   Fax (973)751-3730

Kumar, Mary Ann M., MD {1730340167} FamMed
+ Complete Care Family Medicine
   75 West Red Bank Avenue   Woodbury, NJ 08096   (856)853-2055   Fax (856)848-2879

Kumar, Mehandar, MD {1790082550} OncHem<NJ-STJOSHOS>
+ St. Joseph's Regional Medical Center
   703 Main Street/HemoOnc/3rd Fl   Paterson, NJ 07503   (908)400-5868   mehandarkumar84@gmail.com

Kumar, Monica Puri, MD ObsGyn(90,MA05)<NJ-CHSMRCER>
+ 5 Drinking Brook Road
   Monmouth Junction, NJ 08852

Kumar, Moses, MD {1104052430} RadV&I
+ 132 Linda Lane
   Edison, NJ 08820

Kumar, Nidhi, MD {1124286588} CdvDis, IntrMd(03,NJ06)<NJ-UMDNJ>
+ Drs. Kumar and Kumar
   75 Brunswick Woods Drive/Building L   East Brunswick, NJ 08816   (732)254-1690   Fax (732)613-8525

Kumar, Nirmal A., MD {1538116983} Anesth, PainMd(64,INDI)<NJ-CENTRAST>
+ Liberty Anesthesia & Pain Management
   901 West Main Street/2nd Floor   Freehold, NJ 07728   (732)294-2876   Fax (732)294-2502
+ CentraState Medical Center
   901 West Main Street/Anesth   Freehold, NJ 07728   (732)294-2875

Kumar, Nisha Iyer, MD {1710226568} IntHos, IntrMd(05,INA7Z)
+ Advocare Haddonfield Pediatric Association
   220 North Haddon Avenue   Haddonfield, NJ 08033   (856)429-6719   Fax (856)429-6748

Kumar, Preethi, DO {1205222437} FamMed
+ Medical Institute of New Jersey
   11 Saddle Road   Cedar Knolls, NJ 07927   (973)267-2122   Fax (973)267-3478

Kumar, Puneet, MD {1194968438} FamMed(95,NJ05)<NJ-JFKMED>
+ 136 Chestnut Street
   Dumont, NJ 07628   (917)439-8240   Fax (856)346-6005   punetkumarmd@gmail.com

Kumar, Radha, MD {1174539373} IntrMd(90,INDI)<NJ-JFKMED, NJ-RWJURAH>
+ Edison Medical Associates, LLC
   34-36 Progress Street/Suite A-2   Edison, NJ 08820   (908)226-0600   Fax (908)226-1802

Kumar, Radhika Lingam, MD {1427137470} Ophthl, IntrMd(05,OH06)
+ Eye Surgeons of North Jersey, LLC
   199 Broad Street/Suite 2-B   Bloomfield, NJ 07003   (973)748-3300   Fax (973)748-3802
+ Eye Surgeons of North Jersey, LLC
   27 Baker Avenue   Dover, NJ 07801   (973)748-3300   Fax (973)328-1265

Kumar, Rahul, MD {1861690554} IntrMd<PA-YORK>
+ Cardiac & Arrhythmias Specialist
   905 Allwood Road/Suite 103   Clifton, NJ 07013   (973)778-3111   Fax (973)340-1518

Kumar, Rajat, MD {1356541320} VasNeu, Nrolgy(06,GRN01)<NJ-LOURDMED>
+ Capital Institute for Neurosciences
   2 Capital Way/Suite 456   Pennington, NJ 08534   (609)537-7300   Fax (609)537-7301

Kumar, Ramesh, MD {1114000114} Rheuma(85,INA41)
+ Stafford Medical, P.A.
   1364 Route 72 West/Suite 5   Manahawkin, NJ 08050   (609)597-3416   Fax (609)597-9608

Kumar, Rekha A., MD GenPrc(74,INA04)<NJ-STMRYPAS>
+ St. Mary's Hospital
   350 Boulevard   Passaic, NJ 07055   (973)365-4300

Kumar, Renuka, MD {1598874786} IntrMd(72,INA72)<NJ-VA-LYONS>
+ VA New Jersey Health Care System at Lyons
   151 Knollcroft Road   Lyons, NJ 07939   (908)647-0180   Fax (908)607-6367

Kumar, Ritesh, MD {1699037382} IntrMd<NJ-CHILTON>
+ Chilton Medical Center
   97 West Parkway/Internal Med   Pompton Plains, NJ 07444   (973)831-5000

Kumar, Sadhana, MD {1225065634} IntrMd, Nephro(78,INDI)<NJ-STCLRDOV, NJ-EASTORNG>
+ 362 Parsippany Road/Suite 3A
   Parsippany, NJ 07054   (973)515-0777   Fax (973)515-8243

Kumar, Sanjay, MD {1437120920} IntrMd(90,INA88)
+ Professional Associates of Jackson, LLC
   2105 West County Line Road/Suite 4   Jackson, NJ 08527   (732)367-7575   Fax (732)364-0600

Kumar, Sanjay, MD {1295938496} SrgVas, Surgry(00,DMN01)<NJ-SJHREGMC, NJ-SJRSYELM>
+ Inspira Medical Group Surgical Associates
   1102 East Chestnut Avenue   Vineland, NJ 08360   (856)213-6375   Fax (856)575-4986

Kumar, Tarun, MD {1346235926} IntrMd(82,INDI)<NJ-CLARMAAS>
+ Clara Maass Medical Center
   1 Clara Maass Drive   Belleville, NJ 07109   (973)450-2000

Kumar, Uday, MD {1508886540} InfDis, IntrMd
+ 1553 Route 27/Suite 2100
   Somerset, NJ 08873   (908)429-5755

Kumar, Vinod, MD {1821544115} IntrMd<NJ-STJOSHOS>
+ St. Joseph's Regional Medical Center
   703 Main Street   Paterson, NJ 07503   (973)754-2000

Kumar Shetty, Nagalakshmi Ashok, MD {1710260039} Rheuma
+ Coastal HealthCare
   44 Nautilus Drive/Suite 2A   Manahawkin, NJ 08050   (609)597-4178   Fax (609)597-4387

Kumarasamy, Narmadan Akileswaran, MD {1083900575} RadDia
+ Hackensack Radiology Group, P.A.
   30 Prospect Avenue   Hackensack, NJ 07601   (551)996-2200   Fax (201)489-2812

Kumaresan, Arulnangai, MD {1427102557} OncHem, IntrMd(94,SRI03)<NJ-BAYONNE>
+ Bayonne Medical Center
   29th Street at Avenue E/Hema Oncology   Bayonne, NJ 07002   (201)858-5000   Arul_kumaresan@yahoo.com

Kumari, Kalpana, MD {1477703239} Pedtrc(93,INA54)
+ 908 Oak Tree Road/Suite C
   South Plainfield, NJ 07080   (908)205-0632   Fax (908)205-0629

Kumari, Ruchi, MD {1538486337}<NJ-UMDNJ>
+ University Hospital
   150 Bergen Street   Newark, NJ 07103   (973)972-6056

Kumpta, Shilpa Narsing, MD {1205115607} PedEnd(12,OK01)
+ VMG-Pediatric Endocrinology
   140 East Ridgewood avenue/Suite N280   Paramus, NJ 07652   (201)447-8182   Fax (201)523-9365

Kumta, Jayshree N., MD {1487666269} Pedtrc(91,INA69)<NJ-STBARNMC>
+ St. Barnabas Medical Center
   94 Old Short Hills Road/Pediatrics   Livingston, NJ 07039   (973)322-5000

Kunac, Anastasia, MD {1184948861} SrgCrC, Surgry<NJ-UMDNJ>
+ University Hospital
   150 Bergen Street/Surgery/Criticl   Newark, NJ 07103   (973)972-4900

Kunamneni, Katie Elizabeth, MD {1164620001} IntrMd
+ Windsor Regional Medical Associates, LLC
   300A Princeton-Hightstown Road   East Windsor, NJ 08520   (609)490-0095   Fax (609)490-0091

Kunamneni, Raghu Krishna, MD {1750432720} OncHem, IntrMd(02,GRN01)<NY-LENOXHLL, NJ-JRSYSHMC>
+ Regional Cancer Care Associates, LLC
   4632 US Highway 9   Howell, NJ 07731   (732)367-1535   Fax (732)367-9514

Kung, John S., MD {1497857080} Ophthl, IntrMd(90,NY47)<NY-NYEYEINF, NJ-STPETER>
+ Staten Island Ophthalmology & Academic Eye Center
   192 Summerhill Road   East Brunswick, NJ 08816   (732)257-4900
+ Campus Eye Group & Laser Center
   1700 Whitehorse Hamilton Sq Rd   Hamilton Square, NJ 08690   (732)257-4900   Fax (609)588-9545

Kunjukutty, Felix, MD {1538311154} IntrMd
+ IPC The Hospitalist Company
   220 Ridgedale Avenue/Suite C-2   Florham Park, NJ 07932   (973)538-5844   Fax (973)267-0181

Kunkle, Herbert Lemuel, Jr., MD {1891724076} SrgOrt(79,PA09)
+ Hackensack Meridian Health Orthopedic Surgery
   1173 Beacon Avenue/Suite A   Manahawkin, NJ 08050   (609)250-4101   Fax (609)978-4860

Kuntz, Andrew Frederic, MD {1184784001} SrgOrt, IntCrd(05,VA01)<PA-UPMCPHL>
+ Penn Medicine at Cherry Hill
   409 Route 70 East/Surgery/Ortho   Cherry Hill, NJ 08034   (856)429-1519

Kuntz, George R., MD {1962556233} CritCr, IntrMd(94,NJ06)<NJ-STBARNMC>
+ Lincoln P. Miller, MD, LLC
   1500 Pleasant Valley Way/Suite 201   West Orange, NJ 07052   (973)966-6400   Fax (973)514-1587

Kuo, David, MD {1316910722} IntrMd(93,RI01)<NJ-MORRISTN, NJ-OVERLOOK>
+ Morristown Medical Center Family Medicine
   435 South Street/Suite 350   Morristown, NJ 07960   (973)971-4222   Fax (973)401-2465
+ Internal Medicine Faculty Associates
   435 South Street/Suite 350   Morristown, NJ 07962   (973)971-7165

Kuo, Douglas, DO {1881894285} PhysMd(03,PA77)
+ Rehabilitation Specialists of New Jersey
   505 Goffle Road/Suite 3   Ridgewood, NJ 07450   (201)447-4772   Fax (201)447-4277
+ 370 West Pleasantview Avenue
   Hackensack, NJ 07601   (201)562-2203

Kuo, Eugenia C., MD {1558680561} ObsGyn
+ Physicians for Womens Health
   1124 East Ridgewood Avenue/Suite 105   Ridgewood, NJ 07450   (201)489-2255   Fax (201)489-4799

Kuo, Grace, MD {1932329489} Pedtrc(94,RI01)
+ 2231 Lemoine Avenue
   Fort Lee, NJ 07024   (201)944-1008   Fax (201)242-0029

Kuo, Howard, MD {1811905268} SrgNro, Nrolgy(83,CHN57)<NJ-NWRKBETH, NJ-JFKMED>
+ 505 Plainfield Road
   Edison, NJ 08820   (732)452-1188   Fax (732)452-1168

Physicians by Name and Address

Kuo, Michael, MD {1275881054} IntrMd
+ 26 Rawley Place
Millburn, NJ 07041   (917)580-2393
hsianglung77@yahoo.com

Kupershtein, Ilya, MD {1134379340} SrgSpn
+ Summit Medical Group-Berkeley Heights Campus
1 Diamond Hill Road   Berkeley Heights, NJ 07922
(908)277-8646   Fax (908)790-6576

Kupershtok-Bojko, Aviva Sara, MD {1528162278} Nrolgy, Eplpsy, NroChl(85,ITA17)
+ St. Barnabas Health Care Center
95 Old Short Hills Road   West Orange, NJ 07052   (973)322-4033   Fax (973)322-4416
+ St. Barnabas Institute of Neurology & Neurosurgery
200 South Orange Avenue/Suite 101   Livingston, NJ 07039
(973)322-4033   Fax (973)322-7505

Kupersmith, Eric E., MD {1831271261} IntrMd(95,NJ05)<NJ-COOPRUMC>
+ Cooper University Hospital
One Cooper Plaza/IntMed   Camden, NJ 08103   (856)342-2000

Kupetsky, Erine Allison, DO {1952400012} Dermat
+ One Becca Way
Allentown, NJ 08501

Kupfer, Herschel, MD {1003869470} EmrgMd(02,ISR02)<NJ-TRINIWSC>
+ Team Health East
307 South Evergeen Avenue/Suite 201   Woodbury, NJ 08096   (856)686-4300   Fax (856)848-8536

Kupferberg, Stephen Benjamin, MD {1447365747} Otlryg(92,PA02)
+ Ocean Otolaryngology Associates
54 Bey Lea Road/Suite 3   Toms River, NJ 08753   (732)281-0100   Fax (732)281-0400

Kuponiyi, Cheryl A., MD {1356381198} Pedtrc(82,NIG01)<NJ-ACMCITY, NJ-ACMCMAIN>
+ Island Medical Associates
2626 Tilton Road   Egg Harbor Township, NJ 08234
(609)568-5000   Fax (609)568-5010
+ Island Medical Associates
16 South Rhode Island Ave   Atlantic City, NJ 08401
(609)568-5000   Fax (609)449-8002

Kuponiyi, Olatunji P., MD {1285674010} IntrMd, Addctn(81,NIG01)<NJ-ACMCITY, NJ-ACMCMAIN>
+ Island Medical Associates
2626 Tilton Road   Egg Harbor Township, NJ 08234
(609)568-5000   Fax (609)568-5010
+ Island Medical Associates
16 South Rhode Island Ave   Atlantic City, NJ 08401
(609)568-5000   Fax (609)449-8002

Kuptsow, Scott Warren, DO {1922048941} FamMed(93,PA77)<NJ-VIRTVOOR, NJ-KMHTURNV>
+ Advocare Family Medicine Associates Vineland
602 West Sherman Avenue/Suite B   Vineland, NJ 08360
(856)692-8484   Fax (856)896-3059
+ Advocare Family Medicine Associates Mt. Laurel
3115 Route 38/Suite 200B   Mount Laurel, NJ 08054
(856)692-8484   Fax (856)231-7543
+ Advocare Family Medicine Associates Williamstown
979 North Black Horse Pike   Williamstown, NJ 08360
(856)629-5151   Fax (856)629-0281

Kurani, Amit P., MD {1770707986} Psychy(00,INA65)
+ Center for Family Guidance, PC
765 East Route 70/Building A-101   Marlton, NJ 08053
(856)797-4800   Fax (856)810-0110

Kurani, Devendra, MD {1598875734} Psychy(76,INDI)<NJ-STBARNMC, NJ-CHRIST>
+ Palisades Behavioral Care
221 Palisade Avenue   Jersey City, NJ 07306   (201)656-3116   Fax (201)656-9044

Kuras, Yuri, MD {1841233996} Anesth(89,RUS66)<NJ-STCLRDEN, PA-GSNGER>
+ St. Clare's Hospital-Denville Campus
25 Pocono Road/Anesthesiology   Denville, NJ 07834
(973)625-6000

Kurdali, Basil, MD {1255570925} IntrMd<NJ-NWRKBETH>
+ Newark Beth Israel Medical Center
201 Lyons Avenue/IntrnMed   Newark, NJ 07112   (973)926-8407   Fax (973)926-6130

Kurer, Cheryl C., MD {1245252790} Pedtrc, PedCrd(83,NY47)<NJ-HACKNSK, PA-CHILDHOS>
+ The Pediatric Center for Heart Disease
155 Polifly Road/Suite 106   Hackensack, NJ 07601
(201)487-7617   Fax (201)342-5341
+ CHOP Pediatric & Adolescent Specialty Care Center
707 Alexander Road/Suite 205   Princeton, NJ 08540
(609)520-1717

Kuriakose, Julie Susan, MD {1023242377} AlgyImmn
+ Easton Med
1174 Easton Avenue   Somerset, NJ 08873   (732)354-0159   Fax (732)354-0147

Kuriakose, Marykutty K., MD {1194738369} IntrMd, EmrgMd(77,INA94)<NJ-STPETER>
+ Easton Med
1174 Easton Avenue   Somerset, NJ 08873   (732)354-0159
Fax (732)354-0147

Kurian, Helena, MD {1457580144} IntrMd
+ Hackensack Medical Center-Internal Medicine
30 Prospect Avenue/4 Main/Rm 4621   Hackensack, NJ 07601   (201)996-3664   Fax (551)996-0536

Kurien, Abby V., MD {1982741911} Psychy(92,INA08)<NJ-VAEASTOR>
+ 83 Edgewood Avenue
West Orange, NJ 07052

Kuris, Jay D., MD {1003997453} Psychy(69,LA01)<NJ-UNVMCPRN, NJ-HUNTRDN>
+ 28 Mine Street
Flemington, NJ 08822   (908)788-5551   Fax (908)788-0019
jkuris@aol.com
+ 43 Tamarack Circle
Skillman, NJ 08558   (609)497-1118

Kuriyan, Mercy Achamma, MD {1467538108} BldBnk, PthACl(70,INDI)<NJ-RWJUBRUN>
+ UH- Robert Wood Johnson Med
125 Paterson Street/MEB 232   New Brunswick, NJ 08901
(732)235-7985   Fax (732)235-8124
+ RWJ University Hospital Somerset
110 Rehill Avenue   Somerville, NJ 08876   (732)235-7985
Fax (908)685-2543

Kurkowski, Ellen J., DO {1871720649} EmrgMd
+ Rowan University-School of Osteopathic Medicine
1 Medical Center Drive/Suite 162   Stratford, NJ 08084
(856)566-7050

Kurnick, Warren S., MD {1841290053} Dermat(74,PA01)<NJ-VIRTMHBC>
+ Warren S. Kurnick MD Dermatology Group PA
215 Sunset Road/Suite 102   Willingboro, NJ 08046
(609)871-9500   Fax (609)871-7590
wkurnick@hotmail.com

Kurnik, Brenda R., MD {1730180555} IntrMd, Nephro(78,MO02)<NJ-COOPRUMC>
+ The Cooper Hospital System-Univ Hospital
3 Cooper Plaza/Suite 215   Camden, NJ 08103   (856)342-2439
+ Cooper Cardiology Associates
900 Centennial Boulevard   Voorhees, NJ 08043   (856)342-2439   Fax (856)325-6702
+ Cooper Cardiology Associates
1210 Brace Road/Suite 103   Cherry Hill, NJ 08103
(856)427-7254

Kurnik, Peter B., MD {1396703716} CdvDis, IntrMd(78,MO02)<NJ-COOPRUMC>
+ University Cardiology
3 Cooper Plaza/Room 311   Camden, NJ 08103   (856)342-2034

Kurra, Padmavathy, MD {1205949468} Psychy, PsyGrt(79,INDI)<NJ-RAMAPO>
+ Kurra Associates
15-01 Broadway/Suite 10-B   Fair Lawn, NJ 07410
(201)794-7733   Fax (201)794-6039

Kurtz, Joel H., MD {1205882578} Gastrn, IntrMd(83,NJ06)
+ Gastroenterology Associates
475 State Highway 70   Lakewood, NJ 08701   (732)886-1007   Fax (732)224-8773
+ Gastroenterology Associates
150 Route 37 West/Suite B5   Toms River, NJ 08755
(732)886-1007   Fax (732)244-8773

Kurugundla, Navatha, MD {1497999544} PulDis
+ 2069 Klockner Road
Hamilton, NJ 08690   Fax (609)586-0708

Kurz, Jeremiah S., MD {1124040316} Gastrn, IntrMd(00,NY46)
+ Forest HealthCare Associates, PC
277 Forest Avenue/Suite 200   Paramus, NJ 07652
(201)986-1881   Fax (201)986-1871
+ Drs. Kurz and Rodriguez
318 East Westfield Ave   Roselle Park, NJ 07204   (201)986-1881   Fax (908)245-2384

Kurz, Lisa Beth, MD {1487886875} Pedtrc(09,ISR02)
+ Whole Child Center
690 Kinderkamack Road/Suite 102   Oradell, NJ 07649
(201)634-1600   Fax (201)634-1606

Kushal, Amrita, MD {1679898746} CdvDis
+ Drs. Rudnitzky & Shugar PA
98 James Street/Suite 104   Edison, NJ 08820   (212)434-2170   Fax (212)434-2111

Kushner, Beth Jillian, DO {1972943546} EmrgMd
+ St Joseph's Medical Center Emergency
703 Main Street   Paterson, NJ 07503   (973)754-2000   Fax (973)754-2249

Kushner, Evan G., MD {1538108568} Grtrcs, IntrMd(86,NY15)<NJ-HACKNSK, NJ-VALLEY>
+ Forest HealthCare Associates, PC
277 Forest Avenue/Suite 200   Paramus, NJ 07652
(201)986-1881   Fax (201)986-1871

Kushner, Randy Scott, DO {1437192564} Anesth, AnesPain(84,PA77)<NJ-OURLADY>
+ Our Lady of Lourdes Medical Center
1600 Haddon Avenue/Anesthesiology   Camden, NJ 08103
(856)757-3836

Kushner, Susan C., MD {1093783615} Pedtrc(86,NY15)<NJ-HACKNSK, NJ-VALLEY>
+ Forest Pediatrics PA
299 Forest Avenue   Paramus, NJ 07652   (201)267-0888
Fax (201)483-8874

Kushnir, Alla, MD {1881852267} NnPnMd
+ Cooper Neonatology
One Cooper Plaza   Camden, NJ 08103   (856)342-2265
Fax (856)342-8007

Kushnir, Leon, MD {1003075755} Surgry(04,NY15)<NJ-SJHREGMC, NJ-SJRSYELM>
+ Inspira Medical Group Surgical Associates
1102 East Chestnut Avenue   Vineland, NJ 08360   (856)213-6375   Fax (856)575-4986
leonkushnir@yahoo.com

Kusick, Joseph William, DO {1801116736}<NJ-DEBRAHLC>
+ Deborah Heart and Lung Center
200 Trenton Road   Browns Mills, NJ 08015   (609)893-6610

Kusmaul, Danielle Marie, DO {1467658104} EmrgMd<NJ-KMHSTRAT>
+ Emergency Physician Associates, P.A.
307 South Evergreen Avenue/PO Box 298   Woodbury, NJ 08096   (856)848-3817   Fax (856)848-1431
+ Kennedy Memorial Hospital-University Medical Center
18 East Laurel Road/EmrgMed   Stratford, NJ 08084
(856)346-6000

Kusnetz, Eliot M., MD {1023187945} OccpMd(91,MI01)
+ Total Care Occupational Medicine
370 Campus Drive   Somerset, NJ 08873   (732)748-1900
Fax (732)748-1907
EKUSNETZ@TCOMOCCMED.COM

Kusnierz, Earl I., DO {1902985336} ObsGyn, Gyneco(80,IA75)<NJ-CLARMAAS>
+ Bloomfield Ob-Gyn
350 Bloomfield Avenue/Suite 6   Bloomfield, NJ 07003
(973)743-4748   Fax (973)743-8968

Kusnierz, James L., DO {1932269354} ObsGyn(78,IA75)<NJ-STBARNMC>
+ 855 Grove Street
Irvington, NJ 07111   (973)399-8777   Fax (973)443-0267
Jlkdopa@optonlide.net
+ 81 Northfield Avenue
West Orange, NJ 07052   (973)731-1313

Kusseluk, Eric, MD {1235283367} Dermat(03,PA02)
+ Michele Grodberg, MD & Associates
106 Grand Avenue/Suite 330   Englewood, NJ 07631
(201)567-8884   Fax (201)567-5799

Kussick, Neil J., MD {1245233865} Anesth(93,NJ05)
+ Morris Anesthesia Group, PA
3799 Route 46/Suite 211   Parsippany, NJ 07054   (973)335-1122   Fax (973)335-1448

Kutikov, Jessica K., MD {1114027323} Pedtrc(03,PA01)<NJ-VIRTVOOR, NJ-VIRTMHBC>
+ Virtua Voorhees
100 Bowman Drive/Pediatrics   Voorhees, NJ 08043
(856)325-4421   Fax (856)325-3157
+ Virtua Memorial
175 Madison Avenue/Pediatrics   Mount Holly, NJ 08060
(609)267-0700

Kutko, Martha C., MD {1740251347} Pedtrc(95,NJ05)<NJ-HACKNSK>
+ Hackensack University Medical Center
30 Prospect Avenue/Ped-ICU   Hackensack, NJ 07601
(201)996-2535   Fax (201)996-4398

Kutlu, Hakan M., MD {1164497301} SrgPlstc(88,NY01)<NJ-MORRISTN, NJ-STCLRDEN>
+ 95 Madison Avenue/4th Floor
Morristown, NJ 07960   (973)644-3555   Fax (973)644-3556

Kutner, Donald H., DO {1477522712} Gastrn, IntrMd(77,IA75)<NJ-VALLEY>
+ Gastroenterology Associates of New Jersey
15-01 Broadway/Suite 34   Fair Lawn, NJ 07410   (201)794-6808   Fax (201)797-6238
kutnerdh@aol.com

Kutner, Matthew Alexander, DO {1639469794} Gastrn
+ University Hospital-Doctors Office Center
90 Bergen Street   Newark, NJ 07103   (973)972-2500   Fax (973)972-2510

Kutscher, Austin Harrison, Jr., MD {1467405001} CdvDis, IntrMd(75,NY01)<NJ-HUNTRDN>
+ Hunterdon Cardiovascular Associates
1100 Wescott Drive/Suite G-3 Flemington, NJ 08822
(908)788-6471   Fax (908)788-6460
+ Hunterdon Cardiovascular Associates
1738 Route 31/Suite 210 Clinton, NJ 08809   (908)788-6471   Fax (908)823-9211

Kutscher, Jeffrey J., MD {1801840665} Gastrn, IntrMd(77,OH06)<NJ-VIRTMHBC, NJ-DEBRAHLC>
+ Gastroenterology Consultants of South Jersey
693 Main Street/Suite 2 Lumberton, NJ 08048   (609)265-1700   Fax (609)265-9005
+ Burlington County Endoscopy Center
140 Mount Holly Bypass/Unit 5 Lumberton, NJ 08048
(609)267-1555

Kutzin, Theodore E., MD {1447334370} Anesth(83,MEX03)<NJ-MERIDNHS>
+ Shrewsbury Surgery Center
655 Shrewsbury Avenue Shrewsbury, NJ 07702   (732)450-6000   Fax (732)450-1798

Kuwama, Chika, MD {1275673907} FamMed(89,JAP47)<NJ-ENGLWOOD>
+ Edgewater Family Care Center
725 River Road/Suite 202 Edgewater, NJ 07020   (201)943-4040   Fax (201)941-4599

Kuye, Olabisi O., MD {1447342944} ObsGyn(99,PA12)<NJ-UMDNJ>
+ PO Box 113
Bogota, NJ 07603

Kuyinu, Michael A., MD {1235173568} Pedtrc(76,NIG02)
+ 561 Cranbury Road/Suite A
East Brunswick, NJ 08816   (732)254-1030   Fax (732)254-2055

Kuza, Malgorzata W., MD {1518967496} IntrMd(77,POLA)
+ New Jersey Veterans Memorial Home - Menlo Park
132 Evergreen Road/PO Box 3013 Edison, NJ 08818
(732)452-4225
+ 5 Clinton Lane
Scotch Plains, NJ 07076   (732)452-4225   Fax (732)634-1811

Kuzbari, Oumar, MD {1215124714} RprEnd
+ South Jersey Fertility Center
400 Lippincott Drive Marlton, NJ 08053   (856)282-1231
Fax (856)596-2411

Kuzmick, Peter J., DO {1194751891} IntrMd(80,MO78)<NJ-MONMOUTH>
+ Sea Girt Medical Associates
235 Route 71 Manasquan, NJ 08736   (732)223-4300   Fax (732)223-5273

Kuznetsov, Maryna, MD {1023375474}<NJ-OVERLOOK>
+ Overlook Medical Center
99 Beauvoir Avenue/PO Box 210 Summit, NJ 07902
(908)522-2065

Kuzyshyn, Halyna, MD {1770854499} Rheuma, IntrMd(01,UKR28)<NJ-COOPRUMC>
+ Hackensack Meridian Medical Group
19 Davis Avenue/5th-6th Floor Neptune, NJ 07753
(732)897-3990   Fax (732)897-3997
+ Cooper University Medical Center/Camden
3 Cooper Plaza/Suite 403 Camden, NJ 08103   (732)897-3990   Fax (856)964-1019
+ Cooper University Medical Center/Camden
3 Cooper Plaza/Suite 104 Camden, NJ 07753   (856)342-2000

Kwak, Andrew, MD {1740489418} RadDia
+ Monmouth Medical Imaging
300 Second Avenue/Radiol Long Branch, NJ 07740
(732)923-6806   Fax (732)923-6006

Kwak, James Jihoon, MD {1578552865} FamMed(01,NJ06)<NJ-VIRTUAHS>
+ Kwak Family Medicine
2301 Evesham Road/Suite 505 Voorhees, NJ 08043
(856)520-8718   Fax (856)520-8719

Kwak, Jinhee, MD {1730115585} RadDia, RadNro(99,NY09)<NJ-OURLADY>
+ Our Lady of Lourdes Medical Center
1600 Haddon Avenue/Radiology Camden, NJ 08103
(856)757-3500
+ Radiology Associates of Burlington County
1295 Route 38 West/PO Box 479 Hainesport, NJ 08036
(856)757-3500   Fax (609)261-4180

Kwak, Steve K., MD {1013131705} SrgOrt
+ North Jersey Orthopaedic Specialists
730 Palisade Avenue Teaneck, NJ 07666   (201)353-9000
Fax (201)530-0003
+ North Jersey Orthopaedic Specialists
106 Grand Avenue Englewood, NJ 07631   (201)353-9000
Fax (201)608-0104

Kwapniewski, Agnieszka Monika, MD {1528007457} IntrMd(94,POL03)
+ Internal Medicine Practice LLC
312 Belleville Turnpike/Suite 1 C North Arlington, NJ 07031
(201)997-4040   Fax (201)997-4040

Kwark, Hyun-Soon Ellen, MD {1487730800} PthDrm(82,KORE)<NY-WESTCHMC>
+ Quest Diagnostics Inc.
1 Malcolm Avenue Teterboro, NJ 07608   (201)393-5000
Fax (201)393-6127

Kwartler, Jed A., MD {1164478152} Otlryg, Otolgy, Neutgy(83,NJ05)<NJ-OVERLOOK, NJ-HACKNSK>
+ Summit Medical Group-Berkeley Heights Campus
1 Diamond Hill Road Berkeley Heights, NJ 07922
(908)277-8681   Fax (908)277-8662

Kwee, Darlene J., MD {1891876496} Dermat(83,TX14)<NJ-UNVM-CPRN>
+ Princeton Medical Group, P.A.
419 North Harrison Street Princeton, NJ 08540   (609)924-9300   Fax (609)924-6552
dkwee@patmedia.net
+ Princeton Medical Group PA
2 Research Way/Bldg 2/Suite 302 Monroe Township, NJ 08831   (609)924-9300   Fax (609)655-7466

Kweon, Chang, MD {1023078730} Anesth(01,PA13)
+ Summit Anesthesia Associates, P.A.
33 Overlook Road/Suite 311 Summit, NJ 07901   (908)598-1500   Fax (908)598-0197

Kwok, Elaine, MD {1710423702} Psychy<NJ-TRININPC>
+ Capital Health System/Fuld Campus
750 Brunswick Avenue Trenton, NJ 08638   (609)394-6085
Fax (609)394-6205
+ Trinitas Regional Medical Center-New Point Campus
655 East Jersey Street Elizabeth, NJ 07206   (718)994-7207

Kwon, Alan Fay, MD {1043224108} Anesth(80,CA02)
+ 11 Eves Drive/Suite 170
Marlton, NJ 08053   (856)797-9600   Fax (856)797-9601

Kwon, Albert O., MD {1225298722} SrgC&R, Surgry, IntrMd(05,RI01)
+ North Jersey Colon & Rectal Surgery Associates, LLC.
85 Harristown Road Glen Rock, NJ 07452   (201)689-9100
Fax (201)689-9108
+ Valley Medical Group Colorectal Surgery
1124 East Ridgewood Avenue/Suite 202 Ridgewood, NJ 07450   (201)689-9100   Fax (201)689-9108

Kwon, Alexander K., MD {1770863904} Psychy, PsyAdd(KOR06)
+ Princeton House Behavioral Health- Moorestown
351 New Albany Road Moorestown, NJ 08057   (856)779-2300   Fax (856)779-2988

Kwon, Christopher J., MD {1326029877} Anesth(92,NJ05)<NJ-MORRISTN>
+ Morristown Medical Center
100 Madison Avenue/Anesthesiology Morristown, NJ 07962   (973)971-5548   Fax (201)943-8733

Kwon, Johnny, MD {1164689956} EmrgMd<NJ-JRSYCITY>
+ Jersey City Medical Center
355 Grand Street Jersey City, NJ 07304   (201)915-2000

Kwon, Minho, MD {1548693310} Anesth
+ Hackensack University MC-Anesthesia Dept
30 Prospect Avenue/Room 2703 Hackensack, NJ 07601
(551)996-2419   Fax (201)996-3962

Kwon, Seri, MD {1922501568} FamMed
+ 67 Carriage Drive
Edison, NJ 08820   (908)510-8415

Kwon, Stephen S., MD {1093702359} RadDia(99,NJ06)<NJ-STJOSHOS>
+ Imaging Subspecialists of North Jersey LLC
703 Main Street Paterson, NJ 07503   (973)754-2645

Kwon, Sung, MD {1447458484} Surgry<NJ-HOLYNAME>
+ Holy Name Hospital
718 Teaneck Road Teaneck, NJ 07666   (201)833-3000

Kwon, Sung Wook, MD {1891767497} Surgry, SrgVas(95,NJ05)<NJ-JRSYSHMC>
+ Jersey Coast Vascular Associates
425 Jack Martin Boulevard/Suite 2 Brick, NJ 08724
(732)202-1500   Fax (732)202-1058

Kwon, Yong Min, MD {1528186384} Gastrn, IntrMd(05,AL02)
+ Gastroenterology Group of NJ, PA
123 Highland Avenue/Suite 103 Glen Ridge, NJ 07028
(973)429-8800   Fax (973)748-7076

Kwon, Yong S., MD {1437110780} Anesth(88,TX02)
+ Summit Anesthesia Associates, P.A.
33 Overlook Road/Suite 311 Summit, NJ 07901   (908)598-1500   Fax (908)598-0197
ysk143@aol.com

Kwong, Jenitta, MD {1184033482} Pedtrc, IntrMd(NJ02
+ Princeton Nassau Pediatrics, P.A.
301 North Harrison Street Princeton, NJ 08540   (609)924-5510   Fax (609)924-3577

Kwong, Kelvin Ming-Tak, MD {1184820201} Otlryg(MI07
+ Drs. Kwong and Vella
10 Plum Street/8th Floor New Brunswick, NJ 08901
(732)235-5530   Fax (732)235-8882
+ Center for Healthy Aging
18 Centre Drive/Suite 104 Monroe Township, NJ 08831

(732)235-5530   Fax (732)235-8882

Kycia, Lan Ing, MD {1760500235} PsyCAd, Psychy(92,NJ05)
+ Neurobehavioral Associates LLC
315 East Northfield Road/Suite 3 A Livingston, NJ 07039
(973)716-0833

Kyi, Myint Myint, MD {1003984733} Anesth(91,MYA04)
+ 402 Hartford Drive
Nutley, NJ 07110

Kyin, Robin, MD {1205094281} Anesth(05,NY08)<NJ-HOBUNIMC>
+ Hoboken University Medical Center
308 Willow Avenue/Anesthesia Hoboken, NJ 07030
(201)418-1600

Kyreakakis, Anthony J., MD {1659382349} CdvDis(79,MEXI)<NJ-HOBUNIMC>
+ 604 Wilow Avenue
Hoboken, NJ 07030   (201)659-3311   Fax (201)795-0924

Kyreakakis, George J., MD {1093753170} ObsGyn(79,GREE)<NJ-HOBUNIMC, NJ-PALISADE>
+ 24 Cedar Court
Marlboro, NJ 07746   (732)625-1037

La Couture, Tamara A., MD {1740287721} Radiol, RadThp(94,NJ05)
+ 21st Century Oncology
220 Sunset Road/Suite 4 Willingboro, NJ 08046   (609)877-3064   Fax (609)877-2466

La Forgia, Anthony Pantal, MD {1255324364} Psychy(95,NJ05)
+ 108 Alden Street
Cranford, NJ 07016   (908)497-3975

La Monaca, Anthony G., MD {1982794723} Psychy, PsyFor(90,ITA07)<NJ-JRSYCITY>
+ Jersey City Medical Center
355 Grand Street Jersey City, NJ 07304   (201)915-2000

La Morte, Alfonso M., DO {1215967021} CdvDis(87,NY75)<NJ-KENEDYHS, NJ-KMHSTRAT>
+ Southern New Jersey Cardiac Care Specialists
1020 Laurel Oak Road/Suite 102 Voorhees, NJ 08043
(856)435-8842   Fax (856)435-8665
+ Southern New Jersey Cardiac Care Specialists
151 Fries Mill Road/Suite 101 Turnersville, NJ 08012
(856)435-8842   Fax (856)374-3120

La Motta, Joseph D., MD {1417920968} ObsGyn(90,NJ06)<NJ-VIRTMHBC, NJ-LOURDMED>
+ Cooper University Hospital OBGYN
3 Cooper Plaza/Suite 221 Camden, NJ 08103   (856)325-6600   Fax (856)673-4497

La Porta, Lauren D., MD {1568438471} PsyAdt, Psyphm, Psychy(88,NJ05)<NJ-STJOSHOS>
+ St. Joseph's Regional Medical Center
703 Main Street Paterson, NJ 07503   (973)754-2000   Fax (973)754-4350

La Ratta, John A., DO {1336125574} FamMed(93,PA77)<NJ-VIRTBERL>
+ 23 Harker Avenue
Berlin, NJ 08009   (856)767-0078   Fax (856)767-3662

La Rosa, Niurka, MD {1811150246} Pedtrc(90,PRO05)
+ La Rosa Pediatrics Inc
6900 Park Avenue Guttenberg, NJ 07093   (201)766-0086

La Salle, Michael Drew, MD {1770676397} Urolgy(91,NJ05)<NJ-NWRKBETH, NJ-STBARNMC>
+ New Jersey Center for Prostate Cancer & Urology
255 West Spring Valley Avenue Maywood, NJ 07607
(201)487-8866   Fax (201)487-2602
+ New Jersey Center for Prostate Cancer & Urology
200 South Orange Avenue/Suite 228 Livingston, NJ 07039
(201)487-8866   Fax (973)322-0135
+ Urology & Sexual Health Institute
205 Ridgedale Avenue Florham Park, NJ 07607   (973)443-9200   Fax (973)443-9201

La Voe, Ira Howard, DO {1730126533} Pedtrc(98,PA78)
+ Advocare Woolwich Pediatrics
300 Lexington Road/Suite 200 Woolwich Township, NJ 08085   (856)241-2111   Fax (856)241-2243

Labaczewski, Robert J., DO {1013004902} GenPrc, FamMed(73,PA77)
+ Washington Medical, P.A.
100 Heritage Valley Drive/Suite 2 Sewell, NJ 08080
(856)582-6100   Fax (856)582-0397

Labagnara, James, Jr., MD {1811934714} Otlryg(74,NJ05)<NJ-VALLEY>
+ Otolaryngology Head and Neck Surgery
311 Lexington Avenue Paterson, NJ 07502   (973)942-1300

Laban-Grant, Olgica, MD {1639158462} Eplpsy, Nrolgy, ClNrPh(91,YUG13)
+ Northeast Regional Epilepsy Group
20 Prospect Avenue/Suite 800 Hackensack, NJ 07601
(201)343-6676   Fax (201)343-6689

Labat, Mona Farah, MD {1366530693} PthAClI(82,EGY04)<NJ-OVERLOOK>
+ Overlook Medical Center
99 Beauvoir Avenue/PO Box 210 Summit, NJ 07902
(908)522-2000   Fax (908)522-2320

Physicians by Name and Address

Labbadia, Francesco, MD {1104810092} FamMed(90,NJ06)<NJ-SOMERSET>
+ Martinsville Family Practice
1973 Washington Valley Road Martinsville, NJ 08836 (732)560-9225 Fax (732)560-8095
francescolabbadia@mfpnj.allscriptsdirect.net

Labib, Labib N., DO {1588753206} FamMAdlt(96,NJ75)<NJ-CHRIST, NJ-BAYONNE>
+ Jersey Family Medicine, PC
142 Palisade Avenue/Suite 108 Jersey City, NJ 07306 (201)963-9055 Fax (201)963-9056

Labib, Mina L., MD {1427479872} RadDia
+ University Radiology Group, P.C.
16 Mountain Boulevard Warren, NJ 07059 (908)769-7200 Fax (908)769-9141
+ University Radiology Group, P.C.
579A Cranbury Road East Brunswick, NJ 08816 (908)769-7200 Fax (732)390-1856

Labinson, Robert M., MD {1821149824} IntrMd, EmrgMd(79,NY01)
+ University Emergency Medicine
125 Paterson Street/MEB 104 New Brunswick, NJ 08901 (732)235-8717 Fax (732)235-7379

LaBove, Phillip S., MD {1457333528} Anesth, IntrMd(78,NY01)<NJ-MORRISTN>
+ Anesthesia Associates of Morristown
100 Madison Avenue Morristown, NJ 07960 (973)971-5548 Fax (973)631-8120

Labroli, Melissa D., MD {1437294352} Pedtrc(03,PA02)<NJ-VIRTUAHS, NJ-VIRTVOOR>
+ Advocare Pedi Phys of Burlington Co
693 Main Street/PO Box 367 Lumberton, NJ 08048 (609)261-4058 Fax (609)261-8381
+ Advocare Pedi Phys of Burlington Co
204 Ark Road/Suite 209 Mount Laurel, NJ 08054 (609)261-4058 Fax (856)234-9402

Lacap, Estela Villar, MD {1174511232} Pedtrc(92,PHI01)<NJ-CENTRAST, NJ-JRSYSHMC>
+ Allergy & Pediatric Associates of Jersey Shore
222 Schanck Road/Suite 105 Freehold, NJ 07728 (732)431-3373 Fax (732)303-0172
+ Allergy & Pediatric Associates of Jersey Shore
500 West Kennedy Boulevard Lakewood, NJ 08701 (732)431-3373 Fax (732)905-8773

Lacap, Michael V., MD {1073679502} PhysMd(95,PHI22)
+ Advanced HealthCare
679 Montgomery Street Jersey City, NJ 07306 (201)433-7760

Lacapra, Gina M., MD {1568475911} IntrMd(91,NJ05)
+ Community Health Center at Vauxhall
3 Farrington Street Vauxhall, NJ 07088 (908)598-7950 Fax (908)686-1163

Lacapra, Samuel, MD {1861431702} EmrgMd(91,NJ06)
+ JFK Medical Center
65 James Street Edison, NJ 08820 (732)321-7605

Lacara, Dena L., DO {1790845238} FamMed(02,NJ75)<NJ-MTNSIDE>
+ Town Medical Associates/Verona
271 Grove Avenue/Suite A Verona, NJ 07044 (973)239-2600 Fax (973)239-0482

LaCarrubba Blondin, Lisa, MD {1962589432} FamMed(97,NJ06)
+ AmeriHealth HMO, Inc.
8000 Midlantic Drive/Suite 333 Mount Laurel, NJ 08054 (856)778-6500

Lacava, Paul Vincent, MD {1942399365} IntrMd(96,NY20)<NJ-UNVMCPRN>
+ Princeton Medical Group, P.A.
419 North Harrison Street Princeton, NJ 08540 (609)924-9300 Fax (609)924-6552
+ Princeton Medical Group PA
2 Research Way/Bldg 2/Suite 302 Monroe Township, NJ 08831 (609)924-9300 Fax (609)655-7466

LaCavera, Joseph A., III, DO {1689616344} FamMed(73,PA77)
+ 494 Barrtetts Run Road
Bridgeton, NJ 08302 (856)935-6120 Fax (856)935-2684

Lacay, Edmar Manabat, MD {1821248907} FamMed, IntrMd
+ Cooper Primary Care
390 North Broadway/Suite 100 Pennsville, NJ 08070 (856)678-6411 Fax (856)678-7509
edmar_md@yahoo.com

Lachenal, Edgardo N., MD {1508870890} Anesth, AnesPain, IntrMd(78,PHI01)<NJ-VIRTMHBC>
+ Virtua Memorial
175 Madison Avenue/Anesthesia Mount Holly, NJ 08060 (609)261-1660 Fax (609)261-4454

Lacher, Britt Ilene, MD {1407876337} EmrgMd(95,NJ06)<NJ-STBARNMC>
+ St. Barnabas Medical Center
94 Old Short Hills Road/EmergMed Livingston, NJ 07039 (973)322-5000

Lachman, Leigh Jay, MD {1518032317} Otlryg, SrgPlstc, Ophthl(78,NY06)<NY-CABRINI, NY-NYEYEINF>
+ 65 East Northfield Road
Livingston, NJ 07039 (973)535-2837

Lachman, Reid A., MD {1336174614} Otlryg(81,NY09)
+ Ear, Nose, & Throat Specialists of Morristown LLC
95 Madison Avenue/Suite 105 Morristown, NJ 07960 (973)644-0808 Fax (973)644-9270

Lackman, Richard Daniel, MD {1538197090} SrgOrt(77,PA01)<NJ-COOPRUMC>
+ Cooper University Medical Center/Camden
3 Cooper Plaza/Suite 400 Camden, NJ 08103 (856)361-1754 Fax (856)361-1761

LaCorte, Jared C., MD {1497718209} PedCrd, Pedtrc(96,NY03)<NJ-STBARNMC, NJ-MTNSIDE>
+ Metro Pediatric Cardiology Associates
349 East Northfield Road/Suite 105 Livingston, NJ 07039 (973)597-3333

Lacy, Clifton R., MD {1952511875} CdvDis, IntrMd(79,NJ06)<NJ-RWJUBRUN>
+ UH- Robert Wood Johnson Med
125 Paterson Street/CAB 6200 New Brunswick, NJ 08901 (732)235-6560 Fax (732)235-6530
+ New Jersey Department of Health and Senior Services
50 East State/PO Box 360 Trenton, NJ 08625 (732)235-6560 Fax (609)292-6523

Lacz, Nicole Lynn, MD {1306052246} Radiol, RadDia(04,NJ05)<NJ-OVERLOOK>
+ Summit Medical Group-Berkeley Heights Campus
1 Diamond Hill Road Berkeley Heights, NJ 07922 (908)277-8673 Fax (908)790-6576
+ Montclair Radiology
20 High Street Nutley, NJ 07110 (908)277-8673 Fax (973)284-0269

Ladak, Batul S., MD {1952493967} Pedtrc, PedDvl, OthrSp(79,PAKI)<NJ-STJOSHOS>
+ 50 Market Street/2nd Floor
Saddle Brook, NJ 07663 (201)843-8200 Fax (201)843-8835
+ Hackensack Pediatrics
177 Summit Avenue Hackensack, NJ 07601 (201)843-8200 Fax (201)487-2126

Ladenheim, Hilda S., MD {1316108061}
+ 487 Edward H. Ross Drive
Elmwood Park, NJ 07407

Ladino, John Freddy, MD {1952571515} NnPnMd(COL08)<NJ-CHILTON, NJ-MORRISTN>
+ Somerset Medical Center Neonatology
110 Rehill Avenue Somerville, NJ 08876 (908)685-2473
+ MidAtlantic Neonatology Associates
100 Madison Avenue Morristown, NJ 07962 (908)685-2473 Fax (973)290-7175

Ladocsi, Lewis T., MD {1962574681} ObsGyn, Gyneco(70,NJ05)<NJ-STBARNMC>
+ Associates in Obstetrics Gynecology & Infertility
375 Mount Pleasant Avenue/Suite 202 West Orange, NJ 07052 (973)731-7707 Fax (973)669-0277

Ladoulis, Charles Theodore, MD {1538321609} PthAna, MedCom(64,NY06)<NY-VABRKLYN>
+ Marlboro Gastroenterology PC
50 Franklin Lane/Suite 201/Laboratory Manalapan, NJ 07726 (732)972-6996 Fax (732)972-8610
+ Pathology Solutions, LLC.
246 Industrial Way West/Suite 2 Eatontown, NJ 07724 (732)972-6996 Fax (732)389-5299

Ladov, Norman, MD {1003899063} PsyCAd, Psychy(71,NY46)<NJ-STCLRBOO>
+ 933 Route 23
Pompton Plains, NJ 07444 (973)839-0200 Fax (973)839-4749
+ St. Clare's Hospital-Boonton
130 Powerville Road/Psych Boonton, NJ 07005 (973)316-1800

Laemmle, Patricia C., MD {1891729539} IntrMd(95,NJ06)
+ Associates in Internal Medicine HealthCare Inc
1810 Englishtown Road Old Bridge, NJ 08857 (732)416-6900 Fax (732)416-4823

Lafferty, Kathryn Tatsis, MD {1730145004} Pedtrc(98,PA14)<NJ-VIRTMARL>
+ Advocare The Farm Pediatrics
975 Tuckerton Road/Suite 100 Marlton, NJ 08053 (856)983-6190 Fax (856)983-3805
+ Advocare The Farm Pediatrics
1001 Laurel Oak Boulevard/Suite B Voorhees, NJ 08043 (856)983-6190 Fax (856)782-7404

Lafferty, Keith A., MD {1821091653} EmrgMd
+ Bayfront Emergency Physicians
608 Sunset Boulevard Cape May, NJ 08204

Lafferty, Kristen, MD {1962856302} FamMed<NJ-OVERLOOK>
+ Overlook Medical Center
99 Beauvoir Avenue/PO Box 210 Summit, NJ 07902 (908)522-2000

Lafon, Michael C., MD {1609168715} FamMed(83,FL02)<NJ-UNDRWD>
+ 122 Hopkins Road
Haddonfield, NJ 08033

LaForgia, Sal T., MD {1861579831} Dermat(94,PA13)<NJ-COMMED>
+ Bay Dermatology
780 Route 37 West/Suite 235 Toms River, NJ 08755 (732)557-9300 Fax (732)557-9010

Laganella, Dominic J., DO {1811084791} FamMed, OccpMd(73,PA77)
+ Washington Medical, P.A.
100 Heritage Valley Drive/Suite 2 Sewell, NJ 08080 (856)582-6100 Fax (856)582-0397

Lagarenne, Paul R., MD FamMed(81,DC02)
+ 757 Backhus Estates Road
Glen Gardner, NJ 08826

Lage, Susan Marie, DO {1689784159} IntrMd, Nrolgy(89,NJ75)<NJ-CENTRAST>
+ Central Jersey Neurology Associates
501 Iron Bridge Road/Suite 2 Freehold, NJ 07728 (732)462-7030 Fax (732)308-3562

Lagmay, Merceditas Maria, MD {1457387342} Anesth(88,NY47)<NJ-ACMCMAIN>
+ AtlantiCare Anesthesiology
65 West Jimmie Leeds Road Pomona, NJ 08240 (609)748-7597

Laguduva, Lakshmi Rani Ramasubramanian, MD {1962699330} ObsGyn
+ One to One Female Care, P.A.
111 Madison Avenue/Suite 305 Morristown, NJ 07960 (973)683-1400 Fax (973)683-0700

Lahewala, Sopan, MD {1376910612} IntHos<NJ-JRSYCITY>
+ Jersey City Medical Center
355 Grand Street Jersey City, NJ 07304 (201)915-2431

Lahiri, Devraj, MD {1356393458} IntrMd(98,NJ02)
+ RWJPE Care first
97 Cedar Grove Lane/Suite 203 Somerset, NJ 08873 (732)356-7600 Fax (732)356-7625

Lahiri, Nupur, MD {1477761443} Psychy, FamMed(69,INDI)
+ Life Enhancement Insitute
4105 West City Avenue/Suite 11 Monmouth Junction, NJ 08852 (732)355-1158 Fax (732)355-1157

Lahita, Robert George, MD {1336275288} Rheuma, IntrMd(73,PA02)<NY-SLRRSVLT, NJ-NWRKBETH>
+ St. Joseph's Regional Medical Center
703 Main Street Paterson, NJ 07503 (973)754-2476 Fax (973)754-5475
+ Newark Beth Israel Medical Center
201 Lyons Avenue/Medicine Newark, NJ 07112 (973)754-2476 Fax (973)923-8063

Lahoti, Chitra, MD {1598745960} Pthlgy, PthACll(80,INDI)<NJ-JRSYSHMC, NJ-RIVERVW>
+ Meridian Laboratory Physicians
2517 Highway 35/Building M/Suite 101 Manasquan, NJ 08736 (732)528-7710

Lahoti, Mayank, DO {1255659868} Gastrn
+ Gastroenterology Consultants of South Jersey
693 Main Street/Suite 2 Lumberton, NJ 08048 (609)265-1700 Fax (609)265-9005

Lahr, Robin Joy, DO {1649425356}
+ Rowan University-School of Osteopathic Medicine
1 Medical Center Drive Stratford, NJ 08084 (856)566-6708

Lai, Chia-Lung, MD {1104868454} Anesth(66,CHN9D)<NJ-HUNTRDN>
+ Hunterdon Medical Center
2100 Wescott Drive/Anesthesiology Flemington, NJ 08822 (908)788-6181 Fax (908)788-6145

Lai, Wai-Ling, MD {1083739742} Pedtrc(77,PA13)<NJ-BURDTMLN>
+ 209 South Dennis Road
Cape May Court House, NJ 08210 (609)465-9333 Fax (609)465-9333

Lai, Weil Ron, MD {1154632453} Urolgy
+ Hunterdon Urological Associates
1 Wescott Drive/Suite 101 Flemington, NJ 08822 (908)237-4105 Fax (908)237-4132

Laible, Mark S., MD {1437186681} RadDia, Radiol(78,NY03)<NJ-STBARNMC>
+ St. Barnabas Medical Center
94 Old Short Hills Road/Radiology Livingston, NJ 07039 (973)322-5000

Laikin, Michael Frank, MD {1043383466} Psychy(87,NY19)
+ 60 Bergen Avenue
Kearny, NJ 07032 (201)998-9200 Fax (201)998-9201

Laing, Euton M., MD {1851357081} FamMed(90,NJ06)<NJ-RWJUBRUN, NJ-STPETER>
+ Premier Family Physicians
1527 Route 27 South/Suite 1400   Somerset, NJ 08873
(732)745-9900   Fax (732)246-9910
eutonm@cs.com
+ Premier Family Physicians
5b Auer Court   East Brunswick, NJ 08816   (732)745-9900
Fax (732)651-5950

Laiosa, Catherine Virginia, MD {1518126101} IntrMd<NJ-ENGLWOOD>
+ Leonia Medical Associates, P.A.
25 Rockwood Place/Suite 120   Englewood, NJ 07631
(201)568-3335   Fax (201)568-2450

Lajoie, Lidie M., MD {1932369071}<NJ-UMDNJ>
+ University Hospital
150 Bergen Street/F-102   Newark, NJ 07103   (973)972-6295

Lake, Jeffrey Thomas, DO {1982872784}<NJ-STJOSHOS>
+ St. Joseph's Regional Medical Center Anesthesia
703 Main Street   Paterson, NJ 07503   (973)754-2323   Fax (973)977-9455

Lake, Thomas R., III, MD {1003881277} SrgC&R, Surgry(96,GRN01)<NJ-OCEANMC, NJ-JRSYSHMC>
+ Atlantic Surgical Group, PA
255 Monmouth Road   Oakhurst, NJ 07755   (732)531-5445
Fax (732)531-1776
+ Atlantic Surgical Group, PA
459 Jack Martin Boulevard/Suite 7   Brick, NJ 08724
(732)531-5445   Fax (732)836-1592

Lakhani, Vipul K., MD {1982689303} Ophthl(92,NY08)<NJ-OCEANMC, NJ-COMMED>
+ Lakhanai Eye Associates
202 Route 37 West/Suite 3   Toms River, NJ 08755
(732)244-4322   Fax (732)244-4320
+ Lakhani Eye Associates
1608 Highway 88/Suite 118   Brick, NJ 08724   (732)840-4003
+ Lakhani Eye Associates
399 North Main Street   Manahawkin, NJ 08755   (609)484-0040

Lakhlani, Parul Pravinchandra, MD {1003074097} Anesth<NJ-RBAYPERT>
+ Raritan Bay Medical Center/Perth Amboy Division
530 New Brunswick Avenue/Anesth   Perth Amboy, NJ 08861   (732)442-3700
+ Perth Amboy Anesthesiology PC
530 New Brunswick Avenue   Perth Amboy, NJ 08861
(732)739-5853

Lakin, Jeffrey F., MD {1265474852} SrgHnd, SrgOrt(85,NJ05)
+ 642 Broad Street
Clifton, NJ 07013   (973)365-1139   Fax (973)365-1664

Lakritz, Philip Shev, MD {1699750653} RadV&I, Radiol, RadDia(91,NY46)<NJ-RBAYOLDB, NJ-STPETER>
+ University Radiology Group, P.C.
579A Cranbury Road   East Brunswick, NJ 08816   (732)390-0040   Fax (732)390-1856
+ University Radiology Group, P.C.
483 Cranbury Road   East Brunswick, NJ 08816   (732)390-0040   Fax (732)390-5383
+ University Radiology Group, P.C.
75 Veronica Avenue   Somerset, NJ 08816   (732)246-0060
Fax (732)246-4188

Lakshmi, Vijaya S R, MD {1538162656} Anesth(86,INA5B)<NJ-STMRYPAS>
+ St. Mary's Hospital
350 Boulevard   Passaic, NJ 07055   (973)365-4300

Lal, Devika Sandalee, MD {1609134543} PthAcl, IntrMd(PA13<NJ-RWJUBRUN>
+ RWJ University Hospital New Brunswick
One Robert Wood Johnson Place   New Brunswick, NJ 08901
(732)357-6128

Lal, Victoria Sunil, MD {1881723179} IntrMd, Grtrcs(99,PAK11)
+ 7 Softwood Way
Warren, NJ 07059

Lal, Vikram, DO {1417205279} IntrMd, IntHos(NJ75<NJ-ACMCITY>
+ AtlantiCare Hospitalist Program
1925 Pacific Avenue/8th Floor   Atlantic City, NJ 08401
(609)441-8146   Fax (609)441-8002

Lala, Lekhu K., MD {1912931544} IntrMd, CdvDis(79,BELG)<NJ-VALLEY, NJ-HACKNSK>
+ 541 Cedar Hill Road
Wyckoff, NJ 07481   (201)447-4600   Fax (201)447-9787

Lala, Vinod R., MD {1144259383} PedEnd, Pedtrc, EnDbMt(68,INDI)<NJ-CHRIST>
+ Center for Endocrinology & Diabetes NJ
968 River Road/Suite 203   Edgewater, NJ 07020   (201)224-8328   Fax (201)224-2405
VINOD519@aol.com

Lalani, Omar, MD {1578565966} RadDia, RadV&I(96,MA05)
+ Radiology Associates of Burlington County
1295 Route 38 West/PO Box 479   Hainesport, NJ 08036
(609)261-7017   Fax (609)261-4100

Lalchandani, Mira R., MD {1710246426}
+ University Behavioral HealthCare
183 South Orange Avenue   Newark, NJ 07103   (973)972-4300

Lalcheta, Paresh, MD {1588910343} IntrMd
+ 17 Bridge Pointe Drive
Laurence Harbor, NJ 08879

Lalin, Sean C., MD {1275580128} Ophthl(00,NY01)<NJ-MORRISTN, NY-NYEYEINF>
+ Retina Specialists of New Jersey
330 South Street/Suite 1   Morristown, NJ 07960   (973)871-2020   Fax (973)871-2000
+ Retina Specialists of New Jersey
500 Willow Grove Street/Suite 2   Hackettstown, NJ 07840
(973)871-2020   Fax (973)871-2000
+ Retina Specialists of New Jersey
422 Conventry Drive/2nd Floor   Phillipsburg, NJ 07960
(973)871-2020   Fax (973)871-2000

Lalla, Lalita Raj, MD {1124112149} IntrMd(84,INA69)<NJ-TRENTPSY>
+ Trenton Psychiatric Hospital
Sullivan Way/PO Box 7600   West Trenton, NJ 08628
(609)633-1500

Lalla, Raj N., MD {1770520637} SrgPlstc, SrgCsm, SrgRec(79,INA65)<NJ-CHSFULD, NJ-CHSMRCER>
+ 2051 Klockner Road
Hamilton, NJ 08690   (609)584-8898   Fax (609)584-7825
lallaplasticsurgery@juno.com

Lalla, Sanjay, MD {1295797256} SrgPlstc(91,MA05)
+ 383 Northfield Avenue
West Orange, NJ 07052   (973)324-9455   Fax (973)324-9454
slallamd@aol.com

Lally, Tamkeen, MD {1487941183} PsyGrt
+ Hackensack University Medical Center
30 Prospect Avenue   Hackensack, NJ 07601   (978)982-2300
+ University Behavioral HealthCare
183 South Orange Avenue   Newark, NJ 07103   (973)982-2300

Lam, Adele Dolores, DO {1396863213} EmrgMd
+ 112 Forest Road
Moorestown, NJ 08057

Lam, Allison Christine, MD {1093759235} EmrgMd(94,PA02)<NJ-CLARMAAS>
+ Clara Maass Medical Center
1 Clara Maass Drive/EmrgMed   Belleville, NJ 07109
(973)450-2000
+ Emergency Medical Associates of NJ, P.A.
3 Century Drive   Parsippany, NJ 07054   (973)450-2000
Fax (973)740-9895

Lam, Christopher, MD {1750461976} PsyCAd, Psychy(90,TX13)
+ 45 St. Moritz Lane
Cherry Hill, NJ 08003

Lam, Eleanor Lin, MD {1316166804} EnDbMt, IntrMd(06,PA12)<NJ-VIRTVOOR>
+ Virtua Endocrinology
200 Bowman Drive   Voorhees, NJ 08043   (856)247-7220

Lam, Gloria Fontane, DO {1699038349} IntHos<NJ-KMHSTRAT>
+ Kennedy Memorial Hospital-University Medical Center
18 East Laurel Road   Stratford, NJ 08084   (856)218-5634
Fax (856)218-5664

Lam, Jennifer, MD {1275862328} Pedtrc(06,NY19)
+ UH- Robert Wood Johnson Med
125 Paterson Street/MEB 308   New Brunswick, NJ 08901
(732)828-3000

Lam, Ling Lai, MD {1205832185} RadDia(93,NY45)
+ University Radiology, PA
239 Route 22 East/Suite 302   Green Brook, NJ 08812
(732)968-4899   Fax (732)968-8096
+ University Radiology Group, P.C.
3900 Park Avenue/Suite 107   Edison, NJ 08820   (732)968-4899   Fax (732)548-6290
+ University Radiology Group, P.C.
16 Mountain Boulevard   Warren, NJ 08812   (908)769-7200
Fax (908)769-9141

Lam, Mylan Ngoc, MD {1114915469} OrtSpn, PhysMd(95,TX04)<NJ-KSLRWEST>
+ Kessler Institute for Rehabilitation West Orange
1199 Pleasant Valley Way   West Orange, NJ 07052
(973)731-3600

Lam, Nalini Priya, MD {1780019448} FamMed
+ 15 Mynipoti Court
Piscataway, NJ 08854   (732)221-5281

Lam, Paul C., MD {1609861186} FrtInf, ObsGyn(78,OH06)<NJ-MORRISTN, NJ-STCLRDEN>
+ Drs. Friedel & Lam
1259 US Highway 46 East/Suite 314   Parsippany, NJ 07054
(973)316-9800   Fax (973)316-9805

Lam, Sofia Levin, MD {1376595736} AnesPain(83,ITA13)
+ Pain Control Center of New Jersey
561 Cranbury Road   East Brunswick, NJ 08816   (732)651-1300   Fax (732)651-0375

Lama, Paul Jude, MD {1033130315} Ophthl, IntrMd(89,NY19)<NJ-CLARMAAS>
+ Glaucoma Institute of Northern NJ
87 West Passaic Street   Rochelle Park, NJ 07662   (201)343-3499   Fax (201)343-1799

Lamacchia, Michael A., MD {1528109394} Pedtrc, PedInf(87,ITAL)<NJ-STJOSHOS>
+ St. Joseph's Children's Hospital
703 Main Street/Infectious Dis   Paterson, NJ 07503
(973)754-2549   Fax (973)754-2546

Lamanna, Adolfo C., MD {1215930839} Anesth(81,MEX14)
+ Morris Anesthesia Group, PA
3799 Route 46/Suite 211   Parsippany, NJ 07054   (973)335-1122   Fax (973)335-1448

LaMantia, Anthony P., MD {1013905595} Pedtrc, Allrgy(74,NJ05)<NJ-CENTRAST, NJ-JRSYSHMC>
+ Allergy & Pediatric Associates of Jersey Shore
222 Schanck Road/Suite 105   Freehold, NJ 07728
(732)431-3373   Fax (732)303-0172
+ Allergy & Pediatric Associates of Jersey Shore
500 West Kennedy Boulevard   Lakewood, NJ 08701
(732)431-3373   Fax (732)905-8773

LaMarche, Nelson S., MD {1790752889} CdvDis, IntrMd(83,DOM01)<NJ-JRSYSHMC, NJ-CENTRAST>
+ Monmouth Cardiology Associates, LLC
11 Meridian Road   Eatontown, NJ 07724   (732)663-0300
Fax (732)663-0301
+ Monmouth Cardiology Associates, LLC
222 Schanck Road/Suite 104   Freehold, NJ 07728
(732)663-0300   Fax (732)431-1712

Lamb, David J., MD {1023037959} SrgOrt, SrgSpn(91,PA02)<NJ-VANJHCS>
+ Princeton Orthopaedic Associates, P.A.
325 Princeton Avenue   Princeton, NJ 08540   (609)924-8131   Fax (609)924-8532

Lamb, Marc John, MD {1447273180} SrgHnd, SrgOrt(94,PA02)<NJ-VANJHCS>
+ Princeton Orthopaedic Associates, P.A.
325 Princeton Avenue   Princeton, NJ 08540   (609)924-8131   Fax (609)924-8532
+ Princeton Orthopaedic Associates, P.A.
11 Centre Drive   Jamesburg, NJ 08831   (609)655-4848

Lamba, Renu, MD {1801828330} OncHem, IntrMd, PedHem(88,INA3Z)
+ 473 Broadway/Suie 411
Bayonne, NJ 07002   (201)285-5972

Lamba, Sangeeta, MD {1184702250} IntrMd, EmrgMd(88,INDI)<NJ-UMDNJ>
+ University Hospital
150 Bergen Street/Medicine   Newark, NJ 07103   (973)972-4300

Lambert, Amy L., MD {1457457293} PedOph, Ophthl(87,OH06)
+ Associates in Ophthalmology
22 Old Short Hills Road/Suite 102   Livingston, NJ 07039
(973)992-5200   Fax (973)535-5741

Lambert, George H., MD {1750440228} NnPnMd, Pedtrc(72,IL11)<NJ-RWJUBRUN>
+ RWJ University Hospital New Brunswick
One Robert Wood Johnson Place   New Brunswick, NJ 08901
(732)828-3000

Lambert, Kathryn C., DO {1538149646} FamMed(88,PA77)<NJ-KMHSTRAT>
+ University Hospital-University Family Medicine
42 East Laurel Road/Suite 2100   Stratford, NJ 08084
(856)566-7020   Fax (856)566-6188

Lambert, Rick O., MD {1891739421} EmrgMd, IntrMd(84,NY19)<NJ-STBARNMC>
+ 305 West Grand Avenue/Suite 500
Montvale, NJ 07645   (201)326-4788   Fax (201)649-1798

Lambert-Woolley, Margaret A., MD {1528027984} ObsGyn, IntrMd(86,NJ05)<NJ-RIVERVW, NJ-MONMOUTH>
+ Atlantic Womens Medical Group
240 Wall Street/Suite 300   West Long Branch, NJ 07764
(732)229-1288   Fax (732)728-1487

Lamborne, Nicole Marie, MD {1386671295} ObsGyn(97,NJ06)
+ 2225 East Evesham Road/Suite 105
Voorhees, NJ 08043   (856)325-3575   Fax (856)325-3246

Lambrakis, Christos C., MD {1912988320} Eplpsy, Nrolgy, ClNrPh(93,NY09)
+ Northeast Regional Epilepsy Group
20 Prospect Avenue/Suite 800   Hackensack, NJ 07601
(201)343-6676   Fax (201)343-6689

Lambrinos, Vasilios, MD {1598960551} IntrMd, PulCCr(04,GRN01)<NJ-HACKNSK>
+ Hackensack University Medical Center
30 Prospect Avenue   Hackensack, NJ 07601   (201)996-2000
vlambrinos@hackensackumc.org

Physicians by Name and Address

Lami, Christian John, MD {1598144974} IntHos<NJ-COOPRUMC>
+ Cooper University Hospital
One Cooper Plaza   Camden, NJ 08103   (856)342-3150   Fax (856)968-8418

Lammertse, Thomas E., MD {1811985872} PhysMd(79,OH40)<NJ-KSLRWELK>
+ Kessler Institute for Rehab
201 Pleasant Hill Road   Chester, NJ 07930   (973)584-7500

LaMonica, Christina M, MD {1851399455} Anesth, PedAne(91,MA01)<NJ-STFRNMED>
+ St. Francis Medical Center
601 Hamilton Avenue/CardioThor Anes   Trenton, NJ 08629   (609)599-5306

Lamothe, Maria Elina, MD {1396929295} IntrMd(06,NJ03)
+ 525 Central Avenue/Suite C
Westfield, NJ 07090   (908)389-1910   Fax (908)389-1911
+ Center for Endocrine Health
1121 route 22 west/Suite 205   Bridgewater, NJ 08807   (908)389-1910   Fax (212)249-5628

Lamour, Rytza M., MD {1801983796} Pedtrc, PedEmg(01,MNT01)<NJ-HACKNSK>
+ Hackensack University Medical Center
30 Prospect Avenue   Hackensack, NJ 07601   (201)996-5061   Fax (201)996-3676

Lampariello, James A., MD {1891717294} FamMed(95,NJ05)<NJ-CHILTON>
+ Alps Family Physicians
1500 Alps Road   Wayne, NJ 07470   (973)628-8500   Fax (973)628-7944
+ Carepoint Health
10 Exchange Place   Jersey City, NJ 07302   (201)884-5329

Lampert, Craig, MD {1063403509} OncHem(90,SAF01)
+ Drs. Fein, Porcelli & Richards
75 Veronica Avenue/Suite 201   Somerset, NJ 08873   (732)246-4882   Fax (732)249-5633
+ Regional Cancer Care Associates
111 Union Valley Road/Suite 205   Monroe, NJ 08831   (732)246-4882   Fax (609)395-7955

Lampone, Christina, MD {1841248028} Pedtrc(98,PA09)<NJ-VIRTVOOR, NJ-VIRTMARL>
+ Advocare Marlton Pediatrics
525 Route 73 South   Marlton, NJ 08053   (856)596-3434   Fax (856)596-9110
+ Advocare Township Pediatrics
123 Egg Harbor Road   Sewell, NJ 08080   (856)596-3434   Fax (856)227-5890

Lamprinakos, James P., MD {1710093729} IntrMd(83,MEXI)
+ 363 Neville Street
Perth Amboy, NJ 08861   (732)442-6066   Fax (732)442-4705

Lamprou, Emanuel, Jr., MD {1033104526} Anesth(82,PHI14)
+ Medical Pain Management LLC
2070 Springdale Road/Suite 200   Cherry Hill, NJ 08003   (856)433-8267   Fax (856)375-2251
drlamprou@drlamprou.com

Lamzaky, Xenia G., MD {1518049600} Pedtrc(84,GRN01)<NJ-TRINIWSC>
+ 3112 Lisbon Avenue
Toms River, NJ 08753   (201)725-3971

Lan, Andrew Ente, MD {1003856964} IntrMd(01,NJ06)
+ 400 Tenafly Road/Suite 481
Tenafly, NJ 07670   (201)676-0020   Fax (855)258-4017

Lan, Vivian En-Wei, MD {1619912284} IntrMd(94,NJ47)<NJ-VALLEY>
+ Bergen Medical Associates
466 Old Hook Road/Suite 1   Emerson, NJ 07630   (201)967-8221   Fax (201)967-0340
+ Bergen Medical Associates
1 West Ridgewood Avenue/Suite 301   Paramus, NJ 07652   (201)967-8221   Fax (201)445-4296

LaNatra, Nicole, MD {1538359393} IntrMd, OncHem(02,NY09)
+ Adult Medical Oncology-Hematology LLC
39 Sycamore Avenue   Little Silver, NJ 07739   (732)576-8610   Fax (732)576-8823

Lancefield, Margaret L., MD {1831126754} IntrMd(84,CT01)<NJ-UNVMCPRN>
+ Princeton Medicine
5 Plainsboro Road/Suite 300   Plainsboro, NJ 08536   (609)853-7272   Fax (609)853-7271

Lanciano, Ralph, Jr., DO {1922052588} Ophthl(65,PA77)
+ Wills Eye Surgery Center in Cherry Hill
408 Route 70 East   Cherry Hill, NJ 08034   (856)354-1600   Fax (856)429-7555

Lancman, Marcelo Elias, MD {1609857010} Nrolgy, ClNrPh(84,ARG01)<NY-WHITEPLN, NJ-HACKNSK>
+ Northeast Regional Epilepsy Group
20 Prospect Avenue/Suite 800   Hackensack, NJ 07601   (201)343-6676   Fax (201)343-6689

Land, Stephen M., MD {1558337634} FamMed, Grtrcs, IntrMd(86,NJ06)<NJ-VIRTMHBC>
+ Mt. Laurel Family Physicians
401 Young Avenue/Suite 260   Moorestown, NJ 08057

(856)291-8756   Fax (856)291-8750
+ Avnet Memec
7000 Atrium Way/Suite 6   Mount Laurel, NJ 08054   (856)291-8756   Fax (856)291-6819

Land, Warren K., DO {1952368979} Anesth, PedAne, IntrMd(93,PA77)<NJ-STPETER, NJ-SOMERSET>
+ Anesthesia Consultnts of NJ/Nova Pain
285 Davidson Avenue/Suite 204   Somerset, NJ 08873   (732)271-1400   Fax (732)271-3544

Landa, Joshua, MD {1366647331} SrgSpn, SrgOrt, IntrMd(04,PA01)<NJ-STBARNMC>
+ Landa Spine Center
300 Perrine Road/Suite 333   Old Bridge, NJ 08857   (732)289-9335   Fax (732)289-9336
+ Landa Spine Center
630 East Palisade Avenue   Englewood Cliffs, NJ 07632   (732)289-9335   Fax (201)408-5278
+ Landa Spine Center
680 Broadway/Suite 204   Paterson, NJ 08857   (201)731-3335   Fax (201)408-5278

Landa, Seth E., MD {1912904665} Anesth(86,NY46)<NJ-STMICHL>
+ St. Joseph's Regional Medical Center Anesthesia
703 Main Street   Paterson, NJ 07503   (973)754-2323   Fax (973)977-9455

Landauer, Stephen P., MD {1093747081} Anesth(82,IL02)<NJ-NWTNMEM>
+ 1 Landuer Lane/Suite 19/PO Box 19
Newton, NJ 07860

Landen, Alexandra E., DO {1770733008} Nrolgy, IntrMd(05,NJ75)
+ Capital Institute for Neurosciences
2 Capital Way/Suite 456   Pennington, NJ 08534   (609)537-7300   Fax (609)537-7301

Lander, Jeffrey, MD {1356533889} CdvDis, IntrMd(04,GRN01)<NJ-STBARNMC, NJ-MTNSIDE>
+ Mountainside Family Practice Associates
799 Bloomfield Avenue/Suite 201   Verona, NJ 07044   (973)746-7050   Fax (973)259-3569

Lander, Richard, MD {1093759003} Pedtrc, AdolMd(74,MEX14)<NJ-STBARNMC, NJ-MORRISTN>
+ Essex-Morris Pediatric Group P.A.
203 Hillside Avenue   Livingston, NJ 07039   (973)992-5588   Fax (973)992-1005
+ Essex-Morris Pediatric Group P.A.
34 Elm Street   Morristown, NJ 07960   (973)292-1011

Landers, David Benjamin, MD {1285602383} CdvDis, IntrMd(79,DC02)<NJ-HACKNSK, NJ-HOLYNAME>
+ Bergen Cardiology Associates
292 Columbia Avenue   Fort Lee, NJ 07024   (201)224-0050   Fax (201)224-6061
+ Bergen Cardiology Associates
400 Frank W. Burr Boulevard   Teaneck, NJ 07666   (201)224-0050   Fax (201)692-3263

Landers, Steven Howard, MD {1306864327} FamMed(03,OH06)
+ VNA of Central Jersey Community Health Center, Inc.
176 Riverside Avenue   Red Bank, NJ 07701   (732)221-5109   Fax (732)224-0893

Landesman, Glen S., MD {1558443945} FamMed(88,TX02)<NJ-SOMERSET>
+ Your Doctors Care, PA
71 Route 206 South   Hillsborough, NJ 08844   (908)685-1887   Fax (908)707-0816

Landmann, Dan S., MD {1407043945} Ophthl(05,MA07)<CT-STAMFDH>
+ Eyecare MD of New Jersey
261 James Street/Suite 2-D & 3EL   Morristown, NJ 07960   (973)984-3937   Fax (973)984-0059

Landolfi, Joseph Charles, DO {1033119383} Nrolgy, OncNeu(72,NJ75)<NJ-JFKMED>
+ JFK Neurosciences Institute
65 James Street/Second Floor   Edison, NJ 08818   (732)321-7010   Fax (732)744-5821

Landolfi, Joseph M., MD {1215908470} Ophthl(70,ITAL)<NJ-CLARMAAS>
+ Vision Eye Physicians and Surgeons
567 Franklin Avenue   Belleville, NJ 07109   (973)751-4500   Fax (973)751-3073

Landolfi, Michael Joseph, DO {1356312508} Ophthl(99,NJ75)<NJ-VAEASTOR, NJ-CLARMAAS>
+ Vision Eye Physicians and Surgeons
567 Franklin Avenue   Belleville, NJ 07109   (973)751-4500   Fax (973)751-3073
+ Associated Eye Physicians, P.A.
1033 Clifton Avenue/Suite 107   Clifton, NJ 07013   (973)751-4500   Fax (973)472-4832

Landre, William Joseph, MD {1942223235} EmrgMd, FamMed, IntrMd(65,FRAN)
+ Neighborhood Health Center Newton
238 Spring Street   Newton, NJ 07860   (973)383-7001   Fax (973)383-3088
+ Pathlink, LLC
66 West Gilbert Street/Suite 100   Tinton Falls, NJ 07701

(973)383-7001   Fax (732)212-0061

Lands, Vince Williams, MD {1578905055} SrgOrt
+ Cooper University Hospital
One Cooper Plaza   Camden, NJ 08103   (856)342-2000

Landset, David J., DO {1841229366} Gastrn(82,NY75)<NJ-BURDTMLN>
+ Cape Atlantic Gastroenterology Associates
307 Stone Harbor Boulevard/Suite 5   Cape May Court House, NJ 08210   (609)465-1511   Fax (609)465-5310

Landsman, Howard Scott, DO {1245227826} Otlryg, SrgFPl, OtgyFPlS(99,MO78)<NJ-OCEANMC>
+ ENT & Facial Plastic Surgery Assocs
1608 Route 88/Suite 240   Brick, NJ 08724   (732)458-8575   Fax (732)206-0578

Landzberg, Joel Serge, MD {1730184318} CdvDis, IntrMd(83,NY01)<NJ-HACKNSK, NJ-VALLEY>
+ Westwood Cardiology Associates PA
333 Old Hook Road/Suite 200   Westwood, NJ 07675   (201)664-0201   Fax (201)666-7970
+ Westwood Cardiology Associates PA
20 Prospect Avenue/Suite 810   Hackensack, NJ 07601   (201)664-0201   Fax (201)342-2422

Lane, Elizabeth Lovinger, MD {1932105814} Radiol(90,DC02)<NJ-SOMERSET>
+ University Radiology, PA
239 Route 22 East/Suite 302   Green Brook, NJ 08812   (732)968-4899   Fax (732)968-8096
+ University Radiology Group, P.C.
16 Mountain Boulevard   Warren, NJ 07059   (732)968-4899   Fax (908)769-9141
+ University Radiology Group, P.C.
579A Cranbury Road   East Brunswick, NJ 08812   (732)390-0040   Fax (732)390-1856

Lane, Gregory J., MD {1750488466} SprtMd, SrgArt, SrgOrt(88,PA13)<NJ-JFKMED>
+ Advanced Orthopaedics & Sports Medicine Center, PC
1907 Oak Tree Road/Suite 201   Edison, NJ 08820   (732)548-7332   Fax (732)548-7350

Lane, John F., MD {1497701627} Ophthl(90,DC02)<NJ-OVERLOOK>
+ The Eye Center
65 Mountain Boulevard Ext/Suite 105   Warren, NJ 07059   (732)356-6200   Fax (732)356-0228
+ The Eye Center
213 Stelton Road   Piscataway, NJ 08854   (732)356-6200   Fax (732)752-9492
+ The Eye Center
3900 Park Avenue/Suite 106   Edison, NJ 07059   (732)603-2101

Lane, Stanley R., MD {1124040159} Allrgy, Pedtrc, AlgyImmn(66,NY09)<NJ-VIRTMHBC, NJ-MEMSALEM>
+ Allergy, Asthma & Immunology Management, P.A.
701 East Main Street/Suite 6   Moorestown, NJ 08057   (856)235-2651   Fax (856)231-9812
+ Allergy & Immunology Management PA
330 Salem Woodstown Road/Medical Arts   Salem, NJ 08079   (856)935-8988

Lanese, Stephanie Valentine, MD {1285801894} Pedtrc
+ University Hospital-Cares Institute
42 East Laurel Road/Suite 1100   Stratford, NJ 08084   (856)566-7036   Fax (856)566-6108

Laneve, Anthony, Jr., MD {1255337556} IntrMd(78,NJ05)
+ 275 Paterson Avenue/1st Floor
Little Falls, NJ 07424   (973)785-3334   Fax (973)785-7760
+ Heart & Vascular Associates of Northern Jersey
22-18 Broadway/Suite 201   Fair Lawn, NJ 07410   (973)785-3334   Fax (201)475-5522

Lanez, Carmencita T., MD {1770643959} Psychy(78,PHIL)<NJ-RBAYPERT>
+ 201-205 New Brunswick Ave
Perth Amboy, NJ 08861

Lanez, Charisma Ann, DO {1942637988}
+ Ocean Health Initiatives, Inc.
101 Second Street   Lakewood, NJ 08701   (732)363-6655   Fax (732)363-6656

Lanfranchi, Angela E., MD {1710066956} SrgBst, Surgry(75,DC02)<NJ-SOMERSET, NJ-RWJUBRUN>
+ Surgical Associates of Central NJ
30 Rehill Avenue/Suite 3300   Somerville, NJ 08876   (908)927-8994   Fax (908)927-8995

Lang, Karen Friedman, MD {1174615355} Psychy(90,PA01)
+ 3200 Sunset Avenue/Suite 211
Ocean, NJ 07712   (732)493-3774   Fax (732)493-0499
KFLMD@ARIEM.com

Langan, Abigail E., MD {1154546299} PsyCAd(02,NJ06)<NJ-STJOSHOS>
+ St. Joseph's Regional Medical Center
703 Main Street   Paterson, NJ 07503   (973)754-2000

Langan, Russell, MD {1063646313} SrgOnc
+ Saint Barnabas Medical Center Surgery
94 Old Short Hills Road   Livingston, NJ 07039   (973)322-5995

Lange, David J., MD {1811963150} SrgPlstc(79,MEXI)<NJ-MORRISTN>
+ Peer Group Plastic Surgery Center
124 Columbia Turnpike Florham Park, NJ 07932 (973)822-3000 Fax (973)822-1726

Lange, Michael, MD {1477591196} InfDis, IntrMd, TrpPst(68,ON01)<NJ-STJOSHOS>
+ St. Joseph's Regional Medical Center
703 Main Street/IntMed/InfDis Paterson, NJ 07503 (973)754-2130

Langenfeld, John Eugene, MD {1144399858} Surgry, SrgThr(87,IL01)
+ UH- Robert Wood Johnson Med
125 Paterson Street/MEB 534 New Brunswick, NJ 08901 (732)235-7802 Fax (732)235-7802

Langer, Burton Harris, MD {1861457673} Pedtrc(86,PA01)
+ Advocare, LLC.
402 Lippincott Drive Marlton, NJ 08053 (856)504-8028 Fax (856)504-8029

Langer, Dennis Henry, MD Psychy, PsyCAd(75,DC02)
+ Drs. Langer & Langer
12 Cleveland Lane Princeton, NJ 08540 (609)683-5090

Langer, Marjory Ellen, MD {1750378451} EmrgMd(02,ISR02)<NJ-MTNSIDE, NJ-EASTORNG>
+ Hackensack UMC Mountainside
1 Bay Avenue/EmrgMed Montclair, NJ 07042 (973)429-6000

Langer, Myriam, MD {1255584306} ObsGyn, IntrMd(04,ISR02)
+ Hackensack University Medical Group Montvale
305 West Grand Avenue Montvale, NJ 07645 (201)746-9150 Fax (201)746-9151
+ Hackensack University Medical Group Westwood
250 Old Hook Road Westwood, NJ 07675 (201)746-9150 Fax (201)781-1753
+ Hackensack University Medical Group Emerson
452 Old Hook Road/2nd Floor Emerson, NJ 07645 (201)666-3900 Fax (201)261-0505

Langer, Orli, MD {1528129624} ObsGyn, MtFtMd(01,ISR06)
+ Perinatal Associates
975 Clifton Avenue/Suite 1R Clifton, NJ 07013 (973)614-1171

Langer, Paul D., MD {1538183397} Ophthl, SrgOrb(89,MD07)<NJ-UMDNJ, NJ-HACKNSK>
+ University Ophthalmology Associates
90 Bergen Street/DOC 6100 Newark, NJ 07101 (973)982-2065 Fax (973)972-2068
+ University Ophthalmology Associates
556 Eagle Rock Avenue/Suite 206 Roseland, NJ 07068 (973)722-2108

Langer, Susan F., MD Psychy(75,NY45)
+ Drs. Langer & Langer
12 Cleveland Lane Princeton, NJ 08540 (609)683-5090

Langman, Alex, MD {1619940533} RadDia(97,NY08)<NJ-KIMBALL>
+ Kimball Medical Center
600 River Avenue/Radiology Lakewood, NJ 08701 (732)363-1900 Fax (732)942-5658

Langner, Bruce J., MD {1982779401} Gastrn, IntrMd(76,MEX03)
+ 107 Monmouth Road
West Long Branch, NJ 07764 (732)542-6801 Fax (732)542-1466

Langsner, Alan M., MD {1619966702} PedCrd, Pedtrc, PedCrC(77,MEXI)<NJ-CHDNWBTH, NJ-STBARNMC>
+ Children's Hospital of New Jersey
201 Lyons Avenue/Osborne Terrace Newark, NJ 07112 (973)926-2309

Langston, Kristi Dana, DO {1700015211} Anesth<PA-EXWSTMRL>
+ The Advanced Pulmonary Diagnostic Center
100 Medical Center Way Somers Point, NJ 08244 (954)461-0226 Fax (609)653-3586

Lania-Howarth, Maria, MD {1861574295} Pedtrc, Allrgy(84,NJ05)<NJ-COOPRUMC>
+ Cooper Peds/Children's Regional Ctr
3 Cooper Plaza/Suite 200 Camden, NJ 08103 (856)342-2472 Fax (856)368-8297
+ The Children's Regional Hospital at Cooper Univ Hosp
One Cooper Plaza/Allergy & Immun Camden, NJ 08103 (856)342-2000

Lanka, Himabindu M., MD {1780964825}
+ Cooper University Hospital
One Cooper Plaza Camden, NJ 08103 (856)342-2000

Lankaranian, Dara, MD {1740417385} IntrMd, IntHos(94,IRA09)<NJ-BURDTMLN, NJ-SHOREMEM>
+ Shore Memorial Hospital
1 East New York Avenue/Hospitalist Somers Point, NJ 08244 (609)653-3500 Fax (609)926-4311
+ Cape Hospitalist Associates, P.A.
2 Stone Harbor Boulevard Cape May Court House, NJ 08210 (609)463-2803

Lann, Danielle Erin, MD {1417116682} EnDbMt
+ Hackensack Meridian Medical Group
19 Davis Avenue/5th-6th Floor Neptune, NJ 07753

Lansang, Martin Fidel, MD {1407801269} IntrMd, CritCr, PulDis(02,PHI02)<NJ-HUNTRDN>
+ Pulmonary & Sleep Associates of Hunterdon County
1100 Wescott Drive/Suite G-2 Flemington, NJ 08822 (908)237-1560 Fax (908)806-2529

Lansing, Martha H., MD {1841240785} FamMed(82,OK01)<NJ-CHSFULD, NJ-UNVMCPRN>
+ Capital Health Family Health Center
433 Bellevue Avenue/4th Floor Trenton, NJ 08618 (609)815-2671 Fax (609)815-2672
+ RWJ University Hospital New Brunswick
One Robert Wood Johnson Place New Brunswick, NJ 08901 (609)815-2671 Fax (732)246-8084

Lanteri, Vincent J., MD {1528036670} Urolgy(74,MEXI)<NJ-HACKNSK, NJ-HOLYNAME>
+ New Jersey Center for Prostate Cancer & Urology
255 West Spring Valley Avenue Maywood, NJ 07607 (201)487-8866 Fax (201)487-2602
+ New Jersey Center for Prostate Cancer & Urology
200 South Orange Avenue/Suite 228 Livingston, NJ 07039 (201)487-8866 Fax (973)322-0135

Lanza, Michele R., MD {1558370635} FamMed(02,MNT01)
+ 240 Maple Avenue
Red Bank, NJ 07701 (732)576-1600

Lanza, Paul R., DO {1851320311} FamMed(84,IA75)<NJ-VIRTMHBC, NJ-VIRTBERL>
+ Family Practice of Moorestown
728 Marne Highway/Suite B Moorestown, NJ 08057 (856)235-6600 Fax (856)235-6610
+ Alliance for Better Care PC
520 Stokes Road/Suite D1 Medford, NJ 08055 (856)235-6600 Fax (609)953-8652

Lanza, Raymond, DO {1376518407} Grtrcs, IntrMd(78,IA75)
+ Specialdocs Consultants, Inc.
266 King George Road/Suite F Warren, NJ 07059 (732)893-8150 Fax (732)893-8149

Lanzilotti, Thomas A., MD {1972558484} CdvDis(80,NY08)
+ 5 Route 94/Suite F
Vernon, NJ 07462 (973)827-0844 Fax (973)827-0854
+ Cardiology Associates of Sussex County LLP
222 High Street/Suite 205 Newton, NJ 07860 (973)827-0844 Fax (973)579-6638

Lanzkowsk, Shelley, MD {1992776942} Pedtrc(82,NY20)<NJ-MORRISTN>
+ Morristown Pediatric Associates, LLC
261 James Street/Suite 1-G Morristown, NJ 07960 (973)540-9393 Fax (973)540-1937

Lao, Carlos S., MD {1215907068} IntrMd, OccpMd(65,PHI01)<NJ-CLARMAAS, NJ-JFKMED>
+ Care Station Medical Group
328 St. Georges Avenue Linden, NJ 07036 (908)925-7519 Fax (908)925-2841
+ Care Station Medical Group
456 Prospect Avenue West Orange, NJ 07052 (908)925-7519 Fax (973)731-9881
+ Care Station Medical Group
210 Meadowlands Parkway Secaucus, NJ 07036 (201)348-3636 Fax (201)583-0713

Lao, Jocelyn M., MD {1831105527} Anesth, Pedtrc(84,PHI08)<NJ-CLARMAAS>
+ Clara Maass Medical Center
1 Clara Maass Drive/Anesth Belleville, NJ 07109 (973)450-2000

Lao, Ramon S., MD {1376556647} NuclMd, NucImg(64,PHIL)<NJ-NWRKBETH>
+ Newark Beth Israel Medical Center
201 Lyons Avenue/Nuclr Medicine Newark, NJ 07112 (973)926-7888 Fax (973)923-8232

Lapa, Alan S., MD {1487687794} CdvDis(87,GRNA)<NJ-MTNSIDE>
+ North Jersey Cardiovascular Consultants
329 Belleville Avenue Bloomfield, NJ 07003 (973)748-3800 Fax (973)748-3540

Lapas, Alkies, DO {1790002228} RadNro
+ 75 Passaic Avenue
Belleville, NJ 07109 (973)979-7772

Lapchak, John T., MD {1750363693} Anesth(73,VA04)
+ Anesthesia Associates of Morristown
264 South Street/Suite 2A Morristown, NJ 07960 (973)631-8119

Lapicki, Michael John, DO {1962748863}<NJ-JRSYCITY>
+ Jersey City Medical Center
355 Grand Street Jersey City, NJ 07304 (201)915-2431

Lapicki, Walter S., DO {1346342060} Anesth(85,MO79)<NJ-HUNTRDN>
+ Hunterdon Medical Center
2100 Wescott Drive/Anesth/PainMgmt Flemington, NJ 08822 (908)788-6181 Fax (908)788-6145

Lapidus, Daniel Yitzchok, MD {1770515819} Pedtrc(99,MD01)<NJ-OCEANMC, NJ-COMMED>
+ Pediatric Affiliates, PA
218 Jack Martin Boulevard/Building E-1 Brick, NJ 08724 (732)458-0010 Fax (732)458-9329
+ Pediatric Affiliates, PA
40 Bey Lea Road/Suite B203 Toms River, NJ 08753 (732)458-0010 Fax (732)244-6842
+ Pediatric Affiliates, PA
1616 Route 72 West/Suite 8 Manahawkin, NJ 08724 (609)597-6200 Fax (609)978-1229

Lapidus, Sivia K., MD {1306161278} Pedtrc<NJ-MORRISTN>
+ Pediatric Infectious Disease/Hackensack Univ Med Ctr
30 Prospect Avenue Hackensack, NJ 07601 (201)996-5308 Fax (201)996-9815
+ Morristown Medical Center
100 Madison Avenue Morristown, NJ 07962 (973)971-6000

Lapietra, Alexis Marie, DO {1710290259} EmrgMd(10,NJ75)<NJ-STJOSHOS>
+ St Joseph's Medical Center Emergency
703 Main Street Paterson, NJ 07503 (973)754-2240 Fax (973)754-2249

Lapis, Peter, MD {1164604153} PthACl(80,HUN06)<RI-MEMHOSRI>
+ Accredited Dermatology
111 Water Street Toms River, NJ 08753

Lapman, Peter Grant, MD {1568637858} IntrMd, CdvDis(02,NY09)
+ Atlantic Cardiology LLC
444 Neptune Boulevard/Unit 2 Neptune, NJ 07753 (732)775-5300 Fax (732)775-1737
+ Atlantic Cardiology LLC
22 North Main Street Marlboro, NJ 07746 (732)462-6666
+ Atlantic Cardiology, LLC
27 South Cooks Bridge Road/Suite 216 Jackson, NJ 07753 (848)217-3010

Lappin, Harold S., MD {1457540742} Ophthl(66,NY19)<NJ-HCKTSTWN>
+ 500 Willow Grove Street
Hackettstown, NJ 07840 (908)852-2220 Fax (908)813-0255

Lapsiwala, Pareen Raj, DO {1043631294} FamMed
+ Vanguard Medical Group, P.A.
170 Changebridge Road/Suite C-3 Montville, NJ 07045 (973)575-5540 Fax (973)575-4885

Lapuerta, Pablo, MD {1083313693} IntrMd(89,MA01)
+ Lexicon Pharmaceuticals
350 Carter Road Princeton, NJ 08540

Lara, Jaime F., MD {1992853790} FamMed(79,SPAI)
+ 3A Stanworth Road
Kendall Park, NJ 08824 (732)940-0505

Laraya-Cuasay, Lourdes R., MD {1902875461} PedPul, Pedtrc(63,PHI01)<NJ-MONMOUTH, NJ-COMMED>
+ Monmouth Medical Group Pediatric Specialties
67 Route 37 West Toms River, NJ 08755 (732)557-3541 Fax (732)557-3518
llaraycuasey@barnabashealth.org

Lardizabal, Alfred A., MD {1518051721} CritCr, IntrMd, PulDis(86,PHIL)<NJ-UMDNJ>
+ Global Tuberculosis Institute (GTBI)
225 Warren Street/PO Box 1709/Medicine Newark, NJ 07101 (973)972-8452 Fax (973)972-3268
lardizaa@umdnj.edu

Lardner, Thomas Joseph, MD {1558461251} FamMed, SprtMd, FamMSptM(99,NJ91)
+ RWJPE Hillsborough Primary Care & Sports Med
751 Route 206/Suite 101 Hillsborough, NJ 08844 (908)359-0093
+ RWJ University Hospital Somerset
110 Rehill Avenue Somerville, NJ 08876 (908)685-2200

Largoza, Rosendito S., MD {1750344362} IntrMd, EmrgMd(69,PHIL)<NJ-HOLYNAME>
+ 751 Teaneck Road/Ground Floor
Teaneck, NJ 07666 (201)862-0050 Fax (201)837-0405
rosimd@optonline.net

Lariviere, Aimee T., MD {1154360592} Pedtrc(99,NJ06)<NJ-RWJUBRUN, NJ-UNVMCPRN>
+ Hillsborough Pediatrics
390 Amwell Road/Suite 106 Hillsborough, NJ 08844 (908)431-3100 Fax (908)431-3101

Larkin, Harry, Jr., MD {1821105198} FamMed(88,NJ06)<NJ-SOCEANCO>
+ Island Medical Professional Association
1812 Long Beach Boulevard Ship Bottom, NJ 08008 (609)494-2323 Fax (609)494-4141

Larkin, Jeffrey J., MD {1457359325} RadDia, Radiol(87,PA02)
+ South Jersey Radiology Associates, P.A.
748 Kings Highway West Deptford, NJ 08096 (856)848-4998 Fax (856)853-7362
+ South Jersey Radiology Associates, P.A.
Severan Profess Mews/Suite 105 Sewell, NJ 08080 (856)848-4998 Fax (856)589-6142
+ SJRA South Jersey Radiology Associates, P.A.
113 East Laurel Road Stratford, NJ 08096 (856)566-2552

Physicians by Name and Address

Larkin, Joyce Marie, MD {1831238617} Psychy(87,PA07)
+ Tao Institute of Mind & Body Medicine
1288 Route 73 South/Suite 210   Mount Laurel, NJ 08054   (856)802-6818   Fax (856)802-6878

LaRocca, Sandro, MD {1548267628} SrgOrt(95,PA02)<NJ-UNDRWD>
+ NJ Neck and Back Institute, PC
3131 Princeton Pike   Lawrenceville, NJ 08648   (609)896-0020   Fax (609)896-0041
drlarocca@njnbi.com

Laroche, Harold I., MD {1629060231} FamMed(84,PA01)
+ JFK Medical Center
65 James Street   Edison, NJ 08820   (732)321-7601   Fax (732)744-5614

LaRosa, David F., MD {1871704627} AlgyImmn, IntrMd(00,NY08)
+ Allergic Disease Associates, PC - Forked River
1044 Lacey Road/suite 9   Forked River, NJ 08731   (609)693-5317   Fax (609)693-0351

LaRosa, Jennifer A., MD {1174507024} PulCCr, IntrMd(96,DC01)
+ Morristown Medical Center
100 Madison Avenue   Morristown, NJ 07962   (973)971-5000
+ Newark Beth Israel Medical Center
201 Lyons Avenue/PulmCritCare   Newark, NJ 07112   (973)926-7000

Larose, Jean Eddy, DO {1750529012} IntrMd<NJ-STPETER>
+ St. Peter's University Hospital
254 Easton Avenue   New Brunswick, NJ 08901   (732)745-8600   Fax (732)745-3847

Larrea, Diana Rose, DO {1225460454}
+ University Hospital-University Family Medicine
42 East Laurel Road/Suite 2100   Stratford, NJ 08084   (856)566-6477   Fax (856)566-6188

Larsen, Bartley A., MD {1982600672} RadDia(78,MEX14)<NJ-RWJUHAM>
+ Quakerbridge Radiology Associates
8 Quakerbridge Plaza/Building 8   Mercerville, NJ 08619   (609)890-0033   Fax (609)689-6067

Larsen, Erik Scott, DO {1508841305} SrgOrt, SprtMd(93,NY75)<NJ-COMMED, NJ-KIMBALL>
+ 780 Route 37 West/Suite 330
Toms River, NJ 08755   (732)966-6317   Fax (732)998-8086

Larsen, Johnny R., DO {1417976341} EmrgMd(88,NY75)<NJ-KIMBALL>
+ Kimball Medical Center
600 River Avenue/EmergMed   Lakewood, NJ 08701   (732)363-1900

Larson, Jacqueline Kay, MD {1386996759} PedGst
+ St Joseph's Medical Pediatric Gastroenterology
703 Main Street   Paterson, NJ 07503   (973)754-2000

Larue, Catherine, MD {1558748053} IntrMd
+ Bayside State Prison
4293 Route 47/Med Unit   Leesburg, NJ 08327   (856)785-0040

Larusso, Jennifer Lynn, DO {1932360906} SrgMcr, Dermat, FamMed(01,NJ75)
+ Aesthetic Dermatology, LLC.
771 East Route 70/Suite D-150   Marlton, NJ 08053   (856)596-3393   Fax (856)596-3394

Las, Murray S., MD {1114003928} EnDbMt, IntrMd(75,MA07)
+ Feigin & Las
56 Diamond Springs Road   Denville, NJ 07834   (973)625-1000   Fax (973)625-9122

Lascari, Roland A., MD {1770515918} FamMed(80,ITAL)<NJ-CHILTON>
+ West Milford Medical Center
1485 Union Valley Road   West Milford, NJ 07480   (973)728-1880   Fax (973)728-1559

Lashin, Waleed Sirag, MD {1477590644} Grtrcs, IntrMd(95,EGY04)<NJ-STMRYPAS, NJ-HACKNSK>
+ 1414 Main Avenue
Clifton, NJ 07011   (973)253-6000   Fax (973)253-6009
Wlashin@hotmail.com

Lashley, Susan Leonora, MD {1508935131} ObsGyn(97,NY08)
+ Maternal Fetal Medicine of Practice Associates
11 Overlook Road/Suite LL 102   Summit, NJ 07901   (908)522-3846   Fax (908)522-5557

Laskarzewski, Radhika, MD {1629381025} FamMed(10,STM01)
+ Capital Health Primary Care
4056 Quakerbridge Road/Suite 101   Lawrenceville, NJ 08648   (609)528-9150   Fax (609)528-9151

Lasker, Michelle Rhonda, MD {1073564712} NnPnMd, Pedtrc(85,NJ05)<NJ-VALLEY>
+ The Valley Hospital
223 North Van Dien Avenue   Ridgewood, NJ 07450   (201)447-8000

Lasker, Steven Mark, MD {1437261732} Anesth(85,IL11)
+ Morris Anesthesia Group, PA
3799 Route 46/Suite 211   Parsippany, NJ 07054   (973)335-1122   Fax (973)335-1448

Lasker, Susan J., MD {1043652752} Pedtrc(80,NY09)
+ College of Saint Elizabeth Health Service
2 Convent Road   Morristown, NJ 07960   (973)290-4175   Fax (973)290-4182

Laskey, Richard S., MD {1770676546} SrgPlstc, Otlryg(79,NY46)<NJ-HOBUNIMC, NJ-BAYONNE>
+ 122 Clinton Street/3rd Floor
Hoboken, NJ 07030   (201)795-5103   Fax (201)795-1312
+ 631 Broadway
Bayonne, NJ 07002   (201)858-9800

Laskin, David A., MD {1902905938} IntrMd, Grtrcs(78,PA09)
+ Laskin Internal Medcine
400 Grove Road/PO Box 37   Thorofare, NJ 08086   (856)845-8010   Fax (856)845-9398

Laskow, David A., MD {1689771784} Surgry, SrgTpl(81,NJ06)<NJ-RWJUBRUN>
+ Robert Wood Johnson Transplant Associates, P.A.
10 Plum Street/7th Floor   New Brunswick, NJ 08901   (732)253-3699

Laskowski-Kos, Ursula A., MD {1417188772}<NJ-NWRKBETH>
+ Morristown Medical Center
100 Madison Avenue   Morristown, NJ 07962   (973)971-5000
+ Newark Beth Israel Medical Center
201 Lyons Avenue   Newark, NJ 07112   (973)926-7000

Lasky, Melodee S., MD {1730190133} FamMed(80,PA13)
+ Rutgers Hurtado Health Center
11 Bishop Place   New Brunswick, NJ 08901   (732)932-7402   Fax (732)932-1223

Lasorsa, Antonio G., DO {1093036485}<NJ-VALLEY>
+ The Valley Hospital
223 North Van Dien Avenue   Ridgewood, NJ 07450   (201)447-8000

Lasser, Andrew S., MD {1275665960} RadDia(80,MEXI)<NJ-BERGNMC>
+ 127 Fawn Hill Road
Upper Saddle River, NJ 07458

Lasser, Michael Sidney, MD {1578782223} Urolgy
+ Premier Urology Group, LLC
10 Parsonage Road/Suite 118   Edison, NJ 08837   (732)494-9400   Fax (732)548-3931
+ Premier Urology Group, LLC
570 South Avenue East/Building A   Cranford, NJ 07016   (732)494-9400   Fax (908)497-1633
+ Premier Urology Group, LLC
2 Hospital Plaza/Suite 430   Old Bridge, NJ 08837   (732)494-9400   Fax (732)679-2077

Lastra, Carlos R., MD {1144249137} Nrolgy, Pedtrc, NrlgSpec(84,COL25)<NJ-STPETER>
+ St. Peter's Family Health
123 How Lane   New Brunswick, NJ 08901   (732)745-8600   Fax (732)729-0869
+ St. Peter's University Hospital
254 Easton Avenue/Pediatrics   New Brunswick, NJ 08901   (732)745-8600   Fax (732)745-1632

Lat, Emmanuel A., MD {1417022062} SrgCsm, SrgHnd, SrgPlstc(72,PHIL)<NJ-HACKNSK, NJ-VALLEY>
+ Paramus Plastic Surgery, Skin Care & Laser Center
17 Arcadian Avenue/Suite 103   Paramus, NJ 07652   (201)843-0700   Fax (201)843-0622
paramuspscenter@aol.com

Lateef, Aslam, MD {1679544324} IntrMd, Allrgy, AlgyImmn(98,NJ05)
+ Hamilton Allergy Center
2333 Whitehorse Mercerville Rd/Suite G   Hamilton, NJ 08619   (609)584-9200   Fax (609)584-9299

Latef, Sherif Maurice, MD {1275567810} IntrMd(97,EGY03)
+ 86 Lake Street
Jersey City, NJ 07306

Latif, Madiha, MD {1255644845} IntrMd
+ 89 Fairfax Court
Madison, NJ 07940   (973)647-2866

Latif, Pervaize, MD {1174616064} CdvDis, IntrMd(68,PAK01)<NJ-RBAYOLDB, NJ-RBAYPERT>
+ Clara Barton Cardio-Medical Associates
565 New Brunswick Avenue   Fords, NJ 08863   (732)738-8000   Fax (732)738-1663
+ Clara Barton Cardio-Medical Associates
949 Route 9 North   South Amboy, NJ 08879   (732)738-8000   Fax (732)525-8235

Latif, Saima, MD {1427358712} Psychy(02,NJ05)
+ VA New Jersey Health Care System at Lyons
151 Knollcroft Road   Lyons, NJ 07939   (973)676-1000

Latif, Shahid, MD {1609941764} CdvDis, IntrMd(81,PAKI)<NJ-JFKMED, NJ-RBAYPERT>
+ Clara Barton Cardio-Medical Associates
949 Route 9 North   South Amboy, NJ 08879   (732)525-0390   Fax (732)525-8235
+ Clara Barton Cardio-Medical Associates
565 New Brunswick Avenue   Fords, NJ 08863   (732)525-0390   Fax (732)738-1663
+ Clara Barton Cardio-Medical Associates
78 Amboy Avenue   Metuchen, NJ 08879   (732)548-4365

Latif, Walead, DO {1891738555} Nephro, IntrMd(02,NJ75)<NY-VABRKLYN>
+ American Access Care, LLC.
2401 Morris Avenue/Suite West 112   Union, NJ 07083   (908)686-0123   Fax (908)686-0014

Latimer, Edward A., MD {1194810895} Psychy(85,NJ05)
+ 24 Portland Place
Montclair, NJ 07042   (973)744-1880   Fax (973)746-9575

Latimer, Karen M., MD {1457599615} FamMAdlt(99,NY48)
+ 53 Heights Road
Ridgewood, NJ 07450   (201)857-8589
karenlatimer@mac.com
+ Bergen Volunteer Medical Initiative, Inc.
241 Moore Street/Suite 101   Hackensack, NJ 07601   (201)857-8589   Fax (201)518-8494

Latimore Collier, Sherita Monai, MD {1952346108} IntrMd(96,GA21)
+ Parkside Adolescent and Adult Medical Clinic
1300 Princess Avenue   Camden, NJ 08103   (856)964-5569   Fax (856)964-0744

Latkin, Richard M., MD {1003896218} ObsGyn, Gyneco(63,NY09)<NJ-VALLEY>
+ Women's Total Health-Woodcliff Lake
577 Chestnut Ridge Road/Suite 9   Woodcliff Lake, NJ 07677   (201)391-5770   Fax (201)391-4793

Latorre, Juan J., MD {1336227297} FamMed(84,BRAZ)<NJ-HOBUNIMC>
+ Center for Family Health
122-132 Clinton Street   Hoboken, NJ 07030   (201)418-3100   Fax (201)418-3148

Latorre, Rafael, MD {1629158407} IntrMd(90,SPA11)<NJ-ENGLWOOD, NJ-HACKNSK>
+ Englewood Family Health Center
148 Engle Street   Englewood, NJ 07631   (201)569-1530   Fax (201)569-6022

Latriano, Blaise P., MD {1194779926} CritCr, IntrMd(89,NY08)<NJ-WARREN>
+ Warren Hospital
185 Roseberry Street/CriticalCare   Phillipsburg, NJ 08865   (908)387-6018   Fax (908)859-6813

Lattanzi, Joseph Paul, MD {1538145123} RadOnc(94,WI06)<NJ-SOCEANCO>
+ Southern Ocean County Medical Center
1140 Route 72 West/RadOnc   Manahawkin, NJ 08050   (609)978-2194   Fax (609)978-2843

Latyshev, Yevgeniy, MD {1225342439} CdvDis
+ North Arlington Cardiology Associates
62 Ridge Road   North Arlington, NJ 07031   (201)351-0677   Fax (201)991-2408

Latzko, Karen Marie, DO {1831190909} Urolgy(89,IL76)<NJ-UNVMCPRN>
+ Urology Group of Princeton PA
134 Stanhope Street/Forrestal Village   Princeton, NJ 08540   (609)924-6487   Fax (609)921-7020

Latzko, Michael Patrick, MD {1093940710}<NJ-MONMOUTH>
+ Monmouth Medical Center
300 Second Avenue   Long Branch, NJ 07740   (732)923-6769

Lau, Henry, MD {1316944739} CdvDis, IntrMd(73,TAIW)<NJ-HACKNSK>
+ 211 Essex Street/Suite 403
Hackensack, NJ 07601   (201)646-0044   Fax (201)646-0357

Lau, Ronald, MD {1558466623} FamMed, IntrMd(84,RI01)
+ RWJPE Cranbury Medical Group
557 Cranbury Road/Suite 22   East Brunswick, NJ 08816   (732)613-0500   Fax (732)613-0345

Laub, Edward B., MD {1215974902} IntrMd(76,NJ05)<NJ-CHSFULD, NJ-RWJUHAM>
+ Hamilton Internal Medicine Associates
2055 Klockner Road   Trenton, NJ 08690   (609)586-8060   Fax (609)586-7470

Laub, Glenn W., MD {1417906066} SrgThr, Surgry(81,NH01)<NJ-STFRNMED>
+ St. Francis Medical Center
601 Hamilton Avenue   Trenton, NJ 08629   (609)599-5308   Fax (609)599-5325

Laudadio, Richard Dominick, MD {1386639185} IntrMd(00,MNT01)
+ Summit Medical Group-Berkeley Heights Campus
1 Diamond Hill Road   Berkeley Heights, NJ 07922   (908)273-4300   Fax (908)790-6576

Laudati, Mary, MD {1093779563} Pedtrc(82,ITA01)
+ Gloucester County Pediatrics
849 Cooper Street   Deptford, NJ 08096   (856)848-6346   Fax (856)848-5734

Lauer, Marshall F., MD {1306800859} IntrMd, Addctn(79,MEX03)<NJ-OURLADY, NJ-VIRTVOOR>
+ 414 Hadon Avenue
Collingswood, NJ 08108 (856)854-7800 Fax (856)854-1687
mflauer@hotmail.com
+ Burlington Comprehensive Counseling
75 Washington Street Mount Holly, NJ 08060 (856)854-7800 Fax (609)267-9692

Laufer, Beatrice, MD {1518063577} IntrMd
+ Palisades Medical Center
8100 Kennedy Boulevard North Bergen, NJ 07047 (201)866-6770 Fax (201)866-6771

Laufer, Ilene Caren, MD {1144342569} Pedtrc(90,NJ05)<NJ-HACKNSK, NJ-VALLEY>
+ North Jersey Pediatrics
17-10 Fair Lawn Avenue Fair Lawn, NJ 07410 (201)794-8585 Fax (201)703-9889

Laufer, Samuel J., MD {1114022571} SrgOrt(69,TN06)
+ Pediatric Orthopedic Associates, P.A.
585 Cranbury Road/Suite A East Brunswick, NJ 08816 (732)390-1160 Fax (732)390-8449
+ Pediatric Orthopedic Associates, P.A.
3700 State Route 33 Neptune, NJ 07753 (732)390-1160 Fax (732)897-4205

Laufgraben, Marc Jeffrey, MD {1932146255} EnDbMt, IntrMd(92,MA01)<RI-MEMHOSRI, RI-RIHOSPTL>
+ The Cooper Hospital System-Univ Hospital
3 Cooper Plaza/Suite 215 Camden, NJ 08103 (856)342-2312 Fax (856)968-0735

Laughinghouse, Kenneth, MD {1295720563} IntrMd, Hemato, MedOnc(91,CT01)<NJ-RIVERVW>
+ Regional Cancer Care Associates, LLC
180 White Road Little Silver, NJ 07739 (732)530-8666 Fax (732)530-4139

Lauletta, Maryann Carmella, MD {1659373280} IntrMd(98,PA09)<NJ-KMHTURNV>
+ Internal Medicine Associates of Southern New Jersey
151 Fries Mill Road/Suite 400 Turnersville, NJ 08012 (856)401-9300 Fax (856)374-5805

Laumbach, Robert John, MD {1871716803} FamMed, OccpMd, GPrvMd(97,NJ06)
+ University Hospital-School of Public Health
170 Frelinghuysen Road Piscataway, NJ 08854 (732)445-0123 Fax (732)445-3644

Laumbach, Sonia Caridad G., MD {1841204104} FamMed(99,NJ06)
+ Family Medicine at Monument Square
317 George Street New Brunswick, NJ 08901 (732)235-8993 Fax (732)246-7317

Laureano, Ana Cristina, MD {1740544279} Dermat
+ The Office of Dr Sharon Scherl MD
45 Central Aveue Tenafly, NJ 07670 (201)568-8400 Fax (201)568-8554

Lauredan, Bernier, MD {1639283047} Pedtrc(83,DOMI)<NJ-STBARNMC, NJ-RBAYOLDB>
+ Irvington Pediatric Associates
22 Ball Street/Suite 100 Irvington, NJ 07111 (973)371-1600 Fax (973)372-7677
+ Pedi-Doc, PA
202 Smith Street Perth Amboy, NJ 08861 (732)697-1600

Laurelli, Joseph P., MD {1568678100} Psychy, Addctn(72,NE06)
+ 54 Nathan Drive
Old Bridge, NJ 08857

Laurente, Cristeta A., MD {1558339648} IntrMd(62,PHI01)
+ Laurente Medical Associates
4453 Nottingham Way Hamilton, NJ 08690 (609)587-0119 Fax (609)587-3009

Laurente, Julie Gyi, DO {1750645180}
+ 57 Fourth Street
Hoboken, NJ 07030 (646)338-4796

Laurente, Robert M., MD {1841502937} IntrMd
+ Laurente Medical Associates
4453 Nottingham Way Hamilton, NJ 08690 (609)587-0119 Fax (609)587-3009

Lauricella, Joseph Ned, MD {1316914310} CdvDis, IntrMd(78,MEX14)<NJ-HOLYNAME, NJ-HACKNSK>
+ Bergen Cardiology Associates
292 Columbia Avenue Fort Lee, NJ 07024 (201)224-0450 Fax (201)224-6061
+ Bergen Cardiology Associates
400 Frank W. Burr Boulevard Teaneck, NJ 07666 (201)224-0050 Fax (201)692-3263

Lautenberg, Mitchel Alan, MD {1508833484} Ophthl(93,NJ06)
+ Ocean Eye Institute
601 Route 37 West Toms River, NJ 08755 (732)244-4400 Fax (732)505-2171

Lautenslager, Tara Lee, MD {1114169174} Gastrn
+ Cooper Digestive Health Institute
501 Fellowship Road/Suite 101 Mount Laurel, NJ 08054 (856)642-2133 Fax (856)642-2134

Lauter, Otto Scott, MD {1174512230} IntrMd
+ Chilton Medical Center
97 West Parkway Pompton Plains, NJ 07444 (973)831-5420 Fax (973)831-5183

Lautin, Jeffrey L., MD {1689629875} RadDia, RadV&I(89,NY01)<NJ-NWRKBETH>
+ Millburn Medical Imaging
2130 Millburn Avenue/Suite A-8 Maplewood, NJ 07040 (973)912-0404 Fax (973)912-0444
+ Newark Diagnostic Radiologists, PA
201 Lyons Avenue Newark, NJ 07112 (973)926-7466
+ The Access Center
741 Northfield Avenue/Suite 205 West Orange, NJ 07040 (973)243-9729

Lavaia, Maria A., MD {1538162094} Pedtrc(93,NY08)<NJ-STJOSHOS>
+ Notchview Pediatrics, LLC.
1037 Route 46 East/Suite 201 Clifton, NJ 07013 (973)779-3911 Fax (973)471-2730

LaVan, Frederick B., MD {1003811233} SrgRec(86,PA01)<NJ-KENEDYHS, NJ-UNDRWD>
+ Premier Orthopaedic of South Jersey
1007 Mantua Pike Woodbury, NJ 08096 (856)853-8004 Fax (856)853-8022
+ Plastic and Cosmetic Surgical Group PC of New Jersey
1007 Mantua Pike/Suite B Woodbury, NJ 08096 (856)853-8004 Fax (856)256-7709

Laveman, Lawrence B., MD {1821097908} PedDvl, Pedtrc(89,SPA22)<NJ-BAYONNE, NJ-HOBUNIMC>
+ in Health Associates
15 State Route 15 Lafayette, NJ 07848 (973)579-6700 Fax (973)579-6830
+ St. Mary Community Mental Health Center
506 3rd Street Hoboken, NJ 07030 (201)792-8200

Lavian, Pejman, MD {1871565432} FamMed(99,POL12)
+ Family Medical Care of Clifton
1033 Clifton Avenue/Suite 209 Clifton, NJ 07013 (973)470-8377 Fax (973)470-8534

Lavietes, Marc H., MD {1013001106} IntrMd, PulDis(69,OH06)<NJ-UMDNJ>
+ University Hospital
150 Bergen Street/Room I354 Newark, NJ 07103 (973)972-6058 Fax (973)972-6228
rosemarc@ix.netcom.com

Lavin, Bruce Scott, MD {1497926620} IntrMd, InfDis(82,MD12)
+ 3 John Trout Road
Ringoes, NJ 08551 Fax (908)782-3854

Lavine, Ferne R., MD {1043319155} Otlryg(76,NJ05)<NJ-RWJUBRUN, NJ-STPETER>
+ Ear Nose & Throat Group of Central NJ
2124 Oak Tree Road/2nd floor Edison, NJ 08820 (732)205-1311 Fax (732)205-9648
+ 529 Milltown Road
North Brunswick, NJ 08902 (732)205-1311 Fax (732)246-8256

Lavine, Sean David, MD {1386797868} SrgNro, IntrMd(91,NY20)<NY-NYPRESHS, NY-PRSBCOLU>
+ Neurosurgeons of New Jersey
1200 East Ridgewood Avenue Ridgewood, NJ 07450 (201)824-6131 Fax (212)342-1229

Lavis, James Douglas, DO {1992783609} ObsGyn(74,PA77)<NJ-CHSMRCER>
+ 2 East 14th Street
Ocean City, NJ 08226 (609)602-7969
+ Capital Health System/Mercer Campus
446 Bellevue Avenue Trenton, NJ 08618 (609)394-4000

Lavizzo Mourey, Risa Juanita, MD {1376733998} IntrMd, Grtrcs(79,MA01)
+ Eric B. Chandler Health Center
277 George Street New Brunswick, NJ 08901 (732)235-6700 Fax (732)235-6729

Lavotshkin, Anna Janna, MD {1467560797} IntrMd(75,ISRA)<NJ-HOLYNAME>
+ Drs. Lavotshkin and Znamensky
757 Teaneck Road Teaneck, NJ 07666 (201)833-2288 Fax (201)833-4441

Lavrich, Judith Barbara, MD {1386603769} Ophthl(86,OH41)<NJ-CHSMRCER>
+ Total Eye Care Center
2495 Brunswick Pike/Suite 8 Lawrenceville, NJ 08648 (609)882-8828

Lavrich, Pamela S., MD {1255492310} Anesth(91,NY46)<NJ-VALLEY>
+ The Valley Hospital
223 North Van Dien Avenue Ridgewood, NJ 07450 (201)447-8000

Physicians by Name and Address

Law, Henry, DO {1215161856} Anesth<NJ-KMHTURNV>
+ Rancocas Anesthesiology, PA
700 Route 130 North/Suite 203 Cinnaminson, NJ 08077 (856)829-9345 Fax (856)829-3605

Law, Jeremy P., MD {1790942076} FamMed, IntHos, IntrMd(07,IL06)<NJ-JFKMED>
+ VA New Jersey Health Care System
385 Tremont Avenue/Corporate Office East Orange, NJ 07018 (973)676-1000 Fax (973)676-4226

Law, Kevin F., MD {1558585497} PulDis, SlpDis, CritCr(87,NY19)<NJ-RWJUHAM>
+ 2312 Whitehorse-Mercerville Rd
Trenton, NJ 08619 (609)586-7400 Fax (609)586-7656

Law, Stephen W., DO {1982705778} EmrgMd(94,PA77)<NJ-CLARMAAS, NJ-STBARNMC>
+ Clara Maass Medical Center
1 Clara Maass Drive/EmrgMed Belleville, NJ 07109 (973)450-2000
+ Emergency Medical Associates of NJ, P.A.
3 Century Drive Parsippany, NJ 07054 (973)450-2000 Fax (973)740-9895

Law, William A., MD {1194706192} SrgOrt(88,NY20)<NJ-OCEANMC>
+ Brielle Orthopedics PA
457 Jack Martin Boulevard Brick, NJ 08724 (732)840-7500 Fax (732)840-2088
+ Brielle Orthopedics PA
823 Lacey Road Forked River, NJ 08731 (732)840-7500 Fax (732)840-2088
+ Brielle Orthopedics PA
1301 Route 72 West Manahawkin, NJ 08724 (609)971-7616 Fax (609)971-7639

Lawand, Oussama, MD {1821283623} IntrMd<NJ-UMDNJ>
+ University Hospital
150 Bergen Street Newark, NJ 07103 (973)972-5291

Lawandy, Michael Armia, DO {1134324841} IntrMd, IntHos(05,NJ75)<NJ-STPETER, NJ-VIRTMHBC>
+ Virtua Hospitalist Group Memorial
175 Madison Avenue/2 FL Stokes Mount Holly, NJ 08060 (609)267-0700 Fax (609)914-6182

Lawinski, Richard M., MD {1629073911} Surgry(76,PA13)<NJ-BURDTMLN>
+ 9 Broadway/Suite B
Cape May Court House, NJ 08210 (609)463-1000 Fax (609)463-8301
+ Court House Surgery Center
106 Courthouse South Dennis Rd Cape May, NJ 08204 (609)463-1000 Fax (609)465-8771

Lawit, Alan, MD {1396816468} FamMed, IntrMd(68,PA13)<NJ-UNDRWD>
+ Woodbury Surgical Associates
127 North Broad Street Woodbury, NJ 08096 (856)845-8077 Fax (856)845-1295

Lawler, Gregory James, DO {1083657506} Anesth, PainMd(93,MO79)
+ 6233 JF Kennedy Boulevard
North Bergen, NJ 07047 (201)758-7550 Fax (201)758-7549
+ 1117 US Hwy 46 East/Suite 203
Clifton, NJ 07013 (201)758-7550 Fax (201)758-7549

Lawn, Jennifer Elizabeth, DO
+ Skylands Medical Group PA
26 Gail Court/Suite 2-B Sparta, NJ 07871

Lawrence, David L., MD {1245219989} CdvDis, CarNuc, IntrMd(97,PA02)<NJ-VIRTUAHS, NJ-OURLADY>
+ Associated Cardiovascular Consultants-Lourdes
1 Brace Road/Suite C & F Cherry Hill, NJ 08034 (856)428-4100 Fax (856)428-1517

Lawrence, Denise Antoinette, MD {1659309599} FamMed, IntrMd(88,NY15)<NJ-SOMERSET>
+ Franklin Family Practice PA
29 Clyde Road/Suite 101 Somerset, NJ 08873 (732)873-0330 Fax (732)873-2077
dlawrence13j@hotmail.com

Lawrence, Jeffry Brian, MD {1659662856} PthACl, PthHem, PthCln(79,IL06)
+ Becton Dickinson & Company
1 Becton Drive/Suite 084 Franklin Lakes, NJ 07417 (201)847-6800

Lawrence, John Robert, MD {1144257304} FamMed(02,PA02)
+ Carneys Point Family Practice
341 Shell Road Carneys Point, NJ 08069 (856)299-4600 Fax (856)299-1688

Lawrence, John Todd Rutter, MD {1033279690} SrgOrt<PA-CHILDHOS>
+ CHOP Pediatric & Adolescent Specialty Care Center
1012 Laurel Oak Road/OrtSrg Voorhees, NJ 08043 (856)435-1300 Fax (856)435-0091

Physicians by Name and Address

Lawrence, Naomi, MD {1124100565} Dermat, Surgry, SrgDer(87,LA01)<NJ-COOPRUMC>
+ Cooper Center for Dermatologic Surgery
  10000 Sagemore Drive/Suite 10103 Marlton, NJ 08053 (856)596-3040 Fax (856)596-5651
  lawrence-naomi@cooperhealth.edu
+ The Cooper Hospital System-Univ Hospital
  3 Cooper Plaza/Suite 215 Camden, NJ 08103 (856)342-2439

Lawrie, John A., MD {1134161045} EmrgMd, IntrMd(75,IN20)<NJ-RWJUHAM>
+ Robert Wood Johnson University Hospital at Hamilton
  1 Hamilton Health Place/EmergMed Hamilton, NJ 08690 (609)586-7900 Fax (609)584-6428

Laws-Mobilio, Susan Wendi, DO {1275520579} FamMed(79,PA77)<NJ-KMHCHRRY>
+ Lourdes Medical Associates/Triboro Family Physicians
  1104 Route 130/Suite K Cinnaminson, NJ 08077 (856)786-8010 Fax (856)786-0529
+ Riverton Family Practice
  605 Main Street/Suite 104 Riverton, NJ 08077 (856)786-8010 Fax (856)786-2478

Lawson, Charles Alexander, MD {1457333536} Anesth(89,NY01)<NJ-MORRISTN>
+ Morristown Medical Center
  100 Madison Avenue/Anesthesiology Morristown, NJ 07962 (973)971-5000 Fax (201)943-8733

Lawyer, Edward Zadok, MD {1114189859} EmrgMd(04,IL11)<NJ-HOBUNIMC>
+ Hoboken University Medical Center
  308 Willow Avenue/EmrgMed Hoboken, NJ 07030 (201)418-1000

Laxmi, Sheethal Manipadaga, MD {1316189673} InfDis, IntrMd(03,INA83)<NJ-MONMOUTH>
+ Medical Associates of Marlboro PC
  32 North Main Street Marlboro, NJ 07746 (732)462-4100 Fax (732)462-3798

Lay, Virginia I., MD {1225016892} ObsGyn(85,NJ05)<NJ-CLARMAAS>
+ 36 Newark Avenue/Suite 128
  Belleville, NJ 07109 (973)751-5454 Fax (973)751-1717

Layne, George Stark, MD {1255494258} Psychy, PsyAdd, IntrMd(70,MI01)
+ Center for Family Guidance, PC
  765 East Route 70/Building A-101 Marlton, NJ 08053 (856)797-4800 Fax (856)810-0110

Layne, Trevor J., MD {1124089719} IntrMd, MedOnc(88,GRN01)<NJ-EASTORNG, NJ-NWRKBETH>
+ 354 Main Street
  West Orange, NJ 07052 (973)731-2201

Lazar, Amy D., MD {1568441988} Otlryg, OtgyFPlS(92,IL42)
+ ENT & Allergy Associates-Bridgewater
  245 US Highway 22/3rd Fl/Suite 300 Bridgewater, NJ 08807 (908)722-1022 Fax (908)722-2040
  Alazar@entandallergy.com
+ Raritan Valley Surgery Center
  100 Franklin Square Drive/Suite 100 Somerset, NJ 08873 (908)722-1022 Fax (732)560-5999

Lazar, Eric B., MD {1992701874} Radiol(92,IL06)
+ University Radiology, PA
  239 Route 22 East/Suite 302 Green Brook, NJ 08812 (732)968-4899 Fax (732)968-8096
+ University Radiology Group, P.C.
  3900 Park Avenue/Suite 107 Edison, NJ 08820 (732)968-4899 Fax (732)548-6290
+ University Radiology Group, P.C.
  16 Mountain Boulevard Warren, NJ 08812 (908)769-7200 Fax (908)769-9141

Lazar, Eric L., MD {1558334862} Surgry, PedSrg(89,NY01)<NJ-OVERLOOK, NJ-MORRISTN>
+ Overlook Medical Center
  99 Beauvoir Avenue/PO Box 210 Summit, NJ 07902 (908)522-2000

Lazar, Lorraine M., MD {1043305204} NroChl, NrlgSpec(93,NY47)<NJ-UMDNJ, NY-PRSBWEIL>
+ Northeast Regional Epilepsy Group
  20 Prospect Avenue/Suite 800 Hackensack, NJ 07601 (201)343-6676 Fax (201)343-6689
+ UH-Robert Wood Jhnsn Med Sch
  97 Paterson Street/4th Fl/ChldNeur New Brunswick, NJ 08901

Lazar, Mark H., MD {1679639850} Nrolgy, Elecmy, Acpntr(77,NY19)<NJ-RWJUHAM>
+ The Neurology and Headache Center
  573 Cranbury Road/Suite A5 East Brunswick, NJ 08816 (732)254-5101 Fax (732)254-2640

Lazaroff, Leslie Diann, DO {1386950137} PhysMd(96,NJ75)
+ Water's Edge Healthcare and Rehabilitation Center
  512 Union Street Trenton, NJ 08611 (609)393-8622 Fax (609)393-5409

+ 6 Devon Drive
  Piscataway, NJ 08854 (732)572-5491

Lazarus, Adam Larry, MD {1043264757} EmrgMd(94,PA13)<NJ-VIRTVOOR>
+ Virtua Voorhees
  100 Bowman Drive Voorhees, NJ 08043 (856)247-3000
+ Emergency Physician Associates, P.A.
  307 South Evergreen Avenue/PO Box 298 Woodbury, NJ 08096 (856)247-3000 Fax (856)848-1431

Lazarus, David S., MD {1619018389} IntrMd, PulDis, CritCr(82,NY08)<NJ-HUNTRDN>
+ 1100 Westcott Drive/Suite 301
  Flemington, NJ 08822 (908)237-2358 Fax (908)237-2368

Lazarus, Mark David, MD {1497793657} SrgOrt(88,NJ05)<NJ-ACMCMAIN, NJ-ACMCITY>
+ Rothman Institute
  999 Route 73 North/3rd Fl Marlton, NJ 08053 (856)821-6360 Fax (856)821-6359

Lazarus, Nermin Ahmed, DO {1780668749} FamMed(96,NY75)
+ 100 Brick Road/Suite 210
  Marlton, NJ 08053 (856)596-4470 Fax (856)596-0420

Lazarus, Robert E., MD {1447213392} RadDia(89,PA07)<NJ-SJHREGMC>
+ SJH Regional Medical Center
  1505 West Sherman Avenue Vineland, NJ 08360 (856)641-8000

Lazarus-Wolpov, Dawn E., MD {1609891878} RadDia<NJ-VALLEY>
+ Radiology Associates of Ridgewood, P.A.
  20 Franklin Turnpike Waldwick, NJ 07463 (201)445-8822 Fax (201)447-5053

Lazieh, Janet Tomeh, MD {1730145707} Pedtrc(92,SYRI)
+ Drs. Banschick, Concepcion & Stein
  2500 Lemoine Avenue/Suite 200 Fort Lee, NJ 07024 (201)592-9210 Fax (201)592-6539

Lazo, Angel Amado, Jr., MD {1932168523} IntrMd(84,DOM02)
+ Liberty Medical Associates
  377 Jersey Avenue/Suite 470 Jersey City, NJ 07302 (201)918-2239 Fax (201)918-2243

Lazo Vasquez, Alex F., MD {1023490935}<NJ-MORRISTN>
+ Morristown Medical Center
  100 Madison Avenue Morristown, NJ 07962 (973)971-5000

Lazovitz, David A., MD {1881749083} AdolMd, Pedtrc(71,NY09)
+ 18 Sycamore Drive
  Medford, NJ 08055 (609)457-5590

Lazzara, Elizabeth Wanda, MD {1275540882} Radiol, RadDia, RadNro(89,NY19)
+ University Radiology Group, P.C.
  579A Cranbury Road East Brunswick, NJ 08816 (732)390-0040 Fax (732)390-1856
+ University Radiology Group, P.C.
  483 Cranbury Road East Brunswick, NJ 08816 (732)390-0040 Fax (732)390-5383
+ University Radiology Group, P.C.
  16 Mountain Boulevard Warren, NJ 08816 (908)769-7200 Fax (908)769-9141

Le, Mina Nguyen, MD {1659563955} Otlryg<NJ-BERGNMC>
+ New Bridge Medical Center
  230 East Ridgewood Avenue Paramus, NJ 07652 (201)225-7130 Fax (201)967-4117

Le, Phuong Uyen, DO {1366818783} PhyMPain
+ 499 Cooper Landing Road
  Cherry Hill, NJ 08002 (856)663-7080

Le, Tram N., MD {1912931791} IntrMd(95,NJ06)
+ 170 Linden Avenue
  Oaklyn, NJ 08107 (856)962-8840

Le, Van, MD
+ 201 Marin Boulevard/Suite 1602
  Jersey City, NJ 07302

Le Benger, Jeffrey D., MD {1962404558} Otlryg, SrgHdN, SrgFPlI(84,NY08)<NJ-OVERLOOK, NJ-MORRISTN>
+ Summit Medical Group-Berkeley Heights Campus
  1 Diamond Hill Road Berkeley Heights, NJ 07922 (908)277-8681 Fax (908)277-8662

Le Benger, Kerry S., MD {1982606471} Allrgy, IntrMd, IntMAImm(80,NY08)<NJ-OVERLOOK, NJ-MORRISTN>
+ Summit Medical Group-Berkeley Heights Campus
  1 Diamond Hill Road Berkeley Heights, NJ 07922 (908)273-4300 Fax (908)277-8760

Le Cavalier, Larry Alan, MD {1588661870} RadDia, Radiol(84,IL11)<NJ-STFRNMED>
+ Radiology Affiliates of Central New Jersey, P.A.
  2501 Kuser Road Hamilton, NJ 08691 (609)585-8800 Fax (609)585-1825
+ Radiology Affiliates of Central New Jersey, P.A.
  3120 Princeton Pike Lawrenceville, NJ 08648 (609)585-8800 Fax (609)219-0439

Leach, Thomas A., MD {1114089141} SrgPlstc(85,NJ05)<NJ-UNVMCPRN, NJ-RWJUBRUN>
+ Princeton Center for Plastic Surgery
  932 State Road Princeton, NJ 08540 (609)921-7161 Fax (609)921-6263

Leaf, Daniel Craig, MD {1477710465} Anesth(04,GRN01)<NJ-STBARNMC>
+ St. Barnabas Medical Center
  94 Old Short Hills Road/Anesth Livingston, NJ 07039 (973)322-5000

Leahy, Brendan Hosie, MD {1851657993}<NJ-SJHREGMC>
+ SJH Regional Medical Center
  1505 West Sherman Avenue Vineland, NJ 08360 (856)641-8000

Leary, Jeffrey T., MD {1033314042} SrgOrt
+ North Jersey Orthopaedic Group
  799 Bloomfield Avenue/Suite 111 Verona, NJ 07044 (973)689-6266 Fax (973)689-6264
+ North Jersey Orthopaedic Group
  33 Bleeker Street Millburn, NJ 07041 (973)689-6266 Fax (973)564-8928
+ North Jersey Orthopaedic Group
  246 Hamburg Turnpike/Suite 302 Wayne, NJ 07044 (973)689-6266 Fax (973)689-6264

Leavell, Ellen T., MD {1033288303} EmrgMd, FamMed(75,PA12)
+ 498 Elizabeth Avenue
  Somerset, NJ 08873 (732)735-1897

Leavy, Jeffrey Alan, MD {1548211493} CdvDis(86,IL11)<NJ-VIRTMARL, NJ-KMHCHRRY>
+ Cardiovascular Associates of The Delaware Valley, PA
  1840 Frontage Road Cherry Hill, NJ 08034 (856)795-2227 Fax (856)795-7436
+ Cardiovascular Associates
  210 West Atlantic Avenue Haddon Heights, NJ 08035 (856)795-2227 Fax (856)547-5337
+ Cardiovascular Associates of The Delaware Valley, PA
  525 State Street/Suite 3 Elmer, NJ 08034 (856)358-2363 Fax (856)358-0725

Lebaron, Johnathon Clinton, DO {1548606783} EmrgMd
+ Emergency Medical Associates of NJ, P.A.
  3 Century Drive Parsippany, NJ 07054 (860)377-9780 Fax (973)740-9895

Lebenthal, Mark J., MD {1346240785} CdvDis, IntrMd(76,MEX03)
+ RWJPE Cardiology Associates of Somerset County, P.A.
  487 Union Avenue/Suite A Bridgewater, NJ 08807 (908)722-6410 Fax (908)722-4638

Leber, George B., MD {1275636060} CdvDis, CarNuc, IntrMd(76,NY03)<NJ-ENGLWOOD>
+ Englewood Cardiology Consultants
  177 North Dean Street/Suite 100 Englewood, NJ 07631 (201)569-4901 Fax (201)569-6111

Leber, Ian Brett, MD {1306865092} EmrgMd(97,NJ06)<NJ-CHSMRCER, NJ-CHSFULD>
+ Kimball Medical Center
  600 River Avenue Lakewood, NJ 08701 (732)363-1900

Leber, Sandra Lynn, DO {1144327123} ObsGyn(94,IA75)<NJ-JFKMED, NJ-KMHCHRRY>
+ The University Doctors - UMDNJ -SOM
  570 Egg Harbor Road/Suite C-2 Sewell, NJ 08080 (856)218-0300 Fax (856)589-9487

Lebovic, Daniel M., MD {1033112727} Pedtrc(82,NY15)
+ Pediatric Associates of Central Jersey
  326 Main Street Metuchen, NJ 08840 (732)767-0630 Fax (732)767-3070

Lebovicz, Richard S., MD {1558304220} SrgOrt(79,NY08)<NJ-JFKMED, NJ-STPETER>
+ 908 Oak Tree Road/Suite E
  South Plainfield, NJ 07080 (908)756-9500

Lebovitch, Steve, MD {1396984944} Urolgy
+ Urologic Institute of NJ PA
  277 Forest Avenue/Suite 206 Paramus, NJ 07652 (201)489-8900 Fax (201)489-0877

Lebovitz, Brian Lee, MD {1134173909} Otlryg(94,PA12)<NJ-STCLRDEN>
+ ENT & Allergy Associates of Parsippany
  900 Lanidex Plaza/Suite 300 Parsippany, NJ 07054 (973)394-1818 Fax (973)394-1810
+ ENT & Allergy Associates, LLP
  3219 Route 46 East/Suite 203 Parsippany, NJ 07054 (973)394-1818 Fax (973)394-1810
+ North Jersey Ear Nose Throat and Hearing
  16 Pocono Road/Suite 112 Denville, NJ 07054 (973)625-1818 Fax (973)983-0055

Lebovitz, Philip Lewis, MD {1700875580} CdvDis, IntrMd(66,PA12)<NJ-CHSFULD, NJ-CHSMRCER>
+ Mercer Bucks Cardiology
  3140 Princeton Pike/2nd Floor Lawrenceville, NJ 08648 (609)895-1919 Fax (609)895-1200

Lebovitz, Yaron, MD {1760536981} RadDia(93,NY46)<NJ-STPETER, NJ-RWJUBRUN>
+ University Radiology Group, P.C.
483 Cranbury Road   East Brunswick, NJ 08816   (732)390-0030   Fax (732)390-5383
ylebovitz@aol.com
+ University Radiology Group, P.C.
16 Mountain Boulevard   Warren, NJ 07059   (732)390-0030   Fax (908)769-9141

Lebowitz, Howard Harris, MD {1568483451} IntrMd(90,MA01)<NJ-SPCLMONM, NJ-SPCLKIMB>
+ AcuteCare Health System
500 River Road/Suite 150   Lakewood, NJ 08701   (732)364-0800   Fax (732)364-0846
+ Specialty Hospital at Monmouth
300 Second Avenue/Greenwall 6   Long Branch, NJ 07740   (732)923-5037
+ Specialty Hospital at Kimball
600 River Avenue/4 West   Lakewood, NJ 08701   (732)942-3597

Lebowitz, Jonathan A., MD {1104846377} RadDia(91,NJ06)
+ Princeton Radiology Associates, P.A.
419 North Harrison Street   Princeton, NJ 08540   (609)921-3345   Fax (609)683-8847
+ Princeton Radiology Associates, P.A.
9 Centre Drive   Jamesburg, NJ 08831   (609)921-3345   Fax (609)655-4016
+ University Radiology Group, P.C.
375 Route 206/Suite 1   Hillsborough, NJ 08540   (908)874-7600   Fax (908)874-7052

Lebowitz, Nathaniel Edward, MD {1063418994} CdvDis, IntrMd(91,NY20)<NJ-ENGLWOOD>
+ Advanced Cardiology Institute
2200 Fletcher Avenue/Suite 1   Fort Lee, NJ 07024   (201)461-6200   Fax (201)461-7204
+ Heart and Vascular Institute at EHMC
350 Engle Street/Suite 1000   Englewood, NJ 07631   (201)894-3636

Lebowitz-Naegeli, Nanci L., MD {1699967018} PsyCAd, Psychy(90,CT02)
+ 460 Bloomfield Avenue/Suite 209
Montclair, NJ 07042   (973)744-4900   Fax (973)744-5019

LeBron, Carmen Haydee, MD {1902872468} Pedtrc, IntrMd(01,NJ06)
+ Baby Step Pediatrics
75 Montgomery Street/Suite 401   Jersey City, NJ 07302   (201)600-4306   Fax (800)915-7830
lebronpeds@gmail.com

Lecomte, Jennifer Megan, DO {1104950732} Pedtrc
+ SOM - Department of Internal Medicine
42 East Laurel Road/Suite 3100   Stratford, NJ 08084   (856)566-6845   Fax (856)566-6906

Lecusay, Dario A., Jr., MD {1235103318} FamMed(98,NY15)<NJ-HUNTRDN>
+ Cornerstone Family Practice
9100 Wescott Drive/Suite 103   Flemington, NJ 08822   (908)237-6910   Fax (908)237-6919

Leddy, Timothy P., MD {1538164496} SrgOrt, SrgHnd, OrtS-Hand(96,PA02)<NJ-UNVMCPRN, NJ-STPETER>
+ University Orthopaedic Associates, LLC.
Two Worlds Fair Drive   Somerset, NJ 08873   (732)979-2115   Fax (732)564-9032
+ University Orthopaedic Group
215 Easton Avenue   New Brunswick, NJ 08901   (732)979-2115   Fax (732)545-4011
+ University Orthopaedic Associates, LLC.
211 North Harrison Street   Princeton, NJ 08873   (609)683-7800   Fax (609)683-7875

Leder, David S., MD {1518963263} RadDia, Radiol, IntrMd(89,NJ05)<NJ-RWJUBRUN, NJ-RWJUHAM>
+ Princeton Radiology Associates, P.A.
3674 Route 27   Kendall Park, NJ 08824   (732)821-5563   Fax (732)821-6675
+ Quakerbridge Radiology Associates
8 Quakerbridge Plaza/Building 8   Mercerville, NJ 08619   (732)821-5563   Fax (609)689-6067
+ Quakerbridge Radiology MRI Center at Lawrenceville
21 Lawrenceville-Pennington Rd   Lawrenceville, NJ 08824   (609)895-1500   Fax (609)895-2647

Leder, Robin Ellen, MD {1750437950} GenPrc, Nutrtn(82,NY46)
+ A Better Alternative Medicine Center
235 Prospect Avenue   Hackensack, NJ 07601   (201)525-1155   Fax (201)525-0915

Ledereich, Philip S., MD {1881697373} Otlryg, SrgHdN, OtgyFPlS(89,NY46)<NJ-NWRKBETH>
+ 1033 Clifton Avenue/Suites 204 and 206
Clifton, NJ 07013   (973)470-8266   Fax (973)470-8288
ledereich@optonline.net

Lederman, Jeffrey Craig, DO {1457365660} IntrMd(98,NJ75)
+ Internal Medical Associates of Monmouth
279 Third Avenue/Suite 207   Long Branch, NJ 07740   (732)229-0509   Fax (732)571-0019

Lederman, Steven M., MD {1619944295} CdvDis, IntrMd(74,PA13)
+ The Cardiology Group, P.A.
401 Young Avenue/Suite 275   Moorestown, NJ 08057   (856)291-8855   Fax (856)291-8844
+ The Cardiology Group, P.A.
128 State Highway Route 70/Suite 1-B   Medford, NJ 08055   (856)291-8855   Fax (609)444-5521
+ The Cardiology Group, P.A.
1 Sheffield Drive/Suite 102   Columbus, NJ 08057   (856)291-8855

Ledinh, Thuong, MD {1205936663} FamMed, GenPrc(67,VIE05)
+ Plainfield Family Care Center
38 Watchung Avenue   Plainfield, NJ 07061   (908)769-7881   Fax (908)769-0061
+ Silver Lake Medical
50 Newark Avenue/Suite 205   Belleville, NJ 07109   (973)769-7881   Fax (973)751-2291

Lee, Ada Shuk Chong, MD {1134102858} PedPul, Pedtrc(98,NY08)<NJ-HACKNSK>
+ Joseph M. Sanzari Childrenǽs Hospital
30 Prospect Avenue/WFAN TC375   Hackensack, NJ 07602   (551)996-5207   Fax (551)996-4969

Lee, Ai R., MD {1922038918} Anesth(71,KOR03)<NJ-STMRYPAS>
+ St. Mary's Hospital
350 Boulevard   Passaic, NJ 07055   (973)365-4300   Fax (973)470-3548

Lee, Aland H., MD {1710985742} Anesth(88,MA05)<NJ-VIRTMARL>
+ West Jersey Anesthesia Associates
102-E Center Boulevard   Marlton, NJ 08053   (856)988-6250   Fax (856)988-6270

Lee, Andrew, MD {1619904216} InfDis, IntrMd<NJ-MONMOUTH, NJ-OCEANMC>
+ Infectious Disease Care
1912 State Route 35/Suite 101   Oakhurst, NJ 07755   (732)222-4762   Fax (732)222-4764

Lee, Andrew N., MD {1417162090} PulDis, CritCr, IntrMd(06,NY19)<NJ-VIRTMARL, NJ-VIRTVOOR>
+ Virtua Garden State Pulmonary Associates
520 Lippincott Drive/Suite A   Marlton, NJ 08053   (856)596-9057   Fax (856)596-0837

Lee, Andrew Wen-Tseng, MD InfDis, IntrMd(97,NY20)<PA-TJCNTR>
+ Merck and Company Incorporated
1 Merck Drive/PO Box 100   Whitehouse Station, NJ 08889   (908)423-1000
andrew_wen-tseng_lee@merck.com

Lee, Angie Yookyoung, MD {1568439875} ObsGyn(99,MI01)<CT-YALENHH>
+ 870 Pompton Avenue/Unit A-1
Cedar Grove, NJ 07009   (973)239-3865

Lee, Anna D., MD {1700949401} PhysMd(89,PA09)
+ 59 Westervelt Avenue
Tenafly, NJ 07670

Lee, Anna F., MD {1780625038} IntrMd(88,CHN38)<NJ-RWJUBRUN, NJ-STPETER>
+ 465 Cranbury Road/Suite 202
East Brunswick, NJ 08816   (732)698-9980

Lee, Anthony, MD {1962639567} PhysMd<NJ-KSLRSADB>
+ Kessler Institute for Rehabilitation
300 Market Street   Saddle Brook, NJ 07663   (201)368-6000

Lee, Bong S., MD {1477576395} SrgOrt, SrgHnd(64,KOR01)<PA-CHILDHOS>
+ CHOP Specialty Care Center at Virtua
200 Bowman Drive/2 FL/Suite D-260   Voorhees, NJ 08043   (267)425-5400
+ CHOP Pediatric & Adolescent Specialty Care Center
1012 Laurel Oak Road   Voorhees, NJ 08043   (267)425-5400   Fax (856)435-0091

Lee, Brian, DO {1871754598} Anesth(02,NY75)<NY-MAIMONMC>
+ Hoboken University Medical Center
308 Willow Avenue   Hoboken, NJ 07030   (201)418-1000

Lee, Brian H., MD {1225392178} RadDia
+ Coastal Imaging, LLC
79 Route 37 West/Suite 103   Toms River, NJ 08755   (322)288-3307   Fax (732)276-2325

Lee, Bryant B., MD {1437154960} Otlryg(98,NY19)
+ Summit Medical Group
75 East Northfield Road   Livingston, NJ 07039   (973)436-1435   Fax (973)992-0850

Lee, Chang J., MD {1023049533} Anesth(68,KOR09)<NJ-STMRYPAS>
+ St. Mary's Hospital
350 Boulevard/Anesth   Passaic, NJ 07055   (973)365-4300   Fax (973)779-7385

Lee, Chang Woo, MD {1235152554} IntrMd(91,NY15)<NJ-HOLYNAME, NJ-ENGLWOOD>
+ 464 Hudson Terrace/Suite 100
Englewood Cliffs, NJ 07632   (201)541-6800   Fax (201)541-6924

Lee, Chester C., MD {1912177890} Urolgy(03,DC01)
+ Urologic Specialties PA
177 North Dean Street/Suite 305   Englewood, NJ 07631   (201)569-7777   Fax (201)569-6861

Lee, Chi I., MD {1417924622} EmrgMd, Grtrcs, IntrMd(69,KORE)<NJ-RIVERVW, NJ-BAYSHORE>
+ 717 North Beers Street
Holmdel, NJ 07733   (732)264-4900   Fax (732)739-2201

Lee, Christopher Sang Don, MD {1013901693} Urolgy(96,NJ05)<NJ-SJRSYELM, NJ-KMHTURNV>
+ South Jersey Urology Consultants, LLC
2950 College Drive/Suite 2E   Vineland, NJ 08360   (856)405-0025

Lee, Clara J., MD {1881822369} Pedtrc, IntrMd
+ Riverside Medical Group
200 Main Street   Ridgefield Park, NJ 07660   (201)870-6099   Fax (201)870-6098
drlee@riversidepeds.com

Lee, Dae Woo, MD {1083787295} IntrMd(70,KOR01)
+ 984 Bergen Avenue
North Brunswick, NJ 08902   (732)545-0202   Fax (732)545-5002
Dealee4sky@yahoo.com

Lee, Daniel James, MD {1992799977} SrgCTh, SrgVas(91,NY47)<NJ-CAPITLHS, NJ-CHSFULD>
+ Doctors Dellacroce and Lee
2 Capital Way/Suite 390   Pennington, NJ 08534   (609)818-0040   Fax (609)818-0049

Lee, Daniel Kilho, MD {1811193865} IntrMd(04,GRN01)
+ 449 Mount Pleasant Avenue
West Orange, NJ 07052   (973)992-6487   Fax (973)992-7040

Lee, David Charles, MD {1275633562} Nrolgy, PainMd(83,VA01)
+ South Jersey Neurocare Pain Management
520 Stokes Road/Suite A-4   Medford, NJ 08055   (609)714-7774   Fax (609)714-7775

Lee, David K., MD {1225359847} Ophthl(06,NJ05)<NJ-MONMOUTH>
+ Millennium Eye Care, LLC
500 West Main Street   Freehold, NJ 07728   (732)462-8707   Fax (732)462-1296

Lee, David W., MD {1922144401} FamMed(70,KOR01)<NJ-HOLYNAME, NJ-ENGLWOOD>
+ 1625 Anderson Avenue/Suite 204
Fort Lee, NJ 07024   (201)224-0011   Fax (201)224-8920

Lee, Derek Sai-Wah, MD {1932206521} Otlryg, SrgFPl, OtgyFPlS(92,AZ01)
+ 201 South Livingston Avenue/Suite 1 C
Livingston, NJ 07039   (973)716-9716   Fax (973)716-9738

Lee, Diana, DO {1760794796} Pedtrc, IntrMd(07,ME75)
+ Dr. G. Lee Lerch and Associates
63 North Lakeview Drive/Suite 202   Gibbsboro, NJ 08026   (856)435-6000   Fax (856)782-1667

Lee, Donna J., MD {1972565851} PedEmg, PedPul(93,NJ05)<NJ-HACKNSK>
+ Hackensack University Medical Center
30 Prospect Avenue/PediEmergMed   Hackensack, NJ 07601   (201)996-5207   Fax (201)996-4969

Lee, Dwight E., MD {1285726265} IntrMd, EmrgMd(86,NJ06)<NJ-TRINIWSC>
+ 86 Forrest Hill Road
West Orange, NJ 07052

Lee, Edward G., MD {1558367821} CritCr, IntrMd, PulDis(81,NY20)
+ Adult & Pediatric Allergists of Central Jersey
3 Hospital Plaza/Suite 405   Old Bridge, NJ 08857   (732)679-2525   Fax (732)360-0033

Lee, Edward Howe, MD {1669600326} IntrMd
+ 106 South Dennis Road
Cape May Court House, NJ 08210   (609)465-2710   Fax (609)463-8135

Lee, Edward Sang Keun, MD {1629265657} SrgPlstc(03,DC02)
+ 90 Bergen Street/Suite 7400
Newark, NJ 07103   (973)972-3229   Fax (973)972-8268

Lee, Ellen, MD {1164408597} RadDia(88,NJ06)<NJ-STPETER, NJ-RWJUBRUN>
+ University Radiology Group, P.C.
483 Cranbury Road   East Brunswick, NJ 08816   (732)390-0030   Fax (732)390-5383
+ University Radiology Group, P.C.
10 Plum Street   New Brunswick, NJ 08901   (732)390-0030   Fax (732)249-1208

Lee, Erich Y., MD {1225293392}<NJ-UMDNJ>
+ University Hospital
150 Bergen Street/C320   Newark, NJ 07103   (973)972-5188   Fax (973)972-7429

Lee, Esther Jeehae, MD {1952545162} EnDbMt, IntrMd(05,NY19)<NJ-ENGLWOOD, NJ-HOLYNAME>
+ Valley Medical Group-Endocrinology
947 Linwood Avenue   Ridgewood, NJ 07450   (201)444-5552   Fax (201)444-4490

Physicians by Name and Address

Lee, Frank, MD {1588894398} GenPrc(85,NY09)
+ 13 Main Street
  Bradley Beach, NJ 07720   (732)988-8800

Lee, Fred Suin, MD {1518035807} SrgOrt(91,NY20)
+ Fred Lee MD Orthopaedic Surgery P.C.
  1608 Lemoine Avenue/Suite 204   Fort Lee, NJ 07024
  (201)461-0708   Fax (201)461-9005
  FredSLee@aol.com

Lee, Gene Chiu, MD {1558459883} Pedtrc, NnPnMd(83,MEXI)<NJ-COMMED, NJ-KIMBALL>
+ Drs. Lee and Humphreys
  1479 Route 539/Suite 1 A   Little Egg Harbor, NJ 08087
  (609)296-1900   Fax (609)296-1906

Lee, Gerald J., MD {1982692745} IntrMd(94,PA02)
+ The Park Medical Group
  24 Elm Street   Harrington Park, NJ 07640   (201)784-0123
  Fax (201)784-0065

Lee, Grace Hoyoun, MD {1245494210}<NJ-HOBUNIMC>
+ Hoboken University Medical Center
  308 Willow Avenue   Hoboken, NJ 07030   (201)418-3127
  Fax (201)418-3148

Lee, Hae-Rhi, MD {1891704771} PedCrd, Pedtrc(91,NET01)
+ CHOP Pediatric & Adolescent Specialty Care Center
  707 Alexander Road/Suite 205   Princeton, NJ 08540
  (609)520-1717
+ CHOP Specialty Care Center at Virtua
  200 Bowman Drive/2 FL/Suite D-260   Voorhees, NJ 08043
  (267)425-5400
+ CHOP Pediatric & Adolescent Specialty Care Center
  1012 Laurel Oak Road   Voorhees, NJ 08540   (856)435-0086
  Fax (856)435-0091

Lee, Henry, MD {1447412952} Ophthl, IntrMd(07,NY47)
+ Lee Aesthetic Center, LLC.
  58 Mount Bethel Road/Suite 302   Warren, NJ 07059
  (908)738-1160   Fax (908)738-1170

Lee, Herb, MD {1487745196} Anesth(87,FL02)<NJ-RWJUBRUN>
+ James Street Anesthesia
  102 James Street/Suite 103   Edison, NJ 08820   (732)494-1444   Fax (732)494-7052

Lee, Horton James, MD {1841547007} Pedtrc, EmrgMd<NY-ELMHRST>
+ Newark Beth Israel Medical Center Emergency Medicine
  201 Lyons Avenue   Newark, NJ 07112   (973)926-7240

Lee, Huey J., MD {1871692806} RadDia, RadNro(76,TAIW)<NJ-UMDNJ>
+ University Hospital
  150 Bergen Street/Radiology   Newark, NJ 07103
  (973)972-4202   Fax (973)972-7429
  leehu@umdnj.edu

Lee, Hyejin Robin, MD {1851324792} NnPnMd, Pedtrc(93,NC05)<NJ-HOLYNAME>
+ NICU Associates at Saint Barnabas
  94 Old Short Hills Road   Livingston, NJ 07039   (973)322-5437   Fax (973)322-8833

Lee, Hyok Yop, MD {1902912249} IntrMd, AlgyImmn(79,KOR04)
+ Kang Lee and Lee Allergy/Pediatrics
  2177 Oak Tree Road/Suite 207   Edison, NJ 08820
  (732)767-0955   Fax (732)494-9098

Lee, Hyun K., MD {1437258241} Psychy(69,KOR05)<NJ-VALYONS>
+ VA New Jersey Health Care System at Lyons
  151 Knollcroft Road/Psych   Lyons, NJ 07939   (908)647-0180   Fax (908)604-5251

Lee, Hyun-Soo, MD {1558446674} Dermat(90,NY48)
+ Metro Dermatology
  500 Grand Avenue/Suite 201   Englewood, NJ 07631
  (201)886-9000   Fax (201)917-1299

Lee, Inna, MD {1598955536} Pedtrc(89,RUS37)
+ 620 Anderson Avenue
  Cliffside Park, NJ 07010   (201)840-0101   Fax (201)840-0008
  info@cliffsidepediatrics.com

Lee, Isidore C., MD {1700826856} Anesth(69,KORE)<NJ-RWJUBRUN>
+ Robert Wood Johnson-UMDNJ Anesthesia Group
  125 Paterson Street/CAB 3100   New Brunswick, NJ 08901
  (732)235-7827   Fax (732)235-6131

Lee, Jack C., MD {1083675318} CritCr, IntrMd, PulDis(93,PA09)<NJ-HOLYNAME>
+ Somerset Pulmonary & Critical Care
  245 Union Avenue/Suite 2C   Bridgewater, NJ 08807
  (732)873-8097   Fax (732)873-1827

Lee, Jacob S., MD {1922116029} RadDia, RadNro(98,NY46)<NJ-ACMCITY, NJ-SHOREMEM>
+ Atlantic Medical Imaging, LLC.
  3100 Hingston Avenue   Egg Harbor Township, NJ 08234
  (609)677-9729   Fax (609)646-5369
+ Atlantic Medical Imaging, LLC.
  72 West Jimmie Leeds Road   Galloway, NJ 08205
  (609)677-9729   Fax (609)653-8764
+ Atlantic Medical Imaging, LLC.
  401 Bethel Road   Somers Point, NJ 08234   (609)677-9729

Lee, Jae Young, MD {1629332812} IntrMd
+ Princeton Radiology Associates, P.A.
  419 North Harrison Street   Princeton, NJ 08540   (609)921-3345   Fax (609)683-8847

Lee, James Jeong June, MD {1457335564} Otlryg, OtgyFPIS(97,NY19)
+ Northern Valley ENT
  354 Old Hook Road/Suite 204   Westwood, NJ 07675
  (201)666-8787   Fax (201)358-6686

Lee, James M., Jr., MD {1952509820} SrgOrt(65,NY09)
+ 81 Northfield Avenue/Suite 304
  West Orange, NJ 07052   (973)672-2214   Fax (973)672-1320
  Leesportsmed@gmail.com

Lee, James M., Sr., MD {1356373690} SrgOrt, IntrMd(65,NY09)<NJ-STMICHL>
+ Empire Medical Associates
  5 Franklin Avenue/Suite 302   Belleville, NJ 07109
  (973)759-1221   Fax (973)759-1997
+ Empire Medical Associates
  264 Boyden Avenue   Maplewood, NJ 07040   (973)759-1221   Fax (973)761-7617
+ Empire Medical Associates
  382 West Passaic Avenue   Bloomfield, NJ 07109   (973)338-1900

Lee, James R., MD {1902838253} ObsGyn(89,TX12)
+ 1608 Lemoine Avenue/Suite 201
  Fort Lee, NJ 07024   (201)461-6666   Fax (201)461-7429

Lee, James Wonsang, MD {1073527560} Onclgy, IntrMd, OncHem(83,NY20)<NJ-CHILTON, NJ-VALLEY>
+ Hematology Oncology Associates PA
  175 Madison Avenue/4th Floor   Mount Holly, NJ 08060
  (609)702-1900   Fax (609)702-8455

Lee, Jane Mengchuan, MD {1740377654} Dermat(94,CA02)
+ Advanced Dermatology Center PC
  18 Bridge Street   Metuchen, NJ 08840   (732)635-1200
  Fax (732)635-1266

Lee, Jane S., MD {1962450254} ObsGyn(93,CO02)<NJ-CLARMAAS>
+ Essex Ob/Gyn, LLC
  85 Park Street/1st Floor   Montclair, NJ 07042   (973)259-3888   Fax (973)259-3999
  essexobgyn@earthlink.net

Lee, Jemius Dae, DO {1063826014} EmrgMd<NJ-CHILTON>
+ Chilton Medical Center
  97 West Parkway   Pompton Plains, NJ 07444   (973)831-5447

Lee, Jen Fei, MD {1942244827} SrgHnd, SrgOrt(92,NY47)<NJ-ENGLWOOD, NJ-HOLYNAME>
+ North Jersey Orthopaedic Specialists
  106 Grand Avenue   Englewood, NJ 07631   (201)608-0100
  Fax (201)608-0104
  jenfeilee@aol.com
+ North Jersey Orthopaedic Specialists
  730 Palisade Avenue   Teaneck, NJ 07666   (201)608-0100
  Fax (201)530-0003
+ North Jersey Orthopaedic Specialists
  15 Vervalen Street   Closter, NJ 07631   (201)784-6800   Fax (201)784-6801

Lee, Joan Jean, DO {1639494289} Ophthl(10,NJ75)
+ Freehold Ophthalmology, LLC
  509 Stillwells Corner Road/Suite E-5   Freehold, NJ 07728
  (732)431-9333   Fax (732)431-3312
+ Paul Phillips Eye & Surgery Center
  6 Minneakoning Road/Suite B   Flemington, NJ 08822
  (732)431-9333   Fax (908)968-3239

Lee, Johanna, DO {1588076756}
+ Women's Health Care Group
  870 Palisade Avenue/Suite 301   Teaneck, NJ 07666
  (201)907-0900   Fax (201)907-0229

Lee, John C., MD {1306902903} Anesth(95,MA05)
+ Rancocas Anesthesiology, PA
  700 Route 130 North/Suite 203   Cinnaminson, NJ 08077
  (856)829-9345   Fax (856)829-3605
+ Rancocas Anesthesiology Associates
  700 US Highway 130 North/Suite 203   Cinnaminson, NJ 08077   (856)829-9345

Lee, John Hyung-Il, MD {1154502045} IntCrd(01,KOR01)
+ 747 Shoshone Trail
  Franklin Lakes, NJ 07417

Lee, John Po-Hsiang, MD {1265479570} Anesth(98,DC02)<NJ-VALLEY>
+ Bergen Anesthesia Group, P.C.
  500 West Main Street/Suite 16   Wyckoff, NJ 07481
  (201)847-9320   Fax (201)847-0059

Lee, Johnnie Augustus, MD {1821986006} IntrMd(89,NC01)<CT-STAMFDH>
+ 1070 Hillside Avenue
  Plainfield, NJ 07060   (203)644-0323

Lee, Joo-Young Melissa, MD {1033166582} RadDia(96,NY46)
+ Montclair Breast Center
  37 North Fullerton Avenue   Montclair, NJ 07042   (973)509-1818   Fax (973)509-0532

Lee, Joseph Kim, MD {1124289780} PhysMd(04,NJ06)
+ Reconstructive Orthopedics, P.A.
  401 Young Avenue/Suite 245   Moorestown, NJ 08057
  (609)267-9400   Fax (609)267-9457

Lee, Joseph Sang-Ho, MD {1679839054} IntrMd, Allrgy(90,PA12)
+ 48 Juniper Way
  Basking Ridge, NJ 07920

Lee, Joung Y., MD {1730126848} Radiol, NuclMd, RadV&I(64,KOR09)
+ Medical Park Imaging
  330 Ratzer Road/Suite 6-A   Wayne, NJ 07470   (973)696-5770   Fax (973)633-1204

Lee, Julia Jin-Young, MD {1093813982} Pedtrc, IntrMd(95,PA07)<NY-STANTHNY, MA-ARDHILL>
+ Valley Pediatric Associates, P.A.
  201 East Franklin Turnpike   Ho Ho Kus, NJ 07423   (201)652-6164   Fax (201)652-6485
+ Valley Pediatric Associates PA
  470 North Franklin Turnpike   Ramsey, NJ 07446   (201)652-6164   Fax (201)934-1817

Lee, Jung Du, MD {1114094703} Anesth(66,KOR09)
+ 888 Briarwood Road/P. O. Box 667
  Franklin Lakes, NJ 07417   (973)942-0400

Lee, Jung Hi, MD {1417931494} IntrMd, PsyFor(72,KOR09)<NJ-ANNKLEIN>
+ Ann Klein Forensic Center
  1609 Stuyvesant Avenue/PO Box 7717   West Trenton, NJ 08628   (609)633-0900   Fax (609)633-1312

Lee, Jung S., MD {1093733156} Ophthl(99,MA05)
+ Westwood Ophthalmology Associates
  300 Fairview Avenue/PO Box 698   Westwood, NJ 07675
  (201)666-4014   Fax (201)664-4754

Lee, Kangmin Daniel, MD {1477760353} SrgNro
+ North Jersey Brain and Surgical
  680 Kinderkamack Road/Suite 300   Oradell, NJ 07649
  (201)342-2550   Fax (201)342-7171

Lee, Karen Chang, MD {1780766857} IntrMd(01,GRN01)<NJ-HOLYNAME, NJ-VALLEY>
+ Aspen Medical Associates, P.A.
  1 DeGraw Square   Teaneck, NJ 07666   (201)928-0200
  Fax (201)928-0820

Lee, Karina K., MD {1851732192} IntrMd
+ Princeton Internal Medicine Associates
  281 Witherspoon Street/Suite 220   Princeton, NJ 08542
  (201)788-9132   Fax (609)921-3584
  karina.krystal@gmail.com
+ Urology Group of Princeton PA
  281 Witherspoon Street/Suite 100   Princeton, NJ 08542
  (201)788-9132   Fax (609)921-7020

Lee, Kim Chiu, MD {1912087735} Pedtrc(92,NY08)<NJ-STPETER, NJ-CENTRAST>
+ Best Care Pediatrics
  470 Highway 79/Suite 12   Morganville, NJ 07751
  (732)970-9070   Fax (732)970-9071

Lee, Kristen Kyongae, MD {1942442884} Gastrn, IntrMd(09,NY20)
+ Digestive HealthCare Center
  511 Courtyard Drive/Building 500   Hillsborough, NJ 08844
  (908)218-9222   Fax (908)218-9818

Lee, Kristyna H., MD {1396940334} Dermat
+ Affiliated Dermatologists
  182 South Street/Suite 1   Morristown, NJ 07960   (973)267-0577   Fax (973)439-5401
+ Affiliated Dermatology
  Town Centre 66/Suite 301   Succasunna, NJ 07876
  (973)267-0577   Fax (973)927-7512
+ Affiliated Dermatology
  14 Church Street   Liberty Corner, NJ 07960   (973)267-0300
  Fax (908)604-8544

Lee, Lani Mei, MD {1114200300}
+ 150 14th Street/Apt 303
  Hoboken, NJ 07030   (201)681-6424

Lee, Leonard Young, MD {1457448532} SrgCTh, Surgry(92,NJ06)<NY-PRSBWEIL, NY-METHODST>
+ RWJ University Hospital New Brunswick
  One Robert Wood Johnson Place   New Brunswick, NJ 08901
  (732)235-8725   Fax (732)235-8727
+ Cardiac Surgery Group, P.A.
  20 Prospect Avenue/Suite 900   Hackensack, NJ 07601
  (732)235-8725   Fax (201)343-0609

Lee, Linda K., MD {1225022619} Rheuma, IntrMd(97,IL43)<NJ-OVERLOOK, NJ-MORRISTN>
+ Summit Medical Group-Berkeley Heights Campus
  1 Diamond Hill Road   Berkeley Heights, NJ 07922
  (908)273-4300   Fax (908)673-7241

Lee, Louis Young, MD {1073766143} Anesth, IntrMd(07,NY19)<NJ-ENGLWOOD>
+ Englewood Hospital and Medical Center
  350 Engle Street/Anesthesia   Englewood, NJ 07631
  (201)894-3322

Lee, Madonna Edina, MD {1861787319}<NJ-RWJUBRUN>
+ RWJ University Hospital New Brunswick
One Robert Wood Johnson Place   New Brunswick, NJ 08901   (732)235-7674   Fax (732)235-8372

Lee, Mark, DO {1306144514} FamMAdlt<NJ-PALISADE>
+ Palisades Medical Center
7600 River Road   North Bergen, NJ 07047   (201)854-5000

Lee, Mark Hyon-Min, MD {1174729974} RadDia(02,PA13)<NJ-KMHCHRRY>
+ Radiology Associates of New Jersey
2201 Chapel Avenue West/Suite 106   Cherry Hill, NJ 08002   (856)488-6844   Fax (856)488-6507

Lee, Meichia, MD {1972035384}
+ University Medical Group - General Internal Medicine
125 Paterson Street/Suite 5100A   New Brunswick, NJ 08903   (608)381-5182   Fax (732)235-8935

Lee, Michael Joseph, MD {1528223765} RadDia, Radiol, IntrMd(05,MA07)<NJ-COOPRUMC>
+ Atlantic Medical Imaging, LLC.
44 East Jimmie Leeds Road/Suite 101   Galloway, NJ 08205   (609)677-9729   Fax (609)652-6512
+ The Cooper Health System at Voorhees
900 Centennial Boulevard/Suite B   Voorhees, NJ 08043   (609)677-9729   Fax (856)325-6588

Lee, Mimi Shon, MD {1487668521} RadDia(01,NJ05)<NJ-VAEASTOR>
+ VA New Jersey Health Care System-East Orange Campus
385 Tremont Avenue/Radiology   East Orange, NJ 07018   (973)676-1000

Lee, Nancy, DO {1386859023} FamMed(04,NJ75)
+ Codella Family Practice
1000 Galloping Hill Road/Suite 103   Union, NJ 07083   (908)688-1550   Fax (908)688-1552

Lee, Nellie U., MD {1104034107} CdvDis, IntrMd(66,PHIL)<NJ-HOLYNAME>
+ 190 Euclid Avenue
Ridgefield Park, NJ 07660   (201)440-3366   Fax (201)807-0705
nellieleemd@yahoo.com

Lee, Nelson, DO {1821472630} FamMed
+ Jackson Family Medicine
27 South Cooks Bridge Road/Suite 2-1   Jackson, NJ 08527   (732)367-0166   Fax (732)367-7220

Lee, Patrick C., MD {1356442602} OncHem, EmrgMd, IntrMd(03,NJ06)<NJ-BAYSHORE, NJ-SOMERSET>
+ Monmouth Hematology Oncology Associates PA
100 State Highway 36/Suite 1B   West Long Branch, NJ 07764   (732)222-1711   Fax (732)222-1461

Lee, Peter, MD {1225081334} IntrMd(01,NY48)<NJ-STPETER, NJ-CHSFULD>
+ Princeton Pike Internal Medicine
3100 Princeton Pike/Bldg 3/ 3rd Fl   Lawrenceville, NJ 08648   (609)896-1793   Fax (609)896-1847

Lee, Peter HaeSuk, MD {1205886611} Pedtrc, PedEmg(94,NY08)<NJ-VALLEY>
+ The Valley Hospital
223 North Van Dien Avenue/EmergMed   Ridgewood, NJ 07450   (201)447-8000

Lee, Peter Q., DO {1952728479} EmrgMd
+ Morristown Medical Center Emergency Medicine
100 Madison Avenue   Morristown, NJ 07960   (973)971-7926

Lee, Peter Yen-lai, MD {1871525600} Anesth(00,TX12)<NJ-MTNSIDE>
+ 1300 Clinton Street/Suite 518
Hoboken, NJ 07030

Lee, Peter Yujen, MD {1124101654} Dermat(91,NJ06)<NJ-VIRTMHBC>
+ Advanced Dermatology Center PC
18 Bridge Street   Metuchen, NJ 08840   (732)635-1200   Fax (732)635-1266
+ Moorestown Dermatology Associates
702 East Main Street   Moorestown, NJ 08057   (732)635-1200   Fax (856)235-6566

Lee, Po-Shing, MD {1013112739} PthAClin, PthHem(92,TAI02)
+ Bio-Reference Laboratory, Inc.
481 Edward H. Ross Drive   Elmwood Park, NJ 07407   (201)791-2600   Fax (201)791-1941

Lee, Richard, MD {1225110570} Urolgy(95,NY47)
+ Urologic Specialties PA
177 North Dean Street/Suite 305   Englewood, NJ 07631   (201)569-7777   Fax (201)569-6861

Lee, Richard Thomas, MD {1770621575} IntrMd, OncHem(94,NJ06)
+ Princeton Medical Group, P.A.
419 North Harrison Street   Princeton, NJ 08540   (609)924-9300   Fax (609)924-6552

Lee, Robert, MD {1801180807} Dermat(10,NJ05)
+ SCN Dermatology
2083 Center Avenue/2nd Floor   Fort Lee, NJ 07024   (201)944-3800

+ SCN Dermatology
243 Chestnut Street/3rd Floor   Newark, NJ 07105   (973)522-0300

Lee, Robert Chu-Du, MD {1497830293} IntrMd, PulDis, CritCr(88,NY09)<NY-LINCOLN>
+ Hackensack Sleep & Pulmonary Center
170 Prospect Avenue/Suite 20   Hackensack, NJ 07601   (201)996-0232   Fax (201)996-0095

Lee, Robert Edward, III, MD {1003866542} Ophthl(94,NC07)
+ Erickson, Dreizen & Lee Eye Center
1206 Route 72 West   Manahawkin, NJ 08050   (609)597-8087   Fax (609)597-7192
+ Erickson, Dreizen & Lee Eye Center
730 West Lacey Road/Suite G-07   Forked River, NJ 08731   (609)971-8822

Lee, Robin Ann, MD {1700098100} SrgCrC, Surgry<NJ-STBARNMC>
+ St. Barnabas Medical Center
94 Old Short Hills Road/Surgery   Livingston, NJ 07039   (973)322-5924

Lee, Sang O., MD {1467552257} NuclMd, NucImg(78,KOR04)<NJ-NWRKBETH>
+ Newark Beth Israel Medical Center
201 Lyons Avenue/NuclearMed   Newark, NJ 07112   (973)926-7000   Fax (973)923-8232
solee37me@hotmail.com

Lee, Sang Hyun, MD {1982838587} EmrgMd
+ 86 Hillside Avenue
Tenafly, NJ 07670   (201)723-8883

Lee, Sangwoo, MD {1164476404} Ophthl(98,RI01)<NJ-STMRYPAS>
+ St. Mary's Eye & Surgery Center
540 Bergen Boulevard   Palisades Park, NJ 07650   (201)461-3970   Fax (201)242-9061
slee@dicare.com

Lee, Serena Qi-Qin, MD {1386688083} IntrMd, InfDis, AlgyImmn(77,CHN9D)<NJ-STBARNMC>
+ 1222 US Highway 46
Parsippany, NJ 07054   (973)335-9210   Fax (973)335-9240

Lee, Seung Ho, MD {1770693996} PsyCAd(79,KOR04)
+ Ephatha Mental Health Associates PC
566 Grand Avenue   Ridgefield, NJ 07657   (201)313-8000   Fax (201)313-8002

Lee, Seungho Howard, MD {1144226028} RadNro, Radiol(64,KORE)<NJ-SOMERSET>
+ University Radiology, PA
239 Route 22 East/Suite 302   Green Brook, NJ 08812   (732)968-4899   Fax (732)968-8096

Lee, Shane, MD {1104067651} RadDia
+ Radiology Affiliates of Central New Jersey, P.A.
2501 Kuser Road   Hamilton, NJ 08691   (609)585-8800   Fax (609)585-1825

Lee, Sherrylynn Nacario, MD {1487759130} IntrMd, IntHos(98,PHI10)<NJ-VIRTMHBC, NJ-VIRTMARL>
+ Virtua Marlton Hospital
90 Brick Road/Internal Med   Marlton, NJ 08053   (609)914-6180   Fax (609)914-6182

Lee, Sheue H., MD {1326153586} Hemato, OncHem(73,TAI04)
+ St. Mary's Hospital
350 Boulevard   Passaic, NJ 07055   (973)365-4300
+ 430 Clifton Avenue
Clifton, NJ 07011   (973)365-4300   Fax (973)405-6009

Lee, Shinji S., MD {1699003921} SrgPlstc, GenPrc(90,NY19)
+ 61 Glenwood Road
Englewood, NJ 07631   (201)227-1952

Lee, Song Eun, MD {1972747749} Ophthl
+ Retina Consultants PA
1200 East Ridgewood Avenue/Suite 207   Ridgewood, NJ 07450   (201)612-9600   Fax (201)612-0428

Lee, Soo Gyung, MD {1679508048} IntrMd(98,PA13)
+ North Jersey Orthopaedic Specialists
15 Vervalen Street   Closter, NJ 07624   (201)784-6800   Fax (201)784-6801

Lee, Soomyung, MD {1740246867} Anesth(83,PA14)<NJ-VALLEY>
+ The Valley Hospital
223 North Van Dien Avenue   Ridgewood, NJ 07450   (201)447-8000
soomyung.lee@valleyhealth.com

Lee, Stephen Yong-Taek, MD {1346213907} Ophthl
+ Ophthalmic Partners of New Jersey
775 Route 70 East/Elmwood/Suite F 180   Marlton, NJ 08053   (856)596-1601   Fax (856)983-0396

Lee, Steven Thomas, MD {1538236989} RadDia(93,NY03)<NJ-HCKTSTWN>
+ Hackettstown Regional Medical Center
651 Willow Grove Street/Radiology   Hackettstown, NJ 07840   (908)852-5100

Lee, Sun Hee, MD {1225140403} Pedtrc(67,KOR01)<NJ-ENGLWOOD>
+ 19 Beverly Road
Englewood Cliffs, NJ 07632   (201)944-2858   Fax (201)944-

2872

Lee, Sung Keun, MD {1194764357} FamMed(66,KOR04)<NJ-SOMERSET>
+ 101 Omni Drive
Hillsborough, NJ 08844   (908)359-8251   Fax (908)359-8253
Sungkleemd@patmedia.net

Lee, Sung-Won, MD {1144296492} IntrMd(91,KOR06)
+ Substance Rehab Center
7 Broad Avenue/Suite 203   Palisades Park, NJ 07650   (201)941-2486   Fax (201)941-1577
+ United Medical, P.C.
533 Lexington Avenue   Clifton, NJ 07011   (201)941-2486   Fax (973)546-7707

Lee, Sunjoo, DO {1790858553}<NJ-HOLYNAME>
+ Holy Name Hospital
718 Teaneck Road   Teaneck, NJ 07666   (201)342-1205   Fax (201)342-1259

Lee, Susan, MD {1669695623} Rheuma(02,NY08)<NJ-CENTRAST>
+ Coordinated Health
222 Red Lane   Phillipsburg, NJ 08865   (610)861-8080   Fax (610)849-1013

Lee, Terrance H., MD {1053350389} CdvDis, IntrMd(82,KOR01)
+ Orange Medical Group
310 Central Avenue/Suite 106   East Orange, NJ 07018   (973)674-4542   Fax (973)674-3901
+ New Jersey Medical Group
464 Hudson Terrace/Suite 201   Englewood Cliffs, NJ 07632   (973)674-4542   Fax (201)503-0848

Lee, Terrence Hone Chung, MD {1306817077} RadDia(98,PA09)
+ 7 Yarmouth Road
Chatham, NJ 07928

Lee, Thomas Y., MD {1528084621} Surgry, SrgVas(94,NY19)<NJ-STCLRDEN>
+ Advanced Vascular Associates, PC
131 Madison Avenue/2nd Floor   Morristown, NJ 07960   (973)755-9206   Fax (973)540-9717

Lee, Thomas Yon, MD {1285632950} FamMed(01,NJ02)
+ Mt. Laurel Family Physicians
401 Young Avenue/Suite 260   Moorestown, NJ 08057   (856)291-8756   Fax (856)291-8750

Lee, Ting-Wen An, MD {1194895300} Pedtrc(03,MN04)
+ 579 Franklin Turnpike
Ridgewood, NJ 07450   (201)447-8182

Lee, Tracey-Ann Nadine, MD {1336285832} EmrgMd(95,NY03)<NJ-UNVMCPRN>
+ CentraState Medical Center
901 West Main Street/Emergency   Freehold, NJ 07728   (732)294-2666   Fax (732)431-8267

Lee, Vincent, MD {1881013738} PedRad
+ University Radiology Group, P.C.
483 Cranbury Road   East Brunswick, NJ 08816   (732)390-0030   Fax (732)390-1856

Lee, William, MD {1467419325} Anesth(01,NY08)<NJ-STPETER>
+ Anesthesia Consultnts of NJ/Nova Pain
285 Davidson Avenue/Suite 204   Somerset, NJ 08873   (732)271-1400   Fax (732)271-3543
+ St. Peter's University Hospital
254 Easton Avenue/Anesth   New Brunswick, NJ 08901   (732)745-8600
+ Cares Surgicenter, LLC.
240 Easton Avenue   New Brunswick, NJ 08873   (732)565-5400   Fax (732)296-8677

Lee, William, DO {1962742619}<NJ-NWRKBETH>
+ Newark Beth Israel Medical Center
201 Lyons Avenue   Newark, NJ 07112   (973)926-6671

Lee, Young Jae, MD {1609068659} AnesPain, IntrMd(03,DMN01)<NJ-CENTRAST, NJ-ACMCMAIN>
+ Relievus
2 Eighth Street   Hammonton, NJ 08037   Fax (856)779-0211
+ Relievus
1400 Route 70 East   Cherry Hill, NJ 08034   (888)985-2727

Lee, Young-Il, MD {1578617338} CdvDis, IntrMd(66,KOR04)
+ 2263 St. George Avenue
Rahway, NJ 07065   (732)574-0055   Fax (732)574-1155

Lee Ellis, Nandi T., MD {1376842740} Anesth(07,NY08)<NJ-STMRYPAS>
+ St. Mary's Hospital
350 Boulevard   Passaic, NJ 07055   (973)365-4300   Fax (845)357-5777

Lee-Agawa, Melissa, MD {1831506492} ObsGyn
+ Premier Women's Care
1 Broadway/Suite 301   Elmwood Park, NJ 07407   (201)977-6147   Fax (201)621-0139

Leedom, Karen Ann, MD {1720326458} ObsGyn(05,PA09)
+ Lawrence Ob/Gyn Associates
123 Franklin Corner Road/Suite 214   Lawrenceville, NJ 08648   (609)896-1400   Fax (609)896-3986
+ Lawrence Ob/Gyn Associates
1401 Whitehorse Mercerville Rd   Hamilton, NJ 08619   (609)896-1400   Fax (609)890-2456

Physicians by Name and Address

Leeds, Harold C., MD {1174592901} SrgOrt(71,MA05)
+ Orthopaedic and Joint Reconstruction
22 Old Short Hills Road   Livingston, NJ 07039   (973)533-1050   Fax (973)533-1235

Leeds, Richard S., MD {1962475285} CdvDis, IntrMd(81,NY09)<NJ-SOMERSET, NJ-RWJUBRUN>
+ Medicor Cardiology PA
225 Jackson Street   Bridgewater, NJ 08807   (908)526-8668   Fax (908)231-6781
+ Medicor Cardiology PA
331 US Highway 206/Suite 1A   Hillsborough, NJ 08844   (908)526-8668   Fax (908)431-0808

Leese, Kenneth H., MD {1316964356} Surgry, GenPrc, IntrMd(64,PA09)
+ Our Lady of Lourdes Medical Center
1600 Haddon Avenue/Wound Care   Camden, NJ 08103   (856)546-3900   Fax (856)546-3908

Lefavour, Gertrude S., MD {1841216397} Nephro, IntrMd(70,PA07)<NJ-RWJUBRUN>
+ UMDNJ RWJ Nephrology
125 Paterson Street/Suite 5100-B   New Brunswick, NJ 08901   (732)235-6512   Fax (732)235-6524
+ UH- RWJ Medical School
One Robert Wood Johnson Place   New Brunswick, NJ 08903   (732)235-6512   Fax (732)235-6124
+ Robert Wood Johnson Dialysis Center
117 North Center Drive   North Brunswick, NJ 08901   (732)940-4460

Lefever, Gerald S., MD {1992787071} Anesth(74,IL11)<NJ-MORRISTN>
+ 7 Raskin Road
Morristown, NJ 07960

Leff, Sheryl L., MD {1346355708} RadDia(85,NY09)
+ Imaging Center at Morristown
95 Madison Avenue/Suite 107   Morristown, NJ 07960   (973)984-1111   Fax (973)984-1190

Leff, Steven R., MD {1073586871} Ophthl, VitRet, IntrMd(80,NY01)<NJ-KIMBALL, NJ-RWJUBRUN>
+ UH- Robert Wood Johnson Med
125 Paterson Street   New Brunswick, NJ 08901   (732)235-6333   Fax (732)235-6330
+ Cataract & Laser Institute, P.A.
101 Prospect Street/Suite 102   Lakewood, NJ 08701   (732)235-6333   Fax (732)367-0937
+ Cataract & Laser Institute, P.A.
1527 Route 27/Suite 2600   Somerset, NJ 08901   (732)246-1050   Fax (732)846-1440

Leff, Stuart J., DO {1124000476} IntrMd(78,IA75)<NJ-OVERLOOK>
+ Roselle Park Primary Care
318 Chestnut Street   Roselle Park, NJ 07204   (908)241-4200

Lefkon, Bruce W., MD {1003812975} Urolgy(69,NY08)<NJ-STBARNMC>
+ New Jersey Urology, LLC
741 Northfield Avenue/Suite 206   West Orange, NJ 07052   (973)325-6100   Fax (973)325-1616
+ New Jersey Urology, LLC
700 North Broad Street/Suite 302   Elizabeth, NJ 07208   (973)325-6100   Fax (908)289-0716
+ New Jersey Urology, LLC
375 Mounain Pleasant Ave/Suite 250   West Orange, NJ 07052   (973)323-1300   Fax (973)323-1311

Lefkowitz, Aza, MD {1356341432} DerMOH(96,NY08)<NY-LIJEWSH>
+ Advanced Dermatology, P.C.
1200 East Ridgewood Avenue   Ridgewood, NJ 07450   (201)493-1717   Fax (201)493-1009

Lefkowitz, Heather Rush, MD {1659346518} Nephro(94,NY46)<NJ-NWRKBETH, NJ-STBARNMC>
+ Nephrology Group
111 Northfield Avenue/Suite 311   West Orange, NJ 07052   (973)325-2103   Fax (973)325-2254
+ Nephrology Group
142 Palisade Avenue/Suite 202   Jersey City, NJ 07305   (201)963-1077

Lefkowitz, Jeffrey R., MD {1790757870} Gastrn, IntrMd(82,NY46)<NJ-VALLEY>
+ Medical Multispecialty Associates PA
11-26 Saddle River Road   Fair Lawn, NJ 07410   (201)796-9200   Fax (201)796-7606

Lefkowitz, Miriam, MD {1336223080} IntrMd(98,NJ06)
+ 2204 US Highway 130/Suite C-3
North Brunswick, NJ 08902   (732)821-5151   Fax (732)297-1616

Legaspi, Abbelane S., MD {1497846224} Psychy(75,PHI09)<NJ-TRENTPSY>
+ Trenton Psychiatric Hospital
Sullivan Way/PO Box 7600/Psychiatry   West Trenton, NJ 08628   (609)633-1500

Leger, Pierre R., MD {1366535270} Pedtrc(77,MEX03)<NJ-STBARNMC>
+ Sanford Heights Pediatrics
987 Sanford Place   Irvington, NJ 07111   (973)374-1334   Fax (973)371-2593

Leggat, Christopher Scott, MD {1427196047} Anesth, IntrMd(02,NY15)<NJ-JRSYCITY>
+ Jersey City Medical Center
355 Grand Street/Anesthesia   Jersey City, NJ 07304   (201)915-2405

Leggiero, Nicholas J., DO {1972558534} FamMed(92,MO78)
+ Lakeview Medical Associates
125 US Highway 46   Budd Lake, NJ 07828   (973)691-1111   Fax (973)691-1198

Lehaf, Elias J., MD {1124071030} IntrMd<NJ-BAYSHORE>
+ Bayshore Community Hospital
727 North Beers Street   Holmdel, NJ 07733   (732)739-5981   Fax (732)290-7045

Lehet, Justin Micheal, DO {1831332527} EmrgMd(09,NY75)
+ Emergency Medical Associates of NJ, P.A.
3 Century Drive   Parsippany, NJ 07054   (973)740-0607   Fax (973)740-9895

Lehman, Abraham Reuven, MD {1477797132} Anesth, CarAne, IntrMd(07,ISR02)<NJ-STJOSHOS>
+ St. Joseph's Regional Medical Center Anesthesia
703 Main Street   Paterson, NJ 07503   (973)754-2323   Fax (973)977-9455

Lehman, Frederick, MD {1881621373} IntrMd(81,PHI08)<NJ-COMMED>
+ 307 Route 70/Suite 1A
Lakehurst, NJ 08733   (732)657-8138   Fax (732)657-7747

Lehman, Mark, MD {1073567897} SrgVas, Surgry(80,MEX14)<NJ-CENTRAST>
+ 222 Schanck Road/Suite 100
Freehold, NJ 07728   (732)845-5055   Fax (732)845-1489

Lehman, Ronald Arthur, Jr., MD {1528007358} SrgOrt, SrgSpn(97,PA02)
+ Columbia Grand Orthopaedics
500 Grand Avenue/Suite 101   Englewood, NJ 07631   (201)569-0440   Fax (201)569-4949

Lehmann, Robert Aaron, MD {1750558540}(05,NY48)
+ The Heart Group, PA
654 Broadway   Bayonne, NJ 07002   (201)243-9999   Fax (201)243-9998

Lehnes, Eric G., MD {1396787875} ObsGyn(90,NJ05)<NJ-KIMBALL, NJ-COMMED>
+ Ocean Gynecological & Obstetrical Associates PA
475 Highway 70   Lakewood, NJ 08701   (732)364-8000   Fax (732)364-4601

Lehrer, Luisa E., MD {1992703995} Anesth(86,PA02)<NJ-UNDRWD>
+ West Jersey Anesthesia Associates
102-E Center Boulevard   Marlton, NJ 08053   (856)988-6250   Fax (856)988-6270

Lehrhoff, Bernard J., MD {1336136282} Urolgy(76,NJ05)<NJ-OVERLOOK, NJ-STMICHL>
+ Premier Urology Group, LLC
275 Orchard Street   Westfield, NJ 07090   (908)654-5100   Fax (908)789-8755
+ Premier Urology Group, LLC
659 Kearny Avenue   Kearny, NJ 07032   (908)654-5100   Fax (201)789-8755
+ Premier Urology Group, LLC
1500 Pleasant Valley Road   West Orange, NJ 07090   (973)325-0091   Fax (973)789-8755

Lehrhoff, Sari, MD {1225465834} Psychy<NJ-TRININPC>
+ Trinitas Regional Medical Center-New Point Campus
655 East Jersey Street   Elizabeth, NJ 07206   (732)997-7385

Lehrhoff, Stephanie Rogers, MD {1164681193} Dermat, IntrMd(07,VA04)
+ Advanced Dermatology, Laser, and MOHS Surgery Center
240 East Grove Street   Westfield, NJ 07090   (908)232-6446   Fax (908)232-6447

Lehrman, Mark Leonard, MD {1306809090} IntrMd(74,NJ05)<NJ-VALLEY>
+ 15-01 Broadway/Suite 32
Fair Lawn, NJ 07410   (201)791-6434

Lei, Laura M., MD {1003011065} Anesth
+ Summit Anesthesia Associates, P.A.
33 Overlook Road/Suite 311   Summit, NJ 07901   (908)598-1500   Fax (908)598-0197

Lei, Michaela, DO {1023410701} FamMed
+ Phillips Barber Family Health Center
72 Alexander Avenue   Lambertville, NJ 08530   (609)397-3535   Fax (609)397-0301

Leib, Julie Alison, MD {1851462667} Psychy(96,NJ05)<NJ-MONMOUTH>
+ Ocean Mental Health Services, Inc.
160 Atlantic City Boulevard   Bayville, NJ 08721   (732)349-5550   Fax (732)349-5553
+ Monmouth Medical Center
300 Second Avenue/Psych   Long Branch, NJ 07740   (732)923-6912

Leib, Samantha, MD {1043224140} Pedtrc(99,NJ06)<NJ-STPETER>
+ Union Hill Pediatrics
85 Bridge Plaza Drive   Manalapan, NJ 07726   (732)972-1117   Fax (732)972-0177
+ St. Peter's University Hospital
254 Easton Avenue/Pediatrics   New Brunswick, NJ 08901   (732)745-8600

Leibman, Michael Roy, MD {1518077270} ObsGyn(93,NY46)<NJ-ENGLWOOD, NJ-HOLYNAME>
+ Michael Roy Leibman Ob/Gyn LLC
100 State Street/Suite 1-A   Teaneck, NJ 07666   (201)837-2100   Fax (201)837-2188
+ JFK Medical Center
65 James Street   Edison, NJ 08820   (201)837-2100   Fax (732)906-4961

Leibner, Donald N., MD {1396810214} Allrgy, PedAlg(81,NY08)<NJ-RWJUBRUN, NJ-STPETER>
+ 579-A Cranbury Road/Suite 103
East Brunswick, NJ 08816   (732)390-4900   Fax (732)390-4461

Leibov, Ernest B., MD {1619964996} Psychy, AlcSub, Acpntr(68,RUSS)<NJ-NWTNMEM>
+ Sparta Pain Management Center
350 Sparta Avenue/Building A   Sparta, NJ 07871   (973)729-0224   Fax (973)729-0234   leibov@pol.net

Leibowitz, Evan Howard, MD {1235194986} Rheuma, IntrMd(96,NJ05)<NJ-VALLEY>
+ Prospect Medical Offices, LLC
301 Godwin Avenue   Midland Park, NJ 07432   (201)444-4526   Fax (201)301-1313

Leibowitz, Karen Louise, MD {1043411655} PedGst, Pedtrc, IntrMd<NJ-RWJUBRUN>
+ 107 Cedar Grove Lane/Suite 100
Somerset, NJ 08873   (518)275-9013

Leibowitz, Keith Scott, DO {1134190903} IntrMd, CdvDis(99,NJ75)
+ Lakeland Cardiology Center, P.A.
415 Boulevard   Mountain Lakes, NJ 07046   (973)334-7700   Fax (973)402-5847

Leibowitz, Stacey Bucholtz, MD {1801884853} MedOnc, Hemato, IntrMd(97,MD07)<NJ-MORRISTN>
+ Carol G. Simon Cancer Center
100 Madison Avenue/Suite 4101   Morristown, NJ 07962   (973)538-5210   Fax (973)644-9657   Stacey.leibowitz@ahsys.org

Leibowitz, Steven R., MD {1053323600} Gastrn, IntrMd(85,DC02)<NJ-HACKNSK>
+ Hackensack Gastroenterology Associates
130 Kinderkamack Road/Suite 301   River Edge, NJ 07661   (201)489-7772   Fax (201)489-2544

Leibrandt, Paul N., MD {1205814001} EmrgMd
+ SJ Emergency Physician, PA
175 Madison Avenue   Mount Holly, NJ 08060   (609)914-7046   Fax (609)261-5842

Leibu, Dora, DO {1609271493} FamMed
+ Summit Medical Group-Berkeley Heights Campus
1 Diamond Hill Road   Berkeley Heights, NJ 07922   (908)277-8830   Fax (908)277-8796

Leibu, Dorina, MD {1871536698} Anesth, CarAne(81,ROM09)<NJ-STJOSHCS>
+ St. Joseph's Children's Hospital
703 Main Street/Anesthesia   Paterson, NJ 07503   (973)754-2500
+ St. Joseph's Regional Medical Center Anesthesia
703 Main Street   Paterson, NJ 07503   (973)754-2500   Fax (973)977-9455

Leibu, Rachel Rosenstock, MD {1366582520} IntrMd(92,PA09)<NJ-MORRISTN>
+ Morristown Medical Center
100 Madison Avenue   Morristown, NJ 07962   (973)971-5000   Fax (973)290-2928

Leibu, Tonel, MD {1649249582} IntrMd(84,ROMA)<NJ-VALLEY, NJ-HACKNSK>
+ 16 Arcadian Way
Paramus, NJ 07652   (201)843-4110   Fax (201)843-8810   TONEL@IX.NETCOM.com

Leiby, Alycia A., MD {1871626051} PedGst<NJ-MORRISTN>
+ Morristown Medical Center
100 Madison Avenue/PedGastro   Morristown, NJ 07962   (973)971-5676   Fax (973)290-7365

Leichter, Donald A., MD {1053399303} PedCrd, Pedtrc(80,NY20)<NY-CHLDCOPR, NY-PRSBCOLU>
+ 47 Maple Street/Suite 406
Summit, NJ 07901   (908)522-5566   doc@newjerseypediatriccardiology.com
+ Summit Medical Group
1 Diamond Hill Road/Bensley Pav/2 FL   Berkeley, NJ 07922   (908)522-5566   Fax (908)288-7993

Physicians by Name and Address

Leier, Tim Ulrich, MD {1972777316} Pedtrc, PedSpM, PhyM-SptM(99,GER21)<NJ-MORRISTN, NJ-OVERLOOK>
+ Children's Orthopedic & Sports Medicine Center
261 James Street/Suite 3-C   Morristown, NJ 07960   (973)206-1033   Fax (973)206-1036
+ Children's Orthopedic & Sports Medicine Center
33 Overlook Road/Suite 201   Summit, NJ 07901   (973)206-1033   Fax (973)206-1036

Leifer, Alden, MD {1093740375} Ophthl(81,NY46)
+ Alden Leifer MD and Associates
680 Broadway/Suite 114   Paterson, NJ 07514   (973)862-4713

Leifer, Amy Sarah Budin, MD {1730275173} Pedtrc(98,NY01)<NJ-VALLEY>
+ Valley Pediatric Associates, P.A.
201 East Franklin Turnpike   Ho Ho Kus, NJ 07423   (201)652-1888   Fax (201)652-6485
+ Valley Pediatric Associates PA
470 North Franklin Turnpike   Ramsey, NJ 07446   (201)652-1888   Fax (201)934-1817

Leifer, Bennett P., MD {1760448401} IntrMd, Grtrcs(86,NY15)<NJ-VALLEY>
+ Prospect Medical Offices, LLC
301 Godwin Avenue   Midland Park, NJ 07432   (201)444-4526   Fax (201)301-1313
+ Van Dyk Manor - Ridgewood
304 South Van Dien Avenue   Ridgewood, NJ 07450   (201)444-4526   Fax (201)445-9535

Leighton, Harmony J., DO {1922323120} IntrMd
+ Cardio Medical Group
98 James Street/Suite 313   Edison, NJ 08820   (732)635-1100   Fax (732)635-0918

Leiman, Sher, MD {1841275690} Radiol, Ultsnd, RadDia(68,DC03)<NJ-STPETER, NJ-RWJUBRUN>
+ University Radiology Group, P.C.
483 Cranbury Road   East Brunswick, NJ 08816   (732)390-0030   Fax (732)390-5383
+ University Radiology Group, P.C.
10 Plum Street   New Brunswick, NJ 08901   (732)390-0030   Fax (732)249-1208

Leipsner, George, MD {1073580262} FamMed(66,ITAL)<NJ-HACKNSK>
+ 57 West Pleasant Avenue
Maywood, NJ 07607   (201)488-2111   Fax (201)845-5033
+ Hackensack University Medical Center
30 Prospect Avenue/FamilyMed   Hackensack, NJ 07601   (201)996-2000

Leise, Megan Diane, MD {1326521634} SrgOrt
+ Princeton Orthopaedic Associates, P.A.
325 Princeton Avenue   Princeton, NJ 08540   (609)924-8183   Fax (609)924-8532

Leiser, Aliza Leah, MD {1588789796} GynOnc, ObsGyn(98,NY46)<NY-BETHPETR>
+ Rutgers Cancer Institute of New Jersey
195 Little Albany Street/PO Box 2681   New Brunswick, NJ 08903   (732)235-2465   Fax (732)235-6797

Leisner, William Randolph, MD {1609989045} IntrMd(80,PA02)<NJ-BURDTMLN>
+ Cape Health Solutions, LLC.
650 Town Bank Road   North Cape May, NJ 08204   (609)898-7447   Fax (609)898-1912
+ Cape Regional Physicians Associates
3806 Bayshore Road/Suite 101   North Cape May, NJ 08204   (609)898-7447   Fax (609)898-1912

Leistikow, Kathleen H., MD {1346303906} FamMed(90,MA16)<NJ-OVERLOOK>
+ Westfield Family Practice
563 Westfield Avenue   Westfield, NJ 07090   (908)232-5858   Fax (908)232-0439

Leitao, Mario Mendes, Jr., MD {1225068372} ObsGyn, GynOnc(96,NJ06)<NJ-UMDNJ, NY-SLOANKET>
+ Memorial Sloan-Kettering Cancer Center Basking Ridge
136 Mountain View Boulevard   Basking Ridge, NJ 07920   (908)542-3000   Fax (908)542-3220
+ University Physician Associates
140 Bergen Street/ACC Level C   Newark, NJ 07103   (908)542-3000   Fax (973)972-2739
+ University Hospital
150 Bergen Street/ObGyn   Newark, NJ 07920   (973)972-5554

Leitch, Megan Moran, MD {1457593022} Nrolgy, ClNrPh, IntrMd(08,VT02)<NY-SLRRSVLT>
+ University Hospital-RWJMS Neurology
125 Paterson Street/Suite 4100-6100   New Brunswick, NJ 08901   (732)235-7727   Fax (732)235-7041

Leitman, Mark William, MD {1366485781} Ophthl(71,NY09)
+ 13 Brunswick Woods Drive
East Brunswick, NJ 08816   (732)254-9090   Fax (732)254-4704

Leitner, Robyn R., MD {1659342277} Urolgy(99,NY09)<NJ-OCEANMC, NJ-JRSYSHMC>
+ Drs. Rotolo, Howard, and Leitner

2401 Highway 35   Manasquan, NJ 08736   (732)223-7877   Fax (732)223-7151

Leitner, Stephen J., MD {1669491237} EmrgMd(77,PA09)<NJ-VIRTMHBC>
+ SJ Emergency Physician, PA
175 Madison Avenue   Mount Holly, NJ 08060   (609)267-0700   Fax (609)261-5842

Leitner, Stuart P., MD {1558341735} IntrMd, MedOnc, OncHem(79,NY47)<NJ-STBARNMC>
+ St. Barnabas Medical Center
94 Old Short Hills Road/CancerCtr   Livingston, NJ 07039   (973)322-5000   Fax (973)322-8357
+ St. Barnabas Cancer Center
94 Old Short Hills Road/Suite 1   Livingston, NJ 07039   (973)322-5650

Leizer, Julie M., MD {1780986646}
+ Healthy Woman Ob/Gyn
312 Professional View Drive   Freehold, NJ 07728   (732)431-1616   Fax (732)866-7962

Lekht, Inna, MD {1225312705} Pedtrc
+ Dr. Gittleman & Associates
450 East Kennedy Boulevard   Lakewood, NJ 08701   (732)901-0050   Fax (732)370-2386

Lelyanov, Oleksiy, DO {1356730337} Anesth<NJ-RWJUBRUN>
+ RWJ University Hospital New Brunswick
One Robert Wood Johnson Place   New Brunswick, NJ 08901   (732)828-3000

Lemaire, Anthony, MD {1376700096} SrgCTh, Surgry(01,CT01)<NJ-RWJUBRUN>
+ RWJ University Hospital New Brunswick
One Robert Wood Johnson Place   New Brunswick, NJ 08901   (732)235-6171   Fax (732)235-8963
+ UMDNJ RWJ Vascular Surgery Group
125 Paterson Street/Suite 4100   New Brunswick, NJ 08901   (732)235-6171   Fax (732)235-8538

Lemansky, Alan S., MD {1609813856} EmrgMd, IntrMd(80,NJ06)<NJ-RIVERVW>
+ Riverview Medical Center
1 Riverview Plaza/EmrgMed   Red Bank, NJ 07701   (732)741-2700   Fax (732)224-7498

Lemasters, Patrick Evan, MD {1952535403} Surgry<NY-MTSINAI, NY-MTSINYHS>
+ Summit Medical Group
75 East Northfield Road   Livingston, NJ 07039   (973)436-1530   Fax (908)673-7336
+ Summit Medical Group
6 Brighton Road/2 FL   Clifton, NJ 07012   (973)436-1530   Fax (973)777-5403

Lembert Tezanos, Larissa, MD {1629233515} PthACl
+ New Jersey Urology, LLC
2401 East Evesham Road/Suite F   Voorhees, NJ 08043   (856)673-1600   Fax (856)988-0636

Lempel, Allen L., MD {1578672390} Grtrcs, IntrMd(81,NY09)<NJ-KIMBALL>
+ Ocean County Internal Medicine Associates
1352 River Avenue   Lakewood, NJ 08701   (732)370-5100   Fax (732)901-9240

Lempel, Stephanie J., MD {1588920854}
+ Rutgers- New Jersey Medical School
185 South Orange Avenue/Room F-603   Newark, NJ 07103   (973)972-6015   Fax (973)972-1019

Len, Lucille T., MD {1568494383} FamMed(81,NY47)
+ Center for Family Health, LLC.
431 Route 22 East/Suite 79   Whitehouse Station, NJ 08889   (908)534-5559   Fax (908)534-9166

Lena, Steffi D., DO {1942676457}
+ SOM - Department of Internal Medicine
42 East Laurel Road/Suite 3100   Stratford, NJ 08084   (856)566-6477   Fax (856)566-6906

Lenchur, Peter Michael, MD {1457335309} IntrMd, CdvDis, IntCrd(83,UKR06)<NJ-TRINIWSC, NJ-STBARNMC>
+ 776 East Third Avenue
Roselle, NJ 07203   (908)241-5545   Fax (908)241-5548

Lencina, Leandro H., MD {1285952960}<NJ-UMDNJ>
+ AFC Urgent Care Lyndhurst
560 New York Avenue   Lyndhurst, NJ 07071   (201)831-8125   Fax (201)345-4536

Lencki, Shaun G., MD {1639167562}<NJ-SJHREGMC>
+ SJH Regional Medical Center
1505 West Sherman Avenue   Vineland, NJ 08360   (856)641-7960   Fax (856)641-7645   lenckis@ihn.org

Lendor, E. Cindy, MD ObsGyn(84,PA07)<NJ-CHSMRCER>
+ Drs. Lendor and Evans Murage
1301 Whitehorse Mercerville Rd   Hamilton, NJ 08619   (609)585-9901   Fax (609)585-9919

Lendvai, Ivan, MD {1477537769} Psychy(68,HUNG)
+ University Behavioral Health Care
4326 Route 1 North   Monmouth Junction, NJ 08852   (732)235-5910   Fax (732)235-5644

Leng, Charles Tong-I, MD {1649210147} CdvDis, ClCdEl, IntrMd(94,CA11)<PA-UPMCPHL>
+ 1400 Marlton Pike East
Cherry Hill, NJ 08034   (856)616-2727   charles.leng.md@gmail.com

Lengel, Gary P., MD {1770523938} SrgVas, Surgry, IntrMd(76,PA13)
+ Southern Ocean Medical Center
1100 Route 72 West/Suite 307   Manahawkin, NJ 08050   (609)625-8000   Fax (609)978-8941   Glengelmd@hotmail.com

Lenger, Ellis S., MD {1548368319} Gastrn, IntrMd(79,NY08)<NJ-RWJUBRUN, NJ-STPETER>
+ Lenger and Plumser, MDs, LLC
465 Cranbury Road/Suite 102   East Brunswick, NJ 08816   (732)390-1995   Fax (732)254-4610

Lengner, Marlene, MD {1649206384} PthACl, Pthlgy(64,NE05)<NJ-HACKNSK>
+ Institute for Breast Care
20 Prospect Avenue/Suite 513   Hackensack, NJ 07601   (201)996-2222

Lennon, Christine Marie, MD {1558529982} Anesth
+ 219 Falls Court
Medford, NJ 08055   (646)643-5768

Lennox Thomas, Tricia Lynn, MD {1760423826} Ophthl, IntrMd(99,PA02)<NJ-CHSFULD, NJ-CHSMRCER>
+ Burlington County Eye Physicians
225 Sunset Road   Willingboro, NJ 08046   (609)877-2800   Fax (609)877-1813

Lentine, Nancy, DO {1699869909} FamMed(88,MO78)<NJ-CHILTON>
+ 70 East Main Street/1st Floor
Little Falls, NJ 07424   (973)237-0700   Fax (973)237-0777   nlentinedo@aol.com

Lentini, John Alaric, MD {1164721346} RadDia
+ Kennedy Health System/Cherry Hill Campus
2201 Chapel Avenue West/Radiology   Cherry Hill, NJ 08002   (508)566-4679

Lentnek, Ian Aaron, MD {1104093780} ClCdEl, CdvDis, IntrMd(04,GA01)
+ The Children's Regional Hospital at Cooper Univ Hosp
One Cooper Plaza   Camden, NJ 08103   (856)342-2000

Lentzner, Benjamin Joseph, MD {1356320014} Pedtrc, PedCrd(98,NY09)
+ Rutgers Pediatric Cardiology
125 Paterson Street/CAB 6100   New Brunswick, NJ 08901   (732)235-7905   Fax (732)235-7932

Lenza, Christopher, DO {1598925026} IntrMd(03,NY75)<NJ-RWJUBRUN>
+ RWJ Gastro & Hepatology
125 Paterson Street/CAB 5100B   New Brunswick, NJ 08901   (732)235-7784   Fax (732)235-7792

Leo, Chadwick S., DO {1841527504} Gyneco
+ 185 Howard Avenue
Passaic, NJ 07055

Leo, Mauro Vincenzo, MD {1760457972} ObsGyn(80,ITA07)<NJ-HACKNSK>
+ Hackensack University Medical Center
30 Prospect Avenue/ObsGyn   Hackensack, NJ 07601   (201)996-2000

Leo, Nicole Terese, DO {1952340077} FamMed(00,PA77)<NJ-BURDTMLN>
+ Family Practice Associates of Cape May County PA
210 Route US 9 South/Suite 202   Marmora, NJ 08223   (609)390-0882   Fax (609)390-3511

Leon, Robert John, MD {1063428902} CdvDis, IntrMd(90,NY06)<NJ-HACKNSK>
+ 129 Washington Street/Suite 401
Hoboken, NJ 07030   (201)610-1535   Fax (201)610-1578   rjleonmd@yahoo.com

Leon Wong, Hector J., MD {1457573321} FamMed(81,ECU05)
+ Abbasi Medical Group
1300 Main Avenue/Suite 2-D   Clifton, NJ 07011   (973)851-7818

Leonard, Maurice D., MD {1750334538} Gastrn(82,NY46)<NJ-VIRTMHBC, NJ-DEBRAHLC>
+ Gastroenterology Consultants of South Jersey
693 Main Street/Suite 2   Lumberton, NJ 08048   (609)265-1700   Fax (609)265-9005
+ Burlington County Endoscopy Center
140 Mount Holly Bypass/Unit 5   Lumberton, NJ 08048   (609)267-1555

Leonard, Sara B., MD {1932414620} FamMed(10,ANT02)<NJ-CENTRAST>
+ Drs. Bernardo & Leonard
4255 US Highway 9/Suite B   Freehold, NJ 07728   (732)683-9897   Fax (732)683-9674

Leonardo, Michael H., MD {1023348281} IntrMd(04,PHI33)
+ Allied Medical Associates
510 Hamburg Turnpike   Wayne, NJ 07470   (973)942-6005   Fax (973)442-6009

Physicians by Name and Address

Leone, Anthony J., MD {1073596623} IntrMd, IntMAdMd(80,ITA01)<NJ-OURLADY, NJ-COOPRUMC>
+ 807 Haddon Avenue/Suite 206
Haddonfield, NJ 08033 (856)428-1890 Fax (856)795-4645

Leone, Armand, Jr., MD {1942402052} RadDia, Radiol(82,NY09)
+ 769 Lincoln Avenue
Glen Rock, NJ 07452 Fax (201)444-0803

Leone, Dennis, MD {1235347535} Psychy(83,NJ05)
+ 701 Wiltseys Mill Road/Suite 104
Hammonton, NJ 08037 (609)567-4999 Fax (609)567-4899

Leone, Joseph A., MD {1518053016} SrgPlstc, SrgRec, IntrMd(67,PA09)<NJ-STBARNMC, NJ-JFKMED>
+ 1500 Pleasant Valley Way/Suite 307
West Orange, NJ 07052 (973)324-5333 Fax (973)324-0449

Leone, Mark R., DO {1144295049} FamMed(83,PA77)
+ Voorhees Family Practice
102 West White Horse Road/Suite 102 Voorhees, NJ 08043 (856)783-6200 Fax (856)783-8434

Leonetti, Joyce D., DO {1811086879} OccpMd, GPrvMd, AeroMd(80,PA77)
+ 7 Harker Avenue/Suite 2
Berlin, NJ 08009 (856)767-0017 Fax (856)767-7570

Leong, Kai K., MD {1831118124} Pedtrc, IntrMd(79,SPAI)<NJ-OURLADY>
+ CAMCare Health Corporation
817 Federal Street/Suite 100 Camden, NJ 08103 (856)541-9811 Fax (856)541-4611

Leong, Mila A., MD {1598701971} PedPul, Pedtrc(82,PHIL)<NJ-ACMCMAIN, NJ-ATLANTHS>
+ Pediatric Pulmonary & Asthma Assocs
1750 Zion Road/Suite 107 Northfield, NJ 08225 (609)677-4566 Fax (609)677-6080
+ AtlantiCare Regional Med Ctr/Mainland
65 West Jimmie Leeds Road Pomona, NJ 08240 (609)652-1000

Leong, Perry L., MD {1598744344} IntrMd(92,PA07)<NJ-SOMERSET>
+ Middlesex Medical Care
619 Union Avenue Middlesex, NJ 08846 (732)356-3212 Fax (732)356-5002
middlesexmcare@optonline.net

Leoniak, Steven Michael, MD {1124286851} Otlryg, SrgHdN, IntrMd(NY09)
+ Advanced ENT - Voorhees
200 Bowman Drive/Suite D-285 Voorhees, NJ 08043 (856)602-4000 Fax (856)346-0757
+ Advanced ENT - Willingboro
1113 Hospital Drive/Suite 103 Willingboro, NJ 08046 (856)602-4000 Fax (609)871-0508
+ Advanced ENT - Medford
103 Old Marlton Pike/Suite 219 Medford, NJ 08043 (856)602-4000 Fax (609)953-7146

Leonti, Vincent J., MD {1114903135} FamMed, EmrgMd(81,NY15)<NY-CORNGFP>
+ 134 Franklin Corner Road/Suite 101b
Lawrenceville, NJ 08648 (609)512-1468 Fax (609)512-1546

Leopardi, Nicole Marie, MD {1861624637}
+ Cooper University Hospital Pediatrics/Endocrinology
3 Cooper Plaza/Suite 200 Camden, NJ 08103 (856)342-2001 Fax (856)968-8259

Leopold, Clayton E., MD {1427151711} IntrMd(75,DC02)
+ Complete Care
1814 East Second Street Scotch Plains, NJ 07076 (908)322-6611 Fax (908)322-8665

Leopold, Michael A., MD {1417035361} Psychy(73,PA13)<NJ-UNVMCPRN>
+ 601 Ewing Street/Suite A-12
Princeton, NJ 08540 (609)921-6466
+ Princeton House Behavioral Health - Princeton
905 Herrontown Road Princeton, NJ 08540 (609)921-6466 Fax (609)497-3370
+ Princeton House Behavioral Health - Princeton
741 Mt. Lucas Road Princeton, NJ 08540 (609)497-3343 Fax (609)688-3771

Leopold, Thomas D., MD {1902898737} CdvDis(79,NY19)
+ MedDiag Assocs/Central NJ Cardiology
1511 Park Avenue/Suite 2 South Plainfield, NJ 07080 (908)756-4438 Fax (908)756-9160

LePera, Michael S., MD {1205008588} Surgry(97,VA07)
+ 34 Kentwood Road
Succasunna, NJ 07876
+ Palisades Surgical Associates
1530 Palisade Avenue/Colony Building Fort Lee, NJ 07024 Fax (201)585-0805

Lepis, Carl R., MD {1164438214} ObsGyn(70,ITA01)<NJ-JRSYSHMC, NJ-MONMOUTH>
+ Deal Lake Medical Associates
607 Eighth Avenue Asbury Park, NJ 07712 (732)774-0200 Fax (732)774-1019

Lepis, Michael Alphonse, MD {1972686079} PhysMd(95,GRN01)<NJ-MONMOUTH, NJ-JRSYSHMC>
+ Comprehensive Pain Management
2420 Highway 34 Manasquan, NJ 08736 (732)774-8909 Fax (732)774-8902

Lepore, Frederick E., MD {1710052204} Nrolgy, OphNeu(75,NY45)<NJ-RWJUBRUN>
+ UH- Robert Wood Johnson Med
125 Paterson Street/Neurology New Brunswick, NJ 08901 (732)235-7731 Fax (732)235-7041
leporefe@umdnj.edu

Lequerica, Steve A., MD {1881689495} Nrolgy(81,MA05)<NJ-STJOSHOS>
+ Neurology Group of North Jersey PA
905 Allwood Road/Suite 105 Clifton, NJ 07012 (973)471-3680 Fax (973)471-6360

Lerch, Gordon Lee, Jr., DO {1790885275} Pedtrc(80,PA77)<NJ-VIRTUAHS, NJ-KMHSTRAT>
+ Dr. G. Lee Lerch and Associates
63 North Lakeview Drive/Suite 202 Gibbsboro, NJ 08026 (856)435-6000 Fax (856)782-1667
lerchpeds@comcast.net
+ Dr. G. Lee Lerch and Associates
239 Hurffville Crosskeys Road Sewell, NJ 08080 (856)435-6000 Fax (856)728-0808

Lerer, Daniel Brian, MD {1316066228} RadDia, Radiol, IntrMd(99,NY46)
+ 788 Winthrop Road
Teaneck, NJ 07666 (201)281-0316 Fax (201)836-3194

Lerer, Paul K., MD {1336131176} Gastrn, IntrMd(80,MN08)
+ Medical Diagnostic Associates PA
525 Central Avenue/Suite D Westfield, NJ 07090 (908)232-5333 Fax (908)389-1930
+ Medical Diagnostic Associates, P.A.
MAC, 11 Overlook Road/Suite 100 Summit, NJ 07901 (908)232-5333 Fax (908)273-3125

Leriotis, Theo James, DO {1982043378} EmrgMd<NJ-ACMCITY>
+ AtlantiCare Regional Medical Center/City Campus
1925 Pacific Avenue Atlantic City, NJ 08401 (609)441-8127

Lerma, Pauline Marie Ocampo, MD {1447334172} IntrMd, OncHem, MedOnc(92,PHI29)<NJ-RWJUHAM>
+ Cancer Institute of NJ Hamiltom
2575 Klockner Road Hamilton, NJ 08690 (609)631-6960 Fax (609)631-6888

Lerman, Gabriel Salomon, DO {1609164367} IntrMd<NJ-SJHREGMC>
+ SJH Regional Medical Center
1505 West Sherman Avenue Vineland, NJ 08360 (856)641-8000

Lerman, Nati, MD {1750479937} OncHem, IntrMd(98,ISR01)<NJ-COOPRUMC>
+ Drs. Mehta & Lerman
900 Centiental Boulevard Voorhees, NJ 08043 Fax (856)325-6777
+ Cooper University Medical Center/Camden
3 Cooper Plaza/Suite 215 Camden, NJ 08103 Fax (856)338-9211

Lerner, Amanda Kate, MD {1790043677}<NJ-JRSYSHMC>
+ Jersey Shore University Medical Center
1945 Route 33 Neptune, NJ 07753 (732)775-5500

Lerner, Elliot J., MD {1639166598} RadDia, RadNro(85,RI01)<NJ-VALLEY>
+ Radiology Associates of Ridgewood, P.A.
20 Franklin Turnpike Waldwick, NJ 07463 (201)447-8210 Fax (201)447-8431
ejlmd@bellatlantic.net
+ The Valley Hospital
223 North Van Dien Avenue/Radiology Ridgewood, NJ 07450 (201)447-8000

Lerner, Emanuel D., MD {1275692659} Pedtrc(91,NJ06)<NJ-RWJUBRUN, NJ-STPETER>
+ RWJ University Medical Group/Somerset Pediatrics
1 Worlds Fair Drive/Suite 1 Somerset, NJ 08873 (732)743-5437 Fax (732)564-0212
+ University Medical Group
125 Paterson Street/Suite 5100 New Brunswick, NJ 08901 (732)743-5437 Fax (732)235-6233

Lerner, Kent S., MD {1184821910} SrgOrt, SrgOARec(78,NJ05)<NJ-MTNSIDE>
+ Metropolitan Orthopedics
17 Jauncey Avenue North Arlington, NJ 07031 (201)991-9019 Fax (201)991-0931

Lerner, William A., MD {1417939810} Hemato, IntrMd, Onclgy(77,BELG)<NJ-JRSYSHMC, NJ-OCEANMC>
+ Atlantic Hematology Oncology Associates, L.L.C.
1707 Atlantic Avenue Manasquan, NJ 08736 (732)528-0760 Fax (732)528-0764

Leroy, Christine, MD {1538542949} FamMed
+ St. Joseph's Family Medicine @ Clifton
1135 Broad Street/Suite 201 Clifton, NJ 07013 (973)754-4100 Fax (973)472-9062

Leschhorn, Edwin C., MD {1679553309} PthAcl, Pthlgy(84,DOMI)<NJ-RIVERVW, NJ-JRSYSHMC>
+ Riverview Medical Center
1 Riverview Plaza/Pathology&Lab Red Bank, NJ 07701 (732)530-2347 Fax (732)345-2045
eleschhorn@meridianhealth.com

Leschinsky, Alexandra, MD {1144273277} IntrMd(74,UKRA)<NJ-CENTRAST>
+ EMedical Urgent Care
2 Kings Highway Middletown, NJ 07748 (732)957-0707 Fax (732)957-9852

Lesesne-Ayodeji, Mercedes, MD {1811938293} Pedtrc, AdolMd(76,DC02)
+ Eastside Pediatrics
625 Broadway/1st Floor Paterson, NJ 07514 (973)523-1102 Fax (973)523-7309

Leshner, Stanley B., DO {1972563575} FamMed, IntrMd(72,IL76)<NJ-SJRSYELM, NJ-KENEDYHS>
+ Wedgewood Family Practice Associates PA
302 Hurffville Cross-Keys Road Sewell, NJ 08080 (856)589-4610 Fax (609)589-1624
+ Kennedy Health Systems/Washington Township Campus
435 Hurffville-Cross Keys Road Turnersville, NJ 08012 (856)582-2500

Lesiczka, Adam, MD {1902836919} IntrMd(82,POL02)
+ 42 Locust Avenue
Wallington, NJ 07057 (973)472-2912 Fax (973)472-4235
Adamlesi@verizon.net

Lesko, Cecily A., MD {1558337246} Ophthl(90,NY47)<NJ-STMRY-PAS, NY-MTSINYHS>
+ North Jersey Eye Associates PA
1005 Clifton Avenue Clifton, NJ 07013 (973)472-4114 Fax (973)472-0775
cecilyleskomd@aol.com

Lesko, Richard J., MD {1609865955} EmrgMd, IntrMd(79,NY19)<NJ-OVERLOOK, NJ-MORRISTN>
+ Summit Medical Group-Berkeley Heights Campus
1 Diamond Hill Road Berkeley Heights, NJ 07922 (908)273-4300 Fax (908)790-6524
+ Summit Medical Group
34 Mountain Boulevard/Building B Warren, NJ 07059 (908)273-4300 Fax (908)769-8927

Leslie, Joanne, MD {1265415384} Anesth(83,NY47)<NJ-HACKNSK>
+ Hackensack Anesthesiology Associates
140 Prospect Avenue/Suite 8 Hackensack, NJ 07601 (201)488-0066 Fax (201)488-6769
+ Hackensack University Medical Center
30 Prospect Avenue/Anesth Hackensack, NJ 07601 (201)996-2000
+ Hackensack University MC-Anesthesia Dept
30 Prospect Avenue/Room 2703 Hackensack, NJ 07601 (201)996-2419 Fax (201)996-3962

Leslie, Lori Ann, MD {1972746394} IntrMd
+ John Theurer Cancer Center - HUMC
92 Second Street Hackensack, NJ 07601 (551)996-5900 Fax (201)996-9246

Lesneski, Matthew J., MD {1720240369} Anesth(08,NJ06)
+ Rancocas Anesthesiology, PA
15000 Midlantic Drive/Suite 102 Mount Laurel, NJ 08054 (856)255-5479 Fax (856)393-8691
+ Rancocas Anesthesiology, PA
700 Route 130 North/Suite 203 Cinnaminson, NJ 08077 (856)255-5479 Fax (856)829-3605

Lesniak, Sebastian P., MD {1417252776} Ophthl
+ Matossian Eye Associates
2 Capital Way/Suite 326 Pennington, NJ 08534 (609)882-8833 Fax (609)882-0077

Lesorgen, Philip R., MD {1851342976} ObsGyn, RprEnd(77,MA05)<NJ-HACKNSK, NJ-ENGLWOOD>
+ Women's Fertility Center of NJ
106 Grand Avenue Englewood, NJ 07631 (201)569-6979 Fax (201)569-0269
+ IVF Center
15-01 Broadway Fair Lawn, NJ 07410 (201)569-6979 Fax (201)569-0269
+ Hackensack University Medical Center
30 Prospect Avenue Hackensack, NJ 07631 (201)996-2000

Lespinasse, Antoine Alexandra, MD {1114912052} Pedtrc, NnPnMd(92,HAI01)<NJ-KIMBALL, NJ-COMMED>
+ On-Site Neonatal Partners
1000 Haddonfield-Berlin Road/Suite 210 Voorhees, NJ 08043 (856)782-2212 Fax (856)782-2213

Lespinasse, Pierre Frederic, MD {1023108248} ObsGyn(92,HAI01)<NJ-UMDNJ>
+ 194 Highland Avenue
Montclair, NJ 07042

Lesser, Eric S., MD {1063415487} Pedtrc, NnPnMd(88,NY46)<NJ-STJOSHOS>
+ St Joseph's Medical Center Neonatology
703 Main Street   Paterson, NJ 07503   (973)754-2555   Fax (973)754-2567

Lesser, Gregory Scott, MD {1023096575} Gastrn, IntrMd(99,MNT01)
+ Huntendon Gastroenterology
1100 Wescott Drive/Suite 201   Flemington, NJ 08822   (908)788-4022   Fax (908)788-4066

Lesser, Raymond W., MD {1871538900} Otlryg(81,PA12)
+ Ear Nose & Throat Professional Associates
30 Washington Avenue/Suite E   Haddonfield, NJ 08033   (856)428-9314   Fax (856)428-6149
info@pentadocs.com

Lesserson, Jonathan A., MD {1194764670} Otlryg, PedOto(89,PA01)<NJ-HACKNSK, NJ-CHILTON>
+ ENT & Allergy Associates, LLP
433 Hackensack Avenue/Suite 204   Hackensack, NJ 07601   (201)883-1062   Fax (201)883-9297

Lessig, Marvin A., DO {1144309030} PthAcl(68,PA77)
+ New Jersey Blood Services/New York Blood Center
167 New Street   New Brunswick, NJ 08901   (732)220-7000   Fax (732)220-7199

Lessing, David, MD {1376565747} SrgOrt(78,NY01)
+ Orthopedic Associates of Central Jersey
205 May Street/Suite 202   Edison, NJ 08837   (908)757-1520   Fax (908)769-1388
davidlessingmd@gmail.com
+ Orthopedic Associates of Central Jersey PA
3 Hospital Plaza/Suite 411   Old Bridge, NJ 08857   (908)757-1520   Fax (732)360-0775

Lester, Arthur I., MD {1528028347} Otlryg, IntrMd(70,ITA01)<NJ-CLARMAAS, NJ-STBARNMC>
+ Empire Medical Associates
5 Franklin Avenue/Suite 302   Belleville, NJ 07109   (973)759-1221   Fax (973)759-1997
+ Empire Medical Associates
264 Boyden Avenue   Maplewood, NJ 07040   (973)759-1221   Fax (973)761-7617
+ Empire Medical Associates
382 West Passaic Avenue   Bloomfield, NJ 07109   (973)338-1900

Lester, Jonathan P., MD {1225093602} PhysMd(87,FL03)
+ Comprehensive Spine Care, PA
260 Old Hook Road/Suite 400   Emerson, NJ 07630   (201)634-1811   Fax (201)634-9170

Lestini, Melissa Murray, MD {1689875890} Pedtrc, NnPnMd(02,OH40)<PA-CHILDHOS>
+ CHOP Care Network at Virtua Voorhees Hospital
100 Bowman Drive   Voorhees, NJ 08043   (856)325-3000   Fax (609)261-5842

Leszkowicz, Aditee D., DO {1962492959} Pedtrc(00,NJ75)<NJ-VIRTVOOR, NJ-VIRTUAHS>
+ Advocare Atrium Pediatrics
301 Old Marlton Pike West/Suite 1   Marlton, NJ 08053   (856)988-9101   Fax (856)988-7712
+ Advocare Atrium Pediatrics Cedar Brook
41 South Route 73/Building 1/Suite 101   Hammonton, NJ 08037   (856)988-9101   Fax (609)567-4904

Letizia, Matthew J., DO {1457552457} EmrgMd(03,IL76)<NJ-TRINIWSC>
+ Trinitas Regional Medical Center-Williamson Street
225 Williamson Street/EmrgMed   Elizabeth, NJ 07207   (908)994-5454   Fax (919)425-0478

Leu, Diana S., MD {1447263744} Dermat(02,MA06)<NJ-CHILTON>
+ 601 Hamburg Turnpike/Suite 211
Wayne, NJ 07470   (973)925-7077   Fax (973)925-7078
dianaleu@gmail.com

Leu, James Ping Hsun, MD {1841453677} EnDbMt, IntrMd(03,MA05)
+ 510 Hamburg Turnpike/Suite 201
Wayne, NJ 07470   (973)246-3630   Fax (973)942-1250
+ Complete Endocrinology & Thyroid Center LLC
330 Ratzer Road/Suite D-17   Wayne, NJ 07470   (973)246-3630   Fax (973)832-7489

Leuchten, Lisa, DO {1750667283} EmrgMd<NJ-MTNSIDE>
+ Hackensack UMC Mountainside
1 Bay Avenue   Montclair, NJ 07042   (908)405-8250

Leung, Albert Tao-Man, MD {1982894028} EnDbMt, IntrMd(89,IA02)
+ Merck and Company Incorporated
126 East Lincoln Avenue   Rahway, NJ 07065   (732)594-8164

Leung, Dora Kaman, MD {1659424596} Nrolgy(93,NY01)
+ HSS Paramus Outpatient Center
140 East Ridgewood Avenue/Suite 175-S   Paramus, NJ 07652   (201)796-2255   Fax (201)796-3711

Leung, Jacquelyn Way-Yan, MD {1326925251} FamMed(01,PA02)
+ Drs. Leung & Murphy
196 Speedwell Avenue   Morristown, NJ 07960   (973)539-9580

Leung, Michael Seto, MD {1558305078} IntrMd(99,NJ06)
+ IPC The Hospitalist Company
55 Madison Avenue/Suite 310   Morristown, NJ 07960   (973)993-9536   Fax (973)998-4237

Leung, Samson W., MD {1881619161} Anesth(01,NY08)<NJ-BAYSHORE>
+ Bayshore Community Hospital
727 North Beers Street/Anesthesiology   Holmdel, NJ 07733   (732)739-5900

Leung, Winifred Fong, MD {1619046869} EmrgMd(98,NJ05)<NJ-RWJUBRUN>
+ RWJ University Hospital New Brunswick
One Robert Wood Johnson Place   New Brunswick, NJ 08901   (732)828-3000

Leupold, Kerry Lynn, DO {1164581542} Pedtrc, PedEmg(97,NY75)<NJ-RWJUBRUN>
+ RWJ University Pediatric Emergency Medicine
125 Paterson Street/MEB 342   New Brunswick, NJ 08903   (732)235-7893   Fax (732)235-7077

Leuzzi, Rosemarie Anne, MD {1861574220} IntrMd(89,PA12)
+ Cooper Physician Offices
900 Centennial Boulevard   Voorhees, NJ 08043   (856)325-6770   Fax (856)673-4300

Leva, Ernest G., MD {1144389537} Pedtrc, PedEmg(85,ITA27)<NJ-RWJUBRUN, NJ-STPETER>
+ RWJ University Pediatric Emergency Medicine
125 Paterson Street/MEB 342   New Brunswick, NJ 08903   (732)235-7893   Fax (732)235-9340
+ Union Hill Pediatrics
85 Bridge Plaza Drive   Manalapan, NJ 07726   (732)235-7893   Fax (732)972-0177

Levai, Robert Joseph, MD {1295756120} IntrMd(75,NY03)<NJ-MTNSIDE>
+ Mountainside Medical Group
123 Highland Avenue/Suite 201   Glen Ridge, NJ 07028   (973)748-9246   Fax (973)748-8755

Levan, Anne-Marie, MD {1144402678} FamMGrtc(84,RI01)
+ 29 Trautwein Crescent
Closter, NJ 07624   (201)887-2001

Levan, Ellen, MD {1710960927} IntrMd(90,BLA46)<NY-BETHPETR, NJ-ENGLWOOD>
+ Absolute Medical Care
One Broadway/Suite 301   Elmwood Park, NJ 07407   (201)791-9340   Fax (201)791-9481

LeVan, Maurice X., MD {1770674905} GenPrc(81,FRAN)
+ Woodbine Development Center/NJ Human Services
1175 Dehirsch Avenue   Woodbine, NJ 08270   (609)861-2164   Fax (609)861-2494

Levandowski, Richard, MD {1124175419} FamMed, SprtMd, OstMed(74,NJ06)<NJ-UNVMCPRN, NJ-CHSFULD>
+ Princeton Sports & Family Medicine
3131 Princeton Pike   Lawrenceville, NJ 08648   (609)896-9190   Fax (609)896-3555
r_levandowski@msn.com

Levant, Barry E., MD {1760456016} Grtrcs, IntrMd(76,ITAL)<NJ-CHILTON>
+ 15 Kiel Avenue/Building 2
Kinnelon, NJ 07405   (973)838-4098   Fax (973)838-7628

Levat, Robin H., MD {1174523633} ObsGyn(87,NY19)<NJ-HACKNSK>
+ Prospect Women's Medical Center PA
120 Prospect Avenue   Hackensack, NJ 07601   (201)342-1600   Fax (201)342-2280

Levchook, Christina, MD {1912204447} RadDia, Radiol<NJ-CLARMAAS>
+ Clara Maass Medical Center
1 Clara Maass Drive/Radiology   Belleville, NJ 07109   (973)450-2037

Levenbach, Rachel Shoshana, MD {1902065857} MedOnc
+ Hematology Oncology Associates PA
175 Madison Avenue/4th Floor   Mount Holly, NJ 08060   (609)702-1900   Fax (609)702-8455

Levenberg, Steven, MD {1710977426} IntrMd(79,PA02)<NJ-STFRNMED, NJ-RWJUHAM>
+ Capital Health Primary Care
1445 Whitehorse-Mercerville Ro   Hamilton, NJ 08619   (609)249-6658   Fax (609)249-6659

Leventer, David Benjamin, MD {1578659835} Ophthl(95,NY01)
+ Eye and Face
241 Monmouth Road/Suite 103   West Long Branch, NJ 07764   (732)571-3937   Fax (732)571-1199

Leventhal, Douglas Drew, MD {1508073321} Otlryg, OtgyFPIS(04,NJ06)
+ ENT & Allergy Associates, LLP
690 Kinderkamack Road/Suite 101   Oradell, NJ 07649   (201)722-9850   Fax (201)722-9851

Leventhal, Elaine A., MD {1245302512} IntrMd(74,WI05)<NJ-RWJUBRUN>
+ UH- Robert Wood Johnson Med
125 Paterson Street/CAB/Intrnl Mdcn   New Brunswick, NJ 08901   (732)235-6653

Leventhal, Todd Owen, MD {1609875251} Ophthl(92,MA07)<NJ-OVERLOOK, NJ-SOMERSET>
+ Berkeley Heights Eye Group
571 Central Avenue/Suite 101   New Providence, NJ 07974   (908)464-4600   Fax (908)464-4737
TLeventhal1@verizon.net

Levey, Bryan H., MD {1134119811} Pedtrc(94,NJ05)<NJ-VIRTVOOR>
+ Virtua Voorhees
100 Bowman Drive/Pediatrics   Voorhees, NJ 08043   (856)247-3000

Levey, James Andrew, MD {1316936669} ObsGyn(91,NY03)<NJ-OVERLOOK, NJ-MORRISTN>
+ Summit Medical Group
34 Mountain Boulevard/Building B   Warren, NJ 07059   (908)769-0100   Fax (908)769-8927
+ Summit Medical Group-Berkeley Heights Campus
1 Diamond Hill Road   Berkeley Heights, NJ 07922   (908)769-0100   Fax (908)790-6576

Levey, Stephanie B., MD {1326092115} Ophthl, CrnExD(91,NY03)<NJ-STBARNMC>
+ Cataract & Eye Care Center
16 Pocono Road/Suite 301   Denville, NJ 07834   (973)625-7970   Fax (973)625-9650

Levi, David A., MD {1922248962} RadDia<NY-NSUHMANH>
+ Atlantic Medical Imaging, LLC.
72 West Jimmie Leeds Road   Galloway, NJ 08205   (609)677-9729   Fax (609)653-8764

Levi, Steven A., MD {1902859150} CdvDis(95,PA12)<NJ-COOPRUMC, NJ-OURLADY>
+ Cardiovascular Associates
210 West Atlantic Avenue   Haddon Heights, NJ 08035   (856)546-3003   Fax (856)547-5337
+ Cardiovascular Associates of The Delaware Valley, PA
1840 Frontage Road   Cherry Hill, NJ 08034   (856)546-3003   Fax (856)795-7436
+ Cardiovascular Associates of The Delaware Valley, PA
525 State Street/Suite 3   Elmer, NJ 08035   (856)358-2363   Fax (856)358-0725

Levin, Alexander G., MD {1639105448} Anesth, PainMd(77,BLAR)<NJ-STMRYPAS, NJ-RBAYOLDB>
+ Pain Control Center of New Jersey
561 Cranbury Road   East Brunswick, NJ 08816   (732)651-1300   Fax (732)651-0375

Levin, Barry Edward, MD {1083628200} IntrMd, Nrolgy(67,GA05)<NJ-VAEASTOR>
+ Rutgers- New Jersey Medical School
185 South Orange Avenue/H506   Newark, NJ 07103   (973)972-4300
levin@njms.rutgers.edu

Levin, Bonnie Lorraine, DO {1841371028} FamMed, GenPrc(86,IA75)<NJ-KMHCHRRY>
+ 1020 Kings Highway North/Suite 208
Cherry Hill, NJ 08034   (856)667-3948   Fax (856)321-8328

Levin, Brandt M., MD {1043378979} IntrMd(75,PHI08)<NJ-RWJU-RAH>
+ 100 Commerce Place
Clark, NJ 07066   (732)388-5757   Fax (732)499-8128

Levin, Daniel H., MD {1205850476} CritCr, IntrMd, PulDis(80,NY01)
+ Summit Medical Group Pulmonology
1030 Clifton Avenue/Suite 103   Clifton, NJ 07013   (973)777-7377   Fax (973)777-3806
+ Summit Medical Group
31-00 Broadway   Fair Lawn, NJ 07410   (973)777-7377   Fax (201)796-7020

Levin, David N., MD {1326015199} IntrMd, Nephro(76,NJ05)<NJ-HACKNSK, NJ-HOLYNAME>
+ Nephrology Associates PA
870 Palisade Avenue/Suite 202   Teaneck, NJ 07666   (201)836-0897   Fax (201)836-8042

Levin, Elizabeth H., MD {1588838130} Psychy(79,NY08)<NJ-TRENTPSY, NJ-UMDNJ>
+ University Psychiatric Associates
183 South Orange Avenue/E-F Levels   Newark, NJ 07103   (973)972-2977   Fax (973)972-2979
+ Trenton Psychiatric Hospital
Sullivan Way/PO Box 7600   West Trenton, NJ 08628   (973)972-2977   Fax (609)633-8527

Levin, Francis L., DO {1063453199} EmrgMd(74,PA77)<NJ-KMHSTRAT, NJ-KMHCHRRY>
+ Kennedy Memorial Hospital-University Medical Center
18 East Laurel Road/EmergMed   Stratford, NJ 08084   (856)346-7986

Physicians by Name and Address

Levin, Gary H., MD {1568440592} Gastrn(78,PA01)<NJ-VIRTVOOR, NJ-KMHCHRRY>
+ South Jersey Gastroenterology PA
  406 Lippincott Drive/Suite E   Marlton, NJ 08053   (856)983-1900   Fax (856)983-5110
+ South Jersey Gastroenterology PA
  117 East Laurel Road   Stratford, NJ 08084   (856)983-1900   Fax (856)751-8746
+ South Jersey Gastroenterology PA
  501 Fifth Street/Suite 2   Atco, NJ 08053   (856)753-3066

Levin, Irina, MD {1477749182} FamMed(95,RUSS)<NJ-VIRTMHBC>
+ Advocare Main Street Medical Associates
  714 East Main Street/Suite 1-C   Moorestown, NJ 08057   (856)778-4009   Fax (856)778-4014

Levin, Jacob L., MD {1053390070} CdvDis, IntrMd(78,NY08)<NJ-SHOREMEM>
+ Shore Memorial Hospital
  1 East New York Avenue/Cardiology   Somers Point, NJ 08244   (609)365-3100   Fax (609)365-3165   shorecardio@comcast.net
+ Shore Cardiology Associates PA
  408 Bethel Road/Building D Suite 408   Somers Point, NJ 08244   (609)365-3100   Fax (609)653-2037
+ Penn Medicine Somers Point
  155 Brighton Avenue/Second Floor   Somers Point, NJ 08244   (609)365-3100   Fax (609)365-3165

Levin, Joseph B., MD {1285652149} IntrMd(75,PA09)<NJ-VIRTBERL, NJ-VIRTVOOR>
+ Advocare Main Street Medical Associates
  714 East Main Street/Suite 1-C   Moorestown, NJ 08057   (856)778-4009   Fax (856)778-4014

Levin, Kenneth A., MD {1679534515} Nrolgy(82,IN20)<NJ-VALLEY>
+ Neurology Group of Bergen County
  1200 East Ridgewood Avenue   Ridgewood, NJ 07450   (201)444-0868   Fax (201)444-7363

Levin, Lorin Michelle, MD {1346275591} Pedtrc(00,ISR02)<NJ-MORRISTN, NJ-OVERLOOK>
+ Watchung Pediatrics
  76 Stirling Road/Suite 201   Warren, NJ 07059   (908)755-5437   Fax (908)755-6905
+ Watchung Pediatrics
  346 South Avenue/Suite 3   Fanwood, NJ 07023   (908)755-5437   Fax (908)889-0047
+ Watchung Pediatrics
  225 Millburn Avenue/Suite 301   Millburn, NJ 07059   (973)376-7337   Fax (973)218-6647

Levin, Matthew, MD {1699951210} Psychy(06,PA09)<MA-VAMCBRKT, MA-WSTWDLDG>
+ 623 River Road/Suite 2R
  Fair Haven, NJ 07704   (732)977-8486   Fax (714)443-0202

Levin, Michael Y., DO {1700820669} EmrgMd(99,NY75)<NJ-RIVERVW>
+ Riverview Medical Center
  1 Riverview Plaza/EmergMed   Red Bank, NJ 07701   (732)741-2700   Fax (732)224-7498

Levin, Miles B., MD {1477702124} Pthlgy(04,PA13)<NJ-OVERLOOK>
+ Overlook Medical Center
  99 Beauvoir Avenue/PO Box 210   Summit, NJ 07902   (908)522-6225   Fax (908)522-2320

Levin, Neil, MD {1053343368} CdvDis, IntrMd, IntCrd(84,NY01)<NJ-COOPRUMC>
+ Penn Medicine at Cherry Hill
  1400 East Route 70/Cardiology   Cherry Hill, NJ 08034

Levin, Neil, DO {1487651675} FamMed(76,IA79)<NJ-UNDRWD, NJ-KENEDYHS>
+ Atrium Two Family Practice Associates, P.A.
  468 Hurfville-Crosskeys Road   Sewell, NJ 08080   (856)589-2929   Fax (856)582-1146

Levin, Rafael, MD {1144284134} SrgOrt(98,MD07)<NJ-HACKNSK>
+ Comprehensive Spine Care, PA
  260 Old Hook Road/Suite 400   Emerson, NJ 07630   (201)634-1811   Fax (201)634-9170

Levin, Robin Merle, MD {1659327211} Dermat, IntrMd(96,PA02)<NJ-OURLADY, NJ-KENEDYHS>
+ South Jersey Skin Care & Laser Center
  101 Gaither Drive   Mount Laurel, NJ 08054   (856)810-9888   Fax (856)810-9889

Levin, Sanan L., MD {1730111980} FamMed, IntrMd(76,PA07)<NJ-VIRTMHBC>
+ Advocare Main Street Medical Associates
  714 East Main Street/Suite 1-C   Moorestown, NJ 08057   (856)778-4009   Fax (856)778-4014

Levin, Steven Jonathan, MD {1780777235} FamMed(85,GA05)
+ Eric B. Chandler Health Center
  277 George Street   New Brunswick, NJ 08901   (732)235-7297   Fax (732)235-6726

Levin, Susan Miriam, MD {1932925407408} FamMed(93,NY46)<NJ-VALLEY>
+ Heart & Vascular Associates of Northern Jersey
  22-18 Broadway/Suite 201   Fair Lawn, NJ 07410   (201)475-5050   Fax (201)475-5522
+ H&V Associates MD Partners of Englewood
  50 South Franklin Turnpike/3rd Floor   Ramsey, NJ 07446   (201)475-5050   Fax (201)934-6217

Levin, Todd Philip, DO {1598742629} IntrMd, InfDis(99,IL76)<NJ-KMHSTRAT, NJ-KMHCHRRY>
+ Garden State Infectious Disease Associates
  570 Egg Harbor Road/Suite B-5   Sewell, NJ 08080   (856)566-3190   Fax (856)566-1904
+ Garden State Infectious Diseases Associates, P.A.
  709 Haddonfield Berlin Road   Voorhees, NJ 08043   (856)566-3190   Fax (856)566-1904

Levine, Adam Maxwell, DO {1528267887} IntCrd, IntrMd(07,PA78)
+ Associated Cardiovascular Consultants-Lourdes
  1 Brace Road/Suite C & F   Cherry Hill, NJ 08034   (856)428-4100   Fax (856)428-5748

Levine, Barry Steven, MD {1619040318} SrgOrt, IntrMd(64,IL02)
+ The Orthopedic Group, P.A.
  261 James Street/Suite 3-F   Morristown, NJ 07960   (973)998-5926   Fax (973)538-4957

Levine, Bruce Jay, MD {1255368817} ObsGyn(82,PA01)<NJ-VIRTMHBC>
+ Virtua Phoenix OBGYN
  120 Madison Avenue/Suite B   Mount Holly, NJ 08060   (609)444-5500   Fax (609)444-5501
+ Phoenix Ob-Gyn Associates
  1 Sheffield Drive/Suite 101   Columbus, NJ 08022   (609)444-5500   Fax (609)291-5603
+ Phoenix Ob-Gyn Associates
  110 Marter Avenue/Suite 505   Moorestown, NJ 08060   (856)235-4840   Fax (856)235-3795

Levine, Charles Daniel, MD {1275625022} RadDia(86,NY46)
+ University Radiology Group, P.C.
  579A Cranbury Road   East Brunswick, NJ 08816   (732)390-0040   Fax (732)390-1856

Levine, David B., MD {1295824290} Pedtrc, IntrMd(03,NY19)
+ Summit Medical Group
  560 Springfield Avenue   Westfield, NJ 07090   (908)228-3620

Levine, Deena R., MD {1124218482} Pedtrc
+ Hackensack Univ Medical Center Pediatric Emerg Room
  30 Prospect Avenue   Hackensack, NJ 07601   (201)996-5430   Fax (201)996-3676

Levine, Erika Gaines, MD {1487742508} Dermat(99,NY45)
+ 16 Mountwell Avenue
  Haddonfield, NJ 08033

Levine, Harlan Brett, MD {1922001361} SrgOARec, SrgOrt(98,NY20)<NJ-HACKNSK>
+ Hartzband Center for Hip & Knee Replacement
  10 Forest Avenue   Paramus, NJ 07652   (201)291-4040   Fax (201)291-0440

Levine, Helaine Gale, MD {1609838176} Pedtrc, SprtMd(75,NY46)<NJ-STPETER, NJ-RWJUBRUN>
+ St. Luke's Coventry Family Practice
  755 Memorial Parkway/Suite 300   Phillipsburg, NJ 08865   (908)847-3300   Fax (866)281-6023

Levine, Howard Seth, DO {1578562948} FamMed(87,MO79)<NJ-CHRIST, NJ-BAYONNE>
+ Steinbaum & Levine Associates
  789 Avenue C   Bayonne, NJ 07002   (201)339-2620   Fax (201)339-2785

Levine, Jaime Marissa, DO {1740419704} PhysMd(05,NJ75)<NY-NYURUSK, NY-JTORTHO>
+ JFK Johnson Rehabilitation Institute
  65 James Street   Edison, NJ 08818   (732)906-2644

Levine, Jeffrey, MD {1639137714} Anesth(87,NY46)<NJ-VALLEY>
+ The Valley Hospital
  223 North Van Dien Avenue   Ridgewood, NJ 07450   (201)447-8000

Levine, Jeffrey Pierre, MD {1841379377} FamMed(90,NY47)<NJ-RWJUBRUN>
+ Family Medicine at Monument Square
  317 George Street   New Brunswick, NJ 08901   (732)235-8993   Fax (732)246-7317
+ UH- Robert Wood Johnson Med
  125 Paterson Street/Family Mdcn   New Brunswick, NJ 08901   (732)235-7670

Levine, Jeffrey Richard, MD {1841369261} ObsGyn(83,PA07)<NJ-VIRTBERL, NJ-VIRTVOOR>
+ 2301 Evesham Road/Suite 106
  Voorhees, NJ 08043   (856)770-9436   Fax (856)770-9283

Levine, Jerome Frederic, MD {1023086980} InfDis, IntrMd(76,NY19)<NJ-HACKNSK>
+ Center for Infectious Diseases
  20 Prospect Avenue/Suite 507   Hackensack, NJ 07601   (201)487-4088   Fax (201)489-8930

Levine, Jonathan Marc, MD {1356335558} Otlryg(99,NY09)<NJ-CHILTON>
+ ENT and Facial Plastic Surgeons
  51 Route 23 South/2nd Floor   Riverdale, NJ 07457   (973)831-1220   Fax (973)831-0029

Levine, Lewis Jonathan, MD {1437216777} SrgOrt(92,NJ06)<NJ-STPETER, NJ-RWJUBRUN>
+ Mid Atlantic Orthopedic Associates LLP
  557 Cranbury Road/Suite 10   East Brunswick, NJ 08816   (732)238-8800   Fax (732)238-8246

Levine, Marc Jason, MD {1558339572} SrgOrt, SrgSpn(90,PA02)<NJ-RWJUHAM, NJ-STFRNMED>
+ Trenton Orthopaedic Group
  1225 Whitehorse Mercerville Rd   Trenton, NJ 08619   (609)581-2200   Fax (609)581-1212
+ Trenton Orthopaedic Group
  116 Washington Crossing Road   Pennington, NJ 08534   (609)581-2200   Fax (609)581-1212

Levine, Marc M., MD {1609804418} EmrgMd(83,NJ06)<NJ-COMMED>
+ Community Medical Center
  99 Route 37 West/EmergMed   Toms River, NJ 08755   (732)557-8000

Levine, Martin Scott, DO {1942209218} FamMed, SprtMd(80,MO79)<NJ-BAYONNE, NJ-CHRIST>
+ Steinbaum & Levine Associates
  789 Avenue C   Bayonne, NJ 07002   (201)339-2620   Fax (201)339-2785
+ Portside Medical
  150 Warren Street/Suite 118   Jersey City, NJ 07302   (201)339-2620   Fax (201)309-1300

Levine, Raphael Krevsky, MD {1013122498} SrgOrt(65,PA02)<NJ-ENGLWOOD, NJ-HOLYNAME>
+ Westwood Orthopedic & Sports Medicine PA
  354 Old Hook Road/Suite 103   Westwood, NJ 07675   (201)666-3241   Fax (201)666-6876   www.wog17@aol.com

Levine, Richard Evan, MD {1518096692} Ophthl(85,PA01)<NJ-HOLYNAME>
+ Cliffside Eye Center
  663 Palisade Avenue   Cliffside Park, NJ 07010   (201)941-9400   Fax (201)941-5840

Levine, Richard Marc, MD {1093753816} FamMed, IntrMd(94,PA07)
+ Cherry Hill Family Care & Internal Medicine
  101 Barclay Pavilion West   Cherry Hill, NJ 08034   (856)429-4179   Fax (856)429-3794

Levine, Richard Steven, MD {1982608485} ObsGyn(79,NJ05)<NJ-VALLEY>
+ Valley Center for Women's Health
  550 North Maple Avenue/Suite 102   Ridgewood, NJ 07450   (201)444-4040   Fax (201)444-4473
+ Valley Center for Women's Health
  581 North Franklin Turnpike/2nd Floor   Ramsey, NJ 07446   (201)444-4040   Fax (201)236-5269

Levine, Richard Teddy, MD {1689601791} ObsGyn, Gyneco(76,PA13)<NJ-VIRTMHBC>
+ Virtua Phoenix OBGYN
  120 Madison Avenue/Suite B   Mount Holly, NJ 08060   (609)444-5500   Fax (609)444-5501
+ Phoenix Ob-Gyn Associates
  1 Sheffield Drive/Suite 101   Columbus, NJ 08022   (609)444-5500   Fax (609)291-5603
+ Phoenix Ob-Gyn Associates
  110 Marter Avenue/Suite 505   Moorestown, NJ 08060   (856)235-4840   Fax (856)235-3795

Levine, Robert S., MD {1538190731} Gastrn, IntrMd(87,DC02)<NJ-VALLEY>
+ Bergen Medical Associates
  466 Old Hook Road/Suite 1   Emerson, NJ 07630   (201)967-8221   Fax (201)967-0340
+ Bergen Medical Associates
  1 West Ridgewood Avenue/Suite 301   Paramus, NJ 07652   (201)967-8221   Fax (201)445-4296

Levine, Robert Scott, MD {1801844998} Anesth(87,MEX34)<NJ-KMHSTRAT, NJ-KMHCHRRY>
+ New Jersey Anesthesia Associates, P.C.
  252 Columbia Turnpike/PO Box 0037   Florham Park, NJ 07932   (973)660-9334   Fax (973)660-9779

Levine, Selwyn Eric, MD {1184692105} IntrMd, PulDis, CritCr(82,NY19)<NJ-HOLYNAME, NJ-ENGLWOOD>
+ Holy Name Pulmonary Associates PC
  200 Grand Avenue/Suite 102   Englewood, NJ 07631   (201)871-3636   Fax (201)871-2286
+ Holy Name Pulmonary Associates PC
  8305 Bergenline Avenue   North Bergen, NJ 07047   (201)871-3636   Fax (201)854-0827

Levine, Seth Peter, MD {1386686301} Urolgy(71,MA07)<NJ-CHILTON, NJ-VALLEY>
+ Associates in Urology, PA
  1777 Hamburg Turnpike/Suite 304   Wayne, NJ 07470   (973)616-8400   Fax (973)616-8485

Levine, Sheldon Elliot, MD {1063453322} Allrgy, IntrMd, AlgyImmn(82,ITAL)<NJ-VALLEY>
+ 400 Franklin Turnpike
  Mahwah, NJ 07430   (201)934-1500   Fax (201)934-6655

Levine, Stephanie, DO {1649214818} Pedtrc, GenPrc(88,NY75)<NJ-SOMERSET>
+ Somerset Pediatric Group PA
2345 Lamington Road/Suite 101   Bedminster, NJ 07921   (908)470-1124   Fax (908)470-2845
+ Somerset Pediatric Group PA
155 Union Avenue   Bridgewater, NJ 08807   (908)470-1124   Fax (908)203-8825
+ Somerset Pediatric Group PA
1-C New Amwell Road   Hillsborough, NJ 07921   (908)874-5035   Fax (908)874-3288

Levine, Steven Marc, DO {1891794251} FamMed(78,MO79)<NJ-BAYONNE, NJ-CHRIST>
+ Chatham Family Practice Associates
492 Main Street   Chatham, NJ 07928   (973)635-2432   Fax (973)635-6169
+ Portside Medical
150 Warren Street/Suite 118   Jersey City, NJ 07302   (973)635-2432   Fax (201)309-1300

Levine, Steven Paul, MD {1477672913} Psychy(03,LA01)
+ 1 Palmer Square/Suite 420
Princeton, NJ 08542   (609)430-0500   Fax (609)228-5959

Levine, Stuart Eric, MD {1225057045} SrgOrt(89,NY19)<NJ-STPETER, NJ-RWJUHAM>
+ Princeton Orthopaedic Associates, P.A.
325 Princeton Avenue   Princeton, NJ 08540   (609)924-8131   Fax (609)924-8532

Levine, Zalman, MD {1245335652} ObsGyn, RprEnd, FrtInf(95,NY46)
+ Fertility Institute of New Jersey
400 Old Hook Road/Suite 2-3   Westwood, NJ 07675   (201)666-4200   Fax (201)666-2262

Levinsky, Joseph Judah, MD {1922059476} EmrgMd, Pedtrc, PedEmg(72,PA02)<NJ-JRSYSHMC>
+ EmCare
1945 Route 33   Neptune, NJ 07753   (732)776-4510   Fax (732)776-2329

Levinsky, Liya, MD {1487827630} GenPrc, LeglMd(72,UKR05)
+ 469 Morris Avenue/2nd Floor
Elizabeth, NJ 07208   (908)351-6060   Fax (908)351-5330

Levinson, Barry S., MD {1043301641} OncHem
+ Trinitas Comprehensive Cancer Center
225 Williamson Street   Elizabeth, NJ 07202   (908)964-8772   Fax (908)964-8748

Levinson, Benjamin, MD {1518253137} IntrMd
+ 91 Dead Tree Run Road
Belle Mead, NJ 08502

Levinson, Elizabeth A., MD {1033321229} FamMed
+ Partners in Primary Care
534 Lippincott Drive   Marlton, NJ 08053   (856)985-7373   Fax (856)985-9611

Levinson, Martin L., MD {1699715946} CritCr, PulDis, IntrMd(76,NY20)<PA-UPMCPHL>
+ Penn Medicine at Cherry Hill
409 Route 70 East   Cherry Hill, NJ 08034   (856)429-1519

Levinson, Robert Alan, MD {1366455925} Gastrn, IntrMd(73,NJ05)<NJ-NWRKBETH>
+ Newark Beth Israel Medical Center
201 Lyons Avenue   Newark, NJ 07112   (973)926-7154   Fax (973)923-3825

Levinson, Roy M., MD {1306838800} CritCr, IntrMd, PulDis(80,NY19)<NJ-LOURDMED>
+ Cooper University at Willingboro
218C Sunset Road   Willingboro, NJ 08046   (609)877-0400   Fax (609)877-3542

Levison, Jonathan Andrew, MD {1912900416} SrgVas(92,IL42)<NJ-CLARMAAS, NJ-MTNSIDE>
+ The Cardiovascular Care Group
1401 Broad Street/Suite 1   Clifton, NJ 07013   (973)759-9000   Fax (973)751-3730
+ The Cardiovascular Care Group
433 Central Avenue   Westfield, NJ 07090   (973)759-9000   Fax (908)490-1698

Leviss, Stephen R., MD {1477546315} ObsGyn, Gyneco(67,NY46)
+ Lifeline Medical Associates, LLC
50 Cherry Hill Road/Suite 303   Parsippany, NJ 07054   (973)335-8500   Fax (973)335-8429

Levitas, Andrew S., MD {1265523344} PsyCAd, Psychy, IntrMd(72,NY46)<NJ-KMHCHRRY, NJ-KMHSTRAT>
+ University Hospital-SOM Department of Psychiatry
109 East Laurel Road/First Floor   Stratford, NJ 08084   (856)566-6035   Fax (856)566-6208

Levitch, David, MD {1699770172} Anesth(83,DOM02)<NJ-ACMC-MAIN>
+ AtlantiCare Regional Med Ctr/Mainland
65 West Jimmie Leeds Road/Anesth   Pomona, NJ 08240   (609)652-1000

Levites-Agababa, Elana R., MD {1669793063}
+ CAMCare Health Corporation
817 Federal Street   Camden, NJ 08103   (215)567-2112   Fax (856)541-4611
levites.agababa@gmail.com

Levitsky, Kenneth A., MD {1629045455} SrgOrt(86,MA07)<NJ-HACKNSK, NJ-VALLEY>
+ Garden State Orthopaedic Associates, P.A.
28-04 Broadway   Fair Lawn, NJ 07410   (201)791-4434   Fax (201)791-9377
+ Garden State Orthopaedic Associates, P.A.
33-41 Newark Street   Hoboken, NJ 07030   (201)791-4434   Fax (201)876-5305
+ Garden State Orthopaedic Associates, P.A.
400 Franklin Turnpike   Mahwah, NJ 07430   (201)825-2266   Fax (201)825-9727

Levitsky, Mark K., MD {1962499012} SrgOrt(75,MEX03)
+ 70 Manheim Avenue
Bridgeton, NJ 08302   (856)451-9161   Fax (856)455-8075

Levitt, Alan T., MD {1982666293} IntrMd, PulDis(68,PA09)<NJ-CHSFULD>
+ Pulmonary & Internal Medicine Associates
40 Fuld Street/Suite 201   Trenton, NJ 08638   (609)695-4422   Fax (609)695-4358

Levitt, Cory A., MD {1366769739}
+ West Jersey Anesthesia Associates
102E Centre Boulevard   Marlton, NJ 08053   (856)988-6260   Fax (856)988-6270
cory.levitt@gmail.com

Levitt, Joel W., MD {1174563027} Otlryg, PedOto(79,NJ05)<NJ-STBARNMC, NJ-NWRKBETH>
+ 769 Northfield Avenue/Suite LL2
West Orange, NJ 07052   (973)731-2100   Fax (973)731-2188
+ Short Hills Surgery Center
187 Millburn Avenue/Suite 101   Millburn, NJ 07041   (973)731-2100   Fax (973)671-0557

Levitt, Kimberly Anne, MD {1114123247} FamMed(02,PA02)
+ Capital Health Primary Care
4056 Quakerbridge Road/Suite 101   Lawrenceville, NJ 08648   (609)528-9150   Fax (609)528-9151

Levitt, Michael Joshua, MD {1891979381} OncHem, IntrMd(02,NJ05)
+ Atlantic Hematology Oncology Associates, L.L.C.
1707 Atlantic Avenue   Manasquan, NJ 08736   (732)528-0760   Fax (732)528-0764

Levitt, Myron M., MD {1871578724} Radiol, RadNro(83,NY19)<NJ-RBAYOLDB, NJ-STPETER>
+ University Radiology Group, P.C.
483 Cranbury Road   East Brunswick, NJ 08816   (732)390-0030   Fax (732)390-5383
+ University Radiology Group, P.C.
260 Amboy Avenue   Metuchen, NJ 08840   (732)390-0030   Fax (732)548-3392

Levitt, Robert S., MD {1548344799} ObsGyn(63,PA02)
+ 516 Easton Avenue
Somerset, NJ 08873   (732)828-2600   Fax (732)828-3889

Levitz, Jason Sanford, MD {1689783961} IntrMd, OncHem(99,ISR02)<NJ-MORRISTN>
+ Oncology & Hematology Specialists, PA
23 Pocono Road/Suite 100   Denville, NJ 07834   (973)316-1701   Fax (973)316-1708

Levounis, Petros, MD {1033135538} PsyAdd, Psychy(94,PA07)<NY-SLRRSVLT>
+ 183 South Orange Avenue/Room F-1436
Somers Point, NJ 08244
PetrosLevounis@umdnj.edu

Levy, Andrew Stuart, MD {1386712032} SprtMd, SrgArt(87,PA13)<NJ-OVERLOOK>
+ Center for Advanced Sports Medicine
90 Millburn Avenue/Suite 204   Millburn, NJ 07041   (973)484-6239   Fax (973)484-6804
oblio54@aol.com

Levy, Benjamin D., MD {1992901656} PhysMd(07,NJ05)
+ Spinal & Head Trauma Associates
2040 Sixth Avenue/Suite C   Neptune, NJ 07753   (732)617-9797

Levy, Brahman B., MD {1962536888} Acpntr, FamMed(88,VA04)<NJ-COOPRUMC>
+ Worknet Occupational Medicine
9370 Route 130 North/Suite 200   Pennsauken, NJ 08110   (856)662-0660   Fax (856)662-0798
+ Worknet Occupational Health
37 South White Horse Pike   Stratford, NJ 08084   (856)435-2680

Levy, Brian Leonard, MD {1891813747} EnDbMt, IntrMd(79,MD07)
+ MannKind Corporation
61 South Paramus Road/5th Floor   Paramus, NJ 07652   (201)983-5112

Levy, Daniel S., MD {1639267156} RadDia, Radiol(78,NY09)<NJ-CHILTON>
+ Fair Lawn Diagnostic Imaging
19-04 Fair Lawn Avenue   Fair Lawn, NJ 07410   (201)794-3132   Fax (201)794-6291
+ Chilton Medical Center
97 West Parkway/Radiology   Pompton Plains, NJ 07444   (973)831-5000

Levy, Ian H., DO {1174558084} EnDbMt(87,NY75)<NJ-HOLY-NAME, NJ-VALLEY>
+ 245 East Main Street
Ramsey, NJ 07446   (201)327-5551   Fax (201)327-1440
+ 261 Old Hook Road
Westwood, NJ 07675   (201)327-5551   Fax (201)666-5014

Levy, Jeffrey E., MD {1306880497} Pedtrc, AdolMd(76,MEX03)<NJ-OVERLOOK>
+ 745 Northfield Avenue
West Orange, NJ 07052   (973)731-6400   Fax (973)731-0690

Levy, Jenna, DO {1366464588} ObsGyn(01,NJ75)<NJ-MON-MOUTH>
+ Sunrise Obstetrics & Gynecology
831 Tennent Road   Manalapan, NJ 07726   (732)972-4200   Fax (732)333-4643
+ Sunrise Obstetrics & Gynecology
921 East County Line Road   Lakewood, NJ 08701   (732)987-5950

Levy, Jodi A., MD {1003191305} Pedtrc
+ Rutgers- New Jersey Medical School
185 South Orange Avenue   Newark, NJ 07103   (973)972-0178

Levy, Jodi L., DO {1891780243} IntrMd(01,NY75)<NJ-CHILTON>
+ Chilton Medical Center
97 West Parkway/IntMed   Pompton Plains, NJ 07444   (973)831-5000

Levy, Karen R., MD {1376610444} RadDia
+ Atlantic Medical Imaging, LLC
44 East Jimmie Leeds Road/Suite 101   Galloway, NJ 08205   (609)677-9729   Fax (609)652-6512

Levy, Kirk Jay, MD {1023077393} Nrolgy(93,NY48)<NJ-HACKNSK>
+ Bergen Neurology Consultants
25 Rockwood Place/Suite 110   Englewood, NJ 07631   (201)894-5805   Fax (201)894-1956

Levy, Lauren S., MD {1184611055} Radiol(91,NY08)<NJ-VALLEY>
+ The Valley Hospital
223 North Van Dien Avenue/Radiology   Ridgewood, NJ 07450   (201)447-8000
+ Radiology Associates of Ridgewood, P.A.
20 Franklin Turnpike   Waldwick, NJ 07463   (201)447-8000   Fax (201)447-5053

Levy, Michael Stuart, DO {1104814821} SrgOrt(99,ME75)
+ 807 North Haddon Avenue
Haddonfield, NJ 08033   (856)795-9222   Fax (856)795-0026

Levy, Moshe, MD {1205860889} Pedtrc(96,NY46)
+ Wee Care Pediatrics
831 Tennent Road/Suite A   Manalapan, NJ 07726   (732)536-6222   Fax (732)536-9272
drlevy@optonline.net

Levy, Nat T., MD {1790777225}
+ The Valley Medical Group
140 Chestnut Street/Suite 200   Ridgewood, NJ 07450   (314)721-0862

Levy, Seth Evan, MD {1316980782} IntrMd(96,DC02)
+ Denville Associates of Internal Medicine
16 Pocono Road/Suite 317   Denville, NJ 07834   (973)627-2650   Fax (973)627-8383

Levy, Stephen M., MD {1316947856} CdvDis(88,WIND)<NJ-STBARNMC, NJ-CLARMAAS>
+ Comprehensive Cardiovascular Consultants
299 Madison Avenue/Suite 102   Morristown, NJ 07960   (973)292-1020   Fax (973)292-0564
+ Essex Cardiology Group PC
10 James Street/Suite 130   Florham Park, NJ 07932   (973)292-1020   Fax (973)736-9757

Levy, Stuart J., MD {1245212190} Anesth(79,PA01)<NJ-MORRISTN>
+ 26 Tammy Hill Trail
Randolph, NJ 07869

Levy-Kern, Muriel, MD {1629077797} EnDbMt, IntrMd(85,FRA33)<NJ-BAYSHORE>
+ Saint Peter's Physician Associates
294 Applegarth Road   Monroe Township, NJ 08831   (609)409-1363

Levykh-Chase, Rena E., MD {1215085360} IntrMd(96,NY47)<NJ-VALLEY>
+ Chase Medical Group P.C.
19-21 Fair Lawn Avenue   Fair Lawn, NJ 07410   (201)791-8689   Fax (201)791-2589

Lew, Lai Ping, MD {1134202831} Pedtrc(96,NY47)
+ Notchview Pediatrics, LLC.
1037 Route 46 East/Suite 201   Clifton, NJ 07013   (973)779-3911   Fax (973)471-2730

Physicians by Name and Address

Lewin, Roxanne Marie, MD {1942535406} Psychy, PsyFor(05,GRN01)<NJ-HOBUNIMC, NY-SUNYBRKL>
+ **661 Palisades Avenue/Suite C-2**
  Englewood Cliffs, NJ 07632   (201)500-5864   Fax (201)751-6679
  drrlewin@gmail.com
+ **Ann Klein Forensic Center**
  8 Production Way   Avenel, NJ 07001

Lewin, Sharyn Nan, MD {1083862247} GynOnc, ObsGyn(01,KS02)<NY-SLOANKET>
+ **Holy Name Hospital**
  718 Teaneck Road   Teaneck, NJ 07666   (201)227-6200   Fax (201)227-6209

Lewin, Stacy B., MD {1396745030} Anesth(94,PA02)<NJ-VIRTBERL, NJ-VIRTMARL>
+ **West Jersey Anesthesia Associates**
  102-E Center Boulevard   Marlton, NJ 08053   (856)988-6250   Fax (856)988-6270

Lewinter, Donna Ellen, MD {1053493767} Psychy(89,PA07)
+ **1 Springfield Avenue**
  Summit, NJ 07901   (908)277-6067

Lewis, Alison Dennesha, MD {1669639969} FamMed(07,PA12)
+ **Visiting Nurse Association of Central Jersey**
  1301 Main Street   Asbury Park, NJ 07712   (732)774-6333   Fax (732)774-0313

Lewis, Allan Andrew, MD {1487607859} Anesth(90,PA09)<PA-PENNHOSP>
+ **87 Forrest Hills Drive**
  Voorhees, NJ 08043

Lewis, Beth G., MD {1053362392} IntrMd, ObsGyn(00,NY46)<NJ-STPETER>
+ **St. Peter's University Hospital**
  254 Easton Avenue/MOB2   New Brunswick, NJ 08901   (732)745-8549   Fax (732)745-1339

Lewis, Brent Mckeen, MD {1265886253} EmrgMd
+ **Robert Wood Johnson Emergency Medicine**
  One Robert Wood Johnson Place/MEB 104   New Brunswick, NJ 08901   (732)235-8717

Lewis, Brett Eric, MD {1306010806} RadOnc, Radiol(04,NY46)
+ **John Theurer Cancer Center - HUMC**
  92 Second Street   Hackensack, NJ 07601   (551)996-8704   Fax (551)996-0730

Lewis, Brian S., MD {1487811980} Pedtrc
+ **Maple Avenue Pediatrics**
  23-00 Route 208   Fair Lawn, NJ 07410   (201)797-1900   Fax (201)797-4457

Lewis, David A., MD {1700808938} OtgyFPlS, SrgCsm<NJ-ENGLWOOD, NJ-HOLYNAME>
+ **Englewood Ear Nose & Throat, P.C.**
  216 Engle Street/Suite 101   Englewood, NJ 07631   (201)816-9800   Fax (201)567-1569

Lewis, David Everett, DO {1609218759}
+ **SOM - Department of Internal Medicine**
  42 East Laurel Road/Suite 3100   Stratford, NJ 08084   (856)566-6477   Fax (856)566-6906
+ **Athena Women's Institute for Pelvic Health**
  151 Fries Mill Road/Suite 301   Turnersville, NJ 08012   (856)566-6477   Fax (856)374-2177

Lewis, Frieda Elizabeth, MD {1588692909} ObsGyn(00,NJ05)<NJ-COMMED>
+ **Womens Health Care Associates of Sussex County**
  135 Newton Sparta Road/Suite 201   Newton, NJ 07860   (973)383-8555   Fax (973)383-8424

Lewis, Irwin Holden, MD {1417917238} IntrMd(75,PA01)<NJ-WARREN>
+ **Milford Medical Center**
  207 Strykers Road   Phillipsburg, NJ 08865   (908)995-4125   Fax (908)995-0399

Lewis, Jocelyn A., DO {1700913498} PedHem
+ **Rutgers Cancer Institute of New Jersey**
  195 Little Albany Street/PO Box 2681   New Brunswick, NJ 08903   (732)235-8864   Fax (732)235-8234

Lewis, Lesley Brook, DO {1962687327} Psychy
+ **211 County House Road**
  Sewell, NJ 08080   (856)404-4419

Lewis, Mary Kendra, MD {1801879275} FamMed, Obstet(72,NC07)<NJ-HUNTRDN>
+ **Hunterdon Family Medicine**
  1100 Wescott Drive/Suite 101   Flemington, NJ 08822   (908)788-6535   Fax (908)788-6536

Lewis, Michael Glenn, MD {1295901726} Pedtrc(03,MEX03)
+ **Notchview Pediatrics, LLC.**
  1037 Route 46 East/Suite 201   Clifton, NJ 07013   (973)779-3911   Fax (973)471-2730

Lewis, Michele J., MD {1992894737} Anesth(85,NY08)<NJ-MEADWLND>
+ **Meadowlands Hospital Medical Center**
  55 Meadowlands Parkway   Secaucus, NJ 07096   (201)392-3100

Lewis, Randall Craig, MD {1558445148} EmrgMd(95,OH41)<NJ-OVERLOOK>
+ **Overlook Medical Center**
  99 Beauvoir Avenue/PO Box 210   Summit, NJ 07902   (908)522-2000

Lewis, Shannin Dion, DO {1992940670} PainInvt
+ **Mid Atlantic Pain Specialist**
  2466 East Chestnut Avenue   Vineland, NJ 08361   (610)453-7038

Lewis, Sharol A., MD {1861602930} ObsGyn(85,NJ06)
+ **2 Fawn Ridge Road**
  Lebanon, NJ 08833   (908)236-8920

Lewis, Stephen B., MD {1598708745} PhysMd(90,PA09)
+ **1 Big Barn Road**
  Cranbury, NJ 08512   (856)456-0023

Lewis, Tanya Renee, MD {1831304583} PsyCAd(04,PA09)
+ **Hackensack University Medical Faculty Practice**
  25 East Salem Street   Hackensack, NJ 07601   (201)996-4445   Fax (201)996-5729

Lewis, Thomas Peter, MD {1609961176} IntrMd(76,NY19)<NJ-OVERLOOK>
+ **Drs. Lewis & Jamdar**
  346 South Avenue   Fanwood, NJ 07023   (908)889-4700   Fax (908)889-0867

Lewis, Walter Emmett, III, MD {1285710921} Urolgy(86,NJ05)<NJ-OCEANMC, NJ-COMMED>
+ **Ocean Urology**
  52 Constitution Drive   Monroe, NJ 08831   (732)349-5200   Fax (732)349-5235

Lewis, Walter Michael, MD {1336121417} Anesth(91,NY09)<NJ-MORRISTN>
+ **Morristown Medical Center**
  100 Madison Avenue   Morristown, NJ 07962   (973)971-5000   Fax (201)943-8733

Lewitt, Diana M., DO {1427215953} Pedtrc(06,NJ75)<NJ-KMH-STRAT, NJ-VIRTUAHS>
+ **Dr. G. Lee Lerch and Associates**
  239 Hurffville Crosskeys Road   Sewell, NJ 08080   (856)740-4440   Fax (856)728-0808
+ **Dr. G. Lee Lerch and Associates**
  63 North Lakeview Drive/Suite 202   Gibbsboro, NJ 08026   (856)740-4440   Fax (856)782-1667

Lewko, Michael P., MD {1730121799} IntrMd, Grtrcs, Rheuma(85,NJ06)<NJ-STJOSHOS>
+ **New Jersey Arthritis Osteoporosis Center**
  871 Allwood Road/Suite 1   Clifton, NJ 07012   (973)405-5163   Fax (973)365-8004

Leybel, Boris, MD {1578508685} Nrolgy, PainMd(79,RUSS)<NY-BETHPETR, NY-LICOLLGE>
+ **24-20 Broadway**
  Fair Lawn, NJ 07410   (201)797-8333   Fax (201)797-1977

Leykin, Tanya, MD {1750468971} Pedtrc(86,RUS45)
+ **471 Undercliff Avenue**
  Edgewater, NJ 07020   (201)969-9350   Fax (201)969-9764

Leyson, Jose Flotcante J., MD {1528169539} FrtInf, Urolgy, OthrSp(70,PHIL)<NJ-CHRIST, NJ-VAEASTOR>
+ **Dr. Joven Dungo/NJ Impotence Ctr**
  205 9th Street   Jersey City, NJ 07302   (201)653-1144   Fax (201)653-6104
+ **Westside Medical Associates**
  562 West Side Avenue   Jersey City, NJ 07304   (201)653-1144   Fax (201)434-6715

Leyva-Vega, Melissa, MD {1689734055} Pedtrc, PedGst(03,NY46)
+ **Joseph M. Sanzari Childrens' -Gastro**
  155 Polifly Road/Suite 102   Hackensack, NJ 07601   (551)996-8840   Fax (201)441-9949

Li, Albert C., MD {1700052149} Radiol
+ **University Radiology Group, P.C.**
  483 Cranbury Road   East Brunswick, NJ 08816   (732)390-0030   Fax (732)390-5383
+ **University Radiology Group, P.C.**
  579A Cranbury Road   East Brunswick, NJ 08816   (732)390-0030   Fax (732)390-1856

Li, Annie Hongyan, MD {1548298581} Pedtrc, FamMed(84,CHN21)<NJ-HACKNSK>
+ **1259 Route 46 East/Suite 101**
  Parsippany, NJ 07054   (973)257-8870   Fax (973)257-8871

Li, Cindy Yuk, DO {1265509111} Dermat(93,PA77)
+ **The Dermatology Group, P.C.**
  30 West Century Road/Suite 320   Paramus, NJ 07652   (973)571-2121   Fax (201)986-0702

Li, Dena Yuyun, MD {1083671549} IntrMd(86,CHN1K)<NJ-RWJUBRUN, NJ-JFKMED>
+ **East Brunswick Primary Care, PA**
  F1 Brier Hill Court   East Brunswick, NJ 08816   (732)603-0055   Fax (732)603-8228

Li, Dongchen, MD {1558428920} Anesth(83,CHN57)<NJ-UMDNJ>
+ **University Hospital**
  150 Bergen Street/Anesthesiology   Newark, NJ 07103   (973)972-4300   Fax (973)972-4172
  lido@umdnj.edu

Li, Hua, MD {1700296043} IntrMd<NJ-NWTNMEM>
+ **Newton Medical Center**
  175 High Street   Newton, NJ 07860   (973)579-8321

Li, Jason, DO {1639597370} FamMed
+ **17 Beacon Lane**
  Aberdeen, NJ 07747   (917)843-0287

Li, Jianfeng, MD {1295972735} IntrMd(82,CHN76)<NJ-HACKNSK>
+ **Hackensack University Medical Center**
  30 Prospect Avenue/Rm 4621   Hackensack, NJ 07601   (201)996-3664   Fax (551)996-0536

Li, John Yi-huang, MD {1982678777} Anesth(01,TX13)<NJ-HACKNSK>
+ **Hackensack University Medical Center**
  30 Prospect Avenue/Anesth   Hackensack, NJ 07601   (201)996-2000

Li, Jun, MD {1043324338} PthAcl(99,MD12)<NJ-STCLRDEN, NJ-STCLRDOV>
+ **Hackensack University Medical Center**
  30 Prospect Avenue   Hackensack, NJ 07601   (201)996-4836   Fax (201)996-2156

Li, Kehua, MD {1164488417} Dermat, PthDrm, SrgDer(86,CHN1J)
+ **Advanced Dermatology, P.C.**
  570 Egg Harbor Road/Suite C-1   Sewell, NJ 08080   (856)256-8899   Fax (856)256-8868
+ **Advanced Dermatology, P.C.**
  100 Kings Way East/Suite D-4   Sewell, NJ 08080   (856)256-8899

Li, Leonid, MD {1962460386} PthAcl(75,UKR12)<NJ-STCLRDEN, NJ-HCKTSTWN>
+ **St. Clare's Hospital-Denville Campus**
  25 Pocono Road/Pathology   Denville, NJ 07834   (973)625-6000   Fax (973)983-2367

Li, Lian-Jie, MD {1649259383} Dermat(87,CHN63)
+ **755 Memorial Parkway/Building 204**
  Phillipsburg, NJ 08865   (908)387-1001   Fax (908)387-1195

Li, Lin, MD {1104100049} AlgyImmn, IntrMd(08,NY45)
+ **Center for Asthma & Allergy**
  18 North Third Avenue   Highland Park, NJ 08904   (732)545-0094   Fax (732)545-4087
+ **Center for Asthma & Allergy**
  300 Hudson Street   Hoboken, NJ 07030   (732)545-0094   Fax (201)792-5320
+ **Center for Asthma & Allergy**
  90 Milbum Avenue/Suite 200   Maplewood, NJ 08904   (973)763-5787   Fax (973)763-8568

Li, Liren, MD {1194832683} PsyCAd, Psychy(86,CHN60)
+ **Children's Specialized Hospital**
  3575 Quakerbridge Road   Hamilton, NJ 08619   (609)631-2800   Fax (609)631-2862
+ **Princeton P.C. Clinic**
  1130 Route 202/Units B3 & BA   Raritan, NJ 08869   (609)631-2800   Fax (732)354-4507

Li, Lisa, DO {1851326151} IntrMd(00,PA78)<NJ-STCLRDOV>
+ **St. Clare's Hospital-Dover**
  400 West Blackwell Street/IntMed   Dover, NJ 07801   (973)989-3000   Fax (973)989-3106

Li, Meihong, MD {1407935356} IntrMd(84,CHNA)<NJ-HACKNSK>
+ **Drs. Li and Li**
  98 James Street/Suite 201   Edison, NJ 08820   (732)906-9882   Fax (732)906-9893
  Dr_li@yahoo.com

Li, Ronald W., MD {1760574289} Otlryg, IntrMd(84,NY47)<NJ-UNVMCPRN>
+ **Nassau Ear Nose & Throat**
  2650 US Highway 130   Cranbury, NJ 08512   (609)655-3000   Fax (609)655-3003
+ **Nassau Ear Nose & Throat**
  800 Bunn Drive/Suite 305   Princeton, NJ 08540   (609)655-3000   Fax (609)921-8096

Li, Rongshan, MD {1750335667} PthAna(84,CHN59)
+ **PLUS Diagnostics**
  1200 River Avenue/Suite 10   Lakewood, NJ 08701   (732)901-7575   Fax (732)901-1555

Li, Sean, MD {1386623130} AnesPain
+ **Premier Pain Center**
  160 Avenue at the Commons/Suite 1   Shrewsbury, NJ 07702   (732)380-0200   Fax (732)380-0262

Li, Sharon Mei-Mei, MD {1508894874} Urolgy(94,MA07)<NJ-CHILTON>
+ **Adult and Pediatric Urology Center, P.A.**
  1033 Clifton Avenue   Clifton, NJ 07013   (973)473-5700   Fax (973)473-3367
+ **Adult and Pediatric Urology Center, P.A.**
  2025 Hamburg Turnpike   Wayne, NJ 07470   (973)473-5700   Fax (973)831-0033
+ **Wayne Surgical Center, LLC.**
  1176 Hamburg Pike   Wayne, NJ 07013   (973)709-1900   Fax (973)709-1901

Li, Shing, MD {1184945552} IntrMd
+ **Randolph Medical & Renal Associates**
  121 Center Grove Road/Suite 13-14   Randolph, NJ 07869   (973)361-3737

Li, Suzanne C., MD {1295789147} Pedtrc, PedRhm(85,NY01)<NJ-HACKNSK>
+ Hackensack University Medical Center
30 Prospect Avenue/Pediatrics   Hackensack, NJ 07601
(201)996-5306   Fax (201)996-9815
sli@humed.com

Li, Tong, MD {1245406677} IntrMd(93,CHN19)
+ Primary & Diabetic Care Office
2065 Klockner Road   Hamilton, NJ 08690   (609)586-1001
Fax (609)586-7634
+ Princeton HealthCare System
5 Plainsboro Road/Suite 590   Plainsboro, NJ 08536
(609)586-1001   Fax (609)586-7634

Li, Wei, MD {1073751194} IntHos, IntrMd(96,CHN19)<NJ-MTN-SIDE>
+ Pathlink, LLC
66 West Gilbert Street/Suite 100   Tinton Falls, NJ 07701
(732)212-0060   Fax (732)212-0061

Li, Wei Wei, MD {1720246465} AlgyImmn
+ Comprehensive Allergy and Asthma Care
725 River Road/Suite 208   Edgewater, NJ 07020   Fax (201)840-7808

Li, Xiang, MD {1780762179} IntrMd(84,CHNA)
+ Drs. Li and Li
98 James Street/Suite 201   Edison, NJ 08820   (732)906-9882   Fax (732)906-9893
Drs_li@yahoo.com

Li, Xiaoling, MD {1740617240} IntrMd(83,CHN38)
+ Port Authority Medical Office
241 Erie Street   Jersey City, NJ 07310   (201)216-2012   Fax (201)216-2013

Li, Xin Qin, MD {1124119839} Anesth(82,CHN21)<NJ-JFKMED>
+ James Street Anesthesia
102 James Street/Suite 103   Edison, NJ 08820   (732)494-1444   Fax (732)494-7052

Li, Xuemei, MD {1093022675} IntrMd(93,CHN19)
+ Bristol-Myers Squibb Company
One Squibb Drive   New Brunswick, NJ 08903   (732)905-2640

Li, Yan, MD {1619921442} Pedtrc(86,CHN8A)<NJ-CLARMAAS, NJ-STPETER>
+ Health first Pediatrics
579 Cranbury Road/Suite D   East Brunswick, NJ 08816
(732)698-9080   Fax (732)698-9812

Li, Yong Ming, MD {1124141478} Pthlgy, PthAna, PthCln(82,CHN88)<NJ-WARREN>
+ Warren Hospital
185 Roseberry Street/Pathology   Phillipsburg, NJ 08865
(908)859-6700

Li, Zhexiang, MD {1710929898} IntrMd, Bariat(90,CHN07)<NJ-MORRISTN>
+ Sherry Li, MD PC
171 Ridgedale Avenue/Suite 1-E   Florham Park, NJ 07932
(973)377-3676

Li, Zujun, MD {1689662132} OncHem, IntrMd(84,CHN1J)
+ 14 DeCicco Drive
Raritan, NJ 08869

Liakos, Steven, DO {1295713212} Gastrn(75,IA75)<NJ-VIRTVOOR, NJ-KMHCHRRY>
+ South Jersey Gastroenterology PA
117 East Laurel Road   Stratford, NJ 08084   (856)627-2555
Fax (856)751-8746
+ South Jersey Gastroenterology PA
501 Fifth Street/Suite 2   Atco, NJ 08004   (856)753-3066
+ South Jersey Gastroenterology PA
111 Vine Street   Hammonton, NJ 08084   (609)561-3080
Fax (856)983-5110

Lian, Hanzhou, MD {1881697290} Anesth(86,CHN9D)<NJ-STCLR-DEN>
+ Morris Anesthesia Group, PA
3799 Route 46/Suite 211   Parsippany, NJ 07054   (973)335-1122   Fax (973)335-1448

Liang, Hongyan, MD {1194931568} IntrMd
+ 125 Paterson Street/Room 2500
New Brunswick, NJ 08901   (732)235-7679

Liang, Liang, MD {1437132602} IntrMd(82,CHN11)
+ Med-Care of East Hanover Inc
325 Route 10   East Hanover, NJ 07936   (973)386-1133
Fax (973)386-5522

Liang, Raymond Y., MD {1487626057} IntrMd(78,PA07)<NJ-MTN-SIDE>
+ Hackensack UMC Mountainside
1 Bay Avenue/InternalMed   Montclair, NJ 07042   (973)429-6000

Liang, Songlin, MD {1023195880} PthCyt
+ 46 Carlton Avenue
Piscataway, NJ 08854

Lianos, Elias A., MD {1457377996} IntrMd, Nephro(73,GRE01)
+ Robert Wood Johnson Medical School
51 French Street   New Brunswick, NJ 08901   (732)235-4453   Fax (732)235-6124

+ University Medical Group/UMDNJ
125 Paterson Street/Suite 2200   New Brunswick, NJ 08901   (732)235-4453   Fax (732)235-7677
+ UMDNJ RWJ Nephrology
125 Paterson Street/Suite 5100-B   New Brunswick, NJ 08901   (732)235-6512   Fax (732)235-6524

Liao, Jennifer Ledesma, MD {1770750572} Pedtrc(05,PA09)
+ Colts Neck Pediatrics
26 State Highway 34/Suite 208   Colts Neck, NJ 07722
(732)683-0099

Liao, Pui-Kan, MD {1629043443} PedCrd, IntrMd(75,TAIW)
+ 3 High Oaks Drive
Berkeley Heights, NJ 07922   (908)656-2827   Fax (908)790-9551

Liao, Theresa Hanna, MD {1447354501} IntrMd(96,NJ05)<NJ-NWRKBETH>
+ Newark Beth Israel Medical Center
201 Lyons Avenue/L-4   Newark, NJ 07112   (201)265-8200
Fax (201)265-7645

Liao, Wesley, MD {1871791517}<NJ-VALLEY>
+ Bergen Anesthesia Group, P.C.
500 West Main Street/Suite 16   Wyckoff, NJ 07481
(201)847-9320   Fax (201)847-0059

Liao, Wu-Fei, MD {1538139456} Anesth(75,TAIW)<NJ-NWRK-BETH>
+ Newark Beth Israel Medical Center
201 Lyons Avenue/Anesthesiology   Newark, NJ 07112
(973)926-7143   Fax (201)943-8105

Libby, Joseph Anthony, MD {1861574279} IntrMd(91,NJ06)<NJ-COOPRUMC, NJ-VIRTMARL>
+ Kennedy Health Alliance Vascular Surgery
333 Laurel Oak Road   Voorhees, NJ 08043   (844)542-2273
Fax (856)770-9194

Liberman, Arthur R., MD {1235206830} IntrMd(70,NY01)<NJ-STBARNMC>
+ 895 South Orange Avenue
Short Hills, NJ 07078   (973)379-4251

Libert, Melissa Marie, DO {1033311147} Pedtrc(04,NY75)
+ Plaza Family Care
657 Willow Grove Street/Suite 401   Hackettstown, NJ 07840
(908)850-7800   Fax (908)850-7801
+ Plaza Family Care
245 Main Street/Suite 300 & 302   Chester, NJ 07930
(908)850-7800   Fax (908)879-6738

Liberti, Lorraine M., MD {1922194364} Pedtrc(89,NY01)<NJ-VALLEY>
+ PediatriCare Associates
400 Franklin Turnpike   Mahwah, NJ 07430   (201)529-4545
Fax (201)529-1596
+ PediatriCare Associates
20-20 Fair Lawn Avenue   Fair Lawn, NJ 07410   (201)529-4545   Fax (201)791-3765
+ PediatriCare Associates
901 Route 23 South   Pompton Plains, NJ 07430   (973)831-4545   Fax (973)831-1527

Libis, Zhanna, MD {1659335024} Pedtrc(85,UZB04)<NJ-JFKMED>
+ ABC Pediatrics, LLC.
974 Inman Avenue/Suite 1-A   Edison, NJ 08820   (908)412-8866   Fax (908)412-8363
+ Drs. Meel and Libis
974 Inman Avenue/Suite 1   Edison, NJ 08820   (908)412-8866

Librizzi, Ronald J., DO {1366430324} ObsGyn, MtFtMd(73,PA77)<NJ-VIRTMHBC, NJ-VIRTVOOR>
+ Virtua Maternal Fetal Medicine Center
100 Bowman Drive   Voorhees, NJ 08043   (856)247-3328
Fax (856)247-3276
+ Memorial Maternal Fetal Medicine Center
175 Madison Avenue   Mount Holly, NJ 08060   (609)265-7914
+ Virtua Maternal Fetal Medicine Center
239 Hurffville-Crosskeys Road   Sewell, NJ 08043   (856)341-8300   Fax (856)341-8320

Libster, Boris, DO {1659369122} Gastrn, IntrMd(82,NY75)<NJ-OURLADY, NJ-VIRTVOOR>
+ Allied Gastroenterology Associates
217 White Horse Pike   Haddon Heights, NJ 08035
(856)547-1212   Fax (856)547-6117

Licata, Joseph, Jr., MD {1104895499} Surgry(84,MEX34)<NJ-VALLEY>
+ 245 East Main Street
Ramsey, NJ 07446   (201)327-0220   Fax (201)327-4871

Licata, Thomas C., DO {1811193253} EmrgMd<NJ-KMHSTRAT>
+ Kennedy Memorial Hospital-University Medical Center
18 East Laurel Road   Stratford, NJ 08084   (856)566-7121

Licciardone, Salvatore J., DO {1205889045} FamMed(68,MO79)<NJ-VALLEY>
+ 74 Pascack Road
Park Ridge, NJ 07656   (201)391-4166

Liccini, Mark Stephen, DO {1861562779} Anesth(00,PA77)
+ 31 Wimbledon Way
Marlton, NJ 08053

Licetti, Stephen Charles, DO {1558508192} FamMed(NJ75<NJ-MORRISTN>
+ Hunterdon Family Physicians
111 State Route 31/Suite 111   Flemington, NJ 08822
(908)284-9880   Fax (908)782-4316

Lichnowski, Krzysztof B., MD {1558334458} IntrMd(85,POLA)<NJ-OCEANMC>
+ 204 Jack Martin Boulevard/Suite C 3
Brick, NJ 08724   (732)840-8500   Fax (732)840-7552

Lichtbroun, Alan S., MD {1003855628} Rheuma, IntrMd, Grtrcs(77,NY08)<NJ-RWJUBRUN, NJ-STPETER>
+ Arthritis-Internal Medicine Associates of Middlesex
63 Brunswick Woods Drive   East Brunswick, NJ 08816
(732)613-1900   Fax (732)613-0029
althedoctor@aol.com
+ Robert Wood Johnson Medical School
51 French Street/Clinical   New Brunswick, NJ 08901
(732)235-7619

Lichtenberger, Janice Ann, MD {1730392077} Pedtrc
+ West Park Pediatrics
804 West Park Avenue   Ocean, NJ 07712   (732)531-0010
Fax (732)493-0903

Lichtenstein, David I., MD {1942304969} Ophthl(72,MEX14)<NJ-OVERLOOK, NJ-RBAYPERT>
+ 150 Main Street
Woodbridge, NJ 07095   (732)750-9444   Fax (908)654-3639

Lichtman, Kenneth J., MD {1588857973} Psychy(71,BEL06)
+ Psychiatry Associates
1109 Amboy Avenue   Edison, NJ 08837   (732)549-2220
Fax (732)603-0673

Lichtman, Lisa B., DO {1851371967} FamMed(87,PA77)<NJ-OURLADY, NJ-VIRTVOOR>
+ Holly Oak Family Practice
1 Eves Drive/Suite 109   Marlton, NJ 08053   (856)596-8880
Fax (856)596-8687

Lichtstein, Elliott S., MD {1760487342} IntCrd, CdvDis, IntrMd(81,PA13)<NJ-HACKNSK, NJ-VALLEY>
+ Westwood Cardiology Associates PA
333 Old Hook Road/Suite 200   Westwood, NJ 07675
(201)664-0201   Fax (201)666-7970

Licitra, Edward Joseph, MD {1538139548} MedOnc, IntrMd, OncHem(00,NJ06)<NJ-RWJUBRUN, NJ-STPETER>
+ Regional Cancer Care Associates - Central Jersey Div
454 Elizabeth Avenue/Suite 240   Somerset, NJ 08873
(732)390-7750   Fax (732)390-7725
+ Central Jersey Oncology Center, P.A.
Brier Hill Court/Building J-2   East Brunswick, NJ 08816
(732)390-7750   Fax (732)390-7725
+ Central Jersey Oncology Center, P.A.
205 Easton Avenue   New Brunswick, NJ 08873   (732)828-9570   Fax (732)828-7638

Lieb, Jocelyn Ann, MD {1891945341} Dermat(04,MA07)
+ Skin and Laser Center of NJ LLC
156 Ramapo Valley Road   Mahwah, NJ 07430   (201)500-7525   Fax (201)500-7527

Lieb, Michael D., MD {1770641581} SrgVas, Surgry(07,PA07)
+ Virtua Medford Surgical Group
212 Creek Crossing Boulevard   Hainesport, NJ 08036
(609)267-1004   Fax (609)267-1044

Lieb, Michael D., DO {1609024447}
+ Virtua Surgical Group, PA
1935 Route 70 East   Cherry Hill, NJ 08003   (856)428-7700
Fax (856)424-9120

Lieb, Robert C., MD {1578613766} Psychy(78,DC02)
+ 150 Morristown Road/Suite 20
Bernardsville, NJ 07924   (908)766-1000   Fax (908)766-0100

Lieber, Colette D., MD {1396844163} Dermat(82,PA01)<NJ-VALLEY, NJ-HACKNSK>
+ 400 Franklin Turnpike/Suite 208
Mahwah, NJ 07430   (201)825-0009   Fax (201)825-2622
cliebermd@yahoo.com

Lieberman, Alan Howard, MD {1376629014} Urolgy, IntrMd(71,PA01)<NJ-OCEANMC, NJ-COMMED>
+ Ocean Urology
52 Constitution Drive   Monroe, NJ 08831   (732)349-5200
Fax (732)349-5235

Lieberman, Alexander, III, MD {1821135674} IntrMd(74,PA09)<NJ-ACMCMAIN, NJ-ACMCITY>
+ Atlantic Internal Medicine PA
310 Chris Gaupp Drive/Suite 102   Galloway, NJ 08205
(609)652-9933   Fax (609)652-9955
+ AtlantiCare Regional Med Ctr/Mainland
65 West Jimmie Leeds Road   Pomona, NJ 08240   (609)652-1000

Lieberman, Eric Steven, MD {1275522252} Rheuma, IntrMd(98,NY48)<NJ-OVERLOOK, NJ-MORRISTN>
+ Summit Medical Group-Berkeley Heights Campus
1 Diamond Hill Road   Berkeley Heights, NJ 07922
(908)273-4300   Fax (908)673-7241

Physicians by Name and Address

Lieberman, Jordan A., MD {1750596607} Psychy(89,PA09)<NJ-VIRTMHBC, NJ-HAMPTBHC>
+ Univ Correctional HealthCare-Colpitts
Whittessey Rd & Stuyvesant Ave   Trenton, NJ 08625   (609)292-9700

Lieberman, Kenneth V., MD {1174582951} PedNph, Pedtrc(77,NY46)<NJ-HACKNSK>
+ Hackensack University Medical Center
30 Prospect Avenue/PedsNephrology   Hackensack, NJ 07601   (201)336-8228   Fax (201)996-5397
klieberman@humed.com

Lieberman, Roger D., DO {1376548883} Ophthl(74,MO78)
+ 1601 North 2nd Street/PO Box 1128
Millville, NJ 08332   (856)327-2770   Fax (856)327-9686
mady1942@aol.com

Liebhauser, Catherine A., MD {1497782775} Psychy, PsyFor, PsyGrt(83,MEX03)<NJ-MTNSIDE>
+ 85 Park Street
Montclair, NJ 07042   (973)746-7712   Fax (973)746-7712

Lieblich, Richard M., MD {1811953227} ObsGyn, Gyneco(85,NY19)<NJ-HACKNSK, NJ-HOLYNAME>
+ Tenafly Ob-Gyn Associates PA
2 Dean Drive/2nd Floor   Tenafly, NJ 07670   (201)569-3300   Fax (201)569-7649
+ Cherry Hill Women's Center
502 Kings Highway North   Cherry Hill, NJ 08034   (201)569-3300   Fax (856)667-8304

Liebling, Melissa Schubach, MD {1952386096} Radiol, PedRad(87,NY46)<NJ-HACKNSK>
+ Hackensack Radiology Group, PA/Corporate
130 Kinderkamack Road/Suite 200   River Edge, NJ 07661   (201)488-2660

Liebman, Jared Jason, MD {1760692180} SrgPlstc, Surgry(05,PA02)<PA-ENSTEIN>
+ Cooper Surgical Associates
3 Cooper Plaza/Suite 411   Camden, NJ 08103   (856)342-2270   Fax (856)365-1180

Liebowitz, Stanley, MD {1831271527} SrgOrt(65,NY19)
+ Health East Medical Center
54 South Dean Street   Englewood, NJ 07631   (201)871-4000

Liebross, Ira David, MD {1457359713} FamMed(93,NY48)<NJ-HUNTRDN>
+ Flemington Center for Wellness
32 Church Street   Flemington, NJ 08822   (908)782-0722   Fax (908)782-4460

Liegner, Jeffrey T., MD {1730280314} Ophthl(88,TX13)<NJ-NWTN-MEM>
+ Eye Care Northwest
350 Sparta Avenue   Sparta, NJ 07871   (973)729-5757   Fax (973)729-8322

Lien, Frank W., DO {1003254145}<NJ-MORRISTN>
+ Hackensack University Medical Group Closter
1 Ruckman Road   Closter, NJ 07624   (201)385-6161   Fax (201)385-1671

Lieser, Joan Karen, MD {1689645962} ObsGyn(87,NJ05)<NJ-OVERLOOK>
+ Lourdes Medical Associates
1601 Haddon Avenue   Camden, NJ 08103   (856)757-3700   Fax (856)365-7972

Lifchus Ascher, Rebecca Jean, MD {1407877368} IntrMd, EnDbMt(00,NJ06)<NJ-HUNTRDN>
+ Center for Endocrine Health
1738 Route 31 North/Suite 108   Clinton, NJ 08809   (908)735-3980   Fax (908)735-3981

Liff, Jeremy M., MD {1659638708} Nrolgy, VasNeu(07,NY15)<NY-MTSINAI, NY-MTSINYHS>
+ New Jersey Neurological Specialists
20 Prospect Avenue/Suite 800   Hackensack, NJ 07601   (201)518-7290   Fax (201)604-6428

Lifshitz, Edward I., MD {1902912991} IntrMd, AdolMd(87,NY08)
+ Rutgers University Health Services
110 Hospital Road   Piscataway, NJ 08854   (732)445-3250

Lifson, Donna C., MD {1033176227} IntrMd, PedDvl(87,NJ05)<NJ-KSLRWEST>
+ Kessler Institute for Rehabilitation West Orange
1199 Pleasant Valley Way   West Orange, NJ 07052   (973)731-3600

Liftin, Alan J., MD {1477557304} Dermat, PthDrm(82,NY47)
+ 22 Old Short Hills Road/Suite 103
Livingston, NJ 07039   (973)535-5800   Fax (973)535-9550
aliftin@barnabashealth.org

Ligenza, Claude, MD {1568548709} Pedtrc(86,DOM06)<NJ-VALLEY>
+ Valley Pediatric Associates PA
470 North Franklin Turnpike   Ramsey, NJ 07446   (201)891-7272   Fax (201)934-1817
+ Valley Pediatric Associates, P.A.
201 East Franklin Turnpike   Ho Ho Kus, NJ 07423   (201)891-7272   Fax (201)652-6485

Liggatt, Alexandra B., MD {1437477338}
+ 219 East South Avenue
Westfield, NJ 07090   (816)536-4050
alexliggatt@gmail.com

Liggio, Frank J., MD {1194790535} Pedtrc, SrgOrt(93,NJ05)<NJ-OVERLOOK, NJ-MORRISTN>
+ Frank J. Liggio
194 Main Street   Millburn, NJ 07041   (973)258-1010   Fax (973)258-4030
+ Pediatric Orthopedics, PC
99 Beauvoir Avenue/Suite 750   Summit, NJ 07902   (973)258-1010   Fax (908)522-5519

Light, Francis B., MD {1487753257} Anesth(66,NJ05)<NJ-RWJU-RAH>
+ Robert Wood Johnson University Hospital at Rahway
865 Stone Street/Anesthesiology   Rahway, NJ 07065   (732)381-4200

Lightfoot, Judith A., DO {1922046630} GenPrc(92,PA77)
+ SOM - Department of Internal Medicine
42 East Laurel Road/Suite 3100   Stratford, NJ 08084   (856)566-6845   Fax (856)566-6906
+ Garden State Infectious Diseases Associates, P.A.
709 Haddonfield Berlin Road   Voorhees, NJ 08043   (856)566-6845   Fax (856)783-2193
+ Garden State Infectious Disease Associates
570 Egg Harbor Road/Suite B-5   Sewell, NJ 08084   (856)566-3190   Fax (856)566-1904

Lightner, Angela Nanette, DO {1639603749} ObsGyn<NJ-SJHREGMC>
+ SJH Regional Medical Center
1505 West Sherman Avenue   Vineland, NJ 08360   (856)641-8000

Ligor, David A., DO {1831281815} EmrgMd(94,FL75)<NJ-TRINI-WSC, NJ-TRINIJSC>
+ Raritan Bay Medical Center/Perth Amboy Division
530 New Brunswick Avenue/Emergency   Perth Amboy, NJ 08861   (732)324-5095   Fax (732)324-4995

Ligorski, Morris, MD {1275560005} Anesth, IntrMd(76,MEXI)<NJ-COMMED>
+ Community Medical Center
99 Route 37 West/Anesthesiology   Toms River, NJ 08755   (732)557-8000

Ligot, Jaime L., MD {1457331506} GenPrc, Pthlgy, FamMed(81,PHIL)
+ Newark Department of Health
394 University Avenue/2nd Floor   Newark, NJ 07102   (973)877-6111   Fax (973)733-4328

Ligouri, Adrienne L., MD {1841525813} ObsGyn(07,NY47)
+ CAMCare Health Corporation
817 Federal Street   Camden, NJ 08103   (856)541-9811   Fax (856)541-4611
alf2017@hotmail.com

Ligresti, Dominick Joseph, MD {1598780991} Dermat, IntrMd(78,NY47)<NJ-CLARMAAS, NJ-MTNSIDE>
+ Ligresti Dermatology Associates, P.A.
175 Franklin Avenue/Suite 103   Nutley, NJ 07110   (973)759-6569   Fax (973)759-2562
ligresti@ligrestidermatology.comcastbiz.net

Ligresti, Louise G., MD {1215960232} Hemato, IntrMd, Onclgy(91,NY15)<NJ-CHILTON, NJ-VALLEY>
+ Valley Medical Group-Hematology/Oncology
One Valley Health Plaza   Paramus, NJ 07652   (201)634-5353   Fax (201)986-4702

Ligresti, Rosario Joseph, MD {1235135229} Gastrn, IntrMd(92,NY09)<NJ-HACKNSK>
+ Hackensack Digestive Diseases Associates, P.A.
52 First Street   Hackensack, NJ 07601   (201)488-3003   Fax (201)488-6911

Lijo, Maria Carmen, MD {1538129168} FamMed(84,SPAI)<NJ-MORRISTN>
+ Morris Family Medicine Associates, PA
340 Speedwell Avenue/PO Box 190   Morris Plains, NJ 07950   (973)267-9899   Fax (973)538-3522

Lijtmaer, Hugo N., MD {1669433819} Nrolgy(68,ARG01)<NJ-VALLEY>
+ Neurology Group of Bergen County
1200 East Ridgewood Avenue   Ridgewood, NJ 07450   (201)444-0868   Fax (201)444-7363

Like, Robert C., MD {1306923008} FamMed(79,MA01)
+ UH- Robert Wood Johnson Med
125 Paterson Street/MEB 240   New Brunswick, NJ 08901   (732)235-7662   Fax (732)235-8564
+ Family Medicine at Monument Square
317 George Street   New Brunswick, NJ 08901   (732)235-7662   Fax (732)246-7317

Lilienfeld, Harris C., MD {1447200787} Pedtrc, AdolMd(68,NS01)<NJ-CHSFULD, NJ-CHSMRCER>
+ Delaware Valley Pediatric Associates PA
132 Franklin Corner Road   Lawrenceville, NJ 08648   (609)896-4141   Fax (609)896-3940

Liloia, Peter Anthony, DO {1962601872} FamMed(04,ME75)
+ Premier Health Associates
123 Newton Sparta Road   Newton, NJ 07860   (973)579-6300   Fax (973)579-1524

Lim, Ami Cruz, MD {1346306420} Psychy(78,PHI02)<NJ-NWRK-BETH>
+ Moreines & Goldman PC
577 Westfield Avenue   Westfield, NJ 07090   (908)232-6566

Lim, Anita Tiu, MD {1447278833} NnPnMd, Pedtrc(72,PHI01)<NJ-CHDNWBTH, NJ-UMDNJ>
+ Children's Hospital of New Jersey
201 Lyons Avenue/Osborne Terrace   Newark, NJ 07112   (973)926-7203   Fax (973)926-2332
alim@sbhcs.com

Lim, Betty Bichly, MD {1548322522} Grtrcs(03,NY06)
+ Summit Medical Group
11 Cleveland Place   Springfield, NJ 07081   (973)378-8778   Fax (973)763-1748
+ Summit Medical Group
315 East Northfield Road/Suite 1-E   Livingston, NJ 07039   (973)378-8778   Fax (973)535-1450

Lim, Carlito L., MD {1235216458} IntrMd(87,PHI30)<NJ-ACMCITY, NJ-ACMCMAIN>
+ New Jersey Veterans Memorial Home - Vineland
524 Northwest Boulevard   Vineland, NJ 08360   (856)696-6383

Lim, Fidel Losa, Jr., MD {1962548727} IntrMd(82,PHI20)
+ 119 Ocean Avenue
Jersey City, NJ 07305   (201)200-2626
Flimjr@yahoo.com

Lim, Harold Cinco, MD {1821345687}<NJ-MONMOUTH>
+ Monmouth Medical Center
300 Second Avenue   Long Branch, NJ 07740   (732)923-6537   Fax (732)923-6536

Lim, Jocelyn Marie P., MD {1568516896} IntrMd(88,PHI01)<NY-CABRINI>
+ Hoboken University Medical Center
308 Willow Avenue   Hoboken, NJ 07030   (201)418-1000

Lim, Khengjim, MD {1194169045} Gastrn
+ Advanced Gastroenterology & Nutrition
1100 Wescott Drive/Suite 304   Flemington, NJ 08822   (908)788-4022   Fax (908)788-4066

Lim, Norman Feliz Lopez, MD {1124024401} Pedtrc(75,PHIL)
+ Springfield Pediatrics
190 Meisel Avenue   Springfield, NJ 07081   (973)467-1009   Fax (973)467-7836
+ 161 Halsted Street
East Orange, NJ 07018   (973)465-8590

Lim, Steve S., MD {1548366487} PhysMd(96,NJ05)<NJ-NWTN-MEM, NJ-STCLRDOV>
+ Northwest Rehabiliation Associates PA
400 South Main Street   Wharton, NJ 07885   (973)989-5270   Fax (973)989-5274

Lim, Sungtae, MD {1184626582} RadDia, RadNro(93,NY46)<NJ-VIRTMHBC>
+ Radiology Associates of Burlington County
1295 Route 38 West/PO Box 479   Hainesport, NJ 08036   (609)261-7017   Fax (609)261-4180
+ Virtua Memorial
175 Madison Avenue/Radiology   Mount Holly, NJ 08060   (609)267-0700

Lim, Vicente M., Jr., MD {1275529356} Psychy(84,PHI01)<NJ-MT-CARMEL>
+ Central Jersey Beharioral Health, LLC
216 North Avenue East   Cranford, NJ 07016   (908)272-7500   Fax (908)272-7502

Lima, Francesco W., MD {1679513063} FamMed(91,NJ05)<NJ-MTNSIDE>
+ ImmediCenter/Clifton
1355 Broad Street   Clifton, NJ 07013   (973)778-5566   Fax (973)778-2268
+ ImmediCenter/Totowa
500 Union Boulevard   Totowa, NJ 07512   (973)778-5566   Fax (973)790-6070

Limandri, Giuseppe, MD {1548234628} CdvDis(87,PA09)
+ Comprehensive Cardiovascular Consultants
299 Madison Avenue/Suite 102   Morristown, NJ 07960   (973)292-1020   Fax (973)292-0564

Limaye, Anjali P., MD {1598912875} PthACl, PthCyt(80,INDI)
+ Quest Diagnostics Inc.
1 Malcolm Avenue   Teterboro, NJ 07608   (201)393-5000   Fax (201)393-6127

Lin, Annie, DO {1639566086} FamMed
+ Primary Care Associates of NJ, P.A.
329 Main Road/Suite 101   Montville, NJ 07045   (973)334-9404   Fax (973)334-7615

Lin, Cheng Hsiang, MD {1942287925} Anesth, AnesAddM(69,CHNA)<NJ-CHRIST, NJ-HOBUNIMC>
+ 2023 Center Avenue
Fort Lee, NJ 07024   (201)461-6454   Fax (201)461-7362
+ Hoboken University Medical Center
308 Willow Avenue   Hoboken, NJ 07030   (201)461-6454   Fax (201)418-1570

Lin, Chi-Hsiung, MD {1104863224} IntrMd(76,TAI04)<NJ-TRINI-WSC>
+ 240 Williamson Street/Suite 506
Elizabeth, NJ 07202   (908)965-0234   Fax (908)965-1191

Lin, David, MD {1306227079}<NJ-HACKNSK>
+ Hackensack University Medical Center
30 Prospect Avenue/Main 3682   Hackensack, NJ 07601
(551)996-2331

Lin, David Yih-Min, MD {1558333476} PedOrt, SrgOrt, OthrSp(95,NY47)<NJ-MORRISTN, NJ-STBARNMC>
+ Advocare The Orthopedic Center
218 Ridgedale Avenue/Suite 104   Cedar Knolls, NJ 07927
(973)538-7700   Fax (973)538-9478

Lin, Dennis C., MD {1417955576} RadDia(96,IL11)
+ South Jersey Radiology Associates, P.A.
748 Kings Highway   West Deptford, NJ 08096   (856)848-4998   Fax (856)853-7362
+ South Jersey Radiology Associates, P.A.
Severan Profess Mews/Suite 105   Sewell, NJ 08080
(856)848-4998   Fax (856)589-6142
+ SJRA South Jersey Radiology Associates, P.A.
113 East Laurel Road   Stratford, NJ 08096   (856)566-2552

Lin, Edward Alan, MD {1013234012} SrgOrt<NY-JTORTHO>
+ Kayal Orthopaedic Center, P.C.
784 Franklin Avenue/Suite 250   Franklin Lakes, NJ 07417
(844)281-1783   Fax (201)560-0712

Lin, En-Su, MD {1821170242} Anesth, PainMd(72,TAI07)<NJ-COOPRUMC>
+ Cooper University Hospital
One Cooper Plaza/Anesth   Camden, NJ 08103   (856)342-2919   Fax (856)968-8239

Lin, Erwin, MD {1518927227} RadDia, IntrMd(01,NY15)
+ Radiology Associates of Ridgewood, P.A.
20 Franklin Turnpike   Waldwick, NJ 07463   (201)445-8822
Fax (201)447-5053

Lin, Esson, MD {1689697153} EmrgMd(97,PA12)<NJ-BAYONNE>
+ Bayonne Medical Center
29th Street at Avenue E/EmergMed   Bayonne, NJ 07002
(201)858-5000

Lin, George Szuwei, MD {1518927474} IntrMd, PulDis(96,NJ05)<NJ-HACKNSK>
+ Pulmonary & Medical Associates of Pasack Valley
466 Old Hook Road/Suite 26   Emerson, NJ 07630
(201)261-0821   Fax (201)261-0823

Lin, Giant Chu, MD {1699933044} Otlryg
+ Drs. Aroesty and Lin
400 Valley Road/Suite 105   Mount Arlington, NJ 07856
(973)770-7101   Fax (973)770-7108

Lin, Harry Hui, MD {1538105895} IntrMd(86,CHN57)
+ 201 Bridge Street
Metuchen, NJ 08840   (732)632-8881   Fax (732)632-8050

Lin, Hua, MD {1003839770} PhysMd, Acpntr(82,CHN21)<NJ-HUNTRDN>
+ 10 Fox Chase Turn
Pittstown, NJ 08867   (973)762-8600   Fax (973)762-9006

Lin, Ines Chi-Ying, MD {1982760864} SrgPlstc<PA-CHILDHOS>
+ CHOP Pediatric & Adolescent Specialty Care Center
4009 Black Horse Pike   Mays Landing, NJ 08330   (609)677-7895   Fax (609)677-7835

Lin, Ing-Long, MD {1215110077} IntrMd(69,TAI04)<NJ-COMMED>
+ 495 Lakehurst Road
Toms River, NJ 08753   (732)240-2299

Lin, Janet C., MD {1376545574} InfDis(85,NY09)
+ Infectious Disease Center of New Jersey
22 Old Short Hills Road/Suite 106   Livingston, NJ 07039
(973)535-8355   Fax (973)535-8353
+ Infectious Disease Center of New Jersey
653 Willow Grove Street/Suite 2700   Hackettstown, NJ 07840   (973)535-8355   Fax (973)535-8353

Lin, Jeffrey M., MD {1255641197} Surgry(IL42
+ Atlantic Surgical Group, PA
255 Monmouth Road   Oakhurst, NJ 07755   (732)531-5445
Fax (732)531-1776

Lin, Jian L., MD {1679782817} Anesth(03,NY06)<NJ-CHILTON>
+ Chilton Medical Center
97 West Parkway/Anesth   Pompton Plains, NJ 07444
(973)831-5093

Lin, Judy Mei-Chia, MD {1033123161} IntrMd, Gastrn(98,PA02)
+ Medical Care Institute, P.A.
159 Summit Avenue   Hackensack, NJ 07601   (201)343-7272   Fax (201)343-0228

Lin, Julie Tun-Fang, MD {1467481077} PhysMd, IntrMd(98,NY48)
+ New Jersey Ctr for Orthop Sports Med
150 North Finley Avenue   Basking Ridge, NJ 07920
(908)340-4266   Fax (908)340-4269

Lin, Karen Wei-Ru, MD {1376619908} FamMed(89,NJ06)
+ Family Medicine at Monument Square
317 George Street   New Brunswick, NJ 08901   (732)235-8993   Fax (732)246-6317

Lin, Lei, MD {1104847797} PhysMd(91,CHN4A)<NJ-JFKMED>
+ JFK Medical Center
65 James Street   Edison, NJ 08820   (732)321-7070   Fax (732)321-7330

Lin, Michael Keith, MD {1821199407} IntrMd(97,NJ05)<NJ-VA-LYONS>
+ VA New Jersey Health Care System at Lyons
151 Knollcroft Road   Lyons, NJ 07939   (908)647-0180   Fax (908)604-5218

Lin, Pei-Shiu, MD {1609800226} Otlryg, IntrMd(67,TAI05)
+ RWJPE Bhavani Vietla
2864 Route 27/Suite D   North Brunswick, NJ 08902
(732)966-1703   Fax (732)297-3785

Lin, Qing, MD {1720049091} PthAcl, Pthlgy(88,CHN3B)<NJ-JRSYCITY>
+ Jersey City Medical Center
355 Grand Street   Jersey City, NJ 07304   (201)915-2000

Lin, Renny L., MD {1861543944} Anesth(72,TAI02)<NJ-COMMED>
+ Toms River Anesthesia Associates PC
409 Main Street/2nd Floor   Toms River, NJ 08753
(732)818-7575   Fax (732)818-1567

Lin, Richard M., MD {1316959976} IntrMd, Gastrn(99,NY19)
+ Hackensack Gastroenterology Associates
130 Kinderkamack Road/Suite 301   River Edge, NJ 07661
(201)489-7772   Fax (201)489-2544

Lin, Richie L., MD {1417120932} Dermat(04,NJ05)<NJ-OVER-LOOK>
+ Ravits Margaret MD & Associates
130 Kinderkamack Road/Suite 205   River Edge, NJ 07661
(201)692-0800   Fax (201)488-1582
+ Ravits Margaret MD & Associates
721 Summit Avenue   Hackensack, NJ 07601   (201)692-0800   Fax (201)487-4180

Lin, Ruth Ann, MD {1437264801} IntrMd(98,NY48)
+ 92 Jersey Avenue
Edison, NJ 08820

Lin, Sheldon S., MD {1952475022} SrgOrt, SrgFAk(89,PA02)<NJ-UMDNJ, NJ-OVERLOOK>
+ North Jersey Orthopaedic Institute
33 Overlook Road/MAC L02   Summit, NJ 07901   (908)522-5895   Fax (908)522-2757
+ North Jersey Orthopaedic Institute
90 Bergen Street/DOC 1200   Newark, NJ 07101   (908)522-5895   Fax (973)972-9367

Lin, Shengxi, MD {1114192291} PsyCAd(86,CHN1C)
+ CPC Behavioral HealthCare
270 Highway 35   Red Bank, NJ 07701   (732)842-2000   Fax (732)224-0688
+ CPC Behavioral HealthCare
37 Court Street   Freehold, NJ 07728   (732)842-2000   Fax (732)224-0688

Lin, Shirley H., MD {1366485112} IntrMd, OncHem(73,TAI02)<NJ-COMMED>
+ 20 Hospital Drive/Suite 4
Toms River, NJ 08755   (732)286-0222   Fax (732)286-4225

Lin, Spencer, MD {1962668806} IntrMd
+ PO Box 225
Ridgewood, NJ 07451

Lin, Tatiana Alexeevna, MD {1972530855} Pedtrc(90,BLA02)
+ PediatriCare Associates
20-20 Fair Lawn Avenue   Fair Lawn, NJ 07410   (201)791-4545   Fax (201)791-3765

Lin, Ying, MD {1689647240} IntrMd(96,CHN19)<NJ-JRSYSHMC>
+ Shore Medical Group
2130 Highway 35/Suite 213B   Sea Girt, NJ 08750
(732)974-8668   Fax (732)974-1078

Lin, Ying Bang, MD {1215994181} Anesth(70,TAI06)<NJ-STPETER>
+ St. Peter's University Hospital
254 Easton Avenue/Anesth   New Brunswick, NJ 08901
(732)745-8600
+ Anesthesia Consultnts of NJ/Nova Pain
285 Davidson Avenue/Suite 204   Somerset, NJ 08873
(732)745-8600   Fax (732)271-3543

Lin, Yuhlin, MD {1588641567} Anesth(74,TAI02)<NJ-CHRIST>
+ Christ Hospital
176 Palisade Avenue/Anesthesiology   Jersey City, NJ 07306
(201)795-8200   Fax (201)943-8105

Linares, Hugo Manuel, DO {1013143726} Ophthl
+ Eye Associates
141 Black Horse Pike/Suite 7   Blackwood, NJ 08012
(856)227-6262   Fax (856)227-8830
+ Eye Associates
1401 Route 70 East   Cherry Hill, NJ 08034   (856)227-6262
Fax (856)428-6359

Lind, Eugene Jerome, MD {1811929078} Urolgy(66,NY19)<NJ-JFKMED, NJ-RWJURAH>
+ 1656 Oak Tree Road
Edison, NJ 08820   (732)494-6420   Fax (732)494-5079

Lind, Eugene Joseph, MD {1578570461} Urolgy(74,BELG)<NJ-STBARNMC>
+ Renaissance Medical Group
155 Jefferson Street/Lower Level   Newark, NJ 07105
(973)344-5498   Fax (973)344-6686
+ 41 Wilson Avenue
Newark, NJ 07105   (973)344-5498   Fax (973)344-7171

Lind, Marita Elizabeth, MD {1275503245} Pedtrc(92,PA13)
+ University Hospital-Cares Institute
42 East Laurel Road/Suite 1100   Stratford, NJ 08084
(856)566-7036   Fax (856)566-6108

Lind, Robert Michael, MD {1235244674} IntrMd, EnDbMt(99,NY19)
+ Diabetes & Endocrine Associates of Hunterdon
9100 Westcott Drive/Suite 101   Flemington, NJ 08822
(908)237-6990   Fax (908)237-6995

Lind, Robert S., MD {1609822782} CdvDis(88,VA07)<NJ-HUNTRDN>
+ Hunterdon Cardiovascular Associates
1738 Route 31/Suite 210   Clinton, NJ 08809   (908)823-9200   Fax (908)823-9211
+ Hunterdon Cardiovascular Associates
1100 Wescott Drive/Suite G-3   Flemington, NJ 08822
(908)823-9200   Fax (908)788-6460

Lind, Thomas Eugene, MD {1437129418} Pedtrc(93,PA13)<NJ-KMHSTRAT>
+ Children's Health Associates II LLC
101 Carnie Boulevard   Voorhees, NJ 08043   (856)325-4421
Fax (856)504-8029

Linden, Robert Andor, MD {1932317633} Urolgy(04,PA02)
+ New Jersey Urology, LLC
2401 East Evesham Road/Suite F   Voorhees, NJ 08043
(856)673-1615   Fax (856)763-1617
+ Delaware Valley Urology LLC
63 Kresson Road/Suite 103   Cherry Hill, NJ 08034
(856)673-1615   Fax (856)267-2499
+ Delaware Valley Urology LLC
2003 B Lincoln Drive   Marlton, NJ 08043   (856)985-8000
Fax (856)985-1600

Lindenberg, Erin K., MD {1255447629} Pedtrc(03,MA07)<NJ-ENGLWOOD, NJ-HACKNSK>
+ Tenafly Pediatrics, PA
350 Ramapo Valley Road   Oakland, NJ 07436   (201)651-0404   Fax (201)651-0909

Lindenberg, Noah L., MD {1346311073} IntrMd, OncHem(02,PA09)<NJ-KMHTURNV, NJ-KMHSTRAT>
+ Comprehensive Cancer & Hematology Specialists, P.C.
900 Medical Center Drive/Suite 200   Sewell, NJ 08080
(856)582-0550   Fax (856)582-7640
+ Comprehensive Cancer & Hematology Specialists, P.C.
17 West Red Bank Avenue/Suite 202   Woodbury, NJ 08096
(856)582-0550   Fax (856)848-0958
+ Comprehensive Cancer & Hematology Specialists, P.C.
705 White Horse Road   Voorhees, NJ 08080   (856)435-1777   Fax (856)435-0696

Linder, Earle S., MD {1093704140} Urolgy, IntrMd(80,QU06)<NJ-CHSFULD, NJ-CHSMRCER>
+ Urology Care Alliance
2105 Klockner Road   Hamilton, NJ 08690   (609)588-0770
Fax (609)588-0454

Lindholm, Stephen R., MD {1932190386} SrgOrt, SrgOARec(01,MI01)
+ Restoration Orthopaedics
113 West Essex Street/Suite 201   Maywood, NJ 07607
(201)226-0145   Fax (201)226-0147

Lindner, Marc Isaiah, DO {1891138236}
+ 34 Reynolds Avenue
East Newark, NJ 07029   (973)960-3837
docml87@gmail.com

Lindquist, Lisa A., DO {1477508570} Psychy(89,NJ75)
+ 1 Mall Drive/Suite 920
Cherry Hill, NJ 08002   (856)482-9442   Fax (856)346-1052

Lindsay-O'Reggio, Euldricka B., MD {1013973510} Pedtrc(92,JMA01)<NJ-CHSFULD>
+ Capital Health System/Fuld Campus
750 Brunswick Avenue   Trenton, NJ 08638   (609)394-6000

Lindy, Michael Evan, MD {1386962264} Gastrn<NY-MNTFWEIL>
+ Premier Health Associates
532 Lafayette Road/Suite 100   Sparta, NJ 07871   (973)383-3730   Fax (973)383-2285

Liner, Lisa Hope, MD {1013907799} Pedtrc, IntrMd(00,NET09)<NJ-VIRTVOOR>
+ Virtua Voorhees
100 Bowman Drive/Emerg Med   Voorhees, NJ 08043
(856)772-0798   Fax (856)261-5842

Linet, Leslie S., MD {1528123288} Psychy, PsyCAd, PsyAdd(68,NY46)
+ 2 Trent Road
Monroe Township, NJ 08831   (609)430-9099

Linganna, Sanjay, MD {1740423771} IntrMd(09,GRN01)<PA-TJHSP>
+ Voorhees Specialty Center
443 Laurel Oak Road/Suite 100   Voorhees, NJ 08043
(856)784-7398   Fax (856)784-7357

Physicians by Name and Address

Lingappan, Ahila, MD {1336390624} Ophthl
+ 56 Whyte Drive
Voorhees, NJ 08043
drahila@yahoo.com

Lingaraju, Rajiv, MD {1205150778} Anesth
+ West Jersey Anesthesia Assoc PA
102 Centre Boulevard/Suite East   Marlton, NJ 08053
(856)988-6260   Fax (856)988-6270

Lingasubramanian, Geethanjali, MD {1043408016} Pedtrc, IntrMd(99,INA81)
+ CHOP Newborn and Pediatric Care at UMCPP
One Plainsboro Road/6th Floor   Plainsboro, NJ 08536
(609)853-7626   Fax (609)853-7630

Lingiah, Vivek, MD {1336411453} IntrMd
+ Rutgers- New Jersey Medical School
185 South Orange Avenue/MSB H-538   Newark, NJ 07103
(973)972-5252

Link, Timothy Emerson, MD {1477767705} SrgNro(02,MA07)
+ Neurosurgical Associates of NJ
121 Highway 36 West/Suite 330   West Long Branch, NJ 07764   (732)222-8866   Fax (732)870-6432

Linn, Gary C., MD {1447233416} Urolgy(73,NY20)<NJ-JRSYSHMC, NJ-OCEANMC>
+ Coastal Urology Associates
446 Jack Martin Boulevard   Brick, NJ 08724   (732)840-4300
Fax (732)840-4515

Linn, Steven Craig, MD {1669875407} GPrvMd, IntrMd(88,MD07)<NJ-SJHREGMC>
+ SJH Regional Medical Center
1505 West Sherman Avenue   Vineland, NJ 08360
(856)641-7512   Fax (856)641-7643

Linsenmeyer, Todd A., MD {1992793285} PhysMd, Urolgy(79,HI01)<NJ-KSLRWEST>
+ Kessler Institute for Rehabilitation West Orange
1199 Pleasant Valley Way   West Orange, NJ 07052
(973)731-3600

Lintag, Irene C., MD {1447242987} Pedtrc(75,PHI02)<NJ-UMDNJ>
+ 6 Devonwood Court
Voorhees, NJ 08043

Linz, Stephan M., MD {1740261015} Anesth(92,DC02)<NJ-MORRISTN>
+ Morristown Medical Center
100 Madison Avenue/Anesthesiology   Morristown, NJ 07962   (973)971-5000   Fax (201)943-8733

Liotta, Joseph Anthony, Sr., MD {1669404000} IntrMd(02,GRN01)<NJ-STCLRDOV>
+ 25 Main Street
Sparta, NJ 07871   (973)729-5242   Fax (973)729-0807

Liotti, Joseph B., DO {1093721292} FamMed(86,NJ75)<NJ-MTNSIDE>
+ Fairfield Family Practice
125 Sand Road   Fairfield, NJ 07004   (973)808-9242   Fax (973)244-0585

Liotti, Linda A., DO {1316022965} FamMed(86,NJ75)<NJ-MTNSIDE>
+ Fairfield Family Practice
125 Sand Road   Fairfield, NJ 07004   (973)808-9242   Fax (973)244-0585

Lipani, John David, MD {1275612111} SrgNro(95,ISR02)<NJ-CHSFULD, NJ-CHSMRCER>
+ Princeton Neurological Surgery, P.C.
3836 Quakerbridge Road/Suite 203   Hamilton, NJ 08619
(609)890-3400   Fax (609)890-3410

Lipat, Gregorio A., MD {1790783850} IntrMd, Nephro(68,PHIL)<NJ-JRSYCITY, NJ-CHRIST>
+ 107-123 Pacific Avenue
Jersey City, NJ 07304   (201)200-9984   Fax (201)451-2863
Elipat@aol.com

Lipatov, Yuriy, MD {1851335087} Anesth(81,UKR14)
+ Raritan Bay Medical Center/Perth Amboy Division
530 New Brunswick Avenue   Perth Amboy, NJ 08861   (732)442-3700

Lipert, Zofia J., MD {1831195577} Pedtrc(82,POLA)<NJ-JRSYCITY, NJ-MEADWLND>
+ Total Care Pediatrics in Jersey City
550 Newark Avenue/Suite 200   Jersey City, NJ 07306
(201)714-7902   Fax (201)795-4999
+ Newport Medical Associates
610 Washington Boulevard   Jersey City, NJ 07310
(201)222-1266

Lipetskaia, Lioudmila, MD {1770775470} ObsGyn
+ 6102 Main Street
Voorhees, NJ 08043   (856)325-6622

Lipka, Andrew C., MD {1821199043} Ophthl(82,NY46)<NJ-UNVMCPRN>
+ Ophthalmology Associates
800 Bunn Drive/Suite 301   Princeton, NJ 08540   (609)924-3700   Fax (609)924-4724
+ Brunswick Eye Associates
317 Cleveland Avenue   Highland Park, NJ 08904   (609)924-3700   Fax (732)828-0677
+ University Medical Center of Princeton at Plainsboro
One Plainsboro Road   Plainsboro, NJ 08540   (609)924-3700

Lipkind, Mark Alan, MD {1316922651} Anesth<NJ-CHILTON>
+ Chilton Medical Center
97 West Parkway   Pompton Plains, NJ 07444   (973)831-5000

Lipkowitz, Jeffrey L., MD {1659377729} Ophthl(78,PA13)<NJ-CHSFULD, NJ-CHSMRCER>
+ Delaware Valley Retina Associates
4 Princess Road/Suite 101   Lawrenceville, NJ 08648
(609)896-1414   Fax (609)896-2982
+ Delaware Valley Retina Associates
121 Highway 31 North/Suite 700   Flemington, NJ 08822
(908)806-6191

Lipman, Ted, MD {1932229903} PsyCAd, Psychy(83,CA11)<NJ-STBARBHC>
+ 2 West Northfield Road/Suite 304
Livingston, NJ 07039   (973)535-8512   Fax (973)535-8469

Lipnack, Eric M., DO {1144396987} PhysMd(88,PA77)
+ 3 Muirfield Court
Medford, NJ 08055   Fax (856)784-4379

Liporace, Frank Anthony, MD {1689679722} OrtTrm, SrgOrt(99,NY09)<NY-NYUTISCH>
+ NYU Langon Department of Orthopaedic Surgery
377 Jersey Avenue/Suite 280A   Jersey City, NJ 07302
(201)716-5850   Fax (201)309-2432

Lipp, Alfred J., DO {1821123902} Pedtrc(79,IA75)<NJ-JRSYSHMC, NJ-MONMOUTH>
+ 804 West Park Avenue
Ocean, NJ 07712   (732)775-7337   Fax (732)695-0476

Lipp, Matthew Ivan, MD {1649242868} PhysMd, PainMd(97,MEX03)<NJ-MORRISTN, NJ-STBARNMC>
+ New Jersey Spine Center
40 Main Street   Chatham, NJ 07928   (973)635-0800   Fax (973)635-6254
+ New Jersey Spine Center
1222 Kennedy Boulevard   Bayonne, NJ 07002   (973)635-0800   Fax (973)635-6254
+ New Jersey Spine Center
25 East Willow Street   Millburn, NJ 07928   (973)379-1114   Fax (973)635-6254

Lippe, Scott David, MD {1992766844} Gastrn, IntrMd, Nutrtn(92,NY47)<NJ-BERGNMC, NJ-HACKNSK>
+ 230 East Ridgewood/Suite 6-2
Paramus, NJ 07652   (201)594-0700   Fax (201)225-4702
Doclippemd@aol.com

Lipper, Jeffrey M., MD {1679512891} PulDis, CritCr, IntrMd(83,ROMA)<NJ-SOCEANCO>
+ Stafford Medical, P.A.
1364 Route 72 West/Suite 5   Manahawkin, NJ 08050
(609)597-3416   Fax (609)597-9608
+ Stafford Medical, P.A.
1364 Route 72 West   Manahawkin, NJ 08050   (609)597-3416   Fax (609)597-9608

Lippman, Alan J., MD {1336125509} IntrMd, MedOnc, OncHem(65,PA09)<NJ-MTNSIDE>
+ Essex Hematology-Oncology Group, PA
36 Newark Avenue/Suite 304   Belleville, NJ 07109
(973)751-8880   Fax (973)751-8950

Lippman, Jay Howard, MD {1750378089} IntrMd<NJ-JRSYCITY>
+ Jersey City Medical Center
355 Grand Street   Jersey City, NJ 07304   (201)915-2000

Lipschultz, Todd M., MD {1124197942} SrgHnd, SrgOrt(84,PA01)
+ Premier Orthopaedic of South Jersey
1007 Mantua Pike   Woodbury, NJ 08096   (856)853-8004
Fax (856)853-8022
+ Premier Orthopaedic of South Jersey
522B Lippincott Drive   Marlton, NJ 08053   (856)853-8004
Fax (856)853-7580

Lipset, Shani Lauren, MD {1992752646} FamMed(97,NY15)<NJ-OVERLOOK>
+ Summit Medical Group-Berkeley Heights Campus
1 Diamond Hill Road   Berkeley Heights, NJ 07922
(908)277-8602   Fax (908)790-6576

Lipshutz, Robert L., DO {1740200724} IntrMd(90,PA77)<NJ-ACMCITY, NJ-ACMCMAIN>
+ AtlantiCare Internal Medical Associates
7313 Ventnor Avenue   Ventnor, NJ 08406   (609)441-2199
Fax (609)487-9640
+ Seashore Gardens Living Center
22 West Jimmie Leeds Road   Absecon, NJ 08205   (609)441-2199   Fax (609)404-4841

Lipsitch, Carol E., MD {1891887592} IntrMd(78,CT01)
+ first Care Medical Group
50 Pompton Avenue   Verona, NJ 07044   (973)857-3400
Fax (973)857-7034

Lipsius, Bruce D., MD {1891765434} Nrolgy(72,NY08)<NJ-VIRTMHBC, NJ-VIRTMARL>
+ LMA Neurology Consultants
63 Kresson Road/Suite 101   Cherry Hill, NJ 08034
(856)218-1770   Fax (856)795-3625
+ LMA Neurology Consultants
570 Egg Harbor Road/Suite B-5   Sewell, NJ 08080
(856)218-1770   Fax (856)795-3625

Lipsky, Marvin A., MD {1932198942} Gastrn, IntrMd(81,NY19)<NJ-OVERLOOK>
+ Associates in Digestive Disease
25 Morris Avenue   Springfield, NJ 07081   (973)467-1313
Fax (973)467-3133

Lipson, Adam Craig, MD {1912012071} SrgNro<NJ-OVERLOOK, NJ-TRINIJSC>
+ IGEA Brain & Spine
1057 Commerce Avenue   Union, NJ 07083   (908)688-8800
Fax (908)688-2377

Lipson, David E., MD {1417646575} SrgPlstc, Surgry(71,NY46)<NJ-VALLEY>
+ 23-00 Route 208
Fair Lawn, NJ 07410   (201)797-7770   Fax (201)797-1660
plastic.surgeon@doctor.com

Lipstein, Rebekah Ann, MD {1821243379} Pedtrc(06,MD01)<NY-JACOBIMC>
+ West Park Pediatrics
804 West Park Avenue   Ocean, NJ 07712   (732)531-0010
Fax (732)493-0903
+ West Park Pediatrics
921 East County Line Road/Suite B   Lakewood, NJ 08701
(732)531-0010   Fax (732)370-5550
+ West Park Pediatrics
219 Taylors Mills Road   Manalapan, NJ 07712   (732)577-0088   Fax (732)577-9643

Liptsyn, Tatyana, MD {1891728366} Pedtrc(87,UKR05)<NJ-STBARNMC>
+ St. Barnabas Medical Center
94 Old Short Hills Road/Pediatrics   Livingston, NJ 07039
(973)322-5000

Liquori, Frances, DO {1437234788} FamMed(84,IA75)<NJ-CENTRAST>
+ Howell Family Medicine Center
3701 US Highway 9   Howell, NJ 07731   (732)364-4555
Fax (732)364-9361

Lira, Lorraine Sales, MD {1649354119} Nrolgy(89,PHI01)<NJ-HOLYNAME, NJ-VALLEY>
+ David D. Van Slooten MD, PA
99 Kindermack Road/Suite 307   Westwood, NJ 07675
(201)261-6222   Fax (201)261-4411

Liriano, Monica, MD {1134518426} ObsGyn
+ Women's Care
1044 Main Street   Paterson, NJ 07503   (973)510-2444
Fax (973)278-2818

Lirio, Sixto M., MD {1780683672} FamMed(74,PHI01)<NJ-BURDTMLN>
+ 7 Pershing Avenue
Cape May Court House, NJ 08210   (609)463-0600   Fax (609)463-9477

Lisa, Charles P., MD {1811968316} CdvDis, IntrMd(67,DC02)<NJ-OURLADY, NJ-COOPRUMC>
+ Associated Cardiovascular Consultants, P.A.
1105 Laurel Oak Road/Suite 165   Voorhees, NJ 08043
(856)424-3600   Fax (856)424-7154
+ Associated Cardiovascular Consultants-Lourdes
1 Brace Road/Suite C & F   Cherry Hill, NJ 08034   (856)424-3600   Fax (856)428-5748

Lishko, Olga V., MD {1710940317} IntrMd(88,UKR05)<NJ-VALLEY>
+ 25-15 Fair Lawn Avenue
Fair Lawn, NJ 07410   (201)475-1005   Fax (201)475-1009

Lisik, Chantal Mulan, MD {1275845729}<NJ-OVERLOOK>
+ Overlook Medical Center
99 Beauvoir Avenue/PO Box 210   Summit, NJ 07902
(908)522-2000

Lisko, Trina M., DO {1457471377} PhysMd(04,NJ75)<PA-TMPHOSP>
+ South Jersey Sports Medicine Center
556 Egg Harbor Road/Suite A   Sewell, NJ 08080   (856)589-0650   Fax (856)589-2720

Liss, Donald, MD {1548244395} PhysMd(79,MI07)<NJ-ENGLWOOD, NY-PRSBCOLU>
+ Physical Medicine & Rehabilitation Center
500 Grand Avenue/1st Floor   Englewood, NJ 07631
(201)567-2277   Fax (201)567-7506

Liss, Howard, MD {1801879564} PhysMd, SprtMd, PainMd(77,MI07)<NY-PRSBCOLU, NJ-ENGLWOOD>
+ Physical Medicine & Rehabilitation Center
500 Grand Avenue/1st Floor   Englewood, NJ 07631
(201)567-2277   Fax (201)567-7506
jonlibasci@aol.com
+ Physical Medicine & Rehabilitation Center, PA
1530 Palisade Avenue   Fort Lee, NJ 07024   (201)567-2277
Fax (201)363-8873

Liss, Kenneth A., DO {1033125315} Nephro, IntrMd(90,PA77)<NJ-BAYSHORE, NJ-HLTHSRE>
+ Hypertension & Nephrology Association, PA
6 Industrial Way West/Suite B   Eatontown, NJ 07724
(732)460-1200   Fax (732)460-1211

Physicians by Name and Address

Lissauer, Matthew Eric, MD {1306808019} SrgCrC(NY09
+ RWJMG Acute Care Surgery
 125 Paterson Street/Suite 6300 New Brunswick, NJ 08901 (732)235-7766 Fax (732)235-2964

Lisser, Steven P., MD {1528039773} Ortped, SrgHnd, SrgOrt(87,NY47)<NJ-BAYSHORE, NJ-RIVERVW>
+ Orthopaedic Sports Medicine
 80 Oak Hill Road Red Bank, NJ 07701 (732)741-2313 Fax (732)741-7154

List, James Frank, MD {1619012408} IntrMd, Pedtrc, EnDbMt(96,MN04)
+ Janssen Pharmaceutical Products
 1125 Trenton Harbourton Road Titusville, NJ 08560 (609)730-3100

Lister, Mark Anthony, MD {1043258353} Ophthl, CrnExD(80,MEX14)<NJ-OCEANMC>
+ Mark Anthony Lister MD PA
 1 Clara Maass Drive Belleville, NJ 07109 (973)844-1340 Fax (973)450-5964

Litkouhi, Behrang, MD {1255679916} RadDia
+ Hackensack University Medical Center
 30 Prospect Avenue Hackensack, NJ 07601 (201)996-2000

Litsky, Jason D., DO {1114169539} IntCrd, IntrMd(03,PA77)
+ Monmouth Cardiology Associates, LLC
 222 Schanck Road/Suite 104 Freehold, NJ 07728 (732)431-1332 Fax (732)431-1712
+ Monmouth Cardiology Associates, LLC
 11 Meridian Road Eatontown, NJ 07724 (732)431-1332 Fax (732)663-0301

Litsky, Michelle Badorf, DO {1255535803} Pedtrc, PedPul, IntrMd(07,PA77)<CT-HOSPECL>
+ Monmouth Pediatric Group, P.A.
 272 Broad Street Red Bank, NJ 07701 (732)741-0456 Fax (732)219-9477
+ Monmouth Pediatric Group, P.A.
 3350 Highway 138 Wall, NJ 07719 (732)741-0456 Fax (732)681-6939

Little, James Todd, DO EmrgMd(90,PA77)
+ Urgent Care Now
 712 East Bay Avenue/Suite 22-B Manahawkin, NJ 08050 (609)978-0242 Fax (609)978-0241

Little, Sherrill T., MD {1578555744} RadDia(93,VA04)
+ South Jersey Radiology Associates, P.A.
 748 Kings Highway West Deptford, NJ 08096 (856)848-4998 Fax (856)853-7362
+ South Jersey Radiology Associates, P.A.
 Severan Profess Mews/Suite 105 Sewell, NJ 08080 (856)848-4998 Fax (856)589-6142
+ South Jersey Radiology Associates, P.A.
 100 Carnie Boulevard/Suite B-5 Voorhees, NJ 08096 (856)751-0123 Fax (856)751-0535

Littman, Paul M., DO {1538364369} ObsGyn(03,NY75)<NJ-MORRISTN>
+ Morristown Medical Center
 100 Madison Avenue/Ob/Gyn Morristown, NJ 07962 (973)971-5000
+ Atlantic Health Urology Gyn
 95 Madison Avenue/Suite 204 Morristown, NJ 07960 (973)971-7440
+ Specialty Surgical Center
 380 Lafayette Road/Suite 110 Sparta, NJ 07962 (973)940-3166 Fax (973)940-3170

Litvack, Steven Greg, MD {1588671101} Anesth(82,MEXI)<NJ-LOURDMED>
+ Rancocas Anesthesiology, PA
 700 Route 130 North/Suite 203 Cinnaminson, NJ 08077 (856)829-9345 Fax (856)829-3605

Litvak, Anna Maria, MD {1326319302} MedOnc
+ St. Barnabas Cancer Center
 94 Old Short Hills Road/Suite 1 Livingston, NJ 07039 (973)322-5650

Litvin, Polina L., MD {1669607339}<NJ-STBARNMC>
+ St. Barnabas Medical Center
 94 Old Short Hills Road Livingston, NJ 07039 (818)730-5951

Litvin, Yair, MD {1619954211} EnDbMt, IntrMd(74,ISR01)<NJ-ENGLWOOD, NJ-HOLYNAME>
+ Bergen Medical Associates
 466 Old Hook Road/Suite 1 Emerson, NJ 07630 (201)967-8221 Fax (201)967-0340
+ Bergen Medical Associates
 1 West Ridgewood Avenue/Suite 301 Paramus, NJ 07652 (201)967-8221 Fax (201)445-4296
+ Bergen Medical Associates
 305 West Grand Avenue/Suite 200 Montvale, NJ 07630 (201)391-0071 Fax (201)391-1904

Litvin, Yigal S., MD {1376521476} PedUro, Urolgy(86,CA14)<NJ-JRSYSHMC, NJ-RIVERVW>
+ New Jersey Urologic Institute
 10 Industrial Way East Eatontown, NJ 07724 (732)963-9091 Fax (732)963-9092

Litwin, Jeffrey Sam, MD CdvDis, IntrMd(81,TN07)
+ Executive Health Group, Inc.
 44 Whippany Road Morristown, NJ 07960 (973)540-0177

Litwin, Peter J., MD {1154452712} Psychy(90,NY47)<NJ-RIVERVW, NJ-JRSYSHMC>
+ Riverview Medical Center
 1 Riverview Plaza/Psychiatry Red Bank, NJ 07701 (732)741-2700

Litz, John, Jr., MD {1295949154} ObsGyn(85,NY08)<NJ-VIRTVOOR>
+ 411 Kings Highway South
 Cherry Hill, NJ 08034 (856)429-2441 Fax (856)429-0331

Litz, Steven A., MD {1336182013} Allrgy(79,MEXI)<NJ-UNDRWD, NJ-KENEDYHS>
+ 600 Jessup Road
 Paulsboro, NJ 08066 (609)845-3100 Fax (856)845-1018
+ 2505 East Chestnut Avenue
 Vineland, NJ 08361 (609)696-9596
+ 2301 Eversham Road/Suite 605
 Voorhees, NJ 08066 (856)772-0043

Liu, Andrew Ky, MD {1225061054} Ultsnd<NJ-SJHREGMC>
+ SJH Regional Medical Center
 1505 West Sherman Avenue Vineland, NJ 08360 (856)641-8000

Liu, Bo, MD {1790758357} Anesth(89,CHN21)
+ 100 Julie Drive
 Northfield, NJ 08225

Liu, Charles Li-Chen, MD {1215371224} IntrMd
+ RWJ Hospital Internal Medicine
 One Robert Wood Johnson Place/MEB 486 New Brunswick, NJ 08901 (732)235-8377 Fax (732)235-7427

Liu, Connie Xia, MD {1659566545} FamMed(83,CHN9D)
+ 163 Impatiens Court
 Toms River, NJ 08753
+ 54 Washington Street
 Toms River, NJ 08753 (732)505-0213

Liu, Edmund S., MD {1215032768} Otlryg, OtgyFPlS(96,MA07)<NJ-MTNSIDE>
+ 207 Pompton Avenue
 Verona, NJ 07044 (973)571-1933 Fax (973)571-1904 mailbox@njfaces.com

Liu, Edward Shaoyou, MD {1457449555} PthACl(85,CHN1J)<NJ-CHSMRCER>
+ Capital Health System/Hopewell
 One Capital Way/Pathology Pennington, NJ 08534 (609)303-4019

Liu, Edward Wei Chi, MD {1871587683} InfDis, IntrMd(96,PA14)<NJ-JRSYSHMC, NJ-RIVERVW>
+ Jersey Shore University Medical Center
 1945 Route 33 Neptune, NJ 07753 (732)775-5500
+ Hackensack Meridian Medical Group
 19 Davis Avenue/5th-6th Floor Neptune, NJ 07753 (732)775-5500 Fax (732)897-3997

Liu, Elizabeth Yingxia, MD {1780629931} FamMed(88,CHN9D)
+ 60 Essex Street/Suite 202
 Rochelle Park, NJ 07662 (201)587-8887 Fax (201)587-8869

Liu, James Jingren, MD {1013391457}<NJ-COOPRUMC>
+ Cooper University Hospital
 One Cooper Plaza Camden, NJ 08103 (856)342-2000

Liu, Jenny, MD {1720016108} IntrMd, Nutrtn(87,CHN52)<NJ-VAEASTOR>
+ UniMed Center LLC
 190 Route 18/Suite 202 East Brunswick, NJ 08816 (732)828-9988 Fax (732)828-1010

Liu, Jian, MD {1376718569} IntrMd(93,CHN4A)<NJ-JRSYSHMC>
+ Physican's Home & Health Service
 1532 State Route 33/Suite 202 Neptune, NJ 07753 (732)775-8400 Fax (732)775-8401

Liu, Jun, MD {1528019932} PthACl, Pthlgy(91,CHN38)<NJ-KMHCHRRY>
+ Kennedy Health System/Cherry Hill Campus
 2201 Chapel Avenue West/Pathology Cherry Hill, NJ 08002 (856)488-6500 Fax (856)488-6846

Liu, Kaixuan, MD {1801815287} Anesth, PainInvt, IntrMd(85,CHN76)<NJ-OCEANMC>
+ Atlantic Spine Center
 475 Prospect Avenue/Suite 110 West Orange, NJ 07052 (973)419-0200 Fax (973)419-0223
+ Advanced Spine Surgery Center
 855 Lehigh Avenue Union, NJ 07083 (973)419-0200 Fax (908)557-9438

Liu, Liang, MD {1487759080} PthACl(84,CHN63)
+ BioReference Laboratories
 491-B Edward H. Ross Drive Elmwood Park, NJ 07407 (201)663-9315 Fax (201)791-3758

Liu, Lide, MD {1841224755} FamMed
+ Hunterdon Family Physicians
 111 State Route 31/Suite 111 Flemington, NJ 08822 (908)284-9880 Fax (908)782-4316

Liu, Marcia Nai-Hwa, MD {1144294737} CdvDis, IntrMd(92,PA02)<NJ-CENTRAST, NJ-JRSYSHMC>
+ Monmouth Cardiology Associates, LLC
 222 Schanck Road/Suite 104 Freehold, NJ 07728 (732)431-1332 Fax (732)431-1712
+ Monmouth Cardiology Associates, LLC
 11 Meridian Road Eatontown, NJ 07724 (732)431-1332 Fax (732)663-0301

Liu, Michael, MD {1285600981} Pedtrc(95,PA09)<NJ-CHILTON>
+ Advocare Pediatric Arts
 1403 Route 23 South Butler, NJ 07405 (973)283-2200 Fax (973)283-0406
+ Advocare Pediatric Arts
 1777 Hamburg Turnpike/Suite 103 Wayne, NJ 07470 (973)283-2200 Fax (973)283-0406

Liu, Michelle, MD {1124040548} IntrMd(98,NJ06)<NJ-VALLEY>
+ The Valley Hospital
 223 North Van Dien Avenue Ridgewood, NJ 07450 (201)447-8618 Fax (201)251-3302

Liu, Ming Kong, MD {1205927191} PulDis, IntrMd(85,INDI)<NJ-HOLYNAME>
+ 155 North Washington Avenue
 Bergenfield, NJ 07621 (201)501-0082 Fax (201)501-8859

Liu, Ping, MD {1578723615} IntrMd, IntHos(92,CHN59)<NJ-NWT-NMEM>
+ Capital Health System/Fuld Campus
 750 Brunswick Avenue/Hospitalist Trenton, NJ 08638 (609)815-7887 Fax (609)394-6776
+ Newton Medical Center
 175 High Street/Hospitalist Newton, NJ 07860 (973)383-2863

Liu, Qiang, MD {1780712133} PthACl
+ 36 Brians Circle
 Princeton Junction, NJ 08550 (609)936-0611

Liu, Qinyue, MD {1083753669} Psychy(84,CHN62)<NJ-UMDNJ>
+ 31 Mountain Boulevard/Suite 31W
 Warren, NJ 07059 (908)222-1532 Fax (908)222-1780

Liu, Ren Y., MD {1154437267} Anesth(02,NY08)
+ 11 Gavin Road
 West Orange, NJ 07052

Liu, Renfeng, DO {1942320924} Anesth<NJ-CHSMRCER, NJ-CHS-FULD>
+ Trenton Anesthesiology Associates, PA
 One Capital Way/Second Floor Pennington, NJ 08534 (609)396-4700 Fax (609)396-4900

Liu, Samuel M., MD {1245243013} Ophthl(94,TN05)<NJ-RWJU-RAH, NJ-JFKMED>
+ The Princeton Eye Group
 419 North Harrison Street/Suite 104 Princeton, NJ 08540 (609)921-9437 Fax (609)921-0277
+ The Princeton Eye Group
 1600 Perrinville Road Monroe Township, NJ 08831 (609)921-9437 Fax (609)655-3685
+ The Princeton Eye Group
 900 Eastern Avenue/Suite 50 Somerset, NJ 08540 (732)565-9550 Fax (732)565-0946

Liu, Todd, MD {1396733812} ObsGyn(93,NJ06)<NJ-SOCEANCO>
+ SOMC Medical Group, PC
 1100 Route 72 West/Suite 305 Manahawkin, NJ 08050 (609)978-9841 Fax (609)978-9843

Liu, Xiaoming, MD {1679674816} IntrMd(90,CHN57)
+ Howell Medical Group
 4677 Highway 9 North/Monmouth Plaza Howell, NJ 07731 (732)901-7786 Fax (732)901-4080

Liu, Ying, MD {1720385503} IntrMd(98,CHN59)
+ 220 Hamburg Turnpike/Suite 3
 Wayne, NJ 07470 (973)942-0040 Fax (973)942-4741

Liu, Yiyan, MD {1275558314} Radiol, NuclMd(83,CHN59)<NJ-UMDNJ>
+ University Hospital
 150 Bergen Street/Radiology Newark, NJ 07103 (973)972-4300 Fax (973)972-6954 liuy@umdnj.edu

Liu, Yuyan, MD {1124047592} Anesth(86,CHN57)<NJ-STFRNMED>
+ St. Francis Medical Center
 601 Hamilton Avenue/Anesthesiology Trenton, NJ 08629 (609)599-5000
+ Perth Amboy Anesthesiology PC
 530 New Brunswick Avenue Perth Amboy, NJ 08861 (732)739-5853

Liu, Zach Zhiguang, MD {1134269467} PthACl, PthHem(83,CHNA)
+ Histopathology Services, LLC.
 535 East Crescent Avenue Ramsey, NJ 07446 (201)661-7280 Fax (201)661-7297

Liu-Jarin, Xiaolin, MD {1366692352} PthACl(89,CHN57)
+ Quest Diagnostics Inc.
 1 Malcolm Avenue Teterboro, NJ 07608 (201)393-5000 Fax (201)393-6127

Physicians by Name and Address

Liu-Lee, Yingxue S., MD {1154416410} Pedtrc(86,CHN6D)<NJ-STPETER, NJ-RWJUBRUN>
+ 557 Cranbury Road/Suite 18
  East Brunswick, NJ 08816 (732)390-8780
+ St. Peter's University Hospital
  254 Easton Avenue/Pediatrics New Brunswick, NJ 08901
  (732)745-8600
+ RWJ University Hospital New Brunswick
  One Robert Wood Johnson Place New Brunswick, NJ 08816
  (732)828-3000

Liuzzo, John P., MD {1851329619} IntrMd
+ Mulkay Cardiology Consultants
  9245 Kennedy Boulevard North Bergen, NJ 07047
  (201)567-1703   Fax (201)621-0369

Liva, Bradford C., MD {1669477485} Ophthl(78,MEXI)<NJ-VALLEY, NJ-CLARMAAS>
+ 119 Prospect Street/Suite 1
  Ridgewood, NJ 07450 (201)444-1185   Fax (201)444-1403

Liva, Douglas F., MD {1255447371} Ophthl(81,FL02)<NJ-VALLEY>
+ Liva Eye Center
  1 West Ridgewood Avenue/Suite 101 Paramus, NJ 07652
  (201)444-7770   Fax (201)445-2570

Liva, Jeffrey S., MD {1912963885} OccpMd(84,FL02)<NJ-VALLEY>
+ Preventive PLUS
  1 West Ridgewood Avenue Paramus, NJ 07652 (201)444-3060   Fax (201)447-9338
  info@preventive.com

Liva, Paul A., MD {1245293877} Ophthl(76,MEXI)<NJ-HACKNSK>
+ Hackensack Eye Surgeons
  391 Summit Avenue Hackensack, NJ 07601 (201)342-5191   Fax (201)487-0026

Livelli, Frank D., Jr., MD {1700932761} CdvDis, IntrMd(76,MA01)<NY-NYPRESHS, NY-PRSBCOLU>
+ 311 Oakdene Avenue
  Leonia, NJ 07605 (201)461-5959   Fax (201)461-0839

Livingston, David H., MD {1639197874} SrgCrC, Surgry(81,NY03)<NJ-UMDNJ>
+ University Hospital-Doctors Office Center
  90 Bergen Street/DOC 7100/Surger Newark, NJ 07103
  (973)972-2400   Fax (973)972-2988

Livingston, Denise L., MD {1034436399} EmrgMd<NJ-JRSYSHMC>
+ Jersey Shore University Medical Center
  1945 Route 33/EmergMed Neptune, NJ 07753 (732)775-5500

Livingston, Lawrence I., MD {1003853102} SrgArt, SrgOrt(71,WI06)
+ 21 Philips Parkway/Suite 4
  Montvale, NJ 07645 (201)573-1202   Fax (201)573-8486

Livingston, Wendy E., MD {1073535126} Dermat(88,NY01)
+ Dermatology Associates of Morris PA
  199 Baldwin Road Parsippany, NJ 07054 (973)335-2560
  Fax (973)335-9421
  gqplayaagq@aol.com

Livingstone, Tosan, MD {1861460461} Pedtrc, PedDvl(82,NIG03)<NJ-MORRISTN>
+ Milestones Pediatric Group PA
  11 East Oak Street Oakland, NJ 07436 (201)485-7557
  Fax (201)485-7556

Livornese, Douglas S., MD {1902876915} CritCr, PulDis, IntrMd(90,NJ05)<NJ-JRSYSHMC>
+ Monmouth Pulmonary Consultants
  30 Corbett Way Eatontown, NJ 07724 (732)380-0020
  Fax (732)380-1990

Livote, Joanne, MD {1831342526} IntrMd(94,PA07)<MA-ARDHILL>
+ Novartis Pharmaceuticals Corporation
  59 Route 10 East Hanover, NJ 07936 (973)503-7500

Livshits, Boris M., MD {1962442210} IntrMd(83,RUS06)<NJ-JFKMED, NJ-HACKNSK>
+ Universal Medical Center PC
  239 Avenel Street/Suite 4 Avenel, NJ 07001 (732)602-6192   Fax (732)602-3251
  boris1960@yahoo.com
+ Universal Medical Center PC
  278 Broadway/1st Floor Elmwood Park, NJ 07407
  (732)602-6192   Fax (201)797-8916

Livshits, Larisa L., MD {1982786893} IntrMd(83,RUS06)<NJ-MTNSIDE>
+ Dr's Choice
  1082 St. George Avenue Rahway, NJ 07065 (732)388-4787   Fax (732)388-4380
+ Med-Care of Fairfield, Inc.
  150 Fairfield Road Fairfield, NJ 07004 (973)227-0020

Livstone, Barry J., MD {1295737682} Radiol, RadDia(97,PA12)
+ Radiology Associates of Burlington County
  1295 Route 38 West/PO Box 379 Hainesport, NJ 08036
  (609)261-7017   Fax (609)261-4180

Liwag, Alexander J., MD {1235102575} Pedtrc(98,PHI15)
+ 1079 Roseberry Court
  Morganville, NJ 07751

Lizardo Escano, Therese L., MD {1952792368}
+ 165 Parlin Lane
  Watchung, NJ 07069 (908)757-2149

Lizarraga, Liza Isabel, MD {1518328731} ObsGyn
+ 100 Franklin Street/Apt D206
  Morristown, NJ 07960 (347)449-4758

Lizerbram, Deborah Garber, DO {1295769115} FamMed(85,WV75)
+ Osborn Family Health Center
  1601 Haddon Road Camden, NJ 08103 (856)757-3700
  Fax (856)365-7972

Ljubich, Paul, MD {1578630281} Gastrn(86,NY19)<NJ-ACMCITY, NJ-ACMCMAIN>
+ Jersey Shore Gastroenterology
  108 North Main Street Cape May Court House, NJ 08210
  (609)465-0060
+ Jersey Shore Gastroenterology
  408 Bethel Road/Suite E Somers Point, NJ 08244
  (609)465-0060   Fax (609)926-8578

Llacuna, Florencio, Jr., MD {1710047733} IntrMd(80,PHI10)<NJ-STMRYPAS>
+ 1100 Clifton Avenue/Suite A
  Clifton, NJ 07013 (973)594-8444   Fax (973)773-4491
  Fllacuna@yahoo.com

Llarena, Ramon C., MD {1902858079} EmrgMd, IntrMd(71,PHIL)<NJ-CHRIST>
+ American Physician Services/Hudson HealthCare
  679 Montgomery Street Jersey City, NJ 07306 (201)433-6500   Fax (201)433-8010
+ Christ Hospital
  176 Palisade Avenue Jersey City, NJ 07306 (201)795-8200

Llenado, Jeanne Valencia, DO {1306862602} Surgry, Urolgy(95,NJ75)
+ Cherry Hill Primary and Specialty Care
  457 Haddonfield Road/Suite 110 Cherry Hill, NJ 08002
  (844)542-2273   Fax (856)406-4570

Lloyd, John Mervyn, MD {1457328866} SrgOrt, SprtMd(71,ENGL)<NJ-HACKNSK>
+ Bergen Orthopaedic Surgery and Sports Medicine
  221 Old Hook Road Westwood, NJ 07675 (201)666-0013
  Fax (201)666-0123

Llull Tombo, Rolando, MD {1841562014} IntrMd<NJ-JRSYSHMC>
+ Meridian Medical Associates, P.C.
  1945 Route 33 Neptune, NJ 07753 (732)776-2963   Fax (732)776-3795
  rllulltombo@meridianhealth.com

Lo, Abraham, DO {1568703023} IntrMd<NJ-PALISADE>
+ Palisades Medical Center
  7600 River Road North Bergen, NJ 07047 (510)551-6732

Lo, Hung-Tien, MD {1669518858} Gyneco, ObsGyn(65,TAIW)<NJ-HACKNSK>
+ 211 Essex Street
  Hackensack, NJ 07601 (201)489-3335   Fax (201)599-8971

Lo, Kathy Kai Yee, MD {1306065479} RadOnc, IntrMd(02,PA02)
+ Sparta Cancer Center
  89 Sparta Avenue/Suite 130 Sparta, NJ 07871 (570)504-7210   Fax (570)955-2213
+ Hackettstown Regional Medical Center
  651 Willow Grove Street/Rad Onc Hackettstown, NJ 07840
  (570)504-7210   Fax (908)441-1164

Lo, Pak-Kan A., MD {1780760694} RadDia, Radiol(85,NJ05)<NJ-HCKTSTWN>
+ Hackettstown Regional Medical Center
  651 Willow Grove Street/Radiology Hackettstown, NJ 07840 (908)852-5100   Fax (908)850-6840

Lo, Vivian S., MD {1144381872} ObsGyn(77,PA02)
+ 1553 Route 27/Suite 3500
  Somerset, NJ 08873 (732)828-0102   Fax (732)828-0406
+ Women first Health Center
  520 Pleasant Valley Way West Orange, NJ 07052
  (732)828-0102   Fax (973)669-5722

Lo Buono, Philip J., MD Dermat(71,NJ05)<NJ-JRSYSHMC>
+ 211 Highway 71
  Spring Lake, NJ 07762 (732)499-0167   Fax (732)449-2357
  plobuonomd@verizon.net

Lo Faro, Joseph Rocco, MD {1841282381} EmrgMd(92,DOM17)<NJ-TRINIWSC>
+ Trinitas Regional Medical Center-Williamson Street
  225 Williamson Street/EmrgMed Elizabeth, NJ 07207
  (919)425-1565   Fax (919)425-0478

Lo Presti, Nicholas P., MD {1588790760} Dermat(96,PA02)
+ Dermatology Physicians of South Jersey, P.A.
  112 White Horse Pike Haddon Heights, NJ 08035
  (856)546-5353   Fax (856)546-8711

Lo Verde, Lauren S., MD RadDia, Radiol(87,PA07)<NJ-STFRNMED>
+ Radiology Affiliates of Central New Jersey, P.A.
  2501 Kuser Road Hamilton, NJ 08691 (609)585-8800
  Fax (609)585-1825
+ St. Francis Medical Center
  601 Hamilton Avenue Trenton, NJ 08629 (609)599-5000

Lob, Zev B., DO {1053607820} EmrgMd<NJ-STJOSHOS>
+ St Joseph's Medical Center Emergency
  703 Main Street Paterson, NJ 07503 (973)754-2240   Fax (973)754-2249

Lobel, Gregg P., MD {1679522791} Anesth, PedAne(92,NY47)<NJ-ENGLWOOD>
+ Englewood Hospital and Medical Center
  350 Engle Street/Acute Care Englewood, NJ 07631
  (201)894-3322   Fax (201)871-0619

Lobraico, Dominick, Jr., DO {1649214404} ObsGyn(90,PA77)<NJ-MONMOUTH>
+ West Long Branch Obstetrics & Gynecology
  1019 Broadway West Long Branch, NJ 07764 (732)229-6797   Fax (732)229-6893
+ West Long Branch Obstetrics & Gynecology
  911 East County Line Road/Suite 201 Lakewood, NJ 08701
  (732)364-9299

Locastro, Rosemary H., MD {1952307613} Radiol, RadNuc(75,NY09)<NJ-RWJUHAM>
+ Quakerbridge Radiology Associates
  8 Quakerbridge Plaza/Building 8 Mercerville, NJ 08619
  (609)890-0033   Fax (609)689-6067

Locatelli, Sam Thomas, MD {1932320736} ObsGyn(83,NY09)<NJ-MORRISTN, NJ-STCLRDEN>
+ Total Health Phy Med & Rehab Center
  171 Ridgedale Avenue/Suite A Florham Park, NJ 07932
  (973)377-6327   Fax (973)408-9055

Lockwood, Curtis L., DO {1750380713} Surgry(84,IA75)<NJ-MEMSALEM>
+ General Vascular Surgical Specialists PA
  66 East Avenue Woodstown, NJ 08098 (856)935-2750
  Fax (856)935-0105

Locurcio, Gennaro E., MD {1033286562} FamMed, Hmpthy, Acpntr(76,ITAL)<NY-BETHPETR, NY-STBARNAB>
+ 610 Third Avenue
  Elizabeth, NJ 07202 (908)351-1333   Fax (908)351-3740

Locurto, John, Jr., MD {1487697371} Surgry, SrgCrC(77,ITA01)<NJ-HACKNSK>
+ North Jersey Trauma & Critical Care Associates
  5 Summit Avenue/Suite 105 Hackensack, NJ 07601
  (551)996-2900

Lodhavia, Devang V., MD {1679570634} Nephro, IntrMd(98,INA21)
+ Advocare Nephrology of South Jersey
  300 Sheppard Road Voorhees, NJ 08043 (856)424-7390
  Fax (856)424-7386
+ Advocare Nephrology of South Jersey
  740 Marne Highway/Suite 206 Moorestown, NJ 08057
  (856)424-7390   Fax (856)424-7386
+ Advocare Nephrology of South Jersey
  777 Route 70 East/Suite G101 Marlton, NJ 08043
  (856)424-7390   Fax (856)424-7386

Lodhavia, Jitendra J., MD {1225013600} IntrMd, IntMAdMd(68,INA69)<NJ-HACKNSK>
+ 71 Summit Avenue/Ground Floor
  Hackensack, NJ 07601 (201)488-4420   Fax (201)488-7570

Lodish, Stephanie Renee, MD {1578530267} Pedtrc(96,OH06)
+ Madison Pediatrics
  435 South Street/Suite 200 Morristown, NJ 07960
  (973)822-0003   Fax (973)822-3349

Loeb, Debra M., MD {1760400675} RadDia, Radiol(88,NJ06)<NJ-CENTRAST>
+ Freehold Radiology Group
  901 West Main Street Freehold, NJ 07728 (732)462-4844

Loeb, Paul Norman, DO {1770526048} ObsGyn, Gyneco, IntrMd(83,PA77)<NJ-CHSMRCER, NJ-RWJUBRUN>
+ Lawrence Ob/Gyn Associates
  123 Franklin Corner Road/Suite 214 Lawrenceville, NJ 08648 (609)896-1400   Fax (609)896-3986

Loesberg, Andrew C., MD {1063487726} RadDia, Radiol, RadV&I(89,NJ06)<NJ-HUNTRDN>
+ Hunterdon Medical Center
  2100 Wescott Drive/Radiology Flemington, NJ 08822
  (908)788-6100
+ Hunterdon Radiological Associate
  1 Dogwood Drive Clinton, NJ 08809 (908)788-6100   Fax (908)735-6532
+ Kings Court Imaging Center
  2 Kings Court/Suite 200 Flemington, NJ 08822 (908)806-8600   Fax (908)806-8646

Loesberg, Perry A., MD {1760407670} Anesth(90,DC01)<NJ-STFRNMED>
+ St. Francis Medical Center
  601 Hamilton Avenue/Anesthesiology Trenton, NJ 08629
  (609)599-5140   Fax (609)599-6312

Loewenstein, Robert Elvin, MD {1750475687} EmrgMd(96,NJ05)<NJ-CHRIST>
+ Emergency Medical Associates of NJ, P.A.
  3 Century Drive Parsippany, NJ 07054 (973)740-0607
  Fax (973)740-9895

Loewinger, Lee E., MD {1407939606} IntrMd, CdvDis(03,PA02)
+ 7 Ditzel Farm Court
  Scotch Plains, NJ 07076 (908)347-9756   Fax (908)654-6778

Loewinger, Michael Brian, MD {1477703007} IntrMd(08,PA09)
  + Primary Care NJ
    370 Grand Avenue/Suite 102   Englewood, NJ 07631
    (908)403-2476   Fax (201)816-1265
Lofrumento, Mary Ann, MD {1811194434} Pedtrc(81,PA01)<NJ-MORRISTN>
  + Morristown Medical Center
    100 Madison Avenue/Pediatrics   Morristown, NJ 07962
    (973)971-8686   Fax (973)292-5173
Lofton, Azieb Ghebremedhin, DO {1144229303} ObsGyn(96,NY75)<NJ-MEMSALEM>
  + Westwood Womens Health Center
    600 Jessup Road   West Deptford, NJ 08066   (856)845-4061
    Fax (856)812-2880
Loftus, Frances Ellen, DO {1851381438} PulDis, CritCr, IntrMd(98,NY75)<NJ-ACMCMAIN, NJ-ACMCITY>
  + Atlantic Pulmonary & Critical Care Associates, P.A.
    741 South Second Avenue/Suite A   Galloway, NJ 08205
    (609)748-7300   Fax (609)748-7919
Loftus, James B., MD {1235275504} Anesth(85,NY08)
  + Ocean Endosurgery Center
    129 Route 37 West   Toms River, NJ 08755   (732)606-4440
    Fax (732)797-3963
Logan, Joseph James, DO {1841203775} Anesth(02,PA77)<NY-LAWRENCE>
  + Summit Medical Group-Berkeley Heights Campus
    1 Diamond Hill Road   Berkeley Heights, NJ 07922
    (908)273-4300   Fax (908)790-6576
Loghman-Adham, Mahmoud, MD {1043594120} PedNph(74,FRA26)
  + Hoffman-La Roche Incorporated
    340 Kingsland Street   Nutley, NJ 07110   (973)562-2127
    Fax (908)647-1082
Loghmanee, Cyrus Faz, MD {1831365303} SrgPlstc
  + East Coast Advanced Plastic Surgery
    79 Hudson Street/Suite 700   Hoboken, NJ 07030
    (201)449-1000   Fax (201)399-2433
Logothetis, George Nicholas, MD {1619966223} CdvDis, IntrMd(82,VA01)
  + Cranbury Heart and Lung Associates
    283 Applegarth Road   Monroe, NJ 08831   (609)655-1046
    Fax (609)655-3830
  + 3401 Market Street
    Cranbury, NJ 08512   (609)655-1046
Logothetis, James Nicholas, MD {1740279124} IntrMd, PulDis(77,NJ06)
  + Cranbury Heart and Lung Associates
    283 Applegarth Road   Monroe, NJ 08831   (609)655-1046
    Fax (609)655-3830
LoGrasso, Paul Peter, DO {1134118029} Pthlgy, PthAcl(83,NY75)
  + Diagnostic Pathology Consults
    101 Carnie Boulevard   Voorhees, NJ 08043   (856)325-3170
    Fax (856)325-3164
  + Diagnostic Pathology Consults
    175 Madison Avenue   Mount Holly, NJ 08060   (856)325-3170   Fax (609)261-3751
Loguda, Charles A., MD {1093734113} SrgPlstc, IntrMd(86,NJ05)<NJ-RWJURAH, NJ-OVERLOOK>
  + Associates in Plastic & Aesthetic Surgery
    955 South Springfield Avenue/Suite 105   Springfield, NJ 07081   (908)654-6540   Fax (908)654-6504
  + Associates in Plastic & Aesthetic Surgery
    33 Overlook Road/Suite 411   Summit, NJ 07901   (908)522-0880
  + Associates in Plastic & Aesthetic Surgery
    27 Mountain Boulevard/Suite 9   Warren, NJ 07081
    (908)561-0080
Logue, Raymond J., MD {1376564716} IntrMd(PA13<NJ-COOPRUMC>
  + Cooper University Hospital
    One Cooper Plaza/Hospitalist   Camden, NJ 08103
    (856)342-2000
Loguidice, Vito A., MD {1902893605} SrgOrt, SrgSpn, IntrMd(81,NY15)<NJ-WARREN>
  + Coordinated Health
    222 Red Lane   Phillipsburg, NJ 08865   (610)861-8080   Fax (610)849-1013
Logvinenko, Andrei V., MD {1952348195} PhysMd(81,RUSS)<NJ-ENGLWOOD>
  + Medicine & Rehabilitation, PC
    14-25 Plaza Road/Suite S31   Fair Lawn, NJ 07410
    (201)797-2050   Fax (201)797-2051
Logvinenko, Nina V., MD {1275570335} IntrMd(81,RUSS)<NJ-ENGLWOOD>
  + Medicine & Rehabilitation, PC
    14-25 Plaza Road/Suite S31   Fair Lawn, NJ 07410
    (201)797-2050   Fax (201)797-2051
Loh, Chun Kyu, MD {1598771370} SrgThr, Surgry, IntrMd(68,MN04)<NJ-HOLYNAME>
  + 200 Grand Avenue/Suite 204
    Englewood, NJ 07631   (201)568-8411   Fax (201)568-5357
    chun.loh@mountsinai.org

Loh, Shi, MD {1114009388} IntrMd, OncHem(75,TAI07)<NJ-STMRYPAS>
  + 109 Grand Street/Unit 201
    Hoboken, NJ 07030   (201)659-9027   Fax (201)659-7943
Lohwin, Peter G., MD {1356390280} SrgOrt(82,NJ05)
  + 29 Newton Avenue
    Branchville, NJ 07826   (201)400-6867
Loizidis, Giorgos, MD {1982044277} Rheuma
  + 493 Laurel Oak Road/Suite 130
    Voorhees, NJ 08043   (856)741-0122   Fax (856)741-0121
Lojun, Sharon Lee, MD {1710960216} ObsGyn, GynOnc, IntrMd(88,NY20)
  + AtlantiCare Clinical Associates
    2500 English Creek Avenue   Egg Harbor Township, NJ 08234
    (609)407-2310
Lokchander, Rangaswamy S., MD {1154460269} Gastrn, IntrMd(78,INDI)
  + Ocean Endosurgery Center
    129 Route 37 West   Toms River, NJ 08755   (732)606-4440
    Fax (732)797-3963
Lolis, Margarita Sophia, MD {1881913713}
  + Skin Laser & Surgery Specialists
    20 Prospect Avenue/Suite 702   Hackensack, NJ 07601
    (201)441-9890   Fax (201)441-9893
Loman, Eric, DO {1952662140} Nephro
  + 1617 Route 88 West/Suite 101
    Brick, NJ 08724   (732)458-1903   Fax (732)458-1906
Loman, Jeannette A., DO {1134327109} IntrMd<NJ-OCEANMC>
  + Ocean Medical Center
    425 Jack Martin Boulevard   Brick, NJ 08723   (732)840-2200
Lomax, Kathleen Graham, MD {1356336960} Pedtrc, PedGst, IntrMd(94,TX12)<NY-PRSBCOLU>
  + Just for Kids
    8 Meadowbrook Road   Short Hills, NJ 07078   (973)376-5430   Fax (973)376-5430
  + One Health Plaza
    Basking Ridge, NJ 07920   (862)778-7643
Lomazow, Steven M., MD {1306887880} Nrolgy(76,IL42)<NJ-CLARMAAS, NJ-OVERLOOK>
  + 50 Newark Avenue/Suite 104
    Belleville, NJ 07109   (973)751-5643   Fax (973)751-1322
Lombardi, Adriana, MD {1689938805} Dermat
  + Affiliated Dermatologists
    182 South Street/Suite 1   Morristown, NJ 07960   (973)936-1802   Fax (936)695-1480
  + Advanced Laser & Skin Cancer Center
    870 Palisade Avcenue/Suite 302   Teaneck, NJ 07666
    (973)936-1802   Fax (201)836-4716
Lombardi, Anthony Stephen, Jr., MD {1932259462} SrgPlstc, Surgry(90,NJ05)<NJ-RIVERVW, NJ-JRSYSHMC>
  + Lombardi Plastic Surgery Center
    32 Corbett Way   Eatontown, NJ 07724   (732)460-9555
    Fax (732)460-0699
Lombardi, David D., MD {1144368358} IntrMd(91,NJ06)<NJ-RWJUBRUN, NJ-CENTRAST>
  + Drs. Lombardi & Shetty
    1001 Route 9 North/Suite 106   Howell, NJ 07731
    (732)886-9122   Fax (732)886-5161
Lombardi, Frank T., DO {1437255858} FamMed(03,NY75)
  + Village Medical Center
    207 Strykers Road   Phillipsburg, NJ 08865   (908)859-6568
    Fax (908)859-6697
Lombardi, Joseph S., MD {1801943998} SrgOrt(78,NJ05)<NJ-JFKMED>
  + Edison-Metuchen Orthopedic Group
    10 Parsonage Road/5th Floor/Suite 500   Edison, NJ 08837
    (732)494-6226   Fax (732)494-8762
Lombardi, Joseph V., MD {1184644700} Surgry
  + Cooper Surgical Associates
    3 Cooper Plaza/Suite 411   Camden, NJ 08103   (856)342-2270   Fax (856)365-1180
Lombardi, Paul A., Jr., MD {1679660435} SrgOrt(93,NY46)<NJ-MORRISTN>
  + Tri-County Orthopedics
    160 East Hanover Avenue   Morristown, NJ 07962
    (973)538-2334   Fax (973)829-9174
Lombardi, Robert M., MD {1396892485} SrgHnd, SrgOrt(79,NJ06)<NJ-JFKMED>
  + Edison-Metuchen Orthopedic Group
    10 Parsonage Road/5th Floor/Suite 500   Edison, NJ 08837
    (732)494-6226   Fax (732)494-8762
Lombardi, Susan L., MD {1255371258} EmrgMd, IntrMd(92,NJ05)
  + The Doctors Office Urgent Care
    556 Passaic Avenue   West Caldwell, NJ 07006   (973)808-2273   Fax (973)808-2287
Lombardino, Anthony N., MD {1295861870} Nrolgy(72,NJ05)<NJ-KIMBALL>
  + Kimball Medical Center
    600 River Avenue   Lakewood, NJ 08701   (732)886-4630

Lombardo, Sabato J., MD {1629188495} CdvDis, IntrMd(79,NJ06)<NJ-UMDNJ, NJ-TRINIWSC>
  + Union Medical Associates PA
    1308 Morris Avenue/Suite 101   Union, NJ 07083
    (908)687-8686   Fax (908)687-9694
  + NJ Heart/Elizabeth Office
    240 Williamson Street/Suite 402-406   Elizabeth, NJ 07202
    (908)687-8686   Fax (908)354-0007
Lombardo, Salvatore Antonio, MD {1760440903} Urolgy(00,PA01)
  + Essex Hudson Urology
    256 Broad Street   Bloomfield, NJ 07003   (973)743-4450
    Fax (973)429-9076
  + Essex Hudson Urology
    243 Chestnut Street   Newark, NJ 07105   (973)743-4450
    Fax (973)344-9188
Lombardy, Elyane Emilienne, MD {1992968697} Hemato, IntrMd(70,BEL07)
  + 14 Tillou Road West
    South Orange, NJ 07079   (973)327-4633   Fax (973)327-4633
Lomnitz, Esteban R., MD {1992797740} CdvDis, IntrMd(63,CHIL)
  + Medical Diagnostic Associates, P.A.
    1801 East Second Street/Suite 1   Scotch Plains, NJ 07076
    (908)322-7786   Fax (908)322-0191
  + MedDiag Assocs/Central NJ Cardiology
    1511 Park Avenue/Suite 2   South Plainfield, NJ 07080
    (908)322-7786   Fax (908)756-9160
Lomonaco, Jesse V., DO {1750314274} IntrMd, NeuMus(71,PA77)
  + Garden State Medical Associates
    100 Brick Road/Suite 209   Marlton, NJ 08053   (856)983-2848   Fax (856)985-7645
London, Eric Bart, MD {1144237835} Addctn, Psychy(78,NY09)
  + 42 West Main Street
    Holmdel, NJ 07733   (609)921-0332   Fax (609)921-0339
  + Hunterdon Developmental Center
    40 Pittstown Road/PO Box 4003   Clinton, NJ 08809
    (609)921-0332   Fax (908)730-1338
Long, Ashley Nicole, DO {1043645633} ObsGyn<NJ-SJHREGMC>
  + SJH Regional Medical Center
    1505 West Sherman Avenue   Vineland, NJ 08360
    (856)641-8000
Long, George W., MD {1952360273} IntrMd, Acpntr(84,CHN4D)<NJ-RWJURAH>
  + Qualcare Medi-Center, P.A.
    2 Lincoln Highway/Suite 411   Edison, NJ 08820   (732)396-0777   Fax (732)396-9222
Long, Jessie C., MD {1881871531} Pedtrc(07,PA02)<CT-HOSPSTRA>
  + PediatriCare Associates
    20-20 Fair Lawn Avenue   Fair Lawn, NJ 07410   (201)791-4545   Fax (201)791-3765
Longo, Stacey L., MD {1184799223} PthAcl(93,NJ05)<NJ-BAYSHORE>
  + Bayshore Community Hospital
    727 North Beers Street   Holmdel, NJ 07733   (732)739-5900
Longobardi, Raphael S., MD {1588688303} SprtMd, SrgOrt(90,NY19)<NJ-HACKNSK, NJ-HOLYNAME>
  + University Orthopaedic Center, PA
    433 Hackensack Avenue/Second Floor   Hackensack, NJ 07601   (201)343-1717   Fax (201)343-3217
Longson, Audrey Eve, DO {1841458221} Psychy(07,IL76)
  + Center for Family Guidance, PC
    765 East Route 70/Building A-101   Marlton, NJ 08053
    (856)797-4800   Fax (856)810-0110
Longworth-Gatto, Lisa E., DO {1922276278} Anesth, PainMd(91,NY75)<NY-NASSAUMC>
  + Tri-County Orthopedics
    160 East Hanover Avenue   Morristown, NJ 07962
    (973)538-2334   Fax (973)538-4072
Lontai, Peter, MD {1821192030} IntrMd(78,MEX03)
  + 76 Elmora Avenue
    Elizabeth, NJ 07202   (908)289-4227   Fax (908)289-8871
Loo, Abraham, MD {1578733473} PthAcl
  + Laboratory Medicine Associates, PA
    300 Second Avenue/Dept of Pathology   Long Branch, NJ 07740   (732)923-7352   Fax (732)923-7355
Loo, Deborah, MD {1003012956}<NJ-BAYSHORE>
  + Bayshore Community Hospital
    727 North Beers Street   Holmdel, NJ 07733   (732)739-5900
  + Perth Amboy Anesthesiology PC
    530 New Brunswick Avenue   Perth Amboy, NJ 08861
    (732)739-5853
Lopatynsky, Marta O., MD {1437146560} Ophthl, CrnExD(86,NY03)<NJ-MORRISTN, NJ-BAYONNE>
  + Eyecare MD of New Jersey
    261 James Street/Suite 2-D & 3EL   Morristown, NJ 07960
    (973)984-3937   Fax (973)984-0059
Lopes, Francis, MD {1144318858} FamMed, IntrMd(78,MEX03)<NJ-VIRTVOOR, NJ-OURLADY>
  + 141 South White Horse Pike
    Audubon, NJ 08106   (856)547-8415   Fax (856)547-2438

Physicians by Name and Address

Lopes, James M., MD {1861659476} Surgry, SrgGst, Bariat(04,NY46)<NJ-TRINIWSC, NJ-OVERLOOK>
+ Advanced Surgical Associates LLC
  155 Morris Avenue/2nd Floor   Springfield, NJ 07081   (973)232-2300   Fax (973)232-2301
+ Overlook Medical Center
  99 Beauvoir Avenue/PO Box 210   Summit, NJ 07902   (908)522-2000
+ Trinitas Regional Medical Center-Williamson Street
  225 Williamson Street   Elizabeth, NJ 07081   (908)994-5000

Lopes, Joanne Elizabeth, MD {1679618664} Pedtrc(99,PA09)<NJ-VIRTUAHS>
+ Advocare Cornerstone Pediatrics
  318 North Haddon Avenue/Suite A   Haddonfield, NJ 08033   (856)428-3746   Fax (856)310-0312

Lopes, Joao Alberto, MD {1043268378} SrgCrC, Surgry(98,DMN01)<NJ-OVERLOOK, NJ-TRINIJSC>
+ Advanced Surgical Associates LLC
  155 Morris Avenue/2nd Floor   Springfield, NJ 07081   (973)232-2300   Fax (973)232-2301

Lopes, Melissa M., MD {1003050519} PedAne, IntrMd(04,NJ06)<NJ-MORRISTN>
+ Morristown Medical Center
  100 Madison Avenue/Pedi Anesth   Morristown, NJ 07962   (201)943-5831   Fax (201)943-8733

Lopez, Aurelia P., MD {1528018652} Surgry(78,PHI02)<NJ-STPETER>
+ St. Peter's University Hospital
  254 Easton Avenue/Surgery   New Brunswick, NJ 08901   (732)745-8600

Lopez, Christina Clare, DO {1093973695} Pedtrc
+ Robert Wood Johnson Hospital Pediatrics
  One Robert Wood Johnson Place   New Brunswick, NJ 08901   (732)812-7516
  ccl76@rwjms.rutgers.edu

Lopez, Claudio J., MD {1457365470} Pedtrc(86,DOM16)<NJ-JRSYSHMC, NJ-CENTRAST>
+ Pediatric Health, PA
  4537 Route 9 North   Howell, NJ 07731   (732)367-5717   Fax (732)367-6524
+ Pediatric Health, P.A.
  470 Stillwells Corner Road   Freehold, NJ 07728   (732)367-5717   Fax (732)780-6968
+ Pediatric Health, PA
  23 Kilmer Drive/Building 1 Suite B   Morganville, NJ 07731   (732)972-0900   Fax (732)972-2892

Lopez, David Vincent, MD {1629021399} SrgOrt, SprtMd, IntrMd(99,NJ05)<NJ-BAYSHORE, NJ-RIVERVW>
+ Orthopaedic and Sports Medicine Specialists, Inc.
  200 White Road/Suite 1-C   Little Silver, NJ 07739   (732)888-2100   Fax (732)888-2188

Lopez, Divina Elizabeth, MD {1649598046} Pedtrc, IntrMd(06,DMN01)
+ Children of Joy Pediatrics
  134 Summit Avenue   Hackensack, NJ 07601   (201)525-0077   Fax (201)525-0072

Lopez, Gerardo J., MD {1558337543} ObsGyn(82,MEX09)<NJ-COMMED>
+ Toms River Ob-Gyn Associates PA
  79 Route 37 West/Suite 101   Toms River, NJ 08755   (732)244-9444   Fax (732)244-9468

Lopez, Hector L., Jr., MD {1346446077} PhysMd
+ Northeast Spine & Sports Medicine
  1104 Arnold Avenue   Point Pleasant Beach, NJ 08742   (732)714-0070   Fax (732)714-0188

Lopez, John Pedro Francisco, MD {1255430179} IntrMd, Pedtrc, EmrgMd(96,NY03)<NJ-STPETER>
+ The DoctorsÆ Office Urgent Care of Brick, NJ
  686 Route 70   Brick, NJ 08723   (732)262-8200

Lopez, Jose M., MD {1427150846} IntrMd
+ Eastern Vascular Associates
  16 Pocono Road/Suite 313   Denville, NJ 07834   (973)625-0112   Fax (973)625-0721

Lopez, Juan, MD {1497821250} CdvDis, IntrMd(76,SPA03)<NJ-HOBUNIMC>
+ 35 West Main Street/Suite 101
  Denville, NJ 07834   (201)864-1414
  Juanl3@aol.com

Lopez, Leonardo Nicholas, DO {1588686570} Pedtrc(99,FL75)<NJ-CENTRAST, NJ-JRSYSHMC>
+ Pediatric Health, P.A.
  69 West Main Street   Freehold, NJ 07728   (732)409-3633   Fax (732)409-7133
+ Pediatric Health, P.A.
  470 Stillwells Corner Road   Freehold, NJ 07728   (732)409-3633   Fax (732)780-6968
+ Pediatric Health, PA
  4537 Route 9 North   Howell, NJ 07728   (732)367-5717   Fax (732)367-6524

Lopez, Lina Maria, MD {1861593881} Psychy(94,COL15)
+ Valley Medical Group
  70 Park Avenue   Park Ridge, NJ 07656   (201)930-0900

Fax (201)391-7733

Lopez, Lisa M., MD {1972572394} Pedtrc(00,IL11)
+ Henry J. Austin Health Center
  321 North Warren Street   Trenton, NJ 08618   (609)278-5900   Fax (609)695-3532
+ Passaic Pediatrics PA
  298 Passaic Street   Passaic, NJ 07055   (609)278-5900   Fax (973)249-8110

Lopez, Nicole Melisa Montero, MD {1982999140} SrgOrt
+ Andover Orthopaedic Surgery & Sports
  280 Newton-Sparta Road/Suite 4   Newton, NJ 07860   (973)579-7443   Fax (973)579-5628
+ Premier Health Associates
  89 Sparta Avenue/Suite 100   Sparta, NJ 07871   (973)579-7443   Fax (973)729-3454

Lopez Bernard, Edwin, MD {1730147901} Pedtrc(98,DMN01)<NJ-ACMCMAIN, NJ-ACMCITY>
+ AtlantiCare Special Care Center
  1401 Atlantic Avenue/Suite 2500   Atlantic City, NJ 08401   (609)572-8686   Fax (609)572-6033
+ Mainland Pediatric Association
  741 South Second Avenue/Suite B   Galloway, NJ 08205   (609)572-8686   Fax (609)748-6700

Lopez Canino, Jorge, MD {1184813149}
+ 602 Sargent Road
  River Vale, NJ 07675

Lopez-Allen, Gabriela D., MD Pedtrc(83,PHI08)<NJ-STJOSHOS>
+ 1033 Tabor Road
  Morris Plains, NJ 07950   (973)605-8900

Lopez-Maslak, Edna Retiracion, MD {1396716767} Pedtrc, IntrMd(84,PHI09)<NJ-WESTHDSN>
+ West Hudson Division of Clara Maass Medical Center
  206 Bergen Avenue/Pediatrics   Kearny, NJ 07032   (973)743-0202   Fax (973)743-0777
  erlmaslak@hotmail.com
+ Bloomfield Pediatrics, P.A.
  329 Belleville Avenue/Suite 2   Bloomfield, NJ 07003   (973)743-0202   Fax (973)743-0777

Lopresti, David A., MD {1629012869} Anesth, PainMd, Anes-Pain(87,PA13)<NJ-OURLADY>
+ Reconstructive Orthopedics, P.A.
  570 Egg Harbor Road/Suite C-4   Sewell, NJ 08080   (609)267-9400   Fax (609)267-9457
+ Our Lady of Lourdes Medical Center
  1600 Haddon Avenue   Camden, NJ 08103   (856)757-3839

Lopyan, Kevin S., MD {1114086527} Surgry, SrgVas(82,NJ05)<NJ-MONMOUTH, NJ-BAYSHORE>
+ 142 State Route 35 South/Suite 102-A
  Eatontown, NJ 07724   (732)935-9393   Fax (732)935-0101

Lorber, Julie A., MD {1225245947} SrgC&R, Surgry(OH43)
+ Julie A. Lorber MD PC
  33 Overlook Road/Suite 306   Summit, NJ 07901   (908)273-2886   Fax (908)273-2882
  dr.lorber@gmail.com

Lore, Abigail Leah, MD {1124325063}<NJ-STPETER>
+ St. Peter's University Hospital
  254 Easton Avenue   New Brunswick, NJ 08901   (732)828-0002   Fax (732)828-0153

Lore, Kristen Nicole, DO {1063770568} ObsGyn(NY75)
+ Meridian Medical Group
  514 Bangs Avenue   Asbury Park, NJ 07712   (732)774-0200   Fax (732)774-1019
+ Hackensack Meridian Medical Group Ob/Gyn, Freehold
  3499 Route 9 North/Suite 2B   Freehold, NJ 07728   (732)774-0200   Fax (732)577-8922

Loren, Gary M., MD {1427086040} Anesth, PainInvt(84,PA12)
+ Anesthesia Pain Treatment Center
  1666 Hamilton Avenue/Suite 2   Hamilton, NJ 08629   (609)584-9080   Fax (609)584-0139

Lorenc, Ronald B., MD {1275649691} Otlryg, Otolgy(68,NY09)<NJ-SJERSYHS>
+ 225 Laurel Heights Drive
  Bridgeton, NJ 08302   (856)451-7121   Fax (856)451-7174

Lorenzetti, John D., MD {1568401644} SrgVas, Surgry(81,GRNA)<NJ-ACMCITY, NJ-ACMCMAIN>
+ 2500 English Creek Avenue/Suite 223
  Egg Harbor Township, NJ 08234   (609)677-0088   Fax (609)677-9004

Lorenzo, Judith, MD {1558623181} Pedtrc
+ Ocean Health Initiatives, Inc.
  101 Second Street   Lakewood, NJ 08701   (732)363-6655   Fax (732)363-6656
+ Ocean Health Initiatives, Inc.
  301 Lakehurst Road   Toms River, NJ 08755   (732)363-6655   Fax (732)552-0378
+ Ocean Health Initiatives, Inc.
  333 Haywood Road   Manahawkin, NJ 08701   (609)489-0110   Fax (609)489-0171

Loreti, Michael Earl, MD {1851384283} IntrMd, SprtMd(84,GRN01)
+ Orthopedic Spine and Sports Medicine Center
  2 Forest Avenue   Paramus, NJ 07652   (201)587-1111   Fax (201)587-8192

Lortie, Charles Frederic, MD {1457798134} Dermat(MT01)
+ Affiliated Dermatologists
  182 South Street/Suite 1   Morristown, NJ 07960   (973)267-0300   Fax (973)695-1480

Lorton, Julie Lytton, MD {1073875159} IntrMd
+ Endocrinology Consultants P.C.
  229 Engle Street   Englewood, NJ 07631   (201)678-9995   Fax (201)567-5385

Lory, John Douglas, MD {1750365110} Anesth(93,PA14)
+ 30 River Court/Apt. 2607
  Jersey City, NJ 07310

Losack, Glenn Mark, MD {1689839995} Psychy(81,DOM02)
+ Princeton House Behavioral Health - North Brunswick
  1460 Livingston Avenue   North Brunswick, NJ 08902   (732)435-0202   Fax (732)435-0222

Losada, Mariela, MD {1437142171} PthAna(90,VEN04)
+ Inform Diagnostics
  825 Rahway Avenue   Union, NJ 07083   (732)901-7575   Fax (732)901-1555

Losardo, Anthony A., MD {1982625182} CdvDis, IntrMd(77,NY46)<NJ-VALLEY, NJ-COMMED>
+ Cardiology Associates LLC
  999 McBride Avenue/Suite B-204   West Paterson, NJ 07424   (973)256-5667   Fax (973)256-7758
+ Cardiology Associates LLC
  181 Franklin Avenue/Suite 301   Nutley, NJ 07110   (973)256-5667   Fax (973)667-0561

Losik, Steve Boleslav, MD {1689758567} RadDia(01,MD01)
+ 105 Mountainside View
  Morganville, NJ 07751

Losman, Jacques G., MD {1063552016} SrgThr, SrgVas(68,BEL07)
+ 151 Brentwood Drive
  South Orange, NJ 07079

Losos, Roland Jerzy, MD {1124282033} IntrMd, Grtrcs(92,POL06)
+ Primary Care Physicians Inc.
  155 Park Avenue/Suite 206   Lyndhurst, NJ 07071   (201)933-4700

Lospinuso, Michael Frank, MD {1760461172} SrgOrt, SrgSpn(81,WIND)<NJ-MERIDNHS, NJ-JRSYSHMC>
+ Orthopaedic Institute of Central Jersey
  365 Broad Street   Red Bank, NJ 07701   (732)359-5777   Fax (732)933-0389
  lospinmf@aol.com
+ Orthopaedic Institute of Central Jersey
  2315A Highway 34/Suite D   Manasquan, NJ 08736   (732)359-5777   Fax (732)449-4271
+ Orthopaedic Institute of Central Jersey
  3499 Route 9 North   Freehold, NJ 07701   (732)863-4790   Fax (732)863-4791

Lotan, Roi Meir, MD {1518175637} RadDia(02,IL02)<NJ-STPETER, NJ-RWJUBRUN>
+ University Radiology Group, P.C.
  483 Cranbury Road   East Brunswick, NJ 08816   (732)390-0030   Fax (732)390-5383

Lotano, Ramya, MD {1780766410} CritCr, IntrMd, PulDis(93,GRN01)<NJ-COOPRUMC>
+ Cooper University Medical Center/Camden
  3 Cooper Plaza/Suite 312   Camden, NJ 08103   (856)342-2000   Fax (856)541-3968

Lothe, Prakash S., MD {1164451043} Pedtrc(69,INA00)<NJ-RIVERVW, NJ-MONMOUTH>
+ Pediatric Associates of Shrewsbury PA
  175 Patterson Avenue   Shrewsbury, NJ 07702   (732)741-3280   Fax (732)741-9450

Lotkowski, Susan D., DO {1992738470} Nrolgy(01,PA77)<NJ-MEMSALEM>
+ 95 Woodston Road/Suite D
  Swedesboro, NJ 08085   (856)241-0113   Fax (856)241-1455

Lott, Jason Pelham, MD {1639303373} Dermat(09,PA01)
+ Bayer HealthCare
  100 Bayer Boulevard   Whippany, NJ 07981   (862)404-3000

Lott, Kristen Ellie, MD {1780733667} RadDia(04,NC07)
+ South Jersey Radiology Associates, P.A.
  100 Carnie Boulevard/Suite B-5   Voorhees, NJ 08043   (856)751-0123   Fax (856)751-0535
+ South Jersey Radiology Associates, P.A.
  6650 Browning Road/Suite M14   Pennsauken, NJ 08109   (856)751-0123   Fax (856)661-0686
+ South Jersey Radiology Associates, P.A.
  315 Route 70 East/Suite B   Cherry Hill, NJ 08043   (856)428-4344   Fax (856)428-0356

Lou, William, MD {1306930920} Gastrn, IntrMd(79,NJ06)<NJ-CHSFULD, NJ-RWJUHAM>
+ Ahmad Syed S MD PA
  183 Franklin Corner Road   Lawrenceville, NJ 08648   (609)896-0622   Fax (609)896-0069
+ Drs. Ahmad and Lou
  1607 South Broad Street   Trenton, NJ 08610   (609)393-1870

Loubeau-Magnet, Helene, DO {1902058639} FamMed, IntrMd(05,NY75)<NJ-UNDRWD>
+ Complete Care Family Medicine
75 West Red Bank Avenue   Woodbury, NJ 08096   (856)904-3513   Fax (856)241-3315

Loughlin, Bruce T., DO {1932289899} IntrMd(82,PA77)<NJ-WAY-NEGEN>
+ Wedgewood Primary Care
1055 Hamburg Turnpike/Suite 300   Wayne, NJ 07470   (973)904-1177   Fax (973)904-1166

Loughlin, Jacquelyn S., MD {1720187347} ObsGyn, RprEnd, Frt-Inf(75,NY09)<NJ-HACKNSK, NJ-UMDNJ>
+ University Reproductive Associates, PC
214 Terrace Avenue/2nd Floor   Hasbrouck Heights, NJ 07604   (201)288-6330   Fax (201)288-6331
+ Rutgers- New Jersey Medical School
185 South Orange Avenue   Newark, NJ 07103   (201)288-6330   Fax (973)972-4574

Loughlin-Pherribo, Donna Joyce, DO {1881650703} FamMed(92,PA77)
+ AtlantiCare Family Medicine
120 South White Horse Pike   Hammonton, NJ 08037   (609)561-4211   Fax (609)561-0639

Loughran, Katy, MD {1255853156} PhysMd
+ 740 Marne Highway/Suite 203
Moorestown, NJ 08057   (856)914-1400   Fax (856)914-1444

Louie, Beth G., MD {1205802055} Allrgy, PedAlg, AlgyImmn(75,NY46)<NY-STANTHNY>
+ Warwick Allergy
1 Sears Drive/Fourth Floor   Paramus, NJ 07652   (201)599-0123

Louie, Gina Lin, MD {1093760266} RadDia, RadV&I(88,CA11)<NJ-MONMOUTH>
+ Monmouth Medical Center
300 Second Avenue/Vasc&IntervenRa   Long Branch, NJ 07740   (732)222-5200

Louie, Pearl Maria, MD {1477698355} Psychy(98,NY48)
+ Moreines & Goldman PC
577 Westfield Avenue   Westfield, NJ 07090   (908)232-6566   Fax (908)232-6628

Louis, Marie Edwige, MD {1265472484} FamMed(01,PA09)<NJ-COOPRUMC>
+ Cooper Family Medicine
110 Marter Avenue   Moorestown, NJ 08057   (856)608-8840   Fax (856)722-1898
+ Cooper Family Medicine
1001-F Lincoln Drive West   Marlton, NJ 08053   (856)608-8840   Fax (856)810-1879

Louis, Vely Anthony, MD {1114168382} Anesth
+ Rutgers- New Jersey Medical School
185 South Orange Avenue   Newark, NJ 07103   (973)972-0470

Louis-Jacques, Jocelyne, MD {1306979323} Pedtrc, AdolMd(78,MA05)<NJ-NWRKBETH>
+ 742 Clinton Avenue
Newark, NJ 07108   (973)372-3400

Louissaint, Paraclet S., MD {1164519179} GenPrc, Pedtrc(79,MEX28)<NJ-MEADWLND>
+ Lyons Medical Center LLC
669 Elizabeth Avenue/Partner   Newark, NJ 07112   (973)923-6452   Fax (973)923-1979

Louissaint, Valerie, MD {1578084448} Pedtrc
+ 240 Osborne Terrace
Newark, NJ 07112   (201)320-0464

Louka, Magda F., DO {1013238591}
+ Mountainside Family Practice Associates
799 Bloomfield Avenue/Suite 201   Verona, NJ 07044   (973)746-7050   Fax (973)857-2831

Loutfi, Rania H., MD {1265443618} IntHos, IntrMd(99,LEB01)<NJ-COOPRUMC>
+ Cooper University Hospital
One Cooper Plaza/Hospitalist   Camden, NJ 08103   (856)342-2000

Louvier, Ambra, MD {1679574636} Anesth(82,DC01)
+ 36 Tulane Place
Lincoln Park, NJ 07035

Lovallo, Gregory G., MD {1467515775} Urolgy(01,NJ05)
+ New Jersey Center for Prostate Cancer & Urology
255 West Spring Valley Avenue   Maywood, NJ 07607   (201)487-8866   Fax (201)487-2602
+ New Jersey Center for Prostate Cancer & Urology
200 South Orange Avenue/Suite 228   Livingston, NJ 07039   (201)487-8866   Fax (973)322-0135

Love, Amy Girdler, MD {1841202660} Psychy, IntrMd(88,CT02)
+ Meford Leas
1 Medford Leas Way/Suite 435   Medford, NJ 08055   (609)367-4929   Fax (855)329-1309
amy.lovemd@comcast.net

Love, Larrisha, MD {1477917250} IntrMd
+ University Hospital Medicine
150 Bergen Street/Room I-248   Newark, NJ 07103   (201)895-0502   Fax (973)972-3129

Love, Margaret M., MD {1457523045} PedEmg(05,PA13)
+ 530 Terhune Street
Teaneck, NJ 07666

Love, Thomas Pierce, MD {1114946241} EmrgMd(00,PA02)<NJ-UNDRWD>
+ Inspira Health Network
509 North Broad Street/EmergMed   Woodbury, NJ 08096   (856)845-0100

Loveland-Jones, Catherine Elizabeth, MD {1295996361} SrgBst
+ MS Anderson Cancer Center Cooper
One Cooper Plaza/BreasrSrgy   Camden, NJ 08103   (610)653-3660

Lovenheim, Jay Alon, DO {1770642035} Pedtrc(03,NY75)<NJ-STBARNMC>
+ 173 South Orange Avenue/Suite 1-B
South Orange, NJ 07079   (973)762-3835   Fax (973)762-5538

Loveridge-Lenza, Beth Anne, DO {1043404312} PedGst, Pedtrc(04,NY75)<NJ-JRSYSHMC>
+ Meridian Medical Group - Faculty Practice
61 Davis Avenue/Suite 1   Neptune, NJ 07753   (732)776-4860   Fax (732)776-4867

Loverme, Paul J., MD {1871584029} SrgCsm, SrgRec, SrgBst(78,NJ05)<NJ-MTNSIDE, NJ-STBARNMC>
+ Advanced Aesthetics-Plastic Surgery Center
825 Bloomfield Avenue/Suite 205   Verona, NJ 07044   (973)857-9499   Fax (973)857-9453
drloverme@advanced-aesthetics.com

Lovoulos, Constantinos John, MD {1720268584} Surgry, SrgThr(87,GRE03)<NJ-UMDNJ>
+ University Hospital
150 Bergen Street/Surgery   Newark, NJ 07103   (973)972-3555   Fax (973)972-3510

Low, Ronald Brian, MD {1821086224} Otlryg, Otolgy, SrgHdN(69,IL42)<NJ-HACKNSK>
+ Bergen Ear Nose & Throat Associates PA
20 Prospect Avenue/Suite 909   Hackensack, NJ 07601   (201)489-6520   Fax (201)489-6530
+ Hackensack University Medical Center
30 Prospect Avenue/Otolaryngology   Hackensack, NJ 07601   (201)996-2000

Lowe, Daniel Robert, MD {1932373578} Urolgy(02,NY46)<NJ-HACKNSK, NJ-HOLYNAME>
+ New Jersey Urology, LLC
20 Prospect Avenue/Suite 915   Hackensack, NJ 07601   (201)343-0082   Fax (201)488-1203
+ New Jersey Urology
6 Brighton Road/Suite 108   Clifton, NJ 07012   (201)343-0082   Fax (973)337-1330

Lowe, James G., MD {1528163607} SrgNro(89,PA13)<NJ-ACMC-ITY, NJ-ACMCMAIN>
+ Lowe-Greenwood-Zerbo Spinal Associates
1999 New Road/Suite B   Linwood, NJ 08221   (609)601-6363   Fax (609)601-6364

Lowe, John William, DO {1720233059} FamMed
+ Drs. Zalut and Lowe
1000 White Horse Road/Suite 806   Voorhees, NJ 08043   (856)770-0022   Fax (856)770-9194

Lowe, Samantha B., DO {1447484050} ObsGyn
+ Brescia-Migliaccio Ob/Gyn
609 Washington Street   Hoboken, NJ 07030   (201)659-7700   Fax (201)659-7701

Lowe, William J., III, MD {1831155241} ObsGyn(89,NJ06)
+ Access Obstetrics and Gynecology
190 Greenbrook Road   North Plainfield, NJ 07060   (908)756-6812   Fax (908)756-2525
+ Neighborhood Health Center Plainfield
1700-58 Myrtle Avenue   Plainfield, NJ 07060   (908)756-6812   Fax (908)226-6743
+ St. Peter's Family Health
123 How Lane   New Brunswick, NJ 07060   (732)745-8600   Fax (732)729-0869

Lowell, Barry H., MD {1780735563} CdvDis(82,NY48)<NJ-MOR-RISTN>
+ Morris Heart Associates PA
400 Valley Road/Suite 102   Mount Arlington, NJ 07856   (973)770-7899   Fax (973)770-7840

Lowenstein, Jason E., MD {1932130317} SrgSpn
+ Tri-County Orthopedics
160 East Hanover Avenue   Morristown, NJ 07962   (973)538-2334   Fax (973)829-9174

Lowenstein, Michael Aaron, DO {1629211297} FamMed
+ MedExpress Urgent Care Lodi
184 Essex Street   Lodi, NJ 07644   (201)843-3207   Fax (201)843-3215

Lowenthal, Dennis A., MD {1528050374} MedOnc, IntrMd(79,MA05)<NJ-OVERLOOK>
+ Medical Diagnostic Associates, P.A.
99 Beauvoir Avenue   Summit, NJ 07901   (908)608-0078   Fax (908)608-1504

Lowry, Steven James, MD {1871558783} Surgry, SrgC&R(91,PA07)
+ Ocean Colon & Rectal Surgery
1163 Route 37 West/Building D-2   Toms River, NJ 08753   (732)557-6430

Lowry, Steven Michael, DO {1285637223} FamMed(96,NJ75)
+ Pine Street Family Practice
220 East Pine Street   Williamstown, NJ 08094   (856)629-7436   Fax (856)875-4742

Loya, David Michael, MD {1194794388} SrgOrt(89,IL02)<NJ-STBARNMC>
+ Center for Orthopaedics
1500 Pleasant Valley Way/Suite 101   West Orange, NJ 07052   (973)669-5600   Fax (973)669-0269

Lozano, Rolando, MD {1134195514} Pedtrc, IntrMd(80,PER01)<NJ-STBARNMC, NJ-OVERLOOK>
+ Springfield Pediatrics
190 Meisel Avenue   Springfield, NJ 07081   (973)467-1009   Fax (973)467-7836
+ Springfield Pediatrics
435 Elmora Avenue   Elizabeth, NJ 07208   (973)467-1009   Fax (908)659-9210
+ Springfield Pediatrics
939 Park Avenue   Plainfield, NJ 07081   (908)226-5445   Fax (908)226-5481

Lozito, Deborah A., DO {1134251945} IntrMd(87,PA77)<NJ-VALLEY>
+ Lozito Medical Associates
484 Lafayette Avenue   Hawthorne, NJ 07506   (973)423-4770   Fax (973)423-4816

Lozito, Joseph A., Jr., DO {1821120692} FamMed(77,PA77)<NJ-VALLEY>
+ Lozito Medical Associates
484 Lafayette Avenue   Hawthorne, NJ 07506   (973)423-4770   Fax (973)423-4816

Lozner, Jerrold S., MD {1194714451} SrgThr, SrgVas, Surgry(71,KY02)<NJ-OVERLOOK, NJ-MORRISTN>
+ Summit Medical Group-Berkeley Heights Campus
1 Diamond Hill Road/Grnd Fl   Berkeley Heights, NJ 07922   (908)277-8770   Fax (908)790-6524

Lozovatsky, Michael, MD {1750897880} Psychy
+ 516 Cherry Street/Apt 5D
Elizabeth, NJ 07208   (203)668-2221
+ Veterans Affairs Department Outpatient Clinic
654 East Jersey Street   Elizabeth, NJ 07206   (203)668-2221   Fax (908)994-0131

Lozowski, Thomas E., DO {1104897354} FamMed(97,PA77)<NJ-OCEANMC>
+ Drs. DiChiara and Lozowski
2446 Church Road/Suite 10   Toms River, NJ 08753   (732)255-3636   Fax (732)864-0176

Lu, Andrew Hong, MD {1356890560} IntrMd
+ 318 West Grand Street/Apt 305
Elizabeth, NJ 07202   (510)316-9245

Lu, Brian D., MD MedOnc(00,NY46)
+ 59 Unami Terrace
Westfield, NJ 07090

Lu, Cheh Shiung, DO {1144370057} Anesth, AnesPain(81,WV75)
+ 3 Doris Drive West
Cherry Hill, NJ 08003
Cheh_lu@yahoo.com

Lu, Michael T., MD {1851532600} SrgOrt
+ Garden State Bone & Joint Specialists
1000 Route 9 North/Suite 306   Woodbridge, NJ 07095   (732)283-2663   Fax (732)283-2661

Lu, Phoebe Do, MD {1841495546} Dermat(06,NY19)<NY-VAHAR-BOR>
+ Advanced Dermatology, Laser, and MOHS Surgery Center
240 East Grove Street   Westfield, NJ 07090   (908)232-6446   Fax (908)232-6447

Lu, Rebecca Yun-ru, MD {1144483116} Dermat, IntrMd(05,TX04)
+ Elite Skin
7 Mount Bethel Road/Suite C   Warren, NJ 07059   (908)787-8088   Fax (908)368-8648
+ Advanced Laser & Skin Cancer Center
870 Palisade Avcenue/Suite 302   Teaneck, NJ 07666   (908)787-8088   Fax (201)836-4716

Lu, Sam Chuan, MD {1164803284} EmrgEMed
+ Hackensack Medical Center Emergency Medicine
30 Prospect Avenue/Main 3619   Hackensack, NJ 07601   (551)996-2331   Fax (201)968-1866

Lu, Stanley, MD {1326095688} RadDia, RadNro(99,NY19)<NJ-MONMOUTH>
+ Shrewsbury Diagnostic Imaging, Inc.
1131 Broad Street/Suite 110   Shrewsbury, NJ 07702   (732)578-9640   Fax (732)578-9650

Lu, Ya-Tseng W., MD {1134162431} Anesth, PainMd(86,NJ06)<NY-CMCSTVSI>
+ Anesthesia Consultnts of NJ/Nova Pain
285 Davidson Avenue/Suite 204   Somerset, NJ 08873   (732)271-1400   Fax (732)271-3543

Physicians by Name and Address

Luan, Jennifer X., MD {1588735690} Pedtrc(91,CHN1J)<NJ-CHSM-RCER, NJ-JRSYCITY>
+ Capital Health System/Mercer Campus
446 Bellevue Avenue/Pediatrics   Trenton, NJ 08618
(609)394-4000

Luayon, Joseph Palac, DO {1417999202} IntHos(MO78<NJ-NWT-NMEM>
+ Internal Medicine Consultants
765 State Route 10 East/Suite 201   Randolph, NJ 07869
(973)975-4830   Fax (732)271-1022

Lubansky, Kenneth P., MD {1699749937} IntrMd, PulDis(76,NJ05)<NJ-CHILTON>
+ Atlantic Medical Group
2025 Hamburg Turnpike/Suite D   Wayne, NJ 07470
(973)839-5070   Fax (973)839-0084

Lubas, Andrew S., MD {1932282092} FamMed(83,NJ06)<NJ-STMRYPAS>
+ 379 Ridge Road
North Arlington, NJ 07031   (201)246-0200   Fax (201)246-0668

Lubat, Edward, MD {1396732624} Radiol, NuclMd(82,PA02)<NJ-VALLEY>
+ Radiology Associates of Ridgewood, P.A.
20 Franklin Turnpike   Waldwick, NJ 07463   (201)445-8822   Fax (201)447-5053
+ The Valley Hospital
223 North Van Dien Avenue/Radiology   Ridgewood, NJ 07450   (201)447-8210

Lubin, Hank, MD {1881652691} IntrMd(83,NJ06)<NJ-UNVM-CPRN>
+ Hightstown Medical Associates
186 Princeton Hightstown Road   West Windsor, NJ 08550
(609)443-1150   Fax (609)799-9005

Lubin-Baskin, Alicia F., DO {1801880570} FamMed, IntrMd(90,IA75)<NY-STATNSTH>
+ Avenel Iselin Medical Group
400 Gill Lane   Iselin, NJ 08830   (732)404-1580   Fax (732)404-1594

Lubitz, Sara Elisabeth, MD {1568667855} IntrMd, EnDbMt(03,NJ05)<NJ-RWJUBRUN>
+ University Medical Group - General Internal Medicine
125 Paterson Street/Suite 5100A   New Brunswick, NJ 08903
(732)235-7219   Fax (732)235-8610
lubitzsa@umdnj.edu

Lubkin, Cary L., MD {1083650899} EmrgMd, IntrMd(82,PA02)<NJ-COOPRUMC>
+ Cooper University Hospital
One Cooper Plaza/EemrgMed   Camden, NJ 08103
(856)342-2000

Lublin, Jennifer Caryn, MD {1396710885} ObsGyn, IntrMd(95,NY19)
+ Lifeline Medical Associates
530 Morris Avenue   Springfield, NJ 07081   (973)379-7477   Fax (973)379-9094
lublinj@gmail.com

Lucanie, Anabel, MD {1295736577} IntrMd(86,PRO01)<NJ-VALLEY>
+ Valley Diagnostic Medical Center
581 North Franklin Turnpike   Ramsey, NJ 07446   (201)327-0500   Fax (201)327-8612

Lucanie, Richard, MD {1669473898} IntrMd(88,NY08)<NJ-VALLEY>
+ Valley Diagnostic Medical Center
581 North Franklin Turnpike   Ramsey, NJ 07446   (201)327-0500   Fax (201)327-8612

Lucarelli, Elizabeth Ann, MD {1730381377} ObsGyn(03,PA02)
+ Morristown Medical Center
100 Madison Avenue   Morristown, NJ 07962   (973)971-5000

Lucas, Gem-Estelle Maun, DO {1053496224} Psychy(03,ME75)<NJ-UNIVBHC>
+ Psychiatric Associates of Hunterdon
190 Route 31/Suite 100   Flemington, NJ 08822   (908)788-6654   Fax (908)788-6452

Lucas, Lisa W., DO {1104156769} FamMed(ME75
+ Family Practice of CentraState
901 West Main Street/Suite 106   Freehold, NJ 07728
(732)462-0100   Fax (732)462-0348

Lucas, Michael Joseph, MD {1952315053} Pedtrc(95,NJ06)<NJ-STPETER>
+ St. Peters Pediatric Faculty
123 How Lane   New Brunswick, NJ 08901   (732)745-8419   Fax (732)220-0659

Lucas, Robin S., MD {1841286697} PulDis, CritCr(83,WIND)
+ RWJPE Chest & Intensive Care Medicine
35 Clyde Road/Suite 105   Somerset, NJ 08873   (732)873-9682   Fax (732)873-9683

Lucas, Romeo Augusto, DO {1154576072} ObsGyn
+ Hackensack Meridian Medical Group Ob/Gyn, Freehold
3499 Route 9 North/Suite 2B   Freehold, NJ 07728
(732)577-1199   Fax (732)577-8922

Lucasti, Christopher J., DO {1467447417} InfDis(86,PA77)<NJ-SHOREMEM, NJ-ACMCITY>
+ South Jersey Infectious Disease
730 Shore Road   Somers Point, NJ 08244   (609)927-6662
Fax (609)927-2942

Lucatorto, Anthony J., DO {1760443030} FamMed(92,NY75)<NJ-STCLRDEN, NJ-STCLRDOV>
+ Morris Sussex Family Practice
694 Route 15 South/Suite 103   Lake Hopatcong, NJ 07849
(973)663-8899   Fax (973)663-9511
msfp694@aol.com

Lucciola, Marion, MD {1326361163} Pedtrc(94,ITA01)
+ Kidz Doctor, LLC
11 Overlook Road/Suite 170   Summit, NJ 07901   (908)277-4480   Fax (908)277-4482
+ Cranford Pediatrics
19 Holly Street   Cranford, NJ 07016   (908)277-4480   Fax (908)276-0040

Lucciola, Pompeo Almerico, MD {1659318061} Pedtrc, EmrgMd(94,ITA01)<NJ-OVERLOOK>
+ Summit Medical Group
1 Diamond Hill Road/Bensley Pav/2 FL   Berkeley, NJ 07922
(908)277-8601   Fax (908)277-8706
+ Overlook Medical Center
99 Beauvoir Avenue/PO Box 210   Summit, NJ 07902
(908)277-8601   Fax (908)522-0227

Lucco, Julianne M., MD {1164496147} FamMed(96,NY45)<NJ-HUNTRDN>
+ Delaware Valley Family Health Center
200 Frenchtown Road   Milford, NJ 08848   (908)995-2251
Fax (908)995-2036
+ Hunterdon Medical Center
2100 Wescott Drive/FamilyMed   Flemington, NJ 08822
(908)788-6100

Luceri, Michael Joseph, Jr., DO {1538362371} Pedtrc
+ St Christopher Hospital for Children
100 Kings Way East   Sewell, NJ 08080   (856)582-0644

Luceri, Patricia Marie, DO {1538367198} EnDbMt, IntrMd(07,NJ75)
+ Stratford - Endocrinology
25 East Laurel Road   Stratford, NJ 08084   (856)783-2664
Fax (856)783-8537

Lucerna, Alan Rey Nicolo, DO {1023214178}
+ SOM - Department of Internal Medicine
42 East Laurel Road/Suite 3100   Stratford, NJ 08084
(856)566-6859   Fax (856)566-6906

Lucev, Anthony, MD {1235561796} IntCdTpl
+ 233 Harmon Avenue
Fort Lee, NJ 07024   (201)886-2354

Lucia Ricci, Jodie Italia, MD {1770659005} Ophthl(01,NJ06)<NJ-STBARNMC>
+ Associates in Eye Care
155 Morris Avenue/Suite 302   Springfield, NJ 07081
(973)232-6900   Fax (973)232-6912

Luciani, Richard L., MD {1689789935} ObsGyn(76,NJ05)<NJ-OVERLOOK, NJ-STBARNMC>
+ Millburn Ob-Gyn Associates, P.A.
233 Millburn Avenue   Millburn, NJ 07041   (973)467-9440
Fax (973)376-1680
+ Short Hills Surgery Center
187 Millburn Avenue/Suite 101   Millburn, NJ 07041
(973)467-9440   Fax (973)671-0557

Luciano, Dominick T., MD {1508965237} Anesth(76,NY19)<NJ-RWJURAH>
+ Robert Wood Johnson University Hospital at Rahway
865 Stone Street   Rahway, NJ 07065   (732)381-4200

Luciano, Lisa A., DO {1659392157} PhysMd(91,PA77)<NJ-JFKJHNSN>
+ Shore Rehabilitation Institute
425 Jack Martin Boulevard   Brick, NJ 08724   (732)836-4530
Fax (732)836-4531

Luciano, Pasquale A., DO {1861441966} SrgThr, Surgry(88,PA77)<NJ-OURLADY, NJ-VIRTUAHS>
+ Virtua Surgical Group, PA
1935 Route 70 East   Cherry Hill, NJ 08003   (856)428-7700
Fax (856)424-9120

Lucila, Rafael R., MD {1659318483} FamMed(85,PHIL)
+ Lucila Medical P.C.
780 Allwood Road   Clifton, NJ 07012   (973)249-6202   Fax (973)249-6203

Luckey, Marjorie M., MD {1902800568} EnDbMt, IntrMd(73,GA01)<NJ-STBARNMC>
+ The Osteoporosis and Metabolic Bone Disease Center
200 South Orange Avenue   Livingston, NJ 07039   (973)322-7430   Fax (973)322-7460

Lucking, Jonathan, MD {1366889545} Surgry
+ Associated Colon & Rectal Surgeons PA
3900 Park Avenue/Suite 101   Edison, NJ 08820   (732)494-6640   Fax (732)549-8204

Ludmer, Philip R., MD {1497716435}
+ Princeton Anesthesia Services PC
153 Witherspoon Street   Princeton, NJ 08540

Ludwig, David Aaron, MD {1457855512} PhysMd
+ 1999 New Road/Suite C
Linwood, NJ 08221   (609)601-6140   Fax (609)601-6141

Ludwig, Shelly L., MD {1801860937} Gastrn, IntrMd(74,NY46)<NJ-CENTRAST>
+ 901 West Main Street/MAB/Suite 106
Freehold, NJ 07728   (732)303-3888   Fax (732)414-2292

Ludwig-Cilento, Mary Beth, DO {1235286188} FamMed(89,PA77)<NJ-COMMED, NJ-SOCEANCO>
+ Fischer Family Medicine
1191 Fischer Boulevard   Toms River, NJ 08753   (732)506-7888   Fax (732)506-7766

Ludwin, Fredrick B., DO {1629025218} EmrgMd(81,IA75)<NJ-VIRTVOOR>
+ Emergency Physician Associates, P.A.
307 South Evergreen Avenue/PO Box 298   Woodbury, NJ 08096   (856)848-3817   Fax (856)848-1431
+ Virtua Voorhees
100 Bowman Drive/EmergMed   Voorhees, NJ 08043
(856)247-3000

Lue, Deborah A., MD {1669699823} Surgry(93,NJ05)<NJ-JFKMED>
+ 201 Union Avenue/Suite A-1
Bridgewater, NJ 08807   (908)575-0880   Fax (908)575-0898

Luetke, Brian Scott, DO {1619998481} Anesth
+ Rancocas Anesthesiology, PA
700 Route 130 North/Suite 203   Cinnaminson, NJ 08077
(856)829-9345   Fax (856)829-3605
+ 48 Fox Run Drive
Mount Laurel, NJ 08054

Luff, Ronald David, MD {1336352822} PthACl(73,MD07)<PA-SCRDHRT>
+ Quest Diagnostics Inc.
1 Malcolm Avenue   Teterboro, NJ 07608   (201)393-6007
Fax (201)462-4772

Lugo, Javier J., MD {1508940057} Pedtrc, AdolMd(81,NY46)<NJ-CHILTON>
+ Chilton Medical Center
97 West Parkway   Pompton Plains, NJ 07444   (973)831-5121   Fax (973)831-5458

Lugo, Maria D., MD {1669488375} FamMed, IntrMd(PRO01)
+ Capital Health Primary Care-Bordentown
1 Third Street   Bordentown, NJ 08505   (609)298-2005
Fax (609)815-7814

Lugo, Mirian Dolores, MD {1114127404} Pedtrc(99,PAR01)<NJ-STJOSHOS>
+ L & L Pediatrics
344 Clifton Avenue   Clifton, NJ 07011   (973)435-4545
Fax (973)928-1899
info @ llpeds.com

Luhana, Manish P., MD {1558347641} IntrMd(99,DMN01)
+ Drs. Luhana, Dhirmalani & Patel
239 Baldwin Road/Suite 108   Parsippany, NJ 07054
(973)334-2265   Fax (973)335-9091

Lui, Gene Sing, DO {1669496535} Psychy(02,NY75)<NJ-WARREN>
+ 10 Midland Avenue
Glen Ridge, NJ 07028

Lui, Jackie Zhuojun, MD {1912326810} Pedtrc<NJ-CHDNWBTH>
+ Children's Hospital of New Jersey
201 Lyons Avenue/Osborne Terrace   Newark, NJ 07112
(973)926-7471

Lui, John, MD {1407836364} Anesth(92,MO34)
+ Englewood Anesthesiology
350 Engle Street   Englewood, NJ 07631   (201)894-3238
Fax (201)894-0585
jlui@englewoodhospital.com

Luisi-Purdue, Linda, MD {1427129477} ObsGyn(87,NJ05)<NJ-STBARNMC>
+ Associates in Obstetrics Gynecology & Infertility
375 Mount Pleasant Avenue/Suite 202   West Orange, NJ 07052   (973)731-7707   Fax (973)669-0277
+ Associates in Obstetrics Gynecology & Infertility PA
825 Bloomfield Avenue/Suite 103   Verona, NJ 07044
(973)239-5010

Lujan, Juan Jose, MD {1376777599} SrgThr
+ Strafford Surgical Specialists, P.A.
1100 Route 72 West/Suite 303   Manahawkin, NJ 08050
(609)978-3325   Fax (609)978-3123
+ Monmouth Surgical Specialists
727 North Beers Street   Holmdel, NJ 07733   (609)978-3325
Fax (732)290-7067

Luka, Norman L., MD {1376574129} SrgCdv, SrgThr, Surgry(69,NY45)
+ Overlook Medical Center Wound Healing Center
11 Overlook Road/MAC II, Suite LL 101   Summit, NJ 07901
(908)522-5900   Fax (908)522-5544

Luka, Richard Edward, MD {1447329198} Allrgy, IntMAImm(89,MA05)
+ Consultants in Asthma, Allergy and Immunology
22 Shaw Street   Garfield, NJ 07026   (973)478-5550   Fax (973)478-2290

Physicians by Name and Address

Lukac, Juraj, MD {1013179365} PsyCAd(93,CZE15)
+ Princeton House Behavioral Health - North Brunswick
1460 Livingston Avenue North Brunswick, NJ 08902 (732)435-0202 Fax (732)435-0222

Luke, Brian T., MD {1881826303} ObsGyn(09,NJ05)
+ Tenafly Ob-Gyn Associates PA
2 Dean Drive/2nd Floor Tenafly, NJ 07670 (201)569-3300 Fax (201)569-7649

Luke, Ofure R., MD {1851710784} PhysMd<NJ-JFKJHNSN>
+ JFK Johnson Rehabilitation Institute
65 James Street Edison, NJ 08818 (732)321-7070 Fax (732)321-7330

Luke, Steven, MD {1972597268} FamMed, Pedtrc(82,NY15)<NJ-OVERLOOK, NJ-STBARNMC>
+ Union Pediatric Medical Group, PA
1050 Galloping Hill Road/Suite 200 Union, NJ 07083 (908)688-9900 Fax (908)688-9939

Lukenda, Kevin, DO {1467407759} FamMed(89,NJ75)<NJ-JFKMED>
+ Linden Family Medical Associates
850 North Wood Avenue Linden, NJ 07036 (908)925-9309 Fax (908)925-7910

Lukenda, Robert A., DO {1144470600} FamMed
+ Overlook Family Medicine
33 Overlook Road/Suite 103 Summit, NJ 07901 (908)522-5700 Fax (908)273-8014

Lukof, Amanda Rose, MD {1518223023}<NJ-MONMOUTH>
+ Monmouth Medical Center
300 Second Avenue Long Branch, NJ 07740 (732)222-5200

Luksch, John Richard, DO {1144583188}
+ University Hospital-University Family Medicine
42 East Laurel Road/Suite 2100 Stratford, NJ 08084 (856)566-6477 Fax (856)566-6360

Lum, Kenneth, MD {1033176243} Anesth(82,NY08)
+ Ambulatory Anesthesia Care, PC
1450 Route 22 West Mountainside, NJ 07092 (908)233-2020 Fax (908)233-9322

Lumezanu, Elena Mihaela, MD {1255700858} Rheuma, IntrMd(03,ROM01)
+ Arthritis & Osteoporosis Associates, P.A.
4247 US Highway 9/Building 1 Freehold, NJ 07728 (732)780-7650 Fax (732)780-8817

Lumia, Francis J., MD {1780857631} IntrMd, UtlRQA(67,IL02)<NJ-DEBRAHLC>
+ Deborah Heart and Lung Center
200 Trenton Road Browns Mills, NJ 08015 (609)893-6611 Fax (609)735-1859
lumiaf@deborah.org

Luna, Evangeline A., MD {1881782472} IntrMd, NuclMd, Car-Nuc(77,PHIL)<NJ-RBAYPERT, NJ-RBAYOLDB>
+ Raritan Bay Medical Center/Perth Amboy Division
530 New Brunswick Avenue Perth Amboy, NJ 08861 (732)324-5178 Fax (732)324-4696
+ Raritan Bay Medical Center/Old Bridge Division
One Hospital Plaza Old Bridge, NJ 08857 (732)360-1000

Luna, Luis Freddy, MD {1558453225} IntrMd(98,MA05)
+ 34A Mill Street
Paterson, NJ 07502 (973)341-3782 Fax (973)341-3783
LuisL1@aol.com

Lundberg, John L., MD {1619988169} ObsGyn, IntrMd(88,NY08)
+ Robert Wood Johnson Ob-Gyn Associates
3270 State Route 27/Suite 2200 Kendall Park, NJ 08824 (732)422-8989 Fax (732)422-4526
+ Robert Wood Johnson Ob-Gyn Associates
50 Franklin Lane/Suite 203 Manalapan, NJ 07726 (732)422-8989 Fax (732)536-7118
+ Robert Wood Johnson Ob-Gyn Associates
525 Route 70/Suite B-11 Lakewood, NJ 08824 (732)905-6466 Fax (732)905-6467

Lundholm, Joanne Katherine, MD {1366516544} FamMed(03,MA07)<NJ-SOMERSET>
+ RWJ University Hospital Somerset
110 Rehill Avenue Somerville, NJ 08876 (908)685-2200 Fax (908)685-2891

Lundy, Edward L., DO {1255378360} FamMed(77,PA77)<NJ-UNDRWD>
+ 1017 Market Street
Gloucester City, NJ 08030 (856)456-1042 Fax (856)456-8830

Lunenfeld, Ellen Beth, MD {1841402153} Nephro, IntrMd(02,NJ06)<NJ-RWJUBRUN, NJ-OVERLOOK>
+ Summit Medical Group-Berkeley Heights Campus
1 Diamond Hill Road Berkeley Heights, NJ 07922 (908)273-4300 Fax (908)790-6576
+ Summit Medical Group
95 Madison Avenue Morristown, NJ 07960 (908)273-4300 Fax (973)267-5521

Lunt, David M., MD {1205980646} FamMed(01,NJ05)
+ The Doctor Is in
59 Old Highway 22 Clinton, NJ 08809 (908)730-6363 Fax (908)730-8185

Luo, Chuying, MD {1669451274} IntrMd(88,CHN63)
+ 755 Memorial Parkway/Building 204
Phillipsburg, NJ 08865 (908)387-1001 Fax (908)387-1195

Luo, Hongxiu, MD {1710352554} EnDbMt<NJ-STPETER>
+ St. Peter's University Hospital
254 Easton Avenue New Brunswick, NJ 08901 (732)745-8600 Fax (732)745-3847

Luo, Jane He-Cong, MD {1184648800} Grtrcs(84,CHN4D)
+ VA New Jersey Health Care System at Lyons
151 Knollcroft Road Lyons, NJ 07939 (908)647-0180

Luo, Yan Mei, MD {1255713095}{DMN01}
+ Madison Family Practice
8 Shunpike Road Madison, NJ 07940 (973)377-2610 Fax (973)377-2345

Luongo, Peter A., MD {1376520940} IntrMd(89,PA02)<NJ-VALLEY, NJ-BERGNMC>
+ Valley Medical Group Internal Medicine
1 Sears Drive/Suite 202 Paramus, NJ 07652 (201)262-2333 Fax (201)262-4515

Lupa, Michael David, MD {1942485099} Otlryg
+ Becker ENT
2 Princess Road/Suite East Lawrenceville, NJ 08648 (610)303-5163 Fax (610)303-5164
+ Becker ENT
One Union Street/Suite 203 Robbinsville, NJ 08691 (610)303-5163 Fax (609)436-5741

Luparello, Paul J., MD {1053465112} IntrMd(79,MEXI)<NJ-RIVERVW>
+ Family Practice of CentraState
901 West Main Street/Suite 106 Freehold, NJ 07728 (732)462-0100 Fax (732)462-0348

Lupatkin, William L., MD {1891768156} Pedtrc(74,FL02)<NJ-MORRISTN>
+ Morristown Pediatric Associates, LLC
261 James Street/Suite 1-G Morristown, NJ 07960 (973)540-9393 Fax (973)540-1937
Wllmd@verizon.net

Lupicki, Lucyna K., MD {1669579439} PhysMd(86,POL06)<NJ-BAYSHORE>
+ Drs. Lupicki and Lupicki
200 Perrine Road/Suite 211 Old Bridge, NJ 08857 (732)553-1000 Fax (732)553-1003

Lupicki, Marek R., MD {1508967746} IntrMd(88,POL06)
+ Drs. Lupicki and Lupicki
200 Perrine Road/Suite 211 Old Bridge, NJ 08857 (732)553-1000 Fax (732)553-1003

Lupinska, Malgorzata Teresa, MD {1396791778} Pedtrc, AdolMd(88,POL02)<NJ-HACKNSK>
+ Drs. Lupinska and Rozdeba
42 Locust Avenue Wallington, NJ 07057 (973)777-0090 Fax (973)777-9424

Lupoli, Kristin Anne, MD {1154410082} FamMed(98,NJ05)<NY-STANTHNY>
+ Priority Medical Care
350 Grove Street/Suite 200 Bridgewater, NJ 08807 (908)231-0777 Fax (908)722-6031

Lupovici, Michael, MD {1922089671} Gastrn, Grtrcs, IntrMd(73,NY01)<NJ-UNVMCPRN>
+ M. Lupovici, MD PA
254 Princeton-Hightstown Road East Windsor, NJ 08520 (609)448-7200 Fax (609)448-4607
doc@lupovicimd.com
+ University Medical Center of Princeton at Plainsboro
One Plainsboro Road Plainsboro, NJ 08536 (609)497-4000

Luppescu, Neal E., MD {1548296643} Gastrn(83,NY01)<NJ-SOMERSET>
+ 10 North Gaston Avenue
Somerville, NJ 08876 (908)595-0601 Fax (908)595-0604

Lupski, Donna L., MD {1134109887} Pedtrc(86,NY19)<NJ-OVERLOOK, NJ-MORRISTN>
+ Summit Medical Group-Berkeley Heights Campus
1 Diamond Hill Road Berkeley Heights, NJ 07922 (908)277-8601 Fax (908)277-8706

Lupu, Sarah Ethel Nat, MD {1750678280} Pedtrc(10,NJ06)
+ Chestnut Ridge Pediatrics
595 Chestnut Ridge Road Woodcliff Lake, NJ 07677 (201)391-2020 Fax (201)391-0265

Lupyan, Yan, MD {1841220829} Nrolgy, PainMd(75,BLAR)<NY-NSUHFORS, NJ-RBAYOLDB>
+ 6 Cornwall Court/Suite E
East Brunswick, NJ 08816 (732)257-0003 Fax (732)651-8023

Lurakis, Michael F., DO {1437228178} IntrMd(80,PA77)<NJ-ACMCMAIN>
+ Mercy Medical Associates
1161 Route 50 Mays Landing, NJ 08330 (609)625-7116 Fax (609)625-3275
mercymedical@comcast.net

Luria, Martin J., MD {1477629301} EnDbMt, IntrMd(71,NY19)<NJ-MONMOUTH, NJ-RIVERVW>
+ 170 Morris Avenue/Suite F
Long Branch, NJ 07740 (732)222-8874 Fax (732)222-8584

Lusha, Xhelal Q., MD {1770637977} Pedtrc, GenPrc(63,MAC01)<NJ-HCMEADPS>
+ Hudson County Meadowview Psychiatric Hospital
595 County Avenue/Building 10/GP Secaucus, NJ 07094 (201)319-3660 Fax (201)319-3616

Lusk-Caceres, Christina A., DO {1992090591} FamMSIpM, FamMed, IntrMd(WV75
+ Jersey Shore Sports Medicine Center
51 Davis Avenue/Suite 51-02 Neptune, NJ 07753 (732)776-2433 Fax (732)776-4403

Lustgarten, Jonathan H., MD {1255472940} SrgNro(88,NY01)<NJ-RIVERVW, NJ-JRSYSHMC>
+ Neurosurgeons of New Jersey
121 Highway 36 West/Suite 330 West Long Branch, NJ 07764 (732)963-4631 Fax (732)870-6432
+ Neurosurgeons of New Jersey
530 Lakehurst Road/Suite 308 Toms River, NJ 08755 (732)443-1372

Lustig, Karen C., DO {1326098195} Anesth(85,PA77)
+ 2150 Center Avenue
Fort Lee, NJ 07024

Lustig, Robert Allan, MD {1275569964} RadOnc, RadThp(69,PA02)<NJ-COOPRUMC, PA-CHILDHOS>
+ 21st Century Oncology
220 Sunset Road/Suite 4 Willingboro, NJ 08046 (609)877-3064 Fax (609)877-2466

Lustig, Robert H., DO {1457394652} Gastrn(79,IA75)<NJ-SOMERSET>
+ RWJPE Bridgewater Medical Group
766 Route 202-206/Suite 1 Bridgewater, NJ 08807 (908)722-0808 Fax (908)722-7645

Lustiger, Eliyahu Y., MD {1245604198} EmrgMd(13,NJ06)
+ Robert Wood Johnson Emergency Medicine
One Robert Wood Johnson Place/MEB 104 New Brunswick, NJ 08901 (732)235-4296

Luszcz, Ronald J., DO {1902892821} FamMed(74,IA75)<NJ-NWT-NMEM>
+ Premier Health Associates
202 Route 206 North/Suite A Branchville, NJ 07826 (973)948-5577 Fax (973)728-6487
+ Premier Health Associates
89 Sparta Avenue/Suite 100 Sparta, NJ 07871 (973)948-5577 Fax (973)729-3454

Lutwin Kawalec, Malgorzata S., MD {1093946071} Anesth(01,POL13)<NJ-COOPRUMC>
+ Cooper University Hospital
One Cooper Plaza/Anesth Camden, NJ 08103 (856)968-7334 Fax (856)968-8326

Lutz, Gregory Elmar, MD {1770651044} PhysMd(88,DC02)<NY-SPCLSURG, NJ-UNVMCPRN>
+ Princeton Spine & Sports Physicians
389 Wall Street Princeton, NJ 08540 (609)683-5500 Fax (609)683-0075

Lutz, Joseph S., MD {1245370352} GenPrc, IntrMd(83,GRN01)<NJ-MORRISTN>
+ 211 South Finley Avenue
Basking Ridge, NJ 07920 (908)766-0339 Fax (908)204-9192

Lutz, Mary B., MD {1114064615} Pedtrc(87,DOMI)<NJ-MONMOUTH, NJ-RIVERVW>
+ Doctors Halas & Lutz
2130 Highway 35/Suite 214 Sea Girt, NJ 08750 (732)974-0228 Fax (732)974-7458

Lutz, Philip Edward, MD {1275539645} Anesth(84,GRN01)
+ Montclair Anesthesia Associates PC
185 Fairfield Avenue/Suite 2A West Caldwell, NJ 07006 (973)226-1230 Fax (973)226-1232

Lutzker, Letty Goodman, MD {1922043306} NuclMd, Radiol, RadDia(68,NY46)<NJ-STBARNMC>
+ St. Barnabas Medical Center
94 Old Short Hills Road/Radiology Livingston, NJ 07039 (973)322-5000

Lux, Michael S., MD {1295701688} CdvDis(77,NY19)<NJ-MORRISTN>
+ Associates in Cardiovascular Disease, LLC
211 Mountain Avenue Springfield, NJ 07081 (973)467-0005 Fax (973)912-8989

Luyber, Todd Joseph, DO {1982672960} EmrgMd<NJ-ACMCITY>
+ AtlantiCare Regional Medical Center/City Campus
1925 Pacific Avenue/8th Floor Atlantic City, NJ 08401 (609)345-4000

Lwanga, Juliet R., MD {1346587243} IntrMd(NJ02
+ Advance Hospital Care @ Somerset Medical Center
110 Rehill Avenue Somerville, NJ 08876 (908)429-5833 Fax (908)203-5970

Lyall, Jasleen Kaur, MD {1801117825} Anesth
+ Morris Anesthesia Group, PA
3799 Route 46/Suite 211 Parsippany, NJ 07054 (973)335-1122 Fax (973)335-1448

Physicians by Name and Address

Lygas, Theodore B., MD {1528117207} SrgBst, Surgry, SrgOnc(73,NJ05)<NJ-OCEANMC, NJ-JRSYSHMC>
+ Breast Surgery & Breast Oncology Associates
459 Jack Martin Boulevard   Brick, NJ 08724   (732)458-4600   Fax (732)458-3885
+ Breast Surgery & Breast Oncology Associates
901 West Main Street/Suite 102   Freehold, NJ 07728   (732)303-6310

Lyman, Neil W., MD {1619078367} IntrMd, Nephro(73,NY46)
+ Nephrological Associates, P.A.
83 Hanover Road/Suite 290   Florham Park, NJ 07932   (973)736-2212   Fax (973)736-2989
+ Nephrological Associates PA
206 Belleville Avenue   Bloomfield, NJ 07003   (973)736-2212   Fax (973)259-0396

Lynch, Barrington B., MD {1144424730} IntrMd, Grtrcs(03,DMN01)
+ 205 Morris Turnpike
Randolph, NJ 07869   (973)933-2239

Lynch, Caroline Dorothy, MD {1023242401} ObsGyn(WA04
+ University Medical Group/OBGYN
125 Paterson Street/2nd Floor   New Brunswick, NJ 08901   (732)235-7755   Fax (732)235-6650

Lynch, Claudia, MD {1114451234} Grtrcs
+ first Care Providers LLC
972 Broad Street   Newark, NJ 07102   (973)735-1231

Lynch, David J., MD {1699776781} Surgry(84,PA02)<NJ-UNDRWD>
+ General Vascular Surgical Specialists
17 West Red Bank Avenue/Suite 203   Woodbury, NJ 08096   (856)848-8242   Fax (856)384-6015

Lynch, Jeffrey R., MD {1801894837} Anesth(81,NJ05)<NJ-VIRTMARL>
+ West Jersey Anesthesia Associates
102-E Center Boulevard   Marlton, NJ 08053   (856)988-6250   Fax (856)988-6270

Lynch, Matthew Jude, MD {1609834704} SrgPlstc, SrgRec(96,NJ05)
+ 300-B Princeton Hightstown Rd
Hightstown, NJ 08520

Lynch, Roberta M., MD Radiol(78,DC02)
+ 308 Maple Avenue
Haddonfield, NJ 08033

Lynen, Richard F., MD {1093770950} ObsGyn(90,NJ06)<NJ-HUNTRDN>
+ Affiliates in Obstetrics & Gynecology, P.A.
111 Route 31/Suite 121 2nd FL Bldg B   Flemington, NJ 08822   (908)782-2825   Fax (908)782-0196
+ Affiliates in Obstetrics & Gynecology, P.A.
431 Highway 22 East   Whitehouse, NJ 08888   (908)782-2825   Fax (908)823-1640

Lyons, Andrea Elizabeth, MD {1417922188} RadDia, RadBdI(83,PA07)<NJ-HUNTRDN, NJ-RWJUHAM>
+ Hunterdon Radiological Associate
1 Dogwood Drive   Clinton, NJ 08809   (908)735-4477   Fax (908)735-6532
+ Hunterdon Medical Center
2100 Wescott Drive/Radiology   Flemington, NJ 08822   (908)788-6100
+ Kings Court Imaging Center
2 Kings Court/Suite 200   Flemington, NJ 08809   (908)806-8600   Fax (908)806-8646

Lyons, John S., MD {1972590438} RadDia(80,NY19)<NJ-BERGNMC>
+ 9 Hampton Ridge Court
Old Tappan, NJ 07675

Lyons, Patricia J., MD {1063454189} Nephro, IntrMd
+ Lyons & Chvala Nephrology Associates
730 North Broad Street/Suite 101   Woodbury, NJ 08096   (856)384-0147

Lyons, William J., MD {1831166099} IntrMd, CdvDis(92,DC01)<NJ-HACKNSK>
+ Cardiovascular Consultants of North Jersey
777 Terrace Avenue   Hasbrouck Heights, NJ 07604   (201)288-4252   Fax (201)288-7172

Lytle, Carole F., MD {1205879814} IntrMd(96,NJ06)<NJ-SOMERSET>
+ Summit Medical Group
34 Mountain Boulevard   Warren, NJ 07059   (908)561-8600   Fax (908)561-7265

Lyu, Theodore, MD {1760704803} Ophthl(09,IL42)
+ St. Mary's Eye & Surgery Center
540 Bergen Boulevard   Palisades Park, NJ 07650   (201)461-3970   Fax (201)242-9061

Ma, Manhong, MD {1164472965} Dermat, IntrMd(92,CHN62)<NJ-COMMED, NJ-KIMBALL>
+ Schweiger Dermatology
368 Lakehurst Road/Suite 201   Toms River, NJ 08755   (732)244-4700   Fax (732)731-6134

Ma, Rex Tak Chi, MD {1447270293} PhysMd(98,NY08)<NJ-VAEASTOR>
+ VA New Jersey Health Care System-East Orange Campus
385 Tremont Avenue   East Orange, NJ 07018   (973)676-1000

Ma, Van Kim, MD {1487157699}<NJ-NWRKBETH>
+ Newark Beth Israel Medical Center
201 Lyons Avenue   Newark, NJ 07112   (973)926-7471

Ma, Wei Wei, MD {1063412310} Nrolgy, ClNrPh, NeuMus(83,CHN57)<NJ-JFKMED>
+ JFK Medical Center
65 James Street/Neurology   Edison, NJ 08820   (732)321-7000   Fax (732)632-1584
+ JFK Neurosciences Institute
65 James Street/Second Floor   Edison, NJ 08818   (732)321-7000   Fax (732)632-1669

Ma, Xiaoping, MD {1912946724} Nrolgy(82,CHN76)<NJ-OURLADY>
+ Comprehensive Neurocare Associates, LLC
100 Brick Road/Suite 304   Marlton, NJ 08053   (856)988-9888   Fax (856)988-8866

Ma, Yuhua, MD {1174617179} Psychy(90,CHN59)
+ Princeton House Behavioral Health - Cherry Hill
375 North Kings Highway   Cherry Hill, NJ 08034   (856)779-2300   Fax (856)779-2988

Maaty, Mona, MD {1588891949} Psychy
+ 330 Changebridge Road/Suite 101
Pine Brook, NJ 07058   (973)832-1808

Mabagos, Jerry D., MD {1164458451} Pedtrc, EmrgMd(82,PHIL)<NJ-OCEANMC, NJ-COMMED>
+ 34 Machester Avenue/Suite 201
Forked River, NJ 08731   (609)242-5041   Fax (609)489-4835
+ Pediatric Associates of Brick
525 Route 70/Suite 1C   Brick, NJ 08723   (732)477-1186

Mabanta, Carmelita G., MD {1801879598} Pedtrc
+ 1945 Route 33
Neptune, NJ 07753

Mabanta, Ricardo Y., MD {1730130840} Nrolgy(86,PHIL)<NJ-VIRTVOOR, NJ-VIRTMARL>
+ Center for Neurologic Specialty
12000 Lincoln Drive West/Suite 204   Marlton, NJ 08053   (856)988-3444   Fax (856)988-0553   cnsllc@comcast.net
+ Center for Neurologic Specialty
1173 Beacon Avenue/Suite A   Manahawkin, NJ 08050   (856)988-3444   Fax (609)597-8848
+ Center for Neurologic Specialty
401 Young Avenue/Suite 160   Moorestown, NJ 08053   (856)291-8780   Fax (856)291-8781

Mabrouk, Hanny S., MD {1083872154} Psychy<NJ-UNIVBHC>
+ Univ Correctional HealthCare-Colpitts
Whittesey Rd & Stuyvesant Ave   Trenton, NJ 08625   (609)292-9700

Mabrouk, Tarig, MD {1285114926} IntMAdMd
+ 706 Nottinghill Lane
Hamilton, NJ 08619   (347)410-0422

Mabry, Christian Carl, MD {1063736098} Anesth
+ Robert Wood Johnson-UMDNJ Anesthesia Group
125 Paterson Street/CAB 3100   New Brunswick, NJ 08901   (732)235-7827   Fax (732)235-6131

Mabry, Myra Ann, DO {1306070719} ObsGyn
+ Womens Health Care Associates of Sussex County
135 Newton Sparta Road/Suite 201   Newton, NJ 07860   (973)383-3438   Fax (973)383-8424

Mac, Feminia C., MD {1942386966} Pedtrc, AdolMd(68,PHIL)
+ 18 Ferry Street/Suite 2
Newark, NJ 07105   (973)589-3566   Fax (973)589-1707

Mac Fadden, Wayne, MD {1558500199} Psychy(86,NY06)
+ 14 Hart Lane
Sewell, NJ 08080

Macaione, Alexander, DO {1801861307} Dermat(66,PA77)<NJ-KMHSTRAT, NJ-OURLADY>
+ Macaione and Papa Dermatology Associates
707 White Horse Road/Suite C-103   Voorhees, NJ 08043   (856)627-1900   Fax (856)627-6907

Macalintal, Rose Ann Reyes, MD {1033352950} Pedtrc(05,DMN01)
+ Children of Joy Pediatrics
134 Summit Avenue   Hackensack, NJ 07601   (201)525-0077   Fax (201)525-0072

Macaluso, Charles F., MD {1447385901} IntrMd(71,ITA01)<NJ-STJOSHOS, NJ-WAYNEGEN>
+ Dayspring-Macaluso, MDs
516 Hamburg Turnpike/Suite 5   Wayne, NJ 07470   (973)790-8604   Fax (973)790-1488

MacBride, David G., DO {1992753198} EmrgMd(02,NJ75)<NJ-ACMCITY>
+ AtlantiCare Regional Medical Center/City Campus
1925 Pacific Avenue/EmrgMed   Atlantic City, NJ 08401   (609)345-4000

MacBruce, Daphne Karen, MD {1780966937} CritCr
+ St. Michael's Medical Center
111 Central Avenue   Newark, NJ 07102   (973)877-5491

Maccarone, Joseph L., MD {1447272927} ObsGyn, Gyneco, IntrMd(89,PA09)<NJ-COOPRUMC>
+ Virtua Female Pelvic Medicine
200 Bowman Drive/Suite 325   Voorhees, NJ 08043   (856)247-7420   Fax (856)247-7421

MacCarrick, Matthew Joseph, MD {1245319615} PedCrC, Pedtrc
+ RWJ University Pediatric Critical Care
125 Paterson Street/MEB 343   New Brunswick, NJ 08901   (732)235-7887   Fax (732)235-6609

Macchiavelli, Anthony Joseph, MD {1558389684} IntrMd, IntHos(PA13<NJ-ACMCITY>
+ AtlantiCare Regional Medical Center/City Campus
1925 Pacific Avenue/Internal Med   Atlantic City, NJ 08401   (609)441-8146   Fax (609)441-8002

Maccia, Clement A., MD {1568431351} Allrgy, Pedtrc, IntrMd(71,ITAL)
+ Avenel Iselin Medical Group
400 Gill Lane   Iselin, NJ 08830   (732)404-1580   Fax (732)404-1594
+ Asthma, Sinus & Allergy Centers
19 Holly Street   Cranford, NJ 07016   (732)404-1580   Fax (908)276-7434
+ Child Health Institute of New Jersey
89 French Street/Suite 2300   New Brunswick, NJ 08830   (732)235-6230   Fax (732)235-7419

MacCiocca, Michael J., MD {1700012820} IntrMd<NJ-VIRTMARL>
+ Virtua Marlton Hospital
90 Brick Road   Marlton, NJ 08053   (856)355-6000

Macek, Deanna Z., MD {1508938010} Ophthl(66,CZE01)<NJ-CHILTON, NJ-WAYNEGEN>
+ 2025 Hamburg Tunpike/Suite H
Wayne, NJ 07470   (973)831-0122   Fax (973)616-8402
+ One Cedar Crest Village Lane
Pompton Plains, NJ 07444

Macher, Mark S., MD {1184664187} RadThp, RadOnc(82,DC03)<NJ-JFKMED>
+ JFK Medical Center
65 James Street/Radiology   Edison, NJ 08820   (732)321-7167   Fax (732)906-4915   mmacher@solarishs.org

Machiaverna, Frank E., MD {1427020361} Surgry(80,NJ05)
+ Community Medical Center
99 Route 37 West   Toms River, NJ 08755   (732)557-8193

Machiedo, Christine C., MD {1790895019} IntrMd(71,NJ05)<NJ-VAEASTOR>
+ VA New Jersey Health Care System-East Orange Campus
385 Tremont Avenue   East Orange, NJ 07018   (973)676-1000   Fax (973)676-4226

Machiedo, George W., MD {1629082011} Surgry(71,NJ05)<NJ-VAEASTOR, NJ-UMDNJ>
+ VA New Jersey Health Care System-East Orange Campus
385 Tremont Avenue   East Orange, NJ 07018   (973)676-1000   Fax (973)395-7193

Machler, Brian C., MD {1376676528} Dermat(91,NJ05)<NJ-STBARNMC, NY-NYUTISCH>
+ Center for Dermatology PA
128 Columbia Turnpike/Suite 200   Florham Park, NJ 07932   (973)736-9535   Fax (973)736-2607

MacIver, Barbara Jane, MD {1932545654} Anesth(91,GRN01)
+ 26 Ridge Road
Norwood, NJ 07648   (201)767-2219   Fax (201)767-2219

Mack, Prinze Chan, MD {1609990613} Ophthl(03,NJ05)<PA-JRSYSHOR, NJ-COMMED>
+ Mack Eye Center
445 Brick Boulevard/Suite 203   Brick, NJ 08723   (732)923-9090   Fax (732)923-1772
+ Mack Eye Center
257 Monmouth Road/Building A Suite 100   Oakhurst, NJ 07755   (732)923-9090   Fax (732)695-3200

Mack, Ronald John, MD {1386683894} EmrgMd, OccpMd(69,NJ05)<NJ-NWTNMEM>
+ Newton Medical Center
175 High Street/EmergMed   Newton, NJ 07860   (973)383-2121

Mack, Rose M., DO {1831267152} EmrgMd(97,NJ75)<NJ-STPETER>
+ Phoenix Physician's
225 Williamson Street   Elizabeth, NJ 07202   (908)994-5422

MacKaronis, Anthony C., MD {1801971585} ObsGyn(02,NJ02)
+ Capital Health Women's Group
433 Bellevue Avenue   Trenton, NJ 08618   (609)394-4111   Fax (609)394-4070

MacKenzie, Diane Susan, DO {1316931264} EmrgMd, GenPrc(99,NJ75)
+ The Heart Center of The Oranges
95 Main Street   West Orange, NJ 07052   (973)672-3829

MacKenzie, Shauna, MD {1497157887} Anesth
+ St. Joseph's Regional Medical Center Anesthesia
703 Main Street   Paterson, NJ 07503   (973)754-2000   Fax (973)977-9455

Mackessy, Richard P., MD {1740254564} SrgHnd, SrgOrt, IntrMd(78,NJ05)<NJ-RWJURAH, NJ-TRINIJSC>
+ Union County Orthopaedic Group
210 West St. Georges Avenue/PO Box 330 Linden, NJ 07036 (908)486-1111 Fax (908)583-1034

Mackey, Suzanne Fuller, MD {1972574523} ObsGyn(96,PA12)
+ Wegh Under
2301 Evesham Road/Suite 505 Voorhees, NJ 08043 (856)861-6320 Fax (856)888-2640

Mackey, Timothy Joseph, MD {1750426615} Urolgy(93,VA01)<NJ-VALLEY>
+ Urology Group PA
4 Godwin Avenue Midland Park, NJ 07432 (201)444-7070 Fax (201)444-7228

Mackler, Denise Lynn, MD {1760449631} Anesth, IntrMd(91,NJ06)
+ Anesthesia Consultnts of NJ/Nova Pain
285 Davidson Avenue/Suite 204 Somerset, NJ 08873 (732)271-1400 Fax (732)271-3544

Macklin, Joshua M., MD {1619144284} Anesth<NJ-BAYSHORE>
+ Bayshore Community Hospital
727 North Beers Street Holmdel, NJ 07733 (732)739-5900

Mackuse, Donna M., DO {1821296914} Psychy(86,IA75)
+ 2000 Shore Road/Suite 103
Linwood, NJ 08221 (609)601-7820 Fax (609)601-7822

MacMillan, William Emery, MD {1326015025} ObsGyn, MtFtMd(85,WI05)<NJ-MONMOUTH>
+ UH- Robert Wood Johnson Med
125 Paterson Street/CAB 2140 New Brunswick, NJ 08901 (732)235-8006 Fax (732)235-6650
+ Monmouth Medical Group, P.C.
73 South Bath Avenue Long Branch, NJ 07740 (732)235-8006 Fax (732)870-0119
+ Monmouth Family Center
270 Broadway Long Branch, NJ 08901 (732)923-7100 Fax (732)923-7104

Macri, Michael V., MD {1497864052} FamMed(88,IL42)<NJ-STJOSHOS, NJ-MEADWLND>
+ 10 Fairview Avenue
Westwood, NJ 07675 (201)358-2922 Fax (201)358-9540

Macri, Mirtha J., DO {1760629034} EmrgMd(08,NY75)<NJ-OVER-LOOK>
+ Overlook Medical Center
99 Beauvoir Avenue/PO Box 210 Summit, NJ 07902 (908)400-8951

Madaj, Andrew T., MD {1891116042} FamMed
+ RWJ Physician Enterprise
3 Executive Drive/Suite 400 Somerset, NJ 08873 (732)369-5994 Fax (732)369-5993
+ RWJPE Old Bridge Family Medicine
2107 Highway 516 Old Bridge, NJ 08857 (732)369-5994 Fax (732)463-6071

Madamba, Carlos S., MD {1811994866} Hemato, IntrMd, MedOnc(81,PHI29)<NJ-VIRTBERL, NJ-VIRTMARL>
+ Regional Cancer Care Associates, LLC
200 Bowman Drive/Suite E-125 Voorhees, NJ 08043 (856)424-3311 Fax (856)424-5634
+ The Center for Cancer & Hematologic Disease
856 South White Horse Pike/Suite 4 Hammonton, NJ 08037 (856)424-3311 Fax (609)561-2492
+ The Center for Cancer & Hematologic Disease
609 North Broad Street/Suite 300 Woodbury, NJ 08043 (856)686-1002

Madan, Nandini, MD {1013967934} Pedtrc, PedCrd(88,INA23)<PA-STCHRIS>
+ St. Christopher Care at Washington Township
405 Hurffville-Cross Keys Road Sewell, NJ 08080 (856)582-0644 Fax (856)582-0622

Madan, Pankaj, MD {1285897272} CdvDis<NJ-NWRKBETH>
+ Newark Beth Israel Medical Center
201 Lyons Avenue/D12 Newark, NJ 07112 (973)926-6640 Fax (973)923-7267
pmadan@barnabashealth.org

Madane, Srinivas Janardhan, MD {1750305835} Gastrn, IntrMd(93,INA96)
+ Medical Care Associates
262 Route 10 West Succasunna, NJ 07876 (973)252-1522 Fax (973)252-1422
+ Medical Care Associates
137 Mountain Avenue Hackettstown, NJ 07840 (973)252-1522 Fax (908)852-0614
+ Medical Care Associates
222 High Street Newton, NJ 07876 (973)579-5090 Fax (973)579-4958

Madapati, Indira, MD {1972646487} IntrMd(94,INA39)<NJ-SOMERSET>
+ Medwell Internal Medicine
104 Hickory Corner Road/Suite 201 East Windsor, NJ 08520 (609)371-6100 Fax (609)371-6160
+ RWJ University Hospital Somerset
110 Rehill Avenue/Internal Med Somerville, NJ 08876

(908)685-2200
+ Somerset Valley Rehabilitation and Nursing
1621 Route 22 West Bound Brook, NJ 08520 (908)768-0757 Fax (732)764-9720

Maddaiah, Shaila N., MD {1760594766} Psychy(83,INA28)<NJ-UNIVBHC>
+ University Behavioral Health Care
303 George Street/Suite 200 New Brunswick, NJ 08901 (732)235-6800 Fax (732)235-6187

Maddali, Radhika, MD {1790872638} IntrMd(97,INA47)<NJ-EASTORNG, NJ-STBARNMC>
+ Family Medicine/Pediatricians LLC
310 Central Avenue/Suite 305 East Orange, NJ 07018 (973)678-2900 Fax (973)678-8183
yashk@aol.com

Maddali, Sarala K., MD {1346273323} IntrMd(75,INDI)<NJ-VAEASTOR>
+ VA New Jersey Health Care System-East Orange Campus
385 Tremont Avenue East Orange, NJ 07018 (973)676-1000 Fax (973)395-7003

Maddali, Vani, MD {1588699763} IntrMd(93,INA9Z)
+ 205 South Essex Avenue/First Floor
Orange, NJ 07050 (973)678-6402 Fax (973)678-6443
+ 22 Old Short Hills Road/Suite 104
Livingston, NJ 07039 (973)678-6402 Fax (973)535-3406

Maddalozzo, Gerald Anthony, DO {1851734198} EmrgMd(10,MO78)<NJ-KMHSTRAT>
+ Kennedy Memorial Hospital-University Medical Center
18 East Laurel Road Stratford, NJ 08084 (856)346-7985

Maddalozzo, Wanda K. M., MD {1659534956} Pedtrc(05,DMN01)<NJ-JFKMED>
+ JFK Medical Center
65 James Street Edison, NJ 08820 (732)321-7605 Fax (732)744-5614
+ 125 Paterson Street/Suite 1400
New Brunswick, NJ 08903

Maddatu, Elenito P., MD {1881631729} Pedtrc(87,PHIL)<NJ-OCEANMC>
+ M & M Pediatrics
70 Ramtown-Greenville Rd Howell, NJ 07731 (732)785-0300 Fax (732)785-9420

Maddatu, Rose Mylaine, MD {1417994302} Pedtrc(89,PHIL)<NJ-OCEANMC>
+ M & M Pediatrics
70 Ramtown-Greenville Rd Howell, NJ 07731 (732)785-0300 Fax (732)785-9420

Madden, James M., MD {1891788147} AlgyImmn(87,MEX03)<NJ-SOCEANCO, NJ-COMMED>
+ 400 East Bay Avenue/PO Box 430
Manahawkin, NJ 08050 (609)978-7200 Fax (609)978-9339
+ 302 Candlewood Commons
Howell, NJ 07731 (609)978-7200 Fax (732)886-8215

Maddock, Eric Ryan, DO {1962424473} EmrgMd<NJ-KMHSTRAT>
+ Kennedy Memorial Hospital-University Medical Center
18 East Laurel Road Stratford, NJ 08084 (856)346-7816 Fax (856)346-6385

Madeira, Samuel, Jr., MD {1982609772} CdvDis, IntrMd(74,NY08)<NJ-STFRNMED>
+ St. Francis Medical Center
601 Hamilton Avenue Trenton, NJ 08629 (609)989-0144

Madhavan, Arjun, MD {1265612949} CritCr, PulDis, IntrMd(02,INA2D)<NJ-STPETER>
+ Center for Ambulatory Resources
240 Easton Avenue New Brunswick, NJ 08901 (732)745-8564 Fax (732)745-9156
+ St. Peter's University Hospital
254 Easton Avenue/Pulm Disease New Brunswick, NJ 08901 (732)745-8600

Madhok, Indu, MD {1750470209} Pedtrc(77,INA23)<NJ-CLAR-MAAS, NJ-UMDNJ>
+ 156 Roseville Avenue/Suite 304
Newark, NJ 07107 (973)484-3848 Fax (973)484-5226

Madhwal, Surabhi, MD {1528233418} IntCrd, IntrMd(99,INDI)<NY-MTSINAI, NY-MTSINYHS>
+ Cardiology Consultants
246 Hamburg Turnpike/Suite 201 Wayne, NJ 07470 (973)942-1141 Fax (973)942-1250

Madigan, John D., DO {1427239854} IntrMd, Nephro(03,ME75)<NJ-NWRKBETH, NJ-STBARNMC>
+ Newark Beth Israel Medical Center
201 Lyons Avenue Newark, NJ 07112 (973)926-7000

Madison, Anoja Bala, DO {1154372886} Anesth(00,NJ75)
+ 8 Pepperbush Lane
Moorestown, NJ 08057

Madison, Harry Thomas, DO {1013989334} Psychy(90,PA77)<NJ-OURLADY, NJ-KMHCHRRY>
+ University Hospital-SOM Department of Psychiatry
2250 Chapel Avenue West/Suite 100 Cherry Hill, NJ 08002 (856)482-9000 Fax (856)482-1159

Madison, Joy Hovey, MD {1861643645} FamMed(89,IL11)
+ 15 Wenonah Avenue
Rockaway, NJ 07866

Madison, William A., Jr., DO {1255347365} FamMed(90,NJ75)<NJ-OURLADY>
+ Family Practice Associates
188 Fries Mill Road/Suite N3 Turnersville, NJ 08012 (856)875-8000 Fax (856)875-8494

Madlinger, Robert Vincent, DO {1023180544} Surgry(00,MO78)<NY-LINCOLN>
+ St Joseph's Medical Center Plastic Surgery
703 Main Street Paterson, NJ 07503 (973)754-2413

Madonia, Paul W., MD {1164496188} FamMed, Grtrcs(65,NJ05)<NJ-HUNTRDN>
+ Cornerstone Family Practice
9100 Wescott Drive/Suite 103 Flemington, NJ 08822 (908)237-6910 Fax (908)237-6919

Madonick, Harvey Lloyd, MD {1871530733} EmrgMd, IntrMd(85,PA02)<NJ-COMMED>
+ Community Medical Center
99 Route 37 West/EmergMed Toms River, NJ 08755 (732)557-8000

Madrak, Leslie Nicole, DO {1851363485} Psychy(97,PA77)<NJ-HAMPTBHC>
+ Hampton Behavioral Health Center
650 Rancocas Road/Psychiatry Westampton, NJ 08060 (609)267-7000

Madraswala, Rehman, MD {1477973766} Psychy
+ 551 Park Avenue/Suite 3nC
Scotch Plains, NJ 07076 (908)455-8120 Fax (908)455-8122

Madreperla, Steven Anthony, Jr., MD {1013925254} Ophthl, IntrMd(89,MD07)<NJ-HACKNSK, NJ-VALLEY>
+ Retina Associates of New Jersey, P.A.
5 Franklin Avenue Belleville, NJ 07109 (973)450-5100 Fax (973)450-9494
+ Retina Associates of New Jersey, P.A.
628 Cedar Lane Teaneck, NJ 07666 (973)450-5100 Fax (201)836-6426
+ Retina Associates of New Jersey, P.A.
2952 Vauxhall Road Vauxhall, NJ 07109 (908)349-8155 Fax (908)349-8134

Madrid, Teresa O., MD {1982646295} IntrMd, FamMAdlt(79,PHIL)<NJ-STMICHL>
+ 268 MLK Jr. Boulevard
Newark, NJ 07102 (973)877-5543

Madsen, Melissa L., MD {1922014042} Anesth(93,FL03)<NJ-CHSMRCER, NJ-CHSFULD>
+ Trenton Anesthesiology Associates, PA
One Capital Way/Second Floor Pennington, NJ 08534 (609)396-4700 Fax (609)396-4900

Madubuko, Adaora Gabriellene, MD {1922397025} Pedtrc(05,NIG09)
+ 550 South 19th Street
Newark, NJ 07103 (973)609-6884
agno@doctor.com

Madubuko, Uchenna Anthony, MD {1407122609} Anesth
+ 550 South 19th Street
Newark, NJ 07103 (973)609-6749 Fax (973)877-0989

Madura, Paul P., MD {1144255506} FamMed(80,MO34)<NJ-HUNTRDN>
+ 450 Charlestown Road
Hampton, NJ 08827 (908)537-1042 Fax (908)537-1043
Ppmadura@embarqmail.com

Maeda, Yasuhiro, MD {1871558007} Nrolgy(81,JAPA)<NJ-VAEASTOR>
+ VA New Jersey Health Care System-East Orange Campus
385 Tremont Avenue East Orange, NJ 07018 (973)676-1000

Maenner, Daniel W., DO {1134277619}
+ 6310 Bergenline Avenue
West New York, NJ 07093 (201)869-6220 Fax (201)869-5145

Maestrado, Primo Emnace, MD {1992830400} Anesth, PainMd(99,PHI10)<NJ-MEMSALEM, NJ-VIRTMARL>
+ Memorial Hospital of Salem County
310 Woodstown Road/Anesthesia Salem, NJ 08079 (856)339-6021 Fax (856)935-5420
+ Virtua Marlton Hospital
90 Brick Road/Anesthesia Marlton, NJ 08053 (856)355-6000

Maeuser, Herman L.I., MD {1740264613} Surgry(86,NJ06)<NJ-HUNTRDN>
+ Hunterdon Surgical Associates
1100 Wescott Drive/Suite 302 Flemington, NJ 08822 (908)788-6464 Fax (908)788-6459

Maffei, Mario Stephen, MD {1518956283} FamMed(96,PA13)
+ Tatem Brown Family Practice
2225 East Evesham Road/Suite 101 Voorhees, NJ 08043 (856)795-4330 Fax (856)325-3704

Physicians by Name and Address

Magadan, Silvia Maria, DO {1952361602} Pedtrc(88,NJ75)<NJ-STCLRDEN>
+ Pediatrics of Morris
  16 Pocono Road/Suite 112 Denville, NJ 07834 (973)627-3765   Fax (973)784-4509
+ 35 Green Pond Road/Suite 1A
  Rockaway, NJ 07866   (973)627-3765   Fax (973)625-9424

Magahis, Pacifico Aguila, Jr., MD {1659469005} IntrMd, Gastrn(93,NY47)<NJ-OCEANMC, NJ-SOCEANCO>
+ Coastal Gastroenterology Associates PA
  525 Jack Martin Boulevard/Suite 301 Brick, NJ 08724 (732)840-0067   Fax (732)840-3169

Maganti, Sameera, MD {1972783207} IntrMd(01,INA28)<NJ-RWJUBRUN>
+ Drs. Deka and Ata
  2090 State Route 27/Suite 101 North Brunswick, NJ 08902 (732)979-0035   Fax (908)829-4408

Magarelli, Mary-Lynn, DO {1184760845} EmrgMd(92,NY75)<NJ-STJOSHOS, NY-STBARNAB>
+ St Joseph's Medical Center Emergency
  703 Main Street Paterson, NJ 07503 (973)754-2240 Fax (973)754-2249

Magargle, Jason Kent, DO {1619101797}
+ 1301 Barnesdale Road
  Deptford, NJ 08096   (302)584-5932

Magariello, Mark M., MD {1467491894} EmrgMd, IntrMd(86,MEX14)
+ Emergency Physician Associates, P.A.
  307 South Evergreen Avenue/PO Box 298 Woodbury, NJ 08096 (856)848-3817   Fax (856)848-1431

Magaril, Rhona A., MD {1336114826} ObsGyn(82,FL02)<NJ-OVERLOOK>
+ Lifeline Medical Associates
  530 Morris Avenue Springfield, NJ 07081 (973)379-7477   Fax (973)379-9094

Magasic, Mario V., MD {1376659722} Gastrn, IntrMd(88,DMN01)<NJ-VIRTMARL, NJ-JFKMED>
+ South Jersey Gastroenterology PA
  111 Vine Street Hammonton, NJ 08037 (609)561-3080   Fax (856)983-5110
+ South Jersey Gastroenterology PA
  106 Creek Crossing Hainesport, NJ 08036 (609)561-3080   Fax (856)983-5110
+ South Jersey Gastroenterology PA
  406 Lippincott Drive/Suite E Marlton, NJ 08037 (856)983-1900   Fax (856)983-5110

Magaziner, Allan, DO {1487704896} GenPrc, FamMed(83,IL76)
+ Magaziner Medical Center
  1907 Greentree Road Cherry Hill, NJ 08003 (856)424-8222   Fax (856)424-2599

Magaziner, Edward S., MD {1700842945} PhysMd, PainMd, PhyMPain(85,IL42)<NJ-RWJUBRUN, NJ-STPETER>
+ 2186 Route 27/Suite D
  North Brunswick, NJ 08902 (732)297-2600   Fax (732)297-5770

Magbalon, Domingo, Jr., MD {1417094228} EmrgMd, Surgry(65,PHI08)
+ 1656 Blue Jay Lane
  Cherry Hill, NJ 08003 (856)428-2448

Magera, Michael John, MD {1407899818} Psychy(99,DC02)
+ Hudson Psychiatric Associates, LLC.
  79 Hudson Street/Suite 203 Hoboken, NJ 07030 (201)222-8808   Fax (201)222-8803

Maggio, Vijay, MD {1518954080} Nrolgy
+ 6 Casselberry Way
  Princeton, NJ 08540   Fax (866)634-2766

Maggio, William W., MD {1588623987} SrgNro(81,PA14)
+ Meridian Surgical Associates
  2101 Route 34 South Wall, NJ 07719 (732)974-0003   Fax (732)974-0366
+ JFK Neurosciences Institute
  65 James Street/Second Floor Edison, NJ 08818 (732)974-0003   Fax (732)632-1584

Maghari, Amin, MD {1528209046} Pthlgy, Dermat(00,IRA15)
+ Schweiger Dermatology
  368 Lakehurst Road/Suite 201 Toms River, NJ 08755 (732)244-4700   Fax (732)731-6134
  aminmaghari@dermone.com

Magherini Rothe, Suzanne Aranka, MD {1932140399} ObsGyn(98,NY20)
+ Monmouth Family Health Center Ob/Gyn
  80 Pavilion Avenue Long Branch, NJ 07740 (732)963-0166   Fax (732)229-0299

Maghsood, Shabnam, MD {1649314329} Pedtrc
+ 55 Chelsea Avenue/Apt 405
  Long Branch, NJ 07740

Magid, Marissa, DO {1801238415} ObsGyn
+ Blue River Wellness Health
  695 Broadway Paterson, NJ 07514 (973)321-9342 Fax (973)302-5570

Magidson, Jory G., MD {1669449526} PthAcl, Pthlgy(78,NY01)<NJ-MORRISTN, NJ-OVERLOOK>
+ Morristown Medical Center
  100 Madison Avenue/Path Morristown, NJ 07962 (973)971-5600   Fax (973)290-7370
+ Overlook Medical Center
  99 Beauvoir Avenue/PO Box 210 Summit, NJ 07902 (908)522-2000
+ Morristown Pathology Associates
  100 The American Road/Suite 118 Morris Plains, NJ 07962 (973)867-7298

Magier, Slawomir, MD {1245220177} ObsGyn(87,GER02)<NJ-JFKMED>
+ 1005 Green Street
  Iselin, NJ 08830 (732)283-1075   Fax (732)636-2355

Maglaras, Nicholas C., MD {1336245109} PulDis, IntrMd(87,GRNA)
+ Drs. Maglaras and Brescia
  236 East Westfield Avenue Roselle Park, NJ 07204 (908)245-8222   Fax (908)245-6504

Magliaro, Thomas J., MD {1235287657} ObsGyn, Gyneco(87,NJ06)
+ Saint Peter's Physician Associates
  78 Easton Avenue New Brunswick, NJ 08901 (732)828-3300   Fax (732)937-5739

Magliocco, Melissa Amy, MD {1124190491} IntrMd(99,PA13)<NJ-RWJUBRUN>
+ RWJ University Hospital New Brunswick
  One Robert Wood Johnson Place New Brunswick, NJ 08901 (732)828-3000

Maglione, Theodore James, MD {1932444940}<NJ-RWJUBRUN>
+ RWJ University Hospital New Brunswick
  One Robert Wood Johnson Place New Brunswick, NJ 08901 (973)879-1088

Magnes, Jeffrey B., MD {1164588935} Anesth(84,NY01)<NJ-VALLEY>
+ The Valley Hospital
  223 North Van Dien Avenue Ridgewood, NJ 07450 (201)447-8350

Magness, Rose L., MD {1003863119} ObsGyn(85,PA07)<NJ-VIRTVOOR>
+ Advocare Magness-Stafford Ob-Gyn Associates
  802 Liberty Place Sicklerville, NJ 08081 (856)740-4400   Fax (856)740-4411
+ Advocare Magness-Stafford Ob-Gyn Associates
  1810 Haddonfield Berlin Road Cherry Hill, NJ 08003 (856)740-4400   Fax (856)354-7800

Magnet, Marcus, MD {1740249457} FamMed(98,NJ06)<NJ-UNDRWD>
+ Drs. Magnet & Rogers
  831 Kings Highway/Suite 100 Woodbury, NJ 08096 (856)853-8730   Fax (856)853-8870

Magnus Miller, Leslie, MD {1568022804} Pedtrc
+ 52 Westmount Drive
  Livingston, NJ 07039 (973)740-8933

Magnusen, Mary L., DO {1659340255} FamMed(88,MO78)
+ Skylands Medical Group PA
  5678 Berkshire Valley Road Oak Ridge, NJ 07438 (973)697-0200   Fax (973)383-0448

Magovern, Christopher Jude, MD {1043212434} Surgry, SrgThr(89,TX04)<NJ-MORRISTN, NJ-OVERLOOK>
+ Mid-Atlantic Surgical Associates
  100 Madison Avenue Morristown, NJ 07960 (973)971-7300   Fax (973)984-7019
  christopher.magovern@ahsys.org

Magpantay, Emiliana M., MD {1013054337} ObsGyn(67,PHIL)<NJ-MEADWLND>
+ 330 Grand Street
  Hoboken, NJ 07030 (201)659-7102   Fax (201)659-0160

Magsino, Vicente Martinez, Jr., MD {1255332177} IntrMd(83,PHIL)<NJ-COMMED>
+ 65a Lacey Road
  Whiting, NJ 08759

Maguire, Joseph I., MD Ophthl(83,PA02)
+ Mid Atlantic Retina - Wills Eye Retina Surgeons
  1417 Cantillon Boulevard Mays Landing, NJ 08330 (609)625-0402   Fax (609)625-0788

Maguire, Marcy Frances, MD {1003939646} RprEnd, ObsGyn
+ Reproductive Medicine Associates of New Jersey
  111 Madison Avenue/Suite 100 Morristown, NJ 07962 (973)971-4600   Fax (973)290-8370
+ Reproductive Medicine Associates of New Jersey
  140 Allen Road Basking Ridge, NJ 07920 (973)971-4600   Fax (973)290-8370
+ Reproductive Medicine Associates of New Jersey
  475 Prospect Avenue/Suite 101 West Orange, NJ 07962 (973)325-2229   Fax (973)290-8370

Maguire, Nicole J., DO {1346456076} EmrgMd(03,NY75)<NJ-NWRKBETH>
+ Newark Beth Israel Medical Center
  201 Lyons Avenue/EmrgMed Newark, NJ 07112 (973)926-7000
  nmaguire@sbhcs.com

Maguire, Randall F., MD {1932128980} PthAcl, PthCln(75,PA02)<NJ-LOURDMED>
+ Lourdes Medical Center of Burlington County
  218 Sunset Road Willingboro, NJ 08046 (609)835-2900

Mah, Sue Ann, MD {1386652154} Pedtrc, IntrMd(97,NJ06)<NJ-UNVMCPRN, NJ-SHOREMEM>
+ CHOP Care Network at Princeton Medical Center
  One Plainsboro Road/Pediatrics Plainsboro, NJ 08536 (609)853-7000   Fax (609)497-4173
+ Nemours Dupont Pediatrics
  1925 Pacific Avenue Atlantic City, NJ 08401 (609)853-7000   Fax (609)572-8523

Mahabir, Vishal Shiva, MD {1043532286}
+ 60 Saratoga Drive
  West Windsor, NJ 08550 (703)734-1610
  vishalmahabir@hotmail.com

Mahadass, Pavani, MD {1902825094} Surgry(70,INDI)<NJ-CHS-FULD, NJ-RWJUHAM>
+ Capital Health System/Fuld Campus
  750 Brunswick Avenue Trenton, NJ 08638 (609)394-6000

Mahaga-Ajala, Mark-Robert Oluseyi Ishola, DO {1619471513} ObsGyn<NJ-MORRISTN>
+ Morristown Medical Center
  100 Madison Avenue Morristown, NJ 07962 (973)971-5000

Mahajan, Geeti, MD {1538320510} EnDbMt
+ Hackensack University Medical Group Emerson
  452 Old Hook Road/2nd Floor Emerson, NJ 07630 (201)666-3900   Fax (201)261-0505

Mahajan, Raakhee, MD {1437312139} EmrgMd(05,PA09)
+ 6501 Baltimore Drive
  Marlton, NJ 08053 (908)359-4285

Mahajan, Rohini, MD {1942460266} PhyMHPC(06,NJ05)<NJ-HLTHSRE>
+ HealthSouth Rehabilitation Hospital of New Jersey
  14 Hospital Drive Toms River, NJ 08755 (732)505-5058   Fax (732)818-4817

Mahal, Mona, MD {1720190853} IntrMd, InfDis(88,INA79)<NJ-RWJUBRUN>
+ Eric B. Chandler Health Center
  277 George Street/InfDis New Brunswick, NJ 08901 (732)235-6700   Fax (732)235-6729
  Mahalmo@umdnj.edu
+ RWJ University Hospital New Brunswick
  One Robert Wood Johnson Place New Brunswick, NJ 08901 (732)828-3000

Mahal, Pradeep S., MD {1063551687} Gastrn, MedOnc, IntrMd(74,INDI)<NJ-TRINIWSC, NJ-RWJURAH>
+ 1308 Morris Avenue
  Union, NJ 07083 (908)851-6767   Fax (908)851-0382

Mahal, Sharan S., MD {1851363360} CdvDis, IntrMd(85,INDI)<NJ-MORRISTN, NJ-SOMERSET>
+ CardioMD
  1200 US Highway 22 East/Suite 17 Bridgewater, NJ 08807 (908)864-4027   Fax (908)864-4251
+ CardioMD
  245 Union Avenue/Suite 1A Bridgewater, NJ 08807 (908)864-4027   Fax (908)864-4029

Mahalingam, Banu, MD {1417904509} CdvDis, IntrMd(95,INA04)<NJ-UNVMCPRN>
+ Cardiology Associates of Princeton, P.A.
  731 Alexander Road/Suite 202 Princeton, NJ 08540 (609)921-7456   Fax (609)921-2972
+ Cardiology Associates of Princeton, P.A.
  5 Plainsboro Road/Suite 490 Plainsboro, NJ 08536 (609)921-7456   Fax (609)799-2832

Mahalingam, Rajeshwari Sundaram, MD {1477566222} Pedtrc(94,INDI)<NJ-RWJUBRUN>
+ UH-Robert Wood Jhnsn Med Sch
  97 Paterson Street/Ped - Child Neu New Brunswick, NJ 08901

Mahamitra, Nirandra, MD {1669663217} FamMed, IntrMd(GRN01)
+ Cooper Family Medicine
  141 South Black Horse Pike/Suite 1 Blackwood, NJ 08012 (856)232-6471   Fax (856)232-7028
+ Cooper Family Medicine
  504 White Horse Pike Haddon Heights, NJ 08035 (856)232-6471   Fax (856)546-6686

Mahan, Janet L., MD {1780651448} IntrMd(85,DC03)
+ Ocean County Family Care
400 New Hampshire Avenue   Lakewood, NJ 08701
(732)901-6400   Fax (732)901-0744
+ Ocean County Family Care
2125 Route 88 East   Brick, NJ 08724   (732)901-6400   Fax (732)892-0961

Mahapatro, Darshana, MD {1871531764} PthAna, PthCln, PthCyt(70,INA67)<NJ-DEBRAHLC>
+ PLUS Diagnostics
1200 River Avenue/Suite 10   Lakewood, NJ 08701
(732)901-7575   Fax (732)901-1555
+ Deborah Heart and Lung Center
200 Trenton Road/Path   Browns Mills, NJ 08015   (609)893-6611

Mahapatro, Ramesh C., MD {1679523237} Pthlgy, PthACl, PthCyt(68,INA4Z)<NJ-COMMED, NJ-KIMBALL>
+ Community Medical Center
99 Route 37 West/Pathology   Toms River, NJ 08755
(732)557-8526

Maharaj-Mikiel, Indira Cassandra, MD {1891056164} FamMed
+ Burlington Family Medical Center
666 Madison Avenue   Burlington, NJ 08016   (609)386-0023   Fax (609)386-4648
imaharajmd@gmail.com

Maharaja, Lopa Vijay, MD {1891971305} IntrMd, InfDis(03,DMN01)<NJ-SELSPNNJ>
+ Infectious Diseases Associates
96 Parkway   Rochelle Park, NJ 07662   (201)291-4075
+ Infectious Disease Associates of Northern NJ
255 West Spring Valley/Suite 100   Maywood, NJ 07607
(201)881-0107

Mahdi, Lawrence F., MD {1689607103} CdvDis(82,WIND)<NJ-MTNSIDE>
+ North Jersey Cardiovascular Consultants
329 Belleville Avenue   Bloomfield, NJ 07003   (973)748-3800   Fax (973)748-3540

Mahendrakar, Smita, MD {1083874580} Nephro, IntrMd(01,INA70)
+ 185 South Orange Avenue/MSB I-524
Newark, NJ 07103   (973)972-4100

Maher, Jennifer Lee, DO {1457524050} NnPnMd, Pedtrc, IntrMd(08,PA77)
+ CHOP Care Network at Virtua Voorhees Hospital
100 Bowman Drive   Voorhees, NJ 08043   (856)325-3000   Fax (609)261-5842

Maher, Miriam Ruth, MD {1780689554} IntrMd, Pedtrc(94,NY48)<NJ-MMHKEMBL, NJ-MORRISTN>
+ 130 North Beverwyck Road
Lake Hiawatha, NJ 07034   (973)335-1065   Fax (973)335-2225
+ Summit Medical Group
95 Madison Avenue   Morristown, NJ 07960   (973)335-1065   Fax (973)267-5521

Maheshwari, Vivek, MD {1447232558} Surgry, IntrMd(89,INA23)<NJ-STBARNMC>
+ Professional Associates in Surgery
101 Old Short Hills Road/Suite 206   West Orange, NJ 07052
(973)731-5005   Fax (973)325-6230
+ Professional Associates in Surgery
142 Palisade Avenue/Suite 109   Jersey City, NJ 07306
(201)565-8595

Mahgoub, Hatem Abdelkawi, MD {1932216033} IntrMd(95,EGY05)<NJ-NWTNMEM>
+ Newton Medical Center
175 High Street/Hospitalist   Newton, NJ 07860   (973)383-2121

Mahmood, Afsar, MD {1578719944} PthACl(83,DOM05)
+ Quest Diagnostics Inc.
1 Malcolm Avenue   Teterboro, NJ 07608   (201)393-5698   Fax (201)393-6127

Mahmood, Ashhad, MD {1164657359} PthACl(08,GRN01)<NJ-CLARMAAS>
+ St. Barnabas Medical Center
94 Old Short Hills Road   Livingston, NJ 07039   (973)322-8945

Mahmood, Faisal, MD {1457569196} SrgSpn, SrgOrt, Ortped(05,NJ05)<NJ-WAYNEGEN, NJ-STJOSHOS>
+ North Jersey Orthopaedic Group
246 Hamburg Turnpike/Suite 302   Wayne, NJ 07470
(973)689-6266   Fax (973)689-6264
+ Northeast Spine & Sports Medicine
367 Lakehurst Road   Toms River, NJ 08755   (732)653-1000

Mahmood, Fauzia, MD {1427015619} PsyCAd, Psychy(76,PAKI)<NJ-STCLRBOO>
+ St. Clare's Hospital-Boonton
130 Powerville Road/Psychiatry   Boonton, NJ 07005
(973)316-1982   Fax (973)299-7212

Mahmood, Nader Ahmad, MD {1396906913} IntrMd(08,GRN01)
+ 1040 Main Street/3rd Fl.
Paterson, NJ 07503   (973)321-1670   Fax (973)321-1672

+ Pulmonary & Sleep Associates of Hunterdon County
1100 Wescott Drive/Suite G-2   Flemington, NJ 08822
(973)321-1670   Fax (908)806-2529

Mahmood, Parvez, MD {1174520936} Urolgy(67,PAKI)<NJ-OCEANMC>
+ Mahmood Schor Urology PA
20 Hospital Drive/Suite 15   Toms River, NJ 08755
(732)286-6644   Fax (732)286-9321

Mahmood, Saleem, MD {1700991247} IntrMd(89,PAKI)<NJ-CHRIST, NJ-HOBUNIMC>
+ Dr. Mahmood and Associates
8 Jordan Avenue   Jersey City, NJ 07306   (201)432-5744   Fax (201)432-2729

Mahmood, Shahid, MD {1154340842} Pthlgy, PthCyt, BldBnk(83,PAK15)<NJ-CHILTON>
+ Chilton Medical Center
97 West Parkway/Pathology   Pompton Plains, NJ 07444
(973)831-5000

Mahmood, Tariq, MD {1679521843} Allrgy, IntrMd, Rheuma(71,PAK01)
+ 2333 Morris Avenue/Suite D204
Union, NJ 07083   (908)688-8911   Fax (908)688-8889

Mahmood Arif, Iram, MD {1215059605} IntrMd(97,PAK08)
+ 22 Nestlewood Way
Princeton, NJ 08540

Mahmoud, Ahmad F., MD {1134532708} Otlryg(14,PA01)
+ The Family Center for Otolaryngology
47 Orient Way/Lower Level   Rutherford, NJ 07070
(201)935-5508   Fax (201)465-6088
+ Summit Medical Group
31-00 Broadway   Fair Lawn, NJ 07410   (201)935-5508   Fax (201)796-7020
+ The Family Center for Otolaryngology
6 Brighton Road/Suite 104   Clifton, NJ 07070   (973)470-0282   Fax (201)465-6088

Mahmoud, Ayesha Shabbir, MD {1538185459} Pedtrc
+ Riverside Pediatric Group
506 Broadway   Bayonne, NJ 07002   (201)471-7012   Fax (201)471-7014
+ 10 Exchange Place/15th Floor
Jersey City, NJ 07302   (201)471-7012   Fax (201)603-6688

Mahmoud, Omar M., MD {1467784439} RadOnc, Radiol<NJ-RWJUBRUN>
+ Rutgers Cancer Institute of New Jersey
195 Little Albany Street/PO Box 2681   New Brunswick, NJ 08903   (732)253-3939   Fax (732)253-3952

Mahmud, Hamid, MD {1083662589} IntrMd(87,PAK01)
+ 45 Meadow Run Road
Bordentown, NJ 08505

Mahmud, Hossen, MD {1194387050} IntrMd
+ SNS Rheumatology Associates
2333 Whitehorse Mercerville Rd/Suite J   Trenton, NJ 08619
(609)689-1229

Mahmud, Jamal, MD {1396983532} Psychy(87,PAK01)
+ Psychiatry Consultants
9 Harwood Drive   Voorhees, NJ 08043
+ Pinnacle Behavioral Health Institute
851 Route 73 North/Suite C   Marlton, NJ 08053   Fax (856)267-5824

Mahon, Alyssa Eileen, MD {1235583279}<NJ-NWRKBETH>
+ Newark Beth Israel Medical Center
201 Lyons Avenue   Newark, NJ 07112   (908)433-1860

Mahon, James William, MD {1952390908} Pedtrc, AdolMd(93,NJ05)<NJ-CHILTON>
+ Pediatric Professional Associates PA
330 Ratzer Road/Suite 20   Wayne, NJ 07470   (973)835-5556   Fax (973)628-7942
+ New Jersey Pediatric & Adolescent Care, LLC.
1680 Route 23/Suite 350   Wayne, NJ 07470   (973)835-5556   Fax (973)521-9707

Mahoney, John J., DO {1184660474} Anesth(83,PA77)
+ Hamilton HealthCare Center
3840 Quakerbridge Road/Suite 100   Hamilton, NJ 08619
(609)890-2222   Fax (609)890-0715

Mahoney, Nola T., DO {1235182692} FamMed(83,PA77)
+ 1 Breckenridge Drive
Shamong, NJ 08088

Mahoney, Timothy Hugh, MD {1235303751} CdvDis
+ Electrophysiology Associates, PA
100 Madison Avenue/Suite 5   Morristown, NJ 07962
(973)971-4261   Fax (973)290-7253

Mahpara, Swaleha, MD {1902113772} IntrMd(01,PAK11)
+ 1945 Corlies Avenue
Neptune, NJ 07753   (732)776-4420

Mai, Quynh-Tien, MD {1336403922} Anesth
+ Robert Wood Johnson-UMDNJ Anesthesia Group
125 Paterson Street/CAB 3100   New Brunswick, NJ 08901
(248)881-1985   Fax (732)235-6131

Maiatico, Marcellus A., MD {1508883695} PhysMd(76,NJ05)
+ Pennsville Sports Medicine & Rehabilitation Center
270 South Broadway/PO Box 35   Pennsville, NJ 08070
(856)678-5449   Fax (856)678-3153

Maida, Emanuel M., MD {1114920451} IntrMd(85,ITA24)<NJ-STBARNMC>
+ E. Martin Maida, MD PA
209 South Livingston Avenue/Suite 7   Livingston, NJ 07039
(973)535-2734   Fax (973)535-2810
pmaida1644@aol.com

Maiello, Dominic J., MD {1487628467} IntrMd, Rheuma(81,MO34)<NJ-CHRIST>
+ James G. Sanderson DO Family Practice P.C.
3 Webster Avenue   Jersey City, NJ 07307   (201)798-2900   Fax (201)798-3582

Maier, Dawn Rachel, MD {1750468401} IntrMd(97,NJ06)
+ Virtua Medical Group
401 Route 73/40 Lake Ctr Dr/Ste 201A   Marlton, NJ 08053
(856)355-0340   Fax (856)355-0346

Maier, Herbert S., MD {1780614537} Dermat(67,DC01)<NJ-WAYNEGEN>
+ 220 Hamburg Turnpike
Wayne, NJ 07470   (973)595-6338   Fax (973)595-9446

Maiers, Travis John, MD {1124394820} EmrgMd<NJ-CHSFULD>
+ Capital Health System/Fuld Campus
750 Brunswick Avenue   Trenton, NJ 08638   (609)394-6000

Maiese, Mario L., DO {1528050382} CdvDis(69,IA75)<NJ-VIRTVOOR>
+ South Jersey Heart Group
539 Egg Harbor Road/Suite 1   Sewell, NJ 08080   (856)589-0300   Fax (856)589-1753
sjhg@salu.net
+ South Jersey Heart Group
181 West Whitehorse Pike/Suite 201   Berlin, NJ 08009
(856)589-0300   Fax (856)768-3371

Mailman, Wendy R., MD {1124065081} Anesth(85,PA02)<NJ-MEMSALEM>
+ Memorial Hospital of Salem County
310 Woodstown Road/Anesthesiology   Salem, NJ 08079
(856)935-1000

Mailutha, Karimi, MD {1962602128} Psychy(05,MA01)
+ Atlantic Behavior Health
95 Mount Kemble Avenue/6th floor   Morristown, NJ 07960
(973)971-4456

Maimon, Olga M., MD {1073598850} IntrMd, Gastrn(98,DMN01)<NJ-RBAYOLDB>
+ 758 Route 18 North/Suite 103
East Brunswick, NJ 08816   (732)360-0117   Fax (732)360-1141
omaimon@msn.com
+ 3 Hospital Plaza/Suite 405
Old Bridge, NJ 08857   (732)360-0117   Fax (732)360-0033

Mainero, Michael M., MD {1720090079} Gastrn, IntrMd(85,MEXI)<NJ-CHILTON>
+ Gastroenterology Associates of New Jersey
61 Beaver Brook Road/Suite 301   Lincoln Park, NJ 07035
(973)785-0102   Fax (973)785-0335
+ Gastroenterology Associates of New Jersey
60 Skyline Drive   Ringwood, NJ 07456   (973)785-0102
Fax (973)785-0335
+ Gastroenterology Associates of New Jersey
88 Park Street   Montclair, NJ 07035   (973)233-9559   Fax (973)233-9660

Maio, Theodora J., MD {1013973650} Surgry(74,ITA33)
+ Sall/Myers Medical Associates, PA
100 Hamilton Plaza/Suite 317/3rd Floor   Paterson, NJ 07505
(973)279-2323   Fax (973)279-7551

Maita, Lorraine, MD {1770771016} IntrMd(84,ISR02)<NY-SLR-LUKES, NJ-MORRISTN>
+ Prudential Employee Health Service
213 Washington Street   Newark, NJ 07102   (973)802-6380
Fax (973)802-3182
lorraine.maita@prudential.com

Maitin, Ian B., MD (89,PA02)
+ 1620 Ravenswood Way
Cherry Hill, NJ 08003

Maitland, Ralynne Elizabeth, MD {1285839845} PedEmg, Pedtrc(06,NJ05)<CT-CONCHLD, CT-STMARY>
+ Capital Health System/Fuld Campus
750 Brunswick Avenue/EmergMed   Trenton, NJ 08638
(609)815-7091   Fax (609)815-7886

Maizes, Allen Stuart, MD {1205997202} Anesth(88,NY48)<NY-MAIMONMC>
+ New Jersey Anesthesia Associates, P.C.
252 Columbia Turnpike/PO Box 0037   Florham Park, NJ 07932   (973)660-9334   Fax (973)660-9732

Majchrzak, Tadeusz J., MD {1720061070} FamMed(75,POLA)
+ Vita-Med Family Practice
3000 Kennedy Boulevard/Suite 308   Jersey City, NJ 07306
(201)963-0800   Fax (201)656-6934

Majeed, Asra, MD {1700135472} IntrMd
+ 1702 Fir Court
Somerset, NJ 08873

Physicians by Name and Address

Majeed, Kiran, MD {1447539754}
+ 1900 Frintage Road/Apt 1209
   Cherry Hill, NJ 08034   (516)637-4025
   kiran_md@live.com

Majersky, Stephen P., MD {1215032396} IntrMd(77,ITAL)<NJ-HACKNSK, NJ-HOLYNAME>
+ 255 West Spring Valley Avenue/Suite 2
   Maywood, NJ 07607   (201)368-9212   Fax (201)368-0707

Majid, Abdul, MD {1831287416} IntrMd(92,INA5B)<NJ-STFRN-MED>
+ Trenton Psychiatric Hospital
   Sullivan Way/PO Box 7600   West Trenton, NJ 08628
   (609)633-1502   Fax (609)633-8527

Majid, Mahir J., MD {1568589158} ObsGyn(81,IRAQ)<NJ-MEAD-WLND, NJ-HACKNSK>
+ 7332 John F. Kennedy Boulevard
   North Bergen, NJ 07047   (201)868-9040   Fax (201)868-9041

Majid, Naweed Kamran, MD {1235326612} SrgThr, SrgVas, Surgry(67,PAKI)<NJ-CHILTON, NJ-MTNSIDE>
+ NE Laser Vein Institute, LLC
   257 East Ridgewood Avenue/Suite 302   Ridgewood, NJ 07450   (201)445-4410   Fax (201)444-7594
+ NE Laser Vein Institute, LLC
   230 Sherman Avenue   Glen Ridge, NJ 07028   (973)429-1025
+ NE Laser Vein Institute, LLC
   1031 McBride Avenue   West Paterson, NJ 07450   (973)256-4880

Majid, Saniea Fatima, MD {1932344348} Surgry(02,PAK14)
+ 65 East Northfield Road/Suite K
   Livingston, NJ 07039   (973)704-6161

Majisu, Claire Amume, MD {1144255027} Pedtrc(98,IL02)<NJ-STPETER>
+ University Pediatric Associates PA
   317 Cleveland Avenue   Highland Park, NJ 08904   (732)249-8999   Fax (732)249-7827
+ University Pediatric Associates
   D-1 Brier Hill Court   East Brunswick, NJ 08816   (732)238-3310

Majithia, Meenakshee N., MD {1205858883} Pedtrc(69,INDI)<NJ-CHRIST>
+ 22 Glenwood Avenue
   Jersey City, NJ 07306   (201)451-2330   Fax (201)451-1164

Majmundar, Sapan Haresh, DO {1215272943} IntrMd(NY75<NJ-BAYONNE, NJ-CHRIST>
+ St. Joseph's Regional Medical Center
   703 Main Street/Hospitalist   Paterson, NJ 07503   (973)754-2000

Majumdar, Shikha, MD {1689684383} IntrMd(76,INA9Y)<NJ-CENTRAST, NJ-RBAYOLDB>
+ 3499 Route 9 North/Suite 2C-3
   Freehold, NJ 07728   (732)431-5563   Fax (732)431-5593

Majumdar, Sourav, MD {1629285945} IntrMd(04,INA86)<MA-DEACNASH>
+ UH-Robert Wood Jhnsn Med Sch
   97 Paterson Street   New Brunswick, NJ 08901

Mak, John, MD {1417924168} Anesth, AnesPain(02,NY06)
+ New Jersey Ambulatory Anesthesia Consultants, LLC
   55 Schanck Road/Suite 8-A   Freehold, NJ 07728   (732)431-9544   Fax (732)431-9313

Mak, Mimi, MD {1881025609} IntrMd(11,PA09)<NJ-HUNTRDN>
+ Hunterdon Medical Center
   2100 Wescott Drive/Hospitalist   Flemington, NJ 08822
   (908)788-5486   Fax (908)237-5488

Mak, Sheila Shuk-Yin, DO {1336436211} Pedtrc
+ 328a Sparta Avenue
   Sparta, NJ 07871   (973)729-2197   Fax (973)729-3653

Makadia, Bhaktidevi, MD {1518355262} IntrMd<NJ-JRSYCITY>
+ Jersey City Medical Center
   355 Grand Street   Jersey City, NJ 07304   (201)915-2000

Makadia, Payal Ameesh, MD {1053639229} PedGst<NJ-HACKNSK>
+ Hackensack University Medical Center
   30 Prospect Avenue   Hackensack, NJ 07601   (551)996-2000

Makar, Gamil Lamey Bekheet, MD {1972544815} FamMed, Grtrcs, FamMGrtc(97,EGY05)
+ Valley Medical Associates
   220 Hamburg Turnpike/Suite 9   Wayne, NJ 07470
   (973)826-0068   Fax (973)807-1886
+ Valley Medical Associates
   1700 Route 3 West   Clifton, NJ 07012   (973)826-0068   Fax (973)928-2650

Makar, George A., MD {1023181450} IntrMd, Hepato, Gastrn(00,IA02)<PA-UPMCPHL>
+ Atlantic Gastroenterology Associates, P.A.
   3205 Fire Road/Suite 4   Egg Harbor Township, NJ 08234
   (609)407-1220   Fax (609)407-0220

Makar, Mary Saleeb, MD {1982600367} Ophthl(00,MA01)
+ Soll Eye PC of New Jersey/Cooper Division
   3 Cooper Plaza/Suite 510   Camden, NJ 08103   (856)342-7200   Fax (856)342-6620
+ W. Reed Kindermann, M.D. and Associates
   3001 Chapel Avenue West/Suite 200   Cherry Hill, NJ 08002
   (856)342-7200   Fax (856)667-0661

Makhija, Vasudev N., MD {1740322536} Psychy(75,INA69)<NJ-TRINIWSC, NJ-RWJURAH>
+ 812 Northwood Avenue/Suite 102
   Linden, NJ 07036   (908)486-6666   Fax (908)925-7708

Makhlouf, Jean, MD {1881795912} Pedtrc(74,LEB03)<NJ-ST-BARNMC>
+ Roseland Pediatrics
   556 Eagle Rock Avenue/Suite 106   Roseland, NJ 07068
   (973)228-9190   Fax (973)228-0730

Maki, Junsuke, MD {1184824450} Gastrn, IntrMd(04,NY08)
+ Shore Gastroenterology Associates, P.C.
   1907 Highway 35/Suite 1   Oakhurst, NJ 07755   (732)517-0060   Fax (732)548-7408
+ Shore Gastroenterology Associates, P.C.
   1907 Highway 35/Suite 1   Oakhurst, NJ 07755   (732)517-0060   Fax (732)548-7408
+ Shore Gastroenterology Associates, P.C.
   233 Middle Road   Hazlet, NJ 07730   (732)361-2476

Makimura, Hideo, MD {1063444594} IntrMd(04,NY47)<MA-MA-GENHOS>
+ Merck and Company Incorporated
   126 East Lincoln Avenue   Rahway, NJ 07065   (973)574-4000

Makkapati, Sandhya Rani, MD {1780687806} Anesth(91,INA62)<NJ-STMRYPAS>
+ St. Joseph's Regional Medical Center Anesthesia
   703 Main Street   Paterson, NJ 07503   (973)754-2323   Fax (973)977-9455

Mako, Robert M., DO {1578647491} Anesth(87,NJ75)
+ Ocean Anesthesia Group PA
   1200 Hooper Avenue   Toms River, NJ 08753   (732)797-3890   Fax (732)942-5603

Makowsky, Michael J., MD {1083735104} OccpMd, IntrMd(72,IN20)<NJ-CHSMRCER, NJ-CHSFULD>
+ Corporate Health Center
   832 Brunswick Avenue   Trenton, NJ 08638   (609)695-7471

Makowsky, Tammy B., MD {1790784817} Pedtrc(91,NJ06)<NJ-RWJUBRUN, NJ-STPETER>
+ Healthy Futures Pediatrics
   9 Professional Circle/Suite 107   Colts Neck, NJ 07722
   (732)462-7511   Fax (732)462-2822

Makris, Alex T., MD {1346262748} InfDis, IntrMd(71,KY02)
+ 532 Old Martin Pike/PMB 195
   Marlton, NJ 08053   (856)795-7505   Fax (856)424-4470

Makui, Sheyda, MD {1790066454} FamMed
+ NHCAC Health Center at Passaic
   110 Main Avenue   Passaic, NJ 07055   (973)777-0256   Fax (973)777-3910

Malabanan, Nerissa V., MD {1255428124} Pedtrc(80,PHI08)<NJ-HOBUNIMC, NJ-CHRIST>
+ Progressive Pediatrics
   1222 Kennedy Boulevard   Bayonne, NJ 07002   (201)437-9600   Fax (201)437-9661
+ Progressive Pediatrics
   3196 Kennedy Boulevard   Union City, NJ 07087   (201)437-9600   Fax (201)319-9849

Malagold, Michael, MD {1710976857} CdvDis(75,NY09)
+ Lakeland Cardiology Center, P.A.
   415 Boulevard   Mountain Lakes, NJ 07046   (973)334-7700   Fax (973)402-5847
+ Lakeland Cardiology Center PA
   765 State Route 10/Suite 4   Randolph, NJ 07869   (973)989-2566

Malalis, Carmelita Pingol, MD {1598868523} Pedtrc(64,PHI01)
+ 765 Kennedy Boulevard
   Bayonne, NJ 07002   (201)437-9471   Fax (201)437-1590

Malamut, Jay M., MD {1881682367} Gastrn, IntrMd(81,PA09)<NJ-VIRTMARL>
+ Allied Gastrointestinal Associates
   502 Centennial Boulevard/Suite 3   Voorhees, NJ 08043
   (856)751-2300   Fax (856)751-2333

Malanga, Gerard A., MD {1245275098} PhysMd(87,NJ05)
+ New Jersey Sports Medicine
   197 Ridgedale Avenue/Suite 210   Cedar Knolls, NJ 07927
   (973)998-8301   Fax (973)998-8302

Malantic-Lu, Grace Paula, MD {1679553051} RadDia(96,NJ05)
+ Edison Radiology Group, P.A.
   65 James Street   Edison, NJ 08820   (732)321-7917   Fax (732)737-2968

Malapero, Raymond Joseph, III, MD {1861735326} Anesth(13,NJ05)
+ University Hospital
   150 Bergen Street   Newark, NJ 07103   (973)972-4300

Malaty, Christine B., DO {1477744142} Pedtrc
+ Ivy Pediatrics
   220 Bridge Plaza Drive   Manalapan, NJ 07726   (732)972-9525   Fax (732)972-9055
+ Ivy Pediatrics
   175 North Broadway   South Amboy, NJ 08879   (732)972-9525   Fax (732)852-8816
+ Ivy Pediatrics
   7 Brunswick Woods Drive   East Brunswick, NJ 07726
   (732)432-7337   Fax (732)432-7338

Malave, Esther, MD {1992747885} FamMed(96,NJ06)
+ Center Pediatrics Adolescent & Adult
   12000 Lincoln Drive West/Suite 311   Marlton, NJ 08053
   (856)985-8100   Fax (856)985-0178

Malazarte, Justito B., MD {1851399588} Anesth(82,PHI16)<NJ-STMRYPAS>
+ St. Mary's Hospital
   350 Boulevard   Passaic, NJ 07055   (973)365-4300   Fax (973)779-7385

Malberg, Marc I., MD {1952412694} SrgOrt, SrgOARec, SrgSpn(71,IL06)<NJ-STPETER, NJ-RWJUBRUN>
+ Orthopedic Center of New Jersey
   1527 Route 27/Suite 1300   Somerset, NJ 08873   (732)249-4444   Fax (732)249-6528
   DRMALBERG@BACKNEE.net

Malde, Hiten Maganlal, MD {1336124478} Radiol, RadNro(84,INA67)<NJ-ENGLWOOD, NJ-HACKNSK>
+ Englewood Hospital and Medical Center
   350 Engle Street/Radiology   Englewood, NJ 07631
   (201)894-3412   Fax (201)894-5244
+ Hackensack Radiology Group, P.A.
   30 Prospect Avenue   Hackensack, NJ 07601   (201)894-3412   Fax (201)336-8451

Maldjian, Pierre D., MD {1992813687} RadDia, RadBdl(86,PA09)<NJ-UMDNJ>
+ University Hospital
   150 Bergen Street/Diag Radiology   Newark, NJ 07103
   (973)972-4300   Fax (973)972-7429

Maldonado, Jose O., MD {1932142957} Pedtrc(86,MEX29)<NJ-PALISADE, NJ-STJOSHOS>
+ NHCAC Health Center at West New York
   5301 Broadway/Pedi   West New York, NJ 07093   (201)866-9320   Fax (201)867-9183

Maldonado, Rodolfo, MD {1093823668} IntrMd(94,PER08)
+ 86 New Brunswick Avenue
   Perth Amboy, NJ 08861   (732)826-1609   Fax (732)826-0075

Maldonado, Samuel David, MD {1073842159} Pedtrc(83,HON01)
+ Johnson & Johnson Research & Develop
   920 US Highway Route 202   Raritan, NJ 08869   (908)704-4000

Maldonado-Viera, Lourdes, MD {1932117421} Anesth(88,NY06)<NJ-HUNTRDN>
+ Hunterdon Medical Center
   2100 Wescott Drive/Anesthesiology   Flemington, NJ 08822
   (908)788-6100   Fax (908)788-6361

Malek, Ashraf Hossain, MD {1427194075} Hepato, IntrMd(95,BAN06)<NJ-LOURDEHS>
+ Southern New Jersey Center for Liver Disease
   63 Kresson Road/Suite 105   Cherry Hill, NJ 08034
   (856)796-9340   Fax (856)547-0390

Malek, Sherif, MD {1699716175} IntrMd, Grtrcs(87,EGY04)<NJ-MONMOUTH>
+ Malek Medical Center
   232 Norwood Avenue   West Long Branch, NJ 07764
   (732)222-6637   Fax (732)222-6645

Maleki, Dordaneh, MD {1356378574} Gastrn, Hepato, IntrMd(90,DC01)<NJ-ACMCITY, NJ-ACMCMAIN>
+ 2106 New Road/Unit E-2
   Linwood, NJ 08221
   Dmaleki@comcast.net

Maleki, Kataneh F., MD {1396706651} ClCdEl, IntrMd(92,IRA03)<NJ-RWJUBRUN>
+ Cardio Metabolic Institute
   294 Applegarth Road/Suite F   Monroe Township, NJ 08831
   (609)642-4747   Fax (732)846-7001
+ Cardio Metabolic Institute
   51 Veronica Avenue   Somerset, NJ 08873   (609)642-4747   Fax (732)846-7001
+ 172 Somerset Street/Suite 5
   New Brunswick, NJ 08831   (732)651-1431   Fax (732)257-9922

Maletsky, Mark E., MD {1750478418} SrgOrt(81,NJ05)<NJ-CHILTON>
+ 2025 Hamburg Turnpike/Suite G
   Wayne, NJ 07470   (973)835-3224   Fax (973)835-0779

Maletzky, David Michael, DO {1891736385} IntrMd(98,MO78)<NJ-DEBRAHLC>
+ Deborah Heart and Lung Center
   200 Trenton Road   Browns Mills, NJ 08015   (609)893-6611   Fax (609)893-1213

Maley, Michael Kendrick, MD {1598742736} Ophthl(00,VT02)<NJ-MONMOUTH>
+ Phillips Eye Center
   619 River Drive/Second Floor   Elmwood Park, NJ 07407
   (201)796-2020   Fax (201)796-3644

Malfitano, Laura Anne, DO {1922094242} OrtSHand(99,NJ75)<NJ-SOCEANCO, NJ-COMMED>
+ Brielle Orthopedics PA
457 Jack Martin Boulevard   Brick, NJ 08724   (732)840-7500   Fax (732)840-2088
+ Brielle Orthopedics PA
823 Lacey Road   Forked River, NJ 08731   (732)840-7500   Fax (732)840-2088
+ Brielle Orthopedics PA
1301 Route 72 West   Manahawkin, NJ 08724   (609)971-7616   Fax (609)971-7639

Malhotra, Amisha, MD {1316007792} PedInf, Pedtrc(94,NY03)<NJ-RWJUBRUN>
+ RWJ University Pediatric Infectious Disease
125 Paterson Street/MEB 322   New Brunswick, NJ 08901   (732)235-7894   Fax (732)235-7419
+ Family Medicine at Monument Square
317 George Street   New Brunswick, NJ 08901   (732)235-7894   Fax (732)246-7317

Malhotra, Amit, MD {1982869525} IntrMd, IntHos<NJ-CHRIST, NJ-HOBUNIMC>
+ Christ Hospital
176 Palisade Avenue/Hospitalist   Jersey City, NJ 07306   (201)795-8200
+ Bayonne Medical Center
29th Street at Avenue E/Hospitalist   Bayonne, NJ 07002   (201)858-5000
+ Hoboken University Medical Center
308 Willow Avenue/Hospitalist   Hoboken, NJ 07306   (201)418-1000

Malhotra, Anuj Kumar, MD {1437462926} IntrMd(07,NY15)
+ Princeton Medical Group, P.A.
419 North Harrison Street   Princeton, NJ 08540   (609)924-9300   Fax (609)924-6552
anujmal1980@gmail.com

Malhotra, Chanchal Anand, MD {1184875445} PthACl, PthCyt, PthImm(71,INA7Y)
+ Quest Diagnostics Inc.
1 Malcolm Avenue   Teterboro, NJ 07608   (201)393-5000   Fax (201)393-6127

Malhotra, Gautam, MD {1407879000} PhysMd, Elecmy(01,NJ05)<NJ-VAEASTOR, NJ-VALYONS>
+ VA New Jersey Health Care System-East Orange Campus
385 Tremont Avenue/13thFl/PMRS/Att   East Orange, NJ 07018   (973)676-1000
gautam.malhotra@med.va.gov
+ VA New Jersey Health Care System at Lyons
151 Knollcroft Road   Lyons, NJ 07939   (908)647-0180
+ Overlook Medical Arts Center
33 Overlook Road/Suite 212   Summit, NJ 07018   (908)273-0500   Fax (888)769-6930

Malhotra, Mahamaya, MD {1912074550} Psychy(70,INDI)
+ Partners in Psychiatry, LLP
33 Overlook Road/Suite 212   Summit, NJ 07901   (908)273-6164   Fax (908)277-1439

Malhotra, Pieusha, MD {1932549532} IntrMd<MA-WRCSTMC>
+ New Bridge Medical Center
230 East Ridgewood Avenue   Paramus, NJ 07652   (201)967-4000

Malhotra, Pooja, MD {1376738112}
+ 156 Park Avenue
Dumont, NJ 07628

Malhotra, Rahul, MD {1053626747} Psychy
+ Partners in Psychiatry, LLP
33 Overlook Road/Suite 212   Summit, NJ 07901   (908)273-6164   Fax (908)277-1439

Malhotra, Rakesh, MD {1558302521} IntMHPC, Grtrcs(83,INA86)
+ Garden State Medical Associates
100 Brick Road/Suite 209   Marlton, NJ 08053   (856)983-2848

Malhotra, Sunil Prakash, MD {1063568665} Surgry, SrgVas(97,NY19)<NJ-NWRKBETH>
+ Newark Beth Israel Medical Center
201 Lyons Avenue/Suite L-5   Newark, NJ 07112   (973)926-7000

Mali, Shalini Reddy, MD {1750473286} IntrMd(97,INA5B)<NJ-MTNSIDE>
+ 88 Park Street
Montclair, NJ 07042   (973)746-0009   Fax (973)746-7911

Malicdem, Milagros C., MD {1003879487} NnPnMd, Pedtrc(83,PHI08)<NJ-KMHSTRAT, NJ-KMHTURNV>
+ Kennedy Health Systems/Washington Township Campus
435 Hurffville-Cross Keys Road   Turnersville, NJ 08012   (856)582-2500

Malickel, Jay Varunny, DO {1902893134} FamMed(97,NJ75)<NJ-SJRSYELM>
+ Centerton Family Practice
798 Centerton Road   Elmer, NJ 08318   (856)358-6161   Fax (856)358-0142

Malik, Ankit, DO {1023436433} FamMAdlt<NJ-SHOREMEM>
+ Shore Memorial Hospital
1 East New York Avenue   Somers Point, NJ 08244   (609)653-3500

Malik, Arsalan, MD {1821187626} IntrMd(03,TX12)<NJ-SOMERSET>
+ Advance Hospital Care @ Somerset Medical Center
110 Rehill Avenue   Somerville, NJ 08876   (908)429-5833   Fax (908)203-5970
+ RWJ University Hospital Somerset
110 Rehill Avenue/Hospitalist   Somerville, NJ 08876   (908)685-2200

Malik, Bobby A., MD {1396804712} IntrMd(99,GRN01)<NJ-STJOSHOS>
+ Princeton Medical Care
2050 Route 27/Suite 206   North Brunswick, NJ 08902   (732)821-5511   Fax (732)821-5347

Malik, Chetan, MD {1649246760} PhysMd(96,INA30)<NY-KALBUFLO, NY-ERIECMC>
+ Bogdan Pain Management Services
112 Professional View Drive/Bld 100   Freehold, NJ 07728   (732)577-9126   Fax (732)577-9127

Malik, Farhan, MD {1437572468}
+ Physician Practice Enhancement, LLC
66 West Gilbert Street   Red Bank, NJ 07701   (732)406-4698
fmalik786@gmail.com

Malik, Ghazalah Iqbal, MD {1346595915}
+ 514 Imbrie Place
Morganville, NJ 07751

Malik, Irfan Asim, MD {1679837611} IntrMd<NJ-VIRTMARL>
+ Virtua Marlton Hospital
90 Brick Road   Marlton, NJ 08053   (856)762-1933   Fax (856)762-1777

Malik, Khurram Saleem, MD {1104162767}
+ 867 Pavonia Avenue
Jersey City, NJ 07306   (551)220-0226

Malik, Manish Gulshan, MD {1457555245} CdvDis
+ Penn Specialty Care of Burlington County
200 Campbell Drive/Suite 115   Willingboro, NJ 08046   (609)871-7070   Fax (609)835-4510

Malik, Neveen A., DO {1730370891} PulDis, IntrMd(06,MI12)
+ Kennedy Health Alliance
900 Medical Center Drive/Suite 201   Sewell, NJ 08080   (856)218-2100   Fax (856)218-2101
+ Kennedy Health Alliance Vascular Surgery
333 Laurel Oak Road   Voorhees, NJ 08043   (856)218-2100   Fax (856)770-9194

Malik, Nisha, MD {1013984616} ObsGyn, MtFtMd(89,WI06)<NJ-MONMOUTH>
+ Monmouth Medical Group, P.C.
73 South Bath Avenue   Long Branch, NJ 07740   (732)870-3600   Fax (732)870-0119
+ Monmouth Family Center
270 Broadway   Long Branch, NJ 07740   (732)870-3600   Fax (732)923-7104
+ Barnabas Health Medical Group
166 Morris Avenue/2nd Floor   Long Branch, NJ 07740   (732)263-5024   Fax (732)263-5029

Malik, Parvaiz Akhtar, MD {1871537944} SrgHnd, SrgPlstc, SrgRec(72,PAK11)<NJ-RWJUHAM, NJ-CHSFULD>
+ Plastic Surgery of Central Jersey
1542 Kuser Road/Suite B-2   Hamilton, NJ 08619   (609)585-0044   Fax (609)585-5977
pscj@optimum.net

Malik, Pooja, MD {1568578599} FamMed(98,INA26)<NJ-SJRSYELM>
+ Mullica Hill Medical Associates PC
201 Bridgeton Pike   Mullica Hill, NJ 08062   (856)478-2111   Fax (856)478-4709

Malik, Rajesh, MD {1417997115} IntrMd(96,INA23)
+ Mullica Hill Medical Associates PC
201 Bridgeton Pike   Mullica Hill, NJ 08062   (856)478-2111   Fax (856)478-4709

Malik, Rehan, MD {1235417494} Psychy
+ 4 Belmont Court
Monroe, NJ 08831   (732)900-0060

Malik, Rema, MD {1881960169} Surgry
+ UMDNJ Surgery
185 South Orange Avenue   Newark, NJ 07103   (973)972-5682

Malik, Ritu, MD {1255353512} EnDbMt, IntrMd(97,INA23)<NY-VIAROCHS>
+ Deborah C. Rose Family Chiropractic Center
180 White Road/Suite 205   Little Silver, NJ 07739   (732)842-4111   Fax (732)842-4119

Malik, Rohit, MD {1396944039}
+ Pulmonary and Sleep Physicians
204 Ark Road/Suite 206/Larchmont 1   Mount Laurel, NJ 08054   (856)778-4640   Fax (856)778-0119

Malik, Shoaib, MD {1427312677}<NJ-RWJUHAM>
+ Robert Wood Johnson University Hospital at Hamilton
1 Hamilton Health Place   Hamilton, NJ 08690   (973)251-1081

Malik, Tahseen Rabia, MD {1447561121} FamMed(84,ENG11)
+ Drs. Magnet & Rogers
831 Kings Highway/Suite 100   Woodbury, NJ 08096   (856)853-8730   Fax (856)853-7063

Malik, Tayyaba K., MD {1306956164} Pedtrc(83,PAKI)<NJ-CHRIST>
+ West Side Pediatrics
2749 Kennedy Boulevard   Jersey City, NJ 07306   (201)432-0714   Fax (201)432-0016

Malik, Zeenat Q., MD {1922074509} PedDvl, BhvrMd(90,PAK14)<NJ-CHLSMT>
+ Children's Specialized Hospital
150 New Providence Road   Mountainside, NJ 07092   (908)233-3720   Fax (908)301-5456
+ Children's Specialized Hospital
3575 Quakerbridge Road   Hamilton, NJ 08619   (609)631-2800

Malinverni, Helio J., MD {1174690978} CdvDis, IntrMd(67,BRAZ)<NJ-SOCEANCO>
+ Medical Associates of Ocean County, P.A.
1301 Route 72 West/Suite 300   Manahawkin, NJ 08050   (609)597-6513   Fax (609)597-4593

Malit, Michele Farrah, DO {1528220225} SrgC&R, Surgry(NY75<NJ-BAYSHORE, NJ-RIVERVW>
+ Matawan Surgical Associates
717 North Beers Street/Suite 1-E   Holmdel, NJ 07733   (732)847-3300   Fax (732)739-5295

Malitzky, Susan, MD {1548599822} Pedtrc, IntrMd(09,NY46)<NJ-VALLEYHS>
+ 145 Main Avenue/Suite 203
Passaic, NJ 07055   (973)591-1600   Fax (973)591-1605

Malizia, Robert W., MD {1144426149} EmrgMd(04,PA02)
+ 532 Hudson Street/Unit 2
Hoboken, NJ 07030

Maljian, Meroujan Ardziv, MD {1780888966} Psychy, PsyFor(99,MNT01)
+ University Behavioral HealthCare - UMDNJ
Box 863/Whittlesey Road   Trenton, NJ 08625   (609)341-3093   Fax (609)341-9380

Malkani, Raj S., MD {1245325414} Pedtrc(74,INDI)
+ Rutgers Hurtado Health Center
11 Bishop Place   New Brunswick, NJ 08901   (732)932-7402   Fax (732)932-1223

Malladi, Viswanath, MD {1588845572} IntHos(03,INA1Z)
+ Overlook Medical Center
99 Beauvoir Avenue/PO Box 210   Summit, NJ 07902   (908)522-2000   Fax (973)290-8325
+ IPC The Hospitalist Company
55 Madison Avenue/Suite 310   Morristown, NJ 07960   (908)522-2000   Fax (973)998-4237

Mallamaci, Carmen R., MD {1457314346} Pedtrc(87,NY47)<NJ-PALISADE>
+ NHCAC Health Center at West New York
5301 Broadway   West New York, NJ 07093   (201)866-9320

Mallari, Rolando Q., MD {1598849614} Pedtrc, IntHos, IntrMd(80,PHI02)<NJ-ACMCMAIN, NJ-ACMCITY>
+ AtlantiCare Regional Medical Center/City Campus
1925 Pacific Avenue/Pediatrics   Atlantic City, NJ 08401   (609)345-4000

Mallen, Frederic J., MD {1952373888} Ophthl(74,NY09)<NJ-CHSFULD, NJ-CHSMRCER>
+ 3100 Princeton Pike
Lawrenceville, NJ 08648   (609)896-0101

Malley, Debra S., MD {1447299748} Ophthl(90,MA05)
+ TLC Kremer Cherry Hill LASIK
1800 Chapel Avenue West/Suite 100   Cherry Hill, NJ 08002

Malli, Dipakkumar Purushott, MD {1265410831} IntrMd, PulDis, SlpDis(93,INA20)
+ 140 East Evesham Road
Cherry Hill, NJ 08003   (856)427-4477   Fax (856)427-9199

Malliah, Sangit Bhoosa, MD {1083889620} RadDia(03,NJ05)<NJ-COOPRUMC>
+ The Cooper Hospital System-Univ Hospital
3 Cooper Plaza/Suite 215/Radiology   Camden, NJ 08103   (856)342-2439

Mallik, Aparna, MD {1467487223} Pedtrc, PedDvl, PedNrD(79,INA1K)<NJ-STJOSHOS>
+ St. Joseph's Children's Hospital
703 Main Street/Child Dev   Paterson, NJ 07503   (973)754-2510

Mallipeddi, Harini, MD {1033310586} IntrMd
+ 21 Periwinkle Drive
Monmouth Junction, NJ 08852
+ The Valley Hospital
223 North Van Dien Avenue   Ridgewood, NJ 07450   (201)447-8000

Mallipudi, Rajiv Matthew, MD {1760845747}<NJ-MTNSIDE>
+ Hackensack UMC Mountainside
1 Bay Avenue   Montclair, NJ 07042   (973)429-6000

Physicians by Name and Address

Mallon, Nancy Tyrrell, MD {1912092453} Pedtrc, IntrMd(84,DC02)<NY-PRSBWEIL, NJ-ENGLWOOD>
+ Mountainside Family Practice Associates
  799 Bloomfield Avenue/Suite 201   Verona, NJ 07044   (973)746-7050   Fax (973)857-2831

Mallouhi, Issam, MD {1659312098} IntrMd, EmrgMd(81,SYRI)
+ 1031 McBride Avenue/Suite D-205
  West Paterson, NJ 07424   (973)237-9055   Fax (973)237-9053

Malone, Carolyn Marie, MD {1295900843} RadDia
+ Hackensack Radiology Group, P.A.
  30 Prospect Avenue   Hackensack, NJ 07601   (551)996-2200   Fax (201)489-2812

Malone, Jennie O'Lera, DO {1558569814} FamMed(07,VA75)
+ McGuire Air Force Base/Acute Health Care Clinic
  3458 Neely Road   Trenton, NJ 08641   (609)754-9014   Fax (609)754-9015
+ MedExpress Urgent Care Watchung
  1569 US Highway 22   Watchung, NJ 07069   (609)754-9014   Fax (908)322-2679

Malone, Michael Richard, DO {1194916908} IntrMd, IntHos(FL75<NJ-VIRTMHBC>
+ Virtua Hospitalist Group Memorial
  175 Madison Avenue   Mount Holly, NJ 08060   (609)914-6180   Fax (609)914-6182

Malone, Richard J., DO {1245261460} PhysMd(90,NJ75)<NJ-JFKJHNSN>
+ JFK Johnson Rehabilitation Institute
  65 James Street   Edison, NJ 08818   (732)321-7070   Fax (732)321-7330

Maloney, Marvelle, MD {1063815173} ObsGyn
+ Empire Medical Associates
  264 Boyden Avenue   Maplewood, NJ 07040   (917)403-8057   Fax (973)761-7617

Malovany, Robert J., MD {1255355400} IntrMd, PulDis, SlpDis(70,PA02)<NJ-ENGLWOOD, NJ-HOLYNAME>
+ Bergen Medical Alliance, P.A.
  180 Engle Street   Englewood, NJ 07631   (201)568-8010   Fax (201)568-8936
  rmalovany@bergenmedical.com

Malta, Raymond J., DO {1366481954} EmrgMd(92,NJ75)<NJ-VIRTVOOR>
+ Virtua Voorhees
  100 Bowman Drive/EmergMed   Voorhees, NJ 08043   (856)247-3000

Maltz, Gary S., MD {1114149028} Gastrn, IntrMd(82,NY09)<NJ-RWJUBRUN, NJ-UNVMCPRN>
+ University Medical Group
  125 Paterson Street/Suite 5100   New Brunswick, NJ 08901   (732)235-6968   Fax (732)235-7117

Maltzman, Barry A., MD {1386753648} Ophthl(70,NJ05)
+ Hudson Eye Physicians & Surgeons, LLC
  600 Pavonia Avenue/6th Floor   Jersey City, NJ 07306   (201)963-3937   Fax (201)963-8823

Maludum, Obiora, MD {1972858447} IntrMd<NJ-ACMCITY>
+ AtlantiCare Regional Medical Center/City Campus
  1925 Pacific Avenue   Atlantic City, NJ 08401   (609)441-8146   Fax (609)441-8002

Malzberg, Mark S., MD {1144295817} Radiol, RadBdI(83,IL42)<NJ-HUNTRDN>
+ Hunterdon Radiological Associate
  1 Dogwood Drive   Clinton, NJ 08809   (908)735-4477   Fax (908)735-6532
+ Hunterdon Medical Center
  2100 Wescott Drive/Radiology   Flemington, NJ 08822   (908)788-6100
+ Kings Court Imaging Center
  2 Kings Court/Suite 200   Flemington, NJ 08809   (908)806-8600   Fax (908)806-8646

Mama, Saifuddin Taiyeb, MD {1811906878} ObsGyn(93,PA02)
+ 426 Bridgeboro Road
  Moorestown, NJ 08057

Maman, Arie, MD {1609961408} EnDbMt, IntrMd(74,FRAN)<NJ-RWJUBRUN, NJ-STPETER>
+ Brier Hill Court/Unit D3
  East Brunswick, NJ 08816   (732)613-0707   Fax (732)613-1231
  ariemaman@aol.com

Mamidi, Arunima, MD {1730196478} IntrMd, InfDis(93,INA4D)<NJ-UNVMCPRN, NJ-RWJUHAM>
+ Princeton Infectious Disease Associates, LLC.
  5 Plainsboro Road/Suite 360   Plainsboro, NJ 08536   (609)750-0011   Fax (609)750-0022

Mamji, Salman, MD {1871960013} IntHos<NJ-JRSYCITY>
+ Jersey City Medical Center
  355 Grand Street   Jersey City, NJ 07304   (201)915-2200

Mamkin, Irene, MD {1326210485} PedEnd, Pedtrc, IntrMd(04,GRN01)<NJ-STBARNMC, NJ-NWRKBETH>
+ Children's Hospital of NJ Ped Cntr @ West Orange
  375 Mount Pleasant Avenue/Suite 105   West Orange, NJ 07052   (973)322-6900   Fax (973)322-6999

Mammen, Anish George, MD {1053574277} Gastrn
+ Hackensack Gastroenterology Associates
  130 Kinderkamack Road/Suite 301   River Edge, NJ 07661   (201)489-7772   Fax (201)489-2544
  mammenmd@gmail.com

Mammen-Prasad, Elizabeth K., MD {1366411084} InfDis, Pedtrc, PedInf(84,MNT01)
+ Prime Pediatrics
  50 Union Avenue/Suite 704   Irvington, NJ 07111   (973)373-9600   Fax (732)252-6634

Mammis, Antonios, MD {1417111360} SrgNro(06,NY01)
+ Center for Neurological Surgery UMDNJ
  90 Bergen Street/DOC 8100   Newark, NJ 07103   (973)972-4836   Fax (973)972-2333

Mammone, Joseph F., MD {1518942465} MRImag, RadDia(89,RI01)<NJ-RWJUBRUN, NJ-STPETER>
+ University Radiology Group, P.C.
  483 Cranbury Road   East Brunswick, NJ 08816   (732)390-0030   Fax (732)390-5383
+ University Radiology Group, P.C.
  16 Mountain Boulevard   Warren, NJ 07059   (732)390-0030   Fax (908)769-9141

Mamoun, Sami M., MD {1780620682} SrgPlstc, SrgRec(66,LEB03)<NJ-MORRISTN, NJ-STBARNMC>
+ The Center For Specialized Women's Health
  16 Pocono Road/Suite 103   Denville, NJ 07834   (973)947-9066   Fax (973)947-9056
+ The Center For Specialized Women's Health
  16 Eden Lane   Whippany, NJ 07981   (973)947-9066   Fax (973)947-9056
+ 188 Eagle Rock Avenue/Suite 2A
  Roseland, NJ 07834   (973)226-7565

Man, Jeremy Robert, MD {1104136381} Dermat
+ Skin Laser & Surgery Specialists
  105 Raider Boulevard/Suite 203   Hillsborough, NJ 08844   (201)441-9890   Fax (201)441-9893

Manabat, Eileen Rose, MD {1548380124} Anesth, PainMd
+ ASAP - Advanced Spine and Pain
  2 Eighth Street   Hammonton, NJ 08037   Fax (609)567-8832

Manalis, Helen, DO {1295712347} FamMed(99,PA77)
+ Haddonfield Internal Medicine
  216 Haddon Avenue   Haddon Township, NJ 08108   (856)854-6600   Fax (856)854-6700

Manalo, Rosario Beatriz, MD {1255328936} InfDis, IntrMd(97,PHI09)
+ ID Associates PA/dba ID Care
  765 Route 10 East/Suite 201   Randolph, NJ 07869   (973)989-0068   Fax (973)361-8955
+ ID Associates PA/dba ID Care
  8 Saddle Road   Cedar Knolls, NJ 07927   (973)989-0068   Fax (973)993-5953

Manaqibwala, Ummesalama M., MD PedCrC(09,KEN01)<NJ-JFKMED>
+ JFK Hospital Children's Services
  65 James Street/PedsCritCare   Edison, NJ 08818   (732)321-7000   Fax (732)906-4906

Manara, Louis R., DO {1700893229} RprEnd(76,PA77)
+ 200 A Route 73 North
  Voorhees, NJ 08043   (856)767-0009   Fax (856)767-0009

Manchen, Dennis R., MD {1952383853} FamMed(73,NY08)<NJ-HUNTRDN>
+ Flemington Medical Group, LLC
  200 State Route 31 North/Suite 105   Flemington, NJ 08822   (908)782-5100   Fax (908)782-0290

Mancheno, Mario A., MD {1417041013} Surgry(69,SPA12)<NJ-HOBUNIMC>
+ 89 Columbia Terrace
  Weehawken, NJ 07086   (201)656-8743   Fax (201)680-8884

Manchester, Joseph Matthew, DO {1144660622} EmrgMd
+ St Joseph's Medical Center Emergency
  703 Main Street   Paterson, NJ 07503   (631)433-2255   Fax (973)754-2249

Manchireddy, Suman, MD {1164676037} IntrMd(02,INA19)<NJ-HACKNSK>
+ Hackensack University Medical Center
  30 Prospect Avenue/IntMed   Hackensack, NJ 07601   (201)996-3664   Fax (551)996-0536

Mancuso, Alison M., DO {1861699282} FamMed(07,NJ75)
+ UMDNJ SOM Family Medicine
  141 Ganttown Road   Turnersville, NJ 08012   (856)218-0300

Mancuso, Cathie-Ann, MD {1992115422} IntrMd
+ Matawan Medical Associates
  213 Main Street   Matawan, NJ 07747   (732)566-2363   Fax (732)566-0502

Mand, Christine P., DO {1356382501} IntrMd, Pedtrc(91,NJ75)<NJ-MORRISTN>
+ The Matheny School and Hospital
  Main Street/PO Box 339   Peapack, NJ 07977   (908)234-0011   Fax (908)234-2635

Manda, Jayaprakash, MD {1528298247} IntHos, IntrMd(04,INA97)<NJ-STJOSHOS>
+ St. Joseph's Regional Medical Center
  703 Main Street/Hospitalist   Paterson, NJ 07503   (973)754-2000
+ Heart & Vascular Associates of Northern Jersey
  22-18 Broadway/Suite 201   Fair Lawn, NJ 07410   (973)754-2000   Fax (201)475-5522

Mandadi, Pranathi R., MD {1689695538} IntrMd(99,INA83)
+ Barnabas Health Medical Group
  166 Morris Avenue/2nd Floor   Long Branch, NJ 07740   (732)229-2020   Fax (732)229-2255

Mandal, Aparna, MD {1578594941} IntrMd(91,INA18)<NJ-COMMED, NJ-JRSYCITY>
+ Community Medical Center
  99 Route 37 West/IntMed   Toms River, NJ 08755   (732)557-8000
+ 599 Route 37 West/Suite 2
  Toms River, NJ 08755   (732)557-8000   Fax (732)998-8321

Mandal, Soma, MD {1497701676} IntrMd(97,NY19)<NY-NYUTISCH>
+ Summit Medical Group-Berkeley Heights Campus
  1 Diamond Hill Road   Berkeley Heights, NJ 07922   (908)277-8991   Fax (908)790-6576

Mandala, Ashok R., MD {1629275342} IntrMd, IntHos(01,INA9V)<NJ-VIRTMHBC>
+ Virtua Memorial
  175 Madison Avenue/Hospitalist   Mount Holly, NJ 08060   (609)267-0700

Mandalapu, Padma, MD {1710958624} Pedtrc(88,INDI)
+ Med for Kids
  322 Shore Road   Somers Point, NJ 08244   (609)927-1353
+ Tender Care Pediatrics
  2322 New Road   Northfield, NJ 08225   (609)641-0200

Mandel, Gilbert B., MD {1255374567} IntrMd(67,NY15)
+ Denville Associates of Internal Medicine
  16 Pocono Road/Suite 317   Denville, NJ 07834   (973)627-2650   Fax (973)627-8383

Mandel, Leonid, MD {1710902846} CdvDis, IntHos, IntrMd(03,DMN01)<NJ-COMMED>
+ Cardiology Associates of Morristown
  95 Madison Avenue/Suite 10A   Morristown, NJ 07960   (973)889-9001   Fax (973)889-9051

Mandel, Marc S., MD {1326005521} SrgCrC, Surgry(85,NY46)<NJ-RWJURAH, NJ-OVERLOOK>
+ 11 Overlook Road/Suite 160
  Summit, NJ 07901   (908)598-0966   Fax (908)598-0298

Mandel, Mark S., MD {1194764498} Pedtrc(86,NY48)<NJ-VAL-LEY>
+ Chestnut Ridge Pediatrics
  595 Chestnut Ridge Road   Woodcliff Lake, NJ 07677   (201)391-2020   Fax (201)391-0265

Mandel, Peter C., MD {1730259094} ObsGyn, IntrMd(83,TX13)<NJ-CENTRAST>
+ Women's Physicians & Surgeons
  501 Iron Bridge Road/Suite 10   Freehold, NJ 07728   (732)431-2999   Fax (732)431-2993
+ Women's Physicians & Surgeons
  510 Bridge Plaza Drive   Englishtown, NJ 07726   (732)431-2999   Fax (732)536-4570
+ Women's Physicians & Surgeons
  245A Main Street   Matawan, NJ 07728   (732)566-9466   Fax (732)566-0343

Mandel, Rekha J., MD {1518151463} IntHos<NJ-MONMOUTH>
+ Monmouth Medical Center
  300 Second Avenue   Long Branch, NJ 07740   (732)222-5200
+ Chambers Center
  435 South Street/Suite 160   Morristown, NJ 07960   (973)971-6301

Mandel, Robert, MD {1124108394} Anesth(83,CA14)<NJ-UNVMCPRN>
+ Mercer Dermatology
  3836 Quakerbridge Road/Suite 103   Hamilton, NJ 08619   (609)586-8888   Fax (609)586-0888
  mercerderm@gmail.com

Mandel, Steven S., MD {1184607566} LeglMd, IntrMd(65,MI07)<NJ-STBARNMC>
+ Livingston Medical Associates, LLC.
  449 Mount Pleasant Avenue/First Floor   West Orange, NJ 07052   (973)535-8311   Fax (973)535-1210

Mandelbaum, Bert, MD {1841279924} Pedtrc, AdolMd, IntrMd(97,NJ06)<NJ-UNVMCPRN>
+ Princeton Nassau Pediatrics, P.A.
  301 North Harrison Street   Princeton, NJ 08540   (609)924-5510   Fax (609)924-3577
+ Princeton Nassau Pediatrics, P.A.
  196 Princeton-Hightstown Road   West Windsor, NJ 08550   (609)924-5510   Fax (609)799-2294

Mandelblat, Zarina, MD {1881630770} PhysMd(74,UKR01)<NY-KNGBKJEW>
+ 18 Worlds Fair Drive
Somerset, NJ 08873 (732)271-8010

Mandelker, Eiran Moses, MD {1558340638} RadDia(92,PA01)
+ Coordinated Health
222 Red Lane Phillipsburg, NJ 08865 (610)861-8080 Fax (610)849-1013

Mandell, Ryan S., DO {1598920183} IntrMd
+ 602 Waldorf Road
Marlton, NJ 08053

Manders, Steven M., MD {1457329104} Dermat(88,NJ05)<NJ-COOPRUMC>
+ Heymann, Manders & Green LLC
100 Brick Road/Suite 306 Marlton, NJ 08053 (856)596-0111 Fax (856)596-7194
+ The Cooper Hospital System-Univ Hospital
3 Cooper Plaza/Suite 215 Camden, NJ 08103 (856)342-2439

Mandhle, Pankaja Anil, MD {1316921786} Anesth(83,INA65)<NJ-HACKNSK>
+ Hackensack University Medical Center
30 Prospect Avenue/Anesthesiology Hackensack, NJ 07601 (201)996-2000 Fax (201)488-6769

Mandia, Renita, DO {1851739254} Grtrcs<NY-NYUTISCH>
+ Virtua Voorhees
100 Bowman Drive Voorhees, NJ 08043 (856)247-3000

Mandigo, Grace Kim, MD {1528212511} SrgNro(03,NY01)<NY-SLRRSVLT>
+ St. Joseph's Regional Medical Center
703 Main Street/A-2404 Paterson, NJ 07503 (973)754-3616
+ Neurosurgeons of New Jersey
703 Main Street/Suite A2404 Paterson, NJ 07503 (973)754-3616

Manduley, Robert Alfred, MD {1578542254} PedCrd, Pedtrc(88,NY47)<NJ-STPETER, NY-CHLDCOPR>
+ Rutgers Pediatric Cardiology
125 Paterson Street/CAB 6100 New Brunswick, NJ 08901 (732)235-7905 Fax (732)235-7932

Manevich, Ilya, MD {1093997975} Anesth(03,NJ06)
+ Robert Wood Johnson-UMDNJ Anesthesia Group
1140 Route 72 West Manahawkin, NJ 08050 (609)978-8900

Maneyapanda, Mukundha Belliappa, MD {1578827721} FamMed
+ 1135 Clifton Avenue/Suite 203
Clifton, NJ 07013 (201)396-7616

Manfredonia, Patricia Estrada, MD {1639154180} Pedtrc(01,NJ05)<NJ-JRSYSHMC>
+ Healthy Pediatrics at Old Bridge, LLC
3 Athens Avenue South Amboy, NJ 08879 (732)952-8400 Fax (732)952-8402
info@healthypediatrics.com

Mang, Justin, MD {1780799874} Ophthl(69,PA02)
+ 240 Williamson Street/Suite 505
Elizabeth, NJ 07207 (908)289-0250 Fax (908)289-3713
jmang@comcast.net

Mangahas, Florinda R., MD {1578663514} OccpMd(69,PHI08)<NJ-ESSEXCO>
+ 73 Monroe Avenue
Roseland, NJ 07068 (973)432-1944
+ Essex County Hospital Center
204 Grove Avenue Cedar Grove, NJ 07009 (973)571-2800

Mangal, Rakesh, MD {1356305221} IntrMd, Pedtrc(82,INDI)<NJ-CHSMRCER>
+ 268 Academy Street
Hightstown, NJ 08520 (609)371-2100

Mangalindan, Carmelita C., MD {1285612234} Pedtrc(80,PHI01)<NJ-SJRSYELM, NJ-OURLADY>
+ OLLMC Neonatal Associates
1505 West Sherman Avenue Vineland, NJ 08360 (856)641-4000
+ Our Lady of Lourdes Medical Center
1600 Haddon Avenue/Neonatology Camden, NJ 08103 (856)641-4000 Fax (856)365-7868

Manganaro, David Thomas, MD {1811982200} IntrMd(85,NY08)
+ Manhattan Advanced Medicine
776 Shrewsbury Avenue/Suite 103b Tinton Falls, NJ 07724 (732)383-7310 Fax (732)383-5924
info@mamnyc.com

Manganelli, Douglas M., MD {1184665432} Anesth, AnesPain(85,GRNA)<NJ-KIMBALL>
+ Ocean Anesthesia Group PA
1200 Hooper Avenue Toms River, NJ 08753 (732)797-3890 Fax (732)942-5603

Mangaser, Rhodora D., MD {1881672830} Pedtrc(77,PHIL)<NJ-OURLADY>
+ 600 Somerdale Road
Voorhees, NJ 08043 (856)857-0002 Fax (856)857-0085

Mangia, Anthony J., MD {1750320040} InfDis, IntrMd(82,ITAL)<NJ-CHRIST, NJ-MEADWLND>
+ Mangia Medical Associates
239 Washington Street Jersey City, NJ 07302 (201)521-1100 Fax (201)521-1236
aj239@aol.com

Mangiaracina, Giacomo, MD {1942298427} IntrMd(87,ITAL)<NJ-RWJUHAM>
+ Altus Medical Care
3840 Quakerbridge Road/Suite 206 Mercerville, NJ 08619 (609)890-4200 Fax (609)586-0399

Manginello, Frank P., MD {1053364364} NnPnMd, Pedtrc(73,DC02)<NJ-VALLEY>
+ The Valley Hospital
223 North Van Dien Avenue/Neonatology Ridgewood, NJ 07450 (201)447-8388 Fax (201)447-8616

Mangold, Melissa Beth, DO {1699939561} IntrMd
+ Cooper Perinatology Associates
3 Cooper Plaza/Suite 502 Camden, NJ 08103 (856)968-7433 Fax (856)968-8499

Mangone, Jesse G., DO {1598777112} FamMed, GenPrc(75,PA77)
+ 1117 US Highway 46/Suite 202
Clifton, NJ 07013 (973)614-8484

Mangone, Kevin F., DO {1366675548}<NJ-NWTNMEM>
+ Newton Medical Center
175 High Street Newton, NJ 07860 (973)383-2121

Mangonon, Virgilio D., MD {1356330773} Anesth(72,PHI08)<NJ-BAYONNE>
+ 525 Jack Martin Boulevard/Suite 300
Brick, NJ 08724 (732)840-0067

Mangosing, Emma A., MD {1457357196} Pedtrc(82,PHIL)<NJ-JRSYCITY>
+ Jersey City Medical Center
355 Grand Street Jersey City, NJ 07304 (201)915-2542
+ Total Care Pediatrics in Jersey City
550 Newark Avenue/Suite 200 Jersey City, NJ 07306 (201)915-2542 Fax (201)795-4999

Mangra, Chandra, MD {1336306240} FamMed(96,PHI22)<NJ-STJOSHOS>
+ Care Point Health Associates
1225 McBride Avenue/Suite 200 Little Falls, NJ 07424 (973)850-3391 Fax (973)256-5036

Mangru, Subita S., MD {1043279193} Pedtrc(89,JMAC)<NJ-STBARNMC, NJ-OVERLOOK>
+ Millburn Pediatrics PA
159 Millburn Avenue Millburn, NJ 07041 (973)912-0155 Fax (973)912-8714

Mangsatabam, Ruby, MD {1215379326} Psychy
+ 8 Almond Lane
Edison, NJ 08820 (732)491-3704

Mangubat, Kimberly Mae, MD {1962835207} Pedtrc
+ Cooper University Medical Center/Camden
3 Cooper Plaza Camden, NJ 08103 (856)342-2001

Mangubat, Ofelia R., MD {1073515763} Pedtrc(70,PHIL)<NJ-VIRTVOOR>
+ 2301 Evesham Road/Suite 405
Voorhees, NJ 08043 (856)772-4988 Fax (856)772-2514

Mangunay, Danilo C., MD {1255451225} PhysMd(73,PHI09)
+ 81 Rock Road West
Green Brook, NJ 08812 Fax (908)769-6858

Mangunay, Nora Ramos, MD {1427094309} PsyCAd, Psychy(74,PHI09)<NJ-SUMOAKSH>
+ Summit Oaks Hospital
19 Prospect Street/Psychiatry Summit, NJ 07901 (908)522-7000 Fax (908)522-7098

Mangura, Bonita T., MD {1861586141} IntrMd, PulDis(71,PHIL)<NJ-UMDNJ>
+ Global Tuberculosis Institute (GTBI)
225 Warren Street/PO Box 1709 Newark, NJ 07101 (973)972-6232 Fax (973)972-3832
+ The University Hospital
65 Bergen Street Newark, NJ 07107 (973)972-6232 Fax (973)972-2904

Mangura, Carolina T., MD {1508898073} IntrMd, InfDis(74,PHIL)
+ University Hospital-New Jersey Medical School
30 Bergen Street Newark, NJ 07107 (973)972-4511

Manhoff, Dion T., MD {1063401743} PthCyt, Pthlgy(89,PA13)<NJ-WARREN>
+ Warren Hospital
185 Roseberry Street/Pathology Phillipsburg, NJ 08865 (908)859-6700 Fax (908)859-6849

Mani, Anup S., DO {1033403357} Psychy
+ AtlantiCare Behav Hlth/Hartford
13 North Hartford Avenue Atlantic City, NJ 08401 (609)348-1161

Mani, Ram, MD {1801003199} Nrolgy
+ University Hospital-RWJMS Neurology
125 Paterson Street/Suite 4100-6100 New Brunswick, NJ 08901 (732)235-7733 Fax (732)235-7041

Mani, Shrinidi, MD {1417215823} Pedtrc
+ Riverside Pediatric Group
1111 Hudson Street Hoboken, NJ 07030 (201)942-9320 Fax (201)942-9321

Mani, Srinivasan S., MD {1861489957} Nrolgy(65,INDI)
+ Neurology Consultants of Central Jersey, P.A.
225 May Street/Suite D Edison, NJ 08837 (732)738-8830 Fax (732)738-8831

Maniar, Anoli, MD {1831281682} Otlryg(01,NJ05)
+ Hunterdon Otolaryngology Associates
6 Sand Hill Road/Suite 302 Flemington, NJ 08822 (908)788-9131 Fax (908)788-0945

Maniar, Gina S., DO {1952317570} EmrgMd(94,NY75)<NJ-OCEANMC>
+ Ocean Medical Center
425 Jack Martin Boulevard/EmergMed Brick, NJ 08723 (732)840-2200 Fax (732)389-5395

Maniar, Madhavi N., MD {1497892319} Pedtrc(69,INA20)<NJ-STBARNMC>
+ Drs. Maniar and Nimma
90 Washington Street/Suite 305 East Orange, NJ 07018 (973)676-2492 Fax (973)676-5901

Maniar, Mihir Kishor, DO {1659387264} IntrMd(94,NY75)<NJ-MONMOUTH>
+ Hackensack Meridian Medical Group Primary Care
185 Route 36/Building A Suite 130 West Long Branch, NJ 07764 (848)300-2210 Fax (848)300-2207

Maniar, Payal, MD {1649419193} Pedtrc
+ Drs. Maniar and Nimma
90 Washington Street/Suite 305 East Orange, NJ 07018 (973)676-2492 Fax (973)676-5901

Maniar, Sonali R., MD {1649476946} IntrMd(96,INA5Y)<NJ-STCLRDEN>
+ St. Clare's Hospital-Denville Campus
25 Pocono Road Denville, NJ 07834 (973)625-6000

Manickam, Rajapriya, MD {1285938431}
+ St Joseph's Medical Ctr Internal Med
703 Main Street Paterson, NJ 07503 (973)754-2027 Fax (973)754-3665

Manickavel, Suresh Kumar, MD {1336465061} IntrMd
+ 200 Hospital Plaza/Apt 106
Paterson, NJ 07503 (201)234-9376

Manicone, John A., MD {1518967249} SrgVas, Surgry(89,NJ06)<NJ-NWRKBETH, NJ-STBARNMC>
+ Millburn Surgical Associates
225 Millburn Avenue/Suite 104-B Millburn, NJ 07041 (973)379-5888 Fax (973)912-9757
www.jmanicone@bellatlantic.net

Manigat, Yves J., MD {1477643211} Surgry, Bariat, SrgOnc(68,HAI01)<NJ-OURLADY, NJ-VIRTUAHS>
+ Echelon Medical Center
600 Somerdale Road Voorhees, NJ 08043 (856)429-8445 Fax (856)429-1962
+ Parkside Medical
1300 Princess Avenue Camden, NJ 08103 (856)757-0533

Manigault, Simone A., MD {1417039132} Pedtrc, AdolMd(99,NJ05)<NJ-NWRKBETH>
+ Newark Community Health Center, Inc.
741 Broadway Newark, NJ 07104 (973)675-1900 Fax (973)676-1396
+ JRMC at Malcolm X Shabazz High School
80 Johnson Avenue Newark, NJ 07108 (973)675-1900 Fax (973)623-8938

Maniker, Allen Howard, MD {1275613366} SrgNro(86,MI07)
+ Center for Neurological Surgery UMDNJ
90 Bergen Street/DOC 8100 Newark, NJ 07103 (973)972-2323 Fax (973)972-2333

Manion, William L., MD {1134120801} PthACl, PthFor, PthCln(82,WV01)<NJ-VIRTMHBC, NJ-VIRTUAHS>
+ Virtua Memorial
175 Madison Avenue Mount Holly, NJ 08060 (609)267-0700
+ Diagnostic Pathology Consultants, PA
4 Larsen Park Drive Medford, NJ 08055 (609)261-7095

Manis, Tyler Cory, MD {1346654142}<NJ-STJOSHOS>
+ St. Joseph's Regional Medical Center
703 Main Street Paterson, NJ 07503 (321)217-6797

Maniya, Mariam Z., MD {1598795411} IntrMd(90,PAKI)<NJ-CHS-FULD, NJ-CHSMRCER>
+ 941 Whitehorse Avenue/Suite 5
Trenton, NJ 08610 (609)581-9100 Fax (609)581-7588

Maniya, Zakaria W., MD {1164496832} IntrMd, Nephro(83,PAK11)<NJ-RWJUHAM, NJ-STFRNMED>
+ Zak Maniya, M.D., P.A.
2333 Whitehorse-Mercerville Rd/Suite 4 Mercerville, NJ 08619 (609)890-9111 Fax (609)890-6865

Manji, Faiza, MD {1740697192} IntrMd(11,GRN01)
+ St. Michael's Medical Center
111 Central Avenue Newark, NJ 07102 (973)877-2420 Fax (973)877-2413

Manji, Hussain Mehdi, MD {1760747836} IntrMd<NJ-HACKNSK>
+ Hackensack University Medical Center
30 Prospect Avenue Hackensack, NJ 07601 (551)996-3664

Mankarios, Farag Amin Farag, MD {1912930082} IntrMd(83,EGY04)<NJ-BAYSHORE, NJ-CENTRAST>
+ 410 Route 34/Suite 216
Colts Neck, NJ 07722 (732)863-5515 Fax (732)863-5516

Physicians by Name and Address

Mankikar, Durgesh P., MD {1831116284} Anesth(71,INA67)<NJ-STMRYPAS>
+ St. Mary's Hospital
350 Boulevard/Anesth   Passaic, NJ 07055   (973)365-4300   Fax (973)779-7385

Mankikar, Mohini T., MD {1710908850} Anesth(70,INA00)<NJ-MTNSIDE>
+ 7 Reid Street
West Orange, NJ 07052

Mankikar, Rohan, MD {1851683445}
+ 6 Melanie Manor
East Brunswick, NJ 08816   (732)236-4118   Fax (404)756-1313

Mankowitz, Scott Levi, MD {1922115435} EmrgMd(97,NY08)
+ Hackensack Medical Center Emergency Medicine
30 Prospect Avenue/Main 3619   Hackensack, NJ 07601   (201)996-4614   Fax (201)996-3066

Manlangit, Arsenio C., MD {1124114533} ObsGyn(67,PHIL)<NJ-MORRISTN>
+ 115 Route 46/Bldg D, Suite 27
Mountain Lakes, NJ 07046   (973)263-3165   Fax (973)263-3142

Manlapid, Luis T., MD {1174531032} Pedtrc(71,PHI09)<NJ-JRSYHMC>
+ 700 Candlewood Commons
Howell, NJ 07731   (732)367-3130   Fax (732)901-2539

Mann, Ana Mendes, MD {1487816799} Pedtrc(05,PA13)<NJ-VIRTMHBC, NJ-VIRTVOOR>
+ CHOP Care Network at Virtua
101 Carnie Boulevard   Voorhees, NJ 08043   (856)325-3000

Mann, Dharam P., MD {1063463099} Anesth(94,INA06)<NJ-STJOSHOS>
+ Manchester Surgery Center
1100 Route 70   Whiting, NJ 08759   (732)716-8116   Fax (732)849-1511
+ Garden State Radiation Oncology
512 Lakehurst Road   Toms River, NJ 08755   (732)716-8116   Fax (732)240-9360
+ Garden State Medical Center
780 Highway 37 West/Suite 110   Toms River, NJ 08759   (732)341-3500

Mann, Eric Bryce, MD {1508847930} Ophthl(01,NY45)<NJ-STCLR-DOV, NJ-STCLRDEN>
+ Eye Associates of North Jersey
600 Mount Pleasant Avenue   Dover, NJ 07801   (973)366-1232   Fax (973)366-2960

Mann, Jessica Salas, MD {1790966208} ObsGyn, Gyneco(03,FL03)<PA-JRSYSHOR, NJ-RIVERVW>
+ Reproductive Science Center of New Jersey
234 Industrial Way   Eatontown, NJ 07724   (732)918-2500   Fax (732)918-2504
+ Reproductive Science Center of New Jersey
780 Route 35 West/Suite 150   Toms River, NJ 08755   (732)918-2500   Fax (732)240-3030

Mann, Justin, MD {1710326095} RadOnc
+ Memorial Sloan-Kettering Cancer Center Basking Ridge
136 Mountain View Boulevard   Basking Ridge, NJ 07920   (908)542-3000   Fax (908)542-3220

Mann, Manpreet, MD {1417157033} ObsGyn(04,INDI)
+ JN Obstetrics & Gynecology
370A Market Street   Saddle Brook, NJ 07663   (201)880-8953   Fax (201)880-8955
contact@mannobyn.com

Mann, Nora B., MD {1265532352} Pedtrc(87,NJ05)<NJ-STCLR-DEN>
+ Denville Pediatrics Medical Associates PA
140 East Main Street   Denville, NJ 07834   (973)625-5090   Fax (973)625-8006

Mann, Richard A., MD {1598785883} Nephro, IntrMd(79,NY46)<NJ-RWJUBRUN>
+ Robert Wood Johnson Transplant Associates, P.A.
10 Plum Street/7th Floor   New Brunswick, NJ 08901   (732)253-3699

Mann, Sunita Singh, MD {1437154069} RadNro, RadDia, IntrMd(93,NJ05)<NJ-HLTHSRE>
+ Garden State Medical Center
100 State Route 36/Suite 1C   West Long Branch, NJ 07764   (732)202-3000   Fax (732)849-0015
+ Manchester Surgery Center
1100 Route 70   Whiting, NJ 08759   (732)202-3000   Fax (732)849-1511
+ Garden State Medical Center
1608 New Jersey 88/Suites 102   Brick, NJ 07764   (732)849-0077   Fax (732)849-0015

Manna, Biagio, DO {1881628881} SrgCTh, SrgVas, SrgThr(92,MO79)<NJ-CHSFULD, NJ-CHSMRCER>
+ Mountain View Surgical Associates
1445 Whitehorse-Mercerville Rd   Hamilton, NJ 08691   (609)656-8622   Fax (609)656-8326
cenjer@comcast.net

Mannancheril, Anita, MD {1184962771} FamMed(12,DMN01)
+ Hunterdon Family Medicine
250 Route 28/Suite 100   Bridgewater, NJ 08807   (908)237-4135   Fax (908)237-4136

Mannava, Sumalatha, MD {1477583235} IntrMd(95,INA48)
+ 441 Boulder Drive
Morganville, NJ 07751

Mannheim, Glenn Barry, MD NroChl(83,MEX29)
+ 40 Spruce Street
West Windsor, NJ 08550

Manning, Ana B., MD {1861491623} Radiol, RadDia(78,PRO01)<NJ-VIRTUAHS, NJ-VIRTMHBC>
+ South Jersey Radiology Associates, P.A.
901 Route 168/Suites 301-305   Turnersville, NJ 08012   (856)227-6600   Fax (856)227-8537
+ South Jersey Radiology Associates, P.A.
315 Route 70 East/Suite B   Cherry Hill, NJ 08034   (856)227-6600   Fax (856)428-0356
+ South Jersey Radiology Associates, P.A.
1000 Lincoln Drive East   Marlton, NJ 08012   (856)983-1818   Fax (856)983-3226

Manning, Eric Carlyle, MD {1073535282} IntrMd, Nephro(85,CA19)<NJ-RWJUBRUN, NJ-UNVMCPRN>
+ Montgomery Nephrology & Hypertension
719 Route 206/Suite 100   Hillsborough, NJ 08844   (908)904-9055   Fax (908)904-9069

Manning, Latriece Eileena, DO {1861635203} ObsGyn
+ Pinelands Obstetrics and Gynecology
1617 Route 38   Mount Holly, NJ 08060   (609)261-0240   Fax (609)261-8622

Manning, Michael T., MD {1659538569} Gastrn, IntrMd(75,NY08)
+ St. Gregory The Great Catholic Community Center
4620 Nottingham Way   Hamilton Square, NJ 08690   (609)587-7366

Mannino, Marie L., MD {1790022556} IntrMd(85,ITA17)
+ 91 Mountain Avenue
Hawthorne, NJ 07506

Mannion, Ciaran M., MD {1659309284} Pthlgy, PthACI(90,IRE06)<NJ-HACKNSK>
+ Hackensack University Medical Center
30 Prospect Avenue/Pathology   Hackensack, NJ 07601   (201)996-2000

Mannion, Joseph, MD {1962492009} IntrMd(88,NJ05)<NJ-JRSYSHMC>
+ 123 Main Street
Avon, NJ 07717   (732)775-1400

Manno, Joseph, MD {1578577425} SrgVas, Surgry(82,OK05)<NJ-HACKNSK, NJ-HOLYNAME>
+ North Jersey Surgical Specialists
83 Summit Avenue   Hackensack, NJ 07601   (201)646-0010   Fax (201)646-0600
Jmanno9830@aol.com

Manocchio, Stephen J., MD {1891731766} IntrMd, InfDis(74,MEX14)<NJ-HOBUNIMC, NJ-STMICHL>
+ 400 Grand Street
Hoboken, NJ 07030   (201)656-6054

Manocchio, Teresa, DO {1144212002} Pedtrc, IntrMd(00,NY75)
+ Summit Pediatric Associates
33 Overlook Road/Suite 101   Summit, NJ 07901   (908)273-1112   Fax (908)273-1146
+ Florham Park Pediatrics
195 Columbia Turnpike/Suite 105   Florham Park, NJ 07932   (908)273-1112   Fax (973)845-2883

Manoj, Smitha, MD {1689629560} IntrMd(95,INA76)<NJ-JFKMED, NJ-BAYSHORE>
+ Caring Doctor Medical Center PA
240 Bridge Street   Metuchen, NJ 08840   (732)549-3000   Fax (732)549-3002
info@mycaringdoctor.com

Manor, Einat, MD {1194725200} ObsGyn(00,ISR02)
+ 465 South Street/Suite 103
Morristown, NJ 07960   (973)971-7440   Fax (973)290-7520
+ Atlantic Health Urology Gyn
95 Madison Avenue/Suite 204   Morristown, NJ 07960   (973)971-7440

Manoraj, Vinita, MD {1295781664} IntrMd(95,INA81)<NJ-STJOSHOS>
+ RWJ University Hospital New Brunswick
One Robert Wood Johnson Place   New Brunswick, NJ 08901   (732)937-8777   Fax (732)253-3449

Manoski, Andrew, DO {1194162792} Psychy<NJ-JRSYSHMC>
+ Jersey Shore University Medical Center
1945 Route 33   Neptune, NJ 07753   (732)643-4363   Fax (732)643-4376

Manougian, Ara, MD {1215906599} EnDbMt, IntrMd(72,OK01)<NJ-HACKNSK, NJ-VALLEY>
+ 446 Ridgewood Avenue
Paramus, NJ 07652   (201)265-2184

Manoukian, Aram V., MD {1699847970} Gastrn, IntrMd(84,NY08)
+ RWJ Gastro & Hepatology
125 Paterson Street/CAB 5100B   New Brunswick, NJ 08901   (732)235-7784   Fax (732)235-7792
manoukav@umdnj.edu

Manser, Harry, Jr., DO {1538155007} FamMed(69,PA77)<NJ-VIRTMHBC>
+ Lourdes Medical Associates
501 Delaware Avenue/Suite 1   Roebling, NJ 08554   (609)291-5560   Fax (609)499-0435

Mansfield, Nicole, MD {1942663570}<NJ-COOPRUMC>
+ Cooper University Hospital
One Cooper Plaza   Camden, NJ 08103   (856)342-2351

Manske, Daniel D., MD {1356389860} FamMed(89,NJ06)
+ 154 West Commerce Street
Bridgeton, NJ 08302   (856)459-3500   Fax (856)459-3600

Manson, Florence N., MD {1306891312}
+ CAMCare Health Corporation
817 Federal Street/Pediatrics   Camden, NJ 08103   (856)541-9811   Fax (856)541-4611

Mansoob, Farhana, MD {1780868885} Psychy(93,PAK11)
+ 389 Washington Street/Apt 16-K
Jersey City, NJ 07302

Mansoor, George A., MD {1659377653} Hypten, IntrMd, Nephro(86,JMA01)
+ Merck and Company Incorporated
126 East Lincoln Avenue   Rahway, NJ 07065   (732)574-4000

Mansour, Ali Gaber, MD {1346225885} FamMed(93,EGY05)
+ Care Station
90 Route 22 West   Springfield, NJ 07081   (973)467-2273
+ Care Station Medical Group
456 Prospect Avenue   West Orange, NJ 07052   (973)467-2273   Fax (973)731-9881

Mansour, Ashraf Hakeem, MD {1952402398} IntrMd(84,EGY07)
+ Thalody Medical Associates
240 Williamson Street/Suite 400   Elizabeth, NJ 07207   (908)352-0560   Fax (908)352-4066

Mansour, Ayman M., MD {1124223722} Pedtrc(03,GRN01)
+ Princeton Windsor Pediatrics
88 Princeton Hightstown Road/Suite 103   Princeton Junction, NJ 08550   (609)799-4700   Fax (609)799-4545

Mansour, Esber Hani, MD {1972569374} SrgCrC, Surgry(73,LEBA)<NJ-STBARNMC>
+ Burn Surgeons of Saint Barnabas
94 Old Short Hills Road   Livingston, NJ 07039   (973)322-5924   Fax (973)322-5447

Mansour, Loris N., MD {1710917653} Grtrcs, IntrMd(83,EGY04)<NJ-RAMAPO>
+ Ramapo Ridge Psychiatric Hospital
301 Sicomac Avenue/Geriatrics   Wyckoff, NJ 07481   (201)747-1684

Mansour, Mervat B., MD {1053319962} Nephro, IntrMd(90,EGY05)<NJ-RWJUBRUN>
+ 2 Auer Court/Suite D
East Brunswick, NJ 08816   (732)257-5530   Fax (732)257-5531

Mansouri, Farshad, MD {1689830572} SrgC&R, Surgry, IntrMd(GRN01)
+ Surgical Oncology and Laparoscopy, P.A.
741 Teaneck/Suite B   Teaneck, NJ 07666   (201)833-2888   Fax (201)833-1010
fmansouri1@gmail.com

Manspeizer, Heather Eve, MD {1639305634} Anesth(93,NY47)
+ River Drive Surgery Center
619 River Drive   Elmwood Park, NJ 07407   (201)703-2900

Mansson, Jonas, MD {1144429606} Surgry(DMN01)<NJ-MONMOUTH>
+ Valley Institute for Pain
One Valley Health Plaza/3 FL   Paramus, NJ 07652   (201)634-5690   Fax (201)634-5454

Mansson, Sarah Jane Deleon, DO {1043453616} CdvDis, IntrMd<NJ-DEBRAHLC>
+ Valley Medical Group/Valley Heart Group
1200 East Ridgewood Avenue   Ridgewood, NJ 07450   (201)670-8660   Fax (201)447-1957

Mansuri, Hanif M., MD {1548216393} Surgry(70,INDI)<NJ-BAYSHORE>
+ Bayshore Community Hospital
727 North Beers Street   Holmdel, NJ 07733   (732)264-7444   Fax (732)335-5518

Mansuria, Shetal M., MD {1902883788} ObsGyn(98,FL02)
+ Shetal Mansuria MD, LLC.
22 Old Short Hills Road/Suite 213   Livingston, NJ 07039   (973)535-3800   Fax (973)535-3808

Mantell, Cary Hilton, DO {1417971490} ObsGyn(83,NJ75)<NJ-RWJUHAM, NJ-CHSFULD>
+ Brickner-Mantell Center for Womens' Health, LLC.
1-A Quakerbridge Plaza   Trenton, NJ 08619   (609)689-9991   Fax (609)689-9992

Mantinaos, Mike Konstantinos, MD {1154499168} RadDia(91,PA12)<NJ-HCKTSTWN>
+ Hackettstown Regional Medical Center
651 Willow Grove Street   Hackettstown, NJ 07840   (908)852-5100

Manus, Alan M., DO {1851726152} ObsGyn(74,MO78)<NJ-UNDRWD, NJ-VIRTMARL>
+ Harmony HealthCare for Women, LLC
139 Ganttown Road/PO Box 1109 Turnersville, NJ 08012 (856)232-0050   Fax (856)232-0251
+ Liberty Health, P.A.
630 South White Horse Pike   Hammonton, NJ 08037   (609)567-6043

Manzi, Daniel D., MD {1487636957} Gastrn, IntrMd(78,DC02)<NJ-MTNSIDE>
+ Gastroenterology Health Care PA
799 Bloomfield Avenue/Suite 102   Verona, NJ 07044   (973)857-7600   Fax (973)433-7462

Manzo, Rene Paul, MD {1881630853} RadNro, RadDia(91,NY47)<NJ-STCLRDEN>
+ St. Clare's Hospital-Denville Campus
25 Pocono Road   Denville, NJ 07834   (973)625-6662

Manzoor, Adil, DO {1003200148} FamMed
+ Patient first Urgent Care
641 US Highway Route 130   Hamilton, NJ 08691   (609)568-9383   Fax (609)568-9384

Manzullo, Gregory P., MD {1811009558} IntrMd, MedOnc, Hemato(89,GRNA)<NJ-JRSYSHMC, NJ-OCEANMC>
+ 100 Commons Way/Building A100
Toms River, NJ 08755   (732)818-7561   Fax (732)818-7510

Mao, Cheng-An, MD {1003854761} FamMed, Grtrcs(86,TAIW)<NJ-STJOSHOS>
+ 871 Allwood Road
Clifton, NJ 07012   (862)249-4904   Fax (862)249-4903

Maouelainin, Nina, DO {1710133277} PulCCr, IntrMd(05,PA77)
+ Hunterdon Pulmonary & Critical Care Associates
6 Sand Hill Road/Suite 202   Flemington, NJ 08822   (908)237-1148   Fax (908)237-1749

Mapa, Christopher George, MD {1851527931} IntHos
+ Hackensack Univ Medical Center Hospitalists
30 Prospect Avenue   Hackensack, NJ 07601   (551)996-1548

Mapitigama, Renuka Nilmini, MD {1225149693} IntrMd, PulCCr, PulDis(94,SRI05)<NJ-HACKNSK>
+ American Pulmonary & Sleep Medicine Associates, LLC
One West Ridgewood Avenue/Suite 203   Paramus, NJ 07652   (201)312-5243   Fax (201)444-8560
+ American Pulmonary & Sleep Medicine Associates, LLC
26 Chestnut Ridge Road/Suite 103   Montvale, NJ 07645   (201)313-5243

Mapow, David A., MD {1760642367}
+ 205 Fernwood Court
Mullica Hill, NJ 08062

Mapow, Larry S., MD {1679592992} PthACl, PthFor(74,PA02)<NJ-SJHREGMC>
+ SJH Regional Medical Center
1505 West Sherman Avenue/Path   Vineland, NJ 08360   (856)641-8000

Mapp, Samuel Eugene, MD {1598717795} Surgry(93,GA22)
+ American Physician Services/Hudson HealthCare
679 Montgomery Street   Jersey City, NJ 07306   (201)433-6500   Fax (201)433-8010

Maquilan, Jose March, MD {1619994639} SrgThr, Surgry(72,PHI10)<NJ-OURLADY, NJ-RWJUHAM>
+ Delaware Valley Cardiovascular
1401 Whitehorse Mercerville Rd   Hamilton, NJ 08619   (609)890-2968   Fax (609)752-3036

Mara, Frank J., MD {1437186806} Anesth(80,MEX03)
+ Toms River Anesthesia Associates PC
409 Main Street/2nd Floor   Toms River, NJ 08753   (732)818-7575   Fax (732)818-1567

Marable, Denise Marie, MD {1417684584} Anesth, IntrMd(85,MI07)<NJ-ACMCITY>
+ AtlantiCare Regional Medical Center/City Campus
1925 Pacific Avenue/Anesthesiology   Atlantic City, NJ 08401   (609)345-4000

Marani-Dicovsky, Marcela C., MD {1386727287} IntrMd(90,ARG09)<NJ-STJOSHOS>
+ C. Dicovsky Medical Group LLC
681 Broadway   Paterson, NJ 07514   (973)278-1000   Fax (973)278-1709

Marano, Matthew, Jr., MD {1639912097} Ophthl(78,DC01)<NJ-STMICHL>
+ Marano Eye Care Center
200 South Orange Avenue/Suite 209   Livingston, NJ 07039   (973)322-0102   Fax (973)322-0102   drmatthew@aol.com
+ St. Michael's Medical Center
306 Dr. Martin Luther King Blv   Newark, NJ 07102   (973)877-5534

Marano, Michael A., MD {1972569309} CritCr, Surgry(81,NJ05)<NJ-STBARNMC>
+ Burn Surgeons of Saint Barnabas
94 Old Short Hills Road   Livingston, NJ 07039   (973)322-5924   Fax (973)322-5447

Marasigan, Mariza E., MD {1891767158} Anesth(85,PHI01)<NJ-HACKNSK>
+ Hackensack University Medical Center
30 Prospect Avenue   Hackensack, NJ 07601   (201)996-2000   Fax (201)488-6769
+ Hackensack University MC-Anesthesia Dept
30 Prospect Avenue/Room 2703   Hackensack, NJ 07601   (201)996-2000   Fax (201)996-3962

Maravich, Nick, Jr., MD {1104828599} Radiol(89,PA02)
+ Radiology Associates of Burlington County
1295 Route 38 West/PO Box 479   Hainesport, NJ 08036   (609)261-7017   Fax (609)261-4180

Marcantonio, Eugene E., MD {1053448340} PthAna(84,NY19)<NY-PRSBCOLU>
+ Merck and Company Incorporated
126 East Lincoln Avenue   Rahway, NJ 07065   (732)574-4000

Marcella, Stephen W., MD {1407865694} IntrMd, Pedtrc(83,NY19)<NJ-RWJUBRUN>
+ Eric B. Chandler Health Center
277 George Street/IntMed   New Brunswick, NJ 08901   (732)235-6700   Fax (732)235-6729
+ RWJ University Hospital New Brunswick
One Robert Wood Johnson Place   New Brunswick, NJ 08901   (732)828-3000

Marcelli, Enrico A., DO {1295844348} SrgOrt(81,PA77)<NJ-KMH-STRAT>
+ Reconstructive Orthopedics, P.A.
570 Egg Harbor Road/Suite C-4   Sewell, NJ 08080   (609)267-9400   Fax (609)267-9457

Marcelo, Edmund, DO {1679519359} Anesth(92,PA77)<NJ-VIRTMHBC>
+ Virtua Memorial
175 Madison Avenue/Anesth   Mount Holly, NJ 08060   (609)267-0700

Marchese, Anthony Aristide, DO {1861455867} Pedtrc(01,FL75)<NJ-VIRTVOOR, NJ-VIRTUAHS>
+ Advocare Merchantville Pediatrics
1600 Chapel Avenue/Suite 100   Cherry Hill, NJ 08002   Fax (856)665-3938

Marchese, Michael J., MD {1790768125} RadOnc, RadThp(79,TX04)<NJ-KIMBALL, NJ-OCEANMC>
+ Shore Point Radiation Oncology
900 Route 70   Lakewood, NJ 08701   (732)901-7314   Fax (732)901-5704   mjmmd44@yahoo.com

Marchetti, Michael F., MD {1609810241} EmrgMd(90,NY09)<NJ-BAYSHORE>
+ Bayshore Community Hospital
727 North Beers Street/EmergMed   Holmdel, NJ 07733   (732)739-5924

Marchetto, Paul A., MD {1942248273} SrgOrt(78,MEX03)<NJ-ATLANTHS>
+ Rothman Institute-The Performance Lab
2005 Route 7 East   Cherry Hill, NJ 08003   Fax (856)874-1188
+ Rothman Institute - Voorhees
443 Laurel Oak Road   Voorhees, NJ 08043   (856)821-6360

Marchiano, Dominic Adam, MD {1578594438} ObsGyn, NnPnMd(94,NY19)
+ Clin Health Care Assoc of NJ-Mat/Fetal
2301 Evesham Road/Pav 800/Suite 221   Voorhees, NJ 08043
+ Clin Health Care Assoc of NJ-Mat/Fetal
543 North Broad Street   Woodbury, NJ 08096

Marchildon, Michael B., MD {1447340179} PedSrg, Surgry, SrgCrC(68,CA11)<NJ-VIRTUAHS, NJ-VIRTVOOR>
+ RWJ University Hospital New Brunswick
One Robert Wood Johnson Place   New Brunswick, NJ 08901   (732)235-7821   Fax (732)235-8878
+ Nemours Dupont Pediatrics, Voorhees
443 Laurel Oak Road   Voorhees, NJ 08043   (732)235-7821   Fax (856)309-8556
+ AtlantiCare/Dupont Children's Health Program
2500 English Creek Avenue   Egg Harbor Township, NJ 08901   (609)641-3700   Fax (609)641-3652

Marchione, Victor L., MD {1265540595} PulDis, IntrMd(79,ITAL)
+ 600 Pavonia Avenue/5th Floor
Jersey City, NJ 07306   (201)216-0744   Fax (201)216-0844

Marcilla, Oscar A., MD {1679522486} EmrgMd(94,NY47)<NJ-HOLYNAME, NY-PRSBCOLU>
+ Holy Name Hospital
718 Teaneck Road/EmrgMed   Teaneck, NJ 07666   (201)833-3000
+ The Valley Hospital
223 North Van Dien Avenue/EmrgMed   Ridgewood, NJ 07450   (201)447-8000

Marcinow, Justyna, MD {1447702345} EmrgMd
+ Robert Wood Johnson Emergency Medicine
One Robert Wood Johnson Place/MEB 104   New Brunswick, NJ 08901   (732)235-8717

Marco, James Victor, MD {1720083124} Anesth(97,IL11)<NJ-SOCEANMC>
+ Robert Wood Johnson-UMDNJ Anesthesia Group
1140 Route 72 West   Manahawkin, NJ 08050   (609)978-8900

Marcoff, Leo, MD {1407935398} CdvDis, IntrMd(03,GRN01)<NJ-MORRISTN>
+ Morristown Medical Center
100 Madison Avenue/Gagnon C   Morristown, NJ 07962   (973)971-7416   Fax (973)401-2470

Marcus, Abir Assaad, MD {1467545079} Psychy, PsyAdd, Psythp(92,EGY04)
+ 321 Broad Street
Red Bank, NJ 07701   (732)530-3122

Marcus, Alexander Michael, MD {1992788863} SrgOrt, SrgHnd(97,NY47)
+ Orthopedic Associates of Central Jersey
205 May Street/Suite 202   Edison, NJ 08837   (908)757-1520   Fax (908)769-1388
+ Orthopedic Associates of Central Jersey PA
3 Hospital Plaza/Suite 411   Old Bridge, NJ 08857   (908)757-1520   Fax (732)360-0775

Marcus, Brian F., DO {1235216045} Pedtrc, IntrMd(97,NY75)<NJ-UNVMCPRN>
+ East Windsor Pediatric Group
300B Princeton Hightstown/Suite 201   Hightstown, NJ 08520   (609)448-7300   Fax (609)448-8022

Marcus, Jenna Z., MD {1386871689} GynOnc
+ University Reproductive Association
185 South Orange Avenue/MSB E-506   Newark, NJ 07103   (973)972-5266   Fax (973)972-4574

Marcus, Jennifer, MD {1295834174} Anesth(02,DMN01)<NJ-CLARMAAS>
+ Clara Maass Medical Center
1 Clara Maass Drive/Anesth   Belleville, NJ 07109   (973)450-2000

Marcus, John W., MD {1013075951} ObsGyn, IntrMd(89,IL11)<NJ-VALLEY>
+ John W. Marcus MD
89 North Maple Avenue   Ridgewood, NJ 07450   (201)447-0077   Fax (201)447-3560
+ Lifeline Medical Associates, LLC
2 Sears Drive   Ridgewood, NJ 07450   (201)447-0077   Fax (201)262-9440

Marcus, Linda Susan, MD {1598875619} Dermat(75,NY08)<NJ-VALLEY>
+ 271 Godwin Avenue
Wyckoff, NJ 07481   (201)891-4373   Fax (201)891-0482   sexyderm@verizon.net
+ The Valley Hospital
223 North Van Dien Avenue/Dermatology   Ridgewood, NJ 07450   (201)447-8000

Marcus, Ralph E., MD {1033174677} IntrMd, Rheuma(69,NY46)<NJ-HACKNSK, NJ-HOLYNAME>
+ Rheumatology Associates of North Jersey, PA
1415 Queen Anne Road   Teaneck, NJ 07666   (201)837-7788   Fax (201)837-2077
+ Rheumatology Associates of North Jersey, PA
420 Grand Avenue   Englewood, NJ 07631   (201)837-7788   Fax (201)837-2077
+ Rheumatology Associates of North Jersey, PA
8305A Bergenline Avenue   North Bergen, NJ 07666   (201)837-7788   Fax (201)837-2077

Marcus, Richard W., MD {1548252067} Pedtrc(82,NJ05)<NJ-CLARMAAS>
+ Nutley Pediatric Associates
242 Washington Avenue   Nutley, NJ 07110   (973)667-6676   Fax (973)667-6029   Nutleypeds@aol.com

Marcus, Steven M., MD {1316011588} Pedtrc, PedrMTxy(67,VA04)<NJ-NWRKBETH>
+ New Jersey Poison Center
65 Bergen Street/4th Floor   Newark, NJ 07107   (973)972-9280   Fax (973)972-2679

Marczyk, Stanley C., MD {1346356904} SrgOrt, SrgHnd(91,PA02)<NJ-ACMCMAIN, NJ-SHOREMEM>
+ Shore Orthopedic University Associates
24 Macarthur Boulevard/First Floor   Somers Point, NJ 08244   (609)927-1991   Fax (609)927-4203

Mardam-Bey, Tarek H., MD {1114076437} SrgOrt, PedOrt(72,LEB03)
+ 2 Dean Drive
Tenafly, NJ 07670   (201)569-0061   Fax (201)569-5602

Marella, Gregg G., MD {1922116326} IntrMd(93,PA14)
+ Mendham Medical Group LLP
19 East Main Street/Suite 1   Mendham, NJ 07945   (973)543-6505   Fax (973)543-2967

Marella, Venkata Koteswararao, MD {1083695373} Urolgy(95,INDI)<PA-EASTON, NJ-WARREN>
+ Adult and Pediatric Urology Center, P.A.
1033 Clifton Avenue   Clifton, NJ 07013   (973)473-5700   Fax (973)473-3367

Physicians by Name and Address

Maresca, Michelle Marie, MD {1376746990} PedEnd, Pedtrc(07,NJ06)
+ Hackensack University Medical Center
  30 Prospect Avenue   Hackensack, NJ 07601   (201)996-2000
+ Rutgers- New Jersey Medical School
  185 South Orange Avenue/MSB 456   Newark, NJ 07103   (973)972-1043

Maresca, Phillip A, MD {1437456399} IntrMd
+ Clara Maass Medical Center
  1 Clara Maass Drive   Belleville, NJ 07109   (551)804-9568

Maresca, Warren L., MD {1992726152} CdvDis, IntrMd(78,DC02)<NJ-VALLEY, NJ-STJOSHOS>
+ Cardiology Associates
  4-14 Saddle River Road   Fair Lawn, NJ 07410   (201)794-3987   Fax (201)794-1404
+ Cardiology Associates
  342 Hamburg Turnpike   Wayne, NJ 07470   (973)942-1377
+ Cardiology Associates LLC
  181 Franklin Avenue/Suite 301   Nutley, NJ 07410   (973)667-5511   Fax (973)667-0561

Maressa, Julian M., DO {1275643116} FamMed, FamMAdM(89,FL75)<NJ-VIRTBERL, NJ-VIRTVOOR>
+ Franklin Family Practice
  181 West White Horse Pike/Suite 100   Berlin, NJ 08009   (856)767-6044   Fax (856)767-3518

Marfuggi, Richard A., MD {1134108574} SrgPlstc(76,VT02)<NJ-STCLRDEN>
+ 10 Broadway
  Denville, NJ 07834   (973)377-8950   Fax (973)377-8914

Margallo, Evangeline Cobin, MD {1518096510} Pedtrc(78,PHIL)
+ Advocare Kressville Pediatrics Cherry Hill
  710 Kresson Road   Cherry Hill, NJ 08003   (856)795-3320   Fax (856)795-1213

Margate, Pedro Ramboyong, MD {1528085255} RadDia(68,PHI01)
+ SJH Millville Imaging
  1001 North High Street   Millville, NJ 08332   (856)825-0005   Fax (856)825-5576

Margiotta, Joseph A., MD {1144286337} Anesth(89,NJ06)<NJ-STPETER, NJ-SOMERSET>
+ Anesthesia Consultnts of NJ/Nova Pain
  285 Davidson Avenue/Suite 204   Somerset, NJ 08873   (732)271-1400   Fax (732)271-3543
+ Cares Surgicenter, LLC.
  240 Easton Avenue   New Brunswick, NJ 08901   (732)271-1400   Fax (732)296-8677

Margolin, Gregory, MD {1699908400} ObsGyn
+ Women's Healthcare of Collingswood
  1055 Haddon Avenue   Collingswood, NJ 08108   (856)854-4524   Fax (856)854-8216

Margolin, Michael L., MD {1053316653} Gastrn, IntrMd(82,NY19)<NJ-OVERLOOK, NJ-TRINIWSC>
+ Associates in Gastroenterology of Union County PA
  210 North Avenue East/Suite 2   Cranford, NJ 07016   (908)272-6300   Fax (908)272-6302

Margolin, Susan K., MD {1164455622} Pedtrc(78,NJ06)<NJ-STBARNMC>
+ St. Barnabas Medical Center
  94 Old Short Hills Road/Pediatrics   Livingston, NJ 07039   (973)322-5000

Margolis, Eric Judd, MD {1376545897} Urolgy, IntrMd(90,NY15)<NJ-ENGLWOOD, NJ-HOLYNAME>
+ The Urology Center of Englewood, PA
  663 Palisade Avenue/Suite 304   Cliffside Park, NJ 07010   (201)313-1933   Fax (201)313-9599
+ The Urology Center of Englewood, PA
  300 Grand Avenue/Suite 202   Englewood, NJ 07631   (201)313-1933   Fax (201)816-1777

Margolis, Franklin I., MD {1487727517} Urolgy, IntrMd(95,CA15)<NJ-WARREN>
+ 224 Roseberry Street/Suite 2
  Phillipsburg, NJ 08865   (908)859-9494   Fax (908)213-9203

Margolis, Thomas Ira, MD {1730153461} Ophthl(89,MA01)<NJ-SHOREMEM, NJ-ACMCITY>
+ Retinal & Ophthalmic Consultants, PC
  1500 Tilton Road   Northfield, NJ 08225   (609)646-5200   Fax (609)646-9868
  vitrector@gmail.com
+ Retinal & Ophthalmic Consultants, PC
  2466 East Chestnut Avenue   Vineland, NJ 08360   (609)646-5200   Fax (856)507-0040
+ Retinal & Ophthalmic Consultants, PC
  211 South Main Street/Suite 102   Cape May Court House, NJ 08225   (609)463-4610   Fax (609)463-4616

Margolskee, Dorothy J., MD {1881868891} IntrMd, PulDis(80,MD07)
+ Merck and Company Incorporated
  126 East Lincoln Avenue   Rahway, NJ 07065   (732)574-4000

Margulies, Craig, MD {1912005026} Gastrn(90,PA07)
+ 11 State Road
  Princeton, NJ 08540   (609)497-2770   Fax (609)497-2771

Margulies, Debra Jill, MD {1134177918} EnDbMt, IntrMd(04,NJ06)<NJ-MORRISTN>
+ Summit Medical Group
  95 Madison Avenue   Morristown, NJ 07960   (973)775-5151   Fax (973)267-5521

Margulis, Elynne B., MD {1952468803} ObsGyn(78,NY01)<NJ-OVERLOOK>
+ Associates in OBGYN
  522 East Broad Street   Westfield, NJ 07090   (908)232-4449

Margulis, Stephen J., MD {1689601486} Gastrn, IntrMd(81,RI01)<NJ-VALLEY>
+ Bergen Medical Associates
  466 Old Hook Road/Suite 1   Emerson, NJ 07630   (201)967-8221   Fax (201)967-0340
+ Bergen Medical Associates
  1 West Ridgewood Avenue/Suite 301   Paramus, NJ 07652   (201)967-8221   Fax (201)445-4296

Mari, Arthur D., MD {1902896368} IntrMd(78,ITAL)<NJ-MONMOUTH>
+ 280 Norwood Avenue
  West Long Branch, NJ 07764   (732)222-0031   Fax (732)222-3003

Marian, Valentin Dumitru, MD {1609107549} IntrMd<NJ-JRSYCITY>
+ Jersey City Medical Center
  355 Grand Street/Box 695   Jersey City, NJ 07304   (201)915-2430

Mariani, Chiara, MD {1225222011} PhysMd, IntrMd(99,ITA33)
+ Premier Orthopaedic Associates
  298 South Delsea Drive   Vineland, NJ 08360   (856)690-1616   Fax (856)690-1089

Mariani, John K., DO {1811006885} SrgOrt(81,PA77)<NJ-KMH-TURNV, NJ-KMHCHRRY>
+ Reconstructive Orthopedics, P.A.
  570 Egg Harbor Road/Suite C-4   Sewell, NJ 08080   (609)267-9400   Fax (609)267-9457

Mariano, Domenic L., DO {1457327975} CdvDis(90,FL75)<NJ-MTNSIDE, NJ-STMICHL>
+ Bart De Gregorio MD, LLC.
  946 Bloomfield Avenue   Glen Ridge, NJ 07028   (973)743-1121   Fax (973)743-2627

Mariano-Lau, Elizabeth L., MD {1508807454} Pedtrc(69,PHI08)<NJ-JRSYSHMC>
+ 5140 Route 9 South
  Howell, NJ 07731   (732)364-4141   Fax (732)364-0787

Mariduena, Joseph A., MD {1245506161}
+ Rutgers- New Jersey Medical School
  185 South Orange Avenue/Room F 603   Newark, NJ 07103   (908)380-7578
  jmariduena@hotmail.com

Marin, Adrian Alonso, DO {1083876213} EmrgMd<NJ-STJOSHOS, NJ-STPETER>
+ St Joseph's Medical Center Emergency
  703 Main Street   Paterson, NJ 07503   (973)754-2240   Fax (973)754-2249

Marin, Humberto, MD {1558441287} Psychy(73,COL01)<NJ-RWJUBRUN, NJ-UNIVBHC>
+ University Behavioral Health Care
  303 George Street/Suite 200   New Brunswick, NJ 08901   (732)235-6800   Fax (732)235-6187

Marina, Adele Nabieh, MD {1154508794} Pedtrc(97,SYR01)<NJ-HUNTRDN>
+ Marina Pediatrics
  330 Livingston Avenue/Suite 2aa   New Brunswick, NJ 08901   (732)220-0777   Fax (732)220-0778
+ Hunterdon Pediatric Associates
  6 Sand Hill Road/Suite 202   Flemington, NJ 08822   (732)220-0777   Fax (908)788-5861

Marinas, Virgilio R., MD   RadDia(73,PHI09)
+ 1532 Caroline Lane
  Toms River, NJ 08755

Marini, Robert A., MD {1184656373} PhysMd, PainMd(87,MEXI)<NJ-CLARMAAS>
+ Jersey Rehab, P.A.
  77 Newark Avenue   Belleville, NJ 07109   (973)844-9220   Fax (973)751-0498
+ Jersey Rehab PA
  409 39th Street   Union City, NJ 07087   (973)844-9220   Fax (201)319-1339

Marino, Anthony, Jr., MD {1235187238} PsyCAd, Psychy(81,MEX29)<NJ-CARRIER>
+ Carrier Clinic
  252 Route 601   Belle Mead, NJ 08502   (908)281-1000   Fax (908)281-1660

Marino, Anthony J., Jr., MD {1275564817} NnPnMd, Pedtrc(84,MEX14)<NJ-UNVMCPRN>
+ University Medical Center of Princeton at Plainsboro
  One Plainsboro Road/Neonatology   Plainsboro, NJ 08536   (609)497-4000   Fax (609)497-4420

Marino, Denay L., DO {1215006341} FamMed, IntrMd(87,PA78)<NJ-BURDTMLN>
+ Cape Regional Physicians Associates
  4011 Route 9 South/Suite 201   Rio Grande, NJ 08242   (609)770-7788   Fax (609)770-7774

Marino, Gennaro J., DO {1235197559} EmrgMd(89,IA75)<NJ-CHILTON>
+ Chilton Medical Center
  97 West Parkway/EmrgMed   Pompton Plains, NJ 07444   (973)831-5000

Marino, Joseph Frederick, DO {1962445072} ObsGyn(73,IA75)<NJ-MONMOUTH, NJ-OURLADY>
+ Our Lady of Lourdes Medical Center
  1600 Haddon Avenue/OB/GYN   Camden, NJ 08103   (856)757-3700   Fax (856)668-8479

Marino, Mark, MD {1093759631} ObsGyn(86,GRN01)<NJ-SOCEANCO, NJ-COMMED>
+ Southern Ocean Women's Health
  115 North Lakeshore Drive   Manahawkin, NJ 08050   (609)978-1411
+ Ocean Health Initiatives, Inc.
  301 Lakehurst Road   Toms River, NJ 08755   (609)978-1411   Fax (732)552-0378
+ Ocean Health Initiatives, Inc.
  101 Second Street   Lakewood, NJ 08050   (732)363-6655   Fax (732)363-6656

Marino, Mark T., MD {1508386376} IntrMd, ClnPhm(85,NY03)
+ 49 Wellington Drive
  Long Valley, NJ 07853

Marino, Nicholas A., MD {1821031139} ObsGyn(73,ITA17)<NJ-STJOSHOS>
+ Paterson Community Health Center
  227 Broadway   Paterson, NJ 07501   (973)278-2600   Fax (973)278-5837
+ Paterson Community Health Center
  32 Clinton Street   Paterson, NJ 07522   (973)278-2600   Fax (973)790-7703

Marino, Phyllis E., MD {1417977497} OccpMd, GPrvMd(84,NY09)<NJ-CHILTON, NJ-VALLEY>
+ 15 Essex Road/Suite 5
  Paramus, NJ 07652   (201)291-6135   Fax (201)291-6129

Marino, Richard P., DO {1447221122} IntrMd(91,MO78)<NJ-RIVERVW, NJ-BAYSHORE>
+ Jersey Shore Medical Associates
  734 North Beers Street/Suite U-4   Holmdel, NJ 07733   (732)264-8484   Fax (732)264-4324

Marion, William Joseph, DO {1346226115} FamMed(95,CA22)<NJ-NWTNMEM>
+ Mountain View Family Medicine, LLC
  426 State Route 515   Vernon, NJ 07462   (973)764-5666   Fax (973)764-5778
  drmarion@warwick.net

Mariwalla, Kiran, MD   IntrMd(91,GRN01)<NJ-STCLRDEN>
+ St. Clare's Hospital-Denville Campus
  25 Pocono Road   Denville, NJ 07834   (973)625-6000

Mariyampillai, Joan of Arc J., MD {1417916727} IntrMd(97,INA77)
+ Drs. Mariyampillai and Mariyampillai
  825 Bloomfield Avenue/Suite LL1   Verona, NJ 07044   (973)239-3770   Fax (973)239-3774

Mariyampillai, Marcarious A., MD {1790770279} IntrMd(75,SRI01)<NJ-EASTORNG>
+ Drs. Mariyampillai and Mariyampillai
  825 Bloomfield Avenue/Suite LL1   Verona, NJ 07044   (973)239-3770   Fax (973)239-3774

Marji, Michael Suleiman, MD {1154692077} Anesth
+ St. Michael's Medical Center
  111 Central Avenue   Newark, NJ 07102   (973)877-5034   Fax (973)877-5231
+ St. Joseph's Regional Medical Center Anesthesia
  703 Main Street   Paterson, NJ 07503   (973)877-5034   Fax (973)977-9455

Mark, Arthur K., MD {1629037254} SrgOrt(96,PA13)<NJ-JRSYSHMC, NJ-OCEANMC>
+ Seaview Orthopaedics
  222 Schanck Road/3rd Floor   Freehold, NJ 07728   (732)462-1700   Fax (732)303-8314
+ Seaview Orthopaedics
  1640 Route 88 West   Brick, NJ 08724   (732)462-1700   Fax (732)458-2743
+ Seaview Orthopaedics
  1200 Eagle Avenue   Ocean, NJ 07728   (732)660-6200   Fax (732)660-6201

Mark, Benjamin, MD {1093704199} IntrMd, Nrolgy(76,NJ05)<NJ-MONMOUTH>
+ 279 Third Avenue/Suite 301
  Long Branch, NJ 07740   (732)229-3737   Fax (732)229-5757
  bmarkmd@home.com

Mark, George Edward, MD {1265516488} CdvDis, ClCdEl
+ **Cardiovascular Associates**
210 West Atlantic Avenue Haddon Heights, NJ 08035 (856)546-3003 Fax (856)547-5337
+ **Cardiovascular Associates of The Delaware Valley, PA**
525 State Street/Suite 3 Elmer, NJ 08318 (856)546-3003 Fax (856)358-0725

Mark, Margery H., MD {1679648166} Nrolgy, OthrSp(82,NY08)
+ **University Hospital-RWJMS Neurology**
125 Paterson Street/Suite 4100-6100 New Brunswick, NJ 08901 (732)235-7733 Fax (732)235-7041
+ **UH-Robert Wood Jhnsn Med Sch**
97 Paterson Street/Neurology New Brunswick, NJ 08901

Markatos, Angelo, DO {1447279245} Nephro, IntrMd(99,PA77)<NJ-COMMED, NJ-OCEANMC>
+ **Ocean Renal Associates, P.A.**
210 Jack Martin Boulevard/Suite D-1 Brick, NJ 08724 (732)458-5854 Fax (732)458-8012
+ **Ocean Renal Associates, P.A.**
508 Lakehurst Road/Suite 3 A Toms River, NJ 08755 (732)458-5854 Fax (732)341-4993
+ **Ocean Renal Associates, P.A.**
1301 Route 72 West/Suite 206 Manahawkin, NJ 08724 (609)978-9940 Fax (609)978-9902

Markbreiter, Lance A., MD {1063463016} SrgOrt(88,CT01)<NJ-RIVERVW>
+ **Shore Orthopaedic Group**
35 Gilbert Street South Tinton Falls, NJ 07701 (732)530-1515 Fax (732)747-5433
+ **Shore Orthopaedic Group**
1255 Route 70/Suite 11S Lakewood, NJ 08701 (732)530-1515 Fax (732)942-2311

Markel, David Francis, MD {1548270002} Pedtrc, AdolMd(97,NY01)<NJ-MORRISTN>
+ **Hamburg Pediatrics**
2 Vernon Avenue Hamburg, NJ 07419 (973)827-1918 Fax (800)661-4832

Markenson, Joseph A., MD {1164485637} IntrMd, Rheuma(70,NY08)
+ **HSS Paramus Outpatient Center**
140 East Ridgewood Avenue/Suite 175-S Paramus, NJ 07652 (201)796-2255 Fax (201)796-3711

Marki, Richard E., MD {1184765869} ObsGyn, Gyneco, IntrMd(80,POLA)<NJ-BAYONNE, NJ-OVERLOOK>
+ **United Medical, P.C.**
988 Broadway/Suite 201 Bayonne, NJ 07002 (201)339-6111 Fax (201)339-6333
+ **RejuV Cosmetic Center**
59 Mine Brook Road Bernardsville, NJ 07924 (201)339-6111 Fax (908)630-9619
+ **The Center for Women's Health**
744 Broadway Bayonne, NJ 07002 (201)858-1585 Fax (201)858-0467

Markidan, Yana, MD {1629233903} ObsGyn
+ **Antheia Gynecology**
375 US Highway 130/Suite 103 East Windsor, NJ 08520 (609)448-7800 Fax (609)448-7880

Markley, Daniel James, MD {1790981876} IntrMd, PulCCr(07,NJ06)<NY-MTSINAI, NY-MTSINYHS>
+ **Pulmonary & Allergy Associates**
1 Springfield Avenue Summit, NJ 07901

Markley, Jonathan C., DO {1346455532} Anesth(04,NJ75)<NJ-STJOSHOS, NJ-WAYNEGEN>
+ **St. Joseph's Regional Medical Center Anesthesia**
703 Main Street Paterson, NJ 07503 (973)754-2323 Fax (973)977-9455

Markman Lin, Angela, MD {1437356961}<NJ-MONMOUTH>
+ **Monmouth Medical Center**
300 Second Avenue Long Branch, NJ 07740 (732)923-6795

Markoff, Michael S., MD {1154309672} Pedtrc(82,PA12)<NJ-RIVERVW>
+ **Middletown Pediatrics**
529 Highway 35 Red Bank, NJ 07701 (732)741-9800 Fax (732)758-6367

Markos, Marina Azmy, MD {1891717955} Anesth(85,EGY05)<NJ-JFKMED>
+ **Hamilton Anesthesia Associates**
2119 Highway 33/Suite B Trenton, NJ 08690 (609)581-0770 Fax (609)631-6839

Markou, Theodore Ioannis, MD {1043576309} InfDis
+ **ID Associates PA/dba ID Care**
765 Route 10 East/Suite 201 Randolph, NJ 07869 (973)989-0068 Fax (973)361-8955

Markov, Nikolai Yordanov, DO {1760640502} Surgry(03,NY75)<NJ-RBAYOLDB>
+ **Sterling & SurgiCare**
3 Hospital Plaza/Room 206 Old Bridge, NJ 08857 (732)687-7077 Fax (732)360-0220
+ **Avenel Iselin Medical Group**
400 Gill Lane Iselin, NJ 08830 (732)687-7077 Fax (732)404-1594

Markovitz, Bruce Jay, MD {1144226523} Ophthl(91,PA02)<NJ-COOPRUMC>
+ **Soll Eye PC of New Jersey/Cooper Division**
3 Cooper Plaza/Suite 510 Camden, NJ 08103 (856)342-7200 Fax (856)342-6620

Markovitz, Jacob E., MD {1790873891} ObsGyn(02,NY08)<NJ-ENGLWOOD>
+ **Englewood Women's Health**
25 Rockwood Place/Suite 305 Englewood, NJ 07631 (201)894-0003 Fax (201)894-0006

Markowitz, Charles R., MD {1053302166} Elecmy, PhysMd(86,IL43)<NJ-KIMBALL, NJ-OCEANMC>
+ **485 River Avenue/PO Box 929**
Lakewood, NJ 08701 (732)942-9400 Fax (732)922-1255

Markowitz, David, MD {1841216686} PhysMd(85,GRN01)<NJ-KMHCHRRY, NJ-VIRTVOOR>
+ **104 West Maple Avenue**
Merchantville, NJ 08109 (856)317-0666 Fax (856)317-9116
Davidmarkowitzmd@comcast.net

Markowitz, George Joseph, MD {1497713713} EmrgMd, IntrMd(79,NJ05)<NJ-VALLEY>
+ **The Valley Hospital**
223 North Van Dien Avenue/Emerg Med Ridgewood, NJ 07450 (201)447-8023 Fax (201)447-3201

Markowitz, Rachel Paula, MD {1922071216} Psychy(99,NJ05)<NJ-RIVERVW, NY-BLVUENYU>
+ **Jersey Shore Psychiatric Associates**
3535 Route 66/Building 5/Suite D Neptune, NJ 07753 (732)643-4350 Fax (732)643-4398
+ **Riverview Medical Center**
1 Riverview Plaza/Psychiatry Red Bank, NJ 07701 (732)741-2700

Marks, Caren G., MD {1174507644} Nrolgy, IntrMd(91,IL01)<NJ-CENTRAST>
+ **Linda Cardinale MS Center**
901 West Main Street/Suite 364 Freehold, NJ 07728 (732)294-2505 Fax (732)761-8084

Marks, David Alon, MD {1497854012} Nrolgy, SrgNro(83,SAF02)<NJ-UMDNJ>
+ **University Hospital**
150 Bergen Street/Neurology Newark, NJ 07103 (201)982-7151
+ **Rutgers NJ School of Medicine Neurology**
90 Bergen Street/DOC 5200 Newark, NJ 07103 (201)982-7151 Fax (973)972-5059

Marks, Lloyd Alan, MD {1225091457} PedCrd, Pedtrc(76,MI07)<NJ-NWRKBETH, NJ-CHRIST>
+ **940 South Avenue/Suite A**
Westfield, NJ 07090 (908)789-0512 Fax (908)789-0232
marksnj@erols.com
+ **Spine Care and Rehabilitation**
36 Newark Avenue/Suite 220 Belleville, NJ 07109 (908)789-0512 Fax (973)226-3270
+ **834 Avenue C**
Bayonne, NJ 07090 (201)222-1982 Fax (908)789-0232

Marlys, James P., MD {1386749315} IntrMd(83,DMN01)<NJ-JRSYSHMC, NJ-OCEANMC>
+ **Shore Endocrinology Associates, LLC**
2200 River Road/Suite A Point Pleasant Boro, NJ 08742 (732)892-7300 Fax (732)892-7301

Marmar, Joel L., MD {1356423008} Urolgy, SrgUro(64,PA01)<NJ-COOPRUMC>
+ **Cooper Surgical Associates**
3 Cooper Plaza/Suite 411 Camden, NJ 08103 (856)342-2270 Fax (856)365-1180

Marmol, Jose, Jr., MD {1639229974} IntrMd(72,PHI07)
+ **172 Newark Avenue**
Jersey City, NJ 07302 (201)435-6675 Fax (201)435-7610

Marmolejos, Ginny, MD {1902224033}<NJ-MORRISTN>
+ **Morristown Medical Center**
100 Madison Avenue Morristown, NJ 07962 (973)971-5000

Marmora, James J., MD {1588674956} FamMed(95,NJ05)
+ **East Brunswick Family Practice Associates**
123 Dunhams Corner Road East Brunswick, NJ 08816 (732)254-3300 Fax (732)651-0822

Marmora, Joseph James, MD {1730406760}
+ **Associates in Cardiovascular Disease, LLC**
211 Mountain Avenue Springfield, NJ 07081 (973)467-0005 Fax (973)912-8989

Maro, Robert, Jr., MD {1346284213} Grtrcs, IntrMd(80,PA02)<NJ-VIRTVOOR, NJ-COOPRUMC>
+ **The Maro Group**
27 Covered Bridge Road Cherry Hill, NJ 08034 (856)429-2224 Fax (856)429-1926

Maroldo, Michael G., MD {1760579445} FamMed(74,MI07)<NJ-BURDTMLN>
+ **Cape Health Solutions, LLC.**
650 Town Bank Road North Cape May, NJ 08204 (609)898-7447 Fax (609)898-1912

Maron, Edward M., MD {1275526568} IntrMd(78,MEX03)<NJ-KIMBALL, NJ-COMMED>
+ **Shore Medical Specialists**
500 River Avenue Lakewood, NJ 08701 (732)363-7200 Fax (732)367-4461
+ **Shore Medical Specialists**
9 Hospital Drive Toms River, NJ 08755 (732)363-7200 Fax (732)349-9697

Maron, Norman L., MD SrgOrt(70,NY09)
+ **Orthopedic Associates of Greater Lehigh Valley**
755 Memorial Parkway/Suite 101 Phillipsburg, NJ 08865 (908)859-5585 Fax (908)859-3990

Maron, Scott Michael, MD {1669555074} IntrMd(92,TX04)<NJ-STBARNMC, NJ-MORRISTN>
+ **Maron & Rodrigues Medical Group, LLC.**
10 James Street/Suite 150 Florham Park, NJ 07932 (973)822-2000 Fax (973)822-2001

Marone, Michael L., MD {1598712531} FamMed(68,PA02)<NJ-VIRTVOOR, NJ-VIRTBERL>
+ **707 White Horse Road/Suite C105**
Voorhees, NJ 08043 (856)309-9700 Fax (856)309-9191
Mlmofice@comcast.net

Marotta, Alexander, MD {1720048077} AlgyImmn, Pedtrc(98,PA02)
+ **Allergy & Asthma Comprehensive Care**
541 Cedar Hill Avenue/Suite 8 Wyckoff, NJ 07481 (201)652-6211 Fax (201)652-0321

Marotta, Charles J., MD {1437156882} IntCrd, CdvDis, IntrMd(82,NJ05)
+ **Advanced Cardiology, LLC.**
65 Ridgedale Avenue Cedar Knolls, NJ 07927 (973)401-1100 Fax (973)401-1201
+ **Advanced Cardiology, LLC.**
117 Seber Road/Suite 1-B Hackettstown, NJ 07840 (973)401-1100 Fax (908)979-1493

Marotta, Raymond J., Jr., MD {1588612824} FamMed, Grtrcs, IntrMd(83,NJ05)<NJ-BURDTMLN>
+ **Cape Regional Physicians Associates**
211 North Main Street/Suite 203 Cape May Court House, NJ 08210 (609)536-8272 Fax (609)536-8273

Maroules, Michael, MD {1134221062} OncHem, IntrMd(79,GRE01)
+ **Maroules Hematology Oncology LLC**
1011 Clifton Avenue/Suite 1 Clifton, NJ 07013 (862)591-2002 Fax (862)591-2344

Maroun, Victor, MD {1477564425} EmrgMd(03,NJ05)<NJ-MORRISTN>
+ **Morristown Medical Center**
100 Madison Avenue/EmrgMed Morristown, NJ 07962 (973)971-5000

Marple, Jill Ann, MD {1225022007} PhysMd(01,NH01)
+ **Reconstructive Orthopedics, P.A.**
401 Young Avenue/Suite 245 Moorestown, NJ 08057 (609)267-9400 Fax (609)267-9457

Marquart, Jason D., MD {1386723591} Dermat(00,MD12)<NJ-COOPRUMC>
+ **Cooper Center for Dermatologic Surgery**
10000 Sagemore Drive/Suite 10103 Marlton, NJ 08053 (856)596-3040 Fax (856)596-5651

Marques Baptista, Andreia, MD {1235391285} EmrgMd(05,NJ06)<NJ-RWJUBRUN>
+ **RWJ University Hospital New Brunswick**
One Robert Wood Johnson Place New Brunswick, NJ 08901 (732)828-3000

Marquette, Paul Arthur, MD {1831128727} FamMed(91,PA02)<NJ-JRSYSHMC>
+ **Seabrook Village Medical Center**
3000 Essex Road Tinton Falls, NJ 07753 (732)643-1200 Fax (732)643-2015

Marquinez, Anthony I., MD {1699742551} Nrolgy(91,PHI09)<NJ-HOLYNAME>
+ **Hackensack Neurology Group**
211 Essex Street/Suite 202 Hackensack, NJ 07601 (201)488-1515 Fax (201)488-9471

Marra, Antonio Luigi, DO {1508816281} EmrgMd(00,NJ75)<NJ-OCEANMC>
+ **EmCare**
1945 Route 33 Neptune, NJ 07753 (732)776-4510 Fax (732)776-2329
+ **EmCare**
425 Jack Martin Boulevard Brick, NJ 08724 (732)840-3380

Marrero, Luis C., MD {1124021548} NnPnMd, Pedtrc(87,MEXI)<NJ-STJOSHOS>
+ **St Joseph's Medical Center Neonatology**
703 Main Street Paterson, NJ 07503 (973)754-2555 Fax (973)754-2567

Marrero Figarella, Arturo L., MD {1649225236} PsyCAd, Psychy(80,DOMI)
+ **St. Joseph Medical Center Mental Health Clinic**
56 Hamilton Street Paterson, NJ 07505 (973)754-4771

Physicians by Name and Address

Marrinan, Randy F., MD {1104919109} PhysMd
+ Ridgewood Orthopedic Group, LLC
  85 South Maple Avenue   Ridgewood, NJ 07450   (201)445-2830   Fax (201)445-7471

Marriott, Christine Ryan, MD {1790124394} FamMed(13,NJ06)
+ Capital Health Primary Care-Hamilton
  1445 Whitehorse-Mercerville Rd   Hamilton, NJ 08619   (609)587-6661   Fax (609)587-8503

Marro, Michael Angelo, DO {1639592983} FamMed, Grtrcs(10,FL75)
+ Visiting Nurse Association of Central Jersey
  1301 Main Street   Asbury Park, NJ 07712   (732)774-6333   Fax (732)774-0313

Marroccoli, Barbara A., MD {1306067368} IntrMd(82,NJ06)
+ University Hospital-School of Public Health
  170 Frelinghuysen Road   Piscataway, NJ 08854   (732)445-0123   Fax (732)445-3644

Mars, Audrey Estelle, MD {1295808236} PedDvl, Pedtrc, PedNrD(86,ISR02)<NJ-HUNTRDN>
+ Hunterdon Medical Center
  2100 Wescott Drive/Pediatrics   Flemington, NJ 08822   (908)788-6100   Fax (908)788-2578

Marsh, Anthony William, DO {1083809305}
+ 11 Clifton Terrace
  Weehawken, NJ 07086   (201)865-2882

Marsh, Claire C., MD {1134185176} Psychy(71,PA07)<NJ-CARRIER>
+ Carrier Clinic
  252 Route 601/Psychiatry   Belle Mead, NJ 08502   (908)281-1000

Marsh, Rebecca A., MD {1285773606} InfDis, IntrMd(02,NY19)<NJ-HCKTSTWN, NJ-MORRISTN>
+ ID Associates PA/dba ID Care
  765 Route 10 East/Suite 201   Randolph, NJ 07869   (973)989-0068   Fax (973)361-8955
+ ID Associates PA/dba ID Care
  8 Saddle Road   Cedar Knolls, NJ 07927   (973)989-0068   Fax (973)993-5953

Marshall, Ian, MD {1396760450} Pedtrc, PedEnd(91,SAF02)<NJ-RWJUBRUN>
+ University Hospital-RWJ Medical School
  89 French Street   New Brunswick, NJ 08901   (732)235-9378   Fax (732)235-5002

Marshall, Jessica Lynne, DO {1447561907}
+ 1500 Avenue at Port Imperial
  Weehawken, NJ 07086   (386)316-8802
  jessicamarshall7@gmail.com

Marshall, Lewis West, Jr., MD {1841297223} IntrMd, EmrgMd(83,DC03)<NJ-HOLYNAME>
+ Holy Name Hospital
  718 Teaneck Road/EmergMed   Teaneck, NJ 07666   (201)833-3000

Marshall, Lorraine S., MD {1851418008} Psychy, PsyCAd(96,NY20)<NY-CHLDCOPR>
+ NYU Child Study Center
  411 Hackensack Avenue/7th Floor   Hackensack, NJ 07601

Marshall, Rebecca G., MD {1780655043} Pedtrc, IntrMd(94,PA14)
+ Princeton Nassau Pediatrics, P.A.
  301 North Harrison Street   Princeton, NJ 08540   (609)924-5510   Fax (609)924-3577
+ Princeton Nassau Pediatrics, P.A.
  25 South Route 31   Pennington, NJ 08534   (609)924-5510   Fax (609)745-5320

Marshall, Stefanie N., DO {1184691156} ObsGyn
+ First State Women's Care
  19B West Avenue   Woodstown, NJ 08098   (856)769-3348   Fax (856)769-3987

Marshall-Salomon, Gabrielle S., MD {1710009402} Psychy, PsyCAd(83,NY09)
+ 261 James Street/Suite 3G
  Morristown, NJ 07960   (973)540-1161   Fax (973)540-0716

Marsicano, Joseph G., MD {1881675783} SrgOrt(90,NY15)<NJ-OCEANMC>
+ Brielle Orthopedics PA
  457 Jack Martin Boulevard   Brick, NJ 08724   (732)840-7500   Fax (732)840-2088
+ Brielle Orthopedics PA
  823 Lacey Road   Forked River, NJ 08731   (732)840-7500   Fax (732)840-2088
+ Brielle Orthopedics PA
  1301 Route 72 West   Manahawkin, NJ 08724   (609)971-7616   Fax (609)971-7639

Marta, Peter T., DO {1467464479} Surgry(01,NJ75)
+ Summit Medical Group
  31-00 Broadway   Fair Lawn, NJ 07410   (201)530-5520   Fax (201)796-7020

Marte, Juan M., MD {1437128477} Psychy(86,DOM01)
+ 385 Wagner Court
  Paramus, NJ 07652

Martella, Arthur Thomas, MD {1497799548} SrgCdv, SrgThr(89,PA02)
+ Endocrinology Associates
  1 Brace Road/Suite B   Cherry Hill, NJ 08034   (856)234-0645   Fax (856)234-0498
+ LMA Surgical Associates
  120 White Horse Pike/Suite 103   Haddon Heights, NJ 08035   (856)234-0645   Fax (856)546-3908

Martin, Andrew A., MD {1356413645} IntrMd, CritCr, PulDis(88,NJ05)<NJ-STPETER>
+ Deborah Heart and Lung Center
  200 Trenton Road   Browns Mills, NJ 08015   (609)893-6611   Fax (609)735-1472
+ University Medical Group
  125 Paterson Street/Suite 5100   New Brunswick, NJ 08901   (609)893-6611   Fax (732)235-7117

Martin, Brian McKinley, MD {1124020763} Anesth(01,NY46)<NJ-HOLYNAME>
+ Teaneck Anesthesia Group, P.A.
  718 Teaneck Road   Teaneck, NJ 07666   (201)833-7149   Fax (201)833-6576

Martin, Dean Walter, MD {1780640987} Anesth, IntrMd(93,MA01)<NJ-STPETER>
+ Anesthesia Consultnts of NJ/Nova Pain
  285 Davidson Avenue/Suite 204   Somerset, NJ 08873   (732)271-1400   Fax (732)271-3544

Martin, Erica Nell, MD {1992964142}
+ Princeton Nassau Pediatrics, P.A.
  301 North Harrison Street   Princeton, NJ 08540   (609)924-5510   Fax (609)924-3577

Martin, Gene Joseph, Jr., MD {1366430159} SrgO&M, Surgry(96,NY48)<NJ-VIRTVOOR>
+ 195 Haddon Avenue
  Haddonfield, NJ 08033   (856)429-9097
+ 3012 Dawson Street
  Moorestown, NJ 08057   (856)866-9091
+ 94 Brick Road/Suite 100
  Marlton, NJ 08033   (856)596-9099

Martin, James Furman, MD {1295755486} EmrgMd
+ 7 Buttonwood Lane East
  Rumson, NJ 07760

Martin, Joanne C., MD {1407896608} CdvDis(73,NE06)<NJ-MORRISTN>
+ 457 South Street
  Morristown, NJ 07960   (973)540-1128   Fax (973)984-0416

Martin, Lorraine H., MD {1346281482} Gastrn, IntrMd(68,NE06)<NJ-MORRISTN>
+ 457 South Street
  Morristown, NJ 07960   (973)540-1240   Fax (973)984-0416

Martin, Megan Blake, MD {1750524617} Anesth
+ Hackensack Anesthesiology Associates
  140 Prospect Avenue/Suite 8   Hackensack, NJ 07601   (201)488-0066   Fax (201)488-6769

Martin, Ramelle Dana, MD {1629017280} EmrgMd(00,PA09)<NJ-JFKMED>
+ Emergency Physician Associates, P.A.
  307 South Evergreen Avenue/PO Box 298   Woodbury, NJ 08096   (856)848-3817   Fax (856)848-1431
+ JFK Medical Center
  65 James Street/EmergMed   Edison, NJ 08820   (732)321-7000

Martin, Robert Allen, MD {1487735114} ObsGyn(84,PA02)<NJ-UNVMCPRN>
+ Princeton Medical Group, P.A.
  419 North Harrison Street   Princeton, NJ 08540   (609)924-9300   Fax (609)924-6552
+ Princeton Medical Group PA
  2 Research Way/Bldg 2/Suite 302   Monroe Township, NJ 08831   (609)924-9300   Fax (609)655-7466

Martin, Sheryel Denise, MD {1730291097} Anesth(89,NJ05)
+ 1447 Bally Bunion Drive
  Egg Harbor City, NJ 08215

Martin, Steven W., MD {1295701837} RadDia, RadNro(91,PA02)<NJ-COMMED, NJ-KIMBALL>
+ Community Medical Center
  99 Route 37 West/Radiology   Toms River, NJ 08755   (732)557-8000

Martin, Thomas Reed, MD {1942319686} PulDis
+ Novartis Pharmaceuticals Corporation
  One Health Plaza   East Hanover, NJ 07936   (862)778-1549   Fax (973)781-7387

Martin, William Arthur, DO {1104937903} FamMed, EmrgMd(95,OH75)<NJ-VIRTVOOR>
+ Virtua Voorhees
  100 Bowman Drive/EmergMed   Voorhees, NJ 08043   (856)247-3000

Martin Yeboah, Patrick V., MD {1083683924} Pedtrc(76,GHA01)
+ Bright Futures Pediatrics
  185 Central Avenue/Suite 601   East Orange, NJ 07018   (973)944-1089   Fax (973)866-0023

Martindale, Peter Craig, MD {1609996040} Psychy(72,NY01)<NJ-HACKNSK>
+ 235 Prospect Avenue
  Hackensack, NJ 07601   (201)342-8933   Fax (201)342-2843
  p.martindale2@gte.net

Martinetti, Lorenzo G., MD {1588722318} FamMed(85,NJ06)<NJ-MORRISTN>
+ New Providence Family Practice
  139 South Street/Suite 201   New Providence, NJ 07974   (908)771-9311   Fax (908)771-9302

Martinez, Alan M., MD {1801021720}
+ Jersey Shore CardioThoracic & Vascular Surgery
  234 Industrial Way West/Suite A-103   Eatontown, NJ 07724   (732)918-2500   Fax (848)208-2078
  martinezalan@hotmail.com
+ Eatontown Fertility Clinic
  234 Industrial Way West/Suite A104   Eatontown, NJ 07724   (732)918-2500

Martinez, Armando I., MD {1699809666} SrgOrt, OrtSHand(71,COL06)
+ Concentra Medical Centers
  30 Seaview Drive/Suite 2   Secaucus, NJ 07094   (201)319-1611   Fax (201)319-1233
+ Concentra Medical Centers
  574 Summit Avenue   Jersey City, NJ 07306   (201)319-1611   Fax (201)656-0664

Martinez, Esther G., MD {1588687966} Pedtrc(81,LA01)
+ Kids first
  2006 Salem Road   Burlington, NJ 08016   (609)877-1500   Fax (609)877-4262

Martinez, Frances Aileen, MD {1932165735} ObsGyn
+ Women's Care Center
  3 Cooper Plaza/Suite 301   Camden, NJ 08103   (856)342-2959   Fax (856)968-8568

Martinez, Homar Amador, MD {1003877143} InfDis, IntrMd(85,MEXI)
+ JFK Medical Center
  65 James Street   Edison, NJ 08820   (732)343-1066

Martinez, Humberto L., MD   Psychy(70,PRO01)
+ 82 Eastbrook Drive
  River Edge, NJ 07661   (201)488-3054

Martinez, Ian James, MD {1396176533}
+ Somerset Family Practice
  110 Rehill Avenue   Somerville, NJ 08876   (908)685-2900   Fax (908)685-2891

Martinez, Marcos Manuel, MD {1396052130} SrgOrt(09,NJ05)<NJ-RWJUBRUN>
+ Coordinated Health
  222 Red Lane   Phillipsburg, NJ 08865   (610)861-8080   Fax (610)849-1013

Martinez, Mark, MD {1700140092} EmrgMd
+ Jersey City Medical Center Emergency
  355 Grand Street   Jersey City, NJ 07302   (201)915-2200

Martinez, Miguel E., MD {1558391482} IntrMd, Pedtrc(80,SPA01)
+ Lourdes Medical Associates
  1601 Haddon Avenue   Camden, NJ 08103   (856)757-3700   Fax (856)365-7972
+ The Cooper Hospital System-Univ Hospital
  3 Cooper Plaza/Suite 215   Camden, NJ 08103   (856)757-3700   Fax (856)968-8366

Martinez, Rebecca Marie, DO {1629097340} Anesth(95,WV75)<NJ-NWTNMEM>
+ Newton Medical Center
  175 High Street/Anesthesiology   Newton, NJ 07860   (973)383-2121

Martinez, Richard, MD {1700022316} Anesth<NJ-MTNSIDE>
+ Hackensack UMC Mountainside
  1 Bay Avenue/Anesth   Montclair, NJ 07042   (973)429-6219   Fax (845)357-5777

Martinez, Tiffany Annmarie, DO {1205196573} ObsGyn
+ Ob & Gyn Group of E Brunswick
  172 Summerhill Road/Suite 1   East Brunswick, NJ 08816   (732)254-1500   Fax (732)254-1436

Martinez, Wendy, MD {1265504666} ObsGyn(83,PA13)<NJ-VIRTBERL, NJ-VIRTVOOR>
+ Women's Group for OB/GYN
  2301 Evesham Road/Pav 800/Suite 122   Voorhees, NJ 08043   (856)770-9300   Fax (856)770-9518

Martinez-Arroyo,, Humberto L., MD {1700977535} Psychy
+ 175 Rochelle Avenue/Unit 323
  Rochelle Park, NJ 07662   (201)368-0614   Fax (718)993-0647

Martino, Michael J., MD {1558399030} Gastrn, IntrMd(83,ITAL)
+ Gastroenterology Associates of New Jersey
  1031 McBride Avenue/Suite D-212   Little Falls, NJ 07424   (973)890-1303   Fax (973)890-5609
+ Gastroenterology Associates of New Jersey
  246 Hamburg Turnpike/Suite 203   Wayne, NJ 07470   (973)890-1303   Fax (862)336-9987

Physicians by Name and Address

Martino, Stephen John, MD {1730161654} Nrolgy(98,PA01)<NJ-OCEANMC, NJ-JRSYSHMC>
+ Monmouth Ocean Neurology
1944 State Route 33/Suite 206   Neptune, NJ 07753
(732)774-8282   Fax (732)774-4407
+ Monmouth Ocean Neurology
190 Jack Martin Boulevard/Building B-3   Brick, NJ 08724
(732)774-8282   Fax (732)785-0116

Martins, Damion Antonio, MD {1114954534} IntrMd, SprtMd, IntrSptM(98,DC02)<NJ-MORRISTN>
+ Atlantic Orthopedic Institute
111 Madison Avenue/Suite 400   Morristown, NJ 07960
(973)984-0404   Fax (973)984-2516

Martins, Maria Emilia, MD {1255401733} MtFtMd, ObsGyn(88,NJ06)<NJ-STPETER>
+ University Medical Group/OBGYN
125 Paterson Street/2nd Floor   New Brunswick, NJ 08901
(732)235-6600   Fax (732)235-6627

Martins-Lopes, Maria C., MD {1093969784} MtFtMd, ObsGyn(87,CT02)
+ 117 Truman Drive
Cresskill, NJ 07626

Martinson, Charles F., MD {1548383771} PsyCAd, Psychy, IntrMd(87,NJ05)
+ Alexander Road Associates in Psychiatry & Psychology
707 Alexander Road/Bldg 2 Suite 202   Princeton, NJ 08540
(609)419-0400   Fax (609)419-9200

Martinucci, Stacy M., MD {1982844130} ObsGyn, IntrMd
+ Englewood Women's Health
25 Rockwood Place/Suite 305   Englewood, NJ 07631
(201)894-0003   Fax (201)894-0006

Martucci, Mary T., DO {1568478915} Surgry, SrgOnc(90,PA77)<NJ-CENTRAST>
+ CentraState Medical Center
901 West Main Street   Freehold, NJ 07728   (732)431-2000

Martz, Patricia Ann, MD {1740263300} Surgry(92,IL04)
+ Cape Regional Physicans Associates
217 North Main Street/Suite 104   Cape May Court House, NJ 08210   (609)463-1488   Fax (609)463-4881

Martz, Rebecca Lynn, MD {1164818134} FamMed
+ Endocrinology Associates
740 Marne Highway/Suite 206   Moorestown, NJ 08057
(856)778-4009   Fax (856)234-0498

Maruboyina, Siva Prasad, MD {1265816409} IntrMd
+ St. Michael's Medical Center
111 Central Avenue   Newark, NJ 07102   (862)763-1418
Fax (973)877-5767

Marulendra, Shivaprasad, MD {1205810926} IntrMd, Gastrn(88,INA37)<NJ-CHSMRCER, NJ-RWJUHAM>
+ Hamilton Gastroenterology Group, PC
1374 Whitehorse Hamilton Squar   Trenton, NJ 08690
(609)586-1319   Fax (609)586-1468

Maruri, Krishna K., MD {1790749299} Psychy(78,INDI)<NJ-ESSEXCO>
+ Essex County Hospital Center
204 Grove Avenue/Psychiatry   Cedar Grove, NJ 07009
(973)571-2800   Fax (973)571-2899

Marwaha, Alpana, MD {1043400120}<NJ-JRSYSHMC>
+ Jersey Shore University Medical Center
1945 Route 33   Neptune, NJ 07753   (732)775-5500
+ Meridian Medical Associates, P.C.
1945 Route 33   Neptune, NJ 07753   (732)775-5500   Fax (732)776-3795

Marwaha, Rohit, MD {1528364833} IntrMd<NJ-ACMCITY>
+ AtlantiCare Regional Medical Center/City Campus
1925 Pacific Avenue/Internal Med   Atlantic City, NJ 08401
(609)441-8146

Marwaha, Vijay R., MD {1295750578}
+ Virtua Cardiology Group
2309 East Evesham Road/Suites 201-202   Voorhees, NJ 08043   (856)325-5400   Fax (856)325-5416
+ Brick Cardiovascular Specialists/Brick Office
525 Jack Martin Boulevard/3rd Floor   Brick, NJ 08724
(856)325-5400   Fax (732)206-1563

Marx, Jo-Ann, MD {1285611533} Pedtrc, PedNph(81,DMN01)<NJ-HACKNSK, NJ-CLARMAAS>
+ 1 Wesley Place
North Arlington, NJ 07031   (201)991-0110   Fax (201)991-0070

Marx, Tatyana, MD {1164686960} Nrolgy
+ Drs. Marx and Royce
101 Madison Avenue/Suite 304   Morristown, NJ 07960
(973)292-0999   Fax (973)292-0555

Marza, Lizett Auxiliado, MD {1447232582} IntrMd(89,NIC02)<NJ-RIVERVW, NJ-MONMOUTH>
+ Integrated Medicine Alliance, P.A.
27 Pinckney Road   Red Bank, NJ 07701   (732)747-4600
Fax (732)219-1968
+ Integrated Medical Alliance/IMA Medical Care Center
30 Shrewsbury Plaza   Shrewsbury, NJ 07702   (732)747-4600   Fax (732)542-2992

Marzano, Joseph A., MD {1427052133} Gastrn, IntrMd(91,NJ05)<NJ-RIVERVW>
+ Red Bank Gastroenterology Associates PA
365 Broad Street/Suite 1-E   Red Bank, NJ 07701   (732)842-4294   Fax (732)548-7408

Marzano, Patrick Wayne, DO {1679503254} GenPrc(91,NY75)<NJ-TRINIWSC>
+ Trinitas Regional Medical Center-Williamson Street
225 Williamson Street/Internal Med   Elizabeth, NJ 07207
(908)994-5000

Marzella, Giuseppe, MD {1194866194} Pedtrc, FamMed(89,GRN01)<NJ-MORRISTN>
+ Summit Medical Group
383 Ridgedale Avenue/Suite 8   East Hanover, NJ 07936
(973)887-0200   Fax (973)887-4965

Marzili, Thomas James, MD {1952325334} FamMed(90,NJ06)<NJ-VIRTBERL, NJ-VIRTMARL>
+ 128 Route 70/Suite 13
Medford, NJ 08055   (609)451-2020   Fax (609)451-2021
Contact@DrMarzili.com

Masalia, Gopi V., MD {1528244936}
+ 666 Plainsboro Road
Plainsboro, NJ 08536

Masand, Anjali Narain, MD {1811285570} Nephro
+ North Jersey Nephrology Associates PA
246 Hamburg Turnpike/Suite 207   Wayne, NJ 07470
(973)653-3366   Fax (973)653-3365

Mascarenhas, Daniel A. Neville, MD {1568558906} CdvDis, IntCrd, CarNuc(81,INA69)<NJ-WARREN, NJ-STPETER>
+ Coventry Cardiology Associates
1000 Coventry Drive   Phillipsburg, NJ 08865   (908)859-3800   Fax (908)859-4310

Mascarenhas, Maria R., MD {1780608299} PedGst, Pedtrc(82,INA94)<PA-CHILDHOS>
+ CHOP Pediatric & Adolescent Specialty Care Center
1012 Laurel Oak Road   Voorhees, NJ 08043   (856)435-1300
Fax (856)435-0091

Mascarenhas, Mark Adrian, MD {1841477817} CdvDis, IntrMd(01,PA09)<NY-NYUTISCH>
+ Monmouth Cardiology Associates, LLC
11 Meridian Road   Eatontown, NJ 07724   (732)663-0300
Fax (732)663-0301
+ Monmouth Cardiology Associates, LLC
222 Schanck Road/Suite 104   Freehold, NJ 07728
(732)663-0300   Fax (732)431-1712

Mascarinas, Kristine I., DO {1427288109} EmrgMd<NJ-JFKMED>
+ JFK Medical Center
65 James Street/Emergency   Edison, NJ 08820   (732)321-7601   Fax (732)321-7339
+ St Joseph's Medical Center Emergency
703 Main Street   Paterson, NJ 07503   (732)321-7601   Fax (973)754-2249

Mascaro, Melissa, MD {1154642486} FamMSptM, FamMed(09,GCY01)
+ Hackensack UMC Mountainside
1 Bay Avenue/Fl 3   Montclair, NJ 07042   (973)798-8793
+ Town Medical Associates/Verona
271 Grove Avenue/Suite A   Verona, NJ 07044   (973)798-8793   Fax (973)239-6068

Mascellino, Ann Marie Madaline, MD {1730116690} Nrolgy(96,NJ05)<NJ-WAYNEGEN, NJ-CHILTON>
+ Neurologic Associates
220 Hamburg Turnpike/Suite 16   Wayne, NJ 07470
(973)942-4778   Fax (973)942-7020

Masci, Robert L., MD {1730139619} CdvDis(83,NJ06)<NJ-NWTN-MEM, NJ-MORRISTN>
+ Cardiology Associates of Sussex County LLP
222 High Street/Suite 205   Newton, NJ 07860   (973)579-2100   Fax (973)579-6638

Masciarelli, Anthony, DO {1932109717} Gastrn, IntrMd(87,NJ75)<NJ-KMHCHRRY, NJ-VIRTVOOR>
+ Cape Reg Phys Assoc-Med Commons
217 North Main Street/Suite 102   Cape May Court House, NJ 08210   (609)536-8010   Fax (609)536-8053

Mascio, Christopher Edward, MD {1629023510} SrgThr
+ CHOP Pediatric & Adolescent Specialty Care Center
1012 Laurel Oak Road   Voorhees, NJ 08043   (856)435-1300
Fax (856)435-0091

Masel-Miller, Rachel Jenna, DO {1659764025}
+ Cooper Physicians
1210 Brace Road/Suite 102   Cherry Hill, NJ 08034
(856)428-6616   Fax (856)428-4823

Masella, Robert Michael, MD {1801093737} SrgOrt, SprtMd(03,NJ05)<NJ-RWJUBRUN>
+ North Jersey Orthopaedic Group
246 Hamburg Turnpike/Suite 302   Wayne, NJ 07470
(973)689-6266   Fax (973)689-6264

Masessa, Joseph M., MD {1720115355} Dermat(87,NJ05)<NJ-CHILTON, NJ-STCLRDEN>
+ North Jersey Dermatology Center
35 Green Pond Road   Rockaway, NJ 07866   (973)625-0600
Fax (973)625-0336

+ North Jersey Dermatology Center
7 Oak Ridge Road/Suite 3   Newfoundland, NJ 07435
(973)625-0600   Fax (973)208-8106

Mashburn, Penelope, DO {1154650117} Surgry
+ 2039 Marguerite Street/Flr 2
Fort Lee, NJ 07024   Fax (201)758-2740

Mashru, Pravinkuma K., MD {1457425654} GenPrc, Surgry(72,INDI)
+ Lourdes Medical Center of Burlington County
218 Sunset Road/Suite A   Willingboro, NJ 08046   (609)835-5240

Mashru, Rakesh Pravinkumar, MD {1750318739} SrgOrt, IntrMd(NJ05
+ Cooper Surgical Associates
3 Cooper Plaza/Suite 403   Camden, NJ 08103   (856)342-3113   Fax (856)541-5379

Masia, Alan, MD {1578536264} Pedtrc, AdolMd(80,NY19)
+ Ocean Health Initiatives, Inc.
301 Lakehurst Road   Toms River, NJ 08755   (732)552-0377
Fax (732)552-0378

Maslany, Steven, DO {1821181595} Psychy, PsyGrt, PsyAdd(97,NJ75)<NJ-VALYONS>
+ VA New Jersey Health Care System at Lyons
151 Knollcroft Road   Lyons, NJ 07939   (908)647-0180   Fax (908)604-5251

Maslin, Stuart J., MD {1316935109} FamMed(83,PA02)<NJ-VIRTBERL, NJ-VIRTVOOR>
+ Concentra Medical Centers Urgent Care
817 East Gate Drive/Suite 102   Mount Laurel, NJ 08054
(856)778-1090   Fax (856)778-0801

Maslow, Gregory S., MD {1174549950} SrgOrt(72,PA01)<NJ-UNDRWD, NJ-VIRTMARL>
+ 100 Brick Road/Suite 212
Marlton, NJ 08053   (856)983-8848
+ 1000 Mantua Pike
Woodbury, NJ 08097   (856)983-8848   Fax (856)848-5751

Maso, Kristi Lynn, MD {1841588936}
+ Cooper University Medical Center/Camden
3 Cooper Plaza   Camden, NJ 08103   (856)342-2000

Maso, Martha J., MD {1518968676} Dermat, OccpMd(86,NJ05)
+ Westwood Dermatology
390 Old Hook Road   Westwood, NJ 07675   (201)666-9550
Fax (201)666-1251

Mason, David Craig, DO {1093795478} FamMed, NeuMus(96,NJ75)
+ UMDNJ SOM Family Medicine
310 Creek Crossing Boulevard   Hainesport, NJ 08036
(609)702-7500   Fax (609)702-5928

Mason, Sandra, MD {1265850457} FamMed<NJ-SJHREGMC>
+ SJH Regional Medical Center
1505 West Sherman Avenue   Vineland, NJ 08360
(856)641-7675

Mason, Thornton B. Alexander, II, MD {1811901424} NroChl, Pedtrc(90,VA04)<PA-CHILDHOS>
+ CHOP Specialty Care Center at Virtua
200 Bowman Drive/2 FL/Suite D-260   Voorhees, NJ 08043
(267)425-5400

Mason-Bell, Sharon E., MD {1861523102} PsyCAd, Psychy(82,NJ05)
+ Drs. Bell and Mason-Bell
51 Upper Montclair Plaza/Suite 14   Upper Montclair, NJ 07043   (973)746-9615

Mason-Cederberg, Lauren, MD {1457768178} ObsGyn
+ Shore Area Ob-Gyn
200 White Road/Suite 105   Little Silver, NJ 07739
(732)741-3331

Mason-Eastmond, Tania Alicia, DO {1356362032} Pedtrc(97,OH75)<NJ-NWRKBETH>
+ NHCAC Health Center at West New York
5301 Broadway   West New York, NJ 07093   (201)866-9320
Fax (201)867-9183

Masone, Daniel A., MD {1891766002} IntrMd(70,NE06)
+ 203 Larsens Drive
Denville, NJ 07834

Masone, Patricia A., MD GenPrc(74,MO34)
+ 203 Larsens Drive
Denville, NJ 07834

Masood, Hamid, MD {1689016503} FamMed<NJ-HUNTRDN>
+ Fair Medical Services
1760 Whitehorse Hamilton Squar/Suite 1   Hamilton, NJ 08690   (609)890-8200   Fax (201)331-3637
+ Hunterdon Medical Center
2100 Wescott Drive   Flemington, NJ 08822   (908)788-6100

Masor, Harvey G., MD {1538338199} IntrMd, Hemato(65,NY09)<NJ-NWRKBETH, NJ-STBARNMC>
+ 739 Chancellor Avenue
Irvington, NJ 07111   (973)371-5959   Fax (973)371-0171
hmasor1233@gmail.com

Physicians by Name and Address

Masri, Sammy Ismail, MD {1396770426} IntrMd, SprtMd(00,DMN01)<NJ-HACKNSK>
+ American Orthopedic & Sports Medicine
30 West Century Road/Suite 320   Paramus, NJ 07652
(201)261-0402   Fax (201)261-0587

Masry, Allen Y., MD {1396779054} Psychy, PsyAdd(95,EGY03)<MA-WRCSTST>
+ Ancora Psychiatric Hospital
301 Spring Garden Road   Hammonton, NJ 08037
(609)561-1700
+ Camden County Health Services Center
425 Woodbury Turnersville Rd   Blackwood, NJ 08012
(609)561-1700   Fax (856)374-6790
+ 141 S. Blackhorse Pike
Blackwood, NJ 08037   (617)259-8062

Mass, Alon Y., MD {1447511191} Urolgy
+ Premier Urology Group, LLC
275 Orchard Street   Westfield, NJ 07090   (908)654-5100
Fax (908)789-8755
+ Premier Urology Group, LLC
570 South Avenue East/Building A   Cranford, NJ 07016
(908)654-5100   Fax (908)497-1633
+ Premier Urology Group, LLC
776 East Third Avenue   Roselle Park, NJ 07090   (908)241-5268   Fax (908)241-8755

Mass, Sharon B., MD {1043279292} ObsGyn(93,PA02)
+ Morristown Obstetrics and Gynecology Associates
101 Madison Avenue/Suite 405   Morristown, NJ 07960
(973)267-7272   Fax (973)455-0099

Massabbal, Eltayeb I., MD {1376656488} NnPnMd, Pedtrc(92,SUD01)<NJ-OURLADY>
+ Our Lady of Lourdes Medical Center
1600 Haddon Avenue/Neontlgy   Camden, NJ 08103
(856)757-3500

Massac, Malik Ali, MD {1831528017} IntrMd
+ Patients first
705 Haddonfield Berlin Road   Voorhees, NJ 08043
(856)679-0537   Fax (856)673-0538

Massari, Ronald D., MD {1073510640} CdvDis, IntrMd(88,NJ06)<NJ-NWTNMEM, NJ-MORRISTN>
+ Cardiology Consultants of North Morris, PA
356 US Highway 46/Suite B   Mountain Lakes, NJ 07046
(973)586-3400   Fax (973)586-1916

Massaro, Robert A., MD {1679500482} ObsGyn(83,MNT01)<NJ-MONMOUTH, NJ-RIVERVW>
+ West Long Branch Obstetrics & Gynecology
1019 Broadway   West Long Branch, NJ 07764   (732)229-6797   Fax (732)229-6893
+ Monmouth Family Center
270 Broadway   Long Branch, NJ 07740   (732)229-6797
Fax (732)923-7104

Massler, Dennis J., MD {1982705372} Psychy(73,NJ05)<NJ-STBARNMC>
+ 16 Meadowbrook Road
Boonton, NJ 07005   (973)331-8119   Fax (973)588-4669
relationshrink@optonline.net
+ Living Zen
127 East Mount Pleasant Avenue   Livingston, NJ 07039

Masson, Lalitha, MD {1487762019} ObsGyn(64,INDI)<NJ-CHRIST, NJ-HOBUNIMC>
+ 634 Newark Avenue
Jersey City, NJ 07306

Massoud, Bryan J., MD {1780646232} SrgOrt, IntrMd(91,NJ06)<NJ-VALLEY>
+ Oasis Medical and Wellness
85 Harristown Road/Suite 103   Glen Rock, NJ 07452   Fax (844)366-8900
bfornataro@oasismed.com

Mast, Harold Lee, MD {1396790820} RadDia, RadV&I(85,NJ05)<NJ-NWRKBETH>
+ New Jersey Vein and Cosmetic Surgery Center
741 Northfield Avenue/Suite 105   West Orange, NJ 07052
(973)243-9729   Fax (973)243-9672

Master, Julie, DO {1912044900} CdvDis, IntrMd(03,NY75)<NJ-BAYSHORE, NJ-JRSYSHMC>
+ Barnabas Health Medical Group
166 Morris Avenue/2nd Floor   Long Branch, NJ 07740
(732)263-5024   Fax (732)263-5029
+ Monmouth Heart Specialists
274 Highway 35   Eatontown, NJ 07724   (732)263-5024
Fax (732)440-9404

Master, Kenneth V., MD {1659317949} Psychy, PsyGrt(90,OH41)
+ Master Psychiatric Consulting
2 Whitehorse Pike   Haddon Heights, NJ 08035   (856)310-0042   Fax (856)310-0092
C.master@masterpsych.com

Master, Maria G., MD {1538329396} Psychy
+ 40 Hamilton Avenue
Wayne, NJ 07470   (201)618-3035

Master, Violet S., MD {1609847193} IntrMd(69,INDI)<NJ-ENGLWOOD>
+ 596 Anderson Avenue/Suite 216
Cliffside Park, NJ 07010   (201)943-7246   Fax (201)943-7037

Masters, Martha Meredith, MD {1972948222} EmrgMd<NJ-UMDNJ>
+ University Hospital
150 Bergen Street   Newark, NJ 07103   (973)972-9533

Masterson, Christine, MD {1871536813} ObsGyn(96,NJ05)<NJ-OVERLOOK, NJ-MORRISTN>
+ Summit Medical Group-Berkeley Heights Campus
1 Diamond Hill Road/3rd Fl   Berkeley Heights, NJ 07922
(908)277-8770   Fax (908)219-3011
+ Summit Medical Group
34 Mountain Boulevard/Building B   Warren, NJ 07059
(908)277-8770   Fax (908)769-8927

Masterson, Eileen, MD {1437139375} Grtrcs, IntrMd(84,VA01)<NJ-JRSYSHMC>
+ Jersey Shore University Medical Center
1945 Route 33   Neptune, NJ 07753   (732)776-4302
+ Hackensack Meridian Medical Group
19 Davis Avenue/5th-6th Floor   Neptune, NJ 07753
(732)776-4302   Fax (732)897-3997

Masterson, Margaret, MD {1013005107} PedHem, Pedtrc(82,VA07)<NJ-JRSYSHMC, NJ-RWJUBRUN>
+ Rutgers Cancer Institute of New Jersey
195 Little Albany Street/PO Box 2681   New Brunswick, NJ 08903   (732)235-2465   Fax (732)235-6797
masterma@umdnj.edu
+ Jersey Shore University Medical Center
1945 Route 33/Pedi   Neptune, NJ 07753   (732)235-2465
Fax (732)776-4867

Masterson, Raymond Mark, MD {1720074727} IntrMd(78,PHIL)<NJ-JRSYSHMC, NJ-RIVERVW>
+ Highway 71 & Crescent Place
Sea Girt, NJ 08750   (732)974-0340   Fax (732)974-2854

Masterson, Richard J., MD {1265497895} Surgry(76,MEX14)<NJ-STPETER>
+ St. Peter's University Hospital
254 Easton Avenue/Surgery   New Brunswick, NJ 08901
(732)845-8571   Fax (732)249-5284

Masterson, Robert E., MD {1437167301} Ophthl(68,IRE05)<NJ-MORRISTN>
+ 261 James Street/Suite 2 D
Morristown, NJ 07960   (973)540-1819   Fax (973)540-9706

Masterton, Deirdre C., MD {1235314394} ObsGyn
+ Advanced Obstetrics & Gynecology, LLC
4 Walter E. Foran Boulevard/Suite 302   Flemington, NJ 08822   (908)284-5283   Fax (908)806-3478

Mastrianno, Frank L., MD {1083641955} IntrMd(82,MEX03)<NJ-VALLEY, NJ-HOLYNAME>
+ 466 Old Hook Road/Suite 28
Emerson, NJ 07630   (201)262-0333   Fax (201)634-0976

Mastro, Caroline Briana, MD {1407938780} FamMed(01,PA02)
+ 279 Mathistown Road
Little Egg Harbor, NJ 08087

Mastrokyriakos, Paul, DO {1669401519} EmrgMd(89,MO78)<NJ-OVERLOOK>
+ Overlook Medical Center
99 Beauvoir Avenue/PO Box 210/EmrgMed   Summit, NJ 07902   (908)522-2000   Fax (908)522-0227

Mastromonaco, Denise M., DO {1336399112} Dermat, FamMed(92,IA75)
+ Kennedy Health Alliance
457 Haddonfield Road/Suite 110   Cherry Hill, NJ 08002
(856)406-4091   Fax (856)406-4570

Mastromonaco, Edward Domenick, DO {1821010836} SrgOrt(68,IA75)<NJ-BAYONNE>
+ 696 Avenue C
Bayonne, NJ 07002   (201)339-2284   Fax (201)339-7922

Mastrosimone, Angelo, MD {1801998018} Allrgy(67,MEXI)
+ Allergy & Sinus Center
123 Franklin Corner Road/Suite 105   Lawrenceville, NJ 08648   (609)896-2300   Fax (609)896-2211

Mastroti, Jean-Baptiste J., MD {1093869463} PsyCAd, Psychy(79,VEN07)<NJ-HCMEADPS>
+ Hudson County Meadowview Psychiatric Hospital
595 County Avenue   Secaucus, NJ 07094   (201)319-3660
Fax (201)319-3616

Mastrovitch, Todd Anthony, MD {1477620698} Pedtrc, PedEmg(96,GRNA)<NJ-MONMOUTH>
+ St Joseph's Medical Pedicatic EmerMed
703 Main Street   Paterson, NJ 07503   (973)754-4901

Masud, Avais, MD {1114983541} Nephro, CritCr, IntrMd(85,PAK20)<NJ-OCEANMC, NJ-JRSYSHMC>
+ Shore Nephrology, P.A.
2100 Corlies Avenue/Suite 15   Neptune, NJ 07753
(732)988-8228   Fax (732)774-1528
+ Shore Nephrology, P.A.
1000 West Main Street/Suite 3   Freehold, NJ 07728
(732)988-8228   Fax (732)414-1591
+ Shore Nephrology, PA
27 South Cookbridge Road/Suite 211   Jackson, NJ 07753
(732)987-5990   Fax (732)987-5994

Masullo, Alfredo S., MD {1255518205} Dermat, SrgDer(75,NJ05)<NJ-HACKNSK, NJ-HOLYNAME>
+ Ablative Academic Advanced Aesthetic Institute
120 Prospect Avenue   Hackensack, NJ 07601   (201)488-0707   Fax (201)488-0708
jinxs_laplante@hotmail.com

Matadial, Manjushree, DO {1568542686} EmrgMd, IntrMd(95,MI12)<NJ-STJOSHOS>
+ St. Joseph's Regional Medical Center
703 Main Street/EmergMed   Paterson, NJ 07503
(973)754-2000

Matalkah, Nidal M., MD {1447336771} IntrMd, PulDis, CritCr(90,JORD)<NJ-CHILTON>
+ Drs. Singh & Farhangfar
401 Hamburg Turnpike/Suite 109   Wayne, NJ 07470
(973)595-7456   Fax (973)904-9119

Matalon, Vivienne I., MD {1396858635} Dermat, IntrMd, FamMed(85,CHIL)<NJ-OURLADY, NJ-VIRTMARL>
+ TLC HealthCare
2070 Springdale Road/Suite 100   Cherry Hill, NJ 08003
(856)985-0590   Fax (856)985-2866

Matarese, William A., MD {1962580514} SrgOrt(83,CT02)<NJ-CHILTON, NJ-VALLEY>
+ High Mountain Orthopedics
342 Hamburg Turnpike/Suite 205   Wayne, NJ 07470
(973)595-7779   Fax (973)595-0182
+ Wayne Surgical Center, LLC.
1176 Hamburg Pike   Wayne, NJ 07470   (973)595-7779
Fax (973)709-1901

Matari, Hussein M., MD {1447321476} Radiol, RadDia(81,DOM02)<NJ-HOBUNIMC>
+ Hoboken University Medical Center
308 Willow Avenue   Hoboken, NJ 07030   (201)418-1000
Fax (201)418-1822

Matassa, Daniel Michael, MD {1043552441} IntrMd
+ University Hospital Medicine
150 Bergen Street/Room I-248   Newark, NJ 07103
(973)972-6056   Fax (973)972-3129

Mate, Shrikrishn K., MD {1376646687} Pedtrc(72,INDI)<NJ-OCEANMC, NJ-COMMED>
+ Pediatric Medical Group
525 Jack Martin Boulevard/Suite 102   Brick, NJ 08724
(732)458-1177   Fax (732)458-5942

Matejicka, Anthony V., II, DO {1518917608}<NJ-STBARHCS>
+ St. Barnabas Health Care System
99 Highway 37 West/Comm Medical Center   Toms River, NJ 08755   (732)557-8056
anthony.matejicka@hotmail.com

Matera, James J., DO {1336139732} Nephro, IntrMd(89,IA75)<NJ-CENTRAST>
+ Nephrology Hypertension Associates of Central Jersey
8 Old Bridge Turnpike   South River, NJ 08882   (732)390-4888   Fax (732)390-0255
+ Nephrology Hypertension Associates of Central Jersey
901 West Main Street/Suite 102   Freehold, NJ 07728
(732)625-0707
+ CentraState Medical Center
901 West Main Street   Freehold, NJ 08882   (732)431-2000

Materetsky, Steven H., MD {1497723019} Pedtrc(96,IL42)<NJ-HACKNSK, NJ-VALLEY>
+ Pediatric Specialties PA
90 Prospect Avenue/Suite 1-A   Hackensack, NJ 07601
(201)342-4001   Fax (201)342-9569
+ Pediatric Specialties PA
50 South Franklin Turnpike   Ramsey, NJ 07446   (201)342-4001   Fax (201)934-2947

Materna, Alexander Paul, MD {1669616595}
+ Robert Wood Johnson University Hospital at Hamilton
1 Hamilton Health Place   Hamilton, NJ 08690   (609)586-7900
+ 43 Westview Road
Wayne, NJ 07470

Materna, Thomas W., MD {1356480503} Ophthl(71,NY08)
+ 20 Ferry Street
Newark, NJ 07105   (973)589-0104   Fax (973)589-5084
+ Associated Eye Physicians, P.A.
1033 Clifton Avenue/Suite 107   Clifton, NJ 07013
(973)589-0104   Fax (973)472-4832

Matflerd, Carolynn A., MD {1689887127} Psychy(88,PA02)
+ 63 West Main Street/2nd Floor
Freehold, NJ 07728   (732)409-6220   Fax (732)409-6219

Mathai, Suja John, MD {1356518187} InfDis, IntrMd(02,INA8C)
+ Infectious Disease Consultants
1245 Whitehorse-Mercerville Rd   Mercerville, NJ 08619
(609)581-2000   Fax (609)581-5450

Matharoo, Gurdeep Singh, MD {1972764256} Surgry(08,STM01)<NJ-MONMOUTH>
+ Specialty Surgical Associates
10 Industrial Way East/Suite 104   Eatontown, NJ 07724
(732)389-1331   Fax (732)542-8587

Mathason, Mark David, DO {1669490561} EmrgMd
+ 15 Wood Lark Drive
Mount Laurel, NJ 08054
Mathew, Alexander John, MD {1134219918} IntrMd, CdvDis(00,MNT01)<NJ-COOPRUMC>
+ United Medical, P.C.
988 Broadway/Suite 201   Bayonne, NJ 07002   (201)339-6111   Fax (201)339-6333
+ Cooper University Hospital
One Cooper Plaza   Camden, NJ 08103   (856)342-2000
Mathew, Jacob J., MD {1407160187}<NJ-STJOSHOS>
+ St. Joseph's Regional Medical Center
703 Main Street   Paterson, NJ 07503   (973)754-2000
Mathew, Jocelyn, MD {1124548003} FamMed
+ Dr. De La Cruz and Dhalla
714 Tenth Street   Secaucus, NJ 07094   (201)865-2050   Fax (201)865-0015
Mathew, Joseph, MD {1225197320} CritCr, IntrMd, PulDis(80,INDI)<NJ-BAYSHORE>
+ Medical Associates of Central New Jersey
26 Throckmorton Lane/1st flr.   Old Bridge, NJ 08857   (732)679-9950   Fax (732)679-9956
Mathew, Julie, MD {1013275791} Anesth<NJ-RWJUBRUN>
+ 206 Juniper Court
Somerset, NJ 08873
Mathew, Lovely Sebastian, MD {1043629876} Pedtrc, IntrMd(93,FRAN)
+ Dr. Vijaya Radhakrishna, MD, PC
155 Stelton Road   Piscataway, NJ 08854   (732)752-8442   Fax (732)752-3957
+ Dr. Vinaya Radhakrishna, MD PC
230 State Route 18   East Brunswick, NJ 08816   (732)752-8442   Fax (732)651-1848
Mathew, Mary, MD {1306886577} Pedtrc
+ Williamstown Pediatrics
925-A South Black Horse Pike   Williamstown, NJ 08094   (856)629-9000   Fax (856)629-6440
Mathew, Mini Ann, DO {1255591921} EnDbMt, IntrMd(06,NJ75)
+ Endocrinology Associates of Princeton, LLC
579A Cranberry Road/Suite 101   East Brunswick, NJ 08816   (732)579-6444   Fax (609)896-0079
Mathew, Nisha S., MD {1710012950} EmrgMd<NJ-VIRTVOOR>
+ Team Health East
307 South Evergeen Avenue   Woodbury, NJ 08096   (856)686-4319   Fax (856)848-8536
Mathew, Omana R., MD {1477573657} Pedtrc(82,INDI)<NJ-HOLYNAME>
+ Bergen Pediatric Center PC
167 South Washington Avenue   Bergenfield, NJ 07621   (201)384-8510   Fax (201)384-8511
Mathew, Saritha, MD {1861586349} IntrMd, Grtrcs(96,INDI)
+ Ahmad Syed S MD PA
183 Franklin Corner Road   Lawrenceville, NJ 08648   (609)896-0622   Fax (609)896-0069
Mathew, Seema Alexander, MD {1831389154} Pedtrc
+ 101 Old Short Hills Road/Suite 105
West Orange, NJ 07052   (973)325-1115   Fax (973)325-1186
Mathew, Seena M., MD {1790944536}
+ 2 Caitlin Court
East Hanover, NJ 07936
Mathew, Teena, MD {1568723542} IntrMd<NJ-RBAYPERT>
+ Raritan Bay Medical Center/Perth Amboy Division
530 New Brunswick Avenue   Perth Amboy, NJ 08861   (732)324-5080
Teena.mathew@yahoo.com
Mathew, Thomas, MD {1427035435} Anesth(91,INDI)<NJ-CHRIST>
+ Christ Hospital
176 Palisade Avenue/Anesthesiology   Jersey City, NJ 07306   (201)795-8200   Fax (201)943-8105
Mathew, Tittymol, MD {1114950565} IntrMd(92,INA98)
+ Dover Internal Medicine LLC
530 Lakehurst Road/Suite 307   Toms River, NJ 08755   (732)341-8901   Fax (732)341-8906
Mathews, Cecil, MD {1528078383} InfDis, IntrMd(88,GRN01)
+ Eck, Apelian & Mathews
1056 Stelton Road   Piscataway, NJ 08854   (732)463-0303   Fax (732)463-2289
+ Neighborhood Health Center Plainfield
1700-58 Myrtle Avenue   Plainfield, NJ 07060   (732)463-0303   Fax (908)226-6743
Mathews, Chacko P., MD ObsGyn(71,INDI)
+ 59 Sussex Avenue
Morristown, NJ 07960
Mathews, Jeane M., MD {1912342809}
+ Urgent Care of New Jersey
2090 Route 27   Edison, NJ 08817   (732)662-5657   Fax (732)662-5651
jeanemthomas@gmail.com

Mathews, Jeffrey John, MD {1083825756} Radiol, RadDia, NuclMd(05,NJ06)
+ Radiology Affiliates of Central New Jersey, P.A.
2501 Kuser Road   Hamilton, NJ 08691   (609)585-8800   Fax (609)585-1825
Mathews, Joanne, MD {1336318708} Psychy(97,INA70)
+ Pinnacle Behavioral Health Institute
851 Route 73 North/Suite C   Marlton, NJ 08053   (856)512-8108   Fax (856)267-5824
+ University Hospital-SOM Department of Psychiatry
2250 Chapel Avenue West/Suite 100   Cherry Hill, NJ 08002   (856)512-8108   Fax (856)482-1159
+ 5 Madison Court
Marlton, NJ 08053
Mathews, Jyoti, MD {1053610626} FamMed(07,NJ05)<NJ-BERGNMC>
+ New Bridge Medical Center
230 East Ridgewood Avenue   Paramus, NJ 07652   (201)967-4000   Fax (201)967-7924
+ 450 Island Road/Apt. 122
Ramsey, NJ 07446   (201)686-7340
Mathews, Maju, MD {1508801010} Psychy(96,INA9E)
+ Pinnacle Behavioral Health Institute
851 Route 73 North/Suite C   Marlton, NJ 08053   (856)512-8108   Fax (856)267-5824
Mathews, Robert John, MD {1902060221} IntHos, IntrMd(03,DOM18)<PA-BRYNMAWR>
+ Regional Nephrology Associates
510 Jackson Avenue   Northfield, NJ 08225   (609)383-0200   Fax (609)383-8352
Mathews, Sam, MD {1790054526} EmrgMd
+ St. Michael's Medical Center
111 Central Avenue   Newark, NJ 07102   (201)658-6297
+ 143 Bertha Court
Paramus, NJ 07652   (201)261-1502
Mathias, Claudia Fernandes, MD {1285754721} FamMed(02,NY48)
+ Drs. Vijayakumar & Fernandes
152 Central Avenue   Clark, NJ 07066   (732)382-9700   Fax (732)382-9707
Mathieu, Jacques Jude, MD {1144264250} EnDbMt, GPrvMd, PulDis(77,HAI01)<NJ-GRYSTPSY>
+ Greystone Park Psychiatric Hospital
59 Koch Avenue   Morris Plains, NJ 07950   (973)538-1800
Mathur, Ajay Narain, MD {1053357947} InfDis, IntrMd(01,CT02)<NJ-MONMOUTH, NJ-OCEANMC>
+ Infectious Disease Care
1912 State Route 35/Suite 101   Oakhurst, NJ 07755   (732)222-4762   Fax (732)222-4764
Mathur, Ajit, MD {1124049200} Pedtrc(91,INA9B)<NJ-ACMCITY>
+ Rainbow Pediatrics
2041 US Highway 9   Cape May Court House, NJ 08210   (609)624-9003   Fax (609)624-9002
Mathur, Anjana, MD {1306895982} IntrMd(94,INA76)<NJ-COMMED>
+ 147 Route 37 West
Toms River, NJ 08755   (732)341-8885   Fax (732)341-7408
Mathur, Atish Pratap, MD {1588895064} IntCrd, IntrMd<NJ-HACKNSK>
+ Hackensack University Medical Center
30 Prospect Avenue/Cardiology   Hackensack, NJ 07601   (201)996-2000
Mathur, Mayank, MD {1750591087} Nrolgy(05,NJ05)
+ Neurology Associaates of South Jersey
693 Main Street/Building D   Lumberton, NJ 08048   (609)261-7600   Fax (609)265-8205
+ Advocare Neurology of South Jersey
200-B Route 73 North/Suite 2   Voorhees, NJ 08043   (609)261-7600   Fax (856)335-0406
Mathur, Smita, DO {1184058653} IntHos<NJ-MEADWLND>
+ Meadowlands Hospital Medical Center
55 Meadowlands Parkway   Secaucus, NJ 07096   (201)392-3258
Mathur, Tanisha, MD {1669634671}
+ Valley Rheumatology & Autoimmune Dis
1200 East Ridgewood Avenue   Ridgewood, NJ 07450   (201)389-0096   Fax (201)857-8771
Mathure, Mekhala A., MD {1588942668} IntrMd<NJ-TRINIWSC>
+ Trinitas Regional Medical Center-Williamson Street
225 Williamson Street/Internal Med   Elizabeth, NJ 07207   (908)994-5000
+ Medical Associates of Central New Jersey
26 Throckmorton Lane/1st flr.   Old Bridge, NJ 08857   (908)994-5000   Fax (732)679-9956
Matican, Jeffrey S., MD {1487622247} CdvDis, IntrMd(82,NY09)<NJ-ENGLWOOD, NJ-HACKNSK>
+ 309 Engle Street/Suite 5
Englewood, NJ 07631   (201)503-1920   Fax (201)503-0222
+ Heart and Vascular Institute at EHMC
350 Engle Street/Suite 1000   Englewood, NJ 07631   (201)894-3636
+ Northern New Jersey Cardiology Associates PA

7704 Marine Road   North Bergen, NJ 07631   (201)869-1313   Fax (201)854-7945
Matienzo, Ricardo Martin, MD {1306833660} FamMed(80,CUB06)<NJ-HOBUNIMC>
+ 450 7th Street/Suite LL9
Hoboken, NJ 07030   (201)659-0711   Fax (201)659-4117
Matier, Brian, MD {1942484159} Surgry, SrgC&R(06,GRN01)
+ Ballem Surgical
230 Sherman Avenue/Suite C   Glen Ridge, NJ 07028   (973)744-8585   Fax (973)748-5990
Matin, Nadia, MD {1124298625} Psychy(99,PAK12)<NJ-UMDNJ>
+ VA New Jersey Health Care System-East Orange Campus
385 Tremont Avenue   East Orange, NJ 07018   (973)676-1000
Matjucha, John R., MD {1245326131} EmrgMd(91,IL02)<NJ-NWRKBETH>
+ Newark Beth Israel Medical Center
201 Lyons Avenue   Newark, NJ 07112   (973)926-7000   Fax (610)617-6280
Matkiwsky, Daniel Walter, DO {1841204559} FamMed(97,PA77)
+ Skylands Medical Group PA
406 Route 23/Suite 1   Franklin, NJ 07416   (973)827-2120   Fax (973)827-9445
+ Premier Health Associates
123 Newton Sparta Road   Newton, NJ 07860   (973)827-2120   Fax (973)579-1524
Matkiwsky, Walter, DO {1699789461} FamMed(69,PA77)<NJ-STBARNMC, NJ-OVERLOOK>
+ Hillside Family Practice
100 Hollywood Avenue   Hillside, NJ 07205   (908)353-7949   Fax (908)353-8374
+ Hillside Family Practice
6 North 21st Street   Kenilworth, NJ 07033   (908)353-7949
Matlick, Lonny D., DO {1720088610} Otlryg(81,NJ75)<NJ-BURDTMLN>
+ Drs. Matlick, DeLorio, and Mucci
307 Stone Harbor Boulevard/Suite 3   Cape May Court House, NJ 08210   (609)465-4667   Fax (609)465-9387
Matos, Ninon, MD {1174757256} IntrMd<NJ-OURLADY>
+ Our Lady of Lourdes Medical Center
1600 Haddon Avenue   Camden, NJ 08103   (856)757-3700   Fax (856)365-7972
Matos-Cloke, Susan I., MD {1730107939} IntrMd, GPrvMd(84,NY47)
+ New Bridge Medical Center
230 East Ridgewood Avenue   Paramus, NJ 07652   (201)967-4000
+ Empire Medical Associates
264 Boyden Avenue   Maplewood, NJ 07040   (201)967-4000   Fax (973)761-7617
Matossian, Cynthia, MD {1689635807} Ophthl(81,PA14)<NJ-CAPITLHS>
+ Matossian Eye Associates
2 Capital Way/Suite 326   Pennington, NJ 08534   (609)882-8833   Fax (609)882-0077
+ Matossian Eye Associates
1445 Whitehorse-Mercerville Rd   Hamilton, NJ 08619   (609)882-8833   Fax (609)890-0774
Matossian, Raffee H., MD {1124110119} EmrgMd(76,MEXI)<NJ-TRINIWSC>
+ Trinitas Regional Medical Center-Williamson Street
225 Williamson Street   Elizabeth, NJ 07207   (908)994-5000
Matrale, Michael, DO {1205249174} IntrMd
+ SOM - Department of Internal Medicine
42 East Laurel Road/Suite 3100   Stratford, NJ 08084   (856)566-2753   Fax (856)566-6906
Matsenko, Oxana, MD {1104080076} PsyCAd(97,UKR16)
+ 38-59 Dauria Drive
Fair Lawn, NJ 07410
Matsinger, John Mark, DO {1700827292} IntrMd, IntHos(00,PA77)<NJ-DEBRAHLC, NJ-VIRTMHBC>
+ Virtua Medical Group
401 Route 73/40 Lake Ctr Dr/Ste 201A   Marlton, NJ 08053   (856)355-0340   Fax (856)355-0330
+ Virtua Memorial
175 Madison Avenue/Hospitalist   Mount Holly, NJ 08060   (856)355-0340   Fax (609)914-6182
+ Deborah Heart and Lung Center
200 Trenton Road   Browns Mills, NJ 08053   (609)893-6611
Matsuki, Takashi, MD {1235423195} Psychy<NY-BETHPETR>
+ Edgewater Family Care Center
725 River Road/Suite 202   Edgewater, NJ 07020   (201)943-4040   Fax (201)941-4599
Matta, Jyoti S., MD {1104882588} CritCr, PulDis, IntrMd(92,INDI)<NJ-JRSYCITY, NJ-CHRIST>
+ Liberty Medical Associates
377 Jersey Avenue/Suite 470   Jersey City, NJ 07302   (201)918-2239   Fax (201)918-2243

Physicians by Name and Address

Matta, Paul Gamal, DO {1427014380} ObsGyn, MtFtMd(97,NY75)<NJ-STPETER>
+ Hackensack Meridian Urogynecolgy Medical Group
  19 Davis Avenue/7th Floor   Neptune, NJ 07753   (732)776-3797   Fax (732)776-3796
+ The Perinatal Institute
  1944 State Route 33   Neptune, NJ 07753   (732)776-3797   Fax (732)776-4754

Matta, Rana C., MD {1912311382} Pedtrc(13,LEB06)
+ NuHeights Pediatrics
  2 Brighton Road/Suite 404   Clifton, NJ 07013   (973)250-2970   Fax (973)250-2971
+ NuHeights Pediatrics
  1115 Clifton Avenue/Suite 101   Clifton, NJ 07013   (973)250-2970   Fax (973)250-2971

Mattana, Nina Delman, MD {1538126818} RadDia, RadMam(89,NY46)<NJ-ENGLWOOD>
+ Englewood Radiologic Group PA
  350 Engle Street   Englewood, NJ 07631   (201)894-3000   Fax (201)894-5244
+ Advanced Medical Imaging of North Jersey
  452 Old Hook Road/Suite 301   Emerson, NJ 07630   (201)894-3000   Fax (201)262-2330

Matteace, Frank P., MD {1417925660} IntrMd(84,GRNA)<NJ-COMMED>
+ Drs. Van Wyck & Matteace
  567 Fischer Boulevard   Toms River, NJ 08753   (732)506-6868   Fax (732)506-6879

Mattei, C. Antonia, MD {1346240660} FamMed(92,NC05)<NJ-HUNTRDN>
+ Hunterdon Family Medicine
  1100 Wescott Drive/Suite 101   Flemington, NJ 08822   (908)788-6535   Fax (908)788-6536

Mattel, Stephen F., MD {1336160019} Otlryg, SrgHdN(77,NY19)<NJ-STMRYPAS, NJ-CHILTON>
+ ENT & Allergy Associates, LLP
  1211 Hamburg Turnpike/Suite 205   Wayne, NJ 07470   (973)633-0808   Fax (973)633-8811

Matteo, Diana C., MD {1396066916} RadDia<NJ-COOPRUMC>
+ Cooper University Hospital
  One Cooper Plaza   Camden, NJ 08103   (856)356-4924   Fax (856)356-4793

Mattern, Richard F., MD {1376652073} RadDia(74,NY01)
+ Montclair Radiology
  116 Park Street   Montclair, NJ 07042   (973)746-2525   Fax (973)746-5802
+ Montclair Radiology
  1140 Bloomfield Avenue   West Caldwell, NJ 07006   (973)746-2525   Fax (973)439-6885
+ Montclair Radiology
  20 High Street   Nutley, NJ 07042   (973)284-1881   Fax (973)284-0269

Mattern Palisoc, Kathryn Elizabeth, DO {1750643714}
+ 262 Merritt Avenue/Apt 3
  Bergenfield, NJ 07621
  ktmattern@gmail.com

Matterson, Heideh H., MD {1912148040} NnPnMd<NY-NYUTISCH>
+ On-Site Neonatal Partners
  1000 Haddonfield-Berlin Road/Suite 210   Voorhees, NJ 08043   (856)782-2212   Fax (856)782-2213

Mattes, David G., MD {1336188473} FamMed, EmrgMd, IntrMd(83,ITA17)
+ Drs. Mattes & Collini
  181 High Street   Newton, NJ 07860   (973)383-9898   Fax (973)383-9665

Mattes, Jeffrey A., MD {1104823806} Psychy(72,PA02)
+ Psychopharmacology Research Association of Princeton
  601 Ewing Street/Suite A-12   Princeton, NJ 08540   (609)921-9299   Fax (609)921-1332

Matteson, James R., MD {1497726830} Urolgy(95,MD01)<NJ-HCKTSTWN, NJ-NWTNMEM>
+ Skylands Urology Group
  89 Sparta Avenue/Suite 200   Sparta, NJ 07871   (973)726-7220   Fax (973)726-7230
  jmatteson@skylandsurology.com
+ Skylands Urology Group
  616 Willow Grove Street   Hackettstown, NJ 07840   (973)726-7220   Fax (973)726-7230
+ Specialty Surgical Center
  380 Lafayette Road/Suite 110   Sparta, NJ 07871   (973)940-3166   Fax (973)940-3170

Matthai, William Henry, Jr., MD {1699702597} CdvDis, IntrMd, IntCrd(84,TN05)
+ Penn Cardiac Care Shore Medical Center
  1 East New York Avenue   Somers Point, NJ 08244

Matthews, Calvin C., MD {1376616367} SrgOrt(75,NJ06)<NJ-EASTORNG>
+ East Orange Family Health Center
  240 Central Avenue/Suite 3   East Orange, NJ 07018   (973)674-3500   Fax (973)674-6134
+ East Orange General Hospital
  300 Central Avenue/Orthopedics   East Orange, NJ 07018   (973)672-8400

Matthews, Gail Margaret, MD {1144243775} ObsGyn, MtFtMd, IntrMd(85,VA07)<NJ-VALLEY>
+ Maternal Fetal Medicine Associates
  140 East Ridgewood Avenue/Suite 390S   Paramus, NJ 07652   (201)291-6321   Fax (201)291-6318

Matthews, Jason D., MD {1841404787} Gastrn, IntrMd(00,NY01)
+ Hunterdon Gastroenterology Associates, P.A.
  1100 Wescott Drive/Suite 206-207   Flemington, NJ 08822   (908)483-4000   Fax (908)788-5090
+ Hunterdon Gastroenterology Associates, P.A.
  135 West End Avenue/Suite 204   Somerville, NJ 08876   (908)483-4000   Fax (908)788-5090

Matthews, Lawrence Milbourne, III, MD {1407264294} IntHos<NJ-COOPRUMC>
+ Cooper University Hospital
  One Cooper Plaza   Camden, NJ 08103   (856)342-2000

Matthews, Martha S., MD {1275615825} SrgPlstc(81,PA02)<NJ-COOPRUMC>
+ Cooper Surgical Associates
  3 Cooper Plaza/Suite 411   Camden, NJ 08103   (856)342-2270   Fax (856)365-1180
+ The Cooper Health System at Voorhees
  900 Centennial Boulevard/Suite F   Voorhees, NJ 08043   (856)325-6500
+ Cooper University Medical Center/Camden
  3 Cooper Plaza   Camden, NJ 08103   (856)342-2000

Matthews, Tara Anne, MD {1942226287} Pedtrc(99,GRN01)<NJ-CHLSMT>
+ Children's Specialized Hospital
  150 New Providence Road/Pediatrics   Mountainside, NJ 07092   (908)301-5491   Fax (908)301-5408

Matthews-Brown, Spring R., MD {1093746554} IntrMd(85,NJ05)<NJ-CHSMRCER>
+ Reliance Medical Group, LLC
  25 Scotch Road/Suite 29   Trenton, NJ 08628   (609)771-0404   Fax (609)538-8934

Mattie, James Kenneth, Jr, MD {1710158365}<NJ-MORRISTN>
+ Morristown Medical Center
  100 Madison Avenue   Morristown, NJ 07962   (973)971-5000

Mattina, Charles J., MD {1104890706} CdvDis, CritCr, IntrMd(81,NY19)<NJ-JRSYSHMC, NJ-CENTRAST>
+ Monmouth Cardiology Associates, LLC
  11 Meridian Road   Eatontown, NJ 07724   (732)663-0300   Fax (732)663-0301
+ Monmouth Cardiology Associates, LLC
  222 Schanck Road/Suite 104   Freehold, NJ 07728   (732)663-0300   Fax (732)431-1712

Mattoo, Anju, MD {1114987351} FamMed(88,INDI)
+ Atlantic Medical Group
  116 Millburn Avenue/Suites 105-106   Millburn, NJ 07041   (973)912-8400
+ Diagnostic & Clinical Cardiology
  449 Mount Pleasant Avenue/2nd Floor   West Orange, NJ 07052   (973)912-8400   Fax (973)731-7907

Mattoo, Deepali, MD {1962668145} Pedtrc(96,UKR12)
+ Oak Tree Pediatrics
  111 Park Avenue/2ns Floor   Plainfield, NJ 07060   (908)753-2671   Fax (908)753-1245

Mattox, Scott G., MD {1780685198} RadDia(91,PA13)
+ South Jersey Radiology Associates, P.A.
  748 Kings Highway   West Deptford, NJ 08096   (856)848-4998   Fax (856)853-7362
+ South Jersey Radiology Associates, P.A.
  Severan Profess Mews/Suite 105   Sewell, NJ 08080   (856)848-4998   Fax (856)589-6142
+ South Jersey Radiology Associates, P.A.
  100 Carnie Boulevard/Suite B-5   Voorhees, NJ 08096   (856)751-0123   Fax (856)751-0535

Matula, Joseph John, DO {1649219056} FamMed, EmrgMd(82,IL76)
+ Lockheed Martin Health & Wellness
  199 Borton Landing Road   Moorestown, NJ 08057   (856)733-3336

Matulewicz, Theodore Joseph, MD {1982693917} PthAcl(70,PA09)<NJ-JRSYSHMC>
+ Jersey Shore University Medical Center
  1945 Route 33/Pathology   Neptune, NJ 07753   (732)776-4144   Fax (732)776-4146
  tmatulewicz@meridianhealth.com

Matuozzi, William D., MD {1053391656} Radiol, RadDia(84,NY08)
+ Westfield Imaging Center
  118-122 Elm Street   Westfield, NJ 07090   (908)232-0610   Fax (908)232-7140

Matus, Victorino Managuit, MD {1376653063} Surgry(63,PHI10)
+ 424 Lakehurst Road
  Toms River, NJ 08755   (732)240-0066   Fax (732)240-1327

Matusow, Gary Alan, DO {1033154463} Gastrn, IntrMd(82,PA77)<NJ-SJRSYELM, NJ-MEMSALEM>
+ The Gastroenterology Group of South Jersey
  602 West Sherman Avenue   Vineland, NJ 08360   (856)691-1400   Fax (856)691-7117
+ The Gastroenterology Group of South Jersey
  979 North Blackhorse Pike   Williamstown, NJ 08094   (856)691-1400   Fax (856)691-7117
+ The Gastroenterology Group of South Jersey
  West Front Street/Med Arts Bld   Elmer, NJ 08360   (856)358-2600   Fax (856)691-7117

Matz, Paul Steven, MD {1811945173} Pedtrc(96,NY06)<NJ-VIRTVOOR>
+ Advocare Haddon Pediatric Group
  119 White Horse Pike   Haddon Heights, NJ 08035   (856)547-7300   Fax (856)547-4573

Maugeri, Joseph P., MD {1174578017} ObsGyn, IntrMd(89,NY09)
+ Skylands Medical Group PA
  33 Newton Sparta Road/Suite 6   Newton, NJ 07860   (973)579-3799   Fax (973)579-6859
+ Skylands Medical Group PA
  150 Lakeside Boulevard   Landing, NJ 07850   (973)579-3799   Fax (973)601-1647

Maulion, Christopher Dionisio, MD {1558622340}
+ 1183 Marisa Drive
  Toms River, NJ 08755   (732)773-8492
  cdm304@nyumc.org

Maurer, Kenneth H., MD {1508803727} Grtrcs, IntrMd, Rheuma(68,PA13)<NJ-VIRTUAHS, NJ-VIRTMHBC>
+ Arthritis, Rheumatic & Back Disease Associates
  2309 East Evesham Road/Suite 101   Voorhees, NJ 08043   (856)424-5005   Fax (856)424-4716

Maurer, Philip Mitchell, MD {1093759144} AnesPain, SrgOrt(85,PA02)
+ Aria 3B Orthopaedics, P.C.
  1400 East Route 70/Second Floor   Cherry Hill, NJ 08034

Mauriello, Richard M., DO {1023012952} FamMed(75,PA77)
+ Advocare Berlin Medical Associates
  175 Cross Keys Road/Suite 300A   Berlin, NJ 08009   (856)767-0077   Fax (856)767-6102

Maurizi, Romolo A., MD {1437109030} RadDia, Radiol(82,ITA17)
+ Hudson River Radiology
  547 Summit Avenue   Jersey City, NJ 07306   (201)656-5050   Fax (201)656-0689

Maurrasse, Corazon C., MD {1093785743} Anesth(69,PHI01)<NJ-NWRKBETH>
+ Newark Beth Israel Medical Center
  201 Lyons Avenue/Anesth   Newark, NJ 07112   (973)926-7000   Fax (201)943-8105

Mauti, Joseph M., MD {1609834522} IntrMd(72,ITA17)
+ 1020 Galloping Hill Road
  Union, NJ 07083   (908)964-3700   Fax (908)964-9580

Mautner, Gail H., MD {1053353680} Dermat(91,NY19)<NJ-ST-BARNMC>
+ Millburn Laser Center
  12 East Willow Street   Millburn, NJ 07041   (973)376-8500   Fax (973)376-1820
  gail.mautner@millburnsurgical.com

Mautone, Susan G., MD {1942352448} Pedtrc(78,NJ05)<NJ-UMDNJ>
+ University Hospital
  150 Bergen Street/Pediatrics   Newark, NJ 07103   (973)972-4300   Fax (973)972-7597

Mavani, Bharti N., MD {1124069018} ObsGyn(70,INA74)<NJ-JFKMED, NJ-RWJURAH>
+ Kirit Somabhai Patel, MD PC
  34-36 Progress Street/Suite A-6   Edison, NJ 08820   (908)757-9555   Fax (908)757-2312

Mavani, Nagindas V., MD {1174594066} IntrMd, CdvDis(68,INA33)<NJ-JFKMED, NJ-RWJURAH>
+ Roosevelt Medical
  237 Roosevelt Avenue   Carteret, NJ 07008   (732)541-2141   Fax (732)541-1083
+ 688 Grove Avenue
  Edison, NJ 08820   (732)549-3227

Mavani, Yogini, DO {1326233040} PhysMd(02,NY75)
+ 50 Harrison Street/Suite 212F
  Hoboken, NJ 07030   (201)484-8950   Fax (201)484-8952

Mavasheva, Sofia, MD {1851345995} IntrMd(88,UZB44)<NJ-CHSFULD>
+ Hamilton Internal Medicine Associates
  2055 Klockner Road   Trenton, NJ 08690   (609)586-8060   Fax (609)586-7470

Maximos, Maryann, DO {1942405659}
+ 703 Main Street
  Paterson, NJ 07503   (973)754-2000

Maxwell, Aliona, MD {1841503893} ObsGyn
+ Woman to Woman Obstetrics & Gynecology
  615 Main Street   Toms River, NJ 08753   (732)797-1510   Fax (732)797-2370
  aliona@comcast.net

Physicians by Name and Address

Maxym, Maya, MD {1356531636} Pedtrc<NJ-STBARNMC>
+ St. Barnabas Medical Center
94 Old Short Hills Road   Livingston, NJ 07039   (973)322-5000

May, David Peter, MD {1790786135} Surgry(96,PA13)
+ Shore Physicians Group
2605 Shore Road   Northfield, NJ 08225   (609)365-5300
Fax (609)365-5305

May, Micah Moshe, MD {1487698197} IntrMd(96,PA09)
+ 1100 State Highway North 70
Whiting, NJ 08759   (732)350-0070   Fax (732)350-4439

May, Michael S., MD {1508929175} Pthlgy, PthAcl, PthCyt(83,ISR02)<NJ-TRINIWSC>
+ RWJ University Hospital New Brunswick
One Robert Wood Johnson Place   New Brunswick, NJ 08901
(732)828-3000   Fax (732)235-8124
+ RWJ University Pathology
125 Paterson Street/MEB 212   New Brunswick, NJ 08901
(732)828-3000   Fax (732)418-8445

May, Philip B., MD {1932136892} IntrMd(70,NC01)
+ Hunterdon Developmental Center
40 Pittstown Road/PO Box 4003   Clinton, NJ 08809
(908)735-4031   Fax (908)730-1338

May, Richard Edward, Jr., MD {1073879896} PulDis
+ University Hospital Medicine
150 Bergen Street/Room I-248/Medicine   Newark, NJ 07103   (973)972-6056   Fax (973)972-3129

May, Roberta Russell, DO {1508827379} EmrgMd(98,PA77)<NJ-SHOREMEM>
+ Bayfront Emergency Physicians, P.A.
1 East New York Avenue   Somers Point, NJ 08244
(609)653-3519   Fax (609)653-3247

May-Ortiz, Jennifer L., MD {1316939168} FamMed, IntrMd(00,NY20)
+ Medical Diagnostic Associates, P.A.
MAC, 11 Overlook Road/Suite 100   Summit, NJ 07901
(908)273-1493   Fax (908)273-3125

Maye, Jessica Megan, DO {1629495544} EmrgMd
+ Cooper Univerisry Emergency Physicians
One Cooper Plaza   Camden, NJ 08103   (856)342-2384
Fax (856)968-8272

Mayer, Catharine Carbonetta, MD {1164553426} FamMSptM(95,PA12)
+ Aria 3B Orthopaedics, P.C.
1400 East Route 70/Second Floor   Cherry Hill, NJ 08034

Mayer, Diana R., MD {1770507238} Pedtrc(88,IL42)<NJ-CENTRAST, NJ-JRSYSHMC>
+ Pediatric Health, P.A.
470 Stillwells Corner Road   Freehold, NJ 07728   (732)780-3333   Fax (732)780-6968
+ Pediatric Health, P.A.
69 West Main Street   Freehold, NJ 07728   (732)780-3333   Fax (732)409-7133
+ Pediatric Health, PA
23 Kilmer Drive/Building 1 Suite B   Morganville, NJ 07728   (732)972-0900   Fax (732)972-2892

Mayer, Douglas John, MD {1710906714} EmrgMd(01,DMN01)<NJ-VIRTBERL, NJ-VIRTMHBC>
+ Team Health East
307 South Evergeen Avenue   Woodbury, NJ 08096
(856)686-4319   Fax (856)848-8536
+ SJ Emergency Physician, PA
175 Madison Avenue   Mount Holly, NJ 08060   (856)686-4319   Fax (609)914-6067

Mayer, Marc, DO {1720083132} FamMed(83,IL76)
+ Avenel Iselin Medical Group
400 Gill Lane   Iselin, NJ 08830   (732)404-1580   Fax (732)404-1594

Mayer, Martin P., MD {1831252006} PsyGrt, Psychy(72,NY46)<NJ-RWJURAH>
+ 1503 Saint Georges Avenue
Colonia, NJ 07067   (732)382-1300   Fax (732)382-6923

Mayer, Michael B., MD {1093736878} Otlryg, IntrMd(90,NY46)
+ Summit Medical Group
574 Springfield Avenue   Westfield, NJ 07090   (908)673-7251   Fax (908)673-7265
mmayer@smgnj.com
+ Westfield Ear Nose & Throat Surgical Associates
213 Summit Avenue/Suite 1   Mountainside, NJ 07092
(908)673-7251   Fax (908)233-5776

Mayer, Michelle Saltiel, MD {1962445700} Pedtrc(01,NY08)
+ Chestnut Ridge Pediatrics
595 Chestnut Ridge Road   Woodcliff Lake, NJ 07677
(201)391-2020   Fax (201)391-0265

Mayer, Mitchell F., DO {1639173008} FamMed(85,IL76)
+ Avenel Iselin Medical Group
400 Gill Lane   Iselin, NJ 08830   (732)404-1580   Fax (732)404-1594

Mayer, Oscar Henry, MD {1417970450} PedPul, Pedtrc(95,PA12)<PA-CHILDHOS>
+ CHOP Pediatric & Adolescent Specialty Care Center
1012 Laurel Oak Road   Voorhees, NJ 08043   (856)435-1300
Fax (856)435-0091
+ CHOP Specialty Care Center at Virtua
200 Bowman Drive/2 FL/Suite D-260   Voorhees, NJ 08043
(267)425-5400

Mayer, Tina Marie, MD {1598931420} MedOnc(03,NY20)
+ Rutgers Cancer Institute of New Jersey
195 Little Albany Street/PO Box 2681   New Brunswick, NJ 08903   (732)235-6777   Fax (732)235-2465

Mayerhoff, David I., MD {1861568834} Psychy(83,NY08)<NJ-ESSEXCO, NJ-UMDNJ>
+ Essex County Hospital Center
204 Grove Avenue   Cedar Grove, NJ 07009   (973)571-2800

Maymind, Elina, MD {1538459623}
+ University Hospital-SOM Department of Psychiatry
2250 Chapel Avenue West/Suite 100   Cherry Hill, NJ 08002
(856)482-9000   Fax (856)482-1159

Mayor, Gilbert H., MD {1063653210} IntrMd, Nephro, EnDbMt(65,MI07)
+ Mayor Group
53 School House Lane   Morristown, NJ 07960   (973)206-1936   Fax (973)998-7995

Mayoral, Jorge L., MD {1992798813} PhysMd(81,PRO02)<NJ-LIBERTY, NJ-JRSYCITY>
+ Associates in Rehabilitation Medicine
95 Mount Kemble Avenue   Morristown, NJ 07960
(973)267-2293   Fax (973)226-3144

Mayorga, Mabel, MD {1295115277} EnDbMt
+ The Cooper Hospital System-Univ Hospital
401 Haddon Avenue   Camden, NJ 08103   (856)342-2000
Fax (856)342-2000

Mayorquin, Bertha, MD {1053643361} FamMed
+ 325 Montgomery Street
Jersey City, NJ 07302

Mayrowetz, Burton, MD {1891730354} IntrMd(70,NJ05)<NJ-COMMED>
+ Drs. Mitra & Mayrowetz
368 Lakehurst Road/Suite 207   Toms River, NJ 08755
(732)557-6222   Fax (732)557-6227
bmayrowetz@verizon.net

Mayrowetz, Stanley, MD {1184711400} IntrMd(65,PA09)<NJ-MTNSIDE, NJ-STBARNMC>
+ 8 Brookside Avenue
Caldwell, NJ 07006   (973)228-3333   Fax (973)228-9023

Mays Stovall, Latisse M., MD {1134305667} EmrgEMed
+ 26 McGuire Drive
West Orange, NJ 07052

Mayson, Robert P., MD {1104852219} ObsGyn(83,LIBE)<NJ-CENTRAST, NJ-RWJUHAM>
+ Hamilton OB/GYN Associates @ East Windsor
901 West Main Street/Suite 107   Freehold, NJ 07728
(609)426-0900   Fax (609)426-9014
rpmayson550@aol.com
+ Robert Wood Johnson University Hospital at Hamilton
1 Hamilton Health Place/OB/GYN   Hamilton, NJ 08690
(609)586-7900

Maza, Lauren M., MD {1730150996} IntrMd(93,NY15)<NJ-JFKMED, NJ-RBAYOLDB>
+ Woodbridge Internal Medicine Associates
1000 Route 9 North/Suite 302   Woodbridge, NJ 07095
(732)634-0036   Fax (732)634-9182

Maza, Sharon R., MD {1164507919} CdvDis, IntrMd(81,NY19)
+ 83 Summit Avenue/Rear Suite
Hackensack, NJ 07601   (201)488-1320   Fax (201)488-1596

Mazhar, Noorain, MD {1437538584} IntrMd
+ Capital Health Hospitalist Group
750 Brunswick Avenue   Trenton, NJ 08638   (609)394-6031
Fax (609)394-6299

Maziarz, Anastazja, MD {1629348784} FamMed(09,POL12)
+ Franklin Family Practice PA
29 Clyde Road/Suite 101   Somerset, NJ 08873   (732)873-0330   Fax (732)873-2077
+ RWJPE Primary Care Center at Hillsborough
331 Route 206 North/Suite 2-B   Hillsborough, NJ 08844
(732)873-0330   Fax (908)359-7109

Mazpule, George A., MD {1720306400}
+ 34 John Street/Apt 3c
Bloomfield, NJ 07003   (201)321-4973
george.mazpule@gmail.com

Mazur, Irene, MD {1346405727} PsyCAd(92,UKR28)
+ 17 Molsbury Lane
Millstone Township, NJ 08510   (732)609-0157   Fax (609)259-1592

Mazur, Kimberly L., MD {1649200106} IntrMd(90,NJ05)<NJ-ACMCITY, NJ-ACMCMAIN>
+ AtlantiCare Ambulatory Internal Medicine Clinic
1401 Atlantic Avenue   Atlantic City, NJ 08401   (609)441-8036   Fax (609)572-6021

Mazur, Wieslaw L., MD {1164583175} Anesth(81,POLA)<NJ-STBARNMC>
+ St. Barnabas Medical Center
94 Old Short Hills Road   Livingston, NJ 07039   (973)322-5000

Mazur, Yuri, MD {1255380879} PsyGrt, Psychy(91,UKR01)<NJ-UNIVBHC>
+ University Behavioral Health Care
667 Hoes Lane/Box 1392/Psych   Piscataway, NJ 08854

Mazza, Emilio, MD {1184663239} IntrMd, PulCCr, PulDis(00,NJ06)
+ Virtua Garden State Pulmonary Associates
520 Lippincott Drive/Suite A   Marlton, NJ 08053   (856)596-9057   Fax (856)596-0837

Mazza, Victor Joseph, MD {1841358066} IntrMd(03,GRN01)
+ 240 Cleveland Avenue
Hasbrouck Heights, NJ 07604

Mazzara, Carl Arthur, MD {1174527543} Otlryg(88,NY47)<NJ-BAYSHORE>
+ ENT & Allergy Associates, LLP
485 Route 1 South/Bld B/Suite 350   Iselin, NJ 08830
(732)549-3934   Fax (732)549-7250

Mazzarelli, Anthony Joseph, MD {1033139407} EmrgMd(02,NJ06)<NJ-COOPRUMC>
+ Cooper University Hospital
One Cooper Plaza/EmrgMed   Camden, NJ 08103
(856)342-2000

Mazzarelli, Joanne K., MD {1255495495} IntrMd<NJ-COOPRUMC>
+ Cooper University Hospital
One Cooper Plaza/Drrnce/RmD380   Camden, NJ 08103
(856)342-2000

Mazzei, Elizabeth O'Connell, MD {1902899776} Radiol, RadDia(76,NY09)
+ Bergen Imaging Center
180 North Dean Street   Englewood, NJ 07631   (201)568-4242   Fax (201)568-1298

Mazzella, Carmine A., DO {1326108879} FamMed(92,NY75)<NJ-MTNSIDE>
+ Town Medical Associates/Verona
271 Grove Avenue/Suite A   Verona, NJ 07044   (973)239-2600   Fax (973)239-0482

Mazzella, Fermina Maria, MD {1275522344} PthAna, PthAcl(88,DMN01)<NJ-UMDNJ>
+ University Hospital
150 Bergen Street/Room C-102   Newark, NJ 07103
(973)972-4619   Fax (973)972-3199

Mazziotta, Robert M., MD {1679635007} PthAcl(00,NJ05)<NJ-VALLEY>
+ The Valley Hospital
223 North Van Dien Avenue/Pathology   Ridgewood, NJ 07450   (201)447-8000

Mazziotti, Alexander R., MD {1902996283} IntrMd(78,NJ05)<NJ-VALLEY>
+ 268 Lincoln Avenue
Hawthorne, NJ 07506   (973)423-3335

Mazzocchi, Dominic F., MD {1679546501} IntrMd(81,PRO03)<NJ-OCEANMC>
+ 1401 Beaver Dam Road
Point Pleasant Beach, NJ 08742   (732)295-0808   Fax (732)295-3845
+ Coastal Care Associates
608 Union Avenue   Brielle, NJ 08730   (732)295-0808   Fax (732)528-1245

Mazzoccoli, Vito, MD {1518936053} FamMed, Surgry(87,ITA21)<NJ-STBARNMC, NJ-CLARMAAS>
+ Premier Family Medical, PC
73 Bloomfield Avenue   Caldwell, NJ 07006   (973)403-3200
Fax (973)403-3250
vtmazz@yahoo.com

Mazzochette, John A., MD {1972668358} Psychy(81,DOM03)<NJ-ANCPSYCH>
+ Ancora Psychiatric Hospital
301 Spring Garden Road   Hammonton, NJ 08037
(609)561-1700

Mazzola, Catherine A., MD {1295792380} SrgNro(94,NJ05)<NJ-HACKNSK, NJ-MORRISTN>
+ New Jersey Pediatric Neurosurgical Associates
131 Madison Avenue/Suite 140   Morristown, NJ 07960
(973)326-9000   Fax (973)326-9001
+ New Jersey Pediatric Neurosurgical Associates
385 Prospect Avenue/2nd Floor   Hackensack, NJ 07601
(973)326-9000   Fax (201)996-9301

Mazzone, Jeanae, DO {1871532358} ObsGyn(94,NY75)<NJ-CHILTON>
+ Wayne Surgical Center, LLC.
1176 Hamburg Pike   Wayne, NJ 07470   (973)709-1900
Fax (973)709-1901

Mazzoni, Thomas F., DO {1629192463} OtgyFPlS, OtgyPSHN, OtgyAlgy(02,NJ75)<NJ-STBARNMC, NJ-BAYONNE>
+ Associated Ear Nose & Throat Physicians
505 Chestnut Street   Roselle Park, NJ 07204   (908)241-0200   Fax (908)241-0445
+ Associated Ear Nose & Throat Physicians
778 Kennedy Boulevard   Bayonne, NJ 07002   (908)241-0200   Fax (201)829-1821

Physicians by Name and Address

Mazzuca, Douglas E., DO {1033109848} Ophthl(83,PA77)<NJ-MEMSALEM>
+ Mazzuca Eye and Laser Centers
48 North Broadway   Pennsville, NJ 08070   (856)678-4800   Fax (856)678-3630
+ Mazzuca Eye and Laser Centers
20 Village Center Drive   Swedesboro, NJ 08085   (856)241-8900

Mazzuca, Robert F., DO {1831163237} FamMed(80,PA77)<NJ-VIRTBERL, NJ-VIRTVOOR>
+ 501 Fifth Street/Suite A
Atco, NJ 08004   (856)768-2758   Fax (856)768-8364

Mbachu, Yvonne, MD {1578925962} EmrgMd
+ Cooper Univerisry Emergency Physicians
One Cooper Plaza   Camden, NJ 08103   (856)342-2627   Fax (856)968-8272

Mbianda, Julvet Chepngum, MD {1609398999}<NJ-STFRNMED>
+ St. Francis Medical Center
601 Hamilton Avenue   Trenton, NJ 08629   (601)599-5061

McAbee, Gary Noel, DO {1437232469} NroChl, Pedtrc(80,IA75)<NJ-KMHCHRRY, NJ-COOPRUMC>
+ Cooper Peds/Children's Regional Ctr
3 Cooper Plaza/Suite 200   Camden, NJ 08103   (856)342-2472   Fax (856)368-8297
+ The Children's Regional Hospital at Cooper Univ Hosp
One Cooper Plaza   Camden, NJ 08103   (856)342-2000

McAdam, Kimberly S., DO {1821011784} FamMed, IntrMd(98,NY75)
+ Brigantine Medical Group
353 12th Street South/PO Box 129   Brigantine, NJ 08203   (609)266-7557   Fax (609)266-4450

McAfee, Jacob Seth, MD {1245492735} Otlryg(OH45)
+ Coastal Ear Nose and Throat LLC
1301 Route 72/Suite 340   Manahawkin, NJ 08050   (732)280-7855   Fax (732)280-7815

McAlarney, Lourdes Rupac, MD {1447309059} IntrMd, Grtrcs(91,PHI08)<NJ-JRSYSHMC>
+ 117 Beagle Drive
Manalapan, NJ 07726

McAlarney, Terence, MD {1184773707} Nrolgy(88,FL02)<NJ-CENTRAST>
+ 901 West Main Street/Suite 101
Freehold, NJ 07728   (732)625-8460

McAllister, John Daniel, II, MD {1609877026} RadDia
+ Cape Radiology
4011 Route 9 South/PO Box 244   Rio Grande, NJ 08242   (609)886-0100

McAllister, Michael R., DO {1427048370} Psychy, PsyFor(77,MO78)
+ Hudson County Correctional Center
35 Hackensack Avenue/Psych   Kearny, NJ 07032   (201)395-5600

McAllister, Susan Coutinho, MD {1932120375} IntrMd(03,NJ06)
+ 1040 Stokes Avenue
Collingswood, NJ 08108

McAlpin, Fred, III, DO {1396812632} SprtMd, SrgOrt(93,PA77)<NJ-SJHREGMC, NJ-SJRSYELM>
+ Premier Orthopaedic Associates
298 South Delsea Drive   Vineland, NJ 08360   (856)690-1616   Fax (856)690-1089
+ Premier Orthopaedic Assocs of So NJ
201 Tomlin Station Road/Suite C   Mullica Hill, NJ 08062   (856)690-1616   Fax (856)223-9110

McAnally, James F., MD {1659345395} IntrMd, Nephro(75,NJ05)<NJ-TRINIWSC>
+ 240 Williamson Street/Suite 307
Elizabeth, NJ 07202   (908)994-9200   Fax (908)994-9209

McArthur, Kelly M., DO {1689836926}<NJ-MEADWLND>
+ Meadowlands Hospital Medical Center
55 Meadowlands Parkway   Secaucus, NJ 07096   (201)392-3100

McArthur, Lucas James, MD {1013150077} FamMed
+ 256 Second Avenue
Garwood, NJ 07027   (732)321-7487

McArthur, Marilyn D., MD {1609806181} ObsGyn(76,MA07)<NJ-STBARNMC>
+ Marilyn McArthur MD P.A.
349 East Northfield Road/Suite 212   Livingston, NJ 07039   (973)758-9311   Fax (973)758-1430   Macdoc177@verizon.net

McAuliffe, Vincent J., MD {1306918693} IntrMd, InfDis(73,NY01)
+ Rutgers RWJ Allergy, Immunology and Infectious Group
125 Paterson Street   New Brunswick, NJ 08901   (732)235-7060

McBrearty-Hindson, Ashley, DO {1467894691} IntHos<NJ-ACMCITY>
+ AtlantiCare Regional Medical Center/City Campus
1925 Pacific Avenue   Atlantic City, NJ 08401   (609)345-4000

McBride, Mark J., MD {1609967710} SrgHnd, SrgOrt(80,DC02)<NJ-MORRISTN>
+ Tri-County Orthopedics
160 East Hanover Avenue   Morristown, NJ 07962   (973)538-2334   Fax (973)829-9174

McCabe, Evin Joseph, MD {1710934187} Gastrn, IntrMd(01,NY48)<NY-BETHPETR>
+ Center for Endocrine Health
1121 route 22 west/Suite 205   Bridgewater, NJ 08807   (212)734-8874   Fax (212)249-5628

McCabe, James, III, MD {1790724359} EmrgMd(88,PA02)<NJ-KMHTURNV>
+ Kennedy Health Systems/Washington Township Campus
435 Hurffville-Cross Keys Road   Turnersville, NJ 08012   (856)582-2500   Fax (856)488-6511

McCabe, Johnathan B., MD {1760722489} CdvDis, IntrMd(81,NY46)<NJ-UNVMCPRN>
+ Cardiology Associates of Princeton, P.A.
731 Alexander Road/Suite 202   Princeton, NJ 08540   (609)921-7456   Fax (609)921-2972

McCabe-Bageac, Mary A., MD {1669672283} EmrgMd(88,NY48)<NJ-MONMOUTH>
+ Monmouth Medical Center
300 Second Avenue/EmergMed   Long Branch, NJ 07740   (732)222-5200

McCagg, Caroline O., MD {1346261849} PhysMd(66,CT01)<NJ-JFKJHNSN>
+ JFK Johnson Rehabilitation Institute
65 James Street   Edison, NJ 08818   (732)321-7050   Fax (732)321-7330

McCaig, Misty, MD {1194947663} Pedtrc<NJ-STPETER>
+ St. Peter's University Hospital
254 Easton Avenue   New Brunswick, NJ 08901   (732)745-8600   Fax (732)745-1579

McCain, Donald Andrew, MD {1295801157} Surgry, SrgOnc(91,NY46)<NJ-HACKNSK, NJ-HOLYNAME>
+ Cancer Surgery Associates
20 Prospect Avenue/Suite 603   Hackensack, NJ 07601   (201)342-1010   Fax (201)342-1030

McCans, Kathryn M., MD {1851474886} Pedtrc, PedEmg(91,PA13)<NJ-COOPRUMC>
+ Cooper University Hospital
One Cooper Plaza/Emerg Medicine   Camden, NJ 08103   (856)342-2000

McCarrick, Thomas P., MD {1457411092} FamMed, Grtrcs(82,NY19)<NJ-MTNSIDE, NJ-STBARNMC>
+ Town Medical Associates/Verona
271 Grove Avenue/Suite A   Verona, NJ 07044   (973)239-2600   Fax (973)239-0482

McCarthy, Christopher M., MD {1942421458} EmrgMd, SrgOrt, IntrMd(04,NJ05)
+ Robert Wood Johnson Emergency Medicine
One Robert Wood Johnson Place/MEB 104   New Brunswick, NJ 08901   (732)235-7869

McCarthy, Cornelius Stephen, MD {1801823554} RadDia, RadV&I(89,PA01)<NJ-STBARNMC>
+ St. Barnabas Medical Center
94 Old Short Hills Road   Livingston, NJ 07039   (973)322-5000

McCay, Marissa, MD {1972922441} Pedtrc<NJ-VIRTVOOR>
+ Virtua Voorhees
100 Bowman Drive   Voorhees, NJ 08043   (856)325-3000   Fax (609)261-5842

McClane, Steven J., MD {1770594038}
+ 243 Jefferson Avenue
Haddonfield, NJ 08033   (856)968-8570   Fax (856)365-1180   mcclane-steven@cooperhealth.edu

McCleery, Colleen Marie, MD {1245201391} ObsGyn(95,NJ06)
+ Fox Chase Virtua Health Cancer Center
106 Carnie Boulevard/Suite A   Voorhees, NJ 08043   (856)325-4830   colleenmc1@comcast.net

McCloskey, John R., MD {1881607489} SrgOrt, IntrMd(70,PA02)<PA-CHILDHOS>
+ Shore Orthopedic University Associates
24 Macarthur Boulevard/First Floor   Somers Point, NJ 08244   (609)927-1991   Fax (609)927-4203
+ Shore Orthopedic University Associates
18 East Jimmie Leeds Road   Galloway, NJ 08205   (609)927-1991   Fax (609)927-4203
+ Shore Orthopedic University Associates
9 Stites Avenue   Cape May Court House, NJ 08244   (609)927-1991   Fax (609)927-4203

McCloskey, Ryan C., DO {1467715417}<NJ-STJOSHOS>
+ St. Joseph's Regional Medical Center
703 Main Street   Paterson, NJ 07503   (585)278-3724

McClure, A. Gregory, MD LeglMd, OccpMd(72,PA12)
+ South Jersey Physicians Associates
327 Haddon Avenue   Westmont, NJ 08108   (856)869-0009   Fax (856)869-0008

McCluskey, Tamara B., DO {1801992318} Pedtrc(88,MO79)<NJ-MORRISTN>
+ Morristown Pediatric Associates, LLC
261 James Street/Suite 1-G   Morristown, NJ 07960

(973)540-9393   Fax (973)540-1937

McCoach, Kevin J., MD {1366444002} CdvDis, IntrMd(82,GRN01)
+ Essex Heart Group LLC
1310 Broad Street   Bloomfield, NJ 07003   (973)338-0800   Fax (973)338-1140

McCollum, Brendan Patrick, MD {1942602123} Psychy<NJ-TRININPC>
+ Trinitas Regional Medical Center-New Point Campus
655 East Jersey Street   Elizabeth, NJ 07206   (908)994-7552
+ 19 Holly Street/2nd floor
Cranford, NJ 07016   (908)543-7593

McComb, David Robert, DO {1326018433} Psychy, PsyGrt(98,NJ75)<NJ-VIRTUAHS>
+ 109 West Maple Avenue
Merchantville, NJ 08109   (609)953-5517   Fax (609)953-1135

McConlogue, Joelle Jugant, MD {1861406969} Pedtrc(97,NY01)
+ Princeton Nassau Pediatrics, P.A.
301 North Harrison Street   Princeton, NJ 08540   (609)924-5510   Fax (609)924-3577

McConnell, John C., MD {1154317063} SrgC&R, Surgry(74,NY01)<NJ-VALLEY, NJ-CHILTON>
+ North Jersey Colon & Rectal Surgery Associates, LLC.
191 Hamburg Turnpike   Pompton Lakes, NJ 07442   (973)839-3111   Fax (973)839-2301

McConnell, Julie, MD {1801927199} FamMed(00,FL02)
+ Bergen Medical Associates
466 Old Hook Road/Suite 1   Emerson, NJ 07630   (201)967-8221   Fax (201)634-9647

McCormack, Denise Elizabeth, MD {1225203193} EmrgMd
+ UMDNJ Emergency Medicine
185 South Orange Avenue   Newark, NJ 07103   (347)277-3869

McCormack, Patricia Coppola, MD {1891887543} Dermat(81,NJ06)
+ 822 North Wood Avenue
Linden, NJ 07036   (908)925-8877   info@patriciamccormackmd.com

McCormick, John F., MD {1407863731} PthAcl(70,PA02)<NJ-ACMCITY>
+ AtlantiCare Regional Medical Center/City Campus
1925 Pacific Avenue/Path   Atlantic City, NJ 08401   (609)441-8063

McCormick, John Stuart, MD {1780621813} Radiol, RadDia, Rad-Nuc(91,NY46)<NJ-OVERLOOK, NJ-MORRISTN>
+ Summit Medical Group-Berkeley Heights Campus
1 Diamond Hill Road   Berkeley Heights, NJ 07922   (908)273-4300   Fax (908)790-6524

McCormick, Ryan Charles, MD {1679553861} FamMed(01,NJ05)
+ Partners in Primary Care
534 Lippincott Drive   Marlton, NJ 08053   (856)985-7373   Fax (856)985-9611

McCoy, Chrishonda Curry, MD {1336367119} Ophthl
+ Healthcheck Medical and Eye Center
40 Union Avenue   Irvington, NJ 07111   (973)399-6270

McCoy, Jonathan V., MD {1255351318} EmrgMd<NJ-RWJUBRUN>
+ University Emergency Medicine
125 Paterson Street/MEB 104   New Brunswick, NJ 08901   (732)235-8717   Fax (732)235-7379

McCoy, Lynn, DO {1275706202} EmrgMd(04,NJ75)<NJ-RWJURAH, NJ-TRINIWSC>
+ Trinitas Regional Medical Center-Williamson Street
225 Williamson Street   Elizabeth, NJ 07207   (908)994-5000

McCoy, Susan N., MD {1942362504} Gyneco(74,AL02)<NJ-UNVMCPRN>
+ 601 Ewing Street/Suite C-13
Princeton, NJ 08540   (609)924-6899   Fax (609)924-5759

McCracken, Kevin A., MD {1013944586} SrgOrt, SrgSpn(91,NJ05)
+ Orthopaedic & Spine Institute
45 Mountain Boulevard   Warren, NJ 07059   (908)822-9282   Fax (908)822-9201

McCrosson, Stacy A., MD {1104856251} ObsGyn(92,PA09)<NJ-VIRTVOOR>
+ Cherry Hill Ob/Gyn
150 Century Parkway/Suite A   Mount Laurel, NJ 08054   (856)778-4700   Fax (856)778-1154
+ Cherry Hill Ob/Gyn
777 South White Horse Pike/Suite A-1   Hammonton, NJ 08037   (856)778-4700   Fax (609)561-6309

McCullen, Kristen Michelle, MD {1699981811} Obstet
+ Cherry Hill Ob/Gyn
150 Century Parkway/Suite A   Mount Laurel, NJ 08054   (856)778-4700   Fax (856)778-1154
+ Cherry Hill Ob/Gyn
777 South White Horse Pike/Suite A-1   Hammonton, NJ 08037   (856)778-4700   Fax (609)561-6309

McCullough, Aubrey Susan, DO {1386088995} Otlryg
+ Becker ENT
One Union Street/Suite 203   Robbinsville, NJ 08691   (609)436-5740   Fax (609)436-5741

McDaid, Kevin C., MD {1902004229} SrgOrt(04,PA02)<NJ-MORRISTN>
+ Seaview Orthopaedics
1200 Eagle Avenue   Ocean, NJ 07712   (732)660-6200   Fax (732)660-6201

McDermet, Arthur J., DO {1578542965} FamMed(90,PA77)
+ Virtua Family Medicine - Cooper River
6981 North Park Drive/Suite 200   Pennsauken, NJ 08109   (856)663-4949   Fax (856)663-6076

McDermott, James David, MD {1194079467}
+ 1500 Washington Street/Apt 3 J
Hoboken, NJ 07030   (719)649-4662

McDermott, James P., DO {1255389185} ObsGyn(94,NY75)
+ Ocean Women's Health Care Group
602 Route 72 East/Suite 1   Manahawkin, NJ 08050   (609)978-9870   Fax (609)978-9873

McDermott, Janette H., MD {1942204904} Onclgy, SrgOnc, Surgry(88,NY01)<NJ-STPETER>
+ Somerset Medical Associates
1553 Highway 27/Suite 3100   Somerset, NJ 08873   (732)846-3300   Fax (732)846-3323
+ Cares Surgicenter, LLC.
240 Easton Avenue   New Brunswick, NJ 08901   (732)846-3300   Fax (732)296-8677

McDermott, John P., DO {1386663854} FamMed(89,FL75)<NY-STANTHNY>
+ EmCare
1945 Route 33   Neptune, NJ 07753   (732)776-4510   Fax (732)776-2329

McDermott, Rena, MD {1154508927} IntrMd(05,NY09)
+ ID Associates PA/dba ID Care
105 Raider Boulevard/Suite 101   Hillsborough, NJ 08844   (908)281-0221   Fax (908)281-0940
+ ID Associates PA/dba ID Care
81 Veronica Avenue/Suite 203   Somerset, NJ 08873   (908)281-0221   Fax (732)729-0924

McDevitt, Barbara Ellen, MD {1023034147} Pedtrc, PedEmg, EmrgMd(84,NJ05)<NJ-CHDNWBTH, NJ-MORRISTN>
+ Children's Hospital of New Jersey
201 Lyons Avenue/Osborne Terrace   Newark, NJ 07112   (973)926-7337
bmcdevitt@sbhcs.org
+ Morristown Medical Center
100 Madison Avenue/EmrgMed   Morristown, NJ 07962   (973)971-5000

McDonald, David William, MD {1619167269} Radiol, RadDia, PedRad(02,OH44)<NJ-SPCLMONM, NJ-MONMOUTH>
+ Specialty Hospital at Monmouth
300 Second Avenue/Greenwall 6   Long Branch, NJ 07740   (732)923-5037
+ Monmouth Medical Center
300 Second Avenue/Radiology   Long Branch, NJ 07740   (732)923-5037   Fax (732)923-6006

McDonald, Kathleen L., MD {1346246048} RadDia, NuclMd, RadNuc(76,NJ05)<NJ-RWJUHAM>
+ Quakerbridge Radiology Associates
8 Quakerbridge Plaza/Building 8   Mercerville, NJ 08619   (609)890-0033   Fax (609)689-6067

McDonnell, Elizabeth Lynn, MD {1124036496} ObsGyn(90,MD12)
+ Capital Health System/Hopewell
One Capital Way   Pennington, NJ 08534   (215)915-3559

McDonnell, Matthew, MD {1770785883} SrgOrt
+ University Orthopaedic Associates, LLC.
211 North Harrison Street   Princeton, NJ 08540   (609)683-7800   Fax (609)683-7875
+ University Orthopaedic Associates, LLC.
4810 Belmar Boulevard/Suite 102   Wall, NJ 07753   (609)683-7800   Fax (732)938-5680
+ University Orthopaedic Associates, LLC.
Two Worlds Fair Drive   Somerset, NJ 08540   (732)979-2115   Fax (732)564-9032

McDonnell, Thomas E., MD {1265415129} Anesth(78,IL06)<NJ-MORRISTN>
+ Anesthesia Associates
100 Madison Avenue   Morristown, NJ 07960   (973)971-5548   Fax (973)631-8120

McDonough, Christian P., MD {1194925644} PedCrC(02,GRN01)
+ Robert Wood Johnson-UMDNJ Anesthesia Group
125 Paterson Street/CAB 3100   New Brunswick, NJ 08901   (732)235-7827   Fax (732)235-6131

McDonough, John R., MD {1942285549} FamMed(90,NJ05)<NJ-HUNTRDN>
+ Family Physicians-Hunterdon
2 Kings Court/Suite 203   Flemington, NJ 08822   (908)788-7846   Fax (908)806-6027

McDonough, Kevin J., MD {1518073337} Pedtrc(92,IREL)<NY-CMCSTVSI>
+ City Heights Pediatrics
511 22nd Street   Union City, NJ 07087   (201)866-7740   Fax (201)223-1905

McElroy, Kevin M., DO {1013228386} PhyMPain, IntrMd(05,NJ75)
+ Progressive Spine & Sports Medicine
48 South Franklin Turnpike/Suite 101   Ramsey, NJ 07446   (201)962-9199   Fax (201)962-9198
info@progressivespineandsports.com

McEnrue, James A., MD {1609895465} EmrgMd, IntrMd(75,DC02)<NJ-STBARNMC>
+ St. Barnabas Medical Center
94 Old Short Hills Road   Livingston, NJ 07039   (973)322-5000

McFadden, Christopher Bruce, MD {1164505103} Nephro, IntrMd(96,VA04)<NJ-COOPRUMC, NJ-KMHSTRAT>
+ University Renal Associates
1030 North Kings Highway/Suite 310   Cherry Hill, NJ 08034   (856)667-7266   Fax (856)779-9179
+ The Cooper Hospital System-Univ Hospital
3 Cooper Plaza/Suite 215   Camden, NJ 08103   (856)342-2439

McFadden, Denise C., MD {1063508588} Radiol, RadDia(82,PA02)
+ Montclair Radiology
116 Park Street   Montclair, NJ 07042   (973)746-2525   Fax (973)746-5802
+ Montclair Radiology
20 High Street   Nutley, NJ 07110   (973)746-2525   Fax (973)284-0269

McFadden, Kim Marie, MD {1255372322} EmrgMd(92,NJ06)<NJ-JRSYSHMC>
+ EmCare
1945 Route 33   Neptune, NJ 07753   (732)776-4510   Fax (732)776-2329

McFadden, Robert F., MD {1396753182} Psychy
+ Center for Family Guidance, PC
765 East Route 70/Building A-101   Marlton, NJ 08053   (856)797-4800   Fax (856)810-0110
+ University Hospital-SOM Department of Psychiatry
2250 Chapel Avenue West/Suite 100   Cherry Hill, NJ 08002   (856)797-4800   Fax (856)482-1159

McFadden Parsi, Lovelle, DO {1174787832} Pedtrc(04,NJ75)
+ Lourdes Pediatric Associates
2475 McClellan Avenue/Building B201   Pennsauken, NJ 08109   (856)330-6300   Fax (856)310-0265

McFalls, Susan G., MD {1639199979} Dermat(91,PA02)
+ Advanced Dermatology, Laser, and MOHS Surgery Center
240 East Grove Street   Westfield, NJ 07090   (908)232-6446   Fax (908)232-6447

McFarland, Miles M., MD {1194725218} PthACl(79,PA01)<NJ-VIRTVOOR, NJ-VIRTUAHS>
+ Virtua Voorhees
100 Bowman Drive/Path   Voorhees, NJ 08043   (856)325-3275   Fax (856)325-3164
mmcfarland@virtua.org

McFarlane, Owen R., MD {1205190808} ObsGyn
+ Southern Jersey Family Medical Centers, Inc.
860 South White Horse Pike/Building A   Hammonton, NJ 08037   (609)567-0200   Fax (609)567-1951

McFeely, Erin M., MD {1831104389} Pedtrc
+ Pediatric Health, P.A.
69 West Main Street   Freehold, NJ 07728   (732)409-3633   Fax (732)409-7133

McGarry, Andrew James, MD {1902818610} Nrolgy<NY-STRNGMEM>
+ Cooper University Neurology
1935 Route 70 East   Cherry Hill, NJ 08003   (856)342-2445   Fax (856)964-0504

McGarry, Barbara J., MD {1952462186} FamMed(88,NJ05)<NJ-STPETER, NJ-RWJUBRUN>
+ Family Medicine at Monument Square
317 George Street   New Brunswick, NJ 08901   (732)235-8993   Fax (732)246-7317

McGeady, Rosemary E., MD {1720019581} CdvDis, IntrMd(82,MO34)<NJ-MORRISTN>
+ 124 Woodview Drive
Belle Mead, NJ 08502

McGee, John R., MD {1811991284} IntrMd(89,NJ05)<NJ-BAYONNE>
+ 1160 Kennedy Boulevard/Suite A
Bayonne, NJ 07002   (201)443-8988   Fax (201)443-8986

McGeever, Rose, DO {1518165265} FamMed(06,NJ75)<NJ-OURLADY>
+ LifeCare Physicians, PC of Lawrenceville
4 Princess Road/Suite 209   Lawrenceville, NJ 08648   (609)895-0770   Fax (609)896-1124

McGill, Dennis L., MD {1215970470} EmrgMd(84,NY09)<NJ-RWJUBRUN, NJ-SOMERSET>
+ Robert Wood Johnson Emergency Medicine
One Robert Wood Johnson Place/MEB 104   New Brunswick, NJ 08901   (973)740-0607   Fax (973)740-9895

McGill, Winston, Jr., MD {1093810749} Urolgy(76,NJ05)<NJ-EASTORNG>
+ East Orange Family Health Center
240 Central Avenue/Suite 3   East Orange, NJ 07018   (973)674-3500   Fax (973)674-6134

Mcginley, Thomas Charles, Jr., MD {1144284118} FamMed(92,PA01)
+ St. Luke's Coventry Family Practice
755 Memorial Parkway/Suite 300   Phillipsburg, NJ 08865   (908)454-6303   Fax (866)281-6023

McGinnis, Michael Clifton, MD {1801841358} PthACl(90,NV01)<NJ-CENTRAST>
+ Southwestern Pathology Associates
207 Georgetown Wrightstown Rd   Wrightstown, NJ 08562   (609)723-0070   Fax (609)723-0073
spalaboratory@aol.com
+ PLUS Diagnostics
1200 River Avenue/Suite 10   Lakewood, NJ 08701   (609)723-0070   Fax (732)901-1555
+ CentraState Medical Center
901 West Main Street/Pathology   Freehold, NJ 08562   (732)294-2903   Fax (732)308-1614

McGorty, Francis E., MD {1871557025} IntrMd(91,NJ05)<NJ-VALLEY>
+ Bergen Medical Associates
190 Dayton Street   Ridgewood, NJ 07450   (201)670-7800   Fax (201)670-7720

McGovern, Patrick, Jr., MD {1932174125} SrgVas, Surgry(78,NJ05)<NJ-CHRIST, NJ-BAYONNE>
+ 17 Nardone Place
Jersey City, NJ 07306   (201)656-0646   Fax (201)610-9342
PJMCGO@gmail.com

McGovern, Peter G., MD {1770674004} RprEnd, ObsGyn(86,NY19)<NJ-HACKNSK, NJ-UMDNJ>
+ University Reproductive Associates, PC
214 Terrace Avenue/2nd Floor   Hasbrouck Heights, NJ 07604   (201)288-6330   Fax (201)288-6331

McGovern, Terrance, DO {1164862504} EmrgMd
+ St Joseph's Medical Center Emergency
703 Main Street   Paterson, NJ 07503   (973)754-2918   Fax (973)754-2516

McGowan, John M., MD {1568450237} FamMed(75,PA02)<NJ-HUNTRDN>
+ Hickory Run Family Practice Associates
384 County Road 513   Califon, NJ 07830   (908)832-2125   Fax (908)832-6149

McGowan, Seth A., MD {1932242450} PsyCAd, Psychy(97,NY45)
+ 300 Knickerbocker Road/Suite 3200
Cresskill, NJ 07626   (201)541-8338   Fax (201)541-0338

McGrath, Lynn B., MD {1831137587} SrgCdv, SrgThr, Surgry(74,NF01)<NJ-DEBRAHLC>
+ Deborah Heart and Lung Center
200 Trenton Road   Browns Mills, NJ 08015   (609)893-6611   Fax (609)893-1213

McGrath, Robert C., DO {1912110636} FamMed, PhysMd(80,PA77)
+ Atlantic Spine and Joint Institute
654 West Cuthbert Road   Haddon Township, NJ 08108   (856)528-9838   Fax (856)854-9192

McGrath, Steven Warren, MD {1992091888} AnesPain
+ Rancocas Anesthesiology, PA
15000 Midlantic Drive/Suite 102   Mount Laurel, NJ 08054   (855)727-2465   Fax (856)393-8691

McGrath, Teresa Pirri, DO {1710145081} Pedtrc(04,PA77)<NJ-COOPRUMC>
+ Cooper University Hospital
One Cooper Plaza/Pediatrics   Camden, NJ 08103   (856)342-2000

McGraw, John Daniel, MD {1114913068} FamMed(82,PHI08)<NJ-NWTNMEM>
+ Premier Health Associates
135 Newton Sparta Road   Newton, NJ 07860   (973)579-1000   Fax (973)579-3571
info@mypremierdoctors.com
+ Premier Health Associates
89 Sparta Avenue/Suite 100   Sparta, NJ 07871   (973)579-1000   Fax (973)729-3454

McGroarty, William J., MD {1558367268} RadDia, Radiol, IntrMd(85,NJ05)<NJ-RWJUHAM>
+ Radiology Affiliates of Central New Jersey, P.A.
2501 Kuser Road/Suite 500   Hamilton, NJ 08691   (609)585-8800   Fax (609)585-1825
mfletcher@4rai.com

McGuckin, James Frederick, Jr., MD {1760441760} RadV&I
+ Vascular Access Center
1450 Parkside Avenue/Unit 18   Trenton, NJ 08638   (609)882-1770   Fax (609)882-8406

McGue, Mary Margaret, MD {1629537550} ObsGyn<NJ-MORRISTN>
+ Morristown Medical Center
100 Madison Avenue   Morristown, NJ 07962   (973)971-5000

McGugins Hill, Jennifer Anne, MD {1508865411}
+ Valley Medical Group
70 Park Avenue   Park Ridge, NJ 07656   (212)981-7282   Fax (201)391-7733

Physicians by Name and Address

McGuigan, Kevin, MD {1619050036} PhysMd(86,NJ06)<NJ-ST-LAWRN, NJ-STFRNMED>
+ St. Lawrence Rehabilitation Center
2381 Lawrenceville Road   Lawrenceville, NJ 08648
(609)896-8152   Fax (609)896-4107

McGuire, Thomas M., MD {1932130879} EmrgMd(74,PA09)<NJ-SHOREMEM>
+ Shore Memorial Hospital
1 East New York Avenue/EmergMed   Somers Point, NJ 08244   (609)653-3500

McGuire, Jennifer Lara, MD {1528104783} NrlgSpec<PA-CHILDHOS>
+ CHOP Specialty Care
101 Plainsboro Road   Plainsboro, NJ 08536   (609)452-0825

McGuire, Kimberly Marie, MD {1245271766} Anesth(99,GRN01)<NJ-MTNSIDE>
+ 12 Spruce Drive
Middletown, NJ 07748   (201)725-4148   Fax (732)671-5391

McGuire, Matthew Brian, MD {1780025973}
+ Newton Medical Center
175 High Street   Newton, NJ 07860   (973)383-2121
+ CentraState Family Medicine Residency Practice
1001 West Main Street/Suite B   Freehold, NJ 07728
(973)383-2121   Fax (732)409-2621

McGuire, Patricia L., MD {1730264292} Psychy(80,MI07)
+ 45 North Broad Street/Suite 507
Ridgewood, NJ 07450   (201)445-8004   Fax (201)445-8005

McGuire, Peter A., MD {1801087382} PulDis, CritCr(99,GRN01)
+ 12 Spruce Drive
Middletown, NJ 07748

McHeffey, Dina A., MD {1831137728} IntrMd(94,NJ06)<NJ-MONMOUTH>
+ 188 East Bergen Place/2nd Floor
Red Bank, NJ 07701   (732)842-7000   Fax (732)842-7110

McHugh, Catherine Ann, MD {1528140399} Pedtrc(87,NY48)<NJ-MORRISTN>
+ 106 Main Street
Sparta, NJ 07871   (973)729-7400   Fax (973)729-2201

McHugh, Jennifer L., MD {1033279195} Pedtrc(99,PA14)
+ Cherry Hill Pediatric Group
600 West Marlton Pike   Cherry Hill, NJ 08002   (856)428-5020   Fax (856)216-9433

McIlveen, Stephen J., MD {1619989712} SrgCrt(73,NY19)<NJ-HACKNSK, NJ-VALLEY>
+ One West Ridgewood Avenue/Suite 307
Paramus, NJ 07652   (201)670-6702   Fax (201)447-7098

McInerney, Vincent K., MD {1669496865} SrgOrt(77,NJ05)<NJ-STJOSHOS>
+ New Jersey Orthopaedic Institute
504 Valley Road/Suite 200   Wayne, NJ 07470   (973)694-2690   Fax (973)694-2692
+ St. Joseph's Regional Medical Center
703 Main Street   Paterson, NJ 07503   (201)278-0990

McInnes, Andrew Duncan, MD {1174718035} Pedtrc, PedCrC, PedEmg
+ The Children's Hospital at Saint Peter's University
254 Easton Avenue   New Brunswick, NJ 08901   (732)565-5434   Fax (732)745-0857
+ PO Box 386
Allenwood, NJ 08720   (732)565-5434   Fax (732)745-0857

McInnes, Marcia R., MD {1639138456} Pedtrc(82,PA12)<NJ-MORRISTN, NJ-SOMERSET>
+ 254 Routes 202-206N/PO Box 160
Pluckemin, NJ 07978   (908)234-9777   Fax (908)234-2485

McIntosh, Barbara A., MD {1912956210} EmrgMd(84,NY46)<NJ-HACKNSK>
+ Hackensack Medical Center Emergency Medicine
30 Prospect Avenue/Main 3619   Hackensack, NJ 07601
(201)996-4614   Fax (201)968-1866

McIntosh, Nenita Parrilla, MD {1225145360} OncHem, IntrMd(73,PHI01)<NJ-STFRNMED, NJ-RWJUHAM>
+ Mercer Bucks Hematology Oncology
2 Capital Way/Suite 220   Pennington, NJ 08534   (609)303-0747   Fax (609)303-0771

McIntosh, Violet Merle, MD {1720010929} SrgBst, Surgry, SrgOnc(88,NY08)<NJ-ENGLWOOD>
+ Englewood Hospital and Medical Center
350 Engle Street/Breast Surgery   Englewood, NJ 07631
(201)894-3893   Fax (201)894-3764

McIntyre, Bryan J., DO {1891795068} Anesth(84,MO78)
+ West Jersey Anesthesia Associates
102-E Center Boulevard   Marlton, NJ 08053   (856)988-6250   Fax (856)988-6270

McKay, Cecile M., MD {1013017532} IntrMd(85,NY08)<NJ-TRENTPSY>
+ Trenton Psychiatric Hospital
Sullivan Way/PO Box 7600/Internal Med   West Trenton, NJ 08628   (609)633-1502

McKenna, Cristin, MD {1366636300} PhysMd(03,NJ05)<NJ-KSLRWEST>
+ Kessler Institute for Rehabilitation West Orange
1199 Pleasant Valley Way   West Orange, NJ 07052

(973)731-3600   Fax (973)243-6861

McKenna, Harold V., MD {1609959550} IntrMd(75,MEX03)
+ 305 Main Street
South Amboy, NJ 08879   (732)721-1120   Fax (732)721-2102

McKenna, Michael G., MD {1073556528} RadOnc(88,MA16)<NJ-CHSMRCER, NJ-RWJUBRUN>
+ Rutgers Cancer Institute of New Jersey
195 Little Albany Street/PO Box 2681   New Brunswick, NJ 08903   (732)235-2465   Fax (732)235-6797

McKenna, Tatiana, MD {1376806083}<NJ-CHSFULD>
+ Capital Health System/Fuld Campus
750 Brunswick Avenue   Trenton, NJ 08638   (609)394-6031

McKenzie, Rammurri Anthony, MD {1417224684}
+ Rancocas Anesthesiology, PA
15000 Midlantic Drive/Suite 102   Mount Laurel, NJ 08054
(856)255-5479   Fax (856)393-8691

McKeon, John J., MD {1770688137} SrgOrt, PedOrt(72,NJ05)<NJ-NWRKBETH>
+ Pediatric Orthopedic Associates, P.A.
585 Cranbury Road/Suite A   East Brunswick, NJ 08816
(732)390-1160   Fax (732)390-8449
+ Pediatric Orthopedic Associates, P.A.
3700 State Route 33   Neptune, NJ 07753   (732)390-1160
Fax (732)897-4205

McKeon, John J., MD {1669506580} Anesth(85,DOM10)<NJ-STBARNMC>
+ St. Barnabas Ambulatory Care Center
200 South Orange Avenue   Livingston, NJ 07039   (973)322-7400   Fax (973)322-7685

McKinney, Timothy B., MD {1093741597} Gyneco, UroGyn(87,NJ06)<NJ-KMHSTRAT, NJ-VIRTUAHS>
+ Athena Women's Institute for Pelvic Health
151 Fries Mill Road/Suite 301   Turnersville, NJ 08012
(856)374-1377   Fax (856)374-2177

McLane, Rebecca, MD {1780657916} Pedtrc(97,PA02)
+ Southern Jersey Family Medical
238 East Broadway   Salem, NJ 08079   (856)935-7711   Fax (856)935-9123

McLaughlin, Blaise, MD {1659479020} Anesth(02,NJ05)<NJ-OVERLOOK>
+ Summit Anesthesia Associates, P.A.
33 Overlook Road/Suite 311   Summit, NJ 07901   (908)598-1500   Fax (908)598-0197

McLaughlin, John Patrick, MD {1649653353} Ophthl
+ Horizon Eye Care
4 Village Drive   Cape May Court House, NJ 08210
(609)465-7100   Fax (609)465-7659

McLaughlin, Mark Robert, MD {1053382366} SrgNro(92,VA04)<NJ-UNVMCPRN, NJ-CENTRAST>
+ Princeton Brain & Spine Care LLC
731 Alexander Road/Suite 200   Princeton, NJ 08540
(609)921-9001   Fax (609)921-9055
+ Princeton Brain & Spine Care LLC
190 Route 31N/Suite 300B   Flemington, NJ 08822
(609)921-9001   Fax (908)806-6625

McLaughlin, Michael Joseph, MD {1851845846} SrgPlstc
+ 6 Voorhees Way
Pennington, NJ 08534   (908)938-5099

McLaughlin, Valerie Gail, MD {1861448540} EmrgMd(01,NJ05)<NJ-CENTRAST>
+ CentraState Medical Center
901 West Main Street/EmergMed   Freehold, NJ 07728
(732)431-2000

McLaughlin, Vincent A., MD {1841288321} Gastrn, IntrMd(84,NE06)<NJ-VIRTVOOR>
+ Allied Gastrointestinal Associates
502 Centennial Boulevard/Suite 3   Voorhees, NJ 08043
(856)751-2300   Fax (856)751-2333

McLay, William F., DO {1033133970} FamMed, GenPrc(71,PA77)<NJ-BURDTMLN>
+ 1150 Golf Club Road
Cape May Court House, NJ 08210   (609)465-1984   Fax (609)463-8245

McLean, Edward, Jr., MD {1588654578} SrgCrC, SrgVas, Surgry(73,NY01)
+ Surgical Practice of Rolando Rolandelli, MD
435 South Street/Suite 360   Morristown, NJ 07960
(973)971-7200   Fax (973)290-7521

McLintock, Glenn R., MD {1073590121} IntrMd(95,PA02)
+ Haddonfield Internal Medicine
216 Haddon Avenue   Haddon Township, NJ 08108
(856)854-6600   Fax (856)854-6700

McMahon, Paul Patrick, MD {1720249428} IntrMd<NJ-COOPRUMC>
+ Cooper University Hospital
One Cooper Plaza/Drrance/Ste 222   Camden, NJ 08103
(856)342-3150   Fax (856)968-8418

McMahon, Donald James, DO {1285824839} Gastrn
+ Woodbury Primary and Specialty Care
159 South Broad Street   Woodbury, NJ 08096   (844)542-2273   Fax (856)384-0218

+ The University Doctors - UMDNJ -SOM
570 Egg Harbor Road/Suite C-2   Sewell, NJ 08080
(844)542-2273   Fax (856)589-5082

McMahon, Kerry Rose, MD {1497847339} FamMed(01,NJ05)
+ Franklin Medical Associates
165 State Highway 23   Franklin, NJ 07416   (973)827-5255

McMahon, Mary Ann Patricia, MD {1699773416} IntrMd(00,PA02)<NJ-COOPRUMC, NJ-OURLADY>
+ McMahon Medicine
1305 North Kings Highway/Suite 3   Cherry Hill, NJ 08034
(856)428-9446   Fax (856)428-4330

McMahon, Patrick James, MD {1245423854} Dermat, Pedtrc, IntrMd(05,NY48)<PA-CHILDHOS>
+ CHOP Specialty Care Center at Virtua
200 Bowman Drive/2 FL/Suite D-260   Voorhees, NJ 08043
(267)425-5400

McManus, Edward J., MD {1871569996} InfDis, IntrMd(82,NJ05)<NJ-UNVMCPRN, NJ-RWJUBRUN>
+ ID Associates PA/dba ID Care
765 Route 10 East/Suite 201   Randolph, NJ 07869
(973)989-0068   Fax (973)361-8955
+ ID Associates PA/dba ID Care
8 Saddle Road   Cedar Knolls, NJ 07927   (973)989-0068
Fax (973)993-5953

McManus, Shanda Monique, MD {1487862827} FamMed, IntrMd(96,PA02)
+ Family Practice of Middletown
18 Leonardville Road   Middletown, NJ 07748   (732)671-0860   Fax (732)671-6467

McManus, Stephen William, MD {1750495313} Radiol, RadBdl(96,PA02)<NJ-ACMCMAIN, NJ-ACMCITY>
+ Atlantic Medical Imaging, LLC.
72 West Jimmie Leeds Road   Galloway, NJ 08205
(609)677-9729   Fax (609)653-8764
+ Atlantic Medical Imaging, LLC.
401 Bethel Road   Somers Point, NJ 08244   (609)677-9729
+ Atlantic Medical Imaging, LLC.
421 Route 9 North   Cape May Court House, NJ 08205
(609)463-9500   Fax (609)465-0918

McManus, Susan A., MD {1316941370} SrgBst(79,MEX03)<NJ-STPETER, NJ-HUNTRDN>
+ Somerset Medical Associates
1553 Highway 27/Suite 3100   Somerset, NJ 08873
(732)846-3300   Fax (732)846-3323
+ Cares Surgicenter, LLC.
240 Easton Avenue   New Brunswick, NJ 08901   (732)846-3300   Fax (732)296-8677
+ Medigest Associates P.A.
21 Clyde Road/Suite 102   Somerset, NJ 08873   (732)873-0033

McMaster, Delphine A., MD {1992927529} IntrMd, Rheuma(74,PA13)
+ Hoffman-La Roche Incorporated
340 Kingsland Street/Building 126-T   Nutley, NJ 07110
(973)235-5000   Fax (973)235-2117

McMaster, Michelle, MD {1780905679} Anesth
+ 73 Rugby Place
Woodbury, NJ 08096   (609)680-0199

McMillan, Sean, DO {1689885816} SrgOrt(05,PA77)
+ LMA Professional Orthopaedics
2103 Burlington Mount   Burlington Township, NJ 08016
(609)747-9200   Fax (609)747-1408

McMillan, Tyler, MD {1407202492} IntrMd
+ Cooper University Hospital Hospitalists
One Cooper Plaza/Suite 222/Drrnce   Camden, NJ 08103
(856)342-3150

McMillin, Kendall Lee, DO {1700017399}<NJ-SJHREGMC>
+ SJH Regional Medical Center
1505 West Sherman Avenue   Vineland, NJ 08360
(859)583-7582
kendallmcmillin1@gmail.com

McMurtrie, Robert, Jr., DO {1144269366} PainMd, Anesth(98,PA77)
+ 15000 Midlantic Drive/Suite 110
Mount Laurel, NJ 08054   (856)358-4520

McNab, Theresa Challender, MD {1669497012} NnPnMd(94,VA01)
+ Pediatrix Medical Group
255 Third Avenue   Long Branch, NJ 07740   (732)222-7006

McNair, Timothy P., MD {1831314921} Anesth(03,NY09)<NJ-BAYSHORE>
+ Bayshore Community Hospital
727 North Beers Street/Anesth   Holmdel, NJ 07733
(732)739-5900

McNally, Lauryn Anne, DO {1740519487} ObsGyn<NJ-UNDRWD>
+ Westwood Womens Health Center
600 Jessup Road   West Deptford, NJ 08066   (856)845-4061
Fax (856)812-2880
+ Westwood Womens Center
155 Bridgeton Pike/Suite B   Mullica Hill, NJ 08062
(856)845-4061   Fax (856)812-2880

McNamara, Donna M., MD {1376502237} OncHem, IntrMd(99,IL43)
+ John Theurer Cancer Center - HUMC
92 Second Street   Hackensack, NJ 07601   (201)996-5900   Fax (201)996-9246

McNamara, John Patrick, DO {1760460596} CdvDis, IntrMd(97,PA77)<NJ-DEBRAHLC>
+ Deborah Heart and Lung Center
200 Trenton Road/Cardiology   Browns Mills, NJ 08015   (609)893-6611   Fax (609)893-6038

McNamara, Jonathan, MD {1568889814} IntrMd<NJ-NWRK-BETH>
+ Newark Beth Israel Medical Center
201 Lyons Avenue   Newark, NJ 07112   (973)926-3233

McNamara, Robert E., MD {1083687164} ObsGyn, Obstet(65,DC02)<NJ-TRINIJSC, NJ-TRINIWSC>
+ Womens HealthCare of Union County
950 West Chestnut Street/Suite 102   Union, NJ 07083   (908)688-8545   Fax (908)688-8447

McNeill-Augustine, Roberta Nicole, MD {1477651487} FamMed(00,NY08)
+ Valley Health Medical Group
780 Cedar Lane   Teaneck, NJ 07666   (201)836-7664   Fax (201)836-5710

McPartland, Thomas Girard, MD {1669587622} SrgOrt(01,NJ06)<MA-CHILDRN>
+ Pediatric Orthopedic Associates, P.A.
585 Cranbury Road/Suite A   East Brunswick, NJ 08816   (732)390-1160   Fax (732)390-8449
+ Pediatric Orthopedic Associates, P.A.
3700 State Route 33   Neptune, NJ 07753   (732)390-1160   Fax (732)897-4205

McQueen, Derrick Arnold, MD {1003914748} PedCrC(92,NJ05)<NJ-CHDNWBTH>
+ Children's Hospital of New Jersey
201 Lyons Avenue/Osborne Terrace   Newark, NJ 07112   (973)926-4000   Fax (973)926-6452

McQuilkin, George E., MD {1063457778} ObsGyn(81,NJ05)<NJ-HOBUNIMC, NJ-PALISADE>
+ 129 Washington Street/Suite 200
Hoboken, NJ 07030   (201)795-0501   Fax (201)963-8231

McRae, Valerie A., MD {1922180629} Anesth(93,PA14)<NJ-UMDNJ>
+ Robert Wood Johnson-UMDNJ Anesthesia Group
125 Paterson Street/CAB 3100   New Brunswick, NJ 08901   (732)235-7827   Fax (732)235-6131

McSherry, Kevin Joseph, MD {1336145986} Pedtrc, PedHem(84,NY08)<NJ-MORRISTN>
+ Morristown Medical Center
100 Madison Avenue/EmrgMed   Morristown, NJ 07962   (973)971-5000

McTigue, Maureen A., DO {1285618348} Anesth(90,NJ75)<NJ-HACKNSK>
+ Hackensack University Medical Center
30 Prospect Avenue/Anesthesiology   Hackensack, NJ 07601   (201)996-2000   Fax (201)488-6769

Mead, John Edward, MD {1831165257} Anesth(91,NY15)<NJ-HOBUNIMC, NJ-CHRIST>
+ Hoboken University Medical Center
308 Willow Avenue/Anesthesiology   Hoboken, NJ 07030   (201)418-1000   Fax (201)943-8105

Meadows, Jason Potts, MD {1326335217} IntrMd<NY-SLOAN-KET>
+ SJH Regional Medical Center
1505 West Sherman Avenue   Vineland, NJ 08360   (203)258-2555

Meagher, Richard John, MD {1538107545} SrgNro, Surgry(96,NJ06)
+ The Spine Institute of Southern New Jersey
512 Lippincott Drive   Marlton, NJ 08053   (856)797-9161   Fax (856)797-3637

Mecca, Mauro A., MD {1639227804} IntrMd(76,NY08)<NJ-HACKNSK>
+ 1 South Main Street
Lodi, NJ 07644   (973)778-3303   Fax (973)778-3304
+ Executive Health Group, Inc.
44 Whippany Road   Morristown, NJ 07960   (973)540-0177

Mechanic, Leslie D., MD {1730228891} PthAClf(87,NY06)
+ 3131 Princeton Pike
Lawrenceville, NJ 08648   (609)895-0933

Mechineni, Ashesha, MD {1659784817} IntrMd
+ St Joseph's Medical Ctr Internal Med
703 Main Street   Paterson, NJ 07503   (973)754-2431

Meckael, Dina, MD {1174912950} IntrMd
+ Meridian Medical Associates, P.C.
1945 Route 33   Neptune, NJ 07753   (732)776-2963   Fax (732)776-3795

Medasani, Kiran M., MD {1417251703} IntrMd(07,NET09)
+ 222 South Street
Freehold, NJ 07728   (732)387-7795   Fax (732)387-7796

Medenilla, Rosenio, Jr., MD {1699857011} FamMed(90,PHIL)
+ Family Medicine Center
279 Mathistown Road   Little Egg Harbor, NJ 08087   (609)296-1101
+ Family Medicine Center
1301 Route 72 West/Suite 240   Manahawkin, NJ 08050   (609)296-1101   Fax (609)597-6833

Medepalli, Prasad B., MD {1912941691} CdvDis, IntrMd(70,INA62)<NJ-STJOSHOS>
+ 15-01 Broadway/Suite 38
Fair Lawn, NJ 07410   (201)791-9400

Medford, David J., MD {1023079522} Ophthl(84,NJ05)<NJ-MORRISTN, NJ-STBARNMC>
+ Affiliated Eye Surgeons
405 Northfield Avenue/Suite 206   West Orange, NJ 07052   (973)736-3322   Fax (973)736-7317
+ Affiliated Eye Surgeons
95 Madison Avenue/Suite 400   Morristown, NJ 07960   (973)736-3322   Fax (973)984-5554

Medic, Igor, DO {1154618593}
+ 2141 Route 38/Apt 504 W
Cherry Hill, NJ 08002   (619)850-1254
medic-igor@cooperhealth.edu

Medina, Gladibel, MD {1770597874} Pedtrc(95,NJ06)<NJ-STPETER>
+ St. Peters Pediatric Faculty
123 How Lane   New Brunswick, NJ 08901   (732)745-8419

Medina, Richard A., MD {1598866428} Gastrn, IntrMd(83,NJ05)<NJ-JFKMED>
+ 225 May Street/Suite B
Edison, NJ 08837   (732)549-4747   Fax (732)549-6132

Medina Carcamo, Edwing Gerardo, MD {1184889271} IntrMd
+ The Center for Sleep Medicine at CHS
1445-1401 Whitehorse-Mercervil   Hamilton, NJ 08619   (609)588-5050

Mediratta, Anuj, MD {1457508574} IntrMd<NJ-MORRISTN>
+ Morristown Medical Center
100 Madison Avenue   Morristown, NJ 07962   (973)682-2136   Fax (973)290-8332

Mediterraneo, Susan, MD {1891798351} Pedtrc(87,PHI08)
+ Notchview Pediatrics, LLC.
1037 Route 46 East/Suite 201   Clifton, NJ 07013   (973)779-3911   Fax (973)471-2730

Medlenov, Sergey, DO {1164628392} EmrgMd(05,NJ75)<NJ-KMH-TURNV>
+ Kennedy Health Systems/Washington Township Campus
435 Hurffville-Cross Keys Road   Turnersville, NJ 08012   (856)346-7985

Mednick, Joyce J., MD {1144282369} EmrgMd(70,NY15)<NJ-VALLEY>
+ The Valley Hospital
223 North Van Dien Avenue/EmrgMed   Ridgewood, NJ 07450   (201)447-8000

Medrano, Christina Marie, MD {1033198494} FamMed, IntrMd(01,NET12)
+ Sanofi US-Sanofi-Aventis
55 Corporate Drive/MS 55c-b-100a   Bridgewater, NJ 08807   (908)981-6925   Fax (908)306-9010

Medrano Mendez, Carolina Maria, MD {1538543988}
+ 1084 Kennedy Boulevard/Suite 1
Bayonne, NJ 07002   (908)487-3374

Medunick, David M., DO {1861488736} FamMed(02,PA77)
+ Premier Health Associates
89 Sparta Avenue/Suite 100   Sparta, NJ 07871   (973)729-2121   Fax (973)729-3454

Medunick, Sara Elizabeth, DO {1497742761} FamMed(02,NJ75)
+ Premier Health Associates
272 Route 206 North   Andover, NJ 07821   (973)347-2273   Fax (973)729-3238

Meduru, Pramod, MD {1770683179} GPrvMd, IntrMd
+ 4 Bailey Avenue
Sayreville, NJ 08872

Medvedovsky, Andrew, MD {1649431594} PainInvt
+ Rancocas Anesthesiology, PA
15000 Midlantic Drive/Suite 102   Mount Laurel, NJ 08054   (856)255-5479   Fax (856)393-8691
+ Rancocas Anesthesiology, PA
151 Fries Mill Road/Suite 202   Turnersville, NJ 08012   (856)255-5479   Fax (856)228-7252

Meer, Joel, MD {1740356898} PhysMd(86,NY08)<NJ-NWRKBETH>
+ 119-137 Clifford Street/Suite 101
Newark, NJ 07105   (973)622-0888   Fax (973)622-1610
+ Newark Beth Israel Medical Center
201 Lyons Avenue   Newark, NJ 07112   (973)926-7000

Meer, Shahid B., MD {1346284049} IntrMd, PulDis, SlpDis(84,PAK11)<NJ-CHSMRCER, NJ-CHSFULD>
+ AZZ Medical Associates
1440 Pennington Road/Suite 1   Ewing, NJ 08618   (609)890-1050   Fax (609)890-0950

+ 1601 Whitehorse Mercerville Ro/Suite 4
Trenton, NJ 08619   (609)890-1050   Fax (609)890-0950

Meerson, Maya, MD {1932147352} EmrgMd(00,IL06)<NJ-VIRTVOOR>
+ Virtua Voorhees
100 Bowman Drive/EmrgMed   Voorhees, NJ 08043   (856)247-3000

Meese, Michael Arthur, MD {1588773758} SprtMd, SrgArt, SrgOrt(87,NJ05)<NJ-HACKNSK, NJ-HOLYNAME>
+ 899 Main Street
Hackensack, NJ 07601   (201)968-0508   Fax (201)968-0509

Meeteer, Francis, III, DO {1184670200} FamMed(88,PA77)<NJ-VIRTBERL, NJ-VIRTVOOR>
+ Advocare Family Medicine Associates Mt. Laurel
3115 Route 38/Suite 200B   Mount Laurel, NJ 08054   (856)231-9666   Fax (856)231-7543
+ Advocare Family Medicine Associates Williamstown
979 North Black Horse Pike   Williamstown, NJ 08094   (856)231-9666   Fax (856)629-0281
+ Advocare Family Medicine Associates Vineland
602 West Sherman Avenue/Suite B   Vineland, NJ 08054   (856)692-8484   Fax (856)896-3059

Megahed, Mona, MD {1023229143}
+ 17 Rocky Hill Road
Princeton, NJ 08540

Megariotis, Evangelos, MD {1336144583} SrgOrt(78,NJ05)<NJ-STMRYPAS>
+ 1450 Main Avenue
Clifton, NJ 07011   (973)340-8500   Fax (973)340-4935   Emegariotismd@aol.com
+ St. Mary's Hospital
350 Boulevard/Surgery/Ortho   Passaic, NJ 07055   (973)365-4300
+ Endosurgical Center
999 Clifton Avenue   Clifton, NJ 07011   (973)777-3938   Fax (973)777-6738

Meghadri, Niveditha, MD {1063501872} PsycAd, Psychy(91,INA83)<NJ-UNIVBHC>
+ 295 Pierson Avenue/2nd Floor
Edison, NJ 08837   (732)494-8558

Meglio, Robyn S., MD {1205915634} Gyneco(82,NJ06)<NJ-CLAR-MAAS>
+ 5 Franklin Avenue/Suite 310
Belleville, NJ 07109

Mehalick, Andrew Joseph, DO {1821424102}
+ 311 Renaissance Drive
Pine Hill, NJ 08021   (484)431-1619   andrew.j.mehalick@gmail.com

Mehandru, Sushil K., MD {1366453409} Nephro, IntrMd(72,INDI)<NJ-JRSYSHMC, NJ-BAYSHORE>
+ Drs. Mehandru & Mehandru
1925 Highway 35   Wall, NJ 07719   (732)974-0100   Fax (732)974-0137

Mehandru, Urmila, MD {1811390800} Psychy, IntrMd(72,INDI)
+ Drs. Mehandru & Mehandru
1925 Highway 35   Wall, NJ 07719   (732)974-0100   Fax (732)974-0137

Mehling, Brian MacDermott, MD {1790703965} SrgOrt, SprtMd, OrtTrm(96,OH45)<NJ-HACKNSK, NY-GDSAMMC>
+ Mehling Orthopedics, LLC
214 State Street/Suite 101   Hackensack, NJ 07601   (201)342-7662   Fax (201)342-7663

Mehnert, Janice M., MD {1962617472} MedOnc, IntrMd, Hemato(01,NJ02)<NJ-RWJUBRUN>
+ Rutgers Cancer Institute of New Jersey
195 Little Albany Street/PO Box 2681   New Brunswick, NJ 08903   (732)235-2465   Fax (732)235-6797   mehnerja@umdnj.edu

Mehnert, Michael Joseph, MD {1306927967} PhyMPain, PhysMd(02,NJ06)<NJ-ATLANTHS>
+ Rothman Institute - Egg Harbor Township
2500 English Creek Avenue/Bldg 1300   Egg Harbor Township, NJ 08234   (609)677-7002   Fax (609)677-7000

Mehra, Aditya Chand, MD {1922274141} CdvDis, IntrMd(03,PA09)<NJ-UNVMCPRN>
+ Cardiology Associates of Ocean County PA
495 Jack Martin Boulevard/Suite 2   Brick, NJ 08724   (732)458-7575   Fax (732)458-0874

Mehra, Aruna Sinha, MD   EnDbMt, IntrMd(88,NJ05)
+ 24 Honeyman Road
Basking Ridge, NJ 07920

Mehra, Deepti, MD {1649250697} Pedtrc(88,INA41)
+ Pediatric Group of Central Jersey
200 White Road/Suite 212   Little Silver, NJ 07739   (732)741-5600   Fax (732)345-1001

Mehra, Neeraj, MD {1194705145} FamMed(87,INA41)<NJ-COMMED>
+ Pediatric Group of Central Jersey
200 White Road/Suite 212   Little Silver, NJ 07739   (732)741-5600   Fax (732)345-1001

Physicians by Name and Address

Mehra, Shalini Gupta, MD {1740525294} IntrMd(93,NY48)
+ Parker Family Health Center
211 Shrewsbury Avenue   Red Bank, NJ 07701   (732)212-0777   Fax (732)212-9030

Mehra, Sweeti, MD {1871586735} IntrMd(98,NY48)<NY-SLR-LUKES>
+ Summit Medical Group
85 Woodland Road   Short Hills, NJ 07078   (973)379-4496   Fax (973)376-0357

Mehrotra, Naveen, MD {1295783025} Pedtrc(92,NY48)<NJ-STPETER, NJ-RWJUBRUN>
+ 1315 Stelton Road
Piscataway, NJ 08854   (732)819-8800   Fax (732)819-8801   nmehrotra@pol.net
+ 652 Amboy Avenue
Edison, NJ 08837   (732)819-8800   Fax (732)738-9585
+ Dr. Naveen Mehrotra and Associates
171 Elmora Avenue/3rd Floor   Elizabeth, NJ 08854   (908)289-2239   Fax (908)659-1001

Mehta, Ami A., MD {1932238540} Pedtrc(03,PA09)<NJ-MORRISTN, NJ-STBARNMC>
+ Summit Medical Group-Berkeley Heights Campus
1 Diamond Hill Road   Berkeley Heights, NJ 07922   (908)277-8601   Fax (908)790-6576

Mehta, Amor Ruyintan, MD {1558566471} Nrolgy, ClNrPh(07,NY09)<NY-JTORTHO>
+ 280 US Highway 9 North/Suite 7
Morganville, NJ 07751   (732)856-5999   Fax (732)800-0682
+ Shore Neurology, P.A.
633 Route 37 West   Toms River, NJ 08755   (732)856-5999   Fax (732)240-3114

Mehta, Anila, MD {1619264959} EmrgMd
+ Complete Care Family Medicine
75 West Red Bank Avenue   Woodbury, NJ 08096   (856)853-2055   Fax (856)848-2879

Mehta, Anita Khanna, DO {1467611376} Nrolgy
+ Center for Neurology UMDNJ
166 Lyons Avenue   Newark, NJ 07112   (973)972-2550
+ Rutgers NJ School of Medicine Neurology
90 Bergen Street/DOC 5200   Newark, NJ 07103   (973)972-2550   Fax (973)972-5059

Mehta, Anupama, MD {1518199751}
+ 43 Remington Court
Matawan, NJ 07747   (848)667-1957   anupama.mehta13@gmail.com

Mehta, Archana P., MD {1972764835} AlgyImmn(08,VA04)
+ ENT & Allergy Associates of Parsippany
900 Lanidex Plaza/Suite 300   Parsippany, NJ 07054   (973)394-1818   Fax (973)394-1810
+ ENT & Allergy Associates, LLP
3219 Route 46 East/Suite 203   Parsippany, NJ 07054   (973)394-1818   Fax (973)394-1810
+ ENT & Allergy Associates of Parsippany
900 Lanidex Plaza/Suite 300   Parsippany, NJ 07054   (973)394-1818   Fax (973)394-1810

Mehta, Ariz Ruyintan, MD {1013077395} PhysMd, PainMd, Neu-Mus(03,NY09)
+ Pain & Disability Institute, P.C.
191 Palisade Avenue   Jersey City, NJ 07302   (201)656-4324

Mehta, Avani Shripal, MD {1043415219} RadDia(01,MA07)<NJ-STBARNMC>
+ St. Barnabas Medical Center
94 Old Short Hills Road/Radiology   Livingston, NJ 07039   (973)322-7850

Mehta, Bijal Shah, MD {1306839097} IntrMd(94,FL03)<NJ-MTN-SIDE>
+ Hackensack UMC Mountainside
1 Bay Avenue/Medicine   Montclair, NJ 07042   (973)429-6195

Mehta, Chirag A., MD {1790705820} IntrMd, PulDis, CritCr(00,DMN01)
+ Comprehensive Pulmonary & Critical Care Assoc
96 Millburn Avenue/Suite 200A   Millburn, NJ 07041   (973)763-6800   Fax (973)763-1255   cmehta-md@yahoo.com

Mehta, Deeksha, MD {1366618605}
+ Drs. Seth, Robertson & Seth
310 Central Avenue/Suite 100   East Orange, NJ 07018   (862)520-3104   Fax (973)674-8033   deeksha_15@hotmail.com

Mehta, Deviyani Dilipkumar, MD {1891927158} Nrolgy, IntrMd(98,INA70)
+ Drs. Mehta & Haskins
101 Old Short Hills Road/Suite 401   West Orange, NJ 07052   (973)322-6500   Fax (973)322-6418

Mehta, Eva C., DO {1245557883} IntrMd<NJ-NWRKBETH>
+ Newark Beth Israel Medical Center
201 Lyons Avenue   Newark, NJ 07112   (973)926-7000

Mehta, Harendra U., MD {1104824028} EmrgMd(67,INDI)<NJ-HOBUNIMC>
+ JFK Medical Center
65 James Street   Edison, NJ 08820   (732)321-7668   Fax (732)767-2969

Mehta, Harshna B., MD {1588988505} Pedtrc, AlgyImmn(06,GRN01)<NJ-HOBUNIMC, NJ-ENGLWOOD>
+ ENT and Allergy Associates (ENTA)
79 Hudson Street/Suite 303   Hoboken, NJ 07030   (201)792-1109   Fax (201)792-1145

Mehta, Heeral J., MD {1720303373} Nrolgy
+ Drs. Shah and Mehta
311 Baltimore Street   Phillipsburg, NJ 08865   (908)859-2009   Fax (908)859-3352

Mehta, Hemangini G., MD {1285604645} Anesth(70,INA20)
+ New Jersey Ambulatory Anesthesia Consultants, LLC
55 Schanck Road/Suite 8-A   Freehold, NJ 07728   (732)431-9544   Fax (732)431-9313

Mehta, Hemangini H., MD {1588853626} PhysMd(68,INA67)<NJ-BACHARCH>
+ Bacharach Institute for Rehabilitation
61 West Jimmie Leeds Road   Pomona, NJ 08240   (609)748-5380

Mehta, Jyotsna S., MD {1750531318} ObsGyn(73,INDI)
+ 10 Anderson Road
Bernardsville, NJ 07924   (908)221-1410   Fax (908)221-9304

Mehta, Kartik B., DO {1205123841}
+ Rowan University-School of Osteopathic Medicine
1 Medical Center Drive   Stratford, NJ 08084   (856)566-6708

Mehta, Kumudini U., MD {1225190705} Hemato, PthAcl(72,INA67)
+ Quest Diagnostics Inc.
1 Malcolm Avenue/Path   Teterboro, NJ 07608   (201)393-5000   Fax (201)393-6127

Mehta, Lalit Hargovind, MD {1578526349} FamMed(76,INA2B)
+ Summit Medical Arts Association, LLC.
1201 Summit Avenue   Union City, NJ 07087   (201)974-1311   Fax (201)974-1311

Mehta, Mahesh M., MD {1396859385} Nrolgy, GenPrc(78,INA65)
+ 426 10th Avenue
Paterson, NJ 07514   (973)345-9595   Fax (973)345-6996

Mehta, Monica R., MD {1427099985} PhysMd, PainMd, Orped(70,INDI)<NJ-HOBUNIMC, NJ-CHRIST>
+ Pain & Disability Institute, P.C.
191 Palisade Avenue   Jersey City, NJ 07302   (201)656-4324   Fax (201)656-4019

Mehta, Munira Yusuf, MD {1669704748} CritCr, IntrMd(00,INA5Y)<NJ-KMHTURNV>
+ Robert Wood Johnson University Hospital at Hamilton
1 Hamilton Health Place   Hamilton, NJ 08690   (609)586-7900

Mehta, Nehal L., MD {1679676266} IntrMd, PulCCr, PulDis(97,GRN01)
+ Respacare
489 Union Avenue   Bridgewater, NJ 08807   (732)356-9950   Fax (732)356-9959

Mehta, Nikhilesh D., MD {1083782924} Gastrn, IntrMd(70,INDI)
+ Atlantic Gastroenterology Associates, P.A.
3205 Fire Road/Suite 4   Egg Harbor Township, NJ 08234   (609)407-1220   Fax (609)407-0220

Mehta, Nikunj P., MD {1821017344} IntrMd(78,INDI)<NJ-COMMED>
+ 9 Mule Road/Suite E-14
Toms River, NJ 08755   (732)244-1080   Fax (732)244-1130

Mehta, Nimish Harendra, MD {1396752234} EmrgMd(99,NJ05)<NY-PUTNAMHC>
+ Pegasus Emergency Group
2100 Wescott Drive   Flemington, NJ 08822   (908)788-6183   Fax (908)788-6516

Mehta, Ojas R., DO {1255504031} IntrMd, Nephro(04,NY75)<NJ-RWJUBRUN>
+ Hypertension & Nephrology Specialists, LLC
2 Research Way/Suite 301   Monroe, NJ 08831   (732)521-0800   Fax (732)521-0833
+ Hypertension & Nephrology Specialists, LLC
49 Veronica Avenue/Suite 104   Somerset, NJ 08873   (732)521-0800   Fax (732)521-0833
+ Hypertension & Nephrology Specialists, LLC
601 Ewing Street/Suite C-7   Princeton, NJ 08831   (732)521-0800   Fax (732)521-0833

Mehta, Palak Pranav, MD {1154522167} Grtrcs, IntrMd(00,INA15)<NJ-RWJURAH, NJ-JFKMED>
+ Linden Medical Associates MD PC
540 South Wood Avenue   Linden, NJ 07036   (908)862-2893   Fax (908)862-5810

Mehta, Pallav K., MD {1720126170} OncHem, IntrMd(PA02<NJ-COOPRUMC>
+ Drs. Mehta & Lerman
900 Centienital Boulevard   Voorhees, NJ 08043   Fax (856)325-6777
+ South Jersey Health Care Center
Two Cooper Plaza   Camden, NJ 08103   Fax (856)342-6662

Mehta, Parul J., MD {1154345460} Anesth, Surgry(89,INA67)
+ 821 Wyngate Road
Somerdale, NJ 08083
+ Wills Eye Surgery Center in Cherry Hill
408 Route 70 East   Cherry Hill, NJ 08034   Fax (856)429-7555

Mehta, Pooja S., MD {1801056684} IntrMd<NJ-STJOSHOS>
+ St. Joseph's Regional Medical Center
703 Main Street   Paterson, NJ 07503   (973)754-2000

Mehta, Priti J., MD {1881831469} IntrMd
+ 5 Stanworth Road/Kendall Park
Kendall Park, NJ 08824   (732)297-2343   Fax (732)297-2039

Mehta, Ragini R., DO {1023186624} EmrgMd(94,NJ75)<NJ-CENTRAST>
+ CentraState Medical Center
901 West Main Street/EmergMed   Freehold, NJ 07728   (732)431-2000

Mehta, Rajeev, MD {1730122649} NnPnMd, Pedtrc(78,INDI)<NJ-RBAYPERT>
+ UH- Robert Wood Johnson Med
125 Paterson Street/MEB 238   New Brunswick, NJ 08901   (732)235-7036   Fax (732)235-7075

Mehta, Rajneesh G., MD {1063619294} IntrMd(02,INA20)<NJ-MONMOUTH>
+ Barnabas Health Medical Group
1300 Highway 35 South/Suites 101-103   Ocean, NJ 07712   (732)531-6400   Fax (732)517-0223

Mehta, Rashmi N., MD {1700964137} Psychy(79,INDI)
+ Richard Hall Community Mental Health Center
500 North Bridge Street   Bridgewater, NJ 08807   (908)725-2800   Fax (908)704-1790

Mehta, Rohin, MD {1306067517} PthAna
+ 208 Golf Edge Drive
Westfield, NJ 07090

Mehta, Ruchi, MD {1114177540} Pedtrc<NJ-JRSYSHMC>
+ All Star Pediatrics
106 Broad Street   Bloomfield, NJ 07003   (973)743-1392   Fax (973)743-3707
+ All Star Pediatrics
199 Broad Street/Suite 1-B   Bloomfield, NJ 07003   (973)743-1392   Fax (973)743-3707

Mehta, Sadhana, MD {1386687770} Pedtrc, AdolMd(83,INA69)<NJ-STPETER, NJ-SOMERSET>
+ 498 Union Avenue
Middlesex, NJ 08846   (732)469-4355   Fax (732)469-4392

Mehta, Samir, MD {1003851817} SrgOrt, IntrMd(PA13<PA-UPM-CPHL>
+ Penn Medicine Cherry Hill
1865 Route 70 East/Suite 220   Cherry Hill, NJ 08003   (856)429-1519   Fax (856)427-2933

Mehta, Sanjay, DO {1700084308} Pedtrc(04,NJ75)<NJ-CENTRAST>
+ Central Jersey Emergency Medicine Associates
901 West Main Street   Freehold, NJ 07728   (732)942-2666   Fax (732)431-8267
+ CentraState Medical Center
901 West Main Street/Pedi   Freehold, NJ 07728   (732)431-2000

Mehta, Satish R., MD {1366545402} IntrMd, PulDis(73,INDI)
+ Drs. Mehta and Achar
707 South Orange Avenue   South Orange, NJ 07079   (973)762-4746   Fax (973)762-6862
+ Drs. Mehta and Achar
194 Clinton Avenue   Newark, NJ 07108   (973)762-4746   Fax (973)230-0883

Mehta, Saurabh, MD {1942563994}
+ Cooper University Hospital
One Cooper Plaza   Camden, NJ 08103   (856)342-2000
+ Americare Medical Associates, LLC
445 Whitehorse Avenue/Suite 202   Trenton, NJ 08610   (856)342-2000   Fax (609)585-0309

Mehta, Shiva C., MD {1013310267} Pedtrc, IntrMd(10,GRN01)
+ Summit Medical Group-Berkeley Heights Campus
1 Diamond Hill Road   Berkeley Heights, NJ 07922   (908)277-8601   Fax (908)790-6576
+ Summit Medical Group
574 Springfield Avenue   Westfield, NJ 07090   (908)277-8601   Fax (908)232-0540

Mehta, Siddhart Kumar, MD {1821476003} Nrolgy
+ JFK Neurosciences Institute
65 James Street/Second Floor   Edison, NJ 08818   (732)321-7010   Fax (732)632-1584

Mehta, Sidhartha H., MD {1487969895} IntrMd
+ 131 Passaic Avenue/Unit 6
Nutley, NJ 07110

Mehta, Smita, MD {1043490089} IntrMd(00,OH06)<NY-NYUD-WNTN>
+ Johnson & Johnson
1 Johnson & Johnson/EmpHlth Rm5G32   New Brunswick, NJ 08933   (732)524-3000   Fax (732)828-5493

Mehta, Subhash G., MD {1255312856} IntrMd, FamMed(71,INA87)<NJ-BURDTMLN>
+ 510 Bank Street/Suite 160
Cape May, NJ 08204 (609)884-2121 Fax (609)884-3056
Sgmehta52@hotmail.com
+ 13 Mechanic Street
Cape May Court House, NJ 08210 (609)884-2121 Fax (609)465-2201

Mehta, Sudhir H., MD {1225134661} IntrMd, Nephro(73,INDI)<NJ-HUNTRDN>
+ Somerset Nephrology Associates, P.C.
23 Monroe Street Bridgewater, NJ 08807 (908)722-0106 Fax (908)231-1431
Sudhirm421@optonline.net

Mehta, Sunita, MD {1700846219} Pedtrc(97,GRN01)
+ Lakewood Pediatrics Associates
500 Route 9/3B Lanoka Harbor, NJ 08734 (609)693-8131
+ Lakewood Pediatric Associates
101 Prospect Street/Suite 112 Lakewood, NJ 08701
(609)693-8131 Fax (732)370-0714
+ Lakewood Pediatric Associates
US Highway 9 North Lanoka Harbor, NJ 08734 (609)693-8131 Fax (609)693-3548

Mehta, Taral Divyakant, MD {1043408859} Pedtrc, NnPnMd(86,INA2B)<NJ-ACMCMAIN>
+ AtlantiCare Regional Med Ctr/Mainland
65 West Jimmie Leeds Road/Neonatology Pomona, NJ 08240 (609)652-1000

Mehta, Tejal H., MD {1457642613} Anesth<NJ-RWJUBRUN>
+ Robert Wood Johnson-UMDNJ Anesthesia Group
125 Paterson Street/CAB 3100 New Brunswick, NJ 08901 (732)235-7827 Fax (732)235-6131

Mehta, Uday C., MD {1538135850} Pedtrc, PedNrD, OthrSp(71,INDI)<NJ-CHLSMT>
+ Children's Specialized Hospital
150 New Providence Road Mountainside, NJ 07092 (908)233-3720 Fax (908)301-5456
UMEHTA@childrens-specialized.org

Mehta, Umesh S., MD {1316903818} Psychy(79,INA20)<NJ-CARRIER>
+ Carrier Clinic
252 Route 601/Geriatrics/ECT Belle Mead, NJ 08502
(908)281-1000 Fax (908)281-1423

Mehta, Varsha B., MD {1235229022} Psychy(82,INDI)<NJ-BAYSHORE>
+ 688 North Beers Street/Suite 102
Holmdel, NJ 07733 (732)888-1533

Mehta, Vijay, DO {1942656517} Pedtrc
+ The Cooper Hospital System-Univ Hospital
401 Haddon Avenue Camden, NJ 08103 (856)757-7904 Fax (856)968-9598

Mehta, Vishal, MD {1538353933} Surgry(96,NY09)<NJ-STPETER>
+ 800 Bunn Drive/Suite 303
Princeton, NJ 08540 (732)745-0999 Fax (732)579-4102

Mehta, Vishvesh Mukur, MD {1942243357} Otlryg(00,NY08)<NJ-RBAYOLDB>
+ ENT & Allergy Associates, LLP
485 Route 1 South/Bld B/Suite 350 Iselin, NJ 08830
(732)549-3934 Fax (732)549-7250
+ ENT & Allergy Associates, LLP
3663 Route 9 North/Suite102 Old Bridge, NJ 08857
(732)549-3934 Fax (732)707-3850

Mehta, Vivek M., MD {1114187614} PhysMd(08,GRN01)
+ New Jersey Pain Care Center
44 Route 23 North/Suite 15 B Riverdale, NJ 07457
(973)400-1716 Fax (973)400-1631

Meier, Ronny, MD {1871532200} ObsGyn(72,ISRA)<NJ-HACKNSK, NJ-ENGLWOOD>
+ Drs. Meier and Meier-Ginsberg
35 South Washington Avenue Bergenfield, NJ 07621
(201)385-8350 Fax (201)385-8351
Ronnymeiermd@aol.com

Meier-Ginsberg, Efrat, MD {1578502910} ObsGyn(99,NY46)<NJ-HACKNSK, NJ-HOLYNAME>
+ Drs. Meier and Meier-Ginsberg
35 South Washington Avenue Bergenfield, NJ 07621
(201)385-8350 Fax (201)385-8351

Meigh, Matthew James, DO {1336434208} EmrgMd<NJ-STJOSHOS>
+ St Joseph's Medical Center Emergency
703 Main Street Paterson, NJ 07503 (973)754-2240 Fax (973)754-2249

Meily, Antonio F., Jr., MD {1548281959} IntrMd, NeuMus(81,PHI29)<NJ-KIMBALL, NJ-COMMED>
+ 40 Bey Lea Road/Building B-101
Toms River, NJ 08753 (732)240-9077 Fax (732)240-9227

Meininger, Gary Edward, MD {1558433656} EnDbMt, IntrMd(96,NY19)
+ UH- Robert Wood Johnson Med
125 Paterson Street New Brunswick, NJ 08901 (732)828-3000

Meininger, Michael Eric, MD {1174567010} Gastrn, IntrMd(96,NY19)<NJ-HOLYNAME>
+ Advanced Gastroenterology of Bergen County
140 Sylvan Avenue/Suite 101-A Englewood Cliffs, NJ 07632
(201)945-6564 Fax (201)461-9038

Meinke, Rebecca Lynn, MD {1821256967} Psychy, PsyCAd, IntrMd(06,NJ05)<NJ-UNVMCPRN>
+ Princeton House Behavioral Health- Moorestown
351 New Albany Road Moorestown, NJ 08057 (856)779-2318 Fax (856)608-6941
+ University Medical Center of Princeton at Plainsboro
One Plainsboro Road/Psychiatry Plainsboro, NJ 08536
(609)853-7550

Meirowitz, Robert F., MD {1639179252} Gastrn, IntrMd(84,NY09)<NJ-UNVMCPRN>
+ Princeton Gastroenterology Associates, P.A.
731 Alexander Road/Suite 100 Princeton, NJ 08540
(609)924-1422 Fax (609)924-7473
+ Princeton Endoscopy Center
731 Alexander Road/Suite 104 Princeton, NJ 08540
(609)924-1422 Fax (609)452-1010

Meisel, Mark K., DO {1295830057} FamMed(75,IA75)<NJ-VALLEY>
+ 316 Hamilton Avenue
Glen Rock, NJ 07452 (201)445-8884 Fax (201)445-1932

Meiselas, Karen D., MD {1033382171} Psychy(81,NY09)
+ Integrated Behavioral Care, PA
150 Morristown Road/Plaza 202 Bernardsville, NJ 07924
(908)766-1000 Fax (908)766-0100
+ Integrated Behavioral Care, P.A.
35 Beechwood Road/Suite 3-A & 3-B Summit, NJ 07901
(908)766-1000 Fax (908)598-2408

Meislich, Debrah, MD {1942383989} Pedtrc, PedInf(84,PA01)<NJ-COOPRUMC>
+ Cooper Peds/Children's Regional Ctr
3 Cooper Plaza/Suite 200 Camden, NJ 08103 (856)342-2472 Fax (856)368-8297
+ The Children's Regional Hospital at Cooper Univ Hosp
One Cooper Plaza/InfDisease Camden, NJ 08103
(856)342-2000

Meisner, Errol C., MD {1023000874} IntrMd(63,PA13)<NJ-OVERLOOK>
+ 425 Essex Street
Millburn, NJ 07041 (973)467-0866 Fax (973)467-5485

Meisner, Jay, MD {1982600219} SrgPlstc, Surgry(83,NY47)<NY-BETHPETR, NY-MTSINAI>
+ 680 Kinderkamack Road/Suite 306
Oradell, NJ 07649 (201)483-8880 Fax (201)483-8881

Meisner, Kenneth, MD {1740217850} Surgry(74,SPAI)<NJ-MORRISTN>
+ Northwest Surgical Associates
121 Center Grove Road Randolph, NJ 07869 (973)328-1414 Fax (973)361-1085

Meisner, Patricia Bliss, DO {1932128766} EmrgMd(99,NJ75)<NJ-CHSMRCER, NJ-CHSFULD>
+ Capital Health System/Fuld Campus
750 Brunswick Avenue/EmrgMed Trenton, NJ 08638
(609)394-6000

Mejia, Edgar R., MD {1780645374} Pedtrc(85,COLO)<NJ-STJOSHOS>
+ Kiddie Clinic
760 Market Street Paterson, NJ 07513 (973)523-8083
Fax (973)523-1133
+ 74 Central Avenue
Hackensack, NJ 07601 (973)523-8083 Fax (201)678-9571

Mejia, Gloria, MD {1265692610} Pedtrc(85,COL02)
+ Kiddie Clinic
760 Market Street Paterson, NJ 07513 (973)523-8083
Fax (973)523-1133

Mejia, Joseph Rodrigo, DO {1831362326} PhyMPain, PainInvt(05,WV75)
+ Performance Rehabilitation & Sports Injury Center
459 Watchung Avenue Watchung, NJ 07069 (908)756-2424

Mejias, Erenio, MD {1376603118} IntrMd(77,SPAI)
+ 505 Westfield Avenue
Elizabeth, NJ 07208 (908)354-5461 Fax (908)354-5462

Mekhail, Lilian, MD {1578979720}<NJ-MORRISTN>
+ Morristown Medical Center
100 Madison Avenue Morristown, NJ 07962 (973)971-5000

Mekhjian, Haroutune A., MD {1982810446} Anesth(04,GRN01)<NJ-STJOSHOS>
+ St. Joseph's Regional Medical Center Anesthesia
703 Main Street Paterson, NJ 07503 (973)754-2323 Fax (973)977-9455
+ St. Joseph's Regional Medical Center
703 Main Street/Anesth Paterson, NJ 07503 (973)754-2000

Mekkawy, Ahmed A., MD {1033181680} IntrMd, PulDis(76,EGY16)<NJ-CLARMAAS, NJ-STMRYPAS>
+ 925 Clifton Avenue/Suite 101
Clifton, NJ 07012 (973)778-5070 Fax (973)778-2878

Melamed, Marc S., MD {1033116769} CritCr, IntrMd(77,NY19)<NJ-VALLEY>
+ VMG Respiratory Health & Pulmonary Medicine
1200 East Ridgewood Avenue Ridgewood, NJ 07450
(201)689-7755 Fax (201)689-0521
+ Respiratory Health & Critical Care Associates
1114 Goffle Road/Suite 103 Hawthorne, NJ 07506
(201)689-7755 Fax (973)790-4330
+ The Valley Hospital
223 North Van Dien Avenue Ridgewood, NJ 07450
(201)447-8000

Melamud, Elaine A., MD {1992804553} ObsGyn(97,MA05)
+ 11 Lincoln Boulevard
Clark, NJ 07066 (732)388-1508 Fax (732)388-9040

Melas, Antonia Ana, DO {1326306242} PedCrC<NJ-HACKNSK>
+ Hackensack University Medical Center
30 Prospect Avenue Hackensack, NJ 07601 (551)996-2000

Melchionne Miseo, Christina, MD {1427315068} PedEmg
+ Morristown Medical Center Emergency Medicine
100 Madison Avenue Morristown, NJ 07960 (973)919-5000

Melchiorre, Louis P., Jr., MD {1023096062} Pedtrc(95,PA02)
+ Osborn Family Health Center
1601 Haddon Road Camden, NJ 08103 (856)757-3700
Fax (856)365-7972
+ Lourdes Pediatric Associates
2475 McClellan Avenue/Building B201 Pennsauken, NJ 08109 (856)757-3700 Fax (856)330-6305

Mele, Christopher Mark, MD {1427071067} RadDia(97,NJ05)
+ University Hospital-New Jersey Medical School
30 Bergen Street/Room 1205 Newark, NJ 07107
(973)972-4511

Meleis, Ahmed M., MD {1508132390}
+ 3 Beechwood Grove Court
Holmdel, NJ 07733 (732)888-1363
ahmedmeleis@gmail.com

Meleis, Mohamed E., MD {1396742342} IntrMd(81,EGYP)<NJ-BAYSHORE>
+ Meleis Medical Associates
233 Middle Road/Suite 2 Hazlet, NJ 07730 (732)335-0900
Fax (732)335-8080

Meleka, Matthew, DO {1902283286} IntrMd
+ Jersey Shore University Medical Center
1945 Route 33 Neptune, NJ 07753 (732)775-5500

Melendez, Jody Michael, MD {1639154487} RadDia, Radiol(89,CA02)<NJ-STPETER, NJ-RWJUBRUN>
+ University Radiology Group, P.C.
483 Cranbury Road East Brunswick, NJ 08816 (732)390-0030 Fax (732)390-5383

Melendez Cabrera, Octavio, MD {1770656761} ObsGyn<NJ-HOLYNAME>
+ Women's Health Partners, PC
419 66th Street West New York, NJ 07093 (201)861-9229
Fax (201)861-9272

Melfi, Robert J., MD {1346213998} EnDbMt, IntrMd(83,NY01)<NJ-MORRISTN>
+ Morristown Medical Center
100 Madison Avenue/EndoDiabMt Morristown, NJ 07962
(973)971-5000

Meli, Catherine L., MD {1033188834} Pedtrc(84,ITAL)<NJ-JRSYSHMC>
+ Seashore Pediatrics
1560 Highway 138 West Wall, NJ 07719 (732)449-8592
Fax (732)449-2108

Meli, Gregory M., MD {1649838344} IntrMd(88,ITA17)<NJ-HLTHSRE, NJ-RHBHTNTN>
+ HealthSouth Rehabilitation Hospital of New Jersey
14 Hospital Drive Toms River, NJ 08755 (732)244-3100
+ The Rehab Hosp of Tinton Falls
2 Centre Plaza Tinton Falls, NJ 07724 (732)460-5320

Meli, Lisa A., MD {1841384187} Pedtrc<NJ-VALLEY>
+ Haclensack Bergen Pediatrics
385 Prospect Avenue/Suite 210 Hackensack, NJ 07601
(551)996-9160 Fax (551)996-9165

Melikian, Adrien, MD {1851670129}
+ 7 William Martin Way
Flemington, NJ 08822 (973)669-3294
adrientrent@gmail.com

Melillo, Nicholas G., MD {1033171020} CritCr, IntrMd, PulDis(79,NJ05)<NJ-JFKMED>
+ Middlesex Pulmonary Associates PA
106 James Street Edison, NJ 08820 (732)906-0091 Fax (732)906-0249

Melini, Carlo B., MD {1700932035} Pedtrc, PedDvl(65,PA09)
+ 525 Route 73 South
Marlton, NJ 08053 (856)983-9100 Fax (856)983-9102
kidsmd@aol.com

Physicians by Name and Address

Melisaratos, Darius Paris, MD {1518183938} RadNro, RadDia(87,MA05)
+ Teaneck Radiology Center, LLC.
 699 Teaneck Road   Teaneck, NJ 07666   (201)836-2500   Fax (201)836-0083

Melka, Berhanu Gossaye, MD {1740459874} IntrMd, IntHos(04,ETH03)
+ 5 Raleigh Way
 Freehold, NJ 07728   (617)309-9648

Mellender, Scott Jason, MD {1710135785} Surgry, PainMd, Anesth(01,NY15)<NJ-RWJUBRUN>
+ Robert Wood Johnson-UMDNJ Anesthesia Group
 125 Paterson Street/CAB 3100   New Brunswick, NJ 08901   (732)235-7827   Fax (732)235-6131

Mellendick, George James, MD {1881652824} OccpMd, GPrvMd(74,NJ05)<NJ-HCKTSTWN>
+ Preventive Medicine of NJ Inc
 2 State Route 27/Suite 410   Edison, NJ 08820   (732)906-0016   Fax (732)906-8540
+ Hackettstown Regional Medical Center
 651 Willow Grove Street   Hackettstown, NJ 07840   (908)850-6810

Melli, Jenny, MD {1568690642} IntrMd
+ The Cooper Hospital System-Univ Hospital
 3 Cooper Plaza/Suite 215   Camden, NJ 08103   (856)342-2439

Mellk, Harlan M., MD {1326043647} IntrMd, Nephro(65,PA02)<NJ-STBARNMC, NJ-NWRKBETH>
+ 411 North Ridgewood Road
 South Orange, NJ 07079

Mellody, Sheila M., MD {1770502726}
+ 1005 Riverview Drive
 Brielle, NJ 08730   (732)938-6471
 smmellody@hotmail.com

Mellor, Lisa Marie, MD {1780761387} FamMed(92,NJ06)
+ CentraState Family Medicine Residency Practice
 1001 West Main Street/Suite B   Freehold, NJ 07728   (732)294-2540   Fax (732)294-9328

Mellul, Steven Daniel, DO {1548261605} Ophthl(97,PA77)<NJ-VIRTBERL, NJ-VIRTMARL>
+ Mellul Eye & Facial Plasctic Surgery
 525 Route 73 South/Suite 305A   Marlton, NJ 08053   (856)334-8227   Fax (856)334-8230

Mellul, Victor G., MD {1952331407} Dermat(83,NJ05)<NJ-COOPRUMC, NJ-VIRTVOOR>
+ Dermatology and Skin Care Associates
 200 South Kings Highway   Cherry Hill, NJ 08034   (856)429-9009   Fax (856)429-8400
+ 416 Sicklerville Road
 Sicklerville, NJ 08081   (856)875-8585

Melman, Lora Marie, MD {1689792525} Surgry
+ Advanced Surgical & Bariatrics of NJ, PA
 49 Veronica Avenue/Suite 202   Somerset, NJ 08873   (732)640-5316   Fax (800)689-2361

Melman, Shoshana T., MD {1073564340} Pedtrc, IntrMd(83,PA09)
+ University Hospital-Cares Institute
 42 East Laurel Road/Suite 1100   Stratford, NJ 08084   (856)566-6799   Fax (856)566-6108

Melnick, Gerald J., MD {1760408108} EmrgMd(75,NY06)<NJ-RWJUBRUN, NJ-SOMERSET>
+ Emergency Medical Associates of NJ, P.A.
 3 Century Drive   Parsippany, NJ 07054   (973)740-0607   Fax (973)740-9895

Melnick, Jacob, MD {1619380177} EmrgMd
+ CHCA NJ Emergency at Virtua
 100 Bowman Drive   Voorhees, NJ 08043   (856)247-3000   Fax (609)261-5842

Melnikoff, Barbara, MD {1538232970} ObsGyn(83,ISR02)<NJ-STMRYPAS, NJ-MEADWLND>
+ 123 Franklin Corner Road/Suite 106
 Lawrenceville, NJ 08648

Melograno, Joseph J., DO {1255628707} FamMed, IntrMd(11,NJ75)
+ Morristown Medical Center Family Medicine
 435 South Street/Suite 220-A   Morristown, NJ 07960   (973)971-4222   Fax (973)401-2465

Meloro, Ralph Theodore, MD {1629342670}
+ 13 Mountview Road
 Morris Plains, NJ 07950   (973)539-2447
 ralphmeloro@yahoo.com

Melsky, Lisa, MD {1609950906} IntrMd(87,RUS54)<NJ-WAYNE-GEN>
+ Vita Medical Center
 87 Berdan Avenue   Wayne, NJ 07470   (973)692-9631   Fax (973)692-1112
 lmelsky@optonline.net

Melton, Larry B., MD {1922065812} SrgTpl<NJ-HACKNSK>
+ Hackensack University Medical Center
 30 Prospect Avenue/Trnsplnt   Hackensack, NJ 07601   (551)996-2000
 px64lm@verizon.net

Meltz, Marcy Mencher, MD {1235339722} Anesth(79,NJ06)
+ Digestive Disease Center of New Jersey, LLC
 810 Ryders Lane   East Brunswick, NJ 08816   (732)238-0923   Fax (732)257-0229
+ Ocean Endosurgery Center
 129 Route 37 West   Toms River, NJ 08755   (732)238-0923   Fax (732)797-3963

Meltzer, Alan J., MD {1437126745} Pedtrc(81,NY08)<NJ-MORRISTN, NJ-OVERLOOK>
+ Madison Pediatrics
 435 South Street/Suite 200   Morristown, NJ 07960   (973)822-0003   Fax (973)822-3349

Meltzer, Alfred D., MD {1992707392} Radiol(64,PA09)<NJ-VIRTMHBC>
+ Radiology Associates of Burlington County
 1295 Route 38 West/PO Box 479   Hainesport, NJ 08036   (609)261-7017   Fax (609)261-4180

Meltzer, James Anthony, MD {1548346398} Pedtrc, PedEmg(02,NY46)<NJ-STJOSHOS>
+ St Joseph's Medical Pediactic EmerMed
 703 Main Street   Paterson, NJ 07503   (973)754-2248

Meltzer, Jeffrey I., MD {1437192176} RadOnc, Radiol(72,NY08)<NJ-BURDTMLN, NJ-ACMCMAIN>
+ Cape Regional Medical Center
 2 Stone Harbor Boulevard/Rad Onc   Cape May Court House, NJ 08210   (609)463-2000
+ AtlantiCare Regional Med Ctr/Mainland
 65 West Jimmie Leeds Road/Rad Onc   Pomona, NJ 08240   (609)652-1000

Meltzer, Keith Mitchell, MD {1417939232} Anesth(86,NY08)
+ Red Bank Anesthesia, LLC
 1 Riverview Plaza   Red Bank, NJ 07701   (732)530-2255   Fax (732)450-2620

Meltzer, Michael E., DO {1396784047} FamMed(95,FL75)
+ UMDNJ SOM Family Medicine
 310 Creek Crossing Boulevard   Hainesport, NJ 08036   (609)702-0014   Fax (609)702-7225

Meltzer, Richard B., MD {1366449050} IntrMd(71,SWI01)
+ Barnabas Health Medical Group
 1300 Highway 35 South/Suites 101-103   Ocean, NJ 07712   (732)531-6400   Fax (732)517-0223

Melville, Gordon E., MD {1346246220} Radiol(79,NC01)<NJ-SOMERSET>
+ University Radiology, PA
 239 Route 22 East/Suite 302   Green Brook, NJ 08812   (732)968-4899   Fax (732)968-8096
+ University Radiology Group, P.C.
 3900 Park Avenue/Suite 107   Edison, NJ 08820   (732)968-4899   Fax (732)548-6290
+ University Radiology Group, P.C.
 16 Mountain Boulevard   Warren, NJ 08812   (908)769-7200   Fax (908)769-9141

Melwani, Ramesh D., MD {1174613392} EmrgMd(76,PHI09)
+ PO Box 569
 Franklin Lakes, NJ 07417

Melyokhin, Igor, MD {1336155019} Anesth(80,UKRA)<NY-GOODSAM>
+ Jandee Anesthesiology
 500 North Franklin Turnpike/Suite 206   Ramsey, NJ 07446   (201)962-7282   Fax (201)962-7283

Melzer, Olga Alexandrovna, MD {1740414283} IntrMd(11,RUS32)
+ Obesity Treatment Center
 435 South Street/Suite 330 B   Morristown, NJ 07960   (973)971-7166   Fax (973)290-7518

Memon, Hasan, MD {1447518741} Psychy(12,GRN01)
+ Jersey Shore University Medical Center
 1945 Route 33   Neptune, NJ 07753   (732)775-5500

Memon, Mohammad Khalil, MD {1932101755} IntrMd, CdvDis(69,PAK04)<NJ-JFKMED, NJ-RWJUBRUN>
+ PrimeCare Medical Group
 98 James Street/Suite 300   Edison, NJ 08820   (732)494-6300   Fax (732)494-2490

Memon, Moomal, MD {1538513262} IntrMd
+ AtlantiCare Special Care Center
 54 West Jimmie Leeds Road   Galloway, NJ 08205   (609)404-7300   Fax (609)404-7301

Memon, Mushtaq Ahmed, MD {1780645739} FamMed(90,PAK04)
+ 138 School Street
 Piscataway, NJ 08854

Memon, Nahid, MD {1962427922} IntrMd(93,PAK12)
+ Americare Medical Associates, LLC
 445 Whitehorse Avenue/Suite 202   Trenton, NJ 08610   (609)585-1122   Fax (609)585-0309

Memon, Naureen, MD {1649307091} NnPnMd, Pedtrc, IntrMd(06,NJ02)<NJ-RWJUBRUN>
+ RWJ University Hospital New Brunswick
 One Robert Wood Johnson Place   New Brunswick, NJ 08901   (732)235-5709   Fax (732)235-6609

Memon, Yasmeen Khalique, MD {1114098936} Psychy(84,PAK23)<NJ-MONMOUTH>
+ Monmouth Medical Center
 300 Second Avenue/Psychiatry   Long Branch, NJ 07740   (732)222-5200

Mena, Jessica, DO {1255460275} FamMed
+ Rutgers Hurtado Health Center
 11 Bishop Place   New Brunswick, NJ 08901   (843)832-7402   Fax (732)932-8255

Menack, Michael J., MD {1063455988} Surgry(89,PA09)<NJ-CENTRAST, NJ-COMMED>
+ Advanced Surgical Associates of Central Jersey
 901 West Main Street/MAB Suite 107   Freehold, NJ 07728   (732)303-3837   Fax (732)303-3847

Menacker, Morey J., DO {1629017652} Grtrcs, IntrMd(82,PA77)<NJ-HACKNSK, NJ-VALLEY>
+ Forest HealthCare Associates, PC
 277 Forest Avenue/Suite 200   Paramus, NJ 07652   (201)986-1881   Fax (201)986-1871

Menasha, Joshua Daniel, MD {1295789436} Pedtrc, IntrMd(99,NY47)<NJ-ENGLWOOD, NY-PRSBCOLU>
+ Tenafly Pediatrics, PA
 32 Franklin Street   Tenafly, NJ 07670   (201)569-2400   Fax (201)569-6081
+ Tenafly Pediatrics, PA
 26 Park Place   Paramus, NJ 07652   (201)569-2400   Fax (201)261-8413

Menashe, Richard B., DO {1003989237} GenPrc, FamMed(84,ME75)
+ 15 South Main Street
 Edison, NJ 08837   (732)906-8866   Fax (732)906-0124

Mencel, Peter J., MD {1609858455} IntrMd, MedOnc(82,POL12)<NJ-JRSYSHMC>
+ Atlantic Hematology Oncology Associates, L.L.C.
 1707 Atlantic Avenue   Manasquan, NJ 08736   (732)528-0760   Fax (732)528-0764

Mendel, Howard G., MD {1962444828} Anesth(87,NY48)<NJ-VIRTMHBC>
+ Virtua Memorial
 175 Madison Avenue/Anesthesiology   Mount Holly, NJ 08060   (609)267-0700

Mendelowitz, Paul C., MD {1104830967} PulDis, IntrMd, CritCr(83,DC01)<NJ-HOLYNAME>
+ 42 Whitney Hill
 Park Ridge, NJ 07656

Mendelsohn, Jason, MD {1083118913}
+ Mountainside Family Practice Associates
 799 Bloomfield Avenue/Suite 201   Verona, NJ 07044   (973)746-7050   Fax (973)857-2831

Mendelsohn, Mary E., MD {1720161888} Ophthl, VitRet(89,NY48)<NJ-VALLEY>
+ Woodcliff Lake Ophthalmology
 577 Chestnut Ridge Road   Woodcliff Lake, NJ 07677   (201)782-1700   Fax (201)782-1749

Mendelson, Joel S., MD {1477612950} Allrgy, PedInf, AlgyImmn(82,DOMI)<NJ-NWRKBETH, NJ-OVERLOOK>
+ 1124 Springfield Avenue
 Mountainside, NJ 07092   (908)233-4477   Fax (908)233-3774
+ Newark Beth Israel Medical Center
 201 Lyons Avenue/Allergy/Immun   Newark, NJ 07112   (973)926-8004

Mendelson, Joshua Todd, MD {1265641070} Psychy, Nrolgy
+ Neurology Specialists of Monmouth County
 107 Monmouth Road/Suite 110   West Long Branch, NJ 07764   (732)935-1850   Fax (732)544-0494
+ 1604 Holdbrook Streett
 Oakhurst, NJ 07755

Mendelson, Stuart G., MD {1932175411} Nrolgy(85,NJ05)
+ Neurology Associates
 1140 Bloomfield Avenue/Suite 207   West Caldwell, NJ 07006   (973)227-3344   Fax (973)227-6325

Mendes, John F., MD {1558434803} SrgOrt(76,NY20)<NJ-MTN-SIDE, NJ-STBARNMC>
+ Active Orthopaedics & Sports Medicine
 440 Old Hook Road   Emerson, NJ 07630   (201)358-0707   Fax (201)358-9777
+ Montclair Orthopedic Group PA
 200 Highland Avenue   Glen Ridge, NJ 07028   (201)358-0707   Fax (973)429-2174

Mendez, Jorge G., MD {1356463988} AnesPain, Anesth(03,NJ02)
+ Ivy League Pain Management Center
 9 Crestfield Road   Boonton, NJ 07005   (908)255-6200

Mendez Morales, Alba Nydia, MD {1992914147} Pedtrc
+ 172 Washington Street/Apt 5B
 Bloomfield, NJ 07003

Mendiola, Redentor S., Jr., MD {1710974654} IntrMd, InfDis(93,PHI09)<NJ-OVERLOOK, NJ-MORRISTN>
+ Summit Medical Group-Berkeley Heights Campus
 1 Diamond Hill Road   Berkeley Heights, NJ 07922   (908)273-4300   Fax (908)277-8825

Physicians by Name and Address

Mendis, Kalanie, MD {1407053291} IntrMd, Nephro<NJ-MONMOUTH>
+ Princeton Kidney Care LLC
10 Forrestal Road South/Suite 100   Princeton, NJ 08540
(732)301-4767   Fax (732)626-7600
+ Edison Nephrology Consultants, LLC.
34-36 Progress Street/Suite A-7   Edison, NJ 08820
(732)301-4767   Fax (908)769-0945

Menditto, Darren, DO {1972535516} EmrgMd(01,PA77)<NJ-VIRTVOOR>
+ Virtua Voorhees
100 Bowman Drive/EmrgMed   Voorhees, NJ 08043
(856)247-3000   Fax (856)325-3197

Mendler, James Christopher, MD {1407818032} FamMSptM, IntrMd(94,NJ05)<NJ-VALLEY>
+ 514 Kinderkamack Road
Oradell, NJ 07649   (201)833-3909   Fax (201)833-7073

Mendola, John V., MD {1659388353} IntrMd(72,PA09)
+ Drs. Kaid & Tanwir
2168 Millburn Avenue/Suite 204   Maplewood, NJ 07040
(973)762-3353   Fax (973)762-3370

Mendoza, Adiofel Mark Fidellaga, MD {1144631623} IntrMd<NJ-OVERLOOK>
+ Overlook Medical Center
99 Beauvoir Avenue/PO Box 210   Summit, NJ 07902
(908)522-2000

Mendoza, Concepcion B., MD {1649249707} GenPrc(74,PHI09)
+ Drs. Mendoza & Mendoza
9 Mule Road/Suite E-5   Toms River, NJ 08755   (732)240-3710   Fax (732)240-3783

Mendoza, Justin, DO {1316101389} PhysMd(08,NY75)<NY-JTORTHO>
+ Active Orthopaedics & Sports Medicine
440 Old Hook Road   Emerson, NJ 07630   (201)358-0707   Fax (201)358-9777

Mendoza, Luis, MD {1225011950} Ophthl(65,COL24)<NJ-STJOSHOS>
+ Passaic Vision Center, LLC
289 Monroe Street   Passaic, NJ 07055   (973)473-5151   Fax (973)473-3331

Mendoza, Lynette Maria, DO {1023348596} Surgry<NJ-HOLYNAME>
+ Holy Name Hospital
718 Teaneck Road   Teaneck, NJ 07666   (201)833-3357   Fax (201)541-5972

Mendoza, Narciso D., MD {1972679835} Allrgy, AlgyImmn(74,PHIL)<NJ-COMMED>
+ Drs. Mendoza & Mendoza
9 Mule Road/Suite E-5   Toms River, NJ 08755   (732)240-3710   Fax (732)240-3783
+ 900 Newark Avenue
Forked River, NJ 08731   (732)240-3710   Fax (732)240-3783

Mendoza, Pierre J., MD {1841460821} Urolgy, OthrSp<NJ-JRSYSHMC, NJ-MONMOUTH>
+ Coastal Urology Associates
446 Jack Martin Boulevard   Brick, NJ 08724   (732)840-4300   Fax (732)840-4515
+ Coastal Urology Associates
444 Neptune Boulevard/Suite 3   Neptune, NJ 07753   (732)840-4300   Fax (732)988-8996
+ Coastal Urology Associates
814 River Avenue   Lakewood, NJ 08724   (732)370-2250   Fax (732)901-9119

Mendrinos, Savvas E., MD {1760429070} Pthlgy(94,GREE)<NY-NYUTISCH>
+ Inform Diagnostics
825 Rahway Avenue   Union, NJ 07083   (732)901-7575   Fax (732)901-1555

Mendu, Srinivas, MD {1245235126} IntrMd(84,INA11)<NJ-JFKMED>
+ Garden State Physicians P.C.
10 Jefferson Plaza/Suite 100   Princeton, NJ 08540
(732)274-1274   Fax (732)355-0321
+ Garden State Physicians P.C.
1002 Amboy Avenue   Edison, NJ 08837   (732)274-1274   Fax (732)355-0321
+ Garden State Physicians P.C.
21 Jefferson Plaza   Princeton, NJ 08540   (732)274-1274   Fax (732)355-0321

Menell, Jill Suzanne, MD {1831137876} PedHem, Pedtrc(87,NY08)<NJ-STJOSHOS>
+ St. Joseph Medical Center Pediatric Hematology/Onc
703 Main Street/Xavier-700   Paterson, NJ 07503   (973)754-3230   Fax (973)754-3331

Menendez, Christine M., MD {1669493136} RadDia(95,NJ05)<NJ-MORRISTN>
+ Memorial Radiology Associates
10 Lanidex Plaza West/Suite 125   Parsippany, NJ 07054
(973)503-5700   Fax (973)386-5701

Menet, Scott Douglas, DO {1366547606} EmrgMd(98,PA77)<NJ-ACMCITY, NJ-ACMCMAIN>
+ AtlantiCare Regional Medical Center/City Campus
1925 Pacific Avenue/EmergMed   Atlantic City, NJ 08401
(609)345-4000

Menghetti, Richard A., MD {1235247370} RadDia, Radiol, RadBdl(80,MEXI)<NJ-SHOREMEM, NJ-ACMCITY>
+ Atlantic Medical Imaging, LLC.
72 West Jimmie Leeds Road   Galloway, NJ 08205
(609)677-9729   Fax (609)653-8764
+ Atlantic Medical Imaging, LLC.
401 Bethel Road   Somers Point, NJ 08244   (609)677-9729
+ Atlantic Medical Imaging, LLC.
421 Route 9 North   Cape May Court House, NJ 08205
(609)463-9500   Fax (609)465-0918

Menken, Gregory E., MD {1740283167} NnPnMd(82,NY08)<NJ-STJOSHOS>
+ St. Joseph's Regional Medical Center
703 Main Street/Neonatology   Paterson, NJ 07503
(973)754-2000   Fax (973)754-2567
menkeng@sjhmc.org

Menkin, Serge, MD {1881670784} PhysMd, PainMd, IntrMd(00,GRN01)
+ Petraacco Chiropractic Center, P.A.
311 Newark Avenue   Jersey City, NJ 07302   (201)533-0055   Fax (201)533-0066
+ Holmdel Health Center
670 North Beers Street   Holmdel, NJ 07733   (201)533-0055   Fax (732)757-0824

Menkowitz, Marc Scott, MD {1710179114} SrgOrt(02,PA13)
+ 1131 Broad Street/Suite 201
Shrewsbury, NJ 07702   (732)380-1212

Menon, Aditi Sen, MD {1619125150} PhyMPain(04,NY08)
+ 1740 East 2nd Street
Scotch Plains, NJ 07076   (973)382-5002   Fax (908)322-1120
aditimenon.md@gmail.com

Menon, Divya, MD {1730327834} IntrMd(02,INA3Y)
+ Heart Specialists/Central Jersey
901 West Main Street/Suite 205   Freehold, NJ 07728
(732)866-0800   Fax (732)463-6082
+ Heart Specialists/Central Jersey
901 West Main Street/Suite 205   Freehold, NJ 07728
(732)866-0800   Fax (732)463-6082

Menon, Sujoy, MD {1154556835} RadV&I, IntrMd(08,NJ06)<NJ-CHRIST>
+ Christ Hospital
176 Palisade Avenue/Rad Imag   Jersey City, NJ 07306
(732)447-8095

Mensah, Virginia Akua, MD {1831416403} ObsGyn<RI-WOMINFAN>
+ Eatontown Fertility Clinic
234 Industrial Way West/Suite A104   Eatontown, NJ 07724
(732)918-2500

Mentle, Iris R., MD {1922054022} CdvDis, IntrMd(91,NY48)<NJ-CENTRAST>
+ Heart Specialists/Central Jersey
901 West Main Street/Suite 205   Freehold, NJ 07728
(732)866-0800   Fax (732)463-6082
+ 555 Iron Bridge Road/Suite 16
Freehold, NJ 07728   (732)866-0800   Fax (732)683-1044

Menza, Matthew A., MD {1356429633} Psychy(80,PA13)<NJ-RWJUBRUN>
+ University Behavioral Health Care
671 Hoes Lane/PO Box 1392/Rm D205A   Piscataway, NJ 08855   (732)235-4176   Fax (732)235-5158
+ UH- Robert Wood Johnson Med
125 Paterson Street   New Brunswick, NJ 08901   (732)235-4176   Fax (732)235-7677

Meo, Francis W., MD {1275575011} IntrMd(75,ITAL)<NJ-HACKNSK>
+ 18 Redneck Avenue/Suite 1
Little Ferry, NJ 07643   (201)489-1234

Meoli, Fredrick G., DO {1790970804} Surgry(68,MO78)
+ 87 Harrowgate Drive
Cherry Hill, NJ 08003   Fax (856)424-2128

Meradian, Ara, MD {1184731705} PthAcl(88,SYRI)<NJ-MORRISTN>
+ Morristown Medical Center
100 Madison Avenue   Morristown, NJ 07962   (973)971-5000   Fax (973)290-7370

Merati, Kambiz, MD {1427121581} PthHem, PthAcl(95,IRA01)
+ Bio-Reference Laboratory, Inc.
481 Edward H. Ross Drive   Elmwood Park, NJ 07407
(201)791-2600   Fax (201)791-1941

Mercadante, Zorica Jelisijevic, MD {1285614586} IntrMd(93,NJ05)
+ Barnabas Health Medical Group
166 Morris Avenue/2nd Floor   Long Branch, NJ 07740
(732)263-5024   Fax (732)263-5029
+ 103 Parker Road/Suite B
West Long Branch, NJ 07764   (732)263-5024   Fax (732)923-1772

Mercado, Alex M., MD {1093893232} IntrMd(93,NJ05)<NJ-HCK-TSTWN, NJ-MORRISTN>
+ Washington Family Medicine PC
191 US Highway 206   Flanders, NJ 07836   (973)584-0045   Fax (973)584-0094

Mercado, Donna M., MD {1780682369} FamMed, EmrgMd(76,MEXI)<NJ-HOBUNIMC>
+ 330 Grand Street
Hoboken, NJ 07030   (201)420-1266   Fax (201)420-3374

Mercado, Melissa, DO {1821587270} FamMed<NJ-CHRIST>
+ Christ Hospital
176 Palisade Avenue   Jersey City, NJ 07306   (201)795-8200

Mercedes Salas, Aixell Josefina, MD {1013127372} Pedtrc, IntrMd
+ Advocare DelGiorno Pediatrics
535 South Black Horse Pike   Blackwood, NJ 08012
(856)228-1061   Fax (856)228-1907
+ Tender Care Pediatrics
2322 New Road   Northfield, NJ 08225   (609)641-0200

Mercer, Geraldine O., MD {1588688352} Pthlgy, PthACl, PthCyt(87,NJ05)<NJ-MORRISTN>
+ Morristown Medical Center
100 Madison Avenue/Path   Morristown, NJ 07962
(973)971-5000

Mercer, Stephen Edward, MD {1740449297} PthAna
+ Drs. Kessel & Mercer
1700 White Horse Hamilton Road   Hamilton Square, NJ 08690   (609)890-2600   Fax (609)890-0265

Merchant, Amit, DO {1861623241} PedOrt
+ Hackensack MC Pediatric Orthopedics
30 Prospect Avenue   Hackensack, NJ 07601   (551)996-4334

Merchant, Aziz M., MD {1053595637} Surgry
+ Rutgers- New Jersey Medical School
185 South Orange Avenue   Newark, NJ 07103   (973)972-0072

Merchant, Neepa S., MD {1629120100} FamMed(98,INA5Y)<NJ-SOMERSET>
+ 378 South Branch Road/Suite te 302
Hillsborough, NJ 08844   (908)290-0404   Fax (908)933-0954

Merchant, Prakriti Singh, MD {1447546775}
+ Advanced Gastroenterology Group
1308 Morris Avenue   Union, NJ 07083   (908)851-2770   Fax (908)851-7706

Merchant, Sameer R., MD {1982686077} Anesth(77,INA69)<NJ-MORRISTN>
+ 12 Jacob Arnold Road
Morristown, NJ 07960

Merchant, Yatish B., MD {1598786246} CdvDis, IntrMd(82,INA69)<NJ-ACMCMAIN, NJ-BACHARCH>
+ AtlantiCare Physicians
318 Chris Gaupp Drive/Suite 100   Galloway, NJ 08205
(609)404-9900   Fax (609)404-3653

Mercogliano, Edward A., MD {1285738229} Surgry(71,NJ06)
+ 181 Franklin Avenue/Suite 305
Nutley, NJ 07110   (973)284-0370   Fax (973)667-8547

Mercurio, Carl F., MD {1982601662} SrgOrt(75,ITA01)<NJ-CLAR-MAAS>
+ 36 Newark Avenue/Suite 200
Belleville, NJ 07109   (973)751-3222   Fax (973)751-1040

Mercuro, Tobia J., MD {1851320634} CdvDis, IntrMd, IntCrd(85,NJ06)<NJ-UNVMCPRN>
+ Princeton Interventional Cardiology
800 Bunn Drive/Suite 101   Princeton, NJ 08540   (609)921-2800   Fax (609)921-3499

Mereday, Clifton Samuel, Jr., MD {1366533077} Anesth(92,PA09)
+ James Street Anesthesia
102 James Street/Suite 103   Edison, NJ 08820   (732)494-1444   Fax (732)494-7052

Meredith, Jacob M., MD {1275578122} EmrgMd(78,NC05)<NJ-COMMED, NJ-SOCEANCO>
+ Community Medical Center
99 Route 37 West   Toms River, NJ 08755   (732)557-8060

Meremikwu, Francisca Chinwe, MD {1235150509} ObsGyn(00,NJ06)
+ Newark Community Health Center, Inc.
444 William Street   East Orange, NJ 07017   (973)675-1900   Fax (973)675-4021

Merewitz, Glenn S., MD {1417981614} EmrgMd, IntrMd(77,MD01)<NJ-ACMCMAIN, NJ-ACMCITY>
+ AtlantiCare Regional Med Ctr/Mainland
65 West Jimmie Leeds Road/EmergMed   Pomona, NJ 08240
(609)652-1000
+ AtlantiCare Regional Medical Center/City Campus
1925 Pacific Avenue/EmergMed   Atlantic City, NJ 08401
(609)345-4000

Merikhi, Laleh Afkham, MD {1982865853} Gastrn
+ Monmouth Gastroenterology
142 Route 35   Eatontown, NJ 07724   (732)389-5004   Fax (732)389-1850

Physicians by Name and Address

Meritz, Keith A., MD {1801956974} RadOnc(83,PA07)
+ Cancer Treatment Center
2090 Springdale Road/Suite B   Cherry Hill, NJ 08003
(856)325-2500   Fax (856)751-3243

Merjanian, Lena L., MD {1902076839} ObsGyn(04,NJ06)
+ UH- Robert Wood Johnson Med
125 Paterson Street/CAB/Suite 4200   New Brunswick, NJ 08901   (732)828-3000   Fax (732)235-6650

Merkel, Ira S., MD {1336146125} Gastrn, IntrMd(84,MEX03)<NJ-RWJUBRUN, NJ-STPETER>
+ Digestive Disease Center of New Jersey, LLC
33 Clyde Road/Suite 102   Somerset, NJ 08873   (732)873-9200   Fax (732)873-1699
+ Digestive Disease Center of New Jersey, LLC
810 Ryders Lane   East Brunswick, NJ 08816   (732)873-9200   Fax (732)257-0229

Merkin, Michael D., MD {1669548079} Nrolgy(85,NJ06)<NJ-JFKMED, NJ-RWJURAH>
+ Edison Neurologic Associates
36 Progress Street/Suite B-3   Edison, NJ 08820   (908)757-6633   Fax (908)757-3912

Merkle, Jeffrey, MD {1295721165} IntrMd, Pedtrc(00,NJ06)
+ 254 B Mountain Avenue/Suite 304
Hackettstown, NJ 07840   (908)852-6400   Fax (908)852-6450

Merle, Francois, MD {1912293127} Anesth
+ Hackensack University MC-Anesthesia Dept
30 Prospect Avenue/Room 2703   Hackensack, NJ 07601   (551)996-2419   Fax (201)996-3962

Merle, Nancy, MD {1003921594} FamMed(79,PRO01)
+ Southern Jersey Family Medical Centers Inc.
932 South Main Street   Pleasantville, NJ 08232   (609)383-0880   Fax (609)383-0658
+ Southern Jersey Family Medical Centers, Inc.
860 South White Horse Pike/Building A   Hammonton, NJ 08037   (609)383-0880   Fax (609)567-3492

Merlin, Francky, MD {1740468784} Nephro, IntrMd(79,ARG03)<NJ-STPETER>
+ Excel Medical Care, LLC
1 Williams Road   Kendall Park, NJ 08824   (732)422-0413   Fax (732)422-0439

Merlin, Mark A., DO {1093725822} EmrgMd(94,PA77)<NJ-STMICHL>
+ Drs. Delaney, Merlin & Pourmasiha
66 West Gilbert Street/2nd Floor   Tinton Falls, NJ 07701   (732)212-0051   Fax (732)212-0713

Merlin, Scott, MD {1124244009}
+ 3 Dorothy Avenue
Livingston, NJ 07039

Merlino, John Anthony, III, DO {1811013246} CdvDis, IntrMd, OthrSp(00,NJ75)<NJ-DEBRAHLC>
+ Monmouth Medical Group, P.C
780 Route 37 West/Suite 120   Toms River, NJ 08755   (732)736-5694   Fax (732)244-1860

Merlo, Angela, MD {1851494264} Gastrn, IntrMd, PedGst(82,NY46)<NJ-CAPITLHS, NJ-STPETER>
+ Digestive Health & Nutrition Center
2 Princess Road   Lawrenceville, NJ 08648   (609)896-0800   Fax (609)896-1330
+ Digestive Health & Nutrition Center
1520 Route 130   North Brunswick, NJ 08902   (609)896-0800   Fax (609)896-1330
+ Cares Surgicenter, LLC.
240 Easton Avenue   New Brunswick, NJ 08648   (732)565-5400   Fax (732)296-8677

Mermelstein, Erwin, MD {1538102843} CdvDis, IntrMd(78,NY20)<NJ-RWJUBRUN, NJ-STPETER>
+ Cardiology Associates of New Brunswick
593 Cranbury Road/Suite 2   East Brunswick, NJ 08816   (732)390-3333   Fax (732)967-8770

Mero, Raymond J., DO {1144344649} Psychy(90,ME75)
+ 4 Stone Meadow Road
Annandale, NJ 08801   (908)236-7450

Merola, Rose Mary, MD {1003882606} PedDvl, Pedtrc, Ped-NrD(81,DOM02)<NJ-CHLSMT>
+ Children's Specialized Hospital
150 New Providence Road   Mountainside, NJ 07092   (908)233-3720   Fax (908)301-5456

Merriam, Margaret, DO {1083867147} Surgry
+ LMA Surgical Associates
120 White Horse Pike/Suite 103   Haddon Heights, NJ 08035   (856)546-3900   Fax (856)546-9308

Merriam, Zachary M., DO {1740476563} ObsGyn(07,NY75)
+ Comprehensive Women's Care
401A South Van Brunt Street/Suite 405   Englewood, NJ 07631   (201)871-4346   Fax (201)871-5953

Merz, Daniel Francis, DO {1639378102} EmrgMd(05,NJ75)<NJ-ACMCITY>
+ AtlantiCare Regional Medical Center/City Campus
1925 Pacific Avenue/Emerg Med   Atlantic City, NJ 08401   (609)441-8127   Fax (609)441-8021

Mesa, John Mario, MD {1982783890} SrgRec, IntrMd(01,COL03)
+ Plastic Surgery Center Internationale
89 Valley Road   Montclair, NJ 07042   (973)746-3535   Fax (973)746-4385

Mesad, Salah Mohammed, MD {1053390872} Eplpsy, ClNrPh, Nrolgy(87,GER55)
+ Northeast Regional Epilepsy Group
20 Prospect Avenue/Suite 800   Hackensack, NJ 07601   (201)343-6676   Fax (201)343-6689

Mesham, James R., MD {1609989821} RadDia, RadBdl(82,SAF04)<NJ-ACMCMAIN, NJ-ACMCITY>
+ Atlantic Medical Imaging, LLC.
72 West Jimmie Leeds Road   Galloway, NJ 08205   (609)677-9729   Fax (609)653-8764
+ Atlantic Medical Imaging, LLC.
401 Bethel Road   Somers Point, NJ 08244   (609)677-9729
+ Atlantic Medical Imaging, LLC.
421 Route 9 North   Cape May Court House, NJ 08205   (609)463-9500   Fax (609)465-0918

Meshko, Yanina, MD {1295783421} Pedtrc(84,RUS54)<NJ-STBARNMC, NJ-MORRISTN>
+ Drs. Gruenwald & Comandatore
90 Millburn Avenue/Suite 101   Millburn, NJ 07041   (973)378-7990   Fax (973)378-7991

Meshkov, Steven L., MD {1003812413} RadDia, RadV&I(78,PA13)<NJ-STFRNMED>
+ Radiology Affiliates of Central New Jersey, P.A.
2501 Kuser Road   Hamilton, NJ 08691   (609)585-8800   Fax (609)585-1825
+ Radiology Affiliates of Central New Jersey, P.A.
3120 Princeton Pike   Lawrenceville, NJ 08648   (609)585-8800   Fax (609)219-0439

Mesina, Leon B., MD {1235173428} Pedtrc(84,PHIL)<NJ-RBAYOLDB, NJ-STPETER>
+ Mesina Pediatrics, LLC
2477 Route 516/Suite 202   Old Bridge, NJ 08857   (732)679-0400   Fax (732)679-0445

Meskin, Inna, MD {1548225709} Pedtrc(90,RUSS)<NJ-NWTNMEM>
+ Skylands Pediatrics
328-A Sparta Avenue   Sparta, NJ 07871   (973)729-2197   Fax (973)729-3653
+ Skylands Pediatrics
4 Oxbow Lane/Route 94   Franklin, NJ 07416   (973)729-2197   Fax (973)827-5093

Meskin, Steven J., MD {1851335285} FamMed(90,SAF01)<NJ-KMHTURNV, NJ-UNDRWD>
+ General Practitioners, P.A.
601 North Main Street   Glassboro, NJ 08028   (856)881-1330   Fax (856)881-6982

Meslin, Keith Phillip, MD {1477554780} Surgry, SrgC&R(99,NY09)<NJ-VIRTUAHS, NJ-OURLADY>
+ Virtua Surgical Group, PA
1935 Route 70 East   Cherry Hill, NJ 08003   (856)428-7700   Fax (856)424-9120

Mesnard, William J., MD {1467559617} Rheuma, IntrMd(82,VA04)<NJ-STBARNMC>
+ 116 Millburn Avenue
Millburn, NJ 07041   (973)376-2545   Fax (973)467-4207
+ 6 Sandhill Road
Flemington, NJ 08822   (908)237-1144

Messa, Stephanie Price, MD {1881869188} Anesth(04,SC01)
+ 8 Huxley Court
Marlboro, NJ 07746

Messihi, Jean, MD {1174537419} InfDis, IntrMd(75,LEBA)<NJ-PALISADE, NJ-HOBUNIMC>
+ Carepoint Health Medical Group
331 Grand Street/Ground Floor   Hoboken, NJ 07030   (201)238-2888   Fax (201)656-5989

Messimer, Julie Marie, MD {1649497967} ObsGyn(05,NET09)
+ Donato S. Russo MD LLC
1896 Morris Avenue/Suite 3   Union, NJ 07083   (908)687-8282

Messina, Charles I., MD {1326139072} FamMed(72,MEX14)
+ The Doctor Is in
59 Old Highway 22   Clinton, NJ 08809   (908)730-6363   Fax (908)730-8185

Messina, John Joseph, MD {1922186311} PedCrd, Pedtrc(86,GRNA)<NJ-STJOSHOS>
+ St. Joseph's Children's Hospital
703 Main Street/PediCardiology   Paterson, NJ 07503   (973)754-2529
+ Pediatric Cardiology Associates
1 Broadway/Suite 203   Elmwood Park, NJ 07407   (973)754-2529   Fax (973)569-6270

Messo, Ralph K., Jr., DO {1255309175} IntrMd, Pedtrc(89,ME75)<NJ-CENTRAST>
+ 245A Main Street
Matawan, NJ 07747   (732)765-9500

Messori, Divo Angelo, MD {1366496226} Gastrn
+ Volunteers in Medicine
423 North Route 9   Cape May Court House, NJ 08210   (609)463-2846   Fax (609)463-2830

Mest, Stuart, MD {1720080559} PulDis, CritCr, IntrMd(84,PA14)<NY-SOUTHAMP, NJ-VIRTBERL>
+ Pulmonary & Sleep Associates of SJ, LLC.
811 Sunset Road/Suite 201   Burlington, NJ 08016   (609)298-1776   Fax (609)531-2391

Meszaros, Beata Duli, MD {1811146004} Pedtrc(86,HUN03)<NJ-JFKMED>
+ JFK Medical Center
65 James Street/Children'sServ   Edison, NJ 08820   (732)321-7010   Fax (732)906-4906
moszika@msn.com

Meta, Joubin, DO {1326280058} EmrgMd<NJ-CHRIST>
+ Christ Hospital
176 Palisade Avenue   Jersey City, NJ 07306   (201)795-8200

Meta, Shimbul Shashikant, DO {1326354283} EmrgMd
+ 22 Avenue at Port Imperial/Unit 414
West New York, NJ 07093

Metelitsin, Marina Nikolaevna, MD {1619048238} Psychy(83,UKR12)<NJ-HCMEADPS>
+ Mim Medical PC
11 Mackay Avenue   Paramus, NJ 07652   (201)587-0380   Fax (201)587-0384
+ Hudson County Meadowview Psychiatric Hospital
595 County Avenue   Secaucus, NJ 07094   (201)319-3660

Methvin, Laura, MD {1275066268} IntrMd
+ 110 Somerset Street/Apt 1513
New Brunswick, NJ 08901   (302)377-9359

Metri Mansour, Elie E., MD {1356314280} IntrMd, PulDis(90,LEBA)<NJ-BAYSHORE, NJ-RIVERVW>
+ Central Jersey Pulmonary & Medical Associates
719 North Beers Street/Suites 2E-2F   Holmdel, NJ 07733   (732)264-1001   Fax (732)264-4495

Metro, Wade E., MD {1164473047} Anesth(85,MI07)<NJ-ENGLWOOD>
+ Englewood Hospital and Medical Center
350 Engle Street/Anesthesiology   Englewood, NJ 07631   (201)894-3000   Fax (201)871-0619

Metrus, Nicholas Robert, MD {1356785067} Nrolgy
+ Atlantic Neuroscience Institute at Overlook Hospital
99 Beauvoir Avenue   Summit, NJ 07901   (908)522-5914

Metz, Deborah Lynne, MD {1104987866} FamMed(96,PA02)<NJ-JFKMED>
+ JFK Family Practice Group
65 James Street   Edison, NJ 08818   (732)321-7487   Fax (732)906-4927

Metz, John Patrick, MD {1386705127} FamMed, SprtMd(94,PA02)
+ JFK Family Practice Group
65 James Street   Edison, NJ 08818   (732)321-7488   Fax (732)906-4927

Metz, Rebecca L., MD {1295018133} ObsGyn
+ Durham Women's Center
4 Ethel Road/Suite 402-B   Edison, NJ 08817   (732)287-3643   Fax (973)939-0281

Metzger, Scott E., MD {1730171133} PainMd, Anesth, Anes-Pain(92,MA05)<NJ-RIVERVW, NJ-BAYSHORE>
+ Premier Pain Center
160 Avenue at the Commons/Suite 1   Shrewsbury, NJ 07702   (732)380-0200   Fax (732)380-0124
+ Ultimed HealthCare PC
50 Franklin Lane   Manalapan, NJ 07726   (732)380-0200   Fax (732)972-1026

Meulener, Marc C., MD {1770739633}
+ 768 Springfield Avenue/Unit E-7
Summit, NJ 07901   (908)285-3301

Meusburger, Charles E., MD {1699849505} Psychy(85,ITA17)
+ 3069 English Creek Avenue/Suite 225
Egg Harbor Township, NJ 08234   (609)484-0770   Fax (609)484-0701

Mevs, Stacy Reed, MD {1932249356} FamMed(90,TN07)<NJ-NWRKBETH>
+ Rhomur Medical Services
297 16th Avenue   Newark, NJ 07103   (973)374-3020

Meyer, Ariel, DO {1083887129} Nephro, IntrMd(02,NJ75)<NJ-JRSYSHMC, NJ-OCEANMC>
+ Ocean Renal Associates, P.A.
210 Jack Martin Boulevard/Suite D-1   Brick, NJ 08724   (732)458-5854   Fax (732)458-8012
+ Ocean Renal Associates, P.A.
508 Lakehurst Road/Suite 3 A   Toms River, NJ 08755   (732)458-5854   Fax (732)341-4993
+ Ocean Renal Associates, P.A.
1145 Beacon Avenue/Suite B   Manahawkin, NJ 08724   (609)978-9940   Fax (609)978-9902

Meyer, Carissa Leigh, MD {1831324227} SrgHnd(MA07
+ Active Orthopaedics & Sports Medicine
440 Old Hook Road   Emerson, NJ 07630   (201)358-0707   Fax (201)358-9777

Meyer, Daniel Karl, MD {1306920749} InfDis(93,PA02)
+ The Cooper Hospital System-Univ Hospital
401 Haddon Avenue   Camden, NJ 08103   (856)342-2000

Meyer, Jacqueline Marie, MD {1508853441} IntrMd(00,PA02)<NJ-OVERLOOK>
+ Summit Medical Group-Berkeley Heights Campus
1 Diamond Hill Road/3rd Fl   Berkeley Heights, NJ 07922
(908)277-8683   Fax (908)608-2378

Meyer, Marc Andrew, MD {1467573907} PedAne, Pedtrc, IntrMd(04,NY20)<NJ-HACKNSK>
+ St. Joseph's Regional Medical Center Anesthesia
703 Main Street   Paterson, NJ 07503   (973)754-2323   Fax (973)977-9455

Meyer, Monica Ann, MD {1790759603} FamMed(90,PA02)<NJ-HUNTRDN>
+ Phillips Barber Family Health Center
72 Alexander Avenue   Lambertville, NJ 08530   (609)397-3535   Fax (609)397-0301

Meyer, Monica Lynn, MD {1285638825} ObsGyn(91,NY08)<NJ-VALLEY>
+ The Woman's Group/Bergen Medical Associates
1 West Ridgewood Avenue/Suite 211   Paramus, NJ 07652
(201)251-2323   Fax (201)251-2325
+ The Breslow Center for Plastic Surgery
1 West Ridgewood Avenue/Suite 110   Paramus, NJ 07652
(201)251-2323   Fax (201)444-9277

Meyer, Sarah E., MD {1992962351} Psychy, IntrMd(06,NY20)
+ Sheila Harrington, LCSW
8 Hillside Avenue/Suite 106   Montclair, NJ 07042
(973)509-2371   Fax (973)744-9003

Meyer, Scott Andrew, MD {1518126242} SrgNro(04,RI01)
+ Atlantic Neurosurgical Specialists
310 Madison Avenue/Suite 300   Morristown, NJ 07960
(973)285-7800   Fax (973)285-7839

Meyer, Shira Asekoff, DO {1497799209} Gastrn, IntrMd(02,NY75)<NJ-VALLEY>
+ Family Practice of CentraState
479 Newman Springs Rd/Suite A-101   Marlboro, NJ 07746
(732)780-1601
+ Bergen Medical Associates
466 Old Hook Road/Suite 1   Emerson, NJ 07630   (732)780-1601   Fax (201)967-0340
+ Ocean Health Initiatives, Inc.
301 Lakehurst Road   Toms River, NJ 07746   (732)552-0377   Fax (732)552-0378

Meyer-Grimes, Leslie B., MD {1821133992} FamMed, Bariat, AltnMd(77,MEXI)
+ 259 Brass Castle Road
Oxford, NJ 07863   (908)453-3383   Fax (908)453-3384

Meyerowitz, Jay S., MD {1891892816} Grtrcs, IntrMd(85,MEX34)<NJ-HOLYNAME, NJ-ENGLWOOD>
+ Aspen Medical Associates, P.A.
1 DeGraw Square   Teaneck, NJ 07666   (201)928-0200   Fax (201)928-0820

Meyers, Adam M., DO {1972554426} PhysMd, PainInvt(94,MO78)<NJ-MONMOUTH, NJ-KIMBALL>
+ Seaview Orthopaedics
1200 Eagle Avenue   Ocean, NJ 07712   (732)660-6200   Fax (732)660-6201
+ Seaview Orthopaedics
1640 Route 88 West   Brick, NJ 08724   (732)660-6200   Fax (732)458-2743

Meyers, Lawrence S., MD {1861541146} DrmtPthy, IntrMd(80,PA13)
+ Summit Medical Group-Berkeley Heights Campus
1 Diamond Hill Road   Berkeley Heights, NJ 07922
(908)273-4300   Fax (908)790-6576

Meyers, Marta, MD {1154328755} Hemato, IntrMd(81,PA07)<NJ-MORRISTN>
+ Madison Internal Medicine Associates
95 Madison Avenue/Suite 405   Morristown, NJ 07960
(973)829-9998   Fax (973)829-9991

Meyerson, Steven Jeffrey, MD {1922183573} RadDia(92,NY09)
+ Diagnostic Imaging Center and Group Practice
251 Rochelle Avenue   Rochelle Park, NJ 07662   (201)291-8800   Fax (201)291-1619

Meyler, Zinovy, DO {1689831752} PhysMd, IntrSptM(05,NY75)
+ Princeton Spine and Joint Center
601 Ewing Street/Suite A-2   Princeton, NJ 08540
(609)454-0760   Fax (609)454-0761

Mezera, Megan A., MD {1477865426} RadOnc
+ MD Anderson Cancer Center at Cooper
2 Cooper Plaza   Camden, NJ 08103   (856)735-6119   Fax (856)735-6467

Mezhoudi, Amal, MD {1144393513} FamMed
+ 1203 Bloomfield Street
Hoboken, NJ 07030

Mezic, Edward T., MD {1437218435} IntrMd, PulDis(83,WIND)<NJ-BAYSHORE>
+ Medical Associates of Central New Jersey
26 Throckmorton Lane/1st flr.   Old Bridge, NJ 08857
(732)679-9950   Fax (732)679-9956

Mezzacappa, Peter M., MD {1356363808} Radiol, RadDia(84,NY08)<NJ-CENTRAST>
+ Freehold Radiology Group
901 West Main Street   Freehold, NJ 07728   (732)462-4844
+ CentraState Medical Center
901 West Main Street/Radiology   Freehold, NJ 07728
(732)431-2000

Mgbako, Ambrose O., MD {1629045323} Psychy(72,NIGE)<NJ-EASTORNG, NJ-MTNSIDE>
+ 100 Valley Road
Montclair, NJ 07042   (973)783-8070

Miah, Khorshed Alam, MD {1508811993} Psychy, Psyphm(81,RUS06)<NJ-HACKNSK>
+ Hackensack University Medical Faculty Practice
25 East Salem Street/1st Fl   Hackensack, NJ 07601
(201)996-5950   Fax (201)996-5995

Mian, Asma, MD {1649588229} PsyCAd(09,DMN01)
+ Alexander Road Associates in Psychiatry & Psychology
707 Alexander Road/Bldg 2 Suite 202   Princeton, NJ 08540
(609)419-0400   Fax (609)419-9200

Mian, Bilal A., MD {1700825999} Nrolgy(93,PAKI)
+ Drs. Mian and Mian
310 East Main Street   Somerville, NJ 08876   (908)725-5565
Fax (908)725-2219

Mian, Fawad A., MD {1306006242} Nrolgy
+ 34 Westwood Circle
Edison, NJ 08820

Mian, Nimer F., DO {1518084631} ClNrPh(02,NY75)
+ Drs. Mian and Mian
310 East Main Street   Somerville, NJ 08876   (908)725-5565
Fax (908)725-2219

Mian, Samia Fatima, MD {1033394895} Nephro
+ The Cooper Hospital System-Univ Hospital
3 Cooper Plaza/Suite 215   Camden, NJ 08103   (856)757-7844   Fax (856)757-7778

Mian, Somia Zia, MD {1770787053} Gastrn, IntrMd(01,NJ05)
+ 75 Rockland Road
Trenton, NJ 08638

Miano, Michele A., MD {1245269919} Ophthl(90,PA01)<NJ-VIRTUAHS>
+ Wills Eye Surgery Center in Cherry Hill
408 Route 70 East   Cherry Hill, NJ 08034   (856)354-1600   Fax (856)429-7555
+ Regional Eye Associates
741 Route 70 West   Cherry Hill, NJ 08002   (856)354-1600   Fax (856)795-8688
+ Regional Eye Associates
200 White Horse Pike   Haddon Heights, NJ 08034
(856)547-0200

Miao, Sun, MD {1750314803} IntrMd(82,CHN19)<NJ-ACMC-MAIN, NJ-ACMCITY>
+ 29 South New York Road/Suite 700
Galloway, NJ 08205   (609)404-1823   Fax (609)404-1853

Micabalo, Alvin Francis, DO {1730352576} FamMed(03,NJ75)
+ Rehabilitation Consultation
72 Route 27   Edison, NJ 08820   (732)662-9901   Fax (732)662-9904

Micale, Maria Theresa, DO {1619949252} Pedtrc(96,IA75)<NJ-MONMOUTH>
+ Steppingstone Pediatrics
3350 Highway 138/Building 2/Suite 126   Wall, NJ 07719
(732)280-6455   Fax (732)280-6456

Micale, Philip Louis, MD {1750354346} Gastrn, IntrMd(93,NY19)<NJ-HOLYNAME, NJ-ENGLWOOD>
+ Teaneck Gastroenterology & Endoscopy Center
1086 Teaneck Road/Suite 4-C   Teaneck, NJ 07666
(201)837-9449   Fax (201)578-1699
+ Teaneck Gastroenterology & Endoscopy Center
1086 Teaneck Road/Suite 3-B   Teaneck, NJ 07666
(201)837-9449   Fax (201)837-9544

Micallef, Donald M., MD {1467486365} GenPrc, IntrMd(87,DOMI)<NJ-JRSYSHMC>
+ Wall Family Medical
2130 Highway 35/Building C Suite 324   Sea Girt, NJ 08750
(732)974-8005   Fax (732)974-2117

Miccio, Anthony G., MD {1346280567} FamMed, GenPrc(88,DC01)<NJ-HCKTSTWN, NJ-STCLRDEN>
+ Advocare Family Health at Mt. Olive
183 US Route 206/Suite 1   Flanders, NJ 07836   (973)347-3277   Fax (973)347-3141

Micek Galinat, Laura A., MD {1770583460} FamMed(83,NJ05)
+ Somerset Family Practice
110 Rehill Avenue   Somerville, NJ 08876   (908)685-2900   Fax (908)685-2891

Miceli, James Gerard, MD {1144546706} Rheuma, IntrMd(10,NY46)
+ Rheumatology Associates of North Jersey, PA
1415 Queen Anne Road   Teaneck, NJ 07666   (201)837-7788   Fax (201)837-2077

Miceli, Kurt Phillip, MD {1316155450} Psychy, IntrMd(03,PA09)
+ 1255 Caldwell Road
Cherry Hill, NJ 08034   (856)324-3256   Fax (856)667-1281

Micev, Alan Jordan, MD {1215248349}
+ South Jersey Hand Center
1888 Marlton Pike East/Suite E-F-G   Cherry Hill, NJ 08003
(702)845-3771   Fax (856)489-5631
ajmicev@gmail.com

Micevski, Aleksandar, MD {1114172731} Psychy
+ St Joseph's Medical Center Psychiatry
703 Main Street   Paterson, NJ 07503   (973)754-3295
+ 66d Arcadia Road
Hackensack, NJ 07601

Mich, Robert John, MD {1104810670} CdvDis, IntrMd, IntCrd(79,MD07)<NJ-MORRISTN, NJ-OVERLOOK>
+ Associates in Cardiovascular Disease, LLC
571 Central Avenue/Suite 115   New Providence, NJ 07974
(908)464-4200   Fax (908)464-1332

Michael, Beckie, DO {1346272796} Nephro, IntrMd(89,PA77)
+ Marlton Nephrology and Hypertension
769 East Route 70/Suite C-125   Marlton, NJ 08053
(856)988-8800   Fax (856)988-8804

Michael, Christine R., DO {1053748053}
+ Jersey Shore Monmouth Family Medicine Group
3499 Route 9   Freehold, NJ 07728   (732)625-3166   Fax (732)409-7473

Michael, Hazar, MD {1144392242} Gastrn, IntrMd(92,SYR01)<NY-WINTHROP>
+ Summit Medical Group-Berkeley Heights Campus
1 Diamond Hill Road   Berkeley Heights, NJ 07922
(908)273-4300   Fax (908)790-6576

Michael, Lisa Golomb, MD {1649236993} Pedtrc, IntrMd(99,NY19)<NJ-ENGLWOOD, NJ-HACKNSK>
+ Tenafly Pediatrics, PA
32 Franklin Street   Tenafly, NJ 07670   (201)569-2400   Fax (201)569-6081

Michael, Mark, DO {1528296142} PedCrd<NJ-NWRKBETH>
+ Newark Beth Israel Medical Center
201 Lyons Avenue/Suite L5   Newark, NJ 07112   (973)926-3500

Michael, Patrick M., MD {1235426263} IntrMd<NJ-STJOSHOS>
+ St. Joseph's Regional Medical Center
703 Main Street   Paterson, NJ 07503   (973)754-2431   Fax (973)754-3376

Michael, Rositta, MD {1679655419} Pedtrc(94,INA2X)<NJ-STPETER>
+ Hunterdon Medical Center
2100 Wescott Drive/4 FL/Ped Hospit   Flemington, NJ 08822
(908)788-6100

Michael, Stanley P., MD {1073501284} SrgOrt, SprtMd(78,INA08)<PA-TMPHOSP>
+ Temple University Orthopaedics & Sports Medicine
One Greentree Center/Suite 104   Marlton, NJ 08053
(856)596-0906

Michael, Wedad S., MD {1326137407} IntrMd(74,EGY04)<NJ-SHOREMEM, NJ-BURDTMLN>
+ Somers Medical Care, LLC
1118 Tilton Road   Northfield, NJ 08225   (609)677-5777   Fax (609)677-1711

Michaeli, Danni Z., MD {1164593950} Psychy(90,ISR02)
+ 71 Valley Street/Suite 301
South Orange, NJ 07079   (212)674-2447

Michaels, Jennifer, MD {1629176631} Nrolgy, IntrMd(79,NY48)
+ Center for Neurological Surgery UMDNJ
90 Bergen Street/DOC 8100   Newark, NJ 07103   (973)972-2323   Fax (973)972-2333

Michaels, Lisa A., MD {1982788931} PedHem, Pedtrc(90,VA01)<NJ-RWJUBRUN, NJ-STPETER>
+ Rutgers Cancer Institute of New Jersey
195 Little Albany Street/PO Box 2681   New Brunswick, NJ 08903   (732)235-9854   Fax (732)235-8234
+ RWJ University Hospital New Brunswick
One Robert Wood Johnson Place   New Brunswick, NJ 08901
(732)828-3000

Michaels, Lisa-Ann B., MD {1205027760} Pedtrc, IntrMd(NJ15
+ Milestones Pediatric Group PA
11 East Oak Street   Oakland, NJ 07436   (201)485-7557   Fax (201)485-7556

Michaels, Matthew James, DO {1073776548} IntrMd(08,NY75)<NJ-UMDNJ>
+ University Hospital
150 Bergen Street   Newark, NJ 07103   (973)972-4300

Michaelson, Richard A., MD {1760452528} MedOnc, IntrMd, OncHem(76,PA01)<NJ-STBARNMC>
+ St. Barnabas Medical Center
94 Old Short Hills Road/East Wing   Livingston, NJ 07039
(973)322-5362   Fax (973)322-5044
rmichaelson@sbmcs.com

Michail, Mohsen T., MD {1982607040} AnesPain, PainMd(84,EGY16)
+ Pain Management & Rehab Center, LLC.
1011 Clifton Avenue/Suite 1G   Clifton, NJ 07013   (973)365-0008   Fax (973)365-0004

Physicians by Name and Address

Michalewski, Martin P., MD {1164410643} ObsGyn
+ 601 Sunset Avenue
Asbury Park, NJ 07712 (732)775-7978 Fax (732)988-2545
+ 310 Route 34
Colts Neck, NJ 07722 (732)775-7978 Fax (732)901-0199

Michel, Brian E., MD {1730171893} Nephro(83,NY08)<NY-PRSB-WEIL>
+ Haddon Renal Medical Specialists
401 Kings Highway South/Suite 5 Cherry Hill, NJ 08034
(856)428-8992 Fax (856)428-9614

Michel, Joseph R., MD {1477567980} IntrMd(72,HAIT)<NJ-UN-DRWD>
+ 297 Westwood Drive/Suite 104
Woodbury, NJ 08096 (856)848-1083 Fax (856)848-2271

Michelis, Mary Ann, MD {1710956073} Allrgy, ClnGnt, IntrMd(75,PA12)<NJ-HACKNSK>
+ Center for Healthy Senior Living
360 Essex Street/Suite 401 Hackensack, NJ 07601
(551)996-2065 Fax (551)996-2169

Michelson, Lorelle N., MD {1033107925} SrgPlstc(74,NY08)
+ Lorelle N. Michelson M.D., F.A.C.S., LLC
1590 Anderson Avenue/PH 1 Fort Lee, NJ 07024
(201)871-9808 Fax (201)871-9658
Lmichaelson@nj.rr.com
+ Lorelle N. Michelson M.D., F.A.C.S., LLC
16 Pocono Road/Suite 103 Denville, NJ 07834

Michelson, Marc H., DO {1063404861} IntrMd(86,NY75)<NJ-SJRSYELM>
+ Internal Medicine Associates of Southern New Jersey
151 Fries Mill Road/Suite 400 Turnersville, NJ 08012
(856)401-9300 Fax (856)374-5805

Michner, Richard A., MD {1376527291} ObsGyn(76,MEX03)<NJ-BURDTMLN>
+ Drs. Milio & Michner
214 North Main Street Cape May Court House, NJ 08210
(609)465-2828 Fax (609)465-8617
+ Community Health Care Inc
410 North Route 9 Cape May Court House, NJ 08210
(609)465-0258

Mickey, Kevin J., MD {1538101662} Ophthl, PedOph(86,NJ05)<NJ-STJOSHOS, NJ-CHILTON>
+ Pediatric Ophthalmology of NJ
57 Willowbrook Boulevard/Suite 411 Wayne, NJ 07470
(973)256-4111 Fax (973)256-3719

Mico, Mario R., MD {1730221714} Pedtrc(87,PAR01)
+ Passaic Pediatrics PA
298 Passaic Street Passaic, NJ 07055 (973)249-8100 Fax (973)249-8110
+ Passaic Pediatrics II PA
913 Main Avenue Passaic, NJ 07055 (973)458-8000

Middleton, John R., MD {1891852489} InfDis, IntrMd(70,NJ05)<NJ-RBAYOLDB, NJ-RBAYPERT>
+ Raritan Bay Infectious Disease Consultants
3 Hospital Plaza/Suite 208 Old Bridge, NJ 08857
(732)360-2700 Fax (732)360-2703
+ Raritan Bay Medical Center/Old Bridge Division
One Hospital Plaza/Medicine Old Bridge, NJ 08857
(732)360-1000
+ Raritan Bay Medical Center/Perth Amboy Division
530 New Brunswick Avenue/Medicine Perth Amboy, NJ 08857 (732)442-3700

Midure, Leo L., DO {1336400241}
+ Kennedy Health Systems/Washington Township Campus
435 Hurffville-Cross Keys Road Turnersville, NJ 08012
(856)582-2816

Miedziak, Anita Irmina, MD {1013920867} Ophthl(93,PA07)<NJ-UNVMCPRN>
+ The Princeton Eye Group
419 North Harrison Street/Suite 104 Princeton, NJ 08540
(609)921-9437 Fax (609)921-0277
+ The Princeton Eye Group
1600 Perrinville Road Monroe Township, NJ 08831
(609)921-9437 Fax (609)655-3685
+ The Princeton Eye Group
900 Eastern Avenue/Suite 50 Somerset, NJ 08540
(732)565-9550 Fax (732)565-0946

Miele, Bevon D., MD {1619009099} IntrMd, Nephro(83,ISRA)<NJ-HUNTRDN>
+ 2 Kings Court/Suite 207
Flemington, NJ 08822 (908)806-4466 Fax (908)806-3553

Miele, Ellen H., MD {1154406361} Pedtrc(91,NJ05)<NJ-JRSYSHMC>
+ Spring Lake Pediatrics Associates
613 Warren Avenue Spring Lake, NJ 07762 (732)974-1444
Fax (732)974-1140

Miele, Niel F., MD {1477519502} PedEmg, Pedtrc(86,NY15)<NJ-RWJUBRUN>
+ RWJ University Pediatric Emergency Medicine
125 Paterson Street/MEB 342 New Brunswick, NJ 08903
(732)235-7893 Fax (732)235-9349

Mierlak, Daniel C., MD {1902964828} PsyAdd, Psychy, Psyphm(89,NY08)<NY-PRSBCOLU>
+ 224 Lorraine Avenue
Montclair, NJ 07043 (973)783-3838 Fax (973)783-9185

Migliaccio, Thomas A., MD {1487860359} ObsGyn(98,PA09)<NJ-PALISADE, NJ-HOBUNIMC>
+ Brescia-Migliaccio Ob/Gyn
609 Washington Street Hoboken, NJ 07030 (201)659-7700 Fax (201)659-7701

Miglietta, Mario Adrian, DO {1366405607} EmrgMd(96,NY75)<NJ-HOLYNAME>
+ Holy Name Hospital
718 Teaneck Road/EmergMed Teaneck, NJ 07666
(201)833-3913 Fax (610)617-6280
mmiglietta@holyname.org

Miglietta, Maurizio A., DO {1710973243} SrgTrm, SrgCrC, Surgry(96,NY75)<NJ-HOLYNAME, NJ-PALISADE>
+ Palisades Surgical Associates PC
103 River Road/Suite 101 Edgewater, NJ 07020 (888)320-0922 Fax (888)909-0922

Migliore, Christina, MD {1508883752} PulDis, IntrMd(02,DMN01)<NJ-NWRKBETH>
+ Newark Beth Israel Medical Center
201 Lyons Avenue/C-1 Newark, NJ 07112 (973)926-4430
Fax (973)926-5658
Christina.Migliore@tampabay.rr.com

Migliori, Frank Anthony, MD {1396784021} EmrgMd(01,NJ05)<NJ-RIVERVW>
+ Riverview Medical Center
1 Riverview Plaza/EmergMed Red Bank, NJ 07701
(732)530-2204 Fax (732)224-7498
+ Hazlet Family Care
3253 Route 35 Hazlet, NJ 07730 (732)530-2204 Fax (732)888-7649

Mignone, Robert, DO {1518224153} OtgyFPIS
+ Becker ENT
One Union Street/Suite 203 Robbinsville, NJ 08691
(609)436-5740 Fax (609)436-5741
+ Becker ENT
2 Princess Road/Suite East Lawrenceville, NJ 08648
(609)436-5740 Fax (610)303-5164

Miguel, Eduardo E., MD {1548300734} IntrMd, Rheuma(66,PAR01)
+ Drs. Borchardt & Miguel
200 Grand Avenue/Suite 202 Englewood, NJ 07631
(201)679-2470 Fax (201)300-4384

Miguel, Renato C., MD {1073554549} Anesth(71,PHI02)
+ 100 West Saddle River Road
Saddle River, NJ 07458
rcmiguelmed@aol.com

Miguelino, Bernadette M., MD {1083755482} Pedtrc(79,PHI01)<NJ-RIVERVW, NJ-MONMOUTH>
+ Miguelino and David Pediatrics
717 North Beers Street/Suite 1F Holmdel, NJ 07733
(732)888-0777 Fax (732)888-0880

Miguelino, Ida Alfad, MD {1285614800} Pedtrc(94,NJ06)<NJ-OVERLOOK, NJ-MORRISTN>
+ Summit Medical Group-Berkeley Heights Campus
1 Diamond Hill Road Berkeley Heights, NJ 07922
(908)273-4300 Fax (908)769-2516

Miguez, Priscilla, DO {1114307105} FamMed
+ Maplewood Family Medicine
111 Dunnell Road/Suite 200 Maplewood, NJ 07040
(908)598-6690 Fax (973)762-0840

Mihalyfi, Brigitte E., MD {1740301043} NnPnMd, Pedtrc(83,NJ06)<NJ-UNVMCPRN>
+ CHOP Care Network at Princeton Medical Center
One Plainsboro Road Plainsboro, NJ 08536 (609)853-7000
Fax (609)497-4173

Mihata, Ryan Garner, MD {1760466726} EmrgMd, CritCr, IntrMd(05,MD12)
+ Court House Surgery Center
106 Courthouse South Dennis Rd Cape May, NJ 08204
(609)465-0300 Fax (609)465-8771

Mikadze, Malkhazi, MD {1033150099} Pedtrc, PedEmg(92,GEO02)<NJ-HACKNSK, NJ-STBARNMC>
+ Hackensack University Medical Center
30 Prospect Avenue/Pedi Hackensack, NJ 07601
(201)996-2000
+ St. Barnabas Medical Center
94 Old Short Hills Road/PediEmrg Livingston, NJ 07039
(973)322-5000

Mike, Joseph J., MD {1467453738} Surgry(86,PA02)<NJ-UN-DRWD>
+ General Vascular Surgical Specialists
17 West Red Bank Avenue/Suite 203 Woodbury, NJ 08096
(856)848-8242 Fax (856)384-6015

Mikhail, Fayez A., MD {1770696841} IntrMd(83,EGY04)<NJ-RWJUHAM, NJ-STFRNMED>
+ 2087 Klockner Road
Hamilton, NJ 08690

Mikhail, John David, MD {1205173762}
+ 221 Yorkshire Court
Old Bridge, NJ 08857 (732)654-5035
+ Shore Pulmonary PA
301 Bingham Avenue/Suite B Ocean, NJ 07712 (732)654-5035 Fax (732)775-1212

Mikhail, Magdy H., MD {1629006242} Anesth(83,EGY04)<NJ-CENTRAST>
+ Liberty Anesthesia & Pain Management
901 West Main Street/2nd Floor Freehold, NJ 07728
(732)294-2876 Fax (732)294-2502
+ CentraState Medical Center
901 West Main Street/Anesth Freehold, NJ 07728
(732)431-2000

Mikhail, Maged, MD {1578893608} Pedtrc(99,EGY03)
+ 240 Midland Avenue
South Amboy, NJ 08879 (732)721-6641
drmagedmikhail@yahoo.com

Mikhail, Nagy H., MD {1629015581} Pthlgy, PthAClI(80,EGYP)<NJ-BAYSHORE>
+ Bayshore Community Hospital
727 North Beers Street/Pathology Holmdel, NJ 07733
(732)739-5900

Mikhail, Salwa M., MD {1285785246} Pedtrc(82,EGY04)
+ 85 Brunswick Woods Drive
East Brunswick, NJ 08816 (732)651-0370 Fax (732)651-0372

Mikkilineni, Rao S., MD {1881650273} PulCCr, IntrMd, PulDis(71,INDI)<NJ-JRSYCITY, NJ-MEADWLND>
+ Liberty Medical Associates
377 Jersey Avenue/Suite 470 Jersey City, NJ 07302
(201)918-2239 Fax (201)918-2243

Miklas, Corinne Nicole, DO {1770846404}
+ 900 Medical Center Drive
Sewell, NJ 08080 (717)471-7516
corinnemiklas@gmail.com

Mikulski, Wanda J., MD {1962510727} FamMed(70,POL03)<NJ-MTNSIDE>
+ 1310 Broad Street
Bloomfield, NJ 07003 (973)338-5660 Fax (973)338-0522

Milan, Ronald Kenneth, MD {1841294238} Anesth(88,GRN01)<NJ-BAYSHORE>
+ Bayshore Community Hospital
727 North Beers Street/Anesthesiology Holmdel, NJ 07733
(732)739-5900

Milanes Roberts, Norma B., MD ObsGyn(95,NJ05)
+ 32 Korwel Circle
West Orange, NJ 07052

Milanes-Roberts, Norma, MD {1952488280} ObsGyn(95,NJ05)<NJ-NWRKBETH>
+ NHCAC Health Center at West New York
5301 Broadway West New York, NJ 07093 (201)866-9320
Fax (866)769-7588

Milano, Aubri Marie, DO {1669713566}<NJ-COOPRUMC>
+ Cooper University Hospital
One Cooper Plaza Camden, NJ 08103 (856)757-7904

Milano, Edward L., MD {1447391172} Dermat(89,NY20)<NJ-CHILTON>
+ Wayne Dermatology
10 Route 23 South Wayne, NJ 07470 (973)785-8585 Fax (973)785-8095

Milano, Marc Anthony, MD {1477540219} EmrgMd(01,GRN01)<NJ-STBARNMC, NJ-WAYNEGEN>
+ Emergency Medical Associates of NJ, P.A.
3 Century Drive Parsippany, NJ 07054 (973)740-0607
Fax (973)740-9895

Milano, Michael C., MD {1952401879} ObsGyn, Gyneco(78,NJ05)<NJ-STBARNMC>
+ Associates in Obstetrics Gynecology & Infertility PA
825 Bloomfield Avenue/Suite 103 Verona, NJ 07044
(973)239-5010
+ Associates in Obstetrics Gynecology & Infertility
375 Mount Pleasant Avenue/Suite 202 West Orange, NJ 07052 (973)239-5010 Fax (973)669-0277

Milas, Erica M., DO {1518092428} FamMed
+ Family Health Center of Paulsboro
One West Broad Street Paulsboro, NJ 08066 (856)423-0033 Fax (856)423-4444

Milas, Jerry Peter, DO {1083640809} EmrgMd<NJ-SJHREGMC>
+ SJH Regional Medical Center
1505 West Sherman Avenue Vineland, NJ 08360
(856)641-8000

Milazzo, Carmelo, MD {1760438691} IntrMd, EnDbMt(83,ITAL)<NJ-CHRIST, NJ-HOBUNIMC>
+ 2124 New York Avenue
Union City, NJ 07087 (201)864-6492 Fax (201)864-3207

Milazzo, Salvatore J., Sr, DO {1386763910} FamMed, GenPrc(85,NJ75)
+ PO Box 94
Kenilworth, NJ 07033

Physicians by Name and Address

Milazzo, Vincent J., MD {1144292749} Surgry, SrgVas(85,NJ06)
+ Jersey Coast Vascular Associates
425 Jack Martin Boulevard/Suite 2   Brick, NJ 08724   (732)202-1500   Fax (732)202-1058

Milbauer, James, MD {1598744450} Dermat(82,NY46)
+ 50 Cherry Hill Road
Parsippany, NJ 07054   (973)335-1516   Fax (973)335-5417

Milburn, Christopher Anthony, MD {1609037985} IntrMd, Psychy<PA-TJCNTR>
+ Cooper University Medical Center/Camden
3 Cooper Plaza   Camden, NJ 08103   (856)342-2000

Miles, Liesl Carey, MD {1275713042} IntrMd(09,PA09)<NJ-COOPRUMC>
+ Cooper University Medical Center/Camden
3 Cooper Plaza/Suite 502   Camden, NJ 08103   (856)968-7433   Fax (856)968-8499

Mileto, Vincent F., MD {1275586737} ObsGyn(74,NY09)<NJ-SOMERSET, NY-STPETERS>
+ Somerset Ob-Gyn Associates
215 Union Avenue/Suite A   Bridgewater, NJ 08807   (908)722-2900   Fax (908)722-1856
+ Somerset Ob-Gyn Associates
1 New Amwell Road   Hillsborough, NJ 08844   (908)874-5900

Milgraum, Sandy S., MD {1568498376} Dermat, IntrMd(79,AST06)<NJ-RWJUBRUN>
+ Robert Wood Johnson Medical Group-Dermatology
1 World's Fair Drive/Suite 2400   Somerset, NJ 08873   (732)235-7993   Fax (732)235-7117
+ Academic Dermatology & Laser Surgery Center
81 Brunswick Woods Drive   East Brunswick, NJ 08816   (732)613-0300

Milgrim, Laurence Marc, MD {1255307989} Otlryg(89,NJ05)
+ Northern Jersey Ear, Nose & Throat Associates, PA
44 Godwin Avenue   Midland Park, NJ 07432   (201)445-2900   Fax (201)445-8679
+ Northern Jersey Ear, Nose & Throat Associates, P.A.
1 Degraw Avenue   Teaneck, NJ 07666   (201)445-2900   Fax (201)836-7838

Milic, Milija, MD {1497738843} Anesth(01,DMN01)<NJ-HACKNSK>
+ Hackensack University MC-Anesthesia Dept
30 Prospect Avenue/Room 2703   Hackensack, NJ 07601   (201)996-2419   Fax (201)996-3962

Milicia, Anthony P., MD {1861408155} ObsGyn(80,PA13)
+ 840 Wessex Lane
Somerdale, NJ 08083

Milio, Joseph L., DO {1821072745} ObsGyn(84,NJ75)<NJ-BURDTMLN>
+ Drs. Milio & Michner
214 North Main Street   Cape May Court House, NJ 08210   (609)465-2828   Fax (609)465-8617
+ Community Health Care Inc
410 North Route 9   Cape May Court House, NJ 08210   (609)465-0258

Milite, James Philip, MD {1144210873} Ophthl(90,NY19)<NY-NYEYEINF, NY-BETHPETR>
+ Omni Eye Services
485 Route 1 South/Building A   Iselin, NJ 08830   (732)750-0400   Fax (732)602-0749

Militello, Giuseppe M., MD {1558381681} Dermat, DrmtPthy(02,PA01)
+ Militello Dermatology
6 Brighton Road   Clifton, NJ 07012   (929)242-7056
militello.md@gmail.com
+ Militello Dematology
324 South Avenue East   Westfield, NJ 07090   (908)232-2727

Millar, Kim H., MD {1679729354} Pedtrc(84,TX04)<NJ-UNVMCPRN>
+ Princeton Nassau Pediatrics, P.A.
301 North Harrison Street   Princeton, NJ 08540   (609)924-5510   Fax (609)924-3577
+ Princeton Nassau Pediatrics, P.A.
196 Princeton-Hightstown Road   West Windsor, NJ 08550   (609)924-5510   Fax (609)799-2294

Miller, Aaron Todd, MD {1386802213} FamMed, SrgC&R(94,KY02)
+ Atlantic Colon & Rectal
33 Overlook Road/Suite 412   Summit, NJ 07901   (908)598-0220   Fax (908)598-0415

Miller, Adina Rebecca, MD {1487899480}
+ 394 Warwick Avenue
Teaneck, NJ 07666   (201)894-3322

Miller, Alan Norman, MD {1902902034} Psychy(73,PA09)
+ 123 Greenvale Road
Cherry Hill, NJ 08034

Miller, Alan R., MD {1306813720} SrgOrt, SprtMd(83,NY47)<NJ-HACKNSK>
+ Bergen Orthopaedic Surgery and Sports Medicine
221 Old Hook Road   Westwood, NJ 07675   (201)666-0013   Fax (201)666-0123

Miller, Alan S., MD {1265484562} EmrgMd, InfDis(90,WI06)<NJ-HOLYNAME>
+ Holy Name Hospital
718 Teaneck Road/Emerg Med   Teaneck, NJ 07666   (201)833-3210   Fax (201)833-7090

Miller, Andrea, DO {1649666967} NnPnMd
+ AtlantiCare - Neonatology Department
65 West Jimmie Leeds Road   Pomona, NJ 08240   (609)404-3816   Fax (609)404-3818

Miller, Andrew David, MD {1134388705} GPrvMd, PubHth(79,NY01)
+ HealthCare Quality Strategies
557 Cranbury Road/Suite 21   East Brunswick, NJ 08816   (732)238-5570
amiller.central@hqsi.org

Miller, Andrew Ian, MD {1760439699} Ophthl(98,NY19)
+ 2 Cyprus Lane
Livingston, NJ 07039   (973)376-6333   Fax (973)376-5798

Miller, Andrew John, MD {1134133945} Otlryg, OtgyFPlS(94,TX04)<NJ-JFKMED, NJ-RBAYOLDB>
+ Associates in Plastic Surgery
1150 Amboy Avenue   Edison, NJ 08837   (732)548-3200   Fax (732)548-1919
+ Associates in Plastic Surgery
203 Route 9 South/Marlboro   Englishtown, NJ 07726   (732)617-1800
+ Associates in Plastic Surgery
5 Mountain Boulevard   Warren, NJ 08837   (908)222-8440

Miller, Angela M., MD {1376594853} Dermat(87,AZ01)
+ Drs. Gilson, Orsini & Miller
223 Monmouth Road   West Long Branch, NJ 07764   (732)870-2992   Fax (732)870-2533

Miller, Ann Marie, MD {1619052305} Nrolgy, IntrMd(81,NY08)<NJ-VIRTBERL>
+ 307 South Evergreen Avenue
Woodbury, NJ 08096   (856)848-2088   Fax (856)848-8536

Miller, Anthony Francis, MD {1699001974} RadNro
+ 104 Buckner Avenue
Haddonfield, NJ 08033
afmiller.md@gmail.com

Miller, Arthur H., MD {1033287164} FamMed(80,MEX14)<NJ-RWJUBRUN, NJ-JFKMED>
+ Highland Park Family Practice LLC
505 Raritan Avenue   Highland Park, NJ 08904   (732)393-1331   Fax (732)463-6067

Miller, Benetta L., MD {1316079239} Surgry(82,MA05)<NJ-HOBUNIMC, NJ-CHRIST>
+ Surgical Associates of Hudson County, P.A.
330 Grand Street/Suite 100   Hoboken, NJ 07030   (201)238-2888

Miller, Bruce L., MD {1649278664} Anesth, PainMd(79,WI05)
+ 110 Carnie Boulevard
Voorhees, NJ 08043   (856)325-5800

Miller, Catharine Michele, DO {1932128238} PhysMd(00,NJ75)
+ 5 Chestnut Court
Cedar Grove, NJ 07009

Miller, Charles Luther, MD {1770565251} CdvDis, IntrMd, NuclMd(63,PA13)<NJ-RIVERVW>
+ Integrated Medical Alliance/IMA Medical Care Center
30 Shrewsbury Plaza   Shrewsbury, NJ 07702   (732)542-2124   Fax (732)542-2992

Miller, Christine Venable, MD {1932388220} AnesPain
+ Jersery Shore Anesthesiology
1945 Highway 33   Neptune, NJ 07753   (732)897-0200   Fax (732)897-0263

Miller, Danielle Megan, DO {1154583300} FamMed
+ McGuire Air Force Base/Acute Health Care Clinic
3458 Neely Road   Trenton, NJ 08641   (609)754-9780   Fax (609)754-9015

Miller, David Geoffrey, MD {1083742860} Psychy(80,NJ06)<NJ-STBARNMC>
+ Summit Psychiatric and Counseling Associates
28 Millburn Avenue/Suite 5   Springfield, NJ 07081   (908)218-1770   Fax (973)376-7726

Miller, David Haim, MD {1093714735} Radiol, RadDia(95,MO02)<NJ-VIRTMHBC, NJ-VIRTBERL>
+ South Jersey Radiology Associates, P.A.
100 Carnie Boulevard/Suite B-5   Voorhees, NJ 08043   (856)751-0123   Fax (856)751-0535
+ The Women's Center at Voorhees
100 Carnie Boulevard/Suite A-4   Voorhees, NJ 08043   (856)751-0123   Fax (856)751-5650
+ South Jersey Radiology Associates, P.A.
901 Route 168/Suites 301-305   Turnersville, NJ 08043   (856)227-6600   Fax (856)227-8537

Miller, Denise J., MD SrgOnc, Surgry(78,MO02)
+ 8 Crest Fruit Court
Manalapan, NJ 07726   (732)263-7960   Fax (732)263-7961
mudlj55@gmail.com

Miller, Deon E., DO {1619310570} EmrgMd<NJ-CARONEBA>
+ CareOne at Raritan Bay
530 New Brunswick Avenue/Floor 2 Green   Perth Amboy, NJ 08861   (732)442-3700

Miller, Douglas Andrew, MD {1013034800} RadOnc
+ Shore Radiation Oncology, LLC
425 Jack Martin Boulevard   Brick, NJ 08724   (732)836-4109   Fax (732)836-4036

Miller, Emily S., MD {1902932189} Dermat(78,PA12)<NJ-OURLADY>
+ Dermatology Physicians of South Jersey, P.A.
112 White Horse Pike   Haddon Heights, NJ 08035   (856)546-5353   Fax (856)546-8711

Miller, Eric Jay, MD {1932101961} SrgOnc, SrgBst(85,PA09)<NJ-VIRTMHBC, NJ-VIRTVOOR>
+ Surgical Specialists of New Jersey
668 Main Street/Suite 4   Lumberton, NJ 08048   (609)267-7050   Fax (609)267-7065

Miller, Fred William, III, MD {1811930373} ObsGyn(79,NJ05)<NJ-MTNSIDE, NJ-NWRKBETH>
+ 363 Park Street
Upper Montclair, NJ 07043   (973)783-1550   Fax (973)783-1468

Miller, Gary Stuart, MD {1558488197} Nrolgy, ClNrPh, SlpDis(02,WI06)<NJ-JFKMED>
+ JFK Neurosciences Institute
65 James Street/Second Floor   Edison, NJ 08818   (732)321-7010   Fax (732)744-5873

Miller, George W., Jr., MD {1316942618} Addctn, FamMed(80,NJ05)<NJ-MTNSIDE>
+ Mountainside Family Practice Associates
799 Bloomfield Avenue/Suite 201   Verona, NJ 07044   (973)746-7050   Fax (973)857-2831

Miller, Helene Anne, MD {1477581957} Psychy, AltnMd(93,PA09)<NJ-BERGNMC>
+ Family Psychiatry of North Jersey
351 Evelyn Street   Paramus, NJ 07652   (201)977-2889   Fax (201)977-2890

Miller, Howard M., MD {1992775001} NuclMd, RadDia(70,NY19)<NJ-JFKMED>
+ JFK Medical Center
65 James Street/Radiol/EdisonGp   Edison, NJ 08820   (908)321-7940
+ Edison Radiology Group, P.A.
65 James Street   Edison, NJ 08820   (908)321-7940   Fax (732)737-2968

Miller, Ivan Thomas, MD {1235176512} EmrgMd, IntrMd(97,NY46)
+ St. Barnabas Medical Center
94 Old Short Hills Road   Livingston, NJ 07039   (973)322-5000

Miller, Jane E., MD {1053489849} ObsGyn, RprEnd(78,NY08)<NJ-HOLYNAME>
+ North Hudson IVF
385 Sylvan Avenue   Englewood Cliffs, NJ 07632   (201)871-1999   Fax (201)871-1031

Miller, Janice M., MD {1689994345} FamMed(94,NJ06)
+ 128 Updikes Mill Road
Belle Mead, NJ 08502   (908)874-7720

Miller, Janine D'Amelio, MD {1821291402} Dermat(03,GRN01)
+ Ridgewood ENT and Dermatology
81 North Maple Avenue   Ridgewood, NJ 07450   (201)857-2370   Fax (201)857-2371

Miller, Jason Harris, MD {1679712418} Dermat
+ Drs. Hametz & Picascia
77-55 Schanck Road/Suite B-3   Freehold, NJ 07728   (732)462-9800

Miller, Jeffrey Adam, DO {1184725897} PulDis, IntrMd(87,NY75)<NJ-STBARNMC, NJ-NWRKBETH>
+ Pulmonary and Critical Care Associates
2333 Morris Avenue/Suite B-15   Union, NJ 07083   (908)964-1964   Fax (908)964-6286

Miller, Jeffrey J., DO {1790799443} GenPrc, PhysMd(85,NY75)<NJ-UNVMCPRN, NJ-VANJHCS>
+ Princeton Orthopaedic Associates, P.A.
325 Princeton Avenue   Princeton, NJ 08540   (609)924-8131   Fax (609)924-8532
+ Princeton Neck and Back Institute
727 State Road   Princeton, NJ 08540   (609)924-8131   Fax (609)924-6699

Miller, Jeffrey Karl, MD {1982663969} SrgHnd, SrgOrt, OrtSHand(81,PA12)<NJ-MORRISTN>
+ Hand Surgery & Rehabilitation of North Jersey, P.C.
301 East Hanover Avenue   Morristown, NJ 07960   (973)538-5200
+ Hand Surgery & Rehabilitation of North Jersey, PC
111 Madison Avenue/Suite 302   Morristown, NJ 07960   (973)538-5200
+ Hand Surgery & Rehabilitation of North Jersey, P.C.
2333 Morris Avenue/Suite B-7   Union, NJ 07960   (973)538-5200

Miller, Jessica Schutzbank, MD {1326128737} PhysMd<NJ-RHBHTNTN>
+ The Rehab Hosp of Tinton Falls
2 Centre Plaza   Tinton Falls, NJ 07724   (732)460-5320

339

Physicians by Name and Address

Miller, Katherine H., MD {1871751792} ObsGyn(85,NJ05)<NJ-STPETER, NJ-RWJUBRUN>
+ 42 Reed Drive South
Princeton Junction, NJ 08550

Miller, Kenneth D., MD {1558441238} IntrMd(75,MEX14)<NJ-MORRISTN>
+ 16 Old Brookside Road
Randolph, NJ 07869   (973)895-4000   Fax (973)895-3310

Miller, Kenneth Paul, MD {1043212798} CdvDis, IntrMd, IntCrd(82,NY19)
+ Summit Medical Group Cardiology
62 South Fullerton Avenue   Montclair, NJ 07042   (973)746-8585   Fax (973)746-0088

Miller, Kenneth Scott, MD {1780647081} Ophthl, SrgRef, Catrct(91,IL06)<NJ-STBARNMC>
+ Miller Ophthalmology Associates, LLC
101 Old Short Hills Road/Suite 430   West Orange, NJ 07052   (973)325-3300   Fax (973)325-3320

Miller, Kevin D., MD {1386904969} Anesth
+ Jersery Shore Anesthesiology
1945 Highway 33   Neptune, NJ 07753   (732)897-0200   Fax (732)897-0263

Miller, Lawrence Steven, MD {1447337183} SrgOrt, IntrMd(79,PA02)
+ Cooper Bone and Joint Institute
900 Centennial Boulevard   Voorhees, NJ 08043   (856)325-6677   Fax (856)325-6678

Miller, Lee H., MD {1104811868} Otlryg(71,PA09)<NJ-RWJUHAM>
+ Premier ENT Associates
8 Quakerbridge Plaza   Hamilton, NJ 08619   (609)890-7800   Fax (609)890-6148

Miller, Lesley G., MD {1578976296} AdolMd, Pedtrc, IntrMd(89,NJ05)<NJ-OVERLOOK, NJ-STBARNMC>
+ Westfield Pediatrics, P.A.
532 East Broad Street   Westfield, NJ 07090   (908)232-3445   Fax (908)233-6184

Miller, Leslie Jeanne, MD {1710957477} Radiol(85,NY46)
+ Diagnostic Radiology Associates of Northfield
772 Northfield Avenue   West Orange, NJ 07052   (973)325-0002   Fax (973)325-8140
+ Diagnostic Radiology Associates of Clifton
1339 Broad Street   Clifton, NJ 07013   (973)325-0002   Fax (973)778-4846

Miller, Lincoln Paul, MD {1073574661} InfDis, IntrMd(85,ISRA)
+ 1500 Pleasant Valley Way/Suite 201
West Orange, NJ 07052   (973)966-6400   Fax (973)514-1587

Miller, Lisa Ann B., MD {1609843176} ObsGyn, Gyneco(88,PA09)<NJ-HACKNSK>
+ Excelsior Women's Care
170 Prospect Avenue/Suite 4   Hackensack, NJ 07601   (201)488-2288   Fax (201)488-2298

Miller, Marilyn Ann, MD {1639108988} IntrMd, Nephro(82,NJ05)<NJ-VAEASTOR, NJ-UMDNJ>
+ VA New Jersey Health Care System-East Orange Campus
385 Tremont Avenue   East Orange, NJ 07018   (973)676-1000   Fax (973)395-7026

Miller, Mark I., MD {1144219791} Urolgy(91,NY20)<NJ-OVERLOOK, NJ-WESTHDSN>
+ Premier Urology Group, LLC
275 Orchard Street   Westfield, NJ 07090   (908)654-5100   Fax (908)789-8755
+ Premier Urology Group, LLC
659 Kearny Avenue   Kearny, NJ 07032   (908)654-5100   Fax (201)789-8755
+ Premier Urology Group, LLC
776 East Third Avenue   Roselle Park, NJ 07090   (908)241-5268   Fax (908)241-8755

Miller, Melissa Anne, MD {1639598857} IntrMd(80,NJ06)
+ Health Net of New Jersey
90 Matawan Road   Matawan, NJ 07747   (732)353-7200

Miller, Michael Joseph, MD {1982794707} EnDbMt, IntrMd(81,NY08)<NJ-CLARMAAS, NJ-MTNSIDE>
+ North Essex Medical Association
5 Franklin Avenue/Suite 609   Belleville, NJ 07109   (973)751-1410   Fax (973)751-9422

Miller, Michelle K., MD {1699748699} PedHem(94,MN07)<NJ-MORRISTN>
+ The Valerie Fund Children's Center
33 Overlook Road/Suite 211   Summit, NJ 07901   (908)522-2353   Fax (908)522-0440
michelle.miller@ahsys.org
+ The Valerie Fund Children's Ctr/Goryeb
100 Madison Avenue/Simon 2/Box 70   Morristown, NJ 07962   (973)971-5161

Miller, Mitchell Alan, MD {1245216936} RadDia, IntrMd, Radiol(88,CA11)<NJ-ACMCMAIN, NJ-HACKNSK>
+ AtlantiCare Regional Med Ctr/Mainland
65 West Jimmie Leeds Road   Pomona, NJ 08240   (609)652-1000

+ The Imaging Center
30 South Newman Street   Hackensack, NJ 07601   (609)652-1000   Fax (201)488-5244
+ Hackensack Radiology Group, P.A.
30 Prospect Avenue   Hackensack, NJ 08240   (201)996-2200   Fax (201)336-8451

Miller, Naomi H., MD {1548229461} ObsGyn, Gyneco(86,PA01)<NJ-MORRISTN>
+ Morristown Obstetrics and Gynecology Associates
101 Madison Avenue/Suite 405   Morristown, NJ 07960   (973)267-7272   Fax (973)455-0099
+ Morristown Obstetrics and Gynecology Associates
20 Commerce Boulevard/Unit C   Succasunna, NJ 07876   (973)267-7272   Fax (973)927-7408
+ Morristown Obstetrics & Gynecology Associates
33 Main Street/Suite 220   Chatham, NJ 07960   (973)267-7272   Fax (973)455-0099

Miller, Nicole C., DO {1720303662} PthClLab<NJ-ACMCITY>
+ AtlantiCare Regional Medical Center/City Campus
1925 Pacific Avenue   Atlantic City, NJ 08401   (609)441-8063

Miller, Ralee Ka, MD {1750532503} FamMed(08,PA13)
+ Eric B. Chandler Health Center
277 George Street   New Brunswick, NJ 08901   (732)235-6700   Fax (732)235-6729

Miller, Randall W., DO {1740342575} FamMed(77,MO79)
+ 1170 Clifton Avenue
Clifton, NJ 07013   (973)472-0220   Fax (973)779-5306

Miller, Richard A., MD {1124109319} CritCr, IntrMd, PulDis(83,MEXI)
+ St. Michael's Medical Center
268 MLK Jr. Boulevard/Pulm Disease   Newark, NJ 07102   (973)877-5493   Fax (973)877-2993
+ St. Michael's Medical Center
111 Central Avenue/1st Floor   Newark, NJ 07102   (973)877-5493   Fax (973)877-2993

Miller, Richard Charles, MD {1548262819} ObsGyn(83,DC02)<NJ-STBARNMC>
+ St. Barnabas Medical Center
94 Old Short Hills Road/Ob/Gyn   Livingston, NJ 07039   (973)322-5000

Miller, Robin Jeanne, MD {1932234317} FamMed(86,PA07)
+ Alliance for Better Care, P.C.
130 Lakehurst Road   Browns Mills, NJ 08015   (609)893-3133   Fax (609)893-7972

Miller, Ryan Christopher, MD {1891273629} IntrMd<NJ-COOPRUMC>
+ Cooper University Hospital
One Cooper Plaza   Camden, NJ 08103   (800)826-6737

Miller, Sandra M., MD Pedtrc(88,WIND)
+ 10 Arlene Drive
West Long Branch, NJ 07764

Miller, Sandrene, MD {1912192527} Pedtrc, PedHem(74,JMA01)
+ Irvington Pediatric Associates
22 Ball Street/Suite 100   Irvington, NJ 07111   (973)371-1600   Fax (973)372-7677

Miller, Scott David, MD {1154381184} SrgOrt(84,NY20)<NJ-CHSFULD, NJ-RWJURAH>
+ Lawrence Orthopaedics
4065 Quakerbridge Road   Princeton Junction, NJ 08550   (609)394-3804   Fax (609)989-1550

Miller, Scott Lewis, MD {1316917180} FamMed(90,NJ06)<NJ-VIRTMARL, NJ-VIRTVOOR>
+ Partners in Primary Care
534 Lippincott Drive   Marlton, NJ 08053   (856)985-7373   Fax (856)985-9611

Miller, Shamaal M., MD {1659514511} Anesth<NJ-SJHREGMC>
+ SJH Regional Medical Center
1505 West Sherman Avenue   Vineland, NJ 08360   (856)641-7859   Fax (856)641-7671

Miller, Steven E., DO {1942298096} Pedtrc, IntrMd(85,MO78)<NJ-RIVERVW>
+ Navesink Pediatrics
55 North Gilbert Street/Suite 2101   Tinton Falls, NJ 07701   (732)842-6677   Fax (732)530-2946

Miller, Stuart Henry, MD {1134170293} IntrMd, RadDia, RadV&I(88,OH40)<NJ-CHRIST>
+ Christ Hospital
176 Palisade Avenue/Radiology   Jersey City, NJ 07306   (952)595-1100   Fax (612)294-4903

Miller, Walter P., MD {1851430961} FamMed(78,DC03)<NJ-SOCEANCO>
+ Southern Ocean Primary Care
317 East Main Street   Tuckerton, NJ 08087   (609)296-1336
+ Hackensack Meridian Medical Group
53 Nautilus Drive/Suite 201   Manahawkin, NJ 08050   (609)296-1336   Fax (609)978-8903

Miller, William B., DO {1932332129} CritCr, PulDis, IntrMd(72,PA77)
+ Fox Chase Virtua Health Cancer Center
106 Carnie Boulevard/Suite A   Voorhees, NJ 08043   (856)325-5601

Miller, Yael Spinat, MD {1417959057} Pedtrc(00,NY46)<NJ-STBARNMC, NJ-OVERLOOK>
+ 90 Millburn Avenue
Millburn, NJ 07041   (973)762-8831   Fax (973)378-7991

Miller-Breslow, Anne J., MD {1689629925} SrgHnd, SrgMcr, SrgOrt(83,MA01)<NJ-ENGLWOOD, NJ-HOLYNAME>
+ Englewood Orthopedic Associates
401 South Van Brunt Street   Englewood, NJ 07631   (201)569-2770   Fax (201)569-1774

Miller-Smith, Stacey Ann, MD {1578712956} PhysMd(04,NJ05)<NJ-UNVMCPRN>
+ Princeton Orthopaedic Associates, P.A.
325 Princeton Avenue   Princeton, NJ 08540   (609)924-8131   Fax (609)924-8532
+ Princeton Orthopaedic Associates, P.A.
340 Scotch Road   Ewing, NJ 08628   (609)924-8131   Fax (609)924-8532
+ Princeton Orthopaedic Associates PA
727 State Road   Princeton, NJ 08540

Milligan Milburn, Erin Colleen, MD {1346402922} Pedtrc
+ Advocare Haddonfield Pediatric Assoc
220 Haddon Avenue   Haddonfield, NJ 08033

Millili, John J., MD {1609897198} Surgry(79,PA01)<NJ-UNDRWD>
+ Woodbury Surgical Associates
127 North Broad Street   Woodbury, NJ 08096   (856)845-0500   Fax (856)384-8757

Mills, Lisa Alice, MD {1215052287} OncHem(01,NY08)<NJ-OVERLOOK, NJ-MORRISTN>
+ Summit Medical Group-Berkeley Heights Campus
1 Diamond Hill Road   Berkeley Heights, NJ 07922   (908)273-4300   Fax (908)673-7390

Mills, Orlando F., MD {1043270382} FamMed(84,NJ05)<NJ-CENTRAST>
+ 515 Iron Bridge Road
Freehold, NJ 07728   (732)303-6455   Fax (732)303-6955

Mills, Richard J., MD {1073582813} Nrolgy(82,NJ06)<NJ-JRSYCITY>
+ Carteret Comprehensive Medical Care, P.C.
1175 Roosevelt Avenue   Carteret, NJ 07008   (732)541-2233   Fax (732)541-2234
info@theccmc.com
+ Jersey City Medical Center
355 Grand Street   Jersey City, NJ 07304   (201)915-2000

Mills, Robert, DO {1083027056} FamMed
+ Mt. Laurel Family Physicians
401 Young Avenue/Suite 260   Moorestown, NJ 08057   (856)291-8756   Fax (856)291-8750

Millstein, Jeffrey Howard, MD {1396772281} IntrMd(88,NY15)
+ Penn Medicine at Woodbury Heights
1006 Mantua Pike   Woodbury Heights, NJ 08097   (856)845-8600   Fax (856)845-0535

Milman, Anna, DO {1164450847} FamMed, EmrgMd(97,NJ75)<NJ-VIRTVOOR>
+ Virtua Voorhees
100 Bowman Drive   Voorhees, NJ 08043   (856)247-3000

Milman, Edward, MD {1205823788} RadDia(99,NY08)<NJ-STJOSHOS>
+ Imaging Subspecialists of North Jersey LLC
703 Main Street   Paterson, NJ 07503   (973)754-2645

Milman, Tatyana, MD {1083635403} Ophthl(00,PA01)
+ 4 Penbrook Court
Princeton Junction, NJ 08550

Milne, Charlene E., MD {1952462616} FamMed(89,NJ05)<NJ-JFKMED>
+ JFK Family Practice Group
65 James Street   Edison, NJ 08818   (732)321-7588   Fax (732)906-4927

Milosis, Christine, MD {1790875193} EmrgMd, IntrMd(94,NY08)<NJ-STCLRDEN, NJ-STCLRDOV>
+ 6 Princeton Court
Basking Ridge, NJ 07920

Milov, Seva, MD {1205022746} ObsGyn(89,KAZ05)
+ Pavilion Ob/Gyn AtlantiCare
2500 English Creek Avenue/Suite 214   Egg Harbor Township, NJ 08234   (609)677-7211   Fax (609)677-7210
+ Pavilion Ob/Gyn AtlantiCare
443 Shore Road/Suite 101   Somers Point, NJ 08244   (609)677-7211   Fax (609)611-7210

Milrod, Lewis Martin, MD {1851317572} NroChl, Nrolgy, ClNrPh(85,MA01)
+ 80 State Route 27/Rear Suite
Edison, NJ 08820   (732)548-2724   Fax (732)623-9721

Mimms, Gaines M., MD {1861465072} NnPnMd, Pedtrc(79,BEL07)<NJ-MORRISTN, NJ-STCLRDEN>
+ MidAtlantic Neonatology Associates
100 Madison Avenue   Morristown, NJ 07962   (973)971-5488   Fax (973)290-7175

Min, Dorothy D., MD {1518915131} Nephro, IntrMd(97,VA01)<NJ-VIRTMHBC, NJ-LOURDMED>
+ The Center for Kidney Care
1261 Route 38/Suite A   Hainesport, NJ 08036   (856)222-1975   Fax (856)222-0721

Min, Irene, MD {1760859821} IntrMd<NJ-JRSYCITY>
+ Jersey City Medical Center
355 Grand Street   Jersey City, NJ 07304   (201)915-2000

Mina, Randa Fahim, MD {1174585855} IntrMd(88,EGY09)
+ 2087 Klockner Road
Hamilton, NJ 08690

Minano, Cecilia, MD {1841498714} IntrMd, Gastrn
+ Summit Medical Group
123 Highland Avenue/Suite 103   Glen Ridge, NJ 07028   (973)429-8800   Fax (973)748-7076

Minarich, Michael, MD {1649681321} SrgOnc
+ Cooper Surgical Associates
3 Cooper Plaza/Suite 411   Camden, NJ 08103   (856)342-3012   Fax (856)365-1180

Minassian, Haig, MD {1114986940} Pthlgy, PthACl, PthCyt(82,SYRI)<NJ-RIVERVW, NJ-JRSYSHMC>
+ Riverview Medical Center
1 Riverview Plaza/Path   Red Bank, NJ 07701   (732)741-2700   Fax (732)345-2045

Minaya, Evelyn, MD {1174518286} ObsGyn(90,NY08)<NJ-RIVERVW>
+ Women Caring for Women
43 North Gilbert Street/Suite 8   Tinton Falls, NJ 07701   (732)530-5550   Fax (732)345-8309

Mindich, Bruce Paul, MD {1396714051} SrgThr, Surgry, SrgCdv(72,NY08)<NJ-VALLEY>
+ Valley Columbia Heart Center
223 North Van Dien Avenue   Ridgewood, NJ 07450   (201)447-8377   Fax (201)447-8658

Minerowicz, Christine Marianne, MD {1154440139}
+ 115 Lincoln Avenue
Highland Park, NJ 08904   (908)303-3859
chris.minerowicz@gmail.com

Minett, Danielle Marie, MD {1184944746} EmrgMd(10,NJ06)
+ Emergency Medical Associates of NJ, P.A.
3 Century Drive   Parsippany, NJ 07054   (973)740-0607   Fax (973)740-9895

Minett, Kenneth Matthew, MD {1477780187} EmrgMd
+ Emergency Medical Associates of NJ, P.A.
3 Century Drive   Parsippany, NJ 07054   (973)740-0607   Fax (973)740-9895

Minetti, John J., MD {1720026065} EmrgMd, GenPrc(80,MEXI)<NJ-MONMOUTH>
+ Monmouth Medical Center
300 Second Avenue/EmergMed   Long Branch, NJ 07740   (732)222-5200

Ming, Xue, MD {1346314507} NroChl(84,CHNA)
+ JFK Neurosciences Institute
65 James Street/Second Floor   Edison, NJ 08818   (732)321-7010   Fax (732)744-5873
+ Rutgers NJ School of Medicine Neurology
90 Bergen Street/DOC 5200   Newark, NJ 07103   (732)321-7010   Fax (973)972-5059

Mingin, Todd A., DO {1801241708}<NJ-SJHREGMC>
+ SJH Regional Medical Center
1505 West Sherman Avenue   Vineland, NJ 08360   (856)641-8000

Mingione, Richard A., MD {1154333219} IntrMd(76,PA09)<NJ-ACMCITY, NJ-ACMCMAIN>
+ 4127 Atlantic Avenue
Atlantic City, NJ 08401   (609)347-7135   Fax (609)347-6336

Mingroni, Julius Anthony, DO {1669485751} FamMed(74,PA77)
+ Kennedy Health Alliance
1300 Liberty Place   Sicklerville, NJ 08081   (856)262-8100   Fax (856)885-6859
+ Advocare Berlin Medical Associates
175 Cross Keys Road/Suite 300A   Berlin, NJ 08009   (856)262-8100   Fax (856)767-6102

Minhas, Deepa S., MD {1013979798} Pedtrc(85,INA9B)<NJ-MORRISTN, NJ-STBARNMC>
+ Mendham Pediatric Care
12 West Main Street   Mendham, NJ 07945   (973)543-1996   Fax (973)543-5775

Minhas, Navpreet Singh, MD {1447563754} Pedtrc<NJ-HACKNSK, NJ-HOLYNAME>
+ Primary Care at Oakland
340c Ramapo Valley Road   Oakland, NJ 07436   (973)962-6200   Fax (973)962-0046
+ Riverside Medical Group
714 Tenth Street/Suite 2   Secaucus, NJ 07094   (973)962-6200   Fax (201)656-0093

Minikes, Neil Ira, MD {1629022835} AlgyImmn, PedAlg, Pedtrc(80,NY01)<NJ-ENGLWOOD, NY-PRSBCOLU>
+ Allergy & Asthma Center of Northern New Jersey
500 Piermont Road/Suite 304   Closter, NJ 07624   (201)564-7777   Fax (201)564-7776

Minion, Jason A., MD {1376822023}<NJ-UNIVBHC>
+ University Behavioral Health Care
671 Hoes Lane/PO Box 1392/Rm D325   Piscataway, NJ 08855   (723)235-3344

Minkowitz, Barbara, MD {1154395978} PedOrt(87,NY09)<NJ-MORRISTN, NJ-OVERLOOK>
+ Children's Orthopedic & Sports Medicine Center
261 James Street/Suite 3-C   Morristown, NJ 07960   (973)206-1033   Fax (973)206-1036
+ Children's Orthopedic & Sports Medicine Center
33 Overlook Road/Suite 201   Summit, NJ 07901   (973)206-1033   Fax (973)206-1036

Minn, Joon Hong, MD {1740208602} Radiol, RadDia(97,NY15)
+ Essex Imaging Associates
5 Franklin Avenue/Suite 510   Belleville, NJ 07109   (973)751-2011   Fax (973)751-4456

Minniti, Carl J., Jr., MD {1811993652} Hemato, MedOnc, IntrMd(86,PRO02)<NJ-UNDRWD, NJ-SJSRYELM>
+ The Minniti Center for Medical Oncology & Hematology
174 Democrat Road   Mickleton, NJ 08056   (856)423-0754   Fax (856)423-7508

Minoff, Michael H., MD {1538130604} ObsGyn(82,LA05)<NJ-VIRTMHBC>
+ Minoff Chapman Ob/Gyn
110 Marter Avenue/Suite 504   Moorestown, NJ 08057   (856)642-6580   Fax (856)273-8372

Mintalucci, Dominic J., MD {1114126869} SrgOrt
+ 43 Peters Place
Red Bank, NJ 07701

Mintz, Bruce L., DO {1508834169} IntrMd(80,MO79)<NJ-MORRISTN>
+ Eastern Vascular Associates
16 Pocono Road/Suite 313   Denville, NJ 07834   (973)625-0112   Fax (973)625-0721

Mintz, Jesse M., MD {1912124892} PedNrD, NnPnMd(72,NY01)
+ 10D Auer Court
East Brunswick, NJ 08816   (732)254-7100   Fax (732)254-7474
DRJESSE123@gmail.com

Mintz, Mark I., MD {1649258450} NroChl, Pedtrc, PedNrD(84,NJ05)
+ Ctr for Neurological/Neurodevelopment
250 Haddonfield-Berlin Road/Suite 105   Gibbsboro, NJ 08026   (856)346-0005   Fax (856)784-1799

Mintz, Randy T., MD {1265403984} CdvDis, IntrMd(85,NJ15)<NJ-OURLADY, NJ-COOPRUMC>
+ Virtua Cardiology Group
2309 East Evesham Road/Suites 201-202   Voorhees, NJ 08043   (856)325-5400   Fax (856)325-5416

Mintz, Shari Nan, MD {1730199696} IntrMd, EnDbMt(99,NJ06)
+ North Jersey Endocrine Consultants, LLC
1 Indian Road/Suite 8   Denville, NJ 07834   (973)625-2121   Fax (973)625-8270

Minutillo, Angelo L., MD {1376507871} Pedtrc(82,ITAL)<NJ-UNDRWD, NJ-COOPRUMC>
+ Gloucester County Pediatrics
849 Cooper Street   Deptford, NJ 08096   (856)848-6346   Fax (856)848-5734

Minzter, Ronald M., MD {1861587420} Ophthl, PedOph(87,NJ05)<NJ-CENTRAST>
+ 495 Iron Bridge Road
Freehold, NJ 07728   (732)577-5558   Fax (732)577-5559

Mir, Raema, MD {1508201138} FamMed
+ Partners in Primary Care
141 Route 70 East/Suite E   Marlton, NJ 08053   (856)985-7373   Fax (856)985-9611

Mirabal, Sadie L., DO {1255674008}<NJ-NWRKBETH>
+ Newark Community Health Center, Inc.
741 Broadway   Newark, NJ 07104   (973)675-1900   Fax (973)676-1396
+ Newark Beth Israel Medical Center
201 Lyons Avenue   Newark, NJ 07112   (973)926-7471

Miraglia, Janeen Theresa, DO {1891947412} IntrMd, Pedtrc(06,NY75)
+ PASE HealthCare, PC
225 Millburn Avenue/Suite 303   Millburn, NJ 07041   (973)912-7273   Fax (973)912-7275

Miranda, Chona Santos, MD {1457383549} FamMed(90,PHI01)
+ Miranda Medical Associates
630 Bellevue Avenue   Hammonton, NJ 08037   (856)561-7548   Fax (609)561-7520

Miranda, Claudia Danitza, MD {1639598097} IntrMd
+ Drs. Silverman and Silverman
480 Market Street   Saddle Brook, NJ 07663   (201)845-4048

Miranda, David J., MD {1801276084} EmrgMd
+ Capital Health System/Fuld Emergency
750 Brunswick Avenue   Trenton, NJ 08638   (609)394-6063

Miranda, Irving, MD {1033407879} Surgry
+ University Hospital
150 Bergen Street/E-401   Newark, NJ 07103   (973)972-6591

Miranda, Matilda, MD {1437198215} ObsGyn(00,OH41)
+ Somerset Ob-Gyn Associates
215 Union Avenue/Suite A   Bridgewater, NJ 08807   (908)722-2900   Fax (908)722-1856
+ Somerset Ob-Gyn Associates
1 New Amwell Road   Hillsborough, NJ 08844   (908)874-5900

Miranda, Rosa Josefina, MD {1407826738} Pedtrc(87,DOM04)<NJ-MTNSIDE, NJ-HACKNSK>
+ Children of Joy Pediatrics
134 Summit Avenue   Hackensack, NJ 07601   (201)525-0077   Fax (201)525-0072

Mirani, Gayatri, MD {1942537378} Pedtrc<NJ-HACKNSK, NJ-HOLYNAME>
+ Riverside Medical Group
714 Tenth Street/Suite 2   Secaucus, NJ 07094   (201)863-3346   Fax (201)865-0015

Mirani, Neena M., MD {1275554537} PthACl, PthCyt(71,INA65)<NJ-UMDNJ>
+ University Hospital
150 Bergen Street/Pathology   Newark, NJ 07103   (973)972-4300   Fax (973)972-5724
miraninm@umdnj.edu

Mircea, Cornel, MD {1316055973} IntrMd, Hemato, MedOnc(73,ROM06)<NJ-CLARMAAS, NJ-MTNSIDE>
+ 50 Newark Avenue/Suite 306
Belleville, NJ 07109

Mirchandani, Indu, MD {1881641702} Psychy, PsyGrt(70,INA87)
+ 3 Peach Hill Court
Ramsey, NJ 07446   (201)887-3345

Mirchandani, Jai, MD {1760416283} IntrMd, Gastrn(00,NJ02)
+ Gastroenterologists of Ocean County
477 Lakehurst Road   Toms River, NJ 08755   (732)349-4422   Fax (732)349-5087

Mirchandani, Monica Hargovind, DO {1881607265} Pedtrc
+ 25 Port Imperial Boulevard/Apt 1021
West New York, NJ 07093

Mirchandani, Ratan, MD {1720180730} IntrMd(65,INDI)
+ 304 Central Avenue
Orange, NJ 07050   (609)673-3300   Fax (973)673-5735

Mirchandani, Sunil, MD {1811157381} IntrMd, CdvDis(01,NY19)<NJ-OVERLOOK, NJ-MORRISTN>
+ Summit Medical Group-Berkeley Heights Campus
1 Diamond Hill Road   Berkeley Heights, NJ 07922   (908)273-4300   Fax (908)790-6576

Miric, Slobodan, MD {1710908934} Nrolgy(94,SERB)
+ Dr. Miric Neurology Center
35 West Main Street/Suite 103   Denville, NJ 07834   (973)625-0858   Fax (973)625-0859
contactus@drmiric.org

Mirmadjlessi, Noushin, MD {1891962528} PhysMd
+ Central Pain Institute
3 Cornwall Drive/Suite A   East Brunswick, NJ 08816   (732)698-1000   Fax (732)698-1008

Mirmanesh, John C., MD {1780811034} Pedtrc<NJ-VIRTMARL>
+ Center Pediatrics Adolescent & Adult
12000 Lincoln Drive West/Suite 311   Marlton, NJ 08053   (856)985-8100   Fax (856)985-0178
jmirmanesh@gmail.com

Mirmanesh, Shahin Michael, MD {1679505325} IntrMd(94,DMN01)<NJ-VIRTMARL, NJ-OURLADY>
+ Center for Adult Medicine
12000 Lincoln Drive West/Suite 404-405   Marlton, NJ 08053   (856)985-0203   Fax (856)985-0010
SHAPOURMIR@aol.com

Mirmanesh, Shahram J., MD {1750335360} Pedtrc(83,DMN01)<NJ-VIRTMHBC, NJ-VIRTVOOR>
+ Center for Pediatrics and Adult Medicine
311 The Pavilions at Greentree   Marlton, NJ 08053   (856)985-8100   Fax (856)985-8374
drjay@docmir.com

Mirmanesh, Shapour Steve, MD {1669407375} IntrMd, IntHos(99,SLU01)<NJ-VIRTMARL, NJ-VIRTVOOR>
+ Center for Adult Medicine
12000 Lincoln Drive West/Suite 404-405   Marlton, NJ 08053   (856)985-0203   Fax (856)985-0010

Miron, Mike, MD {1356425128} Ophthl, VitRet(68,ROMA)
+ 40-04 Kilada Court
Fair Lawn, NJ 07410   (201)791-1178

Mirone, Gary Steven, DO {1972653939} Gyneco, UroGyn(01,PA78)<NJ-SJHREGMC>
+ Physicians of Southern New Jersey
2950 College Drive/Suite 2D   Vineland, NJ 08360   (856)641-8680   Fax (856)641-8679

Mirone, Rolande A., DO {1134327786} Pedtrc<NJ-KMHSTRAT, NJ-VIRTUAHS>
+ Pediatric Associates, LLC.
1318 South Main Street   Vineland, NJ 08360   (856)691-8585   Fax (856)691-8489

Physicians by Name and Address

Mirsen, Thomas R., MD {1902980352} Nrolgy, OthrSp(82,NY08)<NJ-COOPRUMC>
+ Cooper University Neurology
1935 Route 70 East   Cherry Hill, NJ 08003   (856)342-2445   Fax (856)964-0504
+ Cooper Physicians Washington Township
1 Plaza Drive/Suite 103/Bunker Hill Pl   Sewell, NJ 08080   (856)342-2445   Fax (856)270-4085

Mirsky, Eric Charles, MD {1447247283} SrgOrt(92,NY19)<NJ-OVERLOOK, NJ-MORRISTN>
+ Summit Medical Group-Berkeley Heights Campus
1 Diamond Hill Road   Berkeley Heights, NJ 07922   (908)273-4300   Fax (908)790-6524

Mirsky, Robert G., MD {1326145111} Ophthl(75,VA04)
+ 745 Northfield Avenue
West Orange, NJ 07052   (973)736-1016   Fax (973)736-4869

Mirson, Sofiya, MD {1386684280} IntrMd(93,RUS81)<PA-ENSTEIN>
+ Dorfner Family Medicine
950 A Chester Avenue/Suite 10   Delran, NJ 08075   (856)764-2500   Fax (856)764-8335

Miryala, Rekha, MD {1942486568} IntrMd(01,INA83)
+ 239 Claremont Avenue/Suite B
Montclair, NJ 07042   (973)338-3300   Fax (973)338-0400

Mirza, Ahmed Anas, MD {1114094711} IntrMd, Grtrcs(92,PAK24)<NJ-UNVMCPRN>
+ Monroe Village Health Care Center
1 David Brainerd Drive   Monroe Township, NJ 08831   (732)521-6400   Fax (732)521-6540
Drmirza2001@yahoo.com
+ Geriatric Associates of New Jersey
666 Plainsboro Road/Suite1318   Plainsboro, NJ 08536   (609)269-8291

Mirza, Babar, MD {1265442875} IntrMd(82,PAKI)
+ Medical Associates of Marlboro
42 Throckmorton Lane/2nd flr   Old Bridge, NJ 08857   (732)607-1111   Fax (732)607-0552
+ Associates in Cardiology and Internal Medicine
790 Amboy Avenue   Perth Amboy, NJ 08861   (732)607-1111   Fax (732)324-8095

Mirza, Bushra F., MD {1679771315}
+ 292 Clinton Road
North Brunswick, NJ 08902   (732)821-7139

Mirza, Ismet Amtul Latif, MD {1538363841} IntrMd(01,PAK08)
+ Geriatric Associates of New Jersey
666 Plainsboro Road/Suite1318   Plainsboro, NJ 08536   (609)269-8291
+ 5 Sanibel Court
Monroe, NJ 08831   (609)619-3091

Mirza, Michael Rohinton, MD {1184043267} EmrgMd
+ Robert Wood Johnson Emergency Medicine
One Robert Wood Johnson Place/MEB 104   New Brunswick, NJ 08901   (732)235-8717

Mirza, Muhammad A., MD {1881677409} IntrMd(95,PAK12)
+ Allied Medical & Diagnostic Services, LLC.
124 Eileen Drive   Cedar Grove, NJ 07009   (973)493-7607

Mirza, Muhammed H., MD {1467450262} IntrMd(81,DOM06)<NJ-JRSYCITY, NJ-CHRIST>
+ 503 Jersey Avenue
Jersey City, NJ 07302   (201)433-1317   Fax (201)433-7919
muhammedhmirza@aol.com
+ 2742 Kennedy Boulevard
Jersey City, NJ 07306   (201)433-1317   Fax (201)433-8365

Mirza, Nadia A., MD {1669678009} Psychy(04,PAK20)
+ University Hospital
150 Bergen Street/Rm C 224   Newark, NJ 07103   (973)972-4300

Mirza, Nadia M., MD {1891021986} Radiol, RadDia(06,NY06)<NJ-STCLRDEN>
+ St. Clare's Hospital-Denville Campus
25 Pocono Road/Radiology   Denville, NJ 07834   (973)983-5261   Fax (201)526-8333

Mirza, Neville M., MD {1558449017} SrgNro(72,INDI)
+ 142 Palisade Avenue/Suite 214
Jersey City, NJ 07306   (201)963-5753   Fax (201)963-5759

Mirza, Nighat, MD {1558306423} GenPrc, Psychy(83,PAKI)
+ 32 Hine Street
Paterson, NJ 07503   (973)523-4100

Mirza, Samina Yasmin, MD {1154689594}
+ University Behavioral HealthCare
183 South Orange Avenue/BHSB E-1447   Newark, NJ 07103   (973)972-4670

Mirza, Zainab Arshad, MD {1134539992} IntrMd
+ Jersey Shore University Medical Center
1945 Route 33   Neptune, NJ 07753   (732)775-5500

Mirzayan, Nadine Kristen, MD {1396016218}
+ St. Joseph's Regional Medical Center Anesthesia
703 Main Street   Paterson, NJ 07505   (973)754-2323   Fax (973)754-3131

Misbin, Michael David, MD {1609950062} Anesth(81,NY03)<NJ-COOPRUMC>
+ Cooper University Hospital
One Cooper Plaza/Anesthesia   Camden, NJ 08103   (856)342-2000

Misher-Harris, Michele, DO {1841276581} Anesth
+ Rancocas Anesthesiology, PA
700 Route 130 North/Suite 203   Cinnaminson, NJ 08077   (856)829-9345   Fax (856)829-3605

Mishik, Anthony N., MD {1699723668} Pedtrc(84,DC02)<NJ-UNDRWD, NJ-KMHTURNV>
+ Advocare West Deptford Pediatrics
1050 Mantua Pike   Wenonah, NJ 08090   (856)468-8330   Fax (856)468-9121
tonymishik@aol.com
+ Advocare West Deptford Pediatrics
19 Village Center Drive   Swedesboro, NJ 08085   (856)468-8330   Fax (856)879-2855
+ Advocare West Deptford Pediatrics
646 Kings Highway   West Deptford, NJ 08090   (856)879-2887   Fax (856)879-2855

Mishkin, Steven K., MD {1093896912} Ophthl(81,NY46)<NJ-CENTRAST, NJ-MONMOUTH>
+ Millennium Eye Care, LLC
500 West Main Street   Freehold, NJ 07728   (732)462-8707   Fax (732)462-1296
+ Millennium Eye Care, LLC
Route 130 & Princeton Road   Hightstown, NJ 08520   (732)462-8707   Fax (609)448-4197
+ Millennium Eye Care, LLC
515 Brick Boulevard/Suite G   Brick, NJ 07728   (732)920-3800   Fax (732)920-5351

Mishler, Ken E., MD {1043279979} Ophthl(72,GA05)<NJ-CHILTON>
+ Eye Associates of Wayne PA
968 Hamburg Turnpike   Wayne, NJ 07470   (973)696-0300   Fax (973)696-0465

Mishra, Arunesh Kumar, MD {1750361671} Psychy, PsyGrt(83,INA57)<NJ-RBAYPERT, NJ-RBAYOLDB>
+ Raritan Bay Medical Center/Perth Amboy Division
530 New Brunswick Avenue/Psych   Perth Amboy, NJ 08861   (732)442-3700   Fax (732)324-5139

Mishra, Monica Shalini, MD {1093013617} RadDia, Radiol, IntrMd(06,NJ06)<NJ-RIVERVW, NJ-BAYSHORE>
+ Riverview Medical Center
1 Riverview Plaza/Diag Radiology   Red Bank, NJ 07701   (732)530-2305
+ Bayshore Community Hospital
727 North Beers Street/Diag Radiology   Holmdel, NJ 07733   (732)530-2305   Fax (732)962-7234

Mishra, Richa, MD {1346400207}
+ 207 Peony Lane
Sewell, NJ 08080

Mishra, Sneha, MD {1427351600} IntHos, IntrMd(05,INA70)
+ Berkeley Internal Medicine
391 Springfield Avenue/Suite 1B   Berkeley Heights, NJ 07922   (908)665-1177   Fax (908)665-8420

Mision, Vicente L., MD {1013937614} Pedtrc(71,PHIL)<NJ-JRSYSHMC>
+ 4057 US Highway 9/Suite 175
Howell, NJ 07731   (732)370-1900   Fax (732)901-0916

Miskimen, Theresa M., MD {1669500950} Psychy, Addctn(90,PRO01)<NJ-UNIVBHC, NJ-RWJUBRUN>
+ University Behavioral Health Care
671 Hoes Lane/PO Box 1392   Piscataway, NJ 08855   (732)235-5500
+ University Behavioral Health Care
303 George Street/Suite 200   New Brunswick, NJ 08901   (732)235-5500   Fax (732)235-6187

Miskin, Chandrabhaga P., MD {1649552688} Pedtrc
+ 2211 Arvell Court
Toms River, NJ 08755

Miskin, Pandurang R., MD {1154371250} Nrolgy(77,INDI)<NJ-COMMED, NJ-OCEANMC>
+ Shore Neurology, PA
1613 Route 88/Suite 3   Brick, NJ 08724   (732)785-3335   Fax (732)785-2599
+ Shore Neurology, P.A.
633 Route 37 West   Toms River, NJ 08755   (732)785-3335   Fax (732)240-3114

Misko, Gary J., Jr., MD {1033213236} IntrMd(94,NJ06)<NJ-RWJUBRUN, NJ-STPETER>
+ PEMCARE
259 Talmadge Road   Edison, NJ 08817   (732)287-6004   Fax (732)287-3575

Miskoff, Jeffrey Aaron, DO {1245232032} IntrMd, PulCCr, PulDis(98,MO78)<NJ-JRSYSHMC, NJ-OCEANMC>
+ Shore Pulmonary PA
2640 Highway 70/Building 6-A   Manasquan, NJ 08736   (732)528-5900   Fax (732)528-0887
+ Shore Pulmonary PA
301 Bingham Avenue/Suite B   Ocean, NJ 07712   (732)528-5900   Fax (732)775-1212
+ Shore Pulmonary PA
1608 Route 88/Suite 117   Brick, NJ 08736   (732)575-1100

Misra, Amit, MD {1750675807} IntrMd<NJ-ACMCITY>
+ AtlantiCare Regional Medical Center/City Campus
1925 Pacific Avenue   Atlantic City, NJ 08401   (609)345-4000

Misra, Amit C., MD {1104060102} PedCrC<NJ-MONMOUTH>
+ Monmouth Medical Center
300 Second Avenue/Pediatrics   Long Branch, NJ 07740   (732)923-7250   Fax (732)923-7255

Misra, Manju, MD {1861552671} Pedtrc, AdolMd(80,INDI)<NJ-STPETER, NJ-RWJUBRUN>
+ 1553 Highway 27/Suite 2500
Somerset, NJ 08873   (732)296-9717   Fax (732)296-9711
mmisramd@yahoo.com

Misra, Neerja, MD {1093824732} IntrMd(78,INDI)
+ Corporate Health Center
832 Brunswick Avenue   Trenton, NJ 08638   (609)695-7471

Misra, Neeti Virendra, MD {1699967323} ObsGyn(92,INA87)<NJ-CENTRAST>
+ Healthy Woman Ob/Gyn
312 Professional View Drive   Freehold, NJ 07728   (732)431-1616   Fax (732)866-7962

Misra, Sanjay, MD {1528096948} IntrMd(82,INA49)<NJ-CENTRAST>
+ Cooper University Hospital
One Cooper Plaza   Camden, NJ 08103   (856)356-4924
+ 17 Holly Drive
East Windsor, NJ 08520

Misthos, Paul, MD {1982645610} IntrMd(84,NY06)
+ Sall/Myers Medical Associates, PA
100 Hamilton Plaza/Suite 317/3rd Floor   Paterson, NJ 07505   (973)279-2323   Fax (973)279-7551

Mistry, Bharati S., MD {1053314468} Anesth(72,INDI)<NJ-STCLRDEN, NJ-STCLRDOV>
+ St. Clare's Hospital-Denville Campus
25 Pocono Road/Anesthesiology   Denville, NJ 07834   (973)625-6000

Mistry, Nirav, MD {1912162066} IntHos, CritCr<NY-NYACKHOS>
+ JFK Medical Center
65 James Street   Edison, NJ 08820   (732)321-7660

Mistry, Tusharkumar N., MD {1053302976} IntrMd(92,INA21)<NJ-RBAYOLDB, NJ-RBAYPERT>
+ 28 Throckmorton Lane
Old Bridge, NJ 08857   (732)679-4200

Mitchel, Jeffrey M., MD {1033126735} CdvDis, IntrMd(74,NY19)<NJ-HACKNSK, NJ-HOLYNAME>
+ 370 Grand Avenue
Englewood, NJ 07631   (201)567-7576   Fax (201)567-8628
+ Heart and Vascular Institute at EHMC
350 Engle Street/Suite 1000   Englewood, NJ 07631   (201)894-3636

Mitchell, Barbara, MD {1629473087} ObsGyn, IntrMd(77,AZ01)
+ 385 State Route 24/Bldg Suite 3-C
Chester, NJ 07930   (908)879-8000   Fax (908)879-1385

Mitchell, Cheryl Marie, MD {1124120811} Ophthl(84,PA01)<NJ-VIRTBERL>
+ 128 Route 70/Suite 2-A/Medford Plaza
Medford, NJ 08055   (609)654-6940   Fax (609)654-5725
C.m.mitchell1@comcast.net

Mitchell, David S., DO {1528179827} GenPrc, IntrMd(89,MO78)<NJ-COMMED>
+ 1151 Church Road
Toms River, NJ 08755   (732)905-8333   Fax (732)503-4823

Mitchell, Joyce Marie, MD {1952407850} EmrgMd, UrgtCr, IntrMd(76,DC02)<NJ-OVERLOOK>
+ Overlook Medical Center
99 Beauvoir Avenue/PO Box 210/EmrgMed   Summit, NJ 07902   (908)522-2000

Mitchell, Lamont Leigh, DO {1831360502} EmrgMd
+ 27 East Chestnut Avenue
Merchantville, NJ 08109

Mitchell, Roger A., Jr., MD {1427275742}
+ Office of The Regional Medical Examiner State of NJ
325 Norfolk Street   Newark, NJ 07103   (973)648-3914   Fax (973)648-3692

Mitchell, William, MD {1548260722} SrgNro(96,CA06)
+ ASAP - Advanced Spine and Pain
3829 Church Road/Suite B   Mount Laurel, NJ 08054   (856)372-9422   Fax (856)409-0393
+ Coastal Spine
4000 Church Road   Mount Laurel, NJ 08054   (856)372-9422   Fax (856)222-0049

Mitchell-Williams, Jocelyn, MD {1730263195} ObsGyn(97,NJ06)
+ Cooper Ob-Gyn
1900 Mount Holly Road/Suite 3-C   Burlington, NJ 08016   (609)835-5570
+ Cooper Faculty Ob/Gyn
1103 Kings Highway North/Suite 201   Cherry Hill, NJ 08034   (609)835-5570   Fax (856)321-0133

Physicians by Name and Address

Mitev, Iliya D., MD {1922299882} FamMed
+ Highlands Family Health Center
61 Frontage Road/Suite 61 Hampton, NJ 08827 (908)735-2594 Fax (908)735-8526

Mithaiwala, Sanaa Saher, DO {1922234004}
+ 6 Vincent Court
Edison, NJ 08820

Mithani, Bharati T., MD {1831275742} Anesth(74,INDI)<NJ-COOPRUMC>
+ The Cooper Health System at Voorhees
900 Centennial Boulevard Voorhees, NJ 08043 (856)325-6500 Fax (856)325-6515

Mithani, Sima, MD {1285875724} AlgyImmn, IntrMd(06,PA13)<NJ-ENGLWOOD>
+ ENT & Allergy Associates, LLP
433 Hackensack Avenue/Suite 204 Hackensack, NJ 07601 (201)883-1062 Fax (201)883-9297
smithani@entandallergy.com

Mithani, Tamanna A., DO {1336382068}<NJ-VIRTMARL>
+ Virtua Marlton Hospital
90 Brick Road Marlton, NJ 08053 (773)732-1172

Mitnick, David Andrew, MD {1720130248} PsyCAd, Psychy(87,NY20)<NY-PRSBWEIL>
+ New Jersey Family Psychiatric Group, P.A.
240 West Passaic Street/Suite 1 Maywood, NJ 07607 (201)880-7575 Fax (201)880-7570

Mitra, Anjali Naz, MD {1487143202} Gyneco
+ University Medical Group/OBGYN
125 Paterson Street/2nd Floor New Brunswick, NJ 08901 (732)235-6375 Fax (732)235-6627

Mitra, Tithi, MD {1124266366} IntrMd(02,INA02)
+ Drs. Mitra & Mayrowetz
368 Lakehurst Road/Suite 207 Toms River, NJ 08755 (732)557-6222 Fax (732)557-6227

Mitrev, Ludmil Vladimirov, MD {1508852153} Anesth(97,NOR01)<NJ-COOPRUMC>
+ Cooper University Hospital
One Cooper Plaza/Radiology Camden, NJ 08103 (856)342-2425 Fax (856)968-8239

Mitskavich, Mary T., MD {1457355117} Otlryg(91,PA12)<NJ-JRSYSHMC>
+ Coastal Ear Nose and Throat LLC
3700 Route 33/Suite 101 Neptune, NJ 07753 (732)280-7855 Fax (732)280-7815
+ Coastal Ear Nose and Throat LLC
1301 Route 72/Suite 340 Manahawkin, NJ 08050 (732)280-7855 Fax (732)280-7815

Mitsos, Stephanie E., MD {1861679516} IntrMd(91,PA01)<NJ-OURLADY>
+ 13 C Route 206
Stanhope, NJ 07874 (973)691-7551 Fax (973)691-7621

Mittal, Manoj Kumar, MD {1720172737} Gastrn, IntrMd(82,INA41)<PA-WARRNGEN, PA-EASTON>
+ 39 Roseberry Street/Hillcrest Plaza
Phillipsburg, NJ 08865 (908)454-4266

Mittal, Satish K., MD {1518912385} IntrMd, PulDis(77,INDI)<NJ-MEMSALEM>
+ 2950 College Drive/Suite 1-C
Vineland, NJ 08360 (856)691-4800 Fax (856)691-4801

Mittal, Shraddha, MD {1265422869} PedEmg, Pedtrc(85,INA72)<NJ-VIRTMHBC, NJ-VIRTVOOR>
+ Children's Health Associates II LLC
101 Carnie Boulevard Voorhees, NJ 08043 (856)325-3000 Fax (609)261-5842
+ Virtua Memorial
175 Madison Avenue/Pediatrics Mount Holly, NJ 08060 (856)325-3000 Fax (609)265-7931
+ Virtua Voorhees
100 Bowman Drive/Pediatrics Voorhees, NJ 08043 (856)247-3921 Fax (856)247-3922

Mittal, Suneet, MD {1477666923} ClCdEl, CdvDis, IntrMd(91,MA05)<NJ-VALLEY>
+ Valley Medical Group-Electrophysiology & Cardiology
223 North Van Dien Avenue Ridgewood, NJ 07450 (201)432-7837 Fax (201)432-7830
+ Valley Medical Group-Electrophysiology & Cardiology
1578 Route 23/Suite 103 Wayne, NJ 07470 (201)432-7837 Fax (201)432-7830

Mittapalli, Kesavarao, MD {1043258023} IntrMd(78,INA11)<NY-YONKRSGH, NJ-HACKNSK>
+ 280 Henry Street
Paramus, NJ 07652 (201)261-0262
+ Hackensack University Medical Center
30 Prospect Avenue/Hospitalist Hackensack, NJ 07601 (201)996-2000

Mittelmann, Eric, MD {1215291240} Nrolgy
+ Progressive Neurology
260 Old Hook Road/Suite 200 Westwood, NJ 07675 (201)546-8510 Fax (201)503-8142

Mitterando, Jeanne G., MD {1083616841} FamMed, IntrMd(97,NJ05)
+ RWJPE Bridgewater Medical Group
766 Route 202-206/Suite 1 Bridgewater, NJ 08807 (908)722-0808 Fax (908)722-7645

Mittman, Roy D., MD {1881653863} SrgOrt(78,NY46)<NJ-JRSYSHMC, NJ-OCEANMC>
+ Seaview Orthopaedics
222 Schanck Road/3rd Floor Freehold, NJ 07728 (732)462-1700 Fax (732)303-8314
+ Seaview Orthopaedics
1640 Route 88 West Brick, NJ 08724 (732)462-1700 Fax (732)458-2743
+ Seaview Orthopaedics
1200 Eagle Avenue Ocean, NJ 07728 (732)660-6200 Fax (732)660-6201

Mitzner, Ann C., MD {1760564876} ObsGyn(92,NY46)<NJ-VALLEY>
+ Valley Medical Group Ob/Gyn in Fairlawn
5-22 Saddle River Road Fair Lawn, NJ 07410 (201)796-2025 Fax (201)796-0587

Mizan, Narmin Farah Hussain, MD {1336316991} RadDia(06,NY08)
+ Robert Wood Johnson University Hospital at Rahway
865 Stone Street Rahway, NJ 07065 (732)381-4200

Mizrachi, Arik, MD {1871744367} PhysMd, PainMd(05,NY03)
+ Princeton Orthopaedic Associates, P.A.
325 Princeton Avenue Princeton, NJ 08540 (609)924-8131 Fax (609)924-8532

Mizrahi, Marc E., MD {1750330452} Anesth(88,NY08)<NJ-ENGLWOOD>
+ Englewood Anesthesiology
350 Engle Street Englewood, NJ 07631 (201)894-3238 Fax (201)894-0585

Mleczko, Joshua, DO {1003298662} FamMed
+ Capital Health Primary Care-Bordentown
1 Third Street Bordentown, NJ 08505 (609)298-2005 Fax (609)324-8267
+ Capital Health Primary Care Columbus
23203 Columbus Road/Suite 1 Columbus, NJ 08022 (609)298-2005 Fax (603)303-4451

Mlynarczyk, Peter J., MD {1144218439} Surgry, CdvDis(69,PA02)
+ Wound Healing & Hyperbaric Medicine
240 Williamson Street/Suite 104 Elizabeth, NJ 07202 (908)994-5480 Fax (908)994-8802

Mmereole, Robert U., MD {1669615308}
+ 6101 Kennedy Boulevard East
West New York, NJ 07093 (412)607-5450
rmmereole@yahoo.com

Moak, Alan Steven, MD {1912939216} CdvDis, IntCrd, IntrMd(72,NY08)<NJ-OURLADY, NJ-COOPRUMC>
+ Penn Medicine at Cherry Hill
1400 East Route 70/Cardiology Cherry Hill, NJ 08034

Moaven, Nader, MD {1831293174} InfDis, IntrMd(88,GRN01)<NJ-CLARMAAS, NJ-WESTHDSN>
+ Empire Medical Associates
5 Franklin Avenue/Suite 302 Belleville, NJ 07109 (973)759-1221 Fax (973)759-1997
+ Empire Medical Associates
264 Boyden Avenue Maplewood, NJ 07040 (973)759-1221 Fax (973)761-7617

Moazami, Delaram, MD {1013182039} IntrMd
+ 433 Bellevue Avenue
Trenton, NJ 08618 (609)815-7374

Moazami, Saman, MD {1578839064} Urolgy
+ Garden State Urology
333 Mount Hope Avenue Rockaway, NJ 07866 (973)895-6636

Mobilio, Joseph N., Jr., DO {1770611865} Psychy(79,PA77)
+ 216 Haddon Avenue
Westmont, NJ 08108 (856)869-9300 Fax (856)869-9011

Mobin Uddin, Omar, MD {1235126327} Ophthl, Glacma(95,OH40)
+ The Glaucoma Institute, PC
10 Plum Street/6th Floor Suite 600 New Brunswick, NJ 08901 (732)546-3910 Fax (480)287-9735

Moccia, Thomas F., DO {1891739686} CdvDis
+ Owens Vergari Unwala Cardiology Associates PC
17 West Red Bank Avenue/Suite 306 Woodbury, NJ 08096 (856)845-6807 Fax (856)845-3760

Mochaver, Sepande, DO {1679735815}
+ 18 Park Avenue
Jersey City, NJ 07302 (310)713-7649
smochaver@yahoo.com

Modarressi, Taher, MD {1811335433} EnDbMt
+ Diabetes & Endocrine Associates of Hunterdon
9100 Westcott Drive/Suite 101 Flemington, NJ 08822 (908)237-6990 Fax (908)237-6995

Modena, Alisa B., MD {1346297298} ObsGyn, MtFtMd(99,NY15)<NJ-VIRTBERL, NJ-VIRTMARL>
+ Memorial Maternal Fetal Medicine Center
175 Madison Avenue Mount Holly, NJ 08060 (609)265-7914
+ Virtua Maternal Fetal Medicine Center
100 Bowman Drive Voorhees, NJ 08043 (609)265-7914
Fax (856)247-3276

Modena, Scott Alan, MD {1659339133} Gastrn, IntrMd(99,NY15)
+ The Gastroenterology Group, PA
103 Old Marlton Pike/Suite 102 Medford, NJ 08055 (609)953-3440 Fax (609)996-4002
+ The Gastroenterology Group, PA
15000 Midlantic Drive/Suite 110 Mount Laurel, NJ 08054 (609)953-3440 Fax (856)996-4007

Modesto, Rosanna A., MD {1306856778} IntrMd(85,DOMI)<NJ-HOLYNAME>
+ 773 Teaneck Road
Teaneck, NJ 07666 (201)837-7662 Fax (201)837-7446

Modi, Chintan, MD {1649506932} Gastrn, IntrMd
+ Drs. Modi & Sarkaria
98 James Street/Suite 200 Edison, NJ 08820 (732)243-9694

Modi, Chirag H., MD {1073894713} IntHos
+ 6 North Drive
East Brunswick, NJ 08816

Modi, Kaushik Chhaganlal, MD {1700886132} CdvDis, IntrMd(81,INDI)<NJ-STBARNMC, NJ-CLARMAAS>
+ Diagnostic & Clinical Cardiology
449 Mount Pleasant Avenue/2nd Floor West Orange, NJ 07052 (973)731-7868 Fax (973)731-7907

Modi, Ketang H., DO {1396736468} RadDia, Radiol, IntrMd(96,NJ75)
+ Fair Lawn Diagnostic Imaging
19-04 Fair Lawn Avenue Fair Lawn, NJ 07410 (201)794-3132 Fax (201)794-6291

Modi, Nita K., MD {1023016771} Anesth(81,INDI)<NJ-STMICHL>
+ St. Michael's Medical Center
111 Central Avenue/Anesthesia Newark, NJ 07102 (973)877-5034 Fax (973)877-5231

Modi, Parag, MD {1336147305} Anesth(93,NJ05)<NJ-VIRTBERL, NJ-VIRTMARL>
+ West Jersey Anesthesia Associates
102-E Center Boulevard Marlton, NJ 08053 (856)988-6250 Fax (856)988-6270

Modi, Tejas J., MD {1912245267} IntrMd(06,INA15)<NJ-STMICHL>
+ St. Michael's Medical Center
111 Central Avenue/Internal Med Newark, NJ 07102 (973)877-5000

Modrzejewska-Kortowska, Malgorz, MD {1427099829} Pedtrc(87,POL17)<NJ-HACKNSK, NJ-HOBUNIMC>
+ Lakeview Pediatrics
266 Lakeview Avenue Clifton, NJ 07011 (973)340-6225 Fax (973)340-0665
lakeviewpediatrics@yahoo.com

Mody, Kalgi, MD {1265741276} Pedtrc, PedCrC(10,GRN01)
+ UH- Robert Wood Johnson Med
125 Paterson Street/CAB 7103 New Brunswick, NJ 08901 (732)828-3000

Mody, Kanika Pravin, MD {1891941449} IntrMd(05,GRN01)
+ 735 Midwood Road
Ridgewood, NJ 07450 (551)804-7679 Fax (201)447-7018

Mody, Kartik D., MD {1770867061} NnPnMd
+ 200 River Park Drive
Raritan, NJ 08869

Mody, Suresh, MD {1437166956} RadDia, RadBdI(80,INA20)<NJ-STMICHL>
+ St. Michael's Medical Center
1036 Amboy Avenue/Media Img Edison, NJ 08837 (973)877-5287
+ Prime Radiology
1036 Amboy Avenue Edison, NJ 08837 (973)877-5287 Fax (732)225-6336

Mody, Sushama, MD {1760682173} IntrMd, Rheuma(01,NY08)
+ 312 Belleville Turnpike/Suite 3a
North Arlington, NJ 07031

Mody, Vipul C., MD {1467417808} IntrMd(94,NJ06)<NJ-SOMERSET>
+ KNJ Hospitalist Group, LLC.
204 South Main Street Manville, NJ 08835 (732)586-9035 Fax (908)213-6618
+ St Luke's Hospitalist Group
185 Roseberry Street Phillipsburg, NJ 08865 (732)586-9035 Fax (484)526-4605

Moeller, Joseph Phillip, DO {1326059270} Nrolgy
+ Community Neurology Associates PC
100 Springdale Road/Suite A-3, 412 Cherry Hill, NJ 08003 (856)616-8777 Fax (856)616-8780

Moeller, Lavinia Paige, DO {1417069931} Surgry(91,IA75)
+ American Physician Services/Hudson HealthCare
679 Montgomery Avenue Jersey City, NJ 07306 (201)433-6500 Fax (201)433-8010

Moerdler, Scott A., MD {1639445083}
+ Rutgers Cancer Institute of New Jersey
195 Little Albany Street/PO Box 2681 New Brunswick, NJ 08903 (732)235-5437 Fax (732)235-6797

Physicians by Name and Address

Moffa, Salvatore M., MD {1861625147} SrgThr(88,DC02)
+ 57 Buckingham Place
Cherry Hill, NJ 08003

Moffett, Shannon, MD {1306085444} EmrgMd<NJ-UMDNJ>
+ University Hospital
150 Bergen Street   Newark, NJ 07103   (973)972-5128   Fax (973)972-6646

Moffitt, Stephen T., MD {1609822840} NnPnMd, Pedtrc(88,NY09)<NJ-CHSMRCER>
+ Capital Health System/Mercer Campus
446 Bellevue Avenue/NICU   Trenton, NJ 08618   (609)394-4239   Fax (609)394-3839

Mofid, Alireza, MD {1366998619} Surgry<NJ-COOPRUMC>
+ Cooper University Hospital
One Cooper Plaza   Camden, NJ 08103   (856)342-2000

Mogan, Glen R., MD {1326015124} Gastrn, IntrMd(75,NY15)
+ Advanced Gastroenterology PA
741 Northfield Avenue/Suite 204   West Orange, NJ 07052   (973)731-8686   Fax (973)731-1911
AGE2493@VERIZON.NET

Moghadam, Faranak E., MD {1770548893}
+ Patient first Urgent Care
630 Mantua Pike   Woodbury, NJ 08096   (856)812-2220   Fax (856)812-2221

Moghe, Vaishali C., MD {1871538520} ObsGyn
+ Ocean Health Initiatives, Inc.
101 Second Street   Lakewood, NJ 08701   (732)363-6655   Fax (732)901-0277

Mogtared, Allen, MD {1104864008} CdvDis, IntrMd(70,NY08)<NJ-DEBRAHLC>
+ Deborah Heart and Lung Center
200 Trenton Road/Cardiology   Browns Mills, NJ 08015   (609)893-1200   Fax (609)735-0175

Mohageb, Salah M., MD {1679599260} IntrMd(90,ALG05)<NJ-VIRTBERL, NJ-VIRTMARL>
+ Virtua Marlton Hospitalist Group
94 Brock Road/Suite 302   Marlton, NJ 08053   (856)355-6730

Mohammadi, Mina, MD {1457331258} IntrMd, PulDis, CritCr(91,INA68)
+ Pulmonary Medical Associates, L.L.P
222 High Street/Suite 102   Newton, NJ 07860   (973)579-5090   Fax (973)579-2994

Mohammed, Ashraf, MD {1811107071} Pedtrc(93,INA2Y)
+ 21 Tufts Road
Clifton, NJ 07013   Fax (973)779-0873

Mohammed, Decca, MD {1679536361} ObsGyn(98,NC05)<NJ-CLARMAAS>
+ Clara Maass Medical Center
1 Clara Maass Drive/Ob/Gyn   Belleville, NJ 07109   (973)450-2000

Mohammed, Nina, MD {1194751016} ObsGyn(90,PA13)<NJ-CHILTON>
+ Associates in Women's Healthcare
1777 Hamburg Turnpike/Suite 202   Wayne, NJ 07470   (973)831-1800   Fax (973)831-8820
+ Associates in Women's Healthcare
1900 Union Valley Road   Hewitt, NJ 07421   (973)831-1800   Fax (973)831-8820
+ Associates in Women's Healthcare
329 Main Road/Suite 101   Montville, NJ 07470   (973)831-1800   Fax (973)831-8820

Mohammed, Raji Hussain, MD {1679961940} PthAcl
+ 1 Washington Avenue/Apt 15-2B
Morristown, NJ 07960   (917)575-0449

Mohan, Janani, MD {1598954604} IntrMd<NJ-STPETER>
+ St. Peter's University Hospital
254 Easton Avenue/Internal Med   New Brunswick, NJ 08901   (732)745-8600

Mohan, Kusum C., MD {1154462604} Pedtrc(72,INA4D)<NJ-MONMOUTH, NJ-RIVERVW>
+ Pediatric Associates of Holmdel, PC
719 North Beers Street/Suite 1E   Holmdel, NJ 07733   (732)739-4414   Fax (732)739-9537

Mohan, Mamatha G., MD {1710016761} IntrMd(01,INA39)
+ Crescent Internal Medicine Group
98 Park Street   Montclair, NJ 07042   (973)783-0800   Fax (973)744-1274

Mohan, Rajani, DO {1851642375}<NJ-CHRIST>
+ Christ Hospital
176 Palisade Avenue   Jersey City, NJ 07306   (201)795-8200

Mohan, Rajesh, MD {1376655507} CdvDis, IntrMd(89,INA92)<NY-CMCSTVSI>
+ Drs. Mohan & Singh
101 Prospect Street/Suite 210   Lakewood, NJ 08701   (732)905-8877   Fax (732)363-4584

Mohan, Vinuta, MD {1740350149} IntrMd(98,NY47)<NY-LINCOLN>
+ St. Francis Medical Center
601 Hamilton Avenue   Trenton, NJ 08629   (609)599-5000

Mohandas, Bhavna, MD {1841414000} CdvDis, IntCrd, IntrMd(02,INA34)
+ Shore Cardiac Center
651 Route 37 West   Toms River, NJ 08755   (732)286-6103   Fax (732)518-5252

Mohankumar, Aditi, MD {1629365440} Otlryg
+ Drs. Aroesty and Lin
400 Valley Road/Suite 105   Mount Arlington, NJ 07856   (973)770-7101   Fax (973)770-7108

Mohapatra, Robert A., MD {1336311661} CdvDis, IntrMd(01,GRN01)<NJ-VIRTMARL, NJ-UNDRWD>
+ Associated Cardiovascular Consultants-Lourdes
1 Brace Road/Suite C & F   Cherry Hill, NJ 08034   (856)428-4100   Fax (856)428-5748

Mohapeloa, Gugu R., MD {1306952635} IntrMd, Rheuma(74,NY06)<NJ-RBAYPERT>
+ 1145 Bordentown Road/Suite 18
Parlin, NJ 08859   (732)727-4700   Fax (732)727-4732

Moharita, Anabella L., MD {1699901371} IntrMd<NJ-UMDNJ>
+ University Hospital-Doctors Office Center
90 Bergen Street/Suite 4400   Newark, NJ 07103   (973)972-1880

Mohazzebi, Cyrus, MD {1144284266} Pedtrc(68,IRAN)<NJ-VIRTVOOR, NJ-KMHTURNV>
+ Advocare Kressville Pediatrics Cherry Hill
710 Kresson Road   Cherry Hill, NJ 08003   (856)795-3320   Fax (856)795-1213
+ Advocare Kressville Pediatrics Sicklerville
431 Sicklerville Road   Sicklerville, NJ 08081   (856)795-3320   Fax (856)875-4042

Mohazzebi, Mahbod, MD {1538319827}
+ Advocare Kressville Pediatrics Cherry Hill
710 Kresson Road   Cherry Hill, NJ 08003   (856)795-3320   Fax (856)795-1213

Mohit-Tabatabai, Mirseyed A., MD {1326153248} MedOnc, Surgry, SrgOnc(74,IRAN)
+ University Hospital-New Jersey Medical School
30 Bergen Street/Room 1207   Newark, NJ 07107   (973)972-4511

Mohiuddin, Fatima A., MD {1518311448} IntrMd<NJ-ACMCITY>
+ AtlantiCare Regional Medical Center/City Campus
1925 Pacific Avenue   Atlantic City, NJ 08401   (609)441-8990

Mohr, Robert Frederick, MD {1205919065} ObsGyn(77,PA09)<NJ-MORRISTN>
+ Lifeline Medical Associates
390 State Route 10/Suite 1   Randolph, NJ 07869   (973)328-1262   Fax (973)328-8576

Mohrin, Carl M., MD {1609848381} IntrMd(78,MEX03)<NJ-HAGEDORN>
+ 552 Charlestown Road
Hampton, NJ 08827

Mohsen, Ekram, DO {1013205400} PhysMd<NJ-HACKNSK>
+ Hackensack University Medical Center
30 Prospect Avenue/Suite 401   Hackensack, NJ 07601   (551)580-3027

Mohsen, Reyad H., MD {1689635286} IntrMd, MedOnc, Hemato(79,EGY04)<NJ-CHILTON, NJ-STJOSHOS>
+ 27 Almadera Drive
Wayne, NJ 07470

Mohsin, Jamil, MD {1306845110} Radiol, NuclMd, RadDia(88,PAK01)<NJ-VIRTMHBC, NJ-VIRTBERL>
+ South Jersey Radiology Associates, P.A.
100 Carnie Boulevard/Suite B-5   Voorhees, NJ 08043   (856)751-0123   Fax (856)751-0535
+ South Jersey Radiology Associates, P.A.
315 Route 70 East/Suite B   Cherry Hill, NJ 08034   (856)751-0123   Fax (856)428-0356
+ The Women's Center at Voorhees
100 Carnie Boulevard/Suite A-4   Voorhees, NJ 08043   (856)751-5522   Fax (856)751-5650

Mohtashemi, Hormoz, MD {1851304562} Gastrn, IntrPrc(64,IRAN)<NJ-WAYNEGEN>
+ 200 Engle Street/Suite 21
Englewood, NJ 07631   (201)608-5284

Moise, Anson Marryshow, MD {1285848739} Anesth
+ St. Joseph's Regional Medical Center Anesthesia
703 Main Street/Anesth   Paterson, NJ 07503   (973)754-2323   Fax (973)977-9455
frances.bruno@mountsinai.org

Moise, Bonard, MD {1578665915} Psychy(87,DOM01)<NJ-HAGEDORN, NJ-VALYONS>
+ Hagedorn Psychiatric Hospital
200 Sanatorium Road   Glen Gardner, NJ 08826   (908)537-2141
BMOISE@pol.net

Moise, Gaetan, MD {1255580858} SrgNro(04,NY01)<NJ-STJOSHOS, NJ-VALLEY>
+ Neurosurgeons of New Jersey
1200 East Ridgewood Avenue   Ridgewood, NJ 07450   (201)824-6131

Moises, Adam U., Jr., DO {1942391651} Anesth(94,NJ75)
+ James Street Anesthesia
102 James Street/Suite 103   Edison, NJ 08820   (732)494-1444   Fax (732)494-7052

Moises, Rodulfo P., Jr., MD {1174560197} Pedtrc(76,PHIL)<NY-STBARNAB, NJ-CHILTON>
+ Allwood Pediatrics
89 Main Street   Paterson, NJ 07505   (973)742-7880
+ Allwood Pediatrics
1040 Clifton Avenue   Clifton, NJ 07013   (973)742-7880   Fax (973)574-8061

Mojares, Dennis C., MD {1548275837} GenPrc, EmrgMd(63,PHIL)
+ Family first Urgent Care & Walk in Medical
1910 State Route 35   Oakhurst, NJ 07755   (732)531-0100   Fax (732)531-0144
decm1@optline.net

Mojares, Gregg E., DO {1760418966} EmrgMd(02,MO78)<NJ-JRSYSHMC>
+ EmCare
1945 Route 33   Neptune, NJ 07753   (732)776-4510   Fax (732)776-2329

Mojares, Richard Alan, MD {1417963505} IntrMd, Pedtrc(97,GRN01)
+ Family first Urgent Care & Walk in Medical
1910 State Route 35   Oakhurst, NJ 07755   (732)531-0100   Fax (732)531-0144

Mojica, Cornelio F., MD {1659359636} Pedtrc, NnPnMd(78,PHI09)<NJ-OURLADY>
+ Our Lady of Lourdes Medical Center
1600 Haddon Avenue/ICN   Camden, NJ 08103   (856)757-3500

Mojica-Itidiare, Jennifer, DO {1508129172}
+ Rowan University-School of Osteopathic Medicine
1 Medical Center Drive/Suite 163   Stratford, NJ 08084   (856)677-6708   Fax (856)566-6222

Mok, Shaffer Randall Shrope, MD {1275878787}
+ The Cooper Hospital System-Univ Hospital
401 Haddon Avenue/E&R 3rd Fl   Camden, NJ 08103   (856)757-7842   Fax (856)968-9587

Mokhashi, Sajida Habib, MD {1669658084} FamMed, FamMGrtc(99,INA2A)<NJ-CENTRAST>
+ UH- Robert Wood Johnson Med
125 Paterson Street/MEB 278   New Brunswick, NJ 08901   (908)685-3732
+ 514 Route 33 West
Millstone, NJ 08535   (908)685-3732   Fax (732)786-0012

Mokrzycki, Mark L., MD {1699731562} ObsGyn, SrgUro, Gyneco(92,PA12)<NJ-STPETER, NJ-CENTRAST>
+ University of Urogynecology of New Jersey
254 Easton Avenue/3 FL/Cares Blg   New Brunswick, NJ 08901   (732)937-6003   Fax (732)249-6140

Molbegott, Debra J., DO {1316978489} Anesth(88,PA77)<NJ-MONMOUTH>
+ Monmouth Medical Center
300 Second Avenue/Anesthesiology   Long Branch, NJ 07740   (732)222-5200

Molbegott, Lester P., MD {1629047410} Anesth, IntrMd, Acpntr(78,NY19)<NJ-MONMOUTH>
+ Monmouth Medical Center
300 Second Avenue/Anesth   Long Branch, NJ 07740   (732)923-6980   Fax (732)923-6977

Molina, Alex Armando, MD {1164442588} EmrgMd(00,NJ06)<NJ-PALISADE>
+ Palisades Emergency Consultants
7600 River Road   North Bergen, NJ 07047   (201)854-5100
+ Palisades Medical Center
7600 River Road/EmrgMed   North Bergen, NJ 07047   (201)854-5000

Molina, Arthur M., MD {1396788618} ObsGyn(81,MEX14)<NJ-KIMBALL, NJ-COMMED>
+ Ocean Gynecological & Obstetrical Associates PA
475 Highway 70   Lakewood, NJ 08701   (732)364-8000   Fax (732)364-4601

Molina, Carlos Guillermo, DO {1225277833} Surgry(05,NJ75)<NJ-KIMBALL, NJ-COMMED>
+ Kimbal Medicall Center
101 Prospect Street/Suite 214   Lakewood, NJ 08701   (732)901-8604   Fax (732)901-8608
+ Barnabas Health Medical Group
731 Lacey Road/Suite 1   Forked River, NJ 08731   (732)901-8604   Fax (609)242-6807

Molina, Leticia K., MD {1558349308} NnPnMd<NJ-OURLADY>
+ Our Lady of Lourdes Medical Center
1600 Haddon Avenue   Camden, NJ 08103   (856)757-3988

Molina, Maria Gregoria, MD {1871627133} PhysMd, PainInvt(86,PHIL)
+ Rehab Partners in Pain Management PC
561 North Church Street   Moorestown, NJ 08057

Molinari, Francis T., MD {1710075452} IntrMd, EmrgMd(77,ITAL)
+ 625 Joralemon Street
Belleville, NJ 07109   (973)759-6698   Fax (973)759-0927

Molinari, Susan P., MD {1720049976} Nrolgy(85,PA12)<NJ-VAL-LEY>
+ Neurology Group of Bergen County
1200 East Ridgewood Avenue   Ridgewood, NJ 07450
(201)444-0868   Fax (201)444-7363

Molinaro, Michael John, MD {1336134600} Dermat(96,NJ05)<NJ-HACKNSK>
+ Westwood Dermatology
390 Old Hook Road   Westwood, NJ 07675   (201)666-9550   Fax (201)666-1251

Molinaro, Michael Louis, MD {1144234634} IntrMd(00,NJ05)<NJ-MTNSIDE>
+ Mountainside Medical Group
123 Highland Avenue/Suite 201   Glen Ridge, NJ 07028
(973)748-9246   Fax (973)748-8755

Molinaro, Thomas Anthony, MD {1386700367} RprEnd, Obs-Gyn(02,NJ05)
+ Reproductive Medicine Associates of New Jersey
140 Allen Road   Basking Ridge, NJ 07920   (908)604-7800   Fax (973)290-8370
+ Reproductive Science Center of New Jersey
234 Industrial Way   Eatontown, NJ 07724   (908)604-7800   Fax (732)918-2504

Molino, Bruno, MD {1265452221} Surgry, SrgCrC, SrgTrm(98,NJ06)<NJ-JRSYCITY>
+ Liberty Surgical Associates
355 Grand Street/TraumaSurgery   Jersey City, NJ 07302
(201)915-2450   Fax (201)915-2192
+ Jersey City Medical Center
355 Grand Street/Surgery   Jersey City, NJ 07304   (201)915-2000

Molino, Richard, MD {1104931831} IntrMd(74,MA07)<NJ-VIRT-MARL, NJ-VIRTVOOR>
+ 303 South Kings Highway/Suite 1
Cherry Hill, NJ 08034   (856)428-2230   Fax (856)428-5075
rm0407@verizon.net

Molisso, Mary Cuellari, DO {1477597698} FamMed, EmrgMd(90,NJ75)<NJ-SOMERSET>
+ Emergency Medical Associates of NJ, P.A.
3 Century Drive   Parsippany, NJ 07054   (973)740-0607   Fax (973)740-9895

Molk, Ian J., MD {1073546636} CdvDis, IntrMd(76,SAF01)
+ Molk Cardiology
4 Ethel Road/Suite 406-A   Edison, NJ 08817   (732)287-2888   Fax (732)287-1176
+ Monk Cardiology
167 Main Street/Suite 1 B   Metuchen, NJ 08840   (732)287-2888   Fax (732)662-9848

Molloy, Thomas J., MD {1154488591} CdvDis, IntrMd(86,NY48)<NJ-HACKNSK, NJ-VALLEY>
+ Summit Medical Group
31-00 Broadway   Fair Lawn, NJ 07410   (201)693-4445   Fax (201)796-7020

Molnar, Eric D., DO {1164866729} FamMed
+ Skylands Medical Group PA
210 Route 94   Columbia, NJ 07832   (908)362-9285   Fax (908)362-7756

Molokwu, Godwin O., MD {1649325333} Gastrn, IntrMd(90,DMN01)
+ 24 Manley Terrace
Maplewood, NJ 07040

Momeni, Reza, MD {1699762435} SrgPlstc(98,PA09)<NJ-OVER-LOOK, NJ-MORRISTN>
+ Summit Medical Group-Berkeley Heights Campus
1 Diamond Hill Road   Berkeley Heights, NJ 07922
(908)273-4300   Fax (908)673-7359

Momi, Anudeep K., DO {1225170954} FamMed(96,PA77)
+ Anu Medical Spa
200 Route 73   Voorhees, NJ 08043   (856)809-0909   Fax (856)809-1919
info@anumedicalspa.com

Momi, Kamaldeep S., MD {1558332957} SrgOrt, SrgSpn(93,PA02)<NJ-VIRTMHBC, NJ-VIRTMARL>
+ Coastal Spine
4000 Church Road   Mount Laurel, NJ 08054   (856)222-4444   Fax (856)222-0049

Momodu, Inua Aitsekegbe, MD {1518067255} PsyCAd, Psychy(88,NIG01)
+ AtlantiCare Clinical Associates
16 South Ohio Avenue   Atlantic City, NJ 08401   (609)441-2104

Momplaisir, Thierry, MD {1255420899} CdvDis, IntrMd
+ LMA CardioThoracic Surgical Services
1 Brace Road/Suite C   Cherry Hill, NJ 08034   (856)470-9029   Fax (856)796-9391
+ South Jersey Heart Group
3001 Chapel Avenue/Suite 101   Cherry Hill, NJ 08002
(856)470-9029   Fax (856)482-7170

Monaco, Carmine D., DO {1124079926} Pedtrc(94,PA77)
+ Cadoro Pediatrics, LLC
750 Route 73 South/Suite 307A   Marlton, NJ 08053
(856)983-9666   Fax (856)983-2662

Monaco, Melissa Garofalo, MD {1588825459} Pedtrc(04,NJ05)<NJ-HACKNSK, NJ-VALLEY>
+ Forest Pediatrics PA
299 Forest Avenue   Paramus, NJ 07652   (201)267-0888   Fax (201)483-8874

Monaco, Robert, MD {1033296504} FamMed, FamMSptM(92,NJ05)<NJ-STPETER, NJ-RWJUBRUN>
+ Rutgers University/Hale Center
1 Scarlet Knight Way   Piscataway, NJ 08854   (732)445-2091   Fax (732)445-2780
+ Family Medicine at Monument Square
317 George Street   New Brunswick, NJ 08901   (732)445-2091   Fax (732)246-7317
+ Rutgers University Health Services
110 Hospital Road   Piscataway, NJ 08854   (732)445-3250

Monaco, Robert A., MD {1124113089} NuclMd, RadDia(71,NJ05)<NJ-OCEANMC>
+ Point Pleasant Radiology Group
1973 State Route 34/Suite E-13   Wall, NJ 07719   (732)974-8011   Fax (732)974-8820

Monaghan, Bruce A., MD {1033117346} SrgHnd, SrgOrt(90,PA01)<NJ-UNDRWD>
+ Advanced Orthopaedic Centers
414 Tatum Street   Woodbury, NJ 08096   (856)848-3880   Fax (856)848-4895

Monahan, Ellen M., MD {1033246897} IntrMd, Pedtrc, PedEmg(90,NJ05)<NJ-UMDNJ, NJ-HACKNSK>
+ University Hospital
150 Bergen Street/PediEmrgMed   Newark, NJ 07103
(973)972-4300   Fax (973)972-5965

Monahan, Lisa Y., DO {1720341464}
+ SOM - Department of Internal Medicine
42 East Laurel Road/Suite 3100   Stratford, NJ 08084
(856)566-2753   Fax (856)566-6906

Monari-Sparks, Mary Joan, MD {1356324263} IntrMd, IntMAdMd(98,PA09)<NJ-COOPRUMC>
+ Cooper Physicians
1103 North Kings Highway/Suite 203   Cherry Hill, NJ 08034
(856)321-1919   Fax (856)321-0206

Monastersky, Bruce Ted, MD {1447231006} Nrolgy(92,NJ05)<NJ-KIMBALL>
+ Neurological Associates of Ocean County PA
40 Bey Lea Road/Suite C103   Toms River, NJ 08753
(732)367-8280   Fax (732)367-1529

Monastyrskyj, Ola A., MD {1467542191} IntrMd(89,MD01)<NJ-MORRISTN>
+ Internal Medicine of Morristown
95 Madison Avenue/Suite A-00   Morristown, NJ 07960
(973)538-1388   Fax (973)538-9501

Monck, Jennefer Erinna, MD {1720019516} Nrolgy, NeuMus, Eplpsy(99,DMN01)
+ Neurologic Associates
220 Hamburg Turnpike/Suite 16   Wayne, NJ 07470
(973)942-4778   Fax (973)942-7020

Mondal, Zahidul Hoque, MD {1427230218} Nephro, IntrMd(06,NY08)<NJ-RWJUBRUN>
+ Robert Wood Johnson Transplant Associates, P.A.
10 Plum Street/7th Floor   New Brunswick, NJ 08901
(732)253-3362

Mondelli, John Anthony, MD {1356340780} CdvDis, IntrMd(94,IL06)<NJ-MORRISTN>
+ Atlantic Cardiology Group LLP
95 Madison Avenue/Suite 300   Morristown, NJ 07960
(973)898-0400   Fax (973)682-9494

Monderer, Renee Shoshana, MD {1225252646} Nrolgy(02,NY46)
+ 308 Rutland Avenue
Teaneck, NJ 07666   (718)920-2260

Mondestin, J. Harry, MD {1730196171} Pedtrc, NnPnMd, IntrMd(77,HAI01)<NJ-CHSMRCER, NJ-RWJUBRUN>
+ 40 Fuld Street/Suite 301
Trenton, NJ 08638   (609)989-9125   Fax (609)989-9706

Mondestin, Myriam A. J., MD {1750370110} ObsGyn(95,PA09)<NJ-OCEANMC, NJ-JRSYSHMC>
+ Princeton Perinatal Institute
3131 Princeton Pike   Lawrenceville, NJ 08648   (609)620-1774   Fax (609)620-1775

Mondoa, Emil I., MD {1124006192} NnPnMd<NJ-OURLADY>
+ Our Lady of Lourdes Medical Center
1600 Haddon Avenue/NeoNatl   Camden, NJ 08103
(856)757-3500

Mondrow, Daniel N., MD {1114999323} CdvDis, CritCr, IntrMd(76,NY08)
+ 280 Main Street
Metuchen, NJ 08840   (732)494-3177   Fax (732)494-0827

Mondshine, Ross T., MD {1588829204} RadDia
+ Montclair Radiology
20 High Street   Nutley, NJ 07110   (973)284-0020   Fax (973)284-6310

Mone, Suzanne Margaret, MD {1376683300} PedCrd<NJ-MORRISTN, NJ-OVERLOOK>
+ Morristown Medical Center
100 Madison Avenue/PedCrd/Bx 50   Morristown, NJ 07962

(973)971-5000

Mongal, Lucretia Sonya, MD {1861620791} FamMed(07,DMN01)
+ Urgent Care of New Jersey
2090 Route 27   Edison, NJ 08817   (732)662-5650   Fax (732)662-5651

Mongeau, Marc Thomas, DO {1053662379} PulDis
+ Kennedy Hospitalist Office
435 Hurffville Cross Keys Road   Turnersville, NJ 08012
(856)513-4124   Fax (856)302-3926

Mongia, Rupa, MD {1427066596} IntrMd, Grtrcs(78,INA65)<NJ-STPETER>
+ Spectrum Medical Associates
3250 State Route 27/Suite 103   Kendall Park, NJ 08824
(732)398-9100   Fax (732)398-9105

Monica, James T., MD {1437270907} OrtSHand(04,NY01)<NJ-STPETER, NJ-RWJUBRUN>
+ University Orthopaedic Associates, LLC.
Two Worlds Fair Drive   Somerset, NJ 08873   (732)979-2115   Fax (732)564-9032
+ University Orthopaedic Associates, LLC.
211 North Harrison Street   Princeton, NJ 08540   (732)979-2115   Fax (609)683-7875

Monica, Kristi Rae, MD {1316151491} Pedtrc(04,MA01)<MA-NWTNWELS, MA-CHILDRN>
+ Princeton Nassau Pediatrics, P.A.
301 North Harrison Street   Princeton, NJ 08540   (609)924-5510   Fax (609)924-3577

Moniem, Howayda A., MD {1750499646} PthAcl(80,EGY04)
+ Laboratory Corporation of America
69 First Avenue   Raritan, NJ 08869

Monka, Ira P., DO {1376588558} FamMed(84,NJ75)<NJ-MORRISTN>
+ Medical Institute of New Jersey
11 Saddle Road   Cedar Knolls, NJ 07927   (973)267-2122   Fax (973)267-3478

Monoky, David John, MD {1073976603} RadNro<NJ-HACKNSK>
+ Hackensack University Medical Center
30 Prospect Avenue   Hackensack, NJ 07601   (201)996-2000   Fax (201)489-4812
+ Hackensack Radiology Group, P.A.
30 Prospect Avenue   Hackensack, NJ 07601   (201)996-2000   Fax (201)336-8451

Monroe, Beatrice, MD {1811981780} IntrMd, EmrgMd(85,HUNG)
+ North Arlington Primary Care Associates, Inc.
25 Locust Avenue   North Arlington, NJ 07031   (201)991-9000   Fax (201)991-9005

Monroy-Miller, Cherry Ann, MD {1790892800} Psychy(86,PHIL)
+ St. Clare's Behavioral Health Center
100 Est Hanover Avenue   Cedar Knolls, NJ 07927
(973)401-2121   Fax (973)401-2140

Monta, Arturo D., MD {1790732089} IntrMd, Nephro(74,PHI09)<NJ-COMMED>
+ 19 Mule Road/Suite C8
Toms River, NJ 08755   (732)244-4777   Fax (732)244-4475
Artdel55@aol.com

Montag, Nathaniel, DO {1033503255} PhysMd
+ Physical Medicine & Rehabilitation Center
500 Grand Avenue/1st Floor   Englewood, NJ 07631
(201)567-2277   Fax (201)567-7506

Montagnino, Joseph W., MD {1013025881} CdvDis, IntrMd(72,NY09)<NJ-VALLEY>
+ 625 Lafayette Avenue
Hawthorne, NJ 07506   (973)238-0055   Fax (973)238-9826

Montalbano, Robert L., MD {1407879976} IntrMd, Pedtrc, EmrgMd(84,ITAL)<NJ-BAYONNE>
+ Bayonne Medical Center
29th Street at Avenue E/EmergMed   Bayonne, NJ 07002
(201)858-5257

Montalvo-Stanton, Evelyn, MD {1609800523} PedPul, Pedtrc(85,NJ05)<NJ-MORRISTN>
+ Pediatric Pulmonology
100 Madison Avenue   Morristown, NJ 07960   (973)971-4142   Fax (973)290-7360

Montana, Barbara E., MD {1326003799} InfDis, IntrMd(87,NY19)
+ Monmouth Family Center
270 Broadway   Long Branch, NJ 07740   (732)923-7100   Fax (732)923-7104

Monte, Lyda Cervantes, MD {1114068236} Psychy(65,PHIL)<NJ-ANCPSYCH>
+ Nueva Vida Behavioral Health Center
427 Market Street   Camden, NJ 08102   (856)338-1995   Fax (856)338-0247

Montefusco, Patrick P., MD {1821032756} Anesth, Surgry(77,DC02)<NJ-RBAYOLDB>
+ JFK Medical Center
65 James Street   Edison, NJ 08820   (732)321-7000

Monteiro, Iona M., MD {1699846527} Pedtrc, PedGst(83,INDI)<NJ-UMDNJ>
+ University Hospital
150 Bergen Street/PdtrcGastrEntro   Newark, NJ 07103
(973)972-4300

Physicians by Name and Address

Monteith, Duane Richard, MD {1194905901} Surgry, SrgThr(02,DC03)
  + Kings Way Primary Care
    100 Kings Way East/Suite D2   Sewell, NJ 08080   (856)716-6598   Fax (856)218-4808
  + Washington Township Thoracic Surgery
    400 Medical Center Drive/Suite F   Sewell, NJ 08080   (856)716-6598   Fax (856)716-6659

Monteleone, Catherine A., MD {1396773248} AlgyImmn(83,NY46)<NJ-RWJUBRUN>
  + University Medical Group
    125 Paterson Street/Suite 5100   New Brunswick, NJ 08901   (732)235-7067   Fax (732)235-7951
  + UH- RWJ Medical School
    One Robert Wood Johnson Place   New Brunswick, NJ 08903   (732)235-7067

Montemurno, Tina Deborah, MD {1003007360} Anesth(02,NY20)<NJ-VALLEY>
  + Bergen Anesthesia Group, P.C.
    500 West Main Street/Suite 16   Wyckoff, NJ 07481   (201)847-9320   Fax (201)847-0059

Montemurro, Daniella, MD {1700152972}<NJ-STBARNMC>
  + St. Barnabas Medical Center
    94 Old Short Hills Road   Livingston, NJ 07039   (973)322-5000

Montemurro, Robert J., MD {1619919651} ObsGyn(89,GRN01)<NJ-STJOSHOS>
  + St. Joseph's Family Health Center
    21 Market Street   Paterson, NJ 07501   (973)754-4200   Fax (973)754-4201

Montero, Gianecarla B., MD {1619173374} Pedtrc
  + 1 Riverview Plaza
    Red Bank, NJ 07701   (815)608-6079

Montero-Cruz, Fergie Ross, DO {1932531548} PhysMd
  + Progressive Spine & Orthopaedics
    440 Curry Avenue/Suite A   Englewood, NJ 07631   (201)227-1299

Montero-Pearson, Per M., MD {1730146127} Surgry(77,SPA04)
  + Cumberland Medical Associates
    1206 West Sherman Avenue   Vineland, NJ 08360   (856)691-8444   Fax (856)691-8325

Montes, Leigh, MD {1699775569} Surgry
  + New Jersey Bariatric Center
    193 Morris Avenue/2nd Floor   Springfield, NJ 07081   (908)481-1270   Fax (908)688-8861

Montes, Myrtho, MD {1023069168} IntrMd(80,NY08)
  + Prudential Employee Health Service
    213 Washington Street   Newark, NJ 07102   (973)802-6380   Fax (973)802-2276

Montezon, Lourdes I., MD {1083699128} Psychy(68,PHI08)<NJ-HAGEDORN>
  + Family Guidance Center of Warren County
    492 State Route 57 West   Washington, NJ 07882   (908)689-1000   Fax (908)689-4529
  + Hagedorn Psychiatric Hospital
    200 Sanatorium Road   Glen Gardner, NJ 08826   (908)537-2141

Montgomery, Catherine P., MD {1013002831} FamMed(90,PA02)<NJ-VIRTMARL, NJ-VIRTVOOR>
  + 2301 East Evesham Road
    Voorhees, NJ 08043   (856)772-1711   Fax (856)772-1758

Montgomery, David H., MD {1124108808} CdvDis, IntrMd, IntCrd(89,NY20)<NJ-VALLEY>
  + Cardiac Associates of North Jersey
    43 Yawpo Avenue/Suite 2   Oakland, NJ 07436   (201)337-0066   Fax (201)337-7417
  + The Valley Hospital
    223 North Van Dien Avenue   Ridgewood, NJ 07450   (201)447-8000

Montgomery, Karyn Mae, MD {1811005135} IntrMd(87,PA02)
  + Jersey Coast Family Medicine
    495 Jack Martin Boulevard/Suite 5   Brick, NJ 08724   (732)458-8000   Fax (732)458-8020

Montgomery, Kenneth D., MD {1922042720} SprtMd, SrgHnd, SrgOrt(90,CA02)<NY-LENOXHLL, NY-NSUHMANH>
  + Tri-County Orthopedics
    160 East Hanover Avenue   Morristown, NJ 07962   (973)538-2334   Fax (973)829-9174

Montgomery, Owen Canterbury, MD {1114982204} ObsGyn(81,PA09)
  + Drexel University Physicians
    400 East Church Street   Blackwood, NJ 08012   (856)228-8066
  + Professional HealthCare for Women
    409 Marlton Pike/Suite 2   Cherry Hill, NJ 08034   (856)424-5656

Monti, Richard A., MD {1750442786} Anesth(87,DMN01)
  + New Jersey Anesthesia Associates, P.C.
    252 Columbia Turnpike/PO Box 0037   Florham Park, NJ 07932   (973)660-9334   Fax (973)660-9779

Monti, Ryan M., MD {1629496880}<NJ-MTNSIDE>
  + Hackensack UMC Mountainside
    1 Bay Avenue   Montclair, NJ 07042   (973)429-6196   Fax (973)429-6575

Monticollo, Gerard M., DO {1376586487} Anesth, PainMd(84,NJ75)<NJ-OURLADY>
  + Our Lady of Lourdes Medical Center
    1600 Haddon Avenue/Anesthesiology   Camden, NJ 08103   (856)757-3500
  + Centennial Surgical Center LLC
    502 Centennial Boulevard/Suite 1   Voorhees, NJ 08043   (856)874-0790

Montiel, Armando A., MD {1649219478} IntrMd, PulDis(80,NY08)<NJ-VIRTBERL, NJ-VIRTMARL>
  + 23 North Whitehorse Pike
    Audubon, NJ 08106   (856)310-0477   Fax (856)310-1835

Montini, Kenneth Michael, MD {1669614921}<NJ-CHSFULD>
  + Capital Health System/Fuld Campus
    750 Brunswick Avenue   Trenton, NJ 08638   (609)815-7532

Montouris, Elaine Alexis, MD {1992878334} IntrMd(86,MNT01)
  + Associates in Plastic & Aesthetic Surgery
    27 Mountain Boulevard/Suite 9   Warren, NJ 07059   (908)757-7557   Fax (732)271-5853

Montuori, James L., DO {1619908555} Radiol, RadDia(95,NY75)<NJ-CHSFULD, NJ-CHSMRCER>
  + Capital Health System/Fuld Campus
    750 Brunswick Avenue   Trenton, NJ 08638   (609)394-6000

Moody, Rumanatha, MD {1891820254} IntrMd, Addctn(75,OH06)
  + Dr's. Choice
    1082 St. George Avenue   Rahway, NJ 07065   (732)388-4787   Fax (732)388-4380
  + The Doctor's In Housecalls
    65 Hawthorne Place/Suite G-2   Montclair, NJ 07042   (973)509-5782

Mookerjee, Anuradha Lele, MD {1902982820} IntrMd(99,INA1Z)<NJ-COOPRUMC>
  + Cooper University Medical Center/Camden
    3 Cooper Plaza   Camden, NJ 08103   (856)342-2000

Moon, Jeremy, MD {1831320605} ObsGyn(05)
  + Brescia-Migliaccio Ob/Gyn
    609 Washington Street   Hoboken, NJ 07030   (201)659-7700   Fax (201)659-7701

Moon, Kyoung, MD Anesth(70,KORE)<NJ-NWRKBETH>
  + Newark Beth Israel Medical Center
    201 Lyons Avenue/Anesthesiology   Newark, NJ 07112   (973)926-7143

Moon, Taewon, MD {1902843972} Otlryg, SrgHdN(85,NJ03)<NJ-ENGLWOOD>
  + 464 Hudson Terrace/Suite 102
    Englewood Cliffs, NJ 07632   (201)503-0066   Fax (201)503-0190

Moondra, Palak, DO {1124267091} Grtrcs, IntrMd(05,NY75)<NJ-STPETER>
  + St. Peter's University Hospital
    254 Easton Avenue   New Brunswick, NJ 08901   (732)565-5432

Mooney, Caroline Mary Esther Banzon, MD {1215977616} IntrMd(98,PHI02)
  + 96 Elm Street
    Tenafly, NJ 07670

Mooney, Kevin K., MD {1285608182} FamMed, Grtrcs(68,ON09)<NJ-HUNTRDN>
  + Phillips Barber Family Health Center
    72 Alexander Avenue   Lambertville, NJ 08530   (609)397-3535   Fax (609)397-0301

Moonka, Neeta K., MD {1578664926} Anesth, Pedtrc(85,PA13)<NJ-ENGLWOOD>
  + Englewood Hospital and Medical Center
    350 Engle Street   Englewood, NJ 07631   (201)894-3000

Moore, Andrew James, MD {1144667247} IntHos, IntrMd<MA-CHACMBR>
  + Cooper University Hospital Hospitalists
    One Cooper Plaza/Suite 222/Drrnce   Camden, NJ 08103   (856)342-3150
  + Cooper Cardiology Associates
    900 Centennial Boulevard   Voorhees, NJ 08043   (856)342-3150   Fax (856)325-6702

Moore, Ann M., MD {1508806282} RadDia(74,MEXI)<NJ-MMHKEMBL, NJ-MORRISTN>
  + Morristown Memorial Hospital/Mt. Kemble Division
    95 Mount Kemble Avenue   Morristown, NJ 07960   (973)971-4758

Moore, Brian J., MD {1952480063} IntrMd(74,MEX14)<NJ-MORRISTN>
  + 1201 Mt. Kemble Avenue
    Morristown, NJ 07960   (908)766-0904   Fax (908)766-5827

Moore, Cheryl Crowley, MD {1356332670} PthAcl, PthCyt, Pthlgy(87,DC02)<NH-WNTWRTH>
  + Inspira Health Network
    509 North Broad Street   Woodbury, NJ 08096   (856)845-0100

Moore, Donnica Lauren, MD {1194157131} Gyneco(86,NY06)
  + Sapphire Women's Health Group, LLC
    3 Saint Bernards Road   Far Hills, NJ 07931   (908)234-2702   Fax (908)234-2703

Moore, Douglas B., MD {1710989116} Radiol(88,CT02)
  + Radiology Associates of Burlington County
    1295 Route 38 West/PO Box 479   Hainesport, NJ 08036   (609)261-7017   Fax (609)261-4180

Moore, Frank Max, MD {1760459374} SrgNro(83,FRAN)<NJ-ENGLWOOD, NY-MTSINAI>
  + Metropolitan Neurosurgery Associates, PA
    309 Engle Street/Suite 6   Englewood, NJ 07631   (201)569-7737   Fax (201)569-1494
    mnasurgerons@hotmail.com

Moore, Michael G., MD {1750328068} SrgOrt(87,TN06)<NJ-HACKNSK, NJ-VALLEY>
  + 171 Franklin Turnpike/Suite 200
    Waldwick, NJ 07463   (201)689-0110   Fax (201)689-0114

Moore, Rebecca Christiane, DO {1558391490} FamMed(03,NJ75)
  + Hammonton Family Medicine Center
    373 South White Horse Pike   Hammonton, NJ 08037   (609)704-0185   Fax (609)704-0195

Moore, Robert P., MD {1356447874} EmrgMd(79,NJ05)<NJ-SOMERSET>
  + Emergency Medical Associates
    110 Rehill Avenue   Somerville, NJ 08876   (908)685-2920   Fax (908)685-2968

Moore, Roger A., MD {1750322822} Anesth, Pedtrc(73,VA01)<NJ-DEBRAHLC>
  + Deborah Heart and Lung Center
    200 Trenton Road   Browns Mills, NJ 08015   (609)893-6611   Fax (609)735-0415
    rogermoore435@yahoo.com

Moore, Ross Edward, MD {1861559155} Anesth(88,TX13)
  + University Hospital-New Jersey Medical School
    30 Bergen Street/ADMC 1205   Newark, NJ 07107   (973)972-0037   Fax (973)972-9355

Moore, Susan Salzberg, MD {1881641900} ObsGyn(91,MI01)
  + Coastal Monmouth Obstetrics & Gynecology
    521 Newman Springs Road/Suite 12   Lincroft, NJ 07738   (732)747-0022   Fax (732)747-0086

Moore, Tarquin Oliver, MD {1992838387} IntrMd
  + Cooper University Medical Center/Camden
    3 Cooper Plaza/Suite 116   Camden, NJ 08103   (856)342-2000   Fax (856)968-8223

Moorthy, Lakshmi Nandini, MD {1326122565} Pedtrc, PedRhm(95,INA23)
  + University Hospital-RWJ Medical School
    89 French Street/CHINJ-1361   New Brunswick, NJ 08901   (732)235-4980   Fax (732)235-5002

Moosvi, Ali R., MD {1093796948} CdvDis, IntrMd(82,INA16)<NJ-JRSYSHMC, NJ-OCEANMC>
  + Shore Cardiology Consultants, LLC
    1640 Route 88/Suite 201   Brick, NJ 08724   (732)840-1900   Fax (732)840-0355
  + Shore Cardiology Consultants, LLC
    3200 Sunset Avenue/Suite 208   Ocean, NJ 07712   (732)840-1900

Moosvi, Mir A., MD {1407949514} Gastrn(74,INDI)
  + 717 North Beers Street/Suite C
    Holmdel, NJ 07733   (732)264-7411   Fax (732)264-1074

Moquete, Manuel J., MD {1568564102} IntrMd, Nephro(86,DOMI)
  + North Jersey Nephrology Associates PA
    246 Hamburg Turnpike/Suite 207   Wayne, NJ 07470   (973)653-3366   Fax (973)653-3365
    mmoquetemd@aol.com

Mor Zilberstein, Lara, MD {1346572260} FamMed(00,ISR02)
  + 15 Engle Street/Suite 305
    Englewood, NJ 07631   (201)731-3150   Fax (201)731-3148

Morabia, Albert, DO {1790164887} IntrMd
  + Jersey Shore University Medical Center
    1945 Route 33   Neptune, NJ 07753   (732)775-5500

Moradi, Bijan Nik, MD {1376863811} CritCr
  + Cooper University Hospital Critical Care
    One Cooper Plaza   Camden, NJ 08103   (202)713-5818   Fax (856)968-8282
    nksprt@hotmail.com

Moradi, Dovid Simcha, MD {1972878239} Gastrn
  + Union County Infectious Disease Group
    240 Williamson Street/Suite 502   Elizabeth, NJ 07207   (908)994-5300   Fax (908)994-5308

Morag, Eyal, MD {1821197666} Radiol, RadV&I, RadDia(94,MA05)
  + University Radiology Group, P.C.
    579A Cranbury Road   East Brunswick, NJ 08816   (732)390-0040   Fax (732)390-1856
  + University Radiology Group, P.C.
    16 Mountain Boulevard   Warren, NJ 07059   (732)390-0040   Fax (908)769-9141

Moraille, Pascale, MD {1407970890} PsyCAd, Psychy(88,PRO02)<NJ-HOBUNIMC>
+ Hoboken University Medical Center
308 Willow Avenue   Hoboken, NJ 07030   (201)418-1000
Moraleda, Jason N., MD {1710949904} FamMed(01,PHI01)
+ Collingswood Medical Center
275 Haddon Avenue   Collingswood, NJ 08108   (856)858-3375   Fax (856)858-3424
Morales, Donna Chelle Viray, DO {1841451291} IntrMd<NJ-MORRISTN>
+ Morristown Medical Center
100 Madison Avenue/Internal Med   Morristown, NJ 07962   (973)971-4179   Fax (973)971-7905
Morales, Fabian Victor, MD {1477785145} EmrgMd, SprtMd(04,NJ05)
+ Pro Form Sports Medicine and Wellness Associates
201 Route 17 North   Rutherford, NJ 07070   (201)549-8846   Fax (201)549-8899
Morales, Jaime A., MD {1588849475} EmrgMd(05,NJ05)<RI-SJFA-TIMA>
+ Emergency Medical Associates of NJ, P.A.
3 Century Drive   Parsippany, NJ 07054   (973)740-0607   Fax (973)740-9895
Morales, Ruben B., MD {1902924467} IntrMd(84,PHI16)
+ 504 Kimberly Drive
Millville, NJ 08332   (856)364-8487
rbm08332@comcast.net
Morales-Mateluna, Carlos Alejandro, MD {1013267285} AlgyImmn(92,COS02)
+ Center for Asthma & Allergy
90 Milbum Avenue/Suite 200   Maplewood, NJ 07040   (973)763-5787   Fax (973)763-8568
Morales-Pelaez, Eileen S., MD {1952436487} Anesth(68,PHI29)<NJ-MEMSALEM>
+ Memorial Hospital of Salem County
310 Woodstown Road/Anesthesiology   Salem, NJ 08079   (856)935-1000
Morales-Ribeiro, Celines, MD {1164672895} Surgry(06,NY06)<NJ-ENGLWOOD>
+ Bergen Laparoscopy & Bariatric, LLC
97 Engle Street   Englewood, NJ 07631   (201)227-5533   Fax (201)227-5537
+ Englewood Hospital and Medical Center
350 Engle Street/Surgery   Englewood, NJ 07631   (201)894-3000
Moran, Christopher John, MD {1548402860} RadV&I
+ Coastal Imaging, LLC
79 Route 37 West/Suite 103   Toms River, NJ 08755   (732)678-0087   Fax (732)276-2325
+ Ocean Medical Center
425 Jack Martin Boulevard/Radiology   Brick, NJ 08723   (732)678-0087   Fax (732)836-4047
Morandi, Joseph T., DO {1245209642} FamMed(94,NY75)<NJ-MORRISTN>
+ 665 Martinsville Road/Suite 218
Basking Ridge, NJ 07920   (908)607-1877   Fax (908)607-1866
Morandi, Michele Meehan, DO {1033186739} FamMed, FamMHPC, IntrMd(94,NY75)<NJ-OVERLOOK, NJ-TRINIJSC>
+ Roselle Park Medical Associates, LLC
744 Galloping Hill Road   Roselle Park, NJ 07204   (908)241-0044   Fax (908)241-0526
Morano, Amy Beth, MD {1881891422} Pedtrc(05,NJ06)<NJ-COMMED, NJ-OCEANMC>
+ Pediatric Affiliates, PA
40 Bey Lea Road/Suite B203   Toms River, NJ 08753   (732)341-0720   Fax (732)244-6842
+ 69 Brookwood Drive
Freehold, NJ 07728
Morato, Ramon V., MD {1295814754} EmrgMd(66,PHIL)<NJ-STCLRDEN>
+ St. Clare's Hospital-Denville Campus
25 Pocono Road/EmergMed   Denville, NJ 07834   (973)625-6000
Moray, Nandini K., MD {1609958131} IntrMd(93,INA9Z)
+ 35-37 Progress Street/Suite AA5
Edison, NJ 08820   (908)546-7070   Fax (908)546-7069
+ Medical Care Associates
209 State Route 18 South   East Brunswick, NJ 08816   (908)546-7070   Fax (732)249-7787
Morchel, Herman George, MD {1154527661} EmrgMd<NJ-HACKNSK>
+ Hackensack Medical Center Emergency Medicine
30 Prospect Avenue/Main 3619   Hackensack, NJ 07601   (201)996-4614   Fax (201)968-1866
Mordan, Eliezer Aurelina, MD {1003886516} EmrgMd(02,NJ02)<NJ-RBAYPERT>
+ Raritan Bay Medical Center/Perth Amboy Division
530 New Brunswick Avenue   Perth Amboy, NJ 08861   (732)442-3700
+ EmCare
1945 Route 33   Neptune, NJ 07753   (732)442-3700   Fax (732)776-2329
Mordecai, Isaac S., MD {1740213693} Dermat(64,GER19)<NJ-ACMCITY, NJ-ACMCMAIN>
+ 1220 Tilton Road
Northfield, NJ 08225   (609)641-2371   Fax (609)641-3650
Mordkovich, Boris, MD {1992915490} SrgPlstc, SrgRec(81,RUS06)
+ Cross Hudson Plastic Surgery
520 Sylvan Avenue/Suite 202   Englewood Cliffs, NJ 07632   (201)751-9490   Fax (201)751-9491
More, Jay, MD {1710980958} SrgNro(87,NY09)<NJ-JFKMED>
+ Neurosurgical Associates of Central Jersey, P.A.
1200 Route 22 East/2nd Floor   Bridgewater, NJ 08807   (732)302-1720   Fax (732)302-1724
+ Raritan Valley Surgery Center
100 Franklin Square Drive/Suite 100   Somerset, NJ 08873   (732)302-1720   Fax (732)560-5999
More, Robert C., MD {1245233899} SprtMd, SrgOrt, NeuMSptM(83,CA14)<NJ-HUNTRDN>
+ MidJersey Orthopaedics, P.A.
8100 Westcott Drive/Suite 101   Flemington, NJ 08822   (908)782-0600   Fax (908)782-7575
+ Hunterdon Orthopaedic Institute, P.A.
80 West End Avenue   Somerville, NJ 08876   (908)182-0600
Morecraft, John A., Jr., MD {1578595526} EmrgMd, IntrMd(79,MEX14)<NJ-STJOSHOS, NJ-NWTNMEM>
+ St. Joseph's Regional Medical Center
703 Main Street/EmergMed   Paterson, NJ 07503   (973)754-2000
Moreines, Robert N., MD {1780722173} Psychy(78,MI20)
+ Moreines & Goldman PC
577 Westfield Avenue   Westfield, NJ 07090   (908)232-6566   Fax (908)232-6628
Morel, Elyse R., MD {1215295316}
+ Virtua Express Urgent Care
401 Young Avenue/Suite 180   Moorestown, NJ 08057   (856)291-8600   Fax (856)291-8615
+ Virtua Express Urgent Care-Voorhees
158 Route 73   Voorhees, NJ 08043   (856)291-8600   Fax (856)246-7231
+ Virtua Immediate Care Center
239 Hurffville Crosskeys Road   Sewell, NJ 08057   (856)341-8200   Fax (856)341-8215
Morelli, Louis C., MD {1801958210} Psychy(84,PA09)<NJ-ACMCITY, NJ-ACMCMAIN>
+ 48 South New York Road/Suite B4
Absecon, NJ 08201   (609)652-5544   Fax (609)748-8415
Morelli, Sara S., MD {1770788481} RprEnd
+ Rutgers- New Jersey Medical School
185 South Orange Avenue/ObsGyn   Newark, NJ 07103   (973)972-4300
Morelos, Joseph C., DO {1861498693} IntrMd(97,FL75)<NJ-OCEANMC, NJ-COMMED>
+ Jersey Shore Medical and Pediatric Associates
1215 Route 70 West/Suite 1005   Lakewood, NJ 08701   (732)942-0888   Fax (732)942-1230
Moreno, Jose G., MD {1487726386} Psychy(74,COL05)
+ 205 Ridgedale Avenue
Florham Park, NJ 07932   (973)966-0072   Fax (973)966-0072
Moreno, Susan I., MD {1750480802} PhysMd, Acpntr, PainMd(86,PA07)<NJ-MEDIPLEX, NJ-UNDRWD>
+ 196 Grove Avenue/Suite E
Thorofare, NJ 08086   (856)845-2323   Fax (856)845-4888
Moreyra, Abel E., MD {1700960499} CdvDis, IntrMd(67,ARGE)
+ UH- Robert Wood Johnson Med
125 Paterson Street   New Brunswick, NJ 08901   (732)235-7208   Fax (732)235-6530
moreyrae@umdnj.edu
+ University Medical Group/Cardiology
125 Paterson Street/CAB-Rm 5200   New Brunswick, NJ 08901   (732)235-7208   Fax (732)235-6530
Morgado, Antonio, MD {1306932249} EnDbMt, IntrMd(84,DOM02)<NJ-PALISADE>
+ Dr Antonio Morgado and Assoc
6045 Kennnedy Boulevard   North Bergen, NJ 07047   (201)453-0322   Fax (201)295-4188
Morgan, Aaron J., MD {1699901389} Dermat(08,NJ05)
+ Morgan Dermatology
1806 Highway 35 South/Suite 105   Belmar, NJ 07719   (732)508-9390   Fax (732)508-9393
Morgan, Allen, MD {1093875965} ObsGyn, RprEnd(86,PHI08)<NJ-JRSYSHMC, NJ-VIRTBERL>
+ Shore Institute for Reproductive Medicine/Shore IVF
475 Route 70/Suite 201   Lakewood, NJ 08701   (732)363-4777   Fax (732)363-2004
+ Shore Institute for Reproductive Medicine/Shore IVF
340 Highway 34/Suite 2-D   Colts Neck, NJ 07722   (732)845-0034
+ Shore Institute for Reproductive Medicine/Shore IVF
775 Route 70 East/Bldg F Suite 120   Marlton, NJ 08701   (856)334-8030   Fax (877)408-7450
Morgan, Benjamin, MD {1538448873} ObsGyn
+ Drs. Morgan and Morgan
1500 Atlantic Avenue/Suite 201   Ocean, NJ 07712   (732)531-1136   Fax (732)531-0177
+ Shore Health Group
525 Highway 70/Suite 2B   Brick, NJ 08723   (732)531-1136   Fax (732)477-4479
+ Shore Health Group
1500 Allaire Avenue/Suite 201   Ocean, NJ 07712   (732)531-1136   Fax (732)531-0177
Morgan, Charles Fisher, MD {1104930460} Ophthl(92,TN05)<NJ-MORRISTN, NJ-STJOSHOS>
+ Pediatric Eye Physicians, PC
95 Madison Avenue/Suite 301   Morristown, NJ 07960   (973)540-8814   Fax (973)540-8556
Morgan, Daniel Robert, MD {1154310811} ObsGyn(99,MNT01)<NJ-BURDTMLN>
+ Atlantic Cape Ob/Gyn
829 Shore Road   Somers Point, NJ 08244   (609)927-3070   Fax (609)927-2553
Morgan, Darlene M., MD {1184699175} ObsGyn(00,IL02)
+ Brick Women's Physicians
1140 Burnt Tavern Road/Suite 2-A   Brick, NJ 08724   (732)202-0700   Fax (732)202-0664
+ Brick Women's Physicians
87 Union Avenue   Manasquan, NJ 08736   (732)202-0700   Fax (732)202-0664
Morgan, Farah Hena, MD {1699966614} IntrMd
+ Cooper Endocrinology Associates
1210 Brace Road/Suite 107   Cherry Hill, NJ 08034   (856)759-3597   Fax (856)795-7590
Morgan, Illiana Alexandrova, MD {1083992416} Anesth(07,DMN01)
+ Jersery Shore Anesthesiology
1945 Highway 33   Neptune, NJ 07753   (732)897-0200   Fax (732)897-0263
Morgan, James Peter, MD {1821164708} IntrMd(91,NE06)<NJ-STBARNMC>
+ M.C. Medical Group
1425 Pompton Avenue/Suite 1-1   Cedar Grove, NJ 07009   (973)785-8686   Fax (973)785-8680
Morgan, John, MD {1710202536} RadDia, Radiol(05,DMN01)<NJ-HOLYNAME>
+ Holy Name Hospital
718 Teaneck Road/Radiology   Teaneck, NJ 07666   (201)833-3280   Fax (201)541-5919
Morgan, Kathleen A., MD {1710985791} Anesth(91,NJ06)<NJ-VIRTBERL, NJ-VIRTMARL>
+ West Jersey Anesthesia Associates
102-E Center Boulevard   Marlton, NJ 08053   (856)988-6250   Fax (856)988-6270
Morgan, Mena M., MD {1861703134} IntrMd
+ 558 Ryders Lane
East Brunswick, NJ 08816
Morgan, Mina Adel, DO {1942610589} Anesth
+ Jersey Shore University Medical Center
1945 Route 33   Neptune, NJ 07753   (732)775-5500
Morgan, Nashaat L., MD {1699742932} IntrMd(89,EGY10)
+ St. Karas Medical
A-2 Brier Hill Court   East Brunswick, NJ 08816   (732)613-5005   Fax (732)613-5004
Morgan, Robert L., MD {1699763730} Pedtrc, IntrMd(82,GRN01)
+ Navesink Pediatrics
55 North Gilbert Street/Suite 2101   Tinton Falls, NJ 07701   (732)842-6677   Fax (732)520-2946
Morgan, Steven A., MD {1609882554} ObsGyn(95,WIND)<NJ-COMMED, NJ-MONMOUTH>
+ 1163 Route 37 West/Suite A-1
Toms River, NJ 08755   (732)736-1331   Fax (732)736-1331
+ Drs. Morgan and Morgan
1500 Atlantic Avenue/Suite 201   Ocean, NJ 07712   (732)736-1331   Fax (732)531-0177
+ Shore Health Group
525 Highway 70/Suite 2B   Brick, NJ 08755   (732)477-4422   Fax (732)477-4479
Morgan, Suzana Emil Anwer, MD {1235378027} IntrMd(09)
+ St. Karas Medical
A-2 Brier Hill Court   East Brunswick, NJ 08816   (732)613-5005   Fax (732)613-5004
Morgan, William A., MD {1700888104} Radiol, RadDia(86,PA13)
+ Radiology Associates of Burlington County
1295 Route 38 West/PO Box 479   Hainesport, NJ 08036   (609)261-7017   Fax (609)261-4180
Morganoff, Abraham D., MD {1366401945} Nrolgy, NeuMus(75,MEX03)<NJ-UMDNJ, NJ-STBARNMC>
+ 5 Mountain Boulevard/Suite 3
Warren, NJ 07059   (908)769-8555
+ 1020 Galloping Hill Road
Union, NJ 07083   (908)769-8555

Physicians by Name and Address

Morganstein, Neil, MD {1568454080} IntrMd, OncHem(98,PA02)
+ Medical Diagnostic Associates, P.A.
99 Beauvoir Avenue   Summit, NJ 07901   (908)608-0078
Fax (908)608-1504

Morganstern, Jill Alison, MD {1265411532} Anesth(01,NY20)
+ 21 Governors Lane
Princeton, NJ 08540

Morgenstern, Alvin Harris, MD {1740284132} Anesth(80,IL43)<NJ-BAYONNE>
+ Bayonne Medical Center
29th Street at Avenue E/Anesth   Bayonne, NJ 07002
(201)858-5000

Morgenstern, Kenneth Eli, MD {1427019207} SrgOrb, SrgFPl(PA01
+ Paul Phillips Eye & Surgery Center
64 Walmart Plaza   Clinton, NJ 08809   (908)735-4100   Fax (908)735-7494
+ Paul Phillips Eye & Surgery Center
6 Minneakoning Road/Suite B   Flemington, NJ 08822
(908)735-4100   Fax (908)968-3239
+ Paul Phillips Eye & Surgery Center
1 Monroe Street   Bridgewater, NJ 08809   (908)526-4588
Fax (908)231-6718

Mori, Mayumi A., MD {1003819905} PedOph(91,NY47)<NJ-HACKNSK>
+ Pediatric Ophthalmology Associates
218 Ridgedale Avenue/Suite 100   Cedar Knolls, NJ 07927
(973)326-8895   Fax (973)326-6805
doctors@pedseyes.com
+ Pediatric Ophthalmology Associates
25-15 Fair Lawn Avenue   Fair Lawn, NJ 07410   (201)791-3166
+ Pediatric Ophthalmology Associates
509 East Broad Street   Westfield, NJ 07927   (908)317-9811
Fax (973)326-6805

Moriarty, Daniel J., MD {1164414850} IntrMd, MedOnc(76,VT02)<NJ-OVERLOOK>
+ Medical Diagnostic Associates, P.A.
99 Beauvoir Avenue   Summit, NJ 07901   (908)608-0078
Fax (908)608-1504

Morin, Joanne M., MD {1528109584} Pedtrc(98,NJ05)<NJ-STBARNMC, NJ-OVERLOOK>
+ Springfield Pediatrics
939 Park Avenue   Plainfield, NJ 07060   (908)226-5445
Fax (908)226-5481
+ Springfield Pediatrics
190 Meisel Avenue   Springfield, NJ 07081   (908)226-5445
Fax (973)467-7836

Morin, Robert J., MD {1346415536} SrgPlstc(04,NY09)
+ 40 Crestwood Place
Hillsdale, NJ 07642

Morino, Tricia Lynn, DO {1881831998} OncHem<NJ-COOPRUMC>
+ Meridian Hematology & Oncology
1100 Route 72 West   Manahawkin, NJ 08050   (609)597-0547   Fax (609)597-8668
+ Cooper University Hospital
One Cooper Plaza   Camden, NJ 08103   (856)342-2000

Moritz, Mark William, MD {1346210648} SrgVas, Phlebgy, IntrMd(77,MD07)<NJ-MORRISTN>
+ Vein Institute of New Jersey
95 Madison Avenue/Suite 109   Morristown, NJ 07960
(973)759-9000   Fax (973)759-2487
+ Vein Institute of New Jersey
532 Lafayette Road   Sparta, NJ 07871
+ Vein Institute of New Jersey
788 Broad Street/US Highway 35   Shrewsbury, NJ 07960

Morkos, Faten Farid, MD {1578578993} Pedtrc(79,EGY03)
+ Newark Community Health Center, Inc.
741 Broadway   Newark, NJ 07104   (973)675-1900   Fax (973)483-3787

Morley, David Matthew Yellin, MD {1063736924}
+ Emergency Medical Associates of NJ, P.A.
3 Century Drive   Parsippany, NJ 07054   (973)740-0607
Fax (973)740-9895

Morley, Laura Balderrama, MD {1801144225} ObsGyn
+ Morristown Obstetrics and Gynecology Associates
101 Madison Avenue/Suite 405   Morristown, NJ 07960
(973)267-7272   Fax (973)455-0099

Morley, Thomas F., DO {1801876305} PulDis, CritCr, SlpDis(79,PA77)<NJ-KMHSTRAT>
+ SOM - Department of Internal Medicine
42 East Laurel Road/Suite 3100   Stratford, NJ 08084
(856)566-6859   Fax (856)566-6952
+ University Doctors
1020 North Kings Highway/Suite 108   Cherry Hill, NJ 08034
(856)566-6859   Fax (856)755-1809
+ University Doctors
570 Egg Harbor Road/Suite C-2   Sewell, NJ 08084
(856)218-0300   Fax (856)589-1793

Morlino, John V., DO {1568400802} FamMed, GenPrc(79,PA77)
+ EMedical Urgent Care
2 Kings Highway   Middletown, NJ 07748   (732)957-0707
Fax (732)957-9852

Morone, John M., MD {1346312774} IntrMd(78,NJ05)<NJ-WAYNEGEN>
+ Drs. Morone and Costello
220 Hamburg Turnpike   Wayne, NJ 07470   (973)942-5230
Fax (973)942-6652

Morone, Teresa Monica, DO {1750337382} EmrgMd, IntrMd(79,PA77)
+ Cross keys Urgent Care
627-B Cross Keys Road   Sicklerville, NJ 08081   (856)728-8700   Fax (856)318-1374

Moront, Barbara Jeanne, MD {1699798009} FamMed(90,DC02)
+ Sunset Road Medical Associates
911 Sunset Road   Burlington, NJ 08016   (609)387-8787
Fax (609)386-8640

Morowitz, William A., MD {1144289315} PulDis, IntrMd(70,IL11)<NJ-OURLADY, NJ-LOURDMED>
+ Pulmonary & Sleep Associates of SJ, LLC.
107 Berlin Road   Cherry Hill, NJ 08034   (856)429-1800
Fax (856)429-1081
+ Pulmonary & Sleep Associates of SJ, LLC.
120 Carnie Boulevard/Suite 3   Voorhees, NJ 08043
(856)429-1800   Fax (856)325-4364
+ Pulmonary & Sleep Associates of SJ, LLC.
750 Route 73 South/Suite 401   Marlton, NJ 08034
(856)375-1288   Fax (856)375-2325

Morr, Edward Simon, MD {1164472130} Anesth(93,NY08)<NJ-VALLEY>
+ The Valley Hospital
223 North Van Dien Avenue   Ridgewood, NJ 07450
(201)447-8000

Morreale, Diego A., MD {1770583098} IntrMd(95,ITA01)
+ Ramtown Medical Center LLC
225 Newtons Corner Road   Howell, NJ 07731   (732)458-9760   Fax (732)458-9762
+ 74 West Shenendoah Road
Howell, NJ 07731

Morreale, Ginja Massey, MD {1700081536} ObsGyn
+ Hackensack Meridian Medical Group Ob/Gyn, Freehold
3499 Route 9 North/Suite 2B   Freehold, NJ 07728
(732)577-1199   Fax (732)577-8922

Morrell, Christopher, MD {1235502485} FamMed
+ 310 Central Avenue
East Orange, NJ 07018   (973)515-8170   Fax (973)242-5234

Morressi, Marc M., MD {1760645030} IntrMd(05,NET09)
+ Van Dyk Manor - Ridgewood
304 South Van Dien Avenue   Ridgewood, NJ 07450
(201)445-8200   Fax (201)445-9535
+ 199 Broad Street/Suite 1 D
Bloomfield, NJ 07003   (973)566-6500

Morris, Craig Madden, MD {1831105113} PsyCAd, Psychy(70,NY46)
+ Care PLUS NJ, Inc. - Fair Lawn Mental Health Center
17-07 Romaine Street   Fair Lawn, NJ 07410   (201)797-2660
Fax (201)797-5025

Morris, Jamie L., MD {1073547840} RprEnd, ObsGyn(92,PA09)<NJ-STBARNMC>
+ Reproductive Medicine Associates of New Jersey
140 Allen Road   Basking Ridge, NJ 07920   (908)604-7800
Fax (973)290-8370
+ Reproductive Medicine Associates of New Jersey
111 Madison Avenue/Suite 100   Morristown, NJ 07962
(908)604-7800   Fax (973)290-8370

Morris, Jason Joseph, DO {1982859898} EmrgMd
+ Rowan University-School of Osteopathic Medicine
1 Medical Center Drive   Stratford, NJ 08084   (609)841-7841

Morris, Jeffrey B., MD {1891733648} EmrgMd, IntrMd(77,PA09)<NJ-VIRTMHBC>
+ SJ Emergency Physician, PA
175 Madison Avenue   Mount Holly, NJ 08060   (609)267-0700   Fax (609)261-5842

Morris, Kathryn E., MD {1407875339} IntrMd(81,PA02)<NJ-UNVMCPRN>
+ Kathryn E. Morris MD, LLC
601 Ewing Street/Suite C-13   Princeton, NJ 08540
(609)924-5753   Fax (609)924-5759

Morris, Kevin Michael, MD {1245201540} Anesth, PainMd(79,ITA22)<NJ-NWRKBETH>
+ Newark Beth Israel Medical Center
201 Lyons Avenue/Anesth   Newark, NJ 07112   (973)926-7000   Fax (201)943-8105

Morris, Mark M., DO {1851390199} Pedtrc, NeuMus(02,ME75)
+ 26 Millburn Avenue
Springfield, NJ 07081   (973)258-1776

Morris, Paul J., DO {1356310692} FamMed(78,IA75)
+ 446 Hackensack Street
Carlstadt, NJ 07072   (201)933-2370   Fax (201)933-6189
morrisdo@aol.com

Morris, Sarah A., MD {1740294966} IntrMd(91,NJ05)<NJ-MONMOUTH>
+ 2-12 Corbett Way
Eatontown, NJ 07724   (732)380-8033   Fax (732)542-0155
+ Internal Medical Associates of Monmouth
279 Third Avenue/Suite 207   Long Branch, NJ 07740
(732)380-8033   Fax (732)571-0019

Morris, Timothy P., DO {1942292578} CdvDis, IntrMd(89,NY75)<NJ-OURLADY>
+ Our Lady of Lourdes Medical Center
1600 Haddon Avenue   Camden, NJ 08103   (856)757-3500
+ South Jersey Heart Group
539 Egg Harbor Road/Suite 1   Sewell, NJ 08080   (856)757-3500   Fax (856)589-1753

Morrison, Daniel H., Jr., MD {1740205962} Otlryg, Otolgy, IntrMd(83,PA13)
+ Daniel H. Morrison Jr.
2500 English Creek Avenue   Egg Harbor, NJ 08234
(609)407-2302   Fax (609)407-2373

Morrison, Daniel Scott, MD {1205895919} EmrgMd(01,NET09)<NJ-RWJUBRUN>
+ University Emergency Medicine
125 Paterson Street/MEB 104   New Brunswick, NJ 08901
(732)235-8717   Fax (732)235-7379
+ RWJ University Hospital New Brunswick
One Robert Wood Johnson Place   New Brunswick, NJ 08901
(732)828-3000

Morrison, Jill S., MD {1184670952} OncHem(91,MA05)<NJ-HOLYNAME>
+ Forte Schleider & Attas MD PA
350 Engle Street/Berrie Building/1 FL   Englewood, NJ 07631
(201)568-5250   Fax (201)568-5358

Morrison, Susan H., MD {1174501886} Allrgy, PedInf, Algy-Immn(81,NJ05)<NJ-CLARMAAS>
+ 36 Newark Avenue/Suite 322
Belleville, NJ 07109   (973)450-0100   Fax (973)450-8088

Morrone, Louis J., MD {1700825841} Ophthl(73,NJ05)
+ 43 Ridge Road
North Arlington, NJ 07031   (201)998-6900   Fax (201)998-7667

Morros, Jay Scott, MD {1184678476} Surgry, EmrgMd(85,MI01)
+ 3 Lamson Lane
Sewell, NJ 08080

Morrow, Franklin A., MD {1962507905} Urolgy(66,NY09)<NJ-RWJURAH, NJ-TRINIWSC>
+ New Jersey Urology, LLC
1600 George Avenue/Suite 202   Rahway, NJ 07065
(732)499-0111   Fax (732)499-0432
+ New Jersey Urology, LLC
700 North Broad Street/Suite 302   Elizabeth, NJ 07208
(732)499-0111   Fax (908)289-0716

Morrow, Todd A., MD {1063418549} Otlryg, SrgFPl(86,PA02)
+ Associates in Otolaryngology
741 Northfield Avenue/Suite 104   West Orange, NJ 07052
(973)243-0600   Fax (973)736-9607
info@tomorrowsface.com
+ Short Hills Surgery Center
187 Millburn Avenue/Suite 101   Millburn, NJ 07041
(973)243-0600   Fax (973)671-0557

Morrow, William J., DO {1831293331} Otlryg, SrgFPl, OtgyF-PIS(89,NJ75)<NJ-SHOREMEM, NJ-BURDTMLN>
+ Drs. Morrow and Syed
715 Bay Avenue   Somers Point, NJ 08244   (609)601-1570
Fax (609)601-1567
+ Drs. Morrow and Syed
601 Route 9 South   Cape May Court House, NJ 08210
(609)601-1570   Fax (609)463-5885

Morse, Anne Marie, DO {1033499207}
+ 60 Wildwood Avenue
West Orange, NJ 07052   (732)279-5960
drannemorse@gmail.com

Morse, Sophie D., MD {1184787723} OncHem, IntrMd(03,NJ06)<NJ-OVERLOOK>
+ Medical Diagnostic Associates, P.A.
99 Beauvoir Avenue   Summit, NJ 07901   (908)608-0078
Fax (908)273-3726

Morsi, Khaled M., MD {1124023601} Anesth, PainInvt(89,EGY05)<NJ-ACMCITY, NJ-ACMCMAIN>
+ AtlantiCare Regional Medical Center/City Campus
1925 Pacific Avenue/Anesthesiology   Atlantic City, NJ 08401
(609)345-4000
+ AtlantiCare Regional Med Ctr/Mainland
65 West Jimmie Leeds Road   Pomona, NJ 08240   (609)652-1000

Morski, Richard S., MD {1588754014} FamMed(81,POL02)<NJ-VALLEY, NJ-CHILTON>
+ North Jersey Family Medicine
19 Yawpo Avenue   Oakland, NJ 07436   (201)337-3412
Fax (201)337-3353

Morsy, Amr Sayed, MD {1447233895} Anesth(92,EGY03)<NJ-HACKNSK>
+ Hackensack Anesthesiology Associates
140 Prospect Avenue/Suite 8   Hackensack, NJ 07601
(201)488-0066   Fax (201)488-6769
+ Hackensack University Medical Center
30 Prospect Avenue/Anesth   Hackensack, NJ 07601
(201)996-2000

Mortensen, Jill, DO {1609816511} FamMed, FamMGrtc(80,IA75)
+ Cumberland Family Medicine Associates
1203 North High Street/Suite A   Millville, NJ 08332
(856)327-0182   Fax (856)327-7381

Morton, John Douglas, MD {1659471720} Gastrn, IntrMd(96,NY15)<NJ-MORRISTN, NJ-STBARNMC>
+ Affiliates in Gastroenterology, P.A.
101 Madison Avenue/Suite 100   Morristown, NJ 07960
(973)455-0404   Fax (973)540-8788

Morton, Kinshasa C., MD {1417157629} FamMed, FamMSptM(DC03)
+ 317 George Street
New Brunswick, NJ 08901   (732)235-7828   Fax (732)246-7317

Morton, Lisa Aseni, MD {1679785786} FamMed, IntrMd(98,NJ05)
+ 403 Route 202 South
Flemington, NJ 08822   (908)782-9123

Mosaddeghi, Mahmood, MD {1659338408} Anesth(94,LA05)<NJ-STPETER, NJ-SOMERSET>
+ Anesthesia Consultnts of NJ/Nova Pain
285 Davidson Avenue/Suite 204   Somerset, NJ 08873
(732)271-1400   Fax (732)271-3543
+ Cares Surgicenter, LLC.
240 Easton Avenue   New Brunswick, NJ 08901   (732)271-1400   Fax (732)296-8677

Mosca, Phillip J., MD {1396767596} Anesth(90,NJ05)<NJ-CHSM-RCER, NJ-CHSFULD>
+ Red Bank Anesthesia, LLC
1 Riverview Plaza   Red Bank, NJ 07701   (732)530-2255   Fax (732)450-2620

Moscato, Michele, DO {1861713422} Gastrn
+ Bergen Medical Associates
466 Old Hook Road/Suite 1   Emerson, NJ 07630   (201)967-8221   Fax (201)967-0340

Mosenthal, Anne Charlotte, MD {1427123629} Surgry, SrgCrC(85,NH01)<NJ-UMDNJ>
+ University Hospital
150 Bergen Street/Surgery/Trauma   Newark, NJ 07103
(973)972-6398   Fax (973)972-7441

Moser, Robert L., MD {1760529267} PthAcl, Pthlgy(78,PA09)<NJ-STFRNMED>
+ Consult Laboratory Systems
3131 Princeton Pike B5/Suite 114   Lawrenceville, NJ 08648
(609)895-1076   Fax (609)896-2030
rmoser@pluto.njcc.com
+ St. Francis Medical Center
601 Hamilton Avenue/Pathology   Trenton, NJ 08629
(609)895-1076   Fax (609)599-6243

Moses, Alan Charles, MD {1922033067} EnDbMt, IntrMd(73,MO02)
+ Novo Nordisk Inc.
100 College Road West   Princeton, NJ 08540   (609)987-5800   Fax (609)921-8082

Moses, Brett Joseph, MD {1427347897} Anesth
+ Anesthesia Consultnts of NJ/Nova Pain
285 Davidson Avenue/Suite 204   Somerset, NJ 08873
(732)271-1400   Fax (732)271-3543
+ Morris Anesthesia Group, PA
3799 Route 46/Suite 211   Parsippany, NJ 07054   (732)271-1400   Fax (973)335-1448

Moses, Brett Lawrence, MD {1326033416} Otlryg(87,PA02)<PA-STMARY, NJ-RWJUBRUN>
+ Premier ENT Associates
8 Quakerbridge Plaza   Hamilton, NJ 08619   (609)890-7800   Fax (609)890-6148

Moses, Eli B., MD {1750515623} Ophthl
+ Corneal Associates of NJ
100 Passaic Avenue/Suite 200   Fairfield, NJ 07004
(973)439-3937   Fax (973)439-3944

Moses, Stuart C., MD {1467553321} Radiol, RadDia, RadNuc(78,NY47)<NJ-CHILTON>
+ Fair Lawn Diagnostic Imaging
19-04 Fair Lawn Avenue   Fair Lawn, NJ 07410   (201)794-3132   Fax (201)794-6291

Moshel, Caroline Rosenberg, MD {1114121340} Ophthl, IntrMd(06,NY19)
+ The Eye Specialists, P.A.
745 Route 202/206/Suite 301   Bridgewater, NJ 08807
(908)231-1110   Fax (908)526-4959

Moshel, Yaron Aharon, MD {1013111830} SrgNro, IntrMd(03,NY08)<NY-BLVUENYU>
+ Atlantic Neurosurgical Specialists
310 Madison Avenue/Suite 300   Morristown, NJ 07960
(973)285-7800   Fax (973)285-7839

Moshet, Osama Mohamed, MD {1225021975} Pedtrc, IntrMd(93,EGY10)
+ Riverside Medical Group
714 Tenth Street/Suite 2   Secaucus, NJ 07094   (201)863-3346   Fax (201)865-0015

Moshiyakhov, Mark, MD {1538293576} CdvDis, IntrMd(01,NY46)<NJ-DEBRAHLC>
+ Deborah Heart and Lung Center
200 Trenton Road   Browns Mills, NJ 08015   (609)893-6611
Fax (609)893-6038
moshiyakhovm@deborah.org

Moshkovich, Marina, MD {1891957379} Psychy(80)
+ Jersey Medical Care, PC
100 Belchase Drive/Suite 101   Matawan, NJ 07747
(732)707-4100   Fax (732)707-4101
+ New Jersey State Prison
861 Second and Cass Street   Trenton, NJ 08611   (732)707-4100   Fax (609)656-8076

Moshkovitch, Vasil Ignatovitch, MD {1326116419} IntrMd(82,DMN01)
+ Barnegat Medical Associates, P.A.
41 Nautilus Drive   Manahawkin, NJ 08050   (609)978-0474
Fax (609)597-6186

Moskovitz, Bruce L., MD {1942457809} InfDis, IntrMd(76,MA05)
+ 613 Heath Court
Lambertville, NJ 08530   (908)927-3305

Moskovitz, Marty J., MD {1669434841} SrgPlstc, Surgry(89,NJ06)<NJ-VALLEY>
+ 140 North Route 17/Suite 105
Paramus, NJ 07652   (201)225-1101

Moskowitz, David H., MD {1063492411} ObsGyn(94,NY46)<NJ-JRSYSHMC, NJ-MONMOUTH>
+ 250 Monmouth Road
Oakhurst, NJ 07755   (732)517-8887   Fax (732)517-1260
+ 1112 Commons Way/Building F
Toms River, NJ 08755   (732)517-8887   Fax (732)349-9756

Moskowitz, David Matthew, MD {1902855638} Anesth, OthrSp(91,NY19)<NJ-ENGLWOOD>
+ Englewood Anesthesiology
350 Engle Street/CrdThrcAnesth   Englewood, NJ 07631
(201)894-3238   Fax (201)871-0619
david.moskowitz@ehmc.com

Moskowitz, Richard L., MD {1689649030} SrgC&R, Surgry(78,PA14)<NJ-MORRISTN>
+ Colon Surgery and Proctology Associates PA
111 Madison Avenue/Suite 312   Morristown, NJ 07960
(973)267-1225   Fax (973)993-9190

Moskowitz, Steven, MD {1003968629} AdolMd, Pedtrc(83,DOM03)
+ The Pediatric Center
556 Central Avenue   New Providence, NJ 07974   (908)508-0400   Fax (908)508-0370

Moskwa, Alexander, Jr., MD {1235193536} SrgOrt, SprtMd(82,MA01)<NJ-UNVMCPRN, NJ-VANJHCS>
+ Princeton Orthopaedic Associates, P.A.
325 Princeton Avenue   Princeton, NJ 08540   (609)924-8131   Fax (609)924-8532
+ Princeton Orthopaedic Associates, P.A.
11 Centre Drive   Jamesburg, NJ 08831   (609)655-4848

Mosquera, Joseph L., MD {1588719587} IntrMd(80,DOM02)<NJ-OVERLOOK>
+ Healthfirst
1 Washington Square   Newark, NJ 07105   Fax (973)344-1988

Mosquera, Maria Cecilia, MD {1750580700} Pedtrc
+ Passaic Pediatrics PA
298 Passaic Street   Passaic, NJ 07055   (973)249-8100   Fax (973)249-8110

Mosquera Charlenea, Claudia, MD {1326377953} ObsGyn
+ Maternal Fetal Medicine Associates
140 East Ridgewood Avenue/Suite 390S   Paramus, NJ 07652
(201)291-6321   Fax (201)291-6318

Moss, Beverly D., MD Pedtrc(93,NJ05)
+ 187 Arlington Avenue
Jersey City, NJ 07305

Moss, Charles M., MD {1134274582} SrgVas, Surgry(67,LA01)<NJ-HACKNSK, NJ-HOLYNAME>
+ Wound Healing & Hyperbaric Medicine
240 Williamson Street/Suite 104   Elizabeth, NJ 07202
(908)994-5480   Fax (908)994-8802

Moss, Edward G., MD {1477583284} Radiol, NuclMd, RadDia(68,PA13)<NJ-COOPRUMC>
+ Cooper University Hospital
One Cooper Plaza/Radiology   Camden, NJ 08103
(856)342-2383   Fax (856)365-0472

Moss, Leonard J., Jr., DO {1417988262} CdvDis, IntrMd(89,ME75)<NJ-MORRISTN>
+ Medical Institute of New Jersey
11 Saddle Road   Cedar Knolls, NJ 07927   (973)267-2122
Fax (973)267-3478

Moss, Pamela F., MD {1902247802} Psychy, PsyCAd(82,PA13)<NJ-HUNTRDN>
+ 111 Route 31
Flemington, NJ 08822   (908)237-4668   Fax (908)237-4607

Moss, Rebecca Anne, MD {1518046762} IntrMd, MedOnc(99,NY01)<NJ-RWJUBRUN, NJ-RWJUHAM>
+ Rutgers Cancer Institute of New Jersey
195 Little Albany Street/PO Box 2681   New Brunswick, NJ 08903   (732)235-2465   Fax (732)235-6797

Moss, Vance Joshaun, MD {1184660433} SrgUro, Urolgy(98,PA13)<NY-DCTRSTAT>
+ Mid-Atlantic Multi-Specialty Surgical Group, L.L.C.
2356 US Highway 9/Suite B6   Howell, NJ 07731   (732)886-2252   Fax (732)886-2260
vjmoss@mamsurg.com

Moss, Vincent Lavaughn, MD {1396799565} SrgTrm, SrgThr, Surgry(98,PA13)<NJ-COMMED>
+ Mid-Atlantic Multi-Specialty Surgical Group, L.L.C.
2356 US Highway 9/Suite B6   Howell, NJ 07731   (732)886-2252   Fax (732)886-2260
vlmoss@msmsurg.com
+ Surgical Practice Associates
98 James Street/Suite 202   Edison, NJ 08820   (732)886-2252   Fax (732)548-7590

Mossoczy-Godyn, Anna M., MD {1730274762} Pedtrc(78,POL02)<NJ-STFRNMED, NJ-CHSFULD>
+ 231 Bordentown Crosswick Road/Unit 2
Bordentown, NJ 08505   (609)298-7204   Fax (609)298-0491

Most, Michael David, MD {1124238316} Surgry, IntrMd(01,ISR06)
+ Summit Medical Group
140 Park Avenue/3rd Floor/Gen Surgery   Florham Park, NJ 07932   (973)404-9980

Moszczynski, Zbigniew, MD {1255431102} Surgry, GenPrc(92,NY19)<NJ-BAYONNE, NJ-CHRIST>
+ 31 West 8th Street
Bayonne, NJ 07002   (201)858-0188   Fax (201)455-8705
+ Short Hills Surgery Center
187 Millburn Avenue/Suite 101   Millburn, NJ 07041
(201)858-0188   Fax (973)671-0557

Motavalli, Lisa S, MD {1497982815} IntrMd(01,NJ06)
+ Princeton Health Medical & Surgical Associates
2 Centre Drive/Suite 200   Monroe, NJ 08831   (609)395-2470   Fax (609)860-5288
+ Princeton Medicine
5 Plainsboro Road/Suite 300   Plainsboro, NJ 08536
(609)395-2470   Fax (609)853-7271
+ Princeton HealthCare Medical Associates
11 Centre Drive/Suite A   Monroe Township, NJ 08831
(609)395-2470   Fax (609)860-5288

Moten, Hadi S., MD {1568605806} AnesPain(09,IL42)
+ Medical Associates of Central New Jersey
26 Throckmorton Lane/1st flr.   Old Bridge, NJ 08857
(732)952-5533   Fax (732)679-9956

Moten, Shirlene Tolbert, MD {1235271040} FamMed
+ Cape Regional Physicians Associates
3806 Bayshore Road/Suite 101   North Cape May, NJ 08204
(609)898-7447   Fax (609)898-1912

Motiwala, Neeta R., MD {1538153531} IntrMd(81,INA67)<NJ-HACKNSK, NJ-HOLYNAME>
+ Bergen Medical Associates
466 Old Hook Road/Suite 1   Emerson, NJ 07630   (201)967-8221   Fax (201)634-9647

Motwani, Sabin B., MD {1699908244} RadOnc(04,CA15)<NJ-RWJUBRUN, NJ-UMDNJ>
+ Rutgers Cancer Institute of New Jersey
195 Little Albany Street/PO Box 2681   New Brunswick, NJ 08903   (732)253-3939   Fax (732)253-3953

Moubarak, Issam F., MD {1639176084} RadDia(95,NJ06)<NJ-RWJUHAM, NJ-STPETER>
+ University Radiology Group, P.C.
579A Cranbury Road   East Brunswick, NJ 08816   (732)390-0040   Fax (732)390-1856
+ University Radiology Group, P.C.
483 Cranbury Road   East Brunswick, NJ 08816   (732)390-0040   Fax (732)390-5383
+ University Radiology Group, P.C.
16 Mountain Boulevard   Warren, NJ 08816   (908)769-7200
Fax (908)769-9141

Mouded, Issam, MD {1629092218} Urolgy(71,SYR01)<NJ-CHRIST, NJ-HOBUNIMC>
+ 255 Route 3 East/Suite 105
Secaucus, NJ 07094   (201)865-1919   Fax (201)865-4309

Moukdad, Jihad S., MD {1235221094} IntrMd(87,MNT01)<NJ-MEADWLND>
+ J. S. Moukdad, MD LLC
1265 Paterson Road   Secaucus, NJ 07094   (201)223-1121
Fax (201)223-1126

Moulayes, Nadra A., DO {1821226242} Surgry
+ 234 Hamburg Tpke/Suite 204
Wayne, NJ 07470   (973)310-0315

Physicians by Name and Address

Mouliswar, Mysore P., MD {1902832066} Grtrcs(81,INA70)
+ New Jersey Division of Developmental Disability
Route 72 East   New Lisbon, NJ 08064   (609)726-1000   Fax (609)894-8430

Mourad, Mohammad Y., MD {1437168663} Nephro(87,SYR01)<NJ-ACMCITY, NJ-ACMCMAIN>
+ AtlantiCare Regional Medical Center/City Campus
1925 Pacific Avenue   Atlantic City, NJ 08401   (609)652-1000

Mouradian, Mary Maral, MD {1750457305} Nrolgy, Rserch, ClnPhm(82,LEB03)
+ University Hospital-RWJMS Neurology
125 Paterson Street/Suite 4100-6100   New Brunswick, NJ 08901   (732)235-7733   Fax (732)235-7041

Mouravskaia, Tatiana Vladimirov, MD {1851481857} IntrMd, InfDis(86,RUSS)<NJ-CLARMAAS>
+ 511 South Orange Avenue
South Orange, NJ 07079   (973)200-3600   Fax (973)821-3651

Mouridy, Gary C., DO {1427045202} EmrgMd, IntrMd(94,MO79)<NJ-SOMERSET>
+ Emergency Medical Associates of NJ, P.A.
3 Century Drive   Parsippany, NJ 07054   (973)740-0607   Fax (973)740-9895

Mousa, Atef, DO {1891006565} IntrMd<NJ-JRSYCITY>
+ Jersey City Medical Center
355 Grand Street   Jersey City, NJ 07304   (201)915-2000

Mousavi, Mohammad Ali, DO {1225398761} NuclMd<NJ-NWRK-BETH>
+ Newark Beth Israel Medical Center
201 Lyons Avenue   Newark, NJ 07112   (973)926-7000

Mousavi, Seyed-Ali, MD {1336184472} RadDia(66,IRAN)<NJ-HOBUNIMC>
+ Hoboken University Medical Center
308 Willow Avenue/Radiology   Hoboken, NJ 07030   (201)418-1000   Fax (201)418-1822

Moussa, Alber Helmy, MD {1740235225} IntrMd(83,EGY04)<NJ-STPETER, NJ-RBAYOLDB>
+ Brunswick Medical Associates Inc
73 Brunswick Woods Drive   East Brunswick, NJ 08816   (732)698-9009   Fax (732)698-1414
drmoussa123@hotmail.com

Moussa, Ghias M., MD {1548341662} CdvDis(79,SYRI)
+ 30 Greenville Avenue
Jersey City, NJ 07305   (201)333-3311   Fax (201)333-4831

Moussa, Ibrahim Abdel, DO {1659382604} CdvDis, IntrMd(03,NY75)
+ Associated Cardiovascular Consultants-Lourdes
1 Brace Road/Suite C & F   Cherry Hill, NJ 08034   (856)323-1232   Fax (856)428-5748

Moussa, Issam, MD {1407933302} IntrMd, CdvDis, IntCrd(87,SYR01)<NY-PRSBCOLU>
+ Robert Wood Johnson Health System
One Robert Wood Johnson Place/MEB 582   New Brunswick, NJ 08903   (732)235-7133   Fax (732)235-8722

Moustafellos, Elaine, MD {1962449207} Pedtrc, PedGst(92,NY08)<NJ-HACKNSK>
+ Joseph M. Sanzari Childrens' -Gastro
155 Polifly Road/Suite 102   Hackensack, NJ 07601   (551)996-8840   Fax (201)441-9949

Moustiatse, Adelia C., MD {1013197573} IntrMd(68,MOL01)<NJ-CHRIST, NJ-HOBUNIMC>
+ A Progressive Longevity Center, LLC
2555 Kennedy Boulevard/Suite 4   Jersey City, NJ 07304   (201)761-0717   Fax (201)761-0787
adeliadrm@verizon.net

Moutier, Christine Y., MD {1962504274} Psychy
+ 36 Stoney Brook Road
Holmdel, NJ 07733

Movshovich, Alexander I., MD {1386659977} Ophthl, IntrMd(78,RUS15)<NY-PRSBWEIL>
+ Movshovich PC
596 Anderson Avenue/Suite 101   Cliffside Park, NJ 07010   (201)943-0022

Movva, Srinivasa R., MD {1699720508} IntrMd(86,INDI)
+ Srinivasa R. Movva MD PC
37 East Washington Avenue   Atlantic Highlands, NJ 07716   (732)291-3430

Moy, Erwin Kar-Leung, MD {1104145986}
+ 21 Cape May Drive
Marlboro, NJ 07746   (732)354-6901

Moy, Jamie Tam, DO {1134514912} FamMed
+ Summit Medical Group-Berkeley Heights Campus
1 Diamond Hill Road   Berkeley Heights, NJ 07922   (908)273-4300   Fax (908)790-6576

Moy, Jonathan M., MD {1124361795} Anesth<NJ-CHRIST>
+ Christ Hospital
176 Palisade Avenue   Jersey City, NJ 07306   (201)795-8200

Moy, Winston C., MD {1225196314} Dermat(81,TAI06)<NJ-STCLRDEN>
+ Drs. Moy and Spinelli
35 West Main Street/Suite 201   Denville, NJ 07834

(973)627-9635   Fax (973)625-7484

Moya-Mendez, Robert F., MD {1659394153} IntrMd, EnDbMt(79,PER04)<NJ-STCLRBOO, NJ-STCLRDEN>
+ 204 Church Street
Boonton, NJ 07005   (973)334-0736   Fax (973)334-2855

Moyle, Henry, MD {1750398939} SrgNro(95,CA14)<NJ-COMMED, NJ-MONMOUTH>
+ Neuerosurgeons of New Jersey
67 Route 37 West/First Floor   Toms River, NJ 08755   (732)443-1372   Fax (732)557-2366
moylhx@gmail.com

Moynihan, Eileen M., MD {1669580353} Rheuma, IntrMd(77,PA13)
+ 52 West Red Bank Avenue/Suite 27
Woodbury, NJ 08096   (856)853-8712   Fax (856)310-1840

Mozafarian, Mona, MD {1417268772}
+ Mountainside Family Practice Associates
799 Bloomfield Avenue/Suite 201   Verona, NJ 07044   (973)746-7050   Fax (973)857-2831

Mravcak, Sally A., MD {1811009657} FamMed(00,NJ06)
+ Vanguard Medical Group, P.A.
127 Montgomery Street   Jersey City, NJ 07302   (201)431-7200   Fax (201)526-0474
+ 123 Church Street
New Brunswick, NJ 08901   (201)431-7200   Fax (732)235-8583

Mroz, Lynne A., MD {1962476325} Anesth(87,PA02)
+ 331 Knoll Top Lane
Haddonfield, NJ 08033

Mucci, Wayne P., DO {1316947211} Otlryg(86,NJ75)<NJ-BURDTMLN>
+ Drs. Matlick, DeLorio, and Mucci
307 Stone Harbor Boulevard/Suite 3   Cape May Court House, NJ 08210   (609)465-4667   Fax (609)465-9387

Muccino, Gary P., MD {1285727529} FamMed(76,MEX14)
+ United Medical, P.C.
533 Lexington Avenue   Clifton, NJ 07011   (973)546-6844   Fax (973)546-7707
schoodicmd@aol.com

Mucha, Samantha Agatha, DO {1770970782} Pedtrc
+ Riverside Medical Group
714 Tenth Street/Suite 2   Secaucus, NJ 07094   (201)863-3346   Fax (201)865-0015

Muddassir, Salman Moazam, MD {1578608220} IntrMd<NJ-STFRNMED>
+ St. Francis Medical Center
601 Hamilton Avenue   Trenton, NJ 08629   (609)599-5000   Fax (609)599-4232

Mudry, Carolyn J., DO {1427013937} IntrMd(02,IA75)
+ Summit Medical Group Internal Medicine
127 Union Street/Suite 101   Ridgewood, NJ 07450   (201)444-5200   Fax (201)444-2399

Muduli, Anjali, MD {1598023210}
+ 205 10th Street/Apt 8V
Jersey City, NJ 07302   (973)970-8416
anjmuduli@gmail.com

Muduli, Hazari, MD {1558333047} Surgry, SrgVas(68,INA25)<NJ-NWTNMEM, NJ-HCKTSTWN>
+ 350 Sparta Avenue/Suite 6-B
Sparta, NJ 07871   (908)850-0028   Fax (908)850-1094

Mueller, Lawrence Peter, MD {1578676771} Surgry<NJ-JRSYSHMC>
+ Jersey Shore University Medical Center
1945 Route 33/Surgery   Neptune, NJ 07753   (732)775-5500   Fax (732)776-3763

Mueller, Loretta L., DO {1912977950} FamMed(88,NJ75)<NJ-OURLADY, NJ-VIRTVOOR>
+ Kennedy Health Alliance
457 Haddonfield Road/Suite 110   Cherry Hill, NJ 08002   (856)406-4091   Fax (856)406-4570
+ Kennedy Health Alliance
80 Tanner Street   Haddonfield, NJ 08033   (856)406-4091   Fax (856)355-0346

Mueller, Nancy L., MD {1124164959} Nrolgy, IntrMd(78,BEL04)<NJ-ENGLWOOD, NJ-HOLYNAME>
+ Institute of Neurological Care
610 East Palisade Avenue   Englewood Cliffs, NJ 07632   (201)569-2282   Fax (201)569-6110

Mueller, Thomas John, MD {1003029836} Urolgy(03,NJ06)<NJ-RWJUBRUN>
+ Delaware Valley Urology LLC
2003 B Lincoln Drive   Marlton, NJ 08053   (856)985-8000   Fax (856)985-1600
+ New Jersey Urology, LLC
2401 East Evesham Road/Suite F   Voorhees, NJ 08043   (856)985-8000   Fax (856)988-0636
+ Delaware Valley Urology LLC
570 Egg Harbor Road/Suite A-1   Sewell, NJ 08053   (856)582-9645   Fax (856)985-4583

Muenzen, Christopher P., MD {1730141821} IntrMd(84,NJ05)<NJ-MORRISTN, NJ-HCKTSTWN>
+ 59 East Mill Road
Long Valley, NJ 07853   (908)876-5300   Fax (908)876-9396

Mufson, Lewis J., MD {1437130622} Gastrn, IntrMd(67,PA09)<NJ-JRSYSHMC, NJ-MONMOUTH>
+ Lewis Jay Mufson MD, PA
8 Thureau Drive   Freehold, NJ 07728   (732)780-1888   Fax (732)780-0148

Mughal, Abdul W., MD {1003877440} IntrMd, OncHem(73,PAK01)<NJ-CHSMRCER>
+ 2097 Klockner Road
Trenton, NJ 08690   (609)588-4747
+ Mercer County Hematology and Oncology PC
40 Fuld Street/Suite 404   Trenton, NJ 08638   (609)588-4747   Fax (609)394-1004

Mughni, Azam, MD {1699199067} Nephro<NY-WOODHULL>
+ Christ Hospital
176 Palisade Avenue   Jersey City, NJ 07306   (201)795-8201

Muglia-Chopra, Christine Ann, MD {1588073159} IntMAImm
+ Hunterdon Otolaryngology Associates
6 Sand Hill Road/Suite 302   Flemington, NJ 08822   (908)788-9131   Fax (908)788-0945

Muhammad, Zaheda, MD {1760766760} ObsGyn(09,NJ05)
+ Liberty Women Ob/Gyn
377 Jersey Avenue/Suite 250   Jersey City, NJ 07302   (201)763-6763   Fax (201)763-6774

Muhr, William, Jr., MD {1174522544} RadDia, Radiol(83,PA09)<NJ-VIRTUAHS, NJ-VIRTMHBC>
+ South Jersey Radiology Associates, P.A.
901 Route 168/Suites 301-305   Turnersville, NJ 08012   (856)227-6600   Fax (856)227-8537
+ South Jersey Radiology Associates, P.A.
807 Haddon Avenue/Suite 5   Haddonfield, NJ 08033   (856)227-6600   Fax (856)616-1125
+ South Jersey Radiology Associates, P.A.
315 Route 70 East/Suite B   Cherry Hill, NJ 08012   (856)428-4344   Fax (856)428-0356

Muhumuza, Catherine, MD {1265534879} NnPnMd, Pedtrc, IntrMd(93,UGA01)<NJ-ACMCMAIN, NJ-ACMCITY>
+ AtlantiCare - Neonatology Department
65 West Jimmie Leeds Road   Pomona, NJ 08240   (609)404-3816   Fax (609)404-3818
+ AtlantiCare Regional Medical Center/City Campus
1925 Pacific Avenue/Neonatology   Atlantic City, NJ 08401   (609)345-4000

Mui, Timothy H., MD {1982869335} FamMed, IntrMd(06,NY01)
+ Cornerstone Family Practice
9100 Wescott Drive/Suite 103   Flemington, NJ 08822   (908)237-6910   Fax (908)237-6919

Mujahid, Anjum, MD {1306811948} Psychy(86,PAK17)<NJ-TRENTPSY>
+ Trenton Psychiatric Hospital
Sullivan Way/PO Box 7600/Psych   West Trenton, NJ 08628   (609)633-1500

Mujic, Lejla, MD {1184659351} EmrgMd(03,NJ06)<NJ-STBARNMC>
+ St. Barnabas Medical Center
94 Old Short Hills Road   Livingston, NJ 07039   (973)322-5000

Mukai, Yuki, MD {1417139759} Psychy, PsyCAd(06,NJ02)
+ Southern Ocean County Hospital
1100 Route 72 West   Manahawkin, NJ 08050   (609)597-4094   Fax (609)978-4442

Mukalian, Gregory G., DO {1659372910} Surgry(85,MO78)<NJ-VIRTMHBC, NJ-LOURDMED>
+ LMA Surgical Specialists - Burlington County
1113 Hospital Drive/Suite 100   Willingboro, NJ 08046   (609)835-5821   Fax (609)835-5827

Mukherjee, Angela, DO {1164718300} Pedtrc<NJ-MORRISTN>
+ Morristown Medical Center
100 Madison Avenue/Pediatrics   Morristown, NJ 07962   (973)971-7802   Fax (973)290-7693

Mukherjee, Robin, DO {1174935811} IntrMd
+ Raritan Family Health Care
901 US Highway 202   Raritan, NJ 08869   (908)253-6640   Fax (908)253-6908

Mukherjee, Shanker, MD {1558340265} Gastrn, IntrMd(80,INA7B)<NJ-WARREN, PA-WARRNGEN>
+ Twin Rivers Gastroenterology Center
755 Memorial Parkway/Suite 202A   Phillipsburg, NJ 08865   (908)859-5400
+ Warren Hospital
185 Roseberry Street   Phillipsburg, NJ 08865   (908)859-6700

Mukherji, Genea, MD {1396038113} FamMed
+ Cornerstone Family Practice
9100 Wescott Drive/Suite 103   Flemington, NJ 08822   (908)237-6910   Fax (908)237-6919

Mukhopadhay, Jayati, MD {1790754125} ObsGyn(71,INA89)
+ 60 Ball Street
Irvington, NJ 07111 (973)374-8889 Fax (973)374-1034
JaySusanta@juno.com
+ 520 Westfield Avenue
Elizabeth, NJ 07208 (908)351-5511

Mulberg, Andrew Evan, MD {1184630808} Pedtrc, PedEmg, PedGst(86,NY47)
+ Cooper Peds/Children's Regional Ctr
6400 Main Street Complex/Gastro Voorhees, NJ 08043
(856)751-9339
+ Cooper University Medical Center/Camden
3 Cooper Plaza/Gastro Camden, NJ 08103 (856)751-9339

Mule, Salvatore, MD {1437577855} FamMed
+ Tatem Brown Family Practice
2225 East Evesham Road/Suite 101 Voorhees, NJ 08043
(856)325-3700 Fax (856)325-3704

Mulford, Gregory J., MD {1083680771} PhysMd(85,NJ06)<NJ-MMHKEMBL>
+ Associates in Rehabilitation Medicine
95 Mount Kemble Avenue Morristown, NJ 07960
(973)267-2293 Fax (973)226-3144

Mulholland, Brendan J., MD {1922080092} FamMed(94,DC02)<NJ-RIVERVW>
+ Red Bank Family Medicine
231 Maple Avenue Red Bank, NJ 07701 (732)842-3050
Fax (732)530-0730
+ 14 East River Road
Rumson, NJ 07760 (732)842-3050 Fax (732)933-1040

Mulholland, Daniel J., MD {1639140841} Ortped, SrgOrt(87,DC02)<NJ-BAYSHORE>
+ Orthopaedic Sports Medicine
80 Oak Hill Road Red Bank, NJ 07701 (732)741-2313
Fax (732)741-7154

Mulkay, Angel J., MD {1013025733} CdvDis, IntrMd(90,DOM02)<NJ-HACKNSK>
+ Mulkay Cardiology Consultants, P.C.
493 Essex Street Hackensack, NJ 07601 (201)996-9244
Fax (201)601-0995
+ Mulkay Cardiology Consultants, P.C.
529 39th Street Union City, NJ 07087 (201)996-9244
Fax (201)601-0995
+ Mulkay Cardiology Consultants, P.C.
15 Ver Valen Street Closter, NJ 07601 (201)996-9244
Fax (201)996-9243

Mullane, Joseph P., MD {1215992664} FamMed(85,DOM08)<NJ-RWJUHAM, NJ-UNVMCPRN>
+ Princeton Occupational Medicine
2271 Highway 33/Suite 109 Hamilton, NJ 08690
(609)584-0117 Fax (609)586-5103

Mullarkey-De Sapio, Cathleen J., MD {1225073505} EnDbMt, IntrMd(84,MA07)
+ Princeton Medical Group, P.A.
419 North Harrison Street Princeton, NJ 08540 (609)924-9300 Fax (609)924-6552
+ Princeton Endocrinology Associates, LLC
10 Forrestal Road South/Suite 106 Princeton, NJ 08540
(609)924-9300 Fax (609)921-3316

Mullarney, Allison Ingrid, DO {1740656024} IntrMd
+ Hospital Medicine Associates
157 Broad Street/Suite 317 Red Bank, NJ 07701
(732)530-2960 Fax (732)530-7446

Mullengada, Krithika, MD {1992785562} IntrMd(96,INA70)<NJ-MORRISTN>
+ Northwest Medical Care LLC
66 Sunset Strip/Suite 407 Succasunna, NJ 07876
(973)252-1676

Mullick, Bharati, MD {1245364314} AdolMd, Pedtrc(67,INA69)<NJ-OVERLOOK, NJ-STBARNMC>
+ 295 Baltusrol Way
Springfield, NJ 07081 (973)467-2644 Fax (973)954-2347

Mullick, Muhammad Azfar, MD {1487925038} IntHos
+ 501 Avalon Drive/Apt 5401
Wood Ridge, NJ 07075

Mulligan, Edward, MD {1881060283} IntHos<NJ-JRSYCITY>
+ Jersey City Medical Center
355 Grand Street Jersey City, NJ 07304 (201)915-2000

Mullin, Guy S., MD {1285680157} Ophthl(92,DC02)
+ Newtown Laser & Eye Institute
4 Princess Road/Suite 202 Lawrenceville, NJ 08648

Mulvey, Lauri D., MD {1326112400} Ophthl(77,MA01)<NJ-UNVMCPRN, PA-CHILDHOS>
+ 213 Nassau Street
Princeton, NJ 08540 (609)924-1661 Fax (609)924-8728
+ CHOP Pediatric & Adolescent Specialty Care Center
707 Alexander Road/Suite 205 Princeton, NJ 08540
(609)520-1717

Mulvihill, Claire A., MD {1417057498} Dermat(88,NY08)<NJ-VA-LYONS>
+ 745 US Highway 202/206/Suite 103
Bridgewater, NJ 08807 (908)393-9755

+ VA New Jersey Health Care System at Lyons
151 Knollcroft Road Lyons, NJ 07939 (908)647-0180

Mulvihill, David J., MD {1417274143} Pedtrc<NJ-RWJUBRUN>
+ MD Anderson Cancer Center at Cooper
2 Cooper Plaza Camden, NJ 08103 (855)632-2667
+ RWJ University Hospital New Brunswick
One Robert Wood Johnson Place New Brunswick, NJ 08901
(855)632-2667 Fax (732)235-6102

Mumneh, Nayla Z., MD {1760489645} AlgyImmn, Allrgy(92,LEB03)<NJ-JFKMED, NJ-RWJURAH>
+ Allergy Treatment Center of New Jersey, Inc.
1000 Route 9 North/Suite 200 Woodbridge, NJ 07095
(732)283-3040 Fax (732)283-3042
+ Allergy Treatment Center of New Jersey, Inc.
1100 Centennial Avenue/Suite 202 Piscataway, NJ 08854
(732)283-3040 Fax (732)762-1770

Mund, Michael L., MD {1457312449} Ophthl, OthrSp(63,NY08)<NJ-STMRYPAS, NJ-STJOSHOS>
+ 1187 Main Avenue/Suite 1F
Clifton, NJ 07011 (973)546-6161 Fax (973)546-1708

Mundassery, Sarala C., MD {1225172638} Psychy(64,INA66)
+ 314-316 East State Street
Trenton, NJ 08608

Munera, Rodolfo A., MD {1154382760} InfDis, IntrMd(84,COLO)<NJ-STMRYPAS>
+ 1001 Clifton Avenue/Suite 1B
Clifton, NJ 07013 (973)472-8000
Rudymu2000@yahoo.com

Mungekar, Mangesh Mohan, MD {1144306069} IntrMd(96,NJ06)<NJ-COOPRUMC>
+ The Cooper Hospital System-Univ Hospital
3 Cooper Plaza/Suite 215/InternalMed Camden, NJ 08103
(856)342-2439

Mungekar, Meaghan, MD {1972760866} Pedtrc(05,NY19)<NY-BETHPETR>
+ Englewood Medical Associates Pediatrics
350 Engle Street Englewood, NJ 07631 (201)585-1261
Fax (201)894-5649

Mungekar, Sagar Sudhir, MD {1174815286} Anesth
+ Robert Wood Johnson-UMDNJ Anesthesia Group
125 Paterson Street/CAB 3100 New Brunswick, NJ 08901
(732)235-6153 Fax (732)235-6131

Munir, Maryam, MD {1093293631} IntrMd<NJ-STFRNMED>
+ St. Francis Medical Center
601 Hamilton Avenue Trenton, NJ 08629 (347)325-0762

Munjal, Ajay K., MD {1972550911} RadDia, Radiol, IntrMd(89,PA09)
+ Center for Diagnostic Imaging
1450 East Chestnut Avenue Vineland, NJ 08360 (856)794-8664 Fax (856)794-2671

Munne, Gisela L., MD {1073556213} IntrMd(88,GRN01)<NJ-CHRIST>
+ PMA Physicians LLC
1 Journal Square Plaza/2nd Floor Jersey City, NJ 07306
(201)216-3030 Fax (201)749-9024

Munoz, Daisy, MD {1336374149} Anesth(09,NJ05)
+ Hackensack University MC-Anesthesia Dept
30 Prospect Avenue/Room 2703 Hackensack, NJ 07601
(201)996-2419 Fax (201)996-3962

Munoz, Francisco, MD {1164484291} IntrMd(81,DOM02)
+ Union Square Medical Associates
824 Elizabeth Avenue Elizabeth, NJ 07201 (908)352-9556
Fax (908)352-9134
doctores@msn.com

Munoz, Guillermo A., DO {1023071669} IntrMd(90,NY75)<NJ-TRINIJSC, NJ-STMICHL>
+ Union Square Medical Associates
824 Elizabeth Avenue Elizabeth, NJ 07201 (908)352-9556
Fax (908)352-3446

Munoz, Raul, MD {1205912128} Anesth(85,PRO01)<NJ-COOPRUMC>
+ Cooper University Hospital
One Cooper Plaza/Anesth Camden, NJ 08103 (856)342-2000

Munoz, Santiago Jose, MD {1578531190} Hepato
+ Capital Health System/Hopewell
One Capital Way/Hepatlgy Pennington, NJ 08534
(609)394-4000

Munoz-Llaverias, Altagracia M., MD {1174624563} Pedtrc(82,DOM01)<NJ-CHRIST>
+ 217 60th Street
West New York, NJ 07093 (201)869-1108
+ NHCAC Health Center at West New York
5301 Broadway West New York, NJ 07093 (201)866-9320

Munoz-Matta, Ana T., MD {1962715540} ObsGyn
+ Physicians for Women
330 Ratzer Road/Suite 7 Wayne, NJ 07470 (973)694-2222
Fax (973)694-7664

Munoz-Silva, Dinohra M., MD {1255462610} PsycAd, Psychy(84,DMN01)
+ 15 Broadway/Suite 206
Cresskill, NJ 07626

Munshi, Pashna N., MD {1770845661} MedOnc
+ UH- RWJ Medical School
One Robert Wood Johnson Place New Brunswick, NJ 08903
(732)235-7678 Fax (732)235-7115
pashna.munshi@gmail.com

Muntazar, Muhammad, MD {1194793836} Anesth<NJ-COOPRUMC>
+ Cooper University Hospital
One Cooper Plaza/Anesth Camden, NJ 08103 (856)342-2000

Munteanu, Katrina M., MD {1114243938} Pedtrc
+ Broadway Pediatric Associates
336 Center Avenue Westwood, NJ 07675 (201)664-7444
Fax (201)666-9476

Munver, Ravi, MD {1891741906} Urolgy(96,NY20)<NJ-HACKNSK>
+ Hackensack University Medical Center
360 Essex Street/Ste 403/Urology Hackensack, NJ 07601
(201)336-8090
+ HUMC Faculty Practice
360 Essex Street/Suite 403 Hackensack, NJ 07601
(201)336-8090 Fax (201)336-8221

Muppala, Sujatha, MD {1275730053}<NJ-MONMOUTH>
+ 906 Oak Tree Road/Suite 106A
South Plainfield, NJ 07080 (908)822-2277 Fax (908)822-1121

Mupparaju, Jyothsna, MD {1861771941}
+ Community Medical Center
99 Route 37 West Toms River, NJ 08755 (732)557-8000
+ 6105 Bainbridge Way
Freehold, NJ 07728 (618)946-9231

Mur, Ahmad A., MD {1801878582} IntrMd(85,PAK01)<NJ-SOMERSET>
+ Ahmad A. Mur MD PA
503 Omni Drive Hillsborough, NJ 08844 (908)595-1199
Fax (866)889-3643

Murachanian, Richard J., MD {1609849249} IntrMd(84,ITA01)
+ 1401 Beaver Dam Road
Point Pleasant Beach, NJ 08742 (732)899-2353 Fax (732)295-3845

Murakata, Linda Ann, MD {1063496271} PthAcl
+ 23 Elm Place
Eatontown, NJ 07724 (856)334-5000

Muralidharan, Soundari, MD {1548363880} IntrMd(82,INA3X)
+ NJ VA/James J Howard Outpatient Clinic
970 Route 70 West Brick, NJ 08724 (732)206-8900 Fax (732)836-6001

Murano, Tiffany Ellyn, MD {1760584015} EmrgMd(96,NY47)<NJ-UMDNJ>
+ University Hospital
150 Bergen Street/EmrgMed Newark, NJ 07103 (973)972-5128 Fax (973)972-6646

Muratschew, Donna M., MD {1548228851} Pedtrc(85,GRN01)<NJ-MORRISTN>
+ Hackensack Pediatrics
177 Summit Avenue Hackensack, NJ 07601 (201)487-8222 Fax (201)487-2126
+ 628 Red Oak Drive
Rivervale, NJ 07675

Murdaco, Francis J., Jr., MD {1962574962} IntrMd, CdvDis(78,NJ05)
+ Holy Name Physicians Associates
255 West Spring Valley Avenue Maywood, NJ 07607
(201)845-6448 Fax (201)845-4321

Murikan, Tom, MD {1699115717}
+ St. Joseph's Family Medicine @ Clifton
1135 Broad Street/Suite 201 Clifton, NJ 07013 (973)754-4100 Fax (973)472-9062

Murillo, Jeremias L., MD {1962438259} InfDis, OthrSp, PedInf(72,PHIL)<NJ-NWRKBETH>
+ Newark Beth Israel Medical Center
201 Lyons Avenue/InfDisease Newark, NJ 07112
(973)926-7000 Fax (973)926-4203

Murillo, Narcisa E., MD {1942282306} IntrMd(86,ECU05)
+ 463 Clifton Avenue
Clifton, NJ 07011 (973)546-2400 Fax (973)546-2441

Murphy, Bernard P., MD {1851362065} SrgOrt(67,NJ05)<NJ-BAYSHORE>
+ Orthopaedic Sports Medicine
80 Oak Hill Road Red Bank, NJ 07701 (732)741-2313
Fax (732)741-7154

Murphy, David M., MD {1275588667} IntrMd, PulDis(65,IREL)<NJ-DEBRAHLC>
+ Deborah Heart and Lung Center
200 Trenton Road/Pulmonary Med Browns Mills, NJ 08015
(609)893-6611 Fax (609)735-1472
murphyd@deborah.org

Physicians by Name and Address

Murphy, Francis Raymond, MD {1063429629} PsyGrt, Psychy, IntrMd(87,MEX34)
+ Center Senior Wellness
 5 North Main Street Medford, NJ 08055 (609)654-0054 Fax (609)288-6784
+ New Jersey Division of Developmental Disability
 Route 72 East New Lisbon, NJ 08064 (609)654-0054 Fax (609)894-8430

Murphy, Guy D., MD {1023191293} ObsGyn(80,NJ05)<NJ-UMDNJ>
+ Drs. Leung & Murphy
 196 Speedwell Avenue Morristown, NJ 07960 (973)539-9580

Murphy, Heather Marie, MD {1376777342} ObsGyn
+ Garden State Obstetrics and Gynecological Associates
 2401 Evesham Road/Suite A Voorhees, NJ 08043 (856)424-3323 Fax (856)424-4994

Murphy, John Charles, MD {1669482428} FamMed(97,NJ05)
+ AstraHealth Urgent & Primary Care
 1100 Centennial Avenue/Suite 104 Piscataway, NJ 08854 (732)981-1111 Fax (732)981-1113
+ AstraHealth Urgent & Primary Care
 95 Hudson Street Hoboken, NJ 07030 (201)464-8888
+ AstraHealth Urgent & Primary Care
 18 Lyons Mall Basking Ridge, NJ 08854 (908)760-8888

Murphy, John W., MD {1740291806} SrgOrt(88,NJ05)<NJ-HCKTSTWN, NJ-MORRISTN>
+ Skylands Orthopaedics PC
 57 US Highway 46/Suite 107 Hackettstown, NJ 07840 (908)813-9700 Fax (908)813-2861
+ Skylands Orthopaedics PC
 1 Robertson Drive/Suite 11 Bedminster, NJ 07921 (908)813-9700 Fax (908)813-2861
+ Emmaus Surgical Center
 57 US Highway 46/Suite 104 Hackettstown, NJ 07840 (908)813-9600 Fax (908)813-9611

Murphy, Kathleen A., MD {1710956982} PedUro, Urolgy(81,NY08)
+ Drs. Murphy & Williams, P.A.
 33 Overlook Road/Suite 412 Summit, NJ 07901 (908)273-7274
+ Drs. Murphy & Williams, P.A.
 867 St. Georges Avenue Rahway, NJ 07065 (732)388-0990
+ Drs. Murphy & Williams, P.A.
 104 North Euclid Avenue Westfield, NJ 07901 (908)232-8416 Fax (908)654-1993

Murphy, Kim, MD {1730143512} IntrMd(01,GRN01)
+ Emergency Medical Offices
 651 West Mount Pleasant Avenue Livingston, NJ 07039 (973)740-9396 Fax (973)251-1165

Murphy, Patricia L., MD {1255336830} CdvDis, IntrMd(89,NY08)<NJ-HACKNSK, NJ-VALLEY>
+ Westwood Cardiology Associates PA
 333 Old Hook Road/Suite 200 Westwood, NJ 07675 (201)664-0201 Fax (201)666-7970
+ Westwood Cardiology Associates PA
 20 Prospect Avenue/Suite 810 Hackensack, NJ 07601 (201)664-0201 Fax (201)342-2422

Murphy, Robert D., MD {1750498556} Pedtrc(77,TN05)<NJ-MONMOUTH>
+ Pediatric & Adolescent Medicine, PA
 223 Monmouth Road West Long Branch, NJ 07764 (732)229-4540 Fax (732)229-8689

Murphy, Robyn C., MD {1083704886} RadDia(92,VA04)<NJ-MORRISTN>
+ Memorial Radiology Associates
 10 Lanidex Plaza West/Suite 125 Parsippany, NJ 07054 (973)503-5700 Fax (973)386-5701
+ Morristown Medical Center
 100 Madison Avenue Morristown, NJ 07962 (973)971-5000

Murphy, Ryan Bruce, MD {1548314263} EmrgMd(02,CT02)<CT-HOSPSTRA>
+ St Joseph's Medical Center Emergency
 703 Main Street Paterson, NJ 07503 (973)754-2240 Fax (973)754-2249

Murphy, Ryan Keith, DO {1396023701} PhysMd(11,ME75)
+ Prospect Medical Offices, LLC
 301 Godwin Avenue Midland Park, NJ 07432 (201)444-4526 Fax (201)301-1313

Murphy, Susan M., MD {1366530016} PedHem(85,NY06)<NJ-STBARNMC, NJ-NWRKBETH>
+ Rutgers Cancer Institute of New Jersey
 195 Little Albany Street/PO Box 2681 New Brunswick, NJ 08903 (732)235-8864 Fax (732)235-8234
+ The Valerie Fund Children's Center
 95 Old Short Hills Road Livingston, NJ 07039 (732)235-8864 Fax (973)322-2856

Murphy, Terri Lee, DO {1750449617} Pedtrc(95,PA77)
+ Pediatric Connection
 135 Jackson Road/Suite B Medford, NJ 08055 (609)654-9961 Fax (609)654-6118

Tanddmurphy@comcast.net

Murr, Peter, MD {1306190665} Ophthl(NJ02<NJ-RWJUBRUN>
+ Santamaria Eye Center
 104 Market Street Perth Amboy, NJ 08861 (732)826-5159 Fax (732)826-2107
+ Santamaria Eye Center
 100 Menlo Park Drive/Suite 408 Edison, NJ 08837 (732)826-5159 Fax (732)767-1871

Murray, Carl Louis, Jr., MD {1447241906} Hemato, MedOnc, IntrMd(79,NJ05)
+ The Doctor's Office
 1 Woodbridge Center/Suite 900 Woodbridge, NJ 07095 (732)965-1050 Fax (732)791-2153
+ The Doctor's Office
 3897 Route 516/Suite 2-C Old Bridge, NJ 08857 (732)965-1050 Fax (732)679-5555

Murray, Elrick A., MD {1972658896} ObsGyn(82,NJ05)
+ 1314 Park Avenue
 Plainfield, NJ 07060 (908)753-0440 Fax (908)753-5107

Murray, Francis, Jr., DO {1316975154} FamMed(74,PA77)<NJ-OURLADY, NJ-KMHSTRAT>
+ 1001 Center Avenue
 Bellmawr, NJ 08031 (856)931-2266 Fax (856)931-5915

Murray, Jeffrey, DO {1922230812} SrgOrt(09,PA77)
+ Reconstructive Orthopedics, P.A.
 570 Egg Harbor Road/Suite C-4 Sewell, NJ 08080 (609)267-9400 Fax (609)267-9457

Murray, Michael Louis, DO {1225212368} GPrvMd, PubHth(86,PA77)
+ Lockheed Martin Health & Wellness
 199 Borton Landing Road/Ms-102-105 Moorestown, NJ 08057 (856)733-3336

Murray, Norma J., MD {1790881472} Pedtrc(80,NJ05)<NJ-HOLYNAME>
+ Holy Name Hospital
 718 Teaneck Road Teaneck, NJ 07666 (201)833-3000 Fax (201)833-4486

Murray, Richard S., MD {1467512913} FamMed, EmrgMd(75,MEX14)<NJ-MTNSIDE>
+ Town Medical Associates/Verona
 271 Grove Avenue/Suite A Verona, NJ 07044 (973)239-2600 Fax (973)239-0482

Murray, Simon D., MD {1093792764} IntrMd(80,PHI08)<NJ-UNVMCPRN>
+ 727 State Road/2nd Floor
 Princeton, NJ 08540 (609)921-7444 Fax (609)921-7443

Murray, Thomas Robert, MD {1942282744} Anesth(83,FL02)<NJ-MORRISTN>
+ Morristown Medical Center
 100 Madison Avenue/Anesthesiology Morristown, NJ 07962 (973)971-5548 Fax (201)943-8733

Murray-Burton, Carolyn I., MD {1366566002} AdolMd, Pedtrc(84,NJ05)
+ 48 Rossmore Place
 Belleville, NJ 07109

Murray-Taylor, Stacey Odell, MD {1437101391} EmrgMd, IntrMd(96,TN07)
+ Emergency Medical Associates of NJ, P.A.
 3 Century Drive Parsippany, NJ 07054 (973)740-0607 Fax (973)740-9895

Murry, Robert L., MD {1780658765} FamMed(02,TX12)<NJ-HUNTRDN>
+ Delaware Valley Family Health Center
 200 Frenchtown Road Milford, NJ 08848 (908)995-2251 Fax (908)995-2036

Murthy, Meena S., MD {1144270281} EnDbMt, Grtrcs, IntrMd(79,INDI)<NJ-STPETER>
+ Thyroid & Diabetes Ctr
 240 Easton Avenue/4th Floor New Brunswick, NJ 08901 (732)745-6667
+ Center for Ambulatory Resources
 240 Easton Avenue/4th Floor New Brunswick, NJ 08901 (732)745-6667 Fax (732)745-9156

Murthy, Sujatha S., MD {1942380191} Anesth(73,INA68)
+ Roxbury Open MRI and Surgical Center
 66 Sunset Strip/Suites 101 & 104 Succasunna, NJ 07876 (973)927-8100 Fax (973)927-2097

Murugesan, Angappan, MD {1003972787} SrgLsr, Surgry, SrgC&R(71,INA04)<NJ-BAYSHORE, NJ-RBAYOLDB>
+ 80 Hazlet Avenue/Suite 7
 Hazlet, NJ 07730 (732)264-2220 Fax (732)264-3090

Musarra, Anthony Mark, MD {1811914476} IntrMd(91,PA02)
+ 216 Lily Road
 Egg Harbor Township, NJ 08234 (609)635-2838

Musat, Dan Laurentiu, MD {1972767192} CdvDis, ClCdEl, IntrMd(96,ROM01)<NJ-VALLEY>
+ Valley Medical Group-Electrophysiology
 970 Linwood Avenue/Suite 102 Ridgewood, NJ 07450 (201)432-7837 Fax (201)432-7830
+ Valley Medical Group-Electrophysiology & Cardiology
 1578 Route 23/Suite 103 Wayne, NJ 07470 (201)432-7837 Fax (201)432-7830

Mushayandebvu, Taonei I., MD {1235148198} ObsGyn, RprEnd, FrtInf(85,ZIMB)<NJ-HACKNSK>
+ 2777 Kennedy Boulevard
 Jersey City, NJ 07306 (201)369-1902

Mushnick, Alan J., MD {1942297866} Gastrn, IntrMd(80,SPAI)<NJ-UNDRWD, NJ-VIRTVOOR>
+ South Jersey Gastrointestinal
 2301 Evesham Road/Suite 110 Voorhees, NJ 08043 (856)772-1600 Fax (856)772-9031
 alanmush@aol.com

**Mushonga, Nyarai Chinyani, MD {1063696763}<NJ-MORRISTN>
+ New Jersey Urology, LLC
 375 Mounain Pleasant Ave/Suite 250 West Orange, NJ 07052 (973)323-1320 Fax (973)323-1311
+ Morristown Medical Center
 100 Madison Avenue Morristown, NJ 07962 (973)971-5000

Mushtaq, Arman, MD {1780190231} IntrMd<NJ-RBAYPERT>
+ Hackensack Meridian Medical Group
 19 Davis Avenue/5th-6th Floor Neptune, NJ 07753 (732)897-3990 Fax (732)897-3997
+ Raritan Bay Medical Center/Perth Amboy Division
 530 New Brunswick Avenue Perth Amboy, NJ 08861 (732)897-3990 Fax (732)324-4669

Mushtaq, Sabina, MD {1326331075} Psychy
+ 40 Conger Street/Apt 810B
 Bloomfield, NJ 07003

Musicant, Joel Marc, MD {1174576052} Gastrn(89,PA09)
+ Gastroenterology Associates
 475 State Highway 70 Lakewood, NJ 08701 (732)886-1007 Fax (732)224-8773

Musico, John J., MD {1639109242} IntrMd(88,GRN01)<NJ-VAEASTOR>
+ NJ VA/James J Howard Outpatient Clinic
 970 Route 70 West Brick, NJ 08724 (732)206-8900
+ VA New Jersey Health Care System-East Orange Campus
 385 Tremont Avenue East Orange, NJ 07018 (973)676-1000

Musser, Erica Lynn, DO {1093922320} Psychy(96,NJ75)
+ South Woods State Prison/NJ Dept of Corrections
 215 South Burlington Road Bridgeton, NJ 08302 (856)459-7000 Fax (856)459-8713

Mussoline, Joseph F., MD {1821084583} Ophthl(81,ITA30)
+ Haddonfield Eye Associates
 320 North Haddon Avenue/Suite B Haddonfield, NJ 08033 (856)429-2199
+ Campus Eye Group & Laser Center
 1700 Whitehorse Hamilton Sq Rd Hamilton Square, NJ 08690 (856)429-2199 Fax (609)588-9545

Mustafa, Diane M., MD {1992088082} ObsGyn
+ Women's Care
 1044 Main Street Paterson, NJ 07503 (973)782-5577

Mustafa, Muhammad A., MD {1932480688} IntrMd<NJ-RWJUBRUN>
+ RWJ University Hospital New Brunswick
 One Robert Wood Johnson Place New Brunswick, NJ 08901 (732)828-3000

Mustafa, Muhammad Usman, MD {1649215989} IntrMd, CdvDis(89,PAK15)
+ Capital Cardiology Associates
 40 Fuld Street/Suite 400 Trenton, NJ 08638 (609)396-1644 Fax (609)394-9526

Mustafa, Rose, MD {1932333101} Surgry
+ Mountain View Surgical Assoicates
 2 Capital Way/Suite 505 Pennington, NJ 08534 (609)537-6700 Fax (609)537-6717

Mustillo, Robert A., MD {1649470295} IntrMd, OccpMd(88,NJ06)
+ Center for Occupational Health
 221 Chestnut Street Newark, NJ 07105 (973)491-2900 Fax (973)491-2901
 robertm@cathedralhealth.org

Muthusamy, Samiappan, MD {1497713184} Gastrn, IntrMd(71,INA77)<NJ-TRINIJSC, NJ-JFKMED>
+ Center for Digestive Diseases
 695 Chestnut Street Union, NJ 07083 (908)688-6565 Fax (908)688-3161
+ EndoSurgi Center of Old Bridge
 42 Throckmorton Lane Old Bridge, NJ 08857 (732)679-8808
+ Center for Digestive Diseases
 1907 Oak Tree Road Edison, NJ 07083

Muthusawmy, Nanda, MD {1699022558} PsyCAd
+ 65 Harristown Road/Suite 101
 Glen Rock, NJ 07452 (201)487-1240
+ Advanced Psychiatric Associates
 65 Harristown Road/Suite 101 Glen Rock, NJ 07452 (201)487-1240

Muthuswamy, Rajeswari, MD {1700844792} PsyCAd, Psychy(96,INA04)<NJ-MORRISTN>
+ Morristown Medical Center
  100 Madison Avenue/Box 28/Psych   Morristown, NJ 07962   (973)971-5000

Muthuswamy, Vijayalakshmi, MD {1124052097} Pedtrc(73,INA68)<NJ-HACKNSK, NJ-VALLEY>
+ Hohokus Pediatrics
  129 Lindenbergh Parkway   Waldwick, NJ 07463   (201)444-9235

Muttana, Renu Devi, MD {1265692552} IntrMd(07,DMN01)
+ BSD Nephrology & Hypertension
  360 Essex Street/Suite 304   Hackensack, NJ 07601   (201)646-0110   Fax (201)646-0219

Mutterperl, Mitchell J., MD {1215972682} IntrMd(81,ITA17)<NJ-BAYONNE>
+ 19 West 33rd Street
  Bayonne, NJ 07002   (201)858-0090   Fax (201)858-1044

Muzones, Santiago, III, MD {1376537241} IntrMd, EmrgMd(89,PHI08)<NJ-RBAYPERT>
+ Raritan Bay Medical Center/Perth Amboy Division
  530 New Brunswick Avenue/InternalMed   Perth Amboy, NJ 08861   (732)442-3700

Mwamuka, Linda, MD {1396139705} IntrMd<NJ-NWRKBETH>
+ Newark Beth Israel Medical Center
  201 Lyons Avenue   Newark, NJ 07112   (973)926-7000

Myers, Khaleah K., MD {1558336008} Anesth(01,MO46)<NJ-TRINIWSC>
+ Trinitas Regional Medical Center-Williamson Street
  225 Williamson Street/Anesthesia   Elizabeth, NJ 07207   (908)994-5204   Fax (908)994-5061

Myers, Scott Elliot, MD {1407839145} IntrMd, Gastrn(82,PA09)
+ Philadelphia Gastroenterology Group, P.C.
  570 Egg Harbor Road/Suite A-2   Sewell, NJ 08080   (856)218-1410   Fax (856)218-0193

Myers, Wendy A., MD {1497876601} Dermat
+ Windsor Dermatology
  59 One Mile Road Extension/Suite G   East Windsor, NJ 08520   (609)443-4500   Fax (609)426-0530
  wmyers@windsordermatology.com

Mykulak, Donald J., MD {1194796540} Urolgy(85,NY08)<NJ-HCKTSTWN, NJ-NWTNMEM>
+ Skylands Urology Group
  89 Sparta Avenue/Suite 200   Sparta, NJ 07871   (973)726-7220   Fax (973)726-7230
  dmykulak@skylandsurology.com
+ Skylands Urology Group
  616 Willow Grove Street   Hackettstown, NJ 07840   (973)726-7220   Fax (973)726-7230
+ Specialty Surgical Center
  380 Lafayette Road/Suite 110   Sparta, NJ 07871   (973)940-3166   Fax (973)940-3170

Myneni, Neelima, MD {1477709962} Anesth<NJ-STBARNMC, NJ-NWRKBETH>
+ St. Barnabas Medical Center
  94 Old Short Hills Road/Anesthesia   Livingston, NJ 07039   (973)322-5512   Fax (973)660-9779
+ New Jersey Anesthesia Associates, P.C.
  30B Vreeland Road/Suite 200   Florham Park, NJ 07932   (973)322-5512   Fax (973)660-9779

Myridakis, Dorothy J., MD {1740335405} PedCrd(84,GRE01)<NJ-STJOSHOS>
+ Pediatric Cardiology Associates
  703 Main Street   Paterson, NJ 07503   (973)754-2572
+ Pediatric Cardiology Associates
  1 Broadway/Suite 203   Elmwood Park, NJ 07407   (973)754-2572   Fax (973)569-6270

Myrow, Ralph E., MD {1649271701} Dermat(66,MA05)<NJ-HACKNSK, NY-NYUTISCH>
+ Westwood Dermatology
  390 Old Hook Road   Westwood, NJ 07675   (201)666-9550   Fax (201)666-1251
  sandymyrow@yahoo.com

Mysh, Dmitry, MD {1033105903} IntrMd, Gastrn(85,RUS37)<NJ-NWTNMEM, NJ-MORRISTN>
+ Sparta Gastroenterology, LLC
  14 Ridgedale Avenue/Suite 128   Cedar Knolls, NJ 07927   (973)579-3174   Fax (973)579-2961

Mysliwiec, Malgorzata Halina, MD {1104192095} IntrMd
+ University Hospital Medicine
  150 Bergen Street/Room I-248   Newark, NJ 07103   (973)972-6056   Fax (973)972-3129

Naadimuthu, Revathi P., MD {1295993731} Ophthl(04,NJ06)
+ Freehold Ophthalmology, LLC
  509 Stillwells Corner Road/Suite E-5   Freehold, NJ 07728   (732)431-9333   Fax (732)431-3312
+ Freehold Ophthalmology, LLC
  20 Hospital Drive   Toms River, NJ 08755   (732)431-9333   Fax (732)505-4322
+ Freehold Ophthalmology, LLC
  202 Jack Martin Boulevard   Brick, NJ 07728   (732)458-5700   Fax (732)458-0693

Naame, Lawrence J., MD {1942303482} SrgOrt, SrgHnd(73,DC02)<NJ-ACMCITY, NJ-ACMCMAIN>
+ Atlantic Bone & Joint Surgeons
  6688 Washington Avenue   Egg Harbor Township, NJ 08234   (609)641-8001   Fax (609)646-1520
+ Volunteers in Medicine
  423 North Route 9   Cape May Court House, NJ 08210   (609)641-8001   Fax (609)463-2830

Naber, Tamim Hani, MD {1578711743} Nephro, IntrMd(03,JOR02)<NJ-ACMCITY, NJ-SHOREMEM>
+ Specialty Medconsultants LLC
  6725 Ventnor Avenue/Suite C   Ventnor City, NJ 08406   (609)350-6780   Fax (609)350-6995

Nabong, Marcelo Yambao, Jr., MD {1669415600} NnPnMd(91,PHI05)<NJ-HACKNSK>
+ Hackensack University Medical Center
  30 Prospect Avenue/NeoPeri   Hackensack, NJ 07601   (201)996-2000   Fax (201)996-3232

Nabulsi, Omar Hisham, MD {1467607978} FamMed, EmrgMd(11,NJ06)
+ Health Consultants of New Jersey
  516 Hamburg Turnpike/Suite 5   Wayne, NJ 07470   (973)925-7770   Fax (973)925-7772
+ Clifton Urgent and Primary Care
  721 Clifton Avenue/Suite 2A   Clifton, NJ 07013   (973)925-7770   Fax (973)779-7906
+ CentraState Family Medicine Residency Practice
  1001 West Main Street/Suite B   Freehold, NJ 07470   (732)294-2540   Fax (732)294-9328

Nachajon, Roberto V., MD {1518908268} PedPul, Pedtrc, SlpDis(86,URU02)<NJ-STJOSHOS, NJ-HOLYNAME>
+ St. Joseph's Regional Medical Center
  703 Main Street/Pulmonology   Paterson, NJ 07503   (973)754-2550   Fax (973)754-2568
+ Pediatric Sub Specialty Outpatient Center
  186 Rochelle Avenue   Rochelle Park, NJ 07662   (973)754-2550   Fax (973)754-2598

Nachbar, James G., MD {1578560629} Ophthl(80,MI01)<NJ-VIRTMHBC>
+ South Jersey Eye Physicians PA
  509 South Lenola Road/Suite 11   Moorestown, NJ 08057   (856)234-0227   Fax (856)727-9518
  nachbar@sjeye.com

Nachevnik, Elina, MD {1396778684} Pedtrc(91,RUS15)<NJ-ST-BARNMC>
+ Kintiroglou Pediatrics
  1500 Pleasant Valley Way/Suite 301   West Orange, NJ 07052   (973)243-0002   Fax (973)243-1227

Nachmann, Marcella Marie, DO {1265479547} Urolgy(91,NY75)
+ New Jersey Urology, LLC
  2401 East Evesham Road/Suite F   Voorhees, NJ 08043   (856)673-1600   Fax (856)988-0636
+ Delaware Valley Urology LLC
  570 Egg Harbor Road/Suite A-1   Sewell, NJ 08080   (856)673-1600   Fax (856)985-4583
+ New Jersey Urology LLC
  2090 Springdale Road/Suite D   Cherry Hill, NJ 08043   (856)751-9010   Fax (856)985-9908

Nachodsky, Denise Marie, MD {1326086026} IntrMd, CdvDis(93,WI06)<NJ-DEBRAHLC, NJ-OURLADY>
+ Deborah Heart and Lung Center
  200 Trenton Road   Browns Mills, NJ 08015   (609)893-6611

Nachtigall, Jonathan C., DO {1790985786} CdvDis
+ 9 Saint Andrews Court
  Westampton, NJ 08060

Nachtigall, Steven Paul, MD {1497808984} IntrMd(79,NY03)<NJ-SHOREMEM>
+ 1015 New Road/Suite C
  Northfield, NJ 08225

Nachwalter, Richard Scott, MD {1194789008} SrgOrt, NeuM-SptM(94,PA12)
+ 131 Madison Avenue/Suite 110
  Morristown, NJ 07960   (973)971-3500   Fax (973)683-0016

Nackman, Gary B., MD {1114096765} SrgVas, Surgry(88,NY03)<NJ-RWJUBRUN>
+ NJ Vein Care
  1037 US Highway 46/Suite 202   Clifton, NJ 07013   (973)778-2222   Fax (973)860-1148

Nadal, Loida C., MD {1588830541} GenPrc(69,PHIL)
+ 26 Magnolia Court
  Piscataway, NJ 08854

Nadaraj, Sumekala, MD {1639198922} Pedtrc, PedCrd(91,INA81)<NJ-STPETER>
+ CHOP Pediatric & Adolescent Specialty Care Center
  1012 Laurel Oak Road   Voorhees, NJ 08043   (856)435-1300   Fax (856)435-0091
+ St. Peter's University Hospital
  254 Easton Avenue/PedCard/2nd Fl   New Brunswick, NJ 08901   (732)745-8538

Nadarajah, Anandhi K., MD {1023308673}
+ Womens Health Care Associates of Sussex County
  135 Newton Sparta Road/Suite 201   Newton, NJ 07860

(973)383-8555   Fax (973)383-8424

Nadarajah, Dayaparan, MD {1063492965} CritCr, IntrMd, PulDis(81,ENG14)<NJ-NWTNMEM, NJ-HCKTSTWN>
+ Pulmonary Medical Associates, L.L.P
  222 High Street/Suite 102   Newton, NJ 07860   (973)579-5090   Fax (973)579-2994
  dayaparan.nadarajah@pmamed.com

Naddelman, Adam Brett, MD {1235118308} Pedtrc, IntrMd(97,NJ06)
+ Princeton Nassau Pediatrics, P.A.
  301 North Harrison Street   Princeton, NJ 08540   (609)924-5510   Fax (609)924-3577
+ Princeton Nassau Pediatrics, P.A.
  196 Princeton-Hightstown Road   West Windsor, NJ 08550   (609)924-5510   Fax (609)799-2294
+ Princeton Nassau Pediatrics, P.A.
  312 Applegarth Road/Suite 104   Monroe Township, NJ 08540   (609)409-5600   Fax (609)409-5610

Nadeau, Pascale, MD {1780846337} CarAne, Anesth(08,PA02)
+ 60 Leonard Drive
  Old Tappan, NJ 07675   (551)404-7766
  pascale.nadeau@gmail.com

Nadeem, Atiya, MD {1811178700} FamMed(95,PAK23)
+ Walk in Medical Center
  1901 Route 130 South   North Brunswick, NJ 08902   (732)658-1102   Fax (732)348-8264

Nadeem, Muhammad, MD {1528580024}<NJ-STFRNMED>
+ St. Francis Medical Center
  601 Hamilton Avenue   Trenton, NJ 08629   (609)599-5061

Nadeem, Shahzinah, MD {1427090794} IntrMd(85,PAK15)
+ Capital Medical Associates
  1235 Whitehorse Mercerville Rd   Trenton, NJ 08619   (609)587-3003   Fax (609)587-4512

Nadel, Lester, MD {1184648826} IntrMd(74,NY19)
+ 63 East Sherbrooke Parkway
  Livingston, NJ 07039

Nadella, Ruchi, MD {1356579841} Psychy(09,NY08)
+ 135 County Road/Suite 2C
  Cresskill, NJ 07626   (201)266-8411

Nader, Kamyar, MD {1528304524}
+ The Cooper Hospital System-Univ Hospital
  401 Haddon Avenue/E&R 3rd Fl   Camden, NJ 08103   (856)342-2000

Nadimintí, Hari, MD {1558520700} Dermat(05,FL02)<NJ-OVER-LOOK, NJ-MORRISTN>
+ Summit Medical Group-Berkeley Heights Campus
  1 Diamond Hill Road   Berkeley Heights, NJ 07922   (908)273-4300   Fax (908)790-6576

Nadiminti, Sheila Gupta, MD {1346482072} CdvDis, IntrMd(06,NY03)
+ United Medical, P.C.
  988 Broadway/Suite 201   Bayonne, NJ 07002   (201)339-6111   Fax (201)339-6333
+ United Medical, P.C.
  612 Rutherford Avenue   Lyndhurst, NJ 07071   (201)339-6111   Fax (201)460-1684
+ United Medical, P.C.
  533 Lexington Avenue   Clifton, NJ 07002   (973)546-6844   Fax (973)546-7707

Nadipuram, Chandrika, MD {1255495123} Psychy(80,INDI)
+ Raritan Bay Mental Health Center
  570 Lee Street   Perth Amboy, NJ 08861   (732)442-1666   Fax (732)442-9512

Nadkarni, Mangala A., MD {1134231863} Nrolgy, Eplpsy(84,INA62)
+ St. Barnabas Institute of Neurology & Neurosurgery
  200 South Orange Avenue/Suite 101   Livingston, NJ 07039   (973)322-7580   Fax (973)322-7505

Nadkarni, Nutan Shirish, MD {1659302578} Pedtrc(87,INA65)
+ 3826 Park Avenue/Suite D
  Edison, NJ 08820   (732)744-9400   Fax (732)516-0608
  Nnadkarni@pol-net

Nadkarni, Swati G., MD {1801975644} FamMed, Grtrcs(91,INDI)
+ Medi Center of Edison
  1813 Oak Tree Road   Edison, NJ 08820   (908)769-9494   Fax (908)755-3833

Nadler, Steven C., MD {1710982210} Gastrn, IntrMd(87,NJ05)<NJ-BAYSHORE, NJ-CENTRAST>
+ Middlesex Monmouth Gastroenterology
  222 Schanck Road/Suite 302   Freehold, NJ 07728   (732)577-1999   Fax (732)845-5356
+ Middlesex Monmouth Gastroenterology
  723 North Beers Street   Holmdel, NJ 07733   (732)264-4253

Nadratowski, Mary Celesta, MD {1356465181} IntrMd(95,DMN01)<NJ-MTNSIDE>
+ Hoffman-La Roche Incorporated
  340 Kingsland Street   Nutley, NJ 07110   (973)235-5000

Naeem, Ambreen, MD {1326120809} Psychy
+ CHOP Pediatric & Adolescent Specialty Care Center
  4009 Black Horse Pike   Mays Landing, NJ 08330   (609)677-7895   Fax (609)677-7835

Physicians by Name and Address

Naeem, Hafiz Saad, MD {1275055758}<NJ-STFRNMED>
+ St. Francis Medical Center
601 Hamilton Avenue   Trenton, NJ 08629   (609)599-5061
Fax (609)599-5061

Naeem, Sana, MD {1922533165} Psychy
+ 66 Westley Road
Old Bridge, NJ 08857   (732)500-8774

Naeem, Sheikh M., MD {1932198538} CdvDis, IntrMd(71,PAK01)
+ Lakeland Cardiology Center, P.A.
415 Boulevard   Mountain Lakes, NJ 07046   (973)334-7700
Fax (973)402-5847

Nafees, Quratulain, MD {1356617542}
+ Hackensack UMC Mountainside
1 Bay Avenue   Montclair, NJ 07042   (973)429-6000
+ 501 Avalon Drive/Unit 5401
Wood Ridge, NJ 07075   (347)339-6873

Naficy, Parvin P., MD {1376569780} Pedtrc(67,IRA01)<NJ-STJOSHOS>
+ Doktor, Alan R.
665 Broadway   Paterson, NJ 07514   (973)278-8885   Fax (973)278-9434

Naftulin, Richard J., DO {1376559708} SrgOrt(74,PA77)<NJ-KENEDYHS, NJ-VIRTUAHS>
+ Cherry Hill Orthopedic Surgeons
PO Box 8285   Cherry Hill, NJ 08002   (856)662-2400   Fax (856)662-5525

Nag, Debashis, MD {1982678983} Pedtrc, PhysMd(94,NJ06)<NJ-HLTHSRE, NJ-COMMED>
+ Atlantic Physical Medicine & Rehab Ctr
9 Hospital Drive/Suite C-25   Toms River, NJ 08755
(732)736-0100   Fax (732)736-0666

Nag Chowdhury, Deepshikha, MD {1255643078}
+ 29 Linden Street/Apt 403
Hackensack, NJ 07601

Naganathan, Srividya, MD {1306805700} Pedtrc(92,INA3D)<NJ-JRSYSHMC>
+ Jersey Shore University Medical Center
1945 Route 33   Neptune, NJ 07753   (732)776-4267   Fax (732)776-3161

Nagarajan, Anuradha, MD {1902071780} Grtrcs, IntrMd(00,INA04)<NJ-VALLEY>
+ The Valley Hospital
223 North Van Dien Avenue   Ridgewood, NJ 07450
(201)447-8000

Nagarakanti, Rangadham, MD {1790836252} IntrMd, CdvDis(99)
+ RWJPE/New Brunswick Cardiology Group, P.A.
75 Veronica Road/Suite 101   Somerset, NJ 08873
(732)247-7444   Fax (732)247-5119
+ RWJPE New Brunswick Cardiology Group, P.A.
15H Briar Hill Court   East Brunswick, NJ 08816   (732)613-9313
+ RWJPE New Brunswick Cardiology Group, P.A.
111 Union Valley Road/Suite 201   Monroe Township, NJ 08873   (609)409-6856   Fax (609)409-6882

Nagarakanti, Sandhya R., MD {1851510390} InfDis
+ 240-F Bridge Street
Metuchen, NJ 08840   (732)514-9624

Nagaria, Neil C., MD {1760401749} IntrMd(01,INA68)
+ Ocean Endosurgery Center
129 Route 37 West   Toms River, NJ 08755   (732)606-4440
Fax (732)797-3963

Nagarsheth, Harish N., MD {1801962311} CdvDis, IntrMd, Grtrcs(74,INA69)<NJ-BAYSHORE, NJ-RBAYOLDB>
+ Nagarsheth MD PA
3B Parlin Drive   Parlin, NJ 08859   (732)238-8500   Fax (732)238-8501

Nagarsheth, Veena H., MD {1881610335} Pedtrc(72,INA15)<NJ-RBAYOLDB, NJ-RBAYPERT>
+ Nagarsheth MD PA
3B Parlin Drive   Parlin, NJ 08859   (732)238-2333   Fax (732)238-8501
vnagarsheth@hotmail.com

Nageen, Farhat, MD {1689694010} Pedtrc(83,PAK20)<NJ-STPETER>
+ 613 Ridge Road
Monmouth Junction, NJ 08852   (732)230-2582   Fax (732)329-0036
+ 666 Plainsboro Road/Bld 100/Ste 1C
Plainsboro, NJ 08536   (732)230-2582   Fax (609)297-5982

Nagel, Isaac R., MD {1831395300} PsyAdd<NJ-STCLRBOO>
+ St. Clare's Hospital-Boonton
130 Powerville Road   Boonton, NJ 07005   (973)316-1800
Fax (973)316-1829

Nagelberg, Henry P., MD {1952307969} Ophthl(86,NY15)<NJ-HUNTRDN>
+ Advanced Eye MDs
1260 State Route 28/Suite 8   Branchville, NJ 08876
(908)253-8686   Fax (908)253-0808

Nagella, Naresh, MD {1497068803} IntrMd(NJ05
+ Robert Wood Johnson-UMDNJ Anesthesia Group
125 Paterson Street/CAB 3100   New Brunswick, NJ 08901
(732)235-7840   Fax (732)235-6511

Nagendra, Parameswar, MD {1881819316} Pedtrc(72,SRI02)<NJ-BAYONNE>
+ Bayonne Medical Center
29th Street at Avenue E/Pediatrics   Bayonne, NJ 07002
(201)858-5000

Nagendra, Shan M., MD {1164533659} Nrolgy, AnesPain(70,SRI02)<NJ-STMRYPAS>
+ 654 Avenue C/Suite 1
Bayonne, NJ 07002   (201)823-3390   Fax (201)823-4420

Nagorna, Malgorzata, MD {1841240413} Pedtrc(90,POL17)<NJ-JRSYCITY, NJ-MEADWLND>
+ Total Care Pediatrics in Jersey City
550 Newark Avenue/Suite 200   Jersey City, NJ 07306
(201)714-7902   Fax (201)795-4999

Nagorny, Wojciech Antoni, MD {1447273701} Anesth(90,POL17)<NJ-HUNTRDN>
+ Hunterdon Medical Center
2100 Wescott Drive/Anesthesiology   Flemington, NJ 08822
(908)788-6100   Fax (908)788-6361

Nagpal, Sangita D., MD {1306890561} Pedtrc(81,INDI)<NJ-CENTRAST>
+ Dr. Nagpal and Assoc
300 Candlewood Commons/PO Box 577   Howell, NJ 07731
(732)370-9600

Nagra, Amandeep Kaur, MD {1225292196} Psychy(02,INA81)
+ University Behavioral HealthCare - UMDNJ
Box 863/Whittlesey Road/Psych   Trenton, NJ 08625
(609)341-3093   Fax (609)341-9380

Nagra, Bipinpreet Singh, MD {1609093590} CdvDis
+ Capital Cardiology Associates
40 Fuld Street/Suite 400   Trenton, NJ 08638   (609)396-1644   Fax (609)394-9526

Nagulapalli, Chaitanya, MD {1093731648} IntrMd(98,INA5B)
+ 2 Millstone Court
Cranbury, NJ 08512   (973)997-1472

Nagy, Aubrie Jacobson, MD {1235111337} IntrMd(TN05
+ Princeton Medicine
5 Plainsboro Road/Suite 300   Plainsboro, NJ 08536
(609)853-7272   Fax (609)853-7271

Nagy, Michael William, MD {1619913746} Surgry, SrgPlstc(96,OH41)
+ Michael W. Nagy MD FACS
2333 Highway 34   Manasquan, NJ 08736   (732)282-0002
Fax (732)282-1522

Nagy, Peter, MD {1952484230} Anesth, PainMd, Acpntr(85,CZE06)<NJ-VALLEY>
+ The Valley Hospital
223 North Van Dien Avenue   Ridgewood, NJ 07450
(201)447-8000

Nagy-Hallet, Andrea, MD {1568684199} PsyAdt, Psychy(89,HUN06)
+ Mt. Carmel Guild/ Behavioral Health System
58 Freeman Street   Newark, NJ 07105   (973)596-4190
Fax (973)639-6583

Nahar, Akash, MD {1700051224}
+ 36 Village Drive
Voorhees, NJ 08043   (215)427-6805

Nahar, Sudha, MD {1164463071} Gastrn, IntrMd(92,INDI)<NJ-STPETER, NJ-RWJUBRUN>
+ 2 Ethel Road/Suite 106-A
Edison, NJ 08817   (732)873-1600   Fax (732)873-1606
+ 17 Clyde Road/Suite 101
Somerset, NJ 08873   (732)873-1600   Fax (732)873-1606
+ Raritan Valley Surgery Center
100 Franklin Square Drive/Suite 100   Somerset, NJ 08817
(732)560-1000   Fax (732)560-5999

Nahas, Arthur G., DO {1447446158} FamMed, SprtMd(76,PA77)<NJ-SHOREMEM>
+ Arthur Medical & Sports Associates
631 Shore Road/Suite 2   Somers Point, NJ 08244
(609)927-6555   Fax (609)653-9133

Nahas, Barbara A., MD {1063515435} IntrMd(81,NJ05)<NJ-STBARNMC>
+ 530 Old Short Hills Road
Short Hills, NJ 07078   (973)379-2700   Fax (973)379-5733

Nahas, Frederick J., MD {1659397297} SrgVas, Surgry(74,PA13)
+ Drs. Schwartz & Nahas
631 Shore Road/PO Box 291   Somers Point, NJ 08244
(609)653-1010   Fax (609)653-9591

Nahas, Ghassan, MD {1700979044} PulDis, IntrMd(68,SYR01)<NJ-MEADWLND>
+ 255 State Route 3 East/Suite 200
Secaucus, NJ 07094   (201)864-2389

Nahass, Ronald G., MD {1023084928} InfDis, IntrMd(82,NJ06)<NJ-SOMERSET, NJ-UNVMCPRN>
+ ID Associates PA/dba ID Care
105 Raider Boulevard/Suite 101   Hillsborough, NJ 08844
(908)281-0221   Fax (908)281-0940
+ ID Associates PA/dba ID Care
81 Veronica Avenue/Suite 203   Somerset, NJ 08873
(908)281-0221   Fax (732)729-0924
+ ID Associates PA/dba ID Care

10 Forrestal Road South/Suite 203   Princeton, NJ 08844
(609)759-2750   Fax (609)919-9700

Nahm, Choong S., MD {1942383484} Otlryg(65,KOR05)<NJ-JRSYSHMC, NJ-OCEANMC>
+ 1551 Highway 138 East
Wall, NJ 07719   (732)280-8822   Fax (732)280-8824

Nahmias, Jeffrey S., MD {1881654036} PulDis, IntrMd(80,NY08)<NJ-NWRKBETH>
+ Pulmonary & Allergy Associates
1 Springfield Avenue/Suite 3-A   Summit, NJ 07901
(908)934-0555   Fax (908)934-0556
+ Newark Beth Israel Medical Center
201 Lyons Avenue/Surgery   Newark, NJ 07112   (908)934-0555   Fax (973)282-0821

Nahmias, Neil Jeffrey, DO {1770656530} Anesth(90,NY75)<NJ-HOLYNAME>
+ Holy Name Hospital
718 Teaneck Road/Anesth   Teaneck, NJ 07666   (201)833-3000   Fax (201)342-1259

Nahum, Kenneth D., DO {1922079904} IntrMd, OncHem(81,NJ75)<NJ-JRSYSHMC, NJ-CENTRAST>
+ Regional Cancer Care Associates, LLC
4632 US Highway 9   Howell, NJ 07731   (732)367-1535
Fax (732)367-9514
+ Kenneth D. Nahum DO PC
1540 Highway 138   Wall, NJ 07719   (732)280-9685

Nahum, Laurie S., MD {1558361295} IntrMd(80,NJ05)<NJ-CHILTON>
+ 2035 Hamburg Turnpike/Suite F
Wayne, NJ 07470   (973)831-9228   Fax (973)831-9856

Naidrich, Shari Ann, MD {1356305304} RadDia(95,NY08)<NJ-ENGLWOOD>
+ Englewood Radiologic Group PA
350 Engle Street   Englewood, NJ 07631   (201)894-3000
Fax (201)894-5244
+ Advanced Medical Imaging of North Jersey
452 Old Hook Road/Suite 301   Emerson, NJ 07630
(201)894-3000   Fax (201)262-2330

Naids, Richard Eric, MD {1700879921} Ophthl
+ Burlington County Eye Physicians
225 Sunset Road   Willingboro, NJ 08046   (609)877-2800
Fax (609)877-1813

Naidu, Salini S., MD {1912167545}
+ 216 Edmonton Court
Livingston, NJ 07039   (215)983-5283

Naidu, Yamini, MD {1801061585} Nrolgy(04,NY15)<NJ-VALLEY>
+ Neurology Group of Bergen County
1200 East Ridgewood Avenue   Ridgewood, NJ 07450
(201)444-0868   Fax (201)444-7363

Naik, Arun Chandrakant, MD {1104887710} Gastrn, IntrMd(85,INA65)<NJ-TRININPC, NJ-RWJURAH>
+ 240 Williamson Street/Suite 507
Elizabeth, NJ 07202   (908)259-1140   Fax (908)259-1144
Aruncn@aol.com

Naik, Komal Desai, DO {1063617082} Nrolgy(02,NY75)<NJ-OVERLOOK, NJ-MORRISTN>
+ Summit Medical Group-Berkeley Heights Campus
1 Diamond Hill Road   Berkeley Heights, NJ 07922
(908)273-4300   Fax (908)790-6524

Naik, Mohit Madan, MD {1215140165} RadDia(02,PA12)
+ Hackensack Radiology Group, PA/Corporate
130 Kinderkamack Road/Suite 200   River Edge, NJ 07661
(201)488-2660
+ Hackensack Radiology Group, P.A.
30 Prospect Avenue   Hackensack, NJ 07601   (201)488-2660   Fax (201)336-8451

Naik, Nalini S., MD {1487734588} Psychy(70,INA20)
+ 5 Kilburn Court
Cherry Hill, NJ 08003

Naik, Purvaja A., DO {1437581444}
+ 3511 Avalon Court
Voorhees, NJ 08043   (973)462-7032

Naik, Ravi, MD {1548433691} Anesth, AnesPain(98,NY08)<NJ-STMRYPAS>
+ 2727 John F. Kennedy Boulevard
Jersey City, NJ 07306   (732)414-9649   Fax (732)553-6120
+ St. Mary's Hospital
350 Boulevard/Anesth   Passaic, NJ 07055   (973)365-4300

Naik, Sameer Sadanand, MD {1952587453}(03,INA69)
+ 18 Hastings Court/Building 8
Fair Lawn, NJ 07410

Naim, Farid A., MD {1578577540} PedEmg, Pedtrc, EmrgEmed(78,AFG01)<NJ-STJOSHOS, NJ-MORRISTN>
+ St Joseph's Medical Pedicatic EmerMed
703 Main Street   Paterson, NJ 07503   (973)754-4901

Naim, Suprema D., MD {1528275807} Pedtrc(85,PHI08)
+ St. Joseph's Regional Medical Center
703 Main Street/Pediatrics   Paterson, NJ 07503   (973)754-2000

Physicians by Name and Address

Naiman, Jeffrey Todd, MD {1629161302} Radiol, RadDia, NuclMd(93,NY01)<NJ-CLARMAAS>
+ Essex Imaging Associates
5 Franklin Avenue/Suite 510   Belleville, NJ 07109   (973)751-2011   Fax (973)751-4456

Naini, Sean, DO {1295765188} IntrMd(01,NJ75)<NJ-RWJUBRUN>
+ Princeton Medicine
5 Plainsboro Road/Suite 300   Plainsboro, NJ 08536   (609)853-7272   Fax (609)853-7271

Nair, Anil Karunakaran, MD {1053570374} SrgNro
+ IGEA Brain & Spine
1057 Commerce Avenue   Union, NJ 07083   (908)688-8800   Fax (908)688-2377

Nair, Nanda K., DO {1265737126} IntrMd<NJ-COOPRUMC>
+ Cooper University Hospital
One Cooper Plaza   Camden, NJ 08103   (856)342-2000

Nair, Prabha J., MD {1174559207} Pedtrc(83,INA34)
+ Community Health Care, Inc.
70 Cohansey Street   Bridgeton, NJ 08302   (856)451-4700   Fax (856)451-0029

Nair, Prathila Karunakaran, MD {1235397373}
+ 79 Birch Street
Ridgefield Park, NJ 07660

Nair, Swapna, MD {1346268521} IntrMd(00,DMN01)
+ Medical Associates of Marlboro PC
32 North Main Street   Marlboro, NJ 07746   (732)462-4100   Fax (732)462-3798
+ Medical Associates of Marlboro, P.C.
3084 State Route 27/Suite 1   Kendall Park, NJ 08824   (732)462-4100   Fax (732)297-7356

Nairn, Sandra J., DO {1134206857} PedEmg, Pedtrc(85,PA77)<NJ-COOPRUMC>
+ Cooper University Hospital
One Cooper Plaza/PediEmerg   Camden, NJ 08103   (856)342-2000

Najafi, Abdul Wahid, MD {1811065634} ObsGyn(71,AFG01)<NJ-CHRIST>
+ 1815 Kennedy Boulevard
Jersey City, NJ 07305   (201)333-5959   Fax (201)333-8335

Najafi, Nawid E., MD {1326258732} FamMed, IntrMd(02,STM01)<NJ-VIRTVOOR>
+ Virtua Internal Medicine-Marlton
601 Route 73 North/Suite 101   Marlton, NJ 08053   (856)429-1910   Fax (856)396-0848
+ Virtua Immediate Care Center
239 Hurffville Crosskeys Road   Sewell, NJ 08080   (856)429-1910   Fax (856)341-8215

Najarian, David James, MD {1760694038} Dermat(03,VA01)
+ 17 Ripplewood Drive
Randolph, NJ 07869

Najarian, Lawrence V., MD {1639271984} Ophthl(82,PA01)<NJ-SOMERSET, NY-NYEYEINF>
+ 400 Main Street/PO Box 103
Bedminster, NJ 07921   (908)781-2020   Fax (908)781-7505
+ 773 Teaneck Road
Teaneck, NJ 07666   (908)781-2020   Fax (201)833-8384

Najarro, Juan Carlos, MD {1710424320} GenPrc
+ 17 Cumberland Court
Somerset, NJ 08873   (305)342-4156

Najib, Nabeel M., MD {1326127879} Pedtrc, Allrgy, PedAlg(84,EGYP)<NJ-PALISADE, NJ-CHRIST>
+ Hudson Pediatrics
6914 Jackson Street   West New York, NJ 07093   (201)662-1520   Fax (201)662-8938

Najjar, Joe E., MD {1659316289} IntrMd(96,LEB01)
+ Crossroads Medical Group
975 Clifton Avenue   Clifton, NJ 07013   (973)778-8666   Fax (973)778-7559

Najjar, Sessine, MD {1497862429} InfDis, IntrMd(74,LEB01)<NJ-STMRYPAS, NJ-VALLEY>
+ Crossroads Medical Group
975 Clifton Avenue   Clifton, NJ 07013   (973)778-8666   Fax (973)778-7559

Najman, Naomi Stein, MD {1215125356} Psychy, PsyCAd, Pedtrc(94,NY46)
+ 163 Engle Street/Building 2
Englewood, NJ 07631   (201)816-0202   Fax (201)837-8938

Najmey, Sawsan S., MD {1225118086} IntrMd, Rheuma(84,JOR01)<NJ-CENTRAST>
+ Midstate Rheumatology Center
900 West Main Street   Freehold, NJ 07728   (732)431-4335   Fax (732)431-4771
+ Midstate Rheumatology Center
508 Lakehurst Road/Suite 1 A   Toms River, NJ 08755   (732)431-4335   Fax (732)818-3320

Najmi, Jamsheed K., MD {1538264676} SrgPlstc, Surgry, SrgRec(69,INDI)<NJ-HUNTRDN>
+ 201 Union Avenue/Building1/Suite B
Bridgewater, NJ 08807   (908)722-6450   Fax (908)722-4107

Najovits, Andrew Joseph, MD {1003139932} CdvDis(04,NY15)
+ Mahwah Medical
10 Franklin Turnpike   Mahwah, NJ 07430   (201)529-0033

Fax (201)529-5913

Nakashian, Michael, MD {1629239645} SrgOrt<NJ-CENTRAST>
+ CentraState Medical Center
901 West Main Street/Bldg.A Suite265   Freehold, NJ 07728   (732)840-7500   Fax (732)041-0451

Nakhate, Vinay Gopal, MD {1386767697} IntrMd(84,INA69)<NJ-SJHREGMC>
+ Vineland Medical Associates/Excel Care Alliance, LLC
1100 East Chestnut Avenue   Vineland, NJ 08360   (856)696-0108   Fax (856)696-0188

Nakhate, Vishakha Vinay, MD {1659380558} Pedtrc(83,INA69)
+ Pediatric Associates, LLC.
1318 South Main Street   Vineland, NJ 08360   (856)691-8585   Fax (856)691-8489

Nakhjo, Shomaf, DO {1184831406} Surgry(05,NY75)
+ 222 High Street/Suite 201
Newton, NJ 07860   (973)383-2222   Fax (973)383-3344
info@advancedsurgerynj.com

Nakhla, Tarek Adib, MD {1205913944} NnPnMd, Pedtrc(87,EGY05)<NJ-COOPRUMC, NJ-OURLADY>
+ The Children's Regional Hospital at Cooper Univ Hosp
One Cooper Plaza   Camden, NJ 08103   (856)342-2000

Nakhleh, Nader John, DO {1598963902} PedPul<NJ-JRSYSHMC>
+ Jersey Shore University Medical Center
1945 Route 33/PedPulm   Neptune, NJ 07753   (732)776-4268

Nakhoda, Zein Khozaim, MD {1235558479} Urolgy
+ Premier Urology Group, LLC
10 Parsonage Road/Suite 118   Edison, NJ 08837   (732)494-9400   Fax (732)548-3931
+ Premier Urology Group, LLC
570 South Avenue East/Building A   Cranford, NJ 07016   (732)494-9400   Fax (908)497-1633
+ Premier Urology Group, LLC
2 Hospital Plaza/Suite 430   Old Bridge, NJ 08837   (732)494-9400   Fax (732)679-2077

Nakra, Neal K., MD {1558561597} PedPul(01,TX13)<NJ-STJOSHOS>
+ St. Joseph's Regional Medical Center
11 Getty Avenue   Paterson, NJ 07503   (973)754-2550
+ St. Joseph's Children's Hospital
703 Main Street   Paterson, NJ 07503   (973)754-2550

Nalaboff, Kenneth Michael, MD {1417902883} Radiol, RadDia(96,ISR02)<NJ-RBAYPERT, NJ-RWJUBRUN>
+ University Radiology Group, P.C.
579A Cranbury Road   East Brunswick, NJ 08816   (732)390-0040   Fax (732)390-1856

Nalbandian, Matthew Martin, MD {1013901842} SrgVas, Surgry(93,NJ05)<NJ-NYUTISCH>
+ Northern Valley Vascular Associates
48 Bi State Plaza/Suite 225   Westwood, NJ 07675   (212)254-6882   Fax (212)254-6886

Nalitt, Beth R., MD {1144210543} IntrMd(85,PA09)<NJ-OVERLOOK, NY-STBARNAB>
+ Summit Medical Group
85 Woodland Road   Short Hills, NJ 07078   (973)315-9075   Fax (973)376-0357
+ Millburn Primary Care LLC
120 Millburn Avenue/Suite 206   Millburn, NJ 07041   (973)315-9075   Fax (973)467-0340

Naljian, Vahe G., MD {1497758585} Anesth(83,DOM03)
+ 21 Orchard Drive
Upper Saddle River, NJ 07458

Nalven, Lisa M., MD {1568409787} BhvrMd, Pedtrc, PedDvl(91,WI05)<NY-CHLDCOPR, NJ-VALLEY>
+ Kireker Center for Child Development
505 Goffle Road   Ridgewood, NJ 07450   (201)447-8151   Fax (201)447-8526

Nam, Daniel, MD {1003850413} IntrMd(98,NY19)
+ 154 Mortimer Avenue
Rutherford, NJ 07070   (201)935-4119

Nam, Sang K., MD {1396807285} Psychy(66,KOR09)
+ 18 Constitution Way
Somerset, NJ 08873

Nambi, Sridhar S., MD {1053388439} EnDbMt, IntrMd(84,INDI)<NJ-STBARNMC, NJ-MORRISTN>
+ Nambi Endocrine Associates LLC
22 Old Short Hills Road/Suite 201   Livingston, NJ 07039   (973)535-8870   Fax (973)535-8818

Nambiar, Sapna Shibhu, MD {1699984583} Pedtrc(02,INA3B)
+ 521 Green Street/Suite 521A
Iselin, NJ 08830   (732)623-9905   Fax (732)983-5484

Namey, Jeffrey Elias, MD {1922067024} CdvDis, IntrMd(96,PA02)
+ The Cardiology Group, P.A.
401 Young Avenue/Suite 275   Moorestown, NJ 08057   (856)291-8855   Fax (856)291-8844
+ The Cardiology Group, P.A.
128 State Highway Route 70/Suite 1-B   Medford, NJ 08055   (856)291-8855   Fax (609)444-5521
+ The Cardiology Group, P.A.
1 Sheffield Drive/Suite 102   Columbus, NJ 08057   (856)291-8855

Namnama, Liborio P., MD {1134559669} Pedtrc(68,PHI07)
+ 133 Hedden Terrace
North Arlington, NJ 07031   (201)998-2573

Nanavati, Farzana Nilesh, MD {1780629592} Nrolgy(99,HUN08)<NJ-VALLEY>
+ Sovereign Medical Group
85 Harristown Road/Suite 104   Glen Rock, NJ 07452   (201)855-8300   Fax (201)857-2541
+ Valley Medical Group
70 Park Avenue   Park Ridge, NJ 07656   (201)855-8300   Fax (201)391-7733

Nanavati, Kartikey Jayendrakumar, MD {1457377475} IntrMd, Grtrcs(73,INA20)<NJ-UNVMCPRN, NJ-STPETER>
+ Hem Care Medical Clinic
6 Agnes Court   Monroe Township, NJ 08831   (609)409-6767   Fax (609)409-6776

Nanavati, Kaushal Kartikey, MD {1427074459} IntrMd, Grtrcs(03,NJ06)<NJ-UNVMCPRN>
+ Hem Care Medical Clinic
6 Agnes Court   Monroe Township, NJ 08831   (609)409-6767   Fax (609)409-6776

Nanavati, Neeraj K., MD {1265724983} Anesth
+ Robert Wood Johnson-UMDNJ Anesthesia Group
125 Paterson Street/CAB 3100   New Brunswick, NJ 08901   (732)937-8841   Fax (732)235-6131

Nanavati, Suketu H., MD {1275562811} CdvDis, IntrMd(69,INDI)<NJ-BURDTMLN>
+ Cape Heart Clinic
2 Village Drive   Cape May Court House, NJ 08210   (609)465-7517   Fax (609)465-2448

Nandakumar, Rajalakshmi, MD {1396855854} IntrMd, InfDis(72,INA37)<NJ-VALYONS>
+ VA New Jersey Health Care System at Lyons
151 Knollcroft Road   Lyons, NJ 07939   (908)647-0180

Nandal, Dharamveer, MD {1215956131} Anesth(92,INA6Z)<NJ-NWRKBETH, NJ-CHSMRCER>
+ Robert Wood Johnson-UMDNJ Anesthesia Group
125 Paterson Street/CAB 3100   New Brunswick, NJ 08901   (732)235-7827   Fax (732)235-6131
+ Newark Beth Israel Medical Center
201 Lyons Avenue/Anesth   Newark, NJ 07112   (973)926-7143

Nandi, Anindita, MD {1669563995} EnDbMt, IntrMd(99,NY47)<NY-PRSBCOLU>
+ Newport Medical Associates
610 Washington Boulevard   Jersey City, NJ 07310   (201)222-1266

Nandigam, Harish, MD {1962650606} Anesth(05,OH06)<NJ-STMICHL>
+ St. Joseph's Regional Medical Center Anesthesia
703 Main Street   Paterson, NJ 07503   (973)754-2323   Fax (973)977-9455

Nandigam, Purna Bindu, MD {1457619421}
+ North Jersey Nephrology Associates PA
246 Hamburg Turnpike/Suite 207   Wayne, NJ 07470   (973)653-3366   Fax (973)653-3365

Nandiwada, Kalpana, MD {1326002965} Anesth, PainMd(90,INA83)<NJ-RBAYPERT>
+ Raritan Bay Medical Center/Perth Amboy Division
530 New Brunswick Avenue/Anesth   Perth Amboy, NJ 08861   (732)442-3700

Nandiwada, Lakshmi P., MD {1477591345} Pedtrc, IntMAdMd(76,INA8Y)<NJ-CENTRAST, NJ-JRSYSHMC>
+ 24 Plaza 9
Manalapan, NJ 07726   (732)431-0505   Fax (732)294-2470

Nandu, Bharat I., MD {1578819652} Psychy(13)<NJ-UNIVBHC>
+ Omni Health Services Inc
85 Raritan Avenue   Highland Park, NJ 08904   (732)227-0070   Fax (732)227-0072

Nanduri, Visala Venkata, MD {1659398386} IntrMd(95,INA39)<NJ-STBARNMC>
+ 315 East Northfield Road/Suite 1 D
Livingston, NJ 07039   (973)992-0658   Fax (973)992-6655

Nanfara, Marcantonio, MD {1326078114} IntrMd(86,ITA01)<NJ-ACMCITY, NJ-ACMCMAIN>
+ first Care LLC
1907 New Road   Northfield, NJ 08225   (609)484-9119   Fax (609)484-9965

Nangia, Arun, MD {1194794099} Nrolgy(81,INDI)
+ 721 Clifton Avenue
Clifton, NJ 07013   (973)471-3730   Fax (973)471-9129

Nanjiani, Aijazali, MD {1639266943} Psychy(77,PAK01)<NJ-BERGNMC, NJ-RAMAPO>
+ Christian Health Care Heritage Manor Nursing Home
301 Sicomac Avenue/Psych   Wyckoff, NJ 07481   (201)848-5200   Fax (201)848-5547
+ Wayne Behavioral Services
401 Hamburg Turnpike/Suite 303   Wayne, NJ 07470   (201)848-5200   Fax (973)790-0671

Physicians by Name and Address

Napiorkowski, Eva M., MD {1699816447} IntrMd(69,POL03)
+ New Jersey Veterans Memorial Home - Menlo Park
132 Evergreen Road/PO Box 3013   Edison, NJ 08818   (732)452-4100

Napoli, Anthony F., Jr., MD {1194789313} Pedtrc(88,PA09)<NJ-VIRTUAHS, NJ-COOPRUMC>
+ Primary Care at Gibbsboro
13 South Lakeview Drive   Gibbsboro, NJ 08026   (856)783-2802   Fax (856)783-2806

Napoli, John D., MD {1962482174} EnDbMt, IntrMd(75,MEXI)<NJ-CLARMAAS, NJ-MTNSIDE>
+ Drs. Seth & Napoli
36 Newark Avenue/Suite 300   Belleville, NJ 07109   (973)759-6896   Fax (973)759-3719
jnapoli@pol.net

Napoli, Joseph C., MD {1587732093} Psychy(72,DC02)
+ 2185 Lemoine Avenue
Fort Lee, NJ 07024   (201)461-0212   Fax (201)461-0362

Napoli, Ralph C., MD {1487614467} SrgFAk(87,CA07)
+ Active Orthopaedics & Sports Medicine
440 Old Hook Road   Emerson, NJ 07630   (201)358-0707   Fax (201)358-9777

Napoli, Salvatore, MD {1891877494} GenPrc(85,PA09)<NJ-HACKNSK>
+ 16 Pocono Road/Suite 117
Denville, NJ 07834   (973)627-1220   Fax (973)627-7834
snapoli@lycos.com
+ 765 Teaneck Road
Teaneck, NJ 07666   (201)833-9294

Napolitana, Elena, MD {1881674943} PhysMd(99,NY06)
+ Rutgers- New Jersey Medical School
185 South Orange Avenue   Newark, NJ 07103   (973)972-4300

Napolitano, Joseph Daniel, MD {1023009131} Ophthl, PedOph(87,NJ06)<NJ-HACKNSK, NJ-RWJUBRUN>
+ Omni Eye Services
485 Route 1 South/Building A   Iselin, NJ 08830   (732)750-0400   Fax (732)602-0749
+ Omni Eye Services
218 State Route 17 North   Rochelle Park, NJ 07662   (732)750-0400   Fax (201)368-0254
+ Omni Eye Services
2200 Route 10 West/Suite 102   Parsippany, NJ 08830   (973)538-7400   Fax (973)538-3007

Napolitano, Massimo M., MD {1316007743} Surgry, SrgVas(84,ITA05)<NJ-HACKNSK, NJ-HOLYNAME>
+ Bergen Surgical Specialists
20 Prospect Avenue/Suite 707   Hackensack, NJ 07601   (201)343-0040   Fax (201)343-2733

Napuli, Maximo C., MD {1992775852} Anesth(68,PHI10)<NJ-NWRKBETH>
+ Newark Beth Israel Medical Center
201 Lyons Avenue/Anesthesiology   Newark, NJ 07112   (973)926-7000   Fax (201)943-8105

Naqi, Muniba, MD {1962631226}<NJ-TRINIWSC>
+ Trinitas Regional Medical Center-Williamson Street
225 Williamson Street   Elizabeth, NJ 07207   (518)253-0253
mnaqi1@gmail.com

Naqui, Mehdi H., MD {1407898927} IntrMd, Nephro(69,INA29)<NJ-STPETER, NJ-UNVMCPRN>
+ Drs. Naqui & Naqui
1574 Route 130 North   North Brunswick, NJ 08902   (732)297-4100   Fax (732)422-7243
Naquimehdi@yahoo.com

Naqui, Nasreen, MD {1558382820} Pedtrc(74,INA74)<NJ-STPETER, NJ-RWJUBRUN>
+ Drs. Naqui & Naqui
1574 Route 130 North   North Brunswick, NJ 08902   (732)297-4100   Fax (732)422-7243

Naqvi, Azeez Fathima, MD {1275593469} Nephro, IntrMd(76,INDI)<NJ-BAYSHORE, NJ-RIVERVW>
+ 875 Poole Avenue/Suite 1
Hazlet, NJ 07730   (732)203-0293   Fax (732)203-0284

Naqvi, Fatima, MD {1740383066} ObsGyn<NJ-STPETER>
+ St. Peter's University Hospital
254 Easton Avenue   New Brunswick, NJ 08901   (732)745-8600

Naqvi, Shabbir Ali, MD {1093927642}
+ 14 Collage Court
Cherry Hill, NJ 08003   (732)890-1121
snaqvi33@gmail.com

Nar, Kishorkumar G., MD {1043273253} PulDis, IntrMd(78,INDI)<NJ-WARREN>
+ Drs. Costacurta & Nar
96A Baltimore Street   Phillipsburg, NJ 08865   (610)258-4337

Naragum, Varun, MD {1457628786} VasNeu
+ Capital Institute for Neurosciences
2 Capital Way/Suite 456   Pennington, NJ 08534   (609)537-7300   Fax (609)537-7301

Naraine, Christopher Anthony, MD {1972505329} ObsGyn(96,PA09)<NJ-RWJUHAM, NJ-SOMERSET>
+ Robert Wood Johnson Ob/Gyn Group
1 Hamilton Health Place   Hamilton, NJ 08690   (609)631-6899   Fax (609)631-6898

Naran, Deepak, MD {1629099783} RadDia(88,INA3C)<NY-CONEY-ISL>
+ AQ Modern Imaging
1921 Oak Tree Road   Edison, NJ 08820   (732)662-1831   Fax (732)662-1833

Narang, Shalu, MD {1134143878} Pedtrc, PedHem(01,GRN01)<NJ-NWRKBETH, NJ-CHDNWBTH>
+ Valerie Fund Childrens Center
201 Lyons Avenue   Newark, NJ 07112   (973)926-7161   Fax (973)282-0395
+ St. Barnabas Medical Center
94 Old Short Hills Road/Pediatrics   Livingston, NJ 07039   (973)322-5000
+ The Valerie Fund Children's Center
95 Old Short Hills Road   Livingston, NJ 07112   (973)322-2800   Fax (973)322-2856

Narang, Sudershan, MD {1033162649} IntrMd, FamMAdlt(64,INA72)<NJ-STMRYPAS, NJ-NWRKBETH>
+ 721 Clifton Avenue
Clifton, NJ 07013   (973)471-9654   Fax (973)471-9576

Narasimhaswamy, Smitha, MD {1679586069} IntrMd(98,INA28)<NJ-SPCLKIMB, NJ-SPCLMONM>
+ Specialty Hospital at Kimball
600 River Avenue/4 West   Lakewood, NJ 08701   (732)942-3597
+ Specialty Hospital at Monmouth
300 Second Avenue/Greenwall 6   Long Branch, NJ 07740   (732)923-5037

Narayanan, Manglam, MD {1447280433} Anesth(76,INA72)<NJ-STMRYPAS, NJ-BERGNMC>
+ New Bridge Medical Center
230 East Ridgewood Avenue/Anesthesia   Paramus, NJ 07652   (973)779-7361   Fax (973)779-7385

Nardi, David A., MD {1285652230} Anesth(85,PA02)<NJ-CHSM-RCER, NJ-CHSFULD>
+ Capital Health System/Mercer Campus
446 Bellevue Avenue/Anesthesiology   Trenton, NJ 08618   (609)394-4000

Nardi, Rebecca A., MD {1518126929} Radiol(07,NY01)
+ University Radiology Group, P.C.
483 Cranbury Road   East Brunswick, NJ 08816   (732)390-0030   Fax (732)390-5383
+ University Radiology Group, P.C.
16 Mountain Boulevard   Warren, NJ 07059   (732)390-0030   Fax (908)769-9141

Nardone, Danielle J., DO {1407838543} IntrMd(96,NJ75)<NJ-RIVERVW, NJ-MONMOUTH>
+ Fair Haven Internal Medicine
569 River Road/Suite 1   Fair Haven, NJ 07704   (732)530-0100   Fax (732)530-5895
dr.nardi@worldnet.att.net

Narinedhat, Ralph, MD {1922248400} ObsGyn<NJ-JRSYSHMC>
+ Jersey Shore University Medical Center
1945 Route 33/ObsGyn   Neptune, NJ 07753   (732)775-5500

Narins, Seth Craig, MD {1356377832} Surgry, IntrMd(98,MA05)
+ Hackensack University Medical Center
20 Prospect Avenue   Hackensack, NJ 07601   (201)996-2608

Nariseti, Chalapathy, MD {1699731083} IntrMd(71,INA4D)<NJ-JRSYCITY, NJ-VALYONS>
+ Liberty Medical Associates
377 Jersey Avenue/Suite 470   Jersey City, NJ 07302   (201)918-2239   Fax (201)918-2243

Narisety, Satya D., MD {1942407861} AlgyImmn(04,NJ05)
+ Allergy Consultants, PA
197 Bloomfield Avenue   Verona, NJ 07044   (973)857-0330   Fax (973)857-0980

Narucki, Wayne Ellis, MD {1902861818} Pedtrc, IntrMd(01,NJ05)
+ Red Wheelbarrow Pediatrics
33 Lincoln Avenue   Rutherford, NJ 07070   (201)340-2468   Fax (201)623-9381
redwheelbarrowpediatrics@gmail.com

Narula, Amar Singh, MD {1811130081} CdvDis
+ Atlantic Cardiology LLC
444 Neptune Boulevard/Unit 2   Neptune, NJ 07753   (732)775-5300   Fax (732)988-9080

Narula, Amarjot S., MD {1396708004} Psychy, PsyGrt(80,INA29)<NJ-VALLEY>
+ 65 North Maple Avenue
Ridgewood, NJ 07450   (201)670-4423   Fax (201)670-1660

Narula, Jiwanjot K., MD {1518158880} IntrMd<NJ-HOBUNIMC>
+ Hoboken University Medical Center
308 Willow Avenue   Hoboken, NJ 07030   (201)418-1000

Narula, Navjot Singh, MD {1578947230} IntHos
+ AtlantiCare Hospitalist Program
1925 Pacific Avenue/8th Floor   Atlantic City, NJ 08401

(609)441-8146   Fax (609)441-8002

Narvaez, Guillermo, Jr., MD {1922110196} Surgry(78,PHI02)<NJ-EASTORNG>
+ Drs. Reyes & Narvaez
135 Bloomfield Avenue/Suite B   Bloomfield, NJ 07003   (973)743-3556   Fax (973)743-3895
gpnarvaez@aol.com

Narvaez, Normita G., MD {1952414849} IntrMd(79,PHI02)
+ Drs. Reyes & Narvaez
135 Bloomfield Avenue/Suite B   Bloomfield, NJ 07003   (973)743-3556   Fax (973)743-3895

Narvel, Wasique Abdulahad, MD {1578501615} FamMed(91,INA70)
+ 2950 College Drive/Suite 1D
Vineland, NJ 08360

Narwani, Vanessa Deepak, MD {1700243813} IntrMd, EnDbMt(13,NJ06)
+ Valley Medical Group-Endocrinology
947 Linwood Avenue   Ridgewood, NJ 07450   (201)444-5552   Fax (201)444-4490

Narymsky, Lyudmila M., MD {1861578841} IntrMd(63,RUSS)<NJ-STJOSHOS>
+ Medical Internists Associates PA
22-18 Broadway/Suite 104   Fair Lawn, NJ 07410   (201)797-4503   Fax (201)797-4270

Nasar, Alan S., MD {1841278116} SrgOrt(00,NJ05)
+ Advanced Orthopedics & Sports Medicine Institute
301 Professional View Drive   Freehold, NJ 07728   (732)720-2555   Fax (732)720-2556

Nascimento, Tome R., MD {1235156100} CdvDis, CritCr, IntrMd(73,BRAZ)<NJ-ACMCMAIN, NJ-SHOREMEM>
+ AtlantiCare Physicians
318 Chris Gaupp Drive/Suite 100   Galloway, NJ 08205   (609)404-9900   Fax (609)404-3653

Naseef, George Salem, III, MD {1053382440} SrgOrt(98,MA05)<NJ-MORRISTN, NJ-STBARNMC>
+ Tri-County Orthopedics
160 East Hanover Avenue   Morristown, NJ 07962   (973)538-0900   Fax (973)538-0909

Naseem, Arif, MD {1295831782} IntrMd(90,PAK11)<NJ-MEADWLND>
+ Frank C. Alario MD Inc
355 Route 9/Suite 2   Bayville, NJ 08721   (732)269-0001   Fax (732)269-9636

Naseem, Rawahuddin, MD {1265759252} Pedtrc
+ CHCA NJ Emergency at Virtua
100 Bowman Drive   Voorhees, NJ 08043   (856)325-3000   Fax (609)261-5842

Nashed, Ashraf H., MD {1700978491} EmrgMd(90,NJ05)<NJ-MORRISTN>
+ Morristown Medical Center
100 Madison Avenue/EmrgMed   Morristown, NJ 07962   (973)971-5000

Nashi, Suhaib G., MD {1467432849} Pedtrc(77,IRQ01)<NJ-MORRISTN>
+ Morristown Pediatric Associates, LLC
261 James Street/Suite 1-G   Morristown, NJ 07960   (973)540-9393   Fax (973)540-1937
s080953@pol.net

Nasiek, Dariusz Jacek, MD {1285636852} Anesth, PainMd(89,POL18)
+ Garden State Pain Control Center, P.A.
1117 Route 46 East/Suite 201   Clifton, NJ 07013   (973)777-5444   Fax (973)777-0304
+ Allied Neurology & Interventional Pain
185 Grand Avenue   Englewood, NJ 07631   (973)777-5444   Fax (201)894-1335

Nasiek, Sara, MD {1043261019} Pedtrc(91,POL03)<NJ-MTNSIDE>
+ Hackensack UMC Mountainside
1 Bay Avenue/Pediatrics   Montclair, NJ 07042   (973)429-6000
+ NHCAC Health Center at Garfield
535 Midland Avenue   Garfield, NJ 07026   (973)429-6000

Nasir Khan, Mohammad Usman, MD {1619102662} SrgVas, Surgry(96,PAK15)<NJ-JRSYSHMC>
+ Meridian Surgical Associates
3700 Route 33/Suite C   Neptune, NJ 07753   (732)212-6590   Fax (732)922-2026

Nasr, John T., MD {1659332591} Nrolgy, ClNrPh(95,LEB03)<NJ-VALLEY>
+ Neurology Group of Bergen County
1200 East Ridgewood Avenue   Ridgewood, NJ 07450   (201)444-0868   Fax (201)444-7363

Nasr, Sherif Abbas, MD {1306814900} PthAcl, Pthlgy, Urolgy(78,EGY05)
+ Si Paradigm, LLC.
690 Kinderkamack Road/Suite 103   Oradell, NJ 07649   (201)599-9044   Fax (201)599-9066
+ Si Paradigm, LLC.
25 Riverside Drive/Suite 2   Pine Brook, NJ 07058   (201)599-9044

Nasra, Magdy A., MD {1467496703} IntrMd(80,EGY04)<NJ-RWJUBRUN, NJ-BAYSHORE>
+ Drs Nasra and Deacon
723 North Beers Street/Suite 2C Holmdel, NJ 07733
(732)888-8255   Fax (732)888-7682
+ Park Place Center
2 Deer Park Drive Monmouth Junction, NJ 08852
(732)888-8255   Fax (732)274-1991

Nassberg, Barton M., MD {1689635187} EnDbMt, IntrMd(79,BEL03)<NJ-BAYSHORE, NJ-RIVERVW>
+ Monmouth Endocrinology Associates
515 Iron Bridge Road Freehold, NJ 07728   (732)780-5885
+ Monmouth Endocrinology Associates
723 North Beers Street Holmdel, NJ 07733   (732)739-0200

Nasseri, Ali, MD {1821045956} ObsGyn, RprEnd(91,MD01)<NJ-VALLEY>
+ The Valley Hospital Fertility Center
140 East Ridgewood Avenue Paramus, NJ 07652
(212)263-7808   Fax (201)634-5503
+ Valley Hospital Fertility Center
One Valley Health Plaza Paramus, NJ 07652   (212)263-7808   Fax (201)634-5503

Nasta, Sucheta M., MD {1760589337} FamMed(70,INA69)<NJ-EASTORNG>
+ Drs. Chatha & Nasta
90 Washington Street/Suite 311 East Orange, NJ 07017
(973)676-7192   Fax (973)676-0525

Nastro, Lawrence J., MD {1013904861} InfDis, IntrMd, PulDis(65,NY08)<NJ-OVERLOOK, NJ-MORRISTN>
+ Summit Medical Group-Berkeley Heights Campus
1 Diamond Hill Road Berkeley Heights, NJ 07922
(908)273-4300   Fax (908)790-6524

Natale, Benjamin P., DO {1326137696} Ophthl(80,IA75)<NJ-HOBUNIMC>
+ Associated Eye Physicians & Surgeons of NJ, P.A.
1050 Galloping Hill Road/Suite 104 Union, NJ 07083
(908)964-7878   Fax (908)964-5434
+ Associated Eye Physicians & Surgeons of NJ, P.A.
724 Jersey Avenue Jersey City, NJ 07302 (908)964-7878 Fax (201)795-9797
+ Associated Eye Physicians & Surgeons of NJ, P.A.
1530 Saint Georges Avenue Rahway, NJ 07083   (732)382-9000   Fax (732)382-7455

Natale, Jessica Ann, DO {1386120780}
+ Summit Medical Group-Berkeley Heights Campus
1 Diamond Hill Road Berkeley Heights, NJ 07922
(908)273-4300   Fax (908)790-6576

Natale-Pereira, Ana M., MD {1215949342} IntrMd(96,NJ05)<NJ-UMDNJ>
+ University Hospital-Doctors Office Center
90 Bergen Street/DOCS 4400 Newark, NJ 07103
(973)972-1880   Fax (973)972-1879
+ 140 Bergen Street/F-Level
Newark, NJ 07103   (973)972-8150

Natalicchio, James Charles, MD {1265409205} PhysMd, PhyM-Pain(98,GRN01)<NJ-HACKNSK>
+ Active Orthopaedics & Sports Medicine
440 Old Hook Road Emerson, NJ 07630 (201)358-0707
Fax (201)358-9777
+ Active Orthopaedics & Sports Medicine
25 Prospect Avenue Hackensack, NJ 07601 (201)358-0707   Fax (201)343-7410

Natanzon, Calvin, MD {1548405129} Nrolgy
+ Summit Medical Group
315 East Northfield Road/Suite 1-E Livingston, NJ 07039
(973)436-4170   Fax (973)535-1450
+ The Heart Group, PA
654 Broadway Bayonne, NJ 07002 (973)436-4170 Fax (201)243-9998

Natarajan, Geetha, MD PthAcl(71,INA77)
+ 2 Berkery Place/P O Box 398
Alpine, NJ 07620

Natarajan, Sekar, MD {1164594354} PulDis, IntrMd<NJ-STMICHL>
+ 142 Palisade Avenue/Suite 213
Jersey City, NJ 07306 (201)653-4247 Fax (201)426-2349

Natarajan, Shobana, MD {1639134394} IntrMd(89,INA04)
+ Goyal & Natarajan MDs LLC
904 Oak Tree Road/Suite M South Plainfield, NJ 07080
(908)757-1414   Fax (908)757-3317
goyalnat2@gmail.com

Natarajan, Usharani, MD {1487620456} InfDis, IntrMd(91,INA85)<NJ-HCKTSTWN, NJ-NWTNMEM>
+ Consultants in Infectious Diseases, PA
25 Lindsley Drive/Suite 110 Morristown, NJ 07960
(972)998-7314   Fax (973)998-7313
+ ID Associates PA/dba ID Care
765 Route 10 East/Suite 201 Randolph, NJ 07869
(972)998-7314   Fax (973)361-8955
+ ID Associates PA/dba ID Care
8 Saddle Road Cedar Knolls, NJ 07960 (973)993-5950
Fax (973)993-5953

Natelli, Anthony A., MD {1740237940} IntrMd, Grtrcs(78,ITA01)<NJ-STJOSHOS>
+ 2035 Hamburg Turnpike
Wayne, NJ 07470 (973)835-2844 Fax (973)835-6955

Natello, Gregory W., DO {1972618874} CdvDis
+ Gagnon Cardiovasular Institute
100 Madison Avenue/Level C Morristown, NJ 07962
(973)971-5597   Fax (973)290-7145

Nath, Ajay, MD {1770549198} Anesth, PedAne, IntrMd(91,NY47)<NJ-STPETER, NJ-SOMERSET>
+ Anesthesia Consultnts of NJ/Nova Pain
285 Davidson Avenue/Suite 204 Somerset, NJ 08873
(732)271-1400   Fax (732)271-3544

Nath, Carl Anthony, MD {1326113564} ObsGyn, MtFtMd(94,NY47)<NJ-HACKNSK>
+ Monmouth Medical Group, P.C.
73 South Bath Avenue Long Branch, NJ 07740 (732)870-3600   Fax (732)870-0119
+ Monmouth Medical Group, P.C.
1 Route 70 Lakewood, NJ 08701 (732)870-3600 Fax (732)901-0199
+ Monmouth Family Center
270 Broadway Long Branch, NJ 07740 (732)923-7100
Fax (732)923-7104

Nath, Mary Madhuri, MD {1427222751} ObsGyn(87,BAN05)<NJ-RBAYPERT, NJ-PALISADE>
+ Palisades Medical Center
7600 River Road/OB/GYN North Bergen, NJ 07047
(201)854-5000
+ Raritan Bay Medical Center/Outpatient
595 New Brunswick Avenue Perth Amboy, NJ 08861
(732)442-7500
+ 516 Lawrie Street
Perth Amboy, NJ 07047 (732)324-4860 Fax (732)324-4861

Nath, Priyanka, MD {1114185576}<NJ-HACKNSK>
+ Hackensack University Medical Center
30 Prospect Avenue Hackensack, NJ 07601   (201)996-2000

Nathan, David Lawrence, MD {1578652517} Psychy(94,PA01)
+ 601 Ewing Street/Suite C-10
Princeton, NJ 08540   (609)688-0400   Fax (609)688-0401

Nathan, Faith E., MD {1235566746} MedOnc, Hemato, IntrMd(86,NJ03)<NJ-KMHTURNV, NJ-VIRTUAHS>
+ 9 West Walnut Avenue
Moorestown, NJ 08057   (856)802-1183

Nathan, Michael D., DO {1578593422} Pedtrc(71,MO79)
+ 280 East 33rd Street
Paterson, NJ 07504   (973)684-0606   Fax (973)684-5575
+ 249 Lexington Avenue
Passaic, NJ 07055   (973)684-0606   Fax (973)473-6886

Nathan, Ponnudurai, MD {1821234972} Anesth(69,SRIL)<NJ-OURLADY>
+ Our Lady of Lourdes Medical Center
1600 Haddon Avenue/Anesthesiology   Camden, NJ 08103
(856)757-3500

Nathan, Ramasamy Swami, MD {1538114566} Gastrn, IntrMd(81,INA47)
+ Gastroenterology Health Care PA
799 Bloomfield Avenue/Suite 102 Verona, NJ 07044
(973)239-8373   Fax (973)239-8403

Nathani, Shujaat Ali, MD {1043229933}<NJ-HAMPTBHC>
+ Hampton Behavioral Health Center
650 Rancocas Road Westampton, NJ 08060 (609)518-2124
san786@yahoo.com

Naticchia, Jennifer M., MD {1588635296} FamMed, SprtMd(92,PA02)<NJ-VIRTVOOR, NJ-VIRTBERL>
+ Virtua Family Medicine Center @Lumberton
1636 Route 38 & Eayrestown Rd. Lumberton, NJ 08048
(609)914-8440   Fax (609)914-8441
+ Kennedy Health Alliance
80 Tanner Street Haddonfield, NJ 08033   (609)914-8440
Fax (856)355-0346

Nativ, Simona Horak, MD {1942448717} Pedtrc, Rheuma, IntrMd(04,ISR02)<NJ-MORRISTN, NJ-OVERLOOK>
+ Morristown Medical Center
100 Madison Avenue/Pedi Rheuma Morristown, NJ 07962
(973)971-4096   Fax (973)290-7177
+ Overlook Medical Center
99 Beauvoir Avenue/PO Box 210 Summit, NJ 07902
(973)971-4096

Naturman, Roy E., MD {1639158041} Anesth(83,MA07)
+ Summit Anesthesia Associates, P.A.
33 Overlook Road/Suite 311 Summit, NJ 07901 (908)598-1500   Fax (908)598-0197

Nau, Allen Reza, DO {1669631404} FamMed, EmrgMd<NJ-CENTRAST>
+ CentraState Medical Center
901 West Main Street/Emerg Med Freehold, NJ 07728
(732)431-2000

Naumova, Alena, MD {1063891265}<NJ-MONMOUTH>
+ Monmouth Medical Center
300 Second Avenue/Room 215 SW Long Branch, NJ 07740
(732)923-6795   Fax (732)923-6793

Navarro, Mark Anthony, MD {1700102316} FamMed(06,PHI08)
+ Ocean County Family Care
2125 Route 88 East Brick, NJ 08724   (732)942-4455   Fax (732)892-0961
mark4navarro@yahoo.com

Navas, Carlene, MD {1427061423} Pedtrc(03,DMN01)<NJ-JFKMED>
+ JFK Medical Center
65 James Street/Pediatrics Edison, NJ 08820   (732)321-7605

Navot, Daniel, MD {1164534277} ObsGyn, RprEnd, IntrMd(78,ISRA)<NY-WESTCHMC, NJ-VALLEY>
+ 30 Creston Avenue
Tenafly, NJ 07670   (201)871-9106   Fax (201)666-2262

Naware, Sanya, MD {1861808313} IntrMd
+ Cooper Physicians
1210 Brace Road/Suite 102 Cherry Hill, NJ 08034
(856)428-6616   Fax (856)428-4823

Nawaz, Yassir, MD {1912139627} CdvDis, IntrMd<NJ-NWRK-BETH>
+ Newark Beth Israel Medical Center
201 Lyons Avenue/Cardiology Newark, NJ 07112
(973)926-6530

Nayak, Bharathi, MD {1912098690} Nrolgy, NeuMSptM, IntrMd(70,INDI)<NJ-CLARMAAS>
+ 350 Bloomfield Avenue/Suite 1
Bloomfield, NJ 07003   (973)680-1200   Fax (973)680-1202
bnayakno1@yahoo.com

Nayak, Shaila V., MD {1891787735} BldBnk, PthAcl(66,INA30)<NJ-JRSYCITY>
+ 32 Vender Lane
Mays Landing, NJ 08330

Nayak, Yeshavanth P., MD {1598870891} IntrMd, PulDis(71,INDI)<NJ-COMMED>
+ Community Pulmonary Assoc PA
20 Hospital Drive/Suite 16 Toms River, NJ 08755
(732)349-5220   Fax (732)914-9668
+ Community Medical Center
99 Route 37 West Toms River, NJ 08755   (732)557-8000

Nayal, Eyad A., MD {1922044924} Nrolgy(89,SYRI)<NJ-WAYNE-GEN, NJ-STJOSHOS>
+ Wayne Neurological Associates
401 Hamburg Turnpike/Suite 208 Wayne, NJ 07470
(973)942-3300   Fax (973)942-0014

Nayar, Amrit P., MD {1821063488} SrgCdv, SrgThr, Surgry(72,INA23)<NJ-KMHSTRAT, NJ-OURLADY>
+ CardioThoracic Surg Specs/Cherry Hill
1245 Brace Road Cherry Hill, NJ 08034   (856)429-7779
Fax (856)429-7455
ANayar1111@aol.com

Nayar, Anju, MD {1649363409} Psychy(78,INA5A)
+ 1245 Brace Road
Cherry Hill, NJ 08034   (856)216-0350   Fax (856)429-7455

Nayar, Devjit Singh, MD {1093787806} Gastrn(99,DMN01)<NJ-JFKMED, NJ-RWJURAH>
+ Gastroenterology Associates of Central Jersey, PA
1921 Oak Tree Road/Suite 101 Edison, NJ 08820
(732)744-9090   Fax (732)744-1592

Nayar, Romesh C., MD {1467493957} Ophthl(76,INA23)
+ 81 Ford Avenue
Wharton, NJ 07885   (973)328-6484   Fax (973)361-5286

Nayee, Sandip Natvarlal, DO {1194041186} RadDia, Radiol(05,NJ75)<PA-STJOBERN>
+ Radiology Affiliates of Central New Jersey, P.A.
2501 Kuser Road Hamilton, NJ 08691   (609)585-8800
Fax (609)585-1825

Naylor, Evan C., MD {1881805968} OncHem, IntrMd(04,NJ05)<NJ-RWJUBRUN, NJ-UNVMCPRN>
+ Meridian Hematology & Oncology
1100 Route 72 West Manahawkin, NJ 08050   (609)597-0547   Fax (609)597-8668
+ RWJ University Hospital New Brunswick
One Robert Wood Johnson Place New Brunswick, NJ 08901
(732)828-3000
+ Rutgers Cancer Institute of New Jersey
195 Little Albany Street/PO Box 2681 New Brunswick, NJ 08050   (732)235-2465   Fax (732)235-6797

Nayman, Defne, MD {1215078472} EmrgMd(91,TUR04)<NY-LDYMRCY>
+ 189 Palisade Avenue/Apt Grnd
Cliffside, NJ 07010

Physicians by Name and Address

Nayyar, Sanjeev, MD {1033193628} IntrMd, Gastrn(84,INA1Z)<NJ-BAYSHORE>
+ 200 Perrine Road/Suite 231
  Old Bridge, NJ 08857   (732)525-0600   Fax (732)525-9777
+ 400 State Street
  Perth Amboy, NJ 08861   (732)525-0600   Fax (732)525-9777
+ May Street Surgi Center
  205 May Street/Suite 103   Edison, NJ 08857   (732)820-4566   Fax (732)661-9619

Nazareth, Joseph M., MD {1174645444} Nrolgy, Pedtrc, NrlgSpec(71,INDI)
+ 350 Bloomfield Avenue/1st Floor
  Bloomfield, NJ 07003   (973)539-9722   Fax (973)539-5087

Nazarian, Ronniel, MD {1972762276} SrgOrt, Surgry(05,NY03)
+ Princeton Orthopaedic Associates, P.A.
  325 Princeton Avenue   Princeton, NJ 08540   (609)924-8131   Fax (609)924-8532

Nazeer, Amjad, MD {1245277599} CdvDis, IntrMd(81,DOM03)<NJ-STCLRDEN, NJ-HOBUNIMC>
+ 22 Howard Boulevard/Suite 103
  Mount Arlington, NJ 07856   (973)398-0870   Fax (973)398-4357

Nazha, Naim T., MD {1730136854} MedOnc(79,SYR01)<NJ-ACMCMAIN, NJ-SHOREMEM>
+ Nazha Cancer Center
  411 New Road   Northfield, NJ 08225   (609)383-6033   Fax (609)383-0064

Nazia, Yasmin, MD {1558769257} Psychy<NJ-RWJUBRUN>
+ RWJ University Hospital New Brunswick
  One Robert Wood Johnson Place   New Brunswick, NJ 08901   (732)828-3000

Nazir, Habib A., MD {1598008948} IntrMd<NJ-NWRKBETH>
+ Newark Beth Israel Medical Center
  201 Lyons Avenue/Pulm&CritCare   Newark, NJ 07112   (732)982-7510

Nazir, Munir A., MD {1639126717} ObsGyn, MtFtMd(71,PAK10)<NJ-NWRKBETH>
+ Newark Beth Israel Medical Center
  201 Lyons Avenue/ObGyn/L2   Newark, NJ 07112   (973)926-4882   Fax (973)923-7497

Nazli, Yasmeen Zuleikha, MD {1952378135} FamMed, Obs-Gyn(84,PAK12)<NY-STJOHNSS>
+ Jewish Renaissance Medical Center
  275 Hobart Street   Perth Amboy, NJ 08861   (732)376-9333   Fax (732)376-0139

Nazmy, Michael, Jr., MD {1881844736} Urolgy(06,NJ05)
+ University Urology Associates of New Jersey
  1374 Whitehorse Hamilton Sq/Suite 101   Hamilton, NJ 08690   (609)581-5900   Fax (609)581-5901

Ndeto, Geoffrey Wambua T., MD {1346266004} Anesth, Anes-Pain(76,KEN01)<NJ-JRSYSHMC>
+ Jersey Shore Anesthesiology Associates
  1945 Route 33/PO Box 397   Neptune, NJ 07754   (732)922-3308   Fax (732)897-0263

Nduaguba, Chiazoka Onyeka, MD {1639330004} Anesth(08,WA04)<NJ-VIRTMARL>
+ West Jersey Anesthesia Associates
  102 East Centre Boulevard   Marlton, NJ 08053   (856)988-6260   Fax (856)988-6270

Ndukwe, Michael Chukwuemeka, MD {1164954566} Pedtrc
+ Rutgers- New Jersey Medical School
  185 South Orange Avenue/MSB F-603   Newark, NJ 07103   (973)972-0740   Fax (973)972-1019

Ndukwe, Nwayieze Chisara, MD {1326381203} Psychy
+ 1924 Essex Avenue
  Linden, NJ 07036   (908)494-0836

Neal, John William, VI, MD {1912293283} SrgOrt
+ UMDNJ-University Hospital
  205 South Orange Avenue   Newark, NJ 07103   (973)972-4520

Neal, Ronald R., MD {1801862024} ObsGyn(74,NJ05)<NJ-COMMED>
+ Toms River Ob-Gyn Associates PA
  79 Route 37 West/Suite 101   Toms River, NJ 08755   (732)244-9444   Fax (732)244-9468

Neal, Wendy, MD {1275543365}
+ Children's Hospital of New Jersey/Newark Beth Israel
  166 Lyons Avenue   Newark, NJ 07112   (973)926-7282   Fax (973)923-2978

Neal, Wendy Patricia, MD
+ 11 Alcott Way
  Succasunna, NJ 07876

Nealis, Justin, MD {1063808103} FamMed<NJ-HUNTRDN>
+ Hunterdon Medical Center
  2100 Wescott Drive   Flemington, NJ 08822   (908)788-6100
+ Hunterdon Family Medicine
  250 Route 28/Suite 100   Bridgewater, NJ 08807   (908)788-6100   Fax (908)237-4136

Neary, Michael J., MD {1144261629} Anesth, CritCr(81,MS01)<NJ-DEBRAHLC>
+ Deborah Heart and Lung Center
  200 Trenton Road/Anesthesiology   Browns Mills, NJ 08015   (609)893-6611   Fax (609)893-1213
+ Alternatives/Princeton Women's Center
  29 Emmons Drive/Suite E-20   Princeton, NJ 08540   (609)514-9191

Necsutu, Simona Camelia, MD {1396949277} FamMed(96,ROM01)<NJ-SJHREGMC>
+ CompleteCare Adult & Specialty Medical Professionals
  1038 East Chestnut Avenue/Suite 110   Vineland, NJ 08360   (856)451-4700

Nedelcu, Dana, MD {1144422163} IntrMd(02,ROM01)<NJ-KIMBALL>
+ Hospital Medicine Associates
  157 Broad Street/Suite 317   Red Bank, NJ 07701   (732)530-2960   Fax (732)530-7446
+ Kimball Medical Center
  600 River Avenue   Lakewood, NJ 08701   (732)363-1900

Nee, Guy, MD {1760429997} IntrMd(90,PA13)<NJ-CHSMRCER>
+ Mercer Internal Medicine, LLC.
  2480 Pennington Road/Suites 104   Pennington, NJ 08534   (609)818-1000   Fax (609)818-9800

Nee, Patricia B., MD {1578606448} FamMed(85,NY06)
+ East Brunswick Family Practice Associates
  123 Dunhams Corner Road   East Brunswick, NJ 08816   (732)254-3300

Needell, Gary S., MD {1477538221} RadDia, Radiol(76,NY03)<NJ-STPETER, NJ-RWJUBRUN>
+ University Radiology Group, P.C.
  483 Cranbury Road   East Brunswick, NJ 08816   (732)390-0030   Fax (732)390-5383
+ University Radiology Group, P.C.
  10 Plum Street   New Brunswick, NJ 08901   (732)390-0030   Fax (732)249-1208

Needle, Michael Neil, MD {1326178443} PedHem, Pedtrc(85,NY08)
+ 1 Gillespie Lane
  Morristown, NJ 07960

Needleman, Jack, MD {1821031626} Pedtrc, GenPrc(74,NY09)<NJ-SOMERSET, NJ-STPETER>
+ Somerset Pediatric Group PA
  155 Union Avenue   Bridgewater, NJ 08807   (908)725-1802   Fax (908)203-8825
+ Somerset Pediatric Group PA
  1390 Route 22 West/Suite 106   Lebanon, NJ 08833   (908)725-1802   Fax (908)236-7557
+ Somerset Pediatric Group PA
  1-C New Amwell Road   Hillsborough, NJ 08807   (908)874-5035   Fax (908)874-3288

Neelgund, Ashwini Kumar, MD {1487869574} Psychy, PssoMd(85,INA97)
+ Stress Care Clinic of New Jersey, LLC
  4122 Route 516/Suite C & D   Matawan, NJ 07747   (732)679-4500   Fax (732)679-4549
  ashwinineelgund@hotmail.com
+ Central Jersey Beharioral Health, LLC
  216 North Avenue East   Cranford, NJ 07016   (732)679-4500   Fax (908)272-7502

Neema, Swarnalatha, MD {1033302120} FamMed, IntrMd(01,INA1R)
+ Community Health Care, Inc.
  319 Landis Avenue/Suites A & B   Vineland, NJ 08360   (856)691-3300   Fax (856)696-0344

Neff, Marc A., MD {1639170137} Surgry(96,PA01)
+ Advocare Associates in General Surgery
  2201 Chapel Avenue West/Suite 100   Cherry Hill, NJ 08002   (856)665-2017   Fax (856)488-6769
+ Advocare Associates in General Surgery
  570 Egg Harbor Road/Suite C-2   Sewell, NJ 08080   (856)665-2017   Fax (856)256-7789
+ Comprehensive Cancer & Hematology Specialists, P.C.
  705 White Horse Road   Voorhees, NJ 08002   (856)435-1777   Fax (856)435-0696

Neff, Pamela Mitra, MD {1770648727} ObsGyn(VA04)
+ Penn Health for Women
  807 Haddon Avenue/Suite 212   Haddonfield, NJ 08033   (856)429-0400   Fax (856)429-8411

Negin, Benjamin Paul, MD {1366477697} IntrMd(04,CT01)
+ Southern Oncology Hematology Associates
  1505 West Sherman Avenue/Suite 101   Vineland, NJ 08360   (856)696-9550   Fax (856)691-1686

Negin, Nathan Samuel, MD {1871520072} IntrMd<NJ-COOPRUMC>
+ Cooper University Hospital
  One Cooper Plaza/Hsplist   Camden, NJ 08103   (856)342-3150   Fax (856)968-8418

Neglia, Janet A., MD {1730303371} EmrgMd(83,MEX29)
+ McCosh Health Center
  Washington Road/McCosh Infirmary   Princeton, NJ 08544   (609)258-5357   Fax (609)258-1355

Negron, Arnaldo E., MD {1659488138} Psychy(90,PRO01)
+ Aroga Behavioral Health of Princeton
  188 Tamarack Circle   Skillman, NJ 08558   (609)279-1339   Fax (609)279-1359

Negron, David, MD {1497799019} EmrgMd(90,NY08)<NJ-HACKNSK>
+ Hackensack Medical Center Emergency Medicine
  30 Prospect Avenue/Main 3619   Hackensack, NJ 07601   (201)996-4614   Fax (201)342-7112
+ Hackensack University Medical Center
  30 Prospect Avenue/EmrgMed   Hackensack, NJ 07601   (201)996-4614   Fax (201)968-1866

Negron, Luis M., MD {1417048521} IntrMd(87,NJ05)
+ LMG Medical Group
  136 North Washington Avenue/Suite 201   Bergenfield, NJ 07621   (201)374-1171   Fax (201)374-1650

Negron-Gonzalez, Maria Alejandra, MD {1457527301} Anesth(97,VEN06)<NJ-RWJUBRUN>
+ Montclair Anesthesia Associates PC
  185 Fairfield Avenue/Suite 2A   West Caldwell, NJ 07006   (973)226-1230   Fax (973)226-1232

Nehmad, Jason Arash, MD {1780920645} IntrMd(10,ANT02)<NJ-JRSYSHMC>
+ Jersey Shore University Medical Center
  1945 Route 33   Neptune, NJ 07753   (732)776-4949
+ Lakewood Medical Associates
  2290 West County Line Road/Suite 101   Jackson, NJ 08527   (732)645-9988
+ Ocean Park Medical Associates
  1900 Highway 35/Suite 200   Oakhurst, NJ 07753   (732)663-0900   Fax (732)663-0901

Nehmer, Steven L., MD {1336248293} SrgOrt, NeuMSptM(80,NJ05)<NJ-OVERLOOK>
+ Dr. Nehmer and Associates
  2121 Morris Avenue   Union, NJ 07083   (908)687-3000   Fax (908)964-0417

Nehra, Anupama, MD {1811935307} IntrMd, Hemato, MedOnc(93,INA6Z)<NJ-JFKMED, NJ-SOMERSET>
+ UMDNJ-University Hospital
  205 South Orange Avenue   Newark, NJ 07103   (973)972-6257   Fax (973)972-2384
+ Somerset Hematology Oncology Associates, P.A.
  30 Rehill Avenue/2nd Floor/Suite 2500   Somerville, NJ 08876   (973)972-6257   Fax (908)927-8706
+ Hematology-Oncology Associates PA - Plainfield
  1314 Park Avenue/Suite 3   Plainfield, NJ 07103   (908)754-0400

Neibart, Richard M., MD {1134120686} SrgThr, Surgry(82,NY47)<NJ-MORRISTN, NJ-JRSYSHMC>
+ Mid-Atlantic Surgical Associates
  100 Madison Avenue   Morristown, NJ 07960   (973)971-7300   Fax (973)984-7019
+ Mid-Atlantic Surgical Associates
  1944 Route 33/Suite 201   Neptune, NJ 07753   (973)971-7300   Fax (732)776-3765

Neibert, John Paul Z., MD {1467493569} IntrMd(89,PHI18)
+ 10 Huron Avenue/Suite 1-L
  Jersey City, NJ 07306   (201)798-6200   Fax (201)798-6207

Neidecker, John Michael, DO {1821289174} FamMed, SprtMd(07,NJ75)<NJ-COOPRUMC>
+ Cooper Bone and Joint Institute
  401 South Kings Highway/Suite 3-A   Cherry Hill, NJ 08003   (856)547-0201   Fax (856)547-0316
+ Cooper Bone and Joint Institute
  900 Centennial Boulevard   Voorhees, NJ 08043   (856)547-0201   Fax (856)325-6678
+ Cooper Bone and Joint Institute
  3 Cooper Plaza/Suite 411   Camden, NJ 08003   (856)673-4500   Fax (856)673-4525

Neidorf, David L., MD {1053334227} FamMed(81,NY48)<NJ-VIRTBERL, NJ-VIRTVOOR>
+ Family Medicine of Lindenwold
  409 East Gibbsboro Road   Lindenwold, NJ 08021   (856)309-0100   Fax (856)309-8827
  dneidorf@comcast.net

Neier, Michelle Dana, MD {1033238571} PedHem, IntrMd(02,NY03)<NJ-MORRISTN, NJ-OVERLOOK>
+ Morristown Medical Center
  100 Madison Avenue/Pediatrics   Morristown, NJ 07962   (973)971-5000
+ Overlook Medical Center
  99 Beauvoir Avenue/PO Box 210   Summit, NJ 07902   (908)522-2000

Neigel, Janet M., MD {1487698163} Ophthl, OthrSp, SrgCsm(81,NJ05)<NJ-STBARNMC, NJ-MORRISTN>
+ Ocul-Facila Surgery
  201 Route 17th North/11th Floor   Rutherford, NJ 07070   (201)549-8847
  janet@eyelid.com
+ Ocul-Facila Surgery
  254 Columbia Turnpike/Suite 200   Florham Park, NJ 07932   (201)549-8847   Fax (973)325-7914

Neilan, Martin J., MD {1912995853} IntrMd(82,MEX03)<NJ-WAY-NEGEN, NJ-CHILTON>
+ 516 Hamburg Turnpike/Suite 13
  Wayne, NJ 07470   (973)790-8585   Fax (973)790-1105

Neilon, Kathleen Mary, DO OthrSp(89,PA77)
+ 7 Wrenfield Drive
  Sewell, NJ 08080

Neiman, Deborah L., MD {1699793547} IntrMd(84,NY09)<NJ-SOMERSET, NJ-MORRISTN>
+ Affiliates in Internal Medicine
  311 Omni Drive   Hillsborough, NJ 08844   (908)281-0632   Fax (908)281-9848
+ Affiliates in Internal Medicine
  49 Route 202   Far Hills, NJ 07931   (908)281-0632   Fax (908)719-1091

Neimark, Matthew A., MD {1609006782} RadDia<NJ-CHSFULD>
+ Capital Health System/Fuld Campus
  750 Brunswick Avenue   Trenton, NJ 08638   (609)815-7532

Neitzel, Kristi M., MD {1801239918} Anesth
+ Kennedy Memorial Hospital-University Medical Center
  18 East Laurel Road   Stratford, NJ 08084   (856)346-6000
+ Rancocas Anesthesiology, PA
  700 Route 130 North/Suite 203   Cinnaminson, NJ 08077   (856)346-6000   Fax (856)829-3605

Nejad, Karan S., MD {1083757744} CdvDis, IntrMd(88,FL02)<NJ-HACKNSK, NJ-HOLYNAME>
+ 20 Prospect Avenue/Suite 809
  Hackensack, NJ 07601   (201)457-3366   Fax (201)457-9050

Nekoranik, Michael G., DO {1578654786} PulDis, IntrMd(86,PA77)
+ St. Luke's Pulmonary Associates
  123B Roseberry Street   Phillipsburg, NJ 08865   (908)847-8852   Fax (908)847-6028

Nekrasova, Irina, MD {1396899753} Psychy(78,RUS06)<NJ-HCMEADPS>
+ Hudson County Meadowview Psychiatric Hospital
  595 County Avenue   Secaucus, NJ 07094   (201)319-3660   Fax (201)319-3616

Nelson, Adin, MD {1073888491} Pedtrc
+ Rutgers- New Jersey Medical School
  185 South Orange Avenue/MSB F585   Newark, NJ 07103   (973)972-9173

Nelson, Andrew L., MD {1497751242} IntrMd, SprtMd, IntrSptM(95,NJ05)<NJ-OCEANMC>
+ Coastal Sports Medicine
  1594 Route 9/Suite 6   Toms River, NJ 08755   (732)349-8888   Fax (732)349-8880
+ Rutgers Hurtado Health Center
  11 Bishop Place   New Brunswick, NJ 08901   (732)349-8888   Fax (732)932-1223

Nelson, Craig A., MD {1184712416} EmrgMd, IntrMd(91,LA01)<NJ-CLARMAAS>
+ Clara Maass Medical Center
  1 Clara Maass Drive/EmergMed   Belleville, NJ 07109   (973)450-2000

Nelson, Elizabeth A., MD {1548552995} Pedtrc
+ Drs. Nelson and Goldin
  541 Clubhouse Court/Unit 3   Union, NJ 07083

Nelson, Geraldine I., MD {1538158589} Pedtrc, AdolMd(65,NY09)<NJ-CHILTON>
+ Pediatric Professional Associates PA
  330 Ratzer Road/Suite 20   Wayne, NJ 07470   (973)835-5556   Fax (973)628-7942
+ New Jersey Pediatric & Adolescent Care, LLC.
  1680 Route 23/Suite 350   Wayne, NJ 07470   (973)835-5556   Fax (973)521-9707

Nelson, Gregory N., Jr., MD {1114174265} SrgOrt
+ Rothman Institute
  999 Route 73 North/3rd Fl   Marlton, NJ 08053   (856)821-6360   Fax (856)821-6359

Nelson, Homer L., MD {1578667044} IntrMd(83,NJ05)
+ US Healthworks of New Jersey
  606 Dowd Avenue   Elizabeth, NJ 07201   (908)527-6334   Fax (908)527-0322

Nelson, Mary Beth, MD {1023197308} Anesth, IntrMd(85,NJ05)<NJ-UNVMCPRN>
+ University Medical Center of Princeton at Plainsboro
  One Plainsboro Road/Anesth   Plainsboro, NJ 08536   (609)497-4329   Fax (609)497-4331
+ Princeton Anesthesia Services PC
  253 Witherspoon Street   Princeton, NJ 08540   (609)497-4329   Fax (609)497-4331

Nelson, Richard Oakleigh, MD {1841287620} IntrMd(85,NY09)<NJ-OVERLOOK, NJ-MORRISTN>
+ Summit Medical Group
  34 Mountain Boulevard/Building B   Warren, NJ 07059   (908)769-0100   Fax (908)769-8927
+ Summit Medical Group-Berkeley Heights Campus
  1 Diamond Hill Road   Berkeley Heights, NJ 07922   (908)769-0100   Fax (908)790-6576
+ Summit Medical Group
  34 Mountain Boulevard   Warren, NJ 07059   (908)561-8600   Fax (908)561-7265

Nelson, Yvonne, MD {1518092055} FamMed(03,NJ05)
+ All Care Family Medicine, LLC
  3 Lincoln Highway/Suite 101   Edison, NJ 08820   (732)494-4500   Fax (732)494-2818

Nelson-Lane, Leigh A., MD {1821356411} Anesth<NJ-RWJUBRUN>
+ RWJ University Hospital New Brunswick
  One Robert Wood Johnson Place   New Brunswick, NJ 08901   (732)212-0051   Fax (732)212-0713

Nemade, Ajay B., MD {1376836874} RadDia
+ Princeton Radiology Associates, P.A.
  3674 Route 27   Kendall Park, NJ 08824   (732)821-5563   Fax (732)821-6675

Nemeh, Elias, MD {1730151416} ObsGyn(77,POLA)
+ 188 Fries Mill Road/Suite N1
  Turnersville, NJ 08012   (856)875-0505   Fax (856)875-9556

Nemeh, Kamila E., MD {1215017843} Pedtrc(79,POLA)
+ 188 Fries Mill Road/Suite N-1
  Turnersville, NJ 08012   (856)875-5767   Fax (856)875-9556

Nemerofsky, Robert Becker, MD {1629061908} SrgPlstc(94,FL02)
+ Nemerofsky Plastic Surgery
  16 Pocono Road/Suite 214   Denville, NJ 07834   (973)784-1024   Fax (973)710-0887
  info@nemerofskyplasticsurgery.com

Nemeth, Laurie Yallowitz, DO {1306856448} FamMed(00,NJ75)
+ Dorfner Family Medicine
  811 Sunset Road/Suite 101   Burlington, NJ 08016   (609)387-9242   Fax (609)387-9408

Nemeth, Nicole Angelina, MD {1699703173} Pedtrc, IntrMd(00,PA01)<NJ-VIRTMHBC>
+ Advocare Pedi Phys of Burlington Co
  204 Ark Road/Suite 209   Mount Laurel, NJ 08054   (856)234-3797   Fax (856)234-9402

Nemetski, Sondra Maureen, MD {1174966816} PedEmg
+ Hackensack Univ Medical Center Pediatric Emerg Room
  30 Prospect Avenue   Hackensack, NJ 07601   (551)996-2870   Fax (201)996-3676

Nemiroff, Richard Lloyd, MD {1891721585} ObsGyn, IntrMd(70,PA02)<PA-UPMCPHL>
+ Penn Medicine at Woodbury Heights
  1006 Mantua Pike   Woodbury Heights, NJ 08097   (856)845-8600   Fax (856)845-0535

Nemirovsky, Dmitry, MD {1518086933} IntrMd, ClCdEl, CdvDis(99,TN05)<NJ-ENGLWOOD, NJ-HOLYNAME>
+ North Jersey Electrophysiology Associates
  350 Engle Street   Englewood, NJ 07631   (201)894-3533
+ North Jersey Electrophysiology Associates
  20 Prospect Avenue/Suite 615   Hackensack, NJ 07601   (201)894-3533   Fax (201)518-8739

Nenna, David Vito, MD {1306945456} SrgHnd, SrgOrt, OrtS-Hand(77,DC02)<NJ-SOMERSET, NJ-HUNTRDN>
+ MidJersey Orthopaedics, P.A.
  8100 Westcott Drive/Suite 101   Flemington, NJ 08822   (908)782-0600   Fax (908)782-7575

Nenninger, Alberto, MD {1750809968}<NJ-OVERLOOK>
+ Overlook Medical Center
  99 Beauvoir Avenue/PO Box 210   Summit, NJ 07902   (908)552-0000

Neno, Rosa M., DO {1407850894} IntrMd(90,MO78)<NJ-BAYONNE>
+ United Medical, P.C.
  988 Broadway/Suite 201   Bayonne, NJ 07002   (201)339-6111   Fax (201)339-6333
+ South Hudson Medical Associates, PA
  19 East 27th Street   Bayonne, NJ 07002   (201)339-6111   Fax (201)339-0506
+ South Hudson Medical Associates PA
  25 McWilliams Place/Suite 402   Jersey City, NJ 07002   (201)217-4227

Neopane, Padam Kumar, MD {1104967488} FamMed, Grtrcs, IntrMd(90,INA97)
+ Erickson Health Medical Group
  1 Cedar Crest Village Drive   Pompton Plains, NJ 07444   (973)831-3540   Fax (973)831-3503

Nepomuceno, Kathleen Chiong, MD {1861463135} Anesth(83,PHI09)<NJ-TRINIWSC>
+ Trinitas Regional Medical Center-Williamson Street
  225 Williamson Street   Elizabeth, NJ 07207   (908)994-5000

Nepp, Mark E., DO {1023037157} EmrgMd, GenPrc(82,NJ75)
+ 19 Furlong Drive
  Cherry Hill, NJ 08003   (856)858-1996

Neri, Linda M., MD {1033256151} Surgry(85,PA09)<NJ-RBAY-OLDB, NJ-JFKMED>
+ 225 May Street/Suite B
  Edison, NJ 08837   (732)738-9292   Fax (732)738-9414
  lindaneri@yahoo.com

Nervi, Stephen James, MD {1487859104} Dermat
+ Dermatology Associates-Livingston
  201 South Livingston Avenue/Suite 1F   Livingston, NJ 07039   (973)994-1170   Fax (973)994-1052
+ Natural Image Skin Center
  108 Bilby Road/Suite 202   Hackettstown, NJ 07840   (973)994-1170   Fax (908)441-2402

Nes, Deana Teplitsky, DO {1851710040} Rheuma
+ Bergen Medical Associates
  466 Old Hook Road/Suite 1   Emerson, NJ 07630   (201)967-8221   Fax (201)967-0340

Neshin, Susan F., MD {1821203316} Addctn, PsyAdd, NrlgAddM(79,MI01)<NJ-EASTORNG>
+ Jersey Shore Addiction Services
  685 Neptune Boulevard/Suite 101   Neptune, NJ 07753

Ness, Seth Lawrence, MD {1013189083} Pedtrc(98,NY46)
+ 10 Marcy Place
  West Orange, NJ 07052

Nestampower, Mindy Lyn, MD {1851476626} Anesth(92,NY03)<NJ-HOLYNAME>
+ Advanced Pain Management of North Jersey LLC
  350 Ramapo Valley Road   Oakland, NJ 07436   (201)644-7700   Fax (201)644-7195

Nesteruk, Tetyana, MD {1598076242} IntrMd<NJ-VIRTVOOR>
+ Virtua Voorhees
  100 Bowman Drive/4th Floor   Voorhees, NJ 08043   (856)247-3000

Netravali, Chitra Arun, MD {1821198177} Pedtrc(72,INA69)<NJ-NWRKBETH>
+ Newark Department of Health and Human Services
  110 William Street/Pediatrics   Newark, NJ 07102   (973)733-4382

Netta, Denise Ann, MD {1508987041} ObsGyn, MtFtMd, IntrMd(93,NJ05)<NJ-MORRISTN, NJ-OVERLOOK>
+ Maternal Fetal Medicine of Practice Associates
  11 Overlook Road/Suite LL 102   Summit, NJ 07901   (908)522-3846   Fax (908)522-5557

Neuberger, Alina P., MD {1346445897} FamMed
+ Concentra Medical Centers
  30 Seaview Drive/Suite 2   Secaucus, NJ 07094   (201)319-1611   Fax (201)319-1233
  alinapc@yahoo.com

Neubrander, James A., MD {1275753063} GenPrc, GPrvMd(75,CA12)
+ 485A US Highway 1 S/Suite 320
  Iselin, NJ 08830

Neugeborn, Ian Scott, MD {1841465010} Anesth<NJ-HACKNSK>
+ Hackensack University Medical Center
  30 Prospect Avenue   Hackensack, NJ 07601   (201)996-2419   Fax (201)996-3962

Neuman, Jane Elaine, MD {1811092695} IntrMd(89,AUS01)<NJ-MONMOUTH>
+ 257 Monmouth Road/Building A Suite 2
  Oakhurst, NJ 07755   (732)222-2021   Fax (732)531-4184

Neuman, Joel David, MD {1164420436} RadDia(86,FL02)
+ Radiology Affiliates of Central New Jersey, P.A.
  2501 Kuser Road   Hamilton, NJ 08691   (609)585-8800   Fax (609)585-1825

Neuman, Steven Scott, MD {1609170430} PhysMd
+ Drs. Neuman & Dambeck
  700 Highway 71/Suite 2   Sea Girt, NJ 08750   (732)974-8100   Fax (732)974-9125

Neumann, Lisa Petriccione, DO {1306809975} FamMed(90,NJ75)
+ 409 Main Street
  Toms River, NJ 08753   (732)974-0700   Fax (732)557-6900

Neusidl, William B., MD {1881637510} Ophthl(84,PA13)<NJ-WARREN, PA-EASTON>
+ Coventry Eye Associates, P.C.
  800 Coventry Drive   Phillipsburg, NJ 08865   (908)859-6055   Fax (908)859-2042
  wneusidl@enter.net
+ Coventry Eye Associates, P.C.
  10 Brass Castle Road   Washington, NJ 07882   (908)859-4268

Neustadt, Charles M., MD {1376714618} Anesth(04,NJ06)
+ Robert Wood Johnson-UMDNJ Anesthesia Group
  125 Paterson Street/CAB 3100   New Brunswick, NJ 08901   (732)235-7827   Fax (732)235-6131

Neustadter, Lawrence M., DO {1629040217} RadDia(81,PA77)<NJ-SJHREGMC>
+ SJH Regional Medical Center
  1505 West Sherman Avenue   Vineland, NJ 08360   (856)641-8000

Physicians by Name and Address

Neuwirth, Safrir, MD {1871519405} ObsGyn, IntrMd(95,NY47)<NJ-CENTRAST>
+ **Women's Physicians & Surgeons**
  501 Iron Bridge Road/Suite 10   Freehold, NJ 07728   (732)431-2999   Fax (732)431-2993
+ **Women's Physicians & Surgeons**
  510 Bridge Plaza Drive   Englishtown, NJ 07726   (732)431-2999   Fax (732)536-4570
+ **Women's Physicians & Surgeons**
  245A Main Street   Matawan, NJ 07728   (732)566-9466   Fax (732)566-0343

Nevado, Jose A., MD {1962571661} Pedtrc, PedCrC(76,PER05)<NJ-UMDNJ>
+ **University Hospital**
  150 Bergen Street/Pediatrics   Newark, NJ 07103   (973)972-4300   Fax (973)972-7597
  nevadoja@umdnj.edu

Neveling, Lance William, DO {1255369369} FamMed(98,NJ75)
+ **Collingwood Family Practice**
  600 Atlantic Avenue   Collingswood, NJ 08108   (856)854-1050   Fax (856)854-5325

Nevin, Marie Eithne, MD {1285718239} EnDbMt, IntrMd(86,NJ05)<NJ-MORRISTN>
+ **Summit Medical Group**
  95 Madison Avenue/Suite B   Morristown, NJ 07960   (973)775-5151   Fax (973)267-5521

Nevins, John J., DO {1316987480} FamMed(87,NY75)<NJ-STPETER, NJ-RWJUBRUN>
+ **Chatham Family Practice Associates**
  492 Main Street   Chatham, NJ 07928   (732)828-5962

Nevins, Sol, MD {1063468965} EmrgMd(74,IL02)<NJ-MORRISTN>
+ **Morristown Medical Center**
  100 Madison Avenue/EmrgMed   Morristown, NJ 07962   (973)971-5000
+ **Emergency Medical Associates of NJ, P.A.**
  3 Century Drive   Parsippany, NJ 07054   (973)971-5000   Fax (973)740-9895

New, Deena R., MD {1114184025} Anesth(04,NY08)<NJ-RBAYPERT>
+ **Raritan Bay Medical Center/Perth Amboy Division**
  530 New Brunswick Avenue/Anesth   Perth Amboy, NJ 08861   (732)442-3700

Newell, Glenn C., MD {1841390150} IntrMd, Nephro(81,DOM02)<NJ-COOPRUMC>
+ **Cooper University Hospital**
  One Cooper Plaza/Hospitalist   Camden, NJ 08103   (856)342-3150   Fax (856)968-8573
+ **Cooper Neurological Institute**
  3 Cooper Plaza/Suite 104   Camden, NJ 08103   (856)342-3150   Fax (856)968-8697

Newkirk, Christine L., MD {1245335058} IntrMd<NJ-VIRTMHBC>
+ **Virtua Memorial**
  175 Madison Avenue   Mount Holly, NJ 08060   (609)267-0700

Newkirk, Kenneth Allen, MD {1750379020} Otlryg, SrgOnc
+ **Coastal Ear Nose and Throat LLC**
  3700 Route 33/Suite 101   Neptune, NJ 07753   (703)282-7074   Fax (732)280-7815
  otorhino66@gmail.com
+ **Coastal Ear Nose and Throat LLC**
  1301 Route 72/Suite 340   Manahawkin, NJ 08050   (703)282-7074   Fax (732)280-7815

Newman, Bernard P., III, MD {1316931744} SrgOrt, SrgSpn(80,NY01)<NJ-HACKNSK>
+ **Orthopedic Spine and Sports Medicine Center**
  2 Forest Avenue   Paramus, NJ 07652   (201)587-1111   Fax (201)587-8192

Newman, Brian F., MD {1053399147} Surgry(80,NY09)<NJ-NWT-NMEM>
+ **Medical & Surgical Specialty Group**
  135 Newton Sparta Road/Suite 201   Newton, NJ 07860   (973)383-6244   Fax (973)383-0573

Newman, Brigitte Jeanne, MD {1487681813} Pedtrc(73,FRAN)<NY-PRSBWEIL>
+ **Tribeca Pediatrics**
  9 McWilliams Place   Jersey City, NJ 07302   (201)706-7175   Fax (201)604-6553

Newman, David M., MD {1639115850} Ophthl(83,PA13)
+ **PO Box 639**
  Millburn, NJ 07041   (973)912-4433

Newman, Frederic R., MD {1164431490} Ophthl(70,NY09)<NJ-VALLEY>
+ **654 Lafayette Avenue**
  Hawthorne, NJ 07506   (973)423-4400   Fax (973)423-5643

Newman, Jared Brad, DO {1093806010} FamMed(00,MO79)<NJ-RWJUBRUN, NJ-UNVMCPRN>
+ **Garden State Heart Care, P.C.**
  333 Forsgate Drive/Suite 205   Jamesburg, NJ 08831   (732)521-1210   Fax (732)521-1239

Newman, Rita Grant, MD {1952649766} AnesCrCr
+ **8 Dale Avenue**
  Pompton Plains, NJ 07444   (973)835-3466   Fax (973)835-3466

Newman, Schuyler, MD {1528002136} Pthlgy, PthACl, PthAna(85,PA02)<MA-ARDHILL>
+ **Histopathology Services, LLC.**
  535 East Crescent Avenue   Ramsey, NJ 07446   (201)661-7280   Fax (201)661-7297

Newman, Sheila F., MD {1578501433} ObsGyn(90,NY19)<NJ-CHILTON>
+ **Valley Health Medical Group**
  759 Hamburg Turnpike/Gynocology   Wayne, NJ 07470   (913)709-0020   Fax (973)709-0201

Newman, Stephen L., MD {1164497129} CritCr, IntrMd, PulDis(77,NY46)<NJ-COMMED>
+ **35 Beaverson Boulevard/Suite 7-C**
  Brick, NJ 08723   (732)920-8022   Fax (732)920-8066

Newman, Suzanne Maria, MD {1558367383} EmrgMd(94,MO46)
+ **Emergency Physician Associates, P.A.**
  307 South Evergreen Avenue/PO Box 298   Woodbury, NJ 08096   (856)848-3817   Fax (856)848-1431

Newrock, William J., MD {1548361660} FamMed(85,ITA07)
+ **Rutgers Hurtado Health Center**
  11 Bishop Place   New Brunswick, NJ 08901   (732)932-7402   Fax (732)932-1223

Newton, Dean A., DO {1164535241} FamMed(89,IA75)
+ **6500 Madison Avenue/Suite 8**
  Merchantville, NJ 08109   (856)910-8889   Fax (856)910-8755

Neyman, Gregory, MD {1093910713} EmrgMd
+ **66 West Gilbert Road**
  Red Bank, NJ 07701

Ng, Alan S., MD {1154525285} PainInvt, PainMd, PhysMd(03,OH06)<NJ-RIVERVW>
+ **670 North Beers Street**
  Holmdel, NJ 07733   (732)847-3163   Fax (732)847-3367

Ng, Arthur F., MD {1053352534} Surgry, SrgThr(88,NY46)<NJ-DEBRAHLC, NJ-COOPRUMC>
+ **Cardiac Surgery Group, P.A.**
  20 Prospect Avenue/Suite 900   Hackensack, NJ 07601   (201)996-2261   Fax (201)343-0609
  Ang@hackensack.org

Ng, Elena M., MD {1730269218} Ophthl, VitRet(83,NY46)<NJ-CENTRAST, NJ-MONMOUTH>
+ **Millennium Eye Care, LLC**
  500 West Main Street   Freehold, NJ 07728   (732)462-8707   Fax (732)462-1296
+ **Millennium Eye Care, LLC**
  Route 130 & Princeton Road   Hightstown, NJ 08520   (732)462-8707   Fax (609)448-4197
+ **Millennium Eye Care, LLC**
  515 Brick Boulevard/Suite G   Brick, NJ 08723   (732)920-3800   Fax (732)920-5351

Ng, Joshua M., MD {1700198777} RadDia
+ **Hackensack Radiology Group, P.A.**
  30 Prospect Avenue   Hackensack, NJ 07601   (201)996-2200   Fax (201)489-2812

Ng, June Hoi Ka, MD {1427551852} ObsGyn<NJ-RWJUBRUN>
+ **RWJ University Hospital New Brunswick**
  One Robert Wood Johnson Place   New Brunswick, NJ 08901   (732)828-3000

Ng, Kevin, MD {1174936736} InfDis
+ **Infectious Disease Physicians PA**
  1001 Briggs Road/Suite 250   Mount Laurel, NJ 08054   (856)866-7466   Fax (856)866-9088

Ng, Manyan, MD {1821027178} Pedtrc(97,NY06)
+ **Advocare Woolwich Pediatrics**
  300 Lexington Road/Suite 200   Woolwich Township, NJ 08085   (856)241-2111   Fax (856)241-2243

Ng, Tommy K., MD {1750345237} CdvDis, IntrMd, IntCrd(83,CHNA)<NJ-DEBRAHLC>
+ **Deborah Heart and Lung Center**
  200 Trenton Road   Browns Mills, NJ 08015   (609)893-6611   Fax (609)735-0175

Ng, Yuk Bing, MD {1760562946}<NJ-UNVMCPRN>
+ **University Medical Center of Princeton at Plainsboro**
  One Plainsboro Road   Plainsboro, NJ 08536   (609)497-4000

Ngai, Ivan Manjun, MD {1053615690} ObsGyn, MtFtMd(07,NY03)
+ **Totowal Maternal Fetal Medicine**
  525 Union Boulevard   Totowa, NJ 07512   (973)904-9778

Ngai, Pakkay, MD {1144273178} Pedtrc, PedPul, SlpDis(95,NY19)<NJ-HACKNSK>
+ **Hackensack University Medical Center**
  30 Prospect Avenue/WFAN Blg/3rd Fl   Hackensack, NJ 07601   (201)996-5207   Fax (201)996-4969

Ngeow, Swee Jian, MD {1952568248} OncHem, IntrMd
+ **Hunterdon Regional Cancer Ctr**
  2100 Wescott Drive   Flemington, NJ 08822   (908)788-6461   Fax (908)788-6412

Nghiem, George T., DO {1245263771} FamMed, IntrMd(92,MO78)
+ **Regional HealthCare Associates**
  5201 West Route 38/Suite 115   Pennsauken, NJ 08109   (856)438-5166   Fax (856)879-2025
  Docgnghiem@yahoo.com

Ngo, Gerald, MD {1326427220} IntrMd
+ **Morristown Medical Center**
  100 Madison Avenue   Morristown, NJ 07962   (973)971-5000

Ngo, Ly Thien, MD {1003077074} IntrMd(NY46<NJ-VIRTBERL, NJ-VIRTMARL>
+ **Virtua Nurosciences**
  200 Bowman Drive/Suite E-385   Voorhees, NJ 08043   (856)247-7770   Fax (856)247-7766

Ngu, Michael Foleng, MD {1215167960} IntHos, InsrMd<NJ-MEMSALEM>
+ **Memorial Hospital of Salem County**
  310 Woodstown Road   Salem, NJ 08079   (856)935-1000

Nguy, Steven Tri, MD {1336249523} IntrMd(94,PA13)<NJ-COOPRUMC>
+ **The Cooper Hospital System-Univ Hospital**
  3 Cooper Plaza/Suite 215   Camden, NJ 08103   (856)342-2439

Nguyen, Ann Phuong Duy, MD {1164415865} EmrgMd, IntrMd(98,QU01)<NJ-HACKNSK>
+ **Hackensack University Medical Center**
  30 Prospect Avenue/Main 3619   Hackensack, NJ 07601   (551)996-3192

Nguyen, Bac Xuan, MD {1295700326} FamMed(98,NH01)<NJ-UNDRWD>
+ **Underwood-Memorial Hospital Family Health Center**
  1120 North Delsea Drive   Glassboro, NJ 08028   (856)582-0500   Fax (856)582-0163
+ **Complete Care Family Medicine**
  75 West Red Bank Avenue/FamResidency   Woodbury, NJ 08096   (856)582-0500   Fax (856)686-5218

Nguyen, Bao D., MD {1871531087} IntrMd, FamMed(74,VIE05)<NJ-VIRTBERL>
+ **2706 Westfield Avenue**
  Camden, NJ 08105   (856)964-2801   Fax (856)964-2080

Nguyen, David Huong, MD {1972808459} PhysMd
+ **Englewood Orthopedic Associates**
  401 South Van Brunt Street   Englewood, NJ 07631   (201)569-2770   Fax (201)569-1774

Nguyen, Han Ngoc, MD {1164606158} IntrMd, InfDis(03,GRN01)<NJ-UMDNJ>
+ **Infectious Disease Associates of Northern NJ**
  255 West Spring Valley/Suite 100   Maywood, NJ 07607   (201)881-0107

Nguyen, Hoan-Vu Tran, MD {1922067909} SrgOrt, Surgry(99,PA13)<NJ-JRSYSHMC, NJ-OCEANMC>
+ **Seaview Orthopaedics**
  1200 Eagle Avenue   Ocean, NJ 07712   (732)660-6200   Fax (732)660-6201
+ **Seaview Orthopaedics**
  1640 Route 88 West   Brick, NJ 08724   (732)660-6200   Fax (732)458-2743

Nguyen, Hung Manh, MD {1942225479} Pedtrc(74,VIE05)<NJ-RBAYOLDB, NJ-RBAYPERT>
+ **760 Amboy Avenue**
  Edison, NJ 08837   (732)661-0966   Fax (732)738-4661

Nguyen, Hung Q., MD {1295890564} Surgry, SrgOnc(90,MO34)<NJ-BAYSHORE>
+ **668 North Beers Street/Suite 101**
  Holmdel, NJ 07733   (732)888-9400   Fax (732)888-9501

Nguyen, Jim A., DO {1346554110} FamMed
+ **70 Greene Street/Apt 3603**
  Jersey City, NJ 07302   (609)335-4985

Nguyen, Jonathan Huy, DO {1285945428} GenPrc
+ **Rowan University-School of Osteopathic Medicine**
  1 Medical Center Drive   Stratford, NJ 08084   (856)566-7121   Fax (856)566-6222

Nguyen, Khanh Q., MD {1235143892} Anesth(90,PA14)<NJ-RIVERVW>
+ **Riverview Medical Center**
  1 Riverview Plaza/Anesthesiology   Red Bank, NJ 07701   (732)741-2700

Nguyen, Maria Bich Thi, DO {1841487485} ObsGyn, SrgLap(NJ75
+ **Rowan SOM Department of Ob/Gyn**
  405 Hurffville-Cross Keys Road   Sewell, NJ 08080   (856)589-1414   Fax (856)256-5772

Nguyen, Matthew Thai-Khang, MD {1922322411} EmrgMd(10,TX04)<RI-SJFATIMA>
+ **Emergency Medical Associates of NJ, P.A.**
  3 Century Drive   Parsippany, NJ 07054   (973)740-0607   Fax (973)740-9895

Nguyen, Steven M., MD {1609166461} FamMed
+ **Allied Medical Associates**
  510 Hamburg Turnpike   Wayne, NJ 07470   (973)942-6005   Fax (973)942-6009

Nguyen, Truc H., MD {1912173980} Ophthl(03,NY15)
+ **Quality Eye Center**
  2020 New Road   Linwood, NJ 08221   (609)927-2020   Fax (609)926-7616

Nia, Hamid Mohammad, MD {1073778429} CdvDis, IntrMd(93,IRA01)<NJ-STJOSHOS>
  + Advanced Cardiovascular Interventions, PA
    20 Prospect Avenue/Suite 615   Hackensack, NJ 07601
    (201)265-5700   Fax (551)996-0774
  + Advanced Cardiovascular Interventions PA
    20-19 Fair Lawn Avenue   Fair Lawn, NJ 07410   (201)265-5700

Niazi, Mohammad Zafar, MD {1639377229} Psychy(97,PAK24)<NJ-BERGNMC>
  + 2 Homested Place
    Bergenfield, NJ 07621

Niazi, Mumtaz A., MD {1528087509} IntrMd(97,PAK24)<NJ-STCLRDEN, NJ-STCLRDOV>
  + 185 South Orange Avenue/MSBH 254
    Newark, NJ 07103   (973)972-5252   Fax (973)972-3144

Niazi, Osama Tariq, DO {1588953285} IntrMd<NJ-UMDNJ>
  + University Hospital
    150 Bergen Street   Newark, NJ 07103   (973)972-6056

Nicastro, Maryann, MD {1891751293} EnDbMt, IntrMd(88,NJ05)<NJ-OVERLOOK>
  + 4 Fieldstone Court
    East Hanover, NJ 07936

Nicholas, Paul George, III, DO {1609898022} FamMed(81,IA75)<NJ-MEMSALEM>
  + 24 East Avenue/PO Box 304
    Woodstown, NJ 08098   (856)769-0900   Fax (856)769-2639

Nicholas, Thomas, MD {1629095237} Anesth, PainInvt(88,MEX03)<NY-CMCSTVSI>
  + Jersey Shore Anesthesiology Associates
    1945 Route 33/PO Box 397   Neptune, NJ 07754   (732)922-3308   Fax (732)897-0263
  + Jersery Shore Anesthesiology
    1945 Highway 33   Neptune, NJ 07753   (732)922-3308   Fax (732)897-0263

Nicholls, Brian Robert, DO {1841244365} EmrgMd(98,NJ75)<NJ-ACMCITY, NJ-ACMCMAIN>
  + AtlantiCare Regional Medical Center/City Campus
    1925 Pacific Avenue/EmergMed   Atlantic City, NJ 08401   (609)345-4000
  + AtlantiCare Regional Med Ctr/Mainland
    65 West Jimmie Leeds Road/EmergMed   Pomona, NJ 08240   (609)652-1000

Nichols, Fred Michael, DO {1982677233} ObsGyn, IntrMd(91,NY75)
  + Womens Total Health LLC
    3317 Route 94   Hamburg, NJ 07419   (973)209-1200   Fax (973)209-1201

Nichols, Rhonda R., MD {1700816360} ObsGyn(77,NJ05)<NJ-JRSYCITY, NJ-MEADWLND>
  + New Margaret Hague Women's Health Institute
    377 Jersey Avenue/Suite 220   Jersey City, NJ 07302   (201)795-9155   Fax (201)795-9157
  + Millburn Professional Group
    187 Millburn Avenue/Suite 3   Millburn, NJ 07041   (973)379-1441

Nickles, Donna E., DO {1063400547} ObsGyn(79,IA75)<NJ-VALLEY>
  + Valley Ob Gyn Associates PA
    80 Eisenhower Drive/Suite 200   Paramus, NJ 07652   (201)843-2800   Fax (201)843-5848

Nickles, Leroy, MD {1710070412} EmrgMd(02,PA14)
  + 257 Wilson Street
    Hackensack, NJ 07601

Nickles, Steven L., DO {1760483051} FamMed(87,IA75)<NJ-VALLEY>
  + Valley Diagnostic Medical Center
    581 North Franklin Turnpike   Ramsey, NJ 07446   (201)327-0500   Fax (201)327-8612

Nicola, Gregory Neal, MD {1396721908} RadDia, RadNro(99,OH06)
  + Hackensack Radiology Group, PA/Corporate
    130 Kinderkamack Road/Suite 200   River Edge, NJ 07661   (201)488-2660
  + Hackensack Radiology Group, P.A.
    30 Prospect Avenue   Hackensack, NJ 07601   (201)488-2660   Fax (201)336-8451

Nicolae, Mona G., MD {1679516991} Psychy, PsyCAd(92)
  + 3 Beechwood Road
    Summit, NJ 07902   Fax (908)363-9977

Nicolai, Michael, MD {1144264029} IntrMd(91,NY09)
  + Denville Associates of Internal Medicine
    16 Pocono Road/Suite 317   Denville, NJ 07834   (973)627-2650   Fax (973)627-8383

Nicolaides, Catherine D., MD {1033415104} Pedtrc(84,PA09)
  + 733 East Route 70
    Marlton, NJ 08053   (856)983-6675   Fax (856)983-5243

Nicolato, Patricia A., DO Surgry(94,MI12)<NJ-DEBRAHLC>
  + Deborah Heart and Lung Center
    200 Trenton Road   Browns Mills, NJ 08015   (609)893-6611

Nicoletta, Marianna, MD {1841523800} Pedtrc<NJ-MORRISTN>
  + Morristown Medical Center
    100 Madison Avenue/Pediatrics   Morristown, NJ 07962   (973)656-6280   Fax (973)290-7495

Nicoll, Anca M., MD {1396832077} IntrMd(65,ROMA)
  + PO Box 419
    West Orange, NJ 07052

Nicoll, Cornelius I., MD {1548364581} SrgOrt(63,ROM01)
  + 33 North Fullerton Avenue
    Montclair, NJ 07042   (973)783-3734   Fax (973)783-0144

Nicolson, Susan C., MD {1255344438} Anesth(76,PA01)<PA-CHILDHOS>
  + CHOP Pediatric & Adolescent Specialty Care Center
    1012 Laurel Oak Road   Voorhees, NJ 08043   (856)435-1300   Fax (856)435-0091

Nicosia, Leonard T., MD {1841246394} ObsGyn(75,MEX03)<NJ-CHILTON>
  + Physicians for Women
    330 Ratzer Road/Suite 7   Wayne, NJ 07470   (973)694-2222   Fax (973)694-7664
  + Wayne Surgical Center, LLC.
    1176 Hamburg Pike   Wayne, NJ 07470   (973)694-2222   Fax (973)709-1901

Nicpon, Christopher B., MD {1588750921} Pedtrc(97,NY03)<NJ-VALLEY>
  + Valley Pediatric Associates PA
    470 North Franklin Turnpike   Ramsey, NJ 07446   (201)891-7272   Fax (201)934-1817
  + Valley Pediatric Associates, P.A.
    201 East Franklin Turnpike   Ho Ho Kus, NJ 07423   (201)891-7272   Fax (201)652-6485

Nidimusili, Amara J., MD {1073935037}
  + 1606 Madaline Drive
    Avenel, NJ 07001

Niedbala, Thomas M., MD {1851390223} RadDia(85,PA09)<NJ-VIRTUAHS, NJ-VIRTMHBC>
  + South Jersey Radiology Associates, P.A.
    901 Route 168/Suites 301-305   Turnersville, NJ 08012   (856)227-6600   Fax (856)227-8537
  + South Jersey Radiology Associates, P.A.
    807 Haddon Avenue/Suite 5   Haddonfield, NJ 08033   (856)227-6600   Fax (856)616-1125
  + South Jersey Radiology Associates, P.A.
    315 Route 70 East/Suite B   Cherry Hill, NJ 08012   (856)428-4344   Fax (856)428-0356

Niedrach, William L., MD {1134190820} Urolgy(84,NY03)
  + New Jersey Urology
    15000 Midlantic Drive/Suite 100   Mount Laurel, NJ 08054   (856)252-1000   Fax (856)985-4582

Niedzwiecki, Stephen Mark, MD {1316961485} Pedtrc(95,NY08)
  + Kids first
    2006 Salem Road   Burlington, NJ 08016   (609)877-1500   Fax (609)877-4262

Nielsen, Earl F., MD {1770550030} IntrMd, Nephro(66,VT02)<NJ-MORRISTN, NJ-STCLRDEN>
  + Internal Medicine Faculty Associates
    435 South Street/Suite 210   Morristown, NJ 07960   (973)971-7165   Fax (973)290-7675

Nielsen, Sarah B., MD {1811081409} Pedtrc, IntrMd(02,NY01)<NJ-VALLEY, NJ-CHILTON>
  + David J. Strader MD, PHD
    799 Bloomfield Avenue/Suite 304   Verona, NJ 07044   (973)618-9990   Fax (973)618-9991

Nielson, Rosemarie, DO {1881128932} IntrMd
  + 557 Adams Avenue/Suite Ff
    Elizabeth, NJ 07201   (646)712-3263

Niemiera, Mark L., MD {1780788109} CdvDis, IntrMd(81,PA09)<NJ-RBAYPERT>
  + 613 Amboy Avenue/Suite 104
    Perth Amboy, NJ 08861   (732)442-1441   Fax (732)442-7684

Nierenberg, Lisa, MD {1184779753} FamMed(79,PA14)<NJ-HUNTRDN>
  + Center for Family Health, LLC.
    431 Route 22 East/Suite 79   Whitehouse Station, NJ 08889   (908)534-5559   Fax (888)256-4023

Nierenberg, Richard J., MD {1477591105} CritCr, EmrgMd, IntrMd(78,CA06)<NJ-HACKNSK>
  + Hackensack University Medical Center
    30 Prospect Avenue/EmrgMed   Hackensack, NJ 07601   (201)996-2300   Fax (201)342-7112

Nieves, David Steiner, MD {1922075068} Dermat(99,PA01)
  + Windsor Dermatology
    59 One Mile Road Extension/Suite G   East Windsor, NJ 08520   (609)443-4500   Fax (609)426-0530   kingdavidonly1@yahoo.com

Nieves, Jeremiah David, MD {1285893578} PhysMd(03,NJ05)<NJ-KSLRWELK>
  + Kessler Institute for Rehab
    201 Pleasant Hill Road/PhysRehab   Chester, NJ 07930   (973)584-7500

Nieves, Luz Celeste, MD {1730447269}<NJ-NWRKBETH>
  + St Joseph's Medical Center Emergency
    703 Main Street   Paterson, NJ 07503   (973)754-2240   Fax (973)754-2249

Niewiadomski, Edward J., MD {1942465646} IntrMd(85,NJ06)<NJ-BURDTMLN>
  + Cape Regional Medical Center
    2 Stone Harbor Boulevard   Cape May Court House, NJ 08210   (609)463-2000

Nigam, Jyoti, MD {1316006315} IntrMd(86,INA43)
  + Medical Associates of Central New Jersey
    26 Throckmorton Lane/1st flr.   Old Bridge, NJ 08857   (732)679-9950   Fax (732)679-9956

Nigro, Mary A., MD {1255311379} OthrSp(80,NJ06)
  + Virtua Berlin
    100 Townsend Avenue   Berlin, NJ 08009   (856)322-3000

Nigro, Peter J., MD OccpMd, FamMed(81,DC02)
  + Merck and Company Incorporated
    1 Merck Drive/PO Box 100/WS1AF-35   Whitehouse Station, NJ 08889   (908)423-1000

Nihalani, Anish B., MD {1447448212} SrgLap, Bariat(00,NJ06)
  + JFK for Life
    98 James Street/Suite 212   Edison, NJ 08820   (732)343-7484

Nihalani, Meena T., MD {1356377261} Pedtrc(75,INAZ6)<NJ-WOODBRDG>
  + Woodbridge Developmental Center
    Rahway Avenue/PO Box 189   Woodbridge, NJ 07095   (732)499-5500   Fax (732)499-5787

Nijhawan, Minakshi, MD {1629088695} IntrMd(89,INA23)<NJ-CENTRAST>
  + 1000 West Main Street
    Freehold, NJ 07728   (732)462-6080   Fax (732)462-8480

Nijhawan, Rohit I., MD {1316237159} Dermat, IntrMd
  + 47 Schindler Court
    Somerset, NJ 08873   (908)240-5937

Nikias, George Andrew, MD {1679585236} Gastrn, IntrMd(89,NY09)<NJ-HACKNSK>
  + Hackensack Gastroenterology Associates
    130 Kinderkamack Road/Suite 301   River Edge, NJ 07661   (201)489-7772   Fax (201)489-2544

Nikodijevic, Vesna, MD {1952497224} Pedtrc(88,SERB)<NJ-MORRISTN, NJ-OVERLOOK>
  + Bernardsville Pediatrics
    40 Morristown Road/Suite 2D   Bernardsville, NJ 07924   (908)766-5960   Fax (866)768-8391
  + Chatham Pediatrics
    12 Parrot Mill Road   Chatham, NJ 07928   (908)766-5960   Fax (973)701-1520

Nikolic, Dejan, MD {1992079750} PthCln<NJ-COOPRUMC>
  + Cooper University Hospital
    One Cooper Plaza   Camden, NJ 08103   (856)356-4924

Niksarli, Kevin K., MD {1376600353} SrgRef, CrnExD, OphthI(93,NY20)<NY-MANHEYE, NY-LENOXHLL>
  + Newsight Laser Center
    2083 Center Avenue/2nd Floor   Fort Lee, NJ 07024

Nillas, Michael S., MD {1649282658} CdvDis, IntrMd(00,GRN01)<NJ-RWJUHAM>
  + Cape Regional Physicians Associates-Cardiology
    217 North Main Street/Suite 205   Cape May Court House, NJ 08210   (609)463-5440   Fax (609)463-9888

Nimchinsky, Esther A., MD {1740485796}
  + 203 West Shearwater Court/Unit 12
    Jersey City, NJ 07305

Nimma, Vijaya, MD {1669573648} Pedtrc(95,INA2Y)
  + Edison Pediatrics
    1802 Oak Tree Road/Suite 101   Edison, NJ 08820   (732)548-3210   Fax (906)548-3966

Nini, Kevin T., MD {1194747964} SrgPlstc, Surgry(84,NJ06)<NJ-STPETER>
  + Plastic Surgery Arts of of New Jersey
    1378 US 206/2nd flr   Skillman, NJ 08558   (609)921-2922   Fax (609)921-0747
  + Plastic Surgery Arts of of New Jersey
    409 Joyce Kilmer Ave./Suite 210   New Brunswick, NJ 08901   (609)921-2922   Fax (732)418-0747

Niranjan, Usha, MD {1396733077} OncHem(77,INA37)<NJ-HCKTSTWN>
  + 108 Bilby Road/Suite 306
    Hackettstown, NJ 07840   (908)813-0790   Fax (908)813-8342

Nirenberg, Elena, MD {1295955219} FamMed(04,PA02)<NJ-VIRTMHBC>
  + Advocare Main Street Medical Associates
    714 East Main Street/Suite 1-C   Moorestown, NJ 08057   (856)778-4009   Fax (856)778-4014

Nisar, Asif, MD {1316911092} IntrMd, Nephro(89,PAK01)<NJ-CHSFULD, NJ-CHSMRCER>
  + Zak Maniya, M.D., P.A.
    2333 Whitehorse-Mercerville Rd/Suite 4   Mercerville, NJ 08619   (609)890-9111   Fax (609)890-6865

Nisar, Asma, MD {1598941007} PsyCAd, Psychy(95,PAK24)<NJ-CARRIER>
  + Carrier Clinic
    252 Route 601   Belle Mead, NJ 08502   (908)281-1000

Physicians by Name and Address

Nisar, Mohammed P., MD {1124114343} IntrMd, MedOnc(65,INDI)<NJ-JFKMED, NJ-VIRTMHBC>
  + Drs. Nisar and Nisar
    1895 Oak Tree Road   Edison, NJ 08820   (732)548-1833   Fax (732)906-3156
  + Drs. Nisar and Nisar
    949 Route 9 North   South Amboy, NJ 08879   (732)721-6260

Nisar, Noor A., MD {1336235571} FamMed(74,INA9A)<NJ-JFKMED>
  + Drs. Nisar and Nisar
    949 Route 9 North   South Amboy, NJ 08879   (732)721-6260
  + Drs. Nisar and Nisar
    1895 Oak Tree Road   Edison, NJ 08820   (732)721-6260   Fax (732)906-3156

Nisar, Sabeeha, MD {1164644597} IntHos, Nephro, IntrMd(95,INA36)<NJ-VIRTMHBC>
  + Virtua Hospitalist Group Memorial
    175 Madison Avenue/1 FL   Mount Holly, NJ 08060   (609)914-6180   Fax (609)914-6182

Nisar, Shiraz Ahmed, MD {1972764314} IntrMd
  + Drs. Nisar and Nisar
    1895 Oak Tree Road   Edison, NJ 08820   (732)548-1833   Fax (732)906-3156

Nishimura, Takashi, MD {1487887881} SrgThr, SrgCTh(03,JAP39)<NY-PRSBWEIL>
  + Robert Wood Johnson Surgery
    One Robert Wood Johnson Place/MEB 596   New Brunswick, NJ 08901   (732)235-7642   Fax (732)235-8727

Nissenbaum, Gerald Aubbie, MD {1144240565} RadDia, NuclMd(70,WI05)<NJ-OURLADY>
  + Our Lady of Lourdes Medical Center
    1600 Haddon Avenue   Camden, NJ 08103   (856)757-3827

Nissenblatt, Michael J., MD {1467441352} MedOnc, OncHem(73,NY01)<NJ-RWJUBRUN, NJ-STPETER>
  + Central Jersey Oncology Center, P.A.
    Brier Hill Court/Building J-2   East Brunswick, NJ 08816   (732)390-7750   Fax (732)390-7725
  + Regional Cancer Care Associates - Central Jersey Div
    454 Elizabeth Avenue/Suite 240   Somerset, NJ 08873   (732)390-7750   Fax (732)390-7725
  + Central Jersey Oncology Center, P.A.
    205 Easton Avenue   New Brunswick, NJ 08816   (732)828-9570   Fax (732)828-7638

Nissirios, Kalliopi, MD {1073927679} Psychy<NJ-BERGNMC>
  + New Bridge Medical Center
    230 East Ridgewood Avenue   Paramus, NJ 07652   (201)967-4000

Nitche, Jason Adam, MD {1700050978} SrgOrt(03,NJ05)
  + Brielle Orthopedics PA
    457 Jack Martin Boulevard   Brick, NJ 08724   (732)840-7500   Fax (732)840-2088
  + Brielle Orthopedics PA
    823 Lacey Road   Forked River, NJ 08731   (732)840-7500   Fax (732)840-2088
  + Brielle Orthopedics PA
    1301 Route 72 West   Manahawkin, NJ 08724   (609)971-7616   Fax (609)971-7639

Nitschmann-Schmoll, Cynthia A., DO {1922144435} FamMed(82,PA77)<NJ-SOCEANCO>
  + Family Medicine Center
    1301 Route 72 West/Suite 240   Manahawkin, NJ 08050   (609)597-7394   Fax (609)597-6833
  + Family Medicine Center
    279 Mathistown Road   Little Egg Harbor, NJ 08087   (609)296-1101

Nitti, David J., MD {1750499158} IntrMd(84,ITA19)<NJ-VALLEY>
  + 179 Lafayette Avenue
    Hawthorne, NJ 07506   (973)427-7243   Fax (973)427-9376

Nitti, Joseph T., MD {1518946128} IntrMd(79,MEXI)<NJ-OCEANMC, NJ-JRSYSHMC>
  + Jersey Shore University Medical Center
    1945 Route 33   Neptune, NJ 07753   (732)776-4790   Fax (732)776-4690

Nitti, Michele, DO {1316008964} FamMed(88,NJ75)<NJ-MTN-SIDE, NJ-MORRISTN>
  + Franklin Pediatrics, PA
    91 South Jefferson Road/Suite 200   Whippany, NJ 07981   (973)538-6116   Fax (973)538-3712
  + Montclair Family Practice
    230 Sherman Avenue/Suite C   Glen Ridge, NJ 07028   (973)538-6116   Fax (973)259-0600
  + Summit Medical Group
    140 Park Avenue/3rd Floor   Florham Park, NJ 07981   (908)273-4300

Nituica, Cristina Magadalena, MD {1710131453} Surgry, WundCr, SrgBst(96,ROM09)<NJ-SJHREGMC, NJ-SJRSYELM>
  + South Jersey HealthCare Breast & General Surgery
    2950 College Drive/Suite 1A   Vineland, NJ 08360   (856)641-8697   Fax (856)507-0233

Nitz, Shelly, MD {1073929956} ObsGyn
  + Valley Center for Women's Health
    581 North Franklin Turnpike/2nd Floor   Ramsey, NJ 07446   (201)236-2100   Fax (201)236-5269

Nitzberg, Richard S., MD {1306818778} SrgVas, Surgry(83,MA01)<NJ-OVERLOOK, NJ-MORRISTN>
  + Summit Medical Group-Berkeley Heights Campus
    1 Diamond Hill Road/4th Fl   Berkeley Heights, NJ 07922   (908)277-8950   Fax (908)673-7350

Niu, Weiwei, MD {1528194719} PthACl, PthHem(85,CHN25)
  + Quest Diagnostics Inc.
    1 Malcolm Avenue   Teterboro, NJ 07608   (201)393-5925   Fax (201)393-6127

Niver, Genghis Erjan, MD {1578747739} OrtSHand
  + Summit Medical Group Orthopedics and Sports Medicine
    140 Park Avenue/2nd Floor   Florham Park, NJ 07932   (973)404-9800   Fax (973)267-7295

Nivera, Noel Taroy, MD {1124034400} IntrMd, Nephro(93,PHI02)<NJ-RIVERVW, NJ-HLTHSRE>
  + Hypertension & Nephrology Association, PA
    6 Industrial Way West/Suite B   Eatontown, NJ 07724   (732)460-1200   Fax (732)460-1211

Niyogi, Sayani, DO {1295092096}
  + Riverside Medical Group
    714 Tenth Street/Suite 2   Secaucus, NJ 07094   (201)293-4030   Fax (201)865-0015

Nizam, Mohammed Farrukh, MD {1326145764} Nrolgy, NrlgSpec(84,PAKI)
  + ENT & Allergy Associates, LLP
    98 James Street/Suite 301   Edison, NJ 08820   (732)494-0100   Fax (732)494-0114
  + ENT & Allergy Associates, LLP
    503 Omni Drive   Hillsborough, NJ 08844   (732)494-0100

Nizam, Zeba S., MD {1598862930} Psychy, PsyGrt(88,PAK11)<NJ-RWJUBRUN>
  + UH-University Behavioral Hlth
    100 Metroplex Drive/Suite 200   Edison, NJ 08817   (732)235-8400   Fax (732)235-8395
  + University Behavioral Health Care
    667 Hoes Lane   Piscataway, NJ 08854

Nizin, Joel S., MD {1972599025} SrgC&R, Surgry, IntrMd(78,DC03)<NJ-CHILTON, NJ-VALLEY>
  + Valley Medical Group Colorectal Surgery
    1124 East Ridgewood Avenue/Suite 202   Ridgewood, NJ 07450   (201)689-9100   Fax (201)689-9108
  + North Jersey Colon & Rectal Surgery Associates, LLC.
    85 Harristown Road   Glen Rock, NJ 07452   (201)689-9100   Fax (201)689-9108

Niziol, John A., MD {1700889268} Pedtrc(72,MD01)
  + Notchview Pediatrics, LLC.
    1037 Route 46 East/Suite 201   Clifton, NJ 07013   (973)779-3911   Fax (973)471-2730

Nkwonta, Joyce O., MD {1467408047} IntrMd(90,NIG03)<NJ-TRINIWSC, NJ-JFKMED>
  + 1314 Park Avenue/Suite 3
    Plainfield, NJ 07060   (908)561-9733   Fax (908)561-8944

Nnaeto, Nkem V., MD {1215999735} Pedtrc(90,NIG02)<NJ-STBARNMC, NJ-NWRKBETH>
  + Universal Pediatrics
    132 Halsted Street   East Orange, NJ 07018   (973)674-0036   Fax (973)674-0322

Nnewihe, Adebola Oyeronke, MD {1154530301} ObsGyn(03,OH06)<NJ-SHOREMEM>
  + 611 New Road
    Northfield, NJ 08225   (609)383-4042   Fax (715)804-5095
  + Reliance Medical Group, LLC.
    22 North Franklin Boulevard   Pleasantville, NJ 08232   (609)383-4042   Fax (609)272-9055
  + Reliance Medical Group, LLC
    331 East Jimmie Leeds Road/Suite 1 & 2   Galloway, NJ 08225   (609)652-6016   Fax (609)652-2406

Nnewihe, Charles Obinna, MD {1760419097} IntrMd, Nephro(03,OH06)<NJ-ACMCITY>
  + Regional Nephrology Associates
    510 Jackson Avenue   Northfield, NJ 08225   (609)383-0200   Fax (609)383-8352

Noah, Jane S., MD {1821068115} ObsGyn(90,PA07)<NJ-VIRTVOOR>
  + Cherry Hill Ob/Gyn
    150 Century Parkway/Suite A   Mount Laurel, NJ 08054   (856)778-4700   Fax (856)778-1154
  + Cherry Hill Ob/Gyn
    777 South White Horse Pike/Suite A-1   Hammonton, NJ 08037   (856)778-4700   Fax (609)561-6309

Noaz, Golam G., MD {1992831929} Pedtrc(70,BAN02)<NJ-JRSYSHMC, NJ-MONMOUTH>
  + Ocean Pediatric Group
    1 Industrial Way West/Suite 1-C   Eatontown, NJ 07724   (732)542-6451   Fax (732)542-1654
  + Ocean Pediatric Group
    2640 Route 70/Suite 1-B   Manasquan, NJ 08736   (732)542-6451   Fax (732)223-5792

Noble, Mary C., MD {1962534404} FamMed, GPrvMd, PubHth(86,NJ06)
  + Capital Health Family Health Center
    433 Bellevue Avenue/4th Floor   Trenton, NJ 08618   (609)815-7296   Fax (609)815-7178

Nobleza, Deanna Jean Dar Juan, MD {1851499586} IntrMd, Psychy(99,NJ06)<NJ-UNIVBHC, NJ-UNVMCPRN>
  + McCosh Health Center
    Washington Road/McCosh Infirmary   Princeton, NJ 08544   (609)258-5357   Fax (609)258-1355

Nocchi, David Martin, MD {1215965942} EmrgMd(97,PA13)<NJ-COOPRUMC>
  + Cooper University Hospital
    One Cooper Plaza/EmrgMed   Camden, NJ 08103   (856)968-7433   Fax (856)968-8499

Noce, Louis Arthur, MD {1669636833} SrgNro(01,NY46)
  + Summit Medical Group
    140 Park Avenue/3rd Floor   Florham Park, NJ 07932   (908)273-4300

Nochlin Soto, David, MD {1457351793} PthNro(72,MEX62)<NJ-JFKMED>
  + JFK Neurosciences Institute
    65 James Street/Second Floor   Edison, NJ 08818   (732)321-7010   Fax (732)205-1477   dnochlin@solarishs.org

Nochumson, Joshua Alan, MD {1740481407} SrgC&R, Surgry, IntrMd(03,TX12)<NJ-CHILTON>
  + Chilton Medical Center
    97 West Parkway/Surgery/ColoRec   Pompton Plains, NJ 07444   (973)831-5063   Fax (973)290-7495

Noel, Christopher Bartlett, MD {1649699547} EmrgMd
  + Cooper Univerisry Emergency Physicians
    One Cooper Plaza   Camden, NJ 08103   (856)342-2000   Fax (856)968-8272

Noel, Gary J., MD {1841456282} PedInf, Pedtrc(80,NY20)<NY-PRSBWEIL, NY-NYPRESHS>
  + 16 Highland Drive
    North Caldwell, NJ 07006

Noff, Tom, MD {1346582277} ClNrPh
  + The Cooper Hospital System-Univ Hospital
    3 Cooper Plaza/Suite 215   Camden, NJ 08103   (856)342-2439   Fax (856)968-8703

Nogueira, John Francis, Jr., MD {1578513743} ClNrPh, Nrolgy(00,NY47)
  + Hackensack Neurology Group
    211 Essex Street/Suite 202   Hackensack, NJ 07601   (201)488-1515   Fax (201)488-9471

Noh, Robert E., MD {1962417303} Urolgy(92,NJ06)
  + Urological Assoc of Central Jersey
    2177 Oak Tree Road   Edison, NJ 08820

Nolan, John P., DO {1932142031} PhysMd, IntrMd(85,NJ75)<NJ-OURLADY>
  + Associated Physiatrists of Southern New Jersey
    1600 Haddon Avenue/Room R-122   Camden, NJ 08103   (856)757-3878   Fax (856)365-4010
  + ASPSNJ The Arthritis Center
    215 East Laurel Road   Stratford, NJ 08084   (856)757-3878   Fax (856)757-3760

Nolan, John P., Jr., MD {1417953258} SrgOrt(82,PA02)<NJ-CHS-FULD, NJ-CHSMRCER>
  + Mercer-Bucks Orthopaedics PC
    3120 Princeton Pike   Lawrenceville, NJ 08648   (609)896-0444   Fax (609)896-1055
  + Mercer-Bucks Orthopaedics, P.C.
    2501 Kuser Road   Hamilton, NJ 08691   (609)896-0444   Fax (609)587-4349

Nolasco, Cesar V., MD {1235112681} Anesth(78,PHI08)<NJ-HACKNSK>
  + Hackensack University MC-Anesthesia Dept
    30 Prospect Avenue/Room 2703   Hackensack, NJ 07601   (201)996-2419   Fax (201)996-3962
  + Hackensack University Medical Center
    30 Prospect Avenue/Anesth   Hackensack, NJ 07601   (201)996-2419   Fax (201)488-6769

Nolasco, Edwin V., MD {1396728424} Anesth(81,PHI08)<NJ-HACKNSK>
  + Hackensack University MC-Anesthesia Dept
    30 Prospect Avenue/Room 2703   Hackensack, NJ 07601   (201)996-2419   Fax (201)996-3962
  + Hackensack University Medical Center
    30 Prospect Avenue/Anesth   Hackensack, NJ 07601   (201)996-2419   Fax (201)488-6769

Noll, Bruce R., MD {1285666537} ObsGyn(74,MEX03)<NJ-BURDTMLN>
  + 108 Mechanic Street
    Cape May Court House, NJ 08210   (609)465-7557   Fax (609)465-9383
  + Court House Surgery Center
    106 Courthouse South Dennis Rd   Cape May, NJ 08204   (609)465-7557   Fax (609)465-8771

Noll, Donald R., DO {1093708067} Grtrcs
+ New Jersey Institute for Successful Aging
42 East Laurel Road/Suite 1800   Stratford, NJ 08084
(856)566-6843   Fax (856)566-6419

Noll, Michael Andrew, MD {1174892178} FamMed, IntrMd(09,DMN01)
+ RWJ University Hospital New Brunswick
One Robert Wood Johnson Place   New Brunswick, NJ 08901
(908)685-3732   Fax (732)235-7001

Nolledo, Michael Teodoro, MD {1154367563} CritCr, PulDis, IntrMd(92,PHI02)<NJ-STPETER, NJ-RWJUBRUN>
+ 15 Dayna Lane
Lawrenceville, NJ 08648

Nolte, Charles Henry, III, DO {1134329865}<NJ-KMHSTRAT>
+ Kennedy Memorial Hospital-University Medical Center
18 East Laurel Road/EmergMed   Stratford, NJ 08084
(856)346-6000

Noor, Emad Roshdy, MD {1043506231} Nrolgy
+ JFK Neurosciences Institute
65 James Street/Second Floor   Edison, NJ 08818   (732)321-7010   Fax (732)632-1584

Noor, Farid A., MD EmrgMd, IntrMd(80,EGYP)
+ 192 Hooton Road
Mount Laurel, NJ 08054

Noor, Fazle Ali, MD {1487817672} Nephro, IntrMd
+ Somerset Nephrology Associates, P.C.
23 Monroe Street   Bridgewater, NJ 08807   (908)722-0106   Fax (908)231-1431

Noorily, Stuart W., MD {1205844453} Ophthl, VitRet, IntrMd(88,MA05)<NJ-HACKNSK, NJ-ENGLWOOD>
+ Retina Associates of New Jersey, P.A.
5 Franklin Avenue   Belleville, NJ 07109   (973)450-5100   Fax (973)450-9494
+ Retina Associates of New Jersey, P.A.
628 Cedar Lane   Teaneck, NJ 07666   (973)450-5100   Fax (201)836-6426
+ Retina Associates of New Jersey, P.A.
1044 Route 23 North/Suite 207   Wayne, NJ 07109
(973)633-9898   Fax (973)633-3892

Noormohamed, Akbar H., MD {1083640965} EmrgMd(89,INDI)<NJ-RBAYOLDB, NJ-RBAYPERT>
+ Raritan Bay Medical Center/Old Bridge Division
One Hospital Plaza/EmrgMed   Old Bridge, NJ 08857
(732)360-1000

Nop, Mallory, MD {1609335769} IntrMd
+ 721 Clifton Avenue/Suite 1C
Clifton, NJ 07013   (973)777-2005

Norden, Richard A., MD {1508902065} Ophthl(80,IL45)<NJ-VALLEY>
+ Norden Laser Eye Associates
1144 East Ridgewood Avenue   Ridgewood, NJ 07450
(201)444-2442

Nordin, Brittany N., DO {1528360203} IntrMd
+ LMA CardioThoracic Surgical Services
1 Brace Road/Suite C   Cherry Hill, NJ 08034   (856)470-9029   Fax (856)796-9391

Nordone, Danielle Suzanne, DO {1699765354} FamMed(02,PA77)
+ Jersey Shore Associates of Internal Medicine
831 Tennent Road   Manalapan, NJ 07726   (732)536-7144   Fax (732)536-7520

Nordstrom, Thomas J., MD {1295796977} SrgOrt(78,NJ06)<NJ-SOMERSET>
+ Orthopedic and Sports Medicine at SMG
215 Union Avenue/Suite B   Bridgewater, NJ 08807
(908)685-8500   Fax (908)685-8009

Noreen, Shahla, MD {1457513525} PthACl, IntrMd(98,PAK08)
+ 977 Feather Bed Lane
Edison, NJ 08820

Nori, Phalgun, MD {1043547656} PhysMd<NJ-KSLRWELK>
+ Kessler Institute for Rehab
201 Pleasant Hill Road   Chester, NJ 07930   (973)252-6368

Noris, Gary L., MD {1952342958} EmrgMd, IntrMd(80,NJ05)<NJ-OCEANMC>
+ EmCare
425 Jack Martin Boulevard   Brick, NJ 08724   (732)840-3380

Norman, Garrett Joseph, III, MD {1376778019}
+ 20 Westmont Avenue
Lavallette, NJ 08735   (732)575-7835

Noroff, Joan P., MD {1962583062} Dermat(73,NY08)
+ Dermatology Affiliates
2954 Kennedy Boulevard/2nd Floor   Jersey City, NJ 07306
(201)653-5555

Noronha, Joaquim L., MD {1710984885} EnDbMt, IntrMd(72,INA69)<NJ-STPETER, NJ-RWJUBRUN>
+ 1553 Route 27/Suite 3000
Somerset, NJ 08873   (732)545-5980

Northridge, Jennifer, MD {1003132853} AdolMd<NJ-HACKNSK>
+ Hackensack University Medical Center
30 Prospect Avenue   Hackensack, NJ 07601   (551)996-2237

Norton, Kevin Patrick, DO {1760461024} FamMed(96,PA77)<NJ-VIRTVOOR>
+ Partners in Primary Care
19 West Main Street   Maple Shade, NJ 08052   (856)779-7386   Fax (856)779-7563

Nosher, John L., MD {1184609141} Radiol, RadDia, RadV&I(71,PA02)<NJ-STPETER, NJ-RWJUBRUN>
+ University Radiology Group, P.C.
483 Cranbury Road   East Brunswick, NJ 08816   (732)390-0030   Fax (732)390-5383
+ UH- Robert Wood Johnson Med
125 Paterson Street/MEB 404   New Brunswick, NJ 08901
(732)390-0030   Fax (732)235-6889
+ University Radiology Group, P.C.
579A Cranbury Road   East Brunswick, NJ 08816   (732)390-0040   Fax (732)390-1856

Nosker, Geoffrey S., MD {1689896110} Anesth<NJ-MONMOUTH>
+ Monmouth Medical Center
300 Second Avenue   Long Branch, NJ 07740   (732)222-5200

Noskin, Olga, MD {1821139502} Nrolgy, VasNeu(02,NY46)
+ Neurology Group of Bergen County
1200 East Ridgewood Avenue   Ridgewood, NJ 07450
(201)444-0868   Fax (201)444-7363

Nosko, Michael G., MD {1801905401} SrgNro(82,ON01)<NJ-RWJUBRUN>
+ UH- Robert Wood Johnson Med
125 Paterson Street/Ste 2100/Chief   New Brunswick, NJ 08901   (732)235-7756   Fax (732)235-7095
nosko@umdnj.edu
+ Rutgers - RWJMS
125 Paterson Street/Suite 2100   New Brunswick, NJ 08901
(732)235-7756   Fax (732)235-7095

Nossa, Robert, MD {1023089554} Dermat(97,NY48)<NJ-MTNSIDE>
+ The Dermatology Group, P.C.
60 Pompton Avenue   Verona, NJ 07044   (973)994-3550   Fax (973)571-2126
rnossa@thedermgroup.com
+ The Dermatology Group, P.C.
44 Route 23 North/Suite 213   Riverdale, NJ 07457
(973)994-3550   Fax (973)839-5751
+ The Dermatology Group, P.C.
30 West Century Road/Suite 320   Paramus, NJ 07044
(973)571-2121   Fax (201)986-0702

Nosseir, Sandy B., MD {1043464704} ObsGyn
+ Jersey Urology Group
403 Bethel Road   Somers Point, NJ 08244   (609)927-8746   Fax (609)601-1406

Notardonato, Henry, MD {1790775146} RadDia, NuclMd(85,ITA01)<NJ-MEADWLND>
+ University Radiology Group, P.C.
483 Cranbury Road   East Brunswick, NJ 08816   (732)390-0030   Fax (732)390-5383

Notari, Teresa V., MD {1104998285} Dermat(91,NY08)<NJ-OVERLOOK, NJ-STBARNMC>
+ 33 Overlook Road/Suite 209
Summit, NJ 07901   (908)598-7200   Fax (908)598-7211

Notaro, Joseph R., MD {1265403307} SrgC&R(86,DC02)
+ Associated Colon & Rectal Surgeons PA
3900 Park Avenue/Suite 101   Edison, NJ 08820   (732)494-6640   Fax (732)549-8204

Notis, Corey M., MD {1255323580} Catrct, Ophthl(88,NJ05)<NJ-STBARNMC, NJ-OVERLOOK>
+ Associates in Eye Care
155 Morris Avenue/Suite 302   Springfield, NJ 07081
(973)232-6900   Fax (973)232-6911
+ Associates in Eye Care
900 Stuyvesant Avenue   Union, NJ 07083   (973)232-6900   Fax (908)687-0139

Notkin, Alicia R., MD {1346428950} IntrMd, Nephro(03,NY19)
+ North Jersey Nephrology Associates PA
246 Hamburg Turnpike/Suite 207   Wayne, NJ 07470
(973)653-3366   Fax (973)653-3365

Noto, Damon Joseph, MD {1255354312} PhysMd(99,NY47)<NJ-HACKNSK>
+ Anti-Aging & Laser Medical Associates
777 Terrace Avenue/Suite 403   Hasbrouck Heights, NJ 07604   (201)288-3777   Fax (201)426-0446
info@aalma.us
+ One West Ridgewood Avenue
Paramus, NJ 07652   (201)251-7725

Noto, Gregory, MD {1801863287} CdvDis, IntrMd(80,DOM02)<NJ-DEBRAHLC, NJ-CENTRAST>
+ Monmouth Cardiology Associates, LLC
222 Schanck Road/Suite 104   Freehold, NJ 07728
(732)431-1332   Fax (732)431-1712
+ Monmouth Cardiology Associates, LLC
11 Meridian Road   Eatontown, NJ 07724   (732)431-1332   Fax (732)663-0301

Notterman, Robyn B., MD {1124008958} Dermat(83,NY20)<NJ-UNVMCPRN>
+ The Princeton Center for Dermatology, LLC
800 Bunn Drive/Suite 201   Princeton, NJ 08540   (609)924-1033   Fax (609)924-7055
rnotterman@yahoo.com

Nouman, Helena, MD {1578519187} Pedtrc(79,CZE02)<NJ-HACKNSK, NJ-ENGLWOOD>
+ Closter Medical Group
200 Closter Dock Road   Closter, NJ 07624   (201)768-3900   Fax (201)768-3840

Novaco, Robert Joseph, MD {1023371952}
+ University Hospital Medicine
150 Bergen Street/Room I-248   Newark, NJ 07103
(973)972-6056   Fax (973)972-3129

Novaes, Denise, MD {1447257225} Pedtrc(84,BRA40)<NJ-PALISADE>
+ 744 Kearny Avenue
Kearny, NJ 07032   (201)955-1015
Dnovasmd@gmail.com

Novak, Caroline J., MD {1659660785} IntrMd
+ Chuback Medical Group
2 Sears Drive/Suite 101   Paramus, NJ 07652   (620)210-8235   Fax (201)261-1776

Novak, Dennis E., MD {1194881094} FamMed(74,NJ06)<NJ-COMMED>
+ Dennis Novak MD PA
1001 Lacey Road/PO Box 780   Forked River, NJ 08731
(609)693-8900   Fax (609)971-2888

Novak, Eva Cesnek, MD {1720313075} FamMed
+ Summit Medical Group
48-50 Fairfield Street   Montclair, NJ 07042   (973)744-8511   Fax (973)744-6356

Novak, Nellie, MD {1649299934} Pedtrc(74,PA07)<NJ-COOPRUMC, NJ-OURLADY>
+ CAMCare Health Corporation
817 Federal Street   Camden, NJ 08103   (856)541-9811   Fax (856)541-4611

Novak, Steven Michael, MD {1356572424} Anesth<NJ-HOLYNAME>
+ Holy Name Hospital
718 Teaneck Road   Teaneck, NJ 07666   (201)833-7149

Noveck, Howard D., MD {1871543389} CdvDis, IntrMd, IntCrd(83,ISR02)
+ Raritan Bay Cardiology Group, P.A.
225 May Street/Suite F   Edison, NJ 08837   (732)738-8855   Fax (732)738-4141
+ Raritan Bay Cardiology Group, P.A.
3 Hospital Plaza/Suite 305   Old Bridge, NJ 08857
(732)738-8855   Fax (732)738-4141
+ Raritan Bay Cardiology Group, P.A.
337 Applegarth Road   Monroe Township, NJ 08837
(609)655-8860   Fax (732)738-4141

Novello, Laura Joyce, MD {1780976332} PedEnd
+ Drs. Barrows and Ostrow
180 Avenue at the Common/Suite 7B   Shrewsbury, NJ 07702   (732)935-7143   Fax (732)935-7245

Novetsky, Akiva Pesach, MD {1811191604} GynOnc
+ University Physician Associates
140 Bergen Street/ACC Level C   Newark, NJ 07103
(973)972-2700   Fax (973)972-2739

Novick, Andrew S., MD {1952356123} RadDia, RadV&I(82,NY47)<NJ-NWRKBETH>
+ Millburn Medical Imaging
2130 Millburn Avenue/Suite A-8   Maplewood, NJ 07040
(973)912-0404   Fax (973)912-0444
+ Newark Diagnostic Radiologists, PA
201 Lyons Avenue   Newark, NJ 07112   (973)926-7466
+ Millburn Medical Imaging
210 West St. Georges Avenue   Linden, NJ 07040   (908)587-0035   Fax (908)587-0037

Noviello, Stephanie Seshagiri, MD Pedtrc(97,LA01)
+ 55 Totten Drive
Bridgewater, NJ 08807

Novik, Edward, MD {1174516157} Anesth(88,UZB02)
+ Union Anesthesia & Pain Management
695 Chestnut Street   Union, NJ 07083   (908)851-7161   Fax (908)851-7536

Novik, Emily, MD {1629411947} Psychy
+ Immediate Care Psychiatric Center, LLC
22 Hill Road   Parsippany, NJ 07054   (973)335-9909   Fax (973)206-2010

Novik, Gerald, MD {1417934597} IntrMd(83,PHI15)<NJ-STFRNMED, NJ-RWJUHAM>
+ 5 Peter Rafferty Drive
Hamilton Square, NJ 08690

Novin, Matthew, DO {1972958072}
+ MedExpress Urgent Care Ledgewood
501 State Route 10   Ledgewood, NJ 07852   (973)584-6751   Fax (973)584-6753

Physicians by Name and Address

Novitt-Moreno, Anne D., MD {1316182058} ClnPhm, Rserch(79,NJ05)
+ 14 Willow Drive
  Chester, NJ 07930 (908)879-2328 Fax (908)879-5009

Novogroder, Michael, MD {1366496572} PedEnd, Pedtrc(69,NY15)<NJ-ENGLWOOD, NY-PRSBCOLU>
+ Metropolitan Pediatric Group
  704 Palisade Avenue Teaneck, NJ 07666 (201)836-4301 Fax (201)836-5110

Novotny, Gregory R., DO {1750315198} IntrMd(87,NJ75)<NJ-ACMCITY, NJ-ACMCMAIN>
+ Woodbine Development Center/NJ Human Services
  1175 Dehirsch Avenue Woodbine, NJ 08270 (609)861-2164 Fax (609)861-2494
+ AtlantiCare Clinical Associates
  2500 English Creek Avenue Egg Harbor Township, NJ 08234 (609)861-2164 Fax (609)407-2311

Novotny, Sherie Lynn, MD {1942218607} PsyCAd, Pedtrc, Psychy(92,PA07)<NJ-UNIVBHC>
+ University Behavioral Health Care
  671 Hoes Lane/PO Box 1392 Piscataway, NJ 08855 (732)235-5500
+ University Behavioral Health Care
  303 George Street/Suite 200 New Brunswick, NJ 08901 (732)235-5500 Fax (732)235-6187

Novy, Donald S., MD {1154323061} IntrMd(76,NY20)<NJ-HUNTRDN>
+ Adult & Adolescent Medical Associates PC
  4 Walter E. Foran Boulevard/Suite 101 Flemington, NJ 08822 (908)782-3204 Fax (908)788-5279

Nowak, Darius Zbigniew, MD {1740200666} IntrMd, EnDbMt(86,POL10)
+ Drs. Czyzewski & Nowak
  515 North Wood Avenue/Suite 302 Linden, NJ 07036 (908)925-3300 Fax (908)925-4300

Nowell, Martha A., MD {1376563973} IntrMd, RadDia, RadNro(78,MA07)<NJ-JFKMED>
+ JFK Medical Center
  65 James Street/Radiology Edison, NJ 08820 (732)321-7000

Nowicki, Noel C., MD {1649295932} IntrMd(75,MEX14)<NJ-MTNSIDE, NJ-KSLRSADB>
+ Apple Acupuncture
  292 Bloomfield Avenue Montclair, NJ 07042 (973)655-1005 Fax (973)655-0095
  undoc@earthlink.net

Nowinowska, Anna, MD {1649372079} Pedtrc(92,POL02)<NJ-JRSYSHMC>
+ EmCare
  1945 Route 33 Neptune, NJ 07753 (732)776-4510 Fax (732)776-2329

Noyan, Earl Lincoln, MD {1447310784} Surgry, SrgLap(97,DC03)<NJ-CENTRAST>
+ Endo-Surgical Associates
  901 West Main Street/Suite 104 Freehold, NJ 07728 (732)761-1740 Fax (732)761-8320
+ CentraState Medical Center
  901 West Main Street Freehold, NJ 07728 (732)431-2000

Nozad, Cyrus H., MD {1457528655} IntrMd, AlgyImmn(05,NY20)
+ The Family Center for Otolaryngology
  47 Orient Way/Lower Level Rutherford, NJ 07070 (201)935-5508 Fax (201)465-6088
+ The Family Center for Otolaryngology
  1265 Paterson Plank Road Secaucus, NJ 07094 (201)935-5508 Fax (201)465-6088
+ The Family Center for Otolaryngology
  6 Brighton Road/Suite 104 Clifton, NJ 07070 (973)470-0282 Fax (201)465-6088

Nu, Than Than, MD {1447233481}
+ 2 State Route 27/Suite 500
  Edison, NJ 08820 (443)397-3707
  bettythanoe@gmail.com

Nucatola, Thomas R., Jr., MD {1407803463} Rheuma, IntrMd(85,NY08)
+ Arthritis Allergy and Immunology
  100 Commerce Place Clark, NJ 07066 (908)301-9800 Fax (908)301-9801

Nucci, Annamaria, MD {1518185198} Psychy, PsyCAd, PsoMd(71,ITAL)
+ 5 Westview Court
  Cedar Grove, NJ 07009 (973)857-2609

Nudelman, Yuliya L., MD {1972700037}<NJ-MONMOUTH>
+ Monmouth Medical Center
  300 Second Avenue Long Branch, NJ 07740 (732)222-5200

Nuesa, Wilson O., IV, MD {1518965268} Anesth(82,PHI14)<NJ-STJOSHOS>
+ St. Joseph's Regional Medical Center Anesthesia
  703 Main Street Paterson, NJ 07503 (973)754-2323 Fax (973)977-9455

Nugent, Grace C., MD {1538275730} IntrMd(89,PA07)
+ Center for Family Guidance, PC
  765 East Route 70/Building A-101 Marlton, NJ 08053 (856)797-4800 Fax (856)810-0110

Nugent, Thomas Rone, MD {1457321044} IntrMd, PulDis, SlpDis(96,PA02)<NJ-OURLADY, NJ-VIRTMARL>
+ Pulmonary & Sleep Associates of SJ, LLC.
  107 Berlin Road Cherry Hill, NJ 08034 (856)429-1800 Fax (856)429-1081
+ Pulmonary & Sleep Associates of SJ, LLC.
  750 Route 73 South/Suite 401 Marlton, NJ 08053 (856)429-1800 Fax (856)375-2325
+ Pulmonary & Sleep Associates of SJ, LLC.
  811 Sunset Road/Suite 201 Burlington, NJ 08034 (609)298-1776 Fax (609)531-2391

Nunez, Aida Rodrigo, MD {1235228537} Psychy(74,PHI05)
+ New Jersey Manufacturers Insurance Group
  301 Sullivan Way/PO Box 1428 West Trenton, NJ 08628 (609)633-1562

Nunez, David A., MD {1750476461} ObsGyn(72,JMA01)
+ 901 Teaneck Road
  Teaneck, NJ 07666 Fax (201)837-7565

Nunez, Elkin Armando, MD {1891973780} IntrMd(05,DMN01)<NJ-MORRISTN>
+ Morristown Medical Center
  100 Madison Avenue/IntMed Morristown, NJ 07962 (973)971-5000

Nunez, Helen Lourdes, MD {1821050816} Pedtrc(98,NJ05)
+ Springfield Pediatrics
  190 Meisel Avenue Springfield, NJ 07081 (973)467-1009 Fax (973)467-7836

Nunez, Jacqueline Denise, MD {1316031313} FamMed(00,NJ05)
+ United Medical, P.C.
  533 Lexington Avenue Clifton, NJ 07011 (973)546-6844 Fax (973)546-7707
+ Doctors' Office Walk-in Urgent Care
  110 East Ridgewood Avenue Paramus, NJ 07652 (973)546-6844 Fax (201)265-1355

Nunez, Venitius D., MD {1407973035} Psychy(75,PHI08)<NJ-SJERSYHS, NJ-LOURDMED>
+ InSight LLC
  765 East Route 70/Bldg A Marlton, NJ 08053 (856)983-9100 Fax (856)810-0110

Nunn, Robert F., MD {1689672917} Ophthl(61,NJ05)<NJ-SHOREMEM>
+ Horizon Eye Care
  9701 Ventnor Avenue Margate City, NJ 08402 (609)822-4242 Fax (609)822-3211
+ Horizon Eye Care
  2401 Bay Avenue Ocean City, NJ 08226 (609)822-4242 Fax (609)399-6284
+ Horizon Eye Care
  4 Village Drive Cape May Court House, NJ 08402 (609)465-7100

Nurenberg, Jeffry Raul, MD {1144396086} Psychy, Psynls, IntrMd(69,MA05)<NJ-MORRISTN, NJ-GRYSTPSY>
+ Morristown Medical Center
  100 Madison Avenue/Psychiatry Morristown, NJ 07962 (973)971-5302
+ Greystone Park Psychiatric Hospital
  59 Koch Avenue/Psychiatry Morris Plains, NJ 07950 (973)538-1800

Nuritdinova, Dilfuza A., MD {1083982789}
+ 18 Covington Court
  East Brunswick, NJ 08816

Nurkiewicz, Stephen A., MD {1093773350} FamMed(86,PA02)
+ Dr. Stephen A. Nurkiewicz and Assoc
  858 South White Horse Pike/Suite B2 Hammonton, NJ 08037 (609)561-2345 Fax (609)561-8969

Nurse-Bey, Hazel Ann, MD {1619190089} FamMAdd, IntrMd(84,NJ05)<NJ-COOPRUMC>
+ Cooper University Hospital
  One Cooper Plaza/Suite 222 Camden, NJ 08103 (856)342-3150 Fax (856)968-8418
  nursebey-hazel@cooperhealth.edu

Nusbaum, Michael Jay, MD {1265460554} Surgry(93,NJ05)<NJ-STBARNMC>
+ Obesity Treatment Centers of New Jersey
  95 Madison Avenue/Suite A-6 Morristown, NJ 07960 (973)998-9833 Fax (973)998-9832

Nuschke, Randell A., MD {1700840758} IntrMd(82,MEX03)<NJ-BURDTMLN>
+ Cape Regional Physicians Associates
  336 96th Street/Suite 1 Stone Harbor, NJ 08247 (609)967-0070 Fax (609)967-0077
+ 9 Broadway/PO Box 130
  Cape May Court House, NJ 08210 (609)967-0070 Fax (609)463-8135

Nussbaum, Nathan Coleman, MD {1760620082} MedOnc
+ 58 Pine Street
  Millburn, NJ 07041 (773)680-3713

Nussbaum, Peter, MD {1972662096} Ophthl(69,NY09)
+ Associates in Ophthalmology
  22 Old Short Hills Road/Suite 102 Livingston, NJ 07039 (973)992-5200 Fax (973)535-5741

Nussey, Richard Hutchins, Jr., DO {1275560161} EmrgMd(97,NJ75)<NJ-BURDTMLN>
+ Cape Regional Medical Center
  2 Stone Harbor Boulevard/EmergMed Cape May Court House, NJ 08210 (609)463-2000 Fax (609)463-2946

Nutanson, Inna, MD {1558522748}
+ 302 High Street/Apt G-42
  Fair Lawn, NJ 07410 (201)835-8246

Nuthakki, Vimala Devi, MD {1861741019} ObsGyn(08,NET09)<NJ-STPETER>
+ Care first OBGYN Group LLC
  1555 Ruth Road/Suite 5 North Brunswick, NJ 08902 (732)398-3939 Fax (732)398-0909
+ Care first OBGYN Group LLC
  666 Plainsboro Road/Suite 432 Plainsboro, NJ 08536 (732)398-3939 Fax (732)398-0909

Nutini, Dennis Neil, MD {1568621134} PhysMd, SprtMd, IntrMd(05,PA09)<MA-SPAULDG>
+ Rothman Institute - Egg Harbor Township
  2500 English Creek Avenue/Bldg 1300 Egg Harbor Township, NJ 08234 (609)677-7002 Fax (609)677-7000
+ Rothman Institute - Manahawkin
  712 East Bay Avenue Manahawkin, NJ 08050

Nutini, Mary Katharine, DO {1306006663} PhysMd, PedReh(05,PA77)
+ Children's Specialized Hospital-Ocean
  94 Stevens Road Toms River, NJ 08755 (732)914-1100

Nuzzo, Roy Michael, MD {1104977453} OthrSp, PedOrt, SrgOrt(70,NY20)<NJ-OVERLOOK>
+ Pediatric Orthopedics, PC
  99 Beauvoir Avenue/Suite 750 Summit, NJ 07902 (908)522-5801 Fax (908)522-5519

Nwankwo, Gloria Obiageli, DO {1134113939} IntrMd, EmrgMd(98,NY75)
+ Pathlink, LLC
  66 West Gilbert Street/Suite 100 Tinton Falls, NJ 07701 (732)212-0060 Fax (732)212-0061

Nwaobasi, Eberechi Ihuoma, MD {1992880215} Pedtrc(01,DC03)<NJ-OVERLOOK>
+ Overlook Medical Center
  99 Beauvoir Avenue/PO Box 210 Summit, NJ 07902 (908)522-2000 Fax (908)522-4066

Nwigwe, Genevieve N., MD {1881968261} IntrMd
+ Neighborhood Health Center Plainfield
  1700-58 Myrtle Avenue Plainfield, NJ 07060 (908)753-6401 Fax (908)226-6743

Nwobu, Uchenna Christian, MD {1619190816} ObGyHPC
+ 4 West Over Terrace
  West Orange, NJ 07052

Nwosu-Nelson, Joel E., MD {1750350682} IntrMd(87,NIGE)<NJ-CENTRAST>
+ 1033 Us Highway 46/Suite 205
  Clifton, NJ 07013 (973)910-8400

Nwotite, Ezinne Ugochi, MD {1457662603} IntrMd, IntHos(NIG02)<NJ-ACMCITY>
+ AtlantiCare Hospitalist Program
  1925 Pacific Avenue/8th Floor Atlantic City, NJ 08401 (609)441-8146 Fax (609)441-8002

Nyajure, Colette, MD {1548669203} IntrMd<NJ-VALLEY>
+ The Valley Hospital
  223 North Van Dien Avenue Ridgewood, NJ 07450 (201)447-8000

Nyaku, Amesika N., MD {1134440647} InfDis<NJ-UMDNJ>
+ University Hospital
  150 Bergen Street/D Level Newark, NJ 07103 (973)972-5111 Fax (973)972-3102

Nyce, Andrew L., MD {1932200466} EmrgMd(96,PA02)<NJ-COOPRUMC>
+ Cooper University Hospital
  One Cooper Plaza Camden, NJ 08103 (856)342-2000

Nychay, Stephen G., MD {1013982586} Dermat, PthDrm, DerMOH(86,LA01)<NJ-HACKNSK>
+ Westwood Dermatology
  390 Old Hook Road Westwood, NJ 07675 (201)666-9550 Fax (201)666-1251

Nyein, Chan Myat Myat, MD {1497024863}
+ Southern Ocean Medical Center
  1100 Route 72 West/Suite 307 Manahawkin, NJ 08050 (917)348-8656 Fax (609)978-8941
  chanmmnyein@gmail.com

Nygaard, Torbjoern G., MD {1417961830} IntrMd, Nrolgy(80,OH06)<NJ-VAEASTOR>
+ VA New Jersey Health Care System-East Orange Campus
385 Tremont Avenue   East Orange, NJ 07018   (973)676-1000   Fax (973)395-7113
+ Rutgers NJ School of Medicine Neurology
90 Bergen Street/DOC 5200   Newark, NJ 07103   (973)676-1000   Fax (973)972-5059

Nyirenda, Thandiwe V., MD {1972705721}<NJ-JRSYCITY>
+ Jersey City Medical Center
355 Grand Street   Jersey City, NJ 07304   (347)933-0690
thandien@hotmail.com

Nyitray, Peter, MD {1093726119} Anesth, AnesPain(96,HUN02)<NJ-HUNTRDN>
+ Hunterdon Medical Center
2100 Wescott Drive/Anesthesiology   Flemington, NJ 08822   (908)788-6100   Fax (908)788-6361

Nyquist, Susan Shoshana, MD {1639314925} Ophthl
+ Center for Eye Care
123 Egg Harbor Road/Suite 300   Sewell, NJ 08080   (856)290-4548   Fax (856)290-4552

Nyunt, Kyaw, MD {1396781175} Anesth(68,MYA04)<NJ-VALLEY>
+ The Valley Hospital
223 North Van Dien Avenue   Ridgewood, NJ 07450   (201)447-8000

Nyunt, Tun, MD {1902817554} IntrMd
+ IPC The Hospitalist Company
55 Madison Avenue/Suite 310   Morristown, NJ 07960   (973)993-9536   Fax (973)998-4237

Nyzio, Joseph Bruno, DO {1609814292} Anesth(00,PA77)<NJ-VIRTMHBC>
+ Burlington Anesthesia Associates
120 Madison Ave/Suite E/PO Box 174   Mount Holly, NJ 08060   (609)261-1660   Fax (609)261-1779

O'Banion, Kathleen S., MD {1295808574} ObsGyn, Gyneco(81,TX12)<NJ-COOPRUMC>
+ Cooper Physicians
1210 Brace Road/Suite 102   Cherry Hill, NJ 08034   (856)428-6616   Fax (856)428-4823

O'Brien, Debra Ann, MD {1780755447} Pedtrc(98,NJ05)
+ TLC Pediatrics
20 White Road/Suite D   Shrewsbury, NJ 07702   (732)741-3400   Fax (732)741-3104

O'Brien, Evan Douglas, MD {1740381185} SrgOrt, SrgSpn(88,PA01)<NJ-UNDRWD>
+ Woodbury Spine
1225 North Broad Street/Suite 3   Woodbury, NJ 08096   (856)845-0707   Fax (856)845-0082

O'Brien, Jonathan Edward, MD {1922233824} ObsGyn<NJ-STBARNMC>
+ St. Barnabas Medical Center
94 Old Short Hills Road   Livingston, NJ 07039   (973)322-5287   Fax (973)322-2309

O'Brien, Joseph Patrick, MD {1689618860} IntrMd(98,NY09)<NJ-STMRYPAS>
+ Summit Medical Group
6 Brighton Road/2 FL   Clifton, NJ 07012   (973)777-7911   Fax (973)777-5403

O'Brien, Katherine Elizabeth, MD {1033159124} ObsGyn(01,NY08)
+ Valley Ob Gyn Associates PA
80 Eisenhower Drive/Suite 200   Paramus, NJ 07652   (201)843-2800   Fax (201)843-5848

O'Brien, Marlene Theresa, MD {1467750422}
+ Jefferson Health Primary & Specialty Care
1A Regulus Drive   Turnersville, NJ 08012   (844)542-2273

O'Brien, Susan Erin, DO {1023332715} EmrgMd<NJ-JRSYCITY>
+ Jersey City Medical Center
355 Grand Street   Jersey City, NJ 07304   (201)915-2000   Fax (973)251-1109

O'Brien, Thomas K., MD {1952322588} IntrMd(83,GRN01)
+ Drs. Guarino & O'Brien
160 Highway 37 West   Toms River, NJ 08755   (732)286-0440   Fax (732)286-2885

O'Brien, Thomas Kevin, MD {1659342889} Pedtrc(97,NJ05)
+ West Park Pediatrics
804 West Park Avenue   Ocean, NJ 07712   (732)531-0010   Fax (732)493-0903
+ West Park Pediatrics
219 Taylors Mills Road   Manalapan, NJ 07726   (732)531-0010   Fax (732)577-9643
+ West Park Pediatrics
921 East County Line Road/Suite B   Lakewood, NJ 07712   (732)370-8500   Fax (732)370-5550

O'Connell, Brendan Garrett, MD {1972763936} Surgry<PA-ABINGTON>
+ Cooper Bone and Joint Institute
3 Cooper Plaza/Suite 411   Camden, NJ 08103   (856)673-4500   Fax (856)673-4525

O'Connell, Frank Michael, MD {1326075490} Anesth, IntrMd, CritCr(85,NY15)<NJ-CHSMRCER, NJ-CHSFULD>
+ AtlantiCare Anesthesiology
65 West Jimmie Leeds Road   Pomona, NJ 08240   (609)748-7597

O'Connell, Joseph J., III, DO {1275573339} GenPrc, EmrgMd(92,NJ75)<NJ-VIRTVOOR>
+ Virtua Voorhees
100 Bowman Drive   Voorhees, NJ 08043   (856)247-3000   Fax (856)325-3197

O'Connell, Mark M., MD {1558365148} CdvDis(85,OH06)<NJ-MONMOUTH>
+ 18 Center Street/Rear Apt.
Rumson, NJ 07760

O'Connor, Andrew, MD {1245297803} EmrgMd(02,NY08)<NJ-RWJUBRUN>
+ University Emergency Medicine
125 Paterson Street/MEB 104   New Brunswick, NJ 08901   (732)235-8717   Fax (732)235-7379

O'Connor, Brandon P., MD {1467624494} FamMed(07,STM01)
+ Montville Primary Care Physicians
137 Main Road   Montville, NJ 07045   (973)402-0025   Fax (973)402-0508

O'Connor, Brian Kevin, MD {1275647216} PedCrd(85,DC02)<NJ-CHDNWBTH, NJ-NWRKBETH>
+ Pediatric Cardiology Associates
1 Broadway/Suite 203   Elmwood Park, NJ 07407   (973)569-6250   Fax (973)569-6270
+ Children's Hospital of New Jersey
201 Lyons Avenue/Osborne Terrace   Newark, NJ 07112   (973)926-2927

O'Connor, David John, MD {1063736510} SrgVas, Surgry(04,FL02)
+ Bergen Surgical Specialists/Hackensack Vascular
211 Essex Street/Suite 102   Hackensack, NJ 07601   (201)487-8882   Fax (201)487-0943

O'Connor, Douglas S., MD {1730174772} RadNro(90,NY08)<NJ-RIVERVW>
+ Red Bank Radiologists, P.A.
200 White Road/Suite 115   Little Silver, NJ 07739   (732)741-9595   Fax (732)741-0985
+ Coastal Imaging, LLC
79 Route 37 West/Suite 103   Toms River, NJ 08755   (732)741-9595   Fax (732)276-2325

O'Connor, James J., III, MD {1477654507} CritCr, PulDis, SlpDis(88,PA02)<NJ-ACMCMAIN, NJ-SHOREMEM>
+ Shore Physicians Group
18 West New York Avenue   Somers Point, NJ 08244   (609)926-1450   Fax (609)926-8419
joconnor@aspsm.net

O'Connor, Mary T., MD {1912920406} RadDia, IntrMd, Rad-Nuc(82,ITA17)
+ Diagnostic Radiology Associates of Cranford
25 South Union Avenue   Cranford, NJ 07016   (908)709-1323   Fax (908)709-1329
+ Diagnostic Radiology Associates of Northfield
772 Northfield Avenue   West Orange, NJ 07052   (908)709-1323   Fax (973)325-8140
+ Diagnostic Radiology Associates of Clifton
1339 Broad Street   Clifton, NJ 07016   (973)778-9600   Fax (973)778-4846

O'Connor, Patrick, MD {1770718710} Anesth(05,PA0)<NJ-VIRT-MARL>
+ Virtua Marlton Hospital
90 Brick Road   Marlton, NJ 08053   (856)355-6000

O'Connor, Patrick Joseph, DO {1326132531} RadDia(99,NJ75)<NJ-OCEANMC>
+ Point Pleasant Radiology Group
1973 State Route 34/Suite E-13   Wall, NJ 07719   (732)974-8011   Fax (732)974-8820
+ Coastal Imaging, LLC
79 Route 37 West/Suite 103   Toms River, NJ 08755   (732)974-8011   Fax (732)276-2325

O'Connor, Robert M., MD FamMed(91,NJ06)
+ Family Medicine at Monument Square
317 George Street   New Brunswick, NJ 08901   (732)235-8993   Fax (732)246-7317

O'Dea, Carol Lynn H., MD {1780859249} Pedtrc, NnPnMd(08,PA14)
+ Lawrenceville School Infirmary
2500 Main Street/PO Box 6011   Lawrenceville, NJ 08648   (609)896-0400

O'Dell, Kimberly Ann, MD {1063573749} FamMed(93,NJ05)
+ Jersey Shore Geriatrics
15 School Road East/Suite 2   Marlboro, NJ 07746   (732)866-9922   Fax (732)866-9970

O'Dell, Xitlalichomiha, DO {1619282985} FamMed, IntrMd(NJ75<NJ-UNDRWD>
+ Inspira Occupational Health
1038 East Chestnut Avenue/Suite 120   Vineland, NJ 08360   (856)507-8548   Fax (856)507-2709

O'Donnell, Carmel Marie, MD {1497754097} IntrMd(96,PA77)
+ Pitman Internal Medicine Associates
410 North Broadway/Suite 1   Pitman, NJ 08071   (856)589-3708   Fax (856)589-2662

O'Donnell, John C., Jr., MD {1194782599} SrgVas, Surgry(72,NJ05)<NJ-SJHREGMC>
+ Surgical Associates of South Jersey
907 North Main Road/Building C   Vineland, NJ 08360   (856)692-7228   Fax (856)692-4155
info@surgiassociates.com

O'Donnell, John Thornton, MD {1205890282} Psychy(82,WV01)<NJ-STCLRBOO>
+ St. Clare's Hospital-Boonton
130 Powerville Road   Boonton, NJ 07005   (973)316-1800

O'Donnell, Lisa-Mary, MD {1487723300} Pedtrc(02,GRN01)
+ Amazing Kids Pediatrics
22 Elm Avenue   Hackensack, NJ 07601   (201)267-0890   Fax (201)343-4635
dro@amazingkidspeds.com

O'Donnell, Mary Theresa, MD {1962473108} IntrMd(94,NY46)<NJ-RBAYOLDB, NJ-JFKMED>
+ Woodbridge Internal Medicine Associates
1000 Route 9 North/Suite 302   Woodbridge, NJ 07095   (732)634-0036   Fax (732)634-9182

O'Donnell, Paul Lawrence, DO {1407825433} SrgVas, Surgry, IntrMd(98,PA77)
+ Cape Regional Physicans Associates
217 North Main Street/Suite 104   Cape May Court House, NJ 08210   (609)463-1488   Fax (609)463-4881

O'Donnell, Robert H., DO {1801836895} ObsGyn(90,MO79)<NJ-ACMCITY, NJ-ACMCMAIN>
+ Drs. O'Donnell and King
1163 Route 37 West/Suite A-2   Toms River, NJ 08755   (732)349-2424   Fax (732)349-8130
+ JFK Medical Center
65 James Street   Edison, NJ 08820   (732)839-9341

O'Donnell, Thomas P., MD {1093756132} Pedtrc(76,PA02)<NJ-VIRTMHBC>
+ Advocare Pedi Phys of Burlington Co
693 Main Street/PO Box 367   Lumberton, NJ 08048   (609)261-4058   Fax (609)261-8381
+ Advocare Pedi Phys of Burlington Co
204 Ark Road/Suite 209   Mount Laurel, NJ 08054   (609)261-4058   Fax (856)234-9402

O'Donnell, Timothy S., DO {1841239050} PulDis, CritCr, UtlRQA(85,NJ75)<NJ-CHILTON, NJ-MORRISTN>
+ Pompton Lakes Pulmonary PC
63 Beaver Brook Road/Suite 301   Lincoln Park, NJ 07035   (973)694-1300   Fax (973)694-1399
polkpul@msn.com

O'Donnell-Mulgrew, Deborah M., DO {1639149123} PsyCAd, Pedtrc, IntrMd(97,NJ75)<NJ-COOPRUMC>
+ University Hospital-Cares Institute
42 East Laurel Road/Suite 1100   Stratford, NJ 08084   (856)566-7036   Fax (856)566-6108

O'Dowd, Thomas J., MD {1598736423} SrgOrt(79,NY20)<NJ-VIRTVOOR, NJ-VIRTBERL>
+ South Jersey Orthopedic Associates PA
502 Centennial Boulevard/Suite 6   Voorhees, NJ 08043   (856)424-8866   Fax (856)424-2665
+ South Jersey Orthopedic Associates PA
901 Route 168/Suite 307   Turnersville, NJ 08012   (856)424-8866   Fax (856)228-1711

O'Driscoll, Margaret Ann, MD Pedtrc(93,NJ05)<NJ-STBARNMC>
+ St. Barnabas Medical Center
94 Old Short Hills Road/Pediatrics   Livingston, NJ 07039   (973)322-5000

O'Flynn, Leisa Diane, DO {1811936289} ObsGyn(00,NJ75)
+ Premier Women's Health of South Jersey
34 Colson Lane   Mullica Hill, NJ 08062   (856)223-1385
+ Premier Women's Health of South Jersey
603 North Broad Street/Suite 300   Woodbury, NJ 08096   (856)223-1385   Fax (856)223-8948
+ Premier Women's Health of South Jersey
340 West Front Street/Suite 201   Elmer, NJ 08062   (856)223-8930   Fax (856)223-8948

O'Grady, John P., MD {1366477283} InfDis(90,NJ05)
+ IPC The Hospitalist Company
220 Ridgedale Avenue/Suite C-2   Florham Park, NJ 07932   (973)538-5844   Fax (973)267-0181

O'Hagan Sotsky, Carol Ann, MD {1710966064} InfDis, IntrMd(82,NY09)<NJ-VALLEY>
+ Ridgewood Infectious Disease Associates
947 Linwood Avenue/Suite 2E   Ridgewood, NJ 07450   (201)447-6468   Fax (201)447-3189

O'Hara, Jennifer Fisk, MD {1457576076} FamMed, IntrMd(04,NJ05)
+ Hunterdon Family Physicians
111 State Route 31/Suite 111   Flemington, NJ 08822   (908)284-9880   Fax (908)782-4316
+ Raritan Family Health Care
901 US Highway 202   Raritan, NJ 08869   (908)284-9880   Fax (908)253-6908

Physicians by Name and Address

O'Hara, Kathleen Patricia, MD {1114970183} SrgCrC, SrgTrm, Surgry(91,DC02)
+ 211 Essex Street/Suite 206
Hackensack, NJ 07601 (201)996-0087 Fax (201)996-0185
KOHARAMD@aol.com

O'Hara, Michael W., DO {1467431536} Anesth, PainMd(90,NJ75)<NJ-CENTRAST>
+ New Jersey Ambulatory Anesthesia Consultants, LLC
55 Schanck Road/Suite 8-A Freehold, NJ 07728 (732)431-9544 Fax (732)431-9313

O'Hare, Kendal Eggers, MD {1831321041} FamMed
+ Tatem Brown Family Practice
2225 East Evesham Road/Suite 101 Voorhees, NJ 08043 (856)795-4330 Fax (856)325-3704

O'Keefe, Arthur A., Jr., MD {1891765269} CdvDis, IntrMd(94,GRNA)<NJ-BAYSHORE>
+ Cardiac Care Center
21 North Gilbert Street Tinton Falls, NJ 07701 (732)741-7400 Fax (732)741-4775

O'Keefe, Mary Clare, MD {1467481846} EmrgMd(89,DC01)<NJ-MONMOUTH>
+ Monmouth Medical Center
300 Second Avenue/EmergMed Long Branch, NJ 07740 (732)222-5200
+ EmCare
1945 Route 33 Neptune, NJ 07753 (732)222-5200 Fax (732)776-2329

O'Laughlin, Richard Lawrence, MD {1023126158} RadDia(85,NJ05)<NJ-ACMCITY, NJ-SHOREMEM>
+ Atlantic Medical Imaging, LLC.
3100 Hingston Avenue Egg Harbor Township, NJ 08234 (609)677-9729 Fax (609)646-5469
+ Atlantic Medical Imaging, LLC.
72 West Jimmie Leeds Road Galloway, NJ 08205 (609)677-9729 Fax (609)653-8764
+ Atlantic Medical Imaging, LLC.
401 Bethel Road Somers Point, NJ 08234 (609)677-9729

O'Mahony, Christopher James, MD {1992023048} Anesth
+ St. Barnabas Medical Center
94 Old Short Hills Road/Anesthesia Livingston, NJ 07039 (973)322-5512 Fax (973)660-9779
+ New Jersey Anesthesia Associates, P.C.
30B Vreeland Road/Suite 200 Florham Park, NJ 07932 (973)322-5512 Fax (973)660-9779

O'Mahony, Lisa, MD {1548296965} Pedtrc(84,PA09)
+ Advocare, LLC.
402 Lippincott Drive Marlton, NJ 08053 (856)504-8028 Fax (856)504-8029

O'Malley, Bernard B., MD {1528088713} RadDia, RadNro, Radiol(85,NY15)<NJ-UNVMCPRN>
+ Princeton Radiology Associates, P.A.
419 North Harrison Street Princeton, NJ 08540 (609)921-3345 Fax (609)683-8847
+ Princeton Radiology Associates, P.A.
3674 Route 27 Kendall Park, NJ 08824 (609)921-3345 Fax (732)821-6675

O'Malley, Michael J., MD {1396976247}
+ Rothman Institute
999 Route 73 North/3rd Fl Marlton, NJ 08053 (856)821-6360 Fax (854)821-6359
mjo.omalley@gmail.com

O'Mara, Adam Graham, DO {1609161512} EmrgMd<NJ-NWRKBETH>
+ Newark Beth Israel Medical Center
201 Lyons Avenue Newark, NJ 07112 (973)926-6671

O'Mara, James M., MD {1093764607} ObsGyn(84,MEX34)<NJ-CHSMRCER>
+ 1450 Parkside Avenue/Suite 20
Trenton, NJ 08638 (609)530-1818

O'Neal, Isaac, MD {1598809626} Pedtrc, IntrMd(80,NJ05)
+ Newark Department of Health and Human Services
110 William Street Newark, NJ 07102 (973)733-5300
+ Paterson Community Health Center
32 Clinton Street Paterson, NJ 07522 (973)733-5300 Fax (973)790-7703

O'Neil, James P., MD {1861469181} CdvDis, IntrMd(71,KS02)<NJ-VIRTMHBC>
+ The Cardiology Group, P.A.
128 State Highway Route 70/Suite 1-B Medford, NJ 08055 (856)291-8855 Fax (609)444-5521
+ The Cardiology Group, P.A.
401 Young Avenue/Suite 275 Moorestown, NJ 08057 (856)291-8855 Fax (856)291-8844
+ Avnet Memec
7000 Atrium Way/Suite 6 Mount Laurel, NJ 08055 (856)291-6818 Fax (856)291-6819

O'Neill, Anna M., MD {1710197421} MtFtMd, ObsGyn, EmrgMd(00,NJ06)
+ St. Christopher Care at Washington Township
405 Hurffville-Cross Keys Road Sewell, NJ 08080 (856)589-1414 Fax (856)589-9487

O'Neill, James P., MD {1699849869} PsyAdt, PsyAdd, NrlgAddM(84,MEX34)<NJ-RWJHLTS>
+ 1540 State route 138/Suite 307
Wall, NJ 07719 (732)280-7555 Fax (732)776-5690

O'Neill, Leon Frederick, IV, DO {1275723736} CdvDis, IntrMd(05,PA77)<NJ-RWJUHAM>
+ Monmouth Cardiology Associates, LLC
11 Meridian Road Eatontown, NJ 07724 (732)663-0300 Fax (732)663-0301
+ Monmouth Cardiology Associates, LLC
222 Schanck Road/Suite 104 Freehold, NJ 07728 (732)663-0300 Fax (732)431-1712

O'Neill, Michael B., MD {1477501782} Pedtrc(69,NJ05)<NJ-NWTNMEM>
+ Skylands Pediatrics
328-A Sparta Avenue Sparta, NJ 07871 (973)729-2197 Fax (973)729-3653
+ Skylands Pediatrics
4 Oxbow Lane/Route 94 Franklin, NJ 07416 (973)729-2197 Fax (973)827-5093

O'Reilly, Colin R., DO {1356671887} PedCrC, PallCr
+ Children's Specialized Hospital
200 Somerset Street New Brunswick, NJ 08901 (732)258-7000
+ The Valerie Fund Children's Ctr/Goryeb
100 Madison Avenue/Simon 2 Morristown, NJ 07962 (732)258-7000 Fax (973)290-7364

O'Reilly, Sara B., DO {1063623205} ObsGyn(04,ME75)<NJ-MORRISTN, NJ-STCLRDEN>
+ Women's Care Source
111 Madison Avenue/Suite 308 Morristown, NJ 07960 (973)285-0400 Fax (973)285-9848
+ Women's Care Source
16 Pocono Road/Suite 309 Denville, NJ 07834 (973)983-7695

O'Reilly, Thomas Christian, MD {1013132141} PsyCAd(03,NJ06)
+ AtlantiCare Behavioral Health/Pact Team A
2511 Fire Road/Suite B-10 Egg Harbor Township, NJ 08234 (609)407-0042 Fax (609)407-0185

O'Shea, Alice P., MD {1912156688} Psychy(83,DOM10)<NJ-ACMCMAIN, NJ-ACMCITY>
+ AtlantiCare Regional Med Ctr/Mainland
65 West Jimmie Leeds Road/Psychiatry Pomona, NJ 08240 (609)652-1000

O'Shea, Joan Frances, MD {1801969357} Surgry, SrgNro(91,NY15)<NJ-VIRTMARL, NJ-VIRTMHBC>
+ The Spine Institute of Southern New Jersey
512 Lippincott Drive Marlton, NJ 08053 (856)797-9161 Fax (856)797-3637

O'Shea, Michelle T., MD {1023040771} Surgry, SrgBst(96,NJ05)<NJ-MORRISTN, NJ-NWTNMEM>
+ Summit Breast Care, LLC.
89 Sparta Avenue/Suite 210 Sparta, NJ 07871 (908)762-0058 Fax (973)729-3194
summitbreastcare@aol.com
+ Summit Breast Care, LLC.
649 Morris Avenue Springfield, NJ 07081 (908)762-0058 Fax (973)258-1153
+ Summit Breast Care/The Connie Dwyer Breast Center
111 Central Avenue Newark, NJ 07871 (908)918-0001 Fax (908)918-0003

Oana, Dan C., MD {1396705406} AdolMd, Pedtrc(78,ROM06)<NJ-STBARNMC>
+ Summit Medical Group
75 East Northfield Road Livingston, NJ 07039 (973)436-1540 Fax (908)673-7336

Oana Soni, Agnes, MD {1306878483} NnPnMd, Pedtrc(78,ROM06)<NJ-STBARNMC>
+ St. Barnabas Medical Center
94 Old Short Hills Road/Neonatology Livingston, NJ 07039 (973)322-5000 Fax (973)322-8833

Oates, Angela Jasmine, MD {1447437868} IntrMd(05,NE06)
+ 8 Bypass Road
Salem, NJ 08079 (856)878-6914

Obade, Thomas P., MD {1356348551} SrgOrt(68,PA12)<NJ-UNDRWD>
+ Advanced Orthopaedic Centers
414 Tatum Street Woodbury, NJ 08096 (856)848-3880 Fax (856)848-4895
+ Advanced Orthopaedic Centers
159 Bridgeton Pike/Building D Mullica Hill, NJ 08062 (856)848-3880 Fax (856)223-0566

Obaid, Nabeel B., MD {1063448504} InfDis, IntrMd(79,EGY03)<NJ-EASTORNG, NJ-PALISADE>
+ 107 Timberline Drive
Wayne, NJ 07470 (973)692-0335 Fax (973)692-0336

Obaid, Sana Hamdan, MD {1619106671} ObsGyn, IntrMd(85,EGY10)
+ 1130 Mcbride Avenue/Suite C
Little Falls, NJ 07424 (973)785-8400 Fax (973)785-8402

Obando, David A., MD {1932109063} PthACl, Pthlgy, PthCln(86,COLO)<NJ-VIRTVOOR>
+ Virtua Voorhees
100 Bowman Drive Voorhees, NJ 08043 (856)247-3000

Obara, Justyna Anna, MD {1174768048} IntrMd, Grtrcs(04,SLU01)<NJ-HACKNSK>
+ CompleteCare Adult & Specialty Medical Professionals
1038 East Chestnut Avenue/Suite 110 Vineland, NJ 08360 (856)451-4700

Obaray, Akbar H., MD {1104863299} CritCr, IntrMd, PulDis(72,INDI)<NJ-RWJUBRUN, NJ-STFRNMED>
+ 2069 Klockner Road
Hamilton, NJ 08690 (609)586-0031 Fax (609)586-0708

Obaze, Ofunne Omo, MD {1386684884} Pedtrc, EmrgMd(84,NIG07)<NJ-JFKMED>
+ Hackensack Univ Medical Center Pediatric Emerg Room
30 Prospect Avenue Hackensack, NJ 07601 (201)996-5430 Fax (201)996-3676

Obeleniene, Rimvida, MD {1073559597} CdvDis, IntrMd(92,LIT02)<NJ-STJOSHOS, NJ-VALLEY>
+ Heart & Vascular Associates of Northern Jersey
1114 Clifton Avenue Clifton, NJ 07013 (973)471-5250
+ Heart & Vascular Associates of Northern Jersey
50 South Franklin Turnpike Ramsey, NJ 07446 (973)471-5250 Fax (201)934-6217
+ Heart & Vascular Associates of Northern Jersey
22-18 Broadway/Suite 201 Fair Lawn, NJ 07013 (201)475-5050 Fax (201)475-5522

Oberdorf, William Eric, DO {1437569431} IntHos<NJ-COOPRUMC>
+ Cooper University Hospital
One Cooper Plaza/Hospitalist Camden, NJ 08103 (856)342-2000

Oberlender, Susan B., MD {1194724575} Radiol, RadDia(86,PA13)<NJ-VIRTVOOR, NJ-VIRTMARL>
+ South Jersey Radiology Associates, P.A.
901 Route 168/Suites 301-305 Turnersville, NJ 08012 (856)227-6600 Fax (856)227-8537
+ South Jersey Radiology Associates, P.A.
315 Route 70 East/Suite B Cherry Hill, NJ 08034 (856)227-6600 Fax (856)428-0356
+ South Jersey Radiology Associates, P.A.
1000 Lincoln Drive East Marlton, NJ 08012 (856)983-1818 Fax (856)983-3226

Oberoi, Mandeep S., MD {1922158542} IntrMd(89,INDI)
+ Central Jersey Health Care Associates
240 Williamson Street/Suite 305 Elizabeth, NJ 07201 (908)354-5353 Fax (908)351-6911

Oberweis, Brandon Scott, MD {1669798419} CdvDis<NY-PRSBCOLU>
+ Cardiology Associates of New Brunswick
593 Cranbury Road/Suite 2 East Brunswick, NJ 08816 (732)390-3333 Fax (732)390-9244

Obi, Manfred K., MD {1467634360} Psychy(78,NIG02)
+ University Behavioral HealthCare
183 South Orange Avenue Newark, NJ 07103

Obianwu, Chike W., MD {1902984909} ObsGyn(84,DMN01)<NJ-VIRTMHBC>
+ Alliance Ob/Gyn Consultants
5045 Route 130 South/Suite 1 Delran, NJ 08075 (856)764-7660 Fax (856)764-5723

Obias, Primabel Villena, MD {1225059579} Nephro, IntrMd(92,PHIL)<NJ-RWJUBRUN, NJ-STPETER>
+ Associated Renal & Hypertension Group, P.C.
7 Cedar Grove Lane/Suite 31 Somerset, NJ 08873 (732)873-1400 Fax (732)960-3444

Obidike, Chika Esther, MD {1740414713} IntrMd
+ Chilton Medical Center
97 West Parkway Pompton Plains, NJ 07444 (973)831-5000 Fax (973)831-5059
chika_obidike@teamhealth.com

Obiefuna, Nkechiyere Angela, MD {1417103417} IntHos
+ 1920 Forest Haven Blvd.
Edison, NJ 08817 (732)710-1214

Obilo, Iwuozo Livinus, MD {1538103825} Pedtrc(86,DOM16)<NY-NYACKHOS>
+ Family Pediatrics, LLC
210 Hamburg Turnpike Wayne, NJ 07470 (973)942-9191 Fax (973)942-7111

Obleada, Clarita N., MD {1538299615} Psychy, PsyCAd(76,PHI30)
+ Catholic Charities Family Service Center
540 US Highway 22 Bridgewater, NJ 08807 (908)722-1881 Fax (908)704-0215

Obleada, Maria C.P., MD {1386754471} Pedtrc(82,PHI01)<NJ-CHSMRCER, NJ-RWJUHAM>
+ 1613 Princeton Avenue
Lawrenceville, NJ 08648 (609)394-9599 Fax (609)394-5511

Obregon, Carlos A., DO {1093785487} CritCr, PulDis, IntrMd(90,NY75)
+ 100A Kings Way West
Sewell, NJ 08080 (856)218-8080 Fax (856)218-8070

Obregon, Raimundo L., MD {1477646362} Otlryg, SrgHdN(72,SPA06)<NJ-TRININPC, NJ-OVERLOOK>
+ 1308 Morris Avenue/Suite 201
Union, NJ 07083 (908)688-8855 Fax (908)688-9282
Drobregon@verizon.net

Obrotka, Thomas M., MD {1649465642} Ophthl(72,MEXI)<NJ-CHILTON>
+ 220 Hamburg Turnpike/Suite 7
Wayne, NJ 07470 (973)904-0271 Fax (973)904-1330

Obuz, Vedat, MD {1255385233} IntrMd(88,TUR03)<NJ-CHSFULD, NJ-CHSMRCER>
+ Lotus Medical Center
40 Fuld Street/Suite 307 Trenton, NJ 08638 (609)278-9700 Fax (609)278-9744
+ Lotus Medical Center
2010 New Albany Road Cinnaminson, NJ 08077 (856)829-5466

Ocasio, Deborah L., MD {1972764983} Psychy(02,MEX03)
+ 213 69th Street/Apt 1
Guttenberg, NJ 07093 (201)892-9118

Ocasio, Maria Elena, MD {1881844330} FamMed, IntrMd(NJ02<NJ-OVERLOOK>
+ Chatham Family Practice Associates
492 Main Street Chatham, NJ 07928 (973)635-2432 Fax (973)635-6169

Ocasio, Robert B., MD {1124054200} IntrMd(94,PRO03)
+ De Persia Medical Group
17 West Red Bank Avenue/Suite 207 Woodbury, NJ 08096 (856)845-0664 Fax (856)845-7602

Ochs, Rachel Catherine, MD {1568624864}
+ 100 The American Road
Morris Plains, NJ 07950 (973)290-1814

Ocken, Stephen M., MD {1598765844} CdvDis, IntrMd(77,NY08)
+ RWJPE Cardiology Associates of Somerset County, P.A.
487 Union Avenue/Suite A Bridgewater, NJ 08807 (908)722-6410 Fax (908)722-4638

Ockrymiek, Steven B., DO {1942757612} Gastrn(77,PA77)
+ US Health Works of New Jersey
16000 Horizon Way/Suite 600 Mount Laurel, NJ 08054 (856)780-9910 Fax (856)780-9911

Oczkos, Patrick, MD {1386208023} Psychy<NJ-BERGNMC>
+ New Bridge Medical Center
230 East Ridgewood Avenue Paramus, NJ 07652 (201)967-4000

Odatalla, Bassam N., MD {1063620060} FamMed
+ St. Joseph's Family Medicine @ Clifton
1135 Broad Street/Suite 201 Clifton, NJ 07013 (973)754-4100 Fax (973)472-9062

Odejobi, Lookman K., MD {1306888789} IntrMd(85,NIG06)
+ Atlantic Shore Medical, PA
2100 Corlies Avenue/Suite 20 Neptune, NJ 07753 (732)776-9776 Fax (732)776-9882

Odell, Tamara Lozier, DO {1356508592} FamMed
+ 1000 Sanger Avenue/Suite 210
Oceanport, NJ 07757 (732)460-1313 Fax (732)460-1333

Odeyemi, Olutunde Olakunle, MD {1730100397} IntrMd(98,NIG05)
+ 7 Radcliffe Drive
Sparta, NJ 07871

Odigboegwu, Joyce Cynthia, MD {1649536194}
+ Mountainside Family Practice Associates
799 Bloomfield Avenue/Suite 201 Verona, NJ 07044 (973)259-3578 Fax (973)857-2831

Odondi, Janet Aoko, MD {1730164302} Anesth(93,KEN01)<NJ-STMRYPAS>
+ St. Mary's Hospital
350 Boulevard/Anesth Passaic, NJ 07055 (973)365-4300 Fax (973)779-7385

Odorczuk, Marzena, MD {1427153527} IntrMd(95,GRN01)<NJ-WAYNEGEN>
+ Totowa Physicians and Surgeons
426 Union Boulevard Totowa, NJ 07512 (973)595-8400 Fax (973)595-8501

Odujebe, Henry A., MD {1487648283} Surgry, EmrgMd(71,IRQ01)<NJ-EASTORNG>
+ Pathlink, LLC
66 West Gilbert Street/Suite 100 Tinton Falls, NJ 07701 (732)212-0060 Fax (732)212-0061
+ East Orange General Hospital
300 Central Avenue East Orange, NJ 07018 (973)672-8400

Odunlami, Henry Bandele, MD {1174570212} Psychy(89,NIG01)<NJ-SOMERSET, NJ-UNVMCPRN>
+ Adams Harris Inc
981 US Highway 22/Suite 200 Bridgewater, NJ 08807 (908)231-0511 Fax (908)231-1115
+ GenPsych
1661 US Highway 22/Suite 200 Bound Brook, NJ 08805 (732)369-6501

Oduye, Adedayo, DO {1942615398}<NJ-MEADWLND>
+ Meadowlands Hospital Medical Center
55 Meadowlands Parkway Secaucus, NJ 07096 (201)392-3258

Oei, Erwin John, MD {1659373421} IntrMd, PulDis(92,NJ06)<NJ-ATLANTHS, NJ-MORRISTN>
+ Pulmonary & Allergy Associates
8 Saddle Road/Suite 101 Cedar Knolls, NJ 07927 (973)267-9393 Fax (973)540-0472
+ Pulmonary & Allergy Associates
1 Springfield Avenue/Suite 3-A Summit, NJ 07901 (973)267-9393 Fax (908)934-0556

Oen, Rose L., MD {1588749048} IntrMd(70,IND10)
+ 781 Kennedy Boulevard
Bayonne, NJ 07002 (201)823-0166 Fax (201)856-4924

Oey, Theresia M., MD {1992725329} Pedtrc(74,IND05)<NJ-STPETER>
+ 75 Monroe Avenue
Belle Mead, NJ 08502

Ofeldt, James D., DO {1700815248} Anesth(89,NJ75)
+ Morris Anesthesia Group, PA
3799 Route 46/Suite 211 Parsippany, NJ 07054 (973)335-1122 Fax (973)335-1448

Ofori Behome, Yaw, MD {1427216746} FamMed
+ 135 South Broadway/Suite A-4
South Amboy, NJ 08879 (732)727-4900 Fax (732)727-4902

Ogbara, Jeffrey, MD {1528112513} IntrMd
+ Cardiovascular Associates of The Delaware Valley, PA
525 State Street/Suite 3 Elmer, NJ 08318 (856)358-2363 Fax (856)358-0725

Ogbeide, Adesuwa, MD {1568958924}
+ JFK Family Practice Group
65 James Street Edison, NJ 08818 (732)321-7487 Fax (732)906-4927

Ogden, Alfred Trecartin, MD {1174795116} SrgNro(00,NY01)
+ Neurosurgeons of New Jersey
1200 East Ridgewood Avenue Ridgewood, NJ 07450 (201)824-6131

Ogden, Neeta Sharma, MD {1467470682} AlgyImmn
+ Madho K. Sharma MD PA
30 Hoy Avenue Fords, NJ 08863 (732)225-9115 Fax (732)225-2814

Ogedegbe, Chinwe, MD {1659365450} EmrgMd(88,NIG05)<NJ-HACKNSK>
+ Hackensack Medical Center Emergency Medicine
30 Prospect Avenue/Main 3619 Hackensack, NJ 07601 (201)996-4614 Fax (201)996-4239
+ Hackensack University Medical Center
30 Prospect Avenue/EmergMed Hackensack, NJ 07601 (201)996-2300

Ogidan, Olabode O., MD {1124096383} Pedtrc(90,NIG07)
+ Vineland Pediatrics
1138 East Chestnut Avenue/Suite 5 Vineland, NJ 08360 (856)692-1108 Fax (609)692-2077

Oglesby, Renita, DO {1548450851}(05,NY75)
+ 70 Union Avenue
Nutley, NJ 07110
+ Horizon Health Center
714 Bergen Avenue Jersey City, NJ 07306 (201)451-6300

Ognibene, Lawrence G., DO {1578631891} Gastrn, IntrMd(90,PA77)<NJ-ACMCITY, NJ-ACMCMAIN>
+ Jersey Shore Gastroenterology
408 Bethel Road/Suite E Somers Point, NJ 08244 (609)926-3330 Fax (609)926-8578
+ Jersey Shore Gastroenterology
108 North Main Street Cape May Court House, NJ 08210 (609)465-0060

Ogolo, Clinton, MD {1730219981} IntrMd(85,NIG07)<NJ-CHSFULD, NJ-CHSMRCER>
+ 1457 Nottingham Way
Trenton, NJ 08609 (609)586-3828 Fax (609)586-9466

Ogon, Bernard Okem, MD {1255509873} FamMed, Grtrcs(99,NIG12)
+ CentraState Family Medicine Residency Practice
1001 West Main Street/Suite B Freehold, NJ 07728 (732)294-1989 Fax (732)294-9328

Oguayo, Kevin Nnaemeka, MD {1477849461} IntrMd
+ Hackensack Medical Center-Internal Medicine
30 Prospect Avenue/4 Main/Rm 4621 Hackensack, NJ 07601 (551)996-3880 Fax (551)996-0949

Ogun, David J., MD {1447350418} IntrMd(93,PA13)<NJ-KIMBALL>
+ Ocean County Internal Medicine Associates
1352 River Avenue Lakewood, NJ 08701 (732)370-5100 Fax (732)901-9240

Ogunbameru, Emilola O., MD {1104830173} Pedtrc, PedEmg, EmrgEMed(90,NIG03)<NJ-STJOSHOS>
+ St Joseph's Medical Pedicatric EmerMed
703 Main Street Paterson, NJ 07503 (973)754-2222
+ St Joseph's Medical Center Emergency
703 Main Street Paterson, NJ 07503 (973)754-2222 Fax (973)754-2249

Ogundare, Tobi M., MD {1376906222} IntrMd<NJ-NWRKBETH>
+ Newark Beth Israel Medical Center
201 Lyons Avenue Newark, NJ 07112 (973)926-7425

Ogunkoya, Adeniyi A., MD {1356432678} IntrMd, Allrgy(81,NY08)<NJ-EASTORNG, NJ-NWRKBETH>
+ Adeniy Ogunkoya, M.D. P.C.
964 Sanford Avenue Irvington, NJ 07111 (973)371-9050 Fax (973)371-2593

Ogunleye, Temitayo A., MD {1891956595} Dermat
+ Penn Medicine at Woodbury Heights
1006 Mantua Pike Woodbury Heights, NJ 08097 (215)662-8060 Fax (856)845-0535

Ogwudu, Ugochukwu Chinweze, MD {1508070061} Surgry, SrgThr(03,MA07)
+ Inspira Medical Group Surgical Associates
1102 East Chestnut Avenue Vineland, NJ 08360 (856)213-6375 Fax (856)575-4986

Oh, David H., MD {1033268321} EmrgMd(95,VA07)<NJ-SOMERSET>
+ Emergency Medical Associates of NJ, P.A.
3 Century Drive Parsippany, NJ 07054 (973)740-0607 Fax (973)740-9895

Oh, Donald, MD {1548321649} Psychy(66,KOR09)
+ 1749 Hooper Avenue/Suite 102
Toms River, NJ 08753 (732)255-9411

Oh, Sangbaek Charles, MD {1578513131} Gastrn, IntrMd(91,NY47)<NJ-MTNSIDE, NJ-CLARMAAS>
+ Montclair Gastroenterology Consultants, LLC
200 Highland Avenue/Suite 10 Glen Ridge, NJ 07028 (973)748-9166 Fax (973)748-1373
scharlesoh@optonline.net

Oh, Youn K., MD {1851458145} Nrolgy, Psychy, IntrMd(64,KOR06)
+ Edison Neurologic Associates
36 Progress Street/Suite B-3 Edison, NJ 08820 (908)757-6633 Fax (908)757-3912

Oh-Park, Moo-Yeon, MD {1760576029} PhysMd, SprtMd(89,KOR04)<NY-MNTFMOSE, NY-MNTFWEIL>
+ Kessler Institute for Rehabilitation West Orange
1199 Pleasant Valley Way West Orange, NJ 07052 (973)243-6943

Ohanian, Heripsime, MD {1134113582} ObsGyn, Dermat(84,FRA06)<NJ-VALLEY, NJ-HACKNSK>
+ Bergen Aesthetics
1 Kalisa Way/Suite 103 Paramus, NJ 07652 (201)265-9042 Fax (201)265-1682

Ohanian, Marc S., MD {1992897185} Anesth(90,NJ05)<NJ-JRSYCITY>
+ Fort Lee Surgery Center
1608 Lemoine Avenue/Suite 101 Fort Lee, NJ 07024 (201)346-1112 Fax (201)346-1885

Ohngemach, Christopher, MD {1033139472} Pedtrc, PedCrC(86,GER16)<NJ-STPETER>
+ St. Peter's University Hospital
254 Easton Avenue/Pediatrics New Brunswick, NJ 08901 (732)745-6684 Fax (732)745-8725

Ohri, Anupam, MD {1902103872} EnDbMt, IntrMd(99,INA07)
+ RWJ University Endocrinology Diabetes & Metabolism
125 Paterson Street/CAB 5100A New Brunswick, NJ 08901 (732)235-7219 Fax (732)235-8610

Ohri, Ranjana, MD {1316931637} Pedtrc(94,NJ05)
+ Union Pediatric Medical Group, PA
1050 Galloping Hill Road/Suite 200 Union, NJ 07083 (908)688-9900 Fax (908)688-9939

Ohri, Renu, MD {1255355533} IntrMd(93,NJ05)<NJ-VAEASTOR, NJ-HACKNSK>
+ VA New Jersey Health Care System-East Orange Campus
385 Tremont Avenue East Orange, NJ 07018 (973)676-1000

Ohsie-Bajor, Linda Hae Eun, MD {1801008354} Ophthl(06,PA02)
+ Eye Care Physicians & Surgeons of New Jersey
2301 Evesham Road/Suite 501-502 Voorhees, NJ 08043 (856)770-0030 Fax (856)770-0840
+ Eye Care Physicians & Surgeons of New Jersey
73 South Main Street Medford, NJ 08055 (856)770-0030 Fax (609)953-2257

Oif, Edward, MD {1730384447} RadDia
+ Lourdes Imaging Associates, PA
1600 Haddon Avenue Camden, NJ 08103 (856)757-3933 Fax (856)668-8436

Ojadi, Vallier Chidiebere, MD {1255370573} Pedtrc(88,NIG02)
+ Family Medicine at Monument Square
317 George Street New Brunswick, NJ 08901 (732)235-8993 Fax (732)246-7317

Ojeabulu, Janet, MD {1013250646}
+ 760 South 15th Street
Newark, NJ 07103 (908)472-4149

Physicians by Name and Address

Oji, Omobola Abiodun, MD {1194880583} FamMed(88,NIG01)
+ 25 Craig Place
North Plainfield, NJ 07060   (908)791-9993
+ Providence Medical Center
119 Gaston Avenue   Somerville, NJ 08876   (908)791-9993   Fax (908)791-9995

Ojiako, Kizito C., MD {1679520431} IntrMd<NJ-SJHREGMC>
+ SJH Regional Medical Center
1505 West Sherman Avenue   Vineland, NJ 08360   (856)641-8000

Ojserkis, Bennett Edward, MD {1619068491} CritCr, Grtrcs, PulDis(79,NY45)<NJ-SHOREMEM, NJ-ACMCMAIN>
+ The Advanced Pulmonary Diagnostic Center
100 Medical Center Way   Somers Point, NJ 08244   (609)653-3467   Fax (609)653-3586

Ojutiku, Oreoluwa Olubukunola, MD {1104004605} RadDia(04,NY46)<NJ-HACKNSK>
+ Hackensack University Medical Center
30 Prospect Avenue/Radiology   Hackensack, NJ 07601   (201)996-2069   Fax (201)996-5116
oreojutiku@gmail.com

Okafor, Anthony Ifechukwu, MD {1306845391} IntrMd, EmrgMd(95,PA09)<NJ-HOBUNIMC>
+ Hoboken University Medical Center
308 Willow Avenue/EmrgMed   Hoboken, NJ 07030   (201)418-1000

Okafor, Chidubem O., DO {1235362963}
+ 73B Maplewood Drive
Maple Shade, NJ 08052

Okafor, Joana O., MD {1285722868} ObsGyn(79,DC03)
+ 484 Main Street
East Orange, NJ 07018   (973)674-6990   Fax (973)674-6680

Okechukwu, Christopher O., MD {1275528143} IntrMd, EmrgMd(88,NIGE)<NJ-NWTNMEM>
+ Newton Medical Center
175 High Street   Newton, NJ 07860   (973)383-2121

Okeke, Ngozi C., MD {1053547745} IntrMd, IntHos(09,NY15)<NJ-ENGLWOOD>
+ Englewood Hospital and Medical Center
350 Engle Street/Hospitalist   Englewood, NJ 07631   (201)894-3364

Okere, Arthur Ezeribe, MD {1790928612} CdvDis(07,MA05)<NY-BETHPETR>
+ Shore Heart Group, P.A.
1820 State Route 33/Suite 4-B   Neptune, NJ 07753   (732)776-8500   Fax (732)776-8946
+ Shore Heart Group, P.A.
555 Iron Bridge Road/Suite 15   Freehold, NJ 07728   (732)776-8500   Fax (732)333-1366
+ Shore Heart Group, P.A.
115 East Bay Avenue   Manahawkin, NJ 07753   (609)971-3300   Fax (609)597-4656

Okezie, Chukueke Tobenna, MD {1235177437} SrgOrt, SrgHnd(92,CT01)<NJ-VALLEY, NJ-STJOSHOS>
+ 351 Evelyn Street/Suite 302
Paramus, NJ 07652   (201)265-3111   Fax (201)265-3117

Okoduwa, Cynthia Onon, MD {1750518056}
+ Rutgers- New Jersey Medical School
185 South Orange Avenue   Newark, NJ 07103   (973)972-4300

Okoh, Gloria Nkiru, MD {1063597441} Pedtrc, IntrMd(91,NIG04)<NJ-CLARMAAS>
+ Dr Gloria Nkiru Okoh and Assoc
163 Belleville Avenue   Belleville, NJ 07109   (973)302-4644   Fax (973)528-2242

Okon, Emmanuel E., MD {1386881993} InfDis, IntrMd(02,NIG02)
+ Lourdes Medical Associates
500 Grove Street/Suite 100   Haddon Heights, NJ 08035   (856)796-9200   Fax (856)547-5570
ufan96@yahoo.com

Okorafor, Nnennaya C., MD {1184816100} Pedtrc, PedInf(88,NIG12)<NJ-CLARMAAS>
+ Dr. Nhennaya Okorafor
1 Clarra Maass Drive   Belleville, NJ 07109   (973)450-2163   Fax (973)844-4180

Okoronkwo, Nneoma O., MD {1770864704}
+ 832 East Main Street
Belleville, NJ 07109
okoronn@njms.rutgers.edu

Okouneva, Evelina, DO {1881836625} NrlgSpec<NJ-CHLSMT>
+ Children's Specialized Hospital
150 New Providence Road   Mountainside, NJ 07092   (908)301-5491   Fax (908)301-5408

Okour, Salman N., MD {1265691505}
+ NJ Best OBGYN
716 Broad Street/Suite 6 A   Clifton, NJ 07013   (973)221-5400   Fax (973)710-0620

Okoya, Jackson A., MD {1174615165} IntrMd(82,GRNA)<NJ-MEADWLND, NJ-HOBUNIMC>
+ Hudson Physicians Associates
40 Union Avenue/Suite 204   Irvington, NJ 07111   (973)416-6981   Fax (973)375-5766

Okoye, Eronmwon, MD {1093293839} Psychy<NJ-TRININPC>
+ Trinitas Regional Medical Center-New Point Campus
655 East Jersey Street   Elizabeth, NJ 07206   (856)885-1297

Okoye, Frederick E., Jr., MD {1306815618} InfDis, IntrMd(84,DMN01)<NJ-STMICHL, NJ-EASTORNG>
+ Sylveric HealthCare Center Inc
642 Broad Street/Suite 7   Clifton, NJ 07013   (973)249-1855   Fax (973)249-1856

Okoye-Okuzu, Enuma I., MD IntrMd, Grtrcs(96,NJ05)
+ Veterans Affairs Clinic
385 Prospect Avenue   Hackensack, NJ 07601   (201)487-1390

Okpala, Augustine C., MD {1124085766} IntrMd(92,NIG02)<NJ-NWTNMEM>
+ Newton Medical Center
175 High Street/IntMed   Newton, NJ 07860   (973)579-8321

Okpala, Nkemamaka Chinenyenwa, MD {1992062749}
+ Goldson Medical Associates
20 Valley Street/Suite 320   South Orange, NJ 07079   (973)313-1113

Okubadejo, Gbolahan, MD {1497947022}
+ 25 Rockwood Place/Suite 335
Englewood, NJ 07631   (877)854-8274   Fax (201)947-0850
+ 32 Marquis Court
Edgewater, NJ 07020   (877)854-8274   Fax (201)947-0850

Okun, Jeffrey, MD {1063730794} Gastrn
+ Summit Medical Group
6 Brighton Road/2 FL   Clifton, NJ 07012   (973)777-7911   Fax (973)777-5403
+ Summit Medical Group
31-00 Broadway   Fair Lawn, NJ 07410   (973)777-7911   Fax (201)796-7020

Okunola, Oladotun A., MD {1073718185} Nrolgy(01,DC03)
+ Neuroscience Center of Northern New Jersey
310 Madison Avenue   Morristown, NJ 07960   (973)285-1446   Fax (973)605-8854

Oladeji, Oluremi O., MD {1508864265} Anesth(85,NIG01)<NJ-STJOSHOS>
+ St. Joseph's Regional Medical Center Anesthesia
703 Main Street   Paterson, NJ 07503   (973)754-2323   Fax (973)977-9455

Olarsch, Richard Gary, DO {1285608745} FamMed(92,FL75)<NJ-BURDTMLN>
+ Wildwood Family Medical Associates
4211 Pacific Avenue   Wildwood, NJ 08260   (609)522-0727   Fax (609)522-2163

Olechowski, George N., MD {1053355347} Anesth(02,NJ05)<NJ-STCLRDEN>
+ Morris Anesthesia Group, PA
3799 Route 46/Suite 211   Parsippany, NJ 07054   (973)335-1122   Fax (973)335-1448

Olegario, Eduardo S., MD {1568426187} Anesth(63,PHI01)<NJ-RBAYPERT, NJ-RBAYOLDB>
+ Raritan Bay Medical Center/Perth Amboy Division
530 New Brunswick Avenue   Perth Amboy, NJ 08861   (732)442-3700

Oleske, James M., MD {1679613830} Immuno, AllmClIm(71,NJ05)
+ Rutgers- New Jersey Medical School
185 South Orange Avenue/Pediatrics   Newark, NJ 07103   (973)972-4300
+ Rutgers- New Jersey Medical School
185 South Orange Avenue/Pediatrics   Newark, NJ 07103   (973)972-4300

Olesnicky, Ludmilla, MD {1275566721} PthAcl, Pthlgy(73,AUS04)<NJ-NWRKBETH>
+ Newark Beth Israel Medical Center
201 Lyons Avenue/Pathology   Newark, NJ 07112   (973)926-7000

Olesnicky, Mark T., MD {1770503617} IntrMd, CdvDis(71,AUS02)<NJ-STBARNMC>
+ 135 Columbia Turnpike/Suite 203
Florham Park, NJ 07932   (973)822-5000   Fax (973)822-3321
molesnicky@earthlink.net

Oliver, Joseph Benton, MD {1992203576}
+ New Bridge Medical Center
230 East Ridgewood Avenue   Paramus, NJ 07652   (201)967-4000
+ University Behavioral HealthCare
183 South Orange Avenue   Newark, NJ 07103   (973)972-6156

Oliver, Mark A., MD {1972609725} IntrMd, VasDis, OthrSp(71,IL42)<NJ-MORRISTN>
+ 182 South Street
Morristown, NJ 07960   (973)538-0165   Fax (973)538-9344

Oliver, Richard D., MD {1811081763} Grtrcs, IntrMd(77,NJ05)<NJ-STJOSHOS, NJ-WAYNEGEN>
+ Medical Internists Associates PA
22-18 Broadway/Suite 104   Fair Lawn, NJ 07410   (201)797-4503   Fax (201)797-4270

Oliveros, Elder A., MD {1851537740} RadDia(04,NJ06)<NJ-RWJUBRUN, NJ-STPETER>
+ University Radiology Group, P.C.
483 Cranbury Road   East Brunswick, NJ 08816   (732)390-0030   Fax (732)390-5383
+ University Radiology Group, P.C.
16 Mountain Boulevard   Warren, NJ 07059   (732)390-0030   Fax (908)769-9141

Olivia, Christopher Todd, MD {1164427241} Ophthl(88,PA09)<NJ-COOPRUMC>
+ Soll Eye PC of New Jersey/Cooper Division
3 Cooper Plaza/Suite 510   Camden, NJ 08103   (856)342-7200   Fax (856)342-6620

Olivieri, Philip J., MD {1831175512} CdvDis, IntrMd(78,NJ06)<NJ-MORRISTN>
+ Atlantic Cardiology Group LLP
8 Tempe Wick Road   Mendham, NJ 07945   (973)543-2288   Fax (973)543-0637
+ Atlantic Cardiology Group LLP
95 Madison Avenue/Suite 300   Morristown, NJ 07960   (973)543-2288   Fax (973)682-9494

Olivieri, William Peter, MD {1083620777} EmrgMd(80,ITAL)<NJ-HCKTSTWN>
+ Hackettstown Regional Medical Center
651 Willow Grove Street/EmergMed   Hackettstown, NJ 07840   (908)850-6800   Fax (856)616-1919

Olivo, Matthew P., MD {1669524088} Dermat(84,GRNA)<NJ-VIRTVOOR, NJ-VIRTBERL>
+ Olivo Dermatology Center
201 Haddon Avenue   Westmont, NJ 08108   (856)854-0300   Fax (856)854-4107

Olivo Mercedes, Yohanna Maria, MD {1639346869} IntrMd(04,DOM14)
+ 111 Central Avenue
Newark, NJ 07102   (973)877-2420   Fax (973)877-2413

Olivo Villabrille, Raquel, MD {1841562593} IntrMd
+ University Hospital
150 Bergen Street   Newark, NJ 07103   (973)972-6000

Olla, Olubukola Opeyemi, MD {1144518481}
+ 22 Rigate Road
Bloomfield, NJ 07003   (201)407-8764
bukola.olla@gmail.com

Oller, Helen Suguitan, MD {1003051251} PhysMd(80,PHI08)
+ 218 Pearsall Avenue
Jersey City, NJ 07305

Oller-Cramsie, Marissa Anne, DO {1528209541} Nrolgy
+ New Jersey Neurological Specialists
20 Prospect Avenue/Suite 800   Hackensack, NJ 07601   (201)518-7290   Fax (201)604-6428

Olmo Durham, Zaida E., MD {1679664007} Pthlgy, PthAClI(80,PRO03)<NJ-STPETER>
+ St. Peter's University Hospital
254 Easton Avenue/Pathology   New Brunswick, NJ 08901   (732)745-8600   Fax (732)220-8595

Oloomiyazdi, Mohammadali, MD {1104810951} Anesth(IRA08)<NJ-HACKNSK>
+ Hackensack University Medical Center
30 Prospect Avenue/Anesthesia   Hackensack, NJ 07601   (201)996-2419   Fax (201)996-3962

Olorunnisola, Moses F., Jr., MD {1467728113} Pedtrc(09,ANT02)<NJ-SOCEANCO>
+ Southern Ocean County Medical Center
1140 Route 72 West   Manahawkin, NJ 08050   (609)597-6405

Olsen, Drew Albert, MD {1215971908} PthAClI, Pthlgy, PthAna(95,NY09)<NJ-HOLYNAME>
+ Holy Name Hospital
718 Teaneck Road/Pathology   Teaneck, NJ 07666   (201)833-3000

Olsen, Janet L., MD {1114901584} Anesth(84,NY01)<NJ-HACKNSK>
+ Hackensack University MC-Anesthesia Dept
30 Prospect Avenue/Room 2703   Hackensack, NJ 07601   (201)996-2419   Fax (201)996-3962
+ Hackensack University Medical Center
30 Prospect Avenue/Anesth   Hackensack, NJ 07601   (201)996-2419   Fax (201)488-6769

Olshanetskiy, Oleg, DO {1861580201} FamMed, OstMed, AeroMd(98,NY75)<NY-BETHKING, NY-PENINSUL>
+ Airport Medical Offices at Newark Liberty
339-1 Airis Drive   Newark, NJ 07114   (973)643-8383
+ 1265 15th Street/Suite 14 G
Fort Lee, NJ 07024   (201)224-5357

Olson, Aubrey M., DO {1962692715} FamMed
+ 713 West Greenman Road
Haddonfield, NJ 08033

Olson, Robert M., MD {1811906704} SrgPlstc, Surgry(74,PA01)<NJ-STPETER, NJ-UNVMCPRN>
+ 213 North Center Drive
North Brunswick, NJ 08902   (732)418-1888   Fax (732)418-1880

Physicians by Name and Address

Olson, Ty James, MD {1174564157} SrgNro(99,NC07)<NJ-MONMOUTH, NJ-RIVERVW>
+ Neurosurgeons of New Jersey
121 Highway 36 West/Suite 330   West Long Branch, NJ 07764   (732)963-4631   Fax (732)870-6342
+ Neurosurgeons of New Jersey
530 Lakehurst Road/Suite 308   Toms River, NJ 08755   (732)443-1372

Olukoya, Olasinbo Atinuke, MD {1912947524} ObsGyn(01,NJ06)<NJ-RWJUHAM, NJ-RBAYPERT>
+ Capital Health Women's Group
433 Bellevue Avenue   Trenton, NJ 08618   (609)394-4111   Fax (609)394-4070

Olweny, Ephrem Odoy, MD {1821272006} Urolgy<NJ-RWJUBRUN>
+ RWJ University Hospital New Brunswick
One Robert Wood Johnson Place   New Brunswick, NJ 08901   (732)235-7775

Omay, Cem S., MD {1053487413} ObsGyn(87,DMN01)
+ Women's Care Source
111 Madison Avenue/Suite 308   Morristown, NJ 07960   (973)285-0400   Fax (973)285-9848

Ombalsky, Joseph, MD {1225023302} ObsGyn(98,NJ06)
+ West Long Branch Obstetrics & Gynecology
1019 Broadway   West Long Branch, NJ 07764   (732)229-6797   Fax (732)229-6893

Ombrellino, Michael, MD {1114997426} Surgry, SrgVas(92,ITA01)
+ Vein Institute of New Jersey
95 Madison Avenue/Suite 109   Morristown, NJ 07960   (973)759-9000   Fax (973)759-2487
+ Vein Institute of New Jersey
532 Lafayette Road   Sparta, NJ 07871
+ Vein Institute of New Jersey
788 Broad Street/US Highway 35   Shrewsbury, NJ 07960

Omesi, Lenore, MD {1457619488} PedHem
+ St. Joseph Medical Center Pediatric Hematology/Onc
703 Main Street   Paterson, NJ 07503   (973)754-3230

Omilian, Karen L., DO {1316053325} Psychy(85,IA75)
+ 388 Pompton Avenue
Cedar Grove, NJ 07009

Omoh, Michael E., MD {1922037746} IntrMd, EmrgMd(85,NIG05)<NJ-STFRNMED, NJ-LOURDMED>
+ Emergency Physician Associates, P.A.
307 South Evergreen Avenue/PO Box 298   Woodbury, NJ 08096   (856)848-3817   Fax (856)848-1431
+ St. Francis Medical Center
601 Hamilton Avenue   Trenton, NJ 08629   (609)599-5000

Omotoso, Babatunji Omolagba, MD {1336146851} Anesth, Pedtrc(84,NIG01)<NJ-MONMOUTH>
+ Monmouth Medical Center
300 Second Avenue/Anesthesiology   Long Branch, NJ 07740   (732)222-5200

Omotoso, Olukemi Yetunde, MD {1871575084} Pedtrc(87,NIG01)
+ Ethel and Raphael Pediatrics Inc
1405 Highway 35 North/Suite 104   Ocean, NJ 07712   (732)663-1161   Fax (732)531-2900

Onat, Esra Samli, MD {1710912902} FamMed(84,TUR01)
+ 25 Lindsley Drive/Suite 105
Morristown, NJ 07960   (973)889-0200   Fax (973)889-3544

Onat, Nermi, MD {1407869985} IntrMd(83,TUR05)
+ 239 Lakeview Avenue
Clifton, NJ 07011   (973)253-9666   Fax (973)253-0088
NONATNJ@aol.com

Ondeyka, Amy Elizabeth, MD {1700144904}<NJ-COOPRUMC>
+ Inspira Urgent Care Glassboro
200 Rowan Boulevard   Glassboro, NJ 08028   (856)582-1500   Fax (856)218-9607

Ong, Alvin C., MD {1992759138} SrgOrt(94,NY48)<NJ-ACMCITY, NJ-ATLANTHS>
+ Rothman Institute - Egg Harbor Township
2500 English Creek Avenue/Bldg 1300   Egg Harbor Township, NJ 08234   (609)677-7002   Fax (609)677-7000
+ Rothman Institute
219 North White Horse Pike   Hammonton, NJ 08037

Ong, Edgardo A., MD {1326199514} CdvDis, IntrMd(71,PHI10)
+ Advanced Cardiology, LLC.
117 Seber Road/Suite 1-B   Hackettstown, NJ 07840   (908)979-1302   Fax (973)401-1201
+ Advanced Cardiology, LLC.
65 Ridgedale Avenue   Cedar Knolls, NJ 07927   (908)979-1302   Fax (973)401-1201

Ong, Phat Vinh, MD {1356546048} Radiol, RadDia, Surgry(00,NY19)
+ Hackensack Radiology Group, P.A.
30 Prospect Avenue   Hackensack, NJ 07601   (201)996-2200   Fax (201)489-2812

Ong, Raquel Sanchez, MD {1972862456} EnDbMt
+ Hackensack Meridian Medical Group
19 Davis Avenue/5th-6th Floor   Neptune, NJ 07753   (732)897-3980   Fax (732)897-3982

Ongcapin, Emelie H., MD {1083795785} PthACl(64,PHIL)<NJ-STBARNMC>
+ St. Barnabas Cancer Center
94 Old Short Hills Road/Pathology   Livingston, NJ 07039   (973)322-5726   Fax (973)322-8917

Ongsiako, Allen R., DO {1790771293} FamMed(91,MO78)<NJ-BAYSHORE>
+ Atlantic Family Medicine LLC
169-B Route 37 West   Toms River, NJ 08755   (732)505-9333

Ongsiako, Maria V., MD {1639262975} PsyGrt, Psychy(82,PHI09)<NJ-RIVERVW>
+ Riverview Medical Center
1 Riverview Plaza/Psych   Red Bank, NJ 07701   (732)741-2700
+ 420-A Bridge Plaza Drive
Manalapan, NJ 07726   (732)617-2222

Onishchuk, Joseph L., DO
+ 18 Roberts Drive
Westampton, NJ 08060

Onopchenko, Alexander, MD {1649296732} Bariat, Surgry(84,PA07)<NJ-ACMCITY, NJ-ACMCMAIN>
+ 2500 English Creek Avenue/Suite 222
Egg Harbor Township, NJ 08234   (609)407-2332

Onufer, Karen Anne, MD {1609891837} EmrgMd(97,NJ06)<NJ-UMDNJ>
+ University Hospital
150 Bergen Street/Suite C-384   Newark, NJ 07103   (973)972-4300   Fax (973)972-2204

Onumah, Neh Johnann, MD {1902040199} Dermat
+ 101 Wenlock Court
Princeton, NJ 08540

Onwochei, Francis, MD {1225404650} IntrMd<NJ-JRSYCITY>
+ Jersey City Medical Center
355 Grand Street   Jersey City, NJ 07304   (201)915-2000

Onwubalili, Ndidiamaka, MD {1851596696} RprEnd
+ Diamond Institute for Infertility & Menopause
89 Millburn Avenue   Millburn, NJ 07041   (973)761-5600   Fax (973)761-5100

Onwudinjo, Adolphus Chukwuelua, MD {1205917978} ObsGyn(79,TN07)
+ Comprehensive Women's Healthcare
220 Hamburg Turnpike/Suite 21   Wayne, NJ 07470   (973)790-8090   Fax (973)790-3198

Onwuka, Aloysius Chukwumuche, MD {1659328987} IntrMd(91,NIG02)
+ Hackensack Meridian Medical Group
19 Davis Avenue/5th-6th Floor   Neptune, NJ 07753   (732)897-3990   Fax (732)897-3997
+ Shore Atlantic Geriatrics
1740 Bayshore Road   Villas, NJ 08251   (732)897-3990   Fax (609)889-1766

Onwuka, Mary N., MD {1649290636} IntrMd, IntHos(89,NIG02)<NJ-ACMCITY>
+ AtlantiCare Regional Medical Center/City Campus
1925 Pacific Avenue   Atlantic City, NJ 08401   (609)345-4000
Onwuka@att.net

Onwuka, William N., MD {1437186590} Pedtrc(88,MEXI)<NJ-ENGLWOOD>
+ 177 North Dean Street/Penthouse Floor
Englewood, NJ 07631   (201)430-7371

Onyeador, Beatrice Ogbonne, MD {1114969870} IntrMd(83,NIG03)<NJ-STMRYPAS, NJ-MTNSIDE>
+ Freedom Medical Clinics
304 Lakeview Avenue   Clifton, NJ 07011   (973)478-8600
Betty@Freedombiotech.com

Oo, Hnin Hnin, MD {1184008021} IntrMd
+ 276 Engle Street/Apt 10 A
Englewood, NJ 07631   (609)321-2680

Oolut, Joseph James, MD {1912913484} IntrMd
+ Vascular Access Center
1450 Parkside Avenue/Unit 18   Trenton, NJ 08638   (609)882-1770   Fax (609)882-8406

Oparaji, Anthony Chibuzor, MD {1285665208} IntrMd(93,NIG02)<NY-NRTHGEN, NY-MTSINAI>
+ Metropolitan Family Health Network
935 Garfield Avenue   Jersey City, NJ 07304   (201)478-5800   Fax (201)475-5814

Opdyke, Karen Stage, MD {1275805079} Psychy(97,PA12)<NJ-VALYONS>
+ VA New Jersey Health Care System at Lyons
151 Knollcroft Road/Psychiatry   Lyons, NJ 07939   (908)647-0180

Opell, M. Brett, MD {1629173679} Urolgy(96,PA02)<NJ-NWRKBETH, NJ-TRININPC>
+ New Jersey Urology, LLC
700 North Broad Street/Suite 302   Elizabeth, NJ 07208   (908)355-3077   Fax (908)289-0716
+ New Jersey Urology, LLC
1600 George Avenue/Suite 202   Rahway, NJ 07065

(908)355-3077   Fax (732)499-0432

Opler, Douglas J., MD {1760717649} Psychy<NY-MNTFMOSE>
+ University Psychiatric Associates
183 South Orange Avenue/E-F Levels   Newark, NJ 07103   (973)972-8254   Fax (973)972-2979

Oppenheim, Jeffrey Charles, MD {1952302259} FamMed, IntrMd(75,NJ06)
+ The University Doctors
100 Century Parkway/Suite 140   Mount Laurel, NJ 08054   (856)380-2400   Fax (856)234-7870

Oppenheim, William C., MD {1649376310} SrgOrt, Ortped(77,IL01)<NJ-HACKNSK>
+ The Joint Institute at Saint Barnabas Medical Center
609 Morris Avenue   Springfield, NJ 07081   (973)379-1991   Fax (973)467-8647

Oppenheimer, Ellen, MD {1841224680} PedEnd, Pedtrc, IntrMd(85,NY46)<NJ-NWRKBETH>
+ Children's Hospital of NJ Ped Cntr @ West Orange
375 Mount Pleasant Avenue/Suite 105   West Orange, NJ 07052   (973)322-6900   Fax (973)322-6999
eoppenheimer@barnabashealth.org

Oppenheimer, Jeffrey Harry, MD {1124082755} SrgNro, IntrMd
+ Anti-Aging & Laser Medical Associates
777 Terrace Avenue/Suite 403   Hasbrouck Heights, NJ 07604   (201)288-3777   Fax (201)426-0446
jomd@advancedhere.com
+ North Jersey Orthopaedic Group
33 Bleeker Street   Millburn, NJ 07041   (201)288-3777   Fax (973)564-8928
+ Ultimed HealthCare PC
50 Franklin Lane   Manalapan, NJ 07604   (732)972-1267   Fax (732)972-1026

Oppenheimer, John Jacob, MD {1639170871} Allrgy, IntrMd(86,PA13)<NJ-MORRISTN, NJ-OVERLOOK>
+ Pulmonary & Allergy Associates
8 Saddle Road/Suite 101   Cedar Knolls, NJ 07927   (973)267-9393   Fax (973)540-0472
+ Pulmonary & Allergy Associates
1 Springfield Avenue/Suite 3-A   Summit, NJ 07901   (973)267-9393   Fax (908)934-0556
+ Pulmonary & Allergy Associates
653 Willow Grove Street   Hackettstown, NJ 07927   (908)850-3338

Oquendo, Sonia I., MD {1295882553} PsycAd, Psychy, PsyFor(83,PRO03)<NJ-HACKNSK>
+ 450 Summit Avenue
Hackensack, NJ 07601   (201)487-9014   Fax (201)487-3403

Or, Drorit, MD {1851533509} ObsGyn
+ 204 Nathaniel Avenue
Cherry Hill, NJ 08003   (856)470-4044

Orafidiya, Yetunde, MD {1891054599} Pedtrc
+ 100 Franklin Street/Apt C206
Morristown, NJ 07960

Oram, Alexis Marissa, MD {1831452598} Pedtrc
+ Ocean Pediatric Group
2640 Route 70/Suite 1-B   Manasquan, NJ 08736   (732)528-8448   Fax (732)223-5792

Oranchak, Deborah J., DO {1225017031} PhysMd(97,NY75)
+ The Neurology and Headache Center
573 Cranbury Road/Suite A5   East Brunswick, NJ 08816   (732)254-5101   Fax (732)254-2640

Oranu, Uzoma, MD {1780943589} IntrMd<NJ-COOPRUMC>
+ Cooper University Hospital
One Cooper Plaza   Camden, NJ 08103   (856)342-2000

Orate-Dimapilis, Christina V., MD {1508831330} IntrMd(97,PHI02)<NJ-COOPRUMC>
+ Cooper University Hospital
One Cooper Plaza/Suite 222/Dorra   Camden, NJ 08103   (856)342-2000

Orbelyan, Gerasim A., MD {1568773711}<NJ-HOBUNIMC>
+ Hoboken University Medical Center
308 Willow Avenue   Hoboken, NJ 07030   (773)263-5052
gorbelyan@gmail.com

Ordene, Kenneth W., MD {1750472205} EnDbMt, IntrMd(77,PA01)<NJ-CENTRAST>
+ Endocrinology Associates of Central NJ
501 Iron Bridge Road/Suite 12   Freehold, NJ 07728   (732)780-0002   Fax (732)308-0117

Ordille, Joseph D., DO {1053354357} FamMed(90,MO79)
+ Center for Family Health/Doctors & Midwives
105 Manheim Avenue/Suite 1   Bridgeton, NJ 08302   (856)455-2700   Fax (856)455-7051

Ordoukhanian, Elsa, MD {1316958101} Dermat(94,PA01)<NJ-ENGLWOOD>
+ Michele Grodberg, MD & Associates
106 Grand Avenue/Suite 330   Englewood, NJ 07631   (201)567-8884   Fax (201)567-5799
elsa.ordoukhanian@ehmc.com

Physicians by Name and Address

Orejola, Wilmo C., MD {1679515878} SrgThr(74,PHIL)<NJ-STJOSHOS>
+ St. Joseph's Regional Medical Center
703 Main Street/CardioDis   Paterson, NJ 07503   (973)754-2000

Orel, Howard N., MD {1548218589} Pedtrc(86,PA01)<NJ-VIRTVOOR, NJ-VIRTMARL>
+ Advocare Marlton Pediatrics
525 Route 73 South   Marlton, NJ 08053   (856)596-3434   Fax (856)596-9110
+ Advocare Township Pediatrics
123 Egg Harbor Road   Sewell, NJ 08080   (856)596-3434   Fax (856)227-5890

Orellana, Katherine Atienza, DO {1265643068} PedGst, Pedtrc<NJ-VALLEY>
+ Drs. Orellana & Volpert
1200 East Ridgewood Avenue/Suite 108   Ridgewood, NJ 07450   (201)389-0815

Orellana Chasi, Pamela, MD {1699157446} FamMed
+ 801 74th Street
North Bergen, NJ 07047   (201)869-5778

Oren, Reva, MD {1831394824} RadOnc, Radiol, RadThp(70,ITAL)
+ Radiation Oncology Associates of North Jersey, P.A.
100 Madison Avenue   Morristown, NJ 07962   (973)971-5329   Fax (973)290-7393

Orenberg, Scott D., DO {1073665485} IntrMd(93,NY75)
+ Marven Wallen & S. Kenneth Jacobson MD PA
1985 Springfield Avenue   Maplewood, NJ 07040   (973)763-5010   Fax (973)761-6980

Origlier, Anthony, MD {1770687071} Ophthl(78,NE06)<NJ-MTNSIDE>
+ Origlieri, Anthony
180 Harrison Avenue   Roseland, NJ 07068   (973)228-8824   Fax (973)228-9482

Origlieri, Catherine Ann, MD {1457585853} Ophthl
+ Hudson Eye Physicians & Surgeons, LLC
600 Pavonia Avenue/6th Floor   Jersey City, NJ 07306   (201)963-3937   Fax (201)963-8823

Orland, Steven M., MD {1861493017} Urolgy, IntrMd(81,NY01)<NJ-RWJUHAM, NJ-CHSFULD>
+ Urology Care Alliance
Two Capital Way/Suite 407   Pennington, NJ 08534   (609)730-1966   Fax (609)730-1166

Orlando, James Frank, MD {1285604207} CdvDis, IntrMd(97,DMN01)<NJ-SOCEANCO, NJ-COMMED>
+ Shore Heart Group, P.A.
1820 State Route 33/Suite 4-B   Neptune, NJ 07753   (732)776-8500   Fax (732)776-8946
+ Shore Heart Group, P.A.
555 Iron Bridge Road/Suite 15   Freehold, NJ 07728   (732)776-8500   Fax (732)333-1366
+ Shore Heart Group, P.A.
115 East Bay Avenue   Manahawkin, NJ 07753   (609)971-3300   Fax (609)597-4656

Orlandoni, Enrico F., DO {1659340107} IntrMd(95,NJ75)
+ Skylands Medical Group PA
174 Edison Road   Lake Hopatcong, NJ 07849   (973)663-1300   Fax (973)663-2848

Orleans, Genevieve Araba, MD {1770632598} Pedtrc(92,GHA02)<NJ-TRINIWSC>
+ Trinitas Regional Medical Center-Williamson Street
225 Williamson Street/Pediatrics   Elizabeth, NJ 07207   (908)994-5000   Fax (908)994-5769

Orlic, Peter Thomas, MD {1659376713} IntrMd(89,NY09)<NJ-MORRISTN>
+ Erickson Health Medical Group
1 Cedar Crest Village Drive   Pompton Plains, NJ 07444   (973)831-3540   Fax (973)831-3503

Orloff, John J., MD EnDbMt, IntrMd(83,VT02)
+ University Medical Group/UMDNJ
125 Paterson Street/Suite 2200   New Brunswick, NJ 08901   (732)235-7647   Fax (732)235-7677

Orlov, Olga, MD {1407813215} Pedtrc, AdolMd(72,UKRA)<NJ-CHILTON, PA-STJORDNG>
+ 508 Hamburg Turnpike/Suite 107
Wayne, NJ 07470   (973)942-0521   Fax (973)942-9542

Orlowicz, Christine Alexis, MD {1417246620} IntrMd<NJ-UMDNJ>
+ University Hospital
150 Bergen Street/Room I-248   Newark, NJ 07103   (973)972-6056

Ornstein, Mark W., MD {1912089681} IntrMd(83,DOMI)<NJ-JRSYSHMC>
+ 43 Main Street
Farmingdale, NJ 07727   (732)449-0914   Fax (732)449-5437

Oropeza, Maria Emilia, MD {1356586796} Pedtrc
+ 5809 Madison Street/Suite 1
West New York, NJ 07093   (917)207-5923   Fax (201)840-0008
mariaemilia45@yahoo.com

Orozco, Fabio R., MD {1306890512} SrgOrt, OrtHKn(93,COL19)<NJ-ACMCITY, NJ-ACMCMAIN>
+ Rothman Institute - Egg Harbor Township
2500 English Creek Avenue/Bldg 1300   Egg Harbor Township, NJ 08234   (609)677-7002   Fax (609)677-7000
+ Rothman Institute - Manahawkin
712 East Bay Avenue   Manahawkin, NJ 08050

Orquiza, Clodualdo Soriano, III, MD {1326040155} Otlryg, OtgyF-PlS(94,PA09)<NJ-ACMCMAIN, NJ-ACMCITY>
+ South Jersey ENT Surgical Associates
2106 New Road/Unit C-9   Linwood, NJ 08221   (609)927-8881   Fax (609)927-8832

Orr, Andrew Philip, MD {1598025033} Psychy
+ 15 Princess Road/Suite EAST
Lawrenceville, NJ 08648   (609)349-7626

Orr, David A., DO {1215016217} CritCr, IntrMd, PulDis(87,NJ75)<NJ-HACKNSK>
+ Hackensack University Medical Group Emerson
452 Old Hook Road/2nd Floor   Emerson, NJ 07630   (201)666-3900   Fax (201)261-0505
+ Northern New Jersey Pulmonary Associates PC
211 Essex Street/Suite 302   Hackensack, NJ 07601   (201)666-3900   Fax (201)498-1312

Orringer, Robert D., MD {1235104019} SrgC&R(75,PA12)<NJ-OVERLOOK>
+ Associates in Colon and Rectal Diseases
231 Millburn Avenue   Millburn, NJ 07041   (973)467-2277   Fax (973)467-1317

Orris, Margie Maria, DO {1518163807}<NJ-KMHSTRAT>
+ Kennedy Memorial Hospital-University Medical Center
18 East Laurel Road   Stratford, NJ 08084   (856)346-7985

Orsini, Anthony J., DO {1225001001} NnPnMd, Pedtrc(90,PA77)<NJ-MORRISTN, NJ-CHILTON>
+ MidAtlantic Neonatology Associates
100 Madison Avenue   Morristown, NJ 07962   (973)971-5488   Fax (973)290-7175

Orsini, James M., MD {1922084185} IntrMd, Onclgy, OncHem(73,ITA01)<NJ-CLARMAAS, NJ-MTNSIDE>
+ Essex Hematology-Oncology Group, PA
36 Newark Avenue/Suite 304   Belleville, NJ 07109   (973)751-8880   Fax (973)751-8950
+ Essex Hematology-Oncology Group, PA
One Bay Avenue/Suite 2   Montclair, NJ 07042   (973)751-8880   Fax (973)744-8340

Orsini, James Michael, MD {1659516813} IntrMd(08,GRN01)<NJ-CLARMAAS>
+ Clara Maass Medical Center
1 Clara Maass Drive/IntMed   Belleville, NJ 07109   (973)450-2000

Orsini, William J., MD {1134170608} Dermat, IntrMd(72,NJ05)<NJ-MONMOUTH>
+ Drs. Gilson, Orsini & Miller
223 Monmouth Road   West Long Branch, NJ 07764   (732)870-2992   Fax (732)870-2533

Ort, Stuart A., MD {1083831325} Otlryg
+ ENT & Allergy Associates, LLP
485 Route 1 South/Bld B/Suite 350   Iselin, NJ 08830   (732)549-3934   Fax (732)549-7250
+ ENT & Allergy Associates, LLP
3663 Route 9 North/Suite102   Old Bridge, NJ 08857   (732)549-3934   Fax (732)707-3850

Ortanez, Iluminado C., MD {1154415222} Psychy(67,PHI09)<NJ-UNVMCPRN>
+ Washington Psychological Services
100 Heritage Valley Road   Sewell, NJ 08080   (856)589-4147   Fax (856)589-3805
+ Princeton House Behavioral Health - Cherry Hill
375 North Kings Highway/StaffPsych   Cherry Hill, NJ 08034   (856)589-4147   Fax (856)779-2988

Ortega, Adela Yrma, MD {1437484631} Psychy
+ 1118 Bluebird Circle
Mays Landing, NJ 08330

Ortega, Diego R., MD {1578793030}<NJ-VIRTVOOR>
+ Virtua Voorhees
100 Bowman Drive   Voorhees, NJ 08043   (862)216-8721
ortega530@gmail.com

Ortega, Eddy A., MD {1104967520} Psychy(81,DOM01)<NJ-ANCPSYCH, NJ-HCMEADPS>
+ Hudson County Meadowview Psychiatric Hospital
595 County Avenue   Secaucus, NJ 07094   (201)319-3660
+ Ancora Psychiatric Hospital
301 Spring Garden Road   Hammonton, NJ 08037   (609)561-1700

Ortega, Jesus Ruben, MD {1386706083} Pedtrc(78,ECU01)<NJ-CLARMAAS, NJ-STBARNMC>
+ Pediatric Center 2000
571 North Sixth Street   Newark, NJ 07107   (973)485-5401   Fax (973)485-1536

Ortega, Rae Lynn, MD {1104047505} EmrgMd(05,TX15)<NJ-OURLADY>
+ Our Lady of Lourdes Medical Center
1600 Haddon Avenue/EmrgMed   Camden, NJ 08103   (856)757-3500

Ortega, Stephanie Lynn Scham, MD {1033202882} EmrgMd(94,MA07)<NJ-STCLRDEN, NJ-STCLRDOV>
+ St. Clare's Hospital-Denville Campus
25 Pocono Road/Emergency   Denville, NJ 07834   (973)625-6000   Fax (973)983-2293

Ortega-Jongco, Anita M., MD {1790778603} IntrMd(68,PHIL)<NJ-STBARNMC, NJ-NWRKBETH>
+ 120 Millburn Avenue/Suite M3
Millburn, NJ 07041   (973)912-8400   Fax (973)912-0099

Orth, Charles Richard, Jr., MD {1750380028} Urolgy(91,PA14)
+ New Jersey Urology, LLC
2401 East Evesham Road/Suite F   Voorhees, NJ 08043   (856)673-1600   Fax (856)988-0636
+ Delaware Valley Urology LLC
17 West Red Bank Avenue/Suite 303   Woodbury, NJ 08096   (856)673-1600   Fax (856)985-4583

Orth, Donald W., MD {1346211075} CdvDis, IntrMd(71,PA01)<NJ-VIRTUAHS, NJ-OURLADY>
+ Associated Cardiovascular Consultants, P.A.
1105 Laurel Oak Road/Suite 165   Voorhees, NJ 08043   (856)424-3600   Fax (856)424-7154
+ Associated Cardiovascular Consultants-Lourdes
1 Brace Road/Suite C & F   Cherry Hill, NJ 08034   (856)424-3600   Fax (856)428-5748

Ortiz, Carlos Arturo, II, MD {1306041116} EmrgMd(03,TX02)<NJ-HACKNSK>
+ Hackensack University Medical Center
30 Prospect Avenue/EmrgMed   Hackensack, NJ 07601   (201)996-2000

Ortiz, Guillermo, MD {1407828445} ObsGyn(86,PRO03)<NJ-STCLRDEN>
+ 294 South Main Street
Wharton, NJ 07885   (973)361-5252   Fax (973)361-6161

Ortiz, Olivia Tanyag, MD {1225191992} IntrMd, InfDis(84,PHI02)
+ Drs. Ortiz, Villanueva and Cruz
1163 Route 37 West/Suite A-1   Toms River, NJ 08755   (732)736-1000   Fax (732)736-8811
+ Drs. Ortiz, Villanueva and Cruz
1255 Route 70/Suite 20-N   Lakewood, NJ 08701   (732)363-4770

Ortiz, Oscar T., MD {1396719662} EnDbMt, IntrMd(83,PHIL)<NJ-COMMED>
+ Drs. Ortiz, Villanueva and Cruz
1163 Route 37 West/Suite A-1   Toms River, NJ 08755   (732)736-1000   Fax (732)736-8811
+ Drs. Ortiz, Villanueva and Cruz
1255 Route 70/Suite 20-N   Lakewood, NJ 08701   (732)363-4770

Ortiz, Thomas R., MD {1750312450} FamMed(81,NJ05)<NJ-CLARMAAS, NJ-NWRKBETH>
+ Forest Hill Family Health Associates, P.A.
465 Mount Prospect Avenue   Newark, NJ 07104   (973)483-3640   Fax (973)483-4895

Ortiz-Evans, Ileana, MD {1053301499} FamMed(97,NJ06)
+ The Doctor Is in
1205 US Highway 22   Phillipsburg, NJ 08865   (908)213-2211   Fax (908)213-9913

Ortman, Matthew Louis, MD {1366582116} CdvDis, CICdEl, IntrMd(MD01)
+ Cooper Cardiology Associates
1210 Brace Road/Suite 103   Cherry Hill, NJ 08034   (856)427-7254

Orwitz, Jonathan Ira, MD {1659486611} Nrolgy(81,PA12)
+ Neurology Associaates of South Jersey
693 Main Street/Building D   Lumberton, NJ 08048   (609)261-7600   Fax (609)265-8205
+ Advocare Neurology of South Jersey
200-B Route 73 North/Suite 2   Voorhees, NJ 08043   (609)261-7600   Fax (856)335-0406

Osei, Charles, MD {1134228927} Pedtrc(90,GHA01)<NJ-NWRKBETH, NJ-STCLRDEN>
+ Newark Beth Israel Medical Center
201 Lyons Avenue/Pediatrics   Newark, NJ 07112   (973)926-7000

Osei Tutu, Ernest Paul, MD {1740250851} IntrMd(84,PA02)
+ 1727 Essex Street/Suite 504
Rahway, NJ 07065   (917)526-9987   Fax (732)382-2832

Osei Tutu, Leslie P., MD {1033313424} Anesth
+ 1727 Essex Street/Unit 504
Rahway, NJ 07065   (732)382-2832

Oser, William, Jr., MD {1548481690} Grtrcs, IntrMd(86,NJ05)<NJ-JFKMED>
+ JFK Medical Center
65 James Street/Med Staff   Edison, NJ 08820   (732)321-7605   Fax (732)549-8532

Osgood, Eric, MD {1427475847} IntrMd<NJ-BURDTMLN>
+ Cape Regional Medical Center
2 Stone Harbor Boulevard   Cape May Court House, NJ 08210   (609)463-2803   Fax (609)463-4991

Osias, Glenn Lawrence, MD {1164422788} IntrMd, Gastrn(94,NJ06)
+ Princeton Gastroenterology Associates, P.A.
  731 Alexander Road/Suite 100   Princeton, NJ 08540
  (609)924-1422   Fax (609)924-7473
+ Princeton Endoscopy Center
  731 Alexander Road/Suite 104   Princeton, NJ 08540
  (609)924-1422   Fax (609)452-1010

Osias, Kimberly Beth, MD {1922006899} IntrMd(95,NY09)<NJ-STFRNMED>
+ Lawrenceville Internal Medicine Associates LLC
  3100 Princeton Pike/Building 4/Suite I   Lawrenceville, NJ 08648   (609)896-0303   Fax (609)896-0308

Osiason, Andrew Wade, MD {1053396929} RadDia, RadBdI(90,PA01)<NJ-HACKNSK>
+ The Imaging Center
  30 South Newman Street   Hackensack, NJ 07601
  (201)488-1188   Fax (201)488-5244
+ New Century Imaging at Oradell
  555 Kinderkamack Road   Oradell, NJ 07649   (201)488-1188
  Fax (201)599-8333
+ Hackensack Radiology Group, P.A.
  30 Prospect Avenue   Hackensack, NJ 07601   (201)996-2200   Fax (201)336-8451

Osinubi, Omowunmi Y., MD {1215080775} OccpMd, Anesth, GPrvMd(88,NIG01)
+ University Hospital-School of Public Health
  170 Frelinghuysen Road   Piscataway, NJ 08854   (732)445-0123   Fax (732)445-3644

Osipuk, Darlene M., MD {1255456927} Psychy(80,NJ06)
+ Darlene Osipuk M.D. P.A.
  420 Boulevard/Suite 106   Mountain Lakes, NJ 07046
  (973)263-8282   Fax (973)263-3141

Osman, Ihsan, MD {1306841283} Pedtrc, AdolMd(66,EGYP)<NJ-RBAYOLDB, NJ-BAYSHORE>
+ Rainbow Medical Associates
  200 Perrine Road/Suite 228   Old Bridge, NJ 08857
  (732)679-6066   Fax (732)679-7177

Osman, Sarah Ann, MD {1053364422} PhysMd, PedReh(94,NJ06)<NJ-MATHENY>
+ The Matheny School and Hospital
  Main Street/PO Box 339   Peapack, NJ 07977   (908)234-0011

Osmanova, Nataliya, MD {1669550901} PsyCAd, Psychy(86,RUS26)
+ Center of Revitalizing Psychiatry, P.C.
  795 Main Street   Hackensack, NJ 07601   (201)488-5161
  Fax (201)488-5162

Osmanovic, Kenan, MD {1396956708} Psychy
+ Somerset Medical Center Psychiatry
  110 Rehill Avenue   Somerville, NJ 08876   (908)685-2200
+ 4 Redcliffe Avenue/Suite 1A
  Highland Park, NJ 08904

Osofsky, Jeffrey Lee, MD {1093789612} CdvDis, IntrMd(92,IL43)<NJ-JRSYSHMC, NJ-CENTRAST>
+ Monmouth Cardiology Associates, LLC
  11 Meridian Road   Eatontown, NJ 07724   (732)663-0300
  Fax (732)663-0301
+ Monmouth Cardiology Associates, LLC
  222 Schanck Road/Suite 104   Freehold, NJ 07728
  (732)663-0300   Fax (732)431-1712

Osofsky, Michael, MD {1376706945} Dermat
+ Westwood Dermatology
  390 Old Hook Road   Westwood, NJ 07675   (201)666-9550
  Fax (201)666-1251

Osorio, Jorge H., MD {1104810936} IntrMd(84,POL06)<NJ-STMICHL>
+ Renaissance Medical Group
  155 Jefferson Street/Lower Level   Newark, NJ 07105
  (973)344-5498   Fax (973)344-6686
+ St. Michael's Medical Center
  268 MLK Jr. Boulevard/Internal Med   Newark, NJ 07102
  (973)877-5000

Ostella, Frank Mario, DO {1821165473} Psychy(95,FL75)
+ UH-University Behavioral Hlth
  100 Metroplex Drive/Suite 200   Edison, NJ 08817
  (732)235-8400   Fax (732)235-8395

Ostrovskaya, Inna Dmytrievna, MD {1558420109} Anesth(85,RUS79)
+ 521 Grandview Terrace
  Leonia, NJ 07605

Ostrovsky, Igor, MD {1487710273} Anesth, AnesPain(80,RUSS)
+ 440 West Street/Suite 302
  Fort Lee, NJ 07024   (718)934-2078   Fax (718)934-1920
  doctor_ostrovsky@yahoo.com

Ostrovsky, Ilya, MD {1275809444} EmrgMd
+ Rutgers- New Jersey Medical School
  185 South Orange Avenue/E609   Newark, NJ 07103
  (973)972-9261

Ostrow, Vlady, DO {1245407337} PedEnd, Pedtrc(03,PA77)
+ Drs. Barrows and Ostrow
  180 Avenue at the Common/Suite 7B   Shrewsbury, NJ 07702   (732)935-7143   Fax (732)935-7245

Ostrum, Donald S., MD {1578563532} Radiol, RadDia(82,PA13)<PA-NZRTH, PA-MRCYSUB>
+ Radiology Affiliates of Central New Jersey, P.A.
  2501 Kuser Road   Hamilton, NJ 08691   (609)585-8800
  Fax (609)585-1825

Ostrum, Gordon J., Jr., MD {1033175005} GenPrc, ObsGyn(76,PA02)<NJ-MEMSALEM>
+ First State Women's Care
  19B West Avenue   Woodstown, NJ 08098   (856)769-3348
  Fax (856)769-3987

Ostrum, Robert Fredric, MD {1366532723} SrgOrt(80,PA13)
+ Cooper Surgical Associates
  3 Cooper Plaza/Suite 411   Camden, NJ 08103   (856)342-2270   Fax (856)365-1180

Ostry, Rachel F., MD {1083615017} Anesth(84,ISR02)
+ 140 Nottingham Drive
  Watchung, NJ 07069   (908)757-5488

Oswald, Mark Anthony, MD {1215935655} FamMed, IntrMd(00,PA02)
+ Community Health Care, Inc.
  265 Irving Avenue   Bridgeton, NJ 08302   (856)451-4700
  Fax (856)863-5732

Oswari, Andrew, MD {1619067071} FamMed(97,CA12)
+ Drs. Chung & Shin
  110 Marter Avenue/Suite 507   Moorestown, NJ 08057
  (856)222-4766   Fax (856)222-1137

Oswari, Daniel, MD {1265506489} FamMed(98,CA12)<NJ-RWJUHAM>
+ Family Practice Associates at Hamilton
  941 Whitehorse Avenue/Suite 3   Hamilton, NJ 08610
  (609)838-7984   Fax (609)838-7986

Otero, Jose Miguel, MD {1194099887}<NJ-TRINIWSC>
+ Trinitas Regional Medical Center-Williamson Street
  225 Williamson Street   Elizabeth, NJ 07207   (908)994-5204

Othman, Essam Abdou, MD {1891897229} IntrMd(79,EGY03)<NJ-TRINIWSC>
+ 700 North Broad Street
  Elizabeth, NJ 07208   (908)436-0022   Fax (908)436-0088

Otrakji, Jean, MD {1154380996} IntrMd, Nephro(72,SYRI)<NJ-BAYSHORE>
+ Nephrology Services Med Group
  721 North Beers Street/Suite 1-F   Holmdel, NJ 07733
  (732)888-9100   Fax (732)888-5515

Ott, Christina Marie, MD {1194160325}
+ Children's Specialized Hospital
  3575 Quakerbridge Road   Hamilton, NJ 08619   (609)631-2811   Fax (609)631-2850

Ott, William Augustine, DO {1063436293} FamMed(93,PA77)<NJ-UNDRWD>
+ Family Health Center of Mullica Hill
  155 Bridgeton Pike/Suite A   Mullica Hill, NJ 08062
  (856)223-0500   Fax (856)223-1098

Otteno, Helen, MD {1710298435} Gyneco<NJ-UMDNJ>
+ University Hospital
  150 Bergen Street/E-401   Newark, NJ 07103   (347)545-9828

Ottley, Anroy K., MD {1457572752} Surgry, SrgTrm(02,GRN01)<NJ-JRSYCITY, NJ-STBARNMC>
+ Jersey City Medical Center
  355 Grand Street/Surgery   Jersey City, NJ 07304   (201)915-2450
  aottley@libertyhcs.org
+ St. Barnabas Medical Center
  94 Old Short Hills Road/Surgery   Livingston, NJ 07039
  (973)322-5000

Ouahchi, Karim, MD {1518030766} Pthlgy
+ 3238 Riverside Station Blvd
  Secaucus, NJ 07094   (509)994-5516
  karimouahchi@yahoo.com

Ouano, Estelita C., MD {1679520449} FamMed(82,PHIL)<NJ-SOMERSET>
+ Priority Medical Care/Family Health Center
  350 Grove Street   Bridgewater, NJ 08807   (908)526-1313
  Fax (908)722-6031

Ouano, Rodolfo C., MD {1568552917} IntrMd(65,PHIL)<NJ-BAYSHORE>
+ 1872 Highway 35/PO Box 755
  South Amboy, NJ 08879   (732)727-7470   Fax (732)525-2204
  rcomdpa@optonline.net

Ould Hammou, Ayesha N. Haque, MD {1093767295} IntrMd(92,PAK14)<NJ-BAYSHORE>
+ The Doctor's Office
  1070 Highway 34/Suite C   Matawan, NJ 07747   (732)290-0300   Fax (732)290-9661

Ourvan, Dorothy R., DO {1154398923} FamMed(84,NY75)<NJ-HACKNSK>
+ Center for Occupational Medicine
  360 Essex Street/Suite 203   Hackensack, NJ 07601
  (201)336-8686   Fax (201)342-3546

Ouw, Willem B., MD {1174671317} FamMed(79,NET08)
+ 79 Lloyd Road
  Montclair, NJ 07042

Ovakimyan, Oxana, MD {1215295704}<NJ-MORRISTN>
+ Barone & Catania Cardiovascular
  786 Mountain Boulevard/Suite 200   Watchung, NJ 07069
  (908)754-0975   Fax (908)754-0260
+ Morristown Medical Center
  100 Madison Avenue   Morristown, NJ 07962   (908)754-0975   Fax (973)898-1600

Ovchinsky, Alexander, MD {1871554469} Otlryg, IntrMd(98,NY08)<NY-LICOLLGE>
+ 1046 South Orange Avenue
  Short Hills, NJ 07078   (973)379-0101   Fax (973)376-6231

Overbeck, Kevin Joseph, DO {1861412421} FamMed, Grtrcs(03,NJ75)
+ New Jersey Institute for Successful Aging
  42 East Laurel Road/Suite 1800   Stratford, NJ 08084
  (856)566-6843   Fax (856)566-6781

Ovnanian, Vagram, MD {1689603573} IntrMd, PulCCr(96,LAT02)<NJ-HACKNSK>
+ Internal Medicine Faculty Practice
  101 Old Short Hills Road/Suite 106   West Orange, NJ 07052
  (973)322-6256   Fax (973)322-6241

Ovsjanikovska, Natalija, MD {1619157237} IntrMd, InfDis(88,LAT03)
+ Paterson Counseling Center
  319-321 Main Street/Internal Med   Paterson, NJ 07505
  (973)523-8316   Fax (973)523-2248

Ow, Cheng H., MD {1245393974} Radiol, RadDia(83,PA01)
+ Montclair Breast Center
  37 North Fullerton Avenue   Montclair, NJ 07042   (973)509-1818   Fax (973)509-0532

Owaid, Nihad Y., MD {1841304607} PhysMd, IntrMd(74,IRAQ)<NY-METHODST, NJ-CHRIST>
+ 591 Summit Avenue/Suite 415
  Jersey City, NJ 07306   (201)963-0200

Owens, Brittany Rose, MD {1427492479} Pedtrc
+ Advocare DelGiorno Pediatrics
  535 South Black Horse Pike   Blackwood, NJ 08012
  (856)228-1061   Fax (856)228-1907

Owens, Jacqueline A., MD {1811007750} Pedtrc(89,NJ05)<NJ-STBARNMC>
+ The Pediatric Group of West Orange, PA
  395 Pleasant Valley Way   West Orange, NJ 07052
  (973)731-6100   Fax (973)731-0612

Owens, John M., MD {1033593911} SrgOrt(89,NY01)<NJ-HOLYNAME, NJ-ENGLWOOD>
+ North Jersey Orthopaedic Specialists
  106 Grand Avenue   Englewood, NJ 07631   (201)608-0100
  Fax (201)608-0104
+ North Jersey Orthopaedic Specialists
  730 Palisade Avenue   Teaneck, NJ 07666   (201)608-0100
  Fax (201)530-0003
+ North Jersey Orthopaedic Specialists
  15 Vervalen Street   Closter, NJ 07631   (201)784-6800   Fax (201)784-6801

Owens, Nefertari Alisha, MD {1922596527} ObsGyn<NJ-COOPRUMC>
+ Cooper University Hospital
  One Cooper Plaza/Suite 221   Camden, NJ 08103   (856)342-2000

Owensby, Jennifer Rita, MD {1942295076} Pedtrc, PedCrC(95,NJ06)
+ UH- Robert Wood Johnson Med
  125 Paterson Street/MEB 338   New Brunswick, NJ 08901
  (732)235-7887   Fax (732)235-6609

Owsiak, Joanne Naamo, MD {1619243417} Anesth(12,IL43)
+ Summit Medical Group
  31-00 Broadway   Fair Lawn, NJ 07410   (201)645-1010
  Fax (201)796-7020
+ Summit Medical Group
  6 Brighton Road/2 FL   Clifton, NJ 07012   (201)645-1010
  Fax (973)777-5403

Owunna, Uzoma I., MD {1457316465} ObsGyn(00,NY47)<NJ-STPETER, NJ-RWJUBRUN>
+ Ob & Gyn Group of E Brunswick
  172 Summerhill Road/Suite 1   East Brunswick, NJ 08816
  (732)254-1500   Fax (732)254-1436

Owusu, Solomon, MD {1487723243} IntrMd(85,GHA01)
+ 550 West Side Avenue
  Jersey City, NJ 07304   (201)432-5300   Fax (201)432-4630

Owusu Boahen, Olivia, MD {1427282631} IntrMd(96,GHA02)
+ CHOP Care Network at Princeton Medical Center
  One Plainsboro Road   Plainsboro, NJ 08536   (609)853-7000
  Fax (609)497-4173

Owusu-Dapaah, Kwabena B., MD {1215091376} EmrgMd, Pedtrc(84,GHA02)
+ 710 Easton Avenue/Suite 1-A
  Somerset, NJ 08873   (732)246-1960   Fax (732)246-3141

Physicians by Name and Address

Oxler, Steven J., MD {1932128063} EmrgMd(73,SC04)<NJ-UN-DRWD>
+ Inspira Health Network
509 North Broad Street/EmrgMed   Woodbury, NJ 08096   (856)845-0100
+ Emergency Physician Associates, P.A.
307 South Evergreen Avenue/PO Box 298   Woodbury, NJ 08096   (856)845-0100   Fax (856)848-1431

Oxman, David J., MD {1538153820} Pedtrc(74,IL42)<NJ-STBARNMC, NJ-OVERLOOK>
+ Union Pediatric Medical Group, PA
1050 Galloping Hill Road/Suite 200   Union, NJ 07083   (908)688-9900   Fax (908)688-9939

Oyejide, Catherine O., MD {1962456178} Psychy<NJ-VIRTVOOR>
+ 69 Tunis Drive
Florham Park, NJ 07932

Oyelese, Kolawole Olayinka, MD {1568407955} ObsGyn(86,NIG01)
+ Maternal Fetal Medicine of Practice Associates
11 Overlook Road/Suite LL 102   Summit, NJ 07901   (908)522-3846   Fax (908)522-5557

Oyetunde, Olasunkanmi Kolawole, MD {1598962722} IntrMd
+ 2274 Fern Terrace
Union, NJ 07083   (908)416-5766   Fax (908)687-6820

Oyeyemi, Jubril Oyekanmi, MD {1003050022} IntHos<NJ-VIRTMHBC>
+ Virtua Memorial
175 Madison Avenue   Mount Holly, NJ 08060   (609)914-6180   Fax (609)914-6182

Oyvin, Vadim, MD {1336114586} Psychy(78,RUS81)<NJ-MT-CARMEL>
+ Mt. Carmel Guild/ Behavioral Health System
1160 Raymond Boulevard/Psych   Newark, NJ 07102   (973)596-4190
+ Center of Revitalizing Psychiatry, P.C.
795 Main Street   Hackensack, NJ 07601   (973)596-4190   Fax (201)488-5162

Oza, Harsha K., MD {1447219290} IntrMd(85,INDI)<NJ-STFRN-MED>
+ RWJ Medical Associates
3100 Quakerbridge Road/Suite 28   Hamilton, NJ 08619   (609)245-7430   Fax (609)245-7432

Oza, Palak, MD {1770725327} ObsGyn
+ Somerset Ob-Gyn Associates
215 Union Avenue/Suite A   Bridgewater, NJ 08807   (908)722-2900   Fax (908)722-1856

Oza, Rohit Madhukar, MD {1205800091} PhysMd, PainMd(99,NJ-HLTHSRE, NJ-COMMED>
+ Summit Medical Group-Berkeley Heights Campus
1 Diamond Hill Road   Berkeley Heights, NJ 07922   (908)273-4300   Fax (908)673-7132
+ Summit Medical Group
34 Mountain Boulevard/Building B   Warren, NJ 07059   (908)273-4300   Fax (908)769-8927

Pabbathi, Pramod, DO {1770690158} Anesth(ME75
+ Anesthesia Consultnts of NJ/Nova Pain
285 Davidson Avenue/Suite 204   Somerset, NJ 08873   (732)271-1400   Fax (732)271-3543

Pablo, Bryan Alcides, MD {1114203239} ObsGyn(10,NJ05)
+ Ob-Gyn Associates of North Jersey
7400 Bergenline Avenue   North Bergen, NJ 07047   (201)869-5488   Fax (201)869-6944

Pabolu, Sangeetha, MD {1093970022} Rheuma<NJ-STPETER>
+ St. Peter's University Hospital
254 Easton Avenue   New Brunswick, NJ 08901   (732)745-8600   Fax (732)745-3847

Pacana, Susan Marie, MD {1497700389} ObsGyn, Obstet(95,PA09)<NJ-CENTRAST>
+ Healthy Woman Ob/Gyn
312 Professional View Drive   Freehold, NJ 07728   (732)431-1616   Fax (732)866-7962

Pace, Enrico, MD {1528066503} Anesth(84,MEXI)<NJ-VIRTUAHS>
+ West Jersey Anesthesia Associates
102-E Center Boulevard   Marlton, NJ 08053   (856)988-6250   Fax (856)988-6270

Pace, Patrick V., MD {1598843898} PsyCAd, Psychy(86,NJ06)<NJ-UNIVBHC>
+ University Behavioral Health Care
671 Hoes Lane/PO Box 1392   Piscataway, NJ 08855   (732)235-5500

Pacheco, Felix Fernando, MD {1033326152} FamMed(00,NJ05)<NJ-VALLEY>
+ Valley Medical Group
140 Route 17 North/Suite 302   Paramus, NJ 07652   (201)444-2646   Fax (201)689-6009

Pacheco-Smith, Sariya Amina, MD {1952316531} Pedtrc(91,NY46)<NJ-CHSMRCER>
+ Henry J. Austin Health Center
321 North Warren Street   Trenton, NJ 08618   (609)278-5900   Fax (609)695-3532

Pacia, Arthur G., MD {1225053846} IntrMd, PulDis(81,PHI01)<NJ-RWJUHAM, NJ-CHSMRCER>
+ Greater Mercer Pulmonary & Medical Assoc PC
445 Whitehorse Avenue/Suite 103   Trenton, NJ 08610   (609)585-0300

Pacific, Scott, MD {1851370290} Anesth(91,NY06)
+ Summit Anesthesia Associates, P.A.
33 Overlook Road/Suite 311   Summit, NJ 07901   (908)598-1500   Fax (908)598-0197

Pack, Jonathan W., MD {1326277104}
+ 3308 High Street
Blackwood, NJ 08012   (856)685-6855

Packer, Michael G., MD {1508832973} PedUro, Urolgy, IntrMd(79,NY01)<NJ-VIRTVOOR>
+ Urology for Children, LLC
120 Carnie Boulevard/Suite 2   Voorhees, NJ 08043   (856)751-7880
+ Urology for Children, LLC
1000 Atlantic Avenue   Camden, NJ 08104   (856)751-7880   Fax (856)751-9133
+ Urology for Children, LLC
239 Hurffville Crosskeys Road   Sewell, NJ 08043   (856)751-7880   Fax (856)751-9133

Packin, Gary S., DO {1457323420} Gyneco, RprEnd(71,PA77)<NJ-VIRTVOOR, NJ-KMHTURNV>
+ South Jersey Fertility Center
570 Egg Harbor Road/Suite B-4   Sewell, NJ 08080

Padamadan, Hosi, MD {1396708657} FamMed(81,INDI)<OH-OSUMEDC>
+ Patient first
2171 Route 70 West   Cherry Hill, NJ 08002   (856)406-0023   Fax (856)406-0024

Padavan, Dean, MD {1649411836} IntrSptM(06,GRN01)
+ Atlantic Orthopedic Institute
111 Madison Avenue/Suite 400   Morristown, NJ 07960   (973)971-6957   Fax (973)984-2516
+ Sparta Health and Wellness Center
89 Sparta Avenue/Suite 120   Sparta, NJ 07871   (973)971-6957   Fax (973)729-1085

Padberg, Frank Thomas, Jr., MD {1982612032} SrgVas, Surgry(73,AR01)<NJ-UMDNJ>
+ University Hospital
150 Bergen Street   Newark, NJ 07103   (973)972-4300
+ University Hospital-Doctors Office Center
90 Bergen Street/Suite 7200   Newark, NJ 07103   (973)972-4300   Fax (973)972-9375

Padder, Farooq Ahmad, MD {1700833449} ClCdEl, CdvDis(81,INA36)<NJ-UNDRWD, NJ-OURLADY>
+ Owens Vergari Unwala Cardiology Associates PC
17 West Red Bank Avenue/Suite 306   Woodbury, NJ 08096   (856)845-6807   Fax (856)845-3760

Padela, Mohammad F., MD {1700855772} Nrolgy(83,PAK11)
+ 721 Clifton Avenue
Clifton, NJ 07013   (973)471-3730   Fax (973)471-9129

Padilla, Adrian, MD {1255618328} IntrMd
+ 465 Mount Prospect
Newark, NJ 07104
+ Center for Remote Medical Management
82 East Allendale Road/Suite 8-A   Saddle River, NJ 07458   (551)697-5399

Padilla, Dominga Sol, MD {1033312541} Pedtrc(00,NJ05)<NJ-VALLEY, NJ-HACKNSK>
+ One West Ridgewood Avenue
Paramus, NJ 07652   (201)689-1939   Fax (201)689-1935

Padilla, Nyree, MD {1164676342} FamMed(04)
+ 345 State Street/Suite B
Perth Amboy, NJ 08861   (732)442-2301   Fax (732)442-2303

Padkowsky, Adrian P., MD {1447559943}
+ University Hospital Medicine
150 Bergen Street/Room I-248   Newark, NJ 07103   (973)972-6056   Fax (973)972-3129

Padkowsky, George O., MD {1497863864} IntrMd(79,DOM02)
+ Stat Medical Services
845 Broadway   Bayonne, NJ 07002   (201)823-8555   Fax (201)823-2979

Padkowsky, Orest, MD {1558479923} IntrMd(79,DOMI)
+ 989 Broadway
Bayonne, NJ 07002   (201)823-8555   Fax (201)823-2979

Padnani, Ashish, MD {1912135583}
+ Surgical Practice of Rolando Rolandelli, MD
435 South Street/Suite 360   Morristown, NJ 07960   (973)971-4179   Fax (973)290-7521

Padron, Celia Z., MD {1013961705} PedGst, Pedtrc, IntrMd(82,DOM03)<NJ-VIRTVOOR>
+ Pediatric Gastroenterology Center
901B Route 73 North   Marlton, NJ 08053   (856)596-6333   Fax (856)596-6655

Padron-Gayol, Maria V., MD {1336168608} PsyCAd, Psychy(69,CUB01)<NJ-TRININPC>
+ 433 - 68th Street
Guttenberg, NJ 07093   (201)861-7639

mpadronmd@hotmail.com
+ Trinitas Regional Medical Center-New Point Campus
655 East Jersey Street/Psychiatry   Elizabeth, NJ 07206   (908)994-5000

Padula, Vincent M., DO {1558397083} Anesth(93,NJ75)<NJ-KMHCHRRY>
+ South Jersey Pain Consultants
525 Route 73 South/Suite 103   Marlton, NJ 08053   (856)797-5777   Fax (856)797-5771

Paduszynski, Adam A., MD {1609869650} FamMed(85,POL08)<NJ-BAYONNE>
+ 20 West 22 Street
Bayonne, NJ 07002   (201)437-7744

Padykula, Anna, MD {1730218066} Pedtrc(78,POL17)<NJ-STCLRDEN>
+ Drs. Padykula and Skripkus
381 Kearny Avenue   Kearny, NJ 07032   (201)991-4824   Fax (201)991-7465

Paez Perez, Yenisleidy, DO {1578947420} EmrgMd
+ St Joseph's Medical Center Emergency
703 Main Street   Paterson, NJ 07503   (786)226-4909   Fax (973)754-2249

Pagan, Juan, MD   IntrMd(85,RI01)
+ 260 Prospect Avenue/Apt 156
Hackensack, NJ 07601

Pagan-Duran, Brenda, MD {1679594436} Ophthl(97,PRO01)<NJ-VAEASTOR>
+ Westwood Ophthalmology Associates
300 Fairview Avenue/PO Box 698   Westwood, NJ 07675   (201)666-4014   Fax (201)664-4754
drbrenda@cox.com

Pagana, Theresa N., MD {1861629388} EmrgMd(09,PA13)
+ Team Health East
307 South Evergeen Avenue/Suite 201   Woodbury, NJ 08096   (856)686-4300   Fax (856)848-8536

Paganessi, Monica A., DO {1255315321} Anesth(91,NJ75)<NJ-HACKNSK>
+ Hackensack University Medical Center
30 Prospect Avenue/Anesthesiology   Hackensack, NJ 07601   (201)996-2419   Fax (201)488-6769

Paganessi, Steven Andrew, MD {1306944079} Anesth(90,NJ05)<NJ-HACKNSK>
+ Hackensack University Medical Center
30 Prospect Avenue/Anesth   Hackensack, NJ 07601   (201)996-2000
+ Short Hills Surgery Center
187 Millburn Avenue/Suite 101   Millburn, NJ 07041   (201)996-2000   Fax (973)671-0557

Pagano, Ann Marie, MD {1679548663} ObsGyn(96,PA09)
+ Brick Women's Physicians
1140 Burnt Tavern Road/Suite 2-A   Brick, NJ 08724   (732)202-0700   Fax (732)202-0664
+ Brick Women's Physicians
87 Union Avenue   Manasquan, NJ 08736   (732)202-0700   Fax (732)202-0664

Pagano, Christine Federline, MD {1891955993} Pedtrc(07,NY09)
+ Tenafly Pediatrics, PA
1135 Broad Street/Suite 208   Clifton, NJ 07013   (973)471-8600   Fax (973)471-3068

Pagano, Francesco P., DO {1538152905} FamMed(85,NY75)<NJ-STJOSHOS, NJ-VALLEY>
+ Drs. Wiener & Pagano
299 Market Street   Saddle Brook, NJ 07663   (201)368-1717   Fax (201)368-9618

Pagano, Joseph James, DO {1891056594} EmrgMd<NH-DRTMTHMC>
+ Rowan University-School of Osteopathic Medicine
1 Medical Center Drive   Stratford, NJ 08084   (856)566-7050

Pagano, Matthew J., MD {1447540661} Urolgy
+ Urology Care Alliance
2 Hospital Plaza/Suite 110   Old Bridge, NJ 08857   (732)972-9000   Fax (732)972-0966

Paghdal, Kapila V., MD {1578724571} DerMOH
+ 13 Hudson Place
Bloomfield, NJ 07003

Pagliaro, Andre J., MD {1902874993} SrgOrt, SrgFAk(88,PA09)<NJ-STFRNMED, NJ-RWJUHAM>
+ Trenton Orthopaedic Group
1225 Whitehorse Mercerville Rd   Trenton, NJ 08619   (609)581-2200   Fax (609)581-1212
+ Trenton Orthopaedic Group
116 Washington Crossing Road   Pennington, NJ 08534   (609)581-2200   Fax (609)581-1212

Pagliaro, Sara Nicole, DO {1679770077} FamMed, IntrMd(06,NJ75)
+ Samaritan HealthCare & Hospice
5 Eves Drive/Suite 300   Marlton, NJ 08053   (856)896-1600   Fax (856)552-3268

Pagnani, Alexander M., MD {1104895606} Urolgy, IntrMd(76,MEXI)<NJ-BURDTMLN, NJ-SHOREMEM>
  + Pagnani, Braga, & Kimmel Urologic Associates PA
    229 Shore Road   Somers Point, NJ 08244   (609)653-4343
    Fax (609)653-2060
    GSPMURO@aol.com
  + Pagnani, Braga, & Kimmel Urologic Associates PA
    222 New Road/Building 700   Linwood, NJ 08221   (609)653-4343   Fax (609)601-9630
  + Pagnani, Braga, & Kimmel Urologic Associates PA
    8 Court House South Dennis Rd   Cape May Court House, NJ 08244   (609)465-4404

Pagulayan, Sylvia R., MD {1568402733} IntrMd(63,PHIL)<NJ-CHRIST, NJ-HOBUNIMC>
  + 8 Baldwin Avenue
    Jersey City, NJ 07304   (201)333-5300   Fax (201)333-5301
  + 332 Martin Luther King Drive
    Jersey City, NJ 07305   (201)333-5300   Fax (201)333-5301

Pahlow, Brian J., DO {1972693349} CdvDis, IntCrd, IntrMd(84,NJ75)<NJ-MEMSALEM>
  + Christiana Care Cardiology Consultants
    499 Beckett Road/Suite 202   Logan Township, NJ 08085   (856)769-3900   Fax (856)769-3903
  + Christiana Care Cardiology Consultants
    125 East Avenue/Suite DSuite D   Woodstown, NJ 08098   (856)769-3900   Fax (856)769-3903

Pahuja, Anil K., MD {1568781573} Surgry
  + Atlantic Shore Surgical Associates
    478 Brick Boulevard   Brick, NJ 08723   (732)701-4848   Fax (732)701-1244

Pai, David Y., MD {1134173222} Nephro(01,NJ05)
  + Mercer Kidney Institute
    40 Fuld Street/Suite 401   Trenton, NJ 08638   (609)599-1004   Fax (609)599-3611

Pai, Prabha B., MD {1407940240} PthACl(73,INDI)<NJ-OVERLOOK>
  + Overlook Medical Center
    99 Beauvoir Avenue/PO Box 210/Patholgy   Summit, NJ 07902   (908)522-2000   Fax (908)522-2320

Pai, Shilpa, MD {1891767166} Pedtrc, IntrMd(01,RI01)
  + RWJ University Medical Group/Somerset Pediatrics
    1 Worlds Fair Drive/Suite 1   Somerset, NJ 08873   (732)743-5437   Fax (732)564-0212

Pai, Sneha, MD {1336484757} Rheuma<NJ-OVERLOOK>
  + Drs. Weinberger & Cannarozzi
    741 Northfield Avenue/Suite 210   West Orange, NJ 07052   (973)630-8950   Fax (973)669-9749

Pai, Usha Laxman, MD {1336131283} PthACl, PthCyt(73,INA14)<NJ-JRSYCITY, NJ-MEADWLND>
  + PLUS Diagnostics
    1200 River Avenue/Suite 10   Lakewood, NJ 08701   (732)901-7575   Fax (732)901-1555

Paige, Cynthia Y., MD {1811900608} FamMed, IntrMd(89,NJ05)<NJ-MTNSIDE, NJ-STBARNMC>
  + University Hospital
    150 Bergen Street/Family Medicine   Newark, NJ 07103   (973)972-4300
  + Affiliated Eye Surgeons
    405 Northfield Avenue/Suite 206   West Orange, NJ 07052   (973)972-4300   Fax (973)736-7317
  + New Jersey Family Practice Center (NJFPC)
    90 Bergen Street/DOC 300/Lower Level   Newark, NJ 07103   (973)972-2111   Fax (973)972-2754

Paige, Melanie Kay, MD {1508929951} Pedtrc(98,NY20)<NJ-HACKNSK, NJ-VALLEY>
  + North Jersey Pediatrics
    17-10 Fair Lawn Avenue   Fair Lawn, NJ 07410   (201)794-8585   Fax (201)703-9889
  + North Jersey Pediatrics
    1010 Clifton Avenue   Clifton, NJ 07013   (201)794-8585   Fax (973)249-1316
  + North Jersey Pediatrics
    1011 Clifton Avenue   Clifton, NJ 07410   (973)249-1231   Fax (973)249-1316

Paik, David, MD {1124294970} NuclMd
  + Memorial Radiology Associates
    10 Lanidex Plaza West/Suite 125   Parsippany, NJ 07054   (973)503-5700   Fax (973)386-5701

Paik, Sung Woo, MD {1316932213} PhysMd(66,KOR06)<NJ-JRSYSHMC, NJ-OCEANMC>
  + 2130 Highway 35/Suite B216
    Sea Girt, NJ 08750   (732)974-0707   Fax (732)974-0569

Paine, Mercedes A., MD {1831319508} PsyCAd, Psychy(88,CHI08)<NJ-HACKNSK>
  + 55 Summit Avenue
    Hackensack, NJ 07601   (201)487-4298

Painter, Michael Wayne, MD FamMed(95,WA04)
  + 409 Village Road East
    Princeton Junction, NJ 08550

Paisner, Raphael, MD {1619041977} Pedtrc(83,NY06)<NJ-MTNSIDE, NJ-STJOSHOS>
  + Montclair Pediatrics
    73 Park Street   Montclair, NJ 07042   Fax (973)746-6772

Paiste, Mark Ronald, DO {1447567979} SrgOrt, OrtSHand(06,PA77)
  + Regional Orthopedic, P.A.
    2201 West Chapel Avenue/PO Box 8566   Cherry Hill, NJ 08002   (856)663-7080   Fax (856)663-4945

Pajaro, Rafael E., MD {1700990637} IntrMd(92,NY09)<NJ-OVERLOOK>
  + Summit Medical Group Orthopedics and Sports Medicine
    140 Park Avenue/2nd Floor   Florham Park, NJ 07932   (973)404-9800   Fax (973)267-7295

Pajoohi, Soheil, MD {1447326806} ObsGyn, Gyneco(69,IRA15)
  + 1373 Broad Street/Suite 308
    Clifton, NJ 07013   (973)473-8269   Fax (973)473-0065

Pak, Hang R., DO {1972638229} Anesth, PainInvt(88,NJ75)<NJ-STBARNMC>
  + St. Barnabas Medical Center
    94 Old Short Hills Road/Anesth   Livingston, NJ 07039   (973)322-5000

Pak, Hong Sik, MD {1427077056} PhysMd(95,NY08)
  + 725 Grand Avenue/Suite 105
    Ridgefield, NJ 07657   (201)840-5065
    drpakpain@yahoo.com

Pak, Jayoung, MD {1053464545} NroChl, Pedtrc, Eplpsy(78,KORE)<NJ-UMDNJ>
  + Rutgers NJ School of Medicine Neurology
    90 Bergen Street/DOC 5200   Newark, NJ 07103   (973)972-5209   Fax (973)972-5059
    pakja@njms.rutgers.edu

Pak-Teng, Carol, MD {1861836827} EmrgMd
  + Jersey City Medical Center Emergency
    355 Grand Street   Jersey City, NJ 07302   (201)915-2200

Pakalnis, Regina, MD {1689645954} Anesth(88,OH43)<NJ-TRINIWSC>
  + Trinitas Regional Medical Center-Williamson Street
    225 Williamson Street/Anesth   Elizabeth, NJ 07207   (908)994-5000

Pakonis, Fiona K., MD {1821163643} Pedtrc(02,GRN01)
  + 54 Devon Road
    Essex Fells, NJ 07021   (201)953-1553
  + Pediatric Associates of West Essex, PA
    3155 Route 10/Suite 104   Denville, NJ 07834   (201)953-1553   Fax (973)361-1842

Pakonis, Gregory Vytautas, MD {1922209717} Anesth(02,GRN01)<NJ-STMICHL>
  + St. Michael's Medical Center
    268 MLK Jr. Boulevard/Anesthesia   Newark, NJ 07102   (973)877-5034   Fax (973)877-5231
  + St. Joseph's Regional Medical Center Anesthesia
    703 Main Street   Paterson, NJ 07503   (973)877-5034   Fax (973)977-9455

Pal, Jayanta Kumar, MD {1992899041} Psychy(88,INA86)
  + Princeton House Behavioral Health - Princeton
    905 Herrontown Road   Princeton, NJ 08540   (609)497-3300   Fax (609)497-3370

Palacios, Alexander L., MD {1093842338} Ophthl(74,SPA15)
  + 201 Bridge Plaza North
    Fort Lee, NJ 07024   (201)944-5522   Fax (201)944-4715
  + 5220 Bergenline Avenue
    West New York, NJ 07093   (201)944-5522   Fax (201)863-6970

Palacios, Robert M., MD {1093891723} SrgOrt, FamMSptM(88,NY46)
  + New Jersey Orthopaedic Institute
    504 Valley Road/Suite 200   Wayne, NJ 07470   (973)694-2690   Fax (973)694-2692

Paladino, Theresa Ann, DO {1649269853} Pedtrc(00,NJ75)
  + Monmouth Pediatric Group, P.A.
    272 Broad Street   Red Bank, NJ 07701   (732)741-0456   Fax (732)219-9477
  + Monmouth Pediatric Group, P.A.
    3350 Highway 138   Wall, NJ 07719   (732)741-0456   Fax (732)681-6939

Paladugu, Madhu Babu, MD {1659532596} IntrMd<NJ-MONMOUTH>
  + Monmouth Medical Center
    300 Second Avenue   Long Branch, NJ 07740   (732)923-6537   Fax (732)923-6536

Palamattam, Jessy R., MD {1265685895} Pedtrc<NJ-VALLEY>
  + The Valley Hospital
    223 North Van Dien Avenue   Ridgewood, NJ 07450   (201)447-8000   Fax (201)447-8491

Palan, Vandana A., MD {1285871681} Nephro, IntrMd(99,INA1P)
  + UMDNJ RWJ Nephrology
    125 Paterson Street/Suite 5100-B   New Brunswick, NJ 08901   (732)235-6512   Fax (732)235-6524
  + 342 West Passaic Avenue
    Rutherford, NJ 07070   (201)893-5845

Palance, Adam L., MD {1205032224} Gastrn, IntrMd(00,IL42)<NJ-HOLYNAME, NJ-ENGLWOOD>
  + Teaneck Gastroenterology & Endoscopy Center
    1086 Teaneck Road/Suite 4-C   Teaneck, NJ 07666   (201)837-9449   Fax (201)578-1699
  + Teaneck Gastroenterology & Endoscopy Center
    1086 Teaneck Road/Suite 3-B   Teaneck, NJ 07666   (201)837-9449   Fax (201)837-9544

Palangio, Kimberly Dawn, MD {1427218429} AlgyImmn<NY-NSUHMANH>
  + Lawrenceville Neurology Center, PA
    3131 Princeton Pike   Lawrenceville, NJ 08648   (609)896-1701   Fax (609)896-3735

Palaniswamy, Guhapriya, MD {1740314053} IntrMd, PulDis, PulCCr(99,INA1C)<NJ-RWJUBRUN>
  + RWJ University Hospital New Brunswick
    One Robert Wood Johnson Place   New Brunswick, NJ 08901   (732)828-3000

Palathingal, Celina G., MD {1184702649} IntrMd(75,INDI)<NJ-ANCPSYCH>
  + Ancora Psychiatric Hospital
    301 Spring Garden Road/IntMed   Hammonton, NJ 08037   (609)561-1700

Palathingal, Rini M., MD {1255440962} IntrMd, Onclgy(91,INA4X)<NJ-HOLYNAME>
  + Combine Hematology Oncology
    210 Palisade Avenue   Jersey City, NJ 07306   (201)963-2213   Fax (201)963-7070

Palayekar, Meena Jayawant, MD {1801060082} ObsGyn(95,INA69)
  + Focus Obstetrics & Gynecology
    1 Ethel Road/Suite 106 B   Edison, NJ 08817   (732)452-9099   Fax (732)287-3301
    mpalayekar@hotmail.com

Palder, Steven B., MD {1417914276} Surgry(80,MD01)<NJ-STPETER>
  + St. Peter's University Hospital
    254 Easton Avenue/Surgery   New Brunswick, NJ 08901   (732)745-8600   Fax (732)249-5284

Palecki, Agnieszka, MD {1205995248} PulDis, CritCr, SlpDis(97,POL10)
  + 848 West Bay Avenue/Unit E
    Barnegat, NJ 08005   (609)660-8100
    agnieszka.palecki@atlanticpulmonary.com

Palecki, Winicjusz, MD {1942240429} Nephro, IntrMd(92,POLA)<NJ-SOCEANCO, NJ-JRSYSHMC>
  + Ocean Renal Associates, P.A.
    508 Lakehurst Road/Suite 3 A   Toms River, NJ 08755   (732)341-4600   Fax (732)341-4993
  + Ocean Renal Associates, P.A.
    210 Jack Martin Boulevard/Suite D-1   Brick, NJ 08724   (732)341-4600   Fax (732)458-8012
  + Ocean Renal Associates, P.A.
    1301 Route 72 West/Suite 206   Manahawkin, NJ 08755   (609)978-9940   Fax (609)978-9902

Palekar, Sadanand S., MD {1275500969} Nephro(82,INDI)<NJ-NWRKBETH>
  + Nephrology Group
    111 Northfield Avenue/Suite 311   West Orange, NJ 07052   (973)325-2103   Fax (973)325-2254

Palermo, Andrea, MD {1972687085} Pedtrc(96,PA77)<NJ-ATLANCHS, NJ-ACMCMAIN>
  + AtlantiCare/Dupont Children's Health Program
    2500 English Creek Avenue   Egg Harbor Township, NJ 08234   (609)641-3700   Fax (609)641-3652
  + AtlantiCare Hospitalist Program
    1925 Pacific Avenue/8th Floor   Atlantic City, NJ 08401   (609)345-4000
  + Nemours Dupont Pediatrics
    1925 Pacific Avenue   Atlantic City, NJ 08234   (609)345-4000   Fax (609)572-8523

Palermo, Angelo David, MD {1700178993} Pedtrc(08,NJ06)<NJ-CHLSMT>
  + Summit Medical Group-Berkeley Heights Campus
    1 Diamond Hill Road   Berkeley Heights, NJ 07922   (908)273-4300   Fax (908)790-6576
  + Children's Specialized Hospital
    200 Somerset Street   New Brunswick, NJ 08901   (732)258-7065

Palermo, Jason, MD {1053561977} CdvDis, IntrMd(03,PA13)<PA-TMPHOSP>
  + Virtua Cardiology Group
    2309 East Evesham Road/Suites 201-202   Voorhees, NJ 08043   (856)325-5400   Fax (856)325-5416
  + Cardiovascular Associates of The Delaware Valley, PA
    525 State Street/Suite 3   Elmer, NJ 08318   (856)325-5400   Fax (856)358-0725

Palermo, Kim Marie, DO {1285840918} IntrMd
  + Internal Medicine Associates of Southern New Jersey
    151 Fries Mill Road/Suite 400   Turnersville, NJ 08012   (856)401-9300   Fax (856)374-5307

Physicians by Name and Address

Paley, Jeffrey Evan, MD {1265604565} IntrMd(95,MA01)<NJ-HACKNSK, NJ-ENGLWOOD>
+ Access Medical Associates PC
177 North Dean Street/Suite 203   Englewood, NJ 07631   (201)503-0833   Fax (201)503-0844
jpaley@accessmedicalassociates.org

Palisoc, Roger Louie, DO {1477815025} FamMed
+ 389 New Bridge Road
Bergenfield, NJ 07621   (201)647-7146

Palit, Kalpana, MD {1386715803} Pedtrc(73,INDI)<NJ-CHSFULD, NJ-CHSMRCER>
+ 3 Parker Road
Plainsboro, NJ 08536

Palkar, Vikram, DO {1376947135} SrgVas<NJ-DEBRAHLC>
+ Deborah Heart and Lung Center
200 Trenton Road   Browns Mills, NJ 08015   (609)893-6611

Palkhiwala, Bharati A., MD {1346313376} Psychy(69,INA6A)<NJ-BERGNMC, NJ-RAMAPO>
+ 748 Fillmore Court
Paramus, NJ 07652   (201)445-0981   Fax (201)670-4294
Bharatipalkhwala@hotmail.com

Pall, Amandeep Kaur, MD {1720222060} InfDis, IntrMd(04,INA07)
+ 2 Eyring Road
Hillsborough, NJ 08844   (732)422-3398   Fax (973)618-5523

Palla, Katharine Theresa, DO {1598828998} IntrMd(93,PA77)
+ 101 Roseland Avenue
Caldwell, NJ 07006   (973)429-6864   Fax (973)521-7888

Palladino, Nicholas G., MD {1639116569} IntrMd(87,MNT01)<NJ-KMHSTRAT, NJ-VIRTVOOR>
+ Advocare Sicklerville Internal Med
485 Williamstown Road   Sicklerville, NJ 08081   (856)237-8100   Fax (856)237-8042

Pallay, Arnold I., MD {1538105960} FamMed(83,MA05)<NJ-STCLRDEN, NJ-CHILTON>
+ Vanguard Medical Group, P.A.
170 Changebridge Road/Suite C-3   Montville, NJ 07045   (973)575-5540   Fax (973)575-4885

Palli, Prameela M., MD {1912987587} Grtrcs, IntrMd(80,INDI)
+ New Jersey Institute for Successful Aging
42 East Laurel Road/Suite 1800   Stratford, NJ 08084   (856)566-6843   Fax (856)566-6781
+ University of Medicine & Dentistry of New Jersey-SOM
42 East Laurel Road/Suite 3200   Stratford, NJ 08084   (856)566-6843   Fax (856)566-6781

Palli, Vasu Motu, DO {1497013619} IntrMd
+ South Jersey Heart Group
3001 Chapel Avenue/Suite 101   Cherry Hill, NJ 08002   (856)482-8900   Fax (856)482-7170

Palli, Vinay Motu, MD {1558776336} IntHos<NJ-COOPRUMC>
+ Cooper University Hospital
One Cooper Plaza   Camden, NJ 08103   (856)342-2000

Pallimulla, Mahipa H., MD {1639124506} ObsGyn(78,RUS15)<NJ-STJOSHOS, NJ-WAYNEGEN>
+ Comprehensive Women's Healthcare
220 Hamburg Turnpike/Suite 21   Wayne, NJ 07470   (973)790-8090   Fax (973)790-3198

Pally, Steven Arthur, DO {1114921079} IntrMd, OstMed(89,IL76)<NJ-STBARNMC, NJ-MORRISTN>
+ 10 James Street/Suite 140
Florham Park, NJ 07932   (973)822-0770   Fax (973)822-2062

Palmer, Barbara A., MD {1427182260} Psychy(84,NY01)<NJ-BERGNMC, NJ-VALLEY>
+ New Bridge Medical Center
230 East Ridgewood Avenue   Paramus, NJ 07652   (201)967-4000

Palmer, Josette C., MD {1104860154} FamMed, IntrMd(93,PA13)<NJ-UNDRWD>
+ Underwood-Memorial Hospital Family Health Center
1120 North Delsea Drive   Glassboro, NJ 08028   (856)582-0500   Fax (856)582-0163

Palmer, Michael Alberto, MD {1710960570} SprtMd, PhysMd, OthrSp(84,ITA17)<NJ-UNVMCPRN, NJ-VANJHCS>
+ Princeton Orthopaedic Associates, P.A.
325 Princeton Avenue/OrthoRehab   Princeton, NJ 08540   (609)924-8131   Fax (609)924-8532
MPalmer@poamd.com

Palmer, Susan M., DO {1346331717} FamMed(87,MO78)
+ ImmediCenter/Clifton
1355 Broad Street   Clifton, NJ 07013   (973)778-5566   Fax (973)778-2268
+ ImmediCenter/Totowa
500 Union Boulevard   Totowa, NJ 07512   (973)778-5566   Fax (973)790-6070
+ ImmediCenter/Bloomfield
557 Broad Street   Bloomfield, NJ 07013   (973)680-8300   Fax (973)743-5601

Palmer, Thalia Christine, MD {1619995081} Anesth<NJ-HACKNSK>
+ Hackensack University Medical Center
30 Prospect Avenue/Suite 2903   Hackensack, NJ 07601   (201)996-2000

Palmer, Victoria R., DO {1164460366} FamMed(94,NJ75)<NJ-HUNTRDN>
+ Highlands Family Health Center
61 Frontage Road/Suite 61   Hampton, NJ 08827   (908)735-2594   Fax (908)735-8526

Palmeri, Barbara A., MD {1215015524} Psychy(77,NC07)<NJ-UNIVBHC>
+ University Behavioral Health Care
671 Hoes Lane/PO Box 1392   Piscataway, NJ 08855   (732)235-5500

Palmieri, Alfred E., MD {1861477655} SrgOrt(73,ITA01)
+ Coast Orthopedic Associates PA
886 Commons Way/Building H   Toms River, NJ 08755   (732)914-8989   Fax (732)914-0262

Palmiery, Ponciano, Jr., MD {1114005329} Pedtrc, AdolMd(67,PHI08)<NJ-STBARNMC>
+ Roseville Pediatric Care Center PA
500 Orange Street/Suite 304   Newark, NJ 07107   (973)483-5529   Fax (973)484-9216
+ Harrison Pediatric Care PA
332 Harrison Avenue   Harrison, NJ 07029   (973)483-5529   Fax (973)481-0754

Palomar, Nicole Liza, MD {1417204645}
+ Women's Health Care Group
870 Palisade Avenue/Suite 301   Teaneck, NJ 07666   (201)907-0900   Fax (201)907-0229

Palomares, Danilo V., MD {1134173065} Pedtrc, AdolMd(74,PHIL)
+ 2743 Kennedy Boulevard
Jersey City, NJ 07306   (201)333-7226   Fax (201)333-5824

Palomares, Kristy Therese Salisbu, MD {1346684701} ObsGyn
+ University Medical Group/OBGYN
125 Paterson Street/2nd Floor   New Brunswick, NJ 08901   (732)235-6632   Fax (732)235-7349

Palomata, Maria Theresa, MD {1821186560} IntrMd(94,PHI01)
+ Subramoni Physicians Associates PA
2091 Klockner Road   Hamilton, NJ 08690   (609)890-9191   Fax (609)586-6163
+ New Jersey Division of Developmental Disability
Route 72 East   New Lisbon, NJ 08064   (609)890-9191   Fax (609)894-8430

Paloni, Stephen Mark, MD {1821012394} Anesth, IntrMd(88,NY48)<NJ-STFRNMED>
+ St. Francis Medical Center
601 Hamilton Avenue/Anesthesia   Trenton, NJ 08629   (609)599-5000   Fax (609)599-6312

Palsky, Glenn S., MD {1104875046} Pedtrc, AdolMd(73,PA14)<NJ-CHSFULD, NJ-CHSMRCER>
+ Delaware Valley Pediatric Associates PA
132 Franklin Corner Road   Lawrenceville, NJ 08648   (609)896-4141   Fax (609)896-3940

Paltrowitz, Irving M., MD {1598738569} Gastrn, IntrMd(69,NY19)<NJ-ENGLWOOD, NJ-HACKNSK>
+ Teaneck Gastroenterology & Endoscopy Center
1086 Teaneck Road/Suite 4-C   Teaneck, NJ 07666   (201)837-9449   Fax (201)578-1699
+ Teaneck Gastroenterology & Endoscopy Center
1086 Teaneck Road/Suite 3-B   Teaneck, NJ 07666   (201)837-9449   Fax (201)837-9544

Paltrowitz, Justin Keith, MD {1194846477} Psychy
+ 60 Grand Avenue
Englewood, NJ 07631

Palumbo, Dante M., DO {1306801030} SrgOrt
+ St. Luke's Orthopedics
755 Memorial Parkway/Suite 201   Phillipsburg, NJ 08865   (908)847-8884   Fax (833)204-9604

Paluzzi, Sandra A., DO {1821099789} InfDis, IntrMd(84,NJ75)
+ LMA Surgical Associates
120 White Horse Pike/Suite 103   Haddon Heights, NJ 08035   (856)795-7505   Fax (856)795-8010

Palyca, Paul, MD {1346545464}
+ UH- RWJ Medical School
One Robert Wood Johnson Place   New Brunswick, NJ 08903   (732)235-5600

Pamaar, Cristina G., MD {1225199268} Anesth(86,PHIL)<NJ-STBARNMC>
+ St. Barnabas Medical Center
94 Old Short Hills Road   Livingston, NJ 07039   (973)322-5000

Pamerla, Mohan Ramkumar, MD {1851605919} IntrMd, IntHos<NJ-JFKMED>
+ JFK Hospitalists
98 James Street/Suite 208   Edison, NJ 08818   (908)731-1981   Fax (732)862-1171

Pamidi, Madhavi, MD {1710987201} IntrMd, CdvDis(90,INA5B)<NJ-STBARNMC, NJ-CLARMAAS>
+ University Medical Group/Cardiology
125 Paterson Street/CAB-Rm 5200   New Brunswick, NJ 08901   (732)235-6561   Fax (732)235-6530
+ New Jersey Cardiology Associates
375 Mount Pleasant Avenue   West Orange, NJ 07052   (732)235-6561   Fax (973)731-8030

Pamintuan, Dominic C., MD {1124034897} IntrMd
+ Fair Haven Internal Medicine
569 River Road/Suite 1   Fair Haven, NJ 07704   (732)530-0100   Fax (732)530-5895

Pampin, Robert J., DO {1740242130} FamMed(91,NY75)
+ Skylands Medical Group PA
33 Newton-Sparta Road/Suite 1   Newton, NJ 07860   (973)383-2244   Fax (973)383-0448

Pamy Perez, Patricia Marcelle, MD {1710116421} EmrgMd
+ 5311 Kennedy Boulevard East/Apt 3
West New York, NJ 07093

Pan, Beiqing, MD {1881910263} OncHem(CHN4D)
+ Somerset Hematology Oncology Associates, P.A.
30 Rehill Avenue/2nd Floor/Suite 2500   Somerville, NJ 08876   (908)927-8700   Fax (908)927-8706

Pan, Jane Chi-Chun, MD {1518113992} Ophthl, IntrMd(03,NY47)
+ Shore Eye Associates
530 Lakehurst Road/Suite 206   Toms River, NJ 08755   (732)341-4733   Fax (732)341-2794
+ Shore Eye Associates
445 Brick Boulevard/Suite 106   Brick, NJ 08723   (732)341-4733   Fax (732)262-0064
+ Shore Eye Associates
550 Route 530/Suite 19   Whiting, NJ 08755   (732)350-3344   Fax (732)350-0093

Pan, Jeff, MD {1972534782} SrgNro(97,NY08)<NJ-JFKMED, NJ-RWJURAH>
+ 1101 Amboy Avenue
Edison, NJ 08837   (732)205-9110   Fax (732)205-9120

Pan, Wilbur James, MD {1477637429} PedHem(94,IL11)<NJ-RWJUBRUN, NJ-JRSYSHMC>
+ Rutgers Cancer Institute of New Jersey
195 Little Albany Street/PO Box 2681   New Brunswick, NJ 08903   (732)235-2465   Fax (732)235-6797

Panagiotou, Demetrios Nicholas, MD {1225284706} CdvDis, IntrMd(NY20
+ Drs. Panagiotou & Panagiotou
1200 East Ridgewood Avenue   Ridgewood, NJ 07450   (201)447-3690   Fax (201)447-3691
+ 255 West Spring Valley Avenue
Maywood, NJ 07607   (201)447-3690   Fax (201)882-6063

Panagiotou, Nicholas D., MD {1316987019} FamMed(78,GRE01)
+ Drs. Panagiotou & Panagiotou
1200 East Ridgewood Avenue   Ridgewood, NJ 07450   (201)447-3690   Fax (201)447-3691

Panah, Daud Mohammad-Masood, MD {1831239649} Psychy(85,AFG01)
+ InSight LLC
765 East Route 70/Bldg A   Marlton, NJ 08053   (856)983-3900   Fax (856)810-0110

Panah, Manizheh Ghaem, MD {1780756049} EnDbMt, IntrMd(67,IRA01)<NJ-WAYNEGEN>
+ M. G. Panah, M.D.
516 Hamburg Turnpike/Suite 11   Wayne, NJ 07470   (973)790-0006   Fax (973)790-0450

Panah, Michael Hormoz, MD {1306828496} Anesth(93,NY03)<NJ-MORRISTN>
+ Morristown Medical Center
100 Madison Avenue/Anesthesiology   Morristown, NJ 07962   (973)971-5000   Fax (201)943-8733

Panaligan, Donato A., MD {1477594273} ObsGyn(73,PHI08)<NJ-STPETER, NJ-RWJUBRUN>
+ F2A Brier Hill Court
East Brunswick, NJ 08816   (732)238-5400   Fax (732)238-9093

Panariello, Anthony L., MD {1215036611} Ophthl(75,NY09)
+ Palisade Eye Associates
203 Palisade Avenue   Jersey City, NJ 07306   (201)653-5722   Fax (201)792-9718

Panayotov, Panayot Panchev, MD {1285691469} PthACl, BldBnk(76,BUL01)<NJ-NWRKBETH>
+ Newark Beth Israel Medical Center
201 Lyons Avenue/Path   Newark, NJ 07112   (973)926-7000   Fax (973)705-8301

Panchal, Neil, DO {1467710756} EmrgMd<NJ-STJOSHOS>
+ Overlook Medical Center
99 Beauvoir Avenue/PO Box 210   Summit, NJ 07902   (908)522-2000
+ St Joseph's Medical Center Emergency
703 Main Street   Paterson, NJ 07503   (908)522-2000   Fax (973)754-2249

Panchal, Rupa Jaydip, MD {1831118819} IntrMd(93,INA15)<NJ-STCLRDOV>
+ St. Clare's Hospital-Dover
400 West Blackwell Street/IntMed   Dover, NJ 07801   (973)989-3000   Fax (973)989-3106

Physicians by Name and Address

Panchani, Mrugesh Chhaganlal, MD {1013213206}<NJ-MONMOUTH>
+ Ocean Renal Associates, P.A.
210 Jack Martin Boulevard/Suite D-1 Brick, NJ 08724 (732)458-5854 Fax (732)458-8012
+ Ocean Renal Associates, P.A.
508 Lakehurst Road/Suite 3 A Toms River, NJ 08755 (732)458-5854 Fax (732)341-4993
+ Monmouth Medical Center
300 Second Avenue Long Branch, NJ 08724 (732)222-5200

Pancu, Ion V., MD {1689765471} Anesth(80,ROM01)
+ 20 Columbia Avenue
Cliffside Park, NJ 07010

Panda, Nirmala, MD {1780692616} Pedtrc(67,INA04)<NJ-VIRTMHBC, NJ-VIRTBERL>
+ Mt. Laurel Pediatric
528 Lippincott Drive Marlton, NJ 08053 (856)983-3899 Fax (856)983-3997

Pande, Chandana, MD {1831509413} IntrMd
+ Hackensack University Medical Group PC
160 Essex Street/Suite 102 Lodi, NJ 07644 (551)996-8111 Fax (551)996-8445

Pande, Sumati, MD {1265465587} Pedtrc, NnPnMd(91,INDI)<NJ-CHDNWBTH, NJ-NWRKBETH>
+ Children's Hospital of New Jersey
201 Lyons Avenue/Osborne Terrace Newark, NJ 07112 (973)926-7203 Fax (973)926-2332

Pandey, Krishna K., MD {1124135314} Pedtrc(83,INA66)<NJ-STMRYPAS, NJ-HACKNSK>
+ DP Pediatrics
142 Totowa Road/Suite 8 Totowa, NJ 07512 (973)904-1000 Fax (973)904-1480

Pandey, Krupa Shah, MD {1255501508} Nrolgy(03,DMN01)
+ Multiple Sclerosis Center
300 Essex Street/Suite 203 Hackensack, NJ 07601 (551)996-8100 Fax (551)996-4140

Pandey, Prasant, MD {1457466518} CdvDis, IntrMd(97,PA14)<PA-LHVLYCED>
+ Coordinated Health
222 Red Lane Phillipsburg, NJ 08865 (610)861-8080 Fax (610)849-1013

Pandey, Rajesh Kumar, MD {1144486200} Rheuma, IntrMd(06,DMN01)
+ Kayal Orthopaedic Center, P.C.
784 Franklin Avenue/Suite 250 Franklin Lakes, NJ 07417 (844)777-0910 Fax (201)560-0712

Pandey, Shivendra, MD {1720044308} Nephro(90,INDI)
+ 2640 Highway 70/Bldg 12/Suite 101B
Manasquan, NJ 08736 (732)223-0008 Fax (732)223-8020

Pandit, Florence A., MD {1699768671} Pedtrc, IntrMd(81,KENY)<NJ-VIRTVOOR, NJ-VIRTMHBC>
+ Mt. Laurel Pediatric
528 Lippincott Drive Marlton, NJ 08053 (856)983-3899 Fax (856)983-3997

Pandit, Paresh B., MD {1386637361} NnPnMd, Pedtrc(80,KEN01)<NJ-VIRTVOOR, NJ-VIRTMHBC>
+ CHOP Care Network at Virtua Voorhees Hospital
100 Bowman Drive Voorhees, NJ 08043 (856)325-3000 Fax (609)261-5842

Pando, Dalia Aurora, MD {1376537100} Pedtrc(85,PER01)
+ Pediatric Care Center
132 Washington Avenue Belleville, NJ 07109 (973)450-0624 Fax (973)450-0626

Panduranga, Satish Chandra, MD {1871564849} RadDia(94,INA68)<NJ-NWRKBETH>
+ 155 State Street
Hackensack, NJ 07601 (201)424-7496 Fax (201)487-5300

Pandya, Dhyanesh C., MD {1114182433} IntrMd
+ KNJ Hospitalist Group, LLC.
204 South Main Street Manville, NJ 08835 (732)586-9035 Fax (908)213-6618
+ St Luke's Hospitalist Group
185 Roseberry Street Phillipsburg, NJ 08865 (732)586-9035 Fax (484)526-4605

Pandya, Dipakkumar P., MD {1265486294} Nrolgy, Eplpsy, ClNrPh(93,INA20)<NJ-STJOSHOS>
+ MidJersey Orthopaedics, P.A.
8100 Westcott Drive/Suite 101 Flemington, NJ 08822 (908)782-0600 Fax (908)782-7575

Pandya, Dipti, MD {1891012662} RadDia, RadMam
+ University Radiology Group, P.C.
483 Cranbury Road East Brunswick, NJ 08816 (732)390-0030 Fax (732)390-5383

Pandya, Ipsit, MD {1356617872} IntrMd<NJ-UMDNJ>
+ PowerBack Rehabilitation
212 Marter Avenue Moorestown, NJ 08057 (856)291-4800

Pandya, Kiritkumar M., MD {1144212598} Urolgy(71,INDI)
+ 101 Prospect Street/Suite 101
Lakewood, NJ 08701 (732)364-2262 Fax (732)364-2262 kiritpandya@hotmail.com

+ 35 Beaverson Boulevard/Suite 1A
Brick, NJ 08723 (732)920-7225

Pandya, Madhukar N., MD {1104804400} CdvDis, IntrMd(77,INDI)<NJ-CHRIST, NJ-JRSYCITY>
+ 20 Lincoln Street
Jersey City, NJ 07307 (201)963-5009 Fax (201)659-5350

Pandya, Manan Kirit, DO {1255695835} IntrMd(10,PA78)
+ Sea Girt Medical Associates
235 Route 71 Manasquan, NJ 08736 (732)223-4300 Fax (732)223-5273
+ The Valley Hospital
223 North Van Dien Avenue Ridgewood, NJ 07450 (201)447-8000

Pandya, Melind Rasik, DO {1396853602} IntrMd, Nephro(99,NJ75)<NJ-BURDTMLN>
+ 15 Village Drive
Cape May Court House, NJ 08210 (609)463-2755
+ Volunteers in Medicine
423 North Route 9 Cape May Court House, NJ 08210 (609)463-2755 Fax (609)463-2830

Pandya, Prashant N., MD {1497738876} LeglMd, IntrMd(92,MI01)<NJ-STBARNMC>
+ Livingston Medical Associates, LLC.
449 Mount Pleasant Avenue/First Floor West Orange, NJ 07052 (973)535-8311 Fax (973)535-1210

Pandya, Shilin R., DO {1952727323} Psychy(10,NJ75)
+ 6550 Delilah Road/Suite 301
Egg Harbor Township, NJ 08234 (609)272-8580 Fax (609)645-7343

Pandya, Shridevi, MD {1336122795} Anesth(93,INA21)<NJ-JFKMED>
+ JFK Medical Center
65 James Street/Anesthesiology Edison, NJ 08820 (732)321-7000

Pandya, Sunandan Anilkumar, MD {1104897487} CdvDis, IntrMd(94,INA15)<NY-NYACKHOS, NY-GOODSAM>
+ Bergen Heart Center
85 Chestnut Ridge Road/Suite 111 Montvale, NJ 07645 (201)444-9913 Fax (201)444-6158

Pandya, Vrunda H., MD {1437324860} Anesth<NJ-ENGLWOOD>
+ Englewood Hospital and Medical Center
350 Engle Street/2 FL Englewood, NJ 07631 (201)871-0684 Fax (201)871-0619
+ 250 Gorge Road/Apt 21a
Cliffside Park, NJ 07010 (732)763-2914

Pane, Carmela R., MD {1780637017} NnPnMd, Pedtrc(84,DC01)<NJ-VALLEY>
+ The Valley Hospital
223 North Van Dien Avenue/Pediatrics Ridgewood, NJ 07450 (201)447-8388 Fax (201)447-8616

Panebianco, Paul S., DO {1801888995} Nephro, IntrMd(74,IA75)
+ Center for Kidney Disease & Hypertension
129 Johnson Road/Suite 4 Turnersville, NJ 08012 (856)374-4440 Fax (856)374-4445
+ Center for Kidney Disease & Hypertension
100 Brick Road/Suite 216 Marlton, NJ 08053 (856)374-4440 Fax (856)374-4445

Panebianco, Robert Antonino, MD {1134129232} CdvDis, CritCr, IntrMd(87,GRN01)<NJ-JFKMED, NJ-RWJUBRUN>
+ RWJPE Heart Specialists of Edison
4 Ethel Road/Suite 406-B Edison, NJ 08817 (732)287-6622 Fax (732)287-2233

Panei, Maryann S., MD {1447252739} Anesth(93,NJ05)<NJ-STCLRDEN>
+ Morris Anesthesia Group, PA
3799 Route 46/Suite 211 Parsippany, NJ 07054 (973)335-1122 Fax (973)335-1448

Panella, Vincent S., MD {1841242393} Gastrn, IntrMd(82,NY09)<NJ-ENGLWOOD, NJ-HOLYNAME>
+ Englewood Endoscopic Assocociates
420 Grand Avenue/Suite 101/Partner Englewood, NJ 07631 (201)569-7044 Fax (201)569-1999

Panem, Cheryl Buensuceso, MD {1215972476} Pedtrc(99,PHI01)
+ NHCAC Health Center at West New York
5301 Broadway West New York, NJ 07093 (201)866-9320 Fax (201)867-9183

Panem, Flordeliz Buensuceso, MD {1770603722} FamMed(99,PHI01)
+ NHCAC Health Center at North Bergen
1116 43rd Street North Bergen, NJ 07047 (201)330-2632 Fax (201)330-2638
+ NHCAC Health Center at West New York
5301 Broadway West New York, NJ 07093 (201)866-9320

Panezai, Fazal R., MD {1710069760} CdvDis, CritCr, Grtrcs(73,PAKI)<NJ-BAYSHORE>
+ 177 Main Street
Matawan, NJ 07747 (732)566-6614 Fax (732)290-9448

Panezai, Spozhmy, MD {1457378945} Nrolgy, ClNrPh, VasNeu(00,NJ06)<NJ-JFKMED>
+ JFK Neurosciences Institute
65 James Street/Second Floor Edison, NJ 08818 (732)321-7010 Fax (732)632-1669

Pang, James, MD {1073994299} Pedtrc<NJ-STBARNMC>
+ St. Barnabas Medical Center
94 Old Short Hills Road Livingston, NJ 07039 (973)322-5000

Pang, Xinzhu, MD {1306919550} PthAna, PthCln, PthACl(82,CHN78)
+ Quest Diagnostics Inc.
1 Malcolm Avenue Teterboro, NJ 07608 (201)393-5000 Fax (201)393-6127

Panganamamula, Uma R., MD {1558326306} ObsGyn(92,INA5B)<NJ-LOURDMED>
+ Community Health Care Inc
484 South Brewster Road Vineland, NJ 08360 (856)696-0300 Fax (856)696-2561
+ Capital Health Family Health Center
433 Bellevue Avenue/4th Floor Trenton, NJ 08618 (856)696-0300 Fax (609)815-7178

Panicker, Usha R., MD {1437131786} EnDbMt, IntrMd(92,NJ15)<NJ-JFKMED, NJ-RWJURAH>
+ 2 Maryland Avenue
Edison, NJ 08820 (732)744-9288 Fax (908)756-8468 Doctor@ushapanickermd.com

Panico, Robert A., MD {1649235896} RadDia
+ Cape Radiology
4011 Route 9 South/PO Box 244 Rio Grande, NJ 08242 (609)886-0477 Fax (609)886-0529

Panitch, Kenneth N., MD {1528038403} FamMed(91,OH06)
+ Advocare Grove Family Medical Associates
132 Grove Street/Suite A Haddonfield, NJ 08033 (856)354-2211 Fax (856)354-6181

Pannullo, Robert Paul, MD {1598724510} PhysMd, PainMd, PhyPMPain(93,MI07)<NJ-CENTRAST, NJ-JRSYSHMC>
+ Orthopaedic Sports Medicine
80 Oak Hill Road Red Bank, NJ 07701 (732)741-2313 Fax (732)741-7154
+ Seaview Orthopaedics
1200 Eagle Avenue Ocean, NJ 07712 (732)741-2313 Fax (732)660-6201
+ University Orthopaedic Associates, LLC.
Two Worlds Fair Drive Somerset, NJ 07701 (732)979-2115 Fax (732)564-9032

Panossian, Alexander M., MD {1699743906} Urolgy(63,LEB03)<NJ-VALLEY>
+ 230 East Ridgewood Avenue/Suite 6-2
Paramus, NJ 07652 (201)447-6117 Fax (201)447-3638

Panse, Ramanand V., MD {1457426322} EmrgMd(84,DOMI)<NJ-JRSYSHMC>
+ EmCare
1945 Route 33 Neptune, NJ 07753 (732)776-4510 Fax (732)776-2329

Pant, Meenakshi, MD {1528290079} ObsGyn
+ University Reproductive Association
185 South Orange Avenue/MSB E-506 Newark, NJ 07103 (973)972-5266 Fax (973)972-4574

Pantagis, Stefanos G., MD {1235212879} Grtrcs, FamMed, IntrMd(94,NJ05)<NJ-HACKNSK, NJ-HOLYNAME>
+ Geriatrics and Longevity Treatment Specialist PC
810 Main Street Hackensack, NJ 07601 (201)633-7375 Fax (201)633-7361

Pantano, Maria V., DO {1841405008} FamMed(04,NJ75)
+ Wood Ridge Medical Associates
245 Valley Boulevard Wood Ridge, NJ 07075 (201)438-5500 Fax (201)438-3363

Pantelick, Julie M., DO {1033303458} IntrMd<NJ-STFRNMED>
+ St. Francis Medical Center
601 Hamilton Avenue/Suite B158 Trenton, NJ 08629 (609)599-5139 Fax (609)599-5047

Pantin, Enrique Jose, MD {1720160427} Anesth(87,VEN04)<NJ-RWJUBRUN>
+ Robert Wood Johnson-UMDNJ Anesthesia Group
125 Paterson Street/CAB 3100 New Brunswick, NJ 08901 (732)235-7827 Fax (732)418-8492

Panucci, Nicholas Joseph, DO {1881175743}
+ Penn Medicine at Cherry Hill
409 Route 70 East Cherry Hill, NJ 08034 (215)755-5700

Panuganti, Sravan, DO {1588045819} Urolgy
+ Rowan University-School of Osteopathic Medicine
1 Medical Center Drive/Suite 162 Stratford, NJ 08084 (856)566-6875

Panush, David, MD {1164407219} Radiol, RadNro(85,NY46)<NJ-HACKNSK>
+ The Imaging Center
30 South Newman Street Hackensack, NJ 07601 (201)488-1188 Fax (201)488-5244
+ New Century Imaging at Oradell
555 Kinderkamack Road Oradell, NJ 07649 (201)488-1188 Fax (201)599-8333
+ Hackensack Radiology Group, P.A.
30 Prospect Avenue Hackensack, NJ 07601 (201)996-2200 Fax (201)336-8451

Physicians by Name and Address

Panza, Nicole, MD {1942698600} Pedtrc
+ Pediatrics Associates
566 Westfield Avenue   Westfield, NJ 07090   (908)233-7171   Fax (908)233-2255

Panza, Robert A., MD {1013074434} Pedtrc(84,ITA17)
+ Pediatrics Associates
566 Westfield Avenue   Westfield, NJ 07090   (908)233-7171   Fax (908)233-2255

Panzner, Elizabeth A., MD {1346234697} Pedtrc, AdolMd(84,MEX14)<NJ-STBARNMC, NJ-OVERLOOK>
+ Union Pediatric Medical Group, PA
1050 Galloping Hill Road/Suite 200   Union, NJ 07083   (908)688-9900   Fax (908)688-9939

Paolicchi, Juliann Marie, MD {1245226059} Pedtrc, ClNrPh, NroChl(88,MD07)
+ Northeast Regional Epilepsy Group
20 Prospect Avenue/Suite 800   Hackensack, NJ 07601   (201)343-6676   Fax (201)343-6689

Paolini, Lawrence, DO {1437263753} Dermat(84,PA77)<NJ-BURDTMLN>
+ 105 North Main Street
Cape May Court House, NJ 08210   (609)465-8788   Fax (609)465-3182
lpaolini@caperegional.com

Paolino, James S., MD {1639192230} Rheuma, IntrMd(66,PA02)<NJ-STBARNMC>
+ 2168 Millburn Avenue/Suite 205
Maplewood, NJ 07040   (973)762-3738   Fax (973)762-7878

Paolucci, Ugo, MD {1265658793} VasNeu
+ University Hospital-RWJMS Neurology
125 Paterson Street/Suite 4100-6100   New Brunswick, NJ 08901   (732)235-7732   Fax (732)235-8115
+ North Jersey Brain and Surgical
680 Kinderkamack Road/Suite 300   Oradell, NJ 07649   (732)235-7732   Fax (201)342-7171

Paonessa, Nina Joanne, DO {1174503197} SrgC&R(98,PA78)
+ 2101 Route 34 South/Suite H
Wall, NJ 07719   (732)282-1500   Fax (732)282-1501

Papa, Christine A., DO {1427023928} Dermat(94,NJ75)
+ Macaione and Papa Dermatology Associates
707 White Horse Road/Suite C-103   Voorhees, NJ 08043   (856)627-1900   Fax (856)627-6907

Papa, Louis, MD {1669439873} Anesth(83,MEXI)
+ Ambulatory Anesthesia Care, PC
1450 Route 22 West   Mountainside, NJ 07092   (908)233-2020   Fax (908)233-9322

Papa, Louis A., DO {1891725610} CdvDis(70,PA77)<NJ-KMHSTRAT, NJ-KENEDYHS>
+ Southern New Jersey Cardiac Care Specialists
1020 Laurel Oak Road/Suite 102   Voorhees, NJ 08043   (856)435-8842   Fax (856)435-8665
+ Southern New Jersey Cardiac Care Specialists
151 Fries Mill Road/Suite 101   Turnersville, NJ 08012   (856)435-8842   Fax (856)374-3120

Papa, Thomas Rowland, DO {1467651935} EmrgMd
+ Kennedy Memorial Hospital-University Medical Center
18 East Laurel Road   Stratford, NJ 08084   (856)346-7985
+ Teamhealth East
307 South Evergreen Avenue   Woodbury, NJ 08096   (856)848-3817

Papa-Molter, Andrea Elisa, DO {1619130499} Psychy<PA-FRIENDS>
+ Pinnacle Behavioral Health Institute
851 Route 73 North/Suite C   Marlton, NJ 08053   (856)512-8108   Fax (856)267-5824

Papa-Rugino, Tommasina, MD {1629050554} Nrolgy(85,NY08)
+ Hackensack Meridian Medical Group
53 Nautilus Drive/Suite 201   Manahawkin, NJ 08050   (609)978-8870   Fax (609)978-8903

Papadakis, Kelly M., MD   IntrMd(97,NJ06)
+ 18 Breckenridge Drive
Shamong, NJ 08088

Papadopoulos, Anthony Jordan, MD {1801852678} Dermat(01,NJ05)
+ 1 Centre Street
Sparta, NJ 07871

Paparone, Basil J., MD {1023129509} Otlryg(68,ITA01)<NJ-SHOREMEM>
+ 72 West Jim Leeds Road
Pomona, NJ 08240   (609)652-6880   Fax (609)748-0889

Paparone, Philip W., DO {1568409159} InfDis, IntrMd, OthrSp(69,MO78)<NJ-ACMCITY, NJ-ACMCMAIN>
+ 72 West Jimmie Leeds Road
Absecon, NJ 08201   (609)652-2240   Fax (609)748-1029

Papastamelos, Athanasios G., DO {1821051277} InfDis, IntrMd(88,NJ75)<NJ-SHOREMEM>
+ 2106 New Road/Suite F-1
Linwood, NJ 08221   (609)926-5451   Fax (609)926-1372

Papastamelos, Caitlin A., MD {1487644589} PedCrC, PedPul, Pedtrc(87,NJ06)<NJ-SHOREMEM>
+ Voorhees Pediatric Facility
1304 Laurel Oak Road   Voorhees, NJ 08043   (856)346-3300

Fax (856)504-8029

Papatheodorou, Dana William, MD {1588957971} IntHos
+ IPC The Hospitalist Company
55 Madison Avenue/Suite 310   Morristown, NJ 07960   (973)993-9536   Fax (973)998-4237

Papish, Steven W., MD {1811985997} Hemato, IntrMd, MedOnc(74,PA01)<NJ-MORRISTN, NJ-MMHKEMBL>
+ Hematology-Oncology Associates of Northern NJ
100 Madison Avenue/PO Box 1089   Morristown, NJ 07962   (973)538-5210   Fax (973)644-9657

Papp, Denes, MD {1619059318} Anesth(81,HUN03)<NJ-RWJUBRUN>
+ Robert Wood Johnson-UMDNJ Anesthesia Group
125 Paterson Street/CAB 3100   New Brunswick, NJ 08901   (732)937-8841   Fax (732)235-6131

Pappagallo, Marco, MD {1720069610} PainMd, Nrolgy(82,ITA17)<NY-JTORTHO>
+ Pain Management Center
11 Overlook Road/MAC 11 Suite B110   Summit, NJ 07901   (917)763-8918   Fax (908)522-6123

Pappalardo, Rebecca A., MD {1699754747} Anesth(91,NJ06)<NJ-ENGLWOOD>
+ Englewood Anesthesiology
350 Engle Street   Englewood, NJ 07631   (201)894-3238   Fax (201)894-0585
+ Englewood Hospital and Medical Center
350 Engle Street/Anesthesiology   Englewood, NJ 07631   (201)894-3000

Pappas, Elena Catherine, DO {1124204425} FamMed(06,NY75)
+ Pappas Family Medical Center
1006 Commons Way/Building G   Toms River, NJ 08755   (732)551-2003   Fax (732)551-2033

Pappas, Gregory A., MD {1235218066} Urolgy(77,MEXI)<NJ-HOBUNIMC, NJ-ENGLWOOD>
+ 4 Main Street/Unit 5, Bldg. F
Edgewater, NJ 07020   (201)969-9700   Fax (201)969-9688

Pappas, Lara, MD {1346498326} PedHem
+ Edison Pediatrics
1802 Oak Tree Road/Suite 101   Edison, NJ 08820   (732)548-3210   Fax (906)548-3966
+ The Children's Hospital at Saint Peter's University
254 Easton Avenue   New Brunswick, NJ 08901   (732)548-3210   Fax (732)418-9708

Pappas, Nadine C., MD {1215984141} SrgBst, Surgry(89,NJ06)<NJ-CLARMAAS, NJ-STBARNMC>
+ 50 Newark Avenue/Suite 308
Belleville, NJ 07109   (973)844-1000   Fax (973)844-4920

Papperman, Thomas W., MD   ObsGyn(84,NY03)<NJ-BURDTMLN, NJ-SHOREMEM>
+ Shore Womans Care
248 Asbury Road   Egg Harbor Township, NJ 08234   (609)927-9777

Pappert, Amy S., MD {1598723884} Dermat(89,NJ06)
+ Robert Wood Johnson Medical Group-Dermatology
1 World's Fair Drive/Suite 2400   Somerset, NJ 08873   (732)235-7993   Fax (732)235-7117

Pappert, Jeffrey Robert, MD {1164695722} IntrMd(03)<NJ-JFKMED>
+ Hudson County Primary Care
377 Jersey Avenue/Suite 590   Jersey City, NJ 07302   (201)763-6313   Fax (201)763-6062

Para, Vijaya L., MD {1699772111} Anesth(92,INA3Y)<NJ-MONMOUTH>
+ Monmouth Medical Center
300 Second Avenue/Anesthesiology   Long Branch, NJ 07740   (732)222-5200

Parada, Joseph A., MD {1508819004} EmrgMd(88,NJ05)
+ Jersey Emergency Specialists, Inc.
185 Roseberry Street   Phillipsburg, NJ 08865   (908)859-6767   Fax (908)859-6812

Paradela, Ephrem Hector, MD {1942227996} IntrMd(91,PHIL)<NJ-ACMCITY, NJ-ACMCMAIN>
+ AtlantiCare Clinical Associates
2500 English Creek Avenue   Egg Harbor Township, NJ 08234   (609)407-2310

Paradiso, Mary J., MD {1033292867} InfDis, IntrMd(90,NJ05)
+ New Jersey Infectious Diseases Associates PA
113 James Street   Edison, NJ 08820   (732)906-1900   Fax (732)906-6666
+ Medical Diagnostic Associates PA
525 Central Avenue/Suite D   Westfield, NJ 07090   (732)906-1900   Fax (908)389-1922

Parag, Yoav, MD {1689848186} RadNro(00,ISR01)<NY-MTSINAI>
+ Advanced Medical Imaging of North Jersey
452 Old Hook Road/Suite 301   Emerson, NJ 07630   (201)262-0001   Fax (201)262-2330

Paragas, Miguela L., MD {1770530545} Pedtrc, GPrvMd, AdolMd(77,PHIL)<NJ-STBARNMC>
+ Paragas Ob-Gyn Associates
312 Belleville Turnpike/Suite 2C   North Arlington, NJ 07031   (201)991-7200   Fax (201)991-1514

Paragi, Prakash Ramaiah, MD {1598992380} Surgry<NJ-STBARNMC>
+ St. Barnabas Medical Center
94 Old Short Hills Road   Livingston, NJ 07039   (973)322-5000

Paragioudakis, Steve J., MD {1265517999} SrgOrt(93,NJ05)<NJ-MONMOUTH>
+ Monmouth Medical Center
300 Second Avenue/OrthoSurgery   Long Branch, NJ 07740   (732)222-5200

Paraiso, Reynaldo S., DO {1477780369} OtgyFPlS<NJ-STBARNMC>
+ St. Barnabas Medical Center
94 Old Short Hills Road   Livingston, NJ 07039   (973)322-8994

Parakh, Shwetambara, MD {1285889766} SrgPlstc
+ Parakh Plastic Surgery
370 Grand Avenue/Suite 202   Englewood, NJ 07631   (201)567-1919   Fax (201)567-1955

Paralkar, Mayur A., MD {1679766232} IntrMd(02,INA1D)
+ The Valley Hospital
223 North Van Dien Avenue   Ridgewood, NJ 07450   (201)447-8000

Paramatmuni, Lakshmi Kantharao, MD {1457468886} IntrMd, Grtrcs(64,INA1L)<NJ-VALYONS>
+ VA New Jersey Health Care System at Lyons
151 Knollcroft Road   Lyons, NJ 07939   (908)647-0180   Fax (908)604-5205

Paranal, Aurora M., MD {1679655344} Psychy(78,PHI01)<NJ-HAGEDORN>
+ Hagedorn Psychiatric Hospital
200 Sanatorium Road   Glen Gardner, NJ 08826   (908)537-2141   Fax (908)537-3100

Parangi, Robert K., MD {1528131281} IntrMd(92,MI01)<NJ-HACKNSK, NJ-BERGNMC>
+ Drs. Parangi and Parangi
9 Yale Court   Paramus, NJ 07652   (201)265-1333   Fax (201)265-6991

Parangi, Sasan M., MD {1255404927} IntrMd(90,NY08)<NJ-VALLEY, NJ-HACKNSK>
+ Drs. Parangi and Parangi
9 Yale Court   Paramus, NJ 07652   (201)265-7564   Fax (201)265-6991
Mparangi@aol.com

Parashurama, Prashant, MD {1851382329} RadDia(98,NY06)<NJ-JFKMED>
+ Edison Radiology Group, P.A.
65 James Street   Edison, NJ 08820   (732)321-7917   Fax (732)737-2968

Parcells, Alexis Lanteri, MD {1659662179}(11,GRN01)
+ 6 Red Oak Drive
Spring Lake, NJ 07762   (201)281-6353

Parcells, Bertrand W., MD {1235494923}<NJ-RWJUBRUN>
+ RWJ University Hospital New Brunswick
One Robert Wood Johnson Place   New Brunswick, NJ 08901   (732)235-7674

Parchment, Alfred B., MD {1073587242} ObsGyn, IntrMd(91,NJ05)<NJ-OCEANMC, NJ-KIMBALL>
+ Brick Women's Physicians
87 Union Avenue   Manasquan, NJ 08736   (732)202-0700   Fax (732)202-0664
drparchment@gmail.com

Parchment, Winsome M., MD {1972598829} ObsGyn(86,NY46)<NJ-MTNSIDE, NJ-UMDNJ>
+ Metropolitan Ob/Gyn, P.A.
1973 Springfield Avenue   Maplewood, NJ 07040   (973)313-2501   Fax (973)313-2505

Parchuri, Hima Bindu, DO {1386843332} FamMed(05,NJ75)
+ Lourdes Medical Associates/Tribro Family Physicians
1104 Route 130/Suite K   Cinnaminson, NJ 08077   (856)786-8010   Fax (856)786-0529

Pardes, Jorge Gustavo, MD {1457349011} RadDia(76,ARG01)<NJ-MONMOUTH>
+ Monmouth Medical Center
300 Second Avenue/Breast Center   Long Branch, NJ 07740   (732)923-7700   Fax (732)923-7710

Pardon, Ilene B., MD {1750452355} Ophthl(93,NY47)
+ Eye Diagnostic Center
3333 Fairmont Avenue   Asbury Park, NJ 07712   (732)988-4000   Fax (732)988-9502
+ Eye Diagnostic Center
525 Route 70   Brick, NJ 08723   (732)988-4000   Fax (732)477-1444
+ Eye Diagnostic Center
258 Broad Street   Red Bank, NJ 07712   (732)530-8500

Pardon, Paul A., MD {1730153321} IntrMd(93,NY09)<NJ-JRSYSHMC>
+ 512 Warren Avenue
Spring Lake, NJ 07762   (732)449-9799   Fax (732)449-7073
+ Jersey Shore Geriatrics
15 School Road East/Suite 2   Marlboro, NJ 07746   (732)449-9799   Fax (732)866-9970

Pare', Jeanne M., MD {1376553032} Rheuma(86,NY08)<NJ-HCKTSTWN>
+ Allergy & Arthritis Associates PA
600 Mount Pleasant Avenue/Suite C   Dover, NJ 07801   (973)989-0500   Fax (973)989-5046
+ Allergy & Arthritis Associates PA
66 Sunset Strip/Suite 207   Succasunna, NJ 07876   (973)989-0500   Fax (973)584-7017

Pareja, Victor Hugo, MD {1184657066} Nrolgy, ClNrPh(89,MEX14)
+ 230 West Jersey Street/Ste 104
Elizabeth, NJ 07202   (908)282-9500   Fax (908)282-9600

Parekh, Jai G., MD {1841222502} Ophthl(93,MA05)<NJ-STJOSHOS, NJ-JFKMED>
+ Eyecare Consultants of New Jersey
1031 McBride Avenue/Suite D-106   West Paterson, NJ 07424   (973)785-2050   Fax (973)785-2423
+ Eyecare Consultants of New Jersey
7 Lincoln Highway   Edison, NJ 08820   (732)516-0099

Parekh, Nili M., MD {1790074433}<NJ-VIRTMHBC>
+ Virtua Memorial
175 Madison Avenue   Mount Holly, NJ 08060   (718)902-6764
parekh.nili@gmail.com

Parekh, Swati Jai Shah, MD {1427087725} Ophthl(93,NJ05)<NJ-STJOSHOS>
+ Eyecare Consultants of New Jersey
1031 McBride Avenue/Suite D-106   West Paterson, NJ 07424   (973)785-2050   Fax (973)785-2423
+ St. Joseph's Regional Medical Center
703 Main Street   Paterson, NJ 07503   (973)754-2275

Parhar, Avtar Singh, MD {1134186489} IntrMd, PulDis(88,MEXI)<NJ-BAYSHORE>
+ Central Jersey Pulmonary Medicine PC
721 North Beers Street/Suite 2-G   Holmdel, NJ 07733   (732)264-7970   Fax (732)264-8858

Pari, Sadhana S., MD {1548331671} Pedtrc(92,INA77)
+ Sadhana Pediatrics, P.C.
49 Veronica Avenue/Suite 101   Somerset, NJ 08873   (732)247-3434   Fax (732)247-1815

Parihar, Jasmit K., DO {1255580601} Anesth(11,NY75)
+ St. Joseph's Regional Medical Center Anesthesia
703 Main Street   Paterson, NJ 07503   (973)754-2790   Fax (973)754-2791

Parihar, Jaspreet Singh, MD {1447563317} Urolgy(09,PA09)<NJ-RWJUBRUN>
+ RWJ University Hospital New Brunswick
One Robert Wood Johnson Place   New Brunswick, NJ 08901   (732)235-7674

Parikh, Amay, MD {1740464924} CritCr, Nephro, IntrMd(05,MA07)
+ University Medical Group
125 Paterson Street/Suite 5100   New Brunswick, NJ 08901   (732)235-6512   Fax (732)235-6124
amay_parikh@rwjuh.edu

Parikh, Anant Parimal, MD {1174819148} Anesth
+ Hackensack University MC-Anesthesia Dept
30 Prospect Avenue/Room 2703   Hackensack, NJ 07601   (551)996-2419   Fax (201)996-3962

Parikh, Ashish Dharnidhar, MD {1821027533} IntrMd(92,FL02)
+ Summit Medical Group-Berkeley Heights Campus
1 Diamond Hill Road   Berkeley Heights, NJ 07922   (908)273-4300   Fax (908)790-6576

Parikh, Bijal Rajendra, MD {1902040850} Anesth
+ New Jersey Anesthesia Associates, P.C.
252 Columbia Turnpike/PO Box 0037   Florham Park, NJ 07932   (973)660-9334   Fax (973)660-9779
bijalparikh@hotmail.com

Parikh, Chaula A., MD {1215023841} Pedtrc(96,INA20)<NJ-MEADWLND, NJ-CHRIST>
+ Riverside Medical Group
714 Tenth Street/Suite 2   Secaucus, NJ 07094   (201)863-3346   Fax (201)865-0015
+ Riverside Pediatric Group
1425 Bloomfield Street   Hoboken, NJ 07030   (201)863-3346   Fax (201)876-3218

Parikh, Chintan Prakash, MD {1124192497} IntrMd(98,INA65)
+ 50 Byrne Court/Suite A
Wayne, NJ 07470   (973)981-4044

Parikh, Chirayu Bharat, DO {1164635033} PsyCAd, Psychy(04,NJ75)
+ Princeton House Behavioral Health - North Brunswick
1460 Livingston Avenue   North Brunswick, NJ 08902   (732)729-3650   Fax (732)435-0222

+ Center for Family Guidance, PC
765 East Route 70/Building A-101   Marlton, NJ 08053   (732)729-3650   Fax (856)810-0110

Parikh, Dhinoj M., MD {1629171020} IntrMd(68,INA4X)<NJ-CHILTON>
+ Atlantic Medical Group
1395 Route 23/Suite 4   Butler, NJ 07405   (973)838-0200   Fax (973)838-1614

Parikh, Dhwani R., MD {1467695692} RadOnc(09,CT02)
+ Rutgers Cancer Institute of New Jersey
195 Little Albany Street/PO Box 2681   New Brunswick, NJ 08903   (732)235-2465   Fax (732)235-6797

Parikh, Gita N., MD {1184728800} Psychy(80,INDI)<NJ-HOBUNIMC, NJ-EASTORNG>
+ 3368 Kennedy Boulevard
Jersey City, NJ 07307   (201)656-8811   Fax (201)656-7215

Parikh, Gunja Paresh, MD {1083935985}
+ 149 Sandpiper Key
Secaucus, NJ 07094   (917)226-9720
gunjaparikh@gmail.com

Parikh, Hiren B., MD {1104874395} IntrMd, IntHos<NJ-ACMCITY>
+ AtlantiCare Hospitalist Program
1925 Pacific Avenue/8th Floor   Atlantic City, NJ 08401   (609)441-8146   Fax (609)441-8002

Parikh, Jayesh K., MD {1932142981} PulDis, IntrMd(86,INDI)<NJ-COMMED, NJ-KIMBALL>
+ Jersey Pulmonary Care, MD PA
9 Hospital Drive/Suite A-18   Toms River, NJ 08755   (732)557-5515   Fax (732)557-5516

Parikh, Manoj R., MD {1972508125} RadDia(75,INDI)
+ Point Pleasant Radiology Group
1973 State Route 34/Suite E-13   Wall, NJ 07719   (732)974-8011   Fax (732)974-8820
+ Lacey Diagnostic Imaging LLC
833 Lacey Road/Suite 2   Forked River, NJ 08731   (732)974-8011   Fax (609)242-2402

Parikh, Meenakshi B., MD {1083630503} Pedtrc(67,INA1G)<NJ-STPETER, NJ-RWJUHAM>
+ 200 Perrine Road/Suite 223
Old Bridge, NJ 08857   (732)727-1818   Fax (732)727-4349

Parikh, Nalini S., MD {1851407951} PthAcl, PthCyt(76,INDI)<NJ-STMICHL>
+ St. Michael's Medical Center
111 Central Avenue   Newark, NJ 07102   (973)877-5202   Fax (973)877-2712

Parikh, Neelesh Vinod, DO {1457386112} EmrgMd(96,MO78)<NJ-VIRTVOOR>
+ Virtua Voorhees
100 Bowman Drive/EmergMed   Voorhees, NJ 08043   (856)247-3000

Parikh, Nikhil S., MD {1336254234} IntrMd(77,INDI)<NJ-ACMCITY, NJ-ACMCMAIN>
+ 2030 New Road
Linwood, NJ 08221   (609)653-0009   Fax (609)653-6648

Parikh, Nitin A., MD {1649337296} IntrMd(79,INA65)<NJ-CHRIST, NJ-HOBUNIMC>
+ 3368 Kennedy Boulevard
Jersey City, NJ 07307   (201)656-8811   Fax (201)656-7215

Parikh, Pallavi M., MD {1639116353} Anesth(76,INDI)<NJ-CENTRAST>
+ Liberty Anesthesia & Pain Management
901 West Main Street/2nd Floor   Freehold, NJ 07728   (732)294-2876   Fax (732)294-2502

Parikh, Payal Dinesh, MD {1972824407}
+ 87 Van Riper Avenue
Rutherford, NJ 07070   (201)893-7299
drparikhzemse@gmail.com
+ UH-RWJ General Internal Medicine
125 Paterson Street/Suite 2300   New Brunswick, NJ 08901   (201)893-7299   Fax (732)235-7114

Parikh, Pratima D., MD {1427023308} IntrMd, IntMAdMd(72,INA21)<NJ-VIRTBERL, NJ-VIRTVOOR>
+ 15 East Taunton Avenue
Berlin, NJ 08009   (856)767-0320   Fax (856)767-3536
+ 777 South White Horse Pike
Hammonton, NJ 08037   (609)567-7444

Parikh, Pujan N., MD {1083156178} IntrMd
+ 2106 New Road/Suite F-1
Linwood, NJ 08221   (904)417-8991

Parikh, Rakesh K., MD {1437177615} Grtrcs, IntrMd(88,INA21)<NJ-JFKMED>
+ Medical Associates of Marlboro
111 James Street   Edison, NJ 08818   (732)452-9700   Fax (732)452-9720
+ Medical Associates of Marlboro PC
32 North Main Street   Marlboro, NJ 07746   (732)452-9700   Fax (732)462-3798

Parikh, Sagar Shailesh, MD {1356570709} PhysMd, PainMd(08,NJ06)<NJ-JFKMED>
+ JFK Medical Center
65 James Street/Pain/Musculo   Edison, NJ 08820   (732)321-7000

Physicians by Name and Address

Parikh, Sahil, MD {1215346812} IntrMd<NJ-RWJUBRUN>
+ RWJ University Hospital New Brunswick
One Robert Wood Johnson Place   New Brunswick, NJ 08901   (732)828-3000

Parikh, Sandip K., MD {1952347619} IntrMd(87,INA21)<NJ-BAYSHORE>
+ 35 Beaverson Boulevard/Suite 6B
Brick, NJ 08723   (732)262-0222   Fax (732)262-0555

Parikh, Sanjiv R., MD {1780762898} Anesth, PainMd, IntrMd(86,INDI)
+ Glen Ridge Surgicenter
230 Sherman Avenue   Glen Ridge, NJ 07028   (973)783-2626   Fax (973)680-4211

Parikh, Shailesh S., MD {1417945445} PhysMd(73,INA20)<NJ-KSLRSADB, NJ-VALLEY>
+ Kessler Institute for Rehabilitation
300 Market Street   Saddle Brook, NJ 07663   (201)368-6043   Fax (201)368-6135

Parikh, Smruti Ashish, MD {1477561249} AlgyImmn, PedAlg, IntrMd(98,CT02)<NJ-STCLRDEN, NJ-MORRISTN>
+ Summit Medical Group
140 Park Avenue/3rd Floor/Allergy   Florham Park, NJ 07932   (973)404-9960

Parikh, Sudha Sudhir, MD {1114200706} Anesth(69,INA20)
+ Wills Surgery Center of Central New Jersey
107 North Center Drive   North Brunswick, NJ 08902   (732)297-8001   Fax (732)297-8007

Parikh, Sudhir Manharlal, MD {1366427585} PedAlg, IntrMd(70,INA20)<NJ-HOBUNIMC>
+ Center for Asthma & Allergy
18 North Third Avenue   Highland Park, NJ 08904   (732)545-0094   Fax (732)545-4087
+ Center for Asthma & Allergy
300 Hudson Street   Hoboken, NJ 07030   (732)545-0094   Fax (201)792-5320
+ Center for Asthma & Allergy
90 Milburn Avenue/Suite 200   Maplewood, NJ 08904   (973)763-5787   Fax (973)763-8568

Parikh, Vasavi Harish, MD {1497761951} Pedtrc(98,DMN01)<NJ-OVERLOOK, NJ-STBARNMC>
+ Warren Pediatrics
34 Mountain Boulevard   Warren, NJ 07059   (908)490-0900   Fax (908)490-0910
warrenpeds@yahoo.com

Parikh, Vidhi J., MD {1275881682}
+ 2141 Route 38/Apt 917 W
Cherry Hill, NJ 08002   (732)318-7249
vipar117@gmail.com

Parikh, Vipul K., MD {1518982958} IntrMd(89,INA15)<NJ-COMMED, NJ-KIMBALL>
+ 601 Route 37 West/Suite 104
Toms River, NJ 08755   (732)240-1100   Fax (732)240-1127

Parinello, Robert M., MD {1467673384} Psychy, PsyCAd(82,ITA17)<NJ-SUMOAKSH>
+ 140 Mountain Avenue
Springfield, NJ 07081   (908)647-9500   Fax (908)647-9000

Paris, Glen Allen, MD {1275594525} Anesth, PainMd(92,NY08)<NJ-OVERLOOK>
+ Summit Anesthesia Associates, P.A.
33 Overlook Road/Suite 311   Summit, NJ 07901   (908)598-1500   Fax (908)598-0197

Parisi, Angela Rosina, MD {1700976511} RadDia(92,NY46)<NJ-MORRISTN>
+ Memorial Radiology Associates
10 Lanidex Plaza West/Suite 125   Parsippany, NJ 07054   (973)503-5700   Fax (973)386-5701
+ Morristown Medical Center
100 Madison Avenue/Radiology   Morristown, NJ 07962   (973)971-5000

Parisi, Danielle, DO {1770731655}
+ CPC Behavioral HealthCare
270 Highway 35   Red Bank, NJ 07701   (516)375-9038   Fax (732)224-0688
danip511@aol.com

Parisi, Frank, MD {1326058587} Ophthl(92,NY46)<NJ-HOLYNAME>
+ The New Jersey Eye Center
1 North Washington Avenue   Bergenfield, NJ 07621   (201)384-7333   Fax (201)384-2564

Parisi, Gerlando V., MD {1265409981} IntrMd(89,MNT01)<NJ-MONMOUTH, NJ-KIMBALL>
+ Monmouth Medical Group, P.C.
223 Monmouth Road   West Long Branch, NJ 07764   (732)229-3838   Fax (732)229-4562

Parisi, Vanessa Marie, DO {1639437825} ObsGyn
+ 181 Franklin Avenue/Suite 101
Nutley, NJ 07110   (973)748-7953

Park, Anne June, DO {1700906815} IntrMd(03,NY75)<NJ-ENGLWOOD>
+ Englewood Hospital and Medical Center
350 Engle Street/Medicine   Englewood, NJ 07631   (201)894-3501   Fax (201)894-5693

Physicians by Name and Address

Park, Byong K., MD {1235104506} IntrMd(78,KORE)<NJ-HACKNSK>
+ United Medical, P.C.
612 Rutherford Avenue   Lyndhurst, NJ 07071   (201)460-0063   Fax (201)460-1684
+ United Medical, P.C.
988 Broadway/Suite 201   Bayonne, NJ 07002   (201)460-0063   Fax (201)339-6333

Park, Charles William, MD {1629179411} Psychy(98,MO03)<NJ-STBARNMC>
+ Associates in Psychiatry
405 Northfield Avenue/Suite 204   West Orange, NJ 07052   (973)325-6120   Fax (973)325-6126

Park, Chong H., MD {1457417180} PainMd, Anesth(73,KOR14)
+ 775 Bloomfield Avenue
Montclair, NJ 07042   (973)509-3401   Fax (973)655-1560

Park, Dong C., MD {1760419147} Anesth(73,KORE)<NJ-COMMED>
+ Community Medical Center
99 Route 37 West/Anesthesiology   Toms River, NJ 08755   (732)505-0278

Park, Henry, MD {1427219807} CritCr
+ Atlantic Neurosurgical Specialists
310 Madison Avenue/Suite 300   Morristown, NJ 07960   (973)285-7800   Fax (973)285-7839

Park, Hyeun Sik, MD {1235226960} CdvDis, IntrMd(99,NY48)<NJ-TRINIWSC, NJ-NWRKBETH>
+ Lakeland Cardiology Center, P.A.
415 Boulevard   Mountain Lakes, NJ 07046   (973)334-7700   Fax (973)334-7116

Park, James Joongchul, MD {1497895056} RadDia, Radiol, OthrSp(99,NY08)<NJ-HOLYNAME>
+ Holy Name Hospital
718 Teaneck Road/Radiology   Teaneck, NJ 07666   (201)833-7023   Fax (201)541-5919

Park, Jane, MD {1700939956} SrgC&R(01,NY15)
+ Atlantic Shore Surgical Associates
478 Brick Boulevard   Brick, NJ 08723   (732)701-4848   Fax (732)701-1244

Park, Jay Hoon, MD {1366478372} EmrgMd(00,DC01)<NJ-TRINIWSC>
+ Trinitas Regional Medical Center-Williamson Street
225 Williamson Street   Elizabeth, NJ 07207   (908)994-5000

Park, Jennifer E., MD {1770674525} Psychy(71,KORE)<NJ-TRENTPSY>
+ Trenton Psychiatric Hospital
Sullivan Way/PO Box 7600   West Trenton, NJ 08628   (609)633-1500

Park, Ji Hae, MD {1205298007} Urolgy
+ 500 First Street
Palisades Park, NJ 07650   (201)240-8599   Fax (201)204-8599

Park, Jin S., MD {1902842057} Nephro, IntrMd(68,KOR06)<NJ-OCEANMC, NJ-SOCEANCO>
+ Ocean Renal Associates, P.A.
210 Jack Martin Boulevard/Suite D-1   Brick, NJ 08724   (732)458-5854   Fax (732)458-8012
+ Ocean Renal Associates, P.A.
508 Lakehurst Road/Suite 3 A   Toms River, NJ 08755   (732)458-5854   Fax (732)341-4993
+ Ocean Renal Associates, P.A.
1301 Route 72 West/Suite 206   Manahawkin, NJ 08724   (609)978-9940   Fax (609)978-9902

Park, John Chonghwan, MD {1255372827} Ophthl(99,NJ06)
+ Edison Ophthalmology Associates
2177 Oak Tree Road/Suite 203   Edison, NJ 08820   (908)822-0070   Fax (908)822-0075

Park, John Jonghyun, MD {1205862075} Anesth, PainMd(94,PA02)
+ South Jersey Spine and Pain Physicians, LLC
310 Egg Harbor Road/Suite B-3   Sewell, NJ 08080   (856)589-4500   Fax (856)589-5380

Park, Jun-Ki, MD {1861713471} Nephro(05,GER25)
+ Edison Nephrology Consultants, LLC.
34-36 Progress Street/Suite A-7   Edison, NJ 08820   (908)769-1440   Fax (908)769-0945

Park, Kee Bum, MD {1891797668}
+ 51 Westview Road
Wayne, NJ 07470

Park, Kenneth Hyun, DO {1609881978} PainMd, Anesth(02,NY75)<NJ-HOLYNAME>
+ Comprehensive Pain Management of NJ
433 Hackensack Avenue/2nd Floor   Hackensack, NJ 07601   (201)487-7246   Fax (201)487-4600
Kpark73@gmail.com
+ Bergen Anesthesia Associates
718 Teaneck Road   Teaneck, NJ 07666   (201)487-7246   Fax (201)833-6576

Park, Kyle Yoonho, MD {1346603388} Rheuma<NJ-RWJUBRUN>
+ RWJ University Hospital New Brunswick
One Robert Wood Johnson Place   New Brunswick, NJ 08901   (732)828-3000

Park, Lisa Lam, MD {1699982868} AdolMd<NJ-MORRISTN>
+ Morristown Medical Center
100 Madison Avenue/AdolMed   Morristown, NJ 07962   (973)971-5000   Fax (973)290-7099

Park, Malsuk, DO {1902890759} EmrgMd(94,NY75)<NJ-RWJU-RAH>
+ Robert Wood Johnson University Hospital at Rahway
865 Stone Street/Emergency Med   Rahway, NJ 07065   (732)381-4200

Park, Mark, MD {1912248683} SrgO&M
+ 260 Old Hook Road/Suite 202
Westwood, NJ 07675   (347)948-8622

Park, Peter Byung, MD {1487609723} RadDia, RadV&I, Radiol(94,NY08)<NJ-MONMOUTH>
+ Vascular & Interventional Specialists, P.C.
300 Perrine Road/Suite 301   Old Bridge, NJ 08857   (732)727-8346   Fax (732)727-8345

Park, Robert Inyeung, MD {1710908595} Otlryg(84,MD01)
+ Ear Nose & Throat Group of Central NJ
2124 Oak Tree Road/2nd floor   Edison, NJ 08820   (732)205-1311   Fax (732)205-9648

Park, Sang T., MD {1508962812} FamMed(68,KORE)<NJ-BURDTMLN>
+ 1 Drumbed Road
Villas, NJ 08251   (609)886-1126   Fax (609)889-9464
Sangpark99@comcast.net

Park, Sarah, DO {1568884617} IntrMd(NY76<NJ-HOLYNAME>
+ Holy Name Hospital
718 Teaneck Road/Internal Med   Teaneck, NJ 07666   (973)594-6650   Fax (201)833-7231

Park, Soo Mi, MD {1780700781} IntrMd(04,NY01)<NY-MTSINAI, NY-MTSINYHS>
+ Mulkay Cardiology Consultants, P.C.
493 Essex Street   Hackensack, NJ 07601   (201)996-9244   Fax (201)996-9243

Park, Steven K., MD {1821086216} IntrMd, Hemato(64,KORE)<NJ-MEMSALEM>
+ 3330 Salem-Woodstown Road/Suite 3
Salem, NJ 08079   (856)935-7757   Fax (856)935-5233

Park, Tae Keun, MD {1093940249} EmrgMd, SprtMd(04,NY20)<NY-NSUHMANH>
+ Pro Form Sports Medicine and Wellness Associates
201 Route 17 North   Rutherford, NJ 07070   (201)549-8846   Fax (201)549-8899

Park, Wonil, MD {1588753842} IntrMd, Nephro(87,KOR01)<NJ-ENGLWOOD>
+ Hanmi Medical Associates
232 Broad Avenue/Suite 208   Palisades Park, NJ 07650   (201)346-0999   Fax (201)346-0118

Park, Yong Il, MD {1154368819} PhysMd, OrtSpn(96,NJ05)<NJ-KSLRWEST>
+ Kessler Institute for Rehabilitation West Orange
1199 Pleasant Valley Way   West Orange, NJ 07052   (973)731-3600
+ South Jersey Sports Medicine Center
556 Egg Harbor Road/Suite A   Sewell, NJ 08080   (973)731-3600   Fax (856)589-2720
+ South Jersey Spine and Pain Physicians, LLC
310 Egg Harbor Road/Suite B-3   Sewell, NJ 07052   (856)589-4500   Fax (856)589-5380

Park, Yong M., MD {1356345722} Anesth(64,KORE)
+ 100 Old Palisade Road/Unit 3203
Fort Lee, NJ 07024

Park, Young, MD {1982645453} Anesth(63,KORE)
+ 83 Schweinberg Drive
Roseland, NJ 07068

Park, Young K., MD {1811905045} InsrMd(67,KORE)
+ Jersey City VA CBOC
115 Christopher Columbus Drive   Jersey City, NJ 07302   (201)435-3055   Fax (201)435-3198

Park, Yung I., MD {1194752725} Anesth(72,KORE)<NJ-COMMED>
+ Toms River Anesthesia Associates PC
409 Main Street/2nd Floor   Toms River, NJ 08753   (732)818-7575   Fax (732)818-1567
+ Community Medical Center
99 Route 37 West/Anesthesiology   Toms River, NJ 08755   (732)240-8040

Parker, Collin Robert, MD {1427431873} Dermat
+ Affiliated Dermatologists
182 South Street/Suite 1   Morristown, NJ 07960   (973)267-0300   Fax (973)984-2670

Parker, Glenn S., MD {1568437739} SrgC&R, Surgry(88,NJ06)<NJ-JRSYSHMC, NJ-OCEANMC>
+ Atlantic Surgical Group, PA
255 Monmouth Road   Oakhurst, NJ 07755   (732)531-5445   Fax (732)531-1776
+ Atlantic Surgical Group, PA
459 Jack Martin Boulevard/Suite 7   Brick, NJ 08724   (732)531-5445   Fax (732)836-1592

Parker, Martin I., MD {1295715688} RadDia, Radiol(70,NY19)<NJ-JFKMED>
+ JFK Medical Center

65 James Street/Radiology   Edison, NJ 08820   (732)321-7917   Fax (732)767-2968
+ Edison Imaging Associates at JFK
60 James Street   Edison, NJ 08820   (732)321-7917   Fax (732)318-3883

Parker, Paul M., MD {1043284466} SrgPlstc, Surgry(77,DC01)<NJ-HACKNSK, NJ-VALLEY>
+ Parker Center for Plastic Surgery
122 East Ridgewood Avenue   Paramus, NJ 07652   (201)967-1212

Parker, Stephen D., DO {1851311674} FamMed, SprtMd(67,MO79)<NJ-STBARNMC>
+ 331 Chestnut Street
Roselle Park, NJ 07204   (908)245-9444   Fax (908)245-8826

Parker, William Andrew, MD {1649280314} RadV&I, Radiol, RadDia(94,NY09)
+ Princeton Radiology Associates, P.A.
419 North Harrison Street   Princeton, NJ 08540   (609)921-3345   Fax (609)683-8847
+ Princeton Radiology Associates, P.A.
9 Centre Drive   Jamesburg, NJ 08831   (609)921-3345   Fax (609)655-4016
+ Princeton Radiology Associates, P.A.
3674 Route 27   Kendall Park, NJ 08540   (732)821-5563   Fax (732)821-6675

Parkes, Lauren H., DO {1689054298} FamMed
+ Jackson Family Medicine
27 South Cooks Bridge Road/Suite 2-1   Jackson, NJ 08527   (732)367-0166   Fax (732)367-7220

Parks, Anthony Lesmore, Jr., MD {1740375898} SrgOrt, SprtMd(96,NY46)<NJ-CLARMAAS, NJ-STMRYPAS>
+ 175 Franklin Avenue/Suite 103
Nutley, NJ 07110   (973)661-1833   Fax (973)661-2270

Parks, Shannon N., DO {1962631457} Psychy(06,ME75)
+ 55 North Gilbert Street/Suite 2203
Tinton Falls, NJ 07701   (732)939-6381
info@drshannonparks.com

Parlavecchio, Joseph G., MD {1558303933} ObsGyn(79,PA02)<NJ-CLARMAAS, NJ-STBARNMC>
+ 1130 US Highway 202/Building D
Raritan, NJ 08869   (908)252-1522   Fax (908)252-4546

Parler, Janet Patricia, MD {1912906835} SrgPlstc, SrgRec(74,MA07)<NJ-JFKMED, NJ-CENTRAST>
+ 20 Albemarle Road
East Brunswick, NJ 08816   (732)390-4470   Fax (732)390-4484
drparler@comcast.net

Parlow, Brittany, MD {1154778892} Pedtrc
+ University Medical Group Pediatrics
125 Paterson Street/MEB 3rd Fl   New Brunswick, NJ 08903   (732)814-7087   Fax (732)235-7345

Parman, Stanley C., MD {1306816152} EmrgMd, IntrMd(78,MO44)<NJ-OVERLOOK, NJ-JFKMED>
+ Care Station
90 Route 22 West   Springfield, NJ 07081   (973)467-2273
+ Care Station Medical Group
328 West St. Georges Avenue   Linden, NJ 07036   (973)467-2273   Fax (908)925-2235
+ Care Station Medical Group
456 Prospect Avenue   West Orange, NJ 07081   (973)731-9881   Fax (973)731-9881

Parmar, Archna S., DO {1578763371} IntrMd<NJ-STPETER>
+ St. Peter's Physicians Associates
1636 Stelton Road/Suite 301   Piscataway, NJ 08854   (732)339-7575
+ Saint PeterÆs Physician Associate
59 Veronica Avenue/Suite 203   Somerset, NJ 08873   (732)937-6008

Parmar, Kiritkumar A., MD {1396813614} IntrMd, Dermat(82,INDI)<NJ-SJHREGMC>
+ Vineland Medical Associates/Excel Care Alliance, LLC
1100 East Chestnut Avenue   Vineland, NJ 08360   (856)696-0108   Fax (856)691-1106

Parmar, Madhu, MD {1417975194} IntrMd(81,INA72)
+ Hackensack Medical Center-Internal Medicine
30 Prospect Avenue/4 Main/Rm 4621   Hackensack, NJ 07601   (201)996-3664   Fax (551)996-0536

Parmar, Pritesh B., MD {1154519403} FamMed(02,DMN01)
+ Forest Hill Family Health Associates, P.A.
465 Mount Prospect Avenue   Newark, NJ 07104   (973)483-3640   Fax (973)483-4895

Parmar, Virendra Pratapsingh, MD {1841328028} Anesth(76,INA7Y)
+ Bergen Anesthesia Associates
718 Teaneck Road   Teaneck, NJ 07666   (201)833-7149   Fax (201)342-1259

Parmett, Steven Russell, MD {1093708919} NuclMd, RadDia, RadNuc(79,MA01)<NJ-NWRKBETH>
+ Newark Diagnostic Radiologists, PA
201 Lyons Avenue   Newark, NJ 07112   (973)926-7466

Parnes, Cindy R., MD {1548289853} ObsGyn, IntrMd(85,TN05)<NJ-HACKNSK>
+ Bergen Ob-Gyn Associates, PA
130 Kinderkamack Road/Suite 300   River Edge, NJ 07661
(201)489-2727   Fax (201)489-5040
+ Drs. Robinson, Parnes & Weinstein
275 Forest Avenue   Paramus, NJ 07652   (201)489-2727
Fax (201)967-9302

Parolie, James M., MD {1831193762} SrgOrt(78,NJ05)<NJ-SOMERSET>
+ Somerset Orthopedic Associates, PA
1081 Route 22 West   Bridgewater, NJ 08807   (908)722-0822   Fax (908)722-6318

Paroulek, George Jiri, MD {1821026782} IntrMd(83,DOM02)
+ Care Station Medical Group
210 Meadowlands Parkway   Secaucus, NJ 07094
(201)348-3636   Fax (201)583-0713

Parowski, Supriya P., DO {1720159940} PhysMd(93,PA77)<NJ-WAYNEGEN>
+ St. Joseph's Wayne Hospital
224 Hamburg Turnpike/Room 714   Wayne, NJ 07470
(973)942-6900   Fax (973)389-4069

Parra, Raul O., MD {1871689968} Urolgy, Surgry(80,SPA02)
+ Holy Name Hospital
718 Teaneck Road   Teaneck, NJ 07666   (201)833-3000
Fax (201)227-6207
+ Regional Cancer Center at Holy Name Medical Center
718 Teaneck Road   Teaneck, NJ 07666   (201)833-3000
Fax (201)541-5988

Parreno, Maritza Georgette, MD {1215048871} EmrgMd, IntrMd(94,NY46)<NJ-STPETER>
+ Ani Orthopaedic Group
200 Perrine Road/Suite 220   Old Bridge, NJ 08857
(732)721-1600   Fax (732)721-1635

Parrillo, Joseph E., MD {1326134487} IntrMd, CdvDis(72,NY20)<NJ-COOPRUMC>
+ Cooper Cardiology Associates
900 Centennial Boulevard   Voorhees, NJ 08043   (856)325-6700   Fax (856)325-6702

Parrish, Andrew, MD {1659789816} EmrgMd
+ Newark Beth Israel Medical Center Emergency Medicine
201 Lyons Avenue/Suite D11   Newark, NJ 07112   (973)926-6671

Parrish, Sherrilynn, MD {1477531382} ObsGyn, Obstet(88,DC03)<NJ-OURLADY>
+ Women's Healthcare of Collingswood
1055 Haddon Avenue   Collingswood, NJ 08108   (856)854-4524   Fax (856)854-8216
+ Lourdes Medical Associates
1055 Haddon Avenue   Collingswood, NJ 08108   (856)854-4524   Fax (856)854-8216

Parron, John Keckhut, MD {1689810731} SprtMd, SrgOrt(05,NJ06)
+ Trokhan Dermatology, LLC.
235 Closter Dock Road   Closter, NJ 07624   (201)767-1908
Fax (201)767-3097

Parsi, Prakasham, MD {1952319352} Pedtrc(89,INA39)
+ 1323 State Route 27/Suite C
Somerset, NJ 08873   (914)354-9844

Partenope, Nicholas A., MD {1033368212} IntrMd(78,NY46)
+ 157 Kensington Avenue
Colonia, NJ 07067

Partnow, Michael J., MD {1467505131} Nrolgy(68,PA12)
+ The Neurological Center
231 Van Sciver Parkway   Willingboro, NJ 08046   (609)871-7500   Fax (609)877-5555

Partrick, Matthew Seamus, MD {1629264007} EmrgMd(03,NC05)<NJ-SOCEANCO, NJ-MORRISTN>
+ Southern Ocean County Medical Center
1140 Route 72 West/EmrgMed   Manahawkin, NJ 08050
(609)597-6011
+ Morristown Medical Center
100 Madison Avenue/EmrgMed   Morristown, NJ 07962
(973)971-5000

Partridge, Joanna Lee, MD {1588707871} SrgPlstc(99,NJ06)<NJ-RWJUBRUN, NJ-UNVMCPRN>
+ 213 North Center Drive
North Brunswick, NJ 08902   (732)297-8090

Partyka, Bronislaw J., MD {1275580292} IntrMd, EmrgMd(78,POLA)<NJ-NWTNMEM>
+ Newton Medical Center
175 High Street/EmergMed   Newton, NJ 07860   (973)383-2121

Partyka, Lukasz Michal, MD {1730344847}
+ 64 Springholm Drive
Berkeley Heights, NJ 07922   (908)494-2442

Parulekar, Manisha Santosh, MD {1285689588} Grtrcs, IntrMd(04,INA65)<NJ-HACKNSK>
+ Hackensack University Medical Center
30 Prospect Avenue/Geriatrics   Hackensack, NJ 07601
(201)996-2503   Fax (201)337-8760
MParulekar@humed.com

+ Center for Healthy Senior Living
5 Summit Avenue/Suite 204   Hackensack, NJ 07601
+ Center for Healthy Senior Living
360 Essex Street/Suite 401   Hackensack, NJ 07601
(551)996-1140   Fax (551)996-0543

Parvez, Ayesha, MD {1710107339} EnDbMt
+ Capital Endocrinology
2 Capital Way/Suite 290   Pennington, NJ 08534   (609)303-4300   Fax (609)303-4301

Parvez, Uzma, MD {1982775714} PhysMd, PainMd, IntrMd(98,PAK15)<NJ-STJOSHOS>
+ St. Joseph's Regional Medical Center
703 Main Street/Phys Rehab   Paterson, NJ 07503
(973)754-2790   Fax (973)754-2791

Parvulescu, Traian D., MD {1265523203} InsrMd, IntrMd(91,ROMA)
+ 116 Littleton Road
Morris Plains, NJ 07950   (973)829-0191   Fax (973)829-1562

Parvus, Britt J., DO {1497926729}
+ 404 Masters Drive
Blackwood, NJ 08012   (215)512-2812

Parziale, Andrew Michael, MD {1346638350}
+ 733-B Cranbury Cross Road
North Brunswick, NJ 08902   (701)274-9539

Parziale, Michael A., MD {1285606657} IntrMd(83,PA09)<NJ-OVERLOOK, NJ-MORRISTN>
+ Summit Medical Group
1 Diamond Hill Road/Bensley Pav/2 FL   Berkeley, NJ 07922
(908)277-8700   Fax (908)288-7993
+ Summit Medical Group
85 Woodland Road   Short Hills, NJ 07078   (908)277-8700
Fax (973)921-0669
+ Atlantic Colon & Rectal
8 Mountain Boulevard   Warren, NJ 07922   (908)769-9111

Pascal, Mark S., MD {1700847373} IntrMd, MedOnc, Surgry(73,PA02)<NJ-HACKNSK, NJ-HOLYNAME>
+ John Theurer Cancer Center - HUMC
92 Second Street   Hackensack, NJ 07601   (201)996-5900
Fax (201)996-9246

Pascarella, Michael Ryan, DO {1043538424} Anesth
+ West Jersey Anesthesia Associates
102E Centre Boulevard   Marlton, NJ 08053   (856)988-6260
Fax (856)988-6270

Pascarelli, Todd D., MD {1316026255} IntrMd(87,WIND)<NJ-HACKNSK>
+ Rochelle Park Medical Center PA
96 Park Way   Rochelle Park, NJ 07662   (201)291-1010
Fax (201)587-0313

Paschkes, Benjamin Neil, DO {1801843701} EmrgMd(00,NY75)
+ Emergency Physician Associates, P.A.
307 South Evergreen Avenue/PO Box 298   Woodbury, NJ 08096   (856)848-3817   Fax (856)848-1431

Pascual, Bolivar, MD {1104882141} Psychy(82,DOM01)
+ Clifton Psychiatric Services
469 Clifton Avenue   Clifton, NJ 07011   (973)253-0266
Fax (973)253-0399
Drbolivarpascual@yahoo.com

Pascual, Rodolfo C., MD {1407857824} SrgThr, Surgry(64,PHI08)<NJ-VIRTUAHS, NJ-OURLADY>
+ Virtua Surgical Group
1935 Route 70 East   Cherry Hill, NJ 08003   (856)428-7700
Fax (856)424-9120
+ Virtua Medford Surgical Group
212 Creek Crossing Boulevard   Hainesport, NJ 08036
(856)428-7700   Fax (609)267-1044

Pascucci, Rocco F., MD {1134117245} Pedtrc(82,WIND)
+ Bethany Pediatrics PA
1 Bethany Road/Building 5/Suite 65   Hazlet, NJ 07730
(732)264-0700   Fax (732)264-1414

Pasia, Eric, MD {1639345713} PhysMd
+ Robalino-Sanghavi, Michelle Marie
120 Eagle Rock Avenue/Suite 154   East Hanover, NJ 07936
(201)447-4772   Fax (862)701-6444

Pasichow, Keith Philip, MD {1366754517} Pedtrc(10,NY47)<NY-LIJEWSH>
+ Gloucester Hospice BAYADA
603 North Broad Street/Suite 301   Woodbury, NJ 08096
(856)845-8220   Fax (888)487-1131

Pasik, Deborah, MD {1992894794} IntrMd, Rheuma(82,NY47)<NJ-MORRISTN>
+ Atlantic Rheumatology & Osteoporosis Associates PA
8 Saddle Road/Suite 202   Cedar Knolls, NJ 07927
(973)984-9796   Fax (973)984-5445

Paskhover, Boris, MD {1952691834} Surgry(11,NY46)<CT-YALENHH>
+ Rutgers University Department of Otolaryngology
9100 Bergen Street/DOC 8100   Newark, NJ 07103
(973)972-2548   Fax (973)972-8567

Paskowski, Elizabeth K., MD {1689676983} ObsGyn, IntrMd(94,NY03)
+ Hackensack University Medical Group Emerson

452 Old Hook Road/2nd Floor   Emerson, NJ 07630
(201)781-1750   Fax (201)781-1753

Pasley, Peter M., MD {1104840503} IntrMd, SprtMd(95,NJ06)
+ Empire Medical Associates
5 Franklin Avenue/Suite 302   Belleville, NJ 07109
(973)759-1221   Fax (973)759-1997
+ Empire Medical Associates
264 Boyden Avenue   Maplewood, NJ 07040   (973)759-1221   Fax (973)761-7617
+ Empire Medical Associates
382 West Passaic Avenue   Bloomfield, NJ 07109   (973)338-1900

Pasquariello, James L., MD {1205873064} CdvDis, IntrMd(78,ITAL)
+ Toms River Medical Group PA
81 Route 37 West/Suite 1   Toms River, NJ 08755   (732)341-0560   Fax (732)341-0574

Pasquariello, James Verniere, MD {1871715169} Surgry<NJ-MORRISTN>
+ Morristown Medical Center
100 Madison Avenue   Morristown, NJ 07962   (973)971-5000

Pasricha, Atul, DO {1326098542} EmrgMd(99,NJ75)<NJ-JRSYSHMC>
+ EmCare
1945 Route 33   Neptune, NJ 07753   (732)776-4510   Fax (732)776-2329

Pass, Mark David, MD {1437156288} IntrMd, Grtrcs(99,BWI01)<NJ-JRSYSHMC, NJ-OCEANMC>
+ Jersey Shore Geriatrics
15 School Road East/Suite 2   Marlboro, NJ 07746
(732)866-9922   Fax (732)866-9970

Passalaqua, Philip Jude, MD {1730167560} Otlryg(95,NC05)<NJ-MONMOUTH, NJ-RIVERVW>
+ ENT and Allergy Associates
1131 Broad Street/Suite 103 Building A   Shrewsbury, NJ 07702   (732)389-3388   Fax (732)389-3389

Passalaris, John Dimitrios, MD {1154351666} IntrMd, CdvDis, CarNuc(94,NY15)<NJ-UNVMCPRN>
+ Princeton Interventional Cardiology
800 Bunn Drive/Suite 101   Princeton, NJ 08540   (609)921-2800   Fax (609)921-3499
+ Princeton Interventional Cardiology
181 North Harrison Street   Princeton, NJ 08540   (609)921-2800   Fax (609)921-3499

Passalaris, Tina Marina, MD {1508951864} IntrMd, MedOnc(92,NY19)<NY-SLOANKET>
+ Memorial Sloan-Kettering Cancer Center Basking Ridge
136 Mountain View Boulevard   Basking Ridge, NJ 07920
(908)542-3000   Fax (908)542-3220

Passannante, Anthony, Jr., MD {1821094558} CdvDis, IntrMd(81,NY47)<NJ-STPETER, NJ-RWJUBRUN>
+ Cardio Metabolic Institute
51 Veronica Avenue   Somerset, NJ 08873   (732)846-7000
Fax (732)846-7001

Passannante, Anthony J., Sr, MD {1407852171} CdvDis(66,NJ05)<NJ-RWJUBRUN, NJ-STPETER>
+ Cardio Metabolic Institute
51 Veronica Avenue   Somerset, NJ 08873   (732)846-7000
Fax (732)846-7001
+ Cardio Metabolic Institute
294 Applegarth Road/Suite F   Monroe Township, NJ 08831
(732)846-7000   Fax (732)846-7001

Passarella, Susan Katherine, DO {1720114416} ObsGyn(04,MO78)
+ North Dover Ob-Gyn Associates
222 Oak Avenue/3rd Floor/Suite 301   Toms River, NJ 08753
(732)914-1919   Fax (732)914-0725
+ North Dover Ob-Gyn Associates
214 Jack Martin Boulevard/Building D-3   Brick, NJ 08723
(732)914-1919   Fax (732)840-9270
+ North Dover Ob-Gyn Associates
442 Lacey Road   Forked River, NJ 08753   (609)971-2999
Fax (609)971-9712

Passariello, Christopher, MD {1427374834} SrgOrt(04,DMN01)<NY-VABRKLYN>
+ Ocean Orthopedic Associates, P.A.
530 Lakehurst Road/Suite 1   Toms River, NJ 08755
(732)349-8454   Fax (732)341-0259

Passi, Rakesh K., MD {1275550915} CdvDis, IntrMd, IntMAdMd(79,INA06)<NJ-RWJUBRUN, NJ-RBAYOLDB>
+ Cardiovascular Health Associates
172 Summerhill Road/Suite 4   East Brunswick, NJ 08816
(732)238-6440   Fax (732)651-1431
+ Cardiovascular Health Associates
400 State Street/Suite 4   Perth Amboy, NJ 08861
(732)238-6440   Fax (732)651-1431

Passi, Vandna, MD {1376840298}
+ 3 Copper Plaza
Camden, NJ 08103   (908)930-7316
vandna.passi@gmail.com

Physicians by Name and Address

Pastena, Anthony M., DO {1659431195} FamMed(94,PA77)<NJ-MTNSIDE, NJ-STBARNMC>
+ 249 Franklin Avenue
Nutley, NJ 07110 (973)542-1106 Fax (973)542-1172
drpastena@optonline.net

Paster, Lauren, MD {1205135548} Nephro
+ Randolph Medical & Renal Associates
121 Center Grove Road/Suite 13-14 Randolph, NJ 07869
(973)361-3737

Paster, Lina Famiglietti, MD {1770568628} RadDia, IntrMd(92,NJ05)<NJ-STPETER, NJ-RWJUBRUN>
+ University Radiology Group, P.C.
483 Cranbury Road East Brunswick, NJ 08816 (732)390-0030 Fax (732)390-5383
+ University Radiology Group, P.C.
579A Cranbury Road East Brunswick, NJ 08816 (732)390-0030 Fax (732)390-1856

Pasternak, Jared A., MD {1336306844} Pedtrc
+ Advocare Laurel Pediatrics
269 Fish Pond Road Sewell, NJ 08080 (856)863-9999 Fax (856)863-9666

Pasternak, Philip Louis, MD {1093761546} AlgyImmn, PedAlg(93,NY46)
+ 911 East County Line Road/Suite 201
Lakewood, NJ 08701 (732)901-4300 Fax (732)901-4337
Dr.Pasternak@yahoo.com
+ 63 Brunswick Woods Drive
East Brunswick, NJ 08816 (732)901-4300 Fax (732)901-4337

Paston, Carrie Zapolin, MD {1235210279} EmrgMd, IntrMd(87,PA02)<NJ-OURLADY>
+ Our Lady of Lourdes Medical Center
1600 Haddon Avenue/Emerg Med Camden, NJ 08103
(856)757-3500

Pastore, AnnaLisa, MD {1003975616}
+ 60 Grand Avenue
Englewood, NJ 07631

Pastore, Domenic J., MD {1710984760} Ophthl(90,PA14)<NJ-BURDTMLN>
+ 605 Route 9 South
Cape May Court House, NJ 08210 (609)465-0404 Fax (609)465-8067
+ Court House Surgery Center
106 Courthouse South Dennis Rd Cape May, NJ 08204
(609)465-0404 Fax (609)465-8771

Pastrano Lluberes, Magna, MD {1548601594} IntrMd(11,DOM11)
+ Forest HealthCare Associates, PC
277 Forest Avenue/Suite 200 Paramus, NJ 07652
(201)986-1881 Fax (201)986-1871

Pasunuri, Ramya Sri, MD {1811934623} IntrMd(94,LAT02)<NJ-NWTNMEM, NJ-STCLRDEN>
+ Newton Medical Center
175 High Street Newton, NJ 07860 (973)383-2121

Pasupuleti, Madhusudan V., MD {1740280874} IntrMd, EmrgMd, Pedtrc(73,INDI)<NJ-RBAYPERT>
+ Raritan Bay Medical Center/Perth Amboy Division
530 New Brunswick Avenue Perth Amboy, NJ 08861
(732)442-3700 Fax (732)324-4995

Pasupuleti, Rao Satyanaray, MD {1891893541} Nrolgy, NroChl(79,INA38)<NJ-CHSFULD, NJ-CHSMRCER>
+ Comprehensive Neurology, LLC.
1245 Whitehorse-Mercerville Rd Hamilton, NJ 08619
(609)585-2666 Fax (609)585-4008

Pasupuleti, Sasikala, MD {1922101732} Psychy(81,INA38)<NJ-ANNKLEIN>
+ Ann Klein Forensic Center
1609 Stuyvesant Avenue/PO Box 7717 West Trenton, NJ 08628 (609)633-0900

Patafio, Onofrio, MD {1568547826} Anesth, IntrMd(82,MEX03)
+ New Jersey Anesthesia Associates, P.C.
252 Columbia Turnpike/PO Box 0037 Florham Park, NJ 07932 (973)660-9334 Fax (973)660-9779

Patankar, Sanjiv Krishna, MD {1255429361} SrgC&R, Surgry(82,INA69)<NJ-RWJUBRUN, NJ-STPETER>
+ Colon and Rectal Surgeons of Central New Jersey
620 Cranbury Road/Suite 111 East Brunswick, NJ 08816
(732)238-2662 Fax (732)613-5359
+ Cares Surgicenter, LLC.
240 Easton Avenue New Brunswick, NJ 08901 (732)238-2662 Fax (732)296-8677

Patankar, Srikanth S., MD {1710048764} Anesth, Pedtrc(84,INA1Z)<NJ-STBARNMC>
+ St. Barnabas Medical Center
94 Old Short Hills Road Livingston, NJ 07039 (973)322-5000

Patashny, Karen M., MD {1265495717} Pedtrc(83,NY06)<NJ-MORRISTN>
+ Advocare West Morris Pediatrics
151 Route 10/Suite 105 Succasunna, NJ 07876 (973)584-0002 Fax (973)584-7107

Patcha, Suparna Dandamudi, MD {1689724643} Pedtrc(91,INDI)<NJ-KIMBALL>
+ Dr. Gittleman & Associates
450 East Kennedy Boulevard Lakewood, NJ 08701
(732)901-0050 Fax (732)370-2386

Patchell, Roy Andrew, MD {1558462093} PsyCAd
+ Capital Health Medical Center Hopewell
Two Capital Way/Suite 380 Pennington, NJ 08534
(609)537-5000 Fax (609)537-5050

Patel, Aarti, MD {1598926651} ClCdEl
+ Hamilton Cardiology Associates
2073 Klockner Road Hamilton, NJ 08690 (609)584-1212
Fax (609)584-0103

Patel, Ajitkumar Gunvantrai, MD {1477510121} Anesth(93,INA21)<NJ-SOMERSET, NJ-STPETER>
+ Anesthesia Consultnts of NJ/Nova Pain
285 Davidson Avenue/Suite 204 Somerset, NJ 08873
(732)271-1400 Fax (732)271-3543
+ Cares Surgicenter, LLC.
240 Easton Avenue New Brunswick, NJ 08901 (732)271-1400 Fax (732)296-8677
+ RWJ University Hospital Somerset
110 Rehill Avenue/Anesth Somerville, NJ 08873 (908)685-2200

Patel, Akhil, MD {1932649860}
+ 88 Maryland Road
Paramus, NJ 07652 (201)207-7647

Patel, Akshar Nilkantha, MD {1548678246}
+ Rutgers Cancer Institute of New Jersey
195 Little Albany Street/PO Box 2681 New Brunswick, NJ 08903 (732)379-2034 Fax (732)235-6797
aksharnpatel@gmail.com

Patel, Akshay D., MD {1396737581} IntrMd(85,INA4X)<NJ-KIMBALL, NJ-COMMED>
+ Shore Medical Specialists
500 River Avenue Lakewood, NJ 08701 (732)363-7200
Fax (732)367-4461
ADPSMS1@yahoo.com
+ Leisure Park Skilled Nursing
1400 Route 70 Lakewood, NJ 08701 (732)363-7200 Fax (732)370-1719
+ Shore Medical Specialists
9 Hospital Drive Toms River, NJ 08701 (732)349-2732
Fax (732)349-9697

Patel, Alka Jashbhai, MD {1790804201} OccpMd, IntrMd(04,INA65)
+ Neighborhood Health Center Plainfield
1700-58 Myrtle Avenue Plainfield, NJ 07060 (908)753-6401 Fax (908)226-6743
+ Concentra Medical Centers
595 Division Street Elizabeth, NJ 07201 (908)753-6401 Fax (908)351-1099

Patel, Alpesh Amrit, MD {1043478118} CdvDis, IntrMd(04,GRN01)
+ CardioMD
1200 US Highway 22 East/Suite 17 Bridgewater, NJ 08807
(908)864-4027 Fax (732)463-5510

Patel, Alpesh Babu, MD {1396969077} IntCrd, CdvDis, NuclMd(00,PA09)<NJ-STPETER, NJ-CENTRAST>
+ 24/7 Heart and Vascular
3084 State Route 27/Suite 5 Kendall Park, NJ 08824 Fax (800)336-7779
+ 24/7 Heart and Vascular
312 Applegarth Road/Suite 207 Monroe, NJ 08831 Fax (800)336-7779
+ 24/7 Heart and Vascular
503 Omni Drive Hillsborough, NJ 08824 Fax (800)336-7779

Patel, Ambarish Ashokkumar, DO {1104938802} FamMed(99,PA78)<NJ-KMHSTRAT, NJ-KMHCHRRY>
+ AAP Family Practice, PC
707 White Horse Road/Suite C-105 Voorhees, NJ 08043
(856)258-4966 Fax (856)258-4972

Patel, Ami R., DO {1811213457} EmrgMd(06,NY75)<NJ-NWRKBETH>
+ Newark Beth Israel Medical Center
201 Lyons Avenue/EmrgMed Newark, NJ 07112 (973)926-7000

Patel, Amish, MD {1699085860} RadDia, IntrMd(06,NJ05)<NJ-HOLYNAME>
+ Holy Name Hospital
718 Teaneck Road/Radiology Teaneck, NJ 07666
(201)833-7268 Fax (201)541-5910

Patel, Amish Thakor, DO {1841460144} IntrMd, CdvDis(04,NJ75)
+ Drs. Chudasama and Patel
1101 Raritan Road Clark, NJ 07066 (732)381-3055 Fax (732)815-9330

Patel, Amit A., MD {1306098827} OncHem(05,GRN01)
+ Hudson Hematology Oncology
377 Jersey Avenue/Suite 160 Jersey City, NJ 07302
(201)333-8248 Fax (201)333-8469

Patel, Amit Arun, MD {1730161316} RadDia, NuclMd(90,PA14)<NJ-BURDTMLN>
+ Cape Regional Medical Center
2 Stone Harbor Boulevard/Radiology Cape May Court House, NJ 08210 (609)463-2000

Patel, Amit H., MD {1346515756} PulDis, IntrMd(08,ANT02)
+ Regional Heart & Lung Associates
207 Court House/S. Dennis Road Cape May Court House, NJ 08210 (609)465-2001 Fax (609)465-8440

Patel, Amit V., MD {1255357257} SrgVas, Surgry(88,NY46)<NJ-NWTNMEM>
+ Advanced Vascular Associates, PC
131 Madison Avenue/2nd Floor Morristown, NJ 07960
(973)755-9206 Fax (973)540-9717
+ Advanced Vascular Associates, PC
222 High Street/Suite 205A Newton, NJ 07860 (973)755-9206 Fax (973)579-6638

Patel, Amol D., DO {1407121874}
+ 11 Patriot Court
Edison, NJ 08820 (732)396-4509
amolpa@gmail.com

Patel, Amrish M., MD {1689683542} Anesth, AnesPain(92,NJ05)
+ Northern Jersey Interventional Pain Specialist P.C.
714 Tenth Street/Suite 6-A Secaucus, NJ 07094 (201)974-1541 Fax (201)974-1581

Patel, Amy, MD {1598264681}
+ Lawrence Ob/Gyn Associates
123 Franklin Corner Road/Suite 214 Lawrenceville, NJ 08648 (609)896-1400 Fax (609)896-3986

Patel, Amy J., MD {1033179619} IntrMd(00,MNT01)
+ 844 Newark Avenue/Suite 2
Jersey City, NJ 07306 (201)222-5202 Fax (201)603-1116

Patel, Amy J., MD {1790274629} ObsGyn
+ University Medical Group/OBGYN
125 Paterson Street/2nd Floor New Brunswick, NJ 08901
(732)235-6375 Fax (732)235-9855

Patel, Anamika K., MD {1700892494} IntrMd, InfDis(98,INA20)
+ Infectious Disease Consultants
1245 Whitehorse-Mercerville Rd Mercerville, NJ 08619
(609)581-2000 Fax (609)581-5450

Patel, Anand, MD {1669911863} Rheuma
+ Princeton Medical Group, P.A.
419 North Harrison Street Princeton, NJ 08540 (609)924-9300 Fax (609)924-6552

Patel, Anik Mayur, MD {1427336429} Gastrn, IntrMd(08,GRN01)
+ Hunterdon Gastroenterology Associates, P.A.
1100 Wescott Drive/Suite 206-207 Flemington, NJ 08822
(908)483-4000 Fax (908)788-5090
+ Hunterdon Gastroenterology Associates, P.A.
135 West End Avenue/Suite 204 Somerville, NJ 08876
(908)483-4000 Fax (908)788-5090

Patel, Anil Jayant, MD {1619053741} Anesth(95,NY08)
+ 466 Old Hook Road/Suite 19
Emerson, NJ 07630 (201)967-2455 Fax (201)634-9647

Patel, Anish Vinit, MD {1952669970} IntrMd
+ Robert Wood Johnson Medical School
51 French Street/Suite 478b New Brunswick, NJ 08901
(469)235-9353

Patel, Anjali Dalal, DO {1891818530} AnesPain, IntrMd(03,NJ75)
+ Clifton Primary Care Center
1111 Clifton Avenue/Suite 204 Clifton, NJ 07013
(973)779-7354 Fax (973)779-7385

Patel, Anjali N., DO {1174844930}
+ 5 Adams Street
Edison, NJ 08820 (732)742-6633
patel.anjali@gmail.com

Patel, Anup H., DO {1194068916} PhyMPain
+ AP Diagnostic Imaging
1692 Oak Tree Road/Suite 1 Edison, NJ 08820 (732)343-6543 Fax (732)906-3675

Patel, Anup Magan, MD {1942391842} IntrMd, Nephro(97,NJ05)<NJ-STBARNMC>
+ St. Barnabas Medical Center
94 Old Short Hills Road/Suite 1 Livingston, NJ 07039
(973)322-5000

Patel, Anuradha P., MD {1306869615} Anesth(78,INDI)<NJ-UMDNJ>
+ University Hospital
150 Bergen Street/Anesthesiology Newark, NJ 07103
(973)972-4300 Fax (973)972-4172
+ University Hospital-New Jersey Medical School
30 Bergen Street/Room 1202 Newark, NJ 07107
(973)972-4511

Patel, Apurva, MD {1831414440} InfDis, IntrMd
+ Infectious Disease Care
1912 State Route 35/Suite 101 Oakhurst, NJ 07755
(732)222-4762 Fax (732)222-4764

Patel, Archana I., MD {1245314913} IntrMd, CdvDis(83,INA65)
+ UH- Robert Wood Johnson Med
125 Paterson Street New Brunswick, NJ 08901 (732)828-3000 Fax (732)235-6530

Patel, Arpit K., MD {1194074591} IntrMd<NJ-RWJUBRUN>
+ RWJ University Hospital New Brunswick
One Robert Wood Johnson Place New Brunswick, NJ 08901
(732)235-8909

Patel, Arpit Nayan, MD {1376930347} Anesth<NJ-RWJUBRUN>
+ RWJ University Hospital New Brunswick
One Robert Wood Johnson Place New Brunswick, NJ 08901
(732)235-3381

Patel, Arti Mahendra, MD {1477811289}<NJ-OCEANMC>
+ Ocean Medical Center
425 Jack Martin Boulevard Brick, NJ 08723 (732)840-2200

Patel, Arti S., MD {1477630978} AnesPain, IntrMd(92,IL06)<NJ-STPETER>
+ Anesthesia Consultnts of NJ/Nova Pain
285 Davidson Avenue/Suite 204 Somerset, NJ 08873
(732)271-1400 Fax (732)271-3543

Patel, Aruna Ghanshyambhai, MD {1225077381} RadOnc(72,INDI)<NJ-COMMED>
+ Community Medical Center
99 Route 37 West Toms River, NJ 08755 (732)557-8000

Patel, Arvind Joitaram, MD {1457464810} Pedtrc
+ Neighborhood Health Center Plainfield
1700-58 Myrtle Avenue Plainfield, NJ 07060 (908)753-6401 Fax (908)753-6401

Patel, Arvind Kumar, MD {1386653319} IntrMd(78,INDI)<NJ-JFKMED, NJ-ACMCITY>
+ Health Med Associates, PC
24 South Carolina Avenue Atlantic City, NJ 08401
(609)345-6000 Fax (609)345-2885
+ Health Med Associates, PC
1080 Stelton Road/First FL Suite 202 Piscataway, NJ 08854
(609)345-6000 Fax (732)985-0552

Patel, Arvind Maganbhai, MD {1770571168} Pedtrc(83,INDI)<NJ-CENTRAST>
+ Allergy & Pediatric Associates of Jersey Shore
222 Schanck Road/Suite 105 Freehold, NJ 07728
(732)431-3373 Fax (732)303-0172

Patel, Arvind Mansukhlal, MD {1134323595} Urolgy(71,INA67)
+ 956 Amboy Avenue
Edison, NJ 08837 (732)738-5151 Fax (732)738-1373
Patelurology@gmail.com

Patel, Ashish Bharat, MD {1083758635} RadOnc, Radiol, IntrMd(03,PA02)<PA-HLYRDMER>
+ South Jersey Health Care Center
Two Cooper Plaza/Radiology Camden, NJ 08103
(856)735-6118 Fax (856)735-6467
+ CUH Cancer & Radiation Oncology Institute
715 Fellowship Road Mount Laurel, NJ 08054 (856)735-6118 Fax (856)638-1188

Patel, Ashish Bhasker, MD {1831366731} IntrMd(01,NY09)<NJ-CENTRAST, NJ-JRSYSHMC>
+ Monmouth Cardiology Associates, LLC
11 Meridian Road Eatontown, NJ 07724 (732)663-0300
Fax (732)663-0301
+ Monmouth Cardiology Associates, LLC
222 Schanck Road/Suite 104 Freehold, NJ 07728
(732)663-0300 Fax (732)431-1712

Patel, Ashish C., MD {1386958189} FamMed, IntrMd(08,DMN01)<NJ-UNDRWD>
+ Inspira Health Network
509 North Broad Street/Fam Med Woodbury, NJ 08096
(609)784-5581

Patel, Ashok Ambalal, MD {1497728745} ClCdEl, CdvDis, IntrMd(90,INA20)<NJ-SOMERSET, NJ-RWJUBRUN>
+ Medicor Cardiology PA
225 Jackson Street Bridgewater, NJ 08807 (908)526-8668
Fax (908)231-6781
+ Medicor Cardiology PA
331 US Highway 206/Suite 1A Hillsborough, NJ 08844
(908)526-8668 Fax (908)431-0808

Patel, Ashok Kantilal, MD {1093809576} PsyGrt, Psychy(79,INA70)
+ Memory and Aging Center
20 Hospital Drive/Suite 12 Toms River, NJ 08755
(732)244-2299 Fax (732)244-5757

Patel, Ashokkumar A., MD {1912940032} IntrMd, FamMed(78,INA20)<NJ-VIRTVOOR, NJ-OURLADY>
+ 300 South Black Horse Pike
Runnemede, NJ 08078 (856)939-6400

Patel, Ashokkumar B., MD {1407862378} GenPrc, FamMed(63,INDI)<NJ-KMHCHRRY>
+ AAP Family Practice, PC
707 White Horse Road/Suite C-105 Voorhees, NJ 08043
(856)258-4966 Fax (856)258-4972
+ 2827 Westfield Avenue
Camden, NJ 08105 (856)258-4966 Fax (856)964-2255

Patel, Ashokkumar J., MD {1275508145} Anesth(79,INA2B)<NJ-BURDTMLN>
+ Cape Regional Medical Center
2 Stone Harbor Boulevard/Anesth Cape May Court House, NJ 08210 (609)463-2000 Fax (609)463-2757

Patel, Ashvin S., MD {1356397079} IntrMd(70,INDI)<NJ-COMMED>
+ 108 Lacey Road/Suite 30
Whiting, NJ 08759 (732)849-0303 Fax (732)849-0860

Patel, Atulkumar V., MD {1659487858} ObsGyn, IntrMd(77,INA69)<NJ-STPETER, NJ-RWJUBRUN>
+ Kirit Somabhai Patel, MD PC
34-36 Progress Street/Suite A-6 Edison, NJ 08820
(908)757-9555 Fax (908)757-2312

Patel, Avanee Kanoo, MD {1578643052} ObsGyn, MtFtMd(02,TX12)<NJ-ENGLEWOOD>
+ Englewood Hospital and Medical Center
350 Engle Street/Antepartum Test Englewood, NJ 07631
(201)894-3669 Fax (201)541-3445

Patel, Bela Ashutosh, MD {1013930304} IntrMd, Grtrcs(95,INA29)<NJ-PALISADE>
+ Palisades Medical Center
7600 River Road/EmrgMed North Bergen, NJ 07047
(201)854-5000

Patel, Bharat K., MD {1699749242} Radiol, RadDia(88,NY15)<NJ-KIMBALL>
+ Kimball Medical Center
600 River Avenue/Radiology Lakewood, NJ 08701
(732)363-1900 Fax (732)942-5658

Patel, Bhavesh, DO {1851659965}
+ SJH Urgent Care, P.C.
201 Tomlin Station Road/Suite B Mullica Hill, NJ 08062
(856)241-2500 Fax (856)241-2511

Patel, Bhavi Ashit, MD {1306850409} IntrMd(91,INA15)
+ OM Medical Care LLC
P.O. Box 6078 Somerset, NJ 08875 (908)866-6310 Fax (732)568-4784
Bhavipatelmd@yahoo.com

Patel, Bhavna K., MD {1205867876} Pedtrc(92,NY19)<NJ-SJER-SYHS>
+ first Step Pediatrics
206 Laurel Heights Drive Bridgeton, NJ 08302 (856)459-2270 Fax (856)459-9674

Patel, Bhupendra C., MD {1639112352} IntrMd, EmrgMd(88,INA53)
+ JFK Medical Center
65 James Street Edison, NJ 08820 (732)321-7601 Fax (732)744-5614

Patel, Bhupendra M., MD {1588728950} PsyGrt, Psychy(64,INA21)<NJ-GRYSTPSY>
+ Greystone Park Psychiatric Hospital
59 Koch Avenue/ClinicalPsych Morris Plains, NJ 07950
(973)538-1800

Patel, Bhupenmra M., MD {1326047655} Radiol, RadDia(74,INA20)<NJ-VIRTMHBC, NJ-VIRTBERL>
+ South Jersey Radiology Associates, P.A.
100 Carnie Boulevard/Suite B-5 Voorhees, NJ 08043
(856)751-0123 Fax (856)751-0535
+ South Jersey Radiology Associates, P.A.
315 Route 70 East/Suite B Cherry Hill, NJ 08034 (856)751-0123 Fax (856)428-0356
+ The Women's Center at Voorhees
100 Carnie Boulevard/Suite A-4 Voorhees, NJ 08043
(856)751-5522 Fax (856)751-5650

Patel, Bhupendrakumar V., MD {1497846109} Anesth, PainMd(82,INA2B)<NJ-UMDNJ>
+ James Street Anesthesia
102 James Street/Suite 103 Edison, NJ 08820 (732)494-1444 Fax (732)494-7052

Patel, Bimal, DO {1174899116} Anesth
+ Metzger Pain Management
170 Avenue At The Commons/Suite 6 Shrewsbury, NJ 07702 (732)380-0200 Fax (732)380-0124

Patel, Bindi Akshay, DO {1225551146} Nrolgy
+ University Hospital-RWJMS Neurology
125 Paterson Street/Suite 4100-6100 New Brunswick, NJ 08901 (732)235-7733 Fax (732)235-7041

Patel, Bipinchand N., MD {1215941315} Pedtrc(74,INA21)<NJ-STPETER>
+ St. Peter's University Hospital
254 Easton Avenue New Brunswick, NJ 08901 (732)745-8600 Fax (732)220-0659

Patel, Chandrakant, MD {1932311073} Anesth(71,INA83)
+ 55 Flint Terrace
Harrington Park, NJ 07640 (201)784-1887 Fax (201)784-1887

Patel, Chandrakant A., MD {1740206655} IntrMd(70,INA20)<NJ-CHRIST>
+ 142 Palisade Avenue/Suite 215
Jersey City, NJ 07306 (201)653-3950 Fax (201)653-8756

Patel, Chandulal Harilal, MD {1306840897} CdvDis, IntrMd(80,INA20)<NJ-WARREN>
+ Easton Cardiovascular Associates
123 Roseberry Street Phillipsburg, NJ 08865 (908)213-3100
eastoncardiovascular@rcn.com

Patel, Chhaya B., DO {1265452841} IntrMd(03,NJ75)<NJ-CHS-FULD>
+ Capital Health System/Fuld Campus
750 Brunswick Avenue Trenton, NJ 08638 (609)394-6000

Patel, Chimanlal J., MD {1841255981} IntrMd(71,INDI)<NJ-SJER-SYHS>
+ 901 Central Avenue/PO Box 698
Minotola, NJ 08341 (856)697-0111
Cjpatelmd@yahoo.com

Patel, Chirag G., MD {1679501084} EmrgMd(00,NJ05)<NJ-HUNTRDN>
+ Hunterdon Medical Center
2100 Wescott Drive/EmergMed Flemington, NJ 08822
(908)788-6100
+ Central Jersey Urgent Care
731 Highway 35/Unit G Ocean, NJ 07712 (908)788-6100
Fax (732)361-0728

Patel, Chirag V., MD {1205940392} Ophthl, IntrMd(01,NJ05)
+ The Retina Group of Princeton
601 Ewing Street/Suite C-17 Princeton, NJ 08540
(609)800-2393
info@pfeye.com
+ Princeton Eye and Ear
5 Plainsboro Road/Suite 510 Plainsboro, NJ 08536
(609)800-2393 Fax (609)716-6900
+ Princeton Flemington Eye Institute
1100 Wescott Drive/Suite 305 Flemington, NJ 08540
(908)237-7037

Patel, Choudhary Balwan S., MD {1003843863}
+ 20 Manor House Court
Cherry Hill, NJ 08003 (508)868-5729
cbspatel@gmail.com

Patel, Dakshesh K., MD {1720202278} Nrolgy(02,NY15)<NJ-UNVMCPRN, NJ-RWJUHAM>
+ Garden State Neurology & Neuro-Oncology, P.C.
100 State Highway 36 East West Long Branch, NJ 07764
(732)229-6200 Fax (732)229-6201
+ Garden State Neurology & Neuro-Oncology, P.C.
9 Hospital Drive/Suite A7 1st Floor Toms River, NJ 08755
(732)229-6200 Fax (732)229-6201

Patel, Dakshkumar B., MD {1497762876} IntrMd(73,INA21)<NJ-CHSFULD, NJ-RWJUHAM>
+ Patel Medical Group
2103 Klockner Road Hamilton Square, NJ 08690
(609)586-4739 Fax (609)588-5314
+ Patel Medical Group PA
1450 Parkside Avenue/Suite 5 Trenton, NJ 08638
(609)586-4739 Fax (609)538-0177

Patel, Deepa N., MD {1689955460} FamMed
+ Medical Associates of Central New Jersey
3F Parlin Drive Parlin, NJ 08859 (732)651-2001 Fax (732)651-2002

Patel, Deepa Samir, MD {1134225162} IntrMd(93,INA21)<NJ-BAYSHORE>
+ SD Medical Corp
2 American Way/Suite 3 Spotswood, NJ 08884 (732)416-0065 Fax (732)416-0053

Patel, Deepak Vaijbhai, MD {1447288378} SrgOrt, IntrMd(83,INA65)
+ Market Street Surgery Center
444 Market Street Saddle Brook, NJ 07663 (201)843-1237
Fax (201)843-9442
bonepatel@yahoo.com

Patel, Deepan N., MD {1912171372} SrgOrt(08,PA02)<NY-JTORTHO, NY-VAHARBOR>
+ North Jersey Orthopaedic Specialists
730 Palisade Avenue Teaneck, NJ 07666 (201)530-1004
Fax (201)530-0003

Patel, Devang G., MD {1558395046} IntrMd, Gastrn(98,NJ05)
+ Center for Gastroenterology & Hepatology
904 Oak Tree Avenue/Suite H South Plainfield, NJ 07080
(908)755-9993 Fax (908)755-9994
+ Access Health Systems
622 Georges Road North Brunswick, NJ 08902 (908)755-9993 Fax (732)828-1713

Patel, Devi, MD {1053670679} IntrMd
+ The Cooper Hospital System-Univ Hospital
3 Cooper Plaza/Suite 215 Camden, NJ 08103 (856)642-2133

Patel, Dharmesh Govind, MD {1487031845} IntrMd<NJ-MORRISTN>
+ Morristown Medical Center
100 Madison Avenue Morristown, NJ 07962 (973)971-4287 Fax (973)290-8325

Patel, Dhirendrakumar A., MD {1487774543} IntrMd(72,INA31)<NJ-MEADWLND, NJ-STMRYPAS>
+ 714 Tenth Street/Suite 6B
Secaucus, NJ 07094 (201)617-8447 Fax (201)617-7838
+ 1236 Route 46 West
Parsippany, NJ 07054 (201)617-8447 Fax (973)335-1880

Physicians by Name and Address

Patel, Dhwani A., DO {1831515105}<NJ-MORRISTN>
+ Morristown Medical Center
  100 Madison Avenue   Morristown, NJ 07962   (973)971-5000

Patel, Dinesh R., MD {1194793125} Pedtrc(83,INA20)<NJ-MORRISTN, NJ-STCLRDEN>
+ 1236 US Highway 46
  Parsippany, NJ 07054   (973)257-0024

Patel, Dineshchandra G., MD {1528139961} Psychy(77,INA53)
+ Union County Psychiatric Clinic, Inc.
  117-119 Roosevelt Avenue   Plainfield, NJ 07060   (908)756-6870   Fax (908)756-5566

Patel, Dipan G., MD {1689939548} AnesPain
+ Garden State Pain Control Center, P.A.
  1117 Route 46 East/Suite 201   Clifton, NJ 07013   (973)777-5444   Fax (973)777-0304

Patel, Dipesh Shashikant, DO {1831504588} FamMed<NY-ARNOTMC>
+ JFK Family Practice Group
  65 James Street   Edison, NJ 08818   (732)321-7487   Fax (732)906-4927

Patel, Divyesh V., MD {1164508008} IntrMd(91,INDI)<NJ-ANCPSYCH>
+ Ancora Psychiatric Hospital
  301 Spring Garden Road/InternalMed   Hammonton, NJ 08037   (609)561-1700   Fax (609)567-7357

Patel, Diptika D., MD {1417949975} IntrMd(77,INDI)<NJ-RBAYOLDB, NJ-RBAYPERT>
+ Dipitka Patel, MD PA
  200 Perrine Road/Suite 227   Old Bridge, NJ 08857   (732)727-4780   Fax (732)727-1989
+ Dipitka Patel, MD PA
  267 Hobart Street   Perth Amboy, NJ 08861   (732)727-4780   Fax (732)826-3121

Patel, Disha, MD {1699919506} IntrMd, SlpDis, IntHos(07,GRN01)
+ The Park Medical Group
  24 Elm Street   Harrington Park, NJ 07640   (201)784-0123   Fax (201)784-0065

Patel, Divya R., MD {1649255738} Anesth(72,INDI)<NJ-STCLRDEN>
+ 4 Coventry Court
  East Hanover, NJ 07936

Patel, Dushyant Rameshchandra, MD {1750330072} IntrMd(95,INA71)
+ 1215 Broadway/Suite 3
  Fair Lawn, NJ 07410   (201)773-6808   Fax (201)773-6862

Patel, Erica, DO {1578823605} Anesth
+ 5 Foxcroft Court
  Voorhees, NJ 08043   (609)790-4437

Patel, Falguni B., MD {1528268299} ObsGyn, UroGyn(98,NY47)<NJ-OVERLOOK>
+ Associates in OBGYN
  522 East Broad Street   Westfield, NJ 07090   (908)232-4449

Patel, Gaurang, MD {1538123542} PulCCr, PulDis, IntrMd(01,DMN01)
+ Associates in Pulmonary Medicine, PA
  16 Pocono Road/Suite 217   Denville, NJ 07834   (973)625-5651
  Gaurang.Patel@earthlink.net
+ Associates in Pulmonary Medicine, PA
  765 State Highway 10 East   Randolph, NJ 07869   (973)625-5651   Fax (973)366-6385
+ RWJ University Hospital Somerset
  110 Rehill Avenue   Somerville, NJ 07834   (908)685-2200

Patel, Gaurang R., MD {1396788980} Pedtrc(99,GRN01)<NJ-JFKMED, NJ-STPETER>
+ Drs. Gaurang R. Patel & Associates
  1503 St Georges Avenue/Suite 205   Colonia, NJ 07067   (732)382-8111   Fax (732)381-0292
+ 1907 Oak Tree Road/Suite 105
  Edison, NJ 08820   (732)382-8111   Fax (732)494-1737

Patel, Gaurav R., MD {1952667867} Anesth
+ Morris Anesthesia Group, PA
  3799 Route 46/Suite 211   Parsippany, NJ 07054   (973)335-1122   Fax (973)335-1448

Patel, Gita R., MD {1396817631} IntrMd(78,INA15)<NJ-SOMERSET>
+ Drs. Patel and Patel
  31 West Somerset Street   Raritan, NJ 08869   (908)722-0035   Fax (908)722-6763

Patel, Gitanjali, MD {1518193366} RadDia
+ University Radiology Group, P.C.
  579A Cranbury Road   East Brunswick, NJ 08816   (732)390-0040   Fax (732)390-1856

Patel, Hansa S., MD {1598867558} Anesth, PainInvt(66,INDI)<NJ-JRSYSHMC>
+ Jersey Shore University Medical Center
  1945 Route 33/Anesth   Neptune, NJ 07753   (732)776-4945   Fax (732)897-0263

Patel, Hardik Bhupendrabhai, MD {1104216688} IntrMd
+ 26 North Ladow Avenue/Apt 13 C
  Millville, NJ 08332   (603)759-9847

Patel, Hareshbhai C., MD {1245208024} Anesth(71,INA20)<NJ-BURDTMLN>
+ Cape Regional Medical Center
  2 Stone Harbor Boulevard   Cape May Court House, NJ 08210   (609)463-2000   Fax (609)463-2757

Patel, Harshad Nathalal, MD {1922115344} AdolMd, IntrMd(67,INDI)
+ Elite Pediatrics
  One Broadway/Suite 303   Elmwood Park, NJ 07407   (201)794-8855   Fax (201)794-6988

Patel, Harshil, MD {1275977555} CdvDis<NY-LUTHERN>
+ Coastal Cardiovascular Consultants, PA
  459 Jack Martin Boulevard/Suite 4   Brick, NJ 08724   (732)458-6200   Fax (732)458-9464

Patel, Hashmukh R., MD {1881895001} IntrMd(83,INA35)<NJ-MEADWLND>
+ Meadowlands Hospital Medical Center
  55 Meadowlands Parkway   Secaucus, NJ 07096   (201)392-3100

Patel, Hasitkumar D., MD {1396022125} IntrMd
+ AtlantiCare Hospitalist Program
  1925 Pacific Avenue/8th Floor   Atlantic City, NJ 08401   (609)441-8146   Fax (609)441-8002

Patel, Hasmukhbha D., MD {1891756789} IntrMd(82,INA53)
+ Excel Care Alliance, LLC
  49 South State Street   Vineland, NJ 08360   (856)696-9697   Fax (856)696-9698
+ Community Health Care, Inc.
  70 Cohansey Street   Bridgeton, NJ 08302   (856)696-9697   Fax (856)451-0029

Patel, Hemali V., DO {1477110591} FamMed
+ SJH Medical Center Family Medicine
  1505 West Sherman Avenue   Vineland, NJ 08360   (856)641-8000

Patel, Hemantkumar G., MD {1932178357} IntrMd, PulDis(80,INDI)<NJ-STBARNMC, NJ-NWRKBETH>
+ West Orange Medical Associates LLC
  91 Main Street/Suite 110   West Orange, NJ 07052   (973)669-0098
+ Berkeley Medical Associates
  2083 Millburn Avenue   Maplewood, NJ 07040

Patel, Hetal, MD {1508800269} EmrgMd(99,NJ05)<NJ-MORRISTN>
+ Morristown Medical Center
  100 Madison Avenue/EmergMed   Morristown, NJ 07962   (973)971-5000

Patel, Hetal Mahendra, MD {1801190962} IntrMd
+ 34 Simpson Avenue
  Edison, NJ 08817   (732)572-0369

Patel, Hetal R., DO {1124334347} FamMed<NJ-CHRIST>
+ Christ Hospital
  176 Palisade Avenue   Jersey City, NJ 07306   (201)795-8200
+ Riverview Medical Center
  1 Riverview Plaza   Red Bank, NJ 07701   (732)741-2700
+ Hospital Medicine Associates
  157 Broad Street/Suite 317   Red Bank, NJ 07306   (732)530-2960   Fax (865)291-3652

Patel, Himanshu K., MD {1619142833} IntrMd(87,INA15)
+ Central Jersey Pediatrics PC
  1553 Ruth Road/Suite 1   North Brunswick, NJ 08902   (732)418-1700   Fax (732)249-9599
+ Central Jersey Pediatrics
  401 Ridge Road/Suite 2   Dayton, NJ 08810   (732)418-1700   Fax (732)249-9599

Patel, Himanshubhai A., MD {1336188622} Pedtrc(87,INA71)<NJ-STPETER, NJ-RWJUBRUN>
+ Central Jersey Pediatrics PC
  1553 Ruth Road/Suite 1   North Brunswick, NJ 08902   (732)418-1700   Fax (732)249-9599
+ Central Jersey Pediatrics
  401 Ridge Road/Suite 2   Dayton, NJ 08810   (732)418-1700   Fax (732)249-9599
+ Princeton Center for Eating Disorders
  One Plainsboro Road   Plainsboror, NJ 08902   (609)853-7575

Patel, Hiren G., MD {1316202823}<NJ-STJOSHOS>
+ St. Joseph's Regional Medical Center
  703 Main Street   Paterson, NJ 07503   (973)754-2431

Patel, Hiren Ramesh, MD {1619089620} RadDia, RadBdI(97,CA11)<NJ-ACMCITY, NJ-SHOREMEM>
+ Atlantic Medical Imaging, LLC.
  72 West Jimmie Leeds Road   Galloway, NJ 08205   (609)677-9729   Fax (609)653-8764
+ Atlantic Medical Imaging, LLC.
  401 Bethel Road   Somers Point, NJ 08244   (609)677-9729
+ Atlantic Medical Imaging, LLC.
  421 Route 9 North   Cape May Court House, NJ 08205   (609)463-9500   Fax (609)465-0918

Patel, Hitendra R., MD {1245314509} Psychy, PsyGrt(96,INA8B)<NJ-TRININPC>
+ Trinitas Regional Medical Center-New Point Campus
  655 East Jersey Street   Elizabeth, NJ 07206   (908)994-5000
+ Amber Court of Assisted Living Community
  1155 East Jersey Street   Elizabeth, NJ 07201

Patel, Hitesh Babubhai, MD {1982652038} IntrMd(00,DMN01)
+ Premier HealthCare Associates, PC
  1631 Route 88 West/Suite A   Brick, NJ 08724   (732)202-7456   Fax (732)202-7459

Patel, Hitesh K., MD {1215959622} Ophthl, IntrMd(93,PA02)
+ Patel Eye Associates
  228 Plainfield Avenue   Edison, NJ 08817   (732)985-5009   Fax (732)985-5155
+ Patel Eye Associates
  3084 State Route 27/Suite 4   Kendall Park, NJ 08824   (732)985-5009   Fax (732)985-5155

Patel, Hitesh Ramesh, MD {1871534305} FamMed(98,NJ06)
+ Primary & Specialty Care at Edison
  10 Parsonage Road/Suite 410   Edison, NJ 08837   (732)452-0680   Fax (732)636-3669

Patel, Indravadan T., MD {1922032879} IntrMd(82,INA2B)<NJ-JFKMED>
+ 2060 Oaktree Road
  Edison, NJ 08820   (732)548-6080   Fax (732)744-0796
  Ipatelmd@yahoo.com

Patel, Indubhai Manibhai, MD {1649477415} IntrMd(85,INA20)
+ Crosskeys Medical Center
  600 Berlin-Crosskeys Road/Unit 102   Sicklerville, NJ 08081   (856)875-5152   Fax (856)875-0313

Patel, Jalpa S., MD {1740695428} IntrMd(03,INA53)
+ Elizabeth Medical Group
  310 New Jersey Avenue   Elizabeth, NJ 07202   (908)351-2222   Fax (908)351-1977

Patel, Jatinchandra Suryakant, DO {1801979901} CdvDis, CarNuc, IntCrd(01,NJ75)
+ Garden State Heart Care, P.C.
  831 Tennent Road/Suite 1-F   Englishtown, NJ 07726   (732)851-4700   Fax (732)851-4703
+ Garden State Heart Care, P.C.
  333 Forsgate Drive/Suite 205   Jamesburg, NJ 08831   (732)851-4700

Patel, Jay, MD {1811286776} RadDia(NJ05
+ 221 High Street/Suite 101
  Newton, NJ 07860   (973)383-1280

Patel, Jay A., DO {1962841452}<NJ-MEADWLND>
+ Meadowlands Hospital Medical Center
  55 Meadowlands Parkway   Secaucus, NJ 07096   (201)392-3100

Patel, Jay Dinesh, MD {1639256696} FamMed, IntrMd(97,NJ05)
+ Elmwood Family Physicians
  777 Route 70 East/Suite G-101   Marlton, NJ 08053   (856)983-9939   Fax (856)983-9936
+ Elmwood Family Physicians
  1529 Route 206/Suite L   Tabernacle, NJ 08088   (856)983-9939   Fax (609)268-7191

Patel, Jay K., MD {1801874045} CdvDis, IntrMd(86,WAL02)<NJ-RWJUHAM, NJ-STFRNMED>
+ Hamilton Cardiology Associates
  2073 Klockner Road   Hamilton, NJ 08690   (609)584-1212   Fax (609)584-0103

Patel, Jayantilal R., MD {1457338253} Psychy(76,INA20)<NJ-ANNKLEIN>
+ Ann Klein Forensic Center
  1609 Stuyvesant Avenue/PO Box 7717   West Trenton, NJ 08628   (609)633-0900

Patel, Jayantkumar N., MD {1447352752} CdvDis, IntrMd(65,INDI)
+ Cardiologist & Intrnest Associates
  211 Essex Street/Suite 104   Hackensack, NJ 07601   (201)489-3888   Fax (201)301-7351

Patel, Jayendra M., MD {1871718775} IntrMd, EmrgMd(80,INDI)
+ Menlo Park Medical Group PA
  111 James Street   Edison, NJ 08820   (732)549-2299   Fax (732)549-2262

Patel, Jayendrakumar N., MD {1023044104} CdvDis, IntrMd(83,INA20)
+ Medical Associates of Marlboro PC
  32 North Main Street   Marlboro, NJ 07746   (732)462-4100   Fax (732)462-3798
+ Medical Associates of Marlboro
  111 James Street   Edison, NJ 08818   (732)462-4100   Fax (732)452-9720

Patel, Jayesh B., MD {1932203171} IntrMd(93,INA5Y)<NJ-OCEANMC>
+ 227 East Somerdale Road
  Somerdale, NJ 08083   (856)784-2626   Fax (856)784-0375

Patel, Jayeshkumar Balu, MD {1760483887} Radiol, RadDia(95,NJ06)
 + South Jersey Radiology Associates, P.A.
  748 Kings Highway   West Deptford, NJ 08096   (856)848-4998   Fax (856)853-7362
 + South Jersey Radiology Associates, P.A.
  100 Carnie Boulevard/Suite B-5   Voorhees, NJ 08043   (856)848-4998   Fax (856)751-0535
 + South Jersey Radiology Associates, P.A.
  315 Route 70 East/Suite B   Cherry Hill, NJ 08096   (856)428-4344   Fax (856)428-0356
Patel, Jayeshkumar Kiritkumar, MD {1316980527} IntrMd(98,INA71)<NJ-BURDTMLN>
 + Cape Regional Medical Center
  2 Stone Harbor Boulevard   Cape May Court House, NJ 08210   (609)463-2803
Patel, Jayeshkumar Shantilal, MD {1962509265} Nephro, IntrMd(91,INA21)<NJ-JRSYCITY>
 + 550 Summit Avenue/Basement
  Jersey City, NJ 07306   (201)209-1802   Fax (201)604-8400
Patel, Jaymica, MD {1235306952} FamMed, IntHos(05,DMN01)<NJ-UNDRWD>
 + Inspira Health Network
  509 North Broad Street/Hospitalist   Woodbury, NJ 08096   (856)686-5396   Fax (856)686-5332
Patel, Jayminkumar R., MD {1548354327} Pedtrc, PedEmg, EmrgMd(82,INDI)<NJ-JRSYCITY, NJ-MEADWLND>
 + NHCAC Health Center at West New York
  5301 Broadway   West New York, NJ 07093   (201)866-9320
 + JFK Medical Center
  65 James Street   Edison, NJ 08820   (201)866-9320   Fax (732)744-5614
Patel, Jayrag Ashwinkumar, MD {1528264215} Ophthl(01,ENG16)
 + Yasgur Eye Associates
  1415 Route 70 East/Suite 404   Cherry Hill, NJ 08034
Patel, Jayshree R., MD {1558542084} Anesth(83,INA21)<NJ-CENTRAST>
 + Liberty Anesthesia & Pain Management
  901 West Main Street/2nd Floor   Freehold, NJ 07728   (732)294-2876   Fax (732)294-2502
Patel, Jharna Mehul, MD {1306335229} ObsGyn
 + University Medical Group/OBGYN
  125 Paterson Street/2nd Floor   New Brunswick, NJ 08901   (732)235-6375   Fax (732)235-9855
Patel, Jigar, MD {1215294657} IntrMd(08,INA8B)<NJ-OVERLOOK>
 + Overlook Medical Center
  99 Beauvoir Avenue/PO Box 210   Summit, NJ 07902   (908)522-2000
Patel, Jigar A., MD {1902018468} CdvDis, IntrMd(01,NJ05)<NJ-SHOREMEM, NJ-BURDTMLN>
 + Mercer Bucks Cardiology
  One Union Street/Suite 101   Robbinsville, NJ 08691   (609)890-6677   Fax (609)890-7292
Patel, Jigar Dhansukh, MD {1619318177} FamMed
 + Capital Health System/Hopewell
  One Capital Way   Pennington, NJ 08534   (800)637-2374
Patel, Jigger, MD {1730573437}
 + Delaware Valley Family Health Center
  200 Frenchtown Road   Milford, NJ 08848   (908)995-2251   Fax (908)995-2036
Patel, Jigna K., MD {1508124025} ObsGyn
 + Palisades Women's Group
  7650 River Road/Suite 230   North Bergen, NJ 07047   (201)868-6755   Fax (201)868-8442
 + 1115 Seventh Street
  North Bergen, NJ 07047   (973)926-4882
Patel, Jignasa, MD {1699867572} IntrMd(92,INA53)
 + Drs. Luhana, Dhirmalani & Patel
  239 Baldwin Road/Suite 108   Parsippany, NJ 07054   (973)334-2265   Fax (973)335-9091
 + 1180 Route 46
  Parsippany, NJ 07054   (973)334-2265   Fax (973)306-3007
Patel, Jitendra K., MD {1316029804} IntrMd(83,INA21)
 + Atlantic Health Center P.C.
  2300 Atlantic Avenue/Suite 1   Atlantic City, NJ 08401   (609)345-9100   Fax (609)345-6114
Patel, Kajal D., DO {1881021509}
 + 209 Europa Court
  Cherry Hill, NJ 08003   (302)423-5248
  kdp302@yahoo.com
Patel, Kalpesh P., DO {1073691226} Pedtrc(02,NY75)<NJ-SOMERSET>
 + RWJ University Hospital Somerset
  110 Rehill Avenue   Somerville, NJ 08876   (908)685-2200   Fax (908)704-3777
Patel, Kalpeshkumar Prahladbhai, MD {1922125038} FamMed(93,INDI)<NJ-JRSYSHMC>
 + Integrated Medicine Alliance, PA.
  363 Highway 36   Port Monmouth, NJ 07758   (732)471-0400   Fax (732)471-7949

 + Howell Jackson Medical Center
  4764 Route 9 South   Howell, NJ 07731   (732)370-3563
 + Parlin Medical Center
  3-F Parlin Drive   Parlin, NJ 07758   (732)651-2001   Fax (732)651-2002
Patel, Kalpeshkumar R., MD {1710182654} IntrMd(01,INA2B)<NJ-MONMOUTH>
 + Cinnaminson Primary & Walk-in Care
  2800 Route 130 North/Suite 102   Riverton, NJ 08077   (856)303-8500   Fax (856)303-8501
Patel, Kamal B., MD {1417997511} EmrgMd(71,INA6A)
 + 1217 Jacksonville Road
  Columbus, NJ 08022
Patel, Kamal Kanubhai, MD {1982692927} IntrMd(90,INA20)<NJ-STCLRDEN>
 + Cobbs Corner Primary Care, P.A.
  1081 Parsippany Boulevard/Suite 102   Parsippany, NJ 07054   (973)917-3555   Fax (973)917-3553
Patel, Karnik, DO {1629458088} IntrMd
 + Hoboken Family Practice
  108 Washington Street   Hoboken, NJ 07030   (201)656-5688   Fax (201)656-8975
Patel, Kartik, DO {1093827834} Ophthl   IntrMd(99,PA77)<NJ-STJOSHOS>
 + 195 Route 46 West/Suite 204
  Mine Hill, NJ 07803   (973)573-9900   Fax (973)537-9901
Patel, Kashmira, MD {1720063498} IntrMd(92,INDI)
 + 3200 Sunset Avenue/Suite 101
  Ocean, NJ 07712   (732)775-1100   Fax (732)775-9165
Patel, Kaushik M., MD {1073596177} RadDia, RadV&I(95,NJ05)<NJ-BURDTMLN, NJ-COOPRUMC>
 + Cape Regional Medical Center
  2 Stone Harbor Boulevard/Radiology   Cape May Court House, NJ 08210   (609)463-2000
Patel, Kavan Girishbhai, MD {1437541406} Gastrn
 + Ocean Family Gastroenterology P.C.
  425 Lakehurst Road   Toms River, NJ 08755   (732)281-1590   Fax (732)281-1593
Patel, Ketan R., MD {1164508867} Pedtrc(90,MEXI)
 + Holly City Pediatrics
  10 East Main Street/Suite A   Millville, NJ 08332   (856)825-5932   Fax (856)825-4819
Patel, Keval V., MD {1023362787} IntrMd<NJ-JRSYSHMC>
 + Jersey Shore University Medical Center
  1945 Route 33/Medicine   Neptune, NJ 07753   (732)776-4483   Fax (732)776-4798
Patel, Keyur Bhupendra, MD {1316149172} RadNro, IntrMd(07,NJ06)
 + University Radiology Group, P.C.
  579A Cranbury Road   East Brunswick, NJ 08816   (732)390-0040   Fax (732)390-1856
  kpatel@univrad.com
 + University Radiology Group, P.C.
  16 Mountain Boulevard   Warren, NJ 07059   (732)390-0040   Fax (908)769-9141
Patel, Killol, MD {1467743286} PulDis, IntrMd
 + Bergen Medical Alliance, P.A.
  180 Engle Street   Englewood, NJ 07631   (201)567-2050   Fax (201)568-8936
Patel, Kinjal M., MD {1538331814} Anesth
 + Cooper Anesthesia Associates
  One Cooper Plaza/Suite 294-B   Camden, NJ 08103   (856)342-2425   Fax (856)968-8239
Patel, Kirit Somabhai, MD {1891727087} ObsGyn, IntrMd(75,INDI)<NJ-JFKMED>
 + 34-36 Progress Street/Suite A-6
  Edison, NJ 08820   (908)757-9555   Fax (908)757-2312
Patel, Kirtikumar J., MD {1588790281} Surgry, IntrMd(70,INA21)
 + JFK Medical Center
  65 James Street/Surgery   Edison, NJ 08820   (732)321-7000
Patel, Kishan Bharat, DO {1720349723} EmrgMd
 + Rowan University-School of Osteopathic Medicine
  1 Medical Center Drive   Stratford, NJ 08084   (856)346-7985   Fax (856)346-6673
Patel, Krishna A., MD {1235166489} Pedtrc(79,INDI)<NJ-WOODBRDG>
 + Hunterdon Developmental Center
  40 Pittstown Road/PO Box 4003   Clinton, NJ 08809   (908)735-4031   Fax (908)730-1340
Patel, Kriya, MD {1598109522}<NJ-OVERLOOK>
 + Overlook Medical Center
  99 Beauvoir Avenue/PO Box 210   Summit, NJ 07902   (908)522-2000
Patel, Kumar R., MD {1194800243} Surgry, SrgVas(70,INDI)<NJ-ENGLWOOD, NJ-VALLEY>
 + 245 East Main Street
  Ramsey, NJ 07446   (201)327-0220
Patel, Kunal Manmohan, MD {1376960591}<NJ-STMICHL>
 + St. Michael's Medical Center
  268 MLK Jr. Boulevard   Newark, NJ 07102   (973)877-5160

Patel, Lopa M., MD {1447268677} IntrMd(02,DMN01)<NJ-NWRKBETH>
 + Newark Beth Israel Medical Center
  201 Lyons Avenue   Newark, NJ 07112   (973)926-7300
Patel, Mahir, MD {1417191917} Dermat
 + The Dermatology Group, P.C.
  347 Mount Pleasant Avenue/Suite 103   West Orange, NJ 07052   (973)571-2121   Fax (973)498-0535
Patel, Maitri, MD {1043398076} IntrMd(98,INA21)
 + Neighborhood Health Center Plainfield
  1700-58 Myrtle Avenue   Plainfield, NJ 07060   (908)753-6401   Fax (908)226-6743
 + Prudent MD
  5 Dundee Avenue   Iselin, NJ 08830   (908)753-6401   Fax (732)218-3933
Patel, Mallik, MD {1548654130} FamMed
 + MedExpress Urgent Care
  124 Washington Avenue   Nutley, NJ 07110   (973)661-0128   Fax (973)667-1453
Patel, Manan Jaykishan, MD {1629070024} RadDia(93,NY20)
 + Radiology Associates of Burlington County
  1295 Route 38 West/PO Box 479   Hainesport, NJ 08036   (609)261-7017   Fax (609)261-4180
Patel, Manish Arvind, DO {1326019175} FamMed(01,NJ75)
 + Lordes Medical Associates
  1900 Mount Holly Road   Burlington Township, NJ 08016   (609)387-0325   Fax (609)387-0149
Patel, Manish B., DO {1962765461}
 + 334 Terrace Avenue
  Jersey City, NJ 07307   (551)655-0953
Patel, Manish Surendra, MD {1013983998} IntrMd(02,NY48)
 + UH- Robert Wood Johnson Med
  125 Paterson Street/Room 2330   New Brunswick, NJ 08901   (732)828-3000   Fax (732)235-7144
Patel, Manish Sureshbhai, MD {1053418459} IntrMd(94,INDI)<NJ-TRINIWSC, NJ-RWJURAH>
 + Union County Pediatrics Group
  817 Rahway Avenue   Elizabeth, NJ 07202   (908)353-5750
Patel, Manisha Saurabh, MD {1568538213} Nephro, IntrMd(84,INDI)<NJ-SOMERSET, NJ-RWJUBRUN>
 + Somerset Nephrology Associates, P.C.
  23 Monroe Street   Bridgewater, NJ 08807   (908)722-0106   Fax (908)231-1431
  kidneydr9@gmail.com
Patel, Manmohan A., MD {1083639512} PulDis(73,INDI)<NJ-CHRIST, NJ-MEADWLND>
 + 55 Meadowlands Parkway
  Secaucus, NJ 07094   (201)216-3055   Fax (201)499-0261
Patel, Manoj, MD {1184898918} IntrMd(01,INA71)
 + Shore Medical Specialists
  500 River Avenue/Suite 140   Lakewood, NJ 08701   (732)363-7200   Fax (732)367-4461
 + Shore Medical Specialists
  500 River Avenue   Lakewood, NJ 08701   (732)363-7200   Fax (732)367-4461
 + Shore Medical Specialists
  9 Hospital Drive   Toms River, NJ 08701   (732)349-2732   Fax (732)349-9697
Patel, Manoj K., MD {1205226784} IntrMd
 + AtlantiCare Regional Medical Center/City Campus
  1925 Pacific Avenue   Atlantic City, NJ 08401   (609)441-8074
Patel, Mansi, MD {1548579519} Pedtrc
 + 7402 A Dane Court
  North Bergen, NJ 07047
Patel, Mayank D., MD {1518985332} Gastrn, IntrMd(79,INDI)
 + 659 New Dover Road
  Edison, NJ 08820   (732)382-0344   Fax (732)382-0340
 + Drs. Patel & Patel
  237 Central Avenue   Jersey City, NJ 07307   (732)382-0344   Fax (201)656-8676
 + Avenel Iselin Medical Group
  400 Gill Lane   Iselin, NJ 08820   (732)404-1580   Fax (732)404-1594
Patel, Mayur Vinod, MD {1649320359} ObsGyn, IntrMd(93,ENG16)
 + 565 Highway 35/Suite 7
  Red Bank, NJ 07701   (732)530-1058   Fax (732)530-1419
Patel, Mayuri, MD {1083057715} EmrgMd
 + Robert Wood Johnson Emergency Medicine
  One Robert Wood Johnson Place/MEB 104   New Brunswick, NJ 08901   (732)235-8717
Patel, Mayuri H., MD {1821265422} IntrMd, CdvDis(96,INA20)<NJ-TRINIWSC>
 + Trinitas Regional Medical Center-Williamson Street
  225 Williamson Street   Elizabeth, NJ 07207   (908)994-5000
Patel, Mayurkumar P., MD {1629207030} Nephro, IntrMd(03,INA2B)<NJ-BAYSHORE, NJ-JRSYSHMC>
 + Drs. Patel & Sharma
  1915 6th Avenue   Neptune, NJ 07753   (732)774-5700   Fax (732)774-7929

Physicians by Name and Address

Patel, Meelan Nick, MD {1801046826}(06,NY09)
+ Princeton Orthopaedic Associates, P.A.
  325 Princeton Avenue Princeton, NJ 08540 (609)924-8131 Fax (609)924-8532

Patel, Meena S., MD {1730128901} IntrMd, Grtrcs(68,INA69)<NJ-STJOSHOS, NJ-WAYNEGEN>
+ 1031 McBride Avenue
  West Paterson, NJ 07424 (973)890-1303 Fax (973)890-5609
+ 14 Oak Ridge Road
  Newfoundland, NJ 07435 (973)890-1303 Fax (973)697-8976

Patel, Meera V., MD {1023348687} FamMed, IntrMd(08,GRN01)
+ Alps Family Physicians
  1500 Alps Road Wayne, NJ 07470 (973)628-8500 Fax (973)628-7944

Patel, Meghal, MD {1457768038}
+ Kirit Somabhai Patel, MD PC
  34-36 Progress Street/Suite A-6 Edison, NJ 08820 (908)757-9555 Fax (908)757-2312

Patel, Mehul Kumar, MD {1376951004} IntrMd(05,MI07)<NJ-ACMCITY>
+ AtlantiCare Hospitalist Program
  1925 Pacific Avenue/8th Floor Atlantic City, NJ 08401 (609)441-8146 Fax (609)441-8002

Patel, Menka Sanghvi, MD {1710307707} Ophthl(13,DC01)
+ Omni Eye Services
  485 Route 1 South/Building A Iselin, NJ 08830 (732)750-0400 Fax (732)602-0749

Patel, Miksha B., MD {1043506025}
+ 6403 Hana Road
  Edison, NJ 08817 (732)819-7272
  miksha.patel@gmail.com

Patel, Minal, MD {1619933306} IntrMd, InfDis(86,ENG07)<NJ-RWJUHAM>
+ Hamilton Cardiology Associates
  2073 Klockner Road Hamilton, NJ 08690 (609)584-1212 Fax (609)584-0103

Patel, Minalkumar Ashokkumar, MD {1083702914} IntrMd, IntHos(95,MA05)
+ 1 Regency Place
  Weehawken, NJ 07086

Patel, Mitesh, MD {1093987034}
+ Rothman Institute - Egg Harbor Township
  2500 English Creek Avenue/Bldg 1300 Egg Harbor Township, NJ 08234 (609)677-6060 Fax (609)677-6061

Patel, Mitul Suresh, MD {1093045197} Surgry
+ 1124 East Ridgewood Avenue/Suite 104
  Ridgewood, NJ 07450

Patel, Mohini Gautam, MD {1720265234} PedGst, Pedtrc, IntrMd(07,NY15)<NJ-MORRISTN, NJ-OVERLOOK>
+ Division of Pediatric GI at Goryeb
  100 Madison Avenue/Box 82/Floor 2 Morristown, NJ 07962 (973)971-5676 Fax (973)290-7365
+ Overlook Medical Center
  99 Beauvoir Avenue/PO Box 210 Summit, NJ 07902 (908)522-8714

Patel, Mona, MD {1477715027} Anesth
+ Morris Anesthesia Group, PA
  3799 Route 46/Suite 211 Parsippany, NJ 07054 (973)335-1122 Fax (973)335-1448

Patel, Mona M., MD {1740257880} PsyCAd, Psychy(85,INA67)<NJ-BERGNMC>
+ 70 Kinderkamack Road/Suite 201
  Emerson, NJ 07630 (201)599-9700 Fax (201)599-3330

Patel, Monika B., MD {1114368974} IntrMd<NJ-COOPRUMC>
+ Cooper University Hospital
  One Cooper Plaza Camden, NJ 08103 (856)342-3150

Patel, Monil K., DO {1336503002}
+ 201 North Hermitage Avenue
  Trenton, NJ 08618 (609)915-4178

Patel, Mukesh D., MD {1063487759} Psychy(80,INA20)<NJ-HUNTRDN>
+ Hunterdon Medical Center
  2100 Wescott Drive Flemington, NJ 08822 (908)788-6654 Fax (908)788-6452
+ Psychiatric Associates of Hunterdon
  190 Route 31/Suite 100 Flemington, NJ 08822 (908)788-6654 Fax (908)788-6452

Patel, Mukesh M., MD {1598740292} IntrMd(80,INA20)<NJ-EASTORNG>
+ 1628 Oak Tree Road
  Edison, NJ 08820 (732)205-9070 Fax (732)205-9165

Patel, Munjal P., MD {1760691406} Surgry, SrgPlstc(99,NJ02)
+ SAMRA Group
  733 North Beers Street/Suite U-1 Holmdel, NJ 07733 (732)739-2100 Fax (732)739-0815
+ SAMRA Group
  300 Perrine Road/Suite 333 & 334 Old Bridge, NJ 08857 (732)739-2100 Fax (732)739-0815

Patel, Nachiket V., MD {1104999036} CdvDis, IntrMd(87,GRN01)<NJ-KIMBALL>
+ Kimball Medical Center
  600 River Avenue Lakewood, NJ 08701 (732)363-1900

Patel, Naishami, DO {1780998807}<NJ-CHRIST>
+ Drs. Viswanathan, Shakir & Patel
  815 Baltimore Avenue Roselle, NJ 07203 (908)245-3446 Fax (908)245-9265

Patel, Namrata, DO {1821366345} EmrgMd
+ 3 Briarwood Way
  North Haledon, NJ 07508

Patel, Napoleon, MD {1548520760}<NJ-MORRISTN>
+ Morristown Medical Center
  100 Madison Avenue Morristown, NJ 07962 (973)971-5152

Patel, Narendra D., MD {1477502193} IntrMd(72,INA37)<NJ-RWJURAH>
+ Drs. Patel and Patel
  2115 Northwood Avenue Linden, NJ 07036 (908)486-0990 Fax (908)925-7745

Patel, Narendra D., MD {1588688501} Psychy, PsyGrt(78,INDI)<NY-ROCKLPSY, NJ-VALLEY>
+ Psychcare PC
  65 North Maple Avenue/Suite 104 Ridgewood, NJ 07450 (201)444-8999 Fax (201)934-3341
  narendrapatelmd@yahoo.com
+ The Valley Hospital
  223 North Van Dien Avenue/Psychiatry Ridgewood, NJ 07450 (201)447-8000

Patel, Narendra K., MD {1386723823} IntrMd, InfDis(74,INDI)
+ 2177 Oak Tree Road/Suite 104
  Edison, NJ 08820 (908)412-1400 Fax (908)490-0038

Patel, Naresh J., DO {1760798797} FamMed(07,NJ75)
+ JFK Medical Center
  65 James Street/Medicine Edison, NJ 08820 (732)321-7000

Patel, Natverlal M., MD {1215045562} Pedtrc(67,INA2B)<NJ-RBAYPERT, NJ-JFKMED>
+ 1817 Oak Tree Road
  Edison, NJ 08820 (732)321-0784
+ 751 Convery Boulevard
  Perth Amboy, NJ 08861 (732)442-6995

Patel, Neha Hector, MD {1750712030} IntrMd(07,INA2I)
+ AtlantiCare Clinical Associates
  2500 English Creek Avenue Egg Harbor Township, NJ 08234 (609)407-2310 Fax (609)407-2311

Patel, Neha Mahendra, MD {1740519859}
+ Arthritis, Rheumatic & Back Disease Associates
  2309 East Evesham Road/Suite 101 Voorhees, NJ 08043 (856)424-5005 Fax (856)424-4716

Patel, Nehul, MD {1174866750} Anesth
+ Jersey Shore Anesthesiology Associates
  1945 Route 33/PO Box 397 Neptune, NJ 07754 (732)897-0200 Fax (732)897-0263

Patel, Nell M., MD {1992993414} SrgC&R(01,NY48)<NJ-RWJUBRUN>
+ UH- Robert Wood Johnson Med
  125 Paterson Street New Brunswick, NJ 08901 (732)828-3000 Fax (732)235-7079

Patel, Nikesh Kirit, MD {1881887800} SrgHnd, SrgPlstc(00,NC05)<NJ-CENTRAST>
+ Drs. Bhasin & Patel
  1001 West Main Street/Suite A Freehold, NJ 07728 (732)637-8444 Fax (732)637-8440

Patel, Nikhil H., MD {1033472170} InsrMd(12,ANTI)<NJ-COOPRUMC>
+ Cooper University Hospital
  One Cooper Plaza Camden, NJ 08103 (856)342-3150
  nikhil.patel@drexelmed.edu

Patel, Nikunjkumar, MD {1174039309} IntrMd<NJ-COMMED>
+ Community Medical Center
  99 Route 37 West Toms River, NJ 08755 (732)781-6428

Patel, Nilesh J., MD {1821095209} Anesth, CritCr(82,INDI)<NJ-MONMOUTH>
+ Monmouth Medical Center
  300 Second Avenue/Anesthesiology Long Branch, NJ 07740 (732)222-5200

Patel, Nilesh J., MD {1649327826} SrgOrt, SrgFak(97,NJ05)<NJ-JFKMED>
+ Edison-Metuchen Orthopedic Group
  10 Parsonage Road/5th Floor/Suite 500 Edison, NJ 08837 (732)494-6226 Fax (732)494-8762

Patel, Nilesh Narendra, DO {1922133248} EmrgMd(03,PA77)<NJ-STJOSHOS>
+ St Joseph's Medical Center Emergency
  703 Main Street Paterson, NJ 07503 (973)754-2240 Fax (973)754-2249

Patel, Nimesh R., MD {1679625785} Anesth(93,NJ05)<NJ-STBARNMC>
+ St. Barnabas Medical Center
  94 Old Short Hills Road Livingston, NJ 07039 (973)322-5000

Patel, Niraj Ranjit, MD {1659327922} Pedtrc, IntrMd(98,GRN01)
+ Summit Medical Group
  383 Ridgedale Avenue/Suite 8 East Hanover, NJ 07936 (973)887-0200 Fax (973)887-4965
+ EMedical Urgent Care
  369 Springfield Avenue Berkeley Heights, NJ 07922 (973)887-0200 Fax (908)464-1091

Patel, Nirav, MD {1467671388} RadDia(04,NY46)
+ Regional Diagnostic Imaging Center
  1505 West Sherman Avenue Vineland, NJ 08360 (856)641-7937 Fax (856)641-7681

Patel, Nish A., MD {1750677993} Anesth<NJ-NWTNMEM>
+ Newton Medical Center
  175 High Street Newton, NJ 07860 (973)383-2121

Patel, Nitesh M., DO {1639360910} Nephro, IntrMd(05,NJ75)<NJ-OURLADY, NJ-KMHCHRRY>
+ Nephrology & Hypertension Associates of New Jersey
  201 Laurel Oak Road/Suite B Voorhees, NJ 08043 (856)566-5478 Fax (856)566-9561

Patel, Nitin Nick, MD {1831327675} Urolgy(05,NJ05)
+ New Jersey Center for Prostate Cancer & Urology
  255 West Spring Valley Avenue Maywood, NJ 07607 (201)487-8866 Fax (201)487-2602
+ New Jersey Center for Prostate Cancer & Urology
  200 South Orange Avenue/Suite 228 Livingston, NJ 07039 (201)487-8866 Fax (973)322-0135

Patel, Nitin Suresh, MD {1194082800} FamMed
+ Hackensack Meridian Medical Group
  19 Davis Avenue/5th-6th Floor Neptune, NJ 07753 (732)897-3990 Fax (732)897-3997

Patel, Niva S., MD {1689865750} Anesth(00,INA20)<MA-BAYSTMC>
+ Morris Anesthesia Group, PA
  3799 Route 46/Suite 211 Parsippany, NJ 07054 (973)335-1122 Fax (973)335-1448

Patel, Palakkumar Kantilal, MD {1053559427} IntrMd
+ Lifeline Primary Care
  662 Commons Way/Bldg 14 Toms River, NJ 08755 (732)279-3681 Fax (732)279-6043

Patel, Pankaj Ambalal, MD {1346264108} PhysMd(92,INA15)
+ 6 Bujak Court
  Bridgewater, NJ 08807

Patel, Pankajkumar Vasantlal, MD {1982614400} IntrMd(81,INA20)
+ OakTree Patient Care
  1941 Oak Tree Road/Suite 203 Edison, NJ 08820 (732)735-0843 Fax (732)516-1255

Patel, Parag Bhailal, MD {1598738858} IntrMd, CdvDis(97,NJ02)<NJ-SOMERSET, NJ-RWJHLTS>
+ Medicor Cardiology PA
  225 Jackson Street Bridgewater, NJ 08807 (908)526-8668 Fax (908)231-6781
+ Medicor Cardiology PA
  331 US Highway 206/Suite 1A Hillsborough, NJ 08844 (908)526-8668 Fax (908)431-0808

Patel, Parag S., MD {1689571646} FamMed, IntrMd(00,GRN01)<NJ-VIRTMARL>
+ Elmwood Family Physicians
  777 Route 70 East/Suite G-101 Marlton, NJ 08053 (856)983-9939 Fax (856)983-9936
+ Elmwood Family Physicians
  1529 Route 206/Suite L Tabernacle, NJ 08088 (856)983-9939 Fax (609)268-7191

Patel, Parag Vishnu, MD {1073597308} IntCrd
+ Drs. Gupta and Patel
  20 Hospital Drive/Suite 12B Toms River, NJ 08755 (732)240-7777 Fax (732)240-7710

Patel, Parini Munjal, MD {1073780854} IntrMd, EnDbMt(99,INA20)
+ 130 Pendleton Place
  Old Bridge, NJ 08857 (732)654-5539

Patel, Parul, MD {1982803474} Pedtrc
+ 45 East 51st Street
  Bayonne, NJ 07002 (732)947-6414

Patel, Pavan, MD {1760748156} IntrMd
+ University Hospital Medicine
  150 Bergen Street/Room I-248 Newark, NJ 07103 (973)972-6056 Fax (973)972-3129

Patel, Payal, MD {1548551385} NroChl(11,TX04)
+ Child Health Institute of New Jersey
  89 French Street/Suite 2300 New Brunswick, NJ 08901 (732)235-6620 Fax (732)235-8766

Patel, Pinakin C., MD {1083634455} IntrMd(78,INDI)<NJ-KIMBALL, NJ-SOCEANCO>
+ Kimball Medical Center
  600 River Avenue Lakewood, NJ 08701 (732)363-1900

Patel, Pooja, MD {1821228644} IntrMd
+ 188 Market Street
  Perth Amboy, NJ 08861 (732)441-4251 Fax (908)351-6911

Patel, Poorvi K., MD {1538101480} NroChl, Nrolgy, Pedtrc(72,INA69)<NJ-STJOSHOS>
+ St. Joseph's Children's Hospital
703 Main Street/Neurology   Paterson, NJ 07503   (973)754-2528
+ Pediatric Sub Specialty Outpatient Center
186 Rochelle Avenue   Rochelle Park, NJ 07662   (973)754-2528   Fax (201)843-6546

Patel, Prabhaker S., MD {1639242852} Psychy(78,INDI)
+ Drs. Barb & Patel
901 Route 168/Suite 101   Turnersville, NJ 08012   (856)228-7577   Fax (856)228-0534
+ New Point Behavioral Health Care
404 Tatum Street   Woodbury, NJ 08096   (856)228-7577   Fax (856)845-0688

Patel, Pradip M., MD {1194044388} IntrMd(95,DMN01)
+ Federal Correctional Institution
5756 Hartford Road   Fort Dix, NJ 08640   (609)723-1100

Patel, Pradip N., MD {1295814747} FamMed(78,INA2B)
+ 657 Blackwood Clementon Rd
Clementon, NJ 08021   (856)566-8325   Fax (856)566-8326

Patel, Prahlad M., MD {1184705535} IntrMd(81,INA21)<NJ-VIRT-BERL, NJ-KENEDYHS>
+ Crosskeys Medical Center
600 Berlin-Crosskeys Road/Unit 102   Sicklerville, NJ 08081   (856)875-5152   Fax (856)875-0313
+ Atlantic Health Center P.C.
2300 Atlantic Avenue/Suite 1   Atlantic City, NJ 08401   (609)345-9100

Patel, Prakruti, MD {1730121716} EmrgMd(94,MI07)<NJ-LOURDMED>
+ Cooper University Hospital
One Cooper Plaza   Camden, NJ 08103   (856)342-2000
+ Lourdes Medical Center of Burlington County
218 Sunset Road/EmergMed   Willingboro, NJ 08046   (609)835-2900

Patel, Prashant A., MD {1316002553} Anesth, AnesPain, IntrMd(02,NJ05)<NJ-MEADWLND, NJ-STMRYPAS>
+ 205 Ridgedale Avenue/1st Floor
Florham Park, NJ 07932   (973)665-2011   Fax (973)867-3677
+ Advanced Pain Management & Spine Health Center
123 Columbia Turnpike/Suite 102-B   Florham Park, NJ 07932   (973)665-2011   Fax (973)867-3677

Patel, Prashant B., MD {1982806915} PulCCr, SlpDis, IntrMd(02,DMN01)<NJ-HUNTRDN>
+ Respacare
489 Union Avenue   Bridgewater, NJ 08807   (732)356-9950   Fax (732)356-9959
+ Hunterdon Pulmonary & Critical Care Associates
6 Sand Hill Road/Suite 202   Flemington, NJ 08822   (732)356-9950   Fax (908)237-1749

Patel, Pratik B., MD {1851397574} CdvDis, IntCrd, IntrMd(97,NJ05)<NJ-RWJUBRUN, NJ-STPETER>
+ Cardio Metabolic Institute
51 Veronica Avenue   Somerset, NJ 08873   (732)846-7000   Fax (732)846-7001
+ Cardio Metabolic Institute
294 Applegarth Road/Suite F   Monroe Township, NJ 08831   (732)846-7000   Fax (732)846-7001

Patel, Pratik Bharat, MD {1902224942} Otlryg(MA01
+ Coastal Ear Nose and Throat LLC
1301 Route 72/Suite 340   Manahawkin, NJ 08050   (732)280-7855   Fax (732)280-7815

Patel, Pratik Surendra, MD {1952321077} IntrMd, PulDis(02,DMN01)<NJ-NWRKBETH>
+ Newark Beth Israel Medical Center
201 Lyons Avenue/Med/Pulmonary   Newark, NJ 07112   (973)926-7000

Patel, Pravinbhal C., MD {1447227970} IntrMd, PulDis(70,INA21)<NJ-STCLRSUS, NJ-NWTNMEM>
+ Route 94/North Church Prof Center
Franklin, NJ 07416   (973)827-2442   Fax (973)827-2669

Patel, Priti P., MD {1760629273} SrgPlstc(06,NJ06)
+ 2345 Lamington Road/Suite 107
Bedminster, NJ 08921   (908)396-6272   Fax (858)925-1769

Patel, Priti S., MD {1275786444} RadOnc(06,NJ05)<NJ-RIVERVW, NJ-JRSYSHMC>
+ Shore Radiation Oncology, LLC
1 Riverview Plaza   Red Bank, NJ 07701   (732)530-2468   Fax (732)836-4036
+ Shore Radiation Oncology, LLC
425 Jack Martin Boulevard   Brick, NJ 08724   (732)530-2468   Fax (732)836-4036

Patel, Pritiben C., MD {1720469828}
+ St Luke's Hospitalist Group
185 Roseberry Street   Phillipsburg, NJ 08865   (484)526-6643   Fax (484)526-4605

Patel, Priya, MD {1477813830}<NJ-MONMOUTH>
+ Monmouth Medical Center
300 Second Avenue   Long Branch, NJ 07740   (732)923-6795   Fax (732)923-6793

Patel, Priya R., MD {1205098597} ObsGyn
+ The Rubino Ob/Gyn Group
101 Old Short Hills Road/Suite 101   West Orange, NJ 07052   (973)736-1100   Fax (973)736-1834

Patel, Priyesh V., MD {1215108188} RadDia, Radiol, IntrMd(07,IL42)
+ Larchmont Medical Imaging
204-210 Ark Road/LMC 1-2   Mount Laurel, NJ 08054   (856)778-8860   Fax (856)866-8102

Patel, Puja, MD {1629451034} FamMed
+ AMG Primary Care at Totowa
650 Union Boulevard/Unit 16   Totowa, NJ 07512   (973)938-5200   Fax (973)938-5191

Patel, Pulin H., MD {1063535664} IntrMd(93,INA15)<NJ-JFKMED, NJ-RBAYPERT>
+ 22 Meridian Road/Unit 10
Edison, NJ 08820   (732)243-9808   Fax (732)791-5765
pulinpat@gmail.com

Patel, Purvee D., MD {1730310509} FamMed, IntrMd(08,POL10)
+ AFC Urgent Care South Plainfield
907 Oak Tree Avenue/Suite H   South Plainfield, NJ 07080   (908)222-3500

Patel, Radhika K., MD {1346555950} Pedtrc(NJ02
+ East Windsor Pediatric Group
300B Princeton Hightstown/Suite 201   Hightstown, NJ 08520   (609)448-7300   Fax (609)448-8022

Patel, Ragin C., MD {1013149277} ObsGyn, Obstet
+ Drs. Desai and Patel
2177 Oak Tree Road/Suite 205   Edison, NJ 08820   (732)549-3700   Fax (732)549-3203

Patel, Rahil, MD {1811023880} FamMed(01,NET12)<NJ-JFKMED, NJ-OVERLOOK>
+ 98 James Street/Suite 105
Edison, NJ 08820   (732)548-0040   Fax (732)548-0042
Rahilpatel@hotmail.com
+ Rutgers- New Jersey Medical School
185 South Orange Avenue/Family Med   Newark, NJ 07103   (973)972-4300

Patel, Rahul, MD {1871956508} RadDia
+ University Radiology Group, P.C.
483 Cranbury Road   East Brunswick, NJ 08816   (327)390-0030   Fax (732)390-5383

Patel, Raj, MD {1457710980} InfDis
+ 701 Stuyvesant Avenue
Irvington, NJ 07111   (973)372-1828

Patel, Rajankuma Popatlal, MD {1396896023} Grtrcs, FamMed, FamMGrtc(93,INA15)<NJ-UMDNJ>
+ Dr. Patel and Associates
1910 Marlton Pike East/Suite 6   Cherry Hill, NJ 08003   (856)751-4831   Fax (856)751-2131

Patel, Rajendra B., MD {1912961947} CdvDis, IntrMd(85,INA21)<NJ-OURLADY, NJ-VIRTVOOR>
+ 320 Route 73
Voorhees, NJ 08043   (856)335-4118   Fax (856)809-2594

Patel, Rajendra Harmanbhai, MD {1649357633} IntrMd, IntCrd, CdvDis(87,INA21)<NJ-RWJUBRUN>
+ 1804 Oak Tree Road/Suite 3
Edison, NJ 08820   (732)494-1991   Fax (732)767-2826

Patel, Rajendra K., MD {1144393950} EmrgMd, IntrMd(74,INDI)<NJ-JRSYSHMC>
+ EmCare
1945 Route 33   Neptune, NJ 07753   (732)776-4510   Fax (732)776-2329

Patel, Rajendrakumar Chimanlal, MD {1265792444} IntHos
+ Drs. Patel and Patel
31 West Somerset Street   Raritan, NJ 08869   (908)722-0035   Fax (908)722-6763

Patel, Rajesh Ishwar, MD {1023125531} RadDia, Radiol(95,PA09)<NY-SLRRSVLT, NJ-ACMCITY>
+ Atlantic Medical Imaging, LLC.
72 West Jimmie Leeds Road   Galloway, NJ 08205   (609)677-9729   Fax (609)653-8764
+ Atlantic Medical Imaging, LLC.
401 Bethel Road   Somers Point, NJ 08244   (609)677-9729
+ Atlantic Medical Imaging, LLC.
421 Route 9 North   Cape May Court House, NJ 08205   (609)463-9500   Fax (609)465-0918

Patel, Rajesh Manharbhai, MD {1003908005} Psychy, PsyAdd(90,INA20)
+ 1466 Ratzer Road
Wayne, NJ 07470

Patel, Rajesh T., DO {1851585863} FamMed(05,NJ75)
+ Family Doctors Associates, Inc.
1416 Park Avenue   Plainfield, NJ 07060   (908)757-6363   Fax (908)754-6807

Patel, Rajiv Arvind, MD {1063434314} IntrMd, CdvDis(96,IN20)
+ 73 Danville Drive
Princeton Junction, NJ 08550

Patel, Rajiv J., DO {1134311756} CdvDis, IntrMd(04,NJ75)
+ Cardiologist & Intrnest Associates
211 Essex Street/Suite 104   Hackensack, NJ 07601   (201)489-3888   Fax (201)301-7351

Patel, Rakesh Bhogilal, MD {1457312589} Otlryg, SrgFPl, SrgRec(95,NJ05)<NJ-HACKNSK>
+ Princeton Eye and Ear
2999 Princeton Pike/2 FL   Lawrenceville, NJ 08648   (609)403-8840   Fax (609)403-8852
+ Princeton Eye and Ear
5 Plainsboro Road/Suite 510   Plainsboro, NJ 08536   (609)403-8840   Fax (609)403-8852
+ 1 West Ridgewood Avenue/Suite 106
Paramus, NJ 08648   (201)445-9915   Fax (201)445-9916

Patel, Rakhee, MD {1124316336} ObsGyn
+ Hudson Digestive Health Center
534 Avenue E/Suite A   Bayonne, NJ 07002   (201)858-8444   Fax (201)858-4260

Patel, Rambhai C., MD {1083790729} IntrMd(70,INDI)<NJ-TRININPC>
+ 224 East Jersey Street
Elizabeth, NJ 07206   (908)351-2442   Fax (908)355-6095
Rambhai@aol.com
+ 182 Ferry Street
Newark, NJ 07104   (908)351-2442   Fax (908)355-6093

Patel, Ramesh L., MD {1437245354} IntrMd(68,INDI)<NJ-EASTORNG>
+ 707 South Orange Avenue
South Orange, NJ 07079   (973)761-6111   Fax (973)761-4990

Patel, Ramiladevi S., MD {1194760447} IntrMd(80,INDI)<NJ-CHRIST>
+ PMA Physicians LLC
1 Journal Square Plaza/2nd Floor   Jersey City, NJ 07306   (201)216-3030   Fax (201)499-0247

Patel, Rasiklal A., MD {1386702181} IntrMd(72,INA2B)<NJ-NWRKBETH, NJ-EASTORNG>
+ 2 Smalley Terrace
Irvington, NJ 07111   (973)371-2543   Fax (973)371-4404

Patel, Ravindra I., MD {1962428169} CdvDis, ClcdEl, Grtrcs(79,INDI)<NJ-BAYSHORE>
+ Associates in Cardiology and Internal Medicine
530 Green Street   Iselin, NJ 08830   (732)283-9473   Fax (732)283-8943
+ Medical Associates of Marlboro
42 Throckmorton Lane/2nd flr   Old Bridge, NJ 08857   (732)283-9473   Fax (732)607-9306

Patel, Ravish Mukesh, MD {1194084756} FamMed
+ Abhijit Chatterjee MD PC
312 Applegarth Road/Suite 207   Monroe Township, NJ 08831   (609)655-2700   Fax (609)655-2565

Patel, Reema Arpit, MD {1346546462}<NJ-RBAYOLDB>
+ Raritan Bay Medical Center/Old Bridge Division
One Hospital Plaza   Old Bridge, NJ 08857   (732)360-1000

Patel, Rekha Arvind, MD {1245255496} Pedtrc, AdolMd(70,INDI)
+ 250 Stelton Road/Suite 4
Piscataway, NJ 08854   (732)752-6633   Fax (732)752-6609

Patel, Rikin Jagdish, DO {1588680359} PhyMPain, PainMd(02,NY75)
+ Mercer-Bucks Orthopaedics PC
3120 Princeton Pike   Lawrenceville, NJ 08648   (609)896-0444   Fax (609)896-1055
+ Mercer-Bucks Orthopaedics, P.C.
2501 Kuser Road   Hamilton, NJ 08691   (609)896-0444   Fax (609)587-4349

Patel, Rima Dipak, MD {1336302447} CdvDis
+ 2218 Broadway/Suite 101
Fair Lawn, NJ 07410   (201)773-0887

Patel, Rita S., MD {1760467674} Radiol, RadNro(92,NY03)<NJ-HACKNSK>
+ The Imaging Center
30 South Newman Street   Hackensack, NJ 07601   (201)488-1188   Fax (201)488-5244
+ New Century Imaging at Oradell
555 Kinderkamack Road   Oradell, NJ 07649   (201)488-1188   Fax (201)599-8333
+ Hackensack Radiology Group, P.A.
30 Prospect Avenue   Hackensack, NJ 07601   (201)996-2200   Fax (201)336-8451

Patel, Ritesh, MD {1356575120} IntrMd(05,INA15)<NJ-COOPRUMC>
+ Cooper University Hospital
One Cooper Plaza/Hospitalist   Camden, NJ 08103   (856)342-3150   Fax (856)968-8418

Patel, Robert Balvant, MD {1275528747} IntrMd(01,GRN01)<NJ-RWJUBRUN>
+ 1 Beekman Road
Kendall Park, NJ 08824

Patel, Rohit Amratlal, MD {1356507727} Surgry, IntrMd(01,INA3D)<NJ-COOPRUMC>
+ Cooper Surgical Associates
3 Cooper Plaza/Suite 403   Camden, NJ 08103   (856)342-2384   Fax (856)541-5379
+ Cooper Surgical Associates
6017 Main Street   Voorhees, NJ 08043   (856)325-6516

Physicians by Name and Address

Patel, Ronak Dilip, MD {1114273893} AnesPain
 + 666 Plainsboro Road/Suite 100
  Plainsboro, NJ 08536 (609)269-4451

Patel, Roshni Dinesh, DO {1932529260} ObsGyn
 + Portside Medical
  150 Warren Street/Suite 118 Jersey City, NJ 07302
  (201)858-8444 Fax (201)309-1300

Patel, Roshni Vinu, MD {1548280571} Pedtrc
 + 571 West Mount Pleasant Avenue
  Livingston, NJ 07039

Patel, Ruchir, MD {1245506625} IntCrd<NJ-HACKNSK>
 + Hackensack University Medical Center
  30 Prospect Avenue Hackensack, NJ 07601 (713)828-3591

Patel, Rupa, MD {1366555450} Urolgy(98,MA05)<NJ-RBAYOLDB, NJ-RBAYPERT>
 + Premier Urology Group, LLC
  10 Parsonage Road/Suite 118 Edison, NJ 08837 (732)494-9400 Fax (732)548-3931
 + Premier Urology Group, LLC
  570 South Avenue East/Building A Cranford, NJ 07016
  (732)494-9400 Fax (908)497-1633
 + Premier Urology Group, LLC
  2 Hospital Plaza/Suite 430 Old Bridge, NJ 08837
  (732)494-9400 Fax (732)679-2077

Patel, Rupert Chandrakant, MD {1063670917} FamMed, IntrMd(05,DMN01)<OH-FHNRTHSD>
 + 524 Bencer Court
  Raritan, NJ 08869 (930)501-4400

Patel, Sachin S., MD {1285024935} IntrMd<NJ-RWJUBRUN>
 + RWJ University Hospital New Brunswick
  One Robert Wood Johnson Place New Brunswick, NJ 08901
  (732)235-8909

Patel, Sagar Y., MD {1649430844} ObsGyn(04,NJ06)<NJ-RIVERVW, NJ-JRSYSHMC>
 + Sagar Y. Patel M.D., F.A.C.O.G.
  100 Commons Way/Suite 260 Holmdel, NJ 07733
  (732)217-3236 Fax (732)217-3327
  sagmd@yahoo.com

Patel, Sameer Ramesh, MD {1063469401} Psychy, Grtrcs(99,MNT01)
 + Mid Atlantic Geriatric Associates
  1205 Route 35 North Ocean, NJ 07712 (732)663-0099
  Fax (732)663-1359

Patel, Samir G., MD {1588659296} IntrMd, EmrgMd(90,INA21)<NJ-RBAYOLDB, NJ-RBAYPERT>
 + 2 American Way/Suite 3
  Spotswood, NJ 08884 (732)416-0065
 + Raritan Bay Medical Center/Old Bridge Division
  One Hospital Plaza Old Bridge, NJ 08857 (732)360-1000

Patel, Samir M., MD {1124058698} Surgry(97,NY46)<NJ-ACMC-MAIN>
 + Salartash Surgical Associates, LLC.
  72 West Jimmie Leeds Road/Suite 1600 Galloway, NJ 08205
  (609)926-5000 Fax (609)926-2020

Patel, Samir Natavar, MD {1649448317} Anesth(04,NY48)<NJ-ENGLWOOD>
 + Anesthesia Consultnts of NJ/Nova Pain
  285 Davidson Avenue/Suite 204 Somerset, NJ 08873
  (732)271-1400 Fax (732)271-3543
 + Englewood Hospital and Medical Center
  350 Engle Street/Anesth Englewood, NJ 07631 (732)271-1400 Fax (201)894-0585
 + Englewood Anesthesiology
  350 Engle Street Englewood, NJ 08873 (201)894-3238
  Fax (201)894-0585

Patel, Samir Popatlal, MD {1407954548} SrgOrt, IntrMd(99,DMN01)<NJ-OVERLOOK, NJ-MORRISTN>
 + Berkeley Internal Medicine
  391 Springfield Avenue/Suite 1B Berkeley Heights, NJ 07922 (908)665-1177 Fax (908)665-8420

Patel, Sandipkumar R., MD {1316225659} IntrMd(INA8B)
 + Shore Medical Specialists
  500 River Avenue/Suite 140 Lakewood, NJ 08701
  (732)363-7200 Fax (732)367-4461

Patel, Sanjeev N., MD {1194803361} IntrMd, CdvDis, CarEch(93,NJ05)
 + The Heart Care Center
  38 Mayhill Street/Suite 1 Saddle Brook, NJ 07663
  (201)843-1019 Fax (201)843-5910

Patel, Sanjiv C., MD {1720113962} FamMed(91,PA02)<NJ-VIRTMHBC>
 + Primary Care of Moorestown
  147 East 3rd Street/Suite 2 Moorestown, NJ 08057
  (856)234-2500 Fax (856)234-3907

Patel, Satishkumar H., MD {1861544405} Psychy(96,INA20)<NJ-UNIVBHC>
 + 35 Beaverson Boulevard/Building 1-D
  Brick, NJ 08723
 + University Behavioral Health Care
  671 Hoes Lane/PO Box 1392/Psych Piscataway, NJ 08855

(732)235-5500

Patel, Saurabh Chandrakant, MD {1790795227} IntrMd(96,DMN01)
 + Universal Industrial Clinic
  99 Madison Street Newark, NJ 07105 (973)344-2929
  Fax (973)344-1239

Patel, Shail, MD {1669887279} Anesth(NJ05<MA-MAGENHOS>
 + JFK Medical Center
  65 James Street/Anesthesiology Edison, NJ 08820
  (732)321-7000

Patel, Shailja, MD {1215272695}<NJ-COOPRUMC>
 + Cooper University Hospital
  One Cooper Plaza Camden, NJ 08103 (856)342-2000

Patel, Shalini Narendra, MD {1104989219} NnPnMd(98,DOM18)<NJ-NWRKBETH>
 + Newark Beth Israel Medical Center
  201 Lyons Avenue/Neontlgy Newark, NJ 07112 (973)926-7000

Patel, Shamik D., DO {1538353206} FamMed
 + Summit Medical Group
  202 Elmer Street Westfield, NJ 07090 (908)228-3675
  Fax (908)654-1053
 + 574 Winchester Avenue
  Union, NJ 07083 (908)451-2856

Patel, Sharad D., MD {1093943631} IntrMd<NJ-COOPRUMC>
 + Cooper University Hospital
  One Cooper Plaza Camden, NJ 08103 (856)342-2000

Patel, Shashikant A., MD {1578555009} RadDia(66,INDI)<NJ-STMICHL>
 + St. Michael's Medical Center
  268 MLK Jr. Boulevard Newark, NJ 07102 (973)877-5287
  Fax (973)877-5275

Patel, Sheenal V., MD {1376806992} AlgyImmn
 + Drs. Boguszz & Weiss
  44 State Route 23 North/Suite 6 Riverdale, NJ 07457
  (973)248-9199 Fax (973)248-9299

Patel, Sheetal V., MD {1316258122} Rheuma, IntrMd<NJ-HACKNSK>
 + Institute for Rheumatic & Autoimmune Diseases
  33 Overlook Road/MAC L01 Summit, NJ 07901 (908)598-7940 Fax (908)598-5447

Patel, Shefali S., MD {1982694857} IntrMd(89,INA20)
 + 1804 Oak Tree Road/Suite 3
  Edison, NJ 08820 (732)494-0080 Fax (732)494-8880

Patel, Shilpa Ashok, MD {1649367129} Pedtrc(95,OH44)<NJ-VALLEY, NJ-HACKNSK>
 + Northern Valley Pediatrics, LLC.
  22 Paris Avenue/Suite 109 Rockleigh, NJ 07647 (201)564-7377 Fax (201)564-7379

Patel, Shital, MD {1467698944} IntrMd(97,NY47)
 + 3 Rivers Edge Drive
  Colts Neck, NJ 07722

Patel, Shivangi, MD {1659568699} IntrMd(04,GRN01)
 + Acute Rehab Unit / Med Ctr Princeton
  One Plainsboro Road/2nd Floor Plainsboro, NJ 08536
  (609)853-7800
 + Intensivists of Toms River, LLC.
  99 Route 37 Toms River, NJ 08755 (609)853-7800 Fax (732)557-8021

Patel, Shivani J., MD {1760761159} Pedtrc(10,GRN01)
 + Notchview Pediatrics, LLC.
  1037 Route 46 East/Suite 201 Clifton, NJ 07013 (973)779-3911 Fax (973)471-2730

Patel, Shodhan J., MD {1457368680} IntrMd(92,INDI)<NJ-CHSFULD, NJ-RWJUHAM>
 + Akshar Medical Group
  1450 Parkside Avenue/Suite 5 Trenton, NJ 08638
  (609)771-1881 Fax (609)538-0177

Patel, Shreya Nalin, MD {1386078814} IntrMd<NJ-MORRISTN>
 + Morristown Medical Center
  100 Madison Avenue Morristown, NJ 07962 (973)971-0126

Patel, Shruti, MD {1952746133} IntrMd
 + My MD Group
  201 North County Line Road Jackson, NJ 08527 (732)901-8880 Fax (732)901-0882

Patel, Sima, MD {1972969350} EnDbMt<NJ-STPETER>
 + St. Peter's Physicians Associates
  1636 Stelton Road/Suite 301 Piscataway, NJ 08854
  (732)339-7575
 + St. Peter's University Hospital
  254 Easton Avenue New Brunswick, NJ 08901 (732)745-8600

Patel, Sizan B., MD {1043655368}<NJ-MONMOUTH>
 + Monmouth Medical Center
  300 Second Avenue Long Branch, NJ 07740 (732)923-6537 Fax (732)923-6536

Patel, Sruti, MD {1750600888} Surgry
 + North Jersey Surgical Specialists
  83 Summit Avenue Hackensack, NJ 07601 (201)646-0010
  Fax (201)646-0600

Patel, Suhas Ramesh, MD {1104844778} IntrMd, Grtrcs(97,DMN01)<NJ-JRSYSHMC, NJ-OCEANMC>
 + Mid Atlantic Geriatric Associates
  1205 Route 35 North Ocean, NJ 07712 (732)663-0099
  Fax (732)663-1359

Patel, Sujal P., MD {1467748301} SrgSpn
 + Oasis Medical and Wellness
  85 Harristown Road/Suite 103 Glen Rock, NJ 07452
  (844)366-8800 Fax (844)366-8900

Patel, Sundip N., MD {1932302635} EmrgMd
 + 132 Wyndmere Road
  Marlton, NJ 08053

Patel, Sunil, MD {1134256936}
 + Prime Heart
  40 Union Avenue/Suite 101 Irvington, NJ 07111
  (973)371-3166

Patel, Sunil Madhusuda, MD {1255354726} CdvDis, CarNuc, IntrMd(94,INA8B)<NJ-TRINIWSC, NJ-JFKMED>
 + Prime Heart
  40 Union Avenue/Suite 101 Irvington, NJ 07111
  (973)371-3166

Patel, Suresh Ishwarlal, MD {1275583130} Pedtrc(80,INDI)
 + 34-36 Progress Street/Suite A1
  Edison, NJ 08820 (908)561-5700 Fax (908)561-5840

Patel, Sureshbhai N., MD {1396785796} IntrMd(80,INA20)<NJ-HACKNSK>
 + 544 Salem Street
  Paramus, NJ 07652

Patel, Swati Hasmukh, MD {1376855908} IntrMd(07,GRN01)<NJ-VIRTMHBC>
 + Hospitalist Group
  175 Madison Avenue Mount Holly, NJ 08060 (609)267-0700

Patel, Taral B., DO {1750743472} Anesth
 + Morris Anesthesia Group, PA
  3799 Route 46/Suite 211 Parsippany, NJ 07054 (973)335-1122 Fax (973)335-1448

Patel, Trupti, MD {1780610667} Pedtrc, GenPrc(01,NJ05)
 + Somerset Pediatric Group PA
  2 World's Fair Drive/Suite 302 Somerset, NJ 08873
  (908)271-7788 Fax (732)271-5151
 + Somerset Pediatric Group PA
  155 Union Avenue Bridgewater, NJ 08807 (908)271-7788
  Fax (908)203-8825

Patel, Tushar R., MD {1205966462} SrgPlstc, Surgry(99,NJ06)
 + The Plastic Surgery Ctr of NJ & Manhat
  535 Sycamore Avenue Shrewsbury, NJ 07702 (732)741-0970 Fax (732)747-2606

Patel, Unnati D., MD {1558523597} Psychy(05,GRN01)
 + Somerset Medical Center Psychiatry
  110 Rehill Avenue Somerville, NJ 08876 (908)685-2200
  Fax (908)231-6144

Patel, Urvish, MD {1750791166} IntHos<NJ-COOPRUMC>
 + Cooper University Hospital
  One Cooper Plaza Camden, NJ 08103 (856)356-4924

Patel, Ushma K., MD {1639378177} ObsGyn(03,NJ06)
 + 8 Farmington Drive
  Marlton, NJ 08053

Patel, Vanita Hitesh, MD {1053502229} ObsGyn(99,INA8B)
 + Atlantic Ob/Gyn Associates
  1631 Route 88 West/Suite A Brick, NJ 08724 (732)202-7458 Fax (732)202-7459

Patel, Varshaben T., MD {1770795207} Pedtrc(98,INA21)
 + 275 Baldwin Road/Suite 101
  Parsippany, NJ 07054 (973)335-1150

Patel, Vijay Ramanikbhai, MD {1922045590} IntrMd(92,INA21)<NJ-RBAYOLDB, NJ-RBAYPERT>
 + 72 State Route 34
  Old Bridge, NJ 08857 (732)952-3800 Fax (732)753-9819

Patel, Vimal Dahya, MD {1932360617} IntrMd(05,NJ05)<NJ-UNVMCPRN>
 + Rutgers Cancer Institute of New Jersey
  195 Little Albany Street/PO Box 2681 New Brunswick, NJ 08903 (732)235-2465 Fax (732)235-6797
 + University Medical Center of Princeton at Plainsboro
  One Plainsboro Road/IntMed Plainsboro, NJ 08536
  (609)497-4000

Patel, Vineshkumar K., MD {1730112632} IntrMd, CdvDis(94,NJ06)<NJ-JRSYSHMC>
 + Atlantic Cardiology in Galloway
  436 Chris Gaupp Drive/Suite 204 Galloway, NJ 08205
  (609)652-0100 Fax (609)652-7616
 + Atlantic Cardiology in Ventor
  6725 Atlantic Avenue/2nd Floor Ventnor, NJ 08406
  (609)822-2006

Patel, Vinodkumar G., MD {1326142597} CdvDis, IntrMd(79,INDI)
 + Drs. Patel & Patel
  237 Central Avenue Jersey City, NJ 07307 (201)798-1616
  Fax (201)656-8676

Patel, Viral D., MD {1760758114} FamMed(11,GCY01)
+ MedExpress Urgent Care Hamilton Square
811 Route 33   Hamilton, NJ 08619   (609)587-8298   Fax (609)587-8570

Patel, Virendra, MD {1508807082} CdvDis, IntrMd(98,GRN01)<NJ-JRSYSHMC, NJ-OCEANMC>
+ Coastal Cardiovascular Consultants, PA
459 Jack Martin Boulevard/Suite 4   Brick, NJ 08724   (732)458-6200   Fax (732)458-9464

Patel, Vishal V., MD {1093781957} FamMed(96,GRN01)<NJ-VALLEY>
+ Firstmed Family HealthCare LLC
637 Route 23 South   Pompton Plains, NJ 07444   (973)859-7277   Fax (862)666-9215
+ Northern Valley Medical Weight Loss Center LLC
244 Livingston Street   Northvale, NJ 07647   Fax (201)768-4569

Patel, Vrunda, MD {1871648014} ObsGyn(85,NY15)<NJ-UNVMCPRN>
+ Princeton Medical Group, P.A.
419 North Harrison Street   Princeton, NJ 08540   (609)924-9300   Fax (609)924-6552

Patel, Yashvantkumar S., MD {1619956687} NnPnMd<NJ-OURLADY>
+ Our Lady of Lourdes Medical Center
1600 Haddon Avenue/Neontlgy   Camden, NJ 08103   (856)757-3500

Patel, Yogesh N., MD {1407110828} IntrMd<NJ-ACMCITY>
+ AtlantiCare Regional Medical Center/City Campus
1925 Pacific Avenue   Atlantic City, NJ 08401   (609)441-8146   Fax (609)441-8002

Patel, Zankhana M., MD {1750642211} ObsGyn
+ Palisades Women's Group
6045 Kennedy Boulevard/Suite B   North Bergen, NJ 07047   (201)868-2630   Fax (201)868-4919

Patel-Cohen, Mital, MD {1619119583} Dermat(09,NY08)
+ Summit Medical Group Florham Park Campus
150 Park Avenue   Florham Park, NJ 07932   (908)273-4300

Patel-Shusterman, Shefali Natavar, MD {1427146596} ObsGyn(99,NY47)<NJ-ENGLWOOD>
+ Englewood Ob/Gyn Associates
370 Grand Avenue   Englewood, NJ 07631   (201)894-9599   Fax (201)894-9192

Paterno, Flavio, MD {1760666507}
+ Liver Transplant & Hepatobiliary Diseases/UMDNJ
140 Bergen Street/ACC Bldg   Newark, NJ 07101   (973)972-7218

Paterno, Jeanette D., MD {1437121068} FamMed(94,NJ06)<NJ-HCKTSTWN, NJ-NWTNMEM>
+ North Warren Medical Associates PC
Route 517/Building B   Hackettstown, NJ 07840   (908)852-0107   Fax (908)850-9160
+ North Warren Medical Associates
155 State Highway 94   Blairstown, NJ 07825   (908)852-0107   Fax (908)362-6984

Paterson, William D., MD {1457386419} Anesth(82,PA02)<NJ-KMHSTRAT>
+ Rancocas Anesthesiology, PA
700 Route 130 North/Suite 203   Cinnaminson, NJ 08077   (856)829-9345   Fax (856)829-3605

Patestos, Chris Anastasios, MD {1780672832} Pedtrc(96,NJ06)
+ Silverton Pediatrics
2446 Church Road   Toms River, NJ 08753   (732)255-7553   Fax (732)255-8901

Pathak, Kunja J., MD {1841330933} ObsGyn(63,INA20)
+ 17 Darkwood Court
Warren, NJ 07059

Pathak, Pinakin J., MD {1679540819} IntrMd(85,INDI)<NJ-STCLRDOV>
+ 400 South Main Street
Wharton, NJ 07885   (973)366-1223

Pathak, Rajiv J., MD {1265528111} IntrMd(83,INA2B)
+ Medical Associates Mount Olive
230 US Route 206/Buildingg 2/Unit 5   Flanders, NJ 07836   (973)584-9669   Fax (973)584-8729

Pathak, Sankalp, MD {1316388234}<NJ-MORRISTN>
+ Morristown Medical Center
100 Madison Avenue   Morristown, NJ 07962   (973)971-5000

Pathak, Sonal, MD {1801020524} EnDbMt, IntrMd
+ Palisades Women's Group
6045 Kennedy Boulevard/Suite B   North Bergen, NJ 07047   (201)453-0322   Fax (201)453-0325

Pathak, Vineeta Jha, MD {1104922939} Pedtrc, PubHth(90,INA3C)<NJ-COMMED, NJ-OCEANMC>
+ 515 Lakehurst Road
Toms River, NJ 08755   (732)244-4416   Fax (732)244-4418

Patharkar, Milind D., MD {1114113891} Anesth, PainMd(01,DMN01)
+ ASAP - Advanced Spine and Pain
1051 West Sherman Avenue   Vineland, NJ 08360   Fax (856)691-0224

+ ASAP - Advanced Spine and Pain
3829 Church Road/Suite B   Mount Laurel, NJ 08054   Fax (856)787-1901

Patil, Kishor K., MD {1487741062} Nrolgy, FamMed(85,INA00)
+ Eastern Neurodiagnostic Associates
2301 Evesham Road/Pav 800/Suite 209   Voorhees, NJ 08043   (856)651-0060   Fax (856)651-0061

Patil, Madhavi Hari, MD {1831399179} PthACl<NJ-JFKMED>
+ JFK Medical Center
65 James Street/Pathlgy   Edison, NJ 08820   (732)321-7680   Fax (732)321-7008

Patil, Meenal Kulkarni, MD {1871640664} AnesPain
+ Reconstructive Orthopedics, P.A.
401 Young Avenue/Suite 245   Moorestown, NJ 08057   (609)267-9400   Fax (609)267-9457
+ The Pain Management Center at Hamilton
2271 Highway 33/Suite 103   Hamilton, NJ 08690   (609)267-9400   Fax (609)890-4090

Patil, Pooja Mittal, MD {1235371865} EmrgMd, IntrMd(05,NY46)<NJ-STPETER>
+ St. Peter's University Hospital
254 Easton Avenue/Emerg Med   New Brunswick, NJ 08901   (732)745-8600

Patil, Sandhya R., MD {1801832183} IntrMd(85,INA69)<NJ-JRSYSHMC, NJ-COMMED>
+ Ace Medical
20 Hospital Drive/Suite 9   Toms River, NJ 08755   (732)914-9955

Patil, Vivek Vinay, MD {1144456484} RadV&I(09,DC01)
+ Freehold Radiology Group
901 West Main Street   Freehold, NJ 07728   (732)462-3302   Fax (732)780-6213

Patil, Vrishali Swanand, MD {1235380767} IntrMd(02,INA3B)
+ IPC The Hospitalist Company
55 Madison Avenue/Suite 310   Morristown, NJ 07960   (973)993-9536   Fax (973)998-4237

Patitucci, Robert S., MD {1902807480} FamMed(82,MEX14)
+ 70 Cornwell Drive
Bridgeton, NJ 08302   (856)455-6770   Fax (856)455-6030

Patnaik, Asit, MD {1831280650} IntrMd
+ 610 Creek Road
Moorestown, NJ 08057
+ Stawicki & Patnaik Medical Associates
1235 Whitehorse Mercerville Rd   Mercerville, NJ 08619   (609)581-5779

Patragnoni, Richard M., DO {1972342422} FamMed(71,IA75)<NJ-VIRTMHBC, NJ-VIRTBERL>
+ Virtua Family Medicine
103 Old Marlton Pike/Suite 103   Medford, NJ 08055   (609)953-7105   Fax (609)953-0042
+ Alliance for Better Care, P.C.
PO Box 1510   Medford, NJ 08055   (609)953-7105   Fax (609)953-8652

Patrawalla, Amee Shirish, MD {1427277821} PulDis, CritCr, IntrMd(00,NY47)<NJ-UMDNJ>
+ University Hospital
150 Bergen Street/Pulm Crtcl Care   Newark, NJ 07103   (973)972-4300

Patrawalla, Shirish C., MD {1245346188} CdvDis, IntrMd(65,INA69)<NJ-STBARNMC, NJ-NWRKBETH>
+ Patrawalla M.D., PA
96 Millburn Avenue/Suite 203   Millburn, NJ 07041   (973)763-4120   Fax (973)763-1713
Patrawalla1@netzero.com

Patricelli, John E., MD {1265498307} Surgry(77,MEX14)<NJ-MEMSALEM>
+ 1 Pointer-Auburn Road
Salem, NJ 08079   (856)935-2424   Fax (856)935-7712

Patrick, Bryan L., MD {1629234653} EmrgMd(87,PA09)<NJ-OCEANMC>
+ 1213 Hemlock Avenue
Sea Girt, NJ 08750

Patrone, Nicole, MD {1417343179} FamMed
+ Summit Medical Group-Berkeley Heights Campus
1 Diamond Hill Road   Berkeley Heights, NJ 07922   (908)273-4300   Fax (908)790-6576

Patrusky, Karen Lynn, MD {1053370262} ObsGyn(93,NY47)<NJ-ENGLWOOD>
+ Comprehensive Women's Care
401A South Van Brunt Street/Suite 405   Englewood, NJ 07631   (201)871-4346   Fax (201)871-5953

Patsis, Michael C., MD {1447312137} SrgPlstc(88,NH01)<NJ-CHILTON, NJ-NWTNMEM>
+ 70 Sparta Avenue/Suite 105
Sparta, NJ 07871   (973)726-4250   Fax (973)726-4260

Pattathil, Jean Catherine, MD {1124103874} IntrMd(96,INA77)
+ William J. McHugh MD PA
240 Williamson Street/Suite 204   Elizabeth, NJ 07202   (908)355-8877   Fax (908)355-0017

Patten-Kline, Nancy H., DO {1295955896} Psychy
+ 304 Newton Avenue/1 FL
Oaklyn, NJ 08107

Patterson, Francis Robert, MD {1477587749} Ortped, SrgOrt(93,NY06)<NJ-HACKNSK, NJ-RWJUBRUN>
+ North Jersey Orthopaedic Institute
90 Bergen Street/DOC 1200   Newark, NJ 07101   (973)972-2153   Fax (973)972-9367
+ North Jersey Orthopedic Institute
20 Prospect Avenue/Suite 901   Hackensack, NJ 07601   (973)972-2153   Fax (201)820-1661
+ University Hospital-Doctors Office Center
90 Bergen Street/Ste 5200   Newark, NJ 07101   (973)972-2500

Patterson, George A., MD {1457368623} FamMed(76,NJ05)
+ 1338 How Lane/Suite 4
North Brunswick, NJ 08902   (732)354-4162   Fax (732)354-3006
drgap1@aol.com

Patterson, Marion Lesley, MD {1194878991} FamMed(96,NJ06)
+ Ocean Health Initiatives, Inc.
101 Second Street   Lakewood, NJ 08701   (732)363-6655   Fax (732)901-0277

Patterson, Raymond Kevin, MD {1336320852} Anesth
+ 112 Sarah Drive
Mickleton, NJ 08056

Patti, James E., MD {1336296441} Ortped, SrgOrt(92,PA12)<NJ-JFKMED>
+ Edison-Metuchen Orthopedic Group
10 Parsonage Road/5th Floor/Suite 500   Edison, NJ 08837   (732)494-6226   Fax (732)494-8762

Patti, Laryssa A., MD {1376909788} EmrgMd
+ Laryssa Patti MD
575 Easton Avenue/Apt 14F   Somerset, NJ 08873   (973)896-8732
+ RWJ University Hospital New Brunswick
One Robert Wood Johnson Place   New Brunswick, NJ 08901   (732)235-8717

Pattner, Austin M., MD {1639150840} IntrMd, Nephro(66,NY15)<NJ-ENGLWOOD, NJ-PALISADE>
+ Drs. Pattner, Grodstein, Fein & Davis
177 North Dean Street/Suite 207   Englewood, NJ 07631   (201)567-0446   Fax (201)567-8775
+ Drs. Pattner, Grodstein, Fein & Davis
8100 Kennedy Boulevard   North Bergen, NJ 07047   (201)868-5905

Patton, Chandler D., MD {1285604868} IntrMd, PulDis, CritCr(85,PA09)<NJ-JRSYSHMC>
+ Monmouth Pulmonary Consultants
30 Corbett Way   Eatontown, NJ 07724   (732)380-0020   Fax (732)380-1990

Patton, Virginia A., MD {1811977234} Anesth(86,NJ05)<NJ-MTNSIDE>
+ 507 New York Boulevard
Sea Girt, NJ 08750

Patwa, Amy Shah, MD {1457512956} EmrgMd
+ Morristown Medical Center Emergency Medicine
100 Madison Avenue   Morristown, NJ 07960   (973)971-8919

Pauch-McNamara, Dorothy Anne, MD {1942294160} FamMed(01,PA02)
+ Hunterdon Family Medicine
1100 Wescott Drive/Suite 101   Flemington, NJ 08822   (908)788-6535   Fax (908)788-6536

Paul, Benoy Krishna, MD {1942366539} Anesth(76,BAN07)<NJ-MEMSALEM>
+ Rancocas Anesthesiology, PA
218 Sunset Road   Willingboro, NJ 08046   (609)835-3069   Fax (609)835-5450

Paul, Karel Joseph, MD {1235225525} IntrMd(97,INA98)<NJ-LOURDMED>
+ Lourdes Medical Center of Burlington County
218 Sunset Road/Suite A/Internal Med   Willingboro, NJ 08046   (609)835-3056   Fax (856)835-3061

Paul, Michael Joseph, DO {1770528754} PhysMd, PainInvt(01,PA77)
+ Coastal Spine
4000 Church Road   Mount Laurel, NJ 08054   (856)222-4444   Fax (856)222-0049

Paul, Sindy M., MD   PubHth, GPrvMd(83,PA13)
+ New Jersey Department of Health and Senior Services
50 East State/PO Box 360/AIDS Prevnt   Trenton, NJ 08625   (609)292-9354   Fax (609)292-6523

Paul, Stephen E., DO {1629075759} FamMed(70,PA77)<NJ-KMHCHRRY, NJ-OURLADY>
+ 111 East Main Street
Maple Shade, NJ 08052   (856)779-9220   Fax (856)779-7890
sepaul@pol.net

Paul, Subroto, MD {1275648933} Surgry, SrgThr(99,MA01)<NY-PRSBWEIL>
+ St. Barnabas Medical Center
94 Old Short Hills Road   Livingston, NJ 07039   (973)322-5195   Fax (973)322-2471

Physicians by Name and Address

Paul Kate, Vasant, MD {1396706453} CdvDis, IntrMd(74,INA6A)<NJ-OCEANMC, NJ-JRSYSHMC>
+ Cardiology Associates of Ocean County PA
  495 Jack Martin Boulevard/Suite 2 Brick, NJ 08724
  (732)458-7575 Fax (732)458-0874
+ Cardiology Associates of Ocean County PA
  500 River Avenue/Suite 220 Lakewood, NJ 08701
  (732)458-7575 Fax (732)458-0874
+ Cardiology Associates of Ocean County PA
  9 Hospital Drive/Suite B8 Toms River, NJ 08724 (732)349-8899 Fax (732)458-0874

Paul Yee, Sabine T., MD {1417278805} FamMed
+ Family Practice of CentraState
  479 Newman Springs Rd/Suite A-101 Marlboro, NJ 07746
  (732)780-1601
+ 1738 State Route 31/Suite 203
  Clinton, NJ 08809 (908)735-7361

Paulin, Cesar M., MD {1801933023} IntrMd(64,PHIL)<NJ-CENTRAST>
+ 1000 West Main Street
  Freehold, NJ 07728 (732)431-1880 Fax (732)866-4268
  omegaisone@aol.com

Paulina, Arthur, Jr., MD {1356311328} IntrMd(75,LA01)<NJ-STBARNMC>
+ 205 Ridgedale Avenue
  Florham Park, NJ 07932 (973)966-0113 Fax (973)966-0176

Paull, Robert M., MD {1427181270} Dermat(83,NJ06)
+ 4 Progress Street/Suite B7
  Edison, NJ 08820 (908)754-0770 Fax (908)754-4137
+ 27 Mountain Boulevard/Suite 7
  Warren, NJ 07059 (908)754-0770 Fax (908)754-7946

Paulo, Jimmy Martins, MD {1013923424} IntrMd(03,DMN01)<NJ-CLARMAAS>
+ Clara Maass Medical Center
  1 Clara Maass Drive/Internal Med Belleville, NJ 07109
  (973)450-2433 Fax (973)450-2434

Paulson, Melyssa Michelle, MD {1144234089} SrgOrt(96,MD01)
+ 867 St. Georges' Avenue
  Rahway, NJ 07065 (732)381-8844

Paulvin, Neil Brian, DO {1285654293} FamMed, Acpntr, IntrMd(00,NJ75)
+ Advanced Orthopedics & Sports Medicine Institute
  301 Professional View Drive Freehold, NJ 07728
  (732)720-2555 Fax (732)720-2556

Pavel, Patricia M., MD {1619106028} ObsGyn, IntrMd(05,NY09)
+ Lumina Women's Care
  401 Hamburg Turnpike/Suite 104 Wayne, NJ 07470
  (973)750-1770 Fax (973)750-1775

Pavelic, Martin Thomas, III, MD {1770825267}
+ Summit Medical Group-Berkeley Heights Campus
  1 Diamond Hill Road Berkeley Heights, NJ 07922
  (908)277-8872 Fax (908)673-7382

Pavell, Jeff Richard, DO {1790769487} PhysMd, PainInvt(94,NY75)<NJ-ENGLWOOD, NY-PRSBCOLU>
+ Physical Medicine & Rehabilitation Center
  500 Grand Avenue/1st Floor Englewood, NJ 07631
  (201)567-2277 Fax (201)567-7506

Pavia, Randyll A., MD {1649240631} Anesth(89,NY09)<NJ-PALISADE>
+ Palisades Medical Center
  7600 River Road/Anesth North Bergen, NJ 07047
  (201)854-5000 Fax (201)854-5772

Pavlak-Schenk, Jayne A., DO {1689664773} GnetMd, IntrMd(84,IA75)
+ NJ Hematology & Oncology Associates
  1608 Route 88 West/Suite 250 Brick, NJ 08724 (732)840-8880 Fax (732)840-3939

Pavlenko, Andriy, MD {1932347440} PthAcl(94,UKR16)<NJ-KMHCHRRY>
+ Kennedy Health System/Cherry Hill Campus
  2201 Chapel Avenue West/Path Cherry Hill, NJ 08002
  (856)488-6500 Fax (856)488-6846

Pavlides, Andreas Constantinos, MD {1992776637} IntrMd, CdvDis(96,PA09)<NJ-OURLADY, NJ-COOPRUMC>
+ Cardiovascular Associates
  210 West Atlantic Avenue Haddon Heights, NJ 08035
  (856)547-0539 Fax (856)547-3178
+ Cardiovascular Associates of The Delaware Valley, PA
  525 State Street/Suite 3 Elmer, NJ 08318 (856)547-0539
  Fax (856)358-0725

Pavlou, George Nicholas, MD {1023014909} Gastrn, IntrMd(86,GRNA)
+ Gastroenterology Associates of New Jersey
  205 Browertown Road/Suite 201 Little Falls, NJ 07424
  (973)812-8120 Fax (973)812-8144
+ Gastroenterology Associates of New Jersey
  88 Park Place Montclair, NJ 07042 (973)812-8120 Fax (973)233-9660
+ Gastroenterology Associates of New Jersey
  19 Yawpo Avenue Oakland, NJ 07424 (973)812-8120
  Fax (973)812-8144

Pavlou, Theophanis A., MD {1871552026} CritCr, IntrMd, PulDis(87,NY09)<NJ-HOLYNAME, NJ-ENGLWOOD>
+ Holy Name Pulmonary Associates PC
  200 Grand Avenue/Suite 102 Englewood, NJ 07631
  (201)871-3636 Fax (201)871-2286

Pavuluri, Srinivas, MD {1255360020} Nrolgy(89,INDI)<NJ-BAYSHORE>
+ 1 Bethany Road/Building 6 Suite 91
  Hazlet, NJ 07730 (732)264-4301 Fax (732)264-1102
+ 205 Bridge Street/Building D
  Metuchen, NJ 08840 (732)264-4301 Fax (732)264-1102

Pawa, Anil K., MD {1942379276} Pedtrc, IntrMd(92,INA92)<NY-BRNXLCON>
+ Drs. Qudsi & Pawa
  27 South Cooks Bridge Road/Suite 2-21 Jackson, NJ 08527
  (732)987-5733 Fax (732)987-5729

Pawa, Sakshi, MD {1508099722} IntrMd
+ Coastal Sports Medicine
  1594 Route 9/Suite 6 Toms River, NJ 08755 (732)349-8888 Fax (732)349-8880

Pawar, Kimmerle A., MD {1114151313}<NJ-STBARNMC>
+ St. Barnabas Medical Center
  94 Old Short Hills Road Livingston, NJ 07039 (973)322-5111
  pawark@emamd.com

Pawar, Rahul Vinay, MD {1487819553}
+ 4 Beech Road
  West Orange, NJ 07052

Pawel, Barbara B., MD {1518973668} Pedtrc, PedEmg, IntrMd(84,NJ05)<NJ-COOPRUMC>
+ Cooper University Medical Center/Camden
  3 Cooper Plaza/Suite 502 Camden, NJ 08103 (856)356-4935
+ Cooper University Hospital
  One Cooper Plaza/Emerg Med Camden, NJ 08103
  (856)968-7337

Pawliw, Myron, MD {1518020296} ObsGyn(78,BELG)<NJ-UNVMCPRN>
+ University Medical Center of Princeton at Plainsboro
  One Plainsboro Road/Ob/Gyn-Suite G Plainsboro, NJ 08536
  (609)924-5363 Fax (609)924-5611

Paxton, Adam Michael, MD {1720286404} ObsGyn(DMN01)
+ Womens Health Care Associates of Sussex County
  135 Newton Sparta Road/Suite 201 Newton, NJ 07860
  (973)383-8555 Fax (973)383-8424
+ Womens Health Care Associates of Sussex County
  123 Route 94/Suite 200 Vernon, NJ 07462 (973)383-8555
  Fax (973)827-4441

Paxton, Laura Anne, MD {1467564146} Rheuma, IntrMd(05,NY15)<NY-HIGHLND>
+ Atlantic Rheumatology & Osteoporosis Associates PA
  8 Saddle Road/Suite 202 Cedar Knolls, NJ 07927
  (973)984-9796 Fax (973)984-5445

Paxton, Timothy X., DO {1356642755} FamMed
+ 10 Foster Avenue/Suite 3A
  Gibbsboro, NJ 08026 (856)761-5840

Payumo, Carmelino C., MD {1306800024} Anesth(69,PHIL)<NJ-RBAYPERT, NJ-RBAYOLDB>
+ Raritan Bay Medical Center/Perth Amboy Division
  530 New Brunswick Avenue/Anesth Perth Amboy, NJ 08861 (732)442-3700

Payumo, Gene Louie, MD {1093906687} IntrMd, Anesth
+ May Street Surgi Center
  205 May Street/Suite 103 Edison, NJ 08837 (732)820-4566 Fax (732)661-9619

Payumo, Paulita C., MD {1225098049} ObsGyn, RprEnd(63,PHIL)<NJ-COMMED>
+ 662 Commons Way/Building 1
  Toms River, NJ 08755 (732)244-8444 Fax (732)244-8444

Paz, Efrain, Jr., DO {1750326534} SrgOrt
+ 449 Hurffville Crosskeys Road/Suite 1
  Sewell, NJ 08080 (856)582-7979

Paz, Rafael E., MD {1235108135} Pedtrc(65,DOM01)
+ 424 River Street
  Paterson, NJ 07524 (973)742-0214 Fax (973)742-3358

Pazwash, Haleh, MD {1902856099} Gastrn, IntrMd(97,NJ05)<NJ-VALLEY>
+ Gastroenterology Associates of New Jersey
  1124 East Ridgewood Avenue/Suite 203 Ridgewood, NJ 07450 (201)523-4141 Fax (201)857-8646

Peace, Nyota Afi, MD {1104923846} ObsGyn(01,SC01)<NJ-MTNSIDE, NJ-OVERLOOK>
+ Metropolitan Ob/Gyn, P.A.
  1973 Springfield Avenue Maplewood, NJ 07040 (973)313-2501 Fax (973)313-2505

Peacock, Kenneth C., MD {1508388257} SrgOrt(78,PA13)
+ Qualmed Evaluations
  523 Fellowship Road/Suite 275 Mount Laurel, NJ 08054
  (856)235-7666

Pearce, Donna Alison, MD {1134134711} Anesth, CritCr(89,NJ05)<NY-MTSNAIQN>
+ St. Joseph's Regional Medical Center Anesthesia

703 Main Street Paterson, NJ 07503 (973)754-2323 Fax (973)977-9455

Pearcy, Cornell, MD {1548482037} IntrMd(83,PA02)<NJ-KMH-STRAT, NJ-VIRTVOOR>
+ 238 Country Club Drive
  Moorestown, NJ 08057 (609)932-1788 Fax (856)295-8114

Peardon, Amy Elizabeth, DO {1548223282} Pedtrc, IntrMd(99,NJ75)<NJ-JRSYSHMC>
+ Bharara Pediatrics, P.C.
  516 Bangs Avenue Asbury Park, NJ 07712 (732)774-0262
  Fax (732)775-8963

Peardon, Nathaniel Andres, DO {1417996604} Urolgy(97,PA77)
+ 2080 State Route 35
  Holmdel, NJ 07733 (732)671-5777 Fax (732)671-3230

Pearlman, Theodore F., MD {1356398812} Ophthl(72,NJ05)<NJ-STCLRDEN>
+ Cataract & Eye Care Center
  16 Pocono Road/Suite 301 Denville, NJ 07834 (973)625-7970 Fax (973)625-9650
  pearlmanoffice@aol.com

Pearlstein, Caryn S., MD {1568439255} PedOph, Ophthl(86,NY48)<NY-STATNRTH, NY-LICOLLGE>
+ Pediatric Eye Care of Monmouth, LLC
  33 Village Court Hazlet, NJ 07730 (732)217-3503 Fax (732)217-3504

Pearson, Gregg Alan, DO {1083645972} FamMed(98,PA77)
+ 369 South White Horse Park
  Waterford, NJ 08089 (609)561-5900 Fax (609)561-8989

Peart, Aubrey George, Jr., MD {1881766236} Gastrn, IntrMd(76,NY47)<NJ-CHSFULD, NJ-RWJUHAM>
+ 1235 Whitehorse Mercerville Rd
  Trenton, NJ 08619 (609)581-5126 Fax (609)737-0962

Pecarsky, Jason Todd, MD {1487660684} IntrMd(97,PA09)<NJ-VIRTVOOR, NJ-VIRTMARL>
+ Advocare Primary Care for Adults
  1401 East Route 70/Suite 16 Cherry Hill, NJ 08034
  (856)427-4180 Fax (856)427-4181

Pecca, Jo Ann Donna, DO {1760542518} FamMed(85,NJ75)
+ Concentra Medical Centers Urgent Care
  817 East Gate Drive/Suite 102 Mount Laurel, NJ 08054
  (856)778-1090 Fax (856)778-9191

Pechet, Taine Tayard, MD {1669415683} Surgry, SrgThr(92,MA01)<PA-PNPRSBYT>
+ Shore Medical Center
  Shore Road and Brighton Avenue Somers Point, NJ 08244

Peck, George C., Jr., MD {1730175951} SrgPlstc(83,MD01)<NJ-HACKNSK>
+ The Peck Center
  776 Northfield Avenue West Orange, NJ 07052 (973)324-2300 Fax (973)324-1421

Peck, Gregory Lance, DO {1316120827} SrgCrC, Surgry, IntrMd(11,NJ75)
+ University Hospital-RWJ Medical School
  89 French Street/3rd Floor New Brunswick, NJ 08901
  (732)235-7766 Fax (732)235-2964
+ UMDNJ RWJ Surgery
  125 Paterson Street/CAB 4th FL 4100 New Brunswick, NJ 08901 (732)235-7766 Fax (732)235-7079

Peck, Richard E., MD {1417943945} Surgry, SrgPlstc(94,NJ05)<NJ-NWTNMEM>
+ The Peck Center
  776 Northfield Avenue West Orange, NJ 07052 (973)324-2300 Fax (973)324-1421

Pecker, Howard M., MD {1154359578} SrgOrt(84,NY09)<NJ-RWJURAH, NJ-JFKMED>
+ Rahway-Edison Orthopaedic Group PA
  867 Saint Georges Avenue Rahway, NJ 07065 (732)381-8844 Fax (732)388-7911

Peckman, Cornelia L., MD {1922087360} Anesth(81,GRNA)<NJ-OVERLOOK, NJ-NWTNMEM>
+ 32 Sparta Road
  Short Hills, NJ 07078 (973)564-8063

Pecora, Andrew L., MD {1770544504} OncHem(83,NJ05)<NJ-HACKNSK>
+ John Theurer Cancer Center - HUMC
  92 Second Street Hackensack, NJ 07601 (201)996-5900
  Fax (201)996-9246
+ Hackensack University Medical Center
  30 Prospect Avenue/HemOnc Hackensack, NJ 07601
  (201)996-2000

Pecora, Andrew Paul, DO {1376637553} FamMed(90,PA77)
+ Associates in Family HealthCare, P.C.
  73 North Maple Avenue/Suite B Marlton, NJ 08053
  (844)542-2273 Fax (856)569-4043

Pecora, Arthur Steven, DO {1023053246} EmrgMd, IntrMd(96,PA77)<NJ-BURDTMLN>
+ Cape Regional Medical Center
  2 Stone Harbor Boulevard/Emerg Med Cape May Court House, NJ 08210 (609)463-2139

Physicians by Name and Address

Pecora, Joseph J., III, DO {1841204666} IntrMd(99,PA78)<NJ-CARRIER, NJ-SOMERSET>
+ Montgomery Medical Associates
  9 Dutchtown Road   Belle Mead, NJ 08502   (908)874-8883   Fax (908)874-3595
+ Carrier Clinic
  252 Route 601/Blake Recovery   Belle Mead, NJ 08502   (908)281-1000

Pecoraro, Michael J., MD {1700861044} SrgHnd, SrgPlstc, Surgry(82,GRNA)<NJ-OCEANMC, NJ-COMMED>
+ Sea Shore Plastic & Hand Surgery Center
  450 Jack Martin Boulevard   Brick, NJ 08724   (732)206-1000
+ Sea Shore Plastic & Hand Surgery Center
  Highway 71/Building 700   Sea Girt, NJ 08750   (732)449-4120

Pecorelli, Nicholas T., MD {1699744755} IntrMd(95,NJ05)<NJ-HACKNSK>
+ Wood Ridge Medical Associates
  245 Valley Boulevard   Wood Ridge, NJ 07075   (201)438-5500   Fax (201)438-3363

Pedalino, Jill Garripoli, DO {1568471472} Pedtrc(03,NJ75)<NJ-HACKNSK>
+ Healthy Kids Pediatrics
  675 Franklin Avenue   Nutley, NJ 07110   (844)437-5455   Fax (862)238-7454
  info@HealthyKidsNJ.com

Peddu, Vijaya, MD {1205875135} Psychy, PsyCAd(92,INA19)<NJ-CARRIER>
+ Carrier Clinic
  252 Route 601   Belle Mead, NJ 08502   (908)281-1000

Pedemonte, Bader Maria, MD {1831282334} Pthlgy, PthACl, PthHem(83,DOMI)<NJ-MORRISTN>
+ 123 Tulip Lane
  Basking Ridge, NJ 07920
+ Morristown Pathology Associates
  100 The American Road/Suite 118   Morris Plains, NJ 07950   (973)867-7298

Pedersen, Daniel A., DO {1790066108} FamMed, IntrMd(NJ75<NJ-SJHREGMC>
+ Pedersen Family Medicine, LLC
  1450 E Chestnut Avenue/Suite 3-D   Vineland, NJ 08361   (856)692-0050   Fax (856)692-0081

Pedersen, Irene A., MD {1932148772} ObsGyn, Gyneco, IntrMd(84,OH06)<NJ-HUNTRDN>
+ Affiliates in Obstetrics & Gynecology, P.A.
  111 Route 31/Suite 121 2nd FL Bldg B   Flemington, NJ 08822   (908)782-2825   Fax (908)782-0196

Pedicini, Joseph P., MD {1194711440} IntrMd(84,MEX14)<NJ-OCEANMC>
+ Ocean Family Care
  800 Route 88/Suite 3   Point Pleasant Beach, NJ 08742   (732)295-0072   Fax (732)295-0224

Pedinoff, Andrew J., MD {1033116801} AlgyImmn, Pedtrc, IntrMd(84,CHIL)
+ Princeton Allergy & Asthma Associates, P.A.
  24 Vreeland Drive   Skillman, NJ 08558   (609)921-2202   Fax (609)924-1468
+ Princeton Allergy & Asthma Associates, P.A.
  1245 Whitehorse Mercerville Rd   Hamilton, NJ 08619   (609)921-2202   Fax (609)924-1468
+ Princeton Allergy & Asthma Associates, P.A.
  666 Plainsboro Road/Building 100-B   Plainsboro, NJ 08558   (609)799-8111   Fax (609)924-1468

Pedowitz, Robert Neil, DO {1851346985} FamMed(99,MO78)
+ Family Practice of CentraState-Jackson
  161 Bartley Road   Jackson, NJ 08527   (732)363-6140   Fax (732)363-6196
+ Family Practice of CentraState
  319 Route 130 North   East Windsor, NJ 08520   (732)363-6140   Fax (609)447-8070

Pedowitz, Walter J., MD {1699748426} SrgOrt, SrgFAk(71,NY08)<NJ-RWJURAH, NJ-TRINIWSC>
+ Union County Orthopaedic Group
  210 West St. Georges Avenue/PO Box 330   Linden, NJ 07036   (908)486-1111   Fax (908)583-1034

Pedra-Nobre, Manuela Gomes, MD {1912939844} Rheuma, IntrMd(84,SPA05)<NJ-UMDNJ>
+ North Jersey Rheumatology Center PA
  577 Westfield Avenue   Westfield, NJ 07090   (908)233-9111   Fax (908)233-9920

Pedro, Helio Fernando, MD {1215983382} Pedtrc, IntrMd, GnetMd(95,GRN01)<NJ-HACKNSK, NJ-UMDNJ>
+ Hackensack University Medical Center
  30 Prospect Avenue/Pediatrics   Hackensack, NJ 07601   (201)996-5264   Fax (201)996-5176
  hpedro@humed.com
+ Liver Transplant & Hepatobiliary Diseases/UMDNJ
  140 Bergen Street/ACC Bldg   Newark, NJ 07101   (973)972-7218
+ Rutgers- New Jersey Medical School
  185 South Orange Avenue   Newark, NJ 07601   (973)972-4300

Pedroza, Lisa Vanchhawng, MD {1235418674} InfDis<NJ-COOPRUMC>
+ Cooper University Hospital
  One Cooper Plaza   Camden, NJ 08103   (856)356-4920

Peek, Erin Heritage, MD {1679772818} EmrgMd<NJ-MORRISTN>
+ Morristown Medical Center
  100 Madison Avenue   Morristown, NJ 07962   (973)971-5007

Peeples, Charles B., MD {1477558518} IntrMd, EmrgMd(81,NY09)<NJ-JRSYSHMC, NJ-MONMOUTH>
+ Eatontown Medical Associates
  158 Wyckoff Road   Eatontown, NJ 07724   (732)544-9500   Fax (732)544-0132

Peeraully, Tasneem, MD {1346516515} Nrolgy
+ Rutgers NJ School of Medicine Neurology
  90 Bergen Street/DOC 5200   Newark, NJ 07103   (973)972-5209   Fax (973)972-5059

Pegher, Matthew David, DO {1588613285} EmrgMd(92,FL75)<NJ-NWTNMEM>
+ Newton Medical Center
  175 High Street/EmrgMed   Newton, NJ 07860   (973)383-2121

Peikin, Steven R., MD {1770655060} Gastrn, IntrMd(74,PA02)<NJ-COOPRUMC, NJ-MEMSALEM>
+ The Cooper Hospital System-Univ Hospital
  401 Haddon Avenue/Gastroenterolog   Camden, NJ 08103   (856)757-7732   Fax (856)968-9564
+ The Cooper Hospital System-Univ Hospital
  3 Cooper Plaza/Suite 215   Camden, NJ 08103   (856)342-2439

Pekala, Bernard A., MD {1083684393} Gyneco, ObsGyn(67,PA09)<NJ-VIRTVOOR, NJ-COOPRUMC>
+ 1305 North Kings Highway/Suite 6
  Cherry Hill, NJ 08034   (856)428-6451   Fax (856)354-9496

Pekala, Raymond T., MD {1033156344} Ophthl(78,PA02)<NJ-OURLADY, NJ-VIRTUAHS>
+ 99 West Gate Drive
  Cherry Hill, NJ 08034   (856)428-1400   Fax (856)428-9358
  Pekala3@covad.net
+ 215 White Horse Pike
  Haddon Heights, NJ 08035   (856)428-1400   Fax (856)547-9138
+ Wills Eye Surgery Center in Cherry Hill
  408 Route 70 East   Cherry Hill, NJ 08034   (856)354-1600   Fax (856)429-7555

Pekar, Aleksandr, MD Anesth(88,BLA01)
+ Advanced Interventional Pain Management
  1176 Hamburg Turnpike   Wayne, NJ 07470   (973)365-4747   Fax (973)365-4596

Pelaez, Linda, MD {1639366362} ObsGyn
+ 1343 Genovese Lane
  Rahway, NJ 07065

Pelavin, Martin D., MD {1386758217} IntrMd(73,NY19)
+ Old Tappan Medical Group PA
  215 Old Tappan Road   Old Tappan, NJ 07675   (201)666-1000   Fax (201)666-4108

Pelavin, Paul Isaac, MD {1114141678} PedEnd, Pedtrc(02,PA01)<NJ-VALLEY>
+ VMG-Pediatric Endocrinology
  140 East Ridgewood avenue/Suite N280   Paramus, NJ 07652   (201)447-8182   Fax (201)523-9365
  pelapa@valleyhealth.com

Pelimskaya, Lutsiya Siliverstovna, MD {1609886902} IntrMd(80,LAT02)<NJ-LOURDMED>
+ Dorfner Family Medicine
  950 South Chester Avenue/Suite A   Delran, NJ 08075   (856)764-2500   Fax (856)764-8335
+ Dorfner Family Medicine
  811 Sunset Road/Suite 101   Burlington, NJ 08016   (856)764-2500   Fax (856)387-9408

Pellecchia, Ralph Joseph, MD {1962527929} ObsGyn(94,NY03)<NJ-JRSYCITY>
+ Metropolitan Family Health Network
  935 Garfield Avenue   Jersey City, NJ 07304   (201)478-5800   Fax (201)478-5850
  Rpellecchia@metrofhn.org

Pellegrino, John M., MD {1730254053} SrgBst, Surgry, SrgOnc(87,NE06)<NJ-JRSYSHMC, NJ-OCEANMC>
+ Breast Surgery & Breast Oncology Associates
  459 Jack Martin Boulevard   Brick, NJ 08724   (732)458-4600   Fax (732)458-3885
+ Breast Surgery & Breast Oncology Associates
  901 West Main Street/Suite 102   Freehold, NJ 07728   (732)303-6310

Pellegrino, Peter Phillip, MD {1053483792} Pedtrc, IntrMd(PA02
+ Princeton Nassau Pediatrics, P.A.
  301 North Harrison Street   Princeton, NJ 08540   (609)924-5510   Fax (609)924-3577
+ Princeton Nassau Pediatrics, P.A.
  25 South Route 31   Pennington, NJ 08534   (609)924-5510   Fax (609)745-5320

Pellegrino, Tara Marie, DO {1043531247} FamMed, IntrMd(10,NJ75)
+ Mt. Laurel Family Physicians
  401 Young Avenue/Suite 260   Moorestown, NJ 08057   (856)291-8756   Fax (856)291-8750

Peller, Alicia S., MD {1548216617} Pedtrc(81,PHIL)<NJ-CHSFULD>
+ Allentown Medical Associates
  163 Burlington Path Road   Cream Ridge, NJ 08514   (609)758-1100   Fax (609)758-3188

Pelletier, Mario E., MD {1457310724} IntrMd, PulDis(77,DOM01)<NJ-PALISADE>
+ 6003 Monroe Place/Suite 1-A
  West New York, NJ 07093   (201)869-6868   Fax (201)869-1819
  Mepno1@aol.com

Pelletier, Ronald Paul, MD {1770538258} Surgry, SrgTpl, PedSrg(87,OH41)<OH-OSUMEDC>
+ Robert Wood Johnson Transplant Associates, P.A.
  10 Plum Street/7th Floor   New Brunswick, NJ 08901   (732)253-3699

Pelletier-Bui, Alexis Elise, MD {1871851857}
+ Cooper University Medical Center/Camden
  3 Cooper Plaza   Camden, NJ 08103   (856)342-2000

Pelliccia, Frances B., MD {1093742793} Pedtrc, IntrMd, AdolMd(85,NJ05)<NJ-JRSYCITY, NJ-MEADWLND>
+ St. Peter's Dorothy B. Hersh Child Protection Center
  123 How Lane   New Brunswick, NJ 08901   (732)448-1000

Pelligra, John, MD {1023057726} ObsGyn, Gyneco(83,GRN01)<NJ-MONMOUTH, NJ-OCEANMC>
+ 2164 Highway 35/Suite D
  Sea Girt, NJ 08750   (732)974-0320   Fax (732)974-1283
+ 3469 Route 9 North
  Howell, NJ 07731   (732)364-6600

Pellman, Elliot J., MD {1235192998} SprtMd, IntrMd, IntrSptM(79,MEX14)<NY-LIJEWSH, NY-MTSINAI>
+ New York Jets Football Club
  1 Jets Drive/MedicalServices   Florham Park, NJ 07932
  epellman@jets.nfl.com

Pellmar, Monte B., MD {1700940954} Acpntr, Nephro, Nrolgy(74,NJ05)<NJ-CENTRAST>
+ 2 Paragon Way/Suite 400
  Freehold, NJ 07728   (732)431-4323   Fax (732)431-4435

Pello, Mark J., MD {1073602546} SrgC&R, Surgry, IntrMd(75,PA02)
+ Cooper Surgical Care at Voorhees
  6015 Main Street/Suite G   Voorhees, NJ 08043   (856)325-6565   Fax (856)325-6555
+ Cooper Surgical Associates
  3 Cooper Plaza/Suite 403   Camden, NJ 08103   (856)325-6565   Fax (856)541-5379

Pello, Scott Jason, MD {1619165867} Nrolgy, PainInvt(06,NJ02)
+ Rancocas Anesthesiology, PA
  15000 Midlantic Drive/Suite 102   Mount Laurel, NJ 08054   (856)255-5479   Fax (856)393-8691
+ Rancocas Anesthesiology, PA
  700 Route 130 North/Suite 203   Cinnaminson, NJ 08077   (856)255-5479   Fax (856)829-3605

Peloro, Concettina M., MD {1174588321} DerMOH, SrgDer, Dermat(93,DC02)
+ Princeton Dermatology Associates
  5 Centre Street/Suite 1-A   Monroe Township, NJ 08831   (609)655-4544   Fax (609)655-2390
  cpeloro@princetonderm.com
+ Princeton Dermatology Associates
  208 Bunn Drive/Suite 1-E   Princeton, NJ 08540   (609)655-4544   Fax (609)683-0298

Pelosi, Marco A., II, MD {1275652745} Gyneco(67,PERU)<NJ-BAYONNE>
+ Pelosi Medical Center
  350 Kennedy Boulevard   Bayonne, NJ 07002   (201)858-1800   Fax (201)858-1002

Pelosi, Marco A., Jr., MD {1063531556} ObsGyn, Gyneco(91,NJ05)<NJ-BAYONNE, NJ-OVERLOOK>
+ Pelosi Medical Center
  350 Kennedy Boulevard   Bayonne, NJ 07002   (201)858-1800   Fax (201)858-1002
  mpelosi3@pelosimedicalcenter.com

Peltz, Hillel, DO {1881622074} EmrgMd(98,FL75)
+ I M E M Clinical Associates LLC
  940 Somerset Avenue   Lakewood, NJ 08701   (732)496-0919   Fax (732)886-5791

Pemberton, Clyde A., MD {1629225594} Psychy(72,WIND)
+ 15 South Ninth Street
  Newark, NJ 07107

Pemberton, Colin Andre, MD {1891935557} IntrMd
+ 500 Orange Street/Suite 1
  Newark, NJ 07107   (973)842-8398

Physicians by Name and Address

Pena, Rafael E., MD {1659307486} IntrMd, ClCdEl, CdvDis(92,COL25)<NJ-BURDTMLN, NJ-SHOREMEM>
+ Mercer Bucks Cardiology
3140 Princeton Pike/2nd Floor   Lawrenceville, NJ 08648   (609)895-1919   Fax (609)895-1200
+ Mercer Bucks Cardiology
One Union Street/Suite 101   Robbinsville, NJ 08691   (609)895-1919   Fax (609)890-7292

Pena Mejia, Jesus A., MD {1174596498} Psychy(79,ELS01)<NJ-TRININPC>
+ Trinitas Regional Medical Center-New Point Campus
655 East Jersey Street/PsychClinic   Elizabeth, NJ 07206   (908)994-5000

Pena Tejada, Gilda, MD {1992828495}
+ 1315 Palisade Avenue
Union City, NJ 07087   (201)865-8900   Fax (201)865-1002

Penaberdiel, Thelma M., MD {1922115013} IntrMd(75,MEX14)
+ Morris County Veterans Service
340 West Hanover Avenue   Morristown, NJ 07960   (973)285-6866   Fax (973)285-6883

Penaloza-Aranibar, Carlos G., MD {1063525319} Surgry, AeroMd(78,SPA05)<NJ-ACMCITY>
+ AtlantiCare Regional Medical Center/City Campus
1925 Pacific Avenue/House Surgeon   Atlantic City, NJ 08401   (609)345-4000

Penberthy, Katherine Ann, MD {1255420667} IntrMd(01,CA02)
+ Cooper Physicians Office
196 Grove Avenue/Suite C/Medicine   Thorofare, NJ 08086   (856)848-7577   Fax (856)848-6554
penberthy-katherine@cooperhealth.edu

Pendino, Alexander M., DO {1851328777} Nrolgy(88,NJ75)<NJ-JRSYSHMC>
+ Hamilton Neurological Associates
3535 Quakerbridge Road/Suite 200   Hamilton, NJ 08619   (609)890-1110   Fax (609)890-1101

Pendse, Vijay K., MD {1528006558} ObsGyn(78,INDI)
+ 293 Broadway
Paterson, NJ 07514   (973)279-3806   Fax (973)279-3202

Penek, John A., MD {1417996562} PulDis, SlpDis, IntrMd(71,NJ05)<NJ-MORRISTN, NJ-STBARNMC>
+ 525 Wanaque Avenue
Pompton Lakes, NJ 07442   (973)616-9500   Fax (973)616-9507
penek5@aol.com
+ 21 Perry Street
Morristown, NJ 07960   (973)616-9500   Fax (973)326-6768

Penera, Norman S., MD {1376593525} IntrMd(87,PHI24)<NJ-VALLEY>
+ Valley Health Medical Group
1114 Goffle Road/Suite 103   Hawthorne, NJ 07506   (973)423-1364   Fax (973)423-0980

Peng, Brian, DO {1538328745} IntrMd, IntHos(08,NY75)<NJ-VIRTMHBC>
+ Virtua Lumberton Family Physicians
1561 Route 38/Suite 6A   Lumberton, NJ 08048   (609)267-2100   Fax (609)267-6921

Peng, Chung J., MD {1902938988} NnPnMd, Pedtrc(78,TAI06)<NJ-MTNSIDE, NY-SAMARIMC>
+ Hackensack UMC Mountainside
1 Bay Avenue/Pediatrics   Montclair, NJ 07042   (973)429-6852
Chungjpeng@aol.com

Peng, Hsin, MD {1215993498} AnesPain, IntrMd(78,TAI05)
+ Anesthesia Consultnts of NJ/Nova Pain
285 Davidson Avenue/Suite 204   Somerset, NJ 08873   (732)271-1400   Fax (732)271-3544

Peng, Minzhong, MD {1508860834} Anesth(84,CHN3B)
+ Peng Consulting Inc.
855 Lehigh Avenue   Union, NJ 07083

Peng, Patricia E., DO {1326096298} Pedtrc(93,IL76)<NJ-MORRISTN, NJ-OVERLOOK>
+ Advocare Sinatra & Peng Pediatrics
169 Minebrook Road   Bernardsville, NJ 07924   (908)766-0034   Fax (908)766-5065

Peng, Victor I., MD {1255688925} FamMed
+ Hunterdon Family Physicians
111 State Route 31/Suite 111   Flemington, NJ 08822   (908)284-9880   Fax (908)782-4316

Penn, Carol A., DO {1265711576} FamMed
+ 72 Harrison Avenue
Red Bank, NJ 07701

Penn, James R., MD {1588094569} IntrMd, Gastrn(12,NJ06)
+ Gastroenterology Consultants PA
205 May Street/Suite 201   Edison, NJ 08837   (732)661-9225   Fax (732)661-9259

Penn-Becoat, Xiomara, MD {1629481023}
+ Kennedy Family Health Services
1 Somerdale Square   Somerdale, NJ 08083   (856)309-7700   Fax (856)566-8944

Pennant, Andria Uzetta, MD {1669585873} ObsGyn(TN07
+ Womens Health Care Associates of Sussex County
135 Newton Sparta Road/Suite 201   Newton, NJ 07860
(973)383-8555   Fax (973)383-8424
+ 101 Main Street/Apt 6
Sparta, NJ 07871

Pennett, Donald T., MD {1689778995} Nrolgy(82,NY08)<NJ-HUNTRDN>
+ 1100 Wescott Drive/Suite 205
Flemington, NJ 08822   (908)788-6555   Fax (908)237-2372

Penney, Robert P., MD {1790773653} ObsGyn(81,MEXI)<NJ-MONMOUTH, NJ-RIVERVW>
+ Ob-Gyn Associates at Holmdel-Shrewsbury
704 North Beers Street   Holmdel, NJ 07733   (732)739-2500   Fax (732)888-2778
+ Ob-Gyn Associates at Holmdel-Shrewsbury
39 Avenue of the Commons   Shrewsbury, NJ 07702   (732)389-0003

Pennington, Demetria, MD {1326000266} Pedtrc(94,NY20)<NJ-STBARNMC>
+ Neighborhood Health Center Plainfield
1700-58 Myrtle Avenue   Plainfield, NJ 07063   (908)753-6401

Pennisi, John Anthony, DO {1154602324}
+ Rowan University-School of Osteopathic Medicine
1 Medical Center Drive   Stratford, NJ 08084   (856)566-6708   Fax (856)566-6222

Pennycooke, Owano M., MD {1013150267} SrgVas, Surgry(03,NJ05)
+ New Jersey Vein and Laser Center
1000 Highway 35 South/Suite 301   Middletown, NJ 07748   (732)784-6550   Fax (732)737-9836

Pennycooke, Shelley-Ann Nicole, DO {1821297938} EmrgMd(NJ75<NJ-KMHSTRAT>
+ Riverview Medical Center
1 Riverview Plaza   Red Bank, NJ 07701   (732)530-2204   Fax (732)224-7498

Penrod, Carey Lynn, DO {1588665947} SrgVas, Surgry(85,PA77)
+ Surgical Specialists of New Jersey
1364 Route 72 West/Suite 5   Manahawkin, NJ 08050   (609)978-0778   Fax (609)978-1377

Pensabeni Jasper, Tiziana, MD {1922059625} IntrMd(90,ITA01)<NJ-STMRYPAS>
+ 1135 Clifton Avenue/Suite 102
Clifton, NJ 07013   (973)778-4440   Fax (973)777-4664

Pensak, Michael J., MD {1942437561} OrtSHand, SrgOrt(09,NY0)
+ Ocean Orthopedic Associates, P.A.
530 Lakehurst Road/Suite 1   Toms River, NJ 08755   (732)349-8454   Fax (732)341-0259

Penso, Desiderio S., MD   Surgry(66,COL24)<NJ-ACMCITY, NJ-ACMCMAIN>
+ 1 Evergreen Road
Linwood, NJ 08221

Penso, S. Desiderio, MD {1376671909} Surgry
+ 1005 North Main Street
Pleasantville, NJ 08232   (609)645-3333

Pentyala, Madhavi, MD {1265490072} IntrMd(99,INDI)<NJ-STBARNMC>
+ Shetal Mansuria MD, LLC.
22 Old Short Hills Road/Suite 213   Livingston, NJ 07039   (973)992-0658   Fax (973)992-6655

Penupatruni, Bharati D., MD {1033150776} GenPrc(76,INA48)<NJ-STPETER>
+ 613 Ridge Road/Suite 104
Monmouth Junction, NJ 08852   (732)329-0071
+ 666 Plainsboro Road/Suite 1005
Plainsboro, NJ 08536   (609)799-3119

Penupatruni, Niranjan K., MD {1053585588} Surgry(74,INA70)<NJ-SOLARIHS>
+ JFK Medical Center
65 James Street   Edison, NJ 08820   (732)321-7000   Fax (732)321-7339

Penzone, Karen Elizabeth, MD {1568413698} Anesth(98,PA14)<NJ-LOURDMED>
+ Lourdes Medical Center of Burlington County
218 Sunset Road/Anesthesiology   Willingboro, NJ 08046   (609)835-2900

Peos, Jennifer Renee, MD {1710986195} IntrMd(96,NJ06)<NJ-STBARNMC>
+ Drs. Gutkin & Peos
349 East Northfield Road/Suite 210   Livingston, NJ 07039   (973)597-1107   Fax (973)597-1407

Pepe, Gary V., MD {1659301117} Pedtrc, FamMAdM(69,ITAL)<NJ-STJOSHOS>
+ High Mountain Health PA
83 Long Hill Road   Little Falls, NJ 07424   (973)785-2440

Pepe, Matthew D., MD {1083653398} SrgOrt, SprtMd(94,DC02)<NJ-ACMCITY, NJ-VIRTUAHS>
+ Rothman Institute - Egg Harbor Township
2500 English Creek Avenue/Bldg 1300   Egg Harbor Township, NJ 08234   (609)677-7002   Fax (609)677-7000
+ Rothman Institute - Voorhees
443 Laurel Oak Road   Voorhees, NJ 08043   (856)821-6360

Pepe, Rosalie, MD {1518965532} InfDis, IntrMd(86,PA02)<NJ-COOPRUMC>
+ EIP Clinic/Early Intervention Program (HIV/AIDS)
3 Cooper Plaza/Suite 513   Camden, NJ 08103   (856)963-3715   Fax (856)635-1052

Pepe, Salvatore, IV, DO {1609809458} EmrgMd, IntrMd(95,IA75)<NJ-COMMED>
+ Community Medical Center
99 Route 37 West/EmergMed   Toms River, NJ 08755   (732)557-8000
+ EmCare
425 Jack Martin Boulevard   Brick, NJ 08724   (732)840-3380

Pepek, Joseph M., MD {1790755304} RadThp
+ Princeton Radiology Associates, P.A.
3674 Route 27/Dept B   Kendall Park, NJ 08824   (732)821-5563   Fax (732)821-6675

Pepen, John Andre, MD {1144462615} SrgCrC
+ Advanced Surgical Associates LLC
155 Morris Avenue/2nd Floor   Springfield, NJ 07081   (972)232-2300   Fax (973)232-2301

Peper, Kathryn, MD {1659452605} Grtrcs, IntrMd(84,NY09)<NJ-MORRISTN>
+ 264 South Street
Morristown, NJ 07960   (973)539-3388   Fax (973)539-3377
+ Family Health Center
200 South Street/Suite 4   Morristown, NJ 07960   (973)889-6800

Pepper, Matthew Philip, MD {1861840456} Pedtrc
+ University Medical Group Pediatrics
125 Paterson Street/MEB 3rd Fl   New Brunswick, NJ 08903   (732)235-7893   Fax (732)235-9340

Peranio, Joanne C., MD {1659389963} Psychy(89,NJ05)<NJ-RAMAPO>
+ 393 Crescent Avenue
Wyckoff, NJ 07481   (201)891-6050   Fax (201)891-4940

Percy, John, Jr., MD {1063440394} Pedtrc(79,FRA11)<NJ-OVERLOOK>
+ Summit Medical Group Pediatrics at Westfield
592B Springfield Avenue   Westfield, NJ 07090   (908)233-8860   Fax (908)301-0265

Percy, Stephen, Jr., MD {1063586485} PedCrC, Pedtrc(90,NJ05)<NJ-HACKNSK, NJ-UMDNJ>
+ Hackensack University Medical Center
30 Prospect Avenue/ViceChair/Pedi   Hackensack, NJ 07601   (201)996-5201   Fax (201)996-3051
spercy@humed.com

Perdomo, Louis Fernando, MD {1669547402} FamMed, IntrMd(88,DOM02)<NJ-HACKNSK, NJ-VALLEY>
+ North Jersey Family Medicine
19 Yawpo Avenue   Oakland, NJ 07436   (201)337-3412   Fax (201)337-3353

Pereira, Audrey P., MD {1922022516} IntrMd(83,INA94)<NJ-VAEASTOR>
+ VA Piscataway CBOC
14 Wills Way/Building 4   Piscataway, NJ 08854   (732)981-8193   Fax (732)818-8194
Audrey.Pereira@med.va.gov

Pereira, Beryl E., MD {1861584724} IntrMd(97,NY46)
+ Bergenfield Internal Medicine
161 North Washington Avenue/Suite A   Bergenfield, NJ 07621   (201)387-6900

Pereira, Michael J., MD {1578675112} RadOnc, RadThp(76,INDI)<NJ-STJOSHOS>
+ St. Joseph's Regional Medical Center
703 Main Street/Radiology   Paterson, NJ 07503   (973)754-2675   Fax (973)754-2677

Pereira, Pedro Miguel, MD {1477512432} IntrMd(96,NJ05)<NJ-HACKNSK>
+ North Jersey Primary Care Associates
9 Post Road/Suite D-7   Oakland, NJ 07436   (201)337-1700   Fax (201)337-1703

Pereira, Sergio F., MD {1417278177}
+ University Hospital-New Jersey Medical School
30 Bergen Street   Newark, NJ 07107   (973)972-4511

Pereira, Stephen G., MD {1669432159} Surgry(91,NJ06)
+ Surgical Associates
90 Prospect Avenue/Room 1D   Hackensack, NJ 07601   (201)343-3433   Fax (201)343-0420

Perelman, Seth I., MD {1811946544} Anesth(89,NY19)<NJ-ENGLWOOD>
+ Englewood Hospital and Medical Center
350 Engle Street/Anesthesiology   Englewood, NJ 07631   (201)894-3238   Fax (201)871-0619
+ Heart and Vascular Institute at EHMC
350 Engle Street/Suite 1000   Englewood, NJ 07631   (201)894-3636

Perera, Santusht A., MD {1942311147} SrgCTh(90,NY47)
+ 142 Palisade Avenue/Suite 202
Jersey City, NJ 07306   (201)876-9119   Fax (973)838-6637

Perera, Sharmalie, MD {1033123153} IntrMd
+ Drs. Badin, De Silva, and Perera
1947 Kennedy Boulevard   Jersey City, NJ 07305   (201)433-4848   Fax (201)946-9292

Perez, Adriana M., MD {1588816045} Pedtrc(00,MEX03)<NJ-HACKNSK>
+ Hackensack University Medical Center
30 Prospect Avenue/Pediatrics   Hackensack, NJ 07601   (201)996-5430   Fax (201)996-5435

Perez, Alejandro, DO {1457674822} IntrMd(09,FL75)
+ 7 Woodlake Drive
Marlton, NJ 08053

Perez, Finucca Renda, MD {1336132174} ObsGyn(99,PA09)
+ Atlantic Cape Ob/Gyn
829 Shore Road   Somers Point, NJ 08244   (609)927-3070   Fax (609)927-2553

Perez, Humberto T., MD {1326121872} GenPrc, FamMed(65,MEXI)
+ 646 Jersey Avenue
Jersey City, NJ 07302   (201)656-5711   Fax (201)656-6354

Perez, James, MD {1770546301} IntrMd(82,DOM02)
+ Union Square Medical Associates
824 Elizabeth Avenue   Elizabeth, NJ 07201   (908)352-9556   Fax (908)352-3446

Perez, Javier Martin, MD {1487694915} Surgry, SrgCrC, SrgAbd(92,MA01)<NJ-RWJUBRUN>
+ Hackensack Surgical Critical Care Physicians
5 Summit Avenue/Suite 105   Hackensack, NJ 07601   (201)996-2900   Fax (201)883-1268

Perez, Jessica, MD {1073748729} PedAne(08,DMN01)<NJ-RWJUBRUN>
+ Robert Wood Johnson-UMDNJ Anesthesia Group
125 Paterson Street/CAB 3100   New Brunswick, NJ 08901   (732)937-8841   Fax (732)418-8492
+ RWJ University Hospital New Brunswick
One Robert Wood Johnson Place   New Brunswick, NJ 08901   (732)828-3000

Perez, Lyla E., MD PthACl, PthFor(72,NICA)
+ Office of The Regional Medical Examiner State of NJ
325 Norfolk Street   Newark, NJ 07103   (973)648-3914   Fax (973)648-3692

Perez, Manuel A., MD {1538126446} Anesth(89,PA01)<NJ-SOMERSET, NJ-STPETER>
+ Anesthesia Consultnts of NJ/Nova Pain
285 Davidson Avenue/Suite 204   Somerset, NJ 08873   (732)271-1400   Fax (732)271-3543

Perez, Marcella, MD {1720474406} FamMed
+ Drs. Stevens and Perez
4 Atno Avenue   Morristown, NJ 07960   (973)267-0002   Fax (973)328-9102

Perez, Maria Esperanza, DO {1346401981} PedGst, Pedtrc(05,NJ75)
+ Division of Pediatric GI at Goryeb
100 Madison Avenue/Box 82   Morristown, NJ 07962   (973)971-5676   Fax (973)290-7365

Perez, Matthew K., MD {1821117847} Ophthl(03,PA02)<NJ-SHOREMEM>
+ Horizon Eye Care
9701 Ventnor Avenue   Margate City, NJ 08402   (609)822-4242   Fax (609)822-3211

Perez, Raul I., MD {1003081076} FamMed(80,CUB07)
+ P & C Medical Group LLC
605 South Broad Street/Unit B   Elizabeth, NJ 07202   (908)659-0075   Fax (908)469-4300

Perez, Reynaldo T., MD {1881660082} Anesth(75,PHIL)<NJ-HOBUNIMC>
+ Hoboken University Medical Center
308 Willow Avenue/Anesthesiology   Hoboken, NJ 07030   (201)418-1000   Fax (201)943-8105

Perez, Ricardo, DO {1841327947} FamMed(00,IL76)<NJ-KMHSTRAT>
+ SOM - Department of Internal Medicine
42 East Laurel Road/Suite 3100   Stratford, NJ 08084   (856)566-6325   Fax (856)566-6377
+ Kennedy Memorial Hospital-University Medical Center
18 East Laurel Road   Stratford, NJ 08084   (856)346-6000

Perez, Robert C., MD {1508262940} Surgry
+ Virtua Medford Surgical Group
212 Creek Crossing Boulevard   Hainesport, NJ 08036   (609)267-1004   Fax (609)267-1044

Perez, Rodemar Albao, MD {1780656272} Psychy(88,PHI08)<NJ-TRININPC, NY-STBARNAB>
+ Union County Jail-Oriscello Correctional Facility
15 Elizabethtown Plaza   Elizabeth, NJ 07201   (908)558-2639
rpmd88@msn.com
+ Trinitas Regional Medical Center-New Point Campus
655 East Jersey Street/Psych   Elizabeth, NJ 07206   (908)994-5000

Perez, Ruben, MD {1346324084} IntrMd(90,CUB03)
+ 525 42nd Street
Union City, NJ 07087   (201)866-2223   Fax (201)866-0449

Perez, Sania Rebecca, MD {1174584890} Pedtrc, IntrMd(98,NY47)
+ PediatriCare Associates
400 Franklin Turnpike   Mahwah, NJ 07430   (201)529-4545   Fax (201)529-1596
+ PediatriCare Associates
20-20 Fair Lawn Avenue   Fair Lawn, NJ 07410   (201)529-4545   Fax (201)791-3765
+ PediatriCare Associates
901 Route 23 South   Pompton Plains, NJ 07430   (973)831-4545   Fax (973)831-1527

Perez, Victoria P., MD {1578673257} IntrMd, PulDis(65,PHIL)
+ 354 Old Hook Road/Suite 105
Westwood, NJ 07675   (201)666-2035   Fax (201)666-5612

Perez, Walter, MD {1255396982} ObsGyn(97,NJ05)
+ Empire Medical Associates
5 Franklin Avenue/Suite 302   Belleville, NJ 07109   (973)759-1221   Fax (973)759-1997
+ Empire Medical Associates
264 Boyden Avenue   Maplewood, NJ 07040   (973)759-1221   Fax (973)761-7617
+ Empire Medical Associates
382 West Passaic Avenue   Bloomfield, NJ 07109   (973)338-1900

Perez Feliz, Ulices Alquimedes, MD {1366619371} IntrMd
+ Shore Memorial Physician Group PC
3320 Simpson Avenue   Ocean City, NJ 08226   (609)814-9550   Fax (609)814-9544

Perez-Steele, Sheila, MD {1407931058} IntrMd, Pedtrc(91,MEXI)
+ West Paterson Family Medical Center
1031 McBride Avenue/Suite D109   West Paterson, NJ 07424   (973)785-4020   Fax (973)785-3186

Pergament, Kathleen Mangunay, DO {1174838130} IntrMd(09)
+ UMDNJ Human Genetics Center
90 Bergen Street/DOC 5400/Suite 4400   Newark, NJ 07101   (973)972-1880   Fax (973)972-1879

Peri, Nityanand, DO {1588019749} IntrMd<NJ-PALISADE>
+ Palisades Medical Center
7600 River Road   North Bergen, NJ 07047   (201)710-2756   Fax (201)758-2740

Periasamy, Jayanthi, MD {1912966573} PsyGrt, Psychy(90,INA04)<NJ-SJERSYHS, NJ-LOURDMED>
+ Center for Family Guidance, PC
765 East Route 70/Building A-101   Marlton, NJ 08053   (856)797-4800   Fax (856)810-0110

Pericic, Romeo, MD {1447286331} Anesth, CarAne(84,CRO01)<NY-WESTCHMC>
+ AtlantiCare Anesthesiology
65 West Jimmie Leeds Road   Pomona, NJ 08240   (609)748-7597

Pericles, John T., DO {1144363250} FamMed(90,NJ75)<NJ-ACMCITY, NJ-BURDTMLN>
+ AtlantiCare Clinical Associates
16 South Ohio Avenue   Atlantic City, NJ 08401   (609)441-2104
+ 5401 Harding Highway/Suite 4
Mays Landing, NJ 08330   (609)441-2104   Fax (609)625-2275

Perilstein, Neil J., MD {1144224510} FamMed(92,DC01)
+ Avenel Iselin Medical Group
400 Gill Lane   Iselin, NJ 08830   (732)404-1580   Fax (732)404-1594

Perin, Patrick V., MD {1093892465} Allrgy(87,GRN01)<NJ-HOLYNAME, NJ-STJOSHOS>
+ St. Joseph's Children's Hospital
703 Main Street/Allrgy/Immnlgy   Paterson, NJ 07503   (973)754-2500
+ 185 Cedar Lane/Suite L2
Teaneck, NJ 07666   (973)754-2500   Fax (201)836-0399

Perin, Robert J., MD {1679564959} Allrgy, Pedtrc, AlgyImmn(74,MEXI)<NJ-UNDRWD, NJ-KMHCHRRY>
+ 2950 College Drive/Suite 2-B
Vineland, NJ 08360   (856)696-5181
rperin@netaxs.com
+ 630 Salem Avenue
Woodbury, NJ 08096   (856)696-5181   Fax (856)845-2512

Perina, Barbara, MD {1174714406} Ophthl, IntrMd(72,NY03)
+ Retina Specialists of New Jersey
330 South Street/Suite 1   Morristown, NJ 07960   (973)871-2020   Fax (973)871-2000

Perisic, Dusan, MD {1073767026} ObsGyn<NJ-HOBUNIMC>
+ Palisades Women's Group
6045 Kennedy Boulevard/Suite B   North Bergen, NJ 07047   (201)868-2630   Fax (201)868-4919

Perkari, Vasantha K., MD {1215032156} IntrMd(78,INDI)<NJ-RIVERVW, NJ-BAYSHORE>
+ 428 Lloyd Road
Aberdeen, NJ 07747   (732)566-7711   Fax (732)566-2482

Perkins, Anthony Ray, MD {1720353725} SrgPlstc(06,QU01)<NJ-COOPRUMC>
+ Cooper University Medical Center/Camden
3 Cooper Plaza/Suite 400   Camden, NJ 08103   (856)356-4935

Perkins, Phyllis M., MD {1326101726} ObsGyn(76,PA13)<NJ-ACMCITY, NJ-ACMCMAIN>
+ Ladies' Choice Ob-Gyn
314 Chris Gaupp Drive/Suite 101   Galloway, NJ 08205   (609)404-1400   Fax (609)404-1430

Perkins, Robert Mark, MD {1992891477} Nephro, IntrMd(00,PA12)
+ Bayer HealthCare
100 Bayer Boulevard   Whippany, NJ 07981   (862)404-3000

Perkins-Waters, Vannette N., MD {1104801430} Anesth, PainMd(86,OK05)<NJ-KENEDYHS, NJ-VIRTUAHS>
+ Professional Pain Management Associates
2007 North Black Horse Pike   Williamstown, NJ 08094   (856)740-4888   Fax (856)740-0558

Perl, Harold, MD {1518906791} NnPnMd, Pedtrc(75,NY46)<NJ-HACKNSK>
+ Hackensack University Medical Center
30 Prospect Avenue/Neonatology   Hackensack, NJ 07601   (201)996-5362   Fax (201)996-3232
HPerl@humed.com

Perl, Louis J., MD {1255423885} RadDia, Radiol(72,MA07)<NJ-OVERLOOK>
+ Westfield Imaging Center
118-122 Elm Street   Westfield, NJ 07090   (908)232-0610   Fax (908)232-7140

Perl, Theodore, MD {1598710378} Ophthl(76,IL42)<NJ-STBARNMC, NJ-MORRISTN>
+ Corneal Associates of NJ
100 Passaic Avenue/Suite 200   Fairfield, NJ 07004   (973)439-3937   Fax (973)439-3944

Perlman, Barry J., MD {1285644948} RadDia(91,MA07)<NJ-UNVMCPRN>
+ Princeton Radiology Associates, P.A.
419 North Harrison Street   Princeton, NJ 08540   (609)921-3345   Fax (609)683-8847

Perlman, Donald Bret, MD {1245236033} AlgyImmn(73,NY47)
+ Associates in Otolaryngology
741 Northfield Avenue/Suite 104   West Orange, NJ 07052   (973)243-0600   Fax (973)736-9607
+ Associates in Otolaryngology
47 Maple Street/Suite 206   Summit, NJ 07901   (908)522-0047

Perlman, Eric S., MD {1326058090} RadDia, RadNuc(85,NY09)<NJ-UNVMCPRN>
+ Princeton Radiology Associates, P.A.
419 North Harrison Street   Princeton, NJ 08540   (609)921-3345   Fax (609)683-8847
+ University Radiology Group, P.C.
375 Route 206/Suite 1   Hillsborough, NJ 08844   (609)921-3345   Fax (908)874-7052
+ Princeton Radiology Associates, P.A.
9 Centre Drive   Jamesburg, NJ 08540   (609)655-1448   Fax (609)655-4016

Perlman, Richard L., MD {1568433084} CdvDis, IntrMd(84,NY09)<NJ-OURLADY, NJ-COOPRUMC>
+ Associated Cardiovascular Consultants, P.A.
1105 Laurel Oak Road/Suite 165   Voorhees, NJ 08043   (856)424-3600   Fax (856)424-7154
+ Associated Cardiovascular Consultants-Lourdes
1 Brace Road/Suite C & F   Cherry Hill, NJ 08034   (856)424-3600   Fax (856)428-5748

Perlmutter, Barbara Lee, MD {1205847399} Grtrcs, IntrMd(76,NJ05)<NJ-HOBUNIMC>
+ 330 Grand Street
Hoboken, NJ 07030   (201)963-5886   Fax (201)432-3608
bl.perlmutter@aol.com
+ Hoboken University Medical Center
308 Willow Avenue/Geriatrics   Hoboken, NJ 07030   (201)963-5886   Fax (201)432-3608

Perlmutter, Harold S., MD {1649204710} Ophthl(64,IL42)<NJ-NWTNMEM>
+ Eye Physicians of Sussex County
183 High Street/Suite 2200   Newton, NJ 07860   (973)383-6345   Fax (973)383-0032

Perlmutter, Mark Alan, MD {1154511012} Urolgy(04,PA12)
+ Drs. Rotolo, Howard, and Leitner
2401 Highway 35   Manasquan, NJ 08736   (732)223-7877   Fax (732)223-7151

Perlov, Marina, MD {1790846772} RadDia(71,RUS01)<NY-LUTHERN>
+ Hudson Radiology Center
657-659 Broadway   Bayonne, NJ 07002   (201)437-3007   Fax (201)437-1418

Perna, David John, MD {1841581899} PhysMd, IntrMd(07,GRN01)
+ 65 East Northfield Road/Suite L
Livingston, NJ 07039   (973)251-2189   Fax (973)486-6186

Pernell, Chris Tonya, MD {1235405127}
+ 80 Berkeley Avenue
Newark, NJ 07104   (973)975-7663

Physicians by Name and Address

Pernelli, David R., MD {1962446344} Ophthl(83,PA09)
+ The Eye Professionals, P.A.
1205 North High Street   Millville, NJ 08332   (856)825-8700   Fax (856)825-8640

Pernice, Mark J., DO {1811940620} FamMed(81,NJ75)<NJ-ACMC-ITY, NJ-ACMCMAIN>
+ 2106 New Road/Suite D-1
Linwood, NJ 08221   (609)927-9545   Fax (609)927-2920

Perno, Joseph R., MD {1689661902} Pedtrc(90,NC07)
+ 14 Innocenzi Drive
Hamilton, NJ 08690

Perocho, Rodolfo R., MD {1316983125} Surgry, EmrgMd(65,PHIL)<NJ-VIRTVOOR>
+ Virtua Voorhees
100 Bowman Drive/Surgery   Voorhees, NJ 08043   (856)247-3000

Peron, Didier L., MD {1184665135} Otlryg, Otolgy, PedOto(70,FRAN)<NJ-MORRISTN, NJ-OVERLOOK>
+ Summit Medical Group
140 Park Avenue/3rd Floor/ENT   Florham Park, NJ 07932   (973)404-9970

Perosi, Joseph J., MD {1649236795} Anesth(80,MEX34)<NJ-STPETER>
+ St. Peter's University Hospital
254 Easton Avenue/Anesthesiology   New Brunswick, NJ 08901   (732)745-8600

Perosi, Nicholas Anthony, MD {1407091374} RadV&I, RadDia(08,DMN01)
+ Coastal Imaging, LLC
79 Route 37 West/Suite 103   Toms River, NJ 08755   (732)678-0087   Fax (732)276-2325
+ Red Bank Radiologists, P.A.
200 White Road/Suite 115   Little Silver, NJ 07739   (732)678-0087   Fax (732)741-0985

Perotte, Schubert, MD {1992752331} EmrgMd(03,NJ06)<NJ-RWJURAH, NY-KINGSTON>
+ Emergency Medical Associates of NJ, P.A.
3 Century Drive   Parsippany, NJ 07054   (973)740-0607   Fax (973)740-9895

Perri, Louis P., MD {1225125255} SrgPlstc, SrgRec(88,NJ06)
+ 474 Hurffville Crosskeys Road/Suite B
Sewell, NJ 08080   (856)582-8900   Fax (856)582-9667

Perril, Rebecca A., DO {1669664298} Pedtrc, AdolMd(04,NY75)
+ Shore Care Pediatrics LLC
4000 Highway 66/Suite 125   Tinton Falls, NJ 07753   (732)922-2105   Fax (732)922-2472
rebeccaperril@shorecarepediatrics.com

Perrino, DinaMarie, DO {1932277332} FamMed(94,NJ75)<NJ-BAYSHORE, NJ-RIVERVW>
+ Drs. Tsompanidis and Perrino Fam Pract
1 Bethany Road/Suite 79   Hazlet, NJ 07730   (732)203-0800   Fax (732)203-9494

Perron, Reed C., MD {1750342697} Nrolgy(66,NY45)<NJ-VALLEY>
+ Neurology Group of Bergen County
1200 East Ridgewood Avenue   Ridgewood, NJ 07450   (201)444-0868   Fax (201)444-7363

Perry, Adam C., MD {1467569947} FamMed(00,PA12)
+ 31 Lafayette Road
Audubon, NJ 08106   (717)856-6050
adperry01@yahoo.com

Perry, Arthur William, MD {1215924519} SrgCsm, SrgPlstc, IntrMd(81,NY03)<NJ-RWJUBRUN, NJ-SOMERSET>
+ Perry Plastic Surgery Center
3055 State Route 27   Franklin Park, NJ 08823   (732)422-9600   Fax (732)422-9606
dr.perry@perryplasticsurgery.com

Perry, Kurt A., MD {1336187681} EmrgMd(77,ITAL)<NJ-MONMOUTH>
+ Monmouth Medical Center
300 Second Avenue/EmergMed   Long Branch, NJ 07740   (732)222-5200

Perry, Luke Daniel, DO {1568954410} Surgry<NJ-SJHREGMC>
+ SJH Regional Medical Center
1505 West Sherman Avenue   Vineland, NJ 08360   (717)440-5577

Perry, Michael David, DO {1023337698} IntrMd(10,PA78)<NJ-DEBRAHLC>
+ Deborah Heart and Lung Center
200 Trenton Road/Internal Med   Browns Mills, NJ 08015   (609)893-1200

Perry, Robin L., MD {1225126378} MtFtMd, ObsGyn(85,NJ06)<NJ-COOPRUMC, NJ-VIRTMHBC>
+ Cooper University Hospital
One Cooper Plaza/Drrnc/Rm 628   Camden, NJ 08103   (856)342-2491

Perry, Russell J., MD {1386671717} FamMed(84,GRN01)<NY-BRNXLFUL, NJ-VALLEY>
+ Valley Health Medical Group
780 Cedar Lane   Teaneck, NJ 07666   (201)836-7664   Fax (201)836-5710

Perry, Ruth Earlene, MD {1174076806} EmrgMd, IntrMd(82,PA13)
+ 218 North Broad Street
Trenton, NJ 08608   (609)256-4555
rperry@trentonhealthteam.org

Persad, Rajendra, MD {1912342361} Hemato, Pthlgy
+ Bio-Reference Laboratory, Inc.
481 Edward H. Ross Drive   Elmwood Park, NJ 07407   (201)791-2600   Fax (201)791-8760

Persichetti, Gregory Blase, DO {1518901925} Dermat, IntrMd(PA78
+ Dermatology Center of Washington Township
100 Kings Way East/Suite A-3   Sewell, NJ 08080   (856)589-3331   Fax (856)589-3416

Persily, Tracy L., DO {1568804912} FamMed(13,NJ76)<NJ-KMHCHRRY>
+ Cherry Hill Primary and Specialty Care
457 Haddonfield Road/Suite 110   Cherry Hill, NJ 08002   (844)542-2273   Fax (856)406-4570

Pertchik, Alan F., MD {1861467664} Nrolgy(70,NY08)<NJ-RIVERVW, NJ-RWJUBRUN>
+ 43 Gilbert Street North/Suite 2
Tinton Falls, NJ 07701   (732)741-3344

Pertschuk, Michael Jeffrey, MD {1609937903} Psychy(72,PA01)<PA-FRIENDS>
+ Eating Disorders Treatment Centers
750 Route 73 South/Suite 104   Marlton, NJ 08053   (856)810-0100   Fax (215)831-2649

Perveen, Mahmoodah, MD {1841206208} IntrMd(86,PAK10)
+ 534 Avenue E/Suite 1-D
Bayonne, NJ 07002   (201)858-8700   Fax (201)436-7825

Perzin, Adam Dean, MD {1104879501} Urolgy(87,NJ05)<NJ-LOURDMED, NJ-VIRTMHBC>
+ New Jersey Urology
243 Route 130/Suite 100   Bordentown, NJ 08505   Fax (856)252-1100
+ New Jersey Urology
15000 Midlantic Drive/Suite 100   Mount Laurel, NJ 08054   Fax (856)985-4582
+ New Jersey Urology
911 Sunset Road   Willingboro, NJ 08505

Pesci, Paula M., MD {1598786337} Psychy(83,MEX14)<NJ-RAMAPO>
+ 139 South Street/Suite 201
New Providence, NJ 07974   (973)615-9217   Fax (973)292-3293

Peshori, Kavita R., MD {1427296235} RadDia
+ Atlantic Medical Imaging, LLC.
72 West Jimmie Leeds Road   Galloway, NJ 08205   (609)677-9729   Fax (609)653-8764

Pesin, Jeffrey L., MD {1205886009} CritCr, IntrMd, PulDis(86,IL42)<NJ-KMHCHRRY>
+ Middlesex Pulmonary Associates PA
106 James Street   Edison, NJ 08820   (732)906-0091   Fax (732)906-0249
+ JFK Family Practice Group
65 James Street   Edison, NJ 08818   (732)906-0091   Fax (732)321-7496

Peska-Mosseri, Jodi L., DO {1518175165} Pedtrc(92,NY75)<NJ-RWJUBRUN, NJ-STPETER>
+ Wee Care Pediatrics
831 Tennent Road/Suite A   Manalapan, NJ 07726   (732)536-6222   Fax (732)536-9272

Peskin, Steven R., MD {1215032263} IntrMd(82,GA05)<NJ-UNVMCPRN>
+ Eric B. Chandler Health Center
277 George Street   New Brunswick, NJ 08901   (732)235-6700   Fax (732)235-6729

Pess, Gary M., MD {1881688794} SrgHnd(81,NY08)<NJ-JRSYSHMC, NJ-BAYSHORE>
+ Central Jersey Hand Surgery
2 Industrial Way West   Eatontown, NJ 07724   (732)542-4477   Fax (732)935-0355
gpess@monmouth.com
+ Central Jersey Hand Surgery
535 Iron Bridge Road   Freehold, NJ 07728   (732)542-4477   Fax (732)431-4770
+ Central Jersey Hand Surgery
780 Route 37 West/Suite 140   Toms River, NJ 07724   (732)286-9000   Fax (732)240-0036

Pesso, Robert S., MD {1730155953} ObsGyn(92,NJ05)<NJ-COMMED>
+ Toms River Ob-Gyn Associates PA
79 Route 37 West/Suite 101   Toms River, NJ 08755   (732)244-9444   Fax (732)244-9468

Petaccio, Claudia Jennifer, MD {1649617325} IntrMd(93,PA09)<NJ-COOPRUMC, NJ-VIRTBERL>
+ 300 East Park Avenue
Haddonfield, NJ 08033

Petcu, Alexandru, MD {1184683146} IntrMd(85,ROMA)<NJ-CENTRAST>
+ 1 Dag Hammarskjold Boulevard
Freehold, NJ 07728   (732)761-1788   Fax (732)761-1323

Peter, Andras, MD {1154344646} IntrMd(84,ROM04)<NJ-RBAYPERT>
+ 1030 St. Georges Avenue
Avenel, NJ 07001   (732)596-1666   Fax (732)596-0158
andy_peter@yahoo.com
+ Raritan Bay Medical Center/Outpatient
595 New Brunswick Avenue   Perth Amboy, NJ 08861   (732)442-9006

Peter, Annie M., MD {1922051317} CdvDis, IntrMd(91,NY09)<NJ-COOPRUMC, NJ-VIRTMARL>
+ Cardiovascular Associates
210 West Atlantic Avenue   Haddon Heights, NJ 08035   (856)546-3003   Fax (856)547-5337
+ Cardiovascular Associates of The Delaware Valley, PA
1840 Frontage Road   Cherry Hill, NJ 08034   (856)546-3003   Fax (856)795-7436
+ Cardiovascular Associates of The Delaware Valley, PA
525 State Street/Suite 3   Elmer, NJ 08035   (856)358-2363   Fax (856)358-0725

Peterka, Ann-Judith, DO {1972628766} IntrMd(87,NJ75)
+ 34 North Highcrest Drive
Hawthorne, NJ 07506

Peters, Albert J., DO {1083773121} ObsGyn, RprEnd(84,PA77)
+ Sher Institutes for Reproductive Med
1 Robertson Drive/Suite 24   Bedminster, NJ 07921

Peters, Bruce W., DO {1326017443} Otlryg, SrgFPl, OtgyFPlS(89,PA77)
+ Ocean Otolaryngology Associates
54 Bey Lea Road/Suite 3   Toms River, NJ 08753   (732)281-0100   Fax (732)281-0400

Peters, Karen R., DO {1609822501} FamMed, GenPrc(89,NJ75)<NJ-HCKTSTWN>
+ Advocare Family Health at Mt. Olive
183 US Route 206/Suite 1   Flanders, NJ 07836   (973)347-3277   Fax (973)347-3141

Peters, Mahafarin P., MD {1639136815} Pedtrc(78,IRA09)<NJ-NWTNMEM>
+ 1919 Bay Boulevard/Unit C25
Seaside Heights, NJ 08751

Peters, Michael A., DO {1811950363} Pedtrc(89,NJ75)<NJ-MORRISTN, NJ-STCLRDEN>
+ Advocare West Morris Pediatrics
151 Route 10/Suite 105   Succasunna, NJ 07876   (973)584-0002   Fax (973)584-7107

Peters, Nancy Castellucci, MD {1043300577} Pedtrc, IntrMd(93,NY09)<NJ-CENTRAST>
+ Family Practice of CentraState
281 Route 34/Suite 813   Colts Neck, NJ 07722   (732)431-2620   Fax (732)431-3707
+ Family Practice of CentraState
479 Newman Springs Rd/Suite A-101   Marlboro, NJ 07746   (732)780-1601
+ Family Practice of CentraState
901 West Main Street/Suite 106   Freehold, NJ 07722   (732)462-0100   Fax (732)462-0348

Petersohn, Jeffrey D., MD {1568499051} PainMd, Anesth, Anes-Pain(84,PA09)<NJ-SHOREMEM>
+ Pain Care, P.C.
199 New Road/Suite 62/63   Linwood, NJ 08221   (609)926-3331   Fax (609)926-3350
JDPMD@aol.com
+ Pain Care, P.C.
3100 Princeton Pike/Building 1/Suite D   Lawrenceville, NJ 08648   (609)926-3331   Fax (609)926-3350

Peterson, Dolores D., MD {1154369346} FamMed(90,NJ05)<NJ-VIRTMHBC>
+ Families first HealthCare
701 East Main Street/Suite 5   Moorestown, NJ 08057   (856)727-0999   Fax (856)727-7997

Peterson, John W., MD {1447202270} InfDis, IntrMd(85,NJ06)<NJ-VIRTUAHS>
+ Infectious Disease Physicians PA
1001 Briggs Road/Suite 250   Mount Laurel, NJ 08054   (856)866-7466   Fax (856)866-9088

Peterson, Lars-Kristofer Nelson, MD {1023336112}<NY-STRNG-MEM>
+ Cooper University Hospital Critical Care
One Cooper Plaza   Camden, NJ 08103   (856)342-2633   Fax (856)968-8282
+ Cooper Univerisry Emergency Physicians
One Cooper Plaza   Camden, NJ 08103   (856)342-2633   Fax (856)968-8272

Peterson, Mary Ann, MD {1801876297} RadDia, Radiol(84,NJ05)<NJ-JFKMED>
+ JFK Medical Center
65 James Street/Radiology   Edison, NJ 08820   (732)321-7917   Fax (732)767-2968

Peterson, Paul, III, DO {1730127564} IntrMd, Nephro, FamMed(79,IA75)
+ Buena Family Practice
1315 Harding Highway/Box 310   Richland, NJ 08350   (856)697-0300   Fax (856)697-8944

Peterson, Thomas Russell, MD {1295800043} SrgNro(76,MA07)<NJ-HOBUNIMC, NJ-STFRNMED>
+ 140 Prospect Avenue/Suite 18
Hackensack, NJ 07601   (201)525-0500   Fax (201)525-1171

Peterson, Vincent Glenn, DO {1487887295}
+ Rowan University-School of Osteopathic Medicine
1 Medical Center Drive   Stratford, NJ 08084   (856)566-6708

Peterson-Deerfield, Laurie Jean, DO {1689676207} Psychy, FamMed(98,FL75)
+ 2301 Evesham Road/Suite 204
Voorhees, NJ 08043   (856)770-0021   Fax (856)770-9521

Petilla-Onorato, Jessica Isabel, MD {1720071541} Grtrcs, IntrMd(91,PHI09)<NY-SLRRSVLT, NY-SLRLUKES>
+ Geriatric Assessment Center
435 South Street/Suite 390   Morristown, NJ 07960   (973)971-7022   Fax (973)290-7046

Petillo, Tina M., DO {1962437244} ObsGyn(83,PA77)<NJ-STBARNMC>
+ 340 East Northfield Road/Suite 2E
Livingston, NJ 07039   (973)533-0001   Fax (973)716-0306

Petit, Anne I., MD {1578615084} ObsGyn(84,PA13)<NJ-ACMCITY, NJ-ACMCMAIN>
+ Ladies' Choice Ob-Gyn
314 Chris Gaupp Drive/Suite 101   Galloway, NJ 08205   (609)404-1400   Fax (609)404-1430

Petivan, Victoria Anne, MD {1457453383} Psychy, IntrMd(89,LA05)<NJ-TRENTPSY>
+ Trenton Psychiatric Hospital
Sullivan Way/PO Box 7600   West Trenton, NJ 08628   (609)633-1502   Fax (609)777-0327

Petracca, Louis J., MD {1073643136} IntrMd, PulDis(77,ITAL)
+ 332 Bloomfield Avenue
Bloomfield, NJ 07003   (973)429-9225   Fax (973)566-0973

Petras, Jennifer Naomi, MD {1417977240} PsyCAd, Pedtrc(01,NY47)<NY-MTSINAI, NY-MTSINYHS>
+ 401A South Brunt Street
Englewood, NJ 07631   (201)894-9011

Petras, Peri Ann, MD {1538136916} Gyneco(80,NY20)<NJ-HACKNSK>
+ Excelsior Women's Care
170 Prospect Avenue/Suite 4   Hackensack, NJ 07601   (201)488-2288   Fax (201)488-2298

Petraske, Alison R., MD {1932127719} ObsGyn(93,MA07)<NJ-UNVMCPRN>
+ Princeton Ob/Gyn
5 Plainsboro Road/Suite 500   Plainsboro, NJ 08536   (609)936-0700   Fax (609)936-0750
+ University Medical Center of Princeton at Plainsboro
One Plainsboro Road/Ob/Gyn   Plainsboro, NJ 08536   (609)497-4000

Petrella, Michael Onofrio, MD {1528001419} Pedtrc, NnPnMd(98,GRN01)<NJ-HACKNSK>
+ Hackensack University Medical Center
30 Prospect Avenue/NeoPeri   Hackensack, NJ 07601   (201)996-2000

Petrides, Joanna, MD {1821496936}
+ University Hospital-SOM Department of Psychiatry
2250 Chapel Avenue West/Suite 100   Cherry Hill, NJ 08002   (856)482-9000   Fax (856)482-1159
+ University Hospital-University Family Medicine
42 East Laurel Road/Suite 2100   Stratford, NJ 08084   (856)482-9000   Fax (856)482-1159

Petriella, Michael R., Jr., MD {1841239449} ObsGyn(72,MD01)<NJ-HACKNSK>
+ 20 Prospect Avenue/Suite 810
Hackensack, NJ 07601   (201)336-8109   Fax (201)336-8112

Petrillo, Jennifer Anne, MD {1568566727} FamMed(97,NY46)
+ Edna Mahan Correctional Fac/Mental Hlt
PO Box 4004   Clinton, NJ 08809   (908)735-7111   Fax (908)730-6788

Petrillo, John A., MD {1215962816} SrgOrt(72,ITAL)<NJ-COMMED, NJ-HLTHSRE>
+ Ocean Orthopedic Associates, P.A.
530 Lakehurst Road/Suite 1   Toms River, NJ 08755   (732)349-8454   Fax (732)341-0259

Petrin, Ziva, MD {1235541475} PhysMd
+ Princeton Spine and Joint Center
256 Bunn Drive/Suite B   Princeton, NJ 08540   (609)454-0760   Fax (609)454-0761

Petrone, Sylvia J., MD {1710943139} Surgry(77,IL43)<NJ-STBARNMC>
+ Burn Surgeons of Saint Barnabas
94 Old Short Hills Road   Livingston, NJ 07039   (973)322-5924   Fax (973)322-5447

Petrosini, Anthony V., MD {1962481499} SrgOrt, SprtMd(91,NY08)<NJ-JRSYSHMC>
+ Orthopaedic Institute of Central Jersey
2315A Highway 34/Suite D   Manasquan, NJ 08736   (732)974-0404   Fax (732)449-4271
+ Orthopaedic Institute of Central Jersey
365 Broad Street   Red Bank, NJ 07701   (732)974-0404   Fax (732)933-1444
+ Orthopaedic Institute of Central Jersey
226 Highway 37 West/Suite 203   Toms River, NJ 08736   (732)240-6060   Fax (732)240-5329

Petroski, Donald, MD {1336132489} Gastrn, Grtrcs, IntrMd(70,PA09)<NJ-LOURDMED>
+ Lourdes Medical Associates
East 1113 Hospital Drive   Willingboro, NJ 08046   (609)835-3624   Fax (609)835-3628
+ GI Consultative Services
805 Cooper Road/Suite 2   Voorhees, NJ 08043   (609)835-3624   Fax (856)424-2218

Petrosyan, Gohar, MD {1366753493} IntrMd<NJ-STJOSHOS>
+ St. Joseph's Regional Medical Center
703 Main Street   Paterson, NJ 07503   (973)754-2000

Petrovani, Mark S., MD {1871758565} FamMed(90,NJ03)
+ Petrovani Family Medicine, PLLC
10 Parker Place   Fords, NJ 08863   (917)858-3293   Fax (914)440-5281

Petrowsky, Deborah, MD {1790129856} PulDis, IntrMd(91,NJ05)<NJ-HUNTRDN>
+ Reflections Center for Skin & Body
299 East Northfield Road   Livingston, NJ 07039   (973)740-2444   Fax (973)740-0070   DPetrowsky@reflectionscenter.com
+ Reflelctions Center for Skin & Body
1924 Washington Valley Road   Martinsville, NJ 08836   (732)356-1666

Petrozzino, Jeffrey, MD {1083852958} NnPnMd<NJ-UNDRWD>
+ Advocare West Deptford Pediatrics
646 Kings Highway   West Deptford, NJ 08096   (856)879-2887   Fax (856)879-2855
+ Inspira Health Network
509 North Broad Street   Woodbury, NJ 08096   (856)845-0100

Petrozzino, Vito A., MD {1366481624} Pedtrc(76,MEX03)<NY-STBARNAB, NJ-OVERLOOK>
+ 15 James Street/Suite 1
Florham Park, NJ 07932   (201)690-5361
+ 349 East Northfield Road/Suite LL2
Livingston, NJ 07039   (201)690-5361   Fax (973)992-2837

Petrucci, James Christopher, DO {1740453471} PedSpM(05,PA77)<NJ-JRSYSHMC>
+ Jersey Shore Sports Medicine Center
51 Davis Avenue/Suite 51-02   Neptune, NJ 07753   (732)776-2433   Fax (732)776-4403

Petrucelli, Janet L., MD {1154404358} PhysMd(02,PA02)
+ Aspen Medical Associates, P.A.
1 DeGraw Square   Teaneck, NJ 07666   (201)928-0200   Fax (201)928-0820

Petrucelli, Marisa Parise, DO {1043506637} Anesth<NJ-NWTN-MEM>
+ Newton Medical Center
175 High Street/Anesthesia   Newton, NJ 07860   (973)383-2121

Petruncio, George J., MD {1689709586} FamMed(83,BWI01)<NJ-UNDRWD, NJ-KMHCHRRY>
+ 188 Fries Mill Road/Suite E-1
Turnersville, NJ 08012   (856)875-7700   Fax (856)262-0428

Petruzzi, Nicholas Joseph, MD {1932360658} IntrMd
+ Atlantic Medical Imaging, LLC.
44 East Jimmie Leeds Road/Suite 101   Galloway, NJ 08205   (609)677-9729   Fax (609)652-6512

Petrychenko, Dmitri, MD {1588644272} AnesPain, Anesth(91,UKR12)<NY-NYUTISCH>
+ Interventional Pain Management Clinic
25 Kilmer Drive/Building 3/Suite 109   Morganville, NJ 07751   (718)336-5123   Fax (718)336-5137   info@freeofpain.org

Pettee, Brett, MD {1356768790} IntrMd
+ Summit Medical Group-Berkeley Heights Campus
1 Diamond Hill Road   Berkeley Heights, NJ 07922   (908)277-8625   Fax (908)608-2378

Petti, Christopher Louis, MD {1285678169} RadDia(93,NY19)
+ Bergen Imaging Center
180 North Dean Street   Englewood, NJ 07631   (201)568-4242   Fax (201)568-1298

Petti, Theodore Andre, MD {1033170121} Psychy, PsyCAd(68,OH06)<NJ-UNIVBHC, NJ-RWJUBRUN>
+ University Behavioral Health Care
671 Hoes Lane/PO Box 1392/Rm D205   Piscataway, NJ 08855   (732)235-4557   Fax (732)235-3923   pettita@umdnj.edu
+ University Behavioral Health Care
303 George Street/Suite 200   New Brunswick, NJ 08901

(732)235-4557   Fax (732)235-6187

Pettigrew, Isabel Hilary, MD {1023098225} FamMed(72,SCOT)<NJ-VIRTMARL, NJ-VIRTVOOR>
+ Endocrinology Associates
740 Marne Highway/Suite 206   Moorestown, NJ 08057   (856)234-0645   Fax (856)234-0498
+ Lourdes Medical Associates
500 Grove Street/Suite 100   Haddon Heights, NJ 08035   (856)234-0645   Fax (856)796-9397

Pettinelli, Damon John, MD {1558477448} Ophthl, IntrMd(PA13
+ LASIK PLUS
351 Evelyn Street/Suite 301   Paramus, NJ 07652   (201)634-1444   Fax (201)634-1555   dpettinelli@lca.com

Pettinelli, Frank P., Jr., DO {1215979307} FamMed(82,PA77)<NJ-VIRTMARL, NJ-VIRTVOOR>
+ Family Practice Medical Associates
3814 Church Road   Mount Laurel, NJ 08054   (856)231-9792   Fax (856)231-9682

Pettis, Larry, MD {1053433276} FamMed(76,CA19)<NJ-STFRN-MED>
+ Addiction Pain Associates
100 Kings Way East/Suite D-3   Sewell, NJ 08080   (856)589-1440   Fax (856)589-4616

Petty, Victoria Morey, MD {1346246725} ObsGyn, IntrMd(PA01
+ Capital Health Medical
2 Capital Way/Suite 356   Pennington, NJ 08534   (609)537-6000   Fax (609)537-6002

Peyser, Irving G., MD {1619915253} Surgry(67,VT02)
+ 3699 US Highway 46
Parsippany, NJ 07054   (973)334-0224   Fax (973)334-0208

Pfisterer, Christine, DO {1245491455} PhysMd
+ Northern Jersey Orthopedic Center PA
870 Palisade Avenue/Suite 205   Teaneck, NJ 07666   (201)836-1663   Fax (201)836-5729

Pfisterer, Dennis James, DO {1669795498} SrgOrt<PA-YORK>
+ Northern Jersey Orthopedic Center PA
870 Palisade Avenue/Suite 205   Teaneck, NJ 07666   (201)836-1663   Fax (201)836-5729

Pfisterer, Dennis L., MD {1063499390} SrgOrt(78,NY46)<NJ-HOLY-NAME>
+ Northern Jersey Orthopedic Center PA
870 Palisade Avenue/Suite 205   Teaneck, NJ 07666   (201)836-1663   Fax (201)836-5729

Pflum, Francis A., Jr., MD {1609939297} SrgOrt(70,NJ05)
+ 550 Newark Avenue/Suite 200
Jersey City, NJ 07306   (201)420-0069

Pflum, Gerald E., MD {1386603066} Otlryg, OtgyFPIS(72,IL43)<NJ-JRSYSHMC, NJ-RIVERVW>
+ 10 Neptune Boulevard
Neptune, NJ 07753   (732)775-1301   Fax (732)775-0507

Phair, Arthur H., MD {1245201441} Ortped, SrgOrt(78,NJ05)<NJ-BAYSHORE>
+ Orthopaedic Sports Medicine
80 Oak Hill Road   Red Bank, NJ 07701   (732)741-2313   Fax (732)741-7154

Phakey, Vishal, DO {1356723084} FamMed
+ Voorhees Primary & Specialty Care
333 Laurel Oak Road   Voorhees, NJ 08043   (844)542-2273   Fax (856)770-9194

Pham, Bich N., MD {1518917178} Pthlgy, PthHem, PthCyt(73,VIE05)<NJ-COMMED>
+ Community Medical Center
99 Route 37 West/Path   Toms River, NJ 08755   (732)557-8141

Pham, Chi H., MD {1912032368} Anesth(74,VIET)<NJ-MEM-SALEM>
+ Memorial Hospital of Salem County
310 Woodstown Road/Anesth   Salem, NJ 08079   (856)935-1000

Pham, Michael Minh, MD {1104091792} Anesth(04,NY47)<NJ-JRSYCITY>
+ Jersey City Medical Center
355 Grand Street/2w 105/Anesth   Jersey City, NJ 07304   (201)915-2000
+ Englewood Surgical Associates
375 Engle Street/Ground Floor   Englewood, NJ 07631   (201)915-2000   Fax (201)894-1022

Pham, Peter H., DO {1063708576} IntHos
+ 29 Silver Brook Drive
Bridgeton, NJ 08302   (609)805-6036

Pham, Vu Linh, MD {1619051885} Anesth(02,PA02)<NJ-COMMED>
+ Morris Anesthesia Group, PA
3799 Route 46/Suite 211   Parsippany, NJ 07054   (973)335-1122   Fax (973)335-1448

Phan, Au Ngoc, MD {1437244852} EmrgMd(99,NJ05)<NJ-STPETER>
+ Brunswick Urgent Care
3185 State Route 27   Franklin Park, NJ 08823

Physicians by Name and Address

Phan, Khanh Bao, DO {1871804328} Pedtrc
+ 1651 Earl Street
Union, NJ 07083 (908)591-9200

Phan, Lily, MD {1871912907} Anesth<NJ-TRINIWSC>
+ Trinitas Regional Medical Center-Williamson Street
225 Williamson Street Elizabeth, NJ 07207 (908)994-5204

Phariss, Bruce Wallace, MD {1255428322} Psychy, PsyAdd, IntrMd(90,NY19)<NY-PRSBWEIL, NY-PRSBCOLU>
+ Sheila Harrington, LCSW
8 Hillside Avenue/Suite 106 Montclair, NJ 07042
(973)509-2371 Fax (973)744-9003

Phatak, Tej Deepak, MD {1841455789} PedRad, Radiol, Pedtrc(02,NY01)<NJ-NWRKBETH>
+ Newark Diagnostic Radiologists, PA
201 Lyons Avenue Newark, NJ 07112 (973)912-4494
Fax (973)282-0911

Phelps, Kristyn Kia, MD {1497917868} IntrMd(03,PA13)
+ Ocean Health Initiatives, Inc.
101 Second Street Lakewood, NJ 08701 (732)363-6655
Fax (732)363-6656

Phen, Huai Lee, MD {1881956381}
+ Tatem Brown Family Practice
2225 East Evesham Road/Suite 101 Voorhees, NJ 08043
(856)795-4330 Fax (856)325-3704

Philip, Abraham Theverthundyil, MD {1447284153} Pthlgy, PthFor, PthACI(78,INA94)
+ Office of The Regional Medical Examiner State of NJ
325 Norfolk Street Newark, NJ 07103 (973)648-3914
Fax (973)648-3692

Philipp, Claire S., MD {1164594206} OncHem, Hemato, IntrMd(78,RI01)<NJ-RWJUBRUN>
+ UMDNJ RWJ Heamtology Oncology
125 Paterson Street/MEB 378 New Brunswick, NJ 08901
(732)235-7682 Fax (732)235-7115

Philips, Jay, MD {1235180878} Pedtrc(77,INA76)<NJ-VALLEY>
+ The Valley Hospital
223 North Van Dien Avenue/Pediatrics Ridgewood, NJ 07450 (201)447-8000 Fax (201)447-8491

Philips, Kaitlyn S., DO {1396151577}<NJ-MORRISTN>
+ Morristown Medical Center
100 Madison Avenue Morristown, NJ 07962 (973)971-5000

Philips-Rodriguez, Dahlia, MD {1831255249} IntrMd(04,CT02)<NY-BETHKING>
+ Summit Medical Group-Berkeley Heights Campus
1 Diamond Hill Road Berkeley Heights, NJ 07922
(908)273-4300 Fax (908)790-6576

Phillips, Anne R., MD {1104015544} Psychy(87,NY48)
+ 8 Turtle Court
Flemington, NJ 08822 (908)812-1028
annerp@comcast.net

Phillips, Bradley John, MD {1104800143} Ophthl(86,NY48)<NY-SUNYBRKL, NJ-RWJUBRUN>
+ Bradley John Phillips MD LLC
1543 Route 27/Suite 23 Somerset, NJ 08873 (732)249-6101 Fax (732)249-6102

Phillips, Hadley H., DO {1629036306} Ophthl(78,MO79)
+ Phillips Eye Center
619 River Drive Elmwood Park, NJ 07407 (201)796-2020
Fax (201)796-2833
+ Hudson Eye Specialists
2201 Bergen Line Avenue/3rd Floor Union City, NJ 07087
(201)601-2020

Phillips, James J., MD {1134220098} ObsGyn(74,MEXI)<NJ-ACMCITY, NJ-ACMCMAIN>
+ Atlantic Ob-Gyn Group PA
501 Bay Avenue/Suite 201 Somers Point, NJ 08244
(609)927-3828 Fax (609)926-8067

Phillips, Keren Amy, MD {1780684951} Pedtrc, AdolMd(96,NY15)
+ Monmouth Family Center
270 Broadway Long Branch, NJ 07740 (732)923-7100
Fax (732)923-7104

Phillips, Michelle Nicole, MD {1629599287} EmrgMd
+ Robert Wood Johnson Emergency Medicine
One Robert Wood Johnson Place/MEB 104 New Brunswick, NJ 08901 (732)235-7883

Phillips, Nancy A., MD {1326166307} ObsGyn, Gyneco(88,NJ06)
+ UMDNJ OBGYN
125 Paterson Street/Suite 4200 New Brunswick, NJ 08901
(732)235-6600 Fax (732)235-6650

Phillips, Nancy L., MD {1215018304} ObsGyn, Obstet(64,PA09)<NJ-COOPRUMC>
+ Cooper Ob/Gyn
3 Cooper Plaza/Suite 300 Camden, NJ 08103 (856)342-2186 Fax (856)968-8575

Phillips, Paul Mathew, MD {1922213107} Ophthl, IntrMd(OH41}
+ Paul Phillips Eye & Surgery Center
1 Monroe Street Bridgewater, NJ 08807 (908)526-4588
Fax (908)231-6718

Phillips, Paul S., MD {1073538153} Ophthl(87,NY48)<NJ-HUNTRDN>
+ Paul Phillips Eye & Surgery Center

6 Minneakoning Road/Suite B Flemington, NJ 08822
(908)824-7144 (908)968-3239
+ Paul Phillips Eye & Surgery Center
64 Walmart Plaza Clinton, NJ 08809 (908)824-7144 Fax
(908)735-7494

Philogene, Clark E., MD {1558462044} IntrMd(90,NY15)<NJ-OVERLOOK>
+ Union Medical Group LLC
2401 Morris Avenue/Suite 101 Union, NJ 07083
(908)688-5000 Fax (908)688-5220

Phinney, Maryann B., MD {1558414979} IntHos(03,NJ06)<NJ-UNVMCPRN>
+ Penn Medicine Princeton Medicine Phys
5 Plainsboro Road/Suite 350 Plainsboro, NJ 08536
(609)853-7220 Fax (609)853-7271
+ Princeton Plainsboro Hospitalists
253 Witherspoon Street/Suite J1 Princeton, NJ 08540 Fax
(609)497-4020

Phung, Michael Hung, MD {1508966219} CdvDis, IntrMd(74,VIE05)<NJ-CHRIST>
+ Drs. Phung and Phung
596 Pavonia Avenue Jersey City, NJ 07306 (201)792-4996
Fax (201)792-9663

Phung, Susan, MD {1548581622} IntrMd, CdvDis(06,PA09)<NJ-STMICHL, NJ-TRINIJSC>
+ Drs. Phung and Phung
596 Pavonia Avenue Jersey City, NJ 07306 (201)792-4996
Fax (201)792-9663

Pi, Justin Jeong-Suk, MD {1427203306} PulDis, SlpDis, IntrMd(05,GRN01)
+ Monmouth Ocean Pulmonary Medicine
901 West Main Street/Suite 160 Freehold, NJ 07728
(732)577-0600 Fax (732)577-6322

Piacentile, Joseph M., MD {1265607410} GenPrc(81,DC02)
+ 25 Angela Court
Woodcliff Lake, NJ 07677

Piantedosi, Benjamin George, MD {1205912144} AdolMd, Pedtrc(82,SPAI)<NJ-UNDRWD>
+ Advocare Woodbury Pediatrics
1050 Mantua Pike/Suite 200 Wenonah, NJ 08090
(856)853-0848 Fax (856)853-1889
+ Advocare Woodbury Pediatrics
340 Front Street/Suite 202 Elmer, NJ 08318 (856)853-0848 Fax (856)358-1889

Piarulli, Michael J., MD {1316926322} GenPrc, IntrMd(83,MEXI)
+ 13 East Delaware Trail
Medford, NJ 08055

Piawa, Dum Livinus, DO {1497076327} IntrMd<NJ-DEBRAHLC>
+ Deborah Heart and Lung Center
200 Trenton Road Browns Mills, NJ 08015 (609)893-1200
Fax (609)893-6038

Picard, Johan Arlenie, MD {1538428578} ObsGyn(09,NY47)
+ Brescia-Migliaccio Ob/Gyn
609 Washington Street Hoboken, NJ 07030 (201)659-7700 Fax (201)659-7701

Picaro, Anthony J., MD {1689710246} FamMed(65,NJ05)<NJ-SOCEANCO>
+ Ocean Medical MD, PA
3003 Long Beach Boulevard Beach Haven, NJ 08008
(609)492-0900 Fax (609)492-1347

Picascia, David D., MD {1306865613} Dermat, IntrMd(82,VA04)<NJ-CENTRAST>
+ Drs. Hametz & Picascia
77-55 Schanck Road/Suite B-3 Freehold, NJ 07728
(732)462-9800

Picascia, Lisa, MD {1104237098}
+ Summit Medical Group
1 Diamond Hill Road/Bensley Pav/2 FL Berkeley, NJ 07922
(908)277-8700 Fax (908)288-7993

Picciano, Anne, MD {1649332081} FamMed(87,PA01)<NJ-JFKMED>
+ JFK Family Practice Group
65 James Street Edison, NJ 08818 (732)321-7487 Fax
(732)906-4927

Picciano, Christina Maria, DO {1518311661}<NJ-RIVERVW>
+ Riverview Medical Center
1 Riverview Plaza Red Bank, NJ 07701 (732)741-2700

Picciano, Laura S., MD {1629040084} IntrMd
+ Drs. Picciano and Alexander
6100 Main Street/Ripa Center Voorhees, NJ 08043
(856)673-4912 Fax (856)938-2077

Picciano, Maria V., MD {1215957246} Ophthl(88,NJ05)
+ Drs. Picciano, Picciano & Sadik
36 Pacific Street Newark, NJ 07105 (973)578-4808 Fax
(973)578-2939

Picciano, Robert, MD {1841210861} IntrMd(88,NJ05)
+ Drs. Picciano, Picciano & Sadik
36 Pacific Street Newark, NJ 07105 (973)578-4808 Fax
(973)578-2939

Picciotti, Brett, DO {1366792616} NeuMus
+ 435 Haddonfield Road
Cherry Hill, NJ 08002 (844)542-2273

+ Kennedy Health Alliance Vascular Surgery
333 Laurel Oak Road Voorhees, NJ 08043 (844)542-2273
Fax (856)770-9194

Picciotti, Christopher David, DO {1912198136}
+ 604 Lagoon Boulevard
Brigantine, NJ 08203

Piccoli, Catherine Welch, MD {1699745901} RadDia
+ South Jersey Radiology Associates, P.A.
100 Carnie Boulevard/Suite B Voorhees, NJ 08043
(856)751-0123 Fax (856)751-0535
+ South Jersey Radiology Associates, P.A.
315 Route 70 East/Suite B Cherry Hill, NJ 08034 (856)751-0123 Fax (856)428-0356
+ South Jersey Radiology Associates, P.A.
901 Route 168/Suites 301-305 Turnersville, NJ 08043
(856)227-6600 Fax (856)227-8537

Piccolo, Christian K, MD {1447485792} IntrMd, Anesth(03,DC01)<NY-PRSBCOLU>
+ New Jersey Pain Consultants
310 Madison Avenue/Suite 301 Morristown, NJ 07960
(212)799-0508 Fax (973)998-9201

Piccone, Dennis L., DO {1578509394} FamMed(76,PA77)<NJ-SHOREMEM>
+ Margate Diagnostic Center
9710 Ventnor Avenue Margate, NJ 08402 (609)822-4800
Fax (609)822-2617

Pichardo, Nelson R., MD {1720110547} IntrMd(76,DOMI)
+ 757 Mount Prospect Avenue
Newark, NJ 07104 (973)510-3518 Fax (973)350-9009
drnelsonpichardo@gmail.com

Pichika, Nirmala, MD {1811056088} IntrMd(98,INA48)<NJ-LOURDMED>
+ Lourdes Medical Center of Burlington County
218 Sunset Road/Suite A/Internal Med Willingboro, NJ
08046 (609)835-3056 Fax (609)835-3061

Pickens, Robert L., MD {1114948007} Urolgy(65,CT01)<NJ-UNVMCPRN, NJ-CAPITLHS>
+ Urology Group of Princeton PA
281 Witherspoon Street/Suite 100 Princeton, NJ 08542
(609)924-6487 Fax (609)921-7020

Pickoff, Robert M., MD {1386762144} CdvDis, IntrMd(79,NY47)<NJ-HUNTRDN, NJ-STPETER>
+ Hunterdon HealthCare System
2100 Wescott Drive Flemington, NJ 08822 (908)788-6100
+ Hunterdon Medical Center
2100 Wescott Drive Flemington, NJ 08822 (908)788-6100
+ Willow Creek Rehabilitation & Care Center
1165 Easton Avenue Somerset, NJ 08822 (732)246-4100
Fax (732)246-3926

Pickover, Lawrence M., MD {1326084310} Gastrn, IntrMd(85,NY19)<NJ-STPETER>
+ 81 Veronica Avenue/Suite 206
Somerset, NJ 08873 (732)846-2777 Fax (732)828-1950
+ Cares Surgicenter, LLC.
240 Easton Avenue New Brunswick, NJ 08901 (732)846-2777 Fax (732)296-8677

Pickrell, Christie Calleo, MD {1992063994} EmrgMd<NJ-NWRKBETH>
+ Newark Beth Israel Medical Center
201 Lyons Avenue Newark, NJ 07112 (973)926-7240

Picone, Frank J., MD {1477502565} Allrgy, AlgyImmn(67,NJ05)<NJ-RIVERVW, NJ-MONMOUTH>
+ Two River Allergy & Asthma Group
709 Sycamore Avenue Tinton Falls, NJ 07701 (732)747-8188 Fax (732)747-5946
info@mdinhale.com

Picone, Maryann, MD {1295888030} Nrolgy(85,NJ05)<NJ-HOLYNAME>
+ MS Center at Holy Name Hospital
718 Teaneck Road Teaneck, NJ 07666 (201)837-0727
Fax (201)837-8504

Picone, Michael J., MD {1629299920} AnesPain, Anesth(02,NJ05)<NJ-SOMERSET>
+ Anesthesia Consultnts of NJ/Nova Pain
285 Davidson Avenue/Suite 204 Somerset, NJ 08873
(732)271-1400 Fax (732)271-3543
+ RWJ University Hospital Somerset
110 Rehill Avenue/Anesthesia Somerville, NJ 08876
(908)685-2200
+ Raritan Valley Surgery Center
100 Franklin Square Drive/Suite 100 Somerset, NJ 08873
(732)560-1000 Fax (732)560-5999

Pidduck, Thomas Charles, MD {1285610998} Ophthl(94,DC02)<NJ-COMMED>
+ Susskind & Almallah Eye Associates, P.A.
20 Mule Road/Focus Center Toms River, NJ 08755
(732)349-5622 Fax (732)349-5625

Pie, Alberto C., MD {1104929397} EmrgMd, FamMed, IntrMd(69,PHI10)
+ 900 Newark Avenue
Forked River, NJ 08731 (609)693-0115

Pie, Cynthia P., MD {1528364809}<NJ-COMMED>
+ Community Medical Center
99 Route 37 West   Toms River, NJ 08755   (609)971-5270
drcindy314@gmail.com

Piech, Richard Frank, MD {1629160361} FamMed(81,MD12)
+ RWJPE Towne Centre Family Care
302 Towne Centre Drive   Hillsborough, NJ 08844
(908)359-8613   Fax (908)874-8509
+ Priority Medical Care
350 Grove Street/Suite 200   Bridgewater, NJ 08807
(908)359-8613   Fax (908)722-6031

Pieczara, Beata Katarzyna, MD {1255444394} IntrMd, Onclgy(93,POL03)<NJ-HOLYNAME>
+ Regional Cancer Center at Holy Name Medical Center
718 Teaneck Road   Teaneck, NJ 07666   (201)227-6008
Fax (201)227-6002

Pieczuro, Barbara Katarzyna, MD {1235105149} Pedtrc(85,POL10)<NJ-HACKNSK>
+ 525 Kipp Street
Teaneck, NJ 07666

Piela, Christina, MD {1992741987} Pedtrc(85,POLA)
+ ABC Pediatric Associates PA
131 Drum Point Road   Brick, NJ 08723   (732)477-8988

Pien, Gary Chai-Li, MD {1841404530} AlgyImmn, Pedtrc(03,RI01)<PA-CHILDHOS>
+ Summit Medical Group-Berkeley Heights Campus
1 Diamond Hill Road   Berkeley Heights, NJ 07922
(908)273-4300   Fax (908)790-6576

Pierce, Brandon Keefe, MD {1417169202} Anesth(05,PA02)<NJ-MEMSALEM>
+ Memorial Hospital of Salem County
310 Woodstown Road/Anesthesia   Salem, NJ 08079
(856)935-5885   Fax (856)935-4757

Pierce, Bruce R., MD {1437159506} ObsGyn(92,VA04)<NJ-CHSFULD, NJ-UNVMCPRN>
+ Delaware Valley Ob/Gyn & Infertility Group, PC
2 Princess Road/Suite C   Lawrenceville, NJ 08648
(609)896-0777   Fax (609)896-3266
+ Delaware Valley Ob/Gyn & Infertility Group, PC
300B Princeton Hightstown Road   East Windsor, NJ 08520
(609)896-0777   Fax (609)443-4506

Pierce, Sean Donovan, MD {1407831415} RadNro(94,MA01)<NJ-HACKNSK>
+ The Imaging Center
30 South Newman Street   Hackensack, NJ 07601
(201)488-1188   Fax (201)488-5244
+ New Century Imaging at Oradell
555 Kinderkamack Road   Oradell, NJ 07649   (201)488-1188
Fax (201)599-8333
+ Hackensack Radiology Group, P.A.
30 Prospect Avenue   Hackensack, NJ 07601   (201)996-2200   Fax (201)336-8451

Pierce, Vincent E., Jr., MD {1285859207} EmrgMd, OccpMd(78,PA01)
+ 1440 Lower Ferry Road
Ewing, NJ 08618   (609)890-4445   Fax (609)890-4447

Piercefield, Dayne Douglas, MD {1003961319}
+ 5240 Oakwood Court
Egg Harbor City, NJ 08215

Pieretti, Gordon Anthony, DO {1881641827} IntrMd(99,NJ75)<NJ-VIRTVOOR, NJ-KMHSTRAT>
+ Advocare Sicklerville Internal Med
485 Williamstown Road   Sicklerville, NJ 08081   (856)237-8100   Fax (856)237-8042

Pieretti, Janice, MD {1154527935} IntrMd, CdvDis(04,NY47)<NY-SPCLSURG, NJ-NWRKBETH>
+ Newark Beth Israel Medical Center
201 Lyons Avenue/Suite L4   Newark, NJ 07112   (973)926-7323   Fax (973)705-3096

Pieri, Danielle, DO {1982866554}
+ Pavilion Ob/Gyn AtlantiCare
2500 English Creek Avenue/Suite 214   Egg Harbor Township, NJ 08234   (609)677-7211   Fax (609)677-7210
danielle.pieri@atlanticare.org

Pierog, Sophie H., MD {1265514517} Pedtrc(63,WI06)<NJ-JRSYCITY>
+ 122 Clinton Street
Hoboken, NJ 07030   (201)418-3129   Fax (201)418-3148

Pierpont, Christopher Edward, MD {1467432864} RadDia, RadV&I(98,NY46)
+ Edison Radiology Group, P.A.
65 James Street   Edison, NJ 08820   (732)321-7917   Fax (732)737-2968

Pierre, Andre M., MD {1932108727} Anesth(77,HAI01)<NJ-VIRTBERL, NJ-VIRTMARL>
+ West Jersey Anesthesia Associates
102-E Center Boulevard   Marlton, NJ 08053   (856)988-6250   Fax (856)988-6270

Pierre, Edeck Saintilien, MD {1083839724} IntHos, IntrMd(02,SLU01)<NJ-CHILTON>
+ Chilton Medical Center
97 West Parkway   Pompton Plains, NJ 07444   (973)831-5000

Pierre, Joelle, MD {1528265279} PedSrg(02,NY47)<NY-VABRKLYN>
+ RWJ University Hospital New Brunswick
One Robert Wood Johnson Place   New Brunswick, NJ 08901
(732)235-7821   Fax (732)235-8878

Pierre, Margarette Rose, MD {1033119367} Pedtrc(90,HAI01)
+ JFK Medical Center
65 James Street   Edison, NJ 08820   (732)321-7000   Fax (732)906-4906
+ La Familia Medical Care
115 Jefferson Avenue   Elizabeth, NJ 07201   (732)321-7000
Fax (908)351-1760

Pierre-Louis, Frantz Junior M., MD {1164733838} InfDis, IntrMd(02,HAI02)
+ People Care Institute
323 Belleville Avenue/Floor 2   Bloomfield, NJ 07003
(973)842-4272   Fax (732)997-3022
+ 9 Burnett Road
Mendham, NJ 07945   (347)232-7297

Pierre-Louis, James, MD {1730226580} Anesth(00,NJ02)<NJ-OVERLOOK>
+ Summit Anesthesia Associates, P.A.
33 Overlook Road/Suite 311   Summit, NJ 07901   (908)598-1500   Fax (908)598-0197

Pierrot, Paul H., MD {1407896053} IntrMd(91,NJ06)<NJ-CHSMRCER, NJ-CHSFULD>
+ Capital Health Primary Care
1230 Parkway Avenue/Suite 203   Ewing, NJ 08628
(609)883-5454   Fax (609)883-2564
+ 941 Whitehorse Avenue/Suite 1
Trenton, NJ 08610   (609)883-5454   Fax (609)581-9300

Pierson, Christopher G., MD {1396701900} CdvDis, IntCrd, IntrMd(89,NY19)<NJ-RIVERVW, NJ-JRSYSHMC>
+ Christopher G. Pierson MD LLC
241 Monmouth Road/Suite 202   West Long Branch, NJ 07764   (732)923-9603   Fax (732)923-9096

Pierson, David Shawn, MD {1003889049} Pedtrc
+ Princeton Nassau Pediatrics, P.A.
301 North Harrison Street   Princeton, NJ 08540   (609)924-5510   Fax (609)924-3577

Pierson, Joseph, Jr., MD {1568442903} Pedtrc, AdolMd(67,MA07)<NJ-UNVMCPRN>
+ Princeton Nassau Pediatrics, P.A.
301 North Harrison Street   Princeton, NJ 08540   (609)924-5510   Fax (609)924-3577
+ Princeton Nassau Pediatrics, P.A.
196 Princeton-Hightstown Road   West Windsor, NJ 08550
(609)924-5510   Fax (609)799-2294

Pietka, Jamie K., MD {1790710333} FamMed<NJ-MORRISTN>
+ Morristown Medical Center
100 Madison Avenue   Morristown, NJ 07962   (973)971-5000

Pietras, Jerome R., DO {1699717637} Urolgy(72,IA75)<NJ-KMHSTRAT, NJ-VIRTUAHS>
+ Delaware Valley Urology LLC
570 Egg Harbor Road/Suite A-1   Sewell, NJ 08080
(856)582-9645   Fax (856)985-4583
+ New Jersey Urology LLC
2090 Springdale Road/Suite D   Cherry Hill, NJ 08003
(856)582-9645   Fax (856)985-9908
+ New Jersey Urology, LLC
2401 East Evesham Road/Suite F   Voorhees, NJ 08080
(856)481-1600   Fax (856)988-0636

Pietrucha, Dorothy M., MD {1598751083} NroChl, Pedtrc, IntrMd(68,NJ05)<NJ-JRSYSHMC>
+ Meridian Pediatric Associates
81 Davis Avenue/Suite 4   Neptune, NJ 07753   (732)776-4551   Fax (732)776-4392
dpietrucha@meridianhealth.com

Piezas, Sylvia M., MD {1730121278} Pedtrc, GenPrc(89,PHI09)<NJ-SOMERSET, NJ-STPETER>
+ Somerset Pediatric Group PA
155 Union Avenue   Bridgewater, NJ 08807   (908)725-1802
Fax (908)203-8825
+ Somerset Pediatric Group PA
2345 Lamington Road/Suite 101   Bedminster, NJ 07921
(908)725-1802   Fax (908)470-2845

Piggee, Mia Christine, MD {1508825928} Pedtrc, IntrMd, IntHos(97,TN07)<NJ-NWTNMEM>
+ Newton Medical Center
175 High Street/Pediatrics   Newton, NJ 07860   (973)383-2121   Fax (973)579-8807
+ Reliance Medical Group, LLC
1325 Baltic Avenue   Atlantic City, NJ 08401   (973)383-2121
Fax (609)441-0953

Pikalov, Andrei A., MD {1033342373} Psychy
+ 5 Honeysuckle Lane
Kinnelon, NJ 07405

Pikus, Igor, MD {1760659528} Anesth, IntrMd(02,GRN01)
+ Morris Anesthesia Group, PA
3799 Route 46/Suite 211   Parsippany, NJ 07054   (973)335-1122   Fax (973)335-1448

Pilcher, Mary Frances, MD {1033352695} Dermat
+ Affiliated Dermatologists
182 South Street/Suite 1   Morristown, NJ 07960   (706)830-6960   Fax (973)695-1480
mary.frances.pilcher@gmail.com

Pilet, Jean-Claude, MD {1750442125} Ophthl(63,HAIT)
+ 78 West Park Avenue/Suite 3
Vineland, NJ 08360   (856)691-6366
+ CompleteCare Adult & Specialty Medical Professionals
1038 East Chestnut Avenue/Suite 110   Vineland, NJ 08360
(856)451-4700

Piliero, Peter James, MD {1972861896} InfDis, IntrMd(89,NY48)
+ Merck and Company Incorporated
1 Merck Drive/PO Box 100   Whitehouse Station, NJ 08889
(908)423-1000

Pilipshen, Stephen J., MD {1467517599} SrgC&R, Surgry(76,NY20)
+ Pilipshen Colon & Rectal Surgical Services
1221 North Church Street/Suite 204   Moorestown, NJ 08057   (856)234-3322   Fax (856)234-3615

Pilla, John D., MD {1447282660} FamMed(84,NJ06)<NJ-SOMERSET>
+ MEDEMERGE
1005 North Washington Avenue   Green Brook, NJ 08812
(732)968-8900   Fax (732)968-4609

Pilla, Timothy S., MD {1023019312} SrgVas, Surgry(82,PA02)<NJ-UNDRWD>
+ General Vascular Surgical Specialists
17 West Red Bank Avenue/Suite 203   Woodbury, NJ 08096
(856)853-7056   Fax (856)384-6015

Pillai, Adip, DO {1841685088} IntrMd<NJ-SJHREGMC>
+ SJH Regional Medical Center
1505 West Sherman Avenue   Vineland, NJ 08360
(856)641-8000

Pillai, Hema R., MD {1144257577} Pedtrc(80,INDI)
+ Sadhana Pediatrics, P.C.
49 Veronica Avenue/Suite 101   Somerset, NJ 08873
(732)247-3434   Fax (732)247-1815

Pillai, Jyoti Ajay, MD {1578513271} Nrolgy
+ Drexel Neurosciences Institute
601 Route 73 North   Marlton, NJ 08053   (215)762-6915
Fax (215)762-6914

Pillai, Renuka, DO {1780634378} EmrgMd(01,NY75)<NJ-OCEANMC>
+ EmCare
1945 Route 33   Neptune, NJ 07753   (732)776-4510   Fax (732)776-2329
+ EmCare
425 Jack Martin Boulevard   Brick, NJ 08724   (732)840-3380

Pillitteri, John, MD {1437166105} Anesth(86,NY08)
+ Jandee Anesthesiology
500 North Franklin Turnpike/Suite 206   Ramsey, NJ 07446
(201)962-7282   Fax (201)962-7283

Pillon, Mark A., MD {1104883313} Anesth, PainMd, OthrSp(87,GRN01)
+ Ambulatory Anesthesia Care, PC
1450 Route 22 West/MedDirector   Mountainside, NJ 07092
(908)233-2020   Fax (908)233-9322

Pilly, Ashok K., MD {1801997523} CdvDis, IntrMd, GenPrc(75,IND)
+ 3662 Delsea Drive
Vineland, NJ 08360   (856)825-8100   Fax (856)825-8711

Pilot, Richard, MD {1124461132} IntrMd(84,GER05)
+ Celgene Corporation
300 Connell Drive/Suite 6000   Berkeley Heights, NJ 07922
(908)673-9000   Fax (908)219-0944

Pina, Liza Miriam, MD {1043541246} Pedtrc(84,HON01)
+ 36 Bluebird Court
Flemington, NJ 08822   Fax (908)237-2871

Pinal, Jose, MD {1013098862} PulDis(74,SPAI)<NJ-HOBUNIMC>
+ 526 42nd Street
Union City, NJ 07087   (201)865-9195   Fax (201)865-4416

Pinal, Laureen, MD {1477940906} FamMed
+ 480 Pompton Avenue
Cedar Grove, NJ 07009   (201)679-3097

Pinchuck, Curt P., MD {1275532871} Psychy(87,NY06)
+ North Jersey Neurofeedback
50 Mount Prospect Avenue/Suite 201   Clifton, NJ 07013
(973)471-4400

Pincus, Jillian R., MD {1376703512} IntrMd, Nephro(74,PA07)
+ 1 Plymouth Road
Chatham, NJ 07928

Pinder, Godfrey C., MD {1891785945} SrgCdv, SrgThr(69,WI06)<NJ-CHILTON>
+ 99 Old Indian Road
West Orange, NJ 07052   (973)731-7441   Fax (973)731-8381
+ 230 Sherman Avenue/Suite B
Glen Ridge, NJ 07028   (973)429-7474
+ 450 North Beverwyck Road
Parsippany, NJ 07052   (973)731-7441

Physicians by Name and Address

Pine, Martin S., MD {1467587485} Allrgy, IntrMd, IntMAImm(70,NY09)
+ Center for Asthma & Allergy
  300 Hudson Street   Hoboken, NJ 07030   (201)792-5900   Fax (201)792-5320
+ Center for Asthma & Allergy
  18 North Third Avenue   Highland Park, NJ 08904   (201)792-5900   Fax (732)545-4087
+ Center for Asthma & Allergy
  90 Milburn Avenue/Suite 200   Maplewood, NJ 07030   (973)763-5787   Fax (973)763-8568

Pineda, Jean, DO {1780627695} ObsGyn(96,NY75)<NJ-STPETER>
+ Somerset Ob-Gyn Associates
  1 New Amwell Road   Hillsborough, NJ 08844   (908)874-5900
+ Somerset Ob-Gyn Associates
  215 Union Avenue/Suite A   Bridgewater, NJ 08807   (908)874-5900   Fax (908)722-1856
+ St. Peter's University Hospital
  254 Easton Avenue/ObGyn   New Brunswick, NJ 08844   (732)745-8600

Pineda, Julita S., MD {1922060011} IntrMd(84,PHI01)<NJ-COMMED, NJ-JRSYSHMC>
+ Physicians for Adults
  681 Route 70   Lakehurst, NJ 08733   (732)657-8111

Pineda, Maria Georgina C., MD Pedtrc(90,PHIL)
+ Pineda Pediatrics
  1608 Route 88 West   Brick, NJ 08724

Pineda, Nonato E., MD {1548229891} IntrMd(84,PHIL)<NJ-JRSYSHMC>
+ Physicians for Adults
  681 Route 70   Lakehurst, NJ 08733   (732)657-8111   Fax (732)657-7828
+ Jersey Shore University Medical Center
  1945 Route 33   Neptune, NJ 07753   (732)775-5500

Pineda, Verne M., MD {1386671287} Gastrn(65,PHIL)
+ 502 Centennial Boulevard/Suite 8
  Voorhees, NJ 08043   (856)772-0111   Fax (856)772-2838

Pineda, Veronica Vargas, DO {1487744223} FamMed(97,NY75)
+ 714-716 Broadway
  Bayonne, NJ 07002

Pinel Villalobos, Silvia P., DO {1023036928} IntrMd(02,NY75)<NJ-MORRISTN>
+ IPC The Hospitalist Company
  220 Ridgedale Avenue/Suite C-2   Florham Park, NJ 07932   (973)538-5844   Fax (973)267-0181

Pineles, Cary L., MD {1760474951} IntrMd(80,NY08)<NJ-KIMBALL, NJ-COMMED>
+ Shore Medical Specialists
  500 River Avenue/Suite 140   Lakewood, NJ 08701   (732)363-7200   Fax (732)363-8183
+ Shore Medical Specialists
  9 Hospital Drive   Toms River, NJ 08755   (732)363-7200   Fax (732)349-9697

Pingol, Carmelo S., MD {1437135738} Psychy(84,PHIL)
+ Mt. Carmel Guild/Behavioral Health
  285 Magnolia Avenue   Jersey City, NJ 07304   (201)395-4819   Fax (201)435-9580

Pinho, Paulo Bandeira, MD {1922006352} IntrMd, Pedtrc(99,NJ05)<NJ-OVERLOOK, NJ-STBARNMC>
+ PASE HealthCare, PC
  225 Millburn Avenue/Suite 303   Millburn, NJ 07041   (973)912-7273   Fax (973)912-7275   pinhomd@pasehealthcare.com

Pinke, Robert S., MD {1437155041} Ophthl(84,NY47)<NJ-STCLRDOV>
+ Roxbury Eye Center, PC
  66 Sunset Strip/Suite 107   Succasunna, NJ 07876   (973)584-4451   Fax (973)584-2099   robertp@roxburyeyecenter.com
+ Mountain Lakes Eye Center
  19 Pocono Road/Suite 212   Denville, NJ 07834   (973)584-4451   Fax (973)584-2099

Pinkerton, Gerald John, DO {1154529881} EmrgMd<NJ-KMHSTRAT>
+ Kennedy Memorial Hospital-University Medical Center
  18 East Laurel Road   Stratford, NJ 08084   (856)346-6000

Pinkhasov, Mark M., DO {1528233756}<NY-VABRKLYN>
+ Palisades Medical Associates
  125 River Road/Suite 103   Edgewater, NJ 07020   (201)969-2111   Fax (201)969-8015

Pinkowsky, Gregory J., MD {1699932137}
+ Center for Orthopaedics
  1500 Pleasant Valley Way/Suite 101   West Orange, NJ 07052   (732)887-8970   Fax (973)669-0269

Pinnelas, David J., MD {1982683025} CdvDis, IntrMd(84,GRNA)<NJ-JRSYSHMC, NJ-COMMED>
+ Shore Heart Group, P.A.
  35 Beaverson Boulevard/Suite 9-B   Brick, NJ 08723   (732)262-4262   Fax (732)262-4317
+ Shore Heart Group, P.A.
  1820 State Route 33/Suite 4-B   Neptune, NJ 07753   (732)262-4262   Fax (732)776-8946
+ Shore Heart Group, P.A.
  555 Iron Bridge Road/Suite 15   Freehold, NJ 08723   (732)308-0774   Fax (732)333-1366

Pinney, Antonia F., MD {1366418170} ObsGyn(97,PA09)<NJ-NWRKBETH>
+ Newark Beth Israel Medical Center
  201 Lyons Avenue/Ob/Gyn   Newark, NJ 07112   (973)926-7000

Pinninti, Narsimha R., MD {1700858222} Psychy(82,INDI)<NJ-OURLADY, NJ-KMHCHRRY>
+ University Hospital-SOM Department of Psychiatry
  2250 Chapel Avenue West/Suite 100   Cherry Hill, NJ 08002   (856)482-9000   Fax (856)482-1159

Pinsky, Abby Michele, MD {1477755957} Surgry, SrgBst(02,FL02)<NJ-JFKMED>
+ 98 James Street/Suite 101
  Edison, NJ 08820   (732)548-8980

Pinsky, Tim A., DO {1518114362} FamMed(86,NY75)
+ 55 State Highway 70 East
  Evesham, NJ 08053   (856)988-7770   Fax (856)988-7638

Pinto, Jamie M., MD {1245457951} Pedtrc<NJ-KMHSTRAT>
+ Kennedy Memorial Hospital-University Medical Center
  18 East Laurel Road/Pediatrics   Stratford, NJ 08084   (856)346-6000

Pinto, Jeffrey Damian, DO {1528258274} OstMed, IntrMd<NJ-VIRTMARL>
+ Virtua Family Medicine
  103 Old Marlton Pike/Suite 103   Medford, NJ 08055   (609)953-7105   Fax (609)953-7110

Pinto, Jose J., DO {1982643045} ObsGyn(88,ME75)<NJ-STBARNMC>
+ New Beginnings Ob/Gyn
  193 Mountain Avenue   Springfield, NJ 07081   (973)218-1579   Fax (973)218-1589

Pinto, Matthew G., DO {1326158783} FamMed, IntrMd(00,PA77)<NJ-VIRTVOOR, NJ-VIRTMARL>
+ Vive Medical Weight Loss & Aesthetics
  10000 Lincoln Drive/Suite 101   Marlton, NJ 08053   (856)968-8483   Fax (856)988-8480

Pinyard, Jeremy Vincent, MD {1689933301} IntHos
+ IPC The Hospitalist Company
  220 Ridgedale Avenue/Suite C-2   Florham Park, NJ 07932   (973)993-9536   Fax (973)267-0181

Pinz, Alexandra, MD {1235166307} Anesth(90,NY09)<NJ-ACMCITY, NJ-ACMCMAIN>
+ AtlantiCare Regional Medical Center/City Campus
  1925 Pacific Avenue   Atlantic City, NJ 08401   (609)345-4000
+ AtlantiCare Regional Med Ctr/Mainland
  65 West Jimmie Leeds Road   Pomona, NJ 08240   (609)652-1000

Pinzon, Amabelle Par, MD {1558561076} FamMed, IntrMd(03,PHI09)
+ Valley Medical Associates
  1700 Route 3 West   Clifton, NJ 07012   (862)249-4901   Fax (973)928-2650
+ Valley Medical Associates
  220 Hamburg Turnpike/Suite 9   Wayne, NJ 07470   (862)249-4901   Fax (973)807-1886

Piotrowski, Linda S., MD {1457572901} Psychy(81,MD07)
+ 4309 Atlantic Brigantine Boule
  Brigantine, NJ 08203

Piotti, Kathryn C., MD {1255566493} PthACl<NJ-MORRISTN>
+ Morristown Medical Center
  100 Madison Avenue   Morristown, NJ 07962   (973)971-5289

Pipan, Mary Ellen, MD {1942216338} Pedtrc, PedDvl(87,VA01)<PA-CHILDHOS>
+ CHOP Pediatric & Adolescent Specialty Care Center
  4009 Black Horse Pike   Mays Landing, NJ 08330   (609)677-7895   Fax (609)677-7835

Piper, Craig S., MD {1114985777} Addctn, NrlgAddM, EmrgMd(76,NJ05)
+ 70 Kensington Drive
  Fort Lee, NJ 07024   (201)346-2086

Piper, George E., DO {1679518567} Psychy(71,PA77)<NJ-KMHCHRRY, NJ-KMHTURNV>
+ 1930 Route 70 East/Suite H-41
  Cherry Hill, NJ 08003   (856)874-1144   Fax (856)874-1144

Piperi, Vincent D., MD {1093226813} IntrMd(78,DC01)
+ 1789 Lincoln Highway/#142
  Edison, NJ 08817

Pirak, Leon, MD {1134190325} Anesth(81,MEX14)<NJ-TRINIWSC>
+ Trinitas Regional Medical Center-Williamson Street
  225 Williamson Street   Elizabeth, NJ 07207   (908)994-5000

Piratla, Lalitha, MD {1841390804} Anesth, PainMd(85,INA48)<NJ-JFKMED>
+ James Street Anesthesia
  102 James Street/Suite 103   Edison, NJ 08820   (732)494-1444   Fax (732)494-7052

Pirigyi, Paul R., MD {1932285897} EmrgMd(75,PA02)<NJ-STPETER>
+ St. Peter's University Hospital
  254 Easton Avenue/EmergMed   New Brunswick, NJ 08901   (732)745-8600   Fax (732)418-1320

Pirogovsky, Victoria, MD {1033186408} Pedtrc(88,UZB04)<NJ-JRSYSHMC>
+ Spring Lake Pediatrics Associates
  613 Warren Avenue   Spring Lake, NJ 07762   (732)974-1444

Pirolli, John A., DO {1639124456} FamMed(81,NJ75)
+ Buena Family Practice
  1315 Harding Highway/Box 310   Richland, NJ 08350   (856)697-0300   Fax (856)697-8944   Bikers5@aol.com

Pirone, Arthur M., MD {1417084112} SrgOrt(81,NY46)
+ Cross County Orthopaedics
  769 Northfield Avenue/Suite LL20   West Orange, NJ 07052   (973)669-9595   Fax (973)669-1050

Pisani, Janet, MD {1548357270} Psychy(81,DC02)
+ Preferred Behavioral Health of New Jersey
  700 Airport Road   Lakewood, NJ 08701   (732)367-4700   Fax (732)364-2253

Pisarenko, Vadim, MD {1609020981} Surgry(03,MN04)
+ 185 Prospect Avenue/Suite 5D
  Hackensack, NJ 07601   (201)546-1729

Pisatowski, Denise Michelle, MD {1669468856} ObsGyn(92,NJ05)<NJ-HUNTRDN>
+ All Women's Healthcare
  1100 Wescott Drive/Suite 105   Flemington, NJ 08822   (908)788-6469   Fax (908)788-6483
+ Affiliates in Obstetrics & Gynecology, P.A.
  111 Route 31/Suite 121 2nd FL Bldg B   Flemington, NJ 08822   (908)788-6469   Fax (908)782-0196
+ Affiliates in Obstetrics & Gynecology, P.A.
  431 Highway 22 East   Whitehouse, NJ 08822   (908)823-1600   Fax (908)823-1640

Pisciotta, Anthony J., MD {1316913015} PhysMd(80,ITAL)<NJ-MMHKEMBL>
+ Associates in Rehabilitation Medicine
  95 Mount Kemble Avenue   Morristown, NJ 07960   (973)267-2293   Fax (973)226-3144

Piscitelli, Janet, MD {1154540789} PthACl, Pthlgy(87,NY08)<NY-MNTFWEIL, NY-MNTFMOSE>
+ Quest Diagnostics Inc.
  1 Malcolm Avenue   Teterboro, NJ 07608   (201)393-5000   Fax (201)393-6127

Piscopiello, Michael, MD {1326000464} CdvDis, IntrMd(00,GRN01)
+ Kivarkis Y. Younan MD PA
  1145 Bordentown Avenue/Suite 10   Parlin, NJ 08859   (732)727-0400   Fax (732)727-1391

Pisera, Donna M., MD {1972501955} Anesth(82,PA09)
+ West Jersey Anesthesia Associates
  102-E Center Boulevard   Marlton, NJ 08053   (856)988-6250   Fax (856)988-6270

Piskun, Andrew, MD {1265583074} SrgOrt(77,NJ06)<NJ-RWJUBRUN, NJ-STPETER>
+ Zemsky & Piskun MD PA
  1132 South Washington Avenue   Piscataway, NJ 08854   (732)752-8484   Fax (732)424-1124

Piskun, Jacob, MD {1427132034} Anesth(96,MNT01)
+ 113 Laredo Drive
  Morganville, NJ 07751

Pistilli, Stephanie Marie, DO {1306243241} ObsGyn
+ Drs. Rhee and Timms
  3 Cooper Plaza/Suite 221   Camden, NJ 08103   (856)342-2965   Fax (856)365-1967

Pistone, Gregory A., MD {1649388398} Dermat, SrgCsm, IntrMd(79,PA14)
+ Gregory A. Pistone MD PC
  601 Route 73 North/Suite 301   Marlton, NJ 08053   (856)988-8080   Fax (856)574-4192   gapistone@drpistone.com

Pistun, Oleksandr, MD {1629374533} IntrMd
+ Hunterdon Pediatric Associates
  6 Sand Hill Road/Suite 202   Flemington, NJ 08822   (908)782-6700   Fax (908)788-5861
+ 1514 Garden Drive/Apt 12
  Ocean, NJ 07712
+ RWJ University Hospital New Brunswick
  One Robert Wood Johnson Place   New Brunswick, NJ 08822   (732)235-7840

Piszcz-Connelly, Malgorzata A., MD {1578651709} IntrMd(84,POL13)
+ Millville Medical Center
  1700 North Tenth Street   Millville, NJ 08332   (856)327-6446   Fax (856)327-0158

Pitchford, Douglas Edward, MD {1255432068} Anesth, PainMd, AnesPain(85,NJ06)<NJ-RWJUHAM>
+ **740 Route 1 North**
    Iselin, NJ 08830   (732)734-1310   Fax (732)264-8131
+ **Perth Amboy Anesthesiology PC**
    530 New Brunswick Avenue   Perth Amboy, NJ 08861   (732)739-5853

Pitchumoni, Suresh Shanker, MD {1083805584} IntrMd, Gastrn(02,NJ06)
+ **Advanced Gastroenterology Associates LLC**
    475 County Road/Suite 201   Marlboro, NJ 07746   (732)370-2220   Fax (732)548-7408
+ **Marlboro Gastroenterology PC**
    50 Franklin Lane/Suite 201   Manalapan, NJ 07726   (732)370-2220   Fax (732)972-8610
+ **CentraState Family Medicine Residency Practice**
    1001 West Main Street/Suite B   Freehold, NJ 07746   (877)442-8829   Fax (732)294-9328

Pitchumoni, Vinita, MD {1598919748} Pedtrc(05)<NJ-JRSYSHMC>
+ **Jersey Shore University Medical Center**
    1945 Route 33/Pediatrics   Neptune, NJ 07753   (732)775-5500

Pitera, Barbara, MD {1912397340} Pedtrc(11,POL12)
+ **14-18 Mandon Place**
    Fair Lawn, NJ 07410   (732)734-8281

Pitera, Matthew J., MD {1225097702} PsyCAd, Psychy(91,NJ05)
+ **1314 Hooper Avenue/Suite C**
    Toms River, NJ 08753

Pitera, Richard, Jr., MD {1215098991} Anesth, OthrSp(91,NJ05)<NJ-STBARNMC>
+ **St. Barnabas Medical Center**
    94 Old Short Hills Road   Livingston, NJ 07039   (973)533-5695

Pitman, Susan Roth, MD {1548378003} ObsGyn(85,IL42)
+ **Pitman and Klachko LLC**
    769 Northfield Avenue/Suite 236   West Orange, NJ 07052   (973)325-5670   Fax (973)325-5677
+ **Short Hills Surgery Center**
    187 Millburn Avenue/Suite 101   Millburn, NJ 07041   (973)325-5670   Fax (973)671-0557

Pitoscia, Thomas, MD {1770586307} IntrMd, IntMAdMd(77,IL01)<NJ-OVERLOOK>
+ **Associates in Primary Care, P.A.**
    25 East Willow Street   Millburn, NJ 07041   (973)379-3069   Fax (973)379-5324

Pitsos, Miltiadis, MD {1407352768} ObsGyn
+ **Chemed Family Health Center**
    1771 Madison Avenue   Lakewood, NJ 08701   (732)364-6666   Fax (732)364-3559

Pitta, Kutumba S., MD {1104885656} PhysMd, Elecmy(70,INA48)<NJ-COMMED>
+ **1868 Hooper Avenue**
    Toms River, NJ 08753   (732)255-1900   Fax (732)255-1940

Pittalwala, Rashida G., MD {1598831984} Pedtrc(94,INA69)<NY-SLRLUKES>
+ **Advocare, LLC.**
    402 Lippincott Drive   Marlton, NJ 08053   (856)504-8028   Fax (856)504-8029

Pittarelli, Lisa A., MD {1730155771} InfDis(94,NJ06)<NJ-UNVM-CPRN, NJ-HCKTSTWN>
+ **ID Associates PA/dba ID Care**
    105 Raider Boulevard/Suite 101   Hillsborough, NJ 08844   (908)281-0221   Fax (908)281-0940
+ **ID Associates PA/dba ID Care**
    81 Veronica Avenue/Suite 203   Somerset, NJ 08873   (908)281-0221   Fax (908)729-0924

Pittman, Robert Hal, MD {1043254535} Gastrn(99,NY19)
+ **Bergen Medical Associates**
    466 Old Hook Road/Suite 1   Emerson, NJ 07630   (201)967-8221   Fax (201)967-0340
+ **Bergen Medical Associates**
    1 West Ridgewood Avenue/Suite 301   Paramus, NJ 07652   (201)967-8221   Fax (201)445-4296

Pivawer, Gabriel, DO {1134175854} RadDia(00,NY75)
+ **Edison Radiology Group, P.A.**
    65 James Street   Edison, NJ 08820   (732)321-7917   Fax (732)737-2968

Pivawer, Lisa S., DO {1750509089} Pedtrc
+ **Kintiroglou Pediatrics**
    1500 Pleasant Valley Way/Suite 301   West Orange, NJ 07052   (973)243-0002   Fax (973)243-1227

Piwowar, Karen, MD {1114345444}
+ **Summit Medical Group**
    48-50 Fairfield Street   Montclair, NJ 07042   (973)744-8511   Fax (973)744-6356
+ **Summit Medical Group**
    75 East Northfield Road   Livingston, NJ 07039   (973)744-8511   Fax (908)673-7336
+ **Summit Medical Group**
    1 Diamond Hill Road/Bensley Pav/2 FL   Berkeley, NJ 07042   (908)277-8700   Fax (908)288-7993

Piwoz, Julia A., MD {1285601682} Pedtrc, PedInf(91,PA09)<NJ-HACKNSK, NJ-HOLYNAME>
+ **Pediatric Infectious Disease/Hackensack Univ Med Ctr**
    30 Prospect Avenue   Hackensack, NJ 07601   (201)996-5308   Fax (201)996-9815

Pizarro, Oscar N., MD {1548321888} IntrMd(72,PHIL)<NJ-HOBUNIMC, NJ-CHRIST>
+ **Westside Medical Associates**
    562 West Side Avenue   Jersey City, NJ 07304   (201)434-7800   Fax (201)434-6715

Pizzano, Richard G., MD {1881621407} Gastrn, IntrMd(69,ITAL)<NJ-MTNSIDE>
+ **135 Bloomfield Avenue**
    Bloomfield, NJ 07003   (973)429-2876   Fax (973)748-0773

Pizzelanti, Donna M., DO {1306928791} FamMed(95,MO78)
+ **Middlebrook Family Practice**
    101 East Union Avenue   Bound Brook, NJ 08805   (732)560-0490   Fax (732)560-3681

Pizzi, Francis Joseph, MD {1326087826} SrgNro, IntrMd(69,NY09)<NJ-HUNTRDN, NJ-STFRNMED>
+ **Neuro-Group PA at Hunterdon Medical Center**
    1100 Wescott Drive/Suite 301   Flemington, NJ 08822   (609)788-6541   Fax (609)788-6519
    JPFISTNER@neurogroup.us
+ **Hunterdon Medical Center**
    2100 Wescott Drive/Surgery/Neuro   Flemington, NJ 08822   (908)788-6100
+ **St. Francis Medical Center**
    601 Hamilton Avenue/Surgery/Neuro   Trenton, NJ 08822   (609)599-5000

Pizzillo, Michael Francis, MD {1740234582} SrgHnd, SrgOrt, OthrSp(92,NY08)<NJ-ENGLWOOD, NJ-HOLYNAME>
+ **Englewood Orthopedic Associates**
    401 South Van Brunt Street   Englewood, NJ 07631   (201)569-2770   Fax (201)569-1774

Pizzutillo, Peter Darrell, MD {1114970597} SrgOrt, PedOrt(70,PA02)<NJ-CHSFULD, NJ-CHSMRCER>
+ **St Chris Care @ Washington Twp**
    100 Kings Way East/Bld C   Sewell, NJ 08080   (215)427-3131   Fax (215)427-5450

Plaine, Suzanne E., DO {1942433511} Pedtrc(06,NJ75)
+ **Meridian Medical Group**
    2130 Route 35/Suite B216   Sea Girt, NJ 08750   (732)974-0228   Fax (732)263-7938

Plakas, Christos, MD {1457593261} PedOrt, Ortped<NJ-MONMOUTH>
+ **Atlantic Pediatric Orthopedics**
    1131 Broad Street/Suite 202   Shrewsbury, NJ 07702   (732)544-9000   Fax (732)544-9099

Plakyda, Derek J., MD {1700882941} Radiol, RadDia(97,NJ06)
+ **Radiology Affiliates of Central New Jersey, P.A.**
    2501 Kuser Road   Hamilton, NJ 08691   (609)585-8800   Fax (609)585-1825
+ **Radiology Affiliates of Central New Jersey, P.A.**
    3120 Princeton Pike   Lawrenceville, NJ 08648   (609)585-8800   Fax (609)219-0439

Planer, Benjamin C., MD {1053358564} NnPnMd, Pedtrc(86,SAF01)<NJ-HACKNSK>
+ **Hackensack University Medical Center**
    30 Prospect Avenue/Neonatology   Hackensack, NJ 07601   (201)996-5362   Fax (201)996-3232
    bplaner@humed.com

Planer, Dorienne Sasto, MD {1851345052} Pedtrc(96,PA02)<NJ-ENGLWOOD, NY-PRSBCOLU>
+ **Metropolitan Pediatric Group**
    704 Palisade Avenue   Teaneck, NJ 07666   (201)836-4301   Fax (201)836-5110

Plasner, Samantha Mara, DO {1346241437} FamMed(02,NJ75)
+ **The University Doctors**
    100 Century Parkway/Suite 140   Mount Laurel, NJ 08054   (856)380-2400   Fax (856)234-7870

Platovsky, Anna, MD {1982966222} Gastrn
+ **Digestive Disease Center of New Jersey, LLC**
    33 Clyde Road/Suite 102   Somerset, NJ 08873   (732)873-9200   Fax (732)873-1699

Platt, Ellen M., DO {1801975842} PsyCAd, Psychy(73,PA77)
+ **Platt Psychiatric Associates, LLC**
    904 Pompton Avenue/Suite B-2   Cedar Grove, NJ 07009   (973)239-4848   Fax (973)239-4704

Platt, Heather L., MD {1922309350} IntrMd<NJ-RWJUBRUN>
+ **RWJ University Hospital New Brunswick**
    One Robert Wood Johnson Place   New Brunswick, NJ 08901   (732)235-7742

Platt, Jennifer, DO {1104061050} Psychy
+ **Platt Psychiatric Associates, LLC**
    904 Pompton Avenue/Suite B-2   Cedar Grove, NJ 07009   (973)239-4848   Fax (973)239-4704

Platt, Marc J., MD {1316954043} Anesth, IntrMd(81,MEX03)<NJ-LOURDMED>
+ **Rancocas Anesthesiology, PA**
    218 Sunset Road   Willingboro, NJ 08046   (609)835-3069   Fax (609)835-5450
+ **Lourdes Medical Center of Burlington County**
    218 Sunset Road/Anesth   Willingboro, NJ 08046   (609)835-2900

Platt, Marvin, MD {1225013170} Radiol, RadDia(64,IL42)<NJ-BAYSHORE, NJ-RBAYPERT>
+ **University Radiology Group, P.C.**
    483 Cranbury Road   East Brunswick, NJ 08816   (732)390-0030   Fax (732)390-5383

Platt, Robert N., MD {1013909803} CdvDis, IntrMd(74,MEXI)<NJ-CHILTON>
+ **West Milford Medical Center**
    1485 Union Valley Road   West Milford, NJ 07480   (973)728-1880   Fax (973)728-1559

Platzman, Robert, DO {1497852966} IntrMd, Grtrcs(99,NY75)<NJ-UNVMCPRN, NJ-RWJUBRUN>
+ **Central Jersey Medicine & Geriatrics, PLLC**
    601 Ewing Street/Suite C7   Princeton, NJ 08540   (609)921-8766   Fax (609)921-0869

Plauka, Alan R., MD {1316954589} IntrMd(84,GRN01)<NJ-TRINI-JSC>
+ **NJ MedCare**
    550 Mount Prospect Avenue   Newark, NJ 07104   (973)482-4697
+ **NJ Heart/Elizabeth Office**
    240 Williamson Street/Suite 402-406   Elizabeth, NJ 07202   (973)482-4697   Fax (908)354-0101

Plaza, Lorna D., MD {1760415210} Pedtrc, Hemato, Rheuma(73,PHIL)
+ **Newark Beth Israel Medical Center**
    201 Lyons Avenue   Newark, NJ 07112   (973)926-7203   Fax (973)926-2332

Pleickhardt, Elizabeth Patricia, DO {1457302093} Pedtrc(02,NY75)
+ **On-Site Neonatal Partners**
    1000 Haddonfield-Berlin Road/Suite 210   Voorhees, NJ 08043   (856)782-2212   Fax (856)782-2213

Pletcher, Beth A., MD {1639243090} ClnGnt, Pedtrc(82,IL01)<NJ-UMDNJ>
+ **University Hospital-Doctors Office Center**
    90 Bergen Street/Suite 5400   Newark, NJ 07103   (973)972-3300   Fax (973)972-3310
    pletchba@umdnj.edu
+ **UMDNJ Center for Human & Molecular Genetics**
    185 South Orange Avenue/MSB F669   Newark, NJ 07101   (973)972-3305

Pliner, Lillian F., MD {1518059351} IntrMd, MedOnc, PallCr(80,NY48)<NJ-UMDNJ, NJ-STBARNMC>
+ **University Hospital**
    150 Bergen Street   Newark, NJ 07103   (973)972-4300
+ **University Hospital-Doctors Office Center**
    90 Bergen Street/DOC 4500   Newark, NJ 07103   (973)972-4300   Fax (973)972-2510
+ **St. Barnabas Medical Center**
    94 Old Short Hills Road   Livingston, NJ 07103   (973)322-5000   Fax (973)322-5666

Ploshchanskaya, Larisa G., MD {1669408944} Nrolgy(70,UKR12)<NJ-HOBUNIMC, NJ-CHRIST>
+ **331 Grand Street**
    Hoboken, NJ 07030   (201)795-9860   Fax (201)296-0603
    lploshchanskaya@nj.rr.com

Ploshnick, Andrea G., MD {1619088945} Pedtrc(89,NJ05)<NJ-MORRISTN, NJ-HCKTSTWN>
+ **Watchung Pediatrics**
    76 Stirling Road/Suite 201   Warren, NJ 07059   (908)755-5437   Fax (908)755-6905
+ **Watchung Pediatrics**
    346 South Avenue/Suite 3   Fanwood, NJ 07023   (908)755-5437   Fax (908)889-0047
+ **Watchung Pediatrics**
    225 Millburn Avenue/Suite 301   Millburn, NJ 07059   (973)376-7337   Fax (973)218-6647

Plotnick, Marc P., MD {1265472476} IntrMd, EmrgMd(87,PA02)<NJ-VIRTVOOR>
+ **Advocare, LLC.**
    402 Lippincott Drive   Marlton, NJ 08053   (856)504-8028   Fax (856)504-8029

Plumer, Robin Susan, DO {1770515942} EmrgMd(83,NJ75)<NJ-VIRTMARL, NJ-VIRTBERL>
+ **Emergency Physician Associates, P.A.**
    307 South Evergreen Avenue/PO Box 298   Woodbury, NJ 08096   (856)848-3817   Fax (856)848-1431

Plumeri, Peter A., DO {1447258777} Gastrn, IntrMd(73,PA77)<NJ-KMHTURNV>
+ **445 Hurffville-Crosskeys Road**
    Sewell, NJ 08080   (856)218-0200   Fax (856)218-0099

Physicians by Name and Address

Plummer, Alice T., MD {1902868268} Psychy(79,DC01)<NJ-RAMAPO>
+ Christian Health Care Counseling Center
301 Sicomac Avenue   Wyckoff, NJ 07481   (201)848-5800   Fax (201)848-5547
+ Christian Health Care Heritage Manor Nursing Home
301 Sicomac Avenue   Wyckoff, NJ 07481   (201)848-5800   Fax (201)848-9758

Plumser, Allan B., MD {1508961681} Gastrn, IntrMd(78,NY09)<NJ-RWJUBRUN, NJ-STPETER>
+ Lenger and Plumser, MDs, LLC
465 Cranbury Road/Suite 102   East Brunswick, NJ 08816   (732)390-1995   Fax (732)254-4610

Plunkett, Lisa A., MD {1114058963} FamMed
+ 62 Redwood Terrace
Flemington, NJ 08822

Plut, Thomas W., DO {1801010723} FamMSptM
+ Lourdes Medical Associates
740 Marne Highway/Suite 102   Moorestown, NJ 08057   (856)234-9006   Fax (856)234-9233

Pluta, Christine Marie, DO {1700833530} FamMed(NJ75
+ Schuylkill Medical Associates, LLC
2681 Quakerbridge Road/Suite B2   Hamilton, NJ 08619   Fax (609)208-3233

Plutchok, Jeffrey J., MD {1851339527} NuclMed, RadDia(91,NJ06)<NJ-STCLRDEN, NJ-STJOSHOS>
+ St. Clare's Hospital-Denville Campus
25 Pocono Road/Radiology   Denville, NJ 07834   (973)625-6000

Pober, Joseph M., MD {1194948703} SrgPlstc, SrgRec(79,MA01)<NY-SLRRSVLT, NY-SLRLUKES>
+ Joseph M. Pober MD FACS PC
400 Old Hook Road/Suite 1-1   Westwood, NJ 07675   (201)722-9700   Fax (201)722-9744
Kerry.bennett@reliantmedicalgroup.org

Pober, Neil J., MD {1386844975} Anesth(93,PA09)
+ 1105 Mount Vernon Court
Marlton, NJ 08053

Poblete, Fredrick M., MD {1508894247} Surgry(98,PHI01)<NJ-RWJUHAM>
+ Poblete Dermatology
1601 Whitehorse-Mercerville Rd/Suite 2   Trenton, NJ 08619   (609)838-9040   Fax (609)838-9042

Poblete, Gwyn Laurice, MD {1295887339} Pedtrc(02,DMN01)
+ Morristown Pediatric Associates, LLC
261 James Street/Suite 1-G   Morristown, NJ 07960   (973)540-9393   Fax (973)540-1937

Poblete, Honesto Madjus, MD {1972761799} SrgVas(99,PHI07)
+ Diabetes and Endocrinology Associates
3525 Quakerbridge Road/Suite 2000   Trenton, NJ 08619   (609)570-2071   Fax (609)689-2614

Poblete, Ronald J., MD {1740271998} InfDis, IntrMd(85,PHI10)<NJ-CHILTON>
+ Poblete Medical Practice PC
289 Market Street/Suite 2   Saddle Brook, NJ 07663   (201)587-9204   Fax (201)587-0623

Poco, Bernardo A., MD {1497749139} IntrMd, EmrgMd(83,PHI14)<NJ-RBAYPERT>
+ JFK Medical Center
65 James Street   Edison, NJ 08820   (732)321-7601   Fax (732)744-5614

Podda, Silvio, MD {1366564460} SrgPlstc, SrgCsm(86,ITA02)<NJ-STJOSHOS>
+ St. Joseph's Children's Hospital
703 Main Street/CraniofacialCtr   Paterson, NJ 07503   (973)754-2213
+ St. Joseph's Regional Medical Center
11 Getty Avenue   Paterson, NJ 07503   (973)754-2413

Poddar, Sameer S., MD {1740591247} IntrMd<NJ-COOPRUMC>
+ Cooper University Hospital
One Cooper Plaza/Dorramce/222   Camden, NJ 08103   (856)342-2000

Podell, Richard N., MD {1790839017} FamMed, IntrMd, Nutrtn(69,MA01)<NJ-OVERLOOK>
+ 11 Overlook Road/Suite 140
Summit, NJ 07901

Podgorski, Edward M., Jr., MD {1316946635} RadDia, Radiol(83,PA02)<NJ-VIRTUAHS, NJ-VIRTMHBC>
+ South Jersey Radiology Associates, P.A.
901 Route 168/Suites 301-305   Turnersville, NJ 08012   (856)227-6600   Fax (856)227-8537
+ South Jersey Radiology Associates, P.A.
807 Haddon Avenue/Suite 5   Haddonfield, NJ 08033   (856)227-6600   Fax (856)616-1125
+ South Jersey Radiology Associates, P.A.
315 Route 70 East/Suite C   Cherry Hill, NJ 08012   (856)428-4344   Fax (856)428-0356

Podkul, Richard L., MD {1083625693} IntrMd(77,ITA17)
+ 1064 Broad Street
Bloomfield, NJ 07003   (973)893-0282   Fax (973)893-0612

Podolsky, Michael Lee, MD {1689631525} ObsGyn
+ Drexel University Physicians
400 East Church Street   Blackwood, NJ 08012   (856)228-8066

Poehling Monaghan, Kirsten L., MD {1780995605}
+ Rothman Institute
999 Route 73 North/3rd Fl   Marlton, NJ 08053   (612)965-8566   Fax (856)821-6359
drkpmonaghan@gmail.com

Poelstra, Beverly A., MD {1659432672} Pedtrc, PedEmg(88,NJ06)<NJ-RWJUBRUN, NJ-STPETER>
+ RWJ University Pediatric Emergency Medicine
125 Paterson Street/MEB 342   New Brunswick, NJ 08903   (732)235-7893   Fax (732)235-9349
+ The Bristol Myers-Squibb Children's Hospital
One Robert Wood Johnson Place   New Brunswick, NJ 08903   (732)253-3300
+ RWJ University Hospital New Brunswick
One Robert Wood Johnson Place   New Brunswick, NJ 08903   (732)828-3000

Pogach, Leonard M., MD {1871509869} EnDbMt, IntrMd(76,PA09)<NJ-VAEASTOR>
+ VA New Jersey Health Care System-East Orange Campus
385 Tremont Avenue   East Orange, NJ 07018   (973)676-1000   Fax (973)395-7111

Pogany, Ursula M., MD {1568450799} Pedtrc(81,NJ06)<NJ-OVERLOOK>
+ Cranford Pediatrics
19 Holly Street   Cranford, NJ 07016   (908)276-6598   Fax (908)276-0040

Pogorelec, Albert Joseph, Jr., DO {1558459487} FamMed(02,MO79)
+ The Integrative Wellness Center
164 Brighton Road   Clifton, NJ 07013   (973)773-2500   Fax (973)773-0508

Pogran, Jessica Rose, DO {1760794010} PsyCAd<NJ-MONMOUTH>
+ Monmouth Medical Center
300 Second Avenue   Long Branch, NJ 07740   (800)300-0628   Fax (732)923-5277

Poiani, George J., MD {1881654754} PulDis, CritCr, IntrMd(81,NJ06)
+ Somerset Pulmonary & Critical Care
245 Union Avenue/Suite 2C   Bridgewater, NJ 08807   (732)873-8097   Fax (732)873-1827

Pokuah, Marian O., MD {1861651093} IntrMd(08,NJ06)<NJ-WARREN>
+ Cooper University Hospital
One Cooper Plaza   Camden, NJ 08103   (856)342-2000
+ Warren Hospital
185 Roseberry Street/Internal Med   Phillipsburg, NJ 08865   (908)859-6700

Polack, Noha, MD {1578530010} Pedtrc(93,NJ05)<NJ-HOBUNIMC>
+ Progressive Pediatrics
3196 Kennedy Boulevard   Union City, NJ 07087   (201)319-9800   Fax (201)319-9849
+ Progressive Pediatrics
1222 Kennedy Boulevard   Bayonne, NJ 07002   (201)319-9800   Fax (201)437-9661

Polakoff, Donald Richard, MD {1407851355} SrgOrt, SrgOARec, OrtHKn(79,NY20)
+ University Hip and Knee Orthopaedic Specialists LLC
111 Union Valley Road/Suite 102   Monroe Township, NJ 08831   (609)655-1818   Fax (609)655-1814
+ Mercer-Bucks Orthopaedics, P.C.
2501 Kuser Road   Hamilton, NJ 08691   (609)655-1818   Fax (609)587-4349

Polam, Sharadha, MD {1780786434} NnPnMd, Pedtrc(93,INA8Y)<NJ-CENTRAST, NJ-RWJHLTS>
+ On-Site Neonatal Partners
1000 Haddonfield-Berlin Road/Suite 210   Voorhees, NJ 08043   (856)782-2212   Fax (856)782-2213

Polcer, Jeffrey D., DO {1942274501} Anesth, PainMd(85,NJ75)<NJ-ACMCITY, NJ-ACMCMAIN>
+ Professional Pain Management Associates
2007 North Black Horse Pike   Williamstown, NJ 08094   (856)740-4888   Fax (856)740-0558

Polczynski, Evette S., MD {1215967963}
+ 46 First Street
Rumson, NJ 07760   (970)403-6174

Polen, Winnie M., DO {1851371330} SrgBst, SrgOnc, Surgry(00,MO79)<NJ-OVERLOOK>
+ Summit Medical Group-Berkeley Heights Campus
1 Diamond Hill Road/Bensley Pav/1FL   Berkeley Heights, NJ 07922   (908)273-4300   Fax (908)790-6576

Polesin, Alena, MD {1679686893} PhysMd, SprtMd, OthrSp(01,NJ06)<NJ-MORRISTN>
+ Tri-County Orthopedics
160 East Hanover Avenue   Morristown, NJ 07962   (973)538-2334   Fax (973)538-4072

Polimeni, Marc David, MD {1861458499} IntrMd(86,GRN01)<NJ-HACKNSK, NJ-HOLYNAME>
+ 481 Kindermack Road
Oradell, NJ 07649   (201)928-0101   Fax (201)599-3131

Polini, Nicole Maria, MD {1033202932} RadDia(01,NJ06)<NJ-STBARNMC>
+ Imaging Consultants of Essex
94 Old Short Hills Road   Livingston, NJ 07039   (973)322-5800   Fax (973)322-5536

Polise, Michael F., DO {1316954845} EmrgMd, FamMed(77,PA77)<NJ-VIRTVOOR>
+ Virtua Voorhees
100 Bowman Drive/EmergMed   Voorhees, NJ 08043   (856)247-3000

Polise, Pamela Ann, MD {1053364554} Anesth(93,PA02)
+ 120 Lafayette Avenue
Haddonfield, NJ 08033

Polisin, Michael J., MD {1871620112} Pedtrc, AdolMd(85,ITA22)
+ Maple Pediatric Associates LLC
47 Maple Street/Suite 107   Summit, NJ 07901   (908)273-5866   Fax (908)273-5811

Politis, Regina, MD {1245224856} Pedtrc(95,GRNA)<NJ-HOBUNIMC, NJ-CHRIST>
+ Drs. Politis and Kaki
3526 Kennedy Boulevard   Jersey City, NJ 07307   (201)653-5933   Fax (201)653-3930

Politsky, Jeffrey Mark, MD {1174620256} Nrolgy, Eplpsy(94,ON06)<NJ-OVERLOOK>
+ NE Regional Epilepsy/Atlantic Neuro
99 Beauvoir Avenue/5th Fl   Summit, NJ 07902   (908)522-4990
+ Northeast Regional Epilepsy Group
20 Prospect Avenue/Suite 800   Hackensack, NJ 07601   (908)522-4990   Fax (201)343-6689

Polizzi, David R., MD {1356349625} FamMed(87,NJ06)<NJ-HUNTRDN>
+ Highlands Family Health Center
61 Frontage Road/Suite 61   Hampton, NJ 08827   (908)735-2594   Fax (908)735-8526

Polizzi, Maria, MD {1679543953} IntrMd, OncHem(94,ITA17)
+ Ramtown Medical Center LLC
225 Newtons Corner Road   Howell, NJ 07731   (732)458-9760   Fax (732)458-9762

Polkampally, Kavitha, MD {1730284746} IntrMd, Grtrcs, PallCr(97,INA16)<NJ-PALISADE>
+ Palisades Medical Center
7600 River Road/House Phys   North Bergen, NJ 07047   (201)854-5000   Fax (856)616-1919

Polkow, Melvin S., MD {1972677169} PulDis, IntrMd(77,NY08)<NJ-HACKNSK>
+ Northern New Jersey Pulmonary Associates PC
211 Essex Street/Suite 302   Hackensack, NJ 07601   (201)498-1311   Fax (201)498-1312

Pollack, Jeffrey S., MD {1336177054} IntrMd(81,DOM21)<NJ-SHOREMEM>
+ Shore Internal Medicine
6044 Harding Highway   Mays Landing, NJ 08330   (609)625-9146   Fax (609)625-7405

Pollack, Joshua David, MD {1174629539} Otlryg(82,NY09)<NJ-WARREN, NJ-HCKTSTWN>
+ 4A Doctors Park Seber Road
Hackettstown, NJ 07840   (908)852-6655
+ 904 Coventry Drive
Phillipsburg, NJ 08865   (908)852-6655   Fax (908)859-6538

Pollack, Marshall S., MD {1366472946} ObsGyn(77,NJ05)<NJ-STBARNMC>
+ Millburn Ob-Gyn Associates, P.A.
233 Millburn Avenue   Millburn, NJ 07041   (973)467-9440   Fax (973)376-1680
+ Short Hills Surgery Center
187 Millburn Avenue/Suite 101   Millburn, NJ 07041   (973)467-9440   Fax (973)671-0557

Pollack, Martin I., MD {1093768384} EmrgMd, IntrMd(83,NY08)
+ 425 Jack Martin Boulevard
Brick, NJ 08724

Pollack, Matthew Scott, MD {1962453001} RadDia, Radiol, IntrMd(81,PA13)<NJ-WARREN>
+ Progressive Physician Associates, Inc.
185 Roseberry Street   Phillipsburg, NJ 08865   (610)868-1100   Fax (610)868-1111

Pollack, Michael A., MD {1992899447} RadDia(98,NY19)
+ Montclair Radiology
20 High Street   Nutley, NJ 07110   (973)284-0020   Fax (973)284-6310

Pollack, Michael Edward, MD {1205832037} SrgOrt, NeuMSptM(97,PA02)<NJ-HUNTRDN>
+ MidJersey Orthopaedics, P.A.
8100 Westcott Drive/Suite 101   Flemington, NJ 08822   (908)782-0600   Fax (908)782-7575
+ Hunterdon Orthopaedic Institute, P.A.
80 West End Avenue   Somerville, NJ 08876   (908)182-0600

Pollack, Shoshannah S., MD {1306800156} Dermat(86,NY46)<NJ-CHILTON>
+ 1777 Hamburg Turnpike/Suite 102
Wayne, NJ 07470 (973)835-1823 Fax (973)831-7585
knealie2002@yahoo.com

Pollak, Joseph A., MD {1952335309} FamMed, Grtrcs, FamM-Grtc(81,NJ05)<NJ-HOBUNIMC>
+ 323 Washington Street
Hoboken, NJ 07030 (201)795-9909 Fax (201)795-9919

Pollak, Kevin Henry, MD {1104979178} Anesth(91,DMN01)
+ Burlington County Endoscopy Center
140 Mount Holly Bypass/Unit 5 Lumberton, NJ 08048 (609)267-1555
+ Digestive HealthCare Center
511 Courtyard Drive/Building 500 Hillsborough, NJ 08844 (609)267-1555 Fax (908)218-9818

Pollak, Michael, MD {1811921273} IntrMd(86,NJ15)<NJ-HOBUNIMC>
+ West River Medical Associates
323 Washington Street Hoboken, NJ 07030 (201)795-9909 Fax (201)795-9919

Pollard, Elizabeth Joan, MD {1952333833} IntHos
+ Virtua Physicians Associates
5 Eaves Drive/Suite 120 A Marlton, NJ 08053

Pollard, Mark Andrew, MD {1437170891} SrgOrt, IntrMd(99,PA09)<NJ-COOPRUMC>
+ Cooper Bone and Joint Institute
900 Centennial Boulevard Voorhees, NJ 08043 (856)325-6677 Fax (856)325-6678
+ Cooper University Orthopedic Trauma
3 Cooper Plaza/Suite 408 Camden, NJ 08103 (856)325-6677 Fax (856)968-8288

Pollaro, Michael Gerard, DO {1487060661}<NJ-MORRISTN>
+ Morristown Medical Center
100 Madison Avenue Morristown, NJ 07962 (973)971-5000

Pollen, Jeffrey Jonah, MD {1235143843} Urolgy(64,SAF01)
+ VA New Jersey Health Care System-East Orange Campus
385 Tremont Avenue East Orange, NJ 07018 (973)676-1000 Fax (973)395-7197

Pollen, Philip C., MD {1245341924} PhysMd(81,GRN01)
+ 3 Athens Avenue
South Amboy, NJ 08879 (732)553-9400 Fax (732)553-1036

Pollock, Jeffrey C., MD {1508894619} Nrolgy(82,GA01)<NJ-OVERLOOK>
+ Vigman and Pollock PA
47 Maple Street/Suite 104 Summit, NJ 07901 (908)277-2722 Fax (908)273-5970

Pollock, Roger G., MD {1023109121} SrgOrt, SrgShr(85,NY01)<NY-PRSBCOLU, NJ-VALLEY>
+ 1 West Ridgewood Avenue/Suite 202
Paramus, NJ 07652 (201)612-9774 Fax (201)612-0103

Polomsky, Marek, MD {1730192071} SrgThr(04,MD01)<NJ-MORRISTN>
+ Mid-Atlantic Surgical Associates
100 Madison Avenue Morristown, NJ 07960 (973)971-7300 Fax (973)984-7019

Polonet, David Russell, MD {1821071911} SrgOrt, OrtTrm, IntrMd(97,NY48)<NJ-CT-BRIDGPRT, NJ-JRSYSHMC>
+ University Orthopaedic Associates, LLC.
Two Worlds Fair Drive Somerset, NJ 08873 (732)979-2115 Fax (732)564-9032
+ University Orthopaedic Associates, LLC.
4810 Belmar Boulevard/Suite 102 Wall, NJ 07753 (732)979-2115 Fax (732)938-5680
+ University Orthopaedic Associates, LLC.
211 North Harrison Street Princeton, NJ 08873 (609)683-7800 Fax (609)683-7875

Polos, Peter George, MD {1285634501} PulDis, IntrMd(86,LA05)<NJ-JFKMED, NJ-OVERLOOK>
+ JFK Neurosciences Institute
65 James Street/Second Floor Edison, NJ 08818 (732)321-7010 Fax (732)632-1584
+ Summit Medical Group-Berkeley Heights Campus
1 Diamond Hill Road Berkeley Heights, NJ 07922 (732)321-7010 Fax (908)790-6576

Polsani, Srujana, MD {1427366350}<NJ-UNVMCPRN>
+ University Medical Center of Princeton at Plainsboro
One Plainsboro Road Plainsboro, NJ 08536 (703)863-9946
srujana_polsani@yahoo.com

Polt, Terry Jane, MD {1942274949} FamMed(98,LA05)<NJ-HUNTRDN>
+ Highlands Family Health Center
61 Frontage Road/Suite 61 Hampton, NJ 08827 (908)735-2594 Fax (908)735-8226

Poltinnikova, Yana M., MD {1114910007} Anesth(91,AZE01)<NJ-PALISADE>
+ Palisades Medical Center
7600 River Road/Anesth North Bergen, NJ 07047 (201)854-5000

Polvino, William James, MD {1063719706} IntrMd(87,NJ06)<NJ-JRSYSHMC>
+ 10 Churchill Downs Drive
Tinton Falls, NJ 07724

Pomerantz, Glenn David, MD {1619247699} IntrMd
+ 56 Twin Oak Road
Short Hills, NJ 07078 (973)218-6373

Pomerantz, Jeffrey David, DO {1376738732} FamMed(86,NJ75)
+ Southern State Correctional Facility
4295 Route 47 Delmont, NJ 08314 (856)785-1300

Pomerantz, Scott Barry, MD {1033186937} Ophthl(86,GA05)<NJ-HACKNSK>
+ 523 Forest Avenue
Paramus, NJ 07652 (201)262-5070 Fax (201)262-5333

Pomeranz, Bruce A., MD {1710975859} PhysMd(89,IL11)<NJ-KSLRWEST, NJ-KSLRSADB>
+ Kessler Institute for Rehabilitation West Orange
1199 Pleasant Valley Way West Orange, NJ 07052 (973)731-3600
+ Kessler Institute for Rehabilitation
300 Market Street Saddle Brook, NJ 07663 (201)587-8500
+ The Valley Hospital
223 North Van Dien Avenue Ridgewood, NJ 07052 (201)447-8000

Pomeroy, Jon K., DO {1942529052}
+ Atlantic Medical Imaging, LLC.
401 Bethel Road Somers Point, NJ 08244 (609)365-6200 Fax (609)365-6201

Pompa, Tiffany, MD {1649558586} OncHem
+ Hope Community Cancer Center LLC
210 South Shore Road/Suite 106-A Marmora, NJ 08223 (609)390-7888 Fax (609)390-2614

Pompeo, Lisa, MD {1265527410} ObsGyn(94,NY48)<NJ-UMDNJ>
+ University Physician Associates
140 Bergen Street/ACC Level C Newark, NJ 07103 (973)972-2700 Fax (973)972-2739

Pompliano, Jennifer Dorothea, DO {1942240098} ObsGyn(99,NJ75)<NJ-MONMOUTH>
+ West Long Branch Obstetrics & Gynecology
1019 Broadway West Long Branch, NJ 07764 (732)229-6797 Fax (732)229-6893
+ West Long Branch Obstetrics & Gynecology
911 East County Line Road/Suite 201 Lakewood, NJ 08701 (732)364-9299

Pompy, Amrita, MD {1225328537} Pedtrc
+ Naveen Mehrotra, MD PC
652 Amboy Avenue Edison, NJ 08837 (732)738-1341 Fax (732)738-9585
amritaa.jha@gmail.com
+ Naveen Mehrotra, MD PC
1315 Stelton Road Piscataway, NJ 08854 (732)738-1341 Fax (732)819-8801

Ponamgi, Suri B., MD {1437155009} SrgPlstc, Surgry(70,INDI)<NJ-HOLYNAME, NJ-HOBUNIMC>
+ 1101 Palisade Avenue
Fort Lee, NJ 07024 (201)224-8831 Fax (201)224-9278

Ponce, Francis B., MD {1912963323} Nrolgy(88,PHI01)<NJ-MONMOUTH, NJ-RIVERVW>
+ Neurology Specialists of Monmouth County
107 Monmouth Road/Suite 110 West Long Branch, NJ 07764 (732)935-1850 Fax (732)544-0494

Ponce, Marie Grace C., MD {1659449973} Pedtrc, PedEmg, ErgMd(89,PHI01)<NJ-STPETER, NJ-UMDNJ>
+ EmCare
1945 Route 33 Neptune, NJ 07753 (732)776-4510 Fax (732)776-2328

Ponce Contreras, Marta R., MD {1942363437} Ophthl(98,GUA03)
+ Eye Care of River Edge
1060 Main Street/Suite 301 River Edge, NJ 07661 (201)489-0096 Fax (201)488-2930

Pond, Charles G., MD {1275674400} Anesth(80,MO34)<NY-PRSB-WEIL>
+ New Jersey Anesthesia Associates, P.C.
252 Columbia Turnpike/PO Box 0037 Florham Park, NJ 07932 (973)660-9334 Fax (973)660-9779

Pond, James M., MD {1538169206} PthAcl, PthCln(90,PA13)<NJ-SHOREMEM>
+ Shore Memorial Hospital
1 East New York Avenue/Pathology Somers Point, NJ 08244 (609)653-3500
+ Coastal Clinical Pathologists
1 East New York Avenue/PO Box 337 Somers Point, NJ 08244 (609)653-3500 Fax (609)926-9056

Pondo, Jaroslaw S., MD {1487665717} IntrMd, PulDis(89,POL14)<NJ-HACKNSK, NJ-STMRYPAS>
+ Jaroslaw S. Pondo MD PC
71 Union Avenue/Suite 107 Rutherford, NJ 07070 (201)896-0050 Fax (201)896-0051
JPONDO.MD@verizon.net

Pondt, Charlesse Maureen, MD {1043479926} IntrMd(08,NJ06)<NJ-JRSYSHMC>
+ Advanced Care Hematology & Oncology Associates
385 Morris Avenue/Suite 100 Springfield, NJ 07081 (973)379-2111 Fax (973)379-2807

Ponnamaneni, Abhilasha Rao, MD {1548574346} FamMed
+ Dorfner Family Medicine
639 Stokes Road/Suite 102 Medford, NJ 08055 (609)654-7556 Fax (609)714-9228

Ponnambalam, Ajit P., MD {1790895548} IntrMd, OncHem(74,SRIL)<NJ-COMMED>
+ 40 Bey Lea Road/Suite B-102
Toms River, NJ 08753 (732)244-4994 Fax (732)244-4226

Ponnambalam, Anil R., MD {1740372911} IntrMd, MedOnc, OncHem(73,SRIL)<NJ-COMMED, NJ-NWRKBETH>
+ 40 Bey Lea Road/Suite B102
Toms River, NJ 08755 (732)244-3300 Fax (732)244-9013

Ponnappa, Gita S., MD {1699972398} IntrMd(97,INA2C)
+ 209 Arlington Avenue
Linwood, NJ 08221

Ponnappan, Ravi Kumar, MD {1558329201} SrgOrt(01,OH40)<NJ-ATLANTHS>
+ Jersey Spine Associates, LLC
710 Centre Street Somers Point, NJ 08244 (609)601-4920 Fax (609)601-4921
appointments@jerseyspineassociates.com

Ponnudurai, Rex N., MD {1639226681} Anesth(71,SRIL)<NJ-UMDNJ>
+ University Hospital
150 Bergen Street/Anesthesiology Newark, NJ 07103 (973)972-4300 Fax (973)972-4172

Ponomarev, Aleksandr, MD {1477726370} Grtrcs
+ Erickson Health Medical Group
1 Cedar Crest Village Drive Pompton Plains, NJ 07444 (973)831-3540 Fax (973)831-3503

Pons, Nieva P., MD {1831200047} IntrMd(71,PHIL)<NJ-RUNNELLS>
+ 5 Copperfield Road
Scotch Plains, NJ 07076 (908)654-5850 Fax (908)654-0363

Pontecorvo, Martin J., DO {1760590251} IntrMd(88,NY75)<NJ-MORRISTN, NJ-OVERLOOK>
+ Associates in Internal Medicine, LLC
1072 Valley Road Stirling, NJ 07980 (908)604-8464 Fax (908)604-2494
+ Associates in Internal Medicine, LLC
248 Columbia Turnpike Florham Park, NJ 07932 (908)604-8464 Fax (973)514-1106

Ponti, Tatyana, MD {1811099005} IntrMd(89,RUS10)<NJ-RIVERVW>
+ 160 White Road/Suite 102
Little Silver, NJ 07739 (732)450-0062 Fax (732)450-0616

Pontoriero, Michael Anthony, MD {1275536765} SrgThr, SrgVas(85,NJ05)<NJ-MTNSIDE, NJ-CLARMAAS>
+ The Cardiovascular Care Group
1401 Broad Street/Suite 1 Clifton, NJ 07013 (973)759-9000 Fax (973)751-3730
+ The Cardiovascular Care Group
433 Central Avenue Westfield, NJ 07090 (973)759-9000 Fax (908)490-1698

Ponzio, Geralyn Michelle, MD {1962484501} IntrMd(01,VT02)<NJ-NWTNMEM>
+ Ponzio Medical Associates
127 Pine Street/Suite 10 Montclair, NJ 07042 (973)783-0073 Fax (973)783-4010
+ Newton Medical Center
175 High Street/Hospitalist Newton, NJ 07860 (973)383-2121

Ponzio, Robert J., DO {1508816661} SrgOrt(87,NJ75)
+ Ponzio Orthopedics
449 Hurffville Crosskeys Road/Suite 1 Sewell, NJ 08080 (856)582-7979 Fax (856)582-4259

Poole, John W., MD {1538173158} Surgry(82,VA01)<NJ-HACKNSK, NJ-HOLYNAME>
+ North Jersey Surgical Specialists
83 Summit Avenue Hackensack, NJ 07601 (201)646-0010 Fax (201)646-0600

Poon, Chiu-Man, MD {1699865832} Pedtrc(77,HKOG)<NJ-STBARNMC, NJ-OVERLOOK>
+ New Jersey Health Care Services, LLC
2780 Morris Avenue/Suite 2A Union, NJ 07083 (908)687-3300 Fax (908)687-4747

Poon, Gilbert B., MD {1265465900} IntrMd(81,DOM01)
+ Morris Medical Associates
3799 Route 46 East/Suite 209 Parsippany, NJ 07054 (973)334-8010 Fax (973)402-9030

Poonawala, Nafisa Z., MD {1700812617} FamMed, GenPrc(78,INA2B)<NJ-WOODBRDG>
+ Woodbridge Developmental Center
Rahway Avenue/PO Box 189 Woodbridge, NJ 07095 (732)499-5500 Fax (732)499-5787

Physicians by Name and Address

Poonia, Amit, MD {1780904359} AnesPain, IntrMd
+ Advanced Interventional Pain Management Center
  20 Cherry Tree Farm Road   Middletown, NJ 07748
  (732)952-5533   Fax (732)707-4732
+ Advanced Interventional Pain Management Center
  204 Eagle Rock Avenue   Roseland, NJ 07068   (732)952-5533   Fax (732)707-4732
+ Advanced Interventional Pain Management Center
  619 Amboy Avenue   Edison, NJ 07748   (732)952-5533   Fax (732)707-4732

Pooran, Nakechand Rai, MD {1841258449} Gastrn, IntrMd(97,GRN01)<NJ-RWJUBRUN>
+ RWJ University Hospital New Brunswick
  One Robert Wood Johnson Place   New Brunswick, NJ 08901
  (732)235-7784   Fax (732)235-7792
+ RWJ Gastro & Hepatology
  125 Paterson Street/CAB 5100B   New Brunswick, NJ 08901
  (732)235-7784   Fax (732)235-7792

Popa, Marcela M., MD {1902964083} IntrMd(89,ROM01)
+ Med-Care of East Rutherford
  245 Park Avenue   East Rutherford, NJ 07073   (201)939-7161   Fax (201)939-4053

Popa, Peter R., MD {1821180860} Anesth, IntrMd(84,ROM05)
+ 500 Grand Avenue
  Englewood, NJ 07631   (201)567-8090

Popa, Vincentiu, MD {1083684401} Anesth(90,ROM01)<NJ-BAYSHORE>
+ Vincentiu Popa Pain Management LLC
  1111 Paulison Avenue   Clifton, NJ 07011   (201)925-0277

Pope, Alan Raymond, MD {1730160391} PulDis, IntrMd, CritCr(80,CT02)<NY-LDYLORDS, NJ-VIRTUAHS>
+ Pulmonary & Sleep Associates of SJ, LLC.
  107 Berlin Road   Cherry Hill, NJ 08034   (856)429-1800   Fax (856)429-1081
+ Pulmonary & Sleep Associates of SJ, LLC.
  750 Route 73 South/Suite 401   Marlton, NJ 08053
  (856)429-1800   Fax (856)375-2325
+ Pulmonary & Sleep Associates of SJ, LLC.
  811 Sunset Road/Suite 201   Burlington, NJ 08034
  (609)298-1776   Fax (609)531-2391

Pope, Ernest J., MD {1073783106} SprtMd, SrgOrt(04,NJ05)
+ Kayal Orthopaedic Center, PC
  385 South Maple Avenue/Suite 206   Ridgewood, NJ 07450
  (201)447-3880   Fax (201)447-9326
+ Kayal Orthopaedic Center, P.C.
  784 Franklin Avenue/Suite 250   Franklin Lakes, NJ 07417
  (201)447-3880   Fax (201)560-0712

Pope, Ronald J., DO {1518993153} FamMed(98,ME75)<NY-COLUMBIA>
+ Wayne Cancer Center LLC
  234 Hamburg Turnpike/Suite 202   Wayne, NJ 07470
  (973)310-0309

Popeck, Paul J., DO {1548292089} FamMed(97,FL75)<NJ-SOMERSET>
+ MEDEMERGE
  1005 North Washington Avenue   Green Brook, NJ 08812
  (732)968-8900   Fax (732)968-4609
+ Linden Family Medical Associates
  850 North Wood Avenue   Linden, NJ 07036   (732)968-8900   Fax (908)925-7910

Popescu, Adrian, MD {1740401066} IntrMd(01,ROM01)<NJ-KMHTURNV>
+ Kennedy Health Systems/Washington Township Campus
  435 Hurffville-Cross Keys Road   Turnersville, NJ 08012
  (856)218-5634   Fax (856)218-5664
+ AtlantiCare Hospitalist Program
  1925 Pacific Avenue/8th Floor   Atlantic City, NJ 08401
  (609)345-4000

Popescu, Anca S., MD {1558459511} Nrolgy(96,ROM09)<NJ-KMHTURNV>
+ Cherry Hill Primary and Specialty Care
  457 Haddonfield Road/Suite 110   Cherry Hill, NJ 08002
  (844)542-2273   Fax (856)406-4570
+ Kennedy Health Systems/Washington Township Campus
  435 Hurffville-Cross Keys Road   Turnersville, NJ 08012
  (844)542-2273   Fax (856)218-5664

Popkave, Arthur H., MD {1023111622} CdvDis(72,PA13)<NJ-WARREN>
+ Coventry Cardiology Associates
  1000 Coventry Drive   Phillipsburg, NJ 08865   (908)859-3800   Fax (908)859-4310

Popkin, Mark D., MD {1225026834} Dermat, IntrMd(85,NY08)<NJ-MORRISTN>
+ Dermatology Consultants of Northern Jersey
  261 James Street/Suite 2-B   Morristown, NJ 07960
  (973)993-1433   Fax (973)993-1176

Popkin, Sara Elizabeth, MD {1770809949} Psychy
+ Alexander Road Associates in Psychiatry & Psychology
  707 Alexander Road/Bldg 2 Suite 202   Princeton, NJ 08540
  (612)968-3706   Fax (609)419-9200
  sara.popkin@gmail.com

Poplawski, Michael, MD {1831437789}<NJ-KMHCHRRY>
+ Kennedy Health System/Cherry Hill Campus
  2201 Chapel Avenue West   Cherry Hill, NJ 08002
  (856)488-6500   Fax (856)922-5109

Poplin, Elizabeth A., MD {1073698767} IntrMd, MedOnc(76,MA16)<NJ-RWJUBRUN>
+ Rutgers Cancer Institute of New Jersey
  195 Little Albany Street/PO Box 2681   New Brunswick, NJ 08903   (732)235-6777   Fax (732)235-8681

Popovich, Joseph F., MD {1063592285} SrgVas, Surgry(87,NJ06)
+ Joseph F. Popovich MD FACS
  159 Palisade Avenue   Jersey City, NJ 07306   (201)217-1110
  Fax (201)217-1130
  popmdpractice@yahoo.com

Poprycz, Walter, MD {1093836041} SrgOrt(74,MA07)<NJ-OURLADY, NJ-VIRTUAHS>
+ Professional Orthopedic Assocs of South Jersey PA
  17 White Horse Pike/Suite 1   Haddon Heights, NJ 08035
  (856)547-2323   Fax (856)547-7932

Porat, Manny David, MD {1629275250} SrgOrt(05,PA13)
+ Reconstructive Orthopedics, P.A.
  200 Bowman Drive/Suite E-100   Voorhees, NJ 08043
  (609)267-9400   Fax (609)267-9457

Porat, Natalie, MD {1902165947} MtFtMd, ObsGyn(11,ISR02)
+ Newark Beth Israel Medical Center
  201 Lyons Avenue   Newark, NJ 07112   (973)919-6166

Porbunderwala, Steven James, MD {1417101502} Surgry
+ Summit Medical Group-Berkeley Heights Campus
  1 Diamond Hill Road   Berkeley Heights, NJ 07922
  (908)273-4300   Fax (908)790-6576
+ Summit Medical Group Florham Park Campus
  150 Park Avenue   Florham Park, NJ 07932   (908)273-4300

Porcaro, Sabina M., MD {1275634636} IntrMd(83,ITAL)<NJ-STBARNMC, NJ-CLARMAAS>
+ 228 North 15th Street
  Bloomfield, NJ 07003   (973)743-3313   Fax (973)743-1136

Porcelli, Marcus P., MD {1972594414} Hemato, IntrMd, MedOnc(83,ITA22)<NJ-STPETER>
+ Drs. Fein, Porcelli & Richards
  75 Veronica Avenue/Suite 201   Somerset, NJ 08873
  (732)246-4882   Fax (732)249-5633
+ Regional Cancer Care Associates
  111 Union Valley Road/Suite 205   Monroe, NJ 08831
  (732)246-4882   Fax (609)395-7955

Poretta, Trina A., DO {1720082092} OncHem(96,NJ75)<NJ-KENEDYHS, NJ-VIRTUAHS>
+ Comprehensive Cancer & Hematology Specialists, P.C.
  900 Medical Center Drive/Suite 200   Sewell, NJ 08080
  (856)582-0550   Fax (856)582-7640
+ Comprehensive Cancer & Hematology Specialists, P.C.
  705 White Horse Road   Voorhees, NJ 08043   (856)582-0550   Fax (856)435-0696
+ Comprehensive Cancer & Hematology Specialists, P.C.
  17 West Red Bank Avenue/Suite 202   Woodbury, NJ 08080
  (856)848-5560   Fax (856)848-0958

Porras, Cornelio J., MD {1255386850} IntrMd, PulDis(87,NY01)
+ Summit Medical Group
  6 Brighton Road/2 FL/Pulmonary   Clifton, NJ 07012
  (973)777-7911   Fax (973)777-5403

Portadin, Robert A., MD {1194743682} ObsGyn, IntrMd(73,NJ05)<NJ-CENTRAST>
+ Women's Physicians & Surgeons
  501 Iron Bridge Road/Suite 10   Freehold, NJ 07728
  (732)431-2999   Fax (732)431-2993
+ Women's Physicians & Surgeons
  510 Bridge Plaza Drive   Englishtown, NJ 07726   (732)431-2999   Fax (732)536-4570
+ Women's Physicians & Surgeons
  245A Main Avenue   Matawan, NJ 07728   (732)566-9466
  Fax (732)566-0343

Portale, Karen Mary, MD {1104876564} EmrgMd(93,NJ06)<NJ-VALLEY>
+ The Valley Hospital
  223 North Van Dien Avenue/Emergency   Ridgewood, NJ 07450   (201)447-8000

Porter, Anne Marisa, MD {1417993627} FamMed
+ 151 South Sixth Street
  Phillipsburg, NJ 08865

Porter, Catherine M., DO {1255606521} Surgry
+ 1014 Central Avenue
  Runnemede, NJ 08078

Porter, David Alexander, MD {1871859371} SprtMd
+ Orthopedic Specialists NJ-Hackensack
  87 Summit Avenue   Hackensack, NJ 07601   (201)489-0022
  Fax (201)489-6991

Porter, David F., DO {1588673180} FamMed, OstMed(78,MI12)<NJ-HOLYNAME>
+ 208 Boulevard/Suite F
  Hasbrouck Heights, NJ 07604   (201)288-0872   Fax (201)288-8180

Porter, James H., MD {1164480380} Pedtrc(87,NJ05)<NJ-NWTNMEM, NJ-MORRISTN>
+ Advocare Sussex County Pediatrics Newton
  39 Newton Sparta Road   Newton, NJ 07860   (973)383-9841   Fax (973)383-7989
+ Advocare Sussex County Pediatrics Montague
  2B Myrtle Drive   Montague, NJ 07827   (973)383-9841
  Fax (973)293-0138

Porter, Joel, MD {1326376278} Ophthl(66,PA01)<NJ-VIRTMARL>
+ Joel Porter MD LLC
  6981 North Park Drive/Suite 101   Pennsauken, NJ 08109
  (856)488-4404   Fax (856)488-5207

Porter, John Maurice, MD {1487735122} SrgCrC, Surgry(85,MD07)<OH-STELIZAB>
+ Cooper Bone and Joint Institute
  3 Cooper Plaza/Suite 411   Camden, NJ 08103   (856)673-4500   Fax (856)673-4525
  porter-john@cooperhealth.edu
+ Cooper University Physician Trauma Center
  One Cooper Plaza   Camden, NJ 08103   (856)342-3014

Porter, Joseph M., MD {1639264393} IntrMd(83,NJ05)<NJ-STJOSHOS>
+ 50 Mount Prospect Avenue/Suite 203
  Clifton, NJ 07013   (973)574-9880   Fax (973)472-1420

Porter, Thomas G., MD {1871555342} Pedtrc(97,NY48)
+ Basking Ridge Pediatric Association
  150 North Finley Avenue   Basking Ridge, NJ 07920
  (908)766-4660   Fax (908)204-9871

Portfolio, Almerindo Gerard, Jr., MD {1669477956} Catrct, Ophthl, IntrMd(78,PA02)<NJ-VALLEY, NY-NYEYEINF>
+ Portfolio Eye Care Associates
  385 South Maple Ave/Suite 101   Glen Rock, NJ 07452
  (201)445-5161   Fax (201)445-7912
  APortfolio@aol.com

Portilla, Diana M., MD {1487769923} IntrMd(95,COL22)
+ 312 Nelson Court
  Edgewater, NJ 07020
+ Englewood Family Health Center
  148 Engle Street   Englewood, NJ 07631   Fax (201)569-6022

Porto, Maura C., DO {1396606516} InfDis
+ Cooper PM & R Assocs
  3 Cooper Plaza/Suite 104   Camden, NJ 08103   (856)963-3518   Fax (856)968-8311

Portugal, Alexander, MD {1215924196} Anesth(75,UKR16)<NJ-PALISADE>
+ Palisades Medical Center
  7600 River Road/Anesth   North Bergen, NJ 07047
  (201)854-5000

Porwal, Anoop, MD {1053373613} PhysMd(89,INA7Y)<NJ-HLTH-SRE, NJ-COMMED>
+ HealthSouth Rehabilitation Hospital of New Jersey
  14 Hospital Drive   Toms River, NJ 08755   (732)244-3100
+ Community Medical Center
  99 Route 37 West   Toms River, NJ 08755   (732)557-8000
+ Anoop Porwal MD, PC
  20 Hospital Drive/Suite 17A   Toms River, NJ 08755
  (732)557-4444

Porwancher, Richard B., MD {1841206521} InfDis(77,IL06)
+ Infectious Disease Consultants
  1245 Whitehorse-Mercerville Rd   Mercerville, NJ 08619
  (609)581-2000   Fax (609)581-5450

Possick, Paul Aaron, MD {1497756431} Dermat(64,MA07)<NJ-HACKNSK, NY-NYUTISCH>
+ Westwood Dermatology
  390 Old Hook Road   Westwood, NJ 07675   (201)666-9550
  Fax (201)666-1251

Post, Ernest M., MD {1558443556} PedEnd, Pedtrc(76,NY15)<NJ-COOPRUMC>
+ Cooper University Hospital Pediatrics/Endocrinology
  3 Cooper Plaza/Suite 200   Camden, NJ 08103   (856)968-8898
+ Cooper Peds/Children's Regional Ctr
  6400 Main Street Complex   Voorhees, NJ 08043   (856)342-2000

Post, Nicole Renee, MD {1740360502} Psychy
+ Center for Family Guidance, PC
  765 East Route 70/Building A-101   Marlton, NJ 08053
  (856)797-4800   Fax (856)810-0110

Post, Robert E., MD {1396826822} FamMed
+ Tatem Brown Family Practice
  2225 East Evesham Road/Suite 101   Voorhees, NJ 08043
  (856)795-4330   Fax (856)325-3704

Postighone, Carl J., DO {1508968991} IntrMd(88,NY75)<NJ-MORRISTN, NJ-OVERLOOK>
+ Associates in Internal Medicine, LLC
  1072 Valley Road   Stirling, NJ 07980   (908)604-8464   Fax (908)604-2494
+ Associates in Internal Medicine, LLC
  248 Columbia Turnpike   Florham Park, NJ 07932   (908)604-8464   Fax (973)514-1106

Potack, Jonathan Zachary, MD {1518004993} IntrMd, Gastrn, Bariat(02,NY47)
+ Bergen Medical Associates
466 Old Hook Road/Suite 1 Emerson, NJ 07630 (201)967-8221 Fax (201)967-0340

Potash, Sarah K., MD {1003920216} ObsGyn(95,NJ06)
+ Summit Medical Group
160 East Hanover Avenue/Suite 101 Cedar Knolls, NJ 07927 (973)605-5090 Fax (973)605-1705

Potashnik, Rashel, MD {1073568176} PhysMd(82,LAT02)
+ Physical Rehabilitation Center LLP
1767 Morris Avenue Union, NJ 07083 (908)624-1050 Fax (908)624-1052

Potestio, Christopher Paul, MD {1558705160} Anesth<NJ-COOPRUMC>
+ Cooper University Hospital
One Cooper Plaza Camden, NJ 08103 (856)356-4924

Potharlanka, Prathibha R., MD {1295761690} IntrMd(99,DMN01)
+ Premier Medicine & Wellness
231 Crosswicks Road/Suite 11 Bordentown, NJ 08505 (609)298-4750

Pothen, Jerrin Thomas, MD {1912168899}<NJ-CLARMAAS>
+ Clara Maass Medical Center
1 Clara Maass Drive Belleville, NJ 07109 (973)450-2000

Potian, Marcelino M., MD {1558418061} Anesth(73,PHI08)<NJ-UMDNJ>
+ University Hospital
150 Bergen Street/Anesthesiology Newark, NJ 07103 (973)972-5254 Fax (973)972-4172
potianmm@umdnj.edu

Potini, Vishnu Choudhary, MD {1013207208} SrgOrt
+ North Jersey Orthopaedic Institute
90 Bergen Street/DOC 7300 Newark, NJ 07103 (973)972-2150

Potluri, Haritha, MD {1225074701} IntrMd, PulDis, CritCr(98,INA2X)
+ Comprehensive Lung Care
1440 How Lane/Suite 2-D North Brunswick, NJ 08902 (732)719-2222 Fax (732)719-2224
Haritha.Potluri@hotmail.com

Potluri, Srinivasa Rao, MD {1427088897} ClNrPh, Nrolgy, IntrMd(94,INA11)<NJ-CHSFULD, NJ-CHSMRCER>
+ Advanced Neurology Center, LLC
676 Route 202-206 North/Suite 2 Bridgewater, NJ 08807 (908)218-1180 Fax (908)218-1718

Potoczek-Salahi, Jolanta, MD {1376532796} FamMed(82,POLA)<NJ-HOBUNIMC>
+ Bayonne Family Practice
391 Kennedy Boulevard Bayonne, NJ 07002 (201)858-4110 Fax (201)858-2240

Potter, Steven D., MD {1679582639} Surgry(90,NJ05)<NJ-CHILTON, NJ-WAYNEGEN>
+ Drs. Potter and Bakosi
287 Boulevard/Suite 1/PO Box 367 Pompton Plains, NJ 07444 (973)839-7400 Fax (973)831-4911

Potter-McQuilkin, Dineasha M., MD {1093021263} ObsGyn
+ 129 Washington Street/Suite 200
Hoboken, NJ 07030 (201)795-0501 Fax (201)963-8231

Pottick-Schwartz, Eliane Amely, MD {1811932247} FamMed(88,ISR01)
+ Valley Health Medical Group
780 Cedar Lane Teaneck, NJ 07666 (201)836-7664 Fax (201)836-5710

Potulski, Frederick J., MD {1659373439} IntrMd, PulDis(79,MEXI)<NJ-JRSYSHMC>
+ Shore Pulmonary PA
2640 Highway 70/Building 6-A Manasquan, NJ 08736 (732)528-5900 Fax (732)528-0887
+ Shore Pulmonary PA
301 Bingham Avenue/Suite B Ocean, NJ 07712 (732)528-5900 Fax (732)775-1212
+ Shore Pulmonary PA
1608 Route 88/Suite 117 Brick, NJ 08736 (732)575-1100

Potylitsina, Yelena, MD {1568592632} Pedtrc(92,UKR16)<NJ-RWJUBRUN>
+ Barnabas Health Medical Group
1270 Highway 35 South/Suite 1 Middletown, NJ 07748 (732)671-1155 Fax (732)671-9630

Poucel, Donna Jeanne, MD {1598876393} EmrgMd(01,PA13)<NJ-SJHREGMC>
+ SJH Regional Medical Center
1505 West Sherman Avenue/EmrgMed Vineland, NJ 08360 (856)641-8000

Poulad, David, MD {1184695090} SrgNro(98,MO34)<NJ-OVERLOOK, NJ-TRINIJSC>
+ IGEA Brain & Spine
1057 Commerce Avenue Union, NJ 07083 (908)688-8800 Fax (908)688-2377

Poulathas, Alexander Steven Simeon, DO {1619914470} IntHos(01,PA77)<NJ-DEBRAHLC>
+ Deborah Heart and Lung Center
200 Trenton Road/Hospitalist Browns Mills, NJ 08015 (609)893-6611 Fax (609)893-1213

Pourmasiha, Niloufar, DO {1689995250} Anesth
+ Drs. Delaney, Merlin & Pourmasiha
66 West Gilbert Street/2nd Floor Tinton Falls, NJ 07701 (732)212-0051 Fax (732)212-0713

Povzhitkov, Igor Moiseyevi, MD {1700924669} Anesth(82,RUS82)
+ North Jersey Surgical Center
520 Sylvan Avenue Englewood Cliffs, NJ 07632 (201)816-1991 Fax (201)632-6403

Powderly, Mary K., MD {1871675322} Gyneco, SrgGyn, AltnMd(84,NJ06)<NJ-SOMERSET>
+ 904 Oak Tree Road/Suite M
South Plainfield, NJ 07080 (908)668-4879 Fax (908)756-8819
+ Total HealthCare for Women
32 Worlds Fair Drive/Suite 201 Somerset, NJ 08873 (908)668-4879 Fax (732)356-1196

Powell, David E., MD {1013902477} CdvDis(90,MA01)
+ Associates in Cardiovascular Disease, LLC
211 Mountain Avenue Springfield, NJ 07081 (973)467-0005 Fax (973)912-8989
+ Mid-Atlantic Cardiology, PA
218 State Route 17 North Rochelle Park, NJ 07662 (973)467-0005 Fax (908)889-5860

Powell, Jeffrey David, DO {1871921551} IntrMd<NJ-SJHREGMC>
+ SJH Regional Medical Center
1505 West Sherman Avenue Vineland, NJ 08360 (610)597-8395

Powell, Kerri Lynette, MD {1891760955} Pedtrc, IntrMd(96,DC03)<NY-STBARNAB>
+ Trinity Pediatrics
430 Morris Avenue/1st Floor Elizabeth, NJ 07208 (908)353-5437 Fax (908)353-0727

Powell, Leonard A., Jr., DO {1750644928}
+ New Jersey Institute for Successful Aging
42 East Laurel Road/Suite 1800 Stratford, NJ 08084 (856)566-6843 Fax (856)566-6781

Power, Rachael Reiko, MD {1215971817} PsyCAd, Psychy(87,ECU04)<NJ-UNIVBHC>
+ University Behavioral HealthCare
183 South Orange Avenue Newark, NJ 07103
+ University Behavioral Health Care
671 Hoes Lane/PO Box 1392 Piscataway, NJ 08855 (732)235-5500

Power, William K., Jr., MD {1205930641} CritCr, Grtrcs, IntrMd(79,MEX03)
+ 730 Lacey Road
Forked River, NJ 08731 (609)693-9240 Fax (609)693-3616
+ Meridian Primary Care
138 Route 9 South Forked River, NJ 08731 (609)693-9240 Fax (609)488-1613

Pozner, Samantha Brooke, MD {1225039670} FamMed(97,PA07)<NJ-OVERLOOK>
+ Springfield Family Practice
11 Overlook Road/Suite 140 Summit, NJ 07901 (908)277-0050 Fax (908)277-0201

Pozzessere, Anthony Samuel, MD {1851642797} Surgry
+ 245 East Main Street/Suite 2
Ramsey, NJ 07446 (201)327-0220 Fax (201)327-4871

Prabhakar, Avinash, MD {1851422885} IntrMd(97,NJ05)<NJ-MEMSALEM>
+ Christiana Care Cardiology Consultants
499 Beckett Road/Suite 202 Logan Township, NJ 08085 (856)769-3900 Fax (856)769-3903

Prabhat, Arvind, MD {1003910472} Otlryg, OtgyPSHN(92,NY20)<CT-WATRBRY, CT-STMARY>
+ ENT and Allergy Associates
1131 Broad Street/Suite 103 Building A Shrewsbury, NJ 07702 (732)389-3388 Fax (732)389-3389

Prabhu, Vasanthi M., MD {1134139801} IntrMd(74,INDI)<NJ-VALYONS>
+ VA New Jersey Health Care System at Lyons
151 Knollcroft Road Lyons, NJ 07939 (908)647-0180 Fax (908)604-5250

Prabhuram, Nagarathna, MD {1891930947} Pedtrc, IntrMd(99,INA97)
+ 2864 Route 27/Suite A
North Brunswick, NJ 08902 (732)331-3046
+ Elizabeth Pediatric Group
701 Newark Avenue/Suite 212 Elizabeth, NJ 07208 (732)331-3046 Fax (908)354-9077

Pradhan, Anuja A., MD {1528260064} InfDis
+ 100 Daibes Court/Apt 1410
Edgewater, NJ 07020 (917)640-0220
docpradhan@gmail.com

Pradhan, Archana, MD {1972684256} ObsGyn(96,NC07)
+ University Medical Group/OBGYN
125 Paterson Street/2nd Floor New Brunswick, NJ 08901 (732)235-6600 Fax (732)235-6627

Pradhan, Basant Kumar, MD {1679965895} PsyCAd, IntrMd(04,INA4E)
+ Cooper Perinatology Associates
3 Cooper Plaza/Suite 502 Camden, NJ 08103 (856)968-7433 Fax (856)968-8499

Pradhan, Kamal M., MD {1538187877}
+ On-Site Neonatal Partners
1000 Haddonfield-Berlin Road/Suite 210 Voorhees, NJ 08043 (517)279-9031 Fax (856)782-2213
1sabkom@gmail.com

Pradhan, Madhura Ravindra, MD {1285640367} Pedtrc, PedNph(91,INA69)<PA-CHILDHOS>
+ CHOP Pediatric & Adolescent Specialty Care Center
1012 Laurel Oak Road Voorhees, NJ 08043 (856)435-1300 Fax (856)435-0091

Pradhan, Prasanna Govind, MD {1841231305} Pedtrc(75,INA21)<NJ-COMMED>
+ 620 West Lacey Road
Forked River, NJ 08731 (609)693-3956 Fax (609)693-7191

Praditpan, Piyapa, MD {1184942773}<NY-PRSBCOLU>
+ Morristown Medical Center
100 Madison Avenue Morristown, NJ 07962 (973)829-4128 Fax (973)898-3914

Prado-Galarza, Neiza L., MD {1689695918} Psychy, PsyGrt, IntrMd(90,PRO02)
+ Central MediPlex
495 Iron Bridge Road/Suite 8 Freehold, NJ 07728 (732)431-8075 Fax (732)431-0307

Pragaspathy, Bhavadarani M., MD {1588870232} Pedtrc, IntrMd(03,NY0)
+ North Brunswick Pediatrics
1598 US Highway 130 North Brunswick, NJ 08902 (732)297-0603 Fax (732)297-2866

Prager, Jason Nicholas, MD {1801047667} Grtrcs, IntrMd(07,NET12)<NJ-MORRISTN>
+ Geriatric Assessment Center
435 South Street/Suite 390 Morristown, NJ 07960 (973)971-5000
+ Morristown Medical Center
100 Madison Avenue/Geriatrics Morristown, NJ 07962 (973)971-5000 Fax (973)290-7675

Prajapati, Binita Prashant, DO {1053324889} FamMed, IntrMd(95,NY75)
+ Valley Health Medical Group
780 Cedar Lane Teaneck, NJ 07666 (201)836-7664 Fax (201)836-5710

Prakash, Ananth N., MD {1437269909} Nephro, IntrMd(71,INA9X)<NJ-STJOSHOS>
+ North Jersey Nephrology Associates PA
246 Hamburg Turnpike/Suite 207 Wayne, NJ 07470 (973)653-3366 Fax (973)653-3365

Prakash, Atul, MD {1427085109} CdvDis, OthrSp(82,INA12)<NJ-STJOSHOS>
+ Cardiac & Arrhythmias Specialist
905 Allwood Road/Suite 103 Clifton, NJ 07013 (973)778-3111 Fax (973)340-1518

Prakash, Kalpana, MD {1740298595} Pedtrc(76,INA7Y)<NJ-STCLRDEN, NJ-MORRISTN>
+ Pediatric Associates
77 Union Street Dover, NJ 07801 (973)366-5236 Fax (973)366-5236

Prakash, Meera V., MD {1306911763} Psychy(78,INA67)
+ North Jersey Developmental Center
169 Minisink Road/PO Box 169/Consltnt Totowa, NJ 07512 (973)256-1700 Fax (973)256-3468

Prakash, Shasha, MD {1417916701} ObsGyn, RprEnd, IntrMd(73,INDI)
+ Hudson Digestive Health Center
534 Avenue E/Suite A Bayonne, NJ 07002 (201)858-8444 Fax (201)858-4260

Prakhina, Boris, MD {1609087659} Anesth(89,RUS02)
+ 33-00 Broadway/Suite 209
Fair Lawn, NJ 07410 (201)796-7666 Fax (201)796-5570

Prasad, Amit, MD {1902067341} CdvDis
+ St. Luke's Cardiology Associates
755 Memorial Parkway Phillipsburg, NJ 08865 (908)859-0514 Fax (908)859-0515

Prasad, Aparna, MD {1457585077} PedCrd<NJ-MORRISTN>
+ Morristown Medical Center
100 Madison Avenue/PedCardio/2nd F Morristown, NJ 07962 (973)971-5996

Prasad, Deepali, MD {1962607952} Nephro
+ Monroe Family Medicine
323 Spotswood Englishtown Road/Suite B Monroe Township, NJ 08831 (732)388-7999 Fax (732)416-0470
+ Drs. Yim & Prasad
913 West Inman Avenue Rahway, NJ 07065 (732)388-7999 Fax (732)388-7992

Prasad, Devineni R., MD {1255418083} Pedtrc(69,INDI)
+ Drs. Amer and Prasad
777 White Horse Pike/Suite E Hammonton, NJ 08037 (609)567-0608 Fax (609)567-1295
Dprasadd@comcast.net

401

Physicians by Name and Address

Prasad, Indra D., MD {1861490377} Hemato, Onclgy(81,INDI)
+ 85 South Harrison Street/Suite 203
  East Orange, NJ 07018   (973)395-1020   Fax (973)395-1030

Prasad, Jitender, MD {1437152501} Anesth(72,INA83)<NJ-STMRYPAS>
+ St. Mary's Hospital
  350 Boulevard   Passaic, NJ 07055   (973)365-4300

Prasad, Kalpana, MD {1174547020} IntrMd(92,INA7B)<NJ-RWJURAH>
+ Robert Wood Johnson University Hospital at Rahway
  865 Stone Street/Internal Med   Rahway, NJ 07065
  (732)381-4200

Prasad, Kamil, MD {1518403989} FamMed
+ JFK Family Practice Group
  65 James Street   Edison, NJ 08818   (732)321-7487   Fax (732)906-4927

Prasad, Keshav, MD {1356379457} FamMed(77,INA49)<NJ-CENTRAST>
+ Monroe Family Medicine
  323 Spotswood Englishtown Road/Suite B   Monroe Township, NJ 08831   (732)723-1000   Fax (732)416-0470

Prasad, Lakshmi, MD {1033165295} IntrMd(95,INDI)
+ Associates in Integrative Medicine
  27 Mountain Boulevard/Suite 9   Warren, NJ 07059
  (908)769-9600   Fax (908)769-9610

Prasad, Nalini, MD {1881787679} Nrolgy(78,INDI)
+ North Bergen Neurology
  8103 Bergenline Avenue   North Bergen, NJ 07047
  (201)758-0660

Prasad, Niloo, MD {1407862519} IntrMd, MedOnc, OncHem(83,INDI)
+ Oncology & Hematology Associates
  2177 Oak Tree Road/Suite 104   Edison, NJ 08820
  (908)755-1165   Fax (908)755-2093

Prasad, Penesetti V., MD {1679511844} CdvDis, IntrMd(73,INA16)<NJ-BAYSHORE>
+ Drs. Prasad and Shah
  717 North Beers Street/PO Box 370   Holmdel, NJ 07733
  (732)264-0210   Fax (732)888-9214

Prasad, Prema, MD {1821034141} FamMed(76,INA47)
+ Concentra Urgent Care at Parsippany
  190 Baldwin Road   Parsippany, NJ 07054   (973)882-0444
  Fax (973)882-3217

Prasad, Sanjiv, MD {1164417523} CdvDis, IntrMd(95,NY09)
+ Associates in Cardiovascular Disease, LLC
  211 Mountain Avenue   Springfield, NJ 07081   (973)467-0005   Fax (973)912-8989

Prasad, Sudhanshu, MD {1982626453} IntrMd(82,INDI)<NJ-RWJURAH>
+ Rahway Medical Associates
  181 Westfield Avenue   Clark, NJ 07066   (732)382-1699

Prasad, Surabhi, MD {1770501603} EnDbMt(86,INDI)
+ 181 Westfield Avenue
  Clark, NJ 07066   (732)382-1699   Fax (732)872-8722
+ 2177 Oak Tree Road
  Edison, NJ 08817   (732)382-1699   Fax (908)755-1165

Prasad, Vijaya, MD {1194752584} Pedtrc, PedEnd(77,INDI)<NJ-STJOSHOS, NJ-VALLEY>
+ St. Joseph's Regional Medical Center
  703 Main Street   Paterson, NJ 07503   (973)754-2000

Prasad, Vineet, MD {1609902493} IntrMd(99,GRN01)
+ 22 Budapest Street
  Monroe Township, NJ 08831

Pratt, Amanda, MD {1063573095} Pedtrc, PedEmg(98,PA07)<NJ-RWJUBRUN>
+ RWJ University Pediatric Emergency Medicine
  125 Paterson Street/MEB 342   New Brunswick, NJ 08903
  (732)235-7893   Fax (732)235-9349
+ RWJ University Hospital New Brunswick
  One Robert Wood Johnson Place   New Brunswick, NJ 08901
  (732)828-3000

Pratt, Michael E., MD {1689855769} EmrgMd(82,IN20)
+ University Hospital-School of Public Health
  170 Frelinghuysen Road   Piscataway, NJ 08854   (732)445-0123   Fax (732)445-3644

Pratt Mccoy, Kia Chriselda, MD {1508892480} IntrMd, IntHos(01,DC03)<NJ-VIRTMHBC, NJ-VIRTMARL>
+ Virtua Hospitalist Group Memorial
  175 Madison Avenue/1 FL   Mount Holly, NJ 08060
  (609)914-6180   Fax (609)914-6182
+ Virtua Hospitalist Group Marlton
  90 Brick Road   Marlton, NJ 08053   (856)355-6730

Pratter, Melvin Richard, MD {1871683565} PulDis, IntrMd, CritCr(73,NY06)<NJ-COOPRUMC>
+ Cooper University Medical Center/Camden
  3 Cooper Plaza/Suite 312   Camden, NJ 08103   (856)342-2407   Fax (856)541-3968
+ The Cooper Health System at Voorhees
  900 Centennial Boulevard/Suite K   Voorhees, NJ 08043
  (856)342-2407   Fax (856)325-6645

Pravda, Douglas J., DO {1427020718} Dermat(73,IA75)<NJ-OVERLOOK>
+ 622 Boulevard
  Kenilworth, NJ 07033   (908)241-3181   Fax (908)241-1669

Prefer, Audrey I., MD {1669417572} ObsGyn, Gyneco(83,NY08)<NJ-MORRISTN>
+ 19 East Main Street
  Mendham, NJ 07945   (973)543-4440   Fax (973)543-3009

Pregenzer, Gerard J., MD {1588671648} ObsGyn, Gyneco, SrgCsm(83,NJ05)<NJ-SOMERSET, NJ-OVERLOOK>
+ Women's Health Care of Warren
  65 Mountain Boulevard Ext/Suite 201   Warren, NJ 07059
  (732)469-9400   Fax (732)469-8192
  whcwarren@aol.com

Pregnar, Joshua Paul, DO {1306107255}<NJ-SJHREGMC>
+ SJH Regional Medical Center
  1505 West Sherman Avenue   Vineland, NJ 08360
  (570)498-0120
  jopregnar@gmail.com

Preis, Keith Victor, MD {1750317301} Nrolgy(95,DMN01)
+ Neurology Associates & Ctr Pain
  1030 North Kings Highway/Suite 200B   Cherry Hill, NJ 08034   (856)482-0030   Fax (856)779-7787
+ Neurology Pain Associates
  222 New Road/Central Park East   Linwood, NJ 08221
  (856)482-0030   Fax (609)601-6009

Preminger, Mark William, MD {1982788691} ClCdEl, IntrMd(85,PA0)<NJ-VALLEY>
+ Valley Medical Group-Electrophysiology & Cardiology
  223 North Van Dien Avenue   Ridgewood, NJ 07450
  (201)432-7837   Fax (201)432-7830
+ Valley Medical Group-Electrophysiology & Cardiology
  1578 Route 23/Suite 103   Wayne, NJ 07470   (201)432-7837   Fax (201)432-7830

Preminger, Michele Lynn, MD {1568577336} ObsGyn, Psychy(87,NY20)
+ Rutgers Hurtado Health Center
  11 Bishop Place   New Brunswick, NJ 08901   (732)932-7402
  Fax (732)932-1223

Prendergast, Nancy C., MD {1023093879} Radiol, RadDia(86,RI01)<NJ-RBAYOLDB>
+ University Radiology Group, P.C.
  483 Cranbury Road   East Brunswick, NJ 08816   (732)390-0030   Fax (732)390-5383

Prendergast, Thomas William, MD {1881617645} SrgCTh, SrgThr(87,PA14)<NJ-NWRKBETH, NJ-STBARNMC>
+ UH- Robert Wood Johnson Med
  125 Paterson Street/MEB 512   New Brunswick, NJ 08901
  (732)235-7810   Fax (732)235-8963
  prendetw@umdnj.edu
+ University Medical Group/Cardiology
  125 Paterson Street/CAB-Rm 5200   New Brunswick, NJ 08901   (732)235-7810   Fax (732)235-7013

Prenner, Jonathan Lawrence, MD {1245203066} Ophthl(98,NY48)<NJ-RWJUBRUN, NJ-KIMBALL>
+ Retina Associates of New Jersey, P.A.
  10 Plum Street/Suite 600   New Brunswick, NJ 08901
  (732)220-1600   Fax (732)220-1603
+ Retina Associates of New Jersey, P.A.
  1200 Route 22 East   Bridgewater, NJ 08807   (732)220-1600
  Fax (908)218-4307
+ Retina Associates of New Jersey, P.A.
  140 Franklin Corner Road   Lawrenceville, NJ 08901
  (609)896-3655   Fax (609)895-0853

Prentice, Hugh J., MD {1669526190} FamMed(87,NJ05)<NJ-HUNTRDN>
+ North Hunterdon Physician Associates
  37 Ruppell Road   Hampton, NJ 08827

Preschel, Samuel Aharon, MD {1063561413} IntrMd, Pedtrc, IntMAdMd(61,FRAN)<NJ-KIMBALL>
+ Osteoporosis Center
  809 River Avenue   Lakewood, NJ 08701   (732)905-9944
  Fax (732)363-3118

Prescott, Theresa Ann, DO {1457404576} Psychy, PsyCAd(94,NJ75)
+ 212 Haddon Avenue/Suite 8
  Haddon Township, NJ 08108   (856)673-0168   Fax (856)673-0169

Presenza, Thomas Jonathan, DO {1013173640} RadDia, PedRad(00,PA77)<NJ-COOPRUMC>
+ Cooper University Hospital
  One Cooper Plaza/Radiology   Camden, NJ 08103
  (856)342-2380   Fax (856)365-0472

Presilla, Alejandro, MD {1902835747} CdvDis, IntrMd(74,SPAI)
+ 322 49th Street
  Union City, NJ 07087   (201)863-0150   Fax (201)863-0444

Press, Howard L., DO {1487692505} FamMed(75,IA75)<NJ-VIRTMHBC, NJ-VIRTMARL>
+ 600 North Route 73/Suite 7A
  Marlton, NJ 08053   (856)985-0558   Fax (856)985-0565
  drpress@covad.net

Press, Lorin R., MD {1720082159} Ophthl(73,NJ05)
+ Edison Ophthalmology Associates
  2177 Oak Tree Road/Suite 203   Edison, NJ 08820
  (908)822-0070   Fax (908)822-0075
+ Edison Eye Group
  7 State Route 27/Suite 101   Edison, NJ 08820   (908)822-0070   Fax (732)549-5869

Pressler, Lee B., MD {1821065483} Urolgy(90,NY09)<NJ-MORRISTN, NJ-STCLRBOO>
+ Morristown Urology Associates
  95 Madison Avenue/Suite 302   Morristown, NJ 07960
  (973)656-0600   Fax (973)656-0200

Pressman, Mark J., MD {1649230673} SrgOrt(87,PA02)<NJ-CHSFULD, NJ-CHSMRCER>
+ Princeton Orthopaedic Associates, P.A.
  325 Princeton Avenue   Princeton, NJ 08540   (609)924-8131   Fax (609)924-8532

Presti, Amy Lynn, MD {1154411320} Pedtrc(99,DC02)
+ MidAtlantic Neonatology Associates
  100 Madison Avenue   Morristown, NJ 07962   (973)971-5488   Fax (973)290-7175

Presti, Jane C., MD {1871802140} Pedtrc(86,DOM11)
+ Pediatrics Associates
  566 Westfield Avenue   Westfield, NJ 07090   (908)233-7171
  Fax (908)233-2255

Presti, Paul Matthew, MD {1710035084} Otlryg(02,DC02)
+ Westfield Ear Nose & Throat Surgical Associates
  213 Summit Road/Suite 1   Mountainside, NJ 07092
  (908)233-5500   Fax (908)233-5776
+ 88 Van Houton Avenue
  Chatham, NJ 07928

Prestifilippo, Christie J., MD {1336129931} IntrMd(97,GRN01)<NJ-MORRISTN>
+ Mendham Medical Group LLP
  19 East Main Street/Suite 1   Mendham, NJ 07945
  (973)543-6505   Fax (973)543-2967

Prestifilippo, Judith A., MD {1518113596} IntrMd(78,ITA01)
+ Novartis Pharmaceuticals Corporation
  59 Route 10   East Hanover, NJ 07936   (973)503-7500

Prestigiacomo, Charles Joseph, MD {1174658272} SrgNro(93,NY01)<NJ-UMDNJ>
+ University Hospital-Doctors Office Center
  90 Bergen Street/DOC 8100   Newark, NJ 07103   (973)972-1163   Fax (973)972-8122

Prestigiacomo, Cynthia R., MD {1730275207} Pedtrc(93,NY01)<NJ-STBARNMC>
+ David J. Strader MD, PHD
  799 Bloomfield Avenue/Suite 304   Verona, NJ 07044
  (973)618-9990   Fax (973)618-9991

Preston, Daniel J., MD {1144295668} IntrMd(81,MEXI)<NJ-STBARNMC>
+ 55 Morris Avenue/Suite 300
  Springfield, NJ 07081   (973)467-5555   Fax (973)467-6779

Prettelt, Adolfo E., MD {1205989241} FamMed, IntrMd(90,COL06)<NJ-COOPRUMC>
+ 123 Egg Harbor Road/Bldg 600 Suite 604
  Sewell, NJ 08080   (856)232-6471   Fax (856)232-7028
+ Cooper Physicians Washington Township
  1 Plaza Drive/Suite 103/Bunker Hill Pl   Sewell, NJ 08080
  (856)232-6471   Fax (856)270-4085

Previti, Francis W., MD {1336165273} SrgVas, Surgry(74,NJ05)<NJ-ACMCITY, NJ-ACMCMAIN>
+ AtlantiCare Cancer Institute
  2500 English Creek Avenue/Building 400   Egg Harbor Township, NJ 08234   (609)677-7700   Fax (609)677-7701
+ Boardwalk Surgical Associates, P.A.
  6725 Ventnor Avenue/Suite C   Ventnor City, NJ 08406
  (609)677-7700   Fax (609)350-6995

Prezioso, Alexander N., MD {1982852034} ObsGyn(81,ITA12)
+ 649 Route 15 South
  Lake Hopatcong, NJ 07849

Price, Ali S., DO {1023117165} EmrgMd(02,PA77)<NJ-VIRTMHBC>
+ Virtua Memorial
  175 Madison Avenue/EmrgMed   Mount Holly, NJ 08060
  (609)267-0700

Price, Andrea Noelle, MD {1477590685} ObsGyn(91,OH06)
+ Women's Center for Integrative Health
  354 Broad Street   Eatontown, NJ 07724   (732)542-3800
  Fax (848)456-4476

Price, Barbara Ellen, MD {1346335114} Nephro, IntrMd(89,MA07)<NJ-STCLRDEN, NJ-MORRISTN>
+ 26 Madison Avenue/Suite 1
  Morristown, NJ 07960   (862)260-9014   Fax (862)260-9094

Price, Craig C., MD {1851313845} IntrMd(86,NJ06)<NJ-UMDNJ>
+ Medical Associates of Marlboro
  42 Throckmorton Lane/2nd flr   Old Bridge, NJ 08857
  (732)607-1111   Fax (732)607-0552

Price, Dennis P., MD {1366503088} EmrgMd(76,PA07)<NJ-UNVMCPRN>
+ University Medical Center of Princeton at Plainsboro
  One Plainsboro Road   Plainsboro, NJ 08536   (609)497-4000

Price, Grant J., MD {1538165410} OthrSp, RadDia, RadV&I(82,RI01)
+ University Radiology, PA
239 Route 22 East/Suite 302   Green Brook, NJ 08812   (732)968-4899   Fax (732)968-8096
+ University Radiology Group, P.C.
3900 Park Avenue/Suite 107   Edison, NJ 08820   (732)968-4899   Fax (732)548-6290
+ University Radiology Group, P.C.
16 Mountain Boulevard   Warren, NJ 08812   (908)769-7200   Fax (908)769-9141

Price, Joel R., MD {1306066279} Psychy(76,ITAL)
+ 159 Millburn Avenue/Suite 2
Millburn, NJ 07041   (973)379-5534   Fax (973)376-4303
+ 223 Bloomfield Street/Suite 120
Hoboken, NJ 07030   (201)420-0811

Price, Judith B., MD {1467582643} PhysMd(86,PA77)<NJ-MMHKEMBL, NJ-MORRISTN>
+ Morristown Memorial Hospital/Mt. Kemble Division
95 Mount Kemble Avenue/PhysMed&Rehab   Morristown, NJ 07960   (973)971-4758
+ South Mountain HealthCare & Rehabilitation Center
2385 Springfield Avenue   Vauxhall, NJ 07088   (973)971-4758   Fax (908)687-4736

Price, Kelly A., MD {1437143336} FamMed(96,NJ06)
+ Martinsville Family Practice
1973 Washington Valley Road   Martinsville, NJ 08836   (732)560-9225   Fax (732)560-8095
kellyprice@mfpnj.allscriptsdirect.net

Price, Letitia, MD {1841426509}
+ 318 Lake Boulevard
Lindenwold, NJ 08021   (609)332-0427
pricelr@gmail.com

Pride, Mikel Jadyne, DO {1477785491} FamMed
+ Springfield Family Practice
11 Overlook Road/Suite 140   Summit, NJ 07901   (908)277-0050   Fax (908)277-0201

Prieto, Debra M., MD {1639175169} Ophthl, PedOph(87,PA01)
+ Friedberg Eye Associates
661 North Broad Street   Woodbury, NJ 08096   (856)845-7968   Fax (856)845-8544

Prieto, Jorge A., MD {1942269931} Gastrn, IntrMd(81,MI01)<NJ-UNDRWD>
+ South Jersey Endoscopy Center
26 East Red Bank Avenue   Woodbury, NJ 08096   (856)848-4464   Fax (856)848-8706
+ Inspira Health Network
509 North Broad Street   Woodbury, NJ 08096   (856)845-0100

Prilutski, Megan A., MD {1598151110} Pedtrc
+ Advocare The Farm Pediatrics
1001 Laurel Oak Boulevard/Suite A   Voorhees, NJ 08043   (856)782-7400   Fax (856)782-7404

Primak, Dmitry, MD {1609860733} Psychy(73,UKRA)<NJ-BERGNMC>
+ 14-25 Plaza Road/Suite 211
Fair Lawn, NJ 07410   (201)796-8008   Fax (201)796-8028
+ New Bridge Medical Center
230 East Ridgewood Avenue/Psychiatry   Paramus, NJ 07652   (201)796-8008   Fax (201)967-4257

Primavera, James Michael, MD {1730154287} PthAcl(93,NY46)<NJ-CLARMAAS>
+ Clara Maass Medical Center
1 Clara Maass Drive/Path   Belleville, NJ 07109   (973)450-2080   Fax (973)844-4976

Primiani, Lisa, MD {1720375439} FamMed, UrgtCr
+ AstraHealth Urgent & Primary Care
564 Broadway   Bayonne, NJ 07002   (201)464-8888
+ AstraHealth Urgent & Primary Care
95 Hudson Street   Hoboken, NJ 07030   (201)464-8888
+ AstraHealth Urgent & Primary Care
18 Lyons Mall   Basking Ridge, NJ 07002   (908)760-8888

Prince, Andrew M., MD {1477639292} Ophthl(81,NY08)<NJ-HACKNSK>
+ 334 Kinderkamack Road
Oradell, NJ 07649   (201)265-9040

Prince, David M., MD {1710982665} Nrolgy(91,NY46)<NJ-ENGLEWOOD>
+ Drs. Rabin, Fremed, Prince, P.C.
700 Palisade Avenue   Englewood Cliffs, NJ 07632   (201)568-3412   Fax (201)568-8249

Prince, Leonie S., MD {1922218569} PsyCAd
+ Center for Family Guidance, PC
765 East Route 70/Building A-101   Marlton, NJ 08053   (732)547-0003   Fax (856)810-0110

Principato, Robert, DO {1922020262} Radiol, RadV&I(85,IA75)<NJ-KMHSTRAT>
+ Kennedy Memorial Hospital-University Medical Center
18 East Laurel Road/Radiology   Stratford, NJ 08084   (856)346-6000

Principe, David Laurence, MD {1417985391} MtFtMd, ObsGyn, IntrMd(91,GRN01)<NJ-STJOSHOS, NJ-HOBUNIMC>
+ Pediatric Cardiology Associates
1 Broadway/Suite 203   Elmwood Park, NJ 07407   (973)569-6264   Fax (973)569-6270

Prineas, Sara L., MD {1376508598} Pedtrc, AdolMd(91,NJ05)
+ Hamilton Pediatric Associates
3 Hamilton Health Place/Suite A   Hamilton, NJ 08690   (609)581-4480   Fax (609)581-5222

Prins, Edward R., MD {1619987905} IntrMd(82,NJ05)<NJ-HACKNSK>
+ Summit Avenue Medical
5 Summit Avenue   Hackensack, NJ 07601   (201)646-0001   Fax (201)646-9101

Prins, Kenneth J., MD {1629056494} IntrMd(72,NJ05)
+ 83 East Bay Avenue
Manahawkin, NJ 08050   (609)597-7100   Fax (609)597-7648

Printz, David A., MD {1912979691} RadDia(83,NY09)
+ Summit Radiological Associates, PA
1811 Springfield Avenue   New Providence, NJ 07974   (908)522-9111

Prinz, Karola Kristina, MD {1437115193} IntrMd(83,NJ06)
+ Prospect Medical Offices, LLC
301 Godwin Avenue   Midland Park, NJ 07432   (201)444-4526   Fax (201)301-1313

Priolo, Steven R., MD {1851311096} Surgry(94,NY08)<NY-MTSINAI, NY-NYHQUEEN>
+ 478 Brick Boulevard
Brick, NJ 08723   (732)701-4848   Fax (732)701-1244

Prior, Francis P., MD {1518952324} CdvDis, IntrMd(82,NY19)<NJ-MTNSIDE, NJ-STBARNMC>
+ Summit Medical Group Cardiology
62 South Fullerton Avenue   Montclair, NJ 07042   (973)746-8585   Fax (973)746-0088
+ Summit Medical Group
75 East Northfield Road   Livingston, NJ 07039   (973)746-8585   Fax (908)673-7336

Prior, Patricia, MD {1861529430} FamMed(89,PA13)
+ Rutgers University Health Services
326 Penn Street   Camden, NJ 08102   (856)225-6005   Fax (856)225-6186
+ Rutgers University Health Services
110 Hospital Road   Piscataway, NJ 08854   (732)445-3250

Priori, Jorge, MD {1396884508} Psychy, PsyGrt(70,BRA02)
+ Cumberland County Guidance Center
2038 Carmel Road/PO Box 808   Millville, NJ 08332   (856)825-6810   Fax (856)327-4281

Pristas, Adrian M., MD {1821088592} PulDis, IntrMd(88,MEX14)<NJ-BAYSHORE, NJ-RIVERVW>
+ 972 State Route 36
Hazlet, NJ 07730   (732)847-3600   Fax (732)847-3602

Prister, James Dmitry, MD {1134466501} IntrMd(10,NJ06)<NJ-RWJUBRUN>
+ RWJ Hospital Internal Medicine
One Robert Wood Johnson Place/MEB 486   New Brunswick, NJ 08901   (732)235-7742   Fax (732)235-7427
+ RWJ University Hospital New Brunswick
One Robert Wood Johnson Place   New Brunswick, NJ 08901   (732)235-7112

Pritchett, Danielle Delores, MD {1518007871} PthAcl(93,MI01)
+ Bio-Reference Laboratory, Inc.
481 Edward H. Ross Drive   Elmwood Park, NJ 07407   (201)791-2600   Fax (201)791-1941

Pritsiolas, James Michael, MD {1063451698} Nephro, IntrMd(99,NY46)<NJ-BAYONNE, NJ-CHRIST>
+ Summit Medical Group
75 East Northfield Road   Livingston, NJ 07039   (908)219-6690   Fax (908)219-6692
+ Summit Medical Group
95 Madison Avenue   Morristown, NJ 07960   (908)219-6690   Fax (973)267-5521
+ Hypertension & Renal Group, P.A.
930 Kennedy Boulevard   Bayonne, NJ 07039   (201)858-1509   Fax (973)994-7085

Pritz, Nicole M., MD {1710299490} Ophthl(09,PA02)
+ Horizon Eye Care
9701 Ventnor Avenue   Margate City, NJ 08402   (609)822-4242   Fax (609)822-3211

Priven, Igor, MD {1518938422} EnDbMt, IntrMd(98,NY48)<NY-BETHKING, NY-NYCOMBRK>
+ 345 US Highway 9 South
Manalapan, NJ 07726   (732)845-2200   Fax (732)845-0154

Pro, Michael James, MD {1639137524} Ophthl
+ Ophthalmic Partners of New Jersey
775 Route 70 East/Elmwood/Suite F 180   Marlton, NJ 08053   (856)596-1601   Fax (856)983-0396

Proban, Rafal, MD {1740430743} Anesth(05,GRN01)
+ Liberty Anesthesia & Pain Management
901 West Main Street/2nd Floor   Freehold, NJ 07728   (732)294-2876   Fax (732)294-2502

Procacci, Pasquale M., MD {1073587580} CdvDis
+ Pasquale M. Procacci MD
119 Augusta Drive   Moorestown, NJ 08057   (856)231-1563   Fax (856)231-1563
pmprocacci@aol.com

Proctor, Asha K., MD {1114919123} ObsGyn(01,NC01)<NJ-CHSFULD, NJ-CHSMRCER>
+ Delaware Valley Ob/Gyn & Infertility Group, PC
2 Princess Road/Suite C   Lawrenceville, NJ 08648   (609)896-0777   Fax (609)896-3266
+ Delaware Valley Ob/Gyn & Infertility Group, PC
300B Princeton Hightstown Road   East Windsor, NJ 08520   (609)896-0777   Fax (609)443-4506

Prodromo, Paul E., MD {1841384260} IntrMd(79,BEL03)<NJ-STPETER, NJ-RWJUBRUN>
+ 510 Georges Road
North Brunswick, NJ 08902   (732)249-3825   Fax (732)249-9330

Profeta, Bernadette Carol, MD {1477579837} Surgry(97,PA02)
+ 22 Lexington Park Road
Sicklerville, NJ 08081

Profeta, Susan B., MD {1194759175} IntrMd(82,NJ05)<NJ-OVERLOOK>
+ Summit Medical Group
11 Cleveland Place   Springfield, NJ 07081   (973)378-8778   Fax (973)783-1748

Profiriu, Alexandru F., MD {1861400541} Psychy
+ 4604 Sagemore Drive
Marlton, NJ 08053

Prokurat, Val, DO {1316109366} Surgry
+ 28 Mulberry Drive
Manalapan, NJ 07726

Prontnicki, Janice L., MD {1346216819} PedDvl, PedNrD(85,NY19)<NJ-CHLSMT, NJ-CHLSOCEN>
+ Children's Specialized Hospital
150 New Providence Road   Mountainside, NJ 07092   (908)233-3720   Fax (908)301-5456
+ Children's Specialized Hospital-Ocean
94 Stevens Road   Toms River, NJ 08755   (732)914-1100

Proper, Michael C., MD {1669443313} CdvDis, IntrMd(67,NY19)<NJ-VIRTMARL, NJ-OURLADY>
+ Associated Cardiovascular Consultants-Lourdes
1 Brace Road/Suite C & F   Cherry Hill, NJ 08034   (856)428-4100   Fax (856)428-1517

Propersi, Marco Egidio, DO {1013297860} IntrMd(08,NY75)<NJ-STJOSHOS>
+ St. Joseph's Regional Medical Center
703 Main Street/Internal Med   Paterson, NJ 07503   (973)754-2000

Proskurovsky, Zoric Lennie, MD {1801138284}<NJ-MTNSIDE>
+ Hackensack UMC Mountainside
1 Bay Avenue   Montclair, NJ 07042   (973)429-6000

Prosperi, Paul William, DO {1952416588} FamMed(95,PA77)<NJ-SOCEANCO>
+ Island Medical Professional Association
1812 Long Beach Boulevard   Ship Bottom, NJ 08008   (609)494-2323

Prosswimmer, Geralyn M., MD {1861466823} Pedtrc(84,NJ06)<NJ-HUNTRDN>
+ Hunterdon Pediatric Associates
6 Sand Hill Road/Suite 202   Flemington, NJ 08822   (908)782-6700   Fax (908)788-5861
+ Hunterdon Pediatric Associates
8 Reading Road/Reading Ridge   Flemington, NJ 08822   (908)782-6700   Fax (908)788-6005

Protano, Marion-Anna E., MD {1972745875} IntrMd(09,NJ06)<NY-MTSINAI, NY-MTSINYHS>
+ Mercer Gastroenterology
2 Capital Way/Suite 487   Pennington, NJ 08534   (609)818-1900   Fax (609)818-1908

Protasis, Liza, MD {1982745451} Pedtrc(91,INA76)<NJ-RIVERVW, NJ-MONMOUTH>
+ Bethany Pediatrics PA
1 Bethany Road/Building 5/Suite 65   Hazlet, NJ 07730   (732)264-0700   Fax (732)264-1414

Protopsaltis, Themistocles Stavros, MD {1245407659} OrtS-Hand(01,NY01)<NY-JTORTHO>
+ 194 Main Street
Millburn, NJ 07041   (212)598-2708

Protter, Randi R., MD {1801906490} IntrMd(94,NJ06)<NJ-UNVMCPRN, NJ-STPETER>
+ 34 Scotch Road/Suite 1
Ewing, NJ 08628   (609)498-7670   Fax (609)385-4150

Proudan, Vladimir Ivanovich, MD {1982862645} IntrMd<PA-GSNGER>
+ Obesity Treatment Center
435 South Street/Suite 330 B   Morristown, NJ 07960   (973)971-7166   Fax (973)290-7518

Prousi, Anthony A., MD {1992934830}
+ Prousi Oral & Facial Surgery
1900 Mount Holly Road/Bldg 500   Burlington, NJ 08016   (609)526-8650   Fax (609)526-8640

Physicians by Name and Address

Provencher, Robert A., DO {1669402152} FamMed(85,NJ75)<NJ-UNDRWD>
+ 296 Kings Highway
Clarksboro, NJ 08020   (856)423-7000   Fax (856)884-0636

Proverbs-Singh, Tracy Ann, MD {1730321662} MedOnc
+ John Theurer Cancer Center - HUMC
92 Second Street   Hackensack, NJ 07601   (551)996-5900   Fax (551)996-8578
+ Regional Cancer Care Center
7650 River Road/2nd Floor   North Bergen, NJ 07047   (212)464-0008

Prowse, Alicia Ann, MD {1104908268} Grtrcs, IntrMd(99,AL02)<NJ-VALLEY>
+ 1 Valley Health Plaza
Paramus, NJ 07652   (201)634-5555   Fax (201)447-5184
+ Valley Medical Group
70 Park Avenue   Park Ridge, NJ 07656   (201)634-5555   Fax (201)391-7733

Pruden, James N., MD {1689680878} EmrgMd, EmrgEMed(79,DC03)<NJ-STJOSHOS>
+ St Joseph's Medical Center Emergency
703 Main Street   Paterson, NJ 07503   (973)754-2240   Fax (973)754-2249

Prugno, Robin Jean, DO {1891148037} ObsGyn
+ Jersey Shore Medical Center Obs/Gyn
3499 US Highway 9/Suite 2B   Freehold, NJ 07728   (732)776-3790   Fax (732)776-4525

Prus, Dina S., MD {1871565887} EnDbMt, IntrMd(92,NY46)<NJ-STBARNMC, NJ-CLARMAAS>
+ Empire Medical Associates
264 Boyden Avenue   Maplewood, NJ 07040   (973)761-5200   Fax (973)761-7617
+ Empire Medical Associates
5 Franklin Avenue/Suite 302   Belleville, NJ 07109   (973)761-5200   Fax (973)759-1997
+ Empire Medical Associates
382 West Passaic Avenue   Bloomfield, NJ 07040   (973)338-1900

Prus Wisniewski, Richard Victor, MD {1558455535} Psychy(91,SAF01)
+ Princeton House Behavioral Health - Princeton
905 Herrontown Road   Princeton, NJ 08540   (609)497-3300   Fax (609)497-3370

Pruzon, Joanna Dawn, DO {1649201112} Ophthl(02,NJ75)
+ Hudson Eye Physicians & Surgeons, LLC
288 Millburn Avenue   Millburn, NJ 07041   (973)912-9100   Fax (973)912-0800
+ Hudson Eye Physicians & Surgeons, LLC
600 Pavonia Avenue/6th Floor   Jersey City, NJ 07306   (973)912-9100   Fax (201)963-8823

Prvulovic, Aleksandar T., MD {1902869779} IntrMd(99,MYA04)<NJ-KSLRSADB>
+ Kessler Institute for Rehabilitation
300 Market Street   Saddle Brook, NJ 07663   (201)587-8500

Prvulovic, Tomi, MD {1831262559} PainInvt, Anesth, PainMd(92,TX16)<NY-STANTHNY, NJ-STCLRDEN>
+ HealthSpine and Anesthesia Institute
197 Ridgedale Avenue/Suite 101C   Cedar Knolls, NJ 07927   Fax (973)292-0772

Pryluck, David Scott, MD {1841495181} RadV&I, RadDia(06,NY19)<PA-UPMCPHL>
+ Radiology Affiliates of Central New Jersey, P.A.
2501 Kuser Road   Hamilton, NJ 08691   (609)585-8800   Fax (609)585-1825

Prystowsky, Barry S., MD {1801976048} Pedtrc(81,NJ05)<NJ-CLARMAAS, NJ-STBARNMC>
+ Prystowsky Medical Associates
562 Kingsland Street   Nutley, NJ 07110   (973)235-0101   Fax (973)667-5716

Prystowsky, Ligaya L., MD {1821071754} Ophthl(81,PHI09)<NJ-EASTORNG, NJ-CLARMAAS>
+ 633 Franklin Avenue
Nutley, NJ 07110   (973)667-4008   Fax (973)667-1655   gaya56@aol.com
+ 310 Central Avenue/Suite 104
East Orange, NJ 07018   (973)667-4008   Fax (973)395-1882

Przybylko, Kira L., MD {1962474841} ObsGyn(93,NJ05)<NJ-CHS-FULD, NJ-CHSMRCER>
+ Lawrence Ob/Gyn Associates
123 Franklin Corner Road/Suite 214   Lawrenceville, NJ 08648   (609)896-1400   Fax (609)896-3986

Przybylski, Gregory J., MD {1740280064} SrgNro, SrgSpn(87,PA02)<NJ-JFKMED>
+ JFK Neurosciences Institute
65 James Street/Second Floor   Edison, NJ 08818   (732)321-7010   Fax (732)632-1669

Psalidas, Panagiotis George, MD {1114907730} Pedtrc, IntrMd(94,NY09)
+ Yee Medicine and Pediatric Associates, P.C.
245 Engle Street/Suite 3   Englewood, NJ 07631   (201)569-9005   Fax (201)569-9080

Pshytycky, Amir, MD {1740470475} PsycCAd, Pedtrc(93,ISR02)<NJ-COOPRUMC>
+ The Children's Regional Hospital at Cooper Univ Hosp
One Cooper Plaza/ChldAdolPsy   Camden, NJ 08103   (856)342-2257

Psillides, Despina, MD {1174758668} Grtrcs, IntrMd(06,NJ06)<NJ-HUNTRDN>
+ The Park Medical Group
24 Elm Street   Harrington Park, NJ 07640   (201)784-0123   Fax (201)784-0065   dpsillides@yahoo.com

Pu, Jessica Lixia, MD {1497949796} Pedtrc, PedHem(84,CHN68)
+ Edison Pediatrics
1802 Oak Tree Road/Suite 101   Edison, NJ 08820   (732)548-3210   Fax (732)228-8416

Pua, Zarah Jane Baysa, MD {1124021449} Pedtrc, NnPnMd(93,PHI09)<NJ-STJOSHOS>
+ St Joseph's Medical Center Neonatology
703 Main Street   Paterson, NJ 07503   (973)754-2555   Fax (973)773-2101

Pucci, Anthony E., DO {1255452447} Surgry(01,NJ75)
+ Advanced Laparoscopic Specialists
61 North Maple Avenue/Suite 205   Ridgewood, NJ 07450   (201)447-2808   Fax (201)447-2809

Pucci, Richard Anthony, DO {1679572739} Bariat, SrgLap(96,IA75)<NY-GOODSAM>
+ Advanced Laparoscopic Specialists
61 North Maple Avenue/Suite 205   Ridgewood, NJ 07450   (201)447-2808   Fax (201)447-2809

Pudinak, Anna, MD {1952665200} FamMed
+ AP Health, LLC
1135 Clifton Avenue/Suite 201   Clifton, NJ 07013   (862)414-3335

Puglisi, Gina Grace, MD {1366472011} IntrMd, IntHos(87,GRN01)<RI-SJFATIMA>
+ Emergency Medical Offices
651 West Mount Pleasant Avenue   Livingston, NJ 07039   (973)740-9396   Fax (973)251-1165

Puing, Alfredo Gonzalo, MD {1841600418} IntrMd<NJ-STPETER>
+ St. Peter's University Hospital
254 Easton Avenue   New Brunswick, NJ 08901   (732)745-8600

Pukenas, Erin W., MD {1205027109} PedAne<NJ-COOPRUMC>
+ Cooper University Hospital
One Cooper Plaza/PediAnesth   Camden, NJ 08103   (856)342-2000

Pukin, Lev, MD {1609849546} RadDia, RadV&I(95,DMN01)<NJ-KIMBALL>
+ Kimball Medical Center
600 River Avenue/Radiology   Lakewood, NJ 08701   (732)363-1900   levster@bogfoot.com

Pulcini, Ashley Elizabeth, DO {1982125662} Pedtrc
+ Navesink Pediatrics
55 North Gilbert Street/Suite 2101   Tinton Falls, NJ 07701   (732)842-6677   Fax (732)530-2946

Pulijaal, Pooja, MD {1053799643} IntHos
+ RWJ University Hospital Hospitalists
One Robert Wood Johnson Place/MEB 256   New Brunswick, NJ 08901   (732)235-6969

Pulinthanathu, Rajiv Rajamohanan, MD {1255540670} PthACI, Pthlgy, IntrMd(95,TUR17)<NJ-STBARNMC>
+ St. Barnabas Medical Center
94 Old Short Hills Road/Pathology   Livingston, NJ 07039   (973)322-5750

Pullatt, Raja C., MD {1477746634} IntrMd, CdvDis(01,INA97)
+ Union County Cardiology Associates, P.A.
1317 Morris Avenue   Union, NJ 07083   (908)964-9370   Fax (908)964-9332

Pullockaran, Janet R., MD {1710120670}
+ 2050 Central Road/Apt 622
Fort Lee, NJ 07024   (609)203-3951   pullocjr@gmail.com

Pulte, Elizabeth Dianne, MD {1417040528} IntrMd(94,TX13)
+ Rutgers- New Jersey Medical School
185 South Orange Avenue/MSB I689   Newark, NJ 07103   (973)972-4300

Pulver, Bradley Lee, MD {1104901537} EmrgMd(96,PA01)<NJ-SOCEANCO>
+ Southern Ocean County Medical Center
1140 Route 72 West/EmrgMed   Manahawkin, NJ 08050   (609)597-6011

Pulver, Deborah Moody, MD {1891011888} Pedtrc
+ The Pediatric Group PA
66 Mount Lucas Road   Princeton, NJ 08540   (609)924-4892   Fax (609)921-9380

Pumariega, Andres Julio, MD {1629065529} Psychy<PA-READING>
+ Cooper Psychiatric Associates
3 Cooper Plaza/Suite 307   Camden, NJ 08103   (856)342-2328   Fax (856)541-6137

Pumill, Rick J., MD {1538164975} CdvDis, IntrMd(84,WIND)<NJ-HACKNSK, NJ-MEADWLND>
+ Cross Country Cardiology
103 River Road/2nd Floor   Edgewater, NJ 07020   (201)941-8100   Fax (201)941-2899
+ Cross Country Cardiology
38 Meadowlands Parkway   Secaucus, NJ 07094   (201)866-5151

Pumo, Jerome, Jr., DO {1558363382} FamMSlpM, UtlRQA, IntrMd(72,IA75)<NJ-STMICHL>
+ 132 Westfield Avenue/Suite 1
Clark, NJ 07066   (732)574-1777   Fax (732)574-2707

Punj, Priti Narula, MD {1154552917} FamMed
+ Princeton Family Care
100 Federal City Road/Suite A   Lawrenceville, NJ 08648   (609)620-1380   Fax (609)771-8991

Punjabi, Kusum A., MD {1376708479} EmrgMd(05,NJ06)<NJ-RWJUBRUN>
+ University Emergency Medicine
125 Paterson Street/MEB 104   New Brunswick, NJ 08901   (732)235-8717   Fax (732)235-7379

Puntambekar, Preeti Vasant, MD {1538336425} Nrolgy, Eplpsy(99,INA4X)
+ Northeast Regional Epilepsy Group
20 Prospect Avenue/Suite 800   Hackensack, NJ 07601   (201)343-6676   Fax (201)343-6689
+ Lawrenceville Neurology Center, PA
3131 Princeton Pike   Lawrenceville, NJ 08648   (201)343-6676   Fax (609)896-3735

Punzalan, Crispino R., MD {1114964699} Anesth(75,PHI09)<NJ-MTNSIDE>
+ 55 Chestnut Street
Nutley, NJ 07110
+ Montclair Anesthesia Associates PC
185 Fairfield Avenue/Suite 2A   West Caldwell, NJ 07006   Fax (973)226-1232

Punzalan, Maria M., MD {1194791517} Anesth(76,PHI01)<NJ-HOBUNIMC>
+ Hoboken University Medical Center
308 Willow Avenue/Anesthesiology   Hoboken, NJ 07030   (201)418-1000   Fax (201)943-8105

Pupo, Louis O., MD {1699751917} Pedtrc(79,SPA06)<NJ-NWTN-MEM, NJ-MORRISTN>
+ 61 Newton Sparta Road
Newton, NJ 07860   (973)579-4604   Fax (973)726-0208

Purani, Gaurav S., MD {1932530953} GenPrc
+ 11 Woodbridge Terrace/Apt C
Woodbridge, NJ 07095   (732)218-7900   pgaurav1983@gmail.com

Purcell, Joseph W., DO {1083676910} FamMed(86,IL76)<NJ-STCLRDEN>
+ Skylands Medical Group PA
150 Lakeside Boulevard   Landing, NJ 07850   (973)398-6300   Fax (973)398-6399
+ Skylands Medical Group PA
174 Edison Road   Lake Hopatcong, NJ 07849   (973)663-1300

Purdy, Adam, MD {1932563582} IntrMd<NJ-OVERLOOK>
+ Overlook Medical Center
99 Beauvoir Avenue/PO Box 210   Summit, NJ 07902   (908)522-2000

Purewal, Baljeet Kaur, MD {1265516355} Ophthl(02,NY08)<NJ-STJOSHOS>
+ Clifton Eye Care
403 Clifton Avenue/Box 2247   Clifton, NJ 07011   (973)546-5700

Puri, Nitin Kumar, MD {1487726287}
+ Cooper University Hospital
One Cooper Plaza   Camden, NJ 08103   (856)342-2000

Puri, Shawn K., MD {1598056293} AnesPain
+ ASAP - Advanced Spine and Pain
1030 Kings Highway North/Suite 200   Cherry Hill, NJ 08034   (888)985-2727

Puri, Sonika, MD {1871757583} Nephro<NJ-RWJUBRUN>
+ RWJ University Hospital New Brunswick
One Robert Wood Johnson Place   New Brunswick, NJ 08901   (732)235-7737

Purisima, Clementino O., MD {1144354788} Surgry, GenPrc(69,PHI01)<NJ-HOBUNIMC>
+ PO box 8126
Union City, NJ 07087   (201)863-5065   Fax (201)934-1383

Purisima, Fely Grecia, MD {1144312737} Pedtrc(69,PHIL)<NJ-HOBUNIMC>
+ PO Box 8126
Union City, NJ 07087   (201)863-5065   Fax (201)934-1383   Fpurisima@aol.com

Pursell, Robert N., MD Nephro(74,ITAL)<NJ-WARREN>
+ Warren Hospital
185 Roseberry Street/Nephrology   Phillipsburg, NJ 08865   (908)859-6700

Purtill, James Joseph, MD {1558300731} SrgOrt(93,PA02)<NJ-ATLANTHS>
+ Rothman Institute - Voorhees
443 Laurel Oak Road   Voorhees, NJ 08043   (856)821-6360

Pushilin, Sergei A., MD {1174884779} OrtTrm
+ University Orthopaedic Associates, LLC.
4810 Belmar Boulevard/Suite 102   Wall, NJ 07753
(732)938-6090   Fax (732)938-5680

Puskas, Roy, MD {1245272665} SrgPlstc(74,MEX03)<NJ-VIRTMHBC, NJ-DEBRAHLC>
+ 737 Main Street/PO Box 498
Lumberton, NJ 08048   (609)267-3552   Fax (609)265-2103

Puskuri, Praneetha, MD {1851581656} IntrMd
+ 22 Reinhart Way
Bridgewater, NJ 08807   (732)309-1040

Putcha, Nitin, DO {1407153265} PhysMd(10,NY75)
+ National Health Rehabilitation
103 River Road/Suite 101   Edgewater, NJ 07020   (201)654-6397

Putcha, Vasundhara, MD {1881799450} PsyAdd, PsyGrt, Psychy(82,INA5B)<NJ-VAEASTOR>
+ St. Clare's Behavioral Health Center
100 Est Hanover Avenue   Cedar Knolls, NJ 07927
(973)401-2121   Fax (973)401-2140

Puthiyathu, Manoj, MD {1649408956} PsyCAd<NJ-BERGNMC>
+ New Bridge Medical Center
230 East Ridgewood Avenue   Paramus, NJ 07652
(201)967-4132

Putnam, Daniel Philip, MD {1427055508} Ophthl(89,TX12)
+ South Jersey Eye Physicians PA
509 South Lenola Road/Suite 11   Moorestown, NJ 08057
(856)234-0222   Fax (856)727-9518

Putterman, Debora, MD {1457436222} Anesth(91,ISR01)<NJ-STJOSHOS, NJ-HOLYNAME>
+ St. Joseph's Regional Medical Center Anesthesia
703 Main Street   Paterson, NJ 07503   (973)754-2323   Fax (973)977-9455

Putukian, Margot, MD {1548343601} IntrMd, SprtMd(89,MA05)
+ McCosh Health Center
Washington Road/McCosh Infirmary   Princeton, NJ 08544
(609)258-5357   Fax (609)258-1355
putukian@princeton.edu

Puvabanditsin, Surasak, MD {1235135880} NnPnMd, Pedtrc(77,THAI)
+ UH- RWJ Medical School
One Robert Wood Johnson Place/MEB 396   New Brunswick, NJ 08903   (732)235-5699   Fax (732)235-6609
+ Robert Wood Johnson University Hospital at Hamilton
1 Hamilton Health Place   Hamilton, NJ 08690   (732)235-5699   Fax (609)584-6439

Puzino, Alan Vincent, MD {1922050582} IntrMd(79,MEX03)
+ Morris Medical Associates
3799 Route 46 East/Suite 209   Parsippany, NJ 07054
(973)263-1499   Fax (973)402-9030

Puzio, Thomas, MD {1609073196} Anesth
+ 375 Engle Street/Second Floor
Englewood, NJ 07631

Pyatov, Yelena V., MD {1003124165} FamMed, Pedtrc, PedHem
+ Advocare Vernon Pediatrics
249 Route 94   Vernon, NJ 07462   (973)827-4550   Fax (973)827-5845

Pyo, Daniel J., MD {1720183999} SrgPlstc(90,NY47)
+ 131 Madison Avenue/Suite 120
Morristown, NJ 07960   (973)540-9055   Fax (973)540-0344

Pyontek, Maria G., DO {1336112390} IntrMd(93,NJ75)<NJ-JRSYSHMC, NJ-OCEANMC>
+ 1725 State Route 35/Suite B
Wall, NJ 07719   (732)681-1063   Fax (732)681-2922

Pyrsopoulos, Nikolaos T., MD {1932131075} Gastrn
+ UMDNJ Division of Gastroenterology & Hepatology
90 Bergen Street/DOC 2100   Newark, NJ 07103   (973)972-5252   Fax (973)972-0752

Pyz, Tadeusz F., MD {1518957109} FamMed(80,POL03)<NJ-STMRYPAS, NJ-MTNSIDE>
+ 379 Main Avenue/Suite 3
Wallington, NJ 07057   (973)779-2277   Fax (973)340-2561
mown379@yahoo.com

Qadir, Abdul, MD {1902809742} Anesth, PainMd, Acpntr(87,PAKI)<NJ-SHOREMEM>
+ Regional Internal Medicine Associates
1004 South New Road   Pleasantville, NJ 08232   (609)652-4141   Fax (609)652-9939
aqadir@paincare.com

Qasim, Mahasin S., MD {1871523530} FrtInf, RprEnd, ObsGyn(88,NJ06)<NJ-JFKMED>
+ Center for Advanced Reproductive Medicine/Fertility
4 Ethel Road/Suite 405A/Co-Director   Edison, NJ 08817
(732)339-9300   (732)339-9400
drqasim@infertilitydocs.com
+ Center for Advanced Reproductive Medicine/Fertility
123 North Union Avenue   Cranford, NJ 07016   (732)339-9300   Fax (908)998-3665
+ Center for Advanced Reproductive Medicine/Fertility
666 Plainsboro Road/Bldg 100/Suite C   Plainsboro, NJ 08817   (609)297-4070   Fax (609)297-4049

Qazi, Rumana Yousef, MD {1922062405} Pedtrc, AdolMd(87,PAK06)<NJ-COMMED>
+ Silverton Pediatrics
2446 Church Road   Toms River, NJ 08753   (732)255-7553
Fax (732)255-8901

Qazi, Sadia Idris, MD {1467491563} IntrMd(94,PAK11)
+ 445 Whitehorse Avenue/Suite 200
Trenton, NJ 08610   (609)581-5502   Fax (609)581-5504

Qian, Fang, MD {1558326769} PthACl(91,CHN57)<NJ-NWRKBETH>
+ Summit Medical Group-Berkeley Heights Campus
1 Diamond Hill Road   Berkeley Heights, NJ 07922
(908)273-4300   Fax (908)790-6576
+ Newark Beth Israel Medical Center
201 Lyons Avenue/Pathology   Newark, NJ 07112
(973)926-7000

Qian, Qiubing, MD {1992709380} Anesth(83,CHN60)
+ 21 Taconic Road
Livingston, NJ 07039   (973)992-1557
joshmaqian@cs.com

Qipo, Alba, MD {1164768461} IntrMd
+ Heart & Vascular Associates of Northern Jersey
22-18 Broadway/Suite 201   Fair Lawn, NJ 07410   (201)490-1217   Fax (201)475-5522

Qiu, William Weiguang, MD {1326012998} RadDia(83,CHN63)<NJ-KIMBALL>
+ Kimball Medical Center
600 River Avenue/Radiology   Lakewood, NJ 08701
(732)363-1900   Fax (732)942-5658

Qu, Peimei, MD {1063431252} IntrMd(90,CHN57)<NJ-SOMERSET>
+ Alliance Medical Associates PC
15 Monroe Street   Bridgewater, NJ 08807   (908)595-6330
Fax (908)595-6331
+ Alliance Medical Associates, PC
15 Monroe Street   Bridgewater, NJ 08807   (908)595-6330
Fax (908)595-6331

Quackenbush, Gail, MD {1245271048} Radiol, PthCyt(88,NC01)
+ Montclair Breast Center
37 North Fullerton Avenue   Montclair, NJ 07042   (973)509-1818   Fax (973)509-0532

Quaglia, Silvio A., MD {1790788313} IntrMd, IntMAdMd(86,MNT01)<NJ-OVERLOOK>
+ Associates in Primary Care, P.A.
25 East Willow Street   Millburn, NJ 07041   (973)379-5055
Fax (973)379-5324

Quan, Matthew Brett, MD {1578535910} Dermat, DerMOH, SrgDer(90,NH01)<NY-NYPRESHS, NJ-STMRYPAS>
+ Dermatology Center of North Jersey
1033 Clifton Avenue   Clifton, NJ 07013   (973)777-6444
Fax (973)777-5277

Quarless, Shelley Ann, DO {1356506422} NuclMd, Radiol(96,IA75)<NJ-UMDNJ>
+ University Hospital
150 Bergen Street/Uh C 320   Newark, NJ 07103   (973)972-4300   Fax (973)972-7429

Quartararo, Louis Gaspar, MD {1467460089} SrgOrt, SrgSpn, SrgTrm(93,NY47)<NJ-HACKNSK, NJ-ATLANTHS>
+ Premier Orthopaedics and Sports Medicine, P.C.
111 Galway Place   Teaneck, NJ 07666   (201)833-9500
Fax (201)862-0095
+ Premier Orthopaedics and Sports Medicine, PC
663 Palisade Avenue/Suite 302   Cliffside Park, NJ 07010
(201)833-9500   Fax (201)943-7308
+ Specialty Surgical Center
380 Lafayette Road/Suite 110   Sparta, NJ 07666   (973)940-3166   Fax (973)940-3170

Quartell, Anthony C., MD {1154424786} ObsGyn(69,NJ05)<NJ-STBARNMC>
+ Dr. Anthony Quartell and Associates
316 Eisenhower Parkway/Suite 202   Livingston, NJ 07039
(973)716-9650   Fax (973)716-9650

Qudah, Yaqeen, MD {1942685375} Surgry<NJ-RWJUBRUN>
+ RWJ University Hospital New Brunswick
One Robert Wood Johnson Place   New Brunswick, NJ 08901
(732)235-7674

Qudsi, Tehsin Riaz, MD {1003852542} Pedtrc, IntrMd(82,PAKI)<NJ-CHLSMT, NJ-COMMED>
+ Drs. Qudsi & Pawa
27 South Cooks Bridge Road/Suite 2-21   Jackson, NJ 08527
(732)987-5733   Fax (732)987-5729

Queler, Seth Robert, MD {1811947187} SrgOrt, SrgFAk(00,IL06)
+ Femino-Ducey Orthopaedic Group
45 Franklin Avenue   Nutley, NJ 07110   (973)751-0111
Fax (973)235-0110

Querimit, Felipe A., Jr., MD {1609980853} Pthlgy, PthACl(63,PHI01)<NJ-HCKTSTWN>
+ 3312 Franklin Lane   Rockaway, NJ 07866

Quest, Donald Oliver, MD {1841342656} SrgNro, IntrMd(70,NY01)<NY-PRSBCOLU, NY-NYPRESHS>
+ Neurosurgeons of New Jersey
1200 East Ridgewood Avenue   Ridgewood, NJ 07450
(201)824-6131

Questelles, Rachael, MD {1780016824} Pedtrc
+ Linden Pediatric Group
517 Rahway Avenue   Elizabeth, NJ 07202   (908)527-1247
Fax (908)354-8822

Quevedo, Jonathan P., MD {1104847631} PhysMd, PainMd(80,NY01)<NJ-JFKMED, NJ-JFKJHNSN>
+ JFK Medical Center
65 James Street/Physiatrist   Edison, NJ 08820   (732)321-7070   Fax (732)744-5833
JQueveDO@Solarishs.org
+ JFK Johnson Rehabilitation Institute
65 James Street/InpatientRehab   Edison, NJ 08818
(732)321-7050

Quezada Reyes, Carlos A., MD {1033123914} FamMed(80,PERU)<NJ-SOMERSET>
+ MEDEMERGE
1005 North Washington Avenue   Green Brook, NJ 08812
(732)968-8900   Fax (732)968-4609

Quiambao, Dante B., MD {1437121266} Anesth(78,PHI01)
+ Ocean Anesthesia Group PA
1200 Hooper Avenue   Toms River, NJ 08753   (732)797-3890   Fax (732)942-5603

Quiba, Ronald C., MD {1356435200} Pedtrc(79,PHIL)<NJ-RBAYPERT, NJ-RIVERVW>
+ SAMRA Pediatrics
300 Perrine Road/Suite 331   Old Bridge, NJ 08857
(732)727-8800   Fax (732)727-0955

Quigley, Craig B., MD {1790763514} FamMed, Grtrcs, SprtMd(81,PA12)<NJ-MEMSALEM>
+ Carneys Point Family Practice
341 Shell Road   Carneys Point, NJ 08069   (856)299-4600
Fax (856)299-1688
Cquigley@christianacare.org

Quigley, Elizabeth A., MD {1649466335} Dermat(05)
+ Memorial Sloan-Kettering Cancer Center Basking Ridge
136 Mountain View Boulevard   Basking Ridge, NJ 07920
(908)542-3400   Fax (908)542-3220
+ 448 Rolling Hills Road
Bridgewater, NJ 08807

Quim, Marinelle De Los Santos, MD {1013249739} Pedtrc
+ Tribeca Pediatrics
9 McWilliams Place   Jersey City, NJ 07302   (201)706-7175
Fax (201)604-6553

Quinlan, Dennis Philip, Jr., MD {1255480919} Surgry, SrgThr(95,NJ05)<NJ-UMDNJ>
+ Capital Surgical Associates
40 Fuld Street/Suite 303   Trenton, NJ 08638   (609)396-2600   Fax (609)396-3600
+ Capital Health Primary Care
832 Brunswick Avenue   Trenton, NJ 08638   (609)396-2600
Fax (609)815-7401

Quinlan, Dennis Philip, Sr, MD {1699701706} IntrMd, Grtrcs(69,NJ05)<NJ-STBARNMC, NJ-VAEASTOR>
+ University Hospital-Doctors Office Center
90 Bergen Street   Newark, NJ 07103   (973)972-2500   Fax (973)972-2510

Quinlan, Jack Francis, Jr., MD {1942460514} CdvDis, InsrMd(02,NJ05)<NJ-SJHREGMC>
+ Wachspress & Rainear Cardiology Associates PA
1076 East Chestnut Avenue   Vineland, NJ 08360   (856)692-7979   Fax (856)794-9479

Quinlan, Liliane Bastos, MD {1104985514} IntrMd, Grtrcs(01,BRA01)
+ Southern Jersey Family Medical Center
1301 Atlantic Avenue   Atlantic City, NJ 08401   (609)572-0000   Fax (609)572-0039
+ Southern Jersey Family Medical Centers, Inc.
860 South White Horse Pike/Building A   Hammonton, NJ 08037   (609)572-0000   Fax (609)567-3492

Quinn, Brian Michael, MD {1811986664} IntrMd, MedOnc(76,NY08)<NJ-HUNTRDN>
+ Hunterdon Regional Cancer Ctr
2100 Wescott Drive   Flemington, NJ 08822   (908)788-6461
Fax (908)788-6412
+ Hunterdon Medical Center
2100 Wescott Drive/Hemat/Oncology   Flemington, NJ 08822   (908)788-6100

Quinn, Graham Earl, MD {1538240163} Ophthl<PA-CHILDHOS>
+ CHOP Pediatric & Adolescent Specialty Care Center
1012 Laurel Oak Road   Voorhees, NJ 08043   (856)435-1300
Fax (856)435-0091

Quinn, Margaret M., MD {1427031533} Grtrcs, IntrMd(80,DC02)<NJ-JRSYSHMC>
+ Jersey Shore University Medical Center
1945 Route 33   Neptune, NJ 07753   (732)775-5500   Fax (732)897-7200

Physicians by Name and Address

Quinones, Ariel, MD {1992715825} FamMed, IntrMd(95,NJ05)
+ Dr. Quinones and Assoc
  38 Elmora Avenue   Elizabeth, NJ 07202   (908)576-8982
  Fax (908)576-8985
+ Spinal Care of Elizabeth
  230 West Jersey Street/Suite 306   Elizabeth, NJ 07202
  (908)576-8982   Fax (908)576-8985

Quinones, Candido P., MD {1164430534} NuclMd, RadBdI(65,DOMI)<NJ-STMICHL>
+ St. Michael's Medical Center
  268 MLK Jr. Boulevard   Newark, NJ 07102   (973)877-5000

Quint, James Douglas, MD {1134448087} Anesth
+ West Jersey Anesthesia Associates
  102E Centre Boulevard   Marlton, NJ 08053   (856)988-6260
  Fax (856)988-6270

Quintana, Jorge D., MD {1326103128} Psychy(82,URU02)<NJ-TRINIWSC>
+ Palisades Behavioral Care
  221 Palisade Avenue   Jersey City, NJ 07306   (201)656-3116
  Fax (201)656-9044
+ 2366 St. Georges Avenue
  Rahway, NJ 07065   (732)381-5700

Quintanilla, Julio Ricardo, MD {1932214467} IntrMd, InfDis(86,PER01)
+ NHCAC Health Center at Passaic
  110 Main Avenue   Passaic, NJ 07055   (973)777-0256   Fax (973)777-3910

Quintero-Solivan, Juliette M., MD {1174684104} Pedtrc, PedEmg(97,NY15)
+ RWJ University Pediatric Emergency Medicine
  125 Paterson Street/MEB 342   New Brunswick, NJ 08903
  (732)235-7893   Fax (732)235-7077

Quirk, Edward, MD {1326023151} AnesAddM
+ Recovery Centers of America at Lighthouse
  5034 Atlantic Avenue   Mays Landing, NJ 08330   (215)728-3714   Fax (215)728-3923

Quiros Rivera, Mercedita, MD {1801917133} FamMed(67,PHI01)
+ 80 Duryea Street
  Newark, NJ 07103   (973)497-4735   Fax (973)497-4753
  Divmer973@yahoo.com

Qumei, Moh'D K. K., MD {1104869825} CritCr, IntrMd, EmrgMd(83,JOR01)<NJ-RIVERVW>
+ Riverview Medical Center
  1 Riverview Plaza/EmrgMed   Red Bank, NJ 07701
  (732)530-2204
+ JFK Medical Center
  65 James Street   Edison, NJ 08820   (732)530-2204   Fax (908)744-5614

Quraishi, Abid Nisar, MD {1982705562} IntrMd(99,NJ05)
+ Drs. Quraishi & Seman
  1 Chopin Court   Jersey City, NJ 07302   (201)333-8111

Quraishi, Faraz, MD {1669762787}
+ University Behavioral HealthCare
  183 South Orange Avenue/Room F-603   Newark, NJ 07103
  (973)972-6015

Quraishi, Huma Asmat, MD {1669543922} PedOto, Otlryg(93,NY47)<NJ-HACKNSK>
+ Hackensack Medical Center-Internal Medicine
  30 Prospect Avenue/4 Main/Rm 4621   Hackensack, NJ 07601   (551)996-5515   Fax (551)996-4499
  hquraishi@hackensackumc.org

Qureshi, Akif Zeshan, MD {1750776209} IntHos
+ Hackensack Univ Medical Center Hospitalists
  30 Prospect Avenue   Hackensack, NJ 07601   (551)996-2000

Qureshi, Hassan I., DO {1669848008} IntrMd
+ 451 Jersey Avenue
  Jersey City, NJ 07302   (732)668-5711

Qureshi, Mohammad Nasar, MD {1174525604} PthAcl, Pthlgy(82,PAK11)<NJ-BAYONNE>
+ QDx Pathology Services
  46 Jackson Drive   Cranford, NJ 07016   Fax (908)272-1478

Qureshi, Nazer, MD {1407978380} SrgNro
+ 901 West Main Street/Suite 267
  Freehold, NJ 07728   (732)333-8702

Qureshi, Shaukat M., MD {1821019373} Urolgy(67,PAK10)<NJ-MEMSALEM>
+ 250 South Broadway
  Pennsville, NJ 08070   (856)678-4452   Fax (856)678-3325
  smqureshi@pol.net
+ MidAtlantic Kidney Stone Center
  100 Brick Road/Suite 103   Marlton, NJ 08053   (856)678-4452   Fax (856)983-6970

Qureshi, Sheeraz Ahmed, MD {1831303106} SrgSpn, SrgOrt(02,MA07)<NY-SPCLSURG>
+ HSS Paramus Outpatient Center
  140 East Ridgewood Avenue/Suite 15-S   Paramus, NJ 07652   (201)796-2255   Fax (201)796-3711

Ra, Daniel, DO {1386881928} Nephro, Pthlgy, IntrMd(08,PA77)
+ Haddon Renal Medical Specialists
  401 Kings Highway South/Suite 5   Cherry Hill, NJ 08034
  (856)428-8992   Fax (856)428-9614

Ra, Michael, DO {1619132123}<NJ-JFKJHNSN>
+ 175 Gunning River Road
  Barnegat, NJ 08005   (609)389-6266   Fax (609)660-0003
+ Northeast Spine & Sports Medicine
  367 Lakehurst Road   Toms River, NJ 08755   (732)653-1000

Raab, Gary W., DO {1972683001} FamMed(85,PA77)
+ 500 Sixth Street
  Ocean City, NJ 08226   (609)399-1862   Fax (609)399-1572

Raab, Rajnik Weerackody, MD {1417953902} SrgNro(97,NY08)<NJ-VALLEY>
+ North Jersey Spine Group
  1680 State Route 23/Suite 250   Wayne, NJ 07470
  (973)633-1132
+ North Jersey Spine Group
  1 West Ridgewood Avenue/Suite 207   Paramus, NJ 07652
  (973)633-1122

Raab, Vicki E., MD {1073600748} Nrolgy(84,TX13)<NJ-RIVERVW>
+ Ethel and Raphael Pediatrics Inc
  1405 Highway 35 North/Suite 104   Ocean, NJ 07712
  (732)663-1161   Fax (732)531-2900

Raacke, Lisa Marie, MD {1346215126} IntrMd(83,DC02)<NY-MTSINAI>
+ Hackensack University Medical Group PC
  160 Essex Street/Suite 102   Lodi, NJ 07644   (551)996-8111
  Fax (551)996-8445

Raad, Michelle L., MD {1114018595} ObsGyn(86,NJ05)<NJ-TRINIWSC>
+ 240 Williamson Street/Suite 503
  Elizabeth, NJ 07202   (908)355-1010   Fax (908)355-5629

Rab, Zia, MD {1548548332} IntCrd
+ Hamilton Cardiology Associates
  2073 Klockner Road   Hamilton, NJ 08690   (609)584-1212
  Fax (609)584-0103

Rabadi, Khalaf E., MD {1285805937} IntrMd(83,PHI08)<NJ-STFRNMED, NJ-RWJUHAM>
+ 2119 Klockner Road/Building 8/Suite 34
  Trenton, NJ 08690   (609)586-6500   Fax (609)586-8694
+ RWJ Medical Associates
  3100 Quakerbridge Road/Suite 28   Hamilton, NJ 08619
  (609)586-6500   Fax (609)245-7432

Rabago-Reyes, Cassandra, MD {1487967972} IntrMd
+ Palisades Medical Center
  8100 Kennedy Boulevard   North Bergen, NJ 07047
  (201)866-6770   Fax (201)866-6771

Rabanal, Marie C., MD {1194883421} Psychy(86,PHI32)<NJ-GRYSTPSY>
+ Greystone Park Psychiatric Hospital
  59 Koch Avenue   Morris Plains, NJ 07950   (973)538-1800

Rabara, Knic Corpuz, DO {1275829939} FamMed, IntrMd
+ Rowan University-School of Osteopathic Medicine
  1 Medical Center Drive   Stratford, NJ 08084   (201)306-6688

Rabbani, Soliman, MD {1720251531} RadDia(76,IRA08)
+ 3 Hawthorne Avenue
  Holmdel, NJ 07733   (732)264-5258   Fax (732)739-9783

Rabbat, Mohamed Salah, MD {1487691200} InfDis, IntrMd(82,EGY04)<NJ-STJOSHOS>
+ St Joseph's Medical Center Infectious Disease
  703 Main Street/Xavier 6   Paterson, NJ 07503   (973)754-2285

Rabie, Glenda, MD {1538126339} FamMed
+ 309 Marlton Avenue
  Camden, NJ 08105   (856)963-5479   Fax (856)963-8457

Rabin, Aaron, MD {1093710949} Nrolgy(76,NY46)<NJ-ENGLWOOD>
+ Drs. Rabin, Fremed, Prince, P.C.
  700 Palisade Avenue   Englewood Cliffs, NJ 07632
  (201)568-3412   Fax (201)568-8249

Rabin, Andrew Michael, MD {1629154984} Radiol, RadDia, RadV&I(81,PA13)
+ University Radiology Group, P.C.
  579A Cranbury Road   East Brunswick, NJ 08816   (732)390-0040   Fax (732)390-1856
+ University Radiology Group, P.C.
  16 Mountain Boulevard   Warren, NJ 07059   (732)390-0040
  Fax (908)769-9141

Rabin, Douglas S., MD {1326156480} RprEnd, Gyneco(77,PA13)<NJ-HACKNSK, NJ-KIMBALL>
+ 33-00 Broadway/Suite 303
  Fair Lawn, NJ 07410   (201)703-9555   Fax (201)475-5678
  doug.rabin@gmail.com

Rabin, Marcie L., MD {1750445680} Nrolgy(06,CA02)<NJ-OVERLOOK>
+ Atlantic Neuroscience Institute at Overlook Hospital
  99 Beauvoir Avenue   Summit, NJ 07901   (908)522-3501
+ Overlook Medical Center
  99 Beauvoir Avenue/PO Box 210   Summit, NJ 07902
  (908)522-3501
+ Atlantic Surgical Oncology
  99 Beauvoir Street   Summit, NJ 07901   (908)522-6429
  Fax (908)598-2392

Rabin-Havt, Sara Schonfeld, MD {1194098509}
+ Lifeline Medical Associates
  530 Morris Avenue   Springfield, NJ 07081   (973)379-7477
  Fax (973)379-9094

Rabines, Alfredo Leonardo, DO {1124311790} EmrgMd(07,PA77)<NJ-JRSYCITY>
+ Jersey City Medical Center
  355 Grand Street   Jersey City, NJ 07304   (201)915-2000
  Fax (973)251-1109

Rabinowitz, Arnold H., MD {1497771455} Pedtrc(79,MEX03)<NJ-HOLYNAME, NJ-ENGLWOD>
+ Madison Avenue Pediatrics
  22 Madison Avenue/3rd floor, Suite 3   Paramus, NJ 07652
  (201)291-9797   Fax (201)291-9798

Rabinowitz, Mitchell, MD {1548211600} RadDia, Radiol, IntrMd(79,NJ06)<NJ-WARREN>
+ Warren Hospital
  185 Roseberry Street/Radiology   Phillipsburg, NJ 08865
  (610)868-1100   Fax (610)868-1111

Rabinowitz, Robert C., MD {1922118850} AdolMd, Pedtrc(74,PA12)<NJ-STBARNMC, NJ-NWRKBETH>
+ The Pediatric Group of West Orange, PA
  395 Pleasant Valley Way   West Orange, NJ 07052
  (973)731-6100   Fax (973)731-0612

Rabinowitz, Robert P., DO {1619983715} Allrgy, AlgyImmn(85,NY75)<NJ-COMMED, NJ-OCEANMC>
+ 462 Lakehurst Road
  Toms River, NJ 08755   (732)341-5403   Fax (732)505-0862
+ Bruce A. De Cotiis, MD, PA
  1673 Highway 88 West   Brick, NJ 08724   (732)458-2000

Rabinowitz, Sidney, MD {1043272081} SrgPlstc, SrgHnd, Surgry(87,NY19)<NJ-HACKNSK, NJ-VALLEY>
+ Sidney Rabinowitz & William K. Boss M.D., P.A.
  305 North Route 17/Suite 3-100A   Paramus, NJ 07652
  (201)967-1100   Fax (201)967-9300

Rabkin, Dimitry, MD {1770675464} Otlryg(90,NY47)<NY-LENOXHLL, NY-MANHEYE>
+ Dimitry Rabkin MD, PC
  19-21 Fairlawn Avenue/2nd Floor   Fair Lawn, NJ 07410
  (201)794-7566

Rabner, Deborah W., MD {1538120845} Dermat(84,IL06)<NJ-MTNSIDE>
+ 1129 Bloomfield Avenue/Suite 205
  West Caldwell, NJ 07006   (973)575-6880   Fax (973)575-1616

Raby, Wilfrid Noel, MD {1518019900} Psychy(93,ON02)
+ 175 Cedar Lane/Suite 7
  Teaneck, NJ 07666   (201)801-0052   Fax (212)568-3832

Racanelli, Joseph Anthony, DO {1801881347} SrgRec(99,PA78)<NJ-EASTORNG>
+ Metamorphosis Plastic Surgery
  9 Madison Avenue   Morristown, NJ 07960   (973)349-0624
  info@drracanelli.com
+ 65 Prospect Street
  Newark, NJ 07105

Racanelli, Vincent J., DO {1427118603} Psychy(87,MO78)
+ 9 Madison Avenue
  Morristown, NJ 07960   (973)539-7476

Racaniello, Angelo R., MD {1962442194} FamMed, EmrgMd(82,DOM02)<NJ-HOBUNIMC>
+ Hoboken University Medical Center
  308 Willow Avenue   Hoboken, NJ 07030   (919)425-1565
  Fax (919)425-0478

Raccuglia, Joseph R., MD {1750328993} FamMed(93,VA07)<NJ-CENTRAST>
+ 4251 US Highway 9 North/Suite 3-A
  Freehold, NJ 07728   (732)780-3744   Fax (732)780-9644

Raccuia, Joseph Salvatore, MD {1013961309} Surgry(84,ITAL)<NY-CMCSTVNY>
+ Hudson Hematology Oncolgny
  377 Jersey Avenue/Suite 160   Jersey City, NJ 07302
  (201)333-8248   Fax (201)333-8469

Racela, Rikki Redona, MD {1023218096} Nrolgy(07,NJ06)<NY-JTORTHO>
+ Bergen Neurology Consultants
  25 Rockwood Place/Suite 110   Englewood, NJ 07631
  (201)894-5805   Fax (201)894-1956

Rachan, Srilatha, MD {1396934436} IntrMd
+ University Hospital-Cares Institute
  42 East Laurel Road/Suite 1100   Stratford, NJ 08084
  (856)566-7036   Fax (856)566-6108

Rachlin, Adrianne, MD {1144595950} ObsGyn
+ 22 Old Short Hills Road
  Livingston, NJ 07039   (973)533-0638

Rachofsky, Edward Lawrence, MD {1316142698} CdvDis, IntCrd, IntrMd(02,NY47)
+ Medicor Cardiology PA
  225 Jackson Street   Bridgewater, NJ 08807   (908)526-8668
  Fax (908)231-6781

Rachoin, Jean Sebastien K., MD {1174796213} IntrMd, Nephro(03,LEB01)<NJ-COOPRUMC>
+ The Cooper Hospital System-Univ Hospital
3 Cooper Plaza/Suite 215/Nephrology   Camden, NJ 08103   (856)342-2439

Rada Banat, Leny M., MD {1598990236} RadDia(88,DMN01)<NJ-STBARNMC, NJ-RIVERVW>
+ Riverview Medical Center
1 Riverview Plaza   Red Bank, NJ 07701   (732)530-2305

Radbel, Jared Michael, MD {1285926469} IntrMd<NJ-RWJUBRUN>
+ RWJ University Hospital New Brunswick
One Robert Wood Johnson Place   New Brunswick, NJ 08901   (732)235-7840   Fax (732)235-7048

Radbill, Keith Philip, DO {1861557795} AnesPain, FamMed, IntrMd(93,PA77)
+ 602 West Maple Avenue/Suite B
Merchantville, NJ 08109   (856)375-1500   Fax (609)482-8024

Radcliff, Nina Singh, MD {1467466813} Anesth
+ AtlantiCare Anesthesiology
65 West Jimmie Leeds Road   Pomona, NJ 08240   (609)748-7597   Fax (609)748-7586

Radevic, Miroslav Rade, MD {1275779894} PthAClf(93,YUG13)
+ Pathology Solutions, Inc.
2-12 Corbett Way   Eatontown, NJ 07724   (732)389-5200

Radhakrishna, Vijaya, MD {1598838708} Pedtrc(70,INA35)
+ 155 Stelton Road
Piscataway, NJ 08854   (732)752-8442   Fax (732)752-3957
+ Dr. Vinaya Radhakrishna, MD PC
230 State Route 18   East Brunswick, NJ 08816   (732)752-8442   Fax (732)651-1848

Radhakrishnan, Indira, MD {1801964663} Anesth(68,INA78)
+ 35 Grandview Place
North Caldwell, NJ 07006

Radhakrishnan, Puthenmadam, MD {1417978677} Pedtrc, IntrMd(82,INA47)<NJ-CHSMRCER>
+ Bellevue Pediatrics
416 Bellevue Avenue/Suite 207   Trenton, NJ 08648   (609)989-9801   Fax (609)989-9896

Radhakrishnan, Radhika, MD {1740387984} Anesth(88,INA47)
+ Robert Wood Johnson-UMDNJ Anesthesia Group
125 Paterson Street/CAB 3100   New Brunswick, NJ 08901   (732)235-7827   Fax (732)235-6131
+ Summit Anesthesia Associates, P.A.
33 Overlook Road/Suite 311   Summit, NJ 07901   (732)235-7827   Fax (908)598-0197

Radic, Rumiana S., MD {1710907654} Psychy(77,BUL01)<NJ-TRENTPSY, NJ-ANCPSYCH>
+ Trenton Psychiatric Hospital
Sullivan Way/PO Box 7600   West Trenton, NJ 08628   (609)633-1500
+ Ocean Mental Health Services, Inc.
160 Atlantic City Boulevard   Bayville, NJ 08721   (609)633-1500   Fax (732)349-0841

Radice, Beverly A., MD {1578629598} IntrMd(83,NJ06)
+ Merrill Lynch HealthCare Services
1300 Merrill Lynch Drive/Ist Floor   Pennington, NJ 08534   (609)274-8879   Fax (609)274-0126

Radin, Audrey A., MD {1134285422} IntrMd(88,NY03)<NJ-MTNSIDE, NJ-STBARNMC>
+ 95 Old Short Hills Road
West Orange, NJ 07052   Fax (973)322-4795

Radjabi Rahat, Amir Reza, MD {1235477290}(01,AUS08)
+ 50 Chelsea Avenue/Apt 332
Long Branch, NJ 07740   (773)391-2826

Radomski, John S., MD {1801874649} Surgry, SrgTpl(81,PA02)<NJ-OURLADY>
+ Our Lady Lourdes Transplant Ctr
1601 Haddon Avenue   Camden, NJ 08103   (856)757-3840

Radoslovich, Glauco A., MD {1598732935} CdvDis, ClCdEl, IntrMd(85,NY01)<NJ-HACKNSK>
+ Electrophysiology Associates
20 Prospect Avenue/Suite 701   Hackensack, NJ 07601   (201)996-2997   Fax (201)996-2571
+ Hackensack University Medical Center
30 Prospect Avenue/Cardiology(EPS)   Hackensack, NJ 07601   (201)996-2287

Radulescu, Raluca Ileana, MD {1447455795} PsyCAd, Psychy, IntrMd(87,ROM01)<NJ-BERGNMC>
+ 140 North Route 17/Suite 330
Paramus, NJ 07652   (201)445-1990   Fax (201)445-1992

Radvinsky, David, MD {1003107178} Surgry
+ Surgical Oncology and Laparoscopy, P.A.
741 Teaneck/Suite B   Teaneck, NJ 07666   (201)833-2888   Fax (201)833-1010

Radwan, Hossam S., MD {1063510014} PedEmg, IntrMd(81,EGY03)<NJ-JRSYCITY, NJ-OCEANMC>
+ EmCare
1945 Route 33   Neptune, NJ 07753   (732)776-4510   Fax (732)776-2329
+ Ocean Medical Center
425 Jack Martin Boulevard   Brick, NJ 08723   (732)776-4510   Fax (732)836-4818
+ 511 New Brunswick Avenue
Perth Amboy, NJ 07753   (732)442-0300

Radwine, Zachary Picker, MD {1265797971} EmrgMd<NJ-CHRIST>
+ Christ Hospital
176 Palisade Avenue   Jersey City, NJ 07306   (201)795-8200

Radzievska, Ludmila Andreevna, MD {1275622656} Psychy, PsyGrt(81,UKR05)
+ New Jersey Division of Developmental Disability
Route 72 East   New Lisbon, NJ 08064   (609)726-1000   Fax (609)894-8430

Rae, Sam, MD {1649277294} IntrMd, Nephro(89,SYRI)<NJ-CHILTON>
+ Suburban Nephrology Group
342 Hamburg Turnpike/Suite 201   Wayne, NJ 07470   (973)389-1119   Fax (973)389-1145
+ Suburban Nephrology Group
1031 McBride Avenue/Suite D-210   Little Falls, NJ 07424   (973)389-1119

Rae, Susan, MD {1437158094} FamMed(89,SYRI)
+ Suburban Nephrology Group
1031 McBride Avenue/Suite D-210   Little Falls, NJ 07424   (973)812-9091   Fax (973)339-9040

Rae-Layne, Norma Alicia, MD {1609950187} ObsGyn(96,IA02)
+ Rae Medical, LLC
59 Main Street/Suite 207   West Orange, NJ 07052   (862)766-5363   Fax (862)766-5363

Rafeq, Zahi, MD {1205981180}
+ Cardiovascular Associates
210 West Atlantic Avenue   Haddon Heights, NJ 08035   (617)459-9274   Fax (856)547-5337
+ Cardiovascular Associates of The Delaware Valley, PA
525 State Street/Suite 3   Elmer, NJ 08318   (617)459-9274   Fax (856)358-0725

Rafer, Ramon V., MD {1114993532} Anesth(76,PHIL)<NJ-HOBUNIMC>
+ Hoboken University Medical Center
308 Willow Avenue/Anesthesiology   Hoboken, NJ 07030   (201)418-1000   Fax (201)943-8105

Raffel, Brian J., DO {1346539236}
+ Robert Wood Johnson-UMDNJ Anesthesia Group
125 Paterson Street/CAB 3100   New Brunswick, NJ 08901   (732)235-7827   Fax (732)235-6131
+ 1408 Clinton Street/Unit 308
Hoboken, NJ 07030   (732)841-8946

Rafferty, William J., MD {1780766790} PthAClf(87,PA13)<NJ-COOPRUMC>
+ Cooper University Hospital
One Cooper Plaza/Path   Camden, NJ 08103   (856)342-2000

Rafiuddin, Shaleeza, MD {1639687940} IntrMd
+ Orion HealthCare
90 Washington Street/Suite 308   East Orange, NJ 07017   (973)677-3300

Rafizadeh, Farhad, MD {1770559064} SrgPlstc, Surgry(75,SWI05)<NJ-MORRISTN, NJ-STBARNMC>
+ 101 Madison Avenue/Suite 105
Morristown, NJ 07960   (973)267-0928   Fax (973)267-6960
drrafizadeh@drrafizadeh.com

Rafizadeh, Mehrad, MD {1790846483} Anesth(77,SWI05)<NJ-STBARNMC>
+ St. Barnabas Medical Center
94 Old Short Hills Road   Livingston, NJ 07039   (973)322-5000

Ragasa, Dante A., MD {1699921544} PthAClf, Pthlgy(70,PHIL)<NJ-VIRTMHBC>
+ Burlington County Health Department
15 Pioneer Boulevard   Westampton, NJ 08060   (609)265-5548

Ragavan, Vijay, MD {1023078433} IntrMd, Grtrcs(74,INA77)<NJ-VAEASTOR>
+ VA New Jersey Health Care System-East Orange Campus
385 Tremont Avenue   East Orange, NJ 07018   (973)676-1000   Fax (973)395-7003

Raghavan, Murli, MD {1679614820} Grtrcs, IntrMd(78,INA1Z)<NY-VIAROCHS>
+ Concentra Medical Centers
30 Seaview Drive/Suite 2   Secaucus, NJ 07094   (201)319-1611   Fax (201)319-1233

Raghavan, Padma, MD {1508826132} IntrMd(77,INDI)<NJ-VAEASTOR>
+ VA New Jersey Health Care System-East Orange Campus
385 Tremont Avenue   East Orange, NJ 07018   (973)676-1000   Fax (973)395-7064

Raghavan, Usha Murli, MD {1427277664} IntrMd(79,INA03)
+ Concentra Medical Centers
375 McCarter Highway   Newark, NJ 07114   (973)643-8601   Fax (973)643-8609

Ragheb, Sameh Makram, MD {1295769404} Psychy(89,EGYP)
+ Care PLUS NJ, Inc. - Mid-Bergen Center
610 Valley Health Plaza   Paramus, NJ 07652   (201)265-8200   Fax (201)265-0366

Ragheb, Sozan L., MD {1336274463} Anesth(83,EGY04)<NJ-RBAYPERT>
+ Raritan Bay Medical Center/Perth Amboy Division
530 New Brunswick Avenue/Anesth   Perth Amboy, NJ 08861   (732)442-3700

Raghu, Shalini Nagarajan, MD {1942355680} Pedtrc, IntrMd(99,INA77)<NJ-JFKMED>
+ JFK Medical Center
65 James Street/Pediatrics   Edison, NJ 08820   (732)321-7010   Fax (732)744-5873

Raghunathan, Susheela I., MD {1144330689} Pedtrc(72,INA29)
+ 1412 Route 130 North
North Brunswick, NJ 08902   (732)821-3211   Fax (732)821-3024

Raghuwanshi, Anita P., MD {1669630109} EnDbMt
+ Cape Regional Physicians Associates
11 Village Drive   Cape May Court House, NJ 08210   (609)465-2273   Fax (609)463-0235

Raghuwanshi, Maya P., MD {1235216557} EnDbMt, IntrMd(75,INDI)<NJ-UMDNJ>
+ Rutgers- New Jersey Medical School
185 South Orange Avenue/Endocrinology   Newark, NJ 07103   (973)972-6171   Fax (973)972-5185
+ University Hospital-Doctors Office Center
90 Bergen Street/Endocrinology   Newark, NJ 07103   (973)972-2500

Ragi, Gangaram, MD {1801906680} Dermat, DerMOH(78,INDI)
+ Advanced Laser & Skin Cancer Center
870 Palisade Avcenue/Suite 302   Teaneck, NJ 07666   (201)836-9696   Fax (201)836-4716
gragi@laserhairremoval.com

Ragland, Raymond, III, MD {1962597328} SrgOrt, SrgHnd(92,PA12)<NY-SLRLUKES>
+ Hand Surgery & Rehabilitation Center of New Jersey
5000 Sagemore Drive/Suite 103   Marlton, NJ 08053   (856)983-4263   Fax (856)983-9362
raymondr@thehanddoctors.com
+ Hand Surgery & Rehabilitation Center of New Jersey
8008 Route 130 North   Delran, NJ 08075   (856)983-4263   Fax (856)764-3561
+ Hand Surgery & Rehabilitation Center of New Jersey
608 North Broad Street/Suite 200   Woodbury, NJ 08053   (856)845-2557   Fax (856)845-8422

Ragone, Daniel, Jr., MD {1922045194} PhysMd(83,GRN01)
+ 3829 Church Road
Mount Laurel, NJ 08054   (856)222-9713   Fax (856)222-9714

Ragone, John P., MD {1184696791} Psychy(87,MEX34)<NJ-STPETER>
+ Catholic Charities Mental Health Center
288 Rues Lane   East Brunswick, NJ 08816   (732)257-6100   Fax (732)651-9834
jr164@msn.com

Ragothaman, Ramesh, MD {1356331482} Pedtrc, IntrMd(89,INA1Z)
+ Mt. Laurel Pediatric
528 Lippincott Drive   Marlton, NJ 08053   (856)983-3899   Fax (856)983-3997

Raguindin, Leah, MD {1053356048} PedEmg, Pedtrc, EmrgPedr(89,GRNA)<NJ-HACKNSK>
+ Hackensack Univ Medical Center Pediatric Emerg Room
30 Prospect Avenue   Hackensack, NJ 07601   (201)996-5430   Fax (201)996-3676
+ Hackensack University Medical Center
30 Prospect Avenue/PediEmergMed   Hackensack, NJ 07601   (201)996-2000

Ragukonis, Thomas P., MD {1992744312} Anesth, PainMd, PainInvt(91,NJ05)
+ Bergen Pain Management
37 West Century Road/Suite 101   Paramus, NJ 07652   (201)634-9000   Fax (201)634-9014
bergenpain@aol.com
+ Integrated Medical Care
5600 Kennedy Boulevard East/Suite 106   West New York, NJ 07093   (201)634-9000   Fax (201)969-9588
+ Columbia Pain Management
950 West Chestnut Street/Suite 101   Union, NJ 07652   (908)688-1100   Fax (908)688-1170

Raguso Failla, Michael Joseph, MD {1497837744} FamMed(96,NY09)<CT-GRENWCH>
+ Family Medicine Center
1301 Route 72 West/Suite 240   Manahawkin, NJ 08050   (609)597-7394   Fax (609)597-6833
+ Family Medicine Center
279 Mathistown Road   Little Egg Harbor, NJ 08087   (609)296-1101

Physicians by Name and Address

Rah, Kang H., MD {1144302852} Anesth, CritCr(68,KOR14)<NJ-RWJUBRUN>
+ Robert Wood Johnson-UMDNJ Anesthesia Group
125 Paterson Street/CAB 3100   New Brunswick, NJ 08901
(732)235-7827   Fax (732)235-6131

Raha, Bandana, MD {1558365239} Pedtrc(75,INA7X)<NJ-HOBUNIMC>
+ Jersey City Pediatrics, PA
550 Newark Avenue/Suite 401   Jersey City, NJ 07306
(201)963-0090   Fax (201)963-0355
Rupakraha@msn.com

Rahal, William J., MD {1053413088} Anesth, PainInvt(91,DOMI)<NJ-JRSYSHMC>
+ Jersey Shore Anesthesiology Associates
1945 Route 33/PO Box 397   Neptune, NJ 07754   (732)922-3308   Fax (732)897-0263
+ Jersery Shore Anesthesiology
1945 Highway 33   Neptune, NJ 07753   (732)922-3308   Fax (732)897-0263

Rahimi, Saum Amir, MD {1366693830} SrgVas<NJ-RWJUBRUN>
+ UMDNJ RWJ Vascular Surgery Group
125 Paterson Street/Suite 4100   New Brunswick, NJ 08901
(732)235-8770   Fax (732)235-8538

Rahman, Abir, DO {1043620040} PhysMd<NJ-WAYNEGEN>
+ St. Joseph's Wayne Hospital
224 Hamburg Turnpike   Wayne, NJ 07470   (973)956-3327

Rahman, Aqsa Fahd, MD {1487944005}
+ 634 South Edge Park Drive
Haddonfield, NJ 08033
aqsabangash@yahoo.com

Rahman, Attique, MD {1538125687} Anesth(01,NJ06)<NJ-STPETER>
+ Anesthesia Consultnts of NJ/Nova Pain
285 Davidson Avenue/Suite 204   Somerset, NJ 08873
(732)271-1400   Fax (732)271-3543
+ Cares Surgicenter, LLC.
240 Easton Avenue   New Brunswick, NJ 08901   (732)271-1400   Fax (732)296-8677

Rahman, Firoz Pushkin, MD {1053351080} Psychy, PsyAdd, IntrMd(88,BAN02)<NJ-UNVMCPRN>
+ Princeton House Behavioral Health - Princeton
905 Herrontown Road   Princeton, NJ 08540   (609)497-3300   Fax (609)497-3370

Rahman, Habeeb U., MD {1114004918} InfDis, IntrMd(89,INA37)<NJ-HOBUNIMC>
+ Hoboken University Medical Center
308 Willow Avenue   Hoboken, NJ 07030   (201)418-1000
+ Center for Family Health
122-132 Clinton Street   Hoboken, NJ 07030   (201)418-1000   Fax (201)418-3148

Rahman, Mahboob Ur, MD {1770511818} IntrMd, Rheuma(82,BAN02)<PA-UPMCPHL>
+ University Physician Associates of New Jersey
125 Paterson Street/CAB 5200   New Brunswick, NJ 08901
(732)235-7217   Fax (732)235-7115

Rahman, Owen R., MD {1104970920} AnesPain(81,PA13)
+ University Hospital-New Jersey Medical School
30 Bergen Street/ADMC 1205   Newark, NJ 07107
(973)972-0037   Fax (973)972-9355

Rahman, Saud Saqib, MD {1063613461} PthAcl
+ Si Paradigm, LLC.
690 Kinderkamack Road/Suite 103   Oradell, NJ 07649
(201)599-9044   Fax (201)599-9066
+ Si Paradigm, LLC.
25 Riverside Drive/Suite 2   Pine Brook, NJ 07058
(201)599-9044

Rahmani, Ghulam Ali, MD {1477823441} IntHos
+ AtlantiCare Hospitalist Program
1925 Pacific Avenue/8th Floor   Atlantic City, NJ 08401
(609)345-4000

Rahmani, Masroor, MD {1144519687} IntrMd<NJ-OVERLOOK>
+ Overlook Medical Center
99 Beauvoir Avenue/PO Box 210   Summit, NJ 07902
(908)522-2000

Rahmanian, Marjan, MD {1033374434}(96,IRA08)<NJ-MTNSIDE>
+ Hackensack UMC Mountainside
1 Bay Avenue   Montclair, NJ 07042   (973)429-6000

Rahmet, Naheed R., MD {1528036472} Pedtrc(82,PAKI)<NJ-JRSYSHMC>
+ Seashore Pediatrics
1560 Highway 138 West   Wall, NJ 07719   (732)449-8592
Fax (732)449-2108

Rahmin, Michael G., MD {1902856313} Gastrn, IntrMd(89,NY19)<NJ-HACKNSK, NJ-VALLEY>
+ Gastrointestinal Associates PA
140 Chestnut Street/Suite 300   Ridgewood, NJ 07450
(201)444-2600   Fax (201)444-9471

Rahulatharan, Rajasingha, MD {1831130202} ObsGyn(69,SRI01)<NJ-CHRIST>
+ 201 Palisade Avenue
Jersey City, NJ 07306   (201)963-2200   Fax (201)963-0011

Rai, Bellipady C., MD {1790799088} NnPnMd, Pedtrc(79,INDI)<NJ-CHDNWBTH, NJ-NWRKBETH>
+ Children's Hospital of New Jersey
201 Lyons Avenue/Osborne Terrace   Newark, NJ 07112
(973)926-7203   Fax (973)926-2332

Rai-Patel, Jitha, MD {1023053402} IntrMd, Gastrn<PA-LNKNAU>
+ Gastroenterology Consultants of South Jersey
693 Main Street/Suite 2   Lumberton, NJ 08048   (609)265-1700   Fax (609)265-9005

Raikin, Steven Mark, MD {1265487623} SrgOrt, SrgFAk(89,SAF01)<NJ-ATLANTHS>
+ Rothman Institute - Voorhees
443 Laurel Oak Road   Voorhees, NJ 08043   (856)821-6360

Raimo, Anthony S., MD {1801136262} Pedtrc
+ 645 Ramapo Valley Road
Oakland, NJ 07436   (201)337-4235

Raimondo, Rick Arthur, MD {1831144138} SrgOrt, SrgFAk(92,NY01)<NJ-VIRTMHBC, NJ-VANJHCS>
+ Reconstructive Orthopedics, P.A.
401 Young Avenue/Suite 245   Moorestown, NJ 08057
(609)267-9400   Fax (609)288-6446
+ Reconstructive Orthopedics, P.A.
243 Route 130/Suite 100   Bordentown, NJ 08505
(609)267-9400   Fax (609)267-9457

Raina, Santosh, MD {1962410159} PthAcl, Pthlgy(74,INA65)
+ 67 Wedgewood Drive
Montville, NJ 07045

Raina, Suresh, MD {1659302453} OthrSp, Surgry(72,INDI)<NJ-UMDNJ>
+ University Hospital
150 Bergen Street/General Surgery   Newark, NJ 07103
(973)972-2400

Rainear, Kristen, DO {1689662165} CdvDis, IntrMd, CarNuc(90,PA77)<NJ-SJHREGMC>
+ Wachspress & Rainear Cardiology Associates PA
1076 East Chestnut Avenue   Vineland, NJ 08360   (856)692-7979   Fax (856)794-9479

Rainville, Harvey Charles, MD {1083843783} Surgry(07,GCY01)
+ Ballem Surgical
230 Sherman Avenue/Suite C   Glen Ridge, NJ 07028
(973)744-8585   Fax (973)748-5990

Raisdana, Behnam, DO {1356695001}<NJ-SJHREGMC>
+ SJH Regional Medical Center
1505 West Sherman Avenue   Vineland, NJ 08360
(856)641-8661   Fax (856)575-4944

Raj, Paarth J., DO {1003224197}<NJ-HACKNSK>
+ Hackensack University Medical Center
30 Prospect Avenue   Hackensack, NJ 07601   (201)996-2000

Raja, Bala Shanmugasundara, MD {1235196668} Anesth(87,INA85)
+ 29 Vista Trail
Wayne, NJ 07470

Raja, Haroon M., MD {1710118229}
+ 2151 Route 38/Apt 1203
Cherry Hill, NJ 08002   (856)342-2406
haroon.raja@gmail.com

Raja, Shashi Ravi, MD {1639102627} IntrMd(94,INDI)
+ Morristown Medical Center
100 Madison Avenue   Morristown, NJ 07962   (973)971-4287   Fax (908)394-2624
+ 757 Route 202/206
Bridgewater, NJ 08807   (973)971-4287   Fax (908)394-2624

Raja, Sreedar V., MD {1821230004} EmrgMd(09,NJ05)
+ Kimball Medical Center
600 River Avenue   Lakewood, NJ 08701   (732)363-1900

Rajagopal, Leena, MD {1396184016}
+ 24 Beacon Way/Apt 1705
Jersey City, NJ 07304   (954)303-5851
leena28@gmail.com

Rajagopalan, Kumar, MD {1023108321} OncHem(87,INA66)
+ Cancer Institute of New Jersey at Cooper
900 Centennial Boulevard/Suite M-2   Voorhees, NJ 08043
(856)325-6750   Fax (856)325-6777

Rajakumar, Nirmala S., MD {1821041294} Psychy, Nrolgy(74,SRI08)<NJ-UMDNJ>
+ University Psychiatric Associates
183 South Orange Avenue/E-F Levels   Newark, NJ 07103
(973)972-2977   Fax (973)972-2979

Rajan, Jennifer Ray, MD {1477509511} Dermat(95,OH40)
+ Alliance Dermatology Associates
3311 Brunswick Pike   Lawrenceville, NJ 08648   (609)799-1600   Fax (609)799-1677

Rajan, Ravi R., MD {1831135078} Urolgy(94,OH40)
+ Urology Care Alliance
3311 Brunswick Pike   Lawrenceville, NJ 08648   (609)895-1991   Fax (609)895-6996

Rajan, Samir, MD {1174719124} Nephro, IntrMd(02,WIN01)
+ Associates in Kidney Disease & Hypertension
2177 Oak Tree Road/Suite 204   Edison, NJ 08820
(908)769-4735   Fax (908)769-4736

Rajan, Shirley M., MD {1902126816} Psychy(10,NJ05)<MA-UMM-LAKE>
+ The Rajan Center for Familiy Wellness, LLC
74 Brunswick Woods Drive   East Brunswick, NJ 08816
(774)314-7797

Rajan, Sivaram Gounder, MD {1073583746} SrgOrt(97,OH06)
+ 211 Essex Street/Suite 101
Hackensack, NJ 07601   (551)999-6433

Rajan-Mohandas, Niranjana, MD {1184633794} Pedtrc(94,NJ05)<NJ-STPETER, NJ-RWJUBRUN>
+ Drs. Rajan-Mohandas and Chow
666 Plainsboro Road/Suite 2000-E   Plainsboro, NJ 08536
(609)799-0068   Fax (609)799-5534

Rajapakse, John S., MD {1639377914} IntrMd(03,GRN01)
+ 495 New Brunswick Avenue
Perth Amboy, NJ 08861   (732)442-4422   Fax (732)442-3577

Rajaram, Arun, MD {1881838993} SrgOrt
+ IGEA Brain & Spine
1057 Commerce Avenue   Union, NJ 07083   (866)467-1770
Fax (908)688-2377
+ Elite Orthopedics & Sports Medicine, P.A.
342 Hamburg Turnpike/Suite 209   Wayne, NJ 07470
(866)467-1770   Fax (973)956-8104
+ Elite Orthopedics & Sports Medicine, P.A.
44 Route 23 North/Suite 3   Riverdale, NJ 07083   (973)513-9646

Rajaram, Sri-Sujanthy, MD {1033209333} CritCr, IntrMd(89,SRIL)<NY-NRTHCBRX>
+ Hackensack Medical Center-Internal Medicine
30 Prospect Avenue/4 Main/Rm 4621   Hackensack, NJ 07601   (551)996-4257   Fax (551)996-0536
+ Windsor Medical Center
339 Princeton-Hightstown Rd/Building B   Hightstown, NJ 08520   (551)996-4257   Fax (609)443-4800

Rajaraman, Karunambal, MD {1346201654} Pedtrc(72,INDI)<NJ-BAYSHORE>
+ 59 Avenue at the Common/Suite 105
Shrewsbury, NJ 07702   (732)544-8899   Fax (732)544-9888

Rajaraman, Ravindran Thirunavu, MD {1487625422} IntrMd, Pedtrc(00,NJ05)<NJ-MONMOUTH>
+ Monmouth Family Center
270 Broadway   Long Branch, NJ 07740   (732)923-7100
Fax (732)923-7104

Rajarathnam, Kavitha, MD {1548518616} Pedtrc
+ 702 Plaza Drive
Woodbridge, NJ 07095   (732)589-8767

Rajaratnam, Ranjit C., MD {1932145943} Psychy, PsyGrt(76,SRI01)<NY-BETHPETR>
+ Bergen County Comprehensive Behavioral Health Care
516 Valley Brook Avenue   Lyndhurst, NJ 07071   (201)935-3322

Rajasekaran, Divya, MD {1891074944}
+ 94 Kline Boulevard
Berkeley Heights, NJ 07922   (732)841-8727
dr2095@gmail.com

Rajasekhar, Hariprem, MD {1083876106}
+ UH- Robert Wood Johnson Med
125 Paterson Street/MEB 343   New Brunswick, NJ 08901
(732)235-7887   Fax (732)235-6609

Rajasekharaiah, Vinutha, MD {1437144979} IntrMd, EmrgMd(93,INA68)<NJ-STCLRDEN, NJ-RIVERVW>
+ Jersey Medical Associates
80 Hazlet Avenue/Suite 10   Hazlet, NJ 07730   (732)264-0400   Fax (732)264-1149
+ Hospital Medicine Associates
157 Broad Street/Suite 317   Red Bank, NJ 07701
(732)264-0400   Fax (732)530-7446

Rajasingham, Jamuna Kandasamy, MD {1073756474} Nrolgy
+ Bergen Neurology Consultants
25 Rockwood Place/Suite 110   Englewood, NJ 07631
(201)894-5805   Fax (201)894-1956

Rajeswaran, Gowri, MD {1144311192} IntrMd, EmrgMd(78,SRI01)<NJ-KIMBALL>
+ Kimball Medical Center
600 River Avenue   Lakewood, NJ 08701   (732)363-1900

Rajiv, Deepa, MD {1891808390} IntrMd(03,INA46)
+ Northern State Prison Corrections Department
168 Frontpage Road/Box 280   Newark, NJ 07106
(973)465-0068

Rajiyah, Gitendra, MD {1083693196} CdvDis, IntrMd(83,SRI01)<NJ-EASTORNG, NJ-NWRKBETH>
+ The Heart Center of The Oranges
310 Central Avenue/Suite 102   East Orange, NJ 07018
(973)395-1550   Fax (973)395-1556
+ The Heart Center of The Oranges
77 Main Street   West Orange, NJ 07052   (973)324-2090
+ The Heart Center of The Oranges
60 Vose Avenue   South Orange, NJ 07018   (973)763-5200

Rajkumar, Aradhana, MD {1730192055} Pedtrc(90,INA83)
+ 3219 Route 46 East
Parsippany, NJ 07054   (973)670-9381

Rajput, Ilyas A., MD {1912961608} CdvDis, IntrMd(74,PAKI)<NJ-ACMCITY, NJ-ACMCMAIN>
+ Med-Com Health Services, P.A.
258 North New Road   Pleasantville, NJ 08232   (609)646-4064   Fax (609)272-8526
+ Med-Com Health Services, PA
76 West Jimmie Leeds Road/Suite 201   Galloway, NJ 08205   (609)646-4064   Fax (609)909-5357

Rajput, Zubeda I., MD {1790746725} IntrMd(76,PAKI)<NJ-ACMCITY, NJ-ACMCMAIN>
+ Med-Com Health Services, P.A.
258 North New Road   Pleasantville, NJ 08232   (609)646-4064   Fax (609)272-8526
+ Med-Com Health Services, PA
76 West Jimmie Leeds Road/Suite 201   Galloway, NJ 08205   (609)646-4064   Fax (609)909-5357

Rajput, Zulfiqar A., MD {1427074285} Psychy(80,PAK16)
+ Brick Psychiatric Services Inc
1541 West Route 88   Brick, NJ 08724   (732)202-0622   Fax (732)202-0620

Raju, Bharat Namburuj, MD {1720217581} FamMed(DMN01)
+ Atlantic Medical Group
1395 Route 23/Suite 4   Butler, NJ 07405   (973)838-0200   Fax (973)838-1614

Raju, Biju, DO {1609163674} FamMed, IntrMd(11,NY75)
+ Pompton Plains Family Health Center
230 West Parkway/Suite 10   Pompton Plains, NJ 07444   (973)835-0800   Fax (973)616-2766

Raju, Govinda S., MD {1740294487} IntrMd, CdvDis(73,INDI)<NJ-VAEASTOR, NJ-VALYONS>
+ VA New Jersey Health Care System-East Orange Campus
385 Tremont Avenue   East Orange, NJ 07018   (973)676-1000

Raju, Pooja Indukuri, MD {1760626774} PulDis, IntrMd(06,NSK03)
+ JFK Medical Center
65 James Street/Sleep Ctr   Edison, NJ 08820   (732)321-7000

Raju, Ramesh K., MD {1013961465} IntrMd(79,INA68)<NJ-JFKMED, NJ-RWJURAH>
+ Metro Medical Associates
870 Green Street   Iselin, NJ 08830   (732)855-9006   Fax (732)326-0095

Raju, Rina M., MD {1538460779} Pedtrc, FamMed(01,INA70)<NJ-HACKNSK, NJ-HOLYNAME>
+ Riverside Medical Group
714 Tenth Street/Suite 2   Secaucus, NJ 07094   (201)863-3346   Fax (201)865-0015
+ Riverside Pediatric Group
506 Broadway   Bayonne, NJ 07002   (201)863-3346   Fax (201)471-7014

Raju, Vijaya L.K., MD {1750465837} ObsGyn(67,INDI)<NJ-UMDNJ>
+ The University Hospital
90 Bergen Street/ObGyn   Newark, NJ 07103   (973)972-2700

Rakhimova, Gulbakhor Alikhonovna, MD {1841594728} Pedtrc(99,TAJ02)
+ Dr. R's Kids
871 Allwood Road/2nd Floor   Clifton, NJ 07012   (973)310-2340
Drrpeds@gmail.com

Rakickas, Jeffrey, MD {1518194349} FamMed
+ MedExpress Urgent Care Cinnaminson
1210 Route 130 North   Cinnaminson, NJ 08077   (856)829-0407   Fax (856)829-0453
jeffrey.rakickas@medexpress.com

Rakitt, Tina Susanne, MD {1124255534} PedGst, Pedtrc, Nutrtn(PA12<NJ-MONMOUTH>
+ Monmouth Medical Group, P.C.
279 Third Avenue/Suite 101   Long Branch, NJ 07740   (732)923-6080   Fax (732)923-6083
+ Monmouth Medical Group Pediatric Specialties
67 Route 37 West   Toms River, NJ 08755   (732)923-6080   Fax (732)557-3518

Rakla, Younus A., MD {1104876499} CdvDis, IntrMd(79,PAK11)<NJ-JFKMED, NJ-NWRKBETH>
+ Cedarbrook Cardiology
902 Oak Tree Avenue/Suite 400   South Plainfield, NJ 07080   (908)756-1703   Fax (908)756-1793

Raklyar, Eduard, MD {1790906006} Dermat(03,NY08)
+ 16 Kinzel Lane
West Orange, NJ 07052

Raklyar, Irina, MD {1356486831} Rheuma, IntrMd(03,NY08)
+ New Jersey Arthritis Osteoporosis Center
871 Allwood Road/Suite 1   Clifton, NJ 07012   (973)405-5163   Fax (973)365-8004

Rakow, Joel I., MD {1326021221} Radiol, RadDia(82,NY46)<NJ-HACKNSK>
+ New Century Imaging at Oradell
555 Kinderkamack Road   Oradell, NJ 07649   (201)599-1311   Fax (201)599-8333

+ The Imaging Center
30 South Newman Street   Hackensack, NJ 07601   (201)599-1311   Fax (201)488-5244
+ Hackensack Radiology Group, P.A.
30 Prospect Avenue   Hackensack, NJ 07649   (201)996-2200   Fax (201)336-8451

Rakowski, Thomas J., MD {1710943436} IntrMd, OncHem(76,NY15)<NJ-VALLEY>
+ Valley Mount Sinai Comprehensive Cancer Care
One Valley Health Plaza   Paramus, NJ 07652   (201)634-5578   Fax (201)986-4702

Raleigh, Elizabeth Ann, DO {1891999637} FamMSptM
+ Phillips Barber Family Health Center
72 Alexander Avenue   Lambertville, NJ 08530   (609)397-3535   Fax (609)397-0301

Ralph, Pamela J., MD {1205953858} PsyCAd(90,TN07)
+ 21 Oriole Way
Moorestown, NJ 08057

Ram, Meryl H., MD {1831182112} IntrMd, MedOnc, OncHem(67,MA01)<NJ-STCLRDEN, NJ-HCKTSTWN>
+ Hematology-Oncology Associates of Northern NJ
3219 US Highway 46/Suite 108   Parsippany, NJ 07054   (973)316-5900   Fax (973)316-5990

Ram, Nand, MD {1992799522} IntrMd(82,MEXI)<NJ-VIRTVOOR>
+ Virtua Voorhees
100 Bowman Drive/Internal Med   Voorhees, NJ 08043   (856)762-1940   Fax (856)762-1777

Rama, Gabriel, MD {1093976797} Pedtrc, PedCrd(08,NJ03)<NY-CHLDCOPR>
+ The Pediatric Center for Heart Disease
155 Polifly Road/Suite 106   Hackensack, NJ 07601   (201)487-7617   Fax (201)342-5341

Rama, Sapna, DO {1316327737} IntrMd<NJ-PALISADE>
+ Palisades Medical Center
7600 River Road   North Bergen, NJ 07047   (201)854-5000

Rama, Sreedevi, MD {1700892510} ObsGyn(89,INA39)<NJ-JFKMED, NJ-STPETER>
+ Focus Obstetrics & Gynecology
4 Ethel Road/Suite 106-B   Edison, NJ 08817   (732)452-9099   Fax (732)287-3301
FOCUSOBGYN@yahoo.com
+ Focus Obstetrics & Gynecology
530 Green Street   Iselin, NJ 08830   (732)452-9099   Fax (732)287-3301

Ramachandra Rao, Vanie Subramanya, MD {1003838723} IntrMd, Grtrcs(96,INA2C)
+ 15A Eatoncrest Drive
Eatontown, NJ 07724   (732)797-2351

Ramachandraiah, Vidya, MD {1982911970} CritCr<NJ-JFKMED>
+ JFK Medical Center
65 James Street   Edison, NJ 08820   (732)321-7660   Fax (732)906-4946

Ramachandran, Jaishree, MD {1508272170} Pedtrc
+ 1 Bellaire Drive
Princeton, NJ 08540   (732)447-4860

Ramachandran, Karthia J., MD {1376585455} EmrgMd, FamMed(74,INDI)<NJ-RIVERVW>
+ Riverside Medical Center
1 Riverview Plaza   Red Bank, NJ 07701   (732)741-2700   Fax (732)224-7498

Ramachandran, Radha, MD {1285730135} EmrgMd(03,INA3D)<NJ-NWRKBETH>
+ 2 Country Lane
Holmdel, NJ 07733

Ramachandran, Reggie, DO {1174933832}<NJ-SJHREGMC>
+ SJH Regional Medical Center
1505 West Sherman Avenue   Vineland, NJ 08360   (856)641-8661   Fax (856)575-4944

Ramachandran, Sudha, MD {1952508293} RadDia, RadNro(04,TX04)<NY-MTSINAI, NY-MTSINYHS>
+ Hackensack Radiology Group, PA/Corporate
130 Kinderkamack Road/Suite 200   River Edge, NJ 07661   (201)488-2660   Fax (201)489-2812

Ramachandran, Usha, MD {1992892285} Pedtrc(91,INA77)<NJ-RWJUBRUN>
+ Eric B. Chandler Health Center
277 George Street/Pedi   New Brunswick, NJ 08901   (732)235-6700   Fax (732)235-6729
+ RWJ University Hospital New Brunswick
One Robert Wood Johnson Place   New Brunswick, NJ 08901   (732)828-3000

Ramadan, Soheir S., MD {1588695530} Pedtrc(77,EGY04)<NJ-STPETER>
+ 380 Davidson Avenue
Somerset, NJ 08873   (732)560-8262   Fax (732)560-1622

Ramadi, Roula Alchaa, MD {1982007571} Pedtrc
+ Elite Pediatrics
One Broadway/Suite 303   Elmwood Park, NJ 07407   (201)794-8855   Fax (201)794-6988

Ramagopal, Maya, MD {1699710137} Pedtrc, PedPul(85,INA66)<NJ-RWJUBRUN>
+ University Hospital-RWJ Medical School
89 French Street/Suite 2218   New Brunswick, NJ 08901   (732)828-3000   Fax (732)235-7707

Ramalingam, Muthulakshmi, MD {1467577940} IntrMd(76,INA37)
+ 40 Fuld Street/Suite 202
Trenton, NJ 08638   (609)656-7701   Fax (609)656-7702

Ramamoorthy, Ravishankar, MD {1801942644} Gastrn, IntrMd(95,NJ05)
+ North Jersey Gastroenterology & Endoscopy Center
1825 State Route 23 South   Wayne, NJ 07470   (973)633-1484   Fax (973)633-7980

Ramamurthy, Kotta M., MD {1528104015} Surgry(64,INDI)
+ 898 Green Street
Iselin, NJ 08830   (732)634-9494   Fax (732)634-4560

Raman, Anoop Manikarnika, MD {1770825242} FamMed
+ Drs. Vijayakumar and Raman
1801 Atlantic Avenue/3rd Floor   Atlantic City, NJ 08401   (609)570-2400   Fax (609)441-7207

Raman, Chidambaram, MD {1063408789} Surgry(76,INA66)<NJ-HOLYNAME, NJ-VALLEY>
+ 1200 East Ridgewood Avenue
Ridgewood, NJ 07450   (201)444-4466   Fax (201)444-6672

Raman, Jennifer Lynne, MD {1104908912} EmrgMd<NJ-VALLEY>
+ The Valley Hospital
223 North Van Dien Avenue   Ridgewood, NJ 07450   (201)447-8000

Raman, Rajesh C., MD {1437135951} Pedtrc
+ Wellness Center Pediatrics LLC
21 Lafayette Road/Suite F   Sparta, NJ 07871   (973)726-4455   Fax (973)726-8445

Ramanadham, Aruna R., MD {1609157692} Pedtrc(77,INDI)
+ 9 Mount Haven Drive
Livingston, NJ 07039

Ramanadham, Smita R., MD {1548464324} Surgry(06,MA07)
+ 2 Cornwall Drive/Unit B2
East Brunswick, NJ 08816   (908)481-3851

Ramanarayanan, Annapurna, MD {1679620033} ObsGyn(70,INDI)
+ 736 Amboy Avenue
Edison, NJ 08837   (732)738-1900   Fax (732)738-0063

Ramanathan, Vivek Sri, MD {1427353630}
+ Southern Ocean Medical Center
1100 Route 72 West/Suite 307   Manahawkin, NJ 08050   (917)434-0814   Fax (609)978-8941
drvivekram@gmail.com

Ramani, Bhavesh Natwarlal, MD {1285054635}<NJ-OVERLOOK>
+ Overlook Medical Center
99 Beauvoir Avenue/PO Box 210   Summit, NJ 07902   (908)522-2000

Ramani, Mohnish N., MD {1942357025} SrgOrt(96,NJ05)<NJ-JFKMED>
+ Edison-Metuchen Orthopedic Group
10 Parsonage Road/5th Floor/Suite 500   Edison, NJ 08837   (732)494-6226   Fax (732)494-8762

Ramanujam, Sailakshmi, MD {1063652642} Psychy
+ Guidance Clinic
39 North Clinton Avenue   Trenton, NJ 08609   (609)394-3202   Fax (609)278-6139

Ramasamy, Dhanasekaran, MD {1689875700} IntrMd, Gastrn(97,INA04)
+ Center for Digestive Diseases
695 Chestnut Street   Union, NJ 07083   (908)688-6565   Fax (908)688-3161

Ramasamy, Kovil Veeraswami, MD {1790765576} Gastrn, IntrMd(09,INA77)<NJ-BAYONNE, NJ-JRSYCITY>
+ Hudson Gastroenterology
534 Avenue E/Suite A   Bayonne, NJ 07002   (201)858-8444   Fax (201)858-4260

Ramasubramani, Anuradha, MD {1437119351} InfDis, IntrMd(93,INA04)<NJ-JRSYSHMC>
+ Drs. Ramasubramani & De Borja
98 James Street/Building F Suite 208   Edison, NJ 08820   (732)514-9624   Fax (732)377-3767

Ramasubramaniam, Nagarani, MD {1861679904} Pedtrc, IntrMd(04,NJ06)<NJ-UMDNJ>
+ Riverside ENT Pediatric Group
324 Palisade Avenue/2nd Floor   Jersey City, NJ 07307   (201)386-1400   Fax (201)386-2343
+ Riverside Medical Group
714 Tenth Street/Suite 2   Secaucus, NJ 07094   (201)386-1400   Fax (201)865-0015

Physicians by Name and Address

Ramaswamy, Kumar K., MD {1285694794} IntrMd(96,INA28)<NJ-SOMERSET>
+ Somerset Health Center
  40 Stirling Road/Suite 208   Watchung, NJ 07069   (908)757-1000   Fax (908)757-0564
+ Somerset Health Center
  425 Amwell Road/Suite 6   Hillsborough, NJ 08844   (908)757-1000   Fax (908)359-2068

Ramaswamy, Preethi V., MD {1750523379} Dermat, IntrMd(08,NH01)
+ Trokhan Dermatology, LLC.
  235 Closter Dock Road   Closter, NJ 07624   (201)767-1908   Fax (201)767-3097
+ Garden State Dermatology
  201 New Jersey 17/11th Floor   Rutherford, NJ 07070   (201)767-1908   Fax (201)623-2999

Ramaswamy, Sunil Rajanna, MD {1376906347} IntrMd
+ Cooper University Hospital Hospitalists
  One Cooper Plaza/Suite 222/Drrnce   Camden, NJ 08103   (856)342-3450   Fax (856)968-8418

Ramay, Mohammad Hanif, MD {1629024005} Psychy, PsyGrp(82,PAKI)<NJ-BERGNMC>
+ New Bridge Medical Center
  230 East Ridgewood Avenue/Psychiatry   Paramus, NJ 07652   (201)967-4000

Rambaran, Hayman Kumar, MD {1639295470} IntrMd, Pedtrc, Addctn(85,DOM19)<NJ-ESSEXCO>
+ Essex County Hospital Center
  204 Grove Avenue   Cedar Grove, NJ 07009   (973)571-2800

Rambaran, Naipaul, MD {1376508036} IntrMd, Pedtrc, FamMed(85,DOM19)<NJ-ESSEXCO>
+ Essex County Hospital Center
  204 Grove Avenue   Cedar Grove, NJ 07009   (973)571-2800   Fax (973)571-2995
+ Daughters of Miriam Center
  155 Hazel Street/PO Box 2698   Clifton, NJ 07011   (973)571-2800   Fax (973)253-5389

Ramchand, Maya, MD {1366654022} GenPrc, IntrMd(84)
+ Smithville Medical Associates
  48 South New York Road/Suite B-3   Galloway, NJ 08205   (609)404-0121   Fax (609)404-0131

Ramchandani, Kishore N., MD {1922053875} Gastrn, IntrMd(74,INA21)
+ May Street Surgi Center
  205 May Street/Suite 103   Edison, NJ 08837   (732)820-4566   Fax (732)661-9619
+ 616 Amboy Avenue
  Woodbridge, NJ 07095   (732)820-4566   Fax (732)750-9667

Ramchandani, Sanjay Mohan, MD {1225009640} ObsGyn(98,NJ05)
+ 37 Hemlock Court
  Hamilton, NJ 08619

Ramdas, Kumar, MD {1780663898} IntrMd(90,RUS61)<NJ-EASTORNG, NJ-NWRKBETH>
+ The Heart Center of The Oranges
  310 Central Avenue/Suite 102   East Orange, NJ 07018   (973)395-1550   Fax (973)395-1556
+ The Heart Center of The Oranges
  60 Vose Avenue   South Orange, NJ 07079   (973)763-5200
+ The Heart Center of The Oranges
  77 Main Street   West Orange, NJ 07018   (973)324-2090

Ramdial, Maria Janine, MD {1720241391} IntrMd(08,DC03)
+ Center for Adult Medicine & Preventive Care
  916-922 Main Avenue/Suite 1-A   Passaic, NJ 07055   (973)773-0334   Fax (973)773-0336

Ramesh, Shruti Chakrabarti, DO {1316257942} Pedtrc(07,PA77)
+ Drs. Gruenwald & Comandatore
  90 Millburn Avenue/Suite 101   Millburn, NJ 07041   (973)378-7990   Fax (973)378-7991

Rametta, Mark J., DO {1114141652} IntrMd(85,MO78)<NJ-CHILTON>
+ Ringwood Medical Associates PA
  52 Skyline Drive   Ringwood, NJ 07456   (973)962-6200   Fax (973)962-0046

Ramieri, Joseph, MD {1164470795} ObsGyn, Gyneco(69,NY09)<NJ-MORRISTN>
+ Morristown Obstetrics and Gynecology Associates
  20 Commerce Boulevard/Unit C   Succasunna, NJ 07876   (973)927-1188   Fax (973)927-7408

Ramirez, Elizabeth, MD {1285716829} ObsGyn, IntrMd(93,DOM02)<NJ-CHRIST, NJ-HACKNSK>
+ Jersey Womens Care Center
  435 Central Avenue   Jersey City, NJ 07307   (201)217-5600
+ 250 Central Avenue
  Jersey City, NJ 07306   (201)217-5600   Fax (201)659-8913
+ 213 Morningside Road
  Paramus, NJ 07307

Ramirez, Epifania L., MD {1013918325} IntrMd(72,PHIL)
+ 1119 Broad Street
  Newark, NJ 07114   (973)824-8226   Fax (973)824-3962

+ 515 Mount Prospect Avenue
  Newark, NJ 07104   (973)497-1933

Ramirez, Rey Natividad, MD {1295960698} SrgOrt
+ Cooper University Orthopedic Trauma
  3 Cooper Plaza/Suite 408   Camden, NJ 08103   (856)968-7845   Fax (856)968-8288

Ramirez, Roberto Hiram, MD {1275950321}<NJ-OVERLOOK>
+ Overlook Medical Center
  99 Beauvoir Avenue/PO Box 210   Summit, NJ 07902   (908)522-2000

Ramirez Chernikova, Anna, MD {1356660476} FamMed
+ Hoboken Integrated Family Medicine LLC
  109 Grand Street   Hoboken, NJ 07030   (201)795-1001   Fax (201)795-1009

Ramirez Pacheco, Luis A., MD {1275604563} PainMd, NrlgPain(75,SPA03)<NJ-GRYSTPSY>
+ 404 32nd Street/Suite 1
  Union City, NJ 07087   (201)758-7530   Fax (201)758-7529

Ramirez-Alexander, Rina M., MD {1881665842} IntrMd(84,NJ06)<NJ-MMHKEMBL, NJ-STCLRDEN>
+ Zufall Health Center
  18 West Blackwell Street   Dover, NJ 07801   (973)328-9100   Fax (973)328-6817

Ramirez-Espinosa, Luz Margarita, MD {1194829069} IntrMd, CdvDis, VasDis(97,COL03)
+ Bristol-Myers Squibb Co. - Occupational Health
  Route 206 & Provinceline Road   Princeton, NJ 08543   (609)252-6529   Fax (609)262-6701

Ramnanan, Terry K., MD {1316973902} Anesth, PainMd(81,JMA01)
+ Interventional Spine & Pain Treatment Center
  PO Box 604   Saddle River, NJ 07458   (973)949-5009   Fax (973)949-5010
  DRRAMNANAN@ISPTC.net

Ramnauth, Subhash C., MD {1043221310} SrgVas, Surgry(96,NC05)
+ Jersey Shore Surgery and Vein Center
  40 Bey Lea Road/Building B/Suite 202   Toms River, NJ 08755   (732)240-4466   Fax (732)240-4451

Ramos, David G.D., MD {1568437382} NnPnMd, Pedtrc(83,PHIL)<NJ-JRSYSHMC>
+ Meridian Medical Group - Faculty Practice
  61 Davis Avenue/Suite 1   Neptune, NJ 07753   (732)776-4860   Fax (732)776-4867
+ Meridian Medical Group - Faculty Practice
  61 Davis Avenue/Suite 1   Neptune, NJ 07753   (732)776-4860   Fax (732)776-4639

Ramos, Joseph, MD {1164442265} Anesth(81,MEXI)<NJ-MTNSIDE>
+ New Jersey Anesthesia Associates PC
  25B Vreeland Road/Suite110/PO Box 0037   Florham Park, NJ 07932   (973)660-9334   Fax (973)660-9732

Ramos, Leonor Vivas, MD {1760440986} FamMed(90,PHI30)<NJ-CHRIST>
+ Center for Family Health
  122-132 Clinton Street   Hoboken, NJ 07030   (201)418-3100   Fax (201)418-3148

Ramos, Maria A., MD {1558428680} IntrMd(88,WIND)<NJ-HACKNSK>
+ 147 Main Street/Suite 5
  Lodi, NJ 07644   Fax (973)777-1088

Ramos, Rafael C., MD {1295774974} Gastrn, IntrMd(67,ARGE)<NJ-PALISADE, NJ-HOLYNAME>
+ Drs. Ramos & Zapiach
  235 60th Street   West New York, NJ 07093   (201)854-4646   Fax (201)854-3203

Ramos, Rey Ferna Pedraza, MD {1124077219} FamMed(90,PHI30)
+ Center for Family Health
  122-132 Clinton Street   Hoboken, NJ 07030   (201)418-3100   Fax (201)418-3148

Ramos, Rosalinda J., MD {1891709598} IntrMd, CdvDis(66,PHI08)
+ Drs. Sanjay & Ramos
  216 Stelton Road/Suite 3B   Piscataway, NJ 08854   (732)752-0051   Fax (732)752-9668

Ramos Bondy, Beatrix Marie, MD {1790035939} CdvDis
+ Gagnon Cardiovasular Institute
  100 Madison Avenue/Level C   Morristown, NJ 07962   (973)971-7416   Fax (973)401-2470

Ramos Velez, Jonathan, MD {1811200199}
+ 330 West Jersey Street/Apt 4c
  Elizabeth, NJ 07202   (917)971-5363
  jorave2014@gmail.com

Ramos-Garcia, Maria D., MD {1477781185}
+ 150 Nathan Boulevard
  Parlin, NJ 08859

Ramos-Genvino, Elizabeth, MD {1699833533} FamMed(96,NJ05)<NJ-MTNSIDE>
+ Summit Medical Group
  48-50 Fairfield Street   Montclair, NJ 07042   (973)744-8511   Fax (973)744-6356

Rampal, Sharan, MD {1578651675} Nrolgy(73,INDI)
+ 60 Landis Avenue
  Bridgeton, NJ 08302   (856)455-6711   Fax (856)455-1979

Rampertab, Saroja Devi, MD {1215995451} Gastrn, IntrMd(98,NY01)<NJ-RWJUBRUN>
+ RWJ Gastro & Hepatology
  125 Paterson Street/CAB 5100B   New Brunswick, NJ 08901   (732)235-7784   Fax (732)235-7792
+ UH- RWJ Medical School
  One Robert Wood Johnson Place/MEB 478   New Brunswick, NJ 08903   (732)235-5600

Ramprasad, Arjun, MD {1992125413} SprtMd
+ Tatem Brown Family Practice
  2225 East Evesham Road/Suite 101   Voorhees, NJ 08043   (856)795-4330   Fax (856)325-3704

Ramprasad, Vatsala, MD {1306936604} Pedtrc, PulDis, PedPul(75,INA2X)<NJ-COOPRUMC>
+ Cooper Peds/Children's Regional Ctr
  3 Cooper Plaza/Suite 200   Camden, NJ 08103   (856)342-2472   Fax (856)368-8297

Ramsetty, Sabena Karina, MD {1659553394} IntrMd(04,NY19)
+ Leonia Medical Associates, P.A.
  25 Rockwood Place/Suite 120   Englewood, NJ 07631   (201)568-3335   Fax (201)568-2450

Ramsey, Matthew Lee, MD {1376571877} SrgOrt(90,NY08)<NJ-ATLANTHS>
+ Rothman Institute - Voorhees
  443 Laurel Oak Road   Voorhees, NJ 08043   (856)821-6360

Ramundo, Giovanni B., MD {1679671481} Anesth(90,PA14)<NJ-STBARNMC>
+ St. Barnabas Medical Center
  94 Old Short Hills Road/Anesth   Livingston, NJ 07039   (973)322-5000
+ Short Hills Surgery Center
  187 Millburn Avenue/Suite 101   Millburn, NJ 07041   (973)322-5000   Fax (973)671-0557

Ramzy, Ayman H., MD {1881700417} Psychy(63,EGYP)<NJ-UNVMCPRN>
+ 154 Tamarack Circle
  Skillman, NJ 08558   (609)924-5250   Fax (609)924-8113
  Ramzy154@aol.com
+ Princeton House Behavioral Health - Princeton
  905 Herrontown Road/Psychiatry   Princeton, NJ 08540   (609)924-5250   Fax (609)497-3370
+ Princeton Center for Eating Disorders
  One Plainsboro Road   Plainsboror, NJ 08558   (609)853-7575

Rana, Badal D., DO {1013365931} Psychy
+ University Hospital-SOM Department of Psychiatry
  2250 Chapel Avenue West/Suite 100   Cherry Hill, NJ 08002   (856)482-9000   Fax (856)482-1159

Rana, Chirag P., MD {1902216419}
+ 26 Wonham Street
  Clifton, NJ 07013   (973)807-8945

Rana, Haris Ishaque, MD {1013125053} CritCr, PulCCr, IntrMd(03,DMN01)
+ St. Peter's University Hospital
  254 Easton Avenue/CaresBldg/Fl4   New Brunswick, NJ 08901   (732)745-8564   Fax (732)745-9156

Rana, Jagpal, MD {1265401061} MtFtMd, ObsGyn(74,INA6Z)<NJ-JFKMED, NJ-NWRKBETH>
+ Perinatal Institute in South Plainfield
  2201 Park Avenue   South Plainfield, NJ 07080   (908)668-8800   Fax (908)668-9469

Rana, Jiten, MD {1518608972} IntrMd, CdvDis(96,PA07)
+ Wachspress & Rainear Cardiology Associates PA
  1076 East Chestnut Avenue   Vineland, NJ 08360   (856)692-7979   Fax (856)794-9479

Rana, Kirtida Dinesh, MD {1013121573} Anesth(04,GRN01)<NJ-STJOSHOS>
+ Morris Anesthesia Group, PA
  3799 Route 46/Suite 211   Parsippany, NJ 07054   (973)335-1122   Fax (973)335-1448

Rana, Meenakshi G., MD {1265747208} IntrMd
+ 11 Pine Street/Apt 236
  Montclair, NJ 07042

Rana, Mukti, MD {1992847024} Pedtrc, PedInf(91,INA68)
+ Lakewood Pediatric Associates
  101 Prospect Street/Suite 112   Lakewood, NJ 08701   (732)363-1424   Fax (732)370-0714

Rana, Najmul, MD {1477569036} IntrMd, CritCr, PulCCr(86,PAK11)
+ Summit Medical Group
  6 Brighton Road/2 FL   Clifton, NJ 07012   (973)777-7911   Fax (973)777-5403
+ Lincoln Park Care Center
  499 Pinebrook Road   Lincoln Park, NJ 07035   (973)777-7911   Fax (973)633-8747
+ Haq Rana, Najm-Ul
  200 Gregory Avenue   Passaic, NJ 07012   (973)473-1970   Fax (973)594-1708

Rana, Nareshkumar G., MD {1336134253} IntrMd(81,INA01)<NJ-CLARMAAS, NJ-MTNSIDE>
  + 733 Bloomfield Avenue
    Bloomfield, NJ 07003   (201)743-7707   Fax (973)743-7808
Rana, Nilesh C., MD {1083660443} IntrMd, Gastrn(70,INDI)<NJ-CHSFULD, NJ-CAPITLHS>
  + Drs. Rana & Roowala
    40 Fuld Street/Suite 302   Trenton, NJ 08638   (609)393-0067   Fax (609)393-4943
Rana, Nimra H., MD {1831392422} IntrMd(98,PAK15)<NJ-COOPRUMC>
  + Cooper University Hospital
    One Cooper Plaza/Hospitalist   Camden, NJ 08103   (856)342-3150   Fax (856)968-8418
Rana, Ramneek, MD {1548680192} ObsGyn
  + Penn Medicine at Cherry Hill
    409 Route 70 East/2nd Floor   Cherry Hill, NJ 08034   (856)795-0587
Rana, Ranjit C., MD {1588617823} IntrMd, IntHos(79,INDI)<NJ-VALLEY, NJ-MEADWLND>
  + The Valley Hospital
    223 North Van Dien Avenue   Ridgewood, NJ 07450   (201)447-8000
Rana, Sanah Ehsan, MD {1013303171} IntrMd<NJ-RIVERVW>
  + Riverview Medical Center
    1 Riverview Plaza   Red Bank, NJ 07701   (732)741-2700
Rana, Sohail Anjum, MD {1679516546} PsyCAd, Psychy(88,PAK01)<NJ-ANCPSYCH>
  + Ancora Psychiatric Hospital
    301 Spring Garden Road   Hammonton, NJ 08037   (609)561-1700   Fax (609)567-7272
Rana, Swetha Basani, MD {1316369820} IntrMd<NJ-STBARNMC>
  + RWJ University Hospital New Brunswick
    One Robert Wood Johnson Place   New Brunswick, NJ 08901   (732)235-7670   Fax (732)235-8313
Rana, Yebarna S., MD {1053399170} CdvDis, IntrMd(72,INA30)
  + 660 Commons Way/Building l
    Toms River, NJ 08755   (732)244-1970
Rana-Mukkavilli, Gopi, MD {1962551242} IntrMd(83,TN07)<NY-NYUTISCH, NY-BLVUENYU>
  + 1 Woodland Court
    West Windsor, NJ 08550   (609)897-9831
    gopirana@pol.net
Ranalli, Jeffery A., DO {1639120462} IntrMd(94,PA77)<NJ-KENEDYHS, NJ-VIRTUAHS>
  + Advocare Sicklerville Internal Medicine Associates
    205 East Laurel Road/1 FL   Stratford, NJ 08084   (856)227-6575   Fax (856)374-9495
  + 1702 Sagemore Drive
    Marlton, NJ 08053
Ranasinghe Rodrigo, Nimalie, MD {1558649681} ObsGyn
  + Rodrigo, Nimalie
    13108 Bainbridge Way   Freehold, NJ 07728   (917)209-2471
    drnimalie@yahoo.com
Ranawat, Anil S., MD {1568653947} SrgOrt(01,NY20)
  + HSS Paramus Outpatient Center
    140 East Ridgewood Avenue/Suite 175-S   Paramus, NJ 07652   (201)796-2255   Fax (201)796-3711
Rand, Victoria Elena, MD {1275743510} IntrMd(91,NY20)
  + Chambers Center
    435 South Street/Suite 160   Morristown, NJ 07960   (973)971-6301
Randall, Jennifer F., MD {1831425180} Gastrn, IntrMd
  + Bergen Medical Associates
    466 Old Hook Road/Suite 1   Emerson, NJ 07630   (201)967-8221   Fax (201)967-0340
  + Bergen Medical Associates
    1 West Ridgewood Avenue/Suite 301   Paramus, NJ 07652   (201)967-8221   Fax (201)445-4296
Randall, Tanya, MD {1932173796} Anesth(92,NY01)<NY-MNTF-MOSE>
  + New Jersey Ambulatory Anesthesia Consultants, LLC
    55 Schanck Road/Suite 8-A   Freehold, NJ 07728   (732)431-9544   Fax (732)431-9313
Randazzo, Ciro Giuseppe, MD {1114116464} SrgNro(03,NJ06)
  + IGEA Brain & Spine
    1057 Commerce Avenue   Union, NJ 07083   (908)688-8800   Fax (908)688-2377
Randazzo, Domenick N., MD {1700862919} IntrMd, CdvDis(90,MA07)<NJ-MORRISTN, NJ-SOMERSET>
  + Atlantic Cardiology Group LLP
    8 Tempe Wick Road   Mendham, NJ 07945   (973)543-2288   Fax (973)543-0637
  + Atlantic Cardiology Group LLP
    95 Madison Avenue/Suite 300   Morristown, NJ 07960   (973)543-2288   Fax (973)682-9494
Randazzo, Jean P., MD {1033215892} IntrMd(90,MA07)<NJ-MORRISTN>
  + Internal Medicine of Morristown
    95 Madison Avenue/Suite A-00   Morristown, NJ 07960   (973)538-1388   Fax (973)538-9501

Randazzo, Vincent T., MD {1407838691} IntrMd(69,PA02)
  + Drs. Randazzo and Tomaino
    225 State Route 35/Suite 102B   Red Bank, NJ 07701   (732)530-3433   Fax (732)758-1953
Randhawa, Preet Mohan Singh, MD {1801816251} IntrMd, CdvDis, IntCrd(92,INDI)<NJ-UMDNJ, NJ-TRINIWSC>
  + NJ Heart/Linden Office
    520 North Wood Avenue   Linden, NJ 07036   (908)354-8900   Fax (908)587-1901
  + NJ Heart/Elizabeth Office
    240 Williamson Street/Suite 402-406   Elizabeth, NJ 07202   (908)354-8900   Fax (908)354-0007
  + Care Station Medical Group
    456 Prospect Avenue   West Orange, NJ 07036   (973)731-6767   Fax (973)731-9881
Randhawa, Smita Devidas, MD {1609971118} FamMed, IntrMd(96,NY03)
  + Cornerstone Family Practice
    9100 Wescott Drive/Suite 103   Flemington, NJ 08822   (908)237-6910   Fax (908)237-6919
Randle, Troy L., DO {1710187513} CdvDis, IntrMd(03,NJ75)
  + LMA CardioThoracic Surgical Services
    1 Brace Road/Suite C   Cherry Hill, NJ 08034   (856)470-9029   Fax (856)796-9391
  + South Jersey Heart Group
    3001 Chapel Avenue/Suite 101   Cherry Hill, NJ 08002   (856)470-9029   Fax (856)482-7170
Randolph, Robert Styles, MD {1508011552} PsyCAd(95,NJ05)<NJ-UNIVBHC>
  + 8 Sunflower Road
    Somerset, NJ 08873   (732)545-6114   Fax (609)298-2554
Rane, Sunanda D., MD {1053348201} Pedtrc(75,INDI)<NJ-WOODBRDG>
  + Woodbridge Developmental Center
    Rahway Avenue/PO Box 189   Woodbridge, NJ 07095   (732)499-5500   Fax (732)499-5787
    dinurane@aol.com
Ranelle, Robert George, DO {1245297399} SrgOrt, IntrMd(82,TX17)
  + Garden State Orthopedics & Sports Medicine
    455 Route 70 West   Cherry Hill, NJ 08002   (609)616-2999   Fax (856)616-1439
Rangam, Tsui H., MD {1245256437} EmrgMd(72,INDI)<NJ-ACMCITY, NJ-ACMCMAIN>
  + AtlantiCare Regional Medical Center/City Campus
    1925 Pacific Avenue/EmergMed   Atlantic City, NJ 08401   (609)345-4000
  + AtlantiCare Regional Med Ctr/Mainland
    65 West Jimmie Leeds Road   Pomona, NJ 08240   (609)652-1000
Ranganathan Chetty, Nirmala, MD {1407022148} IntrMd(02,INA96)
  + 37 Slayback Drive
    Princeton, NJ 08550   (201)281-0601
Rangaraj, Narsimha R., MD {1861402638} IntrMd, IntHos(92,INA5B)<NJ-ACMCITY, NJ-ACMCMAIN>
  + AtlantiCare Regional Medical Center/City Campus
    1925 Pacific Avenue/InternalMed   Atlantic City, NJ 08401   (609)345-4000
Rangaraj, Padmaja, MD {1396990214} IntrMd(91,INA5B)<NJ-SHOREMEM>
  + Shore Memorial Hospital
    1 East New York Avenue/Internal Med   Somers Point, NJ 08244   (609)653-3500   Fax (609)926-4311
Rangasamy, Ajantha, MD {1194882613} IntrMd, Nephro(96,INA81)
  + 256 Prospect Avenue
    Bayonne, NJ 07002
Rangel, Emile I., MD {1598752081} IntrMd(86,NY46)
  + 4501 Palisade Avenue/Apt 10b
    Union City, NJ 07087
Ranginwala, Masood Ahmed, DO {1861521726} EmrgMd(03,NY75)<CT-STAMFDH>
  + The Valley Hospital
    223 North Van Dien Avenue   Ridgewood, NJ 07450   (201)447-8000
Rangwala, Anis F., MD {1992775928} PthACl, Hemato(71,INA69)<NJ-OCEANMC, NJ-JRSYSHMC>
  + Ocean Medical Center
    425 Jack Martin Boulevard/Path   Brick, NJ 08723   (732)840-2200   Fax (732)458-3851
Rangwalla-Malickel, Inciya, DO {1952491250} IntrMd, IntHos(01,FL75)<NJ-COOPRUMC>
  + Cooper University Hospital
    One Cooper Plaza/Dorrance 222   Camden, NJ 08103   (856)342-2000
  + Cooper University Medical Center/Camden
    3 Cooper Plaza   Camden, NJ 08103   (856)342-2000
Ranieri, Joseph N., DO {1851464143} FamMed(91,PA77)<NJ-COOPRUMC>
  + Cooper Physicians Washington Township
    1 Plaza Drive/Suite 103/Bunker Hill Pl   Sewell, NJ 08080

    (856)270-4080   Fax (856)270-4085
Ranieri, William F., DO {1144292665} Psychy(66,PA77)<NJ-KMHCHRRY, NJ-KMHSTRAT>
  + AtlantiCare Behavioral Health/Seaside Counseling
    2021 New Road/Suite 15   Linwood, NJ 08221   (609)927-4200
Ranjini, Mary P., MD {1740292754} IntrMd(74,INA94)<NJ-STPETER>
  + St. Peter's University Hospital
    254 Easton Avenue   New Brunswick, NJ 08901   (732)745-8600   Fax (732)296-8564
Rankin, Laura, MD {1659774255} ObsGyn
  + Rutgers- New Jersey Medical School
    185 South Orange Avenue/E 105   Newark, NJ 07103   (973)972-3574
Ranley, Robert L., MD {1235164013} RadDia, Radiol(70,NJ05)<NJ-NWTNMEM>
  + Sparta Health and Wellness Center
    89 Sparta Avenue/Suite 120   Sparta, NJ 07871   (973)729-0002   Fax (973)729-1085
  + Image Care Centers
    222 High Street/Suite 101   Newton, NJ 07860   (973)729-0002   Fax (973)383-2774
  + Radiologic Associates of Northwest New Jersey
    212 Route 94   Vernon, NJ 07871   (973)827-1961
Ransom, Raymond W., MD {1265573331} Psychy, PsyAdd(67,DC03)
  + 680 Broadway
    Paterson, NJ 07514   (973)970-4707   Fax (973)341-1119
    vihallie@aol.com
  + Paterson Counseling Center
    319-321 Main Street/Psychiatry   Paterson, NJ 07505   (973)970-4707   Fax (973)523-5116
Ranzini, Angela C., MD {1609832575} MtFtMd, ObsGyn(87,VA04)<NJ-STPETER>
  + St. Peter's Family Health
    123 How Lane   New Brunswick, NJ 08901   (732)745-8600   Fax (732)729-0869
  + St. Peter's University Hospital
    254 Easton Avenue/Ob/Gyn   New Brunswick, NJ 08901   (732)745-8600   Fax (732)249-5729
Rao, Anupama J., MD {1417918392} IntrMd(95,INA2X)
  + Primary Care & Preventive Medicine, P.A.
    1479 Route 539/Suite 1 B   Little Egg Harbor, NJ 08087   (609)294-5000   Fax (609)294-5115
Rao, Aruna, MD {1508821489} IntrMd, Grtrcs, EmrgMd(76,INDI)<NJ-STPETER, NJ-RWJUBRUN>
  + 65 Brunswick Woods Drive
    East Brunswick, NJ 08816   (732)238-0543   Fax (732)613-8688
  + University Urgi Care
    1323 Highway 27/Suite 2100   Somerset, NJ 08873   (732)238-0543   Fax (732)412-3123
Rao, Asha Vijendran, MD {1184691255} IntrMd, Nephro(88,INA69)
  + Tinton Falls Community Based Outpatient Clinic
    55 North Gilbert Street   Tinton Falls, NJ 07701   (732)842-4751
Rao, Babar Khan, MD {1447275904} Dermat, PthDrm(83,PAK20)
  + The American Skin and Cancer Center
    25 First Avenue/Suite 113   Atlantic Highlands, NJ 07716   (732)872-2007
  + Robert Wood Johnson Medical Group-Dermatology
    1 World's Fair Drive/Suite 2400   Somerset, NJ 08873   (732)872-2007   Fax (732)235-7117
Rao, Bhavani P., MD {1790887909} Nephro, IntrMd(91,INDI)
  + 904 Oak Tree Road/Suite C
    South Plainfield, NJ 07080   (908)757-6655   Fax (908)757-6653
Rao, Chitharanjan Vithal, MD {1659306835} Nrolgy, ClNrPh(86,INA67)
  + Lawrenceville Neurology Center, PA
    3131 Princeton Pike   Lawrenceville, NJ 08648   (609)896-1701   Fax (609)896-3735
Rao, Gautami Kondamodi, MD {1083795264} Nrolgy, Eplpsy(99,INA96)
  + Northeast Regional Epilepsy Group
    20 Prospect Avenue/Suite 800   Hackensack, NJ 07601   (201)343-6676   Fax (201)343-6689
Rao, Gunjan Pradhan, MD {1841392800} Pedtrc, IntrMd(98,INA69)
  + North Jersey Pediatrics
    17-10 Fair Lawn Avenue   Fair Lawn, NJ 07410   (201)794-8585   Fax (201)703-9889
Rao, Harini, MD {1245486141}<NJ-STJOSHOS>
  + St. Joseph's Regional Medical Center
    703 Main Street   Paterson, NJ 07503   (973)754-2000
Rao, Harshit S., MD {1831205053} PulDis, IntrMd(02,NJ06)<NJ-RWJUBRUN>
  + RWJ University Hospital New Brunswick
    One Robert Wood Johnson Place   New Brunswick, NJ 08901   (732)235-7840

Physicians by Name and Address

Rao, Jayanti Juluru, MD {1528146669} AlgyImmn, IntrMd(01,NJ05)
+ Princeton Allergy & Asthma Associates, P.A.
24 Vreeland Drive   Skillman, NJ 08558   (609)921-2202   Fax (609)924-1468

Rao, Juluru P., MD {1831270990} SrgOrt(68,INDI)
+ 1039 Avenue C
Bayonne, NJ 07002   (201)858-3811   Fax (201)858-2879

Rao, Kavya Madupu, MD {1609139799} NnPnMd, Pedtrc(11,ANT02)<NY-STATNRTH>
+ 158 Wayne Street/Unit 101a
Jersey City, NJ 07302   (917)855-9018
rao.kavya@gmail.com

Rao, Kiran Venkat, MD {1487801403} Gastrn, IntrMd(03,INA28)
+ Premier Health Associates
532 Lafayette Road/Suite 100   Sparta, NJ 07871   (973)383-3730   Fax (973)383-2285

Rao, Maithili V., MD {1366451098} OncHem(99,INA67)
+ Advanced Care Hematology & Oncology Associates
385 Morris Avenue/Suite 100   Springfield, NJ 07081   (973)379-2111   Fax (973)379-2807

Rao, Malini Bhagavathi, MD {1649456005} Anesth(03,INA9Z)<NJ-RWJUBRUN>
+ RWJ University Hospital New Brunswick
One Robert Wood Johnson Place   New Brunswick, NJ 08901   (732)937-8841   Fax (732)418-8492

Rao, Megha N., MD {1629368097} IntrMd<NJ-STPETER>
+ St. Peter's University Hospital
254 Easton Avenue   New Brunswick, NJ 08901   (732)745-8600

Rao, Niranjan V., MD {1851350615} SrgVas, Surgry(76,INA9C)<NJ-STPETER>
+ Central Jersey Surgical Specialists
78 Easton Avenue   New Brunswick, NJ 08901   (732)249-0360   Fax (732)249-0035
+ Cares Surgicenter, LLC.
240 Easton Avenue   New Brunswick, NJ 08901   (732)249-0360   Fax (732)296-8677

Rao, Padmarekha, MD {1093851917} Nrolgy(90,INA04)<NJ-BAYSHORE>
+ 14 Woodard Drive/Suite A
Old Bridge, NJ 08857   (732)360-2888

Rao, Parth Rajeshkumar, MD {1922365568} OncHem
+ St. Barnabas Cancer Center
94 Old Short Hills Road/Suite 1   Livingston, NJ 07039   (973)322-6450

Rao, Pratibha Prasanna, MD {1346231263} IntrMd(95,INA35)<NJ-VALLEY>
+ The Valley Hospital
223 North Van Dien Avenue/IntMed   Ridgewood, NJ 07450   (201)447-8000

Rao, Rajesh Ramchandra, MD {1003842022} PhysMd(91,INA67)<NJ-MMHKEMBL, NJ-MORRISTN>
+ Associates in Rehabilitation Medicine
95 Mount Kemble Avenue   Morristown, NJ 07960   (973)267-2293   Fax (973)226-3144
+ Summit Medical Group
34 Mountain Boulevard/Building B   Warren, NJ 07059   (973)267-2293   Fax (908)769-8927

Rao, Sanjay D., MD {1093851040}
+ 11 Norwich Drive
Lebanon, NJ 08833

Rao, Savitha, MD {1780084590} Psychy<NJ-UNIVBHC>
+ University Behavioral Health Care
671 Hoes Lane/PO Box 1392   Piscataway, NJ 08855   (732)235-4433

Rao, Sheila Yvonne, MD {1831197599} Anesth(94,NJ06)<NJ-STJOSHOS, NJ-WAYNEGEN>
+ St. Joseph's Regional Medical Center Anesthesia
703 Main Street   Paterson, NJ 07503   (973)754-2323   Fax (973)977-9455

Rao, Veena, MD {1841633864} Anesth
+ Trenton Anesthesiology Associates, PA
One Capital Way/Second Floor   Pennington, NJ 08534   (609)396-4700   Fax (609)396-4900

Rao, Vidya J., MD {1477609873} PhysMd(71,INDI)<NJ-BAYSHORE>
+ 25 Winding Ridge Way
Warren, NJ 07059   (732)868-0589

Rao, Vikas Yallapragada, MD {1932349651} Nrolgy
+ Global Neuroscience Institute
750 Brunswick Avenue   Trenton, NJ 08638   (713)662-2940
vikas.rao.md@gmail.com

Rao, Vilayannur Raja Ramachandra, MD {1093742025} Psychy(76,INA4D)<NJ-UNIVBHC>
+ Mercer Behavioral Health Center LLC
1700 Whitehorse Mercerville Rd/Suite 3   Trenton, NJ 08619   (609)689-0800   Fax (609)689-0567

Raoof, Natalia, MD {1871761403} IntrMd, InfDis
+ Raritan Bay Infectious Disease Consultants
3 Hospital Plaza/Suite 208   Old Bridge, NJ 08857   (732)360-2700   Fax (732)360-2703

+ ID Associates PA/dba ID Care
105 Raider Boulevard/Suite 101   Hillsborough, NJ 08844   (732)360-2700   Fax (908)281-0940

Raoof, Nazar, MD {1194742098} IntrMd, InfDis(03,NY47)
+ Raritan Bay Infectious Disease Consultants
3 Hospital Plaza/Suite 208   Old Bridge, NJ 08857   (732)360-2700   Fax (732)360-2703

Raoof, Sidra, MD {1770934432} IntrMd
+ University Medical Group - General Internal Medicine
125 Paterson Street/Suite 5100A   New Brunswick, NJ 08903   (732)235-8909   Fax (732)235-7238

Raouf, Medhat M., MD {1063464246} IntrMd(79,EGYP)<NJ-CHILTON, NJ-VALLEY>
+ Drs. Raouf and Balboul
55 Skyline Drive/Suite 204   Ringwood, NJ 07456   (973)962-4000   Fax (973)962-0640
+ Drs. Raouf and Balboul
508 Hamburg Turnpike/Suite 201   Wayne, NJ 07470   (973)962-4000   Fax (973)942-1360

Rapacon, Magdaleno R., MD {1144212937} Anesth, PedAne(69,PHIL)<NJ-CHILTON>
+ Chilton Medical Center
97 West Parkway/Anesthesiology   Pompton Plains, NJ 07444   (973)831-5000

Rapaport, Jeffrey A., MD {1629161989} Dermat, SrgDer(78,GA05)<NJ-ENGLWOOD, NJ-HOLYNAME>
+ Cosmetic Skin & Surgery Center
333 Sylvan Avenue/Suite 207   Englewood, NJ 07632   (201)227-1567   Fax (201)227-8313

Raphael, Stephen D., MD {1477599702} IntrMd(80,MEXI)<NJ-VIRTVOOR>
+ 303 Haddonfield Berlin Road
Voorhees, NJ 08043   (856)429-6267   Fax (856)429-2445

Rapisarda, Alexander F., MD {1811994692} Gastrn, IntrMd(90,NY03)<NJ-STPETER, NJ-RWJUBRUN>
+ Digestive Disease Center of New Jersey, LLC
33 Clyde Road/Suite 102   Somerset, NJ 08873   (732)873-9200   Fax (732)873-1699
+ Digestive Disease Center of New Jersey, LLC
810 Ryders Lane   East Brunswick, NJ 08816   (732)873-9200   Fax (732)257-0229
+ Cares Surgicenter, LLC.
240 Easton Avenue   New Brunswick, NJ 08873   (732)565-5400   Fax (732)296-8677

Rapp, Brian A., DO {1841591906}<NJ-MORRISTN>
+ Morristown Medical Center
100 Madison Avenue   Morristown, NJ 07962   (973)971-7926

Rapp, Rachel V., MD {1568788354} Pedtrc
+ Mercer County Pediatrics
2113 Klockner Road   Trenton, NJ 08690   (609)586-7887   Fax (609)586-1198

Rappai, James K., MD {1902840556} IntrMd, EmrgMd(81,INDI)<NY-CMCSTVSI>
+ JFK Medical Center
65 James Street   Edison, NJ 08820   (732)321-7605

Rappaport, Brandi Joy, MD {1609835248} FamMed(02,NJ06)<NJ-VIRTMHBC>
+ Lourdes Medical Associates
501 Delaware Avenue/Suite 1   Roebling, NJ 08554   (609)291-5560   Fax (609)499-0435

Rappaport, Delia I., MD {1073545521} Pedtrc(84,ROMA)<NJ-HACKNSK, NJ-VALLEY>
+ Hackensack Bergen Pediatrics
385 Prospect Avenue/Suite 210   Hackensack, NJ 07601   (551)996-9160   Fax (201)487-3009

Rappaport, Liviu I., MD {1629013933} PulDis, IntrMd(84,ROM09)<NJ-CHILTON>
+ Pulmonary Medicine of Wayne
508 Hamburg Turnpike/Suite 202   Wayne, NJ 07470   (973)956-1404   Fax (973)956-1646

Rasa, David V., MD {1437198561} FamMed(81,MEXI)<NJ-STJOSHOS, NJ-WAYNEGEN>
+ Wayne Urgent and Primary Care
246 Hamburg Turnpike/Suite 205   Wayne, NJ 07470   (973)389-1800   Fax (973)636-2734

Raser, Keith A., MD {1881885804} Psychy(86,IL06)
+ 100 Straube Center Boulevard
Pennington, NJ 08534

Rasheed, Fouad Y., MD {1992765226} Pedtrc(75,EGYP)<NJ-HACKNSK>
+ Future Pediatric Group Inc.
240 North 8th Street   Prospect Park, NJ 07508   (973)942-2131   Fax (973)942-2131
futurepediatric2@gmail.com
+ Future Pediatric Group Inc.
1414 Main Street   Clifton, NJ 07011   (973)942-2131   Fax (973)772-6899

Rasheed, Sammar, MD {1669718631} IntrMd, IntHos(06,PAK12)
+ Cooper University Hospital
One Cooper Plaza/Hospitalist   Camden, NJ 08103   (856)342-2000

Rasheed, Syed Adil, MD {1669511036} Psychy(87,PAK12)
+ 506 Hamburg Turnpike/Suite 209
Wayne, NJ 07470   (973)720-9300
+ 12 North State Route 17
Paramus, NJ 07652   (973)720-9300   Fax (201)773-6739

Rashid, Iqbal, MD {1922133040} Anesth(86,PAK20)<NJ-RBAYPERT>
+ Raritan Bay Medical Center/Perth Amboy Division
530 New Brunswick Avenue/Anesth   Perth Amboy, NJ 08861   (732)442-3700

Rashid, Mamoona, MD {1326330861}<NJ-STCLRDOV>
+ St. Clare's Hospital-Dover
400 West Blackwell Street   Dover, NJ 07801   (973)989-3085
monasohail@gmail.com

Rashid, Parveen, MD {1326074022} ObsGyn(71,PAKI)<NJ-VIRTMHBC>
+ Pinelands Obstetrics and Gynecology
1617 Route 38   Mount Holly, NJ 08060   (609)654-4449   Fax (609)261-8622

Rashid, Salman, MD {1649225160} RadDia(95,PAK11)<NJ-MONMOUTH>
+ Shrewsbury Diagnostic Imaging, Inc.
1131 Broad Street/Suite 110   Shrewsbury, NJ 07702   (732)578-9640   Fax (732)578-9650

Rashid, Shahzad, DO {1699967232} PsyGrt, Psychy, IntrMd(02,NJ75)
+ Federal Correctional Institution
5756 Hartford Road   Fort Dix, NJ 08640   (609)723-1100

Rashid, Tasneem J., MD {1205947926} IntrMd, MedOnc, OncHem(80,INA29)
+ 50 Union Avenue
Irvington, NJ 07111   (973)374-4100
+ 2780 Morris Avenue
Union, NJ 07083   (908)687-8741

Rasin, Grigory S., MD {1699800912} Psychy(71,UKRA)
+ Drs. Rasin and Ivanov
2143 Morris Avenue/Suite 3   Union, NJ 07083   (908)686-4145   Fax (908)851-2128

Raska, Anna M.L., MD {1821060377} IntrMd(92,MD07)<NJ-MORRISTN>
+ Internal Medicine Faculty Associates
435 South Street/Suite 210   Morristown, NJ 07960   (973)971-7165   Fax (973)290-7675

Raska, Karel, MD {1740288752} CdvDis(89,MA01)<NJ-MORRISTN>
+ Morristown Cardiology Associates, P.A.
435 South Street/Suite 100   Morristown, NJ 07960   (973)267-3944   Fax (973)455-0399

Raskin, Adam Brett, MD {1225264914} CdvDis
+ Cross Country Cardiology
103 River Road/2nd Floor   Edgewater, NJ 07020   (201)941-8100   Fax (201)941-2899

Raskin, Jeffrey M., MD {1508858879} Gastrn, IntrMd(87,NJ05)<NJ-CHRIST, NJ-ENGLWOOD>
+ Gastroenterology Medical Associates PA
9223 Kennedy Boulevard/Suite D   North Bergen, NJ 07047   (201)868-2849   Fax (201)868-4190
+ Gastroenterology Medical Associates PA
142 Palisades Avenue/Suite 201   Jersey City, NJ 07307   (201)868-2849   Fax (201)792-7812

Raskin, Yosef, MD {1336169663} IntrMd(80,AZE01)
+ 38 Benjamin Ruch Lane
Princeton, NJ 08540

Raslan, Ashraf, MD {1023375649}
+ 57 Sip Avenue/Apt Pha
Jersey City, NJ 07306   (347)944-3960
ashraslan@hotmail.com

Rasmussen, Jeffrey Frank, MD {1609188200}
+ 1 Richmond Street/Apt 1030
New Brunswick, NJ 08901

Raso, Carl L., MD {1306934195} Gastrn, IntrMd(82,GRN01)
+ Ocean Endosurgery Center
129 Route 37 West   Toms River, NJ 08755   (732)606-4440   Fax (732)797-3963

Rasool, Altaf Tahir, MD {1053566257} IntrMd, IntHos<NY-STATNRTH>
+ RWJ University Hospital New Brunswick
One Robert Wood Johnson Place   New Brunswick, NJ 08901   (732)235-8909   Fax (732)235-7238

Rassier, Charles Edgar, Jr., MD {1902025794} Ophthl(01,PA13)<NJ-STBARNMC>
+ Eye Clinic PA
155 Jefferson Street   Newark, NJ 07105   (973)622-2020   Fax (973)817-8666
+ Eye Clinic PA
2333 Morris Avenue/Suite D111   Union, NJ 07083   (973)622-2020   Fax (908)810-9046

Rastgar, Khosrow, MD {1881694909} PthAcl, PthDrm, PthCln(70,IRA09)<NJ-ACMCITY, NJ-ACMCMAIN>
+ AtlantiCare Regional Medical Center/City Campus
1925 Pacific Avenue/Path   Atlantic City, NJ 08401   (609)441-8063   Fax (609)441-2107

Rastogi, Abhijeet A., MD {1114089471} Anesth
+ Virtua Pain and Spine Specialists
404 Creek Crossing Boulevard   Hainesport, NJ 08036   (609)845-3988

Rastogi, Raghav, MD {1780985267}
+ 123 Highland Avenue
Glen Ridge, NJ 07028   (973)748-0678   Fax (973)748-2808

Rastogi, Rishi V., MD {1871681759} EnDbMt, IntrMd(78,INDI)
+ 8 North White Horse Pike/Suite 101
Hammonton, NJ 08037   (609)704-9100

Rastogi, Sadhna, MD {1699714436} IntrMd, InfDis(82,INDI)<NJ-PALISADE, NJ-MEADWLND>
+ Rastogi Medical Associates
524 43rd Street   Union City, NJ 07087   (201)617-8338   Fax (201)868-3235
+ Rastogi Medical Associates
8306 Kennedy Boulevard   North Bergen, NJ 07047   (201)617-8338   Fax (201)868-3235

Rastogi, Sarita, MD {1073501094} Grtrcs, IntrMd(93,INDI)<NJ-HACKNSK>
+ 140 Summit Avenue
Hackensack, NJ 07601   (201)489-8567   Fax (201)489-8565

Rastogi, Surender M., MD {1891741344} IntrMd(79,INDI)<NJ-PALISADE, NJ-CHRIST>
+ Rastogi Medical Associates
8306 Kennedy Boulevard   North Bergen, NJ 07047   (201)868-1333   Fax (201)868-3235
Srastogi@aol.com
+ Rastogi Medical Associates
524 43rd Street   Union City, NJ 07087   (201)868-1333   Fax (201)868-3235

Rastogi, Vijay, MD {1407874886} Surgry(81,INA29)<NJ-WARREN>
+ P'Burg Surgical Professional Associates
755 Memorial Parkway/Suite 105   Phillipsburg, NJ 08865   (484)526-2200   Fax (484)526-2220

Ratakonda, Sridevi, MD {1912907411} RadDia(91,INA62)<NJ-RWJUHAM, NJ-STFRNMED>
+ Hirsch & Ratakonda MD, PA
290 Madison Avenue/Suite 4   Morristown, NJ 07960   (973)538-8181   Fax (973)538-6565

Rathauser, Robert H., MD {1538178330} ObsGyn(79,NY19)<NJ-RWJUBRUN, NJ-STPETER>
+ Robert Wood Johnson Ob-Gyn Associates
50 Franklin Lane/Suite 203   Manalapan, NJ 07726   (732)536-7110   Fax (732)536-7118
+ Robert Wood Johnson Ob-Gyn Associates
525 Route 70/Suite B-11   Lakewood, NJ 08701   (732)536-7110   Fax (732)905-6467

Rathi, Lilly, MD {1912006982} IntrMd(76,INDI)
+ 442 Bordentown Road
South Amboy, NJ 08879   (732)727-6777   Fax (732)422-4129

Rathi, Ravi, MD {1194781013} CdvDis, IntrMd(82,INDI)<NJ-CHILTON>
+ Total Cardiology Care
2035 Hamburg Pike/Suite L   Wayne, NJ 07470   (973)248-0200   Fax (973)248-3455
+ Total Cardiology Care
120 Franklin Street   Jersey City, NJ 07307   (973)248-0200   Fax (201)216-1362

Rathi, Sandeep, MD {1275723348} PhysMd
+ Shore Orthopaedic Group
35 Gilbert Street South   Tinton Falls, NJ 07701   (732)530-1515   Fax (732)747-5433

Rathmann, Allison Marie, DO {1699900704} SrgNro(NY75<NJ-STBARNMC, NJ-HACKNSK>
+ Advanced Neurosurgery Associates
201 Route 17 North/Suite 501   Rutherford, NJ 07070   (201)457-0044   Fax (201)457-0049

Rathnakumar, Charumathi, MD {1023146370} InfDis(93,INA47)
+ Edison Medical Associates, LLC
34-36 Progress Street/Suite A-2   Edison, NJ 08820   (908)226-0600   Fax (908)226-1802
+ 98 James Street/Suite 200
Edison, NJ 08820   (908)226-0600   Fax (732)230-2479

Rathyen, Jill S., MD {1811170764} EmrgMd
+ 171 Colonial Road
Summit, NJ 07901

Ratkalkar, Kishore, MD {1942369947} PulDis, IntrMd(80,INDI)<NJ-BAYSHORE>
+ Medical Associates of Central New Jersey
26 Throckmorton Lane/1st flr.   Old Bridge, NJ 08857   (732)679-9950   Fax (732)679-9956

Ratliff, David Fred, MD {1740569805}(05,NY46)
+ Advanced Orthopedics & Hand Surgery Institute
504 Valley Road/Suite 201   Wayne, NJ 07470   (973)942-1315   Fax (973)942-8724

Ratliff, Henry W., MD {1336185537} Psychy(73,TX12)<NJ-UNVM-CPRN>
+ 601 Ewing Street/Suite A8
Princeton, NJ 08540   (609)921-2689   Fax (609)279-1745
+ Princeton House Behavioral Health - Princeton
905 Herrontown Road   Princeton, NJ 08540   (609)921-2689   Fax (609)497-3370

Ratnathicam, Anjali, DO {1922257252} SrgVas, Surgry, IntrMd(03,MO79)
+ Bergen Surgical Specialists/Hackensack Vascular
211 Essex Street/Suite 102   Hackensack, NJ 07601   (201)487-8882   Fax (201)487-0943

Ratner, Douglas J., MD {1831166156} IntrMd, OccpMd, Grtrcs(81,PA09)<NJ-OVERLOOK>
+ Community Health Center at Vauxhall
3 Farrington Street   Vauxhall, NJ 07088   (908)598-7950   Fax (908)686-1163

Ratner, Lawrence M., MD {1912904152} RadDia, RadNro(79,MO34)<NJ-STFRNMED>
+ Radiology Affiliates of Central New Jersey, P.A.
2501 Kuser Road   Hamilton, NJ 08691   (609)585-8800   Fax (609)585-1825
+ Radiology Affiliates of Central New Jersey, P.A.
3120 Princeton Pike   Lawrenceville, NJ 08648   (609)585-8800   Fax (609)219-0439
+ St. Francis Medical Center
601 Hamilton Avenue/Radiology   Trenton, NJ 08691   (609)599-5000

Rattigan, Meghan Iona, DO {1003116971} ObsGyn(07,PA78)
+ Hackensack Meridian Medical Group Ob/Gyn, Freehold
3499 Route 9 North/Suite 2B   Freehold, NJ 07728   (732)577-1199   Fax (732)577-8922
+ Hackensack Meridian Medical Group Ob/Gyn, Neptune
1828 West Lake Avenue   Neptune, NJ 07753   (732)577-1199   Fax (732)776-4892

Ratush, Edward, MD {1649289646} Psychy(02,MA05)
+ 249 Eighth Street
Jersey City, NJ 07302

Ratzersdorfer, Jonathan, MD {1780977348} ObsGyn
+ Integrative Obstetrics
21 McWilliams Place   Jersey City, NJ 07302   (201)691-8664   Fax (844)886-6072
+ Integrative Obstetrics
358 Beech Street   Hackensack, NJ 07601   (201)691-8664   Fax (201)487-8601

Ratzker, Paul K., MD {1235139700} SrgNro(88,NY46)
+ The Back Institute
700 Rahway Avenue/Suite A-14   Union, NJ 07083   (908)688-1999   Fax (908)688-8180

Rau, Ganesh U., MD {1174671291} Ophthl
+ Palisade Eye Associates
203 Palisade Avenue   Jersey City, NJ 07306   (201)653-5722   Fax (201)792-9718

Rauch, Eden Renee, MD {1336387927} ObsGyn, RprEnd, In-trMd(03,NJ02)
+ Reproductive Medicine Associates of New Jersey
140 Allen Road   Basking Ridge, NJ 07920   (908)604-7800   Fax (973)290-8370

Rausch, Debora Anne, MD {1063411320} InfDis(95,PA02)
+ Delran Family Practice
8008 Route 130/Suite 120   Delran, NJ 08075   (856)764-7997   Fax (856)764-1840

Rauscher, Gregory E., MD {1346244159} SrgPlstc, SrgPHand, Sur-gry(72,NY08)<NJ-HACKNSK, NJ-ENGLWOOD>
+ 20 Prospect Avenue/Suite 600
Hackensack, NJ 07601   (201)488-1036   Fax (201)489-6966
info@drrauscher.com

Raval, Parthiv V., MD {1295712446} IntrMd, Gastrn(89,INA70)<NJ-CHILTON, NJ-VALLEY>
+ 975 Clifton Avenue
Clifton, NJ 07013   (973)614-9700

Raval, Rajendra R., MD {1174684880} Anesth, OthrSp(81,INDI)<NJ-NWRKBETH>
+ Newark Beth Israel Medical Center
201 Lyons Avenue/Anesth   Newark, NJ 07112   (973)926-7000
rajurr@hotmail.com

Raval, Sumul N., MD {1376526673} Nrolgy(90,INA2B)
+ Garden State Neurology & Neuro-Oncology, P.C.
100 State Highway 36 East   West Long Branch, NJ 07764   (732)229-6200   Fax (732)229-6201
+ Garden State Neurology & Neuro-Oncology, P.C.
9 Hospital Drive/Suite A7 1st Floor   Toms River, NJ 08755   (732)229-6200   Fax (732)229-6201

Rave, Arie, MD {1184635377} IntrMd(83,ITAL)<NJ-VALLEY, NJ-HACKNSK>
+ 1250 East Ridgewood Avenue
Ridgewood, NJ 07450   (201)689-1900   Fax (201)447-9011
Medarave@aol.com

Ravella, Supriya, MD {1801165873} Nephro, IntrMd(09,GRN01)<NJ-JFKMED, NJ-UNVMCPRN>
+ Dr. Anu Chaudhry, MD PC
546 Saint Georges Avenue   Rahway, NJ 07065   (732)381-3642   Fax (732)396-4463

Ravelo, Mary Ann, MD {1497809339} Psychy(84,DOM02)<NJ-JRSYCITY>
+ 211 Pennington Avenue
Passaic, NJ 07055   (973)470-3428

Ravi, Anita, MD {1285820555} CdvDis, IntrMd, IntCrd(02,INA47)
+ 102 James Street/Suite 302
Edison, NJ 08820   (818)501-3907

Ravi, Nanjappa, MD {1700800083} IntrMd(69,INDI)
+ 354 Old Hook Road
Westwood, NJ 07675   (201)666-7200   Fax (201)967-8443

Ravi, Radhika, MD {1376570804} Anesth(89,INA5B)<NJ-STJOSHOS, NY-WESTCHMC>
+ St. Joseph's Regional Medical Center
703 Main Street   Paterson, NJ 07503   (973)754-2000   Fax (973)977-9455

Ravichandran, Shoba, MD {1396729430} EnDbMt, IntrMd(87,INA2G)
+ Tinton Falls Community Based Outpatient Clinic
55 North Gilbert Street   Tinton Falls, NJ 07701   (732)842-4751

Ravindra, Sunay B., MD {1982806410} Anesth
+ Morris Anesthesia Group, PA
3799 Route 46/Suite 211   Parsippany, NJ 07054   (973)335-1122   Fax (973)335-1448

Ravindran, Nishal Cholapurath, MD {1669660627} IntrMd(97,INA56)<PA-BLMSBRG, PA-GSNGWYVL>
+ St. Peter's University Hospital
254 Easton Avenue   New Brunswick, NJ 08901   (732)745-8600   Fax (732)745-2980

Ravindran, Wijeyadevendram, MD {1821020330} EmrgMd, SprtMd(74,SRI01)<NJ-COMMED>
+ Community Medical Center
99 Route 37 West/EmrgMed   Toms River, NJ 08755   (732)557-8080

Raviola, Joseph, MD {1356872881} Pedtrc
+ 186 Newman Street
Metuchen, NJ 08840   (732)632-7272

Ravisankar, Shyam Kumar, MD {1700142239}<NJ-STBARNMC>
+ St. Barnabas Medical Center
94 Old Short Hills Road   Livingston, NJ 07039   (973)322-5000

Ravishankar, Indira, MD {1962441873} Pedtrc, NeuMSptM(74,INDI)
+ North Jersey Developmental Center
169 Minisink Road/PO Box 169   Totowa, NJ 07512   (973)256-1700   Fax (973)256-3468

Ravits, Margaret S., MD {1912060708} Dermat(75,FL02)<NY-PRS-BCOLU>
+ Ravits Margaret MD & Associates
721 Summit Avenue   Hackensack, NJ 07601   (201)487-3691   Fax (201)487-4180
+ Ravits Margaret MD & Associates
130 Kinderkamack Road/Suite 205   River Edge, NJ 07661   (201)487-3691   Fax (201)488-1582

Ravulapati, Sravanthi, MD {1538353925} IntrMd, IntHos(04,INA83)
+ Emergency Medical Offices
651 West Mount Pleasant Avenue   Livingston, NJ 07039   (973)740-9396   Fax (973)251-1165

Rawlins, Bernard Alexander, MD {1063523017} SrgOrt, SrgSpn(87,NY20)
+ HSS Paramus Outpatient Center
140 East Ridgewood Avenue/Suite 175-S   Paramus, NJ 07652   (201)796-2255   Fax (201)796-3711

Rawlins, Samantha Geanine, MD {1487875449} ObsGyn(99,DC03)<NJ-MORRISTN>
+ 256 Columbia Turnpike/Suite 212
Florham Park, NJ 07932   (973)377-0440

Ray, Amit H., MD {1033532189} IntrMd<NJ-ACMCITY>
+ AtlantiCare Regional Medical Center/City Campus
1925 Pacific Avenue/Medicine   Atlantic City, NJ 08401   (609)441-8945

Ray, Anjali K., MD {1235228768} FamMed(05,MD01)
+ Cooper Family Medicine
110 Marter Avenue   Moorestown, NJ 08057   (856)608-8840   Fax (856)722-1898

Ray, Debra M., MD {1992809594} OncHem, IntrMd(83,PA09)
+ Monmouth Hematology Oncology Associates PA
100 State Highway 36/Suite 1B   West Long Branch, NJ 07764   (732)222-1711   Fax (732)222-2060
Dmrzyglock@aol.com

Physicians by Name and Address

Ray Jr, Barry Keith, MD {1083785232} Anesth
+ Jersey Shore University Medical Center
1945 Route 33 Neptune, NJ 07753 (732)775-5500

Rayasam, Ramakumar V., MD {1922977666} Otlryg(76,INDI)
+ 207 South 2nd Street
Phillipsburg, NJ 08865 (908)454-2279 Fax (908)454-5404

Rayfield, David Lee, MD {1659461366} SrgPlstc, Surgry(79,TX12)<NJ-ACMCMAIN, NJ-ACMCITY>
+ Feldman-Rayfield Cosmetic Surgery, PA
222 New Road/Suite 6 Linwood, NJ 08221 (609)601-1000 Fax (609)601-1010

Raymond, Gerald M., MD {1700865805} Pedtrc, IntrMd(83,PA14)<NJ-UNVMCPRN>
+ Princeton Nassau Pediatrics, P.A.
301 North Harrison Street Princeton, NJ 08540 (609)924-5510 Fax (609)924-3577
+ Princeton Nassau Pediatrics, P.A.
196 Princeton-Hightstown Road West Windsor, NJ 08550 (609)924-5510 Fax (609)799-2294
+ Princeton Nassau Pediatrics, P.A.
25 South Route 31 Pennington, NJ 08540 (609)745-5300 Fax (609)745-5320

Raymond, Jacques Carol, MD {1407855984} IntrMd(86,HAI01)<NJ-WAYNEGEN>
+ 294 Central Avenue/1st flr.
Orange, NJ 07050 (973)676-6556 Fax (973)676-6543

Raymond, Joshua Joseph, MD {1396751483} FamMed, Grtrcs(96,PA02)<NJ-CENTRAST>
+ Family Practice of CentraState-Jackson
161 Bartley Road Jackson, NJ 08527 (732)363-6140 Fax (732)363-6196

Raymond, Kimberly J., MD {1326213752} FamMed(96,NJ06)
+ Family Practice of CentraState
281 Route 34/Suite 813 Colts Neck, NJ 07722 (732)431-2620 Fax (732)431-3707
info@parkerfamilyhealthcenter.org
+ Parker Family Health Center
211 Shrewsbury Avenue Red Bank, NJ 07701 (732)431-2620 Fax (732)212-9030

Rayner, William J., MD FamMed(75,NY09)
+ 304 Parkville Station Road/Suite 270
Mantua, NJ 08051

Rayudu, Sunita Srinivas, MD {1134137292} IntrMd, Grtrcs(96,INA1L)
+ Care Health Associates
1323 Route 27/Suite G Somerset, NJ 08873 (732)828-0200 Fax (732)828-0300

Raza, Ali Babar, MD {1023304946} IntrMd(10,NET09)
+ Capital Medical Associates
1235 Whitehorse Mercerville Rd Trenton, NJ 08619 (609)498-4142 Fax (609)587-4512

Raza, Mahmooda H., MD {1184778151} Pedtrc(68,PAKI)<NJ-CHSFULD>
+ Kids first
1520 Pennington Road Trenton, NJ 08618 (609)538-8116 Fax (609)538-8364

Raza, Mohammad Aslam, MD {1568516532} IntrMd, Nephro(63,PAKI)<NJ-CHSFULD, NJ-RWJUHAM>
+ 1520 Pennington Road
Trenton, NJ 08618 (609)538-8116

Raza, Mudusar I., MD {1467562371} IntMSlpd
+ 22 Essex Drive
Monmouth Junction, NJ 08852

Raza, Muhammad Rehan, MD {1851607303} CdvDis
+ Cardiology Associates of Ocean County PA
495 Jack Martin Boulevard/Suite 2 Brick, NJ 08724 (732)458-8299 Fax (732)458-0874

Raza, Rubina B., MD {1437188653} IntrMd(81,PAKI)
+ Medical Associates at Hamilton PC
1235 Whitehorse Mercerville Rd Hamilton, NJ 08619 (609)581-9000 Fax (609)585-7228

Raza, Syed Irfan, MD {1790766814} IntrMd, Nephro(90,PAK11)<NJ-HACKNSK, NJ-VALLEY>
+ Bergen Hypertension & Renal Associates PA
44 Godwin Avenue/Suite 301 Midland Park, NJ 07432 (201)447-0013 Fax (201)447-0438
+ Bergen Hypertension & Renal Associates PA
20 Prospect Avenue/Suite 709 Hackensack, NJ 07601 (201)447-0013 Fax (201)678-1072

Raza, Syed Mohsin, MD {1194704585} IntrMd(80,PAK01)
+ 117 Seber Road/Suite 2-B/Doctors' Park
Hackettstown, NJ 07840 (908)684-0684 Fax (908)684-1119

Raza, Syed Mohsin, MD {1407859572} Anesth(88,PAK12)<NJ-STMRYPAS, NY-CROUSE>
+ St. Mary's Hospital
350 Boulevard/Anesthesia Passaic, NJ 07055 (973)365-4300 Fax (845)357-5777

Razak, Hajira Naaz, MD {1700979028} IntrMd(92,INDI)<NJ-TRENTPSY>
+ Trenton Psychiatric Hospital
Sullivan Way/PO Box 7600 West Trenton, NJ 08628 (609)633-1500

Razdan, Dolly, MD {1699859512} RadOnc, Radiol, IntrMd(88,WV01)<NJ-CLARMAAS>
+ Clara Maass Medical Center
1 Clara Maass Drive/Rad Onc Belleville, NJ 07109 (973)450-2270 Fax (973)844-4904

Razi, Parisa, MD {1871557512} Pedtrc(95,DC01)<NJ-COOPRUMC, NJ-OURLADY>
+ Advocare South Jersey Pediatrics Cherry Hill
1949 Route 70 East/Suite 1 & 2 Cherry Hill, NJ 08003 (856)424-6050 Fax (856)424-2943
+ Advocare South Jersey Pediatrics Collingswood
204 White Horse Pike Collingswood, NJ 08107 (856)424-6050 Fax (856)424-2943

Razi, Sadia, MD {1912117052} NnPnMd<NJ-JRSYCITY>
+ Jersey City Medical Center
355 Grand Street Jersey City, NJ 07304 (201)915-2000

Raziano, Joseph Walter, MD {1891734174} EmrgMd, EmrgEMed(96,LA01)<NJ-VIRTVOOR>
+ Teamhealth East
307 South Evergreen Avenue Woodbury, NJ 08096 (856)848-8817
+ Virtua Voorhees
100 Bowman Drive/EmergMed Voorhees, NJ 08043 (856)247-3000

Raziuddin, Mazherunni, MD Anesth(71,INDI)<NJ-HOBUNIMC>
+ 70 Pearl Street
Dumont, NJ 07628

Razvi, Batool, MD {1043555493} IntrMd(10,VA04)
+ Alliance for Better Care, P.C.
130 Lakehurst Road Browns Mills, NJ 08015 (609)893-3133 Fax (609)893-7972
+ Virtual Family Medicine - Mansfield
3242 Route 206/Building A Suite 2 Bordentown, NJ 08505 (609)893-3133 Fax (609)298-4370

Razvi, Sedeq A., MD Otlryg(76,INDI)<NJ-CENTRAST, NJ-RWJUHAM>
+ Center for Ear, Nose, Sinus and Throat Disorders
501 Iron Bridge Road/Suite 11 Freehold, NJ 07728 (732)409-0200 Fax (732)409-0202
+ Center for Ear, Nose, Sinus and Throat Disorders
2333 Whitehorse-Mercerville Rd/Suite 1 Hamilton, NJ 08619 (732)409-0200 Fax (609)890-6935

Razzak, Mannan, MD {1083640627} Pedtrc(98,BAN02)<NJ-UMDNJ, NJ-CHILTON>
+ Woodland Park Pediatrics
205 Browertown Road/Suite 001 Little Falls, NJ 07424 (973)582-0644 Fax (973)582-0605
razzakma@umdnj.edu
+ University Hospital
150 Bergen Street/EmrgMed Newark, NJ 07103 (973)582-0644 Fax (973)972-8276
+ Chilton Medical Center
97 West Parkway Pompton Plains, NJ 07424 (973)831-5394

Razzak, Nadia Mohsin, MD {1710167184} Pedtrc(00,BAN02)
+ Woodland Park Pediatrics
205 Browertown Road/Suite 001 Little Falls, NJ 07424 (973)582-0644 Fax (973)582-0605

Read, John H., MD {1013083849} Urolgy(71,PA02)<NJ-SJRSYELM, NJ-MEMSALEM>
+ Genito Urinary Associates
125 State Street/Suite 4 Elmer, NJ 08318 (856)358-2330
+ Genito Urinary Associates
20 Magnolia Avenue/Suite D Bridgeton, NJ 08302 (856)455-5770

Readie, Jean Eileen, DO {1912011420} EmrgMd(03,NJ75)<NJ-ENGLWOOD>
+ Englewood Hospital and Medical Center
350 Engle Street/EmrgMed Englewood, NJ 07631 (201)894-3000 Fax (201)541-2977

Reardon, Erin Marie, MD {1679668412} EmrgMd(00,NY06)<NJ-STCLRDEN>
+ St. Clare's Hospital-Denville Campus
25 Pocono Road/EmergMed Denville, NJ 07834 (973)625-6000

Rebarber, Andrei, MD {1598723272} ObsGyn, MtFtMd, Ultsnd(67,NY15)<NY-MTSINAI, NJ-VALLEY>
+ The Valley Hospital
223 North Van Dien Avenue Ridgewood, NJ 07450 (201)447-8000

Rebarber, Israel Frank, MD {1538149935} RadDia, Radiol, IntrMd(84,PA09)<NJ-JFKMED>
+ JFK Medical Center
65 James Street/Diag Radiology Edison, NJ 08820 (732)321-7540 Fax (732)632-1674
+ Edison Radiology Group, P.A.
65 James Street Edison, NJ 08820 (732)321-7540 Fax (732)767-2968

Rebba, Bhavana, MD {1043261746} CdvDis, IntrMd(96,INA5B)
+ Raritan Bay Cardiology Group, P.A.
225 May Street/Suite F Edison, NJ 08837 (732)738-8855 Fax (732)738-6949

Rebbecchi, Thomas A., MD {1093896417} EmrgMd(84,PA02)<NJ-COOPRUMC>
+ Cooper University Hospital
One Cooper Plaza/EmergMed Camden, NJ 08103 (856)342-2000

Rebein, Benjamin Harrison, DO {1265743967}<NJ-STJOSHOS>
+ St. Joseph's Regional Medical Center
703 Main Street Paterson, NJ 07503 (973)754-2000

Reboli, Annette C., MD {1457432874} InfDis, IntrMd(81,DC02)<NJ-COOPRUMC>
+ The Cooper Hospital System-Univ Hospital
3 Cooper Plaza/Suite 215 Camden, NJ 08103 (856)342-2439

Rechenberg, Geoffrey Mark, MD {1205009982} Anesth
+ 158 Harcourt Avenue
Bergenfield, NJ 07621
+ Hackensack University MC-Anesthesia Dept
30 Prospect Avenue/Room 2703 Hackensack, NJ 07601 Fax (201)996-3962

Recho, Marielle, MD {1275739799} IntrMd(98,SYR03)
+ Drs. Hanna and Recho
117 State Route 35 Eatontown, NJ 07724 (732)542-4411 Fax (732)542-1070

Recio, Evita I., MD {1194084699} Pedtrc<NJ-NWRKBETH>
+ Newark Beth Israel Medical Center
201 Lyons Avenue Newark, NJ 07112 (973)926-7040

Reda, Frank, MD {1336182716} IntrMd(93,GRN01)
+ 129 Route 37 West/Suite 3
Toms River, NJ 08755 (732)240-2700 Fax (732)240-1304

Reddi, Alluru S., MD {1659460095} IntrMd, Nephro(79,MEX29)<NJ-UMDNJ>
+ University Hospital-Doctors Office Center
90 Bergen Street/DOC 4500 Newark, NJ 07103 (973)972-2500 Fax (973)972-2510

Reddy, Adarsh Surya, MD {1255619037} Psychy<NJ-TRININPC>
+ Trinitas Regional Medical Center-New Point Campus
655 East Jersey Street Elizabeth, NJ 07206 (908)994-7000

Reddy, Anuradha K., MD {1750554341} IntrMd(76,INDI)<NJ-LOURDMED>
+ Lourdes Medical Center of Burlington County
218 Sunset Road Willingboro, NJ 08046 (609)835-2900

Reddy, Aravinda, MD {1497948640} Nephro, IntrMd(01,INA9Z)
+ Drs. Reddy & Cholankeril
240 Williamson Street/Suite 205 Elizabeth, NJ 07202 (908)289-2070 Fax (908)289-4890

Reddy, Chenna G., MD {1306957436} EmrgMd, FamMed(73,INA94)<NJ-CHSMRCER>
+ Emergency Medical Associates of NJ, P.A.
3 Century Drive Parsippany, NJ 07054 (973)740-0607 Fax (973)740-9895

Reddy, Chitra R., MD {1982759676} Pedtrc(70,INDI)<NJ-UMDNJ, NJ-NWRKBETH>
+ University Pediatric Group
90 Bergen Street/DOC 4300 Newark, NJ 07103 (973)972-2100
+ University Hospital
150 Bergen Street/Ambltry Pdtrcs Newark, NJ 07103 (973)972-2100

Reddy, Gerard, MD {1184858524}<NJ-MORRISTN>
+ Memorial Radiology Associates
10 Lanidex Plaza West/Suite 125 Parsippany, NJ 07054 (973)503-5700 Fax (973)386-5701
+ Morristown Medical Center
100 Madison Avenue Morristown, NJ 07962 (973)503-5700

Reddy, Jayant T., MD {1730554965} IntrMd
+ RWJ Hospital Internal Medicine
One Robert Wood Johnson Place/MEB 486 New Brunswick, NJ 08901 (732)235-8377 Fax (732)235-7427

Reddy, Korrapati Shaik Shaval, MD {1245225788} IntrMd, EmrgMd(75,INA9D)<NJ-RBAYPERT>
+ Raritan Bay Medical Center/Perth Amboy Division
530 New Brunswick Avenue Perth Amboy, NJ 08861 (732)442-3700

Reddy, Loveleen, MD {1861789661}
+ The University Hospital
65 Bergen Street Newark, NJ 07107 (973)972-4300 Fax (973)972-2904

Reddy, Manisha S., MD {1114248804} CdvDis, IntrMd(10,NJ05)
+ 36b Henry Street
Somerset, NJ 08873 (848)203-7492
mreddy1286@gmail.com

Reddy, Matt Medapati, MD {1154304285} Anesth(72,INA39)<NJ-HACKNSK>
+ Hackensack University Medical Center
30 Prospect Avenue/Anesthesia Hackensack, NJ 07601 (201)488-0066 Fax (201)488-6769

Reddy, Namrata Polam, MD {1528225646}<NY-BRNXLCON>
+ Edison Pediatrics
1802 Oak Tree Road/Suite 101 Edison, NJ 08820 (732)548-3210 Fax (906)548-3966

Reddy, Narshimha K., MD {1659523660} IntrMd(71,INDI)
+ Drs. Reddy and Reddy
1328 Danchetz Court   Rahway, NJ 07065

Reddy, Nishant P., MD {1780974899}
+ 108 Jackson Street/Unit 3c
Hoboken, NJ 07030   (609)902-5629
nishant144@gmail.com

Reddy, Padmavathi, MD {1952494296} Anesth(74,INA4D)<NJ-TRINIWSC>
+ Trinitas Regional Medical Center-Williamson Street
225 Williamson Street/Anesth   Elizabeth, NJ 07207
(908)994-5000

Reddy, Rajender, MD {1467505784} IntrMd(78,INA39)<NJ-ANCPSYCH>
+ Ancora Psychiatric Hospital
301 Spring Garden Road/Medicine   Hammonton, NJ 08037
(609)561-1700   Fax (609)561-2509

Reddy, Ram K., MD {1972519270} Gastrn, IntrMd(64,INDI)<NJ-CHRIST, NJ-HOBUNIMC>
+ 212 Palisade Avenue
Jersey City, NJ 07306   (201)659-4095

Reddy, Rama R., MD {1386724672} EnDbMt(86,INA04)<NJ-WESTHDSN>
+ Diabetes Associates PC
5 Franklin Avenue/Suite 609   Belleville, NJ 07109
(973)759-1111   Fax (973)759-0894

Reddy, Sadhana K., MD {1043484389} Pedtrc(71,INA39)
+ Drs. Reddy and Reddy
1328 Danchetz Court   Rahway, NJ 07065

Reddy, Seshamma Thikkavarapu, MD {1508020298}
+ 260 Franklin Turnpike/Apt 405
Mahwah, NJ 07430

Reddy, Shanthi Nalamalapu, MD {1194047860} FamMed(91,INA2D)
+ 6 Carri Farm Court
Scotch Plains, NJ 07076

Reddy, Shashidhar Sadda, MD {1285625582} Otlryg(00,LA05)
+ Sparta Health and Wellness Center
89 Sparta Avenue/Suite 220   Sparta, NJ 07871   (973)940-8100   Fax (973)729-7235

Reddy, Sireesha B., MD {1134429111} InfDis
+ ID Associates PA/dba ID Care
765 Route 10 East/Suite 201   Randolph, NJ 07869
(973)989-0068   Fax (973)361-8955
+ ID Associates PA/dba ID Care
8 Saddle Road   Cedar Knolls, NJ 07927   (973)989-0068
Fax (973)993-5953
+ ID Associates PA/dba ID Care
2035 Hamburg Turnpike/Suite F   Wayne, NJ 07869
(973)513-9475   Fax (973)513-9478

Reddy, Sowbhagya Sangam, MD {1346298296} IntrMd(80,INDI)<NY-CMCSTVSI>
+ 79 Stevenson Drive
Marlboro, NJ 07746

Reddy, Srikanth Madadi, MD {1548335243} PsyAdd(96,INA75)<NJ-BERGNMC>
+ New Bridge Medical Center
230 East Ridgewood Avenue/Psychiatry   Paramus, NJ 07652
(201)967-4000

Reddy, Sudershan P., MD {1790791812} Anesth(74,INA83)<NJ-CHSMRCER, NJ-CHSFULD>
+ Trenton Anesthesiology Associates, PA
One Capital Way/Second Floor   Pennington, NJ 08534
(609)396-4700   Fax (609)396-4900

Reddy, Sumitha R., MD {1578742656} IntrMd
+ 6212 Kaitlyn Court
Princeton, NJ 08550

Reddy, Sureka, MD {1427256528} FamMed(99,INA62)<NJ-UNVMCPRN, NJ-CAPITLHS>
+ 362 Morning Glory Drive
Monroe, NJ 08831   (609)529-8802
+ Princeton Family Care
100 Federal City Road/Suite A   Lawrenceville, NJ 08648
(609)529-8802   Fax (609)771-8991

Reddy, Thejaswini K., MD {1396767539} IntrMd(99,DOM10)
+ Drs. Reddy and Reddy
1328 Danchetz Court   Rahway, NJ 07065

Reddy, Uma P., MD {1366437220} IntrMd, EmrgMd(79,INDI)<NJ-CLARMAAS>
+ Clara Maass Medical Center
1 Clara Maass Drive   Belleville, NJ 07109   (973)450-2000

Redel, Henry, MD {1750608642} IntrMd, InfDis(07,ISR05)<NY-NYUTISCH>
+ Highland Park Medical Associates
579A Cranbury Road/Suite 102   East Brunswick, NJ 08816
(732)613-0711   Fax (732)613-5783

Reder, Lorie Jean, MD {1316085467} IntrMd(84,DC02)
+ 44 Whippany Road
Morristown, NJ 07960

Redlich, Adam Daniel, MD {1114986452} SprtMd, OccpMd, FamMSptM(00,NJ06)
+ Aplus Athlete Sports Medicine

38 Robbinsville Allentown Road/Suite A   Robbinsville, NJ 08691   (609)223-2286   Fax (609)223-2286
redlicad@hotmail.com

Redlich, Vijaya Potharlanka, DO {1679786198} FamMed(02,NJ75)<NJ-RWJUHAM>
+ 9 Elisha Drive
Allentown, NJ 08501

Redline, Richard C., MD {1104875772} CdvDis, CritCr, IntrMd(77,VA01)<NJ-NWTNMEM>
+ Cardiology Associates of Sussex County LLP
222 High Street/Suite 205   Newton, NJ 07860   (973)579-2100   Fax (973)579-6638

Redling, Theresa Marie, DO {1295840379} Grtrcs, IntrMd(87,NJ75)<NJ-NWRKBETH, NJ-STBARNMC>
+ The Geriatric Health Center
101 Old Short Hills Road/Suite 302   West Orange, NJ 07052
(973)322-6457   Fax (973)322-6466

Rednor, Jeffrey D., DO {1184648149} FamMed(89,NJ75)<NJ-RWJUHAM, NJ-CHSMRCER>
+ Rednor-Risi Family Medicine Associates, P.C.
1 Washington Boulevard/Suite A   Robbinsville, NJ 08691
(609)448-4353   Fax (609)448-4558

Redondo, Rodolfo C., MD {1639133390} Anesth(73,PHIL)<NJ-WARREN>
+ Warren Hospital
185 Roseberry Street/Anesthesiology   Phillipsburg, NJ 08865   (908)859-6700

Redondo, Teresita Cuyegkeng, MD {1013098714} Pthlgy, PthAna, PthImm(72,PHI02)<NJ-STBARNMC>
+ St. Barnabas Medical Center
94 Old Short Hills Road/Pathology   Livingston, NJ 07039
(973)322-5000

Redstone, Jeremiah Star, MD {1689851172} SrgPlstc(03,NC01)<NY-BETHPETR, NY-NYEYEINF>
+ 200 South Orange Avenue/Suite 107
Livingston, NJ 07039   (212)249-1500   Fax (646)961-4910

Redziniak, Natalie E., MD {1033523022}<NJ-HUNTRDN>
+ Capital Health Primary Care-Bordentown
1 Third Street   Bordentown, NJ 08505   (609)298-2005
Fax (609)324-8267
+ Capital Health Primary Care Columbus
23203 Columbus Road/Suite 1   Columbus, NJ 08022
(609)298-2005   Fax (603)303-4451

Reed, Jean Arlyn Banez, MD {1043418932} Pedtrc(09,NY47)
+ Hackensack Pediatrics
177 Summit Avenue   Hackensack, NJ 07601   (201)487-8222   Fax (201)487-2126
+ 50 Emily Avenue
Nutley, NJ 07110

Reed, Mark K., MD {1538144340} SrgThr, Surgry(83,MN04)<NJ-STBARNMC, NJ-NWRKBETH>
+ St. Barnabas Medical Center
94 Old Short Hills Road   Livingston, NJ 07039   (973)322-5000

Reed, Rebecca Ann, DO {1184687733} Pedtrc(97,PA77)<NJ-VIRTUAHS, NJ-VIRTMHBC>
+ Advocare Medford Pediatric & Adolescent Medicine
520 Stokes Road   Medford, NJ 08055   (609)654-9112   Fax (609)654-7404

Reed, Tony S., MD {1386678787} FamMSptM(00,PA09)<NJ-ACMCITY>
+ AtlantiCare Regional Medical Center/City Campus
1925 Pacific Avenue   Atlantic City, NJ 08401   (609)345-4000

Reed, William E., DO {1649343492} CdvDis, IntrMd(89,IA75)<NJ-SOCEANCO>
+ Medical Associates of Ocean County, P.A.
1301 Route 72 West/Suite 300   Manahawkin, NJ 08050
(609)597-6513   Fax (609)597-4593

Reeder, Jennifer Gordan, MD {1619905379} OncHem, IntrMd(03,NJ03)<NJ-OVERLOOK, NJ-MORRISTN>
+ Summit Medical Group-Berkeley Heights Campus
1 Diamond Hill Road   Berkeley Heights, NJ 07922
(908)277-8890   Fax (908)790-6576

Reedy, Jamie Lynne, MD {1073542569} FamMed(95,NJ06)<NJ-OVERLOOK>
+ Summit Medical Group-Berkeley Heights Campus
1 Diamond Hill Road   Berkeley Heights, NJ 07922
(908)273-4300   Fax (908)790-6576
+ Paramount MedGrou -Westfield FamPract
592 Springfield Avenue   Westfield, NJ 07090   (908)273-4300   Fax (908)301-0883

Reeh, Debora Cummings, DO {1164513982} FamMed(98,NJ75)
+ 701 East Main Street
Moorestown, NJ 08057   (856)296-4303

Reen, Sandeep K., MD {1912284621}
+ 122 Roberts Avenue/1st Floor Apt
Haddonfield, NJ 08033

Reese, Jason, DO {1013358274} CdvDis<NJ-DEBRAHLC>
+ Deborah Heart and Lung Center
200 Trenton Road   Browns Mills, NJ 08015   (609)893-6611

Reeves, Donald Raymond, Jr., MD {1821200403} Psychy, PsyFor(91,TX12)<NJ-UMDNJ>
+ University Psychiatric Associates
183 South Orange Avenue/E-F Levels   Newark, NJ 07103
(973)972-2977   Fax (973)972-2979

Reeves, Lisa Joyce, MD {1154305746} IntrMd(94,PA01)<NY-BETHPETR>
+ The Medical Group of Englewood
140 Grand Avenue   Englewood, NJ 07631   (646)450-7751
info@doctorsintheoffice.com

Refaie, Tarek, MD {1093917874} IntrMd<NJ-STJOSHOS>
+ St. Joseph's Regional Medical Center
703 Main Street   Paterson, NJ 07503   (973)754-2000

Reffler, Marie M., MD {1023257888} Anesth
+ Jersery Shore Anesthesiology
1945 Highway 33   Neptune, NJ 07753   (732)897-0200
Fax (732)897-0263

Reformato, Vincent, MD {1114338050} Anesth
+ Robert Wood Johnson-UMDNJ Anesthesia Group
125 Paterson Street/CAB 3100   New Brunswick, NJ 08901
(732)235-6155   Fax (732)235-7466

Regalman, Elena M., MD {1962581942} IntrMd, Grtrcs(74,RUS15)
+ 401 West Sylvania Avenue/Apt. 6B
Neptune, NJ 07753   (732)245-1563

Regan, Inge Sophia, MD {1831139500} FamMed(93,PA01)<NJ-NWTNMEM>
+ Newton Medical Center
175 High Street/EmrgMed   Newton, NJ 07860   (973)383-2121

Regan, Kasey Calvey, MD {1134331911} Anesth
+ 800 River River Road/Apt. 313
Edgewater, NJ 07020   (201)723-6805

Reger, Donna Pidane, MD {1871518399} IntrMd(95,NJ06)
+ After Hours Family Care
1001 Washington Boulevard   Robbinsville, NJ 08691
(609)448-2401
+ Professional HealthCare Services of Lawrenceville
2500 US Highway 1   Lawrenceville, NJ 08648   (609)448-2401   Fax (609)530-0966

Regevik, Nina K., MD {1548347446} IntrMd(85,DOMI)<NJ-RBAYPERT>
+ Raritan Bay Medical Center/Perth Amboy Division
530 New Brunswick Avenue/IntMed   Perth Amboy, NJ 08861   (732)442-3700   Fax (732)324-4838

Regillo, Carl, MD {1740248038} Ophthl, VitRet(88,MA01)<PA-TJHSP, PA-WILLSEYE>
+ Mid Atlantic Retina - Wills Eye Retina Surgeons
501 Cooper Landing Road   Cherry Hill, NJ 08002   (856)755-1278   Fax (856)755-1223
sclassen@midatlanticretina.com

Regis, Jon M., MD {1508880717} ObsGyn(78,NC01)
+ Absecon Island Centers for Women's Healthcare
4401 Ventnor Avenue   Atlantic City, NJ 08401   (609)344-1836   Fax (609)344-1852
+ Reliance Medical Group, LLC
1325 Baltic Avenue   Atlantic City, NJ 08401   (609)344-1836
Fax (609)441-0953
+ Reliance Medical Group, LLC.
22 North Franklin Boulevard   Pleasantville, NJ 08401
(609)272-9040   Fax (609)272-9055

Rego, Ramon, MD {1033227459} IntrMd(88,MEX03)<NJ-OVERLOOK>
+ Access Medical Associates
3322 Route 22 West/Building 1   Branchburg, NJ 08876
(908)704-0100   Fax (908)704-2237

Regula, Christie Gail, MD {1093949752}
+ Cooper Center for Dermatologic Surgery
10000 Sagemore Drive/Suite 10103   Marlton, NJ 08053
(856)596-3040

Regulapati, Saritha, MD {1942287495} IntrMd(96,INA5B)<NJ-UNVMCPRN>
+ 462 New Road
Monmouth Junction, NJ 08852   Fax (732)274-6777

Rehberg, Joelle Stabile, DO {1477640837} FamMed(97,NJ75)<NJ-STCLRDEN>
+ Montville Primary Care Physicians
137 Main Road   Montville, NJ 07045   (973)402-0025   Fax (973)402-0508

Rehm, Christine M., MD {1033186630} Pedtrc(94,NJ05)
+ Madison Pediatrics
435 South Street/Suite 200   Morristown, NJ 07960
(973)822-0003   Fax (973)822-3349

Rehman, Atiq, MD {1184657645}
+ Endocrinology Associates
1 Brace Road/Suite B   Cherry Hill, NJ 08034   (856)796-9255
Fax (856)234-0498

Rehman, Atta-Ur, MD {1184767931} Psychy, PsyCAdj(92,PAK11)<NJ-HAMPTBHC>
+ Hampton Behavioral Health Center
650 Rancocas Road/Psychiatry   Westampton, NJ 08060
(609)267-7000

Physicians by Name and Address

Rehman, Muhammad Ubaid, MD {1154344786} CritCr, PulDis, EmrgMd(98,PAK11)<NJ-RWJHLTS>
+ 190 Greenbrook Road
  North Plainfield, NJ 07060 (908)899-1549 Fax (206)202-3153

Rehman, Saadia Raza, DO {1316921414} IntrMd(99,NJ75)<NY-BETHPETR>
+ Cooper University Internal Medicine Group
  651 John F. Kennedy Way Willingboro, NJ 08046 (609)835-2838 Fax (609)877-5421

Rehman, Waqas, MD {1750546610} OncHem, IntrMd(07,OH44)
+ Hunterdon Regional Cancer Ctr
  2100 Wescott Drive Flemington, NJ 08822 (908)788-6461 Fax (908)788-6412

Rehor, Francis E., MD {1790947794} IntrMd(05,NY15)<NJ-UNVM-CPRN>
+ Princeton Lifestyle Medicine
  731 Alexander Road/Suite 200 Princeton, NJ 08540 (609)655-3800 Fax (609)655-5203

Rehr, Eric L., MD {1154376879} EmrgMd(87,PA02)<NJ-MONMOUTH>
+ Monmouth Medical Center
  300 Second Avenue/EmergMed Long Branch, NJ 07740 (732)222-5200

Reich, Helene, MD {1669494043} NuclMd, RadDia, RadNuc(88,NJ05)<NJ-CLARMAAS>
+ Clara Maass Medical Center
  1 Clara Maass Drive Belleville, NJ 07109 (973)450-2030 Fax (973)844-4900
+ Essex Imaging Associates
  5 Franklin Avenue/Suite 510 Belleville, NJ 07109 (973)450-2030 Fax (973)751-4456

Reich, Jonathan Makaloa, MD {1659565067} Surgry, Bariat(98,DOM18)<NJ-SOCEANCO, NJ-BAYSHORE>
+ Strafford Surgical Specialists, P.A.
  1100 Route 72 West/Suite 303 Manahawkin, NJ 08050 (609)978-3325 Fax (609)978-3123
+ Monmouth Surgical Specialists
  727 North Beers Street Holmdel, NJ 07733 (609)978-3325 Fax (732)290-7067

Reich, Joseph I., MD {1285795229} Pedtrc, PedEmg(88,NY08)<NJ-RWJUBRUN>
+ RWJ University Pediatric Emergency Medicine
  125 Paterson Street/MEB 342 New Brunswick, NJ 08903 (732)235-7893 Fax (732)235-9349
+ RWJ University Hospital New Brunswick
  One Robert Wood Johnson Place New Brunswick, NJ 08901 (732)828-3000

Reich, Steven M., MD {1043315427} SrgOrt, SrgSpn(86,NY46)<NJ-CENTRAST>
+ Affiliated Orthopaedic Specialists
  2186 Route 27/Suite 1A North Brunswick, NJ 08902 (732)422-1222 Fax (732)422-3636
+ Affiliated Orthopaedic Specialists
  50 Franklin Lane/Suite 102 Manalapan, NJ 07726 (732)617-9500

Reich-Sobel, Debra Gail, DO {1437554463} GenPrc, FamMed(87,ME75)
+ Drs. Reich-Sobel & Schulman
  809 North Wood Avenue Linden, NJ 07036 (908)486-7773 Fax (908)925-4311

Reichard, Kathleen G., DO {1255405874} Pedtrc, PedEmg(93,ME75)<NJ-OVERLOOK>
+ Overlook Medical Center
  99 Beauvoir Avenue/PO Box 210/PediEmrg Summit, NJ 07902 (908)522-2000

Reichard, Peter Seth, MD {1831250554} Anesth(90,NY45)<NJ-STBARNMC>
+ St. Barnabas Medical Center
  94 Old Short Hills Road Livingston, NJ 07039 (973)322-8223

Reichel, Martin, MD {1275534067} Dermat, PthDrm, DerImm(88,NY46)
+ Westwood Dermatology
  390 Old Hook Road Westwood, NJ 07675 (201)666-9550 Fax (201)666-1251

Reicher, Oscar A., MD {1093724593} SrgOrt(79,PA12)<NJ-CHILTON, NJ-VALLEY>
+ SMG Orthopedic Surgery and Sports Medicine Center
  2035 Hamburg Turnpike/Suite D Wayne, NJ 07470 (973)616-0200 Fax (973)616-1792
+ SMG Orthopedic Surgery and Sports Medicine Center
  61 Beaver Brook Road/Suite 201 Lincoln Park, NJ 07035 (973)616-0200 Fax (973)686-9294
+ Chilton Medical Center
  97 West Parkway Pompton Plains, NJ 07470 (973)831-5000

Reichman, Cynthia M., MD {1740289529} Anesth(93,PA09)
+ West Jersey Anesthesia Associates
  102-E Center Boulevard Marlton, NJ 08053 (856)988-6250 Fax (856)988-6270

Reichman, Michael J., MD {1508845124} CdvDis, IntrMd(78,NY46)<NJ-OURLADY, NJ-UNDRWD>
+ Associated Cardiovascular Consultants-Lourdes
  1 Brace Road/Suite C & F Cherry Hill, NJ 08034 (856)428-4100 Fax (856)428-5748
+ Associated Cardiovascular Consultants, P.A.
  730 North Broad Street/Suite 200 Woodbury, NJ 08096 (856)428-4100 Fax (856)251-2344

Reichstein, Michele B., MD Psychy(78,IL42)
+ 20 Trinity Place
  Montclair, NJ 07042 (973)744-3887

Reid, Brittany Michelle, MD {1720341852} Pedtrc
+ On-Site Neonatal Partners
  1000 Haddonfield-Berlin Road/Suite 210 Voorhees, NJ 08043 (856)782-2212 Fax (856)782-2266

Reid, Cheryl Soled, MD {1841291291} GnetMd, ClnGnt, Pedtrc(79,NJ06)
+ Horizon NJ Health
  210 Silvia Street West Trenton, NJ 08628 (609)718-9675 Fax (609)538-1492

Reid, Gillian Salanda, MD {1366843138} FamMed
+ Southern Jersey Medical Center
  651 High Street Burlington City, NJ 08016 (609)386-0775 Fax (609)386-4372

Reid, James Henry, MD {1205870623} SrgOrt(83,PA02)<PA-EASTON>
+ Coordinated Health
  222 Red Lane Phillipsburg, NJ 08865 (610)861-8080 Fax (610)849-1013
  jreid@coordinatedhealth.com

Reid, Jeremy Jackson, MD {1396939252} SrgOrt, IntrMd(07,NY01)
+ Reconstructive Orthopedics, P.A.
  200 Bowman Drive/Suite E-100 Voorhees, NJ 08043 (609)267-9400 Fax (609)267-9457

Reid, Kelly M., MD {1730383290} Psychy(81,DC03)<NJ-ACMCITY, NJ-ACMCMAIN>
+ PO Box 757
  Somers Point, NJ 08244

Reid, Kenneth M., MD {1861421851} Anesth(91,PA09)<NJ-OCEANMC>
+ Ocean Medical Center
  425 Jack Martin Boulevard Brick, NJ 08723 (732)840-2200

Reid, Lisa M., MD {1215041470} Surgry(99,NJ05)
+ Cooper Surgical Associates
  3 Cooper Plaza/Suite 411/Surgery Camden, NJ 08103 (856)342-2270 Fax (856)365-1180

Reid, Phillip Dolivera, MD {1093703969} OncHem, MedOnc(94,CA11)<NJ-RWJUBRUN, NJ-STPETER>
+ Regional Cancer Care Associates - Central Jersey Div
  454 Elizabeth Avenue/Suite 240 Somerset, NJ 08873 (732)390-7750 Fax (732)390-7725
+ Central Jersey Oncology Center, P.A.
  Brier Hill Court/Building J-2 East Brunswick, NJ 08816 (732)390-7750 Fax (732)390-7725
+ Central Jersey Oncology Center, P.A.
  205 Easton Avenue New Brunswick, NJ 08873 (732)828-9570 Fax (732)828-7638

Reid-Duncan, Lucienne Lariane, MD {1629122098} Nrolgy(02,NJ02)
+ AtlantiCare Physician Group Joslin Diabetes Center
  2500 English Creek Avenue/Bldg 800 Egg Harbor Township, NJ 08234 (609)407-2277 Fax (609)272-6306

Reigel, Shawna Ilene, MD {1619900586} FamMed(02,MO34)
+ Complete Care Family Medicine
  75 West Red Bank Avenue Woodbury, NJ 08096 (856)853-2055 Fax (856)848-2879

Reikes, Sanford Todd, MD {1467456384}
+ Summit Medical Group-Berkeley Heights Campus
  1 Diamond Hill Road Berkeley Heights, NJ 07922 (908)273-4300 Fax (908)790-6576
+ Summit Medical Group
  6 Brighton Road/2 FL Clifton, NJ 07012 (908)273-4300 Fax (973)777-5403
+ Summit Medical Group
  95 Madison Avenue Morristown, NJ 07922 (973)267-7673 Fax (973)267-5521

Reilly, Dennis K., DO {1346293503} Anesth
+ West Jersey Anesthesia Associates
  102 East Centre Boulevard Marlton, NJ 08053 (856)988-6260 Fax (856)988-6270

Reilly, Gail G., MD {1235114539} FamMed
+ Parker Family Health Center
  211 Shrewsbury Avenue Red Bank, NJ 07701 (732)212-0777 Fax (732)212-9030
  greilly@parkerhc.com

Reilly, George D., MD {1518006865} Dermat, IntrMd(77,NJ05)<NJ-OVERLOOK>
+ 31-Q Mountain Boulevard
  Warren, NJ 07059 (908)753-7773

Reilly, Mark C., MD {1184701492} SrgOrt, OrtTrm(90,IL42)<NJ-UMDNJ>
+ North Jersey Orthopaedic Institute
  90 Bergen Street/DOC 1200 Newark, NJ 07101 (973)972-0681 Fax (973)972-3897
+ North Jersey Orthopaedic Institute
  33 Overlook Road/MAC L02 Summit, NJ 07901 (973)972-0681 Fax (908)522-2757

Reilly, Megan Eileen, DO {1780687723} FamMed(97,NJ75)
+ Pine Street Family Practice
  220 East Pine Street Williamstown, NJ 08094 (856)629-7436 Fax (856)875-4742

Reilly, Melissa Lynn, DO {1346434081} FamMed(05,NJ75)
+ Premier Health Associates
  272 Route 206 North Andover, NJ 07821 (973)347-2273 Fax (973)729-3238

Reilly, Michael H., MD {1609940246} PthACl, Pthlgy(72,ITAL)<NJ-VALLEY>
+ The Valley Hospital
  223 North Van Dien Avenue/Pathology Ridgewood, NJ 07450 (201)447-8000

Reimer, Jennifer Marie, DO {1558651208} IntrMd(NY75<NJ-OCEANMC>
+ 1515 Richmond Avenue/Suite 3
  Point Pleasant Beach, NJ 08742 (732)295-0072 Fax (732)295-0224
+ Ocean Family Care
  800 Route 88/Suite 3 Point Pleasant Beach, NJ 08742 (732)295-0072 Fax (732)295-0224

Reiner, David M., MD {1598867954} CdvDis, IntrMd(88,IL42)<NJ-HACKNSK, NJ-HOLYNAME>
+ Drs. Wasserman & Reiner
  401 South Van Brunt Street/Suite 402 Englewood, NJ 07631 (201)541-1223 Fax (201)567-1998
+ Heart and Vascular Institute at EHMC
  350 Engle Street/Suite 1000 Englewood, NJ 07631 (201)894-3636

Reiner, Mark J., DO {1942316831} SrgOrt(76,IL76)<NJ-KENEDYHS, NJ-VIRTUAHS>
+ Cherry Hill Orthopedic Surgeons
  PO Box 8285 Cherry Hill, NJ 08002 (856)662-2400 Fax (856)662-5525

Reing, Charles Scot, MD {1629165337} CrnExD, Ophthl(90,NY19)
+ Advanced Eye Care Center PA
  220 Hamburg Turnpike/Suite 7 Wayne, NJ 07470 (973)790-1300 Fax (973)790-5310

Reingold, Stephen Marcus, MD {1770658007} Pedtrc(06,ISR06)
+ Highland Park Pediatrics
  85 Raritan Avenue Highland Park, NJ 08904 (732)246-0202 Fax (732)246-8334

Reinhardt, Rickey R., MD {1730251877} IntrMd, EnDbMt(89,LA05)
+ University Medical Group
  125 Paterson Street/Suite 5100/Cab-A New Brunswick, NJ 08901 (732)235-7993 Fax (732)235-7117

Reinholz, Louis J., Jr., DO {1295796514} EmrgMd(95,PA77)<PA-CHSTNHIL, NJ-OURLADY>
+ Our Lady of Lourdes Medical Center
  1600 Haddon Avenue/EmrgMed Camden, NJ 08103 (856)757-3500

Reinkraut, Jeffrey M., MD {1811079015} ObsGyn(75,NJ06)<NJ-VALLEY>
+ Valley Medical Group Ob/Gyn in Fairlawn
  5-22 Saddle River Road Fair Lawn, NJ 07410 (201)796-2025 Fax (201)796-0587

Reinsdorf, Keith Alan, MD {1174674170} FamMed, SprtMd(97,NJ05)
+ UH- Robert Wood Johnson Med
  125 Paterson Street/MEB 278 New Brunswick, NJ 08901 (732)828-3000 Fax (732)246-7317

Reisen, Charles E., MD {1922113539} NnPnMd, Pedtrc(78,IREL)<NJ-KIMBALL>
+ On-Site Neonatal Partners
  1000 Haddonfield-Berlin Road/Suite 210 Voorhees, NJ 08043 (856)782-2212 Fax (856)782-2213

Reisher, Richard G., DO {1073575791} GenPrc, FamMed(68,MO78)
+ Cedar Bridge Medical Associates
  985 Cedarbridge Avenue Brick, NJ 08723 (732)477-5600 Fax (732)477-1899

Reisler, Scott, MD {1659481133} IntrMd, PulDis, Grtrcs(80,NY46)
+ 1925 State Route 27
  Edison, NJ 08817 (732)985-8937 Fax (732)985-8336 Sreisler@gmail.com

Reisman, Barry M., MD {1598868135} ObsGyn(68,PA02)
+ PO Box 178
  Saddle River, NJ 07458 (201)567-8922 Fax (201)567-8722

Reisman, Jeffrey M., MD {1003843178} Ophthl(91,PA09)<NJ-MORRISTN>
+ Morristown Opthalmology Associates
  261 James Street/Suite 1B Morristown, NJ 07960 (973)267-1113 Fax (973)267-0719

Physicians by Name and Address

Reisner, Colin, MD {1538311311} Allrgy
+ 11 Tamari Court
Randolph, NJ 07869   (973)978-3329

Reisner, Michelle R., MD {1942267158} IntrMd, PallCr, Grtrcs(83,SAFR)<NJ-JRSYCITY>
+ Liberty Medical Associates
377 Jersey Avenue/Suite 470   Jersey City, NJ 07302
(201)918-2239   Fax (201)918-2243
+ Liberty Medical Associates
196 Jewitt Avenue   Jersey City, NJ 07304   (201)332-3354

Reison, Dennis S., MD {1316943483} CdvDis, IntCrd, IntrMd(75,CA11)<NJ-VALLEY>
+ Valley Medical Group/Valley Heart Group
1200 East Ridgewood Avenue   Ridgewood, NJ 07450
(201)670-8660   Fax (201)447-1957

Reiss, Jodi L. W., MD {1760413025} Anesth, IntrMd(95,ISR02)<NJ-RIVERVW>
+ Liberty Ambulatory Surgery Center, LLC
377 Jersey Avenue/Suite 510   Jersey City, NJ 07302
(201)878-3200   Fax (201)878-3201

Reiss, Ronald A., MD {1851498596} FamMed(78,SPA12)<NJ-SOMERSET>
+ 312 US Highway 206
Hillsborough, NJ 08844   (908)359-1345   Fax (908)359-4334

Reissman, David I., MD {1184694945} Gastrn, IntrMd(74,NY46)
+ 2 State Route 27/Suite 311 B
Edison, NJ 08820   (732)549-9495   Fax (732)549-9493

Reiter, Barry A., MD {1215046495} IntrMd, MedOnc, OncHem(69,NY08)
+ Oncology & Hematology Specialists, PA
23 Pocono Road/Suite 100   Denville, NJ 07834   (973)316-1701   Fax (973)316-1708
+ Oncology & Hematology Specialists, PA
100 Madison Avenue/Suite C3402   Morristown, NJ 07960
(973)316-1701   Fax (973)267-2550

Reiter, Mitchell F., MD {1134206444} SrgOrt, SrgSpn(92,FL02)<NJ-UMDNJ>
+ North Jersey Orthopaedic Institute
90 Bergen Street/DOC 1200/Spine Srgry   Newark, NJ 07101
(973)972-0679   Fax (973)972-9367
+ North Jersey Orthopaedic Institute
33 Overlook Road/MAC L02   Summit, NJ 07901   (973)972-0679   Fax (908)522-2757

Reiter, Raymond D., MD {1841447380} PhysMd(82,MEXI)<NY-SPCLSURG>
+ PO Box 182
Franklin Lakes, NJ 07417

Reiter, Stewart Roy, MD {1114077302} Psychy(83,NJ05)<NJ-OVERLOOK>
+ Integrated Behavioral Care, P.A.
35 Beechwood Road/Suite 3-A & 3-B   Summit, NJ 07901
(908)598-2400   Fax (908)598-2408

Reitzen-Bastidas, Shari D., MD {1225173370} Otlryg, GenPrc(04,NY19)
+ Riverside Medical Group
710 Tenth Street   Secaucus, NJ 07094   (201)865-2050
Fax (201)865-0015
+ Riverside Medical Group
255 State Route 3   Secaucus, NJ 07094   (201)865-2050
Fax (201)293-4099

Rejjal, Abdellatif R., MD {1316146541} NnPnMd
+ Somerset Medical Center Neonatology
110 Rehill Avenue   Somerville, NJ 08876   (609)584-6762
Fax (609)584-5917
+ On-Site Neonatal Partners
1000 Haddonfield-Berlin Road/Suite 210   Voorhees, NJ 08043   (609)584-6762   Fax (856)782-2213

Rejowska-Cedrowski, Jolanta M., MD {1285744425} Anesth(77,POL06)<NJ-CLARMAAS>
+ Clara Maass Medical Center
1 Clara Maass Drive   Belleville, NJ 07109   (973)450-2000

Rekant, Mark Spencer, MD {1457388050} SrgOrt, SrgHnd, OrtS-Hand(94,NJ05)
+ South Jersey Hand Center
1888 Marlton Pike East/Suite E-F-G   Cherry Hill, NJ 08003
(856)489-5630   Fax (856)489-5631

Rekant, Stanley I., MD {1154314052} Dermat(69,NY15)<NJ-VIRTVOOR>
+ 600 Somerdale Road/Suite 104
Voorhees, NJ 08043   (856)795-0050
drofskin@yahoo.com
+ 777 South White Horse Pike
Hammonton, NJ 08037   (609)567-0030

Rekedal, Kirby D., MD {1023197969} NnPnMd, Pedtrc(80,MD01)<NJ-MONMOUTH>
+ Monmouth Medical Center
300 Second Avenue   Long Branch, NJ 07740   (732)222-5200

Rekhtman-Sneed, Katya, MD {1396968400} RadDia(05,NY46)<NJ-ENGLWOOD>
+ Englewood Radiologic Group PA
350 Engle Street/Radiology   Englewood, NJ 07631
(201)894-3000   Fax (201)894-5244

Relia, Nitin, MD {1952531857} Nephro, IntrMd(02,INA92)
+ Cumberland Nephrology Associates, PA
1318 South Main Road   Vineland, NJ 08360   (856)205-9900   Fax (856)205-0041

Relkin, Felicia, MD {1720089303} IntrMd, PulDis(87,NY46)<NJ-ENGLWOOD>
+ The Park Medical Group
24 Elm Street   Harrington Park, NJ 07640   (201)784-0123
Fax (201)784-0065
+ The Park Medical Group
274 County Road/Suite A   Tenafly, NJ 07670   (201)784-0123   Fax (201)568-0483

Relvas, Monica De Stefani, MD {1154425593} Pedtrc
+ One Robert Wood Johnson Place
New Brunswick, NJ 08903

Remadevi, Radhika Sekhar, MD {1174720304} IntHos, IntrMd
+ Prime Health Medical LLC.
1129 Bloomfield Avenue/Suite 209   West Caldwell, NJ 07006   (973)500-2686   Fax (973)500-2686

Remde, Alan H., MD {1003865601} FamMed(85,NJ05)
+ St. Luke's Coventry Family Practice
755 Memorial Parkway/Suite 300   Phillipsburg, NJ 08865
(908)847-3300   Fax (866)281-6023

Remer, Paul, MD {1902802283} Ophthl(72,VA04)
+ Quality Eye Center
2020 New Road   Linwood, NJ 08221   (609)927-2020   Fax (609)926-7616
+ Quality Eye Center
315 Route 9 South   Cape May Court House, NJ 08210
(609)465-0100
+ 2500 English Creek Avenue
Egg Harbor Township, NJ 08221

Remick, Kyle Norman, MD {1659315356} Surgry
+ Cooper University Physician Trauma Center
One Cooper Plaza   Camden, NJ 08103   (856)342-3014

Remolina, Carlos, MD {1144398835} IntrMd, PulDis(75,SPAI)
+ 515 North Wood Avenue/Suite 101
Linden, NJ 07036   (908)241-2030   Fax (908)241-5692

Remorca, Carolina U., MD {1548378169} Pedtrc(80,PHI01)<NJ-COMMED, NJ-OCEANMC>
+ Pediatric Medical Group
20 Hospital Drive/Suite 2   Toms River, NJ 08755   (732)341-9333   Fax (732)341-7364

Rempell, Joshua Saul, MD {1417084856} EmrgMd(06,MA01)<MA-MAGENHOS, MA-BRIGWMN>
+ Cooper Univerisry Emergency Physicians
One Cooper Plaza   Camden, NJ 08103   (856)342-2351
Fax (856)968-8272

Rempson, Joseph H., MD {1649217266} PhysMd, IntrMd(90,NY08)<NJ-OVERLOOK, NJ-MORRISTN>
+ Associates in Rehabilitation Medicine
95 Mount Kemble Avenue   Morristown, NJ 07960
(973)267-2293   Fax (973)226-3144

Remsen, Kenneth A., MD {1881688166} Otlryg, SrgFPl, SrgHdN(80,QU01)<NJ-CHILTON>
+ ENT and Facial Plastic Surgeons
51 Route 23 South/2nd Floor   Riverdale, NJ 07457
(973)831-1220   Fax (973)831-0029
+ Wayne Surgical Center, LLC.
1176 Hamburg Pike   Wayne, NJ 07470   (973)831-1220
Fax (973)709-1901

Remstein, Robert Jay, DO {1750483301} IntrMd(81,NY75)<NJ-CHSFULD>
+ Capital Health System/Fuld Campus
750 Brunswick Avenue/Medical Affairs   Trenton, NJ 08638
(609)394-6208   Fax (609)394-6693
+ Capital Health Primary Care
832 Brunswick Avenue   Trenton, NJ 08638   (609)394-6208
Fax (609)815-7401

Ren, Shuyue, MD {1932368990} PthACl<NJ-COOPRUMC>
+ Cooper University Hospital
One Cooper Plaza/Bsmt Room   Camden, NJ 08103
(856)361-1737

Ren, Zhiyong, MD {1275767097}<NJ-ACMCITY>
+ AtlantiCare Regional Medical Center/City Campus
1925 Pacific Avenue   Atlantic City, NJ 08401   (713)459-5302
renzhy@gmail.com

Renda, John A., MD {1447227566} IntrMd(79,PHI08)<NJ-RBAY-OLDB, NJ-RBAYPERT>
+ 200 Perrine Road/Suite 211
Old Bridge, NJ 08857   (732)727-4774   Fax (732)727-4994

Renda, Julie Elaine, DO {1669579983} IntrMd(00,NY75)<NJ-STCLRDOV, NJ-STCLRDEN>
+ 5 Fieldview Road
Andover, NJ 07821

Rengan, Rajagopalan, DO {1003257130}
+ SOM - Department of Internal Medicine
42 East Laurel Road/Suite 3100   Stratford, NJ 08084
(856)566-2753   Fax (856)566-6906

Renjen, Pooja, MD {1891844700} RadDia<NJ-HACKNSK>
+ Hackensack University Medical Center
30 Prospect Avenue/Radiol   Hackensack, NJ 07601
(201)996-4752   Fax (201)996-5116

Renna, Carmen M., MD {1164423398} IntrMd(81,NY46)<NJ-MORRISTN>
+ Madison Internal Medicine Associates
95 Madison Avenue/Suite 405   Morristown, NJ 07960
(973)829-9998   Fax (973)829-9991

Renner, Carl J., MD {1346205705} IntrMd(79,MEXI)<NJ-HACKNSK, NJ-MEADWLND>
+ Heights Medical Associates
288 Boulevard   Hasbrouck Heights, NJ 07604   (201)288-6781   Fax (201)288-2734

Renny, Andrew, MD {1447259957} Gastrn(78,NJ05)<NJ-SHOREMEM>
+ Renny Gastroenterology Assoc PA
222 New Road/Suite 805/Building 8   Linwood, NJ 08221
(609)927-3200   Fax (609)927-9159

Rentala, Manju, MD {1629089719} EmrgMd
+ Emergency Medical Offices
651 West Mount Pleasant Avenue   Livingston, NJ 07039
(973)740-0607   Fax (973)251-1109

Renz, Patricia M., MD {1245265875} IntrMd(84,NJ05)
+ Drs. Scaduto & Renz
223 West Main Street   Boonton, NJ 07005   (973)335-8656
Fax (973)335-8986

Renza, Richard A., DO {1154477479} FamMed, Rheuma(72,PA77)<NJ-BURDTMLN>
+ AtlantiCare Family Medicine
3826 Bayshore Road   North Cape May, NJ 08204
(609)886-3636   Fax (609)886-4880
krisrenza@aol.com
+ AtlantiCare Family Medicine
6410 New Jersey Avenue   Wildwood Crest, NJ 08260
(609)886-3636   Fax (609)522-1516

Renzi, Michael A., DO {1962491241} IntrMd, FamMed(91,PA77)<NJ-COOPRUMC, NJ-VIRTUAHS>
+ Advocare Heights Primary Care
318 White Horse Pike   Haddon Heights, NJ 08035
(856)547-6000   Fax (856)546-3189

Renzi, Vincent Anthony, MD {1760428494} IntrMd(85,MNT01)
+ Renzi Family Medicine
1217 North Church Street/Suite A   Moorestown, NJ 08057
(856)234-2828   Fax (856)234-8931

Repole, Adam N., MD {1619902046} ObsGyn(90,NY08)<NJ-KIMBALL>
+ Ocean Gynecological & Obstetrical Associates PA
475 Highway 70   Lakewood, NJ 08701   (732)364-8000
Fax (732)364-4601

Repudi, Sirisha, MD {1851791075} IntrMd<NJ-RWJUHAM>
+ Robert Wood Johnson University Hospital at Hamilton
1 Hamilton Health Place   Hamilton, NJ 08690   (609)586-7900

Requa, Eric Robert, DO {1164788501} FamMed
+ Virtua Holistic Primary Care
1001 Route 73 North/Lower Level   Marlton, NJ 08053
(844)908-5483   Fax (856)355-7106

Requa, Lindsay Ann, DO {1265799050} Pedtrc<PA-YORK>
+ Advocare Pedi Phys of Burlington Co
693 Main Street/PO Box 367   Lumberton, NJ 08048
(609)261-4058   Fax (609)261-8381

Rescigno, Ronald J., MD {1003835802} Allrgy, Ophthl(87,NJ05)
+ University Hospital-Doctors Office Center
90 Bergen Street/Fl 6, Rm 6166   Newark, NJ 07103
(973)972-9466
resupri@umdnj.edu

Resciniti, Matthew John, DO {1982862231} FamMed
+ Chatham Family Practice Associates
492 Main Street   Chatham, NJ 07928   (973)635-2432   Fax (973)635-6169

Resnick, Jonathan, MD {1497812796} Gastrn, IntrMd(95,NY46)<NJ-VALLEY>
+ Summit Medical Group
31-00 Broadway   Fair Lawn, NJ 07410   (201)625-1977
Fax (201)796-7020

Resnick, Michael B., MD {1003808841} ObsGyn(92,NJ06)
+ Robert Wood Johnson Ob/Gyn Group
1 Hamilton Health Place   Hamilton, NJ 08690   (609)631-6899   Fax (609)631-6898

Resnick, Steven I., MD {1760554323} Psychy(81,NY09)
+ 1000 Herrontown Road
Princeton, NJ 08540   (609)683-0707   Fax (609)683-8322

Physicians by Name and Address

Resnick-Matro, Jennifer Dawn, MD {1265488951} EmrgMd(99,ISR06)<NJ-VIRTVOOR, NJ-JRSYSHMC>
+ Concentra Medical Centers Urgent Care
  817 East Gate Drive/Suite 102 Mount Laurel, NJ 08054 (856)778-1090 Fax (856)778-9191
+ Emergency Physician Associates, P.A.
  307 South Evergreen Avenue/PO Box 298 Woodbury, NJ 08096 (856)778-1090 Fax (856)848-8536
+ Jersey Shore University Medical Center
  1945 Route 33/EmergMed Neptune, NJ 08054 (732)775-5500

Resnikoff, Forrest P., MD {1063491215} Dermat, SrgDer, IntrMd(81,IL42)
+ Center for Dermatologic Care LLC
  170 Avenue of the CMN Shrewsbury, NJ 07702 (732)542-6300 Fax (732)542-6392

Resnikoff, Leonard Barocas, MD {1861496200} RadDia(89,IL42)<NJ-STPETER, NJ-RWJUBRUN>
+ University Radiology Group, P.C.
  260 Amboy Avenue Metuchen, NJ 08840 (732)548-2322 Fax (732)548-3392
+ University Radiology Group, P.C.
  579A Cranbury Road East Brunswick, NJ 08816 (732)548-2322 Fax (732)390-1856

Resnikoff, Michael, MD {1689690786} SrgVas, Surgry(90,NY09)<NJ-MORRISTN, NJ-NWTNMEM>
+ Advanced Vascular Associates, PC
  131 Madison Avenue/2nd Floor Morristown, NJ 07960 (973)755-9206 Fax (973)540-9717

Resnikoff-Gary, Amanda Nicole, MD {1861758633} ObsGyn
+ Integrative Obstetrics
  21 McWilliams Place Jersey City, NJ 07302 (201)691-8664 Fax (844)886-6072
+ Hackensack Hospital Obs/Gyn
  30 Prospect Avenue/4E-90 Hackensack, NJ 07601 (551)996-2000

Respler, Don S., MD {1073581740} Otlryg, PedOto(81,NY47)<NJ-UMDNJ, NJ-HACKNSK>
+ Ear Nose Throat Institute of New Jersey
  2 South Summit Avenue Hackensack, NJ 07601 (201)996-9200 Fax (201)996-9277

Ressler, Steven H., MD {1932135464} Anesth, PainMd(82,MEX14)<NJ-KMHCHRRY, NJ-UNDRWD>
+ South Jersey Pain Consultants
  525 Route 73 South/Suite 103 Marlton, NJ 08053 (856)797-5777 Fax (856)797-5771

Restifo, Robert A., DO {1760483804} PulDis(84,NJ75)<NJ-ATLANTHS, NJ-MORRISTN>
+ Pulmonary & Allergy Associates
  8 Saddle Road/Suite 101 Cedar Knolls, NJ 07927 (973)267-9393 Fax (973)540-0472
+ Pulmonary & Allergy Associates
  1 Springfield Avenue/Suite 3-A Summit, NJ 07901 (973)267-9393 Fax (908)934-0556

Restrepo, Mauricio, MD {1568608370} Pedtrc(00,COL03)<NJ-UMDNJ>
+ 2 East Blackwell Street/Suite 19
  Dover, NJ 07801 (973)620-9924

Restua, Nestor S., MD {1518912179} IntrMd, EmrgMd(82,PHI01)<NJ-CENTRAST>
+ CentraState Medical Center
  901 West Main Street/EmergMed Freehold, NJ 07728 (732)431-2000

Rethy, Kimberly, DO {1295150217}
+ Advanced Otolaryngology Associates
  557 Cranbury Road/Suite 3 East Brunswick, NJ 08816 (732)613-0600 Fax (732)613-0508

Retirado, Allen S., MD {1134114689} EmrgMd(71,PHI09)<NJ-STCLRDEN, NJ-RBAYPERT>
+ St. Clare's Hospital-Denville Campus
  25 Pocono Road/EmrgMed Denville, NJ 07834 (973)625-6000
+ Raritan Bay Medical Center/Perth Amboy Division
  530 New Brunswick Avenue/EmrgMed Perth Amboy, NJ 08861 (732)442-3700

Retirado, Vincent Paul, MD {1104987932} EmrgMd(03,DC02)<NJ-STCLRDEN>
+ St. Clare's Hospital-Denville Campus
  25 Pocono Road/EmrgMed Denville, NJ 07834 (973)625-6000

Reutter, Richard A., MD {1225089923} Pedtrc(72,PA09)
+ 307 Third Avenue
  Long Branch, NJ 07740 (732)870-5175
+ Monmouth Family Center
  270 Broadway Long Branch, NJ 07740 (732)870-5175 Fax (732)923-7204

Reuveni, Michael A., MD {1649273707} Anesth(90,ISR02)<NJ-STMRYPAS>
+ St. Mary's Hospital
  350 Boulevard Passaic, NJ 07055 (973)365-4300

Revankar, Manasi Chandrakant, DO {1619127024} FamMed, IntrMd(07,NY75)
+ St Luke's Hospitalist Group
  185 Roseberry Street Phillipsburg, NJ 08865 (484)526-6643 Fax (484)526-4605

Revesz, Elizabeth, MD {1841519519} Surgry
+ Virtua Breast Specialty Care
  200 Bowman Drive/Suite E-300 Voorhees, NJ 08043 (856)247-7515 Fax (856)247-7525

Revoredo, Fred S., MD {1669588422} FamMed, EmrgMd(94,GRN01)<NY-GOODSAM, NJ-STJOSHOS>
+ Revoredo Medical Affiliates
  425 15th Avenue Paterson, NJ 07504 (973)345-4024 Fax (973)345-4156
  revoredomedical@optonline.net

Rey, Ricardo, MD {1417049131} IntrMd(95,CHI08)
+ Clifton Comprehensive Medical Center
  960 Paulison Avenue Clifton, NJ 07011 (973)773-7713 Fax (973)773-7723

Reydel, Boris, MD {1457394124} Gastrn, IntrMd(82,RUSS)
+ Summit Medical Group
  6 Brighton Road/2 FL Clifton, NJ 07012 (973)777-7911 Fax (973)777-5403

Reyes, Bernadette O., MD {1649287236} IntrMd(78,PHI01)
+ 40 Passaic Avenue
  Passaic, NJ 07055 (973)773-7443 Fax (973)773-1389

Reyes, Christine, MD {1417064908} Psychy, PsyCAd(90,PRO03)
+ Family Connections Inc
  395 South Center Street Orange, NJ 07050 (973)675-3817 Fax (973)673-5782

Reyes, Emmanuel, MD {1174592521} IntrMd(91,PHI29)
+ 1100 Clifton Avenue
  Clifton, NJ 07013 (973)594-8444 Fax (973)773-4491

Reyes, Johan, MD {1750680948} AnesPain<NY-NSUHMANH>
+ Relievus
  1400 Route 70 East Cherry Hill, NJ 08034 (888)985-2727

Reyes, Jonathan Villaroman, MD {1780602177} Pedtrc, EmrgMd(86,PHI28)
+ EmCare
  1945 Route 33 Neptune, NJ 07753 (732)776-4510 Fax (732)776-2329

Reyes, Jose Franco, MD {1396812954} Psychy(91,PHI01)<NJ-ANCPSYCH>
+ 104 Independence Boulevard
  Sicklerville, NJ 08081 (856)885-4529 Fax (856)885-6258

Reyes, Paul H., MD {1497794770} IntrMd, EmrgMd, EmrgEMed(83,PHI09)<NJ-MEMSALEM>
+ Memorial Hospital of Salem County
  310 Woodstown Road/EmergMed Salem, NJ 08079 (856)935-1000

Reyes, Prudencio C., MD {1104903202} EmrgMd, Surgry, EmrgEMed(74,PHIL)<NJ-EASTORNG>
+ Drs. Reyes & Narvaez
  135 Bloomfield Avenue/Suite B Bloomfield, NJ 07003 (973)743-3556 Fax (973)743-3895

Reyes, Reina Duremdes, MD {1376638833} Pedtrc(86,PHI01)<NJ-RWJUHAM, NJ-CHSMRCER>
+ Pediatrics by Night
  1230 Whitehorse Mercerville Ro Hamilton, NJ 08619 (609)581-1700 Fax (609)581-8472

Reyes, Ruby Carina E., MD {1093784050} FamMed(78,PHIL)
+ Adult & Pediatric Allergists of Central Jersey
  1740 Oak Tree Road Edison, NJ 08820 (732)906-1717 Fax (732)906-1781
+ Adult & Pediatric Allergists of Central Jersey
  3 Hospital Plaza/Suite 405 Old Bridge, NJ 08857 (732)906-1717 Fax (732)360-0033

Reyes, Tyrone K., MD {1053463810} Pedtrc, PedEmg(89,NJ05)<NJ-UMDNJ>
+ University Hospital
  150 Bergen Street/Pediatrics Newark, NJ 07103 (973)972-4300 Fax (973)972-5965

Reyman, Lynn D., MD {1043264948} EmrgMd, IntrMd(82,NY19)<NJ-STBARNMC>
+ St. Barnabas Medical Center
  94 Old Short Hills Road/Emergency Livingston, NJ 07039 (973)322-5000

Reyn, Mark, MD {1225064546} IntrMd(74,RUSS)
+ 29-11 Fairlawn Avenue
  Fair Lawn, NJ 07410 (201)794-0940

Reynolds, Daniel, MD {1396162772} EmrgMd
+ CHCA NJ Emergency at Virtua
  100 Bowman Drive Voorhees, NJ 08043 (856)247-2200 Fax (609)261-5842

Reynolds, Matthew Thomas, DO {1366700122} EmrgMd<NJ-NWRKBETH>
+ Newark Beth Israel Medical Center
  201 Lyons Avenue Newark, NJ 07112 (973)926-7000

Reynolds, Nina D., MD {1104895309} ObsGyn(83,NJ05)<NJ-MORRISTN>
+ 33 Main Street/Suite D
  Chatham, NJ 07928

Reynolds, Richard David, MD {1083627822} IntrMd, Ophthl(88,NJ05)<NJ-UNVMCPRN>
+ The Princeton Eye Group
  419 North Harrison Street/Suite 104 Princeton, NJ 08540 (609)921-9437 Fax (609)921-0277
+ The Princeton Eye Group
  1600 Perrinville Road Monroe Township, NJ 08831 (609)921-9437 Fax (609)655-3685
+ The Princeton Eye Group
  900 Eastern Avenue/Suite 50 Somerset, NJ 08540 (732)565-9550 Fax (732)565-0946

Reynolds, Stephanie Marie, DO {1518901024} EmrgMd(00,NY75)<NJ-RIVERVW>
+ Riverview Medical Center
  1 Riverview Plaza/Emerg Med Red Bank, NJ 07701 (732)530-2204 Fax (732)224-7498

Reynon, Melissa A., MD {1447572474} IntrMd
+ Medical Associates of Ocean County, P.A.
  1301 Route 72 West/Suite 300 Manahawkin, NJ 08050 (609)597-6513 Fax (609)597-4593

Rezac, Craig, MD {1730258294} SrgC&R, SrgLap, Surgry(95,ITAL)
+ UH- RWJ Medical School
  One Robert Wood Johnson Place New Brunswick, NJ 08903 (732)235-7920 Fax (732)235-7079
  Rezacc@umdnj.edu
+ UMDNJ RWJ Surgery
  125 Paterson Street/CAB 4th FL 4100 New Brunswick, NJ 08901 (732)235-7920 Fax (732)235-7079

Rezai, Amadi, MD {1487602116} ObsGyn(00,GRN01)
+ Ocean Women's Health Care Group
  602 Route 72 East/Suite 1 Manahawkin, NJ 08050 (609)978-9870 Fax (609)978-9873

Rezai, Fariborz, MD {1942249313} CritCr, PulDis, IntrMd(01,GRN01)<NJ-STBARNMC>
+ St. Barnabas Medical Center
  94 Old Short Hills Road/ICU Livingston, NJ 07039 (973)322-2782 Fax (973)322-8410
  frezai@sbhcs.com
+ Feridoun Rezai MD PC
  550 Newark Avenue/Suite 307 Jersey City, NJ 07306 (973)322-2782 Fax (201)963-6165

Rezai, Feridoun, MD {1467552927} CdvDis, IntrMd(69,IRAN)
+ Feridoun Rezai MD PC
  550 Newark Avenue/Suite 307 Jersey City, NJ 07306 (201)963-8448 Fax (201)963-6165

Rezayat, Combiz, MD {1891954947} SrgVas(03,NY46)
+ The Cardiovascular Care Group
  433 Central Avenue Westfield, NJ 07090 (908)490-1699 Fax (908)490-1698
+ The Cardiovascular Care Group
  1401 Broad Street/Suite 1 Clifton, NJ 07013 (908)490-1699 Fax (973)751-3730

Reznik, Andrea I., MD {1780644641} Nrolgy(77,MA07)<NJ-HUNTRDN, NJ-SOMERSET>
+ 19 Monroe Street/Bldg 2/Suite A
  Bridgewater, NJ 08807 (732)725-4242 Fax (732)725-4006
+ 516 Easton Avenue
  Somerset, NJ 08873 (732)247-7979
+ 1100 Wescott Drive
  Flemington, NJ 08807 (908)806-4970

Reznikov, Boris, DO {1649536608} EmrgMd<NJ-COMMED>
+ Community Medical Center
  99 Route 37 West Toms River, NJ 08755 (732)557-4056

Rezvani, Abas, MD {1003888934} Urolgy, SrgUro, OthrSp(65,IRAN)<NJ-WAYNEGEN, NJ-STJOSHOS>
+ 220 Hamburg Turnpike/Suite 10
  Wayne, NJ 07470 (973)790-1100 Fax (973)790-3138
  abasrezvanimd@aol.com
+ St. Joseph's Wayne Hospital
  224 Hamburg Turnpike/Urology Wayne, NJ 07470 (973)942-6900
+ St. Joseph's Regional Medical Center
  703 Main Street Paterson, NJ 07470 (973)754-2000

Rezvani, Fred F., MD {1104887694} ObsGyn(83,GRN01)<NJ-VALLEY>
+ 119 Prospect Street/Suite 3
  Ridgewood, NJ 07450 (201)444-1600 Fax (201)444-8774

Rezvina, Natalia Y., MD {1023041100} ObsGyn(94,RUS14)<NJ-SOCEANCO>
+ Somers Manor Obstetrics and Gynecology
  599 Shore Road/Suite 101 Somers Point, NJ 08244 (609)926-8353 Fax (609)926-4579

Rhee, Bong Susan, MD {1548300502} Psychy(72,KOR05)
+ 23 White Street
  Shrewsbury, NJ 07702 (732)842-9495

Rhee, Jung L., MD {1295804359} Pedtrc(65,KOR04)<NJ-CHRIST, NJ-HOLYNAME>
+ 69 Center Street
  Englewood Cliffs, NJ 07632 (201)798-1333

Rhee, Kyung-Hwa, MD {1134152390} RadDia<NJ-VALLEY>
+ Radiology Associates of Ridgewood, P.A.
20 Franklin Turnpike Waldwick, NJ 07463 (201)445-8822
Fax (201)447-5053

Rhee, Richard S., MD {1659346112} Nrolgy, PainMd, Acpntr(64,KOR06)<NJ-JRSYSHMC, NJ-RIVERVW>
+ Jersey Shore Neurology Associates PA
1900 Corlies Avenue/Third Floor Neptune, NJ 07753
(732)775-2400 Fax (732)775-5673
drrichardrhee@comcast.net
+ Jersey Shore Neurology Associates PA
222 Jack Martin Boulevard Brick, NJ 08723 (732)840-4666

Rhee, Samuel T., MD {1760416184} SrgPlstc, PlsSHNck(96,NY01)<NJ-UMDNJ>
+ New Jersey Medical School Div Plastic & Hand Surgery
140 Bergen Street/Suite E1620 Newark, NJ 07103
(973)972-8092 Fax (973)972-8268

Rhee, William Choonghee, MD {1033117742} Anesth(99,GRN01)
+ 1332 Ocean Avenue/Unit 7
Sea Bright, NJ 07760
+ Red Bank Anesthesia, LLC
1 Riverview Plaza Red Bank, NJ 07701 Fax (732)450-2620

Rhee, Young Sun Diane, MD {1609847425} PedCrd, Pedtrc(97,NY47)<NJ-MORRISTN>
+ Pediatric Cardiology at The Valley Hospital
205 Robin Road/Suite 100 Paramus, NJ 07652 (201)599-0026 Fax (201)986-1160

Rhim, Richard Dongil, MD {1154588937} SrgSpn, SrgOrt(03,NY19)<NJ-HACKNSK>
+ Active Orthopaedics & Sports Medicine
440 Old Hook Road Emerson, NJ 07630 (201)358-0707
Fax (201)358-9777

Rho, Aloysius Kihyok, MD {1710987334} IntrMd, Gastrn(94,NY08)
+ Princeton Gastroenterology Associates, P.A.
731 Alexander Road/Suite 100 Princeton, NJ 08540
(609)924-1422 Fax (609)924-7473
+ Princeton Endoscopy Center
731 Alexander Road/Suite 104 Princeton, NJ 08540
(609)924-1422 Fax (609)452-1010

Rho, David Samsun, MD {1932106440} Ophthl(89,NY01)<NJ-COOPRUMC>
+ Soll Eye PC of New Jersey/Cooper Division
3 Cooper Plaza/Suite 510 Camden, NJ 08103 (856)342-7200 Fax (856)342-6620

Rho, John I., MD {1366433625} Hypten, Nephro(86,NY08)<NJ-VALLEY, NJ-HACKNSK>
+ Bergen Hypertension & Renal Associates PA
44 Godwin Avenue/Suite 301 Midland Park, NJ 07432
(201)447-0013 Fax (201)447-0438
+ Bergen Hypertension & Renal Associates PA
20 Prospect Avenue/Suite 709 Hackensack, NJ 07601
(201)447-0013 Fax (201)678-1072

Rhoades, Katherine A., MD {1396806766}
+ 1B Cornwall Drive
East Brunswick, NJ 08816 (732)257-0755 Fax (732)257-6177

Rhoades, Walter, Jr., DO {1730152943} Psychy(92,IA75)
+ University Hospital-SOM Department of Psychiatry
2250 Chapel Avenue West/Suite 100 Cherry Hill, NJ 08002
(856)482-9000 Fax (856)482-1159

Rhoads, Frances A., MD {1932129301} Pedtrc(64,ENGL)<NJ-STPETER>
+ St. Peter's Pediatric Faculty Group
123 How Lane New Brunswick, NJ 08901 (732)745-8519

Rhoads, George G., MD {1760614465} PubHth(65,MA01)
+ University Hospital-School of Public Health
170 Frelinghuysen Road/Rm 234, EOHSI Piscataway, NJ 08854 (732)445-0193 Fax (732)445-3644

Rhodes, Michael Eric, MD {1144201302} Anesth
+ 165 Amsterdam Avenue
Passaic, NJ 07055 (973)336-9459 Fax (973)883-0144

Rhodes, Roy Harley, MD {1467564120} PthAna, PthNro, PthAcl(73,CA06)<NJ-RWJUBRUN>
+ RWJ University Pathology
125 Paterson Street/MEB 212 New Brunswick, NJ 08901
Fax (732)418-8445
+ RWJ University Hospital New Brunswick
One Robert Wood Johnson Place New Brunswick, NJ 08901 (732)828-3000

Rhodes, Stancie Christina, MD {1417173659} SrgCrC, Surgry(03,DC01)
+ Pulmonary & Allergy Associates
1 Springfield Avenue/Suite 3-A Summit, NJ 07901
(908)202-6942 Fax (908)934-0556

Rhyme, Timothy L., MD {1992734974} FamMed(93,PA13)<NJ-VIRTBERL, NJ-VIRTVOOR>
+ 1450 East Chestnut Avenue/Suite E
Vineland, NJ 08361

Riabov, Keith A., MD {1417939513} Anesth(91,NJ05)<NJ-MORRISTN>
+ Morristown Medical Center
100 Madison Avenue/Anesthesiology Morristown, NJ 07962 (973)971-5000 Fax (201)943-8733

Riar, Sandeep Singh, MD {1730326133} IntrMd(02,INA6Z)
+ Roosevelt Medical
237 Roosevelt Avenue Carteret, NJ 07008 (732)541-2141
Fax (732)541-1083

Riauba, Linas, MD {1477645273} InfDis(88,LITH)
+ 40 Mitchell Avenue
West Caldwell, NJ 07006 (973)972-7958 Fax (973)972-0303
RiaubaLi@umdnj.edu

Riaz, Adnan, MD {1922523802} EmrgMd
+ Robert Wood Johnson Emergency Medicine
One Robert Wood Johnson Place/MEB 104 New Brunswick, NJ 08901 (732)235-6134

Riaz, Danish, MD {1700172459} FamMed<NJ-STBARNMC>
+ St. Barnabas Medical Center
94 Old Short Hills Road Livingston, NJ 07039 (973)322-5196 Fax (973)322-2281

Riaz, Najeeb, MD {1225073455} PsyCAd(91,PAK11)<NJ-NWRK-BETH>
+ Newark Beth Israel Medical Center
201 Lyons Avenue/Psych Newark, NJ 07112 (973)926-7000
NR7324110@pol.net

Riaz, Omer Junaid, MD {1801006838} Surgry, SrgVas(03,VA04)
+ Advanced Vascular Associates, PC
131 Madison Avenue/2nd Floor Morristown, NJ 07960
(973)755-9206 Fax (973)540-9717

Riba, Ali K., MD {1790767044} PthAcl(87,SYR03)
+ Inform Diagnostics
825 Rahway Avenue Union, NJ 07083 (732)901-7575
Fax (732)901-1555

Ribalta, Marcia, MD {1588611719} Psychy, PsyCAd(79,PRO01)<NJ-STJOSHOS>
+ SJUMC-Harbor House
645 Main Street Paterson, NJ 07503 (973)754-2805
+ St. Joseph's Regional Medical Center
703 Main Street/Psychiatry Paterson, NJ 07503 (973)754-2052

Ribner, Hillel S., MD {1912030123} CdvDis(71,NY19)<NJ-NWRK-BETH>
+ Newark Beth Israel Medical Center
201 Lyons Avenue Newark, NJ 07112 (973)926-7000

Ricanor, Rainier Jude, MD {1598051484}<NJ-CHRIST>
+ Christ Hospital
176 Palisade Avenue Jersey City, NJ 07306 (203)732-7327
Fax (203)732-7185

Ricci, Anthony R., DO SrgOrt, SprtMd(97,NJ75)
+ South Jersey Sports Medicine Center
1004 Haddonfield Road Cherry Hill, NJ 08002 (609)662-7733 Fax (856)662-7727

Ricci, Emily K., MD {1740496835} ObsGyn(06,PA02)<NJ-VIRTVOOR>
+ Garden State Obstetrics and Gynecological Associates
2401 Evesham Road/Suite A Voorhees, NJ 08043
(856)424-3323 Fax (856)424-4994

Ricci, John Anthony, MD {1043383987} FamMed(95,DMN01)
+ Center for Aesthetic and Integrative Medicine
2399 Highway 34/Building A5 Manasquan, NJ 08736
(732)528-5533 Fax (732)528-0360

Ricciardi, Anthony, Jr., MD {1164485314} Pedtrc(76,MEX03)<NJ-CLARMAAS>
+ 161 Halsted Street
East Orange, NJ 07018 (973)678-3133
+ 5 Franklin Avenue/Suite 602
Belleville, NJ 07109 (973)759-7190

Riccioli, Diana L., MD {1073631081} Psychy(88,ITA01)
+ 925 Clifton Avenue
Clifton, NJ 07013 (973)471-5256

Riccobono, Charles A., MD {1215900527} Gastrn, IntrMd(68,ITAL)<NJ-HACKNSK>
+ Center for Healthy Senior Living
360 Essex Street/Suite 401 Hackensack, NJ 07601
(551)996-4220 Fax (551)996-0543

Riccobono, Elizabeth Kay, DO {1952515751} CritCr, Anesth(06,WV75)
+ AtlantiCare Anesthesiology
65 West Jimmie Leeds Road Pomona, NJ 08240 (609)748-7597

Ricculli, Nicholas P., DO {1699751388} CdvDis, IntrMd(85,NJ75)<NJ-MORRISTN>
+ Atlantic Cardiology Group LLP
8 Tempe Wick Road Mendham, NJ 07945 (973)543-2288
Fax (973)543-0637
+ Atlantic Cardiology Group LLP
95 Madison Avenue/Suite 300 Morristown, NJ 07960
(973)543-2288 Fax (973)682-9494

Rice, Daniel, MD {1497266480} EmrgMd
+ Robert Wood Johnson Emergency Medicine
One Robert Wood Johnson Place/MEB 104 New Brunswick, NJ 08901 (732)828-3000

Rice, Daniel A., MD {1861503625} Urolgy(77,MEX03)
+ American Urology Center of NJ
1001 Clifton Avenue Clifton, NJ 07013 (973)779-7231
+ Wayne Surgical Center, LLC.
1176 Hamburg Pike Wayne, NJ 07470 (973)779-7231
Fax (973)709-1901

Rice, Peter Eric, MD {1306871017} SrgC&R, Surgry(83,MA05)<NJ-UMDNJ>
+ University Hospital-Doctors Office Center
90 Bergen Street/DOC 1700/Surgry Newark, NJ 07103
(973)972-2400 Fax (973)972-3562

Rice, Stephen G., MD {1518936954} PedSpM, IntrMd(74,NY19)<NJ-JRSYSHMC>
+ Jersey Shore Sports Medicine Center
51 Davis Avenue/Suite 51-02 Neptune, NJ 07753
(732)776-2433 Fax (732)776-4403
srice@meridianhealth.com
+ Family Health Center
71 Davis Avenue/PO Box 397 Neptune, NJ 07754
(732)776-2433 Fax (732)776-4892

Rice, Stuart Nelson, MD {1366403610} Anesth(80,VT02)<NJ-OVERLOOK>
+ Summit Anesthesia Associates, P.A.
33 Overlook Road/Suite 311 Summit, NJ 07901 (908)598-1500 Fax (908)598-0197

Rich, Stanley E., MD {1548278039} Radiol, RadDia(77,NY09)<NJ-CENTRAST>
+ CentraState Medical Center
901 West Main Street/Radiology Freehold, NJ 07728
(732)294-2946
+ Freehold Radiology Group
901 West Main Street Freehold, NJ 07728 (732)462-4844

Richane, Aberrahmane, MD {1699951467}<NJ-HAMPTBHC>
+ Hampton Behavioral Health Center
650 Rancocas Road Westampton, NJ 08060 (609)267-7000 Fax (609)518-2140

Richard, Merwin Francis, MD {1043233513} CdvDis, IntrMd, Int-Crd(89,INA77)
+ Advanced Garden State Cardiology
550 Newark Avenue/Suite 307 Jersey City, NJ 07306
(201)418-9111 Fax (201)418-9118

Richards, Adam Price, MD {1255363958} Pedtrc, EmrgMd(99,SC01)<NJ-KMHTURNV>
+ Kennedy Health Systems/Washington Township Campus
435 Hurffville-Cross Keys Road Turnersville, NJ 08012
(856)582-2500

Richards, Andrea T., MD {1629293139} NrlgSpec
+ 565 Pierson Street
Westfield, NJ 07090

Richards, Bonnie J., DO {1467627236} FamMed
+ Capital Health Primary Care-Hamilton
1445 Whitehorse-Mercerville Rd Hamilton, NJ 08619
(609)587-6661 Fax (609)587-8503

Richards, Christopher F., MD {1952631715} Psychy(MEX03)
+ Drs. Coira & Richards
851 Franklin Lake Road/Suite 105 Franklin Lakes, NJ 07417
(201)904-2230 Fax (201)904-2232

Richards, David A., MD {1235129396} IntrMd, MedOnc, OncHem(83,ENGL)
+ Drs. Fein, Porcelli & Richards
75 Veronica Avenue/Suite 201 Somerset, NJ 08873
(732)246-4882 Fax (732)249-5633
+ Regional Cancer Care Associates
111 Union Valley Road/Suite 205 Monroe, NJ 08831
(732)246-4882 Fax (609)395-7955

Richards, Patricia T., MD {1003055518} Anesth(82,IL02)
+ 22 Avenue at Port Imperial/Apt 114
West New York, NJ 07093

Richards, Steven Lawrence, MD {1538168489} Urolgy(93,NY46)<NJ-STPETER, NJ-RWJUBRUN>
+ Mid-Jersey Urology
333 Forsgate Drive/Suite 202 Jamesburg, NJ 08831
(732)561-2058 Fax (732)561-2061

Richardson, Celine Anne, MD {1639355423} Surgry(05,NC05)<NJ-HACKNSK>
+ Hackensack University Center
20 Prospect Avenue/Suite 206 Hackensack, NJ 07601

Richardson, Christie, DO {1174184865} Psychy
+ Rowan Medical Psychiatry
100 Century Parkway/Suite 350 Mount Laurel, NJ 08054
(404)889-4990

Richardson, Michael J., MD {1336197060} Anesth, IntrMd(86,CA15)<NJ-STPETER>
+ Anesthesia Consultnts of NJ/Nova Pain
285 Davidson Avenue/Suite 204 Somerset, NJ 08873
(732)271-1400 Fax (732)271-3544

Richardson, Robert W., MD {1033167978} IntrMd(76,MEXI)<NJ-CLARMAAS, NJ-MTNSIDE>
+ 180 Franklin Avenue
Nutley, NJ 07110 (973)667-4568 Fax (973)667-5989

Physicians by Name and Address

Richfield, Eric Karl, MD {1447326632} Nrolgy, PthNro(80,WI06)
+ EOHSI
170 Frelinghuysen Road   Piscataway, NJ 08854   (732)445-3729   Fax (732)445-0131
+ UH- Robert Wood Johnson Med
125 Paterson Street/MEB 222   New Brunswick, NJ 08901   (732)445-3729   Fax (732)235-8124

Richichi, Joann, DO {1023088390} ObsGyn(84,CA22)
+ Obstetrics & Gynecology Associates
239 Hurffville Crosskeys Road   Sewell, NJ 08080   (856)262-8300   Fax (856)262-1635

Richlan, Richard A., MD {1922004118} Anesth(81,MEX14)<NJ-ACMCITY, NJ-ACMCMAIN>
+ Robert Wood Johnson-UMDNJ Anesthesia Group
1140 Route 72 West   Manahawkin, NJ 08050   (609)978-8900
+ Robert Wood Johnson-UMDNJ Anesthesia Group
125 Paterson Street/CAB 3100   New Brunswick, NJ 08901   (609)978-8900   Fax (732)235-6131

Richman, Jesse, MD {1346402872} Ophthl
+ TLC Kremer Cherry Hill LASIK
1800 Chapel Avenue West/Suite 100   Cherry Hill, NJ 08002

Richman, Mitchell S., MD {1518939727} FamMed(82,NY08)<NJ-VIRTMHBC>
+ 91 Peregrine Drive
Voorhees, NJ 08043   (856)264-0541

Richman, Steven D., MD {1982713681} NuclMd, RadDia(71,NY01)
+ Montclair Radiology
20 High Street   Nutley, NJ 07110   (973)284-1881   Fax (973)284-0269
+ Montclair Radiology
1140 Bloomfield Avenue   West Caldwell, NJ 07006   (973)284-1881   Fax (973)439-6885
+ Montclair Radiology
116 Park Street   Montclair, NJ 07110   (973)746-2525   Fax (973)746-5802

Richman, Steven L., DO {1942271077} ObsGyn(81,PA77)<NJ-VIRTMARL, NJ-VIRTBERL>
+ Cherry Hill Ob/Gyn
150 Century Parkway/Suite A   Mount Laurel, NJ 08054   (856)778-4700   Fax (856)778-1154
+ Cherry Hill Ob/Gyn
777 South White Horse Pike/Suite A-1   Hammonton, NJ 08037   (856)778-4700   Fax (609)561-6309

Richmand, David M., MD {1861435885} SrgThr, Surgry, SrgVas(76,MA07)
+ Garden State Surgical Associates
1511 Park Avenue   South Plainfield, NJ 07080   (908)561-9500   Fax (908)561-7162

Richmond, Chad Eric, DO {1659390789} FamMed, EmrgMd(98,NJ75)<NJ-UNDRWD, NJ-KENEDYHS>
+ The University Doctors - UMDNJ -SOM
570 Egg Harbor Road/Suite C-2   Sewell, NJ 08080   (856)218-0300   Fax (856)589-5082
+ Inspira Health Network
509 North Broad Street   Woodbury, NJ 08096   (856)845-0100

Richmond, Daniel B., MD {1851390959} SprtMd, SrgOrt(92,NJ05)<NJ-OVERLOOK>
+ Comprehensive Orthopaedics
235 Millburn Avenue/Suite 102   Millburn, NJ 07041   (973)258-1177   Fax (973)258-1818

Richmond, John Steven, MD {1376591628} RadV&I, Radiol(90,NY08)<NJ-PALISADE>
+ Imaging Consultants of Essex
94 Old Short Hills Road   Livingston, NJ 07039   (973)322-5804   Fax (973)322-5536

Richter, Douglas Martin, MD {1346321767} IntrMd, CdvDis(89,PA02)<NJ-LOURDMED>
+ University Cardiology
3 Cooper Plaza/Room 311   Camden, NJ 08103   (856)342-2034

Richwine, Charles M., IV, DO {1528116795} FamMed(88,PA77)<NJ-ACMCITY, NJ-ACMCMAIN>
+ Drs. Richwine and Richwine
3110 Ocean Heights Avenue/Suite 1   Egg Harbor Township, NJ 08234   (609)927-9555   Fax (609)926-8902

Richwine, Lori T., DO {1518015783} FamMed(89,PA77)<NJ-ACMCITY, NJ-ACMCMAIN>
+ Drs. Richwine and Richwine
3110 Ocean Heights Avenue/Suite 1   Egg Harbor Township, NJ 08234   (609)927-9555   Fax (609)926-8902

Ricigliano, Mark A., DO {1366482630} FamMed, Gastrn(85,NY75)<NJ-OURLADY>
+ Family Care Associates
6705 Park Avenue   Pennsauken, NJ 08109   (856)662-0017   Fax (856)663-3038

Rickerhauser-Krall, Maureen A., MD {1700924727} PedEmg, Pedtrc(82,NJ05)<NJ-UMDNJ>
+ University Hospital
150 Bergen Street/PediEmrgMed   Newark, NJ 07103   (973)972-5139   Fax (973)972-8276

Ricketti, Anthony J., MD {1285680850} AlgyImmn, IntrMd, CritCr(78,PA09)
+ Mercer Allergy and Pulmonary Associates, LLC
1544 Kuser Road/Suite C-6   Trenton, NJ 08619   (609)581-9900   Fax (609)581-9905

Ricketti, Peter Anthony, DO {1013283233} IntMSlpd
+ Mercer Allergy and Pulmonary Associates, LLC
1544 Kuser Road/Suite C-6   Trenton, NJ 08619   (609)581-9900   Fax (609)581-9905

Ricketts, Robyn D., MD {1780623124} Anesth(00,OR02)<NJ-VIRTMARL>
+ Virtua Marlton Hospital
90 Brick Road/Anesth   Marlton, NJ 08053   (856)355-6000

Rickey, Stephanie B., MD {1740380062} Pedtrc(01,PA01)<NJ-VIRTVOOR, NJ-VIRTUAHS>
+ Advocare Atrium Pediatrics
301 Old Marlton Pike West/Suite 1   Marlton, NJ 08053   (856)988-9101   Fax (856)988-7712
+ Advocare Atrium Pediatrics Cedar Brook
41 South Route 73/Building 1/Suite 101   Hammonton, NJ 08037   (856)988-9101   Fax (609)567-4904

Ricks, Ann Marie, MD {1386892545} ObsGyn
+ Summit Medical Group
160 East Hanover Avenue/Suite 101   Cedar Knolls, NJ 07927   (973)605-5090   Fax (973)605-1705

Ricks, Jason D., MD {1932352812} IntrMd
+ Sheppell and Ricks MD
16 Pocono Road/Suite 305   Denville, NJ 07834   (973)627-0555   Fax (973)627-3880

Ricks, Sandy, MD {1255573937} Pedtrc<NJ-MORRISTN>
+ Somerset Pediatric Group PA
3322 Route 22/Suite 1002   Branchburg, NJ 08876   (908)725-5530   Fax (908)223-6559
+ Somerset Pediatric Group PA
2 World's Fair Drive/Suite 302   Somerset, NJ 08873   (908)725-5530   Fax (732)271-5151

Rider, Timothy Eugene, MD {1215998364} FamMed
+ Freeman Integrated Spine & Pain, P.C.
3499 Route 9 North/Suite 2B   Freehold, NJ 07728   (973)893-7246   Fax (973)970-4012

Ridilla, Leonard, Jr., MD {1568468692} FamMed(89,PA02)<NJ-VIRTVOOR>
+ Haddonfield Family Practice PA
15 East Redman Avenue   Haddonfield, NJ 08033   (856)428-1335   Fax (856)428-6334

Ridley, Diane M., MD {1588643746} Anesth(92,NY01)
+ Robert Wood Johnson-UMDNJ Anesthesia Group
125 Paterson Street/CAB 3100   New Brunswick, NJ 08901   (732)235-7827   Fax (732)235-6131

Ridlovsky, Ludmila, MD {1780878181} IntrMd(90,MOL02)<NJ-MONMOUTH>
+ 21 Kilmer Drive/Building 2/Suite A
Morganville, NJ 07751   (732)851-4955   Fax (509)362-9699

Rieber, Michael Harold, MD {1508812330} SrgOrt, NeuMSptM(92,NY09)
+ The Joint Institute at Saint Barnabas Medical Center
609 Morris Avenue   Springfield, NJ 07081   (973)379-1991   Fax (973)467-8647

Riedel, Jacqueline V., DO {1215173513} FamMed
+ Sherwood Family Practice
165 Princeton Avenue   West Deptford, NJ 08096   (856)384-0210   Fax (856)384-0218

Rieder, Michael J., MD {1447256706} RadDia(86,PA01)<NJ-STFRNMED>
+ Radiology Affiliates of Central New Jersey, P.A.
2501 Kuser Road   Hamilton, NJ 08691   (609)585-8800   Fax (609)585-1825
+ Radiology Affiliates of Central New Jersey, P.A.
3120 Princeton Pike   Lawrenceville, NJ 08648   (609)585-8800   Fax (609)219-0439
+ St. Francis Medical Center
601 Hamilton Avenue/Radiology   Trenton, NJ 08691   (609)599-5000

Riedlinger, Gregory M., MD {1639516891}
+ Rutgers Cancer Institute of New Jersey
195 Little Albany Street/PO Box 2681   New Brunswick, NJ 08903   (202)681-2120   Fax (732)235-6797
griedlin@gmail.com

Riegelhaupt, Rona Susan, MD {1770646697} Pedtrc, AdolMed(84,NY47)<NJ-VALLEY, NJ-HACKNSK>
+ North Jersey Pediatrics
17-10 Fair Lawn Avenue   Fair Lawn, NJ 07410   (201)794-8585   Fax (201)703-9889
+ North Jersey Pediatrics
1011 Clifton Avenue   Clifton, NJ 07013   (201)794-8585   Fax (973)249-1316

Rieger, Kenneth J., MD {1275559700} SrgSpn
+ New Jersey Spine Center
40 Main Street   Chatham, NJ 07928   (973)635-0800   Fax (973)635-6254

Rieger, Mark A., MD {1831161751} PedOrt, SrgOrt, IntrMd(83,CT02)
+ Advocare The Orthopedic Center
218 Ridgedale Avenue/Suite 104   Cedar Knolls, NJ 07927   (973)538-7700   Fax (973)538-9478

Rienzo, Francis G., MD {1003887068} IntrMd(88,GRNA)<NJ-JRSYSHMC>
+ 2164 Route 35/Building D
Sea Girt, NJ 08750   (732)974-1877   Fax (732)974-1878

Rienzo, Peter A., MD {1033166285} Anesth, AnesPain(85,GRN01)
+ Orthopaedic Spine Institute
2315 Route 34 South   Manasquan, NJ 08736   (732)974-0404   Fax (732)449-4271

Riesa, Michael, DO {1932462397}<NJ-KMHTURNV>
+ Kennedy Health Systems/Washington Township Campus
435 Hurffville-Cross Keys Road   Turnersville, NJ 08012   (856)218-5634   Fax (856)218-5664

Riesenman, Joseph John, MD {1336101732} FamMed(00,NJ06)
+ Skylands Medical Group PA
5678 Berkshire Valley Road   Oak Ridge, NJ 07438   (973)697-0200   Fax (973)697-6844

Riestra Cortes, Juan L., MD {1841255320} Psychy, PsyGrt(87,NY20)<NJ-MTNSIDE>
+ 70 Park Street
Montclair, NJ 07042   (973)655-9300   Fax (973)439-5780

Riewe, Kathleen O'Day, MD {1851596902} PedHem, Pedtrc, IntrMd(00,MA07)
+ Princeton Nassau Pediatrics, P.A.
25 South Route 31   Pennington, NJ 08534   (609)745-5300   Fax (609)745-5320

Rifai, Aiman, DO {1871534172} SrgOrt(92,NJ75)
+ 1033 Route 46/Suite A-206
Clifton, NJ 07013   (973)594-8500   Fax (973)594-8505

Rifkin, Paul L., MD {1841441250} Hemato, IntrMd, Onclgy(67,DC02)<NJ-TRINIJSC>
+ Visiting Physician Services
23 Main Street/Suite D1   Holmdel, NJ 07733   (732)571-1000   Fax (732)571-1000

Riftine, Julia, MD {1861685216} ObsGyn, IntrMd(03,GRN01)<NJ-MEADWLND>
+ Meadowlands Hospital Medical Center
55 Meadowlands Parkway/Suite 436   Secaucus, NJ 07096   (201)392-3063   Fax (201)392-3069

Rigatti, Damian F., DO {1154311579} FamMed(90,NY75)<NJ-WARREN>
+ Pleasant Run Family Physicians
925 US Highway 202   Neshanic Station, NJ 08853   (908)788-9468   Fax (908)788-5720

Rigatti, Darrell J., MD {1710914411} Pedtrc(86,MEXI)<NJ-MONMOUTH, NJ-RIVERVW>
+ Atlantic Coast Pediatrics
20 White Road   Shrewsbury, NJ 07702   (732)741-4988   Fax (732)741-4979

Riggall, Michael Justin, MD {1164592333} Pedtrc, IntrMd(VA04)
+ Princeton Nassau Pediatrics, P.A.
25 South Route 31   Pennington, NJ 08534   (609)745-5300   Fax (609)745-5320
+ Princeton Nassau Pediatrics, P.A.
196 Princeton-Hightstown Road   West Windsor, NJ 08550   (609)745-5300   Fax (609)799-2294

Riggi, Joseph, DO {1265436638} FamMed(98,NJ75)
+ Avenel Iselin Medical Group
400 Gill Lane   Iselin, NJ 08830   (732)404-1580   Fax (732)404-1594

Riggs, Renee Lisa, DO {1760551998} EmrgMd(02,PA78)<NJ-RWJUBRUN>
+ University Emergency Medicine
125 Paterson Street/MEB 104   New Brunswick, NJ 08901   (732)235-8717   Fax (732)235-7379
+ RWJ University Hospital New Brunswick
One Robert Wood Johnson Place   New Brunswick, NJ 08901   (732)828-3000

Righthand, Richard N., MD {1093738031} IntrMd(85,NY03)<NJ-HACKNSK, NJ-HOLYNAME>
+ 691 Palisade Avenue
Cliffside Park, NJ 07010

Rigoglioso, Camille M., MD {1295909646} IntrMd(86,NJ05)
+ 222 Cedar Lane/Suite 301
Teaneck, NJ 07666   (201)836-4900   Fax (201)836-7141

Rigoglioso, Vincent, MD {1356376719} Gastrn, IntrMd(85,GRNA)<NJ-HACKNSK, NJ-HOLYNAME>
+ Teaneck Gastroenterology & Endoscopy Center
1086 Teaneck Road/Suite 4-C   Teaneck, NJ 07666   (201)837-9449   Fax (201)578-1699

Rigolosi, Robert S., MD {1346240280} IntrMd, Nephro(63,ITA17)<NJ-HOLYNAME, NJ-VALLEY>
+ Holy Name Hospital
718 Teaneck Road/Hemodialysis   Teaneck, NJ 07666   (201)833-3223   Fax (201)833-7090
+ Renal Medicine Associates PA
302 Union Street   Hackensack, NJ 07601   (201)833-3223

Physicians by Name and Address

Rigolosi, Ronald A., MD {1760595888} IntrMd(75,NJ06)<NJ-HOLY-NAME>
+ Riverside Family Care
 4 Hunter Street/Suite 2A   Lodi, NJ 07644   (973)772-8585
 Fax (973)772-8586

Riguerra, Rosalia C., MD {1891886008} IntrMd, EmrgEMed(81,PHI08)<NJ-STJOSHOS>
+ St. Joseph's Regional Medical Center
 703 Main Street   Paterson, NJ 07503   (973)754-2000

Rigueur, Adrienne Brooks, DO {1104022920} EmrgMd(NJ75<NJ-VIRTVOOR>
+ Virtua Voorhees
 100 Bowman Drive/Emerg Med   Voorhees, NJ 08043
 (856)247-3000
+ Emergency Physician Associates, P.A.
 307 South Evergreen Avenue/PO Box 298   Woodbury, NJ 08096   (856)845-3000   Fax (856)848-8536

Rihacek, Gregory S., MD {1114992773} IntrMd, Rheuma(82,NJ06)
+ Arthritis Care Medical Center
 19 Clyde Road/Suite 101   Somerset, NJ 08873   (732)568-0023   Fax (732)568-0159

Rijhsinghani, Sonia J., MD {1831200054} Grtrcs, IntrMd(88,INA87)<NJ-JRSYSHMC, NJ-OCEANMC>
+ 200 Craig Road
 Manalapan, NJ 07726   (732)333-2120   Fax (732)359-1501

Rijhwani, Kiran, MD {1457437121} PthACl(95,INA9B)
+ 20 Vervalen Street
 Norwood, NJ 07648

Rijsinghani, Paresh K., MD {1669407797} Radiol, RadDia(96,NJ05)<NJ-CHSMRCER, NJ-CHSFULD>
+ Capital Health System/Mercer Campus
 446 Bellevue Avenue/Radiology   Trenton, NJ 08618
 (609)394-4000
+ Capital Health System/Fuld Campus
 750 Brunswick Avenue/Radiology   Trenton, NJ 08638
 (609)394-6000

Riley, Cara Ann, MD {1437310836} Anesth<NJ-UNDRWD>
+ Inspira Health Network
 509 North Broad Street   Woodbury, NJ 08096   (856)845-0100

Riley, David J., MD {1265504310} IntrMd, PulDis(68,MD01)<NJ-RWJUBRUN>
+ University Medical Group - General Internal Medicine
 125 Paterson Street/Suite 5100A   New Brunswick, NJ 08903
 (732)235-6511   Fax (732)235-7048

Riley, Roth Leon, MD {1831241264} FamMed
+ 23-08 Maple Avenue
 Fair Lawn, NJ 07410   (201)794-4500   Fax (229)271-3839

Riley-Lowe, Judith E., DO {1497861538} FamMed(03,PA77)
+ Center for Family Health/Doctors & Midwives
 105 Manheim Avenue/Suite 1   Bridgeton, NJ 08302
 (856)455-2700   Fax (856)455-7051

Rilli, Charles F., MD {1639126485} Urolgy(84,NJ05)<NJ-CLAR-MAAS>
+ Essex Hudson Urology
 213 South Frank Rodgers Blvd   Harrison, NJ 07029
 (973)482-7070
+ Essex Hudson Urology
 243 Chestnut Street   Newark, NJ 07105   (973)482-7070
 Fax (973)344-9188
+ Essex Hudson Urology
 256 Broad Street   Bloomfield, NJ 07029   (973)743-4450
 Fax (973)429-9076

Rim, Josephine Myunghi, MD {1023206612} PhysMd, PainMd(95,NY08)
+ 80 Hazlet Avenue/Suite 12
 Hazlet, NJ 07730   (732)379-7773   Fax (732)264-6889

Rimal, Jyotsna, MD {1285714238} Anesth(91,INA02)
+ 24 Country Club Road
 Livingston, NJ 07039

Rimarenko, Seraphim, MD {1003920240} PthACl(79,MEXI)<NJ-HCKTSTWN, NJ-STCLRDEN>
+ St. Clare's Hospital-Denville Campus
 25 Pocono Road   Denville, NJ 07834   (973)625-6718   Fax (973)983-2367
 simrim@aol.com
+ Hackettstown Regional Medical Center
 651 Willow Grove Street   Hackettstown, NJ 07840
 (908)852-5100

Rimmer, Cheryl L., MD {1295784866} PthACl(00,MNT01)
+ 27 Sand Road
 Milltown, NJ 08850

Rimmer, John Joseph, III, DO {1114244787} EmrgMd(05,NY75)<NJ-HOBUNIMC>
+ Hoboken University Medical Center
 308 Willow Avenue/Emerg Med   Hoboken, NJ 07030
 (201)418-1000

Rincon, Fred, MD {1326159443} Nrolgy, VasNeu, CritCre(96,COL23)<NJ-VIRTVOOR>
+ Virtua Voorhees
 100 Bowman Drive/Neurology   Voorhees, NJ 08043
 (856)247-3000

Rinehouse, Jay A., MD {1649237850} Anesth(87,LA01)
+ Ambulatory Anesthesia Care, PC
 1450 Route 22 West   Mountainside, NJ 07092   (908)233-2020   Fax (908)233-9322

Ring, Kenneth S., MD {1225025174} Urolgy, PedUro(85,NY47)<NJ-OVERLOOK, NJ-WESTHDSN>
+ Premier Urology Group, LLC
 275 Orchard Street   Westfield, NJ 07090   (908)654-5100
 Fax (908)654-8021
+ Premier Urology Group, LLC
 659 Kearny Avenue   Kearny, NJ 07032   (908)654-5100
 Fax (201)789-8755
+ Premier Urology Group, LLC
 1500 Pleasant Valley Road   West Orange, NJ 07090
 (973)325-0091   Fax (973)789-8755

Ringel, David M., DO {1598768319} Ophthl(84,NJ75)<NJ-KMH-TURNV, NJ-KMHCHRRY>
+ South Jersey Laser Vision
 101A Kingsway West   Sewell, NJ 08080   (856)582-9507
 Fax (856)582-4472
 dringel@pol.net

Ringwala, Birju H., DO {1497044895}
+ 23 Amberfield Road
 Robbinsville, NJ 08691   (609)529-7999
 birju.ringwala@gmail.com

Ringwelski-Hannan, Anna Ewa, MD {1851583868} EmrgMd(05,IL06)<NJ-MORRISTN>
+ St. Clare's Hospital-Denville Campus
 25 Pocono Road   Denville, NJ 07834   (973)625-6000

Rini, Frank J., MD {1043295884} Ophthl(82,NY01)
+ 595 Chestnut Ridge Road
 Woodcliff Lake, NJ 07677   (201)930-8590

Rink, Lisa Ann, DO {1437101623} IntrMd(95,NJ75)<NJ-VIRTVOOR>
+ Lisa A. Rink Family Medicine, LLC.
 217 White Horse Pike   Haddon Heights, NJ 08035
 (856)672-1115   Fax (856)672-9111

Rinkus, Keith Michael, MD {1750411666} SrgOrt, SrgSpn
+ Orthopaedic Sports Medicine
 80 Oak Hill Road   Red Bank, NJ 07701   (732)741-2313
 Fax (732)741-7154
+ Orthopaedic Sports Medicine & Rehabilitation Center
 25 Kilmer Drive/Building 3/Suite 105   Morganville, NJ 07751
 (732)741-2313   Fax (732)617-5959

Rinnier, Robert Todd, DO {1386962785} Anesth<NJ-COOPRUMC>
+ Cooper University Hospital
 One Cooper Plaza   Camden, NJ 08103   (856)342-2425
 Fax (856)968-8239

Rinvil, Edwine, MD {1386810182} IntrMd(05,NJ05)
+ Capital Health System/Fuld Campus
 750 Brunswick Avenue   Trenton, NJ 08638   (609)394-6000

Riolo, Thomas Antonio, DO {1518260702} PhysMd(10,NY75)<NY-NYUTISCH>
+ Physical Medicine & Rehabilitation Center
 500 Grand Avenue/1st Floor   Englewood, NJ 07631
 (201)567-2277   Fax (201)567-7506

Riordan, Kevin J., MD {1134516060} EmrgMd, FamMed(81,GRN01)<NJ-BURDTMLN>
+ Cape Regional Medical Center
 2 Stone Harbor Boulevard   Cape May Court House, NJ 08210   (609)463-2000   Fax (609)463-2946

Rios, Jose Conrado, MD {1689846123} RadDia, RadNro(04,NY19)<NJ-MORRISTN>
+ Memorial Radiology Associates
 10 Lanidex Plaza West/Suite 125   Parsippany, NJ 07054
 (973)503-5700   Fax (973)386-5701

Rioux, Stephen R., DO {1740209873} FamMed, EmrgMd(86,NJ75)<NJ-UNDRWD>
+ 140 West Tomlin Station Road
 Mickleton, NJ 08056   (856)845-9600

Ripper, Jill Richelle, MD {1245283969} EmrgMd(98,PA02)<NJ-NWRKBETH>
+ Newark Beth Israel Medical Center
 201 Lyons Avenue/EmrgMed   Newark, NJ 07112   (973)926-7000   Fax (610)617-6280

Rippey, Kelly Ann, MD {1275793739} SrgCrC<NJ-HACKNSK>
+ Hackensack University Medical Center
 30 Prospect Avenue   Hackensack, NJ 07601   (201)996-2000
+ Hackensack Surgical Critical Care Physicians
 5 Summit Avenue/Suite 105   Hackensack, NJ 07601
 (201)996-2000   Fax (201)883-1268

Risi, Mark G., DO {1942221957} FamMed(89,NJ75)<NJ-RWJUHAM, NJ-CHSMRCER>
+ Rednor-Risi Family Medicine Associates, P.C.
 1 Washington Boulevard/Suite 7   Robbinsville, NJ 08691
 (609)448-4353   Fax (609)448-4558

Risimini, Robert J., MD {1740365675} Pedtrc, FamMed(68,PA02)<NJ-COOPRUMC>
+ Cooper Family Medicine
 504 White Horse Pike   Haddon Heights, NJ 08035
 (856)546-7990   Fax (856)546-2686

Risin, Michael Simon, MD {1407800808} SrgPlstc(97,MA01)
+ 2 Lincoln Highway/Suite 508
 Edison, NJ 08820   (732)933-8788   Fax (732)933-1536

Rispoli, Frances M., DO {1184832255} PhysMd, SprtMd(92,NY75)
+ Mauti Medical & Sports Medicine Associates
 406 Milltown Road   Springfield, NJ 07081   (973)921-1777
 Fax (973)921-1790
 jmautimd@mautimedical.com

Rispoli, Lauren C., MD {1003801259} Ophthl(89,NJ05)
+ Parsippany Eye Care Associates
 46 Eagle Rock Avenue   East Hanover, NJ 07936   (973)560-1500   Fax (973)560-0419

Riss, Alexander David, DO {1013174507} EmrgMd<NJ-STJOSHOS>
+ St Joseph's Medical Center Emergency
 703 Main Street   Paterson, NJ 07503   (973)754-2240   Fax (973)754-2249

Riss, Martin, DO {1548276827} FamMed(72,MO78)
+ Brick Town Medical
 34 Lanes Mill Road   Brick, NJ 08724   (732)458-0300   Fax (732)458-8449

Rissmiller, David J., DO {1235102443} Psychy(74,PA77)
+ University Hospital-SOM Department of Psychiatry
 2250 Chapel Avenue West/Suite 100   Cherry Hill, NJ 08002
 (856)482-9000   Fax (856)482-1159

Ritch De Herrera, Thaddeus D., MD {1801063714} IntrMd
+ University Hospital-School of Public Health
 170 Frelinghuysen Road/Room 212   Piscataway, NJ 08854
 (732)445-0123   Fax (732)445-3644

Ritchie, Paul Harvey, MD {1568445963} Anesth(99,GRN01)<NJ-HACKNSK>
+ Red Bank Anesthesia, LLC
 1 Riverview Plaza   Red Bank, NJ 07701   (732)530-2255
 Fax (732)450-2620

Ritenour, Kristen J., MD {1043522196}<NJ-VIRTVOOR>
+ Virtua Voorhees
 100 Bowman Drive   Voorhees, NJ 08043   (571)271-1425
 kjrite@gmail.com

Ritota, Perry C., MD {1699762658} SrgPlstc, SrgRec(89,NJ06)<NJ-HACKNSK>
+ 20 Prospect Avenue
 Hackensack, NJ 07601   (201)342-7333   Fax (201)342-4490

Ritsan, Julia B., DO {1730178054} FamMed(01,NY75)
+ Jewish Renaissance Medical Center
 275 Hobart Street   Perth Amboy, NJ 08861   (732)376-9333
 Fax (732)324-5765

Ritsema, Marc E., DO {1942279799} PsyCAd, Psychy(73,MI12)
+ 22 South Holmdel Road
 Holmdel, NJ 07733   (732)946-4086

Ritson, Brenda Marie, MD {1134383086} Pedtrc, IntrMd(06,CT01)<NH-ANDROSGN, NJ-VIRTMARL>
+ CHOP Care Network at Virtua Voorhees Hospital
 100 Bowman Drive   Voorhees, NJ 08043   (856)247-3244
 Fax (609)261-5842

Ritt, Jake Edward, MD {1710297965}
+ Summit Medical Group
 6 Brighton Road/2 FL   Clifton, NJ 07012   (973)777-7911
 Fax (973)777-5403
+ Summit Medical Group
 140 Park Avenue/3rd Floor   Florham Park, NJ 07932
 (973)404-7625

Rittberg, Shannon Bara, DO {1588643944} FamMed(02,NJ75)
+ Center for Aesthetic and Integrative Medicine
 2399 Highway 34/Building A5   Manasquan, NJ 08736
 (732)528-5533   Fax (732)528-0360
+ Wall Family Medical
 2130 Highway 35/Building C Suite 324   Sea Girt, NJ 08750
 (732)528-5533   Fax (732)974-2117
+ 2204 Gramercy Way
 Mount Laurel, NJ 08736

Ritter, Albert W., MD {1821109935} EmrgMd(92,NY09)<NJ-MOR-RISTN>
+ Morristown Medical Center
 100 Madison Avenue   Morristown, NJ 07962   (973)971-5000

Ritter, Jill M., MD {1043272479} Rheuma, IntrMd(89,NY19)<NJ-STBARNMC>
+ Center for Rheumatic & Autoimmune Diseases
 200 South Orange Avenue/Suite 107   Livingston, NJ 07039
 (973)322-7400   Fax (973)322-7420

Rittweger, Edward S., MD {1184621625} RadDia, RadNro(77,NJ05)<NJ-RWJURAH>
+ Red Bank Radiologists, P.A.
 200 White Road/Suite 115   Little Silver, NJ 07739
 (732)741-9595   Fax (732)741-0985
+ Coastal Imaging, LLC
 79 Route 37 West/Suite 103   Toms River, NJ 08755
 (732)741-9595   Fax (732)276-2325
+ Doctors Radiology Center - MRI of Woodbridge
 1500 St. George Avenue/Peach Plaza   Avenel, NJ 07739
 (732)574-1414   Fax (732)574-0845

Physicians by Name and Address

Ritz, Steven Bernard, MD {1205928058} Pedtrc(88,PA01)<NY-NSUHMANH, NY-SOUTHNAS>
+ Nemours Dupont Pediatrics, Voorhees
  443 Laurel Oak Road Voorhees, NJ 08043 (856)309-8508 Fax (856)309-8556
+ AtlantiCare/Dupont Children's Health Program
  2500 English Creek Avenue Egg Harbor Township, NJ 08234 (856)309-8508 Fax (609)641-3652

Riva, Inna, DO {1013327345} FamMed(CA23
+ 206 Washington Street/Suite 1A
  Jersey City, NJ 07302 (408)981-7358 Fax (508)659-8262

Rivas, Jimena, MD {1366811978} ObsGyn
+ Advanced Obstetrics & Gynecology, LLC
  4 Walter E. Foran Boulevard/Suite 302 Flemington, NJ 08822 (908)806-0080 Fax (908)806-8570

Rivas, Manuel A., MD {1093741159} Urolgy(66,MEXI)<NJ-CHS-FULD, NJ-CHSMRCER>
+ 2081 Klockner Road Bldg 4/Suite16
  Trenton, NJ 08690 (609)588-5656 Fax (609)588-9563

Rivell, Crystal Giovanna, DO {1124259460} FamMed
+ Di Lisi Family Medicine LLC
  110 North Woodbury Road Pitman, NJ 08071 (856)589-1212 Fax (856)589-6635
+ Inspira Medical Group
  660 Woodbury Glassboro Road/Suite 26 Sewell, NJ 08080 (856)589-1212 Fax (856)464-1855

Rivera, Adaliz, MD {1508073362} FamMed, IntrMd(05,NJ06)<NJ-COOPRUMC>
+ Cooper University Medical Center/Camden
  3 Cooper Plaza/Suite 502 Camden, NJ 08103 (856)963-6888
+ Cooper Family Medicine
  1865 Harrison Avenue/Suite 1300 Camden, NJ 08103 (856)963-6888 Fax (856)365-0279

Rivera, Alberto R., MD {1639122716} EmrgMd, IntrMd(80,PERU)<NJ-NWTNMEM>
+ Newton Medical Center
  175 High Street/EmergMed Newton, NJ 07860 (973)383-2121

Rivera, Carlos G., MD {1992741326} IntrMd(82,MEX62)
+ 9 Memorial Parkway
  Long Branch, NJ 07740 (732)728-7010 Fax (732)728-0704

Rivera, Edward, MD {1578777439} IntrMd<NJ-LOURDMED>
+ Lourdes Medical Center of Burlington County
  218 Sunset Road/Internal Med Willingboro, NJ 08046 (609)835-3056 Fax (609)835-3061

Rivera, Laura A., MD {1740366640} FamMed(94,NY46)
+ Somerset Health Center
  40 Stirling Road/Suite 208 Watchung, NJ 07069 (908)757-1000 Fax (908)757-0564

Rivera, Leonora M., MD {1518955657} PhysMd(79,PHI29)<NJ-KSLRSADB, NJ-SOMERSET>
+ Kessler Institute for Rehabilitation
  300 Market Street Saddle Brook, NJ 07663 (201)587-8500

Rivera, Loyda I., MD {1235167123} PedCrd, Pedtrc(85,PRO03)<NJ-JRSYSHMC, NJ-CENTRAST>
+ Monmouth Ocean Childrens Heart Center
  3204 Allaire Road Wall, NJ 07719 (732)282-1060 Fax (732)282-1061
+ Monmouth Ocean Childrens Heart Center
  81 Oak Hill Road Red Bank, NJ 07701 (732)282-1060

Rivera, Roger Alberto, Jr., MD {1992940373} Pedtrc(08,NJ05)<NJ-UMDNJ>
+ Building Blocks Pediatric Group
  415 Harrison Avenue Westfield, NJ 07090 (862)955-3183 Fax (862)955-1389

Rivera, Roger Antonio, MD {1538160890} Pedtrc(81,NIC01)<NJ-ENGLWOOD, NJ-HACKNSK>
+ Advanced Pediatrics
  5 Summit Avenue/Suite 203 Hackensack, NJ 07601 (201)343-4800 Fax (201)343-4668

Rivera, Seetha Maneyapanda, MD {1275819732}
+ Building Blocks Pediatric Group
  415 Harrison Avenue Westfield, NJ 07090 (862)955-3183 Fax (862)955-1389

Rivera, Tara Elizabeth, DO {1083669618} FamMed(99,NY75)
+ Princeton Health Medical & Surgical Associates
  401 Ridge Road/Suite 6 Dayton, NJ 08810 (732)329-4800

Rivera, Velmina S., MD {1235120213} Pedtrc, AdolMd, IntrMd(87,PHIL)<NJ-COOPRUMC>
+ Cooper Perinatology Associates
  3 Cooper Plaza/Suite 502 Camden, NJ 08103 (856)356-4935 Fax (856)968-8499
+ Phoenix Ob-Gyn Associates
  110 Marter Avenue/Suite 505 Moorestown, NJ 08057 (856)356-4935 Fax (856)235-3795

Rivera, Yadyra, MD {1346272002} IntrMd, Hemato, MedOnc(92,PRO03)<NJ-HOLYNAME>
+ Holy Name Hospital
  718 Teaneck Road/Cancer Ctr Teaneck, NJ 07666 (201)833-3000

Rivera Curiba, Mary A., MD {1841396504} Rheuma, IntrMd(83,PHI01)
+ 1053 Westfield Avenue
  Rahway, NJ 07065 (732)382-8000 Fax (732)382-2742

Rivera Galindo, Claudia P., MD {1629240668} FamMed(NY46
+ Care Station Medical Group
  456 Prospect Avenue West Orange, NJ 07052 (973)731-6767 Fax (973)731-9881

Rivera-Penera, Maria T., MD {1184671596} Pedtrc, PedGst(87,PHI09)<NJ-STJOSHOS>
+ St. Joseph's Children's Hospital
  703 Main Street/Gstrntrlgy Paterson, NJ 07503 (973)754-2393
+ St. Joseph's Pediatrics DePaul Center
  11 Getty Avenue/2nd Floor Paterson, NJ 07503 (973)754-2727

Rivera-Segarra, Stephanie Denise, MD {1760747356} ObsGyn
+ Tenafly Ob-Gyn Associates PA
  2 Dean Drive/2nd Floor Tenafly, NJ 07670 (201)569-3300 Fax (201)569-7649

Rivers, Colleen Marie, MD {1164669925} EmrgMd
+ Birmingham, Colleen M.
  4b Parmly Street Rumson, NJ 07760

Rivers, Wendy Marie, MD {1215973979} Pedtrc, GenPrc, IntrMd(89,CT01)
+ Princeton Nassau Pediatrics, P.A.
  196 Princeton-Hightstown Road West Windsor, NJ 08550 (609)799-5335 Fax (609)799-2294

Rivlin, Kwan Thanaporn, MD {1427396209} IntrMd, IntHos(08,THA02)<MA-NSSALEM, MA-UNIONNSM>
+ Virtua Hospitalist Group Marlton
  90 Brick Road Marlton, NJ 08053 (856)355-6730

Riyaz, Najmun, MD {1083654651} Psychy(97,INA36)<NJ-UMDNJ>
+ 333 Laurel Oak Road
  Voorhees, NJ 08043 (856)875-6920 Fax (856)429-3826

Rizio, Louis, III, MD {1184645608} SrgOrt, SprtMd, SrgShr(94,NJ03)<NJ-OVERLOOK, NJ-RWJUBRUN>
+ Summit Medical Group
  75 East Northfield Road Livingston, NJ 07039 (973)758-1078 Fax (908)673-7336

Rizk, Nabil Pierre, MD {1578549168} SrgThr, Surgry(92,CT01)
+ Hackensack University Medical Center
  20 Prospect Avenue/Suite 406 Hackensack, NJ 07601 (201)996-5960

Rizk, Naglaa T., MD {1144450826} ObsGyn(96,NJ05)
+ New Bridge Medical Center
  230 East Ridgewood Avenue Paramus, NJ 07652 (201)967-4000

Rizkala, Emad Remond, MD {1255637146} Urolgy, Surgry(05,NY48)
+ Urology Care Alliance
  733 North Beers Street/Suite L-6 Holmdel, NJ 07733 (732)739-2200 Fax (732)739-8988
+ Urology Care Alliance
  2 Hospital Plaza/Suite 110 Old Bridge, NJ 08857 (732)739-2200 Fax (732)972-0966

Rizkalla, Michael H., MD {1477717791} PhysMd(07,DMN01)
+ Performance Spine & Sports Medicine
  9500 K Johnson Boulevard/Suite 1 Bordentown, NJ 08505 (609)817-0050 Fax (609)588-8602
+ Performance Spine & Sports Medicine
  4056 Quakerbridge Road/Suite 111 Lawrenceville, NJ 08648 (609)817-0050 Fax (609)588-8602

Rizkalla, Suzette, MD {1821417528} IntrMd
+ Medical Internists Associates PA
  22-18 Broadway/Suite 104 Fair Lawn, NJ 07410 (201)797-4503 Fax (201)797-4270

Rizvi, Abbas Ali, MD {1437404274}
+ Tatem Brown Family Practice
  2225 East Evesham Road/Suite 101 Voorhees, NJ 08043 (856)795-5330 Fax (856)325-3704

Rizvi, Amir M., MD {1992806129} Psychy(86,PAK24)<NJ-TRENTPSY>
+ Trenton Psychiatric Hospital
  Sullivan Way/PO Box 7600/Psych West Trenton, NJ 08628 (609)633-1500

Rizvi, Anwar Ahmad, MD {1760788061} IntrMd
+ Drs. Rizvi & Rizvi
  151 Jewett Avenue Jersey City, NJ 07304 (201)920-9926

Rizvi, Azam H., MD {1275535668} RadNro(94,NJ06)
+ Radiology Associates of Burlington County
  1295 Route 38 West/PO Box 479 Hainesport, NJ 08036 (609)261-7017 Fax (609)261-4180

Rizvi, Faraz, MD {1760789390} IntrMd(08,STM01)
+ 7360 Clubhouse Circle/Unit 7360
  Egg Harbor, NJ 08215 (201)621-2296

Rizvi, Kashan H., MD {1225308091}
+ Somerset Family Practice
  110 Rehill Avenue Somerville, NJ 08876 (908)685-2900 Fax (908)704-3764

Rizvi, Masood A., MD {1750392197} Gastrn, Grtrcs, IntrMd(68,INDI)<NJ-MTNSIDE, NJ-CLARMAAS>
+ 900 Pompton Avenue/Suite B1
  Cedar Grove, NJ 07009 (973)239-5656 Fax (973)239-4091

Rizvi, Muhammad A., MD {1346277555} IntrMd(01,PAK11)
+ Hope Community Cancer Center LLC
  210 South Shore Road/Suite 106-A Marmora, NJ 08223 (609)390-7888 Fax (609)390-2614

Rizvi, Nazia, MD {1205818135} IntrMd(94,PAK11)
+ Primary HealthCare LLC
  1543 Highway 27/Suite 15 Somerset, NJ 08873 (732)220-0049 Fax (732)354-0486

Rizvi, Sardar Ahmad, MD {1235423948}
+ Drs. Rizvi & Rizvi
  151 Jewett Avenue Jersey City, NJ 07304 (201)912-6877

Rizvi, Syed M., MD {1548371297} IntrMd, CdvDis(64,INA05)<NJ-STMRYPAS>
+ 383 Clifton Avenue
  Clifton, NJ 07011 (973)546-3024 Fax (973)546-4046

Rizvi, Syed Wajih-Ul-Hasan, MD {1275573321} EnDbMt, Nutrtn(86,PAK11)<NJ-RWJUHAM, NJ-SOCEANCO>
+ R Endocrinology
  1100 72 West/Med Arts Pavilion/SOCH Manahawkin, NJ 08050 (609)468-2505
  srizvi@y-endocrinology.com
+ R Endocrinology
  94 Whitehorse-Hamilton Square Hamilton, NJ 08690 (609)468-2505 Fax (609)585-4269

Rizvi, Tariq A., MD {1447277918} IntrMd(90,PAKI)<NJ-STPETER, NJ-RWJUBRUN>
+ Central Jersey Internal Medicine
  75 Veronica Avenue/Suite 204 Somerset, NJ 08873 (732)828-0002 Fax (732)828-7070

Rizwan, Mohammad, MD {1811982648} IntrMd(82,PAK11)
+ Pathlink, LLC
  66 West Gilbert Street/Suite 100 Tinton Falls, NJ 07701 (732)212-0060 Fax (732)212-0061

Rizzetta, Anthony J., DO {1487618427} FamMed, IntrMd(91,PA77)<NJ-BURDTMLN>
+ Cape Regional Medical Center
  2 Stone Harbor Boulevard/Internal Med Cape May Court House, NJ 08210 (609)463-2803 Fax (609)463-4991

Rizzo, Charles C., MD {1285703371} SrgOrt, SprtMd(90,IL42)<NJ-MONMOUTH, NJ-RIVERVW>
+ Shore Orthopaedic Group
  35 Gilbert Street South Tinton Falls, NJ 07701 (732)530-1515 Fax (732)747-5433
+ Shore Orthopaedic Group
  1255 Route 70/Suite 11S Lakewood, NJ 08701 (732)530-1515 Fax (732)942-2311
+ Shore Orthopaedic Group
  1322 Route 72 West Manahawkin, NJ 07701 (609)597-1377 Fax (609)597-0204

Rizzo, David M., DO {1447267208} FamMed(97,NY75)
+ Union Family Medicine
  2300 Vauxhall Road Union, NJ 07083 (908)688-4424

Rizzo, Joseph Alfonso, MD {1659453975} IntrMd(86,NJ06)<NJ-HOLYNAME>
+ Aspen Medical Associates, P.A.
  1 DeGraw Square Teaneck, NJ 07666 (201)928-0200 Fax (201)928-0820

Rizzo, Robert Anthony, MD {1235213000} IntrMd(86,ITAL)<NJ-STJOSHOS>
+ Rizzo Medical Associates
  22-18 Broadway/Suite 102 Fair Lawn, NJ 07410 (201)797-3636 Fax (201)794-9229
+ Heart & Vascular Medical Group
  680 Broadway/Suite 116-A Paterson, NJ 07514 (201)797-3636 Fax (862)264-2386

Rizzo, Thomas F., MD {1194799445} CdvDis, IntrMd(81,MEX34)<NJ-JRSYSHMC, NJ-CENTRAST>
+ Monmouth Cardiology Associates, LLC
  11 Meridian Road Eatontown, NJ 07724 (732)663-0300 Fax (732)663-0301
+ Monmouth Cardiology Associates, LLC
  222 Schanck Road/Suite 104 Freehold, NJ 07728 (732)663-0300 Fax (732)431-1712

Roach, Beth Lynnell, MD {1881612802} PhysMd(94,NJ05)
+ PO Box 940
  Oakhurst, NJ 07755

Roach, Neil A., MD {1114955259} RadDia, Radiol, IntrMd(87,NY01)
+ Heights Imaging Center
  17 White Horse Pike Haddon Heights, NJ 08035 (856)546-1177 Fax (856)546-0666

Roan, Minda Unidad S., MD {1477539740} Pedtrc(78,PHI01)<NJ-ACMCMAIN, NJ-ACMCITY>
+ Kids Care Pediatrics
  6529 Blackhorse Pike Egg Harbor Township, NJ 08234 (609)645-8500 Fax (609)272-8886

Roat, David B., DO {1629137278} Psychy(94,PA77)<NJ-AN-CPSYCH>
  + Ancora Psychiatric Hospital
    301 Spring Garden Road   Hammonton, NJ 08037
    (609)561-1700   Fax (609)561-2509
Robaina, Luis A., MD {1639334923} GenPrc
  + Center for Family Health
    122 Clinton Street   Hoboken, NJ 07030   (201)418-3100
    (201)418-3148
Robalino-Sanghavi, Michelle Marie, MD {1548550072} PhysMd
  + 120 Eagle Rock Avenue/Suite 154
    East Hanover, NJ 07936   (201)447-4772
Robberson, Heather Leigh, MD {1902802739} IntrMd(96,GRN01)<NJ-OCEANMC, NJ-KIMBALL>
  + 475 Route 70
    Lakewood, NJ 08701
Robbins, Inga H., MD {1316988876} CdvDis, IntrMd(88,PA02)
  + Womens Health & Wellness
    2500 English Creek Avenue   Egg Harbor Township, NJ 08234
    (609)677-7776   Fax (609)677-7509
Robbins, Joseph A., DO {1962474767} IntrMd(73,IA75)
  + 451 South Washington Avenue
    Piscataway, NJ 08854   (732)968-8850   Fax (732)968-8855
Robbins, Lisa Ilene, MD {1619005378} Psychy, IntrMd(89,LA01)
  + 127 East Mount Pleasant Avenue
    Livingston, NJ 07039   (973)449-5726   Fax (973)556-1774
Robbins, Steven G., MD {1356446066} SrgOrt(80,MEXI)
  + Center for Orthopaedics
    1500 Pleasant Valley Way/Suite 101   West Orange, NJ 07052   (973)669-5600   Fax (973)669-0269
  + Short Hills Surgery Center
    187 Millburn Avenue/Suite 101   Millburn, NJ 07041
    (973)669-5600   Fax (973)671-0557
Robel, Lindsey, MD {1831500842} Pedtrc
  + Cooper Peds/Children's Regional Ctr
    3 Cooper Plaza/Suite 200   Camden, NJ 08103   (856)342-2001   Fax (856)368-8297
Roberson, Meika Tylese Neblett, MD {1134194954} EmrgMd(98,DC03)<NY-MTSNAIQN>
  + Hoboken University Medical Center
    308 Willow Avenue   Hoboken, NJ 07030   (201)418-1574
Roberti, Maria Isabel, MD {1376580415} Pedtrc, PedNph(83,BRA66)<NJ-STBARNMC, NJ-NWRKBETH>
  + St. Barnabas Medical Center
    94 Old Short Hills Road/Suite 304   Livingston, NJ 07039
    (973)322-5264   Fax (973)322-2315
Roberti, Roberto R., MD {1104811561} CdvDis(83,BRAZ)
  + Associates in Cardiovascular Disease, LLC
    211 Mountain Avenue   Springfield, NJ 07081   (973)467-0005   Fax (973)912-8989
Roberts, Barbara Theresa, MD {1770631822} FamMed, IntrMd(81,PA09)
  + Patients first
    705 Haddonfield Berlin Road   Voorhees, NJ 08043
    (856)679-0537
Roberts, Brian William, MD {1710202122} EmrgMd<NJ-COOPRUMC>
  + Cooper University Hospital
    One Cooper Plaza   Camden, NJ 08103   (856)342-2351
Roberts, David A., MD {1154320273} RadDia, RadV&I(94,PA01)
  + South Jersey Radiology Associates, P.A.
    901 Route 168/Suites 301-305   Turnersville, NJ 08012
    (856)227-6600   Fax (856)227-8537
  + South Jersey Radiology Associates, P.A.
    100 Carnie Boulevard/Suite B-5   Voorhees, NJ 08043
    (856)227-6600   Fax (856)751-0535
  + South Jersey Radiology Associates, P.A.
    315 Route 70 East/Suite B   Cherry Hill, NJ 08012   (856)428-4344   Fax (856)428-0356
Roberts, Kevin W., MD {1609854421} FamMed, SprtMd(82,MA07)<NJ-MEMSALEM>
  + Woodstown Family Practice
    125 East Avenue/Suite C   Woodstown, NJ 08098   (856)769-2800   Fax (856)769-4256
Roberts, Leah Kate, MD {1699081166} EmrgMd, Surgry
  + 944 Hermann Road
    North Brunswick, NJ 08902   (856)816-3808
Roberts, Marc P., MD {1811008402} Pedtrc(73,MEX14)<NJ-CLARMAAS>
  + KidsCare
    495 North 13th Street   Newark, NJ 07107   (973)268-5862
  + Washington Park Medical Associates
    559 Broad Street   Newark, NJ 07102   (973)268-5862   Fax (973)622-6443
Roberts, Paul J., MD {1477664431} Nrolgy(85,CT01)<NJ-NWTN-MEM, NJ-HCKTSTWN>
  + Neuro-Specialists of Morris-Sussex, PA
    369 West Blackwell Street   Dover, NJ 07801   (973)361-7606   Fax (973)361-8942
  + Neuro-Specialists of Morris-Sussex, PA
    350 Sparta Avenue   Sparta, NJ 07871   (973)361-7606   Fax (973)579-9618
  + Neuro-Specialists of Morris-Sussex, PA
    254 Mountain Avenue   Hackettstown, NJ 07801   (908)850-5505   Fax (908)813-8848
Robertson, Janet A., MD {1871649582} IntrMd(84,GRNA)
  + 169 Minebrook Road
    Bernardsville, NJ 07924   (908)766-6110   Fax (908)766-0569
Robertson, John F., Jr., MD {1447401492} FamMed, IntrMd(06,NJ06)
  + Cooper Family Medicine
    141 South Black Horse Pike/Suite 1   Blackwood, NJ 08012
    (856)232-6471   Fax (856)232-7028
Robertson, Joy G., MD {1528135258} Psychy, PsyCAd, IntrMd(86,NH01)<NJ-EASTORNG>
  + Drs. Seth, Robertson & Seth
    310 Central Avenue/Suite 100   East Orange, NJ 07018
    (862)520-3104   Fax (973)674-8033
Robertson, Michelle Williams, MD {1295914430} FamMed(98,RI01)
  + University Hospital-School of Public Health
    170 Frelinghuysen Road   Piscataway, NJ 08854   (732)445-0123   Fax (732)445-3644
Robertson-Hoffmann, Doreen E., MD {1306019567} Psychy(89,NJ06)<NJ-UNIVBHC>
  + 29 Olcott Square/Suite 4
    Bernardsville, NJ 07924
Robin, James Allen, MD {1699724609} IntrMd, Rheuma(68,PA01)<NJ-UNVMCPRN>
  + Hightstown Medical Associates
    186 Princeton Hightstown Road   West Windsor, NJ 08550
    (609)443-1150   Fax (609)799-9005
Robinson, Andrew Tyler, MD {1700228699} Surgry
  + Overlook Surgical Associates
    11 Overlook Road/Suite 160   Summit, NJ 07901   (908)608-9001   Fax (908)608-9030
Robinson, John Michael, DO {1699900191} Obstet
  + 108 Pennsbury Lane
    Deptford, NJ 08096
Robinson, Jonnie M., DO {1679713390} FamMed(99,NY75)
  + RWJPE Old Bridge Family Medicine
    2107 Highway 516   Old Bridge, NJ 08857   (732)952-0626
    Fax (732)463-6071
Robinson, Kimyetta, DO {1578026894}<NJ-OCEANMC>
  + Ocean Medical Center
    425 Jack Martin Boulevard   Brick, NJ 08723   (732)295-6562
Robinson, Lois Pat, MD {1740284017} GnetMd, ObsGyn, IntrMd(78,GA05)<NJ-HACKNSK, NJ-HOLYNAME>
  + Drs. Robinson, Parnes & Weinstein
    275 Forest Avenue   Paramus, NJ 07652   (201)967-9191
    Fax (201)967-9302
Robinson, Mary J., DO {1811967987} PthACl, PthDrm(87,IA75)<NJ-KMHCHRRY>
  + Kennedy Health System/Cherry Hill Campus
    2201 Chapel Avenue West/Pathology   Cherry Hill, NJ 08002
    (856)488-6621   Fax (856)488-6546
  + University of Medicine & Dentistry of New Jersey-SOM
    42 East Laurel Road/Ste3800/Path   Stratford, NJ 08084
    (856)488-6621   Fax (856)566-6176
Robinson, Michael David, MD {1265471874} Psychy, PsyFor(79,MD07)<NJ-MORRISTN>
  + 20 Community Place/4th Floor
    Morristown, NJ 07960   (973)539-8186   Fax (973)539-3687
    MICHAELROBINSONMD@verizon.net
Robinson, Neil H., MD {1801862263} Ophthl(78,LA01)
  + Ocean Eye Institute
    601 Route 37 West   Toms River, NJ 08755   (732)244-4400
    Fax (732)505-2171
Robinson, Patricia Graf, MD {1629000955} ObsGyn, Gyneco, IntrMd(80,OH08)
  + 8 Great Hills Terrace
    Short Hills, NJ 07078   (973)467-0930
Robinson, Sloan A., MD {1144237017} FamMed(76,WI06)<NJ-VIRTMARL>
  + Meetinghouse Family Physicians
    330 East Greentree Road   Marlton, NJ 08053   (856)596-9050   Fax (856)596-0320
Robinson-Gallaro, Bonnie Lee, MD {1518071851} IntrMd, Gastrn(84,MEX34)
  + 668 North Beers Street/Suite 202
    Holmdel, NJ 07733   (732)264-8370   Fax (732)264-8397
Robinton, John E., MD {1750321725} ClNrPh, Nrolgy(78,NY20)<NJ-MTNSIDE>
  + 33 North Fullerton Avenue
    Montclair, NJ 07042   (973)783-6303   Fax (973)783-6303

Robiou, Natalie Genoveva, MD {1144663287} Pedtrc<NJ-UNDRWD>
  + Advocare DelGiorno Pediatrics
    535 South Black Horse Pike   Blackwood, NJ 08012
    (856)228-1061   Fax (856)228-1907
  + Inspira Health Network
    509 North Broad Street   Woodbury, NJ 08096   (856)845-0100
Robison, Kathryn J., MD {1770517377} IntrMd(92,NJ05)<NJ-UNVMCPRN>
  + Princeton Medicine
    5 Plainsboro Road/Suite 300   Plainsboro, NJ 08536
    (609)853-7272   Fax (609)853-7271
Roblejo, Pedro C., MD {1568542249} Urolgy(65,SPAI)
  + 5910 Palisade Avenue
    West New York, NJ 07093   (201)868-0821   Fax (201)868-0160
Roblejo, Peter C., MD {1194772095} Nrolgy(98,NJ05)
  + Roblejo Peter C.
    4 Progress Street/Suite B 4   Edison, NJ 08820   (732)319-6866   Fax (908)834-8033
Robles, Ruth F., MD {1497946446} IntrMd(75,PHI01)
  + 221 Chestnut Street
    Newark, NJ 07105
Robleza, Rolando M., MD {1619998945} FamMed(65,PHIL)<NJ-STCLRBOO>
  + St. Clare's Hospital-Boonton
    130 Powerville Road   Boonton, NJ 07005   (973)316-1800
Roca Piccini, Elsie Isabel, MD {1609937655} Pedtrc(97,NJ06)
  + RWJ University Medical Group/Somerset Pediatrics
    1 Worlds Fair Drive/Suite 1   Somerset, NJ 08873   (732)743-5437   Fax (732)564-0212
Rocamboli, David Charles, DO {1316964752} Anesth(01,NY75)
  + Montclair Anesthesia Associates PC
    185 Fairfield Avenue/Suite 2A   West Caldwell, NJ 07006
    (973)226-1230   Fax (973)226-1232
  + 29 East 29th Street
    Bayonne, NJ 07002
Rocca, Nicole M., MD {1841408796} Dermat(03,NJ05)
  + 121 Ackerson Road
    Blairstown, NJ 07825
  + Natural Image Skin Center
    108 Bilby Road/Suite 202   Hackettstown, NJ 07840   Fax (908)441-2402
Rocereto, Thomas F., MD {1679654008} GynOnc, Gyneco(68,PA01)<NJ-ACMCITY, NJ-ACMCMAIN>
  + Cooper Gynecologic Oncology Associates
    900 Centennial Boulevard/Suite F   Voorhees, NJ 08043
    (856)325-6644
  + Women's Care Center
    3 Cooper Plaza/Suite 301   Camden, NJ 08103   (856)325-6644   Fax (856)968-8575
  + Cooper Ob/Gyn
    3 Cooper Plaza/Suite 300   Camden, NJ 08043   (856)342-2186   Fax (856)968-8575
Roche, Charles Vincent, III, MD {1477680304} IntrMd(04,PA02)<NJ-SHOREMEM>
  + Shore Memorial Hospital
    1 East New York Avenue/Internal Med   Somers Point, NJ 08244   (609)653-3500   Fax (609)926-4311
Roche, Elizabeth Ann, MD {1861452229} Anesth, PainMd(94,NY08)<NJ-VALLEY>
  + Valley Institute for Pain
    One Valley Health Plaza/3 FL   Paramus, NJ 07652
    (201)634-5555   Fax (201)634-5454
  + The Valley Hospital
    223 North Van Dien Avenue/Anesth   Ridgewood, NJ 07450
    (201)447-8000
Roche, Kevin B., MD {1740254606} Pedtrc(84,NJ06)<NJ-HUNTRDN>
  + Hunterdon Pediatric Associates
    537 Route 22 East/3rd Floor   Whitehouse Station, NJ 08889
    (908)823-1100   Fax (908)823-0433
Roche, Kevin Joseph, MD {1760457436} Radiol, PedRad(86,VA07)
  + Hunterdon Radiological Associate
    1 Dogwood Drive   Clinton, NJ 08809   (908)735-4477   Fax (908)735-6532
Roche, Natalie E., MD {1093809170} ObsGyn(80,NY47)<NJ-UMDNJ>
  + University Physician Associates
    140 Bergen Street/ACC Level C   Newark, NJ 07103
    (973)972-2700   Fax (973)972-2739
Rochford, Joseph M., MD {1235233537} Psychy(69,CT01)<NJ-SOMERSET>
  + 407 Omni Drive
    Hillsborough, NJ 08844   (908)359-2312   Fax (908)359-5356
Rock, Joel J., DO {1902997620} Anesth(70,PA77)
  + James Street Anesthesia
    102 James Street/Suite 103   Edison, NJ 08820   (732)494-1444   Fax (732)494-7052

Physicians by Name and Address

Rocksmith, Eugenio Roberto, MD {1225172554} Nrolgy(95,NJ05)<NJ-RHBHSPSJ>
+ Neuro-Rehab Assoc of Southern NJ
  1237 West Sherman Avenue   Vineland, NJ 08360   (856)896-2042   Fax (856)896-2536
+ The Rehabilitation Hospital of South Jersey
  1237 West Sherman Avenue   Vineland, NJ 08360   (856)696-7100

Rodgers, Denise V., MD {1548315278} FamMed, Grtrcs(79,MI20)<NJ-RWJUBRUN>
+ The University Hospital
  65 Bergen Street/Suite 1441   Newark, NJ 07107   (973)972-3645   Fax (973)972-7592
+ Eric B. Chandler Health Center
  277 George Street   New Brunswick, NJ 08901   (973)972-3645   Fax (732)235-6729

Rodino, Maria A., MD {1497820906} EnDbMt, IntrMd(92,NY08)
+ 219 Old Hook Road/Suite 2C
  Westwood, NJ 07675   (201)722-0600   Fax (201)722-0687

Rodis, Angel Victor, MD {1417947094} CritCr, IntrMd, PulDis(86,PHI32)
+ Virtua Garden State Pulmonary Associates
  520 Lippincott Drive/Suite A   Marlton, NJ 08053   (856)596-9057   Fax (856)596-0817

Rodolico, Joseph M., MD {1306049283} Psychy(65,ITA19)<NJ-UNIVBHC>
+ 600 South White Horse Pike
  Hammonton, NJ 08037   (856)825-5072

Rodricks, David Josef, MD {1275579138} SrgOrt, SrgOARec(98,PA02)
+ Brielle Orthopedics PA
  457 Jack Martin Boulevard   Brick, NJ 08724   (732)840-7500   Fax (732)840-2088
+ Brielle Orthopedics PA
  823 Lacey Road   Forked River, NJ 08731   (732)840-7500   Fax (732)840-2088
+ Brielle Orthopedics PA
  1301 Route 72 West   Manahawkin, NJ 08724   (609)971-7616   Fax (609)971-7639

Rodricks, Michael Baltazar, MD {1497732879} AnesCrCr(95,VA01)
+ Anesthesia Consultnts of NJ/Nova Pain
  285 Davidson Avenue/Suite 204   Somerset, NJ 08873   (732)271-1400   Fax (732)271-3544

Rodrigues, Anisha, MD {1174606495} IntrMd(94,INA23)
+ Maron & Rodrigues Medical Group, LLC.
  10 James Street/Suite 150   Florham Park, NJ 07932   (973)822-2000   Fax (973)822-2001

Rodrigues, Anny Elena, MD {1568752467}<NJ-RIVERVW>
+ Riverview Medical Center
  1 Riverview Plaza   Red Bank, NJ 07701   (732)212-0060   Fax (732)212-0061
  antcesmc@gmail.com

Rodrigues, Neesha Ann, MD {1760525133} RadOnc
+ Princeton Radiology Associates, P.A.
  3674 Route 27   Kendall Park, NJ 08824   (732)821-5563   Fax (732)821-6675

Rodrigues, Vanitha J., MD {1396882585} RadDia(94,INA67)<NJ-RWJUBRUN, NJ-TRINIJSC>
+ Sparta Health and Wellness Center
  89 Sparta Avenue/Suite 120   Sparta, NJ 07871   (973)729-0002   Fax (973)729-1085

Rodriguez, Alejandro L., MD {1609877786} SrgCdv, Surgry, SrgThr(88,CT02)<NJ-MORRISTN, NJ-JRSYSHMC>
+ 1 Tennyson Court
  Morristown, NJ 07960

Rodriguez, Andy, MD {1972820330} ClNrPh
+ St. Barnabas Institute of Neurology & Neurosurgery
  200 South Orange Avenue/Suite 101   Livingston, NJ 07039   (973)322-7580   Fax (973)322-7103

Rodriguez, Emmanuel, MD {1023279114} Anesth<NJ-STBARNMC>
+ St. Barnabas Medical Center
  94 Old Short Hills Road   Livingston, NJ 07039   (973)322-5512   Fax (973)322-8165

Rodriguez, Hilton John, MD {1407946635} PsyCAd, Psychy(87,PA09)
+ Cape Counseling Services
  128 Crest Haven Road   Cape May Court House, NJ 08210   (609)465-4100   Fax (609)465-7751
  hrodriguez@eastway.com

Rodriguez, Jaime, MD {1770504573} IntrMd(88,DOM02)<NJ-STMRYPAS>
+ St. Mary's Hospital
  350 Boulevard/Medicine   Passaic, NJ 07055   (973)365-4340

Rodriguez, Lauren C., MD {1598915878} IntrMd
+ Chatham Family Practice Associates
  492 Main Street   Chatham, NJ 07928   (973)635-2432   Fax (973)635-6169

Rodriguez, Liza A., MD {1306877519} Anesth(99,DMN01)<NJ-JRSYCITY>
+ Jersey City Medical Center
  355 Grand Street/Anesthesiology   Jersey City, NJ 07304   (201)915-2000   Fax (201)871-0619

Rodriguez, Maria J., MD {1881882033} Pedtrc(89,DOM15)
+ Mundo Chico Pediatric Associates
  167 Bergenline Avenue   Union City, NJ 07087   (201)590-9490
+ Passaic Pediatrics PA
  298 Passaic Street   Passaic, NJ 07055   (201)590-9490   Fax (973)249-8110

Rodriguez, Marlene V., MD {1093822090} FamMed(81,PRO03)<NJ-SHOREMEM>
+ Southern Jersey Family Medical Center
  1301 Atlantic Avenue   Atlantic City, NJ 08401   (609)572-0000   Fax (609)572-0039
+ Southern Jersey Family Medical Centers, Inc.
  860 South White Horse Pike/Building A   Hammonton, NJ 08037   (609)572-0000   Fax (609)567-3492

Rodriguez, Natalia Maria, MD {1992720742} Ophthl(02,MI07)
+ Marano Eye Care Center
  200 South Orange Avenue/Suite 209   Livingston, NJ 07039   (973)322-0102   Fax (973)322-0102

Rodriguez, Navarra Valencia, MD {1154364081} IntrMd(97,NY01)
+ 1 Stratford Court
  Demarest, NJ 07627

Rodriguez, Pascual B., MD {1245207281} CdvDis, CritCr, IntrMd(79,MA01)<NJ-CENTRAST, NJ-JRSYSHMC>
+ Monmouth Cardiology Associates, LLC
  11 Meridian Road   Eatontown, NJ 07724   (732)663-0300   Fax (732)663-0301
+ Monmouth Cardiology Associates, LLC.
  2102 Corlies Avenue/State Highway 33   Neptune, NJ 07753   (732)663-0300   Fax (732)774-9148

Rodriguez, Ramon Elias, MD {1699832774} Urolgy(95,NY19)
+ P. F. Ioffreda, MD, PA
  1250 Marigold Street   North Brunswick, NJ 08902   (732)545-8259   Fax (732)247-5574

Rodriguez, Reinerio Gerardo, MD {1174750772} FamMed, IntrMd(09,GCY01)
+ Riverside Medical Associates, PA
  225 60th Street   West New York, NJ 07093   (201)869-8888   Fax (201)869-0088

Rodriguez, Ricardo Esteban, MD {1467471821} Gastrn, IntrMd(84,NJ06)<NJ-TRINIWSC, NJ-RWJURAH>
+ Drs. Kurz and Rodriguez
  318 East Westfield Ave   Roselle Park, NJ 07204   (908)245-2229   Fax (908)245-2384

Rodriguez Barea, Hector A., MD {1861487076} Anesth, PedAne(78,MEX03)<NJ-VALLEY>
+ Bergen Anesthesia Group, P.C.
  500 West Main Street/Suite 16   Wyckoff, NJ 07481   (201)847-9320   Fax (201)847-0059

Rodriguez Correa, Daniel Thomas, MD {1356630198} Anesth
+ Rutgers- New Jersey Medical School
  185 South Orange Avenue/MSB E-538   Newark, NJ 07103   (973)972-5007

Rodriguez Montana, Manuel Alejandro, MD {1750637906} Pedtrc
+ Passaic Pediatrics PA
  298 Passaic Street   Passaic, NJ 07055   (973)249-8100   Fax (973)249-8110

Rodriguez-Bostock, Susan M., MD {1750391686} FamMed(96,NJ05)
+ Jackson Family Medicine
  27 South Cooks Bridge Road/Suite 2-1   Jackson, NJ 08527   (732)987-5780   Fax (732)987-5787

Rodriguez-Diaz, Ana M., MD {1710104922} InfDis, IntrMd(83,SPAI)<NJ-STMICHL>
+ 1119 Broad Street
  Newark, NJ 07114   (201)926-6899   Fax (908)352-1036

Rodriguez-Frank, Laura V., MD {1275753436} PsyCAd, Psychy(85,NY20)
+ 225 Franklin Avenue
  Midland Park, NJ 07432   (201)445-7400   Fax (201)447-9553
+ for Keeps
  123 How Lane   New Brunswick, NJ 08901   (201)445-7400   Fax (732)846-5478

Rodriguez-Zierer, Maria Evelyn, MD {1801829239} Pedtrc(84,PHI02)<NJ-HACKNSK, NJ-HOLYNAME>
+ Madison Avenue Pediatrics
  22 Madison Avenue/3rd floor, Suite 3   Paramus, NJ 07652   (201)291-9797   Fax (201)291-9798

Rodriquez, Margaret, MD {1255377909} FamMed(81,NY09)
+ Valley Medical Group of Montvale
  85 Chestnut Ridge Road/Suite 111   Montvale, NJ 07645   (201)930-1700   Fax (201)930-0705

Rodriquez, Victor R., MD Pedtrc(80,PRO03)<NJ-WARREN>
+ Warren Hills Family Health Center
  315 Route 31 South   Washington, NJ 07882   (908)689-0777   Fax (908)835-3037

Roe, Allison Marie Voeks, DO {1497015705}
+ 118 Buckingham Way
  Mount Laurel, NJ 08054

Roehl, Barbara Joan Oppenheim, MD {1962578807} FamMed(01,PA01)
+ Complete Care Family Medicine
  75 West Red Bank Avenue   Woodbury, NJ 08096   (856)853-2055   Fax (856)848-2879

Roehnelt, Alessia Carluccio, MD {1841599651} EnDbMt, IntrMd(11,NJ06)
+ Diabetes Endocrinology Metabolism Specialities PA
  6 Brighton Road/Suite 103   Clifton, NJ 07012   (973)471-2692   Fax (973)470-8188
+ Summit Medical Group Endocrinology
  62 South Fullerton Avenue   Montclair, NJ 07042   (973)471-2692   Fax (973)470-8188

Roehrig, Gregory James, MD {1477562890} SrgOrt(03,MD07)
+ Orthopaedic Institute of Central Jersey
  2315A Highway 34/Suite D   Manasquan, NJ 08736   (732)974-0404   Fax (732)449-4271

Roelke, Marc, MD {1851391429} ClCdEl, CdvDis, InsrMd(87,NY01)<NJ-NWRKBETH, NJ-STBARNMC>
+ New Jersey Cardiology Associates
  375 Mount Pleasant Avenue   West Orange, NJ 07052   (973)731-9442   Fax (973)731-8030
+ New Jersey Cardiology Associates
  201 Lyons Avenue/6th Floor   Newark, NJ 07112   (973)731-9442   Fax (973)923-7267
+ Diagnostic & Clinical Cardiology
  449 Mount Pleasant Avenue/2nd Floor   West Orange, NJ 07052   (973)731-7868   Fax (973)731-7907

Roeloffs, Susan A., MD {1053364489} Pedtrc, PedNrD(84,NJ05)<NJ-MATHENY>
+ The Matheny School and Hospital
  Main Street/PO Box 339   Peapack, NJ 07977   (908)234-0011

Roeltgen, David P., MD {1275551947} Nrolgy, IntrMd(76,MA07)<NJ-BURDTMLN>
+ Shore Physicians Group
  52 East New York Avenue   Somers Point, NJ 08244   (609)365-6202   Fax (609)653-1925
  droeltgen@hotmail.com

Roemheld-Hamm, Beatrix, MD {1992882476} FamMed(79,GERM)
+ Family Medicine at Monument Square
  317 George Street   New Brunswick, NJ 08901   (732)235-8993   Fax (732)246-7317

Roenbeck, Kevin Meehan, MD {1851559033} SrgOrt(04,DC01)
+ Ridgewood Orthopedic Group, LLC
  85 South Maple Avenue   Ridgewood, NJ 07450   (201)445-2830   Fax (201)445-7471

Roesch, Benno George, MD {1700034592} EmrgMd(77,CA06)
+ 241 Main Street
  Hackensack, NJ 07601

Roeske, Jessica L., DO {1972924165} IntrMd<NJ-ACMCITY>
+ AtlantiCare Regional Medical Center/City Campus
  1925 Pacific Avenue   Atlantic City, NJ 08401   (609)441-8908

Roesly, Melissa M., MD {1649250846} FamMed(94,NJ06)
+ Partners in Primary Care
  534 Lippincott Drive   Marlton, NJ 08053   (856)985-7373   Fax (856)985-9611

Roessler, Mark Leonard, DO {1255348900} Otlryg(97,MO78)
+ 55-77 Schanck Road/Suite B-9
  Freehold, NJ 07728   (732)677-3780   Fax (732)677-3782

Roffe, Kenneth A., DO {1689661951} FamMed(88,NY75)<NJ-NWTNMEM>
+ Premier Health Associates
  225 Route 23 South   Hamburg, NJ 07419   (973)209-1550   Fax (973)729-6487

Roffman, Eric Jason, MD {1417079674} Otlryg(02,MA07)<NY-GOODSAM, NY-NYACKHOS>
+ ENT & Allergy Associates, LLP
  690 Kinderkamack Road/Suite 101   Oradell, NJ 07649   (201)722-9850   Fax (201)722-9851
  eroffman@entandallergy.com

Roffman, Jeffrey D., MD {1467415042} Otlryg, OtgyPSHN(68,NY08)<NJ-JRSYSHMC, NJ-BAYSHORE>
+ 43 Gilbert Street North/Suite 5
  Tinton Falls, NJ 07701   (732)747-0900   Fax (732)758-8907
  jroff43@aol.com

Rogachefsky, Arlene S., MD {1235224759} Dermat, DerMOH, SrgLsr(96,NY06)<NJ-HACKNSK>
+ Affiliated Dermatologists
  182 South Street/Suite 1   Morristown, NJ 07960   (973)267-0300   Fax (973)695-1480
+ Affiliated Dermatology
  Town Centre 66/Suite 301   Succasunna, NJ 07876   (973)267-0300   Fax (973)927-7512
+ Affiliated Dermatology
  14 Church Street   Liberty Corner, NJ 07960   (973)267-0300   Fax (908)604-8544

Physicians by Name and Address

Rogal, Gary J., MD {1447250196} CdvDis, IntrMd(78,DC01)<NJ-STBARNMC, NJ-CLARMAAS>
+ New Jersey Cardiology Associates
375 Mount Pleasant Avenue   West Orange, NJ 07052
(973)731-9442   Fax (973)731-8030
+ New Jersey Cardiology Associates
5 Franklin Avenue/Suite 502   Belleville, NJ 07109
(973)731-9442   Fax (973)450-8157

Rogart, Jason Nathaniel, MD {1477648426} Gastrn, Hepato(01,RI01)
+ Capital Health Medical Center Hopewell
Two Capital Way/Suite 380   Pennington, NJ 08534
(609)537-5000   Fax (609)537-5050
+ RWJ Gastro & Hepatology
125 Paterson Street/CAB 5100B   New Brunswick, NJ 08901
(609)537-5000   Fax (732)235-7792

Roger, Marcela Kim, MD {1205063914}<NJ-ACMCITY>
+ AtlantiCare Regional Medical Center/City Campus
1925 Pacific Avenue   Atlantic City, NJ 08401   (609)345-4000

Roger, Scott Kenneth, DO {1972730851}
+ 200 Burning Tree Boulevard
Absecon, NJ 08201

Rogers, Brad S., MD {1538275102} Urolgy, IntrMd(77,PA02)<NJ-CHSFULD, NJ-CHSMRCER>
+ Urology Care Alliance
Two Capital Way/Suite 407   Pennington, NJ 08534
(609)730-1966   Fax (609)730-1166

Rogers, Brian James, MD {1780796805} ObsGyn(94,DC02)<NJ-RIVERVW>
+ Ocean Obstetric and Gynecologic Associates
804 West Park Avenue/Building A   Ocean, NJ 07712
(732)695-2040   Fax (732)493-1640

Rogers, Elisabeth Ann, DO {1033157508} Pedtrc(01,NJ75)
+ Summit Medical Group
34 Mountain Boulevard/Building B   Warren, NJ 07059
(908)769-0100   Fax (908)769-8927

Rogers, James J., DO {1174596944} Nrolgy, Psychy, IntrMd(88,NJ75)
+ University Hospital-SOM Department of Psychiatry
2250 Chapel Avenue West/Suite 100   Cherry Hill, NJ 08002
(856)482-9000   Fax (856)482-1159

Rogers, Jessica Lee, DO {1023243698}<NJ-SJHREGMC>
+ SJH Regional Medical Center
1505 West Sherman Avenue/Box 93   Vineland, NJ 08360
(856)641-8680   Fax (856)641-8679

Rogers, Jody J., MD {1629162888} EmrgMd
+ 4 Meadowbrook Road
Short Hills, NJ 07078

Rogers, Kenneth H., DO {1992723035} PainMd, AnesPain, Anesth(85,NY75)<NJ-UNDRWD, NJ-CAPITLHS>
+ Advanced Pain Consultants, P.A.
326 Route 73   Voorhees, NJ 08043   (856)489-9822   Fax (856)489-9877
+ Advanced Pain Consultants, P.A.
120 Madison Avenue/Suite D   Mount Holly, NJ 08060
(609)267-1707
+ Advanced Pain Consultants, P.A.
1401 Whitehorse Mercerville Rd   Hamilton, NJ 08043
(609)528-8888   Fax (609)584-5151

Rogers, Michael S., MD {1184684268} FamMed, Grtrcs(77,BRAZ)<NJ-UNDRWD>
+ Drs. Magnet & Rogers
831 Kings Highway/Suite 100   Woodbury, NJ 08096
(856)853-8730   Fax (856)853-8870

Rogers, Patrick, DO {1467991471} EmrgMd
+ 40 Florence Avenue
Leonardo, NJ 07737   (732)673-1604

Rogers, Philip S., MD {1174512776} CdvDis(91,NY08)
+ Lakeland Cardiology Center PA
765 State Route 10/Suite 4   Randolph, NJ 07869   (973)989-2566
+ Lakeland Cardiology Center, P.A.
415 Boulevard   Mountain Lakes, NJ 07046   (973)989-2566
Fax (973)334-7116

Rogers, Richard David, III, DO {1306120993}<NJ-MORRISTN>
+ Morristown Medical Center
100 Madison Avenue   Morristown, NJ 07962   (973)971-5000

Rogers-Phillips, Elois G., MD {1174623011} Hemato, MedOnc(70,DC03)<NJ-NWRKBETH>
+ Newark Beth Israel Medical Center
201 Lyons Avenue   Newark, NJ 07112   (973)926-7000
Fax (973)926-9568

Roggemann, Dennis J., MD   CdvDis, IntrMd(76,NY09)
+ Toms River Family Medical Center PA
1028 Hooper Avenue   Toms River, NJ 08753   (732)349-8866

Rogido, Marta R., MD {1518902774} NnPnMd(81,ARG01)<NJ-MORRISTN>
+ MidAtlantic Neonatology Associates
100 Madison Avenue   Morristown, NJ 07962   (973)971-5488   Fax (973)290-7175

Rohani, Pejman, DO {1619134475} SrgTrm(06,CA23)<NY-PENINSUL, NJ-UMDNJ>
+ Salartash Surgical Associates
301 Central Avenue/Suite D   Egg Harbor Township, NJ 08234   (609)926-5000   Fax (609)926-2020
+ Jersey Shore University Medical Center
1945 Route 33/Surgery/Trauma   Neptune, NJ 07753
(609)926-5000   Fax (732)776-4843

Rohani, Sayed M., MD {1083097554} FamMed
+ Hoboken Urgent Care
231 Washington Street   Hoboken, NJ 07030   (201)754-1005   Fax (201)754-1006

Rohatgi, Chand, MD {1457438178} Surgry, SrgBst(94,INDI)<NJ-WARREN, PA-EASTON>
+ Warren Hospital
185 Roseberry Street/Surgery   Phillipsburg, NJ 08865
(908)859-6700
crohatgi@breastcare-surgery.com

Rohatgi, Rajeev, MD {1003810342} CdvDis, IntrMd, CritCr(76,INA30)<NJ-WARREN, PA-EASTON>
+ Easton Cardiovascular Associates
123 Roseberry Street   Phillipsburg, NJ 08865   (908)213-3100

Rohlf, Jane, MD {1194944132} Rserch, IntrMd(75,IA02)<NJ-STFRNMED>
+ St. Francis Medical Center
601 Hamilton Avenue   Trenton, NJ 08629   (609)599-5326

Roitman, Alla, DO {1699093054} IntrMd
+ Valley Health Medical Group
780 Cedar Lane   Teaneck, NJ 07666   (201)836-7664   Fax (201)836-5710

Rojas, Jose, Jr., MD {1629188503} PainMd, Anesth, AnesPain(93,NJ05)<NJ-STMRYPAS, NJ-HOLYNAME>
+ Pain Relief Center of America
211 60th Street/Anesth   West New York, NJ 07093
(201)869-3000   Fax (201)869-3001
+ St. Mary's Hospital
350 Boulevard   Passaic, NJ 07055   (973)365-4300

Rojas, Paulina Elena, MD {1093927089} Pedtrc
+ St. Peter's Pediatric Faculty Group
123 How Lane   New Brunswick, NJ 08901   (732)745-8519
Fax (732)448-0007

Rojas, Veronica Maria, MD {1386707818} PsyCAd, PsyAdt(89,ARG01)<NY-BLVUENYU, NJ-VALLEY>
+ 216 Dayton Street/2nd Floor
Ridgewood, NJ 07450   Fax (201)444-8338

Rojas, Walter Ramiro, MD {1154306330} FamMed(94,MEX14)
+ 531 Mountain Avenue
North Caldwell, NJ 07006

Rojavin, Yuri, MD {1568753945} Surgry(05,PA13)<NJ-CHSFULD>
+ Capital Surgical Associates
40 Fuld Street/Suite 303   Trenton, NJ 08638   (856)342-3012   Fax (609)396-3600
+ Capital Health System/Fuld Campus
750 Brunswick Avenue   Trenton, NJ 08638   (856)342-3012
Fax (609)815-7529
+ Capital Health Primary Care
832 Brunswick Avenue   Trenton, NJ 08638   (609)815-7400
Fax (609)815-7401

Rojer, David Eli, MD {1144293952} Ortped, SrgOrt(97,NY19)<NJ-TRINIWSC, NJ-RWJURAH>
+ Union County Orthopaedic Group
210 West St. Georges Avenue/PO Box 330   Linden, NJ 07036   (908)486-1111   Fax (908)583-1034

Rokhsar, Michael Howard, DO {1578535597} Radiol, RadNro, RadDia(96,NY75)
+ Westfield Imaging Center
118-122 Elm Street   Westfield, NJ 07090   (908)232-0610
Fax (908)232-7140

Rokosz, Gregory J., DO {1013104439} EmrgMd, FamMed(80,IA75)<NJ-STBARNMC>
+ St. Barnabas Medical Center
94 Old Short Hills Road   Livingston, NJ 07039   (973)322-5000   Fax (973)322-8360
GROKOSZ@sbhcs.com

Roksvaag, George E., MD {1205962453} Pedtrc, AdmMgt(78,NJ06)<NJ-HUNTRDN>
+ Hunterdon Medical Center
2100 Wescott Drive/MedMngmnt   Flemington, NJ 08822
(908)788-6100

Rola, David Charles, MD {1861424020} FamMed, IntrMd(81,DMN01)<NJ-COMMED>
+ 26 Azalea Court
Barnegat, NJ 08005   (609)698-2189

Roland, Robert J., DO {1586680458} InfDis, IntrMd, OthrSp(85,MO79)<NJ-OVERLOOK>
+ Overlook Medical Center Wound Healing Center
11 Overlook Road/MAC II, Suite LL 101   Summit, NJ 07901
(908)522-5900   Fax (908)522-5544
Roland1376@aol.com

Rolandelli, Rolando Hector, MD {1457338386} Surgry, SrgC&R(78,ARG01)<NJ-MORRISTN>
+ 435 South Street/Suite 360
Morristown, NJ 07960   (973)971-7200   Fax (973)290-7521

Rolenc, Holly J., MD {1992770226} Pedtrc(00,MNT01)<NJ-OCEANMC, NJ-COMMED>
+ Pediatric Medical Group
525 Jack Martin Boulevard/Suite 102   Brick, NJ 08724
(732)458-1177   Fax (732)458-5942

Rollins, Terry Lee, MD {1235119116} Dermat(99,NJ06)<NJ-KMH-STRAT, NJ-OURLADY>
+ Macaione and Papa Dermatology Associates
707 White Horse Road/Suite C-103   Voorhees, NJ 08043
(856)627-1900   Fax (856)627-6907

Roma, Kevin P., MD {1912939810} EmrgMd(94,NY08)<NJ-RIVERVW>
+ Riverview Medical Center
1 Riverview Plaza/EmergMed   Red Bank, NJ 07701
(732)741-2700   Fax (732)224-7498

Romain, Sharon L., DO {1790987220} FamMed(04,NY75)
+ Valley Health Medical Group
72 Hamburg Turnpike   Riverdale, NJ 07457   (973)835-7290
Fax (973)835-0696
+ Valley Medical Group
140 Route 17 North/Suite 302   Paramus, NJ 07652
(973)835-7290   Fax (201)689-6009

Romald, Jermine Harriet, MD {1710220033} Pedtrc<NJ-MONMOUTH>
+ Monmouth Medical Center
300 Second Avenue   Long Branch, NJ 07740   (732)923-7251

Roman, David, MD {1518036748} IntrMd(85,NJ05)
+ Fair Lawn Medical
15-01 Broadway/Suite 12/AttentionCtr   Fair Lawn, NJ 07410
(201)794-3600

Roman, Jacqueline D., DO {1376785881} ObsGyn(09,PA77)
+ 1300 Highway Route 35
Ocean, NJ 07712   (973)432-7640   Fax (732)517-1359

Roman, Jocelyn, MD {1932355690} Psychy(04,NJ05)
+ Center of Revitalizing Psychiatry, P.C.
795 Main Street   Hackensack, NJ 07601   (201)488-5161
Fax (201)488-5162

Roman, Stephen John, Jr., MD {1265400287} PhysMd, PainMd(97,NJ05)<NJ-RWJUHAM, NJ-STFRNMED>
+ Regene Spine
1230 Whitehorse Mercerville Rd/Suite C   Mercerville, NJ 08619   (609)570-6980   Fax (609)228-5060
+ Regene Spine
197 Ridgedale Avenue/Suite 210   Cedar Knolls, NJ 07927
(973)387-1044

Romanczuk, Bruce J., MD {1427136993} Otlryg(74,PA12)
+ 1172 Beacon Avenue
Manahawkin, NJ 08050   (609)597-7110   Fax (609)597-7113

Romanella, Joseph P., DO {1366413056} IntrMd(90,PA77)<NJ-CENTRAST>
+ Hackensack Meridian Medical Group
195 Route 9 South/Suite 106   Manalapan, NJ 07726
(732)536-7144   Fax (732)536-7520
+ Jersey Shore Associates of Internal Medicine
831 Tennent Road   Manalapan, NJ 07726   (732)536-7144
Fax (732)536-7520
+ Jersey Shore Associates of Internal Medicine
300 Bridge Plaza Drive   Manalapan, NJ 07726   (732)536-7144

Romannikov, Vladimir, MD {1083031173} PhysMd<NJ-KSLR-WELK>
+ Kessler Institute for Rehab
201 Pleasant Hill Road   Chester, NJ 07930   (973)252-6303

Romano, Andrew Leonard, DO {1033153689} IntrMd, IntHos(98,FL75)<NJ-SOCEANCO>
+ Williamsburg Pediatrics
703 Mill Creek Road/Suite D   Manahawkin, NJ 08050
(609)549-6787   Fax (609)756-0870

Romano, Carmen J., MD {1841303799} ObsGyn, Gyneco(75,NJ05)<NJ-STFRNMED>
+ LifeCare Physicians, PC of Lawrenceville
4 Princess Road/Suite 209   Lawrenceville, NJ 08648
(609)895-0770   Fax (609)896-1124

Romano, David L., MD {1215990403} IntrMd, Nephro(80,MEX14)
+ Stuart Homer and Associates, PA
1030 Saint Georges Avenue/Suite 201   Avenel, NJ 07001
(732)602-0244   Fax (732)602-2577

Romano, James A., MD {1255626271} FamMed
+ Samaritan HealthCare & Hospice
5 Eves Drive/Suite 300   Marlton, NJ 08053   (856)596-1600
Fax (856)596-1600

Romano, Joseph P., MD {1831314210} IntrMd, OccpMd(76,DC02)
+ University Hospital-School of Public Health
170 Frelinghuysen Road/EnvOccupMed   Piscataway, NJ 08854   (732)445-0123   Fax (732)445-3644

Physicians by Name and Address

Romano, Kenneth Robert, MD {1124040670} RadDia, Radiol(85,NY06)<NJ-CENTRAST>
+ Freehold Radiology Group
901 West Main Street   Freehold, NJ 07728   (732)462-4844
+ CentraState Medical Center
901 West Main Street/Radiology   Freehold, NJ 07728
(732)431-2000

Romanoff, Nicholas A., MD {1316903313} AlgyImmn, Pedtrc, Allrgy(65,NJ15)<NJ-VIRTVOOR>
+ Professional Allergy Associates, PA
1034 East Route 70   Cherry Hill, NJ 08034   (856)429-4922   Fax (856)429-7780
+ 1750 Zion Road & New Road
Northfield, NJ 08225   (856)429-4922   Fax (609)641-0746

Romanowski, Mark Patrick, MD {1851634018}
+ Capital Health System/Hopewell
One Capital Way   Pennington, NJ 08534   (570)762-8095

Romberger, Charles Frank, MD {1760422752} PthACl, Pthlgy, PthCyt(86,PA13)<NJ-COMMED>
+ Community Medical Center
99 Route 37 West/Pathology   Toms River, NJ 08755   (732)557-8000

Rombough, Gary R., MD {1700860509} SrgOrt, IntrMd(76,NY03)<NJ-MTNSIDE>
+ Glen Ridge Surgicenter
230 Sherman Avenue   Glen Ridge, NJ 07028   (973)746-6844   Fax (973)680-4211

Rome, Sergey, MD {1568431070} Urolgy(97,NY19)<NJ-HACKNSK, NJ-VALLEY>
+ Urologic Institute of NJ PA
277 Forest Avenue/Suite 206   Paramus, NJ 07652
(201)489-8900   Fax (201)489-0877

Romello, Janel B., DO {1265695621} PhysMd
+ 6 Raleigh Court
Holmdel, NJ 07733

Romello, Michael A., MD {1285722900} PhysMd(02,NJ05)
+ Orthopaedic Sports Medicine
80 Oak Hill Road   Red Bank, NJ 07701   (732)741-2313   Fax (732)741-7154

Romero, Alejandro, MD {1538331160} Anesth(04,NY09)
+ 7000 Kennedy Blvd. East/Apt 45-h
Guttenberg, NJ 07093

Romero, Audrey Anita, MD {1942235692} ObsGyn(96,PA09)
+ The Rubino Ob/Gyn Group
101 Old Short Hills Road/Suite 101   West Orange, NJ 07052
(973)736-1100   Fax (973)736-1834
+ The Rubino Ob/Gyn Group
33 Overlook Road   Summit, NJ 07901   (908)522-4558
+ The Rubino Ob/Gyn Group
731 Broadway   Bayonne, NJ 07052   (201)339-3300

Romero, Luis N., MD {1689754152} CdvDis, IntrMd(70,BOL01)<NJ-ACMCITY, NJ-ACMCMAIN>
+ Atlantic Cardiology in Ventor
6725 Atlantic Avenue/2nd Floor   Ventnor, NJ 08406
(609)822-2006
+ Atlantic Cardiology in Galloway
436 Chris Gaupp Drive/Suite 204   Galloway, NJ 08205
(609)822-2006   Fax (609)652-7616

Romero, Luz Ydania, MD {1720027691} Pedtrc(88,DOMI)<NJ-COMMED>
+ 1255 Route 70/Suite 22-S
Lakewood, NJ 08701   (732)364-0041   Fax (732)364-5578

Romero, Melchor D., MD {1720023104} RadDia, Radiol(72,PHI02)
+ University Radiology Group, P.C.
483 Cranbury Road   East Brunswick, NJ 08816   (732)390-0030   Fax (732)390-5383

Romerocaces, Gloria Marcelo, MD {1437248580} Pthlgy, PthACl(79,PHI01)
+ PLUS Diagnostics
1200 River Avenue/Suite 10   Lakewood, NJ 08701
(732)901-7575   Fax (732)901-1555

Romisher, Robert J., DO {1831273317} Anesth(89,FL75)<NJ-COOPRUMC>
+ Cooper University Hospital
One Cooper Plaza/Anesth   Camden, NJ 08103   (856)342-2000

Rommer, James A., MD {1073528634} IntrMd(78,NY20)
+ 349 East Northfield Road
Livingston, NJ 07039   (973)992-2227   Fax (973)535-8643

Rondanina, Richard W., MD {1720064744} IntrMd, Grtrcs(96,HUN07)<NJ-PALISADE>
+ Capital Health Hospitalist Group
750 Brunswick Avenue   Trenton, NJ 08638   (609)815-7887   Fax (609)394-6299

Rondel, Mikhail, MD {1376509596} Surgry, Anesth(89,UKR10)<NJ-STPETER>
+ Anesthesia Consultnts of NJ/Nova Pain
285 Davidson Avenue/Suite 240   Somerset, NJ 08873
(732)271-1400   Fax (732)271-3544

Rondina, Carlo L., MD {1528086444} Radiol, RadDia(81,ITAL)<NJ-CENTRAST>
+ CentraState Medical Center

901 West Main Street/Radiology   Freehold, NJ 07728
(732)294-2946

Rondinella, Louis, MD {1205897188} Otlryg(91,PA01)
+ 647 Shore Road
Somers Point, NJ 08244   (609)601-9055   Fax (609)601-0276

Rondon, Kaylah Christine, MD {1154697712} ObsGyn(NY09)
+ University Consultants in Ob-Gyn & Womens Health
33 Overlook Road/Mac 405   Summit, NJ 07902   (908)608-0300

Ronnen, Ellen A., MD {1003828823} OncHem(99,NY46)<NJ-STPETER, NJ-RWJUBRUN>
+ Regional Cancer Care Associates - Central Jersey Div
454 Elizabeth Avenue/Suite 240   Somerset, NJ 08873
(732)390-7750   Fax (732)390-7725
+ Central Jersey Oncology Center, P.A.
Brier Hill Court/Building J-2   East Brunswick, NJ 08816
(732)390-7750   Fax (732)390-7725
+ Central Jersey Oncology Center, P.A.
205 Easton Avenue   New Brunswick, NJ 08873   (732)828-9570   Fax (732)828-7638

Ronner, Wanda, MD {1417995077} ObsGyn, Gyneco(84,PA13)<NJ-OURLADY>
+ Penn Health for Women
807 Haddon Avenue/Suite 212   Haddonfield, NJ 08033
(856)429-0400   Fax (856)429-8411

Ronsayro, Estrella A., MD {1265729065} GenPrc(74,PHI08)
+ 330 Federal Street
Camden, NJ 08103   (856)225-1975

Roomi, Adil Mohamed, MD {1831146570} EmrgMd(01,PA09)<NJ-VIRTVOOR>
+ Virtua Voorhees
100 Bowman Drive   Voorhees, NJ 08043   (856)247-3000   Fax (856)325-3197

Roomi, Farah, MD {1194903203} FamMed(04,ON01)
+ Community Health Care, Inc.
265 Irving Avenue   Bridgeton, NJ 08302   (856)451-4700   Fax (856)863-5732

Rooney, Michele P., MD {1588668115} ObsGyn(90,NY48)<NJ-VALLEY>
+ Valley Center for Women's Health
581 North Franklin Turnpike/2nd Floor   Ramsey, NJ 07446
(201)236-2100   Fax (201)236-5269

Roosels, Marianne, MD {1487637450} IntrMd(77,BELG)
+ Integrated Medicine Alliance, P.A.
27 Pinckney Road   Red Bank, NJ 07701   (732)747-4600   Fax (732)219-1968

Root, Edward R., MD {1346337912} Pedtrc, PsyCAd, Psychy(73,NY46)
+ Preferred Behavioral Health of New Jersey
700 Airport Road   Lakewood, NJ 08701   (732)367-4700   Fax (732)364-2253

Roowala, Shabbir H., MD {1851330757} IntrMd(71,INDI)<NJ-CHS-FULD, NJ-CAPITLHS>
+ Drs. Rana & Roowala
40 Fuld Street/Suite 302   Trenton, NJ 08638   (609)393-0067   Fax (609)393-4943

Roper, Ashley Annette, MD {1073931945} IntrMd
+ 314 Estate Point Road
Toms River, NJ 08753   (732)903-7540

Roper, Brian K., MD {1134222714} IntrMd(94,NJ05)
+ Physican's Home & Health Service
1532 State Route 33/Suite 202   Neptune, NJ 07753
(732)775-8400   Fax (732)775-8401

Ropiak, Caroline Michelle, MD {1134257470} IntrMd, Pedtrc(04,PA02)<NJ-VIRTVOOR, NJ-VIRTMHBC>
+ Virtua Voorhees
100 Bowman Drive/Hospitalist   Voorhees, NJ 08043
(856)247-3000   Fax (856)504-8029
+ Virtua Hospitalist Group Memorial
175 Madison Avenue   Mount Holly, NJ 08060   (856)247-3000   Fax (609)914-6182

Ropiak, Christopher Robert, MD {1982861654} SrgOrt(05,NY19)<NJ-RWJURAH, NJ-TRINIJSC>
+ Union County Orthopaedic Group
210 West St. Georges Avenue/PO Box 330   Linden, NJ 07036   (908)486-1111   Fax (908)583-1034

Ropiak, Raymond Russell, MD {1265636062} SrgOrt(04,PA02)<NJ-VIRTMHBC, NJ-VIRTUAHS>
+ Reconstructive Orthopedics, P.A.
243 Route 130/Suite 109   Bordentown, NJ 08505
(609)267-9400   Fax (609)267-9457
+ Reconstructive Orthopedics, P.A.
401 Young Avenue/Suite 245   Moorestown, NJ 08057
(609)267-9400   Fax (609)267-9457

Roque, Cesar Ruben, Jr., MD {1063791317} FamMed, IntrMd(10,STM01)
+ Horizon Health Center
714 Bergen Avenue/Fam Med   Jersey City, NJ 07306
(201)451-6300

Roque, Felix Eduardo, MD {1366506495} Anesth, AnesPain(87,DOM15)<NJ-PALISADE, NJ-STMRYPAS>
+ Pain Relief Center
211 60th Street/2nd Floor   West New York, NJ 07093
(201)662-5437   Fax (201)662-7195

Roque Dieguez, Hilda Rosa, MD {1013006592} IntrMd(84,DOMI)<NJ-PALISADE, NJ-HOBUNIMC>
+ 317 60th Street
West New York, NJ 07093   (201)864-0757   Fax (201)861-3126

Roque-Dang, Christine M., DO {1851527543} PhysMd
+ Bergen Medical Associates
466 Old Hook Road/Suite 1   Emerson, NJ 07630   (201)967-8221   Fax (201)967-0340
+ University Hospital-New Jersey Medical School
30 Bergen Street/ADMC1/Rm 101   Newark, NJ 07107
(973)972-5148

Roros, James Gus, MD {1326134917} Surgry, WundCr(93,NJ05)<NJ-SPCLMONM>
+ Specialty Hospital at Monmouth
300 Second Avenue/Greenwall 6   Long Branch, NJ 07740
(732)923-5037

Rorro, Mary C., DO {1417066473} Psychy(95,NJ75)
+ 284 Edinburg Road
Trenton, NJ 08619   (609)587-7001

Ros, Adriana Oksana, DO {1942468392} Dermat(02,NY75)
+ Surgery Associates of North Jersey, P.A.
1100 Clifton Avenue   Clifton, NJ 07013   (973)472-1000
Fax (973)472-1300
+ Dr. Deborah Ruth Spey
101 Old Short Hills Road/Suite 410   West Orange, NJ 07052
(973)472-1000   Fax (973)731-1635

Ros, Oliana R., MD {1942553995}
+ 5 Jordan Court
Long Valley, NJ 07853   (201)747-6145
olianarosmd@gmail.com

Ros, Stephen Joseph, MD {1013320431} SrgOrt(14,NY47)
+ Robert Wood Johnson Orthopedic Surgery
One Robert Wood Johnson Place/MEB 422   New Brunswick, NJ 08901   (732)235-7869

Rosa, Richard A., MD {1396739694} SrgOrt(78,NJ05)<NJ-ST-BARNMC>
+ Center for Orthopaedics
1500 Pleasant Valley Way/Suite 101   West Orange, NJ 07052   (973)669-5600   Fax (973)669-0269
+ Short Hills Surgery Center
187 Millburn Avenue/Suite 101   Millburn, NJ 07041
(973)669-5600   Fax (973)671-0557
+ The Joint Institute at Saint Barnabas Medical Center
609 Morris Avenue   Springfield, NJ 07052   (973)379-1991
Fax (973)467-8647

Rosales, Ramon Javillonar, MD {1457359119} Anesth, IntrMd(83,PHIL)<NJ-STJOSHOS>
+ St. Joseph's Regional Medical Center Anesthesia
703 Main Street   Paterson, NJ 07503   (973)754-2323   Fax (973)754-2791

Rosales Zincone, Jeannette Alicia, MD {1033147780} IntrMd(01,DMN01)<NJ-UMDNJ>
+ 400 West Blackwell Street
Dover, NJ 07801   (973)989-3343

Rosalie, Maria Christina, MD {1609168079} ObsGyn
+ Bergen Medical Associates
466 Old Hook Road/Suite 1   Emerson, NJ 07630   (201)967-8221   Fax (201)967-0340
+ The Woman's Group/Bergen Medical Associates
1 West Ridgewood Avenue/Suite 211   Paramus, NJ 07652
(201)967-8221   Fax (201)251-2325

Rosania, Anthony Russell, MD {1699926782} EmrgMd<NJ-UMDNJ>
+ University Hospital
150 Bergen Street   Newark, NJ 07103   (973)972-4300

Rosario, Imani Jackson, MD {1134384415} Urolgy
+ Rutgers- New Jersey Medical School
185 South Orange Avenue/MSB G538   Newark, NJ 07103
(973)972-4488   Fax (973)972-3892

Rosato, Francis E., MD {1104851898} Surgry(99,PA02)
+ Capital Health Medical
2 Capital Way/Suite 356   Pennington, NJ 08534   (609)537-6000   Fax (609)537-6002

Rosato, Mark G., MD {1972681278} Psychy, PsyCAd(85,ITA17)<NJ-UNIVBHC>
+ University Behavioral Health Care
671 Hoes Lane/PO Box 1392   Piscataway, NJ 08855
(732)235-5500

Roscher, Atilio R., MD {1083667000} FamMed, EmrgMd(73,MEX14)<NJ-WARREN>
+ Jersey Emergency Specialists, Inc.
185 Roseberry Street   Phillipsburg, NJ 08865   (908)859-6767   Fax (908)859-6812

Physicians by Name and Address

Roscioli-Jones, Catherine A., MD {1861460271} Pedtrc, AdolMd(85,PA07)<NJ-VIRTUAHS, NJ-VIRTMHBC>
+ Advocare Medford Pediatric & Adolescent Medicine
520 Stokes Road   Medford, NJ 08055   (609)654-9112   Fax (609)654-7404

Rose, Abigail Lee, MD {1871551275} FamMed(01,PA09)
+ Capital Health Primary Care
4056 Quakerbridge Road/Suite 101   Lawrenceville, NJ 08648   (609)528-9150   Fax (609)528-9151
+ Henry J. Austin Health Center
321 North Warren Street/FamMed   Trenton, NJ 08618   (609)528-9150   Fax (609)695-3532
+ Capital Health Primary Care-Hamilton
1445 Whitehorse-Mercerville Rd   Hamilton, NJ 08648   (609)587-6661   Fax (609)587-8503

Rose, Bruce T., MD {1861420077} IntrMd(97,PA13)
+ Capital Health Primary Care - Princeton
811 Exective Drive   Princeton, NJ 08540   (609)303-4600   Fax (609)303-4601

Rose, Diane, MD {1235299116} Psychy(78,PA01)<NJ-CENTRAST>
+ 224 Taylors Mills Road
Manalapan, NJ 07726   (732)409-0128   Fax (732)409-1131

Rose, Elizabeth, MD {1285650523} Pedtrc, AdolMd(85,NJ06)<NJ-NWRKBETH, NJ-CHDNWBTH>
+ 75 Claremont Road
Bernardsville, NJ 07924   (908)953-8336   Fax (908)953-8339
+ Newark Beth Israel Medical Center
201 Lyons Avenue/Adolescent Medi   Newark, NJ 07112   (908)953-8336
+ Children's Hospital of New Jersey
201 Lyons Avenue/Osborne Terrace   Newark, NJ 07924   (973)926-4000

Rose, Helen M., MD {1588638522} Pedtrc(97,PA13)<NJ-UNVM-CPRN>
+ The Pediatric Group PA
66 Mount Lucas Road   Princeton, NJ 08540   (609)924-4892   Fax (609)921-9380
rose@pedgroup.com

Rose, Henry J., MD {1255395588} IntrMd, PulDis(79,NY05)<NJ-WESTHDSN>
+ 639 Ridge Road
Lyndhurst, NJ 07071   (201)444-1493   Fax (201)939-7196

Rose, John G., MD {1922082627} Urolgy, IntrMd(68,NY20)<NJ-RIVERVW, NJ-BAYSHORE>
+ Urology Associates, P.A.
595 Shrewsbury Avenue/Suite 103   Shrewsbury, NJ 07702   (732)741-5923   Fax (732)741-2759

Rose, Keith Martin, MD {1871514661} IntrMd, PulDis, CritCr(00,NF01)
+ Hackensack University Medical Center
30 Prospect Avenue   Hackensack, NJ 07601   (551)996-4149

Rose, Lane Gruber, MD {1629299615} Psychy, PsyCAd(95,NY47)
+ Jersey Shore Psychiatric Associates
3535 Route 66/Building 5/Suite D   Neptune, NJ 07753   (732)643-4350

Rose, Michael Ian, MD {1225097454} SrgPlstc, Surgry(94,NY19)<NJ-BAYSHORE, NJ-CENTRAST>
+ The Plastic Surgery Ctr of NJ & Manhat
535 Sycamore Avenue   Shrewsbury, NJ 07702   (732)741-0970   Fax (732)747-2606

Rose, Moshe, MD {1982765574} Psychy, PsyCAd, IntrMd(01,OH45)
+ 1195 Highway 70/Suite 2005
Lakewood, NJ 08701   (732)942-2988

Rose, Shelonitda S., MD {1588736631} Hemato, IntrMd(90,INA47)<NJ-RWJUBRUN>
+ University Physician Associates of New Jersey
125 Paterson Street/CAB 5200   New Brunswick, NJ 08901   (732)235-7223   Fax (732)235-7115
rosesh@rwjms.rutgers.edu

Rose, T., MD {1457388498} IntrMd, MedOnc, Hemato(83,INA76)
+ 21 Green Springs Way
Freehold, NJ 07728

Rose, Victoria Summer, MD {1629938231} FamMed
+ AtlantiCare Physician Group
1613 Route 47/Unit G   Rio Grande, NJ 08242   (609)886-5245   Fax (609)886-5873

Roseff, Shelly Anne, MD {1750357877} InfDis, IntrMd(87,PA13)<NJ-UNVMCPRN, NJ-RWJUBRUN>
+ ID Associates PA/dba ID Care
765 Route 10 East/Suite 201   Randolph, NJ 07869   (973)989-0068   Fax (973)361-8955
+ ID Associates PA/dba ID Care
8 Saddle Road   Cedar Knolls, NJ 07927   (973)989-0068   Fax (973)993-5953

Rosefort, Laury, MD {1942575253} IntrMd<NJ-TRINIWSC>
+ Trinitas Regional Medical Center-Williamson Street
225 Williamson Street   Elizabeth, NJ 07207   (908)994-5000

Rosen, Allen D., MD {1659485159} SrgPlstc(83,NY06)<NJ-STBARNMC, NJ-MTNSIDE>
+ Plastic Surgery Group
37 North Fullerton Avenue   Montclair, NJ 07042   (973)233-1933   Fax (973)233-1934

Rosen, Amy T., MD {1548274574} IntrMd(88,NY46)<NJ-HOLYNAME>
+ 865 Teaneck Road/Suite 2
Teaneck, NJ 07666   (201)837-8446   Fax (201)342-1259

Rosen, Arie, MD {1407823404} Otlryg, SrgHdN(79,ISRA)<NJ-UMDNJ, NJ-HACKNSK>
+ Ear Nose Throat Institute of New Jersey
2 South Summit Avenue   Hackensack, NJ 07601   (201)996-9200   Fax (201)996-9277

Rosen, Bruce L., DO {1922158591} Gastrn, IntrMd(84,IA75)<NJ-HOLYNAME, NJ-ENGLWOOD>
+ 200 Engle Street/Suite 26
Englewood, NJ 07631   (201)567-5546   Fax (201)567-2166

Rosen, Chaim E., MD {1619909736} Anesth(78,MEXI)<NJ-VALLEY>
+ The Valley Hospital
223 North Van Dien Avenue   Ridgewood, NJ 07450   (201)447-8000

Rosen, Craig H., MD {1568423135} SrgOrt(79,NY47)
+ 603 North Broad Street
Woodbury, NJ 08096   (856)848-3500   Fax (856)848-1008
+ Premier Orthopaedic of South Jersey
1007 Mantua Pike   Woodbury, NJ 08096   (856)848-3500   Fax (856)853-8022

Rosen, Craig Michael, MD {1073512356} IntCrd, CdvDis(93,NY19)<NJ-MORRISTN>
+ Morristown Cardiology Associates, P.A.
435 South Street/Suite 100   Morristown, NJ 07960   (973)267-3944   Fax (973)455-0399

Rosen, David Michael, MD {1477711349} PulDis(07,PA02)<NJ-VALLEY>
+ Respiratory Health & Critical Care Associates
44 Godwin Avenue/Suite 201   Midland Park, NJ 07432   (201)689-7755   Fax (201)689-0521

Rosen, Ellen Jan, MD {1891895959} IntrMd, Gastrn(93,NY01)
+ 101 Madison Avenue/Suite 100
Morristown, NJ 07960   (973)455-0404

Rosen, Florence E., MD {1053479246} Pedtrc(80,PA01)<NJ-VIRTVOOR>
+ Cherry Hill Pediatric Group
600 West Marlton Pike   Cherry Hill, NJ 08002   (856)428-5020   Fax (856)216-9433

Rosen, Harel D., MD {1295864551} NnPnMd(89,PA02)<PA-RIDDLE>
+ On-Site Neonatal Partners
1000 Haddonfield-Berlin Road/Suite 210   Voorhees, NJ 08043   (856)782-2212   Fax (856)782-2213

Rosen, Ilene Michele, MD {1407871072} IntMSlpd, CritCr, PulDis(93,PA01)<PA-UPMCPHL>
+ Penn Medicine at Cherry Hill
409 Route 70 East/Sleep Center   Cherry Hill, NJ 08034   (856)429-1519

Rosen, Jay S., MD {1477521706} Urolgy(78,MEX14)<NJ-VALLEY, NJ-HACKNSK>
+ Urology Specialty Care
1200 East Ridgewood Avenue   Ridgewood, NJ 07450   (201)444-5988   Fax (201)444-0334
+ SurgiCare of Oradell
555 Kinderkamack Road   Oradell, NJ 07649   (201)444-5988   Fax (201)444-0334
+ SurgiCare Surgical Associates, P.A.
15-01 Broadway/Suites 1 & 3   Fair Lawn, NJ 07450   (201)703-8487   Fax (201)791-6585

Rosen, Jay Stuart, MD {1720139736} FamMed, OccpMd, EmrgMd(73,PA02)<NJ-ESSEXCO>
+ Essex County Hospital Center
204 Grove Avenue/Suite C   Cedar Grove, NJ 07009   (856)467-2009

Rosen, Jeffrey H., MD {1437145059} IntrMd(84,NY09)<NJ-RWJUBRUN, NJ-JFKJHNSN>
+ Park Primary Care Associates
453 Amboy Avenue   Woodbridge, NJ 07095   (732)636-6612   Fax (732)636-8224
wasupdoc@pol.net

Rosen, Kimberly A., MD ObsGyn(96,MA16)<NJ-MORRISTN>
+ 191 North Wyoming Avenue
South Orange, NJ 07079

Rosen, Larry S., MD {1104806868} ObsGyn(79,MEX14)<NJ-VIRTVOOR>
+ Womens Health Associates PA
188 Fries Mill Road/Suite B-1   Turnersville, NJ 08012   (856)629-1400   Fax (856)629-6695
+ Womens Health Associates PA
2301 East Evesham Road/Suite 602   Voorhees, NJ 08043   (856)629-1400   Fax (856)772-9159

Rosen, Lawrence David, MD {1255333050} Pedtrc(93,NY09)<NJ-HACKNSK>
+ Whole Child Center
690 Kinderamack Road/Suite 102   Oradell, NJ 07649   (201)634-1600   Fax (201)634-1606

Rosen, Marc Eliott, DO {1174593271} Surgry(96,CA22)
+ University of Medicine & Dentistry of New Jersey-SOM
42 East Laurel Road/Surgery   Stratford, NJ 08084   (856)566-6000

Rosen, Michael, MD {1730150632} Gastrn, IntrMd(78,PA01)<NJ-OVERLOOK>
+ 116 Millburn Avenue/Suite 211
Millburn, NJ 07041   (973)467-2500

Rosen, Michael David, MD {1881733665} SrgHnd, SrgPlstc, SrgRec(85,PA09)<NJ-JRSYSHMC>
+ 1114 Hooper Avenue
Toms River, NJ 08753   (732)240-6396
+ 1300 Highway 35/Plaza 2
Ocean, NJ 07712   (732)240-6396

Rosen, Neil L., DO {1205863040} FamMed(71,MO79)
+ Preventive Medicine of Monmouth, PC
1029 Sycamore Avenue   Tinton Falls, NJ 07724   (732)876-4917   Fax (732)876-4920

Rosen, Robert M., DO {1275512840} Dermat, DerMOH(86,NY75)<NJ-COMMED>
+ Forked River Dermatology
202 Route 37 West/Suite 6   Toms River, NJ 08755   (609)971-7701   Fax (609)971-3540
+ Aesthetic and Clinical Dermatology
202 Highway 37 West   Toms River, NJ 08755   (732)244-4566

Rosen, Scott Farrell, MD {1265407514} SrgVas, Surgry(93,NY19)<NJ-RWJUBRUN, NJ-STPETER>
+ Highland Park Surgical Associates
31 River Road   Highland Park, NJ 08904   (732)846-9500   Fax (732)846-3931
+ Highland Park Surgical Associates
B2 Brier Hill Court/Suite 3   East Brunswick, NJ 08816   (732)846-9500   Fax (732)238-9697
+ Cares Surgicenter, LLC.
240 Easton Avenue   New Brunswick, NJ 08904   (732)565-5400   Fax (732)296-8677

Rosen, Todd Joshua, MD {1245262880} ObsGyn, MtFtMd, IntrMd(92,NJ05)<NJ-RWJUBRUN, NJ-CENTRAST>
+ UMDNJ OBGYN
125 Paterson Street/Suite 4200   New Brunswick, NJ 08901   (732)235-6600   Fax (732)235-6650
rosentj@rutgers.edu

Rosenbaum, Daniel, MD {1073515706} EnDbMt, IntrMd(86,PA01)<NJ-LOURDMED>
+ Cooper University at Willingboro
218C Sunset Road   Willingboro, NJ 08046   (609)877-0400   Fax (609)877-3542

Rosenbaum, David Herbert, MD {1548307903} Nrolgy(69,NY19)<NY-MTSINAI, NJ-ENGLWOOD>
+ Allied Neurology & Interventional Pain
185 Grand Avenue   Englewood, NJ 07631   (201)894-1313   Fax (201)894-1335
drosenbaummd@gmail.com

Rosenbaum, Jeffrey Mark, MD {1467559823} Otlryg(73,NY03)
+ ENT & Allergy Associates
B-3 Cornwall Drive   East Brunswick, NJ 08816   (732)238-0300   Fax (732)238-4066
+ ENT & Allergy Associates
1543 Route 27/Suite 21   Somerset, NJ 08873   (732)238-0300   Fax (732)873-6853

Rosenbaum, Lee M., MD {1568444362} Anesth(76,NY09)<NJ-MORRISTN>
+ Anesthesia Associates of Morristown
264 South Street/Suite 2A   Morristown, NJ 07960   (973)631-8119

Rosenbaum, Paul, MD {1598999740} Psychy(65,NY46)
+ 658 South Forest Drive
Teaneck, NJ 07666   (201)692-1771

Rosenbaum, Robert L., MD {1285606988} EnDbMt, IntrMd(75,NY01)<NJ-OVERLOOK, NJ-MORRISTN>
+ Summit Medical Group-Berkeley Heights Campus
1 Diamond Hill Road/Endocrine   Berkeley Heights, NJ 07922   (908)277-8667   Fax (908)277-8707

Rosenbaum, Seth David, MD {1942226980} InfDis, IntrMd(99,MEX15)
+ Drs. Rosenbaum & Aufiero
2085 Klockner Road   Hamilton, NJ 08690   (609)587-4122   Fax (609)588-5922
+ RWJ Hamilton/Emergency Services
1 Hamilton Health Place   Hamilton, NJ 08690   (609)587-4122   Fax (609)890-7638

Rosenbaum, Steven B., MD {1689674723} EmrgMd(79,MEX33)<NJ-MTNSIDE>
+ Hackensack UMC Mountainside
1 Bay Avenue/EmrgMed   Montclair, NJ 07042   (973)429-6000

Physicians by Name and Address

Rosenberg, Allison R., DO {1699984328} RadDia<NJ-STBARHCS>
+ Regional Diagnostic Imaging Center
1505 West Sherman Avenue   Vineland, NJ 08360
(856)641-7937   Fax (856)641-7681

Rosenberg, Daniel S., MD {1366465486} PainMd, PhysMd, PhyM-Pain(81,MEX03)<NJ-RWJUBRUN, NJ-CHSMRCER>
+ Physical Medicine and Pain Center
34 Scotch Road   Trenton, NJ 08628   (609)883-0614   Fax (609)883-1606

Rosenberg, Elana Sarah, MD {1255639605} Glacma, Catrct, Ophthl(10,NY19)
+ Omni Eye Services
475 Prospect Avenue   West Orange, NJ 07052   (973)325-6734   Fax (973)325-6738
+ Omni Eye Services
485 Route 1 South/Building A   Iselin, NJ 08830   (973)325-6734   Fax (732)602-0749

Rosenberg, Gary B., MD {1467499186} PsyCAd, Psychy(73,NY08)<NJ-UNIVBHC>
+ University Behavioral Health Care
671 Hoes Lane/PO Box 1392/Psych   Piscataway, NJ 08855   (732)235-5500

Rosenberg, Gene S., MD {1093716219} Urolgy(74,NY19)<NJ-HACKNSK, NJ-HOLYNAME>
+ New Jersey Urology, LLC
20 Prospect Avenue/Suite 915   Hackensack, NJ 07601   (201)343-0082   Fax (201)488-1203
+ New Jersey Urology
6 Brighton Road/Suite 108   Clifton, NJ 07012   (201)343-0082   Fax (973)337-1330

Rosenberg, Jeffrey Steven, MD {1235103870} FamMed, FamM-SptM, IntrMd(94,NY47)<NJ-OVERLOOK>
+ Garden State Orthopaedic Associates, P.A.
28-04 Broadway   Fair Lawn, NJ 07410   (201)791-4434   Fax (201)791-9277
+ Summit Medical Group-Berkeley Heights Campus
1 Diamond Hill Road/1st FL Suite A   Berkeley Heights, NJ 07922   (201)791-4434   Fax (908)790-6576

Rosenberg, Joel W., MD {1861435836} Urolgy(66,NY08)
+ 721 Clifton Avenue
Clifton, NJ 07013   (973)778-7988

Rosenberg, Larry S., MD {1124008651} SrgOrt(84,NY46)
+ Orthopaedic and Sports Specialists
798 South Route 73   West Berlin, NJ 08091

Rosenberg, Leon I., MD {1215941000} Psychy, PsyGrt, PsyFor(78,NY15)
+ Center for Emotional Fitness
One Utah Avenue   Cherry Hill, NJ 08002   (856)857-9500   Fax (856)857-9120
cfef@cfef.com
+ Shore Therapy
310 Chris Gaupp Drive/Suite 105   Galloway, NJ 08205   (856)857-9500   Fax (856)857-9120

Rosenberg, Lori A., DO {1497757363} Pedtrc(98,NY75)<NJ-HOLYNAME>
+ Pedimedica PA
500 Piermont Road/Suite 102   Closter, NJ 07624   (201)784-3200   Fax (201)784-3321

Rosenberg, Mark S., DO {1184622045} EmrgMd(78,PA77)<NJ-HOBUNIMC, NJ-MTNSIDE>
+ St Joseph's Medical Center Emergency
703 Main Street   Paterson, NJ 07503   (973)754-2240   Fax (973)754-2249

Rosenberg, Martin Louis, MD {1306982905} GenPrc
+ Bayer HealthCare
100 Bayer Boulevard   Whippany, NJ 07981   (862)213-8556

Rosenberg, Michael A., MD {1073605069} Pedtrc(87,NJ05)
+ Pediatric Associates, LLC.
1318 South Main Street   Vineland, NJ 08360   (856)691-8585   Fax (856)691-8489

Rosenberg, Michael Eric, MD {1598729626} CrnExD, Ophthl(92,NY19)<NJ-ENGLWOOD, NJ-HACKNSK>
+ Montrose Eye Associates
301 Bridge Plaza North   Fort Lee, NJ 07024   (201)947-5929   Fax (201)947-5507

Rosenberg, Michael L., MD {1275533440} OphNeu, Nrolgy(76,TX04)
+ JFK Neurosciences Institute
65 James Street/Second Floor   Edison, NJ 08818   (732)321-7010   Fax (732)632-1669

Rosenberg, Mitchell C., MD {1477504017} CdvDis(81,RI01)<NJ-KMHCHRRY, NJ-COOPRUMC>
+ Cardiovascular Associates of The Delaware Valley, PA
1840 Frontage Road   Cherry Hill, NJ 08034   (856)795-2227   Fax (856)795-7436
+ Cardiovascular Associates
210 West Atlantic Avenue   Haddon Heights, NJ 08035   (856)795-2227   Fax (856)547-5337
+ Cardiovascular Associates of The Delaware Valley, PA
525 State Street/Suite 3   Elmer, NJ 08034   (856)358-2363   Fax (856)358-0725

Rosenberg, Paul E., MD {1467517151} Psychy(72,PA01)
+ The NJ Center for Short-Term Dynamic Psychotherapy
930 Mount Kemble Avenue   Morristown, NJ 07960   (973)425-1022

Rosenberg, Paul Howard, MD {1447319777} GenPrc, SrgRec(86,PA01)
+ Palisade Plastic Surgery Associates
1567 Palisade Avenue/3rd Floor   Fort Lee, NJ 07024   (201)585-2388   Fax (201)947-2507

Rosenberg, Rhonda Betsy, MD {1104893379} Ophthl(00,NY46)
+ Montrose Eye Associates
301 Bridge Plaza North   Fort Lee, NJ 07024   (201)947-5929   Fax (201)947-5507

Rosenberg, Richard S., MD {1598766636} IntrMd, Nrolgy(81,ISRA)
+ Neuroscience Center of Northern New Jersey
310 Madison Avenue   Morristown, NJ 07960   (973)285-1446   Fax (973)605-8854

Rosenberg, Scott B., MD {1063461614} PulDis, IntrMd(95,PA13)
+ Penn Jersey Pulmonary Associates
52 West Red Bank Avenue/Suite 26   Woodbury, NJ 08096   (856)853-2025   Fax (856)845-8024

Rosenberg, Victor I., MD {1770658502} Surgry
+ NYC Surgical Associates
555 Passiac Avenue   Caldwell, NJ 07006   (212)832-9095

Rosenberg, Zeil Barry, MD {1497797468} Pedtrc, PubHth, GPrvMd(82,CA02)
+ Becton Dickinson & Company
1 Becton Drive/Suite 084   Franklin Lakes, NJ 07417   (201)847-6800

Rosenberg-Henick, Arlene M., MD {1629045539} PedOph, Ophthl(90,NY46)
+ Montrose Eye Associates
301 Bridge Plaza North   Fort Lee, NJ 07024   (201)941-0562   Fax (201)947-5507

Rosenblat, Yoav, MD {1932143740} EmrgMd(98,ISR02)<NJ-STBARNMC>
+ St. Barnabas Medical Center
94 Old Short Hills Road   Livingston, NJ 07039   (973)322-5000

Rosenblatt, Daniel E., MD {1750325395} CritCr, IntrMd(89,PA12)<NJ-JFKMED>
+ JFK Medical Center
65 James Street   Edison, NJ 08820   (732)321-7660
+ RWJ University Hospital New Brunswick
One Robert Wood Johnson Place   New Brunswick, NJ 08901   (732)321-7660   Fax (732)906-4914

Rosenblatt, Jay M., MD {1710989108} RadDia, Radiol(87,NY48)
+ Radiology Associates of Burlington County
1295 Route 38 West/PO Box 479   Hainesport, NJ 08036   (609)261-7017   Fax (609)261-4180

Rosenblatt, Joseph M., DO {1609031715}
+ St Chris Care @ Washington Twp
100 Kings Way East/Bld C   Sewell, NJ 08080   (856)582-0644   Fax (856)582-0622
josephro@gmail.com

Rosenblatt, Joshua S., MD {1780653212} Pedtrc(84,NJ05)<NJ-CHDNWBTH, NJ-NWRKBETH>
+ Newark Beth Israel Medical Center
201 Lyons Avenue/Pediatrics   Newark, NJ 07112   (973)926-7273   Fax (973)705-3148

Rosenbloom, Michael, MD {1508852500} SrgThr
+ Cooper Surgical Associates
3 Cooper Plaza/Suite 411   Camden, NJ 08103   (856)342-2270   Fax (856)365-1180

Rosenblum, Benjamin A., MD {1316904410} Pedtrc(84,PA02)<NJ-VIRTVOOR, NJ-VIRTUAHS>
+ Advocare Atrium Pediatrics
301 Old Marlton Pike West/Suite 1   Marlton, NJ 08053   (856)988-9101   Fax (856)988-7712
+ Advocare Atrium Pediatrics Cedar Brook
41 South Route 73/Building 1/Suite 101   Hammonton, NJ 08037   (856)988-9101   Fax (609)567-4904

Rosenblum, Bruce R., MD {1205864345} SrgNro(82,NY47)<NJ-RIVERVW, NJ-BAYSHORE>
+ 160 Avenue at the Common
Shrewsbury, NJ 07702   (732)460-1522   Fax (732)460-1530

Rosenblum, Howard W., MD {1760485361} Pedtrc(76,NY46)
+ Pediatric Associates of Central Jersey
326 Main Street   Metuchen, NJ 08840   (732)767-0630   Fax (732)767-3070

Rosenblum, Lauren, DO {1841648714} FamMed<NJ-CHRIST>
+ Christ Hospital
176 Palisade Avenue   Jersey City, NJ 07306   (201)795-8201

Rosenblum, Stacy, MD {1639413693} NnPnMd
+ St Joseph's Medical Center Neonatology
703 Main Street   Paterson, NJ 07503   (973)754-2549

Rosenblum, Benjamin Dov, MD {1013930007} RadOnc(01,MA01)<NJ-HOLYNAME>
+ Holy Name Hospital
718 Teaneck Road/Cancer Ctr   Teaneck, NJ 07666   (201)541-6305

Rosenbluth, Jonathan Z., MD {1134107832} IntrMd, MedOnc(99,NJ06)<NJ-SOMERSET, NJ-STPETER>
+ Somerset Hematology Oncology Associates, P.A.
30 Rehill Avenue/2nd Floor/Suite 2500   Somerville, NJ 08876   (908)927-8700   Fax (908)927-8706

Rosenbluth, Richard J., MD {1871552349} Hemato, IntrMd, MedOnc(70,NY19)<NJ-HACKNSK>
+ John Theurer Cancer Center - HUMC
92 Second Street   Hackensack, NJ 07601   (201)996-5900   Fax (201)996-9246

Rosendorf, Eric Robert, MD {1043383995} Gastrn(95,NJ05)<NJ-SOCEANCO>
+ Hackensack Gastroenterology Associates
130 Kinderkamack Road/Suite 301   River Edge, NJ 07661   (201)489-7772   Fax (201)489-2544

Rosenfeld, Cheryl Robyn, DO {1881797215} EnDbMt, IntrMd(91,NY75)<NJ-NWRKBETH>
+ North Jersey Endocrine Consultants, LLC
1 Indian Road/Suite 8   Denville, NJ 07834   (973)625-2121   Fax (973)625-8270

Rosenfeld, David L., MD {1033181342} PedRad, Radiol(67,PA12)<NJ-STPETER, NJ-RWJUBRUN>
+ University Radiology Group, P.C.
483 Cranbury Road   East Brunswick, NJ 08816   (732)390-0030   Fax (732)390-5383

Rosenfeld, David N., MD {1629116371} Psychy(88,NJ06)<NJ-VALLEY>
+ Drs. Rosenfeld & Zisu
265 Ackerman Avenue   Ridgewood, NJ 07450   (201)447-5630   Fax (201)447-0903

Rosenfeld, Jane S., MD {1245232677} CritCr, IntrMd, PulDis(81,NJ06)<NJ-STPETER, NJ-RWJUBRUN>
+ University Medical Group - General Internal Medicine
125 Paterson Street/Suite 5100A   New Brunswick, NJ 08903   (732)235-6968   Fax (732)235-8935

Rosenfeld, Walter D., MD {1376517920} AdolMd, Pedtrc(75,PA13)<NJ-MORRISTN, NJ-OVERLOOK>
+ Morristown Medical Center
100 Madison Avenue/Box 54   Morristown, NJ 07962   (973)971-5199   Fax (973)290-7099
walter.rosenfeld@ahsys.org
+ Adolescent Medicine of MMH
100 Madison Avenue   Morristown, NJ 07960   (973)971-4330

Rosengarten, Herbert H., MD {1912947029} IntrMd(80,NY08)<NJ-CHSFULD>
+ Allentown Medical Associates
163 Burlington Path Road   Cream Ridge, NJ 08514   (609)758-1100   Fax (609)758-3188

Rosenheck, David Mark, MD {1811995046} Gastrn, IntrMd(83,NJ05)<NJ-JFKMED, NJ-RBAYPERT>
+ May Street Surgi Center
205 May Street/Suite 103   Edison, NJ 08837   (732)820-4566   Fax (732)661-9619
+ Gastroenterology Consultants PA
205 May Street/Suite 201   Edison, NJ 08837   (732)820-4566   Fax (732)661-9259
+ Gastroenterology Consultants PA
3 Hospital Plaza/Suite 415   Old Bridge, NJ 08837   (732)360-2282   Fax (732)360-2303

Rosenheck, Justin Philip, DO {1548681679} IntrMd
+ The Cooper Hospital System-Univ Hospital
401 Haddon Avenue/3rd Fl   Camden, NJ 08103   (732)610-9045

Rosenkrantz, Leah Ellen, DO {1689887515} Psychy
+ 12 Marigold Court
Mount Laurel, NJ 08054

Rosenstein, Elliot D., MD {1174585145} Rheuma, Immuno(78,NY47)<NJ-OVERLOOK>
+ Institute for Rheumatic & Autoimmune Diseases
33 Overlook Road/MAC L01   Summit, NJ 07901   (908)598-7940   Fax (908)598-5447
elliot.rosenstein@atlantichealth.org

Rosenstein, Howard P., MD {1710909270} Radiol, RadDia(78,DC01)<NJ-CENTRAST>
+ CentraState Medical Center
901 West Main Street/Radiology   Freehold, NJ 07728   (732)431-2000

Rosenstein, Kenneth Michael, MD {1376792606} Otlryg, IntrMd(07,QU01)<NY-NYEYEINF>
+ Becker Nose & Sinus Center, LLC.
570 Egg Harbor Road   Sewell, NJ 08080   (856)589-6673   Fax (856)589-3443
+ Becker Nose & Sinus Center, LLC.
2301 East Evesham Road/Suite 306   Voorhees, NJ 08043   (856)589-6673   Fax (856)770-0069
+ Becker ENT
2 Princess Road/Suite East   Lawrenceville, NJ 08080   (610)303-5163   Fax (610)303-5164

Rosenstein, Megan Ann, MD {1558528992} Anesth(05,NY48)
+ 33 Overlook Road/Suite 311
Summit, NJ 07901

Rosenstein, Roger G., MD {1114959285} SrgHnd, SrgOrt, OrtS-Hand(75,NY01)<NJ-HACKNSK, NJ-VALLEY>
+ Drs. Rosenstein & Fakharzadeh
22 Madison Avenue/Suite 3-1   Paramus, NJ 07652
(201)587-7767   Fax (201)587-8090

Rosenstock, Adam Seth, MD {1962659912} Surgry(06,PA09)
+ Surgical Associates
90 Prospect Avenue/Room 1D   Hackensack, NJ 07601
(201)343-3433   Fax (201)343-0420

Rosenthal, Adrienne Paula, MD {1467691246} RadDia
+ Radiology Associates of Burlington County
1295 Route 38 West/PO Box 479   Hainesport, NJ 08036
(609)261-7017   Fax (609)261-4180

Rosenthal, Brett Samson, DO {1982687570} IntrMd, Nephro(99,PA77)<NJ-OURLADY, NJ-KMHCHRRY>
+ Haddon Renal Medical Specialists
401 Kings Highway South/Suite 5   Cherry Hill, NJ 08034
(856)428-8992   Fax (856)428-9614

Rosenthal, Lauren Beth, MD {1235394826} Pedtrc, PedCrd(02,NY08)<NJ-MORRISTN, NJ-OVERLOOK>
+ Overlook Medical Center
99 Beauvoir Avenue/PO Box 210   Summit, NJ 07902
(908)522-5340
+ Morristown Medical Center
100 Madison Avenue/Pedi Crtcl Care   Morristown, NJ 07962
(973)971-5996

Rosenthal, Lawrence Stephen, MD {1942359021} Gastrn, IntrMd(01,NY08)
+ Affiliates in Gastroenterology, P.A.
101 Old Short Hills Road/Suite 217   West Orange, NJ 07052
(973)731-4600   Fax (973)731-1477

Rosenthal, Leslie S., MD {1235149022} IntrMd, Grtrcs(82,PA09)<NJ-ACMCITY, NJ-ACMCMAIN>
+ AtlantiCare Internal Medical Associates
7313 Ventnor Avenue   Ventnor, NJ 08406   (609)441-2199
Fax (609)487-9640
+ AtlantiCare Clinical Associates
2500 English Creek Avenue   Egg Harbor Township, NJ 08234
(609)407-2310

Rosenthal, Mark S., MD {1215990858} CdvDis, IntrMd(86,NY46)
+ Cardiology Associates of North Jersey
242 West Parkway   Pompton Plains, NJ 07444   (973)831-7455   Fax (973)831-7585

Rosenthal, Marnie Elyse, DO {1790733921} IntrMd, InfDis(02,ME75)<NJ-JRSYSHMC>
+ Hackensack Meridian Medical Group
19 Davis Avenue/5th-6th Floor   Neptune, NJ 07753
(732)897-3995   Fax (732)897-3997

Rosenthal, Nadine C., MD {1639159742} IntrMd(90,FRA02)
+ Penn Medicine at Woodbury Heights
1006 Mantua Pike   Woodbury Heights, NJ 08097
(856)845-8600   Fax (856)845-0535

Rosenthal, Richard Eugene, DO {1952409724} Radiol, RadDia, IntrMd(79,IA75)<NJ-KMHSTRAT>
+ Magnetic Imaging at Kennedy
900 Medical Center Drive/Suite 101   Sewell, NJ 08080
(856)784-1976   Fax (856)784-2342

Rosenthal, Robert S., MD {1669484341} Psychy, Psythp(81,PA09)
+ 110 Straube Center Boulevard
Pennington, NJ 08534   (609)737-7676   Fax (609)737-6576

Rosenthal, Susan R., MD {1740365634} Pedtrc, PedGst(77,NY47)
+ UH- Robert Wood Johnson Med
125 Paterson Street/MEB 342/Pedi   New Brunswick, NJ 08901   (732)828-3000

Rosenthal, Todd Michael, MD {1831484302} CdvDis
+ Associates in Cardiovascular Disease, LLC
571 Central Avenue/Suite 115   New Providence, NJ 07974
(908)464-4200   Fax (908)464-1332

Rosenwasser, Melvin Paul, MD {1962434720} SrgHnd, SrgOrt(76,NY01)<NY-NYPRESHS, NY-PRSBCOLU>
+ Columbia Grand Orthopaedics
500 Grand Avenue/Suite 101   Englewood, NJ 07631
(201)569-0440   Fax (201)569-4949

Rosenwasser, Robert Hillel, MD {1275553455} SrgNro(79,LA06)<PA-TJHSP>
+ AtlantiCare Regional Medical Center/City Campus
1925 Pacific Avenue/1st Fl/NeuroSrg   Atlantic City, NJ 08401
(609)572-8600

Rosenzweig, Abraham H., MD {1679654891} SrgOrt(76,NJ05)
+ Orthopedic Associates of West Jersey
600 Mount Pleasant Avenue/Suite A   Dover, NJ 07801
(973)989-0888   Fax (973)989-0885

Rosenzweig, Alan, DO {1902883226} FamMed, Grtrcs, FamM-Grtc(78,PA77)<NJ-LOURDMED, NJ-KMHSTRAT>
+ 917 Cinnaminson Avenue
Palmyra, NJ 08065   (856)829-1060   Fax (856)786-4442

Rosenzweig, Debra L., MD {1972671170} ObsGyn(88,GRNA)<NJ-CHILTON>
+ 2035 Hamburg Turnpike/Suite C
Wayne, NJ 07470   (973)616-9395   Fax (973)839-2983

Rosenzweig, Howard J., MD {1861439622} Anesth(86,MEX48)<NJ-STFRNMED>
+ St. Francis Medical Center
601 Hamilton Avenue/Anesthesiology   Trenton, NJ 08629
(609)599-5000

Rosenzweig, Stacey Ann, MD {1265471577} Pedtrc(92,CT01)<NJ-VALLEY>
+ Chestnut Ridge Pediatrics
595 Chestnut Ridge Road   Woodcliff Lake, NJ 07677
(201)391-2020   Fax (201)391-0265

Rosenzweig, Talia S., MD {1952507980} ObsGyn(03,ISR02)
+ Shore Area Ob-Gyn
200 White Road/Suite 105   Little Silver, NJ 07739
(732)741-3331

Rosh, Joel R., MD {1326011255} PedGst, Pedtrc(86,NY46)<NJ-OVERLOOK, NJ-MORRISTN>
+ Overlook Medical Center
99 Beauvoir Avenue/PO Box 210   Summit, NJ 07902
(908)522-2000
+ Division of Pediatric GI at Goryeb
100 Madison Avenue/Box 82   Morristown, NJ 07962
(908)522-2000   Fax (973)290-7365

Rosica, John A., MD {1255404935} EmrgMd, GenPrc(79,MEX14)<NJ-STCLRDEN, NJ-STCLRDOV>
+ St. Clare's Hospital-Denville Campus
25 Pocono Road   Denville, NJ 07834   (973)625-6000   Fax (973)983-2293
+ St. Clare's Hospital-Dover
400 West Blackwell Street   Dover, NJ 07801   (973)989-3000

Rosier, Eric, MD {1790770253} IntrMd(91,MEX34)<NJ-MTNSIDE>
+ Pathlink, LLC
66 West Gilbert Street/Suite 100   Tinton Falls, NJ 07701
(732)212-0060   Fax (732)212-0061

Rosin, Dale, DO {1316283708} Psychy
+ 129 Grove Street
Somerville, NJ 08876   (908)526-5095   Fax (908)218-1588

Rosin, Deborah F., MD {1144224502} Otlryg(89,PA01)
+ ENT & Allergy Associates, LLP
485 Route 1 South/Bld B/Suite 350   Iselin, NJ 08830
(732)549-3934   Fax (732)549-7250

Rosin, Jay Michael, MD {1588744098} Ophthl(92,MI07)<NJ-CENTRAST, NJ-MONMOUTH>
+ Millennium Eye Care, LLC
500 West Main Street   Freehold, NJ 07728   (732)462-8707
Fax (732)462-1296

Rosines, Noam, MD {1316978059} EmrgMd(03,TX04)
+ 26 Hilliard Avenue/Apt 4
Edgewater, NJ 07020

Rosman, Gary A., MD {1548338478} Gastrn(82,NY09)<NJ-ACMCITY, NJ-ACMCMAIN>
+ Atlantic Gastroenterology Associates, P.A.
3205 Fire Road/Suite 4   Egg Harbor Township, NJ 08234
(609)407-1220   Fax (609)407-0220
+ Atlantic Gastroenterology Associates, P.A.
72 West Jimmie Leeds Road/Suite 2600   Galloway, NJ 08205
(609)407-1220   Fax (609)407-0220

Rosman, Jerome D., MD {1073524708} SrgOrt, IntrMd(75,NJ05)<NJ-HCKTSTWN>
+ The Orthopedic Institute of New Jersey
108 Bilby Road/Suite 201   Hackettstown, NJ 07840
(908)684-3005   Fax (908)684-3301
eileenm1@verizon.net
+ The Orthopedic Institute of New Jersey
254-B Mountain Avenue/Suite 201   Hackettstown, NJ 07840
(908)684-3005   Fax (908)684-3301
+ The Orthopedic Institute of New Jersey
222 High Street/Suite 202   Newton, NJ 07840   (908)684-3005   Fax (908)684-3301

Rosner, Bruce P., MD {1518986553} Gastrn, IntrMd(76,PA01)<NJ-STFRNMED>
+ Gastroenterology Associates
2275 Whitehorse-Mercerville Rd   Trenton, NJ 08619
(609)890-0200   Fax (609)890-8335

Rosner, Steven M., MD {1669441929} Rheuma, IntrMd(76,NY09)<NH-MONADNK>
+ Hackensack University Medical Group Emerson
452 Old Hook Road/2nd Floor   Emerson, NJ 07630
(201)666-3900   Fax (201)261-0505

Rosner, William Fredric, MD {1881688141} Radiol, RadDia, IntrMd(75,PA02)<NJ-VIRTVOOR, NJ-VIRTMARL>
+ South Jersey Radiology Associates, P.A.
901 Route 168/Suites 301-305   Turnersville, NJ 08012
(856)227-6600   Fax (856)227-8537
+ South Jersey Radiology Associates, P.A.
315 Route 70 East/Suite B   Cherry Hill, NJ 08034   (856)227-6600   Fax (856)428-0356
+ South Jersey Radiology Associates, P.A.
1000 Lincoln Drive East   Marlton, NJ 08012   (856)983-1818
Fax (856)983-3226

Rosof, Edward, MD {1912955485} Pedtrc(71,PA02)<NJ-VIRTBERL, NJ-VIRTMARL>
+ Advocare Marlton Pediatrics
525 Route 73 South   Marlton, NJ 08053   (856)596-3434
Fax (856)596-9081
+ Advocare Hammonton Pediatrics
856 South Whitehorse Pike   Hammonton, NJ 08037
(856)596-3434   Fax (609)704-8849
+ Advocare Township Pediatrics
123 Egg Harbor Road   Sewell, NJ 08053   (856)227-5437
Fax (856)227-5890

Ross, Ann, MD {1063488997} NnPnMd, Pedtrc(86,CHIL)<NJ-JRSYSHMC>
+ Meridian Medical Group - Faculty Practice
61 Davis Avenue/Suite 1   Neptune, NJ 07753   (732)776-4860   Fax (732)776-4867
+ Meridian Medical Group - Faculty Practice
61 Davis Avenue/Suite 1   Neptune, NJ 07753   (732)776-4860   Fax (732)776-4639

Ross, Carolyn Michelle, MD {1144596156} ObsGyn<NJ-COOPRUMC>
+ Cooper University Hospital
One Cooper Plaza   Camden, NJ 08103   (856)342-2000

Ross, David H., MD {1033113998} OncHem, MedOnc, IntrMd(68,PA13)<NJ-VIRTVOOR, NJ-KENEDYHS>
+ Comprehensive Cancer & Hematology Specialists, P.C.
705 White Horse Road   Voorhees, NJ 08043   (856)435-1777   Fax (856)435-0696
+ Comprehensive Cancer & Hematology Specialists, P.C.
900 Medical Center Drive/Suite 200   Sewell, NJ 08080
(856)435-1777   Fax (856)582-7640
+ Comprehensive Cancer & Hematology Specialists, P.C.
17 West Red Bank Avenue/Suite 202   Woodbury, NJ 08043
(856)848-5560   Fax (856)848-0958

Ross, Douglas A., MD {1518161223} IntrMd(05,GRN01)<NJ-MONMOUTH>
+ Monmouth Medical Center
300 Second Avenue   Long Branch, NJ 07740   (732)222-5200

Ross, Jacqueline, MD {1295055150} AlgyImmn
+ Allergy Partners of New Jersey PC
802 West Park Avenue/Suite 213   Ocean, NJ 07712
(732)695-2555   Fax (732)695-2552
+ Allergy Partners of New Jersey PC
8 Tindall Road   Middletown, NJ 07748   (732)695-2555
Fax (732)671-0144

Ross, Michael Jordan, MD {1659433019} EmrgMd, FamM-SptM(97,NY47)<PA-ENSTEIN>
+ Rothman Institute-The Performance Lab
2005 Route 7 East   Cherry Hill, NJ 08003   Fax (856)874-1188

Ross, Neil E., MD {1548221898} Anesth(86,LA01)
+ Summit Anesthesia Associates, P.A.
33 Overlook Road/Suite 311   Summit, NJ 07901   (908)598-1500   Fax (908)598-0197

Ross, Richard S., MD {1689635948} Catrct, Ophthl, SrgLsr(81,NY71)
+ Richard S. Ross MD PA
445 Hurffville-Cross Keys Road   Sewell, NJ 08080
(856)589-4545   Fax (856)586-6210

Ross, Ronald E., MD {1538472873} SrgThr
+ Mid Atlantic Surgical Associates
200 Trenton Road   Browns Mills, NJ 08015   (973)971-7300
Fax (973)984-7019

Ross, Sarah, MD {1740548502}
+ University Behavioral HealthCare
183 South Orange Avenue   Newark, NJ 07103   (973)972-5401

Ross, Steven E., MD {1730264581} SrgCrC, Surgry, SrgTrm(76,PA02)<NJ-COOPRUMC>
+ Cooper Surgical Associates
3 Cooper Plaza/Suite 411   Camden, NJ 08103   (856)342-2270   Fax (856)365-1180
+ Cooper University Physician Trauma Center
One Cooper Plaza   Camden, NJ 08103   (856)342-3014

Ross, William H., DO {1255392049} IntrMd(85,NY75)
+ 2 Forge Court
Freehold, NJ 07728   (732)780-2881

Ross, William M., MD {1649276387} Radiol, RadDia, RadV&I(79,PA09)<NJ-STFRNMED>
+ Radiology Affiliates of Central New Jersey, P.A.
2501 Kuser Road   Hamilton, NJ 08691   (609)585-8800
Fax (609)585-1825
+ Radiology Affiliates of Central New Jersey, P.A.
3120 Princeton Pike   Lawrenceville, NJ 08648   (609)585-8800   Fax (609)219-0439
+ St. Francis Medical Center
601 Hamilton Avenue/Radiology   Trenton, NJ 08691
(609)599-5000

Physicians by Name and Address

Rossakis, Constantine, MD {1356303390} CdvDis, IntrMd(83,NY19)<NJ-HACKNSK>
+ 357 Prospect Avenue
  Hackensack, NJ 07601 (201)489-3440 Fax (201)489-7920

Rossetos, Ourania S., MD {1396883070} ObsGyn, IntrMd(93,NJ06)<NJ-HOBUNIMC, NJ-CHRIST>
+ Hoboken University Medical Center
  308 Willow Avenue/OB/GYN Hoboken, NJ 07030 (201)418-1000 Fax (855)462-9736

Rossetti-Cartaxo, Annette L., MD {1245288588} Pedtrc(81,MEX03)<NJ-NWTNMEM>
+ Newton Medical Center
  175 High Street/Pediatrics Newton, NJ 07860 (973)383-2121 Fax (973)383-8973

Rossi, Anna Michele, DO {1659593473} Psychy, PsyCAd(96,NJ75)
+ Ann Klein Forensic Center
  8 Production Way Avenel, NJ 07001 (732)574-2250 Fax (732)882-0773

Rossi, Anthony G., MD {1558457192} Otlryg(76,MEXI)
+ 912 Pompton Avenue/Suite A1
  Cedar Grove, NJ 07009 (973)239-5090 Fax (973)239-3579

Rossi, Cynthia Ann, MD {1700915766} FamMed(96,PA07)
+ Milford Medical Center
  207 Strykers Road Phillipsburg, NJ 08865 (908)995-4125

Rossi, Lawrence Nicholas, MD {1093813735} Psychy(71,PA09)<NJ-TRENTPSY>
+ Trenton Psychiatric Hospital
  Sullivan Way/PO Box 7600 West Trenton, NJ 08628 (609)633-1500

Rossi, Regina L., DO {1235186164} IntrMd(91,NJ75)<NJ-CENTRAST>
+ Hackensack Meridian Medical Group
  195 Route 9 South/Suite 106 Manalapan, NJ 07726 (732)536-7144 Fax (732)536-7520
+ Jersey Shore Associates of Internal Medicine
  831 Tennent Road Manalapan, NJ 07726 (732)536-7144 Fax (732)536-7520

Rossi, Roger P., DO {1548281058} PhysMd(89,IA75)<NJ-JFKJHNSN, NJ-JFKMED>
+ JFK Johnson Rehabilitation Institute
  65 James Street Edison, NJ 08818 (732)321-7050 Fax (732)321-7330

Rossi, Wilma Catherine, MD {1558377622} PedEnd, Pedtrc(79,NY08)<PA-CHILDHOS>
+ CHOP Pediatric & Adolescent Specialty Care Center
  1012 Laurel Oak Road Voorhees, NJ 08043 (856)435-1300 Fax (856)435-0091
+ CHOP Pediatric & Adolescent Specialty Care Center
  707 Alexander Road/Suite 205 Princeton, NJ 08540 (609)520-1717

Rossman, Barry R., MD {1811911761} Urolgy(83,MA05)<NJ-UNVMCPRN, NJ-CAPITLHS>
+ Urology Group of Princeton PA
  134 Stanhope Street/Forrestal Village Princeton, NJ 08540 (609)924-6487 Fax (609)921-7020

Rossman, Ian T., MD {1790076404} Pedtrc, NroChl, Psychy(09,NJ02)<NJ-RWJUBRUN>
+ RWJ University Hospital New Brunswick
  One Robert Wood Johnson Place New Brunswick, NJ 08901 (732)235-7883 Fax (732)235-7345

Rossman, Stephen, DO {1346600749}
+ University Physician Associates
  140 Bergen Street/ACC Level D Newark, NJ 07103 (845)304-6969 Fax (973)972-3102

Rossos, Apostolos A., MD {1710074562} Otlryg, OtgyPSHN(81,GRN01)<NJ-CENTRAST>
+ 1542 Kuser Road/Suite B5
  Hamilton, NJ 08619 (609)581-0500 Fax (609)581-2077
+ Center for Ear, Nose, Sinus and Throat Disorders
  501 Iron Bridge Road/Suite 11 Freehold, NJ 07728 (609)581-0500 Fax (732)409-0202

Rossos, Nicholas A., MD {1609962422} IntrMd(75,PHI08)<NJ-RWJUHAM>
+ 619 Farnsworth Avenue
  Bordentown, NJ 08505 (609)298-1673 Fax (609)298-0801

Rossy, Kathleen M., MD {1730341736} Dermat(05,NJ05)
+ The Princeton Center for Dermatology, LLC
  800 Bunn Drive/Suite 201 Princeton, NJ 08540 (609)924-1033 Fax (609)924-7055

Rossy, William H., MD {1548262272} FamMed(78,PRO01)<NJ-JFKMED>
+ PrimeCare Medical Group
  561 Middlesex Avenue Metuchen, NJ 08840 (732)549-9363 Fax (732)603-0397

Rossy, William Henry, IV, MD {1891012183} SrgOrt(10,NJ05)<NY-JTORTHO>
+ Princeton Orthopaedic Associates, P.A.
  325 Princeton Avenue Princeton, NJ 08540 (609)924-8131 Fax (609)924-8532

Rosten, Sloan I., MD {1710987110} RadDia(93,NY45)
+ South Jersey Radiology Associates, P.A.
  748 Kings Highway West Deptford, NJ 08096 (856)848-4998 Fax (856)853-7362
+ South Jersey Radiology Associates, P.A.
  Severan Profess Mews/Suite 105 Sewell, NJ 08080 (856)848-4998 Fax (856)589-6142
+ SJRA South Jersey Radiology Associates, P.A.
  113 East Laurel Road Stratford, NJ 08096 (856)566-2552

Rosvold, David Nelson, MD {1275500852} CdvDis, IntrMd(84,PA14)<NJ-SHOREMEM, NJ-BURDTMLN>
+ Mercer Bucks Cardiology
  3140 Princeton Pike/2nd Floor Lawrenceville, NJ 08648 (609)895-1919 Fax (609)895-1200
+ Mercer Bucks Cardiology
  One Union Street/Suite 101 Robbinsville, NJ 08691 (609)895-1919 Fax (609)890-7292
+ Mercer Bucks Cardiology
  One Union Street/Suite 101 Robbinsville, NJ 08648 (609)890-6677 Fax (609)890-7292

Rosvold, Elizabeth Anne, MD {1558379602} MedOnc, Hemato, OncHem(85,PA14)<NJ-STFRNMED, NJ-RWJUHAM>
+ Mercer Bucks Hematology Oncology
  2 Capital Way/Suite 220 Pennington, NJ 08534 (609)303-0747 Fax (609)303-0771

Roszkowski, Jennifer Rose, DO {1265697528} SlpDis, IntrMd(08,PA77)
+ The Maro Group
  27 Covered Bridge Road Cherry Hill, NJ 08034 (856)429-2224 Fax (856)429-1926

Rota, Anthony P., MD {1770624686} IntrMd(87,PA06)<NJ-UNVMCPRN>
+ Princeton Internal Medicine Associates
  281 Witherspoon Street/Suite 220 Princeton, NJ 08542 (609)921-3362 Fax (609)921-3584
+ Princeton Internal Medicine Associates
  88 Princeton Hightstown Road Princeton Junction, NJ 08550 (609)799-0100

Rotella, Frank A., DO {1801991393} FamMed(70,IA75)<NJ-CHRIST, NJ-MEADWLND>
+ PMA Physicians LLC
  1 Journal Square Plaza/2nd Floor Jersey City, NJ 07306 (201)216-3030 Fax (201)499-0247

Roth, Anne G., DO {1205025574} PedDvl
+ Jersey Shore Child Evaluation Center
  81-04 Davis Avenue Neptune, NJ 07753 (732)776-4178 Fax (732)776-4946

Roth, Daniel Benjamin, MD {1538132352} Ophthl(94,CT01)
+ Retina Associates of New Jersey, P.A.
  10 Plum Street/Suite 600 New Brunswick, NJ 08901 (732)220-1600 Fax (732)220-1603
+ Retina Associates of New Jersey, P.A.
  525 Route 70 West/Suite B-14 Lakewood, NJ 08701 (732)220-1600 Fax (732)363-0403
+ Retina Associates of New Jersey, P.A.
  530 Lakehurst Road/Suite 305 Toms River, NJ 08901 (732)797-3883 Fax (732)797-3886

Roth, Douglas M., DO {1346212057} IntrMd(87,NY75)<NJ-OVERLOOK, NJ-STBARNMC>
+ Summit Medical Group-Berkeley Heights Campus
  1 Diamond Hill Road Berkeley Heights, NJ 07922 (908)273-4300 Fax (908)790-6524
+ Summit Medical Group
  85 Woodland Road Short Hills, NJ 07078 (908)273-4300 Fax (973)921-0669

Roth, Howard Lee, MD {1992966808} RadDia<NJ-COOPRUMC>
+ Cooper University Hospital
  One Cooper Plaza/Radiol Camden, NJ 08103 (856)342-2380 Fax (856)365-0472

Roth, Jonathan A., MD {1215903687} PedUro, Urolgy, IntrMd(94,PA01)<NJ-VIRTVOOR>
+ Urology for Children, LLC
  120 Carnie Boulevard/Suite 2 Voorhees, NJ 08043 (856)751-7880
+ Urology for Children, LLC
  239 Hurffville Crosskeys Road Sewell, NJ 08080 (856)751-7880 Fax (856)751-9133
+ Urology for Children, LLC
  1000 Atlantic Avenue Camden, NJ 08043 (856)751-7880 Fax (856)751-9133

Roth, Jonathan Michael, MD {1831271410} SrgOrt
+ Orthopedic Surgery Center
  1055 Hamburg Turnpike Wayne, NJ 07470 (973)616-0200

Roth, Joseph M., MD {1942238225} Gastrn, IntrMd(81,PA12)<NJ-MEADWLND, NJ-ATLANTHS>
+ Gastroenterology Associates of New Jersey
  71 Union Avenue/Suite 201 Rutherford, NJ 07070 (201)842-0020 Fax (201)842-0010
+ Gastroenterology Associates of New Jersey
  925 Clifton Avenue Clifton, NJ 07013 (201)842-0020 Fax (973)405-6564

Roth, Patrick A., MD {1760459085} SrgNro(87,NY46)
+ North Jersey Brain and Surgical
  680 Kinderkamack Road/Suite 300 Oradell, NJ 07649 (201)342-2550 Fax (201)342-7171

Roth, Robert L., MD {1992878581} Psychy(81,MNT01)<NJ-ANNKLEIN>
+ Ann Klein Forensic Center
  1609 Stuyvesant Avenue/PO Box 7717 West Trenton, NJ 08628 (609)633-0900

Rothbart, Stephen T., MD {1497724876} CdvDis, ClCdEl, IntrMd(77,NJ05)<NJ-NWRKBETH>
+ Newark Beth Israel Medical Center
  201 Lyons Avenue Newark, NJ 07112 (973)926-8590

Rothberg, Michael Steven, MD {1861498628} IntrMd(99,MI07)<NJ-COMMED, NJ-KIMBALL>
+ Ocean County Family Care
  2125 Route 88 East Brick, NJ 08724 (732)892-4548 Fax (732)892-0961

Rothberg, Robert M., MD {1376514497} SrgC&R, Surgry(72,NY19)<NJ-MTNSIDE, NJ-CLARMAAS>
+ 39 South Fullerton Avenue
  Montclair, NJ 07042 (973)744-0550 Fax (973)744-0697

Rothchild, Richard, MD {1073627204} NnPnMd<NJ-UNVMCPRN, PA-CHILDHOS>
+ CHOP Newborn and Pediatric Care at UMCPP
  One Plainsboro Road/6th Floor Plainsboro, NJ 08536 (609)853-7626 Fax (609)853-7630

Rothenberg, Bennett C., MD {1154481281} SrgPlstc, Surgry(86,DC03)
+ 22 Old Short Hills Road
  Livingston, NJ 07039 (973)994-3311 Fax (973)994-7005
+ Short Hills Surgery Center
  187 Millburn Avenue/Suite 101 Millburn, NJ 07041 (973)994-3311 Fax (973)671-0557

Rothenberg, Jerry, MD {1942481551} Hemato, PthACl, PthDrm(64,GA01)
+ New Jersey Dermatopathology Labs
  769 Northfield Avenue West Orange, NJ 07052 (973)669-0141 Fax (973)669-8220

Rothenberg, Nancy A., DO {1326056227} Pedtrc(86,NJ75)
+ Old Tappan Medical Group PA
  215 Old Tappan Road Old Tappan, NJ 07675 (201)666-1000 Fax (201)666-4108
+ Old Tappan Pediatrics
  136 North Washington Avenue Bergenfield, NJ 07621 (201)666-1000 Fax (201)385-4748

Rothenberg, Paul, MD {1912240227} SrgOrt
+ 38 Meadowlands Parkway
  Secaucus, NJ 07094 (551)205-8081

Rothenberg, Richard N., MD {1740356195} ObsGyn(82,PHI08)
+ 16 Pocono Road/Suite 107
  Denville, NJ 07834 (973)627-1400 Fax (973)627-1420

Rothfarb, Steven H., MD {1285674358} RadDia, Radiol, IntrMd(76,NY15)
+ Center for Diagnostic Imaging
  1450 East Chestnut Avenue Vineland, NJ 08360 (856)794-8664 Fax (856)794-2671

Rothfleisch, Jeremy Evan, MD {1790774883} Dermat(97,NY19)<NJ-STPETER>
+ 603 Cranbury Road
  East Brunswick, NJ 08816 (732)545-5366 Fax (732)254-1038

Rothkopf, Michael M., MD {1821137225} IntrMd, Nutrtn, CritCr(79,VA07)<NJ-STBARNMC, NJ-MORRISTN>
+ 95 Madison Avenue/Suite 201
  Morristown, NJ 07960 (973)971-7166 Fax (973)290-7518
+ Metabolic Medicine & Weight Control Center
  1195 Route 70 Lakewood, NJ 08701 (973)971-7166 Fax (973)290-7518
+ Obesity Treatment Center
  435 South Street/Suite 330 B Morristown, NJ 07960 (973)971-7166 Fax (973)290-7518

Rothkopf, Moshe M., MD {1720049588} Ophthl(79,PA09)
+ Garden State Eye Center
  1195 Highway 70 Lakewood, NJ 08701 (732)363-2244 Fax (732)363-1825
+ 1 Plaza Drive
  Toms River, NJ 08757 (732)341-7010

Rothman, Arthur C., MD {1588620298} Nrolgy(85,FL02)<NJ-ENGLWOOD>
+ 440 Curry Avenue
  Englewood, NJ 07631 (201)567-1264 Fax (201)569-9326
+ 211 Essex Street/Suite 405
  Hackensack, NJ 07601 (201)489-7733

Rothman, Craig Michael, MD {1538274170} IntrMd(71,PA01)
+ VA Outpatient Clinic
  Cape May Coast Guard Base Cape May, NJ 08204 (609)898-8700

Rothman, Frederic R., MD {1952360141} Dermat(64,MI01)<NJ-STBARNMC>
+ The Dermatology Group, P.C.
60 Pompton Avenue   Verona, NJ 07044   (973)571-2121   Fax (973)571-2126
+ The Dermatology Group, P.C.
44 Route 23 North/Suite 213   Riverdale, NJ 07457   (973)571-2121   Fax (973)839-5751
+ The Dermatology Group, P.C.
30 West Century Road/Suite 320   Paramus, NJ 07044   (973)571-2121   Fax (201)986-0702
Rothman, Howard C., MD {1134125941} CdvDis, IntrMd(70,OH41)<NJ-ENGLWOOD, NJ-HOLYNAME>
+ Advanced Cardiology Institute
2200 Fletcher Avenue/Suite 1   Fort Lee, NJ 07024   (201)461-6200   Fax (201)461-7204
+ Heart and Vascular Institute at EHMC
350 Engle Street/Suite 1000   Englewood, NJ 07631   (201)894-3636
Rothman, Michael E., MD {1205902129} IntrMd, EmrgMd, FamMed(86,FL02)<NJ-OCEANMC>
+ Ocean Medical Center
425 Jack Martin Boulevard/EmergMed   Brick, NJ 08723   (732)840-2200
Rothman, Murray H., MD {1346349339} Ophthl(74,NY46)<NJ-HACKNSK>
+ 17 West Passaic Avenue
Rutherford, NJ 07070   (201)460-8630   Fax (201)460-9003
Rothschild, Michael Alan, MD {1831132455} Otlryg, PedOto(88,CT01)<NY-MTSINAI, NJ-ENGLWOOD>
+ 163 Engle Street/Suite 1B
Englewood, NJ 07631   (212)996-2995   Fax (212)996-2703
Rothstein, Neil M., MD {1740767955} CdvDis, IntrMd(92,NY46)<NJ-SHOREMEM, NJ-BURDTMLN>
+ Mercer Bucks Cardiology
One Union Street/Suite 101   Robbinsville, NJ 08691   (609)890-6677   Fax (609)890-7292
Rotkowitz, Michael Ian, MD {1649436973} OncHem, IntrMd(GRN01)<PA-CNCREREG>
+ Comprehensive Cancer & Hematology Specialists, P.C.
17 West Red Bank Avenue/Suite 202   Woodbury, NJ 08096   (856)848-5560   Fax (856)848-0958
Rotoli, Domenico, DO {1760700215} IntrMd<NJ-JRSYCITY>
+ Universal Medicine
103 River Road/Suite 101   Edgewater, NJ 07020   (201)308-8995   Fax (201)917-3603
officesupport@universalmedicinenj.com
Rotoli, Giorgio, DO {1790044857} SrgNro
+ SBMC-Institute for Neurosurgery
94 Old Short Hills Road   Livingston, NJ 07039   (973)322-5000
Rotolo, James E., MD {1588635916} Urolgy(84,DC02)
+ Drs. Rotolo, Howard, and Leitner
2401 Highway 35   Manasquan, NJ 08736   (732)223-7877   Fax (732)223-7151
+ Drs. Rotolo and Howard
525 Jack Martin Boulevard/Suite 102   Brick, NJ 08724   (732)206-9830
Rotschild, Tomas, MD {1891751822} NnPnMd, Pedtrc(90,ITA19)<NJ-UNVMCPRN>
+ Somerset Medical Center Neonatology
110 Rehill Avenue   Somerville, NJ 08876   (908)685-2473
+ CHOP Care Network at Princeton Medical Center
One Plainsboro Road   Plainsboro, NJ 08536   (908)685-2473   Fax (609)497-4173
Rotsides, Andreas D., MD {1295799153} IntrMd(84,GRNA)
+ 195 Route 46 West/Suite 200
Mine Hill, NJ 07803   (973)328-1040   Fax (973)328-1544
Rotunda, Roseanne, DO {1730501503} IntrMd
+ 53 Oakley Terrace
Nutley, NJ 07110
Rough, William Alexander, Jr., MD {1013918432} Phlebgy, Surgry(74,NJ05)
+ Surgical Specialists of New Jersey
668 Main Street/Suite 4   Lumberton, NJ 08048   (609)267-7050   Fax (609)267-7065
Rounds, Jacqueline A., DO {1295161628}<NJ-SJHREGMC>
+ SJH Regional Medical Center
1505 West Sherman Avenue   Vineland, NJ 08360   (856)641-8000
Rousseau, Marc Telesphore, MD {1326033838} Anesth, PainMd(81,QU02)<NJ-UNDRWD>
+ Inspira Health Network
509 North Broad Street/Anesth   Woodbury, NJ 08096   (856)845-0100   Fax (856)848-7023
Roussel, Anisha Lanice, MD {1558349597} Pedtrc(99,LA06)<NJ-OURLADY>
+ Osborn Pediatrics
1601 Haddon Avenue   Camden, NJ 08103   (856)757-3700   Fax (856)365-7972

Rousta, Sepideh T., MD {1275513277} PedOph, Ophthl(93,NY48)<NJ-STPETER, NJ-RWJUBRUN>
+ University Children's Eye Center, P.C.
4 Cornwall Court   East Brunswick, NJ 08816   (732)613-9191   Fax (732)613-1139
+ University Children's Eye Center, P.C.
678 Route 202-206 North/Bld 5   Bridgewater, NJ 08807   (732)613-9191   Fax (908)203-9010
+ UH- Robert Wood Johnson Med
125 Paterson Street/Ophthalmology   New Brunswick, NJ 08816   (732)828-3000
Rovner, Aron David, MD {1326010430} SrgOrt(96,NY0)
+ New York Spine and Sports Surgery
190 Midland Avenue   Saddle Brook, NJ 07663   (516)794-2990
+ New York Spine and Sports Surgery
39-40 Broadway   Fair Lawn, NJ 07410   (516)794-2990
Rovner, Joshua Seth, MD {1578765244} SrgSpn, SrgOrt, IntrMd(02,NY08)<NJ-HACKNSK, NJ-HOBUNIMC>
+ Progressive Spine & Orthopaedics
75 Orient Way/Suite 302   Rutherford, NJ 07070   (201)227-1299
jrovnermd@gmail.com
+ Progressive Spine & Orthopaedics
440 Curry Avenue/Suite A   Englewood, NJ 07631   (201)885-4070
Rowan, George Edward, MD {1184663254} Psychy(74,VA01)<NJ-MTCARMEL>
+ Mt. Carmel Guild/ Behavioral Health System
1160 Raymónd Boulevard/Psychiatry   Newark, NJ 07102   (973)596-4190
Rowan, Patrick John, MD {1316090087} Psychy, PsyFor(98,NJ05)<NJ-SOMERSET>
+ RWJ University Hospital Somerset
110 Rehill Avenue   Somerville, NJ 08876   (908)685-2200
Rowan, Philip T., MD {1801896865} Otolgy, Otlryg, IntrMd(90,NY19)<NJ-UNDRWD, NJ-VIRTVOOR>
+ Advanced ENT - Woodbury
620 North Broad Street   Woodbury, NJ 08096   (856)602-4000   Fax (856)848-6029
+ Advanced ENT - Medford
103 Old Marlton Pike/Suite 219   Medford, NJ 08055   (856)602-4000   Fax (609)953-7146
+ Advanced ENT - Cherry Hill
1910 Route 70 East/Suite 3   Cherry Hill, NJ 08096   (856)602-4000   Fax (856)424-4695
Rowe, Jeanne M., MD {1093792368} IntrMd
+ The Advanced Pulmonary Diagnostic Center
100 Medical Center Way   Somers Point, NJ 08244   (609)653-3467   Fax (609)653-3586
Rowe, Norman Maurice, MD {1598788127} SrgPlstc, SrgCsm(92,LA01)<NY-CONEYISL>
+ Rowe Plastic Surgery
333 Broad Street/Suite 1-A   Red Bank, NJ 07701   (732)852-2770   Fax (732)852-2771
Rowe Urquhart, Erica G., MD {1467512350} SrgOrt(00,MD07)<NJ-JRSYCITY, NJ-NWRKBETH>
+ Urquhart Orthopedic Associates
534 Avenue E/Suite 1-B   Bayonne, NJ 07002   (201)436-8289   Fax (201)471-2434
+ Urquhart Orthopedic Associates
609 Morris Avenue   Springfield, NJ 07081   (201)436-8289   Fax (201)471-2434
Rowen, Adam J., MD {1386729325} IntrMd, PulDis(75,NY46)<NJ-TRINIJSC, NJ-RWJURAH>
+ 98 West Jersey Street
Elizabeth, NJ 07202   (908)289-7600   Fax (908)353-7039
Rowland, Sean C., MD {1316962459} IntrMd, EmrgMd(81,MONT)<NJ-COMMED>
+ Community Medical Center
99 Route 37 West/Emerg Medicine   Toms River, NJ 08755   (732)557-8000
Rowlands, Randy R., MD {1417156514} Grtrcs(03,DMN01)<NJ-RBAYOLDB, NJ-RBAYPERT>
+ Monmouth Family Medicine Group
3499 Route 9 North   Freehold, NJ 07728   (732)625-3166   Fax (732)409-7493
Rowley, Scott D., MD {1366402893} MedOnc, Hemato, OncHem(78,MA16)<NJ-HACKNSK>
+ John Theurer Cancer Center - HUMC
360 Essex Street/Suite 303/Transplant   Hackensack, NJ 07601   (201)336-8297   Fax (201)336-8296
+ John Theurer Cancer Center - HUMC
92 Second Street   Hackensack, NJ 07601   (201)336-8297   Fax (551)996-0575
Rowley, Susan Peet, MD {1093781575} PsyAdt, PsyCAd, Addctn(77,NJ06)<NJ-SOMERSET>
+ RWJ University Hospital Somerset
110 Rehill Avenue/Psych   Somerville, NJ 08876   (732)560-1100   Fax (908)575-9572

Roy, Amanda R., MD {1619173341} Anesth(NJ05<NJ-SOMERSET>
+ RWJ University Hospital Somerset
110 Rehill Avenue/Anesthesia   Somerville, NJ 08876   (908)685-2200
+ Anesthesia Consultnts of NJ/Nova Pain
285 Davidson Avenue/Suite 204   Somerset, NJ 08873   (908)685-2200   Fax (732)271-3543
Roy, Arup Kumar, MD {1093884066} IntrMd(76,INA8X)<NJ-ANCPSYCH>
+ Ancora Psychiatric Hospital
301 Spring Garden Road/Internal Med   Hammonton, NJ 08037   (609)561-1700   Fax (609)567-7292
Roy, George A., MD {1205939139} Psychy, PsyAdd(66,ENG25)<NJ-VAEASTOR>
+ VA New Jersey Health Care System-East Orange Campus
385 Tremont Avenue/Psych   East Orange, NJ 07018   (973)676-1000   Fax (973)395-7766
Roy, Manimala, MD {1841355492} PthAClI(79,INDI)<NJ-MTNSIDE>
+ Hackensack UMC Mountainside
1 Bay Avenue/Path   Montclair, NJ 07042   (973)429-6164   Fax (973)429-6992
Roy, Monique S., MD {1295833143} Ophthl(72,FRAN)<NJ-UMDNJ>
+ University Hospital
150 Bergen Street/Ophthalmology   Newark, NJ 07103   (973)972-2065
+ 556 Eagle Rock Avenue
Englewood, NJ 07631   (201)976-2108
Roy, Nicholas E., DO {1619288073}
+ Pulmonary & Sleep Associates of SJ, LLC.
750 Route 73 South/Suite 401   Marlton, NJ 08053   (856)375-1288   Fax (856)375-2325
+ Pulmonary & Sleep Associates of SJ, LLC.
107 Berlin Road   Cherry Hill, NJ 08034   (856)375-1288   Fax (856)429-1081
Roy, Rashmi, MD {1972757458} Surgry(05,NY09)
+ Princeton Surgical Associates, P.A.
5 Plainsboro Road/Suite 400   Plainsboro, NJ 08536   (609)936-9100   Fax (609)936-9700
RRoy@princeton-surgical.com
Roy, Roopa, MD {1437449642}<NJ-UMDNJ>
+ University Hospital
150 Bergen Street   Newark, NJ 07103   (973)972-3555
Roy, Satyajeet, MD {1437116829} IntrMd(93,INA12)
+ Tri-County Medical Associates
120 Millburn Avenue/Suite M3   Millburn, NJ 07041   (973)912-0001   Fax (973)912-0099
Roy, Shailja, MD {1508898594} MedOnc, IntrMd(98,INA26)
+ Southern Oncology Hematology Associates
1505 West Sherman Avenue/Suite 101   Vineland, NJ 08360   (856)696-9550   Fax (856)696-4932
Roy, Vijaykumar, MD {1982688925} OncHem(81,INDI)<NJ-WAYNEGEN, NJ-STJOSHOS>
+ Wayne Hematology-Oncology Associates PA
468 Parish Drive/Suite 4   Wayne, NJ 07470   (973)694-5005   Fax (973)694-5990
WAYNEHEMONC1@AOL.COM
+ Drs. Gandhi and Roy
3665 Kennedy Boulevard   Jersey City, NJ 07306   (973)694-5005   Fax (201)963-7957
Royall, John D., MD {1174519037} IntrMd, PulDis(70,VA01)<NJ-RIVERVW>
+ 108 Avenue Of Two Rivers
Rumson, NJ 07760   (732)747-0591   Fax (732)747-8343
Royce, Roxanne, MD {1952830911} Nrolgy
+ Drs. Marx and Royce
101 Madison Avenue/Suite 304   Morristown, NJ 07960   (973)292-0999   Fax (973)292-0555
Roychowdhury, Sudipta, MD {1821073677} RadDia, Radiol, RadNro(92,IL06)<NJ-RWJUBRUN, NJ-STPETER>
+ University Radiology Group, P.C.
483 Cranbury Road   East Brunswick, NJ 08816   (732)390-0030   Fax (732)390-5383
Roytman, Peter, MD {1407885155} IntrMd, IntHos(89,RUSS)<NJ-MORRISTN, NJ-MMHKEMBL>
+ IPC The Hospitalist Company
220 Ridgedale Avenue/Suite C-2   Florham Park, NJ 07932   (973)538-5844   Fax (973)267-0181
Rozanski, Lawrence T., MD {1770514002} CdvDis, IntrMd(79,DC02)<NJ-KMHSTRAT, NJ-KMHTURNV>
+ Southern New Jersey Cardiac Care Specialists
1020 Laurel Oak Road/Suite 102   Voorhees, NJ 08043   (856)435-8842   Fax (856)435-8665
+ Southern New Jersey Cardiac Care Specialists
151 Fries Mill Road/Suite 101   Turnersville, NJ 08012   (856)435-8842   Fax (856)374-3120
Rozanski, Reuben, MD {1679530588} Dermat(70,MA05)<NJ-MTNSIDE>
+ 200 Highland Avenue
Glen Ridge, NJ 07028   (973)748-9474   Fax (973)748-7880

Physicians by Name and Address

Rozdeba, Christopha H., MD {1013963032} Pedtrc, AdolMd(78,POL02)<NJ-STJOSHOS, NJ-HACKNSK>
+ Drs. Lupinska and Rozdeba
42 Locust Avenue   Wallington, NJ 07057   (973)777-0090   Fax (973)777-9424

Rozdeba, Joseph, MD {1003862368} Urolgy(78,POL02)
+ 42 Locust Avenue
Wallington, NJ 07057   (973)777-0340   Fax (973)777-9424

Rozehzadeh, Rabin, MD {1376508432} FamMed(01,BLZ01)
+ Complete Primary Care
1810 Park Avenue   South Plainfield, NJ 07080   (908)226-1810   Fax (908)226-1833

Rozenbaum, Ilya Maksovich, MD {1831240704} Ophthl(03,NY19)<NY-NYEYEINF>
+ Matossian Eye Associates
2 Capital Way/Suite 326   Pennington, NJ 08534   (609)882-8833   Fax (609)882-0077

Rozenberg, Aleksandr, MD {1306285911} RadDia
+ University Radiology Group, P.C.
483 Cranbury Road   East Brunswick, NJ 08816   (732)390-0030   Fax (732)390-5383

Rozenberg, Larisa, MD {1295934172} FamMed(81,RUS56)
+ Dorfner Family Medicine
811 Sunset Road/Suite 101   Burlington, NJ 08016   (609)387-9242   Fax (609)387-9408

Rozengarten, Kimberly Irene, DO {1801087671} IntRMd(07,PA77)
+ The Maro Group
27 Covered Bridge Road   Cherry Hill, NJ 08034   (856)429-2224   Fax (856)429-1926

Rozengarten, Michael Jacob, MD {1699764498} CdvDis, IntRMd, CICdEI(97,NY08)<NJ-BURDTMLN, NJ-SHOREMEM>
+ Mercer Bucks Cardiology
3140 Princeton Pike/2nd Floor   Lawrenceville, NJ 08648   (609)895-1919   Fax (609)895-1200
+ Mercer Bucks Cardiology
One Union Street/Suite 101   Robbinsville, NJ 08691   (609)895-1919   Fax (609)890-7292

Rozentsvayg, Eka, DO {1255691655} RadDia(06,NJ75)<NJ-HACKNSK>
+ Hackensack University Medical Center
20 Prospect Avenue   Hackensack, NJ 07601   (201)996-2069

Rozman, Anatoly, MD {1386665586} PhysMd
+ 2 Center Plaza
Tinton Falls, NJ 07724   (815)505-4554

Rozmyslowicz, Magdalena Maria, MD {1609821727} Psychy(81,POL03)<NJ-ANCPSYCH>
+ Ancora Psychiatric Hospital
301 Spring Garden Road   Hammonton, NJ 08037   (609)561-1700   Fax (609)567-7292

Rozovsky, Assif, MD {1962507251} Gastrn, IntRMd(88,PA09)<NJ-OCEANMC, NJ-SOCEANCO>
+ Coastal Gastroenterology Associates PA
525 Jack Martin Boulevard/Suite 301   Brick, NJ 08724   (732)840-0067   Fax (732)840-3169

Rozwadowski, Faye M., MD {1801819578}
+ 39 Lansdowne Road
Lakehurst, NJ 08733   (732)961-7630   rozwadof@gmail.com

Rozwadowski, Thomas J., MD {1508917105} EmrgMd(05,DC02)
+ EmCare
1945 Route 33   Neptune, NJ 07753   (732)776-4510   Fax (732)776-2329

Ru, Xun, MD {1114997046} Anesth(83,CHN1J)<NJ-NWRKBETH>
+ Newark Beth Israel Medical Center
201 Lyons Avenue/Anesth   Newark, NJ 07112   (973)926-7000   Fax (201)943-8105

Rubbani, Mariam Shafaq, MD {1801939723} PhysMd, PainMd(98,NY19)<NJ-TRINIWSC>
+ Astra MD PC
550 Bloomfield Avenue   Newark, NJ 07107   (973)483-1500   Fax (973)483-4577

Rubbert-Slawek, Kerstin Anke, MD {1104939818} RadDia, Rad-Nro(92,GER25)
+ Princeton Radiology Associates, P.A.
3674 Route 27   Kendall Park, NJ 08824   (732)821-5563   Fax (732)821-6675

Ruben, Sandhya, MD {1922037761} NnPnMd, Pedtrc(82,INDI)<NJ-STBARNMC>
+ St. Barnabas Medical Center
94 Old Short Hills Road/Pediatrics   Livingston, NJ 07039   (973)322-5000   Fax (973)322-8833

Ruben, Yesudas, MD {1861993016} IntRMd(82,INA75)
+ 19 Sky Top Drive
Denville, NJ 07834

Rubenstein, Andrew F., MD {1730156415} ObsGyn(90,PA09)<NJ-HACKNSK>
+ 82 East Allendale Road/Suite 1-A
Saddle River, NJ 07458   (201)934-5050   Fax (201)934-0056

Rubenstein, Craig Allen, MD {1962441279} EmrgSptM(PA13<NJ-ATLANTHS>
+ Rothman Institute - Voorhees
443 Laurel Oak Road   Voorhees, NJ 08043   (856)821-6360

Rubenstein, Donald G., MD {1912966276} CdvDis, IntRMd, CICdEI(80,LA05)<NJ-STMICHL, NJ-STBARNMC>
+ New Jersey Cardiology Associates
375 Mount Pleasant Avenue   West Orange, NJ 07052   (973)731-9442   Fax (973)731-8030
+ New Jersey Cardiology Associates
5 Franklin Avenue/Suite 502   Belleville, NJ 07109   (973)731-9442   Fax (973)450-8157
+ New Jersey Cardiology Associates
201 Lyons Avenue/6th Floor   Newark, NJ 07052   (973)926-7503   Fax (973)923-7267

Rubenstein, Jennifer, MD {1770902033} FamMed
+ Virtua Family Medicine Center @Lumberton
1636 Route 38 & Eayrestown Rd.   Lumberton, NJ 08048   (609)914-8440   Fax (609)914-8441

Rubenstone, Jay L., DO {1730171505} CdvDis, IntRMd(77,PA77)
+ Associated Cardiovascular Consultants-Lourdes
1 Brace Road/Suite C & F   Cherry Hill, NJ 08034   (856)428-4100   Fax (856)428-5748

Rubia-Sazon, Elvira M., MD {1477711695} Pedtrc(78,PHIL)
+ NHCAC Health Center at West New York
5301 Broadway   West New York, NJ 07093   (201)866-9320

Rubin, Allen J., MD {1831159524} Psychy, Nrolgy, PsyNro(79,IL11)<NJ-COOPRUMC>
+ The Center for Neuropsychiatry, LLC
11009 Lincoln Drive West   Marlton, NJ 08053   (856)985-9851   Fax (856)985-9955

Rubin, Benjamin, MD {1093964157} Anesth(05,NY48)
+ Rutgers- New Jersey Medical School
185 South Orange Avenue/E-538   Newark, NJ 07103   (973)972-0470

Rubin, Elliot H., MD {1689697518} Pedtrc, AdolMd(81,VT02)<NJ-STPETER, NJ-RWJUBRUN>
+ University Pediatric Associates PA
317 Cleveland Avenue   Highland Park, NJ 08904   (732)249-8999   Fax (732)249-7827
+ University Pediatric Associates
D-1 Brier Hill Court   East Brunswick, NJ 08816   (732)238-3310

Rubin, Eric Howard, MD {1003991712} IntRMd, Onclgy, MedOnc(85,FL04)
+ 307 Dolphin Drive
Brigantine, NJ 08203   (201)805-7055   erichrubin@gmail.com

Rubin, Evan Scott, DO {1881750685} OstMed, FamMed(01,NY75)
+ Traditional Osteopathic Medicine
55 North Gilbert Street/Suite 3102   Tinton Falls, NJ 07701   (732)219-8664   Fax (732)383-8799

Rubin, Joshua Adam, MD {1245464783} Anesth
+ Montclair Anesthesia Associates PC
185 Fairfield Avenue/Suite 2A   West Caldwell, NJ 07006   (973)226-1230   Fax (973)226-1232

Rubin, Kenneth J., MD {1699881896} PsyGrt, Psychy(74,NY08)<NJ-MONMOUTH, NJ-HACKNSK>
+ 170 Morris Avenue/Suite D
Long Branch, NJ 07740   (732)870-3535   Fax (732)870-8253
kjr6348@verizon.net

Rubin, Kenneth P., MD {1851344618} Gastrn, IntRMd(75,NJ05)<NY-MTSINAI, NY-MTSINYHS>
+ 142 Palisade Avenue/Suite 202
Jersey City, NJ 07306   (201)656-6060
+ Englewood Endoscopic Assocociates
420 Grand Avenue/Suite 101   Englewood, NJ 07631   (201)656-6060   Fax (201)569-1999

Rubin, Marc R., MD {1598784159} Gastrn, IntRMd(74,NY46)<NJ-STFRNMED, NJ-RWJUHAM>
+ Gastroenterology Associates
2275 Whitehorse-Mercerville Rd   Trenton, NJ 08619   (609)890-0200

Rubin, Mitchell J., MD {1457337826} Nrolgy(81,PA01)
+ Capital Institute for Neurosciences
2 Capital Way/Suite 456   Pennington, NJ 08534   (609)537-7300   Fax (609)537-7301
+ Capital Health System/Fuld Campus
750 Brunswick Avenue   Trenton, NJ 08638   (609)394-6000

Rubin, Seth M., MD {1023070422} ObsGyn(89,NY46)<NJ-HUNTRDN>
+ Advanced Obstetrics & Gynecology, LLC
1390 Route 22 West/Suite 104   Lebanon, NJ 08833   (908)437-1234   Fax (908)437-1227
+ Advanced Obstetrics & Gynecology, LLC
4 Walter E. Foran Boulevard/Suite 320   Flemington, NJ 08822   (908)437-1234   Fax (908)806-8570
+ Advanced Obstetrics & Gynecology, LLC
1100 Wescott Drive   Flemington, NJ 08833   (908)788-6488

Rubin, Sharon, MD {1386667996} CdvDis, IntRMd(90,PA13)<PA-TJHSP>
+ Jefferson HealthCare - Voorhees
443 Laurel Oak Road/Suite 130   Voorhees, NJ 08043

Rubin, Steven F., DO {1992811004} FamMed(84,MO79)<NJ-VALLEY>
+ 805 Minogue Terrace
Paramus, NJ 07652   (201)791-2222   Fax (201)791-7282

Rubinchik, Noemy Aronovici, MD {1912082793} Anesth(89,ROM02)<NJ-HOLYNAME>
+ 583 Mill Run
Paramus, NJ 07652

Rubinetti, Mark J., MD {1699705020} IntRMd(86,GRNA)<NJ-STCLRBOO>
+ 20 Commerce Boulevard/Suite D
Succasunna, NJ 07876   (973)927-2888   Fax (973)927-2807   minj_R@verizon.net

Rubinfeld, David I., MD {1881657393} SrgOrt, NeuMSptM(73,NJ05)
+ 417 West Blackwell Street
Dover, NJ 07801   (973)366-8022   Fax (973)366-3397

Rubinfeld, Julie A., MD {1124000138} Anesth, IntRMd(89,SC04)<NJ-MORRISTN>
+ Anesthesia Associates
100 Madison Avenue   Morristown, NJ 07960   (973)631-8119   Fax (973)631-8120

Rubinfeld, Philip J., MD {1629074091} Anesth, PainMd(81,MEX03)
+ New Jersey Pain Management PA
3130 State Route 10 West/2nd Floor   Denville, NJ 07834   (973)442-9980   Fax (973)442-9984
+ Specialty Surgical Center
380 Lafayette Road/Suite 110   Sparta, NJ 07871   (973)442-9980   Fax (973)940-3170

Rubino, Barry P., MD {1568541027} IntRMd(83,ITA17)<NJ-MONMOUTH>
+ 147 Pavilion Avenue
Long Branch, NJ 07740   (732)229-9417   Fax (732)229-0151

Rubino, Donald J., MD {1992793319} ObsGyn(81,DC02)<NJ-NWT-NMEM>
+ Womens Health Care Associates of Sussex County
135 Newton Sparta Road/Suite 201   Newton, NJ 07860   (973)383-8555   Fax (973)383-8424
+ Womens Health Care Associates of Sussex County
123 Route 94/Suite 200   Vernon, NJ 07462   (973)383-8555   Fax (973)827-4441

Rubino, Gennaro, MD {1194747725} IntRMd(86,DOMI)<NJ-STJOSHOS>
+ Cecere and Rubino Internal Medicine, LLC
1195 Clifton Avenue   Clifton, NJ 07013   (973)471-4004   Fax (973)471-1180

Rubino, Robert J., MD {1285669036} ObsGyn(91,NJ05)<NJ-STBARNMC>
+ The Rubino Ob/Gyn Group
101 Old Short Hills Road/Suite 101   West Orange, NJ 07052   (973)736-1100   Fax (973)736-1834
+ The Rubino Ob/Gyn Group
33 Overlook Road   Summit, NJ 07901   (908)522-4558
+ The Rubino Ob/Gyn Group
731 Broadway   Bayonne, NJ 07052   (201)339-3300

Rubino, Susan Basra, MD {1912948738} IntRMd(94,NJ05)<NJ-STBARNMC>
+ Internal Medicine Faculty Practice
101 Old Short Hills Road/Suite 106   West Orange, NJ 07052   (973)322-6256   Fax (973)322-6241
+ St. Barnabas Medical Center
94 Old Short Hills Road/Assistnt/Med   Livingston, NJ 07039   (973)322-5000

Rubinoff, Mitchell J., MD {1942250345} Gastrn, IntRMd(79,NY47)<NJ-VALLEY>
+ Gastrointestinal Associates PA
140 Chestnut Street/Suite 300   Ridgewood, NJ 07450   (201)444-2600   Fax (201)444-9471

Rubinoff, Susan W., MD {1801821061} RadDia, Radiol(81,NY47)<NJ-HOLYNAME>
+ Radiology Center of Fair Lawn
0-100 28th Street   Fair Lawn, NJ 07410   (201)475-1300   Fax (201)475-1709

Rubinstein, Allen Bernard, DO {1477669232} IntRMd(63,MO78)
+ NJ Heart/Linden Office
520 North Wood Avenue   Linden, NJ 07036   (908)587-9300   Fax (908)587-1901

Rubinstein, Hector T., MD {1992723878} CdvDis, IntRMd(63,ARG01)<NJ-NWRKBETH, NJ-CHRIST>
+ 228 Lafayette Street/5th Floor
Newark, NJ 07105   (973)491-5222   Fax (973)491-0181

Rubinstein, Howard Arthur, MD {1649210303} EmrgMd, IntRMd(92,NJ05)<NJ-RIVERVW>
+ Riverview Medical Center
1 Riverview Plaza/EmergMed   Red Bank, NJ 07701   (732)741-2700   Fax (732)224-7498

Physicians by Name and Address

Rubinstein, Mitchell A., MD {1225081573} Surgry, SrgThr, SrgCTh(84,TX13)<NJ-VALLEY>
+ The Valley Hospital
223 North Van Dien Avenue/Surgery   Ridgewood, NJ 07450   (201)447-8000   Fax (201)447-8658

Rubman, Marc H., MD {1457355927} SprtMd, SrgOrt(87,NY48)<NJ-STCLRDEN, NJ-STCLRDOV>
+ New Jersey Orthopaedics & Sports Medicine, LLC
121 Center Grove Road/Suite 11   Randolph, NJ 07869   (973)366-4411

Ruby, Marianne, MD {1356433528} RprEnd, Gyneco(75,GA05)
+ 307 Stone Harbour Boulevard
Cape May Court House, NJ 08210   (609)465-2525   Fax (609)465-5200

Ruchman, Richard B., MD {1942255450} NuclMd, RadDia(80,MI01)
+ Shrewsbury Diagnostic Imaging, Inc.
1131 Broad Street/Suite 110   Shrewsbury, NJ 07702   (732)578-9640   Fax (732)578-9650

Ruda, Neal, MD {1003804196} Pedtrc(84,ITAL)
+ Bethany Pediatrics PA
1 Bethany Road/Building 5/Suite 65   Hazlet, NJ 07730   (732)264-0700   Fax (732)264-1414

Ruda, William A., MD {1609833524} Anesth, IntrMd(80,NY19)<NJ-SOMERSET, NJ-STPETER>
+ Anesthesia Consultnts of NJ/Nova Pain
285 Davidson Avenue/Suite 204   Somerset, NJ 08873   (732)271-1400   Fax (732)271-3543
+ Cares Surgicenter, LLC.
240 Easton Avenue   New Brunswick, NJ 08901   (732)271-1400   Fax (732)296-8677

Rudd, Jennifer N., MD {1144322611} Gastrn, IntrMd(76,NY05)<NJ-NWRKBETH, NJ-EASTORNG>
+ 90 Washington Street/Suite 213
East Orange, NJ 07017   (973)674-5726   Fax (973)674-5920
Doctorrudd@sprintmail.com

Rudd, Rebecca A., MD {1740253962} FamMed, IntrMd(82,MI07)<NJ-COMMED>
+ Coastal Health Care
1314 Hooper Avenue/Building B   Toms River, NJ 08753   (732)349-4994   Fax (732)341-1717

Rudd, Steven A., MD {1932248184} RadDia, Radiol, IntrMd(88,GA05)
+ Fair Lawn Diagnostic Imaging
19-04 Fair Lawn Avenue   Fair Lawn, NJ 07410   (201)794-3132   Fax (201)794-6291

Ruddock, Heather Ann, MD {1780631846} Pedtrc(93,PA13)
+ Advocare West Deptford Pediatrics
646 Kings Highway   West Deptford, NJ 08096   (856)879-2887   Fax (856)879-2855
+ Advocare West Deptford Pediatrics
19 Village Center Drive   Swedesboro, NJ 08085   (856)879-2887   Fax (856)879-2855

Ruddy, Kathleen T., MD {1356457956} Surgry(89,NJ05)
+ 36 Newark Avenue
Belleville, NJ 07109   (973)450-2710

Ruddy, Michael C., MD {1831138015} CdvDis, Hypten, IntrMd(74,NJ05)<NJ-RWJUBRUN, NJ-UNVMCPRN>
+ Princeton Hypertension-Nephrology
88 Princeton Hightstown Road/Suite 203   Princeton Junction, NJ 08550   (609)750-7330   Fax (609)750-7336

Ruddy, Stephanie Maus, DO {1154676542}<NJ-DEBRAHLC>
+ Deborah Heart and Lung Center
200 Trenton Road   Browns Mills, NJ 08015   (937)723-3248
smausdo@gmail.com

Rudelli, Mercedes N., MD {1124240718} Psychy(70,ARG01)
+ 284 Westview Avenue
Fort Lee, NJ 07024   (201)453-8886

Rudelli, Raul Daniel, MD {1124049671} PthCln, PthAna, PthNro(70,ARG01)<NJ-BAYONNE>
+ 230 60th Street
West New York, NJ 07093

Ruderman, Marvin I., MD {1427129006} Nrolgy(76,NY01)<NJ-STBARNMC, NJ-MTNSIDE>
+ 1099 Bloomfield Avenue
West Caldwell, NJ 07006   (973)439-7000   Fax (973)439-7020

Ruderman, Seth R., MD {1447298161} EmrgMd(80,NY47)<NJ-VIRTMHBC>
+ SJ Emergency Physician, PA
175 Madison Avenue   Mount Holly, NJ 08060   (609)267-0700   Fax (609)261-5842

Ruderman, Todd, DO {1194076307}<NJ-KMHTURNV>
+ Kennedy Health Systems/Washington Township Campus
435 Hurffville-Cross Keys Road   Turnersville, NJ 08012   (856)218-5634   Fax (856)218-5664

Rudge, Trevor M., MD {1730436403}<NJ-UNIVBHC>
+ University Behavioral Health Care
671 Hoes Lane/PO Box 1392   Piscataway, NJ 08855   (732)235-4433

Rudman, David Paul, MD {1821026709} SrgOrt(98,NY15)<NJ-VALLEY>
+ 1124 East Ridgewood Avenue/Suite 201
Ridgewood, NJ 07450   (201)447-1188   Fax (201)447-8935

Rudman, Michael E., MD {1720085145} Anesth(88,PA14)<NJ-MORRISTN>
+ New Jersey Pain Consultants
95 Madison Avenue/Suite 402   Morristown, NJ 07960   (973)971-6824   Fax (973)290-7683
+ New Jersey Pain Consultants
310 Madison Avenue/Suite 301   Morristown, NJ 07960   (973)971-6824   Fax (973)998-9201

Rudner, Elvira, MD {1306189584} Psychy
+ University Psychiatric Associates
183 South Orange Avenue/E-F Levels   Newark, NJ 07103   (973)972-6134   Fax (973)972-1297

Rudnick, Andrew Glenn, MD {1366480352} ClCdEl, CdvDis(99,PA09)
+ Hunterdon Cardiovascular Associates
1100 Wescott Drive/Suite G-3   Flemington, NJ 08822   (908)788-6471   Fax (908)788-6460

Rudnitzky, Elliot M., MD {1215967534} CdvDis, IntrMd(70,PA09)
+ Drs. Rudnitzky & Shugar PA
98 James Street/Suite 104   Edison, NJ 08820   (732)494-6300   Fax (732)494-1028

Rudolph, Herbert J., MD {1871633370} FamMed(85,NJ06)<NJ-KIMBALL>
+ Southern Ocean Primary Care
317 East Main Street   Tuckerton, NJ 08087   (609)296-1336
+ Hackensack Meridian Medical Group
53 Nautilus Drive/Suite 201   Manahawkin, NJ 08050   (609)296-1336   Fax (609)978-8903

Rudolph, Jason Willer, MD {1023052446} Ortped, SrgOrt, IntrMd(93,IL42)<NJ-WARREN>
+ Easton Orthopaedic Group
123 Roseberry Street/Suite A   Phillipsburg, NJ 08865   (908)454-9998   Fax (908)454-9937
eogroup@aol.com
+ Easton Orthopaedic Group
123 A Roseberry Street   Phillipsburg, NJ 08865   (908)454-9998   Fax (908)454-9937

Rudolph, Kafi, DO {1023499340} FamMed
+ Jefferson Health Primary & Specialty Care
1A Regulus Drive   Turnersville, NJ 08012   (844)542-2273

Rudominer, Howard S., MD {1558400390} PsyCAd, Psychy(69,NY08)
+ 59 Springbrook Road
Livingston, NJ 07039   (973)716-9500   Fax (973)992-4449
+ 513 West Mount Pleasant Avenue
Livingston, NJ 07039   (973)716-9500   Fax (973)992-4449

Rudzinskiene, Aliona, MD {1720057540} IntrMd(85,LIT02)<NJ-VALLEY>
+ 19-21 Fair Lawn Avenue
Fair Lawn, NJ 07410   (201)475-4091   Fax (201)475-9473

Rueda, Carlos Alberto, MD {1366490195} Psychy, PsyGrt(90,COL19)<NJ-STJOSHOS>
+ St. Joseph's Regional Medical Center
703 Main Street/Psychiatry   Paterson, NJ 07503   (973)754-2838

Ruedy, Krista R., MD {1417156381} Anesth
+ Anesthesia Consultnts of NJ/Nova Pain
285 Davidson Avenue/Suite 204   Somerset, NJ 08873   (732)271-1400   Fax (732)271-3543

Ruel, Ewa, MD {1023242799} EnDbMt
+ Endocrinology Associates of Princeton, LLC
256 Bunn Drive/Suite D   Princeton, NJ 08540   (609)924-4433   Fax (609)924-4423

Ruff, Lynne H., MD {1952561482} Pedtrc(79,MA01)
+ 8 Lancashire Drive
Princeton Junction, NJ 08550

Ruffin, Judith S., MD {1255523098} ObsGyn
+ Ob-Gyn Care of Southern New Jersey
406 Gibbsboro Road East   Lindenwold, NJ 08021   (856)435-7007   Fax (856)435-7077

Ruffini, Robert A., MD {1407920408} Gastrn, IntrMd(84,PA02)<NJ-STCLRDEN, NJ-STBARNMC>
+ The Medical Group, PA
745 Northfield Avenue   West Orange, NJ 07052   (973)325-0061   Fax (973)325-0219

Ruffo, Scott D., MD {1972611531} CdvDis, IntrMd(94,NY19)
+ Mulkay Cardiology Consultants, P.C.
493 Essex Street   Hackensack, NJ 07601   (201)996-9244   Fax (201)996-9243

Rugel, Jason, DO {1871938704} FamMed<NJ-PALISADE>
+ Palisades Medical Center
7600 River Road   North Bergen, NJ 07047   (201)854-5000

Ruggeri-Weigel, Patricia, MD {1366404527} InfDis, IntrMd(83,GRNA)
+ Medical Assoc of Westfield
324 South Avenue East   Westfield, NJ 07090   (908)233-1444   Fax (908)654-0226

Ruggiero, Michael P., DO {1053367136} EmrgMd(83,IL76)<NJ-ACMCMAIN, NJ-ACMCITY>
+ AtlantiCare Regional Medical Center/City Campus
1925 Pacific Avenue   Atlantic City, NJ 08401   (609)345-4000

Rughani-Shah, Bindoo, MD {1275603151} Pedtrc(85,INDI)
+ 34 Corbett Way
Eatontown, NJ 07724   (732)722-2300

Rugino, Thomas A., MD {1801862172} Pedtrc, PhysMd, PedNrD(85,NY08)<NJ-CHLSOCEN>
+ Children's Specialized Hospital-Ocean
94 Stevens Road/Neurodevelpmnt   Toms River, NJ 08755   (732)914-1100

Rugut, Chloe, MD {1154749299} ObsGyn
+ Lourdes Medical Associates
1601 Haddon Avenue   Camden, NJ 08103   (856)757-3700   Fax (856)580-6498

Ruhl, Kimberly K., MD {1205949567} Dermat(94,PA02)
+ Dr. Deborah Ruth Spey
101 Old Short Hills Road/Suite 410   West Orange, NJ 07052   (973)731-9600   Fax (973)731-1635

Ruiz, David A., MD {1194825570} Psychy(89,VA07)<NJ-STCLRDEN>
+ St. Clare's Health Services
50 Morris Avenue   Denville, NJ 07834   (973)625-7051   Fax (973)625-7110

Ruiz, Frank, MD {1417967019} Gastrn(93,NJ05)
+ Gastroenterology Associates of New Jersey
71 Union Avenue/Suite 201   Rutherford, NJ 07070   (201)842-0020   Fax (201)842-0010
+ Gastroenterology Associates of New Jersey
925 Clifton Avenue   Clifton, NJ 07013   (201)842-0020   Fax (973)405-6564

Ruiz, Restituto Soriano, Jr., MD {1215922661} IntrMd, EmrgMd(86,PHI01)<NJ-NWTNMEM>
+ Newton Medical Center
175 High Street/EmergMed   Newton, NJ 07860   (973)383-2121

Ruiz, Vicente Z., MD {1003090887} Psychy(83,DOMI)
+ 20 78th Street
North Bergen, NJ 07047

Ruiz, Vincent Edward, MD {1306165089} EmrgMd
+ Jersey City Medical Center Emergency
355 Grand Street   Jersey City, NJ 07302

Rukh, Lala, MD {1932419199} FamMed
+ 61 Garfield Avenue
Colonia, NJ 07067

Rukshin, Vladimir B., MD {1760716542} IntrMd, CdvDis(87,RUS01)<NJ-RBAYOLDB>
+ 2433 Highway 516/Suite B
Old Bridge, NJ 08857   (732)617-0033   Fax (866)263-5979

Rullo, Barbara, MD {1629329982} ClnPhm(77,NJ05)
+ 28 Hadley Court
Basking Ridge, NJ 07920

Rumbaugh, Donald W., MD {1720369101} FamMed(84,PA14)<NJ-CHILTON>
+ 620 State Route 23/Suite 1
Pompton Plains, NJ 07444   (973)839-8336   Fax (973)839-8123

Rumberger, John Arthur, MD {1447397419} CdvDis, IntrMd, GPrvMd(78,FL02)
+ The Princeton Longevity Center
136 Main Street   Princeton, NJ 08540   (609)430-0752   Fax (609)430-8470

Ruml, Lisa A., MD {1831160837} IntrMd, OthrSp(88,TX12)
+ PO Box 153
Wharton, NJ 07885   (973)876-5260
LARUML@pol.net

Rundback, John Hugh, MD {1255367280} RadDia, RadV&I(87,NY08)<NJ-HOLYNAME, NJ-CHRIST>
+ Advanced Interventional Radiology Services, LLP
718 Teaneck Road   Teaneck, NJ 07666   (201)227-6210   Fax (201)643-3077
jrundback@airsllp.com
+ Holy Name Hospital
718 Teaneck Road/Radiology   Teaneck, NJ 07666   (201)833-3000

Runfola, James Joseph, MD {1356347488} FamMed(97,NY06)
+ Haddonfield Family Practice PA
15 East Redman Avenue   Haddonfield, NJ 08033   (856)428-1335   Fax (856)428-6334
+ Tatem Brown Family Practice
2225 East Evesham Road/Suite 101   Voorhees, NJ 08043   (856)428-1335   Fax (856)325-3704

Ruocco, Dominic, MD {1134154073} EmrgMd(00,NJ06)<NJ-PALISADE>
+ Palisades Medical Center
7600 River Road/EmrgMed   North Bergen, NJ 07047   (201)295-4000   Fax (201)295-4021

433

Physicians by Name and Address

Ruoff, Mark J., MD {1710949276} SrgOrt(87,NJ05)<NJ-VALLEY>
+ Orthopedic Associates
15-01 Broadway/Suite 20   Fair Lawn, NJ 07410   (201)794-6008   Fax (201)794-6190

Rupani, Bobby Jawahar, MD {1467602367} SrgVas(01,NJ05)
+ 100 Mountain Court
Hackettstown, NJ 07840   (908)852-3301   Fax (908)852-3303

Ruppel, Nicholas James, DO {1679860696} FamMed
+ McGuire Air Force Base/Acute Health Care Clinic
3458 Neely Road   Trenton, NJ 08641   (609)754-9080   Fax (609)754-9015

Ruscito, Bridget Marie, MD {1164412987} Anesth(01,NY15)<NJ-UNVMCPRN, NJ-RWJUHAM>
+ University Medical Center of Princeton at Plainsboro
One Plainsboro Road   Plainsboro, NJ 08536   (609)497-4000

Rushman, John Warren, MD {1528164431} FamMed, EmrgMd, IntrMd(00,NJ05)<NJ-OVERLOOK>
+ Clark Urgent Care
100 Commerce Place   Clark, NJ 07066   (732)499-0606

Rushton, Alan R., MD {1205800166} ClnGnt, Pedtrc(77,IL02)<NJ-HUNTRDN>
+ Hunterdon Pediatric Associates
6 Sand Hill Road/Suite 202   Flemington, NJ 08822   (908)782-6700   Fax (908)788-5861

Ruskey, Elizabeth E., DO {1750463113} FamMed(PA77<NJ-ACMCITY, NJ-ACMCMAIN>
+ Cape Regional Physicians Associates
336 96th Street/Suite 1   Stone Harbor, NJ 08247   (609)967-0070   Fax (609)967-0077

Ruskey, John S., DO {1235174459} EmrgMd(88,PA77)<NJ-BURDTMLN>
+ Cape Regional Medical Center
2 Stone Harbor Boulevard/EmergMed   Cape May Court House, NJ 08210   (609)463-2000   Fax (609)463-2946

Rusli, Melissa K., DO {1558554253} PhysMd, IntrMd<NJ-VALLEY>
+ Daughters of Miriam Center
155 Hazel Street/PO Box 2698   Clifton, NJ 07011   (973)772-3700   Fax (973)253-5389

Rusovici, Arthur, MD {1194966788}
+ Atlantic Cardiology Group LLP
8 Tempe Wick Road   Mendham, NJ 07945   (973)543-2288   Fax (973)543-2608
arusovici1@yahoo.com

Russ, Michelle L., DO {1942561535} Pedtrc
+ Advocare The Farm Pediatrics
1001 Laurel Oak Boulevard/Suite B   Voorhees, NJ 08043   (856)782-7400   Fax (856)782-7404

Russ Meek, Robyn L., DO {1316962780} FamMed(92,NY75)
+ 135 Bloomfield Avenue/Suite D
Bloomfield, NJ 07003

Russell, Carol Mae, DO {1265580096} ObsGyn(01,NY75)<NY-CMCSTVSI, NY-STATNRTH>
+ JFK Medical Center
65 James Street   Edison, NJ 08820   (732)839-9341

Russell, Hortense Patricia, DO {1497089825} FamMed
+ University Hospital-University Family Medicine
42 East Laurel Road/Suite 2100   Stratford, NJ 08084   (856)566-7020   Fax (856)566-6188

Russell, Warren King, MD {1942251467} EmrgMd(89,TX15)<NJ-COMMED>
+ Community Medical Center
99 Route 37 West/EmrgMed   Toms River, NJ 08755   (732)557-8080
+ Jersey Emergency Medicine Specialists
99 Highway 37 West   Toms River, NJ 08755   (732)557-8080

Russell-Brown, Karl E., MD {1477624823} Pedtrc, AdolMd(76,NJ06)<NJ-JFKMED>
+ 203 West 9th Street
Plainfield, NJ 07060   (908)756-5550   Fax (908)756-3072

Russo, Andrea Marie, MD {1396777694} CdvDis, IntrMd(85,NY15)<NJ-ACMCMAIN, NJ-ACMCITY>
+ Cooper Cardiology Associates
900 Centennial Boulevard   Voorhees, NJ 08043   (856)325-6700   Fax (856)325-6702
+ Cooper University Hospital
One Cooper Plaza/Cardiology   Camden, NJ 08103   (856)342-2000

Russo, Armando P., MD {1720008386} ObsGyn(78,MEXI)
+ Cumberland Ob-Gyn PA
1102 East Chestnut Avenue   Vineland, NJ 08360   (856)696-4484   Fax (856)690-1352
+ Cumberland Ob-Gyn, PA
2950 College Drive/Suite 2G   Vineland, NJ 08360   (856)696-4484   Fax (856)696-1694
+ Abulatory Care Center
1133 East Chestnut Avenue   Vineland, NJ 08360   (856)527-0800   Fax (856)507-0824

Russo, Cathy Marie, MD {1992790364} Anesth, PainMd(92,NJ05)<NJ-STBARNMC>
+ New Jersey Anesthesia Associates, P.C.
252 Columbia Turnpike/PO Box 0037   Florham Park, NJ 07932   (973)660-9334   Fax (973)660-9779
+ St. Joseph's Regional Medical Center Anesthesia
703 Main Street   Paterson, NJ 07503   (973)660-9334   Fax (973)977-9455

Russo, David Peter, MD {1588647143} Surgry
+ Cape Regional Physicans Associates
217 North Main Street/Suite 104   Cape May Court House, NJ 08210   (609)463-1488   Fax (609)463-4881

Russo, Donato S., MD {1427073311} ObsGyn(89,IL42)<NJ-STBARNMC>
+ Donato S. Russo MD LLC
1896 Morris Avenue/Suite 3   Union, NJ 07083   (908)687-8282   Fax (908)810-9363

Russo, Eileen Susan, MD {1811072994} CritCr, IntrMd, PulDis(97,DC01)<NJ-STPETER>
+ St. Peter's University Hospital
254 Easton Avenue/Crtcl Care Med   New Brunswick, NJ 08901   (732)745-8600   Fax (732)745-9156

Russo, Frances Jenny, DO {1639357163} FamMed(98,NJ75)
+ Premier Family HealthCare PC
24 Arnett Avenue/Suite 105 First Floor   Lambertville, NJ 08530   (609)397-1775   Fax (609)397-1545

Russo, John A., MD {1346376415} AdolMd, IntrMd(81,MEXI)<NJ-STBARNMC>
+ South Mountain Medical Associates
1500 Pleasant Valley Way/Suite 302   West Orange, NJ 07052   (973)736-8119   Fax (973)736-6818

Russo, Marc William, MD {1073717658} Anesth(06,NY01)<NJ-STMRYPAS>
+ St. Mary's Hospital
350 Boulevard   Passaic, NJ 07055   (973)365-4300

Russo, Mark Joseph, MD {1326289786} SrgCTh(02,NY46)<NJ-NWRKBETH, NJ-STBARNMC>
+ Newark Beth Israel Medical Center
201 Lyons Avenue/Suite G-5   Newark, NJ 07112   (973)926-7905   Fax (973)923-4683
+ St. Barnabas Medical Center
94 Old Short Hills Road   Livingston, NJ 07039   (973)926-8032

Russo, Melchiorre J., MD {1245291277} IntrMd(85,GRN01)
+ Valley Family Care
128 Valley Road   Clifton, NJ 07013   (973)279-5116   Fax (973)279-8899

Russo, Neil J., MD {1235290966} ObsGyn(90,NJ05)<NJ-STBARNMC>
+ Associates in Obstetrics Gynecology & Infertility
375 Mount Pleasant Avenue/Suite 202   West Orange, NJ 07052   (973)731-7707   Fax (973)669-0277

Russo, Ralph E., III, MD {1376510594} CdvDis, IntrMd(85,NJ05)
+ Virtua Cardiology Group
2309 East Evesham Road/Suites 201-202   Voorhees, NJ 08043   (856)325-5400   Fax (856)325-5416
+ The Cardiology Group, P.A.
401 Young Avenue/Suite 275   Moorestown, NJ 08057   (856)325-5400   Fax (856)291-8844
+ The Cardiology Group, P.A.
128 State Highway Route 70/Suite 1-B   Medford, NJ 08043   (856)291-8855   Fax (609)444-5521

Russo, Sandra L., DO {1467404251} FamMed(93,IA75)<NJ-BURDTMLN>
+ 713 Dehirsch Avenue
Woodbine, NJ 08270   (609)861-4241   Fax (609)861-1071

Russo, Steven, MD {1982706503} FamMed, IntrMd(97,NJ06)
+ Premier Family HealthCare PC
24 Arnett Avenue/Suite 105 First Floor   Lambertville, NJ 08530   (609)397-1775   Fax (609)397-1545

Russo, Thomas O., MD {1871581363} ObsGyn(87,NY09)<NJ-VALLEY>
+ Valley Ob Gyn Associates PA
80 Eisenhower Drive/Suite 200   Paramus, NJ 07652   (201)843-2800   Fax (201)843-5848

Russo-Stieglitz, Karen E., MD {1649200239} ObsGyn, IntrMd(93,NJ06)<NJ-CHILTON, NJ-MORRISTN>
+ Maternal Fetal Medicine of Practice Associates
11 Overlook Road/Suite LL 102   Summit, NJ 07901   (908)522-3846   Fax (908)522-5557

Russomano, Salvatore J., MD {1326097874} PhysMd(89,NJ06)<NJ-ACMCITY, NJ-ACMCMAIN>
+ Mid Atlantic Rehabilitation Associates PA
611 New Road   Northfield, NJ 08225   (609)641-2581   Fax (609)641-6901

Russonella, Michael Christopher, DO {1255542486} PedOrt, SrgOrt(03,PA78)
+ North Jersey Orthopaedic & Sports Medicine Institute
6 Brighton Road/Suite 101   Clifton, NJ 07012   (973)340-1940   Fax (973)340-1958
mrussonella@njosmi.com

Russoniello, Alexander P., MD {1497847990} SrgOrt(83,NJ06)
+ New Jersey Orthopaedic Sports & Spine Institute PA
5 Progress Street   Edison, NJ 08820   (908)668-4410   Fax (908)668-0024

Russoniello, Michael A., MD {1356392757} IntrMd, PulDis(78,MEXI)<NJ-STCLRDEN, NJ-STCLRDOV>
+ Associates in Pulmonary Medicine, PA
765 State Highway 10 East   Randolph, NJ 07869   (973)366-6600   Fax (973)366-6385
+ Associates in Pulmonary Medicine, PA
16 Pocono Road/Suite 217   Denville, NJ 07834   (973)625-5651

Rustagi, Anju, MD {1174552806} PhysMd(91,INA69)<NJ-SOMERSET>
+ New Jersey Rehab & Electrodiagnostics PA
15 Monroe Street   Bridgewater, NJ 08807   (908)429-7799   Fax (908)595-6331
+ New Jersey Rehab & Electrodiagnostics, PA
71 Route 206   Hillsborough, NJ 08844   (908)203-0202
+ New Jersey Rehab & Electrodiagnostics, PA
201 Union Avenue/Suite 1A   Bridgewater, NJ 08807   (908)429-7799

Rustemli, Asu, MD {1942452172} CdvDis, IntrMd(98,TUR04)<NY-BRKLNDWN>
+ 25 Mule Road/Suite B2
Toms River, NJ 08755   (917)545-9182

Ruszka, Geza, MD {1831271063} InfDis, IntrMd(80,NJ06)<NJ-OCEANMC>
+ Apogee Medical Group of New Jersey
425 Jack Martin Boulevard   Brick, NJ 08724   (732)836-4817   Fax (732)836-4818

Ruth, Tiffany Karim, MD {1770578221} EmrgMd(96,NJ05)<NJ-RBAYOLDB>
+ Raritan Bay Medical Center/Old Bridge Division
One Hospital Plaza   Old Bridge, NJ 08857   (732)360-1000

Rutigliano, Michael W., MD {1740348077} FamMed(88,NJ05)<NJ-VALLEY>
+ Bergen Medical Associates
1 Sears Drive/Suite 403   Paramus, NJ 07652   (201)261-6061   Fax (201)261-6465

Rutkiewicz, Laura A., MD {1164498093} FamMed(92,DC02)<NJ-VIRTMHBC>
+ Mt. Laurel Family Physicians
401 Young Avenue/Suite 260   Moorestown, NJ 08057   (856)291-8756   Fax (856)291-8750
+ Patient first Urgent Care
641 US Highway Route 130   Hamilton, NJ 08691   (856)291-8756   Fax (609)568-9384

Rutkowska, Ewa, MD {1669428066} Grtrcs, IntrMd(85,POL14)<NJ-HACKNSK>
+ Hackensack University Medical Center
30 Prospect Avenue   Hackensack, NJ 07601   (201)215-2510   Fax (201)343-9823

Rutner, Torin W., MD {1285707273} Surgry(01,NJ05)<NJ-OVERLOOK, NJ-MORRISTN>
+ 552 Westfield Avenue
Westfield, NJ 07090   (908)654-6030   Fax (908)654-8160
+ Union Oral & Maxillofacial Surgery, LLC
261 Springfield Avenue/Suite 203   Berkeley Heights, NJ 07922   (908)464-4664
+ Union Oral & Maxillofacial Surgery, LLC
590 Westfield Avenue   Westfield, NJ 07090   (908)654-6030

Ruvolo, Louis S., MD {1629079942} SrgVas, Surgry(66,IN20)
+ Rancocas Valley Surgical Associates PA
1000 Salem Road/Suite A   Willingboro, NJ 08046   (609)877-1737   Fax (609)877-1589

Ruvolo, Michelle, MD {1407970957} Psychy(67,ROMA)<NJ-BERGNMC>
+ 770 Anderson Avenue/A 11 North
Cliffside Park, NJ 07010

Ruzek, Michael A., DO {1275834830} EmrgMd(10,NJ75)<NJ-MORRISTN>
+ Morristown Medical Center
100 Madison Avenue   Morristown, NJ 07962   (973)971-5000

Ruzicka, Petr O., MD PedSrg(76,MN04)<NJ-RBAYOLDB, NJ-RBAYPERT>
+ UH- Robert Wood Johnson Med
125 Paterson Street/Suite CAB   New Brunswick, NJ 08901   (732)828-3000

Ryan, Catherine S., MD IntrMd, Rheuma(79,MO02)
+ 69 Portland Road
Summit, NJ 07901

Ryan, Christina Marie, MD {1407082902} Pedtrc
+ Goryeb Children's Hospital
100 Madison Avenue   Morristown, NJ 07960   (973)656-6280

Ryan, Colleen A., MD {1154590248} PsyCAd, Psychy(02,IRE03)<MA-CHILDRN>
+ Children's Specialized Hospital
200 Somerset Street/4th Fl   New Brunswick, NJ 08901   (732)797-3824

Ryan, Joseph J., MD {1689649576} Gastrn, Grtrcs, IntrMd(70,NY08)<NJ-MORRISTN>
+ 95 Madison Avenue/Suite 411
Morristown, NJ 07960   (973)971-7022   Fax (973)290-7675

Ryan, Kathleen Lisa, MD {1659356905} CritCr, IntrMd, PulDis(81,MA07)
+ Pulmonary and Sleep Physicians
204 Ark Road/Suite 206/Larchmont 1 Mount Laurel, NJ 08054 (856)778-4640 Fax (856)778-8862

Ryan, Sharon L., MD {1407824691} FamMed, Grtrcs(86,GRNA)<NJ-RWJHLTS>
+ RWJPE Old Bridge Family Medicine
2107 Highway 516 Old Bridge, NJ 08857 (732)952-0626 Fax (732)463-6071

Ryan, Todd C., DO {1720049232} SrgOrt(95,NY75)<NJ-JFKMED>
+ Edison-Metuchen Orthopedic Group
10 Parsonage Road/5th Floor/Suite 500 Edison, NJ 08837 (732)494-6226 Fax (732)494-8762

Ryan, Wanda Dawn, MD {1003825431} EnDbMt, IntrMd(85,NY03)<NJ-HUNTRDN>
+ Center for Endocrine Health
1738 Route 31 North/Suite 108 Clinton, NJ 08809 (908)735-3980 Fax (908)735-3981
+ 1100 Wescott Drive/Suite 301
Flemington, NJ 08822 (908)735-3980 Fax (908)237-2368

Ryave, Steven Samuel, MD {1114961877} EmrgMd(79,PA13)<NJ-RWJUBRUN, NJ-CHSFULD>
+ RWJ University Hospital New Brunswick
One Robert Wood Johnson Place New Brunswick, NJ 08901 (732)937-8550
+ Emergency Medical Associates
110 Rehill Avenue Somerville, NJ 08876 (732)937-8550 Fax (908)685-2968

Ryb, Gabriel E., MD Surgry(87,ARG01)<NJ-ACMCITY, NJ-ACMC-MAIN>
+ AtlantiCare Regional Medical Center/City Campus
1925 Pacific Avenue/Surgery Atlantic City, NJ 08401 (609)345-4000

Rybak, Eli Asher, MD {1306926969} RprEnd, ObsGyn(01,MD07)
+ Reproductive Medicine Associates of New Jersey
140 Allen Road Basking Ridge, NJ 07920 (908)604-7800 Fax (973)290-8370
+ Reproductive Medicine Associates of New Jersey
25 Rockwood Place Englewood, NJ 07631 (908)604-7800 Fax (201)569-8143
+ Reproductive Science Center of New Jersey
234 Industrial Way Eatontown, NJ 07920 (732)918-2500 Fax (732)918-2504

Rybak, Karen J., MD {1114154770} RadDia(03,MD07)
+ Radiology Associates of Ridgewood, P.A.
20 Franklin Turnpike Waldwick, NJ 07463 (201)445-8822 Fax (201)447-5053

Rybalov, Sergey, MD {1386670552} Gastrn, IntrMd(93,UKR12)<NJ-STCLRDEN, NJ-STCLRDOV>
+ Gastroenterology Associates of North Jersey
369 West Blackwell Street Dover, NJ 07801 (973)361-7660 Fax (973)361-0455
+ Gastroenterology Associates of North Jersey
16 Pocono Road/Suite 210 Denville, NJ 07834 (973)361-7660 Fax (973)627-7610

Rybinnik, Igor, MD {1710146386} VasNeu, Nrolgy<NY-LIJEWSH>
+ University Hospital-RWJMS Neurology
125 Paterson Street/Suite 4100-6100 New Brunswick, NJ 08901 (732)235-7733 Fax (732)235-7041

Ryczak, Kristen, MD {1356603872} FamMed(12,PA02)
+ Partners in Primary Care
534 Lippincott Drive Marlton, NJ 08053 (856)985-7373 Fax (856)985-9611

Ryder, Ronald G., DO {1154309532} CdvDis(89,PA77)<NJ-RWJUHAM>
+ Hamilton Cardiology Associates
2073 Klockner Road Hamilton, NJ 08690 (609)584-1212 Fax (609)584-0103

Ryfinski, Eugene A., MD {1073581625} IntrMd(83,MNT01)<NJ-STFRNMED>
+ Ewing Medical Associates
1539 Pennington Road Trenton, NJ 08618 (609)883-4124 Fax (609)883-0031

Rygielski, Jamie Leigh, DO {1033550744}<NJ-MORRISTN>
+ Morristown Medical Center
100 Madison Avenue Morristown, NJ 07962 (973)971-5000

Ryklin, Gennadiy, DO {1730534512} IntrMd<NJ-SJHREGMC>
+ SJH Regional Medical Center
1505 West Sherman Avenue Vineland, NJ 08360 (856)641-8000

Rymond, Claes G., MD {1457321572} EmrgMd, IntrMd(81,NY19)<NY-NYACKHOS, NY-PHELPMEM>
+ Medicon International Corporation
1350 15th Street/Suite 4-H Fort Lee, NJ 07024 (201)224-3688 Fax (201)224-8613

Ryngel, Enrique, MD {1215932280} IntrMd, Nephro(77,ARGE)
+ 302 Harrison Avenue
Harrison, NJ 07029 (973)484-2929 Fax (973)484-4280

Ryu, David Jinsoo, DO {1871780692} Anesth<NJ-HOLYNAME>
+ Holy Name Hospital
718 Teaneck Road Teaneck, NJ 07666 (201)833-7150

Saad, Adam, MD {1891025730} SrgPlstc, Surgry(PA09
+ The Plastic Surgery Center
2500 English Creek Avenue/Suite 605 Egg Harbor Township, NJ 08234 (609)272-7737

Saad, Mohamed Ali, MD {1558344960} Anesth(94,EGY03)
+ Hackensack University MC-Anesthesia Dept
30 Prospect Avenue/Room 2703 Hackensack, NJ 07601 (201)996-2419 Fax (201)996-3962

Saad, Sherif Saad, MD {1730400276}
+ Drs. Saad and Saad
139 Sequoia Drive Berlin, NJ 08009 (856)767-2783 sherifsaad1984@gmail.com

Saad, Walid Y., MD {1164752499} IntrMd
+ 2-10 Linden Avenue
Haddonfield, NJ 08033

Saadeh, Sermin, MD {1245432137} Pedtrc, PedNph(03,JOR02)<NJ-MORRISTN>
+ Morristown Medical Center
100 Madison Avenue/Pediatrics Morristown, NJ 07962 (973)971-5649

Saaraswat, Babita, MD {1891184784} IntrMd
+ 648 Holmdel Road
Hazlet, NJ 07730 (732)693-0050 Fax (732)696-0051

Saaraswat, Vijay, MD {1003800095} IntrMd(92,INA9B)<NY-WYCKOFF>
+ 21 Wooleytown Road
Morganville, NJ 07751

Saba, Ragheda M., MD {1205800885} Pedtrc(80,SYR01)<NJ-MTN-SIDE>
+ Mountainside Family Practice Associates
799 Bloomfield Avenue/Suite 201 Verona, NJ 07044 (973)746-7050 Fax (973)857-2831

Saba, Souheil, MD {1801837182} ObsGyn(78,SYR01)<NJ-STJOSHOS, NJ-MEADWLND>
+ Clifton Medical Group
1003 Main Avenue/Suite 3 C Clifton, NJ 07011 (973)777-9595 Fax (973)777-1311 Sabamd@aol.com

Sabando, Otto F., DO {1821002817} EmrgMd(98,NY75)<NJ-STJOSHOS>
+ St Joseph's Medical Center Emergency
703 Main Street Paterson, NJ 07503 (973)754-2240 Fax (973)754-2249

Sabater, Pilar, MD {1306324586} IntrMd(74,SPA15)<NJ-ENGLWOOD>
+ 201 Bridge Plaza North
Fort Lee, NJ 07024 (201)944-4305 Fax (201)944-4715

Sabates Arnesen, Katrina, MD {1588045298} FamMed
+ 315 State Route 31 South
Washington, NJ 07882 (908)847-3100 Fax (866)276-9292

Sabatini, Louis V., DO {1497716278} EmrgMd, FamMed(87,TX78)<NJ-ACMCITY, NJ-ACMCMAIN>
+ AtlantiCare Regional Medical Center/City Campus
1925 Pacific Avenue/EmergMed Atlantic City, NJ 08401 (609)345-4000
+ AtlantiCare Regional Med Ctr/Mainland
65 West Jimmie Leeds Road/EmergMed Pomona, NJ 08240 (609)652-1000

Sabatino, John C., MD RadDia(95,NJ06)
+ 15 Indian Trail
Medford, NJ 08055

Sabel, Svetlana Lantsman, MD {1124307616} PedGst
+ Children's Hospital of NJ Ped Cntr @ West Orange
375 Mount Pleasant Avenue/Suite 105 West Orange, NJ 07052 (973)322-6900 Fax (973)322-6999

Saber, Mai Said, DO {1538341961} EmrgMd
+ 29 Mountain Avenue
Hawthorne, NJ 07506 (973)949-9222

Saber, Shelley B., MD {1053537472} ObsGyn<NJ-HACKNSK>
+ Hackensack University Medical Center
30 Prospect Avenue/ObsGyn4E90C Hackensack, NJ 07601 (201)996-2755

Sabharwal, Sanjeev, MD {1255418554} SrgOrt(85,INA23)<NJ-RWJUBRUN, NJ-UMDNJ>
+ North Jersey Orthopaedic Institute
90 Bergen Street/DOC 1200 Newark, NJ 07101 (973)972-0244 Fax (973)972-9367

Sabharwal, Tina, MD {1215297981} FamMed, IntrMd(GRN01)
+ Clark Urgent Care
100 Commerce Place Clark, NJ 07066 (732)499-0606

Sabia, Michael, MD {1780881029} Anesth, AnesPain(01,MEX14)
+ 254 Knoll Drive
Blackwood, NJ 08012

Sabido, Michael, MD {1205097383} FamMed, IntrMd(98,CUB05)
+ United Medical, P.C.
533 Lexington Avenue Clifton, NJ 07011 (973)546-6844 Fax (973)546-7707

New Jersey Physicians
Section 1 Name and Practice Address

Sabin, Steven Lloyd, MD {1538266903} Otlryg(92,NJ06)
+ ENT & Allergy Associates
1543 Route 27/Suite 21 Somerset, NJ 08873 (732)873-6863 Fax (732)873-6853
+ ENT & Allergy Associates
B-3 Cornwall Drive East Brunswick, NJ 08816 (732)873-6863 Fax (732)238-4066
+ Raritan Valley Surgery Center
100 Franklin Square Drive/Suite 100 Somerset, NJ 08873 (732)238-0300 Fax (732)560-5999

Sabio, Ivan Alberto, MD {1629047709} IntrMd, Rheuma(97,NY45)<NJ-OCEANMC>
+ 141 Hooper Avenue
Toms River, NJ 08753 (848)223-7120 Fax (732)349-6919

Sabir, Sajjad A., MD {1215033030} IntrMd
+ 2400 McClellan Avenue/Suite E706
Pennsauken, NJ 08109

Sabnani, Indu, MD {1649211921} Hemato, IntrMd, MedOnc(80,INDI)<NJ-NWRKBETH>
+ 2130 Millburn Avenue/Suite C11
Maplewood, NJ 07040 (973)762-7676 Fax (973)762-7677

Sabnani-Nagella, Kavita R., MD {1871523910} IntrMd(95,MA05)
+ Maron & Rodrigues Medical Group, LLC.
10 James Street/Suite 150 Florham Park, NJ 07932 (973)822-2000 Fax (973)822-2001

Sabnis, Vinayak M., MD {1881877421} SrgVas, Surgry(73,INDI)<NJ-BURDTMLN>
+ 301 Stone Harbor Boulevard
Cape May Court House, NJ 08210 (609)465-2221 Fax (609)465-4939
+ Court House Surgery Center
106 Courthouse South Dennis Rd Cape May, NJ 08204 (609)465-2221 Fax (609)465-8771

Sabo, Robert A., MD {1780733618} SrgNro(90,PA02)<NJ-ACMC-ITY, NJ-ACMCMAIN>
+ Coastal Physicians and Surgeons
110 Harbor Lane/Suite A Somers Point, NJ 08244 (609)653-9110 Fax (609)927-3934

Sabogal, Jose Luis, MD {1467424325} IntrMd(94,COL06)
+ Broad Street Medical Associates
201 Route 17/Floor 11 Rutherford, NJ 07070 (973)471-8850 Fax (973)471-5232

Sabzwari, Tabassum Azra, DO {1730418625} ObsGyn(05,NY75)<NJ-TRINIWSC>
+ Preferred Women HealthCare LLC
240 Williamson Street/Suite 405 Elizabeth, NJ 07202 (908)353-5551 Fax (908)353-5052

Sacchetti, Alfred D., MD {1073694014} EmrgMd(79,PA07)<NJ-OURLADY, NJ-ACMCITY>
+ Our Lady of Lourdes Medical Center
1600 Haddon Avenue/EmergMed Camden, NJ 08103 (856)757-3500
+ AtlantiCare Regional Medical Center/City Campus
1925 Pacific Avenue/EmergMed Atlantic City, NJ 08401 (609)345-4000

Sacchieri, Theresa Ann, MD {1578616942} FamMed(02,NJ05)<NJ-HUNTRDN>
+ Annandale Family Practice
56 Payne Road/Suite 21 Lebanon, NJ 08833 (908)238-0100 Fax (908)238-0951

Sacco, Margaret Mary, MD {1831277144} SrgOnc, Surgry, IntrMd(86,PA09)<NJ-CHILTON, NJ-MORRISTN>
+ 33 Overlook Road/Suite 207
Summit, NJ 07901 (908)598-6610 Fax (973)835-9233
+ 350 Main Road/Suite 103
Montville, NJ 07045 (908)598-6610 Fax (973)835-9233

Saccone, Paul Gregori, MD {1407071657} SrgPlstc(87,NJ05)
+ Millburn Surgical Associates
225 Millburn Avenue/Suite 104-B Millburn, NJ 07041 (973)379-5888 Fax (973)912-9757

Saccone, Peter Joseph, DO {1295066181} IntrMd
+ SOM - Department of Internal Medicine
42 East Laurel Road/Suite 3100 Stratford, NJ 08084 (856)566-6859 Fax (856)566-6906

Sachar, Inderpreet, MD {1619141561} IntrMd, Grtrcs(01,NJ05)<NJ-HOLYNAME>
+ 655 Pomander Walk/Suite 239
Teaneck, NJ 07666 (201)836-2990

Sachdeo, Rajesh C., MD {1043232556} Nrolgy(75,INA79)<NJ-STPETER>
+ Princeton Hospital
1 Plainsboro Road/Neuroscience Ca Plainsboro, NJ 08536 (609)853-7530

Sachdev, Rahul, MD {1841228921} ObsGyn, RprEnd, FrtInf(87,NJ05)
+ Center for Advanced Reproductive Medicine/Fertility
4 Ethel Road/Suite 405A Edison, NJ 08817 (732)339-9300 Fax (732)339-9400

Sachdeva, Chander K., MD {1629090915} PhysMd(93,INA23)
+ 7811 Maple Avenue
Merchantville, NJ 08109 (856)488-1212 Fax (856)488-2224

Physicians by Name and Address

Sachdeva, Kush, MD {1750372686} Onclgy, Hemato, MedOnc(90,INA43)<NJ-SJHREGMC, NJ-SJRSYELM>
+ Southern Oncology Hematology Associates
1505 West Sherman Avenue/Suite 101 Vineland, NJ 08360 (856)696-9550 Fax (856)691-1686

Sacher, S. Mark, DO {1871566828} Psychy, PsyCAd(80,IA75)<NJ-ACMCITY>
+ AtlantiCare Behavioral Health/Seaside Counseling
2021 New Road/Suite 15 Linwood, NJ 08221 (609)927-4200
+ University Hospital-SOM Department of Psychiatry
2250 Chapel Avenue West/Suite 100 Cherry Hill, NJ 08002 (609)927-4200 Fax (856)482-1159

Sachinwalla, Eric M., MD {1881997641} IntrMd<NJ-RWJUBRUN>
+ RWJ University Hospital New Brunswick
One Robert Wood Johnson Place New Brunswick, NJ 08901 (732)235-7742

Sachla, Melpomeni, MD {1376612796} Psychy(82,ITA01)
+ 280 Norwood Avenue
West Long Branch, NJ 07764 (732)222-0031 Fax (732)222-3003

Sachs, R. Gregory, MD {1215909874} CdvDis, IntrMd(66,DC02)<NJ-OVERLOOK, NJ-MORRISTN>
+ Summit Medical Group
1 Diamond Hill Road/Bensley Pav/2 FL Berkeley, NJ 07922 (908)277-8700 Fax (908)288-7993

Sachs, Ronald, MD {1336254416} Ophthl, VitRet(88,NY19)<NJ-MORRISTN>
+ 8 Saddle Road/Suite 201
Cedar Knolls, NJ 07927 (973)539-3600 Fax (973)539-7576

Sachs, Seth W., MD {1679512610} Ophthl(78,NY47)<NJ-HACKNSK>
+ 405 Rochelle Avenue
Rochelle Park, NJ 07662 (201)712-5501 Fax (201)712-5505

Sack, Anita D., MD {1306944863} Psychy, PsyFor(81,GRN01)<NJ-TRENTPSY>
+ Trenton Psychiatric Hospital
Sullivan Way/PO Box 7600 West Trenton, NJ 08628 (609)633-1500

Sackman, Scott Marshall, DO {1518901958} Otlryg(84,NY75)<NJ-WARREN>
+ Expert Ear, Nose and Throat Associates
481 Memorial Parkway/Suite 4 Phillipsburg, NJ 08865 (908)387-1500

Sacknowitz, Ivy J., MD {1710980867} Anesth(84,VA04)
+ Advanced Perioperative Medicine, PA
350 Boulevard Passaic, NJ 07055 (973)365-4583

Sacks, Harry Jack, MD {1124310834} PainMd
+ 265 Davidson Avenue/Suite 300
Somerset, NJ 08873

Sacks, Richard, MD {1588649362} SrgOrt(72,TN07)<NJ-COMMED, NJ-KIMBALL>
+ Coast Orthopedic Associates PA
886 Commons Way/Building H Toms River, NJ 08755 (732)914-8989

Sacks, Robert J., DO {1083652960} FamMed(77,IA75)<NJ-VIRTMHBC>
+ Burlington Family Medical Center
666 Madison Avenue Burlington, NJ 08016 (609)386-0023 Fax (609)386-4648

Sackstein, Adam, MD {1396768081} PainMd, Anesth(90,NY08)<NJ-CHSFULD, NJ-STFRNMED>
+ The Pain Management Center at Hamilton
2271 Highway 33/Suite 103 Hamilton, NJ 08690 (609)890-4080 Fax (609)890-4090
+ 1001 Laurel Oak Road/Suite A-2
Voorhees, NJ 08043 (856)566-8600

Sackstein, Stuart A., MD {1285838894} ObsGyn(76,MEXI)<NJ-ACMCITY, NJ-ACMCMAIN>
+ 707 White Horse Pike/Suite A-4
Absecon, NJ 08201 (609)641-7727 Fax (609)641-7769

Sacristan, Carlos, MD {1811971229} GenPrc, FamMed(82,COL24)
+ 17-19 Howe Avenue/PO Box 327
Passaic, NJ 07055 (973)473-4399 Fax (973)473-3039

Saddel, Diana L., DO {1831270610} FamMed(87,NY75)<NJ-OURLADY>
+ 543 Egg Harbor Road
Sewell, NJ 08080 Fax (856)256-2064

Sadegh, Mona, MD {1700225349} Pedtrc(13,NJ05)
+ NuHeights Pediatrics
1115 Clifton Avenue/Suite 101 Clifton, NJ 07013 (973)250-2970 Fax (973)250-2971
+ NuHeights Pediatrics
2 Brighton Road/Suite 404 Clifton, NJ 07013 (973)250-2970 Fax (973)250-2971

Sadeghi, Hooshang, MD {1235275561} Nrolgy(67,IRAN)<NJ-HOBUNIMC>
+ Carepoint Health Medical Group
631 Broadway/3rd Floor Bayonne, NJ 07002 (201)243-0700 Fax (201)243-0377

+ Carepoint Health Medical Group
33 Main Street Chatham, NJ 07928 (201)243-0700 Fax (201)243-0377

Sadeghi Nejad, Hossein, MD {1336118850} Urolgy(89,QU01)<NJ-UMDNJ, NJ-HACKNSK>
+ Center for Male Reproductive Medicine
20 Prospect Avenue/Suite 711 Hackensack, NJ 07601 (201)342-7977 Fax (201)489-0877

Sadek, Ragui W., MD {1235213679} SrgCrC, Surgry(96,EGY05)<NJ-UMDNJ>
+ Advanced Surgical & Bariatrics of NJ, PA
49 Veronica Avenue/Suite 202 Somerset, NJ 08873 (732)640-5316 Fax (800)689-2361
+ Advanced Surgical & Bariatrics of NJ, PA
901 West Main Street/Suite 203 Freehold, NJ 07728 (609)385-0120

Sadi-Ali, Vajeeha, MD {1366730962} IntrMd<NJ-UMDNJ>
+ University Hospital
150 Bergen Street/Rm 446 Newark, NJ 07103 (973)972-1909

Sadik, Aseel, MD {1154348035} CritCr, IntrMd, PulDis(88,NJ05)
+ Drs. Picciano, Picciano & Sadik
36 Pacific Street Newark, NJ 07105 (973)578-4808 Fax (973)578-2939
A.Sadik@mindspring.com

Sadik, Nadia, MD {1295791861} PulDis(84,NJ05)<NJ-ACMCITY, NJ-ACMCMAIN>
+ Atlantic Pulmonary & Critical Care Associates, P.A.
741 South Second Avenue/Suite A Galloway, NJ 08205 (609)748-7300 Fax (609)748-7919

Sadik, Zubaida Y., MD {1639107337} Pedtrc(72,EGYP)<NJ-CENTRAST>
+ Drs. Cato-Varlack & Sadik
495 Iron Bridge Road/Suite 1 Freehold, NJ 07728 (732)577-0047 Fax (732)577-1324

Sadikot, Sean Shabbir, MD {1003075110} PulDis, IntrMd(06,MA05)
+ University Respiratory Medicine, P.A.
75 Summit Avenue Hackensack, NJ 07601 (201)487-4595

Sadimin, Evita T., MD {1366868846} PthACl<NJ-RWJUBRUN>
+ RWJ University Hospital New Brunswick
One Robert Wood Johnson Place New Brunswick, NJ 08901 (732)828-3000

Sadler, Adam D., DO {1295037356} SrgOrt
+ St. Luke's Orthopedics
755 Memorial Parkway/Suite 201 Phillipsburg, NJ 08865 (908)847-8884

Sadler, Daniel L., MD {1871539858} SrgC&R(87,WV01)
+ Central Jersey Colon & Rectal Surgeons
704 Route 202 South Bridgewater, NJ 08807 (908)526-5600 Fax (908)526-5569

Sadler, Michael Alan, MD {1104855733} RadDia(90,MA07)
+ 8 Woodhill Road
Tenafly, NJ 07670

Sadural, Ernani, MD {1902851975} ObsGyn(92,IL06)<NJ-STBARNMC, NJ-CLARMAAS>
+ Contemporary Women's Care
745 Northfield Avenue West Orange, NJ 07052 (973)736-7700 Fax (973)736-8078
+ Contemporary Women's Care
338 Belleville Turnpike Kearny, NJ 07032 (973)736-7700 Fax (201)998-4643

Saedeldine, Imad Khodor, MD {1740227560} IntrMd(86,UKR18)<NJ-STJOSHOS, NJ-WAYNEGEN>
+ Bisan Medical
1040 Main Street/3 FL Paterson, NJ 07503 (973)345-0444 Fax (973)345-0422

Saeed, Mohammed N., MD {1659599256}
+ 169 Spring Valley Road
Paramus, NJ 07652 (908)346-0590

Saeed, Muhammad I., MD {1487806048}
+ 300 Avalon Drive/Apt 3112
Wood Ridge, NJ 07075

Saeed, Qaisra Yasmin, MD {1407829955} CdvDis, IntCrd, IntrMd(94,PAK18)<NJ-CLARMAAS, NJ-NWRKBETH>
+ New Jersey Cardiovascular Care Center
116 Millburn Avenue/Suite 214 Millburn, NJ 07041 (973)218-6000 Fax (973)679-8636
+ The Heart Center of The Oranges
60 Vose Avenue South Orange, NJ 07079 (973)218-6000 Fax (973)761-1049

Saeed, Shamim Jan, MD {1720186455} FamMAdlt, IntrMd(92,PAK23)<NJ-ACMCMAIN, NJ-ACMCITY>
+ Integrated Medical Alliance/IMA Medical Care Center
30 Shrewsbury Plaza Shrewsbury, NJ 07702 (732)542-0002 Fax (732)542-2992

Saeed, Zaid I., DO {1679862270}
+ 43 Juliet Street
New Brunswick, NJ 08901 (718)350-0696
dr.aaidsaeed@gmail.com

Saez Lacy, Deborah A., MD {1245319888} ObsGyn(86,NJ06)
+ Brielle Obstetrics & Gynecology, P.A.

2671 Highway 70/Wall Township Manasquan, NJ 08736 (732)528-6999 Fax (732)528-3397
+ Brielle Obstetrics & Gynecology, P.A.
117 County Line Road Lakewood, NJ 08701 (732)528-6999 Fax (732)942-1919

Safa, Nina, MD {1942357595} IntrMd(98,PA13)<NJ-VALLEY>
+ Sovereign Medical Group
14-01 Broadway/3rd Floor/Suite B Fair Lawn, NJ 07410 (201)855-8455 Fax (201)855-8454

Safar, David S., MD {1548344195} Nrolgy(77,NJ05)<NJ-CHILTON>
+ 2025 Hamburg Turnpike/Suite M-1
Wayne, NJ 07470 (973)839-5005 Fax (973)839-7191

Safaryn, John E., MD {1710069174} Anesth(90,NJ05)<NJ-COOPRUMC>
+ Cooper University Hospital
One Cooper Plaza/Anesthesiology Camden, NJ 08103 (856)342-2000
JSMDZZZZ@msn.com

Safdar, Feroz, MD {1427185511} IntrMd, PulDis(70,PAK01)<NJ-RWJUHAM, NJ-CHSFULD>
+ 3606 Nottingham Way
Trenton, NJ 08690 (609)587-9140 Fax (609)584-9628

Safdar, Mohammad Imran, MD {1982847679} Anesth
+ 118 Elizabeth Avenue
Edison, NJ 08820

Saffran, Bruce Nathan, MD {1124052253} RadNro, Radiol, RadDia(92,OH41)
+ One Queens Court
Columbus, NJ 08022 (609)354-8385

Saffran, Scott Robert, MD {1164420824} Anesth, IntrMd(87,NY09)<NJ-STMICHL>
+ St. Michael's Medical Center
111 Central Avenue/Anesthesia Newark, NJ 07102 (973)877-5034 Fax (973)877-5231
+ St. Joseph's Regional Medical Center Anesthesia
703 Main Street Paterson, NJ 07503 (973)877-5034 Fax (973)977-9455

Safi, Farnaz, MD {1043528029} ObsGyn(06,DMN01)
+ Lawrence Ob/Gyn Associates
123 Franklin Corner Road/Suite 214 Lawrenceville, NJ 08648 (609)896-1400 Fax (609)896-3986

Safirstein, Benjamin Herbert, MD {1073512398} IntrMd, PulDis(65,IL42)
+ Montclair Cardiology Group
123 Highland Avenue/Suite 101 Glen Ridge, NJ 07028 (973)744-9125 Fax (973)744-0280

Safirstein, Jordan Glanzman, MD {1922265495} CdvDis
+ Cardiology Consultants of North Morris, PA
356 US Highway 46/Suite B Mountain Lakes, NJ 07046 (973)586-3400 Fax (973)586-1916

Safran, George F., MD {1316945140} FamMed(85,DMN01)<NJ-HOBUNIMC>
+ Hoboken University Medical Center
308 Willow Avenue Hoboken, NJ 07030 (201)418-1000

Safran, Steven G., MD {1386624864} Ophthl(87,NY08)<NJ-CHSMRCER, NJ-RWJUHAM>
+ 132 Franklin Corner Road/Suite A 1
Lawrenceville, NJ 08648 (609)896-3931 Fax (609)895-1959
safran132@comcast.net
+ New Jersey Surgery Center
1225 Whitehorse Mercerville Rd Trenton, NJ 08619 (609)581-6200

Sagar, Yogesh, MD {1538136510} CdvDis, IntrMd(91,PA09)<NJ-HOLYNAME, NJ-HACKNSK>
+ Bergen Cardiology Associates
400 Frank W. Burr Boulevard Teaneck, NJ 07666 (201)928-2300 Fax (201)692-3263

Sagarwala, Adam, DO {1932426616} SrgVas(09,TX17)<NJ-NWRKBETH>
+ Newark Beth Israel Medical Center
201 Lyons Avenue/Surgery Newark, NJ 07112 (973)926-7000

Sage, Jacob I., MD {1912072109} Nrolgy(72,PA12)<NJ-RWJUBRUN>
+ University Hospital-RWJMS Neurology
125 Paterson Street/Suite 4100-6100 New Brunswick, NJ 08901 (732)235-7733 Fax (732)235-7041
+ RW Johnson University Medical Group Neurology
97 Paterson Street New Brunswick, NJ 08901 (732)235-7733 Fax (732)235-7041

Sagebien, Carlos Alberto, MD {1538142666} SrgOrt, OrtTrm(99,NJ05)<NJ-RWJUBRUN, NJ-JRSYSHMC>
+ University Orthopaedic Associates, LLC.
Two Worlds Fair Drive Somerset, NJ 08873 (732)979-2115 Fax (732)564-9032
+ RWJ University Hospital New Brunswick
One Robert Wood Johnson Place New Brunswick, NJ 08901 (732)828-3000
+ University Orthopaedic Associates, LLC.
211 North Harrison Street Princeton, NJ 08873 (609)683-7800 Fax (609)683-7875

Saggar, Suraj Kumar, DO {1750419958} InfDis, IntrMd(02,PA77)
+ Drs. Seferian and Saggar
200 Grand Avenue/Suite 102   Englewood, NJ 07631   (201)503-0660   Fax (201)503-0685
surajsaggar@hotmail.com

Sagorin, Charles E., MD {1891796769} Hemato, IntrMd, MedOnc(71,NY08)<NJ-MTNSIDE>
+ 127 Pine Street/Suite 6
Montclair, NJ 07042   (973)783-3300   Fax (973)783-1168

Sagransky, David M., MD {1861437717} IntrMd, Rheuma(75,DC02)<NJ-SHOREMEM>
+ 1701 New Road
Linwood, NJ 08221   (609)653-6403   Fax (609)653-8945

Sagullo, Cynthia C., MD {1710944194} ObsGyn(96,PA02)<NJ-VALLEY>
+ Summit Medical Group
31-00 Broadway   Fair Lawn, NJ 07410   (201)530-5475   Fax (201)796-7020
+ Summit Medical Group
19-21 Fair Lawn Avenue   Fair Lawn, NJ 07410   (201)530-5475   Fax (844)262-9607

Sagullo, Nestor M., MD {1306898473} Surgry(63,PHI08)<NJ-PALISADE, NY-GOODSAM>
+ American Physician Services/Hudson HealthCare
679 Montgomery Street   Jersey City, NJ 07306   (201)433-6500   Fax (201)433-8010

Saha, Anita, MD {1063679983} ObsGyn(05,NY46)<NJ-UNVMCPRN>
+ Princeton Medical Group, P.A.
419 North Harrison Street   Princeton, NJ 08540   (609)924-9300   Fax (609)430-9481
+ Princeton Medical Group, P.A.
3 Liberty Street   Plainsboro, NJ 08536   (609)924-9300

Saha, Pavela, MD {1770971954}<NJ-RWJUBRUN>
+ RWJ University Hospital New Brunswick
One Robert Wood Johnson Place   New Brunswick, NJ 08901   (848)391-3514

Sahani, Herneet K., MD {1063672376} EnDbMt, IntrMd(87,INDI)<NJ-CLARMAAS, NJ-MTNSIDE>
+ 539 Bloomfield Avenue
Newark, NJ 07107   (973)497-2420   Fax (973)497-2421

Sahay, Nishi, MD {1417960725} IntrMd(87,INA7B)<NJ-COMMED, NJ-SOCEANCO>
+ Barnegat Medical Associates, P.A.
41 Nautilus Drive   Manahawkin, NJ 08050   (609)978-0474   Fax (609)597-6186
+ Barnegat Medical Associates PA
218 Pocohontas Avenue   Barnegat, NJ 08005   (609)698-3636
+ Barnegat Medical Associates PA
216b Commons Way/Route 37 East   Toms River, NJ 08050   (732)505-9193

Sahay, Rajiv, MD {1508879818} IntrMd(83,INA7B)<NJ-COMMED, NJ-SOCEANCO>
+ Barnegat Medical Associates, P.A.
41 Nautilus Drive   Manahawkin, NJ 08050   (609)978-0474   Fax (609)597-6186
+ Barnegat Medical Associates PA
218 Pocohontas Avenue   Barnegat, NJ 08005   (609)698-3636
+ Barnegat Medical Associates PA
216b Commons Way/Route 37 East   Toms River, NJ 08050   (732)505-9193

Sahlman, Rebecca Lynne, MD {1538194188} RadDia(96,PA09)
+ Kennedy Health System
1099 White Horse Road   Voorhees, NJ 08043   (856)661-5473   Fax (856)661-5473
r.sahlman@kennedyhealth.org

Sahloul, Elsayed Ahmed, MD {1467452565} IntrMd, Hepato(87,EGY05)
+ One Bethany Road/Suite 2
Hazlet, NJ 07730   (732)217-3208

Sahni, Harsha R., MD {1467547232} Allrgy, IntrMd, AlgyImmn(82,INDI)
+ 534 Inman Avenue
Colonia, NJ 07067   (732)388-1221   Fax (732)827-0788

Sahni, Rakesh Kumar, MD {1265636526} CdvDis(77,INDI)
+ Drs. Sahni amd Sahni
53-59 Westfield Avenue   Clark, NJ 07066   (732)396-9500

Sahni, Rana S., MD {1508978271} Otlryg(73,INDI)
+ 534 Inman Avenue
Colonia, NJ 07067   (732)396-9660

Sahni, Ryan, MD {1285018499}
+ Red Bank Family Medicine
231 Maple Avenue   Red Bank, NJ 07701   (732)842-3050   Fax (732)530-0730

Sahni, Sheila, MD {1215251103} CdvDis
+ Drs. Sahni amd Sahni
53-59 Westfield Avenue   Clark, NJ 07066   (732)396-9500   Fax (732)382-1377

Sahni, Sushma, MD {1831199496} IntrMd, GenPrc(76,INDI)<NJ-MEMSALEM>
+ Spotswood Medical Associates PA
498 Main Street   Spotswood, NJ 08884   (732)251-6900   Fax (732)251-5935

Sahoo, Aparna, DO {1528268554} IntrMd, Nephro(02,NY75)<NJ-UNVMCPRN>
+ Allergan
5 Giralda Farms   Madison, NJ 07940   (862)261-7000

Sahoo, Aruna, MD {1235393216} AnesPain(03,MO46)
+ Premier Pain Center
160 Avenue at the Commons/Suite 1   Shrewsbury, NJ 07702   (732)380-0200   Fax (732)380-0124

Sahoo, Madhusmita, MD {1912499377} PsyCAd<NJ-UNIVBHC>
+ University Behavioral Health Care
671 Hoes Lane/PO Box 1392   Piscataway, NJ 08855   (732)235-5256

Sahota, Manpreet S., MD {1265402143} Anesth, IntrMd(83,INDI)<NJ-CHDNWBTH, NJ-NWRKBETH>
+ Children's Hospital of New Jersey
201 Lyons Avenue/Osborne Terrace   Newark, NJ 07112   (908)447-8436   Fax (973)926-8521

Sahu, Anand P., MD {1699782797} IntrMd(64,INDI)
+ Drs. Sahu and Sahu
458 Clifton Avenue   Clifton, NJ 07011   (973)340-7676   Fax (973)340-7770

Sahu, Novneet, MD {1114284585} FamMed
+ Rutgers- New Jersey Medical School
185 South Orange Avenue   Newark, NJ 07103   (973)972-2861

Sahu, Sharad, MD {1164449724} IntrMd(99,GRN01)<NJ-HACKNSK>
+ Drs. Sahu and Sahu
458 Clifton Avenue   Clifton, NJ 07011   (973)340-7676   Fax (973)340-7770

Sahulhameed, Fathima, MD {1205249679} FamMed
+ Summit Medical Group-Berkeley Heights Campus
1 Diamond Hill Road   Berkeley Heights, NJ 07922   (908)273-4300   Fax (908)790-6576
+ Westfield Family Practice
563 Westfield Avenue   Westfield, NJ 07090   (908)273-4300   Fax (908)232-0439

Sai, Priya, MD {1255444329} IntrMd(99,INA76)
+ 209 Dawes Drive
Morganville, NJ 07751
+ Monmouth Medical Group PC
370 Highway 35/Suite 201   Red Bank, NJ 07701   Fax (732)933-0245

Saia, Bryan Edward, DO {1841440377} IntrMd, CdvDis
+ Associated Cardiovascular Consultants-Lourdes
1 Brace Road/Suite C & F   Cherry Hill, NJ 08034   (856)428-4100   Fax (856)428-5748

Saia, John A., DO {1346229911} CdvDis(75,PA77)<NJ-ACMC-MAIN, NJ-ATLANCHS>
+ Associated Cardiovascular Consultants, PA
2 Sindoni Lane   Hammonton, NJ 08037   (609)561-8500   Fax (856)567-0432
+ Associated Cardiovascular Consultants, PA
2500 English Creek Avenue   Egg Harbor Township, NJ 08234   (609)561-8500   Fax (609)569-1896
+ Associated Cardiovascular Consultants-Lourdes
1 Brace Road/Suite C & F   Cherry Hill, NJ 08037   (856)428-4100   Fax (856)428-5748

Said, Joseph, MD {1902171002} OrtSHand, SrgOrt(PA02)
+ Summit Medical Group
574 Springfield Avenue   Westfield, NJ 07090   (908)232-7797   Fax (908)232-0540
+ Summit Medical Group
1 Diamond Hill Road/Bensley Pav/2 FL   Berkeley, NJ 07922   (908)232-7797   Fax (908)288-7993
+ Summit Medical Group Orthopedics and Sports Medicine
140 Park Avenue/2nd Floor   Florham Park, NJ 07090   (973)404-9980   Fax (973)267-7295

Said, Raghad Houfdhi, MD {1659318103} IntrMd, CritCrt(93,IRQ07)<NJ-VALLEY>
+ Hackensack University Medical Center
30 Prospect Avenue/2 Conklin #2501   Hackensack, NJ 07601   (551)996-2379
+ 50 Brown Circle
Paramus, NJ 07652   (201)487-3525

Saidi, James Ali, MD {1194792820} Urolgy(94,TX12)<NJ-MTNSIDE>
+ NJ Urology
799 Bloomfield Avenue/Suite 300   Verona, NJ 07044   (973)746-3322   Fax (973)429-8765

Saieva, Carol E., DO {1538379243} FamMed(87,NY75)<NJ-VALLEY>
+ Bergen Medical Associates
1 Sears Drive/Suite 403   Paramus, NJ 07652   (201)261-6061   Fax (201)261-6465

Saif, Rashida Taher, MD {1538378187} Pedtrc
+ Shankar, Sujatha
77 Brunswick Woods Drive   East Brunswick, NJ 08816   (732)238-6644   Fax (732)238-6550
+ 206 Bridge Street/Bld D
Metuchen, NJ 08840   (732)238-6644   Fax (732)518-3208

Saif, Shazia, MD {1720092141} IntrMd(00,INA29)
+ Linden Medical Associates MD PC
540 South Wood Avenue   Linden, NJ 07036   (908)862-2893   Fax (908)862-5810

Sailam, Vivek Vardha, MD {1386819589} CdvDis, IntrMd(01,DMN01)<NJ-OURLADY, NJ-UNDRWD>
+ Associated Cardiovascular Consultants-Lourdes
1 Brace Road/Suite C & F   Cherry Hill, NJ 08034   (856)428-4100   Fax (856)428-5748
+ Associated Cardiovascular Consultants, P.A.
730 North Broad Street/Suite 200   Woodbury, NJ 08096   (856)428-4100   Fax (856)251-2344

Sailes, Frederick Cortney, MD {1275744450} Surgry
+ Capital Health System/Hopewell
One Capital Way   Pennington, NJ 08534   (609)394-4000

Saini, Amarjit K., MD {1053449421} IntrMd(70,INA9Y)<NJ-RBAYPERT>
+ 956 Amboy Avenue
Edison, NJ 08837   (732)738-9370   Fax (732)738-1373
+ Jewish Renaissance Medical Center
275 Hobart Street   Perth Amboy, NJ 08861   (732)738-9370   Fax (732)376-0139

Saini, Harjinder S., MD {1134147531} IntrMd, Nephro(95,NJ06)<NJ-CHILTON>
+ North Jersey Nephrology Associates PA
246 Hamburg Turnpike/Suite 207   Wayne, NJ 07470   (973)653-3366   Fax (973)653-3365

Saini, Manish K., MD {1730251745} Pedtrc(87,INDI)<NJ-RIVERVW, NJ-JRSYSHMC>
+ Millennium Pediatric Care, PA
1 Riverview Medical Center   Red Bank, NJ 07701   (732)450-2801   Fax (732)450-2802

Saini, Manish Satyaprakash, MD {1962478776} IntrMd, IntHos(95,INA67)<NJ-RIVERVW>
+ Gaetano Medical Associates
1163 Highway 37 West/Suite B1   Toms River, NJ 08755   (732)341-7900   Fax (732)341-4706
+ Riverview Medical Center
1 Riverview Plaza   Red Bank, NJ 07701   (732)741-2700

Saint-Vil, Robert, Jr., DO {1871709642} Psychy, PsyGrt(04,NJ75)<NJ-CARRIER>
+ Carrier Clinic
252 Route 601/Psychiatry   Belle Mead, NJ 08502   (908)281-1000

Saitas, Vasiliki L., MD {1427105428} PthACl, PthCyt(85,GREE)
+ 15-01 Broadway
Fair Lawn, NJ 07410   (201)214-4285   Fax (201)512-1934

Saitta, Jacqueline Danielle, MD {1609026327} ObsGyn
+ 101 Old Short Hills Road
West Orange, NJ 07052   (973)736-1100   Fax (973)736-1834

Saiz Rodriguez, Cristina Margarita, MD {1023219219}
+ Urogynecology & Reconstructive Pelvic Surgery
435 South Street/Suite 370   Morristown, NJ 07960   (973)971-7267

Saiz-Quintana, Maria Elena, MD {1285878272} Psychy(92,CUB06)<NY-BRNXLFUL>
+ 655 East Jersey Street
Elizabeth, NJ 07206   (908)994-7131

Sajous, Jan Bernard, MD {1053597294} RadDia(NY19)
+ South Jersey Radiology Associates, P.A.
748 Kings Highway   West Deptford, NJ 08096   (856)848-4998   Fax (856)853-7362
jsajous@sjra.com
+ South Jersey Radiology Associates, P.A.
100 Carnie Boulevard/Suite B-5   Voorhees, NJ 08043   (856)848-4998   Fax (856)751-0535
+ South Jersey Radiology Associates, P.A.
315 Route 70 East/Suite B   Cherry Hill, NJ 08096   (856)428-4344   Fax (856)428-0356

Sajous, Jocelyne, MD {1609861087} Anesth(85,HAI01)<NJ-HACKNSK>
+ Hackensack University Medical Center
30 Prospect Avenue/Anesth   Hackensack, NJ 07601   (201)996-2000

Sakellaris, Leander D., MD {1194795757} Anesth(86,AUST)<NJ-NWRKBETH>
+ Newark Beth Israel Medical Center
201 Lyons Avenue   Newark, NJ 07112   (973)926-7143   Fax (201)943-8105

Sakowitz, Arthur J., MD {1710955174} PulDis, IntrMd(70,VT02)<NJ-VALLEY>
+ Pulmonary Medicine Associates, P.A.
1 West Ridgewood Avenue   Paramus, NJ 07652   (201)493-0366   Fax (201)493-0379

Physicians by Name and Address

Sakowitz, Barry H., MD {1104894559} PulDis, IntrMd(70,NY08)<NJ-VALLEY>
+ Pulmonary Medicine Associates, P.A.
1 West Ridgewood Avenue Paramus, NJ 07652 (201)493-0366 Fax (201)493-0379

Sakowitz Cohen, Noreen Gail, MD {1700094042} Anesth<NJ-STJOSHOS>
+ St. Joseph's Regional Medical Center Anesthesia
703 Main Street Paterson, NJ 07503 (973)754-2323 Fax (973)977-9455

Sakowski, Jacek, MD {1699774513} AdolMd, Pedtrc(93,POLA)
+ 117 Seber Road/Building 4 Suite C
Hackettstown, NJ 07840 (908)852-8096 Fax (908)852-5012

Sakr, Ashraf M., MD {1679655385} PainMd, Anesth(90,EGY10)<NJ-RWJUBRUN>
+ RWJMG Acute Care Surgery
125 Paterson Street/Suite 6300 New Brunswick, NJ 08901 (732)235-7246 Fax (732)235-2964
+ Spine Institute of North America
300A Princeon Hightstown Road East Windsor, NJ 08520 (732)235-7246 Fax (609)371-9110

Saks, Darren, MD {1952366825} Pedtrc(97,NJ06)<NJ-ENGLWOOD, NJ-HACKNSK>
+ Tenafly Pediatrics, PA
26 Park Place Paramus, NJ 07652 (201)262-1140 Fax (201)261-8413
+ Tenafly Pediatrics, PA
350 Ramapo Valley Road Oakland, NJ 07436 (201)262-1140 Fax (201)651-0909
+ Tenafly Pediatrics, PA
74 Pascack Road Park Ridge, NJ 07652 (201)326-7120 Fax (201)326-7130

Saksena, Rujuta P., MD {1851522197} OncHem(08,PA02)
+ Medical Diagnostic Associates, P.A.
99 Beauvoir Avenue Summit, NJ 07901 (908)608-0078 Fax (908)608-1504
+ Atlantic Surgical Oncology
99 Beauvoir Street Summit, NJ 07901 (908)608-0078 Fax (908)598-2392

Saksena, Sanjeev, MD {1295836294} CdvDis, ClCdEl, IntrMd(74,INDI)
+ Cardiac Eletrophysiology, PA
161 Washington Valley Road/Suite 201 Warren, NJ 07059 (732)302-9988 Fax (732)302-9911
info@eprf.org

Saky, Marie-Therese, MD {1194780320} IntrMd, EnDbMt(89,BEL06)<NJ-MONMOUTH>
+ Ocean Endocrine LLC
1803 State Highway 35/Suite 3 Oakhurst, NJ 07755 (732)663-2900 Fax (732)663-2920

Saladini, Vincent, Jr., MD {1528041936} Anesth(84,NY01)<NJ-HACKNSK>
+ Hackensack University Medical Center
30 Prospect Avenue/Anesth Hackensack, NJ 07601 (201)996-2000 Fax (201)488-6769
+ Hackensack University MC-Anesthesia Dept
30 Prospect Avenue/Room 2703 Hackensack, NJ 07601 (201)996-2000 Fax (201)996-3962

Salah, Hassan H., MD {1356329312} Pedtrc(82,EGY03)<NJ-OURLADY>
+ Our Lady of Lourdes Medical Center
1600 Haddon Avenue/Pediatrics Camden, NJ 08103 (856)757-3500
+ first Step Pediatrics
206 Laurel Heights Drive Bridgeton, NJ 08302 (856)757-3500 Fax (856)459-9674
+ Elmer Pediatrics
525 State Street/Suite 1/PO Box 603 Elmer, NJ 08103 (856)358-5050 Fax (856)358-1141

Salah-Eldin, Alaa A., MD {1548287386} IntrMd, Gastrn(77,EGYP)<NJ-HOBUNIMC, NJ-CHRIST>
+ 550 Summit Avenue/Suite 205
Jersey City, NJ 07306 (201)659-0772 Fax (201)659-6527

Salaki, John S., MD {1669430880} InfDis, IntrMd(71,NJ05)
+ Internal Medicine Faculty Associates
435 South Street/Suite 210 Morristown, NJ 07960 (973)971-7165 Fax (973)290-7675

Salam, Aleya, MD {1730128240} PhyMPain, IntrMd(97,PAK01)
+ MidJersey Orthopaedics, P.A.
8100 Westcott Drive/Suite 101 Flemington, NJ 08822 (908)782-0600 Fax (908)782-7575
+ Hunterdon Orthopaedic Institute, P.A.
80 West End Avenue Somerville, NJ 08876 (908)182-0600

Salam, Misbah U., MD {1396768651} NroChl, Nrolgy, Pedtrc(84,PAKI)<NJ-NWRKBETH, NJ-STBARNMC>
+ Newark Beth Israel Medical Center
201 Lyons Avenue/Pedi Neurology Newark, NJ 07112 (973)926-4813 Fax (973)923-2978

Salamat, Rahat, MD {1629173240} PulCCr<NJ-VALLEY>
+ VMG Respiratory Health & Pulmonary Medicine
1200 East Ridgewood Avenue Ridgewood, NJ 07450 (201)689-7755 Fax (201)689-0521
rahat.salamat@valleymedicalgroup.com

Salamera, Julius Butaran, MD {1548418791}
+ 655 Livingston Street
Elizabeth, NJ 07206 (908)994-7600 Fax (908)994-7599

Salamon, Charbel Georges, MD {1316033483} ObsGyn, UroGyn(98,LEB01)<ME-CALAIS, ME-DOWNEAST>
+ Urogynecology & Reconstructive Pelvic Surgery
435 South Street/Suite 370 Morristown, NJ 07960 (973)971-7267 Fax (973)290-7520
+ Urogynecology & Reconstructive Pelvic Surgery
33 Overlook Road/Suite 409 Summit, NJ 07901 (908)522-7335

Salari, Behnam, DO {1396940037} SrgSpn
+ The Orthopedic Institute of New Jersey
108 Bilby Road/Suite 201 Hackettstown, NJ 07840 (908)684-3005 Fax (908)684-3301
+ The Orthopedic Institute of New Jersey
254-B Mountain Avenue/Suite 201 Hackettstown, NJ 07840 (908)684-3005 Fax (908)684-3301
+ The Orthopedic Institute of New Jersey
222 High Street/Suite 202 Newton, NJ 07840 (908)684-3005 Fax (908)684-3301

Salartash, Alimorad, MD {1710902333} Surgry, SrgAbd, SrgC&R(64,IRAN)<NJ-ACMCITY, NJ-ACMCMAIN>
+ Salartash Surgical Associates
301 Central Avenue/Suite D Egg Harbor Township, NJ 08234 (609)926-5000 Fax (609)926-2020
+ Atlantic Coastal Surgical Center
301 Central Avenue/Suite D Egg Harbor Township, NJ 08234 (609)926-5000 Fax (609)653-6100

Salartash, Khashayar, MD {1457376006} OthrSp, SrgVas, Surgry(92,DC01)<NJ-ACMCMAIN, NJ-SHOREMEM>
+ Salartash Surgical Associates
301 Central Avenue/Suite D Egg Harbor Township, NJ 08234 (609)926-5000 Fax (609)926-2020
+ Salartash Surgical Associates, LLC.
72 West Jimmie Leeds Road/Suite 1600 Galloway, NJ 08205 (609)926-5000 Fax (609)926-2020

Salaru, Gratian, MD {1386710580} PthAcl(95,ROM05)
+ RWJ University Pathology
125 Paterson Street/MEB 212 New Brunswick, NJ 08901 (732)235-8121 Fax (732)235-4661

Salas, A. Peter, MD {1124189030} SrgPlstc, SrgHnd, SrgBst(91,NY09)
+ Aesthetic Plastic Surgery Center
101 Old Short Hills Road/Suite 501 West Orange, NJ 07052 (973)731-2000

Salas, Max, MD {1528088812} PedEnd, Pedtrc(63,MEXI)<NJ-STPETER>
+ St. Peter's University Hospital
254 Easton Avenue/Pedi Endocrinol New Brunswick, NJ 08901 (732)745-8574 Fax (732)514-1956

Salas-Lopez, Debbie, MD {1558396143} IntrMd(96,NJ05)
+ Focus Community Health Center
449 Broad Street Newark, NJ 07102 (973)972-0980 Fax (973)972-0984

Salasin, Robert I., MD {1538183843} Surgry(70,PA02)<NJ-BURDTMLN>
+ Pennsylvania Vascular Associates, PC
8 South Dennis Road Cape May Court House, NJ 08210 (609)465-3939 Fax (609)465-4042

Salazer, Thomas L., MD {1205803152} Hypten, IntrMd, Nephro(89,NY48)<NJ-HOLYNAME, NJ-ENGLWOOD>
+ Nephrology Associates PA
870 Palisade Avenue/Suite 202 Teaneck, NJ 07666 (201)836-0897 Fax (201)836-8042

Salcedo, Elizabeth O., MD {1396840013} IntrMd(84,PHIL)<NJ-CENTRAST, NJ-KIMBALL>
+ Monmouth Medical Group, P.C.
1 Route 70 Lakewood, NJ 08701 (848)222-4690 Fax (848)222-4688
+ 200 Craig Road
Manalapan, NJ 07726 (848)222-4690 Fax (732)625-9202

Salcedo, Glenn A., MD {1386679645} Pedtrc, IntrMd(84,PHIL)<NJ-RIVERVW, NJ-MONMOUTH>
+ Pediatric Associates
9 South Main Street Marlboro, NJ 07746 (732)577-1945 Fax (732)308-3460
bcg221@hotmail.com
+ Pediatric Associates
444 Neptune Boulevard/Suite 4 Neptune, NJ 07753 (732)577-1945 Fax (732)774-4077

Salcedo, Theresa Josue, MD {1447351036} Pedtrc(91,PHI09)
+ 74 Route 9 North
Englishtown, NJ 07726 (732)617-1003 Fax (792)617-1004

Salcone, Mark Anthony, DO {1659563740} Surgry
+ LMA Surgical Associates
120 White Horse Pike/Suite 103 Haddon Heights, NJ 08035 (856)546-3900 Fax (856)546-3908

Saldarini, Candace Tom, MD {1033139811} PsyCAd, Psychy(00,GRN01)
+ Otsuka Pharmaceutical Development
508 Carnegie Center Drive Princeton, NJ 08540 (609)524-6788
ctsaldo@gmail.com

Saldarini, John Christopher, MD {1649361692} IntrMd(00,GRN01)<NJ-STBARNMC, NJ-CLARMAAS>
+ Nephrological Associates, P.A.
83 Hanover Road/Suite 290 Florham Park, NJ 07932 (973)736-2212 Fax (973)736-2989

Saldutti, Gregg M., MD {1952396046} Anesth(90,PA09)<NJ-UNDRWD>
+ Inspira Health Network
509 North Broad Street/Anesthesiology Woodbury, NJ 08096 (856)845-0100 Fax (856)848-7023

Saleeb, Joseph S., MD {1982624581} IntrMd(87,EGY05)<NJ-HOBUNIMC>
+ 3455 J F Kenndy Boulevard
Jersey City, NJ 07307 (201)386-8371

Saleeb, Mariam, MD {1891093829} Nrolgy(06,NY45)
+ Penn Medicine at Woodbury Heights
1006 Mantua Pike Woodbury Heights, NJ 08097 (856)845-8600 Fax (856)845-0535

Saleem, Bushra, MD {1891182382} IntrMd
+ Capital Health Hospitalist Group
750 Brunswick Avenue Trenton, NJ 08638 (609)394-6031 Fax (609)394-6299

Saleem, Mohammed R., MD {1366471872} Surgry(69,INDI)<NJ-CHSFULD, NJ-CHSMRCER>
+ Capital Surgical Associates
40 Fuld Street/Suite 303 Trenton, NJ 08638 (609)396-2600 Fax (609)396-3600

Saleem, Sogra R., MD {1588790323} Pthlgy, PthAcl(69,INDI)<NJ-CENTRAST>
+ CentraState Medical Center
901 West Main Street/Pathology Freehold, NJ 07728 (732)294-2989

Saleemi, Atif, MD {1013274034} FamMed
+ AtlantiCare Urgent Care Center
459 Route 9 South Little Egg Harbor, NJ 08087 (609)296-4014 Fax (609)296-5735

Saleh, Jason Reed, MD {1891953857} SrgOrt(08,NY47)<NY-MTSI-NAI>
+ Professional Orthopaedic Associates
1430 Hooper Avenue/Suite 101 Toms River, NJ 08753 (732)341-6777 Fax (732)349-7722

Saleh, Ramy Alber, DO {1265844054}<NJ-VIRTMARL>
+ Virtua Marlton Hospital
90 Brick Road Marlton, NJ 08053 (856)355-6000

Saleh, Rany Mokhlis, DO {1275606410} CdvDis, IntrMd(02,PA78)
+ Cardiology Center of New Jersey
50 Newark Avenue/Suite 204 Belleville, NJ 07109 (973)450-2158 Fax (973)450-2027

Saleh, Said A., MD {1447236617} Hemato, IntrMd, OncHem(91,JOR01)<NJ-MTNSIDE, NJ-CLARMAAS>
+ Essex Hematology-Oncology Group, PA
36 Newark Avenue/Suite 304 Belleville, NJ 07109 (973)751-8880 Fax (973)751-8950

Salehomoum, Negar Monavar, MD {1013169911} SrgC&R<NJ-RWJUBRUN>
+ RWJ University Hospital New Brunswick
One Robert Wood Johnson Place New Brunswick, NJ 08901 (732)235-7674

Salem, Anasuya, MD {1134267990} PsyFor(92,INDI)
+ 11 Van Dorn Road
Basking Ridge, NJ 07920

Salem, Mohamed M., MD {1861563215} IntrMd, Nephro(76,EGYPT)<NJ-MEMSALEM>
+ Salem Inernal Medicine
316 Merion Avenue Carneys Point, NJ 08069 (856)299-0345 Fax (856)299-9438

Salem, Mohammed Nasser, MD {1336593649}
+ 38 Divan Way
Wayne, NJ 07470 (973)800-8748

Salem, Noel B., MD {1982645065} Grtrcs, IntrMd, Rheuma(72,NY06)<NJ-ENGLWOOD>
+ 385 Sylvan Avenue/Suite 26
Englewood Cliffs, NJ 07632 (201)871-0223 Fax (201)871-1117
+ 285 Engle Street
Englewood, NJ 07631 (201)871-0223 Fax (201)871-1117

Salem, Raja R., MD {1821001272} SrgCrC, Surgry(87,NY47)<NJ-CHSFULD, NJ-CHSMRCER>
+ Capital Surgical Associates
40 Fuld Street/Suite 303 Trenton, NJ 08638 (609)396-2600 Fax (609)396-3600

Salem, Suhail Bakr, MD {1750547030} Gastrn
+ Gastroenterology Med Assocs PA
29 East 29th Street/Suite 71 Bayonne, NJ 07002 (201)795-8596 Fax (201)858-4260

Salerno, Adrienne Lynn, MD {1750563805} FamMed, IntrMd(07,GRN01)
+ Vanguard Medical Group
535 High Mountain Road/Suite 111 North Haledon, NJ 07508 (973)636-9000 Fax (973)636-0913

Salerno, Alexander Gerard, MD {1962476903} IntrMd(98,GRN01)
+ Salerno Medical Associates, LLP
613 Park Avenue East Orange, NJ 07017 (973)672-8573 Fax (973)676-4099

Salerno, Anthony P., MD {1801876222} ObsGyn, IntrMd(80,DC02)<NJ-JFKMED, NJ-OURLADY>
+ Rowan SOM Department of Ob/Gyn
405 Hurffville-Cross Keys Road Sewell, NJ 08080 (856)589-1414 Fax (856)256-5772

Salerno, Christopher J., DO {1194838060} FamMed(97,PA77)
+ Cherry Hill Primary and Specialty Care
457 Haddonfield Road/Suite 110 Cherry Hill, NJ 08002 (844)542-2273 Fax (856)406-4570
+ Dorfner Family Medicine
1 Mainbridge Lane Willingboro, NJ 08046 (844)542-2273 (609)877-0370

Salerno, Simon Anthony, MD {1962455303} SrgNro<NJ-JFKMED>
+ Meridian Surgical Associates
2101 Route 34 South Wall, NJ 07719 (732)974-0003 Fax (732)974-0366

Salerno, Vincent E., MD {1881634202} Hemato, Onclgy(90,ITAL)<NJ-OVERLOOK>
+ Trinitas Comprehensive Cancer Center
225 Williamson Street Elizabeth, NJ 07202 (908)964-8772 Fax (908)964-8748

Salerno, William D., MD {1972683902} CdvDis, CritCr, IntrMd(82,MEXI)<NJ-HACKNSK>
+ The Heart Care Center
38 Mayhill Street/Suite 1 Saddle Brook, NJ 07663 (201)843-1019 Fax (201)843-5910

Sales, Clifford M., MD {1053314005} SrgVas(86,NY47)<NJ-OVERLOOK, NJ-RWJURAH>
+ The Cardiovascular Care Group
433 Central Avenue Westfield, NJ 07090 (908)490-1699 Fax (908)490-1698
+ The Cardiovascular Care Group
25 East Willow Street Millburn, NJ 07041 (973)921-9600
+ The Cardiovascular Care Group
433 Central Avenue Westfield, NJ 07090 (908)490-1699 Fax (908)490-1698

Salese, Joseph Giuseppe, MD {1215945779} IntrMd(75,MEX03)<NJ-STBARNMC, NJ-CLARMAAS>
+ Primary Medical Care
76 Prospect Street Newark, NJ 07105 (973)344-1313 Fax (973)344-1811
+ Primary Medical Care
85 South Jefferson Street Orange, NJ 07050 (973)344-1313 Fax (973)673-0018

Salgado, Fredy R., MD {1235169350} Anesth<NJ-HACKNSK>
+ Hackensack University Medical Center
30 Prospect Avenue Hackensack, NJ 07601 (201)996-2000

Salian Raghava, Preethi, MD {1730573031} Pedtrc<NJ-CHD-NWBTH>
+ Children's Hospital of New Jersey
201 Lyons Avenue/Osborne Terrace Newark, NJ 07112 (973)926-7040

Salib, Hayman Shenoba, MD {1114956067} IntrMd, Hemato, MedOnc(84,EGY05)<PA-EASTON, PA-FOXCAN>
+ 39 Roseberry Street
Phillipsburg, NJ 08865

Saliba, Jehad E., MD {1164480372} PulDis, IntrMd(93,JORD)<NJ-STMICHL>
+ West Hudson Pulmonary Associates
816 Kearny Avenue Kearny, NJ 07032 (201)991-4544 Fax (201)991-8524

Salieb, Lorraine O., MD {1881986263}
+ Cooper Physicians Washington Township
1 Plaza Drive/Suite 103/Bunker Hill Pl Sewell, NJ 08080 (856)270-4080 Fax (856)270-4085

Salim, Shakeel, MD {1912279977} PhyMSptM
+ Reconstructive Orthopedics
994 West Sherman Avenue Vineland, NJ 08360 (609)267-9400 Fax (609)267-9457

Salim, Suhail Mohammed, DO {1851674907} FamMed(10,NY75)
+ CityMD Union Urgent Care
2317 Center Island Route 22 Union, NJ 07083 (201)354-1951 Fax (201)354-1952

Salim, Tamanna Yussouf, MD {1801164074} IntrMd
+ 17 Lenape Drive
Somerset, NJ 08873 (908)400-5041

Salima, Nosheen, MD {1780957530}
+ 25 Colgate Street
Closter, NJ 07624
nosheen.salima@gmail.com

Salimi, Mostafa, MD {1013095009} CdvDis, IntrMd(63,IRAN)
+ Cardiology Consultants
246 Hamburg Turnpike/Suite 201 Wayne, NJ 07470 (973)942-1141 Fax (973)942-7071

Salimi-Ghezelbash, Behzad, MD {1891772935} Anesth(78,IRA09)<NJ-CHRIST, NY-METHODST>
+ Christ Hospital
176 Palisade Avenue Jersey City, NJ 07306 (201)795-8200 Fax (201)943-8105

Salisbury, Jon P., MD {1639233539} FamMed(83,GRNA)
+ Visiting Physician Services
23 Main Street/Suite D1 Holmdel, NJ 07733 (732)571-1000 Fax (732)571-1156

Salizzoni, Jeffrey L., MD {1679655906} IntrMd, PulDis(85,MEXI)<NJ-HOLYNAME, NJ-ENGLWOOD>
+ Aspen Medical Associates, P.A.
1 DeGraw Square Teaneck, NJ 07666 (201)928-0200 Fax (201)928-0820

Salkeld, Charles S., DO {1225031057} Anesth(91,NJ75)<NJ-SHOREMEM>
+ Shore Memorial Hospital
1 East New York Avenue/Anesthesiology Somers Point, NJ 08244 (609)653-3500
+ Access Surgery Center
3205 Fire Road/Suite 3 Egg Harbor, NJ 08234 (609)407-1113

Salley, Pamela R., MD {1003999020} ObsGyn(82,NJ05)
+ Brunswick-Hills Ob/Gyn, PA
751 Route 206/2nd Floor Hillsborough, NJ 08844 (908)725-2510 Fax (908)725-2132

Salloum, Ahmad, MD {1205816717} IntrMd, CdvDis(92,SYR01)
+ Coastal Cardiovascular Consultants, PA
459 Jack Martin Boulevard/Suite 4 Brick, NJ 08724 (732)458-6200 Fax (732)458-9464

Salloum, Azizeh J., MD {1376857177} FamMed
+ Community Health Care, Inc.
1200 North High Street Millville, NJ 08332 (856)451-4700 Fax (856)327-4208

Salloum, Didi, MD {1396700951} ObsGyn(96,NJ05)
+ 1930 Highway 35/Suite 3
Wall Township, NJ 07719 (732)359-7060 Fax (732)359-7058

Salloum, Rafah, MD {1457417040} Rheuma, IntrMd(95,SYR01)
+ Arthritis & Osteoporosis Associates, P.A.
150 Route 37 West Ste A2/Suite A2 Toms River, NJ 08755 (732)414-6001 Fax (732)414-6003

Salm, Allen J., MD {1710977392} IntrMd, PulDis(82,GRNA)
+ Virtua Garden State Pulmonary Associates
520 Lippincott Drive/Suite A Marlton, NJ 08053 (856)596-9057 Fax (856)596-0837

Salman, Zoe Wilson, MD {1306009212} Psychy
+ 212 West Route 38/Suite 105
Moorestown, NJ 08057

Salmieri, Karen Heather, MD {1366606964} Radiol(08,CT01)
+ University Radiology Group, P.C.
579A Cranbury Road East Brunswick, NJ 08816 (732)390-0040 Fax (732)390-1856

Salmon, Barie J., MD {1184090516}<NJ-JRSYCITY>
+ Jersey City Medical Center
355 Grand Street Jersey City, NJ 07304 (201)915-2000

Salmonsen, Mary Beth, DO {1881884401} IntrMd
+ Rowan University-School of Osteopathic Medicine
1 Medical Center Drive/Suite 162 Stratford, NJ 08084 (856)566-7050

Salmun, Luis Marcelo, MD {1245484351} Pedtrc, AlgyImmn(85,ARG01)
+ 1500 Washington Street/Apt 10 L
Hoboken, NJ 07030

Salo, David F., MD {1497803258} EmrgMd, IntrMd(87,NY03)
+ Emergency Medical Offices
651 West Mount Pleasant Avenue Livingston, NJ 07039 (973)740-9396 Fax (973)251-1165

Salo, Ihor, MD {1912132408} IntrMd, Grtrcs(03,UKR25)<NJ-HOBUNIMC>
+ Hoboken University Medical Center
308 Willow Avenue Hoboken, NJ 07030 (201)418-1000

Salob, Peter Andrew, MD {1881646040} Ortped, SrgOrt(95,IL02)<NJ-ENGLWOOD, NJ-HOLYNAME>
+ Englewood Orthopedic Associates
401 South Van Brunt Street Englewood, NJ 07631 (201)569-2770 Fax (201)569-1774

Salomon, Amir, MD {1033181011} RadDia, RadNro(81,QU01)
+ Westfield Imaging Center
118-122 Elm Street Westfield, NJ 07090 (908)232-0610 Fax (908)232-7140

Salomon, Guy, MD {1417932435} Anesth(97,ISR02)<NJ-STMRY-PAS>
+ St. Mary's Hospital
350 Boulevard/Anesthesia Passaic, NJ 07055 (973)365-4480 Fax (845)357-5777

Salomon, Pierre Richard, MD {1134149701} IntrMd(99,MEX14)<NJ-HACKNSK, NJ-JRSYCITY>
+ Summit Medical Group-Berkeley Heights Campus
1 Diamond Hill Road Berkeley Heights, NJ 07922
(201)339-6333 Fax (908)790-6576

Salowe, David Ross, MD {1588622740} Gastrn, IntrMd(86,NJ05)<NJ-VIRTMHBC>
+ The Gastroenterology Group, PA
103 Old Marlton Pike/Suite 102 Medford, NJ 08055 (609)953-3440 Fax (609)996-4002
+ The Gastroenterology Group, PA
15000 Midlantic Drive/Suite 110 Mount Laurel, NJ 08054 (609)953-3440 Fax (856)996-4002

Salsali, Afshin, MD {1841372554} IntrMd, EnDbMt(91,IRA01)
+ RWJ University Endocrinology Diabetes & Metabolism
125 Paterson Street/CAB 5100A New Brunswick, NJ 08901 (732)235-7219 Fax (732)235-8610

Salston, Robert S., MD {1780634626} Pedtrc(77,NY08)<NJ-STPETER, NJ-RWJUBRUN>
+ Pediatric and Adolescent Associates of Central NJ
100 Perrine Road Old Bridge, NJ 08857 (732)316-0900 Fax (732)316-0499

Salter-Lewis, Cynthia, MD {1205007895} IntrMd(95,OH41)<NJ-VIRTMHBC, NJ-KMHSTRAT>
+ 316 US Hwy. 9
Englishtown, NJ 07726 (732)490-5130 Fax (866)567-6614

Saltzman, Erin Alyse, MD {1720033228} EnDbMt
+ Capital Endocrinology
2 Capital Way/Suite 290 Pennington, NJ 08534 (609)303-4300 Fax (609)303-4301

Saltzman, Rushani W., MD {1750588042} Pedtrc<PA-CHILDHOS>
+ CHOP Pediatric & Adolescent Specialty Care Center
1012 Laurel Oak Road Voorhees, NJ 08043 (856)435-1300 Fax (856)435-0091
+ CHOP Pediatric & Adolescent Specialty Care Center
707 Alexander Road/Suite 205 Princeton, NJ 08540 (609)520-1717

Saluja, Gurbir S., MD {1548229081} PedHem, Pedtrc(69,INA30)<NJ-NWTNMEM, NY-STCLARE>
+ Advocare Vernon Pediatrics
249 Route 94 Vernon, NJ 07462 (973)827-4550 Fax (973)827-5845

Saluja, Gurmit Singh, MD {1417916941} Pedtrc(98,IL42)<NJ-MORRISTN, NJ-STCLRDEN>
+ Advocare Vernon Pediatrics
249 Route 94 Vernon, NJ 07462 (973)827-4550 Fax (973)827-5845

Saluja, Ruby, MD {1710994439} IntrMd(98,INA1X)
+ 221 Chestnut Street/Suite 201
Roselle, NJ 07203 (908)241-7922 Fax (908)241-8619

Salvador-Goon, Brenda Mae, MD {1326281767} Pedtrc
+ Navesink Pediatrics
55 North Gilbert Street/Suite 2101 Tinton Falls, NJ 07701 (732)842-6677 Fax (732)530-2946

Salvaji, Madhu, DO {1902851355} IntrMd, CdvDis(93,IL76)
+ The Heart Specialist Group
1216 Route 22 West Mountainside, NJ 07092 (908)654-1200 Fax (908)654-1206

Salvati, Harold Vincent, MD {1063463453} Pedtrc(97,NJ06)<NJ-VIRTUAHS, NJ-VIRTVOOR>
+ Advocare DelGiorno Pediatrics
527 South Black Horse Pike Blackwood, NJ 08012 (856)302-5322 Fax (856)245-7719
+ Advocare DelGiorno Pediatrics
412 Ewan Road Mullica Hill, NJ 08062 (856)302-5322 Fax (856)343-3919

Salvatore, Augusto G., MD {1447212154} IntrMd(83,ITAL)
+ 65 Mountain Boulevard Ext/Suite 209
Warren, NJ 07059 (732)469-7290 Fax (732)469-7917
+ 67 Walnut Avenue/Suite 402
Clark, NJ 07066 (732)469-7290 Fax (732)396-8445

Salvatore, Francis P., Jr., MD {1750328787} EmrgMd(80,PA09)<NJ-ACMCITY, NJ-ACMCMAIN>
+ AtlantiCare Regional Medical Center/City Campus
1925 Pacific Avenue/EmrgMed Atlantic City, NJ 08401 (609)345-4000

Salvatore, Frank Timothy, MD {1215908611} Urolgy(88,DC01)<NJ-NWTNMEM, NJ-HCKTSTWN>
+ Skylands Urology Group
89 Sparta Avenue/Suite 200 Sparta, NJ 07871 (973)726-7220 Fax (973)726-7230
fsalvatore@skylandsurology.com
+ Skylands Urology Group
616 Willow Grove Street Hackettstown, NJ 07840 (973)726-7220 Fax (973)726-7230
+ Specialty Surgical Center
380 Lafayette Road/Suite 110 Sparta, NJ 07871 (973)940-3166 Fax (973)940-3170

Salvatore, Joseph E., Jr., MD {1356401863} Psychy(97,PA09)
+ 20 Nassau Street
Princeton, NJ 08540 (609)252-0777 Fax (609)252-0778

Salvatore, Kate Elizabeth, MD {1578781274} PsyCAd(97,NY47)
+ 3 Woodview Drive
Cranbury, NJ 08512

Physicians by Name and Address

Salvatore, Michelle Lyn, MD {1902988371} ObsGyn(97,NJ06)
+ Cooper Ob-Gyn
1900 Mount Holly Road/Suite 3-C   Burlington, NJ 08016
(609)835-5570

Salvatore, Paolo A., MD {1043516636}
+ 28 Helen Street
Warren, NJ 07059
Paolo30nedo@gmail.com

Salvia, Joseph V., DO {1134157761} PedPul(82,PA77)<NJ-ACMC-ITY, NJ-ACMCMAIN>
+ AtlantiCare/Dupont Children's Health Program
2500 English Creek Avenue   Egg Harbor Township, NJ 08234
(609)641-3700   Fax (609)641-3652

Salvo, Anthony, MD {1841236080} FamMed(89,MEX03)
+ AtlantiCare Family Medicine
120 South White Horse Pike   Hammonton, NJ 08037
(609)561-4211   Fax (609)561-0639

Salvo, John Paul, Jr., MD {1073695458} SrgOrt, SprtMd(94,PA02)<NJ-COOPRUMC>
+ Rothman Institute - Egg Harbor Township
2500 English Creek Avenue/Bldg 1300   Egg Harbor Township, NJ 08234   (609)677-7002   Fax (609)677-7000

Salvo, Victor J., MD {1780658476} OccpMd, IntrMd(84,NY08)<NJ-KIMBALL>
+ Kimball Medical Center
600 River Avenue   Lakewood, NJ 08701   (732)363-1900

Salwitz, James C., MD {1811986706} MedOnc, OncHem(81,NJ06)<NJ-RWJUBRUN, NJ-STPETER>
+ Central Jersey Oncology Center, P.A.
Brier Hill Court/Building J-2   East Brunswick, NJ 08816
(732)390-7750   Fax (732)390-7725
+ Regional Cancer Care Associates - Central Jersey Div
454 Elizabeth Avenue/Suite 240   Somerset, NJ 08873
(732)390-7750   Fax (732)390-7725
+ Central Jersey Oncology Center, P.A.
205 Easton Avenue   New Brunswick, NJ 08816   (732)828-9570   Fax (732)828-7638

Salyer, Robert Harold, DO {1013170554} Pedtrc
+ St Barnabas Medical Center Pediatrics
94 Old Short Hills Road   Livingston, NJ 07039   (808)983-6000

Salz, Alan G., MD {1497845309} Ophthl, IntrMd(81,MA05)
+ The Eye Specialists, P.A.
745 Route 202/206/Suite 301   Bridgewater, NJ 08807
(908)231-1110   Fax (908)526-4959

Salz, David Andrew, MD {1760700355} Ophthl(10,MA05)
+ The Eye Specialists, P.A.
745 Route 202/206/Suite 301   Bridgewater, NJ 08807
(908)231-1110   Fax (908)526-4959

Salzano, Brian Christopher, MD {1366555047} Ophthl(02,NJ05)
+ Salzano Eye Center LLC
526 Bloomfield Avenue   Caldwell, NJ 07006

Salzberg, Felix, MD {1285709519} Psychy(77,AZE01)
+ 1771 Springdale Road
Cherry Hill, NJ 08003

Salzer, Richard L., Jr., MD {1508810300} SprtMd, SrgMcr, SrgOrt(73,MA07)<NJ-ENGLWOOD, NJ-HOLYNAME>
+ Englewood Orthopedic Associates
401 South Van Brunt Street/3 FL   Englewood, NJ 07631
(201)569-2770   Fax (201)569-1774

Salzman, Matthew Scott, MD {1659320935} EmrgMd, IntrMd(01,PA02)<NJ-COOPRUMC>
+ Cooper University Medical Center/Camden
3 Cooper Plaza/Suite 502   Camden, NJ 08103   (856)356-4935
+ Cooper University Hospital
One Cooper Plaza/Emerg Med   Camden, NJ 08103
(856)342-2627

Samaan, Ayman Boushra, MD {1710212642} Anesth(90,EGY05)<NJ-JFKMED>
+ James Street Anesthesia
102 James Street/Suite 103   Edison, NJ 08820   (732)494-1444   Fax (732)494-7052

Samach, Michael A., MD {1861508566} Gastrn, IntrMd(71,NY19)
+ Affiliates in Gastroenterology, P.A.
101 Madison Avenue/Suite 100   Morristown, NJ 07960
(973)455-0404   Fax (973)540-8788

Samad, Ambreen Shariq, MD {1013147131} Pedtrc
+ Henry J. Austin Health Center
112 Ewing Street   Trenton, NJ 08618   (609)396-9600   Fax (609)396-1526

Samad, Arbaz, MD {1831346683}
+ 100 American Road
Morris Plains, NJ 07950   (973)971-6226
arbaz.samad@atlantichealth.org

Samad, Fatima, MD {1447566849}
+ 40 Conger Street
Bloomfield, NJ 07003   (973)337-0925

Samaddar, Soumen, MD {1790004752} FamMed, IntrMd(07,NJ06)
+ Hopewell Family Practice & Sports Medicine
84 Route 31 North/Suite 103   Pennington, NJ 08534

(609)730-1771   Fax (609)730-1274

Samadi, Sharyar Daniel, MD {1124075460} OtIryg, PedOto(96,MD07)<NJ-HACKNSK>
+ Drs. Samadi and Bar-Eli
10 Forest Avenue/Suite 100   Paramus, NJ 07652   (201)996-1505   Fax (201)996-1605
+ Hackensack University Medical Center
20 Prospect Avenue/Ste903/Otolaryn   Hackensack, NJ 07601   (201)996-1505   Fax (201)996-1605

Samaha, Simon J., MD {1144304536} IntrMd(92,LEB01)<NJ-COOPRUMC>
+ Cooper University Hospital
One Cooper Plaza/Ste 222/Dorr   Camden, NJ 08103
(856)342-2000

Samandar, Steve, MD {1639331804} FamMed(07,NET09)
+ Get Well House Call, P.C.
7319 Coventry Court   Riverdale, NJ 07457   (973)370-0052
md@getwellhousecalls.com

Samaniego, Eduardo W., MD {1699930123} FamMed(03,ECUA)
+ 70 Prospect Street
Newark, NJ 07105   (973)344-1313   Fax (973)344-1811

Samanta, Arun K., MD {1356436646} Gastrn, Hepato, SrgTpl(70,INDI)<NJ-UMDNJ>
+ UMDNJ Division of Gastroenterology & Hepatology
90 Bergen Street/DOC 2100   Newark, NJ 07103   (973)972-2343   Fax (973)972-0752
+ Rutgers- New Jersey Medical School
185 South Orange Avenue/RM H-538   Newark, NJ 07103
(973)972-2343   Fax (973)972-3144

Samara, Arafat A., MD {1265739254} ObsGyn<NJ-HACKNSK>
+ Hackensack Hospital Obs/Gyn
30 Prospect Avenue/4E-90   Hackensack, NJ 07601
(201)996-2755

Sambandan, Rama Thirugnana, MD {1063501609} IntrMd(70,INA47)
+ 80 Hazlet Avenue
Hazlet, NJ 07730   (732)264-5253   Fax (732)335-9768

Sambasivan, Roshni D., MD {1841585668} NnPnMd<NJ-UNVM-CPRN>
+ University Medical Center of Princeton at Plainsboro
One Plainsboro Road   Plainsboro, NJ 08536   (609)853-7626
roshnisambasivan@gmail.com

Sambol, Elliot Brett, MD {1336391499} SrgVas, Surgry(07,NJ05)
+ Princeton Surgical Associates, P.A.
5 Plainsboro Road/Suite 400   Plainsboro, NJ 08536
(609)936-9100   Fax (609)936-9700

Sambol, Justin Todd, MD {1376523266} Surgry, SrgThr(97,NJ05)<NJ-UMDNJ>
+ University Hospital
150 Bergen Street/Surgery/F-102   Newark, NJ 07103
(973)972-4300   Fax (973)972-3510
Sambol@umdnj.edu

Sambucci, Deborah A., DO {1518167311} CdvDis, IntrMd(02,NJ75)
+ 512 Middlesex Drive
Moorestown, NJ 08057
+ Cardiovascular Associates of The Delaware Valley, PA
525 State Street/Suite 3   Elmer, NJ 08318   Fax (856)358-0725

Samedi, Vanessa M., MD {1346799152} Pedtrc
+ 25 Shawnee Trail
Denville, NJ 07834   (908)472-5800

Samet, Elliott, MD {1366521536} Pedtrc(81,FRA24)<NJ-HACKNSK>
+ 160 Pennington Avenue
Passaic, NJ 07055   (973)591-1600   Fax (973)591-1605

Samiev, Djamshed, MD {1902245178} IntHos
+ Capital Health Hospitalist Group
750 Brunswick Avenue   Trenton, NJ 08638   (609)394-6031
Fax (609)394-6299

Saminathan, Thamarai, MD {1245268333} PthClLab(78,INA77)<NJ-UNVMCPRN>
+ Pathology Associates of Princeton
253 Witherspoon Street   Princeton, NJ 08540   (609)497-4351   Fax (609)497-4982

Samineni, Sankar Anand, MD {1205131976} IntrMd, IntHos(03,INA1L)<NJ-CHOSHUDC>
+ Children's Hospital of Hudson County
355 Grand Street/Internal Med   Jersey City, NJ 07302
(201)915-2430

Sammarone, Marcello Eliseo, MD {1881755510} Anesth, PainMd(83,ITA26)<NJ-STBARNMC>
+ Advanced Pain Therapy
680 Broadway/Suite 108   Paterson, NJ 07514   (973)294-6228   Fax (800)935-0791

Sammartino, Robert A., DO {1336247451} Nrolgy(90,FL75)
+ 445 Hurffville-Cross Keys/Suite B-8
Sewell, NJ 08080   (856)589-7740   Fax (856)256-0291

Samonte, Catherine Marie, MD {1538459771}
+ Clark Pediatrics LLC
480 Oak Ridge Road   Clark, NJ 07066   (908)463-0928   Fax (732)574-0907

cmsamonte@gmail.com

Sampson, Ruby J., MD {1619982014} Gastrn, IntrMd(83,NJ05)<NY-STBARNAB, NJ-NWRKBETH>
+ 106 Valley Street/Suite 1
South Orange, NJ 07079   (973)313-9300   Fax (973)313-2313

Samra, Asaad H., MD {1285661793} SrgPlstc, SrgHnd(01,NJ06)
+ SAMRA Group
733 North Beers Street/Suite U-1   Holmdel, NJ 07733
(732)739-2100   Fax (732)739-0815
+ Bayshore Wound Care Center
723 North Beers Street/2 West   Holmdel, NJ 07733
(732)497-1611
+ SAMRA Group
300 Perrine Road/Suite 333 & 334   Old Bridge, NJ 07733
(732)739-2100   Fax (732)739-0815

Samra, Fares, MD {1598026148} SrgPlstc
+ SAMRA Group
733 North Beers Street/Suite U-1   Holmdel, NJ 07733
(732)739-2100   Fax (732)739-0815

Samra, Mandeep Singh, MD {1184913865} IntrMd
+ University Hospital Medicine
150 Bergen Street/Room I-248   Newark, NJ 07103
(973)972-6056   Fax (973)972-3129

Samra, Matthew Samuel, DO {1225171382} SrgThr(99,MO79)<NJ-DEBRAHLC>
+ Surgical Specialists of New Jersey
37 Nautilus Drive   Manahawkin, NJ 08050   (609)978-0778
Fax (609)978-1377
+ Deborah Heart and Lung Center
200 Trenton Road   Browns Mills, NJ 08015   (609)978-0778
Fax (609)735-0175

Samra, Said A., MD {1023080140} SrgPlstc, Surgry, SrgHnd(73,SYRI)<NJ-BAYSHORE>
+ SAMRA Group
733 North Beers Street/Suite U-1   Holmdel, NJ 07733
(732)739-2100   Fax (732)739-0815
+ SAMRA Group
300 Perrine Road/Suite 333 & 334   Old Bridge, NJ 08857
(732)739-2100   Fax (732)739-0815

Samra, Salem, MD {1609050939} SrgRec, SrgPHand, IntrMd(06,TX04)
+ SAMRA Group
733 North Beers Street/Suite U-1   Holmdel, NJ 07733
(732)739-2100   Fax (732)727-8039
+ SAMRA Group
300 Perrine Road/Suite 333 & 334   Old Bridge, NJ 08857
(732)739-2100   Fax (732)739-0815

Samra Latif Estafan, Omnia M., MD {1174515902} ObsGyn(98,NJ05)<NJ-RWJUBRUN>
+ Hamilton Women's Health & Wellness Associates
311 White Horse Avenue/Suite D   Hamilton, NJ 08610
(609)589-0185   Fax (609)588-0418
my_doctor@verizon.net

Samsa, Ranka Drazenovic, MD {1962514018} Nephro, IntrMd(86,CRO01)<NJ-MTNSIDE>
+ South Mountain Nephrology
5 Franklin Avenue/Suite 401   Belleville, NJ 07109
(973)450-8999

Samson, Kristine T., MD {1124003272} EmrgMd(00,NY08)<NY-JA-COBIMC>
+ EMedical Urgent Care
2 Kings Highway   Middletown, NJ 07748   (732)957-0707
Fax (732)957-9852

Samson-Bacarro, Edna A., MD {1811024565} ObsGyn(86,PHI21)
+ 44 Pebble Beach Drive
Egg Harbor Township, NJ 08234   (609)927-0647   Fax (609)927-0649

Samson-Daclan, Maria Teresa, MD {1447276043} Psychy(88,PHI21)<NJ-ACMCITY>
+ AtlantiCare Behavioral Health/Pact Team A
2511 Fire Road/Suite B-10   Egg Harbor Township, NJ 08234
(609)407-0042   Fax (609)407-0185
+ AtlantiCare Behavioral Health/Cornerstone
6010 Black Horse Pike   Egg Harbor Township, NJ 08234
(609)407-0042   Fax (609)646-8715
+ AtlantiCare Behav Hlth/Hartford
13 North Hartford Avenue   Atlantic City, NJ 08234
(609)348-1161

Samuel, Anish, MD {1891012332} CdvDis<NJ-STJOSHOS>
+ Heart & Vascular Associates of Northern Jersey
22-18 Broadway/Suite 201   Fair Lawn, NJ 07410   (201)475-5050   Fax (201)475-5522

Samuel, Hala R., MD {1801972989} Pedtrc(89,EGYP)
+ Parkview Pediatrics Group PC
32 Hine Street/Suite 209   Paterson, NJ 07503   (973)345-2420   Fax (973)345-3786

Samuel, Ramez W., MD {1447303417} IntrMd(93,EGY04)<NJ-STCLRDEN>
+ 132 Mckinley Place
Rockaway, NJ 07866

Samuel, Salim, MD {1003892407} Radiol, RadNro(94,PA01)<NJ-RWJUBRUN, NJ-STPETER>
+ University Radiology Group, P.C.
483 Cranbury Road   East Brunswick, NJ 08816   (732)390-0030   Fax (732)390-5383
+ University Radiology Group, P.C.
48 Gilbert Street North   Tinton Falls, NJ 07701   (732)390-0030   Fax (732)530-5848
+ University Radiology Group, P.C.
260 Amboy Avenue   Metuchen, NJ 08816   (732)548-2322   Fax (732)548-3392

Samuel, Shyno, MD {1376027011} FamMed
+ Alnajar Medical PC
89 Hudson Street/Suite 2   Hoboken, NJ 07030   (201)565-2537

Samuel, Steven Alan, MD {1346246600} CdvDis, IntrMd(78,NY46)<NJ-STFRNMED, NJ-RWJUHAM>
+ Mercer Bucks Cardiology
One Union Street/Suite 101   Robbinsville, NJ 08691   (609)890-6677   Fax (609)585-2520

Samuels, Elizabeth E., DO {1487082020}<NJ-SJHREGMC>
+ Patient first
606 Cross Keys Road   Sicklerville, NJ 08081   (856)237-1016
+ SJH Regional Medical Center
1505 West Sherman Avenue   Vineland, NJ 08360   (856)641-8000

Samuels, Francine, MD {1629144084} Pedtrc, PedGst(02,NY20)<NJ-HACKNSK>
+ Joseph M. Sanzari Childrens' -Gastro
155 Polifly Road/Suite 102   Hackensack, NJ 07601   (551)996-8840   Fax (201)441-9949
+ Hackensack University Medical Center
30 Prospect Avenue/Pedi GI   Hackensack, NJ 07601   (201)996-2000

Samuels, Marie Sophia, MD {1740449594} EmrgMd
+ 221 Ross Place/1st Floor
Westfield, NJ 07090

Samuels, Paul Louis, MD {1265421697} RadDia, NuclMd(99,PA13)<NJ-STPETER, NJ-RWJUBRUN>
+ University Radiology Group, P.C.
483 Cranbury Road   East Brunswick, NJ 08816   (732)390-0030   Fax (732)390-5383
+ University Radiology Group, P.C.
16 Mountain Boulevard   Warren, NJ 07059   (732)390-0030   Fax (908)769-9141

Samuels, Steven Charles, MD {1679623797} Psychy, PsyGrt(89,NY06)<NJ-ENGLWOOD>
+ 60 West Ridgewood Avenue/Third Floor
Ridgewood, NJ 07451

San Filippo, Steven Charles, MD {1578991840}<NJ-HUNTRDN>
+ Hunterdon Medical Center
2100 Wescott Drive   Flemington, NJ 08822   (908)788-6160

San Juan, Severiano, Jr., MD {1891701595} Pedtrc(73,PHIL)<NJ-NWRKBETH>
+ 2040 Millburn Avenue/Suite 302
Maplewood, NJ 07040   (973)762-0035   Fax (973)762-0402

Sanakkayala, Nirmala D., MD {1073577870} ObsGyn(70,INDI)<NJ-RIVERVW, NJ-BAYSHORE>
+ 717 North Beers Street
Holmdel, NJ 07733   (732)264-3442   Fax (732)264-0973

Sanandaji, Mehrdad, MD {1376500306} IntrMd(66,CA11)
+ 1124 East Ridgewood Avenue/Suite 103
Ridgewood, NJ 07450   (201)445-9221   Fax (201)612-1439

Sananman, Michael L., MD {1407826514} Nrolgy(64,NY01)
+ Neurological Associates PA
700 North Broad Street/Suite 201   Elizabeth, NJ 07208   (908)354-3994   Fax (908)354-0429

Sancheti, Vinod T., MD {1437176088} IntrMd, Grtrcs(89,INDI)<NJ-COMMED, NJ-MONMOUTH>
+ 25 Mule Road/Unit B8
Toms River, NJ 08755   (732)240-4000   Fax (732)240-1441
+ 307 Route 70/Suite 1-A
Lakehurst, NJ 08733   (732)240-4000   Fax (732)657-7747

Sanchez, Bienvenido, MD {1538277033} IntrMd(85,DOMI)<NJ-HOBUNIMC>
+ Bergenline Medical Center
5005 Bergenline Avenue   West New York, NJ 07093   (201)864-2200   Fax (201)864-9758

Sanchez, Carlos Alfonso, DO {1255624896} FamMed(10,NY75)
+ CityMD Newark Urgent Care
617 Broad Street   Newark, NJ 07102   (862)246-7940   Fax (862)246-7941

Sanchez, Daniel Antonio, MD {1346284148} EmrgMd, Pedtrc(87,DOM11)<NJ-STBARNMC>
+ St. Barnabas Medical Center
94 Old Short Hills Road   Livingston, NJ 07039   (973)322-5000

Sanchez, Daniel Rene, MD {1164482428} Psychy(82,DOM02)<NY-STBARNAB>
+ North Jersey Psychiatry
5912 Palisade Avenue   West New York, NJ 07093   (201)861-0077   Fax (201)861-9595

Dsanchez31@msn.com

Sanchez, Guillermo R., MD {1740299676} PedCrd, Pedtrc(76,NY01)
+ CHOP Pediatric & Adolescent Specialty Care Center
1012 Laurel Oak Road   Voorhees, NJ 08043   (856)435-0086   Fax (856)435-0091
+ Children's Hospital of Phila Cardio
1040 Laurel Oak Road/Suite 1   Voorhees, NJ 08043   (856)435-0086   Fax (856)783-0657
+ CHOP Pediatric & Adolescent Specialty Care Center
707 Alexander Road/Suite 205   Princeton, NJ 08043   (609)520-1717

Sanchez, Hector J., MD {1740231760} Surgry(69,DOMI)<NJ-RWJURAH>
+ Robert Wood Johnson University Hospital at Rahway
865 Stone Street/Surgery   Rahway, NJ 07065   (732)381-4200

Sanchez, Israel L., MD {1205823523} Anesth(81,DOMI)
+ Hamilton Anesthesia and Pain Management
1 Hamilton Health Place   Hamilton, NJ 08690   (609)631-6824   Fax (609)631-6839

Sanchez, John Paul, MD {1720303035} EmrgMd(06,NY46)<NJ-UMDNJ>
+ University Hospital
150 Bergen Street/M-219   Newark, NJ 07103   (973)972-9377   Fax (973)972-6646

Sanchez, Manuel I., MD {1407828999} PsyGrt, Psychy(82,ECUA)<NJ-STMICHL>
+ St. Michael's Medical Center
268 MLK Jr. Boulevard/Psych   Newark, NJ 07102   (973)877-5000

Sanchez, Mauricio Jorge, MD {1215971783} IntrMd, EmrgMd(86,PER01)<NJ-JFKMED>
+ 845 Kearny Avenue
Kearny, NJ 07032   (201)991-1129   Fax (201)991-2799

Sanchez, Miguel A., MD {1497708788} PthAcl, Pthlgy(69,SPAI)<NJ-ENGLWOOD>
+ Englewood Hospital and Medical Center
350 Engle Street/Pathology   Englewood, NJ 07631   (201)894-3423   Fax (201)871-2269

Sanchez, Orestes, MD {1376530857} RadDia, Radiol, RadV&I(79,MEX03)<NJ-STJOSHOS>
+ St. Joseph's Regional Medical Center
703 Main Street/Radiology   Paterson, NJ 07503   (973)754-2645   Fax (973)754-3181
sanchezo@sjhmc.org
+ St. Joseph's Regional MedCtr-Ambulatory Imaging Ctr
1135 Broad Street/3rd Floor/Suite 4   Clifton, NJ 07013   (973)569-9300

Sanchez, Sergio, MD {1962454494} IntrMd(83,DOM04)<NJ-STPETER, NJ-RWJUBRUN>
+ 183 Livingston Avenue
New Brunswick, NJ 08901   (732)846-1900   Fax (732)294-6069
Sergiosanchezmd@yahoo.com

Sanchez Konel, Maria E., MD {1932138880} Pedtrc(80,ECU05)<NJ-STBARNMC>
+ St. Barnabas Medical Center
94 Old Short Hills Road/Pediatrics   Livingston, NJ 07039   (973)322-5000   Fax (973)322-8833

Sanchez Pena, Jose R., MD {1316911282} Grtrcs, IntrMd, PulDis(77,DOM04)
+ 583 Broadway
Paterson, NJ 07514   (973)653-5686   Fax (973)221-8255

Sanchez Trejo, Hernan Alberto, MD {1669887105}<NJ-MORRISTN>
+ Morristown Medical Center
100 Madison Avenue   Morristown, NJ 07962   (973)971-5000

Sanchez-Catanese, Betty, MD {1821055450} IntrMd(83,NY09)
+ 315 East Main Street
Somerville, NJ 08876   (908)722-3442   Fax (908)526-5623

Sancho Mora, Elda P., MD {1003972423} Psychy, PsyFor(91,COS01)<NY-BLVUENYU, NJ-MORRISTN>
+ Morristown Medical Center
100 Madison Avenue   Morristown, NJ 07962   (973)971-5000

Sandau, Roy Lee, DO {1124228788} Surgry, IntrMd
+ Advocare Associates in General Surgery
2201 Chapel Avenue West/Suite 100   Cherry Hill, NJ 08002   (856)665-2017   Fax (856)488-6769
+ Advocare Associates in General Surgery
570 Egg Harbor Road/Suite C-2   Sewell, NJ 08080   (856)665-2017   Fax (856)256-7789
+ Comprehensive Cancer & Hematology Specialists, P.C.
705 White Horse Road   Voorhees, NJ 08002   (856)435-1777   Fax (856)435-0696

Sandberg, Marc Ira, MD {1770557837} EnDbMt, IntrMd(90,PA13)<NJ-HUNTRDN>
+ Diabetes & Endocrine Associates of Hunterdon
9100 Westcott Drive/Suite 101   Flemington, NJ 08822   (908)237-6990   Fax (908)237-6995

Sandeep, Rashmi, MD {1407836711} Pedtrc, AdolMd(93,INA28)<NJ-OCEANMC>
+ Brick Pediatric Group
1301 Route 70   Brick, NJ 08724   (732)892-8700   Fax (732)892-6689

Sanden, Mats Olof, MD {1093730954} Pthlgy, PthAcl(88,SWE04)<NJ-SJHREGMC, NJ-SJRSYELM>
+ SJH Regional Medical Center
1505 West Sherman Avenue/Path   Vineland, NJ 08360   (856)641-8000
+ PLUS Diagnostics
1200 River Avenue/Suite 10   Lakewood, NJ 08701   (856)641-8000   Fax (732)901-1555

Sanders, Linda M., MD {1982639431} Radiol, RadDia(82,PA01)<NJ-STBARNMC>
+ St. Barnabas Medical Center
94 Old Short Hills Road/Radiology   Livingston, NJ 07039   (973)322-5000

Sanders, Paul, MD {1386618387} Anesth(91,NY46)<NJ-HACKNSK>
+ Hackensack University Medical Center
30 Prospect Avenue/Anesthesiology   Hackensack, NJ 07601   (201)996-2000   (201)488-6769
+ Hackensack University MC-Anesthesia Dept
30 Prospect Avenue/Room 2703   Hackensack, NJ 07601   (201)996-2000   Fax (201)996-3962

Sanderson, James Glen, DO {1154328193} FamMed(00,NJ75)<NJ-BAYONNE, NJ-CHRIST>
+ James G. Sanderson DO Family Practice P.C.
3 Webster Avenue   Jersey City, NJ 07307   (201)216-1505   Fax (201)216-8803
+ Carepoint Health Medical Group
1166 Kennedy Boulevard   Bayonne, NJ 07002   (201)216-1505   Fax (201)339-1073

Sanderson, Rhonda, MD {1982627253} ObsGyn(80,PA09)<NJ-OVERLOOK>
+ 8 Mountain Blvd/Suite B
Warren, NJ 07059   (908)754-5775   Fax (908)754-5740

Sandhu, Baldev S., MD {1255458105} SrgPlstc, Dermat(79,SCO05)<NJ-ENGLWOOD, NJ-MEADWLND>
+ 600 Palisade Avenue
Englewood Cliffs, NJ 07632   (201)337-6286
sandhuplas@gmail.com

Sandhu, Basant Singh, MD {1265795744} FamMed
+ Forest HealthCare Associates, PC
277 Forest Avenue/Suite 200   Paramus, NJ 07652   (201)986-1881   Fax (201)986-1871

Sandhu, Bhavna, MD {1841436359} IntrMd<NJ-RWJUBRUN>
+ 1440 How Lane/Suite 2D
North Brunswick, NJ 08902   (732)993-8760
+ RWJ University Hospital New Brunswick
One Robert Wood Johnson Place   New Brunswick, NJ 08901   (732)828-3000

Sandhu, Jagwinder S., MD {1821187691} Psychy, PsyCAd(95,INA03)<NJ-RWJUBRUN, NJ-STPETER>
+ 194 North Harrison Street
Princeton, NJ 08540   (609)751-6607

Sandhu, Mohammad Y., MD {1568405702} CdvDis, IntrMd(70,PAKI)
+ Essex Hudson Cardiology Service
672 Broadway   Bayonne, NJ 07002   (201)339-3710

Sandhu, Narinder, MD {1194021741}<NY-METHODST>
+ United Medical, P.C.
988 Broadway/Suite 201   Bayonne, NJ 07002   (201)339-6111   Fax (201)339-6333

Sandhu, Parminderjeet S., MD {1033298252} Gastrn, IntrMd(77,INA6Z)<NJ-HCKTSTWN>
+ Medical Care Associates
137 Mountain Avenue   Hackettstown, NJ 07840   (908)852-1887   Fax (908)852-0614
+ Medical Care Associates
262 Route 10 West   Succasunna, NJ 07876   (908)852-1887   Fax (908)252-1422

Sandhu, Sarbjit Singh, MD {1760708093} InfDis, IntrMd<NJ-MONMOUTH>
+ ID Associates PA/dba ID Care
105 Raider Boulevard/Suite 101   Hillsborough, NJ 08844   (908)281-0221   Fax (908)281-0890

Sandhu, Sartaj S., MD {1992938039} EnDbMt
+ Advocare DelGiorno Endocrinology
239 Hurffville Cross-Keys Road   Sewell, NJ 08080   (856)728-3636   Fax (856)728-3633

Sandhu, Surinderjeet S., MD {1407839418} Psychy, PsyGrt(82,INDI)
+ Preferred Behavioral Health of New Jersey
700 Airport Road   Lakewood, NJ 08701   (732)367-4700   Fax (732)364-2253

Sandhu, Vineet, MD {1891083127} IntrMd
+ Medical Care Associates
137 Mountain Avenue   Hackettstown, NJ 07840   (908)852-1887   Fax (908)852-0614

Physicians by Name and Address

Sandilya, Vijay Krishna, MD {1801118906} OncHem, IntrMd(02,INA92)
 + AtlantiCare Cancer Institute
  2500 English Creek Avenue/Building 400 Egg Harbor Township, NJ 08234 (609)677-7777 Fax (609)677-7727
 + AtlantiCare Cancer Institute
  106 Courthouse South Dennis Rd Cape May Court, NJ 08210 (609)677-7777 Fax (609)463-3224

Sandler, Leonard Lewis, MD {1184603227} CdvDis, IntrMd(97,PA07)<NJ-SOCEANCO, NJ-COMMED>
 + Shore Heart Group, P.A.
  1820 State Route 33/Suite 4-B Neptune, NJ 07753 (732)776-8500 Fax (732)776-8946
 + Shore Heart Group, P.A.
  35 Beaverson Boulevard/Suite 9-B Brick, NJ 08723 (732)776-8500 Fax (732)262-4317
 + Shore Heart Group, P.A.
  555 Iron Bridge Road/Suite 15 Freehold, NJ 07753 (732)308-0774 Fax (732)333-1366

Sandler, Matthew Jay, MD {1255302915} CdvDis, IntrMd, ClCdEl(86,NY08)<NJ-OURLADY, NJ-COOPRUMC>
 + Associated Cardiovascular Consultants-Lourdes
  1 Brace Road/Suite C & F Cherry Hill, NJ 08034 (856)428-4100 Fax (856)428-0856

Sandler, Rebecca Ellen, MD {1831394527} IntrMd(07,OH40)<NY-NYUTISCH>
 + Summit Medical Group
  6 Brighton Road/2 FL Clifton, NJ 07012 (973)777-7911 Fax (973)777-5403
 + Bergen Medical Associates
  466 Old Hook Road/Suite 1 Emerson, NJ 07630 (973)777-7911 Fax (201)967-0340

Sandor, Earl V., MD {1740377704} Ophthl(80,NY20)<NJ-HACKNSK, NJ-MTNSIDE>
 + 71 Summit Avenue
  Hackensack, NJ 07601 (201)342-0006 Fax (201)342-0038
 + 94 Park Street
  Montclair, NJ 07042 (201)342-0006 Fax (973)746-2453

Sandoval, Marina Penteado, MD {1487978862} DrmtPthy
 + The Dermatology Group, P.C.
  347 Mount Pleasant Avenue/Suite 103 West Orange, NJ 07052 (973)571-2121 Fax (973)498-0535
 + The Dermatology Group, P.C.
  44 Route 23 North/Suite 213 Riverdale, NJ 07457 (973)571-2121 Fax (973)839-5751
 + The Dermatology Group, P.C.
  310 Madison Avenue/Suite 206 Morristown, NJ 07052 (973)571-2121 Fax (973)539-1180

Sandoval, Ramon Antonio, MD {1316032014} IntrMd(76,DOMI)
 + Centro-Ibero-Americano
  406 Mountain Avenue Franklin Lakes, NJ 07417 (973)684-8138
 + Centro Medico Iberoamericano
  416 Park Avenue Paterson, NJ 07501 (973)684-8138 Fax (973)684-0032

Sandoval-Castellanos, Oscar E., MD {1811945595} Psychy(78,COLO)<NJ-MEADWLND>
 + Sandoval, Oscar E
  569 35th Street Union City, NJ 07087 (201)866-6970 Fax (201)866-7144

Sandru, Dan Victor, MD {1548442031} FamMed(99,ROM06)<NJ-CENTRAST>
 + CentraState Medical Center
  901 West Main Street Freehold, NJ 07728 (732)431-2000

Sandy, Lewis G., MD IntrMd(82,MI01)
 + Robert Wood Johnson Foundation
  PO Box 2316 Princeton, NJ 08540 (609)627-5940 Fax (609)452-1865

Sanfilippo, James Arthur, MD {1568596328} SrgOrt(NJ02<NJ-VIRTUAHS, NJ-KENEDYHS>
 + Reconstructive Orthopedics, P.A.
  401 Young Avenue/Suite 245 Moorestown, NJ 08057 (609)267-9400 Fax (609)267-9457

Sang Urai, Chintana, MD {1568425601} EmrgMd<NJ-RBAYPERT>
 + Raritan Bay Medical Center/Perth Amboy Division
  530 New Brunswick Avenue/EmrgMed Perth Amboy, NJ 08861 (732)442-3700

Sangam, Subhasri L., MD {1235391400} NnPnMd, Pedtrc(92,INA1L)
 + 1215 Wessex Place
  Princeton, NJ 08540

Sangavaram, Kristappa, MD {1376635722} Anesth, CritCr, PainMd(70,INA28)
 + Precision Pain Management Center
  303 Molnar Drive/1st Floor Elmwood Park, NJ 07407 (201)796-4007 Fax (201)796-4080

Sanghani, Nipa Vijay, MD {1528204187} Pedtrc, PedEmg<NJ-STPETER>
 + St. Peter's University Hospital
  254 Easton Avenue New Brunswick, NJ 08901 (732)937-6009

Sanghavi, Maya M., MD {1487693255} Gyneco(69,INDI)<NJ-JFKMED>
 + 1550 Park Avenue
  South Plainfield, NJ 07080 (908)757-4448 Fax (908)757-0802

Sanghi, Swathi, MD {1437387016}<NJ-OCEANMC>
 + Ocean Medical Center
  425 Jack Martin Boulevard Brick, NJ 08723 (732)836-4817

Sanghui, Sarika Patel, DO {1851603922} IntrMd
 + 53 Sapphire Lane
  Franklin Park, NJ 08823 (732)690-2698

Sanghvi, Kintur Arvindbhai, MD {1770627200} CdvDis, IntrMd, IntCrd(96,INA8B)<NJ-DEBRAHLC>
 + Deborah Heart and Lung Center
  200 Trenton Road/Cardio Browns Mills, NJ 08015 (609)735-2907

Sanghvi, Shimal H., MD {1689932675} EmrgMd<NJ-JRSYCITY>
 + Jersey City Medical Center
  355 Grand Street/EmergMed Jersey City, NJ 07304 (201)915-2000

Sangosse, Louis V., MD {1487694964} IntrMd, PulDis, CritCr(76,HAI01)<NJ-STBARNMC, NJ-EASTORNG>
 + Louis V. Sangosse MD PA
  745 Northfield Avenue West Orange, NJ 07052 (973)731-0200 Fax (973)325-2244

Sangosse, Marie C., MD {1952358178} IntrMd, OncHem(75,HAIT)<NJ-STBARNMC, NJ-EASTORNG>
 + Louis V. Sangosse MD PA
  745 Northfield Avenue West Orange, NJ 07052 (973)731-0200 Fax (973)325-2244

Sanicola-Johnson, Julie Marie, DO {1235391673} EmrgMd<NJ-STJOSHOS>
 + St. Joseph's Regional Medical Center
  703 Main Street/EmergMed Paterson, NJ 07503 (973)754-2000

Saniewski, Charles A., MD {1336146877} Radiol, RadDia(83,ITAL)<NJ-RWJURAH, NJ-TRINIWSC>
 + Doctors Radiology Center - MRI of Woodbridge
  1500 St. George Avenue/Peach Plaza Avenel, NJ 07001 (732)574-1414 Fax (732)574-0845
 + Red Bank Radiologists, P.A.
  200 White Road/Suite 115 Little Silver, NJ 07739 (732)574-1414 Fax (732)741-0985
 + Coastal Imaging, LLC
  79 Route 37 West/Suite 103 Toms River, NJ 07001 (732)678-0087 Fax (732)276-2325

Sanjay, Priyanka, MD {1619913605} IntrMd(01,INA28)
 + Drs. Sanjay & Ramos
  216 Stelton Road/Suite 3B Piscataway, NJ 08854 (732)662-9959

Sanjuan, Racquel, DO {1295847713} Psychy(98,NJ75)
 + Rutgers Hurtado Health Center
  11 Bishop Place New Brunswick, NJ 08901 (732)932-7402 Fax (732)932-1223

Sankar, Wudbhav Nott, MD {1528128030} SrgOrt, PedOrt<PA-CHILDHOS>
 + CHOP Pediatric & Adolescent Specialty Care Center
  1012 Laurel Oak Road Voorhees, NJ 08043 (856)435-1300 Fax (856)435-0091

Sankary, Howard N., MD {1366481871} SrgTpl
 + Assoicates in Transplan & Surgery
  94 Old Short Hills Road Livingston, NJ 07039

Sankhla, Vijay R., MD {1770516031} Radiol, RadBdI(76,INA65)
 + 1451 Latache Court
  Toms River, NJ 08753

Sankholkar, Kedar Deepak, MD {1053561654} CdvDis, IntrMd(08,NY15)
 + Cardiology Center of North Jersey
  1030 Clifton Avenue Clifton, NJ 07013 (973)778-3777 Fax (973)778-3252

Sannoh, Sulaiman, MD {1740443936} NnPnMd, Pedtrc(95,RUS15)
 + St. Barnabas Health Care System
  99 Highway 37 West/Comm Medical Center Toms River, NJ 08755 (732)557-8070

Sansobrino, Daniel M., MD {1174726491} ObsGyn
 + Associates in Obstetrics Gynecology & Infertility
  375 Mount Pleasant Avenue/Suite 202 West Orange, NJ 07052 (973)731-7707 Fax (973)669-0277

Sant, Manasee Amol, MD {1558520130} Anesth
 + Summit Anesthesia Associates, P.A.
  33 Overlook Road/Suite 311 Summit, NJ 07901 (908)598-1500 Fax (908)598-0197

Santamaria, Jaime, II, MD {1104807015} Ophthl, Catrct, SrgRef(73,NY01)<NY-PRSBCOLU>
 + Santamaria Eye Center
  104 Market Street Perth Amboy, NJ 08861 (732)826-5159 Fax (732)826-2107 drjaime@earthlink.net
 + Santamaria Eye Center
  100 Menlo Park Drive/Suite 408 Edison, NJ 08837

 (732)826-5159 Fax (732)767-1871

Santamaria, Richard G., MD {1568488468} IntrMd(97,PA09)<PA-TJHSP>
 + Voorhees Specialty Center
  443 Laurel Oak Road/Suite 100 Voorhees, NJ 08043 (856)784-7398 Fax (856)784-7357

Santana, Jose O., MD {1497750848} IntrMd(85,PRO03)<NJ-HACKNSK, NJ-COMMED>
 + Hudson Heart Associates
  425 70th Street Guttenberg, NJ 07093 (201)854-0055 Fax (201)854-2633

Santangelo, Donato, III, MD {1720185879} IntrMd(82,GRN01)
 + Alpha Medical
  462 Lake Hurst Road Toms River, NJ 08755 (732)244-3050 Fax (732)244-2556
 + Alpha Medical
  65 Lacey Road/Suite E Whiting, NJ 08759 (732)849-0888

Santangelo, Steven Frank, DO {1255314175} FamMed, IntMAdMd(01,PA77)
 + Virtua Family Medicine - Cooper River
  6981 North Park Drive/Suite 200 Pennsauken, NJ 08109 (856)663-4949 Fax (856)663-6076

Santhanam, Shankar, MD {1982691432} FamMed, IntrMd(00,GRN01)<NJ-OVERLOOK>
 + Family Care Physicians at CPC
  1960 Brunswick Avenue Lawrenceville, NJ 08648 (609)392-6366 Fax (609)581-9082

Santiago, Arthur F., MD {1003860669} IntrMd, Nephro(83,NY20)
 + 307 Grove Street
  Rahway, NJ 07065 (732)382-3390 Fax (732)382-5206

Santiago, Derek W., MD {1649244732} CdvDis(88,NY01)
 + Comprehensive Cardiovascular Consultants
  299 Madison Avenue/Suite 102 Morristown, NJ 07960 (973)292-1020 Fax (973)292-0564
 + Mid-Atlantic Cardiology, PA
  218 State Route 17 North Rochelle Park, NJ 07662 (973)292-1020 Fax (908)889-5860

Santiago, Eddie W., MD {1497796973} IntrMd(98,PA09)
 + West Park Medical, LLC.
  100 Highway 36/Suite 2-K West Long Branch, NJ 07764 (732)531-6600 Fax (732)660-6606

Santiago, Maritza Marie, MD {1689677163} Pedtrc(80,DOM15)
 + Pediatric Associates of Central Jersey
  326 Main Street Metuchen, NJ 08840 (732)767-0630 Fax (732)767-3070

Santiago, Marivic F., MD {1801847462} Pedtrc, PedDvl(94,PHI07)<NJ-VALLEY>
 + UH-Robert Wood Jhnsn Med Sch
  97 Paterson Street/Pediatrics New Brunswick, NJ 08901

Santiago, Teodoro V., MD {1972676534} PulDis, IntrMd(67,PHI29)
 + UH- Robert Wood Johnson Med
  125 Paterson Street/Suite 2300 New Brunswick, NJ 08901 (732)828-3000

Santkovsky, Inna, MD {1821436676}
 + Jersey Shore Medical Center Obs/Gyn
  1945 Route 33 Neptune, NJ 07753 (732)776-3790

Santo Domingo, Jose E., MD {1457381956} NnPnMd, Pedtrc(68,PHI01)<NJ-STBARNMC>
 + St. Barnabas Medical Center
  94 Old Short Hills Road/Pediatrics Livingston, NJ 07039 (973)322-5437 Fax (973)322-8833

Santo Domingo, Norman E., MD {1083677553} Pedtrc(83,PHIL)<NJ-COMMED>
 + 800 Route 9
  Bayville, NJ 08721 (732)269-4100 Fax (732)269-2356

Santolaya, Joaquin, MD {1851338453} MtFtMd(80,SPA04)
 + UH- Robert Wood Johnson Med
  125 Paterson Street/MatFet/2nd Fl New Brunswick, NJ 08901 (732)235-8006 Fax (732)235-7349
 + UMDNJ RWJ Maternal Fetal Medicine
  125 Paterson Street/Suite 4200 New Brunswick, NJ 08901 (732)235-8006 Fax (732)235-6564

Santomauro, Emanuele A., MD {1053485243} CritCr, PulDis, IntrMd(88,WIND)<NJ-HACKNSK>
 + Hackensack University Medical Group PC
  160 Essex Street/Suite 103 Lodi, NJ 07644 (551)996-1370

Santoni, Francesco, MD {1821024696} ClCdEl, CdvDis, IntrMd(90,ITA06)<NY-LENOXHLL>
 + Summit Medical Group
  140 Park Avenue/3rd Floor Florham Park, NJ 07932 (973)404-9900 Fax (908)673-7108

Santora, Arthur Charles, II, MD {1952474520} EnDbMt, IntrMd(78,GA05)
 + UH- Robert Wood Johnson Med
  125 Paterson Street/Clinical New Brunswick, NJ 08901 (732)235-7219
  Art.Santora@attglobal.net

Santoro, Elissa J., MD {1528023405} Surgry, SrgOnc(65,PA07)<NJ-STBARNMC>
+ Breast Care & Treatment Center
200 South Orange Avenue   Livingston, NJ 07039   (973)533-0222   Fax (973)535-1121

Santoro, John J., DO {1245308196} Gastrn(78,PA77)<NJ-ACMC-ITY, NJ-ACMCMAIN>
+ Atlantic Gastroenterology Associates, P.A.
3205 Fire Road/Suite 4   Egg Harbor Township, NJ 08234   (609)407-1220   Fax (609)407-0220
+ Atlantic Gastroenterology Associates, P.A.
72 West Jimmie Leeds Road/Suite 2600   Galloway, NJ 08205   (609)407-1220   Fax (609)407-0220

Santoro, Stephanie Amanda, DO {1609026640} IntrMd(99,PA77)
+ Glendale Family Practice
363A Browning Road/Suite A   Bellmawr, NJ 08031   (856)931-6950   Fax (856)931-6951

Santos, Eduardo V., MD   IntrMd(75,PHIL)
+ 411 North Shore Road
Absecon, NJ 08201

Santos, Francis Parrocho, MD {1518284751} Anesth
+ West Jersey Anesthesia Assoc PA
102 Centre Boulevard/Suite East   Marlton, NJ 08053   (856)988-6260   Fax (856)988-6270

Santos, Frank, MD {1811941651} PsycCAd, Psychy(82,DOM02)
+ 115 River Road/Suite 305
Edgewater, NJ 07020   (201)941-4405   Fax (201)945-8501
drpsych520@aol.com

Santos, Luis A., MD {1205923869} EmrgMd(95,NY15)<NJ-CLAR-MAAS>
+ Clara Maass Medical Center
1 Clara Maass Drive/EmrgMed   Belleville, NJ 07109   (973)450-2000
+ Emergency Medical Associates of NJ, P.A.
3 Century Drive   Parsippany, NJ 07054   (973)450-2000   Fax (973)740-9895

Santos, Norman Verches, MD {1487730719} Surgry(71,PHIL)<NJ-SOMERSET>
+ SA HealthCare Management, LLC
145 Route 46 West/Suite 304   Wayne, NJ 07470   (973)826-8540   Fax (855)834-5434
+ RWJ University Hospital Somerset
110 Rehill Avenue/Surgery   Somerville, NJ 08876   (908)685-2200

Santos, Ray Ryan Crisostomo, MD {1821241381} Pedtrc, IntrMd(05,NJ05)<NJ-CHILTON>
+ Drs Medical Associates
115 Christopher Columbus Drive   Jersey City, NJ 07302   (201)706-3808   Fax (201)369-8032
+ Family Health & Wellness Center
909 Ringwood Avenue   Haskell, NJ 07420   (973)831-6700

Santos, Rodrigo R., MD {1194914556} Surgry(67,PHI01)
+ Haddon Surgical Associates PA
17 White Horse Pike/Suite 6   Haddon Heights, NJ 08035   (856)547-5522   Fax (856)547-0416

Santos, Santos S., MD {1932122421} GenPrc(68,PHI08)<NJ-STCLRBOO>
+ St. Clare's Hospital-Boonton
130 Powerville Road   Boonton, NJ 07005   (973)316-1800   Fax (973)316-1839

Santos Arias, Simon B., MD {1497721062} Surgry(72,DOM01)<NJ-MEADWLND>
+ 410 36th Street/1st Floor
Union City, NJ 07087   (201)863-7744   Fax (201)863-7608

Santos-Borja, Concepcion L., MD {1316988330} Pedtrc(77,PHI01)
+ Riverside ENT Pediatric Group
324 Palisade Avenue/2nd Floor   Jersey City, NJ 07307   (201)386-1400   Fax (201)386-2343
+ NHCAC Health Center at Union City
714 31st Street   Union City, NJ 07087   (201)386-1400   Fax (201)863-2730

Santos-Holgado, Maria C., MD {1164513875} Anesth(92,PHI01)
+ James Street Anesthesia
102 James Street/Suite 103   Edison, NJ 08820   (732)494-1444   Fax (732)494-2152

Sanusi, Akinlabi Adetayo, MD {1790126803}
+ 74 Brunswick Woods Drive
East Brunswick, NJ 08816   (732)306-3887
asanusi@tulane.edu

Sanyal, Sanjukta, MD {1730367293} ClCdEl, IntrMd(06,NY09)<NJ-RWJHLTS>
+ Cardio Care
200 Courtyard Drive/Suite 213   Hillsborough, NJ 08844   (908)725-5200   Fax (908)725-5223
+ Cardio Care
328 Greenbrook Road   Green Brook, NJ 08812   (908)725-5200   Fax (908)725-5223

Sanyal, Saugato, MD {1710931126} IntrMd, CdvDis(87,INA56)<NJ-COOPRUMC, NJ-KMHCHRRY>
+ Cardiovascular Associates
210 West Atlantic Avenue   Haddon Heights, NJ 08035   (856)546-3003   Fax (856)547-5337

Sanyaolu, Rasheed, MD {1790170405} EmrgMd(15,IL11)
+ University Hospital Emergency Medicine
150 Bergen Street   Newark, NJ 07103   (973)972-5128   Fax (973)972-6646

Sanzone, John, MD {1699790980} PedUro, Urolgy(92,NC05)<NJ-CHILTON>
+ Adult and Pediatric Urology Center, P.A.
1033 Clifton Avenue   Clifton, NJ 07013   (973)473-5700   Fax (973)473-3367
+ Adult and Pediatric Urology Center, P.A.
2025 Hamburg Turnpike   Wayne, NJ 07470   (973)473-5700   Fax (973)831-0033
+ Adult and Pediatric Urology Center, P.A.
1031 McBride Avenue/Suite D-108   West Paterson, NJ 07013   (973)256-4038   Fax (973)256-0432

Sapadin, Allen N., MD {1568570661} Dermat(88,NY47)<NJ-HOLYNAME>
+ 370 Summit Avenue
Hackensack, NJ 07601   (201)525-0057   Fax (201)525-0149
drsap@aol.com

Sapanara, Nancy Lauren, MD {1285748418} PthAClr<PA-MRCYFTZG>
+ 33 Technology Drive/2nd Fl
Warren, NJ 07059

Sapega, Alexander, MD {1699783266} SrgOrt, SrgArt, SprtMd(80,PA13)
+ New Jersey Knee & Shoulder Center
1288 Route 73 South/Suite 100   Mount Laurel, NJ 08054   (856)273-8900   Fax (856)802-9772
sapega@kneeandshoulder.md

Saperstein, Jeffrey S., MD {1316057250} Pedtrc(96,NY19)<NJ-STBARNMC>
+ The Pediatric Group of West Orange
395 Pleasant Valley Way   West Orange, NJ 07052   (973)731-6100   Fax (973)731-0612

Saphier, Carl Joseph, MD {1497700173} ObsGyn, MtFtMd, IntrMd(92,HOLYNAME, NJ-ENGLWOOD>
+ Women's Medical Services PA/Women's Ultrasound LLC
498 Engle Street   Englewood, NJ 07631   (201)569-0121   Fax (201)569-6835

Saphier, Douglas Jay, MD {1689960676}
+ Women's Medical Services PA/Women's Ultrasound LLC
498 Engle Street   Englewood, NJ 07631   (201)569-0121   Fax (201)569-6835

Saphier, Nicole Berardoni, MD {1063673671} RadBdl
+ Memorial Sloan Kettering Monmouth
480 Red Hill Road   Middletown, NJ 07748   (848)225-6304

Sapienza, Mark Santo, MD {1619929874} IntrMd, Gastrn(96,IL43)<NJ-HOLYNAME, NJ-ENGLWOOD>
+ Englewood Endoscopic Assocociates
420 Grand Avenue/Suite 101   Englewood, NJ 07631   (201)569-7044   Fax (201)569-1999
mark@marksapienza.com

Sapira, Andrew S., MD {1255431854} EmrgMd(94,NY46)<NJ-JRSYCITY>
+ JFK Medical Center
65 James Street   Edison, NJ 08820   (732)321-7601   Fax (732)744-5614

Sapira, Valdi, MD {1063466456} IntrMd(87,ROM01)<NJ-MEADWLND>
+ Meadowlands Hospital Medical Center
55 Meadowlands Parkway/EmergMed   Secaucus, NJ 07096   (201)392-3100

Saporito, John L., MD {1063516441} Otlryg(79,MEXI)
+ 1131 Broad Street/Suite 102
Shrewsbury, NJ 07702   (732)389-2500   Fax (732)389-2820

Saporito, Robert A., Jr., MD {1326047572} CdvDis, IntrMd, IntCrd(87,GRN01)<NJ-VALLEY, NJ-STJOSHOS>
+ Valley Medical Goup Cardioology Ridgewood
1124 East Ridgewood Avenue   Ridgewood, NJ 07450   (201)689-9400   Fax (201)689-9404

Saporta, Diego, MD {1164423299} Otlryg, Allrgy, OtgyAlgy(79,URUG>
+ Associates in ENT/Allergy
470 North Avenue   Elizabeth, NJ 07208   (908)352-6700   Fax (908)352-6734

Sappal, Baljit S., MD {1124054747} IntrMd(94,INA03)<NJ-LOURDMED>
+ 43 Elizabeth Avenue
Edison, NJ 08820   (732)668-2747

Sapru, Sunil, MD {1235169558} IntrMd(84,INDI)
+ Internal Medicine Faculty Practice
101 Old Short Hills Road/Suite 106   West Orange, NJ 07052   (973)322-6256   Fax (973)322-6241

Saraceno, Leonardo, MD {1306289152} IntrMd
+ Roselle Park Primary Care
318 Chestnut Street   Roselle Park, NJ 07204   (908)241-4200

Saraceno, Libero, MD {1770637928} IntrMd(80,ARG01)<NJ-CLARMAAS, NJ-STBARNMC>
+ Roselle Park Primary Care
318 Chestnut Street   Roselle Park, NJ 07204   (908)241-4200

Saradarian, Kathleen A., MD {1518006675} FamMed(87,NJ05)<NJ-STCLRSUS>
+ Quality Family Practice
22 Wantage Avenue/PO Box 2457   Branchville, NJ 07826   (973)948-4232   Fax (973)948-6712

Saraf, Nirmala, MD {1518986538} Onclgy, OncHem(83,INDI)<NJ-EASTORNG>
+ 310 Central Avenue/Suite 103
East Orange, NJ 07018   (973)395-1500   Fax (973)395-1803

Saraf, Pankhoori, MD {1861771784} OncHem, IntrMd
+ 185 South Orange Avenue
Newark, NJ 07103   (973)972-6257

Saraiya, Biren P., MD {1518173665} OncHem, IntrMd(02,NJ06)<NJ-RWJUHAM, NJ-RWJUBRUN>
+ Rutgers Cancer Institute of New Jersey
195 Little Albany Street/PO Box 2681   New Brunswick, NJ 08903   (732)235-2465   Fax (732)235-7355

Saraiya, Mansi Shah, MD {1942520754} RadDia
+ University Radiology Group, P.C.
579A Cranbury Road   East Brunswick, NJ 08816   (732)390-0040   Fax (732)390-1856

Saraiya, Narendra N., MD {1760553838} Pedtrc, PedHem(72,INA67)<NY-METHODST, NY-LICOLLGE>
+ Union County Pediatrics Group
817 Rahway Avenue   Elizabeth, NJ 07202   (908)353-5750

Saraiya, Neha, MD {1912937582} Pedtrc(01,IL12)
+ 248 Fountayne Lane
Lawrenceville, NJ 08648

Saraiya, Nimit Nitin, MD {1649597733} IntrMd(10,NJ05)<NJ-MTNSIDE>
+ Essex County Infectious Disease
199 Broad Street/Suite 2-C   Bloomfield, NJ 07003   (973)748-4583   Fax (973)748-3243

Saraiya, Piya Vijay, MD {1154520807} RadNro
+ Cooper University Hospital
One Cooper Plaza   Camden, NJ 08103   (856)342-2383   Fax (856)365-9472

Sarayno-Sagge, Perla M., MD {1902805443} Anesth(73,PHIL)<NJ-WARREN>
+ Warren Hospital
185 Roseberry Street/Anesthesiology   Phillipsburg, NJ 08865   (908)859-6700

Sardar, Henry, DO {1427191618} PhysMd, IntrMd(03,NY75)<NY-METHODST>
+ Medical Therapy of New York, PLLC
171 Elmora Avenue   Elizabeth, NJ 07202   (732)654-2407   Fax (347)823-1150

Sardari, Frederic Fereydoun, MD {1871560458} Surgry, SrgThr, CdvDis(88,DC01)<NJ-NWRKBETH>
+ Newark Beth Israel Medical Center
201 Lyons Avenue/Surgery   Newark, NJ 07112   (973)926-7000   Fax (973)923-4683

Sardi, Vincent F., MD {1366411233} Ophthl(88,DC02)
+ Campus Eye Group & Laser Center
1700 Whitehorse Hamilton Sq Rd   Hamilton Square, NJ 08690   (609)587-2020   Fax (609)588-9545

Sareen, Ruchi, MD {1891939203} IntrMd(99,INA21)<NJ-STBARNMC>
+ St. Barnabas Medical Center
94 Old Short Hills Road/Internal Med   Livingston, NJ 07039   (973)722-9022   Fax (801)340-4048

Sarenac, Alexander, MD {1366736241} EmrgMd<NJ-OCEANMC>
+ Ocean Medical Center
425 Jack Martin Boulevard   Brick, NJ 08723   (732)836-4088

sargent, Stephanie Christine, DO {1487656013} IntrMd(02,PA77)
+ Internal Medicine Associates of Southern New Jersey
151 Fries Mill Road/Suite 400   Turnersville, NJ 08012   (856)401-9300   Fax (856)374-5307

Sargent, Thomas G., Jr, DO {1073717468} FamMSptM(07,NY75)
+ Brielle Orthopedics PA
457 Jack Martin Boulevard   Brick, NJ 08724   (732)840-7500   Fax (732)840-2088
+ Brielle Orthopedics PA
823 Lacey Road   Forked River, NJ 08731   (732)840-7500   Fax (732)840-2088
+ Brielle Orthopedics PA
1301 Route 72 West   Manahawkin, NJ 08724   (609)971-7616   Fax (609)971-7639

Saric, Muhamed, MD {1952497257} CdvDis, IntrMd(85,BOSN)<NJ-UMDNJ, NY-NYUTISCH>
+ University Hospital
150 Bergen Street/Medicine   Newark, NJ 07103   (973)972-4300   Fax (973)972-4737

Physicians by Name and Address

Sarier, Kaya K., MD {1164598603} Anesth(91,NJ05)<NJ-HACKNSK>
+ Hackensack University Medical Center
30 Prospect Avenue/Anesthesiology   Hackensack, NJ 07601   (201)996-2000
+ Hackensack University MC-Anesthesia Dept
30 Prospect Avenue/Room 2703   Hackensack, NJ 07601   (201)996-2000   Fax (201)996-3962

Sarigul, Melih B., MD {1215023924} Pedtrc(80,TUR05)<NJ-STJOSHOS, NJ-HACKNSK>
+ Clifton Pediatrics
296 Clifton Avenue/Suite 2   Clifton, NJ 07011   (973)249-8211   Fax (973)249-8611
sarigulmel@worldnet.att.net

Sarkar, Abhishek, MD {1659804961} IntrMd<NJ-RWJUBRUN>
+ RWJ University Hospital New Brunswick
One Robert Wood Johnson Place   New Brunswick, NJ 08901   (732)828-3000

Sarkar, Arunima, MD {1801909866} IntrMd, Grtrcs(93,INA56)
+ 44 Tilghman Drive
Glen Rock, NJ 07452
+ Center for Healthy Senior Living
360 Essex Street/Suite 401   Hackensack, NJ 07601   Fax (551)996-0543

Sarkar, Avik, MD {1528383403}<NJ-RWJUBRUN>
+ RWJ University Hospital New Brunswick
One Robert Wood Johnson Place   New Brunswick, NJ 08901   (732)235-7784
aviksarkar83@gmail.com

Sarkar, Jayati Saha, MD {1275706772} Ophthl(02,INA66)
+ Eyecare MD of New Jersey
261 James Street/Suite 2-D & 3EL   Morristown, NJ 07960   (973)984-3937   Fax (973)984-0059
eyecaremdnj@aol.com

Sarkar, Shubho Ranjan, MD {1932375581} IntrMd, Nephro(94,INA26)<NJ-STCLRDEN, NJ-MORRISTN>
+ Kidney Care
131 Madison Avenue/Suite 3   Morristown, NJ 07960   (973)631-6223   Fax (973)631-6225
+ Nephrology Hypertension Assocs
2 Franklin Place   Morristown, NJ 07960   (973)631-6223   Fax (973)267-3270

Sarkaria, Janak, MD {1356320709} Anesth(67,INDI)
+ Summit Anesthesia Associates, P.A.
33 Overlook Road/Suite 311   Summit, NJ 07901   (908)598-1500   Fax (908)598-0197

Sarkaria, Jasbir S., MD {1447301353} SrgThr, Surgry(68,INDI)
+ Drs. Modi & Sarkaria
98 James Street/Suite 200   Edison, NJ 08820   (732)494-1660   Fax (732)494-2209
+ 1649 Woodland Avenue
Edison, NJ 08820   (732)494-1660   Fax (732)494-2209

Sarker, Tushar, MD {1699935395} Psychy
+ 1143 Gold Pond Court
Voorhees, NJ 08043

Sarkissian, Naver A., MD {1124225693} DrmtPthy<NJ-STBARNMC>
+ St. Barnabas Medical Center
94 Old Short Hills Road   Livingston, NJ 07039   (973)322-5000

Sarkodie, Alex, MD {1598870271} IntrMd, Pedtrc(86,GHA01)
+ 641 Broadway
Paterson, NJ 07514   (862)264-1227   Fax (862)264-1166
Asarkodie@aol.com

Sarkos, Peter Anthony, DO {1174720536} SrgOrt(03,PA77)<NJ-SJHREGMC, NJ-SJRSYELM>
+ Premier Orthopaedic Associates
298 South Delsea Drive   Vineland, NJ 08360   (856)690-1616   Fax (856)690-1089
+ Premier Orthopaedic Assocs of So NJ
201 Tomlin Station Road/Suite C   Mullica Hill, NJ 08062   (856)690-1616   Fax (856)223-9110

Sarlis, Demosthenes N., MD {1407004880}
+ 4000 Riverdale Road
Riverdale, NJ 07457

Sarma, Bani A., MD {1023018132} ObsGyn(93,PA13)<NJ-UNVMCPRN, NJ-CHSFULD>
+ Delaware Valley Ob/Gyn & Infertility Group, PC
2 Princess Road/Suite C   Lawrenceville, NJ 08648   (609)896-0777   Fax (609)896-3266
+ Delaware Valley Ob/Gyn & Infertility Group, PC
300B Princeton Hightstown Road   East Windsor, NJ 08520   (609)896-0777   Fax (609)443-4506

Sarmiento, Samuel I., MD {1891886727} FamMed, FamMAdlt(80,PHI01)<NJ-VIRTBERL, NJ-VIRTVOOR>
+ 901 Route 168
Blackwood, NJ 08012   (856)227-1221   Fax (856)232-9399

Sarnelle, Joseph A., MD {1285648972} CdvDis, IntrMd, Grtrcs(79,MEX03)<NJ-BAYSHORE, NJ-RIVERVW>
+ 812 Poole Avenue/Suite C
Hazlet, NJ 07730   (732)264-3131   Fax (732)264-2141

Sarner, Steven W., MD {1205807930} Psychy(81,GRN01)<NJ-NWTNMEM>
+ Atlantic Behavioral Health at Newton Medical Center
175 High Street   Newton, NJ 07860   (973)383-1533   Fax (973)383-9309

Saro-Nunez, Lilian, MD {1821410192} Nephro
+ BSD Nephrology & Hypertension
360 Essex Street/Suite 304   Hackensack, NJ 07601   (201)646-0110   Fax (201)646-0219

Sarode, Satyeswara K., MD {1720045917} IntrMd, CdvDis(78,INA68)<NJ-STCLRBOO>
+ 1520 Highway 130/Suite 202
North Brunswick, NJ 08902   (732)422-0212   Fax (732)422-0212
sarode@pol.net

Saroff, Alan L., MD {1982658613} CdvDis, IntrMd(65,NY15)<NJ-MTNSIDE, NJ-VALLEY>
+ Montclair Cardiology Group PA
123 Highland Avenue/Suite 302   Glen Ridge, NJ 07028   (973)748-9555   Fax (973)748-2003

Sarokhan, Alan J., MD {1447227194} SrgOrt(77,MA01)
+ Orthopedic Surgical Associates
33 Overlook Road/Suite 201   Summit, NJ 07901   (908)522-4555   Fax (908)522-1128
+ Orthopedic Surgical Associates
10 Mountian Boulevard   Warren, NJ 07059   (908)522-4555   Fax (908)756-6629

Sarokhan, Carol T., MD {1558346304} RadDia(77,MA01)<NJ-STPETER, NJ-RWJUBRUN>
+ University Radiology Group, P.C.
483 Cranbury Road   East Brunswick, NJ 08816   (732)390-0030   Fax (732)390-5383
+ University Radiology Group, P.C.
260 Amboy Avenue   Metuchen, NJ 08840   (732)390-0030   Fax (732)548-3392

Saros, Cathleen Mary, DO {1003054552} FamMed(86,ME75)
+ AFC Urgent Care Paramus
67 East Ridgewood Avenue   Paramus, NJ 07652   (201)899-4765
+ Vanguard Medical Group
535 High Mountain Road/Suite 111   North Haledon, NJ 07508   (201)899-4765   Fax (973)636-0913

Sarraf, Mohammad A., MD {1689648735} IntrMd, PulDis(67,IRAN)
+ Drs. Sarraf and Hebbe
1907 Park Avenue   South Plainfield, NJ 07080   (908)561-1313   Fax (908)561-3917

Sarris, John, MD {1407967177} SrgNro(87,NY03)
+ Coastal Neurosurgery
9 Hospital Drive   Toms River, NJ 08755   (732)341-1881   Fax (732)505-4453
+ Shore Neurology, P.A.
633 Route 37 West   Toms River, NJ 08755   (732)341-1881   Fax (732)240-3114

Sarti, Edward J., MD {1477665586} Otlryg(81,MEXI)<NJ-HACKNSK>
+ The Family Center for Otolaryngology
47 Orient Way/Lower Level   Rutherford, NJ 07070   (201)935-5508   Fax (201)465-6088
+ The Family Center for Otolaryngology
1265 Paterson Plank Road   Secaucus, NJ 07094   (201)935-5508   Fax (201)465-6088
+ The Family Center for Otolaryngology
6 Brighton Road/Suite 104   Clifton, NJ 07070   (973)470-0282   Fax (201)465-6088

Sarti, Evan Edward, DO {1942666211}(NY75
+ The Family Center for Otolaryngology
47 Orient Way/Lower Level   Rutherford, NJ 07070   (201)935-5508   Fax (201)465-6088
+ The Family Center for Otolaryngology
6 Brighton Road/Suite 104   Clifton, NJ 07012   (201)935-5508   Fax (201)465-6088
+ The Family Center for Otolaryngology
1265 Paterson Plank Road   Secaucus, NJ 07070   (201)864-4419   Fax (201)465-6088

Sarvaiya, Ramesh Manjibhai, MD {1578558748} Anesth(79,INA69)<NJ-MEMSALEM>
+ Memorial Hospital of Salem County
310 Woodstown Road/Anesthesiology   Salem, NJ 08079   (856)935-1000

Sarwar, Haroon, MD {1639188949} Rheuma
+ Premier Health Associates
532 Lafayette Road/Suite 100   Sparta, NJ 07871   (973)383-3730   Fax (973)383-2285
+ Premier Health Associates
212 State Route 94/Suite 1-D   Vernon, NJ 07462   (973)383-3730   Fax (973)209-2665
+ Premier Health Associates
123 Newton Sparta Road   Newton, NJ 07871   (973)579-6300   Fax (973)579-1524

Sarwar, Muhammad, MD {1902048168} IntrMd(01,PAK15)<NJ-MONMOUTH, NJ-KMHSTRAT>
+ Kennedy Memorial Hospital-University Medical Center
18 East Laurel Road   Stratford, NJ 08084   (856)566-6845   Fax (856)566-6906
+ Hackensack Medical Center-Internal Medicine
30 Prospect Avenue/4 Main/Rm 4621   Hackensack, NJ 07601   (856)566-6845   Fax (551)996-0536

Sarwar, Samina, DO {1134443013} Nephro
+ JFK Hospitalists
98 James Street/Suite 208   Edison, NJ 08818   (908)731-1981   Fax (732)862-1171

Sasanpour, Majid, MD {1679677918} InfDis, IntrMd(96,IRA13)<NJ-CLARMAAS, NJ-STBARHCS>
+ The Internet Medical Group, P.C.
181 Franklin Avenue/Suite 204   Nutley, NJ 07110   (973)667-8117   Fax (973)667-6642
+ North Arlington Primary Care Associates, Inc.
25 Locust Avenue   North Arlington, NJ 07031   (973)667-8117   Fax (201)955-7467

Sasidhar, Vaidehi, MD {1790756427} FamMed(95,INA48)
+ Monmouth Family Medicine Group
3499 Route 9 North   Freehold, NJ 07728   (732)625-3166   Fax (732)409-7493

Sasinowska, Sylwia, MD {1962829390}<NJ-STFRNMED>
+ St. Francis Medical Center
601 Hamilton Avenue   Trenton, NJ 08629   (609)599-5061   Fax (609)599-6232

Saslo, Christopher R., DO {1275827651} Psychy<NJ-CHSFULD>
+ Capital Health System/Fuld Campus
750 Brunswick Avenue   Trenton, NJ 08638   (609)815-7829

Saslow, Judy G., MD {1922182310} NnPnMd, Pedtrc(79,OH06)<NJ-COOPRUMC>
+ Cooper Neonatology
One Cooper Plaza   Camden, NJ 08103   (856)342-2265   Fax (856)342-8007
+ The Children's Regional Hospital at Cooper Univ Hosp
One Cooper Plaza/2nd floor   Camden, NJ 08103   (856)342-2000

Sasportas, Jonathan Scott, MD {1407942469} Surgry, SrgO&M(95,NJ05)<NJ-RWJUBRUN, NJ-CLARMAAS, NJ-MONMOUTH, NJ-STBARHCS>
+ Oral & Maxillofacial Surgery of Central New Jersey
2303 Whitehorse-Mercerville Rd   Mercerville, NJ 08619   (609)587-2900   Fax (609)587-1749
+ Oral & Maxillofacial Surgery of Central New Jersey
59 One Mile Road   East Windsor, NJ 08520   (609)448-6900
+ Oral & Maxillofacial Surgery of Central New Jersey
601 Ewing Street/Suite A-1   Princeton, NJ 08619   (609)924-6400

Sass, Timothy E., MD {1265573166} IntrMd(85,DC01)
+ Princeton Internal Medicine Associates
281 Witherspoon Street/Suite 220   Princeton, NJ 08542   (609)921-3362   Fax (609)921-3584

Sasso, Michael J., DO {1568469153} Surgry(85,ME75)<NJ-KMHTURNV, NJ-KMHSTRAT>
+ 338 Hurfville Crosskeys Road
Sewell, NJ 08080   (856)589-0600   Fax (856)589-7979

Sasson, Elias, MD {1154392462} Pedtrc(74,NY08)<NJ-JRSYSHMC, NJ-MONMOUTH>
+ West Park Pediatrics
804 West Park Avenue   Ocean, NJ 07712   (732)531-0010   Fax (732)493-0903
+ West Park Pediatrics
219 Taylors Mills Road   Manalapan, NJ 07726   (732)531-0010   Fax (732)577-9643
+ West Park Pediatrics
921 East County Line Road/Suite B   Lakewood, NJ 07712   (732)370-8500   Fax (732)370-5550

Sastic, Daniel Joseph, MD {1235123431} FamMed, IntrMd(80,NY45)
+ Elmer Family Practice
330 Front Street/Suite 4101   Elmer, NJ 08318   (856)358-0770
cheryl.sastic1004@comcast.net

Sastrasinh, Sithiporn, MD {1043324668} Nephro, IntrMd(73,THA03)<NJ-VAEASTOR, NJ-VALYONS>
+ VA New Jersey Health Care System-East Orange Campus
385 Tremont Avenue   East Orange, NJ 07018   (973)676-1000

Sastri, Bhagyalak L., MD {1831133149} IntrMd, IntHos(96,INA4Y)<NJ-OCEANMC>
+ Ocean Medical Center
425 Jack Martin Boulevard/Hospitalist   Brick, NJ 08723   (732)840-2200
+ Sai Inpatient Resources LLC
3626 US Highway 1   Princeton, NJ 08540   (732)840-2200   Fax (609)452-7577

Sastry, Gayathri, MD {1659459949} Psychy, PsyGrt, PsyAdd(81,INDI)<NJ-UMDNJ>
+ 267 Beaufort Avenue
Livingston, NJ 07039   (201)445-2200   Fax (201)445-2204

Sastry, Pillutla V., MD {1457328023} CdvDis, IntrMd(68,INDI)
+ 100 Bentley Avenue
 Jersey City, NJ 07304 (201)433-5678 Fax (201)433-6502
Sathaye, Nirmal, MD {1598865982} PsyGrt, Psychy(79,INA67)<NJ-STBARNMC>
+ Associates in Psychiatry
 405 Northfield Avenue/Suite 204 West Orange, NJ 07052
 (973)325-6120 Fax (973)325-6126
Sathe, Niharika, MD {1255780599}
+ Cooper University Medical Center/Camden
 3 Cooper Plaza/Rm 504 Camden, NJ 08103 (856)342-2312
Sathe, Sadhana S., MD {1881651669} InfDis, IntrMd(64,INA67)
+ 40 Patriots Way
 Somerset, NJ 08873
Sathe, Swati Ajit, MD {1255389177} Nrolgy, IntrMd(97,INA65)<NJ-STJOSHOS>
+ St. Joseph's Regional Medical Center
 703 Main Street/Neurology Paterson, NJ 07503 (973)754-2743 Fax (973)754-3376
+ St. Joseph's Regional MedCtr-Ambulatory Imaging Ctr
 1135 Broad Street/3rd Floor/Suite 4 Clifton, NJ 07013 (973)754-2433
+ Rutgers NJ School of Medicine Neurology
 90 Bergen Street/DOC 5200 Newark, NJ 07503 (973)972-5209 Fax (973)972-5059
Sathya, Bharath, MD {1083842249} IntrMd(09,NJ05)<NJ-RWJUBRUN>
+ RWJ University Hospital New Brunswick
 One Robert Wood Johnson Place New Brunswick, NJ 08901 (732)828-3000
Sathyendra, Vikram Modur, MD {1790986966} SrgOrt<PA-PN-STHRSH>
+ St. Peter's University Hospital
 254 Easton Avenue New Brunswick, NJ 08901 (732)745-8600
Satra, Karin H., MD {1619072303} Dermat, IntrMd(85,NY01)<NJ-VALLEY>
+ North Bergen Dermatologic Group, PA
 400 Route 17 South Ridgewood, NJ 07450 (201)652-4536 Fax (201)652-4906
+ North Bergen Dermatologic Group, PA
 180 Ramapo Valley Road Oakland, NJ 07436 (201)652-4536 Fax (201)337-7710
Sattari, Rouzbeh, MD {1962563510} Anesth, PedAne(92,BEL07)<NJ-STBARNMC>
+ St. Barnabas Medical Center
 94 Old Short Hills Road Livingston, NJ 07039 (973)322-5000
Sattel, Andrew B., MD {1295828853} SrgHnd, SrgOrt(83,PA02)<NJ-VIRTVOOR>
+ Hand Surgery & Rehabilitation Center of New Jersey
 8008 Route 130 North Delran, NJ 08075 (856)764-8804 Fax (856)764-3561
+ Hand Surgery & Rehabilitation Center of New Jersey
 5000 Sagemore Drive/Suite 103 Marlton, NJ 08053 (856)764-8804 Fax (856)983-9362
Sattel, Lisa E., MD Anesth(87,MI20)
+ 8 Deerfield Terrace
 Moorestown, NJ 08057
Sattenspiel, Sigmund Linder, MD {1730177676} OtIryg, SrgFPl, OtgyFPlS(65,MD01)<NJ-BAYSHORE, NJ-CENTRAST>
+ 1050 West Main Street
 Freehold, NJ 07728 (732)780-1333 Fax (732)780-2346
Satwah, Vinay Kumar, DO {1104900448} IntrMd(03,NY75)
+ 3084 Route 27/Suite 11
 Kendall Park, NJ 08824
Satwani, Sunita, MD {1063698116} Pedtrc(98,INA29)
+ 015 Allison Court
 Edison, NJ 08820
Satya, Kumar, MD {1710163357}
+ Hackensack Heart Failure Program
 20 Prospect Avenue Hackensack, NJ 07601 (201)996-4849 Fax (201)996-5703
Sauberman, Roy Burton, MD {1912948142} CdvDis, IntrMd, ClCdEl(90,CT01)<NJ-STBARNMC, NJ-JRSYCITY>
+ Shore Cardiology Consultants, LLC
 579 Main Street Metuchen, NJ 08840 (732)840-1900 Fax (732)840-0355
+ Shore Cardiology Consultants, LLC
 1640 Route 88/Suite 201 Brick, NJ 08724 (732)840-1900 Fax (732)840-0355
Sauchelli, Francis C., MD {1558307934} Anesth(81,MEXI)
+ Bergen Ambulatory Surgery Center
 190 Midland Avenue Saddle Brook, NJ 07663 (973)809-5355 Fax (862)247-8084
+ Paramus Surgical Center
 30 West Century Road/Suite 300 Paramus, NJ 07652 (201)986-9000
Saud, Helmi A., DO {1811928286} IntrMd(94,MI12)<NJ-STFRN-MED, NJ-JFKMED>
+ St. Francis Medical Center
 601 Hamilton Avenue Trenton, NJ 08629 (609)599-5000 Fax (609)599-6385
Sauer, Mark Victor, MD {1770644783} ObsGyn, RprEnd, FrtInf(80,IL11)<NY-PRSBCOLU>
+ UMDNJ OBGYN
 125 Paterson Street/Suite 4200 New Brunswick, NJ 08901 (732)235-7628 Fax (732)235-6650
Sauer, Scott Thomas, MD {1336149145} SrgFAk, SrgOrt
+ Coordinated Health
 222 Red Lane Phillipsburg, NJ 08865 (610)861-8080 Fax (610)849-1013
Sauers, Paul W., DO {1649272071} CdvDis, IntrMd(71,PA77)<NJ-MEMSALEM>
+ 298 Bianca Avenue
 Carneys Point, NJ 08069 (856)299-0002 Fax (856)299-6169
Sauerwein, Anthony G., MD {1750340857} CdvDis, IntrMd(87,PA12)
+ The Cardiology Group, P.A.
 401 Young Avenue/Suite 275 Moorestown, NJ 08057 (856)291-8855 Fax (856)291-8844
+ The Cardiology Group, P.A.
 128 State Highway Route 70/Suite 1-B Medford, NJ 08055 (856)291-8855 Fax (609)444-5521
+ The Cardiology Group, P.A.
 1 Sheffield Drive/Suite 102 Columbus, NJ 08057 (856)291-8855
Saul, Howard Marc, DO {1730185968} GynOnc, ObsGyn(83,IA75)<NJ-VIRTBERL, NJ-VIRTMARL>
+ Marlton Gynecologic Oncology
 750 Route 73 South/Suite 309A & 310A Marlton, NJ 08053 (856)334-5550
Saul, Jared Michael, MD {1093780777} RadNro, RadDia(96,NJ06)
+ Hunterdon Radiological Associate
 1 Dogwood Drive Clinton, NJ 08809 (908)735-4477 Fax (908)735-6532
Saulino, Patrick F., MD {1043282551} CdvDis, IntrMd(81,DC02)<NJ-MORRISTN, NJ-SOMERSET>
+ 3322 Route 22 West
 Branchburg, NJ 08876 (908)231-0041 Fax (908)231-0048
Saulon, Winston B., MD {1538199542} Anesth(91,PHI08)<NJ-STJOSHOS>
+ St. Joseph's Regional Medical Center Anesthesia
 703 Main Street Paterson, NJ 07503 (973)754-2323 Fax (973)977-9455
Saunders, Alan M., MD {1255337135} RadDia, Radiol(87,NY03)<NJ-JFKMED, NJ-SOMERSET>
+ University Radiology, PA
 239 Route 22 East/Suite 302 Green Brook, NJ 08812 (732)968-4899 Fax (732)968-8096
+ Bridgewater Imaging Center-Associated Radiologists
 201 Union Avenue/Building 2/Suite G Bridgewater, NJ 08807 (732)968-4899 Fax (908)725-8335
+ University Radiology Group, P.C.
 3900 Park Avenue/Suite 107 Edison, NJ 08812 (732)548-6800 Fax (732)548-6290
Saunders, Craig Raymond, MD {1821065400} SrgThr, Surgry, CdvDis(70,IA02)<NJ-NWRKBETH>
+ Newark Beth Israel Medical Center
 201 Lyons Avenue/Surgery Newark, NJ 07112 (973)926-7000 Fax (973)923-4683
Saunders, Eric Monroe, MD {1699730937} Ophthl(96,MD07)<NJ-VALLEY>
+ Ridgewood Ophthalmology PC
 1200 East Ridgewood Avenue Ridgewood, NJ 07450 (201)612-0044 Fax (201)612-9446
Saunders, Kyauna Sharae, MD {1659534477} Pedtrc<OH-COLM-BCHL>
+ Ocean Health Initiatives, Inc.
 101 Second Street Lakewood, NJ 08701 (732)363-6655 Fax (732)363-6656
Saunders, Peter J., MD {1235303454} PthACl
+ The Advanced Pulmonary Diagnostic Center
 100 Medical Center Way Somers Point, NJ 08244 (609)653-3500 Fax (609)653-3586
Saur, David P., MD {1932161569} Nrolgy(68,MO34)
+ 507 Westfield Avenue
 Westfield, NJ 07090 (908)232-1365
Savage, Danielle S., MD {1891084083} IntrMd(11,NY46)<NJ-MMHKEMBL>
+ Internal Medicine of Morristown
 95 Madison Avenue/Suite A-00 Morristown, NJ 07960 (973)538-1388 Fax (973)292-6438
Savaille, Juanito E., DO {1467885061} IntrMd(11,NJ75)
+ Salerno Medical Associates, LLP
 613 Park Avenue East Orange, NJ 07017 (973)672-8573 Fax (973)676-4099
Savarese, Joseph, MD {1700200953} IntHos<NJ-COMMED>
+ Southern Ocean Medical Center
 1100 Route 72 West/Suite 307 Manahawkin, NJ 08050 (609)597-6011 Fax (609)978-8941
+ Community Medical Center
 99 Route 37 West Toms River, NJ 08755 (732)557-8000
+ Shore Hospitalists Associates
 100 Medical Center Way Somers Point, NJ 08050 (609)653-3500 Fax (609)926-4799
Savarese, Vincent William, MD {1033325444} EnDbMt
+ Endocrine Associates of Southern Jersey
 703 East Main Street/Suite 5 Moorestown, NJ 08057 (856)727-0900 Fax (856)231-8428
Savary, Khalil William, MD {1699061416} PedPul
+ UMDNJ Pediatric Pulmonary
 90 Bergen Street/DOC 5200 Newark, NJ 07103 (973)972-5779 Fax (973)972-5895
Savatsky, Gary J., MD {1508859935} SprtMd, SrgOrt(75,NY01)<NJ-HACKNSK>
+ Orthopedic Spine and Sports Medicine Center
 2 Forest Avenue Paramus, NJ 07652 (201)587-1111 Fax (201)587-8192
Savatta, Domenico James, MD {1366439192} Urolgy, IntrMd(97,NY48)<NJ-NWRKBETH, NJ-OVERLOOK>
+ New Jersey Urology, LLC
 741 Northfield Avenue/Suite 206 West Orange, NJ 07052 (973)325-6100 Fax (973)325-1616
 dsavatta@roboticsurgeon.com
+ New Jersey Urology, LLC
 700 North Broad Street/Suite 302 Elizabeth, NJ 07208 (973)325-6100 Fax (908)289-0716
+ New Jersey Urology, LLC
 375 Mounain Pleasant Ave/Suite 250 West Orange, NJ 07052 (973)323-1300 Fax (973)323-1311
Savci, Sariye, MD {1760660559} ObsGyn(02,TUR20)
+ 106 Grand Avenue/Suite 300
 Englewood, NJ 07631 (201)308-8282 Fax (201)308-8283
Savera, Adnan Tabrez, MD {1811078892} PthAna(91,PAK11)
+ 36 Townsend Drive
 Florham Park, NJ 07932
Saviano, George J., MD {1295808889} CdvDis, IntrMd, IntCrd(77,NY09)
+ Cardio Intervent of Ctrl Jersey
 465 Cranbury Road/Suite 201 East Brunswick, NJ 08816 (732)613-1988 Fax (732)651-7734
Saviano, Nicole, MD {1992062103} PthACl
+ 19 Woodfield Lane
 Saddle River, NJ 07458 (201)236-1844
Savino, Leonard, MD {1447277991} CdvDis, IntrMd(77,NY09)<NJ-STJOSHOS, NJ-CLARMAAS>
+ Cardiology Associates LLC
 181 Franklin Avenue/Suite 301 Nutley, NJ 07110 (973)667-5511 Fax (973)667-0561
+ Cardiology Associates LLC
 312 Belleville Turnpike North Arlington, NJ 07031 (973)667-5511 Fax (973)667-0561
Savla, Jayshree Sameer, MD {1598963456} NnPnMd
+ Somerset Medical Center Neonatology
 110 Rehill Avenue Somerville, NJ 08876 (908)685-2473
Savon, Joseph J., MD {1285740639} Gastrn(87,NJ06)<NJ-VIRTU-AHS, NJ-KENEDYHS>
+ South Jersey Gastroenterology PA
 111 Vine Street Hammonton, NJ 08037 (609)561-3080 Fax (856)983-5110
+ South Jersey Gastroenterology PA
 106 Creek Crossing Hainesport, NJ 08036 (609)561-3080 Fax (856)983-5110
+ South Jersey Gastroenterology PA
 406 Lippincott Drive/Suite E Marlton, NJ 08053 (856)983-1900 Fax (856)983-5110
Savopoulos, Andreas A., MD {1972660496} IntrMd, OncHem, Onclgy(74,GREE)
+ 401 Pleasant Valley Way
 West Orange, NJ 07052 (973)669-5931 Fax (973)669-7342
Savransky, Ernest, MD {1912032293} Nephro
+ 225 Highway 35 North/Suite 204
 Red Bank, NJ 07701 (732)747-5048 Fax (732)747-5037
Sawaged, Khalid S., DO {1003850314} ObsGyn(93,MO79)
+ 671 Mount Prospect Avenue/Suite A
 Newark, NJ 07104 (973)497-9611 Fax (973)497-9621
Sawczuk, Ihor Steven, MD {1225084825} Urolgy(79,PA07)<NJ-HACKNSK, NY-PRSBCOLU>
+ HUMC Faculty Practice
 360 Essex Street/Suite 403 Hackensack, NJ 07601 (201)336-8090 Fax (201)336-8221
Sawhney, Ramesh Kumar, MD {1942244256} Anesth, PainMd(81,MEX03)
+ Anesthesia Group of Orange, PA
 45 Oak Bend Road West Orange, NJ 07052 (973)763-3350 Fax (973)763-3355
Sawicki, John M., DO FamMed(81,MO79)<NJ-ENGLWOOD>
+ 178 Blanch Avenue
 Harrington Park, NJ 07640 (201)768-3301

Physicians by Name and Address

Sawin, Stephen Wooten, MD {1821062456} ObsGyn, RprEnd(91,NY45)<NJ-ACMCITY>
+ South Jersey Fertility Center
400 Lippincott Drive Marlton, NJ 08053 (856)282-1231 Fax (856)596-2411
+ South Jersey Fertility Center
2500 English Creek Avenue/Suite 225 Egg Harbor Township, NJ 08234

Saxena, Amita, MD {1831299866} IntrMd(76,INA9B)
+ 1100 Westcott Drive/Suite G-2
Flemington, NJ 08822 (908)806-6275 Fax (908)806-2891

Saxena, Arjun, MD {1003934530} SrgOrt
+ Trenton Orthopaedic Group
1225 Whitehorse Mercerville Rd Trenton, NJ 08619 (609)581-2200 Fax (609)581-1212
+ Trenton Orthopaedic Group
116 Washington Crossing Road Pennington, NJ 08534 (609)581-2200 Fax (609)581-1212

Saxena, Mark, MD {1871745042} IntrMd(05,DC03)<NJ-RWJUBRUN>
+ UH- RWJ Medical School
One Robert Wood Johnson Place New Brunswick, NJ 08903 (732)828-3000

Saxena, Neil, MD {1013151117} CdvDis, IntrMd(03,NJ05)
+ Capital Health-Heart Care Specialists
2 Capital Way/Suite 385 Pennington, NJ 08534 (609)303-4838 Fax (609)303-4835
+ Capital Health-Heart Care Specialists
1445 Whitehorse-Mercerville Rd Hamilton, NJ 08619 (609)303-4838 Fax (609)303-4835

Saxena, Rachna Vidiasagar, DO {1043251283} EmrgMd(01,NJ75)<NJ-ENGLWOOD>
+ Englewood Hospital and Medical Center
350 Engle Street Englewood, NJ 07631 (204)984-3000 Fax (610)617-6280

Saxena, Shilpa M., MD {1023291333} FamMed(99,INA16)
+ Concentra Medical Centers
574 Summit Avenue/4th Fl Jersey City, NJ 07306 (201)656-7678 Fax (201)656-0664

Say, Irene Sy, MD {1285990804}
+ Rutgers NJ School of Medicine Neurology
90 Bergen Street/DOC 5200 Newark, NJ 07103 (973)972-5209 Fax (973)972-5059
irene.say24@gmail.com

Saybolt, Matthew Douglas, MD {1841519709} IntrMd
+ Monmouth Cardiology Associates, LLC
11 Meridian Road Eatontown, NJ 07724 (732)663-0300 Fax (732)663-0301

Sayde, William M., MD {1295964708} SrgOrt
+ The Orthopedic Institute of New Jersey
108 Bilby Road/Suite 201 Hackettstown, NJ 07840 (908)684-3005 Fax (908)684-3301
+ The Orthopedic Institute of New Jersey
254-B Mountain Avenue/Suite 201 Hackettstown, NJ 07840 (908)684-3005 Fax (908)684-3301
+ The Orthopedic Institute of New Jersey
380 Lafayette Road/Route 15 Sparta, NJ 07840 (908)684-3005 Fax (908)684-3301

Sayed, Durr-E-shahwaar, DO {1821228263} FamMed(09,CA22)<NJ-UNDRWD>
+ Inspira Medical Group
200 Rowan Boulevard Glassboro, NJ 08028 (856)582-0500 Fax (856)582-0163

Sayed, Saquib Bashir, MD {1609054360} Psychy(87,INA4X)
+ 4 Turtle Hollow Court
Sicklerville, NJ 08081

Sayeed, Zarina Shaikh, MD {1386807907} Otlryg(FL02<NJ-STCLR-BOO, NJ-RBAYOLDB>
+ ENT & Allergy Associates of Parsippany
900 Lanidex Plaza/Suite 300 Parsippany, NJ 07054 (973)394-1818 Fax (973)394-1810
+ ENT & Allergy Associates, LLP
3219 Route 46 East/Suite 203 Parsippany, NJ 07054 (973)394-1818 Fax (973)394-1810

Sayegh, Rockan, MD {1427466754} EmrgMd
+ Hackensack Medical Center Emergency Medicine
30 Prospect Avenue/Main 3619 Hackensack, NJ 07601 (551)996-3192 Fax (201)968-1866

Sayo Lim, Carina P., MD {1215014436} IntrMd(88,PHI05)
+ New Jersey Veterans Memorial Home - Vineland
524 Northwest Boulevard Vineland, NJ 08360 (856)405-4200

Saypol, David C., MD {1568455640} Urolgy(77,NY19)
+ Morristown Urology Associates PC
261 James Street/Suite 1A Morristown, NJ 07960 (973)539-1050 Fax (973)538-6111

Sbarra, Michael A., MD {1073582011} ObsGyn, Gyneco(86,ITA01)<NJ-HACKNSK>
+ 20 Prospect Avenue/Suite 705
Hackensack, NJ 07601 (201)488-0409 Fax (201)488-8333

Scaccia, Frank J., MD {1891793204} Otlryg, OtgyFPIS(85,NC05)<NJ-BAYSHORE>
+ 70 East Front Street/Third Floor
Red Bank, NJ 07701 (732)747-5300 Fax (732)747-9922

Scaduto, Philip M., MD {1710912332} IntrMd, Grtrcs(83,NJ05)<NJ-STCLRDEN>
+ Drs. Scaduto & Renz
223 West Main Street Boonton, NJ 07005 (973)335-8656 Fax (973)335-8986

Scafidi, Richard F., MD {1083898076} RadDia, Radiol(03,PA09)
+ Radiology Affiliates of Central New Jersey, P.A.
2501 Kuser Road Hamilton, NJ 08691 (609)585-8800 Fax (609)585-1825

Scala, Peter L., MD {1659432391} Anesth(92,NJ06)
+ New Jersey Anesthesia Associates, P.C.
252 Columbia Turnpike/PO Box 0037 Florham Park, NJ 07932 (973)660-9334 Fax (973)660-9779

Scalea, Donald D., MD {1285705962} Psychy(79,NY15)
+ Drs. Scalea & Belt
100 Northfield Avenue West Orange, NJ 07052 (973)731-1535 Fax (973)731-5782

Scalera, John V., MD {1326009192} Urolgy(80,NJ05)<NJ-ACMC-MAIN, NJ-ACMCITY>
+ 3205 Fire Road/Suite 1
Egg Harbor Township, NJ 08234 (609)484-7557 Fax (609)484-0939

Scales, James, Jr., MD {1811948920} SrgOrt(79,NJ06)<NJ-NWTN-MEM>
+ Andover Orthopaedic Surgery & Sports
280 Newton-Sparta Road/Suite 4 Newton, NJ 07860 (973)579-7443 Fax (973)579-5628
+ Andover Orthopaedic Surgery & Sports
452 Route 206 Montague, NJ 07827 (973)579-7443 Fax (973)293-7581

Scali, Victor, DO {1164479895} EmrgMd(80,PA77)<NJ-VIRTVOOR>
+ Virtua Voorhees
100 Bowman Drive Voorhees, NJ 08043 (856)247-3000

Scalia, Joseph A., DO {1346257508} FamMed(94,NJ75)
+ Advanced Primary Care LLC
346 South Avenue/Suite 6 Fanwood, NJ 07023 (908)889-8700 Fax (908)889-7799

Scalia, Joseph Frank, DO {1477560670} FamMed(96,NY75)
+ Raritan Family Health Care
901 US Highway 202 Raritan, NJ 08869 (908)253-6640 Fax (908)253-6908

Scalia, Peter D., MD {1285633321} SrgThr, Surgry, IntrMd(83,NJ05)
+ Jersey Shore CardioThoracic & Vascular Surgery
234 Industrial Way West/Suite A-103 Eatontown, NJ 07724 (848)208-2055 Fax (848)208-2078

Scally, Monique, DO {1780714618} CdvDis, IntrMd(00,PA77)<NJ-BURDTMLN>
+ Cape Regional Physicians Associates-Cardiology
217 North Main Street/Suite 205 Cape May Court House, NJ 08210 (609)463-5440 Fax (609)463-9888

Scanlin, Thomas Francis, Jr., MD {1619066636} PedPul, Pedtrc(71,PA01)<PA-CHILDHOS>
+ Child Health Institute of New Jersey
89 French Street/Suite 2300 New Brunswick, NJ 08901 (732)235-7899 Fax (732)235-7077

Scannapiego, Saveren, MD {1346236668} Ophthl(71,ITAL)<NJ-UMDNJ>
+ Klein & Scannapiego MD PA
230 West Jersey Street Elizabeth, NJ 07202 (908)289-1166 Fax (908)352-4752
+ Paterson Eye Associates
100 Main Street Paterson, NJ 07505 (908)289-1166 Fax (973)278-7207

Scappaticci, John, Jr., DO {1063448603} FamMed(86,IA75)<NJ-VIRTMHBC, NJ-KMHSTRAT>
+ Alliance for Better Care, PC/Mount Holly Division
1613 Route 38 Lumberton, NJ 08048 (609)261-3716 Fax (609)261-5507
+ Alliance for Better Care, P.C.
PO Box 1510 Medford, NJ 08055 (609)261-3716 Fax (609)953-8652

Scardella, Anthony T., MD {1659313609} CritCr, IntrMd, PulDis(77,NY15)<NJ-STPETER, NJ-RWJUBRUN>
+ UH- Robert Wood Johnson Med
125 Paterson Street/MEB 568 New Brunswick, NJ 08901 (732)235-6305 Fax (732)235-7242

Scardigli, Dennis Michael, MD {1457663072} IntrMd(76,PA13)<NJ-OURLADY>
+ NaltrexZone, LLC.
1 South Centre Street/Suite 201 Merchantville, NJ 08109 (856)663-4447 Fax (856)488-6380

Scarfi, Catherine Anne, MD {1003038027} PedEmg, Pedtrc(99,GRN01)
+ 4 Oxford Road
Caldwell, NJ 07006

Scarlett, Franklin H., MD {1528129384} FamMed(76,PA09)<NJ-VIRTBERL, NJ-VIRTVOOR>
+ 6012 Westfield Avenue/1st Floor
Pennsauken, NJ 08110 (856)966-3466

Scarmato, Albert Clark, Jr., DO {1194040402} Anesth
+ Liberty Anesthesia & Pain Management
901 West Main Street/2nd Floor Freehold, NJ 07728 (732)294-2876 Fax (732)294-2502

Scarpa, Nicholas P., MD {1770523433} IntrMd, Rheuma(80,NJ05)
+ Arthritis Center of New Jersey
600 Pavonia Avenue/5th Floor Jersey City, NJ 07306 (201)216-3050 Fax (201)499-0254

Scasta, David L., MD {1083638084} Psychy, PsyFor(77,TX04)
+ Independent Psychiatric Services
115 Commons Way Princeton, NJ 08540 (609)274-9330 Fax (609)279-9336

Scatliffe, Kristen Denise, MD {1194086694}
+ 5665 Kennedy Blvd./Apt 522
North Bergen, NJ 07047 (305)458-0945
scatlikd@gmail.com

Scattergood, Emily D., MD {1740327121} RadDia, PedRad(00,PA13)<PA-STCHRIS>
+ One Cooper Plaza
Camden, NJ 08103 (856)342-2380 Fax (856)365-0472

Scerbo, Ernest John, MD {1245399187} IntrMd(74,MEXI)
+ 3100 Broadway
Fair Lawn, NJ 07410 (201)796-0038
+ Hackensack University Medical Center
30 Prospect Avenue Hackensack, NJ 07601 (551)996-3006

Scerbo, Jessica, MD {1659607562} Pedtrc, PedHem(05,GRN01)
+ Pediatrix Medical Group
255 Third Avenue Long Branch, NJ 07740 (732)222-7006

Scevola Dattoli, Angela, MD {1417191651} FamMed<NJ-HUNTRDN>
+ Hunterdon Medical Center
2100 Wescott Drive Flemington, NJ 08822 (908)788-6100

Schaaf, H. William, MD {1609872837} SrgOrt
+ Rothman Institute
999 Route 73 North/3rd Fl Marlton, NJ 08053 (856)821-6360 Fax (267)339-3761

Schaaff, Robert P., MD {1457435372} Anesth(92,NJ05)<NJ-MERIDNHS>
+ Shrewsbury Surgery Center
655 Shrewsbury Avenue Shrewsbury, NJ 07702 (732)450-6000 Fax (732)450-1798

Schaar, Dale G., MD {1568547768} MedOnc(97,NJ06)<NJ-RWJUBRUN>
+ Rutgers Cancer Institute of New Jersey
195 Little Albany Street/PO Box 2681 New Brunswick, NJ 08903 (732)235-2465 Fax (732)235-6797

Schachter, Laurence Howard, MD {1932120367} Anesth<NJ-STFRNMED>
+ St. Francis Medical Center
601 Hamilton Avenue/Anesthesia Trenton, NJ 08629 (609)599-5000 Fax (609)599-6312

Schachter, Meri, MD {1356305650} Psychy(69,NY09)<NJ-VALLEY>
+ 124 Woodvale Road
Glen Rock, NJ 07452 (201)445-0220 Fax (201)445-6099

Schachter, Nora Claudia, MD {1801179304} IntrMd
+ IPC The Hospitalist Company
55 Madison Avenue/Suite 310 Morristown, NJ 07960 (973)993-9536 Fax (973)998-4237

Schachter, Norbert, MD {1285792747} Ophthl(64,NY46)<NJ-MTNSIDE>
+ 547 Valley Road/Suite 1
Montclair, NJ 07043 (973)783-6446 Fax (973)783-6448
nschachter@yahoo.com

Schachter, Todd, DO {1295727121} SrgC&R, FamMed(84,NJ75)<NJ-KMHTURNV, NJ-KMHSTRAT>
+ Advocare Sterling Medical Associates Sewell
202B Kings Way West Sewell, NJ 08080 (856)582-7900 Fax (856)582-7479
+ Advocare Sterling Medical Associates Somerdale
300 South Warwick Road Somerdale, NJ 08083 (856)582-7900 Fax (856)435-7073

Schackman, Paul E., MD {1144216342} CdvDis, IntrMd(75,WI06)
+ Union County Cardiology Associates, P.A.
1317 Morris Avenue Union, NJ 07083 (908)964-9370 Fax (908)964-9332

Schactman, Brian, MD {1942240551} IntrMd(95,VA04)
+ Summit Medical Group
6 Brighton Road/2 FL Clifton, NJ 07012 (973)777-7911 Fax (973)777-5400

Schaebler, David L., MD {1235143926} OncHem, IntrMd(88,PA02)<NJ-CHSFULD, NJ-CHSMRCER>
+ Mercer Bucks Hematology Oncology
2 Capital Way/Suite 220 Pennington, NJ 08534 (609)303-0747 Fax (609)303-0771

Schaechter, Jason D., MD {1275793366} Anesth
+ 5 Manchester Way
Pine Brook, NJ 07058

Schaefer, Robert M., MD {1972599595} ObsGyn(80,PA02)<NJ-STPETER, NJ-RWJUBRUN>
+ **680 Easton Avenue/Suite 2**
Somerset, NJ 08873   (732)846-9080   Fax (732)846-0171
rschaefermd@verizon.net
+ **330 Livingston Avenue**
New Brunswick, NJ 08901   (732)846-9080   Fax (732)846-0171

Schaefer, Sarah Stuart, MD {1427014182} Surgry, SrgOnc(89,NY19)<NJ-STBARNMC>
+ **Breast Care & Treatment Center**
200 South Orange Avenue   Livingston, NJ 07039   (973)533-0222   Fax (973)535-1121

Schaefer, Kathleen M., DO {1629174172} ObsGyn(00,PA77)<NJ-COOPRUMC>
+ **Cooper University Medical Center/Camden**
3 Cooper Plaza/Suite 221/ObGyn   Camden, NJ 08103   (856)342-2000

Schaeffer, Mark A., MD {1194866087} IntrMd(84,NY09)<NJ-UNVMCPRN>
+ **800 Bunn Drive/Suite 302**
Princeton, NJ 08540   (609)921-1680   Fax (609)921-1438

Schaer, David H., MD {1205892809} CdvDis, IntrMd(81,CA18)
+ **Cardiology Associates of New Brunswick**
593 Cranbury Road/Suite 2   East Brunswick, NJ 08816   (732)390-3333   Fax (732)390-9244

Schaer, Teresa McKinley, MD {1639116395} Grtrcs, IntrMd(81,CA18)<NJ-STPETER>
+ **The Cardio-Thoracic Surgical Group PA**
12 Stults Road/Suite 123   Dayton, NJ 08810   (732)230-3272   Fax (732)230-3309

Schafer, Laura, MD {1558523555} PsyCAd, Psychy(83,CT01)
+ **20 Nassau Street/Suite 301**
Princeton, NJ 08542   (609)683-9795   Fax (609)683-4050

Schaffer, Ashley Marie, MD {1588045769} Pedtrc
+ **Notchview Pediatrics, LLC.**
1037 Route 46 East/Suite 201   Clifton, NJ 07013   (201)452-5030   Fax (973)471-2730

Schaffer, Julie Votava, MD {1760473342} Dermat(00,CT01)<NY-NYUTISCH>
+ **155 Polifly Road/Suite 101**
Hackensack, NJ 07601   (551)996-8697   Fax (201)441-9963

Schaffer, Scott R., MD {1013940717} Otlryg, PedOto, OtgyFPIS(83,PA07)<NJ-COOPRUMC, NJ-VIRTVOOR>
+ **The ENT Specialty Center, PC**
2500 English Creek Avenue   Egg Harbor Township, NJ 08234   (856)489-3113   Fax (856)874-0128
+ **Advocare ENT Specialty Center**
88 South Lakeview Drive/Building 1   Gibbsboro, NJ 08026   (856)489-3113   Fax (856)435-9112

Schaffzin, David Marc, MD {1275582587} SrgC&R, Surgry(97,PA02)<NJ-VIRTUAHS>
+ **Virtua Surgical Group, PA**
1935 Route 70 East   Cherry Hill, NJ 08003   (856)428-7700   Fax (856)424-9120

Schafranek, William, MD {1982815635} CdvDis, IntrMd(01,NJ05)
+ **Hunterdon Cardiovascular Associates**
1100 Wescott Drive/Suite G-3   Flemington, NJ 08822   (908)788-1710   Fax (908)788-1716

Schaible, Derek D., MD {1194779819} EmrgMd
+ **38 Wilshire Drive**
Tinton Falls, NJ 07724

Schainker, Bruce Allan, MD {1609802560} PthAClI, Pthlgy, PthCyt(75,MO02)<NJ-HOLYNAME>
+ **Holy Name Hospital**
718 Teaneck Road/Pathology   Teaneck, NJ 07666   (201)833-3000

Schair, Barry David, MD {1023289774} CdvDis, IntrMd(02,NY08)
+ **Cardiology Consultants**
246 Hamburg Turnpike/Suite 201   Wayne, NJ 07470   (973)942-1141   Fax (973)942-1250

Schairer, Janet Lynn, MD {1275524548} Pedtrc(99,PA09)<NJ-JRSYSHMC, NJ-KIMBALL>
+ **Jersey Shore University Medical Center**
1945 Route 33/Pediatrics   Neptune, NJ 07753   (732)776-4270   Fax (732)776-3161
+ **Kent Plaza Pediatrics**
4780 Route 9 South   Howell, NJ 07731   (732)776-4270   Fax (732)886-6292

Schalet, Bennett David, DO {1437159902} CdvDis(87,IA75)
+ **95 Madison Avenue**
Morristown, NJ 07960   (973)898-1200   Fax (973)898-1496
+ **369 West Blackwell Street**
Dover, NJ 07801   (973)537-0300

Schalet, Michael Alan, DO {1275679649} Gastrn(79,IA75)
+ **95 Madison Avenue/Suite B01**
Morristown, NJ 07960   (973)267-6474   Fax (973)267-9494

Schaller, Richard J., MD {1154308708} EmrgMd, GPrvMd(90,PA14)<NJ-OVERLOOK>
+ **Complete Care**
1814 East Second Street   Scotch Plains, NJ 07076   (908)322-6611   Fax (908)322-8665

rjschaller@worldnet.att.net

Schaller, Richard Vincent, Jr., MD {1659530459} Surgry, SrgC&R(04,GRN01)<NJ-LOURDMED>
+ **LMA Surgical Specialists - Burlington County**
1113 Hospital Drive/Suite 100   Willingboro, NJ 08046   (609)835-5821   Fax (609)835-5827

Scham, Arnold, MD {1063481307} PainMd, Psychy(65,NY08)<NJ-VALLEY>
+ **169 Dayton Street/Suite 2**
Ridgewood, NJ 07450
+ **The Valley Hospital**
223 North Van Dien Avenue/Psychiatry   Ridgewood, NJ 07450   (201)447-8000

Schamban, Neil Eric, MD {1144273335} EmrgMd, PedEmg(95,PA07)<NJ-NWRKBETH>
+ **Newark Beth Israel Medical Center**
201 Lyons Avenue/EmrgMed   Newark, NJ 07112   (973)926-7000   Fax (610)617-6280

Schanzer, Barry M., MD {1053456509} Ophthl, OphNeu(91,NY19)<NJ-JFKMED>
+ **Advanced Ophthalmology Center**
1812 Oak Tree Road   Edison, NJ 08820   (732)548-0700   Fax (732)494-5059
+ **Omni Eye Services**
485 Route 1 South/Building A   Iselin, NJ 08830   (732)548-0700   Fax (732)602-0749
+ **Omni Eye Services**
218 State Route 17 North   Rochelle Park, NJ 08820   (201)368-2444   Fax (201)368-0254

Schanzer, Robert Joseph, MD {1114923661} CdvDis, IntrMd(95,NY46)<NJ-JFKMED, NJ-NWRKBETH>
+ **One Ethel Road/Suite 106-D**
Edison, NJ 08817   (732)650-0040   Fax (732)650-0045

Scharf, Henry J., MD {1063516169} Gastrn, IntrMd(78,NY46)<NJ-SOMERSET>
+ **51 Veronica Avenue**
Somerset, NJ 08873   (732)545-0002   Fax (732)979-2262
DRHANK123@AOL.COM

Scharf, Jeffrey I., MD {1568402642} ObsGyn(75,PA09)<NJ-CHSMRCER, NJ-RWJUHAM>
+ **Capital Health System/Mercer Campus**
446 Bellevue Avenue   Trenton, NJ 08618   (609)394-4000
+ **Brickner-Mantell Center for Womens' Health, LLC.**
1-A Quakerbridge Plaza   Trenton, NJ 08619   (609)394-4000   Fax (609)689-9992

Scharf, Richard C., DO {1861439481} Otlryg(86,MO78)
+ **Associated Ear Nose & Throat Physicians**
505 Chestnut Street   Roselle Park, NJ 07204   (908)241-0200   Fax (908)241-0445
+ **Associated Ear Nose & Throat Physicians**
778 Kennedy Boulevard   Bayonne, NJ 07002   (908)241-0200   Fax (201)829-1821

Scharfman, Robert M., MD {1700990801} Ophthl(89,NY09)<NJ-RWJUBRUN, NJ-RBAYOLDB>
+ **Atlantic Medical Eye Care**
3 Hospital Plaza/Suite 310   Old Bridge, NJ 08857   (732)607-0555   Fax (732)607-0555

Schauer, Joseph W., III, MD {1801861828} FamMed(81,PA02)<NJ-JRSYCITY, NJ-KIMBALL>
+ **Farmingdale Family Practice**
43 Main Street   Farmingdale, NJ 07727   (732)938-6471   Fax (732)938-3563

Schaumberger, David Andrew, MD {1093771339} Pedtrc, IntrMd(98,NY47)<NJ-ENGLWOOD, NJ-HACKNSK>
+ **Tenafly Pediatrics, PA**
32 Franklin Street   Tenafly, NJ 07670   (201)569-2400   Fax (201)569-6081
+ **Tenafly Pediatrics, PA**
74 Pascack Road   Park Ridge, NJ 07656   (201)569-2400   Fax (201)326-7130

Schechter, Alan Lance, MD {1710097829} Dermat(89,FL02)<NJ-RBAYOLDB, NY-MTSINYHS>
+ **Drs. Schechter and Silbret**
26 Plaza 9 Road   Manalapan, NJ 07726   (732)303-1500   Fax (732)303-0033
alsmdphd@aol.com

Scheer, Linda B., MD RadDia(88,NY47)
+ **Image Care Centers**
222 High Street/Suite 101   Newton, NJ 07860   (973)729-0002   Fax (973)383-2774

Scheets, Kristen Joanna, DO {1437359296} EmrgMd(04,NJ75)<NJ-VIRTBERL>
+ **7 Pinecrest Drive**
Medford, NJ 08055

Scheff, Elizabeth Anne, MD {1114930880} ObsGyn(02,NJ05)
+ **Healthy Woman Ob/Gyn**
312 Professional View Drive   Freehold, NJ 07728   (732)431-1616   Fax (732)866-7962

Schehr-Kimble, Danielle Jessica, DO {1952370736} FamMed, OstMed(01,MO79)
+ **Portside Medical**
150 Warren Street/Suite 118   Jersey City, NJ 07302

(201)309-3000   Fax (201)309-1300
+ **Steinbaum & Levine Associates**
789 Avenue C   Bayonne, NJ 07002   (201)309-3000   Fax (201)339-2785

Scheibelhoffer, John J., MD {1194764712} Otlryg, SrgHdN, SrgFPI(89,NJ02)<NJ-CHILTON, NJ-WAYNEGEN>
+ **ENT & Allergy Associates, LLP**
1211 Hamburg Turnpike/Suite 205   Wayne, NJ 07470   (973)633-0808   Fax (973)633-8811

Scheick, Jennifer Theresa, MD {1396984134} PhysMd, IntrMd(05,PA09)<NJ-OCEANMC>
+ **Shore Rehabilitation Institute**
425 Jack Martin Boulevard   Brick, NJ 08724   (732)836-4530
+ **1933 State Route 35/Suite 105-286**
Wall Township, NJ 07719   (609)992-6414

Scheid, Edward Herbert, Jr., MD {1124102652} SrgNro(98,PA02)<NY-STPETERS>
+ **Summit Medical Group**
140 Park Avenue/3rd Floor   Florham Park, NJ 07932   (908)273-4300

Schein, Aviva B., MD {1740275411} Pedtrc(97,NY46)<NY-MAIMONMC, NJ-ENGLWOOD>
+ **Tenafly Pediatrics, PA**
1135 Broad Street/Suite 208   Clifton, NJ 07013   (973)471-8600   Fax (973)471-3068
+ **Tenafly Pediatrics, PA**
32 Franklin Street   Tenafly, NJ 07670   (973)471-8600   Fax (201)569-6081

Scheiner, Edward David, DO {1184690315} OtgyFPIS, Otlryg, SrgPIstc(76,PA77)<NJ-KMHSTRAT, NJ-KMHCHRRY>
+ **Advanced ENT - Voorhees**
200 Bowman Drive/Suite D-285   Voorhees, NJ 08043   (856)602-4000   Fax (856)346-0757
+ **Advanced ENT - Washington Township**
239 Hurffville Crosskeys Road   Sewell, NJ 08080   (856)602-4000   Fax (856)629-3391
+ **Advanced ENT - Haddonfield**
11A Laurel Road East   Stratford, NJ 08043   (856)602-4000   Fax (856)346-0757

Scheiner, Marc A., MD {1245268077} IntrMd, ClCdEl, CdvDis(93,NY46)
+ **Cardiology Associates of New Brunswick**
593 Cranbury Road/Suite 2   East Brunswick, NJ 08816   (732)390-3333   Fax (732)390-9244

Scheinthal, Stephen M., DO {1790765196} PsyAdt, PsyGrt, Psychy(91,NJ75)<NJ-KMHSTRAT, NY-LDYLORDS>
+ **New Jersey Institute for Successful Aging**
42 East Laurel Road/Suite 1800   Stratford, NJ 08084   (856)566-6843   Fax (856)566-6781
+ **University of Medicine & Dentistry of New Jersey-SOM**
42 East Laurel Road   Stratford, NJ 08084   (856)566-6843   Fax (856)566-6781
+ **University Hospital-SOM Department of Psychiatry**
2250 Chapel Avenue West/Suite 100   Cherry Hill, NJ 08084   (856)482-9000   Fax (856)482-1159

Schell, Harold S., Jr., MD {1245247709} Surgry, SrgBst(70,MA05)<NJ-CHSMRCER>
+ **Capital Health System/Mercer Campus**
446 Bellevue Avenue/GenSrgry/Attndg   Trenton, NJ 08618   (609)392-8100   Fax (609)695-6202
hsschell@hotmail.com
+ **Mountain View Surgical Associates**
1445 Whitehorse-Mercerville Rd   Hamilton, NJ 08691   (609)392-8100   Fax (609)528-8875
+ **Mountain View Surgical Assocaites**
2 Capital Way/Suite 505   Pennington, NJ 08618   (609)656-8844   Fax (609)656-8845

Schell, Paul Lee, MD {1770570541} ObsGyn(66,IL43)<NJ-LOURDMED, NJ-VIRTMHBC>
+ **Advocare Burlington County Obstetrics & Gynecology**
1000 Salem Road/Suite B   Willingboro, NJ 08046   (609)871-2060   Fax (609)871-5478
+ **Burlington County Ob-Gyn**
8008 Route 130 N/Suite 320   Delran, NJ 08075   (609)871-2060   Fax (856)764-0103
+ **Burlington County Ob-Gyn**
210 Ark Road/Suite 216   Mount Laurel, NJ 08046   (856)778-2060   Fax (856)778-8182

Schellato, Teodora A., DO {1184839698}
+ **100 Pheasant Fields Lane**
Moorestown, NJ 08057   (267)253-1150
schellato@gmail.com

Scheller, Tracey Frances, MD {1912095092} ObsGyn(97,TX14)
+ **300 Grand Avenue/Suite 201**
Englewood, NJ 07631   (201)731-3178   Fax (201)731-3179
doctor@tracyschellermd.com

Schenk, Richard S., MD {1578538039} SrgOrt, OrtTrm(84,NJ05)
+ **Atlantic Orthopedic Associates**
91 South Jefferson Road/Suite 201   Whippany, NJ 07981   (973)599-9779   Fax (973)599-1179

447

Physicians by Name and Address

Schenker, Samuel D., MD {1750327326} Nrolgy(77,SPA05)<NJ-COMMED, NJ-KIMBALL>
+ Pain Institute of Central Jersey and Neurology
388 Lakehurst Road   Toms River, NJ 08755   (732)341-2822   Fax (732)341-7087

Schenkman, Andrew C., MD {1659344869} NnPnMd, Pedtrc(76,CHI04)<NJ-MORRISTN, NJ-OVERLOOK>
+ MidAtlantic Neonatology Associates
100 Madison Avenue   Morristown, NJ 07962   (973)971-5488   Fax (973)290-7175

Scher, Daniel A., MD {1912946583} Otlryg(98,PA07)<NJ-CHILTON, NJ-WAYNEGEN>
+ ENT & Allergy Associates, LLP
1211 Hamburg Turnpike/Suite 205   Wayne, NJ 07470   (973)633-0808   Fax (973)633-8811
+ Wayne Surgical Center, LLC.
1176 Hamburg Pike   Wayne, NJ 07470   (973)633-0808   Fax (973)709-1901

Scher, Richard M., DO {1043205313} IntrMd, MedOnc(83,NJ75)<NJ-VIRTMHBC, NJ-RIVERVW>
+ Regional Cancer Care Associates, LLC
180 White Road   Little Silver, NJ 07739   (732)530-8666   Fax (732)530-4139

Scherer, Susan Denys, MD {1750350815} Pedtrc(97,TX13)
+ Madison Pediatrics
435 South Street/Suite 200   Morristown, NJ 07960   (973)822-0003   Fax (973)822-3349

Scherl, Jonathan Daniel, MD {1376510248} SrgOrt(91,PA01)<NJ-HACKNSK>
+ 440 Curry Avenue/Suite A
Englewood, NJ 07631   (201)569-4443   Fax (201)569-1987

Scherl, Michael P., MD {1801894183} Otlryg, SrgHdN(82,NY03)<NJ-ENGLWOOD>
+ Northern Valley ENT
163 Engle Street/Suite 1B   Englewood, NJ 07631   (201)569-6789   Fax (201)569-6709
+ Northern Valley ENT
354 Old Hook Road/Suite 204   Westwood, NJ 07675   (201)569-6789   Fax (201)358-6686

Scherl, Sharon, MD {1770515595} Dermat(88,NY09)<NJ-ENGLWOOD>
+ The Office of Dr Sharon Scherl MD
45 Central Aveue   Tenafly, NJ 07670   (201)568-8400   Fax (201)568-8554

Scherling, Richard H., DO {1902993215} IntrMd(72,IA75)<NJ-CHILTON>
+ 33 Yawpo Ave/Suite 1
Oakland, NJ 07436   (973)831-1444   Fax (973)831-9609

Schettino, Michael Christopher, MD {1497872824} IntrSptM
+ Penn Medicine at Cherry Hill
409 Route 70 East   Cherry Hill, NJ 08034   (856)429-1519

Scheuch, John R., MD {1144283235} Urolgy(81,GRNA)<NJ-HACKNSK, NJ-HOLYNAME>
+ 870 Palisade Avenue
Teaneck, NJ 07666   (201)836-6060   Fax (206)339-9130
+ 30 Prospect Avenue/Suite 717
Hackensack, NJ 07601   (201)343-9010

Scheuermann, Richard Ernest, MD {1073547428} FamMed(82,BWI01)<NJ-KMHTURNV>
+ Pineland Plaza Family Practice
617 Stokes Road/Suite 9   Medford, NJ 08055   (609)953-8080   Fax (609)953-2133

Schewitz, Gail, MD {1609820844} Pedtrc(80,IL01)<NJ-ENGLWOOD, NJ-HACKNSK>
+ Metropolitan Pediatric Group
704 Palisade Avenue   Teaneck, NJ 07666   (201)836-4301   Fax (201)836-5110
+ Metropolitan Pediatric Group
570 Piermont Road/17 Closter Commons   Closter, NJ 07624   (201)836-4301   Fax (201)768-7316

Schiano, Catherine Jean, DO {1649233347} FamMed(87,NJ75)<NJ-STPETER, NJ-RWJUHAM>
+ Central Jersey Family Physicians
754 State Highway 18 North/Suite 107   East Brunswick, NJ 08816   (732)257-1171   Fax (732)257-2618

Schiavi, Jonathan Michael, MD {1710273602} RadDia
+ Radiation Oncology Associates of North Jersey, P.A.
100 Madison Avenue   Morristown, NJ 07962   (856)889-7863   Fax (973)290-7393

Schiavone, Joseph Adriano, MD {1326042698} CdvDis, IntrMd, IntCrd(85,GRNA)<NJ-WARREN>
+ Easton Cardiovascular Associates
123 Roseberry Street   Phillipsburg, NJ 08865   (908)213-3100
+ Warren Hospital
185 Roseberry Street   Phillipsburg, NJ 08865   (908)859-6700

Schiavone, Ronald L., DO {1225075096} GenPrc, FamMed(77,PA77)
+ Drs. Heck & Schiavone
416 Haddon Avenue   Collingswood, NJ 08108   (856)858-1240

+ Drs. Heck & Schiavone
222 Gibbsboro Road   Clementon, NJ 08021   (856)858-1240   Fax (856)784-0258

Schiavone-Forlenza, Maria, MD {1790927465} GynOnc<NJ-HOLYNAME>
+ Holy Name Hospital
718 Teaneck Road   Teaneck, NJ 07666   (201)833-3000

Schiebert, Steven S., DO {1205042546} SrgOrt, SrgSpn(07,NY75)
+ Ultimed HealthCare PC
50 Franklin Lane   Manalapan, NJ 07726   (732)972-1267   Fax (732)972-1026

Schiers, Kelly Anne, DO {1528268521} PulDis, IntrMd
+ Kennedy Hospitalist Office
435 Hurffville Cross Keys Road   Turnersville, NJ 08012   (856)513-4124   Fax (856)302-5932
+ Kennedy Health Alliance Vascular Surgery
333 Laurel Oak Road   Voorhees, NJ 08043   (856)513-4124   Fax (856)770-9194

Schiff, Matthew M., MD {1134259831} Psychy, PsyCAd(68,NY08)<NJ-CENTRAST>
+ 170 Morris Avenue
Long Branch, NJ 07740   (732)870-6260   Fax (732)870-0105

Schiff, Robert Michael, MD {1730442898} RadV&I<NH-DRTMTHMC>
+ Monmouth Medical Imaging
300 Second Avenue   Long Branch, NJ 07740   (732)923-6806   Fax (732)923-6216

Schiffenhaus, Elizabeth, MD {1720440563} EmrgMd
+ 5 Newberry Court
Medford, NJ 08055   (609)760-1704

Schiffman, Erica R., MD {1013041631} PsyFor, Psychy(82,NY46)<NJ-BERGNMC>
+ St. Joseph's Regional Medical Center
703 Main Street/Psychiatry   Paterson, NJ 07503   (973)754-2000

Schiffman, Jonathan Samson, MD {1528068830} Pedtrc, PedCrC(97,PA02)<NJ-JFKMED>
+ 192 High Street
Passaic, NJ 07055   (973)472-0365   Fax (973)472-1007

Schiffman, Joshua M., MD {1881954170}
+ 24 Pitney Street
West Orange, NJ 07052   (973)879-4266   joshschiffman25@gmail.com

Schiffman, Lawrence Adam, DO {1386622397} Dermat(00,NJ75)
+ 10 Heritage Court
Demarest, NJ 07627

Schiffman, Philip L., MD {1992894265} CritCr, IntrMd, PulDis(72,NY08)
+ Pulmonary & Intensive Care Specialists of NJ
593 Cranbury Road   East Brunswick, NJ 08816   (732)613-8880   Fax (732)613-0077

Schiffmiller, Moshe Y., MD {1295007847}
+ University Behavioral HealthCare
183 South Orange Avenue   Newark, NJ 07103   (973)972-0470

Schiller, Andrew P., MD {1841219607} EmrgMd(81,NJ06)
+ Emergency Medical Associates of NJ, P.A.
3 Century Drive   Parsippany, NJ 07054   (973)740-0607   Fax (973)740-9895

Schiller, Arnold Laurence, DO {1285745984} EmrgMd(96,IA75)<NJ-SJHREGMC>
+ SJH Regional Medical Center
1505 West Sherman Avenue/EmrgMed   Vineland, NJ 08360   (856)641-8000

Schiller, Jeffrey D., MD {1710989470} Ophthl, SrgPlstc(79,NJ05)<NY-DCTRSTAT, NJ-JFKMED>
+ 101 Old Short Hills Road/Suite 430
West Orange, NJ 07052   (973)228-7760   info@beautifuleyes.com
+ 98 James Street/Suite 207
Edison, NJ 08820   (732)494-2766

Schiller, Terence G., MD {1710921697} IntrMd(95,NJ05)<NJ-VIRTVOOR, NJ-VIRTBERL>
+ The Maro Group
27 Covered Bridge Road   Cherry Hill, NJ 08034   (856)429-2224   Fax (856)429-1926

Schimenti, Robert J., MD {1326007428} CdvDis, IntrMd(90,NJ05)
+ The Cardiology Group, P.A.
401 Young Avenue/Suite 275   Moorestown, NJ 08057   (856)291-8855   Fax (856)291-8844
+ The Cardiology Group, P.A.
128 State Highway Route 70/Suite 1-B   Medford, NJ 08055   (856)291-8855   Fax (609)444-5521
+ The Cardiology Group, P.A.
1 Sheffield Drive/Suite 102   Columbus, NJ 08057   (856)291-8855

Schimler, Michael Edward, MD {1205835030} EmrgMd, IntrMd(84,DOM02)<NJ-BAYONNE>
+ JFK Medical Center
65 James Street   Edison, NJ 08820   (732)321-7605   Fax (732)744-5614

Schindel, Leonard J., MD {1811023930} IntrMd, Grtrcs(82,MEXI)<NJ-RBAYOLDB, NJ-RBAYPERT>
+ Leanard J. Schindel MD PC
28 Plaza 9   Manalapan, NJ 07726   (732)303-0700   Fax (732)303-9633

Schindelheim, Adam M., MD {1003961368} PhysMd(02,NY15)
+ 38 Wilson Place
Closter, NJ 07624

Schineller, Tanya M., MD {1821234808} Psychy(IRE02)<NJ-RIVERVW>
+ Riverview Medical Center
1 Riverview Plaza/LL-1   Red Bank, NJ 07701   (732)530-2478   Fax (732)224-3910   TSchineller@meridianhealth.com

Schirripa, Joseph V., MD {1609804384} Nephro, IntrMd(01,NJ05)<NJ-COMMED, NJ-JRSYSHMC>
+ Ocean Renal Associates, P.A.
210 Jack Martin Boulevard/Suite D-1   Brick, NJ 08724   (732)458-5854   Fax (732)458-8012
+ Ocean Renal Associates, P.A.
508 Lakehurst Road/Suite 3 A   Toms River, NJ 08755   (732)458-5854   Fax (732)341-4993
+ Ocean Renal Associates, P.A.
1301 Route 72 West/Suite 206   Manahawkin, NJ 08724   (609)978-9940   Fax (609)978-9902

Schlachter, Scott M., DO {1346213386} Gastrn, IntrMd(91,MO78)<NJ-JRSYSHMC, NJ-OCEANMC>
+ Coastal Gastroenterology Associates PA
525 Jack Martin Boulevard/Suite 301   Brick, NJ 08724   (732)840-0067   Fax (732)840-3169

Schlachter, Steven A., MD {1679537633} Pedtrc, AdolMd(71,DC01)<NJ-COMMED>
+ Silverton Pediatrics
2446 Church Road   Toms River, NJ 08753   (732)255-7553   Fax (732)255-8901

Schlakman, Martin D., MD {1144413873} Psychy(92,NJ05)<NJ-JFKMED>
+ Psychiatry Associates
1109 Amboy Avenue   Edison, NJ 08837   (732)549-2220   Fax (732)603-0673

Schlam, Everett W., MD {1033183629} FamMed(86,NJ06)
+ Mountainside Family Practice Associates
799 Bloomfield Avenue/Suite 201   Verona, NJ 07044   (973)746-7050   Fax (973)857-2831

Schlecker, Burton A., MD {1891710182} PedUro, Urolgy(81,NY19)<NJ-CHILTON, NJ-MTNSIDE>
+ Adult and Pediatric Urology Center, P.A.
2025 Hamburg Turnpike   Wayne, NJ 07470   (973)831-0011   Fax (973)831-0033
+ Adult and Pediatric Urology Center, P.A.
1031 McBride Avenue/Suite D-108   West Paterson, NJ 07424   (973)831-0011   Fax (973)256-0432
+ Adult and Pediatric Urology Center, P.A.
1033 Clifton Avenue   Clifton, NJ 07470   (973)473-5700   Fax (973)473-3367

Schleicher, Lori R., MD {1518036540} IntrMd, OncHem(02,NY45)<NJ-NWRKBETH>
+ Newark Beth Israel Medical Center
201 Lyons Avenue/IntMed   Newark, NJ 07112   (973)926-7000

Schleicher, Pooja K V, MD {1366765554}
+ 92 Overlook Drive
Clinton, NJ 08809

Schleider, Michael A., MD {1508810474} Hemato, IntrMd, MedOnc(69,PA01)<NJ-ENGLWOOD, NJ-HOLYNAME>
+ Forte Schleider & Attas MD PA
350 Engle Street/Berrie Building/1 FL   Englewood, NJ 07631   (201)568-5250   Fax (201)568-5358

Schleifer, Steven J., MD {1548331838} Psychy(75,NY47)<NJ-UMDNJ>
+ University Hospital
150 Bergen Street/Psychiatry   Newark, NJ 07103   (973)972-5023   Fax (973)972-8305   schleife@umdnj.edu

Schlenker, Clinton James, DO {1538461306} FamMed
+ Rowan University-School of Osteopathic Medicine
1 Medical Center Drive   Stratford, NJ 08084   (856)566-6477

Schlesinger, Esther M., MD {1447341722} Psychy, PsyCAd(88,NJ05)
+ Catholic Charities Mental Health Center
288 Rues Lane   East Brunswick, NJ 08816   (732)257-6100   Fax (732)651-9834
+ Catholic Charities Mental Health Center
319 Maple Street   Perth Amboy, NJ 08861   (732)324-8200
+ Catholic Charities Mental Health Center
26 Safran Avenue   Edison, NJ 08816   (732)246-1149

Schlesinger, Fred H., MD {1447257803} Radiol, RadDia, IntrMd(87,DC01)<NJ-RWJUHAM>
  + Princeton Radiology Associates, P.A.
    3674 Route 27   Kendall Park, NJ 08824   (732)821-5563   Fax (732)821-6675
  + Quakerbridge Radiology Associates
    8 Quakerbridge Plaza/Building 8   Mercerville, NJ 08619   (732)821-5563   Fax (609)689-6067
  + Quakerbridge Radiology MRI Center at Lawrenceville
    21 Lawrenceville-Pennington Rd   Lawrenceville, NJ 08824   (609)895-1500   Fax (609)895-2647

Schlesinger, James M., MD {1295753317} Anesth(89,NY19)
  + 619 River Drive
    Elmwood Park, NJ 07407   (800)738-1659   Fax (704)871-2128

Schlesinger, Mark D., MD {1528041688} Anesth(82,NJ06)<NJ-HACKNSK>
  + Hackensack University MC-Anesthesia Dept
    30 Prospect Avenue/Room 2703   Hackensack, NJ 07601   (201)996-2419   Fax (201)996-3962
  + Hackensack University Medical Center
    30 Prospect Avenue/Anesth   Hackensack, NJ 07601   (201)996-2419   Fax (201)488-6769

Schlesinger, Scott D., MD {1538149943} RadNro, Radiol(83,OH44)<NJ-RWJUBRUN, NJ-RBAYOLDB>
  + University Radiology Group, P.C.
    483 Cranbury Road   East Brunswick, NJ 08816   (732)390-0030   Fax (732)390-5383
  + University Radiology Group, P.C.
    260 Amboy Avenue   Metuchen, NJ 08840   (732)390-0030   Fax (732)548-3392
  + University Radiology Group, P.C.
    16 Mountain Boulevard   Warren, NJ 08816   (908)769-7200   Fax (908)769-9141

Schlesinger-Kamelgard, Naomi, MD {1457424020} Rheuma, IntrMd(90,ISRA)<NJ-UMDNJ>
  + UMDNJ RWJ Rheumatology
    125 Paterson Street/MEB 474   New Brunswick, NJ 08903   (732)235-7217   Fax (732)235-7238

Schlessel, David R., MD {1962478826} CdvDis, IntrMd(90,NY19)<NJ-OURLADY, NJ-VIRTVOOR>
  + Associated Cardiovascular Consultants, P.A.
    1105 Laurel Oak Road/Suite 165   Voorhees, NJ 08043   (856)424-3600   Fax (856)424-7154
  + Associated Cardiovascular Consultants-Lourdes
    1 Brace Road/Suite C & F   Cherry Hill, NJ 08034   (856)424-3600   Fax (856)428-5748

Schlessinger, Leslie D., MD {1780683912} IntrMd(72,MA01)<NJ-MORRISTN>
  + 45 Baileys Mill Road
    Basking Ridge, NJ 07920   (908)303-1374
    Les195@verizon.net

Schlisserman, David A., MD {1275583072} Ophthl(71,DC03)<NJ-OCEANMC>
  + Freehold Ophthalmology, LLC
    202 Jack Martin Boulevard   Brick, NJ 08724   (732)458-5700   Fax (732)458-0693
    mschliss@aol.com
  + Freehold Ophthalmology, LLC
    20 Hospital Drive   Toms River, NJ 08755   (732)458-5700   Fax (732)505-4322
  + Freehold Ophthalmology, LLC
    509 Stillwells Corner Road/Suite E-5   Freehold, NJ 08724   (732)431-9333   Fax (732)431-3312

Schlitt, Mark George, MD {1023071073} Pedtrc(89,PA02)<NJ-VIRTUAHS>
  + Advocare Haddon Pediatric Group
    119 White Horse Pike   Haddon Heights, NJ 08035   (856)547-7300   Fax (856)547-4573

Schlitt, Meghan Ann, MD {1215323092} Pedtrc
  + PediatriCare Associates
    20-20 Fair Lawn Avenue   Fair Lawn, NJ 07410   (201)791-4545   Fax (201)791-3765

Schlitt, Michael T., MD {1639133168} Pedtrc(87,PA02)<NJ-VIRTUAHS>
  + Advocare Haddon Pediatric Group
    119 White Horse Pike   Haddon Heights, NJ 08035   (856)547-7300   Fax (856)547-4573

Schlitt, Stephanie N., MD {1811951486} Pedtrc(94,MA07)<NJ-VIRTVOOR>
  + Advocare Haddon Pediatric Group
    119 White Horse Pike   Haddon Heights, NJ 08035   (856)547-7300   Fax (856)547-4573

Schlogl, Jeffrey G., MD {1184915191} EmrgMd
  + EmCare
    425 Jack Martin Boulevard   Brick, NJ 08724   (732)840-3380

Schloo, Betsy L., MD {1679514137} PthAcl(79,PA13)<NJ-DEBRAHLC>
  + Deborah Heart and Lung Center
    200 Trenton Road   Browns Mills, NJ 08015   (609)893-6611   Fax (609)893-1213

Schlossberg, Hope R., MD {1558320150} ObsGyn(93,NJ06)<NJ-ENGLWOOD, NJ-HACKNSK>
  + Comprehensive Women's Care
    401A South Van Brunt Street/Suite 405   Englewood, NJ 07631   (201)871-4346   Fax (201)871-5953

Schlussel, Richard N., MD {1497809784} Urolgy, PedUro(86,NY46)<NJ-ENGLWOOD, NY-CHLDWEIL>
  + Englewood Hospital and Medical Center
    350 Engle Street/5 W Med Suites   Englewood, NJ 07631   (201)894-3690   Fax (201)894-5264

Schmalz, William Francis, Jr., MD {1689852428} GenPrc(04,GRN01)
  + first Care Medical Group
    750 Valley Brook Avenue   Lyndhurst, NJ 07071   (201)896-0900   Fax (201)896-2726

Schmaus, Peter Howard, MD {1801880232} PhysMd, PhyM-Pain(85,NY47)<NJ-HACKNSK>
  + Orthopedic Spine and Sports Medicine Center
    2 Forest Avenue   Paramus, NJ 07652   (201)587-1111   Fax (201)587-8192

Schmell, Eric Brad, MD {1316927726} RadDia(94,NY09)
  + Edison Radiology Group, P.A.
    65 James Street   Edison, NJ 08820   (732)321-7167   Fax (732)906-4915

Schmelzer, John F., DO {1457454647} Dermat(68,PA77)<NJ-OCEANMC>
  + Drs. Schmelzer & Caruso
    4 Bypass Road/Suite 104   Salem, NJ 08079   (856)983-4646   Fax (856)983-4760
  + Drs. Schmelzer & Caruso
    427 Egg Harbor Road   Sewell, NJ 08080   (856)589-2267

Schmid, Daniel B., MD {1386844660} SrgPlstc, SrgBst(07,IL06)
  + Plastic Surgery Center of New Jersey at SMG
    131 Madison Avenue/Suite 120   Morristown, NJ 07960   (973)540-9055

Schmid, George F., MD {1568426559} IntrMd(80,NJ05)
  + 714 South White Horse Pike
    Audubon, NJ 08106   (856)547-6151   Fax (856)547-3477

Schmidheiser, Mark Andrew, MD {1104896349} Anesth(94,PA09)<NJ-LOURDMED>
  + AtlantiCare Anesthesiology
    65 West Jimmie Leeds Road   Pomona, NJ 08240   (609)748-7597

Schmidling, Michael John, MD {1518942408} Radiol, RadV&I, RadDia(97,NJ06)<NJ-RBAYPERT, NJ-RBAYOLDB>
  + Atlantic Medical Imaging, LLC.
    72 West Jimmie Leeds Road   Galloway, NJ 08205   (609)677-9729   Fax (609)653-8764
  + Atlantic Medical Imaging, LLC.
    401 Bethel Road   Somers Point, NJ 08244   (609)677-9729
  + Atlantic Medical Imaging, LLC.
    421 Route 9 North   Cape May Court House, NJ 08205   (609)463-9500   Fax (609)465-0918

Schmidt, Alvin M., MD {1275640187} IntrMd(78,SPA02)<NJ-STBARNMC>
  + 741 Northfield Avenue
    West Orange, NJ 07052   (973)325-0006   Fax (973)736-8964

Schmidt, Carol L., MD {1790764074} FamMed(86,OH45)<NJ-VIRTBERL, NJ-VIRTVOOR>
  + Partners in Primary Care
    239 Hurffville Crosskeys Road   Sewell, NJ 08080   (856)881-1940

Schmidt, Courtland M., Jr., MD {1578536124} Glacma, Ophthl(85,MI07)
  + Wills Eye Surgery Center in Cherry Hill
    408 Route 70 East   Cherry Hill, NJ 08034   (856)354-1600   Fax (856)429-7555

Schmidt, Hans J., MD {1033276845} SrgAbd, Surgry(91,NJ05)<NJ-HACKNSK>
  + Advanced Laparoscopic Associates
    81 Route 4 West/Suite 401/35 Plaza   Paramus, NJ 07652   (201)646-1121   Fax (201)646-1110
    drhschmidt@yahoo.com
  + Paramus Surgical Center
    30 West Century Road/Suite 300   Paramus, NJ 07652   (201)986-9000

Schmidt, John August, Jr., MD {1164752002} Immuno, IntrMd(76,PA01)
  + 709 Seventh Avenue
    Belmar, NJ 07719   (732)282-8166   Fax (732)280-0147

Schmidt, Kenneth A., MD {1932163219} Anesth, IntrMd(79,NY47)<NJ-VALLEY>
  + The Valley Hospital
    223 North Van Dien Avenue   Ridgewood, NJ 07450   (201)447-8000

Schmidt, Michael H., MD {1710951348} Gastrn, IntrMd(85,IL42)<NJ-HOLYNAME, NJ-ENGLWOOD>
  + Teaneck Gastroenterology & Endoscopy Center
    1086 Teaneck Road/Suite 4-C   Teaneck, NJ 07666   (201)837-9449   Fax (201)578-1699
  + Teaneck Gastroenterology & Endoscopy Center
    1086 Teaneck Road/Suite 3-B   Teaneck, NJ 07666   (201)837-9449   Fax (201)837-9544

Schmidt, Ryan Bausch, MD {1073951687} IntrMd
  + Cooper University Medical Center/Camden
    3 Cooper Plaza   Camden, NJ 08103   (856)342-2000

Schmitt, David J., MD {1730153594} FamMed(92,NJ05)<NJ-HUNTRDN>
  + Phillips Barber Family Health Center
    72 Alexander Avenue   Lambertville, NJ 08530   (609)397-3535   Fax (609)397-0301

Schmoll, Todd C., DO {1942346432} FamMed(92,PA77)<NJ-SOCEANCO>
  + Ocean Medical MD, PA
    3003 Long Beach Boulevard   Beach Haven, NJ 08008   (609)492-0900   Fax (609)492-1347

Schmucker, Linda N., MD {1952395212} Radiol, RadBdl(90,PA09)<NJ-VIRTVOOR, NJ-VIRTMARL>
  + South Jersey Radiology Associates, P.A.
    901 Route 168/Suites 301-305   Turnersville, NJ 08012   (856)227-6600   Fax (856)227-8537
  + South Jersey Radiology Associates, P.A.
    315 Route 70 East/Suite B   Cherry Hill, NJ 08034   (856)227-6600   Fax (856)428-0356
  + South Jersey Radiology Associates, P.A.
    1000 Lincoln Drive East   Marlton, NJ 08012   (856)983-1818   Fax (856)983-3226

Schnall, Bruce M., MD {1154328748} PedOph, Ophthl(83,PA13)
  + 1000 White Horse Road/Suite 106
    Voorhees, NJ 08043   (856)772-9090   Fax (856)772-1460

Schneebaum, Katherine, MD {1518949643} FamMed(00,NY46)
  + Chapel Hill Family Medicine
    100 Village Court/Suite 302   Hazlet, NJ 07730   (732)758-0048   Fax (732)758-0052

Schneid, Sharona, MD {1225051535} EmrgMd(02,NY48)<NJ-PALISADE>
  + Palisades Medical Center
    7600 River Road/EmrgMd   North Bergen, NJ 07047   (201)854-5000

Schneider, Allen J., MD {1477536597} Pedtrc, IntrMd(72,PA01)<NJ-UNVMCPRN>
  + Princeton Nassau Pediatrics, P.A.
    301 North Harrison Street   Princeton, NJ 08540   (609)924-5510   Fax (609)924-3577
  + Princeton Nassau Pediatrics, P.A.
    196 Princeton-Hightstown Road   West Windsor, NJ 08550   (609)924-5510   Fax (609)799-2294

Schneider, Barbara P., MD {1144307257} Surgry(77,NY03)<NJ-COMMED>
  + 9 Hospital Drive
    Toms River, NJ 08755   (732)244-2060   Fax (732)914-8712

Schneider, Benjamin Mark, MD {1548406465} RadDia(04,NJ06)
  + Summit Radiological Associates, PA
    1811 Springfield Avenue   New Providence, NJ 07974   (908)522-9111

Schneider, Daniel Paul, MD {1891840781} Nrolgy(03,NY06)<NY-PRSBCOLU>
  + University Hospital-RWJMS Neurology
    125 Paterson Street/Suite 4100-6100   New Brunswick, NJ 08901   (732)235-7733   Fax (732)235-7041

Schneider, Henry E., MD {1295705143} IntrMd, PthAcl, Pthlgy(75,PA09)<NJ-OCEANMC, NJ-RIVERVW>
  + Meridian Laboratory Physicians
    2517 Highway 35/Building M/Suite 101   Manasquan, NJ 08736   (732)528-7710

Schneider, Katherine Ann, MD {1902885940} FamMed(95,NY01)
  + AtlantiCare Health Plans, Inc.
    1001 South Grand Street/PO Box 941   Hammonton, NJ 08037

Schneider, Lisa Frances, MD {1154527141} SrgPlstc(07,NY01)
  + The Plastic Surgery Ctr of NJ & Manhat
    535 Sycamore Avenue   Shrewsbury, NJ 07702   (732)741-0970   Fax (732)747-2606

Schneider, Martin S., MD {1063592574} CrnExD, Ophthl(81,NY46)<NJ-CENTRAST, NJ-MONMOUTH>
  + Millennium Eye Care, LLC
    500 West Main Street   Freehold, NJ 07728   (732)462-8707   Fax (732)462-1296
  + Millennium Eye Care, LLC
    Route 130 & Princeton Road   Hightstown, NJ 08520   (732)462-8707   Fax (609)448-4197
  + Millennium Eye Care, LLC
    515 Brick Boulevard/Suite G   Brick, NJ 07728   (732)920-3800   Fax (732)920-5351

Schneider, Mona, MD {1356438329} PsyCAd, Psychy, Psynls(75,ITA01)
  + 74 Large Avenue
    Hillsdale, NJ 07642   (201)666-6676
    mschneider@aim.com

Physicians by Name and Address

Schneider, Rhonda R., MD {1063404333} Dermat, IntrMd(85,NY08)<NJ-MORRISTN>
+ Dermatology Consultants of Northern Jersey
   261 James Street/Suite 2-B   Morristown, NJ 07960   (973)993-1433   Fax (973)993-1176

Schneider, Samuel, MD {1972620391} IntrMd, Psychy, NrlgAddM(75,PA14)
+ 33 State Road
   Princeton, NJ 08540   (609)924-3980   Fax (609)924-1256

Schneider, Stephen, MD {1912001033} SrgOrt(72,MEX14)
+ Raritan Valley Orthopedic Surgery
   515 Church Street   Bound Brook, NJ 08805   (732)469-6160   Fax (732)469-6436
+ Raritan Valley Surgery Center
   100 Franklin Square Drive/Suite 100   Somerset, NJ 08873   (732)469-6160   Fax (732)560-5999

Schneider, Stephen H., MD {1972688752} EnDbMt(72,NJ06)<NJ-RWJUBRUN>
+ RWJ University Hospital New Brunswick
   One Robert Wood Johnson Place   New Brunswick, NJ 08901   (732)235-7751   Fax (732)235-7096
   schneide@umdnj.edu

Schneider, Wayne R., MD {1619916244} FamMed(94,NJ05)
+ Family Practice Associates of Cape May County PA
   210 Route US 9 South/Suite 202   Marmora, NJ 08223   (609)390-0882   Fax (609)390-3511

Schneiderman, Joyce F., MD {1891805305} IntrMd(79,QU01)<NJ-RWJUBRUN>
+ UH-RWJ General Internal Medicine
   125 Paterson Street/Suite 2300   New Brunswick, NJ 08901   (732)235-7145   Fax (732)235-7144
+ Eric B. Chandler Health Center
   277 George Street/IntMed   New Brunswick, NJ 08901   (732)235-7145   Fax (732)235-6729

Schneiderman, Steven, MD {1366415960} Gastrn, IntrMd(84,NY08)<NJ-JRSYSHMC>
+ Atlantic Coast Gastroenterology
   1944 Corlies Avenue/Suite 205   Neptune, NJ 07753   (732)776-9300   Fax (732)776-8059
+ Atlantic Coast Gastroenterology
   1640 Route 88 West/Suite 202   Brick, NJ 08724   (732)776-9300   Fax (732)458-8529

Schneiderman, Todd Aron, MD {1801879895} Otlryg, IntrMd(92,PA12)<NJ-SOMERSET>
+ 215 Union Avenue/Suite C
   Bridgewater, NJ 08807   (908)725-5050   Fax (908)333-4145

Schneidkraut, Jason S., MD {1639337884} OrtTrm(06,NY46)<NJ-COOPRUMC>
+ Elite Orthopedics & Sports Medicine, P.A.
   342 Hamburg Turnpike/Suite 209   Wayne, NJ 07470   (973)956-8100   Fax (973)956-8104
+ Elite Orthopedics & Sports Medicine, P.A.
   44 Route 23 North/Suite 3   Riverdale, NJ 07457   (973)513-9646
+ Elite Orthopedics & Sports Medicine, P.A.
   1035 Route 46 East/Suite G-2   Clifton, NJ 07470   (973)513-9646

Schnell, John Raymond, MD {1316902513} SrgOrt, IntrMd(91,NY45)<NJ-RWJUHAM, NJ-STFRNMED>
+ Trenton Orthopaedic Group
   1225 Whitehorse Mercerville Rd   Trenton, NJ 08619   (609)581-2200   Fax (609)581-1212
+ Trenton Orthopaedic Group
   116 Washington Crossing Road   Pennington, NJ 08534   (609)581-2200   Fax (609)581-1212

Schnitzer, Robert E., MD {1578539466} Ophthl(77,NJ05)
+ 20 Sunrise Court
   Toms River, NJ 08753   (732)255-8115   Fax (732)505-2171

Schnitzlein, Robert, MD {1629057757} PsyCAd, Psychy(91,NJ05)
+ 3186 Route 27/Suite 204
   Kendall Park, NJ 08824   (732)940-6117

Schnur, Rhonda E., MD {1023114592} GnetMd, Pedtrc, ClnGnt(81,TX04)<NJ-COOPRUMC, NJ-VIRTVOOR>
+ The Children's Regional Hospital at Cooper Univ Hosp
   One Cooper Plaza/Med Genetics   Camden, NJ 08103   (856)342-2000

Schnurr, Deborah G. P., MD {1932112133} IntrMd(99,GRN01)
+ 5 Franklin Avenue/Suite 410
   Belleville, NJ 07109   (973)751-6610   Fax (973)759-1155

Schob, Clifford J., MD {1992704092} SrgOrt, SprtMd(82,NJ06)<NJ-OVERLOOK, NJ-STBARNMC>
+ Comprehensive Orthopaedics
   235 Millburn Avenue/Suite 102   Millburn, NJ 07041   (973)258-1177   Fax (973)258-1818

Schoen, Arnold Paul, MD {1164493532} IntrMd(94,NY46)<NJ-HACKNSK>
+ 151 Prospect Avenue/Suite 8 C
   Hackensack, NJ 07601   (201)488-4914   Fax (201)488-4355

Schoenfeld, Allan H., MD {1194791541} Ophthl(73,MEX14)
+ Ocean Eye Institute
   601 Route 37 West   Toms River, NJ 08755   (732)244-4400   Fax (732)505-2171

Schoenfeld, Mark R., MD {1699702019} Anesth, Radiol, IntrMd(79,MEX03)<NJ-TRINIJSC>
+ New Beginnings Ob/Gyn
   55 Morris Avenue/Suite 204   Springfield, NJ 07081   (973)232-5391   Fax (973)232-5392

Schoenlank, Casey R., MD {1043659725} PhysMd<NJ-SHOREREH>
+ Shore Rehabilitation Institute
   425 Jack Martin Boulevard   Brick, NJ 08724   (732)836-4504   Fax (732)836-4532

Schofield, Neal B., MD {1053400119} Psychy(74,NY08)
+ Princeton House Behavioral Health - Princeton
   905 Herrontown Road/Psychiatry   Princeton, NJ 08540   (609)497-3300   Fax (609)497-3370

Schoifet, Scott D., MD {1871532572} SrgOrt, OrtHKn(83,NY01)<NJ-VIRTMHBC, NJ-VIRTUAHS>
+ Reconstructive Orthopedics, P.A.
   243 Route 130/Suite 100   Bordentown, NJ 08505   (609)267-9400   Fax (609)267-9457
+ Reconstructive Orthopedics, P.A.
   401 Young Avenue/Suite 245   Moorestown, NJ 08057   (609)267-9400   Fax (609)267-9457

Scholl, Seth David, DO {1245262922} PhysMd(01,NY75)
+ Coastal Spine
   4000 Church Road   Mount Laurel, NJ 08054   (856)222-4444   Fax (856)222-0049

Scholz, Peter M., MD {1255400719} SrgCdv, SrgThr, Surgry(70,SWI01)<NJ-RWJUBRUN>
+ UH- RWJ Medical School
   One Robert Wood Johnson Place   New Brunswick, NJ 08903   (732)235-7642   Fax (732)235-7013
   scholz@umdnj.edu

Schonfeld, Steven M., MD {1639156813} RadNro, Radiol(78,NY47)<NJ-STPETER, NJ-RWJUBRUN>
+ University Radiology Group, P.C.
   483 Cranbury Road   East Brunswick, NJ 08816   (732)390-0030   Fax (732)390-5383

Schonfield, Leah R., DO {1265530208} IntrMd, Pedtrc(88,IA75)<NJ-STCLRDEN>
+ The Family Medical Center at Dover
   375 East McFarland Street   Dover, NJ 07801   (973)366-5859   Fax (973)366-0026

Schooff, Mary Lieder, MD {1841318201} Psychy(86,MI07)
+ CENTRA Comprehensive Psychotherapy
   5000 Sagemore Drive/Suite 205   Marlton, NJ 08053   (856)983-3866   Fax (856)985-8148

Schopfer, Carl L., DO {1285677492} FamMed, GenPrc(76,PA77)<NJ-SJRSYELM, NJ-KMHTURNV>
+ 115 South Delsea Drive/PO Box 565
   Clayton, NJ 08312   (856)881-0010   Fax (856)881-0157

Schor, Joshua David, MD {1578639514} Grtrcs, IntrMd(85,CT01)<NJ-STBARNMC>
+ Daughters of Israel Pleasant Valley Home
   1155 Pleasant Valley Way   West Orange, NJ 07052   (973)731-5100   Fax (973)736-7698

Schor, Martin J., MD {1295733582} Urolgy(68,NY15)
+ Mahmood Schor Urology PA
   20 Hospital Drive/Suite 15   Toms River, NJ 08755   (732)286-6644   Fax (732)286-9321

Schorr, Ethlynn Susan, MD {1780664599} Dermat, SrgDer(81,NY08)<NY-MTSINAI, NY-BETHPETR>
+ TKL Research, Inc.
   4 Forest Avenue   Paramus, NJ 07652   (201)587-0500   Fax (201)587-0209
   e_schorr@msn.com

Schorr, Ian M., MD {1114917515} Ophthl(69,NY06)<NJ-STCLR-DOV, NJ-HCKTSTWN>
+ Eye Associates of North Jersey
   600 Mount Pleasant Avenue   Dover, NJ 07801   (973)366-1232   Fax (973)366-2960
   eyefix@hotmail.com

Schorr, Pesach Daniel, MD {1619311800}<NJ-STBARNMC>
+ St. Barnabas Medical Center
   94 Old Short Hills Road   Livingston, NJ 07039   (973)322-5000

Schottenfeld, Mark A., MD {1538238233} SrgOrt, SrgOARec(67,IL42)
+ 3 Progress Street/Suite 106
   Edison, NJ 08820   (908)222-8858   Fax (908)222-8857
+ Central Jersey Medical Diagnostics
   1005 North Washington Avenue   Green Brook, NJ 08812   (908)222-8858   Fax (732)752-0772

Schrader, Patricia A., MD {1033139779} SrgCrC, Surgry(87,PA09)<NJ-JRSYCITY>
+ Jersey City Medical Center
   355 Grand Street/Surgery   Jersey City, NJ 07304   (201)915-2000   Fax (201)915-2192

Schrader-Barile, Nicole Annette, MD {1215058128} Otlryg(98,GER07)
+ Glasgold Group for Plastic Surgery
   31 River Road   Highland Park, NJ 08904   (732)846-6540   Fax (732)846-8231

+ 256 Bunn Drive/Suite B
   Princeton, NJ 08540   (609)279-0009
+ Becker ENT
   2 Princess Road/Suite East   Lawrenceville, NJ 08904   (610)303-5163   Fax (610)303-5164

Schrag, Sherwin Phan, MD {1295928737} Surgry, SrgCrC(01)<NJ-JRSYCITY>
+ Jersey City Medical Center
   355 Grand Street/Surgical ICU   Jersey City, NJ 07304   (201)915-2000   Fax (201)369-5315

Schram, Adriann Susie, MD {1265419634} RadDia(99,NJ05)<NJ-RWJUBRUN, NJ-STPETER>
+ University Radiology Group, P.C.
   483 Cranbury Road   East Brunswick, NJ 08816   (732)390-0030   Fax (732)390-5383
+ University Radiology Group, P.C.
   16 Mountain Boulevard   Warren, NJ 07059   (732)390-0030   Fax (908)769-9141

Schram, Amy Elizabeth, DO {1396781076} FamMed(03,NY75)<NJ-OVERLOOK>
+ Springfield Family Practice
   11 Overlook Road/Suite 140   Summit, NJ 07901   (908)277-0050   Fax (908)277-0201

Schran, Mary Ann, MD {1609877281} IntrMd(87,MA01)
+ The Park Medical Group
   24 Elm Street   Harrington Park, NJ 07640   (201)784-0123   Fax (201)784-0065
+ Plaza Regency at Park Ridge
   120 Noyes Drive   Park Ridge, NJ 07656   (201)784-0123   Fax (201)505-0483

Schreck, David M., MD {1346213782} EmrgMd, IntrMd, IntHos(80,IL43)<NJ-OVERLOOK>
+ Summit Medical Group-Berkeley Heights Campus
   1 Diamond Hill Road   Berkeley Heights, NJ 07922   (908)273-4300   Fax (908)908-2778
+ Overlook Medical Center
   99 Beauvoir Avenue/PO Box 210   Summit, NJ 07902   (908)522-2000

Schreiber, Marie F., DO {1144249087} EmrgMd(94,NY75)
+ Emergency Medical Offices
   651 West Mount Pleasant Avenue   Livingston, NJ 07039   (973)740-9396   Fax (973)251-1165

Schreiber, Martha L., MD {1114002722} Surgry(77,NJ06)<NJ-JRSYSHMC>
+ Kashlan & Schreiber
   1540 Highway 138/Suite 201   Wall, NJ 07719   (732)280-0020   Fax (732)681-0261

Schreiber, Thomas J., MD {1497887889} PsyCAd, Psychy(74,NY20)
+ 111 Dean Drive
   Tenafly, NJ 07670   (201)567-3112   Fax (201)567-7760

Schreibman, Barbara A., MD {1992741656} EmrgMd(83,MEX14)<NJ-ENGLWOOD>
+ Englewood Hospital and Medical Center
   350 Engle Street/Emerg Med   Englewood, NJ 07631   (201)984-3000   Fax (610)617-6280

Schreibman, Stephen M., MD {1659480929} MedOnc, IntrMd, OncHem(69,NY08)
+ Oncology & Hematology Specialists, PA
   23 Pocono Road/Suite 100   Denville, NJ 07834   (973)316-1701   Fax (973)316-1708
+ Oncology & Hematology Specialists, PA
   100 Madison Avenue/Suite C3402   Morristown, NJ 07960   (973)316-1701   Fax (973)267-2550

Schreyer, Raymond S., MD {1518976745} Nephro, IntrMd(78,PA09)<NJ-SHOREMEM, NJ-ACMCMAIN>
+ Regional Nephrology Associates
   510 Jackson Avenue   Northfield, NJ 08225   (609)383-0200   Fax (609)383-8352

Schriber, Andrew David, MD {1801871173} PulDis, IntrMd, PulCCr(96,OH06)<NJ-VIRTUAHS>
+ Pulmonary and Sleep Physicians
   204 Ark Road/Suite 206/Larchmont 1   Mount Laurel, NJ 08054   (856)778-4640   Fax (856)778-8862

Schrift, David S., MD {1316168230} EmrgMd<NJ-COOPRUMC>
+ Cooper University Hospital
   One Cooper Plaza/CrCareMed   Camden, NJ 08103   (856)342-2000

Schroeder, Donald C., MD {1245266212} RadDia(86,NJ05)
+ Tri County MRI & Diagnostic Radiology
   97 Main Street   Chatham, NJ 07928   (973)635-2000   Fax (973)635-1749

Schroeder, Gregory D., MD {1770816134} SrgOrt
+ Rothman Institute
   999 Route 73 North/3rd Fl   Marlton, NJ 08053   (856)821-6360   Fax (856)821-6359

Schroeder, Mary E., MD {1578714549} Surgry, AnesCrCr(07,MI20)
+ University Hospital-RWJ Medical School
   89 French Street/AcuteCr   New Brunswick, NJ 08901   (732)828-3000

Schuitema, Henry R., DO {1992737175} EmrgMd(90,PA77)<NJ-KMHSTRAT>
+ Kennedy Memorial Hospital-University Medical Center
18 East Laurel Road/EmergMed Stratford, NJ 08084 (856)346-7816 Fax (856)346-6385

Schulder-Katz, Micol, MD {1760683023} EnDbMt, IntrMd(04,NY46)
+ Diabetes Endocrinology Metabolism Specialities PA
6 Brighton Road/Suite 103 Clifton, NJ 07012 (973)471-2692 Fax (973)470-8188
+ Diabetes Endocrinology Metabolism Specialities PA
870 Palisade Avenue/Suite 203 Teaneck, NJ 07666 (973)471-2692 Fax (201)836-3571

Schulhafer, Edwin P., MD {1205886785} Allrgy, IntrMd, AlgyImmn(83,NJ06)<NJ-SOMERSET, NJ-OVERLOOK>
+ Allergy, Asthma & Sinus Center of New Jersey
724 Courtyard Drive Hillsborough, NJ 08844 (908)252-1050 Fax (908)252-1055

Schulhof, Zev, MD {1487723136} SrgO&M(03,NY47)
+ North Jersey Oral and Maxillofacial Surgery
315 Cedar Lane/2nd Floor Teaneck, NJ 07666 (201)692-7737 Fax (201)287-9716

Schulman, Jared E., MD {1386840858} SrgOrt, OccpMd(04,NY09)
+ Meridian Occupational Health
2441 Route33/Suite A Neptune, NJ 07753 (732)776-4251

Schulman, Joseph M., DO {1992745061} FamMed, Grtrcs(89,NJ75)<NJ-TRINIJSC, NJ-OVERLOOK>
+ Drs. Reich-Sobel & Schulman
809 North Wood Avenue Linden, NJ 07036 (908)486-7773 Fax (908)925-4311

Schulman, William M., MD {1396788550} Surgry(74,PA02)<NJ-KIMBALL, NJ-COMMED>
+ Lakewood Surgical Group PA
901 West Main Street/Suite 107 Freehold, NJ 07728 (732)363-0044 Fax (732)905-5845
LSG23458@aol.com
+ Lakewood Surgical Group
9 Hospital Drive Toms River, NJ 08755 (732)363-0044 Fax (732)341-4338

Schulner, Kenneth D., MD {1417900614} CdvDis, IntrMd(77,WI06)<NJ-LOURDMED>
+ 220 Sunset Road/Suite 2B
Willingboro, NJ 08046 (609)871-4487 Fax (609)871-4491

Schultes, Arthur H., DO {1235163817} FamMed, OccpMd(80,PA77)<NJ-UNDRWD, NJ-KMHTURNV>
+ General Practitioners, P.A.
601 North Main Street Glassboro, NJ 08028 (856)881-1330 Fax (856)881-6982
+ General Practitioners, P.A.
601 North Main Street Glassboro, NJ 08028 (856)881-1330 Fax (856)881-6982

Schultes, Katherine Anne, MD {1861735987}<NJ-UNDRWD>
+ Inspira Health Network
509 North Broad Street Woodbury, NJ 08096 (856)853-2001

Schultz, Alan E., MD {1972510428} SrgOrt, SprtMd(73,MEX03)
+ 516 Hamburg Turnpike/Suite 2
Wayne, NJ 07470 (973)595-1444 Fax (973)595-8777

Schultz, Atara Batsheva, MD {1912112731} EnDbMt, IntrMd(04,MA01)<NY-MTSINAI>
+ Diabetes Endocrinology Metabolism Specialities PA
6 Brighton Road/Suite 103 Clifton, NJ 07012 (973)471-2692 Fax (973)470-8188
atara.schultz@mssm.edu
+ Diabetes Endocrinology Metabolism Specialities PA
870 Palisade Avenue/Suite 203 Teaneck, NJ 07666 (973)471-2692 Fax (201)836-3571

Schultz, Charles Martin, MD {1962580910} Otlryg(71,ITAL)<NJ-STCLRDEN>
+ ENT & Allergy Associates, LLP
3219 Route 46 East/Suite 203 Parsippany, NJ 07054 (973)394-1818 Fax (973)394-1810

Schultz, Edward Joseph, MD {1366659898} EmrgMd(04,GRN01)
+ 35 Madison Avenue
Flemington, NJ 08822

Schultz, Gail, MD {1578524823} Anesth(89,IL01)<NJ-OVERLOOK>
+ Summit Anesthesia Associates, P.A.
33 Overlook Road/Suite 311 Summit, NJ 07901 (908)598-1500 Fax (908)598-0197

Schultz, Pamela Sue, MD {1720335037} ObsGyn
+ University Medical Group/OBGYN
125 Paterson Street/2nd Floor New Brunswick, NJ 08901 (732)235-7785 Fax (732)235-6627

Schultz, Robert A., MD {1265491369} SrgOrt(78,NY20)<NJ-HACKNSK, NJ-VALLEY>
+ Garden State Orthopaedic Associates, P.A.
28-04 Broadway Fair Lawn, NJ 07410 (201)791-4434 Fax (201)791-9377
+ Garden State Orthopaedic Associates, P.A.
33-41 Newark Street Hoboken, NJ 07030 (201)791-4434 Fax (201)876-5305
+ Garden State Orthopaedic Associates, P.A.
400 Franklin Turnpike/Suite 112 Mahwah, NJ 07410 (201)825-2266 Fax (201)825-9727

Schulze, Ruth J., MD {1538149752} ObsGyn(83,NY48)<NJ-VALLEY>
+ Women's Total Health-Woodcliff Lake
577 Chestnut Ridge Road/Suite 9 Woodcliff Lake, NJ 07677 (201)391-5770 Fax (201)391-4793

Schumacher, Hermann Christian, MD {1013123587} Nrolgy(85,GER01)<NJ-CHSFULD>
+ Capital Institute for Neurosciences
2 Capital Way/Suite 456 Pennington, NJ 08534 (609)537-7300 Fax (609)537-7301
+ Capital Health System/Fuld Campus
750 Brunswick Avenue/Neurology Trenton, NJ 08638 (609)394-6000

Schumacher, William Delmar, DO {1801857677} EmrgMd(95,PA77)<NJ-ACMCITY, NJ-ACMCMAIN>
+ AtlantiCare Regional Medical Center/City Campus
1925 Pacific Avenue/EmergMed Atlantic City, NJ 08401 (609)345-4000
+ AtlantiCare Regional Med Ctr/Mainland
65 West Jimmie Leeds Road/EmergMed Pomona, NJ 08240 (609)652-1000

Schuman, Richard M., MD {1952344277} OncHem, IntrMd(80,PA09)
+ Regional Cancer Care Specialists
34-36 Progress Street/Suite B-2 Edison, NJ 08820 (908)757-9696 Fax (908)757-9721

Schuman, Robert J., MD {1003958588} Psychy(84,PA02)
+ Ocean Mental Health Services, Inc.
160 Atlantic City Boulevard Bayville, NJ 08721 (732)349-5550 Fax (732)349-0841
+ CPC Behavioral HealthCare
1 Highpoint Center Way Morganville, NJ 07751 (732)349-5550 Fax (732)591-2516

Schuman, Robert W., MD {1689774713} Gastrn, IntrMd(89,NC07)
+ Affiliates in Gastroenterology, P.A.
101 Old Short Hills Road/Suite 217 West Orange, NJ 07052 (973)731-4600 Fax (973)731-1477

Schumeister, Robert S., MD {1700935186} Psychy(90,NY46)
+ 285 Engle Street
Englewood, NJ 07631 (201)569-1133 Fax (201)569-1822

Schupner, Kathleen A., MD {1982609616} EmrgMd(82,MI07)<NJ-HUNTRDN>
+ Hunterdon Medical Center
2100 Wescott Drive/EmergMd Flemington, NJ 08822 (908)788-6100

Schuricht, Alan Leslie, MD {1114925005} Surgry
+ Penn Medicine at Cherry Hill
409 Route 70 East Cherry Hill, NJ 08034 (856)429-1519

Schuss, Steven A., MD {1720030679} Pedtrc(79,NY46)<NJ-ENGLEWOOD, NJ-HACKNSK>
+ Teaneck Pediatric Associates PA
197 Cedar Lane Teaneck, NJ 07666 (201)836-7171 Fax (201)928-4227

Schuster, Joseph C., MD {1386694362} IntrMd(81,NY03)<NJ-HACKNSK, NJ-HOLYNAME>
+ 175 Cedar Lane
Teaneck, NJ 07666 (201)692-7766 Fax (201)692-9876

Schuster, Mark Brian, DO {1851595565} IntrMd(03,NJ75)<NJ-OURLADY, NJ-KMHCHRRY>
+ Nephrology & Hypertension Associates of New Jersey
201 Laurel Oak Road/Suite B Voorhees, NJ 08043 (856)566-5478 Fax (856)566-9561

Schuster, Meike, DO {1316175904} MtFtMd
+ UMDNJ RWJ Maternal Fetal Medicine
125 Paterson Street/Suite 4200 New Brunswick, NJ 08901 (908)247-5323 Fax (732)235-6564

Schuster, Michael Charles, MD {1215091269} Rheuma(02,WI05)
+ Arthritis, Rheumatic & Back Disease Associates
2309 East Evesham Road/Suite 101 Voorhees, NJ 08043 (856)424-4005 Fax (856)424-4716

Schutzer, Steven E., MD {1518166883} Allrgy, ClnGnt, IntrMd(79,NY20)<NJ-UMDNJ>
+ University Hospital
150 Bergen Street/Allergy/Immnlgy Newark, NJ 07103 (201)982-4872

Schuyler, Andrew P., MD {1952576258} FamMed(76,NY20)
+ ImmediCenter/Bloomfield
557 Broad Street Bloomfield, NJ 07003 (973)680-8300 Fax (973)743-5601
+ Aetna, Inc.
55 Lane Road Fairfield, NJ 07004 (973)575-5600

Schwab, Joseph V., MD {1013081280} Pedtrc(90,NJ05)<NJ-UMDNJ, NJ-NWRKBETH>
+ University Pediatric Group
90 Bergen Street/DOC 4300 Newark, NJ 07103 (973)972-2100
+ University Hospital
150 Bergen Street/Ambltry Pdtrcs Newark, NJ 07103 (973)972-2100

Schwab, Kenneth S., MD {1649347444} Gastrn, IntrMd(87,FL04)<NJ-ACMCITY, NJ-ACMCMAIN>
+ Jersey Shore Gastroenterology
408 Bethel Road/Suite E Somers Point, NJ 08244 (609)926-3330 Fax (609)926-8578
+ Jersey Shore Gastroenterology
108 North Main Street Cape May Court House, NJ 08210 (609)465-0060

Schwab, Maria Divina G., MD {1659403061} GnetMd, ClnGnt, Pedtrc(90,PHI02)<NJ-UMDNJ>
+ 183 South Orange Avenue
Newark, NJ 07103 (973)972-3817 Fax (973)972-0812

Schwab, Richard M., MD {1639132970} EmrgMd(77,CA06)<NJ-HOLYNAME>
+ Holy Name Hospital
718 Teaneck Road/Emerg Medicine Teaneck, NJ 07666 (201)833-3213 Fax (610)617-6280
schwab@holyname.org

Schwanwede, Jacqueline M., MD {1881681138} CdvDis, IntrMd(95,NJ06)
+ Consultants in Cardiology
741 Northfield Avenue/Suite 205 West Orange, NJ 07052 (973)467-1544 Fax (973)467-9586

Schwarcz, Aron Isaac, MD {1881822518} CdvDis, CarEch, IntrMd(06,NY47)
+ Cardiovascular Associates of North Jersey
25 Rockwood Place/Suite 440 Englewood, NJ 07631 (201)568-3690 Fax (201)568-3667
+ Cardiovascular Associates of North Jersey
1555 Center Avenue Fort Lee, NJ 07024 (201)568-3690 Fax (201)568-3667

Schwartz, Andrew Robert, MD {1467438259} InfDis, IntrMd(65,NY08)
+ Virtua Internal Medicine & Senior Care
301 Lippincott Drive/Suite 410 Marlton, NJ 08053 (856)840-4534 Fax (856)234-4640

Schwartz, Bennett K., MD {1902860364} Dermat(VT02<NJ-VIRTVOOR>
+ 2301 Evesham Road/Suite 403
Voorhees, NJ 08043 (856)772-2221 Fax (856)772-0936

Schwartz, Carolyn L., MD {1265415962} Dermat(94,NY48)<NJ-ENGLWOOD>
+ 135 Kinnelon Road/Suite 103
Kinnelon, NJ 07405 (973)838-1771 Fax (973)492-2858

Schwartz, Daniel I., MD {1609835487} Pedtrc(81,NJ05)<NJ-VALLEY>
+ Broadway Pediatric Associates
336 Center Avenue Westwood, NJ 07675 (201)664-7444 Fax (201)666-9476
dis@nic.com

Schwartz, Daniel Richard, MD {1558333112} CdvDis, IntCrd, IntrMd(84,MO02)<NJ-OVERLOOK, NJ-MORRISTN>
+ Summit Medical Group
1 Diamond Hill Road/Bensley Pav/2 FL Berkeley, NJ 07922 (908)277-8700 Fax (908)288-7993
+ Summit Medical Group
140 Park Avenue/3rd Floor/Cardiology Florham Park, NJ 07932 (973)404-9900

Schwartz, David N., MD {1770580524} Otlryg, Otolgy, IntrMd(82,MA05)<NJ-VIRTVOOR, NJ-UNDRWD>
+ Advanced ENT - Woodbury
620 North Broad Street Woodbury, NJ 08096 (856)602-4000 Fax (856)848-6029
+ Advanced ENT - Voorhees
200 Bowman Drive/Suite D-285 Voorhees, NJ 08043 (856)602-4000 Fax (856)946-1747
+ Advanced ENT - Medford
103 Old Marlton Pike/Suite 219 Medford, NJ 08096 (856)602-4000 Fax (609)953-7146

Schwartz, Diane C., MD {1861400764} IntrMd(92,NY08)<NJ-VALLEY>
+ Old Tappan Medical Group PA
215 Old Tappan Road Old Tappan, NJ 07675 (201)666-1000 Fax (201)666-4108

Schwartz, Eric, MD {1447266028} Gastrn(89,ISR02)
+ Corporate Health Center
832 Brunswick Avenue Trenton, NJ 08638 (609)815-7400 Fax (609)815-7401

Schwartz, Eric Ian, MD {1174551071} Radiol, RadDia(96,PA02)<NJ-CHSFULD>
+ Capital Health System/Fuld Campus
750 Brunswick Avenue/Radiology Trenton, NJ 08638 (609)394-6000
+ Capital Health Primary Care
832 Brunswick Avenue Trenton, NJ 08638 (609)394-6000 Fax (609)815-7401

Schwartz, Fredric Ira, MD {1124123039} Pedtrc, PedEmrg(93,NY46)<NJ-STBARNMC>
+ St. Barnabas Medical Center
94 Old Short Hills Road/PediEmrgMed Livingston, NJ 07039 (973)322-5000

Physicians by Name and Address

Schwartz, Gary D., MD {1366443780} IntrMd(89,MNT01)<NJ-HACKNSK>
+ 20 Prospect Avenue/Suite 516
Hackensack, NJ 07601 (201)488-8989 Fax (201)996-5765

Schwartz, Jay Harris, MD {1932201613} RadV&I, Surgry(94,PA02)
+ Drs. Schwartz & Nahas
631 Shore Road/PO Box 291 Somers Point, NJ 08244
(609)653-1010 Fax (609)653-9591

Schwartz, Jeffrey G., MD {1023016052} CdvDis, CarNuc(94,NY20)<NJ-MORRISTN>
+ Morristown Cardiology Associates, P.A.
435 South Street/Suite 100 Morristown, NJ 07960
(973)267-3944 Fax (973)455-0399

Schwartz, Joseph Jay, MD {1538185491} EnDbMt, IntrMd(98,NY46)<NJ-ENGLWOOD, NJ-HOLYNAME>
+ Endocrinology Consultants P.C.
229 Engle Street Englewood, NJ 07631 (201)567-3674
Fax (201)567-5385

Schwartz, Joseph T., DO {1225052111} FamMed(81,PA77)<NJ-BURDTMLN>
+ 10 Village Drive
Cape May Court House, NJ 08210 (609)463-0900 Fax (609)465-2363

Schwartz, Joshua J., MD {1992748800} Anesth(83,PA07)<NJ-VIRTMHBC>
+ Burlington Anesthesia Associates
120 Madison Ave/Suite E/PO Box 174 Mount Holly, NJ 08060 (609)261-1660 Fax (609)261-1779
+ Virtua Memorial
175 Madison Avenue Mount Holly, NJ 08060 (609)267-0700

Schwartz, Lauren Faith, MD {1144239286} SrgNro, IntrMd(92,PA13)<NJ-JRSYSHMC, NJ-OCEANMC>
+ The Center for Advanced Neurosurgery
20 Prospect Avenue/Suite 811 Hackensack, NJ 07601
(201)781-5964 Fax (201)881-0700

Schwartz, Lawrence A., DO {1538184858} Allrgy, PedAlg, Algy-Immn(90,FL75)<NJ-ACMCITY, NJ-ACMCMAIN>
+ Atlantic Allergy & Asthma Center PC
408 Bethel Road/Suite D-1 Somers Point, NJ 08244
(609)653-6676 Fax (609)653-8828
+ Atlantic Allergy & Asthma Center PC
76 West Jimmie Leeds Road/Suite 402 Galloway, NJ 08205
(609)653-6676 Fax (609)653-8828

Schwartz, Louis E., MD {1699764563} RadOnc, Pedtrc, IntrMd(74,NY08)<NJ-OVERLOOK, NJ-HACKNSK>
+ Radiation Oncology at Overlook Medical Center
33 Overlook Road/MAC 1 Suite L-05 Summit, NJ 07901
(908)522-2871 Fax (908)522-5628

Schwartz, Malcolm, MD {1083601033} Urolgy(72,NJ05)<NJ-OVERLOOK, NJ-WESTHDSN>
+ Premier Urology Group, LLC
570 South Avenue East/Building A Cranford, NJ 07016
(908)603-4200 Fax (908)497-1633
+ Premier Urology Group, LLC
659 Kearny Avenue Kearny, NJ 07032 (908)603-4200 Fax (201)789-8755
+ Premier Urology Group, LLC
275 Orchard Street Westfield, NJ 07016 (908)654-5100 Fax (908)789-8755

Schwartz, Malcolm S., DO {1801851076} PedEnd, Pedtrc(67,IA75)<NJ-MONMOUTH>
+ Pediatric Endocrine, LLC.
133 Pavilion Avenue Long Branch, NJ 07740 (732)923-1170 Fax (732)923-1176

Schwartz, Mark, MD {1659796183} IntrMd<NJ-RWJUBRUN>
+ Princeton Medicine
5 Plainsboro Road/Suite 300 Plainsboro, NJ 08536
(609)853-7272 Fax (609)853-7271

Schwartz, Mark Glen, MD {1184690042} SrgOrt(84,NY47)
+ Burlington County Orthopaedic Specialists, PA
204 Ark Road/Suite 105 Mount Laurel, NJ 08054
(856)235-7080 Fax (856)273-6384

Schwartz, Mark Lawrence, DO {1164436325} PhyMPain, FamMed, NeuMSptM(93,NY75)<NJ-VALLEY, NJ-HACKNSK>
+ 293 Passaic Street
Passaic, NJ 07055 (201)783-0780 Fax (201)664-0853

Schwartz, Mark Robert, MD {1760453567} Surgry(83,PA09)<NJ-JRSYSHMC, NJ-MONMOUTH>
+ Atlantic Surgical Group, PA
255 Monmouth Road Oakhurst, NJ 07755 (732)531-5445 Fax (732)531-1776
+ Atlantic Surgical Group, PA
459 Jack Martin Boulevard/Suite 7 Brick, NJ 08724
(732)531-5445 Fax (732)836-1592

Schwartz, Marlan K., MD {1497741581} ObsGyn(86,NC05)<NJ-SOMERSET>
+ Tri-County Ob-Gyn Associates, PA
24 Stelton Road/Suite C Piscataway, NJ 08854 (732)968-4444 Fax (732)968-1675

Schwartz, Melanie Schrader, MD {1447434535} ObsGyn
+ Princeton Medical Group, P.A.
419 North Harrison Street Princeton, NJ 08540 (609)924-9300 Fax (609)430-9481

Schwartz, Michael, MD {1457649865} Anesth
+ Cooper Anesthesia Associates
One Cooper Plaza/Suite 294-B Camden, NJ 08103
(856)342-2000 Fax (856)968-8239

Schwartz, Mitchell S., MD {1174594089} Gastrn, IntrMd(83,NY46)<NJ-JRSYSHMC, NJ-CENTRAST>
+ Shore Gastroenterology Associates, P.C.
1907 Highway 35/Suite 1 Oakhurst, NJ 07755 (732)517-0060 Fax (732)548-7408
+ Shore Gastroenterology Associates, P.C.
1907 Highway 35/Suite 1 Oakhurst, NJ 07755 (732)517-0060 Fax (732)548-7408
+ Shore Gastroenterology Associates, P.C.
233 Middle Road Hazlet, NJ 07755 (732)361-2476

Schwartz, Robert Allen, MD {1548354566} Dermat, Immuno(74,NY09)<NJ-UMDNJ>
+ University Hospital-Doctors Office Center
90 Bergen Street/Dermatology Newark, NJ 07103
(973)972-2500

Schwartz, Robert B., DO {1023019270} IntrMd(73,IA75)<NJ-KMH-TURNV>
+ Internal Medicine Associates of Southern New Jersey
151 Fries Mill Road/Suite 400 Turnersville, NJ 08012
(856)401-9300 Fax (856)374-5805

Schwartz-Chevlin, Jill F., MD {1295767911} IntrMd(93,NY46)<NJ-JRSYSHMC, NJ-UNVMCPRN>
+ Princeton Home & Primary Care, PC
8 Marian Drive Princeton Junction, NJ 08550 (609)936-0958 Fax (609)785-5555
frontdesk@princetonhomedoc.com

Schwartz-Eisdorfer, Barbara Harriet, MD {1063417723} Ophthl, SrgRef, SrgLsr(94,NY46)
+ Edison Eye Group
7 State Route 27/Suite 101 Edison, NJ 08820 (732)494-6720 Fax (732)549-5869
+ Edison Ophthalmology Associates
2177 Oak Tree Road/Suite 203 Edison, NJ 08820
(732)494-6720 Fax (908)822-0075

Schwartzberg, Paul Marc, DO {1619936960} Pedtrc(93,PA77)
+ Madison Pediatrics
435 South Street/Suite 200 Morristown, NJ 07960
(973)822-0003 Fax (973)822-3349

Schwartzer, Thomas A., MD {1649297110} IntrMd(93,NJ05)<NJ-STPETER>
+ Central Jersey Internal Medicine
75 Veronica Avenue/Suite 204 Somerset, NJ 08873
(732)828-0002 Fax (732)828-7070

Schwartzman Lane, Roberta, MD {1700928942} IntrMd, Psychy(83,NJ06)
+ 225 Millburn Avenue/Suite 210
Millburn, NJ 07041

Schwarz, Alexandra, MD {1215413216} FamMed
+ 406 Cardinal Lane
Bedminster, NJ 07921 (908)432-9442

Schwarz, Karl O., MD {1124188412} Pthlgy, PthNro, PthFor(75,ISR02)<NJ-RWJUBRUN, NJ-STPETER>
+ St. Peter's University Hospital
254 Easton Avenue/Path/5th Fl New Brunswick, NJ 08901
(732)745-8534 Fax (732)220-8595

Schwarz, Michael L., MD {1952349763} CdvDis, IntrMd(88,NJ05)
+ 201 Route 17/Floor 11
Rutherford, NJ 07070 (973)779-0019 Fax (973)320-4080

Schwarz, Naomi S., MD {1364446473} RadDia<NJ-RWJUHAM>
+ JFK Medical Center
65 James Street Edison, NJ 08820 (732)321-7000

Schwarz, Rachelle, DO {1487093472} FamMed
+ Hackensack University Medical Center
20 Prospect Avenue/Suite 715 Hackensack, NJ 07601
(201)342-1877

Schwarz, Scott A., MD {1902068612} CdvDis, IntrMd(04,NJ05)<NJ-MORRISTN, NJ-NWTNMEM>
+ Cardiology Associates of Sussex County LLP
222 High Street/Suite 205 Newton, NJ 07860 (973)579-2100 Fax (973)579-6638

Schwarz, Warrren, MD {1437155223} Radiol, RadV&I, RadDia(77,PA13)
+ University Radiology, PA
239 Route 22 East/Suite 302 Green Brook, NJ 08812
(732)968-4899 Fax (732)968-8096
+ University Radiology Group, P.C.
16 Mountain Boulevard Warren, NJ 07059 (732)968-4899 Fax (908)769-9141

Schwarz-Miller, Jan, MD {1467420851} OccpMd, IntrMd(84,ISR02)<NJ-MORRISTN, NJ-MTNSIDE>
+ Atlantic Health System
475 South Street Morristown, NJ 07960 (973)660-3579 Fax (973)660-9116

Schwarzman, Marc I., MD {1780627661} Urolgy, IntrMd(80,PA01)<NJ-UNVMCPRN, NJ-RWJUBRUN>
+ Urology Care Alliance
60 Mount Lucas Road/Suite 500 Princeton, NJ 08540
(609)497-3400

Schweickert, Adam Joseph, MD {1174709885}
+ 88 Morgan Street/Apt 4703
Jersey City, NJ 07302 (419)509-0100
aschweickert@gmail.com

Schweiger, Bruce Daniel, MD {1407958481} Psychy, PsyCAd(70,NY46)<NJ-CARRIER>
+ Central Jersey Beharioral Health, LLC
216 North Avenue East Cranford, NJ 07016 (908)272-7500 Fax (908)272-7502

Schweiker, Olga, MD {1437396280}
+ The Cooper Hospital System-Univ Hospital
3 Cooper Plaza/Suite 215 Camden, NJ 08103 (856)342-2439 Fax (856)966-0735

Schweitzer, Justin Stephen, DO {1386894129} FamMed
+ Associates in Family HealthCare, P.C.
73 North Maple Avenue/Suite B Marlton, NJ 08053
(844)542-2273 Fax (856)569-4043

Schweitzer, Richard Joseph, MD {1194746560} FamMed(99,NJ05)
+ Mountain Lakes Medical Center-Urgent Care
100 Route 46 East/Bldg B/ Suite 204 Mountain Lakes, NJ 07046 (973)917-3200 Fax (973)917-3201

Schwika, John T., DO {1699786798} IntrMd, Nephro(01,NJ75)<NJ-SHOREMEM, NJ-ATLANCHS>
+ Advocare, LLC.
402 Lippincott Drive Marlton, NJ 08053 (856)504-8028 Fax (856)504-8029

Schwoeri, Linda J., MD {1336488576}
+ University Hospital-SOM Department of Psychiatry
2250 Chapel Avenue West/Suite 100 Cherry Hill, NJ 08002
(856)482-9000 Fax (856)482-1159

Sciales, Christopher W., MD {1316965007} Dermat(88,NY46)<NJ-STBARNMC>
+ Dermatology Associates-Warren
122 Mount Bethel Road Warren, NJ 07059 (908)756-7999 Fax (908)756-8017
+ Dermatology Associates-Livingston
201 South Livingston Avenue/Suite 1F Livingston, NJ 07039
(908)756-7999 Fax (973)994-1052

Sciamanna, Mary Ann, DO {1801876016} Acpntr(91,MO78)
+ Marlton Pain Control and Acupuncture Center
525 Route 73/Suite 301 Marlton, NJ 08053 (856)596-1005 Fax (856)596-5870
drsciamanna@verizon.net

Scian, John P., MD {1306807854} ObsGyn(83,NJ05)<NJ-CHILTON>
+ Drs. Scian & Scian Ob/Gyn Associates
16 Pompton Avenue Pompton Lakes, NJ 07442 (973)831-6866 Fax (973)831-9639

Scian, Joseph A., MD {1093776551} ObsGyn(77,ITA16)<NJ-CHILTON, NJ-VALLEY>
+ Drs. Scian & Scian Ob/Gyn Associates
16 Pompton Avenue Pompton Lakes, NJ 07442 (973)831-6866 Fax (973)831-9639

Sciancalepore, Justin, DO {1659784072} IntrMd
+ Rowan University-School of Osteopathic Medicine
1 Medical Center Drive/Suite 162 Stratford, NJ 08084
(856)566-6708

Sciarappa, Lorette J., MD {1578651790} Pedtrc(91,NJ05)
+ Spring Lake Pediatrics Associates
613 Warren Avenue Spring Lake, NJ 07762 (732)974-1444 Fax (732)974-1140

Sciarra, Michael A., DO {1811035280} Gastrn, IntrMd(91,NJ75)<NJ-HOLYNAME, NJ-PALISADE>
+ Riverview Gastroenterology
968 River Road/Suite 200 Edgewater, NJ 07020 (201)969-2111 Fax (201)969-8015
RIVERVIEWGI@aol.com
+ Palisades Medical Associates
125 River Road/Suite 103 Edgewater, NJ 07020 (201)969-2111 Fax (201)969-8015

Scibetta, Maria T., MD {1194779454} IntrMd(90,NJ06)<NJ-VALLEY>
+ Valley Medical Group
470 North Franklin Turnpike Ramsey, NJ 07446 (201)327-8765 Fax (201)327-8496

Scilaris, Thomas Anastasios, MD {1619073368} SrgOrt(93,DC02)<NY-BETHPETR, NY-LENOXHLL>
+ Health East Medical Center
54 South Dean Street Englewood, NJ 07631 (201)568-6850

Scillia, Anthony James, MD {1518151547} SprtMd
+ New Jersey Orthopaedic Institute
504 Valley Road/Suite 200 Wayne, NJ 07470 (973)694-2690 Fax (973)694-2692

Scimeca, Gregory H., MD {1730285651} Ophthl(85,PA02)
+ Burlington County Eye Physicians
225 Sunset Road Willingboro, NJ 08046 (609)877-2800 Fax (609)877-1813

Scimone, Anthony, MD {1932174737} Psychy(94,NJ05)<NJ-NWT-NMEM>
+ **Atlantic Behavioral Health at Newton Medical Center**
    175 High Street   Newton, NJ 07860   (973)383-1533   Fax (973)383-9309

Scinas, Athanasios, MD {1922000207} Anesth(92,GRN01)
+ **550 Newark Avenue/5th Floor**
    Jersey City, NJ 07305   (201)795-0205

Scivoletti, Peter D., MD {1437182581} IntrMd(74,PA09)<NJ-VALLEY>
+ **760 Paramus Road**
    Paramus, NJ 07652   (201)445-1819   Fax (201)445-3203

Scivoletti Polan, Nicole Anne, DO {1699098095} PulDis, IntrMd(07,PA77)
+ **Cherry Hill Primary and Specialty Care**
    457 Haddonfield Road/Suite 110   Cherry Hill, NJ 08002   (844)542-2273   Fax (856)406-4570
+ **Kennedy Health Alliance**
    900 Medical Center Drive/Suite 201   Sewell, NJ 08080   (844)542-2273   Fax (856)218-2101
+ **Penn Jersey Pulmonary Associates**
    52 West Red Bank Avenue/Suite 26   Woodbury, NJ 08002   (856)853-2025   Fax (856)845-8024

Sclafani, Michael A., MD {1366421703} SrgOrt, SprtMd(88,NY09)<NJ-JRSYSHMC>
+ **Orthopaedic Institute of Central Jersey**
    2315A Highway 34/Suite D   Manasquan, NJ 08736   (732)974-0404   Fax (732)449-4271
+ **Orthopaedic Institute of Central Jersey**
    226 Highway 37 West/Suite 203   Toms River, NJ 08755   (732)974-0404   Fax (732)240-5329
+ **Orthopaedic Institute of Central Jersey**
    365 Broad Street   Red Bank, NJ 08736   (732)933-4300   Fax (732)933-1444

Sclafani, Steven, MD {1831176254} SrgOrt(91,NY09)
+ **Atlantic Orthopedic Institute**
    111 Madison Avenue/Suite 400   Morristown, NJ 07960   (973)971-6898   Fax (973)984-2516

Scofield, Lisa E., MD {1386601672} Pedtrc, AdolMd(90,NJ05)<NJ-STJOSHOS>
+ **Willowbrook Pediatrics**
    57 Willowbrook Boulevard/Suite 421   Wayne, NJ 07470   (973)754-4025   Fax (973)754-4044

Scognamiglio, Michael F., MD {1316901671} Anesth(81,NY48)<NJ-VALLEY>
+ **The Valley Hospital**
    223 North Van Dien Avenue   Ridgewood, NJ 07450   (201)337-3318
+ **Bergen Anesthesia Group, P.C.**
    500 West Main Street/Suite 16   Wyckoff, NJ 07481   (201)337-3318   Fax (201)847-0059

Scola, Michael Anthony, MD {1245228295} OncHem, IntrMd(93,TX04)
+ **Hematology-Oncology Associates of Northern NJ**
    100 Madison Avenue/PO Box 1089   Morristown, NJ 07962   (973)538-5210   Fax (973)644-9657

Scolamiero, Amedeo J., MD {1467523407} FamMed(77,ITA01)<NJ-MTNSIDE, NJ-CLARMAAS>
+ **Med-Care of Fairfield, Inc.**
    150 Fairfield Road   Fairfield, NJ 07004   (973)227-0020   Fax (973)808-3320

Scolamiero, John C., MD {1780766600} IntrMd(82,ITA01)<NJ-STJOSHOS, NJ-MTNSIDE>
+ **Med-Care of East Rutherford**
    245 Park Avenue   East Rutherford, NJ 07073   (201)939-7161   Fax (201)939-4053
    Jcs@medcarenj.com

Scolnick, David, MD {1306850888} EmrgMd, IntrMd(80,ROMA)<NJ-HCKTSTWN>
+ **Hackettstown Regional Medical Center**
    651 Willow Grove Street/Emerg Med   Hackettstown, NJ 07840   (908)850-6800   Fax (908)850-6896

Scolnick, Ita, MD {1194768580} Pedtrc, AdolMd(80,ROM06)<NJ-MORRISTN, NJ-STCLRDEN>
+ **447 State Route 10/Suite 16**
    Randolph, NJ 07869   (973)361-2860   Fax (973)361-3419

Scoopo, Frederic J., MD {1750382818} PulDis, IntrMd, Pedtrc(88,CT02)<NJ-MORRISTN, NJ-OVERLOOK>
+ **Pulmonary & Allergy Associates**
    8 Saddle Road/Suite 101   Cedar Knolls, NJ 07927   (973)267-9393   Fax (973)540-0472
+ **Pulmonary & Allergy Associates**
    1 Springfield Avenue/Suite 3-A   Summit, NJ 07901   (973)267-9393   Fax (908)934-0556

Scoppetuolo, Michael, Jr., MD {1801876081} IntrMd, MedOnc, OncHem(79,IL42)<NJ-STBARNMC, NJ-MTNSIDE>
+ **94 Old Short Hills Road/Suite 201**
    Livingston, NJ 07039   (973)322-5735
+ **The Center for Hospice Care Inc.**
    3 High Street   Glen Ridge, NJ 07028   (973)429-0300
+ **Essex Hematology-Oncology Group, PA**
    36 Newark Avenue/Suite 304   Belleville, NJ 07039

        (973)751-8880   Fax (973)751-8950

Scopulovic-Nikolic, Biljana, MD {1508029042} IntrMd(99,YUG13)
+ **Palisades Medical Center**
    8100 Kennedy Boulevard   North Bergen, NJ 07047   (201)866-6770   Fax (201)866-6771

Scott, Charles A., MD {1992773436} Pedtrc(77,IL06)<NJ-VIRTUAHS, NJ-VIRTMHBC>
+ **Advocare Medford Pediatric & Adolescent Medicine**
    520 Stokes Road   Medford, NJ 08055   (609)654-9112   Fax (609)654-7404

Scott, George John, DO {1699755710} FamMed(97,NJ75)
+ **University Hospital-University Family Medicine**
    42 East Laurel Road/Suite 2100   Stratford, NJ 08084   (856)566-7020   Fax (856)566-6188

Scott, Martin J., DO {1578562211} FamMed(81,NJ75)<NJ-RWJUHAM, NJ-UNVMCPRN>
+ **Martin J. Scott D.O. and Associates**
    2312 Whitehorse Mercerville Rd   Mercerville, NJ 08619   (609)890-6363   Fax (609)588-5225

Scott, Nancy Michelle, MD {1700029139} Anesth(05,DC03)<NJ-UMDNJ>
+ **Hackensack Anesthesiology Associates**
    140 Prospect Avenue/Suite 8   Hackensack, NJ 07601   (201)488-0066   Fax (201)488-6769
+ **Hackensack University MC-Anesthesia Dept**
    30 Prospect Avenue/Room 2703   Hackensack, NJ 07601   (201)488-0066   Fax (201)996-3962

Scott, Peter J., MD {1588638480} Pedtrc(87,NJ05)<NJ-STPETER, NJ-RWJUBRUN>
+ **Hunterdon Pediatric Associates**
    537 Route 22 East/3rd Floor   Whitehouse Station, NJ 08889   (908)823-1100   Fax (908)823-0433

Scott, Richard J., MD {1972665776} Ortped, SrgOrt(82,PA01)<NJ-BAYSHORE>
+ **Orthopaedic Sports Medicine**
    80 Oak Hill Road   Red Bank, NJ 07701   (732)741-2313   Fax (732)741-7154

Scott, Richard Thomas, Jr., MD {1700810553} RprEnd, ObsGyn, FrtInf(83,VA01)<NJ-STBARNMC>
+ **Reproductive Medicine Associates of New Jersey**
    111 Madison Avenue/Suite 100   Morristown, NJ 07962   (973)971-4600   Fax (973)290-8370

Scott, Robert D., MD {1710999230} IntrMd(93,IL02)
+ **1163 Route 37 West/Building B-3**
    Toms River, NJ 08755   (732)557-9012   Fax (732)557-9015

Scott, Sabriya Carolyn, MD {1124297619} FamMed, Grtrcs, IntrMd(06,PA09)
+ **Neighborhood Health Center Phillipsburg**
    427-429 South Main Street   Phillipsburg, NJ 08865   (908)454-4600   Fax (908)454-3619

Scott, Sandra Renita, MD {1467554758} EmrgMd(94,TX04)<NJ-UMDNJ>
+ **University Hospital**
    150 Bergen Street/EmrgMed   Newark, NJ 07103   (973)972-4300   Fax (973)972-6646
+ **University Hospital-New Jersey Medical School**
    30 Bergen Street/ADMC 12 1205   Newark, NJ 07107   (973)972-4511

Scott, Tiffany Lynn, MD {1356515597} Pedtrc
+ **Watchung Pediatrics**
    76 Stirling Road/Suite 201   Warren, NJ 07059   (908)755-5437   Fax (908)755-6905

Scott, Winston J., MD {1780729921} Ophthl(79,NJ06)<NJ-EAST-ORNG>
+ **310 Central Avenue/Suite 206**
    East Orange, NJ 07018   (973)674-1070   Fax (973)674-0219
    Scottmd160@aol.com

Scotti, Angelo T., MD {1669535829} IntrMd, EmrgMd, InfDis(65,PA01)<NJ-BAYSHORE>
+ **180 White Road/Suite 211**
    Little Silver, NJ 07739   (732)747-4007   Fax (732)747-8497

Scotti, Daniel M., MD {1801809173} Radiol, SrgVas(73,PA02)<NJ-OURLADY, NJ-LOURDMED>
+ **Our Lady of Lourdes Medical Center**
    1600 Haddon Avenue/Radiology   Camden, NJ 08103   (856)757-3500
    scottid@lourdesnet.org
+ **Lourdes Medical Center of Burlington County**
    218 Sunset Road   Willingboro, NJ 08046   (609)835-2900

Scranton, Richard E., MD {1083672661} IntrMd(94,TN20)<MA-BRIGWMN, MA-VAMCWRX>
+ **Pacira Pharmaceuticals**
    5 Slyvan Way   Parsippany, NJ 07054   (973)254-3560

Scriffignano, Marla, MD {1134408669} ObsGyn
+ **708 Sip Street/Suite 4A**
    Union City, NJ 07087

Scrimenti, Michael P., MD {1164516704} Nrolgy, Hdache, Elecmy(80,NJ05)
+ **400 Franklin Turnpike**
    Mahwah, NJ 07430   (201)818-9100

Scro, Joseph Salvatore, MD {1649271909} Anesth(93,NJ05)<NJ-CHILTON>
+ **Chilton Medical Center**
    97 West Parkway/Anesthesiology   Pompton Plains, NJ 07444   (973)831-5000

Scuderi, Steven A., MD {1366421661} IntrMd(83,NY45)<NJ-VIRTMHBC>
+ **Virtua Medford Medical Center**
    128 Route 70   Medford, NJ 08055   (609)953-7111   Fax (609)953-1544

Seabron-Rambert, Cheryl, MD {1518916139} Anesth(87,NY08)<NJ-COOPRUMC>
+ **Cooper University Hospital**
    One Cooper Plaza/Anesth   Camden, NJ 08103   (856)342-2000
    seabron-rambert-cher@cooperhealth.edu

Sealove, Brett Andrew, MD {1528239050} CdvDis(02,IL42)<NJ-JRSYSHMC, NJ-MONMOUTH>
+ **Monmouth Cardiology Associates, LLC**
    11 Meridian Road   Eatontown, NJ 07724   (732)663-0300   Fax (732)663-0301
+ **Monmouth Cardiology Associates, LLC**
    222 Schanck Road/Suite 104   Freehold, NJ 07728   (732)663-0300   Fax (732)431-1712

Seaman, Eric K., MD {1548266414} Urolgy(89,NY19)
+ **New Jersey Urology, LLC**
    741 Northfield Avenue/Suite 206   West Orange, NJ 07052   (973)325-6100   Fax (973)325-1616
+ **New Jersey Urology, LLC**
    700 North Broad Street/Suite 302   Elizabeth, NJ 07208   (973)325-6100   Fax (908)289-0716
+ **New Jersey Urology, LLC**
    375 Mounain Pleasant Ave/Suite 250   West Orange, NJ 07052   (973)323-1300   Fax (973)323-1311

Seares, Petronilo, Jr., MD {1831135110} IntrMd(77,PHI08)<NJ-KIMBALL, NJ-OCEANMC>
+ **Drs. Seares and Bautista-Seares**
    35 Beaverson Boulevard/Building 7   Brick, NJ 08723   (732)262-2400   Fax (732)262-3883

Seaver, Philip, Jr., MD {1588647192} SrgVas, SrgThr, Phlebgy(74,PA02)<NJ-STBARNMC>
+ **Vein Center of North Jersey**
    248 Columbia Turnpike/Suite 1   Florham Park, NJ 07932   (973)408-8346   Fax (973)408-8350
    info@NorthJerseyVeinCenter.com

Sebastian, Clifford Cecil, MD {1164409538} IntCrd, CdvDis, IntrMd(99,NY03)
+ **Lawrence Charles Antonucci MD LLC**
    415 Route 24/Suite E   Chester, NJ 07930   (908)879-1500   Fax (908)879-1515
+ **95 Madison Avenue/Suite B01**
    Morristown, NJ 07960   (973)984-2222

Sebastian, Cyrus T., MD {1457617680}
+ **Inpatient Medical Associates**
    99 Beauvoir Avenue   Summit, NJ 07901

Sebastian, Ely M., MD {1407494998} SrgTpl
+ **Our Lady Lourdes Transplant Ctr**
    1601 Haddon Avenue   Camden, NJ 08103   (856)757-3840

Sebastian, Jodi Komoroski, MD {1023292307} Rheuma, IntrMd(00,IL43)
+ **Atlantic Rheumatology & Osteoporosis Associates PA**
    8 Saddle Road/Suite 202   Cedar Knolls, NJ 07927   (973)984-9796   Fax (973)984-5445

Sebastian, Suniti, MD {1194733139} IntrMd, Grtrcs(86,INA34)<NJ-STBARNMC>
+ **Veterans Affairs Department Outpatient Clinic**
    654 East Jersey Street   Elizabeth, NJ 07206   (908)994-0120   Fax (908)994-0131

Sebrow, Osher S., MD {1659335958} Ophthl, CrnExD, SrgRef(79,NY46)<NJ-HACKNSK, NJ-VALLEY>
+ **Sebrow Laser Vision**
    23-00 Route 208 South   Fair Lawn, NJ 07410   (201)797-7978   Fax (201)796-3937
    drsebrow@sebrowlaservision.com

Sebti, Rani, MD {1396712584} InfDis, IntrMd(91,MOR02)<NJ-HACKNSK>
+ **Center for Infectious Diseases**
    20 Prospect Avenue/Suite 507   Hackensack, NJ 07601   (201)487-4088   Fax (201)489-8930

Seck, Thomas F., MD {1083733687} FamMed, OthrSp, OccpMd(83,NJ06)
+ **Concentra Managed Care**
    135 Raritan Center Parkway   Edison, NJ 08837   (732)225-5454   Fax (732)417-0003

Seckin, Ali Inanc, MD {1497738801} PainMd, Anesth(96,TUR16)<NJ-HACKNSK>
+ **Hackensack University Medical Center**
    30 Prospect Avenue/Anesthesiology   Hackensack, NJ 07601   (201)996-2000   Fax (201)488-6769

Physicians by Name and Address

Seckler, Mark M., MD {1063479194} SrgOrt, SprtMd(86,NY47)<NJ-JRSYSHMC>
+ 2444 Route 34 North
Manasquan, NJ 08736   (732)528-4407   Fax (732)528-4525

Secoy, John Walton, MD {1023093564} Anesth, PainMd(88,GRN01)<NJ-MTNSIDE>
+ Montclair Anesthesia Associates PC
185 Fairfield Avenue/Suite 2A   West Caldwell, NJ 07006   (973)226-1230   Fax (973)226-1232
+ Hackensack UMC Mountainside
1 Bay Avenue/Anesthesia   Montclair, NJ 07042   (973)429-6000

Seda, Evelyn R., MD {1164609608} IntrMd(81,MA05)
+ Ferraro Medical Associates
414 Broadway   Paterson, NJ 07501   (973)742-1761   Fax (973)742-2033

Sedacca, Paul Jack, MD {1982688115} IntrMd, GenPrc, SrgLsr(76,MEX14)
+ 1910 Route 70/The Atrium/Suite 10
Cherry Hill, NJ 08003   (856)424-3350

Sedarat, Ali, MD {1366409310} Gastrn, IntrMd(80,IRA01)<NJ-HACKNSK>
+ Medical Care Institute, P.A.
159 Summit Avenue   Hackensack, NJ 07601   (201)343-7272   Fax (201)343-0228

Sedarat, Alireza, MD {1629133913} Gastrn
+ Medical Care Institute, P.A.
159 Summit Avenue   Hackensack, NJ 07601   (201)343-7272   Fax (201)343-0228

Sedarous, Mary, MD {1114187465} Nrolgy(07,DMN01)<NJ-JRSYSHMC, NJ-OCEANMC>
+ Monmouth Ocean Neurology
190 Jack Martin Boulevard/Building B-3   Brick, NJ 08724   (732)785-0114   Fax (732)785-0116
+ Monmouth Ocean Neurology
1944 State Route 33/Suite 206   Neptune, NJ 07753   (732)785-0114   Fax (732)774-4407

Sedgh, Raymond, MD {1013353218}
+ Mountainside Family Practice Associates
799 Bloomfield Avenue/Suite 201   Verona, NJ 07044   (973)746-7050   Fax (973)857-2831

Sednev, Dmytro V., MD {1356909337} IntrMd
+ St. Michael's Medical Center
111 Central Avenue   Newark, NJ 07102   (973)877-5000

Sedutto, Joseph Mario, MD {1851485734} Anesth(01,NY08)
+ Jersery Shore Anesthesiology
1945 Highway 33   Neptune, NJ 07753   (732)897-0200   Fax (732)897-0263

Sedutto, Paulina Magdalena, MD {1679735005}
+ 1806 Carriage Hill Drive
Belmar, NJ 07719

See, Manuel T., MD {1538125190} Pedtrc(72,PHI01)<NJ-STJOSHOS>
+ St. Joseph's Family Health Center
21 Market Street   Paterson, NJ 07501   (973)754-4200   Fax (973)754-4259

Seedhom, Magdi Ebrahim, MD {1174717698} AnesCrCr(91,EGY03)
+ 411 South Livingston Avenue
Livingston, NJ 07039   (201)792-1183

Seeger, Douglas H., MD {1306884044} SrgO&M(03,PA01)
+ 992 Mantua Pike/Suite 302
Woodbury Heights, NJ 08097   (856)845-1341   Fax (856)384-9067

Seelagan, Davindra, MD {1225251077} RadDia
+ Radiology Affiliates of Central New Jersey, P.A.
2501 Kuser Road   Hamilton, NJ 08691   (609)585-8800   Fax (609)585-1825

Seelagy, Marc M., MD {1336195056} CritCr, IntrMd, PulDis(86,IL02)
+ Allergy and Pulmonary Associates
1542 Kuser Road/Suite B-7   Trenton, NJ 08619   (609)581-1400   Fax (609)585-5234
+ Snoring and Sleep Apnea Center Mercer County
1401 Whitehorse Mercerville Rd   Hamilton, NJ 08619   (609)581-1400   Fax (609)584-5144

Seelall, Vijay Harpal, MD {1821219171} PulDis, CritCr, IntrMd(00,NY09)<NY-BLVUENYU>
+ Atlantic Sleep & Pulmonary Associates
300 Madison Avenue/Suite 201   Madison, NJ 07940   (973)822-2772   Fax (973)822-2773

Seeley, Brian T., DO {1275897118} FamMed
+ Drs. Zalut and Lowe
1000 White Horse Road/Suite 806   Voorhees, NJ 08043   (844)542-2273   Fax (856)770-9194

Seem, Eric H., MD {1386627792} Anesth(94,NY09)<NJ-HACKNSK>
+ Hackensack Anesthesiology Associates
140 Prospect Avenue/Suite 8   Hackensack, NJ 07601   (201)488-0066   Fax (201)488-6769
+ Hackensack University MC-Anesthesia Dept
30 Prospect Avenue/Room 2703   Hackensack, NJ 07601   (201)488-0066   Fax (201)996-3962

Seeni, Aysha, MD {1942333885} IntrMd
+ Goyal & Natarajan MDs LLC
904 Oak Tree Road/Suite M   South Plainfield, NJ 07080   (908)757-1414
+ Geriatric Associates of New Jersey
666 Plainsboro Road/Suite1318   Plainsboro, NJ 08536   (609)269-8291

Seenivasan, Meena, MD {1255308185} InfDis, IntrMd(93,INA77)<NJ-SOMERSET, NJ-UNVMCPRN>
+ ID Associates PA/dba ID Care
105 Raider Boulevard/Suite 101   Hillsborough, NJ 08844   (908)281-0221   Fax (908)281-0940
+ ID Associates PA/dba ID Care
81 Veronica Avenue/Suite 203   Somerset, NJ 08873   (908)281-0221   Fax (732)729-0924

Seenivasan, Thangamani, MD {1083665053} Surgry, SrgOnc(85,INA77)<NJ-SOMERSET, NJ-STPETER>
+ Breast Cancer Prevention Institute
30 Rehill Avenue/Suite 3400   Somerville, NJ 08876   (908)725-2400   Fax (908)927-8990

Seery, Christopher M., MD {1790793925} Ophthl, IntrMd(84,NJ05)<NJ-HACKNSK>
+ Retina Associates of New Jersey, P.A.
5 Franklin Avenue   Belleville, NJ 07109   (973)450-5100   Fax (973)450-9494
+ Retina Associates of New Jersey, P.A.
2952 Vauxhall Road   Vauxhall, NJ 07088   (973)450-5100   Fax (908)349-8134

Seethamraju, Harish, MD {1417037847} PulDis
+ Newark Beth Israel Medical Center
201 Lyons Avenue/Suite C-1   Newark, NJ 07112   (973)926-4430   Fax (973)926-5658

Seferian, Mihran A., MD {1821198805} IntrMd, InfDis(87,EGY03)<NJ-HOLYNAME>
+ Drs. Seferian and Saggar
200 Grand Avenue/Suite 102   Englewood, NJ 07631   (201)503-0660   Fax (201)503-0685

Seftel, Allen D., MD {1538187653} Urolgy(84,NY08)
+ Cooper Surgical Associates
3 Cooper Plaza/Suite 411   Camden, NJ 08103   (856)342-2270   Fax (856)365-1180

Segal, Arthur M., MD {1568532018} Psychy(71,PA02)
+ CPC Behavioral HealthCare
270 Highway 35   Red Bank, NJ 07701   (732)842-2000   Fax (732)224-0688
+ CPC Behavioral HealthCare
37 Court Street   Freehold, NJ 07728   (732)842-2000   Fax (732)780-5157

Segal, Avni, MD {1225325087} ObsGyn(11,DMN01)
+ Virtua Phoenix OBGYN
120 Madison Avenue/Suite B   Mount Holly, NJ 08060   (609)444-5500   Fax (609)444-5501
+ Virtua Phoenix OBGYN
3242 Route 206   Bordentown, NJ 08505   (609)444-5500   Fax (609)444-5606
+ Virtua Obstetrics & Gynecology
401 Young Avenue   Moorestown, NJ 08060   (856)291-8865   Fax (856)291-8880

Segal, Elana Tova, MD {1013938661} Dermat, IntrMd(01,NJ06)<NJ-KENEDYHS>
+ Dermatology Center of Washington Township
100 Kings Way East/Suite A-3   Sewell, NJ 08080   (856)589-3331   Fax (856)589-3416

Segal, Eric B., MD {1770736530} PedNrD, NroChl(05,NY46)<NY-PRSBCOLU>
+ Northeast Regional Epilepsy Group
20 Prospect Avenue/Suite 800   Hackensack, NJ 07601   (201)343-6676   Fax (201)343-6689

Segal, Ilia, MD {1699866871} IntrMd, PulDis, CritCr(70,LIT41)<NJ-BAYONNE, NJ-STBARNMC>
+ Pulmonary and Critical Care Associates
2333 Morris Avenue/Suite B-15   Union, NJ 07083   (908)964-1964   Fax (908)964-6286
+ Pulmonary and Critical Care Associates
534 Avenue East   Bayonne, NJ 07002   (201)858-1021

Segal, Jeffrey Loren, MD {1780652990} ObsGyn, UroGyn, IntrMd(97,PA02)<NJ-STBARNMC, NJ-CLARMAAS>
+ Summit Medical Group
315 East Northfield Road/Suite 1-E   Livingston, NJ 07039   (973)535-3200   Fax (973)535-1450

Segal, Joshua Howard, MD {1710997101} ObsGyn, IntrMd(99,NY08)<NJ-RWJUBRUN>
+ Robert Wood Johnson Ob-Gyn Associates
3270 State Route 27/Suite 2200   Kendall Park, NJ 08824   (732)422-8989   Fax (732)422-4526
+ Robert Wood Johnson Ob-Gyn Associates
50 Franklin Lane/Suite 203   Manalapan, NJ 07726   (732)422-8989   Fax (732)536-7118
+ Robert Wood Johnson Ob-Gyn Associates
525 Route 70/Suite B-11   Lakewood, NJ 08824   (732)905-6466   Fax (732)905-6467

Segal, Lawrence David, DO {1659311215} FamMed, EmrgMd(96,NJ75)<NJ-LOURDMED>
+ Emergency Physician Associates, P.A.
307 South Evergreen Avenue/PO Box 298   Woodbury, NJ 08096   (856)848-3817   Fax (856)848-1431

Segal, Leigh G., MD {1679593644} Rheuma, IntrMd(91,GA05)
+ Richard. D. Gordon, MD PA
2121 Klockner Road   Hamilton, NJ 08690   (609)587-9898   Fax (609)584-1774

Segal, Melissa Anne, MD {1518974849} Pedtrc(96,PA01)<NJ-HOLYNAME, NJ-VALLEY>
+ Hecht and Segal MDs
171 Franklin Turnpike/Suite 110   Waldwick, NJ 07463   (201)612-5100   Fax (201)612-4499

Segal, Michael H., DO {1982643128} FamMed
+ Michael H. Segal DO PC
50 Fairfield Road   Fairfield, NJ 07004   (973)808-5550

Segal, Michele Robyn, MD {1316084189} Pedtrc, AdolMd(01,NY48)<NJ-CLARMAAS, NJ-MTNSIDE>
+ 187 Washington Avenue/Suite 2D
Nutley, NJ 07110   (973)235-9449   Fax (973)235-0434

Segal, Robert Eric, MD {1265408264} InfDis, IntrMd(96,NY20)<NJ-RWJUBRUN, NJ-MORRISTN>
+ ID Associates PA/dba ID Care
81 Veronica Avenue/Suite 203   Somerset, NJ 08873   (732)729-0920   Fax (732)729-0924
+ ID Associates PA/dba ID Care
105 Raider Boulevard/Suite 101   Hillsborough, NJ 08844   (732)729-0920   Fax (908)281-0940

Segal, Saya, MD {1669679940} ObsGyn(05,TX12)
+ UMDNJ RWJ Surgery
125 Paterson Street/CAB 4th FL 4100   New Brunswick, NJ 08901   (732)235-7920   Fax (732)235-7079

Segal, Shiri Nicole, MD {1649429739} IntrMd
+ New Bridge Medical Center
230 East Ridgewood Avenue   Paramus, NJ 07652   (201)967-4000
+ 71 Marvin Lane
Piscataway, NJ 08854   (201)835-7720

Segal, Thalia R., MD {1467751255} RprEnd
+ 296 Durie Avenue
Closter, NJ 07624   (646)577-5120

Segal, William Nathan, MD {1881694974} Gastrn(90,PA01)
+ Princeton Gastroenterology Associates, P.A.
731 Alexander Road/Suite 100   Princeton, NJ 08540   (609)924-1422   Fax (609)924-7473
+ Princeton Endoscopy Center
731 Alexander Road/Suite 104   Princeton, NJ 08540   (609)924-1422   Fax (609)452-1010

Segaram, Gnana, MD {1407864044} Anesth(69,SRI02)<NJ-LOURDMED>
+ Rancocas Anesthesiology, PA
218 Sunset Road   Willingboro, NJ 08046   (609)835-3069   Fax (609)835-5450
+ Rancocas Anesthesiology, PA
700 Route 130 North/Suite 203   Cinnaminson, NJ 08077   (609)835-3069   Fax (856)829-3605

Segaram, Sandira V., MD {1508813346} IntrMd(74,SRI01)<NJ-NWTNMEM, NJ-HCKTSTWN>
+ 653 Willow Grove Street/Suite 1600
Hackettstown, NJ 07840   (908)813-2888   Fax (908)813-2521
sandi50@verizon.net

Segarra, Michael L., MD {1891805909} Pedtrc(76,CT02)<NJ-STPETER, NJ-RWJUBRUN>
+ North Brunswick Pediatrics
1598 US Highway 130   North Brunswick, NJ 08902   (732)297-0603   Fax (732)297-2866

Seger, James E., DO {1346667003}<NJ-MORRISTN>
+ Morristown Medical Center
100 Madison Avenue   Morristown, NJ 07962   (973)971-5000

Segovia, Fernando, MD {1073518411} CdvDis, IntrMd(84,MEX55)<NJ-HACKNSK, NJ-MEADWLND>
+ Cross Country Cardiology
103 River Road/2nd Floor   Edgewater, NJ 07020   (201)941-8100   Fax (201)941-2899
+ Cross Country Cardiology
38 Meadowlands Parkway   Secaucus, NJ 07094   (201)866-5151

Seguerra, Eliezer Montero, Jr., MD {1316162621} PthAcl(99,PHI26)<NJ-STMICHL>
+ St. Michael's Medical Center
268 MLK Jr. Boulevard   Newark, NJ 07102   (973)877-5000

Sehdev, Harish Mohan, MD {1841228442} NnPnMd, ObsGyn(91,PA01)
+ Clin Health Care Assoc of NJ-Mat/Fetal
2301 Evesham Road/Pav 800/Suite 224   Voorhees, NJ 08043
+ Clin Health Care Assoc of NJ-Mat/Fetal
110 Marter Avenue   Moorestown, NJ 08057

Sehdev, Jasjit Singh, MD {1972984334} AnesPain
+ Cooper University Medical Center/Camden
3 Cooper Plaza/Suite 314 Camden, NJ 08103 (856)963-6770

Sehdev, Michele S., MD ObsGyn(92,PA02)
+ Cooper Ob/Gyn
4 Plaza Drive/Suite 403/Bunker Hill Pl Sewell, NJ 08080 (856)270-4020 Fax (856)270-4022
+ Cooper Ob/Gyn
3 Cooper Plaza/Suite 300 Camden, NJ 08103 (856)270-4020 Fax (856)968-8575

Sehgal, Arun, MD {1326017799} IntrMd(88,INA07)<NJ-VALLEY>
+ 27 South Franklin Turnpike/Suite 201
Ramsey, NJ 07446 (201)818-6800 Fax (201)825-9537

Sehgal, Evan D., MD {1982671871} CdvDis, IntCrd, IntrMd(82,NY01)<NJ-HACKNSK>
+ Cardiovascular Consultants of North Jersey
777 Terrace Avenue Hasbrouck Heights, NJ 07604 (201)288-4252 Fax (201)288-7172

Sehgal, Geeta, DO {1114915543} ObsGyn, IntrMd(97,ME75)
+ 179 High Street
Newton, NJ 07860 (973)383-4500 Fax (973)383-8943

Sehgal, Saroj, MD {1871512616} IntrMd, PulDis(72,INA92)<NJ-NWRKBETH>
+ 1023 South Orange Avenue
Newark, NJ 07106 (973)761-4455 Fax (973)789-8403

Sehgal, Shaley Prem, MD {1508059411} PsyCAd
+ Bartky HealthCare Center, LLC
One Springfield Avenue/Suite 1B Summit, NJ 07901 (908)273-1189
+ Bartky HealthCare Center, LLC
513 West Mount Pleasant Avenue Livingston, NJ 07039 (908)273-1189 Fax (973)533-1305

Sehgel, Robert R., DO {1619230307} IntrMd
+ Patient first Urgent Care
641 US Highway Route 130 Hamilton, NJ 08691 (609)568-9383 Fax (609)568-9384

Seibel, David L., MD {1669574364} GenPrc(74,PA13)
+ 3268 North Delsea Drive
Vineland, NJ 08360 (856)696-3908 Fax (856)563-1918

Seibel Seamon, Jolene S., MD {1063546067} MtFtMd, ObsGyn(PA12<NJ-VIRTMHBC, NJ-VIRTVOOR>
+ Virtua Maternal Fetal Medicine Center
100 Bowman Drive Voorhees, NJ 08043 (856)247-3328 Fax (856)247-3276
+ Memorial Maternal Fetal Medicine Center
175 Madison Avenue Mount Holly, NJ 08060 (609)265-7914

Seibert, Henry Edward, MD {1629093133} EmrgMd
+ AtlantiCare Hospitalist Program
1925 Pacific Avenue/8th Floor Atlantic City, NJ 08401 (609)441-8127

Seibt, R. Stephen, MD {1275578890} Dermat, SrgDer(76,MN04)<NY-SLRRSVLT, NY-PRSBCOLU>
+ 92 Old Northfield Road
West Orange, NJ 07052 (973)736-5354 Fax (973)736-8854

Seid, Ira A., MD {1215941794} EmrgMd(81,MEX03)<NJ-HCKTSTWN, NJ-JFKMED>
+ Hackettstown Regional Medical Center
651 Willow Grove Street/EmrgMed Hackettstown, NJ 07840 (908)852-5100 Fax (856)616-1919

Seidel, Benjamin Joseph, DO {1790071215} PhysMd(11,ME75)
+ Kessler Institute for Rehabilitation
300 Market Street/Suite 1 Saddle Brook, NJ 07663 (201)368-6000

Seiden, Jeffrey A., MD {1942330980} EmrgPedr
+ CHOP Care Network at Virtua Voorhees Hospital
100 Bowman Drive Voorhees, NJ 08043 (856)325-3000 Fax (609)261-5842

Seidenberg, Keith B., MD {1588623631} Ophthl(90,NY01)<NJ-VALLEY>
+ 600 Godwin Avenue
Midland Park, NJ 07432 (201)447-9101 Fax (201)447-9103

Seidenstein, Ari Douglas, MD {1902040546} SrgOrt, SrgOARec(04,NJ06)<NJ-HACKNSK, NJ-HOLYNAME>
+ Hartzband Center for Hip & Knee Replacement
10 Forest Avenue Paramus, NJ 07652 (201)291-4040 Fax (201)291-0440

Seidenstein, Michael Kenneth, MD {1285682260} SrgOrt, IntrMd(70,NY09)<NJ-NWRKBETH>
+ 81 Northfield Avenue
West Orange, NJ 07052 (973)736-8080 Fax (973)736-8471
+ Newark Rehabilitation Center
638 Mount Prospect Avenue Newark, NJ 07104 (973)736-8080 Fax (973)481-1338

Seidman, Barry R., MD {1437157641} Urolgy(78,NY47)<NJ-OVERLOOK>
+ 33 Overlook Road/Suite 408
Summit, NJ 07901 (908)219-4479 Fax (908)219-4647

barrys7@verizon.net
+ 8 Mountain Boulevard
Warren, NJ 07059 (908)561-6691

Seidner, Michael David, MD {1891746145} ObsGyn, SrgLsr(82,MEX03)<NJ-HACKNSK>
+ Aesthetic & Reconstructive Surgery
113 Essex Street/Suite 202 Maywood, NJ 07607 (201)488-1700 Fax (201)488-1404
+ Aesthetic & Reconstructive Surgery
1033 Route 46 East/Suite 101 Clifton, NJ 07013 (201)488-1700 Fax (973)779-7920

Seigel, Mark J., MD {1366438178} ObsGyn(80,DC01)<NJ-CENTRAST>
+ Back, Seigel & Goldstein, MD, PA
501 Iron Bridge Road Freehold, NJ 07728 (732)431-1807 Fax (732)409-2777
mark1.siegel@mountsinai.org
+ Back, Seigel & Goldstein, MD PA
4200 Route 9 South Howell, NJ 07731 (732)431-1807 (732)409-2777

Seigelstein, Nina, MD {1619056819} ObsGyn(92,NY06)<NJ-RIVERVW>
+ Riverview Medical Center
1 Riverview Plaza/Ob/Gyn Red Bank, NJ 07701 (732)741-2700 Fax (732)530-8754

Seigerman, Daniel Allan, MD {1275777591} SrgOrt, OrtSHand
+ 620 Essex Street/Suite 202
Harrison, NJ 07029 (888)900-9262

Seigerman, Howard M., MD {1205823028} Radiol, RadNro(88,NY46)<NJ-VALLEY>
+ Radiology Associates of Ridgewood, P.A.
20 Franklin Turnpike Waldwick, NJ 07463 (201)445-8822 Fax (201)447-5053
+ The Valley Hospital
223 North Van Dien Avenue/Radiology Ridgewood, NJ 07450 (201)447-8000

Seinfeld, Fredric I., MD {1275582728} SrgCdv, SrgThr, Surgry(76,NY06)<NJ-STFRNMED>
+ St. Francis Medical Center
601 Hamilton Avenue/Surgery/CardiTh Trenton, NJ 08629 (609)599-5308 Fax (609)599-5325

Sekel, James James, DO {1497779623} FamMed(94,NY75)<NJ-OURLADY>
+ Virtua Family Medicine of Washington Township
239 Hurffville Crosskeys Road Sewell, NJ 08080 (856)341-8181 Fax (856)881-2071

Sekiya, Steven T., DO {1700985314} FamMed(00,NY75)<NJ-CLARMAAS, NY-MTSINYHS>
+ Ligresti Dermatology Associates, P.A.
175 Franklin Avenue/Suite 103 Nutley, NJ 07110 (973)759-6569 Fax (973)759-2562

Selan, Jeffrey Craig, MD {1134480205} IntCrd
+ Monmouth Cardiology Associates, LLC
11 Meridian Road Eatontown, NJ 07724 (732)663-0300 Fax (732)663-0301

Selby, Ronald M., MD {1154407047} SrgOrt, SprtMd(79,MEX03)<NJ-STPETER, NJ-RWJUBRUN>
+ 330 Livingston Avenue/Suite 3
New Brunswick, NJ 08901 (732)846-4900 Fax (732)846-4901

Seldes, Richard Meyer, MD {1023030830} SrgOrt, SrgRec(94,PA01)
+ 401 Hackensack Avenue/10th Floor
Hackensack, NJ 07601 (201)343-3999

Selevany, Muhammad Tahir, MD {1588758809} IntrMd, Hepato, InfDis(76,IRAQ)
+ Selevany Medical Group
397 Haledon Avenue/Suite 104 Haledon, NJ 07508 (973)595-1122 Fax (973)595-7711

Seliem, Ahmed, MD {1104187368} IntrMd<NJ-NWRKBETH>
+ Newark Beth Israel Medical Center
201 Lyons Avenue Newark, NJ 07112 (973)926-7000

Seligsohn, Audrey Lynn, DO {1194787911} Ophthl(97,NJ75)<NJ-MORRISTN>
+ Affiliated Eye Surgeons
405 Northfield Avenue/Suite 206 West Orange, NJ 07052 (973)736-3322 Fax (973)736-7317
+ Affiliated Eye Surgeons
95 Madison Avenue/Suite 400 Morristown, NJ 07960 (973)736-3322 Fax (973)984-5554

Selina, Elena V., MD {1700191582} IntrMd(02,RUS33)
+ Smithville Medical Associates
48 South New York Road/Suite B-3 Galloway, NJ 08205 (609)404-0121 Fax (609)404-0131

Selinger, Sharon E., MD {1447337415} EnDbMt, IntrMd(81,NY20)<NJ-OVERLOOK>
+ Sharon E. Selinger MD PA
1 Springfield Avenue/Suite 1A Summit, NJ 07901 (908)273-8300 Fax (908)273-8807

Selke, Melissa D., MD {1669488367} FamMed, IntrMd(95,TX04)<NJ-STPETER>
+ Dr. Melissa D. Selke and Associates
390 Amwell Road/Bldg 4/Suite 405 Hillsborough, NJ 08844 (908)281-1199 Fax (908)281-4311

Sell, Neelam K., MD {1417936824} Pedtrc(00,VA04)<PA-CHILDHOS>
+ Monmouth Medical Group, P.C.
255 Third Avenue/SH 001 Long Branch, NJ 07740 (732)923-7790
+ Drs. Sell and Baxi
507 4th Avenue Asbury Park, NJ 07712 (732)774-5600

Sell, Samantha Dawn, DO {1053546606} GenPrc
+ McGuire Air Force Base/Acute Health Care Clinic
3458 Neely Road Trenton, NJ 08641 (609)754-9014 Fax (609)754-9015

Seltzer, Gregory Ian, MD {1194901553} IntrMd(03,NJ06)
+ 485 Williamstown Road/Suite J
Sicklerville, NJ 08081 (856)237-8045 Fax (856)237-8047

Seltzer, Lawrence G., MD {1417983412} Radiol, RadDia(89,NJ06)
+ Breast Health Center of Ridgewood, P.C.
385 South Maple Avenue Ridgewood, NJ 07450 (201)670-4550 Fax (201)670-7812
+ Tri County MRI & Diagnostic Radiology
97 Main Street Chatham, NJ 07928 (201)670-4550 Fax (973)635-1749

Seltzer, Ronni Lee, MD {1871526798} Psychy, PsyFor(77,IL42)
+ Ronni Lee Seltzer M.D., P.A.
15 Engle Street/Suite 101A Englewood, NJ 07631 (201)894-0505 Fax (201)894-5593

Selvaggi, Thomas A., MD {1083664197} AlgyImmn, Diagns, IntrMd(89,PA07)<NJ-HACKNSK>
+ Hackensack Allergy & Asthma Center
211 Essex Street/Suite 205 Hackensack, NJ 07601 (201)343-6673 Fax (201)343-7555

Selvam, Nirmala, MD {1356534028} IntrMd, Grtrcs(90,INA85)
+ New Jersey Institute for Successful Aging
42 East Laurel Road/Suite 1800 Stratford, NJ 08084 (856)566-6843 Fax (856)566-6781
+ University of Medicine & Dentistry of New Jersey-SOM
42 East Laurel Road/Suite 3200 Stratford, NJ 08084 (856)566-6843 Fax (856)566-6781

Selvaraj, Kavitha, MD {1023080181} IntrMd(94,INA68)
+ 350 Sparta Avenue/Suite B6b
Sparta, NJ 07871 (973)729-9122 Fax (973)729-3358

Selvaraj, Sundararajan, MD {1891956207} IntrMd
+ Hackensack Medical Center-Internal Medicine
30 Prospect Avenue/4 Main/Rm 4621 Hackensack, NJ 07601 (201)996-3664 Fax (551)996-0536

Seman, Ahmed B., MD {1942538715} IntrMd
+ Drs. Quraishi & Seman
1 Chopin Court Jersey City, NJ 07302 (201)434-2675

Semanczuk, William Paul, MD {1720061146} Anesth(99,NJ05)<NJ-HACKNSK>
+ Hackensack University Medical Center
30 Prospect Avenue/Anesthesiology Hackensack, NJ 07601 (201)996-2000 Fax (201)488-6769
+ Hackensack University MC-Anesthesia Dept
30 Prospect Avenue/Room 2703 Hackensack, NJ 07601 (201)996-2000 Fax (201)996-3962

Semar, David P., MD {1619021045} Psychy(87,MNT01)<NJ-VALLEY>
+ 148 West Saddle River Road
Saddle River, NJ 07458 (201)694-1543

Sembrano, Eduardo U., Jr., MD {1326017567} PedPul(84,PHI02)<NJ-MONMOUTH>
+ Monmouth Medical Group, P.C.
279 Third Avenue/Suite 604 Long Branch, NJ 07740 (732)222-4474 Fax (732)222-4472

Semel, William J., MD {1588624167} AdolMd, Pedtrc(63,NY09)<NJ-STBARNMC>
+ Summit Medical Group
75 East Northfield Road Livingston, NJ 07039 (973)436-1540 Fax (908)673-7336

Semet, Elliot C., MD {1710951280} SrgHnd, SrgOrt(92,NJ05)
+ 2446 Church Road/Suite 2A
Toms River, NJ 08753 (732)279-1100 Fax (732)279-1130

Semmler, Helaina D., MD {1982698254} Radiol, NuclMd, RadNuc(96,NJ05)<NJ-VIRTMHBC, NJ-VIRTBERL>
+ South Jersey Radiology Associates, P.A.
100 Carnie Boulevard/Suite B-5 Voorhees, NJ 08043 (856)751-0123 Fax (856)751-0535
+ South Jersey Radiology Associates, P.A.
315 Route 70 East/Suite B Cherry Hill, NJ 08034 (856)751-0123 Fax (856)428-0356
+ The Women's Center at Voorhees
100 Carnie Boulevard/Suite A-4 Voorhees, NJ 08043 (856)751-5522 Fax (856)751-5650

Semple, Camille Eleanor, DO {1871541938} ObsGyn(97,NJ75)
+ Access Women's ObGyn
215 Sunset Road/Suite 204 Willingboro, NJ 08046 (609)871-6800 Fax (609)871-9399

Physicians by Name and Address

Sen, Ajanta, DO {1033309513} IntrMd, InfDis(04,NJ75)
+ 82 Lincoln Avenue
Piscataway, NJ 08854

Sen, Rik Supriya, MD {1346354586} RadDia(89,INA4X)<NJ-UNVMCPRN>
+ Princeton Radiology Associates, P.A.
253 Witherspoon Street   Princeton, NJ 08540   (609)497-4310   Fax (609)497-4989
+ Princeton Radiology Associates, P.A.
419 North Harrison Street   Princeton, NJ 08540   (609)497-4310   Fax (609)683-8847
+ Princeton Radiology Associates, P.A.
9 Centre Drive   Jamesburg, NJ 08540   (609)655-1448   Fax (609)655-4016

Sen, Shuvendu, MD {1780860684} NuclMd, IntrMd(93,INA8X)
+ Raritan Bay Medical Center/Perth Amboy Division
530 New Brunswick Avenue   Perth Amboy, NJ 08861
(732)324-5080   Fax (732)324-3150
shuvendusen57@gmail.com

Sen, Sourav, MD {1417617693} IntrMd<NJ-STJOSHOS>
+ Heart & Vascular Associates of Northern Jersey
22-18 Broadway/Suite 201   Fair Lawn, NJ 07410   (201)490-1217   Fax (201)475-5522
+ St. Joseph's Regional Medical Center
703 Main Street   Paterson, NJ 07503   (973)754-2000

Sen, Surjya, MD {1144293663} Anesth, PainMd(02,NJ05)<NJ-HACKNSK>
+ Hackensack University Medical Center
30 Prospect Avenue/Anesth   Hackensack, NJ 07601
(201)996-2000   Fax (201)488-6769

Sen, Urmi, MD {1457543837} NuclMd, IntrMd(06,NY08)<CT-BRADMEM, NY-MTSINAI>
+ Newark Beth Israel Medical Center
201 Lyons Avenue   Newark, NJ 07112   (973)926-7000

Sen Gupta, Surupa, MD {1104138221}
+ UH- Robert Wood Johnson Med
125 Paterson Street/MEB 596   New Brunswick, NJ 08901
(732)235-7674

Sen Hightower, Indrani, MD {1952410458} Nrolgy(99,NJ06)
+ Bromley Neurology, P.C.
739 South White Horse Pike/Suite 1   Audubon, NJ 08106
(856)546-2300   Fax (856)546-2301
+ Woodbury Neurology Associates
17 West Red Bank Avenue/Suite 204   Woodbury, NJ 08096
(856)546-2300   Fax (856)845-5405

Senaldi, Eric M., MD {1881801900} BldBnk, PthACl(84,MEXI)<NJ-HACKNSK>
+ The Blood Center of New Jersey
45 South Grove Street   East Orange, NJ 07018   (973)676-4700   Fax (973)676-4933

Senator, Laura Julie, MD {1740360020} Pedtrc(90,NY45)
+ Pedi Health Medical Associates
720 Route 202-206 North/Suite 4   Bridgewater, NJ 08807
(908)722-5444   Fax (908)722-5071

Senatore, Peter Joseph, MD {1194719039} SrgC&R, Surgry(82,MD07)<MA-SSHREHOS>
+ Frank & Edith Scarpa Regional Cancer
1505 West Sherman Avenu/Suite B   Vineland, NJ 08360
(856)641-8635   Fax (856)641-8636
+ Inspira Colon and Rectal Surgery
155 Bridgeton Pike/Suite C   Mullica Hill, NJ 08062
(856)641-8635   Fax (856)641-8635

Sender, Slawomir, MD {1366603441}<NJ-VAEASTOR>
+ VA New Jersey Health Care System-East Orange Campus
385 Tremont Avenue   East Orange, NJ 07018   (973)676-1000

Senekjian, Elizabeth K., MD {1790726032} Psychy, ObsGyn(74,PA07)
+ 20 Nassau Street/Suite 250SW
Princeton, NJ 08542   (609)279-9228
+ 56 South Main Street/Suite C
Stockton, NJ 08559

Senese, Karen, MD {1881767390} PsyCAd(92,GRN01)
+ 520 Main Street
Toms River, NJ 08753   (732)557-4147   Fax (732)557-4147

Senese, Susan A., DO {1992809198} FamMed(91,PA77)<NJ-ACMCITY, NJ-ACMCMAIN>
+ Richard Stockton State College of New Jersey
Jimmie Leeds Road   Pomona, NJ 08240   (609)652-4701

Senft, Carl Joseph, MD {1275611345} IntrMd, Ophthl(95,NC05)
+ Jersey Shore Eye Associates
1809 Corlies Avenue/Suite 1   Neptune City, NJ 07753
(732)774-5566   Fax (732)988-7574

Sengupta, Ranjita, MD {1043368749} CdvDis
+ RWJPE Cardiology Associates of Somerset County, P.A.
487 Union Avenue/Suite A   Bridgewater, NJ 08807
(908)722-6410   Fax (908)722-4638

Sengupta, Shyamashree, MD {1477662013} MtFtMd, ObsGyn(77,INA7B)<NJ-STPETER, NJ-RWJUBRUN>
+ High Risk Pregnancy Center of New Jersey PC
1 Auer Court/Suites A & B   East Brunswick, NJ 08816
(732)390-1020   Fax (732)390-8035
+ High Risk Pregnancy Center of New Jersey PC
908 Oak Tree Road/Suite M & N   South Plainfield, NJ 07080
(732)390-1020   Fax (908)753-2473

Sennett, Jane M., DO {1780622043} EmrgMd(93,NJ75)<NJ-MONMOUTH, NJ-RWJURAH>
+ EMedical Urgent Care
2 Kings Highway   Middletown, NJ 07748   (732)957-0707   Fax (732)957-9852
+ EMedical Urgent Care
369 Springfield Avenue   Berkeley Heights, NJ 07922
(732)957-0707   Fax (908)464-1091

Sensakovic, John W., MD {1871670927} InfDis, IntrMd(77,NJ05)<NJ-STMICHL, NJ-JFKMED>
+ 113 James Street
Edison, NJ 08820   (732)549-3449   Fax (732)741-2599

Senzer, Richard P., MD {1508961772} IntrMd(85,GRN01)<NJ-HCKTSTWN>
+ 279 State Route 32 South/Suite 1
Washington, NJ 07882   (908)689-8246   Fax (908)689-8202

Seo, Christina J., MD {1730384686} SrgC&R(01)<NJ-VALLEY>
+ Drs. White & Waxenbaum
216 Engle Street/Suite 203   Englewood, NJ 07631
(201)567-7615   Fax (201)567-8033
+ Drs. White & Waxenbaum
127 Union Street/Suite 112   Ridgewood, NJ 07450
(201)567-7615   Fax (201)493-1718

Sepede, Jennifer, DO {1225441405} FamMed
+ The University Doctors
100 Century Parkway/Suite 140   Mount Laurel, NJ 08054
(856)380-2400   Fax (856)234-7870

Sequeira, Sophia Almeida, MD {1760860753} Pedtrc<NJ-MORRISTN>
+ Morristown Medical Center
100 Madison Avenue   Morristown, NJ 07962   (973)971-7550   Fax (973)290-2388

Serafino, Vincent Joseph, MD {1497799183} Pedtrc(81,DOM02)<NJ-BAYONNE>
+ Drs. Serafino & Dahrouj
834 Avenue C   Bayonne, NJ 07002   (201)339-4222   Fax (201)339-4498

Serban, Valeria, MD {1306942933} Nrolgy, NeuMus(92,ROM06)
+ New Jersey Institute for Successful Aging
42 East Laurel Road/Suite 1800   Stratford, NJ 08084
(856)566-6843   Fax (856)566-6419

Serbes, Sinan, MD {1871841882} FamMed(80,TURK)
+ 152 Division Avenue
Garfield, NJ 07026   (973)772-7579

Seretis, George J., DO {1144208968} FamMed(94,PA77)<NJ-MEMSALEM>
+ Seretis Care Family Practice
499 Beckett Road/Suite 201-B   Swedesboro, NJ 08085
(856)467-6400   Fax (856)467-1033

Sergi, Thomas J., MD {1205820438} RadDia(80,DC02)<NJ-VIRTUAHS, NJ-VIRTVOOR>
+ South Jersey Radiology Associates, P.A.
315 Route 70 East/Suite B   Cherry Hill, NJ 08034   (856)428-4344   Fax (856)428-0356
+ South Jersey Radiology Associates, P.A.
901 Route 168/Suites 301-305   Turnersville, NJ 08012
(856)428-4344   Fax (856)227-8537
+ South Jersey Radiology Associates, P.A.
807 Haddon Avenue/Suite 5   Haddonfield, NJ 08034
(856)616-1130   Fax (856)616-1125

Sergie, Ziad, MD {1427217173}
+ Monmouth Cardiology Associates, LLC
11 Meridian Road   Eatontown, NJ 07724   (732)663-0300   Fax (732)663-0301

Seril, Darren Neil, MD {1174728679} IntrMd, Gastrn(07,NJ06)
+ RWJ Gastro & Hepatology
125 Paterson Street/CAB 5100B   New Brunswick, NJ 08901
(732)235-7784   Fax (732)235-7792

Serletti, Joseph Michael, MD {1770513822} SrgPlstc(82,NY45)<NY-STRNGMEM>
+ Virtua Primary Care
401 Young Avenue/Suite 260   Moorestown, NJ 08057
(856)291-8920   Fax (856)291-8922

Serrano, Camilo Francisco, MD {1780744250} Psychy(85,HON01)<NJ-MEMSALEM>
+ HealthCare Commons Inc.
500 Pennsville-Auburn Road   Carneys Point, NJ 08069
(856)299-3200   Fax (856)299-7183

Serrano, Jesus Canoza, MD {1225283401} IntrMd
+ 140 Pleasant Avenue
Englewood, NJ 07631   (201)783-7033

Sersanti, John Paul, MD {1003882697} IntrMd, FamMed(97,IL43)
+ 3 Plaza Drive/Suite 10
Toms River, NJ 08757   Fax (732)797-0644

Sesana, Georgina Maria, MD {1285930958}<NJ-STJOSHOS>
+ St. Joseph's Regional Medical Center Anesthesia
703 Main Street   Paterson, NJ 07503   (973)754-2323   Fax (979)754-2791

Seshadri, Kapila, MD {1740375989} Pedtrc, PedDvl(82,INA72)
+ Children's Specialized Hospital
10 Plum Street/6th Floor   New Brunswick, NJ 08901
(732)258-7253
+ Child Health Institute of New Jersey
89 French Street/Suite 2300   New Brunswick, NJ 08901
(732)258-7253   Fax (732)235-6620

Seshadri, Mahalakshmi, MD {1861419830} FamMed, EmrgMd(93,INA77)
+ Medical Center at Budd Lake
125 US Highway 46   Budd Lake, NJ 07828   (973)691-9400   Fax (973)691-3283

Sestito, Joseph, Jr., MD {1235156159} Anesth(84,NJ06)
+ 41 Buena Vista Avenue
Rumson, NJ 07760   (732)741-4230
+ Red Bank Anesthesia, LLC
1 Riverview Plaza   Red Bank, NJ 07701   (732)741-4230   Fax (732)450-2620

Seth, Amit Kumar, MD {1316196165} EnDbMt, IntrMd(06,GRN01)<NJ-CLARMAAS, NJ-NWRKBETH>
+ Drs. Seth & Napoli
36 Newark Avenue/Suite 300   Belleville, NJ 07109
(973)759-6896   Fax (973)759-3719
jnapoli@pol.net
+ Drs. Seth, Robertson & Seth
310 Central Avenue/Suite 100   East Orange, NJ 07018
(973)759-6896   Fax (973)674-8033
+ 622 Eagle Rock Avenue/Suite G-4
West Orange, NJ 07109   (973)736-0081   Fax (973)736-3785

Seth, Sarwan K., MD {1295765527} IntrMd, FamMAdlt(68,INA82)
+ Drs. Seth, Robertson & Seth
310 Central Avenue/Suite 100   East Orange, NJ 07018
(862)520-3104   Fax (973)674-8033

Sethi, Chitra, MD {1558473231} Pedtrc(65,INA05)<NJ-MEADWLND, NJ-PALISADE>
+ 513 Anderson Avenue
Cliffside Park, NJ 07010   (201)945-3354   Fax (201)945-4751

Sethi, Mohammad Awais, MD {1174595037} PsyGrt(92,PAK02)<NJ-TRININPC>
+ Trinitas Regional Medical Center-New Point Campus
655 East Jersey Street/Psych   Elizabeth, NJ 07206
(908)994-5000

Sethi, Ripka, MD {1942220306} IntrMd(02,DMN01)<NJ-STBARNMC>
+ St. Barnabas Medical Center
94 Old Short Hills Road   Livingston, NJ 07039   (973)322-5000

Sethi, Ruchi S., MD {1699726323} CdvDis, IntrMd(96,IL06)<NJ-HACKNSK>
+ Bergen Invasive Cardiovascular Consultants
211 Essex Street/Suite 306   Hackensack, NJ 07601
(201)343-2050   Fax (201)343-4512

Sethi, Shalini K., MD {1861747438} FamMed
+ 184 Plainsboro Road
Cranbury, NJ 08512   (609)655-1269

Sethi, Virender, MD {1205875002} CdvDis, IntrMd, IntCrd(64,INDI)<NJ-HACKNSK>
+ Bergen Invasive Cardiovascular Consultants
211 Essex Street/Suite 306   Hackensack, NJ 07601
(201)343-2050   Fax (201)343-4512

Setoguchi Iwata, Soko, MD {1336583061} IntrMd
+ RWJ Gastro & Hepatology
125 Paterson Street/CAB 5100B   New Brunswick, NJ 08901
(732)235-7784   Fax (732)235-7792

Setoodeh, Farhad, MD {1174678916} PthACl, PthCln, PthCyt(71,IRA01)<NJ-STMRYPAS>
+ St. Mary's Hospital
350 Boulevard   Passaic, NJ 07055   (973)365-4300

Setton, Ellen E., MD {1750352977} Pedtrc(83,NY08)<NJ-JRSYSHMC, NJ-MONMOUTH>
+ West Park Pediatrics
804 West Park Avenue   Ocean, NJ 07712   (732)531-0010   Fax (732)493-0903
+ West Park Pediatrics
219 Taylors Mills Road   Manalapan, NJ 07726   (732)531-0010   Fax (732)577-9643
+ West Park Pediatrics
921 East County Line Road/Suite B   Lakewood, NJ 07712
(732)370-8500   Fax (732)370-5550

Setty, Arathi Radhakrishna, MD {1528035938} Rheuma, IntrMd(01,NY15)<MA-MTAUBURN>
+ Institute for Rheumatic & Autoimmune Diseases
33 Overlook Road/MAC L01   Summit, NJ 07901   (908)598-7940   Fax (908)598-5447

Setty, Rajendra P., MD {1407943830} PedGst
+ Cooper Peds/Children's Regional Ctr
3 Cooper Plaza/Suite 200   Camden, NJ 08103   (856)342-2472   Fax (856)368-8297

Setya, Amit, DO {1417969270} EmrgMd(02,NJ75)<NJ-KIMBALL>
+ Kimball Medical Center
  600 River Avenue/EmrgMed   Lakewood, NJ 08701
  (732)363-1900
+ Emergency Medical Associates of NJ, P.A.
  3 Century Drive   Parsippany, NJ 07054   (732)363-1900
  Fax (973)740-9895

Setya, Shilpy, MD {1013109925} Pedtrc<NJ-STBARNMC>
+ St. Barnabas Medical Center
  94 Old Short Hills Road   Livingston, NJ 07039   (973)322-5690

Seungdamrong, Aimee Malunda, MD {1952431355} ObsGyn, RprEnd(00,TX12)
+ Damien Fertility Partners
  655 Shrewsbury Avenue/Suite 300   Shrewsbury, NJ 07702
  (732)758-6511   Fax (732)758-1048
+ Hoboken University Medical Center
  308 Willow Avenue   Hoboken, NJ 07030   (201)418-1000

Severe, Monique Marie, MD {1477604189} PedEmg(89,NY06)<NY-LICOLLGE>
+ St Joseph's Medical Pediatic EmerMed
  703 Main Street   Paterson, NJ 07503   (973)754-4901

Sevrin, Amanda Hope, MD {1033393129} IntrMd<NJ-COOPRUMC>
+ Cooper University Hospital
  One Cooper Plaza/Internal Med   Camden, NJ 08103
  (856)795-7505   Fax (856)795-8010
  Sevrin-amanda@cooperhealth.edu

Sewell, Grant, MD {1063897023} FamMed
+ CentraState Family Medicine Residency Practice
  1001 West Main Street/Suite B   Freehold, NJ 07728
  (732)294-2540   Fax (732)409-2621

Sewell, Myron L., MD IntrMd(81,PA02)
+ Southern Jersey Medical Center
  651 High Street   Burlington City, NJ 08016   (609)386-0775
  Fax (609)747-8864
  myrsew@msn.com

Sexauer, William Patrick, MD {1992728869} PulDis, CritCr(84,NJ05)
+ UH- RWJ Medical School
  One Robert Wood Johnson Place   New Brunswick, NJ 08903
  (732)235-5600

Sexton, Thomas Francis, DO {1184604563} IntrMd(96,PA77)<NJ-KMHTURNV>
+ Kennedy Health Systems/Washington Township Campus
  435 Hurffville-Cross Keys Road   Turnersville, NJ 08012
  (856)218-5634   Fax (856)218-5664

Seybert, John, Jr., MD {1144300260} Anesth(88,NJ06)<NJ-UNVM-CPRN>
+ University Medical Center of Princeton at Plainsboro
  One Plainsboro Road/Anesthesiology   Plainsboro, NJ 08536
  (609)497-4000

Seydafkan, Shabnam, MD {1477056679} IntrMd
+ 233 Hillside Avenue
  Paramus, NJ 07652   (470)270-3267

Seymour, Carmela, MD {1164543120} ObsGyn(89,NY08)
+ Valley Medical Group Ob/Gyn in Fairlawn
  5-22 Saddle River Road   Fair Lawn, NJ 07410   (201)796-2025   Fax (201)796-0587

Seymour, Christopher R., MD {1154436400} ObsGyn(89,NY08)<NJ-OVERLOOK, NJ-STBARNMC>
+ Millburn Ob-Gyn Associates, P.A.
  233 Millburn Avenue   Millburn, NJ 07041   (973)467-9440
  Fax (973)467-2567
+ Short Hills Surgery Center
  187 Millburn Avenue/Suite 101   Millburn, NJ 07041
  (973)467-9440   Fax (973)671-0557

Sforza, Frank J., MD {1639241151} FamMed(86,NY15)<NJ-HUNTRDN>
+ North Hunterdon Physician Associates
  37 Ruppell Road   Hampton, NJ 08827

Sgambati, Theodore P., Jr., MD {1053398602} IntrMd(86,ITA17)<NJ-VALLEY, NJ-BERGNMC>
+ Valley Medical Group Internal Medicine
  1 Sears Drive/Suite 202   Paramus, NJ 07652   (201)262-2333   Fax (201)262-4515

Sgambelluri, Carol E., MD {1255363701} FamMed(88,NJ05)<NJ-SOMERSET>
+ MEDEMERGE
  1005 North Washington Avenue   Green Brook, NJ 08812
  (732)968-8900   Fax (732)968-4609

Sgroi, Donald A., MD {1063469237} ObsGyn(74,MEX03)<NJ-WAYNEGEN, NJ-STJOSHOS>
+ Lumina Women's Care
  401 Hamburg Turnpike/Suite 104   Wayne, NJ 07470
  (973)750-1770   Fax (973)750-1775
+ Wayne Surgical Center, LLC.
  1176 Hamburg Pike   Wayne, NJ 07470   (973)750-1770
  Fax (973)709-1901

Shaaban, Hamid Salim, MD {1578854618} OncHem, InfDis, IntrMd(04,GRN01)<NJ-STMICHL>
+ St. Michael's Medical Center
  111 Central Avenue/Hema Oncology   Newark, NJ 07102
  (973)877-5000
  hamidshaaban@gmail.com

Shaari, Christopher M., MD {1003088675} Otlryg(91,NY03)<NJ-HACKNSK, NJ-HOBUNIMC>
+ 20 Prospect Avenue/Suite 712
  Hackensack, NJ 07601   (201)342-8060   Fax (201)546-1536
+ The Doctors Shaari
  413 60th Street   West New York, NJ 07093   (201)342-8060
  Fax (201)867-5566

Shaari, Jeffrey M., MD {1891742342} Otlryg(01,NY19)
+ The Doctors Shaari
  413 60th Street   West New York, NJ 07093   (201)867-5557
  Fax (201)867-5566

Shabazz, Shakeilla Lavern, MD {1205118361} FamMed
+ Virtua Holistic Primary Care
  1001 Route 73 North/Lower Level   Marlton, NJ 08053
  (856)355-7110   Fax (856)355-7112

Shaber, Marc L., MD {1639151129} IntrMd(94,NJ05)<NJ-UNVM-CPRN>
+ Flemington Medical Group, LLC
  200 State Route 31 North/Suite 105   Flemington, NJ 08822
  (908)782-5100   Fax (908)782-0290

Shabo, Jessica E., MD {1275869612} PsyCAd
+ 675 Pascack Road
  Paramus, NJ 07652

Shack, Evan Tyler, MD {1932193166} Radiol, RadBdI(96,PA01)<NJ-VIRTMHBC, NJ-VIRTBERL>
+ South Jersey Radiology Associates, P.A.
  100 Carnie Boulevard/Suite B-5   Voorhees, NJ 08043
  (856)751-0123   Fax (856)751-0535
+ South Jersey Radiology Associates, P.A.
  315 Route 70 East/Suite B   Cherry Hill, NJ 08034   (856)751-0123   Fax (856)428-0356
+ The Women's Center at Voorhees
  100 Carnie Boulevard/Suite A-4   Voorhees, NJ 08043
  (856)751-5522   Fax (856)751-5650

Shad, Abdur Rauf, MD {1225124738} IntrMd, PulCCr, PulDis(90,PAK11)
+ 8 Sherwood Drive
  Mountain Lakes, NJ 07046

Shad, Yasar, MD {1851651442} IntrMd<NJ-VIRTMARL>
+ Virtua Marlton Hospital
  90 Brick Road/Internal Med   Marlton, NJ 08053   (856)981-3426
  dryasirshad@yahoo.com

Shadiack, Edward Charles, Jr., DO {1245339779} FamMed(81,NJ75)
+ 1200 NE Central Avenue/Suite 2
  Seaside Park, NJ 08752   (732)830-4884

Shafa, Eiman, MD {1215258462} SrgOrt
+ MidJersey Orthopaedics, P.A.
  8100 Westcott Drive/Suite 101   Flemington, NJ 08822
  (908)782-0600   Fax (908)782-7575

Shafaie, Farrokh, MD {1679581524} SrgPlstc(73,IRAN)<NJ-OVERLOOK, NJ-STBARNMC>
+ Med-FEM Aesthetic Surgery Center
  33 Overlook Road/Suite 302   Summit, NJ 07901   (908)522-1777   Fax (908)522-3051

Shafey, Moustafa Hassan, MD {1164574463} Psychy(77,EGY05)<NJ-CENTRAST>
+ CentraState Medical Center
  901 West Main Street/Psychiatry   Freehold, NJ 07728
  (732)294-2857
+ Freehold Psychiatric Associates
  901 West Main Street/Suite 103   Freehold, NJ 07728
  (732)303-5281

Shaffer, Brian L., MD {1447247689} IntrMd(85,BEL12)<NJ-STFRN-MED, NJ-RWJUHAM>
+ 133 Franklin Corner Road/2nd Floor
  Lawrenceville, NJ 08648   (609)436-5900   Fax (609)452-0222

Shaffer, Jaclyn, MD {1225545452} EmrgSptM
+ 67 Wellington Place
  Burlington, NJ 08016   (609)670-1176   Fax (609)670-1176

Shaffer, Liba C., MD {1700123189} Surgry(01,LA01)
+ 525 Albin Street
  Teaneck, NJ 07666

Shaffrey, Thomas Andrew, MD {1518993443} FamMed, IntrMd(93,PA12)
+ 3322 US Highway 22/Suite 1350
  Branchburg, NJ 08876   (732)595-2525   Fax (908)595-1012

Shafi, Heather Claire, MD {1750640470} Pedtrc
+ PediatriCare Associates
  20-20 Fair Lawn Avenue   Fair Lawn, NJ 07410   (201)791-4545   Fax (201)791-3709

Shafi, Mohammad, MD {1184627937} SrgOrt(63,PAK01)<NJ-JFKMED>
+ Central Jersey Orthopaedic Specialists PA
  1907 Park Avenue/Suite 102   South Plainfield, NJ 07080
  (908)561-3400   Fax (908)769-5308

Shafiq, Saima, MD {1306001441} Psychy, PsyCAd(94,PAK11)<NJ-STCLRDEN>
+ St. Clare's Health Services
  50 Morris Avenue   Denville, NJ 07834   (973)625-7051

Shafqat, Uzma Zohra, MD {1386855849} EnDbMt, IntrMd(99,PAK18)
+ Montclair Endocrine Associates
  123 Highland Avenue/Suite 301   Glen Ridge, NJ 07028
  (973)744-3733   Fax (973)707-5821

Shafritz, Randy, MD {1962476663} SrgVas, Surgry(90,PA02)<NJ-RWJUBRUN, NJ-UMDNJ>
+ University Medical Group/Vascular Surgery
  One Robert Wood Johnson Place/MEB 541   New Brunswick, NJ 08901   (732)235-7816   Fax (732)235-8538
+ 18 Centre Drive/Suite 203
  Monroe Township, NJ 08831   (609)655-0691

Shah, Ajay S., MD {1144486523} IntrMd(93,INA4Y)
+ Medical Health Center
  1270 State Highway 35   Middletown, NJ 07748   (732)615-3900   Fax (732)615-0865
+ Monmouth Heart Specialists
  274 Highway 35   Eatontown, NJ 07724   (732)615-3900
  Fax (732)440-9404

Shah, Ajit M., MD {1851333793} IntrMd, Nephro(68,INDI)<NJ-STBARNMC, NJ-MTNSIDE>
+ Essex Medical and Nephrology
  539 Bloomfield Avenue   Newark, NJ 07107   (973)566-9900
  Fax (973)566-6692

Shah, Amisha A., MD {1629394879} Pedtrc(10,PA14)
+ Princeton Nassau Pediatrics, P.A.
  301 North Harrison Street   Princeton, NJ 08540   (609)658-6911   Fax (609)924-3577
  parikh.amisha@gmail.com

shah, Amisha M., MD {1235458498} Pedtrc, IntrMd(10,NY19)
+ Princeton Nassau Pediatrics, P.A.
  312 Applegarth Road/Suite 104   Monroe Township, NJ 08831   (609)409-5600   Fax (609)409-5610
+ Princeton Nassau Pediatrics, P.A.
  196 Princeton-Hightstown Road   West Windsor, NJ 08550
  (609)409-5600   Fax (609)799-2294

Shah, Amit A., MD {1992025852} Anesth(10,NJ05)
+ Christ Hospital
  176 Palisade Avenue/Anesthesia   Jersey City, NJ 07306
  (201)795-8200

Shah, Amy Mehta, DO {1679898266} Pedtrc(06,PA77)
+ 27 Douglass Drive
  Princeton, NJ 08540

Shah, Anand Subhash, MD {1558849406} IntrMd(12,IN20)
+ CentraState Family Medicine Residency Practice
  1001 West Main Street/Suite B   Freehold, NJ 07728
  (732)294-2540   Fax (732)409-2621

Shah, Angana Nayan, MD {1891795563} Ophthl(98,PA02)<NJ-CHSFULD, NJ-HUNTRDN>
+ Princeton Eye and Ear
  2999 Princeton Pike/2 FL   Lawrenceville, NJ 08648
  (609)403-8840   Fax (609)403-8852
+ Paul Phillips Eye & Surgery Center
  64 Walmart Plaza   Clinton, NJ 08809   (609)403-8840   Fax (908)735-7494
+ Paul Phillips Eye & Surgery Center
  6 Minneakoning Road/Suite B   Flemington, NJ 08648
  (908)824-7144   Fax (908)968-3239

Shah, Anish Pravin, MD {1699790436} IntrMd, Nephro(98,DMN01)
+ American Access Care
  207 South Kings Highway/Suite 2   Cherry Hill, NJ 08034
  (856)616-8600   Fax (856)616-8601

Shah, Ankit Prafulbhai, MD {1972741957} Nephro, IntrMd(04,INA21)
+ Ocean Renal Associates, P.A.
  1145 Beacon Avenue/Suite B   Manahawkin, NJ 08050
  (609)978-9940   Fax (609)978-9902
+ Ocean Renal Associates, P.A.
  508 Lakehurst Road/Suite 3 A   Toms River, NJ 08755
  (609)978-9940   Fax (732)341-4993

Shah, Ankur, MD {1346554870} RadDia
+ Atlantic Medical Imaging, LLC.
  421 Route 9 North   Cape May Court House, NJ 08210
  (609)677-9729   Fax (609)465-0918

Shah, Anuj Raju, MD {1922274190} IntrMd, CarEch(03,INA15)
+ Center for Adult Medicine & Preventive Care
  293 Passaic Street   Passaic, NJ 07055   (973)773-0334   Fax (973)773-0336
+ Apex Heart & Vascular Care
  124 Gregory Avenue/Suite 203   Passaic, NJ 07055
  (973)773-0334   Fax (973)916-0027
+ Mulkay Cardiology Consultants
  550 Summit Avenue/Bsmt   Jersey City, NJ 07055
  (201)996-9244   Fax (201)996-9243

Shah, Apeksha, MD {1689930257} Gastrn<NJ-COOPRUMC>
+ Cooper University Hospital
  One Cooper Plaza   Camden, NJ 08103   (856)342-2000

Physicians by Name and Address

Shah, Apurva Surendra, MD {1053538280} SrgOrt, OrtSHand
+ Virtua Health and Wellness Center
200 Bowman Drive   Voorhees, NJ 08043   (734)945-2478
apurva.shah@aya.yale.edu

Shah, Arvind P., MD {1588694335} Pedtrc(68,INA21)<NJ-OVERLOOK>
+ 1272 Central Avenue
Westfield, NJ 07090   (908)654-3525   Fax (908)654-3541
Apshah1272@yahoo.com

Shah, Asha Dinesh, MD {1811103567} Urolgy(05,OH44)<NJ-HCMEADPS>
+ Children's Hospital of Hudson County
355 Grand Street/Suite 280   Jersey City, NJ 07302
(201)915-2450   Fax (201)915-2192

Shah, Ashish R., MD {1003880329} Pedtrc, PedPul(89,IN20)<NJ-MORRISTN, NJ-CHILTON>
+ Pediatric Pulmonology
100 Madison Avenue   Morristown, NJ 07960   (973)971-4142   Fax (973)290-7360

Shah, Ashish Vinaychandra, MD {1104245232} EnDbMt
+ St. Luke's Diabetes & Endocrinology
755 Memorial Parkway/Suite 302 A   Phillipsburg, NJ 08865
(908)847-2050   Fax (866)449-5832

Shah, Asit K., MD {1184676223} SrgOrt(99,PA02)<NJ-ENGLWOOD, NJ-HOLYNAME>
+ Englewood Orthopedic Associates
401 South Van Brunt Street   Englewood, NJ 07631
(201)569-2770   Fax (201)569-1774
asitshahmd@yahoo.com

Shah, Asma Aftab, MD {1427122084} IntrMd(89,PAK20)
+ Lourdes Medical Center of Burlington County
218 Sunset Road/Suite A   Willingboro, NJ 08046   (609)835-2900
ashmaaftab@yahoo.com

Shah, Avnee, MD {1750600656}
+ The Dermatology Group, P.C.
347 Mount Pleasant Avenue/Suite 205   West Orange, NJ 07052   (973)571-2121   Fax (973)498-0512

Shah, Azam, DO {1659535045} Anesth
+ 35 Beaumont Place
Mount Holly, NJ 08060

Shah, Bankim, MD {1790151116} IntrMd
+ 32 Wakefield Place
Caldwell, NJ 07006   (347)241-5713

Shah, Bankim D., MD {1609899632} IntrMd(74,INA87)<NJ-COMMED>
+ 56A Schoolhouse Road
Whiting, NJ 08759   (732)849-0501
+ Drs Shah and Shah
25 Mule Road/Suite B4   Toms River, NJ 08755   (732)849-0501   Fax (732)341-0072

Shah, Bharti C., MD {1164401261} ObsGyn(64,INA21)<NJ-JFKMED, NJ-RBAYOLDB>
+ 481 Grove Avenue
Edison, NJ 08820   (732)549-1777   Fax (732)494-8354

Shah, Bharti K., MD {1770646101} Pedtrc(75,SCO05)
+ 190 Greenbrook Road
North Plainfield, NJ 07060   (908)756-6426

Shah, Bindi, DO {1902084791} Psychy(99,NJ75)
+ Wellness Services @ Montclair State University
1 Normal Avenue   Upper Montclair, NJ 07043   (973)655-7051   Fax (973)655-6977

Shah, Chandravadan I., MD {1881654168} ObsGyn(82,INA20)<NJ-NWRKBETH>
+ Newark Beth Israel Medical Center
201 Lyons Avenue/Ob/Gyn   Newark, NJ 07112   (973)926-7342   Fax (973)705-8650
+ Ocean Health Initiatives, Inc.
301 Lakehurst Road   Toms River, NJ 08755   (973)926-7342   Fax (732)552-0378
+ Ocean Health Initiatives, Inc.
101 Second Street   Lakewood, NJ 07112   (732)363-6655   Fax (732)363-6656

Shah, Chetan K., DO {1518971936} IntrMd, Nephro(95,TX78)
+ Shore Kidney & Hypertension Specialists
13 Mechanic Street   Cape May Court House, NJ 08210
(609)678-1816   Fax (609)465-2201

Shah, Chetan S., MD {1750306734} Otlryg(93,NJ06)<NJ-CHSM-RCER, NJ-UNVMCPRN>
+ Princeton Eye and Ear
2999 Princeton Pike/2 FL   Lawrenceville, NJ 08648
(609)403-8840   Fax (609)403-8852
+ Princeton Eye and Ear
5 Plainsboro Road/Suite 510   Plainsboro, NJ 08536
(609)403-8840   Fax (609)403-8852

Shah, Chirag H., DO {1225257199} IntrMd, CdvDis(00,NJ75)<NJ-STPETER, NJ-RWJUBRUN>
+ Cardio Metabolic Institute
51 Veronica Avenue   Somerset, NJ 08873   (732)846-7000   Fax (732)846-7001
+ Cardio Metabolic Institute
294 Applegarth Road/Suite F   Monroe Township, NJ 08831

(732)846-7000   Fax (732)846-7001

Shah, Chirag J., MD {1396986881} PedAne, Anesth(06,GRN01)<NJ-UMDNJ>
+ University Hospital
150 Bergen Street/Anesth   Newark, NJ 07103   (973)972-0470

Shah, Chirag M., MD {1053345629} Hemato, MedOnc, IntrMd(92,INA2B)<NJ-UMDNJ>
+ Advanced Cancer Care of New Jersey
40 Bey Lea Road/Suite B102   Toms River, NJ 08753
(732)244-3380   Fax (732)244-9013

Shah, Chirag N., MD {1982613741} EmrgMd(02,NY08)<NJ-RWJUBRUN>
+ University Emergency Medicine
125 Paterson Street/MEB 104   New Brunswick, NJ 08901
(732)235-8717   Fax (732)235-7379
+ RWJ University Hospital New Brunswick
One Robert Wood Johnson Place   New Brunswick, NJ 08901
(732)828-3000

Shah, Chirag S., MD {1174550818} Ophthl(97,NJ06)<NJ-CHSM-RCER>
+ Princeton Eye and Ear
2999 Princeton Pike/2 FL   Lawrenceville, NJ 08648
(609)403-8840   Fax (609)403-8852

Shah, Chirag Vijaykumar, MD {1922161421} PulDis(00,MO46)<NJ-ATLANTHS, NJ-MORRISTN>
+ Pulmonary & Allergy Associates
8 Saddle Road/Suite 101   Cedar Knolls, NJ 07927
(973)267-9393   Fax (973)540-0472
+ Pulmonary & Allergy Associates
1 Springfield Avenue/Suite 3-A   Summit, NJ 07901
(973)267-9393   Fax (908)934-0556

Shah, Darsit, MD {1083718456} Otlryg, OtgyPSHN(91,PA07)<NJ-MONMOUTH>
+ ENT and Allergy Associates
1131 Broad Street/Suite 103 Building A   Shrewsbury, NJ 07702   (732)389-3388   Fax (732)389-3389

Shah, Debra Stahl, MD {1487754180} Pedtrc(87,PA14)<NJ-HUNTRDN>
+ Hunterdon Pediatric Associates
6 Sand Hill Road/Suite 202   Flemington, NJ 08822
(908)782-6700   Fax (908)788-5861

Shah, Deepak O., MD {1831258607} CdvDis, IntrMd(76,INA65)<NJ-CHRIST, NJ-JRSYCITY>
+ 143 Palisade Avenue
Jersey City, NJ 07306   (201)792-2727   Fax (201)653-3420

Shah, Deepali A., DO {1356521587} IntrMd(06,IL76)<NJ-KSLR-WEST>
+ Kessler Institute for Rehabilitation West Orange
1199 Pleasant Valley Way   West Orange, NJ 07052
(973)993-9536

Shah, Dhanvanti B., MD {1023037116} FamMed(74,INDI)<NJ-COMMED>
+ Drs Shah and Shah
25 Mule Road/Suite B4   Toms River, NJ 08755   (732)341-0020   Fax (732)341-0072

Shah, Dhiren, MD {1548627102} IntrMd
+ 1101 Westminster Boulevard
Parlin, NJ 08859   (848)203-1145
+ Ocean Pulmonary Associates PA
457 Jack Martin Boulevard/Suite 4   Brick, NJ 08724
(848)203-1145   Fax (732)840-6444

Shah, Dhiren A., MD {1356337810} IntrMd, SlpDis, CritCr(95,INA8B)<NJ-COMMED>
+ Ocean Pulmonary Associates PA
3 Plaza Drive/Suite 2   Toms River, NJ 08757   (732)341-1380
Fax (732)505-9296

Shah, Dhwani B., MD {1144386632} Psychy(03,NJ06)
+ 20 Nassau Street/Suite 202
Princeton, NJ 08540   (609)924-9222
dhwanishahmd@gmail.com
+ Princeton University
307 Nassau Hall/StaffPsychtrst   Princeton, NJ 08544
(609)258-3000

Shah, Dilip A., MD {1689728040} Psychy(77,INDI)<NJ-CHRIST, NJ-HOBUNIMC>
+ 721 Clifton Avenue/Clifton Med Pl
Clifton, NJ 07013   (973)471-8888   Fax (973)778-7851
+ 142 Palisade Avenue/Suite 210
Jersey City, NJ 07306   (201)963-0827

Shah, Dina B., MD {1255348587} Psychy(72,INA15)
+ 32 Hansen Drive
Edison, NJ 08820   (908)753-0100   Fax (908)668-0777

Shah, Dinesh K., MD {1477659191} EmrgMd, IntrMd(84,INA15)<NJ-BAYSHORE>
+ Bayshore Community Hospital
727 North Beers Street/Emerg Medicine   Holmdel, NJ 07733   (732)739-5924
din1957@aol.com

Shah, Dipal, MD {1356607576} Ophthl
+ 1432 51st Street
North Bergen, NJ 07047   (551)358-8655

Shah, Faisal Majeed, MD {1093915852} RadDia, IntrMd(05,GRN01)
+ Shore Imaging
1166 River Avenue/Suite 102   Lakewood, NJ 08701
(732)364-9565   Fax (732)364-1908

Shah, Falguni Samir, MD {1265452932} PedInf, Pedtrc(91,INA20)<NJ-STBARNMC>
+ St. Barnabas Medical Center
94 Old Short Hills Road   Livingston, NJ 07039   (973)322-5000

Shah, Harish H., MD {1619952181} OncHem(70,INA20)<NJ-STJOSHOS>
+ Wayne Hematology-Oncology Associates PA
468 Parish Drive/Suite 4   Wayne, NJ 07470   (973)694-5005
Fax (973)694-5990
waynehemonc1@aol.com

Shah, Hemangini R., DO {1336162015} RadOnc, Radiol, IntrMd(94,NJ75)<NJ-SOCEANCO>
+ Southern Ocean County Medical Center
1140 Route 72 West/Radiology   Manahawkin, NJ 08050
(609)978-2194   Fax (609)978-2843

Shah, Hemant R., MD {1104863258} NuclMd, Radiol, FamMed(66,INA69)<NJ-MEADWLND, NJ-HOBUNIMC>
+ 297 Central Avenue
Jersey City, NJ 07307   (201)420-7373

Shah, Hetal Subodh, MD {1497784094} FamMed, IntrMd(00,OH45)
+ Elmwood Family Physicians
777 Route 70 East/Suite G-101   Marlton, NJ 08053
(856)983-9939   Fax (856)983-9936
+ Elmwood Family Physicians
1529 Route 206/Suite L   Tabernacle, NJ 08088   (856)983-9939   Fax (609)268-7191

Shah, Himani, MD {1831399674} IntrMd<NJ-STPETER>
+ St. Peter's University Hospital
254 Easton Avenue   New Brunswick, NJ 08901   (732)745-8600

Shah, Himanshu P., MD {1578666764} PulDis(83,INDI)
+ Comprehensive Pulmonary & Critical Care Assoc
96 Millburn Avenue/Suite 200A   Millburn, NJ 07041
(973)763-6800   Fax (973)761-1255

Shah, Himanshu Shirish, MD {1104833276} Ophthl, IntrMd(88,NJ06)
+ Patel Eye Associates
228 Plainfield Avenue   Edison, NJ 08817   (732)985-5009
Fax (732)985-5155
+ Patel Eye Associates
3084 State Route 27/Suite 4   Kendall Park, NJ 08824
(732)985-5009   Fax (732)985-5155

Shah, Hinna Ehsanullah, MD {1083911598} Psychy<NJ-TRININPC>
+ Trinitas Regional Medical Center-New Point Campus
655 East Jersey Street/6th Floor   Elizabeth, NJ 07206
(908)994-7207

Shah, Hitesh M., MD {1215136114} EmrgMd<NJ-TRINIWSC>
+ Trinitas Regional Medical Center-Williamson Street
225 Williamson Street/Emerg Med   Elizabeth, NJ 07207
(609)516-7599

Shah, Ila A., MD {1245208545} Nrolgy(75,INA15)<NJ-WARREN>
+ Drs. Shah and Mehta
311 Baltimore Street   Phillipsburg, NJ 08865   (908)859-2009   Fax (908)859-3352

Shah, Ila H., MD {1235340092} Psychy(71,INA26)<NJ-ESSEXCO>
+ The first Occupational Center of New Jersey
391 Lakeside Avenue/PsychConsultant   Orange, NJ 07050
(973)672-5800   Fax (973)672-0065
info@ocnj.org
+ North Jersey Developmental Center
169 Minisink Road/PO Box 169   Totowa, NJ 07512
(973)672-5800   Fax (973)256-3468
+ Essex County Hospital Center
204 Grove Avenue   Cedar Grove, NJ 07050   (973)571-2800

Shah, Jatin, MD {1417201567}<NJ-STPETER>
+ St. Peter's University Hospital
254 Easton Avenue   New Brunswick, NJ 08901   (732)930-1087

Shah, Jay Pravinkumar, MD {1043294499} Psychy<NJ-STCLRBOO>
+ St. Clare's Hospital-Boonton
130 Powerville Road   Boonton, NJ 07005   (973)316-1800

Shah, Jigisha Tanmay, MD {1891950770}
+ Valley Health Medical Group
780 Cedar Lane   Teaneck, NJ 07666   (201)836-7664   Fax (201)836-5710

Shah, Kalpana N., MD {1619906153} Anesth(71,INA20)<NJ-OCEANMC>
+ Ocean Medical Center
425 Jack Martin Boulevard/Anesth   Brick, NJ 08723
(732)840-2200

Shah, Kalpeshkumar Kanaiyalal, MD {1184141293}
+ St. Michael's Medical Center
111 Central Avenue   Newark, NJ 07102   (973)877-5000

Shah, Kamalesh R., MD {1891780912} IntrMd(84,INDI)<NJ-MEADWLND, NJ-CHRIST>
+ Summit Medical Arts
9225 John F Kennedy Boulevard   North Bergen, NJ 07047   (201)453-2800

Shah, Kamlesh Manher, MD {1811094204} Gastrn, IntrMd(99,NJ06)
+ Ocean Endosurgery Center
129 Route 37 West   Toms River, NJ 08755   (732)606-4440   Fax (732)797-3963
+ 9 Mule Road/Suite E-15
Toms River, NJ 08755   (732)606-4440   Fax (732)914-9088

Shah, Kavitha, MD {1881974574}
+ St. Joseph's Family Medicine @ Clifton
1135 Broad Street/Suite 201   Clifton, NJ 07013   (973)754-4100   Fax (973)472-9062

Shah, Kekul Bharat, MD {1467493718} Ophthl, IntrMd(98,NJ06)
+ Delaware Valley Retina Associates
4 Princess Road/Suite 101   Lawrenceville, NJ 08648   (609)896-1414   Fax (609)896-2982
+ Delaware Valley Retina Associates
121 Highway 31 North/Suite 700   Flemington, NJ 08822   (908)806-6191

Shah, Kishori Praful, MD {1225009111} Anesth(69,INDI)
+ SurgiCare of Central Jersey
40 Stirling Road   Watchung, NJ 07069   (908)769-8000   Fax (908)769-4139

Shah, Komal Saurabh, MD {1942388228} Psychy(93,INDI)<NJ-UNIVBHC>
+ UH-University Behavioral Hlth
100 Metroplex Drive/Suite 200   Edison, NJ 08817   (732)235-8443   Fax (732)235-3485

Shah, Kumar, MD {1457613952} RadDia
+ University Radiology Group, P.C.
579A Cranbury Road   East Brunswick, NJ 08816   (732)390-0040   Fax (732)390-1856

Shah, Kusum J., MD {1255337242} Anesth(71,INA20)
+ 7 Jennie Court
Cedar Grove, NJ 07009

Shah, Lata R., MD {1790843258} Pedtrc(75,INA67)<NJ-JFKMED>
+ 1804 Oak Tree Road/Suite 2
Edison, NJ 08820   (732)549-0051   Fax (732)549-3305

Shah, Leena P., MD {1386613156} ObsGyn, MtFtMd(84,INDI)<NJ-MORRISTN, NJ-OVERLOOK>
+ Atlantic Maternal Fetal Medicine
435 South Street/Suite 380   Morristown, NJ 07960   (973)971-7080   Fax (973)290-8312
+ Maternal Fetal Medicine of Practice Associates
11 Overlook Road/Suite LL 102   Summit, NJ 07901   (973)971-7080   Fax (908)522-5557

Shah, Lesha Dilip, MD {1497075295}
+ 156 Rolling Hills Road
Clifton, NJ 07013   (973)777-3920
lesha.shah@gmail.com

Shah, Lopa Suryakant, MD {1801893292} Anesth(88,INA65)<NJ-MONMOUTH>
+ Monmouth Medical Center
300 Second Avenue/Anesthesiology   Long Branch, NJ 07740   (732)222-5200

Shah, Madhavi, MD {1316059033} Pedtrc(71,INA20)<NJ-CLARMAAS, NJ-MTNSIDE>
+ All Star Pediatrics
199 Broad Street/Suite 1-B   Bloomfield, NJ 07003   (973)743-1392   Fax (973)743-3707

Shah, Mahendra Govindlal, MD {1780690818} Anesth, AnesPain(78,INA9Y)<NJ-CHSMRCER, NJ-CHSFULD>
+ Trenton Anesthesiology Associates, PA
One Capital Way/Second Floor   Pennington, NJ 08534   (609)396-4700   Fax (609)396-4900

Shah, Mahesh Maneklal, MD {1053451492} ObsGyn, Gyneco(68,INA21)
+ 19 Holly Street
Cranford, NJ 07016   (908)276-2778
+ 366 Vail Avenue
Piscataway, NJ 08854   (732)968-4502

Shah, Mala T., MD {1013179894} RadDia
+ Montclair Radiology
116 Park Street   Montclair, NJ 07042   (973)746-2525   Fax (973)746-5802

Shah, Manish, MD {1962792986} Anesth<PA-PNSTHRSH>
+ Rancocas Anesthesiology, PA
15000 Midlantic Drive/Suite 102   Mount Laurel, NJ 08054   (856)255-5479   Fax (856)393-8691

Shah, Manish A., MD {1669670071} IntrMd(04,STM01)<NJ-STPETER>
+ 1330 Route 206 South
Skillman, NJ 08558   (732)305-0444   Fax (732)645-7909

Shah, Mansi R., MD {1679093413} GenPrc
+ 1100 Parsippany Boulevard/Suite 209
Parsippany, NJ 07054   (973)452-1513

Shah, Maya M., MD {1285734301} Hemato, IntrMd, MedOnc(80,INDI)<NJ-NWRKBETH, NJ-STBARNMC>
+ Newark Beth Israel Medical Center
201 Lyons Avenue   Newark, NJ 07112   (973)926-7000   Fax (973)926-9568

Shah, Mayuri N., MD {1417993254} Pedtrc(73,INA65)<NJ-HACKNSK>
+ Hackensack University Medical Center
30 Prospect Avenue/Pediatrics   Hackensack, NJ 07601   (201)996-2000

Shah, Megha, MD {1437393352} OncHem
+ Hunterdon Regional Cancer Ctr
2100 Wescott Drive   Flemington, NJ 08822   (908)788-6461   Fax (908)788-6412

Shah, Mehul D., DO {1447577028} Anesth(10,FL75)
+ Morris Anesthesia Group, PA
3799 Route 46/Suite 211   Parsippany, NJ 07054   (973)335-1122   Fax (973)335-1448

Shah, Mehul N., MD {1427119247} Gastrn, IntrMd(81,INA20)<NJ-STMICHL, NJ-CLARMAAS>
+ 116 Millburn Avenue
Millburn, NJ 07041   (973)376-2121   Fax (973)371-0171
+ 614 Franklin Avenue
Nutley, NJ 07110   (973)376-2121   Fax (973)667-0535

Shah, Milind Narendra, MD {1538361290} IntrMd, OccpMd(99,NJ05)
+ Schering Plough Research Institute
2000 Galloping Hill Road   Kenilworth, NJ 07033   (908)298-2820   Fax (908)298-2834

Shah, Mubina, MD {1790960920} FamMed(90,PAK11)<NJ-RWJUBRUN>
+ My Family Practice Associates
37 South Main Street   Manville, NJ 08835   (908)722-9333   Fax (908)722-9990

Shah, Mukesh Chinubhai, MD {1801867395} IntrMd(93,INA21)<NJ-KIMBALL, NJ-OCEANMC>
+ Professional Associates of Jackson, LLC
2105 West County Line Road/Suite 4   Jackson, NJ 08527   (732)367-7575   Fax (732)364-0600
shahkalpan@hotmail.com
+ Point Pleasant Medical Group
1010 Beaverdam Road   Point Pleasant Beach, NJ 08742   (732)367-7575   Fax (732)892-8266

Shah, Nalini Arvindkumar, MD {1841376274} OncHem, IntrMd(77,INA67)
+ Total Cardiology Care
120 Franklin Street   Jersey City, NJ 07307   (201)653-8403   Fax (201)714-9336

Shah, Nalini D., MD {1184765513} IntrMd(73,INA69)<NJ-STJOSHOS, NJ-WAYNEGEN>
+ 415 21st Avenue
Paterson, NJ 07513   (973)345-2142   Fax (973)345-1626
NShahMD@yahoo.com
+ St. Joseph's Regional Medical Center
703 Main Street   Paterson, NJ 07503   (973)754-2000
+ Passaic Valley Hospice
783 Riverview Drive   Totowa, NJ 07513   (973)256-4636

Shah, Namrata Jinesh, MD {1508962044} ObsGyn(92,INA69)
+ Island Reproductive Services
3000 Hadley Road/Suite 2-C   South Plainfield, NJ 07080   (732)662-5499   Fax (908)412-9910
+ Island Reproductive Services
1817 Oak Tree Road   Edison, NJ 08820
+ Eric B. Chandler Health Center
277 George Street   New Brunswick, NJ 07080   (732)235-6700   Fax (732)235-6729

Shah, Neel Praful, MD {1952545691} Urolgy, IntrMd(05,NJ06)
+ Anthony J. Catanese MD
315 East Main Street   Somerville, NJ 08876   (908)722-6900   Fax (908)722-6699

Shah, Neena Manharlal, DO {1366644379} EmrgMd(94,NJ75)<NJ-STMICHL>
+ St. Michael's Medical Center
268 MLK Jr. Boulevard/Emergency   Newark, NJ 07102   (973)877-5500
neenams@pol.net

Shah, Neha Naresh, MD {1518912559} Pedtrc, EmrgMd(99,MNT01)<NJ-CENTRAST>
+ CentraState Medical Center
901 West Main Street/EmergMed   Freehold, NJ 07728   (732)431-2000

Shah, Nehabahen V., MD {1932388931} IntrMd(99,INA21)
+ 2141 Oaktree Road
Edison, NJ 08820   (732)516-0707   Fax (732)516-0088

Shah, Nehaben Ketankumar, MD {1194928879} IntrMd(93,INA20)
+ AstraHealth Urgent & Primary Care
1100 Centennial Avenue/Suite 104   Piscataway, NJ 08854   (732)981-1111   Fax (732)981-1113

Shah, Neil J., MD {1194084053} IntrMd(INA8B)
+ 216 B Davey Street
Bloomfield, NJ 07003   (201)673-7781

drneilshah87@gmail.com

Shah, Nihar N., MD {1356605018} IntrMd<NJ-STJOSHOS>
+ St. Joseph's Regional Medical Center
703 Main Street   Paterson, NJ 07503   (973)754-2000

Shah, Nihir Biharilal, MD {1346332194} CdvDis, IntrMd(88,NJA21)<NJ-STPETER, NJ-RWJUBRUN>
+ Heart and Vascular Institute of Central NJ
317 George Street/Suite 440   New Brunswick, NJ 08901   (732)994-3278   Fax (800)732-0366
+ Heart and Vascular Institute of Central NJ
98 James Street/Suite 314   Edison, NJ 08820   (732)994-3278   Fax (732)549-2853
+ Heart and Vascular Institute of Central NJ
333 Forsgate Drive/Suite 202   Jamesburg, NJ 08901   (732)994-3278   Fax (800)732-0366

Shah, Nilay Ramesh, MD {1154372621} Nrolgy, ClNrPh(98,GRN01)
+ 14-01 Broadway/Suite 3
Fair Lawn, NJ 07410   (201)279-6340   Fax (201)279-6341

Shah, Nima M., MD {1083954606} ObsGyn
+ Drs. Rhee and Timms
3 Cooper Plaza/Suite 221   Camden, NJ 08103   (856)342-2965   Fax (856)365-1967

Shah, Nimit Ashwinbhai, MD {1386975894} IntHos
+ 811 Fox Run Drive
Plainsboro, NJ 08536   (281)217-7839

Shah, Nina M., MD {1982064176} Pedtrc<NJ-JRSYSHMC>
+ Jersey Shore University Medical Center
1945 Route 33   Neptune, NJ 07753   (201)919-6796

Shah, Niranjan S., MD {1184662470} CdvDis, IntrMd(74,INA4X)<NJ-BAYSHORE>
+ Drs. Prasad and Shah
717 North Beers Street/PO Box 370   Holmdel, NJ 07733   (732)264-0210   Fax (732)888-9214

Shah, Nirav K., MD {1477505329} SrgNro
+ Princeton Brain & Spine Care LLC
731 Alexander Road/Suite 200   Princeton, NJ 08540   (609)921-9001   Fax (609)921-9055
+ Princeton Brain & Spine Care LLC
190 Route 31N/Suite 300B   Flemington, NJ 08822   (609)921-9001   Fax (908)806-6625

Shah, Nirav M., MD {1720299340} PulDis, CritCr(03,AZ02)<NJ-CENTRAST, NJ-KIMBALL>
+ Monmouth Ocean Pulmonary Medicine
901 West Main Street/Suite 160   Freehold, NJ 07728   (732)577-0600   Fax (732)577-6332
+ Monmouth Ocean Pulmonary Medicine
886 River Avenue   Lakewood, NJ 08701   (732)577-0600   Fax (732)360-0336
+ Monmouth Ocean Pulmonary Medicine
312 Applegarth Road   Monroe Township, NJ 07728   (609)409-0029

Shah, Nita K., MD {1538139399} Nephro, IntrMd(86,INDI)
+ Modern Nephrology & Transplant, LLC
767 Northfield Avenue   West Orange, NJ 07052   (973)992-9022   Fax (973)992-9024

Shah, Niva, DO {1366837288} Pedtrc<NJ-MORRISTN>
+ Morristown Medical Center
100 Madison Avenue   Morristown, NJ 07962   (973)971-5000

Shah, Nrupa, MD {1407998784} IntrMd(96,NJ06)<NJ-STFRNMED>
+ St. Francis Medical Center
601 Hamilton Avenue   Trenton, NJ 08629   (609)599-5000   Fax (609)599-6232

Shah, Pallav N., DO {1386633212} RadNro, RadDia(99,NY75)
+ Cooper University Medical Center/Camden
3 Cooper Plaza   Camden, NJ 08103   (856)342-2383

Shah, Pallavi Devendra, MD {1497929673} IntrMd(73,INA87)<NJ-GRYSTPSY>
+ 165 Morris Turnpike
Randolph, NJ 07869   (973)895-2529

Shah, Paresha Snehal, MD {1134168776} AlgyImmn, Allrgy, Pedtrc(83,INA65)<NJ-MEMSALEM>
+ Allergy & Asthma Care Center
901 Route 168/Suite 504   Turnersville, NJ 08012   (856)227-5700   Fax (856)227-9800

Shah, Parul Samir, MD {1730424805} Psychy(93,INA53)<NJ-VALYONS>
+ VA New Jersey Health Care System at Lyons
151 Knollcroft Road/PTSD Psych   Lyons, NJ 07939   (908)647-0180   Fax (908)604-5288
Parul.Shah2@va.gov

Shah, Payal A., MD {1962406504} ObsGyn(99,GRN01)<NJ-HOLYNAME, NJ-HACKNSK>
+ Women's Health Care Group
870 Palisade Avenue/Suite 301   Teaneck, NJ 07666   (201)907-0900   Fax (201)907-0229

Shah, Pooja, MD {1477953123} IntrMd
+ 1964 Oak Tree Road
Edison, NJ 08820   (732)635-0050

Physicians by Name and Address

Shah, Pradip A., MD {1437175155} IntrMd, InfDis(80,INA67)<NJ-JFKMED, NJ-RWJURAH>
+ 680 Broadway/Suite 506
Paterson, NJ 07514 (973)553-5872 Fax (732)635-0051
drpshah635@yahoo.com
+ 1964 Oak Tree Road
Edison, NJ 08820 (973)553-5872 Fax (732)635-0051

Shah, Pradip S., MD {1326059320} IntrMd, Grtrcs(82,INA20)
+ Crane's Mill - Oak Health Center
459 Passaic Avenue West Caldwell, NJ 07006 (973)276-3026 Fax (973)276-7881

Shah, Praful M., MD {1306065156} IntrMd(68,INA02)
+ 520 North Wood Avenue
Linden, NJ 07036

Shah, Prafulla R., MD {1407899602} Anesth(74,INDI)<NJ-STCLRSUS, NJ-WESTHDSN>
+ St. Clare's Hospital-Sussex
20 Walnut Street/Anesthesiology Sussex, NJ 07461
(973)702-2600

Shah, Pranav N., MD {1144215963} RadDia(92,NJ06)<NJ-RIVERVW>
+ Red Bank Radiologists, P.A.
200 White Road/Suite 115 Little Silver, NJ 07739
(732)741-9595 Fax (732)741-0985
+ Coastal Imaging, LLC
79 Route 37 West/Suite 103 Toms River, NJ 08755
(732)741-9595 Fax (732)276-2325

Shah, Pritesh J., MD {1114121175} Psychy, PsyGrt(85,INA20)<NJ-HOLYNAME>
+ 354 Old Hook Road
Westwood, NJ 07675 (201)358-0400 Fax (201)358-6114

Shah, Priyank P., MD {1285946988}
+ 249 Belleville Avenue/Apt 21 B
Bloomfield, NJ 07003 (862)591-4954
priyank_221084@yahoo.com

Shah, Purviben R., MD {1295049039} IntrMd<NJ-VIRTMHBC>
+ Virtua Memorial
175 Madison Avenue Mount Holly, NJ 08060 (609)261-7486 Fax (609)914-6182

Shah, Rahul V., MD {1235242934} SrgOrt(05,NJ02)<NJ-SJHREGMC, NJ-SJRSYELM>
+ Premier Orthopaedic Associates
298 South Delsea Drive Vineland, NJ 08360 (856)690-1616 Fax (856)690-1089
+ Premier Orthopaedic Assocs of So NJ
201 Tomlin Station Road/Suite C Mullica Hill, NJ 08062
(856)690-1616 Fax (856)223-9110

Shah, Rajeev Rajat, MD {1043264849} Pedtrc(96,NY46)<NJ-CHSMRCER>
+ Capital Health System/Mercer Campus
446 Bellevue Avenue Trenton, NJ 08618 (609)394-4000

Shah, Rajen S., MD {1356378434} IntrMd, Gastrn(78,INA21)<NJ-EASTORNG>
+ Drs. Shah & Shah
1060 Broad Street Newark, NJ 07102 (973)642-0280
Fax (973)642-0047
Rajsanshah@gmail.com

Shah, Rajiv K., MD {1912108291} Surgry(94,INA15)
+ LifeCare Physicians, PC of Hamilton
1225 Whitehorse Mercerville Rd Trenton, NJ 08619
(609)581-6060 Fax (609)581-9561

Shah, Rameshchan H., MD {1376536946} Anesth(72,INA20)<NJ-STCLRSUS, NJ-WESTHDSN>
+ St. Clare's Hospital-Sussex
20 Walnut Street/Anesthesiology Sussex, NJ 07461
(973)702-2600
+ West Hudson Division of Clara Maass Medical Center
206 Bergen Avenue/Anesthesiology Kearny, NJ 07032
(201)955-7000

Shah, Rasesh Pravin, MD {1437159407} Otlryg(00,NJ05)
+ Advanced ENT - Willingboro
1113 Hospital Drive/Suite 103 Willingboro, NJ 08046
(856)602-4000 Fax (609)871-0508
+ Advanced ENT - Woodbury
620 North Broad Street Woodbury, NJ 08096 (856)602-4000 Fax (856)848-6029
+ Advanced ENT - Washington Township
239 Hurffville Crosskeys Road Sewell, NJ 08046 (856)602-4000 Fax (856)629-3391

Shah, Rehan A., MD {1386895688} Rheuma, IntrMd(04,PAK26)
+ 2239 Whitehorse Mercerville Ro/Suite 1
Hamilton, NJ 08619 (609)838-9700 Fax (609)838-9702

Shah, Reza A., DO {1891740080} Surgry(93,NJ75)<NJ-CHSFULD, NJ-CAPITLHS>
+ 2063 Klockner Road
Hamilton, NJ 08690 (609)586-9788 Fax (609)586-1232
+ Mercer Surgical Group
2063 Klockner Road/Suite 1 Hamilton, NJ 08690
(609)586-9788 Fax (609)588-5970

Shah, Rohitkumar I., MD {1558308668} IntrMd(81,INDI)
+ 297 Central Avenue
Jersey City, NJ 07307 (201)420-7373 Fax (201)795-0606

Shah, Ruchir Nikunjbihari, MD {1922081082} PedAne, Anesth(97,INA15)<NJ-HACKNSK>
+ Hackensack University MC-Anesthesia Dept
30 Prospect Avenue/Room 2703 Hackensack, NJ 07601
(201)996-2419 Fax (201)996-3962

Shah, Sachin Jitendra, MD {1497798201} EmrgMd(98,PA07)<NJ-JRSYCITY, NY-WESTCHMC>
+ Emergency Medical Associates of NJ, P.A.
3 Century Drive Parsippany, NJ 07054 (973)740-0607
Fax (973)740-9895

Shah, Sachin K., MD {1265665228} Anesth
+ Gagliano Medical Group
50 Mount Prospect Avenue/Suite 209 Clifton, NJ 07013
(862)238-8250 Fax (862)238-8255

Shah, Saira, MD {1013265826} IntrMd<NJ-JRSYCITY>
+ Jersey City Medical Center
355 Grand Street/Medicine/3rd Fl Jersey City, NJ 07304
(201)915-2000

Shah, Samir, MD {1821094194} Otlryg(96,NY08)<NJ-HCKTSTWN>
+ Advanced ENT - Haddonfield
130 North Haddon Avenue Haddonfield, NJ 08033
(856)602-4000 Fax (856)429-1284
+ Advanced ENT - Mount Laurel
204 Ark Road/Building 1/Suite 102 Mount Laurel, NJ 08054
(856)602-4000 Fax (856)946-1747
+ Advanced ENT - Voorhees
1307 White Horse Road Voorhees, NJ 08033 (856)602-4000 Fax (856)346-0480

Shah, Samir D., MD {1083691000} PulDis, CritCr, IntrMd(91,INA20)<NJ-NWTNMEM>
+ Premier Health Associates
123 Newton Sparta Road Newton, NJ 07860 (973)579-6300 Fax (973)579-1524

Shah, Samir M., MD {1205197480}<NY-STONYBRK>
+ Anesthesia Consultnts of NJ/Nova Pain
285 Davidson Avenue/Suite 204 Somerset, NJ 08873
(732)271-1400 Fax (732)271-3543

Shah, Samir Nalin, MD {1659544716} IntrMd, Nephro(03,NJ06)<NJ-VIRTMHBC, NJ-LOURDMED>
+ The Center for Kidney Care
1261 Route 38/Suite A Hainesport, NJ 08036 (856)222-1975 Fax (856)222-0721

Shah, Sandeep K., MD {1225314966} PedCrC(07,INA87)<NJ-JFKMED>
+ JFK Medical Center
65 James Street/PedsCritCare Edison, NJ 08820 (732)321-7000 Fax (732)906-4906

Shah, Sandhya R., MD {1770513376} IntrMd(80,INA71)<NJ-NWRKBETH>
+ Drs. Shah & Shah
1060 Broad Street Newark, NJ 07102 (973)642-0280
Fax (973)642-0047
Docshahs@gmail.com

Shah, Sanjay R., MD {1568624302} Nephro, Grtrcs, IntrMd(96,INA71)
+ North Jersey Nephrology Associates PA
246 Hamburg Turnpike/Suite 207 Wayne, NJ 07470
(713)294-7344 Fax (973)653-3365

Shah, Sapna V., MD {1932490877} Pedtrc(11,NJ05)
+ PediatriCare Associates
901 Route 23 South Pompton Plains, NJ 07444 (973)831-4545 Fax (973)831-1527
+ PediatriCare Associates
20-20 Fair Lawn Avenue Fair Lawn, NJ 07410 (973)831-4545 Fax (201)791-3765

Shah, Satish P., MD {1730129826} Radiol, RadDia, IntrMd(67,INA65)<NJ-SJHREGMC>
+ Center for Diagnostic Imaging
1450 East Chestnut Avenue Vineland, NJ 08360 (856)794-8664 Fax (856)794-2671

Shah, Satyam Ashvinkumar, MD {1265691471} IntHos<NJ-OURLADY>
+ Our Lady of Lourdes Medical Center
1600 Haddon Avenue/Internal Med Camden, NJ 08103
(856)757-3500 Fax (856)668-8479

Shah, Sejal Gohel, MD {1104981000} IntrMd(01,DC01)
+ Franklin Medical Center
514 Route 33 West/Suite 6 Millstone Township, NJ 08535
(732)851-7007 Fax (732)786-0012

Shah, Shailaja K., MD {1750464491} PsyGrt, Psychy, IntrMd(89,INA67)<NJ-CARRIER>
+ Behavioral HealthCare Consultants, LLC.
407 Omni Drive Hillsborough, NJ 08844 (732)689-3832
Shaila@bhcc-MD.com
+ Carrier Clinic
252 Route 601/GeriatricPsy Belle Mead, NJ 08502
(732)689-3832 Fax (908)281-1301

Shah, Shailen Ramesh, MD {1982799359} AlgyImmn
+ Allergy & Asthma Consultants of NJ, P.A.
9004 Lincoln Drive West/Suite B Marlton, NJ 08053
(856)596-3100 Fax (856)596-3133

+ Allergy & Asthma Consultants of NJ, P.A.
110 South Dennisville Road Cape May Court House, NJ 08210 (856)596-3100 Fax (856)596-3133

Shah, Shailen S., MD {1982692836} ObsGyn, MtFtMd(91,PA02)<NJ-VIRTVOOR, NJ-VIRTMHBC>
+ Virtua Maternal Fetal Medicine Center
100 Bowman Drive Voorhees, NJ 08043 (856)247-3328
Fax (856)247-3276
+ Memorial Maternal Fetal Medicine Center
175 Madison Avenue Mount Holly, NJ 08060 (609)265-7914

Shah, Shaili Niranjan, MD {1730408048} AlgyImmn
+ Princeton Allergy & Asthma Associates, P.A.
24 Vreeland Drive/Suite 1 Skillman, NJ 08558 (609)921-2202 Fax (609)924-1468

Shah, Shamji K., MD {1588631626} SrgCdv, SrgThr, CdvDis(73,INA69)<NJ-NWRKBETH, NJ-STBARNMC>
+ 96 Millburn Avenue/Suite 200 A
Millburn, NJ 07041 (973)313-0011 Fax (973)763-1569

Shah, Shazia M., DO {1801810528} IntrMd(96,NY75)<NJ-STFRNMED>
+ St. Francis Medical Center
601 Hamilton Avenue/Assistant Trenton, NJ 08629
(609)599-5000 Fax (609)599-5000
doc2nj@aol.com
+ Elite Internal Medicine, PA
601 Hamilton Avenue/Hospitalist Trenton, NJ 08629 Fax (609)599-5391

Shah, Shefali A., DO {1578525432} FamMed(93,NY75)
+ Skylands Medical Group PA
150 Lakeside Boulevard Landing, NJ 07850 (973)398-6300
Fax (973)398-6399

Shah, Shilpan H., MD {1508061623} IntrMd(98,INA20)<NJ-MONMOUTH>
+ Monmouth Medical Center
300 Second Avenue/IntMed Long Branch, NJ 07740
(732)222-5200

Shah, Shital R., MD {1417992447} RadDia(01,NJ05)
+ Sparta Health and Wellness Center
89 Sparta Avenue/Suite 120 Sparta, NJ 07871 (973)729-0002 Fax (973)729-1085

Shah, Shrenik G., MD {1053352732} IntrMd(78,INA20)<NJ-MTNSIDE, NJ-STJOSHOS>
+ 55 West Passaic Avenue
Bloomfield, NJ 07003 (973)338-8059 Fax (973)338-6013
Shrenikgsman@yahoo.com

Shah, Shruti A., MD {1114158755} Anesth(97,INA87)
+ Robert Wood Johnson-UMDNJ Anesthesia Group
125 Paterson Street/CAB 3100 New Brunswick, NJ 08901
(732)235-7246 Fax (732)235-6131

Shah, Smita S., MD {1790847903} CritCr, IntrMd, PulDis(80,INA69)
+ Comprehensive Pulmonary & Critical Care Assoc
96 Millburn Avenue/Suite 200A Millburn, NJ 07041
(973)763-6800 Fax (973)763-1255

Shah, Snehal, MD {1417123605} Psychy, IntrMd(07,DMN01)<NJ-NWRKBETH>
+ Newark Beth Israel Medical Center
201 Lyons Avenue/Psychiatry Newark, NJ 07112
(732)207-1205

Shah, Sonal Ashwin, DO {1336285899} Pedtrc(03,AZ02)
+ Union Hill Pediatrics
85 Bridge Plaza Drive Manalapan, NJ 07726 (732)972-1117 Fax (732)972-0177

Shah, Subhadra Sundaram, MD {1922023001} Dermat, DerMOH(00,PA02)
+ Dermatology Associates of Morris PA
199 Baldwin Road Parsippany, NJ 07054 (973)335-2560
Fax (973)335-9421

Shah, Sudha S., MD {1144257213} Anesth(69,INA67)<NJ-ACMCITY, NJ-ACMCMAIN>
+ AtlantiCare Regional Medical Center/City Campus
1925 Pacific Avenue/Anesthesiology Atlantic City, NJ 08401
(609)345-4000
+ AtlantiCare Regional Med Ctr/Mainland
65 West Jimmie Leeds Road Pomona, NJ 08240 (609)652-1000

Shah, Suken H., MD {1891709564} Radiol, RadV&I(00,PA02)<NJ-NWRKBETH>
+ Newark Beth Israel Medical Center
201 Lyons Avenue/Attending Phys Newark, NJ 07112
(973)926-7000

Shah, Suketu Rajina, MD {1124050570} EnDbMt(01,NJ05)
+ 4 Progress Street/Suite B-6
Edison, NJ 08820 (908)222-2658

Shah, Sulay Hiteshkumar, MD {1386075224} IntHos<NJ-ACMCITY>
+ AtlantiCare Regional Medical Center/City Campus
1925 Pacific Avenue Atlantic City, NJ 08401 (609)441-8146 Fax (609)441-8002

Physicians by Name and Address

Shah, Sumit Pravinkumar, MD {1346439213} Ophthl, VitRet, IntrMd(05,NJ05)
+ Retina Associates of New Jersey, P.A.
10 Plum Street/Suite 600   New Brunswick, NJ 08901   (732)220-1600   Fax (732)220-1603
+ Retina Associates of New Jersey, P.A.
2 Industrial Way West   Eatontown, NJ 07724   (732)220-1600   Fax (732)389-2788
+ Retina Associates of New Jersey, P.A.
525 Route 70 West/Suite B-14   Lakewood, NJ 08901   (732)363-2396   Fax (732)363-0403

Shah, Sweta, MD {1003203118} FamMed
+ Drs Shah and Shah
25 Mule Road/Suite B4   Toms River, NJ 08755   (732)341-0020   Fax (732)341-0072

Shah, Talaxi D., MD {1982703500} Psychy(63,INA79)
+ 33 Overlook Road/Suite 404
Summit, NJ 07901   (908)522-3099   Fax (908)522-3299
TEDSHAH@gmail.com

Shah, Tanmaya Chetan, MD {1659590792} Radiol(02,NJ05)<MA-MAGENHOS>
+ South Jersey Radiology Associates, P.A.
100 Carnie Boulevard/Suite B-5   Voorhees, NJ 08043   (856)374-4031   Fax (856)751-0535
+ South Jersey Radiology Associates, P.A.
315 Route 70 East/Suite B   Cherry Hill, NJ 08034   (856)374-4031   Fax (856)428-0356
+ South Jersey Radiology Associates, P.A.
901 Route 168/Suites 301-305   Turnersville, NJ 08043   (856)227-6600   Fax (856)227-8537

Shah, Taral Jobanputra, MD {1659670123} IntrMd(07,GRN01)
+ 6507 Hana Road
Edison, NJ 08817   (848)667-3795
+ AtlantiCare Physician Group Joslin Diabetes Center
2500 English Creek Avenue/Bldg 800   Egg Harbor Township, NJ 08234   (848)667-3795   Fax (609)272-6306

Shah, Tarun J., MD {1053385484} Allrgy, Pedtrc(84,INA21)<NJ-JRSYSHMC, NJ-COMMED>
+ 1539 State Route 138
Belmar, NJ 07719
tjshah@pol.net
+ 200 Perrine Road/Suite 226
Old Bridge, NJ 08857   (732)681-8141
+ 525 Jack Martin Boulevard
Brick, NJ 07719   (732)840-9100

Shah, Trishna Kirit, MD {1699163337} Anesth
+ Robert Wood Johnson-UMDNJ Anesthesia Group
125 Paterson Street/CAB 3100   New Brunswick, NJ 08901   (732)235-7827   Fax (732)235-6131

Shah, Udayan Kanaiyalal, MD {1386734317} Otlryg(92,MA05)
+ CHOP Pediatric & Adolescent Specialty Care Center
1012 Laurel Oak Road   Voorhees, NJ 08043   (856)435-1300   Fax (856)435-0091

Shah, Umang Lalit, MD {1750514154} CdvDis, IntCrd<NJ-HACKNSK>
+ Hackensack University Medical Center
30 Prospect Avenue   Hackensack, NJ 07601   (865)230-2827
umangshah@yahoo.com

Shah, Ushma R., MD {1841453818} IntrMd(08,GRN01)
+ Robert Wood Johnson-UMDNJ Anesthesia Group
125 Paterson Street/CAB 3100   New Brunswick, NJ 08901   (732)235-7827   Fax (732)235-6131

Shah, Usman Ali, MD {1215255310}<NJ-RWJUBRUN>
+ RWJ University Hospital New Brunswick
One Robert Wood Johnson Place   New Brunswick, NJ 08901   (732)828-3000

Shah, Utpal S., MD {1225066491} Pedtrc, AdolMd(98,DMN01)<NJ-UNVMCPRN>
+ East Windsor Pediatric Group
300B Princeton Hightstown/Suite 201   Hightstown, NJ 08520   (609)448-7300   Fax (609)448-8022

Shah, Vinay R., MD {1356358709} ObsGyn(83,INDI)<NJ-HACKNSK>
+ 985 Paulison Avenue
Clifton, NJ 07011   (973)471-2000   Fax (973)773-8553

Shah, Vinaychandra B., MD {1750340519} FamMed(72,INA69)<NJ-BAYSHORE>
+ 702 North Beers Street
Holmdel, NJ 07733   (732)264-8788   Fax (732)264-8323

Shah, Vinnie Pooja, MD {1992970578} Ophthl(07,NY20)
+ Summit Medical Group-Berkeley Heights Campus
1 Diamond Hill Road   Berkeley Heights, NJ 07922   (908)277-8682   Fax (908)277-8694

Shah, Vipul V., MD {1104976455} PhysMd, IntrMd(85,MEXI)
+ Medical Care Associates
262 Route 10 West   Succasunna, NJ 07876   (973)252-1522   Fax (973)252-1422
+ Medical Care Associates
137 Mountain Avenue   Hackettstown, NJ 07840   (973)252-1522   Fax (908)852-0614

Shah, Viral Jagdishbhai, MD {1336318344} EnDbMt(95,INA2B)<NY-WESTCHSQ>
+ Endocrine Associates
30 West Century Drive/Suite 255   Paramus, NJ 07652   (201)444-4363   Fax (201)444-6590

Shah, Vrinda B., MD {1922264795} Pedtrc(90,INA69)<NJ-CENTRAST>
+ 100 Professional Drive/Suite 101
Freehold, NJ 07728   (732)866-9300   Fax (732)866-9747

Shah, Yashica Manish, MD {1538112727} ObsGyn(98,NJ06)
+ Lifeline Medical Associates, LLC
16 Pocono Road/Suite 105   Denville, NJ 07834   (973)831-2777   Fax (973)831-2780

Shahab, Farhang, MD {1265429005} RadDia, Radiol(64,IRA01)<NJ-COMMED>
+ Community Medical Center
99 Route 37 West/Radiology   Toms River, NJ 08755   (732)557-8000   Fax (732)557-2064

Shahabuddin, Saiham, MD {1295078145} IntrMd<NY-ELMHRST>
+ 600 River Avenue
Lakewood, NJ 08701   (732)942-5721

Shahamat, Morteza, MD {1154429959} IntrMd, Pthlgy(70,IRA01)<NJ-VALLEY>
+ 400 Franklin Turnpike/Suite 104
Mahwah, NJ 07430   (201)995-1005   Fax (201)995-1007

Shahane, Manoj Raghunath, MD {1891755666} Anesth(90,INA69)<NJ-OVERLOOK, NJ-TRINIWSC>
+ Overlook Medical Center
99 Beauvoir Avenue/PO Box 210   Summit, NJ 07902   (908)522-2000

Shahar, Yoel S., MD {1033359740} Surgry, SrgPlstc(73,ISR01)
+ Shahar Cosmetic Surgery Center
370 Grand Avenue   Englewood, NJ 07631   (201)871-0855

Shahateet, Omar, MD {1922379957}
+ Specialty Medconsultants LLC
6725 Ventnor Avenue/Suite C   Ventnor City, NJ 08406   (609)350-6780   Fax (609)350-6995

Shahbandi, Matthew, MD {1912969379} Urolgy(95,MA05)<NJ-CHILTON, NJ-HACKNSK>
+ Adult and Pediatric Urology Center, P.A.
1033 Clifton Avenue   Clifton, NJ 07013   (973)473-5700   Fax (973)473-3367
mshahbandi@hotmail.com
+ Adult and Pediatric Urology Center, P.A.
2025 Hamburg Turnpike   Wayne, NJ 07470   (973)473-5700   Fax (973)831-0033
+ Adult and Pediatric Urology Center, P.A.
1031 McBride Avenue/Suite D-108   West Paterson, NJ 07013   (973)256-4038   Fax (973)256-0432

Shaheen, Zafar A., MD {1982641239} CdvDis, IntrMd(73,INA70)
+ 498 Union Avenue
Middlesex, NJ 08846   (732)297-8651   Fax (732)469-6103

Shahi, Chandreshwar N., MD {1063412484} CdvDis, IntrMd(83,INDI)
+ CardioMD
1200 US Highway 22 East/Suite 17   Bridgewater, NJ 08807   (908)864-4027   Fax (908)864-4029
+ CardioMD
245 Union Avenue/Suite 1A   Bridgewater, NJ 08807   (908)864-4027   Fax (908)864-4029

Shahid, Muhammad Salman, MD {1609138908}(15,NY46)
+ 44 Hampshire Drive
Plainsboro, NJ 08536   (609)799-6410
shahidmsal@gmail.com

Shahid, Nasar Mahmood, MD {1891940938} PhysMd(85,PAK10)<NY-NYPRESHS, NY-PRSBCOLU>
+ 179 CEDAR LN
Teaneck, NJ 07666   (201)907-5094

Shahidi, Hosseinali, MD {1326074030} Pedtrc, PedEmg, EmrgMd(71,IRA09)<NJ-UMDNJ>
+ University Hospital
150 Bergen Street/EmrgMed   Newark, NJ 07103   (973)972-4300   Fax (973)972-6646

Shahinian, Toros S., MD {1831231380} IntrMd(69,AUS08)
+ 349 East Northfield Road
Livingston, NJ 07039   (973)994-0007   Fax (973)994-3656

Shahmehdi, Seyed Akhtar, MD {1356521439} FamMed
+ 10 Hluchy Road
Robbinsville, NJ 08691

Shahsamand, Zabi Z., MD {1831353655} Anesth, IntrMd<NJ-MTNSIDE>
+ Hackensack UMC Mountainside
1 Bay Avenue/Anesthesia   Montclair, NJ 07042   (973)429-6982   Fax (845)357-5777

Shaigany, Nina N., MD {1033172861} Pedtrc(98,MD01)<NJ-VIRTUAHS>
+ Advocare Haddon Pediatric Group
119 White Horse Pike   Haddon Heights, NJ 08035   (856)547-7300   Fax (856)547-4573

Shaikh, Hafeza, DO {1235320870} CdvDis, IntrMd(NY75
+ South Jersey Heart Group
1113 Hospital Drive/Suite 202   Willingboro, NJ 08046   (609)835-3550   Fax (609)835-3557
+ South Jersey Heart Group
3001 Chapel Avenue/Suite 101   Cherry Hill, NJ 08002   (609)835-3550   Fax (856)482-7170

Shaikh, Hamadullah Ghafoor, MD {1306365200}<NJ-STFRNMED>
+ St. Francis Medical Center
601 Hamilton Avenue   Trenton, NJ 08629   (609)599-5000

Shaikh, Junaid Rasheed, MD {1598042970} PthFor(80,PAK11)
+ 90 Changebridge Road
Montville, NJ 07045   (973)220-0172   Fax (973)331-0880
jrshaikhmd@aol.com
+ Union County Medical Examiner Office
300 North Avenue East/Deputy ME   Westfield, NJ 07090   (908)654-9893

Shaikh, Najmussaha M., MD Psychy(69,INDI)
+ Rutgers Hurtado Health Center
11 Bishop Place   New Brunswick, NJ 08901   (732)932-7402   Fax (732)932-1223

Shaikh, Nasir Hussain A., MD {1861440281} FamMed(94,INDI)<NJ-UNVMCPRN, NJ-RWJUHAM>
+ Princeton Family Care
100 Federal City Road/Suite A   Lawrenceville, NJ 08648   (609)620-1380   Fax (609)771-8991

Shaikh, Sahil R., DO {1114309077}<NJ-BURDTMLN>
+ Cape Regional Medical Center
2 Stone Harbor Boulevard   Cape May Court House, NJ 08210   (609)463-2803   Fax (609)463-4991

Shaikh, Tasneem, MD {1336228550} Psychy(88,PAKI)<NJ-SOMERSET>
+ RWJ University Hospital Somerset
110 Rehill Avenue   Somerville, NJ 08876   (908)685-2200

Shaiman, Alan, MD {1619065059} RadOnc(80,PA07)<NJ-CHRIST, NJ-NWRKBETH>
+ Christ Hospital
176 Palisade Avenue/RadOnc   Jersey City, NJ 07306   (201)795-8252
+ Sovereign Oncology, LLC
20 Woodridge Avenue   Hackensack, NJ 07601   (201)795-8252   Fax (201)880-7585
+ Sovereign Oncology, LLC.
631 Grand Street   Jersey City, NJ 07306   (201)942-3999   Fax (201)942-3998

Shajenko, Lydia, MD {1841289634} Nrolgy, ClNrPh(97,CT02)
+ Riverfront Medical Associates
725 River Road/Suite 55   Edgewater, NJ 07020   (646)712-1635   Fax (866)267-8173

Shakarjian, Jo-Ann, MD {1225115769} ObsGyn(90,NY09)<NJ-VALLEY, NJ-HACKNSK>
+ Women's Health at Hackettstown
108 Bilby Road/Suite 305   Hackettstown, NJ 07840   (908)813-8877   Fax (908)813-9984

Shakarshy, Jack, MD {1851304299} Radiol, RadBdI(84,NY19)<NJ-ACMCITY, NJ-ACMCMAIN>
+ Atlantic Medical Imaging, LLC.
72 West Jimmie Leeds Road   Galloway, NJ 08205   (609)677-9729   Fax (609)653-8764
+ Atlantic Medical Imaging, LLC.
401 Bethel Road   Somers Point, NJ 08244   (609)677-9729
+ Atlantic Medical Imaging, LLC.
421 Route 9 North   Cape May Court House, NJ 08205   (609)463-9500   Fax (609)465-0918

Shaker, Ashraf F., MD {1235159658} EmrgMd, IntrMd(90,EGY04)
+ 125 Hudson Avenue
Ridgefield Park, NJ 07660   (973)365-4489   Fax (201)440-0311

Shaker, David, DO {1396130365}
+ Drs. Shaker and Shaker
38 Summit Avenue/Suite 1   Hackensack, NJ 07601   (201)343-6360   Fax (201)343-6367

Shaker, Elhamy I., MD {1285665695} IntrMd(78,EGY03)<NJ-HOLYNAME, NJ-HACKNSK>
+ 147 Cedar Lane
Teaneck, NJ 07666   (201)287-1010   Fax (201)287-9049

Shaker, Mina, MD {1770977852}
+ Drs. Shaker and Shaker
38 Summit Avenue/Suite 1   Hackensack, NJ 07601   (201)343-6360   Fax (201)343-6367

Shaker, Safwat I., MD {1144246042} IntrMd(82,EGY03)<NJ-HACKNSK>
+ Drs. Shaker and Shaker
38 Summit Avenue/Suite 1   Hackensack, NJ 07601   (201)343-6360   Fax (201)343-6367

Shaker, Taylor, MD {1215390083} FamMed
+ Valley Medical Group
43 Yawpo Avenue/Suite 3   Oakland, NJ 07436   (201)337-9600

Shakiba, Khashayar, MD {1114121571} ObsGyn
+ Physicians for Women
330 Ratzer Road/Suite 7   Wayne, NJ 07470   (973)694-2222   Fax (973)694-7664

Physicians by Name and Address

Shakibai, Nader, MD {1881685147} IntrMd, Nephro(99,CT02)
+ 145 Prospect Street/2nd Fl
Ridgewood, NJ 07450   (201)621-7101   Fax (201)447-1190

Shakir, Aarefa H., MD {1295942548} FamMed(00,INA1P)
+ Drs. Viswanathan, Shakir & Patel
815 Baltimore Avenue   Roselle, NJ 07203   (908)245-3446   Fax (908)245-9265

Shakir, Ahmar, DO {1861451452} SrgOrt(96,NJ75)
+ Lawrence Orthopaedics
4065 Quakerbridge Road   Princeton Junction, NJ 08550   (609)394-3804   Fax (609)989-1550

Shakir, Huzaifa Abbas, MD {1437290707} SrgThr, Surgry(99,MA05)<NJ-STMRYPAS>
+ St. Mary's Hospital
350 Boulevard   Passaic, NJ 07055   (973)365-4300

Shaknovsky, Thomas J., DO {1568690014} Surgry<NJ-PALISADE>
+ Palisades Medical Center
7600 River Road   North Bergen, NJ 07047   (201)854-5000

Shakov, Emil, MD {1790928521} Surgry, IntrMd(04,BWI01)<NJ-BAYSHORE, NJ-OCEANMC>
+ The Plastic Surgery Center
501 Stillwells Corner Road/Suite 9   Freehold, NJ 07728   Fax (732)358-0524
shakovmd@gmail.com

Shakov, Rada, MD {1831308303} Gastrn, Hepato, IntrMd(04,BWI01)
+ Ocean Endosurgery Center
129 Route 37 West   Toms River, NJ 08755   (732)606-4440   Fax (732)797-3963
+ 501 Iron Bridge Road/Suite 9
Freehold, NJ 07728   (732)333-3747

Shalem, Lena Hourwitz, MD {1730441676} EnDbMt
+ Diabetes Endocrinology Metabolism Specialities PA
6 Brighton Road/Suite 103   Clifton, NJ 07012   (973)471-2692   Fax (973)470-8188
+ Summit Medical Group
1 Diamond Hill Road/Bensley Pav/2 FL   Berkeley, NJ 07922   (973)471-2692   Fax (908)288-7993

Shalit, Stuart L., DO {1861421281} ObsGyn(90,FL75)<NJ-VIRTMHBC>
+ Virtua Phoenix OBGYN
120 Madison Avenue/Suite B   Mount Holly, NJ 08060   (609)444-5500   Fax (609)444-5501
+ Phoenix Ob-Gyn Associates
1 Sheffield Drive/Suite 101   Columbus, NJ 08022   (609)444-5500   Fax (609)291-5603
+ Phoenix Ob-Gyn Associates
110 Marter Avenue/Suite 505   Mooorestown, NJ 08060   (856)235-4840   Fax (856)235-3795

Shalts, Edward, MD {1518035732} Psychy, IntrMd(82,RUS79)<NJ-MEADWLND>
+ Meadowlands Hospital Medical Center
55 Meadowlands Parkway/2nd Floor   Secaucus, NJ 07096   (646)301-2578   Fax (201)510-0820

Shamash, Felix S., MD {1871694570} SrgVas, Surgry(81,NY19)<NJ-KIMBALL, NJ-OCEANMC>
+ Surgeon Associates
26 Pine Boulevard   Lakewood, NJ 08701   (732)364-1010   Fax (732)364-1991

Shamash, Steven Baroukh, DO {1780841312} OrtSHand
+ Garden State Orthopaedic Associates, P.A.
28-04 Broadway   Fair Lawn, NJ 07410   (201)791-4434   Fax (201)791-9257

Shami, Joseph G., MD {1144259649} Gastrn, IntrMd(78,ITAL)<NJ-STJOSHOS, NJ-WAYNEGEN>
+ Gastroenterology Associates of New Jersey
205 Browertown Road/Suite 204   Little Falls, NJ 07424   (973)812-5230   Fax (973)812-5235
+ Gastroenterology Diagnostics of Northern New Jersey
205 Browertown Road/Suite 102   West Paterson, NJ 07424   (973)812-5230   Fax (973)890-1097
+ St. Joseph's Regional Medical Center
703 Main Street/Div. Chief Gast   Paterson, NJ 07424   (973)754-2000

Shami, Msallam M., MD RadDia(89,SYR01)
+ 202 Goldmine Lane/PO Box 258
Old Bridge, NJ 08857

Shami, Samar, MD {1598822389} PthDrm, DrmtPthy(88,SYR01)
+ Dermatopathology Institute of New Jersey
225 Highway 35/Suite 201   Red Bank, NJ 07701   (732)450-0820   Fax (732)450-0823

Shamilov, Maasi Don, MD {1528073491} Psychy, PsyCAd(86,RUSS)<NJ-LOURDMED, NJ-STPETER>
+ Center for Family Guidance, PC
765 East Route 70/Building A-101   Marlton, NJ 08053   (856)983-3900   Fax (856)810-0110

Shamim, Ferheen, MD {1659683894} PhysMd(NY03
+ The Orthopedic Institute of New Jersey
108 Bilby Road/Suite 201   Hackettstown, NJ 07840   (908)684-3005   Fax (908)684-3301
+ The Orthopedic Institute of New Jersey
254-B Mountain Avenue/Suite 201   Hackettstown, NJ 07840   (908)684-3005   Fax (908)684-3301
+ The Orthopedic Institute of New Jersey
222 High Street/Suite 202   Newton, NJ 07840   (908)684-3005   Fax (908)684-3301

Shamim, Rehan Syed, MD {1730314485} SprtMd(09,NJ06)
+ The Orthopedic Institute of New Jersey
108 Bilby Road/Suite 201   Hackettstown, NJ 07840   (908)684-3005   Fax (908)684-3301
+ The Orthopedic Institute of New Jersey
254-B Mountain Avenue/Suite 201   Hackettstown, NJ 07840   (908)684-3005   Fax (908)684-3301
+ The Orthopedic Institute of New Jersey
222 High Street/Suite 202   Newton, NJ 07840   (908)684-3005   Fax (908)684-3301

Shamim, Syed Q., MD {1811985047} Gastrn, IntrMd(74,INDI)<NJ-STPETER, NJ-RWJUHAM>
+ Drs. Shamim and Shamim
1283 State Highway 27   Somerset, NJ 08873   (732)745-9025   Fax (732)545-3423

Shamim, Tasneem F., MD {1518987791} Ophthl(81,NJ06)
+ Drs. Shamim and Shamim
1283 State Highway 27   Somerset, NJ 08873   (732)745-9025   Fax (732)545-3423

Shammas, James T., MD {1295796134} Nrolgy(90,NY47)<NJ-VALLEY>
+ Neurology Group of Bergen County
1200 East Ridgewood Avenue   Ridgewood, NJ 07450   (201)444-0868   Fax (201)444-7363

Shammash, Jonathan Baruch, MD {1518055896} IntrMd, GPrvMd(92,PA01)<NJ-ENGLWOOD>
+ Englewood Hospital and Medical Center
350 Engle Street/Medicine   Englewood, NJ 07631   (201)894-3329   Fax (201)894-0839

Shammout, Jumana Sa'ad, MD {1174663231} Pedtrc, PedGst(92,JOR01)
+ Joseph M. Sanzari Childrens' -Gastro
155 Polifly Road/Suite 102   Hackensack, NJ 07601   (551)996-8840   Fax (201)441-9949

Shamoon, Fayez E., MD {1528053477} CdvDis, IntrMd(81,JOR01)<NJ-STMICHL>
+ St. Michael's Medical Center
268 MLK Jr. Boulevard/Bldg B/5th Fl   Newark, NJ 07102   (973)877-5160
Billing@shamoon.com

Shampain, Lawrence R., MD {1881789816} PsyCAd, Psychy(82,PA09)<NJ-UNIVBHC, NJ-SOMERSET>
+ 32 Wernik Place/Suite B
Metuchen, NJ 08840   (732)548-1600   Fax (732)548-4591
lshamp@optonline.net
+ University Behavioral Health Care
671 Hoes Lane/PO Box 1392/Psych   Piscataway, NJ 08855   (732)235-5785
+ RWJ University Hospital Somerset
110 Rehill Avenue/Psych   Somerville, NJ 08840   (908)685-2200

Shams, Setareh, MD {1003176462}<NJ-MONMOUTH>
+ Monmouth Medical Center
300 Second Avenue   Long Branch, NJ 07740   (732)923-6795   Fax (732)923-6793

Shamshad, Munaza, MD {1336186386} FamMed(90,PAK14)
+ 359 Mount Lucas Road
Princeton, NJ 08540

Shamsi, Mahmood A., MD {1437202561} Grtrcs, IntrMd, OccpMd(80,EGYP)
+ 1273 Bound Brook Road/Suite 10
Middlesex, NJ 08846   (732)563-6630   Fax (732)563-6733
mashamsi@yahoo.com

Shamsi, Zahira B., MD {1962501304} Grtrcs, IntrMd(81,EGY04)
+ Mahmood A. Shamsi, MD, PA
1273 Bound Brook Road/Suite 10   Middlesex, NJ 08846   (732)563-6630   Fax (732)563-6733

Shan, Yizhi, MD {1730590530} Surgry
+ RWJMG Acute Care Surgery
125 Paterson Street/Suite 6300   New Brunswick, NJ 08901   (732)235-5114   Fax (732)235-2964

Shanahan, Andrew J., MD {1881635084} CdvDis, IntrMd(89,WI06)<NJ-RWJUBRUN, NJ-UNVMCPRN>
+ Cardiology Associates of Princeton, P.A.
731 Alexander Road/Suite 202   Princeton, NJ 08540   (609)921-7456   Fax (609)921-2972
+ Cardiology Associates of Princeton, P.A.
5 Plainsboro Road/Suite 490   Plainsboro, NJ 08536   (609)921-7456   Fax (609)799-2832

Shanahan, Eileen Marie, MD {1083642508} PthAcl, PthAna(88,NJ06)<NJ-UNVMCPRN>
+ University Medical Center of Princeton at Plainsboro
One Plainsboro Road/Anatm/Clnc Path   Plainsboro, NJ 08536   (609)497-4000   Fax (609)497-4982

Shanahan-Prendergast, Kelsey, MD {1164818860} IntrMd<NJ-OVERLOOK>
+ Overlook Medical Center
99 Beauvoir Avenue/PO Box 210   Summit, NJ 07902   (908)522-6414

Shanbhag, Suhas R., MD {1144292004} Psychy(69,INDI)<NJ-TRININPC>
+ Trinitas Regional Medical Center-New Point Campus
655 East Jersey Street/Psych   Elizabeth, NJ 07206   (908)994-5000

Shander, Aryeh, MD {1578541942} Anesth, CritCr, IntrMd(77,VT02)<NJ-ENGLWOOD>
+ Englewood Anesthesiology
350 Engle Street/Anesthesiology   Englewood, NJ 07631   (201)894-3238   Fax (201)894-0585
ashander@englewoodhospital.com
+ Englewood Hospital and Medical Center
350 Engle Street/Anesthesiology   Englewood, NJ 07631   (201)894-3000

Shane, Steven A., DO {1689667578} Anesth, PainMd, Anes-Pain(78,IA75)
+ Union Anesthesia & Pain Management
695 Chestnut Street   Union, NJ 07083   (908)851-7161   Fax (908)851-7536

Shang, Xiaozhou, MD {1063673432} Psychy(85,PA09)<NJ-SJERSYHS>
+ South Woods State Prison/NJ Dept of Corrections
215 South Burlington Road   Bridgeton, NJ 08302   (856)459-7000
+ Center for Family Guidance, PC
765 East Route 70/Building A-101   Marlton, NJ 08053   (856)459-7000   Fax (856)810-0110

Shanik, Robert A., MD {1306864962} Pedtrc(74,VA04)<NJ-COMMED, NJ-KIMBALL>
+ Pediatric Affiliates, PA
40 Bey Lea Road/Suite B203   Toms River, NJ 08753   (732)341-0720   Fax (732)244-6842
+ Pediatric Affiliates, PA
400 Madison Avenue   Lakewood, NJ 08701   (732)341-0720   Fax (732)364-9292
+ Pediatric Affiliates, PA
1616 Route 72 West/Suite 8   Manahawkin, NJ 08753   (609)597-6200   Fax (609)978-1229

Shankar, Kala, MD {1942416763} ObsGyn, Obstet(96,INA67)
+ Ocean Health Initiatives, Inc.
301 Lakehurst Road   Toms River, NJ 08755   (732)552-0377   Fax (732)552-0378
+ Ocean Health Initiatives, Inc.
101 Second Street   Lakewood, NJ 08701   (732)552-0377   Fax (732)363-6656

Shankar, Ramamurthy R., MD {1730115122} PedEnd
+ 135 Park Avenue
Verona, NJ 07044

Shankar, Sujatha, MD {1508810268} Pedtrc(92,INA68)
+ 77 Brunswick Woods Drive
East Brunswick, NJ 08816   (732)238-6644   Fax (732)238-6550
+ 208 Bridge Street/Bld D
Metuchen, NJ 08840   (732)238-6644   Fax (732)518-3208

Shanker, Mukesh J., MD {1750376141} CdvDis, IntrMd(82,GRN01)<NJ-SHOREMEM, NJ-ACMCMAIN>
+ PO Box 1201
Absecon, NJ 08201   (609)653-1611   Fax (609)653-9352

Shanker, Soma, MD {1093884157} Anesth(89,INDI)<NJ-STBARNMC>
+ St. Barnabas Medical Center
94 Old Short Hills Road   Livingston, NJ 07039   (973)322-5000
sshanker@njanesthesia.com

Shanley, Frank M., DO {1588617708} CdvDis, IntrMd(75,PA77)
+ 124 East Main Street/Suite 106
Denville, NJ 07834   (973)627-6901   Fax (973)627-5657

Shanmugam, Revathi, MD {1457445033} Psychy(68,INA04)
+ 123 Abbie Court
Guttenberg, NJ 07093

Shao, John Han, MD {1336302199} CdvDis, IntrMd(01,PA13)
+ North Jersey Cardiovascular Consultants
329 Belleville Avenue   Bloomfield, NJ 07003   (973)748-3800   Fax (973)748-3540
+ North Jersey Cardiovascular Consultants
96 Millburn Avenue/Suite 200B   Millburn, NJ 07041   (973)748-3800   Fax (973)762-1946

Shapiro, Barry E., DO {1316949720} CdvDis, IntrMd(85,NY75)<NJ-SJERSYHS>
+ South Jersey Cardiology PC
1203 North High Street/Suite B   Millville, NJ 08332   (856)293-7466   Fax (856)293-7472
+ Cardiovascular Associates of The Delaware Valley, PA
525 State Street/Suite 3   Elmer, NJ 08318   (856)293-7466   Fax (856)358-0725

Shapiro, Deborah Lee, MD {1306869078} Rheuma, IntrMd(86,IL06)<NY-METROHOS, NY-MTSNAIQN>
+ 663 Palisade Avenue
Cliffside Park, NJ 07010

Physicians by Name and Address

Shapiro, Dein M., MD {1548202443} FamMed, Acpntr(76,DC02)<NJ-HUNTRDN>
+ 3461 Route 22 East
Somerville, NJ 08876 (908)534-6271 Fax (908)526-4495
+ Hunterdon Family Medicine
250 Route 28/Suite 100 Bridgewater, NJ 08807 (908)534-6271 Fax (908)237-4136

Shapiro, Eugene, MD {1811124746} Pedtrc
+ Delaware Valley Pediatric Associates PA
132 Franklin Corner Road Lawrenceville, NJ 08648 (609)896-4141 Fax (609)896-3940

Shapiro, Gary I., MD {1386610228} FamMed(93,PA12)<NJ-VIRTMHBC>
+ Mt. Laurel Family Physicians
401 Young Avenue/Suite 260 Moorestown, NJ 08057 (856)291-8756 Fax (856)291-8750

Shapiro, Jason, MD {1457346165} GenPrc<NJ-CLARMAAS>
+ Clara Maass Medical Center
1 Clara Maass Drive Belleville, NJ 07109 (973)450-2000

Shapiro, Jeffrey L., MD {1558408682} Anesth(03,PA09)<NJ-KENEDYHS>
+ Rancocas Anesthesiology, PA
700 Route 130 North/Suite 203 Cinnaminson, NJ 08077 (856)829-9345 Fax (856)829-3605

Shapiro, Leonid, MD {1992754634} Anesth, IntrMd(86,LAT02)
+ 790 Bloomfield Avenue
Clifton, NJ 07012 (201)448-4100

Shapiro, Marion D., DO {1326264409} EmrgMd(81,PA77)<NJ-STBARNMC>
+ St. Barnabas Medical Center
94 Old Short Hills Road/EmergMed Livingston, NJ 07039 (973)322-5000

Shapiro, Mark, MD {1720246309} SrgThr, Surgry(05,NY47)
+ VPS Thoracic Surgery
One Valley Health Plaza Paramus, NJ 07652 (201)634-5722 Fax (201)634-5381

Shapiro, Mark L., MD {1447215710} Radiol, RadDia(88,NY08)<NJ-ENGLWOOD>
+ Englewood Radiologic Group PA
350 Engle Street Englewood, NJ 07631 (201)894-3000 Fax (201)894-5244
+ Advanced Medical Imaging of North Jersey
452 Old Hook Road/Suite 301 Emerson, NJ 07630 (201)894-3000 Fax (201)262-2330

Shapiro, Michael Eliot, MD {1023052149} SrgTpl, Surgry(77,NY45)<NJ-HACKNSK>
+ Hackensack University Medical Center
30 Prospect Avenue/OrganTransplant Hackensack, NJ 07601 (201)996-2867 Fax (201)498-0148
mshapiro@humed.com

Shapiro, Paul, DO {1821155441} FamMed(80,MO79)<NJ-VIRTMHBC>
+ Alliance for Better Care, P.C.
130 Lakehurst Road Browns Mills, NJ 08015 (609)893-3133 Fax (609)893-7972

Shapiro, Sofia, MD {1265581714} IntrMd(90,RUS06)<NJ-STBARNMC>
+ 511 South Orange Avenue
South Orange, NJ 07079 (973)763-8950 Fax (973)763-5216

Shapiro, Stephen R., MD {1295773570} Gastrn, IntrMd(69,IL42)<NJ-STPETER, NJ-SOMERSET>
+ Gastromed HealthCare, PA
25 Monroe Street Bridgewater, NJ 08807 (908)231-1999 Fax (908)231-1612
+ Gastromed HealthCare PA
203 Towne Centre Drive Hillsborough, NJ 08844 (908)359-1639

Shapiro, Tyler Kenneth, MD {1497047609} EmrgMd
+ Cooper Univerisry Emergency Physicians
One Cooper Plaza Camden, NJ 08103 (856)342-2000 Fax (856)968-8272

Shapnik, Bella, MD {1467462416} IntrMd(86,MOL02)
+ Drs. Shapnik & Gurtovy
2150 Center Avenue/Suite 1-B Fort Lee, NJ 07024 (201)461-2444 Fax (201)461-7148

Shapren, Kristen Marie, MD {1225147358} Pedtrc(95,PA13)<NJ-OVERLOOK, NJ-STBARNMC>
+ Summit Medical Group Pediatrics at Westfield
592B Springfield Avenue Westfield, NJ 07090 (908)233-8860 Fax (908)301-0265

Sharaan, Mona El-Sayed, MD {1730392002} PthCyt, PthACl(85,EGY03)
+ PLUS Diagnostics
1200 River Avenue/Suite 10 Lakewood, NJ 08701 (732)901-7575 Fax (732)901-1555

Sharafi, Khalida, MD {1144289398} ObsGyn(95,NJ06)
+ Morristown Obstetrics and Gynecology Associates
20 Commerce Boulevard/Unit C Succasunna, NJ 07876 (973)927-1188 Fax (973)927-7408

Sharahy, Tatiana, MD {1598889248} IntrMd(89,RUS33)
+ 1144 East Ridgewood Avenue
Ridgewood, NJ 07450 (201)445-9969

Sharan, Kanu Priya, MD {1033129234} OncHem, IntrMd(96,INA72)<NJ-COOPRUMC>
+ Cooper University Medical Center/Camden
3 Cooper Plaza/Suite 215 Camden, NJ 08103 (856)963-2439 Fax (856)338-9211

Share, David Seth, MD {1750330015} Nephro, IntrMd(87,PA13)<NJ-VIRTMHBC, NJ-LOURDMED>
+ The Center for Kidney Care
1261 Route 38/Suite A Hainesport, NJ 08036 (856)222-1975 Fax (856)222-0721

Share, Lisa J., MD {1609899434} Pedtrc(95,PA09)
+ Harborview KidsFirst
505 Bay Avenue Somers Point, NJ 08244 (609)927-4235 Fax (609)927-5590
+ Harborview Smithville
48 South New York Road/Route 9 Smithville, NJ 08205 (609)927-4235 Fax (609)748-3067
+ Harborview KidsFirst Cape May
1315 Route 9 South Cape May Court House, NJ 08244 (609)465-6100 Fax (609)465-1539

Shareef, Kishwar I., MD {1659348142} IntrMd(91,PAK11)
+ 447 Route 10 East/Suite 15
Randolph, NJ 07869 Fax (973)442-3017

Sharer, Leroy Ralph, Jr., MD {1245265081} PthNro, PthACl, PthAna(69,NY20)<NJ-UMDNJ>
+ University Hospital
150 Bergen Street/Path Newark, NJ 07103 (973)972-4770 Fax (973)972-5933

Sharetts, Scott R., MD {1437202116} Nrolgy(77,PA13)<NJ-LOURDMED, NJ-VIRTMARL>
+ The Neurological Center
231 Van Sciver Parkway Willingboro, NJ 08046 (609)871-7500 Fax (609)877-5555

Shargorodsky, Josef, MD {1669719381} IntrMd<NJ-RWJUBRUN>
+ Coastal Ear Nose and Throat LLC
3700 Route 33/Suite 101 Neptune, NJ 07753 (732)280-7855 Fax (732)280-7815
jshargor@gmail.com
+ Coastal Ear Nose and Throat LLC
1301 Route 72/Suite 340 Manahawkin, NJ 08050 (732)280-7855 Fax (732)280-7815

Shariati, Amir, MD {1386842136} ObsGyn
+ Atlantic Health Urology Gyn
95 Madison Avenue/Suite 204 Morristown, NJ 07960 (973)971-7440

Shariati, Nasseredin, MD {1861486623} InfDis, IntrMd(72,IRA01)
+ 2345 Lamington Road/Unit 103
Bedminster, NJ 07921 (908)234-2295 Fax (908)234-0579

Shariati, Nazly M., MD {1992770168} SrgThr(95,OH41)<NJ-NWRKBETH, NJ-MORRISTN>
+ Newark Beth Israel Medical Center
201 Lyons Avenue Newark, NJ 07112 (973)926-7000

Sharif, Uzma M., MD {1053394098} NroChl, Nrolgy, Eplpsy(90,PAK11)
+ CHOP Specialty Care Center at Virtua
200 Bowman Drive/2 FL/Suite D-260 Voorhees, NJ 08043 (267)425-5400

Shariff, Haji Mohammed, MD {1144247131} SrgThr, Surgry, IntrMd(72,INA5B)<NJ-STFRNMED>
+ St. Francis Medical Center
601 Hamilton Avenue/Suite 109 Trenton, NJ 08629 (609)599-5307 Fax (609)599-5325

Shariff, Yasmeen K., MD {1427003920} RadDia(93,PA13)<NY-LDYLORDS, NJ-UNVMCPRN>
+ Shrewsbury Diagnostic Imaging, Inc.
1131 Broad Street/Suite 110 Shrewsbury, NJ 07702 (732)578-9640 Fax (732)578-9650

Sharim, Iradj, MD {1790739423} IntrMd(70,IRA01)<NJ-CHSFULD, NJ-STFRNMED>
+ Drs. Sharim & Zubair
40 Fuld Street/Suite 402 Trenton, NJ 08638 (609)393-4911 Fax (609)394-6770

Sharkey, Charles John, DO {1104835040} FamMed(02)<NJ-VIRTVOOR, NJ-KMHTURNV>
+ Advocare Family Medicine Associates Williamstown
979 North Black Horse Pike Williamstown, NJ 08094 (856)629-5151 Fax (856)629-0281
+ Advocare Family Medicine Associates Mt. Laurel
3115 Route 38/Suite 200B Mount Laurel, NJ 08054 (856)629-5151 Fax (856)231-7543
+ Advocare Family Medicine Associates Vineland
602 West Sherman Avenue/Suite B Vineland, NJ 08094 (856)692-8484 Fax (856)896-3059

Sharma, Aadya, MD {1255751723}
+ Rockaway Family Medicine Associates
333 Mount Hope Avenue Rockaway, NJ 07866 (973)895-6601 Fax (973)895-5324

Sharma, Adity, MD {1861653826} IntrMd
+ Central Pain Institute
3 Cornwall Drive/Suite A East Brunswick, NJ 08816 (732)698-1000 Fax (732)698-1008
adityasharmamd@gmail.com

Sharma, Akanksha D., MD {1568441640} Anesth, PainMd(92,INA72)
+ Summit Anesthesia Associates, P.A.
33 Overlook Road/Suite 311 Summit, NJ 07901 (908)598-1500 Fax (908)598-0197

Sharma, Amita K., MD {1881929032} PedNph, Pedtrc, IntrMd(05,INA23)<NJ-VIRTMHBC>
+ Virtua Memorial
175 Madison Avenue/Pediatrics Mount Holly, NJ 08060 (609)945-2565

Sharma, Amrita, MD {1073535332} Psychy(94,INDI)<NJ-VAEASTOR>
+ VA New Jersey Health Care System-East Orange Campus
385 Tremont Avenue East Orange, NJ 07018 (973)676-1000

Sharma, Anil K., MD {1730137878} IntrMd(89,INDI)
+ Spine & Pain Centers
303 West Main Street/Lower Level Freehold, NJ 07728 (732)345-1180 Fax (732)530-4476
+ Spine & Pain Centers
1430 Hooper Avenue/Suite 205 Toms River, NJ 08753 (732)345-1180 Fax (732)473-9574
+ Spine & Pain Centers
655 Shrewbury Avenue/Suite 202 Shrewsbury, NJ 07728 (732)345-1180 Fax (732)530-4476

Sharma, Anil Kumar, MD {1255372892} IntrMd(86,INA1X)
+ 3 Plaza Drive/Suite 4
Toms River, NJ 08757 (732)473-0025 Fax (732)473-0087

Sharma, Anjali, DO {1548393549} Pedtrc<NJ-CHSMRCER>
+ Capital Health System/Mercer Campus
446 Bellevue Avenue Trenton, NJ 08618 (609)394-4000

Sharma, Anupa, DO {1669719381} IntrMd<NJ-RWJUBRUN>
+ RWJ University Hospital New Brunswick
One Robert Wood Johnson Place New Brunswick, NJ 08901 (732)828-3000

Sharma, Anuradha, MD {1780094003} IntrMd
+ Jersey Shore University Medical Center
1945 Route 33 Neptune, NJ 07753 (732)775-5500

Sharma, Archana, DO {1598923096} Pedtrc(04,ME75)
+ Rutgers Cancer Institute of New Jersey
195 Little Albany Street/PO Box 2681 New Brunswick, NJ 08903 (732)235-8864 Fax (732)235-6797

Sharma, Ashok K., MD {1497804405} CdvDis, IntrMd(74,INA07)<NJ-VALLEY>
+ Drs. Sharma and Sharma
400 Franklin Turnpike/Suite 102 Mahwah, NJ 07430 (201)934-5700 Fax (201)934-5560

Sharma, Bhudev, MD {1477555100} CdvDis, IntrMd(75,INA30)<NJ-JFKJHNSN, NJ-JFKMED>
+ PrimeCare Medical Group
98 James Street/Suite 300 Edison, NJ 08820 (732)548-2523 Fax (732)549-8827
+ JFK Johnson Rehabilitation Institute
65 James Street Edison, NJ 08818 (732)321-7050

Sharma, Deepa, DO {1457519001} FamMed
+ Maplewood Family Medicine
111 Dunnell Road/Suite 200 Maplewood, NJ 07040 (908)598-6690 Fax (973)762-0840

Sharma, Ekta, MD {1932527082}
+ Mountainside Family Practice Associates
799 Bloomfield Avenue/Suite 201 Verona, NJ 07044 (973)259-3563 Fax (973)259-3569

Sharma, Gaurav S., MD {1710276605} Surgry
+ Virtua Primary Care
401 Young Avenue/Suite 260 Moorestown, NJ 08057 (856)291-8920 Fax (856)291-8922

Sharma, Hemlata, MD {1538472378}<NJ-HACKNSK>
+ Hackensack University Medical Center
30 Prospect Avenue Hackensack, NJ 07601 (551)996-2000

Sharma, Indu, MD {1386793313} IntrMd, Hemato, Onclgy(76,INA59)<NJ-JRSYSHMC, NJ-VALLEY>
+ Drs. Sharma and Sharma
400 Franklin Turnpike/Suite 102 Mahwah, NJ 07430 (201)934-5700 Fax (201)934-5560

Sharma, Indu, MD {1982692265} IntrMd, Nephro(82,INA5Z)<NJ-JRSYSHMC, NJ-RIVERVW>
+ Drs. Patel & Sharma
1915 6th Avenue Neptune, NJ 07753 (732)774-5700 Fax (732)774-7929

Sharma, Jyoti, MD {1609276443} Surgry
+ 400 Riverfront Boulevard/Apt 419
Elmwood Park, NJ 07407 (203)257-6272
jsharma25@gmail.com

Physicians by Name and Address

Sharma, Keerti, MD {1255437794} Grtrcs, IntrMd(93,INDI)<NJ-MORRISTN>
+ Geriatric Assessment Center
435 South Street/Suite 390   Morristown, NJ 07960
(973)971-7022
+ Morristown Medical Center Family Medicine
435 South Street/Suite 350   Morristown, NJ 07960
(973)971-7022   Fax (973)401-2465

Sharma, Lokesh, MD {1154397198} IntrMd(90,INA23)
+ VNA of Central Jersey Community Health Center, Inc.
176 Riverside Avenue   Red Bank, NJ 07701   (732)695-4652
Fax (732)224-0893

Sharma, Madho K., MD {1134111883} IntrMd, PulDis, CritCr(66,INA07)
+ Madho K. Sharma MD PA
30 Hoy Avenue   Fords, NJ 08863   (732)225-9115   Fax (732)225-2814
Madhosharma@yahoo.com
+ Sharma and Sharma MDs
974 Inman Avenue   Edison, NJ 08820   (732)225-9115   Fax (908)757-0942

Sharma, Madhulika Brahm, MD {1033294202} Psychy, PsyCAd(93,INA15)<NJ-UNIVBHC>
+ University Behavioral Health Care
671 Hoes Lane/PO Box 1392   Piscataway, NJ 08855
(732)235-5500

Sharma, Meena R., MD {1992801237} IntrMd, IntHos(98,NJ06)<NJ-COOPRUMC, NJ-MEDIPLEX>
+ Cooper University Hospital
One Cooper Plaza/Medicine   Camden, NJ 08103   (856)342-3150   Fax (856)968-8573

Sharma, Naresh Durgaprasad, MD {1033180831} Anesth(73,INDI)<NJ-MEMSALEM>
+ Memorial Hospital of Salem County
310 Woodstown Road/Anesthesiology   Salem, NJ 08079
(856)935-1000

Sharma, Neha, MD {1417442062} ObsGyn<NJ-JRSYCITY>
+ Jersey City Medical Center
355 Grand Street   Jersey City, NJ 07304   (845)287-3859

Sharma, Niti, DO {1154640472} EmrgMd(06,NJ75)
+ Pathlink, LLC
66 West Gilbert Street/Suite 100   Tinton Falls, NJ 07701
(732)212-0060   Fax (732)212-0061

Sharma, Nivedita, MD {1932134855} IntrMd(96,INA9B)
+ My MD Group
201 North County Line Road   Jackson, NJ 08527   (732)901-8880   Fax (732)901-0882

Sharma, Priti, MD {1225398639} Pedtrc<NJ-STPETER>
+ St. Peter's University Hospital
254 Easton Avenue   New Brunswick, NJ 08901   (732)745-8600

Sharma, Puja, MD {1225364821} FamMed(07,STM01)
+ Hackensack Meridian Medical Group
195 Route 9 South/Suite 106   Manalapan, NJ 07726
(732)536-7144   Fax (732)536-7520
+ Meridian Primary Care
831 Tennent Road/Suite D   Manalapan, NJ 07726
(732)536-7144   Fax (732)536-7520

Sharma, Puneeta, MD {1215030143} IntrMd(00,INA35)
+ The Valley Hospital
223 North Van Dien Avenue   Ridgewood, NJ 07450
(201)381-1317

Sharma, Pushpendra, MD {1558422964} IntrMd, Grtrcs(87,INA9Y)
+ Preakness Pediatrics Associates
150 Hinchman Avenue/Suite 4   Wayne, NJ 07470
(973)595-6996   Fax (973)595-6706

Sharma, Raj Kumar, MD {1033120316} NnPnMd<PA-TJCNTR>
+ OLLMC Neonatal Associates
1600 Haddon Avenue   Camden, NJ 08103   (856)757-3500
Fax (856)365-7868
info@lourdesnet.org

Sharma, Rajendra M., MD {1487760872} IntrMd, Nephro(71,INA92)
+ 319 North Eighth Street
Vineland, NJ 08360   (856)692-6034   Fax (859)794-2002

Sharma, Rajinder, MD {1356357438} Surgry(65,INA36)<NJ-STPETER, NJ-RWJUBRUN>
+ JFK Medical Center
65 James Street   Edison, NJ 08820   (732)321-7000   Fax (732)767-2961

Sharma, Rakesh, MD CritCr, PulDis, IntrMd(87,INA03)<NJ-VALLEY>
+ 27 South Franklin Turnpike/Suite 202
Ramsey, NJ 07446   (201)785-8899   Fax (201)785-8869
Rakesh.Sharma@comcast.net
+ NJ Heart/Elizabeth Office
240 Williamson Street/Suite 402-406   Elizabeth, NJ 07202
(201)785-8899   Fax (908)354-0007

Sharma, Rakesh B., MD {1396824157} Pedtrc, NnPnMd(98,INA87)<NJ-COOPRUMC>
+ The Children's Regional Hospital at Cooper Univ Hosp
One Cooper Plaza   Camden, NJ 08103   (856)342-2000

Sharma, Rakesh Somabhai, MD {1447353792} IntrMd(93,INA20)<NJ-GRYSTPSY>
+ Greystone Park Psychiatric Hospital
59 Koch Avenue/Internal Med   Morris Plains, NJ 07950
(973)538-1800

Sharma, Ranita, MD {1578675625} IntrMd, MedCom(93,INA70)
+ RWJ University Hospital New Brunswick
One Robert Wood Johnson Place   New Brunswick, NJ 08901
(732)828-3000   Fax (732)235-8313
+ Eric B. Chandler Health Center
277 George Street   New Brunswick, NJ 08901   (732)828-3000   Fax (732)235-6729

Sharma, Rashi, MD {1972986917} IntrMd<NJ-RWJUBRUN>
+ RWJ University Hospital New Brunswick
One Robert Wood Johnson Place   New Brunswick, NJ 08901
(732)235-7708   Fax (732)235-7951

Sharma, Ravinder, MD {1306947999} CdvDis, IntrMd(78,INDI)<NJ-RWJUBRUN>
+ 153 Livingston Avenue
New Brunswick, NJ 08901   (732)745-1100   Fax (732)296-1883

Sharma, Rekha, MD {1447251616} IntrMd(80,INA9B)<NJ-EASTORNG>
+ 701 Newark Avenue
Elizabeth, NJ 07206   (908)282-0474   Fax (908)282-0475
Sharmar@comcast.net

Sharma, Ritu, MD {1205008414} IntrMd<NJ-HACKNSK, NJ-HOLYNAME>
+ Drs Medical Associates
115 Christopher Columbus Drive   Jersey City, NJ 07302
(201)706-3808   Fax (201)369-8032

Sharma, Sanjiv Kumar, MD {1285607739} Grtrcs, IntrMd(93,INDI)<NJ-COMMED, NJ-KIMBALL>
+ 9 Mule Road/Suite E-8
Toms River, NJ 08755   (732)341-6070   Fax (732)341-6077

Sharma, Sarika, MD {1821042771} CdvDis, IntrMd(79,INA05)<NJ-HOLYNAME, NJ-HACKNSK>
+ 211 Essex Street/Suite 301
Hackensack, NJ 07601   (201)343-8757   Fax (201)343-9161
+ 2 Dean Drive/Suite 3N
Tenafly, NJ 07670   (201)567-0200

Sharma, Shelly, MD {1538465760}
+ University Behavioral HealthCare
183 South Orange Avenue/Suit 547 E   Newark, NJ 07103
(973)476-3905

Sharma, Shivani, MD {1376704627} IntrMd(99,INA26)
+ RWJPE Dayton Medical Group
12 Stults Road/Suite 121   Dayton, NJ 08810   (732)329-8600   Fax (609)395-7519
+ Arvind K. Doshi, MD PA
906 Oak Tree Road/Suite K   South Plainfield, NJ 07080
(732)329-8600   Fax (908)822-1121

Sharma, Siddharth, MD {1528018991} EmrgMd(97,NJ05)<NJ-VALLEY, NJ-CHILTON>
+ The Valley Hospital
223 North Van Dien Avenue   Ridgewood, NJ 07450
(201)447-8000

Sharma, Silky, MD {1083974166} IntrMd(06,SLU01)
+ Acute Rehab Unit / Med Ctr Princeton
One Plainsboro Road/2nd Floor   Plainsboro, NJ 08536
(609)853-5600

Sharma, Smriti, MD {1508817008} IntrMd, Pedtrc(89,INA7Y)<NJ-CHSFULD, NJ-CHSMRCER>
+ Capital Health Primary Care-Hamilton
1445 Whitehorse-Mercerville Rd   Hamilton, NJ 08619
(609)587-6661   Fax (609)587-8503

Sharma, Sonia, MD {1336595925} FamMed
+ AtlantiCare Family Medicine
219 North White Horse Pike/Suite 101   Hammonton, NJ 08037   (609)561-4211   Fax (609)561-0639

Sharma, Surendra M., MD {1982629184} CdvDis, IntrMd(68,INDI)
+ 147 Hamilton Avenue
Passaic, NJ 07055   (973)594-0808   Fax (973)594-0508
+ Drs. Sharma and Castilla
293 Passaic Street   Passaic, NJ 07055   (973)594-0808   Fax (973)365-1229
+ 151 48th Street
Union City, NJ 07055   (201)223-2263   Fax (201)223-2293

Sharma, Swati, MD {1396768438} IntrMd, EnDbMt(00,NJ05)
+ North Jersey Endocrine Consultants, LLC
1 Indian Road/Suite 8   Denville, NJ 07834   (973)625-2121
Fax (973)625-8270
+ 2 Waters Edge Road
Morristown, NJ 07960   (973)813-3013

Sharma, Tarun K., MD {1033138029} IntrMd(98,GRN01)<NJ-STCLRDEN>
+ 195 Highway 46/Suite 100
Mine Hill, NJ 07803   (973)366-7300   Fax (973)306-3043
+ The Center For Specialized Women's Health
16 Pocono Road/Suite 103   Denville, NJ 07834   (973)366-

7300   Fax (973)947-9056

Sharma, Uma, MD {1881658052} EmrgMd, FamMed, IntrMd(66,INDI)<NJ-STJOSHOS>
+ St. Joseph's Regional Medical Center
703 Main Street   Paterson, NJ 07503   (973)754-2000

Sharma, Usha, MD {1467444935} FamMed(69,INA07)
+ Sharma and Sharma MDs
974 Inman Avenue   Edison, NJ 08820   (908)561-0183   Fax (908)757-0942
+ Madho K. Sharma MD PA
30 Hoy Avenue   Fords, NJ 08863   (908)561-0183   Fax (732)225-2814

Sharma, Veena, MD {1265403943} Anesth(70,INA23)<NJ-HACKNSK>
+ Hackensack University MC-Anesthesia Dept
30 Prospect Avenue/Room 2703   Hackensack, NJ 07601
(201)996-2419   Fax (201)996-3962
+ Hackensack University Medical Center
30 Prospect Avenue/Anesth   Hackensack, NJ 07601
(201)996-2419   Fax (201)488-6769

Sharo, Ronald J., MD {1396769014} RadDia, Radiol(92,NJ05)<NJ-STBARNMC>
+ St. Barnabas Medical Center
94 Old Short Hills Road   Livingston, NJ 07039   (973)322-5000

Sharobeem, Andrew Mena, DO {1629389382} IntrMd(10,NY75)
+ Arthritis & Osteoporosis Associates, P.A.
4247 US Highway 9/Building 1   Freehold, NJ 07728
(732)410-6844   Fax (732)780-8817

Sharon, David J., MD {1730299041} IntrMd, MedOnc, OncHem(77,NY09)<NJ-MONMOUTH>
+ Monmouth Hematology Oncology Associates PA
100 State Highway 36/Suite 1B   West Long Branch, NJ 07764   (732)222-1711   Fax (732)571-2043
+ Monmouth Medical Center
300 Second Avenue/Cancer Ctr   Long Branch, NJ 07740
(732)222-5200

Sharon, Jill Israel, DO {1033115530} Pedtrc(02,PA78)
+ Fresh Future
100 Craig Road/Floor 2   Manalapan, NJ 07726   (732)409-1446

Sharon, Yoram, DO {1649202193} IntrMd(96,NY75)<NJ-SOMERSET>
+ MEDEMERGE
1005 North Washington Avenue   Green Brook, NJ 08812
(732)968-8900   Fax (732)968-4609

Sharp, Frank J., III, MD {1861465338} SrgVas, Surgry(85,NJ05)<NJ-JRSYSHMC>
+ Jersey Coast Vascular Associates
425 Jack Martin Boulevard/Suite 2   Brick, NJ 08724
(732)202-1500   Fax (732)202-1058

Sharp, Harry Walton, DO {1235231044} FamMed, IntrMd(73,IA75)<NJ-UNDRWD, NJ-KMHSTRAT>
+ Winslow Primary Care Associates, PC
524 Williamstown Road/Suite A   Sicklerville, NJ 08081
(856)728-1181   Fax (856)728-1182

Sharrar, William G., MD {1235235516} Pedtrc(66,PA01)<NJ-COOPRUMC>
+ Cooper Peds/Children's Regional Ctr
3 Cooper Plaza/Suite 200   Camden, NJ 08103   (856)342-2472   Fax (856)368-8297
sharrar.william@cooperhealth.edu
+ Cooper Peds/Children's Regional Ctr
6400 Main Street Complex   Voorhees, NJ 08043   (856)342-2000
+ The Children's Regional Hospital at Cooper Univ Hosp
One Cooper Plaza/Pediatrics   Camden, NJ 08103
(856)342-2000

Shastri, Jay Gautam, DO {1477758720} Nephro, IntrMd(02,NY75)<NJ-SHOREMEM, NJ-ATLANCHS>
+ Regional Nephrology Associates
510 Jackson Avenue   Northfield, NJ 08225   (609)383-0200
Fax (609)383-8352

Shastri, Shefali Mavani, MD {1316152861} ObsGyn, RprEnd(02,NJ02)
+ Reproductive Medicine Associates of New Jersey
81 Veronica Avenue/Suite 101   Somerset, NJ 08873
(732)220-9060   Fax (732)220-1164

Shastry, Jyothsna S., MD {1811013675} IntrMd, OccpMd(71,INA69)
+ Concentra Managed Care
135 Raritan Center Parkway   Edison, NJ 08837   (732)225-5454   Fax (732)417-0003

Shatkin, Bennett J., MD {1336146695} CdvDis, IntrMd(80,IL02)<NJ-SJHREGMC>
+ Shatkin Cardiology
1051 West Sherman Avenue   Vineland, NJ 08360
(856)691-8070   Fax (856)691-8074
+ 9901 Seapointe Boulevard/Suite 604
Wildwood Crest, NJ 08260   (609)774-5372

Shatkin, Jason Alan, MD {1669529202} IntrMd, PulDis, SlpDis(95,NY46)<NJ-VALLEY>
+ Physician Specialists of New Jersey
1 Sears Drive/Suite 306   Paramus, NJ 07652   (201)830-2287   Fax (201)830-2286

Shats, Daniel, MD {1710005970} Gastrn, IntrMd(06,DMN01)<NJ-COOPRUMC>
+ Cooper University Hospital
One Cooper Plaza   Camden, NJ 08103   (856)342-2000
+ Cooper Digestive Health Institute
501 Fellowship Road/Suite 101   Mount Laurel, NJ 08054   (856)342-2000   Fax (856)642-2134

Shatz, Matthew Jay, MD {1447251020} Anesth(87,PA12)<NJ-PALISADE>
+ Palisades Medical Center
7600 River Road/Anesth   North Bergen, NJ 07047   (201)854-5000

Shatzkes, Joseph Aaron, MD {1427218239} IntrMd, CdvDis, CarNuc(08,NY08)
+ Englewood Cardiology Consultants
177 North Dean Street/Suite 100   Englewood, NJ 07631   (201)569-4901   Fax (201)569-6111
+ Englewood Cardiology Consultants
220 Livingston Street   Northvale, NJ 07647   (201)569-4901

Shavelson, Robert P., MD {1730173584} ObsGyn, IntrMd(86,NY47)<NJ-JRSYSHMC>
+ Tinton Falls Medical Associates
4057 Asbury Avenue/Suite 14   Neptune, NJ 07753   (732)922-1222   Fax (732)922-7708

Shaw, Brian Richard, DO {1578890570} IntrMd
+ Virtua Cardiology Group
2309 East Evesham Road/Suites 201-202   Voorhees, NJ 08043   (856)325-5400   Fax (856)325-5416

Shaw, Daniel A., MD {1891789731} SprtMd, SrgOrt(89,MI01)<NJ-OVERLOOK, NJ-RWJURAH>
+ Westfield Orthopedic Group
541 East Broad Street   Westfield, NJ 07090   (908)232-3879   Fax (908)232-5789

Shaw, Donia Renee, MD {1952360455} ObsGyn(96,NJ05)
+ Morristown Obstetrics and Gynecology Associates
20 Commerce Boulevard/Unit C   Succasunna, NJ 07876   (973)927-1188   Fax (973)927-7408
+ Morristown Obstetrics and Gynecology Associates
101 Madison Avenue/Suite 405   Morristown, NJ 07960   (973)927-1188   Fax (973)455-0099

Shaw, Jennifer Robin, MD {1407005291} Psychy, PsyNro(84,ON10)
+ 24 Sherwood Road
Short Hills, NJ 07078   (973)376-0202   Fax (973)218-1347

Shaw, Richard Amedeo, DO {1467646604} IntrMd
+ Medical Group Associates
190 North Evergreen Avenue/Suite 102   Woodbury, NJ 08096   (856)845-8010   Fax (856)845-9398

Shaw, Wayne, MD {1407017908} IntrMd
+ Southern Jersey Family Medical Centers, Inc.
600 Pemberton-Browns Mills Rd   Pemberton, NJ 08068   (609)894-1100   Fax (609)894-1110

Shaw Brachfeld, Jennifer L., MD {1306885579} Pedtrc, PedDvl(89,CT02)<NJ-MORRISTN, NJ-OVERLOOK>
+ Touchpoint Pediatrics
17 Watchung Avenue   Chatham, NJ 07928   (973)665-0900   Fax (973)665-0901

Shazly, Amin, MD {1780024117} Anesth
+ Cooper Anesthesia Associates
One Cooper Plaza/Suite 294-B   Camden, NJ 08103   (856)968-7330   Fax (856)968-8250

Shcherba, Marina, DO {1902064975} OncHem, IntrMd(07,NJ75)
+ Memorial Sloan Kettering Monmouth
480 Red Hill Road   Middletown, NJ 07748   (848)225-6119   Fax (201)691-6685

Shea, Caitlin M., DO {1801183702} FamMed(11,WV75)
+ Premier Health Associates
89 Sparta Avenue/Suite 100   Sparta, NJ 07871   (973)729-2121   Fax (973)729-3454

Sheaffer, Carol M., MD {1548355647} Psychy, PsyCAd(74,PA07)
+ 10 Wexford Drive
Lawrenceville, NJ 08648   (856)924-1320   Fax (856)924-1806

Shearin, Jonathan Winkworth, MD {1295050847}
+ Rothman Institute
999 Route 73 North/3rd Fl   Marlton, NJ 08053   (202)374-8400   Fax (856)821-6359
jwshearin@gmail.com

Shears-Bethke, Tracey M., MD {1073549333} IntrMd(94,NJ06)<NJ-CHSMRCER, NJ-VIRTMHBC>
+ Besen-Goldstein Medical Associates PC
1000 Birchfield Drive/Suite 1004   Mount Laurel, NJ 08054   (856)866-1557   Fax (856)231-7955

Sheehan, Christine, DO {1821063629} Pedtrc, EmrgMd(97,NJ75)<NJ-VIRTBERL, NJ-VIRTMARL>
+ CHOP Care Network at Virtua Voorhees Hospital
100 Bowman Drive   Voorhees, NJ 08043   (856)247-3244

Fax (609)261-5842

Sheehan, Lori A., MD {1720242456} Nrolgy
+ Underwood Neurology
155 Bridgeton Pike/Suite A   Mullica Hill, NJ 08062   (856)467-4432   Fax (856)467-5959

Sheekey, Owen, Jr., MD {1639188865} IntrMd(74,PA09)
+ Owen Sheekey MD LLC
1138 East Chestnut Avenue/Suite 8A   Vineland, NJ 08360   (856)696-2245   Fax (856)696-8052

Sheen, Eun H., MD {1255316675} PedAlg, IntrMd(75,KOR03)
+ Center for Asthma & Allergy
18 North Third Avenue   Highland Park, NJ 08904   (732)545-0094   Fax (732)545-4087
+ Center for Asthma & Allergy
300 Hudson Street   Hoboken, NJ 07030   (732)545-0094   Fax (201)792-5320
+ Center for Asthma & Allergy
90 Milburn Avenue/Suite 200   Maplewood, NJ 08904   (973)763-5787   Fax (973)763-8568

Sheen, Jerry, MD {1851344915} InfDis(01,GRN01)
+ ID Associates PA/dba ID Care
105 Raider Boulevard/Suite 101   Hillsborough, NJ 08844   (908)281-0221   Fax (908)281-0940
+ ID Associates PA/dba ID Care
81 Veronica Avenue/Suite 203   Somerset, NJ 08873   (908)281-0221   Fax (732)729-0924

Sheetz, Maurice Saunders, MD {1902832157} PulDis, IntrMd(83)
+ Cumberland Medical Associates
1206 West Sherman Avenue   Vineland, NJ 08360   (856)462-6250   Fax (856)691-8325

Sheffer, Emily Hope, MD {1770678039} EmrgMd(99,DC01)<NY-BRNXLCON>
+ 480 Washington Boulevard
Jersey City, NJ 07310

Sheffy, Ohad, MD {1295087005} FamMed
+ 20 Lewis Street/Apt 403
Rahway, NJ 07065   (732)397-8988

Sheft, Stanley A., MD {1285662072} Otlryg, SrgFPl(84,NJ06)<NJ-HUNTRDN>
+ Hunterdon Otolaryngology Associates
6 Sand Hill Road/Suite 302   Flemington, NJ 08822   (908)788-9131   Fax (908)788-0945
ssheft@hunterdonent.com

Shehadeh, Abbas A., MD {1215900774} CdvDis, IntrMd(87,ROMA)
+ Abbas Shehadeh Cardiology & Internal Medicine
443 Northfield Avenue/Suite 301   West Orange, NJ 07052   (973)731-0203   Fax (973)731-0017

Shehata, Ahmed Abdelhalim, MD {1497717516} IntrMd, Gastrn(85,EGY03)<NJ-VIRTVOOR, NJ-VIRTMARL>
+ Professional Gastroenterology Associates, PA
1939 Route 70 East/Suite 250   Cherry Hill, NJ 08002   (856)429-4433   Fax (856)424-6732

Shehata, Sanaa K., MD {1235203423} Anesth(90,EGY04)<NJ-RBAYPERT>
+ 8 Witherspoon Way
Marlboro, NJ 07746
+ Raritan Bay Medical Center/Perth Amboy Division
530 New Brunswick Avenue   Perth Amboy, NJ 08861   (732)442-3700

Sheiban, Tuti Fareen, MD {1245291285} UroGyn, Gyneco(01,LA01)<NJ-VALLEY>
+ 625 Franklin Turnpike/Suite 3
Ridgewood, NJ 07450   (201)447-3100   Fax (201)447-3400

Sheikh, Afzal J., MD {1265465348} Anesth, AnesPain(77,INA4X)<NJ-STMRYPAS>
+ Garden State Pain Control Center, P.A.
1117 Route 46 East/Suite 201   Clifton, NJ 07013   (973)777-5444   Fax (973)777-0304

Sheikh, Ednan Salahuddin, MD {1013128016} AnesPain, IntrMd(05,PA02)
+ New Jersey Pain & Spine
1040 Main Street/Suite 301   Paterson, NJ 07503   Fax (201)215-6992
+ New Jersey Pain & Spine
333 Grand Street   Jersey City, NJ 07302   Fax (201)215-6992

Sheikh, Emran Salahuddin, MD {1043259898} SrgPHand(96,PA02)<NJ-ACMCITY, NJ-ATLANTHS>
+ Drs. Sheikh & Weber
201 Route 17 North   Rutherford, NJ 07070   (201)549-8860   Fax (201)549-8861

Sheikh, Muzamil Wamiq, MD {1437370848} IntrMd
+ St Joseph's Medical Center Pulmonary
703 Main Street   Paterson, NJ 07512   (973)754-2000

Sheikh, Selim U., MD {1992921811} IntrMd(81,BAN02)<NJ-RWJUHAM>
+ 2312 Whitehorse-Mercerville Rd
Hamilton, NJ 08619   (609)586-6244   Fax (609)586-6221
Selimsheikhmd@aol.com

Sheikh, Shuja, MD {1811383755} Nrolgy
+ Preventive Medicine & Community Health
185 South Orange Avenue/MSB F-506   Newark, NJ 07101   (973)972-5209   Fax (973)972-7625

Sheikh, Sirajuddin, MD {1184831455} FamMAdM, Pedtrc, IntrMd(67,PAK01)
+ AZZ Medical Associates
1440 Pennington Road/Suite 1   Ewing, NJ 08618   (609)890-1050   Fax (609)890-0950

Sheikh, Usman, MD {1598184079} Anesth<NJ-HOLYNAME>
+ Holy Name Hospital
718 Teaneck Road   Teaneck, NJ 07666   (201)833-3000

Sheikh, Wasif M., MD {1205066149}
+ 200 Centennial Avenue
Piscataway, NJ 08854   (708)833-2356

Sheil, Christina A., MD {1619531142} FamMed(90,NJ06)
+ 103 Hidden Lake Drive
North Brunswick, NJ 08902

Sheinman, Marc Daniel, DO {1215377486} IntrMd
+ Carepoint Health Bayonne Med Center
29 East 29th Street   Bayonne, NJ 07002   (201)858-5000

Shekhtman, Yevgenia, MD {1508000787} SrgNro
+ JFK Neurosciences Institute
65 James Street/Second Floor   Edison, NJ 08818   (732)321-7010   Fax (732)744-5873

Shelchkov, Dmitry A., MD {1023128402} Anesth
+ 122 Cedar Road
Mullica Hill, NJ 08062

Sheldon, Howard A., DO {1124343728} FamMed(74,PA77)<NJ-VIRTMARL, NJ-KMHSTRAT>
+ Greentree Family Medical Associates
55 Lakeview Drive North/Suite A   Gibbsboro, NJ 08026   (856)985-5655   Fax (856)985-1895

Sheldon, Lynne T., DO {1942525530} FamMed(74,PA77)<NJ-VIRTMARL, NJ-KMHSTRAT>
+ Greentree Family Medical Associates
55 Lakeview Drive North/Suite A   Gibbsboro, NJ 08026   (856)985-5655   Fax (856)985-1895

Shell, Roger A., MD {1518927425} CdvDis, IntrMd(77,NJ06)<NJ-RWJUBRUN, NJ-STPETER>
+ Cardiology Associates of New Brunswick
593 Cranbury Road/Suite 2   East Brunswick, NJ 08816   (732)390-3333   Fax (732)390-9244

Shelmet, John J., MD {1770699480} EnDbMt, IntrMd(81,NJ06)<NJ-UNVMCPRN>
+ 3131 Princeton Pike 2B/Suite 104
Lawrenceville, NJ 08648   (609)896-8050   Fax (609)896-3053

Shembede, Dwarkanath Sonaji, MD {1720045008} RadDia(82,INA69)<NJ-ENGLWOOD>
+ Englewood Radiologic Group PA
350 Engle Street   Englewood, NJ 07631   (201)894-3000   Fax (201)894-5244
+ Advanced Medical Imaging of North Jersey
452 Old Hook Road/Suite 301   Emerson, NJ 07630   (201)894-3000   Fax (201)262-2330

Shen, Calvin T., MD {1255304028} NnPnMd, Pedtrc(85,NY08)<NJ-MORRISTN, NJ-OVERLOOK>
+ MidAtlantic Neonatology Associates
100 Madison Avenue   Morristown, NJ 07962   (973)971-5488   Fax (973)290-7175

Shen, Edred Vig-Ny, MD {1154302024} IntrMd, Acpntr(94,NJ06)
+ 2253 South Avenue
Scotch Plains, NJ 07076   (908)654-1500   Fax (908)654-7391

Shen, Edward, MD {1093973174} Anesth
+ Drs. Shen and Shen
219 South Broad Street   Elizabeth, NJ 07202   (201)877-0518   Fax (908)352-6181

Shen, Ein-Yuan A., MD {1265536544} IntrMd, CritCr, PulDis(69,TAI07)<NJ-NWRKBETH, NJ-STBARNMC>
+ 40 Union Avenue/Suite 201
Irvington, NJ 07111   (201)372-6663   Fax (973)372-0322

Shen, Hongxie, MD {1316107006} FamMed
+ Drs Husain and Shen
5 West Chestnut Avenue   Merchantville, NJ 08109   (856)665-9424

Shen, Jeffrey Jou, MD {1801998141} IntrMd(99,NJ05)
+ Veterans Affairs Clinic
385 Prospect Avenue   Hackensack, NJ 07601   (201)487-1390

Shen, Jung-San, MD {1053411272} IntrMd, PulDis(68,TAI07)
+ Drs. Shen and Shen
219 South Broad Street   Elizabeth, NJ 07202   (908)352-5927   Fax (908)352-6181

Shen, Lijing, MD {1962432542} IntrMd(89,CHN19)<NJ-RWJURAH, NJ-JFKMED>
+ 906 Inman Avenue
Edison, NJ 08820   (732)382-2762   Fax (732)382-0845

Shen, Mengmeng, MD {1891085718} Anesth
+ 46 Merlot Court
Monroe, NJ 08831   (732)379-1783

Physicians by Name and Address

Shen, Rhuna, MD {1114089729} CdvDis, IntCrd, IntrMd(98,INA9B)
+ Morris Heart Associates PA
  400 Valley Road/Suite 102   Mount Arlington, NJ 07856
  (973)770-7899   Fax (973)770-7840

Shen, Tingliang, MD {1972777894} PthACl(82,CHN40)<PA-TM-PHOSP, NJ-MEADWLND>
+ PLUS Diagnostics
  1200 River Avenue/Suite 10   Lakewood, NJ 08701
  (732)901-7575   Fax (732)901-1555

Shen Schwarz, Susan C., MD {1649330895} Pthlgy, PedPth, PthACl(71,HKOG)<NJ-STPETER, NJ-RWJUBRUN>
+ St. Peter's University Hospital
  254 Easton Avenue/Box 591/Pathlgy   New Brunswick, NJ 08901   (732)745-8600   Fax (732)220-8595
+ RWJ University Hospital New Brunswick
  One Robert Wood Johnson Place   New Brunswick, NJ 08901
  (732)828-3000

Sheng, Huaibao, MD {1942299516} PthACl, Pthlgy(83,CHN5D)<NY-CMCSTVSI>
+ Pathology Solutions, LLC.
  246 Industrial Way West/Suite 2   Eatontown, NJ 07724
  (732)389-5200   Fax (732)389-5299

Shenk, Kristina Suzanne, MD {1821330713} Pedtrc
+ 333 15th Street/2nd Floor
  Hoboken, NJ 07030   (201)482-9770

Shenk, Suzanne H., DO {1447352364} IntrMd(87,MI12)<NJ-STFRNMED>
+ St. Francis Medical Center
  601 Hamilton Avenue   Trenton, NJ 08629   (609)599-5000

Shenker, Bennett Steven, MD {1427082429} FamMed(02,NJ05)
+ CentraState Family Medicine Residency Practice
  1001 West Main Street/Suite B   Freehold, NJ 07728
  (732)294-2540   Fax (732)294-9328

Shenoi, Shanthi Ramesh, MD {1831102680} Pedtrc(80,INA28)<NJ-HOLYNAME>
+ Holy Name Hospital
  718 Teaneck Road/Pediatrics   Teaneck, NJ 07666
  (201)833-3000

Shenouda, Magdy L., MD {1982684767} IntrMd(82,EGY04)<NJ-JRSYSHMC>
+ 1820 Route 33/Suite 4-A
  Neptune, NJ 07753   (732)775-4138   Fax (732)775-4158
+ 1729 Belmar Blvd
  Belmar, NJ 07719   (732)775-4138   Fax (732)775-4158

Shenoy, Mangalore Shantheri, MD {1457688285} Nephro, IntHos
+ Warren Hospital
  185 Roseberry Street   Phillipsburg, NJ 08865   (347)933-2771

Shenoy, Nigel Arvind, MD {1245451848} PhysMd<NJ-VAEASTOR>
+ VA New Jersey Health Care System-East Orange Campus
  385 Tremont Avenue   East Orange, NJ 07018   (973)676-1000

Shepherd, Annemarie Fernandes, MD {1356669279} IntrMd(10,NJ06)
+ Memorial Sloan-Kettering Cancer Center Basking Ridge
  136 Mountain View Boulevard   Basking Ridge, NJ 07920
  (908)542-3000   Fax (908)542-3220

Sheppard, Lisa Marie, MD {1083673479} RadDia, RadNro, Radiol(87,PA02)
+ Pink Breast Center
  680 Broadway/Barnet Medical Plaza   Paterson, NJ 07514
  (973)977-6662   Fax (973)341-1128
+ Radiology Affiliates of Central New Jersey, P.A.
  2501 Kuser Road   Hamilton, NJ 08691   (973)977-6662
  Fax (609)585-1825

Sheppard, Sherry Manon, MD {1871893917} IntrMd<NJ-UMDNJ>
+ University Hospital
  150 Bergen Street/I 248   Newark, NJ 07103   (973)972-6056

Sheppell, Arthur L., MD {1871698274} IntrMd, Grtrcrs(81,FRA07)<NJ-STCLRDEN>
+ Sheppell and Ricks MD
  16 Pocono Road/Suite 305   Denville, NJ 07834   (973)627-0555   Fax (973)627-3880

Shepperly, David C., MD {1740452929} OccpMd, IntrMd(88,CO02)
+ ID Associates PA/dba ID Care
  105 Raider Boulevard/Suite 101   Hillsborough, NJ 08844
  (908)281-0221   Fax (908)281-0940
+ ID Associates PA/dba ID Care
  81 Veronica Avenue/Suite 203   Somerset, NJ 08873
  (908)281-0221   Fax (732)729-0924

Sheps, Michal R., DO {1427223106}
+ 16 Beech Road
  Englewood, NJ 07631   (201)406-6404
  michalsheps@gmail.com

Sher, Ellen R., MD {1710961602} Allrgy, IntrMd, AlgyImmn(86,DC02)
+ Allergy Partners of New Jersey PC
  802 West Park Avenue/Suite 213   Ocean, NJ 07712
  (732)695-2555   Fax (732)695-2552

ersher@pol.net
+ Allergy Partners of New Jersey PC
  8 Tindall Road   Middletown, NJ 07748   (732)695-2555
  Fax (732)671-0144

Sher, Leo, MD {1891844189} Psychy
+ 1600 Center Avenue/Apt 4C
  Fort Lee, NJ 07024

Sher, Michael Laurence, MD {1336149707} IntrMd(94,NY09)<NJ-OCEANMC, NJ-KIMBALL>
+ 74 Brick Boulevard/Suite 115
  Brick, NJ 08723   (732)920-8001   Fax (732)920-8004

Sher, Peter Mitchell, MD {1053304717} FamMed(96,PA13)
+ Lakeview Medical Associates
  125 US Highway 46   Budd Lake, NJ 07828   (973)691-1111
  Fax (973)691-1198

Sherbany, Ariel A., MD {1972729499} Nrolgy, Pedtrc, NrlgSpec(79,NY19)
+ 20 Prospect Avenue/Suite 705
  Hackensack, NJ 07601   (201)488-8570

Shere, Amar, MD {1982066387}<NJ-HACKNSK>
+ Hackensack University Medical Center
  30 Prospect Avenue   Hackensack, NJ 07601   (551)996-2000

Sheren, Lorne B., MD {1699744219} Anesth, IntrMd(77,NY08)
+ 1 Miller Road
  New Vernon, NJ 07976   (973)714-6777   Fax (973)377-9754

Sherer, Clark B., MD {1629048541} InfDis, IntrMd(82,NY03)<NJ-TRINIWSC>
+ Trinitas Regional Medical Center-Williamson Street
  225 Williamson Street   Elizabeth, NJ 07207   (908)994-5000
  Fax (908)355-9583

Sherer, Stephen B., MD {1730156829} CdvDis, IntrMd(75,ITA01)<NJ-HACKNSK, NJ-HOLYNAME>
+ 714 Bergen Boulevard
  Ridgefield, NJ 07657   (201)945-3022   Fax (201)945-5604

Sherif, Ajfar, MD {1316331804} FamMed
+ 415 West Saint Georges Avenue
  Linden, NJ 07036   (973)259-3563   Fax (908)486-2016

Sheris, Steven Jay, MD {1629062187} IntrMd, CdvDis(88,NJ06)
+ Associates in Cardiovascular Disease, LLC
  571 Central Avenue/Suite 115   New Providence, NJ 07974
  (908)464-4200   Fax (908)464-1332
+ Associates in Cardiovascular Disease, LLC
  29 South Street   New Providence, NJ 07974   (908)464-4200   Fax (908)464-1332

Sherman, Anthony, MD {1235235524} IntrMd(83,PA09)<NJ-VIRTVOOR>
+ Cooper Physicians
  1103 North Kings Highway/Suite 203   Cherry Hill, NJ 08034
  (856)321-1919   Fax (856)321-0206

Sherman, Glenn Stewart, MD {1720066558} ObsGyn(91,NY03)<NJ-NWTNMEM>
+ 222 High Street/Suite 201
  Newton, NJ 07860   (973)300-3200   Fax (973)579-5777

Sherman, Henry M., MD {1922334457} IntrMd(71,NJ05)
+ Eva's Village Medical Clinic
  393 Main Street   Paterson, NJ 07501   (973)523-6220

Sherman, Jennifer Ann, DO {1891755179} Pedtrc, AlgyImmn(99,PA77)
+ Summit Medical Group
  19-21 Fair Lawn Avenue   Fair Lawn, NJ 07410   (201)414-5095   Fax (855)256-7256

Sherman, Joyce, MD   Radiol(92,NY48)<NJ-STBARNMC>
+ St. Barnabas Medical Center
  94 Old Short Hills Road/Radiology   Livingston, NJ 07039
  (973)322-5000

Sherman, Mark David, MD {1417095142} SrgVas, Srgry, IntrMd(74,FL02)<NJ-VALLEY>
+ Valley Medical Group of Montvale
  85 Chestnut Ridge Road/Suite 111   Montvale, NJ 07645
  (201)444-1775   Fax (201)930-8509
  Sherm670@aol.com

Sherman, Michael Bruce, MD {1124019930} AlgyImmn, PedAlg, IntrMd(90,NY46)<NJ-RIVERVW, NJ-CENTRAST>
+ Allergy & Asthma Center, PC
  15 South Main Street   Marlboro, NJ 07746   (732)303-8787
  Fax (732)303-7870
+ Allergy & Asthma Center, PC
  1 Bethany Road/Suite 11   Hazlet, NJ 07730   (732)303-8787
  Fax (732)739-8740

Sherman, Neil David, MD {1487684551} Urolgy(98,NY09)<NJ-UMDNJ>
+ Premier Urology Group, LLC
  10 Parsonage Road/Suite 118   Edison, NJ 08837   (732)494-9400   Fax (732)548-3931
+ Premier Urology Group, LLC
  570 South Avenue East/Building A   Cranford, NJ 07016
  (732)494-9400   Fax (908)497-1633
+ Premier Urology Group, LLC
  2 Hospital Plaza/Suite 430   Old Bridge, NJ 08837
  (732)494-9400   Fax (732)679-2077

Sherman, Richard A., MD {1902826209} IntrMd, Nephro(75,NY46)<NJ-RWJUBRUN>
+ UMDNJ RWJ Nephrology
  125 Paterson Street/Suite 5100-B   New Brunswick, NJ 08901   (732)235-6512   Fax (732)235-6124
+ UH- Robert Wood Johnson Med
  125 Paterson Street/MEB 408B   New Brunswick, NJ 08901
  (732)235-6512   Fax (732)235-6124
+ Robert Wood Johnson Dialysis Center
  117 North Center Drive   North Brunswick, NJ 08901
  (732)940-4460

Sherman, Rimma L., MD {1659438992} IntrMd(81,AZE01)<NJ-STBARNMC>
+ Integrative Medicine of New Jersey
  101 Old Short Hills Road/Suite 214   West Orange, NJ 07052
  (973)736-5300   Fax (973)597-1157
  Rimmashermanmedical@yahoo.com

Sherman, Ronna S., MD {1780826859}
+ Summit Medical Group-Berkeley Heights Campus
  1 Diamond Hill Road   Berkeley Heights, NJ 07922
  (908)273-4300   Fax (908)790-6576

Sherrow, Keith Ira, MD {1225130701} IntrMd(87,NY08)<NJ-STPETER>
+ Monroe Internal Medicine
  1600 Perineville Road   Monroe Township, NJ 08831
  (609)655-1945   Fax (609)655-1967

Sherry, Stephen H., MD {1497856629} EnDbMt, IntrMd(76,CT02)<NJ-MTNSIDE>
+ Montclair Endocrine Associates
  123 Highland Avenue/Suite 301   Glen Ridge, NJ 07028
  (973)744-3733   Fax (973)707-5821

Shersher, David Daniel, MD {1831345461} Surgry
+ Women's Care Center
  3 Cooper Plaza/Suite 301   Camden, NJ 08103   (856)342-2959   Fax (856)968-8575

Shertz, Wendy T., MD {1518028307} PedPth, PthACl(80,PA09)<NJ-MONMOUTH>
+ Laboratory Medicine Associates, PA
  300 Second Avenue/Dept of Pathology   Long Branch, NJ 07740   (732)923-7362   Fax (732)923-7355

Shestak, Aleksandr, MD {1801848981} IntrMd(83,UKR13)
+ 21 Demarest Drive
  Manalapan, NJ 07726

Sheth, Amarish Rasiklal, MD {1376550665} Pedtrc(70,INA6Y)<NJ-CHSFULD, NJ-CHSMRCER>
+ 1544 Kuser Road/Suite C-1
  Hamilton, NJ 08619   (609)585-2200   Fax (609)581-6994

Sheth, Anish A., MD {1336235191} IntrMd, Gastrn(01,RI01)
+ Princeton Gastroenterology
  5 Plainsboro Road/Suite 260   Plainsboro, NJ 08536
  (609)853-7204   Fax (609)853-6386

Sheth, Arpita A., MD {1144512369} InfDis, IntrMd(06,INA21)
+ Infectious Disease Center of New Jersey
  22 Old Short Hills Road/Suite 106   Livingston, NJ 07039
  (973)535-8355   Fax (973)535-8353

Sheth, Manoj Indubhai, MD {1427295963} Pedtrc
+ Ocean Medical Center
  425 Jack Martin Boulevard/Emergency   Brick, NJ 08723
  (732)840-2200
+ JFK Medical Center
  65 James Street/Emergency   Edison, NJ 08820   (732)321-7000

Sheth, Meetkumar Tusharbhai, MD {1164680500} IntrMd(05)<NJ-NWRKBETH>
+ Heart & Vascular Associates of Northern Jersey
  22-18 Broadway/Suite 201   Fair Lawn, NJ 07410   (201)490-1217   Fax (201)475-5522
+ St. Joseph's Regional Medical Center
  703 Main Street   Paterson, NJ 07503   (973)754-2000

Sheth, Milan Pravin, MD {1710077573} RadDia(99,NJ05)<NJ-MORRISTN>
+ Memorial Radiology Associates
  10 Lanidex Plaza West/Suite 125   Parsippany, NJ 07054
  (973)503-5700   Fax (973)386-5701

Sheth, Naitik D., MD {1134417587} IntrMd
+ Nephrology Associates PA
  870 Palisade Avenue/Suite 202   Teaneck, NJ 07666
  (201)836-0897   Fax (201)836-8042

Sheth, Nidhir Ras, MD {1902859184} Gastrn, IntrMd(96,GRN01)
+ Gastroenterology Consultants of South Jersey
  693 Main Street/Suite 2   Lumberton, NJ 08048   (609)265-1700   Fax (609)265-9005
+ Burlington County Endoscopy Center
  140 Mount Holly Bypass/Unit 5   Lumberton, NJ 08048
  (609)267-1555

Sheth, Nila A., MD {1780752998} Psychy
+ 1544 Kuser Road/Suite C1
  Hamilton, NJ 08619   (609)585-2200   Fax (609)585-2206

Sheth, Sameer Anil, MD {1891821286} SrgNro(05,CA14)
+ Neurosurgeons of New Jersey
  1200 East Ridgewood Avenue   Ridgewood, NJ 07450
  (201)824-6131

Sheth, Sharvil U., MD {1598900177}
+ Rutgers- New Jersey Medical School
185 South Orange Avenue/MSB G-520   Newark, NJ 07103
(973)972-4300

Sheth, Surendra C., MD {1205880432} FamMed, Pedtrc(70,INDI)
+ 526 Lippincott Drive
Marlton, NJ 08053   (856)985-3700   Fax (856)985-8476
Suren44@msn.com

Shetty, Phyllis J., MD {1730245333} Anesth(75,INA09)<NJ-LOURDMED>
+ Rancocas Anesthesiology, PA
700 Route 130 North/Suite 203   Cinnaminson, NJ 08077
(856)829-9345   Fax (856)829-3605

Shetty, Sanjay, MD {1821011453} CdvDis, IntrMd(96,INA68)
+ Womens Health & Wellness
2500 English Creek Avenue   Egg Harbor Township, NJ 08234
(609)677-7776   Fax (609)677-7509

Shetty, Vinod J., MD {1366580581} IntrMd(92,NY15)<NJ-CENTRAST>
+ Drs. Lombardi & Shetty
1001 Route 9 North/Suite 106   Howell, NJ 07731
(732)886-9122   Fax (732)886-5161

Shetty, Vyshali S., MD {1134279201} IntrMd, IntHos(99,INA37)
+ JFK Medical Center - Muhlenberg Campus
Park Avenue & Randolph Road   Plainfield, NJ 07061
(908)668-2000   Fax (908)668-3149
+ JFK Medical Center
65 James Street   Edison, NJ 08820   (908)668-2000   Fax (721)909-2070

Shetzline, Michael Anthony, MD Gastrn, IntrMd(91,OH40)
+ Novartis Pharmaceuticals Corporation
One Health Plaza   East Hanover, NJ 07936   (862)778-8081
Fax (973)781-6504

Shevelev, Irene, MD {1477639615} Pedtrc(77,UKRA)<NJ-VALLEY>
+ Valley Pediatric Associates PA
470 North Franklin Turnpike   Ramsey, NJ 07446   (201)891-7272   Fax (201)934-1817
+ Valley Pediatric Associates, P.A.
201 East Franklin Turnpike   Ho Ho Kus, NJ 07423   (201)891-7272   Fax (201)652-6485

Shi, Yong, MD {1134278526} Grtrcs, IntrMd(84,CHN1K)
+ 10 Witherspoon Way
Marlboro, NJ 07746   (732)245-6461   Fax (732)303-0997

Shiau, Horngfu, MD {1104828474} Anesth(70,TAI05)<NJ-STCLRDEN>
+ St. Clare's Hospital-Denville Campus
25 Pocono Road   Denville, NJ 07834   (973)625-6000

Shieh, Frederick, MD {1801918917} Gastrn, IntrMd
+ Summit Medical Group
75 East Northfield Road   Livingston, NJ 07039   (973)436-1408   Fax (973)436-1762

Shieh, Luke, MD {1154697142} Pedtrc
+ Advocare Kressville Pediatrics Cherry Hill
710 Kresson Road   Cherry Hill, NJ 08003   (856)795-3320   Fax (856)795-1213

Shieh, Paul Y., MD {1376745828} RadDia(01,RI01)<NJ-COMMED>
+ Community Medical Center
99 Route 37 West/Radiology   Toms River, NJ 08755
(732)557-8151   Fax (732)557-2064

Shields, David S., MD {1205828365} Gastrn, IntrMd(89,NJ06)<NJ-SJERSYHS>
+ 2950 West Sherman Avenue/Suite 2A
Vineland, NJ 08360   (856)691-1129   Fax (856)691-1229

Shields, Jack M., MD {1730119934} IntrMd(76,MEX03)
+ 20 Magnolia Avenue
Bridgeton, NJ 08302   (856)455-8833   Fax (856)453-8358

Shields, Mary Susan, MD {1760803456} AlgyImmn, Pedtrc, IntrMd(77,PA13)
+ 402 Tidal Drive
Beach Haven, NJ 08008   (609)494-1599

Shields, Stephen Damien, MD {1548480858} EmrgMd(04,GRN01)<NJ-NWRKBETH>
+ Newark Beth Israel Medical Center
201 Lyons Avenue/EmrgMed   Newark, NJ 07112   (973)926-7000

Shienbaum, Alan J., DO {1811967904} PthCyt(94,PA77)
+ Kennedy Health System/Cherry Hill Campus
2201 Chapel Avenue West   Cherry Hill, NJ 08002
(856)488-6506   Fax (856)488-6846

Shiff, Steven J., MD {1235344938} Gastrn, IntrMd(84,PA01)
+ Forest Research Institute, Inc
Plaza V/28th Floor   Jersey City, NJ 07311   (201)427-8000

Shifrin, Alexander L., MD {1346624116} Surgry, EnDbMt, OthrSp(92,RUSS)<NJ-JRSYSHMC>
+ Jersey Shore University Medical Center
1945 Route 33/PO Box 397/Surg   Neptune, NJ 07753
(732)775-5500   Fax (732)776-2763

Shih, Duen S., MD {1629055637} Anesth, IntrMd(69,TAI07)<NJ-CHRIST, NJ-HOBUNIMC>
+ Christ Hospital
176 Palisade Avenue/Anesthesia   Jersey City, NJ 07306
(201)795-8200

+ Hoboken University Medical Center
308 Willow Avenue/Anesthesia   Hoboken, NJ 07030
(201)418-1570
+ 600 Pavonia Avenue
Jersey City, NJ 07306   (973)564-8159   Fax (973)543-3308

Shih, Eunhee, MD {1972562700} Pedtrc, AdolMd(00,NJ06)<NJ-OVERLOOK, NJ-STBARNMC>
+ The Pediatric Center
556 Central Avenue   New Providence, NJ 07974   (908)508-0400   Fax (908)508-0370

Shih, Henry Tsong-Ir, MD {1932165404} Pedtrc(97,PA01)<NJ-STPETER, NJ-RWJUBRUN>
+ 100 Perrine Road
Old Bridge, NJ 08857   (732)316-0405   Fax (732)316-0499

Shih, Richard D., MD {1811931413} EmrgMd(88,PA02)<NJ-MORRISTN>
+ Morristown Medical Center
100 Madison Avenue/Emergency   Morristown, NJ 07962
(973)971-8919

Shih, Yangyu Steven, MD {1396722427} Anesth(88,TAIW)<NJ-CHRIST>
+ Morris Anesthesia Group, PA
3799 Route 46/Suite 211   Parsippany, NJ 07054   (973)335-1122   Fax (973)335-1448

Shihabuddin, Bashar Sami, MD {1922261452} Pedtrc<NJ-NWRKBETH>
+ Newark Beth Israel Medical Center
201 Lyons Avenue   Newark, NJ 07112   (973)926-7000

Shihabuddin, Lina Sami, MD {1528014925} Psychy, PsyGrt(89,LEB03)
+ Center for Geriatric Health Care
156 Lyons Avenue   Newark, NJ 07112   (973)926-8491
Fax (973)923-6599

Shikiar, Steven Paul, MD {1437174026} Surgry(88,NY46)<NJ-PALISADE>
+ General Surgery Practice of Northern New Jersey
140 Grand Avenue   Englewood, NJ 07631   (201)541-7940
Fax (201)541-7942
sshikiar@njsurgery.com
+ General Surgery Practice of Northern New Jersey
6701 Bergenline Avenue   West New York, NJ 07093
(201)541-7940   Fax (201)541-7942

Shilad, Aiman K., MD {1992750715} ObsGyn(00,GRN01)
+ Blue River Women's Health
680 Broadway/Suite 506   Paterson, NJ 07514   (973)500-2399

Shiller, David P., MD {1073554697} EmrgMd(89,CT02)<NJ-KMH-TURNV>
+ Kennedy Health Systems/Washington Township Campus
435 Hurffville-Cross Keys Road   Turnersville, NJ 08012
(856)582-2500   Fax (856)582-2712

Shim, Mark Inbo, MD {1104836352} CdvDis, IntrMd(83,KOR04)<NY-LUTHERN, NY-BRKLNDWN>
+ Cardiology Consultants of Englewood Cliffs, PC
700 East Palisade Avenue/1st Floor   Englewood Cliffs, NJ 07632   (201)569-1800

Shim, Zae U., MD {1750397121} Pedtrc(64,KORE)<NJ-SJHREGMC>
+ 1000 North High Street
Millville, NJ 08332   (856)327-0016   Fax (856)327-5264

Shimelfarb, Marianna Borkovskaya, MD {1275842452} FamMed(07,NM01)
+ Summit Medical Group
48-50 Fairfield Street   Montclair, NJ 07042   (973)744-8511
Fax (973)744-6356

Shimoni, Noaa, MD {1144433921} FamMed, IntrMd(04,NJ05)
+ University Hospital-Doctors Office Center
90 Bergen Street/Suite 1750   Newark, NJ 07103   (973)972-8219   Fax (973)972-0018

Shin, David, MD {1558320994} Urolgy(97,NY20)
+ HUMC Faculty Practice
360 Essex Street/Suite 403   Hackensack, NJ 07601
(201)336-8090   Fax (201)336-8222

Shin, Dongwook, MD {1083005151} PulDis, IntrMd(70,KOR04)
+ Hackensack Gastroenterology Associates
130 Kinderkamack Road/Suite 301   River Edge, NJ 07661
(201)567-0633   Fax (201)489-2544

Shin, Helen Theresa, MD {1396799433} Dermat, PedDrm(95,NY20)<NJ-HACKNSK>
+ Hackensack University Medical Center
30 Prospect Avenue/Dermatology   Hackensack, NJ 07601
(201)996-2000

Shin, Jacob, MD {1003221763} RadOnc(14,MA05)<NY-SLOANKET>
+ Memorial Sloan Kettering Monmouth
480 Red Hill Road/Radiation Onc   Middletown, NJ 07748
(848)225-6000

Shin, John Jung Hoon, MD {1477577682} IntrMd, EnDbMt(97,GRN01)<NJ-VAEASTOR>
+ 154 Panorama Drive
Edgewater, NJ 07020   (201)676-2245
+ VA New Jersey Health Care System-East Orange Campus
385 Tremont Avenue   East Orange, NJ 07018   (973)676-

1000

Shin, Jong Tae, DO {1992966717} FamMSptM
+ Drs. Chung & Shin
110 Marter Avenue/Suite 507   Moorestown, NJ 08057
(856)222-4766   Fax (856)222-1137

Shin, Kyun, MD {1346238771} Psychy(67,KOR14)
+ 130 Maple Avenue/Suite 5C
Red Bank, NJ 07701   (732)747-0513

Shin, Kyung Hee, MD {1386662492} Anesth(64,KOR04)
+ River Drive Surgery Center
619 River Drive/Anesth   Elmwood Park, NJ 07407
(800)738-1659   Fax (704)871-2128

Shin, Mira, MD {1659334498} PhysMd, PhyMPain, IntrMd(00,NET09)
+ 2050 Center Avenue/Suite 425
Fort Lee, NJ 07024   (201)261-1000   Fax (201)261-1188

Shin, Nara Chi Sun, MD {1952333494} EmrgMd, IntrMd(02,CT01)<PA-TJHSP, PA-TJFMETHD>
+ McCosh Health Center
Washington Road/McCosh Infirmary   Princeton, NJ 08544
(609)258-5357   Fax (609)258-1355

Shin, Peter Young, MD {1194917963} IntrMd(05,NY01)<NJ-ENGLWOOD>
+ 350 Engle Street/Suite 5265
Englewood, NJ 07631   (201)894-3364

Shin, Pheodora L., MD {1326020355} Anesth, Pedtrc(89,IL06)<NJ-MORRISTN>
+ Morristown Medical Center
100 Madison Avenue/Anesthesiology   Morristown, NJ 07962   (973)971-5000   Fax (201)943-8733

Shin, Seulkih, MD {1023437092} IntrMd
+ The Park Medical Group
24 Elm Street   Harrington Park, NJ 07640   (201)784-0123
Fax (201)784-0065

Shin, Seung Hoon, MD {1831422260} SrgTrm
+ Meridian Trauma Associates PC
1945 State Route 33   Neptune, NJ 07754   (327)764-9497

Shin, Young H., MD Pedtrc(64,KOR07)
+ 50 Park Avenue
Paterson, NJ 07501   (973)278-9800

Shinde, Tejas Shashikant, MD {1164495909} Radiol(99,NY19)<NJ-MONMOUTH>
+ Shrewsbury Diagnostic Imaging, Inc.
1131 Broad Street/Suite 110   Shrewsbury, NJ 07702
(732)578-9640   Fax (732)578-9650
+ Monmouth Medical Center
300 Second Avenue   Long Branch, NJ 07740   (732)222-5200

Shindle, Michael Kenneth, MD {1952578627} SrgOrt, SprtMd(04,MD07)
+ Summit Medical Group Orthopedics and Sports Medicine
140 Park Avenue/2nd Floor   Florham Park, NJ 07932
(973)404-9800   Fax (973)267-1737

Shindler, Daniel M., MD {1114003613} CdvDis, IntrMd(79,SPA02)
+ UH- Robert Wood Johnson Med
125 Paterson Street/MEB 575   New Brunswick, NJ 08901
(732)235-7855   Fax (732)235-8722
+ University Medical Group/Cardiology
125 Paterson Street/CAB-Rm 5200   New Brunswick, NJ 08901   (732)235-7855   Fax (732)235-6530

Shindler, Maria Danielle, MD {1265739619} Anesth(07,TN07)
+ Hackensack University MC-Anesthesia Dept
30 Prospect Avenue/Room 2703   Hackensack, NJ 07601
(201)996-2419   Fax (201)996-3962

Shioleno, Charles A., MD {1245230804} CdvDis, IntrMd(77,DC02)<NJ-MORRISTN>
+ Atlantic Cardiology Group LLP
8 Tempe Wick Road   Mendham, NJ 07945   (973)543-2288
Fax (973)543-0637
+ Atlantic Cardiology Group LLP
95 Madison Avenue/Suite 300   Morristown, NJ 07960
(973)543-2288   Fax (973)682-9494

Shirazi, Michael E., MD {1326289679} RadDia(05,NJ05)
+ East Orange General Hospital
300 Central Avenue   East Orange, NJ 07018   (973)672-8400

Shirguppi, Renu, MD {1982966941} EmrgMd<NJ-CHSFULD>
+ Capital Health System/Fuld Campus
750 Brunswick Avenue   Trenton, NJ 08638   (609)537-6171
Fax (609)537-6184

Shirley, Lauren, DO {1699092312} EmrgMd(10,MO79)
+ 384 Hampshire Court
Wyckoff, NJ 07481   (201)230-1764

Shiroff, Adam Michael, MD {1346376365} Surgry, SrgCrC(02,NJ06)<NJ-RWJUBRUN>
+ Child Health Institute of New Jersey
89 French Street/Suite 2300   New Brunswick, NJ 08901
(732)235-7766   Fax (732)235-2964
+ UH- Robert Wood Johnson Med
125 Paterson Street/Suite 4100   New Brunswick, NJ 08901
(732)235-7766   Fax (732)235-7079

Shirolawala, Pankaj Ramanlal, MD {1003882523}

Physicians by Name and Address

IntrMd(83,INA21)<NJ-RBAYPERT, NJ-JFKMED>
+ 609 Amboy Avenue/Suite 101
Perth Amboy, NJ 08861 (732)442-2211 Fax (732)326-0517
Shirolawala@verizon.com

Shiu, David, DO {1649546458}<NJ-NWRKBETH>
+ Newark Beth Israel Medical Center
201 Lyons Avenue/Medicine Newark, NJ 07112 (973)926-7425

Shivashankar, Keshavamurthy, MD {1811050404} IntCrd, IntrMd(76,INA9A)<NJ-CLARMAAS, NJ-NWRKBETH>
+ Drs. Keshav & Shivashankar
140 Belmont Avenue/Suite 102 Belleville, NJ 07109 (973)751-7870 Fax (973)751-7875

Shklar, David Lewis, MD {1124040407} IntrMd(98,NY46)<NJ-COOPRUMC>
+ Cooper University Hospital
One Cooper Plaza/Hospitalist Camden, NJ 08103 (856)342-3150 Fax (856)968-8418

Shkolnaya, Tatyana, MD {1497729842} Pedtrc(90,UKRA)<NJ-JRSYSHMC, NJ-MONMOUTH>
+ Candlewood Pediatrics
1540 State Route 138/Suite 105 Wall, NJ 07719 (732)280-3100 Fax (732)280-3103
TSPPEDIATRICS@optonline.net

Shlien, Robert D., MD {1154322246} Gastrn(82,DC01)<NJ-CHILTON>
+ Gastrointestinal Group of North Jersey
1777 Hamburg Turnpike/Suite 101 Wayne, NJ 07470 (973)839-6400 Fax (973)839-7083
robert.shlien@gmail.com
+ Wayne Surgical Center, LLC.
1176 Hamburg Pike Wayne, NJ 07470 (973)839-6400 Fax (973)709-1901

Shluper, Victoria, MD {1639238884} Pedtrc(99,NY09)
+ 101 Madison Avenue/Suite 103
Morristown, NJ 07960 (973)644-9000 Fax (973)644-9282

Shmulevich, Mark, MD {1417053125} PhysMd(00,DMN01)
+ 12 Millie Lane
East Hanover, NJ 07936

Shmuts, Rachel Lauren, MD {1821230079}
+ University Hospital-SOM Department of Psychiatry
2250 Chapel Avenue West/Suite 100 Cherry Hill, NJ 08002 (856)482-9000 Fax (856)482-1159

Shmuts, Robert Jaron, DO {1427203694} Gastrn, IntrMd(08,NJ75)
+ 1113 Hospital Drive/Suite 305
Willingboro, NJ 08046 (856)835-3624 Fax (856)835-3628

Shnaidman, Vivian T., MD {1174706618} Psychy, PsyFor, IntrMd(88,ISR02)
+ Jersey Forensic Consulting, LLC.
10 Vreeland Drive/Suite 103 Skillman, NJ 08558 (609)910-1715 Fax (609)964-1700
VIVIAN.T@RCN.COM

Shnaps, Yitzchak, MD {1275757171} Psychy(80,ISR01)
+ 41 Tamarack Circle
Skillman, NJ 08558 (609)921-7878 Fax (609)921-0112

Shnayder, Eric, MD {1861477465} Ophthl(97,PA07)<NJ-STBARNMC>
+ Eric Shnayder MD PC
11 Kiel Avenue/2nd Floor Kinnelon, NJ 07405 (973)838-7722 Fax (973)838-3579

Shnayderman, Aleksandr, DO {1881656353} Psychy(99,NY75)<NJ-TRINIWSC, NJ-TRININPC>
+ Trinitas Regional Medical Center-New Point Campus
655 East Jersey Street Elizabeth, NJ 07206 (908)994-5000

Shneidman, Paul S., MD {1962435925} Nrolgy(80,NY46)
+ Drexel Neurosciences Institute
1600 Haddon Avenue Camden, NJ 08103 (844)464-6387 Fax (215)239-3037

Shoen, Steven Lloyd, MD {1629159694} SrgHnd, SrgPlstc, Surgry(85,NY46)<NJ-RBAYOLDB, NJ-RWJUBRUN>
+ 222 Bridge Street/Building E
Metuchen, NJ 08840 (732)632-6090 Fax (732)632-6094

Shoenfeld, Richard B., MD {1033164553} Radiol, RadDia(76,FRA10)<NJ-NWRKBETH>
+ New Jersey Vein and Cosmetic Surgery Center
741 Northfield Avenue/Suite 105 West Orange, NJ 07052 (973)243-9729 Fax (973)243-9674

Shoengold, Stuart D., MD {1689689275} Urolgy(76,NJ05)<NJ-NWRKBETH, NJ-STBARNMC>
+ Essex Urology Associates/UGNJ
225 Millburn Avenue/Suite 304 Millburn, NJ 07041 (973)218-9400 Fax (973)218-9420
+ Short Hills Surgery Center
187 Millburn Avenue/Suite 101 Millburn, NJ 07041 (973)218-9400 Fax (973)671-0557
+ New Jersey Urology, LLC
700 North Broad Street/Suite 302 Elizabeth, NJ 07041 (908)289-3666 Fax (908)289-0716

Sholevar, Darius P., MD {1093794729} CdvDis, ClCdEl, IntrMd(88,PA02)<NJ-OURLADY, NJ-VIRTUAHS>
+ Associated Cardiovascular Consultants-Lourdes
1 Brace Road/Suite C & F Cherry Hill, NJ 08034 (856)428-4100 Fax (856)428-5748

Sholevar, Ghodrat Pirooz, MD {1649324955}
+ Nueva Vida Behavioral Health Center
427 Market Street Camden, NJ 08102 (856)338-1995 Fax (856)338-0247

Shoman, Adam Mohamed, MD {1316987670} ObsGyn, IntrMd(94,EGY05)<NJ-HACKNSK>
+ 93-95 Hudson Street
Hoboken, NJ 07030 (201)342-7002 Fax (201)342-7055
+ 155 Polifly Road/Suite 207
Hackensack, NJ 07601 (201)342-7002 Fax (201)342-7055
+ 610 Washington Boulevard
Jersey City, NJ 07030 (201)342-7002 Fax (201)342-7055

Shomo, Marcia Rosenberg, MD {1366464489} Radiol, RadDia(86,PA09)
+ Atlantic Medical Imaging
455 Jack Martin Boulevard Brick, NJ 08724 (732)223-9729 Fax (732)840-6459

Shoner, Lawrence Gene, MD {1255452132} IntrMd, OccpMd(81,PRO03)
+ Monmouth Medical Center
300 Second Avenue Long Branch, NJ 07740 (732)222-5200

Shonowo, Owobamishola Adanma, MD {1114966157} ObsGyn(99,TX02)<NJ-RBAYOLDB>
+ SAS OBGYN
565 New Brunswick Avenue Fords, NJ 08863 (848)203-3520 Fax (848)203-3627
drshonowo@sasobgyn.com

Shoor, Priya, MD {1700143559} RadDia
+ Imaging Consultants of Essex
94 Old Short Hills Road Livingston, NJ 07039 (977)322-8945 Fax (973)322-5536

Shor, Raida, MD {1679661839} Pedtrc, AdolMd(67,RUS54)<NJ-VALLEY>
+ 545 Island Road
Ramsey, NJ 07446 (201)818-8810 Fax (201)818-9233

Shore, Michael W., MD {1932100641} Psychy, PsyAdd, Addctn(80,PA13)
+ 1500 North Kings Highway/Suite 106
Cherry Hill, NJ 08034 (856)428-8190 Fax (856)428-8182
Michaelwshoremd@comcast.net

Shore, Robin L., DO {1689623670} EmrgMd(90,FL75)<NJ-WAYNEGEN>
+ St. Joseph's Wayne Hospital
224 Hamburg Turnpike/EmergMed Wayne, NJ 07470 (973)942-6900

Shore, Ronald Andrew, DO {1649272915} Anesth(88,MO78)<NJ-STCLRDEN>
+ Morris Anesthesia Group, PA
3799 Route 46/Suite 211 Parsippany, NJ 07054 (973)335-1122 Fax (973)335-1448

Shorshtein, Alexander, MD {1215950399} Anesth(03,NJ05)
+ Hackensack University MC-Anesthesia Dept
30 Prospect Avenue/Room 2703 Hackensack, NJ 07601 (201)996-2419 Fax (201)996-3962

Shoshani, Shai, MD {1609195726} FamMed
+ 46 Union Avenue
Cresskill, NJ 07626 (201)431-5115 Fax (201)399-7697

Shoshilos, Anna G., DO {1427025980} ObsGyn, IntrMd(95,NY75)<NJ-NWRKBETH>
+ Martinsville Women's Health
96 Linwood Plaza/Suite 374 Fort Lee, NJ 07024 (973)699-6765
+ Newark Beth Israel Medical Center
201 Lyons Avenue/Suite L-4 Newark, NJ 07112 (973)699-6765 Fax (973)705-8650

Shoulson, Shana S., MD {1992807945} FamMed(94,NJ06)
+ Piscataway Dunellen Family Practice
24 Stelton Road/Suite A Piscataway, NJ 08854 (732)424-0440 Fax (732)424-0443

Shovlin, Jane Ann, MD {1336192723} IntrMd, IntMAdMd(94,NJ05)<NJ-CHSFULD>
+ Capital Health System/Fuld Campus
750 Brunswick Avenue Trenton, NJ 08638 (609)815-7887 Fax (609)394-6776

Shovlin, Joseph Peter, MD {1861450710} Ophthl(87,NJ05)<NJ-UNVMCPRN>
+ Outlook Eyecare
100 Canal Pointe Boulevard/Suite 100 Princeton, NJ 08540 (609)279-9500 Fax (609)279-0150
+ Outlook Eyecare
5 Centre Drive/1B Monroe Township, NJ 08831 (609)279-9500 Fax (609)409-2718

Shraga, Alexander, MD {1265460604} Dermat, IntrMd(98,MD07)<NJ-UNVMCPRN>
+ Adult and Pediatric Dermatology, LLC.
385 Route 18 South/Suite C East Brunswick, NJ 08816 (732)390-1883 Fax (732)907-1711

Shrager, Brian L., MD {1588761936} Surgry, IntrMd(99,PA02)<NJ-MORRISTN, NY-MTSINAI>
+ 16 Pocono Road/Suite 208
Denville, NJ 07834 (862)267-0388 Fax (862)267-0387

Shrayber, Yelena Y., DO {1922038199} FamMed, IntrMd(00,NY75)
+ Cherry Hill Primary and Specialty Care
457 Haddonfield Road/Suite 110 Cherry Hill, NJ 08002 (844)542-2273 Fax (856)406-4570
+ Kennedy Health Alliance Vascular Surgery
333 Laurel Oak Road Voorhees, NJ 08043 (844)542-2273 Fax (856)770-9194

Shraytman, Arkadiy, DO {1932103355} FamMed(97,NY75)<NJ-BAYONNE>
+ Clifton Urgent and Primary Care
721 Clifton Avenue/Suite 2A Clifton, NJ 07013 (973)777-7727 Fax (973)779-7906

Shrem, Leslie Allen, MD {1598768442} Anesth(84,PHI08)
+ Surgical Center at Cedar Knolls
197 Ridgedale Avenue Cedar Knolls, NJ 07927 (973)292-0700

Shridharani, Kanan Vasant, MD {1639266729} IntrMd(91,NY47)
+ Summit Medical Group-Berkeley Heights Campus
1 Diamond Hill Road Berkeley Heights, NJ 07922 (908)277-8683 Fax (908)608-2378

Shrivastava, Abhishek, MD {1285842096} RadDia, Radiol(04,NJ02)<NJ-RWJURAH>
+ Robert Wood Johnson University Hospital at Rahway
865 Stone Street/Radiology Rahway, NJ 07065 (952)595-1100 Fax (612)294-4903

Shrivastava, Arpita G., MD {1831350925} EmrgMd(04,NJ05)<NJ-JFKMED>
+ JFK Medical Center
65 James Street Edison, NJ 08820 (732)321-7605 Fax (732)744-5614

Shriver, Amy Rubin, MD {1164665998} Gastrn, IntrMd(09,NJ06)
+ Princeton Gastroenterology Associates, P.A.
731 Alexander Road/Suite 100 Princeton, NJ 08540 (609)924-1422 Fax (609)924-7473

Shroff, Ninad A., MD {1558377754} EmrgMd, EmrgEMed(98,NJ06)<NJ-STJOSHOS>
+ St Joseph's Medical Center Emergency
703 Main Street Paterson, NJ 07503 (973)754-2222 Fax (973)754-2249

Shroff, Punita, MD {1962829903}
+ Hackensack University Medical Center
30 Prospect Avenue Hackensack, NJ 07601 (201)996-2000

Shroff, Shilpa Anilkumar, MD {1245338391} IntHos, IntrMd(00,GRN01)<NJ-OVERLOOK, NJ-MORRISTN>
+ IPC The Hospitalist Company
55 Madison Avenue/Suite 310 Morristown, NJ 07960 (973)993-9736 Fax (973)998-4237
+ Overlook Medical Center
99 Beauvoir Avenue/PO Box 210 Summit, NJ 07902 (908)522-2000

Shroff, Yogini J., MD {1396814877} Pthlgy, PthACl(66,INDI)<NJ-CHRIST>
+ Christ Hospital
176 Palisade Avenue/Path Jersey City, NJ 07306 (201)795-5963 Fax (201)795-8118

Shroyer, Stephen J., MD {1588600340} Pedtrc(80,MEX03)<NJ-JRSYSHMC>
+ 1420-1/2 Schoolhouse
Wall, NJ 07753 (732)280-0660 Fax (732)681-1264

Shtern, Tatiana, MD {1730133802} Pedtrc(93,RUSS)<NJ-VALLEY, NJ-HACKNSK>
+ 22 Madison Avenue/Suite 101
Paramus, NJ 07652 (201)712-1599 Fax (201)712-7996
Dshtern@yahoo.com

Shteynberg, Elena, MD {1922043116} Pedtrc, IntrMd(91,UKR16)
+ Somerset Pediatric Group PA
2345 Lamington Road/Suite 101 Bedminster, NJ 07921 (908)470-1124 Fax (908)470-2845

Shtindler, Feliks, MD {1053330035} IntrMd(89,UKR08)<NJ-STCLRDOV, NJ-STCLRDEN>
+ 35-E Elizabeth Street
New Brunswick, NJ 08901 (732)238-3800 Fax (732)238-2883

Shua Haim, Joshua Roy, MD {1073554879} Grtrcs, IntrMd(84,ISR02)<NJ-JRSYSHMC>
+ Mid Atlantic Geriatric Associates-Ocean, P.A.ac
1043 Route 70 West/Unit C3 Lakehurst, NJ 08733 (732)657-6100 Fax (732)657-0111
+ Mid Atlantic Geriatric Associates
1205 Route 35 North Ocean, NJ 07712 (732)657-6100 Fax (732)663-1359

Shubeck, Caroline A., MD {1508956905} IntrMd(81,IL42)
+ St. Anne Villa
190 Park Avenue Florham Park, NJ 07932 (973)292-6555

Shubert, Roy Alan, II, MD {1992750293} EmrgMd(96,PA02)<NJ-VIRTMHBC>
+ Virtua Memorial
175 Madison Avenue/EmergMed   Mount Holly, NJ 08060   (609)267-0700   Fax (609)914-6067

Shubhakar, Vishwanath, MD {1750612131} IntrMd<NJ-MORRISTN>
+ Morristown Medical Center
100 Madison Avenue/Internal Med   Morristown, NJ 07962   (973)971-5526   Fax (973)290-8325

Shufler, Daniel E., MD {1598731085} Gastrn, IntrMd(80,PA09)<NJ-MEMSALEM, NJ-COOPRUMC>
+ 48 North Broadway/Suite D
Pennsville, NJ 08070   (856)678-5252   Fax (856)678-2333

Shugar, Ronald A., MD {1164452462} Gastrn, IntrMd(69,NY09)<NJ-JFKMED, NJ-RWJURAH>
+ Drs. Rudnitzky & Shugar PA
98 James Street/Suite 104   Edison, NJ 08820   (732)494-6300   Fax (732)494-1028

Shukla, Apexa Nilesh, MD {1730393547}
+ 329 Goffle Road
Ridgewood, NJ 07450   (201)857-4140

Shukla, Ashish, MD {1366674889}
+ Heart Specialists/Central Jersey
901 West Main Street/Suite 205   Freehold, NJ 07728   (732)866-0800   Fax (732)463-6082
azshukla@gmail.com

Shukla, Chirag S., MD {1164520854} Nrolgy, Psychy, VasNeu(93,INA2B)<NJ-CHSMRCER>
+ Capital Institute for Neurosciences
2 Capital Way/Suite 456   Pennington, NJ 08534   (609)537-7300   Fax (609)537-7301
+ Capital Institute for Neurosciences
1445 Whitehorse Mercerville Rd   Hamilton, NJ 08619   (609)537-7300   Fax (609)537-7301

Shukla, Gunjan Jayendrabhai, MD {1861487431} ClCdEl, CdvDis, IntrMd(96,INA20)
+ Electrophysiology Associates
20 Prospect Avenue/Suite 701   Hackensack, NJ 07601   (201)996-2997   Fax (201)996-2571
gunjanshukla@hotmail.com

Shukla, Kishorchandra S., MD {1417016650} Pedtrc(71,INA71)<NJ-GRYSTPSY>
+ 1144 Sussex Turnpike
Randolph, NJ 07869

Shukla, Mrudula S., MD {1285671651} ObsGyn(66,INA69)
+ Bergen Women Ob-Gyn Associates
92 Hillside Avenue   Tenafly, NJ 07670

Shukla, Nilesh B., MD {1710058334} Gastrn, IntrMd(96,NY03)
+ Salvatore Focella, MD LLC
1 West Ridgewood Avenue/Suite 203   Paramus, NJ 07652   (201)652-8800   Fax (201)444-8560

Shukla, Nimisha J., MD {1801981386} Pedtrc(85,INA69)<NJ-JFKMED, NJ-STPETER>
+ 1802 Oak Tree Avenue
Edison, NJ 08820   (732)548-3210   Fax (732)906-3966

Shukla, Paresh Parashar, MD {1477618767} IntrMd(85,DOMI)<NJ-PALISADE, NJ-HOBUNIMC>
+ Integrated Physicians of NJ
316-20th Street   Union City, NJ 07087   (201)866-8626   Fax (201)866-2556

Shukla, Rajesh, MD {1184626772} IntrMd(94,INA69)<NJ-NWTNMEM>
+ 175 High Street
Newton, NJ 07860   (973)579-8419

Shukla, Sandhya, MD {1821220336} Gastrn
+ Atlantic Coast Gastroenterology
1640 Route 88 West/Suite 202   Brick, NJ 08724   (732)485-8300   Fax (732)458-8529

Shulkin, David J., MD {1225012883} IntrMd(86,PA09)<NY-BETHPETR, NY-BETHKING>
+ Morristown Medical Center
100 Madison Avenue   Morristown, NJ 07962   (973)971-5450

Shulman, Gayle S., MD {1689615510} Ophthl(84,NJ05)<NJ-HOBUNIMC>
+ 2255 Kennedy boulevard
Jersey City, NJ 07304   (201)433-8484   Fax (201)994-1404

Shulman, Leon H., MD {1477599348} EnDbMt, IntrMd(86,NJ06)
+ Drs. Agrin and Shulman
78 Easton Avenue   New Brunswick, NJ 08901   (732)545-1065   Fax (732)545-1063
+ Drs. Agrin & Shulman
245 Union Avenue/Suite 2B   Bridgewater, NJ 08807   (732)545-1065   Fax (908)231-1324

Shulman, Lois E., MD {1134151392} ObsGyn(78,DC01)<NJ-STPETER, NJ-RWJUBRUN>
+ 1553 Route 27/Suite 2400
Somerset, NJ 08873   (732)246-4000   Fax (732)246-0368

Shulman, Michael, MD {1194915884} Anesth(05,DMN01)
+ Hackensack University MC-Anesthesia Dept
30 Prospect Avenue/Room 2703   Hackensack, NJ 07601   (201)996-2419   Fax (201)996-3962
+ 88 Mounthaven Drive
Livingston, NJ 07039   (973)758-0803

Shulman, Oleg M., MD {1578530473} Anesth, PainMd(81,LAT02)<NJ-CHILTON>
+ Chilton Medical Center
97 West Parkway/Anesthesiology   Pompton Plains, NJ 07444   (973)831-5000

Shulman, Sabra W., MD {1306932702} Pedtrc, AdolMd(84,NY19)<NJ-RWJUBRUN, NJ-STPETER>
+ Mid Jersey Pediatrics
33 Brunswick Woods Drive   East Brunswick, NJ 08816   (732)257-4330   Fax (732)257-1177
+ Mid Jersey Pediatrics
25 Kilmer Drive/Building 3/Suite 107   Morganville, NJ 07751   (732)257-4330   Fax (732)972-1677

Shulman, Yale C., MD {1114946142} Urolgy(76,NY46)<NJ-CHRIST, NJ-ENGLWOOD>
+ Shulman Urology
2255 Kennedy Boulevard   Jersey City, NJ 07304   (201)433-1057   Fax (201)435-2716
ycshulman@gmail.com
+ Shulman Urology
807 Kennedy Boulevard   Bayonne, NJ 07002   (201)339-5799
+ Shulman Urology
163 Engle Street   Englewood, NJ 07304

Shulruff, Stuart E., MD {1871590448} CdvDis, IntrMd(78,IL02)<NJ-MORRISTN, NJ-HCKTSTWN>
+ Cardiology Consultants of North Morris, PA
356 US Highway 46/Suite B   Mountain Lakes, NJ 07046   (973)586-3400   Fax (973)586-1916

Shultz, Lisa Ann, MD {1811901903} Nrolgy, Psychy(00,NY46)<NJ-CHSFULD>
+ Capital Health System/Fuld Campus
750 Brunswick Avenue/Neurology   Trenton, NJ 08638   (609)394-6000

Shumko, John Zachary, MD {1295739571} PhysMd(92,NJ05)<NJ-STBARNMC>
+ St. Barnabas Ambulatory Care Center
200 South Orange Avenue   Livingston, NJ 07039   (973)322-7600   Fax (973)322-7685

Shupper, Peter Joseph, MD {1578902284} PhyMPain
+ Center for Pain Management
294 State Street/Suite 1   Hackensack, NJ 07601   (201)488-7246   Fax (201)488-3790

Shustik, Ofer Josef, MD {1750304937} FamMed
+ Coordinated Health
222 Red Lane   Phillipsburg, NJ 08865   (610)861-8080   Fax (610)849-1013

Shute, Amy L., MD {1700969532} FamMed(85,NJ06)<NJ-SOMERSET>
+ RWJPE Towne Centre Family Care
302 Towne Centre Drive   Hillsborough, NJ 08844   (908)359-8613   Fax (908)874-8509

Shypula, Gregory J., MD {1902869720} Hemato, Onclgy, OncHemat(81,POLA)<NJ-RBAYOLDB, NJ-JFKMED>
+ Gregory Shypula MD PA
1030 St. Georges Avenue/Suite 307   Avenel, NJ 07001   (732)750-1200   Fax (732)602-4044
+ Gregory Shypula MD PA
2045 Route 35 South/Suite 202   South Amboy, NJ 08879   (732)750-1200   Fax (732)602-4044

Sia, Dominic Chionglo, MD {1720362635} Pedtrc
+ 2215 Royal Oaks Drive
Toms River, NJ 08753

Sia, Valerie May Gumban, MD {1699080499} Pedtrc(93,PHI02)
+ Silverton Pediatrics
2446 Church Road   Toms River, NJ 08753   (732)255-7553   Fax (732)255-8901

Sicat, Jon F., DO {1972552230} IntrMd, Pedtrc(94,NY75)<NJ-NWRKBETH>
+ Newark Beth Israel Medical Center
201 Lyons Avenue/OstheoMedEdu   Newark, NJ 07112   (973)926-7472   Fax (973)923-8063

Sicherman, Harlan J., MD {1952320103} CdvDis, IntrMd(71,PA09)
+ 1338 How Lane
North Brunswick, NJ 08902

Sicherman, Hervey S., MD {1083713853} SrgOrt(68,MA07)<NJ-CHILTON>
+ Advanced Orthopaedic Associates
1777 Hamburg Turnpike/Suite 301   Wayne, NJ 07470   (973)839-5700   Fax (973)616-4343

Sichrovsky, Tina Claudia, MD {1558567206} ClCdEl, CdvDis, IntrMd(98,AUS07)<NY-SLRLUKES, NJ-VALLEY>
+ Valley Medical Group-Electrophysiology
970 Linwood Avenue/Suite 102   Ridgewood, NJ 07450   (201)432-7837   Fax (201)432-7830
+ Valley Medical Group-Electrophysiology & Cardiology
223 North Van Dien Avenue   Ridgewood, NJ 07450   (201)432-7837   Fax (201)432-7830

Siciliano, Janice M., DO {1689612129} FamMed, IntrMd(86,NJ75)<NJ-JRSYSHMC>
+ Wall Family Medical
2130 Highway 35/Building C Suite 324   Sea Girt, NJ 08750   (732)974-8005   Fax (732)974-8020
+ Wall Family Medical
500 Candlewood Commons   Howell, NJ 07731   (732)974-8005   Fax (732)364-7713

Siciliano, Louis J., MD {1760487250} Anesth(92,PA13)<NJ-SOCEANCO>
+ Southern Ocean County Medical Center
1140 Route 72 West/Anesth   Manahawkin, NJ 08050   (609)597-6011

Siciliano, Mary J., DO {1205834454} FamMed(92,ME75)<NJ-WARREN>
+ St. Luke's Coventry Family Practice
755 Memorial Parkway/Suite 300   Phillipsburg, NJ 08865   (908)847-3300   Fax (866)281-6023

Sidali, Mustafa M., DO {1811982762} InfDis, IntrMd(95,NJ75)
+ Prime Care Medical Group
55-59 Washington Avenue   Belleville, NJ 07109   (973)207-0640

Siddiq, Syed A., MD {1578501565} IntrMd(84,PAK11)
+ 190 Greenbrook Road
North Plainfield, NJ 07060   (908)756-5206   Fax (908)756-5214

Siddiqi, Asim, MD {1396004438}
+ 468 Forest Avenue
Paramus, NJ 07652   (973)919-2788
asim2334@yahoo.com

Siddiqi, Faisal Khursheed, MD {1861676678} CdvDis, IntrMd
+ Associated Cardiovascular Consultants-Lourdes
1 Brace Road/Suite C & F   Cherry Hill, NJ 08034   (856)428-4100   Fax (856)428-5748

Siddiqi, Kashif Inam, MD {1619166774} Anesth
+ UH- Robert Wood Johnson Med
125 Paterson Street/Suite 5123   New Brunswick, NJ 08901   (732)828-3000   Fax (732)235-3520

Siddiqi, Tariq S., MD {1861431942} SrgNro(73,PAK11)<NJ-VIRTVOOR>
+ 1 Sheppard Road/Suite 900
Voorhees, NJ 08043   (856)751-6600   Fax (856)751-5556
tsiddiqimd@aol.com

Siddique, Mahbubur Rahman, MD {1013168467} IntrMd(BAN02)<NJ-COOPRUMC>
+ Cooper University Hospital
One Cooper Plaza/Internal Med   Camden, NJ 08103   (856)342-3150   Fax (856)968-8573

Siddique, Mahmood I., DO {1700976073} IntrMd, PulCCr, SlpDis(91,IL76)<NJ-RWJUBRUN, NJ-STFRNMED>
+ Sleep & Wellness Medical Associates
3836 Quakerbridge Road/Suite 206   Hamilton, NJ 08619   (609)587-9944   Fax (609)587-9955
info@sleep-wellness.org

Siddique, Muhammad Neaman, MD {1497784920} Pedtrc, IntrMd(87,PAKI)<NJ-JFKMED, NJ-BAYONNE>
+ Bayonne Medical Care LLC
415 Avenel Street/Suite A   Avenel, NJ 07001   (732)750-1180   Fax (732)750-1182

Siddiqui, Afzaal Ahmad, MD {1255467064} Anesth, PainMd, AnesPain(82,NY75)<NJ-STMRYPAS>
+ Garden State Endoscopy & Surgery Center
1000 Galloping Hill Road   Kenilworth, NJ 07033   (908)241-8900

Siddiqui, Arshad Uddin, MD {1033257712} Psychy
+ 1691 US Highway 9/CN 2025
Toms River, NJ 08754

Siddiqui, Asma, MD {1639187503} PhysMd, IntrMd(97,SLU01)
+ Innovative Pain Care Center
415 Avenel Street   Avenel, NJ 07001   (732)636-7888   Fax (732)636-7887

Siddiqui, Durdana Aamir, MD {1699911297} IntrMd, IntHos(PAK22)<NJ-ACMCITY>
+ AtlantiCare Hospitalist Program
1925 Pacific Avenue/8th Floor   Atlantic City, NJ 08401   (609)441-8146   Fax (609)441-8002

Siddiqui, Farhan A., MD {1770905176}<NJ-TRININPC>
+ Trinitas Regional Medical Center-New Point Campus
655 East Jersey Street   Elizabeth, NJ 07206   (908)994-7325

Siddiqui, Imtiazuddin M., MD {1851477186} Psychy(75,INA83)<NJ-CHILTON>
+ Drs. Siddiqui and Siddiqui
510 Hamburg Turnpike/Suite E-106   Wayne, NJ 07470   (973)904-3161   Fax (973)904-3163

Siddiqui, Kamran, MD {1801206396} IntHos
+ Jersey Shore University Medical Center
1945 Route 33   Neptune, NJ 07753   (732)775-5500

Siddiqui, Maaz M., MD {1366707317}
+ 252 Washington Valley Road
Randolph, NJ 07869   (267)838-0642

Physicians by Name and Address

Siddiqui, Mohammed Ahmer, MD {1861759516}<NJ-HOBUNIMC>
+ Hoboken University Medical Center
  308 Willow Avenue   Hoboken, NJ 07030   (201)418-3127

Siddiqui, Muhammad Rehan, MD {1669549309} Pedtrc(98,DOM18)<NJ-STJOSHOS>
+ St. Joseph's Family Health Center
  21 Market Street   Paterson, NJ 07501   (973)754-4200   Fax (973)754-4201

Siddiqui, Muhammad U., MD {1841619632}<NJ-ENGLWOOD>
+ Englewood Hospital and Medical Center
  350 Engle Street   Englewood, NJ 07631   (201)894-3000

Siddiqui, Nafeesa, MD {1225107121} Psychy(77,INDI)<NJ-CHILTON>
+ Drs. Siddiqui and Siddiqui
  510 Hamburg Turnpike/Suite E-106   Wayne, NJ 07470   (973)904-3161   Fax (973)904-3163

Siddiqui, Rehan, MD {1871736397} Psychy<NJ-TRININPC>
+ St Joseph's Medical Center Psychiatry
  703 Main Street   Paterson, NJ 07503   (973)754-5525

Siddiqui, Rehma, MD {1992961502} Pedtrc<NJ-STJOSHOS>
+ St. Joseph's Regional Medical Center
  703 Main Street   Paterson, NJ 07503   (973)754-2543
+ St. Joseph's Pediatrics DePaul Center
  11 Getty Avenue/2nd Floor   Paterson, NJ 07503   (973)754-2727

Siddiqui, Sabeen A., MD {1760701320} Pedtrc(03,PAK11)
+ East Windsor Pediatric Group
  300B Princeton Hightstown/Suite 201   Hightstown, NJ 08520   (609)448-7300   Fax (609)448-8022

Siddiqui, Shahida, MD {1669549655} Psychy, IntrMd(68,INA83)
+ 10 Southard Street
  Trenton, NJ 08609   (609)394-3202   Fax (609)278-6139

Siddiqui, Sheraz U., MD {1730333188} FamMed
+ UH- Robert Wood Johnson Med
  125 Paterson Street/MEB 256   New Brunswick, NJ 08901   (908)685-3732   Fax (732)235-7001

Siddiqui, Waqar Ahmed, MD {1699840314} PsyCAd, Psychy(88,PAK11)<NJ-JFKMED>
+ Behavioral Medicine Associates, P.A.
  1550 Park Avenue/Suite 102   South Plainfield, NJ 07080   (908)561-6851   Fax (908)561-6863
+ 10 Station Place/Suite 16
  Metuchen, NJ 08840   (732)494-1770

Siddiqui, Zehra, DO {1578740197} Pedtrc(01,MO79)
+ SAMRA Pediatrics
  300 Perrine Road/Suite 331   Old Bridge, NJ 08857   (732)727-8800   Fax (732)727-0955

Sidebotham, Helen Lee, MD {1245210491} RadOnc, IntrMd(93,PA02)
+ Memorial Sloan-Kettering Cancer Center Basking Ridge
  136 Mountain View Boulevard   Basking Ridge, NJ 07920   (908)542-3000   Fax (908)542-3220
  sideboth@optonline.net

Siderits, Richard H., MD {1043378805} PthACl(85,DMN01)<NJ-RWJUHAM>
+ Robert Wood Johnson University Hospital at Hamilton
  1 Hamilton Health Place   Hamilton, NJ 08690   (609)584-6741   Fax (609)584-6439

Sidhom, Ibrahim W., MD {1851301220} Hemato, MedOnc, OncHem(81,EGYP)
+ Drs. Behman & Sidhom
  48 Pulaski Avenue   Carteret, NJ 07008   (732)541-5595   Fax (732)541-1451

Sidhu, Gurpreet Singh, MD {1255641163} IntrMd(07,BLZ01)
+ Lawrence Charles Antonucci MD LLC
  415 Route 24/Suite E   Chester, NJ 07930   (908)879-1500   Fax (908)879-1515

Sidhu, Gursimar K., MD {1063651735} Anesth(07,BLZ01)
+ St. Joseph's Regional Medical Center Anesthesia
  703 Main Street   Paterson, NJ 07503   (973)754-2323   Fax (973)977-9455

Sidhu, Harpreet, MD {1346271756} Grtrcs, IntrMd(91,INA07)<NJ-UNVMCPRN, NJ-RWJUBRUN>
+ Merwick Care & Rehabilitation Center
  100 Plainsboro Road   Plainsboro, NJ 08536   (609)759-6000
+ Hamilton Continuing Care Center
  1059 Old Trenton Road   Hamilton Square, NJ 08690   (609)759-6000   Fax (609)890-7183
+ The Millhouse Nursing Home
  325 Jersey Street   Trenton, NJ 08536   (609)394-3400   Fax (609)396-5378

Sidhu, Loveleen, MD {1790707750} IntrMd, Grtrcs(95,INA82)
+ 263 Patriot Hill Drive
  Basking Ridge, NJ 07920

Sidler, Bonnie Beryl, MD {1538166368} IntrMd, EnDbMt(87,QU01)
+ The Joslin Center for Diabetes
  200 South Orange Avenue/2nd Floor   Livingston, NJ 07039   (973)322-7200   Fax (973)322-7250

Sidor, Michael Louis, MD {1851405880} SrgShr, SrgOrt, SrgArt(87,PA13)
+ New Jersey Knee & Shoulder Center
  1288 Route 73 South/Suite 100   Mount Laurel, NJ 08054   (856)273-8900   Fax (856)802-9772
  sidor@kneeandshoulder.md

Sidwa, Robert Joshua, DO {1093911893} EmrgMd
+ 29 Country Walk
  Cherry Hill, NJ 08003

Sidwa, Robert M., DO {1528090586} EmrgMd(94,PA77)<NJ-UNDRWD>
+ Inspira Health Network
  509 North Broad Street/EmergMed   Woodbury, NJ 08096   (856)845-0100

Sieber, James Curtis, MD {1477535417} Anesth(92,CT02)<NJ-MORRISTN>
+ Morristown Medical Center
  100 Madison Avenue   Morristown, NJ 07962   (973)971-5000   Fax (201)943-8733

Siebert, Charles F., Jr., MD {1285881433} Pthlgy, PthFor(92,NJ05)
+ Cape May County - Medical Examiner
  1175 Dehirsch Avenue   Woodbine, NJ 08270   (609)861-3355   Fax (609)861-5814

Siefring, Robert P., MD {1598861791} ObsGyn(80,MEX14)<NJ-VIRTMHBC>
+ Cooper Ob-Gyn
  1900 Mount Holly Road/Suite 3-C   Burlington, NJ 08016   (609)835-5570

Siegal, John D., MD {1992746630} Urolgy(82,PA01)<NJ-OVERLOOK, NJ-STBARNMC>
+ Summit Medical Group-Berkeley Heights Campus
  1 Diamond Hill Road   Berkeley Heights, NJ 07922   (908)273-4300   Fax (908)790-6524

Siegal, Scott L., DO {1164416590} CdvDis, IntrMd(90,MO78)
+ Associated Cardiovascular Consultants-Lourdes
  1 Brace Road/Suite C & F   Cherry Hill, NJ 08034   (856)428-4100   Fax (856)428-5748
+ South Jersey Heart Group
  3001 Chapel Avenue/Suite 101   Cherry Hill, NJ 08002   (856)428-4100   Fax (856)482-7170
+ South Jersey Heart Group
  539 Egg Harbor Road/Suite 1   Sewell, NJ 08034   (856)589-0300   Fax (856)589-1753

Siegel, Amy Judith, DO {1992736680} ObsGyn(97,PA77)<NJ-VIRTMHBC>
+ Penn Medicine Department of Ob/Gyn - Medford
  103 Old Marlton Pike/Suite 101   Medford, NJ 08055
+ Pinelands Obstetrics and Gynecology
  1617 Route 38   Mount Holly, NJ 08060   Fax (609)261-8622

Siegel, Amy Michele, MD {1396787388} ObsGyn(91,NY19)<NJ-VALLEY>
+ Bergen Womens HealthCare LLC
  1 Sears Drive/2 FL   Paramus, NJ 07652   (201)225-2555   Fax (201)225-2532

Siegel, Andrew L., MD {1144293499} Urolgy, IntrMd(81,IL42)
+ New Jersey Center for Prostate Cancer & Urology
  255 West Spring Valley Avenue   Maywood, NJ 07607   (201)342-6600   Fax (201)342-4222

Siegel, Arthur David, MD {1912121534} IntrMd, IntMAdMd(87,GRN01)
+ Essex Health Care
  195 First Avenue   Newark, NJ 07107   (973)483-5551   Fax (973)484-0331

Siegel, Brian Keith, MD {1477555977} Surgry, SrgCrC, SrgTrm(97,NY09)<NJ-MORRISTN, NY-WESTCHMC>
+ Morristown Medical Center
  100 Madison Avenue   Morristown, NJ 07962   (973)971-5000
  brian.siegel@atlantichealth.org

Siegel, David Samuel Dicapua, MD {1457310815} MedOnc, IntrMd, OncHem(86,NY19)<NJ-MORRISTN>
+ John Theurer Cancer Center - HUMC
  92 Second Street   Hackensack, NJ 07601   (201)336-8704   Fax (551)996-0582
  DSiegel@humed.com
+ Center for Healthy Senior Living
  360 Essex Street/Suite 401   Hackensack, NJ 07601   (201)336-8704   Fax (551)996-0543

Siegel, Eric Scott, MD {1275578262} Dermat, IntrMd(93,NY08)
+ Millburn Laser Center
  12 East Willow Street   Millburn, NJ 07041   (973)376-8500   Fax (973)376-1820

Siegel, Francine Michelle, MD {1285621078} ObsGyn(96,PA13)<NJ-VIRTMHBC, NJ-LOURDMED>
+ Advocare Burlington County Obstetrics & Gynecology
  1000 Salem Road/Suite B   Willingboro, NJ 08046   (609)871-2060   Fax (609)871-3535
+ Burlington County Ob-Gyn
  8008 Route 130 N/Suite 320   Delran, NJ 08075   (609)871-2060   Fax (856)764-0103
+ Burlington County Ob-Gyn
  210 Ark Road/Suite 216/Larchmont II   Mount Laurel, NJ 08046   (856)778-2060   Fax (856)778-8182

Siegel, Harvey P., DO {1588723746} FamMed(70,MO79)
+ Roxbury Family Primary Care
  66 Sunset Strip/Suite 400   Succasunna, NJ 07876   (973)584-9984   Fax (973)584-9954

Siegel, Howard Ira, MD {1649268129} IntrMd, Gastrn(85,NJ06)<NJ-OURLADY, NJ-VIRTUAHS>
+ Allied Gastroenterology Associates
  217 White Horse Pike   Haddon Heights, NJ 08035   (856)547-1212   Fax (856)547-6117

Siegel, Ira B., MD {1285602060} Anesth, IntrMd(84,NY48)
+ 3800 New York Avenue
  Union City, NJ 07087   (201)617-8600   Fax (216)617-8601

Siegel, Jeffrey Alan, MD {1427000728} SrgOrt(95,NY46)
+ The Orthopedic Group, P.A.
  50 Cherry Hill Road   Parsippany, NJ 07054   (973)263-2828   Fax (973)263-3243
+ Associated Orthopaedics
  654 Broadway   Bayonne, NJ 07002   (973)263-2828   Fax (201)436-8110
+ The Orthopedic Group, P.A.
  261 James Street/Suite 3-F   Morristown, NJ 07054   (973)538-0029   Fax (973)538-4957

Siegel, Jerome Harold, MD {1992735443} Gastrn, IntrMd(60,GA01)
+ Center for Endocrine Health
  1121 route 22 west/Suite 205   Bridgewater, NJ 08807   (212)734-8874   Fax (212)249-5628

Siegel, Joseph K., MD {1043266729} Gyneco(63,IL42)<NJ-MORRISTN, NJ-STCLRDEN>
+ Drs. Siegel & Siegel
  16 Pocono Road/Suite 107   Denville, NJ 07834   (973)586-8400   Fax (973)586-4206

Siegel, Mark Eric, MD {1053494021} PedCrC, Pedtrc(93,DC02)<NJ-HACKNSK>
+ Hackensack University Medical Center
  30 Prospect Avenue/Pediatrics   Hackensack, NJ 07601   (201)336-8335

Siegel, Norman H., MD {1255338323} Hemato, IntrMd, MedOnc(65,PA12)<NJ-VIRTBERL, NJ-VIRTMARL>
+ Regional Cancer Care Associates, LLC
  200 Bowman Drive/Suite E-125   Voorhees, NJ 08043   (856)424-3311   Fax (856)424-5634
+ The Center for Cancer & Hematologic Disease
  856 South White Horse Pike/Suite 4   Hammonton, NJ 08037   (856)424-3311   Fax (609)561-2492
+ The Center for Cancer & Hematologic Disease
  609 North Broad Street/Suite 300   Woodbury, NJ 08043   (856)686-1002

Siegel, Scott S., MD {1629035217} Anesth, PedAne, Pedtrc(86,PA07)<NJ-STPETER>
+ Anesthesia Consultnts of NJ/Nova Pain
  285 Davidson Avenue/Suite 204   Somerset, NJ 08873   (732)271-1400   Fax (732)271-3543

Siegel, Sheera Karch, MD {1285686626} EnDbMt, IntrMd(96,NY46)<NJ-MORRISTN>
+ Drs. Siegel and Kissin
  10 James Street/Suite 140   Florham Park, NJ 07932   (973)665-8100   Fax (973)665-8097

Siegel, Stacey, MD {1952339905} RadDia(88,NY09)<NJ-HOLYNAME>
+ Holy Name Hospital
  718 Teaneck Road/Diag Radiology   Teaneck, NJ 07666   (201)833-3000
+ University Hospital-New Jersey Medical School
  30 Bergen Street/Radiology   Newark, NJ 07107   (973)972-4511

Siegel, Stacey Beth, DO {1578504890} Gyneco(96,NY75)<NJ-STCLRDEN, NJ-MORRISTN>
+ Drs. Siegel & Siegel
  16 Pocono Road/Suite 107   Denville, NJ 07834   (973)586-8400   Fax (973)586-4206

Siegel, Wayne Douglas, MD {1063409191} Gastrn, IntrMd, Hepato(86,NY15)<NJ-CHRIST, NJ-PALISADE>
+ Ctr for Gastro and Liver Disease LLC
  255 Route 3 East/Suite 210   Secaucus, NJ 07094   (201)866-2400   Fax (201)866-0444
  hip2hep4u@aol.com
+ Ctr for Gastro and Liver Disease LLC
  214-216 Palisade Avenue   Jersey City, NJ 07306   (201)866-2400   Fax (201)866-0444

Siegel-Robles, Deborah S., MD {1821172495} IntrMd(84,MEX03)
+ Capital Health Primary Care - Princeton
  811 Exective Drive   Princeton, NJ 08540   (609)303-4600   Fax (609)303-4601

Siegel-Stein, Francine M., MD {1235233248} Pedtrc(79,NY09)
+ 497 Cumberland Street
  Englewood, NJ 07631   (201)569-1729
+ 263 Arch Road
  Englewood, NJ 07631   (201)569-1729

Siegelman, Gary M., MD {1386904159} IntrMd(86,IL11)<NJ-ACMCITY>
+ AtlantiCare Regional Medical Center/City Campus
1925 Pacific Avenue   Atlantic City, NJ 08401   (609)345-4000

Siegert, Elisabeth A., MD {1255437182} Grtrcs, IntrMd(87,NJ06)<NJ-COOPRUMC>
+ The Evergreens
309 Bridgeboro Road   Moorestown, NJ 08057   (856)439-2069   Fax (856)439-2078

Siegfried, Richard Norman, MD {1366522682} PainInvt, Anesth(87,NY08)<NJ-STCLRDOV, NJ-PALISADE>
+ 540 Lafayette Road/Second Floor
Sparta, NJ 07871   (973)746-5216   Fax (973)746-5216
info@siegfriedmd.com
+ 400 West Blackwell Street
Dover, NJ 07801   (973)746-5216   Fax (973)796-5216
+ Specialty Surgical Center
380 Lafayette Road/Suite 110   Sparta, NJ 07871   (973)940-3166   Fax (973)940-3170

Sieler, Shawn D., MD {1457446916} SrgOrt, SprtMd(91,NJ06)<NJ-CENTRAST>
+ Affiliated Orthopaedic Specialists
2186 Route 27/Suite 1A   North Brunswick, NJ 08902   (732)422-1222   Fax (732)422-3636
+ Affiliated Orthopaedic Specialists
50 Franklin Lane/Suite 102   Manalapan, NJ 07726   (732)617-9500

Sieminski, Douglas Peter, DO {1922066125} FamMed(03,NY75)
+ Skylands Medical Group PA
33 Newton-Sparta Road/Suite 1   Newton, NJ 07860   (973)383-2244   Fax (973)383-0448

Siemons, Gary O., MD {1427059930} SrgC&R, Surgry(80,VA01)<NJ-VIRTVOOR>
+ Colon & Rectal Surgical Associates of South Jersey
502 Centennial Boulevard/Suite 5   Voorhees, NJ 08043   (856)429-8030   Fax (856)428-2718

Siems, Nicole Mary, DO {1639404973} ObsGyn<NJ-UNVMCPRN>
+ Princeton Ob/Gyn
5 Plainsboro Road/Suite 500   Plainsboro, NJ 08536   (609)936-0700   Fax (609)936-0750

Siepser, Stuart L., MD {1306809314} CdvDis, IntrMd, CarNuc(68,NY19)<NJ-CHILTON>
+ Cardiology Associates of North Jersey
242 West Parkway   Pompton Plains, NJ 07444   (973)831-7455   Fax (973)831-7585

Sierocki, John S., MD {1487792354} MedOnc, IntrMd(73,PA09)<NJ-UNVMCPRN>
+ Princeton Medical Group, P.A.
419 North Harrison Street   Princeton, NJ 08540   (609)924-9300   Fax (609)924-6552
+ Princeton Medical Group PA
2 Research Way/Bldg 2/Suite 302   Monroe Township, NJ 08831   (609)924-9300   Fax (609)655-7466

Sierra, Nancy, MD {1083609846} EmrgMd, IntrMd(89,NJ06)<NJ-STMICHL>
+ St. Michael's Medical Center
111 Central Avenue/Emerg Med   Newark, NJ 07102   (973)877-5000

Sifonios, Anthony N., MD {1598906984} AnesPain
+ Rutgers- New Jersey Medical School
185 South Orange Avenue   Newark, NJ 07103   (973)972-5007

Sifri, Ziad Charles, MD {1205905031} SrgCrC, Surgry(95,QU01)<NJ-UMDNJ>
+ University Hospital
150 Bergen Street/ER/TraumaUnit   Newark, NJ 07103   (973)972-4900   Fax (973)972-7441

Sigler, Aaron Charles, DO {1215294947}<NJ-STBARNMC>
+ St. Barnabas Medical Center
94 Old Short Hills Road   Livingston, NJ 07039   (973)322-5000

Sijuwade, Atinuke Oluwaseyi, MD {1477907996} IntrMd<NJ-JRSYSHMC>
+ Jersey Shore University Medical Center
1945 Route 33   Neptune, NJ 07753   (732)776-3170

Sikand, Seema, MD {1114023041} IntrMd(96,GRN01)<NJ-COOPRUMC>
+ The Cooper Hospital System-Univ Hospital
401 Haddon Avenue/Room 282   Camden, NJ 08103   (856)342-2000
+ The Cooper Hospital System-Univ Hospital
3 Cooper Plaza/Suite 215   Camden, NJ 08103   (856)342-2439

Sikand, Vandna, MD   ObsGyn, Gyneco(FL04<NJ-CENTRAST>
+ 5 Scobeyville Drive
Colts Neck, NJ 07722   (732)580-9234   Fax (732)542-1019
vandnamd@yahoo.com

Sikand, Vikram Singh, MD {1487652251} Pedtrc, IntrMd(97,GRN01)<NJ-HOBUNIMC>
+ Hoboken University Medical Center
308 Willow Avenue   Hoboken, NJ 07030   (201)418-1000

Sikand, Vinay, MD {1568499374} IntrMd, PulDis(89,INA1Z)
+ Dover Pulmonary Associates PA
508 Lakehurst Road/Suite 1 A   Toms River, NJ 08755   (732)244-5864   Fax (732)244-3326
vinay.sikand@kentpulmonaryllc.com

Sikorski, Kristen Melissa, MD {1194792991} AlgyImmn, IntrMd(98,GRN01)
+ Princeton Allergy & Asthma Associates, P.A.
24 Vreeland Drive   Skillman, NJ 08558   (609)921-2202   Fax (609)924-1468
+ Princeton Allergy & Asthma Associates, P.A.
1245 Whitehorse Mercerville Rd   Hamilton, NJ 08619   (609)921-2202   Fax (609)924-1468
+ Princeton Allergy & Asthma Associates, P.A.
666 Plainsboro Road/Building 100-B   Plainsboro, NJ 08558   (609)799-8111   Fax (609)924-1468

Sikowitz, David J., MD {1083700306} Psychy(89,GRN01)<NJ-RIVERVW>
+ Riverview Medical Center
1 Riverview Plaza   Red Bank, NJ 07701   (732)741-2700
+ David J. Sikowitz MD
41 Reckless Place   Red Bank, NJ 07701   (732)610-0824

Silacci, John Truman, MD {1356668784}
+ Emergency Medical Associates of NJ, P.A.
3 Century Drive   Parsippany, NJ 07054   (973)740-0607   Fax (973)740-9895

Silber, Danuta, MD {1083710123} IntrMd, EnDbMt(69,POL08)<NJ-NWRKBETH, NJ-BAYONNE>
+ 740 Kennedy Boulevard
Bayonne, NJ 07002   (201)858-0848   Fax (201)858-1106

Silber, David Joseph, DO {1760748537} CdvDis
+ Hackensack University Medical Center
20 Prospect Avenue/Suite 201   Hackensack, NJ 07601   (551)996-4849

Silber, Judy G., MD {1144223686} Dermat(78,NY08)<NJ-MEADWLND>
+ Drs. Silber & Tanzer
992 Clifton Avenue   Clifton, NJ 07013   (973)365-1800   Fax (973)777-0380

Silber, Michael B., DO {1871705855} Anesth(00,PA77)<NJ-HUNTRDN>
+ Hunterdon Medical Center
2100 Wescott Drive/Anesth   Flemington, NJ 08822   (908)788-6100

Silberberg, Jeffrey M., MD {1922101161} Hemato, MedOnc, IntrMd(78,NY19)<NJ-CENTRAST, NJ-BAYSHORE>
+ Monmouth-Middlesex Hematology/Oncology
326 Professional View Drive   Freehold, NJ 07728   (732)431-8400   Fax (732)431-0114
jmsilberberg@aol.com
+ Regional Cancer Care Associates, LLC
723 North Beers Street   Holmdel, NJ 07733   (732)431-8400   Fax (732)739-4438

Silberman, Marc Richard, MD {1215964846} FamMed, FamMSptM(98,NJ06)
+ Complete Care
1814 East Second Street   Scotch Plains, NJ 07076   (908)322-6611   Fax (908)322-8665

Silberstein, Stuart L., MD {1982787321} IntrMd, PulDis(72,NY47)<NJ-HOLYNAME, NJ-ENGLWOOD>
+ S. L. Silverstein MD LLC
180 North Dean Street   Englewood, NJ 07631   (201)871-8366   Fax (201)871-8356

Silbert, Glenn R., MD {1275530404} Ophthl(79,NY01)<NJ-HACKNSK>
+ 316 State Street
Hackensack, NJ 07601   (201)342-8115   Fax (201)342-3257

Silbert, Paul J., MD {1568433993} Nrolgy(71,PA02)<NJ-JRSYSHMC>
+ 2100 Corlies Avenue/Suite 10
Neptune, NJ 07753   (732)776-8866   Fax (732)776-8550

Silbret, Lisa Michele, MD {1407968233} Dermat(95,NY46)
+ Drs. Schechter and Silbret
26 Plaza 9 Road   Manalapan, NJ 07726   (732)303-1500   Fax (732)303-0033

Silen, Ramon S., MD {1134151988} Surgry(64,PHI02)
+ Clifton Urgent Family Care
1117 Route 46 East/Suite 301   Clifton, NJ 07013   (973)779-4242   Fax (973)779-0146

Siliunas, Vytas B., DO {1275534497} Otlryg, SrgFPl, OtgyAlgy(80,IL76)<NJ-ACMCMAIN, NJ-ACMCITY>
+ South Jersey ENT Surgical Associates
2106 New Road/Unit C-9   Linwood, NJ 08221   (609)927-8881   Fax (609)927-8832

Silk, Maanasi Puranik, DO {1598929895} ObsGyn
+ AtlantiCare Physician Group
2500 English Creek Avenue   Egg Harbor Township, NJ 08234   (609)909-0200   Fax (609)909-0267

Silkov, Andrey, MD {1598922981} IntrMd<NJ-CLARMAAS>
+ Clara Maass Medical Center
1 Clara Maass Drive   Belleville, NJ 07109   (973)450-2000

Silodor, Scott W., MD {1053392258} Ophthl(90,PA02)<NJ-CHILTON>
+ Eye Associates of Wayne PA
968 Hamburg Turnpike   Wayne, NJ 07470   (973)696-0300   Fax (973)696-0465

Silva, Francisco, MD {1548529282} Pedtrc, IntrMd<NJ-MORRISTN>
+ Florham Park Pediatrics
195 Columbia Turnpike/Suite 105   Florham Park, NJ 07932   (973)437-8300   Fax (973)845-2883
+ Summit Pediatric Associates
33 Overlook Road/Suite 101   Summit, NJ 07901   (973)437-8300   Fax (908)273-1146

Silva, Lourdes G., DO {1952545840} Psychy, IntrMd(06,PA78)
+ 3 Penn Plaza East
Newark, NJ 07105   (973)364-2152   Fax (973)364-2020

Silva, Raul R., MD {1568523173} PsycCAd, Psychy, IntrMd(83,DMN01)<NY-BLVUENYU>
+ 80 Broadway/Suite 2D
Cresskill, NJ 07626   (201)218-1380
RaulSilvaMD@gmail.com

Silva, Waldemar E., MD {1740332980} IntrMd(82,MA01)<NJ-CHILTON>
+ 488 Newark Pompton Turnpike
Pompton Plains, NJ 07444   (973)835-9100   Fax (973)835-5328

Silva-Karcz, Linda, MD {1699743229} ObsGyn(00,GRN01)
+ 118 Banta Avenue
Garfield, NJ 07026

Silva-Khazaei, Maria Lourders, MD {1588646400} Nephro, IntrMd(86,DOM02)
+ 240 Williamson Street/Suite 405
Elizabeth, NJ 07207   (908)353-2064   Fax (908)353-5052

Silveira, Diosely De Castro, MD {1427223791} Nrolgy, IntrMd(83,BRA04)
+ JFK Neurosciences Institute
65 James Street/Second Floor   Edison, NJ 08818   (732)321-7950   Fax (732)632-1584

Silver, Arielle S., MD {1083623763} Rheuma
+ Arthritis, Rheumatic & Back Disease Associates
2309 East Evesham Road/Suite 101   Voorhees, NJ 08043   (856)424-5005   Fax (856)424-4716

Silver, Barry C., MD {1659343549} Dermat(72,VA04)<NJ-OVERLOOK, NJ-MORRISTN>
+ Advanced Dermatology, P.C.
33 Overlook Road/MAC 1/Suite 405   Summit, NJ 07901
+ Advanced Dermatology, P.C.
1200 East Ridgewood Avenue   Ridgewood, NJ 07450   Fax (201)493-1009

Silver, Bennett, MD {1689715294} PsycCAd, Psychy(74,NY08)<NJ-HOBUNIMC>
+ B. Silver, MD & G. Kaplan, MD, PA
535 Morris Avenue   Springfield, NJ 07081   (973)376-1020   Fax (973)376-0802

Silver, David Foster, MD {1134279052} ObsGyn, GynOnc(92,PA02)<PA-STLKBTHL, NJ-WARREN>
+ St. Luke's Cardiology Associates
755 Memorial Parkway   Phillipsburg, NJ 08865   (908)859-0514   Fax (908)859-0515

Silver, Jordan, MD {1336536705} IntHos, IntrMd(DMN01)<NJ-ACMCITY>
+ AtlantiCare Regional Medical Center/City Campus
1925 Pacific Avenue/Hospitalist   Atlantic City, NJ 08401   (609)441-8146   Fax (609)441-8002

Silver, Seth M., MD {1750381521} SprtMd, SrgOrt(83,DC02)
+ Reconstructive Orthopedics
994 West Sherman Avenue   Vineland, NJ 08360   (609)267-9400   Fax (609)267-9457

Silver, Stephen G., MD {1932293255} SrgOrt(94,NY09)<NY-LENOXHLL, NY-BETHPETR>
+ Active Orthopaedics & Sports Medicine
25 Prospect Avenue   Hackensack, NJ 07601   (201)343-2277   Fax (201)343-7410

Silver, Steven Eric, MD {1114970225} CdvDis(97,PA02)<NJ-OURLADY, NJ-COOPRUMC>
+ Cardiovascular Associates of The Delaware Valley, PA
1840 Frontage Road   Cherry Hill, NJ 08034   (856)795-2227   Fax (856)795-7436
+ Cardiovascular Associates
210 West Atlantic Avenue   Haddon Heights, NJ 08035   (856)795-2227   Fax (856)547-5337
+ Cardiovascular Associates of The Delaware Valley, PA
525 State Street/Suite 3   Elmer, NJ 08034   (856)358-2363   Fax (856)358-0725

Silverberg, Fred Marshall, MD {1922055201} ObsGyn(80,VA04)<NJ-MORRISTN>
+ 33 Main Street/Suite 200
Chatham, NJ 07928   (973)635-2299   Fax (973)635-8187

Physicians by Name and Address

Silverberg, Michael S., MD {1699770412} GenPrc, FamMed(73,NY08)
+ The Doctor Is in
  59 Old Highway 22 Clinton, NJ 08809 (908)730-6363 Fax (908)730-8185

Silverberg, Miriam Shayna, MD {1487620522} Rheuma, IntrMd(98,ON01)
+ Rheumatology Associates of North Jersey, PA
  1415 Queen Anne Road Teaneck, NJ 07666 (201)837-7788 Fax (201)837-2077
+ Rheumatology Associates of North Jersey, PA
  420 Grand Avenue Englewood, NJ 07631 (201)837-7788 Fax (201)837-2077
+ Rheumatology Associates of North Jersey, PA
  8305A Bergenline Avenue North Bergen, NJ 07666 (201)837-7788 Fax (201)837-2077

Silverbrook, Robert M., DO {1083665558} IntrMd(85,MO78)<NJ-RWJUHAM, NJ-CHSMRCER>
+ 606 A North Victoria Avenue
  Ventnor City, NJ 08406 (609)334-4445
+ Robert Wood Johnson University Hospital at Hamilton
  1 Hamilton Health Place Hamilton, NJ 08690 (609)586-7900

Silverman, Abby Robin, MD {1659471381} Pedtrc(97,NY48)<NJ-STBARNMC, NJ-ATLANTHS>
+ The Pediatric Group of West Orange, PA
  395 Pleasant Valley Way West Orange, NJ 07052 (973)731-6100

Silverman, Brian S., DO {1487617726} EmrgMd(79,PA77)<NJ-HOLYNAME>
+ Holy Name Hospital
  718 Teaneck Road/EmergMed Teaneck, NJ 07666 (201)833-3000

Silverman, Cary M., MD {1124011325} Ophthl(82,NJ05)<NJ-STBARNMC, NJ-UMDNJ>
+ Parsippany Eye Care Associates
  46 Eagle Rock Avenue East Hanover, NJ 07936 (973)560-1500 Fax (973)560-0419

Silverman, Farrel Keith, DO {1063708436}
+ Rowan University-School of Osteopathic Medicine
  1 Medical Center Drive Stratford, NJ 08084 (856)566-6708
+ Virtua Primary Care
  1201 New Road/Suite 150a Linwood, NJ 08221 (609)788-3338

Silverman, Jesse A., MD {1619991304} SrgOrt(73,NJ05)
+ 33 Oak Lane
  Mountain Lakes, NJ 07046

Silverman, Lawrence Andrew, MD {1336113653} PedEnd(87,NJ06)<NJ-MORRISTN, NJ-OVERLOOK>
+ Morristown Medical Center
  100 Madison Avenue/Box 53 Morristown, NJ 07962 (973)971-4340 Fax (973)290-7367

Silverman, Mathew Joshua, DO {1043271984} IntrMd(98,PA77)
+ Drs. Silverman and Silverman
  480 Market Street Saddle Brook, NJ 07663 (201)845-4048 Fax (201)845-3982

Silverman, Michael Evan, MD {1114976412} IntrMd, EmrgMd(93,NY09)<NJ-MORRISTN>
+ Morristown Medical Center
  100 Madison Avenue/EmrgMed Morristown, NJ 07962 (800)290-5309 Fax (803)434-4354

Silverman, Mitchell S., MD {1043378292} EnDbMt, IntrMd(80,NC07)<NY-STBARNAB, NJ-NWRKBETH>
+ Summit Medical Group
  75 East Northfield Road Livingston, NJ 07039 (973)436-1450 Fax (908)964-5718

Silverman, Philip, DO {1710941190} IntrMd(72,MO79)<NJ-HACKNSK>
+ Drs. Silverman and Silverman
  480 Market Street Saddle Brook, NJ 07663 (201)845-4048 Fax (201)845-3982

Silverman, Robert S., MD {1881759169} Anesth, PainMd, AnesPain(93,OH44)<NJ-VALLEY>
+ Valley Institute for Pain
  One Valley Health Plaza/3 FL Paramus, NJ 07652 (201)634-5555 Fax (201)634-5454
+ The Valley Hospital
  223 North Van Dien Avenue/Anesth Ridgewood, NJ 07450 (201)447-8000

Silverman, Russell V., DO {1013170083} FamMed, GPrvMd(70,PA77)
+ 110 East Maryland Avenue
  Somers Point, NJ 08244

Silverman, Warren, MD {1831203991} OccpMd, IntrMd, OthrSp(78,NY03)
+ Access Health Systems
  622 Georges Road North Brunswick, NJ 08902 (732)951-8000

Silvers, Lawrence W., MD {1932142098} SrgVas, Surgry(76,NY03)<NJ-KIMBALL, NJ-COMMED>
+ Lakewood Surgical Group PA
  901 West Main Street/Suite 107 Freehold, NJ 07728 (732)363-0044 Fax (732)905-5845
+ Lakewood Surgical Group
  9 Hospital Drive Toms River, NJ 08755 (732)363-0044 Fax (732)341-4338

Silverstein, Gary S., MD {1942207030} RadDia(78,NY03)<NJ-STFRNMED>
+ Radiology Affiliates of Central New Jersey, P.A.
  2501 Kuser Road Hamilton, NJ 08691 (609)585-8800 Fax (609)585-1825
+ St. Francis Medical Center
  601 Hamilton Avenue/Radiology Trenton, NJ 08629 (609)599-5000

Silverstein, Jeffrey I., MD {1871530170} Urolgy(85,NY08)<NJ-BAYSHORE>
+ 495 Iron Bridge Road
  Freehold, NJ 07728 (732)683-1617 Fax (732)683-1619
+ 565 Highway 35
  Red Bank, NJ 07701 (732)933-1800

Silverstein, Leonard, MD {1639138571} Allrgy, PedAlg(87,NC07)
+ Allergy and Asthma Specialists
  82 East Allendale Road/Suite 7-B Saddle River, NJ 07458 (201)236-8282 Fax (201)236-0138
+ Allergy and Asthma Specialists
  51 State Route 23 Riverdale, NJ 07457 (201)236-8282 Fax (973)831-7422

Silverstein, Mark Michael, MD {1962518084} Anesth(79,ITAL)<NJ-COMMED>
+ Community Medical Center
  99 Route 37 West/Anesth Toms River, NJ 08755 (732)557-8000

Silverstein, Michael P., MD {1255587366} Nrolgy
+ Hackensack Neurology Group
  211 Essex Street/Suite 202 Hackensack, NJ 07601 (201)488-1515 Fax (201)488-9471

Silverstein, Niki A., MD {1669478731} Ophthl(77,NY08)
+ Silverstein Eye Group
  408 Main Street Chester, NJ 07930 (908)879-7297 Fax (908)879-4798

Silverstein, Rodger H., MD {1063418192} Ophthl(78,NY09)
+ 198 North Road
  Chester, NJ 07930 (908)879-7297

Silverstein, Wendy Beth, MD {1336108422} Anesth(86,NY19)<NJ-VALLEY, NY-PRSBCOLU>
+ The Valley Hospital
  223 North Van Dien Avenue Ridgewood, NJ 07450 (201)847-9403 Fax (201)847-0059

Sim, Andrew R., MD {1912295122} Anesth(11,GRN01)
+ Morris Anesthesia Group, PA
  3799 Route 46/Suite 211 Parsippany, NJ 07054 (973)335-1122 Fax (973)335-1448

Sim, Herena, MD {1104909167} IntrMd(94,NJ06)<NJ-VALLEY>
+ Valley Diagnostic Medical Center
  581 North Franklin Turnpike Ramsey, NJ 07446 (201)327-0500 Fax (201)327-8612

Sim, Sang Eui, MD {1902845464} RadOnc, IntrMd, Radiol(97,NJ06)<NJ-MONMOUTH>
+ Monmouth Medical Center
  300 Second Avenue Long Branch, NJ 07740 (732)923-6890 Fax (732)923-6896

Sim, Vasiliy, MD {1093141780} Surgry<NY-BROOKDAL>
+ University Hospital-RWJ Medical School
  89 French Street/Rm 3265 New Brunswick, NJ 08901 (732)828-3000

Simandl, Susan Lynn, MD {1831130079} CdvDis, IntrMd(87,NJ06)<NY-VANORTH>
+ The Heart Group, PA
  161 Millburn Avenue Millburn, NJ 07041 (973)467-4220 Fax (973)467-9889

Simela, Tanasha, DO {1538321997} Dermat
+ Dermatology & Laser Center of Northern New Jersey
  347 Mount Pleasant Avenue/Suite 205 West Orange, NJ 07052 (973)571-2121 Fax (973)498-0569

Simigiannis, Helen, MD {1366497265} ObsGyn, Obstet(99,DMN01)
+ Antheia Gynecology
  375 US Highway 130/Suite 103 East Windsor, NJ 08520 (609)448-7800 Fax (609)448-7880

Simkhayev, Lev Samsonovi, MD {1578563243} IntrMd(81,RUS15)<NJ-RBAYOLDB>
+ 758 State Route 18/Suite 103-B
  East Brunswick, NJ 08816 (732)360-9996 Fax (732)360-1141

Simmerano, Rocco Anthony, MD {1518973296} SrgOrt(99,NJ05)<NJ-STCLRDEN, NJ-STCLRSUS>
+ Morris County Orthopaedic Group
  109 US Highway 46 East Denville, NJ 07834 (973)625-1221 Fax (973)625-1594

Simmers, Richard C., DO {1831337013} Pedtrc(69,PA77)
+ St. Christopher Care at Washington Township
  405 Hurffville-Cross Keys Road Sewell, NJ 08080 (856)582-0033 Fax (856)582-2305

Simmers-Dabinett, Donna Lee, DO {1841215340} EmrgMd(02,PA77)<NJ-KMHSTRAT>
+ Kennedy Memorial Hospital-University Medical Center
  18 East Laurel Road/EmrgMed Stratford, NJ 08084 (856)346-7816 Fax (856)346-6385

Simmons, Marc Z., MD {1841208386} RadDia(86,NY15)<NJ-UMDNJ>
+ Memorial Sloan-Kettering Cancer Center Basking Ridge
  136 Mountain View Boulevard Basking Ridge, NJ 07920 (908)542-3000 Fax (908)542-3220

Simoes, Sonia C., MD {1346406600} IntrMd(04,DMN01)
+ University Renal and Hypertension Consultants LLC
  390 New York Avenue Newark, NJ 07105 (973)755-1585 Fax (973)344-3525

Simoes De Carvalho, Victor L., MD {1164408613} Radiol, RadDia(90,KS02)<NJ-RWJUBRUN, NJ-STPETER>
+ University Radiology Group, P.C.
  483 Cranbury Road East Brunswick, NJ 08816 (732)390-0030 Fax (732)390-5383
+ University Radiology Group, P.C.
  579A Cranbury Road East Brunswick, NJ 08816 (732)390-0030 Fax (732)390-1856
+ University Radiology Group, P.C.
  10 Plum Street New Brunswick, NJ 08816 (732)249-4410 Fax (732)249-1208

Simon, Abraham M., DO {1669686044} Anesth, PedAne(03,NY75)
+ Anesthesia Consultnts of NJ/Nova Pain
  285 Davidson Avenue/Suite 204 Somerset, NJ 08873 (732)271-1400 Fax (732)271-3543

Simon, Alan David, MD {1316946270} IntCrd, CdvDis, FamMSptM(90,NY19)<NJ-VALLEY>
+ Valley Medical Goup Cardioology Ridgewood
  1124 East Ridgewood Avenue Ridgewood, NJ 07450 (201)689-9400 Fax (201)689-9404

Simon, Andrew L., MD {1992767388} Urolgy(82,NY09)<NJ-OCEANMC, NJ-JRSYSHMC>
+ 459 Jack Martin Boulevard/Suite 3
  Brick, NJ 08724 (732)840-0900 Fax (732)840-0912
+ 900 Route 70
  Lakewood, NJ 08701

Simon, Clifford J., MD {1487668299} IntrMd, PulDis(73,NY20)<NJ-ENGLWOOD, NJ-HOLYNAME>
+ Bergen Medical Alliance, P.A.
  180 Engle Street Englewood, NJ 07631 (201)567-2050 Fax (201)568-8936

Simon, Daniel Ross, MD {1619135738} Urolgy(05,NJ05)<NJ-HOLYNAME, NJ-ENGLWOOD>
+ The Urology Center of Englewood, PA
  663 Palisade Avenue/Suite 304 Cliffside Park, NJ 07010 (201)313-1933 Fax (201)313-9599
+ The Urology Center of Englewood, PA
  300 Grand Avenue/Suite 102 Englewood, NJ 07631 (201)313-1933 Fax (201)816-1777

Simon, Daniel W., MD {1013997428} RadDia, RadV&I(91,NY46)
+ Edison Radiology Group, P.A.
  65 James Street Edison, NJ 08820 (732)321-7917 Fax (732)737-2968

Simon, Eddy, MD {1851385058} IntrMd(86,MEXI)
+ 2091 Millburn Avenue/Suite 401
  Maplewood, NJ 07040 (973)275-1970 Fax (973)275-1971
+ JFK Medical Center
  65 James Street Edison, NJ 08820 (973)275-1970 Fax (732)744-5614

Simon, Egbert A., MD {1699864439} IntrMd, EmrgMd(83,CUBA)<NJ-HOBUNIMC, NJ-BAYSHORE>
+ IPC The Hospitalist Company
  55 Madison Avenue/Suite 310 Morristown, NJ 07960 (973)993-9536 Fax (973)998-4237

Simon, Elisabeth M., MD {1649360405} Pedtrc, AdolMd(90,DMN01)<NJ-RWJUBRUN, NJ-STPETER>
+ Mid Jersey Pediatrics
  33 Brunswick Woods Drive East Brunswick, NJ 08816 (732)257-4330 Fax (732)257-1177

Simon, Elizabeth R., DO {1467788703} IntrMd
+ Riverside Medical Group
  6045 Kennedy Boulevard/Suite A North Bergen, NJ 07047 (201)861-4443 Fax (201)861-0941

Simon, Jeffrey Hayden, MD {1861651077} Psychy, PsyCAd, PsyAdd(03,NSKT)
+ 800 Kings Highway North/Suite 506
  Cherry Hill, NJ 08003 (856)685-6510 Fax (856)382-7695

Simon, Jessica, MD {1659651099} Dermat
+ Windsor Dermatology
  59 One Mile Road Extension/Suite G East Windsor, NJ 08520 (609)443-4500 Fax (609)426-0530

Simon, Jonathan M., MD {1578626636} Rheuma, IntrMd(78,NY19)<NJ-MTNSIDE>
+ 1018 Broad Street
  Bloomfield, NJ 07003 (973)338-3383 Fax (973)338-1177

Simon, Marc L., DO {1619013778} Surgry(78,PA77)
+ 16 Pocono Road/Suite 311
 Denville, NJ 07834 (973)627-4227 Fax (973)729-0003
Simon, Michael J., MD {1538185657} IntrMd(89,NJ06)<NJ-STPETER, NJ-RWJUBRUN>
+ Carepoint Health Medical Group
 53 Main Street Sayreville, NJ 08872 (732)254-6200 Fax (732)254-7803
Simon, Mitchell Lyle, MD {1225014780} RadDia, PedRad(98,PA09)<NJ-RWJUBRUN, NJ-STPETER>
+ University Radiology Group, P.C.
 483 Cranbury Road East Brunswick, NJ 08816 (732)390-0030 Fax (732)390-5383
+ University Radiology Group, P.C.
 10 Plum Street New Brunswick, NJ 08901 (732)390-0030 Fax (732)249-1208
+ University Radiology Group, P.C.
 16 Mountain Boulevard Warren, NJ 08816 (908)769-7200 Fax (908)769-9141
Simon, Paul J., DO {1417908468} Pthlgy, PthAClˈ(82,IL76)<NJ-COMMED, NJ-KIMBALL>
+ Community Medical Center
 99 Route 37 West/Path Toms River, NJ 08755 (732)557-8000
Simon, Purabi Mehta, DO {1073566469} EmrgMd(02,NY75)
+ Pathlink, LLC
 66 West Gilbert Street/Suite 100 Tinton Falls, NJ 07701 (732)212-0060 Fax (732)212-0061
Simon, Richard M., DO {1932206349} FamMed(63,PA77)<NJ-VIRTVOOR, NJ-KMHSTRAT>
+ Wolfe-Simon Associates
 511 Kings Highway North Cherry Hill, NJ 08034 (856)667-1654 Fax (856)482-8057
Simon, Riya Jose, DO {1740570688} EmrgMd<NJ-STPETER>
+ St. Peter's University Hospital
 254 Easton Avenue New Brunswick, NJ 08901 (732)745-8600
+ JFK Medical Center
 65 James Street Edison, NJ 08820 (732)745-8600 Fax (732)744-5614
Simon, Robert B., MD {1992901052} Urolgy(01,NJ05)<NJ-ENGLWOOD, NJ-HOLYNAME>
+ The Urology Center of Englewood, PA
 663 Palisade Avenue/Suite 304 Cliffside Park, NJ 07010 (201)313-1933 Fax (201)313-9599
+ The Urology Center of Englewood, PA
 300 Grand Avenue/Suite 102 Englewood, NJ 07631 (201)313-1933 Fax (201)816-1777
Simon, Robert T., MD {1538242037} IntrMd(86,NJ05)
+ 20 Hospital Drive/Suite 8
 Toms River, NJ 08755 (732)281-0530 Fax (732)281-0534
Simon, Segun V., MD {1194956490} Nephro, IntrMd<NJ-NWRKBETH, NJ-CLARMAAS>
+ 2130 Millburn Avenue/Suite C-3
 Maplewood, NJ 07040 (973)996-2727 Fax (973)763-2558
Simon, Shari Kim, DO {1104992825} IntrMd(91,IA75)
+ Patient first
 606 Cross Keys Road Sicklerville, NJ 08081 (856)237-1016
Simon, Susan M. C., MD {1093704777} IntrMd(96,MA05)<NJ-OVERLOOK>
+ Summit Medical Group
 560 Springfield Avenue Westfield, NJ 07090 (908)228-3610
Simone, Charles B., MD {1821019662} RadOnc, MedOnc, Nutrtn(75,NJ06)
+ 123 Franklin Corner Road/Suite 108
 Lawrenceville, NJ 08648 (609)896-2646 Fax (609)885-1515
Simone, Jill B., MD {1558515395} Pedtrc(73,MEX14)
+ NJ Dept of Human Services/Ofc of Managed Health Care
 PO Box 712/MedAssistance Trenton, NJ 08625 (609)588-2705
Simone, Philip M., MD {1952372468} FamMed(97,NJ06)<NJ-JRSYSHMC>
+ Toms River Family Medical Center PA
 1028 Hooper Avenue Toms River, NJ 08753 (732)349-8866
Simonetti, John M., MD {1396850665} ObsGyn(92,NJ05)
+ Millburn Ob-Gyn Associates, P.A.
 233 Millburn Avenue Millburn, NJ 07041 (973)467-9440 Fax (973)467-2567
+ Short Hills Surgery Center
 187 Millburn Avenue/Suite 101 Millburn, NJ 07041 (973)467-9440 Fax (973)671-0557
Simonetti, Michael, MD {1306073218} EmrgMd(05,NY08)<NJ-VALLEY>
+ The Valley Hospital
 223 North Van Dien Avenue Ridgewood, NJ 07450 (201)447-8000
Simonian, Armen John, MD {1972566263} Gastrn, IntrMd(91,NJ06)<NJ-CHSMRCER>
+ Mercer Gastroenterology
 2 Capital Way/Suite 487 Pennington, NJ 08534 (609)818-1900 Fax (609)818-1908
Simonian, Carla Daria, MD {1649238528} ObsGyn(96,PA09)<NJ-HACKNSK>
+ Bergen Surgical Specialists
 20 Prospect Avenue/Suite 707 Hackensack, NJ 07601 (201)343-0040 Fax (201)343-2733
Simonian, Gregory T., MD {1528017944} SrgVas, Surgry(92,NJ05)
+ Bergen Surgical Specialists
 20 Prospect Avenue/Suite 707 Hackensack, NJ 07601 (201)343-0040 Fax (201)343-2733
+ Bergen Surgical Specialists/Hackensack Vascular
 211 Essex Street/Suite 102 Hackensack, NJ 07601 (201)343-0040 Fax (201)487-0943
Simons, Grant Russell, MD {1568532927} CdvDis, OthrSp, ClCdEl(90,NC07)<NJ-ENGLWOOD>
+ North Jersey Electrophysiology Associates
 20 Prospect Avenue/Suite 615 Hackensack, NJ 07601 (201)472-3627 Fax (201)518-8739
+ Englewood Hospital and Medical Center
 350 Engle Street/CardElectrophys Englewood, NJ 07631 (201)894-3000
+ Heart and Vascular Institute at EHMC
 350 Engle Street/Suite 1000 Englewood, NJ 07601 (201)894-3636
Simons, Robert Mark, MD {1194821967} Surgry(91,PA02)<NJ-COOPRUMC>
+ The Cooper Hospital System-Univ Hospital
 3 Cooper Plaza/Suite 215 Camden, NJ 08103 (856)342-2439 Fax (856)365-1180
+ Cooper Surgical Associates
 3 Cooper Plaza/Suite 411 Camden, NJ 08103 (856)342-2439 Fax (856)365-1180
Simonson, Leslie J., MD {1831262252} FamMed, FamMAdlt(87,PHIL)<NJ-MEADWLND, NJ-OVERLOOK>
+ 415 43rd Street
 Union City, NJ 07087 (201)583-1600 Fax (201)583-1114
Simonson, Marc H., MD {1902973589} RadDia(82,PHI18)
+ Diagnostic Medical Imaging of NJ
 415 43rd Street Union City, NJ 07087 (201)867-9002 Fax (201)867-2004
Simotas, Christopher J., MD {1932351137} Pedtrc(04,NJ05)<NJ-UMDNJ>
+ UMDNJ Human Genetics Center
 90 Bergen Street/DOC 5400 Newark, NJ 07101 (973)972-3300
Simpkins, Nancy M., MD {1891876280} IntrMd(84,IL42)<NJ-STBARNMC>
+ 124 East Mount Pleasant Avenue
 Livingston, NJ 07039 (973)992-6864 Fax (973)992-8005
Simpson, Alan J., MD {1093728412} Radiol, NuclMd, RadDia(68,NC05)<NJ-ACMCITY, NJ-ACMCMAIN>
+ Atlantic Medical Imaging, LLC.
 72 West Jimmie Leeds Road Galloway, NJ 08205 (609)677-9729 Fax (609)653-8764
+ Atlantic Medical Imaging, LLC.
 401 Bethel Road Somers Point, NJ 08244 (609)677-9729
+ Atlantic Medical Imaging, LLC.
 421 Route 9 North Cape May Court House, NJ 08205 (609)463-9500 Fax (609)465-0918
Simpson, Alyson Beth, MD {1538288162} Pedtrc(04,IL06)<NJ-VIRTVOOR>
+ Virtua Voorhees
 100 Bowman Drive Voorhees, NJ 08043 (856)247-3000
Simpson, Thomas E., MD {1326139007} Surgry, SrgAbd, SrgC&R(76,NY19)<NJ-BAYONNE, NJ-CHRIST>
+ 124 West 32nd Street
 Bayonne, NJ 07002 (201)339-2332 Fax (201)339-2465
Simpson, Timothy E., MD {1255469904} CdvDis(88,NY08)
+ Cardiac Medical Associates PA
 920 Main Street Hackensack, NJ 07601 (201)342-7733 Fax (201)342-7998
Sinatra, Frank A., MD {1306894274} GenPrc, Pedtrc(83,MONT)<NJ-MORRISTN, NJ-OVERLOOK>
+ Advocare Sinatra & Peng Pediatrics
 169 Minebrook Road Bernardsville, NJ 07924 (908)766-0034 Fax (908)766-5065
Sinatra, Melanie A., MD {1043245954} Ophthl(91,NY08)<NJ-VALLEY>
+ Drs. The & Sinatra
 348 Summit Avenue Hackensack, NJ 07601 (201)343-9300
Sinclair, George Lawrence, III, MD {1225437031}
+ Center for Neurological Surgery UMDNJ
 90 Bergen Street/DOC 8100 Newark, NJ 07103 (973)972-7404 Fax (973)972-2333
Sinclair, Melissa Renee, DO {1285977025} Pedtrc
+ Somerset Pediatric Group PA
 2 World's Fair Drive/Suite 302 Somerset, NJ 08873 (732)271-7788 Fax (732)271-5151
Sindoni, Frank W., MD {1689724395} ObsGyn(78,NJ05)<NJ-SHOREMEM>
+ Atlantic Cape Ob/Gyn
 829 Shore Road Somers Point, NJ 08244 (609)927-3070 Fax (609)927-2553
Sinensky, Gary B., MD {1376585067} Gastrn, IntrMd(78,NY46)<NJ-HOBUNIMC>
+ 24-28 Merchant Street
 Newark, NJ 07105 (973)344-4787 Fax (973)344-3755
Singal, Dinesh K., MD {1548266125} CdvDis, IntrMd, IntCrd(83,INA30)<NJ-RWJUBRUN, NJ-STPETER>
+ Cardio Metabolic Institute
 51 Veronica Avenue Somerset, NJ 08873 (732)846-7000 Fax (732)846-7001
+ Cardio Metabolic Institute
 294 Applegarth Road/Suite F Monroe Township, NJ 08831 (732)846-7000 Fax (732)846-7001
Singal, Presh, MD {1609861301} IntrMd(99,DMN01)
+ NJ VA/James J Howard Outpatient Clinic
 970 Route 70 West Brick, NJ 08724 (732)206-8900
Singer, Beth Carol, MD {1033182514} Pedtrc(98,NY19)<NJ-OVERLOOK, NJ-MORRISTN>
+ Summit Medical Group
 34 Mountain Boulevard/Building B Warren, NJ 07059 (908)769-0100 Fax (908)769-8927
+ Summit Medical Group-Berkeley Heights Campus
 1 Diamond Hill Road Berkeley Heights, NJ 07922 (908)769-0100 Fax (908)790-6576
Singer, Eileen M., DO {1538191432} EmrgMd(81,IA75)<NJ-VIRTVOOR>
+ Virtua Voorhees
 100 Bowman Drive/EmrgMed Voorhees, NJ 08043 (856)247-3000
Singer, Elizabeth Kara, MD {1669418703} EmrgMd, IntrMd(94,NY08)<NJ-ENGLWOOD>
+ Englewood Hospital and Medical Center
 350 Engle Street/EmrgMed Englewood, NJ 07631 (201)894-3440 Fax (201)894-3446
Singer, Eric Alan, MD {1144334467} Urolgy(03,DC02)
+ Robert Wood Johnson-UMDNJ Anesthesia Group
 125 Paterson Street/CAB 3100 New Brunswick, NJ 08901 (732)235-7827 Fax (732)235-6131
Singer, Judith C. J., MD {1750467593} Anesth(93,NY08)<NJ-HOLYNAME>
+ Bergen Anesthesia Associates
 718 Teaneck Road Teaneck, NJ 07666 (201)833-7149 Fax (201)342-1259
+ Holy Name Hospital
 718 Teaneck Road/Anesthesiology Teaneck, NJ 07666 (201)833-3000
Singer, Mark Andrew, MD {1235136789} RadDia, Radiol(92,NJ06)
+ Doctors Radiology Center - MRI of Woodbridge
 1500 St. George Avenue/Peach Plaza Avenel, NJ 07001 (732)574-1414 Fax (732)574-0845
+ Coastal Imaging, LLC
 79 Route 37 West/Suite 103 Toms River, NJ 08755 (732)574-1414 Fax (732)276-2325
+ Red Bank Radiologists, P.A.
 200 White Road/Suite 115 Little Silver, NJ 07001 (732)741-9595 Fax (732)741-0985
Singer, Robert A., MD {1396716825} CdvDis, IntrMd(87,NY08)<NJ-ACMCMAIN, NJ-OURLADY>
+ Virtua Cardiology Group
 2309 East Evesham Road/Suites 201-202 Voorhees, NJ 08043 (856)325-5400 Fax (856)325-5416
Singer, Roberto, MD {1982604864} IntrMd, Nephro(68,ARG01)<NJ-HOLYNAME, NJ-VALLEY>
+ Holy Name Hospital
 718 Teaneck Road Teaneck, NJ 07666 (201)833-3223 Fax (201)833-7090
+ Renal Medicine Associates PA
 302 Union Street Hackensack, NJ 07601 (201)833-3223 Fax (201)646-0365
Singer, Samuel, MD {1083871933} Nrolgy(07,NY46)<NY-PRSBWEIL>
+ John Theurer Cancer Center - HUMC
 92 Second Street Hackensack, NJ 07601 (201)996-5900 Fax (201)996-9246
Singer-Granick, Carol Joyce, MD {1538185871} Pedtrc, PedEnd(78,MA05)<NJ-UMDNJ>
+ Rutgers- New Jersey Medical School
 185 South Orange Avenue/Pedi/MSBF 576 Newark, NJ 07103 (973)972-2189 Fax (973)972-1565
 singercj@umdnj.edu
Singh, Ajay B., MD {1518417203} IntrMd, Nephro(83,PA02)<NJ-UNVMCPRN>
+ 6 Bradford Court
 West Windsor, NJ 08550
Singh, Amandeep, MD {1922356898} IntrMd
+ United Medical, P.C.
 988 Broadway/Suite 201 Bayonne, NJ 07002 (201)339-6111 Fax (201)339-6333

Physicians by Name and Address

Singh, Amita, MD {1316153844} Pedtrc(92,INA3C)<NJ-STMICHL>
+ Oak Tree Pediatrics
  111 Park Avenue/2ns Floor   Plainfield, NJ 07060   (908)753-2671   Fax (908)753-1245

Singh, Amrinder, MD {1174963078} Nrolgy
+ JFK Neurosciences Institute
  65 James Street/Second Floor   Edison, NJ 08818   (732)321-7010   Fax (732)632-1584

Singh, Amrita Kaur, MD {1740457324} IntrMd
+ Heart & Vascular Associates of Northern Jersey
  22-18 Broadway/Suite 201   Fair Lawn, NJ 07410   (201)475-5050   Fax (201)475-5522

Singh, Anil Kumar, MD {1023214897} IntrMd(05,PAK11)<NJ-NWRKBETH>
+ Newark Beth Israel Medical Center
  201 Lyons Avenue/Internal Med   Newark, NJ 07112   (973)926-2164

Singh, Anita J., MD {1033347018} EmrgMd, IntrMd(GRN01)<NJ-OVERLOOK>
+ Summit Medical Group-Berkeley Heights Campus
  1 Diamond Hill Road   Berkeley Heights, NJ 07922   (908)277-8880   Fax (908)790-6576

Singh, Anup, MD {1245225242} PedNph, Pedtrc(85,PHI32)<NY-STATNRTH, NY-STATNSTH>
+ The Children's Hospital at Saint Peter's University
  254 Easton Avenue   New Brunswick, NJ 08901   (732)565-5489

Singh, Archana, MD {1902139561} PedPul<NJ-STPETER>
+ St. Peter's University Hospital
  254 Easton Avenue   New Brunswick, NJ 08901   (732)745-8600   Fax (732)214-0314

Singh, Arun J., DO {1649367566} EmrgMd(95,NJ75)<NJ-COMMED>
+ EmCare
  425 Jack Martin Boulevard   Brick, NJ 08724   (732)840-3380

Singh, Avtar, MD {1568547677} IntrMd, PulDis(74,INA29)
+ Drs. Singh & Farhangfar
  401 Hamburg Turnpike/Suite 109   Wayne, NJ 07470   (973)595-7456   Fax (973)904-9119

Singh, Bharat, MD {1245295922} CdvDis, IntrMd(72,INDI)
+ Drs. DiGioia & Singh
  1971 Kennedy Boulevard   Jersey City, NJ 07305   (201)432-5222   Fax (201)333-2503

Singh, Bikramjit, MD {1033156591} Nephro, Hypten, IntrMd(92,INA5Z)<NJ-RBAYPERT, NJ-RBAYOLDB>
+ Carteret Medical Center
  606 Roosevelt Avenue   Carteret, NJ 07008   (732)541-6521   Fax (732)541-0060
+ North Edison Family Practice Group
  35-37 Progress Street/Suite A-3   Edison, NJ 08820   (732)541-6521   Fax (908)668-4848

Singh, Chandandeep, MD {1992264782} IntrMd<NJ-MORRISTN>
+ Morristown Medical Center
  100 Madison Avenue   Morristown, NJ 07962   (973)971-5000

Singh, Chetna, MD {1144246273} EmrgMd(94,INA49)<NJ-COMMED>
+ Community Medical Center
  99 Route 37 West/Emerg Med   Toms River, NJ 08755   (732)557-8000

Singh, David, MD {1962655654} RadDia(03,NY15)<NJ-CHRIST, NJ-HOLYNAME>
+ Christ Hospital
  176 Palisade Avenue   Jersey City, NJ 07306   (518)852-8114
  dsinghmd@hotmail.com

Singh, Gagandeep, MD {1629252614} Psychy, PsyCAd(04,NJ06)
+ 43 Linwood Drive
  Monroe Township, NJ 08831

Singh, Harmeet, MD {1639197437} IntrMd, CritCr, PulDis(82,INA9B)
+ 1 West Ridgewood Avenue/Suite 108
  Paramus, NJ 07652
  H.Singh@yahoo.com

Singh, Harshpal, MD {1437317567} SrgNro<NY-MTSINAI, NY-MTSINYHS>
+ North Jersey Brain and Surgical
  680 Kinderkamack Road/Suite 300   Oradell, NJ 07649   (201)342-2550   Fax (201)342-7171

Singh, Iqbal K., MD {1558456608} IntrMd(76,INA40)
+ Drs. Singh & Singh
  19 Holly Street/Suite 8   Cranford, NJ 07016   (908)276-3132   Fax (908)931-0842

Singh, Ishita, MD {1760773352} EnDbMt
+ St. Luke's Diabetes & Endocrinology
  755 Memorial Parkway/Suite 302 A   Phillipsburg, NJ 08865   (484)526-7200   Fax (866)449-5832

Singh, Jagjeet, MD {1740456755} Anesth, PainMd, PhyMSptM(05,GRN01)
+ Morris Anesthesia Group, PA
  3799 Route 46/Suite 211   Parsippany, NJ 07054   (973)335-1122   Fax (973)335-1448

Singh, Jasvinder, MD {1003867219} Ophthl(69,INA72)<NJ-OVERLOOK>
+ The Eye Center
  3900 Park Avenue/Suite 106   Edison, NJ 08820   (732)603-2101
+ Healthcheck Medical and Eye Center
  40 Union Avenue   Irvington, NJ 07111   (973)399-6270
+ The Eye Center
  213 Stelton Road   Piscataway, NJ 08820   (732)752-9090   Fax (732)752-9492

Singh, Jaya, MD {1104005552} IntrMd
+ Advance Hospital Care @ Somerset Medical Center
  110 Rehill Avenue   Somerville, NJ 08876   (908)429-5833   Fax (908)203-5970

Singh, Jyotsana, MD {1629363007} IntrMd
+ Virtua Family Medicine of Washington Township
  239 Hurffville Crosskeys Road   Sewell, NJ 08080   (856)341-8181   Fax (856)341-8180

Singh, Luvkarnjit, MD {1063795284}<NJ-MORRISTN>
+ Morristown Medical Center
  100 Madison Avenue   Morristown, NJ 07962   (973)971-4336

Singh, Malwinder, MD {1871558791} CritCr, PulDis, IntrMd(89,INA93)<NJ-VALLEY>
+ Fair Lawn Dental Associates
  25-15 Fair Lawn Avenue/Apt 102   Fair Lawn, NJ 07410   (201)797-8464
+ Endocrinology & Diabetes Associates, LLC
  333 Old Hook Road/Suite 103   Westwood, NJ 07675   (201)797-8464   Fax (201)820-4647

Singh, Manik, MD {1871765826} FamMed, SprtMd(DMN01)
+ North Jersey Orthopaedic & Sports Medicine Institute
  6 Brighton Road/Suite 101   Clifton, NJ 07012   (973)340-1940   Fax (973)340-1958

Singh, Manish Kumar, MD {1982712063} Nrolgy, PainMd(92,INA6C)<NJ-BURDTMLN>
+ 12 Village Drive
  Cape May Court House, NJ 08210   (609)465-7780   Fax (609)465-7891

Singh, Manjula, MD {1609046374} Anesth, AnesPain(92,INA7B)
+ Garden State Medical Center
  1608 New Jersey 88/Suites 102   Brick, NJ 08724   (732)849-0077   Fax (732)849-0015
+ Garden State Medical Center
  780 Highway 37 West/Suite 110   Toms River, NJ 08755   (732)341-3500
+ Garden State Medical Center
  100 State Route 36/Suite 1C   West Long Branch, NJ 08724   (732)202-3000   Fax (732)849-0015

Singh, Manoj Kumar, MD {1790913804} Surgry, IntrMd(91,NF01)<OH-WCHSTRMD>
+ Professional Associates in Surgery
  101 Old Short Hills Road/Suite 206   West Orange, NJ 07052   (973)731-5005   Fax (973)325-6230

Singh, Maulshree, MD {1427250703} FamMed
+ Advocare Aygen Pediatrics and Adult Care
  530 East Main Street   Chester, NJ 07930   (908)879-4300   Fax (908)879-8956

Singh, Millee, DO {1306004262} CdvDis
+ Penn Medicine Somers Point
  155 Brighton Avenue/Second Floor   Somers Point, NJ 08244   (609)365-3100   Fax (609)365-3168

Singh, Mohinder P., MD {1770677726} IntrMd(76,INA13)
+ Drs. Singh & Singh
  19 Holly Street/Suite 8   Cranford, NJ 07016   (908)276-3132   Fax (908)931-0842

Singh, Mukesh Kumar, MD {1679555189} Grtrcs, IntrMd(81,INDI)<NY-MTSINAI, NJ-COMMED>
+ University Geriatrics & Internal Medicine Associates
  1553 Highway 27/Suite 2100-2300   Somerset, NJ 08873   (732)418-0589   Fax (732)418-9428

Singh, Narpinder, MD {1518039791} CdvDis, IntrMd(89,INA5Z)
+ Coventry Cardiology Associates
  1000 Coventry Drive   Phillipsburg, NJ 08865   (908)859-3800   Fax (908)859-4310

Singh, Novia, MD {1356738835} IntHos
+ Cooper University Hospital Hospitalists
  One Cooper Plaza/Suite 222/Drrnce   Camden, NJ 08103   (856)342-3150

Singh, Padmakshi, MD {1912187881} IntrMd(03,INA46)<NJ-STMICHL>
+ St. Michael's Medical Center
  111 Central Avenue   Newark, NJ 07102   (973)877-5000

Singh, Pritpaul, MD {1164717807} Psychy
+ Medical Care Associates
  262 Route 10 West   Succasunna, NJ 07876   (973)252-1522   Fax (973)252-1422
+ Medical Care Associates
  137 Mountain Avenue   Hackettstown, NJ 07840   (973)252-1522   Fax (908)852-0614

Singh, Priyanka, MD {1013112911} IntrMd(03,INA1Z)<NJ-STPETER>
+ South Plainfield Primary Care
  2509 Park Avenue/Suite 1A   South Plainfield, NJ 07080   (908)668-8290   Fax (908)561-4914

Singh, Rachana, MD {1568494888} RadOnc(98,NJ06)<NJ-COOPRUMC>
+ Cooper University Hospital
  One Cooper Plaza/RadOnc   Camden, NJ 08103   (856)342-2000

Singh, Rajendra Sant, MD {1548410525} PthAna, PthDrm(92,INA21)
+ 19 Louis Drive
  Montville, NJ 07045   (973)415-7698
  skinpathology@gmail.com

Singh, Rajkumar R., MD {1932262102} Psychy, IntrMd(76,INA6Z)
+ Freehold Diagnostic & Treatment Center
  18 Throckmorton Street   Freehold, NJ 07728   (732)845-8220   Fax (732)845-8221
+ Monmouth Medical Center
  75 North Bath Avenue   Long Branch, NJ 07740   (732)845-8220   Fax (732)923-5277

Singh, Rashpal, MD {1285629014} PulDis, IntrMd, SlpDis(98,INDI)
+ Roosevelt Medical
  237 Roosevelt Avenue   Carteret, NJ 07008   (732)541-2141   Fax (732)541-1083

Singh, Rohini, MD {1437393600} PedHem
+ Hackensack Meridian Medical Group
  19 Davis Avenue/5th-6th Floor   Neptune, NJ 07753   (732)897-3400   Fax (732)897-3481

Singh, Samundar K., MD {1982691895} Anesth(70,INA32)<NJ-PALISADE>
+ Palisades Medical Center
  7600 River Road/Anesth   North Bergen, NJ 07047   (201)854-5000

Singh, Sapna, MD {1306934864} IntrMd(96,UZB03)
+ North Jersey Urgent Care
  344 Prospect Avenue/Suite 1A   Hackensack, NJ 07601   (201)646-9700

Singh, Sarabjit, MD {1114050846} PsyCAd, Psychy, IntrMd(96,INA92)
+ Center for Family Guidance, PC
  765 East Route 70/Building A-101   Marlton, NJ 08053   (856)983-3900   Fax (856)797-4785

Singh, Sarva D., MD {1760574651} IntrMd(78,INA12)<NJ-STMRYPAS, NJ-STJOSHOS>
+ Clifton Primary Care Center
  1111 Clifton Avenue/Suite 204   Clifton, NJ 07013   (973)779-9500   Fax (973)779-8900

Singh, Satyendra Pratap, MD {1811907108} IntrMd(91,INA96)<NY-DCTRSTAT>
+ Drs. Mohan & Singh
  101 Prospect Street/Suite 210   Lakewood, NJ 08701   (732)905-8877   Fax (732)363-4584

Singh, Shilpi, MD {1871970160}<NJ-RBAYPERT>
+ Medicare Internal Medicine
  100 Lakeview Drive/Suite 2   Jamesburg, NJ 08831   (402)280-2010

Singh, Sukhdeep, MD {1316328834} ObsGyn(PA0<PA-HHN-MANN>
+ Shah, Vinay R.
  985 Paulison Avenue   Clifton, NJ 07011   (973)471-2000   Fax (973)773-8553

Singh, Sukhjeet, DO {1851690200} IntrMd(11,NJ75)<NJ-UMDNJ>
+ Cooper University Hospital
  One Cooper Plaza/3rd FLSuite 377   Camden, NJ 08103   (856)342-2000

Singh, Sunil K., MD {1841229382} IntrMd, Nrolgy, PainMd(80,INDI)<NJ-SHOREMEM, NJ-BURDTMLN>
+ Neurology, Headache & Pain Relief Center
  1801 New Road   Linwood, NJ 08221   (609)653-3055   Fax (609)653-8469
  skup56@aol.com

Singh, Supreet, MD {1659530921} RadDia, Radiol(03,NJ02)<NJ-HOBUNIMC, NJ-CHRIST>
+ Hoboken University Medical Center
  308 Willow Avenue/Radiology   Hoboken, NJ 07030   (201)418-1827   Fax (201)418-1822
  supreet22@gmail.com
+ Christ Hospital
  176 Palisade Avenue/Radiology   Jersey City, NJ 07306   (201)795-8200
+ Bayonne Medical Center
  29th Street at Avenue E/Radiology   Bayonne, NJ 07030   (201)858-5000

Singh, Surbparkash Kaur, MD {1891966024} Pedtrc(04,NJ05)
+ Matheny Medical Center
  65 Highland Avenue   Peapack, NJ 07977

Singh, Vandana, DO {1033321815} IntrMd, Rheuma(01,CA23)
+ Atlantic Rheumatology & Osteoporosis Associates PA
  8 Saddle Road/Suite 202   Cedar Knolls, NJ 07927   (973)984-9796   Fax (973)984-5445

Singh, Varinder M., MD {1093883597} CdvDis, IntCrd, IntrMd(87,INA82)<NJ-JFKMED, NJ-RBAYPERT>
+ Central Jersey Cardiology
215 Bridge Street/Bld E   Metuchen, NJ 08840   (732)452-0400   Fax (732)452-0450

Singh, Vijay, MD {1174786297} Rheuma, InsrMd(98,UKR12)
+ Arthritis Osteoporosis & Rheumatology Associates
123 Egg Harbor Road/Suite 804   Sewell, NJ 08080   (856)302-0500   Fax (856)302-0504
+ Arthritis Osteoporosis & Rheumatology Associates
2059 Briggs Road/Suite 306   Mount Laurel, NJ 08054   (856)302-0500   Fax (856)924-6061

Singh, Vijayant, MD {1881821429} IntrMd
+ 29 East 269th Street
Bayonne, NJ 07002   (201)858-6519

Singh-Mohapatra, Sherry, MD {1528020062} IntrMd(00,GRN01)
+ 147 Renaissance Drive
Cherry Hill, NJ 08003

Singhal, Monisha, MD {1093883209} IntrMd(90,INA05)
+ St. Joseph's Regional Medical Center
703 Main Street   Paterson, NJ 07503   (973)754-2431   Fax (973)754-3376
singhalm@sjhmc.org

Singhal, Pratap C., MD {1164477303} FamMed, EmrgMd(64,INDI)<NJ-CLARMAAS, NJ-STMICHL>
+ 431 Washington Avenue
Belleville, NJ 07109   (973)759-2241

Singhal, Shalabh, MD {1699976498} CdvDis, IntrMd(03,NY15)
+ Mercer Bucks Cardiology
One Union Street/Suite 101   Robbinsville, NJ 08691   (609)890-7292   Fax (609)890-7292

Singla, Ruchika, MD {1508980590} IntrMd
+ 34 Tiloru Road
South Orange, NJ 07079

Singman, Bradford A., MD {1164513354} Dermat(86,NY08)<NJ-VALLEY>
+ 14-23 River Road
Fair Lawn, NJ 07410   (201)794-6000   Fax (201)794-7223

Sinha, Anita, MD {1528479359} Pedtrc
+ Pediatrix Medical Group
1505 West Sherman Avenue/MSO-Box 104   Vineland, NJ 08360   (856)845-0100   Fax (302)651-4945

Sinha, Anjali, DO {1447435334} PhysMd(06,PA78)
+ Dr. Vinod K. Sinha, MD, PA
260 Hobart Street   Perth Amboy, NJ 08861   (732)442-6464   Fax (732)442-6367

Sinha, Anubha, MD {1730107145} Gastrn, IntrMd(98,DMN01)<NJ-HUNTRDN>
+ Hunterdon Digestive Health Specialists, P.A.
170 Route 31/Suite 5/HunterdonProfPl   Flemington, NJ 08822   (908)788-8200   Fax (908)788-8207
Amarsinha@verizon.net

Sinha, Anubha, MD {1639349939} IntrMd(01,WIN01)
+ 7 Allison Court
Edison, NJ 08820

Sinha, Anushua, MD {1255374526} IntrMd, Pedtrc(92,MA01)
+ Rutgers- New Jersey Medical School
185 South Orange Avenue/MSB F506   Newark, NJ 07103   (973)972-4422   Fax (973)972-7625

Sinha, Ashok Kumar, MD {1477501062} IntrMd(77,INA7B)<NJ-KIMBALL, NJ-COMMED>
+ Drs. Kumar and Kumar
75 Brunswick Woods Drive/Building L   East Brunswick, NJ 08816   (732)254-1450   Fax (732)613-8525
+ 25 Mule Road/Suite B-10
Toms River, NJ 08755   (732)254-1450   Fax (732)505-9913

Sinha, Binod K., MD {1134293723} Urolgy, IntrMd(75,INDI)<NJ-OVERLOOK, NJ-EASTORNG>
+ Urology Care Alliance
4 Progress Street/Suite A-9   Edison, NJ 08820   (908)754-9280   Fax (908)754-9287
+ Urology Care Alliance
81 Veronica Avenue/Suite 205   Somerset, NJ 08873   (908)754-9280   Fax (908)754-9287

Sinha, Binod P., MD {1932201662} Anesth, PainMd, AnesPain(74,INDI)
+ Garden State Pain Control Center, P.A.
1117 Route 46 East/Suite 201   Clifton, NJ 07013   (973)777-5444   Fax (973)777-0304

Sinha, Dev, MD {1447542469}
+ 3 Helene Avenue
Edison, NJ 08820   (732)986-0496

Sinha, Gopal K., MD {1306887997} FamMed, IntrMd(65,INA88)<NJ-RBAYOLDB, NJ-RBAYPERT>
+ Durham Medical Center
2 Ethel Road/Suite 206-C   Edison, NJ 08817   (732)650-0009   Fax (732)650-1976
gksinha@aol.com

Sinha, Jyoti, MD {1205164134} PedGst, Pedtrc(02,GRN01)
+ 1303 State Route 27
Somerset, NJ 08873   (732)246-4727   Fax (732)246-0982

+ Summit Medical Group
34 Mountain Boulevard/Building B   Warren, NJ 07059   (732)246-4727   Fax (908)769-8927

Sinha, Karabi, MD {1841519006} PthACl, PthFor(71,INA86)<NJ-CENTRAST>
+ CentraState Medical Center
901 West Main Street/Pathology   Freehold, NJ 07728   (732)294-2549   Fax (732)308-1614

Sinha, Kavita, MD {1710043179} Nrolgy, Pedtrc, NroChl(82,INDI)
+ Neuroscience Associates
31-A Mountain Boulevard   Warren, NJ 07059   (908)822-1030   Fax (908)822-1299

Sinha, Kumar Gautam, MD {1194919340} SrgSpn
+ University Spine Center
504 Valley Road/Second Floor/Suite 203   Wayne, NJ 07470   (973)686-0700   Fax (973)686-0701

Sinha, Meena, MD {1376531186} IntrMd(66,INA7B)
+ 55 Henderson Road
Kendall Park, NJ 08824   (732)821-0592

Sinha, Neil, MD {1932433703} Anesth, PainMd(07,NJ05)
+ Garden State Pain Control Center, P.A.
1117 Route 46 East/Suite 201   Clifton, NJ 07013   (973)777-5444   Fax (973)777-0304
+ 155 New Brunswick Avenue
Perth Amboy, NJ 08861   (973)777-5444   Fax (973)777-0304

Sinha, Prabhat Kumar, MD {1013988286} IntrMd(92,INDI)<NJ-COMMED, NJ-KIMBALL>
+ 20 Hospital Drive/Suite 3
Toms River, NJ 08755   (732)341-9900

Sinha, Sharmila, MD {1083817522} Psychy
+ 24 Paddock Drive
Plainsboro, NJ 08536

Sinha, Sudir K., MD {1912011883} IntrMd, CritCr(81,INA61)<NJ-HACKNSK, NJ-HOLYNAME>
+ Sudir K Sinha MD PC
333 Old Hook Road/Suite 5   Westwood, NJ 07675   (201)599-8440   Fax (201)599-8427

Sinha, Sugiti, MD {1548206329} Nrolgy(82,INA49)<NJ-JFKMED>
+ 2177 Oak Tree Road/Suite 104
Edison, NJ 08820   (908)754-2400   Fax (908)755-2093

Sinha, Taru, MD {1750461232} FamMed(92,INA72)
+ CentraState Family Medicine Residency Practice
1001 West Main Street/Suite B   Freehold, NJ 07728   (732)294-2540   Fax (732)294-9328

Sinha, Vinod K., MD {1619035037} CritCr, IntrMd, PulDis(74,INA10)<NJ-RBAYPERT, NJ-RWJURAH>
+ 260 Hobart Street
Perth Amboy, NJ 08861   (732)442-6464   Fax (732)442-6367
vinodsinha@gmail.com

Sinha, Virteeka, MD {1912211277} EmrgPedr
+ Rutgers- New Jersey Medical School
185 South Orange Avenue   Newark, NJ 07103   (973)972-1973

Siniakowicz, Robert Miroslaw, MD {1689776122} IntrMd(91,POLA)
+ Hamilton Medical Group
2275 State Route 33/Suite 301   Hamilton Square, NJ 08690   (609)586-6006

Sinkoff, Michael Richard, DO {1720227002} IntHos, IntrMd(08,NJ75)<NJ-VIRTVOOR, NJ-VIRTMHBC>
+ Virtua Voorhees
100 Bowman Drive/Hospitalist   Voorhees, NJ 08043   (856)247-2594   Fax (856)244-8259

Sinner, Scott William, MD {1144296161} InfDis, IntrMd(98,PA09)<OH-CLERMONT>
+ ID Associates PA
411 Courtyard Drive   Hillsborough, NJ 08844   (908)725-2522

Sinofsky, Francine E., MD {1427013432} ObsGyn, IntrMd(81,NJ06)<NJ-MONMOUTH>
+ University Medical Group/OBGYN
125 Paterson Street/2nd Floor   New Brunswick, NJ 08901   (732)235-6600   Fax (732)235-6650

Sinquee, Dianne M., MD {1871658724} PedCrC, Pedtrc(82,JMA01)<NJ-UMDNJ>
+ University Hospital
150 Bergen Street/PICU   Newark, NJ 07103   (973)972-3784   Fax (973)972-7597

Sinvhal, Ranjeeta Mukul, MD {1053581264} IntrMd(96,INA26)<NJ-STJOSHOS, NJ-STCLRDEN>
+ 9 Treetops Court
Princeton, NJ 08540   (732)422-3839
+ St. Joseph's Regional Medical Center
703 Main Street   Paterson, NJ 07503   (973)754-2000

Sio, Reymond Guieb, MD {1710944533} Anesth(88,PHI07)<NJ-STPETER>
+ Anesthesia Consultnts of NJ/Nova Pain
285 Davidson Avenue/Suite 204   Somerset, NJ 08873   (732)271-1400   Fax (732)271-3543

Physicians by Name and Address

+ Cares Surgicenter, LLC.
240 Easton Avenue   New Brunswick, NJ 08901   (732)271-1400   Fax (732)296-8677

Sion, Armi T., MD {1427017953} Pedtrc(77,PHI01)<NJ-WARREN>
+ New Beginnings Pediatrics
755 Memorial Parkway/Suite 115   Phillipsburg, NJ 08865   (908)454-3737   Fax (908)454-0402

Sioss, Robert G., MD {1962688689} IntrMd(78,NJ06)
+ 19 Lavender Drive
Piscataway, NJ 08854   (732)805-9225

Sipio, James C., MD {1467451732} Surgry, Urolgy(81,PA13)
+ New Jersey Urology, LLC
2401 East Evesham Road/Suite F   Voorhees, NJ 08043   (856)673-1600   Fax (856)988-0636

Sipzner, Robert J., MD {1467491589} IntrMd, Nephro(82,NY19)<NJ-STBARNMC, NJ-BAYONNE>
+ Hypertension & Renal Group, P.A.
22 Old Short Hills Road/Suite 212   Livingston, NJ 07039   (973)994-4550   Fax (973)994-7085
+ Hypertension & Renal Group, P.A.
930 Kennedy Boulevard   Bayonne, NJ 07002   (973)994-4550   Fax (973)994-7085

Siragusa, Joseph, MD {1376957761} Psychy
+ 5 Pascack Road
Woodcliff Lake, NJ 07677   (914)424-5702   Fax (201)343-4391

Sirajuddin, Syed K., MD {1710114301} FamMed
+ Riverside Pediatric Group
506 Broadway   Bayonne, NJ 07002   (201)471-7015   Fax (201)471-7014
+ Riverside Medical Group
710 Tenth Street   Secaucus, NJ 07094   (201)471-7015   Fax (201)865-0015

Sirchio, Kevin J., DO {1417973512} EmrgMd(95,NY75)<NJ-KIMBALL>
+ Kimball Medical Center
600 River Avenue   Lakewood, NJ 08701   (732)363-1900

Sireci, John Bernard, DO {1306880737} EmrgMd(99,PA77)
+ Emergency Physician Associates, P.A.
307 South Evergreen Avenue/PO Box 298   Woodbury, NJ 08096   (856)848-3817   Fax (856)848-1431

Sireci, Joseph, DO {1659313005} FamMed(98,PA77)<NJ-KMHCHRRY>
+ 475 Old Malton Pike West/Suite 5
Marlton, NJ 08053   (856)702-6700   Fax (856)702-6701

Sireci, Steven N., Jr., MD {1174744916} NuclMd, Radiol, RadNuc(84,NJ05)<NJ-HOLYNAME>
+ Holy Name Hospital
718 Teaneck Road/Radiology   Teaneck, NJ 07666   (201)833-3000

Siri, Matthew A., MD {1659433845} Anesth(03,NJ06)<NJ-KMHCHRRY, NJ-KMHSTRAT>
+ Rancocas Anesthesiology, PA
700 Route 130 North/Suite 203   Cinnaminson, NJ 08077   (856)829-9345   Fax (856)829-3605

Siricilla, Mamatha, MD {1487967576}
+ 318 Cobble Creek Circle
Cherry Hill, NJ 08003   (304)216-0611
msiricilla@gmail.com

Sirisinahal, Sudhamshu, DO {1124382080}
+ 1011 Azalea Drive
North Brunswick, NJ 08902   (732)305-6752
ssirisin@drexelmed.edu

Sirken, Steven M., DO {1689762775} FamMed(89,NY75)<NJ-KMHCHRRY>
+ 401 Cooper Landing Road/Suite C-22
Cherry Hill, NJ 08002   (856)779-7779   Fax (856)779-7790

Sirkin, Michael S., MD {1194759589} SrgOrt, OrtTrm(91,NJ05)<NJ-RWJUBRUN, NJ-UMDNJ>
+ North Jersey Orthopaedic Institute
90 Bergen Street/DOC 1200   Newark, NJ 07101   (973)972-0681   Fax (973)972-9367

Sirna, Paul William, MD {1548220387} Pedtrc(96,GRN01)<NJ-STBARNMC>
+ Park Avenue Pediatrics
36 Park Avenue   Verona, NJ 07044   (973)239-7001   Fax (973)239-8867

Sirover, William D., MD {1265538904} IntrMd
+ The Cooper Hospital System-Univ Hospital
401 Haddon Avenue/Room 283   Camden, NJ 08103   (856)342-2000

Sisbarro, Susan E., MD {1205040789} Anesth(05,GRN01)<NJ-STJOSHOS>
+ Montclair Anesthesia Associates PC
185 Fairfield Avenue/Suite 2A   West Caldwell, NJ 07006   (973)226-1230   Fax (973)226-1232
+ 1125 Maxwell Lane/Suite 722
Hoboken, NJ 07030   (973)449-7655

Siskind, Jonathan B., DO {1073802898} Anesth
+ James Street Anesthesia
102 James Street/Suite 103   Edison, NJ 08820   (732)494-1444   Fax (732)494-7052

Physicians by Name and Address

Sison, Antonio, MD {1346232204} ObsGyn(86,PA07)<NJ-RWJUHAM>
+ Robert Wood Johnson Ob/Gyn Group
1 Hamilton Health Place   Hamilton, NJ 08690   (609)631-6899   Fax (609)631-6898

Sison, Edwin Ruan Racela, MD {1598925380} Anesth(MA07
+ Robert Wood Johnson-UMDNJ Anesthesia Group
125 Paterson Street/CAB 3100   New Brunswick, NJ 08901   (732)235-7827   Fax (732)235-6131

Sison, Genevieve Yvonne, MD {1912193632} Pedtrc(04,DMN01)<NJ-NWTNMEM, NJ-MORRISTN>
+ Advocare Sussex County Pediatrics Newton
39 Newton Sparta Road   Newton, NJ 07860   (973)383-9841   Fax (973)383-7989
+ Advocare Sussex County Pediatrics Montague
2B Myrtle Drive   Montague, NJ 07827   (973)383-9841   Fax (973)293-0138

Sison, Raymund Vincent Sebastian, MD {1598023152} InfDis, IntrMd
+ St. Michael's Medical Center
111 Central Avenue/Medical Educ   Newark, NJ 07102   (201)920-9948

Sisskin, Mark I., MD {1922071505} IntrMd(81,SPA06)<NJ-JRSYSHMC>
+ Shore Health Group
3200 Sunset Avenue/Suite 100   Asbury Park, NJ 07712   (732)774-4114   Fax (732)774-6869

Sisti, Michael Brian, MD {1649209008} SrgNro, IntrMd(81,NY01)
+ Neurosurgeons of New Jersey
1200 East Ridgewood Avenue   Ridgewood, NJ 07450   (201)824-6131

Sitahal-Dhaniram, Sasha, MD {1902166051} IntrMd<NJ-NWRKBETH>
+ Newark Beth Israel Medical Center
201 Lyons Avenue   Newark, NJ 07112   (973)926-7828   Fax (973)926-8216

Sitoy, Fernando R., MD {1629182654} Pedtrc(65,PHI10)
+ 1100 Centennial Avenue/Suite 204
Piscataway, NJ 08854   (732)529-6330   Fax (732)529-6332

Sitrin, Edith S., MD {1417155516} IntrMd(89,NJ06)
+ Bristol-Myers Squibb Company
One Squibb Drive/Building 137   New Brunswick, NJ 08903   (732)227-5549   Fax (732)227-3550

Sitt, Hal, MD {1376958108} Pedtrc
+ Riverside Pediatrics
714 Tenth Street   Secaucus, NJ 07094   (551)257-7038   Fax (201)552-2358

Siu, Albert, MD {1063668895} Nephro, IntrMd(05,NET12)<NJ-STJOSHOS>
+ Center for Nephrology & Hypertension
526 Bloomfield Avenue/Suite 104   Caldwell, NJ 07006   (973)226-0500   Fax (973)226-7221
CenterForNephrology@hotmail.com

Siu, Dwayne Winfred, DO {1073549135} CdvDis, ClCdEl, IntrMd(86,NJ75)
+ Cardiology Associates of New Brunswick
593 Cranbury Road/Suite 2   East Brunswick, NJ 08816   (732)390-3333   Fax (732)390-9244
dwaynesiu@hotmail.com

Siu, Gilbert, DO {1801062443} PhysMd
+ 203 Hidden Drive
Blackwood, NJ 08012

Siu, Karleung, MD {1649417437} OncHem, IntrMd(05,NY08)
+ Summit Medical Group Florham Park Campus
150 Park Avenue   Florham Park, NJ 07932   (908)273-4300

Siu, Larry K., MD {1972765675} Gastrn, IntrMd(08,NY08)
+ Affiliates in Gastroenterology, P.A.
101 Old Short Hills Road/Suite 217   West Orange, NJ 07052   (973)731-4600   Fax (973)731-1477
+ Affiliates in Gastroenterology, P.A.
101 Madison Avenue/Suite 100   Morristown, NJ 07960   (973)731-4600   Fax (973)540-8788

Sivalingam, Arunan, MD {1700850179} Ophthl(85,NJ06)<NJ-VIRTUAHS>
+ Mid Atlantic Retina - Wills Eye Retina Surgeons
1417 Cantillon Boulevard   Mays Landing, NJ 08330   (609)625-0402   Fax (609)625-0788

Sivalingam, Varunan, MD {1578501128} Ophthl(88,NJ06)<NJ-VIRTMHBC>
+ 103 Old Marlton Pike/Suite 203
Medford, NJ 08055   (609)654-1770   Fax (609)654-2320
drvarunan@hotmail.com

Sivanesan, Swarna Priya, MD {1104024165} Dermat
+ Family Dermatology
901 West Main Street   Freehold, NJ 07728

Sivaprasad, Rajagopalan, MD {1699713354} InfDis, IntrMd(67,INA08)<NJ-MONMOUTH>
+ PO Box 240
Oakhurst, NJ 07755   (732)842-5272   Fax (732)244-1005

Sivaraaman, Kartik, MD {1962651026} Nrolgy, Eplpsy<PA-TJHSP>
+ University Hospital-RWJMS Neurology
125 Paterson Street/Suite 4100-6100   New Brunswick, NJ 08901   (732)235-7733   Fax (732)235-7041

Sivaraju, Kannan, MD {1659508687} IntrMd, Grtrcs(97,INA85)
+ Town Medical Associates/Verona
271 Grove Avenue/Suite A   Verona, NJ 07044   (973)239-2600   Fax (973)239-0482

Sivaraman, Priya, MD {1952398588} FamMed
+ Alps Family Physicians
1500 Alps Road   Wayne, NJ 07470   (973)628-8500   Fax (973)628-7944

Sivaraman, Sivashankar, MD {1922259514} IntrMd(02,INA1Z)
+ Atlantic Pulmonary & Critical Care Associates, P.A.
741 South Second Avenue/Suite A   Galloway, NJ 08205   (609)748-7300   Fax (609)748-7919

Sivasubramanian, Hema, MD {1093078248} FamMed
+ Millburn Family Practice
33 Bleeker Street/Suite 104   Millburn, NJ 07041   (973)379-3051

Sivendra, Shan, MD {1538154307} IntrMd(89,INA70)<NJ-STBARNMC>
+ St. Barnabas Medical Center
94 Old Short Hills Road   Livingston, NJ 07039   (201)322-5000

Sivendran, Meera, MD {1245551779} Dermat, IntrMd(10,PA02)
+ The Dermatology Group, P.C.
347 Mount Pleasant Avenue/Suite 205   West Orange, NJ 07052   (973)571-2121

Sivitz, Adam B., MD {1508872631} Pedtrc, PedEmg(01,PA13)<NJ-NWRKBETH>
+ Newark Beth Israel Medical Center
201 Lyons Avenue   Newark, NJ 07112   (973)926-2484   Fax (973)282-0562

Sivitz, Jennifer Nicole, MD {1023096450} PedEnd(02,NY09)<NJ-NWRKBETH, NJ-STBARNMC>
+ Pediatric Endocrinology & Diabetes at St. Barnabas
200 South Orange Avenue/1st Floor   Livingston, NJ 07039   (973)322-7337   Fax (973)322-7504

Siyamwala, Munaf M., MD {1992941900} IntrMd, IntHos(06)<NJ-SOCEANCO, NJ-STMICHL>
+ St. Michael's Medical Center
111 Central Avenue/Internal Med   Newark, NJ 07102   (973)877-2420
+ Southern Ocean County Medical Center
1140 Route 72 West/Internal Med   Manahawkin, NJ 08050   (973)877-2420   Fax (609)978-3113

Sjolund, Paula A., DO {1659323731} IntrMd(91,NJ75)<NJ-UNVMCPRN>
+ 75 Washington Avenue
Milltown, NJ 08850   (732)828-1175

Sjovall, Frances, DO {1811082373} FamMed(92,IA75)<NJ-JRSYSHMC, NJ-CHILTON>
+ Doctors MediCenter
835 Roosevelt Avenue/Plaza 12/Suite 4A   Carteret, NJ 07008   (732)969-2240   Fax (732)969-2152

Sjovall, William J., Jr., DO {1649293986} Pedtrc(96,FL75)<NJ-STBARNMC>
+ St. Barnabas Medical Center
94 Old Short Hills Road/Pediatrics   Livingston, NJ 07039   (973)322-5000

Skaf, Robert A., MD {1497727051} RprEnd, ObsGyn(73,SYR01)<NJ-VIRTMHBC, NJ-ACMCMAIN>
+ South Jersey Fertility Center
400 Lippincott Drive   Marlton, NJ 08053   (856)282-1231   Fax (856)596-2411
+ South Jersey Fertility Center
2500 English Creek Avenue/Suite 225   Egg Harbor Township, NJ 08234

Skalla, Matthew T., MD {1619908142} Radiol, RadDia(90,NY47)<NJ-NWTNMEM>
+ Sparta Health and Wellness Center
89 Sparta Avenue/Suite 120   Sparta, NJ 07871   (973)729-0002   Fax (973)729-1085
+ Image Care Centers
222 High Street/Suite 101   Newton, NJ 07860   (973)729-0002   Fax (973)383-2774
+ Radiologic Associates of Northwest New Jersey
212 Route 94   Vernon, NJ 07871   (973)827-1961

Skalsky, Susan E., MD {1265605919} AdolMd, Pedtrc, IntrMd(72,NY09)
+ Wellness Services @ Montclair State University
1 Normal Avenue   Upper Montclair, NJ 07043   (973)655-7051   Fax (973)655-6977

Skariah, Jody, MD {1386064855} FamMed
+ Medical Diagnostic Associates PA
525 Central Avenue/Suite D   Westfield, NJ 07090   (908)232-5333   Fax (908)389-1922
+ 1801 East Second Street/Suite 2
Scotch Plains, NJ 07076   (908)322-0190

Skarimbas, Alicia C., MD {1245239490} FamMed(01,PA12)
+ Primary Care NJ
370 Grand Avenue/Suite 102   Englewood, NJ 07631   (201)567-3370   Fax (201)816-1265

Skarinsky, Evgenya, MD {1093715120} PthACl, PthCln(69,UKR25)<NJ-VIRTVOOR, NJ-VIRTMHBC>
+ Virtua Voorhees
100 Bowman Drive   Voorhees, NJ 08043   (856)247-3000
+ Virtua Family Health Center
1000 Atlantic Avenue   Camden, NJ 08104   (856)247-3000   Fax (856)246-3528
+ Virtua Memorial
175 Madison Avenue   Mount Holly, NJ 08043   (609)267-0700

Skeehan, Christopher J., MD {1831164318} FamMed, IntrMd(76,MEXI)<NJ-CENTRAST>
+ Family Practice of CentraState
319 Route 130 North   East Windsor, NJ 08520   (609)426-1555   Fax (609)447-8070
+ Family Practice of CentraState
281 Route 34/Suite 813   Colts Neck, NJ 07722   (609)426-1555   Fax (732)431-3707
+ Family Practice of CentraState
901 West Main Street/Suite 106   Freehold, NJ 08520   (732)462-0100   Fax (732)462-0348

Skeete-Jackson, Kalia Nicole, MD {1699086793} CdvDis<NJ-BERGNMC>
+ New Bridge Medical Center
230 East Ridgewood Avenue   Paramus, NJ 07652   (201)967-4000   Fax (201)967-4117

Skerker, Robert Scott, MD {1912944539} PhysMd(86,MA16)
+ Wound Healing Program at Morristown Medical Center
435 South Street/Suite 320   Morristown, NJ 07960   (973)971-4550

Skiba, Chester John, Jr., MD {1063431005} IntrMd, EmrgMd(83,MNT01)<NJ-HCKTSTWN>
+ Hackettstown Regional Medical Center
651 Willow Grove Street   Hackettstown, NJ 07840   (908)850-6800   Fax (856)616-1919

Skillinge, David D., DO {1992769913} FamMed, IntrMd(95,PA77)
+ Delaware Valley Family Health Center
200 Frenchtown Road   Milford, NJ 08848   (908)995-2251   Fax (908)995-2036

Skinner, Dirk E., MD {1265530091} Nrolgy(79,PA09)
+ 1138 East Chestnut Avenue/Building 7-B
Vineland, NJ 08360   (856)691-8383   Fax (856)691-9505
+ 212 North Main Street
Cape May Court House, NJ 08210   (609)465-4747

Sklar, Jeffrey, MD {1083658520} Anesth(81,GRN01)<NJ-BERGNMC>
+ 700 Queen Anne Road
Teaneck, NJ 07666

Sklower, Jay A., DO {1871530154} FamMed(71,MO78)<NJ-CHRIST, NJ-JRSYCITY>
+ PMA Physicians LLC
1 Journal Square Plaza/2nd Floor   Jersey City, NJ 07306   (201)216-3030   Fax (201)499-0247

Skobac, Edward A., MD {1285607671} IntrMd(80,NJ05)<NJ-VIRTVOOR, NJ-KMHCHRRY>
+ University Doctors
2301 East Evesham Road/Suite 202   Voorhees, NJ 08043   (856)770-1305   Fax (856)770-1732

Skoczylas, Stanley J., MD {1992760011} ObsGyn(73,MEX03)<NJ-HCKTSTWN, NJ-MORRISTN>
+ 32 Nancy Terrace
Hackettstown, NJ 07840   (908)852-7100   Fax (908)813-1067

Skole, Kevin S., MD {1568431914} Gastrn, IntrMd(00,PA02)<NJ-RWJUBRUN, NJ-STPETER>
+ Princeton Medicine
5 Plainsboro Road/Suite 300   Plainsboro, NJ 08536   (609)853-7272   Fax (609)853-7271

Skolnick, Bruce A., MD {1700831831} CdvDis, IntrMd, IntCrd(90,NJ05)<NJ-CHILTON, NJ-VALLEY>
+ Cardiology Center of North Jersey
1030 Clifton Avenue   Clifton, NJ 07013   (973)778-3777   Fax (973)778-3252
+ Wayne Primary Care, P.A.
508 Hamburg Turnpike/Suite 102   Wayne, NJ 07470   (973)778-3777   Fax (973)595-6414

Skolnick, Cary I., MD   SrgOrt(77,NE06)<NJ-CENTRAST>
+ Medico-Legal Evaluations, PA
50 Franklin Lane/Suite 201   Manalapan, NJ 07726   (732)972-4771   Fax (732)972-8610

Skolnick, Helen Sharlene, MD {1962409755} Allrgy, Pedtrc, AlgyImmn(94,NJ06)
+ Princeton Allergy & Asthma Associates, P.A.
24 Vreeland Drive   Skillman, NJ 08558   (609)921-2202   Fax (609)924-1468
+ Princeton Allergy & Asthma Associates, P.A.
1245 Whitehorse Mercerville Rd   Hamilton, NJ 08619   (609)921-2202   Fax (609)924-1468
+ Princeton Allergy & Asthma Associates, P.A.
666 Plainsboro Road/Building 100-B   Plainsboro, NJ 08558   (609)799-8111   Fax (609)924-1468

Skolnick, Justin S., DO {1598963266}
+ Rowan University-School of Osteopathic Medicine
  1 Medical Center Drive/Suite 162   Stratford, NJ 08084
  (856)566-7121   Fax (856)566-6222

Skolnick, Lawrence M., MD {1871566737} NnPnMd, Pedtrc(72,NY19)<NJ-MORRISTN, NJ-OVERLOOK>
+ MidAtlantic Neonatology Associates
  100 Madison Avenue   Morristown, NJ 07962   (973)971-5488   Fax (973)290-7175

Skop, Neal Franklin, MD {1144269408} CdvDis
+ Cardiovascular Associates
  210 West Atlantic Avenue   Haddon Heights, NJ 08035
  (856)546-3003   Fax (856)547-5337
+ Cardiovascular Associates of The Delaware Valley, PA
  525 State Street/Suite 3   Elmer, NJ 08318   (856)546-3003   Fax (856)358-0725

Skorenko, Kenneth R., MD {1790727279} ObsGyn(82,NJ05)<NJ-MONMOUTH>
+ West Long Branch Obstetrics & Gynecology
  1019 Broadway   West Long Branch, NJ 07764   (732)229-6797   Fax (732)229-6893
+ West Long Branch Obstetrics & Gynecology
  911 East County Line Road/Suite 201   Lakewood, NJ 08701
  (732)364-9299

Skotzko, Christine Ellen, MD {1336227669} Psychy, IntrMd(88,NY45)<NJ-HUNTRDN>
+ Psychiatric Associates of Hunterdon
  190 Route 31/Suite 100   Flemington, NJ 08822   (908)788-6654   Fax (908)788-6452
+ Hunterdon Medical Center
  2100 Wescott Drive/Physiatry   Flemington, NJ 08822
  (908)788-6100

Skrelja, Valerie, MD {1124106380} IntrMd(02,OH40)<NJ-OVERLOOK, NJ-MORRISTN>
+ Summit Medical Group-Berkeley Heights Campus
  1 Diamond Hill Road/3rd Floor   Berkeley Heights, NJ 07922
  (908)277-8683   Fax (908)790-6524

Skripak, Justin Michael, MD {1437205929} PedAlg, Pedtrc(01,NJ05)
+ ENT & Allergy Associates, LLP
  690 Kinderkamack Road/Suite 101   Oradell, NJ 07649
  (201)722-9850   Fax (201)722-9851

Skripkus, Aldona J., MD {1316055148} Pedtrc(66,PA07)<NJ-CLARMAAS, NJ-STMICHL>
+ Drs. Padykula and Skripkus
  381 Kearny Avenue   Kearny, NJ 07032   (201)991-4824
  Fax (201)991-7465

Skroce, Linda C., MD {1093718314} Pedtrc, NnPnMd(90,NJ06)<NJ-STJOSHOS>
+ St Joseph's Medical Center Neonatology
  703 Main Street   Paterson, NJ 07503   (973)754-2555   Fax (973)754-2567

Skrzynski, Angela Anita, DO {1407141385} FamMed
+ Virtua Holistic Primary Care
  1001 Route 73 North/Lower Level   Marlton, NJ 08053
  (856)355-7115   Fax (856)355-7116

Skrzypczak, Jan L., MD {1962665620} RadV&I
+ Ocean Medical Center
  425 Jack Martin Boulevard   Brick, NJ 08723   (732)840-2200
+ Coastal Imaging, LLC
  79 Route 37 West/Suite 103   Toms River, NJ 08755
  (732)840-2200   Fax (732)276-2325

Skrzypczak, Marek J., MD {1205818689} IntrMd(84,POL08)<NJ-JFKMED>
+ Healthpro Medical Center
  1500 Saint Georges Avenue   Avenel, NJ 07001   (732)669-9191   Fax (732)669-9899

Skurnick, Blanche Jacqueline, MD {1609989110} IntrMd(90,NJ05)
+ The Heart Center of The Oranges
  310 Central Avenue/Suite 102   East Orange, NJ 07018
  (973)395-1550   Fax (973)395-3711

Skylizard, Loki, MD {1326110081} SrgThr, Surgry(01,MI01)<NJ-MONMOUTH>
+ Barnabas Health Medical Group
  166 Morris Avenue/2nd Floor   Long Branch, NJ 07740
  (732)263-5024   Fax (732)263-5029

Slaby, Andrew Edmund, MD {1295892321} Psychy(68,NY01)<NY-LENOXHLL, NJ-OVERLOOK>
+ 50-E New England Avenue
  Summit, NJ 07901   (908)277-2950   Fax (908)277-6964
  aeslaby@aol.com

Slama, Robert D., MD {1528030384} CdvDis, IntrMd(71,PA13)<NJ-OVERLOOK, NJ-MORRISTN>
+ Summit Medical Group-Berkeley Heights Campus
  1 Diamond Hill Road   Berkeley Heights, NJ 07922
  (908)273-4300   Fax (908)790-6524

Slamovits, Thomas L., MD {1689717712} Ophthl(75,OH40)<NY-MNTFMOSE, NJ-HACKNSK>
+ Retina Associates of New Jersey, P.A.
  628 Cedar Lane   Teaneck, NJ 07666   (201)837-7300   Fax (201)836-6426

Slankard, Marjorie L., MD {1306938337} Allrgy, IntrMd, IntMAImm(71,MO03)<NY-PRSBCOLU, NY-NYPRESHS>
+ 1200 East Ridgewood Avenue
  Ridgewood, NJ 07450   (201)670-8100

Slasky, Shira E., MD {1821258591} RadNro(02,NY46)<NJ-UMDNJ>
+ University Hospital
  150 Bergen Street/Rm C-320/Rad   Newark, NJ 07103
  (973)972-4300

Slater, Gregg Matthew, MD {1578717732} RadDia, Radiol, RadNro(03,MD07)
+ University Radiology Group, P.C.
  579A Cranbury Road   East Brunswick, NJ 08816   (732)390-0040   Fax (732)390-1856
+ University Radiology Group
  2100 Route 33/Neptune City Med Bld   Neptune, NJ 07753
  (732)390-0040   Fax (732)502-0368
+ University Radiology Group
  900 West Main Street   Freehold, NJ 08816   (732)462-1900   Fax (732)462-1848

Slater, James P., MD {1841292232} Surgry, SrgThr(90,OH06)<NJ-MORRISTN, NJ-JRSYSHMC>
+ Mid-Atlantic Surgical Associates
  100 Madison Avenue   Morristown, NJ 07960   (973)971-7300   Fax (973)984-7019
  james.slater@ahsys.org

Slater, John G., MD {1699731125} Pedtrc(74,MA01)<NJ-VALLEY, NJ-ENGLWOOD>
+ Tenafly Pediatrics, PA
  26 Park Place   Paramus, NJ 07652   (201)262-1140   Fax (201)261-8413
+ Tenafly Pediatrics, PA
  32 Franklin Street   Tenafly, NJ 07670   (201)262-1140   Fax (201)569-6081

Slater, Shakira L., MD {1861718546} FamMed
+ Mountainside Family Practice Associates
  799 Bloomfield Avenue/Suite 201   Verona, NJ 07044
  (973)746-7050   Fax (973)857-2831

Slater-Myer, Linda Paige, MD {1063477735} NnPnMd, Pedtrc
+ Cooper Neonatology
  One Cooper Plaza   Camden, NJ 08103   (856)342-2265
  Fax (856)342-8007

Slatkin, Ava, MD {1346439973} IntrMd(82,PHI08)
+ Schering Plough Research Institute
  2000 Galloping Hill Road   Kenilworth, NJ 07033   (908)298-2820   Fax (908)298-2834

Slaven, Timothy M., DO {1043215288} CdvDis, IntrMd(93,IL76)
+ Atlantic Medical Imaging, LLC.
  219 North White Horse Pike   Hammonton, NJ 08037
  (609)573-5077   Fax (609)652-8258
+ AtlantiCare Physician Group
  712 East Bay Avenue/Suite 19   Manahawkin, NJ 08050
  (609)573-5077   Fax (609)597-0746

Slavick, Harris D., MD {1699872234} Urolgy(69,IL06)<NJ-SJERSYHS>
+ 1317 South Main Road/Suite 2 A
  Vineland, NJ 08360   (856)691-2225   Fax (856)691-7726
  h.slavick@comcast.net

Slavin, Anna, MD {1417934712} Pedtrc(96,NY46)<NJ-MORRISTN>
+ Princeton Medical Group, P.A.
  419 North Harrison Street   Princeton, NJ 08540   (609)924-9300   Fax (609)924-6552
+ Morristown Medical Center
  100 Madison Avenue/Box 157 Simon 3   Morristown, NJ 07962   (609)924-9300   Fax (973)401-2465

Slavin, Kevin A., MD {1205803624} PedInf, ClnPhm(93,CA14)<NJ-HACKNSK, NJ-HOLYNAME>
+ Hackensack University Medical Center
  30 Prospect Avenue/PedilnfDis   Hackensack, NJ 07601
  (201)996-2000   Fax (201)996-9815

Slavin, Stuart F., MD {1134188402} Pedtrc(96,NY46)<NJ-VALLEY>
+ Touchpoint Pediatrics
  17 Watchung Avenue   Chatham, NJ 07928   (973)665-0900
  Fax (973)665-0901

Slawek, Joseph E., MD {1629070016} Radiol(91,PA02)
+ Radiology Associates of Burlington County
  1295 Route 38 West/PO Box 479   Hainesport, NJ 08036
  (609)261-7017   Fax (609)261-4180

Slazak, Katherine L., MD {1255356218} RadDia, Radiol(84,NY09)<NJ-STBARNMC>
+ St. Barnabas Medical Center
  94 Old Short Hills Road/Radiology   Livingston, NJ 07039
  (973)322-5000

Sleavin, Harold J., MD {1164471686} Pedtrc(82,ITA01)
+ 551 Westwood Avenue
  Long Branch, NJ 07740   (732)229-7480

Sleman, Ingy Hanna, MD {1164877510} RadDia
+ 70 Boatworks Drive
  Bayonne, NJ 07002   (781)249-6270

Slep, Borys, MD {1255442661} EmrgMd(74,POLA)<NJ-CHRIST>
+ Christ Hospital
  176 Palisade Avenue/EmrgMed   Jersey City, NJ 07306
  (201)795-8200

Sless, Dana E., DO {1184615973} Pedtrc(98,PA77)<NJ-ACMCITY>
+ Brighton Pediatrics PA
  2829 Atlantic Avenue   Atlantic City, NJ 08401   (609)348-4813

Slevin, Kieran Anthony, MD {1588693675} Anesth, AnesPain, IntrMd(98,IRE12)<NJ-VIRTBERL, NJ-VIRTMARL>
+ Virtua Pain and Spine Specialists
  404 Creek Crossing Boulevard   Hainesport, NJ 08036
  (609)845-3988

Slim, Jihad, MD {1366411076} InfDis, IntrMd(80,LEB01)<NJ-STMICHL>
+ St. Michael's Medical Center
  268 MLK Jr. Boulevard   Newark, NJ 07102   (973)364-2682
  Fax (973)364-1430

Sliwinski, Stanley John, MD {1467504464} ObsGyn(75,WI06)<NJ-CHSMRCER>
+ Capital Health System/Mercer Campus
  446 Bellevue Avenue   Trenton, NJ 08618   (609)394-4000

Sliwowska, Anna, MD {1972921351} FamMed
+ Drs. Tran and Sliwowska
  317 George Street   New Brunswick, NJ 08901   (732)235-6972

Sliwowski, Martha S., MD {1942300462} Pedtrc(90,UKR05)<NJ-HACKNSK, NJ-STJOSHOS>
+ Prime Care Pediatrics
  42 Locust Avenue/Suite 5   Wallington, NJ 07057   (973)473-4033   Fax (973)473-2988

Sliwowski, Stanislaw, MD {1003914706} Pedtrc(78,POL14)<NJ-STJOSHOS, NJ-HACKNSK>
+ Prime Care Pediatrics
  42 Locust Avenue/Suite 5   Wallington, NJ 07057   (973)473-4033   Fax (973)473-2988

Sloan, Kim W., MD {1255505541} SrgArt, SrgOrt, IntrMd(73,MA05)
+ Glen Ridge Surgicenter
  230 Sherman Avenue   Glen Ridge, NJ 07028   (201)393-9333   Fax (973)680-4211

Sloan, Victor S., MD {1700969771} Rheuma(89,NY09)<NJ-RWJUHAM>
+ UH- RWJ Medical School
  One Robert Wood Johnson Place   New Brunswick, NJ 08903
  (732)235-7702   Fax (732)235-7238
+ UH- Robert Wood Johnson Med
  125 Paterson Street/5th Fl   New Brunswick, NJ 08901
  (732)235-7702   Fax (732)235-6526

Sloan, William C., MD {1578750204} Gastrn, IntrMd(65,PA01)<NJ-MORRISTN>
+ Affiliates in Gastroenterology, P.A.
  101 Old Short Hills Road/Suite 217   West Orange, NJ 07052
  (973)731-4600   Fax (973)731-0525
+ Affiliates in Gastroenterology, P.A.
  101 Madison Avenue/Suite 100   Morristown, NJ 07960
  (973)731-4600   Fax (973)540-8788

Sloane, Amy Johnson, MD {1922364785} IntHos<NJ-UNDRWD>
+ Inspira Health Network
  509 North Broad Street   Woodbury, NJ 08096   (856)845-0100   Fax (302)651-5954

Slomovitz, Brian Matthew, MD {1306885512} ObsGyn, GyOnc(98,NJ05)<NJ-MORRISTN>
+ Morristown Medical Center
  100 Madison Avenue   Morristown, NJ 07962   (973)971-5900   Fax (973)290-7257
+ Carol G. Simon Cancer Center
  33 Overlook Road/Suite LL 102   Summit, NJ 07901
  (973)971-6100

Slone, Helen L., MD {1285639732} EnDbMt(87,GRN01)
+ 1601 North 2nd Street/Suite D-3
  Millville, NJ 08332   (856)293-0305   Fax (856)293-8058

Slota, Yuriy E., MD {1689994766}
+ 277 Lafayette Avenue/Unit A
  Cliffside Park, NJ 07010   (347)885-1759
  yuriy_slota@yahoo.com

Slotoroff, Howard, MD {1184663403} Urolgy(68,IL42)<NJ-ACMCMAIN>
+ 72 West Jimmie Leeds Road/Suite 1600
  Galloway, NJ 08205   (609)652-6876   Fax (609)652-5277
+ AtlantiCare Regional Med Ctr/Mainland
  65 West Jimmie Leeds Road   Pomona, NJ 08240   (609)652-1000

Slotoroff, Jon W., DO {1760565071} IntrMd(75,PA77)<NJ-ACMCITY, NJ-ACMCMAIN>
+ Seashore Medical Associates
  48 Ansley Boulevard   Pleasantville, NJ 08232   (609)641-1077   Fax (609)641-1023

Slupchynskyj, Oleh Swatuslav, MD {1811942220} Otlryg, SrgHdN, SrgFPl(91,NY09)<NY-NYEYEINF>
+ Short Hills Surgery Center
  187 Millburn Avenue/Suite 101   Millburn, NJ 07041
  (973)671-0555   Fax (973)671-0557

Physicians by Name and Address

Slusser, Jonathan, DO {1750644704} IntrMd(12,PA77)<NJ-KMH-TURNV>
+ Jefferson Health Primary & Specialty Care
 1A Regulus Drive Turnersville, NJ 08012 (844)542-2273
+ Voorhees Primary & Specialty Care
 333 Laurel Oak Road Voorhees, NJ 08043 (844)542-2273 Fax (856)770-9194
+ Rowan University-School of Osteopathic Medicine
 1 Medical Center Drive Stratford, NJ 08012 (856)677-6708 Fax (856)566-6222

Slutsky, Jay B., DO {1871857136}
+ 612 Second Street/Apt 2-l
 Hoboken, NJ 07030 (516)395-3413

Small, Daniel Alan, MD {1528030186} ObsGyn, IntrMd(82,PA01)<NJ-CHSMRCER>
+ Lawrence Ob/Gyn Associates
 123 Franklin Corner Road/Suite 214 Lawrenceville, NJ 08648 (609)896-1400 Fax (609)896-3986

Small, Stephen Edward, DO {1518956002} SrgPlstc(98,PA77)
+ Ocean Plastic Surgery P.A.
 413 Lakehurst Road/Suite 301 Toms River, NJ 08755 (732)255-7155 Fax (732)255-7455
 oceanplasticsurgery@verizon.net
+ 1301 Route 72 West/Suite 260
 Manahawkin, NJ 08050

Small, Tzvi, MD {1033188461} SrgPlstc, Surgry(94,NY19)<NJ-HACKNSK, NJ-VALLEY>
+ Bergen Plastic Surgery
 275 Forest Avenue/Suite 202 Paramus, NJ 07652 (201)599-1500 Fax (201)599-1501

Smart, Frank W., MD {1275571341} CdvDis, ClCdEl(85,LA05)<NJ-MORRISTN, NJ-OVERLOOK>
+ Morristown Medical Center
 100 Madison Avenue/Cardio Morristown, NJ 07962 (973)971-5000
+ Overlook Medical Center
 99 Beauvoir Avenue/PO Box 210/Cardio Summit, NJ 07902 (908)522-2000

Smeal, Brian C., MD {1720194442} Surgry(89,PA02)
+ 105 Bshop Road
 Mullica Hill, NJ 08062

Smeglin, Anthony G., MD {1992739668} IntrMd, CdvDis, IntCrd(03,NY09)<NJ-VIRTUAHS, NJ-OURLADY>
+ Associated Cardiovascular Consultants-Lourdes
 1 Brace Road/Suite C & F Cherry Hill, NJ 08034 (856)428-4100 Fax (856)428-5748

Smelkinson, Ann E., MD {1487731972} Grtrcs, IntrMd(81,ISR02)
+ 2650 Route 130 & Dey Road
 Cranbury, NJ 08512 (609)860-8000 Fax (609)860-8004

Smergel, Henry, MD {1144284399} Pedtrc(79,DC02)<NJ-OURLADY, NJ-VIRTUAHS>
+ Advocare Haddonfield Pediatric Association
 220 North Haddon Avenue Haddonfield, NJ 08033 (856)429-6719 Fax (856)429-6748

Smialowicz, Chester R., MD {1003857467} InfDis, IntrMd(67,MO34)<NJ-DEBRAHLC>
+ Deborah Heart and Lung Center
 200 Trenton Road Browns Mills, NJ 08015 (609)893-6611 Fax (609)677-1306

Smick, Robert J., DO {1720013196} FamMed, OccpMd(93,PA77)<NJ-SJHREGMC>
+ SJH Regional Medical Center
 1505 West Sherman Avenue Vineland, NJ 08360 (856)641-7595 Fax (856)641-7913

Smighelschi, Corina Daniela, MD {1427345446} IntrMd(09,DMN01)<NJ-NWRKBETH>
+ 1767 Morris Avenue/Suite 115
 Union, NJ 07083 (908)258-7405 Fax (908)258-7406
+ Newark Beth Israel Medical Center
 201 Lyons Avenue/Internal Med Newark, NJ 07112 (908)258-7405 Fax (973)924-7255

Smilen, Scott Walter, MD {1811985518} ObsGyn, GynOnc(88,NY19)<NY-NYUTISCH, NJ-VALLEY>
+ 577 Chestnut Ridge Road/Suite 9
 Woodcliff Lake, NJ 07677

Smires, Harvey E., Jr., MD {1407872369} SrgOrt, IntrMd(83,NY01)<NJ-UNVMCPRN, NJ-VANJHCS>
+ Princeton Bone & Joint
 5 Plainsboro Road/Suite 100 Plainsboro, NJ 08536 (609)750-1600 Fax (609)750-1611

Smith, Abigail, MD {1326467838}
+ McGuire Air Force Base/Acute Health Care Clinic
 3458 Neely Road Trenton, NJ 08641 (609)754-9780 Fax (609)754-9015

Smith, Adam Powell, MD {1639598436} Surgry
+ Surgical Associates
 90 Prospect Avenue/Room 1D Hackensack, NJ 07601 (201)343-3433 Fax (201)343-0420

Smith, Arien Javon, MD {1023277829} SrgNro(03,CT01)<NY-IMCBRKLN>
+ Brain & Spine Institute of NY & NJ
 25 Kennedy Boulevard/Suite 850 East Brunswick, NJ 08816

(732)875-3814 Fax (732)354-0091

Smith, Arvin P., MD {1629008032} Radiol, RadDia(69,NY46)<NJ-STCLRDEN>
+ St. Clare's Hospital-Denville Campus
 25 Pocono Road/Radiology Denville, NJ 07834 (973)625-6000

Smith, Brian L., MD {1538179452} Surgry, GenPrc(80,MEX03)<NY-STATNRTH>
+ Jonathan Alan Wang DO LLC
 290 Madison Avenue/Suite 2 A Morristown, NJ 07960 (973)285-1999 Fax (973)359-8979

Smith, Charlene M., MD {1790876787} RadDia, Radiol, NuclMd(81,PA09)<NJ-OURLADY>
+ Our Lady of Lourdes Medical Center
 1600 Haddon Avenue/Radiology Camden, NJ 08103 (856)757-3500

Smith, Cheryl E., MD {1194863324} Pthlgy, PthDrm(76,PA13)
+ Cheryl E. Smith MD, P.C.
 15 East High Street/Suite M Glassboro, NJ 08028 (856)881-0665 Fax (856)881-1449

Smith, Corey Kamahl, MD {1699724237} EmrgMd(02,NJ06)<NJ-JRSYSHMC, NJ-RWJURAH>
+ EmCare
 1945 Route 33 Neptune, NJ 07753 (732)776-4510 Fax (732)776-2329

Smith, Daniel Brian J., MD {1477510873} Anesth(01,NJ06)<NJ-STPETER>
+ Anesthesia Consultnts of NJ/Nova Pain
 285 Davidson Avenue/Suite 204 Somerset, NJ 08873 (732)271-1400 Fax (732)271-3543
+ Cares Surgicenter, LLC.
 240 Easton Avenue New Brunswick, NJ 08901 (732)271-1400 Fax (732)296-8677

Smith, Daniel Humphreys, MD {1326009382} GynOnc, ObsGyn, Surgry(72,MA01)<NJ-HOLYNAME>
+ John Theurer Cancer Center - HUMC
 20 Prospect Avenue/Suite 703 Hackensack, NJ 07601 (201)996-5900
+ Holy Name Hospital
 718 Teaneck Road/CancerCtr/2ndFl Teaneck, NJ 07666 (201)996-5900 Fax (201)227-6295

Smith, David E., MD {1700088952} PhysMd(03,NJ05)
+ Hamilton HealthCare Center
 3840 Quakerbridge Road/Suite 100 Hamilton, NJ 08619 (609)890-2222 Fax (609)890-0715
 drdavidesmith@yahoo.com

Smith, David J., MD {1912085465} Ophthl(71,WI06)<NJ-ACMCITY, NJ-ACMCMAIN>
+ Drs. Dunn & Smith
 4807 Atlantic Avenue Ventnor, NJ 08406 (609)823-8488 Fax (609)823-1787
+ Drs. Dunn & Smith
 4 East Jimmie Leeds Road/Suites 1-2 Galloway, NJ 08205 (609)652-6100

Smith, Dominic, MD {1578982757}
+ Summit Medical Group-Berkeley Heights Campus
 1 Diamond Hill Road Berkeley Heights, NJ 07922 (908)273-4300 Fax (908)673-7336

Smith, Donard Scott, MD {1790290740} EmrgMd
+ 139 Elmwood Avenue
 Ho Ho Kus, NJ 07423 (201)241-0544 Fax (201)445-7317

Smith, Donna M., MD {1275584054} ObsGyn(80,MA05)
+ 2040 Millburn Avenue/Suite 306
 Maplewood, NJ 07040 (973)762-2479 Fax (973)313-1605

Smith, Ebben Will, MD {1043248941} IntrMd(99,NY47)<NJ-HOLYNAME>
+ Primary Care NJ
 370 Grand Avenue/Suite 102 Englewood, NJ 07631 (201)567-3370 Fax (201)816-1265

Smith, Elton John, MD {1679526784} Psychy
+ Center for Family Guidance, PC
 765 East Route 70/Building A-101 Marlton, NJ 08053 (856)797-4800 Fax (856)810-0110

Smith, Eric Brandon, MD {1982666939} SrgOrt
+ Rothman Institute
 999 Route 73 North/3rd Fl Marlton, NJ 08053 (856)821-6360 Fax (856)821-6359

Smith, Franz Omar Desric, MD {1942503610} Surgry<NJ-STBARNMC>
+ St. Barnabas Medical Center
 94 Old Short Hills Road Livingston, NJ 07039 (973)322-8945

Smith, George Philip, MD {1205801982} SrgHnd, SrgPlstc, Surgry(94,NY46)<NY-METHODST>
+ 272-274 High Street
 Perth Amboy, NJ 08861 (732)826-0111 Fax (732)826-2111

Smith, Glenda Ruth, MD {1477554418} RadOnc<NJ-SJHREGMC>
+ SJH Regional Medical Center
 1505 West Sherman Avenue/RadOnclgy Vineland, NJ 08360 (856)641-7920 Fax (856)641-7915

Smith, Jacqueline Marie, MD {1255643615} ObsGyn(08,SC01)
+ NJ Best OBGYN
 716 Broad Street/Suite 6 A Clifton, NJ 07013 (973)221-3122 Fax (973)574-1008

Smith, Jade, DO {1366845968} ObsGyn
+ Ob/Gyn and Infertility Services of Northern NJ
 721 Clifton Avenue/Suite 1A Clifton, NJ 07013 (201)957-7547 Fax (973)471-2112

Smith, James Randolph, MD {1124052410} IntrMd, SlpDis(88,NJ05)<NJ-HCKTSTWN, NJ-MORRISTN>
+ Morristown Memorial Sleep Disorder Center
 95 Mount Kemble Avenue Morristown, NJ 07960 (973)971-4567
+ 98 Route 46 West/Village Green Annex
 Budd Lake, NJ 07828 (973)426-8484

Smith, Jason Anthony, DO {1578724324} CdvDis, IntrMd
+ Associated Cardiovascular Consultants-Lourdes
 1 Brace Road/Suite C & F Cherry Hill, NJ 08034 (856)428-4100 Fax (856)428-5748

Smith, Jason Anthony, MD {1780818047} PhysMd(09,NJ05)
+ Associates in Rehabilitation Medicine
 95 Mount Kemble Avenue Morristown, NJ 07960 (973)267-2293 Fax (973)226-3144
+ Coordinated Health
 222 Red Lane Phillipsburg, NJ 08865 (973)267-2293 Fax (610)849-1013

Smith, Jeffrey Todd, DO {1659366904} IntrMd(02,MO78)
+ Haskell Towne Medical LLC
 1141 Ringwood Avenue/Suite 7 Haskell, NJ 07420 (973)835-6777

Smith, Jillian Corbett, MD {1508009325} EmrgMd(NJ06<NJ-COOPRUMC>
+ Cooper University Hospital
 One Cooper Plaza/Emerg Med Camden, NJ 08103 (856)342-2351

Smith, John Edmund, Jr., MD {1275521361} OncHem, MedOnc, IntrMd(87,MEX48)
+ Starr Hematology & Medical Oncology Associates
 755 Memorial Parkway/Suite 102 Phillipsburg, NJ 08865 (908)454-0370 Fax (908)454-9858

Smith, John P., DO {1043389869} CdvDis, IntrMd(73,PA77)<NJ-VALLEY, NJ-NWRKBETH>
+ 15-01 Broadway/Suite 4
 Fair Lawn, NJ 07410 (201)794-6505

Smith, Jonathan, MD {1912994740} Radiol, RadV&I(82,NY19)<NJ-VALLEY>
+ Radiology Associates of Ridgewood, P.A.
 20 Franklin Turnpike Waldwick, NJ 07463 (201)445-8822 Fax (201)447-5053
+ The Valley Hospital
 223 North Van Dien Avenue/Radiology Ridgewood, NJ 07450 (201)447-8000

Smith, Joseph Arthur, MD {1366524761} FamMed(82,NY15)<NJ-SOMERSET>
+ Your Doctors Care, PA
 71 Route 206 South Hillsborough, NJ 08844 (908)685-1887 Fax (908)707-0816

Smith, Justin Kerry, MD {1609295187} Anesth
+ Bergen Anesthesia Group PC
 223 North Van Dien Avenue Ridgewood, NJ 07450 (201)847-9320 Fax (201)847-0059

Smith, Kenneth, Jr., DO {1760431209} Anesth, CritCr(96,NJ75)<NJ-UNDRWD>
+ Inspira Health Network
 509 North Broad Street/Anesth Woodbury, NJ 08096 (856)845-0100

Smith, Kindra Renee, MD {1083634406} FamMed, IntrMd(01,NJ03)
+ Patient first
 4000 Route 130/Bldg. C Delran, NJ 08075 (856)705-0685 Fax (856)705-0686

Smith, Leon G., Jr., MD {1467454751} MtFtMd, ObsGyn(85,DC02)<NJ-STBARNMC>
+ St. Barnabas Medical Center
 94 Old Short Hills Road/Ob/Gyn Livingston, NJ 07039 (973)322-5000 Fax (973)322-2309

Smith, Leslie Robert, MD Dermat, PthDrm(67,MI07)
+ 1176 Karin Street
 Vineland, NJ 08360 (856)691-1737

Smith, Liam R., MD {1699935098} Surgry
+ Princeton Surgical Associates, P.A.
 5 Plainsboro Road/Suite 400 Plainsboro, NJ 08536 (609)936-9100 Fax (609)936-9200
 LSmith@princeton-surgical.com

Smith, Michael Adam, MD {1134392343} Pedtrc<NJ-ENGLWOOD, NJ-HACKNSK>
+ Tenafly Pediatrics, PA
 32 Franklin Street Tenafly, NJ 07670 (201)569-2400 Fax (201)569-6081

Smith, Monika, DO {1508913872} EmrgMd
+ 512 Washington Terrace
 Audubon, NJ 08106

Smith, Peter Lloyd, MD {1861497224} RadDia(87,MO02)
+ Comprehensive Cardiovascular Consultants
299 Madison Avenue/Suite 102 Morristown, NJ 07960
(973)292-1020 Fax (973)292-0564

Smith, Robert Charles, MD {1316922784} Urolgy, IntrMd(89,NY01)<NJ-RIVERVW, NJ-BAYSHORE>
+ Urology Associates, P.A.
595 Shrewsbury Avenue/Suite 103 Shrewsbury, NJ 07702
(732)741-5923 Fax (732)741-2759

Smith, Robert T., MD {1902844251} RadDia, Radiol(70,SC01)<NJ-COOPRUMC>
+ Cooper University Hospital
One Cooper Plaza/Radiology Camden, NJ 08103
(856)342-2000

Smith, Sharon Marie, MD {1659349066} ObsGyn(93,NJ05)<NJ-ACMCMAIN, NJ-ACMCITY>
+ 1 Highway 70
Lakewood, NJ 08701 (848)222-4689

Smith, Shrita Marie, MD {1801139522}
+ 1516 Hiawatha Avenue
Hillside, NJ 07205 (862)452-3489
smith.shrita@gmail.com
+ Coordinated Health
222 Red Lane Phillipsburg, NJ 08865 (862)452-3489 Fax (610)849-1013

Smith, Simon N., DO {1740532613} IntrMd(09,PA78)<NJ-DEBRAHLC>
+ Deborah Heart and Lung Center
200 Trenton Road Browns Mills, NJ 08015 (609)893-6611

Smith, Stephanie, MD {1326369968} FamMed(10,GRN01)
+ Town Medical Associates/Verona
271 Grove Avenue/Suite A Verona, NJ 07044 (973)239-6500 Fax (973)239-0482

Smith, Stephen Marshall, MD {1104875814} InfDis, IntrMd(89,CT01)<NJ-STBARNMC, NJ-STMICHL>
+ ID Associates PA
189 Eagle Rock Avenue Roseland, NJ 07068 (973)980-0195 Fax (973)774-1920
btopy@idcare.com

Smith, Tara Marie, MD {1548352628} PedCrC, Pedtrc, IntrMd(85,STM01)<NJ-COOPRUMC>
+ Cooper University Hospital
One Cooper Plaza/Pediatrics Camden, NJ 08103
(856)968-9575

Smith, Terri L., MD {1417043894} Pedtrc(91,NJ05)<NJ-HOLYNAME, NJ-ENGLWOOD>
+ 307 East Madison Avenue
Dumont, NJ 07628 (201)530-0551 Fax (201)530-0553

Smith-Dipalo, Tracy A., MD {1851371835} IntrMd(84,NJ05)<NJ-CHILTON>
+ Physicians Health Alliance
28 Jackson Avenue Pompton Plains, NJ 07444 (973)835-2575 Fax (973)835-0531

Smith-Elfant, Stacy A., MD {1164470787} Pedtrc(89,NJ06)<NJ-OURLADY, NJ-COOPRUMC>
+ Advocare Atrium Pediatrics
301 Old Marlton Pike West/Suite 1 Marlton, NJ 08053
(856)988-9101 Fax (856)988-7712

Smith-Martin, Kimberley Yvette, MD {1679648646} PhysMd, PainMd, PhyMPain(99,PA13)<NJ-SJHREGMC, NJ-SJRSYELM>
+ Premier Orthopaedic Associates
298 South Delsea Drive Vineland, NJ 08360 (856)690-1616 Fax (856)690-1089
+ Premier Orthopaedic Assocs of So NJ
201 Tomlin Station Road/Suite C Mullica Hill, NJ 08062
(856)690-1616 Fax (856)223-9110

Smithers, Wilda I., MD {1811922032} IntrMd(82,NJ05)<NJ-KIMBALL>
+ 1166 River Avenue/Suite 210
Lakewood, NJ 08701 (732)367-8272 Fax (732)367-3693

Smithson, Sarah, MD {1477966307} ObsGyn<NJ-MONMOUTH>
+ Monmouth Medical Center
300 Second Avenue/Rm 215 SW Long Branch, NJ 07740
(732)923-6795

Smok, Jeffrey Thomas, MD {1033168232} Anesth(97,WV02)<NJ-ENGLWOOD>
+ Englewood Anesthesiology
350 Engle Street Englewood, NJ 07631 (201)894-3238
Fax (201)894-0585

Smolarz, Brian Gabriel, MD {1467632349} EnDbMt, IntrMd(NY03<NJ-UNVMCPRN>
+ Concierge Endocrinology
38 Robbinsville Allentown Road Robbinsville, NJ 08691
(609)250-2766 Fax (877)991-8162

Smolinsky, Adi, MD {1831352889} ObsGyn(03,HUN03)<NJ-STPETER>
+ Ob-Gyn Associates at Holmdel-Shrewsbury
704 North Beers Street Holmdel, NJ 07733 (732)739-2500
Fax (732)888-2778

Smolinsky, Ciaran, MD {1699279893} ObsGyn
+ Cooper University Hospital OBGYN
3 Cooper Plaza/Suite 221 Camden, NJ 08103 (908)268-9228 Fax (856)968-8575

Smoller, Alison Brett, DO {1730384884} Pedtrc, PedDvl(02,MO78)<NY-BLVUENYU>
+ 1806 Highway 35/Suite 107
Oakhurst, NJ 07755

Smotkin-Tangorra, Margarita, DO {1477673341} PedEnd, Pedtrc
+ Meridian Medical Group - Faculty Practice
61 Davis Avenue/Suite 1 Neptune, NJ 07753 (732)776-4860 Fax (732)776-4867
+ Meridian Practice Insitute-Pediatrics
1944 State Route 33/Suite 204 Neptune, NJ 07753
(732)776-4860 Fax (732)776-4867

Smotrich, Gary A., MD {1588683098} SrgPlstc, SrgBst, SrgHnd(82,CT02)<NJ-CHSFULD, NJ-CHSMRCER>
+ Lawrenceville Plastic Surgery
3131 Princeton Pike Lawrenceville, NJ 08648 (609)896-2525 Fax (609)896-2639
drsmotrich@lawrencevilleplasticsurgery.com

Smukler, Naomi R., MD {1417185547}<NJ-OVERLOOK>
+ Overlook Medical Center
99 Beauvoir Avenue/PO Box 210 Summit, NJ 07902
(908)522-2000

Smuro, Daniel J., MD {1407927296} Radiol, RadDia(72,PA09)<NJ-MONMOUTH>
+ Monmouth Radiologists, PA
279 Third Avenue Long Branch, NJ 07740 (732)222-7676
Fax (732)229-1863

Snady, Harry Walter, Jr., MD {1144322801} Gastrn, IntrMd(77,NY19)<NJ-HOBUNIMC, NY-MTSINYHS>
+ GastroCare
96 Hudson Street Hoboken, NJ 07030 (201)659-8200
gastrocare@gastrocare.info
+ GastroCare
5600 Kennedy Boulevard West New York, NJ 07093
(201)902-9500

Snead Poellnitz, Stephanie E., MD {1962572073} Psychy(73,PA02)<NJ-ACMCITY, NJ-ACMCMAIN>
+ AtlantiCare Behavioral Health/Pact Team A
2511 Fire Road/Suite B-10 Egg Harbor Township, NJ 08234
(609)407-0042 Fax (609)407-0185

Snellings, Richard Barton, MD {1750546982} RadDia<NJ-UMDNJ>
+ University Hospital
150 Bergen Street/C 320 Newark, NJ 07103 (973)972-4300

Snepar, Richard A., MD {1881664522} InfDis, IntrMd(76,NY20)
+ Highland Park Medical Associates
579A Cranbury Road/Suite 102 East Brunswick, NJ 08816
(732)613-0711 Fax (732)613-5783

Snepar, Rory B., DO {1609161322}
+ Atlantic Shore Surgical Associates
478 Brick Boulevard Brick, NJ 08723 (732)447-3904 Fax (732)701-1244
rorysnepar@gmail.com

Snieckus, Peter J., MD {1306818166} RadDia, Radiol(82,NJ05)<NJ-OVERLOOK>
+ Westfield Imaging Center
118-122 Elm Street Westfield, NJ 07090 (908)232-0610
Fax (908)232-7140
+ Summit Radiology Associates
99 Beauvoir Avenue Summit, NJ 07901 (908)522-2066

Snyder, Craig Adam, MD {1427008945} IntrMd, IntCrd, CdvDis(95,NY48)
+ Raritan Bay Cardiology Group, P.A.
225 May Street/Suite F Edison, NJ 08837 (732)738-8855
Fax (732)738-4141
+ Raritan Bay Cardiology Group, P.A.
3 Hospital Plaza/Suite 305 Old Bridge, NJ 08857
(732)738-8855 Fax (732)738-4141
+ Raritan Bay Cardiology Group, P.A.
337 Applegarth Road Monroe Township, NJ 08837
(609)655-8860 Fax (732)738-4141

Snyder, David L., MD {1750387718} PsyGrt, Psychy, PsyCAd(80,PA09)
+ Snyder Behavioral Health
509 South Lenola Road/Suite 4A Moorestown, NJ 08057
(856)439-9300 Fax (856)727-9337

Snyder, Harvey A., MD {1003869488} CdvDis, IntCrd(76,MD07)<NJ-COOPRUMC, NJ-VIRTBERL>
+ Cardiovascular Associates
210 West Atlantic Avenue Haddon Heights, NJ 08035
(856)546-3003 Fax (856)547-5337
+ Cardiovascular Associates of The Delaware Valley, PA
1840 Frontage Road Cherry Hill, NJ 08034 (856)546-3003
Fax (856)795-7436
+ Cardiovascular Associates of The Delaware Valley, PA
525 State Street/Suite 3 Elmer, NJ 08035 (856)358-2363
Fax (856)358-0725

Snyder, Hugh David, MD {1376535591} FamMed(95,NJ05)
+ Springfield Family Practice
11 Overlook Road/Suite 140 Summit, NJ 07901 (908)277-0050 Fax (908)277-0201

Snyder, Kenneth R., MD {1558378976} FamMed(90,NY09)
+ RWJPE Primary Care Center at Hillsborough
331 Route 206 North/Suite 2-B Hillsborough, NJ 08844
(908)685-2528 Fax (908)359-7109

Snyder, Laura Jean, MD {1184654766} EmrgMd, PedEmg(96,NJ06)
+ Family Medicine at Monument Square
317 George Street New Brunswick, NJ 08901 (732)235-8993 Fax (732)246-7317

Snyder, Michael T., MD {1871580639} ObsGyn(89,NY19)<NJ-LOURDMED, NJ-VIRTMHBC>
+ Advocare Burlington County Obstetrics & Gynecology
1000 Salem Road/Suite B Willingboro, NJ 08046
(609)871-2060 Fax (609)871-3535
+ Burlington County Ob-Gyn
8008 Route 130 N/Suite 320 Delran, NJ 08075 (609)871-2060 Fax (856)764-0103
+ Burlington County Ob-Gyn
210 Ark Road/Suite 216 Mount Laurel, NJ 08046
(856)778-2060 Fax (856)778-8182

Snyder, Natali P., DO {1770894925} EmrgMd
+ 38 Dublin Lane
Cherry Hill, NJ 08003

Snyder, Randall William, III, MD {1295729598} RadV&I, Radiol(94,NY19)<NJ-VIRTUAHS, NJ-VIRTMHBC>
+ South Jersey Radiology Associates, P.A.
315 Route 70 East/Suite B Cherry Hill, NJ 08034 (856)428-4344 Fax (856)428-0356
+ South Jersey Radiology Associates, P.A.
1000 Lincoln Drive East Marlton, NJ 08053 (856)428-4344
Fax (856)983-3226
+ South Jersey Radiology Associates, P.A.
807 Haddon Avenue/Suite 5 Haddonfield, NJ 08034
(856)616-1130 Fax (856)616-1125

Snyder, Ronald David, MD {1962405340} SrgOrt(91,PA01)<NJ-VALLEY>
+ 22 Madison Avenue/Suite 6
Paramus, NJ 07652 (201)342-4100 Fax (201)342-6250

Snyder, Samuel Jay, MD {1568439305} SrgOrt, SprtMd(83,NY20)<NJ-VALLEY>
+ Garden State Surgical Center, L.L.C.
28-06 Broadway Fair Lawn, NJ 07410 (201)475-8940
Fax (201)475-8944
+ Garden State Orthopaedic Associates, P.A.
28-04 Broadway Fair Lawn, NJ 07410 (201)475-8940
Fax (201)791-9377
+ Garden State Orthopaedic Associates, P.A.
33-41 Newark Street Hoboken, NJ 07410 (201)876-5300
Fax (201)876-5305

So, Hee Young, MD {1215080270} Psychy(70,KOR06)<NJ-JRSYCITY>
+ Ocean Mental Health Services, Inc.
160 Atlantic City Boulevard Bayville, NJ 08721 (732)349-5550 Fax (732)349-0841

So, Kenneth Chan-Lee, MD {1528448461}<NJ-COOPRUMC>
+ Cooper University Hospital
One Cooper Plaza Camden, NJ 08103 (856)342-3150

Soares-Velez, Javier Ignacio, MD {1275854747}
+ 788 Shrewsbury Avenue/Bldg 1/Suite 103
Tinton Falls, NJ 07724 (787)557-6061

Sobel, David Charles, MD {1730181173} IntrMd(76,NY08)<NJ-BAYSHORE, NJ-RIVERVW>
+ Old Bridge Primary Care
300 Perrine Road/Suite 324 Old Bridge, NJ 08857
(732)753-9890 Fax (732)753-9893

Sobel, Gail M., MD {1477533750} ObsGyn(90,NJ05)<NJ-VALLEY>
+ Women's Total Health-Woodcliff Lake
577 Chestnut Ridge Road/Suite 9 Woodcliff Lake, NJ 07677
(201)391-5770 Fax (201)391-4793

Sobel, Janine M., MD {1528143930} Psychy(81,NY19)
+ 2301 Evesham Road/Suite 304
Voorhees, NJ 08043 (856)772-9404 Fax (856)795-8063

Sobel, Mark, MD {1629124722} SrgOrt(87,OH06)
+ 25 First Avenue/Suite 110
Atlantic Highlands, NJ 07716 (732)291-4085 Fax (732)291-4086
info@msobelmd.com

Sobel, Mark A., MD {1326115700} SrgOrt(80,NY19)<NJ-VIRTMARL>
+ Sobel & Zell Orthopaedic Associates
525 Route 73 South/Suite 303 Marlton, NJ 08053
(856)596-0555 Fax (856)596-7658

Sobelman, Joseph S., MD {1023123650} Nrolgy(82,MEX03)
+ Neurology & Neurodiagnostics, P.A.
22 Old Short Hills Road/Suite 106 Livingston, NJ 07039
(973)994-1123 Fax (973)994-7158
Jssmd@comcast.net

Soberano, Wilfredo T., MD {1588703102} Psychy(84,PHI32)<NJ-HCMEADPS>
+ Hudson County Meadowview Psychiatric Hospital
595 County Avenue Secaucus, NJ 07094 (201)319-3660

Physicians by Name and Address

Sobers-Brown, Karen D., MD {1023047982} EmrgMd(91,PA09)<NJ-KMHSTRAT>
+ Kennedy Memorial Hospital-University Medical Center
18 East Laurel Road/EmergMed Stratford, NJ 08084 (856)346-7985 Fax (856)346-6539

Soble, Toby K., MD {1184658494} FamMed(91,PA02)<NJ-VIRTBERL, NJ-VIRTMARL>
+ Family Practice Associates of Voorhees
805 Cooper Road/Suite 3 Voorhees, NJ 08043 (856)751-1777 Fax (856)751-8090

Sobol, Igor Leonidovich, MD {1992858112} Nrolgy(79,RUS03)<NJ-JFKMED, NJ-RBAYPERT>
+ General Neurology Headache
2 Lincoln Highway/Suite 509 Edison, NJ 08820 (732)767-1500 Fax (732)767-0090

Sobol, Marina B., MD {1841344694} Nrolgy(79,RUS03)
+ General Neurology Headache
2 Lincoln Highway/Suite 509 Edison, NJ 08820 (732)767-1500 Fax (732)767-0090

Sobrepena, Jose S.M., MD {1932178209} Anesth(82,PHI20)<NJ-MTNSIDE>
+ 31 Point Pleasant Road
Hopatcong, NJ 07843

Sobti, Rimmi, MD {1801915483} IntrMd(91,INDI)
+ 511 Lakehurst Road
Toms River, NJ 08755 (732)797-0007 Fax (732)797-0063

Sobti, Sanjiv, MD {1245235050} CdvDis(80,INDI)
+ Cardiology Consultants
368 Lakehurst Road/Suite 301 Toms River, NJ 08755 (732)240-1048 Fax (732)240-3464
+ Cardiology Consultants
63-C Lacey Road Whiting, NJ 08759 (732)240-1048 Fax (732)350-7054

Soda, Michael, MD {1811911340} Surgry, SrgVas(72,MEX03)
+ 195 Route 46 West/Suite 201
Mine Hill, NJ 07803 (973)328-0160 Fax (973)328-4097

Sodagum, Lakshmi Lavanya, MD {1265421283} IntrMd, Nephro(98,INA62)<NJ-NWTNMEM, NJ-HCKTSTWN>
+ The Renal Care Clinic, P.C.
67 High Street/Suite 102 Newton, NJ 07860 (973)579-5009 Fax (973)579-3009
Lsodagum@hotmail.com
+ The Renal Care Clinic, P.C.
655 Willow Grove Street/Suite 2700 Hackettstown, NJ 07840 (973)579-5009 Fax (973)579-3009

Sodha, Amee, MD {1548687569} IntrMd<NJ-NWRKBETH>
+ Newark Beth Israel Medical Center
201 Lyons Avenue Newark, NJ 07112 (973)926-3233

Sodhi, Ajit S., MD {1750474656} CdvDis, IntrMd(78,INA07)
+ Clara Barton Cardio-Medical Associates
78 Amboy Avenue Metuchen, NJ 08840 (732)548-4365
+ Clara Barton Cardio-Medical Associates
565 New Brunswick Avenue Fords, NJ 08863 (732)548-4365 Fax (732)738-1663

Sodhi, Jasdeep Singh, MD {1922246396} IntrMd<NJ-VIRTMHBC>
+ Virtua Memorial
175 Madison Avenue Mount Holly, NJ 08060 (609)914-6180 Fax (609)914-6182

Sodhi, Jitendra, MD {1598702953} SrgCdv, SrgThr(79,INA8Z)<NJ-DEBRAHLC>
+ Deborah Heart and Lung Center
200 Trenton Road Browns Mills, NJ 08015 (609)893-6611 Fax (609)893-1213
jsodhi@yahoo.com

Sodhi, Sarab, MD {1184091779}<NJ-COOPRUMC>
+ Cooper University Hospital
One Cooper Plaza/Kelemen 152 Camden, NJ 08103 (856)342-2500

Sodhi, Surinder K., MD {1871599423} Pedtrc(75,INDI)
+ Urgent Health Care Center
719 Route 22 West North Plainfield, NJ 07060 (908)561-4300 Fax (908)561-4340
+ Total Care Pediatrics in Jersey City
550 Newark Avenue/Suite 200 Jersey City, NJ 07306 (908)561-4300 Fax (201)795-4999
+ Horizon Health Center
714 Bergen Avenue Jersey City, NJ 07060 (201)451-6300

Sofair, Jane Brown, MD {1811946494} Psychy, IntrMd(80,NY19)<NJ-MORRISTN, CT-HALLBRK>
+ 597 Springfield Avenue
Summit, NJ 07901 (973)292-0960 Fax (908)634-6138

Soffen, Deborah A.S., MD Pedtrc(85,NY19)<NJ-UNVMCPRN>
+ 631 Lake Drive
Princeton, NJ 08540

Soffen, Edward M., MD {1841200706} RadOnc(86,PA13)<NJ-CENTRAST>
+ CentraState Medical Center
901 West Main Street/RadOncology Freehold, NJ 07728 (732)303-5290
+ Princeton Radiation Oncology Center
9 Centre Drive/Suite 115 Jamesburg, NJ 08831 (732)303-5290 Fax (609)655-5725

Soffer, Jeffrey, MD {1659438596} ObsGyn(75,DC03)<NJ-OVERLOOK>
+ Associates in OBGYN
522 East Broad Street Westfield, NJ 07090 (908)232-4449
Jcschneider@partners.org

Soffer, Mark Jay, MD {1497722060} IntCrd, CdvDis, IntrMd(78,NY01)<NJ-STFRNMED, NJ-RWJUHAM>
+ Mercer Bucks Cardiology
One Union Street/Suite 101 Robbinsville, NJ 08691 (609)890-6677 Fax (609)890-7292

Sohagia, Amitkumar Bhikhalal, MD {1447456306} Gastrn(00,INA20)<PA-WARRNGEN>
+ Twin Rivers Gastroenterology Center
755 Memorial Parkway/Suite 202A Phillipsburg, NJ 08865 (908)859-5400

Sohaib, Muhammad, MD {1679972905} IntHos
+ AtlantiCare Hospitalist Program
1925 Pacific Avenue/8th Floor Atlantic City, NJ 08401 (609)345-4000

Sohmer, Kenette K., MD {1700840204} Ophthl(68,KY12)<NJ-HUNTRDN>
+ Branchburg Eye Physicians
3461 Route 22 Somerville, NJ 08876 (908)526-5424 Fax (908)707-8054

Sohn, Theresa J. H., MD {1801835467} Allrgy, AlgyImmn(94,NJ05)<NJ-CHILTON, NJ-WAYNEGEN>
+ ENT & Allergy Associates, LLP
1211 Hamburg Turnpike/Suite 205 Wayne, NJ 07470 (973)633-0808 Fax (973)633-8811

Sojka, Leslie W., MD {1477609634} IntrMd(80,CT01)<NJ-CENTRAST>
+ Family Practice of CentraState
901 West Main Street/Suite 106 Freehold, NJ 07728 (732)462-0100 Fax (732)462-0348
+ Family Practice of CentraState
281 Route 34/Suite 813 Colts Neck, NJ 07722 (732)462-0100 Fax (732)431-3707
+ Family Practice of CentraState
319 Route 130 North East Windsor, NJ 07728 (609)426-1555 Fax (609)447-8070

Sokalsky, Brian Edward, DO {1881872828} FamMSptM(05,NJ75)
+ Jersey Shore Sports Medicine
801 Central Avenue Ocean City, NJ 08226 (609)545-8553 Fax (609)545-8706
info@jerseyshoresportsmedicine.com

Sokel, Andrew H., MD {1255336541} FamMed(81,NY08)<NJ-CHSFULD, NJ-UNVMCPRN>
+ Plainsboro Family Physicians
666 Plainsboro Road Plainsboro, NJ 08536 (609)275-8100 Fax (609)275-6133

Sokkar, Rita, DO {1013414580} FamMed
+ Phillips Barber Family Health Center
72 Alexander Avenue Lambertville, NJ 08530 (609)397-3535 Fax (609)397-0301

Sokol, David B., MD {1235163833} MedOnc, Hemato, IntrMd(90,MD07)<NJ-UNVMCPRN>
+ University Medical Center of Princeton at Plainsboro
One Plainsboro Road/Medicine Plainsboro, NJ 08536 (609)497-4116 Fax (609)497-4992
+ Princeton Medicine
5 Plainsboro Road/Suite 300 Plainsboro, NJ 08536 (609)497-4116 Fax (609)853-7271

Sokol, Deborah Klein, MD {1417975749} Gastrn, IntrMd(90,NY19)<NJ-STFRNMED, NJ-RWJUHAM>
+ 1315 Whitehorse Mercerville Rd
Hamilton, NJ 08619 (609)750-3040 Fax (609)683-6912

Sokol, Levi Olatokunbo, MD {1053436808} RadDia, RadNuc, Radiol(04,NY01)
+ University Radiology Group, P.C.
483 Cranbury Road East Brunswick, NJ 08816 (732)390-0040 Fax (732)390-5383
+ University Radiology Group, P.C.
16 Mountain Boulevard Warren, NJ 07059 (732)390-0040 Fax (908)769-9141

Sokol, Michael C., MD {1396000246} GPrvMd, IntrMd(93,PA02)
+ 34 Princeton Court
Basking Ridge, NJ 07920 (201)280-9225

Sokol, Shima C., MD {1447489489} OrtSHand
+ Trokhan Dermatology, LLC.
235 Closter Dock Road Closter, NJ 07624 (201)767-1908 Fax (201)767-3097

Sokolova, Anna, MD {1295717247} Anesth(74,LAT02)
+ 30 Bonnell Lane
Randolph, NJ 07869 (973)540-5548

Sokolovskaya, Evgeniya, DO {1306164918}<NJ-MONMOUTH>
+ Monmouth Medical Center
300 Second Avenue Long Branch, NJ 07740 (732)923-6537

Solages, Joseph, MD {1407893365} Pedtrc(71,HAI01)
+ 1510 Park Avenue
South Plainfield, NJ 07080 (908)754-2739 Fax (908)226-1386

Solaimanzadeh, Sima, MD {1629203401} PhysMd
+ Complete Primary Care
1810 Park Avenue South Plainfield, NJ 07080 (908)226-1810 Fax (908)226-1833

Solanki, Dhenu G., MD {1376849893} FamMed(08,NJ06)<NJ-HUNTRDN, NY-MTSINAI>
+ Hunterdon Medical Center
2100 Wescott Drive/FamMed Flemington, NJ 08822 (908)788-6100

Solanki, Pallavi S., MD {1760681530} CdvDis, IntrMd(92,INA9B)<OH-OSUMEDC>
+ 185 South Orange Avenue/MSB I-578
Newark, NJ 07103 (973)972-4731 Fax (973)972-8927

Solanki, Rashminkumar R., MD {1578840492} Psychy
+ Immediate Care Psychiatric Center, LLC
22 Hill Road Parsippany, NJ 07054 (973)335-9909 Fax (973)335-9910

Solanky, Mukesh, MD {1003883836} Nrolgy(92,INDI)
+ Hackensack Neurology Group
211 Essex Street/Suite 202 Hackensack, NJ 07601 (201)488-1515 Fax (201)488-9471

Solas, John R., DO {1144246521} EmrgMd(95,IA75)<NJ-CHSFULD, NJ-CHSMRCER>
+ Kimball Medical Center
600 River Avenue Lakewood, NJ 08701 (732)363-1900

Soleymani, Taraneh, MD {1558677385} IntrMd
+ Summit Medical Group
140 Park Avenue/3rd Floor Florham Park, NJ 07932 (973)404-7880 Fax (973)285-7629

Solhkhah, Ramon, MD {1245255702} PsyAdd, PsyCAd, Psychy(93,NY09)<NJ-JRSYSHMC>
+ Jersey Shore University Medical Center - Psychiatry
1200 Jumping Brook Road Neptune, NJ 07753 (732)643-4356 Fax (732)643-4378
+ Jersey Shore University Medical Center
1945 Route 33/Psych Neptune, NJ 07753 (732)643-4356 Fax (732)643-4378

Soliman, Alaaeldin Abdalla Ali, MD {1053346866} PulDis, CritCr, IntrMd(83,EGY04)<NJ-COMMED>
+ Intensivists of Toms River, LLC.
99 Route 37 Toms River, NJ 08755 (732)557-8000 Fax (732)557-8021

Soliman, Hesham S., MD {1275596355} InfDis, IntrMd(88,DMN01)<NJ-LOURDMED>
+ Soliman Medical Associates
2400 Whitehorse Mercerville Rd Hamilton, NJ 08619 (609)587-4778 Fax (609)587-1202

Soliman, Isaac K., MD {1760876767}<NJ-MTNSIDE>
+ Hackensack UMC Mountainside
1 Bay Avenue Montclair, NJ 07042 (973)429-6196 Fax (973)429-6575

Soliman, Ishak G., MD {1578505509} FamMed(87,EGY03)<NJ-STMRYPAS>
+ Passaic Primary Care Physicians
140 Passaic Ave Passaic, NJ 07055 (973)777-8900 Fax (973)777-8929

Soliman, Monir Louis Hanna, MD {1154358604} IntrMd, OncHem(80,EGY04)
+ Regional Cancer Care Associates, LLC
4632 US Highway 9 Howell, NJ 07731 (732)367-1535 Fax (732)367-9514

Soliman, Yasser S., MD {1982667531} FamMed, IntrMd(90,NJ06)<NJ-CHSFULD>
+ Soliman Medical Associates
2400 Whitehorse Mercerville Rd Hamilton, NJ 08619 (609)587-4778 Fax (609)587-1202

Solina, Alann R., MD {1629150339} Anesth(86,GRN01)<NJ-RWJUBRUN>
+ Robert Wood Johnson-UMDNJ Anesthesia Group
125 Paterson Street/CAB 3100 New Brunswick, NJ 08901 (732)937-8841 Fax (732)235-6131

Solis, Maria S., MD {1235235995} RadDia, Radiol(78,MEX03)<NJ-COOPRUMC>
+ Cooper University Hospital
One Cooper Plaza Camden, NJ 08103 (856)342-2000

Solis, P. Ariel, MD {1033139464} SrgThr(67,NICA)<NJ-BAYSHORE, NJ-RIVERVW>
+ 80 Hazlet Avenue/Suite 8
Hazlet, NJ 07730 (732)739-5222 Fax (732)739-3983

Solis, Roberto A., MD {1376650754} PulCCr, IntrMd(88,GRN01)
+ Pulmonary & Critical Care Associates of Northern NJ
205 Browertown Road/Suite 202-203 West Paterson, NJ 07424 (973)785-7515 Fax (973)785-2205
Rasolis429@pol.net

Solish Gittens, Allison, MD {1023315819} RadDia
+ Cooper University Hospital Diagnostic Radiology
One Cooper Plaza/Suiate B23 Camden, NJ 08103 (856)342-2588

Solitro, Matthew Joseph, MD {1306870555} Nephro, IntrMd(01,PA12)<NJ-DEBRAHLC, NJ-VIRTMHBC>
+ The Center for Kidney Care
1261 Route 38/Suite A   Hainesport, NJ 08036   (856)222-1975   Fax (856)222-0721

Solitro, Tamara Stolz, MD {1811106669} IntrMd(CT02<PA-TJHSP>
+ Jefferson HealthCare - Voorhees
443 Laurel Oak Road   Voorhees, NJ 08043   (856)784-7398   Fax (856)784-7357

Soll, Stephen Matthew, MD {1114924701} Ophthl(88,IL42)<NJ-COOPRUMC>
+ Soll Eye PC of New Jersey/Cooper Division
3 Cooper Plaza/Suite 510   Camden, NJ 08103   (856)342-7200   Fax (856)342-6620

Sollitto, Robert B., MD {1740237627} SrgFPl, SrgDer, DerMOH(90,PA01)
+ 2 Van Buren Road
Voorhees, NJ 08043   (856)770-0800   Fax (856)770-4996

Solof, Arnold J., MD {1871561829} Pedtrc(76,PA09)
+ Vineland Pediatrics
1138 East Chestnut Avenue   Vineland, NJ 08360   (856)692-1108   Fax (609)692-2077

Solomon, Edward Mark, MD {1174525406} Ophthl(68,MA07)<NJ-VALLEY>
+ 85 South Maple Avenue
Ridgewood, NJ 07450   (201)444-3010   Fax (201)444-8071

Solomon, Edward Martin, MD {1033155320} RadDia(81,PA01)<NJ-STCLRDEN>
+ St. Clare's Hospital-Denville Campus
25 Pocono Road/Radiology   Denville, NJ 07834   (973)625-6000

Solomon, Jason S., MD {1992902035} RadDia(98,PA13)
+ 816 Witherspoon Way
Mullica Hill, NJ 08062

Solomon, Jennifer, MD {1073552766} FamMed(02,CT01)<NJ-MTNSIDE>
+ Drs. Carson & Solomon
203 Passaic Avenue   Passaic, NJ 07055   (973)767-2640   Fax (973)767-2641

Solomon, Leah F., MD {1093724031} IntrMd(02,NJ05)
+ PO Box 45
Mendham, NJ 07945

Solomon, Michael I., MD {1437125010} IntrMd(78,NY46)<NJ-OVERLOOK>
+ 123 Millburn Avenue
Millburn, NJ 07041   (973)376-1244

Solomon, Richard Jay, MD {1639148927} IntrMd(84,PHI32)<NJ-STBARNMC, NJ-NWRKBETH>
+ 2130 Millburn Avenue
Maplewood, NJ 07040   (973)763-5770   Fax (973)762-5411

Solomon, Robert Alan, MD {1306987227} SrgNro(80,MD07)<NY-PRSBCOLU>
+ Neurosurgeons of New Jersey
1200 East Ridgewood Avenue   Ridgewood, NJ 07450   (201)824-6131

Solomon, Robert B., MD {1376602805} Grtrcs, IntrMd(77,NY08)<NJ-TRININPC, NJ-OVERLOOK>
+ Roselle Park Medical Associates, LLC
744 Galloping Hill Road   Roselle Park, NJ 07204   (908)241-0044   Fax (908)241-0526

Solomon, Sheldon D., MD {1699712810} Grtrcs, IntrMd, Rheuma(64,PA13)<NJ-VIRTBERL, NJ-VIRTMARL>
+ Arthritis, Rheumatic & Back Disease Associates
2309 East Evesham Road/Suite 101   Voorhees, NJ 08043   (856)424-5005   Fax (856)424-4716

Solomon, Stuart R., DO {1467492744} EmrgMd(76,IA75)
+ Team Health East
307 South Evergeen Avenue   Woodbury, NJ 08096   (856)848-2088   Fax (856)848-8536

Solomon-Bergen, Peggy A., MD {1689623621} AdolMd, Pedtrc(82,NJ05)<NJ-ACMCITY, NJ-ACMCMAIN>
+ Bergen Medical Group PC
24 Wilson Drive   Northfield, NJ 08225

Solomonov, Mikhail, MD {1225095672} Anesth
+ Pain Management and Anesthesiology
8 Saddle Road/Suite 204   Cedar Knolls, NJ 07927   (973)998-7868   Fax (973)998-7883

Solonick, Douglas M., MD {1063498368} RadDia, Radiol(79,NY09)<NJ-RWJUBRUN, NJ-STPETER>
+ University Radiology Group, P.C.
483 Cranbury Road   East Brunswick, NJ 08816   (732)390-0030   Fax (732)390-5383
+ University Radiology Group, P.C.
10 Plum Street   New Brunswick, NJ 08901   (732)390-0030   Fax (732)249-1208

Soloveychik, Natalya, DO {1235320300} RadDia(03,PA78)<PA-UPMCMRCY, NJ-CHSFULD>
+ Capital Health System/Fuld Campus
750 Brunswick Avenue   Trenton, NJ 08638   (609)394-6000

Soloway, Peter H., MD {1396752242} RadDia(81,GRN01)
+ Hudson Radiology Center
657-659 Broadway   Bayonne, NJ 07002   (201)437-3007   Fax (201)437-1418

Soloway, Stephen, MD {1609997873} IntrMd, Rheuma(88,MNT01)
+ Arthritis & Rheumatology Assoc of South Jersey
2848 South Delsea Drive/Suite 2-C   Vineland, NJ 08360   (856)794-9090   Fax (856)794-3058
+ Arthritis & Rheumatology Assoc of South Jersey
524 Williamstown Road/Suite A   Sicklerville, NJ 08081   (856)794-9090   Fax (856)794-3058

Solt, Veronika, MD {1861504359} Psychy, IntrMd(83,HUN06)
+ 1122 Rte 22 West
Mountainside, NJ 07092   (908)654-7501

Soltys, Remigiusz, MD {1538587845} IntrMd<NJ-TRINIWSC>
+ Trinitas Regional Medical Center-Williamson Street
225 Williamson Street   Elizabeth, NJ 07207   (908)994-5000

Som, Sumit, MD {1104082353} IntrMd<NJ-TRINIWSC>
+ Advanced Cardiology, LLC.
65 Ridgedale Avenue   Cedar Knolls, NJ 07927   (973)401-1100   Fax (973)401-1201
+ Trinitas Regional Medical Center-Williamson Street
225 Williamson Street/Medicine   Elizabeth, NJ 07207   (908)994-5000

Somar, Rohan, MD {1568556751} EmrgMd(90,NY47)<NJ-STCLRDEN>
+ St. Clare's Hospital-Denville Campus
25 Pocono Road   Denville, NJ 07834   (973)625-6000

Somasundaram, Manamadurai R., MD {1730133307} Pedtrc(77,INA85)<NJ-COMMED, NJ-UNVMCPRN>
+ Family Health Center/Community Medical Center
301 Lakehurst Road   Toms River, NJ 08755   (732)557-3304   Fax (732)557-3952
+ Child Health Associates
666 Plainsboro Road/Suite 1300   Plainsboro, NJ 08536   (732)557-3304   Fax (609)750-1523

Somberg, Eric D., MD {1245330232} SrgCdv, SrgThr(74,NY46)<NJ-HACKNSK>
+ Cardiac Surgery Group, P.A.
20 Prospect Avenue/Suite 900   Hackensack, NJ 07601   (201)996-2261   Fax (201)343-0609

Somer, Nancy C., MD {1023096302} IntrMd(91,NJ06)
+ Park Primary Care Associates
453 Amboy Avenue   Woodbridge, NJ 07095   (732)636-6612   Fax (732)636-8224

Somer, Robert A., MD {1285725267} IntrMd, OncHem(97,NY48)
+ The Cooper Hospital System-Univ Hospital
3 Cooper Plaza/Suite 215   Camden, NJ 08103   (856)963-3572   Fax (856)338-9211
+ Cancer Institute of New Jersey at Cooper
900 Centennial Boulevard/Suite M-2   Voorhees, NJ 08043   (856)963-3572   Fax (856)325-6777

Somera-Uy, Constancia L., MD {1508935248} Pedtrc, PedNph(67,PHI02)<NJ-UMDNJ, NJ-CHRIST>
+ University Hospital-Doctors Office Center
90 Bergen Street/Doc 5100/Pedi   Newark, NJ 07103   (973)972-5779   Fax (973)972-5895

Somers, Joann, MD {1821177064} ObsGyn(82,FL04)<NJ-STBARNMC>
+ 22 Old Short Hills Road/Suite 204
Livingston, NJ 07039   (973)533-0638   Fax (973)535-6244

Somma, Edward A., MD {1316954563} IntrMd(85,DMN01)
+ Union County HealthCare Associates
400 Westfield Avenue   Elizabeth, NJ 07208   (908)620-3800   Fax (908)620-3243
+ Union County HealthCare Associates
689 Inman Avenue   Colonia, NJ 07067   (908)620-3800   Fax (732)381-0070

Sommer, Lacy Louise, MD {1891089033} IntrMd
+ Heymann, Manders & Green LLC
100 Brick Road/Suite 306   Marlton, NJ 08053   (856)596-0111   Fax (856)596-7194

Sommers, Daniel, MD {1366497307} EmrgMd<PA-GRNDVIEW>
+ 1210 Route 130 North/Suite 1438
Cinnaminson, NJ 08077

Sommers, Gara M., MD {1508801432} GynOnc, ObsGyn(81,NY19)<NJ-HOBUNIMC, NJ-CHRIST>
+ 718 Teaneck Road
Teaneck, NJ 07666   (201)833-1027   Fax (201)833-3282

Somogyi, Steven G., MD {1558468090} IntrMd(83,ITA07)<NJ-RBAYOLDB, NJ-RBAYPERT>
+ 613 Amboy Avenue/L101
Perth Amboy, NJ 08861   (732)826-6859   Fax (732)826-6790
Somogyi.staff@yahoo.com

Son, Andrew, MD {1265608996} Anesth<NJ-RWJURAH>
+ Robert Wood Johnson University Hospital at Rahway
865 Stone Street   Rahway, NJ 07065   (732)381-6303

Son, Chang Bae, MD {1063493898} Dermat(01,QU01)
+ The Dermatology Group, P.C.
44 Route 23 North/Suite 213   Riverdale, NJ 07457   (973)571-2121   Fax (973)839-5751
+ The Dermatology Group, P.C.
30 West Century Road/Suite 320   Paramus, NJ 07652   (973)571-2121   Fax (201)986-0702
+ The Dermatology Group, P.C.
310 Madison Avenue/Suite 206   Morristown, NJ 07457   (973)571-2121   Fax (973)539-1180

Son, In K., MD {1497815518} Psychy(71,KOR04)<NJ-GRYSTPSY>
+ 2 First Street
Englewood Cliffs, NJ 07632   (201)947-6342

Son, Kyoung J., MD {1376642132} Anesth(77,KOR06)<NJ-RWJURAH>
+ Robert Wood Johnson University Hospital at Rahway
865 Stone Street/Anesthesiology   Rahway, NJ 07065   (732)381-4200

Sonatore, Carol, DO {1629028501} PhysMd, NeuMus, PainMd(97,NY75)<NJ-UNVMCPRN>
+ HealthSouth Rehabilitation Hospital of New Jersey
14 Hospital Drive   Toms River, NJ 08755   (732)244-3100

Sonavane, Vidya Kiran, MD {1922292911} Pedtrc
+ Drs. Sonavane and Benoy
1503 Saint Georges Avenue/Suite 205   Colonia, NJ 07067   (732)382-8111   Fax (732)381-0292
+ 1817 Oak Tree Road
Edison, NJ 08820   (732)516-1010

Sonbol, Sherif A., MD {1851358667} Anesth(90,EGY09)<NJ-SOMERSET, NJ-STPETER>
+ Anesthesia Consultnts of NJ/Nova Pain
285 Davidson Avenue/Suite 204   Somerset, NJ 08873   (732)271-1400   Fax (732)271-3543

Sondhi, Manu, MD {1659311751} IntrMd, EmrgMd(90,INA30)
+ Sanofi US-Sanofi-Aventis
55 Corporate Drive/Comparative Eff   Bridgewater, NJ 08807

Sondhi, Nidhi, DO {1306189956} Anesth
+ Metzger Pain Management
170 Avenue At The Commons/Suite 6   Shrewsbury, NJ 07702   (732)380-0200   Fax (732)380-0124

Song, Agatha Bockja, MD {1992925507} IntrMd(78,GER24)
+ 8 Devonshire Way
Jackson, NJ 08527

Song, Erica Yoon-Jung, MD {1881645489} ObsGyn(97,NY19)<NY-NYUDWNTN, NY-NYUTISCH>
+ Englewood Ob Gyn Women's Group
286 Engle Street   Englewood, NJ 07631   (201)569-6190   Fax (201)569-6940

Song, Frederick Suh, MD {1427265131} SrgOrt(03,PA02)<NJ-UNVMCPRN>
+ Princeton Orthopaedic Associates, P.A.
325 Princeton Avenue   Princeton, NJ 08540   (609)924-8131   Fax (609)924-8532

Song, Haodong, MD {1285704486} Nrolgy, Elecmy(90,CHN4A)<NJ-RBAYOLDB, NJ-RBAYPERT>
+ 2698 Highway 516/Suite D
Old Bridge, NJ 08857   (732)707-3771   Fax (732)707-3772
+ Raritan Bay Medical Center/Old Bridge Division
One Hospital Plaza   Old Bridge, NJ 08857   (732)360-1000

Song, Hongya, MD {1295756625} IntrMd(85,CHN1J)
+ 239 New Road/Building B, Suite 105
Parsippany, NJ 07054   (973)727-9654

Song, Hung S. William, MD {1629077276} IntrMd, Grtrcs(92,NJ05)<NJ-HACKNSK>
+ Omni Health Professionals, LLC
337 Market Street/Suite 1   Saddle Brook, NJ 07663   (201)368-3800   Fax (201)368-9787

Song, Kimberly J., MD {1962720425}<NJ-UMDNJ>
+ University Hospital
150 Bergen Street/Suite E-401   Newark, NJ 07103   (973)972-4417

Song, Maria H., MD {1013216985} FamMed<NJ-RWJUBRUN>
+ Premier Health Associates
225 Route 23 South   Hamburg, NJ 07419   (973)209-1550   Fax (973)209-4832

Song, Mi-Hae, MD {1144665423} ObsGyn(NY08
+ University Medical Group/OBGYN
125 Paterson Street/2nd Floor   New Brunswick, NJ 08901   (732)235-7755   Fax (732)235-7349

Song, Michael M., MD {1104925080} Anesth, PainMd(91,CA06)
+ Jandee Anesthesiology
500 North Franklin Turnpike/Suite 206   Ramsey, NJ 07446   (201)962-7282   Fax (201)962-7283

Song, Sang Ho, DO {1952386518} PhyMPain, PhysMd, IntrMd(00,NJ75)
+ Avenel Iselin Medical Group
400 Gill Lane   Iselin, NJ 08830   (732)404-1580   Fax (732)404-1594
+ 241 Forsgate Drive/Suite 107
Jamesburg, NJ 08831   (732)404-1580   Fax (732)906-0124

Song, Woo Kwang, MD {1922008879} Gastrn, IntrMd(81,MD01)
+ 1458 West Landis/Suite 1
Vineland, NJ 08360   (856)691-2552   Fax (856)691-8885

Soni, Dhiren D., DO {1629021548} Anesth(94,FL75)<NJ-ACMCMAIN>
+ AtlantiCare Regional Med Ctr/Mainland
65 West Jimmie Leeds Road   Pomona, NJ 08240   (609)652-1000

Physicians by Name and Address

Soni, Monika K., MD {1386692192} Anesth
+ 36 Locust Drive
Summit, NJ 07901

Soni, Poonam, MD {1598850760} IntrMd(98,INA72)<NJ-SOCEANCO>
+ Drs Soni & Soni
697 Millcreek Road/Suite 1 Manahawkin, NJ 08050
(609)597-5699 Fax (609)597-5722

Soni, Shikhar, MD {1730128968} IntrMd(97,INA23)
+ Drs Soni & Soni
697 Millcreek Road/Suite 1 Manahawkin, NJ 08050
(609)597-5699 Fax (609)597-5722

Sonnenberg, Edith, MD {1740452903} IntrMd, InfDis(02,NJ06)
+ ID Associates PA/dba ID Care
105 Raider Boulevard/Suite 101 Hillsborough, NJ 08844
(908)281-0221 Fax (908)281-0940

Sonnenberg, Frank A., MD {1093880759} IntrMd(80,CA14)<NJ-RWJUBRUN>
+ University Medical Group - General Internal Medicine
125 Paterson Street/Suite 5100A New Brunswick, NJ 08903
(732)235-6968 Fax (732)235-8935

Sonnenblick, Howard C., MD {1336202241} Pedtrc, AdolMd(88,ISR02)<NJ-VALLEY>
+ North Jersey Pediatrics
17-10 Fair Lawn Avenue Fair Lawn, NJ 07410 (201)794-8585 Fax (201)703-9889
+ North Jersey Pediatrics
1010 Clifton Avenue Clifton, NJ 07013 (201)794-8585
Fax (973)249-1316

Sonyey, Alexandra Yevgenyevna, MD {1659539492} IntrMd, InfDis(96,RUS01)<NJ-RWJUBRUN>
+ RWJ University Hospital New Brunswick
One Robert Wood Johnson Place New Brunswick, NJ 08901
(732)828-3000

Sood, Amit, MD {1447493820} SrgOrt(09,WI06)
+ Kayal Orthopaedic Center, P.C.
784 Franklin Avenue/Suite 250 Franklin Lakes, NJ 07417
(844)281-1783 Fax (201)560-0712

Sood, Delcine Ann, DO {1417148362} IntrMd, CdvDis
+ Penn Medicine Somers Point
155 Brighton Avenue/Second Floor Somers Point, NJ 08244
(609)365-3100 Fax (609)365-3165

Sood, Jasen, DO {1053725960}
+ Patient first Urgent Care
641 US Highway Route 130 Hamilton, NJ 08691 (609)568-9383 Fax (609)568-9384

Sood, Mohit, DO {1972737385} SrgRec, Surgry
+ Shore Physicians Group
2605 Shore Road Northfield, NJ 08225 (609)653-4535
Fax (609)365-5301

Sood, Monica, MD {1346447794} Anesth(00,INA6Z)<NJ-JRSYCITY>
+ Jersey City Medical Center
355 Grand Street Jersey City, NJ 07304 (201)915-2405

Sood, Rahul, DO {1861625279} PainInvt(05,PA78)<NJ-RWJUBRUN>
+ New Bridge Medical Center
230 East Ridgewood Avenue Paramus, NJ 07652
(973)779-7361 Fax (973)779-7385

Sood, Ravi, MD {1184874968} NuclMd(79,INA3Z)
+ 100 Middlesex Boulevard/Apt. 118
Plainsboro, NJ 08536

Sood, Rohit, MD {1427293117} Anesth
+ 18 Overhill Drive
North Brunswick, NJ 08902 (732)658-1078

Sood, Supriya G., MD {1587373886} Dermat
+ Cornerstone Family Practice
9100 Wescott Drive/Suite 103 Flemington, NJ 08822
(908)237-6910 Fax (908)237-6919

Sopeju, Temilola Adedayo, MD {1033406673} Pedtrc
+ Ocean Health Initiatives, Inc.
101 Second Street Lakewood, NJ 08701 (732)363-6655
Fax (732)901-0557

Soper, Robert Earl, DO {1811926678} EmrgMd, AeroMd(91,WV75)<NJ-MEMSALEM>
+ Patient first
606 Cross Keys Road Sicklerville, NJ 08081 (856)237-1016
+ Memorial Hospital of Salem County
310 Woodstown Road/EmergMed Salem, NJ 08079
(856)935-1000

Sophias, Olympia Margaret, DO {1174961403}
+ 32 Starlight Drive
Morristown, NJ 07960 (727)457-6231
olympia.potaris@atlantichealth.org

Sophocles, Maria E., MD {1932344967} ObsGyn(91,PA02)
+ 225 Hun Road
Princeton, NJ 08540

Sordo, Sarah, MD {1669575403} IntrMd(92,CUB06)<NJ-CHSFULD, NJ-RWJUHAM>
+ Capital Health Primary Care
2 Capital Way/Suite 359 Pennington, NJ 08534 (609)303-4440 Fax (609)303-4441

Soremekun Salami, Olutoyin M., MD {1992867188} Anesth
+ Rancocas Anesthesiology, PA
700 Route 130 North/Suite 203 Cinnaminson, NJ 08077
(856)829-9345 Fax (856)829-3605

Sorensen, Barbara J., MD {1841214160} Anesth(84,NY08)
+ Kennedy Surgical Center
540 Egg Harbor Road Sewell, NJ 08080 (856)218-4900

Sorensen, Mark R., MD {1053383877} CdvDis, IntrMd, CritCr(80,MD07)<NJ-BURDTMLN>
+ Cape Shore Cardiology
211 South Main Street/Suite 205 Cape May Court House, NJ 08210 (609)463-0800 Fax (609)463-0957

Sori, Alan J., MD {1790724342} CritCr, SrgTrm, Surgry(84,NJ05)<NJ-STJOSHOS>
+ St. Joseph Medical Center Surgery
703 Main Street Paterson, NJ 07503 (973)754-2460

Soriano, Aida N., MD {1043281124} CritCr, IntrMd, PulDis(76,PHIL)<NJ-SOMERSET>
+ Somerset Pulmonary & Critical Care
245 Union Avenue/Suite 2C Bridgewater, NJ 08807
(732)873-8097 Fax (732)873-1827

Soriano, Brian J., MD {1154337285} Anesth(97,DMN01)<NJ-CENTRAST>
+ CentraState Medical Center
901 West Main Street/Anesthesiology Freehold, NJ 07728
(732)431-2000

Soriano, Bruce V., MD {1861400475} IntrMd(77,MEX03)
+ 171 Amboy Avenue
Metuchen, NJ 08840 (732)603-2220

Soriano, Jaime R., MD {1205928017} Surgry, SrgVas(69,PHI02)
+ 50 Union Avenue/Suite 506
Irvington, NJ 07111 (973)374-3200 Fax (973)399-0081

Soriano, John G., MD {1861472292} Gastrn, IntrMd(81,MEX03)<NJ-STCLRDEN, NJ-MORRISTN>
+ Morris County Gastroenterology Associates
16 Pocono Road/Suite 201 Denville, NJ 07834 (973)627-4430 Fax (973)586-2336

Soriano, Myrna Lopez, MD {1639199383} EnDbMt, IntrMd(75,PHI01)<NJ-CHSFULD, NJ-CHSMRCER>
+ Primary & Diabetic Care Office
2065 Klockner Road Hamilton, NJ 08690 (609)586-1001
Fax (609)586-7634

Sorkin, Greg Charles, DO {1083792410} EmrgMd(01,ME75)<NJ-STMICHL>
+ Pathlink, LLC
66 West Gilbert Street/Suite 100 Tinton Falls, NJ 07701
(732)212-0060 Fax (732)212-0061

Sorkin, Norman S., MD {1265415897} RadDia, RadV&I, Radiol(82,NJ05)<NJ-RBAYOLDB, NJ-STPETER>
+ University Radiology Group, P.C.
483 Cranbury Road East Brunswick, NJ 08816 (732)390-0030 Fax (732)390-5383
+ University Radiology Group, P.C.
75 Veronica Avenue Somerset, NJ 08873 (732)390-0030
Fax (732)246-4188
+ University Radiology Group, P.C.
260 Amboy Avenue Metuchen, NJ 08816 (732)548-2322
Fax (732)548-3392

Sornaraj, Amutha Arularasi, MD {1659685519} FamMed(96,INA2X)<NJ-UNDRWD>
+ South Jersey Family Medicine Associates
608 North Broad Street/Suite 100 Woodbury, NJ 08096
(856)848-1307 Fax (856)848-1682
amuthasornaraj@yahoo.com

Sorokin, Evan Scott, MD {1619960325} Surgry, SrgPlstc, SrgRec(98,PA09)<NJ-UNDRWD, NJ-VIRTUAHS>
+ Delaware Valley Plastic Surgery, P.A.
1734 Marlton Pike East Cherry Hill, NJ 08003 (856)872-4158 Fax (856)751-7700

Sorokin, Jeffrey J., MD {1992793590} Gastrn, IntrMd(68,NY08)
+ Gastroenterology Associates
100 Brick Road/Suite 216 Marlton, NJ 08053 (856)596-5559 Fax (856)596-5373
jsorokin@pol.net

Soroko, Theresa A., MD {1407829526} InfDis, IntrMd(84,GRN01)
+ Essex County Infectious Diseases
199 Broad Street/Suite 2-A Bloomfield, NJ 07003
(973)748-4583 Fax (973)748-3243

Soroush, Azam, MD {1720057318} Pedtrc, PedGst(88,IRAN)<NJ-JRSYSHMC>
+ Meridian Medical Group - Faculty Practice
61 Davis Avenue/Suite 1 Neptune, NJ 07753 (732)776-4860 Fax (732)776-4867
+ Jersey Shore University Medical Center
1945 Route 33/Pediatrics Neptune, NJ 07753 (732)775-5500

Sorrentino, Mark David, MD {1104907088} PedCrC
+ 65 Commerce Wat
Hackensack, NJ 07601

Sorvino, Damian W., MD {1962436964} Otlryg, Otolgy(87,NY08)
+ Ear, Nose, & Throat Specialists of Morristown LLC
95 Madison Avenue/Suite 105 Morristown, NJ 07960

(973)644-0808 Fax (973)644-9270

Sorvino, Noel R., MD {1831171248} Pedtrc(85,NY08)<NJ-MORRISTN>
+ 59 East Mill Road
Long Valley, NJ 07853 (908)876-4900 Fax (908)876-1089

Sosin, Beth L., MD {1679815922} ObsGyn
+ South Orange Ob/Gyn & Infertility Group
106 Valley Street South Orange, NJ 07079 (973)763-4334
Fax (973)763-4355

Sosland, Morton D., MD {1861575003} PsyCAd, Psychy(00,PA02)
+ 1924 Cardinal Lake Drive
Cherry Hill, NJ 08003

Sosnow, Meg W., MD {1730294703} Psychy(99,NY19)
+ 332 Springfield Avenue
Summit, NJ 07901 (908)277-1990

Sossong, Duane G., DO {1720021488} IntrMd(84,IL76)<NJ-STCLRDEN>
+ 765 Route 10 East
Randolph, NJ 07869 (973)366-1789 Fax (973)366-6201

Sostre, Samiris, MD {1265596647} Psychy(93,NY06)<NJ-STMRYPAS>
+ 450 Summit Avenue
Hackensack, NJ 07601 (201)487-9104

Sostre, Samuel Oliver, MD {1477729374} Psychy(98,MA05)
+ 450 Summit Avenue
Hackensack, NJ 07601 (201)562-2088

Sostre-Oquendo, Shirley, MD {1710121991}
+ 450 Summit Avenue
Hackensack, NJ 07601 (201)294-1245

Sotelo, Julio E., MD {1639282908} IntrMd, Nephro, Hypten(64,PERU)<NY-PRSBWEIL, NJ-HOLYNAME>
+ 563 Queen Anne Road
Teaneck, NJ 07666 (201)836-7031 Fax (201)836-1859

Sotillo, Melissa Maria, MD {1184613077} ObsGyn(00,NY08)<NJ-NWTNMEM>
+ Dr. G's Weightloss & Wellness
147 Woodport Road Sparta, NJ 07871 (973)726-0801
Fax (973)726-0802
+ Womens Health Care Associates of Sussex County
135 Newton Sparta Road/Suite 201 Newton, NJ 07860
(973)726-0801 Fax (973)383-8424

Sotiriadis, John, MD {1659578664} Gastrn(04,IL42)<NJ-HOLYNAME>
+ Drs. Caride and Sotiriadis
9226 Kennedy Boulevard/Suite A North Bergen, NJ 07047
(201)869-9500 Fax (201)869-9501

Soto, David Rodolfo, MD {1386885382} RadV&I
+ Vascular Acess Center West Orange
347 Mount Pleasant Avenue West Orange, NJ 07052
(917)405-8859
davidrsoto@gmail.com

Soto, Haydee M., MD {1184626764} IntrMd, Pedtrc(93,NJ05)<NJ-OVERLOOK, NJ-MORRISTN>
+ Summit Medical Group-Berkeley Heights Campus
1 Diamond Hill Road Berkeley Heights, NJ 07922
(908)273-4300 Fax (908)277-8779

Soto, Norberto Luke, MD {1003875063} SrgPlstc(99,NJ05)
+ Advanced Aesthetic Associates
106 Grand Avenue/Suite 490 Englewood, NJ 07631
(201)816-0040 Fax (201)945-4255

Soto Moise, Olga Bienvenida, MD {1750483210} PsyGrt, Psychy(88,DOM11)
+ Tinton Falls Community Based Outpatient Clinic
55 North Gilbert Street Tinton Falls, NJ 07701 (732)842-4751

Soto Perello, Jose Manuel, MD {1801842398} Psychy(78,DOM01)
+ 516 51st Street
West New York, NJ 07093 (201)864-4897 Fax (201)864-4871

Soto-Pereira, Angelica Maria, MD {1902034960} Pedtrc(06,COLO)
+ NuHeights Pediatrics
1115 Clifton Avenue/Suite 101 Clifton, NJ 07013
(973)250-2970 Fax (973)250-2971
+ NuHeights Pediatrics
2 Brighton Road/Suite 404 Clifton, NJ 07013 (973)250-2970 Fax (973)250-2971

Sotolongo, Anays M., MD {1285779124} CritCr, PulDis, IntrMd(92,NY06)<NJ-RWJUBRUN>
+ UH- Robert Wood Johnson Med
125 Paterson Street/Rm 5100 New Brunswick, NJ 08901
(732)828-3000

Sotsky, Gerald, MD {1134192552} CdvDis, IntrMd, CritCr(81,NY47)<NJ-VALLEY>
+ Valley Medical Group/Valley Heart Group
1200 East Ridgewood Avenue Ridgewood, NJ 07450
(201)670-8660 Fax (201)447-1957

Sotsky, Mark I., MD {1922070150} CdvDis, IntrMd(80,NY47)<NY-STBARNAB, NY-LDYMRCY>
+ Valley Medical Group/Valley Heart Group
1200 East Ridgewood Avenue Ridgewood, NJ 07450
(201)670-8660 Fax (201)447-1957

Physicians by Name and Address

Souayah, Nizar, MD {1558402032} Nrolgy(90,TUN01)<NJ-UMDNJ>
+ Rutgers NJ School of Medicine Neurology
90 Bergen Street/DOC 5200   Newark, NJ 07103   (973)972-5209   Fax (973)972-5059
souayani@njms.rutgers.edu

Soucier, Ronald J., DO {1184667693} IntrMd(82,MO78)
+ AtlantiCare Physician Group
2500 English Creek Avenue   Egg Harbor Township, NJ 08234   (609)909-0200   Fax (609)909-0267

Souidi, Anasse, MD {1114193984} IntrMd<NJ-CHSFULD>
+ Capital Health System/Fuld Campus
750 Brunswick Avenue/Medicine   Trenton, NJ 08638   (609)394-6143

Soukiazian, Sevak, MD {1407809742} EmrgMd, EmrgEMed(91,IRA03)
+ JFK Medical Center
65 James Street   Edison, NJ 08820   (732)321-7000

Sourial, Hany A., MD {1427027200} IntrMd(81,EGY05)
+ Physicians Practice at New Bridge Med Ctr
230 East Ridgewood Avenue   Paramus, NJ 07652   (201)225-4700   Fax (201)225-4702
+ Christian Health Care Heritage Manor Nursing Home
301 Sicomac Avenue   Wyckoff, NJ 07481   (201)225-4700   Fax (201)848-9758

Sous, Manal Ann, MD {1255434312} Psychy(88,EGY04)<NJ-RAMAPO>
+ 637 Wyckoff Avenue
Wyckoff, NJ 07481   (201)848-0700   Fax (201)848-0677
+ Christian Health Care Heritage Manor Nursing Home
301 Sicomac Avenue   Wyckoff, NJ 07481   (201)848-0700   Fax (201)848-9758

Sousa, David, MD {1891954434} IntrMd<NY-MTSINAI, NY-MTSINYHS>
+ Pulmonary & Allergy Associates
1 Springfield Avenue   Summit, NJ 07901

Sousa, Rolando Cristobal, MD {1144277211} Pedtrc, IntrMd(90,PANA)
+ Hackensack University Medical Center
20 Prospect Avenue/Suite 905   Hackensack, NJ 07601   (973)222-4653   Fax (646)304-3194

Soussan, Elie R., MD {1891958674} ObsGyn(06,ISR02)
+ A Woman's Place
34 Sycamore Avenue   Little Silver, NJ 07739   (732)747-9310   Fax (732)747-9320

South, Harry L., MD {1780817205} CdvDis
+ Hamilton Cardiology Associates
2073 Klockner Road   Hamilton, NJ 08690   (609)584-1212   Fax (609)584-0103

Southern, Darrell Loren, MD {1548268907} AlgyImmn, Pedtrc, IntrMd(71,NY01)
+ Princeton Allergy & Asthma Associates, P.A.
24 Vreeland Drive   Skillman, NJ 08558   (609)921-2202   Fax (609)924-1468
+ Princeton Allergy & Asthma Associates, P.A.
1245 Whitehorse Mercerville Rd   Hamilton, NJ 08619   (609)921-2202   Fax (609)924-1468
+ Princeton Allergy & Asthma Associates, P.A.
666 Plainsboro Road/Building 100-B   Plainsboro, NJ 08558   (609)799-8111   Fax (609)924-1468

Southgate, Theodore J., MD {1730156217} SrgThr, Surgry, CritCr(80,MI01)<NJ-NWRKBETH>
+ New Jersey Cardiology Associates
201 Lyons Avenue/6th Floor   Newark, NJ 07112   (973)926-7749   Fax (973)923-4683

Souto, Henry Lee, DO {1518078211} EmrgMd(94,NJ75)<NJ-ACMCITY, NJ-ACMCMAIN>
+ Shore Memorial Hospital
1 East New York Avenue   Somers Point, NJ 08244   (609)653-3500
+ AtlantiCare Emergency Services
600 South White Horse Pike   Hammonton, NJ 08037   (609)561-1589

Sowemimo, Fiolakemi O., MD {1063673200} IntrMd(06,CT02)<NJ-CENTRAST>
+ CentraState Medical Center
901 West Main Street/Suite 103   Freehold, NJ 07728   (732)252-6688   Fax (732)761-9705

Sowemimo, Oluseun Akande, MD {1780609628} Surgry(95,NIG03)<NJ-CENTRAST>
+ CentraState Medical Center
901 West Main Street/Suite 207   Freehold, NJ 07728   (732)431-2000

Soyombo, Aderemi B., MD {1649437856} CdvDis
+ Heart & Vascular Associates of Northern Jersey
22-18 Broadway/Suite 201   Fair Lawn, NJ 07410   (201)475-5050   Fax (201)475-5522

Sozzi, Roberto S., MD {1326160128} Psychy(71,ARG06)
+ 1187 Main Avenue/Auite 3
Clifton, NJ 07011   (973)458-8380

Spagnuola, Christopher J., MD {1831158815} SrgOrt(96,NJ05)<NJ-MONMOUTH, NJ-OCEANMC>
+ Seaview Orthopaedics
1200 Eagle Avenue   Ocean, NJ 07712   (732)660-6200   Fax (732)660-6201
+ Seaview Orthopaedics
222 Schanck Road/3rd Floor   Freehold, NJ 07728   (732)660-6200   Fax (732)303-8314

Spagnuolo, Vincent J., MD {1487621090} CdvDis, IntrMd(80,NJ05)
+ The Cardiology Group, P.A.
1 Sheffield Drive/Suite 102   Columbus, NJ 08022   (856)291-8855
+ The Cardiology Group, P.A.
128 State Highway Route 70/Suite 1-B   Medford, NJ 08055   (856)291-8855   Fax (609)444-5521
+ The Cardiology Group, P.A.
401 Young Avenue/Suite 275   Moorestown, NJ 08022   (856)291-8855   Fax (856)291-8844

Spalla, Thomas Christopher, MD {1174732200} Otlryg, SrgHdN, IntrMd<NJ-COOPRUMC>
+ Cooper University Medical Center/Camden
3 Cooper Plaza/Suite 104   Camden, NJ 08103   (856)342-2000
+ Cooper Surgical Associates
3 Cooper Plaza/Suite 403   Camden, NJ 08103   (856)342-2000   Fax (856)541-5379

Spallin, Danielle Marie, DO {1063770055}
+ 115 Old Short Hills Road/Apt 364
West Orange, NJ 07052   (914)262-5664
dspallin@gmail.com

Spano-Brennan, Liana Marie, DO {1740466861} IntrMd
+ Summit Medical Group
1 Diamond Hill Road/Bensley Pav/2 FL   Berkeley, NJ 07922   (908)277-8700   Fax (908)288-7993
+ Summit Medical Group
67 Walnut Avenue/Suite 202   Clark, NJ 07066   (908)277-8700   Fax (732)388-1330

Sparagna, Angelo, III, MD {1518961986} FamMed, IntrMd(74,NJ05)<NJ-SHOREMEM>
+ Shore Physician Group
401 Bethel Road   Somers Point, NJ 08244   (609)365-6200   Fax (609)365-6201

Sparano, Anthony Michael, MD {1992861850} Otlryg, SrgRec(02,IL43)<NJ-JRSYSHMC>
+ 2331 Highway 34/Building 1 Suite 118
Manasquan, NJ 08736   (732)280-3223   Fax (732)280-2626

Spariosu, Magdalena, MD {1467472050} Psychy, PssoMd(96,ROM05)
+ 1301 Wall Street West/Apt 6210
Lyndhurst, NJ 07071

Spates, Stephen Thomas, MD {1740251495} Dermat, DerMOH(97,IA02)<NJ-MTNSIDE>
+ The Dermatology Group, P.C.
60 Pompton Avenue   Verona, NJ 07044   (973)571-2121   Fax (973)571-2126
+ The Dermatology Group, P.C.
44 Route 23 North/Suite 213   Riverdale, NJ 07457   (973)571-2121   Fax (973)839-5751
+ The Dermatology Group, P.C.
30 West Century Road/Suite 320   Paramus, NJ 07044   (973)571-2121   Fax (201)986-0702

Speaker, Olenka Matkiwsky, DO {1417989880} Dermat(92,PA77)
+ 315 East Northfield Road/Suite 2 A
Livingston, NJ 07039   (973)535-3200

Spears, Myriam, DO {1770841322}<NJ-NWRKBETH>
+ Newark Beth Israel Medical Center
201 Lyons Avenue   Newark, NJ 07112   (973)926-7000

Spechler, Floyd F., MD {1073556189} Ophthl(71,PA02)<NJ-COOPRUMC>
+ 1802 Berlin Road
Cherry Hill, NJ 08003   (856)354-1717   Fax (856)354-2031

Specter, Richard L., MD {1316128291} Nephro, IntrMd(02,NJ02)
+ Haddon Renal Medical Specialists
401 Kings Highway South/Suite 5   Cherry Hill, NJ 08034   (856)428-8992   Fax (856)428-9614

Specthrie, Leon Kotler, MD {1043295520} Anesth(90,NY01)<NJ-STCLRDEN, NY-MTSINAI>
+ St. Clare's Hospital-Denville Campus
25 Pocono Road   Denville, NJ 07834   (973)625-6000

Spector, Edward D., MD {1730197260} EmrgMd(95,NJ05)<NJ-HUNTRDN>
+ Pegasus Emergency Group
2100 Wescott Drive   Flemington, NJ 08822   (908)788-6183   Fax (908)788-6516

Spector, Elisabeth, MD {1598765638} FamMed(97,NJ06)
+ Somerset Family Practice
110 Rehill Avenue   Somerville, NJ 08876   (908)685-2900   Fax (908)685-2891

Spector, Janet, MD {1114949674} RadDia, Radiol(92,NY46)<NJ-CENTRAST>
+ Freehold Radiology Group
901 West Main Street   Freehold, NJ 07728   (732)462-4844
+ CentraState Medical Center
901 West Main Street/Radiology   Freehold, NJ 07728   (732)431-2000

Spector, Randy A., DO {1700857794} FamMed(84,NY75)
+ 124 North Beverwyce Road
Lake Hiawatha, NJ 07034   (973)334-1660   Fax (973)334-5471

Spector, Sean David, MD {1891175436} ObsGyn
+ Cooper University Hospital Obstetrics & Gynecology
One Cooper Plaza   Camden, NJ 08103   (800)826-6737

Spedick, Michael J., MD {1720054836} IntrMd, Ophthl, PedOph(78,NJ06)
+ Ocean Eye Institute
601 Route 37 West   Toms River, NJ 08755   (732)244-4400   Fax (732)505-2171

Speer, Robert R., DO {1811900210} GenPrc, Rheuma(71,PA77)<NJ-BURDTMLN>
+ Harbor Medical Associates
9301 3rd Avenue   Stone Harbor, NJ 08247   (609)368-1613   Fax (609)368-6775

Speert, Tory, DO {1972843548} PainInvt
+ University Hospital-Doctors Office Center
90 Bergen Street/DOC 3203   Newark, NJ 07103   (973)972-7085

Speesler, Matthew J., MD {1861428880} Pedtrc, FamMed(80,MEX55)
+ Pediatric Center of Somerset, LLC
7 Cedar Grove Lane/Suite 34   Somerset, NJ 08873   (732)764-0004   Fax (732)960-2301
kidsdoc@gmx.com
+ Alternative Integrated Medical Services, LLC
150-A Tices Lane   East Brunswick, NJ 08816   (732)764-0004   Fax (732)238-6194

Speez, Nancy Sprague, MD {1962581009} PhysMd(88,NY09)
+ Sall/Myers Medical Associates, PA
100 Hamilton Plaza/Suite 317/3rd Floor   Paterson, NJ 07505   (973)279-2323   Fax (973)279-7551

Spektor, Vadim Y., MD {1144381542}<NJ-NWRKBETH>
+ Newark Beth Israel Medical Center
201 Lyons Avenue   Newark, NJ 07112   (973)926-8510
vspektor@yahoo.com

Spellman, Charles L., DO {1932187895} IntrMd(94,NY75)
+ PO Box 150
Long Branch, NJ 07740   (732)222-0180

Spence, Abraham M., MD {1407018575} Urolgy
+ Jersey Urology Group
403 Bethel Road   Somers Point, NJ 08244   (609)927-8746   Fax (609)601-1406

Spence, Richard Kevin, MD {1801122205} SrgVas, Surgry(71,DC01)
+ 1828 Cardinal Lake Drive
Cherry Hill, NJ 08003   Fax (856)428-9282

Spencer, Kristen Renee, DO {1720400906}
+ RWJ Hospital Internal Medicine
One Robert Wood Johnson Place/MEB 486   New Brunswick, NJ 08901   (732)235-8377   Fax (732)235-7427

Spensieri, Diana Patricia, MD {1740360569} Pedtrc, IntrMd(85,DMN01)
+ Skylands Pediatrics
328-A Sparta Avenue   Sparta, NJ 07871   (973)729-2197   Fax (973)729-3653
+ Skylands Pediatrics
4 Oxbow Lane/Route 94   Franklin, NJ 07416   (973)729-2197   Fax (973)827-5093

Sperandio, Peter G.N., MD {1679571657} Anesth(89,PA02)<NJ-VIRTBERL, NJ-VIRTMARL>
+ West Jersey Anesthesia Associates
102-E Center Boulevard   Marlton, NJ 08053   (856)988-6250   Fax (856)988-6270

Sperber, Steven J., MD {1740258680} InfDis(82,NY19)<NJ-HACKNSK>
+ Center for Infectious Diseases
20 Prospect Avenue/Suite 507   Hackensack, NJ 07601   (201)487-4088   Fax (201)489-8930

Spergel, Jonathan Michael, MD {1043226996} AlgyImmn, Pedtrc(92,NY47)<NJ-UNVMCPRN, PA-CHILDHOS>
+ CHOP Pediatric & Adolescent Specialty Care Center
707 Alexander Road/Suite 205   Princeton, NJ 08540   (609)520-1717

Sperling, Brian Lee, DO {1013122977} Urolgy, Surgry(04,PA77)
+ Hunterdon Urological Associates
121 Highway 31/Suite 1200   Flemington, NJ 08822   (908)782-0019   Fax (908)782-0630
+ Hunterdon Somerset Medical Office Building
1121 Route 22/Suite 202   Bridgewater, NJ 08807   (908)782-0019

Sperling, Danny S., MD {1245255249} RadDia, Radiol(99,PRO03)
+ Sports Medicine & Orthopedic Center
349 East Northfield Avenue/Suite 120   Livingston, NJ 07039   (973)369-7202   Fax (973)740-2003

Physicians by Name and Address

Sperling, Howard J., MD {1356442909} FamMed(80,MEXI)
+ Drs. Sperling & Sperling
 162 South New York Road/Suite B-3 Galloway, NJ 08205 (609)748-8200 Fax (609)748-9200

Sperling, Michael James, MD {1518222108} IntrMd(12,DMN01)
+ Drs. Sperling & Sperling
 162 South New York Road/Suite B-3 Galloway, NJ 08205 (609)748-8200 Fax (609)748-9200
 michael.j.sperling@gmail.com

Sperling, Shari Yaffa, DO {1649509126} Dermat, FamMed(05,NY75)
+ 71 Union Avenue/Suite 108
 Rutherford, NJ 07070 (201)804-8900 Fax (201)804-8901

Sperrazza, James Christopher, MD {1518924083} Anesth, PedAne(94,PA02)<NJ-STPETER>
+ Anesthesia Consultnts of NJ/Nova Pain
 285 Davidson Avenue/Suite 204 Somerset, NJ 08873 (732)271-1400 Fax (732)271-3543

Spertus, Silvana H., DO {1891719555} Anesth(89,NY75)
+ Montclair Anesthesia Associates PC
 185 Fairfield Avenue/Suite 2A West Caldwell, NJ 07006 (973)226-1230 Fax (973)226-1232

Spetko, Nicholas, III, MD {1235121047} IntrMd(86,MEX03)
+ 1650 Route 35/Suite 1
 Middletown, NJ 07748 (732)957-0313 Fax (732)957-0631

Spevetz, Antoinette, MD {1770699472} CritCr, IntrMd, PulDis(93,PA09)<NJ-COOPRUMC>
+ Cooper University Hospital
 One Cooper Plaza/Critical Care Camden, NJ 08103 (856)342-2000
 antoinette.spevetz@cooperhealth.edu

Spey, Deborah Ruth, MD {1417975640} Dermat(92,NY01)
+ Dr. Deborah Ruth Spey
 101 Old Short Hills Road/Suite 410 West Orange, NJ 07052 (973)731-9600 Fax (973)731-1635

Spicuzza, Eric Gerald, DO {1629505680}<NJ-SJHREGMC>
+ SJH Regional Medical Center
 1505 West Sherman Avenue Vineland, NJ 08360 (856)641-8000

Spiegel, David Andrew, MD {1568544963} PedOrt(90,NC07)<PA-CHILDHOS>
+ CHOP Pediatric & Adolescent Specialty Care Center
 1012 Laurel Oak Road Voorhees, NJ 08043 (856)435-1300 Fax (856)435-0091

Spiel, Douglas J., MD {1013059716} PainInvt, RadDia(91,NY08)
+ Dr. Spiel and Associates
 1921 Oak Tree Road Edison, NJ 08820 (732)548-2000

Spielberg, Joel A., MD {1881692788} Ophthl, IntrMd(73,BEL04)<NJ-ACMCITY, NJ-ACMCMAIN>
+ Horizon Eye Care
 76 West Jimmie Leeds Road Galloway, NJ 08205 (609)652-0300 Fax (609)652-0730
 drspielberg@horizoneyecare.com
+ Horizon Eye Care
 9701 Ventnor Avenue Margate City, NJ 08402 (609)652-0300 Fax (609)822-3211
+ Horizon Eye Care
 655 Route 72 Manahawkin, NJ 08205 (609)597-0666

Spielholz, Kathi Melanie, MD {1518012699} Pedtrc, IntrMd(88,NJ05)
+ 172 Halsted Street
 East Orange, NJ 07018 (973)678-3133 Fax (973)678-6305

Spielman, Charles C., MD {1851549356} CdvDis<NJ-ACMCMAIN>
+ AtlantiCare Regional Med Ctr/Mainland
 65 West Jimmie Leeds Road/Cardiology Pomona, NJ 08240 (609)652-1000

Spielman, Joel H., MD {1568555019} SrgOrt, SrgSpn(86,NY46)
+ Orthopedic Associates of West Jersey
 600 Mount Pleasant Avenue/Suite A Dover, NJ 07801 (973)989-0888 Fax (973)989-0885

Spier, Bernard C., MD {1871578468} Ophthl(81,NJ05)<NJ-STBARNMC>
+ Northern New Jersey Eye Institute
 71 Second Street South Orange, NJ 07079 (973)763-2203 Fax (973)762-9449
+ Northern New Jersey Eye Institute
 616 Bloomfield Avenue West Caldwell, NJ 07006 (973)763-2203 Fax (973)762-9449
+ Eric Shnayder MD PC
 11 Kiel Avenue/2nd Floor Kinnelon, NJ 07079 (973)838-7722 Fax (973)838-3579

Spierer, Robert, MD {1750466975} EmrgMd, FamMed, Grtrcs(71,NY46)<NJ-JFKMED, NJ-RWJUBRUN>
+ Monroe Medical Group
 78 West Railroad Avenue Jamesburg, NJ 08831 (609)395-1900 Fax (609)395-1010

Spiler, Ira J., MD {1790876142} EnDbMt, IntrMd(71,NY46)<NJ-RBAYPERT, NJ-RWJUBRUN>
+ 3 Hospital Plaza/Suite 307
 Old Bridge, NJ 08857 (732)360-1122 Fax (732)360-2725

Spina, Laurie J., MD {1760469712} Anesth(87,NY03)
+ Morris Anesthesia Group, PA
 3799 Route 46/Suite 211 Parsippany, NJ 07054 (973)335-1122 Fax (973)335-1448

Spinapolice, Joseph A., DO {1063678670} GenPrc(73,PA77)
+ 596 Anderson Avenue/Suite 104
 Cliffside Park, NJ 07010 (201)840-6600 Fax (201)840-6620

Spinelli, Nancy Ann, DO {1376555847} Dermat(97,OK79)<NY-STBARNAB>
+ Drs. Moy and Spinelli
 35 West Main Street/Suite 201 Denville, NJ 07834 (973)627-9635 Fax (973)625-7484
+ 574 Franklin Avenue
 Franklin Lakes, NJ 07417 (201)773-0845

Spinnell, Mitchell Kyle, MD {1194763177} Gastrn, IntrMd(91,NY06)<NJ-HOLYNAME>
+ Advanced Gastroenterology of Bergen County
 140 Sylvan Avenue/Suite 101-A Englewood Cliffs, NJ 07632 (201)945-6564 Fax (201)461-9038

Spinnickie, Anthony O., MD {1639113608} SrgOrt(01,NJ06)
+ 91 South Jefferson Road
 Whippany, NJ 07981

Spinosi, Maryjeanne, DO {1326018805} FamMed, IntrMd(86,PA77)<NJ-UNDRWD>
+ Sicklerville Family Care
 570 Egg Harbor Road Sewell, NJ 08080 (856)723-8100 Fax (856)723-8107

Spira, Etan, MD {1003011891} Gastrn, IntrMd(07,NY19)
+ North Jersey Gastroenterology Associates PA
 5 Franklin Avenue/Suite 109 Belleville, NJ 07109 (973)759-7240 Fax (973)759-7243

Spira, Robert S., MD {1902877525} Gastrn, IntrMd(75,NY19)<NJ-HOLYNAME, NJ-MTNSIDE>
+ North Jersey Gastroenterology Associates PA
 741 Northfield Avenue/Suite 101 West Orange, NJ 07052 (973)736-1991 Fax (973)736-9377
+ North Jersey Gastroenterology Associates PA
 5 Franklin Avenue/Suite 109 Belleville, NJ 07109 (973)736-1991 Fax (973)759-7243

Spirn, Benjamin David, MD {1417941592} Ophthl(00,NY47)
+ Franklin H. Spirn MD Inc
 1656 Oaktree Road/Suite 3 Edison, NJ 08820 (732)549-8080 Fax (732)549-0528

Spirn, Franklin H., MD {1710948674} Ophthl(67,NY06)<NJ-RWJURAH, NJ-JFKMED>
+ Franklin H. Spirn MD Inc
 1656 Oaktree Road/Suite 3 Edison, NJ 08820 (732)549-8080 Fax (732)549-0528

Spiro, Scott A., MD {1093896250} SrgPlstc, Surgry(88,NJ05)
+ Spiro Plastic Surgery LLC
 101 Old Short Hills Road/Suite 510 West Orange, NJ 07052 (973)736-5907 Fax (973)736-4987

Spiteri, Andrew, MD {1366439788} Anesth(90,NY48)<NJ-RWJUHAM>
+ Robert Wood Johnson University Hospital at Hamilton
 1 Hamilton Health Place/Anesth Hamilton, NJ 08690 (609)586-7900 Fax (609)631-6839

Spiteri, Isaac Daniel, MD {1740454115} Anesth(03,GRN01)<NJ-MORRISTN>
+ Morristown Medical Center
 100 Madison Avenue/Anesth Morristown, NJ 07962 (973)971-5000

Spiteri, Sharon, MD {1104874148} Pedtrc(00,GRN01)<NJ-MORRISTN>
+ Drs. Gruenwald & Comandatore
 90 Millburn Avenue/Suite 101 Millburn, NJ 07041 (973)378-7990 Fax (973)378-7991

Spitzer, Ayelet, DO {1568804359} IntMHPC
+ Valley Hospital Palliative Care
 One Valley Health Plaza Paramus, NJ 07652 (201)634-5699 Fax (201)986-4702
+ The Valley Hospital
 223 North Van Dien Avenue Ridgewood, NJ 07450 (201)634-5699 Fax (201)447-8014

Spivack, Talya R., MD {1417151549} CdvDis, IntrMd(07,PA02)
+ Virtua Cardiology Group
 2309 East Evesham Road/Suites 201-202 Voorhees, NJ 08043 (856)325-5400 Fax (856)325-5416

Spivak, Dana, MD {1285642934} FamMed(99,MI01)<NY-BRKLNDWN>
+ Spivak , Dana
 137 Park Avenue/Unit 1 Hoboken, NJ 07030

Spivak, Michael, DO {1063484970} Radiol, RadDia(66,MO79)
+ Radiology Associates of Burlington County
 1295 Route 38 West/PO Box 479 Hainesport, NJ 08036 (609)261-7017 Fax (609)261-4180

Spodik, Boris, DO {1366525701} Anesth
+ Hamilton Anesthesia Associates
 2119 Highway 33/Suite B Trenton, NJ 08690 (609)581-5303
 Bspodik@gmail.com

Sporn, Aaron A., MD {1568535243} SrgOrt(78,NY01)
+ 8 Quakerbridge Plaza/MedArt
 Mercerville, NJ 08619 (609)587-4600 Fax (609)586-9702

Sportelli, Domenick J., DO {1952613598}<NJ-UNIVBHC>
+ University Behavioral Health Care
 671 Hoes Lane/PO Box 1392 Piscataway, NJ 08855 (732)235-4433

Spotnitz, Alan J., MD {1164591640} SrgThr, Surgry(70,NY01)
+ UH- Robert Wood Johnson Med
 125 Paterson Street/CAB Suite 4100 New Brunswick, NJ 08901 (732)235-7800 Fax (732)235-7013
 spotnitz@umdnj.edu

Sprance, Henry Ernest, MD {1447239959} ObsGyn, GynOnc(85,NY09)<NJ-JRSYSHMC, NJ-OCEANMC>
+ Jersey Shore University Medical Center
 1945 Route 33 Neptune, NJ 07753 (732)775-5500

Sprankle, Steven Michael, DO {1801043146} CdvDis, IntrMd(08,PA78)<NJ-DEBRAHLC>
+ Deborah Heart and Lung Center
 200 Trenton Road/Cardiology Browns Mills, NJ 08015 (609)893-1200 Fax (609)893-6038

Sprenger, Alice Q., MD {1083689442} RadDia, RadNuc, Radiol(79,NJ06)<NJ-HUNTRDN>
+ Hunterdon Radiological Associate
 1 Dogwood Drive Clinton, NJ 08809 (908)735-4477 Fax (908)735-6532

Sprigman, Charles Jeffrey, III, DO {1730105388} FamMed, EmrgMd(98,NJ75)
+ SJH Urgent Care, P.C.
 201 Tomlin Station Road/Suite B Mullica Hill, NJ 08062 (856)241-2500 Fax (856)241-2511

Springer, Stuart Ira, MD {1538173067} SrgOrt, IntrMd(70,NY09)<NY-JTORTHO>
+ Ultimed HealthCare PC
 50 Franklin Lane Manalapan, NJ 07726 (732)972-1267 Fax (732)972-1026

Sproch, Amy Lee, MD {1538289921} Psychy(98,PA02)
+ 376 Farwood Road
 Haddonfield, NJ 08033

Sprott, Kendell R., MD {1063567659} Pedtrc(77,NJ05)<NJ-UMDNJ>
+ University Hospital-Doctors Office Center
 90 Bergen Street/DOC 4100 Newark, NJ 07103 (973)972-0543 Fax (973)972-0388

Sproule, William Joseph, MD {1578774394}<NJ-CHSFULD>
+ Capital Health System/Fuld Campus
 750 Brunswick Avenue Trenton, NJ 08638 (609)394-6000

Spruell, Joshua Lyn, MD {1326209693} Anesth<NJ-MONMOUTH>
+ Monmouth Medical Center
 300 Second Avenue/Suite 251 Long Branch, NJ 07740 (732)923-6769

Squillante, Christian Michael, MD {1720212467} OncHem
+ MD Anderson Cancer Center at Cooper
 2 Cooper Plaza Camden, NJ 08103 (855)632-2667

Squillaro, Anthony J., MD {1740289875} SrgCdv, SrgThr, Surgry(85,NJ05)<NJ-JRSYSHMC, NJ-OCEANMC>
+ Jersey Shore CardioThoracic & Vascular Surgery
 234 Industrial Way West/Suite A-103 Eatontown, NJ 07724 (848)208-2055 Fax (848)208-2078
 jsctvsurgi@aol.com

Squires, Leslie S., MD {1790885457} IntrMd, CdvDis(81,PA02)<NJ-VIRTMHBC>
+ Delran Family Practice
 8008 Route 130/Suite 120 Delran, NJ 08075 (856)764-7997 Fax (856)764-1840

Squires, Sandra, MD {1720057946} Psychy(88,NY09)<NJ-NWTNMEM>
+ in Health Associates
 15 State Route 15 Lafayette, NJ 07848 (973)579-6700 Fax (973)579-6830
+ Atlantic Behavioral Health at Newton Medical Center
 175 High Street Newton, NJ 07860 (973)579-6700 Fax (973)383-9309

Srapyan, Aram, MD {1033652607} Urolgy(08,ARM27)
+ Capital Health System/Fuld Campus
 750 Brunswick Avenue Trenton, NJ 08638 (609)394-6000

Sree, Aruna, MD {1780881813} InfDis, IntrMd(00,INA83)
+ Drs. Ramasubramani & De Borja
 98 James Street/Building F Suite 208 Edison, NJ 08820 (732)514-9624 Fax (732)377-3767
+ National Alliance On Mental Illness - NAMI NJ
 1562 Route 130 North Brunswick, NJ 08902 (732)514-9624 Fax (732)940-0355

Sreedharan, Raman R., MD {1922023852} Pedtrc<PA-CHILDHOS>
+ CHOP Pediatric & Adolescent Specialty Care Center
 1012 Laurel Oak Road Voorhees, NJ 08043 (856)435-1300 Fax (856)435-0091
+ CHOP Pediatric & Adolescent Specialty Care Center
 4009 Black Horse Pike Mays Landing, NJ 08330 (856)435-1300 Fax (609)677-7835

Sreepada, Gangadhar S., MD {1801842893} Otlryg, OtgyFPlS(00,NJ05)<NJ-CHILTON, NJ-WAYNEGEN>
+ ENT & Allergy Associates, LLP
1211 Hamburg Turnpike/Suite 205 Wayne, NJ 07470 (973)633-0808 Fax (973)633-8811
+ Wayne Surgical Center, LLC.
1176 Hamburg Pike Wayne, NJ 07470 (973)633-0808 Fax (973)709-1901

Srichai, Manakan Betsy, MD {1396772299} Nephro, IntrMd(98,WV01)
+ Associated Renal & Hypertension Group, P.C.
7 Cedar Grove Lane/Suite 31 Somerset, NJ 08873 (732)873-1400 Fax (732)960-3444

Sridar, Buvaneswari, MD {1528634306} IntrMd(95)
+ RWJBH Primary Care Eatontown
145 Wyckoff Road/Suite 301 Eatontown, NJ 07724 (732)222-0180 Fax (732)935-1590
+ Integrated Medicine Alliance, P.A.
27 Pinckney Road Red Bank, NJ 07701 (732)222-0180 Fax (732)460-9848

Sridhara, Bangalore S., MD {1063482636} CdvDis, IntrMd(83,INA68)<NY-GOODSAM, NY-NYACKHOS>
+ Bergen Heart Center
85 Chestnut Ridge Road/Suite 111 Montvale, NJ 07645 (201)444-9913 Fax (201)444-6158

Sridharan, Ashwin, MD {1598044273} OncHem
+ Robert Wood Johnson Medical School
51 French Street/MEB 378 New Brunswick, NJ 08901 (845)323-9512

srikanth, Rashmi, MD {1386073427} FamMed(11,NJ06)
+ Capital Health Primary Care
2330 Route 33/Suite 107 Robbinsville, NJ 08691 (609)303-4400 Fax (609)303-4401
+ Capital Health Primary Care Columbus
23203 Columbus Road/Suite 1 Columbus, NJ 08022 (609)303-4400 Fax (603)303-4451

Srinivas, Abhishek, MD {1821394362} RadV&I<NJ-CHSFULD>
+ Capital Health System/Fuld Campus
750 Brunswick Avenue Trenton, NJ 08638 (609)394-6000

Srinivas, Shanthi, MD {1164446811} IntrMd, Hemato(82,INA04)<NJ-VAEASTOR, NJ-JRSYSHMC>
+ VA New Jersey Health Care System-East Orange Campus
385 Tremont Avenue East Orange, NJ 07018 (973)676-1000 Fax (973)395-7096

Srinivasan, Anand, MD {1912929969} IntrMd(98,GRN01)
+ The Park Medical Group
24 Elm Street Harrington Park, NJ 07640 (201)784-0123 Fax (201)784-0065
METRO86@AOL.COM

Srinivasan, Deepak, MD {1467465831} Anesth, IntrMd, IntCrd(90,PA12)
+ 11-10 5th Street
Fair Lawn, NJ 07410 (201)312-7682

Srinivasan, Geetha, MD {1801937727} IntrMd(90,INDI)
+ Princeton Internal Medicine Associates
281 Witherspoon Street/Suite 220 Princeton, NJ 08542 (609)921-3362 Fax (609)921-3584

Srinivasan, McDonald T., MD {1659415834} Surgry, EmrgMd(65,INA77)<NJ-ENGLWOOD, NJ-STJOSHOS>
+ Englewood Hospital and Medical Center
350 Engle Street Englewood, NJ 07631 (201)894-3000

Srinivasan, Rekha, MD {1093061632} Psychy<NJ-UNIVBHC>
+ University Behavioral Health Care
671 Hoes Lane/PO Box 1392/Rm D-409 Piscataway, NJ 08855 (732)235-3923

Srinivasan, Shankar, MD {1093855728} PsyCAd(01,JMA01)
+ Immediate Care Psychiatric Center LLC
28 Hill Road/Suite A Parsippany, NJ 07054 (973)335-9909 Fax (973)335-0010
lcpsych@verizon.net

Srinivasan-Mehta, Jaya, MD {1962648832} PedRhm
+ St. Joseph's Children's Hospital
703 Main Street/Rm X609 Paterson, NJ 07503 (973)754-2535 Fax (973)754-3389

Srisethnil, Pudchong, MD {1770690315} IntrMd, EnDbMt(72,THA03)
+ 342 Hamburg Turnpike/Suite 107
Wayne, NJ 07470 (973)790-6260

Srivastav, Sushmita, MD {1548591340} IntrMd<NJ-STPETER>
+ Margaret McLaughlin McCarrick Care Center
15 Dellwood Lane Somerset, NJ 08873 (732)545-4200 Fax (732)846-1089

Srivastava, Nilam, MD {1053511824} IntrMd<NJ-STPETER>
+ St. Peter's University Hospital
254 Easton Avenue New Brunswick, NJ 08901 (732)745-8600 Fax (732)745-2980

Srivastava, Sushama, MD {1245344886} IntrMd(81,INA67)<NJ-NWRKBETH, NJ-STBARNMC>
+ Beth Prime Care
166 Lyons Avenue/Ground Floor Newark, NJ 07112 (973)926-3535 Fax (973)926-6111

Srivastava, Tulika Sinha, MD {1598796963} PsyCAd(91,INA13)
+ Vantage Health System
93 West Palisade Avenue Englewood, NJ 07631 (201)567-0500 Fax (201)567-9335

Srulowitz, Allen Judah, MD {1033495015} EmrgMd(11,NY46)
+ St. Michael's Medical Center
268 MLK Jr. Boulevard Newark, NJ 07102 (973)877-5500

St. Fleur, Rose Martine, MD {1346264934} Pedtrc(02,NY45)<NJ-JRSYSHMC>
+ Jersey Shore University Medical Center
1945 Route 33/Pediatrics Neptune, NJ 07753 (732)776-4267 Fax (732)776-2344

St. George, Dustin, MD {1093177495}<NJ-NWRKBETH>
+ Newark Beth Israel Medical Center
201 Lyons Avenue Newark, NJ 07112 (512)733-4981

St. Jean, Monika Kulkarni, MD {1578542734} Anesth(99,DC01)<NJ-ENGLWOOD>
+ Englewood Hospital and Medical Center
350 Engle Street/Anesthesiology Englewood, NJ 07631 (201)894-3000 Fax (201)871-0619

St. John, Thomas A., MD {1710941851} SrgOrt, IntrMd(95,NY48)
+ Hunterdon Orthopaedic Institute, P.A.
80 West End Avenue Somerville, NJ 08876 (908)182-0600
+ MidJersey Orthopaedics, P.A.
8100 Westcott Drive/Suite 101 Flemington, NJ 08822 (908)182-0600 Fax (908)782-7575

St. Victor, Ruth Alleen, DO {1639364896} ObsGyn(06,NY75)
+ 84 Ellington Street
East Orange, NJ 07017

Sta. Maria, Emilia Navarro, MD {1750329710} Pedtrc(87,PHI02)
+ Premier Pediatric Care, LLC
670 North Beers Street Holmdel, NJ 07733 (732)335-3434 Fax (732)335-3436
+ 883 Poole Avenue/Suite 5
Hazlet, NJ 07730 (732)335-3434 Fax (732)335-3436

Staab, Victoriya S., MD {1104064971} PedSrg<NJ-RWJUBRUN>
+ Meridian Pediatric Surgical Associates
4 Industrial Way W/Suite 100 Eatontown, NJ 07724 (732)935-0407 Fax (732)935-0757

Staats, Nancy Elizabeth, MD {1265412688} Anesth(89,MI20)
+ Monmouth Gastroenterology
142 Route 35 Eatontown, NJ 07724 (732)389-5004 Fax (732)389-1850

Staats, Peter Sean, MD {1013909340} Anesth, PainMd, AnesPain(89,MI01)<NJ-RIVERVW>
+ Premier Pain Center
160 Avenue at the Commons/Suite 1 Shrewsbury, NJ 07702 (732)380-0200 Fax (732)380-0124

Stabile, Daniel, MD {1841384757} Anesth, IntrMd, PainInvt(87,NY09)
+ 300 Rock Oak Road
Freehold, NJ 07728 (732)863-9349
dtm725@optonline.net

Stabile, John R., MD {1043344716} GenPrc, IntrMd(76,MEX03)<NJ-CHSFULD>
+ Capital Health Primary Care
1401 Whitehorse Mercerville Ro Hamilton, NJ 08619 (609)689-5760 Fax (609)689-5759
+ Stabile Medical Associates
1755 Klockner Road Trenton, NJ 08619 (609)689-5760 Fax (609)587-0211

Stabile, John R., MD {1225042278} Ophthl(76,NY09)<NJ-ENGLWOOD, NJ-HOLYNAME>
+ Tenafly Eye Associates, PA
111 Dean Drive/Suite 2 Tenafly, NJ 07670 (201)567-5995 Fax (201)567-1354

Stabile, Marissa Jimenez, DO {1487925509}
+ Family Medicine at Monument Square
317 George Street New Brunswick, NJ 08901 (732)235-8993 Fax (732)246-7317

Stabile, Michael C., MD {1265665798} FamMed(08,STM01)
+ Stabile Medical Associates
1755 Klockner Road Trenton, NJ 08619 (609)838-7940 Fax (609)587-0211
+ Capital Health Primary Care
1401 Whitehorse Mercerville Ro Hamilton, NJ 08619 (609)838-7940 Fax (609)689-5759

Stabile, Richard J., MD {1588750673} RadOnc, RadThp(71,NY09)<NJ-MTNSIDE>
+ Hackensack UMC Mountainside
1 Bay Avenue/Radiation Onco Montclair, NJ 07042 (973)429-6096 Fax (973)429-6749
richardstabile@ahsys.org
+ Montclair Radiology
20 High Street Nutley, NJ 07110 (973)429-6096 Fax (973)284-0269
+ Montclair Radiology
1140 Bloomfield Avenue West Caldwell, NJ 07042 (973)439-9729 Fax (973)439-6885

Stable, Joaquin Jose, MD {1790985026} Psychy
+ The Cooper Hospital System-Univ Hospital
401 Haddon Avenue/Psychy/3rd F Camden, NJ 08103 (856)342-2000

Stack, Jay I., MD {1245325026} Nephro, IntrMd(76,PA01)<NJ-MORRISTN, NJ-STCLRDEN>
+ Nephrology Hypertension Assocs
2 Franklin Place Morristown, NJ 07960 (973)267-7673 Fax (973)267-3270
+ Summit Medical Group
1 Diamond Hill Road/Bensley Pav/2 FL Berkeley, NJ 07922 (973)267-7673 Fax (908)288-7993
+ Summit Medical Group
95 Madison Avenue Morristown, NJ 07960 (973)775-5151 Fax (908)673-7336

Stack, Thomas Joseph, III, DO {1891808572} FamMed(91,NJ75)
+ 170 Changebridge Road/Building A-3
Montville, NJ 07045 (973)808-3200

Stackhouse, Lisa A., DO {1083835599} FamMed, Psychy(81,NJ75)
+ Moorestown Behavioral Medicine
509 South Lenola Road/Suite 4A Moorestown, NJ 08057 (856)439-9300 Fax (856)439-1190

Stackhouse, Thomas G., MD {1578659082} SrgHnd, SrgOrt, IntrMd(79,NY01)<NJ-VIRTBERL, NJ-VIRTMARL>
+ Reconstructive Orthopedics, P.A.
200 Bowman Drive/Suite E-100 Voorhees, NJ 08043 (609)267-9400 Fax (609)267-9457
+ 773 Route 70 East/Suite E-100
Marlton, NJ 08053 (609)267-9400 Fax (856)396-0621

Stafford, Patricia T., MD {1285672543} ObsGyn(89,PA09)<NJ-VIRTVOOR>
+ Advocare Magness-Stafford Ob-Gyn Associates
802 Liberty Place Sicklerville, NJ 08081 (856)740-4400 Fax (856)740-4411
+ Advocare Magness-Stafford Ob-Gyn Associates
1810 Haddonfield Berlin Road Cherry Hill, NJ 08003 (856)740-4400 Fax (856)354-8780

Stagliano, Robert A., DO {1134158108} GenPrc, FamMed(76,PA77)<NJ-VIRTBERL, NJ-VIRTMARL>
+ Collingwood Family Practice
600 Atlantic Avenue Collingswood, NJ 08108 (856)854-1050 Fax (856)854-2453

Stagnaro-Green, Alex Stewart, MD {1124052048} EnDbMt, IntrMd(83,NY47)<NY-MTSINAI, NJ-UMDNJ>
+ University Hospital-Doctors Office Center
90 Bergen Street/Suite 4500 Newark, NJ 07103 (973)972-2500

Stahl, Gary E., MD {1962500983} NnPnMd, Pedtrc(77,NY45)<NJ-COOPRUMC>
+ Cooper Neonatology
One Cooper Plaza Camden, NJ 08103 (856)342-2265 Fax (856)342-8007
stahl-gary@cooperhealth.edu
+ The Children's Regional Hospital at Cooper Univ Hosp
One Cooper Plaza/NICU/5 Dorrance Camden, NJ 08103 (856)342-2000

Stahl, Rosalyn E., MD {1770536005} Pthlgy, PthCyt, PthAcl(76,NY46)<NJ-ENGLWOOD>
+ Englewood Hospital and Medical Center
350 Engle Street/Path Englewood, NJ 07631 (201)894-3422 Fax (201)871-2269
Rosalyn.Stahl@EHMC.com

Stahl, Roslyn Marie, MD {1104944859} Ophthl, Catrct(04,NY08)
+ Eye Care and Surgery Center
10 Mountain Boulevard Warren, NJ 07059 (908)754-4800 Fax (908)754-4803
+ Eye Care and Surgery Center
517 Route 1 South/Suite 1100 Iselin, NJ 08830 (908)754-4800 Fax (732)636-7497
+ Eye Care and Surgery Center
592 Springfield Avenue Westfield, NJ 07059 (908)789-8999 Fax (908)789-1379

Staiger, Melinda J., MD {1467469866} RadDia, OthrSp(80,NY19)<NJ-MONMOUTH>
+ Monmouth Medical Center
300 Second Avenue/J.W. Breast Ctr Long Branch, NJ 07740 (732)222-5200

Stailey-Sims, Mary Katherine, DO {1538198346} Pedtrc(98,PA77)<NJ-KMHTURNV>
+ Kennedy Health Systems/Washington Township Campus
435 Hurffville-Cross Keys Road Turnersville, NJ 08012 (856)582-2816 Fax (856)582-2712

Stambaugh, Michael D., MD {1407841190} RadOnc(94,PA02)
+ 21st Century Oncology
17 West Red Bank Avenue Woodbury, NJ 08096 (856)848-7374 Fax (856)848-5855
+ 21st Century Oncology
130 Carnie Boulevard Voorhees, NJ 08043 (856)848-7374 Fax (856)424-0055
+ 21st Century Oncology
220 Sunset Road/Suite 4 Willingboro, NJ 08096 (609)877-3064 Fax (609)877-2466

Physicians by Name and Address

Stamos, Bruce Dumont, MD {1669453650} SprtMd, SrgOrt(97,PA09)
+ Brielle Orthopedics PA
  457 Jack Martin Boulevard Brick, NJ 08724 (732)840-7500 Fax (732)840-2088
+ Brielle Orthopedics PA
  823 Lacey Road Forked River, NJ 08731 (732)840-7500 Fax (732)840-2088
+ Brielle Orthopedics PA
  1301 Route 72 West Manahawkin, NJ 08724 (609)971-7616 Fax (609)971-7639

Stanell, William P., MD {1164496279} ObsGyn(92,PA09)<NJ-CHSMRCER>
+ Lawrence Ob/Gyn Associates
  123 Franklin Corner Road/Suite 214 Lawrenceville, NJ 08648 (609)896-1400 Fax (609)896-3986

Stanford, Brian J., DO {1811095979} Hemato, Pthlgy, PthACl(90,FL75)<NJ-SOMERSET, NJ-STPETER>
+ RWJ University Hospital Somerset
  110 Rehill Avenue/Pathology Somerville, NJ 08876 (908)685-2200 Fax (908)704-3756

Stanford, Paulette D., MD {1801967740} Pedtrc, AdolMd(75,NJ05)<NJ-UMDNJ>
+ University Hospital-Doctors Office Center
  90 Bergen Street/DOC 4300/Pedi Newark, NJ 07103 (973)972-2100 Fax (973)972-2102

Staniaszek, Alina B., MD {1316960792} Psychy, PsyCAd(89,POL02)
+ 301 Route 9
  Englishtown, NJ 07726 (732)617-1400 Fax (732)617-2176

Stanisce, Luke Thomas, MD {1790348803} Surgry
+ Cooper Surgical Associates
  3 Cooper Plaza/Suite 411 Camden, NJ 08103 (732)770-8484 Fax (856)365-1180

Stanislaus, Galen P., MD {1902820178} Grtrcs, IntrMd(81,NY08)<NJ-VAEASTOR>
+ VA New Jersey Health Care System-East Orange Campus
  385 Tremont Avenue East Orange, NJ 07018 (973)676-1000

Stankiewicz, Danuta, MD {1982925376} FamMed, IntrMd(07,NET12)
+ Valley Medical Group Family Practice
  560 Essex Street/Suite 3 Rochelle Park, NJ 07662 (201)243-3152 Fax (201)843-3197

Stankovits, Lawrence Matthew, MD {1861440737} SrgOrt, PedOrt(99,OH41)<NJ-MONMOUTH>
+ Atlantic Pediatric Orthopedics
  1131 Broad Street/Suite 202 Shrewsbury, NJ 07702 (732)544-9000 Fax (732)544-9099

Stanley, Linda, MD {1376761262} ObsGyn, OthrSp(77,PA01)<NJ-OURLADY, NJ-VIRTVOOR>
+ Reliance Medical Group, LLC
  331 East Jimmie Leeds Road/Suite 1 & 2 Galloway, NJ 08205 (609)652-6016 Fax (609)652-2406

Stanley, Lorna Maria, MD {1700971959} Psychy(78,CHI04)<NJ-UNVMCPRN>
+ Princeton House Behavioral Health - Princeton
  905 Herrontown Road/Psychiatry Princeton, NJ 08540 (609)497-3300 Fax (609)497-3370

Stansbury, Frederick H., DO {1699098251} IntrMd
+ Eastern Vascular Associates
  16 Pocono Road/Suite 313 Denville, NJ 07834 (973)625-0112 Fax (973)625-0721

Stanzione, Steven, MD {1134111859} IntrMd, MedOnc(66,NJ05)<NJ-OVERLOOK>
+ Medical Diagnostic Associates, P.A.
  1801 East Second Street/Suite 1 Scotch Plains, NJ 07076 (908)322-7786 Fax (908)322-2924

Stapleton, George S., MD {1912176827} EmrgMd(05,NY01)<NJ-UMDNJ>
+ Emergency Medical Associates of NJ, P.A.
  3 Century Drive Parsippany, NJ 07054 (973)740-0607 Fax (973)740-9895

Starcic-Herrera, Sandra, DO {1770570632} Anesth, IntrMd(00,NJ75)<NJ-VALLEY>
+ Bergen Anesthesia Group, P.C.
  500 West Main Street/Suite 16 Wyckoff, NJ 07481 (201)847-9320 Fax (201)847-0059
+ The Valley Hospital
  223 North Van Dien Avenue/Anesth Ridgewood, NJ 07450 (201)847-9403

Starer, Yvette R., MD {1407812779} Pedtrc, IntrMd(88,NY46)<NJ-ENGLWOOD, NJ-HACKNSK>
+ Tenafly Pediatrics, PA
  32 Franklin Street Tenafly, NJ 07670 (201)569-2400 Fax (201)569-6081
+ Tenafly Pediatrics, PA
  301 Bridge Plaza North Fort Lee, NJ 07024 (201)569-2400 Fax (201)592-6350

Staritz, Amy, MD {1427168145} FamMed
+ Advocare Heights Primary Care
  318 White Horse Pike Haddon Heights, NJ 08035

(856)547-6000 Fax (856)546-3189

Stark, Ira R., DO {1710987854} RadDia(78,PA77)
+ Able Imaging
  2051 Springdale Road Cherry Hill, NJ 08003 (856)424-2929 Fax (856)424-6111

Stark, Richard C., MD {1093782369} IntrMd(79,NJ05)<NJ-VAEASTOR, NJ-VALYONS>
+ VA New Jersey Health Care System-East Orange Campus
  385 Tremont Avenue East Orange, NJ 07018 (973)676-1000

Stark, Zohar, MD {1952367385} SrgOrt(76,ITA03)<NJ-OURLADY>
+ 703 Whitehorse Road/Suite 4
  Voorhees, NJ 08043 (856)346-8686 Fax (856)435-4363

Starke, John James, Jr., DO {1982963021} EmrgMd
+ Newark Beth Israel Medical Center Emergency Medicine
  201 Lyons Avenue/Suite D11 Newark, NJ 07112 (973)926-6671 Fax (973)282-0562

Starker, Isaac, MD {1932175536} SrgPlstc(81,NY19)
+ Peer Group Plastic Surgery Center
  124 Columbia Turnpike Florham Park, NJ 07932 (973)822-3000 Fax (973)822-1726

Starker, Lee Fahey, MD {1710161807}{DMN01}<CT-YALENHH>
+ Atlantic Surgical Oncology
  100 Madison Avenue Morristown, NJ 07960 (973)971-7111 Fax (973)397-2901
+ Atlantic Surgical Oncology
  99 Beauvoir Street Summit, NJ 07901 (973)971-7111 Fax (908)598-2392

Starker, Paul M., MD {1659376747} Surgry(80,NY01)<NJ-OVERLOOK>
+ Overlook Surgical Associates
  11 Overlook Road/Suite 160 Summit, NJ 07901 (908)608-9001 Fax (908)608-9030

Starkey, Lawrence Paul, MD EmrgMd, FamMed(83,DOMI)
+ 40 Windward Way
  Red Bank, NJ 07701

Starkman, Harold S., MD {1518931120} PedEnd, Pedtrc(76,NY46)<NJ-MORRISTN, NJ-OVERLOOK>
+ Morristown Medical Center
  100 Madison Avenue/Pedi Endo Morristown, NJ 07962 (973)971-4340

Starkman, Moishe, MD {1871609149} FamMed(86,PA13)
+ Patient first
  4000 Route 130/Bldg. C Delran, NJ 08075 (856)705-0685 Fax (856)705-0686
+ 163 US Highway 130/Suite 1B
  Bordentown, NJ 08505 Fax (609)291-8359
+ Patient first Urgent Care
  641 US Highway Route 130 Hamilton, NJ 08075 (609)568-9383 Fax (609)568-9384

Staroselsky, Galina, MD {1013092949} Psychy, PsyGrt, IntrMd(81,RUSS)
+ The Psychiatric Group at Princeton
  1000 Herrontown Road Princeton, NJ 08540 (609)751-3740 Fax (609)921-7897

Starosta, Daria Marie, DO {1063465094} EmrgMd
+ Jersey Emergency Specialists, Inc.
  185 Roseberry Street Phillipsburg, NJ 08865 (908)859-6769

Starr, Cynthia D., MD {1710957824} OncHem, IntrMd(67,IL42)<NJ-WARREN>
+ Starr Hematology & Medical Oncology Associates
  755 Memorial Parkway/Suite 102 Phillipsburg, NJ 08865 (908)454-0370 Fax (908)454-9858

Starr, Gail E., MD {1558346569} RadDia(90,PA01)<NJ-HACKNSK>
+ Hackensack University Medical Center
  30 Prospect Avenue/Radiol Hackensack, NJ 07601 (201)996-4752 Fax (201)996-5116
+ New Century Imaging at Oradell
  555 Kinderkamack Road Oradell, NJ 07649 (201)996-4752 Fax (201)599-8333

Starr, Harriette L., MD {1487984886} Pedtrc
+ McNeil Pediatrics
  1125 Trenton Harbourton Road Titusville, NJ 08560

Starrett-Keller, Cheryl Michelle, MD {1952544983} Anesth
+ Rancocas Anesthesiology, PA
  700 Route 130 North/Suite 203 Cinnaminson, NJ 08077 (856)829-9345 Fax (856)829-3605

Stas, Sameer, MD {1871541185} IntrMd, EnDbMt(96,SYR01)
+ Premier Health Associates
  123 Newton Sparta Road Newton, NJ 07860 (973)579-6300 Fax (973)579-1524

Stathopoulos, Labrini, MD {1780887273} Pedtrc(95,NY08)<NJ-HOLYNAME, NJ-ENGLWOOD>
+ 160 Terrace Street
  Haworth, NJ 07641

Stave, Jeffrey R., DO {1386625309} IntrMd(73,IA75)<NJ-BERGNMC, NJ-BURDTMLN>
+ One Enterprise Drive/Suite A
  Cape May Court House, NJ 08210 (609)465-9980 Fax (609)465-9982

Stavrellis, Steve John, MD {1669573861} Pedtrc(68,GRE01)<NJ-KIMBALL, NJ-COMMED>
+ Lakewood Pediatric Associates
  101 Prospect Street/Suite 112 Lakewood, NJ 08701 (732)363-5599 Fax (732)370-0714
+ Lakewood Pediatric Associates
  US Highway 9 North Lanoka Harbor, NJ 08734 (732)363-5599 Fax (609)693-3548
+ Lakewood Pediatrics Associates
  500 Route 9/3B Lanoka Harbor, NJ 08701 (609)693-8131

Stawicki, Jesse J., DO {1497732598} IntrMd(83,ME75)<NJ-CHSFULD>
+ Stawicki & Patnaik Medical Associates
  1235 Whitehorse Mercerville Rd Mercerville, NJ 08619 (609)581-5586 Fax (609)581-5779

Stayer, Catherine C., MD {1487876025} PsyCAd, Psychy(95,GER16)
+ 36 Drakes Corner Road
  Princeton, NJ 08540 (609)924-2028 Fax (609)924-2028 DR.STAYER@yahoo.com

Stebbins, Michael G., MD {1619975489} RadDia(78,FL04)<NJ-RWJUHAM>
+ Quakerbridge Radiology Associates
  8 Quakerbridge Plaza/Building 8 Mercerville, NJ 08619 (609)890-0033 Fax (609)689-6067

Stechna, Sharon Beth, MD {1407940091} ObsGyn(94,NY15)<NY-PRSBWEIL, NJ-RWJUBRUN>
+ Eric B. Chandler Health Center
  277 George Street/ObGyn New Brunswick, NJ 08901 (732)235-6700 Fax (732)235-6729

Steck, William M., MD {1003944414} ObsGyn, Gyneco(72,MEX14)<NJ-STBARNMC, NJ-MEADWLND>
+ 1115 Summit Avenue
  Union City, NJ 07087 (201)866-1440
+ IMMC Health
  737 Northfield Avenue West Orange, NJ 07052 (201)866-1440 Fax (973)544-8911

Stecker, Steven, MD {1346335874} SrgOrt, SprtMd(93,NY09)
+ Orthopedic Associates of West Jersey
  600 Mount Pleasant Avenue/Suite A Dover, NJ 07801 (973)989-0888 Fax (973)989-0885

Steckler, Robert E., MD {1669496717} Urolgy, PedUro(85,NY03)<PA-STCHRIS>
+ St. Christopher Care at Washington Township
  405 Hurffville-Cross Keys Road Sewell, NJ 08080 (856)582-0644 Fax (856)582-0622

Steckowych, Jayde Mary, MD {1477542389} OtgyFPlS, Otlryg, IntrMd(81,PHI08)<NJ-VALLEY, NJ-CHILTON>
+ 21 Franklin Turnpike/Suite 11
  Mahwah, NJ 07430 (201)642-4002 Fax (201)642-4003 mail@TriCountyEnt.com

Stedman, Martin J., MD {1144396672} Urolgy(66,NY09)
+ 7332 Kennedy Boulevard
  North Bergen, NJ 07047 (201)662-0900 Fax (201)662-9622

Steeger, Joseph R., MD {1255386595} IntrMd, PulDis(83,PA07)
+ Allergy and Pulmonary Associates
  1542 Kuser Road/Suite B-7 Trenton, NJ 08619 (609)581-1400 Fax (609)585-5234

Steel, Ann Elizabeth, MD {1912009713} Psychy
+ Garden State Behavioral Health South
  2 Eves Drive/Suite 104 Marlton, NJ 08053 (856)797-8777
+ Center for Family Guidance, PC
  765 East Route 70/Building A-101 Marlton, NJ 08053 (856)797-8777 Fax (856)797-4785
+ Life Counseling Services
  118 Ellis Avenue Haddonfield, NJ 08053 (856)216-7560

Steel, R. Knight, MD {1699713834} Grtrcs, IntrMd(65,NY01)<NJ-HACKNSK>
+ Hackensack University Medical Center
  30 Prospect Avenue/Geriatrics Hackensack, NJ 07601 (201)996-2503 Fax (201)883-0870
+ Center for Healthy Senior Living
  360 Essex Street/Suite 401 Hackensack, NJ 07601 (201)996-2503 Fax (551)996-0543
+ Center for Healthy Senior Living
  360 Essex Street/Suite 401 Hackensack, NJ 07601 (551)996-1140 Fax (551)996-0543

Steele, Cindy S., MD {1134138266} PedHem, Pedtrc(81,ITAL)<NJ-HACKNSK>
+ Tomorrow's Children's Inst/HUMC
  30 Prospect Avenue/WFAN - PC 116 Hackensack, NJ 07601 (201)996-5437 Fax (201)487-7340 csteele@humed.com

Steenland, Richard H., MD {1326119579} Anesth(83,NJ05)<NJ-JRSYSHMC>
+ Jersey Shore Anesthesiology Associates
  1945 Route 33/PO Box 397 Neptune, NJ 07754 (732)922-3308

Steer, Robert L., MD {1801821657} ObsGyn(86,NY20)<NJ-MORRISTN>
+ Advanced Ob Gyn Associates
60 Franklin Street   Morristown, NJ 07960   (973)993-1919   Fax (973)993-5562

Stefaniwsky, Andrew B., MD {1811061807} Gastrn, IntrMd(77,NJ06)<NJ-STBARNMC, NJ-OVERLOOK>
+ The Medical Group, PA
745 Northfield Avenue   West Orange, NJ 07052   (973)325-0061   Fax (973)325-0219

Stefanovich, Michael Vladimir, MD {1396753604} Psychy(85,GER32)<NJ-ENGLWOOD>
+ Englewood Hospital and Medical Center
350 Engle Street/Psychiatry   Englewood, NJ 07631   (201)894-3000
Mstefanovich@verizon.net

Steffe, Thomas J., MD {1962407221} SrgPlstc, SrgRec(88,PA13)<NJ-KENEDYHS, NJ-UNDRWD>
+ Plastic and Cosmetic Surgical Group PC of New Jersey
1007 Mantua Pike/Suite B   Woodbury, NJ 08096   (856)256-7705   Fax (856)256-7709

Stegman, Daniel Ychac, MD {1740251040} Ophthl, IntrMd(87,VEN04)<NJ-STJOSHCS, NJ-STJOSHOS>
+ Clifton Eye Care
1016 Main Street   Clifton, NJ 07011   (973)546-5700   Fax (973)546-8898
dys853@aol.com
+ Clifton Eye Care
245 Engle Street   Englewood, NJ 07631   (973)546-5700   Fax (201)568-4233

Stegmuller, Joseph A., DO {1093793911} FamMed(92,PA77)<NJ-OURLADY>
+ Osborn Family Health Center
1601 Haddon Road   Camden, NJ 08103   (856)547-3111   Fax (856)365-7972

Stehman, Glenn R., DO {1457419053} CdvDis(79,PA77)<NJ-OURLADY, NJ-VIRTUAHS>
+ 15 Dutchtown Road
Voorhees, NJ 08043   (856)753-8062   Fax (856)753-3241

Steighner, Kathleen Marie, MD {1275504334} ObsGyn(85,PA01)<NJ-VIRTVOOR, NJ-VIRTBERL>
+ Garden State Obstetrics and Gynecological Associates
2401 Evesham Road/Suite A   Voorhees, NJ 08043   (856)424-3323   Fax (856)424-4994

Steigman, Elliot G., MD {1407923584} Urolgy(75,NY08)<NJ-CHRIST>
+ 142 Palisade Avenue/Suite 211
Jersey City, NJ 07306   (201)435-2244   Fax (201)222-7733
Esteigman@hotmail.com

Stein, Aaron A., MD {1487644548} CdvDis, IntrMd(79,NY08)<NJ-PALISADE, NJ-ENGLWOOD>
+ Drs. Kelly & Stein
One Marine Road/Suite 100   North Bergen, NJ 07047   (201)869-1313   Fax (201)854-7945
nnjca@optonline.net

Stein, Alan David, MD {1952730442} IntrMd(98,PA01)
+ Medcosm, LLC.
1604 Crown Point Lane   Cherry Hill, NJ 08003   (856)795-0573

Stein, Bernardo, MD {1861416158} IntrMd, Grtrcs(75,BEL07)<NJ-VAEASTOR>
+ VA New Jersey Health Care System-East Orange Campus
385 Tremont Avenue   East Orange, NJ 07018   (973)676-1000

Stein, Beth, MD {1710146865} Nrolgy<NJ-STJOSHOS>
+ St. Joseph's Regional Medical Center
703 Main Street/Neurology   Paterson, NJ 07503   (973)754-2433   Fax (973)754-2410

Stein, Elliott M., MD {1508851965} CdvDis, IntrMd(64,PA02)
+ Associates in Cardiovascular Disease, LLC
211 Mountain Avenue   Springfield, NJ 07081   (973)467-0005   Fax (973)912-8989

Stein, Harmon Charles, MD {1588624357} Ophthl(79,NY09)<NJ-CHSMRCER, NJ-CHSFULD>
+ Total Eye Care Center
2495 Brunswick Pike/Suite 8   Lawrenceville, NJ 08648   (609)882-8828
+ Campus Eye Group & Laser Center
1700 Whitehorse Hamilton Sq Rd   Hamilton Square, NJ 08690   (609)882-8828   Fax (609)588-9545

Stein, Howard A., DO {1619141140} FamMed, UtlRQA(85,FL75)<NJ-CENTRAST>
+ CentraState Medical Center
901 West Main Street/Medical   Freehold, NJ 07728   (732)294-2962

Stein, Howard Larry, MD {1427047182} SrgPlstc, SrgHnd(77,MEX03)<NJ-JRSYSHMC, NJ-RBAYOLDB>
+ 4257 Route 9 North
Freehold, NJ 07728   (732)462-5800   Fax (732)462-8963
plastics97@aol.com

Stein, Irving H., DO {1225109366} Radiol, RadDia(67,PA77)
+ Monmouth Radiologists, PA
279 Third Avenue   Long Branch, NJ 07740   (732)222-7676   Fax (732)229-1863

Stein, Lawrence B., MD {1306946447} Gastrn, IntrMd(65,MN04)<NJ-MORRISTN>
+ Affiliates in Gastroenterology, P.A.
101 Old Short Hills Road/Suite 217   West Orange, NJ 07052   (973)731-4600   Fax (973)731-1477
+ Affiliates in Gastroenterology, P.A.
101 Madison Avenue/Suite 100   Morristown, NJ 07960   (973)731-4600   Fax (973)540-8788
+ Affiliates in Gastroenterology, P.A.
101 Madison Avenue/Suite 102   Morristown, NJ 07052   (973)410-0960   Fax (973)455-1671

Stein, Lynne H., MD {1700850336} PsyCAd, Psychy(79,NY19)
+ Burlington Youth and Family Services
79 Chestnut Street   Lumberton, NJ 08048   (609)518-5470

Stein, Mark Herbert, MD {1417039074} Anesth(85,NJ05)<NJ-RWJUBRUN>
+ Robert Wood Johnson-UMDNJ Anesthesia Group
125 Paterson Street/CAB 3100   New Brunswick, NJ 08901   (732)937-8841   Fax (732)235-6131

Stein, Mark Nathan, MD {1568549319} OncHem, IntrMd(98,NY09)<NJ-RWJUBRUN>
+ Rutgers Cancer Institute of New Jersey
195 Little Albany Street/PO Box 2681   New Brunswick, NJ 08903   (732)235-2465   Fax (732)235-6797

Stein, Meryl Yvonne, MD {1770590648} NeuMSptM, Elecmy, Acpntr(99,NJ02)
+ South Jersey Sport & Spine
525 Route 73 North/Suite 104   Marlton, NJ 08053   (856)874-9777   Fax (856)874-9444

Stein, Michael Alan, MD {1578812848} IntCrd
+ 110 Lazarus Drive
Ledgewood, NJ 07852   (862)251-4345

Stein, Peter Paris, MD {1831264506} IntrMd, EnDbMt(81,PA01)
+ University Medical Group - General Internal Medicine
125 Paterson Street/Suite 5100A   New Brunswick, NJ 08903   (732)235-7219   Fax (732)235-8935

Stein, Shani, MD {1023207263} Psychy
+ 59 Westminster Avenue
Bergenfield, NJ 07621

Stein, Steven J., MD {1275576084} Anesth(92,MO02)
+ 31 Pleasant Avenue
Passaic, NJ 07055

Steinbach, Gary B., MD {1285797712} ObsGyn(80,NJ05)<NJ-JFKMED>
+ Durham Women's Center
4 Ethel Road/Suite 402-B   Edison, NJ 08817   (732)287-3643   Fax (732)287-3406

Steinbaum, Deborah Paige, MD {1619938313} Pedtrc(99,CT01)<NJ-VALLEY, NJ-HACKNSK>
+ PediatriCare Associates
20-20 Fair Lawn Avenue   Fair Lawn, NJ 07410   (201)791-4545   Fax (201)791-3765

Steinbaum, Norman F., MD {1881611333} Ophthl(63,VA01)
+ Pascack Valley Ophthalmology Associates
400 Old Hook Road   Westwood, NJ 07675   (201)664-8989   Fax (201)664-5106

Steinbeck, Wayne E., MD {1265534978} ObsGyn, RprEnd(82,NJ06)<NJ-JFKMED, NJ-STPETER>
+ Obstetrical & Gynecological Group of Metuchen, PA
73 Amboy Avenue   Metuchen, NJ 08840   (732)548-0698   Fax (732)548-3087

Steinberg, Dale Louise, DO {1427047703} Pedtrc(84,NJ75)<NJ-CLARMAAS>
+ 50 Newark Avenue/Suite 102
Belleville, NJ 07109   (973)450-8700   Fax (973)450-5168

Steinberg, David N., MD {1023033131} Psychy, PsyCAd, PsyNro(88,NY46)
+ 940 Main Street
Hackensack, NJ 07601   (201)487-2273

Steinberg, David Richard, MD {1285662783} OrtSHand, IntrMd(84,PA01)<PA-UPMCPHL>
+ Penn Medicine at Cherry Hill
409 Route 70 East/Surgery/Hand   Cherry Hill, NJ 08034   (856)429-1519

Steinberg, Edward, MD {1720012131} Psychy(81,RUS16)<NJ-CARRIER, NJ-UNIVBHC>
+ Princeton House Behavioral Health - North Brunswick
1460 Livingston Avenue   North Brunswick, NJ 08902   (732)435-0202   Fax (732)435-0222

Steinberg, Evan L., MD {1790787646} IntrMd, PulDis, CritCr(82,NY19)<NJ-VALLEY>
+ 407 Faletti Circle
River Vale, NJ 07675   (201)358-9365   Fax (201)358-9367

Steinberg, Frederic, DO {1750489662} Obstet, RprEnd, ObsGyn(64,PA77)<NJ-VIRTMHBC>
+ Cooper Ob-Gyn
1900 Mount Holly Road/Suite 3-C   Burlington, NJ 08016   (609)835-5570

Steinberg, Jay Mitchell, DO {1720294069} SrgThr(98,NY75)<NJ-VIRTUAHS, NJ-OURLADY>
+ Washington Township Thoracic Surgery
400 Medical Center Drive/Suite F   Sewell, NJ 08080   (856)716-6598   Fax (856)716-6659
+ Kings Way Primary Care
100 Kings Way East/Suite D2   Sewell, NJ 08080   (856)716-6598   Fax (856)218-4808
+ Voorhees Primary & Specialty Care
333 Laurel Oak Road   Voorhees, NJ 08080   (844)542-2273   Fax (856)770-9194

Steinberg, Joel S., MD {1477650638} VasDis, IntrMd(76,PA13)
+ Angiology Associates
113 North Frontenac Avenue   Margate City, NJ 08402

Steinberg, Jonathan S., MD {1194729822} CdvDis, ClCdEl, IntrMd(80,NY47)<NJ-VALLEY, NY-SLRLUKES>
+ Summit Medical Group
140 Park Avenue/3rd Floor   Florham Park, NJ 07932   (973)404-7880

Steinberg, Joseph, MD {1659367209} Urolgy, PedUro(92,IL06)<NJ-STCLRDEN>
+ Adult & Pediatric Urology Group PA
261 James Street/Suite 1-A   Morristown, NJ 07960   (973)539-0333   Fax (973)539-8909

Steinberg, Melissa S., MD {1225078868} Ophthl(87,NY46)<NJ-JRSYCITY>
+ 212 Main Avenue
Passaic, NJ 07055   (973)471-8400   Fax (973)473-7442
Mfsteinb@yahoo.com
+ Jersey City Medical Center
355 Grand Street   Jersey City, NJ 07304   (973)471-8400   Fax (201)915-2475

Steinberg, Michael Barry, MD {1134162233} IntrMd(94,NJ06)<NJ-RWJUBRUN>
+ UH-RWJ General Internal Medicine
125 Paterson Street/Suite 2300   New Brunswick, NJ 08901   (732)235-7122   Fax (732)235-7144

Steinberg, Michael L., MD {1114908811} Radiol(90,NJ05)<NJ-WAYNEGEN>
+ Point View Radiology Associates
246 Hamburg Turnpike/Suite 101   Wayne, NJ 07470   (973)904-0404   Fax (973)904-0423
+ Red Bank Radiologists, P.A.
200 White Road/Suite 115   Little Silver, NJ 07739   (973)904-0404   Fax (732)741-0985

Steinberg, Susanne Inez, MD {1427279462} Psychy, IntrMd(79,QU01)
+ Princeton House Behavioral Health- Moorestown
351 New Albany Road   Moorestown, NJ 08057   (215)287-2961   Fax (856)608-6941

Steinberg, Vitaly G., MD {1457560864} Psychy(91,UKR11)
+ Bayside State Prison
4293 Route 47/Med Unit/Psych   Leesburg, NJ 08327   (856)785-9371   Fax (856)785-1586
STEINBVG@yahoo.com

Steinberger, Alfred A., MD {1326015926} SrgNro(76,NY01)<NJ-ENGLWOOD, NY-MTSINAI>
+ Metropolitan Neurosurgery Associates, PA
309 Engle Street/Suite 6   Englewood, NJ 07631   (201)569-7737   Fax (201)569-1494
abo1651@aol.com

Steineke, Thomas C., MD {1477553782} SrgNro(96,MD07)
+ JFK Neurosciences Institute
65 James Street/Second Floor   Edison, NJ 08818   (732)321-7010   Fax (732)632-1584

Steinel, Lisa A., MD {1639232739} Pedtrc, AdolMd(91,NY19)<NJ-VALLEY>
+ North Jersey Pediatrics
17-10 Fair Lawn Avenue   Fair Lawn, NJ 07410   (201)794-8585   Fax (201)703-9889
+ The Valley Hospital
223 North Van Dien Avenue/Pediatrics   Ridgewood, NJ 07450   (201)447-8000

Steiner, Federico A., MD {1598828527} SrgThr, Surgry(97,NY19)<NJ-MORRISTN, NJ-OVERLOOK>
+ North Jersey Thoracic Surgical Associates, P.C.
100 Madison Avenue/PO Box 1348   Morristown, NJ 07962   (973)644-4844   Fax (973)644-4776

Steiner, Kenneth D., MD {1659498020} EmrgMd, GenPrc(79,TN06)
+ Primary & Specialty Care at Edison
10 Parsonage Road/Suite 410   Edison, NJ 08837   (732)452-0680   Fax (732)636-3669

Steiner, Zachary John, DO {1801043013} SrgVas
+ 509 First Street/Apt 2
Hoboken, NJ 07030

Steinfeld, Jason Israel, MD {1003800848} Ophthl, SrgRef(99,PA14)<NJ-BAYSHORE, NJ-RIVERVW>
+ Ophthalmic Physicians of Monmouth PA
733 North Beers Street/Suite U-4   Holmdel, NJ 07733   (732)739-0707   Fax (732)739-6722

Physicians by Name and Address

Steinhardt, Amelia L., DO {1477645190} FamMed(85,NY75)<NJ-MTNSIDE>
+ first Care Medical Group
  50 Pompton Avenue   Verona, NJ 07044   (973)857-3400   Fax (973)857-7034

Steinig, Jeffrey Daniel, MD {1447347455} RadDia
+ Radiology Affiliates of Central New Jersey, P.A.
  2501 Kuser Road   Hamilton, NJ 08691   (609)585-8800   Fax (609)585-1825

Steinlight, Sasha Juli, MD {1881756252} FamMed
+ Family Medicine at Monument Square
  317 George Street   New Brunswick, NJ 08901   (732)235-8993   Fax (732)246-7317

Steinman, Edward A., MD {1073517470} Anesth(80,TX13)<NJ-BAYONNE>
+ Bayonne Medical Center
  29th Street at Avenue E   Bayonne, NJ 07002   (201)858-5000

Steinman, Natasha Margolin, MD {1689685778} Dermat(94,NY19)<NJ-HOLYNAME>
+ Michele Grodberg, MD & Associates
  106 Grand Avenue/Suite 330   Englewood, NJ 07631   (201)567-8884   Fax (201)567-5799

Steinman, Sharon A., MD {1114901436} IntrMd, IntHos(97,NJ05)<NJ-JRSYSHMC>
+ Jersey Shore University Medical Center
  1945 Route 33/Med/Hospitalist   Neptune, NJ 07753   (732)776-4420   Fax (732)776-3795
+ Meridian Medical Associates, P.C.
  1945 Route 33   Neptune, NJ 07753   (732)776-4420   Fax (732)776-3795

Steinschneider, Mitchell, MD {1629032016} NroChl, ClNrPh, Psychy(84,NY46)
+ Neurology Group of Bergen County
  1200 East Ridgewood Avenue   Ridgewood, NJ 07450   (201)444-0868   Fax (201)444-7363

Steinway, Mitchell I., MD {1538129861} SrgOrt(76,NY08)
+ 323 Washington Street
  Hoboken, NJ 07030   (201)963-9597   Fax (201)963-0034

Stella, Nunzio R., MD {1326266644} Otlrgy, OtgyFPIS(74,MEX14)
+ 1901 Hooper Avenue/Suite C
  Toms River, NJ 08753   (732)255-2933   Fax (732)255-2657

Stella, Stefano M., MD {1033114475} ObsGyn(81,DMNA)<NJ-HOLYNAME, NJ-PALISADE>
+ 71 Union Avenue/Suite 101
  Rutherford, NJ 07070   (201)935-1111   Fax (201)935-0549   drstella@live.com
+ 3196 Kenney Boulevard/Box 10
  Union City, NJ 07087   (201)935-1111

Stemmer, Shlomo Marc, MD {1336234780} ObsGyn, UroGyn(88,ISRA)<NJ-VIRTVOOR, NJ-COOPRUMC>
+ 807 Haddon Avenue/Suite 207
  Haddonfield, NJ 08033   (856)428-6355   Fax (856)428-6388

Stenn, Judit O., MD {1407823669} Dermat(81,CT02)
+ Windsor Dermatology
  59 One Mile Road Extension/Suite G   East Windsor, NJ 08520   (609)443-4500   Fax (609)426-0530

Stennett, Richard A., MD {1982686952} Anesth, CritCr(90,NY01)<NJ-MORRISTN>
+ Morristown Medical Center
  100 Madison Avenue/Anesthesiology   Morristown, NJ 07962   (973)971-5000   Fax (201)943-8733

Stepanyuk, Olena, MD {1861690380} IntrMd(94,UKR02)
+ ED Medical Associates
  140 Grand Avenue   Englewood, NJ 07631   (201)569-9010   Fax (201)569-9063

Stephen, Infanta Anusha, MD {1114019072} Nrolgy(93,SRI03)<NJ-HCKTSTWN, NJ-NWTNMEM>
+ Neuro-Specialists of Morris-Sussex, PA
  369 West Blackwell Street   Dover, NJ 07801   (973)361-7606   Fax (973)361-8942
+ Neuro-Specialists of Morris-Sussex, PA
  254 Mountain Avenue   Hackettstown, NJ 07840   (973)361-7606   Fax (908)813-8848
+ Neuro-Specialists of Morris-Sussex, PA
  350 Sparta Avenue   Sparta, NJ 07801   (973)579-1089   Fax (973)579-9618

Stephen, Priya Chachikutty, MD {1447228986} Pedtrc(00,MA05)
+ Capital Emergency Physicians & Associates
  One Capital Way   Pennington, NJ 08534   (609)303-4000   Fax (609)815-7894

Stephenson, Derek Allen, MD {1740441443} Surgry(04,GA21)
+ ESA South Jersey Bariatrics
  1103 West Sherman Avenue   Vineland, NJ 08360   (856)362-5259   Fax (856)405-6978

Stephenson, Karen Rosemarie, MD {1770531873} EmrgMed, Pedtrc, IntrMd(95,NJ06)<NJ-STMRYPAS>
+ St. Mary's Hospital
  350 Boulevard/Emerg Med   Passaic, NJ 07055   (973)365-4489   Fax (973)916-2032

Stephenson, Ruth Deborah, DO {1063649051}
+ UMDNJ OBGYN
  125 Paterson Street/Suite 4200   New Brunswick, NJ 08901   (732)235-6600   Fax (732)235-6650

Sterio, Mara, MD {1215939822} Pedtrc(76,SERB)
+ Drs. Gruenwald & Comandatore
  90 Millburn Avenue/Suite 101   Millburn, NJ 07041   (973)378-7990   Fax (973)378-7991

Sterling, J. Barton, MD {1053478180} Dermat(00,NJ06)<NJ-JRSYSHMC>
+ 215 Morris Avenue/1st Floor
  Spring Lake, NJ 07762   (732)449-3005   Fax (732)449-5110

Sterling, Joshua, MD {1477007722} Surgry
+ Robert Wood Johnson Medical School
  51 French Street   New Brunswick, NJ 08901   (723)235-7673

Sterling, Karen Sohria, MD {1114295918} FamMed
+ 425-70th Street
  Guttenberg, NJ 07093   (201)854-0055

Sterling, Michelle Gold, MD {1497957252} RadNro
+ Radiology Affiliates of Central New Jersey, P.A.
  2501 Kuser Road   Hamilton, NJ 08691   (609)585-8800   Fax (609)585-1825

Sterling-Jean, Yolette, MD {1578517785} Hemato, IntrMd, OncHem(86,HAI01)<NJ-UMDNJ>
+ University Physician Associates
  140 Bergen Street/ACC Level F   Newark, NJ 07103   (973)972-8087   Fax (973)972-6651

Sterman, Harris Robert, MD {1528014750} SrgCsm, SrgPlstc(85,NY08)<NJ-HOLYNAME, NY-MNTFWEIL>
+ 870 Palisade Avenue/Suite 304
  Teaneck, NJ 07666   (201)836-4111   Fax (201)836-3571   hsterman@pol.net
+ Wayne Surgical Center, LLC.
  1176 Hamburg Pike   Wayne, NJ 07470   (201)836-4111   Fax (973)709-1901

Sterman, Lance M., MD {1851491922} EmrgMd, FamMed(71,BEL04)
+ 16 Woodland Drive
  East Windsor, NJ 08520   (609)448-1569

Sterman, Paul Lawrence, MD {1699714899} IntrMd, Nephro(99,NY19)
+ Hypertension & Nephrology Specialists, LLC
  2 Research Way/Suite 301   Monroe, NJ 08831   (732)521-0800   Fax (732)521-0833
+ Hypertension & Nephrology Specialists, LLC
  49 Veronica Avenue/Suite 104   Somerset, NJ 08873   (732)521-0800   Fax (732)521-0833
+ Hypertension & Nephrology Specialists, LLC
  601 Ewing Street/Suite C-7   Princeton, NJ 08831   (732)521-0800   Fax (732)521-0833

Stern, Alan G., MD {1497744666} CdvDis, IntrMd(70,PA13)<NJ-CHSFULD, NJ-CHSMRCER>
+ Mercer Bucks Cardiology
  3140 Princeton Pike/2nd Floor   Lawrenceville, NJ 08648   (609)895-1919   Fax (609)895-1200

Stern, Julie Beth, MD {1598923245} FamMed(05,MEX03)<NJ-CENTRAST>
+ 2352 Route 9 South
  Howell, NJ 07731   (732)625-7900   Fax (732)625-7990

Stern, Lorraine C., MD {1225290281} SrgOrt(08,DC01)<NJ-CHILTON>
+ Advanced Orthopedics & Hand Surgery Institute
  504 Valley Road/Suite 201   Wayne, NJ 07470   (973)942-1315   Fax (973)942-8724

Stern, Marcel, MD {1053329748} GenPrc, IntrMd, EmrgMd(79,ROM06)<NJ-ACMCMAIN, NJ-ACMCITY>
+ Health Med Associates, PC
  1080 Stelton Road/First FL Suite 202   Piscataway, NJ 08854   (732)985-2552   Fax (732)985-0552
+ Health Med Associates, PC
  24 South Carolina Avenue   Atlantic City, NJ 08401   (732)985-2552   Fax (609)345-2885
+ US Healthworks
  16 Ethel Road   Edison, NJ 08854   (732)248-0088   Fax (732)248-4408

Stern, Peter, MD {1902959331} EmrgMd, IntrMd(89,FRA02)
+ The Doctor's Inn Medical Center
  171 Lake Street   Ramsey, NJ 07446   (201)785-0011

Stern, Stephanie Klein, MD {1295829513} Psychy(90,NY48)
+ 320 Raritan Avenue/Suite 201
  Highland Park, NJ 08904   (732)985-3500   Fax (732)985-3544   sksternmd@comcast.net

Sternschein, Michael J., MD {1467626275} SrgCsm, SrgLsr, SrgPlstc(76,NY01)<NJ-VALLEY>
+ Ridgewood Plastic Surgery Center
  1200 East Ridgewood Avenue   Ridgewood, NJ 07450   (201)444-1188   Fax (201)612-0840

Sterry, Thomas Patrick, MD {1306932058} SrgPlstc(95,NY48)<NY-MTSINAI>
+ Med-FEM Aesthetic Surgery Center
  33 Overlook Road/Suite 302   Summit, NJ 07901   (908)522-1777   Fax (908)522-3051   thomas.sterry@mountsinai.org

Stettner, Lisa G., DO {1639242712} Pedtrc(87,ME75)
+ 120 Millburn Avenue/Suite M1
  Millburn, NJ 07041

Steuer, Jeffrey K., MD {1447261458} SrgOrt(84,NY19)<NJ-HOLYNAME>
+ Eastern Orthopedic Associates
  222 Cedar Lane/Suite 120   Teaneck, NJ 07666   (201)836-5332   Fax (201)836-4002

Stevens, Amy W., MD {1578609541} Dermat, IntrMd(89,NY01)
+ North Bergen Dermatologic Group, PA
  400 Route 17 South   Ridgewood, NJ 07450   (201)652-4536   Fax (201)652-4906
+ North Bergen Dermatologic Group, PA
  180 Ramapo Valley Road   Oakland, NJ 07436   (201)652-4536   Fax (201)337-7710

Stevens, Hilary Kristin, MD {1760712004} FamMed
+ Drs. Stevens and Perez
  4 Atno Avenue   Morristown, NJ 07960   (973)267-0002   Fax (973)328-9102

Stevens, John M., MD {1336116524} IntrMd(80,NJ05)<NJ-VAEASTOR>
+ VA New Jersey Health Care System-East Orange Campus
  385 Tremont Avenue/Admin   East Orange, NJ 07018   (973)676-1000   Fax (973)395-7010

Stevens, Lisa Deborah, MD {1497765589} Gastrn, IntrMd(93,NY20)<NJ-CHILTON>
+ Gastrointestinal Group of North Jersey
  1777 Hamburg Turnpike/Suite 101   Wayne, NJ 07470   (973)839-6400   Fax (973)839-7083
+ Wayne Surgical Center, LLC
  1176 Hamburg Pike   Wayne, NJ 07470   (973)839-6400   Fax (973)709-1901

Stevens, Susan H., MD FamMed(81,PHI08)
+ 290 South Livingston Avenue/1st Floor
  Livingston, NJ 07039   (973)716-9000

Stewart, David M., MD {1417916131} Gastrn, IntrMd(69,NY19)<NJ-VALLEY, NJ-HACKNSK>
+ 297 Hillsdale Avenue
  Hillsdale, NJ 07642   (201)666-2110   Fax (201)666-4243

Stewart, Judly Pierre, MD {1265613632} Anesth(03,NY08)<NJ-JFKMED>
+ James Street Anesthesia
  102 James Street/Suite 103   Edison, NJ 08820   (732)494-1444   Fax (732)494-7052
+ JFK Medical Center
  65 James Street/Anesth   Edison, NJ 08820   (732)494-1444   Fax (732)494-7052

Stewart, Michael Starbin, MD {1588712467} PsyCAd(94,NJ05)<NJ-JRSYCITY>
+ Jersey City Medical Center
  355 Grand Street/Psychiatry   Jersey City, NJ 07304   (201)915-2000

Stewart, Peter Jeremy, MD {1255302592} SrgCrC, Surgry(83,WI05)<NJ-HACKNSK>
+ Hackensack University Medical Center
  30 Prospect Avenue/Trauma Service   Hackensack, NJ 07601   (201)996-2000   Stewartpa@comcast.net
+ Hackensack Surgical Critical Care Physicians
  5 Summit Avenue/Suite 105   Hackensack, NJ 07601   (201)996-2000   Fax (201)883-1268

Stewart, Richard Allen, DO {1669422911} ObsGyn, Obstet(87,MO78)<NJ-STPETER>
+ St. Peter's Family Health
  123 How Lane   New Brunswick, NJ 08901   (732)745-8600   Fax (732)729-0869
+ St. Peter's University Hospital
  254 Easton Avenue/ObGyn   New Brunswick, NJ 08901   (732)745-8600

Stidd, David A., MD {1538368428} Surgry<NJ-ACMCITY>
+ AtlantiCare Regional Medical Center/City Campus
  1925 Pacific Avenue/1st Floor   Atlantic City, NJ 08401   (609)572-8600   Fax (609)572-8667

Stiefel, Gregory Gene, DO {1649267881} FamMed(97,NJ75)<NJ-SJRSYELM>
+ SJH Urgent Care, P.C.
  201 Tomlin Station Road/Suite B   Mullica Hill, NJ 08062   (856)241-2500   Fax (856)241-2511

Stiefel, Jay A., DO {1780600338} EmrgMd, IntrMd(86,NY75)<NJ-UNDRWD, NJ-VIRTVOOR>
+ Inspira Health Network
  509 North Broad Street/EmergMed   Woodbury, NJ 08096   (856)845-0100

Stiefel, Laurence N., MD {1205891173} Pedtrc(90,NY46)<NJ-ENGLWOOD, NJ-HACKNSK>
+ Tenafly Pediatrics, PA
  26 Park Place   Paramus, NJ 07652   (201)262-1140   Fax (201)261-8413

Stiefel, Michael Fred, MD {1427111681} SrgNro<PA-UPMCPHL>
+ Capital Institute for Neurosciences
2 Capital Way/Suite 456 Pennington, NJ 08534 (609)537-7300 Fax (609)537-7301

Stieg, Frederic C., MD {1952330276} FamMed, PainMd(72,NY08)
+ 3535 Quakerbridge Road
Trenton, NJ 08619 (609)584-6262 Fax (609)890-1101

Stier, Kyle Thomas, MD {1669406427} PhysMd(02,NJ05)<NJ-UNVMCPRN, NJ-VANJHCS>
+ Princeton Orthopaedic Associates, P.A.
325 Princeton Avenue Princeton, NJ 08540 (609)924-8131 Fax (609)924-8532

Stifelman, Michael Drew, MD {1750375564} Urolgy, SrgLap, IntrMd(93,NY46)
+ HUMC Faculty Practice
360 Essex Street/Suite 403 Hackensack, NJ 07601 (201)894-3645 Fax (201)336-8221

Stiffler, Kyle M., MD {1164577227} Psychy(85,CHIL)
+ Catholic Charities-Delaware Mental Health Services
25 Ikea Drive Westampton, NJ 08060 (609)267-9339

Stillerman, Charles Blair, MD {1477628667} SrgNro, OrtSpn, SrgSpn(IL43)
+ Atlantic Neurosurgical Specialists
310 Madison Avenue/Suite 300 Morristown, NJ 07960 (973)285-7800 Fax (973)285-7839
+ Atlantic Neurosurgical Specialists
3700 Route 33 Neptune, NJ 07753 (732)455-8225

Stillman, Jonathon S., MD {1174649289} Gastrn
+ North Jersey Gastroenterology & Endoscopy Center
1825 State Route 23 South Wayne, NJ 07470 (973)633-1484 Fax (973)633-7980

Stillman, Richard I., MD {1194782030} Anesth, PainMd(85,VA01)
+ Surgical Center at Millburn
37 Willow Street Millburn, NJ 07041 (973)912-8111 Fax (973)912-0181

Stillo, Joseph V., MD {1063483204} PhysMd(84,SC01)<NJ-HLTHSRE>
+ Kare Rehabilitation
14 Hospital Drive Toms River, NJ 08755 (732)818-4756 Fax (732)793-8784

Stillwell, Paul C., MD {1750473658} IntrMd(88,MEX03)<NJ-CHSFULD, NJ-CHSMRCER>
+ Drs. Stillwell & Hohl
1423 Pennington Road Trenton, NJ 08618 (609)882-8080 Fax (609)882-8433

Stirling, Jeffrey E., MD {1114924669} Radiol, RadV&I, RadDia(88,NY48)<NJ-TRINIWSC, NJ-RWJUBRUN>
+ University Radiology Group, P.C.
483 Cranbury Road East Brunswick, NJ 08816 (732)390-0030 Fax (732)390-5383
+ Trinitas Regional Medical Center-Williamson Street
225 Williamson Street Elizabeth, NJ 07207 (732)390-0030 Fax (732)390-1856

Stitik, Todd P., MD {1356361349} Elecmy, PainMd, PhysMd(88,PA01)<NJ-UMDNJ>
+ University Hospital-Doctors Office Center
90 Bergen Street/Ste 3100 Newark, NJ 07103 (973)972-2802 Fax (973)972-2825
+ Rutgers-Department of Physical Med
183 South Orange Ave/Suite F-1555 Newark, NJ 07101 (973)972-3606

Stivala, Adam, MD {1467738617}<NJ-TRININPC>
+ Trinitas Regional Medical Center-New Point Campus
655 East Jersey Street Elizabeth, NJ 07206 (908)994-7325

Stoch, Sharon Rachel, MD {1811092984} IntrMd(95,NY20)<NJ-OVERLOOK>
+ Summit Medical Group
34 Mountain Boulevard Warren, NJ 07059 (908)561-8600 Fax (908)561-7265
+ Summit Medical Group-Berkeley Heights Campus
1 Diamond Hill Road Berkeley Heights, NJ 07922 (908)561-8600 Fax (908)790-6576

Stock, Ilana Rose, MD {1770939662} Pedtrc
+ Tenafly Pediatrics, PA
350 Ramapo Valley Road Oakland, NJ 07436 (201)651-0404 Fax (201)651-0909
+ Tenafly Pediatrics, PA
32 Franklin Street Tenafly, NJ 07670 (201)651-0404 Fax (201)569-6081

Stock, Jerrold M., MD {1225100662} EnDbMt, IntrMd(68,IL02)<NJ-MORRISTN>
+ 2 Luth Terrace
West Orange, NJ 07052

Stockham, Chad Eric, MD {1053575209} IntrMd
+ Princeton Medical Group, P.A.
419 North Harrison Street Princeton, NJ 08540 (609)924-9300 Fax (609)430-9481

Stoev, Borislav Georgiev, DO {1457536203} EmrgMd(06,MO79)
+ 16 Red Oak Street
Monroe, NJ 08831

Stoicescu, Lavinia D., MD {1285904003} Pedtrc, IntrMd(02,ROM01)
+ Specialdocs Consultants, Inc.
266 King George Road/Suite F Warren, NJ 07059 (908)647-8843 Fax (908)647-3001

Stoler, Alexander, MD {1720014400} InfDis(87,RUSS)
+ Rutgers- New Jersey Medical School
185 South Orange Avenue Newark, NJ 07103 (973)972-4300

Stoller, Jill S., MD {1457306391} Pedtrc(86,NY47)<NJ-VALLEY>
+ Chestnut Ridge Pediatrics
595 Chestnut Ridge Road Woodcliff Lake, NJ 07677 (201)391-2020 Fax (201)391-0265

Stoller, Seth Ryan, MD {1467408583} Nrolgy, IntrMd(00,NJ06)
+ Pain Management Center
11 Overlook Road/MAC 11 Suite B110 Summit, NJ 07901 (908)522-2808 Fax (908)522-6123

Stoller, Steven M., MD {1114942398} SrgOrt, SprtMd(77,MEX03)<NJ-VALLEY>
+ American Orthopedic & Sports Medicine
30 West Century Road/Suite 320 Paramus, NJ 07652 (201)261-0402 Fax (201)261-0587
StevenStollerMD@yahoo.com

Stolman, Lewis Peter, MD {1396749321} Dermat, IntrMd(65,ON05)<NJ-STBARNMC>
+ Dermatology & Laser Center of Northern New Jersey
347 Mount Pleasant Avenue/Suite 205 West Orange, NJ 07052 (973)740-0101 Fax (973)740-0103

Stom, Mary C., MD {1750494019} IntrMd, Nephro(74,PA07)<NJ-OURLADY>
+ Haddon Renal Medical Specialists
401 Kings Highway South/Suite 5 Cherry Hill, NJ 08034 (856)428-8992 Fax (856)428-9614

Stone, Chester I., MD {1992797369} Urolgy(71,NJ05)
+ 66 Sunset Strip/Suite 300
Succasunna, NJ 07876 (973)927-3388 Fax (973)927-2590
+ Specialty Surgical Center
380 Lafayette Road/Suite 110 Sparta, NJ 07871 (973)927-3388 Fax (973)940-3170

Stone, Frederick J., MD {1336183920} Pthlgy(73,IL06)<NJ-RBAYPERT>
+ Raritan Bay Medical Center/Perth Amboy Division
530 New Brunswick Avenue Perth Amboy, NJ 08861 (732)324-5165 Fax (732)324-4811
fstone@rbmc.org

Stone, Jane E., MD {1114968781} CdvDis, IntrMd(77,PA01)<NJ-VALLEY>
+ 163 Engle Street
Englewood, NJ 07631 (201)569-2520 Fax (201)569-8703

Stone, Jay H., MD {1710961024} CdvDis, IntrMd, IntCrd(84,GRN01)<NJ-COMMED, NJ-JRSYSHMC>
+ Shore Cardiac Institute
367 Lakehurst Road Toms River, NJ 08755 (732)473-0158 Fax (732)473-0033

Stone, Mark J., MD {1710928478} EmrgMd(88,NJ05)
+ AtlantiCare Urgent Care Center
2500 English Creek Avenue Egg Harbor Township, NJ 08234 (609)407-2273

Stone, Paul A., MD {1932101664} OncHem, IntrMd(92,PA13)<NJ-LOURDMED>
+ Cooper University at Willingboro
218C Sunset Road Willingboro, NJ 08046 (609)877-0400 Fax (609)877-3542

Stoneham, John L., III, MD {1982650644} Urolgy(88,NY09)<NJ-SOCEANCO, NJ-COMMED>
+ Urologic Health Center of New Jersey
67 Route 37 West/Building 2/Suite 1 Toms River, NJ 08755 (732)914-1300 Fax (732)914-0849
+ Urologic Health Center of New Jersey
63C Lacey Road Whiting, NJ 08759 (732)914-1300 Fax (732)350-7054
+ Urologic Health Center of New Jersey
949 Lacey Road Forked River, NJ 08755 (609)242-6930 Fax (609)242-6932

Stoner, Edward D., MD {1467427450} IntrMd(81,CHIL)<NJ-MONMOUTH, NJ-CENTRAST>
+ Family Practice of CentraState
479 Newman Springs Rd/Suite A-101 Marlboro, NJ 07746 (732)780-1601
+ Family Practice of CentraState
901 West Main Street/Suite 106 Freehold, NJ 07728 (732)780-1601 Fax (732)462-0348
+ Family Practice of CentraState
281 Route 34/Suite 813 Colts Neck, NJ 07746 (732)431-2620 Fax (732)431-3707

Stoopack, Paul Mitchell, MD {1073559931} Gastrn, IntrMd(79,NY19)
+ Pavonia Gastroenterology
600 Pavonia Avenue/3rd Floor Jersey City, NJ 07306 (201)216-3065 Fax (201)499-0250

Storch, Kenneth J., MD {1841285954} IntrMd, Nutrtn, EnDbMt(79,NY08)<NJ-OVERLOOK, NJ-MORRISTN>
+ Storch Nutritional Medical Assoc
147 Columbia Turnpike/Suite 308 Florham Park, NJ 07932

Storch, Marc I., MD {1376659466} IntrMd, Rheuma(87,ISR02)<NJ-HUNTRDN>
+ 1100 Wescott Drive/Suite 106
Flemington, NJ 08822 (908)284-9221 Fax (908)237-2366

Story-Roller, Elizabeth, MD {1558770925}
+ University Medical Group - General Internal Medicine
125 Paterson Street/Suite 5100A New Brunswick, NJ 08903 (732)235-6968 Fax (732)235-8935

Stotland, Mira, MD {1104023837} Dermat(06,NY08)
+ 206 Shearwater Court West/Apt 45
Jersey City, NJ 07305

Stoupakis, George, MD {1235103243} IntrMd, IntCrd, CdvDis(98,GRN01)
+ 5 Summit Avenue/Suite 200
Hackensack, NJ 07601 (201)343-7001 Fax (201)343-7232

Stowe, Arthur Chester, Jr., MD {1376682856} Gastrn, IntrMd(89,NC01)<NJ-WESTHDSN>
+ Balwin Medical Associates
377 Jersey Avenue/Suite 50 Jersey City, NJ 07302 (201)332-4110 Fax (201)332-4122

Stoyko, Zoryana, MD {1346689049} OncHem
+ Nazha Cancer Center
411 New Road Northfield, NJ 08225 (609)383-6033 Fax (609)383-1548
+ Nazha Cancer Center Galloway
436 Chris Craupp Drive/Suite 101 Galloway, NJ 08205 (609)383-6033 Fax (609)652-2004

Stoytchev, Hristo Vassilev, MD {1023277290} IntrMd
+ IPC The Hospitalist Company
55 Madison Avenue/Suite 310 Morristown, NJ 07960 (973)993-9536 Fax (973)998-4237

Strader, David J., MD {1306931787} Pedtrc(83,NC07)<NJ-STBARNMC>
+ David J. Strader MD, PHD
799 Bloomfield Avenue/Suite 304 Verona, NJ 07044 (973)618-9990 Fax (973)618-9991

Strain, Janet E., MD {1750358966} CdvDis, IntrMd, IntCrd(77,NY46)<NJ-VALLEY>
+ Valley Medical Goup Cardioology Ridgewood
1124 East Ridgewood Avenue Ridgewood, NJ 07450 (201)689-9400 Fax (201)689-9404

Strain, Jeffrey Witt, MD {1629036272} Surgry(92,OH06)<NJ-ENGLWOOD, NJ-HOLYNAME>
+ Bergen Laparoscopy & Bariatric, LLC
97 Engle Street Englewood, NJ 07631 (201)227-5533 Fax (201)227-5537

Strair, Roger Kurt, MD {1174625347} Hemato, IntrMd, MedOnc(81,NY46)<NJ-RWJUBRUN>
+ Rutgers Cancer Institute of New Jersey
195 Little Albany Street/PO Box 2681 New Brunswick, NJ 08903 (732)235-6044 Fax (732)235-8098
strairrk@umdnj.edu

Straker, Michael J., MD {1194773440} ObsGyn(99,NY47)<NJ-CLARMAAS, NJ-STBARNMC>
+ 359 Centre Street/Suite 1
Nutley, NJ 07110 (973)667-1500 Fax (973)667-0324
+ Clara Maass Medical Center
1 Clara Maass Drive/ObGyn Belleville, NJ 07109 (973)450-2000

Strakhan, Marianna, MD {1144489022} OncHem, IntrMd(02,ISR02)<NY-JACOBIMC>
+ Summit Medical Group
6 Brighton Road/2 FL Clifton, NJ 07012 (973)471-0981 Fax (973)777-5403
+ Summit Medical Group
31-00 Broadway Fair Lawn, NJ 07410 (973)471-0981 Fax (201)796-7020
+ Summit Medical Group-Berkeley Heights Campus
1 Diamond Hill Road Berkeley Heights, NJ 07012 (908)277-8890 Fax (908)790-6576

Stramandi, Danielle Nicole, MD {1831419399} FamMAdlt, IntrMd(08,DMN01)
+ Princeton Sports & Family Medicine
3131 Princeton Pike Lawrenceville, NJ 08648 (609)896-9190 Fax (609)896-3555

Strand, Barbara G., MD {1801858899} Pedtrc(85,NY01)
+ Advocare West Morris Pediatrics
151 Route 10/Suite 105 Succasunna, NJ 07876 (973)584-0002 Fax (973)584-7107

Strand, Calvin L., MD {1154323533} MedMcb, PthACl(65,MN04)<NJ-JRSYCITY>
+ PLUS Diagnostics
1200 River Avenue/Suite 10 Lakewood, NJ 08701 (732)901-7575 Fax (732)901-1555
+ Jersey City Medical Center
355 Grand Street/Path Jersey City, NJ 07304 (732)901-7575 Fax (201)915-2377

Physicians by Name and Address

Stranges, Douglas M., DO {1225475825}
+ Rowan University-School of Osteopathic Medicine
  1 Medical Center Drive Stratford, NJ 08084 (856)346-7985

Straseskie, Ryan Kenneth, MD {1023436268} FamMed
+ Primary Care at Oakland
  340c Ramapo Valley Road Oakland, NJ 07436 (973)962-6200 Fax (973)962-0046
+ Ringwood Medical Associates PA
  52 Skyline Drive Ringwood, NJ 07456 (973)962-6200 Fax (973)962-0046

Strassberg, David M., MD {1235165085} Gastrn, IntrMd(74,NY08)<NJ-VALLEY>
+ Valley Medical Group
  470 North Franklin Turnpike Ramsey, NJ 07446 (201)327-8765 Fax (201)327-8496
  dstrassbergmd@aol.com

Strassberg, Joshua A., MD {1932260353} SrgOrt
+ Advocare The Orthopedic Center
  218 Ridgedale Avenue/Suite 104 Cedar Knolls, NJ 07927 (973)538-7700 Fax (973)538-9478

Strater, Sharon, MD {1336190743} EmrgMd(95,NJ05)<NJ-HACKNSK>
+ Hackensack University Medical Center
  30 Prospect Avenue/EmrgMed Hackensack, NJ 07601 (201)996-2300

Strauch, Joseph M., MD Dermat(69,DC02)
+ Route 27 & Parsonage Road
  Edison, NJ 08837 (732)549-2448

Strauchler, Irving D., MD {1184630907} SrgOrt, SrgHnd(73,NY46)<NJ-STBARNMC, NJ-MTNSIDE>
+ Eastern Surgical Associates PA
  1099 Bloomfield Avenue West Caldwell, NJ 07006 (973)882-0600 Fax (973)882-0602

Strauchler, Roberta A., MD {1972519700} Ophthl(76,NY46)<NJ-MTNSIDE, NJ-STBARNMC>
+ Eastern Surgical Associates PA
  1099 Bloomfield Avenue West Caldwell, NJ 07006 (973)882-0600 Fax (973)882-0602

Strauss, Alexander Sangor, MD {1396946869} Psychy, NrlgSptM, NrlgSpec(05,IL06)
+ CENTRA Comprehensive Psychotherapy
  5000 Sagemore Drive/Suite 205 Marlton, NJ 08053 (856)983-3866 Fax (856)985-8148
  drstrauss@alexstraussmd.com

Strauss, Andrea L., MD {1033251632} SrgPlstc(83,PA14)<NJ-SOMERSET>
+ Plastic Surgical Associates
  11 Monroe Street Somerville, NJ 08876 (908)725-4600 Fax (908)725-4603
  info@plasticsurgicalassociatesnj.com

Strauss, Bernard S., MD {1356347223} Urolgy(64,NY46)<NJ-STBARNMC>
+ New Jersey Urology, LLC
  741 Northfield Avenue/Suite 206 West Orange, NJ 07052 (973)325-6100 Fax (973)325-1616

Strauss, Danielle Savitsky, MD {1336378736} Ophthl(09,NY47)<NY-NYUTISCH>
+ Omni Eye Services
  485 Route 1 South/Building A Iselin, NJ 08830 (732)750-0400 Fax (732)602-0749
+ The Eye Care Ctr of New Jersey
  108 Broughton Avenue Bloomfield, NJ 07003 (732)750-0400 Fax (732)743-6577

Strauss, Eric A., MD {1073535134} Dermat(96,PA01)
+ Dermatology Associates of Morris PA
  199 Baldwin Road Parsippany, NJ 07054 (973)335-2560 Fax (973)335-9421

Strauss, Eric D., MD {1912093428} SrgHnd, SrgOrt(81,NY19)<NJ-VIRTMARL, NJ-VIRTMHBC>
+ Hand Surgery & Rehabilitation Center of New Jersey
  5000 Sagemore Drive/Suite 103 Marlton, NJ 08053 (856)983-4263 Fax (856)983-9362
+ Hand Surgery & Rehabilitation Center of New Jersey
  608 North Broad Street/Suite 200 Woodbury, NJ 08096 (856)983-4263 Fax (856)983-9362
+ Hand Surgery & Rehabilitation Center of New Jersey
  8008 Route 130 North Delran, NJ 08053 (856)764-8804 Fax (856)764-3561

Strauss, Ira M., MD {1225006927} IntrMd, Nephro(78,MEX03)<NJ-JRSYSHMC>
+ Shore Nephrology, P.A.
  2100 Corlies Avenue/Suite 15 Neptune, NJ 07753 (732)988-8228 Fax (732)774-1528
+ Shore Nephrology, P.A.
  35 Beaverson Boulevard Brick, NJ 08723 (732)988-8228 Fax (732)451-0071
+ The Hernia Center
  495 Iron Bridge Road/Suite 3 Freehold, NJ 07753 (732)462-5995 Fax (732)845-1002

Strauss, Richard Charles, MD {1750315867} SrgNro(86,MD01)<NJ-SJRSYELM, NJ-SJERSYHS>
+ 2950 College Drive/Suite 1A
  Vineland, NJ 08360 (856)507-0600 Fax (856)507-0233

Strauss, Scott R., DO {1811986391} FamMed(97,FL75)<NJ-SOMERSET>
+ MEDEMERGE
  1005 North Washington Avenue Green Brook, NJ 08812 (732)968-8900 Fax (732)968-4609

Strauss, Walter D., MD {1235152356} IntrMd, PulDis(78,NY46)<NJ-VAEASTOR>
+ VA New Jersey Health Care System-East Orange Campus
  385 Tremont Avenue East Orange, NJ 07018 (973)676-1220

Straw, Simone A., MD {1861486821} Pedtrc(95,NJ05)<NJ-TRINIJSC>
+ Union Pediatric Medical Group, PA
  1050 Galloping Hill Road/Suite 200 Union, NJ 07083 (908)688-9900 Fax (908)688-9939

Straznicky, Pavel, MD {1093866626} SrgHnd, Surgry(75,NY09)<CT-BRADMEM, CT-BRISTOL>
+ Fitcare Corporation
  291 Franklin Avenue Wyckoff, NJ 07481 (201)847-0119 Fax (201)847-0871

Strazzella, William D., DO {1639245343} IntrMd, PulDis(83,NY75)<NJ-JRSYSHMC>
+ Community Pulmonary Assoc PA
  20 Hospital Drive/Suite 16 Toms River, NJ 08755 (732)349-5220 Fax (732)557-6032

Strazzeri, Mia Domenica, DO {1306856612} FamMed
+ Dorfner Family Medicine
  811 Sunset Road/Suite 101 Burlington, NJ 08016 (609)387-9242 Fax (609)387-9408

Streeks, Nicole N., MD {1386083004} Pedtrc
+ Pediatrix Medical Group
  1505 West Sherman Avenue/MSO-Box 104 Vineland, NJ 08360 (856)845-0100 Fax (302)651-4945

Streicher, James Tabb, MD {1295716561} Anesth(97,PA01)<NJ-MORRISTN>
+ Morristown Medical Center
  100 Madison Avenue/Anesthesiology Morristown, NJ 07962 (973)971-5000 Fax (201)943-8733

Streit, Steven, MD {1467476861} IntrMd, Acpntr(78,MEX03)<NJ-KIMBALL, NJ-CENTRAST>
+ 4710 Route 9
  Howell, NJ 07731 (732)367-5330 Fax (732)367-4394

Strell, Robert Frederic, MD {1336228279} PhysMd(94,ISR02)
+ 317 Willow Avenue
  Hoboken, NJ 07030 (201)222-0082 Fax (201)222-6799

Strenger, Keith David, MD {1942245352} PainMd, AnesPain(98,IL42)
+ 1750 Zion Road/Suite 210
  Northfield, NJ 08225 (609)415-0415 Fax (609)241-1935

Stricker, Howard, DO {1083662621} FamMed, FamMAdlt(64,PA77)<NJ-HOLYNAME>
+ Holy Name Physician Network
  143 Anderson Avenue Fairview, NJ 07022 (201)945-1400 Fax (201)945-4441
  Howsthedoc@aol.com

Stricoff, Alan L., DO {1386620011} IntrMd(00,NY75)
+ Johnson & Johnson
  1 Johnson & Johnson/EmpHlth Rm5G32 New Brunswick, NJ 08933 (732)524-3000 Fax (732)828-5493

Strizhevsky, Marina A., DO {1235386574} EnDbMt, IntrMd(02,NY75)
+ United Medical, P.C.
  612 Rutherford Avenue Lyndhurst, NJ 07071 (201)460-0063 Fax (201)460-1684
+ United Medical, P.C.
  533 Lexington Avenue Clifton, NJ 07011 (201)460-0063 Fax (973)546-7707

Strobeck, John Edward, MD {1215936299} CdvDis, IntrMd(74,OH41)<NJ-VALLEY>
+ The Heart and Lung Center
  22-18 Broadway Fair Lawn, NJ 07410 (201)773-8925 Fax (201)773-8886

Strobel, Ronald E., MD {1952360240} CdvDis, IntrMd(85,NY08)<NJ-HOLYNAME, NJ-ENGLWOOD>
+ 200 Grand Avenue/Suite 202
  Englewood, NJ 07631 (201)541-1220 Fax (201)541-4005
+ Heart and Vascular Institute at EHMC
  350 Engle Street/Suite 1000 Englewood, NJ 07631 (201)894-3636

Stroh, Jack A., MD {1356347066} CdvDis, IntCrd(84,NY46)<NJ-RWJUBRUN, NJ-STPETER>
+ RWJPE/New Brunswick Cardiology Group, P.A.
  75 Veronica Road/Suite 101 Somerset, NJ 08873 (732)247-7444 Fax (732)247-5119
+ RWJPE New Brunswick Cardiology Group, P.A.
  111 Union Valley Road/Suite 201 Monroe Township, NJ 08831 (732)247-7444 Fax (609)409-6882
+ RWJPE New Brunswick Cardiology Group, P.A.
  15H Briar Hill Court East Brunswick, NJ 08873 (732)613-9313

Strom, Karl William, MD {1831249275} Surgry, SrgBrtc(98,GRN01)<NJ-BAYSHORE, NJ-SOCEANCO>
+ Strafford Surgical Specialists, P.A.
  1100 Route 72 West/Suite 303 Manahawkin, NJ 08050 (609)978-3325 Fax (609)978-3123
+ Monmouth Surgical Specialists
  727 North Beers Street Holmdel, NJ 07733 (609)978-3325 Fax (732)290-7067

Strong, Gusti Lickfield, DO {1245405125} FamMed(90,PA77)<NJ-VIRTMHBC>
+ 25 Masters Circle
  Marlton, NJ 08053

Strongwater, Allan, MD {1932283314} PedOrt(78,IL01)<NY-MAIMONMC, NY-JTORTHO>
+ St. Joseph's Regional Medical Center
  703 Main Street Paterson, NJ 07503 (973)754-2000

Strony, John Thomas, MD {1699942912} IntrMd, CdvDis(80,PA13)
+ 2015 Galloping Hill Road
  Kenilworth, NJ 07033 (908)740-3747 Fax (908)740-2143

Strozeski, Janet E., MD {1497945398} Psychy(03,NJ06)
+ Care PLUS NJ, Inc. - Fair Lawn Mental Health Center
  17-07 Romaine Street Fair Lawn, NJ 07410 (201)797-2660 Fax (201)797-5025

Strozuk-McDonough, Stephanie, MD {1114967049} Pedtrc, AdolMd(98,GRN01)<NJ-RWJUBRUN>
+ Child Health Institute of New Jersey
  89 French Street/Suite 2300 New Brunswick, NJ 08901 (732)235-6230 Fax (732)235-8766

Struble, Dale W., MD {1790848125} IntrMd(76,NJ05)
+ 125 Brigantine Boulevard
  Waretown, NJ 08758

Struble, Eric Michael, MD {1477879740}
+ Capital Health-Heart Care Specialists
  2 Capital Way/Suite 385 Pennington, NJ 08534 (609)303-4838 Fax (609)303-4835

Struby, Christopher, DO {1174903256} IntrMd
+ Internal Medicine Associates
  201 Laurel Heights Drive/Suite 201 Bridgeton, NJ 08302 (856)455-4800 Fax (856)455-0650

Strumeyer, Alan D., MD {1952325821} Urolgy, IntrMd(88,DC02)<NJ-NWRKBETH, NJ-STBARNMC>
+ Essex Urology Associates/UGNJ
  225 Millburn Avenue/Suite 304 Millburn, NJ 07041 (973)218-9400 Fax (973)218-9420
+ New Jersey Urology, LLC
  1600 George Avenue/Suite 202 Rahway, NJ 07065 (973)218-9400 Fax (732)499-0432
+ New Jersey Urology, LLC
  375 Mounain Pleasant Ave/Suite 250 West Orange, NJ 07041 (973)323-1300 Fax (973)323-1311

Strumkovsky, Lyalya Olga, MD {1134491327} IntrMd<NY-MTVERNON>
+ MEDEMERGE
  1005 North Washington Avenue Green Brook, NJ 08812 (732)968-8900 Fax (732)968-5607

Strutin, Millard D., MD {1598798654} SrgCrC, Surgry(81,ITA17)
+ Northwest Surgical Associates
  121 Center Grove Road Randolph, NJ 07869 (973)328-1414 Fax (973)361-1085

Stuart, Jennifer Marie, MD {1477962520} EmrgMd
+ Hackensack Medical Center Emergency Medicine
  30 Prospect Avenue/Main 3619 Hackensack, NJ 07601 (551)996-2000 Fax (201)968-1866

Studint, Erika B., MD {1730288259} IntrMd, Pedtrc(94,NY03)<NJ-STCLRDEN>
+ The Family Medical Center at Dover
  375 East McFarland Street Dover, NJ 07801 (973)366-5859 Fax (973)366-0026

Stuebben, Kurt C., MD {1356361133} Psychy(90,PA12)<NJ-UNVMCPRN>
+ 144Tamarack Circle
  Skillman, NJ 08558 (609)921-9293
+ Princeton House Behavioral Health - Princeton
  905 Herrontown Road Princeton, NJ 08540 (609)921-9293 Fax (609)497-3370

Stueben, Benjamin L., MD {1306103437} PthAcl(11,GRN01)
+ St. Barnabas Medical Center
  94 Old Short Hills Road Livingston, NJ 07039 (973)322-5752

Stuffo, Kathryn, DO {1316280043} Pedtrc
+ 1303 Liberty Place
  Sicklerville, NJ 08081 (856)885-4584 Fax (856)885-4896

Stulbach, Harry Bruce, MD {1760490452} RadDia(82,NY47)<NJ-STBARNMC>
+ St. Barnabas Medical Center
  94 Old Short Hills Road Livingston, NJ 07039 (973)322-5800

Stump, James Basil, MD {1437146834} Anesth(01,MD01)<NJ-CENTRAST>
+ Liberty Anesthesia & Pain Management
901 West Main Street/2nd Floor   Freehold, NJ 07728   (732)294-2876   Fax (732)294-2502

Stumpo, Patrick P., DO {1336295260} Psychy(83,PA77)
+ 228 Wayne Avenue
Haddonfield, NJ 08033   (609)463-0099

Sturr, Marianne, DO {1407941867} PhysMd, OrtSpn(91,OH75)<NJ-ACMCMAIN, NJ-BACHARCH>
+ Lowe-Greenwood-Zerbo Spinal Associates
1999 New Road/Suite B   Linwood, NJ 08221   (609)601-6363   Fax (609)601-6364

Sturt, Cindy, MD {1073838173} Surgry(01,NY15)
+ Vein Institute of New Jersey
95 Madison Avenue/Suite 109   Morristown, NJ 07960   (973)759-9000   Fax (973)759-2487

Stutman, Robin Eugenia, MD {1346412392} InfDis<NJ-COOPRUMC>
+ Cooper University Hospital
One Cooper Plaza   Camden, NJ 08103   (856)342-3150   Fax (856)968-8418

Style, Daniel J., DO {1386638377} FamMed(85,IA75)<NJ-VIRTVOOR, NJ-KENEDYHS>
+ Style Family Medicine
1 Britton Place/Suite 12   Voorhees, NJ 08043   (856)772-1880   Fax (856)770-0718
+ Style Family Medicine
502 Hillside Terrace   Pennsauken, NJ 08110   (856)772-1880   Fax (856)633-5158

Style, Stuart D., DO {1538153523} FamMed(90,PA77)<NJ-VIRTBERL, NJ-VIRTVOOR>
+ Style Family Medicine
1 Britton Place/Suite 12   Voorhees, NJ 08043   (856)772-1880   Fax (856)770-0718
+ Style Family Medicine
502 Hillside Terrace   Pennsauken, NJ 08110   (856)772-1880   Fax (856)633-5158

Stylman, Jay Ira, MD {1760414700} Surgry(83,NY09)
+ 847 Kearny Avenue
Kearny, NJ 07032   (201)991-0041   Fax (201)991-5305
JSTYLMAN1@msn.com

Su, Hsiu, MD {1518130442} RadDia, OthrSp(04,NY19)
+ Advanced Medical Imaging of North Jersey
452 Old Hook Road/Suite 301   Emerson, NJ 07630   (201)262-0001   Fax (201)262-2330
+ Memorial Radiology Associates
10 Lanidex Plaza West/Suite 125   Parsippany, NJ 07054   (201)262-0001   Fax (973)386-5701

Su, Lan, MD {1093128191}
+ 72 Dorchester Drive
Basking Ridge, NJ 07920
randisu@gmail.com

Su, Melissa, MD {1801834858} IntrMd(87,MI20)<NJ-BAYSHORE>
+ Bayshore Medical Group
1128 Campus Drive   Morganville, NJ 07751   (732)972-0660   Fax (732)972-1061
+ Bayshore Community Hospital
727 North Beers Street/Internal Med   Holmdel, NJ 07733   (732)739-5900

Su, Michael Yu-Man, MD {1104870427} Ophthl(02,PA09)
+ Ophthalmic Consultants of New Jersey, Inc.
620 Cranbury Road/Suite 205   East Brunswick, NJ 08816   (732)708-3937   Fax (609)228-5120

Su, Mu, MD {1669675153} PthCyt<NJ-STBARNMC>
+ St. Barnabas Medical Center
94 Old Short Hills Road   Livingston, NJ 07039   (973)322-2772   Fax (973)322-8917

Su, Sherwin Leu, MD {1144532698} SrgOARec
+ High Mountain Orthopedics
342 Hamburg Turnpike/Suite 205   Wayne, NJ 07470   (973)595-7779   Fax (973)595-0182

Su, Tze-Jung, MD {1306932017} IntrMd(04,NY48)
+ 15 Paulin Boulevard
Leonia, NJ 07605   (212)238-7479

Suaco, Benjamin S., MD {1083601488} Anesth(82,PHIL)
+ Hamilton Anesthesia and Pain Management
1 Hamilton Health Place   Hamilton, NJ 08690   (609)631-6824   Fax (609)631-6839

Suapengco-Samonte, Dulce Hernandez, MD {1356417075} NnPnMd, Pedtrc(76,PHI09)
+ Clark Pediatrics LLC
480 Oak Ridge Road   Clark, NJ 07066   (732)574-9444   Fax (732)574-0907

Suaray, Khalil M., MD {1578567160} CdvDis(91,DC01)
+ Medical Health Center
1270 State Highway 35   Middletown, NJ 07748   (732)671-3836   Fax (732)671-1930
+ University Cardiology Group
125 Paterson Street/MEB 578   New Brunswick, NJ 08901   (732)671-3836   Fax (732)235-8722

Suaray, Mafudia Abibatu, MD {1831414424} FamMed<NJ-RWJUBRUN>
+ RWJ University Hospital New Brunswick
One Robert Wood Johnson Place   New Brunswick, NJ 08901   (732)235-7660

Suarez, Edwin, MD {1831230507} Gastrn, IntrMd(85,PRO01)
+ Drs. Suarez & Suarez
360 Bloomfield Avenue   Caldwell, NJ 07006   (973)226-8464   Fax (973)226-3750

Suarez, Kathryn Reynes Novak, MD {1275625410} ObsGyn(93,DC02)<NJ-COOPRUMC>
+ Cooper Faculty Ob/Gyn
127 Church Road/Suite 200   Marlton, NJ 08053   (856)983-5691   Fax (856)983-5763
+ Cooper Faculty Ob/Gyn
1103 Kings Highway North/Suite 201   Cherry Hill, NJ 08034   (856)983-5691   Fax (856)321-0133

Suarez, Lisbet D., MD {1063856318} IntrMd<NJ-OVERLOOK>
+ Overlook Medical Center
99 Beauvoir Avenue/PO Box 210/Medicine   Summit, NJ 07902   (908)522-2000

Suarez, Lynette G., MD {1689736993} Gastrn, IntrMd(86,DC03)<NJ-NWRKBETH, NJ-MTNSIDE>
+ Drs. Suarez & Suarez
360 Bloomfield Avenue   Caldwell, NJ 07006   (973)226-8464   Fax (973)226-3750

Suarez, Melissa Lehn, DO {1942511837} ObsGyn
+ Kennedy Family Health Services
1 Somerdale Square   Somerdale, NJ 08083   (856)309-7700   Fax (856)566-8944

Suarez, Militza E., MD {1477652196} InfDis, IntrMd(81,MEX27)<NJ-RWJUBRUN>
+ Eric B. Chandler Health Center
277 George Street   New Brunswick, NJ 08901   (732)235-6700   Fax (732)235-6729

Suarez, Norka J., MD {1043329014} Radiol, RadDia(86,NY47)
+ South Mountain Imaging
120 Millburn Avenue   Millburn, NJ 07041   (973)376-0900   Fax (973)376-0010
+ Imaging Center at Morristown
95 Madison Avenue/Suite 107   Morristown, NJ 07960   (973)376-0900   Fax (973)984-1190

Suarez, Ronald V., MD {1245539261} PthFor, Pthlgy(81,NJ06)
+ Morris County Medical Examiner
PO Box 900   Morristown, NJ 07963   (973)829-8270

Suarez, Teresa, MD {1376643981} ObsGyn(73,NY46)<NJ-ENGLWOOD>
+ Women Physicians Ob-Gyn Associates
300 Grand Avenue/Suite 102   Englewood, NJ 07631   (201)569-5151   Fax (201)569-9193

Suatengco, Jose Ramon, MD {1518932615} Gastrn, IntrMd(83,PHI09)
+ Ocean Endosurgery Center
129 Route 37 West   Toms River, NJ 08755   (732)606-4440   Fax (732)797-3963

Subbarayan, Srividhya, MD {1548297971} IntrMd(93,INA1C)
+ 666 Plainsboro Road/Suite 2000B
Plainsboro, NJ 08536   (609)799-1100   Fax (609)799-1189

Subendra-Konini, Logithya, MD {1447520200}
+ Somerset Family Practice
110 Rehill Avenue   Somerville, NJ 08876   (908)685-2900   Fax (908)704-3764

Subramaniam, Cristin Devika, MD {1295978278} Ophthl(09,IL06)
+ Bayshore Ophthalmology, LLC.
719 North Beers Street   Holmdel, NJ 07733   (732)264-6464   Fax (732)264-5114

Subramanian, Gomathy, MD {1922066182} IntrMd(98,POL03)
+ Summit Internal Medicine, LLC
33 Overlook Road/Suite LO6   Summit, NJ 07901   (908)522-0050   Fax (908)516-2946

Subramanian, Govindammal N., MD {1154357101} Pedtrc(78,INA77)
+ Neighborhood Health Center Plainfield
1700-58 Myrtle Avenue   Plainfield, NJ 07060   (908)753-6401   Fax (908)226-6743

Subramanian, Kavitha, MD {1174661110} IntrMd(98,INA81)
+ 53 Heatherhill Road
Cresskill, NJ 07626   (201)374-4120

Subramanian, Srilakshmi, MD {1013172170} FamMed
+ 611 Limelight Court
Edison, NJ 08820
+ 400 US Highway 130
East Windsor, NJ 08520   Fax (609)443-8781

Subramanian, Subhashini, MD {1043486129} Pedtrc, PedCrd(99,INA66)<NY-STRNGMEM>
+ The Pediatric Center for Heart Disease
155 Polifly Road/Suite 106   Hackensack, NJ 07601   (201)487-7617   Fax (201)342-5341

Subramanyam, Sujata, MD {1437144243} IntrMd, Nephro, EmrgMd(81,INA02)<NJ-RBAYPERT>
+ Raritan Bay Medical Center/Perth Amboy Division
530 New Brunswick Avenue   Perth Amboy, NJ 08861   (732)442-3700

Subramoni, Jaya, MD {1912077728} Anesth(67,INA34)<NJ-UNVMCPRN>
+ University Medical Center of Princeton at Plainsboro
One Plainsboro Road/Anesthesiology   Plainsboro, NJ 08536   (609)497-4000

Subramoni, Venkateswar, MD {1316009822} FamMed, SprtMd, FamMAdlt(67,INA34)<NJ-STFRNMED>
+ Subramoni Physicians Associates PA
2091 Klockner Road   Hamilton, NJ 08690   (609)890-9191   Fax (609)586-6163

Subrati, Rahman Ryan, MD {1932479094}
+ Montville Primary Care Physicians
137 Main Road   Montville, NJ 07045   (973)402-0025   Fax (973)402-0508

Suche, Kara J., MD {1740495167} PhysMd(03,PA09)
+ Advanced Physical Medicine Center
222 Bergen Boulevard/Suite 8   Fairview, NJ 07022   (201)945-1156   Fax (201)946-0012

Suchin, Elliot Jay, MD {1285683532} Nephro, IntrMd(95,NY20)<NJ-VIRTMHBC, NJ-LOURDMED>
+ The Center for Kidney Care
1261 Route 38/Suite A   Hainesport, NJ 08036   (856)222-1975   Fax (856)222-0721

Suchin, Karen Rebecca, MD {1326132150} Dermat, SrgDer(97,PA01)
+ Haddonfield Dermatology Associates
24 West Kings Highway   Haddonfield, NJ 08033   (856)795-1341   Fax (856)795-5034
ksuchin@comcast.net

Suchy, Matthew Robert, DO {1114293875} Anesth
+ Morris Anesthesia Group, PA
3799 Route 46/Suite 211   Parsippany, NJ 07054   (973)335-1122   Fax (973)335-1448

Suckno, Lee J., MD {1316947419} Psychy(80,NJ05)<NJ-STCLRBOO, NJ-STCLRDEN>
+ 170 East Main Street/Suite 202
Rockaway, NJ 07866   (973)627-8915

Suczewski, Edward J., MD {1952458903} IntrMd(82,POLA)
+ Drs. Suczewski & Suczewski
323 Avenue E/Corner 25th St   Bayonne, NJ 07002   (201)339-8600   Fax (973)839-3653

Suczewski, Thomas J., MD {1750424180} IntrMd(82,NJ05)<NJ-BAYONNE>
+ Drs. Suczewski & Suczewski
323 Avenue E/Corner 25th St   Bayonne, NJ 07002   (201)339-8600   Fax (201)339-2894

Suda, Abhay K., MD {1962454967} EnDbMt, Grtrcs, IntrMd(72,INA25)<NJ-CHILTON>
+ Kinnelon Medical & Pediatric Associates
170 Kinnelon Road/Suite 28   Kinnelon, NJ 07405   (973)838-1717   Fax (973)838-1775

Suda, Anjuli, MD {1467404434} Pedtrc(74,INA67)<NJ-CHILTON>
+ Kinnelon Medical & Pediatric Associates
170 Kinnelon Road/Suite 28   Kinnelon, NJ 07405   (973)838-7650   Fax (973)838-1775

Suddeth, James N., MD {1992812275} FamMed, Grtrcs(84,MD01)<NJ-SOCEANCO>
+ Island Medical Professional Association
1812 Long Beach Boulevard   Ship Bottom, NJ 08008   (609)494-2323   Fax (609)494-4141

Sudhakar, Telechery A., MD {1568491405} Nephro, IntrMd(72,INA09)<NJ-CHSFULD, NJ-RWJUHAM>
+ Mercer Kidney Institute
40 Fuld Street/Suite 401   Trenton, NJ 08638   (609)599-1004   Fax (609)599-3611

Sudheendra, Preeti Khetarpal, MD {1750517785}
+ South Jersey Health Care Center
Two Cooper Plaza   Camden, NJ 08103   (856)735-6260   Fax (856)342-6662
preetikmd@gmail.com

Sudhindra, Ramakrishna R., MD {1164413076} IntrMd, MedOnc, OncHem(70,INA68)<NJ-SJHREGMC, NJ-SJRSYELM>
+ Southern Oncology Hematology Associates
1505 West Sherman Avenue/Suite 101   Vineland, NJ 08360   (856)696-9550   Fax (856)691-1686

Sudjono-Santoso, Dewi S., MD {1053342865} Pedtrc, AdolMd(86,INDO)<NJ-CHSMRCER, NJ-RWJUBRUN>
+ Pediatrics by Night
1230 Whitehorse Mercerville Ro   Hamilton, NJ 08619   (609)581-1700   Fax (609)581-8472

Sudler, Joy D., MD {1538319447} IntrMd, EnDbMt(86,NJ06)
+ 28 Cottage Lane
Springfield, NJ 07081   (973)376-1210   Fax (973)376-1242

Sudol, Robert R., MD {1154424182} IntrMd(83,NJ05)<NJ-ACMCITY, NJ-ACMCMAIN>
+ 408 East Jimmie Leeds Road
Absecon, NJ 08201   (609)652-6947   Fax (609)748-9075

Physicians by Name and Address

Suede, Samuel, MD {1164503116} CdvDis, IntrMd(86,NY08)<NJ-ENGLWOOD, NJ-HOLYNAME>
+ Cardiovascular Associates of North Jersey
  25 Rockwood Place/Suite 440 Englewood, NJ 07631
  (201)568-3690   Fax (201)568-3667
  Smoothmd@aol.com
+ Cardiovascular Associates of North Jersey
  1555 Center Avenue Fort Lee, NJ 07024 (201)568-3690
  Fax (201)568-3667

Suell, Jeffrey, MD {1154777449} Pedtrc
+ Robert Wood Johnson Hospital Pediatrics
  One Robert Wood Johnson Place/MEB 308 New Brunswick, NJ 08901 (908)472-8733

Suffin, Arthur Lee, MD {1205876612} ObsGyn(68,NY19)<NJ-CHILTON>
+ Physicians for Women
  330 Ratzer Road/Suite 7 Wayne, NJ 07470 (973)694-2222
  Fax (973)694-7664
+ Wayne Surgical Center, LLC.
  1176 Hamburg Pike Wayne, NJ 07470 (973)694-2222
  Fax (973)709-1901

Suffin, Daniel Matthew, DO {1881853802} PulDis, IntrMd(04,NJ75)<NJ-STMICHL>
+ VMG Respiratory Health & Pulmonary Medicine
  1200 East Ridgewood Avenue Ridgewood, NJ 07450
  (201)689-7755   Fax (201)689-0521

Suffin, Stephen Chester, MD {1609993088} PthAcl(72,CA14)
+ 76 Albert Court
  Parsippany, NJ 07054

Sugar, Nina S., MD {1457561292} PsyCAd, Psychy(88,ISR02)
+ 589 Franklin Turnpike
  Ridgewood, NJ 07450 (201)670-7370
+ William D. Becker MD and Associates
  589 Franklin Turnpike/Suite 11 Ridgewood, NJ 07450
  (201)670-4075

Sugarman, Lynn B., MD {1588620462} Pedtrc, IntrMd(77,MA01)<NJ-ENGLWOOD, NJ-HACKNSK>
+ Tenafly Pediatrics, PA
  32 Franklin Street Tenafly, NJ 07670 (201)569-2400 Fax (201)569-6081
+ Tenafly Pediatrics, PA
  26 Park Place Paramus, NJ 07652 (201)569-2400 Fax (201)261-8413

Sugarmann, William M., MD {1982727880} Surgry(92,CT02)<NJ-SOMERSET>
+ Surgical Associates of Central NJ
  30 Rehill Avenue/Suite 3300 Somerville, NJ 08876
  (908)927-8994   Fax (908)927-8995

Suh, Jason W., MD {1538491212} OncHem, IntrMd(07,GRN01)
+ Valley Mount Sinai Comprehensive Cancer Care
  One Valley Health Plaza Paramus, NJ 07652 (201)634-5578 Fax (201)986-4702

Suh, Jin Suk, MD {1649299975} IntrMd, InfDis, HivAid(92,RI01)<NY-SLRLUKES>
+ St Joseph's Medical Center Infectious Disease
  703 Main Street/Xavier 6 Paterson, NJ 07503 (973)754-2256

Suh, Matthew Yongwon, MD {1720085707} Surgry(03,NY08)<NY-MTSINAI>
+ 16 Pocono Road/Suite 208
  Denville, NJ 07834 (646)397-4068   Fax (646)351-0893
+ 222 High Street/Suite 206
  Newton, NJ 07860 (646)397-4068

Suh, Se Young, MD {1215355425} EnDbMt<NJ-ENGLWOOD>
+ Englewood Hospital and Medical Center
  350 Engle Street Englewood, NJ 07631 (201)894-3000

Sujovolsky, Jeannette A., DO {1821179904} FamMed(01,NY75)
+ NHCAC Health Center at North Bergen
  1116 43rd Street North Bergen, NJ 07047 (201)330-2632
  Fax (201)330-2638

Sukhavasi, Sujatha, MD {1164605663} Anesth(99,INA8Y)<NJ-STMRYPAS>
+ St. Mary's Hospital
  350 Boulevard/Anesth Passaic, NJ 07055 (973)365-4300
  Fax (845)357-5777

Sukkarieh, Troy Z., MD {1003913815} Urolgy(00,NY47)<NJ-COOPRUMC>
+ Central Jersey Urology Associates LLC
  23 Kilmer Drive/Suite C/Building 1 Morganville, NJ 07751
  (732)972-9000   Fax (732)972-0966
+ Urology Care Alliance
  2 Hospital Plaza/Suite 110 Old Bridge, NJ 08857
  (732)972-9000   Fax (732)972-0966
+ Urology Care Alliance
  733 North Beers Street/Suite L-6 Holmdel, NJ 07751
  (732)739-2200   Fax (732)739-8988

Sulaj, Donjeta, MD {1477799807}<NJ-ENGLWOOD>
+ Englewood Hospital and Medical Center
  350 Engle Street Englewood, NJ 07631 (201)894-3364

Suldan, Dora I., MD {1831137918} Pedtrc(91,MA05)<NJ-HOLY-NAME, NJ-ENGLWOOD>
+ Pedimedica PA
  870 Palisade Avenue/Suite 201 Teaneck, NJ 07666
  (201)692-1661   Fax (201)692-9219

Suldan, Zalman Lewis, MD {1922007574} IntrMd, Nephro(00,NY20)
+ BSD Nephrology & Hypertension
  360 Essex Street/Suite 304 Hackensack, NJ 07601
  (201)646-0110   Fax (201)646-0219

Sule, Harsh Prakash, MD {1699721969} EmrgMd, IntrMd(99,IL11)
+ University Hospital
  150 Bergen Street/Emerg Med Newark, NJ 07103
  (973)972-9377

Suleiman, Addi, MD {1518262088} IntrMd<NJ-TRINIWSC>
+ Trinitas Regional Medical Center-Williamson Street
  225 Williamson Street Elizabeth, NJ 07207 (908)422-1774

Sulewski, Agnieszka, DO {1598971335} EmrgMd(06,NJ75)
+ EmCare
  1945 Route 33 Neptune, NJ 07753 (732)776-4510 Fax (732)776-2329

Suliaman, Fawzi A., MD {1508186909} AlgyImmn, Pedtrc, IntrMd(74,IRQ01)
+ Center for Asthma & Allergy
  18 North Third Avenue Highland Park, NJ 08904
  (732)545-0094   Fax (732)545-4087
+ Center for Asthma & Allergy
  300 Hudson Street Hoboken, NJ 07030 (732)545-0094
  Fax (732)792-5320
+ Center for Asthma & Allergy
  90 Milbum Avenue/Suite 200 Maplewood, NJ 08904
  (973)763-5787   Fax (973)763-8568

Sullivan, Anastassia D., MD {1801299938} EmrgMd
+ Hackensack Medical Center Emergency Medicine
  30 Prospect Avenue/Main 3619 Hackensack, NJ 07601
  (201)996-2000   Fax (201)968-1866

Sullivan, Bessie M., MD {1427147453} Allrgy, IntrMd, Rheuma(67,PA07)
+ Arthritis Allergy and Immunology
  100 Commerce Place Clark, NJ 07066 (908)301-9800
  Fax (908)301-9801

Sullivan, Brendan Patrick, MD {1174521140} CdvDis, IntrMd(98,GRN01)<NJ-CHILTON>
+ 1135 Clifton Avenue/Suite 206
  Clifton, NJ 07013 (973)777-3286 Fax (973)777-0435
+ Chuback Medical Group
  2 Sears Drive/Suite 101 Paramus, NJ 07652 (973)777-3286 Fax (201)261-1776

Sullivan, Edwin J., DO {1477580306} Urolgy(70,PA77)
+ Saddle Brook Medical Center
  449 Market Street/Suite B Saddle Brook, NJ 07663
  (201)843-7942   Fax (201)712-7902

Sullivan, Gregory F., MD {1851398911} CdvDis, IntrMd(66,NY19)
+ Drs. Sullivan and Sullivan
  1117 Route 46 East Clifton, NJ 07013 (973)779-1221
  Fax (973)778-6014

Sullivan, Jared Martin, MD {1225128952} ObsGyn(00,NET09)
+ Drs. Sullivan and Sullivan
  1117 Route 46 East Clifton, NJ 07013 (973)779-1221
  Fax (973)778-6014

Sullivan, Michael C., MD {1588827174} Surgry
+ Hackensack Meridian Medical Group Surgery
  19 Davis Avenue/Hope Tower 2nd Floor Neptune, NJ 07753
  (732)776-4770   Fax (732)776-3763
+ Hackensack Meridian Medical Group Surgery
  3 Hospital Plaza/Suite 206 Old Bridge, NJ 08857
  (732)776-4770   Fax (732)776-3763
+ Northern Monmouth County Medical Associates
  100 Commons Way/Suite 150 Holmdel, NJ 07753
  (732)776-4770   Fax (732)776-3763

Sullivan, Patrick O., DO {1154536738} EmrgMd
+ 61 Timbercrest Drive
  Sewell, NJ 08080

Sullivan, Sean Dominick, DO {1407146699}<NJ-UMDNJ>
+ University Hospital
  150 Bergen Street Newark, NJ 07103 (973)973-4300

Sullivan, Timothy Patrick, MD {1154408011} Otlryg(73,DC01)<NJ-RIVERVW, NJ-BAYSHORE>
+ 19 North Rivers Edge Drive
  Little Silver, NJ 07739 (732)530-7799

Sullivan, Timothy Patrick, MD {1417944562} Ophthl(78,NY08)
+ Somerset Hills Eye Care Center & Optical Shop
  2345 Lamington Road/Suite 110 Bedminster, NJ 07921
  (908)766-4834   Fax (908)234-9183

Sullivan-Miller, Julia Ann, MD {1386651339} Ophthl(99,LA01)<NJ-JFKMED>
+ Associates in Ophthalmology
  1150 Amboy Avenue Edison, NJ 08820 (732)548-3200
  Fax (732)548-1919
+ Associates in Ophthalmology
  203 Route 9 South Marlboro, NJ 07746 (732)617-1800

Sultan, Ahmed Said, DO {1437443322} Anesth
+ St. Joseph's Regional Medical Center Anesthesia
  703 Main Street Paterson, NJ 07503 (973)754-2499 Fax (973)977-9455

Sultan, Richard I., DO {1295700359} NroChl, Nrolgy(83,NY75)<NJ-JRSYSHMC>
+ Jersey Shore Neurology Associates PA
  1900 Corlies Avenue/Third Floor Neptune, NJ 07753
  (732)775-2400   Fax (732)775-5673
+ Jersey Shore Neurology Associates PA
  222 Jack Martin Boulevard Brick, NJ 08723 (732)840-4666
+ Jersey Shore Child Evaluation Center
  81-04 Davis Avenue Neptune, NJ 07753 (732)776-4178
  Fax (732)776-4946

Sultan, Ronald R., MD {1962403147} Surgry(73,NY19)<NJ-CHRIST, NJ-BAYONNE>
+ 11 Swayze Street
  West Orange, NJ 07052 (973)434-3305 Fax (973)669-5955
  ronaldsultan@gmail.com
+ 2255 Kennedy Boulevard
  Jersey City, NJ 07304 (201)434-3300

Sultan, Saima, MD {1740493634} Grtrcs, IntrMd(99,PAK18)
+ 212 Lozier Terrace
  River Edge, NJ 07661

Sultan, Sharmeen, DO {1649270687} EmrgMd(99,NJ75)<NJ-MTN-SIDE>
+ Hackensack UMC Mountainside
  1 Bay Avenue/EmrgMed Montclair, NJ 07042 (973)429-6000

Sultan, Wamiq S., MD {1699873463} Nephro, IntrMd(90,PAK11)<NJ-MEMSALEM, NJ-COOPRUMC>
+ University Renal Associates
  310 Woodstown Road Salem, NJ 08079 (856)878-1500
  Fax (856)878-1600
+ The Cooper Hospital System-Univ Hospital
  401 Haddon Avenue/Suite 280 Camden, NJ 08103
  (856)757-7844

Sultana, Meher, MD {1619969128} IntrMd, InfDis(99,INDI)<NJ-ATLANTHS>
+ Medical Diagnostic Associates PA
  525 Central Avenue/Suite D Westfield, NJ 07090
  (908)232-5333   Fax (908)389-1933
+ Atlantic Health System
  475 South Street Morristown, NJ 07960 (973)660-3100

Sultana, Noushin, MD {1083979249} EmrgMd<NJ-JRSYCITY>
+ Jersey City Medical Center
  355 Grand Street Jersey City, NJ 07304 (201)915-2000

Sultana, Rumana, MD {1215274949} MedOnc, IntrMd(03,BAN06)
+ Aly Internal Medicine/Hematology Oncology
  883 Poole Avenue/Suite 4 Hazlet, NJ 07730 (732)203-9500 Fax (732)203-0851

Sultana, Tanjim, MD {1427314996}
+ 870 Palisade Avenue
  Teaneck, NJ 07666 (201)836-0847 Fax (201)836-0897

Sultana, Yasmeen, MD {1730442658} InfDis, IntrMd(98,INA3Y)
+ 11 Godwin Place
  Clifton, NJ 07013 (201)563-5651

Sumarokov, Alina, MD {1417110693} Pedtrc(05,NY08)<NJ-ENGLWOOD, NJ-HACKNSK>
+ Tenafly Pediatrics, PA
  350 Ramapo Valley Road Oakland, NJ 07436 (201)651-0404 Fax (201)651-0909
+ Tenafly Pediatrics, PA
  26 Park Place Paramus, NJ 07652 (201)651-0404 Fax (201)261-8413

Sumas, Maria Elaina, MD {1174577027} SrgNro(89,DC02)<PA-CARLSLE>
+ 46 Shalebrook Drive
  Morristown, NJ 07960

Sumathisena, Sena, MD {1013951227} CdvDis(66,INDI)<NJ-DEBRAHLC>
+ Deborah Heart and Lung Center
  200 Trenton Road/Cardiology Browns Mills, NJ 08015
  (609)893-1200   Fax (609)735-0175

Sumers, Anne R., MD {1518921501} Catrct, Glacma, Ophthl(83,OH41)<NJ-VALLEY>
+ Ridgewood Ophthalmology PC
  1200 East Ridgewood Avenue Ridgewood, NJ 07450
  (201)612-0044   Fax (201)612-9446

Sumerson, Jeffrey Marc, MD {1073566303} InfDis, IntrMd(96,PA02)
+ Infectious Disease Physicians PA
  1001 Briggs Road/Suite 250 Mount Laurel, NJ 08054
  (856)866-7466   Fax (856)866-9088

Summa, Geraldine M., MD {1932171691} Pedtrc(84,NY09)<NJ-OVERLOOK, NJ-MORRISTN>
+ Summit Medical Group-Berkeley Heights Campus
  1 Diamond Hill Road Berkeley Heights, NJ 07922
  (908)273-4300   Fax (908)790-6524
+ Summit Medical Group
  34 Mountain Boulevard/Building B Warren, NJ 07059
  (908)273-4300   Fax (908)769-8927

Summers, Michael Edward, DO {1134469232} IntrMd<NJ-DEBRAHLC>
+ Deborah Heart and Lung Center
200 Trenton Road   Browns Mills, NJ 08015   (609)893-6611
Summersgill, Richard Blair, MD {1174520845} FamMed(78,PA02)<NJ-VIRTMHBC>
+ Moorestown Family Practice, PC
301 North Church Street/Suite 101   Moorestown, NJ 08057
(856)234-2101
Summerville, Gregg Paul, MD {1982604922} EmrgMd(90,PA02)<NJ-CHILTON>
+ St Joseph's Medical Center Emergency
703 Main Street   Paterson, NJ 07503   (973)754-2240   Fax (973)754-2249
Sumski, Jessica Lynn, MD {1568775856}<NJ-UNVMCPRN>
+ University Medical Center of Princeton at Plainsboro
One Plainsboro Road   Plainsboro, NJ 08536   (609)853-9792
Sun, Andrew N., MD {1497744619} ObsGyn(96,PA09)
+ Shore Area Ob-Gyn
200 White Road/Suite 105   Little Silver, NJ 07739
(732)741-3331   Fax (732)741-5119
Sun, Harry, MD {1225058738} SrgTpl<NJ-STBARNMC>
+ St. Barnabas Medical Center
94 Old Short Hills Road/RenalTransplt   Livingston, NJ 07039
(973)322-5000
Sun, Jidong, MD {1033158282} PhysMd(87,CHN19)<NJ-JRSYSHMC, NJ-BAYSHORE>
+ Union Medical, LLC
2182 Morris Avenue   Union, NJ 07083   (908)851-2666
+ Bayshore Rehab Medicine, PC
721 North Beers Street/Suite 1-B   Holmdel, NJ 07733
(732)888-3300
+ Jidong Sun MD
1542 Kuser Road/Suite B3   Trenton, NJ 07083   (732)888-3300   Fax (732)888-3116
Sun, Karen Hong Xue, MD {1558307900} IntrMd(84,CHN57)<NJ-SOMERSET>
+ Alliance Medical Associates, PC
15 Monroe Street   Bridgewater, NJ 08807   (908)595-6330
Fax (908)595-6331
Sun, Li, DO {1952663718} SrgOrt<NJ-PALISADE>
+ Palisades Medical Center
7600 River Road   North Bergen, NJ 07047   (201)854-5000
Sun, Lu Amy, MD {1720525827} IntrMd, EnDbMt, ClnPhm(82,CHN62)
+ 55 Corporate Drive
Bridgewater, NJ 08807   (215)622-5386
Sun, Lydia Lijuan, MD {1578744041} IntrMd(90,CHN57)<NJ-UNVMCPRN>
+ Riverdel Medical Practice
302 Clay Street   Riverside, NJ 08075   (856)461-7755
Sun, Nancy, MD {1538365408} Ophthl(07,NJ06)
+ University Children's Eye Center, P.C.
4 Cornwall Court   East Brunswick, NJ 08816   (732)613-9191   Fax (732)613-1139
+ University Children's Eye Center, P.C.
678 Route 202-206 North/Bld 5   Bridgewater, NJ 08807
(732)613-9191   Fax (908)203-9010
Sun, Qi, MD {1518063049} IntrMd, IntHos(88,CHN4A)<NJ-ACMCITY, NJ-ACMCMAIN>
+ AtlantiCare Clinical Associates
16 South Ohio Avenue   Atlantic City, NJ 08401   (609)441-2104
+ AtlantiCare Regional Medical Center/City Campus
1925 Pacific Avenue   Atlantic City, NJ 08401   (609)345-4000
Sun, Qiang, MD {1548227820} RadDia(99,OH06)<NY-PRSBCOLU>
+ Medical Park Imaging
330 Ratzer Road/Suite 6-A   Wayne, NJ 07470   (973)696-5770   Fax (973)633-1204
Sun, Stephen, MD (96,NJ05)
+ 17 Alpaugh Drive
Asbury, NJ 08802
Sun, Sung Wook, MD {1932125994} IntrMd(94,KOR06)<NJ-ENGLWOOD>
+ Dr. Sun and Associates
200 Grand Avenue/Suite 203   Englewood, NJ 07631
(201)944-3115   Fax (866)278-0484
Sun, Xinlai, MD {1053335976} PthHem, PthAcl(84,CHN07)<NJ-NWRKBETH>
+ Newark Beth Israel Medical Center
201 Lyons Avenue/Suite EL-4/Path   Newark, NJ 07112
(973)926-7000   Fax (973)705-8301
Sun, Xiu, MD {1649405473}<NJ-STBARNMC>
+ St. Barnabas Medical Center
94 Old Short Hills Road   Livingston, NJ 07039   (973)322-5000
Sun, Ye Ming Jimmy, MD {1427226109} Psychy(86,CHN60)
+ University Psychiatric Associates
183 South Orange Avenue/E-F Levels   Newark, NJ 07103
(973)972-8259   Fax (973)972-8305
sunye@umdnj.edu

+ University Behavioral HealthCare
183 South Orange Avenue   Newark, NJ 07103
Sun, Yun Lynn, MD {1659471217} Nrolgy(84,CHN57)
+ Virtua Nurosciences
200 Bowman Drive/Suite E-385   Voorhees, NJ 08043
(856)247-7770   Fax (856)247-7766
Sunaryo, Francis P., MD {1730287491} PedGst, Pedtrc(71,IND05)<NJ-NWRKBETH>
+ Newark Beth Israel Medical Center
201 Lyons Avenue/PediGastroenter   Newark, NJ 07112
(973)926-7000   Fax (973)705-3148
Sundaram, Ashany, MD {1124310404} FamMed
+ Care Station Medical Group
328 West St. Georges Avenue   Linden, NJ 07036   (908)925-2273   Fax (908)467-5385
Sundaram, Kanaga N., MD {1922151935} Gastrn, Hepato, Immuno(67,INDI)<NJ-MORRISTN, NJ-OVERLOOK>
+ Allergy and Clinical Immunology Center
2333 Morris Avenue/Suite D13   Union, NJ 07083
(908)688-1330   Fax (908)964-0991
+ Allergy and Clinical Immunology Center
29 Columbia Turnpike/Suite 202   Florham Park, NJ 07932
(908)688-1330   Fax (973)377-2775
+ Allergy and Clinical Immunology Center
40 Morristown Road/Suite A   Bernardsville, NJ 07083
(908)766-6608   Fax (908)766-7991
Sundaram, Palanisamy S., MD {1114010477} Pedtrc(69,INDI)<NJ-NWRKBETH>
+ 860 Grove Street
Irvington, NJ 07111   (973)399-8650   Fax (973)533-4470
Sundaram, Punidha, MD {1730275751} IntrMd, InfDis(93,INA77)
+ 50 Center Street
Ramsey, NJ 07446
Sundaram, Raghunand, MD {1760555007} Pedtrc(94,INA9Z)
+ 817 Rahway Avenue
Elizabeth, NJ 07202   (908)355-7365   Fax (908)355-2452
+ 103 James Street/Suite 303
Edison, NJ 08820   (908)355-7365   Fax (732)662-3299
Sundaram, Savitri, MD {1386700409} Psychy(70,INA21)
+ 195 Route 46 West/Suite 200
Mine Hill, NJ 07803   (973)328-7772   Fax (973)361-0066
Sundaram, Subramoni, MD {1811075005} IntrMd, Nephro(70,INDI)<NJ-HCKTSTWN>
+ 195 Route 46 West/Suite 101
Mine Hill, NJ 07803   (973)361-2550   Fax (973)361-0066
Sundaram, Uma, MD {1841247186} Pedtrc, NnPnMd(76,INDI)<NJ-OCEANMC, NJ-CENTRAST>
+ Ocean Medical Center
425 Jack Martin Boulevard   Brick, NJ 08723   (732)840-3305
Fax (732)785-8830
umasundarammd@yahoo.com
+ Uma Sundaram MD FAAP LLC
1541 Highway 88 West/Suite B   Brick, NJ 08724   (732)840-3305   Fax (732)458-6265
Sundaram, Usha K., MD {1568513539} Allrgy(72,NJ05)<NJ-STBARNMC>
+ Allergy and Clinical Immunology Center
29 Columbia Turnpike/Suite 202   Florham Park, NJ 07932
(973)377-4112   Fax (973)377-2775
+ Allergy and Clinical Immunology Center
40 Morristown Road/Suite A   Bernardsville, NJ 07924
(973)377-4112   Fax (908)766-7991
+ Allergy and Clinical Immunology Center
2333 Morris Avenue/Suite D13   Union, NJ 07932
(908)688-1330   Fax (908)964-0991
Sundararajan, Subha V., MD {1770741084} Gastrn
+ Red Bank Gastroenterology Associates PA
365 Broad Street/Suite 1-E   Red Bank, NJ 07701   (732)842-4294   Fax (732)842-3248
ssundararajan@rbgastro.com
Sunday, James Michael, MD {1316945132} SrgOrt
+ Coordinated Health
222 Red Lane   Phillipsburg, NJ 08865   (610)861-8080   Fax (610)849-1013
Sunderam, Darshi, MD {1679597280} IntrMd(75,SRI01)
+ Drs. Sunderam and Sunderam
310 Central Avenue/Suite 102   East Orange, NJ 07018
(973)266-9111   Fax (973)266-1227
Sunderam, Gnana, MD {1164446761} Grtrcs, IntrMd, PulDis(72,SRIL)<NJ-STBARNMC>
+ Drs. Sunderam and Sunderam
310 Central Avenue/Suite 102   East Orange, NJ 07018
(973)266-9111   Fax (973)266-1227
Sunderram, Jagadeeshan, MD {1780929899} CritCr, IntrMd, PulDis(88,INDI)
+ UH- Robert Wood Johnson Med
125 Paterson Street/MEB 568   New Brunswick, NJ 08901
(732)235-7840   Fax (732)235-7048
Jagadeeshan.Sunderam@rwjuh.edu
Sundhar, Joshua Bharat, MD {1760623193} IntrMd, Rheuma(06,HUN04)
+ Arthritis, Rheumatic & Back Disease Associates

2309 East Evesham Road/Suite 101   Voorhees, NJ 08043
(856)424-5005   Fax (856)424-4716
Sundheim, John M., MD {1093795015} Grtrcs, IntrMd(73,PA02)<NJ-COMMED>
+ 1433 Hooper Avenue/Suite 230
Toms River, NJ 08753   (732)818-6800
Sundick, Scott Adam, MD {1649449687} SrgVas(05,ISR06)
+ The Cardiovascular Care Group
433 Central Avenue   Westfield, NJ 07090   (908)490-1699
Fax (973)759-2487
Sundstrom, David C., MD {1346246832} SrgNro(84,NY46)<NJ-CHILTON, NJ-VALLEY>
+ North Jersey Spine Group
1680 State Route 23/Suite 250   Wayne, NJ 07470
(973)633-1132
+ North Jersey Spine Group
1 West Ridgewood Avenue/Suite 207   Paramus, NJ 07652
(973)633-1122
Sung, Boram, MD {1235373010} AdolMd
+ Mid Jersey Pediatrics
33 Brunswick Woods Drive   East Brunswick, NJ 08816
(732)257-4330   Fax (732)257-1177
Sung, Diana, MD {1114285129} PthAcl
+ Morristown Medical Center Pathology
100 Madison Avenue   Morristown, NJ 07960   (973)971-5600   Fax (973)290-7370
Sung, Edward L., MD {1821004011} ObsGyn(67,VA04)<NJ-ACMC-MAIN, NJ-ACMCITY>
+ Coastal Obstetrics & Gynecology Associates PA
72 West Jimmie Leeds Road/Suite 2500   Pomona, NJ 08240
(609)652-6600   Fax (609)652-1267
Sunkavalli, Anupama, MD {1669676375} ObsGyn, IntrMd(GRN01)<NJ-STBARHCS, NJ-COMMED>
+ Ocean Women's Health Care Group
602 Route 72 East/Suite 1   Manahawkin, NJ 08050
(609)978-9870   Fax (609)978-9873
canupama@yahoo.com
Sunkavalli, Paul Venugopal, MD {1841288495} Pedtrc(99,SLU01)
+ Meridian Pediatrics - Manahawkin
1100 Route 72 West/Suite 306B   Manahawkin, NJ 08050
(609)978-3910   Fax (609)978-3912
Sunkavalli, Sunitha Aluri, MD {1760467781} RadDia(94)<NJ-HACKNSK>
+ Hackensack University Medical Center
30 Prospect Avenue/Radiol   Hackensack, NJ 07601
(201)996-2069   Fax (201)996-5116
Sunwoo, Daniel, MD {1811959034} PhysMd
+ Spinal & Head Trauma Associates
1123 Campus Drive West   Morganville, NJ 07751
(732)617-9797   Fax (732)617-8899
Supe Dzidic, Dana, MD {1679511208} PulDis, IntrMd(86,CRO01)
+ JFK Medical Center
65 James Street   Edison, NJ 08820   (732)321-7000
+ Princeton Health Medical & Surgical Associates
2 Centre Drive/Suite 200   Monroe, NJ 08831   (732)321-7000   Fax (609)860-5288
Surace, Anthony, MD {1053348128} Anesth(98,GRN01)<NJ-MTNSIDE>
+ Summit Anesthesia Associates, P.A.
33 Overlook Road/Suite 311   Summit, NJ 07901   (908)598-1500   Fax (908)598-0197
+ Hackensack UMC Mountainside
1 Bay Avenue/Anesth   Montclair, NJ 07042   (973)429-6000
Surahio, Ali R., MD {1558764910} Psychy<NJ-TRININPC>
+ Trinitas Regional Medical Center-New Point Campus
655 East Jersey Street   Elizabeth, NJ 07206   (908)994-7207
Surakanti, Sujani Ganga, MD {1568549137} IntrMd, OncHem, MedOnc(02,NM01)
+ Rutgers Cancer Institute of New Jersey
195 Little Albany Street/PO Box 2681   New Brunswick, NJ 08903   (732)235-2465   Fax (732)235-7355
Surana, Gautam C., MD {1437144391} IntrMd, EmrgMd(73,INA16)<NJ-TRINIWSC>
+ 520 Westfield Avenue/Suite 305
Elizabeth, NJ 07208   (908)351-4511
Surapanani, Devi, MD {1215963673} IntrMd(93,INA64)<NJ-HUNTRDN>
+ Hunterdon Medical Center
2100 Wescott Drive   Flemington, NJ 08822   (908)788-6100
Fax (908)237-5488
Surapaneni, Padmaja, MD {1881776193} IntrMd, Grtrcs(93,INA96)<NJ-HACKNSK>
+ Holy Name Medical Partners Office
15 Anderson Street   Hackensack, NJ 07601   (201)487-3355
Fax (201)487-0960
Surapaneni, Purus Hotham N., MD {1467401596} IntrMd(87,INDI)<NJ-VALLEY>
+ 27 South Franklin Turnpike/Suite 2
Ramsey, NJ 07446   (201)818-0960   Fax (201)825-9537
pnsurapaneni@gmail.com

Physicians by Name and Address

Sureja, Dhaval, MD {1033434436} Nephro
+ Warren Hospital
185 Roseberry Street Phillipsburg, NJ 08865 (908)859-6700

Suresh, Tejas, MD {1679836365}
+ 199 Pierce Street/Apt 938
Somerset, NJ 08873
tejassuresh@gmail.com

Surgan, Matthew Louis, MD {1871798579} EnDbMt(01,NJ05)
+ Endocrinology Associates of New Jersey
9 Auer Court/Suite A East Brunswick, NJ 08816 (732)390-6666 Fax (732)390-7711

Surgan, Victoria, MD {1073603007} NroChl, ClNrPh<NJ-STPETER>
+ St. Peter's University Hospital
254 Easton Avenue/PediNeurology New Brunswick, NJ 08901 (732)339-7870 Fax (732)745-1632

Suri, Nipun, MD {1548558877} IntrMd<NJ-UMDNJ>
+ University Hospital
150 Bergen Street Newark, NJ 07103 (973)972-2179 Fax (973)972-1141

Suri, Ritu, MD {1972696409} FamMed, Grtrcs, FamMGrtc(92,INA72)<NJ-HOLYNAME, NJ-VALLEY>
+ Dr. Ritu Suri and Associates
245 Engle Street Englewood, NJ 07631 (201)569-5330 Fax (201)871-9722

Surikov, Vadim Michailovich, DO {1962529586} FamMed(96,NY75)
+ Integrated HealthCare Group
5600 Kennedy Boulevard/Suite 102 West New York, NJ 07093 (201)866-3100

Surks, Howard K., MD {1841222379} CdvDis(89,NY46)<MA-NEMEDCEN, MA-LAWRMEM>
+ 115 Wells Street
Westfield, NJ 07090

Surmeli, Sedat M., MD {1457306029} ObsGyn(94,PA09)<NJ-STBARNMC, NJ-CLARMAAS>
+ Contemporary Women's Care
338 Belleville Turnpike Kearny, NJ 07032 (201)991-3838 Fax (201)998-4643
+ Contemporary Women's Care
745 Northfield Avenue West Orange, NJ 07052 (201)991-3838 Fax (973)736-8078

Surow, Jason B., MD {1619968997} Otlryg, PedOto(82,PA01)<NJ-VALLEY, NJ-HOLYNAME>
+ ENT & Allergy Associates, LLP
690 Kinderkamack Road/Suite 101 Oradell, NJ 07649 (201)722-9850 Fax (201)722-9851

Surowitz, Clara Pauline, MD {1881817278} ObsGyn(ISR05)<NJ-MONMOUTH>
+ Lakewood Obstetrics and Gynecology
1001 Route 9 North/Suite 107 Howell, NJ 07731 Fax (732)994-4245

Surrey, Christine Marie, DO {1972583540} Grtrcs, IntrMd(97,NJ75)
+ Lighhouse Hospice
1040 Kings Highway/Suite 100 Cherry Hill, NJ 08034 (856)414-1155 Fax (856)414-1313

Surti, Daxa Bhupendra, MD {1598719684} Pedtrc(77,INA2B)<NJ-PALISADE>
+ NHCAC Health Center at Jersey City
324 Palisade Avenue Jersey City, NJ 07306 (201)459-8888 Fax (201)459-8872
+ NHCAC Health Center at West New York
5301 Broadway West New York, NJ 07093 (201)866-9320

Surya, Babu V., MD {1164525382} Urolgy(75,INA04)<NJ-BAYSHORE>
+ 670 North Beers Street/Bldg 4
Holmdel, NJ 07733 (732)888-8737 Fax (732)888-3738

Surya, Girija S., MD {1073607321} SrgThr, SrgCdv, IntrMd(75,INA04)<NJ-BAYSHORE, NJ-RBAYOLDB>
+ Vein Center for Women Inc.
670 North Beers Street/Suite 2 Holmdel, NJ 07733 (732)290-1100 Fax (732)254-1558
admin@veincenterforwomen.com
+ Vein Center for Women Inc.
646 Route 18/Suite 103/Building A East Brunswick, NJ 08816 (732)290-1100 Fax (732)254-1558

Susi, Brian Dievendorf, MD {1922079862} CdvDis
+ 101 Jefferson Street
Hoboken, NJ 07030 (201)443-8988

Sussman, Barry C., MD {1801881487} SrgVas, Surgry(73,NY19)<NJ-ENGLWOOD, NJ-HOLYNAME>
+ Englewood Surgical Associates
375 Engle Street/Ground Floor Englewood, NJ 07631 (201)894-0400 Fax (201)894-1022
+ Heart and Vascular Institute at EHMC
350 Engle Street/Suite 1000 Englewood, NJ 07631 (201)894-3636

Sussman, Cindy Pearsall, MD {1659536555} EmrgMd(82,PA07)
+ Henry J. Austin Health Center
321 North Warren Street Trenton, NJ 08618 (609)278-5900 Fax (609)695-3532

Sussman, David O., DO {1407898406} Urolgy(85,ME75)<NJ-KMH-TURNV>
+ New Jersey Urology, LLC
2401 East Evesham Road/Suite F Voorhees, NJ 08043 (856)673-1600 Fax (856)988-0636
+ Delaware Valley Urology LLC
570 Egg Harbor Road/Suite A-1 Sewell, NJ 08080 (856)673-1600 Fax (856)985-4583

Sussman, Emily Melissa, DO {1407239064} IntrMd<NJ-COOPRUMC>
+ Cooper University Hospital
One Cooper Plaza Camden, NJ 08103 (856)342-2000

Sussman, Jay I., MD {1851368062} CdvDis, IntrMd(81,NY47)
+ The Cardiology Group, P.A.
401 Young Avenue/Suite 275 Moorestown, NJ 08057 (856)291-8855 Fax (856)291-8844
+ The Cardiology Group, P.A.
128 State Highway Route 70/Suite 1-B Medford, NJ 08055 (856)291-8855 Fax (609)444-5521
+ The Cardiology Group, P.A.
1 Sheffield Drive/Suite 102 Columbus, NJ 08057 (856)291-8855

Sussman, Jonathan S., MD {1194779801} IntrMd, CdvDis, ClCdEI(98,NY46)<NJ-MORRISTN>
+ Morristown Medical Center
100 Madison Avenue Morristown, NJ 07962 (973)971-5000 Fax (973)290-7253

Sussman, Robert, MD {1831190990} CritCr, IntrMd, PulDis(81,NY46)<NJ-ATLANTHS, NJ-MORRISTN>
+ Pulmonary & Allergy Associates
1 Springfield Avenue/Suite 3-A Summit, NJ 07901 (908)934-0555 Fax (908)934-0556
R.Sussman@gmail.com.com
+ Pulmonary & Allergy Associates
8 Saddle Road/Suite 101 Cedar Knolls, NJ 07927 (908)934-0555 Fax (973)540-0472

Sussmann, Amado Ross, MD {1780880096} RadBdI, RadDia
+ University Radiology Group, P.C.
579A Cranbury Road East Brunswick, NJ 08816 (732)390-0040 Fax (732)390-1856

Sutain, Nathaniel, MD {1720025299} PhyMPain(02,NY19)<NJ-RWJURAH, NJ-TRINIJSC>
+ Union County Orthopaedic Group
210 West St. Georges Avenue/PO Box 330 Linden, NJ 07036 (908)486-1111 Fax (908)583-1034

Sutaria, Hasmukhbha N., MD {1366408056} Nrolgy(71,INA20)
+ 40 Union Avenue/Suite 206
Irvington, NJ 07111 (973)373-1196 Fax (973)373-1197

Sutaria, Perry Maganlal, MD {1063405157} Urolgy, OthrSp(92,NY20)<NJ-MORRISTN, NY-STCLARE>
+ Morristown Urology Associates PC
261 James Street/Suite 1A Morristown, NJ 07960 (973)539-1050 Fax (973)538-6111

Sutaria, Samir Hasmukh, MD {1083677579} IntrMd, Nephro(99,DMN01)
+ Associates in Kidney Disease & Hypertension
2177 Oak Tree Road/Suite 204 Edison, NJ 08820 (908)769-4735 Fax (908)769-4736
Samsuts@yahoo.com

Sutherland, Jewelle R., MD {1861482440} PulDis, IntrMd(89,PA13)
+ Virtua Garden State Pulmonary Associates
520 Lippincott Drive/Suite A Marlton, NJ 08053 (856)596-9057 Fax (856)596-0837

Sutherland, John R., MD {1134159742} ObsGyn(83,ITA12)<NJ-COMMED, NJ-MONMOUTH>
+ North Dover Ob-Gyn Associates
222 Oak Avenue/3rd Floor/Suite 301 Toms River, NJ 08753 (732)914-1919 Fax (732)914-0725
+ North Dover Ob-Gyn Associates
442 Lacey Road Forked River, NJ 08731 (732)914-1919 Fax (609)971-9712
+ North Dover Ob-Gyn Associates
214 Jack Martin Boulevard/Building D-3 Brick, NJ 08753 (732)840-3900 Fax (732)840-9270

Sutker, Burton, MD {1073540183} RadDia, Radiol(82,NY19)<NJ-STCLRDEN, NJ-STCLRDOV>
+ St. Clare's Hospital-Denville Campus
25 Pocono Road/Radiology Denville, NJ 07834 (973)625-6000

Sutter, David Brand, MD {1487639191} IntrMd(73,DC02)<NJ-VALLEY>
+ David Brand Sutter MD PA
638 Summit Avenue Franklin Lakes, NJ 07417 (201)848-1731

Sutter, Garrett Gerald, MD {1801834338} EmrgMd<NJ-CHSFULD>
+ Capital Health System/Fuld Campus
750 Brunswick Avenue Trenton, NJ 08638 (609)394-6000

Sutter, John I., MD {1407848575} Pedtrc, AdolMd(78,PHIL)<NJ-STJOSHOS, NJ-HACKNSK>
+ NuHeights Pediatrics
1115 Clifton Avenue/Suite 101 Clifton, NJ 07013

(973)250-2970 Fax (973)250-2971
jisutter@optonline.net
+ NuHeights Pediatrics
2 Brighton Road/Suite 404 Clifton, NJ 07013 (973)250-2970 Fax (973)250-2971

Suzuki, Ron Yks, MD {1750476396} FamMed(99,MNT01)<NJ-UN-VMCPRN, NJ-CHSFULD>
+ Suzuki Medical Associates, PA
11 Schalks Crossing Road Plainsboro, NJ 08536 (609)275-5700

Svider, Peter, MD {1821436304} Otlryg
+ Bergen Medical Associates
466 Old Hook Road/Suite 1 Emerson, NJ 07630 (201)967-8221 Fax (201)967-0340

Svigals, Paul J., MD {1265452684} RadV&I
+ 200 Century Parkway/Suite East
Mount Laurel, NJ 08054 (856)482-2800 Fax (856)482-9399

Swajian, Mary, DO {1407923774} PhysMd(79,PA77)<NJ-HACKNSK>
+ 381 Park Street/Suite 1-A
Hackensack, NJ 07601 (201)487-9790 Fax (201)487-9791

Swaminathan, Anangur P., MD {1104885417} Surgry(66,INDI)<NJ-JFKMED, NJ-RBAYPERT>
+ Comprehensive Surgical Associates
225 May Street/Suite A Edison, NJ 08837 (732)346-5400 Fax (732)346-5404

Swaminathan, Shobha, MD {1275564411} IntrMd, InfDis(96,INA26)<NJ-UMDNJ>
+ University Physician Associates
140 Bergen Street/ACC Level D Newark, NJ 07103 (973)972-4071 Fax (973)972-3102

Swamy, Aldonia A., MD {1568577146} Psychy(65,PHI01)
+ 400 Perrine Road/Suite 404
Old Bridge, NJ 08857 (732)727-3723

Swan, Alexander Mynt, MD {1346218856} IntrMd, Nephro(87,MYAN)
+ 1030 Saint Georges Avenue
Avenel, NJ 07001 (732)750-5555 Fax (732)750-5550

Swan, Kenneth Girvan, Jr., MD {1518035625} SrgOrt(00,NY20)
+ University Orthopaedic Associates, LLC.
Two Worlds Fair Drive Somerset, NJ 08873 (732)979-2115 Fax (732)564-9032
+ Brunswick Orthopaedic Associates, P.C.
252 Bridge Street/Building G Metuchen, NJ 08840 (732)321-9700
+ Brunswick Orthopaedic Associates, P.C.
303 George Street/Suite 105 New Brunswick, NJ 08873 (732)846-6100 Fax (732)846-6113

Swanson, Jonathan Raymond, MD {1588878128}
+ MidAtlantic Neonatology Associates
100 Madison Avenue Morristown, NJ 07962 (973)971-5488 Fax (973)290-7175

Swartz, Harry M., MD {1629059522} FamMed(56,PA02)<NJ-RIVERVW>
+ Drs. Swartz & Swartz
138 Cherry Tree Farm Road Middletown, NJ 07748 (732)671-3313 Fax (732)671-8513

Swartz, Jennifer L., DO PthAna, PthFor(95,IA75)
+ Bergen County Medical Examiner's Office
351 East Ridgewood Avenue Paramus, NJ 07652 (201)634-2940 Fax (201)634-2950

Swartz, Joel David, MD {1942231279} RadDia, RadNro, IntrMd(75,DC01)
+ Open Air MRI
430 Memorial Parkway/Suite 2 Phillipsburg, NJ 08865 (908)213-3600

Swartz, Stephen Jay, MD {1245211705} IntrMd, Grtrcs(83,IL42)<NJ-RIVERVW>
+ Drs. Swartz & Swartz
138 Cherry Tree Farm Road Middletown, NJ 07748 (732)671-3313 Fax (732)671-8513

Swarup, Subir, DO {1093954372} IntrMd<NJ-OURLADY>
+ Our Lady of Lourdes Medical Center
1600 Haddon Avenue Camden, NJ 08103 (856)757-3500 Fax (856)668-8479

Swatski, Michael A., MD {1881618809}
+ CAMCare Health Corporation
817 Federal Street Camden, NJ 08103 (610)664-4503 Fax (856)541-4611

Swayne, Kathleen Amy, MD {1316105406} Pedtrc(05,NJ05)<NJ-JRSYSHMC>
+ Pediatric Health, P.A.
69 West Main Street Freehold, NJ 07728 (732)409-3633 Fax (732)409-7133
+ Pediatric Health, PA
4200 Route 9 South Howell, NJ 07731 (732)409-3633 Fax (732)905-5502
+ Pediatric Health, PA
23 Kilmer Drive/Building 1 Suite B Morganville, NJ 07728 (732)972-0900 Fax (732)972-2892

Swayne, Lawrence C., MD {1699872788} RadDia, Radiol(79,NJ06)<NJ-MORRISTN>
+ Memorial Radiology Associates
10 Lanidex Plaza West/Suite 125   Parsippany, NJ 07054   (973)503-5700   Fax (973)386-5701

Swe, Yuzana, MD {1760888366} Pedtrc<NJ-UNDRWD>
+ Inspira Health Network
509 North Broad Street   Woodbury, NJ 08096   (856)845-0100

Sweberg, Warren A., MD {1285729566} Pedtrc, AdolMd(71,NY08)<NJ-STPETER, NJ-RWJUBRUN>
+ Mid Jersey Pediatrics
33 Brunswick Woods Drive   East Brunswick, NJ 08816   (732)257-4330   Fax (732)257-1177
+ Mid Jersey Pediatrics
25 Kilmer Drive/Building 3/Suite 107   Morganville, NJ 07751   (732)257-4330   Fax (732)972-1677

Swedlund, Anne P., MD {1972503597} Gastrn, IntrMd(81,IL02)
+ Princeton Center for Plastic Surgery
932 State Road   Princeton, NJ 08540   (609)921-7161   Fax (609)921-6263

Swee, David E., MD {1740367127} FamMed(75,NS01)<NJ-STPETER>
+ Family Medicine at Monument Square
317 George Street   New Brunswick, NJ 08901   (732)235-8993   Fax (732)246-7317

Sweeney, Ralph, Jr., MD {1801875067} SrgOrt(73,DC02)<NJ-TRINIJSC>
+ New Jersey Spine Group
1122 South Avenue W   Westfield, NJ 07090   (908)232-2700   Fax (908)232-3763

Sweeney, Robert L., DO {1023088242} EmrgMd, Pedtrc(81,NJ75)<NJ-JRSYSHMC>
+ EmCare
1945 Route 33   Neptune, NJ 07753   (732)776-4510   Fax (732)776-2329

Sweeting, Robert, MD {1710062294} IntrMd(84,MA05)<NJ-BERGNMC>
+ New Bridge Medical Center
230 East Ridgewood Avenue/Medicine   Paramus, NJ 07652   (201)967-4000   rsweeting@bergenregional.com

Sweidan, Safwan A., MD {1578644860} FamMed, IntrMd(82,SYR01)<NJ-STJOSHOS>
+ C. Dicovsky Medical Group LLC
681 Broadway   Paterson, NJ 07514   (973)278-1000   Fax (973)278-1709

Sweinhart, Marty Dawn, MD {1447359963} FamMed, IntrMd(93,NJ06)
+ Advocare Dover Family Medicine
369 West Blackwell Street   Dover, NJ 07801   (973)620-9000   Fax (973)891-1457

Swibinski, Edward T., MD {1700844784} EnDbMt, IntrMd(75,NY09)
+ Cooper Endocrinology Associates
1210 Brace Road/Suite 107   Cherry Hill, NJ 08034   (856)795-3597   Fax (856)795-7590

Swidryk, John P., MD {1689656043} FamMed(72,NJ05)
+ 403 River Road
Fair Haven, NJ 07704   (732)842-6727   Fax (732)842-7901

Swidryk, John Paul, MD {1740277516} Radiol, FamMed, RadDia(92,NY09)<NJ-COMMED, NJ-SOCEANCO>
+ Community Medical Center
99 Route 37 West/Radiology   Toms River, NJ 08755   (732)557-8000   Fax (732)557-2064
+ Coastal Imaging, LLC
79 Route 37 West/Suite 103   Toms River, NJ 08755   (732)557-8000   Fax (732)276-2325

Swift, Joanne, MD {1174595342} ObsGyn(86,PA02)<NJ-VIRTBERL, NJ-VIRTVOOR>
+ Garden State Obstetrics and Gynecological Associates
2401 Evesham Road/Suite A   Voorhees, NJ 08043   (856)424-3323   Fax (856)424-4994

Swigar, Mary E., MD {1659483188} Psychy, PssoMd, Psyphm(66,PA13)<NJ-RWJUBRUN>
+ UH- Robert Wood Johnson Med
125 Paterson Street/Ste 2200/ClAcBl   New Brunswick, NJ 08901   (732)235-7647   Fax (732)235-7677   swigar@umdnj.edu
+ University Medical Group/UMDNJ
125 Paterson Street/Suite 2200   New Brunswick, NJ 08901   (732)235-7647   Fax (732)235-7677

Swinger, Alan Bennett, DO {1215971502} Anesth(87,PA77)<NJ-OCEANMC>
+ Ocean Medical Center
425 Jack Martin Boulevard   Brick, NJ 08723   (732)840-2200

Switenko, Zenon M., DO {1538250881} FamMed(89,NJ75)<NJ-VIRTMHBC>
‡ Lourdes Medical Associates/Triboro Family Physicians
1104 Route 130/Suite K   Cinnaminson, NJ 08077   (856)786-8010   Fax (856)786-0529

Sy, Marjorie Grace Teng, MD {1568697605}<NJ-STBARNMC>
+ St. Barnabas Medical Center
94 Old Short Hills Road   Livingston, NJ 07039   (973)322-8945

Sy, Nena L., MD {1225031370} Anesth(65,PHI01)
+ 10 Audubon Drive
Denville, NJ 07834   (973)625-3492

Sy, Pacita C., MD {1861474256} IntrMd(85,PHI01)
+ 196 Jackmartin Boulevard/Suite A-2
Brick, NJ 08724   (732)458-4045   Fax (732)458-4979

Sy-Te, Emilie, MD {1316959075} PedDvl, Pedtrc, IntrMd(94,PHI02)
+ Center for Children with Special Needs
953 Garfield Avenue   Jersey City, NJ 07304   (201)915-2059   Fax (201)915-2551

Syed, Amer K., MD {1023214418} IntrMd, Hypten(98,PAK01)<NJ-JRSYCITY, NJ-HOBUNIMC>
+ Lutheran Senior Life at Jersey City
377 Jersey Avenue/Suite 310   Jersey City, NJ 07302   (609)599-5433

Syed, Faraz A., DO {1033264817} Anesth
+ 300 Home Street
Teaneck, NJ 07666

Syed, Kirin K., DO {1770895864} Urolgy
+ Rowan University-School of Osteopathic Medicine
1 Medical Center Drive   Stratford, NJ 08084   (856)566-6708

Syed, Sameera Mukaram, MD {1992887574} FamMed(97)
+ 43 Moorsgate Circle
Hightstown, NJ 08520

Syed, Saqib Abdul, MD {1699849067} Psychy(89,PAK11)<NJ-ANCPSYCH>
+ Ancora Psychiatric Hospital
301 Spring Garden Road   Hammonton, NJ 08037   (609)561-1700

Syed, Saquiba, MD {1639164486} EmrgMd, IntrMd(96,PAK01)<NJ-MTNSIDE>
+ Alpine Medical Associates, P.C.
634 Summit Avenue   Jersey City, NJ 07307   (201)897-7700   Fax (201)217-9455
+ Alpine Medical Associates, P.C.
2727 Kennedy Boulevard   Jersey City, NJ 07306   (201)897-7700   Fax (201)222-9392
+ Alpine Medical Associates, P.C.
303 Grand Street/Suite G   Jersey City, NJ 07307   (201)897-7800   Fax (201)516-2577

Syed, Tariqshah Muhammad, MD {1811054703} CdvDis, IntrMd(99,PAK18)
+ Cardiovascular Associates of Teaneck
954 Teaneck Road   Teaneck, NJ 07666   (201)833-2300   Fax (201)833-7600

Syed, Wajiha F., MD {1144385071} Psychy<NJ-JRSYCITY>
+ Jersey City Medical Center
355 Grand Street   Jersey City, NJ 07304   (201)915-2000

Syed, Zainab, MD {1275883456} IntrMd
+ Heart & Vascular Associates of Northern Jersey
22-18 Broadway/Suite 201   Fair Lawn, NJ 07410   (201)475-5050   Fax (201)475-5522

Syed, Zareen Taj, MD {1497959696} FamMed(INA2Y)
+ Union County HealthCare Associates
4 Adams Street   Clark, NJ 07066   (732)381-3441   Fax (732)381-8225
+ Union County HealthCare Associates
999 Raritan Road   Clark, NJ 07066   (732)381-3441   Fax (732)381-3733
+ Union County HealthCare Associates
400 Westfield Avenue   Elizabeth, NJ 07066   (908)620-3800   Fax (908)620-3243

Syed, Zubair, DO {1437253929} Otlryg, SrgFPl(95,NY75)<NJ-BURDTMLN, NJ-SHOREMEM>
+ Drs. Morrow and Syed
601 Route 9 South   Cape May Court House, NJ 08210   (609)463-5888   Fax (609)463-5885
+ Drs. Morrow and Syed
715 Bay Avenue   Somers Point, NJ 08244   (609)463-5888   Fax (609)601-1567

Syed-Naqvi, Samina Altaf, MD {1306998752} IntrMd(86,PAK15)
+ 415 Avenel Street/Suite B
Avenel, NJ 07001   (732)634-4300   Fax (732)634-4302

Sylvester, Claudine M., MD {1033263744} ObsGyn(96,DC01)
+ Women first Health Center
520 Pleasant Valley Way   West Orange, NJ 07052   (973)325-0087   Fax (973)669-5722

Symington, Peter Anthony, MD {1629064837} IntrMd(96,PA02)
+ The Park Medical Group
220 Livingston Street/Suite 202   Northvale, NJ 07647   (201)768-9090   Fax (201)768-9009
+ The Park Medical Group
24 Elm Street   Harrington Park, NJ 07640   (201)768-9090   Fax (201)784-0065

Syracuse, Donald C., MD {1275525578} SrgCdv, SrgThr, Surgry(73,NY01)<NJ-MTNSIDE, NJ-CLARMAAS>
+ The Cardiovascular Care Group
1401 Broad Street/Suite 1   Clifton, NJ 07013   (973)759-9000   Fax (973)751-3730
+ The Cardiovascular Care Group
433 Central Avenue   Westfield, NJ 07090   (973)759-9000   Fax (908)490-1698

Syritsyna, Olga, MD {1346689262} Nrolgy
+ Salem Medical Group - Pennsville
181 North Broadway/Suite 3   Pennsville, NJ 08070   (856)678-9002   Fax (856)678-4027

Sysel, Irene A., MD IntrMd, MedOnc(91,NE05)
+ PharmaNet Development Group
504 Carnegie Center   Princeton, NJ 08540   (609)951-6800   Fax (609)520-3054

Szallasi, Arpad, MD {1801959317} PthAcl, Hemato(84,HUN01)<NJ-MONMOUTH>
+ Monmouth Medical Center
300 Second Avenue/Pathology   Long Branch, NJ 07740   (732)222-5200   Fax (732)229-0245

Szapiel, Susan V., MD {1316954555} Nrolgy(84,IL01)<NJ-NWRKBETH>
+ Newark Beth Israel Medical Center
201 Lyons Avenue/BldG-3/Attndng   Newark, NJ 07112   (973)926-8088   Fax (973)926-8571

Szatko, Miroslaw, MD {1780822411} EmrgMd<NJ-COOPRUMC>
+ Cooper University Hospital
One Cooper Plaza   Camden, NJ 08103   (856)342-2000

Szawlewicz, Stephen A., MD {1811953789} Pedtrc(70,PA02)<NJ-VIRTMARL>
+ Advocare The Farm Pediatrics
975 Tuckerton Road/Suite 100   Marlton, NJ 08053   (856)983-6190   Fax (856)983-3805
+ Advocare The Farm Pediatrics
1001 Laurel Oak Boulevard/Suite B   Voorhees, NJ 08043   (856)983-6190   Fax (856)782-7404

Szawlewicz, Stephen J., MD {1023103884} IntrMd(97,PA02)<NJ-COOPRUMC>
+ Cooper University Medical Center/Camden
3 Cooper Plaza   Camden, NJ 08103   (856)342-2000

Szczech, Emily C., DO {1801181938}<NJ-STJOSHOS>
+ St. Joseph's Regional Medical Center
703 Main Street   Paterson, NJ 07503   (973)754-2490

Szczech, Kazimierz M., MD {1821037805} Anesth(81,POLA)
+ Clifton-Wallington Medical Group
1033 Clifton Avenue/Suite 210   Clifton, NJ 07013   (973)473-4400   Fax (973)473-6822
+ Wayne Surgical Center, LLC.
1176 Hamburg Pike   Wayne, NJ 07470   (973)473-4400   Fax (973)709-1901

Szczurek, Linda J., DO {1073703492} Surgry(05,NY75)
+ Advocare Associates in General Surgery
2201 Chapel Avenue West/Suite 100   Cherry Hill, NJ 08002   (856)665-2017   Fax (856)488-6769
+ Advocare Associates in General Surgery
570 Egg Harbor Road/Suite C-2   Sewell, NJ 08080   (856)665-2017   Fax (856)256-7789
+ Professional Gastroenterology Associates, PA
1939 Route 70 East/Suite 250   Cherry Hill, NJ 08002   (856)429-4433   Fax (856)424-6732

Sze, Michael Shu Shin, MD {1710914031} ObsGyn
+ SOMC Medical Group, PC
1100 Route 72 West/Suite 305   Manahawkin, NJ 08050   (609)978-9841   Fax (609)978-9843

Szeeley, Pamela J., MD {1043305808} Psychy(83,PA12)
+ Cooper Psychiatric Associates
3 Cooper Plaza/Suite 307   Camden, NJ 08103   (856)342-2328   Fax (856)541-6137

Szema, Katherine Fang, MD {1841363660} PedAlg, IntrMd(95,PA02)<NJ-MONMOUTH, NJ-RIVERVW>
+ ENT and Allergy Associates
1131 Broad Street/Suite 103 Building A   Shrewsbury, NJ 07702   (732)389-3388   Fax (732)389-2387

Szenics, Jonathan M., MD OccpMd(81,NJ06)
+ Corporate Health Center
832 Brunswick Avenue   Trenton, NJ 08638   (609)695-7471

Szenkiel, Grazyna, MD {1710051743} IntrMd(77,POLA)<NJ-RBAYPERT, NJ-JFKMED>
+ 469 Cornell Street
Perth Amboy, NJ 08861   (732)442-2159   Fax (732)442-1233
+ 676 Amboy Avenue
Woodbridge, NJ 07095   (732)442-2159   Fax (732)634-0146

Szeto, Oliver Jo-Yang, MD {1487861365} PthACl(05,MA07)
+ Histopathology Services, LLC.
535 East Crescent Avenue   Ramsey, NJ 07446   (201)661-7280   Fax (201)661-7297

Physicians by Name and Address

Szewczyk-Szczech, Krystyna H., MD {1871532895} IntrMd(80,POL06)<NJ-STMRYPAS>
+ Clifton-Wallington Medical Group
  60 Main Avenue   Wallington, NJ 07057   (973)471-3555
+ Clifton-Wallington Medical Group
  1033 Clifton Avenue/Suite 210   Clifton, NJ 07013   (973)471-3555   Fax (973)473-4547

Szgalsky, Joseph Brian, MD {1689653644} FamMed, Grtrcs, IntrMd(85,PA02)<NJ-UNDRWD>
+ Inspira Medical Group
  200 Rowan Boulevard   Glassboro, NJ 08028   (856)582-0500   Fax (856)582-0163

Szikman, Howard Shawn, DO {1285609644} Radiol, RadDia, RadBdI(98,FL75)<NJ-HUNTRDN>
+ Hunterdon Medical Center
  2100 Wescott Drive/Radiology   Flemington, NJ 08822   (908)788-6100

Szmak, Lauren, MD {1932661071} PhysMd
+ 29 Thrumont Road
  West Caldwell, NJ 07006   (973)303-5267

Szpalski, Caroline, MD {1114379864} SrgPlstc
+ St Joseph's Medical Center Plastic Surgery
  703 Main Street   Paterson, NJ 07503   (973)754-2413

Szpiech, Maria, MD {1730325515} EnDbMt, IntrMd(90,POL03)
+ Stratford - Endocrinology
  25 East Laurel Road   Stratford, NJ 08084   Fax (856)783-8537

Szteinbaum, Edward M., MD {1063506293} Psychy, PsyAdd, PsyFor(79,COL05)<NJ-CARRIER>
+ 330 North Harrison Street/Suite 1
  Princeton, NJ 08540   (609)921-3666
+ UH- RWJ Medical School
  One Robert Wood Johnson Place   New Brunswick, NJ 08903   (732)235-5600

Sztejman, Eric S., MD {1255386355} IntrMd, PulDis(00,NET09)<NJ-VIRTUAHS, NJ-VIRTVOOR>
+ Virtua Garden State Pulmonary Associates
  520 Lippincott Drive/Suite A   Marlton, NJ 08053   (856)596-9057   Fax (856)596-0837

Szuchman, Mario, MD {1144221573} Pedtrc(76,SPA05)<NJ-STBARNMC, NJ-MTNSIDE>
+ Zufall Health Center
  18 West Blackwell Street   Dover, NJ 07801   (973)328-9100   Fax (973)328-6817

Szucs, Paul Andrew, MD {1497704696} EmrgMd, EmrgUHyM(89,CA02)<NJ-MORRISTN>
+ Morristown Medical Center
  100 Madison Avenue   Morristown, NJ 07962   (800)290-5309   Fax (803)434-4354

Szulazkowski, Wojciech Wadim, MD {1316916315} Psychy(86,POL17)<NJ-CARRIER>
+ Carrier Clinic
  252 Route 601/Psych   Belle Mead, NJ 08502   (908)281-1000

Szulc, Magdalena, MD {1144553660} IntrMd(00,POL12)<NJ-ACMCITY>
+ AtlantiCare Regional Medical Center/City Campus
  1925 Pacific Avenue/Hospitalist   Atlantic City, NJ 08401   (609)441-8146   Fax (609)441-8002

Szwed, Stanley A., MD {1629023478} CdvDis, IntrMd, IntCrd(82,GRN01)<NJ-STMRYPAS, NJ-HACKNSK>
+ 925 Clifton Avenue/Suite 108
  Clifton, NJ 07013   (973)471-6200   Fax (973)471-6221
  stashsz@aol.com

Szydlowski, Ellen Gayle, MD {1174641054} Pedtrc<PA-CHILDHOS>
+ CHOP Care Network at Virtua Voorhees Hospital
  100 Bowman Drive   Voorhees, NJ 08043   (856)325-3000   Fax (609)261-5842

Szylit, Jo-Ann, MD {1134102106} Dermat, IntrMd(78,NY48)<NJ-CHILTON>
+ 135 Kinnelon Road/Suite 103
  Kinnelon, NJ 07045   (973)838-1771   Fax (973)492-2858

Szymanski, Jesse, MD {1194142323} IntrMd<NJ-NWRKBETH>
+ Newark Beth Israel Medical Center
  201 Lyons Avenue   Newark, NJ 07112   (973)926-7000

Tabachnick, John Frederick, MD {1639174139} FamMed, IntrMd(79,NY47)<NJ-OVERLOOK>
+ Westfield Family Practice
  563 Westfield Avenue   Westfield, NJ 07090   (908)232-5858   Fax (908)232-0439

Tabaksblat, Martin Yaron, MD {1437326550} CdvDis(08,NY48)<NY-SLRLUKES>
+ Cardiology Associates of North Jersey
  242 West Parkway   Pompton Plains, NJ 07444   (973)831-7455   Fax (973)831-7585

Tabbarah, Khalid Zuhayr, MD {1962524975} Nrolgy
+ Center for Neurological Surgery UMDNJ
  90 Bergen Street/DOC 8100   Newark, NJ 07103   (973)972-2323   Fax (973)972-2333
  kzt2@njms.rutgers.edu

Tabije, Kevin, DO {1164710463} PhyMPain
+ Performance Rehabilitation & Sports Injury Center
  459 Watchung Avenue   Watchung, NJ 07069   (908)756-2424   Fax (908)756-2447

Taboada, Javier Gustavo, MD {1780731802} Nrolgy, Psychy(66,PER05)
+ 2000 Hamilton Avenue
  Trenton, NJ 08619   (609)587-3333

Taclob, Erlinda V., MD {1184647273} IntrMd(67,PHI10)
+ Main Medical Associates
  100 Main Street   Paterson, NJ 07505   (973)523-0317   Fax (973)684-8590

Taclob, Lowell T., MD {1164446209} IntrMd, Nephro(67,PHI10)
+ Main Medical Associates
  100 Main Street   Paterson, NJ 07505   (973)523-0317   Fax (973)684-8590

Taclob, Michelle Maria, MD {1619131398} IntrMd<NJ-STJOSHOS>
+ Main Medical Associates
  100 Main Street   Paterson, NJ 07505   (973)523-0317   Fax (973)684-8590

Tacopina, Teresa Anne, MD {1205813672} IntrMd, Gastrn(02,GRN01)<NJ-COMMED>
+ Ocean Endosurgery Center
  129 Route 37 West   Toms River, NJ 08755   (732)606-4440   Fax (732)797-3963

Tadi, Kiranmayi, MD {1366689382} IntrMd<NJ-VIRTMHBC>
+ Virtua Memorial
  175 Madison Avenue   Mount Holly, NJ 08060   (609)267-6200   (609)914-6182

Tadisina, Vani, MD {1487881413} IntHos<NJ-OVERLOOK>
+ Overlook Medical Center
  99 Beauvoir Avenue/PO Box 210   Summit, NJ 07902   (866)251-0094   Fax (908)598-2337

Tadros, Carmen E. G., MD {1659438943} IntrMd(90,EGY16)
+ Saint Peter's Physician Associate
  59 Veronica Avenue/Suite 203   Somerset, NJ 08873   (732)745-8600

Tadros, Dalia Anwar, MD {1497702187} IntrMd(96,EGY04)<NJ-HACKNSK>
+ Hackensack University Medical Center
  30 Prospect Avenue   Hackensack, NJ 07601   (201)215-2510   Fax (201)343-9823
+ Regent Care Center
  50 Polifly Road   Hackensack, NJ 07601   (201)215-2510   Fax (201)487-3835

Tadros, Mahfouz M., MD {1720129810} Surgry(70,EGY03)<NJ-HOLYNAME>
+ PO Box 156
  Demarest, NJ 07627   (201)794-7878   Fax (201)567-8118

Tadros, Monica, MD {1144231515} Otlryg(00,PA02)
+ 300 Grand Avenue/Suite 104
  Englewood, NJ 07631   (201)408-5430   Fax (201)408-5437

Tadros, Wagih F., MD {1578680708} IntrMd, FamMed(76,EGY04)
+ East Brunswick Medical Associates PA
  63 West Prospect Avenue   East Brunswick, NJ 08816   (732)651-8118   Fax (732)651-9797

Tadrous, Kathreen Tharwat, MD {1043501265}
+ University Behavioral HealthCare
  183 South Orange Avenue   Newark, NJ 07103

Taffet, Berton, MD {1366430209} SrgOrt, IntrMd(78,NY46)<NJ-MORRISTN>
+ Atlantic Orthopedic Institute
  111 Madison Avenue/Suite 400   Morristown, NJ 07960   (973)984-0404   Fax (973)984-2516

Taffet, Robert, MD {1598708505} SprtMd, SrgOrt, IntrMd(88,NY46)
+ Cross keys Medical & Dental
  600 Berlin Cross Keys Road   Sicklerville, NJ 08081   (856)629-9770   Fax (856)629-9771

Tagayun, Myrna B., MD {1205872785} Nrolgy, IntrMd, Addctn(66,PHI01)
+ Comprehensive Medical Therapeutics
  1360 Clifton Avenue/Suite 275   Clifton, NJ 07012   (973)773-7800   Fax (973)253-0213
  electronstagmography@yahoo.com

Tager, Patricia, MD {1841240637} Dermat(94,FL02)<NJ-COMMED, NJ-KIMBALL>
+ Schweiger Dermatology
  67 Lacey Road   Whiting, NJ 08759   (732)849-4410   Fax (732)849-4421
+ Accredited Dermatology
  525 Route 70 West/Suite A1   Lakewood, NJ 08701   (732)849-4410   Fax (732)370-1526
+ Schweiger Dermatology
  712 East Bay Avenue/Suite 19   Manahawkin, NJ 08759   (609)597-5850   Fax (609)597-9667

Tagle, Lauren, MD {1841785672} FamMAdlt
+ Get Clare
  137 High Street/Suite 2 A   Mount Holly, NJ 08060   (609)474-0120

Tagle, Raymundo T., MD {1942227376} IntrMd, EmrgMd(75,PHI08)<NJ-VIRTVOOR>
+ Virtua Voorhees
  100 Bowman Drive/EmergMed   Voorhees, NJ 08043   (856)247-3000

Tagni, Carine-Ange, MD {1851759591} ObsGyn
+ Drs. Rhee and Timms
  3 Cooper Plaza/Suite 221   Camden, NJ 08103   (856)342-2965   Fax (856)365-1967

Tagore, Ammundeep Singh, MD {1710245667}<NJ-NWRKBETH>
+ Newark Beth Israel Medical Center
  201 Lyons Avenue   Newark, NJ 07112   (973)926-6671   Fax (973)282-0562

Taguba Madrid, Leslie Catherine, MD {1801885389} IntrMd
+ 1163 Route 37 West/Bldg A1
  Toms River, NJ 08755

Tah, Peter A., MD {1548254428} ObsGyn, IntrMd(90,TN07)
+ 930 Clifton Avenue/Suite 104
  Clifton, NJ 07013   (973)405-6333   Fax (973)754-4298

Taha, Abdallah R., MD {1992887962} CdvDis, Surgry(69,EGY03)
+ 1815 Kennedy Boulevard
  Jersey City, NJ 07305   (201)860-9121   Fax (201)433-2586

Taha, Firas Abdallah, MD {1073752382} Eplpsy, NroChl, ClNrPh(05,DMN01)<NY-NYUTISCH>
+ Northeast Regional Epilepsy Group
  20 Prospect Avenue/Suite 800   Hackensack, NJ 07601   (201)343-6676   Fax (201)343-6689

Taha, Nora, MD {1962632695} PhysMd, IntrMd(NJ02
+ Spine Center
  106 Grand Avenue/Suite 220   Englewood, NJ 07631   (201)503-1900   Fax (201)503-1901

Taha, Salah H., MD {1659434595} SrgVas, Surgry(72,EGY03)
+ 550 Summit Avenue/Suite 203
  Jersey City, NJ 07306   (201)659-0536   Fax (201)659-0405

Taher, Reza, MD {1518230176}
+ 200 Hospital Plaza/Apt 604
  Paterson, NJ 07503   (818)317-2244

Tahil, Fatimah Ann, MD {1225096555} Psychy, PssoMd(86,PHI02)<NJ-OVERLOOK>
+ Overlook Medical Center
  99 Beauvoir Avenue/PO Box 210/Psych   Summit, NJ 07902   (908)522-2000

Tahmoush, Albert J., MD {1801819115} Nrolgy, ClNrPh(67,MA07)<NJ-UMDNJ, NJ-SJERSYHS>
+ AtlantiCare Physician Group Joslin Diabetes Center
  2500 English Creek Avenue/Bldg 800   Egg Harbor Township, NJ 08234   (609)407-2277   Fax (609)272-6306

Tahzib, Munirih Nura, MD {1437233921} AlgyImmn, Pedtrc, Allrgy(95,NET04)
+ Center for Asthma and Allergy
  546 Westfield Avenue   Westfield, NJ 07090   (908)232-1565   Fax (908)232-9301
+ Hoboken University Medical Center
  308 Willow Avenue   Hoboken, NJ 07030   (201)418-1000

Tai, Mustafa, MD {1689023152} Psychy<NJ-UNIVBHC>
+ University Behavioral Health Care
  671 Hoes Lane/PO Box 1392/Suite D409   Piscataway, NJ 08855   (732)235-4295

Tai, Qing, MD {1093750069} PhysMd, PainMd, PhyMPain(87,CHN62)<NJ-STPETER, NJ-SOMERSET>
+ Center for Pain Management
  635 East Main Street   Bridgewater, NJ 08807   (908)231-1131   Fax (908)231-1132

Tai, Richard W., MD {1164521175} ObsGyn(77,JMA01)
+ 1945 Morris Avenue/Suite 1
  Union, NJ 07083   (908)964-7676   Fax (908)686-0434

Tai, Stephen Jay, MD {1689870073} Otlryg
+ Advocare ENT Specialty
  406 Lippincott Drive   Marlton, NJ 08053   (215)563-1085

Tai, Victoria Chih-Chuang, MD {1790720050} ObsGyn<PA-JEANES>
+ Ob-Gyn Specialists
  157 Route 73   Voorhees, NJ 08043   (856)874-1114   Fax (856)874-9555

Tailor, Amit, MD {1861431041} IntrMd(00,DMN01)<NJ-HACKNSK>
+ Tailor Associates LLC
  455 Union Avenue   Rutherford, NJ 07070   (201)933-7611   Fax (201)933-7622
  Mdtailor@comcast.net

Tailor, Unnati, DO {1912920158} FamMed, IntrMd(03,NY75)<NJ-SOCEANCO, PA-DUBOIS>
+ Stafford Medical, P.A.
  1364 Route 72 West   Manahawkin, NJ 08050   (609)597-3416   Fax (609)597-9608
+ Plaza Family Care
  657 Willow Grove Street/Suite 401   Hackettstown, NJ 07840   (609)597-3416   Fax (908)850-7801

Physicians by Name and Address

Tairu, Oluwole Ayodeji, MD {1912133109} RadDia, Radiol(08)<NJ-UMDNJ>
+ University Hospital-Doctors Office Center
90 Bergen Street/Suite C   Newark, NJ 07103   (973)972-2161   Fax (973)972-2307

Taitel, Janice Beth, MD {1306937172} Pedtrc, IntrMd(91,MA01)<NJ-STCLRDEN>
+ Zufall Health Center
18 West Blackwell Street/Pediatrics   Dover, NJ 07801   (973)328-9100   Fax (973)328-6817

Taitsman, James P., MD {1659330975} SrgOrt, IntrMd(73,NY45)<NJ-CHSFULD, NJ-CHSMRCER>
+ Associated Ortho & Sports Med
123 Franklin Corner Road/Suite 114   Lawrenceville, NJ 08648   (609)896-0707   Fax (609)896-2227
JIMTAITSMAN@COMCAST.NE

Taitt, Beverley B., MD {1801829916} IntrMd(79,DC03)<NJ-VAEASTOR>
+ VA New Jersey Health Care System-East Orange Campus
385 Tremont Avenue   East Orange, NJ 07018   (973)676-1000

Takahashi, Eric Michael, DO {1326229188} IntrMd, IntHos(04,FL75)
+ Emergency Medical Associates of NJ, P.A.
3 Century Drive   Parsippany, NJ 07054   (973)740-0607   Fax (973)740-9895

Takhalov, Yuriy, MD {1841515392} CritCr
+ Carepoint Health Bayonne Med Center
29 East 29th Street   Bayonne, NJ 07002   (917)575-8884

Takla, Magdy F.G., MD {1396771283} Anesth(81,EGY05)<NJ-ACMCITY, NJ-ACMCMAIN>
+ AtlantiCare Regional Medical Center/City Campus
1925 Pacific Avenue/Anesthesiology   Atlantic City, NJ 08401   (609)345-4000
+ AtlantiCare Regional Med Ctr/Mainland
65 West Jimmie Leeds Road   Pomona, NJ 08240   (609)652-1000

Takla, Sarwat S., MD {1316907983} IntrMd(84,EGY04)<NJ-HOBUNIMC, NJ-CHRIST>
+ Quality Medical Services, LLC
1163 Route 37 West/Suite C1   Toms River, NJ 08755   (732)281-8580   Fax (732)551-2075

Takvorian, Sylva A., MD {1366419145} IntrMd(00,NJ05)<NJ-HACKNSK>
+ 20 Prospect Avenue/Suite 516
Hackensack, NJ 07601   (201)215-2510
+ Center for Occupational Medicine
360 Essex Street/Suite 203   Hackensack, NJ 07601   (201)215-2510   Fax (201)342-3546

Takyi, Michele, MD {1619465473} Pedtrc
+ University Medical Group Pediatrics
125 Paterson Street/MEB 3rd Fl   New Brunswick, NJ 08903   (732)235-7345

Tal, Moty N., MD {1710951355} ObsGyn(76,NY46)<NJ-MONMOUTH, NJ-JRSYSHMC>
+ 590 West Kennedy Boulevard
Lakewood, NJ 08701   (732)370-1111
+ 1300 State Route 35/Suite 201
Asbury Park, NJ 07712   (732)517-8899

Talamati, Jayanthi, MD {1114091949} IntrMd
+ 64 Oakland Mills Road
Manalapan, NJ 07726   (732)462-8189

Talamayan, Randy P. C., MD {1407826399} IntrMd, IntMAdM(93,PHI01)<NJ-OCEANMC, NJ-KIMBALL>
+ Jersey Shore Medical and Pediatric Associates
1215 Route 70 West/Suite 1005   Lakewood, NJ 08701   (732)942-0888   Fax (732)942-1230
+ Ocean County Family Care
2125 Route 88 East   Brick, NJ 08724   (732)942-0888   Fax (732)892-0961

Talangbayan, Leizle E., MD {1023023462} RadDia(01,PA09)
+ Monmouth Medical Imaging
300 Second Avenue   Long Branch, NJ 07740   (732)923-6806   Fax (732)923-6006
+ 100 Marine Terrace
Long Branch, NJ 07740

Talansky, Marvin L., MD {1295807782} Ophthl(73,SC01)<NJ-JRSYSHMC, NJ-MONMOUTH>
+ Eye Diagnostic Center
3333 Fairmont Avenue   Asbury Park, NJ 07712   (732)988-4000   Fax (732)988-9502
Talansky@gmail.com
+ Eye Diagnostic Center
525 Route 70   Brick, NJ 08723   (732)988-4000   Fax (732)477-1444

Talat, Afnan, MD {1740718220} FamMed(14,GRN01)
+ CityMD Union Urgent Care
2317 Center Island Route 22   Union, NJ 07083   (201)354-1951   (201)354-1952

Talati, Amita N., MD {1306911979} PsyGrt, Psychy(79,INA69)
+ Rosato & Talati MD PA
2301 Evesham Road/Suite 108   Voorhees, NJ 08043

(856)770-1300   Fax (856)770-8331

Talati, Sapan Nitinbhai, MD {1083862601}
+ Advanced Cardiology, LLC.
65 Ridgedale Avenue   Cedar Knolls, NJ 07927   (973)401-1100   Fax (973)401-1201

Talavera, Jose Galang, MD {1538380811} Urolgy(00)
+ Summit Medical Group
202 Elmer Street   Westfield, NJ 07090   (908)228-3675   Fax (908)654-1053

Talavera, Joyce R., MD {1003860040} OncHem, MedOnc, IntrMd(96,MA07)<NJ-OVERLOOK>
+ Summit Medical Group
552 Westfield Avenue   Westfield, NJ 07090   (908)654-3377   Fax (908)654-4044

Talbo, Norma B., MD {1316097918} Psychy(68,PHI01)<NJ-ESSEXCO>
+ Essex County Hospital Center
204 Grove Avenue/Psychiatry   Cedar Grove, NJ 07009   (973)571-2800

Talbot, Lori C., MD {1013930023} FamMed(84,VA04)<NJ-SJERSYHS>
+ South Cumberland Medical Associates
215 Back Neck Road   Bridgeton, NJ 08302   (856)451-4414   Fax (856)451-2052

Talbot, Susan M., MD {1942252291} IntrMd, MedOnc, Hemato(90,AST02)<NJ-NWRKBETH>
+ Newark Beth Israel Medical Center
201 Lyons Avenue/Cancer Ctr   Newark, NJ 07112   (973)926-7000

Taliadouros, George S., MD {1790722155} ObsGyn, RprEnd(75,GRE01)<NJ-VIRTMHBC, NJ-COOPRUMC>
+ Delaware Valley Institute of Fertility & Genetics
6000 Sagemore Drive/Suite 6102   Marlton, NJ 08053   (856)988-0072   Fax (856)988-0056
+ Delaware Valley Institute of Fertility & Genetics
2950 College Drive/Suite 2B   Vineland, NJ 08360   (856)988-0072   Fax (609)794-3058
+ Delaware Valley Institute of Fertility & Genetics
3100 Princeton Pike/Building 4/Suite D   Lawrenceville, NJ 08053   (609)895-0088

Tallia, Alfred F., MD {1043397441} FamMed(78,NJ06)<NJ-RWJUBRUN, NJ-STPETER>
+ UH- Robert Wood Johnson Med
125 Paterson Street/MEB 288   New Brunswick, NJ 08901   (732)235-6029   Fax (732)246-8084
+ Family Medicine at Monument Square
317 George Street   New Brunswick, NJ 08901   (732)235-6029   Fax (732)246-7317

Talon, Dennis J., MD {1225193451} Nephro, IntrMd(90,PHI09)<NJ-NWTNMEM, NJ-STBARNMC>
+ Kidney Specialty Clinic, PA
222 High Street/Suite 206   Newton, NJ 07860   (973)300-1289   Fax (973)300-9573

Talone, Albert A., DO {1235235623} GenPrc(75,MO78)
+ Sunset Road Medical Associates
911 Sunset Road   Burlington, NJ 08016   (609)387-8787   Fax (609)386-8640

Talotta, Nicholas Joseph, Jr., MD {1104999390} EmrgMd(04,PA02)<NJ-SHOREMEM>
+ Bayfront Emergency Physicians, P.A.
1 East New York Avenue   Somers Point, NJ 08244   (609)653-3519   Fax (609)653-3247
+ Cross keys Urgent Care
627-B Cross Keys Road   Sicklerville, NJ 08081   (609)653-3519   Fax (856)318-1374

Talwar, Jotica, MD {1720056377} PthHem, PthACl(90,INA23)
+ Bio-Reference Laboratory, Inc.
481 Edward H. Ross Drive   Elmwood Park, NJ 07407   (201)791-2600   Fax (201)791-1941

Talwar, Sumit, MD {1679752547} OncHem(05,INA23)
+ Hudson Hematology Oncology
377 Jersey Avenue/Suite 160   Jersey City, NJ 07302   (201)333-8248   Fax (201)333-8469

Tam, Elizabeth, MD {1295121853} IntHos<NJ-HACKNSK>
+ Hackensack University Medical Center
30 Prospect Avenue   Hackensack, NJ 07601   (551)996-2000

Tam, Tiffanie, MD {1083033179} ObsGyn<NJ-STBARNMC>
+ St. Barnabas Medical Center
94 Old Short Hills Road   Livingston, NJ 07039   (408)455-7787

Tamas, Ecaterina F., MD {1396992301} PthACl(92,ROM05)
+ Quest Diagnostics Inc.
1 Malcolm Avenue   Teterboro, NJ 07608   (201)393-5000   Fax (201)393-6127

Tamashausky, Shaun R., DO {1164616876} EmrgMd(07,NJ75)
+ Team Health East
307 South Evergeen Avenue   Woodbury, NJ 08096   (856)686-4319   Fax (856)848-8536

Tamaska, Wayne G., DO {1962459180} EmrgMd, IntrMd(92,ME75)<NJ-KMHSTRAT>
+ Kennedy Memorial Hospital-University Medical Center

18 East Laurel Road/EmergMed   Stratford, NJ 08084   (856)346-7985   Fax (856)346-6539

Tamburello, Anthony C., III, MD {1487649364} Psychy, PsyFor(00,VA01)
+ South Woods State Prison/NJ Dept of Corrections
215 South Burlington Road   Bridgeton, NJ 08302   (856)459-7000
tamburac@umdnj.edu

Tamburello, Traci Ann, DO {1013911486} FamMed(99,NJ75)<NJ-RBAYPERT>
+ Jewish Renaissance Medical Center
275 Hobart Street   Perth Amboy, NJ 08861   (732)376-9333   Fax (732)376-0139

Tamburrino, Joseph F., MD {1073840377} SrgPlstc
+ Prestige Institute for Plastic Surgery
1605 East Evesham Road/Suite 201   Voorhees, NJ 08043   (856)304-1114   Fax (267)454-7196

Tameem, Murtuza, MD {1851741284} IntHos<NJ-STJOSHOS>
+ St. Joseph's Regional Medical Center
703 Main Street   Paterson, NJ 07503   (973)754-2000

Tamimi, Omar A., MD {1932148327} Gastrn, IntrMd(87,GRN01)
+ Gastroenterologists of Ocean County
477 Lakehurst Road   Toms River, NJ 08755   (732)349-4422   Fax (732)349-5087

Tammana, Swarna, DO {1235239013} FamMed
+ Hunterdon Family Physicians
111 State Route 31/Suite 111   Flemington, NJ 08822   (908)284-9880   Fax (908)782-4316

Tammaro, Yolanda Rose, MD {1598927477} Surgry(06,NY47)<NJ-OCEANMC>
+ Ocean Medical Center
425 Jack Martin Boulevard/Surgery   Brick, NJ 08723   (732)212-6391

Tamres, David Michael, MD {1780682492} IntrMd(96,NY47)
+ Summit Medical Group
140 Park Avenue/3rd Floor/Internal Med   Florham Park, NJ 07932   (973)404-7880

Tan, Christina Geok-Beng, MD IntrMd(96,NY47)
+ New Jersey Department of Health and Senior Services
50 East State/PO Box 360   Trenton, NJ 08625   (609)292-9354   Fax (609)292-6523

Tan, Edgardo L., MD {1356402952} FamMed, Pedtrc(73,PHI30)
+ 314 First Avenue
Elizabeth, NJ 07206   (908)353-5280

Tan, Elizabeth Listiani, MD {1346210077} RadBdl, RadDia, Radiol(93,NY03)
+ Larchmont Medical Imaging
204-210 Ark Road/LMC 1-2   Mount Laurel, NJ 08054   (856)778-8860   Fax (856)866-8102

Tan, Gary K., DO {1366734717}
+ 604 Lincoln Drive
Voorhees, NJ 08043   (412)477-3667
gtan93@midwestern.edu

Tan, Jianyou, MD {1790712271} PthACl, PthDrm(85,CHN07)<NJ-HACKNSK>
+ 145 Lawrence Drive
Short Hills, NJ 07078   (973)517-6928
tanj03@yahoo.com

Tan, John J., MD {1659450377} Otlryg(65,NY46)<NJ-MTNSIDE>
+ 77 Park Street
Montclair, NJ 07043   (973)746-4855   Fax (973)746-5305

Tan, Kong L., MD {1184667289} PthACl, Pthlgy(70,IND10)<NJ-RBAYPERT>
+ Raritan Bay Medical Center/Perth Amboy Division
530 New Brunswick Avenue   Perth Amboy, NJ 08861   (908)324-5172   Fax (732)324-4811

Tan, Lamberto A., MD {1023022159} Psychy(72,PHI09)<NJ-JRSYSHMC, NJ-COMMED>
+ Ocean Mental Health Services, Inc.
160 Atlantic City Boulevard   Bayville, NJ 08721   (732)349-5550   Fax (732)349-0841

Tan, Leong Hean, MD {1902996788} IntrMd, Gastrn, Hepato(67,TAI02)<NJ-HCKTSTWN>
+ 121 Shelley Drive/Suite 1D
Hackettstown, NJ 07840   (908)852-0900   Fax (908)850-8730
leonheantan@yahoo.com

Tan, Madeline P., MD {1720068414} Pedtrc(85,PHI21)
+ Ventnor Pediatric Center, LLC
6601 Ventnor Avenue/Suite 14   Ventnor City, NJ 08406   (609)487-6507   Fax (609)487-6508

Tan, Manuel R., MD {1962415471} EmrgMd(69,PHI01)<NJ-RWJURAH>
+ Robert Wood Johnson University Hospital at Rahway
865 Stone Street   Rahway, NJ 07065   (732)381-4200

Tan, Martin H., MD {1457442162} Anesth, PainMd(84,IND05)<NJ-UMDNJ>
+ James Street Anesthesia
102 James Street/Suite 103   Edison, NJ 08820   (732)494-1444   Fax (732)494-7052

Physicians by Name and Address

Tan, Mary Catherine D., MD {1740471366} Pedtrc(00,PHI01)<NJ-COMMED, NJ-OCEANMC>
+ Pediatric Affiliates, PA
40 Bey Lea Road/Suite B203   Toms River, NJ 08753   (732)341-0720   Fax (732)244-6842

Tan, Pilar O., MD {1194875724} IntrMd(65,PHI09)
+ 860 Park Avenue
Elizabeth, NJ 07208   (908)351-8840   Fax (908)351-1431

Tan, Royland C., MD {1124026893} Anesth(77,PHI09)<NJ-STMICHL>
+ St. Michael's Medical Center
268 MLK Jr. Boulevard/Anesth   Newark, NJ 07102   (973)877-5034   Fax (973)877-5231
+ St. Joseph's Regional Medical Center Anesthesia
703 Main Street   Paterson, NJ 07503   (973)877-5034   Fax (973)977-9455

Tan, Vicente G., MD {1447330253} Pedtrc, NnPnMd(71,PHI01)<NJ-CHRIST, NJ-HOBUNIMC>
+ Pediatric Care P.A.
3342 Kennedy Boulevard   Jersey City, NJ 07307   (201)653-8999   Fax (201)653-4477

Tan, Virak, MD {1841373438} SrgOrt, OrtSHand(94,PA01)
+ North Jersey Orthopaedic Institute
90 Bergen Street/DOC 1200   Newark, NJ 07101   (973)972-8240   Fax (973)972-9367
+ UMDNJ Dept of Orthopaedics
90 Bergen Street/DOC 1200   Jersey City, NJ 07305   (973)972-2150

Tan, William W., MD {1134297880} CdvDis, IntrMd(64,IND01)
+ 90 North Street
Bayonne, NJ 07002   (201)858-2604

Tanaka, Sho, MD {1881011138} Anesth
+ Robert Wood Johnson-UMDNJ Anesthesia Group
125 Paterson Street/CAB 3100   New Brunswick, NJ 08901   (732)235-7827   Fax (732)235-6131

Tanase, Anca, MD {1497920292}
+ 146 Saddleback Court
Sparta, NJ 07871   (973)512-3964   Fax (973)512-3962   anca88t@yahoo.com

Tancer, Nancy Kaplan, MD {1114124070} Psychy, PsyCAd(84,NJ05)
+ 1 Dewolf Road/Suite 3
Old Tappan, NJ 07675   (201)767-9399   Fax (201)767-3105

Tancer, Richard B., DO {1588677629} FamMed(84,PA77)<NJ-HOLYNAME>
+ 18 Redneck Avenue
Little Ferry, NJ 07643   (201)641-3115   Fax (201)641-3116

Tanchel, Mark E., MD {1598762676} Gastrn, IntrMd(94,MA07)<NJ-HACKNSK>
+ Hackensack Digestive Diseases Associates, P.A.
52 First Street   Hackensack, NJ 07601   (201)488-3003   Fax (201)488-6911

Tandon, Pooja, MD {1922377258} PsyGrt
+ Memory and Aging Center
20 Hospital Drive/Suite 12   Toms River, NJ 08755   (732)244-2299   Fax (732)244-5757

Tandon, Prabhat Kumar, MD {1245265941} EnDbMt, IntrMd(94,INA23)<NJ-WARREN, PA-EASTON>
+ Open Air MRI
430 Memorial Parkway/Suite 2   Phillipsburg, NJ 08865   (908)213-3600

Tandon, Raj, MD {1396736690} Otlryg, IntrMd(96,NY01)<NY-NYEYEINF, NJ-HACKNSK>
+ ENT and Allergy Associates (ENTA)
79 Hudson Street/Suite 303   Hoboken, NJ 07030   (201)792-1109   Fax (201)792-1145   rtandon@entandallergy.com

Taneja, Deepak, DO {1396911921} FamMed(94,NY75)
+ 43 Main Street
Farmingdale, NJ 07727   (732)938-6471

Taneja, Indra, MD {1952475113} Pedtrc(73,INDI)<NJ-UMDNJ, NJ-NWRKBETH>
+ University Hospital
150 Bergen Street/Ambltry Pdtrcs   Newark, NJ 07103   (973)972-2100

Taneja, Monica M., MD {1164584355} Anesth
+ 63 White Road
Shrewsbury, NJ 07702

Taneja, Uttama, DO {1649271065} Pedtrc(95,NY75)<NJ-HACKNSK, NJ-VALLEY>
+ Pedimedica PA
43 Yawpo Avenue/Suite 9   Oakland, NJ 07436   (201)405-0800   Fax (201)337-5585

Taneli, Tolga, MD {1386729457} Psychy, PsyCAd(94,TUR20)<NJ-UMDNJ>
+ 66 Maple Avenue/Suite 3
Morristown, NJ 07960   (973)671-1259

Tang, Daniel Di, MD {1770648321} Pthlgy(85,CHN38)<NJ-MTN-SIDE>
+ Hackensack UMC Mountainside
1 Bay Avenue/Path   Montclair, NJ 07042   (973)429-6164   Fax (973)429-6992

Tang, Godffery R., MD {1932174257} IntrMd(94,PA02)
+ 90 Woodlake Drive
Marlton, NJ 08053

Tang, Lin-Lan, MD {1083637896} Pedtrc, AdolMd(84,NY06)
+ 27 Mountain Boulevard/Suite 2
Warren, NJ 07059   (908)756-6767   Fax (908)756-5320

Tang, Linda Yinglin, MD {1700059185} Gastrn, IntrMd(03,ON05)
+ Premier Health Associates
532 Lafayette Road/Suite 100   Sparta, NJ 07871   (973)383-3730   Fax (973)383-2285
+ Premier Health Associates
89 Sparta Avenue/Suite 100   Sparta, NJ 07871   (973)383-3730   Fax (973)729-3454

Tang, Xiaoyin, MD {1437128568} Rheuma, IntrMd(84,CHN1B)<NJ-JRSYSHMC>
+ Hackensack Meridian Medical Group
19 Davis Avenue/5th-6th Floor   Neptune, NJ 07753   (732)897-3985   Fax (732)897-3982

Tang, Yen-Shin Daisy, MD {1528296829} Pedtrc
+ Kintiroglou Pediatrics
1500 Pleasant Valley Way/Suite 301   West Orange, NJ 07052   (973)243-0002   Fax (973)243-1227

Tang, Ying Margie, MD {1730478520} Gastrn
+ Medical Diagnostic Associates PA
525 Central Avenue/Suite C   Westfield, NJ 07090   (908)233-0895

Tangco, Evacueto P., MD {1154367225} FamMed(67,PHI01)
+ 302 Clay Street
Riverside, NJ 08075   (856)461-7755   Fax (856)461-2699

Tangorra, Matthew, DO {1609985597} Gastrn, IntrMd(01,KY13)<NY-MTSINYHS>
+ Atlantic Coast Gastroenterology
1640 Route 88 West/Suite 202   Brick, NJ 08724   (732)458-8300   Fax (732)458-8529
+ Atlantic Coast Gastroenterology
1944 Corlies Avenue/Suite 205   Neptune, NJ 07753   (732)458-8300   Fax (732)776-8059

Tangreti, Nicholas W., MD {1235195363} Anesth(83,NJ05)<NJ-STPETER>
+ Anesthesia Consultnts of NJ/Nova Pain
285 Davidson Avenue/Suite 204   Somerset, NJ 08873   (732)271-1400   Fax (732)271-3543
+ St. Peter's University Hospital
254 Easton Avenue/Anesth   New Brunswick, NJ 08901   (732)745-8600
+ Cares Surgicenter, LLC.
240 Easton Avenue   New Brunswick, NJ 08873   (732)565-5400   Fax (732)296-8677

Tank, Hasmukh C., MD {1508801945} Anesth(96,INA20)<NJ-BUR-DTMLN>
+ Toms River Anesthesia Associates PC
409 Main Street/2nd Floor   Toms River, NJ 08753   (732)818-7575   Fax (732)818-1567

Tank, Lisa Kaushal, MD {1811943897} IntrMd, Grtrcs(96,INA2B)<NJ-HACKNSK>
+ Center for Healthy Senior Living
360 Essex Street/Suite 401   Hackensack, NJ 07601   (551)996-1140   Fax (551)996-0543

Tank, Niti, MD {1184825879} RadDia(06,NJ05)
+ Kennedy Health System/Cherry Hill Campus
2201 Chapel Avenue West   Cherry Hill, NJ 08002   (856)488-6500

Tank, Renuka H., MD {1063430627} Psychy(76,INA00)
+ Ocean Mental Health Services, Inc.
160 Atlantic City Boulevard   Bayville, NJ 08721   (732)349-5550   Fax (732)349-0841

Tankha, Pavan, DO {1881854842} Anesth(NJ75
+ Garden State Pain Control Center, P.A.
1117 Route 46 East/Suite 201   Clifton, NJ 07013   (973)777-5477   Fax (973)777-0304

Tannenbaum, Alan K., MD {1588747521} CdvDis(73,MEX03)<NJ-RWJUBRUN>
+ Monroe Cardiology LCC
18 Centre Drive/Suite 205   Monroe Township, NJ 08831   (609)395-7600   Fax (609)395-7559
+ UH- Robert Wood Johnson Med
125 Paterson Street/Cardiology   New Brunswick, NJ 08901   (732)235-6561

Tanner, Fritzi Alma, MD {1326140013} Pedtrc(92,NJ06)
+ first Step Pediatrics
206 Laurel Heights Drive   Bridgeton, NJ 08302   (856)459-2270   Fax (856)459-9674

Tanner-Sackey, Fritzi A., MD Pedtrc(92,NJ06)<NJ-RIVERVW>
+ Wee Care Pediatrics
831 Tennent Road/Suite A   Manalapan, NJ 07726   (732)536-6222   Fax (732)536-9272

Tansey, William Austin, III, MD {1649242306} CdvDis, IntrMd(70,NY01)<NJ-OVERLOOK, NJ-MORRISTN>
+ Summit Medical Group
85 Woodland Road   Short Hills, NJ 07078   (973)379-4496   Fax (973)921-0669

+ Summit Medical Group-Berkeley Heights Campus
1 Diamond Hill Road   Berkeley Heights, NJ 07922   (973)379-4496   Fax (908)790-6576

Tantawi, Mahnaz Chand, MD {1699823328} IntrMd(00,NJ06)
+ Saddle Brook Medical Center
449 Market Street/Suite B   Saddle Brook, NJ 07663   (201)712-7900   Fax (201)712-7902

Tantawi, Mohamed Asem, MD {1114945888} Pedtrc(00,NJ05)<NJ-HACKNSK, NJ-STJOSHOS>
+ Hackensack Pediatrics
177 Summit Avenue   Hackensack, NJ 07601   (201)487-8222   Fax (201)487-2126

Tantawi, Mona M., MD {1104873272} Pedtrc, AdolMd(72,EGY03)<NJ-HACKNSK>
+ Hackensack Pediatrics
177 Summit Avenue   Hackensack, NJ 07601   (201)487-8222   Fax (201)487-2126

Tanuos, Hanan A., MD {1235160300} Pedtrc(91,EGY04)<NJ-UMDNJ, NJ-STBARNMC>
+ University Hospital-Doctors Office Center
90 Bergen Street/DOC 4100   Newark, NJ 07103   (973)972-0543   Fax (973)972-0388
+ University Pediatric Group
90 Bergen Street/DOC 4300   Newark, NJ 07103   (973)972-2100

Tanwir, Anjum, MD {1144320128} CdvDis, IntrMd(02,DMN01)
+ Drs. Kaid & Tanwir
2168 Millburn Avenue/Suite 204   Maplewood, NJ 07040   (973)762-3353   Fax (973)762-3370

Tanzer, Floyd R., MD {1780687228} Dermat, IntrMd(73,NY08)<NJ-MEADWLND, NJ-STJOSHOS>
+ Drs. Silber & Tanzer
992 Clifton Avenue   Clifton, NJ 07013   (973)365-1800   Fax (973)777-0380

Tanzer, Ira D., MD {1215080163} Urolgy(74,NJ05)<NJ-CHRIST, NJ-HACKNSK>
+ New Jersey Urology Associates, PA
110 Meadowlands Parkway   Secaucus, NJ 07094   (201)867-1297   Fax (201)867-4165

Tao, Feng, MD {1285621748} IntrMd, RadDia(84,CHN1K)<NJ-STJOSHOS>
+ St. Joseph's Regional Medical Center
703 Main Street/InternalMed   Paterson, NJ 07503   (973)754-2000

Tao, Jiangchuan, MD {1679895676}
+ Si Paradigm, LLC.
690 Kinderkamack Road/Suite 103   Oradell, NJ 07649   (631)965-3750   Fax (201)599-9066   taojiangchuan@yahoo.com
+ Si Paradigm, LLC.
25 Riverside Drive/Suite 2   Pine Brook, NJ 07058   (201)599-9044

Tao, Jimmy Ziming, MD {1689955288} Pthlgy<NJ-COMMED>
+ Community Medical Center
99 Route 37 West/Pthlgy   Toms River, NJ 08755   (917)536-8084   ziming_t@yahoo.com

Tao, Ying, MD {1265402812} Nrolgy(82,CHN3B)
+ Neurological Associates PA
700 North Broad Street/Suite 201   Elizabeth, NJ 07208   (908)354-3994   Fax (908)354-0429

Taormina, Vincent J., MD {1538161922} Radiol(78,PA01)<NJ-SOCEANCO, NJ-VIRTMHBC>
+ Radiology Associates of Burlington County
1295 Route 38 West/PO Box 479   Hainesport, NJ 08036   (609)261-7017   Fax (609)261-4180

Tapia, Alfredo J., MD {1194013516} EmrgMd
+ 13 Franklin Place/Bldg 7E
Morristown, NJ 07960

Tapia, Susana, MD {1255565214} IntrMd<NJ-UMDNJ>
+ University Hospital
150 Bergen Street/UH H-245   Newark, NJ 07103   (973)972-5672   Fax (973)972-0365

Tapliga, Eduard Constantin, MD {1356302483} IntrMd(90,ROM01)<NJ-OCEANMC>
+ Ocean Medical Center
425 Jack Martin Boulevard   Brick, NJ 08723   (732)840-2200

Tapnio, Cezar B., MD {1619985975} EmrgMd, IntrMd(81,PHI09)<NJ-JRSYSHMC>
+ EmCare
1945 Route 33   Neptune, NJ 07753   (732)776-4510   Fax (732)776-2329

Tapper, Ben R., DO {1174566608} OstMed, EmrgMd(85,IL76)<NJ-LOURDMED>
+ Emergency Physician Associates, P.A.
307 South Evergreen Avenue/PO Box 298   Woodbury, NJ 08096   (856)848-3817   Fax (856)848-1431
+ St Joseph's Medical Center Emergency
703 Main Street   Paterson, NJ 07503   (856)848-3817   Fax (973)754-2249

Taragin, Benjamin H., MD {1326005554} RadDia, PedRad(99,NY46)<NJ-STJOSHOS>
+ St. Joseph's Regional Medical Center
703 Main Street/Radiology   Paterson, NJ 07503   (973)754-2000

Taragin, Michael S., MD {1013995349} Anesth(88,NY08)
+ Morris Anesthesia Group, PA
3799 Route 46/Suite 211   Parsippany, NJ 07054   (973)335-1122   Fax (973)335-1448

Tarantino, David P., MD {1285666859} Anesth<NJ-BURDTMLN>
+ Cape Regional Medical Center
2 Stone Harbor Boulevard   Cape May Court House, NJ 08210   (609)463-2183   Fax (609)463-2931

Tarantino, Debra R., MD {1952477986} SrgC&R, Surgry(94,NY06)<NJ-OVERLOOK>
+ Associates in Colon and Rectal Diseases
231 Millburn Avenue   Millburn, NJ 07041   (973)467-2277   Fax (973)467-4037
+ Short Hills Surgery Center
187 Millburn Avenue/Suite 101   Millburn, NJ 07041   (973)467-2277   Fax (973)671-0557

Tarasenko, Anthony J., MD InsrMd, IntrMd, OccpMd(75,MEX03)
+ 68 Kent Place Boulevard
Summit, NJ 07901   (908)277-2135
+ Concentra Medical Centers
595 Division Street/FAA Exam   Elizabeth, NJ 07201   (908)277-2135   Fax (908)351-1099
+ Concentra Medical Centers
116 Corporate Boulevard/Suite E   South Plainfield, NJ 07901   (908)757-1424   Fax (908)757-5678

Tarasov, Ethan A., MD {1760488068} RadDia, RadV&I, Radiol(81,NY45)<NJ-RWJUHAM, NJ-STFRNMED>
+ Radiology Affiliates of Central New Jersey, P.A.
2501 Kuser Road   Hamilton, NJ 08691   (609)585-8800   Fax (609)585-1825
+ Radiology Affiliates of Central New Jersey, P.A.
3120 Princeton Pike   Lawrenceville, NJ 08648   (609)585-8800   Fax (609)219-0439
+ St. Francis Medical Center
601 Hamilton Avenue/Radiology   Trenton, NJ 08691   (609)599-5000

Tarchichi, Tony R., MD {1275738411} Pedtrc, IntrMd(NJ05
+ Family Health & Wellness Center
43 Conforti Avenue/Apt 45   West Orange, NJ 07052   (973)481-6700

Tarditi, Daniel John, DO {1386672467} IntrMd, CdvDis(01,NJ75)<NJ-COOPRUMC, NJ-OURLADY>
+ Cardiovascular Associates of The Delaware Valley, PA
570 Egg Harbor Road/Suite B-1   Sewell, NJ 08080   (856)582-2000   Fax (856)582-2061
+ Cardiovascular Associates of The Delaware Valley, PA
525 State Street/Suite 3   Elmer, NJ 08318   (856)582-2000   Fax (856)358-0725

Tardos, Jonathan George, MD {1235391038} CdvDis, IntrMd(07,NY47)
+ RWJPE/New Brunswick Cardiology Group, P.A.
75 Veronica Road/Suite 101   Somerset, NJ 08873   (732)247-7444   Fax (732)247-5119

Tareco, Jennifer M., MD {1184626327} PedOrt, SrgOrt, NeuM-SptM(92,MD07)<NJ-HUNTRDN>
+ St. Barnabas Ambulatory Care Center
200 South Orange Avenue   Livingston, NJ 07039   (973)322-7600   Fax (973)322-7685

Targino, Marcelo Cordeiro, MD {1821054362} IntrMd, OccpMd, GPrvMd(02,FL04)<MA-CHACMBR, NH-EXETER>
+ Johnson & Johnson
1 Johnson & Johnson/EmpHlth Rm5G32   New Brunswick, NJ 08933   (732)524-3000   Fax (732)828-5493

Tarina, Dana Ileana, MD {1952375743} IntrMd(91,ROM01)<NJ-JRSYSHMC>
+ Jersey Shore University Medical Center
1945 Route 33/AcademicOffice   Neptune, NJ 07753   (732)776-4420   Fax (732)776-3795
+ Hackensack Meridian Medical Group
19 Davis Avenue/5th-6th Floor   Neptune, NJ 07753   (732)776-4420   Fax (732)897-3997

Tariq, Samreen, MD {1164803714} FamMed
+ 622 Broadway
Bayonne, NJ 07002   (201)436-2800   Fax (201)436-1353

Tarlow, Mordechai M., MD {1992762017} Dermat(01,NY46)
+ Advanced Dermatology & Skin Surgery
456 Chesnut Street/Suite 201   Lakewood, NJ 08701   (732)905-9200   Fax (732)905-4470

Tarng, George W., MD {1013204023} IntrMd
+ Hudson Internal Medicine
744 Broadway   Bayonne, NJ 07002   (201)436-8888

Tarr, William Ellsworth, Jr., MD {1285833814} PthAClt(79,MD01)
+ Quest Diagnostics Inc.
1 Malcolm Avenue   Teterboro, NJ 07608   (201)393-5000   Fax (201)393-6127

Tartacoff, Randy S., MD {1508829110} EmrgMd(80,NY47)<NJ-HOLYNAME>
+ Holy Name Hospital
718 Teaneck Road/EmergMed   Teaneck, NJ 07666   (201)833-3913   Fax (201)833-0795

Tartaglia, Marco, MD {1093753516} IntrMd(79,ITAL)
+ 244 Park Avenue
Caldwell, NJ 07006   (973)857-7131

Tartakovsky, Irina, MD {1982685103} IntrMd(93,NY03)<NJ-ENGLWOOD>
+ Drs. Pattner, Grodstein, Fein & Davis
177 North Dean Street/Suite 207   Englewood, NJ 07631   (201)567-0446   Fax (201)567-8775

Tartini, Albert, MD {1346240298} IntrMd, Nephro(84,GRN01)<NJ-HOLYNAME, NJ-VALLEY>
+ Renal Medicine Associates PA
400 Franklin Turnpike/Suite 208   Mahwah, NJ 07430   (201)825-3322
+ Renal Medicine Associates PA
302 Union Street   Hackensack, NJ 07601   (201)825-3322   Fax (201)646-0365
+ Renal Medicine Associates PA
718 Teaneck Road   Teaneck, NJ 07430   (201)833-3223

Tarulli, Andrew William, MD {1700872561} Nrolgy(01,NY19)<NJ-OVERLOOK>
+ Overlook Medical Center
99 Beauvoir Avenue/PO Box 210   Summit, NJ 07902   (908)522-5697   Fax (908)522-6123
+ Atlantic Surgical Oncology
99 Beauvoir Street   Summit, NJ 07901   (908)522-5697   Fax (908)598-2392

Tasca, Philip, MD {1780668764} PhysMd(99,PA13)<NJ-ENGLWOOD>
+ Physical Medicine & Rehabilitation Center
500 Grand Avenue/1st Floor   Englewood, NJ 07631   (201)567-2277   Fax (201)567-7506

Tase, Douglas Sheperd, MD {1750389292} SrgOrt
+ Cooper University Orthopedic Trauma
3 Cooper Plaza/Suite 408   Camden, NJ 08103   (856)968-7354   Fax (856)968-8288

Tasharofi, Kamran, MD {1174595466} IntrMd(00,DMN01)<NJ-TRINIWSC, NJ-RWJURAH>
+ Union County HealthCare Associates
2005 St. Georges Avenue   Rahway, NJ 07065   (732)381-3740   Fax (732)215-4344
+ Union County HealthCare Associates
400 Westfield Avenue   Elizabeth, NJ 07208   (732)381-3740   Fax (908)620-3243

Tashjian, Audrey Brigitta, MD {1518939495} ObsGyn(92,PA01)<NJ-CHSFULD, NJ-CHSMRCER>
+ Lawrence Ob/Gyn Associates
123 Franklin Corner Road/Suite 214   Lawrenceville, NJ 08648   (609)896-1400   Fax (609)896-3986

Taskin, Metin, MD {1518032820} PthAClt(87,TUR03)<NJ-VALLEY>
+ The Valley Hospital
223 North Van Dien Avenue/Pathology   Ridgewood, NJ 07450   (201)447-8000

Tassakis, Tom A., MD {1689760951} Gastrn, IntrMd(88,GRNA)<NJ-SJRSYELM>
+ Southern Gastroenterology Assoc
1317 South Main Road/Building 1/Unit C   Vineland, NJ 08360   (856)691-1910   Fax (856)691-8330
+ S Gastroenterology Assoc of NJ
1005 Kings Highway/PO Box 62   Swedesboro, NJ 08085   (856)691-1910   Fax (856)467-9747
+ S. Gastroenterology Associates
350 Front Street/Suite 2401   Elmer, NJ 08360   (856)358-2083   Fax (856)467-9747

Tassan, Robert F., MD {1578596508} MedOnc, IntrMd(99,NJ06)<NJ-VALLEY>
+ Regional Cancer Center Associates
250 Old Red Hook Road/Suite 301   Westwood, NJ 07675   (201)383-4840   Fax (201)383-4824

Tatarowicz, Roman J., MD {1942228911} ObsGyn(88,GRN01)<NJ-CHSFULD, NJ-CHSMRCER>
+ Henry J. Austin Health Center
321 North Warren Street   Trenton, NJ 08618   (609)278-5900   Fax (609)695-3532

Tatz, Mark A., MD {1972546489} Anesth(78,MEXI)<NJ-VIRTMHBC>
+ Virtua Memorial
175 Madison Avenue/Anesthesiology   Mount Holly, NJ 08060   (609)267-0700   Fax (609)261-4801   MTATZ@virtua.org
+ Burlington Anesthesia Associates
120 Madison Ave/Suite E/PO Box 174   Mount Holly, NJ 08060   (609)267-0700   Fax (609)261-1779

Taub, Katherine Susan, MD {1689874901} NrlgSpec(05,DC02)<PA-CHILDHOS>
+ CHOP Pediatric & Adolescent Specialty Care Center
1012 Laurel Oak Road   Voorhees, NJ 08043   (856)435-1300   Fax (856)435-0091
+ CHOP Specialty Care Center at Virtua
200 Bowman Drive/2 FL/Suite D-260   Voorhees, NJ 08043   (267)425-5400

Taub, William H., MD {1992759757} Gastrn(83,NY15)<NJ-VIRTMHBC, NJ-DEBRAHLC>
+ Gastroenterology Consultants of South Jersey
693 Main Street/Suite 2   Lumberton, NJ 08048   (609)265-1700   Fax (609)265-9005
+ Burlington County Endoscopy Center
140 Mount Holly Bypass/Unit 5   Lumberton, NJ 08048   (609)267-1555

Taubman, Bruce Melvin, MD {1982762167} Pedtrc, IntrMd(72,NY46)
+ Cherry Hill Pediatric Group
600 West Marlton Pike   Cherry Hill, NJ 08002   (856)428-5020   Fax (856)216-9433

Taubman, Jessica, MD {1053630178} FamMed
+ 235 Hudson Street/Unit 1112
Hoboken, NJ 07030

Tauro, Joseph C., MD {1477662567} SrgOrt, SrgOARec(83,NJ05)
+ Ocean County Sports Medicine Ctr
9 Hospital Drive   Toms River, NJ 08755   (732)341-6226   Fax (732)341-3247

Tauro, Victor, MD {1770557761} IntrMd(81,GRN01)
+ Comprehensive Medical Associates
411 Route 9/Suite 6   Lanoka Harbor, NJ 08734   (609)971-1711   Fax (609)971-3390

Taus, Lynne F., MD {1376544064} RadDia(84,IL43)
+ Radiology Affiliates of Central New Jersey, P.A.
2501 Kuser Road   Hamilton, NJ 08691   (609)585-8800   Fax (609)585-1825
+ Radiology Affiliates Imaging
3625 Quakerbridge Road   Hamilton, NJ 08619

Tavani, Denis A., MD {1114959939} IntrMd(81,PA07)<NJ-MEM-SALEM>
+ 309 Salem-Woodstown Road/Route 45
Salem, NJ 08079   (856)935-0567   Fax (856)935-7576

Tavarez, Laura, MD {1053675397}
+ 6035 Park Avenue/Apt 319
West New York, NJ 07093   (201)937-3840

Tavel, Stacey C., MD {1477514933} Pedtrc, IntrMd(01,NY19)
+ Summit Medical Group-Berkeley Heights Campus
1 Diamond Hill Road   Berkeley Heights, NJ 07922   (908)273-4300   Fax (908)790-6576

Tavill, Michael A., MD {1417030792} Otlryg, PedOto(91,OH06)
+ ENT and Allergy Associates
1131 Broad Street/Suite 103 Building A   Shrewsbury, NJ 07702   (732)389-3388   Fax (732)389-3389

Tavorath, Ranjana, MD {1013251073} MedOnc, IntrMd(83,INA72)
+ Novartis Pharmaceuticals Corporation
One Health Plaza   East Hanover, NJ 07936   (862)778-4118   Fax (973)781-6504

Taw, Julie, MD {1518987338} IntrMd(98,NY46)<NJ-ENGLWOOD>
+ Englewood Hospital and Medical Center
350 Engle Street   Englewood, NJ 07631   (201)894-3000

Tawadrous, Alfred Rezk, MD {1437237773} PainMd(78,EGY16)<NJ-KMHCHRRY, NJ-RWJUBRUN>
+ Neurology Associates & Ctr Pain
1030 North Kings Highway/Suite 200B   Cherry Hill, NJ 08034   (856)482-0030   Fax (856)779-7787
+ Neurology Associates & Ctr Pain
1030 North Kings Highway/Suite 200A   Cherry Hill, NJ 08034   (856)482-0030   Fax (856)779-7787

Tawadrous, Hanan K., MD {1346554060} PedNph(90,EGY04)
+ St. Joseph's Children's Hospital
703 Main Street   Paterson, NJ 07503   (973)754-2570

Tawde, Darshana Prafullaraj, MD {1548338080} IntrMd
+ Middlesex Medical Group
225 May Street/Suite E   Edison, NJ 08837   (732)661-2020   Fax (732)661-2022

Tawfik, Hany Wahba, MD {1821308925} IntrMd(84,EGY16)
+ 2087 Klockner Road
Hamilton, NJ 08690   (609)587-2300

Tawfik, Isaac H., MD {1073612990} IntrMd, CdvDis, EmrgMd(03,PA13)
+ Etheridge Family Medicine LLC
81 Veronica Avenue/Suite 202   Somerset, NJ 08873   (908)812-4460   Fax (732)263-5029
+ Monmouth Heart Specialists
274 Highway 35   Eatontown, NJ 07724   (908)812-4460   Fax (732)440-9404

Tayal, Rajiv, MD {1134457898} IntrMd<NJ-CHDNWBTH>
+ Children's Hospital of New Jersey
201 Lyons Avenue/Osborne Terrace   Newark, NJ 07112   (973)926-7213
+ Cardiac Care
1314 Park Avenue/Suite 9   Plainfield, NJ 07060   (973)926-7213   Fax (908)222-8762

Physicians by Name and Address

Taylor, Christopher, MD {1780678243} Radiol, RadBdI, IntrMd(99,NJ06)
+ University Radiology Group, P.C.
579A Cranbury Road East Brunswick, NJ 08816 (732)390-0040 Fax (732)390-1856
+ University Radiology Group
2100 Route 33/Neptune City Med Bld Neptune, NJ 07753 (732)390-0040 Fax (732)502-0368
+ University Radiology Group
900 West Main Street Freehold, NJ 08816 (732)462-1900 Fax (732)462-1848

Taylor, Clifford A., MD {1467544361} Psychy(78,MA01)<NJ-MORRISTN>
+ The Center for Psychiatry & Psycho-Oncology
261 James Street/Unit 2-E L Morristown, NJ 07960 (973)540-1656 Fax (973)540-1889

Taylor, Cody Wolfson, MD {1114372075} EmrgMd
+ Hackensack Medical Center Emergency Medicine
30 Prospect Avenue/Main 3619 Hackensack, NJ 07601 (551)996-2000 Fax (201)968-1866

Taylor, David L., MD {1871593947} Urolgy(79,MI01)<NJ-MORRISTN>
+ Adult & Pediatric Urology Group PA
261 James Street/Suite 1-A Morristown, NJ 07960 (973)539-0333 Fax (973)539-8909

Taylor, Douglas A., MD {1093735284} IntrMd, InfDis(87,GHA01)<NJ-EASTORNG, NJ-MTNSIDE>
+ 60 Evergreen Place/Suite 302
East Orange, NJ 07018 (973)395-3700 Fax (973)395-3717

Taylor, Greg Michael, DO {1306826797} FamMed(01,NJ75)<NJ-OURLADY, NJ-KMHSTRAT>
+ Jefferson Health Primary & Specialty Care
1A Regulus Drive Turnersville, NJ 08012 (844)542-2273
+ Kennedy Health Alliance
80 Tanner Street Haddonfield, NJ 08033 (844)542-2273 Fax (856)355-0346

Taylor, Guy Adrian, MD {1619959608} Anesth(93,NY06)<NJ-MORRISTN>
+ Morristown Medical Center
100 Madison Avenue/Anesth 112 Morristown, NJ 07962 (973)971-5000 Fax (201)943-8733

Taylor, Howard, MD {1932193117} Otlryg, Otolgy, PedOto(76,NY01)<NJ-CHILTON>
+ ENT and Facial Plastic Surgeons
51 Route 23 South/2nd Floor Riverdale, NJ 07457 (973)831-1220 Fax (973)831-0029
+ Wayne Surgical Center, LLC.
1176 Hamburg Pike Wayne, NJ 07470 (973)831-1220 Fax (973)709-1901

Taylor, Jamie Latiolais, MD {1437217767} Anesth(02,LA05)
+ University Hospital-RWJ Medical School
89 French Street New Brunswick, NJ 08901 (732)828-3000

Taylor, Jeff Thomas, MD {1841290194} CdvDis, IntrMd, IntCrd(93,NY08)
+ Cardio Care
200 Courtyard Drive/Suite 213 Hillsborough, NJ 08844 (908)725-5200 Fax (908)725-5223
+ Cardio Care
328 Greenbrook Road Green Brook, NJ 08812 (908)725-5200 Fax (908)725-5223

Taylor, Jennifer, MD {1760838148} Psychy<NJ-TRININPC>
+ Trinitas Regional Medical Center-New Point Campus
655 East Jersey Street Elizabeth, NJ 07206 (908)994-5000

Taylor, John M., MD {1457322554} SrgRec, SrgPlstc, Surgry(88,PA01)<NJ-MONMOUTH, NJ-JRSYSHMC>
+ Allure Plastic Surgery Center
48 Pavilion Avenue Long Branch, NJ 07740 (732)483-1800 Fax (732)483-1622

Taylor, Marian L., MD {1235222787} IntrMd(83,NJ05)
+ 1813 Oak Tree Road
Edison, NJ 08820 (732)287-6362 Fax (732)287-4339

Taylor, Michael, MD {1245632058} IntrMd
+ Cooper University Medical Center/Camden
3 Cooper Plaza Camden, NJ 08103 (856)342-2000

Taylor, Robert L., MD {1063464808} SrgC&R, Surgry(70,DC01)
+ 25 East Willow Street
Millburn, NJ 07041 (973)467-5605 Fax (973)379-5324

Taylor, Robert Roland, MD {1629075593} GynOnc, SrgGyn(85,MD12)<NJ-STBARNMC, NJ-MORRISTN>
+ Gynecologic Cancer and Pelvic Surgery, LLC
101 Old Short Hills Road/Suite 400 West Orange, NJ 07052 (973)243-9300 Fax (973)325-8254

Taylor, Tanisha K., MD {1154366805} IntrMd, OccpMd, EnvnMd(01,NY09)
+ Corporate Health Center
832 Brunswick Avenue Trenton, NJ 08638 (609)695-7471 Fax (609)393-5272

Tchabo, Nana Eleonore, MD {1851508436} GynOnc, ObsGyn(00,RI01)<NJ-MORRISTN>
+ Morristown Medical Center
100 Madison Avenue/CancerCtr Morristown, NJ 07962

(973)971-5000 Fax (973)290-7257

Tchikindas, Olga M., MD {1508997552} Psychy
+ 33 Coppervail Court
Princeton, NJ 08540
+ Global Medical Institutes, LLC
256 Bunn Drive/Suite 6 Woodslands Bldg Princeton, NJ 08540 Fax (609)921-3620

Tchorbajian, Kourkin, MD {1730278904} Ophthl(80,FRA38)<NJ-HOBUNIMC>
+ Associated Eye Physicians & Surgeons of NJ, P.A.
1050 Galloping Hill Road/Suite 104 Union, NJ 07083 (908)964-7878 Fax (908)964-5434
+ Associated Eye Physicians & Surgeons of NJ, P.A.
724 Jersey Avenue Jersey City, NJ 07302 (908)964-7878 Fax (201)795-9797
+ Associated Eye Physicians & Surgeons of NJ, P.A.
1530 Saint Georges Avenue Rahway, NJ 07083 (732)382-9000 Fax (732)382-7455

Teasley, Melanie, MD {1528157682} Psychy(81,NJ06)<NJ-UNVM-CPRN>
+ 3 Benedek Road
Princeton, NJ 08540 (609)921-2113
+ Princeton House Behavioral Health - North Brunswick
1460 Livingston Avenue North Brunswick, NJ 08902 (609)921-2113 Fax (732)435-0222

Tecson, Maria Vida Tupaz, MD {1518043470} IntrMd(84,PHI22)
+ 116 Millburn Avenue/Suite 207
Millburn, NJ 07041

Tedeschi, John B., MD {1477517605} Pedtrc(93,PA09)<NJ-VIRTU-AHS, NJ-COOPRUMC>
+ Advocare South Jersey Pediatrics Cherry Hill
1949 Route 70 East/Suite 1 & 2 Cherry Hill, NJ 08003 (856)424-6050 Fax (856)424-2943
+ Advocare South Jersey Pediatrics Collingswood
204 White Horse Pike Collingswood, NJ 08107 (856)424-6050 Fax (856)424-2943
+ Advocare Hammonton Pediatrics
856 South Whitehorse Pike Hammonton, NJ 08003 (609)704-8848 Fax (609)704-8849

Tedeschi, John M., MD {1194879156} Pedtrc(64,NE06)<NJ-VIRTU-AHS, NJ-COOPRUMC>
+ Advocare South Jersey Pediatrics Cherry Hill
1949 Route 70 East/Suite 1 & 2 Cherry Hill, NJ 08003 (856)424-6050 Fax (856)424-2943
+ Advocare South Jersey Pediatrics Collingswood
204 White Horse Pike Collingswood, NJ 08107 (856)424-6050 Fax (856)424-2943
+ Advocare Hammonton Pediatrics
856 South Whitehorse Pike Hammonton, NJ 08003 (609)704-8848 Fax (609)704-8849

Teehan, Edwin P., MD {1366491532} Surgry, SrgVas(88,NJ05)<NJ-CHILTON>
+ 510 Hamburg Tpke/Suite 205
Wayne, NJ 07470 Fax (973)290-3198

Tehranirad, Mohammad, MD {1356516082} IntHos, IntrMd(00,IRA16)<NJ-MTNSIDE>
+ Hackensack UMC Mountainside
1 Bay Avenue/Hospitalist Montclair, NJ 07042 (973)429-6000

Teicher, Mark, MD {1689620353} CdvDis, IntrMd(84,NY46)<NJ-CHILTON, NJ-VALLEY>
+ Cardiology Center of North Jersey
1030 Clifton Avenue Clifton, NJ 07013 (973)778-3777 Fax (973)778-3252

Teichholz, Louis E., MD {1457308165} CdvDis, IntrMd(66,MA01)<NJ-HACKNSK, NY-MTSINAI>
+ Hackensack University Medical Center
30 Prospect Avenue/Cardio/Rm4655 Hackensack, NJ 07601 (201)996-2314 Fax (201)996-4909

Teichman, Amanda Liane, MD {1609215029} SrgTrm
+ UH- Robert Wood Johnson Med
125 Paterson Street New Brunswick, NJ 08901 (732)828-3000

Teichman, Ronald F., MD {1336151471} IntrMd, OccpMd(83,NY09)<NJ-EASTORNG>
+ 4 Forest Drive
West Orange, NJ 07052

Teitelbaum, Jonathan Evan, MD {1831154475} Pedtrc, PedGst, Nutrtn(93,PA01)<NJ-MONMOUTH>
+ Monmouth Medical Center
300 Second Avenue/Pediatrics Long Branch, NJ 07740 (732)923-6080

Teitelman, Karen Lynn Bottone, DO {1225114499} Psychy(97,NJ75)<NJ-SJERSYHS, NJ-LOURDMED>
+ Center for Family Guidance, PC
765 East Route 70/Building A-101 Marlton, NJ 08053 (856)797-4800 Fax (856)810-0110

Teja, Paul Gregory, DO {1316943012} SrgOrt, SprtMd(96,NJ75)<NJ-HCKTSTWN>
+ The Orthopedic Institute of New Jersey
108 Bilby Road/Suite 201 Hackettstown, NJ 07840 (908)684-3005 Fax (908)684-3301

+ The Orthopedic Institute of New Jersey
66 Sunset Strip/Suite 400 Town Center Succasunna, NJ 07876 (908)684-3005 Fax (908)684-3301
+ The Orthopedic Institute of New Jersey
222 High Street/Suite 202 Newton, NJ 07840 (908)684-3005 Fax (908)684-3301

Tejeda, Carlos Alberto, MD {1851342703} IntrMd(00,DOM01)<NJ-STJOSHOS, NJ-STMRYPAS>
+ Center for Adult Medicine & Preventive Care
916-922 Main Avenue/Suite 1-A Passaic, NJ 07055 (973)773-0334 Fax (973)773-0336
Carlostejedamd@gmail.com
+ Center for Adult Medicine & Preventive Care
293 Passaic Street Passaic, NJ 07055 (973)773-0334 Fax (973)773-0336

Tekleyohannes, Girmay Haile, MD {1164689055} PedHem, Pedtrc
+ 500 Kings Court
Woodbridge, NJ 07095

Teklezgi, Semhar, DO {1578982955} IntrMd
+ The Advanced Pulmonary Diagnostic Center
100 Medical Center Way Somers Point, NJ 08244 (609)653-3500 Fax (609)653-3586

Tekriwal, Mahesh Kumar, MD {1801841226} CdvDis, IntrMd(79,INDI)
+ Stafford Medical, P.A.
1364 Route 72 West/Suite 5 Manahawkin, NJ 08050 (609)597-3416 Fax (609)597-9608
+ Stafford Medical, P.A.
1364 Route 72 West Manahawkin, NJ 08050 (609)597-3416 Fax (609)597-9608

Telfeyan, Celeste A., DO {1699732719} Anesth(80,PA77)<NJ-VALLEY>
+ The Valley Hospital
223 North Van Dien Avenue Ridgewood, NJ 07450 (201)447-8000

Teli, Kunal J., MD {1295041671} CdvDis
+ 200 Hospital Plaza/Apt 507
Paterson, NJ 07503 (973)851-9072

Tell, Alan Michael, MD {1194883454} Otlryg(78,MEX03)<NJ-HACKNSK>
+ 140 Prospect Avenue/Suite 7
Hackensack, NJ 07601 (201)487-2777 Fax (201)487-1369

Tello Valcarcel, Carlos A., MD {1518978063} SrgVas, Surgry(77,PER01)
+ Drs. Tello Valcarcel & Calderon
356 Totowa Avenue Paterson, NJ 07502 (973)904-0100 Fax (973)595-8286

Tempera, Patrick G., MD {1508830050} Gastrn, IntrMd, SrgC&R(86,GRN01)<NJ-OVERLOOK, NJ-SOMERSET>
+ Advanced Gastroenterology Group
1308 Morris Avenue Union, NJ 07083 (908)851-2770 Fax (908)851-7706

Tempesta, Sabrina L., DO {1821298795} IntrMd(04,NJ75)
+ Bergen Medical Associates
305 West Grand Avenue/Suite 200 Montvale, NJ 07645 (201)391-0071 Fax (201)391-1904
+ Bergen Medical Associates
466 Old Hook Road/Suite 1 Emerson, NJ 07630 (201)391-0071 Fax (201)967-0340

Temple, Julia K., MD {1063783769} Psychy(87,LA01)
+ 1000 Herrontown Road
Princeton, NJ 08540 (609)430-0522 Fax (609)430-0649

Tenaglia, Nicholas Charles, MD {1194938217} EmrgMd(03,PA02)<NJ-MEADWLND>
+ Meadowlands Hospital Medical Center
55 Meadowlands Parkway Secaucus, NJ 07096 (201)392-3100

Tench, Mavola L., MD {1013958875} FamMed(93,PA13)<NJ-KMHTURNV, NJ-KENEDYHS>
+ Kennedy Family Health Center
445 Hurffville Crosskeys Road Sewell, NJ 08080 (856)262-1900
+ Kennedy Family Health Services
1 Somerdale Square Somerdale, NJ 08083 (856)262-1900 Fax (856)566-8944

Tendler, Craig L., MD {1093058851} PedHem, Pedtrc(84,NY47)<NY-MTSINAI>
+ 920 Route 202
Raritan, NJ 08869 (908)927-4772

Tendler, Jay M., MD {1700804838} Anesth(81,WI06)
+ River Drive Surgery Center
619 River Drive Elmwood Park, NJ 07407 (201)703-2900

Tendler, Michael R., MD {1003873928} Gastrn, IntrMd(86,NJ06)<NJ-CENTRAST>
+ Advanced Gastroenterology Associates LLC
475 County Road/Suite 201 Marlboro, NJ 07746 (732)370-2220 Fax (732)548-7408
+ Advanced Gastroenterology Associates LLC
403 Candlewood Commons/Building 4 Howell, NJ 07731 (732)370-2220 Fax (732)548-7408

Tenenzapf, Mark J., MD {1467450247} RadDia, Radiol, IntrMd(78,NY08)<NJ-RWJUHAM>
+ **Princeton Radiology Associates, P.A.**
  3674 Route 27   Kendall Park, NJ 08824   (732)821-5563   Fax (732)821-6675
+ **Quakerbridge Radiology Associates**
  8 Quakerbridge Plaza/Building 8   Mercerville, NJ 08619   (732)821-5563   Fax (609)689-6067
+ **Quakerbridge Radiology MRI Center at Lawrenceville**
  21 Lawrenceville-Pennington Rd   Lawrenceville, NJ 08824   (609)895-1500   Fax (609)895-2647

Tener, Trilby Jo, MD {1972682268} ObsGyn(95,PA07)
+ **145 Route 46 West**
  Wayne, NJ 07470

Tengson, Roger C., Jr., MD {1326094921} Pedtrc(87,PHIL)<NJ-STJOSHOS>
+ **32 Hines Street**
  Paterson, NJ 07503   (973)742-0046
+ **St. Joseph's Regional Medical Center**
  641 Main Street/Pediatrics   Paterson, NJ 07503   (973)754-2580

Tennen, Elad, MD {1700221561} FamMSptM
+ **Orthopaedic Institute of Central Jersey**
  2315A Highway 34/Suite D   Manasquan, NJ 08736   (732)974-0404   Fax (732)449-4271

Tennenbaum, Steven Y., MD {1124041827} PedUro, PedSrg(84,NY46)<NY-CHLDCOPR, NY-MNTFWEIL>
+ **Castle Connolly Medical, LTD.**
  699 Teaneck Road/Suite 103   Teaneck, NJ 07666   (201)645-3362   Fax (201)692-1363

Tenner, Bruce S., DO {1841244332} CdvDis(88,NJ75)
+ **Toms River Medical Group PA**
  81 Route 37 West/Suite 1   Toms River, NJ 08755   (732)341-0560   Fax (732)341-0574

Tenner, Jeffrey P., DO {1235134784} Surgry(84,NJ75)<NJ-BUR-DTMLN>
+ **Cape Regional Physicans Associates**
  217 North Main Street/Suite 104   Cape May Court House, NJ 08210   (609)463-1488   Fax (609)463-4881

Tenorio, Grace Cipres, MD {1114951134} Pthlgy
+ **Robert Wood Johnson University Hospital**
  51 French Street/MEB-234B/Pthlgy   New Brunswick, NJ 08903

Tentler, Aleksey, MD {1922269414} Pedtrc, IntrMd(08,NY45)<NJ-UMDNJ>
+ **University Hospital-Doctors Office Center**
  90 Bergen Street/Suite 4400   Newark, NJ 07103   (973)972-1880   Fax (888)768-5044

Teodoro, Paul C., MD {1720177405} FamMed(79,MEX34)<NJ-MEADWLND, NJ-HOBUNIMC>
+ **422 Grand Street**
  Hoboken, NJ 07030   (201)866-6666   Fax (201)656-6667

Teper, Ariel Abel, MD PedPul, Pedtrc(90,ARG01)<NY-JACOBIMC>
+ **Sanofi US-Sanofi-Aventis**
  55 Corporate Drive   Bridgewater, NJ 08807

Tepler, Harold George, MD {1073505376} Gastrn, IntrMd(88,NY46)<NJ-PALISADE, NJ-CHRIST>
+ **Gastroenterology Medical Associates PA**
  9223 Kennedy Boulevard/Suite D   North Bergen, NJ 07047   (201)868-2849   Fax (201)868-4190
+ **Gastroenterology Medical Associates PA**
  142 Palisades Avenue/Suite 201   Jersey City, NJ 07307   (201)868-2849   Fax (201)792-7812

Teplinsky, Eleonora, MD {1477871474} IntrMd, MedOnc(09,MA07)
+ **Valley Mount Sinai Comprehensive Cancer Care**
  One Valley Health Plaza/Suite C211   Paramus, NJ 07652   (201)634-5578   Fax (201)986-4702

Tepper, Drew I., MD {1982992913} Psychy(11,PA13)
+ **University Behavioral Health Care**
  671 Hoes Lane/PO Box 1392/D325   Piscataway, NJ 08855   (732)235-4433   Fax (732)235-4649

Tepper, Howard N., MD {1336168442} SrgPlstc, IntrMd(75,NY46)<NJ-OVERLOOK, NJ-CHLSMT>
+ **Associates in Plastic & Aesthetic Surgery**
  955 South Springfield Avenue/Suite 105   Springfield, NJ 07081   (908)654-6540   Fax (908)654-6504
+ **Associates in Plastic & Aesthetic Surgery**
  33 Overlook Road/Suite 411   Summit, NJ 07901   (908)522-0880
+ **Associates in Plastic & Aesthetic Surgery**
  27 Mountain Boulevard/Suite 9   Warren, NJ 07081   (908)561-0080

Tepper, Richard Eric, MD {1396768354} SrgPlstc, SrgHnd(94,NY19)<NJ-OVERLOOK, NJ-STBARNMC>
+ **Associates in Plastic & Aesthetic Surgery**
  955 South Springfield Avenue/Suite 105   Springfield, NJ 07081   (908)654-6540   Fax (908)654-6504

Tepper, Steven Ari, DO {1790948016} IntrMd(08,PA77)<NJ-VIRTVOOR>
+ **Virtua Voorhees**
  100 Bowman Drive/Hospitalist   Voorhees, NJ 08043

  (856)247-2594   Fax (856)247-2597

Tepper, Suzanne, MD {1760778633} FamMed
+ **Medical Institute of New Jersey**
  11 Saddle Road   Cedar Knolls, NJ 07927   (973)267-2122   Fax (973)267-3478

Tepper Levine, Shawn, DO {1174742704} OstMed, NeuMus(00,FL75)
+ **20 Heathcote Road/PO Box 142**
  Kingston, NJ 08528   (609)924-0496   Fax (609)945-2535

Ter, Suat E., MD RadDia(87,ASTL)
+ **6 Saddle Horn Drive**
  Cherry Hill, NJ 08003

Teraguchi, Kari Jane, MD {1073685095} Pedtrc(98,OH06)<NY-NY-ACKHOS, NY-GOODSAM>
+ **Progressive Pediatrics**
  3196 Kennedy Boulevard   Union City, NJ 07087   (201)319-9800   Fax (201)319-9849
+ **Progressive Pediatrics**
  1222 Kennedy Boulevard   Bayonne, NJ 07002   (201)319-9800   Fax (201)437-9661

Teran Vargas, Rafael Antonio, MD {1962658187} IntrMd
+ **Hackensack Medical Center-Internal Medicine**
  30 Prospect Avenue/4 Main/Rm 4621   Hackensack, NJ 07601   (201)996-3664   Fax (551)996-0536

Terens, William L., MD {1013020189} FrtInf, Urolgy(86,NY19)
+ **Premier Urology Group, LLC**
  10 Parsonage Road/Suite 118   Edison, NJ 08837   (732)494-9400   Fax (732)548-3931
+ **Premier Urology Group, LLC**
  2 Hospital Plaza/Suite 430   Old Bridge, NJ 08857   (732)494-9400   Fax (732)679-2077
+ **Premier Urology Group, LLC**
  570 South Avenue East/Building A   Cranford, NJ 08837   (908)603-4200   Fax (908)497-1633

Teresh, Michelle A., MD {1942585948} Pedtrc
+ **Pediatric Health, P.A.**
  470 Stillwells Corner Road   Freehold, NJ 07728   (732)780-3333   Fax (732)780-6968

Terk, Alyssa Robyn, MD {1386697118} Otlryg, Surgry(01,NY09)
+ **St Christopher Hospital for Children**
  100 Kings Way East   Sewell, NJ 08080   (856)582-0644   Fax (856)582-0622

Terlizzi, Joseph P., MD {1811208390} Surgry
+ **UH- Robert Wood Johnson Med**
  125 Paterson Street   New Brunswick, NJ 08901   (732)235-6096

Termini, Joseph F., MD {1699741538} FamMed, IntrMd(78,PA14)<NJ-VIRTMHBC>
+ **Mt. Laurel Family Physicians**
  401 Young Avenue/Suite 260   Moorestown, NJ 08057   (856)291-8756   Fax (856)291-8750

Terranova, Lauren M., DO {1821363292} PhyMSptM
+ **Ridgewood Orthopedic Group, LLC**
  85 South Maple Avenue   Ridgewood, NJ 07450   (201)445-2830   Fax (201)445-7471

Terranova, Matthew Patrick, Jr DO {1245546142} IntrMd(PA77)
+ **RWJPE Cranbury Medical Group**
  557 Cranbury Road/Suite 22   East Brunswick, NJ 08816   (732)613-0500   Fax (732)613-0345

Terranova, Robert J., DO {1871538330} Nrolgy(71,PA77)<NJ-SOCEANCO>
+ **Hackensack Meridian Medical Group**
  53 Nautilus Drive/Suite 201   Manahawkin, NJ 08050   (609)978-8870   Fax (609)978-8903

Terrany, Ben, MD {1578528592} Gastrn, IntrMd(88,MEXI)<NJ-MONMOUTH, NJ-JRSYSHMC>
+ **Shore Gastroenterology Associates, P.C.**
  1907 Highway 35/Suite 1   Oakhurst, NJ 07755   (732)517-0060   Fax (732)548-7408
+ **Shore Gastroenterology Associates, P.C.**
  1907 Highway 35/Suite 1   Oakhurst, NJ 07755   (732)517-0060   Fax (732)548-7408
+ **Shore Gastroenterology Associates, P.C.**
  233 Middle Road   Hazlet, NJ 07755   (732)361-2476

Terregino, Carol A., MD {1265681035} IntrMd, EmrgMd(86,NJ05)
+ **RWJ Medical School Univ of Med**
  675 Hoes Lane   Piscataway, NJ 08854   (732)235-4565   Fax (732)235-5078

Terrels, Mary Ellen, DO {1033290606} FamMed(84,PA77)<NJ-ACMCITY, NJ-ACMCMAIN>
+ **AtlantiCare Regional Medical Center/City Campus**
  1925 Pacific Avenue/FamMed   Atlantic City, NJ 08401   (609)441-8959

Terrence, Christopher, Jr., MD {1326064346} Nrolgy(70,PA12)<NJ-VAEASTOR, NJ-VALYONS>
+ **VA New Jersey Health Care System-East Orange Campus**
  385 Tremont Avenue   East Orange, NJ 07018   (973)676-1000   Fax (973)676-4226
+ **VA New Jersey Health Care System at Lyons**
  151 Knollcroft Road   Lyons, NJ 07939   (908)647-0180

Physicians by Name and Address

Terreri, Michael Robert, Jr., MD {1184937716} Anesth(09,NJ06)<PA-TJCNTR>
+ **Morris Anesthesia Group, PA**
  3799 Route 46/Suite 211   Parsippany, NJ 07054   (973)335-1122   Fax (973)335-1448

Terrigno, Donato A., MD {1760593461} EmrgMd(80,MEXI)<NJ-SJHREGMC, NJ-SJERSYHS>
+ **SJH Regional Medical Center**
  1505 West Sherman Avenue/EmrgMed   Vineland, NJ 08360   (856)641-8000

Terrigno, Nicole, MD {1679985097} IntHos<NJ-COOPRUMC>
+ **Cooper University Hospital**
  One Cooper Plaza   Camden, NJ 08103   (856)342-2000

Terrigno, Rocco Felice, MD {1477975720}
+ **The Cooper Hospital System-Univ Hospital**
  401 Haddon Avenue/E&R 3rd Fl   Camden, NJ 08103   (856)757-7842
+ **Cooper Cardiology Associates**
  900 Centennial Boulevard   Voorhees, NJ 08043   (856)757-7842   Fax (856)325-6702

Terrin, Bruce N., MD {1528090081} PedHem, Pedtrc(78,NY19)<NJ-HACKNSK, NJ-VALLEY>
+ **Haclensack Bergen Pediatrics**
  385 Prospect Avenue/Suite 210   Hackensack, NJ 07601   (551)996-9160   Fax (201)487-3009
+ **Tomorrow's Children's Inst/HUMC**
  30 Prospect Avenue/WFAN - PC 116   Hackensack, NJ 07601   (201)996-5437

Terrone, Dom A., MD {1750383048} ObsGyn(93,NJ05)<NJ-ST-BARNMC>
+ **St. Barnabas Medical Center**
  94 Old Short Hills Road/Ob/Gyn   Livingston, NJ 07039   (973)322-5000   Fax (973)322-2309

Terry, Alon, MD {1942464128} IntrMd
+ **Summit Medical Group-Berkeley Heights Campus**
  1 Diamond Hill Road   Berkeley Heights, NJ 07922   (908)273-4300   Fax (908)790-6576

Terry, Bernard, MD {1134125875} Radiol, RadDia(72,NY47)
+ **University Radiology, PA**
  239 Route 22 East/Suite 302   Green Brook, NJ 08812   (732)968-4899   Fax (732)968-8096

Terry, Charles M., MD {1497837538} PhysMd, Acpntr, SprtMd(94,PA09)<NJ-STLAWRN>
+ **St. Lawrence Rehabilitation Center**
  2381 Lawrenceville Road   Lawrenceville, NJ 08648   (609)896-8152   Fax (609)896-4107

Terushkin, Vitaly, MD {1699099671} Dermat
+ **Dermatology & Skin Cancer Center**
  55 North Gilbert Street   Tinton Falls, NJ 07701   (732)747-5500   Fax (732)747-1212
  vitaly.terushkin@gmail.com

Terwes, Estella, MD {1104831551} CdvDis, GenPrc(72,MEXI)
+ **906 Summit Avenue/Ground Floor**
  Jersey City, NJ 07307   (201)653-0330
  estella@TELL-ALL.com

Tesfaye, Melaku, MD {1245659028} IntrMd<NJ-HACKNSK>
+ **Hackensack University Medical Center**
  30 Prospect Avenue/Rm 3619   Hackensack, NJ 07601   (551)996-3192

Tesfaye, Melaku Berhanu, MD {1417390527}<NJ-STBARNMC>
+ **St. Barnabas Medical Center**
  94 Old Short Hills Road   Livingston, NJ 07039   (973)322-5000

Tesher, Harris Brandon, MD {1639338205} PulDis, CritCr
+ **Holy Name Pulmonary Associates PC**
  200 Grand Avenue/Suite 102   Englewood, NJ 07631   (201)871-3636   Fax (201)871-2286
+ **Holy Name Pulmonary Associates PC**
  8305 Bergenline Avenue   North Bergen, NJ 07047   (201)871-3636   Fax (201)854-0827

Tesoriero, Laura M., MD {1457368573} FamMed(92,PA07)<NJ-COMMED>
+ **Our Family Practice**
  1899 State Highway 88   Brick, NJ 08723   (732)840-8177   Fax (732)840-2195

Tesoro, Louis J., MD {1982773461} Pedtrc(85,CT01)<NJ-UNVM-CPRN>
+ **The Pediatric Group PA**
  66 Mount Lucas Road   Princeton, NJ 08540   (609)924-4892   Fax (609)921-9380
  tesoro@pedgroup.com

Tessema, Abiy Meaza, MD {1962769737}<NJ-STBARNMC>
+ **St. Barnabas Medical Center**
  94 Old Short Hills Road   Livingston, NJ 07039   (888)724-7123

Testa, David A., DO {1326198490} FamMed(97,MO78)
+ **524 Clifton Avenue**
  Clifton, NJ 07011   (973)478-3556   Fax (973)478-3544

Testa, Joseph M., MD {1891739025} EmrgMd, IntrMd(88,NJ06)<NJ-WAYNEGEN>
+ **St. Joseph's Wayne Hospital**
  224 Hamburg Turnpike   Wayne, NJ 07470   (973)942-6900

New Jersey Physicians
Section 1 Name and Practice Address

Physicians by Name and Address

Testaiuti, Mark A., MD {1316919517} SrgNro, SrgSpn(89,PA09)<NJ-VIRTUAHS, NJ-UNDRWD>
  + Coastal Spine
    4000 Church Road Mount Laurel, NJ 08054 (856)222-4444 Fax (856)222-0049

Tetelbom, Miriam, MD {1598927956} PsyCAd(88,BRA96)
  + 1806 Highway 35/Suite 303
    Oakhurst, NJ 07755 (732)503-9812 Fax (732)303-9901
    Drtetelbom@gmail.com

Tetteh, Shirley S., MD {1639303175} Pedtrc<NJ-STPETER>
  + St. Peter's University Hospital
    254 Easton Avenue/MOB 3 New Brunswick, NJ 08901 (732)745-7600

Tew, Beverly Ellen, MD {1669661062} Gyneco
  + Cooper University Medical Center/Camden
    3 Cooper Plaza/Suite 221 Camden, NJ 08103 (856)342-2000

Tewari, Sanjay Om, MD {1326021742} Anesth(99,DMN01)<NJ-HACKNSK>
  + Hackensack University Medical Center
    30 Prospect Avenue/Anesthesia Hackensack, NJ 07601 (201)996-2000

Tewfik, George L., MD {1407182660} Anesth<NJ-STBARNMC>
  + St. Barnabas Medical Center
    94 Old Short Hills Road/Anesthesia Livingston, NJ 07039 (973)322-5512 Fax (973)322-8165
  + New Jersey Anesthesia Associates, P.C.
    30B Vreeland Road/Suite 200 Florham Park, NJ 07932 (973)322-5512 Fax (973)660-9779
  + University Hospital
    150 Bergen Street Newark, NJ 07039 (973)972-5007

Tha, Teemu, MD {1366752792} ObsGyn(10,PA02)
  + Garden State Obstetrics and Gynecological Associates
    2401 Evesham Road/Suite A Voorhees, NJ 08043 (856)424-3323 Fax (856)424-4994

Thacker, Sunil Rajan, MD {1053455345} SrgOrt(98,NJ05)
  + Edison Orthopedic Institute
    3 Progress Street/Suite 106 Edison, NJ 08820 (732)494-1050 Fax (732)494-5424

Thadhani, Ramchand, MD {1619035342} FamMed(85,PAKI)<NJ-ACMCMAIN, NJ-ACMCITY>
  + Smithville Medical Associates
    48 South New York Road/Suite B-3 Galloway, NJ 08205 (609)404-0121 Fax (609)404-0131

Thakar, Opal V., MD {1659792802}
  + Meridian Medical Group
    552 Westwood Avenue Long Branch, NJ 07740 (732)222-7800

Thaker, Jayeshkumar, MD {1417951815} Anesth(90,INDI)<NJ-BAYSHORE>
  + Robert Wood Johnson-UMDNJ Anesthesia Group
    125 Paterson Street/CAB 3100 New Brunswick, NJ 08901 (732)235-7827 Fax (732)235-6131

Thakkar, Priyesh Tarunkumar, DO {1689683815} IntrMd(99,PA77)<NJ-SHOREMEM, NJ-ATLANCHS>
  + Regional Nephrology Associates
    510 Jackson Avenue Northfield, NJ 08225 (609)383-0200 Fax (609)383-8352

Thakkar, Shivani, MD {1841546389} Anesth<NJ-OVERLOOK>
  + Overlook Medical Center
    99 Beauvoir Avenue/PO Box 210 Summit, NJ 07902 (908)522-2000

Thakker, Manoj Mangaldas, MD {1679550297} Ophthl(99,NY47)
  + Retinal & Ophthalmic Consultants, PC
    1500 Tilton Road Northfield, NJ 08225 (609)646-5200 Fax (609)646-9868
  + Retinal & Ophthalmic Consultants, PC
    2466 East Chestnut Avenue Vineland, NJ 08360 (609)646-5200 Fax (856)507-0040
  + 719 North Beers Street/Suite 2G
    Holmdel, NJ 08225 (732)739-3937 Fax (732)739-3225

Thakker, Priya Sambandan, MD {1538359633} Dermat(03,VT02)<NJ-JRSYSHMC>
  + Corederm Dermatology and Cosmetic Center
    246 Hamburg Turnpike/Suite 306 Wayne, NJ 07470 (973)956-0500 Fax (973)956-0522
  + Cosmetic & Dermatologic Surgery Associates, LLC
    719 North Beers Street/Suite 2-G Holmdel, NJ 07733 (973)956-0500 Fax (732)739-3225

Thakur, Jagdish G., MD {1083616353} Anesth(73,INA69)
  + Morris Anesthesia Group, PA
    3799 Route 46/Suite 211 Parsippany, NJ 07054 (973)335-1122 Fax (973)335-1448

Thakur, Ranjana, MD {1780732552} IntrMd(85,INA9B)
  + 105 Raider Boulevard/Suite 102
    Hillsborough, NJ 08844 (908)431-9911 Fax (908)431-9937

Thakur, Shivani, MD {1487913026} FamMed
  + Highlands Family Health Center
    61 Frontage Road/Suite 61 Hampton, NJ 08827 (908)735-2594 Fax (908)735-8526

Thakur, Shubhangi J., MD {1144322355} IntrMd(76,INDI)<NJ-JFKMED>
  + 1856 Oak Tree Road
    Edison, NJ 08820 (732)548-9119 Fax (732)906-7820

Thal, Stephen Wayne, DO {1811022288} RadDia, RadBdl(71,MO78)<PA-MRCYSUB>
  + Radiology Affiliates of Central New Jersey, P.A.
    2501 Kuser Road Hamilton, NJ 08691 (609)585-8800 Fax (609)585-1825

Thalasila, Anuradha, MD {1013058957} IntrMd, OncHem(96,INA48)
  + 2 Dimisa Drive
    Holmdel, NJ 07733

Thalassinos, Antonios, DO {1043288566} IntrMd, Anesth(99,PA77)<NJ-ACMCITY>
  + AtlantiCare Regional Medical Center/City Campus
    1925 Pacific Avenue Atlantic City, NJ 08401 (609)345-4000

Thalayur, Keerti, MD {1194047068}
  + Advocare West Deptford Pediatrics
    646 Kings Highway West Deptford, NJ 08096 (856)879-2887 Fax (856)879-2855
  + The Cooper Hospital System-Univ Hospital
    3 Cooper Plaza/Suite 215 Camden, NJ 08103 (856)342-2001

Thaler, Adam M., DO {1386887461} Anesth(09,OH75)
  + Virtua Memorial
    175 Madison Avenue Mount Holly, NJ 08060 (609)261-1660 Fax (609)261-4454

Thalody, George V., MD {1679634778} IntrMd, Nephro(73,SWI07)
  + Thalody Medical Associates
    240 Williamson Street/Suite 400 Elizabeth, NJ 07207 (908)352-0560 Fax (908)352-4066

Thalody, Lucyamma, MD {1790892941} IntrMd(69,INA16)
  + Thalody Medical Associates
    240 Williamson Street/Suite 400 Elizabeth, NJ 07207 (908)352-0560 Fax (908)352-4066

Thalody, Nina George, MD {1295979607}
  + Thalody Medical Associates
    240 Williamson Street/Suite 400 Elizabeth, NJ 07207 (908)432-8140 Fax (908)352-4066

Thalody, Usha George, MD {1740472885} IntrMd(02,INA97)
  + Thalody Medical Associates
    240 Williamson Street/Suite 400 Elizabeth, NJ 07207 (908)352-0560 Fax (908)352-4066

Thamburaj, Ravi Daniel, DO {1760503205} Pedtrc(02,OH75)<NJ-NWRKBETH>
  + Newark Beth Israel Medical Center
    201 Lyons Avenue Newark, NJ 07112 (973)926-7000 Fax (973)923-2441

Thame, Craig H., MD {1790760734} RadDia(93,NJ05)<NJ-HACKNSK>
  + New Century Imaging at Oradell
    555 Kinderkamack Road Oradell, NJ 07649 (201)599-1311 Fax (201)599-8333

Thamman, Prem, MD {1609837905} IntrMd(64,INA8Z)<NJ-HACKNSK>
  + Lodi Internists
    361 Garibaldi Avenue Lodi, NJ 07644 (973)773-3556 Fax (973)773-2337

Thamman, Vijay K., MD {1790746097} CdvDis, IntrMd(63,INA23)<NJ-HACKNSK>
  + Lodi Internists
    361 Garibaldi Avenue Lodi, NJ 07644 (973)773-3556 Fax (973)773-2337

Thani, Suresh R., MD {1265496806} ObsGyn, Gyneco(77,JMA01)<NJ-STBARNMC, NJ-NWRKBETH>
  + Professional Ob-Gyn
    566 Nye Avenue Irvington, NJ 07111 (973)399-9155 Fax (973)399-3936

Thapar, Garima, MD {1689963464} EnDbMt(08,INA70)
  + Endocrinology Associates
    1 Brace Road/Suite B Cherry Hill, NJ 08034 (856)470-9029 Fax (856)428-4053

Thatcher, Jacob Bryce, DO {1992263438} Urolgy
  + 1 Medical Center Drive/Suite 162
    Stratford, NJ 08084 (856)566-6946

Thaung, Diana W., MD {1689985368}<NJ-MONMOUTH>
  + Monmouth Medical Center
    300 Second Avenue/SW251 Long Branch, NJ 07740 (732)923-6769

Thawabi, Mohammad, MD {1356730881} IntrMd<NJ-NWRKBETH>
  + Newark Beth Israel Medical Center
    201 Lyons Avenue/Internal Med Newark, NJ 07112 (201)815-3339

Thawani, Kalpana, MD {1033148259} IntrMd, IntHos(93,UZB03)<NJ-KMHSTRAT>
  + Osborn Family Health Center
    1601 Haddon Road Camden, NJ 08103 (856)757-3700 Fax (856)668-8479

The, Andrew Hong-Siang, MD {1467602201} IntrMd
  + Samuel HS The MD, PA
    130 Orient Way/Suite BB Rutherford, NJ 07070 (201)438-6916 Fax (201)438-4227

The, Arlene H., MD {1790835106} Ophthl
  + Drs. The & Sinatra
    348 Summit Avenue Hackensack, NJ 07601 (201)343-9300

The, Samuel H., MD {1588637292} IntrMd, PulDis(69,IND10)<NJ-HACKNSK>
  + Samuel HS The MD, PA
    130 Orient Way/Suite BB Rutherford, NJ 07070 (201)438-6916 Fax (201)438-4227
  + Samuel HS The MD, PA
    33 East Century Road Paramus, NJ 07652 (201)438-6916 Fax (201)265-3646

The, Tiong Gwan, MD {1790819951} PedCrC, Pedtrc(84,WIN01)<NJ-STPETER, NJ-CENTRAST>
  + St. Peter's University Hospital
    254 Easton Avenue/Pediatrics New Brunswick, NJ 08901 (732)745-8600 Fax (732)745-0857
    ttheccanat@saintpetersuh.com

Theccanat, Stephen M., MD {1831261288} Psychy(87,INA94)<NJ-MONMOUTH>
  + Monmouth Medical Center
    300 Second Avenue/Psychiatry Long Branch, NJ 07740 (732)222-5200

Theivanayagam, Kalyani, MD {1598878910} IntrMd(95,GRN01)<NJ-EASTORNG>
  + Drs. Ganesh and Theivanayagam
    24 Park Avenue West Orange, NJ 07052 (973)669-8181 Fax (973)669-1687

Thek, Wesley K., MD {1275562837} EmrgMd(94,VA04)
  + Am/PM Walk in Urgent Care Center
    19 South Washington Avenue Bergenfield, NJ 07621 (201)387-0177 Fax (201)387-0114
    md@ampmwalkinurgentcare.com

Thekumparampil, Rani Koshy, MD {1588922389}<NJ-NWRK-BETH>
  + Newark Beth Israel Medical Center
    201 Lyons Avenue Newark, NJ 07112 (973)926-7040 Fax (973)926-6452

Then, Ryna K., MD {1427346303}
  + Cooper University Cardiology
    3 Cooper Plaza/Suite 320 Camden, NJ 08103 (856)968-8349

Theocharides, Thomas, MD {1528014412} ObsGyn(80,QU06)<NJ-MONMOUTH>
  + Ocean Obstetric and Gynecologic Associates
    804 West Park Avenue/Building A Ocean, NJ 07712 (732)695-2040 Fax (732)493-1640

Theophilopoulos, Constantine G., MD NnPnMd, Pedtrc(92,FL03)
  + On-Site Neonatal Partners
    1000 Haddonfield-Berlin Road/Suite 210 Voorhees, NJ 08043 (727)271-5650 Fax (856)782-2213
    dtheophi@tampabay.rr.com

Thepmankorn, Pidok, MD {1073508438} EmrgMd, Hemato, IntrMd(68,JAP89)<NJ-HOBUNIMC>
  + 30 Copeland Road
    Denville, NJ 07834 (973)361-4467

Therattil, Maya Rose, MD {1306930664} PhysMd, OrtSpn, IntrMd(98,INA94)<NY-MNTFWEIL, NY-MNTFMOSE>
  + St. Lawrence Rehabilitation Center
    2381 Lawrenceville Road Lawrenceville, NJ 08648 (609)896-8152

Therrien, Philip J., MD {1043315401} PedOrt, SrgOrt(84,MA16)<NJ-RWJUBRUN, NJ-CHLSMT>
  + Pediatric Orthopedic Associates, P.A.
    585 Cranbury Road/Suite A East Brunswick, NJ 08816 (732)390-1160 Fax (732)390-8449
  + Pediatric Orthopedic Associates, P.A.
    3700 State Route 33 Neptune, NJ 07753 (732)390-1160 Fax (732)897-4205
  + Children's Specialized Hospital
    150 New Providence Road/PediOrtho Mountainside, NJ 08816 (908)233-3720

Theune, Lillian J., DO {1053383869} IntrMd(93,PA77)<NJ-HCK-TSTWN, NJ-MORRISTN>
  + Plaza Family Care
    657 Willow Grove Street/Suite 401 Hackettstown, NJ 07840 (908)850-7800 Fax (908)850-7801
  + Plaza Family Care
    245 Main Street/Suite 300 & 302 Chester, NJ 07930 (908)879-6738

Thiagarajah, Christopher Krishan, MD {1952435919} Ophthl(02,DC03)
  + Eye Care and Surgery Center
    592 Springfield Avenue Westfield, NJ 07090 (908)789-8999 Fax (908)789-1379

Physicians by Name and Practice Address

Thierman, David H., MD {1265429732} RadDia(79,PA07)<NJ-STJOSHOS>
+ St. Joseph's Regional MedCtr-Ambulatory Imaging Ctr
1135 Broad Street/3rd Floor/Suite 4   Clifton, NJ 07013   (973)569-6300
+ Imaging Subspecialists of North Jersey LLC
703 Main Street   Paterson, NJ 07503   (973)754-2645

Thimmaiah, Manavattir B., MD {1841360138} Psychy(68,INA28)<NJ-STJOSHOS>
+ St. Joseph's Regional Medical Center
703 Main Street/Psych   Paterson, NJ 07503   (973)754-2000

Thind, Narinder K., MD {1396725586} ObsGyn(79,NJ05)<NJ-JRSYSHMC>
+ 1540 Route 138/Suite 103
Wall, NJ 07719   (732)280-2700   Fax (732)280-2785
nthind@aol.com

Thind, Pritinder K., MD {1467457614} NuclMd, RadDia, IntrMd(94,NJ05)<NJ-JRSYSHMC>
+ University Radiology Group, P.C.
579A Cranbury Road   East Brunswick, NJ 08816   (732)390-0040   Fax (732)390-1856
+ University Radiology Group
2100 Route 33/Neptune City Med Bld   Neptune, NJ 07753   (732)390-0040   Fax (732)502-0368
+ University Radiology Group
900 West Main Street   Freehold, NJ 08816   (732)462-1900   Fax (732)462-1848

Thirugnanam, Saraswathi, MD {1649250903} IntrMd(73,INDI)<NJ-RWJUHAM, NJ-CHSMRCER>
+ 2544 Nottingham Way
Trenton, NJ 08619   (609)588-9500   Fax (609)588-9595

Thirumavalavan, Vallur S., MD {1346283009} IntrMd(77,INA84)<NJ-JRSYCITY>
+ University Geriatrics & Internal Medicine Associates
1553 Highway 27/Suite 2100-2300   Somerset, NJ 08873   (732)301-2628   Fax (732)377-3319

Thirunahari, Nandan R., MD {1437462835} IntrMd
+ 206 Millburn Avenue/Apt 7B
Millburn, NJ 07041

Thiruwilwamala, Parvathy S., MD {1023056819} IntrMd(96,INDI)<NJ-STBARNMC>
+ St. Barnabas Medical Center
94 Old Short Hills Road   Livingston, NJ 07039   (973)322-5000

Tholany, Jason Joseph, MD {1922234616} Radiol, RadV&I
+ 40 Constitution Way/Suite 102
Jersey City, NJ 07305
jason.tholany@gmail.com

Thomas, Abraham S., MD {1275619611} Pedtrc(90,INA34)<NJ-STJOSHCS>
+ Pediatric Associates of Paterson
675 Broadway   Paterson, NJ 07514   (973)523-1213   Fax (973)881-7661
abethomas@worldnet.att.net
+ West Orange Pediatrics
81 Northfield Avenue/Suite 101   West Orange, NJ 07052   (973)324-5437

Thomas, Alan E., MD {1891767554} Pedtrc(92,PRO03)<NJ-OVERLOOK, NJ-MORRISTN>
+ Summit Medical Group-Berkeley Heights Campus
1 Diamond Hill Road   Berkeley Heights, NJ 07922   (908)277-8601   Fax (908)277-8706
+ Summit Medical Group
34 Mountain Boulevard/Building B   Warren, NJ 07059   (908)277-8601   Fax (908)769-8927

Thomas, Alapatt Porinchu, MD {1386601060} IntrMd(73,INA56)<NJ-NWRKBETH>
+ Tri-County Medical Associates
120 Millburn Avenue/Suite M3   Millburn, NJ 07041   (973)912-0001   Fax (973)912-0099
+ Tri-County Medical Associates
1945 Morris Avenue/Suite B   Union, NJ 07083   (973)912-0001   Fax (908)686-2637

Thomas, Alphonsa, DO {1922419779}<NJ-OCEANMC>
+ Ocean Medical Center
425 Jack Martin Boulevard   Brick, NJ 08723   (732)836-4504   Fax (732)836-4532

Thomas, Ann C., MD {1639300247} FamMed(08,GRN01)
+ Summit Medical Group
560 Springfield Avenue   Westfield, NJ 07090   (908)228-3610

Thomas, Antonio, MD {1902833684} Pedtrc, PedEmg(94,NJ05)<NJ-HACKNSK>
+ Hackensack Univ Medical Center Pediatric Emerg Room
30 Prospect Avenue   Hackensack, NJ 07601   (201)996-5430   Fax (201)996-3676
+ Hackensack University Medical Center
30 Prospect Avenue/Pediatrics   Hackensack, NJ 07601   (201)996-2000
+ 1907 Park Avenue/Suite 103
South Plainfield, NJ 07601   (908)561-2333   Fax (908)561-2443

Thomas, Brian David, MD {1386694891} IntrMd(00,NJ06)<NJ-UNVMCPRN>
+ Windsor Regional Medical Associates, LLC
300A Princeton-Hightstown Road   East Windsor, NJ 08520   (609)490-0095   Fax (609)490-0091

Thomas, Carole E., MD {1083666333} Nrolgy(90,PA02)<NJ-VIRTMHBC, NJ-VIRTBERL>
+ Neurology Associaates of South Jersey
693 Main Street/Building D   Lumberton, NJ 08048   (609)261-7600   Fax (609)265-8205
+ Advocare Neurology of South Jersey
200-B Route 73 North/Suite 2   Voorhees, NJ 08043   (609)261-7600   Fax (856)335-0406

Thomas, Cherryl L., MD {1134113640} IntrMd(86,NY08)
+ Advancing Wellness LLC
18 Centre Drive/Suite 205   Monroe Township, NJ 08831   (732)658-1375   Fax (732)658-1376
+ Advancing Wellness LLC
1445 Route 130   North Brunswick, NJ 08902   (732)658-1375   Fax (732)658-1376

Thomas, Chris, MD {1437594660} PhysMd
+ Performance Rehabilitation & Sports Injury Center
459 Watchung Avenue   Watchung, NJ 07069   (908)754-1960

Thomas, Dianne, MD {1669689360} Pedtrc(88,JMA01)
+ 165 State Street/Suite 2
Hackensack, NJ 07601   (201)457-1500   Fax (201)457-1501
diannethomasmd@gmail.com

Thomas, Elsa, MD {1801878491} IntrMd(01,PA07)<MA-BIDMCEST, MA-BIDMCWST>
+ Internal Medicine Faculty Associates
435 South Street/Suite 210   Morristown, NJ 07960   (973)971-7165   Fax (973)290-7675

Thomas, Eric David, MD {1528378072} IntrMd(08,GRN01)<NJ-STMICHL, NJ-CLARMAAS>
+ Comprehensive Women's Healthcare
44 Ridge Road   North Arlington, NJ 07031   (201)991-2880   Fax (201)991-0027
+ North Arlington Primary Care Associates, Inc.
25 Locust Avenue   North Arlington, NJ 07031   (201)991-2880   Fax (201)991-9005

Thomas, George, MD {1841392537} Anesth<NJ-STMRYPAS>
+ St. Mary's Hospital
350 Boulevard   Passaic, NJ 07055   (973)365-2840   Fax (845)357-5777

Thomas, Isabelle Marie B., MD {1164527644} Dermat(83,FRA24)<NJ-VAEASTOR>
+ VA New Jersey Health Care System-East Orange Campus
385 Tremont Avenue/Dermatology   East Orange, NJ 07018   (973)676-1000

Thomas, Jessy Joykutty, MD {1437387586} FamMed, IntrMd(09,DC03)<NJ-BAYSHORE, NJ-RIVERVW>
+ Riverside Medical Group Bayonne
432 Broadway   Bayonne, NJ 07002   (201)471-7015   Fax (201)471-7017

Thomas, Jhibu, MD {1659578797} IntrMd(03,HUN01)
+ Urgent Care - Hamilton
2222 New Jersey 33/Suite H   Hamilton, NJ 08690   (609)890-4100   Fax (609)890-4189

Thomas, Jodi, MD {1912003765} PhysMd(96,NY15)<NJ-STCLRDOV, NJ-NWTNMEM>
+ 41 Watchung Plaza/Suite 155
Montclair, NJ 07042   (973)928-8909   Fax (973)928-8928

Thomas, Jolly, MD {1790862100} Pedtrc, AdolMd(91,INA9A)
+ 18 Morris Avenue/Suite 2A
Springfield, NJ 07081   (973)379-4300   Fax (973)379-4302

Thomas, Kathleen, MD {1417031873} AlgyImmn, PedAlg(75,INA76)<NJ-CLARMAAS, NJ-TRINIJSC>
+ 206 Bergen Avenue/Suite 202
Kearny, NJ 07032   (201)246-7500   Fax (201)246-7501
+ 695 Chestnut Street
Union, NJ 07083   (201)246-7500   Fax (908)933-0112

Thomas, Kornelia, MD {1134500051}<NJ-SOMERSET>
+ RWJ University Hospital Somerset
110 Rehill Avenue   Somerville, NJ 08876   (908)685-2800

Thomas, Kurt Florian P., MD {1043274350} OrtSpn
+ Neuroscience Institute
30 Prospect Avenue   Hackensack, NJ 07601   (314)706-6488

Thomas, Mark Allen Voltis, DO {1043391618} IntrMd(95,PA77)<NJ-VIRTMHBC>
+ Virtua Memorial
175 Madison Avenue/InternalMed   Mount Holly, NJ 08060   (609)267-0700

Thomas, Mary Kathleen, MD {1417081068} Pedtrc(02,IL42)
+ NuHeights Pediatrics
1115 Clifton Avenue/Suite 101   Clifton, NJ 07013   (973)250-2970   Fax (973)250-2971
+ NuHeights Pediatrics
2 Brighton Road/Suite 404   Clifton, NJ 07013   (973)250-2970   Fax (973)250-2971

Thomas, May A., MD {1902830763} Grtrcs, IntrMd(81,PA13)<NJ-COOPRUMC>
+ Cooper University Medical Center/Camden
3 Cooper Plaza   Camden, NJ 08103   (856)342-2000
+ Cooper Senior Health Care Center
1210 Brace Road/Suite 109   Cherry Hill, NJ 08034   (856)342-2000   Fax (856)428-0050
+ The Cooper Hospital System-Univ Hospital
3 Cooper Plaza/Suite 215   Camden, NJ 08103   (856)342-2439

Thomas, Melissa Dias, MD {1538337423} PedCrC, Pedtrc(94,BRA37)<NJ-MORRISTN>
+ Morristown Medical Center
100 Madison Avenue/Pedi Crtcl Care   Morristown, NJ 07962   (973)971-7550

Thomas, Miriam, MD {1760525257} Pedtrc(92,INDI)
+ Pediatrics of Morris
16 Pocono Road/Suite 112   Denville, NJ 07834   (973)627-6010   Fax (973)625-9424

Thomas, Montrae C., MD {1124071840} AdolMd, Pedtrc(76,NJ05)<NJ-MTNSIDE, NJ-STBARNMC>
+ Park Avenue Pediatric Associates
485 Park Avenue   Orange, NJ 07050   (973)672-2770   Fax (973)672-7009

Thomas, Pauline A., MD {1871569699} Pedtrc(77,CT01)<NJ-OVERLOOK, NJ-MORRISTN>
+ Preventive Medicine & Community Health
185 South Orange Avenue/MSB F-506   Newark, NJ 07101   (973)972-9384   Fax (973)972-7625
thomasp1@umdnj.edu
+ Summit Medical Group-Berkeley Heights Campus
1 Diamond Hill Road   Berkeley Heights, NJ 07922   (973)972-9384   Fax (908)219-3045

Thomas, Prashant Jacob, MD {1285999094} RadDia<NJ-UMDNJ>
+ University Hospital
150 Bergen Street/Suite C-318   Newark, NJ 07103   (973)972-4300

Thomas, Samuel Charles, III, MD {1881653228} PedCrC, Pedtrc, IntrMd(93,PA09)<NJ-COOPRUMC>
+ Cooper University Hospital
One Cooper Plaza/Pediatrics   Camden, NJ 08103   (856)356-4935

Thomas, Sara S., MD {1659596653} Psychy(78,INDI)
+ 416 Bellevue Avenue/Suite 404
Trenton, NJ 08618   (609)278-6100
+ 721 W. Kennedy Boulevard/Room 4
Lakewood, NJ 08701   (732)431-3990

Thomas, Seymour W., MD {1831279546} FamMed(93,NJ05)<NJ-STJOSHOS>
+ Comprehensive Women's Healthcare
424 Clifton Avenue   Clifton, NJ 07011   (973)340-3700   Fax (973)340-4668

Thomas, Shilpa Ani, MD {1205359346} IntrMd<NJ-ENGLWOOD>
+ Englewood Hospital and Medical Center
350 Engle Street   Englewood, NJ 07631   (201)894-3000

Thomas, Sumi Varghese, MD {1528353547} PthAClI, PthCyt(03,INA19)
+ One Robert Wood Johnson Place/MEB 212
New Brunswick, NJ 08901   (732)235-8120

Thomas, Sunil Raj, MD {1427362698}
+ Capital Endocrinology
2 Capital Way/Suite 290   Pennington, NJ 08534   (609)303-4300   Fax (609)303-4301

Thomas, Susheela, MD {1619939642} Pedtrc, IntrMd(78,INA65)<NJ-STCLRDEN, NJ-MORRISTN>
+ Advocare Pediatric Arts
1403 Route 23 South   Butler, NJ 07405   (973)283-2200   Fax (973)283-0406
+ Advocare Pediatric Arts
1777 Hamburg Turnpike/Suite 103   Wayne, NJ 07470   (973)283-2200   Fax (973)283-0406

Thomas, Teresa E., MD {1417976531} IntrMd(88,NY45)
+ Eastern Medical Associates PC
101 Prospect Street/Suite 212   Lakewood, NJ 08701   (732)886-9400   Fax (732)905-7719

Thomas, Tijo, DO {1033577101}
+ St. Michael's Medical Center
111 Central Avenue   Newark, NJ 07102   (973)877-5000

Thomas, Timmy, MD {1508203720} OccpMd
+ EOHSI
170 Frelinghuysen Road/Rm 212   Piscataway, NJ 08854   (848)445-6071

Thomas, Tina Theresa, MD {1619104213} Surgry
+ 20 Prospect Avenue/Suite 408
Hackensack, NJ 07601   (551)996-2625   Fax (551)996-2021

Thomas, Tom, MD {1871501643} Otlryg, SrgHdN, IntrMd(05,DC03)
+ Leonard B. Kahn Head and Neck Cancer Institute
100 Madison Avenue   Morristown, NJ 07960   (973)971-7355   Fax (973)290-7393

Physicians by Name and Address

Thomas, Vinoo Sebastian, MD {1780709220} Anesth(02,NY15)<NY-MTSINAI>
+ Metropolitan Neurosurgery Associates, PA
309 Engle Street/Suite 6   Englewood, NJ 07631   (201)569-7737   Fax (201)569-1494

Thomas-Patterson, Denne Michelle, MD {1386797603}
+ Virtua Express Urgent Care-Voorhees
158 Route 73   Voorhees, NJ 08043   (610)564-4297   Fax (856)246-7231

Thompson, Dawn Dorel, MD Pedtrc(96,CA06)<NJ-HUNTRDN, NJ-STPETER>
+ RWJ University Pediatric Emergency Medicine
125 Paterson Street/MEB 342   New Brunswick, NJ 08903   (732)235-7044   Fax (732)235-9340
+ RWJ University Hospital Somerset
110 Rehill Avenue   Somerville, NJ 08876   (732)235-7044   Fax (908)231-6194

Thompson, Elizabeth Ann, MD {1023125234} EmrgMd(02,PA09)<NJ-VIRTMHBC>
+ Virtua Memorial
175 Madison Avenue/EmergMed   Mount Holly, NJ 08060   (609)267-0700   Fax (609)914-6067

Thompson, Flavius Mark, MD {1871667097} ObsGyn(73,RUS54)
+ 149 Bristol Court
Lakewood, NJ 08701   (732)905-6560   Fax (732)363-8284

Thompson, Matthew, MD {1902997760} Anesth(92,NJ06)
+ James Street Anesthesia
102 James Street/Suite 103   Edison, NJ 08820   (732)494-1444   Fax (732)494-7052

Thompson, Nicole, DO {1083977862} IntHos<NJ-KMHTURNV>
+ Kennedy Health Systems/Washington Township Campus
435 Hurffville-Cross Keys Road   Turnersville, NJ 08012   (856)218-5634   Fax (856)218-5664

Thompson, Peter N., MD {1326013509} SrgVas, Surgry(85,NJ05)<NJ-ACMCITY, NJ-ACMCMAIN>
+ AtlantiCare Regional Medical Center/City Campus
1925 Pacific Avenue/Trauma Unit   Atlantic City, NJ 08401   (609)441-8023   Fax (609)441-8178

Thompson, Robert M., MD {1760480909} SrgThr, Surgry(79,ITA23)<NJ-JRSYSHMC>
+ Jersey Shore CardioThoracic & Vascular Surgery
234 Industrial Way West/Suite A-103   Eatontown, NJ 07724   (848)208-2055   Fax (848)208-2078
+ Jersey Shore CardioThoracic & Vascular Surgery
301 Bingham Avenue/Suite A   Ocean, NJ 07712   (848)208-2055   Fax (732)988-7852

Thompson, Roger McLachlan, MD {1376526442} FamMed(82,NJ05)<NJ-RIVERVW, NJ-BAYSHORE>
+ Family Practice of Middletown
18 Leonardville Road   Middletown, NJ 07748   (732)671-0860   Fax (732)671-6467
+ Integrated Medical Alliance/IMA Medical Care Center
30 Shrewsbury Plaza   Shrewsbury, NJ 07702   (732)671-0860   Fax (732)542-2992

Thompson, Stacy Ellen, DO {1912134289} Pedtrc
+ Drs. Gruenwald & Comandatore
90 Millburn Avenue/Suite 101   Millburn, NJ 07041   (973)378-7990   Fax (973)378-7991

Thompson, Stephanie M, MD {1568669075} ObsGyn(06,NC01)
+ Rutgers- New Jersey Medical School
185 South Orange Avenue/Box 506   Newark, NJ 07103   (973)972-4300

Thomsen, Kathleen M., MD {1215067392} FamMed, OthrSp(89,NJ05)
+ 252 West Delaware Avenue
Pennington, NJ 08534   (609)818-9700   Fax (609)818-9811

Thomsen, Stephen, MD {1992373760} Nephro, IntrMd(77,ITA17)<NJ-CHRIST, NJ-MTNSIDE>
+ Hudson Essex Nephrology
510 31st Street   Union City, NJ 07087   (201)866-3322   Fax (201)866-2289
+ Hudson Essex Nephrology
123 Highland Avenue/Suite G-2   Glen Ridge, NJ 07028   (201)866-3322   Fax (973)866-2289

Thomson, Fani Jacqueline, DO {1013176247} PhysMd, PainInvt, IntrMd(03,NY75)<NJ-VALLEY, NY-MTSINAI>
+ Valley Institute for Pain
One Valley Health Plaza/3 FL   Paramus, NJ 07652   (201)634-5555   Fax (201)634-5454

Thomson, Mary Jo G., DO {1982670618} FamMed(89,PA77)<NJ-MORRISTN>
+ Blair Medical Associates PA
261 James Street/Suite 2A   Morristown, NJ 07960   (973)539-2468   Fax (973)539-7699

Thongrod, Sumena C., DO {1245479724} Anesth(05,NY75)<NJ-HACKNSK>
+ Hackensack University Medical Center
30 Prospect Avenue   Hackensack, NJ 07601   (201)996-2000
+ Hackensack University MC-Anesthesia Dept
30 Prospect Avenue/Room 2703   Hackensack, NJ 07601

(201)996-2000   Fax (201)996-3962

Thopcherla, Manjula, MD {1598782930} IntrMd, Grtrcs(90,INA39)
+ Shore Medicine, LLC
1255 Highway 70/Suite 24S   Lakewood, NJ 08701   (732)730-0020   Fax (732)730-0035
myerra@yahoo.com

Thoppil, Anoop Jose, MD {1508344128} IntMAdMd<NJ-STFRNMED>
+ St. Francis Medical Center
601 Hamilton Avenue/IntrMed   Trenton, NJ 08629   (609)949-3213

Thorell, Erik Christopher, DO {1215247820} FamMed
+ Penn Medicine at Cherry Hill
409 Route 70 East   Cherry Hill, NJ 08034   (856)427-4336

Thorne, Robert Bruce, MD {1912115791} PhysMd, PallCr, IntrMd(80,NJ06)
+ 7000 Kennedy Boulevard East/Suite 21E
West New York, NJ 07093   (201)210-8235   Fax (201)210-8235

Thornhill, Marsha Lynne, MD {1578648366} Anesth(87,NY01)<NJ-HOLYNAME>
+ Bergen Anesthesia Associates
718 Teaneck Road   Teaneck, NJ 07666   (201)833-7149   Fax (201)342-1259
+ Holy Name Hospital
718 Teaneck Road   Teaneck, NJ 07666   (201)833-3000

Thornton, Robin W., MD {1164465027} Anesth(85,GA21)
+ Burlington Anesthesia Associates
120 Madison Ave/Suite E/PO Box 174   Mount Holly, NJ 08060   (609)261-1660   Fax (609)261-1779

Thorp, Andrea Rita, DO {1023039500} Pedtrc(95,PA77)
+ Harborview KidsFirst
505 Bay Avenue   Somers Point, NJ 08244   (609)927-4235   Fax (609)927-5590
+ Harborview KidsFirst Cape May
1315 Route 9 South   Cape May Court House, NJ 08210   (609)927-4235   Fax (609)465-1539
+ Harborview Smithville
48 South New York Road/Route 9   Smithville, NJ 08244   (609)748-2900   Fax (609)748-3067

Thorpe, Michelle Lynn, MD {1891956843} Psychy(08,DMN01)
+ B. Silver, MD & G. Kaplan, MD, PA
535 Morris Avenue   Springfield, NJ 07081   (201)787-1148   Fax (973)376-0802
michellethorpe@optonline.net
+ St. Mary's Residential Home
33 Mineral Springs   Passaic, NJ 07055   (973)773-3005
+ St. Mary's Hospital - Behavioral Health Services
530 Main Avenue   Passaic, NJ 07081   (973)470-3056

Thosani, Maya K., MD {1528248747} Dermat(04,NJ03)
+ The American Skin and Cancer Center
25 First Avenue/Suite 113   Atlantic Highlands, NJ 07716   (732)872-2007

Thota, Sreevani, MD {1912232695} IntrMd
+ Total Cardiology Care
120 Franklin Street   Jersey City, NJ 07307   (201)216-9791   Fax (201)216-1362

Thrower, Albert B., MD {1083663173} SrgOrt, IntrMd(77,PA09)<NJ-OVERLOOK>
+ Summit Medical Group
574 Springfield Avenue   Westfield, NJ 07090   (908)673-7227   Fax (908)232-0540
abtmd@comcast.net

Thukkaram, Kavitha, MD {1003854282} IntrMd(98,INA04)<NJ-RBAYPERT, NJ-RWJURAH>
+ Prime Medical Care LLC
212 Bridge Street   Metuchen, NJ 08840   (732)632-1700   Fax (732)632-1704

Thum, Robert G., MD {1265492102} IntrMd, PulDis(80,MEX03)<NJ-HACKNSK>
+ Pulmonary & Medical Associates of Pasack Valley
466 Old Hook Road/Suite 26   Emerson, NJ 07630   (201)261-0821   Fax (201)261-0823

Thumar, Adeep Bhagvanji, MD {1245425495} Surgry
+ Summit Medical Group-Berkeley Heights Campus
1 Diamond Hill Road   Berkeley Heights, NJ 07922   (908)273-4300   Fax (908)790-6576
+ Summit Medical Group
315 East Northfield Road/Suite 1-E   Livingston, NJ 07039   (908)273-4300   Fax (973)535-1450
+ Summit Medical Group Florham Park Campus
150 Park Avenue   Florham Park, NJ 07922   (908)273-4300

Thur, Paul C., MD {1801895073} Urolgy(99,NY09)<NJ-UNDRWD, NJ-OURLADY>
+ New Jersey Urology, LLC
2401 East Evesham Road/Suite F   Voorhees, NJ 08043   (856)673-1600   Fax (856)988-0636
+ Delaware Valley Urology LLC
17 West Red Bank Avenue/Suite 303   Woodbury, NJ 08096   (856)673-1600   Fax (856)985-4583
+ New Jersey Urology LLC

2090 Springdale Road/Suite D   Cherry Hill, NJ 08043   (856)751-9010   Fax (856)985-9908

Tibaldi, Kim Nguyen, MD {1346309531} Nephro, IntrMd(99,NY08)<NJ-STBARNMC>
+ St. Barnabas Medical Center Renal Transplant Center
94 Old Short Hills Road   Livingston, NJ 07039   (973)322-5065

Tibb, Amit Singh, MD {1811914856} IntrMd(00,INA87)<NY-VAS-SAR>
+ VMG Respiratory Health & Pulmonary Medicine
1200 East Ridgewood Avenue   Ridgewood, NJ 07450   (201)689-7755   Fax (201)689-0521
+ Respiratory Health & Critical Care Associates
44 Godwin Avenue/Suite 201   Midland Park, NJ 07432   (201)689-7755   Fax (201)689-0521
+ Valley Health System
223 North Van Dien Avenue   Ridgewood, NJ 07450   (201)447-8000

Tiedemann, Richard N., MD {1952394132} Surgry, IntrMd(65,NJ05)
+ 1100 Rahway Road
Scotch Plains, NJ 07076   (908)625-8036   Fax (908)754-5907

Tiedrich, Allan D., MD {1174690242} PhysMd(77,DC03)
+ 1304 South Avenue
Plainfield, NJ 07062   (732)769-7999   Fax (732)469-5816

Tiefenbrunn, Larry J., MD {1336118025} Pedtrc, AdolMd(82,NY46)<NJ-STPETER, NJ-RWJUBRUN>
+ Tiefenbrunn & Fortin Pediatrics, PA
503 Cranbury Road   East Brunswick, NJ 08816   (732)390-8400   Fax (732)390-8970

Tien, Huey-Chung, MD {1720010820} NnPnMd, Pedtrc(76,TAI05)<NJ-STBARNMC>
+ NICU Associates at Saint Barnabas
94 Old Short Hills Road   Livingston, NJ 07039   (973)322-5437   Fax (973)322-8833

Tieng, Fortunata T., MD {1386605921} IntrMd, Nephro(71,PHI10)
+ 91 Main Street
Paterson, NJ 07505   (973)278-3800

Tierney, Kevin J., MD {1205135761} EmrgMd(11,NJ05)
+ St. Clare's Hospital-Denville Campus
25 Pocono Road   Denville, NJ 07834   (908)461-1486

Tierney, Peter C., MD {1467524405} FamMed(83,VA01)<NJ-CHS-FULD, NJ-UNVMCPRN>
+ Plainsboro Family Physicians
666 Plainsboro Road   Plainsboro, NJ 08536   (609)275-8100   Fax (609)275-6133

Tiesi, Gregory J., MD {1942464003}
+ 3312 Hudson Avenue/Apt 5J
Union City, NJ 07087

Tievsky, Erika Fiorella, DO {1902225584} IntrMd
+ Valley Medical Group
140 Route 17 North/Suite 302   Paramus, NJ 07652   (201)444-2646   Fax (201)689-6009

Tiger, Arthur H., MD {1154483063} SrgOrt, IntrMd(64,NY19)
+ Orthopedic Associates of West Jersey
600 Mount Pleasant Avenue/Suite A   Dover, NJ 07801   (973)989-0888   Fax (973)989-0885
ateegs@aol.com
+ 8 Glenbrook Drive
Mendham, NJ 07945   (201)826-3948

Tiger, Eric Harvey, MD {1689787871} Radiol, RadBdl(87,PA13)<NJ-ACMCMAIN, NJ-ACMCITY>
+ Atlantic Medical Imaging, LLC.
72 West Jimmie Leeds Road   Galloway, NJ 08205   (609)677-9729   Fax (609)653-8764
+ Atlantic Medical Imaging, LLC.
401 Bethel Road   Somers Point, NJ 08244   (609)677-9729
+ Atlantic Medical Imaging, LLC.
421 Route 9 North   Cape May Court House, NJ 08205   (609)677-9729   Fax (609)652-6270

Tijani, Hakeem Gbolahan, MD {1376777631} PulDis, CritCr, IntrMd
+ 0072 34th Street
Fair Lawn, NJ 07410   (201)417-0450

Tikoo, Ravinder Kumar, MD {1780713255} Nrolgy(91,IA02)
+ Summit Medical Arts
9225 John F Kennedy Boulevard   North Bergen, NJ 07047   (201)869-2707

Tiku, Moti L., MD {1780758763} Rheuma, IntrMd, Immuno(67,INDI)
+ University Geriatrics & Internal Medicine Associates
1553 Highway 27/Suite 2100-2300   Somerset, NJ 08873   (732)301-2628   Fax (732)377-3319
+ UH- Robert Wood Johnson Med
125 Paterson Street   New Brunswick, NJ 08901   (732)301-2628   Fax (732)235-6482

Tilak, Samir Shripad, MD {1760443519} RadDia(95,MA05)<NJ-OURLADY>
+ South Jersey Radiology Associates, P.A.
748 Kings Highway   West Deptford, NJ 08096   (856)848-4998   Fax (856)853-7362
+ South Jersey Radiology Associates, P.A.
Severan Profess Mews/Suite 105   Sewell, NJ 08080   (856)848-4998   Fax (856)589-6142
+ South Jersey Radiology Associates, P.A.
100 Carnie Boulevard/Suite B-5   Voorhees, NJ 08096   (856)751-0123   Fax (856)751-0535

Tilak, Vasanti A., MD {1699700443} Anesth(80,INA26)<NJ-UMDNJ>
+ University Physician Associates
140 Bergen Street/ACC Level C   Newark, NJ 07103   (973)972-2700   Fax (973)972-2739

Tilara, Amy N., MD {1477711794} IntrMd, Gastrn<NY-PRSBWEIL>
+ Advanced Gastroenterology Associates LLC
475 County Road/Suite 201   Marlboro, NJ 07746   (646)713-7284   Fax (732)548-7408
+ Advanced Gastroenterology Associates LLC
403 Candlewood Commons/Building 4   Howell, NJ 07731   (646)713-7284   Fax (732)548-7408

Tillack, Lindsey Ann, MD {1285947911} EmrgMd<NJ-STJOSHOS>
+ St Joseph's Medical Center Emergency
703 Main Street   Paterson, NJ 07503   (973)754-2240   Fax (973)754-2249

Tillem, Michael P., MD {1215113311} IntrMd(80,MEX03)<NJ-STBARNMC, NJ-NWRKBETH>
+ 70 Wilkshire Boulevard
Randolph, NJ 07869   (973)895-4372   Fax (973)895-3568

Tilluckdharry, Natasha S., MD {1104138775}
+ 140 Mayhill Street/Apt 429
Saddle Brook, NJ 07663   (908)967-7279

Tilson, Morris A., MD {1851363964} IntrMd(79,MEX34)<NJ-VALLEY, NY-ARDNHILL>
+ Sovereign Medical Group
85 Harristown Road/Suite 104   Glen Rock, NJ 07452   (201)855-8300   Fax (201)857-2541

Timins, Julie K., MD {1881776185} RadDia, NuclMd(71,PA02)
+ 20 Footes Lane
Morristown, NJ 07960   (973)267-7847
+ Hirsch & Ratakonda MD, PA
290 Madison Avenue/Suite 4   Morristown, NJ 07960   (973)267-7847   Fax (973)538-6565

Timmapuri, Ajaz J., MD {1215983143} FamMed(69,INDI)
+ 2061 Klockner Road
Hamilton, NJ 08690   (609)890-1002   Fax (609)890-6207

Timmapuri, Sarah L., MD {1356392088} IntrMd, CdvDis(91,IL06)<NJ-HACKNSK>
+ Bergen Invasive Cardiovascular Consultants
211 Essex Street/Suite 306   Hackensack, NJ 07601   (201)343-2050   Fax (201)343-4512

Timmerman, Lori D., DO {1780848051} Surgry
+ Salem Medical Group
4 Bypass Road/Suite 101   Salem, NJ 08079   (215)498-6267   Fax (856)935-4382
lorianddaniel@gmail.com

Timms, Brian Daniel, DO {1811955875} IntrMd(03,NJ75)<CT-HARTFRD>
+ AtlantiCare Ambulatory Internal Medicine Clinic
1401 Atlantic Avenue/Suite 2600   Atlantic City, NJ 08401   (609)572-6055   Fax (609)572-6021

Timms, Diane De Lisi, DO {1083874069} ObsGyn, MtFtMd(04,NJ75)<NJ-COOPRUMC>
+ Drs. Rhee and Timms
3 Cooper Plaza/Suite 221   Camden, NJ 08103   (856)342-2965   Fax (856)365-1967

Tindoc, Lorelane Pagulayan, MD {1003012410} FamMed
+ Lucila Medical P.C.
780 Allwood Road   Clifton, NJ 07012   (973)249-6202   Fax (973)249-6203

Ting, Leon L., MD {1740242791} CritCr, PulDis, IntrMd(97,NY08)<NJ-HACKNSK>
+ University Respiratory Medicine, P.A.
75 Summit Avenue   Hackensack, NJ 07601   (201)487-4595   Fax (201)487-0641

Tinianow, Lloyd N., MD {1114983756} NnPnMd<NJ-KMHSTRAT>
+ Kennedy Memorial Hospital-University Medical Center
18 East Laurel Road   Stratford, NJ 08084   (856)346-6208

Tinkelman, Brad J., MD {1730133158} Hdache, Nrolgy(92,PA07)
+ 11 Saddlehorn Drive
Cherry Hill, NJ 08003

Tintea, Petru Ion, MD {1124041587} Psychy(74,ROM01)<NJ-VAEASTOR>
+ VA New Jersey Health Care System-East Orange Campus
385 Tremont Avenue   East Orange, NJ 07018   (973)676-1000

Tinti, Meredith Sarah, MD {1003900952} Surgry, SrgCrC, SrgTrm(00,PA09)<NJ-RWJUBRUN>
+ UH- Robert Wood Johnson Med
125 Paterson Street/Ste 4100/Srgry   New Brunswick, NJ 08901   (732)828-3000
+ UH- RWJ Medical School
One Robert Wood Johnson Place   New Brunswick, NJ 08903   (732)235-5600

Tintorer, Christine C., MD {1114101409} Psychy(04,NJ03)
+ Monmouth Medical Center
75 North Bath Avenue   Long Branch, NJ 07740   (732)923-8500   Fax (732)923-5277

Tiongco, Judith Perlas, MD {1669591491} IntrMd(92,PHI02)<NJ-OVERLOOK>
+ Maron & Rodrigues Medical Group, LLC.
10 James Street/Suite 150   Florham Park, NJ 07932   (973)822-2000   Fax (973)822-2001
+ Associates in Primary Care, P.A.
25 East Willow Street   Millburn, NJ 07041   (973)822-2000   Fax (973)379-5324

Tiosecco, Jennifer Anne, MD {1306801667} NnPnMd, Pedtrc, IntrMd(98,PHI09)<NJ-STPETER>
+ AtlantiCare - Neonatology Department
65 West Jimmie Leeds Road   Pomona, NJ 08240   (609)404-3816   Fax (609)404-3818

Tipermas, Alan, MD {1306984844} Psychy(80,NC07)
+ 815 Executive Drive
Princeton, NJ 08540   (609)252-9919   Fax (609)252-0023

Tirmal, Viraj Vijay, MD {1164608568} IntrMd, IntHos(03,JMA01)<NJ-VIRTVOOR>
+ Advocare, LLC.
402 Lippincott Drive   Marlton, NJ 08053   (856)504-8028   Fax (856)504-8029

Tirmazi, Syed Jawad H, MD {1073656419} Psychy<NJ-TRENTPSY>
+ Trenton Psychiatric Hospital
Sullivan Way/PO Box 7600   West Trenton, NJ 08628   (609)633-1501

Tirri, Carmelina, MD {1710919253} Pedtrc, IntrMd(95,NJ05)<NJ-HACKNSK, NJ-VALLEY>
+ Milestones Pediatric Group PA
11 East Oak Street   Oakland, NJ 07436   (201)485-7557   Fax (201)485-7556
melinat@optonline.net

Tirunahari, Vijaya Latha, MD {1942221940} IntrMd, PulDis, CritCr(92,INA39)
+ Pulmonary Internists, PA
2 Lincoln Highway/Suite 301   Edison, NJ 08820   (732)549-7380   Fax (732)548-8216
+ Pulmonary Internists, PA
3 Hospital Plaza/Suite 205   Old Bridge, NJ 08857   (732)360-2255

Tiruvury, Hemavarna, MD {1942436340} InfDis, IntrMd(04,INA83)<NJ-STBARNMC, NJ-OVERLOOK>
+ Middlesex Infectious Diseases
200 Perrine Road/Suite 229   Old Bridge, NJ 08857   (732)910-6961   Fax (908)325-1940
tiruvurymd@gmail.com

Tisch, Bruce H., MD {1932117629} FrtInf, ObsGyn(70,ITA01)<NJ-HACKNSK, NJ-ENGLWOOD>
+ Ob-Gyn Associates of Englewood
177 North Dean Street/Suite 208   Englewood, NJ 07631   (201)569-0200   Fax (201)569-8287

Tischler, Charles D., MD {1376557850} SrgCrC, Surgry(75,NJ05)<NJ-VAEASTOR, NJ-UMDNJ>
+ VA New Jersey Health Care System-East Orange Campus
385 Tremont Avenue/Surgry   East Orange, NJ 07018   (973)676-1000   Fax (973)675-3238

Tisdale, Avian L., MD {1740297076} Pedtrc, EmrgMd, IntHos(06,DMN01)<NJ-KMHTURNV, NJ-ACMCITY>
+ Kennedy Health Systems/Washington Township Campus
435 Hurffville-Cross Keys Road   Turnersville, NJ 08012   (856)346-7985
+ AtlantiCare Regional Medical Center/City Campus
1925 Pacific Avenue   Atlantic City, NJ 08401   (609)441-8087
+ Nemours Dupont Pediatrics
1925 Pacific Avenue   Atlantic City, NJ 08012   (609)345-4000   Fax (609)572-8523

Tishuk, Pavel, MD {1205088572} Nrolgy, IntrMd(89,BLA02)
+ Neurologic Arts Associated, LLC.
183 High Street/Suite 1200   Newton, NJ 07860   (973)300-0579   Fax (973)300-5535

Tismenetsky, Mikhail, MD {1205029212} PthAClp(02,MI07)<NJ-ENGLWOOD>
+ Englewood Pathologists
350 Engle Street   Englewood, NJ 07631   (201)894-3420   Fax (201)871-2269
+ Englewood Hospital and Medical Center
350 Engle Street/Path   Englewood, NJ 07631   (201)894-3000

Titton, Barry Sheldon, MD {1053654186} ObsGyn(73,PA07)<NJ-ACMCITY, NJ-ACMCMAIN>
+ 7503 Bayshore Drive
Margate City, NJ 08402   (609)822-7030   Fax (609)487-0740

Titton, Ross Lewis, MD {1144220799} RadDia, RadV&I(96,FL02)
+ South Jersey Radiology Associates, P.A.
748 Kings Highway   West Deptford, NJ 08096   (856)848-4998   Fax (856)853-7362
+ South Jersey Radiology Associates, P.A.
Severan Profess Mews/Suite 105   Sewell, NJ 08080   (856)848-4998   Fax (856)589-6142
+ SJRA South Jersey Radiology Associates, P.A.
113 East Laurel Road   Stratford, NJ 08096   (856)566-2552

Titus, Benny Elizabeth, MD {1316923683} Psychy(93,INA87)
+ 901 Coventry Center
Phillipsburg, NJ 08865

Titus, Puthanpura J., MD Psychy(64,INDI)
+ 12 Serpentine Drive
Clinton, NJ 08809   (908)638-4161

Tiu, Evelyn Venzon, MD {1750335253} IntrMd, InfDis(88,PHI32)<NJ-SHOREMEM, NJ-BURDTMLN>
+ Infectious Disease Physicians PA
1001 Briggs Road/Suite 250   Mount Laurel, NJ 08054   (856)866-7466   Fax (856)866-9088

Tiu, Gladys Tompar, MD {1871810788} Psychy(DMN01)<NJ-UNIVBHC>
+ University Medical Group/UMDNJ
125 Paterson Street/Suite 2200   New Brunswick, NJ 08901   (732)235-7647   Fax (732)235-7677

Tiwari, Ramrakshah, MD {1801833710} EmrgMd, IntrMd(89,NJ05)<NJ-VIRTVOOR>
+ Virtua Voorhees
100 Bowman Drive/EmergMed   Voorhees, NJ 08043   (856)247-3000

Tiyyagura, Satish Reddy, MD {1457501363} ClCdEl, CdvDis, CarNuc(99,PA02)<NY-MTSINAI, NJ-STJOSHOS>
+ Heart & Vascular Associates of Northern Jersey
22-18 Broadway/Suite 201   Fair Lawn, NJ 07410   (201)475-5050   Fax (201)475-5522
satish.nyc@gmail.com

Tizio, Steven Christopher, MD {1285809541}
+ Atlantic Surgical Group, PA
255 Monmouth Road   Oakhurst, NJ 07755   (732)531-5445   Fax (732)531-1776
tiziomd06@gmail.com

Tjionas, Harisios, DO {1326456880}<NJ-MONMOUTH>
+ Monmouth Medical Center
300 Second Avenue   Long Branch, NJ 07740   (732)222-5200
harisios.tjionas@gmail.com

Tjoumakaris, Fotios P., MD {1720035926} SrgOrt
+ Penn Medicine at Cherry Hill
409 East Route 70   Cherry Hill, NJ 08034

Tkach-Chubay, Irina, MD {1598866550} ObsGyn(81,MOL02)
+ Totowa Ob/Gyn
525 Union Boulevard   Totowa, NJ 07512   (973)790-1117   Fax (973)790-1143

Tlamsa, Aileen P., MD {1134485493} IntrMd
+ Leonia Medical Associates, P.A.
25 Rockwood Place/Suite 120   Englewood, NJ 07631   (201)568-3335   Fax (201)568-2450

To, Jennifer Q., DO {1053675546}<NJ-STJOSHOS>
+ St. Joseph's Regional Medical Center
703 Main Street   Paterson, NJ 07503   (973)754-2000

Tobe, Edward H., DO {1487728663} Psychy(72,MO79)
+ 1001-B Greentree Exec Campus
Marlton, NJ 08053   (856)983-4940   Fax (856)983-3408

Tobia, Anthony Michael, MD {1932287257} IntrMd, Psychy(96,GRN01)<NJ-UNIVBHC, NJ-RWJUBRUN>
+ University Behavioral Health Care
671 Hoes Lane/PO Box 1392   Piscataway, NJ 08855   (732)235-5500
+ RWJ Medical School Univ of Med
675 Hoes Lane   Piscataway, NJ 08854   (732)235-5500   Fax (732)235-4430

Tobia, Dennis A., MD {1295801330} Gastrn, IntrMd(71,ITA01)
+ 123 Highland Avenue
Glen Ridge, NJ 07028   (973)744-2939   Fax (973)680-8230

Tobias, Daniel Henry, MD {1508830746} GynOnc, ObsGyn(92,MO46)<NJ-MORRISTN, NJ-OVERLOOK>
+ Carol G. Simon Cancer Center
100 Madison Avenue/Suite 4101   Morristown, NJ 07962   (973)971-5900   Fax (973)290-7257
+ Carol G. Simon Cancer Center
33 Overlook Road/Suite LL 102   Summit, NJ 07901   (973)971-6100

Tobias, David A., MD {1932227246} FamMed, GPrvMd(92,NJ05)
+ Priority Medical Care/Family Health Center
350 Grove Street   Bridgewater, NJ 08807   (908)526-1313   Fax (908)722-6031
+ Concentra Medical Centers
560 Broad Street   Newark, NJ 07102   (908)526-1313   Fax (973)643-3657

Physicians by Name and Address

Tobias, Geoffrey Wayne, MD {1326145939} Otlryg, SrgHdN(73,MA07)<NJ-ENGLWOOD>
+ 214 Engle Street
Englewood, NJ 07631 (201)567-6770 Fax (201)567-7966
info@rhinoplasty.com

Tobias-Quiroz, Aurea Bautista, MD {1174665491} Pedtrc, IntrMd(64,PHI01)
+ Children of Joy Pediatrics
134 Summit Avenue Hackensack, NJ 07601 (201)525-0077 Fax (201)525-0072

Tobiasson, Mary M., DO {1265744072} IntrMd<NJ-NWRKBETH>
+ Newark Beth Israel Medical Center
201 Lyons Avenue Newark, NJ 07112 (732)747-6190

Tobin, Matthew Steven, MD {1366425332} Urolgy(90,NY01)<NJ-JRSYSHMC, NJ-OCEANMC>
+ Atlantic Coast Urology
1944 Corlies Avenue/Suite 101 Neptune, NJ 07753 (732)840-6606 Fax (732)840-6601
+ Atlantic Coast Urology
525 Jack Martin Boulevard/Suite 304 Brick, NJ 08723 (732)840-6606 Fax (732)840-6601

Toci, Gregory R., Sr., DO {1386624849} AlgyImmn, Allrgy, Ped-Alg(93,PA77)<NJ-VIRTUAHS, NJ-OURLADY>
+ Advocare Allergy & Asthma
54 East Main Street Marlton, NJ 08053 (856)988-0570 Fax (856)988-0303
+ Advocare Allergy & Asthma
409 Kings Highway South Cherry Hill, NJ 08034 (856)988-0570 Fax (856)988-0303
+ Advocare Allergy & Asthma
239 Hurffville Crosskeys Road Sewell, NJ 08053 (856)988-0570 Fax (856)988-0303

Todd, Mary Beth, DO {1407933260} MedOnc, IntrMd(78,OK79)<NJ-RWJUBRUN>
+ Johnson & Johnson Pharmaceuticals Research
700 US Highway Route 202/PO Box 300 Raritan, NJ 08869 (908)927-3506 Fax (908)927-3800

Todd, William Upton, IV, MD {1245452499} ImmCLa, IntrMd(05,PA13)<NJ-ACMCITY>
+ AtlantiCare Regional Medical Center/City Campus
1925 Pacific Avenue/Pathology Atlantic City, NJ 08401 (609)441-8063 Fax (609)441-2107

Toder, Stephen Paul, MD {1679671861} Radiol, RadDia(76,NY19)
+ Woodland Radiology
743 Northfield Avenue West Orange, NJ 07052 (973)669-5200

Todi, Neelam T., MD {1427084268} OncHem, MedOnc, IntrMd(96,PA02)<NJ-VALLEY>
+ Summit Medical Group
6 Brighton Road/2 FL Clifton, NJ 07012 (973)471-0981 Fax (973)777-5403
+ Summit Medical Group
31-00 Broadway Fair Lawn, NJ 07410 (973)471-0981 Fax (201)796-3711

Todt, Mark J., MD {1477595064} IntrMd(86,NJ05)<NJ-VIRTVOOR, NJ-VIRTBERL>
+ Drs. Damereau, Todt & Dructor
1401 Marlton Pike East/Suite 26 Cherry Hill, NJ 08034 (856)479-9400 Fax (856)281-9913

Toffey, Lisa H., MD {1699763920} IntrMd(88,NH01)<NJ-OVERLOOK>
+ Summit Internal Medicine, LLC
33 Overlook Road/Suite LO6 Summit, NJ 07901 (908)522-0050 Fax (908)516-2946

Toft, Maria Campos, MD {1659445724} Pedtrc(83,PA14)<NJ-UMDNJ, NJ-NWRKBETH>
+ Newark Community Health Center, Inc.
741 Broadway Newark, NJ 07104 (973)675-1900 Fax (973)676-1396
+ University Hospital
150 Bergen Street/Ambltry Pdtrcs Newark, NJ 07103 (973)675-1900 Fax (973)972-2102

Tohfafarosh, Nilofer J., MD {1053672865} FamMed
+ Patient first Urgent Care
641 US Highway Route 130 Hamilton, NJ 08691 (609)568-9383 Fax (609)568-9384

Tohme, Jacques Fuad, MD {1831166982} EnDbMt, IntrMd(74,LEB03)<NJ-VALLEY>
+ Endocrine Associates
30 West Century Drive/Suite 255 Paramus, NJ 07652 (201)444-4363 Fax (201)444-6590

Toidze, Tamara V., MD {1942581616} ObsGyn(93,GEO02)
+ CAMCare Health Corporation
817 Federal Street Camden, NJ 08103 (856)541-2229 Fax (856)964-0597

Tokat, Ikbal, MD {1770723652} Pedtrc(98,TUR19)
+ NuHeights Pediatrics
1115 Clifton Avenue/Suite 101 Clifton, NJ 07013 (973)250-2970 Fax (973)250-2971
+ NuHeights Pediatrics
2 Brighton Road/Suite 404 Clifton, NJ 07013 (973)250-2970 Fax (973)250-2971

Tokazewski, Jeffrey Thomas, MD {1932139094} FamMed(98,NJ06)
+ PennCare South Jersey Family Medicine
55 Lakeview Drive North/Suite A Gibbsboro, NJ 08026 (856)783-1777 Fax (856)783-8519
+ PennCare South Jersey Family Medicine
55 Haddonfield-Berlin Road/Route 561 Gibbsboro, NJ 08026 (856)783-1777
+ Family Medicine Gibbsboro
63 North Lakeview Drive/Suite 201 Gibbsboro, NJ 08026 (856)783-1777

Tolea, Marilena, MD {1659521342}<NJ-HUNTRDN>
+ Hunterdon Medical Center
2100 Wescott Drive Flemington, NJ 08822 (908)788-6100 Fax (908)788-6361

Tolentino, Eduardo D., MD {1568432086} Anesth(72,PHI09)<NJ-NWRKBETH>
+ Newark Beth Israel Medical Center
201 Lyons Avenue/Anesth Newark, NJ 07112 (973)926-7000 Fax (973)282-3285

Tolentino, Ernesto A., MD {1396808143} SrgOrt, SprtMd(68,DC03)<NJ-CHRIST, NJ-JRSYCITY>
+ Drs. Tolentino & Irving MD PA
600 Pavonia Avenue/7th Floor Jersey City, NJ 07306 (201)216-9300 Fax (201)216-0091

Tolentino, John G., MD {1548289523} Pedtrc, GenPrc(77,PHI08)
+ Primary Care & Pediatrics
10 Palisade Avenue Bergenfield, NJ 07621 (201)385-9810 Fax (201)385-9812

Tolentino, Pablito L., MD {1629084785} Anesth(63,PHI08)<NJ-CHSFULD, NJ-CHSMRCER>
+ Trenton Anesthesiology Associates, PA
One Capital Way/Second Floor Pennington, NJ 08534 (609)396-4700 Fax (609)396-4900

Tolentino-Dela Cruz, Milagros P., MD {1518978816} Pedtrc, NnPnMd(71,PHI08)<NJ-TRINIWSC>
+ Trinitas Regional Medical Center-Williamson Street
225 Williamson Street/Neonatology Elizabeth, NJ 07207 (908)994-5000
+ Rutgers- New Jersey Medical School
185 South Orange Avenue/Neonatology Newark, NJ 07103 (973)972-4300

Tolerico, Christopher S., MD {1982627451} FamMed, EmrgMd(86,NJ06)<NJ-BAYONNE>
+ Bayonne Medical Center
29th Street at Avenue E/EmrgMed Bayonne, NJ 07002 (201)858-5257

Toliver, Clifford W., MD {1942215306} ObsGyn, Gyneco(76,NJ05)<NJ-EASTORNG>
+ 310 Central Avenue/Suite 201
East Orange, NJ 07018 (973)676-6207 Fax (973)676-3974

Toliver, Tiffany Elizabeth Marie, MD {1538459698} FamMed
+ Southern Jersey Family Medical Center
1301 Atlantic Avenue Atlantic City, NJ 08401 (609)572-0000 Fax (609)572-0039
+ Southern Jersey Family Medical Centers Inc.
1125 Atlantic Avenue Atlantic City, NJ 08401 (609)572-0000 Fax (609)348-1157

Toller-Artis, Erin Corrine, DO {1881965051} AlgyImmn, Pedtrc, IntrMd(10)<PA-ARHTRRDL, NJ-COOPRUMC>
+ Allergy & Asthma Care, P.C.
213 North Haddon Avenue Haddonfield, NJ 08033 (856)795-5600 Fax (856)795-6644
+ Allergy & Asthma Care, P.C.
2301 East Evesham Road/Suite 207 Voorhees, NJ 08043 (856)795-5600 Fax (856)795-6644

Toloui, Gerald J., MD {1144202599} RadDia, NuclMd(69,IRA01)<NJ-BURDTMLN>
+ Cape Radiology
4011 Route 9 South/PO Box 244 Rio Grande, NJ 08242 (609)886-0100

Tolston, Evelyn, MD {1528066834} IntrMd, AlgyImmn, ImmAsm(82,UKR25)<NY-NYUTISCH, NY-BETHPETR>
+ Allergy & Immunology
19-21 Fairlawn Avenue Fair Lawn, NJ 07410 (201)791-9779

Tom, Valerie, MD {1295820470} Pedtrc, IntrMd(97,NJ05)<NJ-STBARNMC, NJ-ATLANTHS>
+ Touchpoint Pediatrics
17 Watchung Avenue Chatham, NJ 07928 (973)665-0900 Fax (973)665-0901

Toma, Cornelius, MD {1003966482} IntrMd(63,ROM01)<NJ-CHSMRCER>
+ 8 Quakerbridge Plaza
Trenton, NJ 08619 (609)586-9666 Fax (609)586-6847

Toma, Wadie, MD {1821163437} IntrMd, Rheuma(82,EGY04)
+ Center for Arthritis & Rheumatology
904 Oak Tree Road/Suite J South Plainfield, NJ 07080 (732)869-1002 Fax (732)869-1012
+ Center for Arthritis & Rheumatism
3 Hospital Plaza/Suite 409 Old Bridge, NJ 08857 (732)869-1002 Fax (732)869-1012
+ Center for Arthritis & Rheumatology
3350 Route 138/Suite 212 Wall, NJ 07080 (732)235-7217

Tomaino, Jeanne, MD {1629050760} EmrgMd, IntrMd(84,DMN01)<NJ-KIMBALL, NJ-RIVERVW>
+ Drs. Randazzo and Tomaino
225 State Route 35/Suite 102B Red Bank, NJ 07701 (732)530-3433 Fax (732)758-1953

Tomaino, Alfred C., MD {1033292883} PhysMd(94,NJ05)<NJ-COOPRUMC>
+ Cinnaminson Center
1700 Wynwood Drive Cinnaminson, NJ 08077 (856)755-1616 Fax (856)755-0098

Tomar, Raghuraj S., MD {1467412858} IntrMd(81,INA30)
+ Excel Care Alliance, LLC
49 South State Street Vineland, NJ 08360 (856)696-9697 Fax (856)696-9698
+ Community Health Care, Inc.
319 Landis Avenue/Suites A & B Vineland, NJ 08360 (856)696-9697 Fax (856)696-0344

Tomaro, Robert, Jr., MD {1972586162} ObsGyn(87,MEX03)<NJ-JRSYSHMC, NJ-MONMOUTH>
+ Hackensack Meridian Medical Group Ob/Gyn, Wall
1924 Route 35/Suite 5 Wall, NJ 07719 (732)974-8404 Fax (732)974-8904
bt2811@aol.com
+ Monmouth County Associates
4788 US Highway 9 Howell, NJ 07731 (732)974-8404 Fax (732)905-1919

Tomasco, Thomas Joseph, MD {1982618104} Nephro, IntrMd, Grtrcs(85,BWI01)
+ 524 Jessica Lane
Brick, NJ 08724 (732)456-1971

Tomasello, Nicholas James, DO {1881036192} EmrgMd
+ Rowan University-School of Osteopathic Medicine
1 Medical Center Drive/Suite 162 Stratford, NJ 08084 (856)566-6708

Tomasino, Garrett M., DO {1881906527}
+ AtlantiCare Regional Medical Center/City Campus
1925 Pacific Avenue Atlantic City, NJ 08401 (609)441-8127

Tomasso, Robert A., MD {1730101882} FamMed, IntrMd(93,ITAL)<NJ-SOMERSET>
+ RWJPE Primary Care Raritan
34 East Somerset Street Raritan, NJ 08869 (908)685-2532 Fax (908)685-2542

Tomasso, Tara, MD {1225122401} FamMed(98,NJ06)
+ 612 Glassboro Road
Woodbury Heights, NJ 08097 (856)845-0323 Fax (856)845-4322

Tomasuolo, Vincent A., MD {1053317701} CritCr, IntrMd, PulDis(87,GRN01)<NJ-COMMED, NJ-KIMBALL>
+ LTR Pulmonary
552 Commons Way Toms River, NJ 08755 (732)286-9700 Fax (732)286-9722

Tomaszewski, Charles S., MD {1295794642} Urolgy(83,IL01)
+ Associated Urologists LLC
1255 Route 70 Lakewood, NJ 08701 (732)364-1664 Fax (732)364-1667

Tomaszewski, Jeffrey John, MD {1710166244} Urolgy, Surgry(06,PA02)<NJ-COOPRUMC>
+ Cooper Perinatology Associates
3 Cooper Plaza/Suite 502 Camden, NJ 08103 (856)342-3113 Fax (856)968-8499
+ 127 Church Road/Suite 400
Marlton, NJ 08053
+ The Cooper Health System at Voorhees
900 Centennial Boulevard/Suite G Voorhees, NJ 08103 (856)342-3113 Fax (856)325-6555

Tomberg, Ryan, MD {1336534676}<NJ-JRSYSHMC>
+ Jersey Shore University Medical Center
1945 Route 33 Neptune, NJ 07753 (732)776-4203 Fax (732)776-4774

Tomkovich, Kenneth R., MD {1447272919} RadDia, RadV&I, Radiol(93,NJ05)<NJ-CENTRAST>
+ CentraState Medical Center
901 West Main Street/Radiology Freehold, NJ 07728 (732)431-2000
+ Freehold Radiology Group
901 West Main Street Freehold, NJ 07728 (732)462-4844

Tomlinson-Phelan, Michelle Ann, DO {1801859517} FamMed, IntrMd(87,NJ75)<NJ-STPETER, NJ-RWJUBRUN>
+ Central Jersey Family Physicians
754 State Highway 18 North/Suite 107 East Brunswick, NJ 08816 (732)257-1171 Fax (732)257-2618

Tomlinson-Phelan, Tracy Michelle, MD {1700091709} ObsGyn, MtFtMd(01,MO02)
+ Central Jersey Family Physicians
754 State Highway 18 North/Suite 107 East Brunswick, NJ 08816 (732)257-1171 Fax (732)257-2618

Tomor, Esther M., MD {1427325810} IntrMd
+ 124 Halsey Street/Third Floor
Newark, NJ 07102

Tomovic, Senja, MD {1255568846}
+ Bergen Ear Nose & Throat Associates PA
20 Prospect Avenue/Suite 909   Hackensack, NJ 07601
(201)489-6520   Fax (201)489-6530

Tompkins, Marianne J., DO {1881763951} Anesth(85,NJ75)<NJ-STBARNMC>
+ St. Barnabas Medical Center
94 Old Short Hills Road   Livingston, NJ 07039   (973)322-5000

Ton, Mimi Nu, MD {1033178355} PedGst(98,NY19)<NJ-CHD-NWBTH, NJ-STBARNMC>
+ St. Barnabas Ambulatory Care Center
200 South Orange Avenue/Pediatrics   Livingston, NJ 07039
(973)322-7600   Fax (973)322-7685
+ 28 West Third Street/Apt 1419
South Orange, NJ 07079

Tong, Fumin, MD {1699091918} Nrolgy
+ Neurology Group of Bergen County
1200 East Ridgewood Avenue   Ridgewood, NJ 07450
(201)444-0868   Fax (201)444-5716
ftong@neurobergen.com

Tong, Shiwei, MD {1407810468} Pedtrc(85,CHNA)<NJ-STPETER>
+ 666 Plainsboro Road/Suite 1005
Plainsboro, NJ 08536   (609)275-6810   Fax (609)275-8862

Tong, Yeow C., MD {1710072301} IntrMd(71,SIN02)
+ 1098 Stelton Road
Piscataway, NJ 08854   (732)572-5950   Fax (732)572-6384

Tonnessen, Glen E., MD {1154387389} CdvDis, IntrMd(87,GRN01)
+ Hunterdon Cardiovascular Associates
1100 Wescott Drive/Suite G-3   Flemington, NJ 08822
(908)788-6471   Fax (908)788-6460
+ Hunterdon Cardiovascular Associates
1738 Route 31/Suite 210   Clinton, NJ 08809   (908)788-6471   Fax (908)823-9211

Tonzola, Anthony M., MD {1871658971} Surgry(72,NJ05)<NJ-RWJURAH, NJ-OVERLOOK>
+ 1503 Saint Georges Avenue
Colonia, NJ 07067   (732)382-0880   Fax (732)382-2657

Tonzola, Richard F., MD {1669465100} Nrolgy(73,NJ05)<NJ-STCLRDEN>
+ Central Morris Neurology
170 East Main Street/Suite 6   Rockaway, NJ 07866
(973)625-8888   Fax (973)625-7877

Toohey, Kristina, MD {1003392929} IntHos<NJ-STCLRDEN>
+ St. Clare's Hospital-Denville Campus
25 Pocono Road   Denville, NJ 07834   (973)989-3085

Toome, Birgit K., MD {1891788121} Dermat(86,NJ05)
+ Advanced Dermatology, Laser & Cosmetic Center
2466 East Chestnut Avenue   Vineland, NJ 08361   (856)691-3442   Fax (856)691-6582
btoome@aol.com

Toomey, Kathleen, MD {1720087752} Hemato, IntrMd, MedOnc(78,ITA01)<NJ-RWJUBRUN, NJ-SOMERSET>
+ Somerset Hematology Oncology Associates, P.A.
30 Rehill Avenue/2nd Floor/Suite 2500   Somerville, NJ 08876   (908)927-8700   Fax (908)927-8706

Toor, Khadija T., MD {1225290919} PedGst
+ 38 Meadowlands Parkway/Suite 205
Secaucus, NJ 07094   (551)257-7039

Toor, Saddad Zafar, MD {1649253998} CdvDis, IntrMd(03,PA09)
+ Cardiology Consultants
246 Hamburg Turnpike/Suite 201   Wayne, NJ 07470
(973)942-1141   Fax (973)942-1250

Topalian, Simon Kevork, MD {1225084353} IntrMd, IntCrd, CdvDis(98,LEB01)<NJ-COOPRUMC>
+ Cooper University Hospital
One Cooper Plaza/Cardiology   Camden, NJ 08103
(856)342-2000

Topalovic, Pavle, MD {1144399791} FamMed(66,SER03)<NJ-CHILTON>
+ 220 Hamburg Turnpike/Suite 20
Wayne, NJ 07470   (973)956-1121   Fax (973)595-8997

Topf, Andrew Irwin, MD {1669473971} Anesth, PainMd(86,NY15)<NJ-CHILTON>
+ Chilton Medical Center
97 West Parkway/PainMedicine   Pompton Plains, NJ 07444
(973)831-5000

Topfer, Steven Alan, DO {1033192455} Anesth(87,PA77)<NJ-HACKNSK>
+ Hackensack Anesthesiology Associates
140 Prospect Avenue/Suite 8   Hackensack, NJ 07601
(201)488-0066   Fax (201)488-6769
+ Hackensack University MC-Anesthesia Dept
30 Prospect Avenue/Room 2703   Hackensack, NJ 07601
(201)488-0066   Fax (201)996-3962

Topiel, Martin S., MD {1336191154} InfDis, IntrMd(79,NY19)<NJ-VIRTMHBC>
+ Infectious Disease Physicians PA
1001 Briggs Road/Suite 250   Mount Laurel, NJ 08054

(856)866-7466   Fax (856)866-9088

Topilow, Arthur A., MD {1538141387} Hemato, IntrMd, MedOnc(67,NY09)<NJ-JRSYSHMC>
+ Atlantic Hematology Oncology Associates, L.L.C.
1707 Atlantic Avenue   Manasquan, NJ 08736   (732)528-0760   Fax (732)528-0764

Topilow, Judith F., MD {1932170248} Pedtrc(67,NY09)<NJ-MONMOUTH, NJ-JRSYSHMC>
+ West Park Pediatrics
804 West Park Avenue   Ocean, NJ 07712   (732)531-0010
Fax (732)493-0903
+ West Park Pediatrics
219 Taylors Mills Road   Manalapan, NJ 07726   (732)531-0010   Fax (732)577-9643
+ West Park Pediatrics
921 East County Line Road/Suite B   Lakewood, NJ 07712
(732)370-8500   Fax (732)370-5550

Topol, Howard Ira, MD {1003016569} Pedtrc, IntrMd(06,NJ05)<NJ-VIRTVOOR, NJ-VIRTBERL>
+ CHOP Care Network at Virtua Voorhees Hospital
100 Bowman Drive   Voorhees, NJ 08043   (856)325-3000
Fax (609)261-5842
+ Virtua Memorial
175 Madison Avenue/Pediatrics   Mount Holly, NJ 08060
(856)325-3000   Fax (609)265-7931

Toporowski, Beverly Christine, MD {1972524551} FamMed
+ Virtua Family Medicine - Cooper River
6981 North Park Drive/Suite 200   Pennsauken, NJ 08109
(856)663-4949   Fax (856)663-6076

Topoulos, Arthur Peter, MD {1952331944} IntrMd, VasDis, RadV&I(92,GER25)
+ Penn Medicine at Cherry Hill
1400 East Route 70   Cherry Hill, NJ 08034
+ Penn Medicine at Woodbury Heights
1006 Mantua Pike   Woodbury Heights, NJ 08097   Fax (856)845-0535

Topper, Leonid Lev, MD {1851487193} Nrolgy, NroChl(88,LIT02)
+ The Heart Group, PA
654 Broadway   Bayonne, NJ 07002   (201)243-9999   Fax (201)243-9998
+ Summit Medical Group
34 Mountain Boulevard/Building B   Warren, NJ 07059
(201)243-9999   Fax (908)769-8927
+ Summit Medical Group
315 East Northfield Road/Suite 1-E   Livingston, NJ 07002
(973)535-3200   Fax (973)535-1450

Toppmeyer, Deborah Lynn, MD {1114004975} IntrMd, Onclgy, MedOnc(85,NY03)<NJ-RWJUBRUN>
+ Rutgers Cancer Institute of New Jersey
195 Little Albany Street/PO Box 2681   New Brunswick, NJ 08903   (732)235-9692   Fax (732)235-7493
+ RWJ University Hospital New Brunswick
One Robert Wood Johnson Place   New Brunswick, NJ 08901
(732)828-3000

Toran, Stephen A., MD {1982626206} Anesth(91,NY08)<NJ-RIVERVW>
+ Riverview Medical Center
1 Riverview Plaza/Anesthesiology   Red Bank, NJ 07701
(732)741-2700

Torbus, Andrzej Peter, MD {1699070441}<NJ-OVERLOOK>
+ Warren Primary Care
23 Mountain Boulevard   Warren, NJ 07059   (908)598-7970
Fax (908)322-4989
+ Overlook Medical Center
99 Beauvoir Avenue/PO Box 210   Summit, NJ 07902
(908)522-2000

Torchia, Michele A., MD {1336125558} ObsGyn(86,NJ05)
+ Community Health Care Inc
484 South Brewster Road   Vineland, NJ 08360   (856)696-0300   Fax (856)696-2561

Tordella, Joseph R., DO {1003901950} AeroMd, OccpMd, AlcSub(76,PA77)<NJ-ACMCITY, NJ-BURDTMLN>
+ Air, Land & Sea, LLC
Atlantic City International Ai   Egg Harbor Township, NJ 08234   (609)272-9333   Fax (609)272-9338

Torigian, Christine V., MD {1154351286} IntrMd(96,NJ05)
+ Mt. Holly Internal Medicine
409 Marlton Pike East/Suite 2   Cherry Hill, NJ 08034

Torine, Ilana J., DO {1477660264} NnPnMd
+ Meridian Medical Group - Faculty Practice
61 Davis Avenue/Suite 1/Neontlgy   Neptune, NJ 07753
(732)776-4524   Fax (732)776-4639

Tormenti, Matthew J., MD {1831396357} SrgNro<NJ-CENTRAST>
+ CentraState Medical Center
901 West Main Street/Suite 267   Freehold, NJ 07728
(732)333-8702   Fax (732)333-8703

Toro Echague, Bernardo J., MD {1083687461} IntrMd(83,BEL07)
+ 45 South Avenue West
Cranford, NJ 07016   (908)709-1212   Fax (908)709-1584

Torok, Geza, MD {1902815988} FamMed, FamMAdlt(76,HUN01)
+ Medigest Associates P.A.
21 Clyde Road/Suite 102   Somerset, NJ 08873   (732)873-

0033

Torpey, Brian M., MD {1841277985} SrgOrt(89,DC02)<NJ-JRSYSHMC, NJ-MONMOUTH>
+ Professional Orthopaedic Associates
776 Shrewsbury Avenue/Suite 201   Tinton Falls, NJ 07724
(732)530-4949   Fax (732)530-3618
+ Professional Orthopaedic Associates
1430 Hooper Avenue/Suite 101   Toms River, NJ 08753
(732)530-4949   Fax (732)349-7722
+ Professional Orthopaedic Associates
303 West Main Street   Freehold, NJ 07724   (732)530-4949
Fax (732)577-0036

Torre, Arthur J., MD {1083669709} PedAlg, UndsMd(70,NJ05)
+ 25 Hollywood Avenue
Fairfield, NJ 07004   (973)882-0880   Fax (973)882-9539

Torre, Sabino Richard, MD {1518967165} CdvDis, IntCrd, IntrMd(85,NY06)<NJ-STBARNMC, NJ-STMICHL>
+ New Jersey Cardiology Associates
375 Mount Pleasant Avenue   West Orange, NJ 07052
(973)731-9442   Fax (973)731-8030

Torre, Steven, MD {1154716744} IntrMd
+ Jersey Shore University Medical Center
1945 Route 33   Neptune, NJ 07753   (732)775-5500

Torrei, Payam G., MD {1376867150} RadDia(05,NJ06)
+ University Radiology Group, P.C.
483 Cranbury Road   East Brunswick, NJ 08816   (732)390-0030   Fax (732)390-5383
+ University Radiology Group, P.C.
16 Mountain Boulevard   Warren, NJ 07059   (732)390-0030
Fax (908)769-9141

Torrens, Javier I., MD {1578555298} IntrMd, EnDbMt(91,MA05)<NJ-UMDNJ>
+ Center for Endocrine Health
1738 Route 31 North/Suite 108   Clinton, NJ 08809
(908)735-3980   Fax (908)735-3981

Torrente, Jessica, MD {1669513099} RadDia
+ Montclair Radiology
20 High Street   Nutley, NJ 07110   (973)661-4674   Fax (973)284-0269

Torres, Alexander, DO {1629310396} EmrgMd
+ Newark Beth Israel Medical Center Emergency Medicine
201 Lyons Avenue   Newark, NJ 07112   (973)926-6671

Torres, Catherine P., MD {1457306557} IntrMd, EnDbMt(91,PHI02)<NJ-HACKNSK, NJ-HOLYNAME>
+ Diabetes Endocrinology Metabolism Specialities PA
6 Brighton Road/Suite 103   Clifton, NJ 07012   (973)471-2692   Fax (973)470-8188
+ Diabetes Endocrinology Metabolism Specialities PA
870 Palisade Avenue/Suite 203   Teaneck, NJ 07666
(973)471-2692   Fax (201)836-3571

Torres, Florinda L., MD {1932308905} GenPrc, FamMed(64,PHI01)<NJ-LOURDMED>
+ Rancocas Occupational Center
2103 Mt. Holly Road   Burlington, NJ 08016   (609)747-1891

Torres, Jonathan William, DO {1124251939} FamMed(09,NJ75)
+ University Pain Care Center
42 East Laurel Road/Suite 1700   Stratford, NJ 08084
(856)566-7010   Fax (856)566-6956

Torres, Joseph Charles, MD {1881696821} RadDia, IntrMd(92,PA09)
+ Kennedy Health System/Cherry Hill Campus
2201 Chapel Avenue West   Cherry Hill, NJ 08002
(856)661-5454   Fax (856)661-5470

Torres, Maria Elissa, MD {1629189048} Psychy, Nrolgy(01,NJ05)<NJ-STJOSHOS, NJ-WAYNEGEN>
+ St. Joseph's Regional Medical Center
703 Main Street/Psych   Paterson, NJ 07503   (973)754-2000

Torres, Mariela, MD {1780889642} EmrgMd
+ 65 Fulton Street
East Orange, NJ 07017   (201)259-7353
+ Hoboken Urgent Care
231 Washington Street   Hoboken, NJ 07030   (201)259-7353   Fax (201)754-1006
+ Newark Beth Israel Medical Center Emergency Medicine
201 Lyons Avenue   Newark, NJ 07017   (973)926-7240

Torres, Mary Jane Buenaseda, MD {1407899636} Pedtrc(99,PHI01)
+ M & M Pediatrics
70 Ramtown-Greenville Rd   Howell, NJ 07731   (732)785-0300   Fax (732)785-9420

Torres, Omar, MD {1477578607} Dermat(99,PRO01)
+ Affiliated Dermatologists
182 South Street/Suite 1   Morristown, NJ 07960   (973)267-0300   Fax (973)695-1480
+ Affiliated Dermatology
Town Centre 66/Suite 301   Succasunna, NJ 07876
(973)267-0300   Fax (973)927-7512

Torres, Stephanie A., DO {1497152219} Pedtrc
+ 5564 Snyder Avenue
Millville, NJ 08332   (732)668-2240

Physicians by Name and Address

Torres, Theresa M., MD {1326155466} Pedtrc, IntrMd(94,NJ05)<NJ-CHILTON, NJ-VALLEY>
+ Wyckoff Pediatric
  219 Everett Avenue   Wyckoff, NJ 07481   (201)891-4777   Fax (201)891-3823

Torres Cruz, Joshua, MD {1861638439} EmrgMd<NJ-COOPRUMC>
+ Cooper University Hospital
  One Cooper Plaza/EmergMed   Camden, NJ 08103   (856)342-2000

Torres Isasiga, Julian Andres, MD {1912277419} InfDis(06,COL06)<NJ-ENGLWOOD>
+ Leonia Medical Associates, P.A.
  25 Rockwood Place/Suite 120   Englewood, NJ 07631   (201)568-3335   Fax (201)568-2450

Torres-Soto, Eileen Mariette, MD {1700828647} Pedtrc(97,NJ05)
+ 792 Arrow Lane
  Ridgewood, NJ 07450

Torrey, Margaret Jennings, MD {1174576722} RadOnc, Radiol(92,NY08)<NJ-VALLEY, NY-NYUTISCH>
+ The Valley Hospital
  223 North Van Dien Avenue   Ridgewood, NJ 07450   (201)447-8220

Torsiello, Michael J., MD {1750343968} SrgPlstc, SrgRec(75,MEX03)<NJ-HOBUNIMC, NJ-HACKNSK>
+ North Jersey Plastic Surgery Associates
  290 Lafayette Avenue   Hawthorne, NJ 07506   (201)444-2999   Fax (201)444-2947

Tortora, Matthew J., MD {1184841900} PthACl<NJ-STBARNMC>
+ St. Barnabas Medical Center
  94 Old Short Hills Road   Livingston, NJ 07039   (973)322-5763

Tortosa Nacher, Rafael M., MD {1477607851} Psychy, Nrolgy(70,SPA08)<NJ-MTCARMEL, NJ-HAGEDORN>
+ Mt. Carmel Guild/ Behavioral Health System
  1160 Raymond Boulevard   Newark, NJ 07102   (973)596-3857

Toruner, Gokce, MD {1467797282} GnetCy
+ Rutgers- New Jersey Medical School
  185 South Orange Avenue/MSB F-647   Newark, NJ 07103   (201)618-2160

Toscano, Andrew, MD {1063783318} CritCr<NJ-MORRISTN>
+ Morristown Medical Center
  100 Madison Avenue   Morristown, NJ 07962   (973)656-6280

Toscano-Zukor, Amy M., DO {1821269341} EnDbMt, IntrMd(03,NJ75)<NJ-OVERLOOK, NJ-MORRISTN>
+ Summit Medical Group-Berkeley Heights Campus
  1 Diamond Hill Road   Berkeley Heights, NJ 07922   (908)277-8667   Fax (908)790-6576

Tosiello, Lorraine Lerma, MD {1659350171} IntrMd(81,NY08)
+ Visiting Nurse Association of Central Jersey
  1301 Main Street   Asbury Park, NJ 07712   (732)774-6333   Fax (732)774-0313
+ 123 Woodland Avenue
  Westfield, NJ 07090

Tossounian, Nora Zabel, MD {1184662777} IntrMd(95,MD07)<NJ-HACKNSK>
+ Hackensack UMC-Internal Medicine
  20 Prospect Avenue/Suite 613   Hackensack, NJ 07601   (551)996-8111   Fax (551)996-8445

Toth, Patrick J., MD {1346225216} RadDia(82,CT01)<NJ-HACKNSK>
+ The Imaging Center
  30 South Newman Street   Hackensack, NJ 07601   (201)488-1188   Fax (201)488-5244
+ New Century Imaging at Oradell
  555 Kinderkamack Road   Oradell, NJ 07649   (201)488-1188   Fax (201)599-8333
+ Hackensack Radiology Group, P.A.
  30 Prospect Avenue   Hackensack, NJ 07601   (201)996-2200   Fax (201)336-8451

Toturgul, David T., MD {1487813036} Pedtrc
+ Gym Spa Medical Center
  1806 Highway 35/Suite 106   Oakhurst, NJ 07755   (855)496-7721   Fax (855)496-7721

Tourkova, Marina, MD {1386790038} PsyGrt, Psychy, Psythp(81,UKR08)
+ Center of Revitalizing Psychiatry, P.C.
  795 Main Street   Hackensack, NJ 07601   (201)488-5161   Fax (201)488-5162
  mtourkova@RevitalizingPsychiatry.com

Tovmasian, Lucy Tamar, MD {1679808562} ObsGyn
+ Holy Name Physician Network
  420 Grand Avenue/Suite 202   Englewood, NJ 07631   (201)871-4040   Fax (201)871-7326

Tozzi, John Michael, MD {1093794539} SrgOrt, SprtMd, SrgOARec(83,IL42)<NJ-JRSYSHMC>
+ Orthopaedic Institute of Central Jersey
  2315A Highway 34/Suite D   Manasquan, NJ 08736   (732)974-0404   Fax (732)974-2653

+ Orthopaedic Institute of Central Jersey
  365 Broad Street   Red Bank, NJ 07701   (732)974-0404   Fax (732)933-1444
+ Orthopaedic Institute of Central Jersey
  226 Highway 37 West/Suite 203   Toms River, NJ 08736   (732)240-6060   Fax (732)240-5329

Tozzi, Robert J., MD {1811943020} PedCrd(83,NJ05)<NJ-HACKNSK>
+ Hackensack University Medical Center
  30 Prospect Avenue/Pedi Cardiology   Hackensack, NJ 07601   (201)996-2000
+ The Pediatric Center for Heart Disease
  155 Polifly Road/Suite 106   Hackensack, NJ 07601   (201)996-2000   Fax (201)342-5341

Traba, Christin M., MD {1326284977} Pedtrc
+ 34 West 31st Street
  Bayonne, NJ 07002   (201)388-3537
+ 150 Bergen Street
  Newark, NJ 07103   (973)972-5632

Trabold, Lucille A., MD {1518914688} RadOnc(91,NY08)<NJ-JFKMED>
+ JFK Medical Center
  65 James Street/Rad/Onc   Edison, NJ 08820   (732)321-7167   Fax (732)906-4915

Traboulsi, Rana, MD {1144453010} InfDis, IntrMd(01,LEB05)
+ LMA Surgical Associates
  120 White Horse Pike/Suite 103   Haddon Heights, NJ 08035   (856)795-7505   Fax (856)546-3908
+ Infectious Diseases Consultants of N.J., PA
  102 White Horse Pike   Haddon Heights, NJ 08035   (856)795-7505   Fax (856)795-8010

Tracey, Gregory Joseph, MD {1821017617} FamMed(90,DOMI)<NJ-HOBUNIMC>
+ Elan Medical Associates
  79 Hudson Street/Suite 500   Hoboken, NJ 07030   (201)653-7450   Fax (201)653-8266
  Elanmedical079@gmail.com

Tracy, Bridget, MD {1366670473} IntrMd, PallCr(09,NY0)
+ Meridian Medical Group-Palliative Care
  1 Riverview Plaza   Red Bank, NJ 07701   (732)268-8470   Fax (732)268-8459

Tracy, Toby William, DO {1316029689} FamMed(98,PA77)
+ Family Medicine Center
  279 Mathistown Road   Little Egg Harbor, NJ 08087   (609)296-1101

Trader, Catherine R., DO {1689722001} FamMed(90,NJ75)<NJ-NWTNMEM>
+ 8 Lenape Road
  Andover, NJ 07821   (973)786-0235   Fax (973)786-0315

Traeger, Eveline C., MD {1326016304} NroChl, NrlgSpec(84,NY06)<NJ-CHLSMT, NJ-CHLSOCEN>
+ Children's Specialized Hospital
  150 New Providence Road/PediNeurology   Mountainside, NJ 07092   (908)233-3720
+ Children's Specialized Hospital-Ocean
  94 Stevens Road   Toms River, NJ 08755   (732)914-1100

Traficante, Allen, MD {1023254539} InsrMd(79,NY09)
+ Drs. Dapas and Traficante
  2 Joanna Way   Chatham, NJ 07928   (973)635-6547   Fax (973)635-5826

Traflet, Robert F., MD {1609982073} RadDia, Radiol(83,NJ05)
+ Magnetic Resonance of New Jersey
  410 Centre Street   Nutley, NJ 07110   (973)661-2000
+ New Jersey Magnetic Resonance of Oradell
  550 Kinderkamack Road   Oradell, NJ 07649   (201)599-8100

Trager, Mark A., MD {1013097153} Anesth(82,NY09)<NJ-UNVM-CPRN>
+ University Medical Center of Princeton at Plainsboro
  One Plainsboro Road/Anesthesiology   Plainsboro, NJ 08536   (609)497-4000

Train, William Walker, MD {1457559759}
+ 11 Cooper Avenue/Unit 211
  Long Branch, NJ 07740   (732)267-3805
  williamtrain@gmail.com

Traisak, Pamela, MD {1679734503} Rheuma
+ Cooper Physician Offices
  900 Centennial Boulevard   Voorhees, NJ 08043   (856)325-6770   Fax (856)673-4510

Tramontana, Anthony F., MD {1639114093} RadDia(76,MEX14)<NJ-MEADWLND, NJ-JRSYCITY>
+ Meadowlands Hospital Medical Center
  55 Meadowlands Parkway/Radiology   Secaucus, NJ 07096   (201)392-3100

Tran, Bao Chau Minh, MD {1558501320} Anesth, IntrMd(05,NJ06)<NJ-STMRYPAS>
+ RejuV Aesthetic Gynecology
  285 Durham Avenue/Suite 1A, Bldg. 6   South Plainfield, NJ 07080   (732)338-0228
+ St. Mary's Hospital
  350 Boulevard/Anesthesia   Passaic, NJ 07055   (973)365-4300

Tran, Baohuong Nguyen, DO {1396004644} ObsGyn<NJ-NWRK-BETH>
+ Newark Beth Israel Medical Center
  201 Lyons Avenue/ObsGyn   Newark, NJ 07112   (973)926-4882

Tran, Dan-Thuy V., MD {1629181896} AnesPain, Anesth(01,NY03)<NJ-MONMOUTH>
+ Monmouth Medical Center
  300 Second Avenue/Anesth   Long Branch, NJ 07740   (732)222-5200

Tran, Duc T., MD {1073518684} Radiol, RadDia(90,NJ06)
+ 530 Lakehurst Road
  Toms River, NJ 08753

Tran, Kevin, MD {1992265623} Pedtrc<NJ-CHDNWBTH>
+ Children's Hospital of New Jersey
  201 Lyons Avenue/Osborne Terrace   Newark, NJ 07112   (408)726-3437

Tran, Ly-Le, MD {1972748283} IntrMd(83,NC05)
+ Novartis Pharmaceuticals Corporation
  One Health Plaza   East Hanover, NJ 07936   (862)778-8081   Fax (973)781-6504

Tran, Minh Q., MD {1194059386}<NJ-STJOSHOS>
+ St. Joseph's Regional Medical Center
  703 Main Street   Paterson, NJ 07503   (973)754-2000

Tran, Thai Thi, MD {1528562337}
+ Drs. Tran and Sliwowska
  317 George Street   New Brunswick, NJ 08901   (732)235-6972

Tran, Thomas Hien Dieu, MD {1912922790} Radiol, RadDia(97,TN05)<NJ-ACMCITY, NJ-SHOREMEM>
+ Atlantic Medical Imaging, LLC.
  72 West Jimmie Leeds Road   Galloway, NJ 08205   (609)677-9729   Fax (609)653-8764
+ Atlantic Medical Imaging, LLC.
  401 Bethel Road   Somers Point, NJ 08244   (609)677-9729
+ Atlantic Medical Imaging, LLC.
  421 Route 9 North   Cape May Court House, NJ 08205   (609)463-9500   Fax (609)465-0918

Tran, Trong D., MD {1376543157} Ophthl(99,NY20)<NJ-VIRTMHBC>
+ South Jersey Eye Physicians PA
  509 South Lenola Road/Suite 11   Moorestown, NJ 08057   (856)234-0222   Fax (856)727-9518
+ South Jersey Eye Physicians PA
  25 Homestead Drive/Suite A   Columbus, NJ 08022   (856)234-0222   Fax (609)291-1972

Tran, Vincent Phuong, DO {1245284074} FamMed(01,IL76)<NJ-BAYSHORE>
+ The Doctor's Office
  1070 Highway 34/Suite C   Matawan, NJ 07747   (732)290-0300   Fax (732)290-9661

Tran-Hoppe, Ngoc Quynh T., MD {1336104298} ObsGyn(99,NJ06)<NJ-STPETER>
+ Family Practice & Gynecology
  273 Durham Avenue   South Plainfield, NJ 07080   (908)561-9900   Fax (908)561-6650
+ Middlesex County Public Health
  586 Jersey Avenue   New Brunswick, NJ 08901   (732)565-3788

Trani, Jose Luis, MD {1750544599} SrgVas<NJ-COOPRUMC>
+ Cooper University Hospital
  One Cooper Plaza   Camden, NJ 08103   (856)342-2143   Fax (856)342-3299

Traquina, Diana Nogueira, MD {1669533766} PedOto, Otlryg(84,CT01)<NJ-RWJUBRUN>
+ University Otolaryngology Associates
  181 Somerset Street/PediOtolaryng   New Brunswick, NJ 08901   (732)247-2401   Fax (732)247-6920
+ RWJ University Hospital New Brunswick
  One Robert Wood Johnson Place   New Brunswick, NJ 08901   (732)828-3000

Trastman-Caruso, Elyse Randi, MD {1104974864} Ophthl(04,NY46)
+ Ocean Eye Institute
  601 Route 37 West   Toms River, NJ 08755   (732)244-4400   Fax (732)505-2171
+ Wills Eye Surgery Center in Cherry Hill
  408 Route 70 East   Cherry Hill, NJ 08034   (732)244-4400   Fax (856)429-7555

Tratenberg, Mark Adam, DO {1780812461} Rheuma
+ Atlantic Health Weight & Wellness Center @ MMC
  435 South Street/Suite 220-B   Morristown, NJ 07960   (973)540-9198   Fax (973)540-1614

Trattner, Lauren Beth, DO {1033150339} EmrgMd(95,NY75)<NJ-RIVERVW>
+ Riverview Medical Center
  1 Riverview Plaza/EmrgMed   Red Bank, NJ 07701   (732)741-2700   Fax (732)224-7498

Traub, Michael Lawrence, MD {1366513749} ObsGyn, RprEnd(02,PHI15)<NY-STATNRTH, NY-STATNSTH>
+ Island Reproductive Services
 3000 Hadley Road/Suite 2-C   South Plainfield, NJ 07080
 (908)412-9909   Fax (908)412-9910

Trauffer, Patrice, MD {1841257953} ClnGnt, NnPnMd, ObsGyn
+ Mercer Maternal Fetal Specialty Group
 One Capital Way   Pennington, NJ 08534   (609)537-7262
 Fax (609)537-6070
+ Mercer Maternal Fetal Specialty Group
 750 Brunswick Avenue   Trenton, NJ 08638   (609)537-7262
 Fax (609)394-6316

Trautman, Natalie, MD {1558818021} Anesth
+ Cooper Anesthesia Associates
 One Cooper Plaza/Suite 294-B   Camden, NJ 08103
 (856)342-2000   Fax (856)968-8239

Treadwell, Kenneth, Jr., MD {1659347086} ObsGyn(77,NY45)<NJ-NWRKBETH, NJ-RBAYOLDB>
+ 1387 Clinton Avenue
 Irvington, NJ 07111   (973)372-1441   Fax (973)372-6019
 ktjrmd@aol.com
+ Raritan Obstetrical Associates
 485 New Brunswick Avenue/Suite 100   Perth Amboy, NJ 08861   (732)324-4290

Treiman, Arthur M., MD {1932280526} FamMed(90,PA02)<NJ-COOPRUMC>
+ Cooper Family Medicine
 141 South Black Horse Pike/Suite 1   Blackwood, NJ 08012
 (856)232-6471   Fax (856)227-4383
 Arthurtreiman@comcast.net

Treiser, Susan L., MD {1740492990} ObsGyn, RprEnd(83,DC02)<NJ-CENTRAST>
+ Reproductive Medicine Associates of New Jersey
 81 Veronica Avenue/Suite 101   Somerset, NJ 08873
 (732)220-9060   Fax (732)220-1164
+ IVF New Jersey
 495 Iron Bridge Road/Suite 10   Freehold, NJ 07728
 (732)220-9060   Fax (732)577-6510

Trend, Carolyn Cozine, MD {1457395220} Pedtrc(00,NJ06)
+ Somerset Pediatric Group PA
 2345 Lamington Road/Suite 101   Bedminster, NJ 07921
 (908)470-1124   Fax (908)470-2845

Trenton, Adam James, DO {1720249923} Psychy
+ University Medical Group/UMDNJ
 125 Paterson Street/Suite 2200   New Brunswick, NJ 08901
 (732)235-7647   Fax (732)235-7677

Trespalacios, Vanessa Nadia, MD {1053339945} IntrMd(99,DOM02)<NJ-MORRISTN>
+ St. Barnabas Ambulatory Care Center
 200 South Orange Avenue/Suite 112   Livingston, NJ 07039
 (973)322-7838   Fax (973)322-7842

Trespicio, Rogelio T., MD {1194886739} Anesth(66,PHI10)<NJ-STBARNMC>
+ St. Barnabas Medical Center
 94 Old Short Hills Road   Livingston, NJ 07039   (973)322-5000

Tresvalles, Monette M., MD {1962586396} IntrMd, OncHem(91,PHI01)
+ Monette M. Tresvalles MD LLC
 65 Lacey Road/Suite D   Whiting, NJ 08759   (732)716-1000
+ Monette M. Tresvalles MD LLC
 651 Route 37 West   Toms River, NJ 08755   (732)716-1000

Treworgy, Jordan, MD {1144627100}<NJ-HACKNSK>
+ Hackensack University Medical Center
 30 Prospect Avenue   Hackensack, NJ 07601   (551)996-2000

Tria, Alfred J., Jr., MD {1760593404} SrgOARec(72,MA01)<NJ-STPETER, NJ-RWJUBRUN>
+ Orthopedic Center of New Jersey
 1527 Route 27/Suite 1300   Somerset, NJ 08873   (732)249-4444   Fax (732)249-6528

Tribuna, Joseph, MD {1215970447} FamMed(90,NY08)<NJ-OVERLOOK>
+ Chatham Family Practice Associates
 492 Main Street   Chatham, NJ 07928   (973)635-2432   Fax (973)635-6169

Tridico, Tanner Joseph, MD {1376581215} IntrMd(03,LA06)<NJ-CHSFULD>
+ Princeton Medical Group, P.A.
 419 North Harrison Street   Princeton, NJ 08540   (609)924-9300   Fax (609)430-9481

Trifiletti, Rosario R., MD {1518997659} Nrolgy, Pedtrc(86,MD07)
+ 545 Island Road/Suite 1D
 Ramsey, NJ 07446   (201)236-3876   Fax (201)236-3888

Triggs, Cynthia Bilsly, MD {1578613170} Pedtrc(03,NY09)<NY-BLVUENYU>
+ Bergen West Pediatric Center, PA
 541 Cedar Hill Avenue   Wyckoff, NJ 07481   (201)652-0300
 Fax (201)444-6209

Trigiani, Charles J., DO {1538233721} Psychy, PsyCAd(79,PA77)<NJ-HAMPTBHC>
+ Hampton Behavioral Health Center

 650 Rancocas Road   Westampton, NJ 08060   (609)267-7000   Fax (609)518-2150

Trikha, Rupan, MD {1003033689} Ophthl, IntrMd(03,NJ05)
+ Retina Consultants
 39 Sycamore Avenue   Little Silver, NJ 07739   (732)530-7730   Fax (732)530-3837

Trim, George G., MD {1154379881} ObsGyn(84,DMN01)<NJ-COMMED>
+ Ocean Women's Health Care Group
 602 Route 72 East/Suite 1   Manahawkin, NJ 08050
 (609)978-9870   Fax (609)978-9873
+ 34 Manchester Avenue/Suite 105
 Forked River, NJ 08731   (609)978-9870   Fax (609)489-4651

Trimor, Fay Ann I., MD {1922138015} Pedtrc<NJ-VIRTVOOR>
+ Virtua Voorhees
 100 Bowman Drive   Voorhees, NJ 08043   (856)247-3000
 Fax (856)325-3157

Trinh, Diem Thi, MD {1407077829} Dermat(97,MI01)
+ Ravits Margaret MD & Associates
 130 Kinderkamack Road/Suite 205   River Edge, NJ 07661
 (201)692-0800   Fax (201)488-1582

Trinidad, Altagracia A., MD {1407870611} Pedtrc(83,PA13)<NJ-NWRKBETH>
+ Newark Department of Health and Human Services
 110 William Street   Newark, NJ 07102   (973)733-5300

Trinidad, Jennilee A., MD {1952629925} IntHos, IntrMd(09,DMN01)
+ IPC The Hospitalist Company
 55 Madison Avenue/Suite 310   Morristown, NJ 07960
 (973)993-9536   Fax (973)998-4237

Triola, Victoria, DO {1124000112} FamMed(97,NJ75)
+ Chapel Hill Family Medicine
 100 Village Court/Suite 302   Hazlet, NJ 07730   (732)758-0048   Fax (732)758-0052

Triolo, Diane Cecilia, MD {1710166228} Nephro, IntrMd(07,NY09)<NY-VANORTH>
+ North Jersey Nephrology Associates PA
 246 Hamburg Turnpike/Suite 207   Wayne, NJ 07470
 (973)653-3366   Fax (973)653-3365

Triolo, Joseph, MD {1649267402} RadDia, Radiol(89,PA02)<NJ-COMMED>
+ Community Medical Center
 99 Route 37 West/Radiology   Toms River, NJ 08755
 (732)557-8000   Fax (732)557-2064

Triolo, Michael James, MD {1447439955} RadDia, IntrMd(07,NY09)<NY-VANORTH>
+ 79 New Street
 Englewood Cliffs, NJ 07632

Triolo, Paul, MD {1821056151} FamMed(89,PA02)<NJ-COMMED>
+ Dover Family Medicine, P.A.
 2292 Clover Hill Lane   Toms River, NJ 08755   (732)323-0100   Fax (732)818-9741

Tripathi, Harsha M., MD {1194735969} IntrMd(73,INA15)
+ Neighborhood Health Center Plainfield
 1700-58 Myrtle Avenue/AdultMed   Plainfield, NJ 07060
 (908)753-6401   Fax (908)226-6740
+ 491 New Brunswick Avenue
 Perth Amboy, NJ 08861   (732)324-8033

Tripathi, Mohan Sanjay, MD {1194080168}<NJ-RWJUBRUN>
+ RWJ University Hospital New Brunswick
 One Robert Wood Johnson Place   New Brunswick, NJ 08901
 (732)235-7865

Tripathi, Neeta, MD {1164492385} IntrMd, CdvDis(88,INA05)<NJ-RWJUHAM>
+ Hamilton Cardiology Associates
 2073 Klockner Road   Hamilton, NJ 08690   (609)584-1212
 Fax (609)584-0103

Tripathi, Tushar Mahesh, MD {1417171992} SrgVas, Surgry(00,PA02)
+ Comprehensive Vascular Care, PA
 111 Union Valley Road/Suite 202   Monroe Township, NJ 08831   (732)305-6444   Fax (732)305-6445
 comprehensive vascularcare@gmail.com

Trivedi, Amit, MD {1386701282} Surgry(93,NY48)<NJ-HACKNSK>
+ Advanced Laparoscopic Associates
 81 Route 4 West/Suite 401/35 Plaza   Paramus, NJ 07652
 (201)646-1121   Fax (201)646-1110
+ Paramus Surgical Center
 30 West Century Road/Suite 300   Paramus, NJ 07652
 (201)986-9000

Trivedi, Anuja, DO {1750708103}<NJ-CHSFULD>
+ Capital Health System/Fuld Campus
 750 Brunswick Avenue   Trenton, NJ 08638   (609)394-6000

Trivedi, Avani P., DO {1376878512} Anesth(05,NJ75)<NJ-HOLYNAME>
+ Teaneck Anesthesia Group, P.A.
 718 Teaneck Road   Teaneck, NJ 07666   (201)833-7149
 Fax (201)833-6576

Physicians by Name and Address

Trivedi, Darshini, DO {1912294265} EmrgMd<NJ-JRSYSHMC>
+ Jersey Shore University Medical Center
 1945 Route 33   Neptune, NJ 07753   (732)775-5500

Trivedi, Deep B., MD {1750394771} Urolgy, IntrMd(06,NY48)
+ Urology Care Alliance
 2 Princess Road/Suite J   Lawrenceville, NJ 08648
 (609)895-1991   Fax (609)895-6996
 deeptrivedi33@gmail.com

Trivedi, Keyur Chandrakant, MD {1356422943} Anesth<NJ-COOPRUMC>
+ Cooper University Hospital
 One Cooper Plaza   Camden, NJ 08103   (856)342-2000

Trivedi, Malti S., MD {1902911092} Radiol, RadNuc(72,INA53)<NJ-UMDNJ>
+ 388 St Cloud Avenue
 West Orange, NJ 07052

Trivedi, Manish Niranjan, MD {1760785414} InfDis
+ Manish N Trivedi MD
 208 West Whitehorse Pike   Pomona, NJ 08240   (609)652-2256   Fax (609)652-8023
 Mtrivedimd@yahoo.com

Trivedi, Manoj M., MD {1003964420} Grtrcs, IntrMd(84,INA71)<NJ-OVERLOOK, NJ-MORRISTN>
+ 802 Old Springfield Avenue
 Summit, NJ 07901   Fax (908)273-1435

Trivedi, Maulik Mahesh, MD {1023108941} EmrgMd(96,DC03)<NJ-WAYNEGEN>
+ St. Joseph's Wayne Hospital
 224 Hamburg Turnpike/EmrgMed   Wayne, NJ 07470
 (973)942-6900
+ Emergency Medical Associates of NJ, P.A.
 3 Century Drive   Parsippany, NJ 07054   (973)942-6900
 Fax (973)740-9895

Trivedi, Niranjan G., MD {1558306886} CdvDis, IntrMd(73,RUSS)<NJ-ACMCITY, NJ-ACMCMAIN>
+ 208 Whitehorse Pike/PO Box 907
 Pomona, NJ 08240   (609)652-1120   Fax (609)652-8023

Trivedi, Nirmal I., MD {1841697109} Psychy(11,GRN01)
+ Trinitas Regional Medical Center-New Point Campus
 655 East Jersey Street   Elizabeth, NJ 07206   (908)994-5000

Trivedi, Prabhas Arunbhai, MD {1902856834} Dermat(81,INDI)<NJ-COMMED, NJ-KIMBALL>
+ Schweiger Dermatology
 368 Lakehurst Road/Suite 201   Toms River, NJ 08755
 (732)244-4700   Fax (732)731-6134
+ Schweiger Dermatology
 67 Lacey Road   Whiting, NJ 08759   (732)244-4700   Fax (732)849-4421
+ Accredited Dermatology
 525 Route 70 West/Suite A1   Lakewood, NJ 08755
 (732)370-3003   Fax (732)370-1526

Trivedi, Raksha A., MD {1659452712} IntrMd(82,INDI)
+ PO Box 7717
 West Trenton, NJ 08628

Trivedi, Seeta, MD {1295962728} MedOnc, IntrMd
+ Somerset Hematology Oncology Associates, P.A.
 30 Rehill Avenue/2nd Floor/Suite 2500   Somerville, NJ 08876   (908)927-8700   Fax (908)927-8706

Trivedi, Shivang M., MD {1912907312} IntrMd, CdvDis(91,INA21)
+ RWJPE Cardiology Associates of Somerset County, P.A.
 487 Union Avenue/Suite A   Bridgewater, NJ 08807
 (908)722-6410   Fax (908)722-4638

Trnovski, Stefan, MD {1902832991} Anesth(88,MAC01)
+ Columbia Anesthesia Associates
 37 West Century Road/Suite 101   Paramus, NJ 07652
 (201)634-9000   Fax (201)634-9014
+ Paramus Surgical Center
 30 West Century Road/Suite 300   Paramus, NJ 07652
 (201)986-9000

Trobliger, Robert William, MD {1548597156} PsyNro
+ Northeast Regional Epilepsy Group
 20 Prospect Avenue/Suite 800   Hackensack, NJ 07601
 (201)343-6676   Fax (201)343-6689

Trocki, Ira M., MD {1235296088} SrgPlstc, Otlryg(75,IL43)
+ Trocki Plastic Surgery Center
 631 Tilton Road/PO Box 865   Northfield, NJ 08225
 (609)645-3000   Fax (856)645-0253

Trofa, Andrew F., MD {1679981708} InfDis, IntrMd(82,PHI01)
+ South Jersey Infectious Disease
 730 Shore Road   Somers Point, NJ 08244   (609)927-6662
 Fax (609)927-2942

Trogan, Igor, MD {1982650453} Pedtrc, IntrMd(00,CT01)
+ Ivy Pediatrics
 220 Bridge Plaza Drive   Manalapan, NJ 07726   (732)972-9525   Fax (732)972-9055
+ Ivy Pediatrics
 175 North Broadway   South Amboy, NJ 08879   (732)972-9525   Fax (732)852-8816
+ Ivy Pediatrics
 7 Brunswick Woods Drive   East Brunswick, NJ 07726
 (732)432-7337   Fax (732)432-7338

509

Physicians by Name and Address

Trokhan, Eileen Q., MD {1447214804} Dermat(02,NY47)
+ Trokhan Dermatology, LLC.
235 Closter Dock Road   Closter, NJ 07624   (201)767-1908   Fax (201)767-3097
derm@trokhan.com

Trokhan, Shawn Edward, MD {1710168588} SrgOrt(05,OH06)
+ Trokhan Dermatology, LLC.
235 Closter Dock Road   Closter, NJ 07624   (201)767-1908   Fax (201)767-3097

Trom, Andrew, DO {1285044289} EmrgMd<NJ-UNDRWD>
+ Inspira Health Network
509 North Broad Street   Woodbury, NJ 08096   (856)845-0100

Trom, Kristen Elizabeth, DO {1164858700}<NJ-SJHREGMC>
+ Family Health Center of Mullica Hill
155 Bridgeton Pike/Suite A   Mullica Hill, NJ 08062   (856)223-0500   Fax (856)223-1098

Troncoso, Alexis B., MD {1154307106} EmrgMd(75,ITA17)<NJ-RWJUBRUN>
+ Emergency Medical Associates of NJ, P.A.
3 Century Drive   Parsippany, NJ 07054   (973)740-0607   Fax (973)740-9895

Troncoso, Alexis B., II, MD {1528186194} EmrgMd, EmrgEMed(04,NJ05)<NJ-MORRISTN>
+ Morristown Medical Center
100 Madison Avenue/EmrgMed   Morristown, NJ 07962   (973)971-5000
+ Emergency Medical Associates of NJ, P.A.
3 Century Drive   Parsippany, NJ 07054   (973)971-5000   Fax (973)740-9895

Tronolone, William, MD {1750348660} Anesth(86,NY01)<NJ-STPETER, NJ-SOMERSET>
+ Anesthesia Consultnts of NJ/Nova Pain
285 Davidson Avenue/Suite 204   Somerset, NJ 08873   (732)271-1400   Fax (732)271-3543

Trontell, Marie C., MD {1053486662} PulDis, IntrMd(76,NJ06)<NJ-RWJUBRUN>
+ UH-Robert Wood Jhnsn Med Sch
97 Paterson Street/Rm 118/MedEdu   New Brunswick, NJ 08901

Trooskin, Stanley Zachary, MD {1174684161} Surgry, SrgCrC, OthrSp(75,PA12)
+ UMDNJ RWJ Surgery
125 Paterson Street/CAB 4th FL 4100   New Brunswick, NJ 08901   (732)235-7920   Fax (732)235-7079

Tropea, Joseph N., DO {1013028729} OncHem
+ Lourdes Medical Associates Hematology Oncology
101 Burrs Road/Suite C   Westampton, NJ 08060   (609)702-7550   Fax (609)702-1277
+ Lourdes Medical Associates Hematology Oncology
1 Brace Road/Suite B   Cherry Hill, NJ 08034   (609)702-7550   Fax (609)702-1277

Trotta, Celia V., MD {1891007142} Psychy<NJ-JRSYCITY>
+ Jersey City Medical Center
355 Grand Street   Jersey City, NJ 07304   (201)915-2000

Trotta, Nicholas C., MD {1811967474} Ophthl(64,TN05)<NJ-MEADWLND, NJ-BERGNMC>
+ 17-15 Maple Avenue/Suite 1
Fair Lawn, NJ 07410   (201)398-0077   Fax (201)398-0042

Trotz, Christopher R., MD {1215025283} FamMed(96,JMA01)<NJ-UNDRWD, NJ-KENEDYHS>
+ Evergreen Medical
40 Elm Avenue/Suite 3   Woodbury Heights, NJ 08097   (856)853-5888   Fax (856)853-5913
admin@njfamilypractice.com
+ South Jersey Family Medicine Associates
608 North Broad Street/Suite 100   Woodbury, NJ 08096   (856)853-5888   Fax (856)848-1682

Troum, Richard M., DO {1609805027} Gastrn(85,PA77)<NJ-BURDTMLN>
+ Cape Atlantic Gastroenterology Associates
307 Stone Harbor Boulevard/Suite 5   Cape May Court House, NJ 08210   (609)465-1511   Fax (609)465-5310
+ Court House Surgery Center
106 Courthouse South Dennis Rd   Cape May, NJ 08204   (609)465-1511   Fax (609)465-8771

Trovato, Matthew J., MD {1528157617} SrgPlstc
+ 2400 Hudson Terrace/Apt 6-i
Fort Lee, NJ 07024

Trowers, Reynold L., MD {1811080575} IntrMd, EmrgMd(79,RI01)<NY-HARLEM>
+ 110 Passaic Avenue
Passaic, NJ 07055   (347)386-6176   Fax (212)939-4130

Troyanovich, Esteban F., MD {1679590020} IntrMd(01,NJ05)<NJ-COOPRUMC>
+ Cooper University Hospital
One Cooper Plaza/Hospitalist   Camden, NJ 08103   (856)342-3150   Fax (856)968-8418

Trudo, Frank J., MD {1225013584} PulDis(90,NY03)
+ Pulmonary and Sleep Physicians
204 Ark Road/Suite 206/Larchmont 1   Mount Laurel, NJ 08054   (856)778-4640   Fax (856)778-8862

True, Robert Henry, Jr., MD {1790894848} DerHar, FamMed, SrgRec(73,QU01)
+ TRUE & Dorin Medical Group, P.C.
51 JFK Parkway/Suite 115   Short Hills, NJ 07078   (973)218-2447

Trujillo-Carvalho, Cecilia J., MD {1770842809} ObsGyn
+ Palisades Women's Group
6045 Kennedy Boulevard/Suite B   North Bergen, NJ 07047   (201)868-2630   Fax (201)868-4919
+ Palisades Women's Group
7650 River Road/Suite 230   North Bergen, NJ 07047   (201)868-2630   Fax (201)868-8442

Trusky, Diana E., MD {1245238294} Dermat(75,NY46)<NJ-RIVERVW, NJ-BAYSHORE>
+ Associated Dermatologists
92 Half Mile Road   Red Bank, NJ 07701   (732)219-0700   Fax (732)224-0750

Truxal, Brian A., MD {1891759940} Pedtrc(77,TN05)<NJ-MONMOUTH>
+ Pediatric & Adolescent Medicine, PA
223 Monmouth Road   West Long Branch, NJ 07764   (732)229-4540   Fax (732)229-8689
+ Monmouth Family Center
270 Broadway   Long Branch, NJ 07740   (732)229-4540   Fax (732)923-7104

Trzeciak, Stephen Walter, MD {1124109723} CritCr, EmrgMd, IntrMd(96,WI05)<NJ-COOPRUMC>
+ Cooper University Hospital
One Cooper Plaza/CritCare   Camden, NJ 08103   (856)342-2000

Tsafos, Vassilios, MD {1902195217} Anesth(11,NY03)
+ Morris Anesthesia Group, PA
3799 Route 46/Suite 211   Parsippany, NJ 07054   (973)335-1122   Fax (973)335-1448

Tsai, Anderson F., MD {1083602858} IntrMd(70,TAI04)<NJ-BAYSHORE>
+ Drs. Abrina & Tsai
319 Main Street/Suite B4   Keansburg, NJ 07734   (732)787-0568   Fax (732)787-0270

Tsai, Fu-Li, MD {1417084294} IntrMd, Nephro, OthrSp(77,TAI05)
+ 182 Franklin Avenue
Ridgewood, NJ 07450   (201)599-9719   Fax (201)664-9164
tsaimdot@yahoo.com

Tsai, Henry K., MD {1063480010} RadOnc(02,MA01)<NJ-CENTRAST>
+ Princeton Radiation Oncology
901 West Main Street   Freehold, NJ 07728   (732)303-5290   Fax (732)303-5299
+ Princeton Radiology Associates, P.A.
3674 Route 27   Kendall Park, NJ 08824   (732)303-5290   Fax (732)821-6675
+ Princeton Radiology Associates, P.A.
9 Centre Drive   Jamesburg, NJ 07728   (609)655-1448   Fax (609)655-4016

Tsai, Joseph C., MD {1871595330} Radiol(85,NC07)<NJ-VIRTMHBC>
+ Radiology Associates of Burlington County
1295 Route 38 West/PO Box 479   Hainesport, NJ 08036   (609)261-7017   Fax (609)261-4180

Tsai, Joyce, MD {1447513213} Nrolgy
+ Progressive Neurology
260 Old Hook Road/Suite 200   Westwood, NJ 07675   (201)546-8510   Fax (201)503-8142

Tsai, Jung-Tsung, MD {1669496931} SrgVas, Surgry(71,TAI06)
+ 60 Elmora Avenue
Elizabeth, NJ 07202   (908)355-7659   Fax (908)355-7722

Tsai, Philip Henry, MD {1245346113} Hemato, IntrMd, MedOnc(80,NY15)<NY-MTSINAI>
+ 185 Cedar Lane/Suite L-1
Teaneck, NJ 07666   (201)836-5144   Fax (201)836-8210

Tsai, Steve Chun-Hung, MD {1386849719} IntrMd, CdvDis(02,NJ05)
+ Rutgers- New Jersey Medical School
185 South Orange Avenue/MSB I-536   Newark, NJ 07103   (973)972-8320
+ VA New Jersey Health Care System
385 Tremont Avenue/Corporate Office   East Orange, NJ 07018   (973)972-8320   Fax (973)676-4226

Tsai, Yan-San, MD {1265590392} ObsGyn, GynOnc(65,CHNA)<NJ-STCLRDEN>
+ The Center For Specialized Women's Health
16 Pocono Road/Suite 103   Denville, NJ 07834   (973)947-9066   Fax (973)947-9056
+ The Center For Specialized Women's Health
16 Eden Lane   Whippany, NJ 07981   (973)947-9066   Fax (973)947-9056

Tsairis, Peter, MD {1811034606} Nrolgy(65,NY20)<NJ-MORRISTN>
+ Tri-County Orthopedics
160 East Hanover Avenue   Morristown, NJ 07962   (973)538-2334   Fax (973)829-9174

Tsakrios, Charles N., Jr., MD {1699860932} Ophthl(77,GRE03)<NJ-VALLEY>
+ 89 North Maple Avenue/Suite 3
Ridgewood, NJ 07450   (201)445-1991   Fax (201)445-4827

Tsang, Kock-Yen, MD {1821149741} CdvDis(72,TAI01)
+ Community Medical Center Department of Cardiology
20 Hospital Drive/Suite 1   Toms River, NJ 08755   (732)240-6688   Fax (732)240-5757

Tsang, Patricia Chiu-Wun, MD {1952365769} PthACl, Hemato, GntMMPty(92,MA05)<NJ-NWRKBETH>
+ Newark Beth Israel Medical Center
201 Lyons Avenue/Path   Newark, NJ 07112   (973)926-7431   Fax (973)282-0495

Tsangalidis, Eirini, MD {1578874319} FamMed
+ Overlook Family Medicine
33 Overlook Road/Suite 103   Summit, NJ 07901   (908)522-5700   Fax (908)273-8014

Tsao, Francis, MD {1487790085} Otlryg, SrgHdN(83,PA01)<NY-METROHOS, NY-METHODST>
+ Otolaryngology Head and Neck Surgery
311 Lexington Avenue   Paterson, NJ 07502   (973)942-1300

Tsao, Julie Ching Yen, MD {1316171473} Nrolgy, Psychy
+ Northeast Regional Epilepsy Group
20 Prospect Avenue/Suite 800   Hackensack, NJ 07601   (201)343-6676   Fax (201)343-6689

Tsao, Lawrence, MD {1376682393} PthACl, Hemato(01,NY08)
+ Quest Diagnostics Inc.
1 Malcolm Avenue   Teterboro, NJ 07608   (201)393-5934   Fax (201)393-6127

Tsao, Peter Dean, DO {1083663777} EmrgMd(02,AZ02)<NJ-VIRTMHBC>
+ Virtua Memorial
175 Madison Avenue/EmrgMed   Mount Holly, NJ 08060   (609)267-0700

Tsarouhas, Louis, MD {1417945825} FamMed(87,NJ06)<NJ-RWJUHAM>
+ Tsarouhas Medical, LLC
2999 Princeton Pike/Suite 3   Lawrenceville, NJ 08648   (609)882-9333   Fax (609)882-1026
tsarmed@aol.com

Tsay, Donald, MD {1962586321} IntrMd, Pedtrc(97,NY46)<NJ-CHILTON, NJ-NWTNMEM>
+ J&J Pediatrics
97 West Parkway   Pompton Plains, NJ 07444   (973)831-5454
dtsay73@yahoo.com

Tse, James T.C., MD {1023190691} Anesth(86,NE05)<NJ-RWJUBRUN>
+ Robert Wood Johnson-UMDNJ Anesthesia Group
1140 Route 72 West   Manahawkin, NJ 08050   (609)978-8900
+ Robert Wood Johnson-UMDNJ Anesthesia Group
125 Paterson Street/CAB 3100   New Brunswick, NJ 08901   (609)978-8900   Fax (732)235-6131

Tselniker, Maryana, MD {1871993154} FamMed
+ RWJ Medical Associates
3100 Quakerbridge Road/Suite 28   Hamilton, NJ 08619   (609)245-7430   Fax (609)245-7432

Tseng, Grace N., MD {1457778896}<NJ-UNVMCPRN>
+ St. Francis Medical Center
601 Hamilton Avenue/Room B-158   Trenton, NJ 08629   (609)599-5061   Fax (609)599-6232
+ Patient first Urgent Care
641 US Highway Route 130   Hamilton, NJ 08691   (609)599-5061   Fax (609)568-9384

Tseng, William P., MD {1861436305} Anesth, PainMd(70,CHNA)<NJ-BERGNMC>
+ Essex Specialized Surgery Institute
475 Prospect Avenue   West Orange, NJ 07052

Tsenovoy, Petr Leonidovich, MD {1558507178} CdvDis, IntrMd(96,RUS81)<NJ-MEADWLND>
+ 19 Mohawk Avenue
Norwood, NJ 07648   (201)392-3588
+ Meadowlands Hospital Medical Center
55 Meadowlands Parkway/Cardiology   Secaucus, NJ 07096   (201)392-3100

Tsigonis, Natalie, DO {1659301836} FamMed(92,NJ75)<NJ-KMHSTRAT>
+ Salem Medical Group
95 Woodstown Road/Suite B   Swedesboro, NJ 08085   (856)832-7359   Fax (856)832-4381

Tsimring, Yuliya, DO {1114433786}<NJ-JRSYSHMC>
+ Jersey Shore University Medical Center
1945 Route 33   Neptune, NJ 07753   (732)776-4267   Fax (732)776-2344

Tsiouris, Simon John, MD {1114085040} IntrMd, InfDis(98,MD07)<NJ-VALLEY>
+ Ridgewood Infectious Disease Associates
947 Linwood Avenue/Suite 2E   Ridgewood, NJ 07450   (201)447-6468   Fax (201)447-3189

Tsirogiannis, Vasiliky, MD {1316296544} IntHos, IntrMd(01,SLU01)<NJ-MEADWLND>
+ Meadowlands Hospital Medical Center
55 Meadowlands Parkway/Internal Med   Secaucus, NJ 07096   (201)392-3228   Fax (201)392-3228

Tsomos, Evangelia, MD {1134178122} EmrgMd(95,NY15)<NJ-VALLEY>
+ The Valley Hospital
223 North Van Dien Avenue/EmergMed   Ridgewood, NJ 07450   (201)447-8000

Tsompanidis, Antonios A.J., DO {1679646608} FamMed, OstMed(94,NJ75)<NJ-BAYSHORE, NJ-RIVERVW>
+ Drs. Tsompanidis and Perrino Fam Pract
1 Bethany Road/Suite 79   Hazlet, NJ 07730   (732)203-0800   Fax (732)203-9494

Tsong, Shirley W., MD {1306835327} ObsGyn(98,NJ06)
+ 180 White Road/Suite 209
Little Silver, NJ 07739   (732)842-0673   Fax (732)842-7352
+ Drs. Karoly, Kaskiw, Hammond & Jacoby
1 Bethany Road/Building 2/Suite 31   Hazlet, NJ 07730

Tsui, Elaina Y., MD {1912201765}
+ University Hospital-RWJ Medical School
89 French Street/Rm 3268   New Brunswick, NJ 08901   (732)828-3000

Tsveniashvili, Liya Vladimirovna, MD {1275566564} InfDis(91,GEO02)<NJ-STBARNMC>
+ St. Barnabas Medical Center
94 Old Short Hills Road/Internal Med   Livingston, NJ 07039   (973)322-5055

Tsyganov, Igor Vlademer, MD {1720081540} Anesth(83,RUS33)<NJ-SHOREMEM>
+ Shore Memorial Hospital
1 East New York Avenue/Anesthesia   Somers Point, NJ 08244   (609)653-3500
ivtmd@hotmail.com

Tsyvine, Daniel, MD {1245420330} CdvDis(05,MA05)<NJ-NWRK-BETH>
+ Newark Beth Israel Medical Center
201 Lyons Avenue/MSB/Rm I-538   Newark, NJ 07112   (973)926-7000

Tu, Chun, MD {1811316060} IntrMd
+ Summit Medical Group-Berkeley Heights Campus
1 Diamond Hill Road   Berkeley Heights, NJ 07922   (908)273-4300   Fax (908)790-6576

Tuason, Dominick Anthony, MD {1588867790} SrgOrt(05,PA01)
+ Pediatric Orthopedic Associates, P.A.
585 Cranbury Road/Suite A   East Brunswick, NJ 08816   (732)390-1160   Fax (732)390-8449

Tubilleja, Joala Martha Perez, DO {1235440819}
+ 1601 Haddon Avenue
Camden, NJ 08103   (856)757-3700   Fax (856)365-7972

Tubilleja, Nina Lapidario, MD {1144291196} IntrMd(90,PHIL)<NJ-COMMED>
+ Nina L. Tubilleja MD PC
403 Penn Avenue North   Forked River, NJ 08731   (609)971-9392   Fax (609)971-8232

Tuboku-Metzger, Folarin Deloris, MD {1306881602} IntrMd(97,NY09)<NJ-BAYSHORE>
+ 150 Cherry Tree Farm Road
Middletown, NJ 07748   (732)320-9196   Fax (866)476-1624

Tucci, Mauro A., III, MD {1619156445} IntrMd(85,DMN01)<NJ-STPETER, NJ-RWJUBRUN>
+ Medical Associates of New Brunswick
8 Auer Court/Suites C & D   East Brunswick, NJ 08816   (732)254-2216   Fax (732)254-1027

Tuchin, Terry A., MD {1467545178} Psychy(67,NJ05)<NJ-VALLEY>
+ 55-A East Ridgewood Avenue/Suite 6
Ridgewood, NJ 07450   (201)444-3131
tatmd@idt.net

Tuck, Michelle Patran, MD {1871562173} Pedtrc, AdolMd(98,NJ05)<NJ-STPETER, NJ-RWJUBRUN>
+ Tiefenbrunn & Fortin Pediatrics, PA
503 Cranbury Road   East Brunswick, NJ 08816   (732)390-8400   Fax (732)390-8970

Tucker, Bradford S., MD {1598871162} SrgOrt, SprtMd(97,NJ06)<NJ-ACMCITY, NJ-ACMCMAIN>
+ Rothman Institute - Egg Harbor Township
2500 English Creek Avenue/Bldg 1300   Egg Harbor Township, NJ 08234   (609)677-7002   Fax (609)677-7000
+ Rothman Institute
219 North White Horse Pike   Hammonton, NJ 08037

Tucker, Burton Stanley, MD {1932191665} IntrMd, Nephro(66,IL42)<NJ-OVERLOOK, NJ-MORRISTN>
+ Medical Diagnostic Associates PA-Nephrology
1511 Park Avenue/3rd Floor   South Plainfield, NJ 07080   (908)757-4544   Fax (908)757-2427
+ Medical Diagnostic Associates PA
384 Shunpike Road   Chatham, NJ 07928   (908)757-4544   Fax (973)377-4117
+ Medical Diagnostic Associates PA
525 Central Avenue/Suite D   Westfield, NJ 07080   (908)232-5333   Fax (908)389-1922

Tucker, Kimberly Victoria, MD {1023308988} SprtMd
+ Atlantic Sports Health at Bridgewater
720 US Highway 202-206   Bridgewater, NJ 08807   (908)722-2033   Fax (908)707-8344

Tucker, Richard G., DO {1376514448} ObsGyn(74,PA77)<NJ-LOURDEHS, NJ-VIRTMHBC>
+ 115 Union Mill Road
Mount Laurel, NJ 08054   (856)778-8622   Fax (856)727-1854
+ 85 Nautilus Drive
Manahawkin, NJ 08050   (609)597-8260

Tucker, Tiffany, MD {1396156931} Pedtrc
+ The Children's Regional Hospital at Cooper Univ Hosp
One Cooper Plaza   Camden, NJ 08103   (856)342-2001

Tuckman, Drew E., MD {1063459105} SrgHnd, SrgPlstc(74,IN20)<NJ-CHILTON, NJ-WAYNEGEN>
+ 30 West Century Road/Suite 220
Paramus, NJ 07652   (201)986-1010
drewet@msn.com

Tufankjian, Dearon K., DO {1902804792} Radiol, RadDia(96,PA77)<NJ-SJHREGMC, NJ-SJERSYHS>
+ Quakerbridge Radiology Associates
8 Quakerbridge Plaza/Building 8   Mercerville, NJ 08619   (609)890-0033   Fax (609)689-6067
+ SJH Regional Medical Center
1505 West Sherman Avenue/Radiology   Vineland, NJ 08360   (856)641-8000

Tufankjian, Lisa Gruszka, DO {1912999749} ObsGyn(96,PA77)
+ Robert Wood Johnson Ob/Gyn Group
1 Hamilton Health Place   Hamilton, NJ 08690   (609)631-6899   Fax (609)631-6898

Tugman, Catherine K., MD {1932122942} FamMed(84,VA07)<NJ-SJERSYHS>
+ South Cumberland Medical Associates
215 Back Neck Road   Bridgeton, NJ 08302   (856)451-4414   Fax (856)451-2052

Tuladhar, Swosty, MD {1437593035} IntrMd
+ Summit Medical Group
1 Diamond Hill Road/Bensley Pav/2 FL   Berkeley, NJ 07922   (908)277-8640   Fax (908)288-7993
+ Summit Medical Group
31-00 Broadway   Fair Lawn, NJ 07410   (908)277-8640   Fax (201)796-7020

Tullo, Nicholas G., MD {1982603239} CdvDis, ClCdEl, IntrMd(82,NY15)
+ Consultants in Cardiology
741 Northfield Avenue/Suite 205   West Orange, NJ 07052   (973)467-1544   Fax (973)530-3554

Tully, Lisa Anita, MD {1043485055} CdvDis, IntrMd(08,NJ06)
+ Atlantic Cardiology Group LLP
8 Tempe Wick Road   Mendham, NJ 07945   (973)543-2288   Fax (973)543-0637

Tully, Nicole S., MD {1437337813} FamMed(05,NJ05)
+ 130 Garden Street
Hoboken, NJ 07030

Tulman, Alan Bruce, MD {1972563740} Gastrn, IntrMd(74,NY19)<NJ-VIRTUAHS, NJ-KENEDYHS>
+ South Jersey Gastroenterology PA
406 Lippincott Drive/Suite E   Marlton, NJ 08053   (856)983-1900   Fax (856)983-5110
+ South Jersey Gastroenterology PA
807 Haddon Avenue/Suite 205   Haddonfield, NJ 08033   (856)983-1900   Fax (856)983-5110
+ South Jersey Gastroenterology PA
111 Vine Street   Hammonton, NJ 08053   (609)561-3080   Fax (856)983-5110

Tulsyan, Nirman, MD {1447323118} SrgVas(99,NJ05)<NJ-MORRISTN, NJ-STCLRDEN>
+ Advanced Vascular Associates, PC
131 Madison Avenue/2nd Floor   Morristown, NJ 07960   (973)755-9206   Fax (973)540-9717

Tulsyan, Vasudha, MD {1962692376} Pedtrc, NnPnMd(98,INDI)<NJ-NWRKBETH>
+ Newark Beth Israel Medical Center
201 Lyons Avenue/Suite C-10   Newark, NJ 07112   (973)926-7203   Fax (973)926-2332
vasudhatulsyan@yahoo.com

Tuma, Augustine Lavelle, MD {1205874815} IntrMd(83,NIGE)
+ Mountain View Surgical Associates
1445 Whitehorse-Mercerville Rd   Hamilton, NJ 08691   (609)392-8100   Fax (609)695-6202

Tuma, Gary Alan, MD {1083707541} SrgPlstc, Surgry(96,PA02)<NJ-CHSFULD, NJ-CHSMRCER>
+ Mountain View Surgical Assocaites
2 Capital Way/Suite 505   Pennington, NJ 08534   (609)537-7000   Fax (609)537-7070

Tuma, Victor B., MD {1659385888} Pedtrc(69,PA02)<NJ-JFKMED>
+ Metuchen Pediatric Associates
215 Amboy Avenue   Metuchen, NJ 08840   (732)549-7364   Fax (732)549-6017
metuchen.pediatrics@verizon.net

Tumaliuan, Janet Ang, MD {1346219912} Allrgy, Pedtrc, Algy-Immn(85,PHI21)<NJ-OCEANMC, NJ-COMMED>
+ Bruce A. De Cotiis, MD, PA
1673 Highway 88 West   Brick, NJ 08724   (732)458-2000

Tumillo, John G., Jr., MD {1568467058} Anesth(92,NJ05)<NJ-SOCEANCO>
+ 16 North 9th Street
Surf City, NJ 08008

Tummala, Sumalatha, MD {1083727382} IntrMd(92,INA11)<NJ-CHSMRCER, NJ-RWJUHAM>
+ Princeton Professional Bldg
251 Princeton-Hights Road   Hightstown, NJ 08520   (609)918-0333   Fax (609)918-0336

Tunc, Feza Sevket, MD {1144208588} Radiol, RadNuc(95,PA07)<NJ-STPETER, NJ-RWJUBRUN>
+ University Radiology Group, P.C.
483 Cranbury Road   East Brunswick, NJ 08816   (732)390-0030   Fax (732)390-5383
+ University Radiology Group, P.C.
105 Raider Boulevard/Suite 101   Hillsborough, NJ 08844   (732)390-0030   Fax (908)359-9273
+ University Radiology Group, P.C.
16 Mountain Boulevard   Warren, NJ 08816   (908)769-7200   Fax (908)769-9141

Tunde-Agbede, Oluwafisayo, MD {1881195881} ObsGyn<NJ-MORRISTN>
+ Morristown Medical Center
100 Madison Avenue   Morristown, NJ 07962   (917)993-2353

Tung, Cindy Wei-Yi, MD {1932152261} Pedtrc(99,NY47)<NJ-HACKNSK, NJ-HOLYNAME>
+ Drs. Baydar, Davidson & Tung
370 Grand Avenue/Suite 203   Englewood, NJ 07631   (201)568-3262   Fax (201)569-2634

Tung, John Yu, MD {1194832311} Pedtrc, PedGst(87,ENG25)<NJ-ATLANCHS>
+ South Jersey Pediatric Gastroenterology LLC
5429 Harding Highway/Suite 302   Mays Landing, NJ 08330   (609)625-8688   Fax (609)641-3652
Tungj@yahoo.com

Tunia, Krzysztof Stanislaw, MD {1922171065} GenPrc(86,POLA)
+ Pediatric Health Center
54 Plauderville Avenue/Suite 1   Garfield, NJ 07026   (973)772-0262   Fax (973)253-2067

Tunuguntla, Hari Siva Gurun, MD {1285842310} Urolgy
+ UMDNJ RWJ Surgery
125 Paterson Street/CAB 4th FL 4100   New Brunswick, NJ 08901   (732)235-7774   Fax (732)235-6042

Tunuguntla, Renuka, MD {1740401413} Grtrcs<NJ-HUNTRDN>
+ Hunterdon Medical Center
2100 Wescott Drive/Geriatric   Flemington, NJ 08822   (908)788-6100

Tuppo, Ehab E., MD {1053310524} IntrMd(95,MI20)<NJ-KMH-STRAT, NJ-VIRTVOOR>
+ Hawthorne Family Practice
1083 Goffle Road   Hawthorne, NJ 07506   (973)427-2421   Fax (973)427-5892

Tuppo, Enas Elias, MD {1346240215} FamMed(95,MI07)<NJ-VALLEY>
+ Hawthorne Family Practice
1083 Goffle Road   Hawthorne, NJ 07506   (973)427-2421   Fax (973)427-6205

Turbin, Roger Eric, MD {1710905161} Ophthl(93,MO02)
+ University Hospital-Doctors Office Center
90 Bergen Street/6th Fl/Ophthl   Newark, NJ 07103   (973)972-2209   Fax (973)972-1244

Turcanu, Dumitru Sabin, MD {1841513173} NnPnMd<NJ-UNVM-CPRN>
+ CHOP Newborn Care at Princeton
253 Witherspoon Street   Princeton, NJ 08540   (609)497-4415   Fax (609)497-4173

Turcios, Nelson L., MD {1407914633} PedPul, Pedtrc(73,ELS01)<NJ-STPETER, NJ-RWJUBRUN>
+ Pediatric Pulmonology/Asthma Institute
282 East Main Street   Somerville, NJ 08876   (908)526-5212   Fax (908)526-5477
nlturcios@gmail.com
+ Pediatric Pulmonology/Asthma Institute
579 Cranbury Road/Suite A   East Brunswick, NJ 08816   (908)526-5212   Fax (908)526-5477

Turenne Kolpan, Laurie Kathleen, MD {1619945177} FamMed(98,NJ06)
+ Delaware Valley Family Health Center
200 Frenchtown Road   Milford, NJ 08848   (908)995-2251   Fax (908)995-2036

Physicians by Name and Address

Turi, Zoltan G., MD {1548341142} CdvDis, IntrMd(74,NY01)<NJ-RWJUBRUN>
+ RWJ University Hospital New Brunswick
One Robert Wood Johnson Place   New Brunswick, NJ 08901   (856)795-6874   Fax (856)795-8071
+ UH- Robert Wood Johnson Med
125 Paterson Street/MEB 582   New Brunswick, NJ 08901   (856)795-6874   Fax (732)235-8722

Turizo, Maria Cecilia, MD {1083836944} Pedtrc(97,COL03)<NJ-STJOSHOS>
+ Integral Pediatrics
1255 Broad Street/Suite 105   Bloomfield, NJ 07003   (973)233-5494   Fax (973)233-5492

Turkel-Parrella, David, MD {1225233141} VasNeu, Nrolgy(07,NJ05)
+ Interventional Neuro Associates, LLC
777 Terrace Avenue/Suite 401   Hasbrouck Heights, NJ 07604   (201)387-1957   Fax (201)351-0656

Turkish, Jennifer M., MD {1801937123} FamMed(05)<NJ-RBAY-OLDB>
+ Hackensack Meridian Medical Group-Primary Care
3 Hospital Plaza/Suite 200   Old Bridge, NJ 08857   (732)360-4085   Fax (732)360-4086

Turkish, Jonathan Lee, MD {1851446272} ObsGyn(99,DMN01)
+ Obstetrical & Gynecological Group of Perth Amboy P A
511 New Brunswick Avenue   Perth Amboy, NJ 08861   (732)826-3600   Fax (732)826-5183

Turner, Craig S., DO {1538109640} EmrgMd, FamMed(87,NJ75)<NJ-VIRTMHBC>
+ SJ Emergency Physician, PA
175 Madison Avenue   Mount Holly, NJ 08060   (609)267-0700   Fax (609)261-5842

Turner, Ellen K., MD {1376542357} InfDis, IntrMd(97,NJ06)
+ Infectious Diseases Consultants of N.J., PA
102 White Horse Pike   Haddon Heights, NJ 08035   (856)795-7505   Fax (856)795-8010

Turner, Garth M., MD {1689870933} Nrolgy
+ Summit Medical Group-Berkeley Heights Campus
1 Diamond Hill Road   Berkeley Heights, NJ 07922   (908)273-4300   Fax (908)790-6576

Turner, James William, III, MD {1245424159} IntrMd(76,NJ05)<NJ-STMRYPAS>
+ Internal Medicine Associates of North Jersey, PA
842 Clifton Avenue/Suite 2   Clifton, NJ 07013   (973)472-3331   Fax (973)472-7847

Turner, Mitchell S., MD {1285858894} Dermat(82,NY08)
+ Union Dermatology Center
1945 Morris Avenue   Union, NJ 07083   (908)688-7546   Fax (908)688-8894

Turner, Nicoletta A., MD {1255442414} IntrMd(95,NJ05)
+ Burlington Medical Center
640 Beverly Rancocas Road   Willingboro, NJ 08046   (609)835-9555   Fax (609)835-2313

Turner, Peter E., MD {1053301184} Pedtrc, Anesth, PedDvl(77,CT02)<NJ-COOPRUMC>
+ Cooper University Medical Center/Camden
3 Cooper Plaza/Suite 200   Camden, NJ 08103   (856)342-2000   Fax (856)342-2472

Turnier, Auguste P., MD {1225076326} Gastrn, IntrMd(86,PA07)<NJ-VIRTUAHS>
+ Drs. Ackerman & Turnier
501 Haddon Avenue/Suite 9   Haddonfield, NJ 08033   (856)428-6024   Fax (856)216-1558
+ Drs. Ackerman & Turnier
2301 Evesham Road/Suite 401   Voorhees, NJ 08043   (856)428-6024   Fax (856)216-1558

Turtel, Lawrence S., MD {1487725933} Ophthl, PedOph(86,NY01)<NJ-JRSYSHMC>
+ Eye Diagnostic Center
3333 Fairmont Avenue   Asbury Park, NJ 07712   (732)988-4000   Fax (732)988-9502
+ Eye Diagnostic Center
525 Route 70   Brick, NJ 08723   (732)988-4000   Fax (732)477-1444
+ Eye Diagnostic Center
258 Broad Street   Red Bank, NJ 07712   (732)530-8500

Turtel, Penny S., MD {1609847730} Gastrn, IntrMd(86,NY20)<NJ-JRSYSHMC, NJ-MONMOUTH>
+ Shore Gastroenterology Associates, P.C.
1907 Highway 35/Suite 1   Oakhurst, NJ 07755   (732)517-0060   Fax (732)548-7408
+ Shore Gastroenterology Associates, P.C.
1907 Highway 35/Suite 1   Oakhurst, NJ 07755   (732)517-0060   Fax (732)548-7408
+ Shore Gastroenterology Associates, P.C.
233 Middle Road   Hazlet, NJ 07755   (732)361-2476

Turturea, Jennifer Megan, DO {1861915381}
+ 2200 Route 66/Suite 5
Neptune, NJ 07753   (732)775-0013   Fax (732)775-3513

Turtz, Alan R., MD {1811083991} SrgNro(86,PA07)
+ Cooper Surgical Associates
3 Cooper Plaza/Suite 411   Camden, NJ 08103   (856)342-2270   Fax (856)365-1180

Turyan, Hach Vladimir, MD {1548366453} PthAcl(83,AZE01)
+ 239 Wedgewood Drive
Paramus, NJ 07652   Fax (201)262-0859

Tusheva, Marija, MD {1629480033} IntHos
+ AtlantiCare Hospitalist Program
1925 Pacific Avenue/8th Floor   Atlantic City, NJ 08401   (609)441-8146

Tussey, Natalie Belle, MD {1922145689} FamMed<PA-CHESTRCT>
+ Naval Air Engineering Station
Lansdowne Road/Building 39   Lakehurst, NJ 08733   (732)323-7111   Fax (732)323-7095

Tutela, Arthur C., MD {1144257155} Ophthl(01,GRN01)
+ Arthur C. Tutela MD, PA
347 Mount Pleasant Avenue/Suite 101   West Orange, NJ 07052   (973)669-1240   Fax (973)669-8190

Tutela, John Paul, MD {1477878205} Surgry, SrgPlstc(05,NJ05)
+ 200 South Orange Avenue/Suite 170
Livingston, NJ 07039   (973)727-9275   Fax (973)629-1707

Tutela, Rocco Robert, Jr., MD {1306979208} Surgry, SrgCrC(00,NET09)<NJ-RWJUBRUN, NJ-STPETER>
+ Highland Park Surgical Associates
31 River Road   Highland Park, NJ 08904   (732)846-9500   Fax (732)846-3931
+ Highland Park Surgical Associates
B2 Brier Hill Court/Suite 3   East Brunswick, NJ 08816   (732)846-9500   Fax (732)238-9697
+ Cares Surgicenter, LLC.
240 Easton Avenue   New Brunswick, NJ 08904   (732)565-5400   Fax (732)296-8677

Tuzzeo, Salvatore T., MD {1275697682} SrgVas, Surgry(72,MEX03)
+ 122 Marsellos Place
Garfield, NJ 07026   Fax (973)546-8379

Twardzik, Jennifer Lynn, DO {1619065075} IntrMd(97,PA77)<NJ-ACMCMAIN, NJ-ACMCITY>
+ AtlantiCare Clinical Associates
2500 English Creek Avenue   Egg Harbor Township, NJ 08234   (609)407-2310   Fax (609)407-2311

Tweddel, George K., III, MD {1013928647} ObsGyn(90,NY19)<NJ-SOMERSET, NJ-OVERLOOK>
+ Roseland Ob/Gyn Services
27 Mountain Boulevard/Suite 6   Warren, NJ 07059   (908)561-1102   Fax (908)561-1105

Twersky, Harris A., DO {1669402822} FamMed, Grtrcs, IntrMd(77,PA77)<NJ-OURLADY, NJ-VIRTMARL>
+ Advocare, LLC.
402 Lippincott Drive   Marlton, NJ 08053   (856)782-3300   Fax (856)504-8029

Twisdale, Donna R., MD {1659430692} ObsGyn(77,NJ05)
+ Durham Women's Center
4 Ethel Road/Suite 402-B   Edison, NJ 08817   (732)287-3643   Fax (732)287-3406

Tydings, John D., MD {1750430260} SrgSpn(84,NY03)<NJ-UNVM-CPRN, NJ-CHSFULD>
+ Central Jersey Spine Associates, PA
123 Franklin Corner Road/Suite 109   Lawrenceville, NJ 08648   (609)896-3131   Fax (609)896-4103
ifixbax@pol.net

Tye, Joann Li Yen, MD {1982982583} ObsGyn
+ New Beginnings Ob/Gyn
193 Mountain Avenue   Springfield, NJ 07081   (973)218-1579   Fax (973)218-1589

Tyerech, Sangeeta K., MD {1356347504} RadOnc(92,NJ06)<NJ-STFRNMED>
+ St. Francis Medical Center
601 Hamilton Avenue/RadOnc   Trenton, NJ 08629   (609)599-5000   Fax (609)599-5000
+ Radiology Affiliates of Central New Jersey, P.A.
2501 Kuser Road   Hamilton, NJ 08691   (609)599-5000   Fax (609)585-1825

Tyler, Grace Tung, MD {1700152899}
+ Primary Care at Gibbsboro
13 South Lakeview Drive   Gibbsboro, NJ 08026   (856)783-2802   Fax (856)783-2806

Tyler, James Ralph, MD {1548273956} Anesth(66,DC03)
+ Wills Surgery Center of Central New Jersey
107 North Center Drive/Anesthesia   North Brunswick, NJ 08902   (732)297-8001   Fax (732)297-8007

Tyler, Matthew D., MD {1891052437} EmrgMd
+ Cooper Univerisry Emergency Physicians
One Cooper Plaza   Camden, NJ 08103   (856)342-2000   Fax (856)968-8272

Tyndall, Alina, MD {1720233315} FamMed(06,NJ05)
+ T and D Medical Associates
1036 North Broad Street   Hillside, NJ 07205   (908)409-2121   Fax (908)409-2119

Tyree, Laura Lynne, MD {1598737256} ObsGyn, IntrMd(99,NJ05)<NJ-OURLADY>
+ Osborn Family Health Center
1601 Haddon Road/OB/GYN   Camden, NJ 08103   (856)757-3700   Fax (856)365-7972

Tyrie, Leslie S., MD {1205162435} Surgry<NJ-UMDNJ>
+ University Hospital
150 Bergen Street/Trauma Ctr   Newark, NJ 07103   (973)972-0559

Tyris, Nickolas M., MD {1821309154}
+ 2 Doral Court
Marlton, NJ 08053   (856)874-6190
nick.tyris@gmail.com

Tyrrell, John A., DO {1164441978} EmrgMd, GenPrc(81,IA75)
+ Overlook Emerg Svcs Union Camp
1000 Galloping Hill Road   Union, NJ 07083

Tyshkov, Michael, MD {1902882038} PedGst, Pedtrc(77,RUSS)<NY-STATNRTH, NJ-OVERLOOK>
+ Children's SubSpecialty Center
33 Overlook Road/Suite 207   Summit, NJ 07901   (908)273-2300   Fax (908)273-4320
TYSHKOV@comcast.net

Tyson, Sydney L., MD {1639113665} Ophthl(87,MA01)
+ Eye Associates
251 South Lincoln Avenue   Vineland, NJ 08361   (856)691-8188   Fax (856)691-0421
+ Eye Associates
1401 Route 70 East   Cherry Hill, NJ 08034   (856)691-8188   Fax (856)428-6359
+ Eye Associates
141 Black Horse Pike/Suite 7   Blackwood, NJ 08361   (856)227-6262   Fax (856)227-8830

Tzeng, Alice Chaw, MD {1821025040} PhysMd(98,NJ05)
+ Associates in Rehabilitation Medicine
95 Mount Kemble Avenue   Morristown, NJ 07960   (973)267-2293   Fax (973)226-3144

Tzeng, Bowen Chi, MD {1952591760} FamMed
+ 195 Forest Avenue
Paramus, NJ 07652   (201)261-0379

Tzeng, Jausheng, MD {1275584864} PthAcl(96,NJ06)<NY-ELMHRST, NJ-ENGLWOOD>
+ Englewood Hospital and Medical Center
350 Engle Street/Pathology   Englewood, NJ 07631   (201)894-3000

Tzorfas, Scott D., MD {1780654061} Nrolgy(90,NJ05)<NJ-SHOREMEM, NJ-BURDTMLN>
+ 160 Shore Road
Somers Point, NJ 08244   (609)653-9595   Fax (609)653-9898
+ 15 Village Drive
Cape May Court House, NJ 08210   (609)653-9595   Fax (609)463-9899

Ubele, Deborah Anne, DO {1689985806} FamMed
+ Kennedy Health Alliance
1300 Liberty Place   Sicklerville, NJ 08081   (856)262-8100   Fax (856)885-6859

Ubhi, Damanpreet K., MD {1346410560} InfDis
+ ID Associates PA/dba ID Care
765 Route 10 East/Suite 201   Randolph, NJ 07869   (973)989-0068   Fax (973)361-8955
+ ID Associates PA/dba ID Care
8 Saddle Road   Cedar Knolls, NJ 07927   (973)989-0068   Fax (973)993-5953

Ucheagwu, Hyacinth Emenike, MD {1245420678} Pedtrc
+ 129 Jewett Avenue
Jersey City, NJ 07304

Ucheya, Blessing C., MD {1649415472} IntrMd<NJ-VIRTMHBC>
+ Virtua Memorial
175 Madison Avenue   Mount Holly, NJ 08060   (609)914-6180   Fax (609)914-6182

Uczkowska, Alicja Teresa, MD {1245288091} Pedtrc(82,POL08)<NJ-HACKNSK, NJ-NWTNMEM>
+ Pediatric Health Center
54 Plauderville Avenue/Suite 1   Garfield, NJ 07026   (973)772-0262   Fax (973)772-0265
+ Newton Medical Center
175 High Street   Newton, NJ 07860   (973)383-2121

Udani, Chandrakan I., MD {1518974229} FamMed, GenPrc(71,INA67)<NJ-SHOREMEM>
+ 5548 Asbury Avenue
Ocean City, NJ 08226   (609)399-1519   Fax (609)398-4712
+ 707 White Horse Pike/Suite E2
Absecon, NJ 08201   (609)646-0020

Udani, Neil P., MD {1003835232} IntrMd, IntHos(01,DMN01)<NJ-KNDRMRRS>
+ Kindred Hospital-New Jersey Morris County
400 West Blackwell Street   Dover, NJ 07801   (973)989-3085

Udani, Rajen I., MD {1245224039} PulDis, IntrMd, CritCr(80,INA67)<NJ-BURDTMLN>
+ Sleep & Respiratory Care
17 Court House South Dennis Ro   Cape May Court House, NJ 08210   (609)465-2646   Fax (609)465-7330
+ Sleep & Respiratory Care
318 South Chris Gaupp Drive   Galloway, NJ 08205   (609)465-2646   Fax (609)404-3653

Physicians by Name and Address

Udasco, Jocelynda O., MD {1376623116} Psychy(80,PHI01)<NJ-UNIVBHC>
+ University Behavioral HealthCare
183 South Orange Avenue   Newark, NJ 07103
Udascojo@umdnj.edu

Udasin, Gary E., MD {1043411804} IntrMd, OccpMd(82,NY08)
+ Schering Plough Research Institute
2000 Galloping Hill Road   Kenilworth, NJ 07033   (908)298-2820   Fax (908)298-2834
geudasin@spcorp.com

Udasin, Iris G., MD {1629114913} OccpMd, IntrMd, GPrvMd(82,NY08)<NJ-RWJUBRUN>
+ University Hospital-School of Public Health
170 Frelinghuysen Road   Piscataway, NJ 08854   (732)445-0123   Fax (732)445-0127
+ EOHSI Clinical Center - UMDNJ
681 Frelinghuysen Road   Piscataway, NJ 08855   (732)445-0123   Fax (732)445-0131
+ UH- RWJ Medical School
One Robert Wood Johnson Place   New Brunswick, NJ 08854   (732)418-8466   Fax (732)418-8126

Uddin, Nihat, MD {1841431269} Anesth
+ 21 Eisele Avenue
Ocean, NJ 07712

Uddin, Sarah T., DO {1104262948} FamMed(PA77)
+ Valley Medical Group
43 Yawpo Avenue/Suite 3   Oakland, NJ 07436   (201)337-9600

Uderman, Howard David, MD {1841335262} ClnPhm, IntrMd(78,PA13)
+ Chemed Family Health Center
1771 Madison Avenue   Lakewood, NJ 08701   (732)364-2144   Fax (732)364-3559

Udeshi, Hansa S., MD {1659476935} ObsGyn(65,INA69)
+ 1445 Route 130 South
North Brunswick, NJ 08902   (732)821-8550   Fax (732)821-1449

Udoh, Adaora Ngozi, MD {1225152283} ObsGyn(03,DC03)
+ Regional Women's Health Management
227 Laurel Road/Suite 300   Voorhees, NJ 08043   (856)669-6050   Fax (856)651-0792
info@rwhm.org

Udovenko, Olga, MD {1477962835} GenPrc<NJ-MEADWLND>
+ Meadowlands Hospital Medical Center
55 Meadowlands Parkway   Secaucus, NJ 07096   (201)392-3100

Uduaghan, Victor Aboiye, MD {1326198003} Pedtrc, PedCrC(95,NIG07)<NJ-UMDNJ>
+ University Hospital
150 Bergen Street/PICU   Newark, NJ 07103   (973)972-3784   Fax (973)972-7597

Udvarhelyi, Ian Steven, MD {1053413724} IntrMd(83,MD07)
+ AmeriHealth HMO, Inc.
8000 Midlantic Drive/Suite 333   Mount Laurel, NJ 08054   (856)778-6500

Ufondu, Ebele E., MD {1003979048} IntrMd(86,NIG01)<NJ-CHSMRCER, NJ-RWJUHAM>
+ Ebele Medical Associates
941 Whitehorse Avenue/Suite 14   Hamilton, NJ 08610   (609)581-4800   Fax (609)581-9980

Uglialoro, Adele Marie, MD {1295813095}
+ 34 Vinton Road
Madison, NJ 07940   (917)880-8312
adele87@hotmail.com

Ugoeke, Nene Linda, MD {1285926840}<NJ-JRSYSHMC>
+ Jersey Shore University Medical Center
1945 Route 33   Neptune, NJ 07753   (732)775-5500

Ugorec, Igor, MD {1790875961} Nrolgy, IntrMd(87,LIT02)<NY-PRSBWEIL>
+ Atlantic Neurosurgical Specialists
310 Madison Avenue/Suite 300   Morristown, NJ 07960   (973)285-7800   Fax (973)285-7839

Ugras, Steven A., MD {1649414541} SrgHnd(04,NJ06)
+ Hand & Wrist Surgery of NJ
140 Route 17 North/Suite 323   Paramus, NJ 07652   (201)483-9555   Fax (201)331-7003
+ Hand & Wrist Surgery of NJ
601 Hamburg Turnpike/Suite 101   Wayne, NJ 07470   (201)483-9555   Fax (201)331-7003

Ugras Rey, Sandra S., DO {1992758932} EmrgMd(01,NJ75)
+ Clifton Comprehensive Medical Center
960 Paulison Avenue   Clifton, NJ 07011   (973)773-7713   Fax (973)773-7723

Uhm, Kyudong, MD {1740222454} Hemato, IntrMd, MedOnc(69,KOR04)
+ North Jersey Hematology Oncology Group
1117 Route 46/Suite 205   Clifton, NJ 07013   (973)471-0981   Fax (973)471-5818

Uhrik, Eric Joseph, DO {1942330998} Nrolgy, GenPrc(89,ME75)
+ Neurology Consultants of Central Jersey, P.A.
225 May Street/Suite D   Edison, NJ 08837   (732)738-8830   Fax (732)738-8831

Ujire, Manasa P., MD {1063679413}
+ LMA Transplant Nephrology
1601 Haddon Avenue   Camden, NJ 08103   (856)757-3840

Ukazu, Adanna C., MD {1154612760} ObsGyn
+ Rutgers- New Jersey Medical School
185 South Orange Avenue/Room E506   Newark, NJ 07103   (973)972-5266

Uko, Smart E., MD {1679669048} NnPnMd, Pedtrc<NJ-OURLADY>
+ Our Lady of Lourdes Medical Center
1600 Haddon Avenue   Camden, NJ 08103   (856)757-3500   Fax (856)365-7868

Ukonu, Ugochukwu, MD {1639586845} FamMed<NY-GDSAMMC>
+ Red Bank Primary Care Center
188 East Bergen Place/Suite 302   Red Bank, NJ 07701   (732)219-6620   Fax (732)219-6225

Ukraincik, Miro, MD {1114029659} Pedtrc(93,CROA)<NJ-KIMBALL>
+ Dr. Gittleman & Associates
450 East Kennedy Boulevard   Lakewood, NJ 08701   (732)901-0050   Fax (732)370-2386

Ukrainski, Gerald J., MD {1477532992} CdvDis, IntrMd(79,NY20)<NJ-ACMCMAIN, NJ-ATLANCHS>
+ Associated Cardiovascular Consultants, PA
2 Sindoni Lane   Hammonton, NJ 08037   (609)561-8500   Fax (856)567-0432
+ Associated Cardiovascular Consultants, PA
2500 English Creek Avenue   Egg Harbor Township, NJ 08234   (609)561-8500   Fax (609)569-1896
+ Associated Cardiovascular Consultants-Lourdes
1 Brace Road/Suite C & F   Cherry Hill, NJ 08037   (856)428-4100   Fax (856)428-5748

Ukrainskyj, Motria O., MD {1396791703} Surgry, SrgBst(86,NY09)<NJ-STJOSHOS>
+ St. Mary's Hospital
350 Boulevard/Suite 100   Passaic, NJ 07055   (973)365-4100

Ulep, Shirley Dollaga, MD {1740245133} Pedtrc(94,PHI15)
+ Silverton Pediatrics
2446 Church Road   Toms River, NJ 08753   (732)255-7553   Fax (732)255-8901

Ulke, Taner A., DO {1528478138} FamMed<NJ-SJHREGMC>
+ SJH Regional Medical Center
1505 West Sherman Avenue   Vineland, NJ 08360   (856)641-8000

Ulker Sarokhan, Erol E., MD {1083633283} Urolgy(78,MEX03)<NJ-CLARMAAS, NJ-STBARNMC>
+ Urology Consultants
7 Colonial Way   Chatham, NJ 07928   (973)759-6180   Fax (973)759-2006
rockdoc96@aol.com

Ulloque, Rory Alexander, MD {1407127343} FamMed
+ Family Medicine at Monument Square
317 George Street   New Brunswick, NJ 08901   (732)235-8993   Fax (732)246-7317
+ UH- Robert Wood Johnson Med
125 Paterson Street/MEB 278   New Brunswick, NJ 08901   (732)235-8993   Fax (732)235-7001
+ PromptMD Urgent Care Center
309 First Street   Hoboken, NJ 08901   (201)222-8411   Fax (201)222-8711

Umakanthan, Suganthini, MD {1609973346} IntrMd(89,SRIL)<NJ-NWRKBETH>
+ Newark Beth Israel Medical Center
201 Lyons Avenue/Geriatrics   Newark, NJ 07112   (973)926-8491

Umali, Alma B., MD {1720161680} EmrgMd, Pedtrc, EmrgEMed(65,PHI01)<NJ-STMRYPAS, NJ-CHILTON>
+ St. Mary's Hospital
350 Boulevard/Pediatrics   Passaic, NJ 07055   (973)365-4300
+ Chilton Medical Center
97 West Parkway/Pediatrics   Pompton Plains, NJ 07444   (973)831-5000

Umali, Winston Caraos, MD {1740395433} Pedtrc(94,PHI02)<NJ-CHRIST>
+ Winston C. Umali MD PC
395 Danforth Avenue   Jersey City, NJ 07305   (201)209-9007   Fax (201)432-5142

Umali Pamintuan, Maria Angela T., MD {1164631537} PedCrd(00,PHI30)<NJ-JRSYSHMC>
+ Alpert Zales & Castro Pediatric Cardiology, PA
1623 Route 88/Suite A/PO Box 1719   Brick, NJ 08723   (732)458-9666   Fax (732)458-0840
+ Alpert Zales & Castro Pediatric Cardiology, PA
2 Apple Farm Road/PO Box 4176   Middletown, NJ 07748   (732)458-9666   Fax (732)458-0840

Umanoff, Michael D., MD {1902804438} Anesth(81,MEX33)<NJ-STJOSHOS>
+ St. Joseph's Regional Medical Center Anesthesia
703 Main Street   Paterson, NJ 07503   (973)754-2323   Fax (973)977-9455

Umer, Muhammad S., MD {1548237704} IntrMd(90,PAKI)<NJ-HACKNSK, NJ-HOLYNAME>
+ Internal Medicine PA
155 Cedar Lane   Teaneck, NJ 07666   (201)836-4248   Fax (201)836-5420

Umeukeje, Judith N., MD {1710936448} Pedtrc(97,NIG02)<NJ-STCLRDEN>
+ St. Clare's Hospital-Denville Campus
25 Pocono Road   Denville, NJ 07834   (973)983-5750

Undavia, Samir Suresh, MD {1811130057} OtgyFPIS, OtgyPSHN, Otlryg(05,NY09)
+ Princeton Eye and Ear
2999 Princeton Pike/2 FL   Lawrenceville, NJ 08648   (609)403-8840   Fax (609)403-8852
+ Princeton Eye and Ear
5 Plainsboro Road/Suite 510   Plainsboro, NJ 08536   (609)403-8840   Fax (609)403-8852

Underberg-Davis, Sharon J., MD {1942286232} PedRad, Radiol(88,MA01)<NJ-RWJUBRUN, NJ-STPETER>
+ University Radiology Group, P.C.
483 Cranbury Road   East Brunswick, NJ 08816   (732)390-0030   Fax (732)390-5383
+ University Radiology Group, P.C.
16 Mountain Boulevard   Warren, NJ 07059   (732)390-0030   Fax (908)769-9141

Ung, Kenneth H., MD {1730189804} ObsGyn(93,PA13)<NJ-CHSMRCER, NJ-UNVMCPRN>
+ Delaware Valley Ob/Gyn & Infertility Group, PC
2 Princess Road/Suite C   Lawrenceville, NJ 08648   (609)896-0777   Fax (609)896-3266
+ Delaware Valley Ob/Gyn & Infertility Group, PC
300B Princeton Hightstown Road   East Windsor, NJ 08520   (609)896-0777   Fax (609)443-4506

Unger, Jeffrey S., MD {1104864487} Gastrn, IntrMd(94,MA05)<NJ-SOMERSET>
+ Gastromed HealthCare, PA
25 Monroe Street   Bridgewater, NJ 08807   (908)231-1999   Fax (908)231-1612

Ungerleider, Deborah L., MD {1437118544} Pedtrc(85,NJ06)<NJ-VALLEY>
+ 44 Godwin Avenue/Suite 100
Midland Park, NJ 07432   (201)444-8389   Fax (201)444-2309

Unni, Nisha, MD {1366619579} IntrMd
+ 705 Yosko Drive
Edison, NJ 08817

Unson, Enrique Miguel S., MD {1487077350}
+ 100 Hiram Square/Apt 519
New Brunswick, NJ 08901   (609)356-3492
vinounson@gmail.com

Untawale, Vasundhara G., MD {1548426935} Pthlgy, PthACl(70,INA3A)
+ Quest Diagnostics Inc.
1 Malcolm Avenue   Teterboro, NJ 07608   (201)393-5122   Fax (201)393-6127

Unterman, Michael I., MD {1033114194} Radiol, RadV&I, RadDia(78,NY09)<NJ-OCEANMC>
+ Open MRI of Wall
1975 Route 34   Wall, NJ 07719   (732)974-8060
+ Lacey Diagnostic Imaging LLC
833 Lacey Road/Suite 2   Forked River, NJ 08731   (732)974-8060   Fax (609)242-2402
+ Coastal Imaging, LLC
79 Route 37 West/Suite 103   Toms River, NJ 07719   (732)678-0087   Fax (732)276-2325

Unuigbe, Augustine Aigbovbioise, MD {1902118383} IntrMd
+ Drs. Unuigbe and Unuigbe
118 Peach Tree Lane   Egg Harbor Township, NJ 08234

Unuigbe, Florence, MD {1710257571} IntrMd
+ Drs. Unuigbe and Unuigbe
118 Peach Tree Lane   Egg Harbor Township, NJ 08234   (609)457-2769

Unwala, Ashfaque A., MD {1861447260} CdvDis, IntrMd(83,IL01)
+ Owens Vergari Unwala Cardiology Associates PC
17 West Red Bank Avenue/Suite 306   Woodbury, NJ 08096   (856)845-6807   Fax (856)845-3760

Upadhyay, Anu, MD {1801974118} PsyCAd, PsyAdt(92,INA95)<NJ-UNIVBHC>
+ University Behavioral Health Care
671 Hoes Lane/PO Box 1392/Psych   Piscataway, NJ 08855   (732)235-5500

Upadhyay, Hinesh Natwarlal, MD {1144632944} IntrMd(05,INA53)<NJ-JFKMED>
+ JFK Medical Center
65 James Street/Internal Med   Edison, NJ 08820   (732)321-7935
+ Pulmonary Internists, PA
2 Lincoln Highway/Suite 301   Edison, NJ 08820   (732)321-7935   Fax (732)548-8216

Physicians by Name and Address

Upadhyay, Shivanck, MD {1376815647} CritCr
+ St. Joseph's Regional Medical Center Anesthesia
  703 Main Street   Paterson, NJ 07503   (973)754-2323   Fax (973)754-3376

Upadhyaya, Hitendrakumar C., MD {1902912561} IntrMd, OncHem(83,INDI)<NJ-JRSYCITY, NJ-BAYONNE>
+ Colanta Hematology & Oncology Center
  564 Broadway/1st Floor   Bayonne, NJ 07002   (201)823-3107   Fax (201)437-4979
  info@colantahomc.com
+ Jersey City Medical Center
  355 Grand Street   Jersey City, NJ 07304   (201)823-3107   Fax (201)915-2192
+ United Medical, P.C.
  988 Broadway/Suite 201   Bayonne, NJ 07002   (201)339-6111   Fax (201)339-6333

Upadya, Padmaja Koppal, MD {1518965045} Anesth(97,INDI)<NJ-STJOSHOS>
+ St. Joseph's Regional Medical Center Anesthesia
  703 Main Street   Paterson, NJ 07503   (973)754-2323   Fax (973)977-9455

Uppal, Jaspreet Singh, MD {1346507548}
+ 49 Fela Drive
  Parlin, NJ 08859   (732)306-3181
  juppalmd@gmail.com

Uppal, Muhammad S., MD {1144589730} IntrMd<NJ-JRSYCITY>
+ Jersey City Medical Center
  355 Grand Street   Jersey City, NJ 07304   (201)915-2000

Uppal, Parveen, MD {1215905070} CdvDis, IntrMd, IntCrd(84,INDI)<NJ-BAYSHORE, NJ-RIVERVW>
+ Heart Care Center/Parveen Uppal LLC
  80 Hazlet Avenue/Suite 3   Hazlet, NJ 07730   (732)888-7901   Fax (732)888-7905

Uppal, Rajiv, MD {1508804345} Gastrn, IntrMd, Pedtrc(82,INDI)<NJ-MONMOUTH, NJ-RIVERVW>
+ Monmouth Gastroenterology
  142 Route 35   Eatontown, NJ 07724   (732)389-5004   Fax (732)389-1850
+ Monmouth Gastroenterology
  142 State Route 35 South/Suite 103   Eatontown, NJ 07724

Uppal, Vijay L., MD {1124004411} Radiol, RadDia(70,INA82)<NJ-STPETER, NJ-RWJUBRUN>
+ University Radiology Group, P.C.
  483 Cranbury Road   East Brunswick, NJ 08816   (732)390-0030   Fax (732)390-5383
+ University Radiology Group, P.C.
  260 Amboy Avenue   Metuchen, NJ 08840   (732)390-0030   Fax (732)548-3392

Uppaluri, Lakshmi P., MD {1629198783} Pedtrc, PedPul
+ University Hospital-RWJ Medical School
  89 French Street/2nd Floor   New Brunswick, NJ 08901   (732)235-7899   Fax (732)235-7077
  UppaluriL@umdnj.edu

Uppuluri, Pranay C., MD {1396991451}
+ 79 Beeachwood Avenue
  Edison, NJ 08837   (732)791-2972

Uram, Martin, MD {1396781506} Ophthl(77,PA09)
+ Retina Consultants
  39 Sycamore Avenue   Little Silver, NJ 07739   (732)530-7730   Fax (732)530-3837

Urban, Scott Michael, DO {1952348930} EmrgMd(98,PA77)<NJ-ACMCITY, NJ-ACMCMAIN>
+ AtlantiCare Regional Medical Center/City Campus
  1925 Pacific Avenue/EmergMed   Atlantic City, NJ 08401   (609)345-4000
+ AtlantiCare Regional Med Ctr/Mainland
  65 West Jimmie Leeds Road/EmergMed   Pomona, NJ 08240   (609)652-1000

Urbano, Frank Louis, MD {1184711921} IntrMd(94,NJ05)<NJ-COOPRUMC, NJ-VIRTMHBC>
+ Cooper University Hospital
  One Cooper Plaza   Camden, NJ 08103   (856)342-2000

Urbina, Emily Anne, MD {1457595118} Psychy
+ 115 Old Short Hills Road/Apt 374
  West Orange, NJ 07052   (561)598-9834

Urena, Julio H., MD {1356302186} IntrMd(76,DOM01)
+ 40 Union Avenue
  Clifton, NJ 07011   (973)574-0010   Fax (973)574-0031

Uretsky, Seth, MD {1194823856} CdvDis, IntrMd(01,NY19)
+ Gagnon Cardiovasular Institute
  100 Madison Avenue/Level C   Morristown, NJ 07962   (973)971-5597   Fax (973)290-7145

Uretsky, Stephen H., MD {1235188798} Ophthl(77,DC01)<NJ-ACMCMAIN, NJ-ACMCITY>
+ Coastal Jersey Eye Center
  2021 New Road/Suite 6   Linwood, NJ 08221   (609)927-3373   Fax (609)927-4041
+ Coastal Jersey Eye Center
  101 Courthouse-South Dennis Rd   Cape May Court House, NJ 08210   (609)465-7926
+ Court House Surgery Center
  106 Courthouse South Dennis Rd   Cape May, NJ 08221

(609)465-0300   Fax (609)465-8771

Urkowitz, Alan L., DO {1689634263} FamMed(86,IA75)<NJ-SJRSYELM, NJ-KENEDYHS>
+ Wedgewood Family Practice Associates PA
  302 Hurffville Cross-Keys Road   Sewell, NJ 08080   (856)589-4610   Fax (609)589-1624

Urman, Alina, DO {1871908525} IntrMd<NJ-PALISADE>
+ Palisades Medical Center
  7600 River Road   North Bergen, NJ 07047   (201)854-5713

Urman, Felix, MD {1902844210} Dermat(01,NY03)
+ Academic Dermatology Inc
  75 Veronica Avenue/Suite 205   Somerset, NJ 08873   (732)246-9900   Fax (732)246-9902

Urquhart, Marc Wayne, MD {1235208794} SrgOrt, SrgHnd, SprtMd(93,MD07)<NJ-MEADWLND, NJ-STBARNMC>
+ Urquhart Orthopedic Associates
  534 Avenue E/Suite 1-B   Bayonne, NJ 07002   (201)436-8289   Fax (201)471-2434
+ Urquhart Orthopedic Associates
  609 Morris Avenue   Springfield, NJ 07081   (201)436-8289   Fax (201)471-2434

Urquhart, Megan C., DO {1982834768} EmrgMd<NJ-SJHREGMC>
+ SJH Regional Medical Center
  1505 West Sherman Avenue   Vineland, NJ 08360   (856)641-8000

Urrutia, Ellen E., MD {1629046388} IntrMd, CdvDis(87,GRNA)<NJ-STMICHL, NJ-HACKNSK>
+ Bart De Gregorio MD, LLC.
  946 Bloomfield Avenue   Glen Ridge, NJ 07028   (973)743-1121   Fax (973)743-2627

Urs, Krishna J., MD {1366484768}<NJ-JFKMED>
+ JFK Medical Center
  65 James Street   Edison, NJ 08820   (732)321-7000   Fax (732)321-7330

Ursani, Sekander A., MD EmrgMd(73,PAK04)<NJ-VIRTBERL, NJ-ACMCITY>
+ 722 Moonraker Court
  Smithville, NJ 08205

Usal, Hakan Marc, MD {1396732954} SrgPlstc, SrgMcr, IntrMd(86,TUR01)
+ Usal Cosmetic Surgery, P.C.
  305 Route 17 South   Paramus, NJ 07652   (201)967-9200   Fax (201)967-8300

Usgaonker, Susrut R., DO {1730520073} IntrMd(13,WV75)
+ The Valley Hospital
  223 North Van Dien Avenue   Ridgewood, NJ 07450   (201)447-8618

Usiene, Irmute, MD {1588862221}<NJ-BERGNMC>
+ New Bridge Medical Center
  230 East Ridgewood Avenue   Paramus, NJ 07652   (201)967-4000

Usiskin, Keith S., MD {1023215225} EnDbMt, IntrMd(84,NJ06)
+ 3 Ogden Road
  Mendham, NJ 07945   (973)267-9099

Usman, Mohammed Haris Umer, MD {1265622195} IntrMd, CdvDis, IntCrd(PAK11)<PA-MRCYFTZG>
+ Monmouth Heart Specialists
  274 Highway 35   Eatontown, NJ 07724   (732)440-7336   Fax (732)440-9404

Usmani, Aniqa, MD {1457649451} Psychy
+ 5 Creekside Trail
  Delran, NJ 08075

Usmani, Qaisar H., MD {1548364896} IntrMd, Rheuma(86,PAKI)
+ SNS Rheumatology Associates
  2333 Whitehorse Mercerville Rd/Suite J   Trenton, NJ 08619   (609)689-1229

Ussery-Kronhaus, Kelly G., MD {1285731745} FamMed(02,DMN01)
+ Jersey Coast Family Medicine
  495 Jack Martin Boulevard/Suite 5   Brick, NJ 08724   (732)458-8000   Fax (732)458-8020

Uthappa, Machia M., MD {1124098678} IntrMd(86,INA37)<NJ-JFKJHNSN>
+ Mid Jersey Medical Associates
  1 Ethel Road/Suite 107b   Edison, NJ 08817   (732)287-2020   Fax (732)287-2071

Utkewicz, Mark D., MD {1356420517} EmrgMd(87,NJ05)<NJ-SOMERSET>
+ Emergency Medical Associates of NJ, P.A.
  3 Century Drive   Parsippany, NJ 07054   (973)740-0607   Fax (973)740-9895

Utpat, Sandeepa Makarand, MD {1205864899} InfDis, IntrMd(94,INA39)<NJ-OCEANMC>
+ Infectious Disease Associates
  2360 Route 9 South   Howell, NJ 07731   (732)905-6635   Fax (732)905-6643

Utrankar, Deepti Sameer, MD {1033200746} Anesth(91,INA67)
+ James Street Anesthesia
  102 James Street/Suite 103   Edison, NJ 08820   (732)494-1444   Fax (732)494-7052

Utreras, Juan S., MD {1518906270} IntrMd(97,ECU01)<NJ-COOPRUMC>
+ Cooper Perinatology Associates
  3 Cooper Plaza/Suite 502   Camden, NJ 08103   (856)356-4935   Fax (856)968-8499
+ Cooper Physicians Office
  196 Grove Avenue/Suite C   Thorofare, NJ 08086   (856)356-4935   Fax (856)848-6554

Uustal, Heikki, MD {1952328635} PhysMd(84,VT02)<NJ-JFKMED, NJ-JFKJHNSN>
+ JFK Medical Center
  65 James Street/Phys Med&Rehab   Edison, NJ 08820   (908)321-7070   Fax (732)321-7330
+ JFK Johnson Rehabilitation Institute
  65 James Street   Edison, NJ 08818   (732)321-7050

Uy, Loreta M., MD {1164447587} Pedtrc, AdolMd(85,PHI10)
+ Internet Medical Group, P.C.
  66 Somme Street   Newark, NJ 07105   (973)589-7337   Fax (973)589-1905
  Loreta.uy@verizon.net

Uy, Vena, MD {1770691032} ObsGyn(68,PHI08)
+ 142 Palisade Avenue/Suite 102
  Jersey City, NJ 07306   (201)653-0506   Fax (201)653-6229

Uychich, Priscilla M., DO {1962623868} IntrMd(91,IA75)
+ 290 Market Street
  Elmwood Park, NJ 07407   (201)796-0866   Fax (201)475-1554

Uzbay, Lisa Ann, MD {1619004934} ObsGyn(93,NY48)<NJ-HCKTSTWN>
+ Women's Health at Hackettstown
  108 Bilby Road/Suite 305   Hackettstown, NJ 07840   (908)813-8877   Fax (908)813-9984

Uzoaru, Charles O., MD {1659317709} ObsGyn(77,PA01)
+ 112 South Munn Avenue
  East Orange, NJ 07018   (973)674-0053
  info@eastorangewomenservices.com

Uzun, Nagehan, DO {1073872727}<NJ-HLTHSRE>
+ HealthSouth Rehabilitation Hospital of New Jersey
  14 Hospital Drive   Toms River, NJ 08755   (609)686-8000

Vacca, Michael John, MD {1174676944} Pedtrc, IntrMd(72,ITA01)<NJ-CHILTON>
+ Advocare Pediatric Arts
  1403 Route 23 South   Butler, NJ 07405   (973)283-2200   Fax (973)283-0406
+ Advocare Pediatric Arts
  1777 Hamburg Turnpike/Suite 103   Wayne, NJ 07470   (973)283-2200   Fax (973)283-0406

Vaccaro, Carl Anthony, DO {1528245461} IntrMd(05,PA78)<NJ-JRSYSHMC>
+ Cape Health Solutions, LLC.
  650 Town Bank Road   North Cape May, NJ 08204   (609)884-3680   Fax (609)884-3649

Vaccaro, Carmine A., MD {1871560243} IntrMd(70,ITA28)<NJ-JRSYSHMC>
+ 804 West Park Avenue/Building B
  Ocean, NJ 07712   (732)493-4100   Fax (732)493-3302
+ 19 Cambridge Way
  Ocean, NJ 07712   (732)922-1656

Vaccaro, John J., MD {1861463267} SrgPlstc, IntrMd(73,MEX03)<NJ-HACKNSK, NY-KINGSCO>
+ 202 Route 37 West/Suite 1-A
  Toms River, NJ 08755   (732)914-2100

Vaccaro, John J., MD {1083682017} Nrolgy, Elecmy(92,VA07)<NJ-MTNSIDE, NJ-CLARMAAS>
+ Neurological Consultants
  230 Sherman Avenue/Suite K   Glen Ridge, NJ 07028   (973)743-9555   Fax (973)743-7663
+ Neurological Consultants
  1100 Clifton Avenue   Clifton, NJ 07013   (973)743-9555   Fax (973)743-7663

Vaclavik, John Philip Charles, MD {1548467137} ObsGyn(04,GRN01)<NJ-MONMOUTH>
+ Monmouth Medical Center
  300 Second Avenue   Long Branch, NJ 07740   (732)222-5200

Vaclavik, Peter Svatopluk, MD {1922043579} PedAne, Anesth(02,NJ06)<NJ-JRSYSHMC>
+ Jersey Shore Anesthesiology Associates
  1945 Route 33/PO Box 397   Neptune, NJ 07754   (732)897-0200   Fax (732)897-0263

Vadada, Kiran, MD {1497912489} PhysMd, IntrMd
+ Spine Center
  106 Grand Avenue/Suite 220   Englewood, NJ 07631   (201)503-1900   Fax (201)503-1901

Vadakara, Laisa L., MD {1558371930} IntrMd(89,INA68)<NJ-CHSMRCER, NJ-RWJUHAM>
+ Vadakara Internal Medicine
  2117 Klockner Road   Hamilton, NJ 08690   (609)584-1001   Fax (609)584-0404

Vadakara, Lukose Simon, MD {1255340345}
IntrMd(90,INA98)<NJ-CHSMRCER, NJ-RWJUHAM>
+ Vadakara Internal Medicine
2117 Klockner Road   Hamilton, NJ 08690   (609)584-1001
Fax (609)584-0404

Vadali, Rajyalaks Vaidehi, MD {1134129448}
Pedtrc(88,INA5B)<NJ-JFKMED, NJ-NWRKBETH>
+ Rainbow Medical Associates
200 Perrine Road/Suite 228   Old Bridge, NJ 08857
(732)679-0660   Fax (732)679-7177
+ Rainbow Medical Associates
2177 Oak Tree Drive   Edison, NJ 08818   (732)679-0660

Vadde, Kavitha, MD {1184641003} Radiol, RadDia(94,MA07)<NJ-ENGLWOOD>
+ Englewood Radiologic Group PA
350 Engle Street   Englewood, NJ 07631   (201)894-3000
Fax (201)894-5244
+ Advanced Medical Imaging of North Jersey
452 Old Hook Road/Suite 301   Emerson, NJ 07630
(201)894-3000   Fax (201)262-2330

Vadehra, Vivek Kumar, MD {1073602793} IntrMd(95,NJ05)
+ University Hospital-New Jersey Medical School
30 Bergen Street/Room 1207   Newark, NJ 07107
(973)972-4511   Fax (973)972-9355

Vadhavkar, Aarti Sanjeev, MD {1003076373} Anesth
+ Capital Health System/Hopewell
One Capital Way/Anesthesia   Pennington, NJ 08534
(609)394-4000

Vagadia, Neha R., DO {1649326463}
+ Virtua Garden State Pulmonary Associates
520 Lippincott Drive/Suite A   Marlton, NJ 08053   (856)596-9057   Fax (856)596-8897
nvagadia@virtua.org

Vagaonescu, Tudor Dumitru, MD {1417031170} IntrMd, CdvDis, IntCrd(86,ROM06)<NY-LENOXHLL>
+ University Cardiology Group
125 Paterson Street/MEB 578   New Brunswick, NJ 08901
(732)235-7855   Fax (732)235-8722
+ University Cardiology Group
125 Paterson Street/Suite 5200   New Brunswick, NJ 08901
(732)235-7855   Fax (732)235-6530

Vaghasiya, Rick Parsotam, MD {1275776098} Nephro, IntrMd
+ Kidney & Hypertension Center of Central Jersey
23 Clyde Road/Suite 101   Somerset, NJ 08873   (732)873-9500   Fax (732)873-0261
+ Kidney & Hypertension Center of Central Jersey
1 Eastern Avenue   Somerville, NJ 08876   (732)873-9500

Vaiana, Paul, MD {1073523627} IntrMd(83,MEX29)
+ 216 Palmer Street
Elizabeth, NJ 07202   (908)352-4477   Fax (908)355-1202

Vaidhyanathan, Ketaki, MD {1992904445} Psychy<NJ-MTNSIDE>
+ Hackensack UMC Mountainside
1 Bay Avenue   Montclair, NJ 07042   (973)429-6260

Vaidya, Ami P., MD {1982678413} GynOnc, ObsGyn(99,NY01)<NJ-RWJUBRUN>
+ John Theurer Cancer Center - HUMC
92 Second Street/GynOncology   Hackensack, NJ 07601
(201)996-5373   Fax (551)996-0572

Vaidya, Darshan C., MD {1609000199} Dermat
+ Princeton Dermatology Associates
5 Centre Street/Suite 1-A   Monroe Township, NJ 08831
(609)655-4544   Fax (609)655-2390
dvaidya83@gmail.com

Vaidya, Kamini P., MD {1316005531} PthAcl, PthCyt(72,INDI)<NJ-HOBUNIMC>
+ Hoboken University Medical Center
308 Willow Avenue/Path   Hoboken, NJ 07030   (201)418-1000   Fax (201)418-1983

Vaidya, Ketankumar N., MD {1487688586} IntrMd, Grtrcs(95,INA8B)
+ 2149 Woodbridge Avenue
Edison, NJ 08817   (732)985-2151   Fax (732)985-0650

Vaidya, Pranaychan J., MD {1659322204} CdvDis, IntrMd, IntCrd(71,INA20)<NJ-HACKNSK>
+ Bergen Invasive Cardiovascular Consultants
211 Essex Street/Suite 306   Hackensack, NJ 07601
(201)343-2050   Fax (201)343-4512

Vaillant, Juan Guillermo, MD {1063509651} Dermat(71,CHI02)
+ 40 Throckmorton Lane
Old Bridge, NJ 08857   (732)679-0222

Vakar, Emil, DO {1518274273} Psychy(NY75
+ Riverview Medical Center
1 Riverview Plaza/Psychiatry   Red Bank, NJ 07701
(732)741-2700

Vakil, Rupesh M., MD {1043466535} PulCCr, CritCr, IntrMd(05,DMN01)
+ VMG Respiratory Health & Pulmonary Medicine
1200 East Ridgewood Avenue   Ridgewood, NJ 07450
(201)689-7755   Fax (201)689-0521
+ Respiratory Health & Critical Care Associates
1114 Goffle Road/Suite 103   Hawthorne, NJ 07506

(201)689-7755   Fax (973)790-4330

Vakil, Vidya S., MD {1356453880} Pedtrc, AdolMd(75,INA75)<NJ-UNVMCPRN, NJ-CHSMRCER>
+ 666 Plainsboro Road
Plainsboro, NJ 08536   (609)275-0729   Fax (609)275-3875

Vakili, Babak, MD {1184705501} UroGyn, ObsGyn(97,PA02)<NJ-COOPRUMC>
+ University Urogynecology Associates
6012 Piazza at Main Street   Voorhees, NJ 08043   (856)325-6622   Fax (856)325-6522
+ Women's Care Center
3 Cooper Plaza/Suite 301   Camden, NJ 08103   (856)325-6622   Fax (856)968-8575

Valane, Honora W., MD {1669689964} Surgry(76,NJ05)<NJ-JFKMED>
+ JFK Medical Center
65 James Street/Surgery   Edison, NJ 08820   (732)321-7668

Valarezo, Vanessa C., MD {1891239034}
+ Lifeline Medical Associates, LLC
50 Cherry Hill Road/Suite 303   Parsippany, NJ 07054
(973)335-8500   Fax (973)335-8429

Valcarcel, Raul, MD {1831223510} IntrMd(87,PRO01)<NJ-SOMERSET>
+ Monroe Medical Associates, P.A.
685 Avon Drive   East Windsor, NJ 08520   (609)918-0330
Fax (609)918-0331

Valdellon, Alejandro M., MD {1306829379} EmrgMd(66,PHI01)<NJ-ANNKLEIN>
+ Ann Klein Forensic Center
1609 Stuyvesant Avenue/PO Box 7717   West Trenton, NJ 08628   (609)633-0900

Valdes, Michael E., MD {1760441414} SrgPlstc, SrgCsm, SrgBst(75,NY01)<NJ-STCLRDOV, NJ-STCLRDEN>
+ 101 Gibraltar Drive/Suite 3E
Morris Plains, NJ 07950   (973)984-2121   Fax (973)984-2119

Valdesuso, Gladys M., MD {1467665554} IntrMd(84,NJ05)
+ McCosh Health Center
Washington Road/McCosh Infirmary   Princeton, NJ 08544
(609)258-5357   Fax (609)258-1355

Valdez, Napoleon A., MD {1760548770} SrgOrt(66,PHI08)<NJ-VALLEY>
+ 39-04 Broadway/Suite 101
Fair Lawn, NJ 07410   (201)791-0033   Fax (201)791-0411

Valdivieso, Julio, MD {1306834080} NnPnMd, Pedtrc(75,PER08)<NY-SOUTHNAS, NJ-UMDNJ>
+ University Hospital
150 Bergen Street/Neonatology   Newark, NJ 07103
(973)972-4300

Valdivieso, Yaira Michelle, MD {1578746327} Pedtrc(05,COS02)<NJ-STJOSHOS>
+ Riverside Pediatric Group
4201 New York Avenue   Union City, NJ 07087   (201)601-9515   Fax (201)601-9516

Valencia, Maria Linda, MD {1487716312} Pedtrc(71,PHI01)<NJ-CHSFULD, NJ-CHSMRCER>
+ Mercer County Pediatrics
2113 Klockner Road   Trenton, NJ 08690   (609)586-7887
Fax (609)586-1198

Valencia, Maria R., MD {1598725087} Anesth, FamMed(74,PHI01)<NJ-UNDRWD>
+ Inspira Health Network
509 North Broad Street   Woodbury, NJ 08096   (856)845-0100   Fax (856)853-9334

Valencia, Rafael L., MD {1518045525} Pedtrc(74,PHI01)
+ 146 Haddonfield Berlin Road/Suite 102
Gibbsboro, NJ 08026   (856)435-6530   Fax (856)435-3206

Valentin-Torres, Melanie Rouse, MD {1366721698} IntrMd
+ ID Associates PA/dba ID Care
765 Route 10 East/Suite 201   Randolph, NJ 07869
(973)989-0068   Fax (973)361-8955

Valentino, Steven John, DO {1366400798} SrgOrt(82,PA77)
+ South Jersey Sports Medicine Center
556 Egg Harbor Road/Suite A   Sewell, NJ 08080   (856)589-0650   Fax (856)589-2720

Valenza, Joseph P., MD {1316935372} PhysMd, PainMd(92,NY06)<NJ-KSLRSADB, NJ-KSLRWELK>
+ Kessler Institute for Rehabilitation
300 Market Street   Saddle Brook, NJ 07663   (201)587-8500
+ Kessler Institute for Rehab
201 Pleasant Hill Road   Chester, NJ 07930   (973)584-7500
+ Kessler Institute for Rehabilitation West Orange
1199 Pleasant Valley Way   West Orange, NJ 07663
(973)731-3600

Valenzuela, Julie Y., MD {1386751014}<NJ-UMDNJ>
+ University Hospital
150 Bergen Street   Newark, NJ 07103   (201)381-0222
julie.son0@gmail.com

Valenzuela, Rolando Gabriel, MD {1275794885} EmrgMd
+ University Hospital-New Jersey Medical School
30 Bergen Street/ADMC Rm 1110   Newark, NJ 07107
(973)972-9261

Physicians by Name and Address

Valerian, Christopher, DO {1841462058} FamMed(94,NY75)<NJ-HOBUNIMC>
+ Center for Family Health
122-132 Clinton Street   Hoboken, NJ 07030   (201)418-3100   Fax (201)418-3148

Valeus, Pierre Rigens, MD {1306021027} IntHos<NJ-VIRTMHBC>
+ Virtua Memorial
175 Madison Avenue   Mount Holly, NJ 08060   (609)267-0700

Valinoti, Anne Marie, MD {1801852579} IntrMd(91,NY01)<NJ-VALLEY>
+ Prospect Medical Offices, LLC
301 Godwin Avenue   Midland Park, NJ 07432   (201)444-4526   Fax (201)301-1313

Valiveti, Sailaja Devi, MD {1053320275} PsyGrt, Psychy(91,INA8Y)
+ Kurra Associates
15-01 Broadway/Suite 10-B   Fair Lawn, NJ 07410
(201)794-7733   Fax (201)794-6039

Valko, Peter C., MD {1528003159} EmrgMd, IntrMd(84,MEXI)
+ Integrated Medical Alliance/IMA Medical Care Center
30 Shrewsbury Plaza   Shrewsbury, NJ 07702   (732)542-0002   Fax (732)542-2992

Vallabhaneni, Purnima, MD {1316945645} IntrMd(94,INA1L)<NJ-STPETER>
+ Medical Associates of Marlboro, P.C.
3084 State Route 27/Suite 1   Kendall Park, NJ 08824
(732)821-0873   Fax (732)297-7356
+ Medical Associates of Marlboro PC
32 North Main Street   Marlboro, NJ 07746   (732)821-0873
Fax (732)462-3798

Vallar, Robert V., MD {1750350609} Ophthl(85,NY08)<NJ-VALLEY, NJ-MTNSIDE>
+ Retina Consultants PA
1200 East Ridgewood Avenue/Suite 207   Ridgewood, NJ 07450   (201)612-9600   Fax (201)612-0428
+ Retina Consultants PA
39 South Fullerton Avenue   Montclair, NJ 07042   (973)783-7830

Vallario, Michael J., MD {1073597001} IntrMd(77,MEX03)<NJ-MORRISTN>
+ Parsippany Medical Group
50 Cherry Hill Road/Suite 204   Parsippany, NJ 07054
(973)299-1400   Fax (973)299-9011

Vallee, Michael F., DO {1215098868} Anesth(85,NY75)<NJ-STBARNMC>
+ St. Barnabas Medical Center
94 Old Short Hills Road   Livingston, NJ 07039   (973)322-5000

Vallejo, Edgardo C., MD {1518050467} IntrMd(72,PHI01)
+ 240 Williamson Street/Suite 502
Elizabeth, NJ 07202   (908)352-1173   Fax (908)352-0665

Vallejo, Jose A., MD {1851439418} Psychy(96,PER01)<NJ-ANCPSYCH>
+ Ancora Psychiatric Hospital
301 Spring Garden Road   Hammonton, NJ 08037
(609)561-1700

Vallejo, Phyu P., MD {1295802247} Psychy(82,MYA04)<NJ-ANCPSYCH>
+ Ancora Psychiatric Hospital
301 Spring Garden Road   Hammonton, NJ 08037
(609)561-1700
+ 5 Chambord Lane
Voorhees, NJ 08043

Vallone, Paul J., MD {1790893998} SrgPlstc, SrgRec(81,GRN01)<NJ-HCKTSTWN, NJ-NWTNMEM>
+ PO Box 619
Florham Park, NJ 07932   (973)366-3005
+ 369 West Blackwell Street
Dover, NJ 07801   (973)366-3005
+ 350 Sparta Avenue
Sparta, NJ 07932   (973)366-3005

Valskys, Rytis, MD {1285634337} AnesPain, IntrMd(89,LIT02)
+ 1187 Main Avenue/1d
Clifton, NJ 07011   (201)984-2294   Fax (201)984-2348
+ Immediate Care, PC
621 Kennedy Boulevard   North Bergen, NJ 07047
(201)984-2294   Fax (201)325-0385

Valthaty, Rebekah, MD {1366758898} ObsGyn
+ Ocean Health Initiatives, Inc.
301 Lakehurst Road   Toms River, NJ 08755   (732)552-0377
Fax (732)552-0378

Valvano, Amanda A., DO {1023249331} IntrMd(09,PA78)
+ 1450 East Chestnut Avenue/Suite 3-A
Vineland, NJ 08361   (856)794-8700   Fax (856)794-2752

Van Beever, Jordan Grant, MD {1306087705} Anesth<NJ-HACKNSK>
+ Hackensack University Medical Center
30 Prospect Avenue   Hackensack, NJ 07601   (201)488-0066

Physicians by Name and Address

Van Boxtel, Benjamin, MD {1962727644}
+ Mid-Atlantic Surgical Associates
  100 Madison Avenue Morristown, NJ 07960 (973)971-7300 Fax (973)984-7019

Van Deerlin, Peter G., MD {1629040365} RprEnd, Gyneco(90,MO02)<NJ-ACMCITY>
+ South Jersey Fertility Center
  400 Lippincott Drive Marlton, NJ 08053 (856)282-1231 Fax (856)596-2411
+ South Jersey Fertility Center
  2500 English Creek Avenue/Suite 225 Egg Harbor Township, NJ 08234

Van Dien, Craig, MD {1750623112} PhysMd<NJ-JFKJHNSN>
+ JFK Johnson Rehabilitation Institute
  65 James Street Edison, NJ 08818 (732)321-7070 Fax (732)321-7330

Van Engel, Daniel R., MD {1912968165} Nrolgy(73,NY15)<NJ-VALLEY>
+ Neurology Group of Bergen County
  1200 East Ridgewood Avenue Ridgewood, NJ 07450 (201)444-0868 Fax (201)444-7363

Van Gelderen, Jeffrey Thomas, MD {1275791386} SprtMd
+ Orthopaedic Sports Medicine
  80 Oak Hill Road Red Bank, NJ 07701 (732)741-2313 Fax (732)936-8445

Van Grouw, Brian P., DO {1669433165} SrgOrt(89,NJ75)<NJ-VALLEY>
+ 44 Godwin Avenue
  Midland Park, NJ 07432 (201)444-5770 Fax (201)444-3746

Van Hise, Aaron C., DO {1265618920} CarNuc, IntCrd, IntrMd(05,NY75)<NJ-NWRKBETH, NJ-DEBRAHLC>
+ Deborah Heart and Lung Center
  200 Trenton Road/Cardiology Browns Mills, NJ 08015 (609)735-2907 Fax (609)735-1858
+ Garden State Heart Care, P.C.
  831 Tennent Road/Suite 1-F Englishtown, NJ 07726 (609)735-2907 Fax (732)851-4703
+ Garden State Heart Care, P.C.
  333 Forsgate Drive/Suite 205 Jamesburg, NJ 08015 (732)851-4700

Van Hook, Jeffrey E., DO {1295935054} CdvDis, IntrMd(04,NJ75)<NJ-ATLANCHS>
+ Atlantic Cardiology in Galloway
  436 Chris Gaupp Drive/Suite 204 Galloway, NJ 08205 (609)652-0100 Fax (609)652-7616
+ Atlantic Cardiology in Ventor
  6725 Atlantic Avenue/2nd Floor Ventnor, NJ 08406 (609)822-2006

Van Horn, Lawrence G., Jr., MD {1780631036} ObsGyn(97,NJ05)<NJ-JRSYSHMC>
+ Hackensack Meridian Medical Group
  1900 Route 35/Suite 100 Oakhurst, NJ 07755 (732)663-0030 Fax (732)663-0882

Van Houten-Sauter, Lee A., DO {1508869553} FamMed(91,PA77)
+ Pine Street Family Practice
  220 East Pine Street Williamstown, NJ 08094 (856)629-7436 Fax (856)875-4742

Van Hoven, Anne Marie, MD {1821048307} EnDbMt, IntrMd(99,NJ06)<NJ-STPETER>
+ St. Peter's University Hospital
  254 Easton Avenue New Brunswick, NJ 08901 (732)745-8600 Fax (732)249-0969
+ Thyroid & Diabetes Ctr
  240 Easton Avenue/4th Floor New Brunswick, NJ 08901 (732)745-6667

Van Inwegen, Jeffrey R., MD {1003876996} Ophthl(91,NJ05)<NJ-VALLEY>
+ New Jersey Regional Eye Care, PA
  245 East Main Street Ramsey, NJ 07446 (201)327-3006 Fax (201)327-0720
  Ocudocs@hotmail.com

Van Kooy, Mark A., MD {1508854605} FamMed(80,NJ05)<NJ-VIRTMHBC>
+ Virtua Family Medicine Center @Lumberton
  1636 Route 38 & Eayrestown Rd. Lumberton, NJ 08048 (609)914-8440 Fax (609)914-8441

Van Patten, Yancy L., DO {1750536033} FamMed
+ Capital Health Primary Care-Bordentown
  1 Third Street Bordentown, NJ 08505 (609)298-2005 Fax (609)324-8267

Van Pelt, Lindsay A., MD {1689962250}<NJ-MORRISTN>
+ Chilton Medical Center
  97 West Parkway Pompton Plains, NJ 07444 (973)831-5000
+ Morristown Medical Center
  100 Madison Avenue Morristown, NJ 07962 (973)831-5000 Fax (973)290-7202

Van Pelt, Stephen Robert, MD {1306103635} EmrgMd<NJ-MORRISTN>
+ Morristown Medical Center
  100 Madison Avenue/EmergMed Morristown, NJ 07962

(973)971-5000

Van Raalte, Heather Michelle, MD {1285660183} UroGyn, SrgGyn, Gyneco(01,TN05)<NJ-UNVMCPRN>
+ Princeton Urogynecology
  10 Forrestal Road South/Suite 205 Princeton, NJ 08540 (609)924-2230 Fax (609)924-5006

Van Slooten, David D., MD {1639521218} Nrolgy, ClNrPh(84,NJ05)<NJ-HOLYNAME, NJ-VALLEY>
+ David D. Van Slooten MD, PA
  99 Kinderamack Road/Suite 307 Westwood, NJ 07675 (201)261-6222 Fax (201)261-4411

Van Uitert, Craig E., MD {1720003833} Pthlgy, PthAcl(80,GA05)<NJ-UNVMCPRN>
+ University Medical Center of Princeton at Plainsboro
  One Plainsboro Road/Pathology Plainsboro, NJ 08536 (609)497-4351

Van Volkenburgh, Robert John, MD {1518034669} EmrgMd(96,IL06)<NJ-RWJUBRUN>
+ RWJ University Hospital New Brunswick
  One Robert Wood Johnson Place New Brunswick, NJ 08901 (732)828-3000

Van Wyck, William Louis, MD {1629184205} IntrMd(01,GRN01)
+ Drs. Van Wyck & Matteace
  567 Fischer Boulevard Toms River, NJ 08753 (732)506-6868 Fax (732)506-6879

Vanam, Kamalakar Rao, MD {1386688968} EmrgMd(84,INDI)<NY-WYCKOFF, NY-CMCSTVSI>
+ JFK Medical Center
  65 James Street Edison, NJ 08820 (732)321-7605 Fax (732)744-5614

Vanbeek, Stephen, MD {1437648417} IntrMd
+ Rutgers- New Jersey Medical School
  185 South Orange Avenue/Rm 547 Newark, NJ 07103 (973)972-0470

Vanderwerken, Suzanne W., MD {1881677490} FamMed(87,PA02)<NJ-UNDRWD>
+ Complete Care Family Medicine
  75 West Red Bank Avenue Woodbury, NJ 08096 (856)853-2055 Fax (856)848-2879

Vandyck-Acquah, Marian M., MD {1790752798} CdvDis, IntrMd(94,GHA01)<NJ-HOLYNAME>
+ Bergen Cardiology Associates
  400 Frank W. Burr Boulevard Teaneck, NJ 07666 (201)928-2300 Fax (201)692-3263

Vangurp, James Mark, Jr., DO {1881107498} PthAcl
+ 25 Raymond Place
  Hawthorne, NJ 07506 (551)999-3079

Vangvanichyakorn, Kamtorn, MD {1699704825} NnPnMd, Pedtrc(74,THA01)<NJ-STBARNMC>
+ St. Barnabas Medical Center
  94 Old Short Hills Road/NeoPeri Livingston, NJ 07039 (973)322-5000 Fax (973)322-8833

VanHise, Tara Hungspruke, DO {1124213418} FamMed(05,NY75)
+ Capital Health Primary Care-Bordentown
  1 Third Street Bordentown, NJ 08505 (609)298-2005 Fax (609)324-8267

Vankawala, Sonya, DO {1386057438} Pedtrc<NJ-COOPRUMC>
+ Cooper University Hospital
  One Cooper Plaza Camden, NJ 08103 (856)342-2000

Vankawala, Viren Rameshchandra, MD {1063441145} CdvDis, IntrMd(93,INA53)
+ AtlantiCare Physicians
  318 Chris Gaupp Drive/Suite 100 Galloway, NJ 08205 (609)404-9900 Fax (609)404-3653

Vankouwenberg, Emily, MD {1396004677} SrgPlstc
+ UMDNJ RWJ Surgery
  125 Paterson Street/CAB 4th FL 4100 New Brunswick, NJ 08901 (732)235-7865 Fax (732)235-7079

Vanna, Stephen C., MD {1598716623} Nrolgy(65,NJ05)<NJ-VIRTMARL, NJ-VIRTVOOR>
+ Neurological Regional Associates
  504 Route 38 East Maple Shade, NJ 08052 (856)866-0466 Fax (856)727-1483

Vannoy, Dioscora R., MD {1114015146} Pedtrc, AdolMd(63,PHI08)<NJ-NWRKBETH>
+ 15 Main Street
  Orange, NJ 07050 (973)677-3344 Fax (973)677-0097

Vannozzi, Brian Michael, MD {1649330580} SrgOrt(03,PA01)<NJ-UNVMCPRN>
+ Princeton Orthopaedic Associates, P.A.
  325 Princeton Avenue Princeton, NJ 08540 (609)924-8131 Fax (609)924-8532

Vanston, Vincent J., MD {1851385744}
+ Cooper University Medical Center/Camden
  3 Cooper Plaza/Suite 506 Camden, NJ 08103 (856)968-7003
  jvanston@gmail.com

Vantuono, Rosanne, MD {1306864194} PhysMd(88,NJ05)<NJ-SHOREREH, NJ-OCEANMC>
+ PO Box 143
  Manasquan, NJ 08736 (732)223-5227

+ Laurelton Village
  475 Jack Martin Boulevard Brick, NJ 08724 (732)223-5227 Fax (732)458-2674

Vara, Manjula L., MD {1932143112} Pthlgy, PthAna, PthCyt(74,INA65)<NJ-TRINIWSC>
+ PLUS Diagnostics
  1200 River Avenue/Suite 10 Lakewood, NJ 08701 (732)901-7575 Fax (732)901-1555

Varadarajan, Sushila, MD {1720003676} Pthlgy, PthAcl(67,INA3X)<NJ-SJHREGMC, NJ-SJRSYELM>
+ SJH Regional Medical Center
  1505 West Sherman Avenue/Path Vineland, NJ 08360 (856)641-8000 Fax (856)641-7623

Varadarajan, Vijayaiaxmi, MD {1114949310} Anesth(75,INA5B)<NJ-RIVERVW>
+ Red Bank Anesthesia, LLC
  1 Riverview Plaza Red Bank, NJ 07701 (732)530-2255 Fax (732)450-2620
+ Riverview Medical Center
  1 Riverview Plaza Red Bank, NJ 07701 (732)741-2700

Varallo, Gerardo, Jr., DO {1821044496} IntrMd, Nephro(01,MO78)<NJ-KMHSTRAT, NJ-KMHTURNV>
+ Nephrology & Hypertension Associates of New Jersey
  201 Laurel Oak Road/Suite B Voorhees, NJ 08043 (856)566-5478 Fax (856)566-9561

Varallo, Marisa R., MD {1285965806}
+ Carepoint Health Bayonne Med Center
  29 East 29th Street Bayonne, NJ 07002 (646)220-9136
  marvar614@aol.com

Varano, Catherine Alano, MD {1588740443} FamMed, IntrMd(83,NJ06)
+ 470A Hwy 202/206 North
  Bedminster, NJ 07921 (908)781-7171 Fax (908)781-7172

Varas, Elizabeth A., MD {1740369511} Psychy(88,NJ05)<NJ-BERGNMC>
+ Care PLUS NJ, Inc. - Mid-Bergen Center
  610 Valley Health Plaza Paramus, NJ 07652 (201)265-8200 Fax (201)265-0366

Varbaro, Gian Stefano, MD {1952463101} IntrMd, IntHos(00,NY19)<CT-STVNCNT>
+ New Bridge Medical Center
  230 East Ridgewood Avenue Paramus, NJ 07652 (201)225-7130 Fax (201)967-4117

Vardy, Michael D., MD {1710925078} ObsGyn, UroGyn, GynOnc(92,ISR02)<NJ-ENGLWOOD>
+ Englewood Hospital and Medical Center
  350 Engle Street/Urogynecology Englewood, NJ 07631 (201)894-3000
  dr.vardy@gmail.com

Vare, Christopher, MD {1558688986} FamMed
+ Columbus Family Physicians
  23659 Columbus Road/Suite 4 Columbus, NJ 08022 (609)238-3304 Fax (609)289-7091

Vare, Katie Marie, MD {1699932558} Pedtrc(07,NJ05)
+ 66 Country Squire Lane
  Marlton, NJ 08053
+ Advocare DelGiorno Pediatrics
  527 South Black Horse Pike Blackwood, NJ 08012 Fax (856)245-7719

Varela, Linda Florence, MD {1629178116} EmrgMd<NJ-NWRKBETH>
+ Newark Beth Israel Medical Center
  201 Lyons Avenue/EmergMed Newark, NJ 07112 (973)926-6671 Fax (610)617-6280

Varela, Luis Fernando, MD {1982633327} EmrgMd<NJ-HACKNSK>
+ Hackensack University Medical Center
  30 Prospect Avenue Hackensack, NJ 07601 (201)996-2000 Fax (201)968-1866

Varela, Rebecca A., MD {1265460208} PainMd, Anesth(92,NJ05)<NJ-UNVMCPRN>
+ Princeton HealthCare System
  253 Witherspoon Street Princeton, NJ 08540
+ University Medical Center of Princeton at Plainsboro
  One Plainsboro Road/Anesthesiology Plainsboro, NJ 08536 (609)497-4371
+ Pain Management of New Jersey
  40 Stirling Road Watchung, NJ 08540 (908)803-4762 Fax (908)668-8244

Varevice-McAndrew, Susan, MD {1457372369} FamMed, IntrMd(95,NJ03)<NJ-VIRTVOOR, NJ-KMHCHRRY>
+ Virtua Family Medicine
  1605 Evesham Road/Suite 100 Voorhees, NJ 08043 (856)741-7100 Fax (856)424-2629
+ Advocare Sicklerville Internal Med
  485 Williamstown Road Sicklerville, NJ 08081 (856)741-7100 Fax (856)237-8042

Vargas, Myra Theresa, MD {1285683573} Nephro, IntrMd(88,NY46)<NJ-VIRTMHBC, NJ-LOURDMED>
+ The Center for Kidney Care
  1261 Route 38/Suite A Hainesport, NJ 08036 (856)222-1975 Fax (856)222-0721

Varghese, Betsy Mathew, MD {1437449691} IntrMd(11,PA13)
+ 186 Rochelle Avenue
Rochelle Park, NJ 07662   (551)996-9230   Fax (551)996-9240

Varghese, Joby, DO {1508063033} EmrgMd, Pedtrc, IntrMd(03,PA77)<NJ-VIRTBERL, NJ-VIRTMARL>
+ Emergency Physician Associates, P.A.
307 South Evergreen Avenue/PO Box 298   Woodbury, NJ 08096   (856)848-2088   Fax (856)848-8536
+ Virtua Voorhees
100 Bowman Drive/EmergMed   Voorhees, NJ 08043   (856)247-3000

Varghese, Juliet George, MD {1831333210} IntHos<NJ-WARREN>
+ Warren Hospital
185 Roseberry Street   Phillipsburg, NJ 08865   (908)859-6611

Varghese, Mathew, MD {1407884125} IntrMd
+ 136 North Washington Avenue/Suite 203
Bergenfield, NJ 07621   (201)374-1718   Fax (201)374-1719
+ ENT & Allergy Associates, LLP
98 James Street/Suite 301   Edison, NJ 08820   (201)374-1718   Fax (732)549-7250

Varghese, Rebecca M., MD {1275563934} IntrMd(88,INA56)
+ Valley Medical Group of Montvale
85 Chestnut Ridge Road/Suite 111   Montvale, NJ 07645   (201)930-1700   Fax (201)930-0705

Varghese, Sajini S., DO {1427196641} Psychy
+ HealthCare Commons Inc.
500 Pennsville-Auburn Road   Carneys Point, NJ 08069   (856)299-3200   Fax (856)299-7183

Varghese, Sarah, MD {1417182577} EnDbMt
+ Endocrinology Associates
1 Brace Road/Suite B   Cherry Hill, NJ 08034   (856)234-0645   Fax (856)234-0498

Varghese, Sarat J., MD {1104261106} FamMed(09,POL06)
+ Bayonne Medical Center
29th Street at Avenue E   Bayonne, NJ 07002   (201)858-5000

Varghese, Sherin V., MD {1225202955} Anesth
+ Jersery Shore Anesthesiology
1945 Highway 33   Neptune, NJ 07753   (732)897-0200   Fax (732)897-0263

Varghese, Teena P., MD {1427455833} PhysMd
+ Spinal & Head Trauma Associates
1123 Campus Drive West   Morganville, NJ 07751   (732)617-9797   Fax (732)617-8899

Varghese, Vibu, MD {1316340979} IntrMd<NJ-STJOSHOS>
+ St. Joseph's Regional Medical Center
703 Main Street   Paterson, NJ 07503   (201)490-1217

Varkey, Ciby B., MD {1407014350} FamMed(04,POL06)
+ Burlington Family Medical Center
666 Madison Avenue   Burlington, NJ 08016   (609)386-0023   Fax (609)386-4648

Varkey, Sarah Hema, MD {1346303047} IntrMd, IntHos(98,INA1C)
+ St Luke's Hospitalist Group
185 Roseberry Street   Phillipsburg, NJ 08865   (484)526-6643   Fax (484)526-4605
+ JFK Hospitalists
98 James Street/Suite 208   Edison, NJ 08818   (484)526-6643   Fax (732)862-1171

Varma, Ajay Medavaram, MD {1841482106} AnesPain, IntrMd(99,ENG08)<NJ-BAYSHORE>
+ Gramercy Pain Center
2124 Route 35 South   Holmdel, NJ 07733   (732)788-0349   Fax (877)211-6276
ajayvarma14@hotmail.com

Varma, Deepti Sagar, MD {1760792402} PsyCAd
+ 10 Georjean Drive
Holmdel, NJ 07733

Varma, Gurbachan K., MD {1932251329} Psychy(68,INA67)<NJ-BAYSHORE>
+ 721 North Beers Street/Suite 1-A
Holmdel, NJ 07733   (732)264-7803   Fax (732)739-4408

Varma, Medavaram Vikram, MD {1871525006} EmrgMd(97,ENG19)<NJ-COMMED>
+ Community Medical Center
99 Route 37 West   Toms River, NJ 08755   (732)557-8000

Varma, Mekhla, MD {1760723191} Pedtrc, Rheuma(04,INA69)
+ Tribeca Pediatrics
9 McWilliams Place   Jersey City, NJ 07302   (201)706-7175   Fax (201)604-6553

Varma, Raghunandan Medavaram, DO {1851489231} EmrgMd(95,NJ75)<NJ-STCLRDEN>
+ St. Clare's Hospital-Denville Campus
25 Pocono Road/EmergMed   Denville, NJ 07834   (973)625-6000

Varma, Sanjay, MD {1760593487} Psychy(92,NJ05)<NJ-UNVM-CPRN>
+ Princeton House Behavioral Health - Princeton
905 Herrontown Road/Psychiatry   Princeton, NJ 08540   (609)497-3300   Fax (609)497-3370

Varma, Seema N., MD {1588820708} OncHem, IntrMd(02,INA5Y)
+ Medical Associates of Marlboro PC
32 North Main Street   Marlboro, NJ 07746   (732)462-4100   Fax (732)462-3798
+ Medical Associates of Marlboro
111 James Street   Edison, NJ 08818   (732)462-4100   Fax (732)452-9720

Varma, Shubha, MD {1437220795} Surgry, SrgVas(90,INA23)
+ 33 Magnolia Avenue
Tenafly, NJ 07670

Varner, Philip T., DO {1336111939} IntrMd(95,NJ75)<NJ-BURDTMLN>
+ Cape Regional Medical Center
2 Stone Harbor Boulevard   Cape May Court House, NJ 08210   (609)463-2803   Fax (609)463-4991

Varoqua, Sabah, MD {1740264498}
+ Crossroads Medical Group
975 Clifton Avenue   Clifton, NJ 07013   (973)778-8666   Fax (973)778-7559

Varrell, James R., MD {1689779043} PsyCAd, Psychy, IntrMd(89,NJ06)<NJ-ACMCITY, NJ-ACMCMAIN>
+ InSight LLC
765 East Route 70/Bldg A   Marlton, NJ 08053   (856)983-3900   Fax (856)797-4785

Varriano, Anthony, MD {1598770026} IntrMd, EmrgMd(91,NY03)<NJ-BERGNMC>
+ New Bridge Medical Center
230 East Ridgewood Avenue/EmrgMed   Paramus, NJ 07652   (201)967-4000

Varshavski, Mikhail, DO {1548680986} FamMed<NJ-OVERLOOK>
+ Chatham Family Practice Associates
492 Main Street   Chatham, NJ 07928   (973)635-2432   Fax (973)635-6169
+ Overlook Medical Center
99 Beauvoir Avenue/PO Box 210   Summit, NJ 07902   (908)522-2000

Varshneya, Nikita, MD {1275551103} CdvDis, IntrMd(94,INDI)
+ 29 Broadway
Clark, NJ 07066   (732)396-0080

Vasani, Devang, MD {1760757330} RadDia(07,NJ06)
+ University Radiology Group, P.C.
483 Cranbury Road   East Brunswick, NJ 08816   (732)390-0030   Fax (732)390-5383
+ University Radiology Group, P.C.
16 Mountain Boulevard   Warren, NJ 07059   (732)390-0030   Fax (908)769-9141

Vascan, Andreea Carmen, MD {1962598003} IntrMd(96,ROM01)
+ Internal Medicine Faculty Associates
435 South Street/Suite 210   Morristown, NJ 07960   (973)971-7165   Fax (973)290-7675

Vaseghi, Moein Faghih, MD {1003892779} NuclMd, CarNuc(97,ITA22)
+ 24 Sentinel Drive
Basking Ridge, NJ 07920

Vasen, Arthur Philip, MD {1134188113} SrgOrt, SrgHnd(90,NJ06)<NJ-JRSYSHMC, NJ-OCEANMC>
+ Seaview Orthopaedics
222 Schanck Road/3rd Floor   Freehold, NJ 07728   (732)462-1700   Fax (732)303-8314
+ Seaview Orthopaedics
1640 Route 88 West   Brick, NJ 08724   (732)462-1700   Fax (732)458-2743
+ Seaview Orthopaedics
1200 Eagle Avenue   Ocean, NJ 07728   (732)660-6200   Fax (732)660-6201

Vasena Marengo, Maria Jose, MD {1417201021} Pedtrc
+ Hawthorne Pediatrics
330 Lafayette Avenue   Hawthorne, NJ 07506   (973)841-5112

Vasilakis, Vasileios, MD {1255623153} Surgry<NJ-MORRISTN>
+ Morristown Medical Center
100 Madison Avenue   Morristown, NJ 07962   (973)971-5684

Vasiliades, Thalia, DO {1912075185} FamMed(01,NJ75)
+ Allied Medical Associates
510 Hamburg Turnpike   Wayne, NJ 07470   (973)942-6005   Fax (973)442-6009

Vasilov, Anatoliy I., MD {1982832291} Psychy, PsyAdd(99,CMRN)
+ Princeton House Behavioral Health - Princeton
905 Herrontown Road   Princeton, NJ 08540   (609)497-2640   Fax (609)497-2641

Vasireddi, Srinivas S., MD {1417986167} Gastrn, IntrMd(89,INDI)<NJ-BAYSHORE, NJ-JFKMED>
+ Advanced Digestive Center
205 Bridge Street/Bridgepointe Bldg D   Metuchen, NJ 08840   (732)200-3535   Fax (732)444-3611
vasiboy@comcast.net
+ Advanced Digestive Center
21 Jefferson Plaza   Princeton, NJ 08540   (732)200-3535   Fax (732)355-0321

Vasireddy, Hemalatha, MD {1053397224} IntrMd, OncHem(96,INA8Y)<NJ-CLARMAAS, NJ-MTNSIDE>
+ Essex Hematology-Oncology Group, PA
36 Newark Avenue/Suite 304   Belleville, NJ 07109   (973)751-8880   Fax (973)751-8950
+ Essex Hematology-Oncology Group, PA
One Bay Avenue/Suite 2   Montclair, NJ 07042   (973)751-8880   Fax (973)744-8340

Vasisht, Bhupesh, MD {1114924487} SrgPlstc, SrgPHand(95,NJ06)<NJ-KMHCHRRY, NJ-VIRTUAHS>
+ South Shore Plastic Surgery
1307 White Horse Road/Suite E-501   Voorhees, NJ 08043   (856)784-2639   Fax (856)784-2659

Vasishta, Shiva G., MD {1932269982} Nrolgy(76,INA26)<NJ-VIRTVOOR>
+ Virtua Voorhees
100 Bowman Drive   Voorhees, NJ 08043   (856)247-3000

Vaskul, Roksolana, MD {1215098520} Anesth(90,UKR30)<NJ-ST-BARNMC>
+ St. Barnabas Medical Center
94 Old Short Hills Road   Livingston, NJ 07039   (973)322-5000

Vasoya, Amita P., DO {1992785406} PulDis, IntrMd(95,NJ75)
+ SOM - Department of Internal Medicine
42 East Laurel Road/Suite 3100   Stratford, NJ 08084   (856)566-6859   Fax (856)566-6906

Vasquez, Wendelly Judith, MD {1093044588} ObsGyn<NJ-JRSYSHMC>
+ Jersey Shore University Medical Center
1945 Route 33   Neptune, NJ 07753   (732)776-3790

Vassallo, Frank A., DO {1396818753} PsyCAd, Psychy(87,NJ75)
+ 801 Route 73 North
Marlton, NJ 08053   (856)983-7100

Vassallo, Michael Anthony, DO {1093729204} Anesth(91,NY75)
+ 40 Stirling Road
Watchung, NJ 07069   (908)769-0912

Vassallo, Sheryl Lisa, MD {1225281470} Pedtrc(05,GRN01)
+ 82 Miami Trail
Rockaway, NJ 07866

Vassalluzzo, Pasquale D., MD {1861498560} FamMed(71,ITA17)
+ 78 Virginia Drive
Atco, NJ 08004   (856)336-2842   Fax (215)725-3619
weightman43@hotmail.com

Vasselli, Anthony J., MD {1578559845} Urolgy(79,NY09)
+ 299 Witherspoon Street
Princeton, NJ 08542   (609)252-0575   Fax (609)252-0871

Vassilidze, Teimouraz V., MD {1649299553} Anesth(72,RUS06)<NJ-TRINIWSC>
+ Trinitas Regional Medical Center-Williamson Street
225 Williamson Street/Anesthesiology   Elizabeth, NJ 07207   (908)994-5000

Vaswani, Khimya I., MD {1043431430} IntrMd(72,INA00)
+ 18 Bernadette Court
Springfield, NJ 07081

Vaswani, Vijay, MD {1194785956} Surgry(95,TX04)<NJ-RWJUHAM, NJ-STFRNMED>
+ 311 Whitehorse Avenue/Suite C
Hamilton, NJ 08610   (609)585-3900   Fax (609)585-3365

Vates, Thomas S., III, MD {1447258637} PedUro, Urolgy(89,DC02)<NJ-MONMOUTH, NJ-STPETER>
+ Pediatric Urology Associates PC
557 Cranbury Road/Suite 4   East Brunswick, NJ 08816   (732)613-9144   Fax (732)613-5121

Vattasseril, Renjy, MD {1093748089} Gastrn, IntrMd(02,HUN04)<NJ-MEMSALEM>
+ Cape Reg Phys Assoc-Med Commons
217 North Main Street/Suite 102   Cape May Court House, NJ 08210   (609)536-8010   Fax (609)536-8053

Vaughn, Anita C., MD {1578503942} IntrMd(79,DC03)
+ Newark Community Health Center
101 Ludlow Street   Newark, NJ 07114   (973)565-0355   Fax (973)565-0461
+ 85 South Harrison Street/Suite 201
East Orange, NJ 07018   (973)565-0355   Fax (862)252-9399

Vaughn, Michelle Marie, MD {1982766184} Anesth(03,MI20)<PA-UPMCPHL>
+ Rancocas Anesthesiology, PA
700 Route 130 North/Suite 203   Cinnaminson, NJ 08077   (856)829-9345   Fax (856)829-3605

Vause, Sandra E., MD {1720150600} Dermat, SrgCsm(82,PA02)<NJ-MEMSALEM>
+ Schweiger Dermatology
200 Tilton Road/Suite 5   Northfield, NJ 08225   (609)400-3910
+ Vause Dermatology Cosmetic Surgery Associates
545 Beckett Road/Suite 101   Logan Township, NJ 08085   (609)400-3910   Fax (856)241-3969

Vavilathota, Jayachandra Babu, MD {1942455746}
+ Beth Israel Medical Center
201 Lyons Avenue   Newark, NJ 07112

Physicians by Name and Address

Vaydovsky, Joseph, MD {1609800564} ObsGyn(01,GRN01)<NJ-RBAYPERT>
+ 485 New Brunswick Avenue
Perth Amboy, NJ 08861   (732)324-4290   Fax (732)324-4293

Vaysberg, Yevgeniy, MD {1225189251} IntrMd, FamMed(93,UKR01)
+ Visiting Physician Services
23 Main Street/Suite D1   Holmdel, NJ 07733   (732)571-1000   Fax (732)571-1156

Vaz, Richard, DO {1790762706} IntrMd(94,NJ75)<NJ-NWTN-MEM>
+ Premier Health Associates
123 Newton Sparta Road   Newton, NJ 07860   (973)579-6300   Fax (973)579-1524

Vazir, Amanullah A., MD {1033283759} PulDis, IntrMd(87,GRN01)
+ 999 McBride Avenue/Suite 201-B
Little Falls, NJ 07424   (973)256-0287   Fax (973)256-2876

Vazirani, Minal, MD {1124183017} Pedtrc, IntrMd(02,NJ05)
+ Integrative Health and Wellness, P.A.
200 South Orange Avenue   Livingston, NJ 07039   (973)322-7007   Fax (973)322-7436

Vazirani, Tina A., MD {1598965071} Gastrn, IntrMd(07,NJ05)
+ Advanced Gastroenterology Associates LLC
475 County Road/Suite 201   Marlboro, NJ 07746   (732)370-2220   Fax (732)548-7408
+ Advanced Gastroenterology Associates LLC
403 Candlewood Commons/Building 4   Howell, NJ 07731   (732)370-2220   Fax (732)548-7408

Vazquez, Franklyn, MD {1699724872} Surgry, Bariat(89,NJ05)
+ 716 Broad Street/Suite 2-E
Clifton, NJ 07013   (973)777-7978

Vazquez, Jose S., MD {1427142520} Psychy(77,MEX03)<NJ-UNVMCPRN>
+ Princeton House Behavioral Health - Princeton
905 Herrontown Road   Princeton, NJ 08540   (609)497-3300   Fax (609)497-3370

Vazquez, Oscar, MD {1063608875} SrgOrt(03,MD07)<NJ-HACKNSK>
+ Active Orthopaedics & Sports Medicine
440 Old Hook Road   Emerson, NJ 07630   (201)358-0707   Fax (201)358-9777
drvazquez@activeorthopedic.com
+ Active Orthopaedics & Sports Medicine
25 Prospect Avenue   Hackensack, NJ 07601   (201)358-0707   Fax (201)343-7410

Vazquez, Pablo, MD {1811280175} PhyMPain
+ Atlas Spine Interventional Medicine
8901 Kennedy Boulevard/Suite 1-W   North Bergen, NJ 07047   (201)430-2022   Fax (201)243-7261

Vazquez Falcon, Luis Enrique, MD {1134132871} IntrMd(92,CUB08)
+ Primary Care Medical Group
450 Bergen Street   Harrison, NJ 07029   (973)484-6900   Fax (973)484-0029

Vecchi, Anthony R., MD {1477935229} IntrMd
+ Summit Medical Group-Berkeley Heights Campus
1 Diamond Hill Road   Berkeley Heights, NJ 07922   (908)273-4300   Fax (908)673-7336

Vecchio, Lisa C., MD {1285778449} Pedtrc, AdolMd(90,SPAI)
+ Drs. Albanese and Vecchio
20 Valley Street   South Orange, NJ 07079   (973)762-2606   Fax (973)762-4515

Vecchione, Edward J., DO {1760440929} IntrMd(74,PA77)<NJ-CLARMAAS, NJ-MTNSIDE>
+ The Internet Medical Group, P.C.
181 Franklin Avenue/Suite 204   Nutley, NJ 07110   (973)667-8117   Fax (973)667-6642

Vece, Lorrie J., MD {1770585689} AdolMd, Pedtrc(89,GRN01)<NJ-HOLYNAME, NJ-HACKNSK>
+ 185 Cedar Lane/Suite U-4
Teaneck, NJ 07666   (201)836-1919   Fax (201)836-5693

Veder, Liana, MD {1447265244} FamMed
+ NJ VA/James J Howard Outpatient Clinic
970 Route 70 West   Brick, NJ 08724   (732)836-6033

Vedula, Ramya S., DO {1851591622} IntrMd
+ Princeton Medical Group, P.A.
419 North Harrison Street   Princeton, NJ 08540   (609)924-9300   Fax (609)924-6552

Veerappan, Sutharsanam, MD {1972568780} NnPnMd, Pedtrc(81,INA3X)<NJ-HUNTRDN, NJ-STPETER>
+ Hunterdon Medical Center
2100 Wescott Drive   Flemington, NJ 08822   (908)788-6100
+ St. Peter's University Hospital
254 Easton Avenue   New Brunswick, NJ 08901   (908)788-6100   Fax (732)745-1902

Veeraraghavan, Gowri, MD {1619900883} IntrMd(00,INA96)<NJ-HUNTRDN>
+ Hunterdon Medical Center
2100 Wescott Drive/AdltHospitalist   Flemington, NJ 08822   (908)237-5486   Fax (908)237-5488

Veeraswamy, Pramila, MD {1376560110} InfDis, IntrMd(90,INA97)<NY-ELMHRST>
+ St. Peter's University Hospital
254 Easton Avenue/Medicine   New Brunswick, NJ 08901   (732)745-8600
+ Saint Peter's Physician Associates
294 Applegarth Road   Monroe Township, NJ 08831   (609)409-1363
+ St. Peter's Adult Family Health Center
123 How Lane   New Brunswick, NJ 08901   (732)745-6642

Vefali, Huseng, MD {1083901227} IntCrd, IntrMd(10,GRN01)
+ St. Michael's Medical Center
111 Central Avenue   Newark, NJ 07102   (973)877-5000

Vega, Andres, MD {1700292851} FamMed
+ Center for Adult Medicine & Preventive Care
916-922 Main Avenue/Suite 1-A   Passaic, NJ 07055   (973)773-0334   Fax (973)773-0336
+ Wayne Primary Care
468 Parish Drive/Suite 1   Wayne, NJ 07470   (973)773-0334   Fax (973)305-8157
+ Waldwick Urgent Care & Primary Care
71 Crescent Avenue   Waldwick, NJ 07055   (201)445-1700   Fax (201)445-1701

Vega, Dennis, MD {1750571253} SrgThr, Surgry(01,NY47)<NJ-STJOSHOS>
+ St. Joseph's Regional Medical Center
703 Main Street/Surgery/Thorac   Paterson, NJ 07503   (646)265-8510

Vega, Teresa, MD {1942367198} SrgOrt(78,SPAI)<NJ-JFKMED>
+ Edison-Metuchen Orthopedic Group
10 Parsonage Road/5th Floor/Suite 500   Edison, NJ 08837   (732)494-6226   Fax (732)494-8762

Vega, Vivian, MD {1962434274} ObsGyn, IntrMd(85,DC03)
+ Premier Women's Health of South Jersey
603 North Broad Street/Suite 300   Woodbury, NJ 08096   (856)223-8930   Fax (856)223-8948
+ Premier Women's Health of South Jersey
340 West Front Street/Suite 201   Elmer, NJ 08318   (856)223-8930   Fax (856)223-8948
+ Premier Women's Health of South Jersey
34 Colson Lane   Mullica Hill, NJ 08086   (856)223-1385

Vehra, Ijaz R., MD {1720192032} CdvDis, IntrMd(81,PAK01)<NJ-STJOSHOS, NJ-VALLEY>
+ Heart & Vascular Associates of Northern Jersey
22-18 Broadway/Suite 201   Fair Lawn, NJ 07410   (201)475-5050   Fax (201)475-5522
+ Heart & Vascular Associates of Northern Jersey
1114 Clifton Avenue   Clifton, NJ 07013   (973)471-5250
+ Heart & Vascular Associates of Northern Jersey
50 South Franklin Turnpike   Ramsey, NJ 07410   (201)934-0046   Fax (201)934-6217

Vekhnis, Betty, MD {1871548206} PhysMd(84,LAT02)
+ Physical Rehabilitation Center LLP
1767 Morris Avenue   Union, NJ 07083   (908)624-1050   Fax (908)624-1052

Veksler, Boris, MD {1073792594} Anesth
+ Robert Wood Johnson-UMDNJ Anesthesia Group
125 Paterson Street/CAB 3100   New Brunswick, NJ 08901   (732)235-7827   Fax (732)235-6131

Vekteris, Gerald E., DO {1366463853} Pedtrc(88,MO78)<NJ-ACMCMAIN, NJ-ACMCITY>
+ Harborview KidsFirst
505 Bay Avenue   Somers Point, NJ 08244   (609)927-4235   Fax (609)927-5590
+ Harborview KidsFirst Cape May
1315 Route 9 South   Cape May Court House, NJ 08210   (609)927-4235   Fax (609)465-1539
+ Harborview Smithville
48 South New York Road/Route 9   Smithville, NJ 08244   (609)748-2900   Fax (609)748-3067

Velasco, Antonio Quiachon, DO {1053519702} PulCCr, CritCr, IntrMd(04,PA79)
+ Pulmonary & Sleep Associates of SJ, LLC.
107 Berlin Road   Cherry Hill, NJ 08034   (856)429-1800   Fax (856)429-1081
+ Pulmonary & Sleep Associates of SJ, LLC.
750 Route 73 South/Suite 401   Marlton, NJ 08053   (856)429-1800   Fax (856)375-2325
+ Pulmonary & Sleep Associates of SJ, LLC.
811 Sunset Road/Suite 201   Burlington, NJ 08034   (609)298-1776   Fax (609)531-2391

Velasco, Brenda Raquel, MD {1548422405} Gastrn(03,NY47)
+ 94 Orlando Drive
Sicklerville, NJ 08081

Velasco, Mauricio, MD {1508848979} IntrMd(00,NJ05)
+ Cardio-Med Services
3196 Kennedy Boulevard/3rd Floor   Union City, NJ 07087   (201)974-0077
+ Cardio-Med Services
635 Broadway   Paterson, NJ 07514   (973)742-6266

Velasco, Reynaldo, MD {1720042906} Pedtrc(82,NJ05)<NJ-VIRTUAHS, NJ-COOPRUMC>
+ Advocare South Jersey Pediatrics Collingswood
204 White Horse Pike   Collingswood, NJ 08107   (856)424-6050   Fax (856)424-2943
+ Advocare South Jersey Pediatrics Cherry Hill
1949 Route 70 East/Suite 1 & 2   Cherry Hill, NJ 08003   (856)424-6050   Fax (856)424-2943

Velasco, Sonia C., MD {1013014521} IntrMd(67,PHI09)
+ 172 Newark Avenue
Jersey City, NJ 07302   (201)332-4727   Fax (201)332-4157

Velayadikot, Deepa Nandankumar, MD {1437176880} IntrMd(94,INA69)<NJ-COOPRUMC>
+ Cooper University Hospital
One Cooper Plaza/Hsplist   Camden, NJ 08103   (856)342-2000

Velazquez, Danitza M., MD {1225452964} Pedtrc
+ RWJ Medical School Univ of Med
675 Hoes Lane   Piscataway, NJ 08854   (732)235-7883

Veldanda, Ashokvardhan R., MD {1780630764} FamMed(85,INDI)
+ Stafford Medical, P.A.
1364 Route 72 West   Manahawkin, NJ 08050   (609)339-2008   Fax (609)597-9608

Velez, Alberto A., MD {1972699544} SrgOrt(63,PHI01)<NJ-BAYSHORE, NJ-CENTRAST>
+ Medical Specialists
1000 West Main Street   Freehold, NJ 07728   (732)431-1686   Fax (732)845-3350

Velez, Corazon S., MD {1669578910} Pedtrc(64,PHI08)<NJ-CENTRAST>
+ Medical Specialists
1000 West Main Street   Freehold, NJ 07728   (732)431-1686   Fax (732)845-3350

Velez, Henry, MD {1487762803} IntrMd, PulDis(76,NY09)<NJ-VALLEY>
+ 19-20 Fair Lawn Avenue
Fair Lawn, NJ 07410   (201)794-6411   Fax (201)794-2117

Velez, Isabel Odeida, MD {1992194906} Pedtrc
+ Progressive Pediatrics
3196 Kennedy Boulevard   Union City, NJ 07087   (201)319-9800   Fax (201)319-9849

Velicheti, Kavitha, MD {1033310404} NroChl, ClNrPh, Pedtrc(95,INA48)
+ JFK Neurosciences Institute
65 James Street/Second Floor   Edison, NJ 08818   (732)321-7950   Fax (732)632-1584
+ 25 Clyde Road/Suite 201
Somerset, NJ 08873

Velickovic, Marina, MD {1215066857} Pedtrc(90,SER02)<NJ-CHLSMT>
+ Children's Specialized Hospital
150 New Providence Road   Mountainside, NJ 07092   (908)233-3720

Velivis, Leticia, MD {1619384450} Psychy<NJ-UNIVBHC>
+ University Behavioral Health Care
671 Hoes Lane/PO Box 1392   Piscataway, NJ 08855   (732)235-4433

Vella, Joseph Bayer, MD {1073888434} OtgyFPIS
+ Drs. Kwong and Vella
10 Plum Street/8th Floor   New Brunswick, NJ 08901   (732)235-5530   Fax (732)235-8882

Vella, Joseph M., MD {1982797023} PthACl<NY-STRNGMEM>
+ Histopathology Services, LLC.
535 East Crescent Avenue   Ramsey, NJ 07446   (201)661-7280   Fax (201)661-7297

Vellas, Elaine, MD {1649362377} SrgPlstc, OccpMd(81,NE05)
+ first Care Medical Group
750 Valley Brook Avenue   Lyndhurst, NJ 07071   (201)896-0900   Fax (201)896-2726
+ first Care Medical Group
50 Pompton Avenue   Verona, NJ 07044   (201)896-0900   Fax (973)857-7034

Velmahos, Vasilios, MD {1013000355} IntrMd, InfDis(86,DOM08)
+ New Jersey Infectious Diseases Associates PA
113 James Street   Edison, NJ 08820   (732)906-1900   Fax (732)906-6666

Veloso, Corazon M., MD {1861443855} FamMed(82,PHI10)<NJ-HOBUNIMC>
+ NHCAC Health Center at Union City
714 31st Street   Union City, NJ 07087   (201)863-7077   Fax (201)863-2730

Veloudios, Angela, MD {1265571459} Ophthl, IntrMd(84,NY15)
+ Eye Care Physicians & Surgeons of New Jersey
73 South Main Street   Medford, NJ 08055   (609)654-6140   Fax (609)953-2257
+ Eye Care Physicians & Surgeons of New Jersey
2301 Evesham Road/Suite 501-502   Voorhees, NJ 08043   (609)654-6140   Fax (856)770-0840
+ Eye Care Physicians & Surgeons of New Jersey
1701 Wynwood Drive   Cinnaminson, NJ 08055   (856)829-0600   Fax (856)829-2832

Velpari, Sudarshan, MD {1235450263} IntrMd
+ Grove Medical Associates
129 Newark Avenue   Jersey City, NJ 07302   (201)451-8867   Fax (201)451-2819

Velpari, Sugirdhana, MD {1437449675} Gastrn<NJ-STPETER>
+ St. Peter's University Hospital
254 Easton Avenue   New Brunswick, NJ 08901   (732)745-8600
+ Saint PeterÆs Physician Associate
59 Veronica Avenue/Suite 203   Somerset, NJ 08873   (732)937-6008

Vemula, Rahul, MD {1053572024} SrgPlstc(08,NJ02)
+ Michael W. Nagy MD FACS
2333 Highway 34   Manasquan, NJ 08736   (732)282-0002   Fax (732)282-1522

Venanzi, Michael V., MD {1417038373} ObsGyn(77,MEX03)<NJ-MORRISTN, NJ-STCLRDEN>
+ Lifeline Medical Associates
390 State Route 10/Suite 1   Randolph, NJ 07869   (973)328-1262   Fax (973)328-8576
+ Lifeline Medical Associates
550 West Main Street   Boonton, NJ 07005   (973)328-7019

Vender, Lydia A., DO {1669563755} Psychy, PsyCAd, IntrMd(89,NJ75)<NJ-KMHTURNV, NJ-KMHSTRAT>
+ University Hospital-Cares Institute
42 East Laurel Road/Suite 1100   Stratford, NJ 08084   (856)566-7036   Fax (856)566-6108
+ University Hospital-SOM Department of Psychiatry
109 East Laurel Road/First Floor   Stratford, NJ 08084   (856)566-7036   Fax (856)566-6208

Venditti, Marilouise, MD {1427142686} Psychy, PsyFor(85,DMN01)<NJ-ACMCITY, NJ-ACMCMAIN>
+ AtlantiCare Regional Medical Center/City Campus
1925 Pacific Avenue/Psychiatry   Atlantic City, NJ 08401   (609)345-4000
+ AtlantiCare Regional Med Ctr/Mainland
65 West Jimmie Leeds Road/Psychiatry   Pomona, NJ 08240   (609)652-1000

Venezia, Sara, DO {1114364585} RadDia
+ University Radiology Group, P.C.
579A Cranbury Road   East Brunswick, NJ 08816   (732)390-0040   Fax (732)390-1856

Venkataraman, Ravi Kumar, MD {1194755173} Anesth, PainMd(84,INA92)
+ 211 Pennington Avenue
Passaic, NJ 07055   (973)470-3598   Fax (973)470-3548
+ Pain Centers of America
1060 Clifton Avenue   Clifton, NJ 07013   (973)470-3598   Fax (608)571-1035

Venkatasubramanian, Anuradha, MD {1992720866} NroChl(92,INA81)<PA-CHILDHOS>
+ UH-Robert Wood Jhnsn Med Sch
97 Paterson Street/Neurology   New Brunswick, NJ 08901

Venkatesulu, Sunder, MD {1437148210} CdvDis, IntrMd(89,PA02)<NJ-CHSMRCER, NJ-BURDTMLN>
+ Mercer Bucks Cardiology
3140 Princeton Pike/2nd Floor   Lawrenceville, NJ 08648   (609)895-1919   Fax (609)895-1200

Venkatraman, Guha K., MD {1356517593}
+ St. Barnabas Institute of Neurology & Neurosurgery
200 South Orange Avenue/Suite 101   Livingston, NJ 07039   (973)322-7580   Fax (973)322-7103

Ventrella, Gerard, MD {1639157068} FamMed(89,NJ06)<NJ-SJRSYELM>
+ Elmer Family Practice, P.C.
330 West Front Street/P.O. Box 577   Elmer, NJ 08318   (856)358-0770   Fax (856)358-0108

Ventrella, Samuel M., MD {1114986213} CdvDis, IntrMd(91,PA02)
+ The Cardiology Group, P.A.
401 Young Avenue/Suite 275   Moorestown, NJ 08057   (856)291-8855   Fax (856)291-8844
+ The Cardiology Group, P.A.
128 State Highway Route 70/Suite 1-B   Medford, NJ 08055   (856)291-8855   Fax (609)444-5521
+ The Cardiology Group, P.A.
1 Sheffield Drive/Suite 102   Columbus, NJ 08057   (856)291-8855

Ventriglia, Warren J., MD {1518993245} EmrgMd, OccpMd(81,PA02)<NJ-BURDTMLN>
+ Cape Regional Medical Center
2 Stone Harbor Boulevard/EmergMed   Cape May Court House, NJ 08210   (609)463-2000   Fax (609)463-2946

Ventura, Evelyn Ortiz, MD {1952487985} Pedtrc, IntrMd(95,DC02)
+ Horizon Health Center
714 Bergen Avenue   Jersey City, NJ 07306   (201)451-6300
+ Passaic Pediatrics II PA
913 Main Avenue   Passaic, NJ 07055   (973)458-8000

Ventura, Kenilia, MD {1306226360}<NJ-ACMCITY>
+ AtlantiCare Regional Medical Center/City Campus
1925 Pacific Avenue/Medicine   Atlantic City, NJ 08401

(305)720-3311

Ventura, William Raphael, MD {1134197973} Anesth, IntrMd(81,GRN01)<NJ-STJOSHOS>
+ St. Joseph's Regional Medical Center
703 Main Street/Anesthesia   Paterson, NJ 07503   (973)754-2000

Venugopal, Narasimhal, MD {1093883316} IntrMd(65,INA37)<NJ-SJHREGMC>
+ Vineland Medical Associates/Excel Care Alliance, LLC
1100 East Chestnut Avenue   Vineland, NJ 08360   (856)696-0108   Fax (856)691-1106

Venugopal, Roshni L., MD {1639327612} SrgCrC
+ University Hospital-Doctors Office Center
90 Bergen Street/DOC 7100   Newark, NJ 07103   (973)972-2400   Fax (973)972-2988

Venuti, John David, DO {1487668398} FamMed(96,PA77)
+ Family Practice Associates
188 Fries Mill Road/Suite N3   Turnersville, NJ 08012   (856)875-8000   Fax (856)875-8494

Venuti, Robert L., DO {1548274442} FamMed(85,PA77)<NJ-OURLADY>
+ Family Practice Associates
188 Fries Mill Road/Suite N3   Turnersville, NJ 08012   (856)875-8000   Fax (856)875-8494
rvenuti@comcast.net

Vera, Ariel Eduardo, MD {1386908259} EmrgMd
+ Morristown Medical Center
100 Madison Avenue   Morristown, NJ 07962   (973)971-5007

Vera, Luis Fernando, MD {1578764963} GenPrc(83,ECU03)
+ Virtua Berlin
100 Townsend Avenue   Berlin, NJ 08009   (856)322-3000

Verde, Michael Joseph, MD {1891910832} PhysMd
+ Northeast Spine & Sports Medicine
367 Lakehurst Road   Toms River, NJ 08755   (732)573-6235   Fax (732)504-7676

Verde, Valerie Sylvia, MD {1902936032} Psychy, PsyCAd(95,IN20)
+ New Bridge Services Inc.
390 Main Road   Montville, NJ 07045   (973)316-9333   Fax (973)316-5790

Verdesca, James A., MD {1528032497} CdvDis(90,NJ05)
+ Comprehensive Cardiovascular Consultants
299 Madison Avenue/Suite 102   Morristown, NJ 07960   (973)292-1020   Fax (973)292-9405

Verdi, Michelle Diane, DO {1144251224} Pedtrc(98,PA77)<NJ-OCEANMC, NJ-COMMED>
+ Pediatric Affiliates, PA
3508 Route 9 South   Howell, NJ 07731   (732)905-9166   Fax (732)905-9380
+ Pediatric Affiliates, PA
40 Bey Lea Road/Suite B203   Toms River, NJ 08753   (732)905-9166   Fax (732)244-6842
+ Pediatric Affiliates, PA
218 Jack Martin Boulevard/Building E-1   Brick, NJ 08731   (732)458-0010   Fax (732)458-9329

Verdon, John J., Jr., MD {1750461927} Addctn, Psychy, PsyAdd(85,DC02)<NJ-RIVERVW, NJ-MONMOUTH>
+ 234 Maple Avenue
Red Bank, NJ 07701   (732)842-9468   Fax (732)842-0666
JJVerdon@comcast.net

Verdoni, John A., MD {1225108566} IntrMd(74,MEX03)
+ 11 Centre Drive/Suite A
Jamesburg, NJ 08831   (609)655-3990   Fax (609)655-2190

Verea, Jorge L., MD {1164469540} IntrMd(83,MEX03)<NJ-PALISADE, NJ-CHRIST>
+ 6500 Broadway
West New York, NJ 07093   (201)864-3456   Fax (201)869-7224
laurarodang@hotmail.com
+ NHCAC Health Center at West New York
5301 Broadway   West New York, NJ 07093   (201)866-9320
+ NHCAC Health Center at North Bergen
1116 43rd Street   North Bergen, NJ 07093   (201)330-2632   Fax (201)330-2638

Verea, Vickie, MD {1558505925} Anesth(08,NJ03)<NY-NYUTISCH>
+ Short Hills Surgery Center
187 Millburn Avenue/Suite 101   Millburn, NJ 07041   (201)214-5236   Fax (973)671-0557

Verga, Barbara Jean, MD {1952364358} Pedtrc, PedGst(95,NY15)<NJ-MORRISTN, NJ-OVERLOOK>
+ Division of Pediatric GI at Goryeb
100 Madison Avenue/Box 82   Morristown, NJ 07962   (973)971-5676   Fax (973)290-7365

Verga, Diane G., MD {1770626111} Grtrcs, IntrMd(85,NJ05)<NJ-HACKNSK>
+ 13-21 Plaza Road
Fair Lawn, NJ 07410   (201)791-2900   Fax (201)791-3241

Vergano, Sefton Cappi, MD {1427266717} EnDbMt, IntrMd(04,PA13)
+ Endocrinology Associates of Princeton, LLC
168 Franklin Corner Road   Lawrenceville, NJ 08648

(609)896-0075   Fax (609)896-0079

Vergara, Jesus Roberto, MD {1699752642} IntrMd(81,PHIL)
+ Premier Health Associates
123 Newton Sparta Road   Newton, NJ 07860   (973)579-6300   Fax (973)579-1524

Vergara, Manuel Salvador, MD {1487638268} Nrolgy(88,COL25)<NJ-UNVMCPRN, NJ-CHSFULD>
+ Lawrenceville Neurology Center, PA
3131 Princeton Pike   Lawrenceville, NJ 08648   (609)896-1701   Fax (609)896-3735

Vergara, Rebecca B., MD {1396894143} Pthlgy, PthACl(81,PHI02)<NJ-NWTNMEM>
+ Newton Medical Center
175 High Street/Pathology   Newton, NJ 07860   (973)383-2121   Fax (973)383-1249

Vergari, John, Jr., MD {1609815976} CdvDis, IntrMd(80,NY09)
+ Owens Vergari Unwala Cardiology Associates PC
17 West Red Bank Avenue/Suite 306   Woodbury, NJ 08096   (856)845-6807   Fax (856)845-3760

Vergilio, Cory D., MD {1841203940} Gastrn, IntrMd(89,NJ05)
+ Consultants in Digestive Diseases, P.C.
319 East Main Street/Suite B   Somerville, NJ 08876   (908)203-0900   Fax (908)203-0990

Verma, Anjali, MD {1619905445} NnPnMd, Pedtrc(79,INA05)<NJ-CENTRAST, NJ-LOURDMED>
+ Somerset Medical Center Neonatology
110 Rehill Avenue   Somerville, NJ 08876   (908)685-2473

Verma, Archana, MD {1770894040} Pedtrc, PedEmg
+ CHCA NJ Emergency at Virtua
100 Bowman Drive   Voorhees, NJ 08043   (856)247-3244   Fax (609)261-5842

Verma, Madhoolika, MD {1568656270} Pedtrc<NJ-RBAYPERT>
+ Raritan Bay Medical Center/Perth Amboy Division
530 New Brunswick Avenue   Perth Amboy, NJ 08861   (732)442-3700

Verma, Parveen Kaur, DO {1639149495} EnDbMt, IntrMd(99,NJ75)<NJ-CHSFULD, NJ-CHSMRCER>
+ Endocrinology Associates
1 Brace Road/Suite B   Cherry Hill, NJ 08034   (856)234-0645   Fax (856)234-0498

Verma, Rajiv, MD {1144237645} PedCrd, Pedtrc(84,ZAM01)<NJ-NWRKBETH>
+ Newark Beth Israel Medical Center
201 Lyons Avenue/PediCardiology   Newark, NJ 07112   (973)926-3500   Fax (973)926-8206
RVERMA@SBHCS.com

Verma, Renuka, MD {1518907773} PedInf, Pedtrc(86,INA8Z)<NJ-MONMOUTH>
+ Monmouth Medical Group, P.C.
279 Third Avenue/Suite 604   Long Branch, NJ 07740   (732)222-4474   Fax (732)222-4472
+ Monmouth Family Center
270 Broadway   Long Branch, NJ 07740   (732)222-4474   Fax (732)923-7104

Verma, Siddharth, DO {1285892463} IntHos, IntrMd(06,NJ75)<NY-METHODST>
+ 185 South Orange Avenue/MSB H-538
Newark, NJ 07103   (973)972-5252   Fax (973)972-3144

Verma, Vijayendra Kishore, MD {1275585846} CdvDis, IntrMd, IntCrd(99,NET09)<NJ-OURLADY, NJ-VIRTUAHS>
+ Cardiovascular Associates
210 West Atlantic Avenue   Haddon Heights, NJ 08035   (856)546-3003   Fax (856)547-5337
+ Cardiovascular Associates of The Delaware Valley, PA
525 State Street/Suite 3   Elmer, NJ 08318   (856)546-3003   Fax (856)358-0725

Vermani, Prathiba, MD {1942636626} FamMed<NJ-JFKMED>
+ JFK Medical Center
65 James Street   Edison, NJ 08820   (732)321-7605   Fax (732)744-5614

Vermeulen, Meagan Wega, MD {1255311627} FamMed, IntrMd(99,PA09)<NJ-UNDRWD>
+ The University Doctors - UMDNJ -SOM
570 Egg Harbor Road/Suite C-2   Sewell, NJ 08080   (856)218-0300   Fax (856)589-5082

Verner, Edwina D., MD {1457303919} Pedtrc(77,MA07)<NJ-NWRKBETH, NJ-STBARNMC>
+ Bright Futures Pediatrics
185 Central Avenue/Suite 601   East Orange, NJ 07018   (973)944-1089   Fax (973)866-0023

Vernon, Gerald Michael, DO {1790851061} FamMed(95,NJ75)
+ South Jersey Health & Wellness Center
1919 Greentree Road   Cherry Hill, NJ 08003   (856)761-8100   Fax (856)761-8107

Vernon, Lisa S., MD {1447223128} ObsGyn(02,TN07)
+ 85 Nautilus Drive/Suite A
Manahawkin, NJ 08050   (609)807-1414   Fax (609)382-0707
+ SOMC Medical Group, P.C.
730 Lacey Road/Suite G-08   Forked River, NJ 08731   (609)807-1414   Fax (609)242-5437

Physicians by Name and Address

Vernon, Paul L., MD {1649273038} Ophthl(77,PA09)
+ 2026B Briggs Road
Mount Laurel, NJ 08054 (856)235-1211 Fax (856)231-1149

Verona, Paul T., MD {1255324406} RadDia(81,GRN01)<NJ-EASTORNG>
+ East Orange General Hospital
300 Central Avenue/Radiology East Orange, NJ 07018 (973)672-8400

Verrecchia, Courtney, MD {1588112411} Pedtrc
+ Cooper Peds/Children's Regional Ctr
3 Cooper Plaza/Suite 200 Camden, NJ 08103 (856)342-2001 Fax (856)368-8297

Verret, Joseph M., MD {1861464364} Psychy(78,HAI01)<NJ-STJOSHOS>
+ St. Joseph's Regional Medical Center
703 Main Street/Psychiatry Paterson, NJ 07503 (973)754-2000
Verretj@sjhmc.org

Verrico, Tracy B., DO {1205898830} ObsGyn(01,NJ75)
+ Summit Medical Group
31-00 Broadway Fair Lawn, NJ 07410 (201)530-5475 Fax (201)796-7020

Versi, Ebrahim Eboo, MD {1184732406} Gyneco(80,ENG03)<MA-BRIGWMN, MA-MAGENHOS>
+ Urigen Pharmaceuticals
675 US Highway 1/Suite B206 North Brunswick, NJ 08902 (732)640-0160

Verzosa, Oscar E., MD {1396844148} IntrMd(72,PHI09)
+ 240 Williamson Street/Suite 403
Elizabeth, NJ 07202 (908)289-6996 Fax (201)943-8733

Vesole, David H., MD {1790773356} IntrMd, Hemato, MedOnc(84,IL06)<NJ-HACKNSK>
+ John Theurer Cancer Center - HUMC
92 Second Street/Co-Div Chief Hackensack, NJ 07601 (551)996-8704 Fax (551)996-0582
+ John Theurer Cancer Center - HUMC
360 Essex Street/Suite 303 Hackensack, NJ 07601 (551)996-8704 Fax (551)996-0582

Vessa, Paul P., MD {1508863663} SrgOrt, SrgSpn(85,NJ06)<NJ-HACKNSK, NJ-HCKTSTWN>
+ Somerset Orthopedic Associates, PA
1081 Route 22 West Bridgewater, NJ 08807 (908)722-0822 Fax (908)722-6318
+ Spine Surgery Associates MD PC
PO Box 323 Pluckemin, NJ 07978 (908)532-0576

Vester, John W., MD {1902826605} Nrolgy, SrgNro(73,DC02)<NJ-UNVMCPRN, NJ-HUNTRDN>
+ Capital Institute for Neurosciences
2 Capital Way/Suite 456 Pennington, NJ 08534 (609)537-7300 Fax (609)537-7301

Vetrano, Joseph S., MD {1861414294} Psychy(70,NY09)
+ 43 West Front Street/Suite 14B
Red Bank, NJ 07701 (732)747-0963 Fax (732)747-0963
+ Booker Behavioral Health Center
661 Shrewsbury Avenue Shrewsbury, NJ 07702 (732)747-0963 Fax (732)345-3401

Vetrano, Stephen J., DO {1770527459} EmrgMd, EmrgEMed(98,NJ75)<NJ-OURLADY>
+ Our Lady of Lourdes Medical Center
1600 Haddon Avenue/Emerg Med Camden, NJ 08103 (856)757-3803

Vets, Steve Michael, DO {1790944601} EmrgMd(06)
+ 61 Route 24
Chester, NJ 07930

Vetter, Paul L., MD {1457328064} ObsGyn(92,NJ06)<NJ-OCEANMC>
+ Brick Women's Physicians
1140 Burnt Tavern Road/Suite 2-A Brick, NJ 08724 (732)202-0700 Fax (732)202-0664
+ Brick Women's Physicians
87 Union Avenue Manasquan, NJ 08736 (732)202-0700 Fax (732)202-0664

Vettori, David John, DO {1609183474} MtFtMd, ObsGyn
+ Virtua Memorial
175 Madison Avenue Mount Holly, NJ 08060 (609)267-0700

Veysman, Boris D., MD {1891846234} EmrgMd<NJ-RWJUBRUN>
+ Robert Wood Johnson Emergency Medicine
One Robert Wood Johnson Place/MEB 104 New Brunswick, NJ 08901
+ University Emergency Medicine
125 Paterson Street/MEB 104 New Brunswick, NJ 08901 Fax (732)235-7379

Vialotti, Charles P., Jr., MD {1205861366} RadOnc, Radiol(71,NY09)<NJ-HOLYNAME>
+ Holy Name Hospital
718 Teaneck Road/RadOncology Teaneck, NJ 07666 (201)833-3000 Fax (201)541-0305

Vicente, Virgilio C., MD {1780790998} Pedtrc(78,PHI01)<NJ-CHRIST, NJ-JRSYCITY>
+ Ironbound Pediatrics P.C

155 Jefferson Street/Suite 3 Newark, NJ 07105 (973)466-0300 Fax (973)466-1117

Vichnevetsky, Simon, MD {1427020197} EmrgMd(80,BEL07)<NJ-CHSFULD>
+ Capital Health System/Fuld Campus
750 Brunswick Avenue/EmrgMed Trenton, NJ 08638 (609)394-6063

Vick, James W., MD {1336145465} FamMed, Grtrcs(79,PA02)<NJ-VIRTBERL, NJ-VIRTMARL>
+ Haddonfield Family Practice PA
15 East Redman Avenue Haddonfield, NJ 08033 (856)428-1335 Fax (856)428-6334

Vickery, Donna R., MD {1255373841} FamMed(87,NJ05)<NJ-SUMOAKSH>
+ Summit Oaks Hospital
19 Prospect Street/FamMed Summit, NJ 07901 (330)758-4515 Fax (330)758-5121

Victor, Carl H., MD {1538107719} IntrMd, EnDbMt(74,NY09)<NJ-CHSFULD, NJ-CHSMRCER>
+ West Trenton Medical Associates
1230 Parkway Avenue/Suite 203 Trenton, NJ 08638 (609)883-5454 Fax (609)883-2565

Victor, Frank Charles, MD {1275624256} Dermat(03,NJ02)
+ Robert Wood Johnson Medical Group-Dermatology
1 World's Fair Drive/Suite 2400 Somerset, NJ 08873 (732)235-7993 Fax (732)235-7117
+ Shore Dermatology at Brielle Hills
2640 Highway 70/Building 5/Suite 200 Manasquan, NJ 08736 (732)235-7993 Fax (732)528-5262
+ The American Skin and Cancer Center
25 First Avenue/Suite 113 Atlantic Highlands, NJ 08873 (732)872-2007

Victor, Isaac L., MD {1073678280} ObsGyn, Gyneco(90,NJ05)<NJ-STBARNMC, NJ-OVERLOOK>
+ Union & Cranford Ob/Gyn & Infertility Group
1323 Stuyvesant Avenue Union, NJ 07083 (908)686-4334 Fax (908)686-1744
+ Union & Cranford Ob/Gyn & Infertility Group
118 South Avenue East Cranford, NJ 07016 (908)276-7333
+ Union & Cranford Ob/Gyn & Infertility Group
349 Valley Street South Orange, NJ 07083 (973)763-4334

Vida, Jay A., DO {1831195601} IntrMd(91,MO78)<NJ-KIMBALL, NJ-COMMED>
+ Ocean County Family Care
2125 Route 88 East Brick, NJ 08724 (732)892-4548 Fax (732)892-0961
+ Ocean County Family Care
9 Mule Road Toms River, NJ 08755 (732)892-4548 Fax (732)818-7775

Vidal, Heidi Robin, MD {1942367032} PsyCAd, Psychy(94,NJ06)
+ New Point Behavioral Health Care
404 Tatum Street Woodbury, NJ 08096 (856)845-8050 Fax (856)845-0688
+ 101 Route 130 South/Grant/Suite 425
Cinnaminson, NJ 08077 (856)845-8050 Fax (888)819-1363

Vidal, Jennifer Lyn, DO {1649565201} Pedtrc
+ Harrison Pediatric Care PA
332 Harrison Avenue Harrison, NJ 07029 (973)484-4584 Fax (973)481-0754

Vidal Burke, Angela M., MD {1902068075} FamMed
+ Hillside Family Practice
100 Hollywood Avenue Hillside, NJ 07205 (908)353-7949 Fax (908)353-8374

Vidal-Phelan, Johanna Maria, MD {1326076134} Pedtrc, IntrMd(01,NJ06)
+ Kids first
2006 Salem Road Burlington, NJ 08016 (609)877-1500 Fax (609)877-4262

Vidaver, Patrick S., MD {1295718518} Anesth(93,TN05)<NJ-HACKNSK>
+ Hackensack University Medical Center
30 Prospect Avenue/Anesthesiology Hackensack, NJ 07601 (201)996-2419 Fax (201)488-6769
+ Hackensack University MC-Anesthesia Dept
30 Prospect Avenue/Room 2703 Hackensack, NJ 07601 (201)996-2419 Fax (201)996-3962

Videtti, Nicholas A., MD {1699861658} Psychy(85,GRN01)<NJ-VALLEY>
+ 127 Union Street
Ridgewood, NJ 07450 (201)444-1255 Fax (201)251-9551

Vieira, Pedro, MD {1730111535} SrgPlstc, Surgry(00,NJ05)
+ Contemporary Plastic Surgery LLC
579A Cranbury Road/Suite 202 East Brunswick, NJ 08816 (732)254-1919 Fax (732)254-0703

Vierheilig, Jacqueline M., MD {1649388133} InfDis, IntrMd(85,ARG02)<NJ-CHILTON, NJ-STJOSHOS>
+ 333 Godwin Avenue
Midland Park, NJ 07432 (201)445-6669

Vietla, Bhavani Durga, MD {1831137215} IntrMd(92,INDI)<NJ-RWJUBRUN, NJ-STPETER>
+ RWJPE Bhavani Vietla
2864 Route 27/Suite D North Brunswick, NJ 08902 (732)297-4272 Fax (732)297-3785

Vigario, Jose C., DO {1487691929} Grtrcs, IntrMd(92,NY75)<NJ-STPETER>
+ Princeton Health Medical & Surgical Associates
2 Centre Drive/Suite 200 Monroe, NJ 08831 (609)395-2470 Fax (609)860-5288

Viggiano, Joseph T., MD {1568499200} RadNuc, RadDia(90,NJ05)<NJ-STBARNMC>
+ St. Barnabas Medical Center
94 Old Short Hills Road/Radiology Livingston, NJ 07039 (973)322-5000

Vigman, Melvin P., MD {1427094226} Nrolgy(64,PA09)<NJ-OVERLOOK>
+ Vigman and Pollock PA
47 Maple Street/Suite 104 Summit, NJ 07901 (908)277-2722 Fax (908)273-5970

Vigorita, John F., MD {1205928777} Pedtrc, AdolMd, IntrMd(74,MEX03)<NJ-OVERLOOK>
+ Summit Pediatric Associates
33 Overlook Road/Suite 101 Summit, NJ 07901 (908)273-1112 Fax (908)273-1146
+ Florham Park Pediatrics
195 Columbia Turnpike/Suite 105 Florham Park, NJ 07932 (908)273-1112 Fax (973)845-2883

Vij, Angela, MD {1073887501} IntrMd
+ Hackensack Medical Center-Internal Medicine
30 Prospect Avenue/4 Main/Rm 4621 Hackensack, NJ 07601 (551)996-3500 Fax (551)996-0536

Vij, Raman L., MD {1295723443} PhysMd(72,INDI)<NJ-KSLR-WEST>
+ Kessler Institute for Rehabilitation West Orange
1199 Pleasant Valley Way West Orange, NJ 07052 (973)731-3600

Vijay-Sharma, Mayuri, MD {1326236308} IntrMd
+ 10 Salrit Avenue
Waldwick, NJ 07463 (201)670-4451

Vijayakumar, Asha M., MD {1043389083} IntrMd(85,INA67)
+ Drs. Vijayakumar & Fernandes
152 Central Avenue Clark, NJ 07066 (732)382-9700 Fax (732)382-9707

Vijayakumar, Ashvin, MD {1659782464} IntrMd
+ Drs. Vijayakumar and Raman
1801 Atlantic Avenue/3rd Floor Atlantic City, NJ 08401 (609)570-2400 Fax (609)441-7207

Vijayakumar, Chellappan, MD {1457393167} CdvDis, IntrMd(78,INA77)<NJ-OCEANMC, NJ-JRSYSHMC>
+ Cardiology Associates of Ocean County PA
495 Jack Martin Boulevard/Suite 2 Brick, NJ 08724 (732)458-7575 Fax (732)458-0874

Vijayan, Radhika, MD {1215972179} Pedtrc(75,INA94)<NJ-HACKNSK>
+ Hackensack Univ Medical Center Pediatric Emerg Room
30 Prospect Avenue Hackensack, NJ 07601 (201)996-5430 Fax (201)996-3676
+ Hackensack University Medical Center
30 Prospect Avenue Hackensack, NJ 07601 (201)996-2000

Vijayanathan, Thurairasa, MD {1205808813} Radiol, RadDia(63,SRIL)<NJ-JRSYCITY, NJ-STMICHL>
+ 11 Highfield Terrace
North Caldwell, NJ 07006

Vijayaraghavan, Swathi, MD {1467610493} Nrolgy, IntrMd(08,PA02)
+ Center for Neurologic Specialty
401 Young Avenue/Suite 160 Moorestown, NJ 08057 (856)291-8780 Fax (856)291-8781
+ Virtua Nurosciences
200 Bowman Drive/Suite E-385 Voorhees, NJ 08043 (856)291-8780 Fax (856)247-7766
+ Neurology Associaates of South Jersey
693 Main Street/Building D Lumberton, NJ 08057 (609)261-7600 Fax (609)265-8205

Vijaysadan, Viju, MD {1538110754} Pedtrc, IntrMd(95,INA76)
+ Kinnelon Medical & Pediatric Associates
170 Kinnelon Road/Suite 28 Kinnelon, NJ 07405 (973)838-7650 Fax (973)838-1775

Vikner, Lin M., MD {1053310151} ObsGyn(82,CHN07)<NJ-HACKNSK, NJ-VALLEY>
+ 11 Fairlawn Street
Ho Ho Kus, NJ 07423

Viksjo, Michael Joseph, MD {1508028770} Gastrn, IntrMd(03,NY06)
+ 414 Manchester Way
Wyckoff, NJ 07481 (201)482-4674

Physicians by Name and Address

Viksman, Michael Y., MD {1972668747} Allrgy, IntrMd, Algy-Immn(72,RUSS)<NJ-RIVERVW, NJ-BAYSHORE>
+ The Allergy & Asthma Group
717 North Beers Street/Suite 2 A   Holmdel, NJ 07733
(732)739-0660   Fax (732)739-1406
+ The Allergy & Asthma Group
368 Lakehurst Road/Suite 304   Toms River, NJ 08755
(732)739-0660   Fax (732)349-0117
+ The Allergy & Asthma Group
100 Craig Road/Suite 204   Manalapan, NJ 07733
(732)303-9101   Fax (732)683-1070

Vila, Maria N., DO {1255534673} FamMed(04,NJ75)<NJ-VALLEY>
+ Absolute Medical Care
One Broadway/Suite 301   Elmwood Park, NJ 07407
(201)791-9340   Fax (201)791-9481

Vilenskaya, Irina, MD {1518064567} IntrMd(84,EST01)<NJ-MONMOUTH>
+ 127 Pavilion Avenue
Long Branch, NJ 07740   (732)222-1133   Fax (732)222-9345

Vilko, Naomi R., MD {1780701391} Psychy, PsySex, Psyphm(75,NY09)
+ 419 North Harrison Street/Suite 206
Princeton, NJ 08540   (609)924-3225   Fax (609)921-7533
naomivilko@msn.com

Villa, John J., DO {1144309147} PulDis, SlpDis, IntrMd(89,NJ75)<NJ-HACKNSK>
+ Hackensack University Medical Group PC
160 Essex Street/Suite 103   Lodi, NJ 07644   (551)996-1370

Villabona, Beatriz, MD {1144286725} Pedtrc(86,COL01)<NJ-PALISADE>
+ NHCAC Health Center at West New York
5301 Broadway   West New York, NJ 07093   (201)866-9320
+ St. Joseph's Family Health Center
21 Market Street   Paterson, NJ 07501   (201)866-9320
Fax (973)754-4201
+ Ocean Health Initiatives, Inc.
301 Lakehurst Road/Pediatric   Toms River, NJ 07093
(732)552-0377   Fax (732)552-0378

Villafane, Eric, MD {1871557686} PedAne, Anesth(01,FL03)<NY-STATNRTH>
+ Red Bank Anesthesia, LLC
1 Riverview Plaza   Red Bank, NJ 07701   (732)530-2255
Fax (732)450-2620

Villafania, Zenaida S., MD {1144396755} Anesth(67,PHI01)<NJ-NWTNMEM>
+ Newton Medical Center
175 High Street/Anesthesiology   Newton, NJ 07860
(973)383-2121

Villafranca, Manuel V., MD {1992759955} Psychy(71,PHIL)<NJ-SUMOAKSH>
+ Summit Oaks Hospital
19 Prospect Street/Psych   Summit, NJ 07901   (330)758-4515   Fax (330)758-5121
+ 220 Lenox Avenue
Westfield, NJ 07090   (330)758-4515   Fax (908)232-4520

Villamayor, Carlos Pestelos, MD {1356349336} Anesth(99,PA01)
+ West Jersey Anesthesia Associates
102-E Center Boulevard   Marlton, NJ 08053   (856)988-6250   Fax (856)988-6270

Villamayor, Rosemarie Cruz, MD {1336179407} FamMed(99,PA02)
+ PennCare South Jersey Family Medicine
55 Haddonfield-Berlin Road/Route 561   Gibbsboro, NJ 08026   (856)783-1777
+ Family Medicine Gibbsboro
63 North Lakeview Drive/Suite 201   Gibbsboro, NJ 08026
(856)783-1777

Villani, Michael A., MD {1457323040} RadDia, RadV&I(81,MEX14)<NJ-SJHREGMC>
+ SJH Regional Medical Center
1505 West Sherman Avenue   Vineland, NJ 08360
(856)641-8000

Villanobos, Rey T., MD {1023049558} IntrMd, EnDbMt(90,PHI10)<NJ-STPETER>
+ 9 Clyde Road/Suite 102
Somerset, NJ 08873   (732)828-2030   Fax (732)828-2043
rtvillamd@yahoo.com

Villanueva, Dioscoro T., MD {1346299401} SrgThr, Surgry(64,PHI08)<NJ-VIRTUAHS, NJ-OURLADY>
+ Virtua Surgical Group, PA
1935 Route 70 East   Cherry Hill, NJ 08003   (856)428-7700
Fax (856)424-9120

Villanueva, Erika, MD {1861718223} EnDbMt
+ Capital Endocrinology
2 Capital Way/Suite 290   Pennington, NJ 08534   (609)303-4300   Fax (609)303-4301

Villanueva, Norma I., MD {1003925850} EmrgMd<NJ-HUNTRDN>
+ Hunterdon Medical Center
2100 Wescott Drive   Flemington, NJ 08822   (908)788-6100

Villanueva, Ronald Banaag, MD {1508838434} EnDbMt, IntrMd(93,PHI02)
+ Drs. Ortiz, Villanueva and Cruz
1163 Route 37 West/Suite A-1   Toms River, NJ 08755
(732)736-1000   Fax (732)736-8811
+ Drs. Ortiz, Villanueva and Cruz
1255 Route 70/Suite 20-N   Lakewood, NJ 08701   (732)363-4770

Villare, Anthony W., MD {1114954054} FamMed(82,DOM03)<NJ-UNDRWD>
+ 560 Mantua Avenue
Paulsboro, NJ 08066   (856)423-5466

Villare, Robert C., MD {1124012273} SrgThr, SrgVas, Surgry(82,MNT01)<NJ-UNDRWD, NJ-MEMSALEM>
+ Vanguard Group, LLC
113 Westwood Hill   Woodbury, NJ 08096   (856)848-4131
Fax (856)848-4131

Villasis, Cynthia Dancel, MD {1598718579} Pedtrc, NnPnMd(72,PHI02)
+ AtlantiCare - Neonatology Department
65 West Jimmie Leeds Road   Pomona, NJ 08240   (609)404-3816   Fax (609)404-3818

Villegas, Noah, MD {1780950261} Psychy
+ University Behavioral HealthCare
183 South Orange Avenue   Newark, NJ 07103   (973)972-4678

Villegas, Robert A., MD {1508885534} Anesth, CritCr, IntrMd(85,NY01)
+ 130 West Pleasant Avenue/Suite 334
Maywood, NJ 07607   (201)957-1090

Villongco, Raymond Manzano, MD {1962420281} IntrMd, Grtrcs(89,PHI01)<NY-MTSINAI>
+ 381 Teaneck Road/Suite 1
Teaneck, NJ 07666   (201)836-4228   Fax (201)357-2150

Villota, Francisco Javier, MD {1194825661} IntrMd(86,MEX22)<NJ-STFRNMED>
+ St. Francis Medical Center
601 Hamilton Avenue/InternalMed   Trenton, NJ 08629
(609)599-5000

Viloria, Edermiro, MD {1447364922} IntrMd(75,DOM01)<NY-BETHPETR>
+ American Physician Services/Hudson HealthCare
679 Montgomery Street   Jersey City, NJ 07306   (201)433-6500   Fax (201)433-8010

Vincent, Michael G., MD {1902872385} GenPrc, IntrMd(75,NJ05)
+ Plaza West Diagnostic and Treatment Center
1475 Bergen Boulevard/Plaza West   Fort Lee, NJ 07024
(201)585-8105   Fax (201)585-9862

Vine, John E., MD {1720044670} DerMOH, SrgDer, SrgCsm(92,RI01)<NJ-UNVMCPRN, NJ-RWJUBRUN>
+ Dermatology and Skin Surgery Center of Princeton
5 Plainsboro Road/Suite 460   Plainsboro, NJ 08536
(609)799-6222   Fax (609)799-6555
johnevinemd@earthlink.net

Vinekar, Ajanta S., MD {1780792929} Psychy, PsyGrt, IntrMd(83,INA67)<NJ-SOMERSET>
+ 666 Plainsboro Road/Suite 2
Plainsboro, NJ 08536   (609)936-9444   Fax (609)897-9189
avinekar@comcast.net

Vingan, Roy David, MD {1356318950} SrgNro(85,NY08)
+ North Jersey Brain and Surgical
680 Kinderkamack Road/Suite 300   Oradell, NJ 07649
(201)342-2550   Fax (201)342-7171

Vinluan, Ghia Lynn M., MD {1861628513}
+ 7112 Park Avenue/Aptt 405
North Bergen, NJ 07047   (858)200-6405
glvinluan@gmail.com

Vinnakota, Radha I., MD {1184718306} Otlryg, Otolgy(72,INA35)
+ 27 Mountain Boulevard/Suite 1
Warren, NJ 07059   (908)753-2662   Fax (908)753-2633

Vinnakota, Rao V., MD {1295716157} Pedtrc(68,INA8Y)<NJ-SOMERSET, NJ-OVERLOOK>
+ 27 Mountain Boulevard/Suite 1
Warren, NJ 07059   (908)753-2662   Fax (908)753-2633
vinnakota@doctor.com
+ 49 Brant Avenue
Clark, NJ 07066   (908)753-2662   Fax (732)381-5350

Vinod, Arundhati Hrishikesh, MD {1407804610} ObsGyn(67,INDI)<NJ-HACKNSK>
+ Summit OBGYN LLC
331 Summit Avenue   Hackensack, NJ 07601   (201)457-2300   Fax (201)457-1715

Vinod, Jeevan, MD {1992941587} Gastrn(06,GRN01)<NY-LENOXHLL>
+ Hudson Surgeons
142 Palisade Avenue/Suite 108   Jersey City, NJ 07306
(201)795-8596   Fax (201)795-3550

Vinod, Sheela U., MD {1730336959} PthACl, PthCyt, Pthlgy(73,INA69)
+ Quest Diagnostics Inc.
1 Malcolm Avenue   Teterboro, NJ 07608   (201)393-5000
Fax (201)393-6127

Vinokur, Anna, DO {1841345907} Pedtrc(01,NY75)<NJ-CHILTON>
+ Chilton Medical Center
97 West Parkway   Pompton Plains, NJ 07444   (973)831-5120   Fax (973)831-5342

Vintayen, Enrico V., MD {1003103706} Nrolgy
+ Hudson Neurosciences, PC
605 Broadway   Bayonne, NJ 07002   (201)339-6531   Fax (201)339-6536
enrico8279@yahoo.com

Vintzileos, Anthony M., MD {1538234612} MtFtMd, ObsGyn(75,GRE01)<NJ-STPETER>
+ University Medical Group/OBGYN
125 Paterson Street/2nd Floor   New Brunswick, NJ 08901
(732)235-6600   Fax (732)235-6627

Vinuela, Andres, MD {1649539479} Psychy
+ Palisades Behavioral Care
221 Palisade Avenue   Jersey City, NJ 07306   (646)799-0088
Fax (201)656-3116

Vira, Indu N., MD {1013962968} IntrMd(74,INA20)<NJ-EASTORNG>
+ 202 Stuvesant Avenue
Newark, NJ 07106   (973)374-8807   Fax (973)374-9580
+ Oak Tree Medical Group
1628 Oak Tree Road   Edison, NJ 08820   (732)205-9576

Viradia, Jayant K., MD {1881616084} Anesth, IntrMd(80,INA20)
+ Shore Outpatient Surgicenter LLC
360 Highway 70   Lakewood, NJ 08701   (732)942-9835

Viradia, Manish Bhikhabhai, MD {1457345324} Nrolgy(93,INA20)<NJ-HUNTRDN>
+ MidJersey Orthopaedics, P.A.
8100 Westcott Drive/Suite 101   Flemington, NJ 08822
(908)782-0600   Fax (908)782-7575

Virani, Zahra N., MD {1023387354} FamMed<NJ-RWJUBRUN>
+ RWJ University Hospital New Brunswick
One Robert Wood Johnson Place   New Brunswick, NJ 08901
(732)235-8964   Fax (732)235-6309

Viray, Ruth Mariel, MD {1699802397} Pedtrc
+ Advocare Kressville Pediatrics Cherry Hill
710 Kresson Road   Cherry Hill, NJ 08003   (856)795-3320
Fax (856)795-1213

Virk, Hartaj Singh, MD {1568626877} IntrMd, CdvDis(99,INA1H)
+ Heart & Vascular Associates of Northern Jersey
22-18 Broadway/Suite 201   Fair Lawn, NJ 07410   (201)475-5050   Fax (201)475-5522

Virk, Jaskirat Singh, MD {1053603100} Radiol
+ Hackensack University Medical Center
30 Prospect Avenue/Radiology   Hackensack, NJ 07601
(201)996-2000

Viroja, Yogesh V., MD {1174515753} Grtrcs, IntrMd(80,INA20)<NJ-WARREN>
+ 755 Memorial Parkway/Suite 203
Phillipsburg, NJ 08865   (908)859-4446   Fax (908)859-1569

Visci, Denise, MD {1922150549} Pedtrc(83,PRO02)<NJ-STBARNMC, NJ-OVERLOOK>
+ The Pediatric Center
556 Central Avenue   New Providence, NJ 07974   (908)508-0400   Fax (908)508-0370

Visci, John J., MD {1013975499} AdolMd, Pedtrc(83,MEX03)<NJ-MORRISTN, NJ-OVERLOOK>
+ Advocare Sinatra & Peng Pediatrics
169 Minebrook Road   Bernardsville, NJ 07924   (908)766-0034   Fax (908)766-5065

Visco, Alexander Joseph, MD {1205968310} PhysMd, PhyM-SptM(02,NJ05)<NY-SLOANKET, NY-PRSBCOLU>
+ 510 43rd Street
Weehawken, NJ 07086

Visconti, Raymond, Jr., MD {1972542025} IntrMd(91,NJ05)<NJ-VALLEY>
+ Valley Health Medical Group
72 Hamburg Turnpike   Riverdale, NJ 07457   (973)835-7290
Fax (973)835-0696

Viscuso, Maria B., MD {1518971068} IntrMd, FamMed(79,ITA17)<NJ-WESTHDSN, NJ-CLARMAAS>
+ 8 Hedden Terrace
North Arlington, NJ 07031   (201)991-5353

Viscuso, Ronald L., MD {1467553172} IntrMd, Nephro(68,ITA17)<NJ-MTNSIDE, NJ-CLARMAAS>
+ Nephrological Associates, P.A.
83 Hanover Road/Suite 290   Florham Park, NJ 07932
(973)736-2212   Fax (973)736-2989
+ Nephrological Associates PA
206 Belleville Avenue   Bloomfield, NJ 07003   (973)736-2212   Fax (973)259-0396

Vishwanath, Sahana, MD {1871726901} IntrMd(08)
+ Advocare Allergy & Asthma
54 East Main Street   Marlton, NJ 08053   (856)988-0570
Fax (856)988-0303

Physicians by Name and Address

Viswambharan, Ajay, MD {1275649998} RadDia, RadNro, RadBdI(91,NY20)<NJ-ACMCITY, NJ-SHOREMEM>
+ Atlantic Medical Imaging, LLC.
  72 West Jimmie Leeds Road   Galloway, NJ 08205   (609)677-9729   Fax (609)653-8764
+ Atlantic Medical Imaging, LLC.
  401 Bethel Road   Somers Point, NJ 08244   (609)677-9729
+ Atlantic Medical Imaging, LLC.
  421 Route 9 North   Cape May Court House, NJ 08205   (609)463-9500   Fax (609)465-0918

Viswanath, Dilip Banad, MD {1528019262} CdvDis(93,NY03)<NJ-OURLADY, NJ-KMHTURNV>
+ Cardiovascular Associates
  210 West Atlantic Avenue   Haddon Heights, NJ 08035   (856)546-3003   Fax (856)547-5337
+ Cardiovascular Associates of The Delaware Valley, PA
  1840 Frontage Road   Cherry Hill, NJ 08034   (856)546-3003   Fax (856)795-7436
+ Cardiovascular Associates of The Delaware Valley, PA
  525 State Street/Suite 3   Elmer, NJ 08035   (856)358-2363   Fax (856)358-0725

Viswanathan, Amrutha, MD {1033154679} IntrMd(78,INDI)<NJ-VAEASTOR>
+ VA New Jersey Health Care System-East Orange Campus
  385 Tremont Avenue/Internal Med   East Orange, NJ 07018   (973)676-1000
  amrutha.viswa@gmail.com

Viswanatha, Kallahalli V., MD {1437194123} Grtrcs, IntrMd(71,INDI)<NJ-VAEASTOR>
+ VA New Jersey Health Care System-East Orange Campus
  385 Tremont Avenue   East Orange, NJ 07018   (973)676-1000

Viswanathan, Anjali, MD {1366415192} IntrMd(00,RI01)<NJ-TRINIJSC>
+ Drs. Viswanathan, Shakir & Patel
  815 Baltimore Avenue   Roselle, NJ 07203   (908)245-3446   Fax (908)245-9265

Viswanathan, Revathi, MD {1659419109} Pedtrc(76,INA1X)
+ 122 Market Street
  Passaic, NJ 07055   (973)473-6916

Visweswaran, Gautam Karteek, MD {1528293354} IntrMd(07)<PA-PNSTHRSH>
+ Newark Beth Israel Medical Center
  201 Lyons Avenue   Newark, NJ 07112   (932)925-7852   Fax (973)282-0839

Vital, Michelle Maria, MD {1386612380} Pedtrc(97,INDI)
+ Osborn Family Health Center
  1601 Haddon Road   Camden, NJ 08103   (856)757-3700   Fax (856)365-7972

Vitale, Carl J., MD {1588621007} CdvDis, IntrMd(79,DOM02)<NJ-TRINIWSC>
+ Suburban Heart Group, P.A.
  1000 Galloping Hill Road/Suite 107   Union, NJ 07083   (908)964-7333   Fax (908)687-7855
  CarlVitale@hotmail.com

Vitale, Diana Rodrigues, MD {1043525439} ObsGyn
+ 502 Valley Road/Suite 106
  Wayne, NJ 07470   (973)696-3567   Fax (973)696-1921

Vitale, Joseph, MD {1205845427} IntrMd(77,NJ05)<NJ-STJOSHOS, NJ-WAYNEGEN>
+ West Paterson Family Medical Center
  154 Union Avenue   Paterson, NJ 07502   (973)942-3618
+ West Paterson Family Medical Center
  1031 McBride Avenue/Suite D109   West Paterson, NJ 07424   (973)785-4020

Vitale, Joseph Thomas, MD {1780965905} FamMed(ANT02)
+ West Paterson Family Medical Center
  1031 McBride Avenue/Suite D109   West Paterson, NJ 07424   (973)785-4020

Vitale, Lidia F., MD {1316909625} ObsGyn(90,NY09)<NJ-HUNTRDN>
+ Advanced Obstetrics & Gynecology, LLC
  1100 Wescott Drive   Flemington, NJ 08822   (908)788-6488
+ Advanced Obstetrics & Gynecology, LLC
  1390 Route 22 West/Suite 104   Lebanon, NJ 08833   (908)788-6488   Fax (908)437-1227
+ Advanced Obstetrics & Gynecology, LLC
  4 Walter E. Foran Boulevard/Suite 302   Flemington, NJ 08822   (908)806-0080   Fax (908)806-8570

Vitanzo, Peter Charles, MD {1831139401} FamMSptM(96,PA13)<NJ-ATLANTHS>
+ Rothman Institute - Voorhees
  443 Laurel Oak Road   Voorhees, NJ 08043   (856)821-6530

Vitenson, Jack H., MD {1982673489} Urolgy(65,NY09)<NJ-HACKNSK, NJ-UMDNJ>
+ Urologic Institute of NJ PA
  277 Forest Avenue/Suite 206   Paramus, NJ 07652   (201)489-8900   Fax (201)489-0877

Vitievsky, Alexander Michael, MD {1447250303} Nephro, IntrMd(93,UKR18)<NJ-HOLYNAME, NJ-VALLEY>
+ Renal Medicine Associates PA
  302 Union Street   Hackensack, NJ 07601   (201)646-0414   Fax (201)646-0365
+ Renal Medicine Associates PA
  400 Franklin Turnpike/Suite 208   Mahwah, NJ 07430   (201)825-3322
+ Holy Name Hospital
  718 Teaneck Road/Hemodialysis   Teaneck, NJ 07601   (201)833-3000

Vitievsky, Ellen, MD {1366547135} IntrMd(93,UKR18)<NJ-HOLYNAME>
+ Integrated HealthCare Group
  5600 Kennedy Boulevard/Suite 102   West New York, NJ 07093   (201)866-3100

Vitoc, Camelia S., MD {1225269970} FamMed<NJ-VIRTVOOR>
+ The Maro Group
  27 Covered Bridge Road   Cherry Hill, NJ 08034   (856)429-2224   Fax (856)429-1926

Vitola, Carl A., DO {1922021138} FamMed(78,MO78)<NJ-KENEDYHS, NJ-VIRTVOOR>
+ Drs. Vitola & Kernis
  900 Route 168/Suite C3   Turnersville, NJ 08012   (856)374-0430   Fax (856)374-0048

Vitolo, John, MD {1922074616} SrgOrt, SprtMd(84,NJ05)<NJ-STCLRDEN, NJ-MORRISTN>
+ Skyview Orthopedic Associates
  540 Lafayette Road/Suite D   Sparta, NJ 07871   (973)300-1553   Fax (973)383-6236
+ Skyview Orthopedic Associates
  540 Lafayette road/Suite D   Sparta, NJ 07871   (973)300-1553   Fax (973)383-6236
+ Specialty Surgical Center
  380 Lafayette Road/Suite 110   Sparta, NJ 07871   (973)940-3166   Fax (973)940-3170

Vitolo, Joseph Glen, MD {1730353814} Psychy, Addctn, GenPrc(77,MEX55)
+ 27 Hillsborough Drive
  Monroe, NJ 08831   (732)583-8554   Fax (732)583-8554

Vittal, Melba G., MD {1184709974} Anesth(72,INA2A)<NJ-HOLYNAME>
+ Holy Name Hospital
  718 Teaneck Road/Anesthesiology   Teaneck, NJ 07666   (201)833-6570   Fax (201)833-6576

Vitting, Kevin E., MD {1598762148} Nephro, IntrMd(82,NJ06)<NJ-STJOSHOS, NJ-CHILTON>
+ Suburban Nephrology Group
  342 Hamburg Turnpike/Suite 201   Wayne, NJ 07470   (973)389-1119   Fax (973)389-1145
+ Suburban Nephrology Group
  1031 McBride Avenue/Suite D-210   Little Falls, NJ 07424   (973)389-1119

Vivar-Aguirre, Jorge Luis, MD {1003249319}<NJ-ENGLWOOD>
+ Englewood Hospital and Medical Center
  350 Engle Street/Medicine   Englewood, NJ 07631   (201)984-3664

Vives, Michael J., MD {1568549871} SrgOrt, SrgSpn(95,PA01)<NJ-UMDNJ>
+ North Jersey Orthopaedic Institute
  90 Bergen Street/DOC 1200   Newark, NJ 07101   (973)972-8240   Fax (973)972-9367

Vizzone, Jerald P., DO {1861617623} SrgOrt(89,MO78)
+ 242 Claremont Avenue
  Montclair, NJ 07042   (973)783-1444   Fax (973)783-7755

Vizzoni, Hiedi Taylor, MD {1326012774} FamMed(97,PA09)<NJ-CENTRAST>
+ Capital Health Primary Care-Bordentown
  1 Third Street   Bordentown, NJ 08505   (609)298-2005   Fax (609)324-8267

Vizzoni, Joseph Anthony, MD {1982678330} IntrMd(97,PA09)<NJ-CENTRAST>
+ Family Practice of CentraState
  901 West Main Street/Suite 106   Freehold, NJ 07728   (732)462-9622   Fax (732)780-0014

Vlad, Luigina D., MD {1982601720} EnDbMt, IntrMd(87,ROMA)<NJ-STBARNMC>
+ 65 East Northfield Road/Suite E
  Livingston, NJ 07039   (973)422-9400   Fax (973)422-9495

Vlad, Tudor Jon, MD {1740469485} IntrMd(01,ROM01)<NJ-KMHTURNV>
+ Kennedy Hospitalist Office
  435 Hurffville Cross Keys Road   Turnersville, NJ 08012   (856)513-4124   Fax (856)302-5932
+ Kennedy Health Alliance Vascular Surgery
  333 Laurel Oak Road   Voorhees, NJ 08043   (856)513-4124   Fax (856)770-9194

Vladu, Ana Daniela, MD {1851524722} IntrMd
+ 148 Riveredge Road/8 Garden Place
  Tinton Falls, NJ 07724

Vladu, Cristian, MD {1033151451} IntrMd(97,ROM01)
+ 230 Neptune Boulevard
  Neptune, NJ 07753

Vlahos, Aristotelis E., MD {1184694028} CdvDis, IntrMd, IntCrd(88,GRNA)<NJ-BAYSHORE>
+ Cardiac Care Center
  21 North Gilbert Street   Tinton Falls, NJ 07701   (732)741-7400   Fax (732)741-4775

Vlasica, Katherine, DO {1568674273} EmrgMd(03,NY75)
+ St Joseph's Medical Center Emergency
  703 Main Street   Paterson, NJ 07503   (973)754-2240   Fax (973)754-2249

Vo, Eleanor B., MD {1447580451} Psychy<NJ-VAEASTOR>
+ 19 Farm Lane/PO Box 51
  Roosevelt, NJ 08555

Vo, Ha, MD {1962849497} Pedtrc
+ East Windsor Pediatric Group
  300B Princeton Hightstown/Suite 201   Hightstown, NJ 08520   (609)448-7300   Fax (609)448-8022

Vo, Hung Nam, MD {1972923076} IntrMd<NJ-RWJUBRUN>
+ RWJ University Hospital New Brunswick
  One Robert Wood Johnson Place   New Brunswick, NJ 08901   (732)235-7827

Voca, Ioan Bogdan, MD {1497747281} Anesth(96,ROM09)<NJ-CHILTON>
+ Chilton Medical Center
  97 West Parkway/Anesthesiology   Pompton Plains, NJ 07444   (973)831-5000

Voddi, Swetha Devi, MD {1033245311} FamMed(01,INA68)
+ Snoring and Sleep Apnea Center Mercer County
  1401 Whitehorse Mercerville Rd   Hamilton, NJ 08619   (609)584-5150   Fax (609)584-5144

Vogdes, Tara Ann, DO {1386601649} FamMed(98,PA77)<NJ-BURDTMLN>
+ Cape Regional Physicians Associates
  336 96th Street/Suite 1   Stone Harbor, NJ 08247   (609)967-0070   Fax (609)967-0077

Vogel, David P., MD {1396854824} PulDis, IntrMd(87,DC02)
+ Allergy and Pulmonary Associates
  1542 Kuser Road/Suite B-7   Trenton, NJ 08619   (609)581-1400   Fax (609)585-5234
  davidpvogel@yahoo.com

Vogel, Laurie D., MD EmrgMd, IntrMd(83,MEXI)
+ 7 Manor Drive
  Warren, NJ 07059

Vogel, Mark F., MD {1811947138} EmrgMd(81,DC02)<NJ-VALLEY>
+ The Valley Hospital
  223 North Van Dien Avenue/EmergMed   Ridgewood, NJ 07450   (201)447-8000

Vogel, Martin Joseph, MD {1780811877} AnesPain<NJ-STBARNMC>
+ St. Barnabas Medical Center
  94 Old Short Hills Road   Livingston, NJ 07039   (973)322-5512   Fax (973)322-8165

Vogel, Mitchell, MD {1891799771} Ophthl(91,PA13)<NJ-STMRYPAS, NJ-OVERLOOK>
+ New Jersey Vision Associates
  124 Gregory Avenue/Suite 104   Passaic, NJ 07055   (973)779-0808   Fax (973)471-1929
  njvision@optimum.net
+ Omni Eye Services
  485 Route 1 South/Building A   Iselin, NJ 08830   (973)779-0808   Fax (732)750-1507

Vogiatzidakis, Sophia I., DO {1447663547} ObsGyn
+ Rowan SOM Department of Ob/Gyn
  405 Hurffville-Cross Keys Road   Sewell, NJ 08080   (856)589-1414   Fax (856)256-5772

Voinov, Luba A., MD {1407015761} Anesth(07,NJ06)<NJ-MORRISTN>
+ Morristown Medical Center
  100 Madison Avenue/Anesthesia   Morristown, NJ 07962   (201)943-5831   Fax (201)943-8733

Vojnyk, Charlene Louise, MD {1104300086} Nephro
+ Dr. Anu Chaudhry, MD PC
  546 Saint Georges Avenue   Rahway, NJ 07065   (732)381-3642   Fax (732)396-4463

Volchonok, Oleg, MD {1275571945} Gastrn, IntrMd(86,RUSS)<NJ-VIRTVOOR, NJ-KMHCHRRY>
+ 1060 North Kings Highway/Suite 113
  Cherry Hill, NJ 08034   (856)779-7110   Fax (856)779-9431

Voleti, Vinod Babu, MD {1245452804} Ophthl, IntrMd(07,NY01)
+ Retina Associates of New Jersey, P.A.
  5 Franklin Avenue   Belleville, NJ 07109   (973)450-5100   Fax (973)450-9494
+ Retina Associates of New Jersey, P.A.
  2952 Vauxhall Road   Vauxhall, NJ 07088   (973)450-5100   Fax (908)349-8134
+ Retina Associates of New Jersey, P.A.
  182 South Street/Suite 5   Morristown, NJ 07109   Fax (973)605-5807

Volfson, Ariy, MD {1306008446} Gastrn, IntrMd(07,NY03)
+ Gastroenterology Associates of New Jersey
  88 Park Street   Montclair, NJ 07042   (973)233-9559   Fax (973)233-9660
+ Gastroenterology Associates of New Jersey
  1124 East Ridgewood Avenue/Suite 203   Ridgewood, NJ 07450   (973)233-9559   Fax (201)857-8646
+ Gastroenterology Associates of New Jersey
  1031 McBride Avenue/Suite D-212   Little Falls, NJ 07042   (973)890-1303   Fax (973)890-5609

Volk, Yuri, MD {1265562862} Gastrn, IntrMd(88,RUSS)
+ 193 US Highway 9/Suite 1 C
  Englishtown, NJ 07726   (732)637-8334   Fax (732)252-9404

Volkov, Anatoly, MD {1760411748} Anesth(97,NJ05)<NJ-VALLEY>
+ The Valley Hospital
  223 North Van Dien Avenue   Ridgewood, NJ 07450   (201)447-8000

Volokhov, Alexey, MD {1780656157} IntrMd(84,RUS77)
+ Primary Care NJ
  370 Grand Avenue/Suite 102   Englewood, NJ 07631   (201)569-8786   Fax (201)816-1265

Volosin, Kent Joseph, MD {1760418479} CdvDis, IntrMd(80,NC05)<NJ-ACMCMAIN, NJ-ACMCITY>
+ Penn Medicine at Cherry Hill
  1400 East Route 70/Cardiology   Cherry Hill, NJ 08034
+ Associated Cardiovascular Consultants, P.A.
  1105 Laurel Oak Road/Suite 165   Voorhees, NJ 08043   Fax (856)424-7154

Volpe, Anthony P., MD {1801900824} IntrMd(81,MEX03)
+ 466 Old Hook Road/Suite 14
  Emerson, NJ 07630   (201)262-6485   Fax (204)262-9419

Volpe, John Anthony, DO {1063460624} Allrgy, Gastrn(83,IA75)
+ The Gastroenterology Group, PA
  103 Old Marlton Pike/Suite 102   Medford, NJ 08055   (609)953-3440   Fax (609)996-4002
+ The Gastroenterology Group, PA
  15000 Midlantic Drive/Suite 110   Mount Laurel, NJ 08054   (609)953-3440   Fax (856)996-4002

Volpe, Lorraine, MD {1982633622} Anesth(86,NY09)
+ Englewood Anesthesiology
  350 Engle Street   Englewood, NJ 07631   (201)894-3238   Fax (201)871-0619

Volpe, Michael Anthony, MD {1568435089} Urolgy(94,NY08)<NJ-OVERLOOK, NJ-MORRISTN>
+ Summit Medical Group-Berkeley Heights Campus
  1 Diamond Hill Road   Berkeley Heights, NJ 07922   (908)273-4300   Fax (908)277-8909

Volpert, Diana, MD {1356317572} Pedtrc, PedGst(87,ISR02)<NJ-VALLEY>
+ Drs. Orellana & Volpert
  1200 East Ridgewood Avenue/Suite 108   Ridgewood, NJ 07450   (201)389-0815

Volpicella-Levy, Susan L., DO {1821062977} FamMed(87,NY75)<NJ-VALLEY>
+ 261 Old Hook Road
  Westwood, NJ 07675   (201)666-9600   Fax (201)666-5014
+ The Valley Hospital
  223 North Van Dien Avenue/Medicine   Ridgewood, NJ 07450   (201)447-8000

Volshteyn, Boris, MD {1033107669} SrgRec(95,MO03)
+ Atlantic Surgical Associates
  2 Lincoln Highway/Suite 508   Edison, NJ 08820   (732)641-3350   Fax (732)333-6324
  drv@plasticsurgerynewyorknewjersey.com
+ Atlantic Surgical Associates
  107 Monmouth Road/Suite 102   West Long Branch, NJ 07764   (732)641-3350   Fax (732)333-6324

Volskaya, Svetlana, MD {1265610885} Psychy(83,UKR05)<NJ-HAGEDORN>
+ Hagedorn Psychiatric Hospital
  200 Sanatorium Road   Glen Gardner, NJ 08826   (908)537-2141   Fax (908)537-3186

Volvovsky, Alexander, MD {1013100098} RadDia
+ Summit Medical Group
  1 Diamond Hill Road/Bensley Pav/2 FL   Berkeley Heights, NJ 07922   (908)277-8673   Fax (908)288-7993

Von Der Schmidt, Edward, III, MD {1043302110} SrgNro(84,NJ05)
+ 330 North Harrison Street/Suite 4
  Princeton, NJ 08540   (609)924-3614   Fax (609)924-3528

von Poelnitz, Audrey E., MD {1558369579} CdvDis, IntrMd(79,PA01)<NJ-MORRISTN>
+ Morristown Cardiology Associates, P.A.
  435 South Street/Suite 100   Morristown, NJ 07960   (973)267-3944   Fax (973)455-0399

Von Poelnitz, Michael, MD {1407088818} Psychy(75,GERM)
+ PO Box 87
  Mendham, NJ 07945

Von Roemer, Marc, MD {1841200862} Ophthl(93,NJ05)
+ Invision, Inc.
  One Route 70   Lakewood, NJ 08701   (732)905-5600
  drmarc@hotmail.com

Von Suskil, Kurt E., MD {1750317889} FamMed(87,NJ06)<NJ-MONMOUTH>
+ Sea Girt Medical Associates
  235 Route 71   Manasquan, NJ 08736   (732)223-4300   Fax (732)223-5273

Vona, Cynthia E., MD {1831253749} IntrMd(85,DC02)
+ Pansophy Medical Consultants, LLC
  150 Wild Dunes Way   Jackson, NJ 08527   (908)415-1242

VonBose, Michael J., MD {1386879443} EmrgEMed(78,GER16)<NJ-STMICHL>
+ St. Michael's Medical Center
  111 Central Avenue   Newark, NJ 07102   (973)877-5500   Fax (973)877-5690

Vongviphut, Don, DO {1003356684} GenPrc
+ McGuire Air Force Base/Acute Health Care Clinic
  3458 Neely Road   Trenton, NJ 08641   (609)754-9080   Fax (609)754-9015

Vonroth, William, Jr., MD {1215902317} SrgOrt(71,NJ05)<NJ-MTNSIDE>
+ Glen Ridge Surgicenter
  230 Sherman Avenue   Glen Ridge, NJ 07028   (973)783-6363   Fax (973)680-4211

Vora, Amit V., MD {1295999142} Ophthl(08,NJ06)
+ Eye Physicians of Sussex County
  183 High Street/Suite 2200   Newton, NJ 07860   (973)383-6345   Fax (973)383-0032

Vora, Bhupendra N., MD {1538232434} Ophthl(65,INA67)<NJ-CHRIST>
+ 142 Palisade Avenue
  Jersey City, NJ 07306   (201)656-7171   Fax (201)656-1611

Vora, Jaimini Neeraj, MD {1760773808} PthACl(93,INA8B)<NY-NYUTISCH>
+ 2001 Green Hollow Drive
  Iselin, NJ 08830

Vora, Kajol, MD {1780157370} PhyMNMus
+ 425 Washington Boulevard/Apt 2012
  Jersey City, NJ 07310   (772)480-9938

Vora, Naginadas M., MD {1558386144} Surgry(72,INA21)<NJ-MEMSALEM>
+ 294 East Main Street/PO Box 311
  Penns Grove, NJ 08069   (856)299-4808   Fax (856)299-4809
+ Memorial Hospital of Salem County
  310 Woodstown Road/Surgery   Salem, NJ 08079   (856)935-1000

Vora, Parag V., MD {1326270661}
+ CHOP Care Network at Virtua Voorhees Hospital
  100 Bowman Drive   Voorhees, NJ 08043   (215)868-4080   Fax (609)261-5842

Vora, Shobhana B., MD {1922217199} Psychy(64,INA69)
+ 142 Palisade Avenue
  Jersey City, NJ 07306

Voremberg, Sandra R., MD {1689656225} Pedtrc(89,NJ06)<NJ-OVERLOOK, NJ-STBARNMC>
+ 120 Millburn Avenue/Suite M-1
  Millburn, NJ 07041   (973)218-0707   Fax (973)218-0177
  drsandyv@aol.com
+ Summit Medical Group
  1 Diamond Hill Road/Bensley Pav/2 FL   Berkeley, NJ 07922   (973)218-0707   Fax (908)288-7993

Vorobyev, Leonid A., MD {1245259431} Psychy, Acpntr(85,RUS15)
+ Jersey Medical Care, PC
  100 Belchase Drive/Suite 101   Matawan, NJ 07747   (732)707-4100   Fax (732)707-4101

Voros, Stephen C., MD {1528080355} Anesth(92,NJ05)<NJ-CHSMRCER, NJ-CHSFULD>
+ Trenton Anesthesiology Associates, PA
  One Capital Way/Second Floor   Pennington, NJ 08534   (609)396-4700   Fax (609)396-4900

Vosatka, Robert J., MD {1700085883} ClnGnt, NnPnMd, Pedtrc(87,NY19)
+ Advocare West Morris Pediatrics
  151 Route 10/Suite 105   Succasunna, NJ 07876   (973)584-0002   Fax (973)584-7107
+ 12 Forge Road
  Kinnelon, NJ 07405

Vosburgh, Evan, MD {1518955517} Hemato, IntrMd, Onclgy(82,NY03)<CT-YALENHH>
+ Bayer HealthCare Corporation
  PO Box 1000   Montville, NJ 07045

Voskoboynik, Diana, MD {1598965766} Pedtrc, PedEmg(05,NY03)<NY-JACOBIMC, NJ-VALLEY>
+ The Valley Hospital
  223 North Van Dien Avenue/PediEmrgMed   Ridgewood, NJ 07450   (201)447-8000

Vosough, Cyrus R., MD {1194729475} PhysMd, PhyMPain(94,NJ06)
+ 510 Hamburg Turnpike
  Wayne, NJ 07470   (973)595-0063   Fax (973)720-0408

Vosough, Khashayar, MD {1487692299} ObsGyn(93,NJ05)
+ Comprehensive Women's Healthcare
  220 Hamburg Turnpike/Suite 21   Wayne, NJ 07470   (973)790-8090   Fax (973)790-3198

Vosseller, James Turner, MD {1326244799} SrgOrt(04,DC02)<NY-SPCLSURG>
+ Columbia Grand Orthopaedics
  500 Grand Avenue/Suite 101   Englewood, NJ 07631   (201)569-0440   Fax (201)569-4949

Vossler, Cathleen M., MD {1811063381} EmrgMd(92,NY15)<NJ-UNVMCPRN>
+ University Medical Center of Princeton at Plainsboro
  One Plainsboro Road/EmergMed   Plainsboro, NJ 08536   (609)497-4000

Vossough, Sima, MD {1861415911} Gastrn, IntrMd(88,NJ06)<NJ-VAEASTOR, NJ-VANJHCS>
+ VA New Jersey Health Care System-East Orange Campus
  385 Tremont Avenue/Med/GI   East Orange, NJ 07018   (973)676-1000   Fax (973)395-7076

Vossough, Soheila, MD {1144379504} CritCr, IntrMd(87,NJ05)<NJ-STMRYPAS>
+ Park Avenue Medical Associates
  30 Park Avenue/Suite 202   Lyndhurst, NJ 07071   (201)438-5900   Fax (201)438-5980

Voudouris, Apostolos Athanasios, MD {1902842446} CdvDis, ClCdEl, IntrMd(98,NY48)
+ Bart De Gregorio MD, LLC.
  946 Bloomfield Avenue   Glen Ridge, NJ 07028   (973)743-1121   Fax (973)743-2627

Voyack, Michael John, DO {1003896028} FamMed, IntrMd(83,PA77)
+ Cooper Family Medicine
  1001-F Lincoln Drive West   Marlton, NJ 08053   (856)810-1800   Fax (856)810-1879

Vozos, Frank J., MD {1154457539} Surgry(74,GRE01)
+ 26 Burnt Mill Circle
  Oceanport, NJ 07757

Vrablik, Robert H., MD {1699871517} PhysMd(91,NJ05)<NJ-NWTNMEM, NJ-STCLRDEN>
+ Northwest Rehabiliation Associates PA
  400 South Main Street   Wharton, NJ 07885   (973)989-5270   Fax (973)989-5274
+ Newton Medical Center
  175 High Street   Newton, NJ 07860   (973)989-5270   Fax (973)383-9869

Vu, Hung Quoc, MD {1669582409} Radiol, RadDia, RadBdI(94,PA13)<NJ-ACMCMAIN, NJ-ACMCITY>
+ Atlantic Medical Imaging, LLC.
  72 West Jimmie Leeds Road   Galloway, NJ 08205   (609)677-9729   Fax (609)653-8764
+ Atlantic Medical Imaging, LLC.
  401 Bethel Road   Somers Point, NJ 08244   (609)677-9729
+ Atlantic Medical Imaging, LLC.
  421 Route 9 North   Cape May Court House, NJ 08205   (609)463-9500   Fax (609)465-0918

Vudarla, Neelima, MD {1598945412} IntHos
+ Rowan University-School of Osteopathic Medicine
  1 Medical Center Drive/Suite 3100   Stratford, NJ 08084   (856)566-7050

Vujic, Dragomir M., MD {1295710739} Anesth(87,PA02)<NJ-HCKTSTWN>
+ Montclair Anesthesia Associates PC
  185 Fairfield Avenue/Suite 2A   West Caldwell, NJ 07006   (973)226-1230   Fax (973)226-1232

Vukasin, Alexander P., MD {1659392546} Urolgy(89,CT01)<NJ-UNVMCPRN, NJ-CAPITLHS>
+ Urology Group of Princeton PA
  281 Witherspoon Street/Suite 100   Princeton, NJ 08542   (609)924-6487   Fax (609)921-7020
+ Urology Group of Princeton PA
  134 Stanhope Street/Forrestal Village   Princeton, NJ 08540   (609)924-6487   Fax (609)921-7020

Vukic, Mario, MD {1043287865} Nrolgy, ClNrPh(98,NY48)<NJ-HACKNSK, NJ-HOLYNAME>
+ Hackensack Neurology Group
  211 Essex Street/Suite 202   Hackensack, NJ 07601   (201)488-1515   Fax (201)488-9471
  mvukic@nyc.rr.com

Vuong, Charlotte Hwa, MD {1770823049} Dermat
+ 636 Morris Turnpike/Suite 2H
  Short Hills, NJ 07078   (973)232-6245   Fax (973)232-6247

Vuotto, Angela Marie, DO {1811147556} PsyFor(00,NJ75)
+ 122 North Third Street
  Hammonton, NJ 08037

Vuppala, Gulab, MD {1912950387} IntrMd, EmrgMd(72,INDI)<NJ-RBAYPERT>
+ Raritan Bay Medical Center/Perth Amboy Division
  530 New Brunswick Avenue   Perth Amboy, NJ 08861   (732)442-3700

Vyas, Hema, MD {1619160892} Psychy
+ 6 Paragon Way
  Freehold, NJ 07728   (732)303-9900

Physicians by Name and Address

Vyas, Mihir, DO {1235422171}
+ 68 Hilltop Road
Howell, NJ 07731 (732)642-9425
vyas810@gmail.com

Vyas, Nishant, MD {1700294535} IntrMd<NJ-OVERLOOK>
+ Overlook Medical Center
99 Beauvoir Avenue/PO Box 210 Summit, NJ 07902
(908)522-6414

Vyas, Rajiv Krishnakant, MD {1376757435} Psychy(85,GRN01)
+ 215 South Burlington Road
Bridgeton, NJ 08302 (856)459-7224

Vyas, Shefali, MD {1780676056} Pedtrc, PedNph, IntrMd(91,INA21)<NJ-STBARNMC>
+ Drs. Vyas & Bridges
101 Old Short Hills Road/Suite 505 West Orange, NJ 07052
(973)322-6767 Fax (973)322-6780

Vypritskaya, Ekaterina Anatolyevna, MD {1790952299} IntrMd
+ Corporate Health Center
832 Brunswick Avenue Trenton, NJ 08638 (609)695-7471
Fax (609)815-7401
+ Capital Health Family Health Center
433 Bellevue Avenue/4th Floor Trenton, NJ 08618
(609)695-7471 Fax (609)815-7178

Wachman, Jill, MD {1750703492} IntrMd(90,NY15)
+ 21H Nobhill
Roseland, NJ 07068 (732)730-1877

Wachsberg, Ronald H., MD {1982636759} RadDia, Radiol(83,QU01)<NJ-UMDNJ>
+ University Hospital
150 Bergen Street/Level C/Radio Newark, NJ 07103
(973)972-5188 Fax (973)972-7429

Wachtel, Jessica F., MD {1396011573}<NJ-NWRKBETH>
+ Newark Beth Israel Medical Center
201 Lyons Avenue Newark, NJ 07112 (973)926-7000

Wachtel, Zev, MD {1770581217} Anesth(83,DOMI)<NJ-STMICHL>
+ St. Joseph's Regional Medical Center Anesthesia
703 Main Street Paterson, NJ 07503 (973)754-2323 Fax (973)977-9455

Waciega, Mark, MD {1346295482} EmrgMd, Anesth(83,PA02)<NJ-CENTRAST>
+ CentraState Medical Center
901 West Main Street/Emerg Medicine Freehold, NJ 07728
(732)294-2667

Wade, Mark J., MD {1962782474} Pedtrc(FL03)
+ Jewish Renaissance Medical Center
275 Hobart Street Perth Amboy, NJ 08861 (732)376-9333
Fax (732)376-0139

Wadehra, Ramneet, DO {1205031614} CdvDis, IntrMd(08,NJ75)
+ Associated Cardiovascular Consultants-Lourdes
1 Brace Road/Suite C & F Cherry Hill, NJ 08034 (856)428-4100 Fax (856)428-5748

Wadhwa, Aruna, MD {1093795593} FamMed, Grtrcs(87,INA72)
+ New Jersey Institute for Successful Aging
42 East Laurel Road/Suite 1800 Stratford, NJ 08084
(856)566-6843 Fax (856)566-6781

Wadhwa, Dom P., MD {1548361637} IntrMd(82)
+ 215 East Camden Avenue/Suite H-13
Moorestown, NJ 08057

Wadhwa, Namrata, MD {1144263260} PainMd, AnesPain(91,INA23)<NJ-OURLADY, NJ-LOURDMED>
+ Our Lady of Lourdes Medical Center
1600 Haddon Avenue/Anesthesia Camden, NJ 08103
(856)757-3500

Wadhwa, Rajesh, MD {1801945381} IntrMd(83,INA1Z)<NJ-RWJUBRUN, NJ-STPETER>
+ Wholehealth-Continental Clinic
Suite 136/Terminal C Newark, NJ 07114 (973)681-1700
Fax (973)681-1189

Wadlinger, Rebecca, DO {1124304282}<NJ-PALISADE>
+ Palisades Medical Center
7600 River Road North Bergen, NJ 07047 (201)854-5000

Waggoner, Thomas E., I, DO {1891083812} CdvDis<NJ-DEBRAHLC>
+ Deborah Heart and Lung Center
200 Trenton Road Browns Mills, NJ 08015 (609)893-6611

Wagh, Anju M., MD {1033171178} EmrgMd, Pedtrc, PedEmg(91,INDI)<NJ-VALLEY>
+ The Valley Hospital
223 North Van Dien Avenue Ridgewood, NJ 07450
(201)447-8000

Wagle, Priya Jennifer, MD {1770585762} Otlryg(98,NY48)<NJ-ACMCMAIN, NJ-ACMCITY>
+ South Jersey ENT Surgical Associates
2106 New Road/Unit C-9 Linwood, NJ 08221 (609)927-8881 Fax (609)927-8832

Wagle, Sharad D., MD {1801011283} Psychy, PsycAd(72,INA67)<NJ-HOLYNAME>
+ Holy Name Hospital
718 Teaneck Road/Psych Teaneck, NJ 07666 (201)833-3000 Fax (201)541-5962

Wagman, Raquel Tamara, MD {1982641015} Onclgy, RadOnc, RadThp(95,MI01)<NJ-STBARNMC>
+ St. Barnabas Medical Center
94 Old Short Hills Road/Rad/Onc Livingston, NJ 07039
(973)322-5000 Fax (973)322-5648

Wagmiller, Jennifer Ann, MD {1649289364}<NJ-STBARNMC>
+ St. Barnabas Medical Center
94 Old Short Hills Road Livingston, NJ 07039 (973)322-5000

Wagner, Claudia Anne, MD {1982631677} FamMed(88,NY47)
+ Westfield Family Practice
563 Westfield Avenue Westfield, NJ 07090 (908)232-5858
Fax (908)232-0439
+ Summit Medical Group-Berkeley Heights Campus
1 Diamond Hill Road Berkeley Heights, NJ 07922
(908)232-5858 Fax (908)790-6576

Wagner, Craig R., DO {1326033572} Anesth(87,NJ75)<NJ-UNDRWD>
+ Inspira Health Network
509 North Broad Street Woodbury, NJ 08096 (856)845-0100

Wagner, Robert Austin, MD {1205907086} Nrolgy(99,PA09)
+ Neurologic Associates
220 Hamburg Turnpike/Suite 16 Wayne, NJ 07470
(973)942-4778 Fax (973)942-7020

Wagner, Rudolph S., MD {1366484222} PedOph, Ophthl(78,NJ05)<NJ-STBARNMC>
+ 1 Clara Maass Drive
Belleville, NJ 07109 (973)751-1702 Fax (973)450-5964
+ Institute of Ophthalmology & Visual Science
556 Eagle Rock Avenue/Suite 206 Roseland, NJ 07068
(973)751-1702 Fax (973)226-4010

Wagner, Scott Erik, MD {1356452064} EmrgMd(99,PA02)<NJ-SJHREGMC>
+ SJH Regional Medical Center
1505 West Sherman Avenue/EmergMed Vineland, NJ 08360 (856)641-8000

Wagner, Wendy Joan, MD {1609832179} ObsGyn(97,CT02)<NJ-STPETER, NJ-RWJUBRUN>
+ Lifetime Ob/Gyn
378 South Branch Road/Suite 403 Hillsborough, NJ 08844
(908)369-0970 Fax (908)369-0216
+ Womens Health Care Associates of Sussex County
135 Newton Sparta Road/Suite 201 Newton, NJ 07860
(908)369-0970 Fax (973)383-8424

Wagreich, Allison Robin, MD {1083855332} GynOnc, ObsGyn(99,NY08)<NJ-MORRISTN>
+ Morristown Medical Center
100 Madison Avenue/Suite 109 Morristown, NJ 07962
(973)971-5900 Fax (973)290-7257

Wagshul, Adam David, MD {1831164300} SrgOrt(96,MD01)
+ The Orthopedic Group, P.A.
261 James Street/Suite 3-F Morristown, NJ 07960
(973)538-0029 Fax (973)538-4957
+ The Orthopedic Group, P.A.
50 Cherry Hill Road Parsippany, NJ 07054 (973)538-0029
Fax (973)263-3243

Wahba, Janette M., MD {1659331114} Pedtrc, AdolMd(70,EGY03)<NJ-CLARMAAS>
+ 525 Ridge Road
Lyndhurst, NJ 07071 (201)935-5512 Fax (201)935-1914

Wahba, Magdy A., MD {1497871546} PulDis, IntrMd, CritCr(77,EGY04)<NJ-CHILTON>
+ 401 Hamburg Turnpike/Suite 310
Wayne, NJ 07470 (973)790-5300
+ PO Box 665
Ridgewood, NJ 07451

Wahdat, Razwana, DO {1104238856} EmrgMd
+ Kennedy Mem Hospital Emergency Medicine
18 East Laurel Road Stratford, NJ 08084 (856)346-7985

Wain, Nadeem, MD {1538555479} IntHos<NJ-MTNSIDE>
+ Hackensack UMC Mountainside
1 Bay Avenue Montclair, NJ 07042 (732)801-6350

Wainen, Glen P., MD {1831100999} SrgOrt(92,NJ05)<NJ-HCKTSTWN, NJ-MORRISTN>
+ Skylands Orthopaedics PC
57 US Highway 46/Suite 107 Hackettstown, NJ 07840
(908)813-9700 Fax (908)813-2861
+ Skylands Orthopaedics PC
230 West Parkway/Unit 10 Pompton Plains, NJ 07444
(908)813-9700 Fax (908)813-2861
+ Emmaus Surgical Center
57 US Highway 46/Suite 104 Hackettstown, NJ 07840
(908)813-9600 Fax (908)813-9611

Waintraub, Stanley Eli, MD {1609835586} Hemato, IntrMd, MedOnc(77,NY09)<NJ-HACKNSK, NJ-HOLYNAME>
+ John Theurer Cancer Center - HUMC
92 Second Street Hackensack, NJ 07601 (201)996-5900 Fax (201)996-9246

Wainwright Edwards, Marsha, MD {1194980789} EmrgMd(08,NJ05)
+ 4209 Bishops View Circle
Cherry Hill, NJ 08002

Wajcberg, Estela, MD {1356599294} IntrMd(95)<NJ-TRINIWSC>
+ Montgomery Medical Associates
9 Dutchtown Road Belle Mead, NJ 08502 (908)874-8883
Fax (908)874-3595

Wajnberg, Alexander, MD {1215962618} CdvDis, IntrMd(81,NY08)
+ 3 Hospital Plaza/Suite 417
Old Bridge, NJ 08857 (732)360-1169 Fax (732)360-2526

Waksman, Howard Kenneth, MD {1427050103} PulDis, IntrMd(88,MA05)
+ Pulmonary & Intensive Care Specialists of NJ
593 Cranbury Road East Brunswick, NJ 08816 (732)613-8880 Fax (732)613-0077

Walcott, Adrian B., MD {1124110226} Pedtrc(90,NJ05)<NJ-STBARNMC>
+ Agape Pediatric Center LLC
185 Central Avenue/Suite 401 East Orange, NJ 07018
(973)673-6311 Fax (973)673-6511
adrian@apc.pcc.com

Walczyszyn, Bartosz Adam, MD {1376833723}
+ NJ Hematology & Oncology Associates
1608 Route 88 West/Suite 250 Brick, NJ 08724 (732)840-8880 Fax (732)840-3939

Walden, Philip Louis, Jr., MD {1790714137} EmrgMd(95,NJ05)<NJ-HACKNSK>
+ Hackensack University Medical Center
30 Prospect Avenue/EmergMed Hackensack, NJ 07601
(201)996-2300 Fax (201)342-7112

Waldman, Brett Andrew, MD {1407192289}<NJ-COOPRUMC>
+ Cooper University Hospital
One Cooper Plaza Camden, NJ 08103 (856)342-2000

Waldman, Ilan, MD {1871711655} Urolgy(02,DC01)
+ New Jersey Urologic Institute
10 Industrial Way East Eatontown, NJ 07724 (732)963-9091 Fax (732)963-9092
+ New Jersey Urologic Institute
25 Kilmer Drive/Building 3/Suite 214 Morganville, NJ 07751
(732)536-8880

Waldman, Steven Paul, MD {1861416364} AnesPain, IntrMd(83,NY08)
+ Atlas Spine Interventional Medicine
8901 Kennedy Boulevard/Suite 1-W North Bergen, NJ 07047 (201)243-2022 Fax (201)243-7261
+ Hudson Crossing Surgery Center
2 Executive Drive Fort Lee, NJ 07024 (201)243-2022 Fax (201)292-3165

Waldor, Philip Arthur, MD {1841443140} Surgry(76,PA13)
+ 210 East Berkshire Avenue
Linwood, NJ 08221

Waldron, Frederick Andrew, MD {1528053337} EmrgMd(98,NJ05)<NJ-NWRKBETH>
+ Newark Beth Israel Medical Center
201 Lyons Avenue/EmrgMed Newark, NJ 07112 (973)926-7000

Waldron, John R., DO {1154356343} IntrMd(78,PA77)<NJ-VIRTMHBC>
+ Advocare Medford Station Internal Medicine
69 North Main Street Medford, NJ 08055 (609)953-9000
Fax (609)953-9696

Waldron, Robert John, MD {1558634824} Pedtrc
+ 536 Ocean Terrace
Normandy Beach, NJ 08739 (732)793-0186

Waldron, Winifred Marie, MD {1750355939} FamMed(96,VT02)<NJ-HUNTRDN>
+ Charlestown Medical Associates
140 Boulevard Washington, NJ 07882 (908)689-3200
Fax (908)689-8295

Waldstreicher, Joanne, MD {1285770826} EnDbMt, IntrMd(87,MA01)
+ Johnson & Johnson Development Corporation
410 George Street New Brunswick, NJ 08901 (732)524-2115 Fax (732)247-5309

Walia, Jasjit S., MD {1477573814} IntrMd, CdvDis(92,INA41)<NJ-UMDNJ, NJ-TRINIWSC>
+ NJ Heart/Elizabeth Office
240 Williamson Street/Suite 402-406 Elizabeth, NJ 07202
(908)354-8900 Fax (908)354-0077
jw@njheart.net

Walia, Kulbir Singh, MD {1982690715} AnesPain(92,INDI)
+ Premier Pain Center
160 Avenue at the Commons/Suite 1 Shrewsbury, NJ 07702
(732)380-0200 Fax (732)380-0262

Walimbe, Mona S,, MD {1275730871} EnDbMt, IntrMd(07,PA12)
+ Drs. Chon & Chon
435 South Street/Suite 230-A Morristown, NJ 07960
(973)971-6480 Fax (973)290-7435

Walk, Zem, MD {1043310907} ObsGyn(68,BEL07)<NJ-STBARNMC>
+ Associates in Obstetrics Gynecology & Infertility
375 Mount Pleasant Avenue/Suite 202 West Orange, NJ 07052 (973)731-7707 Fax (973)669-0277

Physicians by Name and Address

Walker, Bridget Ann, DO {1932268802} IntrMd
+ Schuylkill Medical Associates, LLC
2681 Quakerbridge Road/Suite B2   Hamilton, NJ 08619
Fax (609)208-3233

Walker, Camille D., MD {1114981172} NnPnMd, ObsGyn, MtFtMd(89,NY47)
+ 519 South Orange Avenue
South Orange, NJ 07079   (973)313-2550   Fax (973)313-2550
+ Children's Hospital of New Jersey
201 Lyons Avenue/Osborne Terrace   Newark, NJ 07112
(973)313-2550   Fax (201)309-4519

Walker, John A., MD {1407876709} IntrMd, Nephro(76,NY08)<NJ-RWJUBRUN>
+ UMDNJ RWJ Nephrology
125 Paterson Street/Suite 5100-B   New Brunswick, NJ 08901   (732)235-6512   Fax (732)235-6124
+ UH- RWJ Medical School
One Robert Wood Johnson Place   New Brunswick, NJ 08903
(732)235-6512   Fax (732)235-6124

Walker, John S., DO {1013974500} Anesth(90,NY75)<NJ-SOMERSET, NJ-STPETER>
+ Anesthesia Consultnts of NJ/Nova Pain
285 Davidson Avenue/Suite 204   Somerset, NJ 08873
(732)271-1400   Fax (732)271-3543
+ Cares Surgicenter, LLC.
240 Easton Avenue   New Brunswick, NJ 08901   (732)271-1400   Fax (732)296-8677

Walker, Paul A., DO {1922077056} FamMed, IntrMd(87,IA75)<NJ-STFRNMED>
+ Ewing Medical Associates
1539 Pennington Road   Trenton, NJ 08618   (609)883-4124
Fax (609)883-1909

Walker, Richard Nathaniel, DO {1497892996} Ophthl(03,NJ75)
+ Randolph Eyecare Center
477 Route 10 East   Randolph, NJ 07869   (973)328-1311

Walker, Ryan D., MD {1457675589} PedOto
+ Advanced ENT - Voorhees
200 Bowman Drive/Suite D-285   Voorhees, NJ 08043
(856)602-4000   Fax (856)842-5109

Walker, Tracy Lynne, MD {1003836123} CdvDis, IntrMd(99,DMN01)
+ Bergen Medical Associates
466 Old Hook Road/Suite 1   Emerson, NJ 07630   (201)967-8221   Fax (201)967-0340

Walks, Pauline Angela, MD {1063434447} Pedtrc(80,NY46)<NY-LICOLLGE>
+ Newark Community Health Center, Inc.
741 Broadway   Newark, NJ 07104   (973)675-1900   Fax (973)676-1396
+ Irvington Community Health Center
1148-1150 Springfield Avenue   Irvington, NJ 07111
(973)675-1900   Fax (973)372-4534

Wall, Robert M., MD {1477543247} CdvDis, IntrMd(82,NJ05)
+ Lakeland Cardiology Center, P.A.
415 Boulevard   Mountain Lakes, NJ 07046   (973)334-7700
Fax (973)402-5847
+ Lakeland Cardiology Center PA
765 State Route 10/Suite 4   Randolph, NJ 07869   (973)989-2566

Wallace, David Morrow, MD {1336116656} MtFtMd, NnPnMd, ObsGyn(80,PA09)<NJ-MONMOUTH>
+ Monmouth Medical Group, P.C.
73 South Bath Avenue   Long Branch, NJ 07740   (732)870-3600   Fax (732)870-0119
+ Monmouth Medical Center
300 Second Avenue/Ob/Gyn Rm215 SW   Long Branch, NJ 07740   (732)870-3600   Fax (732)923-6793
+ Monmouth Family Center
270 Broadway   Long Branch, NJ 07740   (732)923-7100
Fax (732)923-7104

Wallace, Derrick I., MD {1114900362} Otlryg(96,NY47)
+ North Jersey Ear, Nose and Throat Associates, Inc.
187 Washington Avenue/Suite 2   Nutley, NJ 07110
(973)235-0090   Fax (973)235-0090

Wallace, Stephen Gary, MD {1144255498} IntrMd, OncHem(93,SAF02)<NJ-VIRTMHBC>
+ Hematology Oncology Associates PA
175 Madison Avenue/4th Floor   Mount Holly, NJ 08060
(609)702-1900   Fax (609)702-8455

Wallace, Theresa C., MD {1801842091} FamMed(92,PA02)<NJ-MTNSIDE, NJ-MORRISTN>
+ Summit Medical Group
95 Madison Avenue   Morristown, NJ 07960   (973)267-1010   Fax (973)267-5521

Wallach, Bruce H., MD {1649256066} Hemato, Onclgy, IntrMd(84,MEX34)
+ Regional Cancer Care Specialists
34-36 Progress Street/Suite B-2   Edison, NJ 08820
(908)757-9696   Fax (908)757-9721

Wallach, Carl B., MD {1962593947} Gastrn, IntrMd(85,FL02)
+ Affiliates in Gastroenterology, P.A.
101 Old Short Hills Road/Suite 217   West Orange, NJ 07052
(973)731-4600   Fax (973)731-1477
+ Affiliates in Gastroenterology, P.A.
101 Madison Avenue/Suite 100   Morristown, NJ 07960
(973)731-4600   Fax (973)540-8788

Wallach, Jonathan Brett, MD {1851640700} RadOnc<NY-MNTFMOSE>
+ St. Peter's University Hospital
254 Easton Avenue   New Brunswick, NJ 08901   (732)745-8590

Wallach, Sara L., MD {1144279779} Grtrcs, IntrMd(80,NY08)<NJ-STFRNMED>
+ St. Francis Medical Center
601 Hamilton Avenue/Geriatrics   Trenton, NJ 08629
(609)599-5050   Fax (609)599-4318

Wallen, Mark C., MD {1366416901} PsyAdd, Psychy, NrlgAddM(75,NJ05)<NJ-KMHCHRRY, NJ-OURLADY>
+ University Hospital-SOM Department of Psychiatry
2250 Chapel Avenue West/Suite 100   Cherry Hill, NJ 08002
(856)482-9000   Fax (856)482-1159
+ Rowan Medical Department of Psychiatry
42 Laurel Road East/Suite 3610   Stratford, NJ 08084
(856)482-9000   Fax (856)482-1159

Waller, Alfonso Hillman, MD {1326219577} CdvDis, IntrMd(06,GRN01)
+ 90 Bergen Street/Suite 3500
Newark, NJ 07103   (973)972-2573   Fax (973)972-4695

Waller, Leon H., DO {1497847131} Dermat, IntrMd(76,IL76)<NJ-CLARMAAS, NJ-MTNSIDE>
+ first Care Medical Group
50 Pompton Avenue   Verona, NJ 07044   (973)857-3400
Fax (201)896-2627
+ first Care Medical Group
750 Valley Brook Avenue   Lyndhurst, NJ 07071   (973)857-3400   Fax (201)896-2726

Wallis, Joseph J., DO {1285672154} ObsGyn(70,PA77)
+ Lifeline Medical Associates, LLC
600 Mount Pleasant Avenue   Dover, NJ 07801   (973)989-9000   Fax (973)989-8225

Wallner, Paul E., DO {1952468233} RadOnc(68,PA77)<NJ-COOPRUMC>
+ 21st Century Oncology
220 Sunset Road/Suite 4   Willingboro, NJ 08046   (609)877-3064   Fax (609)877-2466

Walmsley, Konstantin, MD {1730156456} Urolgy(97,TN05)<NJ-MTNSIDE>
+ NJ Urology
799 Bloomfield Avenue/Suite 300   Verona, NJ 07044
(973)746-3322   Fax (973)429-8765

Walor, David Michael, MD {1770569063} RadDia, PedRad(99,NY01)
+ University Radiology Group, P.C.
483 Cranbury Road   East Brunswick, NJ 08816   (732)390-0030   Fax (732)390-5383
+ University Radiology Group, P.C.
260 Amboy Avenue   Metuchen, NJ 08840   (732)390-0030   Fax (732)548-3392

Walsh, Brian W., MD {1720022528} EmrgMd(02,MO03)<NJ-MORRISTN>
+ Morristown Medical Center
100 Madison Avenue   Morristown, NJ 07962   (973)971-5000

Walsh, Christina M., MD {1285629550} Hemato, IntrMd, MedOnc(77,DC02)<NJ-RIVERVW>
+ Regional Cancer Care Associates, LLC
180 White Road   Little Silver, NJ 07739   (732)530-8666
Fax (732)530-7911

Walsh, Courtney A., DO {1528326600}
+ 306 Courtney Way
Mount Laurel, NJ 08054   (585)764-2516
caileen17@gmail.com

Walsh, Kathleen S., MD {1851374045} ObsGyn(94,NJ05)<NJ-JRSYSHMC>
+ Hackensack Meridian Medical Group Ob/Gyn, Wall
1924 Route 35/Suite 5   Wall, NJ 07719   (732)974-8404
Fax (732)974-8904
+ Monmouth County Associates
4788 US Highway 9   Howell, NJ 07731   (732)974-8404
Fax (732)905-1919

Walsh, Kelly Anne, DO {1114191699} FamMed(97,NY75)
+ UMDNJ Student Health Services
249 University Avenue   Newark, NJ 07102   (973)353-5231
Fax (973)353-1390

Walsh, Kristen Anne, MD {1902021173} Pedtrc(00,MO03)<NJ-OVERLOOK, NJ-HCKTSTWN>
+ Plaza Family Care
657 Willow Grove Street/Suite 401   Hackettstown, NJ 07840
(908)850-7800   Fax (908)850-7801
+ Plaza Family Care
245 Main Street/Suite 300 & 302   Chester, NJ 07930
(908)850-7800   Fax (908)879-6738

Walsh, Liron, MD {1417117490} Nephro<NJ-NWRKBETH>
+ Newark Beth Israel Medical Center
201 Lyons Avenue   Newark, NJ 07112   (973)926-7000

Walsh, Rhonda M., MD {1477735280} Urolgy
+ Summit Medical Group
315 East Northfield Road/Suite 1-E   Livingston, NJ 07039
(973)436-1070   Fax (973)992-1220

Walsh, Rowan Frank, MD {1629197371} Pedtrc, PedCrd(97,IRE02)<NJ-NWRKBETH, NY-MTSINAI>
+ Newark Beth Israel Medical Center
201 Lyons Avenue/L-5   Newark, NJ 07112   (973)926-3500
Fax (973)926-8206
+ Children's Hospital of NJ Ped Cntr @ West Orange
375 Mount Pleasant Avenue/Suite 105   West Orange, NJ 07052   (973)926-3500   Fax (973)322-6999

Walsh, Susan M., MD {1205845039} IntrMd(81,NJ05)
+ Neighborhood Health Center Plainfield
1700-58 Myrtle Avenue   Plainfield, NJ 07060   (908)753-6401   Fax (908)226-6743

Walsh, Sussannah Savitri, MD {1548411895} ObsGyn(04,NJ05)
+ Cumberland Ob-Gyn, PA
2950 College Drive/Suite 2G   Vineland, NJ 08360
(856)696-4484   Fax (856)696-1694

Walsky, Robert S., MD {1174595417} SrgLap, SrgVas, SrgBst(69,KY02)<NJ-HOLYNAME, NJ-ENGLWOOD>
+ Robert S. Walsky MD, P.A.
452 Old Hook Road/Suite 302   Emerson, NJ 07630
(201)967-1105   Fax (201)967-1272

Walsman, Scott Michael, MD {1215172994} Ophthl
+ Hudson Eye Physicians & Surgeons, LLC
600 Pavonia Avenue/6th Floor   Jersey City, NJ 07306
(201)963-3937   Fax (201)963-8823

Walter, Briza V., MD {1942632088} ObsGyn<NJ-MORRISTN>
+ Morristown Medical Center
100 Madison Avenue/ObsGyn/1st Fl   Morristown, NJ 07962
(973)908-3368

Walter, Robert J., MD {1649254632} Psychy(82,NJ05)
+ Barnabas Health Behavior Health Networ
1 Clara Maass Drive   Belleville, NJ 07109   (973)450-2205

Walters, Richard Lawrence, DO {1982856928} Gastrn, IntrMd
+ Kennedy Health Alliance Vascular Surgery
333 Laurel Oak Road   Voorhees, NJ 08043   (844)542-2273
Fax (856)770-9194

Walters, Samuel Roy, MD {1144368606} IntrMd(71,DC03)
+ 701 State Rt 440/Suite 33
Jersey City, NJ 07304   (201)435-4558   Fax (201)435-4588

Walzman, Daniel Ezra, MD {1407823727} SrgNro(98,NJ06)
+ North Jersey Brain and Surgical
680 Kinderkamack Road/Suite 300   Oradell, NJ 07649
(201)342-2550   Fax (201)342-7171

Wanalista, David Michael, DO {1497789077} IntrMd, Rheuma(98,PA77)
+ Cumberland Medical Associates
1206 West Sherman Avenue   Vineland, NJ 08360
(856)691-8444   Fax (856)691-8325

Wanat, Francis E., MD {1134173586} CdvDis, IntrMd(63,MA05)<NJ-MTNSIDE, NJ-VALLEY>
+ Montclair Cardiology Group PA
123 Highland Avenue/Suite 302   Glen Ridge, NJ 07028
(973)748-9555   Fax (973)748-2003

Wancier, Zisalo, MD {1205962297} Psychy(65,COL25)
+ Palisades General Hospital Mental Health Center
7101 Kennedy Boulevard   North Bergen, NJ 07047
(201)854-0500

Wang, Ai-Lan, MD {1487646444} IntrMd, AlgyImmn(85,NY09)<NJ-STBARNMC, NJ-UMDNJ>
+ 349 East Northfield Road/Suite 106
Livingston, NJ 07039   (973)533-9255   Fax (973)535-9081

Wang, Aijuan, MD {1992850820} Pedtrc(83,CHN67)
+ 2 State Route 27/Suite 500
Edison, NJ 08820   (732)516-9868   Fax (732)516-9869

Wang, Andy Chun Yao, MD {1922263979} NnPnMd<PA-ENSTEIN>
+ On-Site Neonatal Partners
1000 Haddonfield-Berlin Road/Suite 210   Voorhees, NJ 08043   (856)782-2212   Fax (856)782-2213

Wang, Annie Pai, DO {1437597648} Pedtrc
+ University Medical Group Pediatrics
125 Paterson Street/MEB 3rd Fl   New Brunswick, NJ 08903
(732)235-7883   Fax (732)235-6609

Wang, Belle, MD {1194790550} ObsGyn, IntrMd(91,NY47)<NJ-VALLEY>
+ Ob-Gyn Associates of Bergen County, PA
680 Kinderkamack Road/Suite 204   Oradell, NJ 07649
(201)391-5443   Fax (201)391-8019

Wang, Candace, MD {1487202354}
+ 128 Bobolink Court
Wayne, NJ 07470

Wang, Cecilia S., MD {1083780753} Psychy(83,CHN2B)<NJ-ENGLWOOD, NJ-CHILTON>
+ 2035 Hamburg Turnpike/Suite M
Wayne, NJ 07470   (973)839-2945   Fax (973)839-1244

Physicians by Name and Address

Wang, Changzhen, MD {1518969872} Anesth(98,CHN2D)<NJ-STCLRDEN>
+ St. Clare's Hospital-Denville Campus
25 Pocono Road   Denville, NJ 07834   (973)625-6000

Wang, Cheng-Teng, MD {1235237280} EmrgMd(99,NJ06)<NJ-JRSYCITY>
+ Jersey City Medical Center
355 Grand Street/EmrgMed   Jersey City, NJ 07304
(201)915-2000

Wang, Danny, MD {1619962578} CdvDis, IntrMd(85,NY46)
+ Guarino & Chen PA
35-37 Progress Street/Suite B2   Edison, NJ 08820
(908)754-9292   Fax (908)754-3358

Wang, David Alexander, MD {1447504089} FamMed(10,MA07)
+ HSS Paramus Outpatient Center
140 East Ridgewood Avenue/Suite 175-S   Paramus, NJ 07652   (201)796-2255   Fax (201)796-3711

Wang, Di, MD {1427270362}<NJ-STBARNMC>
+ St. Barnabas Medical Center
94 Old Short Hills Road   Livingston, NJ 07039   (973)322-5000

Wang, Edward, MD {1598789794} Anesth(84,POLA)<NJ-HUNTRDN>
+ Hunterdon Medical Center
2100 Wescott Drive/Anesthesiology   Flemington, NJ 08822
(908)788-6100   Fax (908)788-6361

Wang, George Cho-Ching, MD {1669507588} Grtrcs, IntrMd(01,NY08)
+ Premier Health Associates
89 Sparta Avenue/Suite 100   Sparta, NJ 07871   (973)729-2121   Fax (973)729-3454

Wang, Hongling, MD {1205995172} PthCyt, PthACl(92,CHN63)<NJ-BAYSHORE>
+ Bayshore Community Hospital
727 North Beers Street/Pathology   Holmdel, NJ 07733
(732)739-5847

Wang, Jean C., MD {1588761548} IntrMd(82,GRN01)
+ Alpha Medical
462 Lake Hurst Road   Toms River, NJ 08755   (732)255-7570
Fax (732)244-2556

Wang, Jian, MD {1356402093} FamMed(85,CHN1J)<NJ-VALYONS>
+ VA New Jersey Health Care System at Lyons
151 Knollcroft Road/Extended Care   Lyons, NJ 07939
(908)647-0180

Wang, Jianfeng, MD {1922395664}
+ 132B Cedar Lane
Highland Park, NJ 08904   (617)680-4609
jw904@rwjms.rutgers.edu

Wang, Jonathan Alan, DO {1467580142} IntrMd, FamMed(89,NY75)
+ Jonathan Alan Wang DO LLC
290 Madison Avenue/Suite 2 A   Morristown, NJ 07960
(973)285-1999   Fax (973)359-8979

Wang, Ju Lin, MD {1730461765} SrgCrC(05,GRN01)
+ 27 North 6th Avenue
Highland Park, NJ 08904

Wang, Kyu Sung, MD {1518037340} IntrMd, Nephro(75,KOR04)<NJ-ENGLWOOD, NJ-HOLYNAME>
+ 1033 Palisade Avenue
Fort Lee, NJ 07024   (201)224-6800   Fax (201)224-6804

Wang, Lan, MD {1306828447} Pthlgy, PthACl(93,CHN63)<NJ-CHILTON>
+ Chilton Medical Center
97 West Parkway   Pompton Plains, NJ 07444   (973)831-5000

Wang, Le, MD {1528277852} IntrMd, OncHem
+ Nazha Cancer Center
411 New Road   Northfield, NJ 08225   (609)383-6033   Fax (609)383-0064

Wang, Linda, MD {1073540787} Pedtrc(94,NY03)
+ Tenafly Pediatrics, PA
74 Pascack Road   Park Ridge, NJ 07656   (201)326-7120
Fax (201)326-7130

Wang, Ling, MD {1629373808} Anesth<NJ-STFRNMED>
+ St. Francis Medical Center
601 Hamilton Avenue   Trenton, NJ 08629   (609)599-5000

Wang, Luoquan, MD {1972683472} PthAna(82,CHN96)<NY-MNTFMOSE>
+ Bio-Reference Laboratory, Inc.
481 Edward H. Ross Drive   Elmwood Park, NJ 07407
(201)791-2600   Fax (201)791-1941

Wang, Mei-Hui, MD {1821067232} IntrMd(90,NY48)<NJ-RWJUBRUN, NJ-STPETER>
+ Mei-Hui Wang MD, LLC
1 Clyde Road/Suite 101   Somerset, NJ 08873   (732)565-7770   Fax (732)565-7771
+ Advanced Surgical & Bariatrics of NJ, PA
49 Veronica Avenue   Somerset, NJ 08873   (732)565-7770
Fax (800)689-2361

Wang, Monty H.S., MD {1346322914} Anesth(78,TAI05)<NJ-RWJUBRUN>
+ Robert Wood Johnson-UMDNJ Anesthesia Group
125 Paterson Street/CAB 3100   New Brunswick, NJ 08901
(732)235-7827   Fax (732)418-8492

Wang, Paul Xinze, MD {1720003940} IntrMd, FamMed, ImmAsm(84,CHN96)<NJ-HOLYNAME, NJ-HACKNSK>
+ 235 Prospect Avenue/Suite LD
Hackensack, NJ 07601   (201)343-4250   Fax (201)343-7779
xzwangmd@hotmail.com

Wang, Qi, MD {1427147420} Pthlgy, PthACl(86,CHNA)<NJ-STPETER>
+ St. Peter's University Hospital
254 Easton Avenue/Path   New Brunswick, NJ 08901
(732)745-8534

Wang, Qian, MD {1417151473} IntrMd, Grtrcs(97,CHN8A)
+ Princeton Medicine
5 Plainsboro Road/Suite 300   Plainsboro, NJ 08536
(609)853-7272   Fax (609)853-7271

Wang, Qin, MD {1972530012} Anesth
+ AtlantiCare Anesthesiology
65 West Jimmie Leeds Road   Pomona, NJ 08240   (609)748-7088

Wang, Qing, MD {1306086152} PthHem<NJ-UMDNJ>
+ University Hospital
150 Bergen Street   Newark, NJ 07103   (973)972-4619
Fax (973)972-3199

Wang, Robert L., MD {1043219876} CdvDis, IntrMd(83,NY47)<NJ-HCKTSTWN>
+ Cardiology Consultants of North Morris, PA
356 US Highway 46/Suite B   Mountain Lakes, NJ 07046
(973)586-3400   Fax (973)586-1916

Wang, Rui, MD {1942576954} MedOnc
+ Memorial Sloan Kettering Bergen
225 Summit Avenue   Montvale, NJ 07645   (201)775-7445

Wang, Sandy, DO {1154562551} EmrgMd(05,CA22)<NJ-TRINI-WSC>
+ Trinitas Regional Medical Center-Williamson Street
225 Williamson Street   Elizabeth, NJ 07207   (908)994-5000

Wang, Shuang, MD {1447548052} IntrMd
+ Southern Jersey Family Medical
238 East Broadway   Salem, NJ 08079   (856)935-7711   Fax (856)935-9123

Wang, Steven Q., MD {1265511968} DerMOH
+ Memorial Sloan-Kettering Cancer Center Basking Ridge
136 Mountain View Boulevard   Basking Ridge, NJ 07920
(908)542-3000   Fax (908)542-3220

Wang, Steven S., MD {1982021309}
+ 336 West Passaic Street/4th Floor
Rochelle Park, NJ 07662   (201)291-1010

Wang, Trent Peng, DO {1023332566} OncHem
+ University Hospital Medicine
150 Bergen Street/Room I-248   Newark, NJ 07103
(973)972-6056   Fax (973)972-3129

Wang, Wayne, MD {1528403086} Anesth
+ Summit Anesthesia Associates, P.A.
33 Overlook Road/Suite 311   Summit, NJ 07901   (908)598-1500   Fax (908)598-0197

Wang, Wei, MD {1902813876} PsyCAd, Psychy(87,CHN59)<NY-PRSBWEST, NY-UNTYPKRG>
+ NHCAC Health Center at West New York
5301 Broadway   West New York, NJ 07093   (201)866-9320
Fax (201)330-3825

Wang, Weizheng William, MD {1952491854} Gastrn, IntrMd(83,CHN69)<NJ-OVERLOOK, NJ-UMDNJ>
+ UMDNJ Division of Gastroenterology & Hepatology
90 Bergen Street/DOC 2100   Newark, NJ 07103   (973)972-2343   Fax (973)972-0752
+ University Hospital-Doctors Office Center
90 Bergen Street   Newark, NJ 07103   (973)972-2343   Fax (973)972-0752
+ Rutgers- New Jersey Medical School
185 South Orange Avenue/MSB H514   Newark, NJ 07103
(973)972-4300

Wang, Wenjing, MD {1508051012} PthCyt, PthACl(89,CHN3A)
+ 166 Smoke Rise Road
Basking Ridge, NJ 07920

Wang, Xiangbing, MD {1831264456} EnDbMt(83,CHN07)<NJ-STPETER>
+ RWJ University Endocrinology Diabetes & Metabolism
125 Paterson Street/CAB 5100A   New Brunswick, NJ 08901
(732)235-7219   Fax (732)235-8610
+ St. Peter's University Hospital
254 Easton Avenue   New Brunswick, NJ 08901   (732)745-8600

Wang, Xuan, MD {1578706032} PthAna, DrmtPthy(87)
+ Pathology Solutions, LLC
246 Industrial Way West/Suite 2   Eatontown, NJ 07724
(732)389-5200   Fax (732)389-5299

Wang, Yize Richard, MD {1053576207} Gastrn
+ Cooper Digestive Health Institute
501 Fellowship Road/Suite 101   Mount Laurel, NJ 08054
(856)642-2133   Fax (856)642-2134

Wang, Yue He, MD {1225143134} FamMed(86,CHN57)<NJ-STFRNMED>
+ UH- Robert Wood Johnson Med
125 Paterson Street/MEB 288   New Brunswick, NJ 08901
(908)685-3732   Fax (732)235-7001

Wang, Yue-He, MD {1669549903} FamMed(83,CHN50)
+ Family Medical Care
1130 Route 202/Unit B3   Raritan, NJ 08869   (908)393-6263
Fax (908)393-6263

Wang, Yvette, DO {1972846574} IntrMd
+ Kennedy Hospitalist Office
435 Hurffville Cross Keys Road   Turnersville, NJ 08012
(856)513-4124   Fax (856)302-5932

Wang, Zhimin, MD {1942295787} IntrMd, EmrgMd(82,CHN21)<NJ-RBAYPERT>
+ Raritan Bay Medical Center/Perth Amboy Division
530 New Brunswick Avenue   Perth Amboy, NJ 08861
(732)442-3700

Wang-Epstein, Christina C., MD {1861591984} IntrMd(99,CHN57)<NJ-STPETER, NJ-RWJUBRUN>
+ Central Jersey Internal Medicine
75 Veronica Avenue/Suite 204   Somerset, NJ 08873
(732)828-0002   Fax (732)828-0153
+ Central Jersey Internal Medicine
111 Union Valley Road/Suite 203   Monroe, NJ 08831
(732)828-0002   Fax (609)655-2253

Wangenheim, Paul M., MD {1437146792} CdvDis, IntrMd(82,NJ05)
+ Consultants in Cardiology
741 Northfield Avenue/Suite 205   West Orange, NJ 07052
(973)467-1544   Fax (973)467-9586

Wanich, Niya, MD {1043402357} AlgyImmn, Pedtrc(02,IL06)
+ Englewood Ear Nose & Throat, P.C.
216 Engle Street/Suite 101   Englewood, NJ 07631
(201)816-9800   Fax (201)567-1569

Wanich, Tony Suchai, MD {1477754752} SrgOrt, SprtMd, IntrMd(02,MA07)<NY-SPCLSURG>
+ High Mountain Orthopedics
342 Hamburg Turnpike/Suite 205   Wayne, NJ 07470
(973)595-7779   Fax (973)595-0182

Waninger, Kevin N., MD {1740244219} FamMed, SprtMd<PA-STLKBTHL>
+ Coordinated Health
222 Red Lane   Phillipsburg, NJ 08865   (610)861-8080   Fax (610)849-1013

Wannamaker, Megan, DO {1750643557}<NJ-PALISADE>
+ St. Joseph's Wayne Hospital
224 Hamburg Turnpike/Hospitalist   Wayne, NJ 07470
(973)956-3357

Wappel, Michael A., MD {1356315873} CdvDis, IntCrd, IntrMd(81,IL45)<NJ-CENTRAST, NJ-JRSYSHMC>
+ Monmouth Cardiology Associates, LLC
11 Meridian Road   Eatontown, NJ 07724   (732)663-0300
Fax (732)663-0301
+ Monmouth Cardiology Associates, LLC
222 Schanck Road/Suite 104   Freehold, NJ 07728
(732)663-0300   Fax (732)431-1712

Waqar, Anum Khan, DO {1578950317} IntrMd
+ Summit Medical Group-Berkeley Heights Campus
1 Diamond Hill Road   Berkeley Heights, NJ 07922
(908)273-4300   Fax (908)790-6576

Waqar, Shaan M., MD {1205135472} AlgyImmn
+ ENT & Allergy Associates, LLP
485 Route 1 South/Bld B/Suite 350   Iselin, NJ 08830
(732)549-3934   Fax (732)549-7250

Waran, Sandy P., MD {1750477071} NroChl, Nrolgy(68,SRI01)<NJ-MORRISTN>
+ Advocare Pediatric Neurology Associates
25 Lindsley Drive/Suite 205   Morristown, NJ 07960
(973)993-8777   Fax (973)993-8577

Waran, Shantha P., MD {1184662819} Radiol, RadDia(71,SRI01)<NJ-STCLRDEN, NJ-STCLRDOV>
+ St. Clare's Hospital-Denville Campus
25 Pocono Road/Radiology   Denville, NJ 07834   (973)625-6000
+ St. Clare's Hospital-Dover
400 West Blackwell Street   Dover, NJ 07801   (973)989-3000

Warchaizer, Susan J., MD {1699986224} ObsGyn(93,ISR02)<NJ-UNVMCPRN>
+ Rider University Student Health Center
2083 Lawrenceville Road   Lawrenceville, NJ 08648
(609)896-5060
+ 10 Earle Lane
Princeton, NJ 08540   (609)279-2970

Ward, David S., MD {1215927058} Srugry(94,NJ06)<NJ-MORRISTN>
+ Surgical Practice of Rolando Rolandelli, MD
435 South Street/Suite 360   Morristown, NJ 07960
(973)971-7200   Fax (973)290-7521

Ward, Patrice Taylor, DO FamMed(90,PA77)
+ Healthward Inc
 300 Collins Avenue   Moorestown, NJ 08057
Ward, Wendy Allison, MD {1326088253} Anesth(89,NY47)
+ Advanced Gastroenterology of Bergen County
 140 Sylvan Avenue/Suite 101-A   Englewood Cliffs, NJ 07632
 (201)945-6564   Fax (201)461-9038
Wardeh, Ghassan Louis, MD {1255332789} PulDis, IntrMd(89,IRQ04)
+ Wayne Medical Care, PA
 342 Hamburg Turnpike/Suite 101   Wayne, NJ 07470
 (973)942-4140   Fax (973)942-5070
+ 714 Tenth Street
 Secaucus, NJ 07094   (973)942-4140   Fax (973)579-1524
Warden, Mary Jane, MD {1780767087} Surgry, SrgBst(78,NJ05)<NJ-HACKNSK>
+ Hackensack University Medical Center
 20 Prospect Avenue/Surgery/Breast   Hackensack, NJ 07601
 (201)336-8777   Fax (201)996-3279
Warden, Todd M., MD {1417196544} EmrgMd(79,IL06)
+ 549 Delaware Street
 Deptford, NJ 08096   Fax (856)845-7460
Ware, Steven M., MD {1437126430} Urolgy(74,NJ05)<NJ-HCK-TSTWN>
+ Garden State Urology
 282 US Highway 46   Denville, NJ 07834   (973)895-6636
 Fax (973)895-5327
+ Associates in Pediatric & Adult Urology
 20 Commerce Boulevard/Suite D   Succasunna, NJ 07876
 (973)895-6636   Fax (973)927-6831
+ Associates in Pediatric & Adult Urology
 653 Willow Grove Street   Hackettstown, NJ 07834
 (908)684-4670
Wargo, Heather Carol, MD {1841261534} Urolgy(95,PA01)
+ New Jersey Urology
 773 Route 70 East/Building H-120   Marlton, NJ 08053
+ New Jersey Urology
 15000 Midlantic Drive/Suite 100   Mount Laurel, NJ 08054
 Fax (856)985-4582
Wargovich, Raymond M., MD {1588605067} CritCr, IntrMd(80,PA02)<NJ-DEBRAHLC>
+ Deborah Heart and Lung Center
 200 Trenton Road/Cardiology   Browns Mills, NJ 08015
 (609)893-6611   Fax (609)893-1213
 wargovichr@deborah.org
Warmuth, Ingrid P., MD {1811942717} Dermat(87,GER22)<NJ-SJERSYHS>
+ Dr. Warmuth Skin Care Center
 350 Front Street/Suite 2101   Elmer, NJ 08318   (856)358-1500   Fax (856)358-1117
Warner, Matthew J., MD {1598779324} EmrgMd(03,NJ06)<NJ-SJHREGMC, NJ-SJRSYELM>
+ SJH Regional Medical Center
 1505 West Sherman Avenue/EmrgMed   Vineland, NJ 08360
 (856)641-8000
+ SJH Bridgeton Health Center
 333 Irving Avenue/EmrgMed   Bridgeton, NJ 08302
 (856)575-4500
Warner, Sharon D., MD {1417008871} IntrMd(78,NY08)<NJ-VIRTVOOR, NJ-KMHCHRRY>
+ 119 East Laurel Road
 Stratford, NJ 08084
Waronker-Silverstein, Amy S., MD {1912905779} InsrMd(91,PA09)
+ Endocrine Associates of Southern Jersey
 703 East Main Street/Suite 5   Moorestown, NJ 08057
 (856)727-0900   Fax (856)231-8428
Warren, Beth Ann, DO {1942612585} EmrgMd
+ Virtua Camden
 1000 Atlantic Avenue   Camden, NJ 08104   (856)246-3000
 Fax (856)246-3061
Warren, Karma Brown, MD {1962497776} EmrgMd(01,NJ05)<NJ-UMDNJ>
+ University Hospital
 150 Bergen Street   Newark, NJ 07103   (973)972-4300
Warren, Ronald L., MD {1306808555} IntrMd, PulDis(68,PA01)<NJ-CHSFULD>
+ Pulmonary & Internal Medicine Associates
 40 Fuld Street/Suite 201   Trenton, NJ 08638   (609)695-4422   Fax (609)695-4358
Warren, Ronald M., MD {1477680742} SrgPlstc(84,IL42)
+ 2000 Academy Drive/Ste 200
 Mount Laurel, NJ 08054   (856)727-0030   Fax (856)727-9701
Warren, Stephen W., MD {1063492577} RadDia, Radiol(73,NY47)<NJ-RBAYOLDB, NJ-TRINIJSC>
+ University Radiology Group, P.C.
 483 Cranbury Road   East Brunswick, NJ 08816   (732)390-0030   Fax (732)390-5383
+ University Radiology Group, P.C.
 260 Amboy Avenue   Metuchen, NJ 08840   (732)390-0030

 Fax (732)548-3392
Warren, Wendy B., MD {1992707293} MtFtMd, ObsGyn(82,NY20)<NJ-STBARNMC>
+ St. Barnabas Medical Center
 94 Old Short Hills Road/Suite 402   Livingston, NJ 07039
 (973)322-5000   Fax (973)322-2309
Warshal, David Philip, MD {1326144940} ObsGyn, GynOnc(86,PA14)<NJ-ACMCITY>
+ Cooper Gynecologic Oncology Associates
 900 Centennial Boulevard/Suite F   Voorhees, NJ 08043
 (856)325-6644   Fax (856)325-6643
 warshal-david@cooperhealth.edu
+ Women's Care Center
 3 Cooper Plaza/Suite 301   Camden, NJ 08103   (856)325-6644   Fax (856)968-8575
Warshauer, Bruce L., MD {1831112689} Dermat(77,NH01)
+ 2424 Bridge Avenue
 Point Pleasant Beach, NJ 08742   (732)295-0100   Fax (732)295-0741
Warshauer, Jeffrey M., DO {1558360222} SrgOrt(89,PA77)
+ Infinity Orthopedics
 1450 Route 22 West/Suite 200   Mountainside, NJ 07092
 (908)364-7801   Fax (908)222-2757
+ Infinity Orthopedics
 3 Progress Street/Suite 106   Edison, NJ 08820   (908)364-7801   Fax (908)222-2757
Warshaw, Abraham Lee, MD {1952484776} EmrgMd(88,NY08)<NY-NRTHGEN, NJ-NWRKBETH>
+ Newark Beth Israel Medical Center
 201 Lyons Avenue   Newark, NJ 07112   (973)926-7000
Warta, Melissa Hayward, MD {1083660278} Surgry(03,NJ02)
+ St. Joseph Medical Center Surgery
 703 Main Street   Paterson, NJ 07503   (973)754-2490
Waseem, Mehnaz, MD {1174810873} Psychy<NJ-BERGNMC>
+ New Bridge Medical Center
 230 East Ridgewood Avenue   Paramus, NJ 07652
 (201)967-4132
Waseem, Samrah, MD {1295022051}<NJ-BERGNMC>
+ New Bridge Medical Center
 230 East Ridgewood Avenue   Paramus, NJ 07652
 (201)967-4132
Waseem, Sarwat, MD {1033186200} IntrMd(91,PAK11)
+ Internal Medicine PA
 155 Cedar Lane   Teaneck, NJ 07666   (201)836-4247   Fax (201)836-5420
Wasenda, Erika Joy, MD {1548584428} ObsGyn
+ 435 South Street/Suite 409
 Morristown, NJ 07960   (858)657-8435   Fax (858)657-6828
Washington, Judy C., MD {1588612121} FamMed(83,TN07)<NJ-STPETER, NJ-RWJUBRUN>
+ Overlook Family Medicine
 33 Overlook Road/Suite 103   Summit, NJ 07901   (908)522-5700   Fax (908)273-8014
Washington, Monica Michaelle, MD {1346655578} ObsGyn<NJ-STPETER>
+ St. Peter's University Hospital
 254 Easton Avenue   New Brunswick, NJ 08901   (732)745-8600
Wasilewski, Stan J., MD {1841240132} CdvDis, IntrMd, ClCdEl(87,MA07)
+ Raritan Bay Cardiology Group, P.A.
 225 May Street/Suite F   Edison, NJ 08837   (732)738-8855   Fax (732)738-4141
+ Raritan Bay Cardiology Group, P.A.
 3 Hospital Plaza/Suite 305   Old Bridge, NJ 08857
 (732)738-8855   Fax (732)738-4141
+ Raritan Bay Cardiology Group, P.A.
 337 Applegarth Road   Monroe Township, NJ 08837
 (609)655-8860   Fax (732)738-4141
Waskin, Hetty Anne, MD {1447424759} IntrMd, InfDis(78,MI01)
+ Schering-Plough Research Global Clinical Development
 2015 Galloping Hill Road/K-15-3-3395   Kenilworth, NJ 07033   (908)298-4000
Wasleski, Karen J., MD {1417106782} FamMed(92,PA07)<NJ-VIRTMHBC>
+ Mt. Laurel Family Physicians
 401 Young Avenue/Suite 260   Moorestown, NJ 08057
 (856)291-8756   Fax (856)291-8750
Wason, Suman, MD {1811324304} ClnPhm, Pedtrc, Txclgy(75,ENG02)
+ 45 Summit Drive
 Basking Ridge, NJ 07920
Wassef, Mariam Gamal, DO {1033475249}
+ Dr. Mariam G. Wassef and Associates
 74 Brunswick Woods Drive   East Brunswick, NJ 08816
 (732)947-8084   Fax (201)256-4101
+ 550 Newark Avenue/Suite 207
 Jersey City, NJ 07306   (732)947-8084   Fax (201)256-4101
+ University Hospital Medicine
 150 Bergen Street/Room I-248   Newark, NJ 08816
 (973)972-6056   Fax (973)972-3129

Wassef, Michael Karim, MD {1962715334} Anesth(10,NJ05)
+ Morris Anesthesia Group, PA
 3799 Route 46/Suite 211   Parsippany, NJ 07054   (973)335-1122   Fax (973)335-1448
Wassef, Tamer William, MD {1255654752} Psychy
+ 424 Baldwin Avenue
 Jersey City, NJ 07306   (848)667-5225
Wassef, Wagih G., MD {1588760094} IntrMd(80,EGY03)
+ Montville Park Physician Associates
 150 River Road/Suite N-1   Montville, NJ 07045   (973)263-9900   Fax (973)263-9919
Wasser, Kenneth B., MD {1881670321} Rheuma, IntrMd(77,OH06)<NJ-RIVERVW, NJ-MONMOUTH>
+ 43 Gilbert Street North/Suite 7
 Tinton Falls, NJ 07724   (732)530-7999   Fax (732)530-7998
Wasser, Keri Nicole, MD {1629272273} Psychy(03,NY19)<NJ-MORRISTN>
+ Morristown Medical Center
 100 Madison Avenue/Psych   Morristown, NJ 07962
 (973)971-4700   Fax (973)290-7614
Wasser, Samuel H., MD {1457352791} SrgVas, Surgry(83,DC01)
+ Rancocas Valley Surgical Associates PA
 1000 Salem Road/Suite A   Willingboro, NJ 08046
 (609)877-1737   Fax (609)877-1589
Wasserman, Alan, MD {1770584468} GenPrc(70,ITA01)
+ Open MRI of North Jersey
 160 Market Street   Saddle Brook, NJ 07663   (201)587-8755
 Fax (201)587-8838
 Alanwasserman2@aol.com
Wasserman, Barry N., MD {1659378248} Ophthl, IntrMd(92,NJ05)
+ 100 Canal Point Boulevard/Suite 112
 Princeton, NJ 08540   (609)243-8711   Fax (609)243-0199
 drwasserman@barrywasserman.com
Wasserman, Carrie Brooke, MD {1255567285} OncHem, IntrMd(03,ENG29)
+ John Theurer Cancer Center - HUMC
 92 Second Street   Hackensack, NJ 07601   (917)974-9027
 Fax (718)250-6493
Wasserman, Elen, DO {1437490463}
+ 20 Raymond Avenue
 Rutherford, NJ 07070   (201)933-8964
 elenwasserman@gmail.com
Wasserman, Eric Jonathan, MD {1962500918} EmrgMd(96,NY47)<NJ-JRSYCITY, NJ-NWRKBETH>
+ Newark Beth Israel Medical Center
 201 Lyons Avenue   Newark, NJ 07112   (973)926-8589
Wasserman, Ethan Jeffrey, MD {1811104292} IntrMd, OncHem(02,PA02)<NJ-RWJUBRUN>
+ Cancer Institute of NJ Hamiltom
 2575 Klockner Road   Hamilton, NJ 08690   (609)631-6960
 Fax (609)631-6888
+ UH- RWJ Medical School
 One Robert Wood Johnson Place   New Brunswick, NJ 08903
 (732)235-5600
+ Rutgers Cancer Institute of New Jersey
 195 Little Albany Street/PO Box 2681   New Brunswick, NJ 08690   (732)235-2465   Fax (732)235-6797
Wasserman, Gary D., MD {1518049832} Urolgy(85,LA01)<NJ-ENGLWOOD, NJ-HOLYNAME>
+ The Urology Center of Englewood, PA
 663 Palisade Avenue/Suite 304   Cliffside Park, NJ 07010
 (201)313-1933   Fax (201)313-9599
Wasserman, Jared Mark, MD {1194923847} Otlryg(02,NY47)
+ ENT & Allergy Associates, LLP
 433 Hackensack Avenue/Suite 204   Hackensack, NJ 07601
 (201)883-1062   Fax (201)883-9297
 Jwasserman@entandallergy.com
Wasserman, Kenneth H., MD {1932112760} IntrMd(79,NY46)<NJ-ENGLWOOD, NJ-HOLYNAME>
+ Drs. Wasserman & Reiner
 401 South Van Brunt Street/Suite 402   Englewood, NJ 07631   (201)567-1140   Fax (201)567-1998
Wasserstrom, William R., MD {1194755686} Nrolgy(74,MI01)
+ Brier Hill Court/Unit F1
 East Brunswick, NJ 08816   (732)238-0804   Fax (732)651-8790
Wassner, Jesse V., MD {1154394906} IntrMd(87,NJ05)<NJ-HACKNSK>
+ Physicians Health Alliance
 1777 Hamburg Turnpike/Suite 205   Wayne, NJ 07470
 (973)248-1440   Fax (973)248-1448
Wasti, Naila H., MD {1740230051} IntrMd(88,PAK11)<NJ-CHSFULD>
+ Capital Health Primary Care
 4056 Quakerbridge Road/Suite 101   Lawrenceville, NJ 08648   (609)528-9150   Fax (609)528-9151
+ East Windsor Family Practice
 569 Abbington Drive/Suite 6   East Windsor, NJ 08520
 (609)528-9150   Fax (609)448-8370

Physicians by Name and Address

Wasty, Najam, MD {1841247343} CdvDis, IntrMd, IntCrd(77,PAK01)<NJ-NWRKBETH, NJ-BAYONNE>
+ Newark Beth Israel Medical Center
201 Lyons Avenue Newark, NJ 07112 (973)926-8592 Fax (973)923-8859

Waters, John S., MD {1659345411} FamMed, Grtrcs(81,NC05)<NJ-HUNTRDN>
+ Phillips Barber Family Health Center
72 Alexander Avenue Lambertville, NJ 08530 (609)397-3535 Fax (609)397-0301

Waters, Renee M., MD {1063463172} Anesth(93,PA07)<NJ-COOPRUMC>
+ Rancocas Anesthesiology, PA
700 Route 130 North/Suite 203 Cinnaminson, NJ 08077 (856)829-9345 Fax (856)829-3605

Watson, John A., MD {1962662312} Urolgy(02,NJ05)
+ Urology Care Alliance
2105 Klockner Road Hamilton, NJ 08690 (609)588-0770 Fax (609)588-0454

Watson, Marc C., MD {1578605929} SrgVas, Surgry(72,MA05)
+ 6 Pompton Avenue/Suite 11
Cedar Grove, NJ 07009 (973)571-9170 Fax (973)571-9174

Watson, Marcia G., DO {1447458153} IntrMd(04,NJ75)
+ SOM - Department of Internal Medicine
42 East Laurel Road/Suite 3100 Stratford, NJ 08084 (856)566-6859 Fax (856)566-6906

Watson, Richard A., MD {1487694543} Urolgy(68,DC02)<NJ-UMDNJ, NJ-HACKNSK>
+ Rutgers- New Jersey Medical School
185 South Orange Avenue/Rm G536 Newark, NJ 07103 (973)972-4300

Watson, Richard I., MD {1003814039} CdvDis, IntrMd(77,MA07)<NJ-MORRISTN>
+ Morristown Cardiology Associates, P.A.
435 South Street/Suite 100 Morristown, NJ 07960 (973)267-3944 Fax (973)455-0399

Watson, Todd A., MD {1750400826} Anesth(01,MA05)<NJ-MORRISTN>
+ Anesthesia Associates of Morristown
264 South Street/Suite 2A Morristown, NJ 07960 (973)631-8119
+ Morristown Medical Center
100 Madison Avenue/Anesth Morristown, NJ 07962 (973)971-5000

Wattamwar, Anoop Suresh, MD {1952628372} RadNro(IL06<NJ-HACKNSK>
+ Hackensack Radiology Group, PA/Corporate
130 Kinderkamack Road/Suite 200 River Edge, NJ 07661 (201)488-2660
+ Hackensack Radiology Group, P.A.
30 Prospect Avenue Hackensack, NJ 07601 (201)488-2660 Fax (201)336-8451
+ Hackensack University Medical Center
30 Prospect Avenue Hackensack, NJ 07661 (201)996-2000 Fax (201)489-2812

Watters, Nathan Paul, MD {1275976250}
+ Cherry Hill Ob/Gyn
150 Century Parkway/Suite A Mount Laurel, NJ 08054 (856)778-4700 Fax (856)778-1154

Watts, David C., MD {1699730234} SrgPlstc, Surgry(87,PA02)<NJ-SJERSYHS, NJ-MEMSALEM>
+ 1051 West Sherman Avenue/Suite 2-A
Vineland, NJ 08360 (856)691-0200 Fax (856)691-5984
dcwatts52@comcast.net

Watts, Helena B., MD {1801865720} IntrMd, PulDis(86,MA01)
+ Center for Adult Medicine
1051 West Sherman Avenue/Suite 2-A Vineland, NJ 08360 (856)205-1770 Fax (856)691-5984

Wawer-Chubb, Allison Kristen, DO {1639338494} Pedtrc(05,PA77)
+ Monmouth Pediatric Group, P.A.
272 Broad Street Red Bank, NJ 07701 (732)741-0456 Fax (732)219-9477

Wawrzyniak, Zygmunt T., MD {1720187859} IntrMd(75,POL03)<NJ-RWJURAH>
+ 911 North Wood Avenue
Linden, NJ 07036 (908)925-7425 Fax (908)925-6520
zwawrzyniak@verizon.net

Wax, Craig M., DO {1124072285} FamMed, OstMed(94,NY75)<NJ-KMHTURNV, NJ-SJRSYELM>
+ 155 North Main Street
Mullica Hill, NJ 08062 (856)478-4780 Fax (856)478-0789

Wax, Martin Bruce, MD {1033267893} Ophthl
+ 41 Branch Road
Far Hills, NJ 07931

Wax, Michael B., MD {1255306296} IntrMd, MedOnc, OncHem(77,PA07)<NJ-OVERLOOK, NJ-STBARNMC>
+ Summit Medical Group-Berkeley Heights Campus
1 Diamond Hill Road Berkeley Heights, NJ 07922 (908)277-8890 Fax (908)673-7390

Waxenbaum, Steven I., MD {1952373466} SrgC&R, Surgry(88,NJ06)<NJ-VALLEY, NJ-ENGLWOOD>
+ Drs. White & Waxenbaum
216 Engle Street/Suite 203 Englewood, NJ 07631 (201)567-7615 Fax (201)567-8033
+ Drs. White & Waxenbaum
127 Union Street/Suite 112 Ridgewood, NJ 07450 (201)567-7615 Fax (201)493-1718

Waxler, Jennifer L., DO {1881637924} EmrgMd(90,PA77)<NJ-MONMOUTH>
+ Monmouth Medical Center
300 Second Avenue/EmergMed Long Branch, NJ 07740 (732)222-5200

Waxman, Harvey Louis, MD {1073545414} CdvDis, ClCdEl, IntrMd(74,NY47)
+ Penn Medicine at Cherry Hill
1400 East Route 70/Cardiology Cherry Hill, NJ 08034
+ Penn Cardiac Care Shore Medical Center
1 East New York Avenue Somers Point, NJ 08244

Waxman, Howard S., MD {1104874668} Pedtrc(81,PA07)<NJ-VIRTVOOR, NJ-VIRTUAHS>
+ Advocare Marlton Pediatrics
525 Route 73 South Marlton, NJ 08053 (856)596-3434 Fax (856)596-9110
+ Advocare Hammonton Pediatrics
856 South Whitehorse Pike Hammonton, NJ 08037 (856)596-3434 Fax (609)704-8849

Waxman, Mark S., MD {1396719894} Gastrn, IntrMd(78,NY08)<NJ-CLARMAAS>
+ 312 Bellevue Turnpike/Suite 1B
North Arlington, NJ 07031 (201)997-6776 Fax (201)997-6610
markwaxman@rwjbh.org

Waxman, Robert N., MD {1467422105} RadDia(93,NY19)
+ Diagnostic Radiology Associates of Northfield
772 Northfield Avenue West Orange, NJ 07052 (973)325-0002 Fax (973)325-8140
+ Diagnostic Radiology Associates of Clifton
1339 Broad Street Clifton, NJ 07013 (973)325-0002 Fax (973)778-4846
+ Diagnostic Radiology Associates of Cranford
25 South Union Avenue Cranford, NJ 07052 (908)709-1323 Fax (908)709-1329

Wayman, Bernard R., III, MD {1821069584} FamMed(89,PA02)<NJ-JRSYSHMC>
+ Toms River Family Medical Center PA
1028 Hooper Avenue Toms River, NJ 08753 (732)349-8866 Fax (732)349-7842

Wayslow, Alfred J., DO {1902879828} Psychy(92,ME75)
+ Camden County Health Services Center
20 N Woodbury-Turnersville Rd Blackwood, NJ 08012 (856)374-6600 Fax (856)374-6436
+ University Hospital-SOM Department of Psychiatry
2250 Chapel Avenue West/Suite 100 Cherry Hill, NJ 08002 (856)374-6600 Fax (856)482-1159

Wazeka, April Natasha, MD {1548234784} Pedtrc, PedPul, SlpDis(96,WA04)<NJ-MORRISTN, NJ-OVERLOOK>
+ Pediatric Pulmonology
100 Madison Avenue Morristown, NJ 07960 (973)971-4242 Fax (973)290-7360
+ Overlook Medical Center
99 Beauvoir Avenue/PO Box 210 Summit, NJ 07902 (908)522-2000

Weaner, Scott Michael, DO {1922084219} Nrolgy
+ 2275 Whitehorse Mercerville Rd/Suite 5
Mercerville, NJ 08619 (609)584-8588 Fax (609)584-7806

Webb, James A., MD {1972522977} IntrMd(83,DOMI)
+ 1280 Yardville-Allentown
Allentown, NJ 08501 (609)259-3635 Fax (609)259-9508

Webber, Seth Michael, MD {1982675153} Gastrn, IntrMd(91,PA09)<NJ-RBAYOLBD, NJ-JFKMED>
+ Woodbridge Internal Medicine Associates
1000 Route 9 North/Suite 302 Woodbridge, NJ 07095 (732)634-0036 Fax (732)634-9182
+ May Street Surgi Center
205 May Street/Suite 103 Edison, NJ 08837 (732)634-0036 Fax (732)661-9619

Weber, Barry Joseph, MD {1487648218} IntrMd, PulDis(66,DC01)<NJ-CLARMAAS, NJ-MTNSIDE>
+ Respiratory Disease Associates PA
200 Highland Avenue/Suite 100 Glen Ridge, NJ 07028 (973)746-7474 Fax (973)743-0265

Weber, Carolyn Harding, MD {1972567816} Pedtrc(01,PA12)<NJ-COOPRUMC, NJ-VIRTUAHS>
+ Advocare South Jersey Pediatrics Collingswood
204 White Horse Pike Collingswood, NJ 08107 (856)424-6050 Fax (856)424-2943
lmknight@challc.net
+ Advocare South Jersey Pediatrics Cherry Hill
1949 Route 70 East/Suite 1 & 2 Cherry Hill, NJ 08003 (856)424-6050 Fax (856)424-2943

Weber, Charles A., MD {1144213042} IntrMd, Rheuma(81,MEXI)<NJ-JRSYSHMC>
+ 3350 Highway 138/Suite 115
Wall Township, NJ 07719 (732)988-5030 Fax (732)988-5301

Weber, Jason Stuart, MD {1689638520} Pedtrc(01,PA12)<NJ-VIRTUAHS, NJ-COOPRUMC>
+ Advocare South Jersey Pediatrics Cherry Hill
1949 Route 70 East/Suite 1 & 2 Cherry Hill, NJ 08003 (856)424-6050 Fax (856)424-2943
+ Advocare South Jersey Pediatrics Collingswood
204 White Horse Pike Collingswood, NJ 08107 (856)424-6050 Fax (856)424-2943

Weber, Renata Vanja, MD {1790855815} SrgPlstc, SrgHnd(94,NY19)<NY-MNTFWEIL>
+ Drs. Sheikh & Weber
201 Route 17 North Rutherford, NJ 07070 (201)549-8860 Fax (201)549-8861

Weber, Vance J., MD {1548255904} CdvDis, IntrMd(76,NY15)
+ Associates in Cardiovascular Disease, LLC
211 Mountain Avenue Springfield, NJ 07081 (973)467-0005 Fax (973)912-8989

Wechsler, Marius A., MD {1952348864} Pedtrc(85,NJ06)<NJ-VIRTMHBC>
+ Advocare Pedi Phys of Burlington Co
693 Main Street/PO Box 367 Lumberton, NJ 08048 (609)261-4058 Fax (609)261-8381
+ Advocare Pedi Phys of Burlington Co
204 Ark Road/Suite 209 Mount Laurel, NJ 08054 (609)261-4058 Fax (856)234-9402

Wedmid, Alexei, MD {1134387343} Urolgy<NY-MTSINAI>
+ Urology Group of Princeton PA
134 Stanhope Street/Forrestal Village Princeton, NJ 08540 (609)924-6487 Fax (609)921-7020
+ Urology Group of Princeton PA
281 Witherspoon Street/Suite 100 Princeton, NJ 08542 (609)924-6487 Fax (609)921-7020

Weeks, Alicia, MD {1629199591} IntrMd(03,NJ06)
+ Arthritis, Rheumatic & Back Disease Associates
2309 East Evesham Road/Suite 101 Voorhees, NJ 08043 (856)424-5005 Fax (856)424-4716

Weeks, Daniel J., III, DO {1801837174} EmrgMd(91,NJ75)<NJ-KMHTURNV, NJ-BURDTMLN>
+ Kennedy Health Systems/Washington Township Campus
435 Hurffville-Cross Keys Road Turnersville, NJ 08012 (856)582-2816 Fax (856)582-2712
dweeks@pol.net

Weems, Lela Demilo, MD {1184618373} Anesth(97,MI01)
+ Montclair Anesthesia Associates PC
185 Fairfield Avenue/Suite 2A West Caldwell, NJ 07006 (973)226-1230 Fax (973)226-1232
+ 80 Plymouth Street
Montclair, NJ 07042 (973)226-1230 Fax (973)337-8219

Wehbe, Anthony, DO {1275731986} IntrMd, IntHos<NJ-KMHTURNV>
+ Kennedy Health Systems/Washington Township Campus
435 Hurffville-Cross Keys Road Turnersville, NJ 08012 (856)218-5634 Fax (856)218-5664

Wehbe Saloukhan, Cristin, MD {1184177602} ObsGyn
+ 88 Clifton Place/Unit 411
Jersey City, NJ 07304 (786)616-9882

Wehmann, Robert E., MD {1528035763} EnDbMt, IntrMd(74,NY03)<NJ-VALLEY, NJ-HACKNSK>
+ PO Box 65
Hillsdale, NJ 07642 (201)666-1400 Fax (201)664-8705

Wei, Catherine, MD {1902346224} IntrMd<NJ-RWJUBRUN>
+ RWJ University Hospital New Brunswick
One Robert Wood Johnson Place New Brunswick, NJ 08901 (732)235-7739

Wei, Fong, MD {1811082563} IntrMd, Nephro(67,MA07)<NJ-UNVMCPRN>
+ Princeton Medical Group, P.A.
419 North Harrison Street Princeton, NJ 08540 (609)924-9300 Fax (609)924-6552
+ Princeton Medical Group PA
2 Research Way/Bldg 2/Suite 302 Monroe Township, NJ 08831 (609)924-9300 Fax (609)655-7466

Wei, Grant, MD {1083647457} EmrgMd(02,RI01)<NJ-RWJUBRUN>
+ University Emergency Medicine
125 Paterson Street/MEB 104 New Brunswick, NJ 08901 (732)235-8717 Fax (732)235-7379

Wei, Pan-Son, MD {1457359994} Anesth(72,TAI07)<NJ-STMICHL>
+ St. Michael's Medical Center
268 MLK Jr. Boulevard/Anesthesiology Newark, NJ 07102 (973)877-5000

Wei, Ronald Shaw, MD {1588601306} Psychy(00,NJ05)<NJ-ES-SEXCO>
+ Essex County Hospital Center
204 Grove Avenue/Psych   Cedar Grove, NJ 07009   (973)571-2800
+ University Behavioral HealthCare
183 South Orange Avenue   Newark, NJ 07103

Wei, Tzong-Jer, MD {1730263799} Pedtrc, NnPnMd(78,TAIW)<NJ-UMDNJ>
+ University Hospital
150 Bergen Street/NICU   Newark, NJ 07103   (973)972-5610   Fax (973)972-7158

Weidman, Joshua A., MD {1891759684} ObsGyn(84,NY08)<NJ-VALLEY>
+ Drs Weidman and Kintzing
841 Franklin Avenue/Suite 5   Franklin Lakes, NJ 07417   (201)891-8811   Fax (201)891-9010
+ Bergen-Passaic Women's Health
2024 Macopin Road/Suite D   West Milford, NJ 07480   (201)891-8811   Fax (973)728-7707

Weidner, James R., MD {1164468815} Pedtrc(92,PA13)<NJ-VIRTVOOR, NJ-VIRTUAHS>
+ Advocare Cornerstone Pediatrics
318 North Haddon Avenue/Suite A   Haddonfield, NJ 08033   (856)428-3746   Fax (856)310-0312

Weidner, Melissa, MD {1902123615} PedGst
+ Robert Wood Johnson Medical School
51 French Street/MEB 303   New Brunswick, NJ 08901   (732)235-5192

Weigel, Peter J., MD {1043272768} IntrMd(86,NJ05)<NJ-OVERLOOK, NJ-RWJURAH>
+ Medical Assoc of Westfield
324 South Avenue East   Westfield, NJ 07090   (908)233-1444   Fax (908)654-0226

Weil, Irina Lisker, MD {1457748410} FamMed<NJ-HUNTRDN>
+ Hunterdon Medical Center
2100 Wescott Drive   Flemington, NJ 08822   (908)788-6160

Wein, Joshua Lewis, MD {1346353422} Urolgy(96,NY08)
+ Premier Urology Group, LLC
10 Parsonage Road/Suite 118   Edison, NJ 08837   (732)494-9400   Fax (732)548-3931
+ Premier Urology Group, LLC
570 South Avenue East/Building A   Cranford, NJ 07016   (732)494-9400   Fax (908)497-1633
+ Premier Urology Group, LLC
2 Hospital Plaza/Suite 430   Old Bridge, NJ 08837   (732)494-9400   Fax (732)679-2077

Weinar, Marvin A., MD {1114023363} FamMed(82,NJ06)
+ Lourdes Medical Associates
200 Campbell Drive/Suite 102   Willingboro, NJ 08046   (609)877-4545   Fax (609)877-5129

Weinberg, Fredrick M., MD {1578603692} CdvDis(78,NY08)<NJ-UNVMCPRN, NJ-RWJUBRUN>
+ 193 North Harrison Street
Princeton, NJ 08540   (609)683-1180   Fax (609)683-4598

Weinberg, Harvey I., MD {1598771172} Dermat(69,NY06)<NY-PRSBCOLU>
+ Dermatology Associates of Morris PA
199 Baldwin Road   Parsippany, NJ 07054   (973)335-2560   Fax (973)335-9421

Weinberg, Howard M., DO {1851383483} CdvDis, IntrMd(87,NY75)<NJ-JFKMED, NJ-VIRTBERL>
+ South Jersey Heart Group
539 Egg Harbor Road/Suite 1   Sewell, NJ 08080   (856)589-0300   Fax (856)589-1753

Weinberg, Kenneth R., MD {1033119094} EmrgMd(80,GRN01)<NJ-HOLYNAME>
+ Holy Name Hospital
718 Teaneck Road/EmrgMed   Teaneck, NJ 07666   (201)833-3210

Weinberg, Martin R., MD {1043288608} Ophthl(79,VA07)<NJ-ENGLWOOD, NJ-HACKNSK>
+ 405 Cedar Lane/Suite 5
Teaneck, NJ 07666   (201)836-8333   Fax (201)836-7301

Weinberg, Richard M., MD {1477632305} AdmMgt, PulDis, CritCr(70,NY03)<NJ-CHILTON>
+ Chilton Medical Center
97 West Parkway   Pompton Plains, NJ 07444   (973)831-5000
richard_weinberg@chiltonmemorial.org

Weinberg, Ronald M., MD {1881618684} Grtrcs, IntrMd(78,MEX03)<NJ-MONMOUTH>
+ Internal Medical Associates of Monmouth
279 Third Avenue/Suite 207   Long Branch, NJ 07740   (732)229-0509   Fax (732)571-0019
+ Internal Medical Associates of Monmouth
219 Taylors Mills Road   Manalapan, NJ 07726   (732)229-0509   Fax (732)462-1290
+ Monmouth Family Center
270 Broadway   Long Branch, NJ 07740   (732)923-7100   Fax (732)923-7104

Weinberger, Adrian, MD {1730208257} OccpMd, IntrMd(84,ROM05)
+ Concentra Medical Centers
30 Seaview Drive/Suite 2   Secaucus, NJ 07094   (201)319-1611   Fax (201)319-1233

Weinberger, Andrew Bruce, MD {1871531533} Rheuma, IntrMd(70,NY19)<NJ-STBARNMC>
+ Drs. Weinberger & Cannarozzi
741 Northfield Avenue/Suite 210   West Orange, NJ 07052   (973)630-8950   Fax (973)669-9749

Weinberger, Barry I., MD {1124060108} NnPnMd, Pedtrc(87,NY46)
+ UMDNJ RWJ Neonatal-Perinatal
125 Paterson Street/MEB 312   New Brunswick, NJ 08901   (732)235-5684   Fax (732)235-6609

Weinberger, Daniela, MD {1487871141} IntrMd, OccpMd(85,ROM05)
+ Automatic Data Processing
1 ADP Boulevard/Medical   Roseland, NJ 07068   (973)974-5757   Fax (973)974-3348

Weinberger, George I., MD {1447238639} Dermat(73,NJ05)
+ 190 Greenbrook Road
North Plainfield, NJ 07060   (908)561-8070   Fax (908)561-8071

Weinberger, George T., DO {1124062625} FamMed, Grtrcs, IntrMd(67,MO79)
+ Palisades Medical Center
705B Anderson Avenue   Cliffside Park, NJ 07010   (201)861-1851   Fax (201)861-1853

Weinberger, Michael Kalman, MD {1477501468} Anesth, IntrMd, PainMd(93,NY01)<NY-LENOXHLL>
+ Bloomberg Health Center
100 Business Park drive   Princeton, NJ 08542   (609)279-4860   Fax (609)279-4850

Weinberger, Sharon Melissa Seltzer, MD {1134360746} PedCrd
+ Rutgers Pediatric Cardiology
125 Paterson Street/CAB 6100   New Brunswick, NJ 08901   (732)235-7905   Fax (732)235-7932

Weine, Douglas Matthew, MD {1336307305} Gastrn, IntrMd(04,NY20)<NJ-RIVERVW>
+ Red Bank Gastroenterology Associates PA
365 Broad Street/Suite 1-E   Red Bank, NJ 07701   (732)842-4294   Fax (732)548-7408

Weine, Gary R., MD {1164428611} IntrMd(76,NY20)<NJ-MORRISTN>
+ Madison Internal Medicine Associates
95 Madison Avenue/Suite 405   Morristown, NJ 07960   (973)829-9998   Fax (973)829-9991

Weiner, Alison L., MD {1346310349} Psychy(86,IL42)<NJ-NWRKBETH>
+ 31 South Fullerton Avenue/Floor 3
Montclair, NJ 07042   (973)655-0012   Fax (973)655-0010
+ Newark Beth Israel Medical Center
201 Lyons Avenue/Psychiatry   Newark, NJ 07112   (973)926-7026

Weiner, Barry, MD {1922180348} IntrMd, Nephro(63,NY08)
+ 109 Pacific Avenue
Jersey City, NJ 07304   (201)434-0008   Fax (204)451-2863

Weiner, Barry C., MD {1932160991} Dermat(87,NY08)<NJ-KIMBALL>
+ All-County Dermatology
4535 Highway 9 North   Howell, NJ 07731   (732)363-0100   Fax (732)363-3071

Weiner, Brian C., MD {1982653671} Gastrn, IntrMd(81,NY08)<NJ-RWJUBRUN, NJ-CENTRAST>
+ Marlboro Gastroenterology PC
50 Franklin Lane/Suite 201   Manalapan, NJ 07726   (732)972-6996   Fax (732)972-8610
drweiner@optonline.net

Weiner, Francine L., MD {1952504599} Nrolgy(86,IL01)
+ Neurology Associates & Ctr Pain
1030 North Kings Highway/Suite 200B   Cherry Hill, NJ 08034   (856)482-0030   Fax (856)779-7787

Weiner, Joseph Paul, MD {1174819577} RadOnc(11,NJ05)
+ Rutgers Cancer Institute of New Jersey
195 Little Albany Street/PO Box 2681   New Brunswick, NJ 08903   (732)235-2465   Fax (732)235-6797

Weiner, Leonard D., MD {1952571085} IntrMd, Nephro(03,NJ05)
+ Jersey Coast Nephrology & Hypertension Associates
1541 Route 88/Suite A   Brick, NJ 08724   (732)836-3200   Fax (732)836-3201

Weiner, Monica B., MD {1295743912} Pedtrc(01,NY46)
+ University Hospital-Cares Institute
42 East Laurel Road/Suite 1100   Stratford, NJ 08084   (856)566-7036   Fax (856)566-6108

Weiner, Peter R., MD {1972691814} InfDis, IntrMd(81,DC02)
+ 96 Millburn Avenue/Suite 200A
Millburn, NJ 07041   (908)686-7542   Fax (973)334-4253

Weiner, Samuel David, MD {1346220555} FamMed, IntrMd(01,PA02)<NJ-VIRTVOOR, NJ-VIRTMARL>
+ Virtua Family Medicine
1605 Evesham Road/Suite 100   Voorhees, NJ 08043

(856)741-7100   Fax (856)424-2629

Weiner, Sharon M., MD {1316918618} CritCr(85,NJ06)
+ Monmouth Pulmonary Consultants
30 Corbett Way   Eatontown, NJ 07724   (732)380-0020   Fax (732)380-1990

Weiner, Steven Martin, MD {1053393942} Anesth(88,NY03)<NJ-MORRISTN>
+ Morristown Medical Center
100 Madison Avenue/Anesthesiology   Morristown, NJ 07962   (973)971-5000   Fax (201)943-8733

Weingart, Brian M., DO {1871826784} IntrMd<NJ-VIRTVOOR>
+ Virtua Voorhees
100 Bowman Drive   Voorhees, NJ 08043   (856)762-1940   Fax (856)762-1777

Weingarten, Harvey S., MD {1629159892} FamMed, IntrMd(81,MEX02)
+ 3270 State Route 27
Kendall Park, NJ 08824   (732)422-2400   Fax (732)463-6087

Weingarten, Michael P., DO {1831382548} FamMed(71,IL76)
+ 814 Heritage Road
Cinnaminson, NJ 08077
+ University Doctors Family Practice
100 Centruy Parkway/Suite 140   Mount Laurel, NJ 08054   (856)667-9054

Weinrauch, Michael L., MD {1992778856} CdvDis, IntrMd(89,NY47)<NJ-OVERLOOK, NJ-STBARNMC>
+ Associates in Cardiovascular Disease, LLC
211 Mountain Avenue   Springfield, NJ 07081   (973)467-0005   Fax (973)912-8989
+ Associates in Cardiovascular Disease, LLC
29 South Street   New Providence, NJ 07974   (973)467-0005   Fax (908)464-1332

Weinreb, Barry D., MD {1720083710} Allrgy, Pedtrc(82,ISRA)<NJ-MORRISTN, NJ-STCLRBOO>
+ Allergy & Asthma Associates of North Jersey
261 James Street/Suite 1D   Morristown, NJ 07960   (973)267-3646   Fax (973)335-3319
+ Allergy & Asthma Associates of North Jersey
1160 Parsippany Boulevard/Suite 200   Parsippany, NJ 07054   (973)267-3646   Fax (973)335-3319

Weinroth, Heidi J., MD {1598713752} Pedtrc(94,MA07)<NJ-VIRTVOOR, NJ-VIRTMARL>
+ Cooper Family Medicine
110 Marter Avenue   Moorestown, NJ 08057   (856)608-8840   Fax (856)722-1898
+ Cooper Pediatrics
110 Marter Avenue/Bldg. 500, Suite 505   Moorestown, NJ 08057   (856)608-8840   Fax (856)536-1402

Weinschenk, Robert C., MD {1962445155} SrgOrt(79,NJ05)<NJ-NWTNMEM>
+ Andover Orthopaedic Surgery & Sports
280 Newton-Sparta Road/Suite 4   Newton, NJ 07860   (973)579-7443   Fax (973)579-5628
+ Andover Orthopaedic Surgery & Sports
452 Route 206   Montague, NJ 07827   (973)579-7443   Fax (973)293-7581

Weinshenker, Naomi Joyce, MD {1295951960} PsyAdt, PsyCAd(89,PA01)
+ 925 Clifton Avenue/Suite 103
Clifton, NJ 07013   (973)471-4448   Fax (973)471-5157
Naomi.Weinshenker@yahoo.com

Weinstein, Benjamin, MD {1215101928} IntrMd(76,NJ06)<NJ-CENTRAST>
+ CentraState Medical Center
901 West Main Street/Medical Dir   Freehold, NJ 07728   (732)294-2780
bweinste@centrastate.com

Weinstein, Craig M., MD {1083716104} Anesth(78,NJ05)<NJ-RWJUBRUN>
+ University Surgical Center
561 Cranbury Road/Anesthesia   East Brunswick, NJ 08816   (732)390-4300   Fax (732)390-0556
wb2boi1@verizon.net

Weinstein, David M., MD {1275509671} Pedtrc, IntrMd(84,NJ05)<NJ-CHILTON>
+ Advocare Pediatric Arts
1403 Route 23 South   Butler, NJ 07405   (973)283-2200   Fax (973)283-0406
+ Advocare Pediatric Arts
1777 Hamburg Turnpike/Suite 103   Wayne, NJ 07470   (973)283-2200   Fax (973)283-0406

Weinstein, Dora Hagar Foa, MD {1497920110} Dermat, IntrMd(89,NY20)
+ 34 West Shore Road
Mountain Lakes, NJ 07046

Weinstein, Jack S., MD {1124045612} Psychy(66,NJ05)
+ Union County Psychiatric Clinic, Inc.
117-119 Roosevelt Avenue   Plainfield, NJ 07060   (908)756-6870   Fax (908)756-5566

Physicians by Name and Address

Weinstein, Joseph R., MD {1437231826} FamMed(82,NJ06)<NJ-SOMERSET>
+ Your Doctors Care, PA
  71 Route 206 South Hillsborough, NJ 08844 (908)685-1887 Fax (908)707-0816

Weinstein, Larry, MD {1306839733} SrgHnd, SrgPlstc(80,NY47)<NJ-STBARNMC, NJ-OVERLOOK>
+ Plastic Surgery Associates
  385 Route 24/Suite 3-K Chester, NJ 07930 (908)879-2222 Fax (908)876-8993
  info@docweinstein.com
+ Plastic Surgery Associates
  33 Overlook Road Summit, NJ 07901 (908)522-3232

Weinstein, Mark E., MD {1528274040} Pedtrc
+ 40 Gray Street
  Montclair, NJ 07042

Weinstein, Mark J., MD {1376549576} IntrMd(85,NJ06)<NJ-CHSMRCER>
+ Princeton Pike Internal Medicine
  3100 Princeton Pike/Bldg 3/ 3rd Fl Lawrenceville, NJ 08648 (609)896-1793 Fax (609)896-1847

Weinstein, Melissa A., DO {1194727271} ObsGyn(96,NY75)<NJ-HACKNSK, NJ-HOLYNAME>
+ Drs. Robinson, Parnes & Weinstein
  275 Forest Avenue Paramus, NJ 07652 (201)967-9191 Fax (201)967-9302

Weinstein, Melvin P., MD {1609941228} InfDis, IntrMd, MedMcb(70,DC01)<NJ-RWJUBRUN>
+ Rutgers RWJ Allergy, Immunology and Infectious Group
  125 Paterson Street New Brunswick, NJ 08901 (732)235-7060

Weinstein, Rita, MD {1033109046} Dermat(69,NY19)<NJ-STPETER, NJ-RWJUBRUN>
+ 603 Cranbury Road
  East Brunswick, NJ 08816 (732)545-5366 Fax (732)254-1038

Weinstock, Brett Michael, MD {1356753883} Ophthl
+ Friedberg Eye Associates
  661 North Broad Street Woodbury, NJ 08096 (856)845-7968 Fax (856)845-8544

Weinstock, Lisa R., MD {1871506485} Radiol, RadDia(88,NY08)<NJ-UMDNJ>
+ Breast Health Center of Ridgewood, P.C.
  385 South Maple Avenue Ridgewood, NJ 07450 (201)670-4550 Fax (201)670-7812

Weinstock, Murray, MD {1275531204} CdvDis, IntrMd(65,MA05)<NJ-HACKNSK>
+ Hackensack UMG
  150 Overlook Avenue Hackensack, NJ 07601 (201)489-5999 Fax (201)489-1898

Weinstock, Perry J., MD {1841396009} CdvDis(85,NJ05)
+ University Cardiology
  3 Cooper Plaza/Room 311 Camden, NJ 08103 (856)342-2034 Fax (856)342-6608
+ Cooper Cardiology Associates
  900 Centennial Boulevard Voorhees, NJ 08043 (856)342-2034 Fax (856)325-6702
+ Cooper Cardiology Associates
  1210 Brace Road/Suite 103 Cherry Hill, NJ 08103 (856)427-7254

Weintraub, Bernard M., MD {1922000934} Nrolgy, IntrMd(67,PA13)
+ Neurologic Arts Associated, LLC.
  183 High Street/Suite 1200 Newton, NJ 07860 (973)300-0579 Fax (973)300-5535

Weintraub, Steve L., DO {1619033529} SprtMd, IntrSptM(89,NY75)<NJ-CHSFULD, NJ-OCEANMC>
+ Sports Medicine of New Jersey
  475 County Road 520/Suite 101 Marlboro, NJ 07746 (732)946-2100 Fax (732)463-6070

Weisband, Ira David, DO {1255460382} SrgOrt, IntrMd(71,MO04)
+ 875 Cox Road
  Moorestown, NJ 08057 (856)778-0544 Fax (856)778-5906

Weisberg, Lawrence Stephen, MD {1235235128} Nephro, IntrMd(81,PA13)<NJ-COOPRUMC>
+ Cooper University Medical Center/Camden
  3 Cooper Plaza/Suite 314 Camden, NJ 08103 (856)342-2439 Fax (856)757-7778
+ The Cooper Hospital System-Univ Hospital
  401 Haddon Avenue/Room 286 Camden, NJ 08103 (856)342-2439 Fax (856)757-7803
+ Cooper Cardiology Associates
  1210 Brace Road/Suite 103 Cherry Hill, NJ 08103 (856)427-7254

Weisberg, William R., MD {1679643597} GenPrc, EmrgMd, IntrMd(82,PA14)<NJ-BURDTMLN>
+ Cape Regional Medical Center
  2 Stone Harbor Boulevard/EmrgMed Cape May Court House, NJ 08210 (609)463-2000
+ Cape Urgent Care
  900 Route 109 Cape May, NJ 08204 (609)463-2000 Fax (609)884-4377

Weisberger, James D., MD {1336289578} IntrMd, Pthlgy(83,PA01)
+ Bio-Reference Laboratory, Inc.
  481 Edward H. Ross Drive Elmwood Park, NJ 07407 (201)791-2600 Fax (201)791-1941

Weisbrot, Frederick J., MD {1164540019} Nrolgy(73,WI06)<NJ-STMICHL>
+ 190 Eagle Rock Avenue
  Roseland, NJ 07068 (973)226-9003 Fax (201)997-2041

Weisbrot, Joshua, MD {1720221484} CdvDis
+ Morristown Cardiology Associates, P.A.
  435 South Street/Suite 100 Morristown, NJ 07960 (973)267-3944 Fax (973)455-0399

Weisburg, Rhoda S., MD {1508895947} EmrgMd, IntrMd(72,PA09)<NJ-HACKNSK>
+ Hackensack University Medical Center
  30 Prospect Avenue/IntMed Hackensack, NJ 07601 (201)996-2000 Fax (201)968-1866

Weisel, Arthur S., MD {1194795815} Radiol, RadDia(73,NY47)
+ Diagnostic Radiology Associates of Hackensack
  433 Hackensack Avenue/Lower Lobby Hackensack, NJ 07601 (201)488-1144 Fax (201)488-0853
+ Diagnostic Radiology Associates of Northfield
  772 Northfield Avenue West Orange, NJ 07052 (201)488-1144 Fax (973)325-8140
+ Diagnostic Radiology Associates of Clifton
  1339 Broad Street Clifton, NJ 07601 (973)778-9600 Fax (973)778-4846

Weisen, Steven Fred, MD {1598702623} CdvDis, IntrMd(96,NY46)<NY-PRSBCOLU>
+ Morristown Cardiology Associates, P.A.
  435 South Street/Suite 100 Morristown, NJ 07960 (973)267-3944 Fax (973)455-0399

Weisensel, Joseph Daniel, DO {1811096522}
+ 3 Sparrowbush Road
  Upper Saddle River, NJ 07458 (347)612-7776
  Joseph.Weisensel@gmail.com

Weiser, Jessica Ann, MD {1619172541} Dermat(07,NY46)
+ Dermatology Associates of Morris PA
  199 Baldwin Road Parsippany, NJ 07054 (973)335-2560 Fax (973)335-9421

Weiser, Mitchell M., MD {1417920836} IntrMd, CdvDis(97,NY46)<NJ-VALLEY>
+ Valley Medical Group/Valley Heart Group
  1200 East Ridgewood Avenue Ridgewood, NJ 07450 (201)670-8660 Fax (201)447-1957

Weiser, Paul J., MD {1104822451} Radiol, RadDia(71,NY46)
+ Radiology Affiliates of Central New Jersey, P.A.
  2501 Kuser Road Hamilton, NJ 08691 (609)585-8800 Fax (609)585-1825
+ Radiology Affiliates of Central New Jersey, P.A.
  3120 Princeton Pike Lawrenceville, NJ 08648 (609)585-8800 Fax (609)219-0439

Weiser, Sheldon, DO {1184730210} Psychy(65,PA77)
+ 289 Market Street
  Saddle Brook, NJ 07663 (201)843-1248 Fax (201)843-5999

Weisfogel, Gerald M., MD {1063458180} CdvDis, IntrMd(70,NY08)
+ Cardiovascular Health Associates
  2050 State Route 27/Suite 205 North Brunswick, NJ 08902 (732)821-5511 Fax (732)821-5347

Weisfuse, Judith E., MD {1669447165} IntrMd, OncHem(78,PA07)<NJ-OVERLOOK, NJ-MORRISTN>
+ Summit Medical Group-Berkeley Heights Campus
  1 Diamond Hill Road Berkeley Heights, NJ 07922 (908)273-4300 Fax (908)790-6524

Weisgras, Josef Mordechay, MD {1700857463} IntrMd(81,MEX29)<NJ-HOLYNAME>
+ Excelcare
  375 South Washington Avenue Bergenfield, NJ 07621 (201)384-0036 Fax (201)384-7304

Weisholtz, Steven J., MD {1053318964} InfDis, IntrMd(78,PA01)<NJ-ENGLWOOD, NJ-HOLYNAME>
+ Leonia Medical Associates, P.A.
  25 Rockwood Place/Suite 120 Englewood, NJ 07631 (201)568-3335 Fax (201)568-2450

Weisman, David Seth, MD {1952406316} SrgOrt(86,NJ06)<NJ-RWJUBRUN, NJ-STPETER>
+ Pediatric Orthopedic Associates, P.A.
  585 Cranbury Road/Suite A East Brunswick, NJ 08816 (732)390-1160 Fax (732)390-8449
+ Pediatric Orthopedic Associates, P.A.
  3700 State Route 33 Neptune, NJ 07753 (732)390-1160 Fax (732)897-4205

Weisman, Harlan Frederick, MD {1619147410} IntrMd, CdvDis(79,MD01)
+ 17 Stout Road
  Princeton, NJ 08540

Weisman, Tamara K., DO Psychy(97,NY75)
+ 1259 Route 46 East
  Parsippany, NJ 07054 (973)299-9919

Weiss, Aaron R., DO {1013945708} Pedtrc, PedHem(99,PA77)<NJ-RWJUBRUN>
+ Rutgers Cancer Institute of New Jersey
  195 Little Albany Street/PO Box 2681 New Brunswick, NJ 08903 (732)235-2465 Fax (732)235-6797

Weiss, Christopher A., DO {1538189568} Pedtrc, AdolMd(96,FL75)<NJ-ENGLWOOD, NJ-HACKNSK>
+ Washington Avenue Pediatrics
  95 North Washington Avenue Bergenfield, NJ 07621 (201)384-0300 Fax (201)384-9518
  caweiss@yahoo.com

Weiss, Daniel E., MD {1982810610} EmrgMd(04,NJ05)<NJ-JFKMED>
+ JFK Medical Center
  65 James Street/EmrgMed Edison, NJ 08820 (732)321-7601
+ Emergency Physician Associates, P.A.
  307 South Evergreen Avenue/PO Box 298 Woodbury, NJ 08096 (732)321-7601 Fax (856)848-1431

Weiss, Darryl S., MD {1306836309} Dermat(86,VA04)<NJ-VALLEY>
+ 23-00 Route 208 South
  Fair Lawn, NJ 07410 (201)797-7770 Fax (201)797-1660

Weiss, Eliezer, MD {1891939187} Gastrn
+ NJ Gastro LLC
  24 Merchant Street Newark, NJ 07105 (973)645-0000

Weiss, Emmanuel M., MD {1538226360} CdvDis, IntrMd(80,ROM06)
+ Medical Specialties of New Jersey
  842 Clifton Avenue/Suite 4 Clifton, NJ 07013 (973)777-2440 Fax (973)777-1848
+ Rutgers- New Jersey Medical School
  185 South Orange Avenue/Clinical Newark, NJ 07103 (973)972-4300

Weiss, Evan A., DO {1417013012} Anesth
+ Rancocas Anesthesiology, PA
  700 Route 130 North/Suite 203 Cinnaminson, NJ 08077 (856)829-9345 Fax (856)829-3605

Weiss, Fred Harvey, MD {1659318210} PedCrd, Pedtrc(71,NY09)<PA-PNSTHRSH>
+ St. Christopher Care at Washington Township
  405 Hurffville-Cross Keys Road Sewell, NJ 08080 (856)582-0644 Fax (856)582-0622

Weiss, Gabriella Antionette, MD {1558437251} InfDis, IntrMd(79,ROM09)<NJ-STMRYPAS>
+ Medical Specialties of New Jersey
  842 Clifton Avenue/Suite 4 Clifton, NJ 07013 (973)777-2440 Fax (973)777-1848

Weiss, Gerson, MD {1013002872} RprEnd, ObsGyn(64,NY19)<NJ-UMDNJ>
+ University Reproductive Associates, PC
  214 Terrace Avenue/2nd Floor Hasbrouck Heights, NJ 07604 (201)288-6330 Fax (201)288-6331

Weiss, Gony Alexandra, MD {1912150517} Psychy, PsycAd(04,ISR02)
+ ADHD, Mood & Behavior Center of New Jersey
  210 Malapardis Road Cedar Knolls, NJ 07927 (973)605-5000
+ Park West Associates
  33 Plymouth Street/Suite 104 Montclair, NJ 07042 (973)605-5000 Fax (973)509-1446

Weiss, Howard C., MD {1154364164} IntrMd, OccpMd, GPrvMd(83,NY47)
+ 9 Franklin Street/Suite 2
  Morristown, NJ 07960 (973)898-1770 Fax (973)898-0030

Weiss, Jeffrey A., MD {1215215835} IntHos<NJ-STMRYPAS>
+ Medical Specialties of New Jersey
  842 Clifton Avenue/Suite 4 Clifton, NJ 07013 (973)777-2440 Fax (973)777-1848

Weiss, Jeffrey Gregg, MD {1366625162} Pedtrc, Allrgy(97,PA09)<NJ-CHILTON, NJ-VALLEY>
+ Drs. Bogusz & Weiss
  44 State Route 23 North/Suite 6 Riverdale, NJ 07457 (973)248-9199 Fax (973)248-9299

Weiss, Jennifer Ellen, MD {1487608337} Pedtrc, PedRhm(98,GRN01)<NJ-HACKNSK>
+ Hackensack University Medical Center
  30 Prospect Avenue/Pediatrics Hackensack, NJ 07601 (201)996-5306 Fax (201)996-9815

Weiss, Kerry I., MD {1477518306} NnPnMd(80,PHI09)<NJ-HUNTRDN>
+ Hunterdon Medical Center
  2100 Wescott Drive/Neonatology Flemington, NJ 08822 (908)788-6100

Weiss, Kyle Matthew, DO {1902219702} PhysMd<NJ-JFKMED>
+ JFK Medical Center
  65 James Street Edison, NJ 08820 (732)321-7070 Fax (732)321-7330

Weiss, Lynne S., MD {1003924903} PedNph, Pedtrc(74,PA09)
+ Child Health Institute of New Jersey
89 French Street/Suite 2300   New Brunswick, NJ 08901
(732)235-7880   Fax (732)235-6620

Weiss, Maurice D., MD {1659350882} CdvDis, IntrMd, IntCrd(88,NY08)<NJ-JRSYSHMC, NJ-COMMED>
+ Shore Heart Group, P.A.
1820 State Route 33/Suite 4-B   Neptune, NJ 07753
(732)776-8500   Fax (732)776-8946
+ Shore Heart Group, P.A.
35 Beaverson Boulevard/Suite 9-B   Brick, NJ 08723
(732)776-8500   Fax (732)262-4317
+ Shore Heart Group, P.A.
555 Iron Bridge Road/Suite 15   Freehold, NJ 07753
(732)308-0774   Fax (732)333-1366

Weiss, Mitchell F., MD {1982643458} RadOnc, Radiol(98,IL02)<NJ-MONMOUTH>
+ Monmouth Medical Center
300 Second Avenue   Long Branch, NJ 07740   (732)222-5200

Weiss, Ned Martin, MD {1093736522} EnDbMt(80,PA09)<NJ-UNVMCPRN>
+ Princeton Endocrinology Associates, LLC
10 Forrestal Road South/Suite 106   Princeton, NJ 08540
(609)921-1511   Fax (609)921-3316

Weiss, Nofit, MD {1861443467} ObsGyn, IntrMd(95,NY46)
+ 440 Curry Avenue/Suite C
Englewood, NJ 07631   (201)408-4810   Fax (201)567-3269

Weiss, Richard Lee, MD {1053343376} CdvDis, IntrMd(84,PA09)<NJ-VIRTVOOR, NJ-VIRTMARL>
+ Penn Medicine at Cherry Hill
1400 East Route 70/Cardiology   Cherry Hill, NJ 08034
+ Penn Medicine at Woodbury Heights
1006 Mantua Pike/Cardiology   Woodbury Heights, NJ 08097
Fax (856)845-0535

Weiss, Richard S., DO {1568568459} FamMed(80,PA77)
+ Kennedy Health Alliance
457 Haddonfield Road/Suite 110   Cherry Hill, NJ 08002
(856)406-4091   Fax (856)406-4570

Weiss, Robert Edward, MD {1669541157} Onclgy, Urolgy(85,NY19)<NJ-RWJUBRUN>
+ Rutgers Cancer Institute of New Jersey
195 Little Albany Street/PO Box 2681   New Brunswick, NJ 08903   (732)235-6777   Fax (732)235-6797
+ RWJ University Hospital New Brunswick
One Robert Wood Johnson Place   New Brunswick, NJ 08901
(732)235-6777   Fax (732)235-6042

Weiss, Robert Jay, MD {1033203260} OccpMd, IntrMd(76,NY08)
+ Adult and Child Dermatology Center
1721 East Main Street   Millville, NJ 08332   (856)825-3023
+ Adult and Child Dermatology Center
8 Village Drive   Cape May Court House, NJ 08210
(856)825-3023   Fax (609)624-1281
+ Adult and Child Dermatology Center
3324 Simpson Avenue   Ocean City, NJ 08332   (609)398-0290

Weiss, Robert Joseph, Sr., MD {1427239532} Dermat, IntrMd(76,MI20)
+ Adult and Child Dermatology Center
8 Village Drive   Cape May Court House, NJ 08210
(609)465-4477   Fax (609)624-1281

Weiss, Ronald D., MD {1215047386} IntrMd(88,NJ05)
+ The Doctor Is in
6701 Bergenline Avenue   West New York, NJ 07093
(201)758-9100   Fax (201)758-9511

Weiss, Stanley H., MD {1093910085} Epdmlg, PubHth, IntrMd(78,MA01)
+ University Hospital-New Jersey Medical School
30 Bergen Street/ADMC6/Ste 1614   Newark, NJ 07107
(973)972-4623
weiss@umdnj.edu

Weiss, Steven Jay, MD {1841269867} Allrgy, IntrMd, AlgyImmn(82,IL42)<NJ-STBARNMC, NY-MTSINAI>
+ Allergy, Asthma & Immunology PA
209 South Livingston Avenue   Livingston, NJ 07039
(973)992-4171   Fax (973)992-6325
+ Allergy, Asthma & Immunology PA
381 Chestnut Street   Union, NJ 07083   (973)992-4171
Fax (908)688-4416

Weiss Baker, Marissa Beth, DO {1972544062} Pedtrc(99,PA77)<NJ-KMHTURNV>
+ Advocare Woolwich Pediatrics
300 Lexington Road/Suite 200   Woolwich Township, NJ 08085   (856)241-2111   Fax (856)241-2243
+ Kennedy Health Systems/Washington Township Campus
435 Hurffville-Cross Keys Road   Turnersville, NJ 08012
(856)241-2111   Fax (856)582-2712

Weiss-Bloom, Leslie J., MD {1750455978} Anesth(86,NY47)<NJ-HACKNSK>
+ Hackensack University MC-Anesthesia Dept
30 Prospect Avenue/Room 2703   Hackensack, NJ 07601
(201)996-2419   Fax (201)996-3962

+ Hackensack University Medical Center
30 Prospect Avenue/Anesth   Hackensack, NJ 07601
(201)996-2000

Weissbach, Debra D., MD {1689696742} Pedtrc(81,NY19)<NJ-VIRTMHBC>
+ CHOP Primary Care Mount Laurel
3201 Marne Highway   Mount Laurel, NJ 08054   (856)829-5545   Fax (856)829-9268

Weissman, Allan Mark, MD {1063546208} Anesth, AnesPain(90,NY46)<NY-LICOLLGE>
+ 351 Terhune Avenue
Passaic, NJ 07055

Weissman, Andrew J., MD {1376675637} CdvDis, IntrMd
+ Cardiovascular Associates of North Jersey
25 Rockwood Place/Suite 440   Englewood, NJ 07631
(201)568-3690   Fax (201)568-3667
+ Cardiovascular Associates of North Jersey
1555 Center Avenue   Fort Lee, NJ 07024   (201)568-3690
Fax (201)568-3667

Weissman, Barry J., MD {1639103500} Pedtrc(75,ITA01)<NJ-HACKNSK, NJ-VALLEY>
+ Haclensack Bergen Pediatrics
385 Prospect Avenue/Suite 210   Hackensack, NJ 07601
(551)996-9160   Fax (551)996-9165

Weissman, Evan Laird, DO {1033209804} Pedtrc(95,NY75)<NY-NSUHMANH>
+ Tenafly Pediatrics, PA
32 Franklin Street   Tenafly, NJ 07670   (201)569-2400   Fax (201)569-6081

Weissman, Lauren, MD {1821217191} RprEnd
+ South Jersey Fertility Center
400 Lippincott Drive   Marlton, NJ 08053   (856)282-1231
Fax (856)596-2411

Weissman, Michelle S., MD {1174682603} NnPnMd(02,ISR02)<MA-NEMEDCEN>
+ St Joseph's Medical Center Neonatology
703 Main Street   Paterson, NJ 07503   (973)754-2555

Weissman, Paul S., MD {1063478469} Gastrn, IntrMd(82,NJ05)<NJ-JRSYCITY>
+ Liberty Medical Associates
377 Jersey Avenue/Suite 470   Jersey City, NJ 07302
(201)918-2239   Fax (201)918-2243
+ Jersey City Medical Center
355 Grand Street/Gastro/2 West   Jersey City, NJ 07304
(201)915-2000

Weissman, Tanya, MD {1497709638} PhysMd(02,NJ06)
+ Comprehensive Rehabilitation
69 Brunswick Woods Drive   East Brunswick, NJ 08816
(732)238-0080   Fax (732)238-0070

Weissmann, David J., MD {1740348424} PthAcl, Pthlgy(89,PA09)<NJ-RWJUBRUN>
+ RWJ University Pathology
125 Paterson Street/MEB 212   New Brunswick, NJ 08901
Fax (732)418-8445
+ RWJ University Hospital New Brunswick
One Robert Wood Johnson Place   New Brunswick, NJ 08901
(732)828-3000

Weissmann, Murray H., MD {1285614602} RadDia, Radiol, NuclMd(73,NY47)<NJ-JFKMED>
+ Edison Radiology Group, P.A.
65 James Street   Edison, NJ 08820   (732)321-7917   Fax (732)737-2968
+ JFK Medical Center
65 James Street/Radiology   Edison, NJ 08820   (732)321-7000

Weiswasser, Jonathan M., MD {1285617308} Surgry, SrgVas(93,NY19)
+ Vascular Associates of New Jersey
200 South Orange Street   Livingston, NJ 07039

Weitz, Robert D., DO {1154399913} Pedtrc(86,NJ75)<NJ-VIRTU-AHS, NJ-VIRTMHBC>
+ Advocare Medford Pediatric & Adolescent Medicine
520 Stokes Road   Medford, NJ 08055   (609)654-9112   Fax (609)654-7404

Weitzman, Richard Brian, MD IntrMd(95,NY19)<NJ-HACKNSK>
+ 766 Albemarle Street
Wyckoff, NJ 07481

Weitzman, Robert H., MD {1699791962} IntrMd, PulDis(66,NJ05)<NJ-OVERLOOK>
+ 216 Thelma Terrace
Linden, NJ 07036

Weitzman, Stephen M., MD {1063580876} Anesth, CdvDis(78,NY01)<NJ-HACKNSK>
+ GMS Anesthesia Associates
100 Prospect Avenue   Hackensack, NJ 07601   (201)487-8557
+ Hackensack University MC-Anesthesia Dept
30 Prospect Avenue/Room 2703   Hackensack, NJ 07601
(201)487-8557   Fax (201)996-3962

Weizman, Howard B., MD {1033190103} Nephro, IntrMd(82,NY46)<NJ-VALLEY, NJ-HACKNSK>
+ Bergen Hypertension & Renal Associates PA
44 Godwin Avenue/Suite 301   Midland Park, NJ 07432
(201)447-0013   Fax (201)447-0438
+ Bergen Hypertension & Renal Associates PA
20 Prospect Avenue/Suite 709   Hackensack, NJ 07601
(201)447-0013   Fax (201)678-1072

Welber, Mark R., DO {1285654244} EmrgMd(90,NJ75)<NJ-STBARNMC>
+ St. Barnabas Medical Center
94 Old Short Hills Road   Livingston, NJ 07039   (973)322-5000

Welch, James W., MD {1659583003} Psychy(79,TX13)
+ 50 North Franklin Turnpike/Suite 105
Ho Ho Kus, NJ 07423   (201)251-0435

Weldon, Stacey Bidigare, MD {1073648325} EmrgMd(04,BWI01)<CT-STAMFDH, NJ-UNDRWD>
+ Inspira Health Network
509 North Broad Street   Woodbury, NJ 08096   (856)845-0100

Welish, Steven Jay, MD {1639147325} CdvDis, IntrMd(86,VT02)<NJ-HOLYNAME, NJ-HACKNSK>
+ Holy Name Hospital
718 Teaneck Road   Teaneck, NJ 07666   (201)530-7917
Fax (201)357-8217

Weller, Alan Scott, MD {1760426555} Pedtrc, IntrMd(92,PA13)<NJ-RWJUBRUN>
+ University Hospital-RWJ Medical School
89 French Street/Suite 2205   New Brunswick, NJ 08901
(732)235-7981   Fax (732)235-9340

Wellner, Robert Leo, DO {1790862977} AnesPain, Anesth(00,PA77)
+ 10 Forrestal Road South/Suite 209
Princeton, NJ 08540
+ Robert Wood Johnson-UMDNJ Anesthesia Group
125 Paterson Street/CAB 3100   New Brunswick, NJ 08901
Fax (732)235-6131

Wells, Evelyn Ruth, MD {1962459313} EmrgMd(98,DC03)<NJ-JRSYSHMC>
+ EmCare
1945 Route 33   Neptune, NJ 07753   (732)776-4510   Fax (732)776-2329

Wells, Lawrence, MD {1275622391} SrgOrt(85,CA02)<PA-CHILDHOS>
+ CHOP Specialty Care Center at Virtua
200 Bowman Drive/2 FL/Suite D-260   Voorhees, NJ 08043
(267)425-5400

Wells-Roth, David S., MD {1366576845} SrgNro(00,DC01)<NY-PRSBWEIL>
+ Atlantic Neurosurgical Specialists
310 Madison Avenue/Suite 300   Morristown, NJ 07960
(973)285-7800   Fax (973)285-7839

Welsh, John W., DO {1982706909} IntrMd, Pedtrc, FamMed(69,PA77)<NJ-SHOREMEM, NJ-ACMCMAIN>
+ 513 Tilton Road
Northfield, NJ 08225   (609)645-7770   Fax (609)645-7966

Welsh, Terrence Mathew, MD {1821231135} Anesth, PainMd(06,NY19)
+ New Jersey Pain Consultants
310 Madison Avenue/Suite 301   Morristown, NJ 07960
(973)998-9200   Fax (973)998-9201
+ New Jersey Pain Consultants
175 Morristown Road/Suite 202   Basking Ridge, NJ 07920
(908)630-0175

Welsh, Theresa M., MD {1013971894} Pedtrc(83,PA02)<NJ-OURLADY, NJ-VIRTUAHS>
+ Advocare Haddonfield Pediatric Association
220 North Haddon Avenue   Haddonfield, NJ 08033
(856)429-6719   Fax (856)429-6748

Welt, Alan J., MD {1699854364} ObsGyn(77,NJ05)<NJ-OCEANMC>
+ Brielle Obstetrics & Gynecology, P.A.
2671 Highway 70/Wall Township   Manasquan, NJ 08736
(732)528-6999   Fax (732)528-3397
+ Brielle Obstetrics & Gynecology, P.A.
117 County Line Road   Lakewood, NJ 08701   (732)528-6999   Fax (732)942-1919

Wen, Fang, MD {1184945131}
+ 150 Grant Street
Haworth, NJ 07641   (858)334-5991

Wendel, Ian William, DO {1780902627}
+ 219 Willow Avenue/Apt 3f
Hoboken, NJ 07030

Weng, Francis Liu, MD {1457442378} IntrMd, Nephro(97,NY01)<NJ-STBARNMC>
+ St. Barnabas Medical Center Renal Transplant Center
94 Old Short Hills Road   Livingston, NJ 07039   (973)322-5065   Fax (973)322-8930

Physicians by Name and Address

Wenger, Christopher D., DO {1861650772} IntrMd, CdvDis(06,PA77)
+ **South Jersey Heart Group**
  3001 Chapel Avenue/Suite 101 Cherry Hill, NJ 08002 (856)755-1173 Fax (856)667-6588
+ **Rowan University-School of Osteopathic Medicine**
  1 Medical Center Drive Stratford, NJ 08084 (856)566-7050

Wenger, Peter Christopher, MD {1396066627} PhyMSptM
+ **Princeton Sports & Family Medicine**
  3131 Princeton Pike Lawrenceville, NJ 08648 (609)896-9190 Fax (609)896-3555

Wenger, Peter N., MD {1396759429} Pedtrc, PedInf(89,NJ05)<NJ-UMDNJ>
+ **The Children's Hospital at Saint Peter's University**
  254 Easton Avenue New Brunswick, NJ 08901 (732)745-8538

Wengerter, Kurt Richard, MD {1265491880} SrgVas, Surgry(80,NY08)<NJ-ENGLWOOD, NJ-HOLYNAME>
+ **Bergen Thoracic & Vascular Associates PC**
  25 Rockwood Place/Suite 330 Englewood, NJ 07631 (201)408-5195 Fax (201)408-2485

Wenokor, Cornelia B. C., MD {1851409528} Radiol, OthrSp(90,GER53)<NJ-UMDNJ>
+ **University Hospital**
  150 Bergen Street/Radiology Newark, NJ 07103 (973)972-4300 Fax (973)972-2307

Wenzler, Danya J., MD {1154511244} IntrMd, InfDis(04,NJ05)<NJ-STCLRDOV, NJ-MORRISTN>
+ **ID Associates PA/dba ID Care**
  765 Route 10 East/Suite 201 Randolph, NJ 07869 (973)989-0068 Fax (973)361-8955
+ **ID Associates PA/dba ID Care**
  8 Saddle Road Cedar Knolls, NJ 07927 (973)989-0068 Fax (973)993-5953

Wer Arrivillaga, Santiago, MD {1083049282}
+ **St. Peter's Adult Family Health Center**
  123 How Lane New Brunswick, NJ 08901 (732)745-6642

Werbel, Sarah A., MD {1063500775} IntrMd(99,NJ05)
+ **Lawrenceville Internal Medicine Associates LLC**
  3100 Princeton Pike/Building 4/Suite I Lawrenceville, NJ 08648 (609)896-0303 Fax (609)896-0308

Werber, John Frank, MD {1417275520} IntrMd, CdvDis(03,NY0)<NJ-RWJUBRUN>
+ **Heart Specialists/Central Jersey**
  901 West Main Street/Suite 205 Freehold, NJ 07728 (732)866-0800 Fax (732)463-6082
+ **RWJ University Hospital New Brunswick**
  One Robert Wood Johnson Place New Brunswick, NJ 08901 (732)828-3000

Werbitt, Warren, DO {1275595035} Gastrn, IntrMd(66,IA75)<NJ-OURLADY, NJ-VIRTBERL>
+ **Professional Gastroenterology Associates, PA**
  1939 Route 70 East/Suite 250 Cherry Hill, NJ 08002 (856)429-4433 Fax (856)424-6732
+ **Professional Gastroenterology Associates, PA**
  188 Fries Mill Road/Suite M4 Turnersville, NJ 08012 (856)429-4433 Fax (856)424-6732

Werkmeister, Lindsay, MD {1467847962}<NJ-NWRKBETH>
+ **Newark Beth Israel Medical Center**
  201 Lyons Avenue Newark, NJ 07112 (612)695-0732

Werman, Richard Evan, DO {1992786578} RadDia(95,FL75)
+ **Cape Radiology**
  4011 Route 9 South/PO Box 244 Rio Grande, NJ 08242 (609)886-0477 Fax (609)886-0529

Werner, Marie D., MD {1962660621} ObsGyn, RprEnd(08,NJ06)
+ **Reproductive Medicine Associates of New Jersey**
  140 Allen Road Basking Ridge, NJ 07920 (908)604-7800 Fax (973)290-8370

Werner, Philip M., MD {1073682399} Psychy(64,NJ05)
+ **310 Madison Avenue/Suite 220**
  Morristown, NJ 07960 (973)538-2055 Fax (973)540-8849

Werner, Robert L., DO {1174558225} IntrMd(81,NJ75)<NJ-HCK-TSTWN>
+ **500 Willow Grove Street**
  Hackettstown, NJ 07840 (908)850-3377 Fax (908)850-3124

Werring, John Andrew, MD {1366428971} Radiol(98,DC01)
+ **59 Madison Avenue**
  Summit, NJ 07901

Wertenteil, Mark Elliot, MD {1922067180} IntrMd(94,NY19)<NJ-VALLEY>
+ **Radburn Medical Associates**
  20-20 Fair Lawn Avenue/Suite 104 Fair Lawn, NJ 07410 (201)703-0202 Fax (201)703-1231

Werthaim, Ofer Avi, MD {1548234941} IntrMd(85,MEX03)<NJ-RWJUBRUN>
+ **Doctor's Care Center**
  597 Cranbury Road/Suite A East Brunswick, NJ 08816 (732)238-6800 Fax (732)238-9696

Wertheim, Mordecai, MD {1518088202} IntrMd(81,MEX14)
+ **321 Summit Avenue**
  Hackensack, NJ 07601

Wertheimer, David Eliot, MD {1821040486} CdvDis, IntrMd(79,IL43)
+ **801 Franklin Avenue/Second FL Suite 2**
  Franklin Lakes, NJ 07417 (201)853-4923

Wertheimer, Robert M., MD {1972692598} Ophthl, IntrMd(92,NY46)<NJ-MTNSIDE, NJ-STBARNMC>
+ **Essex Eye Physicians, LLC**
  195 Fairfield Avenue/Suite 4B West Caldwell, NJ 07006 (973)228-4990 Fax (973)228-4464
+ **Essex Eye Physicians, LLC**
  213 Park Street Montclair, NJ 07042 (973)228-4990 Fax (973)744-1233

Wesley, Carl Christopher, MD {1568673788} Anesth(05,PA02)<PA-TJCNTR>
+ **Hackensack University MC-Anesthesia Dept**
  30 Prospect Avenue/Room 2703 Hackensack, NJ 07601 (201)996-2419 Fax (201)996-3962

Wesley, Louis A., MD {1114937398} ObsGyn, IntrMd(83,NC01)<NJ-ACMCMAIN, NJ-ACMCITY>
+ **Reliance Medical Group, LLC**
  331 East Jimmie Leeds Road/Suite 1 & 2 Galloway, NJ 08205 (609)652-6016 Fax (609)652-2406

Weslow, Renee G., MD {1932134608} CdvDis, IntrMd(87,GRNA)<NJ-HACKNSK>
+ **425 Livingston Street/Suite 1**
  Norwood, NJ 07648 (201)784-0071 Fax (207)784-2662

Wessner, Scott Richard, DO {1972899607}
+ **St Joseph's Medical Center Plastic Surgery**
  703 Main Street Paterson, NJ 07503 (973)754-2490

Wesson, Michael F., MD {1760437321} RadOnc, Radiol(83,VA01)<NJ-VALLEY>
+ **Valley Radiation Oncology Associates**
  One Valley Health Plaza Paramus, NJ 07652 (201)634-5403

West, Beryl E., MD {1639279169} FamMed, IntrMd(84,NJ05)
+ **925 Belvidere Avenue**
  Plainfield, NJ 07060

West, Gerald, DO {1447205067} Otlryg(67,MO78)<NJ-STFRN-MED>
+ **Associated Ear Nose & Throat Physicians**
  505 Chestnut Street Roselle Park, NJ 07204 (908)241-0200 Fax (908)241-0445
+ **Associated Ear Nose & Throat Physicians**
  778 Kennedy Boulevard Bayonne, NJ 07002 (908)241-0200 Fax (201)829-1821

West, Helen T., MD {1598720179} PsyGrt, Psychy(90,NIGE)<NJ-HAGEDORN>
+ **Hagedorn Psychiatric Hospital**
  200 Sanatorium Road Glen Gardner, NJ 08826 (908)537-2141 Fax (908)537-3187

Westerband, Julio V., MD (74,PRO01)
+ **1224 Briar Way**
  Fort Lee, NJ 07024 (714)679-2332 jvwortho@hotmail.com

Westerberg, Dyanne Pergolino, DO {1215911987} FamMed(83,PA77)<NJ-COOPRUMC>
+ **Cooper Family Medicine**
  3156 River Road Camden, NJ 08105 (856)963-0126 Fax (856)365-0279
+ **The Cooper Hospital System-Univ Hospital**
  401 Haddon Avenue/FamMed Camden, NJ 08103 (856)342-2000

Westover, Thomas, MD {1972609899} MtFtMd, ObsGyn(88,NJ05)<NJ-COOPRUMC>
+ **Cooper University Medical Center/Camden**
  3 Cooper Plaza/OB/GYN Camden, NJ 08103 (856)342-2000

Westreich, Laurence M., MD {1164523056} Psychy(88,MN04)<NJ-MTNSIDE>
+ **Park West Associates**
  33 Plymouth Street/Suite 104 Montclair, NJ 07042 (973)509-1444 Fax (973)509-1446

Westrich, David J., MD {1396752044} Anesth(85,NY01)<NJ-VALLEY>
+ **The Valley Hospital**
  223 North Van Dien Avenue/Anesth Ridgewood, NJ 07450 (201)447-8000

Westrol, Michael Steven, MD {1184977936} EmrgMd<NJ-ACMCITY>
+ **AtlantiCare Regional Medical Center/City Campus**
  1925 Pacific Avenue/8th Floor Atlantic City, NJ 08401 (609)441-8127

Wetjen, Thomas F., DO {1427005750} EmrgMd, IntrMd(00,NJ75)<NJ-KMHSTRAT>
+ **Kennedy Memorial Hospital-University Medical Center**
  18 East Laurel Road/EmrgMed Stratford, NJ 08084 (856)346-7985

Wetli, Charles Victor, MD PthAcl, PthFor(69,MO34)
+ **PO Box 398**
  Alpine, NJ 07620

Wetstein, Lewis, MD {1790774230} Surgry, SrgThr(73,SPA15)<NJ-COMMED, NJ-OCEANMC>
+ **143 South Street**
  Freehold, NJ 07728 (732)780-9270 Fax (732)780-2107 lewiswetstein@yahoo.com

Wetzler, Merrick Jay, MD {1396716239} PhysMd, SprtMd, SrgOrt(86,PA13)
+ **South Jersey Orthopedic Associates PA**
  502 Centennial Boulevard/Suite 6 Voorhees, NJ 08043 (856)424-8866 Fax (856)424-2665 mjwetz@aol.com
+ **South Jersey Orthopedic Associates PA**
  901 Route 168/Suite 307 Turnersville, NJ 08012 (856)424-8866 Fax (856)228-1711

Wexler, Amy R., MD {1306843404} Ophthl, PedOph(84,NY46)<NJ-MEMSALEM>
+ **South Jersey Eye Physicians PA**
  509 South Lenola Road/Suite 11 Moorestown, NJ 08057 (856)234-0222 Fax (856)727-9518
+ **South Jersey Eye Physicians PA**
  103 Old Marlton Pike/Suite 216 Medford, NJ 08055 (856)234-0222 Fax (609)714-8759
+ **South Jersey Eye Physicians PA**
  25 Homestead Drive/Suite A Columbus, NJ 08057 (609)298-0888 Fax (609)291-1972

Wexler, David E., MD {1386637254} Gastrn, IntrMd(80,NJ05)<NJ-RWJURAH>
+ **727 Raritan Road/Suite 101**
  Clark, NJ 07066 (732)499-8000 Fax (732)396-9413
+ **Health Care Associates PA**
  999 Raritan Road Clark, NJ 07066 (732)499-8000 Fax (732)396-9413

Wexler, Jeffrey A., MD {1326086141} RadDia, Radiol(78,TX04)<NJ-STCLRDEN>
+ **St. Clare's Hospital-Denville Campus**
  25 Pocono Road/Radiology Denville, NJ 07834 (973)625-6000
+ **Magnetic Imaging of Morris**
  402 Boulevard/Suite 103 Mountain Lakes, NJ 07046 (973)402-9111

Wey, Philip D., MD {1083630339} SrgPlstc(86,RI01)<NJ-RWJUBRUN>
+ **Plastic Surgery Arts of of New Jersey**
  409 Joyce Kilmer Ave./Suite 210 New Brunswick, NJ 08901 (732)418-0709 Fax (732)418-0747
+ **Plastic Surgery Arts of of New Jersey**
  1378 US 206/2nd flr Skillman, NJ 08558 (732)418-0709 Fax (609)921-0747

Whalen, Joanna Hallmark, DO {1336453745} EmrgMd<NJ-STJOSHOS>
+ **St Joseph's Medical Center Emergency**
  703 Main Street Paterson, NJ 07503 (973)754-2240 Fax (973)754-2249

Whalen, Kathryn, MD {1720229479} Anesth
+ **Rutgers- New Jersey Medical School**
  185 South Orange Avenue Newark, NJ 07103 (973)972-0470

Whang, Gene, MD {1235269234} ObsGyn, Gyneco(91,IL01)<NJ-WARREN>
+ **Hunterdon Developmental Center**
  40 Pittstown Road/PO Box 4003 Clinton, NJ 08809 (908)735-4031 Fax (908)730-1338

Whang, Ihn Young, MD {1235137787} Anesth(91,KOR05)<NJ-STJOSHOS>
+ **St. Joseph's Regional Medical Center Anesthesia**
  703 Main Street Paterson, NJ 07503 (973)754-2323 Fax (973)754-2791

Whang, Inwhan, MD {1790716066} RadDia, Radiol(83,GA01)
+ **Wayne Urgent and Primary Care**
  246 Hamburg Turnpike/Suite 205 Wayne, NJ 07470 (973)595-1300 Fax (973)790-7398 c.whang@highmountainhealth.com

Whang, John, MD {1861471310} IntrMd, CdvDis(93,NY01)
+ **24 Woodland Avenue**
  Mountain Lakes, NJ 07046 (973)334-2880 Fax (973)588-3339
+ **Comprehensive Cardiovascular Consultants**
  299 Madison Avenue/Suite 102 Morristown, NJ 07960 (973)334-2880 Fax (973)292-0564

Whang, Matthew I.S., MD {1295883312} Urolgy(87,NY01)
+ **Modern Urology**
  1001 Pleasant Valley Way West Orange, NJ 07052 (973)669-8448 Fax (973)669-9536
+ **New Jersey Urology, LLC**
  700 North Broad Street/Suite 302 Elizabeth, NJ 07208 (973)669-8448 Fax (908)289-0716

Whang, Phil Joo, MD {1326166802} Psychy, PsyGrt(02,NJ06)
+ **20 Washington Place/3rd Floor**
  Newark, NJ 07102 (973)645-3042 Fax (201)781-0773

Wheatley, Harold M., MD {1154394963} Ophthl, VitRet(94,MD04)<NJ-RWJUBRUN, NJ-KIMBALL>
+ Retina Associates of New Jersey, P.A.
10 Plum Street/Suite 600   New Brunswick, NJ 08901
(732)220-1600   Fax (732)220-1603
+ Retina Associates of New Jersey, P.A.
98 James Street/Suite 209   Edison, NJ 08820   (732)220-1600   Fax (732)906-1883
+ Retina Associates of New Jersey, P.A.
1200 Route 22 East   Bridgewater, NJ 08901   (908)218-4303   Fax (908)218-4307

Wheeler, Ralph B., MD {1194706895} Radiol, RadDia(91,NJ06)
+ Point View Radiology Associates
246 Hamburg Turnpike/Suite 101   Wayne, NJ 07470
(973)904-0404   Fax (973)904-0423

Whetstone, Abigail Sarah, DO {1437599610}
+ Jersey Shore Medical Center Obs/Gyn
1945 Route 33   Neptune, NJ 07753   (732)776-3790   Fax (732)776-4525

Whipple, D. Sandra, MD Dermat(76,PA01)
+ Dermatology Physicians of South Jersey, P.A.
112 White Horse Pike   Haddon Heights, NJ 08035
(856)546-5353   Fax (856)546-8711

White, Christian Paul, DO {1629276746} Psychy(07,NJ75)
+ New Jersey Institute for Successful Aging
42 East Laurel Road/Suite 1800   Stratford, NJ 08084
(856)566-6843   Fax (856)566-6781

White, Deborah A., DO {1679702682} ObsGyn(09,ME75)
+ Kennedy Family Health Services
1 Somerdale Square/Bld A   Somerdale, NJ 08083
(856)309-7700   Fax (856)566-8944

White, Edward C., MD {1558383786} Urolgy(78,MEX03)<NJ-RWJUBRUN, NJ-STPETER>
+ 4 Auer Court/Suite A B
East Brunswick, NJ 08816   (732)390-4447

White, Evelyn W., MD {1134197395} ObsGyn(89,GA01)
+ St. Joseph's Family Health Center
21 Market Street   Paterson, NJ 07501   (973)754-4200   Fax (973)754-4298
+ St. Joseph's DePaul Center ObsGyn
11 Getty Avenue   Paterson, NJ 07503   (973)754-4200

White, Harvey L., MD {1952459018} Psychy(64,NY09)<NY-SLRRSVLT, NJ-HACKNSK>
+ 163 Engle Street/Building 5
Englewood, NJ 07631   (201)894-0594

White, Joseph A., DO {1467539379} GenPrc, Acpntr, FamMed(92,IA75)
+ 215 East Laurel Road/Suite 202
Stratford, NJ 08084   (856)783-0204   Fax (856)783-9606

White, Kevin S., DO {1740485887} SrgOrt(03,NJ75)<NJ-HCKTSTWN>
+ The Orthopedic Institute of New Jersey
108 Ridge Road/Suite 201   Hackettstown, NJ 07840
(908)684-3005   Fax (908)684-3301
+ The Orthopedic Institute of New Jersey
33 Newton Sparta Road/Unit 2   Newton, NJ 07860
(908)684-3005   Fax (908)684-3301
+ The Orthopedic Institute of New Jersey
222 High Street/Suite 202   Newton, NJ 07840   (908)684-3005   Fax (908)684-3301

White, Melvin C., MD {1851498588} ClCdEl, CdvDis, IntrMd(76,PA09)
+ Atlantic Heart Rhythm Center
415 Chris Gaupp Drive/Suite C   Galloway, NJ 08205
(609)748-7580   Fax (609)748-7574

White, Robert M., MD {1427155167} RadDia, RadNro(84,PA01)<NJ-OURLADY, NJ-COOPRUMC>
+ Lourdes Imaging Associates, PA
218-A Sunset Road   Willingboro, NJ 08046   (609)835-3070   Fax (609)835-3190
+ Lourdes Imaging Associates, PA
1600 Haddon Avenue   Camden, NJ 08103   (609)835-3070   Fax (856)668-8436

White, Ronald A., MD {1154393056} SrgC&R, Surgry(81,MA05)<NJ-ENGLWOOD, NJ-VALLEY>
+ Drs. White & Waxenbaum
216 Engle Street/Suite 203   Englewood, NJ 07631
(201)567-7615   Fax (201)567-8033
+ Drs. White & Waxenbaum
127 Union Street/Suite 112   Ridgewood, NJ 07450
(201)567-7615   Fax (201)493-1718

White, Sanford F., MD {1609966076} ObsGyn(78,NY09)<NJ-STPETER, NJ-RWJUBRUN>
+ B 4 Cornwall Court
East Brunswick, NJ 08816   (732)698-1115   Fax (732)698-1366

White, Thomas M., DO {1598745028} CdvDis(89,IA75)<NJ-OCEANMC, NJ-JRSYSHMC>
+ Coastal Cardiovascular Consultants, PA
459 Jack Martin Boulevard/Suite 4   Brick, NJ 08724
(732)458-6200   Fax (732)458-9464

+ Coastal Cardiovascular Consultants, PA
1930 Highway 35/Suite 3   Wall, NJ 07719   (732)458-6200   Fax (732)974-8609

Whiteman, Martin, DO {1588633903} Nrolgy(89,NY75)<NJ-KIMBALL>
+ 217 Falling Oaks Road
Toms River, NJ 08753   (732)206-5531

Whiteru, Uvie Christina, MD {1114366044} Anesth
+ Hoboken University Medical Center
308 Willow Avenue   Hoboken, NJ 07030   (201)418-1000

Whiting, Philip Howard, DO {1568450658} FamMed(00,ME75)
+ Virtua Family Health Center
1000 Atlantic Avenue   Camden, NJ 08104   (856)246-3542   Fax (856)246-3528

Whitley, Markus A., MD {1740281013} NuclMd, RadDia(84,NY01)
+ South Jersey Radiology Associates, P.A.
748 Kings Highway   West Deptford, NJ 08096   (856)848-4998   Fax (856)853-7362
+ South Jersey Radiology Associates, P.A.
Severan Profess Mews/Suite 105   Sewell, NJ 08080
(856)848-4998   Fax (856)589-6142
+ SJRA South Jersey Radiology Associates, P.A.
113 East Laurel Road   Stratford, NJ 08096   (856)566-2552

Whitley, Ronda M., MD {1043650278} IntrMd(95,TN07)
+ One Path Plaza/Concourse
Jersey City, NJ 07306   (201)216-6696   Fax (201)216-6694

Whitley-Williams, Patricia, MD {1639230543} PedInf, Pedtrc(75,MD07)<NJ-RWJUBRUN>
+ UH- Robert Wood Johnson Med
125 Paterson Street/MEB 306   New Brunswick, NJ 08901
(732)235-7894   Fax (732)235-7419
+ RWJ University Hospital New Brunswick
One Robert Wood Johnson Place   New Brunswick, NJ 08901
(732)235-7894

Whitman, Eric David, MD {1609840636} Surgry, IntrMd(85,PA14)<NJ-MORRISTN, NJ-OVERLOOK>
+ Atlantic Surgical Oncology
100 Madison Avenue   Morristown, NJ 07960   (973)971-7111   Fax (973)397-2901

Whitman, Marc S., MD {1386780195} InfDis, IntrMd(88,NJ06)<NJ-CHSFULD, NJ-CHSMRCER>
+ Capital Health Infectious Disease Specialists
40 Fuld Street/Suite 305   Trenton, NJ 08638   (609)394-6338   Fax (609)394-6328
+ Early Intervention Services
413 Hillcrest Avenue/Bldg. 413   Trenton, NJ 08618
(609)538-0025

Whitman, Sarah Marie, MD {1659422103} Psychy, IntrMd(87,NY45)
+ Rowan University Student Health Center
201 Mullica Hill Road   Glassboro, NJ 08028   (856)256-4333   Fax (856)256-4427

Whitney, Julie Sherman, DO {1568555357} Pedtrc, PedEmg, EmrgEMed(00,NY75)<NJ-COOPRUMC>
+ Dr Julie Sherman Whitney and Assoc
325 Marlton Pike East   Cherry Hill, NJ 08034   (856)528-5370
+ Cooper University Hospital
One Cooper Plaza/PediEmrgMed   Camden, NJ 08103
(856)342-2000

Whittingham, Jennifer J., MD {1487881298} Anesth(94,NJ06)<NJ-WARREN>
+ Warren Hospital
185 Roseberry Street/Anesth   Phillipsburg, NJ 08865
(908)859-6700

Whittington, Wendy Louise, MD {1639145238} Pedtrc(90,NJ05)<NJ-NWTNMEM, NJ-MORRISTN>
+ Wellness Center Pediatrics LLC
21 Lafayette Road/Suite F   Sparta, NJ 07871   (973)726-4455   Fax (973)726-8445

Whitworth, Jeffrey Michael, MD {1144269440} Dermat, DerHar, DerMOH(93,OK01)
+ Atlantic Dermatology Associates LLC
1031 McBride Avenue/Suite D-203   Little Falls, NJ 07424
(973)256-6350   Fax (973)256-7388
+ Atlantic Dermatology Associates LLC
110 Passaic Avenue/1st Floor   Passaic, NJ 07055   (973)256-6350   Fax (973)256-7388

Whyte, Peta-Gaye Kenisha, DO {1598268526} Pedtrc
+ University Medical Group Pediatrics
125 Paterson Street/MEB 3rd Fl   New Brunswick, NJ 08903
(732)235-7883   Fax (732)235-7345

Wichman, Paul H., MD {1760534879} IntrMd(79,MEX14)
+ 39 Maple Avenue
Netcong, NJ 07857   (973)347-4121   Fax (973)347-1545

Widdess-Walsh, Peter Patrick, MD {1316055742} Nrolgy, ClNrPh(98,IRE03)<NJ-STBARNMC>
+ St. Barnabas Institute of Neurology & Neurosurgery
200 South Orange Avenue/Suite 101   Livingston, NJ 07039
(973)322-7580   Fax (973)322-7505

Widman, David, MD {1821168816} Rheuma, IntrMd(75,MA01)<NJ-MORRISTN>
+ Atlantic Health Weight & Wellness Center @ MMC
435 South Street/Suite 220-B   Morristown, NJ 07960
(973)540-9198   Fax (973)540-1614

Widmann, Mark Dennis, MD {1982674248} SrgThr, Surgry(87,CT01)
+ North Jersey Thoracic Surgical Associates, P.C.
100 Madison Avenue/PO Box 1348   Morristown, NJ 07962
(973)644-4844   Fax (973)644-4776

Widmann, Roger Franklin, MD {1649298977} PedOrt, SrgOrt, IntrMd(89,CT01)
+ HSS Paramus Outpatient Center
140 East Ridgewood Avenue/Suite 175-S   Paramus, NJ 07652   (201)796-2255   Fax (201)796-3711

Widroff, Jacob S., MD {1376764928}
+ 1803 Jason Drive
Cinnaminson, NJ 08077   (914)582-6218
jacobwidroff@yahoo.com

Widuri, Srie, MD {1548525066}
+ 8 Vauxhall Road
East Brunswick, NJ 08816   (732)698-2798
wids2012@gmail.com

Wieder, Robert, MD {1073692208} IntrMd, MedOnc, OncHem(83,NY47)<NJ-UMDNJ>
+ University Hospital
150 Bergen Street   Newark, NJ 07103   (973)972-5108   Fax (973)972-8390
+ 330 South Chestnut Street
Westfield, NJ 07090

Wiederholz, Matthias Heinz, MD {1336327279} PhysMd(03,NJ06)
+ Performance Spine & Sports Medicine
4056 Quakerbridge Road/Suite 111   Lawrenceville, NJ 08648   (609)588-8600   Fax (609)588-8602

Wiederhorn, Noel M., MD {1093716359} Pedtrc(69,NY09)<NJ-VALLEY, NJ-HACKNSK>
+ Pedimedica PA
43 Yawpo Avenue/Suite 9   Oakland, NJ 07436   (201)405-0800   Fax (201)337-5585

Wiederkehr, Michael, MD {1396759783} Dermat(98,MD07)
+ Center for Dermatology & Skin Surgery, LLC
1 West Ridgewood Avenue/Suite 103   Paramus, NJ 07652
(201)857-4200   Fax (201)857-4199

Wiedermann, Joseph Gad, MD {1952334542} CdvDis, IntrMd, IntCrd(84,NY01)<NJ-JRSYSHMC, NJ-HACKNSK>
+ Interventional Cardiovascular Associates, P.A.
2 Sears Drive   Paramus, NJ 07653   (201)996-1444   Fax (201)646-9204

Wien, Frederic E., MD {1639141054} Gastrn, Grtrcs, IntrMd(78,BELG)<NJ-HACKNSK, NJ-VALLEY>
+ Wien Medical Group
30 West Century Road/Suite 240   Paramus, NJ 07652
(201)265-7001   Fax (201)265-7078
+ Wien Medical Group
625 Broadway   Paterson, NJ 07514   (201)265-7001   Fax (973)742-2297

Wiener, Craig B., MD {1801886148} ObsGyn, IntrMd(88,NJ05)<NJ-VALLEY, NJ-HACKNSK>
+ 555 Kindermack Road/Suite 5
Oradell, NJ 07649   (201)262-0075   Fax (201)262-9440

Wiener, Ethan Saul, MD {1184614968} Pedtrc, PedEmg(96,PA12)<NJ-MORRISTN>
+ Morristown Medical Center
100 Madison Avenue/EmrgMed   Morristown, NJ 07962
(973)971-5000

Wiener, Howard E., MD {1831226307} Pedtrc(71,NY46)<NJ-STPETER, NJ-RWJUBRUN>
+ New Brunswick Pediatric Group, P.A.
1300 How Lane   North Brunswick, NJ 08902   (732)247-1510   Fax (732)247-8885

Wiener, Jaclyn Faye, DO {1295053056} Pedtrc
+ Summit Medical Group
75 East Northfield Road/Pediatrics   Livingston, NJ 07039
(973)436-1540   Fax (908)673-7336

Wiener, Michael I., DO {1922091370} FamMed(77,PA77)<NJ-VALLEY>
+ Drs. Wiener & Pagano
299 Market Street   Saddle Brook, NJ 07663   (201)368-1717   Fax (201)368-9618

Wierzbicki, Jonathan Edmund, MD {1104801331} FamMed, IntrMd(97,PA13)<NJ-HUNTRDN>
+ Premier Family Medicine
5 Walter East Foran Boulevard   Flemington, NJ 08822
(908)824-7179   Fax (908)824-7684

Physicians by Name and Address

Wiesen, Mark, MD {1053367912} EnDbMt, IntrMd(75,NY01)<NJ-HACKNSK, NJ-HOLYNAME>
+ Diabetes Endocrinology Metabolism Specialities PA
  870 Palisade Avenue/Suite 203   Teaneck, NJ 07666   (201)836-5655   Fax (201)836-3571
+ Diabetes Endocrinology Metabolism Specialities PA
  6 Brighton Road/Suite 103   Clifton, NJ 07012   (201)836-5655   Fax (973)470-8188

Wiesen, Robert S., MD {1437103678} IntrMd, Gastrn(00,ISR02)
+ Gastromed HealthCare, PA
  25 Monroe Street   Bridgewater, NJ 08807   (908)231-1999   Fax (908)231-1612
+ Gastromed HealthCare PA
  203 Towne Centre Drive   Hillsborough, NJ 08844   (908)359-1639

Wiggins, Ernest Flowers, III, MD {1972759025} RadDia, RadV&I(02,PA09)<NJ-MONMOUTH>
+ Monmouth Medical Center
  300 Second Avenue/Radiology   Long Branch, NJ 07740   (732)222-5200

Wignayaratne, Kanagarayer R., MD {1891856027} IntrMd, PthACl(67,SRI02)<NJ-BAYONNE>
+ Drs. Wignarajan and Wignarajan
  875 Kennedy Boulevard   Bayonne, NJ 07002   (201)339-1035   Fax (201)858-3350

Wignarajan, Nadika V., MD {1386877819} IntrMd
+ Drs. Wignarajan and Wignarajan
  875 Kennedy Boulevard   Bayonne, NJ 07002   (201)339-1035   Fax (201)858-3350

Wijaya, Don H., MD {1295008373} Psychy
+ St. Francis Medical Center
  601 Hamilton Avenue   Trenton, NJ 08629   (609)599-5180

Wijayaratne, Madhavi, MD {1568570679} Pedtrc(86,SRI01)<NJ-CLARMAAS>
+ 5 Franklin Avenue/Suite 409
  Belleville, NJ 07109   (973)751-1112

Wilcenski, Michael A., MD {1164415733} Anesth, AnesPain(91,NY08)
+ Union Anesthesia & Pain Management
  695 Chestnut Street   Union, NJ 07083   (908)851-8602   Fax (908)851-8758

Wilchfort, Samuel D., MD CdvDis, IntrMd(75,NY46)
+ 125 Madison Avenue
  Englewood, NJ 07631

Wilcox, Ellis I., MD {1497829634} IntrMd, PulDis(83,GRN01)<NJ-HOBUNIMC, NJ-MEADWLND>
+ Hudson Physicians Associates
  40 Union Avenue/Suite 204   Irvington, NJ 07111   (973)416-6981   Fax (973)375-5766

Wilczynski, Frank L., DO {1992876023} FamMed(77,PA77)
+ Concentra Medical Centers Urgent Care
  817 East Gate Drive/Suite 102   Mount Laurel, NJ 08054   (856)778-1090   Fax (856)778-9191

Wild, David Marc, MD {1013112671} CdvDis, IntrMd(02,NJ02)
+ Cardiovascular Associates of Teaneck
  954 Teaneck Road   Teaneck, NJ 07666   (201)833-2300   Fax (201)833-7600

Wild, William A., DO {1700820396} EmrgMd(99,PA77)<NJ-OURLADY>
+ Our Lady of Lourdes Medical Center
  1600 Haddon Avenue/EmrgMed   Camden, NJ 08103   (856)757-3500

Wilderman, Michael Jeffrey, MD {1497802938} Surgry, SrgVas(01,PA01)
+ Bergen Surgical Specialists
  20 Prospect Avenue/Suite 707   Hackensack, NJ 07601   (201)343-0040   Fax (201)343-2733

Wilding, Todd Meredith, MD {1992927859} Addctn, Psychy(84,NY06)
+ 7 Macculloch Avenue/2nd Floor
  Morristown, NJ 07960   (973)644-3550   Fax (973)644-3557

Wildman, Joseph M., MD {1114995941} OncHem, IntrMd(71,NY19)
+ 65 East Northfield Road/Suite A
  Livingston, NJ 07039   (973)422-0023   Fax (973)422-0033

Wilen, Daniel, DO {1154702363}<NJ-COOPRUMC>
+ Cooper University Hospital
  One Cooper Plaza   Camden, NJ 08103   (856)342-3150

Wiley, Joan C., DO {1235384405} PulDis, IntrMd(08,NJ75)
+ Kennedy Hospitalist Office
  435 Hurffville Cross Keys Road   Turnersville, NJ 08012   (856)513-4124   Fax (856)302-5932
+ Kennedy Health Alliance Vascular Surgery
  333 Laurel Oak Road   Voorhees, NJ 08043   (856)513-4124   Fax (856)770-9194

Wiley, Olga V., MD {1184994253} FamMed, IntrMd(10,NJ05)
+ Primary & Specialty Care at Edison
  10 Parsonage Road/Suite 410   Edison, NJ 08837   (732)452-0680   Fax (732)636-3669

Wilgucki, John D., DO {1457418642} Ophthl(87,ME75)
+ 1500 Saint Georges Avenue/Unit D
  Avenel, NJ 07001   (732)388-3030   Fax (732)388-3528

Wilkenfeld, Craig, MD {1194828905} CdvDis, CarNuc, IntrMd(86,NY19)<NJ-ENGLWOOD>
+ Englewood Cardiology Consultants
  177 North Dean Street/Suite 100   Englewood, NJ 07631   (201)569-4901   Fax (201)569-6111
+ Englewood Cardiology Consultants
  200 Grand Avenue/Suite 202   Englewood, NJ 07631   (201)569-4901

Wilkerson, Eric Christopher, MD {1841556396} Dermat
+ Hackensack University Medical Center
  20 Prospect Avenue/Suite 702   Hackensack, NJ 07601   (201)441-9890

Wilkerson, Zachary, DO {1194166215} EmrgMd<NJ-SJHREGMC>
+ SJH Regional Medical Center
  1505 West Sherman Avenue   Vineland, NJ 08360   (856)641-8000

Wilkes, Adam L., MD {1407828460}
+ 411 Society Hill Boulevard
  Cherry Hill, NJ 08003   (856)325-0351
  awilkesmd@gmail.com

Wilkes, Kristen, MD {1043553738} EmrgMd<NJ-JRSYCITY>
+ Jersey City Medical Center
  355 Grand Street   Jersey City, NJ 07304   (201)915-2000

Wilkin, Daniel James, DO {1922092121} FamMed(02,PA77)
+ Bergen Primary Care Associates
  680 Kinderkamack Road/Suite 205   Emerson, NJ 07630   (201)262-0608   Fax (201)262-8689

Wilkins, Charles E., MD {1609828383} SrgOrt(65,PA02)<NJ-VIRTVOOR>
+ 146 Lakeview Drive/Suite 301
  Gibbsboro, NJ 08026   (856)784-1111   Fax (856)784-1132

Wilkins, John J., DO {1154438786} Psychy(86,MO78)<NJ-HAMPTBHC, NJ-CAPITLHS>
+ Hampton Behavioral Health Center
  650 Rancocas Road   Westampton, NJ 08060   (609)267-7000

Wilkins, Kirsten Bass, MD {1811968548} Surgry, SrgC&R(94,MD07)<NJ-JFKMED>
+ Associated Colon & Rectal Surgeons PA
  3900 Park Avenue/Suite 101   Edison, NJ 08820   (732)494-6640   Fax (732)549-8204
+ Associated Colon & Rectal Surgeons, PA
  One Penn Plaza/Ferren Mall-Lower Level   New Brunswick, NJ 08901   (973)679-4664

Wilkinson, Edmund, DO {1912987389} IntrMd(93,NJ75)<NJ-KMHTURNV>
+ Kennedy Health Systems/Washington Township Campus
  435 Hurffville-Cross Keys Road   Turnersville, NJ 08012   (856)218-5634

Wilks, Michelle Anne, MD {1689737082} FamMed(00,NY46)<NJ-JFKMED>
+ JFK Family Practice Group
  65 James Street   Edison, NJ 08818   (732)321-7488   Fax (732)906-4927

Willard, Mary A., MD {1336138007} FamMed(75,PA07)<NJ-VIRTVOOR>
+ Tatem Brown Family Practice
  2225 East Evesham Road/Suite 101   Voorhees, NJ 08043   (856)795-4330   Fax (856)325-3704

Willard, Scott David, MD {1497047096} PedRad
+ Nemours Dupont Pediatrics
  325 Route 70 East   Cherry Hill, NJ 08034   (856)309-8508   Fax (856)309-8556

Willems-Plakyda, Michele C., MD {1437222478} Pedtrc, Ped-Dvl(97,NJ06)<NJ-HUNTRDN>
+ Hunterdon Medical Center
  2100 Wescott Drive/Dev Pediatrics   Flemington, NJ 08822   (908)788-6100   Fax (908)788-2578

Willenborg, Ronald, MD {1801897897} FamMed(77,NJ05)
+ 543 Valley Road
  Upper Montclair, NJ 07043   (973)746-6466   Fax (973)746-0312

Willett, Laura R., MD {1821163452} IntrMd(83,CA02)
+ UH- Robert Wood Johnson Med
  125 Paterson Street/CAB/Intrnl Mdcn   New Brunswick, NJ 08901   (732)235-6968

Williams, Alice, MD {1619235843} Ophthl
+ Eye Associates
  251 South Lincoln Avenue   Vineland, NJ 08361   (856)691-8188   Fax (856)691-0421

Williams, Arnold A., MD {1588801518}<NJ-COMMED, NJ-ST-BARNMC>
+ St. Barnabas Behavioral Health Center
  1691 US Highway 9   Toms River, NJ 08755   (732)886-4474
+ Community Medical Center
  99 Route 37 West/Emerg Med   Toms River, NJ 08755   (732)886-4474   Fax (732)557-4015

Williams, Celia, DO {1881989770} Pedtrc(NY75<NJ-HACKNSK, NJ-HOLYNAME>
+ Riverside Medical Group
  714 Tenth Street/Suite 2   Secaucus, NJ 07094   (201)863-3346   Fax (201)865-0015
+ Riverside Medical Group
  200 Main Street   Ridgefield Park, NJ 07660   (201)863-3346   Fax (201)870-6098

Williams, Delores J., MD {1235263120} ObsGyn(81,PA02)<NJ-CHSFULD, NJ-CHSMRCER>
+ Williams Medical Associates
  1245 Whitehorse Mercerville Rd   Trenton, NJ 08619   (609)581-8111   Fax (609)581-4673

Williams, Dione M., MD {1356437693} Otlryg, Otolgy(82,IL06)<NJ-NWRKBETH, NJ-EASTORNG>
+ 1787 Springfield Avenue
  Maplewood, NJ 07040   (973)761-8700   Fax (973)761-5942

Williams, Edward G., Jr., MD {1306831623} CdvDis, IntrMd(64,NY01)
+ Union County Cardiology Associates, P.A.
  1317 Morris Avenue   Union, NJ 07083   (908)964-9370   Fax (908)964-9332

Williams, Edwin Rae, MD {1497714083} EmrgMd(89,NC05)
+ Virtua Immediate Care Center
  239 Hurffville Crosskeys Road   Sewell, NJ 08080   (856)341-8200   Fax (856)341-8215

Williams, Eric James, MD {1699718064} IntrMd(96,NJ05)
+ Capital Health Primary Care
  1230 Parkway Avenue/Suite 203   Ewing, NJ 08628   (609)883-5454   Fax (609)883-2564
+ West Trenton Medical Associates
  1230 Parkway Avenue/Suite 203   Trenton, NJ 08638   (609)883-5454   Fax (609)883-2565

Williams, Errol Baldwin, MD {1366456519} CdvDis(90,MA05)<NJ-MTNSIDE>
+ Cardiovascular Health Associates of New Jersey LLC
  799 Bloomfield Avenue/Suite 112   Verona, NJ 07044   (973)239-2323   Fax (973)239-7556

Williams, Estelle Vaughns, MD {1336168004} EmrgMd(99,NJ06)
+ 190 Grove Street
  Montclair, NJ 07042

Williams, Fred W., MD {1679565782} ObsGyn(78,MA05)<NJ-CHSMRCER, NJ-CHSFULD>
+ 1450 Parkside Avenue/Suite 10
  Trenton, NJ 08638   (609)406-1250   Fax (609)406-1249
  DrFred8519@prodigy.net

Williams, Frederick M., MD IntrMd(78,DC03)
+ Concentra Medical Centers
  210 Benigno Boulevard   Bellmawr, NJ 08031   (856)931-0691   Fax (856)931-9253

Williams, James R., MD {1497753594} InfDis, IntrMd(80,DC03)
+ Kennedy Wound Care Center
  2211 Chapel Avenue West/Suite 404   Cherry Hill, NJ 08002   (856)922-5010   Fax (856)922-0515

Williams, Jeffrey Franklin, MD {1225007438} Surgry, Urolgy(95,NJ06)
+ NJ Urology
  799 Bloomfield Avenue/Suite 300   Verona, NJ 07044   (973)429-0462   Fax (973)429-8765
+ Drs. Murphy & Williams, P.A.
  104 North Euclid Avenue   Westfield, NJ 07090   (973)429-0462   Fax (908)654-1993
+ Drs. Murphy & Williams, P.A.
  33 Overlook Road/Suite 412   Summit, NJ 07044   (908)273-7274

Williams, Jill M., MD {1366542565} Psychy, PsyAdd(93,NJ06)<NJ-UNIVBHC>
+ University Behavioral Health Care
  671 Hoes Lane/PO Box 1392/D339   Piscataway, NJ 08855   (732)235-5500   Fax (732)235-4277

Williams, John A., MD {1720092109} PsyAdd, Psychy(86,TX15)<NJ-VALYONS>
+ VA New Jersey Health Care System at Lyons
  151 Knollcroft Road/Psych   Lyons, NJ 07939   (908)647-0180   Fax (908)604-5251

Williams, John Michael, MD {1457389678} Dermat, IntrMd(99,PA09)
+ The Skin Care and Surgery Center
  33 Overlook Road/Suite 202   Summit, NJ 07901   (908)598-1300   Fax (908)598-1301

Williams, John Morgan, MD {1538167663} SrgOrt
+ Coordinated Health
  222 Red Lane   Phillipsburg, NJ 08865   (610)861-8080   Fax (610)849-1013

Williams, Juliette Marie, MD {1174777429} FamMed
+ St. Mary Center for Family Health
  122-132 Clinton Street   Hoboken, NJ 07030   (201)418-3126   Fax (201)418-3148

Williams, Karen Lynn, MD {1710911391} FamMed(04,IN20)
+ Hickory Run Family Practice Associates
  384 County Road 513   Califon, NJ 07830   (908)832-2125   Fax (908)832-6149

Williams, Keith Patrick, MD {1487684973} MtFtMd, ObsGyn(79,WIN01)
+ Rowan SOM Department of Ob/Gyn
405 Hurffville-Cross Keys Road Sewell, NJ 08080 (856)589-1414 Fax (856)256-5772

Williams, Kristina, MD {1922426485} Obstet
+ Ripa Center for Women's Health & Wellness
6100 Main Street Voorhees, NJ 08043 (856)325-6600 Fax (856)673-4497

Williams, Krystle Michelle, MD {1477782118} PhysMd<NJ-JFKMED>
+ JFK Medical Center
65 James Street Edison, NJ 08820 (732)321-7000

Williams, Marcus L., MD {1467526525} CdvDis, IntrMd, IntCrd(82,DC01)<NJ-CHILTON, NJ-VALLEY>
+ Cardiac Associates of North Jersey
43 Yawpo Avenue/Suite 2 Oakland, NJ 07436 (201)337-0066 Fax (201)337-7417
+ 10-14 Saddle River Road
Fair Lawn, NJ 07410 (201)337-0066 Fax (201)703-1100

Williams, Perry Swintz, MD {1932177268} RadOnc(89,NY09)<NJ-WESTHDSN, NJ-CHILTON>
+ 15 North 5th Street/Suite 104
Saddle Brook, NJ 07663 (732)901-7314 Fax (732)901-5704

Williams, Raashan Carlos, MD {1851310726} IntrMd, IntCrd, CdvDis(99,PA13)<NJ-CHRIST, NJ-MEADWLND>
+ Raashan Carlos Williams MD FACC LLC
120 48th Street Union City, NJ 07087 (201)758-8000 Fax (201)758-8003
+ Total Cardiology Care
120 Franklin Street Jersey City, NJ 07307 (201)758-8000 Fax (201)216-1362

Williams, Richard A., MD {1699755520} Surgry(71,MI07)<NJ-BAYONNE>
+ 964 Avenue C
Bayonne, NJ 07002 (201)437-2772 Fax (201)437-4372

Williams, Robert H., Jr., MD {1457409492} FamMed, EmrgMd(77,PA02)<NJ-ACMCITY>
+ Williams Family Practice
415 Chris Gaupp Drive Galloway, NJ 08205 (609)652-2033 Fax (609)652-3318

Williams, Robert M., MD {1467469171} FamMed, Grtrcs, SprtMd(80,VA01)<NJ-VIRTVOOR>
+ 100 Kingston Avenue
Barrington, NJ 08007 (856)547-1177 Fax (856)547-2509

Williams, Shauna F., MD {1306008859} ObsGyn(02,NJ05)
+ Rutgers- New Jersey Medical School
185 South Orange Avenue Newark, NJ 07103 (973)972-5262 Fax (973)972-4574

Williams, Stephen Joseph, MD {1184690190} IntrMd, InfDis(98,MO03)<NJ-STCLRDOV, NJ-STCLRDEN>
+ ID Associates PA/dba ID Care
765 Route 10 East/Suite 201 Randolph, NJ 07869 (973)989-0068 Fax (973)361-8955
+ ID Associates PA/dba ID Care
8 Saddle Road Cedar Knolls, NJ 07927 (973)989-0068 Fax (973)993-5953

Williams, Tanishia Alise, MD {1861625907} PedNrD
+ 3575 Quakerbridge Road
Trenton, NJ 08619 (732)258-7065

Williams-Martin, Pamela Y., MD {1831312065} Psychy, PssoMd(91,NJ05)<NJ-NWRKBETH>
+ Mental Health Clinic of Passaic
111 Lexington Avenue Passaic, NJ 07055 (973)471-8006 Fax (973)471-1630
+ Newark Beth Israel Medical Center/School Services
21 Uitman Street Newark, NJ 07103 (973)824-0806

Williams-Phillips, Jacqueline A., MD {1043371966} PedCrC, Pedtrc, IntrMd(87,NY09)<NJ-RWJUBRUN>
+ RWJ University Hospital New Brunswick
One Robert Wood Johnson Place New Brunswick, NJ 08901 (732)235-7900

Williamson, Judith S., MD {1114019676} IntrMd, Grtrcs(86,DC02)<NJ-CHSMRCER>
+ Capital Health Medical Group
One Capital Way Pennington, NJ 08534 (609)303-4000

Williamson, Shirnett Karean, MD {1083785042} RadOnc(91,DC03)<NJ-CHSMRCER>
+ Capital Health Radiation Oncology Department
One Capital Way Pennington, NJ 08534 (609)304-4244 Fax (609)303-4156

Willis, Alexander R., MD {1073878088}<NJ-MONMOUTH>
+ Monmouth Medical Center
300 Second Avenue Long Branch, NJ 07740 (732)923-6784 Fax (732)923-7247

Willis, Andrew Albert, MD {1154412187} SrgOrt, SprtMd(97,NY01)
+ Tri-County Orthopedics
160 East Hanover Avenue Morristown, NJ 07962 (973)538-2334 Fax (973)829-9174

Willis, Karen Christine, MD {1699830547} Pedtrc(02,OH41)<MA-NEMEDCEN>
+ Morristown Medical Center
100 Madison Avenue Morristown, NJ 07962 (973)971-7550 Fax (973)290-2388

Willis, Kenneth W., MD {1356431696} Psychy(78,NH01)<NJ-UNVMCPRN>
+ Eating Disorder Center of Princeton
168 Tamarack Circle Skillman, NJ 08558 (609)497-1560 Fax (609)497-7670
SKIMD111@aol.com

Willis, Kevin, MD {1174510937} RadDia(98,NJ06)<NJ-COMMED, NJ-SOCEANCO>
+ Community Medical Center
99 Route 37 West/Radiology Toms River, NJ 08755 (732)557-8000 Fax (732)557-2064
+ Coastal Imaging, LLC
79 Route 37 West/Suite 103 Toms River, NJ 08755 (732)557-8000 Fax (732)276-2325

Willis, Rudolph C., MD {1104887819} FamMed(82,NJ06)<NJ-EASTORNG>
+ 12 Krotik Place
Irvington, NJ 07111 (973)373-3000

Willis, Stephen Laird, MD {1629139076} Gastrn, IntrMd(98,NJ06)
+ Advanced Gastroenterology & Nutrition
1100 Wescott Drive/Suite 304 Flemington, NJ 08822 (908)788-4022 Fax (908)788-4066
+ Advanced Gastroenterology & Nutrition
1738 Route 31 North/Suite 108 Clinton, NJ 08809 (908)788-4022 Fax (908)788-4066

Willis, William John, MD {1700882180} Anesth(88,MNT01)
+ 15 Fox Run
Sparta, NJ 07871
+ Montclair Anesthesia Associates PC
185 Fairfield Avenue/Suite 2A West Caldwell, NJ 07006 Fax (973)226-1232

Willman, Kelly Marie, MD {1013177153} SrgCrC, Surgry(05,NY15)<NJ-ACMCITY>
+ AtlantiCare Regional Medical Center/City Campus
1925 Pacific Avenue/Surgery/Trauma Atlantic City, NJ 08401 (609)441-8023 Fax (609)441-8178

Willman, Margaret A., DO {1376604222} Psychy(77,MI12)
+ Drenk Behavioral Health Center
795 Woodlane Road/Suite 301 Mount Holly, NJ 08060 (609)267-1377 Fax (609)265-9268

Willner, Joseph Harrison, MD {1295703312} Nrolgy(70,NY19)<NJ-MEADWLND, NJ-HACKNSK>
+ Bergen Neurology Consultants
25 Rockwood Place/Suite 110 Englewood, NJ 07631 (201)894-5805 Fax (201)894-1956
jwillner@email.com

Willoughby, Ronald P., DO {1477582823} FamMed(84,PA77)<NJ-VIRTMHBC, NJ-KMHSTRAT>
+ Alliance for Better Care, P.C.
130 Lakehurst Road Browns Mills, NJ 08015 (609)893-3133 Fax (609)893-7972
+ Alliance for Better Care, P.C.
PO Box 1510 Medford, NJ 08055 (609)893-3133 Fax (609)953-8652

Willsie, Philip S., DO {1669710638}
+ Kennedy Hospitalist Office
435 Hurffville Cross Keys Road Turnersville, NJ 08012 (856)513-4124 Fax (856)302-5932
+ SOM - Department of Internal Medicine
42 East Laurel Road/Suite 3100 Stratford, NJ 08084 (856)513-4124 Fax (856)566-6952

Wilmot, Peter Clifford, DO {1093766875} Pedtrc, PedGst(99,PA78)<NJ-MORRISTN, NJ-OVERLOOK>
+ Overlook Medical Center
99 Beauvoir Avenue/PO Box 210 Summit, NJ 07902 (908)522-2000
+ Division of Pediatric GI at Goryeb
100 Madison Avenue/Box 82 Morristown, NJ 07962 (908)522-2000 Fax (973)290-7365

Wilmott, Annette Lynne, DO {1982011250} Pedtrc(PA78)
+ Monmouth Pediatric Group, P.A.
272 Broad Street Red Bank, NJ 07701 (732)741-0456 Fax (732)219-9477

Wilsey, Stephanie, MD {1700204617} EmrgMd
+ Cooper Univerisry Emergency Physicians
One Cooper Plaza Camden, NJ 08103 (856)342-2000 Fax (856)968-8272

Wilson, Alyson Nicole, DO {1184941833} EmrgMd<NJ-COOPRUMC>
+ Cooper University Hospital
One Cooper Plaza Camden, NJ 08103 (856)342-2000

Wilson, Bruce Leonard, MD {1457667487} CdvDis
+ Hamilton Cardiology Associates
2073 Klockner Road Hamilton, NJ 08690 (609)584-1212 Fax (609)584-0103

Wilson, David A., MD {1942238423} Radiol, NuclMd, RadDia(92,NJ05)<NJ-STBARNMC>
+ St. Barnabas Medical Center
94 Old Short Hills Road/Radiology Livingston, NJ 07039 (973)322-5000

Wilson, Donna E., DO {1740309582} OstMed, IntrMd(04,PA78)
+ Cape Atlantic Internal Medicine
518A Sea Isle Boulevard Ocean View, NJ 08230 (609)624-0070 Fax (609)624-0078

Wilson, Dorian J., MD {1700811494} Surgry, SrgTpl(82,NJ05)<NJ-UMDNJ>
+ Liver Transplant & Hepatobiliary Diseases/UMDNJ
140 Bergen Street/ACC Bldg Newark, NJ 07101 (973)972-7218

Wilson, Francis P., DO {1982669214} FamMed(73,MO79)<NJ-OCEANMC>
+ Cedar Bridge Medical Associates
985 Cedarbridge Avenue Brick, NJ 08723 (732)477-5600 Fax (732)477-1899

Wilson, George F., MD {1417056276} Psychy(68,NY09)<NJ-UNVMCPRN>
+ Princeton House Behavioral Health - Princeton
905 Herrontown Road Princeton, NJ 08540 (609)688-3714 Fax (609)497-2680

Wilson, Howard Marc, MD {1578590162} FamMed(76,SPA15)
+ Patient Centered Medical Associates PA
89 Valley Road Montclair, NJ 07042 (973)746-3400 Fax (973)746-6214

Wilson, James Ashley, II, MD {1467483750} ObsGyn, Gyneco(80,PA02)
+ Shore Physicians Group
213 West Avenue Ocean City, NJ 08226 (609)399-0700 Fax (609)399-0033
+ Shore Physicians Group
2605 Shore Road Northfield, NJ 08225 (609)399-0700 Fax (609)365-5301

Wilson, John Goss, Jr., MD {1124291612} GynOnc, ObsGyn, IntrMd(74,MEX03)<NJ-VIRTBERL, NJ-VIRTVOOR>
+ NaltrexZone, LLC.
1 South Centre Street/Suite 201 Merchantville, NJ 08109 (856)663-4447 Fax (856)488-6380

Wilson, John J., MD {1902855455} RadOnc(01,PA01)<NJ-VIRTVOOR>
+ Fox Chase Virtua Health Cancer Center
106 Carnie Boulevard/Suite A Voorhees, NJ 08043 (856)325-4830
+ Radiology Associates of Burlington County
1295 Route 38 West/PO Box 479 Hainesport, NJ 08036 (856)325-4830 Fax (609)261-4180

Wilson, John Joseph, MD {1861559528} Anesth(87,BWI01)<NJ-HUNTRDN>
+ Hunterdon Medical Center
2100 Wescott Drive/Anesthesia Flemington, NJ 08822 (908)788-6181 Fax (908)788-6145

Wilson, Justin B., MD {1831161850} IntrMd(87,DOM02)
+ Greystone Park Psychiatric Hospital
59 Koch Avenue/Internal Med Morris Plains, NJ 07950 (973)538-1800 Fax (973)889-8486

Wilson, Lynn Marie, DO {1619298973} FamMed(10,PA77)
+ Morristown Medical Center Family Medicine
435 South Street/Suite 220-A Morristown, NJ 07960 (973)971-4222 Fax (973)290-7050

Wilson, Sylvia V., MD {1457303174} Nrolgy(64,PA07)<NJ-JRSYSHMC>
+ 2 Smith Road/PO Box 4556
Toms River, NJ 08754 (732)341-3371 Fax (732)914-2011

Wilson, Vasthi Christensen, MD {1760548556} RadOnc(99,ENG09)<PA-PENNHOSP, NJ-SHOREMEM>
+ AtlantiCare Cancer Institute
2500 English Creek Avenue/Building 400 Egg Harbor Township, NJ 08234 (609)677-7777 Fax (609)677-7727
+ Shore Memorial Hospital
1 East New York Avenue/Rad Onc Somers Point, NJ 08244 (609)653-3500

Wilson Smith, Robin Renee', DO {1487747283} ObsGyn(99,NJ75)
+ Cooper Ob/Gyn
3 Cooper Plaza/Suite 300 Camden, NJ 08103 (856)342-2186 Fax (856)968-8575

Wilt, Jessie Swain, MD {1386723328} PulDis, IntrMd(96,NJ06)
+ Summit Medical Group-Berkeley Heights Campus
1 Diamond Hill Road Berkeley Heights, NJ 07922 (908)277-8674 Fax (908)277-8927

Wimalawansa, Sunil J., MD {1194811042} IntrMd, EnDbMt, OrtOst(75,SRI02)<NJ-RWJUBRUN>
+ UH- RWJ Medical School
One Robert Wood Johnson Place New Brunswick, NJ 08903 (732)235-7224 Fax (732)235-8610

Wimmer, Angela M., MD {1669427944} ObsGyn(94,NJ06)<NJ-ST-BARNMC, NJ-CLARMAAS>
+ Contemporary Women's Care
745 Northfield Avenue   West Orange, NJ 07052   (973)736-7700   Fax (973)736-8078
+ Contemporary Women's Care
338 Belleville Turnpike   Kearny, NJ 07032   (973)736-7700   Fax (201)998-4643

Wimmers, Eric Geoffrey, MD {1326373812} Surgry
+ The Plastic Surgery Ctr of NJ & Manhat
535 Sycamore Avenue   Shrewsbury, NJ 07702   (732)741-0970   Fax (732)747-2606

Win, Sithu, MD {1932427945} Pedtrc<NJ-HACKNSK, NJ-HOLY-NAME>
+ Riverside Medical Group
714 Tenth Street/Suite 2   Secaucus, NJ 07094   (201)863-3346   Fax (201)865-0015

Winant, John, Jr., MD {1235196262} Allrgy, Pedtrc, AlgyImmn(75,OH41)<NJ-UNVMCPRN>
+ 8 Quakerbridge Plaza
Trenton, NJ 08619   (609)890-8782   Fax (609)890-0025
Hsantos-martins@partners.org

Winarsky, Eric L., MD {1144303421} Otlryg(76,BEL03)<NJ-JRSYSHMC>
+ Eric Winarsky MD LLC
1131 Broad Street/Suite 102   Shrewsbury, NJ 07702   (732)389-2500   Fax (732)389-2820

Winchman, Heidi K., MD {1265418727} Radiol, RadDia(84,NY08)<NJ-STPETER, NJ-RWJUBRUN>
+ University Radiology Group, P.C.
483 Cranbury Road   East Brunswick, NJ 08816   (732)390-0030   Fax (732)390-5383
+ University Radiology Group, P.C.
10 Plum Street   New Brunswick, NJ 08901   (732)390-0030   Fax (732)249-1208

Windsor, Stephen J., MD {1902885122} OncHem(86,WIND)<NJ-MONMOUTH, NJ-JRSYSHMC>
+ Adult Medical Oncology-Hematology LLC
39 Sycamore Avenue   Little Silver, NJ 07739   (732)576-8610   Fax (732)576-8823

Winell, Jennifer Jo, MD {1548300817} PedOrt, SrgOrt(96,NY19)<NY-MNTFMOSE, NY-MNTFWEIL>
+ CHOP Specialty Care Center at Virtua
200 Bowman Drive/2 FL/Suite D-260   Voorhees, NJ 08043   (267)425-5400
+ CHOP Pediatric & Adolescent Specialty Care Center
1012 Laurel Oak Road   Voorhees, NJ 08043   (267)425-5400   Fax (856)435-0091

Winer, Steven A., MD {1194764126} IntrMd(82,GRN01)<NJ-VALLEY, NJ-HACKNSK>
+ Forest HealthCare Associates, PC
277 Forest Avenue/Suite 200   Paramus, NJ 07652   (201)986-1881   Fax (201)986-1871
+ The Valley Hospital
223 North Van Dien Avenue   Ridgewood, NJ 07450   (201)447-8000

Winetsky, Daniel Eric, MD {1023378312}
+ 1100 Woodbridge Road
Rahway, NJ 07065   (215)760-6307

Winfield, Barbara A., DO {1992898720} FamMed(96,NJ75)
+ 2301 East Evesham Road/Suite 102
Voorhees, NJ 08043
Bwinfield@yahoo.com

Winfield, Steven S., MD {1790858165} Ophthl(82,MI01)
+ 200 Gregory Avenue
Passaic, NJ 07055   (973)778-8439   Fax (973)777-1143

Winfree, Christopher Jules, MD {1013064948} Nrolgy, SrgNro(96,NY01)
+ Neurosurgeons of New Jersey
1200 East Ridgewood Avenue   Ridgewood, NJ 07450   (201)824-6131

Winfrey, Chris, MD {1093001588}
+ 1 Market Street/Apt 360
Camden, NJ 08102   (501)541-9255
chriswinfrey99@yahoo.com

Wingfield, Edward Anthony, MD {1164606034} IntrMd<NJ-RWJUHAM>
+ Hamilton Cardiology Associates
2073 Klockner Road   Hamilton, NJ 08690   (609)584-1212   Fax (609)584-0103

Winikoff, Stephen P., MD {1578561031} Anesth, Pedtrc(82,IL42)<NJ-STJOSHOS>
+ St. Joseph's Children's Hospital
703 Main Street/Anesthesiology   Paterson, NJ 07503   (973)754-2323   Fax (973)977-9455
Winikofs@SJHMC.org

Winikor, Jared, MD {1952644452} Pedtrc
+ Princeton Nassau Pediatrics, P.A.
301 North Harrison Street   Princeton, NJ 08540   (609)924-5510   Fax (609)924-3577

Wininger, Eric Amiel, MD {1750489340} EnDbMt, IntrMd(99,NY19)<NJ-CENTRAST>
+ Endocrinology Associates of Central NJ
501 Iron Bridge Road/Suite 12   Freehold, NJ 07728   (732)780-0002   Fax (732)308-0117

Wininger, Jon G., MD {1417915943} Dermat(73,NY47)<NJ-RWJU-RAH, NJ-RBAYOLDB>
+ Central Jersey Skin Care Associates, PA
1125 St. Georges Avenue   Rahway, NJ 07065   (732)499-0440   Fax (732)499-0225
+ Central Jersey Skin Care Associates, PA
260 Hobart Street   Perth Amboy, NJ 08861   (732)442-2700

Winn, Robert Jerald, MD {1629096821} FamMed
+ 575 Haddon Avenue/Unit 1
Collingswood, NJ 08108   (856)656-6859   Fax (856)240-1102

Winn, Terrance T., MD {1538336557} AnesPain, IntrMd(03,NY15)
+ Angel Pain Management
3 Hospital Plaza/Suite 313   Old Bridge, NJ 08857   (732)360-1800   Fax (732)360-1807

Winne, Richard P., Jr., MD {1134125743} Anesth, PainMd(87,NJ05)<NJ-MORRISTN>
+ New Jersey Pain Consultants
95 Madison Avenue/Suite 402   Morristown, NJ 07960   (973)971-6824   Fax (973)290-7683
+ New Jersey Pain Consultants
310 Madison Avenue/Suite 301   Morristown, NJ 07960   (973)971-6824   Fax (973)998-9201

Winograd, Barbara H., MD {1750442216} PsyCAd, Psychy(87,NJ06)
+ 320 Amboy Avenue/Suite 1
Metuchen, NJ 08840   (732)548-0482   Fax (732)548-2942

Winograd, Jonathan Isaac, DO {1023038346} EmrgMd(99,PA77)<NJ-STBARNMC>
+ St. Barnabas Medical Center
94 Old Short Hills Road/Emerg Med   Livingston, NJ 07039   (973)322-5000
+ Emergency Medical Associates of NJ, P.A.
3 Century Drive   Parsippany, NJ 07054   (973)322-5000   Fax (973)740-9895

Winston, Maryana, MD {1396838132} Pedtrc(99,GRN01)<NJ-VALLEY>
+ 128 Spring Hill Circle
Wayne, NJ 07470

Winter, Howard J., MD {1689676454} Surgry, SrgC&R(74,NY46)<NJ-VIRTUAHS>
+ Regional Surgical Associates
502 Centennial Boulevard/Suite 7   Voorhees, NJ 08043   (856)596-7440   Fax (856)596-6723

Winter, Ivan David, MD {1265788053} AdmMgt, IntrMd(84,MEXI)
+ 9226 Kennedy Boulevard/Flr 2
North Bergen, NJ 07047   (201)863-3055   Fax (201)863-5744

Winter, Jonathan M., MD {1922028950} Dermat, IntrMd(84,NY46)<NJ-KMHTURNV>
+ Dermatology Center of Washington Township
100 Kings Way East/Suite A-3   Sewell, NJ 08080   (856)589-3331   Fax (856)589-3416
jonathan.winter@addictionpain.com

Winter, Rebecca Cooper, MD {1407016280} PedRad(08,PA02)
+ Radiology Affiliates of Central New Jersey, P.A.
2501 Kuser Road   Hamilton, NJ 08691   (609)585-8800   Fax (609)585-1825

Winter, Robin O., MD {1295896157} FamMed, Grtrcs(78,NY46)
+ JFK Family Practice Group
65 James Street/FamPrc   Edison, NJ 08818   (732)321-7487   Fax (732)906-4927

Winters, Brian Seth, MD {1740456318} SrgFAk
+ Rothman Institute - Egg Harbor Township
2500 English Creek Avenue/Bldg 1300   Egg Harbor Township, NJ 08234   (609)677-6060   Fax (609)677-6061

Winters, Jayshree P., MD {1568556884} Psychy, Nrolgy(73,INA21)
+ Christian Health Care Heritage Manor Nursing Home
301 Sicomac Avenue   Wyckoff, NJ 07481   (201)848-5200   Fax (201)848-9758
+ 71 Andrea Court
Paramus, NJ 07652   (201)652-5120

Winters, Richard Allan, MD {1114092236} Psychy(72,NY09)
+ 29 North Farview Avenue
Paramus, NJ 07652   (201)843-4944   Fax (201)265-7647
winterz2@aol.com

Winters, Richard M., MD {1215996012} SrgPlstc(90,CT02)<NJ-HACKNSK>
+ Cohen/Winters Aesthetic & Reconstructive Surgery
113 West Essex Street/Suite 202   Maywood, NJ 07607   (201)487-3400   Fax (201)487-2481
+ Aesthetic and Reconstructive Surgeons
20 Prospect Avenue/Suite 501   Hackensack, NJ 07601   (201)487-3400

Winters, Stephen L., MD {1548291131} ClCdEl, CdvDis(79,NY47)<NJ-MORRISTN, NJ-OVERLOOK>
+ Morristown Medical Center
100 Madison Avenue/CardElct   Morristown, NJ 07962   (973)971-4261   Fax (973)290-7253
stephen.winters@atlantichealth.org

Winzelberg, Neal J., MD {1689764466} Gastrn, IntrMd(84,NY08)<NJ-OCEANMC, NJ-SOCEANCO>
+ Coastal Gastroenterology Associates PA
525 Jack Martin Boulevard/Suite 301   Brick, NJ 08724   (732)840-0067   Fax (732)840-3169
+ Ocean Medical Center
425 Jack Martin Boulevard/Med/Gastro   Brick, NJ 08723   (732)840-2200

Wirtshafter, David Glenn, MD {1225035785} Radiol, RadDia(89,NJ06)
+ Red Bank Radiologists, P.A.
200 White Road/Suite 115   Little Silver, NJ 07739   (732)741-9595   Fax (732)741-0985
+ Coastal Imaging, LLC
79 Route 37 West/Suite 103   Toms River, NJ 08755   (732)741-9595   Fax (732)276-2325
+ Doctors Radiology Center - MRI of Woodbridge
1500 St. George Avenue/Peach Plaza   Avenel, NJ 07739   (732)574-1414   Fax (732)574-0845

Wirtshafter, Karen A., MD {1184717142} Otlryg(86,NJ06)<NJ-STCLRDEN>
+ ENT & Allergy Associates of Parsippany
900 Lanidex Plaza/Suite 300   Parsippany, NJ 07054   (973)394-1818   Fax (973)394-1810
+ ENT & Allergy Associates, LLP
3219 Route 46 East/Suite 203   Parsippany, NJ 07054   (973)394-1818   Fax (973)394-1810

Wisda, Catherine L., MD {1699717975} Ophthl, IntrMd(82,NJ05)<NJ-SJRSYELM>
+ Wisda Eye Center, P.A.
1318 South Main Road   Vineland, NJ 08360   (856)692-8008   Fax (856)692-8044
Caccesewisdaeye@comcast.net
+ Wisda Eye Center, P.A.
340 Front Street   Elmer, NJ 08318   (856)692-8008   Fax (856)358-3953

Wise, Jeffrey B., MD {1760698716} Otlryg(01,NY20)
+ 1680 Route 23/Suite 100
Wayne, NJ 07470   (973)305-1400

Wise, Richard Bryan, MD {1619971520} Ophthl(96,ON01)<NJ-SHOREMEM, NJ-ACMCITY>
+ 54 West Jimmie Leeds Road/Unit 15
Galloway, NJ 08205   Fax (609)652-7759

Wise, Susannah S., MD {1568571768} Surgry(97,NJ05)
+ UMDNJ RWJ Surgery
125 Paterson Street/CAB 4th FL 4100   New Brunswick, NJ 08901   (732)235-7920   Fax (732)235-7079

Wiser-Estin, Mindy Ellen, MD {1407904063} ObsGyn(91,CT01)
+ Shore Area Ob-Gyn
200 White Road/Suite 105   Little Silver, NJ 07739   (732)741-3331   Fax (732)741-5119

Wisniewski, Robert E., MD {1487610416} ObsGyn(77,PA02)
+ First State Women's Care
19B West Avenue   Woodstown, NJ 08098   (856)769-3348   Fax (856)769-3987

Wisotsky, Burton J., MD {1972594083} Ophthl(90,NY46)<NJ-ENGLWOOD, NY-NYEYEINF>
+ Omni Eye Services
485 Route 1 South/Building A   Iselin, NJ 08830   (732)750-0400   Fax (732)602-0749
+ Omni Eye Services
218 State Route 17 North   Rochelle Park, NJ 07662   (732)750-0400   Fax (201)368-0254

Wisotsky, David H., MD {1124084405} Pedtrc, IntrMd(74,NY46)<NJ-ENGLWOOD, NJ-HACKNSK>
+ Tenafly Pediatrics, PA
32 Franklin Street   Tenafly, NJ 07670   (201)569-2400   Fax (201)569-6081
+ Tenafly Pediatrics, PA
1135 Broad Street/Suite 208   Clifton, NJ 07013   (201)569-2400   Fax (973)471-3068

Wisotsky, Lisa L., MD {1780669119} PhysMd(90,NY46)<NJ-ENGLWOOD>
+ Physical Medicine & Rehabilitation Center
500 Grand Avenue/1st Floor   Englewood, NJ 07631   (201)567-2277   Fax (201)567-7506

Wisser, Jamie R., MD {1114069671} SrgPlstc(86,PA07)<NJ-CHSFULD, NJ-CHSMRCER>
+ East Windsor Medical Commons
300A Princeton Hightstown Road   East Windsor, NJ 08520   (609)426-9200   Fax (609)426-9211

Wistreich, Sarah J., DO {1518237452} FamMed
+ 1401 Whitehorse Mercerville Ro
Hamilton, NJ 08619   (609)588-5059   Fax (609)528-8868

Physicians by Name and Address

Witham, Marie-Grace, DO {1164496519} FamMed(94,NY75)<NJ-STBARNMC, NJ-WAYNEGEN>
+ VA New Jersey Health Care System
385 Tremont Avenue/Corporate Office   East Orange, NJ 07018   (973)676-1000   Fax (973)676-4226
+ Care Station Medical Group
456 Prospect Avenue   West Orange, NJ 07052   (973)676-1000   Fax (973)731-9881

Witkowska, Renata A., MD {1043203474} AlgyImmn, IntrMd(92,POL12)
+ Center for Asthma & Allergy
18 North Third Avenue   Highland Park, NJ 08904   (732)545-0094   Fax (732)545-4087
+ Center for Asthma & Allergy
300 Hudson Street   Hoboken, NJ 07030   (732)545-0094   Fax (201)792-5320
+ Center for Asthma & Allergy
90 Milbum Avenue/Suite 200   Maplewood, NJ 08904   (973)763-5787   Fax (973)763-8568

Witkowski, Mary E., MD {1023006095} ObsGyn(93,NJ05)
+ Ob-Gyn Associates at Holmdel-Shrewsbury
39 Avenue of the Commons   Shrewsbury, NJ 07702   (732)389-0003
+ Ob-Gyn Associates at Holmdel-Shrewsbury
704 North Beers Street   Holmdel, NJ 07733   (732)389-0003   Fax (732)888-2778

Witlin, Richard S., MD {1063459212} Ophthl(75,NY46)<NJ-CENTRAST>
+ The Witlin Center for Advanced Eye Care
557 Cranbury Road/Suite 6   East Brunswick, NJ 08816   (732)698-9300   Fax (732)625-0107
r.witlin@aol.com
+ Community Eye Consultants
501 Lakehurst Road   Toms River, NJ 08755   (732)698-9300   Fax (732)625-0107
+ The Witlin Center for Advanced Eye Care
21 Perry Street   Morristown, NJ 08816   (973)285-9300   Fax (732)625-0107

Witmer, George Robert, III, MD {1659397610} IntrMd(00,NY45)<NJ-VIRTMARL, NJ-VIRTVOOR>
+ Jefferson HealthCare - Voorhees
443 Laurel Oak Road/Suite 130   Voorhees, NJ 08043   (856)784-7398   Fax (856)784-7357

Witt, Virginia Marie, MD {1689673923} FamMed, IntrMd(97,NC07)<NJ-CHRIST, NJ-BAYONNE>
+ Hoboken Integrated Family Medicine LLC
109 Grand Street   Hoboken, NJ 07030   (201)795-1001   Fax (201)795-1009

Witte, Arnold S., MD {1477504546} Nrolgy(77,MA07)<NJ-CHSMRCER, NJ-CHSFULD>
+ Capital Institute for Neurosciences
2 Capital Way/Suite 456   Pennington, NJ 08534   (609)537-7300   Fax (609)537-7301
+ Mercer Neurology
2 Princess Road/Suite 2F   Lawrenceville, NJ 08648   (609)537-7300   Fax (609)895-1006

Wittenborn, John Richard, MD {1629145115} Nrolgy, SrgNro(73,MO02)<NJ-SOMERSET>
+ 215 Union Avenue
Bridgewater, NJ 08807   (908)927-0342   Fax (609)261-7199

Witter, Theodore O., MD {1386656577} ObsGyn(75,NY06)
+ New Margaret Hague Women's Health Institute
377 Jersey Avenue/Suite 220   Jersey City, NJ 07302   (201)795-9155   Fax (201)795-9157

Wixted, William M., MD {1336188572} Urolgy(72,PA02)<NJ-SHOREMEM>
+ Shore Memorial Hospital
1 East New York Avenue/Urology   Somers Point, NJ 08244   (609)653-3500

Wjasow, Christina, MD {1689612186} IntrMd, ClCdEl(98,NY46)<NJ-DEBRAHLC>
+ Deborah Heart and Lung Center
200 Trenton Road/Cardiology   Browns Mills, NJ 08015   (609)893-6611   Fax (609)735-0175

Wnek, Gary E., MD {1205875184} Anesth, AnesPain(83,MEX29)<NJ-OURLADY>
+ Our Lady of Lourdes Medical Center
1600 Haddon Avenue   Camden, NJ 08103   (856)757-3500

Wnorowski, Brian R., MD {1780669101} Ophthl, IntrMd(89,NJ05)
+ Shore Eye Associates
530 Lakehurst Road/Suite 206   Toms River, NJ 08755   (732)341-4733   Fax (732)341-2794
Phaco@optonline.net
+ Shore Eye Associates
445 Brick Boulevard/Suite 106   Brick, NJ 08723   (732)341-4733   Fax (732)262-0064
+ Shore Eye Associates
550 Route 530/Suite 19   Whiting, NJ 08755   (732)350-3344   Fax (732)350-0093

Wofsy, Alice, MD {1265493423} EmrgMd, IntrMd(84,NJ05)
+ 300 Lexington Road/Suite 220
Woolwich Township, NJ 08085   (856)241-2227   Fax (856)241-2110

Wohler, Alexander M., MD {1699928580} SrgThr<NJ-STJOSHOS>
+ St. Joseph's Regional Medical Center
703 Main Street/CT Surgery   Paterson, NJ 07503   (973)754-2486   Fax (973)754-2975

Wohler, Anh Van, MD {1699113928}<NJ-ENGLWOOD>
+ Englewood Hospital and Medical Center
350 Engle Street   Englewood, NJ 07631   (201)894-3000

Wohlfarth, Erik, MD {1124446729} Anesth
+ Bergen Anesthesia Group PC
223 North Van Dien Avenue   Ridgewood, NJ 07450   (201)847-9320   Fax (201)847-0059

Wohlstadter, Sanford W., MD {1649268616} ObsGyn(81,WEST)<NJ-MONMOUTH, NJ-RIVERVW>
+ Ob-Gyn Associates at Holmdel-Shrewsbury
704 North Beers Street   Holmdel, NJ 07733   (732)739-2500   Fax (732)888-2778
sanman1100@worldnet.att.net
+ Ob-Gyn Associates at Holmdel-Shrewsbury
39 Avenue of the Commons   Shrewsbury, NJ 07702   (732)389-0003

Wojnarska-Alvarez, Gabriela, MD {1023256559} Nephro, IntrMd
+ Kessler Rehabilitation Center
221 West Grand Avenue/Suite 105   Montvale, NJ 07645   (201)794-8989

Wojno Oranski, Alexander, DO {1457318206} CritCr, PulDis, IntrMd(94,ME75)<NJ-MTNSIDE>
+ Advanced Urology Associates, P.C.
1600 Saint Georges Avenue/Suite 111   Rahway, NJ 07065   (732)388-2422   Fax (732)388-1706

Wold, Robert E., MD {1306831482} Radiol, RadDia(86,NJ06)<NJ-RIVERVW>
+ Red Bank Radiologists, P.A.
200 White Road/Suite 115   Little Silver, NJ 07739   (732)741-9595   Fax (732)741-0985
+ Coastal Imaging, LLC
79 Route 37 West/Suite 103   Toms River, NJ 08755   (732)741-9595   Fax (732)276-2325

Wolenski, Matthew J., MD {1275542623} SrgFak, SrgOrt(NJ05)
+ Brielle Orthopedics PA
457 Jack Martin Boulevard   Brick, NJ 08724   (732)840-7500   Fax (732)840-2088
+ Brielle Orthopedics PA
823 Lacey Road   Forked River, NJ 08731   (732)840-7500   Fax (732)840-2088
+ Brielle Orthopedics PA
1301 Route 72 West   Manahawkin, NJ 08724   (609)971-7616   Fax (609)971-7639

Wolf, Andreas, MD {1073519336} CdvDis, IntCrd, IntrMd(86,GER23)<NJ-STFRNMED, NJ-RWJURAH>
+ Mercer Bucks Cardiology
One Union Street/Suite 101   Robbinsville, NJ 08691   (609)890-6677   Fax (609)890-7292

Wolf, Barry Z., MD {1447274402} IntrMd, PulDis, CritCr(82,NY19)<NJ-RWJUBRUN, NJ-RWJURAH>
+ Pulmonary Internists, PA
2 Lincoln Highway/Suite 301   Edison, NJ 08820   (732)549-7380   Fax (732)548-8216
bzwolf98@aol.com
+ Pulmonary Internists, PA
3 Hospital Plaza/Suite 205   Old Bridge, NJ 08857   (732)360-2255

Wolf, Edward J., MD {1881696185} MtFtMd, ObsGyn(84,DC02)<NJ-STBARNMC>
+ St. Barnabas Medical Center
94 Old Short Hills Road/Ob/Gyn   Livingston, NJ 07039   (973)322-5000   Fax (973)322-2309

Wolf, James H., MD {1497743876} Grtrcs, IntrMd(74,NY19)<NJ-MORRISTN>
+ Mendham Medical Group LLP
19 East Main Street/Suite 1   Mendham, NJ 07945   (973)543-6505   Fax (973)543-2967

Wolf, Mary Campion, MD {1700128725} Pedtrc
+ Goryeb Children's Hospital
100 Madison Avenue   Morristown, NJ 07960   (973)971-6900

Wolf, Michael Jacob, MD {1457558660} Pedtrc, FamMSptM(07,PA01)<PA-CHILDHOS>
+ St. Christopher Care at Washington Township
405 Hurffville-Cross Keys Road   Sewell, NJ 08080   (856)582-0644   Fax (856)582-0622

Wolf Greene, Susan Amy, MD {1427102110} FrtInf, Gyneco, RprrEnd(84,NY47)
+ University Reproductive Associates, PC
214 Terrace Avenue/2nd Floor   Hasbrouck Heights, NJ 07604   (201)288-6330   Fax (201)288-6331

Wolfe, Jeffrey S., MD {1447248935} Pedtrc(74,NJ05)<NJ-MONMOUTH, NJ-CENTRAST>
+ Allergy & Pediatric Associates of Jersey Shore
222 Schanck Road/Suite 105   Freehold, NJ 07728   (732)431-3373   Fax (732)303-0172
doctorsail@msn.com
+ Allergy & Pediatric Associates of Jersey Shore
500 West Kennedy Boulevard   Lakewood, NJ 08701   (732)431-3373   Fax (732)905-8773

Wolfe, Taida J., MD {1548494875} ObsGyn
+ 761 Mosswood Avenue
Orange, NJ 07050   (201)506-2065
hatshepsutmd@gmail.com

Wolfeld, Michael Brent, MD {1225297229} SrgPlstc(03,NY08)<NY-LENOXHLL, NY-MANHEYE>
+ Wolfeld Plastic Surgery
25 Prospect Avenue/2nd Floor   Hackensack, NJ 07601   (201)500-7050

Wolff, Alan H., MD {1548210016} Allrgy, IntrMd(84,MD01)<NJ-SOMERSET>
+ Allergy Center of Warren
5 Mountain Boulevard/Suite 3   Warren, NJ 07059   (908)755-5335

Wolff, David E., MD {1699971200} Psychy(89,DC01)
+ 2290 West County Line Road/Suite 105
Jackson, NJ 08527   (732)675-3451

Wolff, Jeffrey G., MD {1306886104} Psychy(82,NY08)<NJ-MORRISTN>
+ 59 Franklin Street/Suite 2
Morristown, NJ 07960   (973)540-1720   Fax (973)540-1820

Wolfman, Brian P., MD {1336309673} IntrMd
+ 525 Jack Martin Boulevard/Suite 300
Brick, NJ 08724   (732)840-0067

Wolfman, Marc R., MD {1174521355} Gastrn(74,MEX03)
+ Gastroenterology Consultants PA
205 May Street/Suite 201   Edison, NJ 08837   (732)661-9225   Fax (732)661-9259
+ May Street Surgi Center
205 May Street/Suite 103   Edison, NJ 08837   (732)661-9225   Fax (732)661-9619

Wolfson, Alexander, MD {1659466266} Anesth(02,NY06)<NJ-UNVMCPRN>
+ University Medical Center of Princeton at Plainsboro
One Plainsboro Road/Anesthesia   Plainsboro, NJ 08536   (609)497-4000

Wolfson, Keith Richard, MD {1417047275} CdvDis, IntrMd(01,PA02)<NJ-BURDTMLN, NJ-SHOREMEM>
+ Mercer Bucks Cardiology
3140 Princeton Pike/2nd Floor   Lawrenceville, NJ 08648   (609)895-1919   Fax (609)895-1200
+ Penn Cardiac Care Mercer Bucks
2 Capitol Way/Suite 487A   Pennington, NJ 08534

Wolfson, Natasha Susan, MD {1326226515} RadDia(03,NY06)<NJ-STPETER, NJ-RWJUBRUN>
+ University Radiology Group, P.C.
483 Cranbury Road   East Brunswick, NJ 08816   (732)390-0030   Fax (732)390-5383
+ University Radiology Group, P.C.
105 Raider Boulevard/Suite 101   Hillsborough, NJ 08844   (732)390-0030   Fax (908)359-9273
+ University Radiology Group, P.C.
75 Veronica Avenue   Somerset, NJ 08816   (732)246-0060   Fax (732)246-4188

Wolinsky, Steven I., MD {1548531882} IntrMd
+ 4 Prospect Street
Highlands, NJ 07732

Wolk, Eric Todd, DO {1871765453} EmrgMd<NJ-ACMCITY>
+ AtlantiCare Regional Medical Center/City Campus
1925 Pacific Avenue/EmergMed   Atlantic City, NJ 08401   (609)345-4000

Wolk, Larry A., MD SrgThr, Surgry(76,PA09)
+ Memorial Hospital of Salem County
310 Woodstown Road   Salem, NJ 08079   (856)935-1000

Wolkomir, Alfred F., MD {1447217427} SrgC&R, Surgry(81,GRN01)<NJ-JRSYSHMC, NJ-BAYSHORE>
+ 205 Maple Avenue
Red Bank, NJ 07701   (732)219-9699   Fax (732)219-0208
+ 1820 Route 33
Neptune, NJ 07753   (732)775-2125

Wolkstein, David S., MD {1528122033} SrgOrt(65,NJ05)<NJ-STBARNMC>
+ 2333 Morris Avenue
Union, NJ 07083   (908)964-8550

Wollman, Carol A., MD {1831344019} RadDia(91,MA07)
+ Breast Health Center of Ridgewood, P.C.
385 South Maple Avenue   Ridgewood, NJ 07450   (201)670-4550   Fax (201)670-7812

Wolodiger, Fred A., MD {1073511085} SrgVas, Surgry(80,NY08)<NJ-ENGLWOOD, NJ-HOLYNAME>
+ Englewood Surgical Associates
375 Engle Street/Ground Floor   Englewood, NJ 07631   (201)894-0400   Fax (201)894-1022
+ Heart and Vascular Institute at EHMC
350 Engle Street/Suite 1000   Englewood, NJ 07631   (201)894-3636

Physicians by Name and Address

Wolpert, Joshua D., MD {1740253996} Pedtrc(92,OH06)<NJ-OCEANMC>
+ Joshua D. Wolpert MD LLC
  87 Union Avenue   Manasquan, NJ 08736   (732)292-9044   Fax (732)292-9055

Wolstein, Jesse, MD {1710372008}<NJ-MORRISTN>
+ Morristown Medical Center
  100 Madison Avenue   Morristown, NJ 07962   (973)971-5000

Woltz, Ayanna Rashea, MD {1699714915} ObsGyn(99,NJ05)
+ Somerset Ob-Gyn Associates
  215 Union Avenue/Suite A   Bridgewater, NJ 08807   (908)722-2900   Fax (908)722-1856
+ Somerset Ob-Gyn Associates
  1 New Amwell Road   Hillsborough, NJ 08844   (908)874-5900

Womack, Jason Peter, MD {1497875249} FamMed, FamM-SptM(04,NJ06)
+ Family Medicine at Monument Square
  317 George Street   New Brunswick, NJ 08901   (732)235-8993   Fax (732)246-7317

Womack, Meghan E., MD {1164646683} EmrgMd
+ 4151 Squankum Allenwood Road
  Wall Township, NJ 07731

Won, Bokran, MD {1023049194} RadDia(92,PA09)<NJ-MONMOUTH>
+ Monmouth Medical Center
  300 Second Avenue/Radiology   Long Branch, NJ 07740   (732)222-5200

Won, Peter Arm-Woo, MD {1821035445} PhysMd(79,KOR04)<NJ-MMHKEMBL, NJ-OVERLOOK>
+ 24 Wernik Place/Suite East
  Metuchen, NJ 08840   (908)412-0900   Fax (732)662-3306
+ 285 Durham Avenue/Suite 1-B
  South Plainfield, NJ 07080   (908)412-0900

Wondisford, Frederic Edward, MD {1992885636} EnDbMt, IntrMd(83,OH44)<MA-BIDMCEST>
+ RWJ University Endocrinology Diabetes & Metabolism
  125 Paterson Street/CAB 5100A   New Brunswick, NJ 08901   (732)235-7219   Fax (732)235-8610

Wong, Aubrey S., DO {1073827663} FamMed<NJ-CHRIST>
+ Christ Hospital
  176 Palisade Avenue   Jersey City, NJ 07306   (201)795-8201

Wong, Austin Henry, MD {1700832573} PedCrd, Pedtrc(97,NY46)<NJ-HACKNSK>
+ The Pediatric Center for Heart Disease
  155 Polifly Road/Suite 106   Hackensack, NJ 07601   (201)487-7617   Fax (201)342-5341
  awong@hackensackumc.org

Wong, Casey, MD {1104143148} CdvDis
+ Princeton Medical Group, P.A.
  419 North Harrison Street   Princeton, NJ 08540   (609)924-9300   Fax (609)430-9481

Wong, Charissa J., MD {1780783498} Ophthl
+ Berkeley Heights Eye Group
  571 Central Avenue/Suite 101   New Providence, NJ 07974   (908)464-4600   Fax (908)464-4737

Wong, Christopher K., MD {1275508392} IntrMd(94,NJ05)<NJ-UNVMCPRN, NJ-CENTRAST>
+ Family Practice of CentraState
  319 Route 130 North   East Windsor, NJ 08520   (609)426-1555   Fax (609)447-8070

Wong, Dennis, MD {1669544433} Psychy(80,MEX03)
+ CPC Behavioral HealthCare
  270 Highway 35   Red Bank, NJ 07701   (732)842-2000   Fax (732)224-0688

Wong, Gabriel Ho Yu, MD {1194759225} Otlryg, OtgyPSHN, OtgyFPIS(00,NJ06)<NJ-VIRTUAHS>
+ Advocare ENT Specialty Center
  88 South Lakeview Drive/Building 1   Gibbsboro, NJ 08026   (856)435-9100   Fax (856)435-9112

Wong, Geoffrey, MD {1811916745} SrgVas
+ Garden State Surgical Associates
  1511 Park Avenue   South Plainfield, NJ 07080   (908)561-9500   Fax (908)561-7162

Wong, Henry Chen, MD {1598769994} Anesth(87,VA04)
+ Morris Anesthesia Group, PA
  3799 Route 46/Suite 211   Parsippany, NJ 07054   (973)335-1440   Fax (973)335-1446

Wong, James Robert, MD {1053350777} Onclgy, RadOnc, IntrMd(86,MA01)
+ Radiation Oncology Associates of North Jersey, P.A.
  100 Madison Avenue   Morristown, NJ 07962   (973)971-5329   Fax (973)290-7393

Wong, Jeanne, MD {1316941792} Anesth(70,MYA01)<NJ-EASTORNG>
+ East Orange General Hospital
  300 Central Avenue/Anesth   East Orange, NJ 07018   (973)672-8400

Wong, Jiyoung, DO {1336527555} IntrMd<NJ-STMRYPAS>
+ St. Mary's Hospital
  350 Boulevard   Passaic, NJ 07055   (973)365-4300

Wong, Jonathan Wane, MD {1881662401} Pedtrc(97,NY46)<NJ-HACKNSK, NJ-VALLEY>
+ Pediatric Specialties PA
  90 Prospect Avenue/Suite 1-A   Hackensack, NJ 07601   (201)342-4001   Fax (201)342-9569
+ Pediatric Specialties PA
  50 South Franklin Turnpike   Ramsey, NJ 07446   (201)342-4001   Fax (201)934-2947

Wong, Judy, MD {1972538882} EmrgMd<NJ-ENGLWOOD>
+ Englewood Hospital and Medical Center
  350 Engle Street   Englewood, NJ 07631   (201)984-3000   Fax (610)617-6280

Wong, Karen Clark, MD {1760496707} Pedtrc(97,NJ05)<NJ-KIMBALL>
+ Dr. Gittleman & Associates
  450 East Kennedy Boulevard   Lakewood, NJ 08701   (732)901-0050   Fax (732)370-2386

Wong, Kristin G., MD {1932360112} Pedtrc, IntrMd(08,KS02)<NJ-UMDNJ>
+ University Hospital
  150 Bergen Street/Suite H-245   Newark, NJ 07103   (973)972-5672

Wong, Michael Y., MD {1295748002} Ophthl, IntrMd(78,NY03)<NJ-UNVMCPRN>
+ The Princeton Eye Group
  419 North Harrison Street/Suite 104   Princeton, NJ 08540   (609)921-9437   Fax (609)921-0277
+ The Princeton Eye Group
  1600 Perrinville Road   Monroe Township, NJ 08831   (609)921-9437   Fax (609)655-3685
+ The Princeton Eye Group
  900 Eastern Avenue/Suite 50   Somerset, NJ 08540   (732)565-9550   Fax (732)565-0946

Wong, Patrick, MD {1508250705} FamMed
+ 10 Parsonage Road/Suite 410
  Edison, NJ 08837   (732)795-6130   Fax (732)463-5535

Wong, Peter J., MD {1154493070} CdvDis, IntrMd(80,NY46)
+ 601 Pavonia Avenue/Suite 301
  Jersey City, NJ 07306   (201)217-7999   Fax (201)217-7997

Wong, Que-Chi V., MD {1558314641} FamMed, Grtrcs, FamM-Grtc(00,NJ06)
+ 3322 Avalon Court
  Voorhees, NJ 08043

Wong, Richard H., MD {1427061266} Ophthl, IntrMd(79,NJ05)<NJ-UNVMCPRN>
+ The Princeton Eye Group
  419 North Harrison Street/Suite 104   Princeton, NJ 08540   (609)921-9437   Fax (609)921-0277
+ The Princeton Eye Group
  1600 Perrinville Road   Monroe Township, NJ 08831   (609)921-9437   Fax (609)655-3685
+ The Princeton Eye Group
  900 Eastern Avenue/Suite 50   Somerset, NJ 08540   (732)565-9550   Fax (732)565-0946

Wong, Robert L., MD {1003981648} IntrMd, Rheuma(80,MA07)
+ UH- Robert Wood Johnson Med
  125 Paterson Street/MEB 483   New Brunswick, NJ 08901   (732)235-7702   Fax (732)235-6526
+ Family Medicine at Monument Square
  317 George Street   New Brunswick, NJ 08901   (732)235-7702   Fax (732)246-7317

Wong, Sarah, MD {1932498607} Surgry
+ Drs. Wong and Ilonzo
  20 Prospect Avenue   Hackensack, NJ 07601   (551)996-2000

Wong, Serena Tsan-Lai, MD {1881689511} IntrMd, Hemato, MedOnc(01,NY01)<NJ-RWJUBRUN, NJ-RBAYOLDB>
+ Rutgers Cancer Institute of New Jersey
  195 Little Albany Street/PO Box 2681   New Brunswick, NJ 08903   (732)235-9692   Fax (732)235-4321

Wong, So Mui, MD {1659554012} ObsGyn(92,NY08)<NJ-JFKMED>
+ SM Wong, MD LLC
  8 Brant Avenue   Clark, NJ 07066   (732)388-3338   Fax (732)388-3278

Wong, Stephen, MD {1942293881} Nrolgy(00,NC07)
+ University Hospital-RWJMS Neurology
  125 Paterson Street/Suite 4100-6100   New Brunswick, NJ 08901   (732)235-7733   Fax (732)235-7041
+ RW Johnson University Medical Group Neurology
  97 Paterson Street   New Brunswick, NJ 08901   (732)235-7733   Fax (732)235-7041

Wong, Sze Ho, MD {1093158743} Glacma
+ World Class LASIK
  28 Throckmorton Lane/Suite 103   Old Bridge, NJ 08857   (732)679-6100   Fax (732)673-6703

Wong, Tracie Mei Han, MD {1619185675} PedGst, Nutrtn(00,NY19)<NJ-HACKNSK>
+ Joseph M. Sanzari Childrens' -Gastro
  155 Polifly Road/Suite 102   Hackensack, NJ 07601   (551)996-8840   Fax (201)441-9949

Wong, Wilbur P., MD {1487640306} FamMed(94,NJ05)<NJ-VAEASTOR>
+ 108th Medical Group Air National Guard
  3466 Neely Road/87 Amds/sgpo   Trenton, NJ 08641   (609)754-9361
+ VA New Jersey Health Care System-East Orange Campus
  385 Tremont Avenue   East Orange, NJ 07018   (973)676-1000
+ McGuire Air Force Base/Acute Health Care Clinic
  3458 Neely Road   Trenton, NJ 08641   (609)754-9014   Fax (609)754-9015

Wong Duran, Elizabeth, MD {1407917597} Pedtrc(86,PER08)<NJ-STPETER>
+ Children Health Center
  55 West Union Avenue   Bound Brook, NJ 08805   (732)564-0044   Fax (732)469-4650

Wong Liang, Ruth C., MD {1306810551} IntrMd(78,PA13)<NJ-MTNSIDE>
+ Hackensack UMC Mountainside
  1 Bay Avenue/IntMed   Montclair, NJ 07042   (973)429-6195

Woo, Daniel Hee-Suk, MD {1750360103} Anesth(95,NJ06)<NJ-OVERLOOK, NJ-TRINIWSC>
+ Summit Anesthesia Associates, P.A.
  33 Overlook Road/Suite 311   Summit, NJ 07901   (908)598-1500   Fax (908)598-0197
+ New Jersey Bariatric Center
  193 Morris Avenue/2nd Floor   Springfield, NJ 07081   (908)598-1500   Fax (908)688-8861

Woo, James K., MD {1861420598} FamMed, FamMGrtc(90,VA04)<NJ-CHILTON, NJ-STJOSHOS>
+ Wayne Medical Care, PA
  342 Hamburg Turnpike/Suite 101   Wayne, NJ 07470   (973)942-4140   Fax (973)942-5070

Woo, Judy, MD {1093759938} NroChl, Pedtrc(85,NY47)
+ Bergen Passaic Pediatric Neurology
  17-15 Maple Avenue/Suite 203   Fair Lawn, NJ 07410   (201)796-9500   Fax (201)796-9509

Woo, Melissa Lee Mei, MD {1376679027} PedEnd(03,NH01)
+ Morristown Medical Pediatric Endocrinology
  100 Madison Avenue   Morristown, NJ 07960   (973)971-4340   Fax (973)290-7367

Woo, Thomas Hyunsop, MD {1619942802} RadDia, RadV&I(95,MI01)
+ Hunterdon Radiological Associate
  1 Dogwood Drive   Clinton, NJ 08809   (908)735-4477   Fax (908)735-6532

Wood, Jessica R., DO {1821183344} Pedtrc(03,PA77)
+ Navesink Pediatrics
  55 North Gilbert Street/Suite 2101   Tinton Falls, NJ 07701   (732)842-6677   Fax (732)530-2946

Wood, Kevin C., MD {1134428998} OncHem(11,KS02)
+ Valley Medical Group-Hematology/Oncology
  One Valley Health Plaza   Paramus, NJ 07652   (201)634-5578   Fax (201)986-4702

Wood, Margaret Diana, MD {1336137223} CdvDis, IntHos, IntrMd(87,PA07)<NJ-LOURDMED>
+ Lourdes Medical Center of Burlington County
  218 Sunset Road/Internal Med   Willingboro, NJ 08046   (609)835-2900   Fax (856)566-6906

Wood, Robert H., MD {1245351634} Pthlgy, PthAcl(78,PA01)<NJ-CHSMRCER, NJ-CHSFULD>
+ Capital Health System/Mercer Campus
  446 Bellevue Avenue/Path/Laboratory   Trenton, NJ 08618   (609)394-4021   Fax (609)394-4685
+ Capital Health System/Fuld Campus
  750 Brunswick Avenue/Path/Laboratory   Trenton, NJ 08638   (609)394-6095
+ Capital Health System/Hopewell
  One Capital Way/Pathology   Pennington, NJ 08618   (609)303-4019   Fax (609)394-4685

Wood, Sterling Harbert, DO {1982788816} Anesth(88,MO79)<NJ-MERIDNHS>
+ Shrewsbury Surgery Center
  655 Shrewsbury Avenue   Shrewsbury, NJ 07702   (732)450-6000   Fax (732)450-1798

Woodham, Philip G., MD {1174667836} IntrMd(96,PA13)<NJ-HACKNSK>
+ Hackensack University Medical Center
  20 Prospect Avenue/Suite 715   Hackensack, NJ 07601   (201)881-0721   Fax (201)881-0725

Woodriffe, Philipa G., MD {1174597694} Surgry(76,NY01)<NJ-BAYSHORE>
+ 1029 Sycamore Avenue
  Tinton Falls, NJ 07724   (732)542-4228   Fax (732)542-2423

Woods, Barrett I., MD {1073774386} SrgOrt(08,PA12)
+ Rothman Institute - Egg Harbor Township
  2500 English Creek Avenue/Bldg 1300   Egg Harbor Township, NJ 08234   (609)677-6060   Fax (609)677-6061

Woods, Krystina L., MD {1679734925} IntrMd, InfDis(08,DMN01)
+ Stat Medical Services
  845 Broadway   Bayonne, NJ 07002   (201)858-2930   Fax (201)858-2910

Woods, Peter Albert, Jr., DO {1649321381}<NJ-CHRIST>
+ Christ Hospital
176 Palisade Avenue   Jersey City, NJ 07306   (201)795-8765   Fax (201)795-8685
peter.woods@carepointhealth.org

Woodward, Ralph P., MD {1093965196} InfDis, IntrMd(86,MEXI)<NJ-STMICHL>
+ St. Michael's Medical Center
268 MLK Jr. Boulevard   Newark, NJ 07102   (973)877-5000

Woodward, Shelly W., MD {1093965022} PhysMd(87,MD01)
+ 111 Cemetery Road
Blairstown, NJ 07825   Fax (908)459-4509

Woolbright, William Charles, MD {1407155161} PedHem
+ St. Joseph Medical Center Pediatric Hematology/Onc
703 Main Street   Paterson, NJ 07503   (973)754-2000

Woolrich, Andrew G., MD {1619062940} Dermat(89,NY09)<NY-LENOXHLL, NJ-HOLYNAME>
+ Dermatology Center
363 Grand Avenue   Englewood, NJ 07631   (201)568-6977   Fax (201)568-7567

Woolverton, Kahra, MD {1821503350} PhysMd
+ 1372 Route 9/Bldg 2
Toms River, NJ 08755   (732)240-9296   Fax (732)240-9297

Wooton, Robert P., Jr., MD {1821046681} IntrMd(90,NJ05)<NJ-UMDNJ, NJ-HACKNSK>
+ Summit Medical Group
6 Brighton Road/2 FL   Clifton, NJ 07012   (973)777-7911   Fax (973)777-5403

Worden, Douglas L., MD {1144266685} Otlryg(90,NY09)<NJ-HUNTRDN>
+ Hunterdon Otolaryngology Associates
6 Sand Hill Road/Suite 302   Flemington, NJ 08822   (908)788-9131   Fax (908)788-0945

Work, Adam Nicholas, MD {1467794826} GenPrc
+ McGuire Air Force Base/Acute Health Care Clinic
3458 Neely Road   Trenton, NJ 08641   (609)754-9080   Fax (609)754-9015

Woroch, Bohdar O., MD {1902983471} CdvDis, IntrMd(73,SPA22)
+ 349 East Northfield Road/Suite 202
Livingston, NJ 07039

Woroch, Paul, MD {1083081392} IntrMd
+ Mountainside Medical Group
123 Highland Avenue/Suite 201   Glen Ridge, NJ 07028   (973)748-9246   Fax (973)748-8755

Woroch, Peter Michael, MD {1255687067} ObsGyn
+ 799 Bloomfield Avenue/Suite 301
Verona, NJ 07044   (973)748-7953   Fax (201)523-9550

Worth, David A., MD {1861406902} Rheuma(71,NY45)<NJ-OVERLOOK>
+ 2376 Morris Avenue
Union, NJ 07083   (908)686-6616   Fax (908)686-5806

Worth, Richard Lowell, MD {1871710624} Psychy, PsyCAd(99,NJ06)<NY-BLVUENYU, NJ-SJERSYHS>
+ Center for Family Guidance, PC
765 East Route 70/Building A-101   Marlton, NJ 08053   (856)797-4800   Fax (856)810-0110

Worth, Robert Harry, MD {1588749303} Anesth(99,ISR06)
+ Holy Name Hospital
718 Teaneck Road   Teaneck, NJ 07666   (201)833-3000

Wortzel, Jay V., MD {1841327129} GenPrc, EmrgMd(80,NY19)
+ 240 Monmouth Road
Oakhurst, NJ 07755   (732)531-7711   Fax (732)531-3669

Woska, Scott Corey, MD {1326098351} PhysMd, PainMd, OthrSp(97,NJ06)<NJ-MONMOUTH>
+ Shore Orthopaedic Group
35 Gilbert Street South   Tinton Falls, NJ 07701   (732)530-1515   Fax (732)747-5433
+ Shore Orthopaedic Group
1255 Route 70/Suite 11S   Lakewood, NJ 08701   (732)530-1515   Fax (732)942-2311
+ Shore Orthopaedic Group
1322 Route 72 West   Manahawkin, NJ 07701   (609)597-1377   Fax (609)597-0204

Wosu, Carolee Ngozi, MD {1255493417} Pedtrc(01,NJ05)<NJ-HACKNSK, NJ-HOLYNAME>
+ Riverside Medical Group
714 Tenth Street/Suite 2   Secaucus, NJ 07094   (201)863-3346   Fax (201)865-0015

Wreiole, August L., DO {1942247333} IntrMd(76,PA77)
+ 422 Morris Avenue/Suite 4
Long Branch, NJ 07740

Wright, Camylla Dimetruss, DO {1407281322} EmrgMd
+ SJH Emergency Medicine
1505 West Sherman Avenue   Vineland, NJ 08360   (856)641-8000   Fax (888)395-8975

Wright, Christopher, MD {1790003267}
+ 140 Bergen Street/Suite G1680
Newark, NJ 07103   (973)972-4488

Wright, Craig, MD {1285942268} Ortped
+ New Jersey Orthopaedic Institute
504 Valley Road/Suite 200   Wayne, NJ 07470   (973)626-3203   Fax (973)694-2692

wright3@gmail.com

Wright, Deborah Sue, MD {1619060902} FamMed(89,PA02)<NJ-HUNTRDN>
+ Hunterdon Family Physicians
111 State Route 31/Suite 111   Flemington, NJ 08822   (908)284-9880   Fax (908)782-4316

Wright, Douglas G., MD {1568497469} SrgOrt(NY09)
+ Hackensack Meridian Health Orthopedic Surgery
1173 Beacon Avenue/Suite A   Manahawkin, NJ 08050   (609)250-4101   Fax (609)997-8486

Wright, Erin Armstead, MD {1023147006} Pedtrc(05,PA09)<NJ-COOPRUMC>
+ Cooper Peds/Children's Regional Ctr
3 Cooper Plaza/Suite 200   Camden, NJ 08103   (856)342-2472   Fax (856)368-8297

Wright, Evan Michael, DO {1447426457} AeroMd(08,PA77)
+ CentraState Family Medicine Residency Practice
1001 West Main Street/Suite B   Freehold, NJ 07728   (732)294-2540   Fax (732)409-2621

Wright, Toni Rene, MD {1154417830} EmrgMd(90,DC03)<NJ-RWJURAH>
+ Robert Wood Johnson University Hospital at Rahway
865 Stone Street/EmergMed   Rahway, NJ 07065   (732)381-4200

Wright-Cadet, Yvonne, MD {1679524128} ObsGyn(86,NY20)<NJ-NWRKBETH>
+ Yvonne Wright-Cadet MD PC
2130 Milburn Avenue/Suite C 14   Maplewood, NJ 07040   (973)313-2550   Fax (973)313-0250

Wrigley, Steven N., MD {1356475263} EmrgMd, NeuMus(80,SPA13)<NJ-COMMED>
+ 368 Lakehurst Road/Suite 206
Toms River, NJ 08755   (732)557-9980   Fax (732)557-9985

Wroblewski, Edward A., MD {1891774402} CdvDis, IntrMd(68,PA02)<NJ-ACMCMAIN, NJ-ATLANCHS>
+ Associated Cardiovascular Consultants, PA
2 Sindoni Lane   Hammonton, NJ 08037   (609)561-8500   Fax (856)567-0432
+ Associated Cardiovascular Consultants, PA
2500 English Creek Avenue   Egg Harbor Township, NJ 08234   (609)561-8500   Fax (609)569-1896
+ Associated Cardiovascular Consultants-Lourdes
1 Brace Road/Suite C & F   Cherry Hill, NJ 08037   (856)428-4100   Fax (856)428-5748

Wroblewski, Henry M., MD {1730181785} PhysMd, PhyM-Pain(84,GRN01)
+ St. Barnabas Ambulatory Care Center
200 South Orange Avenue   Livingston, NJ 07039   (973)322-7700

Wrone, David A., MD {1043276108} Dermat(96,CA11)<NJ-UNVMCPRN>
+ Princeton Dermatology Associates
1950 State Route 27/Suite A   North Brunswick, NJ 08902   (732)297-8866   Fax (732)821-0626
+ Princeton Dermatology Associates
208 Bunn Drive/Suite 1-E   Princeton, NJ 08540   (732)297-8866   Fax (609)683-0298

Wruble, Steven J., MD {1861613531} PsyCAd(87,TN06)
+ 1250 East Ridgewood Avenue
Ridgewood, NJ 07450   (201)444-7794   Fax (201)444-7371

Wry, Ann M., MD {1013964204} IntrMd(89,VA07)<NJ-HACKNSK>
+ Ann Wry MD LLC
114 Essex Street/2nd Floor   Rochelle Park, NJ 07662   (201)368-0201   Fax (201)368-0346
annwry@aol.com

Wry, Philip C., MD SrgCrC, Surgry(OH43<NJ-COOPRUMC>
+ 306 East Main Street
Moorestown, NJ 08057

Wu, Albert B., MD {1669415675} PsyGrt(00,IL06)<NJ-UMDNJ, NJ-UNIVBHC>
+ University Psychiatric Associates
183 South Orange Avenue/E-F Levels   Newark, NJ 07103   (973)972-2977   Fax (973)972-2979
+ University Behavioral Health Care
671 Hoes Lane/PO Box 1392   Piscataway, NJ 08855   (732)235-5500

Wu, Brenda Yunqing, MD {1255406443} ClNrPh, Nrolgy, Psychy(90,CHN21)
+ 90 Paterson Street/Suite 100
New Brunswick, NJ 08901   (732)258-0061   Fax (732)993-9497
+ Northeast Regional Epilepsy Group
290 Madison Avenue/Building 5 2nd FL   Morristown, NJ 07960   (201)343-6676
+ NE Regional Epilepsy/Atlantic Neuro
99 Beauvoir Avenue/5th Fl   Summit, NJ 08901   (908)522-4990

Wu, Chi M., MD {1497720551} PhysMd, Acpntr, PainMd(85,PA07)<NJ-HLTHSRE, NJ-COMMED>
+ Multi-Med Associates, PC
9 Mule Road/Suite E-6   Toms River, NJ 08755   (732)505-5050   Fax (732)505-9979

+ HealthSouth Rehabilitation Hospital of New Jersey
14 Hospital Drive   Toms River, NJ 08755   (732)244-3100

Wu, Chia F., MD {1497800312} CdvDis, IntrMd(69,TAI02)
+ 35 Park Avenue
West Orange, NJ 07052   (973)325-3445   Fax (973)325-3507

Wu, Daniel C., MD {1114052693} Anesth<NJ-HCKTSTWN>
+ Hackettstown Regional Medical Center
651 Willow Grove Street   Hackettstown, NJ 07840   (908)852-5100

Wu, David Sweghsien, MD {1871533844} Urolgy(96,MD07)
+ Essex Hudson Urology
256 Broad Street   Bloomfield, NJ 07003   (973)743-4450   Fax (973)429-9076
+ Essex Hudson Urology
243 Chestnut Street   Newark, NJ 07105   (973)743-4450   Fax (973)344-9188
+ Essex Hudson Urology
213 South Frank Rodgers Blvd   Harrison, NJ 07003   (973)482-7070

Wu, Dee Dee Yui, MD {1871640334} Rheuma, IntrMd(98,NJ06)
+ HSS Paramus Outpatient Center
140 East Ridgewood Avenue/Suite 175-S   Paramus, NJ 07652   (201)796-2255   Fax (201)796-3711
deedeewu9001@hotmail.com

Wu, Donald T., MD {1033178413} PhysMd(89,PA07)<NJ-MEDIPLEX, NJ-VIRTUAHS>
+ Marlton Rehabilitation Hospital
92 Brick Road   Marlton, NJ 08053   (856)988-4103
Donteew@hotmail.com

Wu, Duoping, MD {1568556306} Anesth(86,CHN21)<NJ-HACKNSK>
+ Hackensack University Medical Center
30 Prospect Avenue   Hackensack, NJ 07601   (201)996-2000   Fax (201)488-6769

Wu, Eddie S., DO {1215182332}
+ Premier Orthopaedic Associates
298 South Delsea Drive   Vineland, NJ 08360   (856)690-1616   Fax (856)690-1089

Wu, Eileen Pey Chi, MD {1689822769} Anesth<NJ-MORRISTN>
+ Morristown Medical Center
100 Madison Avenue   Morristown, NJ 07962   (973)971-5000   Fax (201)943-8733

Wu, Elain, DO {1134583461} IntrMd<NJ-OVERLOOK>
+ Overlook Medical Center
99 Beauvoir Avenue/PO Box 210   Summit, NJ 07902   (908)522-2000

Wu, Frances Y., MD {1952302838} FamMed(84,RI01)<NJ-SOMERSET>
+ Somerset Family Practice
110 Rehill Avenue   Somerville, NJ 08876   (908)685-2900   Fax (908)685-2891

Wu, Hen-Vai, MD {1043219983} Hemato, IntrMd, MedOnc(72,TAI02)<NJ-SOMERSET, NJ-STPETER>
+ Somerset Hematology Oncology Associates, P.A.
30 Rehill Avenue/2nd Floor/Suite 2500   Somerville, NJ 08876   (908)927-8700   Fax (908)927-8706
susan.zhcenter@yahoo.com

Wu, Irene Y., MD {1881859957} FamMed(05,NJ06)
+ Visiting Nurse Association of Central Jersey
1301 Main Street   Asbury Park, NJ 07712   (732)774-6333   Fax (732)774-0313

Wu, Jack Chen-Jen, MD {1588624977} FamMed(68,TAIW)<NJ-VIRTMARL, NJ-VIRTBERL>
+ Drs. Wu and Wu
219 Highland Avenue   Westville, NJ 08093   (856)456-1881   Fax (856)456-3959

Wu, Jason Jon, DO {1598024507} IntrMd
+ The Orthopedic Institute of New Jersey
108 Bilby Road/Suite 201   Hackettstown, NJ 07840   (908)684-3005   Fax (908)684-3301
+ The Orthopedic Institute of New Jersey
254-B Mountain Avenue/Suite 201   Hackettstown, NJ 07840   (908)684-3005   Fax (908)684-3301
+ The Orthopedic Institute of New Jersey
222 High Street/Suite 202   Newton, NJ 07840   (908)684-3005   Fax (908)684-3301

Wu, Jeffrey P., MD {1902051394} Anesth, PedAne(06,NY19)<NJ-JRSYSHMC>
+ Jersey Shore Anesthesiology Associates
1945 Route 33/PO Box 397   Neptune, NJ 07754   (732)776-4896   Fax (732)776-2442
+ Jersey Shore University Medical Center
1945 Route 33/Anesthesia   Neptune, NJ 07753   (732)776-4896   Fax (732)776-2442

Wu, Jing, MD {1124126776} Anesth(82,CHN21)<NJ-HACKNSK>
+ Hackensack University Medical Center
30 Prospect Avenue/Anesthesiology   Hackensack, NJ 07601   (201)996-2000

Physicians by Name and Address

Wu, Jung-Faug, MD {1760469761} Anesth, AnesAddM(67,TAI07)<NJ-CHRIST>
+ Christ Hospital
176 Palisade Avenue/Anesthesiology   Jersey City, NJ 07306   (201)795-8200   Fax (201)943-8105

Wu, Justine Peen, MD {1790897379} FamMed(00,NJ05)
+ Family Medicine at Monument Square
317 George Street   New Brunswick, NJ 08901   (732)235-8993   Fax (732)246-7317
wuju1@umdnj.edu

Wu, Karen, MD {1487718946} Pedtrc, AdolMd(92,NY01)<NJ-VALLEY, NJ-HACKNSK>
+ North Jersey Pediatrics
1010 Clifton Avenue   Clifton, NJ 07013   (973)249-1231   Fax (973)249-1316
+ North Jersey Pediatrics
17-10 Fair Lawn Avenue   Fair Lawn, NJ 07410   (973)249-1231   Fax (201)703-9889

Wu, Kevin, DO {1043274228} FamMed(99,NJ75)
+ Drs. Wu and Wu
219 Highland Avenue   Westville, NJ 08093   (856)456-1881   Fax (856)456-3959

Wu, Margaret J., MD {1033384250}<NJ-STMRYPAS>
+ St. Mary's Hospital
350 Boulevard   Passaic, NJ 07055   (973)365-4300   Fax (845)357-5777

Wu, Melissa S., MD {1770927477} Anesth
+ Robert Wood Johnson-UMDNJ Anesthesia Group
125 Paterson Street/CAB 3100   New Brunswick, NJ 08901   (732)235-7827   Fax (732)235-6131

Wu, Nan, MD {1073903142}
+ Cooper Surgical Associates
3 Cooper Plaza/Suite 411   Camden, NJ 08103   (856)342-3012   Fax (856)365-1180

Wu, Peter, MD {1144382383} Anesth(02,NY46)<NJ-VALLEY>
+ Bergen Anesthesia Group, P.C.
500 West Main Street/Suite 16   Wyckoff, NJ 07481   (201)847-9320   Fax (201)847-0059
+ 800 Madison Avenue
Morristown, NJ 07960

Wu, Peywen, MD {1366533150} Pedtrc(99,NJ06)
+ Basking Ridge Pediatric Association
150 North Finley Avenue   Basking Ridge, NJ 07920   (908)766-4660   Fax (908)204-9871

Wu, Shiann J., MD {1437261161} Pedtrc(64,TAIW)<NJ-VIRTVOOR, NJ-JFKMED>
+ Advocare Berlin Medical Associates
175 Cross Keys Road/Suite 300A   Berlin, NJ 08009   (856)767-0077   Fax (856)767-6102

Wu, Timothy, MD {1619179686} SrgVas, Surgry(03,NY08)<NJ-UMDNJ>
+ University Hospital-Doctors Office Center
90 Bergen Street/Suite 7200   Newark, NJ 07103   (973)972-9371   Fax (973)972-0002

Wu, Yan, MD {1831191550} IntrMd, EnDbMt(87,CHN19)<NJ-LOURDMED, NJ-VIRTMHBC>
+ Capital Endocrinology
2 Capital Way/Suite 290   Pennington, NJ 08534   (609)303-4300   Fax (609)303-4301

Wu, Yihui Yvonne, MD {1922069301} PthACl(84,CHN4D)<NJ-WAYNEGEN>
+ St. Joseph's Wayne Hospital
224 Hamburg Turnpike   Wayne, NJ 07470   (973)956-3589   Fax (973)942-1884

Wujciak, Michael P., MD {1760560106} SrgOrt(77,NJ05)<NJ-CLARMAAS>
+ 181 Franklin Avenue
Nutley, NJ 07110   (973)667-8414   Fax (973)667-8547

Wulach, Sandra H., MD {1215014899} Psychy(75,NY09)
+ West Bergen Mental Health Care
120 Chestnut Street   Ridgewood, NJ 07450   (201)444-3550   Fax (201)652-1613

Wulkan, Sheryl Lynn, MD {1710991765} IntrMd, IntrSptM(85,NY48)
+ Universal Industrial Clinic
99 Madison Street   Newark, NJ 07105   (973)344-2929   Fax (973)344-1239

Wunsh, Stuart Eugene, MD {1588630271} Ophthl(63,NY20)<NJ-STMRYPAS, NY-MTSINYHS>
+ North Jersey Eye Associates PA
1005 Clifton Avenue   Clifton, NJ 07013   (973)472-4114   Fax (973)472-0775
sewunshmd@aol.com

Wurmser, Eric A., MD {1033128921} SrgPlstc(70,NY47)<NJ-RIVERVW, NJ-BAYSHORE>
+ 225 Highway 35 North/Suite 102
Red Bank, NJ 07701   (732)747-5353   Fax (732)747-5535

Wurtzel, David, MD {1063441566} Pedtrc, PainMd(80,MEX14)<NJ-VIRTVOOR>
+ Virtua Voorhees
100 Bowman Drive/Pediatrics   Voorhees, NJ 08043   (856)247-3000

Wurzel, Bernard Samuel, MD {1295749679} FamMed(70,NY08)
+ 405 Northfield Avenue/Suite 203
West Orange, NJ 07052   (973)736-8645   Fax (973)736-1914

Wurzer, James C., MD {1659311934} RadOnc(94,PA13)<NJ-BURDTMLN, NJ-ACMCMAIN>
+ Cape Regional Medical Center
2 Stone Harbor Boulevard   Cape May Court House, NJ 08210   (609)463-2000
+ AtlantiCare Regional Med Ctr/Mainland
65 West Jimmie Leeds Road/RadOncology   Pomona, NJ 08240   (609)652-1000
+ Shore Memorial Hospital
1 East New York Avenue/RadOncology   Somers Point, NJ 08210   (609)653-3500

Wuu, Zukwung, MD {1720034101} Anesth(91,KS02)<NJ-CHSMRCER, NJ-CHSFULD>
+ Trenton Anesthesia Associates, PA
One Capital Way/Second Floor   Pennington, NJ 08534   (609)396-4700   Fax (609)396-4900

Wyche Bullock, Tara Lynette, MD {1720008931} FamMed(01,NJ05)
+ Family Health Center of Mullica Hill
155 Bridgeton Pike/Suite A   Mullica Hill, NJ 08062   (856)223-0500   Fax (856)223-1098

Wydo, Salina Marie, MD {1801058136} Surgry
+ Cooper Surgical Associates
3 Cooper Plaza/Suite 411   Camden, NJ 08103   (856)342-3341   Fax (856)365-1180

Wymer, Edwin Anthony, DO {1912975996} Pedtrc
+ Ocean Pediatric Group PA
1C Industrial Way West   Eatontown, NJ 07724

Wynkoop, Walter Alan, MD {1992774657} PulDis, IntrMd, SlpDis(95,PA13)<NJ-OCEANMC, NJ-COMMED>
+ Ocean Pulmonary Associates PA
457 Jack Martin Boulevard/Suite 4   Brick, NJ 08724   (732)840-4200   Fax (732)840-6444
+ Ocean Pulmonary Associates PA
3 Plaza Drive/Suite 2   Toms River, NJ 08757   (732)840-4200   Fax (732)505-9296
+ Ocean Pulmonary Associates PA
70 Lacey Road/Irish Branch Mall   Whiting, NJ 08724   (732)350-4777

Wynn, Laurence, MD {1962623389} IntrMd, GPrvMd, PubHth(73,PHI09)
+ Hudson County Correctional Center
35 Hackensack Avenue   Kearny, NJ 07032   (201)395-5600

Wynne, Brenna, MD {1235156258} EmrgMd(03,PA0)
+ Cooper Univerisry Emergency Physicians
One Cooper Plaza   Camden, NJ 08103   (856)342-2351   Fax (856)968-8272

Wynne, Peter J., MD {1720178593} Radiol, RadNro(90,NJ05)<NJ-MORRISTN>
+ Memorial Radiology Associates
10 Lanidex Plaza West/Suite 125   Parsippany, NJ 07054   (973)503-5700   Fax (973)386-5701

Wysocki, Julianne M., DO {1124255203} EmrgMd
+ Rowan University-School of Osteopathic Medicine
1 Medical Center Drive   Stratford, NJ 08084   (856)566-6708

Xagoraris, Andreas E., MD {1609848977} Anesth(93,NJ06)<NJ-HACKNSK>
+ Hackensack University Medical Center
30 Prospect Avenue/Anesthesiology   Hackensack, NJ 07601   (201)996-2000   Fax (201)488-6769

Xavier, Geralda A., MD {1275619322} EmrgMd(01,NJ02)
+ JFK Medical Center
65 James Street/Emergency   Edison, NJ 08820   (732)321-7000

Xenachis, Cristina Z., MD {1497819940} EnDbMt, IntrMd(80,ROMA)<NJ-BAYSHORE, NJ-RIVERVW>
+ Downtown Osteoporosis Center, Inc.
158 Main Street/Suite 100   Matawan, NJ 07747   (732)765-1166   Fax (732)765-0027

Xia, Wenlang, MD {1578508693} Nrolgy, NroChl, NrlgSpec(87,CHN40)<NJ-STJOSHOS>
+ St. Joseph's Regional Medical Center
703 Main Street/Neurology   Paterson, NJ 07503   (973)754-2000

Xiao, Danhua, MD {1649538141}
+ Atlantic Health Metabolic Center
33 Overlook Road/Suite 208   Summit, NJ 07901   (908)598-6517   Fax (908)522-5789

Xiao, Han, MD {1194705533} MedOnc, IntrMd(84,CHN21)<NY-SLOANKET>
+ Memorial Sloan-Kettering Cancer Center Basking Ridge
136 Mountain View Boulevard   Basking Ridge, NJ 07920   (908)542-3000   Fax (908)542-3220

Xie, Bingru, MD {1487802690} Hepato, IntrMd(02,CHN57)
+ New Jersey Digestive Disease Associates
239 New Road/A106   Parsippany, NJ 07054   (973)287-7055   Fax (973)362-4619

+ New Jersey Digestive Disease Associates
211 Bridge Street/Bldg. D   Metuchen, NJ 08840   (973)287-7055   Fax (732)362-4619
+ University Hospital
150 Bergen Street   Newark, NJ 07054   (973)972-4300

Xie, Jinghui, MD {1760659809} AnesPain, IntrMd(95,CHN19)
+ Advanced Interventional Pain Management Center
20 Cherry Tree Farm Road   Middletown, NJ 07748   (732)952-5533   Fax (732)707-4732
+ Advanced Interventional Pain Management Center
204 Eagle Rock Avenue   Roseland, NJ 07068   (732)952-5533   Fax (732)707-4732
+ Advanced Interventional Pain Management Center
619 Amboy Avenue   Edison, NJ 07748   (732)952-5533   Fax (732)707-4732

Xie, Linjun, MD {1639242928} PthACl, IntrMd(83,CHN07)
+ Pathology Solutions, LLC.
246 Industrial Way West/Suite 2   Eatontown, NJ 07724   (732)389-5200   Fax (732)389-5299

Xiong, Ming, MD {1487714077} Anesth(87,CHN40)<NJ-UMDNJ>
+ University Hospital
150 Bergen Street/Anesth   Newark, NJ 07103   (973)972-5006   Fax (973)972-4172

Xiong, Wen, MD {1447408216} Rheuma, IntrMd(94,CHN17)<NJ-NWRKBETH>
+ Humane Center for Arthritis and Rheumatism
2424 Morris Avenue/Suite 110   Union, NJ 07083   (908)688-1288   Fax (908)688-1588

Xu, Lin, MD {1386671071} IntrMd(82,CHN57)<NJ-BAYSHORE>
+ 1 Bethany Road & Route 35
Hazlet, NJ 07730   (732)888-1203   Fax (732)888-1204
+ Menlo Park Medical Group PA
111 James Street   Edison, NJ 08820   (732)888-1203   Fax (732)549-2262

Xu, Qian, MD {1386923415} PhysMd
+ Premier Orthopaedics and Sports Medicine, PC
663 Palisade Avenue/Suite 302   Cliffside Park, NJ 07010   (201)833-9500   Fax (201)862-0095

Xu, Wei, MD {1861690570} PhysMd(85,CHN2A)<NJ-ATLANTHS>
+ Rothman Institute - Egg Harbor Township
2500 English Creek Avenue/Bldg 1300   Egg Harbor Township, NJ 08234   (609)677-7002   Fax (609)677-7000

Xu, Weizhen, MD {1881787604} PedEnd, Pedtrc, PhysMd(87,CHN4A)<NJ-VIRTVOOR, NJ-COOPRUMC>
+ The Children's Hospital at Saint Peter's University
254 Easton Avenue/MOB Third Floor   New Brunswick, NJ 08901   (732)745-8574   Fax (732)514-1956

Yablonsky, Thaddeus M., MD {1194815977} RadDia, Radiol(90,NJ06)<NJ-MORRISTN>
+ Memorial Radiology Associates
10 Lanidex Plaza West/Suite 125   Parsippany, NJ 07054   (973)503-5700   Fax (973)386-5701
+ Morristown Medical Center
100 Madison Avenue/Radiology   Morristown, NJ 07962   (973)971-5000

Yaccarino, Pasquale J., MD {1427020742} IntrMd(77,ITA01)<NY-STANTHNY>
+ 6 Church Street/Box 920
Vernon, NJ 07462   (973)764-5155   Fax (973)764-9929

Yacoub, Magdy Yousef, MD {1144251869} Anesth(75,EGY09)<NJ-MTNSIDE>
+ Hackensack UMC Mountainside
1 Bay Avenue/Anesthesia   Montclair, NJ 07042   (973)429-6982

Yacoub, Mounzer H., MD {1992091573} ObsGyn
+ 399 Hoover Avenue/Suite 1
Bloomfield, NJ 07003   (201)572-7000   Fax (973)566-0866

Yadalla, Vanitha S., MD {1093702961} IntrMd(98,GRN01)<NJ-JRSYSHMC>
+ 3350 Route 138 West/Bldg. 2 Suite 128
Wall, NJ 07719   (732)280-2727   Fax (732)280-1147

Yadav, Jagdish P., MD {1447207014} IntrMd(83,INA8Z)<NJ-COOPRUMC, NJ-SJHREGMC>
+ Cooper University Medical Center/Camden
3 Cooper Plaza/Internal Med   Camden, NJ 08103   (856)356-4935
+ SJH Regional Medical Center
1505 West Sherman Avenue/Internal Med   Vineland, NJ 08360   (856)641-8000

Yadav, Priyanka Singh, DO {1063633402} Pedtrc, SlpDis(03,NY75)
+ RWJPE Primary Care Center at Hillsborough
331 Route 206 North/Suite 2-B   Hillsborough, NJ 08844   (908)685-2528   Fax (908)359-7109
+ 331 Us Highway 206
Hillsborough, NJ 08844   (908)685-2528   Fax (908)231-6148

Yager, Scott, MD {1669522595} IntrMd(89,FL02)<NJ-RBAYOLDB, NJ-RBAYPERT>
+ 4 Cornwall Drive/Suite 201
East Brunswick, NJ 08816   (732)432-7040   Fax (732)432-7183

Physicians by Name and Address

Yahav, Eric Kfir, MD {1013156686} ObsGyn
+ Cooper University Medical Center/Camden
3 Cooper Plaza   Camden, NJ 08103   (856)342-2000

Yakobashvili, David, MD {1265420137} IntrMd(91,GEO02)
+ 81 Veronica Avenue/Suite 203
Somerset, NJ 08873   (732)545-3080

Yakoby, Jordan M., MD {1811364375}<NJ-COOPRUMC>
+ Cooper University Hospital
One Cooper Plaza   Camden, NJ 08103   (800)826-6737

Yakubov, Boris, MD {1518934645} IntrMd(82,UZB44)
+ NJ VA/James J Howard Outpatient Clinic
970 Route 70 West   Brick, NJ 08724   (732)206-8900
boriscobi@yahoo.com

Yalamanchi, Geeta, MD {1235210352} IntrMd
+ 245 Union Avenue/Suite 2 A
Bridgewater, NJ 08807   (908)450-7735   Fax (908)450-7737

Yalamanchi, Krishan, MD {1205804291} Pedtrc, PedNrD(81,INA66)<NJ-CHLSMT>
+ Children's Specialized Hospital
150 New Providence Road/Brain Injury   Mountainside, NJ 07092   (908)233-3720
Kyalamanchi@childrens-specialized.org

Yalamanchili, Praveen K., MD {1982841920} SrgOrt(06,NJ06)
+ Seaview Orthopaedics
1200 Eagle Avenue   Ocean, NJ 07712   (732)660-6200   Fax (732)660-6201

Yallowitz, Joseph, MD {1013967439} EmrgMd, IntrMd(89,MEX14)<NJ-VALLEY>
+ The Valley Hospital
223 North Van Dien Avenue/EmergMed   Ridgewood, NJ 07450   (201)447-8000

Yama, Asher Z., MD {1972605210} Anesth, CritCr, IntrMd(87,NY46)<NJ-RWJUBRUN>
+ University Surgical Center
561 Cranbury Road/Anesthesia   East Brunswick, NJ 08816   (201)342-1205   Fax (201)342-1259

Yamane, Michael H., MD {1487694501} IntrMd(81,CA02)<NJ-CHSMRCER>
+ Mercer Internal Medicine, LLC.
2480 Pennington Road/Suites 104   Pennington, NJ 08534   (609)818-1000   Fax (609)818-9800

Yamin, Edward, MD {1225077506} EmrgMd(92,DOMI)<NJ-HACKNSK>
+ Hackensack Medical Center Emergency Medicine
30 Prospect Avenue/Main 3619   Hackensack, NJ 07601   (201)996-4614   Fax (201)342-7112
+ Hackensack University Medical Center
30 Prospect Avenue/EmergMed   Hackensack, NJ 07601   (201)996-4614   Fax (201)968-1866

Yampaglia, Joseph P., MD {1386649879} Anesth(82,MEX02)<NJ-SOCEANCO>
+ Southern Ocean County Medical Center
1140 Route 72 West/Anesthesiology   Manahawkin, NJ 08050   (609)597-6011

Yamusah, Emmanuel N., MD {1134346901} MedOnc, Hemato, IntrMd(83,GRN01)
+ Zara Cancer Medicine
634 Broadway   Paterson, NJ 07514   (973)279-2616   Fax (973)279-0399

Yanagida, Roh, MD {1104059880}<NJ-NWRKBETH>
+ Newark Beth Israel Medical Center
201 Lyons Avenue   Newark, NJ 07112   (310)614-9614
ryanagida@barnabashealth.org

Yanamadula, Dinash Kumar, MD {1578507893} PainInvt
+ Universal Industrial Clinic
99 Madison Street   Newark, NJ 07105   (973)344-2929   Fax (973)344-1239
+ Drs. Desai & Yanamadula
123 Franklin Corner Road/Suite 104   Lawrenceville, NJ 08648   (973)344-2929   Fax (609)512-1674

Yang, Anthony, MD {1902953268} EmrgMd(94,NY08)<NJ-RWJUBRUN>
+ RWJ University Hospital New Brunswick
One Robert Wood Johnson Place   New Brunswick, NJ 08901   (732)828-3000

Yang, Arvin S., MD {1255549481} OncHem, IntrMd(05,NJ06)<MA-BIDMCEST>
+ Bristol-Myers Squibb Co. - Occupational Health
Route 206 & Provinceline Road   Princeton, NJ 08543   (609)252-7194

Yang, Ben Ming-Chien, MD {1407858814} RadDia(93,NY19)<NJ-VIRTMHBC>
+ Radiology Associates of Burlington County
1295 Route 38 West/PO Box 479   Hainesport, NJ 08036   (609)261-7017   Fax (609)261-4180

Yang, Bin, MD {1740320233} OccpMd, Psychy(87,CHN52)<NJ-VAEASTOR>
+ VA New Jersey Health Care System-East Orange Campus
385 Tremont Avenue   East Orange, NJ 07018   (973)676-1000

+ 30 Ten Broek Court
Bridgewater, NJ 08807

Yang, Charles, MD {1679736706} RadBdI<NY-STONYBRK>
+ University Radiology Group, P.C.
579A Cranbury Road   East Brunswick, NJ 08816   (732)390-0040   Fax (732)390-1856
+ University Radiology Group, P.C.
16 Mountain Boulevard   Warren, NJ 07059   (732)390-0040   Fax (908)769-9141

Yang, Clement, MD {1225050636} RadDia<NJ-HACKNSK>
+ Hackensack University Medical Center
30 Prospect Avenue   Hackensack, NJ 07601   (201)996-2200   Fax (201)489-2812
+ Hackensack Radiology Group, P.A.
30 Prospect Avenue   Hackensack, NJ 07601   (201)996-2200   Fax (201)336-8451

Yang, Dingming, MD {1235219734} PthAcl(82,CHN87)<NJ-RWJUHAM>
+ Robert Wood Johnson University Hospital at Hamilton
1 Hamilton Health Place/Pathology   Hamilton, NJ 08690   (609)586-7900

Yang, Domingo Berzamin, Jr, MD {1518286939}(01,PHI08)
+ Valley Medical Associates
1700 Route 3 West   Clifton, NJ 07012   (862)249-4901   Fax (973)928-2650

Yang, Hee Kon, MD {1174559280} Surgry, SrgVas(89,IL01)<NY-SSWESTCH>
+ 464 Hudson Terrace/Suite 101
Englewood Cliffs, NJ 07632   (201)567-7747   Fax (201)567-3916

Yang, Jingduan, MD {1356566905} Psychy(84,CHN43)
+ Tao Institute of Mind & Body Medicine
1288 Route 73 South/Suite 210   Mount Laurel, NJ 08054   (856)802-6888   Fax (856)802-6878

Yang, John Y., MD {1659322766} Nrolgy(72)<NJ-VIRTUAHS, NJ-VIRTMARL>
+ Neurological Regional Associates
504 Route 38 East   Maple Shade, NJ 08052   (856)866-0466   Fax (856)727-1483
neuroreg@snip.net

Yang, Jun, MD {1730164542} IntrMd(91,CHN4A)<NJ-COOPRUMC>
+ Cooper University Hospital
One Cooper Plaza/Hsplist   Camden, NJ 08103   (856)342-2000

Yang, Jun, MD {1730166414} Allrgy
+ Center for Asthma & Allergy
2566 Nottingham Way   Trenton, NJ 08610   (609)587-3041   Fax (609)587-9347

Yang, Kenneth E., MD {1114985595} Ophthl(91,NJ05)<NJ-RWJUBRUN>
+ Chen, Kenneth E.
C-5 Cornwall Court   East Brunswick, NJ 08816   (732)257-5767   Fax (732)238-3777

Yang, Lihua, MD {1245495928} IntrMd
+ Allergy Better Care
22 Old Short Hills Road/Suite 110   Livingston, NJ 07039   (973)602-9860   Fax (646)926-0360

Yang, Rayson C., MD {1841301637} CdvDis
+ Shore Heart Group, P.A.
1820 State Route 33/Suite 4-B   Neptune, NJ 07753   (732)776-8500   Fax (732)776-8946
+ Shore Heart Group, P.A.
115 East Bay Avenue   Manahawkin, NJ 08050   (732)776-8500   Fax (609)597-4656
+ Shore Heart Group, P.A.
555 Iron Bridge Road/Suite 15   Freehold, NJ 07753   (732)308-0774   Fax (732)333-1366

Yang, Rebecca Chaohua, MD {1891895827} Surgry, SrgBst(93,MD01)<NJ-ATLANTHS>
+ Atlantic Breast Associates
11 Overlook Road/Suite LL-102   Summit, NJ 07901   (908)598-6576

Yang, Roger S., MD {1376540831} RadDia(92,IL06)
+ University Radiology, PA
239 Route 22 East/Suite 302   Green Brook, NJ 08812   (732)968-4899   Fax (732)968-8096
+ University Radiology Group, P.C.
3900 Park Avenue/Suite 107   Edison, NJ 08820   (732)968-4899   Fax (732)548-6290
+ University Radiology Group, P.C.
16 Mountain Boulevard   Warren, NJ 08812   (908)769-7200   Fax (908)769-9141

Yang, Sherry, MD {1225076961} PedOph, Ophthl(96,NY19)<NJ-CHILTON, NJ-HACKNSK>
+ Pediatric Ophthalmology of NJ
57 Willowbrook Boulevard/Suite 411   Wayne, NJ 07470   (973)256-4111   Fax (973)256-3719
drsherry@yahoo.com

Yang, Tianzhong, MD {1255521753}<NJ-MTNSIDE>
+ Dedicated Primary Care
239 Claremont Avenue   Montclair, NJ 07042   (973)893-5317   Fax (973)893-5321

Yang, Xiao Yan, MD {1356370886} PthAcl(83,CHN4C)<NJ-HACKNSK>
+ Hackensack University Medical Center
30 Prospect Avenue/Pathology   Hackensack, NJ 07601   (201)996-2000

Yang, Yulong, MD {1013392919} IntrMd
+ 2083 Center Avenue/Suite 2 A
Fort Lee, NJ 07024

Yang, Zhaomin, MD {1629153168} Anesth, PainInvt(84,CHNA)<NJ-JRSYSHMC>
+ Jersey Shore University Medical Center
1945 Route 33/Anesthesiology   Neptune, NJ 07753   (732)775-5500   Fax (732)897-0263
+ Jersery Shore Anesthesiology
1945 Highway 33   Neptune, NJ 07753   (732)775-5500   Fax (732)897-0263

Yang-Novellino, Sue Y., DO {1740593920} FamMed, IntrMd(NJ75)
+ Collingswood Osteopathic Medicine
504 White Horse Pike   Collingswood, NJ 08107   (856)425-2577   Fax (856)282-5610
collingswoodosteomed@gmail.com

Yangala, Ravi, MD {1144216755} Nrolgy, IntrMd(85,INA8Y)
+ Shore Physicians Group
52 East New York Avenue   Somers Point, NJ 08244   (609)365-6202   Fax (609)653-1925

Yangala, Sridevi, MD {1114174687} IntrMd(90,INA83)<NJ-SHOREMEM>
+ Shore Hospitalists Associates
100 Medical Center Way   Somers Point, NJ 08244   (609)653-3500   Fax (609)926-4799
+ Shore Memorial Hospital
1 East New York Avenue/Internal Med   Somers Point, NJ 08244   (609)653-3500   Fax (609)926-4311

Yangchen, Tenzing, MD {1972845410} PsyCAd
+ University Psychiatric Associates
183 South Orange Avenue/E-F Levels   Newark, NJ 07103   (973)972-4818   Fax (973)972-2979

Yankovitch, Pierre, MD {1275567356} IntrMd<NJ-SHOREMEM>
+ Shore Hospitalists Associates
100 Medical Center Way   Somers Point, NJ 08244   (609)653-3500   Fax (609)926-4799
+ Shore Memorial Hospital
1 East New York Avenue/Internal Med   Somers Point, NJ 08244   (609)653-3500   Fax (609)926-4311

Yankus, Wayne A., MD {1376502484} Pedtrc, IntrMd(75,MEX14)<NJ-VALLEY>
+ 358 Evergreen Place
Ridgewood, NJ 07450   (201)637-3569

Yanni, Baher S., MD {1053409219} PainMd, Anesth(99,EGY03)
+ Spine Institute of North America
300A Princeon Hightstown Road   East Windsor, NJ 08520   (609)337-6496   Fax (609)371-9110
+ Spine Institute of North America
777 East Route 70   Evesham, NJ 08053   (609)337-6496   Fax (609)371-9110
+ Spine Institute of North America
385 Cranbury Road   East Brunswick, NJ 08520   (609)337-6496   Fax (609)371-9110

Yanoschak, Jennifer Lee, MD {1255300778} Nrolgy, VasNeu(97,PA07)
+ Associated Cardiovascular Consultants, P.A.
1105 Laurel Oak Road/Suite 165   Voorhees, NJ 08043   (856)424-3600   Fax (856)424-7154
+ Neurology Associaates of South Jersey
693 Main Street/Building D   Lumberton, NJ 08048   (856)424-3600   Fax (609)265-8205
+ Advocare Neurology of South Jersey
200-B Route 73 North/Suite 2   Voorhees, NJ 08043   (856)335-0400   Fax (856)335-0406

Yanovskaya, Liliya, MD {1851329411} Anesth(78,EST01)
+ Meredian Medical PC
412 Pleasant Valley Way/Suite 201   West Orange, NJ 07052   (973)731-9707   Fax (973)731-9709
Liliya54@yahoo.com

Yanovskiy, Anatoliy M., MD {1922029800} Psychy(83,UZB44)<CT-STAMFDH>
+ Princeton House Behavioral Health - Princeton
905 Herrontown Road   Princeton, NJ 08540   (609)497-3300   Fax (609)497-3370

Yanow, Jennifer Hannah, MD {1942402599} AnesPain(04,NY46)
+ Infinity Orthopedics
1450 Route 22 West/Suite 200   Mountainside, NJ 07092   (917)270-7677   Fax (908)222-2757
+ The New Jersey Pain Management Institute
49 Veronica Avenue/Suite 102   Somerset, NJ 08873   (917)270-7677   Fax (732)745-8318

Yao, Daniel Duan, MD {1275512634} Anesth(00,VA01)<NJ-OVERLOOK>
+ Summit Anesthesia Associates, P.A.
33 Overlook Road/Suite 311   Summit, NJ 07901   (908)598-1500   Fax (908)598-0197

Physicians by Name and Address

Yao, Kevin Chi-Kai, MD {1407971542} SrgNro(97,NY01)<NJ-ENGLWOOD, NY-MTSINYHS>
+ Metropolitan Neurosurgery Associates, PA
  309 Engle Street/Suite 6   Englewood, NJ 07631   (201)569-7737   Fax (201)569-1494
  kevin.yao@mssm.edu
+ Metropolitan Neurosurgery Associates, PA
  142 Palisades Avenue   Jersey City, NJ 07306   (201)653-2112

Yao, Siu-Long, MD {1902029309} MedOnc, OncHem(90,CT01)
+ Merck and Company Incorporated
  126 East Lincoln Avenue/Box 2000   Rahway, NJ 07065   (732)574-4000

Yao, Su-Lin G., MD {1982630877} Anesth(94,NY48)<NJ-ACMC-MAIN>
+ AtlantiCare Anesthesiology
  65 West Jimmie Leeds Road   Pomona, NJ 08240   (609)748-7597

Yap, Joseph Jim Estrella, MD {1427024637} Anesth(83,PHI16)<NJ-HOBUNIMC>
+ Hoboken University Medical Center
  308 Willow Avenue/Anesthesiology   Hoboken, NJ 07030   (201)418-1000   Fax (201)943-8105

Yap, Wilson C., MD {1588638563} IntrMd(90,PHIL)<NJ-KIMBALL>
+ 525 Route 70 West/Suites 9-10
  Lakewood, NJ 08701   (732)730-8074   Fax (732)730-8076
  wkyapunagi@yahoo.com
+ Kimball Medical Center
  600 River Avenue   Lakewood, NJ 08701   (732)363-1900

Yaqub, Zunera, MD {1285836296} FamMed(00,PAK01)
+ Internal Medicine of Morristown
  95 Madison Avenue/Suite A-0   Morristown, NJ 07960   (973)538-1388   Fax (973)538-9501

Yarian, David L., MD {1497728299} Ophthl, VitRet(74,MO02)<NJ-RWJUBRUN, NJ-JFKMED>
+ Retina Associates of New Jersey, P.A.
  98 James Street/Suite 209   Edison, NJ 08820   (732)906-1887   Fax (732)906-1883
+ Retina Associates of New Jersey, P.A.
  140 Franklin Corner Road   Lawrenceville, NJ 08648   (732)906-1887   Fax (609)895-0853
+ Retina Associates of New Jersey, P.A.
  1200 Route 22 East   Bridgewater, NJ 08820   (908)218-4303   Fax (908)218-4307

Yarlagadda, Vivek, MD {1669836854} IntrMd<NJ-ACMCITY>
+ AtlantiCare Regional Medical Center/City Campus
  1925 Pacific Avenue   Atlantic City, NJ 08401   (609)441-8990

Yaros, Michael J., MD {1154327708} Ophthl(79,PA13)<NJ-VIRTVOOR, NJ-VIRTMARL>
+ Advanced Eyecare and Laser Center
  619 West Clements Bridge Road   Runnemede, NJ 08078   (856)939-9111   Fax (856)939-9650
  eyescraper@aol.com
+ Advanced Eyecare and Laser Center
  100 Brace Road   Cherry Hill, NJ 08034   (856)939-9111   Fax (856)939-9650
+ Advanced Eyecare and Laser Center
  124 East White Horse Pike   Berlin, NJ 08078   (856)767-2500   Fax (856)939-9650

Yarramneni, Akhila, MD {1679657605} SrgThr
+ Skillman CardioThoracic Surgery, LLC.
  25 Dogwood Lane   Skillman, NJ 08558   (908)281-6608   Fax (908)829-3330

Yarus, Christine V., MD {1942330584} IntrMd(87,NJ05)<NJ-VAEASTOR>
+ VA New Jersey Health Care System-East Orange Campus
  385 Tremont Avenue   East Orange, NJ 07018   (973)676-2830

Yasgur, Lee H., MD {1225118771} Ophthl, SrgLsr, IntrMd(77,PA09)<NJ-VIRTBERL, NJ-VIRTMARL>
+ Yasgur Eye Associates
  1415 Marlton Pike East/Suite 404   Cherry Hill, NJ 08034   (856)429-0997   Fax (856)429-4799
  Drleeyasgur@comcast.net
+ Yasgur Eye Associates
  206 North Blackhorse Pike   Runnemede, NJ 08078   (856)429-0997   Fax (856)312-1106
+ Virtua Voorhees
  100 Bowman Drive/Ophthalmology   Voorhees, NJ 08043   (856)247-3000

Yashar, Alyson Gail, MD {1639252794} Ophthl(93,NY19)<NJ-HACKNSK, NJ-VALLEY>
+ Woodcliff Lake Ophthalmology
  577 Chestnut Ridge Road   Woodcliff Lake, NJ 07677   (201)782-1700   Fax (201)782-1749

Yasin, Sami F., MD {1316007651} InfDis, IntrMd(85,DOMI)<NJ-STCLRSUS, NY-STANTHNY>
+ 199 Route 284
  Sussex, NJ 07461   (973)875-7121   Fax (973)875-7123

Yassin, Mahmoud M., MD {1922387620} Pedtrc(76,EGY06)<NJ-COMMED>
+ 115 Lacey Road/PO Box 537
  Forked River, NJ 08731   (609)971-0010
+ 1193 Beacon Avenue
  Manahawkin, NJ 08050   (609)597-7799

Yatrakis, Nicholas D., MD {1316993876} IntrMd, OthrSp(74,GRE01)<NJ-OVERLOOK, NJ-MORRISTN>
+ Summit Medical Group
  560 Springfield Avenue   Westfield, NJ 07090   (908)228-3610
+ Summit Medical Group-Berkeley Heights Campus
  1 Diamond Hill Road   Berkeley Heights, NJ 07922   (908)228-3610   Fax (908)790-6576

Yau, Assumpta K., MD {1831156660} Anesth(75,HKOG)<NJ-STPETER>
+ Anesthesia Consultnts of NJ/Nova Pain
  285 Davidson Avenue/Suite 204   Somerset, NJ 08873   (732)271-1400   Fax (732)271-3544

Yavorsky, John M., DO {1265594402} IntrMd(91,NJ75)<NJ-OVERLOOK>
+ Associates in Internal Medicine
  91 Center Street   Garwood, NJ 07027   (908)789-0626   Fax (908)789-3123

Yazdi, Mondana S., MD {1174602288} Pedtrc(91,TN20)<NJ-CHILTON, NJ-VALLEY>
+ Wyckoff Pediatric
  219 Everett Avenue   Wyckoff, NJ 07481   (201)891-4777   Fax (201)891-3823

Yazgi, Nabil M., MD {1144337908} Nrolgy, IntrMd(79,SYR01)
+ 401 Hamburg Turnpike/Suite 102
  Wayne, NJ 07470   (973)790-1180   Fax (973)790-0712

Ye, Dongjiu, MD {1598980948} PthACl
+ 49 Finnigan Avenue/Apt K-07
  Saddle Brook, NJ 07663

Ye, Michelle, MD {1265504062} PthACl(86,CHNA)<NJ-NWRKBETH>
+ Newark Beth Israel Medical Center
  201 Lyons Avenue/Pathology   Newark, NJ 07112   (973)926-7000

Ye, Sheng H., MD {1740203520} IntrMd, Grtrcs(85,CHNA)<NJ-HOLYNAME, NJ-ENGLWOOD>
+ Primary Care NJ
  370 Grand Avenue/Suite 102   Englewood, NJ 07631   (201)567-3370   Fax (201)816-1265

Ye, Xiaodan, MD {1700802212} IntrMd(84,CHN4A)<NJ-VIRTMHBC>
+ Virtua Memorial
  175 Madison Avenue   Mount Holly, NJ 08060   (609)267-0700

Ye, Xueming, MD {1427088566} Psychy, PsyCAd(88,CHN59)<NJ-RWJUBRUN>
+ Princeton Neurological Surgery, P.C.
  3836 Quakerbridge Road/Suite 203   Hamilton, NJ 08619   (609)890-3400   Fax (609)890-3410
+ University Hospital-New Jersey Medical School
  30 Bergen Street/Clinical Psych   Newark, NJ 07107   (973)972-4511

Yeager, Richard J., MD {1356675367} IntrMd(71,NY20)<NJ-OCEANMC>
+ 200 Bergen Avenue
  Mantoloking, NJ 08738   Fax (732)776-4690

Yee, Mary, MD {1881628246} Pedtrc(81,INA13)<NJ-JRSYSHMC>
+ Pediatric Associates
  9 South Main Street   Marlboro, NJ 07746   (732)577-1945   Fax (732)308-3460
+ Pediatric Associates
  444 Neptune Boulevard/Suite 4   Neptune, NJ 07753   (732)577-1945   Fax (732)774-4077

Yee, Mei-Ling, MD {1669408704} Ophthl(82,NJ05)
+ 142 Palisades Avenue/Suite 208
  Jersey City, NJ 07306   (201)795-2020   Fax (201)222-5125
  drmei-ling@gmail.com

Yee, Sau Yan, MD {1740288570} IntrMd, Pedtrc, EmrgMd(92,NY09)<NJ-ENGLWOOD, NJ-HOLYNAME>
+ Yee Medicine and Pediatric Associates, P.C.
  245 Engle Street/Suite 3   Englewood, NJ 07631   (201)569-9005   Fax (201)569-9080
+ Center for Remote Medical Management
  82 East Allendale Road/Suite 8-A   Saddle River, NJ 07458   (551)697-5399

Yegen, Lonna K., MD {1184625501} Pedtrc(72,NY19)<NJ-HOLYNAME, NJ-ENGLWOOD>
+ Pedimedica PA
  500 Piermont Road/Suite 102   Closter, NJ 07624   (201)784-3200   Fax (201)784-3321

Yegya-Raman, Sivaraman, MD {1558353326} CdvDis, IntrMd(75,INA66)<NJ-LOURDEHS, NJ-KENEDYHS>
+ Associated Cardiovascular Consultants-Lourdes
  1 Brace Road/Suite C & F   Cherry Hill, NJ 08034   (856)428-4100   Fax (856)428-5748

+ South Jersey Heart Group
  539 Egg Harbor Road/Suite 1   Sewell, NJ 08080   (856)428-4100   Fax (856)589-1753

Yeh, Janet Tristine, MD {1386873289}<NJ-MORRISTN>
+ Morristown Medical Center
  100 Madison Avenue   Morristown, NJ 07962   (973)971-4336   Fax (973)290-7350

Yeh, Jesson S.T., MD {1003043100}
+ Holy Name Hospital
  718 Teaneck Road/Emergency   Teaneck, NJ 07666   (201)833-3210   Fax (201)833-7226
+ 459 Utah Street
  Paramus, NJ 07652

Yeh, Shao-Chun, DO {1720368079} FamMed, Grtrcs
+ Advocare, LLC.
  402 Lippincott Drive/Geriatrics   Marlton, NJ 08053   (856)762-1933   Fax (856)762-1777

Yeh, Shihlong, MD {1376975805} AnesPain
+ University Medical Group
  125 Paterson Street/Suite 5100   New Brunswick, NJ 08901   (732)235-7246   Fax (732)235-7117

Yeh, Timothy Stephen, MD {1851404560} Pedtrc, PedCrC(76,CA19)<NJ-STBARNMC>
+ St. Barnabas Medical Center
  94 Old Short Hills Road/Room 414A   Livingston, NJ 07039   (973)322-5691   Fax (973)322-5504

Yehl, Mary Ann Mclaughlin, DO {1003958604}
+ Atlantic Womens Medical Group
  240 Wall Street/Suite 300   West Long Branch, NJ 07764   (732)229-1288   Fax (732)728-1487

Yelchur, Anuradha, MD {1417032855} IntrMd(91,INDI)
+ 8 Queens Pass
  Colts Neck, NJ 07722   (732)308-4396
  madhuschintala@hotmail.com
+ INSTACARE Medical Center
  71 Main Street   South River, NJ 08882   (732)308-4396   Fax (732)254-8484

Yeldandi, Aruna G., MD {1255479028} IntrMd, Nephro(80,INA29)<NJ-EASTORNG>
+ 310 Central Avenue/Suite 109
  East Orange, NJ 07018   (973)677-1999   Fax (973)677-1998
  Arunayeldandi@hotmail.com

Yellayi, Priya A., MD {1073596276} FamMed(87,INDI)
+ Tinton Falls Community Based Outpatient Clinic
  55 North Gilbert Street   Tinton Falls, NJ 07701   (732)842-4751

Yellin, Michael Jay, MD {1164741641} IntrMd, Rheuma(84,NY08)
+ Celldex Therapeutics
  222 Cameron Drive   Phillipsburg, NJ 08865   (908)454-7120
  myellin@celldextherapeutics.com

Yellin, Tova G., MD {1356307201} Pedtrc(80,NY01)<NJ-VALLEY>
+ Maple Avenue Pediatrics
  23-00 Route 208   Fair Lawn, NJ 07410   (201)797-1900   Fax (201)797-4457

Yemini, Matan, MD {1255415345} OthrSp, RprEnd(77,ISR01)<NJ-CLARMAAS>
+ Diamond Institute for Infertility & Menopause
  89 Millburn Avenue   Millburn, NJ 07041   (973)761-5600   Fax (973)761-5100

Yen, Gary L., MD {1356383566} PhyMPain(00,DMN01)
+ Advanced Wellness
  17 North Main Street   Marlboro, NJ 07746   (732)431-2155   Fax (732)931-2889
  gyen@advanced-wellness.net

Yen, Ya-Tang, MD {1952374530} CdvDis, IntrMd(70,TAI02)<NJ-BAYSHORE>
+ Holmdel Cardiology and Internal Medicine Associates
  733 North Beers Street/Suite L2   Holmdel, NJ 07733   (732)264-4020   Fax (732)264-1292

Yenicay, Altan Omer, MD {1780653964} Anesth
+ The Bergen Anesthesia Group, PC
  500 West Main Street   Wyckoff, NJ 07481

Yenukashvili, Nana R., MD {1447460712} Pedtrc(84,RUS15)
+ Pedimedica PA
  810 Abbott Boulevard/Suite 101   Fort Lee, NJ 07024   (201)224-3200   Fax (201)224-4045

Yepez, Humberto R., MD {1932122272} Surgry(68,ECU01)
+ 88 Congress Street
  Newark, NJ 07105   (973)344-4772

Yeretsian, Rita A., MD {1710184437}(03,PA12)
+ Summit Radiological Associates, PA
  1811 Springfield Avenue   New Providence, NJ 07974   (908)522-9111

Yeretsky, Yelena, DO {1144329830} IntrMd, Dermat(99,NY75)<NJ-CLARMAAS, NY-MTSINYHS>
+ Ligresti Dermatology Associates, P.A.
  175 Franklin Avenue/Suite 103   Nutley, NJ 07110   (973)759-6569   Fax (973)759-2562

Physicians by Name and Address

Yero, Sergio Alberto, MD {1538382718} PsyAdd, Psychy(74,CUB08)
+ Advanced Psychiatric Associates
65 Harristown Road/Suite 101 Glen Rock, NJ 07452 (201)487-1240

Yeroushalmi, Parviz K., MD {1609968742}(85,IRA04)
+ 121 North Church Street
Moorestown, NJ 08057 (856)217-9995 Fax (856)234-7200
yeroushalm@aol.com

Yerovi, Luis A., Jr., MD {1598822942} ObsGyn(89,NJ05)<NJ-CLARMAAS>
+ 91 Congress Street/2nd Floor
Newark, NJ 07105 (973)344-7676 Fax (973)690-5109
Yerovijrmd@gmail.com
+ NJ Best OBGYN
716 Broad Street/Suite 6 A Clifton, NJ 07013 (973)344-7676 Fax (973)574-1008

Yerovi, Maria D., MD {1356429807} Pedtrc(91,NJ05)<NJ-MORRISTN, NJ-STBARNMC>
+ 399 Hoover Avenue/Suite 4
Bloomfield, NJ 07003 (973)429-2120 Fax (973)429-2181

Yerramalli, Sitamahala M., MD {1780676759} IntrMd, Hemato, Grtrcs(77,INA83)<NJ-EASTORNG>
+ 36 Newark Avenue/Sutie 304
Belleville, NJ 07109 (973)378-9889 Fax (973)378-9233

Yerramilli, Ramalakshmi V., MD {1275546160} Pedtrc(70,INA48)<NJ-STPETER, NJ-RWJUBRUN>
+ Livingston Pediatrics
345 Livingston Avenue New Brunswick, NJ 08901 (732)246-7171 Fax (732)246-8974
rvmd@Livingstonpediatrics.com

Yeshou, Dima, MD {1124287412} EnDbMt, IntrMd(02,SYR02)<NJ-VALLEY>
+ 12-04 Saddle River Road
Fair Lawn, NJ 07410 (201)773-8710 Fax (201)773-8711
+ New Bridge Medical Center
230 East Ridgewood Avenue Paramus, NJ 07652 (201)773-8710 Fax (201)225-4702

Yeum, Sandy H., MD {1487762050} ObsGyn(99,PA09)<NJ-CLARMAAS>
+ Clara Maass Medical Center
1 Clara Maass Drive/ObGyn Belleville, NJ 07109 (973)450-2000
+ Short Hills Surgery Center
187 Millburn Avenue/Suite 101 Millburn, NJ 07041 (973)450-2000 Fax (973)671-0557

Yeung, Cindy S., DO {1356356141} Psychy, GenPrc(01,NY75)<NJ-UNIVBHC>
+ 75 Amberly Court
Franklin Park, NJ 08823

Yeung, Wilbert Derek, MD {1871711218} PsyCAd, Psychy(04,NJ06)
+ 728 Brushwood Court
Somerset, NJ 08873

Yevdokimova, Oksana, MD {1437290772} FamMed(93,UKR11)<NJ-WARREN>
+ Warren Hills Family Health Center
315 Route 31 South Washington, NJ 07882 (908)689-0777 Fax (908)835-3037

Yevelenko, Olga, MD {1366701872}<NJ-NWRKBETH>
+ Newark Beth Israel Medical Center
201 Lyons Avenue Newark, NJ 07112 (973)926-7040

Yi, Bryan Sang, MD {1689832248} RadDia
+ University Radiology Group, P.C.
483 Cranbury Road East Brunswick, NJ 08816 (732)390-0040 Fax (732)390-1856

Yi, Helen Huafang, MD {1124091061} Psychy(83,CHN2C)<NJ-KMHCHRRY>
+ University Hospital-SOM Department of Psychiatry
2250 Chapel Avenue West/Suite 100 Cherry Hill, NJ 08002 (856)482-9000 Fax (856)482-1159

Yi, Lusia Sang-suk, DO {1740424035} Dermat(PA77)
+ Alliance Dermatology Associates
3311 Brunswick Pike Lawrenceville, NJ 08648 (609)799-1600 Fax (609)799-1677

Yi, Peter I., MD {1457499618} Hemato, IntrMd, MedOnc(84,NY20)
+ Princeton Medical Group, P.A.
419 North Harrison Street Princeton, NJ 08540 (609)924-9300 Fax (609)924-8398
+ Princeton Medical Group PA
2 Research Way/Bldg 2/Suite 302 Monroe Township, NJ 08831 (609)924-9300 Fax (609)655-7466

Yia, Grace Mercado, MD {1457327983} Pedtrc(86,PHI01)<NJ-RIVERVW>
+ Complete Care Pediatrics LLC
723 North Beers Street Holmdel, NJ 07733 (732)264-3344 Fax (732)264-1699

Yiengpruksawan, Anusak, MD {1023184918} SrgOnc, Surgry(78,JAP10)<NJ-VALLEY>
+ One Valley Health Plaza
Paramus, NJ 07652 (201)634-5438 Fax (201)634-5352

Yih, Melissa Christina, MD {1992973036} RprEnd, ObsGyn(95,VT02)<NJ-RWJUHAM, NJ-STPETER>
+ Reproductive Medicine Associates of New Jersey
140 Allen Road Basking Ridge, NJ 07920 (908)604-7800 Fax (973)290-8370

Yim, Frances D., MD {1073573713} PulDis, IntrMd(67,ITA09)<NJ-RWJURAH>
+ Drs. Yim & Prasad
913 West Inman Avenue Rahway, NJ 07065 (732)388-7999 Fax (732)388-7992

Yim, Hoi-Wing Susanna, MD {1013358134} IntrMd
+ St. Michael's Medical Center
111 Central Avenue Newark, NJ 07102 (973)877-5000

Yim, Simon D., MD {1225225519} Urolgy(77,SWI05)
+ 1166 Street George Avenue
Avenel, NJ 07001 (732)636-6113 Fax (732)636-1006

Yim, Yoori W., MD {1730125196} Anesth(95,KOR01)
+ Ambulatory Surgical Center of Union County
950 West Chestnut Street/Suite 200 Union, NJ 07083 (908)688-2700 Fax (908)688-7424
+ Paramus Surgical Center
30 West Century Road/Suite 300 Paramus, NJ 07652 (201)986-9000

Yin, Chun Hui, MD {1346204583} Pedtrc(99,NY19)<NJ-STBARNMC, NJ-OVERLOOK>
+ Drs. Patel & Patel
237 Central Avenue Jersey City, NJ 07307 (201)656-2999 Fax (201)656-8676

Ying, Yu-Lan Mary, MD {1205091527} Otlryg, IntrMd(03,NY48)
+ Rutgers NJ School of Medicine Neurology
90 Bergen Street/DOC 5200 Newark, NJ 07103 (973)972-4588 Fax (973)972-5059

Ying Chang, Jean S., MD {1386670800} PsyCAd, Psychy(92,LA01)<NJ-STCLRDEN>
+ St. Clare's Health Services
50 Morris Avenue Denville, NJ 07834 (973)625-7009 Fax (972)625-7128

Yocom, Steven S., DO {1730272550} Surgry, SrgNro(93,PA77)<NJ-COOPRUMC>
+ The Cooper Hospital System-Univ Hospital
3 Cooper Plaza/Suite 215/Surgery Camden, NJ 08103 (856)342-2439 Fax (856)968-8222
+ Cooper Surgical Associates
3 Cooper Plaza/Suite 411 Camden, NJ 08103 (856)342-2439 Fax (856)365-1180

Yodice, Paul Carmine, MD {1912975078} IntrMd, CritCr(89,NY09)<NJ-STBARNMC>
+ St. Barnabas Medical Center
94 Old Short Hills Road Livingston, NJ 07039 (973)322-5000 Fax (973)322-8564

Yoganathan, Thil, MD {1851316442} Anesth, CritCr(67,SRI01)<NJ-STJOSHOS, NJ-NYUTISCH>
+ St. Joseph's Regional Medical Center
703 Main Street/CardiacAnesth Paterson, NJ 07503 (973)754-2320 Fax (973)754-2381
yoganatt@sjhmc.org

Yohannan, Wendy S., MD {1932356946} PthACl, PthCyt(85,NY48)
+ Quest Diagnostics Inc.
1 Malcolm Avenue Teterboro, NJ 07608 (201)393-5000 Fax (201)393-6127

Yon, Katherine Sunhee, MD {1700999091} Pedtrc(01,KOR08)
+ Southern Jersey Family Medical Centers Inc.
932 South Main Street Pleasantville, NJ 08232 (609)383-0880 Fax (609)383-0658

Yonclas, Elaine Marie, MD {1760483200} PhyMHPC, IntrMd(00,NY08)
+ 41 Watchung Avenue/Suite 510
Montclair, NJ 07043 (973)255-1155

Yonclas, Peter Philip, MD {1265453518} PhysMd(99,NJ05)<NJ-UMDNJ>
+ University Hospital-Doctors Office Center
90 Bergen Street/DOC 7100 Newark, NJ 07103 (973)972-2400 Fax (973)972-2988
+ Rutgers-Department of Physical Med
183 South Orange Ave/Suite F-1555 Newark, NJ 07101 (973)972-3606

Yong, Jinghong, MD {1285696559} Anesth(87,CHN4A)<NJ-COOPRUMC>
+ Cooper University Hospital
One Cooper Plaza/Anesth Camden, NJ 08103 (856)342-2000

Yoo, Daniel J., MD {1053490268} SrgOrt, SrgShr(01,ON01)
+ Advanced Shoulder, Knee & Orthopedics Clinic
669 Broad Avenue/Suite 201 Ridgefield, NJ 07657 (201)735-5779 Fax (201)735-5887
comments@advancedshoulderknee.com

Yoo, Eun Y., MD {1558481861} Anesth(72,KOR05)<NJ-MEADWLND>
+ Meadowland Anesthesia Associates
55 Meadowlands Parkway/Suite 1 Secaucus, NJ 07094 (201)392-3211 Fax (201)392-3110

Yoo, Hojun, MD {1528048055} CdvDis, IntCrd(94,NJ05)<NJ-JRSYSHMC, NJ-OCEANMC>
+ Coastal Cardiovascular Consultants, PA
1930 Highway 35/Suite 3 Wall, NJ 07719 (732)974-8800 Fax (732)974-8609
+ Coastal Cardiovascular Consultants, PA
459 Jack Martin Boulevard/Suite 4 Brick, NJ 08724 (732)974-8800 Fax (732)458-9464

Yoo, Nina, MD {1548612328} ObsGyn<NJ-STPETER>
+ St. Peter's University Hospital
254 Easton Avenue/MOB Rm 4350 New Brunswick, NJ 08901 (732)565-5415

Yoo, Sang W., MD {1508977943} Psychy(71,KOR05)<NJ-MTNSIDE>
+ 245 Hillside Avenue
Nutley, NJ 07110 (973)667-8800 Fax (973)284-1100

Yoo, Susan S., MD {1134527298} Pedtrc(89,NY03)<NJ-VALLEY>
+ Drs. Albanese and Vecchio
20 Valley Street South Orange, NJ 07079 (973)762-2606 Fax (973)762-4515

Yook, Soonjae, MD {1952316309} IntrMd(69,KOR04)<NJ-VAEASTOR>
+ VA New Jersey Health Care System-East Orange Campus
385 Tremont Avenue East Orange, NJ 07018 (973)676-1000 Fax (973)395-7003

Yoon, Eui-Sun L., MD {1700944790} Psychy, PsyGrt(75,KOR03)
+ 599 Franklin Avenue/Suite 11
Ridgewood, NJ 07450 (201)444-9199 Fax (201)444-9121

Yoon, Hyukjun, MD {1871859074} RadDia
+ University Radiology Group, P.C.
579A Cranbury Road East Brunswick, NJ 08816 (732)390-0040 Fax (732)390-1856

Yoon, Ji Ae, MD {1033539986} IntrMd<NJ-UMDNJ>
+ University Hospital
150 Bergen Street/Suite H245 Newark, NJ 07103 (973)972-5672

Yoon, Kyung In, MD {1669729810} EmrgMd
+ Family Medicine at Monument Square
317 George Street New Brunswick, NJ 08901 (908)235-7252 Fax (732)246-7317

Yoon, Sora, MD {1679771935}<NJ-BAYSHORE>
+ Bayshore Community Hospital
727 North Beers Street/Anesth Holmdel, NJ 07733 (732)739-5900

Yoon, Young Dug, MD {1043232788} EmrgMd(93,NY48)<NJ-HUNTRDN>
+ Hunterdon Medical Center
2100 Wescott Drive/EmrgMed Flemington, NJ 08822 (908)788-6100 Fax (856)616-1919

Yoon-Flannery, Kahyun, DO {1871889386} SrgOnc
+ Kennedy Health Alliance
900 Medical Center Drive/Suite 201 Sewell, NJ 08080 (856)218-2100 Fax (856)218-2101

Yoong, Michael P., MD {1972564227} FamMed, GenPrc, IntrMd(72,MAL01)
+ 1 Heron Lane
Millville, NJ 08332 (856)825-4120 Fax (856)825-4120

Yorio, David S., DO {1487759171} FamMed, FamMAdM, IntrMd(02,NJ75)<NJ-SOMERSET>
+ Valley Medical Associates
220 Hamburg Turnpike/Suite 9 Wayne, NJ 07470 (973)826-0068 Fax (973)807-1886

Yorke, Eric R., MD {1437105079} Pedtrc, GenPrc(82,NY01)<NJ-SOMERSET, NJ-STPETER>
+ Somerset Pediatric Group PA
2345 Lamington Road/Suite 101 Bedminster, NJ 07921 (908)470-1124 Fax (908)470-2845
+ Somerset Pediatric Group PA
1390 Route 22 West/Suite 106 Lebanon, NJ 08833 (908)470-1124 Fax (908)236-7557
+ Somerset Pediatric Group PA
1-C New Amwell Road Hillsborough, NJ 07921 (908)874-5035 Fax (908)874-3288

Yoslov, Michael D., DO {1780653956} Nephro, IntrMd(91,IA75)<NJ-MEMSALEM>
+ Nephrology & Hypertension Associates of NJ
1206 West Sherman Avenue Vineland, NJ 08360 (856)692-0673 Fax (856)692-1460

Yosry, Mohamed Hussein, MD {1932170651} PsyGrt, Psychy(79,EGY03)<NJ-JRSYSHMC>
+ 40 Bey Lea Road/Suite B201
Toms River, NJ 08753 (732)240-5544 Fax (732)240-1180

You, Jerome H., MD {1316149073} Anesth(03,NJ06)
+ Hackensack UMC Mountainside
1 Bay Avenue Montclair, NJ 07042 (973)429-6000

You, Ruoxu, MD {1154300515} Anesth(90,CHNA)<NJ-OVERLOOK>
+ Summit Anesthesia Associates, P.A.
33 Overlook Road/Suite 311 Summit, NJ 07901 (908)598-1500 Fax (908)598-0197

Physicians by Name and Address

You, Yimei, MD {1487909339}
+ 22 Whitney Road
  Short Hills, NJ 07078 (973)564-5968
  yym.yym@gmail.com

Youmans, David Carey, MD {1285747998} RadV&I, Radiol, RadDia(94,CA02)<NJ-UNVMCPRN>
+ Princeton Radiology Associates, P.A.
  419 North Harrison Street Princeton, NJ 08540 (609)921-3345 Fax (609)683-8847
+ Princeton Radiology Associates, P.A.
  9 Centre Drive Jamesburg, NJ 08831 (609)921-3345 Fax (609)655-4016
+ University Radiology Group, P.C.
  375 Route 206/Suite 1 Hillsborough, NJ 08540 (908)874-7600 Fax (908)874-7052

Younan, K. George, MD {1568442648} CdvDis, IntrMd(70,LEB01)<NJ-BAYSHORE>
+ Kivarkis Y. Younan MD PA
  1145 Bordentown Avenue/Suite 10 Parlin, NJ 08859 (732)727-0400 Fax (732)727-1391
+ Drs. Younan and Younan
  717 North Beers Street Holmdel, NJ 07733 (732)888-1115

Younan, Shaddy Kivarkis, MD {1881665693} IntrMd, CdvDis(99,NJ05)<NJ-BAYSHORE>
+ Kivarkis Y. Younan MD PA
  1145 Bordentown Avenue/Suite 10 Parlin, NJ 08859 (732)727-0400 Fax (732)727-1391
+ Drs. Younan and Younan
  717 North Beers Street Holmdel, NJ 07733 (732)888-1115

Younan, Zyad, MD {1114147220} IntrMd, CdvDis, ClCdEl(00,GRN01)
+ Kivarkis Y. Younan MD PA
  1145 Bordentown Avenue/Suite 10 Parlin, NJ 08859 (732)727-0400 Fax (732)727-1391

Younes, Desiree Marie, MD {1396970208} CdvDis
+ Cardiology Associates of Princeton, P.A.
  731 Alexander Road/Suite 202 Princeton, NJ 08540 (609)921-7456 Fax (609)921-2972

Younes, Elie, MD {1801908751} CdvDis, IntrMd(74,LEB01)<NJ-BAYSHORE>
+ 246 Main Street
  South Amboy, NJ 08879 (732)721-1660 Fax (732)721-9682

Young, Alexis Livingston, MD {1659539443} Dermt
+ Forest HealthCare Associates, PC
  277 Forest Avenue/Suite 200 Paramus, NJ 07652 (201)986-1881 Fax (201)986-1871

Young, Annamarie C., DO {1548374036} FamMed(78,PA77)<NJ-BURDTMLN>
+ 4204 Landis Avenue
  Sea Isle City, NJ 08243 (609)263-7111 Fax (609)263-0519

Young, Faith M., MD {1760400451} Hemato, Onclgy, IntrMd(82,MA01)
+ 2 Cooper Plaza/Suite 3200
  Camden, NJ 08103 (856)735-6309 Fax (856)382-6455

Young, George William, DO {1568667392} PhysMd, AnesPain, FamMed(02,PA77)
+ Rothman Institute
  219 North White Horse Pike Hammonton, NJ 08037

Young, Jill F., DO {1558398859} FamMed, IntrMd(03,PA77)<NJ-CHSMRCER>
+ Capital Health Primary Care
  4056 Quakerbridge Road/Suite 101 Lawrenceville, NJ 08648 (609)528-9150 Fax (609)528-9151

Young, Jill S., DO {1003818360} Anesth(91,NJ75)
+ Morris Anesthesia Group, PA
  3799 Route 46/Suite 211 Parsippany, NJ 07054 (973)335-1122 Fax (973)335-1448

Young, Jimmie, MD {1326087032} IntrMd(81,NJ05)
+ CAMCare Health Corporation
  2610 Federal Street Camden, NJ 08104 (856)635-0212

Young, Joseph M., MD {1871579102} Psychy(84,PHI01)<NJ-NWTNMEM>
+ Catholic Community Services
  1160 Raymond Boulevard Newark, NJ 07102 (973)596-4190

Young, Karen D., MD {1114091923} FamMed, IntrMd(94,VA01)<NJ-MTNSIDE>
+ Maplewood Family Medicine
  111 Dunnell Road/Suite 200 Maplewood, NJ 07040 (908)598-6690 Fax (973)762-0840

Young, Kristopher F., DO {1669693875} IntrMd, CdvDis(03,PA77)<NJ-DEBRAHLC>
+ Capital Health-Heart Care Specialists
  2 Capital Way/Suite 385 Pennington, NJ 08534 (609)303-4838 Fax (609)303-4835
+ Capital Health-Heart Care Specialists
  1445 Whitehorse-Mercerville Rd Hamilton, NJ 08619 (609)303-4838 Fax (609)303-4835

Young, Marc, MD {1083706808} Ophthl(81,NY45)
+ Drs. Kresloff and Young
  900 Haddon Avenue/Suite 102 Collingswood, NJ 08108

  (856)854-4242 Fax (856)854-3585
  myoung@gmail.com

Young, Marie Lisette, MD {1902852817} Anesth(79,DC03)<PA-PENNHOSP>
+ Wills Eye Surgery Center in Cherry Hill
  408 Route 70 East Cherry Hill, NJ 08034 (856)354-1600 Fax (856)429-7555

Young, Matthew John, DO {1306023122} EmrgMd(04,PA77)<PA-ARHTRRDL>
+ Emergency Physician Associates, P.A.
  307 South Evergreen Avenue/PO Box 298 Woodbury, NJ 08096 (856)582-2816 Fax (856)848-1431

Young, Melissa G., MD {1831174739} EnDbMt, IntrMd(93,PHI02)
+ Mid-Atlantic Endocrinology & Diabetes Associates
  555 Iron Bridge Road/Suite 18 Freehold, NJ 07728 (732)409-6233 Fax (732)409-6414

Young, Michael Anthony, MD {1750587713} Anesth, PainMd(99,DC03)<NJ-MTNSIDE>
+ Hackensack UMC Mountainside
  1 Bay Avenue/Anesthesia Montclair, NJ 07042 (973)429-6991 Fax (845)357-5777

Young, Patricia A., MD {1336112994} IntrMd(81,NJ05)<NJ-JRSYSHMC>
+ Shore Medical Group
  2130 Highway 35/Suite 213B Sea Girt, NJ 08750 (732)974-8668 Fax (732)974-1078

Young, Sarah M., MD {1952480717} Psychy(87,NJ06)<NJ-UNIVBHC>
+ UH-University Behavioral Hlth
  100 Metroplex Drive/Suite 200 Edison, NJ 08817 (732)235-8400 Fax (732)235-8395

Young, Sophia C., MD {1427054451} RadDia, RadNro(81,PA02)<NJ-RWJUHAM, NJ-STFRNMED>
+ Radiology Affiliates of Central New Jersey, P.A.
  2501 Kuser Road Hamilton, NJ 08691 (609)585-8800 Fax (609)585-1825
+ Radiology Affiliates of Central New Jersey, P.A.
  3120 Princeton Pike Lawrenceville, NJ 08648 (609)585-8800 Fax (609)219-0439
+ St. Francis Medical Center
  601 Hamilton Avenue/Radiology Trenton, NJ 08691 (609)599-5000

Young, Steven Eugene, MD {1093715369} Hemato, Onclgy, IntrMd(89,PHI01)
+ Somerset Hematology Oncology Associates, P.A.
  30 Rehill Avenue/2nd Floor/Suite 2500 Somerville, NJ 08876 (908)927-8700 Fax (908)927-8706

Young, Tiffany, DO {1932365319} ObsGyn(03,NY75)
+ Ocean Health Initiatives, Inc.
  101 Second Street Lakewood, NJ 08701 (732)363-6655 Fax (732)363-6656
+ Ocean Health Initiatives, Inc.
  301 Lakehurst Road Toms River, NJ 08755 (732)363-6655 Fax (732)552-0378

Young, William P., MD {1346263597} IntrMd(83,TN07)<NJ-COOPRUMC, NJ-VIRTBERL>
+ 23 Warwick Road South
  Lawnside, NJ 08045 (856)547-8348 Fax (856)310-1977

Young, Yvette S., MD {1477560233} Pedtrc<NJ-VALLEY>
+ The Valley Hospital
  223 North Van Dien Avenue Ridgewood, NJ 07450 (201)447-8000

Youngerman, Neil L., MD {1770527749} Pedtrc, GenPrc(82,GA05)<NJ-SOMERSET, NJ-STPETER>
+ Somerset Pediatric Group PA
  1-C New Amwell Road Hillsborough, NJ 08844 (908)874-5035 Fax (908)874-3288
+ Somerset Pediatric Group PA
  155 Union Avenue Bridgewater, NJ 08807 (908)874-5035 Fax (908)203-8825
+ Somerset Pediatric Group PA
  1390 Route 22 West/Suite 106 Lebanon, NJ 08844 (908)236-9500 Fax (908)236-7557

Youngren, Kjell A., MD {1386702868} Urolgy(94,NY01)
+ New Jersey Urology, LLC
  741 Northfield Avenue/Suite 206 West Orange, NJ 07052 (973)325-6100 Fax (973)325-1616
+ New Jersey Urology, LLC
  700 North Broad Street/Suite 302 Elizabeth, NJ 07208 (973)325-6100 Fax (908)289-0716
+ New Jersey Urology, LLC
  375 Mounain Pleasant Ave/Suite 250 West Orange, NJ 07052 (973)323-1300 Fax (973)323-1311

Youngren, Sonya Jitendra, MD {1821062076} ObsGyn(97,NJ05)
+ Summit Medical Group
  75 East Northfield Road Livingston, NJ 07039 (973)436-1410 Fax (973)379-4724
+ Women first Health Center
  520 Pleasant Valley Way West Orange, NJ 07052 (973)436-1410 Fax (973)669-5722

Youngworth, Lynda A., MD {1073677225} Ophthl(78,NY08)<NJ-MTNSIDE>
+ 615 Pompton Avenue
  Cedar Grove, NJ 07009 (973)857-2000 Fax (973)857-7036

Younus, Mohammad A., MD {1700114931}
+ 360 Essex Street/Suite 302
  Hackensack, NJ 07601 (551)996-2065 Fax (551)996-2169

Yousef, Javed Muhammad, MD {1700823655} Grtrcs, IntrMd(85,PAK01)<NJ-HACKNSK, NJ-VALLEY>
+ Forest HealthCare Associates, PC
  277 Forest Avenue/Suite 200 Paramus, NJ 07652 (201)986-1881 Fax (201)986-1871

Yousef, Mona E., MD {1447262472} ObsGyn(72,EGY03)<NJ-RWJUBRUN>
+ 161 Livingston Avenue
  New Brunswick, NJ 08902 (732)249-0011 Fax (732)249-0075

Yousef, Nadia P., MD {1053654343} Nephro
+ North Jersey Nephrology Associates PA
  246 Hamburg Turnpike/Suite 207 Wayne, NJ 07470 (973)653-3366 Fax (973)653-3365

Yousif, Abdalla M., MD {1912009879} IntrMd(81,SUD01)<NJ-RBAYPERT>
+ Raritan Bay Medical Center/Perth Amboy Division
  530 New Brunswick Avenue/MedEdu Perth Amboy, NJ 08861 (732)442-3700
  abdallayousif@hotmail.com

Yousry, Ahmed Sameh, MD {1750317418} ObsGyn(92,EGY05)<NJ-HACKNSK>
+ Hackensack University Medical Center
  30 Prospect Avenue/Ob/Gyn Hackensack, NJ 07601 (201)996-2000

Youssef, Ashraf Fouad Kam, MD {1821083064} RadOnc, Radiol, IntrMd(83,EGY04)<NJ-VIRTVOOR, NJ-UNDRWD>
+ Chilton Medical Center
  97 West Parkway/Radiology Pompton Plains, NJ 07444 (856)342-2300 Fax (856)365-8504

Youssef, Caroline, MD {1598214280} Pedtrc
+ 2119 Route 88
  Brick, NJ 08724 (732)899-0008 Fax (732)899-0447

Youssef, Hatim Fathi, DO {1376754903} IntrMd, PulCCr(02,NJ75)<NJ-UNVMCPRN>
+ University Medical Center of Princeton at Plainsboro
  One Plainsboro Road Plainsboro, NJ 08536 (609)497-4000
+ Respiratory & Sleep Specialists, LLC.
  3546 State Route 27 Kendall Park, NJ 08824 (609)497-4000 Fax (877)632-3456

Youssef, Iman Shawki, MD {1386679942} Nrolgy, ClNrPh, SlpDis(85,EGY05)<NJ-BACHARCH, NJ-SHOREMEM>
+ Neurology Consultants of South Jersey LLC
  76 West Jimmy Leeds Road/Suite 503 Galloway, NJ 08205 (609)652-7820 Fax (609)748-7825
  Iman@duamail.com

Youssef, Jan Samir, MD {1386680635} Otlryg(99,NJ05)<NJ-CLARMAAS, NJ-CHRIST>
+ New Margaret Hague Women's Health Institute
  377 Jersey Avenue/Suite 220 Jersey City, NJ 07302 (201)795-9155 Fax (201)795-9157
+ Ear Nose and Throat Center of New Jersey, P.A.
  115 Franklin Avenue Nutley, NJ 07110 (201)795-9155 Fax (973)773-9525

Youssef, Maher A., MD {1982670063} IntrMd(77,EGY05)<NJ-CENTRAST>
+ 215 Gordons Corner Road
  Manalapan, NJ 07726 (732)446-6240 Fax (732)446-7766

Youssef, Michael Elias, MD {1497753727} Anesth(80,SYR02)
+ 12 North Wickom Drive
  Westfield, NJ 07090 (908)654-7961
  NETYOUSSEF@AOL.COM

Youssef, Nader Namir, MD {1275507436} PedGst, Pedtrc(90,DMN01)<NJ-MORRISTN, NJ-OVERLOOK>
+ Digestive HealthCare Center
  511 Courtyard Drive/Building 500 Hillsborough, NJ 08844 (908)218-9222 Fax (908)218-9818

Youssef, Nasser Ibrahim, MD {1063490860} SrgTpl, SrgVas(85,SYR02)<NJ-OURLADY>
+ Our Lady Lourdes Transplant Ctr
  1601 Haddon Avenue Camden, NJ 08103 (856)757-3840

Youssef, Oliver S., MD {1801826219} Otlryg, OtgyFPIS(95,NJ05)
+ Ear Nose and Throat Center of New Jersey, P.A.
  115 Franklin Avenue Nutley, NJ 07110 (973)773-9250 Fax (973)773-9525

Youssef, Rafik Z., MD {1083705214} Psychy(79,EGY04)<NJ-RAMAPO>
+ Ramapo Ridge Psychiatric Hospital
  301 Sicomac Avenue Wyckoff, NJ 07481 (201)560-9973 Fax (201)425-4063

Youssef-Bessler, Manal Farouk, MD {1649236027} IntrMd, InfDis(92,EGY03)
+ Infectious Disease Center of New Jersey
22 Old Short Hills Road/Suite 106   Livingston, NJ 07039
(973)535-8355   Fax (973)535-8353
+ Infectious Disease Center of New Jersey
653 Willow Grove Street/Suite 2700   Hackettstown, NJ 07840   (973)535-8355   Fax (973)535-8353

Youssouf, Andrew Joseph, MD {1003130006} EmrgMd<NJ-MORRISTN>
+ Morristown Medical Center
100 Madison Avenue/EmergMed   Morristown, NJ 07962
(973)971-7926

Yousuf, Saad, MD {1477814960}<NJ-NWRKBETH>
+ Newark Beth Israel Medical Center
201 Lyons Avenue   Newark, NJ 07112   (973)926-7425   Fax (973)926-6130

Yrad, Jonathan Proces Flores, MD {1053330647} Surgry(92,PHI18)
+ Atlantic Shore Surgical Associates
478 Brick Boulevard   Brick, NJ 08723   (732)701-4848   Fax (732)701-1244

Ysique, Jacqueline Rosa, MD {1437568086}
+ Capital Health Family Health Center
433 Bellevue Avenue/4th Floor   Trenton, NJ 08618
(609)278-5900   Fax (609)815-7178

Yu, Byung H., MD {1386683092} IntrMd(93,IL42)<NJ-SOCEANCO>
+ Stafford Medical, P.A.
1364 Route 72 West/Suite 5   Manahawkin, NJ 08050
(609)597-3416   Fax (609)597-9608
+ Stafford Medical, P.A.
1364 Route 72 West   Manahawkin, NJ 08050   (609)597-3416   Fax (609)597-9608

Yu, Cha J., MD {1093899320} Psychy
+ Warren Hospital
185 Roseberry Street   Phillipsburg, NJ 08865   (908)859-6782   Fax (908)859-6821

Yu, Channing, MD {1518036672} IntrMd(03,MA01)
+ Daiichi Sankyo, Inc.
211 Mount Airy Road   Basking Ridge, NJ 07920   (732)590-5923

Yu, Daniel Kwang-Jin, MD {1750325494} EmrgMd(96,PA07)<NJ-BAYSHORE>
+ Bayshore Community Hospital
727 North Beers Street/Emergency   Holmdel, NJ 07733
(732)739-5900

Yu, David H., MD {1548262447} Anesth(86,TX14)
+ PO Box 907
Englewood Cliffs, NJ 07632

Yu, Deborah, MD {1073811220} SrgPlstc(02,DC02)
+ 40 West Beechcroft Road
Short Hills, NJ 07078   (212)431-0155
deborahyumd@gmail.com

Yu, Edgar L., MD {1780628222} Anesth(81,PHIL)<NJ-NWTNMEM>
+ Newton Medical Center
175 High Street/Anesthesiology   Newton, NJ 07860
(973)383-2121

Yu, Fei, MD {1790727444} IntrMd(82,CHN57)<NJ-HACKNSK, NJ-ENGLWOOD>
+ 385 Sylvan Avenue Route 9 West/Room 25
Englewood Cliffs, NJ 07632   (201)567-0686   Fax (201)567-2060

Yu, Henry K., MD {1891892972} IntrMd(82,GRN01)
+ Alpha Medical
462 Lake Hurst Road   Toms River, NJ 08755   (732)244-3050   Fax (732)244-2556
+ Alpha Medical
65 Lacey Road/Suite E   Whiting, NJ 08759   (732)849-0888

Yu, Lawrence Sikyong, MD {1063455574} Radiol, RadNro(94,NY46)<NJ-STCLRDEN>
+ St. Clare's Hospital-Denville Campus
25 Pocono Road/Radiology   Denville, NJ 07834   (973)625-6000

Yu, Nenita L., MD {1104980457} IntrMd(65,PHI08)<NJ-GRYSTPSY>
+ Greystone Park Psychiatric Hospital
59 Koch Avenue   Morris Plains, NJ 07950   (973)538-1800

Yu, Thomas C., MD {1538156310} RadDia, RadV&I(93,NJ06)<NJ-COMMED, NJ-SOCEANCO>
+ Community Medical Center
99 Route 37 West/Radiology   Toms River, NJ 08755
(732)557-8000   Fax (856)770-1515
+ Coastal Imaging, LLC
79 Route 37 West/Suite 103   Toms River, NJ 08755
(732)557-8000   Fax (732)276-2325

Yu, William C., MD {1407852056} Pedtrc(82,PHI01)<NJ-JRSYCITY, NJ-MEADWLND>
+ Jersey City Medical Center
355 Grand Street   Jersey City, NJ 07304   (201)915-2455
+ Total Care Pediatrics in Jersey City
550 Newark Avenue/Suite 200   Jersey City, NJ 07306

(201)915-2455   Fax (201)795-4999
+ Newport Medical Associates
610 Washington Boulevard   Jersey City, NJ 07304
(201)222-1266   Fax (201)626-4548

Yu, Xiaolin, MD {1861717779} IntrMd(10,VA04)<NJ-ATLANCHS, NJ-MORRISTN>
+ Morristown Medical Center
100 Madison Avenue/Suite 96   Morristown, NJ 07962
(973)971-4287

Yu, Yao, MD {1386915122} RadOnc
+ Memorial Sloan Kettering Monmouth
480 Red Hill Road   Middletown, NJ 07748   (482)256-4358

Yu, Yin Tat, MD {1750482501} PainMd, Anesth(01,DMN01)<NJ-SOCEANCO>
+ University Pain Associates
462 Lakehurst Road/Suite A   Toms River, NJ 08755
(732)244-9020   Fax (732)244-2902

Yu, Yun S., MD {1548288731} Anesth(75,KOR05)<NJ-KSLRSADB>
+ River Drive Surgery Center
619 River Drive   Elmwood Park, NJ 07407   (800)738-1659   Fax (704)871-2128

Yu Chen, Robert P., MD {1447276233} Grtrcs, FamMed(96,PA02)<NJ-HOBUNIMC>
+ CentraState Family Medicine Residency Practice
1001 West Main Street/Suite B   Freehold, NJ 07728
(732)294-2540   Fax (732)294-9328
+ Hazlet Family Care
3253 Route 35   Hazlet, NJ 07730   (732)294-2540   Fax (732)888-7649

Yuan, Ann Lee, MD {1578507158} EmrgMd(84,NJ06)<NJ-WAYNE-GEN>
+ St. Joseph's Wayne Hospital
224 Hamburg Turnpike   Wayne, NJ 07470   (973)942-6900

Yuan, Cai, MD {1881782886} Psychy(82,CHN19)<NJ-SJERSYHS, NJ-LOURDMED>
+ Center for Family Guidance, PC
765 East Route 70/Building A-101   Marlton, NJ 08053
(856)797-4800   Fax (856)810-0110

Yuan, Carol Jia-Luh, MD {1528221850} PulCcr, PulDis, IntrMd(05,NY46)
+ Hunterdon Pediatric Associates
6 Sand Hill Road/Suite 202   Flemington, NJ 08822
(908)782-6700   Fax (908)788-5861
+ Hunterdon Pediatric Associates
8 Readng Road/Reading Ridge   Flemington, NJ 08822
(908)782-6700   Fax (908)788-6005

Yuan, Rui Rong, MD {1558693606} MedOnc(83,CHN1J)
+ 4 Horizon Road/Unit 620
Fort Lee, NJ 07024   (201)224-6627

Yucel, Cengiz, MD {1144526674} Pedtrc, IntrMd(91,TUR12)
+ Natural Pediatrics
155 Polifly Road/Suite 204   Hackensack, NJ 07601
(201)525-0214   Fax (201)525-0217
dryucel@naturalpediatric.com

Yucht, Justin A., DO {1912299579}
+ 15 Lafayette Lane
Cherry Hill, NJ 08003   (610)328-8830
justinyucht@gmail.com

Yudd, Anthony P., MD {1699751172} NuclMd, Radiol, RadNuc(79,NJ06)<NJ-STPETER, NJ-RWJUBRUN>
+ University Radiology Group, P.C.
483 Cranbury Road   East Brunswick, NJ 08816   (732)390-0030   Fax (732)390-5383
+ University Radiology Group, P.C.
16 Mountain Boulevard   Warren, NJ 07059   (732)390-0030   Fax (908)769-9141

Yudd, Michael, MD {1497762975} IntrMd, Nephro(80,ITA01)<NJ-VAEASTOR>
+ VA New Jersey Health Care System-East Orange Campus
385 Tremont Avenue/Nephrology   East Orange, NJ 07018
(973)676-1000   Fax (973)395-7078

Yudin, Joel S., DO {1730155805} FamMed, Grtrcs(83,MI12)<NJ-VIRTMHBC>
+ Mt. Laurel Family Physicians
401 Young Avenue/Suite 260   Moorestown, NJ 08057
(856)291-8756   Fax (856)291-8750

Yueh, Janet Han, MD {1821232133} SrgPHand(09,MA01)
+ Cohen/Winters Aesthetic & Reconstructive Surgery
113 West Essex Street/Suite 202   Maywood, NJ 07607
(201)487-3400   Fax (201)487-2481

Yuen, Sharon Shue, MD {1316973738} Pedtrc, FamMed(93,NY48)<NJ-CENTRAST>
+ Best Care Pediatrics
470 Highway 79/Suite 12   Morganville, NJ 07751
(732)970-9070   Fax (732)970-9071

Yufit, Pavel Vladimirovich, MD {1093984890} SrgOrt(04,NY19)
+ Mehling Orthopedics, LLC
214 State Street/Suite 101   Hackensack, NJ 07601
(201)342-7662   Fax (201)342-7663

Yulo, John A., MD {1821102054} AnesPain
+ 701 White Horse Road/Suite 1
Voorhees, NJ 08043

Yum, Sun Young, MD {1649480385} Psychy(02,KOR04)
+ University Behavioral HealthCare
183 South Orange Avenue/BHSB E-1428   Newark, NJ 07103
(973)972-1050

Yun, Haenam, MD {1013077874} Pedtrc(86,DOM15)<NJ-HOLY-NAME>
+ 110 Broad Avenue/Suite S-7
Palisades Park, NJ 07650   (201)945-4002   Fax (201)945-4140

Yun, Hyungkoo, MD ObsGyn(73,KOR04)
+ 425 Egret Lane
Secaucus, NJ 07094

Yun, Sung K., MD {1003833682} ObsGyn(86,DOM02)<NJ-MEADWLND>
+ Gene Medical Group
464 Hudson Terrace/Suite 203   Englewood Cliffs, NJ 07632
(201)567-7725   Fax (201)567-5255

Yung Poon, Karen York-Mui, MD {1801986005} IntrMd(76,HKOG)<NJ-STJOSHOS>
+ Paterson Community Health Center
227 Broadway   Paterson, NJ 07501   (973)278-2600   Fax (973)278-5837

Yuppa, Frank R., MD {1912994484} RadDia, RadNro(81,NJ05)<NJ-STJOSHOS>
+ St. Joseph's Regional MedCtr-Ambulatory Imaging Ctr
1135 Broad Street/3rd Floor/Suite 4   Clifton, NJ 07013
(973)569-6300
+ Imaging Subspecialists of North Jersey LLC
703 Main Street   Paterson, NJ 07503   (973)754-2645

Yurchenco, Peter, MD {1033277710} PthACl, PthAna(76,NY46)<NJ-RWJUBRUN>
+ RWJ Medical School Univ of Med
675 Hoes Lane   Piscataway, NJ 08854   (732)463-4674

Yurcisin, Basil Michael, II, MD {1003062050} Surgry
+ Garden State Bariatrics and Wellness Center LLC
225 Millburn Avenue/Suite 204   Millburn, NJ 07041
(973)218-1990   Fax (973)629-1274

Yussaf, Shiraz, MD {1134448251} FamMed(06,INA9X)
+ Care Point Health Associates
1225 McBride Avenue/Suite 200   Little Falls, NJ 07424
(973)256-5557   Fax (973)256-5036

Yusupov, Albert A., DO {1639518178}
+ 517 Lindberg Avenue/2nd Fl
Cliffside Park, NJ 07010   (917)843-5080

Zaatreh, Megdad M., MD {1285719591} Nrolgy, IntrMd(94,JOR01)
+ Epilepsy Neurology Group
901 West Main Sreet/Suite 203   Freehold, NJ 07728
(732)414-8585   Fax (732)875-0509
njepilepsy@gmail.com

Zabar, Benjamin, MD {1497046650} EmrgMd<NY-SLRRSVLT>
+ Hackensack Medical Center Emergency Medicine
30 Prospect Avenue/Main 3619   Hackensack, NJ 07601
(201)996-4614   Fax (201)968-1866

Zabek Gallegos, Joanna M., MD {1669420519} Pedtrc(88,POL08)<NJ-VALLEY>
+ Ridgewood Pediatrics LLC
265 Ackerman Avenue/Suite 204   Ridgewood, NJ 07450
(201)444-3309   Fax (201)444-3349

Zabinski, Stephen J., MD {1417960063} SrgArt, SrgOrt(91,NY01)<NY-SPCLSURG>
+ Shore Orthopedic University Associates
24 Macarthur Boulevard/First Floor   Somers Point, NJ 08244   (609)927-1991   Fax (609)927-4203
+ Shore Orthopedic University Associates
18 East Jimmie Leeds Road   Galloway, NJ 08205   (609)927-1991   Fax (609)927-4203
+ Shore Orthopedic University Associates
9 Stites Avenue   Cape May Court House, NJ 08244
(609)927-1991   Fax (609)927-4203

Zablocki, Chana Shira, MD {1760633556} FamMed
+ Neighborhood Health Center Plainfield
1700-58 Myrtle Avenue   Plainfield, NJ 07060   (908)753-6401   Fax (908)226-6743
+ Faith Family Health Care
400 West Front Street/Suite B   Plainfield, NJ 07060
(908)753-6401   Fax (908)822-9701

Zablocki, Lisa R., MD {1760432694} Pedtrc(77,NY46)<NJ-RWJUBRUN>
+ University Pediatric Associates PA
317 Cleveland Avenue   Highland Park, NJ 08904   (732)249-8999   Fax (732)249-7827
+ University Pediatric Associates
D-1 Brier Hill Court   East Brunswick, NJ 08816   (732)238-3310

Zablow, Andrew Ira, MD {1477500528} RadOnc, Radiol(81,MEX14)
+ Garden State Urology
16 Eden Lane   Whippany, NJ 07981   (973)240-2178   Fax (973)947-9055

Physicians by Name and Address

Zablow, Bruce Charles, MD {1285618843} RadNro, Radiol, IntrMd(75,NY08)
+ North Jersey Brain and Surgical
  680 Kinderkamack Road/Suite 300   Oradell, NJ 07649   (201)342-2550   Fax (201)342-7171

Zaboski, Michael R., MD {1043302946} IntrMd, EmrgMd(87,GRN01)
+ William J. McHugh MD PA
  240 Williamson Street/Suite 204   Elizabeth, NJ 07202   (908)355-8877   Fax (908)355-0017

Zabrodina, Yanina V., MD {1235174673} Anesth(89,UKR05)
+ Morris Anesthesia Group, PA
  3799 Route 46/Suite 211   Parsippany, NJ 07054   (973)335-1122   Fax (973)335-1448

Zaccaria, Alan, MD {1154316123} SrgPlstc, Surgry, SrgRec(86,NJ06)<NJ-JRSYSHMC, NJ-MONMOUTH>
+ 180 White Road/Suite 102
  Little Silver, NJ 07739   (732)530-8565   Fax (732)530-4788

Zacchei, Anthony Christopher, MD {1902912660} Ophthl
+ TLC Kremer Cherry Hill LASIK
  1800 Chapel Avenue West/Suite 100   Cherry Hill, NJ 08002

Zachariah, Teena, MD {1477815702} Nephro, IntrMd<NJ-ENGLWOOD, NJ-HOLYNAME>
+ Drs. Pattner, Grodstein, Fein & Davis
  177 North Dean Street/Suite 207   Englewood, NJ 07631   (201)567-0446   Fax (201)567-8775

Zacharias, Daniel, MD {1598730368} FamMed, EmrgMd, GenPrc(78,IL42)
+ 7 Short Hills Avenue
  Short Hills, NJ 07078   (973)912-0006   Fax (973)912-0007   daniel@danielzacharias.com
+ Just for Kids
  8 Meadowbrook Road   Short Hills, NJ 07078   (973)912-0006   Fax (973)376-5430

Zachary, Samuel, DO {1700090289} Anesth(05,NY75)<NJ-STJOSHOS>
+ Liberty Anesthesia & Pain Management
  901 West Main Street/2nd Floor   Freehold, NJ 07728   (732)294-2876   Fax (732)294-2502

Zack, Brian Gary, MD {1346444106} FamMed, Pedtrc(76,NC07)
+ 14 Hageman Lane
  Princeton, NJ 08540   (609)306-6256   Fax (609)924-8354

Zacks, Eran Sol, MD {1982760526} CdvDis, ClCdEI, IntrMd(01,CA11)<NJ-BURDTMLN, NJ-SHOREMEM>
+ Mercer Bucks Cardiology
  3140 Princeton Pike/2nd Floor   Lawrenceville, NJ 08648   (609)895-1919   Fax (609)895-1200

Zaeeter, Wissam Sabri, MD {1801191408}
+ Cooper Perinatology Associates
  3 Cooper Plaza/Suite 502   Camden, NJ 08103   (856)968-7433   Fax (856)968-8499

Zaeh, Douglas H., MD {1790754794} IntrMd(81,NJ05)<NJ-MTNSIDE>
+ Hackensack UMC Mountainside
  1 Bay Avenue   Montclair, NJ 07042   (973)429-6196   Fax (973)429-6575

Zafar, Ahsan U., MD {1962430595} Radiol, NuclMd, IntrMd(66,PAK01)
+ Capitol Open MRI
  2000 South Broad Street   Trenton, NJ 08610   (609)695-0085   Fax (609)695-4289

Zafar, Fateen D., MD {1811080641} IntrMd(00,GRN01)<NJ-COOPRUMC>
+ Cooper University Medical Center/Camden
  3 Cooper Plaza/Suite 215   Camden, NJ 08103   (856)342-2000   Fax (856)966-0735

Zafar, Jabbar Ben, DO {1649214495} FamMed, IntrMd(90,NY75)<NJ-CHSFULD>
+ Capital Health Family Health Center
  433 Bellevue Avenue/4th Floor   Trenton, NJ 08618   (609)815-7296   Fax (609)815-7178

Zafarani, Amy Jo, DO {1679884308} ObsGyn
+ Ocean Health Initiatives, Inc.
  101 Second Street   Lakewood, NJ 08701   (732)363-6655   Fax (732)363-6656

Zager, Robert, MD {1417021650} Hemato, IntrMd, MedOnc(68,NY20)<NJ-MTNSIDE>
+ Hackensack UMC Mountainside
  1 Bay Avenue/2ndFl/Suite 1   Montclair, NJ 07042   (973)429-6000   Fax (973)259-3554   bzager@viconet.com

Zaghloul, Nibal Ahmad, MD {1447251764} Pedtrc, PedHem(97,LEB03)<NJ-STPETER>
+ St. Peter's University Hospital
  254 Easton Avenue/Pediatrics   New Brunswick, NJ 08901   (732)745-6674   Fax (732)418-9708

Zaharko, Wendy, MD   GenPrc(84,GRN01)
+ Worknet Occupational Medicine
  510 Heron Drive/Suite 108   Bridgeport, NJ 08014   (856)467-8550   Fax (856)467-3361

Zahka, Karym, MD {1447576533} ObsGyn
+ NHCAC Health Center at West New York
  5301 Broadway   West New York, NJ 07093   (201)866-9320

Zahos, Peter A., MD {1356305049} SrgNro(90,DC01)<NJ-JFKMED>
+ Sovereign Medical Group
  555 Kinderkamack Road/Suite D   Oradell, NJ 07649   (201)855-8467

Zahran, Ali Abdelrahman, MD {1992782940} InfDis, IntrMd(86,EGY04)<NJ-STJOSHOS>
+ St. Joseph's Regional Medical Center
  703 Main Street   Paterson, NJ 07503   (973)754-4327
+ St. Joseph's Comprehensive Care Center
  160 Market Street   Paterson, NJ 07501   (973)754-4701

Zaider, Arik, MD {1962478917} IntrMd, Rheuma(97,NY01)<NJ-VALLEY>
+ Prospect Medical Offices, LLC
  301 Godwin Avenue   Midland Park, NJ 07432   (201)444-4526   Fax (201)301-1313

Zaidi, Sajjad, MD {1750452546} PsyCAd, Psychy(80,INA39)<NJ-CENTRAST>
+ Freehold Child Diagnostic Center, Inc.
  501 Iron Bridge Road   Freehold, NJ 07728   (732)761-1900   Fax (732)761-2388

Zaidi, Shaquib Ahmed, MD {1740215300}
+ 320 Eighth Street/Unit 7
  Lakewood, NJ 08701   (727)748-6154   szaidi22@gmail.com

Zaidi, Syed Arif Raza, MD {1982675476} Psychy(84,PAK11)<NJ-JRSYCITY, NJ-HACKNSK>
+ Bergen Psychiatric Asoociates PC
  294 State Street/Suite 2   Hackensack, NJ 07601   (201)342-4004   Fax (201)342-4208

Zaim, Sina, MD {1073579033} ClCdEI, CdvDis, IntrMd(81,NY20)<NJ-NWRKBETH>
+ 255 West Spring Valley Avenue
  Maywood, NJ 07607   (201)546-8746   Fax (800)549-5893

Zaina, Samir A., MD {1699906354} FamMed(04,RUS33)<NJ-HOLYNAME>
+ 991 Main Street/Suite 2-A
  Paterson, NJ 07503   (862)336-1200   Fax (862)236-1202

Zaino, Christian, MD {1437477411} SrgHnd
+ The Orthopedic Institute of New Jersey
  218 Ridgedale Avenue/Suite 202   Cedar Knolls, NJ 07927   (908)684-3005   Fax (908)684-3301
+ The Orthopedic Institute of New Jersey
  108 Bilby Road/Suite 201   Hackettstown, NJ 07840   (908)684-3005   Fax (908)684-3301

Zairis, Ignatios S., MD {1760519151} Surgry, SrgVas, SrgThr(73,GRE01)<NJ-ENGLWOOD, NJ-HOLYNAME>
+ 741 Teaneck Road
  Teaneck, NJ 07666   (201)837-8282   Fax (201)837-0016

Zaitsev, Alexander Alexeevic, MD {1588635791} Anesth, IntrMd(91,RUS15)<NJ-TRINIWSC>
+ Trinitas Regional Medical Center-Williamson Street
  225 Williamson Street/Anesthesia   Elizabeth, NJ 07207   (908)944-5204

Zaitz, Jennifer, DO {1205031911} EnDbMt, IntrMd(07,NY75)<NJ-BAYSHORE, NJ-RIVERVW>
+ Northern Monmouth County Medical Associates
  100 Commons Way/Suite 100   Holmdel, NJ 07733   (732)450-2940   Fax (732)450-2942
+ Rutgers- New Jersey Medical School
  185 South Orange Avenue/MSB I-588   Newark, NJ 07103   (973)972-6171

Zajac, Anna T., MD {1578794335} FamMed(POL02)<NJ-SOMERSET>
+ RWJPE Primary Care Center at Hillsborough
  331 Route 206 North/Suite 2-B   Hillsborough, NJ 08844   (908)685-2528   Fax (908)359-7109

Zajfert, Michael S., MD {1740581263} Psychy(06,GCY01)<NJ-HACKNSK, NJ-MTNSIDE>
+ Hackensack UMC Mountainside
  1 Bay Avenue/Physiatry   Montclair, NJ 07042   (973)429-6813   Fax (973)680-7715
+ Intensivists of Toms River, LLC.
  99 Route 37   Toms River, NJ 08755   (973)429-6813   Fax (732)557-8021

Zajkowski, Edward Joseph, MD {1770580938} Pedtrc(71,NY15)<NJ-ENGLWOOD, NJ-HOLYNAME>
+ Teaneck Pediatric Associates PA
  197 Cedar Lane   Teaneck, NJ 07666   (201)836-7171   Fax (201)928-4227

Zak, Madeline, DO {1811042955} Surgry(72,IA75)<NJ-BAYONNE>
+ 839 Avenue A
  Bayonne, NJ 07002   (201)437-0400   Fax (201)437-6607

Zakharchenko, Svetlana, DO {1174820302} EmrgMd, IntrMd(08,PA77)<NJ-HACKNSK>
+ Hackensack University Medical Center
  30 Prospect Avenue/EmrgMd/3rd Fl   Hackensack, NJ 07601   (201)996-3192

Zaki, Isaac Kamal, MD {1114211190} FamMed, IntrMd<NJ-HOBUNIMC>
+ first Urgent Medical Care
  3175 Route 10 East/Suite 500   Denville, NJ 07834   (973)891-1213   Fax (973)891-1216

Zaki, Merajuddin, MD {1770692378} Hmpthy, IntrMd, Nephro(83,AFGH)<NJ-COMMED>
+ 1160 Highway 37 West/Suite D2
  Toms River, NJ 08755   (732)240-0033

Zakir, Ramzan Muhammad, MD {1659579274} CdvDis, IntrMd(01,DMN01)
+ Heart and Vascular Institute of Central NJ
  317 George Street/Suite 440   New Brunswick, NJ 08901   (732)994-3278   Fax (800)732-0366
+ Heart and Vascular Institute of Central NJ
  98 James Street/Suite 314   Edison, NJ 08820   (732)994-3278   Fax (732)549-2853
+ Heart and Vascular Institute of Central NJ
  333 Forsgate Drive/Suite 202   Jamesburg, NJ 08901   (732)994-3278   Fax (800)732-0366

Zaklama, Joanne A., MD {1457586752} NnPnMd<NY-PRSBCOLU>
+ Hackensack Univ Medical Center Pediatric Emerg Room
  30 Prospect Avenue/Don Imus 218   Hackensack, NJ 07601   (551)996-5362   Fax (201)996-3676

Zaklama, Selvia G., MD {1336126473} Anesth(76,EGY04)<NJ-CHRIST>
+ Christ Hospital
  176 Palisade Avenue/Anesthesiology   Jersey City, NJ 07306   (201)795-8200   Fax (201)943-8105

Zaky, Mark, MD {1780950675}
+ Family Practice of Middletown
  18 Leonardville Road   Middletown, NJ 07748   (732)671-0860   Fax (732)671-6467

Zaldivar, Marjel L., DO {1497900971} Pedtrc
+ Essex-Morris Pediatric Group P.A.
  203 Hillside Avenue   Livingston, NJ 07039   (973)992-5588   Fax (973)992-1005

Zales, Vincent R., MD {1992772693} PedCrd, Pedtrc(81,DOMI)<NJ-CENTRAST, NJ-NWRKBETH>
+ Alpert Zales & Castro Pediatric Cardiology, PA
  1623 Route 88/Suite A/PO Box 1719   Brick, NJ 08723   (732)458-9666   Fax (732)458-0840   VZalesfam@aol.com
+ Alpert Zales & Castro Pediatric Cardiology, PA
  2 Apple Farm Road/PO Box 4176   Middletown, NJ 07748   (732)458-9666   Fax (732)458-0840

Zaleska, Violetta, MD {1497821227} AlgyImmn, Pedtrc(90,POL13)<NY-LICOLLGE>
+ PO Box 4184
  Clifton, NJ 07012

Zaleski, Theodore G., MD {1053399493} SrgOrt(74,DC02)
+ 212 Jack Martin Boulevard No
  Brick, NJ 08724   (732)840-0446   Fax (732)840-0491

Zalewitz, Jodi Michelle, MD {1124124458} Pedtrc, AdolMd(01,ISR02)<NJ-STPETER>
+ St. Peter's University Hospital
  254 Easton Avenue/Pediatrics   New Brunswick, NJ 08901   (732)745-8600

Zalkin, Michael I., MD {1831186626} ObsGyn(77,MEX03)<NJ-LOURDMED, NJ-VIRTMHBC>
+ Advocare Burlington County Obstetrics & Gynecology
  1000 Salem Road/Suite B   Willingboro, NJ 08046   (609)871-2060   Fax (609)871-3535
+ Burlington County Ob-Gyn
  8008 Route 130 N/Suite 320   Delran, NJ 08075   (609)871-2060   Fax (856)764-0103
+ Burlington County Ob-Gyn
  210 Ark Road/Suite 216   Mount Laurel, NJ 08046   (856)778-2060   Fax (856)778-8102

Zalkowitz, Alan, MD {1760487938} Rheuma, IntrMd(70,BEL04)<NJ-VALLEY>
+ Kayal Orthopaedic Center, P.C.
  784 Franklin Avenue/Suite 250   Franklin Lakes, NJ 07417   (844)777-0910   Fax (201)891-2146

Zalman, Richard, MD {1841227915} Anesth(87,PA09)<NJ-ACMC-ITY, NJ-ACMCMAIN>
+ AtlantiCare Regional Medical Center/City Campus
  1925 Pacific Avenue/Anesthesiology   Atlantic City, NJ 08401   (609)345-4000

Zalut, David S., MD {1649276320} FamMed(82,PA07)<NJ-VIRTVOOR, NJ-VIRTMARL>
+ Voorhees Primary & Specialty Care
  333 Laurel Oak Road   Voorhees, NJ 08043   (844)542-2273   Fax (856)770-9194
+ Drs. Zalut and Lowe
  1000 White Horse Road/Suite 806   Voorhees, NJ 08043   (844)542-2273   Fax (856)770-9194

Zaman, Aamir, MD {1659524702} MedOnc, IntrMd(84,PAK01)<NJ-ENGLWOOD>
+ 1035 US Highway 46/Suite 202
  Clifton, NJ 07013   (973)777-2212   Fax (973)777-0469

Zaman, Taimur, MD {1871542886} Nrolgy, IntrMd(83,PAK01)<NJ-NWRKBETH, NJ-PALISADE>
 + Jefferson Health Primary & Specialty Care
  1A Regulus Drive   Turnersville, NJ 08012   (844)542-2273
 + Kennedy Health Systems/Washington Township Campus
  435 Hurffville-Cross Keys Road   Turnersville, NJ 08012
  (844)542-2273   Fax (856)218-5664
Zamani, Mohammad, MD {1972514743} Pedtrc(67,IRA01)<NJ-STMRYPAS>
 + 424 Clifton Avenue
  Clifton, NJ 07011   (973)778-1236   Fax (973)778-9650
Zambetti, Eileen F., MD {1750474995} Radiol, RadDia(80,NY01)<NY-JACOBIMC, NJ-ENGLWOOD>
 + Englewood Radiologic Group PA
  350 Engle Street   Englewood, NJ 07631   (201)894-3000
  Fax (201)894-5244
Zambrano, Rosario M., MD {1659328839} Pedtrc(92,NJ05)<NJ-STBARNMC>
 + Essex Pediatrics
  26 Baldwin Street   East Orange, NJ 07017   (973)672-1212
  Fax (973)672-2722
Zamecki, Andrzej M., MD {1043289564} Anesth(72,POL03)<NJ-VALLEY>
 + The Valley Hospital
  223 North Van Dien Avenue   Ridgewood, NJ 07450
  (201)447-8000
 + Bergen Anesthesia Group, P.C.
  500 West Main Street/Suite 16   Wyckoff, NJ 07481
  (201)447-8000   Fax (201)847-0059
Zamel, Laith Naser, MD {1336467844} IntHos<NJ-JRSYSHMC>
 + Jersey Shore University Medical Center
  1945 Route 33   Neptune, NJ 07753   (732)775-5500
 + Meridian Medical Associates, P.C.
  1945 Route 33   Neptune, NJ 07753   (732)775-5500   Fax (732)776-3795
Zamel, Yaacov B., MD {1184659237} PedPul(96,ISR02)<NJ-OCEANMC>
 + Ocean Medical Center
  425 Jack Martin Boulevard   Brick, NJ 08723   (732)840-2200
Zamir, Zafar, MD {1336123058} Gastrn, IntrMd(83,PAK11)
 + Hamilton Gastroenterology Group, PC
  1374 Whitehorse Hamilton Squar   Trenton, NJ 08690
  (609)586-1319   Fax (609)586-1468
Zamora, Violeta C., MD {1265571640} Psychy, PsyCAd(63,PHI01)<NJ-JRSYCITY>
 + Liberty Behavioral Health
  395 Grand Avenue   Jersey City, NJ 07302   (201)915-2278
  Fax (201)915-2838
Zampella, Edward J., MD {1821055914} SrgNro, PedNrD, PainMd(82,AL02)<NJ-OVERLOOK, NJ-ATLANTHS>
 + Atlantic Neurosurgical Specialists
  310 Madison Avenue/Suite 300   Morristown, NJ 07960
  (973)285-7800   Fax (973)285-7839
 + Overlook Medical Center
  99 Beauvoir Avenue/PO Box 210   Summit, NJ 07902
  (908)522-2000
 + Short Hills Surgery Center
  187 Millburn Avenue/Suite 101   Millburn, NJ 07960
  (973)671-0555   Fax (973)671-0557
Zampino, Dominick J., DO {1972690998} IntrMd, IntHos(91,PA77)<NJ-ACMCITY, NJ-ACMCMAIN>
 + Atlantic Internal Medicine PA
  310 Chris Gaupp Drive/Suite 102   Galloway, NJ 08205
  (609)652-9933
 + AtlantiCare Regional Medical Center/City Campus
  1925 Pacific Avenue/Medicine   Atlantic City, NJ 08401
  (609)345-4000
 + AtlantiCare Regional Med Ctr/Mainland
  65 West Jimmie Leeds Road/Medicine   Pomona, NJ 08205
  (609)652-1000
Zanchelli Astran, Gina M., DO {1033274196} PthAcl(02,TX17)
 + Hunterdon HealthCare System
  2100 Wescott Drive   Flemington, NJ 08822   (908)788-6100
Zand, Perry H., MD {1023196250} Psychy(68,KY02)<NJ-KMHCHRRY>
 + 620 North Broad Street/2nd Floor
  Woodbury, NJ 08096   (856)848-6188
 + Kennedy Health System/Cherry Hill Campus
  2201 Chapel Avenue West   Cherry Hill, NJ 08002
  (856)848-6188   Fax (856)429-4212
Zander, Judith W., MD IntrMd(80,NY09)
 + 3 Saint Moritz Lane
  Cherry Hill, NJ 08003
Zandieh, Shadi, MD {1326320870}
 + Physician Practice Enhancement, LLC
  66 West Gilbert Street   Red Bank, NJ 07701   (732)212-0060   Fax (732)212-0061
  sz94978@gmail.com
Zang, Rachel M., MD {1699192781}<NJ-COOPRUMC>
 + Cooper University Hospital
  One Cooper Plaza   Camden, NJ 08103   (856)342-3278

Zangaladze, Andro T., MD {1255358602} Nrolgy, ClNrPh, IntrMd(87,GEO02)<NJ-VIRTBERL, NJ-VIRTMARL>
 + Woodbury Neurology Associates
  17 West Red Bank Avenue/Suite 204   Woodbury, NJ 08096
  (856)853-1133   Fax (856)845-5405
  azangaladze@virtua.org
Zangara, Joseph Anthony, MD {1447240254} Gastrn, IntrMd(93,NJ05)<NJ-CHILTON>
 + North Jersey Gastroenterology & Endoscopy Center
  1825 State Route 23 South   Wayne, NJ 07470   (973)633-1484   Fax (973)633-7980
Zanger, Diane Rachel, MD {1760488696} CdvDis
 + Advanced Cardiology Institute
  2200 Fletcher Avenue/Suite 1   Fort Lee, NJ 07024
  (201)461-6200   Fax (201)461-7204
Zanger, Ron, MD {1255424099} IntrMd, Nephro(81,NY46)
 + University Renal Associates
  1030 North Kings Highway/Suite 310   Cherry Hill, NJ 08034
  (856)667-7266   Fax (856)779-9179
  Zqib3@aol.com
Zanjanian, M. H. Amir, MD {1144264508} AlgyImmn, Pedtrc(65,IRA01)<NJ-STMRYPAS>
 + Allergy & Asthma Consultants
  930 Clifton Avenue   Clifton, NJ 07013   (973)471-9191
  Fax (973)470-9858
Zanna, Martin Thomas, MD PubHth, GPrvMd(73,MN04)
 + NJ Human Services
  12D Quakerbridge Plaza   Mercerville, NJ 08619   (609)588-6561
Zanni, Robert L., MD {1982669529} PedPul, Pedtrc(77,MEX03)<NJ-MONMOUTH, NJ-CHLSMT>
 + Monmouth Medical Group, P.C.
  279 Third Avenue/Suite 604   Long Branch, NJ 07740
  (732)222-4474   Fax (732)222-4472
Zanotti Cavazzoni, Sergio Luis, MD {1497848238} CritCr, IntrMd(95,PAR01)<NJ-COOPRUMC>
 + Cooper University Hospital
  One Cooper Plaza/CrtclCare   Camden, NJ 08103   (856)342-2000
Zaontz, Mark R., MD {1346216710} PedUro, Urolgy(79,DC02)<NJ-VIRTVOOR>
 + Urology for Children, LLC
  120 Carnie Boulevard/Suite 2   Voorhees, NJ 08043
  (856)751-7880
 + Urology for Children, LLC
  239 Hurffville Crosskeys Road   Sewell, NJ 08080   (856)751-7880   Fax (856)751-9133
 + Urology for Children, LLC
  1000 Atlantic Avenue   Camden, NJ 08043   (856)751-7880
  Fax (856)751-9133
Zapanta, Rex A., MD {1013975515} Pedtrc(76,PHI01)<NJ-JRSYSHMC, NJ-CENTRAST>
 + 1021 Bennetts Mills Road
  Jackson, NJ 08527   (732)364-6333   Fax (732)364-4160
Zapanta, Vicente T., MD {1285660290} Otlryg, OtgyPSHN(68,PHI08)
 + 340 Ernston Road
  Parlin, NJ 08859   (732)727-5114   Fax (732)721-7221
Zapiach, Leonidas, MD {1528014594} Gastrn, IntrMd(68,ARG02)<NJ-CHRIST, NJ-HOLYNAME>
 + Drs. Ramos & Zapiach
  235 60th Street   West New York, NJ 07093   (201)854-4646
  Fax (201)854-3203
Zapiach, Luis Alberto, MD {1609954890} SrgRec, SrgHnd
 + Art Plastic Surgery
  1 West Ridgewood Avenue/Suite 302   Paramus, NJ 07652
  (201)251-6622   Fax (201)251-6626
Zapiach, Mauricio, MD {1831260777}
 + Drs. Ramos & Zapiach
  235 60th Street   West New York, NJ 07093   (201)854-4646
  Fax (201)854-3203
Zapolanski, Alex, MD {1457320186} SrgThr, Surgry(73,ARG01)<NJ-VALLEY>
 + Valley Columbia Heart Center
  223 North Van Dien Avenue   Ridgewood, NJ 07450
  (201)447-8377   Fax (201)447-8658
  Azapolanski@mac.com
Zapolanski, Tamar, MD {1457524076}
 + Valley Medical Group
  70 Park Avenue   Park Ridge, NJ 07656   (201)930-0900
  Fax (201)391-7733
Zaputowycz, Larysa, MD {1275652208} Rheuma, IntrMd(83,DOM02)<NJ-CHILTON>
 + Larysa Zaputowycz
  1500 Pleasant Valley Way   West Orange, NJ 07052
  (973)261-1470   Fax (973)651-0197
 + Bergen Medical Associates
  466 Old Hook Road/Suite 1   Emerson, NJ 07630   (973)261-1470   Fax (201)967-0340
Zara, Graciano L., MD {1225188543} IntrMd, InfDis(76,PHI01)<NJ-RWJUBRUN>
 + Doctors Home Care

1445 Route 130 South   North Brunswick, NJ 08902
(732)390-8161   Fax (732)390-6110
Zarah, Jake P., MD {1356585681}
 + 60 Derwent Avenue
  Verona, NJ 07044
Zarbin, Marco A., MD {1376641423} Ophthl(84,MD07)<NJ-UMDNJ>
 + University Hospital-Doctors Office Center
  90 Bergen Street/Ophth/DOC6100   Newark, NJ 07103
  (973)972-2065   Fax (973)972-2068
  zarbin@umdnj.edu
 + Institute of Ophthalmology & Visual Science
  556 Eagle Rock Avenue/Suite 206   Roseland, NJ 07068
  (973)972-2065   Fax (973)228-7477
Zaretsky, Craig Lawrence, MD {1841304623} Surgry(99,MEX14)<NJ-VIRTMHBC, NJ-VIRTMARL>
 + Virtua Surgical Group, PA
  1935 Route 70 East   Cherry Hill, NJ 08003   (856)428-7700
  Fax (856)424-9120
Zarkua, Kristina, MD {1871956227}
 + Capital Health Hospitalist Group
  750 Brunswick Avenue   Trenton, NJ 08638   (609)394-6031
  Fax (609)394-6299
Zarny, Steven David, MD {1689642126} RadOnc(95,NY08)<NJ-JFKMED>
 + JFK Medical Center
  65 James Street/Rad/Oncology   Edison, NJ 08820
  (732)321-7167   Fax (732)906-4915
Zarrabi, Shabnam, DO {1346566114}
 + 4307 Michael Lane
  Voorhees, NJ 08043   (856)770-9252
  zarrabsh@gmail.com
Zarrabi, Yasaman, DO {1427232420} Pedtrc, PedAlg, PedDrm(07,NJ75)<NJ-HOBUNIMC>
 + Riverside Pediatric Group
  609 Washington Street/Ground Floor   Hoboken, NJ 07030
  (201)706-8488   Fax (201)706-8489
 + Riverside Pediatric Group
  1425 Bloomfield Street   Hoboken, NJ 07030   (201)706-8488   Fax (201)876-3218
Zarrella, Geoffrey Carl, DO {1891873865} CdvDis, IntrMd(01,PA77)
 + South Jersey Heart Group
  3001 Chapel Avenue/Suite 101   Cherry Hill, NJ 08002
  (856)482-8900   Fax (856)482-7170
 + South Jersey Heart Group
  539 Egg Harbor Road/Suite 1   Sewell, NJ 08080   (856)482-8900   Fax (856)589-1753
Zarro, Christopher M., MD {1730223298} SrgOrt, SrgSpnc(02,NJ05)<NJ-STBARNMC, NJ-CLARMAAS>
 + Spine Care and Rehabilitation
  200 South Orange Ave./Suite 180   Livingston, NJ 07039
  (973)226-2725   Fax (973)226-3270
 + Spine Care and Rehabilitation
  36 Newark Avenue/Suite 220   Belleville, NJ 07109
  (973)226-2725   Fax (973)226-3270
 + St. Barnabas Ambulatory Care Center
  200 South Orange Avenue   Livingston, NJ 07039   (973)226-2725   Fax (973)226-3270
Zarroli, Hannah J., MD {1063497279} FamMed(02,OH41)
 + Virtua Medford Medical Center
  128 Route 70   Medford, NJ 08055   (609)953-7111   Fax (609)953-1544
Zarubin, Vadim, MD {1790188050} OncHem
 + Hudson Hematology Oncology
  377 Jersey Avenue/Suite 160   Jersey City, NJ 07302
  (201)333-8248   Fax (201)333-8469
Zarzour, Hekmat Khodr, MD {1609001130} RadNro
 + 445 Hurffville Crosskeys Road
  Sewell, NJ 08080   (856)256-7591
Zarzuela, Arminia T., MD {1851458210} NnPnMd, Pedtrc(74,PHI29)
 + 1 Holmes Court
  Bridgewater, NJ 08807
Zaslavsky, Alexander, MD {1245474568} Anesth
 + 185 South Orange Avenue/MSB 1-538
  Newark, NJ 07103   (973)972-0284
Zaslavsky, Alexandr, MD {1003090275} IntrMd
 + Patient first
  2171 Route 70 West   Cherry Hill, NJ 08002   (856)406-0023
  Fax (856)406-0024
Zathureczky, Izabella K., MD {1174513345} IntrMd(80,ROMA)<NJ-CHSFULD, NJ-CHSMRCER>
 + 3100 Princeton Pike/Building 4/Suite K
  Lawrenceville, NJ 08648   (609)895-8103   Fax (609)895-8105
Zauber, Neil P., MD {1164581534} Hemato, IntrMd(71,MD07)<NJ-STBARNMC>
 + Drs. Chu & Zauber
  22 Old Short Hills Road/Suite 108   Livingston, NJ 07039
  (973)533-9299   Fax (973)992-7648

Physicians by Name and Address

Zaubler, Thomas S., MD {1578532172} Psychy, PssoMd(91,NY46)<NJ-MORRISTN>
+ Morristown Medical Center
100 Madison Avenue/Psychiatry Morristown, NJ 07962 (973)971-5366 Fax (973)290-5166
thomas.zaubler@atlantichealth.org

Zauk, Adel M., MD {1669475174} NnPnMd, Pedtrc(81,BEL06)<NJ-STJOSHOS, NJ-HOBUNIMC>
+ St. Joseph's Regional Medical Center
703 Main Street/Neonatology Paterson, NJ 07503 (973)754-2555 Fax (973)754-2567

Zavala, Ramon E., MD {1811925597} IntrMd(84,ARG08)<NJ-VANJHCS>
+ VA Outpatient Clinic/Hamilton
3635 Quakerbridge Road/Suite 10 Trenton, NJ 08619 (609)570-6600
+ Presbyterian Homes & Services, Inc.
300 Meadow Lakes Hightstown, NJ 08520

Zaveri, Sarla J., MD {1821168774} ObsGyn(70,INA45)
+ 1031 McBride Avenue/Suite D-206
West Paterson, NJ 07424 (973)785-2131 Fax (973)785-3336
+ NJ Best OBGYN
716 Broad Street/Suite 6 A Clifton, NJ 07013 (973)785-2131 Fax (973)574-1008

Zavotsky, Jeffry, MD {1164481354} Surgry(91,NJ05)<NJ-STPETER>
+ Central Jersey Surgical Specialists
78 Easton Avenue New Brunswick, NJ 08901 (732)249-0360 Fax (732)249-0035
+ Cares Surgicenter, LLC.
240 Easton Avenue New Brunswick, NJ 08901 (732)249-0360 Fax (732)296-8677

Zawahir, Fawzia, MD {1184790941} Pedtrc, FamMed(03,INA3D)
+ 91 Knickerbocker Road
Tenafly, NJ 07670

Zawahir, Shamila Balkis, MD {1497958441} PedGst
+ Englewood Medical Associates Pediatrics
350 Engle Street Englewood, NJ 07631 (201)608-2775 Fax (201)894-5286

Zawid, Joseph, MD {1396717260} FamMed, GPrvMd, IntrMd(71,NJ05)
+ Absecon Family Practice
310 New Jersey Avenue/PO Box 568 Absecon, NJ 08201 (609)646-7131 Fax (609)646-7161

Zawodniak, Leonard J., MD {1144225202} RadDia, RadNro, IntrMd(86,NJ06)<NJ-JRSYSHMC>
+ University Radiology Group, P.C.
579A Cranbury Road East Brunswick, NJ 08816 (732)390-0040 Fax (732)390-1856
+ University Radiology Group
2100 Route 33/Neptune City Med Bld Neptune, NJ 07753 (732)390-0040 Fax (732)502-0368
+ University Radiology Group
900 West Main Street Freehold, NJ 08816 (732)462-1900 Fax (732)462-1848

Zayan, Eman, MD {1518192715}
+ 431 Westview Place
Fort Lee, NJ 07024 (978)505-8632

Zayoud, Rajaa M., MD {1033110853} FamMed(91,SYR01)
+ JFK Family Practice Group
65 James Street Edison, NJ 08818 (732)321-7605 Fax (732)744-5614

Zazzali, Albert John, MD {1942318126} Ophthl(93,NJ05)
+ 670 Franklin Avenue
Nutley, NJ 07110 (973)844-0511

Zazzali, George N., MD {1568596773} PhysMd(89,MEXI)<NJ-MTNSIDE>
+ Independent Medical Group
670 Franklin Avenue/Suite A Nutley, NJ 07110 (973)667-8493

Zazzali, Kathleen Mary, DO {1750522611} IntrMd<NJ-DEBRAHLC>
+ Deborah Heart and Lung Center
200 Trenton Road Browns Mills, NJ 08015 (609)893-6611

Zazzali, Peter G., MD {1528136603} IntrMd, PulCCr(90,NJ05)<NJ-MTNSIDE>
+ Independent Medical Group
670 Franklin Avenue/Suite A Nutley, NJ 07110 (973)667-8493
+ Independent Medical Group
235 Washington Avenue Belleville, NJ 07109 (973)667-8493 Fax (973)759-5041

Zbar, Lloyd I. S., MD {1275504813} Otlryg, Otolgy, SrgHdN(64,ON05)<NJ-MTNSIDE>
+ 200 Highland Avenue
Glen Ridge, NJ 07028 (973)744-2424 Fax (973)743-3111

Zbar, Ross Ian Seth, MD {1912996885} SrgPlstc, Otlryg(92,CT05)
+ 200 Highland Avenue
Glen Ridge, NJ 07028 (973)744-4800 Fax (973)743-4800

Zdorovyak, Mina, MD {1881608859} EmrgMd, IntrMd, EmrgEMed(71,UZB44)<NJ-STJOSHOS>
+ St. Joseph's Regional Medical Center
703 Main Street Paterson, NJ 07503 (973)754-2000

Zeb, Marta R., MD {1760406136} Pedtrc(97,DOM08)<NJ-CENTRAST, NJ-JRSYSHMC>
+ Pediatric Health, P.A.
470 Stillwells Corner Road Freehold, NJ 07728 (732)780-3333 Fax (732)780-6968
+ Pediatric Health, PA
4537 Route 9 North Howell, NJ 07731 (732)780-3333 Fax (732)367-6524
+ Pediatric Health, PA
23 Kilmer Drive/Building 1 Suite B Morganville, NJ 07728 (732)972-0900 Fax (732)972-2892

Zecca, Tina Concetta, DO {1790753630} Allrgy, Pedtrc, AlgyImmn(91,NJ75)<NJ-MONMOUTH>
+ Allergy & Asthma Associates of Monmouth County
200 White Road/Suite 205 Little Silver, NJ 07739 (732)741-8222 Fax (732)741-6217
TINOCH@OPTONLINE.COM

Zechowy, Allen C., MD {1023088648} Elecen, RadNro, Nrolgy(74,MD04)<NJ-VIRTMHBC, NJ-VIRTMARL>
+ LMA Neurology Consultants
63 Kresson Road/Suite 101 Cherry Hill, NJ 08034 (856)795-2000 Fax (856)795-3625
+ LMA Neurology Consultants
570 Egg Harbor Road/Suite B-5 Sewell, NJ 08080 (856)795-2000 Fax (856)795-3625

Zechowy, Racine B., MD {1679669618} Pedtrc(93,ISR02)<NJ-SJHREGMC, NJ-SJRSYELM>
+ Advocare Greentree Pediatrics
127 Church Road/Suite 800 Marlton, NJ 08053 (856)988-7899 Fax (856)988-9499
+ Osborn Pediatrics
1601 Haddon Avenue Camden, NJ 08103 (856)988-7899 Fax (856)365-7972

Zedie, Nishat, MD {1477644821} Anesth, NnPnMd, Pedtrc(72,PAK10)
+ Metro Anesthesia, LLC
561 Cranbury Road East Brunswick, NJ 08816 (732)390-4300 Fax (732)390-9046

Zee, Pamela A., MD {1831282672} IntrMd(98,NJ06)<NJ-COOPRUMC>
+ The Cooper Hospital System-Univ Hospital
3 Cooper Plaza/Suite 215 Camden, NJ 08103 (856)342-2439 Fax (856)966-0735

Zefren, Jacob M., MD {1053584185} IntrMd, MedOnc(75,MO34)
+ Hoffman-La Roche Incorporated
340 Kingsland Street/Bldg 719 Nutley, NJ 07110 (973)235-5000 Fax (973)562-3563

Zegar, Melissa, DO {1255760492}
+ 901 Route 202
Raritan, NJ 08869 (908)253-6640

Zeh, Catherine A., MD {1063463636} FamMed
+ Atlantic Medical Care Primary Care
3322 Route 22/Suite 1204 Branchburg, NJ 08876 (908)378-7227 Fax (908)252-0127

Zeibeq, John Paul, MD {1821250341}
+ Pulmonary & Allergy Associates
1 Springfield Avenue Summit, NJ 07901 (908)934-0555
jzeibeq@yahoo.com

Zeiberg, Andrew S., MD {1447252838} Radiol, RadDia(90,DC01)
+ Radiology Associates of Burlington County
1295 Route 38 West/PO Box 479 Hainesport, NJ 08036 (609)261-7017 Fax (609)261-4180

Zeidwerg, David Martin, DO {1245450998} Nrolgy(90,ME75)<NJ-ACMCITY>
+ AtlantiCare Regional Medical Center/City Campus
1925 Pacific Avenue/Neurology Atlantic City, NJ 08401 (609)345-4000

Zeiger, Jill M., MD {1609924372} EmrgMd(93,NJ05)<NJ-SOMERSET>
+ Emergency Medical Associates
110 Rehill Avenue Somerville, NJ 08876 (908)685-2920 Fax (908)685-2968

Zeitels, Jerrold R., MD {1457371957} SrgPlstc, SrgHnd, IntrMd(80,IL02)<NJ-OVERLOOK, NJ-RWJURAH>
+ Associates in Plastic & Aesthetic Surgery
955 South Springfield Avenue/Suite 105 Springfield, NJ 07081 (908)654-6540 Fax (908)654-6504
+ Associates in Plastic & Aesthetic Surgery
33 Overlook Road/Suite 411 Summit, NJ 07901 (908)522-0880
+ Associates in Plastic & Aesthetic Surgery
27 Mountain Boulevard/Suite 9 Warren, NJ 07081 (908)561-0080

Zeldin, Gillian Ann, MD {1598918807} IntrMd, Gastrn(91,NJ06)
+ 30 Eagle Ridge Way
West Orange, NJ 07052

Zeldina, Elina, MD {1659563815} ObsGyn
+ Valley Center for Women's Health
550 North Maple Avenue/Suite 102 Ridgewood, NJ 07450 (201)444-4040 Fax (201)444-4473

Zeldis, Jerome B., MD {1144567686} Gastrn, IntrMd(78,CT01)
+ Celgene Global Health
86 Morris Avenue Summit, NJ 07901 (732)673-9613 Fax (732)673-9001

Zelener, Marina L., DO {1396943031} Grtrcs, IntrMd(03,NY75)
+ IPC The Hospitalist Company
55 Madison Avenue/Suite 310 Morristown, NJ 07960 (973)993-9536 Fax (973)998-4237

Zelikson, Irina Yelyanovn, DO {1942210380} FamMed(99,NY75)
+ 44 Catherine Court
Laurence Harbor, NJ 08879

Zelinger-Bernhaut, Shani, I, MD {1063977874} PhysMd
+ Jewish Home at Rockleigh
10 Link Drive Northvale, NJ 07647 (291)784-1414

Zelinski, Jay Michael, DO {1184806309} IntrMd, Gastrn(85,NJ75)<NJ-BAYONNE, NJ-CHRIST>
+ 350 JFKennedy Boulevard
Bayonne, NJ 07002 (201)243-0445 Fax (201)858-1002
+ Bayonne Medical Center
29th Street at Avenue E Bayonne, NJ 07002 (201)858-5000

Zelinsky, Catherine Marie, MD {1134184369} Pedtrc, AdolMd(94,NJ06)<NJ-CHSMRCER>
+ Hamilton Pediatric Associates
3 Hamilton Health Place/Suite A Hamilton, NJ 08690 (609)581-4480 Fax (609)581-5222

Zelkowitz, Marc, MD {1609134576} IntrMd, Nephro
+ Drs. Abramovici, Jan & Zelkowitz
140 Grand Avenue/Suite B Englewood, NJ 07631 (201)567-5787 Fax (201)567-7652

Zell, Brian Kirk, MD {1669570891} SrgOrt(80,DC02)<NJ-VIRTMARL>
+ Sobel & Zell Orthopaedic Associates
525 Route 73 South/Suite 303 Marlton, NJ 08053 (856)596-0555 Fax (856)596-7658

Zelondzhev, Vladislav, DO {1639307945}
+ University Hospital-SOM Department of Psychiatry
2250 Chapel Avenue West/Suite 100 Cherry Hill, NJ 08002 (856)482-9000 Fax (856)482-1159

Zelop, Carolyn M., MD {1376541458} MtFtMd, ObsGyn, Ultsnd(87,MA07)<NJ-VALLEY>
+ Maternal Fetal Medicine Associates
140 East Ridgewood Avenue/Suite 390S Paramus, NJ 07652 (201)291-6321 Fax (201)291-6318

Zeltser, Eugene, MD {1215948617} Nephro, IntrMd(01,NY47)<NJ-STJOSHOS, NJ-WAYNEGEN>
+ Suburban Nephrology Group
342 Hamburg Turnpike/Suite 201 Wayne, NJ 07470 (973)389-1119 Fax (973)389-1145
+ Suburban Nephrology Group
1031 McBride Avenue/Suite D-210 Little Falls, NJ 07424 (973)389-1119

Zeman, David, MD {1104049741} Psychy, PsyGrt(89,NY08)
+ 29 North Livingston Avenue
Livingston, NJ 07039 (973)953-8580 Fax (973)740-9362

Zembrzuski, Andrzej Jan, MD {1700888054} Anesth(83,POL17)<NJ-STCLRDEN, NJ-STCLRDOV>
+ St. Clare's Hospital-Denville Campus
25 Pocono Road/Anesthesiology Denville, NJ 07834 (973)625-6000

Zemel, Mathias, MD {1649381310} Dermat(80,NY47)
+ 675 Broadway
Paterson, NJ 07514 (973)279-1232 Fax (973)279-5001

Zemel, Nathan, MD {1629102421} PhysMd(82,MEX03)
+ 50 Park Place/Suite 1542
Newark, NJ 07102 (973)642-1034 Fax (973)642-0538

Zemel, Suzanne, MD {1467507681} IntrMd(77,NJ05)
+ Newark Orthopedic & Neurologic
50 Park Place/Suite 1542 Newark, NJ 07102 (973)622-7274
Suzannezemelmd@aol.com

Zemsky, Lewis M., MD {1699826339} SrgOrt(71,MI07)<NJ-RWJUHAM, NY-STPETERS>
+ Zemsky & Piskun MD PA
1132 South Washington Avenue Piscataway, NJ 08854 (732)752-8484 Fax (732)424-1124
LZAP1132@msn.com

Zenack, Alissa Hayley, DO {1427005768} Pedtrc, IntrMd(99,ME75)<NJ-HACKNSK>
+ Top Notch Pediatrics, LLC
899 Main Street Hackensack, NJ 07601 (201)820-4600 Fax (201)820-4597
ahzenack2000@yahoo.com

Zenenberg, Robert D., DO {1245331834} IntrMd, Nephro(95,PA77)<NJ-MTNSIDE>
+ Nephrological Associates, P.A.
83 Hanover Road/Suite 290 Florham Park, NJ 07932 (973)736-2212 Fax (973)736-2989
+ Nephrological Associates PA
206 Belleville Avenue Bloomfield, NJ 07003 (973)736-2212 Fax (973)259-0396

Physicians by Name and Address

Zeng, Yu Grace, MD {1013118637} RadDia(03,NY19)
+ Hunterdon Radiological Associate
1 Dogwood Drive   Clinton, NJ 08809   (908)735-4477   Fax (908)735-6532

Zenn, Juliane Janis, MD {1316159866} Psychy(84,NY46)
+ 265 Cedar Lane
Teaneck, NJ 07666   (201)836-8392
+ 467 Springfield Avenue
Summit, NJ 07901   (908)277-1254

Zerbo, Erin Alexandra, MD {1992900732} PsyAdd, IntrMd(07,NY19)
+ University Behavioral HealthCare
183 South Orange Avenue/Suite F-1542   Newark, NJ 07103   (973)972-1661

Zerbo, Joseph R., DO {1023021672} SrgOrt(83,IA75)<NJ-BURDTMLN>
+ Lowe-Greenwood-Zerbo Spinal Associates
1999 New Road/Suite B   Linwood, NJ 08221   (609)601-6363   Fax (609)601-6364

Zerykier, Gisela B., MD {1275735615} PsyAdt, PsyCAd, Psynls(80,BELG)
+ 932 Ridgeway Street
Teaneck, NJ 07666   (201)862-0056   Fax (201)862-0867

Zetkulic, Marygrace M., MD {1669422762} IntrMd(95,NJ05)<NJ-STPETER>
+ Saint PeterÆs Physician Associate
59 Veronica Avenue/Suite 203   Somerset, NJ 08873   (732)937-6008

Zeveloff, Susan R., MD {1821108937} IntrMd, Nephro(80,MA05)<NJ-HOBUNIMC, NJ-HACKNSK>
+ 136 North Washington Avenue/Suite 102
Bergenfield, NJ 07621   (201)387-2040   Fax (201)385-9308

Zevin, Ronald A., MD {1386716389} ObsGyn, Gyneco(65,MA05)<NJ-NWRKBETH>
+ 50 Union Avenue/Suite 303
Irvington, NJ 07111   (973)372-8844   Fax (973)372-6687

Zhai, Elaine, DO {1093057432}
+ 32 Riker Hill Road
Livingston, NJ 07039   (646)761-6957
elaizhai@gmail.com

Zhang, Alex Xun, MD PthACl, PthFor(86,CHN19)
+ Office of The Regional Medical Examiner State of NJ
325 Norfolk Street   Newark, NJ 07103   (973)648-3914   Fax (973)648-3692

Zhang, Christina Ting, DO {1417193384} EmrgMd(05,IA75)
+ Phoenix Physician's
225 Williamson Street   Elizabeth, NJ 07202   (908)994-5422

Zhang, Hailing, MD {1346331675} Psychy(89,CHN19)<NJ-MTNSIDE>
+ 215 Union Avenue/Suite E
Bridgewater, NJ 08807   (908)685-0556   Fax (908)685-0480

Zhang, Hailing, MD {1225273030} PthHem(94,CHN5A)<NJ-CHILTON>
+ Chilton Medical Center
97 West Parkway/Path   Pompton Plains, NJ 07444   (973)831-5046

Zhang, Hao, MD {1568732527} IntrMd
+ Yong Kang Medical PLLC
2 Ethol Road/Suite 203c   Edison, NJ 08817   (732)662-1100   Fax (732)662-1153

Zhang, Huayan, MD {1497785828} Pedtrc(91,CHN19)<PA-CHILDHOS>
+ 5 Windsor Drive
Voorhees, NJ 08043

Zhang, Lanjing, MD {1245499888} PthACl, IntrMd(00,CHN59)<NJ-UNVMCPRN>
+ Pathology Associates of Princeton
One Plainsboro Road   Plainsboro, NJ 08536   (609)853-6834   Fax (609)853-6801

Zhang, Lei, MD {1821149659} ClNrPh, Nrolgy(86,CHN19)
+ Comprehensive Neurology, LLC.
1245 Whitehorse-Mercerville Rd   Hamilton, NJ 08619   (609)585-2666   Fax (609)585-4008

Zhang, Li, MD {1013089457} Pedtrc(82,CHNA)<NJ-HACKNSK, NJ-HOLYNAME>
+ 232 Belleville Turnpike
Kearny, NJ 07032   (201)998-3020   Fax (201)998-0021

Zhang, Linda, MD {1831358381} Ophthl(08,MI01)
+ The Eye Center
65 Mountain Boulevard Ext/Suite 105   Warren, NJ 07059   (732)356-6200   Fax (732)356-9257
drlinda@comcast.com

Zhang, Mei, MD {1457306045} RadOnc(85,CHN40)
+ 72c West Front Street
Red Bank, NJ 07701

Zhang, Miaoying, MD {1932446374} IntrMd(10,NJ06)
+ PrimeCare Medical Group
561 Middlesex Avenue   Metuchen, NJ 08840   (732)549-9363   Fax (732)603-0397

Zhang, Qi, MD {1184751240} PthACl(82,CHN42)<NJ-PALISADE>
+ Palisades Medical Center
7600 River Road/Path   North Bergen, NJ 07047   (201)854-5000

Zhang, Shehui, MD {1730154733} Anesth(83,CHN68)
+ 47 Farmhaven Avenue
Edison, NJ 08820

Zhang, Tianshu, MD {1790851541} Nrolgy(84,CHNA)
+ 227 Bridge Street
Metuchen, NJ 08840   (732)632-8858   Fax (732)632-8861
+ 10 North Gaston Avenue
Somerville, NJ 08876   (908)231-0154

Zhang, Vincent, MD {1104263698} ObsGyn
+ Atlantic Cape Ob/Gyn
829 Shore Road   Somers Point, NJ 08244   (609)927-3070   Fax (609)927-2553

Zhang, Xiaowei, MD {1356378517} IntrMd(88,CHN40)<NJ-WOODBRDG, NJ-BAYSHORE>
+ Woodbridge Developmental Center
Rahway Avenue/PO Box 189   Woodbridge, NJ 07095   (732)499-5500   Fax (732)499-5787

Zhang, Yan Chun, MD {1841363520} Nrolgy, OthrSp(84,CHN21)<NJ-OVERLOOK, NJ-STMICHL>
+ Suburban Neurology, PC
111 East Northfield road   Livingston, NJ 07039   (973)992-9819   Fax (973)535-9819

Zhang, Yiqiu, MD {1194961219} PthACl, PthDrm(87,CHN4A)
+ Quest Diagnostics Inc.
1 Malcolm Avenue   Teterboro, NJ 07608   (201)393-5000   Fax (201)393-6127

Zhao, Lin, MD {1770516726} Anesth(87,CHN57)
+ Institute of Ophthalmology & Visual Science
556 Eagle Rock Avenue/Suite 206   Roseland, NJ 07068   (973)228-2771   Fax (973)228-7477

Zhao, Rong, MD {1356607436} Anesth
+ Jersery Shore Anesthesiology
1945 Highway 33   Neptune, NJ 07753   (732)897-0200   Fax (732)897-0263

Zheng, Fangfei, MD {1982098802} IntrMd
+ 25 Manor Drive
Morristown, NJ 07960   (917)617-4843

Zheng, Jing-Sheng, MD {1992784565} IntrMd, CdvDis(84,CHN64)<NJ-VIRTVOOR, NJ-VIRTMARL>
+ Associated Cardiovascular Consultants, PA
2 Sindoni Lane   Hammonton, NJ 08037   (609)561-8500   Fax (856)567-0432
+ Associated Cardiovascular Consultants, PA
2500 English Creek Avenue   Egg Harbor Township, NJ 08234   (609)561-8500   Fax (609)569-1896
+ Associated Cardiovascular Consultants-Lourdes
1 Brace Road/Suite C & F   Cherry Hill, NJ 08037   (856)428-4100   Fax (856)428-5748

Zheng, Lin, MD {1598095747}<NJ-COOPRUMC>
+ Cooper University Hospital
One Cooper Plaza/Drrnce 222   Camden, NJ 08103   (856)342-2000   Fax (856)968-8418
zhenglintj18@gmail.com

Zheng, Min, MD {1013905074} Pthlgy, PthACl(85,CHN67)<NJ-JRSYSHMC>
+ Jersey Shore University Medical Center
1945 Route 33/Pathology   Neptune, NJ 07753   (732)776-4148

Zheng, Shao, MD {1376680042} Pedtrc(92,CHN9D)
+ 1681 State Route 27
Edison, NJ 08817   (732)985-0666

Zheng, Xin, MD {1124285283} IntrMd(99,CHN4A)
+ 20 Livingston Avenue/Apt 705
New Brunswick, NJ 08901

Zheng, Yining, MD {1053394593} PhysMd(83,CHN4A)
+ Associates in Rehabilitation Medicine
95 Mount Kemble Avenue   Morristown, NJ 07960   (973)267-2293   Fax (973)226-3144

Zhivago, Eileen Ann, MD {1821258492} PsyCAd
+ Advanced Psychiatric Associates
211 Essex Street/Suite 204   Hackensack, NJ 07601   (201)487-1240   Fax (201)487-1241
eileenzhivagomd@gmail.com
+ Advanced Psychiatric Associates
65 Harristown Road/Suite 101   Glen Rock, NJ 07452   (201)487-1240

Zhong, Hua, MD {1376749432} PthACl<NJ-COMMED>
+ Laboratory Medicine Associates, PA
300 Second Avenue/Dept of Pathology   Long Branch, NJ 07740   (732)923-7380   Fax (732)923-7355
+ Community Medical Center
99 Route 37 West/Pathology   Toms River, NJ 08755   (732)235-8058

Zhou, Ben Yuan, MD {1124005277} Anesth(82,CHN07)<NJ-CHRIST>
+ Christ Hospital
176 Palisade Avenue/Anesth   Jersey City, NJ 07306   (201)795-8200   Fax (201)943-8105

Zhou, Henry Haifeng, MD {1356319016} Anesth(82,CHN21)<NJ-VALLEY>
+ Bergen Anesthesia Group, P.C.
500 West Main Street/Suite 16   Wyckoff, NJ 07481   (201)847-9320   Fax (201)847-0059
+ The Valley Hospital
223 North Van Dien Avenue   Ridgewood, NJ 07450   (201)447-8000

Zhou, Jie, MD {1154323491} Anesth(88,CHN57)<NJ-STCLRDEN>
+ St. Clare's Hospital-Denville Campus
25 Pocono Road/Anesth   Denville, NJ 07834   (973)625-6000

Zhou, Lingbin, MD {1528097060} Anesth(84,CHN57)<NJ-OCEANMC>
+ Ocean Medical Center
425 Jack Martin Boulevard   Brick, NJ 08723   (732)840-2200

Zhou, Linqiu, MD {1932128717} PhyMPain, PainMd(84,CHN34)
+ Professional Pain Associates
730 North Broad Street/Suite 205   Woodbury, NJ 08096   (856)202-5331

Zhou, Ren, MD {1942257290} IntrMd(88,CHN4A)
+ 233 Bridge Street
Metuchen, NJ 08840   (732)906-8662   Fax (732)906-8602

Zhu, Binghua, MD {1851547889} IntrMd(85,CHN96)<NJ-STBARNMC>
+ 493 Morris Avenue
Springfield, NJ 07081   (973)379-5980   Fax (908)481-1888

Zhu, Ching, MD {1962404202} Anesth(84,CHN21)<NJ-STCLRDEN>
+ St. Clare's Hospital-Denville Campus
25 Pocono Road   Denville, NJ 07834   (973)625-6000

Zhu, Gord Guo, MD {1407115157}<NJ-COOPRUMC>
+ Cooper University Hospital
One Cooper Plaza   Camden, NJ 08103   (856)342-2622

Zhu, Yun, MD {1750318820} Anesth
+ 102 Marshall Drive
Egg Harbor Township, NJ 08234

Zhuang, Sen Hong, MD IntrMd, MedOnc(92,CHN21)
+ Johnson & Johnson Research & Develop
920 US Highway Route 202   Raritan, NJ 08869   (908)704-4000

Zhukova, Irina, DO {1790811107} IntrMd(03,NY75)
+ Med-Care of Fairfield, Inc.
150 Fairfield Road   Fairfield, NJ 07004   (973)227-0020

Zhuravkov, Alexander, MD {1306881784} Anesth(79,BLA02)
+ Columbia Anesthesia Associates
37 West Century Road/Suite 101   Paramus, NJ 07652   (201)634-9000   Fax (201)634-9014
+ Paramus Surgical Center
30 West Century Road/Suite 300   Paramus, NJ 07652   (201)986-9000

Zhuravsky, Ruslan, DO {1861780173} OtgyFPIS(11,FL75)
+ Coastal Ear Nose and Throat LLC
1301 Route 72/Suite 340   Manahawkin, NJ 08050   (732)280-7855   Fax (732)280-7815
+ 1001 US Hwy. 9/Suite 107
Howell, NJ 07731   (732)280-7855   Fax (732)851-1131
+ SOM - Department of Internal Medicine
42 East Laurel Road/Suite 3100   Stratford, NJ 08050   (856)566-6859   Fax (856)566-6906

Zia, Shahzad S., MD {1023314408} IntrMd(10,DMN01)<NJ-ACMC-ITY>
+ AtlantiCare Regional Medical Center/City Campus
1925 Pacific Avenue/Internal Med   Atlantic City, NJ 08401   (609)345-4000

Zia, Ziaulhaq, MD {1134154776} IntrMd, Nephro(81,MNT01)<NJ-COMMED>
+ 56B Schoolhouse Road
Whiting, NJ 08759   (732)350-7900
+ 651 Route 37 West
Toms River, NJ 08753   (732)349-0001

Ziccardi, Vincent Bernard, MD {1942262548} SrgO&M(93,PA12)
+ 110 Bergen Street/Rm B854
Newark, NJ 07103   (973)972-7462   Fax (973)972-7322

Zicherman, Barry A., MD {1649250440} Radiol, RadDia(67,NY46)<NJ-STPETER, NJ-RWJUBRUN>
+ University Radiology Group, P.C.
483 Cranbury Road   East Brunswick, NJ 08816   (732)390-0030   Fax (732)390-5383
+ University Radiology Group, P.C.
10 Plum Street   New Brunswick, NJ 08901   (732)390-0030   Fax (732)249-1208

Ziegler, Brenda L., DO {1073581419} FamMed, IntrMd(94,IA75)
+ Rockaway Family Medicine Associates
333 Mount Hope Avenue   Rockaway, NJ 07866   (973)895-6601   Fax (973)895-5324

Physicians by Name and Address

Ziegler, William Francis, DO {1649265307} FrtInf, RprEnd(90,IA75)<NJ-JRSYSHMC, NJ-MONMOUTH>
+ Reproductive Science Center of New Jersey
  234 Industrial Way Eatontown, NJ 07724 (732)918-2500 Fax (732)918-2504
+ Reproductive Science Center of New Jersey
  780 Route 35 West/Suite 150 Toms River, NJ 08755 (732)918-2500 Fax (732)240-3030
+ Eatontown Fertility Clinic
  234 Industrial Way West/Suite A104 Eatontown, NJ 07724 (732)918-2500

Zielinski, Glenn D., DO {1457324303} Psychy(92,NJ75)<NJ-ACMC-MAIN, NJ-ACMCITY>
+ University Hospital-SOM Department of Psychiatry
  2250 Chapel Avenue West/Suite 100 Cherry Hill, NJ 08002 (856)482-9000 Fax (856)482-1159
+ AtlantiCare Behavioral Health/Seaside Counseling
  2021 New Road/Suite 15 Linwood, NJ 08221 (609)927-4200

Ziemke, Karen Sue, MD {1467474536} Pedtrc, AlgyImmn, Allrgy(89,NJ06)<NJ-STBARNMC, NJ-MTNSIDE>
+ 745 Northfield Avenue/Suite 4
  West Orange, NJ 07052 (973)716-0041 Fax (973)716-0042
  kziemke@pol.net

Zieniuk, Gregory J., MD {1811139710} Pedtrc<NJ-VIRTVOOR>
+ CHOP Care Network at Virtua Voorhees Hospital
  100 Bowman Drive Voorhees, NJ 08043 (856)325-3000 Fax (609)261-5842

Zierer, Kenneth G., MD {1417978883} Gastrn, IntrMd, Pedtrc(88,NJ05)
+ Gastroenterology Associates of New Jersey
  71 Union Avenue/Suite 201 Rutherford, NJ 07070 (201)842-0020 Fax (201)842-0010
+ Gastroenterology Associates of New Jersey
  925 Clifton Avenue Clifton, NJ 07013 (201)842-0020 Fax (973)405-6564

Ziering, Thomas S., MD {1902854870} FamMed(87,NJ05)
+ 1201 Mount Kemble Ave./Suite 2D
  Morristown, NJ 07960 (908)221-1919 Fax (908)221-0404
  info@drtomziering.com

Zigadlo, Tatyana, MD {1356349187} FamMed(98,GRN01)<NJ-HOBUNIMC>
+ Hoboken University Medical Center
  308 Willow Avenue Hoboken, NJ 07030 (201)418-1000

Zilber, Eugenia, MD {1841209673} IntrMd(82,RUS55)
+ Old Bridge Primary Care
  300 Perrine Road/Suite 324 Old Bridge, NJ 08857 (732)753-9890 Fax (732)753-9893
  ezilber@hotmail.com

Zilpert, Marina, MD {1861754772}
+ Princeton House Behavioral Health - North Brunswick
  1460 Livingston Avenue North Brunswick, NJ 08902 (732)729-3600 Fax (732)435-0222
  mzilpert@princetonhcs.org
+ CPC Behavioral HealthCare
  270 Highway 35 Red Bank, NJ 07701 (732)729-3600 Fax (732)224-0688

Zimering, Mark B., MD {1740202704} EnDbMt, IntrMd(84,NY46)<NJ-VALYONS>
+ VA New Jersey Health Care System at Lyons
  151 Knollcroft Road/IntMed/EDM Lyons, NJ 07939 (908)647-0180 Fax (908)604-5248

Zimmer, Gary David, MD {1053368407} EmrgMd, IntrMd(97,NY20)
+ Emergency Physician Associates, P.A.
  307 South Evergreen Avenue/PO Box 298 Woodbury, NJ 08096 (856)848-3817 Fax (856)848-1431

Zimmer, Ross Randall, MD {1750313078} IntCrd, CdvDis(89,PA13)<NJ-ACMCITY>
+ Penn Medicine at Cherry Hill
  1400 East Route 70/Cardiology Cherry Hill, NJ 08034

Zimmerman, Anahita, MD {1760571483} IntrMd(04,GA01)
+ Vanguard Medical Group, P.A.
  170 Changebridge Road/Suite C-3 Montville, NJ 07045 (973)575-5540 Fax (973)575-5548

Zimmerman, Aphrodite Marta, MD {1932303583} Psychy<NJ-OVERLOOK>
+ Overlook Medical Center
  99 Beauvoir Avenue/PO Box 210 Summit, NJ 07902 (908)522-2857

Zimmerman, Barry L., DO {1467433912} Nrolgy(83,NY75)<NJ-KIMBALL>
+ Neurological Associates of Ocean County PA
  40 Bey Lea Road/Suite C103 Toms River, NJ 08753 (732)367-8280 Fax (732)367-1529

Zimmerman, Daniel J., MD {1801919741} EmrgMd, IntrMd(82,NY08)
+ Addiction Pain Associates
  100 Kings Way East/Suite D-3 Sewell, NJ 08080 (856)589-1440 Fax (856)589-4616
  Drz1947@yahoo.com

Zimmerman, Deena R., MD {1033376041} Pedtrc(88,NY46)
+ 1020 Phelps Road
  Teaneck, NJ 07666

Zimmerman, Gail B., MD {1548385537} IntrMd(88,NY01)
+ 519 Main Avenue
  Bay Head, NJ 08742 (732)899-9440

Zimmerman, Gregg E., MD {1790766228} Urolgy(00,NY48)<NJ-STCLRDEN, NJ-STCLRDOV>
+ Morris Urology
  16 Pocono Road/Suite 205 Denville, NJ 07834 (973)627-0060 Fax (973)627-6821
+ Morris Urology
  195 Route 46/Suite 100 Mine Hill, NJ 07803 (973)627-0060 Fax (973)627-6821

Zimmerman, Jerald R., MD {1255384624} PhysMd(82,IL11)<NJ-KSLRWEST, NJ-ENGLWOOD>
+ Kessler Institute for Rehabilitation West Orange
  1199 Pleasant Valley Way West Orange, NJ 07052 (973)731-3600
+ Englewood Hospital and Medical Center
  350 Engle Street/RehabMed Englewood, NJ 07631 (201)894-3707
+ Primary Care NJ
  370 Grand Avenue/Suite 102 Englewood, NJ 07052 (201)567-3370 Fax (201)816-1265

Zimmerman, Jill Robin, MD {1144242355} RadDia(93,NY46)<NJ-VALLEY>
+ Radiology Associates of Ridgewood, P.A.
  20 Franklin Turnpike Waldwick, NJ 07463 (201)445-8822 Fax (201)447-5053

Zimmerman, John M., MD {1528036217} CdvDis(78,NY09)<NJ-HACKNSK>
+ Electrophysiology Associates
  20 Prospect Avenue/Suite 701 Hackensack, NJ 07601 (201)996-2997 Fax (201)996-2571
+ Hackensack University Medical Center
  30 Prospect Avenue/Cardiology(EPS) Hackensack, NJ 07601 (201)996-2287

Zimmerman, Joshua M., MD {1265414312} SrgOrt(87,DC02)
+ Orthopedic Associates of Central Jersey
  205 May Street/Suite 202 Edison, NJ 08837 (908)757-1520 Fax (908)769-1388
+ Orthopedic Associates of Central Jersey PA
  3 Hospital Plaza/Suite 411 Old Bridge, NJ 08857 (908)757-1520 Fax (732)360-0775

Zimmerman, Lisa M., MD {1427085653} IntrMd, Grtrcs(87,VA04)
+ 776 Shrewsbury Avenue/Suite 103
  Tinton Falls, NJ 07724 (732)440-4782
+ Family Wellness Center
  1680 State Route 35 Middletown, NJ 07748 (732)440-4782 Fax (732)706-1078

Zimmerman, Mark I., MD {1447251509} CritCr, PulDis, IntrMd(85,NY19)<NJ-OVERLOOK, NJ-MORRISTN>
+ Pulmonary & Allergy Associates
  1 Springfield Avenue/Suite 3-A Summit, NJ 07901 (908)934-0555 Fax (908)934-0556
+ Pulmonary & Allergy Associates
  8 Saddle Road/Suite 101 Cedar Knolls, NJ 07927 (908)934-0555 Fax (973)540-0472

Zimmerman, Patrick Whaley, MD {1538489315} EmrgMd<NJ-MORRISTN>
+ Morristown Medical Center
  100 Madison Avenue/Emerg Med Morristown, NJ 07962 (973)971-5044

Zimmerman, Ronald Lee, MD {1437157476} PhysMd, IntrMd
+ Primary Care NJ
  370 Grand Avenue/Suite 102/Phys Rehab Englewood, NJ 07631 (201)567-3370 Fax (201)816-1265

Zimmerman, Stanley R., MD {1639124399} IntrMd(75,NY46)
+ RWJPE Internal Medicine North Brunswick
  2300 Route 27 North Brunswick, NJ 08902 (732)821-5656 Fax (732)821-7743

Zimmerman, Thomas, Jr., MD {1154539492} IntrMd, Nrolgy, EmrgMd(86,NJ05)<NJ-RWJUBRUN>
+ 230 Mendham Road
  Bernardsville, NJ 07924 (201)368-5031 Fax (908)766-4870
  t.r.zimmerman@att.net
+ Johnston McGregor LLC
  80 Morristown Road/Suite 302 Bernardsville, NJ 07924 (908)766-0750

Zimmerman-Bier, Barbie L., MD {1669407110} Pedtrc, PedDvl(86,NY08)<NJ-STPETER>
+ St. Peter's University Hospital
  254 Easton Avenue/Pediatrics New Brunswick, NJ 08901 (732)745-8600
  bzimmerbanbier@saintpetersuh.com

Zimmermann, Carol E., MD {1124007588} Anesth(68,NM01)
+ Summit Anesthesia Associates, P.A.
  33 Overlook Road/Suite 311 Summit, NJ 07901 (908)598-1500 Fax (908)598-0197

Zimmermann, Laura Senn, MD {1407893530} ObsGyn(99,NY19)<NJ-OVERLOOK, NJ-MORRISTN>
+ Summit Medical Group
  574 Springfield Avenue/2nd flr Westfield, NJ 07090 (908)389-6391 Fax (908)232-0540
+ Summit Medical Group-Berkeley Heights Campus
  1 Diamond Hill Road/Wittman 3rd Fl Berkeley Heights, NJ 07922 (908)389-6391 Fax (908)228-3617

Zimmermann, Susanne W., MD {1083685747} FamMed(89,NJ06)<NJ-JRSYSHMC>
+ Jersey Shore Internal Medicine
  241 Monmouth Road/Suite 102 West Long Branch, NJ 07764 (732)263-7965 Fax (732)263-7962
+ Wall Family Medical
  500 Candlewood Commons Howell, NJ 07731 (732)263-7965 Fax (732)364-7713

Zimmern, Andrea, MD {1669641296} Surgry, SrgC&R(77,NY09)<NJ-TRINIWSC>
+ Trinitas Regional Medical Center-Williamson Street
  225 Williamson Street/Surgery Elizabeth, NJ 07207 (908)994-8449

Zincone, John Peter, MD {1881700888} Psychy, PsyFor(00,DMN01)
+ St. Clare's Behavioral Health Center
  100 Est Hanover Avenue Cedar Knolls, NJ 07927 (973)401-2121 Fax (973)401-2140

Zinda, Ashley Beth, DO {1588978506} IntrMd<NJ-DEBRAHLC>
+ Deborah Heart and Lung Center
  200 Trenton Road Browns Mills, NJ 08015 (609)893-6611

Zingler, Barry M., MD {1508808601} Gastrn, IntrMd(85,NJ06)<NJ-ENGLWOOD, NJ-HOLYNAME>
+ Advanced Gastroenterology of Bergen County
  140 Sylvan Avenue/Suite 101-A Englewood Cliffs, NJ 07632 (201)945-6564 Fax (201)461-9038

Zingrone, Denise Michele, DO {1821193558} IntrMd
+ 30 Kay Drive
  Hammonton, NJ 08037

Zingrone, Joseph Peter, DO {1619923109} IntrMd, Nephro(99,NJ75)<NJ-KMHCHRRY, NJ-KMHSTRAT>
+ Nephrology & Hypertension Associates of New Jersey
  201 Laurel Oak Road/Suite A Voorhees, NJ 08043 (856)566-5478 Fax (856)566-9561

Zinman, James Douglas, MD {1578591467} Urolgy(96,NY19)<NJ-CHILTON>
+ Adult and Pediatric Urology Center, P.A.
  1033 Clifton Avenue Clifton, NJ 07013 (973)473-5700 Fax (973)473-3367
+ Adult and Pediatric Urology Center, P.A.
  2025 Hamburg Turnpike Wayne, NJ 07470 (973)473-5700 Fax (973)831-0033
+ Wayne Surgical Center, LLC.
  1176 Hamburg Pike Wayne, NJ 07013 (973)709-1900 Fax (973)709-1901

Zinn, Andrew P., MD {1366632432} CdvDis
+ Cardiovascular Associates
  210 West Atlantic Avenue Haddon Heights, NJ 08035 (856)546-3003 Fax (856)547-5337
+ Cardiovascular Associates of The Delaware Valley, PA
  525 State Street/Suite 3 Elmer, NJ 08318 (856)546-3003 Fax (856)358-0725

Zinsky, Paul J., MD {1164402673} ObsGyn(86,PA12)<NJ-VIRTMARL, NJ-VIRTVOOR>
+ Womens Health Associates PA
  2301 East Evesham Road/Suite 602 Voorhees, NJ 08043 (856)772-2066 Fax (856)772-9159
+ Womens Health Associates PA
  188 Fries Mill Road/Suite B-1 Turnersville, NJ 08012 (856)772-2066 Fax (856)629-6695

Zinterhofer, Louis J., MD {1629134457} PthACl, PthChm, PthRso(67,LA01)<NJ-MONMOUTH>
+ Laboratory Medicine Associates PA
  279 Third Avenue/Suite 204 Long Branch, NJ 07740 (732)229-8494
+ Monmouth Medical Center
  300 Second Avenue/Path Long Branch, NJ 07740 (732)229-8494 Fax (732)923-7355

Zinzuwadia, Shreni Natoo, MD {1629233275} EmrgMd(03,NJ05)<NJ-UMDNJ>
+ University Hospital
  150 Bergen Street/Room C-370/Emrg Newark, NJ 07103 (973)972-4300

Ziolo, Gregory Michael, MD {1972503001} IntrMd, CdvDis(91,POL02)<NJ-MORRISTN>
+ 95 Madison Avenue/Suite B-01
  Morristown, NJ 07960 (973)898-1220 Fax (973)898-1496

Ziolo, Malgorzata Maria, MD {1528129483} IntrMd(91,POL02)
+ 415 Parsippany Road
  Parsippany, NJ 07054 (973)884-0666 Fax (973)560-9166

Ziontz, Kristy L., DO {1629235502} EmrgMd(04,NJ75)
+ St Joseph's Medical Center Emergency
  703 Main Street Paterson, NJ 07503 (973)754-2240 Fax (973)754-2249

Zipagan, James Talamayan, MD {1467554527} EmrgMd(70,PHI01)<NJ-ACMCITY, NJ-ACMCMAIN>
+ AtlantiCare Regional Medical Center/City Campus
1925 Pacific Avenue/EmergMed Atlantic City, NJ 08401 (609)345-4000

Zipp, Christopher Paul, DO {1811949076} FamMed(02,NJ75)<NJ-MORRISTN>
+ Morristown Medical Center Family Medicine
435 South Street/Suite 220-A Morristown, NJ 07960 (973)971-4222 Fax (973)290-7050

Zirkman, Daniel M., MD {1881663755} IntrMd, Nephro(86,TX13)<NJ-JRSYSHMC, NJ-CENTRAST>
+ 495 Iron Bridge Road/Suite 4
Freehold, NJ 07728 (732)866-9988 Fax (732)866-9998

Zirvi, Monib Ahmad, MD {1457307464} Dermat(00,NY20)<NJ-OVERLOOK, NJ-MORRISTN>
+ Summit Medical Group-Berkeley Heights Campus
1 Diamond Hill Road Berkeley Heights, NJ 07922 (908)769-0100 Fax (908)790-6524
+ Summit Medical Group
34 Mountain Boulevard/Building B Warren, NJ 07059 (908)769-0100 Fax (908)769-8927

Zisa, Salvatore Anthony, Jr., MD {1376877977} Anesth
+ St. Joseph's Regional Medical Center Anesthesia
703 Main Street Paterson, NJ 07503 (973)754-2323 Fax (973)977-9455

Zisis, Eletherios G., MD {1659384584} SrgThr, SrgVas, Surgry(73,GRE01)<NJ-EASTORNG>
+ 24 Park Avenue
West Orange, NJ 07052 (973)669-0878
+ East Orange Family Health Center
240 Central Avenue/Suite 3 East Orange, NJ 07018 (973)669-0878 Fax (973)674-6134

Ziskind, Daniela Michele, MD {1093973919} Pedtrc
+ Children's Hospital of Phila Cardio
1040 Laurel Oak Road/Suite 1 Voorhees, NJ 08043 (856)783-0287 Fax (856)783-0657

Zisu, Traian A., MD {1639293103} Psychy, Grtrcs(90,ROMA)<NJ-VALLEY>
+ Drs. Rosenfeld & Zisu
265 Ackerman Avenue Ridgewood, NJ 07450 (201)447-5630 Fax (201)447-0903

Zitnay, Christopher G., MD {1033199815} EnDbMt
+ Cape Regional Physicians Associates
11 Village Drive Cape May Court House, NJ 08210 (609)465-2273 Fax (609)463-0236

Zito, Frederick J., MD {1043205081} RadDia(90,NJ05)<NJ-RIVERVW>
+ Red Bank Radiologists, P.A.
200 White Road/Suite 115 Little Silver, NJ 07739 (732)741-9595 Fax (732)741-0985
+ Coastal Imaging, LLC
79 Route 37 West/Suite 103 Toms River, NJ 08755 (732)741-9595 Fax (732)276-2325

Ziyaaudhin, Kappukalar A., MD {1033101035} IntrMd(69,INA85)<NJ-EASTORNG>
+ 186 West Market Street/Suite 211
Newark, NJ 07103 (973)623-9011 Fax (973)624-1208

Zlotnick, Matthew Phillip, MD {1043276090} Anesth(01,IL42)<NJ-MONMOUTH>
+ Monmouth Medical Center
300 Second Avenue/Anesthesia Long Branch, NJ 07740 (732)923-6980 Fax (732)923-6977

Zloza, Donna Lynn, MD {1154529840}
+ Newark Community Health Center, Inc.
741 Broadway Newark, NJ 07104 (973)675-1900 Fax (973)676-1396
dzloza@gmail.com

Znamensky, Addi, MD {1619137494} IntrMd
+ Drs. Lavotshkin and Znamensky
757 Teaneck Road Teaneck, NJ 07666 (201)833-2288 Fax (201)833-4441

Zodda, David F., MD {1588976443} EmrgMd(10,DMN01)
+ Hackensack Medical Center Emergency Medicine
30 Prospect Avenue/Main 3619 Hackensack, NJ 07601 (551)996-4614 Fax (551)996-4239

Zodiatis, Alexander Demetrius, DO {1972655322} AdolMd(03,NY75)
+ Totowa Pediatric Group, P.A.
290 Union Boulevard/Suite 2 Totowa, NJ 07512 (973)595-0600 Fax (973)595-0206
+ Totowa Pediatric Group, P.A.
400 West Blackwell Street Dover, NJ 07801 (973)595-0600 Fax (973)989-3651

Zodiatis, Paras Jayant, DO {1699890830} Anesth(03,NY75)<NJ-STJOSHOS>
+ St. Joseph's Regional Medical Center Anesthesia
703 Main Street Paterson, NJ 07503 (973)754-2323 Fax (973)977-9455

Zoeller, Garrett Keith, MD {1255532669} PedSrg
+ New Jersey Pediatric Neurosurgical Associates
131 Madison Avenue/Suite 140 Morristown, NJ 07960 (973)326-9000 Fax (973)326-9001

Zohny, Jeahad, MD {1376703140} Pedtrc
+ Advocare Sussex County Pediatrics Newton
39 Newton Sparta Road Newton, NJ 07860 (973)383-9841 Fax (973)383-7989

Zolli, Christine L., MD {1720066087} Ophthl(70,NY08)
+ New Jersey Eye Physicians & Surgeons
16 Ferry Street Newark, NJ 07105 (973)344-0023

Zollner, Paula G., MD {1831116656} Pedtrc(88,NJ06)<NJ-UNVM-CPRN, NJ-CHSMRCER>
+ The Pediatric Group PA
66 Mount Lucas Road Princeton, NJ 08540 (609)924-4892 Fax (609)921-9380

Zolty, Ronald, MD {1023108701} IntCrd(90,SWI04)
+ 1260 West Laurelton Parkway
Teaneck, NJ 07666

Zomorodi, Ali, MD {1679601348} Psychy(68,IRA01)<NJ-CARRIER>
+ 407 Omni Drive
Hillsborough, NJ 08844 (908)359-3779 Fax (908)359-5356

Zomorodi-Ardebili, Waldburg M., MD {1619003597} Psychy, Psy-Grt(70,SWI04)<NJ-UNIVBHC>
+ Catholic Charities Mental Health Center
288 Rues Lane East Brunswick, NJ 08816 (732)257-6100 Fax (732)651-9834

Zonn, Svetlana, MD {1013948199} Pedtrc(77,UZB02)<NJ-STPETER>
+ 1024 Park Avenue/Suite 6-C
Plainfield, NJ 07060 (908)755-7773
Svetlanazoon@yahoo.com
+ Dr. Svetlana Zonn and Associates
776 Amboy Avenue/Suite 201 Edison, NJ 08837 (732)661-0030

Zorba, Yildiz, MD {1760856439} IntrMd
+ Hackensack Medical Center Internal Medicine
385 Prospect Avenue Hackensack, NJ 07601 (551)996-9140 Fax (551)996-9144

Zoretic, Stephen N., MD {1295703890} Urolgy(75,MEX03)<NJ-HACKNSK, NJ-VALLEY>
+ Urology Specialty Care, P.A.
555 Kindermack Road/Suite D Oradell, NJ 07649 (201)834-1890 Fax (201)834-1898
pocroat2@aol.com

Zornitzer, Matthew Howard, MD {1972538999} SprtMd
+ Center for Orthopaedics
1500 Pleasant Valley Way/Suite 101 West Orange, NJ 07052 (973)669-5600 Fax (973)669-0269

Zornitzer, Michael R., MD {1033275813} Psychy(71,NY08)<NJ-STBARNMC>
+ 2 West Northfield Road/Suite 305
Livingston, NJ 07039 (973)992-6090 Fax (973)992-1383
mzornitzer@aol.com

Zorrilla, Lilian, MD {1861545105} IntrMd, EnDbMt(84,NY09)<NJ-STCLRDOV>
+ Zufall Health Center
18 West Blackwell Street/Internal Med Dover, NJ 07801 (973)328-9100 Fax (973)328-6817

Zozzaro, Michael A., MD {1659535433}(06,NJ06)
+ The Family Center for Otolaryngology
47 Orient Way/Lower Level Rutherford, NJ 07070 (201)935-5508 Fax (201)465-6088
+ The Family Center for Otolaryngology
1265 Paterson Plank Road Secaucus, NJ 07094 (201)935-5508 Fax (201)465-6088
+ The Family Center for Otolaryngology
6 Brighton Road/Suite 104 Clifton, NJ 07070 (973)470-0282 Fax (201)465-6088

Zrada, Stephen Eugene, MD {1407852676} IntrMd, MedOnc, OncHem(95,PA09)
+ Regional Cancer Care Associates, LLC
200 Bowman Drive/Suite E-125 Voorhees, NJ 08043 (856)424-3311 Fax (856)424-5634
+ The Center for Cancer & Hematologic Disease
856 South White Horse Pike/Suite 4 Hammonton, NJ 08037 (856)424-3311 Fax (609)561-2492
+ The Center for Cancer & Hematologic Disease
609 North Broad Street/Suite 300 Woodbury, NJ 08043 (856)686-1002

Zu, James Shanwei, MD {1083787824} Nrolgy(83,CHN07)<NJ-JFKMED, NJ-RWJURAH>
+ 2 Lincoln Highway/Suite 468
Edison, NJ 08820 (908)756-5733 Fax (908)756-4483
quann2004@hotmail.com

Zuazua-Pacillo, Maria Cristina, MD {1972619591} FamMed(00,KS02)<NJ-KMHSTRAT>
+ Family Health Center of Mullica Hill
155 Bridgeton Pike/Suite A Mullica Hill, NJ 08062 (856)223-0500 Fax (856)223-1098
+ Alliance for Better Care, P.C.
PO Box 1510 Medford, NJ 08055 (856)223-0500 Fax (609)953-8652

Zuback, Joseph R., DO {1447287354} Radiol, RadNro(89,NJ75)<NJ-VAEASTOR>
+ VA New Jersey Health Care System-East Orange Campus
385 Tremont Avenue East Orange, NJ 07018 (973)676-1000

Zubair, Faiza, DO {1114189941}
+ 42 Kingsberry Drive
Somerset, NJ 08873

Zubair, Khurram, MD {1730134826} IntrMd(89,PAKI)<NJ-CHS-FULD>
+ Drs. Sharim & Zubair
40 Fuld Street/Suite 402 Trenton, NJ 08638 (609)393-4911 Fax (609)394-6770
+ Capital Health Primary Care
832 Brunswick Avenue Trenton, NJ 08638 (609)393-4911 Fax (609)815-7401

Zubair, Mohammad A., MD {1003872268} IntrMd, PulDis(85,DMN01)<NJ-JFKMED, NJ-NWRKBETH>
+ 400 Osborne Terrace/Suite L4
Newark, NJ 07112 (973)926-8203
+ Woodbridge Sleep Disorders Center
900 Woodbridge Center Drive Woodbridge, NJ 07095 (973)926-8203 Fax (732)636-7060

Zuber, Janie Anne, MD {1619108453} Pedtrc
+ Children's Specialized Hospital
200 Somerset Street New Brunswick, NJ 08901 (732)258-7038

Zuber, Nicole Alexandra, MD {1407017932}
+ 201 Railroad Avenue/Apt 301
East Rutherford, NJ 07073 (973)943-0408
nicole.zuber.md@gmail.com

Zuberi, Faizah, MD {1992703466} Anesth(90,PAKI)<NJ-STBARNMC>
+ St. Joseph's Regional Medical Center Anesthesia
703 Main Street Paterson, NJ 07503 (973)754-2323 Fax (973)977-9455

Zuberi, Jamshed A., MD {1558456137} SrgCrC, Surgry<NJ-STJOSHOS>
+ St. Joseph Medical Center Surgery
703 Main Street Paterson, NJ 07503 (973)754-2490

Zubowski, Robert I., MD {1558425561} SrgPlstc, Surgry(83,MEX03)<NJ-HACKNSK, NJ-VALLEY>
+ Robert Zubowski MD Ctr Cosmetic/Recon
1 Sears Drive Paramus, NJ 07652 (201)261-7550 Fax (201)261-7515

Zucconi, Adam J., DO {1770837833} FamMed<NJ-SJHREGMC>
+ Premier Orthopaedic Associates
298 South Delsea Drive Vineland, NJ 08360 (856)690-1616 Fax (856)690-1089
+ SJH Regional Medical Center
1505 West Sherman Avenue Vineland, NJ 08360 (856)641-8000

Zucconi, Nicole Christina, DO {1053651398} FamMed<NJ-SJHREGMC>
+ SJH Regional Medical Center
1505 West Sherman Avenue Vineland, NJ 08360 (856)641-8000

Zuck, Glenn M., DO {1568552966} SrgOrt, SprtMd(85,NJ75)<NJ-SHOREMEM>
+ Pace Orthopedics & Sports Medicine
547 New Road Somers Point, NJ 08244 (609)927-9200 Fax (609)927-1616

Zucker, Ira I., MD {1730160870} Gastrn, IntrMd(81,IL42)<NJ-VALLEY>
+ Hackensack University Medical Group Emerson
452 Old Hook Road/2nd Floor Emerson, NJ 07630 (201)666-3900 Fax (201)261-0505

Zucker, Mark J., MD {1356319180} CdvDis, IntrMd, SrgTpl(81,IL06)<NJ-NWRKBETH, NJ-STBARNMC>
+ Newark Beth Israel Medical Center
201 Lyons Avenue/HeartTrnspltPgm Newark, NJ 07112 (973)926-7205 Fax (973)923-8993
mzucker@barnabashealth.org
+ Morristown Medical Center
100 Madison Avenue/Level C Morristown, NJ 07962 (973)971-4179

Zucker, Scott W., MD {1285697748} Pedtrc(81,NY48)<NJ-VALLEY, NJ-STJOSHOS>
+ PediatriCare Associates
20-20 Fair Lawn Avenue Fair Lawn, NJ 07410 (201)791-4545 Fax (201)791-3765
+ PediatriCare Associates
400 Franklin Turnpike Mahwah, NJ 07430 (201)791-4545 Fax (201)529-1596
+ PediatriCare Associates
901 Route 23 South Pompton Plains, NJ 07410 (973)831-4545 Fax (973)831-1527

Zuckerbrod, Jacqueline E., DO {1942391974} FamMed(85,MO78)<NJ-KIMBALL, NJ-CENTRAST>
+ Drs. Axelrad & Zuckerbrod
4774 Route 9 South Howell, NJ 07731 (732)363-6222 Fax (732)363-9203

Physicians by Name and Address

Zuckerbrot, Rachel Aryella, MD {1184774069} Pedtrc, PsyCAd(97,NY46)
+ 214 Engle Street/Suite 23
Englewood, NJ 07631 (917)538-6034

Zuckerman, Gary B., MD {1174672463} PedCrC, Allrgy(86,NY08)<NJ-RWJUBRUN>
+ Central NJ Allergy Asthma Associates
3084 State Route 27/Suite 6 Kendall Park, NJ 08824
(732)821-0595 Fax (732)821-1174

Zuker-Silberberg, Dora D., MD {1629253604} Anesth<NJ-RWJUBRUN>
+ Robert Wood Johnson-UMDNJ Anesthesia Group
125 Paterson Street/CAB 3100/Anesth New Brunswick, NJ 08901 (732)235-7827 Fax (732)235-6131

Zukerman, Louis Steven, MD {1326015306} CdvDis, IntrMd(81,IL05)<NJ-CENTRAST, NJ-JRSYSHMC>
+ Monmouth Cardiology Associates, LLC
222 Schanck Road/Suite 104 Freehold, NJ 07728
(732)431-1332 Fax (732)431-1712
+ Monmouth Cardiology Associates, LLC
11 Meridian Road Eatontown, NJ 07724 (732)431-1332 Fax (732)663-0301

Zukoff, David S., MD {1023089778} CdvDis, IntrMd(87,MEX34)<NJ-BAYSHORE>
+ Cardiac Care Center
21 North Gilbert Street Tinton Falls, NJ 07701 (732)741-7400 Fax (732)741-4775

Zukoff, Paul B., MD {1891858569} IntrMd(86,PA02)<NJ-OVERLOOK>
+ New Providence Internal Medical Associates
571 Central Avenue/Suite 112 New Providence, NJ 07974
(908)464-7300 Fax (908)464-7350

Zukowski, Christopher W., DO {1407826746} FamMed, SprtMd(80,MO78)
+ Meridian Occupational Health
150 Airport Road/Suite 100 Lakewood, NJ 08701
(732)942-9550 Fax (732)942-9554

Zulueta, Erica, DO {1396973525} Anesth<NJ-STBARNMC>
+ St. Barnabas Medical Center
94 Old Short Hills Road Livingston, NJ 07039 (973)322-5512

Zuniga, Gina, MD {1346295342} ObsGyn(99,NY45)<NJ-STBARNMC, NJ-CLARMAAS>
+ Contemporary Women's Care
745 Northfield Avenue West Orange, NJ 07052 (973)736-7700 Fax (973)736-8078

Zuniga, Joseph Michael Romilla, MD {1063675064} Surgry, SrgVas(06,PHI29)<MA-NEMEDCEN>
+ Virtua Surgical Group, PA
1935 Route 70 East Cherry Hill, NJ 08003 (856)428-7700 Fax (856)424-9120

Zuniga, Rina De Guzman, MD {1043565179} IntrMd
+ Virtua Internal Medicine-Marlton
601 Route 73 North/Suite 101 Marlton, NJ 08053
(856)429-1910 Fax (856)396-0848

Zurada, Joanna Magdalena, MD {1285953570} Dermat(06,NY01)
+ Dermatology Center of North Jersey
1033 Clifton Avenue Clifton, NJ 07013 (973)777-6444
Fax (973)777-5277
+ 71 Union Avenue/Suite 108
Rutherford, NJ 07070 (973)777-6444 Fax (201)804-8901

Zurkovsky, Avivit Gizzele, MD {1104229285}
+ 325 Garfield Avenue
Oakhurst, NJ 07755 (201)873-4176
dravivit@yahoo.com

Zurkovsky, Eugene, MD {1831343045} Surgry(02,ISR02)
+ Atlantic Shore Surgical Associates
478 Brick Boulevard Brick, NJ 08723 (732)701-4848 Fax (732)701-1244

Zurlo, John V., MD {1750318051} Radiol, RadDia(95,NJ05)<NJ-STBARNMC, NJ-UMDNJ>
+ St. Barnabas Medical Center
94 Old Short Hills Road/Radiology Livingston, NJ 07039
(973)322-5000

Zwerin, Glenn A., MD {1235264854} Grtrcs(82,NJ06)<NJ-MONMOUTH>
+ Monmouth Medical Center
300 Second Avenue/Geriatrics Long Branch, NJ 07740
(732)222-5200

Zwick, Annette E., MD {1306833710} Anesth(87,OH06)
+ Hamilton Anesthesia and Pain Management
1 Hamilton Health Place Hamilton, NJ 08690 (609)631-6824 Fax (609)631-6839

Zwil, Alexander S., MD {1861540601} Psychy, PsyGrt(84,PA13)
+ 61 Jimmie Leeds Road
Pomona, NJ 08240

Zwitiashvili, Robert, MD {1841346392} IntrMd, Nephro(70,RUS37)
+ 335 Harmon Cove Tower/Suite 335
Secaucus, NJ 07094 (973)278-8818
+ Passaic County Medical Care
124 Gregory Avenue Passaic, NJ 07055 (973)278-8818

Fax (973)471-9240

Zwolska-Demczuk, Barbara A., MD {1114997053} Anesth(73,POL10)<NJ-NWRKBETH>
+ Newark Beth Israel Medical Center
201 Lyons Avenue Newark, NJ 07112 (973)926-7000
Fax (201)943-8105

Zylberger, David A., MD {1043307127} Anesth, AnesPain(91,NY09)<NY-PRSBWEIL, NY-PRSBCOLU>
+ New Jersey Anesthesia Associates, P.C.
30B Vreeland Road/Suite 200 Florham Park, NJ 07932
(973)660-9334 Fax (973)660-9779

Physicians by Town and Medical Specialty

**Physicians Alphabetically
by Town and Medical Specialty**
(Primary Practice Town and Specialty)

New Jersey
　　Section 2

**Physicians Alphabetically
by Town and Medical Specialty**
(Primary Practice Town and Primary Medical Speicalty)

Aberdeen
Cardiovascular Disease
Adler,Eric David,MD
Family Medicine
Li,Jason,DO
Internal Medicine
Guirguis,Nagy Nimr,MD
Perkari,Vasantha K.,MD
Neurology
Daniel,Joshua,MD
Psychiatry
Awad,Maher Bekheet,MD
Awad,Sahar Fathi,MD
Bennett,Robert J.,MD
Green,Anthony J.,MD

Absecon
Cardiovascular Disease
Shanker,Mukesh J.,MD
Family Medicine
Zawid,Joseph,MD
General Practice
Jhaveri,Bharat J.,MD
Infectious Disease
Paparone,Philip W.,DO
Internal Medicine
Catalina,Gabriel Richard,DO
Driscoll,Eric Joseph,DO
Fiorentino,Diego M.,DO
Khan-Jaffery,Kaniz F.,MD
Santos,Eduardo V.,MD
Sudol,Robert R.,MD
Obstetrics & Gynecology
Carfagno,Salvatore Jr.,DO
Sackstein,Stuart A.,MD
Physical Medicine & Rehab
Khan,Naheed A.,MD
Psychiatry
Kammiel,Rita R.,MD
Morelli,Louis C.,MD
Radiology
Dauito,Ralph,MD
Surgery (General)
Del Rosario,Michael Patrick,MD

Allendale
Internal Medicine
Hershman,Jerald B.,MD

Allenhurst
Forensic Psychiatry
Dengrove,Robert S.,MD
Physical Medicine & Rehab
Fernicola,Richard G.,MD

Allentown
Dermatology
Kupetsky,Erine Allison,DO
Emergency Medicine
Krivoshik,Mark P.,MD
Family Medicine
Byrnes,Curtis W.,DO
Redlich,Vijaya Potharlanka,DO
Internal Medicine
Webb,James A.,MD

Alpine
Anatomic/Clinical Pathology
Natarajan,Geetha,MD
Wetli,Charles Victor,MD

Andover
Family Medicine
Medunick,Sara Elizabeth,DO
Reilly,Melissa Lynn,DO
Trader,Catherine R.,DO
Internal Medicine
Renda,Julie Elaine,DO

Annandale
Dermatologic Surgery
Abel,Carter Grant,MD
Family Medicine
Imran,Uzma,MD
Internal Medicine
Espinoza,Andrey,MD
Psychiatry
Mero,Raymond J.,DO

Asbury Park
Family Medicine
Dhar,Gargi,MD
Khandelwal,Anil,MD
Lewis,Alison Dennesha,MD
Marro,Michael Angelo,DO
Wu,Irene Y.,MD

Internal Medicine
Chinnici,Angelo A.,MD
Sisskin,Mark I.,MD
Tosiello,Lorraine Lerma,MD
Obstetrics & Gynecology
Herron,Garland Ella,MD
Lepis,Carl R.,MD
Lore,Kristen Nicole,DO
Michalewski,Martin P.,MD
Oncological Surgery
Kohli,Manpreet K.,MD
Ophthalmology
Berg,Bruce R.,MD
Chiang,Peter Keh-dah,MD
Pardon,Ilene B.,MD
Talansky,Marvin L.,MD
Turtel,Lawrence S.,MD
Pediatrics
Baxi,Nilay Manojkumar,MD
Kharod,Sudhakar J.,MD
Peardon,Amy Elizabeth,DO
Physical Medicine & Rehab
Brustein,Fredric,MD

Atco
Family Medicine
Mazzuca,Robert F.,DO
Vassalluzzo,Pasquale D.,MD
Internal Medicine
Campbell,Colin A.,DO
Pain Medicine
Davis,Kara Alison,MD

Atlantic City
Anatomic Pathology
Bansal,Meenakshi,MD
Dantas,Bruno Felipe,MD
Anatomic/Clinical Pathology
Hamel,Marianne,MD
McCormick,John F.,MD
Rastgar,Khosrow,MD
Anesthesiology
Crompton,Thomas F.,MD
Droney,Timothy J. III,MD
Marable,Denise Marie,MD
Morsi,Khaled M.,MD
Pinz,Alexandra,MD
Shah,Sudha S.,MD
Takla,Magdy F.G.,MD
Zalman,Richard,MD
Child & Adolescent Psychiatry
Momodu,Inua Aitsekegbe,MD
Clinical & Lab Immunology
Todd,William Upton IV,MD
Clinical Pathology/Laboratory
Miller,Nicole C.,DO
Colon & Rectal Surgery
Aarons,William Jr.,MD
Emergency Medicine
Acunto,Brian Anthony,DO
Becher,John W.,DO
Donaldson,James Kenneth,DO
Dubin,Reva,MD
Farnsworth,Marie N.,MD
Hawkins,Nancy S.,MD
Khatiwala,Manisha P.,MD
Khebzou,Zaki,MD
Leriotis,Theo James,DO
Luyber,Todd Joseph,DO
MacBride,David G.,DO
Menet,Scott Douglas,DO
Merz,Daniel Francis,DO
Nicholls,Brian Robert,DO
Rangam,Tsui H.,MD
Ruggiero,Michael P.,DO
Sabatini,Louis V.,DO
Salvatore,Francis P. Jr.,MD
Schumacher,William Delmar,DO
Seibert,Henry Edward,MD
Urban,Scott Michael,DO
Westrol,Michael Steven,MD
Wolk,Eric Todd,DO
Zipagan,James Talamayan,MD
Family Med-Sports Medicine
Reed,Tony S.,MD
Family Medicine
Bisk,Bradley A.,DO
Castro-Chevere,Nancy Ann,MD
Corrales,Michelle D.,MD
Delice,Anael Destin Jr.,MD
Digenio,Ines Elena,MD
Fog,Edward Roland,DO

Holder,Sarah Schell,DO
Keiner,Lisa R.,DO
Pericles,John T.,DO
Raman,Anoop Manikarnika,MD
Rodriguez,Marlene V.,MD
Terrels,Mary Ellen,DO
Toliver,Tiffany E.,MD
General Practice
Giamporcaro,Steven J.,MD
Gynecology
De Stefano,Joseph L.,MD
Hospitalist
Abbasi,Danish P.,MD
Abella-Ramirez,Katherine,MD
Ahmad,Israr,MD
Baby,Benesa,MD
Bakr,Mohamed Mokhtar,MD
Dhaliwal,Harleen,MD
Huma,Sabahath,MD
Iqbal,Javid,MD
Jaleel,Syed,MD
McBrearty-Hindson,Ashley,DO
Narula,Navjot Singh,MD
Rahmani,Ghulam Ali,MD
Shah,Sulay Hiteshkumar,MD
Silver,Jordan,MD
Sohaib,Muhammad,MD
Tusheva,Marija,MD
Infectious Disease
Bayer,Deborah D.,MD
Internal Medicine
Ahmad,Naheed Kaleem,MD
Alexander,Karen Elizabeth,MD
Alexander,Mark P.,MD
Asghar,Sheba,MD
Ashraf,Afia,MD
Bane,Susan H.,MD
Barzaga,Ricardo A.,MD
Belete,Senayit Girma,MD
Bernardo,Gregory,MD
Collins,Gregory C.,MD
Ghetia,Ditina,MD
Hasni,Syed Shayan Ahmed,MD
Hinkle,Mary Katrina,MD
Hocbo,Aileen Aileen,MD
Hussain,Arif,MD
Hussain,Asiya,MD
Infantolino,Edward,MD
Kelly,Brendan S.,DO
Lal,Vikram,DO
Macchiavelli,Anthony Joseph,MD
Maludum,Obiora,MD
Marwaha,Rohit,MD
Mazur,Kimberly L.,MD
Mingione,Richard A.,MD
Misra,Amit,MD
Mohiuddin,Fatima A.,MD
Nwotite,Ezinne Ugochi,MD
Onwuka,Mary N.,MD
Parikh,Hiren B.,MD
Patel,Arvind Kumar,MD
Patel,Hasitkumar D.,MD
Patel,Jitendra K.,MD
Patel,Manoj K.,MD
Patel,Mehul Kumar,MD
Patel,Yogesh N.,MD
Quinlan,Liliane Bastos,MD
Rangaraj,Narsimha R.,MD
Ray,Amit H.,MD
Roeske,Jessica L.,DO
Siddiqui,Durdana Aamir,MD
Siegelman,Gary M.,MD
Sun,Qi,MD
Szulc,Magdalena,MD
Thalassinos,Antonios,DO
Timms,Brian Daniel,DO
Vijayakumar,Ashvin,MD
Yarlagadda,Vivek,MD
Zia,Shahzad S.,MD
Neonatal-Perinatal Medicine
Celestial,Rommel M.,MD
Escareal,Myrna S.,MD
Nephrology
Degapudi,Bhargavi,MD
Kessler,Alex,DO
Mourad,Mohammad Y.,MD
Neurology
Zeidwerg,David Martin,DO
Obstetrics & Gynecology
Irvis,Kenneth M.,MD
Regis,Jon M.,MD

Physicians by Town and Medical Specialty

Pathology
Can,Seyit A.,MD
Pediatrics
Davenport,Leamon L.,DO
Lopez Bernard,Edwin,MD
Mallari,Rolando Q.,MD
Sless,Dana E.,DO
Psychiatry
Borden,Doris Rita,MD
Corvari,Steven Joseph,MD
Gomez,Arturo A.,MD
Isaacson,Brian Eric,MD
Mani,Anup S.,DO
Venditti,Marilouise,MD
Surgery (General)
Almendras,Nole E.,MD
Penaloza-Aranibar,Carlos G.,MD
Ryb,Gabriel E.,MD
Stidd,David A.,MD
Surgical Critical Care
Dudick,Catherine A.,MD
Willman,Kelly Marie,MD
Trauma Surgery
Ali,Ayoola O.,MD
Vascular Neurology
Guterman,Jonathan Glenn,MD
Vascular Surgery
Thompson,Peter N.,MD

Atlantic Highlands
Dermatology
Thosani,Maya K.,MD
Internal Medicine
De Noia,Anthony Philip,MD
Movva,Srinivasa R.,MD
Orthopedic Surgery
Sobel,Mark,MD

Audubon
Cardiovascular Disease
Crawford,Jeffrey R.,DO
Emergency Medicine
Smith,Monika,DO
Family Medicine
Bromley,William II,DO
Lopes,Francis,MD
Perry,Adam C.,MD
Internal Medicine
Montiel,Armando A.,MD
Schmid,George F.,MD
Neurology
Sen Hightower,Indrani,MD
Psychiatry
Doria,Marie E.,MD

Avalon
Emergency Medicine
Alspach,Charlotte A.,MD
Internal Medicine
Hierholzer,Paul D.,DO

Avenel
Dermatology
Cerbone,Joseph Eugene,MD
Diagnostic Radiology
Singer,Mark Andrew,MD
Gastroenterology
Duhl,Jozsef S.,MD
Hematology
Kulper,Bernard J.,MD
Shypula,Gregory J.,MD
Internal Medicine
Homer,Stuart M.,MD
Livshits,Boris M.,MD
Peter,Andras M.,MD
Romano,David L.,MD
Skrzypczak,Marek J.,MD
Swan,Alexander Myint,MD
Syed-Naqvi,Samina Altaf,MD
Neurological Radiology
Fontana,Leo John,MD
Obstetrics & Gynecology
Kline,Philip E.,MD
Ophthalmology
Wilgucki,John D.,DO
Pediatrics
Basit,Nauman A.,MD
Siddique,Muhammad Neaman,MD
Physical Medicine & Rehab
Siddiqui,Asma,MD
Psychiatry
De Crisce,Dean M.,MD
Rossi,Anna Michele,DO

555

New Jersey Physicians
Section 2 Town and Medical Specialty

Physicians by Town and Medical Specialty

Avenel (cont)
Radiology
Saniewski, Charles A., MD
Urology
Yim, Simon D., MD

Avon
Internal Medicine
Mannion, Joseph, MD

Barnegat
Anesthesiology
Frank, Howard, MD
Family Medicine
Rola, David Charles, MD
Internal Medicine
Desai, Amee B., MD
Pediatrics
Czar, Elizabeth Erin, DO
Feldman, Kira, MD
Pulmonary Disease
Palecki, Agnieszka, MD

Barrington
Family Medicine
Williams, Robert M., MD
Ophthalmology
Kamerling, Joseph M., MD

Basking Ridge
Clinical Pharmacology
Rullo, Barbara, MD
Wason, Suman, MD
Cytopathology
Wang, Wenjing, MD
Dermatology
Haliasos, Helen C., MD
Quigley, Elizabeth A., MD
Diagnostic Radiology
Hernandez, Allyn, MD
Simmons, Marc Z., MD
Emergency Medicine
Amalfitano, Christopher, MD
Milosis, Christine, MD
Endocrinology
Mehra, Aruna Sinha, MD
Family Medicine
Morandi, Joseph T., DO
Fertility/Infertility
Darder, Michael C., MD
Forensic Psychiatry
Salem, Anasuya, MD
General Practice
Lutz, Joseph S., MD
General Preventive Medicine
Dessio, Whitney Charnell, MD
Sokol, Michael C., MD
Hematology Oncology
Chalasani, Sree Bhavani, MD
Internal Medicine
Chartash, Elliot Keith, MD
Dawson, Cleve R., MD
Gaito, Andrea D., MD
Gerhard, Harvey, MD
Gorsky, Mila, MD
Kachirayan, Vasanthi, MD
Lee, Joseph Sang-Ho, MD
Passalaris, Tina Marina, MD
Schlessinger, Leslie D., MD
Shepherd, Annemarie Fernandes, MD
Sidhu, Loveleen, MD
Yu, Channing, MD
MOHS Micrographic Skin Cancer
Wang, Steven Q., MD
Mammography
Aboody, Linda R., MD
Medical Oncology
Fan, Pang-Dian, MD
Hamilton, Audrey May, MD
Xiao, Han, MD
Neurology
Gavrilovic, Igor T., MD
Nuclear Medicine
Vaseghi, Moein Faghih, MD
Obstetrics & Gynecology
Doherty, Leo Francis, MD
Fagan, Linda Nadine, MD
Hong, Kathleen H., MD
Jurema, Marcus W., MD
Kim, Julia G., MD
Leitao, Mario Mendes Jr., MD
Rauch, Eden Renee, MD
Werner, Marie D., MD
Orthopedic Surgery
Blank, Peter Bradley, DO
Pathology
Pedemonte, Bader Maria, MD
Pediatrics
Coyne, Christine Ann, MD
Kerrigan, Margot I., MD
Kohn, Jocelyn Cramer, MD
Porter, Thomas G., MD
Wu, Peywen, MD
Physical Medicine & Rehab
Lin, Julie Tun-Fang, MD
Plastic Surgery
Evdokimow, David Z., MD
Radiation Oncology
Mann, Justin, MD
Sidebotham, Helen Lee, MD
Reproductive Endocrinology
Bohrer, Michael K., MD
Costantini-Ferrando, Maria F., MD
Drews, Michael Robert, MD
Klimczak, Amber, MD
Molinaro, Thomas Anthony, MD
Morris, Jamie L., MD
Rybak, Eli Asher, MD
Yih, Melissa Christina, MD
Surgery (General)
Capko, Deborah M., MD

Bay Head
Internal Medicine
Zimmerman, Gail B., MD

Bayonne
Anatomic/Clinical Pathology
Hudacko, Rachel Mary, MD
Anesthesiology
Alekseyeva, Irina, MD
Ancevska Taneva, Natasa, MD
Canals-Ferrat, Pedro, MD
Fersel, Jordan S., MD
Hanna, Mamdouh Soliman, MD
Hashemi, Zaher Mohammad Said, MD
Klein, Ira A., MD
Morgenstern, Alvin Harris, MD
Steinman, Edward A., MD
Cardiovascular Disease
Elkind, Barry M., MD
Hefferan, James J., MD
Nadiminti, Sheila Gupta, MD
Sandhu, Mohammad Y., MD
Tan, William W., MD
Critical Care Medicine
Takhalov, Yuriy, MD
Dermatology
Kopec, Anna V., MD
Diagnostic Radiology
Chandiwala-Mody, Priti, DO
Perlov, Marina, MD
Sleman, Ingy Hanna, MD
Soloway, Peter H., MD
Emergency Medicine
Bessette, Michael John, MD
Coccaro, John A., MD
Istvan, David Joseph, MD
Lin, Esson, MD
Endocrinology
Goykhman, Stanislav, MD
Family Medicine
Chiara, Bianca A., MD
Diaz, Francisco J., MD
George-Vickers, Jonelle, DO
Katsman, Tatyana, DO
Levine, Howard Seth, DO
Levine, Martin Scott, DO
Paduszynski, Adam A., MD
Pineda, Veronica Vargas, DO
Potoczek-Salahi, Jolanta, MD
Primiani, Lisa, MD
Sirajuddin, Syed K., MD
Tariq, Samreen, MD
Thomas, Jessy Joykutty, MD
Tolerico, Christopher S., MD
Varghese, Sarat J., MD
Gastroenterology
Hahn, John C., MD
Ramasamy, Kovil Veeraswami, MD
Salem, Suhail Bakr, MD
General Practice
Desai, Bankimchandra D., MD
Geriatrics
Brown, Mitchell L., MD
Gynecology
Pelosi, Marco A. II, MD
Hematology Oncology
Iyengar, Arjun D., MD
Kumaresan, Arulnangai, MD
Lamba, Renu, MD
Hospitalist
Khan, Irfana B., MD
Internal Medicine
Acharya, Saurav, MD
Agpaoa, Ulysses V., MD
Akhtar, Shahnaz, MD
Black, Ellen M., MD
Brooks, Ira M., MD
Burghauser, Alan H., MD
Byrd, Lawrence H., MD
Cabral, Cesar A. Sr., MD
Cadoo, Lisa K.A., MD
Cardiello, Gary P., MD
Chavez, Rowland, MD
Condo, Dominick, MD
Dedousis, John Jr., MD
Engel, Margaret A., MD
Florino, Guy Michael, MD
Guittari, Nicholas S., MD
Haque, Nadeem U., MD
Herscu, Joseph I., MD
Hoffman, Mark Andrew, MD
Iyengar, Devarajan P., MD
Khalid, Khaula, DO
Mathew, Alexander John, MD
McGee, John R., MD
Montalbano, Robert L., MD
Mutterperl, Mitchell J., MD
Neno, Rosa M., DO
Oen, Rose L., MD
Padkowsky, George O., MD
Padkowsky, Orest, MD
Perveen, Mahmoodah, MD
Rangasamy, Ajantha, MD
Sheinman, Marc Daniel, DO
Silber, Danuta, MD
Singh, Amandeep, MD
Singh, Vijayant, MD
Suczewski, Edward J., MD
Suczewski, Thomas J., MD
Tarng, George W., MD
Upadhyaya, Hitendrakumar C., MD
Wignarajan, Kanagarayer R., MD
Wignarajan, Nadika V., MD
Woods, Krystina L., MD
Zelinski, Jay Michael, DO
Nephrology
Choudhry, Hammad S., MD
Gupta, Shabnam, MD
Neurology
Charles, James A., MD
Kapoor, Ashish, MD
Kapoor, Vinod, MD
Nagendra, Shan M., MD
Sadeghi, Hooshang, MD
Topper, Leonid Lev, MD
Vintayen, Enrico V., MD
Neuropathology
Ferrer, Gerrard F. A., DO
Obstetrics & Gynecology
Marki, Richard E., MD
Patel, Rakhee, MD
Pelosi, Marco A. Jr., MD
Prakash, Shasha, MD
Ophthalmology
Gurland, Keith G., MD
Orthopedic Surgery
Augustin, Jeffrey Franck, MD
Mastromonaco, Edward Domenick, DO
Rao, Juluru P., MD
Rowe Urquhart, Erica G., MD
Urquhart, Marc Wayne, MD
Pain Medicine
Huish, Stephen H., DO
Ibrahim, Joseph G., MD
Pediatrics
Aly, Sayed Raafat M., MD
Mahmoud, Ayesha Shabbir, MD
Malabanan, Nerissa V., MD
Malalis, Carmelita Pingol, MD
Nagendra, Parameswar, MD
Patel, Parul, MD
Serafino, Vincent Joseph, MD
Traba, Christin M., MD
Physical Medicine & Rehab
Chaudhary, Yasmeen Amjad, MD
Psychiatry
Aftel, Scott, MD
Gewolb, Eric B., MD
Jacoby, Jacob Herman, MD
Radiation Oncology
Baron, Joseph, MD
Radiology
Castillo, Luciano Jr., MD
Surgery (General)
Moszczynski, Zbigniew, MD
Simpson, Thomas E., MD
Williams, Richard A., MD
Zak, Madeline, DO
Urology
Goldman, Gerald A., MD
Katz, Herbert I., MD
Kerr, Eric S., MD

Bayville
Emerg Medicine-Pediatric
Iledan, Liesl P., MD
Internal Medicine
Alario, Frank C., MD
Ingato, Steven P., MD
Naseem, Arif, MD
Pediatrics
Santo Domingo, Norman E., MD
Psychiatry
Bengali, Sakina H., MD
Fabila, Jocelyn E., MD
Kolipakam, Vani S., MD
Leib, Julie Alison, MD
Schuman, Robert J., MD
So, Hee Young, MD
Tan, Lamberto A., MD
Tank, Renuka H., MD

Beach Haven
Allergy & Immunology
Shields, Mary Susan, MD
Family Medicine
Picaro, Anthony J., MD
Schmoll, Todd C., DO
Orthopedic Surgery
Khaleel, Abdul R., MD

Bedminster
Arthroscopic Surgery
France, Matthew P., MD
Family Medicine
Schwarz, Alexandra, MD
Varano, Catherine Alano, MD
Infectious Disease
Shariati, Nasseredin, MD
Internal Medicine
Bonaventura, Lisa M., MD
Campbell, Arthur Scott, MD
Garg, Anju, MD
Obstetrics & Gynecology
Bosin, Corey S., MD
Hersh, Judith Ellen, MD
Peters, Albert J., DO
Ophthalmology
Najarian, Lawrence V., MD
Sullivan, Timothy Patrick, MD
Orthopedic Surgery
Chan, Peter S., MD
Otolaryngology
Janjua, Tanveer Ahmed, MD
Pediatrics
Agathis, Allyson, MD
Ebel, Keren Zahav, MD
Fischer, John F., MD
Levine, Stephanie, DO
Shteynberg, Elena, MD
Trend, Carolyn Cozine, MD
Yorke, Eric R., MD
Plastic Surgery
Patel, Priti P., MD

Belle Mead
Cardiovascular Disease
McGeady, Rosemary E., MD
Child & Adolescent Psychiatry
Marino, Anthony Jr., MD
Nisar, Asma, MD
Family Medicine
Doctoroff, Ella, DO
Gopalam, Mrunalini, MD
Miller, Janice M., MD
Infectious Disease
Holowinsky, Mary I., MD

Internal Medicine
Levinson, Benjamin, MD
Pecora, Joseph J. III, DO
Wajcberg, Estela, MD
Pediatrics
Evans, Barbara J. Marcelo, MD
Oey, Theresia M., MD
Psychiatry
Dragert, Robert Joseph, DO
Marsh, Claire C., MD
Mehta, Umesh S., MD
Peddu, Vijaya, MD
Saint-Vil, Robert Jr., DO
Szulaczkowski, Wojciech Wadim, MD

Belleville
Adolescent Medicine
Murray-Burton, Carolyn I., MD
Allergy
Morrison, Susan H., MD
Anatomic/Clinical Pathology
De Leon, Essel Marie B., MD
Primavera, James Michael, MD
Anesthesiology
Bada, Laureto Jr., MD
Choi, Bong H., MD
Cizmar, Stephan, MD
Concepcion, Cleo L., MD
De Trespalacios, Jose A., DO
Eisele, Joseph Carl, DO
Gerges, Maged Moussa, MD
Khan, Muhammad B.H., MD
Lao, Jocelyn M., MD
Marcus, Jennifer, MD
Rejowska-Cedrowski, Jolanta, MD
Breast Surgery
Pappas, Nadine C., MD
Cardiovascular Disease
Criscito, Mario A., MD
Saleh, Rany Mokhlis, DO
Dermatology
Eastern, Joseph S., MD
Diagnostic Radiology
Acosta, Robert G., MD
Heimann, James A., MD
Levchook, Christina, MD
Emergency Medicine
Ciccone, Antonio, DO
Dib, Joe Elias, MD
Fontanetta, John Anthony, MD
Futterman, Noah D., DO
Giles, Robert A., MD
Lam, Allison Christine, MD
Law, Stephen W., DO
Nelson, Craig A., MD
Santos, Luis A., MD
Endocrinology
Miller, Michael Joseph, MD
Napoli, John D., MD
Reddy, Rama R., MD
Seth, Amit Kumar, MD
Family Medicine
Cerritelli, John A., MD
Gould, Peter L., MD
Hilderbrand, Rene Francis, DO
Singhal, Pratap C., MD
Gastroenterology
Spira, Etan, MD
General Practice
Shapiro, Jason, MD
Gynecology
Meglio, Robyn S., MD
Hematology
Saleh, Said A., MD
Infectious Disease
Admani, Ariff, MD
Johnson, Edward S., MD
Moaven, Nader, MD
Sidali, Mustafa M., DO
Internal Medicine
Ardolino, Joseph M., MD
Beggs, Donald James, MD
Beresford, Dianne Walker, MD
Christiana, William A., MD
Chun, Kye S., MD
Colon, German R., MD
Conti, John A., MD
D'Aconti, John S., DO
De Franco, Penny E., MD
Dealmeida, Patrick, DO
Eswarapu, Srinivasa, MD
Feehan, Brian Patrick, DO
Fernandes, Jaxon James, MD
Gamss, Jonathan, MD
Gandhi, Senthamara, MD
Gialanella, Craig David, MD
Houng, Mindy S., MD
Johnson, Timothy David, MD
Kaul, Sameer, MD
Klughaupt, Stanley, MD
Kumar, Tarun, MD
Lippman, Alan J., MD
Maresca, Phillip A, MD
Mircea, Cornel, MD
Molinari, Francis T., MD
Orsini, James M., MD
Orsini, James Michael, MD
Pasley, Peter M., MD
Paulo, Jimmy Martins, MD
Reddy, Uma P., MD
Schnurr, Deborah G. P., MD
Silkov, Andrey, MD
Vasireddy, Hemalatha, MD
Yerramalli, Sitamahala M., MD
Interventional Cardiology
Shivashankar, Keshavamurthy, MD
Nephrology
Keshav, Gayithri R., MD
Keshav, Roger, MD
Samsa, Ranka Drazenovic, MD
Neurological Radiology
Lapas, Alkies, DO
Neurology
Deluca, Matthew J., MD
Lomazow, Steven M., MD
Nuclear Medicine
Reich, Helene, MD
Obstetrics & Gynecology
Cicalese, Gerard R., MD
Devalla, Meena, MD
Esiely, Mohamed A., MD
Jain, Ratnam, MD
Lay, Virginia I., MD
Mohammed, Decca, MD
Perez, Walter, MD
Yeum, Sandy H., MD
Occupational Medicine
Danko, Doris Julia, MD
Ophthalmology
Brooks, Nneka Offor, MD
Eichler, Joel D., MD
Landolfi, Joseph M., MD
Landolfi, Michael Joseph, DO
Lister, Mark Anthony, MD
Madreperla, Steven A. Jr., MD
Noorily, Stuart W., MD
Seery, Christopher M., MD
Voleti, Vinod Babu, MD
Orthopedic Surgery
Greifinger, David J., MD
Lee, James M. Sr., MD
Mercurio, Carl F., MD
Otolaryngology
Lester, Arthur I., MD
Pathology
Benedetti, Robert C., MD
Pediatric Ophthalmology
Wagner, Rudolph S., MD
Pediatrics
Cozzini, Nancy, MD
Khatib, Amira, MD
Okoh, Gloria Nkiru, MD
Okorafor, Nnennaya C., MD
Pando, Dalia Aurora, MD
Steinberg, Dale Louise, DO
Wijayaratne, Madhavi, MD
Physical Medicine & Rehab
Almentero, Felix Antonio, MD
Gangemi, Edwin Michael, MD
Gangemi, Frederick D., MD
Hajela, Shailendra, MD
Psychiatry
Ahmad, Raheela, MD
Barness, Michael, MD
Dalgetty, Donna Earnice, MD
Istafanous, Rafik Monir, MD
Walter, Robert J., MD
Radiation Oncology
Blank, Kenneth Robert, MD
Borofsky, Karen Esther, MD
Devereux, Corinne K., MD
Razdan, Dolly, MD
Radiology
Fusco, Joseph M., MD
Minn, Joon Hong, MD
Naiman, Jeffrey Todd, MD
Surgery (General)
Amirata, Edwin A., MD
Bonitz, Joyce A., MD
Brautigan, Robert Anthony, MD
Ruddy, Kathleen T., MD
Urology
Ciccone, Michael Paul, MD
Ciccone, Patrick N., MD
Delgaizo, Anthony, MD

Bellmawr
Family Medicine
Murray, Francis Jr., DO
Internal Medicine
Howe, Joseph H., MD
Santoro, Stephanie Amanda, DO
Williams, Frederick M., MD

Belmar
Allergy
Shah, Tarun J., MD
Dermatology
Morgan, Aaron J., MD
Immunology
Schmidt, John August Jr., MD
Vascular Surgery
Frasco, Franklin J., MD

Belvidere
Family Medicine
Bernard, John V., MD
Fritz, John Patrick, DO

Bergenfield
Anesthesiology
Rechenberg, Geoffrey Mark, MD
Emergency Medicine
Thek, Wesley K., MD
Family Medicine
Palisoc, Roger Louie, DO
Internal Medicine
De Gennaro, Michael A., MD
Desai, Foram R., MD
Diamond, Paul M., MD
Jiu, Wun-Ye, MD
Negron, Luis M., MD
Pereira, Beryl E., MD
Varghese, Mathew, MD
Weisgras, Josef Mordechay, MD
Zeveloff, Susan R., MD
Nephrology
Benson, Payam, MD
Obstetrics & Gynecology
Meier, Ronny, MD
Meier-Ginsberg, Efrat, MD
Ophthalmology
Bauza, Alain Michael, MD
Dello Russo, Jeffrey, MD
Parisi, Frank, MD
Pediatrics
Friedman, Howard Michael, MD
Kaye, Shana Malka, MD
Mathew, Omana R., MD
Tolentino, John G., MD
Weiss, Christopher A., DO
Psychiatry
Baron, Ann R., MD
Niazi, Mohammad Zafar, MD
Stein, Shani, MD
Pulmonary Disease
Liu, Ming Kong, MD

Berkeley
Cardiovascular Disease
Sachs, R. Gregory, MD
Schwartz, Daniel Richard, MD
Diagnostic Radiology
Volvovsky, Alexander, MD
Internal Medicine
Bose, Konika Paul, MD
Kole, Alison S., MD
Parziale, Michael A., MD
Spano-Brennan, Liana Marie, DO
Tuladhar, Swosty, MD
Pediatrics
Gatoulis, Maria K., MD
Lucciola, Pompeo Almerico, MD
Surgery (General)
Bell, Robert Lawrence, MD

Berkeley Heights
Adolescent Medicine
Bender, Michelle Anne, MD
Allergy
Le Benger, Kerry S., MD
Allergy & Immunology
Khedkar, Meera, MD
Anatomic/Clinical Pathology
Qian, Fang, MD
Breast Surgery
Addis, Diana Medina, MD
Polen, Winnie M., DO
Cardiovascular Disease
Beamer, Andrew D., MD
Kothavale, Avinash Annash, MD
Slama, Robert D., MD
Dermatology
Abbasi, Naheed R., MD
Goldfaden, Isabel, MD
Gruber, Gabriel G., MD
Kim, Sam, MD
Nadiminti, Hari, MD
Zirvi, Monib Ahmad, MD
Dermatology: Dermatopathology
Meyers, Lawrence S., MD
Emergency Medicine
Drivas, Antonios, MD
Kennedy, Kevin J., MD
Kothari, Rajesh Suryakant, DO
Lesko, Richard J., MD
Schreck, David M., MD
Singh, Anita J., MD
Endocrinology
Batacchi, Zona Olivia, MD
Rosenbaum, Robert L., MD
Toscano-Zukor, Amy M., DO
Family Medicine
Deitz, Ruth Ellen Thisbe, MD
El Zein, Lama, MD
Leibu, Dora, DO
Lipset, Shani Lauren, MD
Moy, Jamie Tam, DO
Patrone, Nicole, MD
Reedy, Jamie Lynne, MD
Sahulhameed, Fathima, MD
Gastroenterology
Barrison, Adam F., MD
Belladonna, Joseph A., MD
Ben-Menachem, Tamir, MD
Brown, William Howard, MD
Gillin, James Scott, MD
Klein, Roger Scott, MD
Michael, Hazar, MD
General Practice
Ghanbari, Cecilia W., MD
Hematology Oncology
Mills, Lisa Alice, MD
Reeder, Jennifer Gordan, MD
Hospitalist
Banda, Pragati, MD
Desai, Nicky, MD
Mishra, Sneha, MD
Infectious Disease
Karim, Anjum Hasan, MD
Nastro, Lawrence J., MD
Internal Medicine
Abramson, Marla Lyn, MD
Arif, Orooj, MD
Bass, Jon Lawrence, MD
Bauman, Jeffrey Michael, MD
Berardi, Richard Jr., DO
Boni, Christopher M., DO
Cajulis, Michelle C., MD
Camacho, Ricardo Miguel, MD
Cheung, Deborah Jee Hae, MD
Cirangle, Lori Beth, MD
Colucio, Peter M., MD
Dokko, John Hoon, DO
Feinberg, Craig Harlan, MD
Goldman-Gorelov, Victoria, MD
Harjani, Vashdeo Daulat, MD
Jeereddy, Bhavani, MD
Kapur, Sakshi, MD
Laudadio, Richard Dominick, MD
Mandal, Soma, MD
Mendiola, Redentor S. Jr., MD
Meyer, Jacqueline Marie, MD
Mirchandani, Sunil, MD
Parikh, Ashish Dharnidhar, MD
Pettee, Brett, MD
Philips-Rodriguez, Dahlia, MD

Physicians by Town and Medical Specialty

Berkeley Heights (cont)
Internal Medicine
Pilot, Richard, MD
Roth, Douglas M., DO
Salomon, Pierre Richard, MD
Shridharani, Kanan Vasant, MD
Skrelja, Valerie, MD
Soto, Haydee M., MD
Terry, Alon, MD
Tu, Chun, MD
Vecchi, Anthony R., MD
Waqar, Anum Khan, DO
Wax, Michael B., MD
Weisfuse, Judith E., MD
Interventional Cardiology
Juliano, Nickolas Daniel, MD
Nephrology
Lunenfeld, Ellen Beth, MD
Neurological Surgery
Beyerl, Brian David, MD
Neurology
Cohen, Eric R., DO
Coohill, Lisa Marie, MD
Naik, Komal Desai, DO
Turner, Garth M., MD
Obstetrics & Gynecology
Forrester, Dara Lynn, MD
Masterson, Christine, MD
Oncological Surgery
Cunningham, John David, MD
Gumbs, Andrew Alexander, MD
Ophthalmology
Bazargan Lari, Hamed, MD
Gurwin, Eric B., MD
Hsueh, Linda, MD
Khalil, Monica B., MD
Shah, Vinnie Pooja, MD
Orthopedic Surgery
Garberina, Matthew J., MD
Mirsky, Eric Charles, MD
Patel, Samir Popatlal, MD
Orthopedics
Corona, Joseph T., MD
Otolaryngology
Burstein, David Harris, MD
Eden, Avrim Reuben, MD
Gnoy, Alexander Roman, MD
Gurey, Lowell Evan, MD
Kwartler, Jed A., MD
Le Benger, Jeffrey D., MD
Otology
Cooper, David M., MD
Pediatric Anesthesia
Bilenker, Michael Evan, DO
Pediatric Cardiology
Liao, Pui-Kan, MD
Pediatrics
Dardanello, Marnie Cambria, MD
Hermann, Daniel Eric, MD
Kemeny, Alexa C., MD
Kornfeld, Howard Neil, MD
Lupski, Donna L., MD
Mehta, Ami A., MD
Mehta, Shiva C., MD
Miguelino, Ida Alfad, MD
Palermo, Angelo David, MD
Summa, Geraldine M., MD
Tavel, Stacey C., MD
Thomas, Alan E., MD
Physical Med & Rehab-Pain Med
Freed, Brian, DO
Physical Medicine & Rehab
Atalla, Sara N., DO
Khademi, Allen Mansour, MD
Oza, Rohit Madhukar, MD
Plastic & Reconstructive Srgy
Joseph, Jain, MD
Plastic Surgery
Hyans, Peter, MD
Momeni, Reza, MD
Psychiatry
Huang, Bei Barbara, MD
Pulmonary Disease
Wilt, Jessie Swain, MD
Radiation Oncology
Gabel, Molly Mary, MD
Radiology
Berman, Erika Jacobs, MD
Dodge, Sarah Ann, MD
Lacz, Nicole Lynn, MD
McCormick, John Stuart, MD
Rheumatology
Flowers, Shari Carla, MD
Kennish, Lauren M., MD
Lee, Linda K., MD
Lieberman, Eric Steven, MD
Spinal Surgery
Kupershtein, Ilya, MD
Surgery (General)
Porbunderwala, Steven James, MD
Thumar, Adeep Bhaguanji, MD
Thoracic Surgery
Lozner, Jerrold S., MD
Urology
Blitstein, Jeffrey, MD
Siegal, John D., MD
Volpe, Michael Anthony, MD
Vascular Surgery
Nitzberg, Richard S., MD

Berlin
Family Medicine
Costa, Richard C., DO
Galezniak, John, DO
Gigliotti, David T., DO
Hassman, David R., DO
Hassman, Joseph M., DO
Hassman, Michael A., DO
La Ratta, John A., DO
Maressa, Julian M., DO
Mauriello, Richard M., DO
General Practice
Vera, Luis Fernando, MD
Internal Medicine
Chugh, Rajinder P., MD
Parikh, Pratima D., MD
Occupational Medicine
Leonetti, Joyce D., DO
Ophthalmology
Dorfman, Neil H., MD
Other Specialty
Nigro, Mary A., MD
Pediatrics
Wu, Shiann J., MD
Psychiatry
Ahmed, Aisha I., MD
Hossain, Shawn Isteak, DO

Bernardsville
Adolescent Medicine
Visci, John J., MD
Family Medicine
Kaftal, Sergiusz I., MD
General Practice
Sinatra, Frank A., MD
Internal Medicine
Costea-Misthos, Maria A., MD
Dixon, Rosina B., MD
Robertson, Janet A., MD
Zimmerman, Thomas Jr., MD
Obstetrics & Gynecology
Mehta, Jyotsna S., MD
Pediatrics
Ganek, Ellen Beth, MD
Nikodijevic, Vesna, MD
Peng, Patricia E., DO
Rose, Elizabeth, MD
Psychiatry
Lieb, Robert C., MD
Meiselas, Karen D., MD
Robertson-Hoffmann, Doreen E., MD

Beverly
Family Medicine
Dow, William A., MD

Blackwood
Anesthesiology
Sabia, Michael, MD
Family Medicine
Adewunmi, Kafilat, DO
Fisicaro, Tamara Marie, MD
Gecys, Gintare T., DO
Horvath Matthews, Jessica E., MD
Mahamitra, Nirandra, MD
Robertson, John F. Jr., MD
Sarmiento, Samuel I., MD
Treiman, Arthur M., MD
General Practice
Banks, Frank M., DO
Internal Medicine
Deshields, Michael S., MD
Doshi, Ila H., MD
Frisoni, Lorenza, MD
Jain, Sneh, MD
Jehangir, Waqas, MD
Obstetrics & Gynecology
Croff, William J., DO
Delvadia, Dipak R., DO
Montgomery, Owen Canterbury, MD
Ophthalmology
Linares, Hugo Manuel, DO
Other Specialty
Corson-Diaz, Cathy Lynn, MD
Diaz Jimenez, Jose Eduardo, MD
Pediatrics
Del Giorno, Joseph John, MD
Delgiorno, John Michael, MD
George, Cyriac, DO
Iacobucci, Audrey J., MD
Mercedes Salas, Aixell J., MD
Owens, Brittany Rose, MD
Robiou, Natalie Genoveva, MD
Salvati, Harold Vincent, MD
Physical Medicine & Rehab
Siu, Gilbert, DO
Psychiatry
Ashraf, Mohammad, MD
Aslam, Masood, MD
Bolarinwa, Isiaka A., MD
Wayslow, Alfred J., DO

Blairstown
Dermatology
Rocca, Nicole M., MD
Physical Medicine & Rehab
Woodward, Shelly W., MD

Bloomfield
Anatomic/Clinical Pathology
Borbon-Reyes, Araceli O., MD
Cardiovascular Disease
Horowitz, Michael S., MD
Lapa, Alan S., MD
Mahdi, Lawrence F., MD
McCoach, Kevin J., MD
Shao, John Han, MD
Emergency Medicine
Reyes, Prudencio C., MD
Endocrinology
Dorcely, Brenda, MD
Family Medicine
Basista, Michael P., MD
Bhatia, Hemlata, MD
Garcia Marotta, Ylonka, MD
Hyatt, Gayon Marie, MD
Kerlegrand, Pascale, MD
Mikulski, Wanda J., MD
Russ Meek, Robyn L., DO
Schuyler, Andrew P., MD
Gastroenterology
Bajwa, Mohammad Ayub, MD
Celebre, Louis J., MD
Devito, Fiore J., MD
Pizzano, Richard G., MD
Infectious Disease
Pierre-Louis, Frantz Junior, MD
Soroko, Theresa A., MD
Internal Medicine
Abdelshahid, Mounir Y., MD
Barbier, Andrea, DO
Bhalodia, Manish V., MD
De Juliis, Aurora, MD
Kelly, John V. Jr., MD
Narvaez, Normita G., MD
Petracca, Louis J., MD
Podkul, Richard L., MD
Porcaro, Sabina M., MD
Rana, Nareshkumar G., MD
Saraiya, Nimit Nitin, MD
Shah, Neil J., MD
Shah, Shrenik G., MD
MOHS Micrographic Skin Cancer
Paghdal, Kapila V., MD
Nephrology
Coyle, Raluca, MD
Neurology
Nayak, Bharathi, MD
Nazareth, Joseph M., MD
Obstetrics & Gynecology
Kusnierz, Earl I., DO
Yacoub, Mounzer H., MD
Ophthalmology
D'Amato, Anthony P., MD
Ditkoff, Jonathan W., MD
Glatt, Herbert L., MD
Gould, Joshua Mark, DO
Jackson, Kurt T., MD
Kallina, Lauren A., MD
Kumar, Radhika Lingam, MD
Pediatric Infectious Diseases
Cooper, Roger W. Jr., MD
Pediatrics
Cheng, Guo-Pao, MD
Colyer-Aversa, Lori A., MD
Flynn, Sean A., MD
Kastner, Theodore A., MD
Kellum, Sandra, MD
Mehta, Ruchi, MD
Mendez Morales, Alba Nydia, MD
Shah, Madhavi, MD
Turizo, Maria Cecilia, MD
Yerovi, Maria D., MD
Psychiatry
Guanci, Nicole Alexis, MD
Mushtaq, Sabina, MD
Radiation Oncology
Kagan, Eduard, MD
Rheumatology
Simon, Jonathan M., MD
Surgery (General)
Colavita, Donato A., MD
Narvaez, Guillermo Jr., MD
Urology
Caruso, Robert Peter, MD
Franzoni, David Fred, MD
Hsieh, Kuang-Yiao, MD
Lombardo, Salvatore Antonio, MD
Wu, David Sweghsien, MD

Bloomingdale
Internal Medicine
Jaaj, Hedoneia C., MD

Bloomsbury
Geriatric Psychiatry
Caruso, Edward Francis, MD

Bogota
Obstetrics & Gynecology
Kuye, Olabisi O., MD

Boonton
Addiction Psychiatry
Bajwa, Ghulam Murtaza, MD
Nagel, Isaac R., MD
Anesthesiology
Caruthers, Samuel Grenville, MD
Anesthesiology: Pain Medicine
Mendez, Jorge G., MD
Child & Adolescent Psychiatry
Mahmood, Fauzia, MD
Family Medicine
Robleza, Rolando M., MD
General Practice
Santos, Santos S., MD
Internal Medicine
Hammerman, Louis, MD
Moya-Mendez, Robert F., MD
Renz, Patricia M., MD
Scaduto, Philip M., MD
Obstetrics & Gynecology
Dibenedetto, Robert J., MD
Ophthalmology
Ahmad, Arlene, MD
Psychiatry
Ilardi, Jeffrey Michael, MD
Jalan, Suman L., MD
Massler, Dennis J., MD
Shah, Jay Pravinkumar, MD

Bordentown
Anatomic/Clinical Pathology
Deluzio, Antonio John, DO
Diagnostic Radiology
Daniels, Richard John, MD
Family Med-Sports Medicine
Konakondla, Krishna, MD
Family Medicine
Breig, Jason Anthony, MD
Carty, Robert W., MD
Chen, Timothy, MD
Devers, Paul Dix, MD
Flynn, Jamie, DO
Garbarini Carty, Elyse, MD
Hughes, Janey Ballin, DO
Jimma, Lulu A., MD
Lugo, Maria D., MD
Mleczko, Joshua, DO
Van Patten, Yancy L., DO
VanHise, Tara Hungspruke, DO

Vizzoni,Hiedi Taylor,MD
General Practice
Addis,David J.,MD
Internal Medicine
Chokshi,Seema Patel,MD
Frascella,Rosemary C.,MD
Mahmud,Hamid,MD
Potharlanka,Prathibha R.,MD
Rossos,Nicholas A.,MD
Ophthalmology
Caci,Jerry A.,MD
Orthopedic Surgery
Farrell,Joseph E.,DO
Gray,John Michael,MD
Jain,Rajesh K.,MD
Ropiak,Raymond Russell,MD
Scholfet,Scott D.,MD
Pediatrics
Mossoczy-Godyn,Anna M.,MD
Physical Medicine & Rehab
Karam,Christopher S.,MD
Rizkalla,Michael H.,MD
Urology
Asroff,Scott Wayne,MD
Goldlust,Robert W.,MD
Perzin,Adam Dean,MD

Bound Brook
Child & Adolescent Psychiatry
Ismail,Mona S. A.,MD
Family Medicine
Goldman,Frieda Shepsel,MD
Pizzelanti,Donna M.,DO
Internal Medicine
Byra,William M.,MD
Ehrlich,Harold B.,MD
Orthopedic Surgery
Schneider,Stephen,MD
Pediatrics
Jalil,Kiran,MD
Wong Duran,Elizabeth,MD
Psychiatry
Borton,Miriam A.,MD
Cortez,Jacqueline M.,MD
Friedman,Ella,MD

Bradley Beach
General Practice
Lee,Frank,MD

Branchburg
Allergy & Immunology
Fox,James A.,MD
Cardiovascular Disease
Saulino,Patrick F.,MD
Critical Care Medicine
Arno,Louis J.,MD
Dermatology
Fox,Alissa B.,MD
Emergency Medicine
Goldberg,Lon E.,DO
Family Medicine
Donetz,Pamela Suzanne,MD
Gujjula,Prashanthi,MD
Shaffrey,Thomas Andrew,MD
Zeh,Catherine A.,MD
Internal Medicine
Rego,Ramon,MD
Obstetrics & Gynecology
Andrin,Margaret,MD
Horowitz,Alyssa G.,MD
Ophthalmology
Nagelberg,Henry P.,MD
Pediatrics
Housam,Ryan Ann,MD
Ricks,Sandy,MD

Branchville
Family Medicine
Luszcz,Ronald J.,DO
Saradarian,Kathleen A.,MD
Internal Medicine
De Paola,Anthony A.,DO
Orthopedic Surgery
Lohwin,Peter G.,MD

Brick
Adolescent Medicine
Condren,Eileen,DO
Allergy
De Cotiis,Bruce A.,MD
Tumaliuan,Janet Ang,MD
Anatomic/Clinical Pathology
Baron-Gabriel,Icynth M.,MD

Coletta,Umberto,MD
Krumerman,Martin Saul,MD
Rangwala,Anis F.,MD
Anesthesiology
Barone,Frank Anthony,MD
Bean,David E.,MD
Gantner,Mark,MD
Higgins,James Martin,MD
Jasper,Gabriele P.,MD
Mangonon,Virgilio D.,MD
Reid,Kenneth M.,MD
Shah,Kalpana N.,MD
Singh,Manjula,MD
Swinger,Alan Bennett,DO
Zhou,Lingbin,MD
Breast Surgery
Lygas,Theodore B.,MD
Pellegrino,John M.,MD
Cardiovascular Disease
Ahmad,Tanveer,MD
Apolito,Renato A.,MD
Cohen,Todd S.,DO
Komorowski,Thomas W.,MD
Mehra,Aditya Chand,MD
Moosvi,Ali R.,MD
Patel,Harshil,MD
Patel,Virendra,MD
Paul Kate,Vasant,MD
Pinnelas,David J.,MD
Raza,Muhammad Rehan,MD
Vijayakumar,Chellappan,MD
White,Thomas M.,DO
Colon & Rectal Surgery
Park,Jane,MD
Critical Care Medicine
Newman,Stephen L.,MD
Dermatology
Abel,Mark,MD
Diagnostic Radiology
Alcasid,Lino M.,MD
Cardo,Amelia J.,MD
Dillon,Richard Lansing,MD
Jain,Chandru U.,MD
Kaplan,Sheldon B.,MD
Karmel,Mitchell I.,MD
Emergency Medicine
Abe,Minako,MD
Darocki,Mark,MD
Gronsky,Rudolph Edward,DO
Haroun,Sandra,MD
Kathuria,Richa,MD
Kaufer,Michael Jason,MD
Maniar,Gina S.,DO
Noris,Gary L.,MD
Pollack,Martin I.,MD
Sarenac,Alexander,MD
Schlogl,Jeffrey G.,MD
Singh,Arun J.,DO
Family Med-Sports Medicine
Sargent,Thomas G. Jr,DO
Family Medicine
Alcasid,Ninfa A.,MD
Carolan,Owen J.,MD
Cascarina,Michael A.,MD
Eapen,Prema Mary,MD
Fung,Kent C.,MD
Konigsberg,David,DO
Kronhaus,Kenneth E.,MD
Navarro,Mark Anthony,MD
Riss,Martin,DO
Tesoriero,Laura M.,MD
Ussery-Kronhaus,Kelly G.,MD
Veder,Liana,MD
Wilson,Francis P.,DO
Foot & Ankle Surgery
Wolenski,Matthew J.,MD
Forensic Psychiatry
Baum,Raymond M.,MD
Gastroenterology
Aaron,Bernard M.,MD
Boss,David T.,MD
Cerefice,Mark L.,MD
Hiley,Paul C.,MD
Rozovsky,Assif,MD
Schlachter,Scott M.,DO
Shukla,Sandhya,MD
Tangorra,Matthew,DO
Winzelberg,Neal J.,MD
General Practice
Reisher,Richard G.,DO

Geriatrics
Boyan,William P.,MD
Hand Surgery
Pecoraro,Michael J.,MD
Hematology
Amin,Girish S.,MD
Hospitalist
Botu,Devi Prasad,MD
Infectious Disease
Ruszka,Geza,MD
Internal Medicine
Abbas,Shahida M.,MD
Abidi,Mutahir Ali,MD
Afiniwala,Swara,MD
Allen,Luzmary,DO
Babayev,Lily L.,MD
Bautista-Seares,Jessica M.,MD
Chiu,Kenny,MD
DeDona,Anna,DO
DeVita,Michael G.,DO
Donkor,Lawrence Tawiah,MD
Edelman,Carrie Allysia,MD
Georgy,Mary Sarah,MD
Gross,Tiberiu A.,MD
Gudapati,Raghu,MD
Hansalia,Riple Jayamtilal,MD
Hasan,Bassam I.,MD
Heacock,James K.,MD
Ilkhanizadeh,Ladan,MD
Infantolino,John A.,MD
Ital,Rosa,MD
Jain,Vishal K.,MD
Jarahian,George Jr.,MD
Karam,Edmund Thomas,MD
Kaur,Sundip,MD
Kianfar,Hormoz,MD
Lichnowski,Krzysztof B.,MD
Loman,Jeannette A.,DO
Lopez,John Pedro Francisco,MD
Magahis,Pacifico Aguila Jr.,MD
Montgomery,Karyn Mae,MD
Muralidharan,Soundari,MD
Musico,John J.,MD
Parikh,Sandip K.,MD
Patel,Hitesh Babubhai,MD
Rothberg,Michael Steven,MD
Rothman,Michael E.,MD
Salloum,Ahmad,MD
Sastri,Bhagyalak L.,MD
Seares,Petronilo Jr.,MD
Sher,Michael Laurence,MD
Singal,Presh,MD
Sy,Pacita C.,MD
Tapliga,Eduard Constantin,MD
Vida,Jay A.,DO
Weiner,Leonard D.,MD
Wolfman,Brian P.,MD
Yakubov,Boris,MD
Interventional Cardiology
Escandon,Pedro J.,MD
Medical Genetics
Pavlak-Schenk,Jayne A.,DO
Medical Oncology
Agrawal,Apurv,MD
Nephrology
Albanese,Joseph J.,DO
Brouder,Daniel J.,MD
Bruno,Robert,DO
DePalma,John Anthony,DO
Dounis,Harry James,DO
Ellis,Stephen J.,MD
Haider,Nadeem Z.,MD
Iglesias,Jose Ignacio,DO
Jain,Keshani,MD
Kapoor,Rajat,DO
Loman,Eric,DO
Markatos,Angelo,DO
Meyer,Ariel,DO
Park,Jin S.,MD
Schirripa,Joseph V.,MD
Tomasco,Thomas Joseph,MD
Neurological Radiology
Jain Lakhani,Neelu,MD
Neurology
Barcas,Peter P.,DO
Escandon,Sandra L.,MD
Miskin,Pandurang R.,MD
Sedarous,Mary,MD
Obstetrics & Gynecology
Benecki,Theresa R.,MD
Ketelaar,Pieter J.,MD

Morgan,Darlene M.,MD
Pagano,Ann Marie,MD
Patel,Vanita Hitesh,MD
Vetter,Paul L.,MD
Ophthalmology
Mack,Prinze Chan,MD
Schlisserman,David A.,MD
Orthopedic Surgery
Bogdan,Joseph P.,MD
Hebela,Nader M.,MD
Katt,Brian Matthew,MD
Law,William A.,MD
Marsicano,Joseph G.,MD
Nitche,Jason Adam,MD
Rodricks,David Josef,MD
Zaleski,Theodore G.,MD
Orthopedic-Hand Surgery
Malfitano,Laura Anne,DO
Otolaryngology
Brandeisky,Thomas E.,DO
Landsman,Howard Scott,DO
Pediatric Cardiology
Alpert,Mitchel B.,MD
Castro,Elsa Imelda,MD
Umali Pamintuan,Maria Angela,MD
Zales,Vincent R.,MD
Pediatric Pulmonology
Zamel,Yaacov B.,MD
Pediatrics
Almazan,Gerald C.,MD
Caputo,Enza P.,MD
Charles,Diane Isaacson,MD
Chin,Stephanie Elaine,MD
Collado,Maria R.,MD
Gallardo,Mary Rose Ramos,MD
Katsoulis-Emnace,Maria G.,MD
Kraynock,John,MD
Lapidus,Daniel Yitzchok,MD
Mate,Shrikrishn K.,MD
Piela,Christina,MD
Pineda,Maria Georgina C.,MD
Rolenc,Holly J.,MD
Sandeep,Rashmi,MD
Sheth,Manoj Indubhai,MD
Sundaram,Uma,MD
Youssef,Caroline,MD
Physical Medicine & Rehab
Barshikar,Surendra S.,MD
Chen,Suann S.,MD
Esquieres,Raymond Edel,MD
Freeman,Ted Lawrence,DO
Kanarek,Samantha Leigh,DO
Luciano,Lisa A.,DO
Scheick,Jennifer Theresa,MD
Schoenlank,Casey R.,MD
Psychiatry
Bhashyam,Vinod Rao,MD
Clark,Kristen S.,MD
Patel,Satishkumar H.,MD
Rajput,Zulfiqar A.,MD
Pulmonary Critical Care
Alcasid,Patrick J.,MD
Pulmonary Disease
Kamel,Emad R.,MD
Kerr,Brian S.,MD
Wynkoop,Walter Alan,MD
Radiation Oncology
Kaufman,Nathan,MD
Miller,Douglas Andrew,MD
Radiology
Connors,Diane,MD
Feeney,Charlee Wallis,DO
Koven,Marshall B.,MD
Shomo,Marcia Rosenberg,MD
Sports Medicine
Stamos,Bruce Dumont,MD
Surgery (General)
Aquino,Rainier,MD
Becker,Stephen A.,MD
Bhandari,Tarun,MD
Cappadona,Charles Richard,MD
Cluley,Scott R.,MD
Houlis,Nicholas J.,DO
Huang,Kevin,MD
Kamath,Ashwin S.,MD
Kelly,Francis J.,MD
Kwon,Sung Wook,MD
Milazzo,Vincent J.,MD
Pahuja,Anil K.,MD
Priolo,Steven R.,MD
Tammaro,Yolanda Rose,MD

Physicians by Town and Medical Specialty

Brick (cont)
Surgery (General)
Yrad, Jonathan Proces Flores, MD
Zurkovsky, Eugene, MD
Urology
Burzon, Daniel Todd, MD
Chapman, John Robert, MD
Fam, Mina, MD
Kim, Chong M., MD
Linn, Gary C., MD
Mendoza, Pierre J., MD
Simon, Andrew L., MD
Vascular & Intrvntnal Radiology
Skrzypczak, Jan L., MD
Vascular Surgery
Chu, Tun S., MD
Jain, Vikalp, MD
Kaufman, Jarrod Peter, MD
Sharp, Frank J. III, MD

Bridgeport
Emergency Medicine
Harris, Brian E., MD
General Practice
Zaharko, Wendy, MD

Bridgeton
Cardiovascular Disease
Baptist, Gladwyn D., MD
Dermatology
Fenichel, Stefan, MD
Family Medicine
Ballas, Christopher Thomas, MD
Bear, John G., MD
Bear, Michelle H., DO
Copare, Fiore J., MD
De Biaso, Tracy A., MD
Kohler, Frank R., DO
LaCavera, Joseph A. III, DO
Manske, Daniel D., MD
Ordille, Joseph D., DO
Oswald, Mark Anthony, MD
Patitucci, Robert S., MD
Riley-Lowe, Judith E., DO
Roomi, Farah, MD
Talbot, Lori C., MD
Tugman, Catherine K., MD
Hospitalist
Pham, Peter H., DO
Internal Medicine
Ahmed, Ilyas, MD
Bagan, Stanley L., MD
Candelore, Joseph Timothy Jr., DO
Hanna, Ekram Labeb, MD
Hatzantonis, John Emanuel, MD
Hoey, Stephen E., DO
Ismail, Elham Mohamed, MD
Jimenez-Silva, Jeanette, MD
Shields, Jack M., MD
Struby, Christopher, DO
Nephrology
De Priori, Elis Maria, MD
Neurology
Rampal, Sharan, MD
Orthopedic Surgery
Levitsky, Mark K., MD
Otolaryngology
Lorenc, Ronald B., MD
Pediatrics
De Leonardis, John A., MD
Fleischer, Gilbert E., MD
Harris, Jazmine A., MD
Kim, Joh W., MD
Nair, Prabha J., MD
Patel, Bhavna K., MD
Tanner, Fritzi Alma, MD
Psychiatry
Friel, David M., MD
Musser, Erica Lynn, DO
Shang, Xiaozhou, MD
Tamburello, Anthony C. III, MD
Vyas, Rajiv Krishnakant, MD
Surgery (General)
Haq, Imran Ul, MD
Iqbal, Nauveed, MD
Urology
Diaz, Jose F., MD
Vascular Surgery
Khan, Aftab A., MD

Bridgewater
Allergy & Immunology
Camacho-Halili, Marie M., MD

Cardiovascular Disease
Ahn, Joe Kyuhyun, MD
Cheng, Chao T., MD
Cheng, Shiow-Jane L., MD
Chew, Paul H., MD
Friedman, Glenn T., MD
Georgeson, Steven E., MD
Hall, Jason O., MD
Ivanov, Alexander, MD
Kulkarni, Rachana A., MD
Lebenthal, Mark J., MD
Leeds, Richard S., MD
Mahal, Sharan S., MD
Ocken, Stephen M., MD
Patel, Alpesh Amrit, MD
Rachofsky, Edward Lawrence, MD
Sengupta, Ranjita, MD
Shahi, Chandreshwar N., MD
Child & Adolescent Psychiatry
Hagino, Owen Rinzo, MD
Clinical Cardiac Elctrphyslgy
Frenkel, Daniel, MD
Patel, Ashok Ambalal, MD
Clinical Neurophysiology
Potluri, Srinivasa Rao, MD
Colon & Rectal Surgery
Sadler, Daniel L., MD
Critical Care Medicine
Lee, Jack C., MD
Soriano, Aida N., MD
Dermatology
Agarwal, Smita, MD
Mulvihill, Claire A., MD
Endocrinology
Agrin, Richard Joel, MD
Aurand, Lisa Ann, MD
Family Medicine
Boguslavsky, David, MD
Del Valle, Mario James, DO
Gora, Jill Suzanne, MD
Gubbi, Smitha Ayodhyarama, MD
Hamilton, Kathryn Diane, MD
Klein, Martin Edward, MD
Kripsak, John P., DO
Lupoli, Kristin Anne, MD
Mannancheril, Anita, MD
Medrano, Christina Marie, MD
Mitterando, Jeanne G., MD
Ouano, Estelita C., MD
Tobias, David A., MD
Gastroenterology
Lustig, Robert H., DO
Shapiro, Stephen R., MD
Unger, Jeffrey S., MD
Internal Medicine
Garcia, Calixto G., DO
Irakam, Surya Prakash, MD
Khan, Amber Manzoor, MD
Mehta, Nehal L., MD
Mehta, Sudhir H., MD
Patel, Parag Bhailal, MD
Puskuri, Praneetha, MD
Qu, Peimei, MD
Sondhi, Manu, MD
Sun, Karen Hong Xue, MD
Sun, Lu Amy, MD
Trivedi, Shivang M., MD
Wiesen, Robert S., MD
Yalamanchi, Geeta, MD
Neonatal-Perinatal Medicine
Zarzuela, Arminia T., MD
Nephrology
Daskalakis, Nikki, MD
Noor, Fazle Ali, MD
Patel, Manisha Saurabh, MD
Neurological Surgery
Chimenti, James M., MD
More, Jay, MD
Neurology
Reznik, Andrea I., MD
Wittenborn, John Richard, MD
Obstetrics & Gynecology
Bernstein, Sambra H., MD
Errico, Carmine P., MD
Mileto, Vincent F., MD
Miranda, Matilda, MD
Oza, Palak, MD
Woltz, Ayanna Rashea, MD
Ophthalmology
Faigenbaum, Steven J., MD
Moshel, Caroline Rosenberg, MD

Phillips, Paul Mathew, MD
Salz, Alan G., MD
Salz, David Andrew, MD
Orthopedic Surgery
Bhandutia, Amit Ketan, MD
Hiramoto, Harlan E., MD
Nordstrom, Thomas J., MD
Parolie, James M., MD
Vessa, Paul P., MD
Other Specialty
Choi, Mingi, MD
Otolaryngology
Fenster, Gerald F., MD
Hekiert, Adrianna Maria, MD
Lazar, Amy D., MD
Schneiderman, Todd Aron, MD
Otolaryngology-Facial Plastic
Abraham, Mena, DO
Burachinsky, Dennis Andrew, DO
Pediatric Pulmonology
Teper, Ariel Abel, MD
Pediatrics
Abraham, Daniel J., MD
Calimlim, Grace T., MD
Chennapragada, Ravi S., MD
Dionne-McCracken, Laura, MD
Ferrante, Robyn, MD
Jain, Ami J., MD
Jessel, Nele, MD
Needleman, Jack, MD
Noviello, Stephanie Seshagiri, MD
Piezas, Sylvia M., MD
Senator, Laura Julie, MD
Physical Medicine & Rehab
Kanuri, Kavitha, MD
Patel, Pankaj Ambalal, MD
Rustagi, Anju, MD
Tai, Qing, MD
Plastic Surgery
Najmi, Jamsheed K., MD
Psychiatry
Antohina, Alena, MD
Goldfine, Yvette Bernice, MD
Mehta, Rashmi N., MD
Obleada, Clarita N., MD
Odunlami, Henry Bandele, MD
Zhang, Hailing, MD
Pulmonary Critical Care
Patel, Prashant B., MD
Pulmonary Disease
Poiani, George J., MD
Rheumatology
Abdel-Megid, Ahmed Mahmoud, MD
Sports Medicine
Tucker, Kimberly Victoria, MD
Surgery (General)
Lue, Deborah A., MD

Brielle
Infectious Disease
Kleinfeld, David I., MD

Brigantine
Family Medicine
McAdam, Kimberly S., DO
Internal Medicine
Chaikin, Harry L., MD
Dunn, Michael Joseph, MD
Gabros, David E., MD
Glasser, Barry D., MD
Rubin, Eric Howard, MD
Ophthalmology
Di Marco, Eugene M., DO
Psychiatry
Piotrowski, Linda S., MD

Browns Mills
Anatomic/Clinical Pathology
Schloo, Betsy L., MD
Anesthesiology
Dateshidze, Konstantin, MD
Guarini, Vincent, MD
Khawaja, Hasan Sajjad, MD
Moore, Roger A., MD
Neary, Michael J., MD
Cardiovascular Disease
Altimore, David, MD
Amico, Frank Joseph Jr., DO
Buchanan, David J., DO
Bullock Palmer, Renee Patrice, MD
Corbisiero, Raffaele, MD
Evans, Matthew, DO
Ferlise, Kathleen M., MD

Fish, Frank H., MD
Garabedian, J. Andre, DO
McNamara, John Patrick, DO
Mogtader, Allen, MD
Moshiyakhov, Mark, MD
Ng, Tommy K., MD
Reese, Jason, DO
Sanghvi, Kintur Arvindbhai, MD
Sprankle, Steven Michael, DO
Sumathisena, Sena, MD
Waggoner, Thomas E. I, DO
Cardiovascular Surgery
Boris, Walter J., DO
Cane, Michael Elliot, MD
McGrath, Lynn B., MD
Sodhi, Jitendra, MD
Critical Care Medicine
Wargovich, Raymond M., MD
Emergency Medicine
Ganguly, Tarun, DO
Family Medicine
Miller, Robin Jeanne, MD
Shapiro, Paul, DO
Willoughby, Ronald P., DO
Hospitalist
Poulathas, Alexander S., DO
Infectious Disease
Aboujaoude, Rania Nassif, MD
Smialowicz, Chester R., MD
Internal Medicine
Christian, Sangita-Ann Justin, MD
Godfrey, John Trevor, DO
Huynh, Nha T., DO
Lumia, Francis J., MD
Maletzky, David Michael, DO
Martin, Andrew A., MD
Murphy, David M., MD
Nachodsky, Denise Marie, MD
Perry, Michael David, DO
Piawa, Dum Livinus, DO
Razvi, Batool, MD
Smith, Simon N., DO
Summers, Michael Edward, DO
Wjasow, Christina, MD
Zazzali, Kathleen Mary, DO
Zinda, Ashley Beth, DO
Nuclear Cardiology
Van Hise, Aaron C., DO
Pulmonary Disease
Brar, Navdeep K., MD
Cajulis, Marivi Ora, MD
Surgery (General)
Burns, Paul Gerard, MD
Nicolato, Patricia A., DO
Thoracic Surgery
Ross, Ronald E., MD
Vascular Surgery
Chang, Kane L., MD
Kamath, Vijay, MD
Palkar, Vikram, DO

Budd Lake
Family Medicine
Hoey, Kathleen Marie, MD
Leggiero, Nicholas J., DO
Seshadri, Mahalakshmi, MD
Sher, Peter Mitchell, MD
Internal Medicine
Brett, Brian P., MD

Burlington
Emergency Medicine-Sports Med
Shaffer, Jaclyn, MD
Family Medicine
Cumarasamy, Thayalan K., MD
Cynn, Jhin J., MD
Griffin, Amanda, MD
Maharaj-Mikiel, Indira C., MD
Moront, Barbara Jeanne, MD
Nemeth, Laurie Yallowitz, DO
Rozenberg, Larisa, MD
Sacks, Robert J., DO
Strazzeri, Mia Domenica, DO
Varkey, Ciby B., MD
General Practice
Blank, Andrew Jay, DO
Brandt-Park, Nicole, MD
Talone, Albert A., DO
Torres, Florinda L., MD
Internal Medicine
Aliferova, Tatyana N., MD
Butt, Saeed Ahmed, MD

Dorfner,Scott M.,DO
Jordan,Daniel Robert,MD
Kamra,Roopama,MD
Obstetrics
Steinberg,Frederic,DO
Obstetrics & Gynecology
Mitchell-Williams,Jocelyn,MD
Salvatore,Michelle Lyn,MD
Siefring,Robert P.,MD
Pediatrics
Arnaud-Turner,Denise Marie,MD
Berg,Jodi Liebman,MD
Bonett,Deirdre Maria,MD
Gould,Carolyn L.,MD
Harbist,Noel Rebecca,MD
Hickey,John Selano Jr.,MD
Horten,James,MD
Martinez,Esther G.,MD
Niedzwiecki,Stephen Mark,MD
Vidal-Phelan,Johanna Maria,MD
Pulmonary Disease
Mest,Stuart,MD

Burlington City
Family Medicine
D'Guerra,Mignon Marie,MD
Reid,Gillian Salanda,MD
Internal Medicine
Sewell,Myron L.,MD
Pediatrics
Aiello,Kathleen Kuykendall,MD
Graham,April Danielle,DO

Burlington Township
Family Medicine
Patel,Manish Arvind,DO
Orthopedic Surgery
Eakin,David Eugene,DO
McMillan,Sean,DO

Butler
Endocrinology
Covello,Lucy F.,MD
Family Medicine
Kielar,Francis,MD
Infectious Disease
Abdul Shafi,Samya B.,MD
Internal Medicine
Hawruk,Elizabeth A.,MD
Parikh,Dhinoj M.,MD
Pediatrics
Blecherman,Sarah W.,MD
Horowitz,Deborah L.,MD
Liu,Michael,MD
Thomas,Susheela,MD
Vacca,Michael John,MD
Weinstein,David M.,MD

Caldwell
Child & Adolescent Psychiatry
Cammarata,Sandra,MD
Emergency Medicine
Izakov,Natalya B.,DO
Family Medicine
Aquilio,Ernest J.,DO
Hauter,Moneef S.,MD
Mazzoccoli,Vito,MD
Gastroenterology
Suarez,Edwin,MD
Suarez,Lynette G.,MD
Internal Medicine
Mayrowetz,Stanley,MD
Palla,Katharine Theresa,DO
Shah,Bankim,MD
Tartaglia,Marco,MD
Nephrology
Siu,Albert,MD
Ophthalmology
Salzano,Brian Christopher,MD
Pediatric Emergency Medicine
Scarfi,Catherine Anne,MD
Plastic Surgery
Agresti,Robert J.,DO
Surgery (General)
Rosenberg,Victor I.,MD

Califon
Family Medicine
Byrd,Raymond J.,MD
Jaskolski,Joseph A.,MD
McGowan,John M.,MD
Williams,Karen Lynn,MD

Camden
Adolescent Medicine
Acquavella,Anthony Peter,MD

Brown,Robert Theodore,MD
Allergy
Cline,Douglas C.,MD
Knowles,William O.,MD
Anatomic Pathology
Haupt,Helen M.,MD
Anatomic/Clinical Pathology
Enriquez,Miriam Lynn,MD
Holdbrook,Thomas,MD
Joneja,Upasana,MD
Kocher,William D.,MD
Rafferty,William J.,MD
Ren,Shuyue,MD
Anesthesiology
Armstrong,James M.,MD
Bolkus,Kelly Ann,DO
Burden,Amanda R.,MD
Cassotis,Maria,DO
Deal,Edward R.,DO
Deangelis,Matthew Michael,DO
Desai,Ronak G.,DO
Dippo,Grace E.,MD
Ganguly,Kingsuk,MD
Ghaul,Mark R.,MD
Goldberg,Michael E.,MD
Gollotto,Michael R.,DO
Gourkanti,Bharathi,MD
Gratz,Irwin,DO
Habib,Fatimah,MD
Hasher-Mascoveto,Wendy M.,DO
Hirsh,Robert Alan,MD
Hsu,George Chiahung,MD
Hughes,Wray,DO
Khan,Asim Haleem,MD
Kushner,Randy Scott,DO
Lin,En-Su,MD
Lutwin Kawalec,Malgorzata S.,MD
Misbin,Michael David,MD
Mitrev,Ludmil Vladimirov,MD
Monticollo,Gerard M.,DO
Munoz,Raul,MD
Muntazar,Muhammad,MD
Nathan,Ponnudurai,MD
Patel,Kinjal M.,MD
Potestio,Christopher Paul,MD
Rinnier,Robert Todd,DO
Romisher,Robert J.,DO
Safaryn,John E.,MD
Schwartz,Michael,MD
Seabron-Rambert,Cheryl,MD
Shazly,Amin,MD
Trautman,Natalie,MD
Trivedi,Keyur Chandrakant,MD
Wnek,Gary E.,MD
Yong,Jinghong,MD
Anesthesiology: Critical Care
Ben-Jacob,Talia K.,MD
Anesthesiology: Pain Medicine
Beelitz,John Darren,MD
Brennan,Mark D.,MD
Sehdev,Jasjit Singh,MD
Breast Surgery
Koniges,Frank C.,MD
Loveland-Jones,Catherine E.,MD
Cardiovascular Disease
Aji,Janah I.,MD
Cartwright,Travante Mcnae,MD
Cotto,Maritza,MD
Dadhania,Manish Suresh,MD
Gessman,Lawrence J.,MD
Ginsberg,Fredric L.,MD
Heintz,Kathleen M.,DO
Javed,Omair,MD
Khan,Mubashar H.,MD
Kurnik,Peter B.,MD
Morris,Timothy P.,DO
Weinstock,Perry J.,MD
Child & Adolescent Psychiatry
Cagande,Consuelo Corazon,MD
Pradhan,Basant Kumar,MD
Pshytycky,Amir,MD
Child (Pediatric) Neurology
Gonzalez Monserrate,Evelyn,MD
McAbee,Gary Noel,DO
Clinical Neurophysiology
Noff,Tom,MD
Clinical Pathology
Nikolic,Dejan,MD
Colon & Rectal Surgery
Kann,Brian Robert,MD
Kawata,Michitaka,MD

Critical Care Medicine
Bekes,Carolyn E.,MD
Charron,Mariane,MD
Dellinger,Richard Phillip,MD
Dettmer,Matthew Robert,MD
Gerber,David R.,DO
Gray,Edward Harlan,DO
Green,Adam Godfrey,MD
Kreidy,Mazen Pierre,MD
Lotano,Ramya,MD
Moradi,Bijan Nik,MD
Spevetz,Antoinette,MD
Trzeciak,Stephen Walter,MD
Zanotti Cavazzoni,Sergio L.,MD
Dermatology
Ghazi,Elizabeth Rose,MD
Diagnostic Radiology
Abujudeh,Hani H.,MD
Baraldi,Raymond Lawrence Jr.,MD
Barshay,Veniamin,MD
Bhimani,Chandni,DO
DeStefano,Michael William,MD
Gefen,Ron,MD
Greatrex,Kathleen Mae V.,MD
Hanono,Joseph A.,MD
Huang,Hoi Pan,MD
Ives,Elizabeth Payne,MD
Jarrett,Vincent A.,DO
Khorrami,Cyrus,MD
Klifto,Eugene J.,DO
Kovacs,James E.,DO
Kwak,Jinhee,MD
Malliah,Sangit Bhoosa,MD
Matteo,Diana C.,MD
Nissenbaum,Gerald Aubbie,MD
Oif,Edward,MD
Presenza,Thomas Jonathan,DO
Roth,Howard Lee,MD
Scattergood,Emily D.,MD
Smith,Charlene M.,MD
Smith,Robert T.,MD
Solis,Maria S.,MD
Solish Gittens,Allison,MD
Emerg Medicine-Pediatric
Drago,Lisa Anne Marie,DO
Emergency Medicine
Bartimus,Holly A.,MD
Baumann,Brigitte Monika,MD
Bendesky,Brad S.,MD
Bergquist,Harveen Bal,MD
Bhamidipati,Anita,MD
Byrne,Richard George,MD
Carnevale,Shawn A.,DO
Carroll,Gerard Gregori,MD
Cassidy-Smith,Tara Nicole,MD
Cesarine,Joseph,MD
Chansky,Michael,MD
Chase,Rachel Eisenbrock,DO
Chien,Christina H.,MD
Damuth,Emily K.,MD
Delvecchio,Joanna Catherine,MD
Dillon,John J.,MD
Disandro,Daniel G.,MD
Eldrich,Samuel Reich,MD
Fernandes,Michael Alexandre,MD
Filippone,Lisa M.,MD
Forde Baker,Jenice M.,MD
Freeze,Brian,MD
Greenman,Rachelle A.,MD
Guerrera,Angela Dixon,MD
Haroz,Rachel,MD
Hennessey,Adam S.,DO
Hong,Rick,MD
Hummel,Joseph C.,DO
Jarecki,Jennifer A.,DO
Jaworski,Alison,MD
Jensen,Sharone Lynn,MD
Jones,Christopher Warren,MD
Karagiannis,Paul,MD
Kilgannon,Jennifer Hope,MD
Kirchhoff,Michael Anthony,MD
Lubkin,Cary L.,MD
Maye,Jessica Megan,DO
Mazzarelli,Anthony Joseph,MD
Mbachu,Yvonne,MD
Nocchi,David Martin,MD
Noel,Christopher Bartlett,MD
Nyce,Andrew L.,MD
Ortega,Rae Lynn,MD
Paston,Carrie Zapolin,MD
Patel,Prakruti,MD
Rebbecchi,Thomas A.,MD

Reinholz,Louis J. Jr.,DO
Rempell,Joshua Saul,MD
Roberts,Brian William,MD
Sacchetti,Alfred D.,MD
Salzman,Matthew Scott,MD
Schrift,David S.,MD
Shapiro,Tyler Kenneth,MD
Smith,Jillian Corbett,MD
Szatko,Miroslaw,MD
Torres Cruz,Joshua,MD
Tyler,Matthew D.,MD
Vetrano,Stephen J.,DO
Warren,Beth Ann,DO
Wild,William A.,DO
Wilsey,Stephanie,MD
Wilson,Alyson Nicole,DO
Wynne,Brenna,MD
Endocrinology
Laufgraben,Marc Jeffrey,MD
Mayorga,Mabel,MD
Family Med- Addiction Medicine
Nurse-Bey,Hazel Ann,MD
Family Medicine
Bascelli,Lynda Marie,MD
Baston,Kaitlan,MD
Bhalodia,Amit Maganlal,DO
Bialecki,Rosemarie,DO
Brenner,Jeffrey Craig,MD
Brooks,Julius A. Jr.,MD
Colopinto,Christopher F.,DO
Dinks-Brown,Shantay M.,DO
Enyeribe,Chioma J.,MD
Fesnak,Susan Gail,DO
Figliola,Robin A.,DO
Franks,Ralph Robert Jr.,DO
Gitler,Steven F.,DO
Goldis,Michael E.,DO
Kim,Kyur Gsook Cho,MD
Kleeman,Jeffrey A.,DO
Lizerbram,Deborah Garber,DO
Prior,Patricia,MD
Rabie,Glenda,MD
Rivera,Adaliz,MD
Stegmuller,Joseph A.,DO
Westerberg,Dyanne Pergolino,DO
Whiting,Philip Howard,DO
Gastroenterology
DeSipio,Joshua Peter,MD
Griech-McCleery,Cynthia,MD
Peikin,Steven R.,MD
Shah,Apeksha,MD
Shats,Daniel,MD
General Practice
Ronsayro,Estrella A.,MD
Geriatrics
Akhter,Rowsonara,MD
Greenberg,Alan,MD
Thomas,May A.,MD
Gynecology
Tew,Beverly Ellen,MD
Hematology
Brus,Christina R.,MD
Young,Faith M.,MD
Hematology Oncology
Bhattacharya,Prianka,MD
Budak-Alpdogan,Tulin,MD
Georges,Peter T.,MD
Hageboutros,Alexandre,MD
Kesselheim,Howard I.,DO
Koch,Marjan Leoni,MD
Sharan,Kanu Priya,MD
Squillante,Christian Michael,MD
Hematopathology
Allen,Ashleigh,MD
Hospitalist
Adarkwa,Agnes,MD
Anter,Afaf A.,DO
Ausaf,Sadaf,MD
Bazergui,Christopher,DO
Contino,Krysta Marie,MD
Divilov,Vadim,MD
Doktor,Katherine Leigh,MD
Ibekwe,Ola,MD
Kabadi,Rajesh Mahesh,MD
Kamalu,Okebugwu,MD
King,Cecile Carol-Ann,MD
Lami,Christian John,MD
Loutfi,Rania H.,MD
Matthews,Lawrence M. III,MD
Moore,Andrew James,MD
Oberdorf,William Eric,DO

Physicians by Town and Medical Specialty

Camden (cont)

Hospitalist
- Palli, Vinay Motu, MD
- Patel, Urvish, MD
- Shah, Satyam Ashvinkumar, MD
- Singh, Novia, MD
- Terrigno, Nicole, MD

Infectious Disease
- Baxter, John D., MD
- Fraimow, Henry S., MD
- Gabriel, Nathaniel F., MD
- Kim, Rose, MD
- Meyer, Daniel Karl, MD
- Pedroza, Lisa Vanchhawng, MD
- Pepe, Rosalie, MD
- Porto, Maura C., DO
- Reboli, Annette C., MD
- Stutman, Robin Eugenia, MD

Insurance Medicine
- Patel, Nikhil H., MD

Internal Medicine
- Abouzgheib, Wissam B., MD
- Abraham, Aney M., MD
- Amin, Naeem Muhammad, MD
- Aplin, Kara Stanig, MD
- Arapurakal, Rajiv, MD
- Atkuri, Rajeshwari Venkata, MD
- Badr, Samer, MD
- Bajaj, Jasmeet Singh, MD
- Bakhshi, Aditya, MD
- Barrington, Dorrie-Susan A., MD
- Borra, Gayatri D., MD
- Butt, Kambiz Reza, MD
- Calder, Nicholas, MD
- Cerceo, Elizabeth Ann, MD
- Chasanov, William M. II, DO
- Chaudhry, Kunal, MD
- Coleman, Ashley J., DO
- Cooke, Jacqueline P., MD
- De La Torre, Pola, MD
- Dragomir, Dan, MD
- Elbaum, Philip, MD
- Fabius, Daniel, DO
- Fan, Lu, MD
- Farajallah, Awny Sb, MD
- Farmer, Alka Rajesh, MD
- Fix, Cecilia Crane, MD
- Gandhi, Snehal V., MD
- Gordon, Marilyn L., MD
- Grana, Generosa, MD
- Gue, Jean B., MD
- Gupta, Ravi, MD
- Hagans, Iris, MD
- Hanes, Douglas James, MD
- Haroldson, Kathryn, MD
- Headly, Anna, MD
- Helmer, Diana Lynn, MD
- Henry, Camille Angela Nicole, MD
- Holtsclaw, John David, MD
- Hwee, Lillian, DO
- Kaplun, Olga, MD
- Kass, Jonathan Eliot, MD
- Khrizman, Polina, MD
- Kim, Nami, DO
- Kothari, Raksha Anil, MD
- Kumar, Anand, MD
- Kupersmith, Eric E., MD
- Kurnik, Brenda R., MD
- Latimore Collier, Sherita M., MD
- Logue, Raymond J., MD
- Mangold, Melissa Beth, DO
- Martinez, Miguel E., MD
- Matos, Ninon, MD
- Mazzarelli, Joanne K., MD
- McMackin, Paul Patrick, MD
- McMillan, Tyler, MD
- Melli, Jenny, MD
- Milburn, Christopher Anthony, MD
- Miles, Liesl Carey, MD
- Miller, Ryan Christopher, MD
- Misra, Sanjay, MD
- Mookerjee, Anuradha Lele, MD
- Moore, Tarquin Oliver, MD
- Mungekar, Mangesh Mohan, MD
- Nair, Nanda K., DO
- Negin, Nathan Samuel, MD
- Newell, Glenn C., MD
- Nguy, Steven Tri, MD
- Nguyen, Bao D., MD
- Oranu, Uzoma, MD
- Orate-Dimapilis, Christina V., MD
- Patel, Devi, MD
- Patel, Monika B., MD
- Patel, Ritesh, MD
- Patel, Sharad D., MD
- Poddar, Sameer S., MD
- Pokuah, Marian O., MD
- Rachoin, Jean Sebastien K., MD
- Ramaswamy, Sunil Rajanna, MD
- Rana, Nimra H., MD
- Rangwalla-Malickel, Inciya, DO
- Rasheed, Sammar, MD
- Richter, Douglas Martin, MD
- Rosenheck, Justin Philip, DO
- Samaha, Simon J., MD
- Schmidt, Ryan Bausch, MD
- Sevrin, Amanda Hope, MD
- Sharma, Meena R., MD
- Shklar, David Lewis, MD
- Siddique, Mahbubur Rahman, MD
- Sikand, Seema, MD
- Singh, Sukhjeet, DO
- Sirover, William D., MD
- Somer, Robert A., MD
- Sussman, Emily Melissa, MD
- Swarup, Subir, DO
- Szawlewicz, Stephen J., MD
- Taylor, Michael, MD
- Thawani, Kalpana, MD
- Topalian, Simon Kevork, MD
- Troyanovich, Esteban F., MD
- Urbano, Frank Louis, MD
- Utreras, Juan S., MD
- Velayadikot, Deepa Nandakumar, MD
- Yadav, Jagdish P., MD
- Yang, Jun, MD
- Young, Jimmie, MD
- Zafar, Fateen D., MD
- Zee, Pamela A., MD

Maternal & Fetal Medicine
- Feld, Steven M., MD
- Fischer, Richard L., MD
- Perry, Robin L., MD
- Westover, Thomas, MD

Medical Genetics
- Schnur, Rhonda E., MD

Medical Oncology
- Devereux, Linda, MD

Neonatal-Perinatal Medicine
- Anwar, Muhammad Usman, MD
- Bautista, Amelia B., MD
- Bhat, Vishwanath, MD
- Brandsma, Erik, MD
- Crawford, Carolyn S., MD
- Fabia, Candida M., MD
- Fernandes, Margaret C., MD
- Kushnir, Alla, MD
- Massabbal, Eltayeb I., MD
- Molina, Leticia K., MD
- Mondoa, Emil I., MD
- Nakhla, Tarek Adib, MD
- Patel, Yashvantkumar S., MD
- Saslow, Judy G., MD
- Sharma, Raj Kumar, MD
- Slater-Myer, Linda Paige, MD
- Stahl, Gary E., MD
- Uko, Smart E., MD

Nephrology
- Chakravarty, Arijit, MD
- Kasama, Richard K., MD
- Kline, Jason Andrew, MD
- Mian, Samia Fatima, MD
- Weisberg, Lawrence Stephen, MD

Neurological Radiology
- Saraiya, Piya Vijay, MD
- Shah, Pallav N., DO

Neurological Surgery
- Goldman, Howard Warren, MD
- Turtz, Alan R., MD

Nuclear Diagnostic Radiology
- Hardy, Caitlin Judith, MD

Nuclear Medicine
- Grabski, Karsten, MD

Obstetrics
- Diaz, Yanirys, MD

Obstetrics & Gynecology
- Askia, Gyasi Abena, DO
- Aves, Cindy, MD
- Bahora, Masuma, MD
- Barnea, Eytan R., MD
- Bilbao, Michelle Cifone, DO
- Bruckler, Paula A., DO
- Cardonick, Elyce Hope, MD
- Chang, Eric, DO
- Chang, Leona, DO
- Chen, Peter Jen-Chih, MD
- Christophe, Kathleen Mary, MD
- Deary, Michael J., MD
- Desimone, Dennis Charles, DO
- Dinh, Tuan A., MD
- Elshoreya, Hazem Mohamed, MD
- Frattarola, Michael A., MD
- Fuseini, Nurain M., MD
- Hall, Bianca Elena, DO
- Hernandez, Marcia Lynn, DO
- Hewlett, Guy Stewart, MD
- Hyman, Francine, MD
- Iyer, Neel Subramanian, DO
- Khandelwal, Meena, MD
- Kim, Yon Sook, MD
- Knights, Jayci Elenor, MD
- La Motta, Joseph D., MD
- Lieser, Joan Karen, MD
- Ligouri, Adrienne L., MD
- Marino, Joseph Frederick, DO
- Martinez, Frances Aileen, MD
- Owens, Nefertari Alisha, MD
- Phillips, Nancy L., MD
- Pistilli, Stephanie Marie, MD
- Ross, Carolyn Michelle, MD
- Rugut, Chloe, MD
- Schaeffer, Kathleen M., DO
- Shah, Nima M., MD
- Smolinsky, Ciaran, MD
- Spector, Sean David, MD
- Tagni, Carine-Ange, MD
- Timms, Diane De Lisi, DO
- Toidze, Tamara V., MD
- Tyree, Laura Lynne, MD
- Wilson Smith, Robin Renee', MD
- Yahav, Eric Kfir, MD

Oncological Surgery
- Minarich, Michael, MD

Ophthalmology
- Coleman, Colleen Marie, MD
- Driver, Paul J., MD
- Makar, Mary Saleeb, MD
- Markovitz, Bruce Jay, MD
- Olivia, Christopher Todd, MD
- Rho, David Samsun, MD
- Soll, Stephen Matthew, MD

Orthopedic Surgery
- De Jesus, Dino Nicol Enanoza, DO
- Freeland, Erik Christopher, DO
- Fuller, David Alden, MD
- Gutowski, Christina, MD
- Kim, Tae Won Benjamin, MD
- Lackman, Richard Daniel, MD
- Lands, Vince Williams, MD
- Mashru, Rakesh Pravinkumar, MD
- Ostrum, Robert Fredric, MD
- Ramirez, Rey Natividad, MD
- Tase, Douglas Sheperd, MD

Otolaryngology
- Spalla, Thomas Christopher, MD

Pain Medicine
- Wadhwa, Namrata, MD

Pathology
- Behling, Kathryn C., MD
- Bierl, Charlene, MD
- Camacho, Jeanette M., MD
- Fitzpatrick, Brendan Thomas, MD
- Kim, Hoon, MD

Pediatric Anesthesia
- Pukenas, Erin W., MD

Pediatric Critical Care
- Briglia, Francis A., MD
- DaSilva, Shonola Samuel, MD
- Smith, Tara Marie, MD
- Thomas, Samuel Charles III, MD

Pediatric Emergency Medicine
- Harris, Elliott Michael, MD
- Nairn, Sandra J., DO

Pediatric Endocrinology
- Post, Ernest M., MD

Pediatric Gastroenterology
- Farhath, Sabeena, MD
- Isola, Kimberly Jean, MD
- Setty, Rajendra P., MD

Pediatric Otolaryngology
- Barrese, James L., MD

Pediatric Surgery
- Hoelzer, Dennis James, MD

Pediatrics
- Acosta, Ramon, MD
- Aghai, Zubairul Hasan, MD
- Ashong, Emmanuel F., MD
- Badolato, Kevin Arthur, MD
- Burton, Monica L., MD
- Buttress, Sharon M., MD
- Churlin, Donna M., MD
- Coren, Jennifer B., DO
- Douglass-Bright, April M., MD
- Dye, Autumn J., DO
- Feingold, Anat Rachel, MD
- Feldman-Winter, Lori, MD
- Fish, Michelle Leigh Karam, DO
- Gormley, Jillian, DO
- Graessle, William R., MD
- Green, Patricia, MD
- Grossman, Sandra Lynn, MD
- Gupta, Monika, MD
- Hussain, Mohammed Jawaad, MD
- Imaizumi, Sonia O., MD
- Johnson, Karen Teresa, DO
- Karmilovich, Beth Ann, DO
- Kline, David M., DO
- Knoflicek, Lisa E., MD
- Krol, Anna, MD
- Lania-Howarth, Maria, MD
- Leong, Kai K., MD
- Mangubat, Kimberly Mae, MD
- McCans, Kathryn M., MD
- McGrath, Teresa Pirri, DO
- Mehta, Vijay, DO
- Meislich, Debrah, MD
- Melchiorre, Louis P. Jr., MD
- Mojica, Cornelio F., MD
- Mulvihill, David J., MD
- Novak, Nellie, MD
- Pawel, Barbara B., MD
- Ramprasad, Vatsala, MD
- Rivera, Velmina S., MD
- Robel, Lindsey, MD
- Roussel, Anisha Lanice, MD
- Salah, Hassan H., MD
- Sharma, Rakesh B., MD
- Sharrar, William G., MD
- Tucker, Tiffany, MD
- Turner, Peter E., MD
- Vankawala, Sonya, DO
- Verrecchia, Courtney, MD
- Vital, Michelle Maria, MD
- Wright, Erin Armstead, MD

Physical Medicine & Rehab
- Anthony, William P., MD
- Cohen, Stephen Jonathan, MD
- DiMarco, Jack Peter, MD
- Khona, Nithyashuba B., MD
- Nolan, John P., DO

Plastic Surgery
- Brown, Arthur Samuel, MD
- Buckley, Karen Marie, MD
- Liebman, Jared Jason, MD
- Matthews, Martha S., MD
- Perkins, Anthony Ray, MD

Psychiatry
- Aguilar, Francis, MD
- Ayala, Omar, MD
- Clements, David IV, MD
- Dimaio, Andrea Lynne, DO
- Elman, Igor, MD
- Gogineni, Rama Rao, MD
- Iftekhar, Ruksana, MD
- Monte, Lyda Cervantes, MD
- Pumariega, Andres Julio, MD
- Stable, Joaquin Jose, MD
- Szeeley, Pamela J., MD

Pulmonary Critical Care
- Kennedy-Little, Dawn Marie, DO

Pulmonary Disease
- Abou-Rayan, Mohamed Magdy, MD
- Akers, Stephen M., MD
- Boujaoude, Ziad C., MD
- Pratter, Melvin Richard, MD

Radiation Oncology
- Ahlawat, Stuti, MD
- Asbell, Sucha Order, MD
- Dragun, Anthony E., MD
- Eastwick, Gary, MD
- Henson, Clarissa F., MD
- Hughes, Lesley Ann, MD
- Kramer, Noel Melitta, DO
- Mezera, Megan A., MD

Patel,Ashish Bharat,MD
Singh,Rachana,MD
Radiology
Articolo,Glenn Anthony,MD
Bobrow,Michael L.,MD
Brody,Joshua David,DO
Della Peruta,Joseph,MD
Jacoby,James Howard,MD
Kaplan,Carol Ellen,MD
Kerner,Sheldon P.,DO
Moss,Edward G.,MD
Scotti,Daniel M.,MD
Surgery (General)
Ahmad,Nadir,MD
Atabek,Umur M.,MD
Awad,Nadia Amal,MD
Barth,Nadine,MD
Bea,Vivian Jolley,MD
Bird,Dorothy Waterbury,MD
Bowen,Frank Winslow III,MD
Brill,Kristin Lynne,MD
Chopra,Vinod Kumar,MD
Duncan,Beth R.,MD
Fox,Nicole M.,MD
Goldenberg-Sandau,Anna,DO
Harris,William Matthew,MD
Hendershott,Karen Jean,MD
Hong,Young Ki,MD
Leese,Kenneth H.,MD
Lombardi,Joseph V.,MD
Mofid,Alireza,MD
O'Connell,Brendan Garrett,MD
Patel,Rohit Amratlal,MD
Radomski,John S.,MD
Reid,Lisa M.,MD
Remick,Kyle Norman,MD
Shersher,David Daniel,MD
Simons,Robert Mark,MD
Stanisce,Luke Thomas,MD
Wydo,Salina Marie,MD
Yocom,Steven S.,DO
Surgical Critical Care
Axelrad,Alexander,MD
Porter,John Maurice,MD
Ross,Steven E.,MD
Thoracic Surgery
Highbloom,Richard Yale,MD
Rosenbloom,Michael,MD
Transplant Surgery & Medicine
Guy,Stephen Reed,MD
Sebastian,Ely M.,MD
Youssef,Nasser Ibrahim,MD
Trauma Surgery
Burns,Richard Kent,MD
Egodage,Tanya,MD
Hazelton,Joshua Paul,DO
Urology
Bernhard,Peter Howard,MD
Krisch,Evan B.,MD
Marmar,Joel L.,MD
Seftel,Allen D.,MD
Tomaszewski,Jeffrey John,MD
Vascular & Intrvntnal Radiology
Akinyemi,Michael Omobolaji,MD
Broudy,Joseph Benjamin,MD
De Cotiis,Dan A.,MD
Vascular Surgery
Alexander,James B.,MD
Trani,Jose Luis,MD
Cape May
Emergency Medicine
Carlin,Teresa Mary,MD
Cramer,Kenneth E.,MD
Lafferty,Keith A.,MD
Mihata,Ryan Garner,MD
Family Medicine
Koskinen,Kjersti,MD
Internal Medicine
Mehta,Subhash G.,MD
Rothman,Craig Michael,MD
Orthopedic Surgery
Anapolle,David M.,MD
Psychiatry
Dick,Charles,MD
Cape May Court House
Anesthesiology
Barth,Holli Ami,MD
Dragon,Greg R.,MD
Patel,Ashokkumar J.,MD
Patel,Hareshbhai C.,MD
Tarantino,David P.,MD

Cardiovascular Disease
Boriss,Michael N.,DO
Burhanna,Amy Scally,MD
Nanavati,Suketu H.,MD
Nillas,Michael S.,MD
Scally,Monique,DO
Sorensen,Mark R.,MD
Child & Adolescent Psychiatry
Rodriguez,Hilton John,MD
Dermatology
Paolini,Lawrence,DO
Weiss,Robert Joseph Sr.,MD
Developmental Pediatrics
Hackford,Robert R.,MD
Diagnostic Radiology
Capecci,Louis J.,MD
Garrett,Paul R.,MD
Patel,Amit Arun,MD
Patel,Kaushik M.,MD
Shah,Ankur,MD
Emergency Medicine
Banfield,Kimberly Ann,DO
Bridge-Jackson,Teresa A.,MD
Cascarino,Raymond Patrick,DO
Cimino,Robert,MD
Coletta,Domenic Jr.,MD
Dudnick,Michael,DO
Nussey,Richard Hutchins Jr.,DO
Pecora,Arthur Steven,DO
Riordan,Kevin J.,MD
Ruskey,John S.,DO
Ventriglia,Warren J.,MD
Endocrinology
Raghuwanshi,Anita P.,MD
Zitnay,Christopher G.,MD
Family Medicine
Corrado,Peter M.,DO
Crowley,Elizabeth Ann,MD
Deignan,Dianna T.,MD
Jain,Manoj Prakash,MD
Koskinen,Jason Alexander,DO
Lirio,Sixto M.,MD
Marotta,Raymond J. Jr.,MD
McLay,William F.,DO
Rizzetta,Anthony J.,DO
Schwartz,Joseph T.,DO
Gastroenterology
Beitman,Robert G.,MD
Landset,David J.,DO
Ljubich,Paul,MD
Masciarelli,Anthony,DO
Troum,Richard M.,DO
Vattasseril,Renjy,MD
General Practice
Weisberg,William R.,MD
Hematology
Gandhi,Vijaykumar K.,MD
Infectious Disease
Hansen,Eric Andrew,DO
Internal Medicine
Aversa,Jeffrey Martin,MD
Childs,Arthur L.,DO
Gandhi,Shveta V.,DO
Hong,John S.,MD
Lee,Edward Howe,MD
Niewiadomski,Edward J.,MD
Osgood,Eric,MD
Pandya,Melind Rasik,DO
Patel,Jayeshkumar Kiritkumar,MD
Shah,Chetan K.,DO
Stave,Jeffrey R.,DO
Varner,Philip T.,DO
Neurology
Edwards,Jillian,DO
Singh,Manish Kumar,MD
Obstetrics & Gynecology
Michner,Richard A.,MD
Milio,Joseph L.,DO
Noll,Bruce R.,MD
Ophthalmology
Altman,Brian,MD
Caruso,Michael J.,DO
McLaughlin,John Patrick,MD
Pastore,Domenic J.,MD
Otolaryngology
DeLorio,Nicola Anne,DO
Matlick,Lonny D.,DO
Mucci,Wayne P.,DO
Syed,Zubair,DO
Pathology
Jurasinski,Craig M.,MD

Pediatrics
Cavaliere,Ava A.,DO
Deliz,Yasmin D.,DO
Dierkes,Thomas F.,DO
Flick,Jeffrey L.,DO
Freund,William Roy,DO
Lai,Wai-Ling,MD
Mathur,Ajit,MD
Psychiatry
Blackinton,Charles H.,MD
Hankin,William H.,MD
Harrison,David E.,DO
Pulmonary Disease
Bradway,William R.,DO
Komansky,Henry J.,DO
Patel,Amit H.,MD
Udani,Rajen I.,MD
Radiation Oncology
Cassir,Jorge F.,MD
Cho,David Shen,MD
Meltzer,Jeffrey I.,MD
Wurzer,James C.,MD
Surgery (General)
Attiya,Rafael,MD
Falivena,Richard Peter,DO
Lawinski,Richard M.,MD
Martz,Patricia Ann,MD
Russo,David Peter,MD
Salasin,Robert I.,MD
Tenner,Jeffrey P.,DO
Vascular Surgery
O'Donnell,Paul Lawrence,DO
Sabnis,Vinayak M.,MD
Carlstadt
Family Medicine
Morris,Paul J.,DO
Nuclear Medicine
Dakhel,Mahmoud,MD
Carneys Point
Cardiovascular Disease
Sauers,Paul W.,DO
Family Medicine
Lawrence,John Robert,MD
Quigley,Craig B.,MD
Internal Medicine
Salem,Mohamed M.,MD
Neurology
Fernandez,Maria Elmina,MD
Graham,Dennis C.,DO
Psychiatry
Serrano,Camilo Francisco,MD
Varghese,Sajini S.,DO
Carteret
Family Medicine
Anderson-Wright,Phyllis,DO
Kindzierski,Michael A.,DO
Sjovall,Frances,DO
Hematology
Sidhom,Ibrahim W.,MD
Internal Medicine
Behman,Daisy M.,MD
Behman,Tamer Abdelmonam,MD
Darvish,Arash,MD
Goraya,Sukhjender,MD
Kalika,Sanna,MD
Mavani,Nagindas V.,MD
Riar,Sandeep Singh,MD
Nephrology
Singh,Bikramjit,MD
Neurology
Behman,Haidy Mankarios,MD
Mills,Richard J.,MD
Pulmonary Disease
Singh,Rashpal,MD
Cedar Grove
Anesthesiology
Shah,Kusum V.,MD
Child & Adolescent Psychiatry
Platt,Ellen M.,DO
Dermatology
Cohen,Alan Polan,MD
Cunningham,Ellen Elizabeth,MD
Farley-Loftus,Rachel L.,MD
Kandula,Swetha,MD
Family Medicine
Pinal,Laureen,MD
Rosen,Jay Stuart,MD
Gastroenterology
Rizvi,Masood A.,MD

General Practice
Eltaki,Madiha Ahmed,MD
Internal Medicine
Chaturvedi,Ratan B.,MD
Huang,Kuei-Huang,MD
Mirza,Muhammad A.,MD
Morgan,James Peter,MD
Rambaran,Hayman Kumar,MD
Rambaran,Naipaul,MD
Obstetrics & Gynecology
Lee,Angie Yookyoung,MD
Ophthalmology
Youngworth,Lynda A.,MD
Otolaryngology
Rossi,Anthony G.,MD
Physical Medicine & Rehab
Miller,Catharine Michele,DO
Plastic Surgery
Berlet,Anthony C.,MD
Psychiatry
Maruri,Krishna K.,MD
Mayerhoff,David I.,MD
Nucci,Annamaria,MD
Omilian,Karen L.,DO
Platt,Jennifer,DO
Talbo,Norma B.,MD
Wei,Ronald Shaw,MD
Pulmonary Disease
Dikengil,Yahya Mete,MD
Urology
Agarwal,Saurabh,MD
Vascular Surgery
Watson,Marc C.,MD
Cedar Knolls
Addiction Psychiatry
Putcha,Vasundhara,MD
Allergy
Oppenheimer,John Jacob,MD
Allergy & Immunology
Graffino,Donatella B.,MD
Anatomic/Clinical Pathology
Alfonso,Flores,MD
Anesthesiology
Shrem,Leslie Allen,MD
Solomonov,Mikhail,MD
Cardiovascular Disease
Feitell,Leonard A.,MD
Godkar,Darshan,MD
Moss,Leonard J. Jr.,DO
Child & Adolescent Psychiatry
Hubsher,Merritt S.,MD
Critical Care Medicine
Capone,Robert Anthony,MD
Dimitry,Edward Jr.,MD
Family Medicine
Dave,Bijal A.,MD
Gellerstein,Alan Stuart,MD
Gibbions,James Vernon Jr.,MD
Gopin,Joan M.,MD
Kumar,Preethi,DO
Monka,Ira P.,DO
Tepper,Suzanne,MD
Gastroenterology
Dalena,John Michael,MD
Hand Surgery
Zaino,Christian,MD
Infectious Disease
Burstin,Stuart J.,MD
Internal Medicine
Fuchs,Eliyahu Elliot,MD
Hussain,Adnan,MD
James,David Joel,MD
Mysh,Dmitry,MD
Oei,Erwin John,MD
Pasik,Deborah,MD
Singh,Vandana,DO
Som,Sumit,MD
Interventional Cardiology
Marotta,Charles J.,MD
Obstetrics & Gynecology
Chu,Mary M.,MD
Kuchera,James Joseph,MD
Kuchera,Michael W.,MD
Potash,Sarah K.,MD
Ricks,Ann Marie,MD
Ophthalmology
Sachs,Ronald,MD

Physicians by Town and Medical Specialty

Cedar Knolls (cont)
Orthopedic Surgery
D'Agostini,Robert J.,MD
Decter,Edward M.,MD
Goldman,Robert T.,MD
Hunt,Stephen A.,MD
Strassberg,Joshua A.,MD
Pain Medicine-Interventional
Prvulovic,Tomi,MD
Pediatric Ophthalmology
Mori,Mayumi A.,MD
Pediatric Orthopedics
Bloom,Tamir,MD
Friedman,Samara,MD
Lin,David Yih-Min,MD
Rieger,Mark A.,MD
Pediatric Pulmonology
Kohn,Gary Lawrence,MD
Physical Med & Rehab-Sports Med
Dona,Samuel Torres Jr.,MD
Physical Medicine & Rehab
Bowen,Jay E.,DO
Dunn,Kevin B.,MD
Malanga,Gerard A.,MD
Psychiatry
Barnas,Matthew Edward,MD
Monroy-Miller,Cherry Ann,MD
Weiss,Gony Alexandra,MD
Zincone,John Peter,MD
Pulmonary Critical Care
Epstein,Matthew D.,MD
Pulmonary Disease
Restifo,Robert A.,DO
Scoopo,Frederic J.,MD
Shah,Chirag Vijaykumar,MD
Radiology
Goodman,Jonathan L.,DO
Rheumatology
Paxton,Laura Anne,MD
Sebastian,Jodi Komoroski,MD

Changewater
Dermatology
Errickson,Carla V.,MD

Chatham
Adolescent Medicine
Estrada,Elsie C.,MD
Anesthesiology
Blumenfeld,Daniel J.,MD
Dermatology
Breslauer,Lisa Marie,MD
Diagnostic Radiology
Gelber,Lawrence J.,MD
Kingsly,Jill H.,MD
Lee,Terrence Hone Chung,MD
Schroeder,Donald C.,MD
Family Medicine
Baker,Janice E.,MD
Cirello,Joseph Anthony,MD
Gruber,Amy D.,MD
Holland,Elbridge T. Jr.,MD
Levine,Steven Marc,DO
Nevins,John J.,DO
Ocasio,Maria Elena,MD
Resciniti,Matthew John,DO
Tribuna,Joseph,MD
Varshavski,Mikhail,DO
Gastroenterology
Franzese,John,MD
Insurance Medicine
Traficante,Allen,MD
Internal Medicine
Collins,Neal,MD
Pincus,Jillian R.,MD
Rodriguez,Lauren C.,MD
Medical Oncology
Hirawat,Samit,MD
Neurology
Dorflinger,Ernest Edward Jr.,MD
Obstetrics & Gynecology
Ganitsch,Christine A.,MD
Reynolds,Nina D.,MD
Silverberg,Fred Marshall,MD
Orthopedic Surgery
Alapatt,Michael F.,MD
Dorsky,Steven G.,MD
Pain Medicine
Gerstman,Brett A.,MD
Pediatrics
Corpuz,Danielle M.,MD
Shaw Brachfeld,Jennifer L.,MD

Slavin,Stuart F.,MD
Tom,Valerie,MD
Physical Med & Rehab-Pain Med
Allen Artiglere,Kara D.,DO
Physical Medicine & Rehab
Lipp,Matthew Ivan,MD
Psychiatry
DeMilio,Lawrence T.,MD
Dorsky,Seth Michael,MD
Spinal Surgery
Clark-Schoeb,James Scott,MD
Rieger,Kenneth J.,MD
Urology
Ulker Sarokhan,Erol E.,MD

Cherry Hill
Addiction Psychiatry
Wallen,Mark C.,MD
Allergy & Immunology
Graziano,Linda M.,MD
Romanoff,Nicholas A.,MD
Anatomic/Clinical Pathology
Gao,Hong-Guang,MD
Godyn,Janusz J.,MD
Liu,Jun,MD
Pavlenko,Andriy,MD
Robinson,Mary J.,DO
Anesthesiology
Carr,Alan D.,DO
Grosh,Taras,MD
Heyman,David Mark,DO
Kerner,Michael B.,DO
Lamprou,Emanuel Jr.,MD
Lu,Cheh Shiung,DO
Young,Marie Lisette,MD
Anesthesiology: Critical Care
Flaxman,Alexander,MD
Anesthesiology: Pain Medicine
Maurer,Philip Mitchell,MD
Puri,Shawn K.,MD
Reyes,Johan,MD
Cardiothoracic Surgery
Derivaux,Christopher Charles,MD
Cardiovascular Disease
Akhigbe,Kelvin Osagie,DO
Akula,Devender Nagarajan,MD
Bauer,Hans Henry Jr.,MD
Bhavsar,Jignesh,MD
Blaber,Reginald J.,MD
Burke,Gary C.,DO
Chaudhry,Nasser A.,MD
Cohen,Ronald A.,DO
Dickstein,Richard A.,MD
Duffy,Kevin James Jr.,MD
Dunham,Rozy D.,MD
Fertels,Scott H.,DO
Fox,Steven N.,MD
Friedman,Terry David,MD
Fuhrman,Mitchell J.,MD
Gelernt,Mark D.,MD
Godin,Willis Eugene,DO
Gomberg,Richard M.,DO
Hamaty,John N.,DO
Harkins,Michael J.,MD
Hollenberg,Steven M.,MD
Horwitz,Jerome M.,DO
Kernis,Steven J.,MD
Khatiwala,Jayesh Ramesh,MD
Khaw,Kenneth,MD
Klodnicki,Walter E.,MD
Kothari,Anil G.,MD
Lawrence,David L.,MD
Leavy,Jeffrey Alan,MD
Mohapatra,Robert A.,MD
Momplaisir,Thierry,MD
Moussa,Ibrahim Abdel,MD
Ortman,Matthew Louis,MD
Proper,Michael C.,MD
Randle,Troy L.,DO
Reichman,Michael J.,MD
Rosenberg,Mitchell C.,MD
Rubenstone,Jay L.,DO
Sailam,Vivek Vardha,MD
Sandler,Matthew Jay,MD
Sholevar,Darius P.,MD
Siddiqi,Faisal Khursheed,MD
Siegal,Scott L.,MD
Silver,Steven Eric,MD
Smith,Jason Anthony,DO
Wadehra,Ramneet,DO
Yegya-Raman,Sivaraman,MD
Zarrella,Geoffrey Carl,DO

Cardiovascular Surgery
Kuchler,Joseph A.,MD
Martella,Arthur Thomas,MD
Nayar,Amrit P.,MD
Child & Adolescent Psychiatry
Denbo,Nancy J.,MD
Gurak,Randall B.,MD
Sosland,Morton D.,MD
Colon & Rectal Surgery
Berg,David Adam,MD
Cody,William C.,MD
Deleon,Miguel L.,MD
El Badawi,Khaled Iqbal,MD
Schaffzin,David Marc,MD
Critical Care Medicine
Baumgarten,Steven S.,MD
Horowitz,Ira David,MD
Cytopathology
Shienbaum,Alan J.,DO
Dermatology
DeCosmo,Michael J.,DO
Mastromonaco,Denise M.,DO
Matalon,Vivienne I.,MD
Mellul,Victor G.,MD
Diagnostic Radiology
Barzel,Eyal,MD
Bufalino,Kevin Thomas,MD
Curtis,Paul A.,MD
De Laurentis,Joseph,MD
Depersia,Lori Angela,MD
Desai,Vishal,MD
Dheer,Sachin,MD
Fazekas,Jessica Eden,DO
Germaine,Pauline,DO
Goodworth,Gregory J.,MD
Haney,James Joseph III,MD
Kramer,Neil Robert,MD
Lee,Mark Hyon-Min,MD
Lentini,John Alaric,MD
Sergi,Thomas J.,MD
Stark,Ira R.,DO
Tank,Niti,MD
Ter,Suat E.,MD
Torres,Joseph Charles,MD
Electroencephalography
Zechowy,Allen C.,MD
Emergency Medicine
Bernhardt,Jarrid,DO
Caravello,Andrew Benedetto,DO
Demangone,Dawn Adele,MD
Dileonardo,Francesca,MD
Feld,Ross J.,DO
Hall,Philip Isaac,DO
Hinchliffe,Susan,MD
Magbalon,Domingo Jr.,MD
Nepp,Mark E.,DO
Ross,Michael Jordan,MD
Sidwa,Robert Joshua,DO
Snyder,Natali P.,DO
Wainwright Edwards,Marsha,MD
Endocrinology
Anand,Rishi Dev,MD
Barone,Gregory John,DO
Bhat,Geetha K. G.,MD
Haddad,Ghada,MD
Jennings,Anthony S.,MD
Kaufman,Steven Todd,MD
Kaul,Shailja,MD
Swibinski,Edward T.,MD
Thapar,Garima,MD
Varghese,Sarah,MD
Verma,Parveen Kaur,DO
Facial Plastic Surgery
Hughes,Susan M.,MD
Family Med-Adult Medicine
Fish,Gabrielle A.,DO
Family Med-Sports Medicine
Duprey,Kevin M.,DO
Kimmel,Craig S.,MD
Family Medicine
Bidigare,Susan Ann,MD
Bieler,Bert Michael,MD
Chen,Anna,MD
Chung,Lynn S.,MD
Costa,Ralph F.,MD
De Prince,Daniel III,DO
DiMaio,Robert D.,DO
Finan,Cathleen M.,DO
Finan-Duffy,Colleen M.,DO
Fine,Manette K.,DO
Forman,Lawrence S.,DO

Greenberg,Scott Ross,MD
Gurrieri,John E.,MD
Hanley,Thomas T.,MD
Kocinski,Michael Stephen I,DO
Kopp Mulberg,F. Elyse,DO
Levin,Bonnie Lorraine,DO
Levine,Richard Marc,MD
Mueller,Loretta L.,DO
Neidecker,John Michael,DO
Persily,Tracy L.,DO
Salerno,Christopher J.,DO
Shrayber,Yelena Y.,DO
Simon,Richard M.,DO
Sirken,Steven M.,DO
Vernon,Gerald Michael,DO
Vitoc,Camelia S.,MD
Weiss,Richard S.,MD
Gastroenterology
Berberian,Brian,MD
Volchonok,Oleg,MD
Werbitt,Warren,DO
General Practice
Goldsmith,Joyce,MD
Jensen,Edwin A.,DO
Magaziner,Allan,DO
Geriatrics
Abelow,Gerald G.,MD
Hasbun,William Miguel,MD
Maro,Robert Jr.,MD
Patel,Rajankuma Popatlal,MD
Surrey,Christine Marie,DO
Gynecology
Pekala,Bernard A.,MD
Hand Surgery
Ames,Elliot L.,DO
Bednar,John M.,MD
Headache
Tinkelman,Brad J.,MD
Hematology Oncology
Alley,Evan Wayne,MD
Goldberg,Jack,MD
Hepatology
Elgenaidi,Hisham,MD
Malek,Ashraf Hossain,MD
Hospitalist
Kashif,Soofia,MD
Kotturi,Vijendra B.,MD
Infectious Disease
Alessi,Paul J.,DO
Williams,James R.,MD
Internal Medicine
Ali,Tuba Muhammad,MD
Antonelli,William M.,DO
Avetian,Garo Charles,DO
Bastien,Arnaud,MD
Chen,Shwu-Miin Y.,MD
Damerau,Keith R.,MD
Dey,Chaitali,MD
Driscoll,Michael Joseph,DO
Dructor,Lisa Ann,DO
Epelboim Feldman,Joyce,MD
Favata,Elissa A.,MD
Galabi,Michael,MD
Gerber,Steven Lewis,MD
Gerber,Susan Marie,MD
Gooberman,Bruce D.,MD
Halickman,Isaac J.,MD
Hanna,Gamil Sabet Fawzy,MD
Jafry,Behjath,MD
Josephson,Tina M.,MD
Kalu,Eke N.,MD
Kemps,Anton P.,MD
Kirby,John A.,MD
Klausman,Kenneth Barry,MD
Malli,Dipakkumar Purushott,MD
McMahon,Mary Ann Patricia,MD
Molino,Richard,MD
Monari-Sparks,Mary Joan,MD
Morgan,Farah Hena,MD
Naware,Sanya,MD
Nordin,Brittany N.,DO
Nugent,Thomas Rone,MD
Palli,Vasu Motu,MD
Pecarsky,Jason Todd,MD
Rosenthal,Brett Samson,DO
Rozengarten,Kimberly Irene,MD
Saia,Bryan Edward,MD
Schiller,Terence G.,MD
Shah,Anish Pravin,MD
Shehata,Ahmed Abdelhalim,MD
Sherman,Anthony,MD

Singh-Mohapatra,Sherry,MD
Smeglin,Anthony G.,MD
Stein,Alan David,MD
Stom,Mary C.,MD
Todt,Mark J.,MD
Torigian,Christine V.,MD
Wenger,Christopher D.,DO
Zander,Judith W.,MD
Zanger,Ron,MD
Zaslavsky,Alexandr,MD
Interventional Cardiology
Levine,Adam Maxwell,DO
Neonatal-Perinatal Medicine
Chawla,Harbhajan Singh,MD
Nephrology
Bodiwala,Brijesh Shreyas,DO
Butani,Savita M.,MD
McFadden,Christopher Bruce,MD
Michel,Brian E.,MD
Ra,Daniel,DO
Specter,Richard L.,MD
Neurology
Abrams,Russell I.,MD
Burakgazi Dalkilic,Evren,MD
Campellone,Joseph V. Jr.,MD
Colcher,Amy,MD
Ingala,Erin Einbinder,MD
Janoff,Larry Stewart,DO
Lipsius,Bruce D.,MD
McGarry,Andrew James,MD
Mirsen,Thomas R.,MD
Moeller,Joseph Phillip,DO
Popescu,Anca S.,MD
Preis,Keith Victor,MD
Rogers,James J.,DO
Weiner,Francine L.,MD
Neuromusculoskeletal Med & OMM
Picciotti,Brett,DO
Obstetrics & Gynecology
Arole,Chidinma N.,MD
Benett,Jodi A.,DO
Borromeo,Rita Gonzalez,MD
Burke,Gerald V.,MD
Glass,Phillip,MD
Hunter,Robert L.,MD
Kaufman,Susan I.,DO
Khosla,Jayasree,MD
Litz,John Jr.,MD
O'Banion,Kathleen S.,MD
Or,Drorit,MD
Rana,Ramneek,MD
Occupational Medicine
Chorney,Jeffrey R.,MD
Ophthalmology
Andrew,Mark S.,MD
Bannett,Gregg A.,DO
Cohen,Avraham N.,MD
Goel,Ravi Desh,MD
Ho,Allen C.,MD
Hsu,Jason,MD
Kaplan,Barnard A.,MD
Kindermann,Wilfred Reed,MD
Lanciano,Ralph Jr.,DO
Malley,Debra S.,MD
Miano,Michele A.,MD
Patel,Jayrag Ashwinkumar,MD
Pekala,Raymond T.,MD
Regillo,Carl,MD
Richman,Jesse,MD
Spechler,Floyd F.,MD
Yasgur,Lee H.,MD
Orthopedic Surgery
Barr,Lawrence I.,DO
Beaver,Andrew Bradley,MD
Booth,Robert Emrey Jr.,MD
Clements,David H. III,MD
Dubowitch,Stuart G.,DO
Gleimer,Barry S.,DO
Gleimer,Jeffrey Robert,DO
Gordon,Stuart Leon,MD
Hopkins,Leigh Hastings,MD
Hume,Eric Lynn,MD
Jacoby,Sidney Mark,MD
Kahn,Marc L.,MD
Kahn,Steven H.,DO
Naftulin,Richard J.,DO
Paiste,Mark Ronald,DO
Ranelle,Robert George,DO
Reiner,Mark J.,MD
Rekant,Mark Spencer,MD
Ricci,Anthony R.,DO

Tjoumakaris,Fotios P.,MD
Orthopedics
Kane,Patrick Martin,MD
Otolaryngology
Busch,Scott L.,DO
Hall,Patrick J.,MD
Otolaryngology-Facial Plastic
Corrado,Anthony Charles,DO
Pain Medicine
Band,Ricard Louis,MD
Korn,Barry Allen,DO
Tawadrous,Alfred Rezk,MD
Pediatric Radiology
Willard,Scott David,MD
Pediatrics
Ayres,Julie Clarke,MD
Baldino,Anna Rita,DO
Chase,Melissa Sussman,DO
Ehrlich,Jerry S.,MD
Gargiulo,Katherine Anne,MD
Harris,Esther R.,MD
Ibay,Maria Lourdes D.,MD
Kaplan,Leonard F.,MD
Kothari,Nita H.,MD
Marchese,Anthony Aristide,DO
Margallo,Evangeline Cobin,MD
McHugh,Jennifer L.,MD
Mohazzebi,Cyrus,MD
Razi,Parisa,MD
Rosen,Florence E.,MD
Shieh,Luke,MD
Taubman,Bruce Melvin,MD
Tedeschi,John B.,MD
Tedeschi,John M.,MD
Viray,Ruth Mariel,MD
Weber,Jason Stuart,MD
Whitney,Julie Sherman,DO
Physical Med & Rehab-Pain Med
Le,Phuong Uyen,DO
Physical Medicine & Rehab
Bodofsky,Elliot B.,MD
Citta-Pietrolungo,Thelma J.,DO
Gupta,Rajan S.,MD
Plastic Surgery
Back,Lyle M.,MD
Brownstein,Gary M.,MD
Davis,Steven L.,DO
Gatti,John E.,MD
Psychiatry
Ager,Mary Ann Michelle,MD
Ager,Steven A.,MD
Aronowitz,Jeffrey S.,DO
Baez,Rafael M.,MD
Ball,Roberta R.,DO
Blackburn,Lisa D.,MD
Blum,Lawrence D.,MD
Chen,Yirong,MD
Dabrow,Jennifer,DO
Denysenko,Lex,MD
Faden,Justin B.,DO
Friedman,Michael J.,DO
Gulab,Nazli E.,MD
Hauser,Adam Dankner,MD
Heard,Delano R.,DO
Islam,Mohammed Nazrul,MD
Ivanov,Ilya,DO
Kaldany,Herbert A.,DO
Khan,Aneela,MD
Khan,Munaza Anwar,MD
Lindquist,Lisa A.,DO
Ma,Yuhua,MD
Madison,Harry Thomas,DO
Miceli,Kurt Phillip,MD
Miller,Alan Norman,MD
Naik,Nalini S.,MD
Nayar,Anju,MD
Pinninti,Narsimha R.,MD
Piper,George E.,DO
Rana,Badal D.,DO
Rhoades,Walter Jr.,DO
Rissmiller,David J.,DO
Rosenberg,Leon I.,MD
Salzberg,Felix,MD
Shore,Michael W.,MD
Simon,Jeffrey Hayden,MD
Yi,Helen Huafang,MD
Zielinski,Glenn D.,DO
Pulmonary Critical Care
Velasco,Antonio Quiachon,DO
Pulmonary Disease
Crookshank,Aaron David,MD

Dostal,Courtney Lynne,DO
Hamaty,Edward G. Jr.,DO
Morowitz,William A.,MD
Pope,Alan Raymond,MD
Scivoletti Polan,Nicole Anne,DO
Radiation Oncology
Dicker,Adam P.,MD
Hirsh,Alina Z.,MD
Kornmehl,Carol,MD
Meritz,Keith A.,MD
Radiology
Barber,Locke W.,DO
Di Marcangelo,Mark T.,DO
Sleep Disorders Medicine
Roszkowski,Jennifer Rose,DO
Sports Medicine
Bartolozzi,Arthur Robert,MD
Surgery (General)
Acholonu,Emeka Joseph,MD
Bedi,Ashish,MD
Cohen,Larry W.,DO
Costabile,Joseph P.,MD
Fakulujo,Adeshola D.,MD
Franckle,William C. IV,MD
Iyer,Malini,MD
Llenado,Jeanne Valencia,DO
Meoli,Fredrick G.,DO
Meslin,Keith Phillip,MD
Neff,Marc A.,MD
Sandau,Roy Lee,DO
Sorokin,Evan Scott,MD
Szczurek,Linda J.,DO
Zaretsky,Craig Lawrence,MD
Zuniga,Joseph Michael R.,MD
Thoracic Surgery
Davis,Paul K.,MD
Luciano,Pasquale A.,DO
Moffa,Salvatore M.,MD
Pascual,Rodolfo C.,MD
Villanueva,Dioscoro T.,MD
Urology
Biester,Robert J.,MD
Chow,Shih-Han,MD
Fallick,Mark Lawrence,MD
Keeler,Louis L. III,MD
Vascular & Intrvntnal Radiology
Snyder,Randall William III,MD
Vascular Surgery
Andrew,Constantine T.,MD
Bak,Yury,DO
Field,Charles K.,MD
Spence,Richard Kevin,MD
Chester
Cardiovascular Disease
Antonucci,Lawrence Charles,MD
Clinical Pharmacology
Novitt-Moreno,Anne D.,MD
Dermatology
Geller,Jay D.,MD
Emergency Medicine
Vets,Steve Michael,DO
Family Medicine
Singh,Maulshree,MD
Hand Surgery
Weinstein,Larry,MD
Internal Medicine
Chanin,Alan H.,MD
Davis,Glenn A.,MD
Sidhu,Gurpreet Singh,MD
Interventional Cardiology
Sebastian,Clifford Cecil,MD
Obstetrics & Gynecology
Mitchell,Barbara,MD
Ophthalmology
Hirschfeld,James M.,MD
Hoye,Vincent Joseph III,MD
Silverstein,Niki A.,MD
Silverstein,Rodger H.,MD
Pediatrics
Aygen,Kadri M.,MD
Aygen,Zehra Zeynep,MD
Physical Medicine & Rehab
Georgekutty,Jason,DO
Lammertse,Thomas E.,MD
Nieves,Jeremiah David,MD
Nori,Phalgun,MD
Romannikov,Vladimir,MD
Reproductive Endocrinology
Dlugi,Alexander M.,MD

Cinnaminson
Anesthesiology
Andalft,Anthony C.,MD
Assiamah,Andrew Aboagye,MD
Bowie,Lester J.,MD
Chun,John Y.,MD
Cypel,David,MD
Daniels,James W. III,MD
Feinerman,Larry Robert,MD
Goldberg,Marc B.,MD
Gordon,Jeffrey,MD
Gray,Terence Bay,MD
Halevy,Jonathan D.,MD
Kor,Danuta C.,MD
Law,Henry,DO
Lee,John C.,MD
Litvack,Steven Greg,MD
Luetke,Brian Scott,DO
Misher-Harris,Michele,DO
Paterson,William D.,MD
Shapiro,Jeffrey L.,MD
Shetty,Phyllis J.,MD
Siri,Matthew A.,MD
Soremekun Salami,Olutoyin M.,MD
Starrett-Keller,Cheryl M.,MD
Vaughn,Michelle Marie,MD
Waters,Renee M.,MD
Weiss,Evan A.,DO
Emergency Medicine
Sommers,Daniel,MD
Family Medicine
Laws-Mobilio,Susan Wendi,DO
Parchuri,Hima Bindu,DO
Rakickas,Jeffrey,MD
Switenko,Zenon M.,DO
Weingarten,Michael P.,DO
Ophthalmology
Dante,Karen L. Fung,MD
Physical Medicine & Rehab
Tomaio,Alfred C.,MD
Clark
Allergy
Sullivan,Bessie M.,MD
Cardiovascular Disease
Aliasgharpour,Farzin M.,MD
Chudasama,Lalji S.,MD
Sahni,Rakesh Kumar,MD
Sahni,Sheila,MD
Varshneya,Nikita,MD
Endocrinology
Prasad,Surabhi,MD
Family Med-Sleep Medicine
Pumo,Jerome Jr.,DO
Family Medicine
Beams,Michael E.,DO
Gilsenan,Michele T.,DO
Kowalenko,Karen F.,DO
Kowalenko,Thomas Alex,DO
Mathias,Claudia Fernandes,MD
Rushman,John Warren,MD
Sabharwal,Tina,MD
Syed,Zareen Taj,MD
Gastroenterology
Wexler,David E.,MD
Internal Medicine
Acocella,Michael A.,DO
Banayat,Geronimo Jr.,MD
Barry,Peter Francis,DO
Chudasama,Neelesh Lalji,MD
Ford,Stephen D.,MD
Goldstein,Alan F.,MD
Hwang,Cheng-Hong,DO
Kang,David H.,MD
Kornicki,Janusz S.,MD
Kudryk,Alexander B.,MD
Levin,Brandt M.,MD
Patel,Amish Thakor,DO
Prasad,Sudhanshu,MD
Vijayakumar,Asha M.,MD
Neonatal-Perinatal Medicine
Suapengco-Samonte,Dulce H.,MD
Obstetrics & Gynecology
Beauchamp,Jeffrey Thomas,MD
Blum,Richard Howard,MD
Hoebich,Karen A.,MD
Melamud,Elaine A.,MD
Wong,So Mui,MD
Ophthalmology
Inverno,Anthony J.,MD
Jacobs,Miriam,MD

Physicians by Town and Medical Specialty

Clark (clark)
Orthopedic Surgery
Bercik,Robert J.,MD
Rheumatology
Nucatola,Thomas R. Jr.,MD

Clarksboro
Family Medicine
Provencher,Robert A.,DO
Forensic Pathology
Feigin,Gerald A.,MD

Clayton
Family Medicine
Schopfer,Carl L.,DO

Clementon
Family Medicine
Patel,Pradip N.,MD
General Practice
Heck,Gary X.,DO

Cliffside
Emergency Medicine
Nayman,Defne,MD

Cliffside Park
Acupuncture
Desai,Aruna A.,MD
Anesthesiology
Pancu,Ion V.,MD
Cataract
Arturi,Frank C.,MD
Dermatology
Hershenbaum,Esther,MD
Diagnostic Radiology
Dhanani,Harsha Narendra,MD
Emergency Medicine
Chouake,Benjamin S.,MD
Family Medicine
Cirignano,Barbara M.,MD
Weinberger,George T.,DO
Gastroenterology
Fishbein,Susan,MD
General Practice
Spinapolice,Joseph A.,DO
Internal Medicine
Friedman,Bernard,MD
Hamada,Murray S.,MD
Joseph,Merab,MD
Korenfeld,Alexander,MD
Korenfeld,Yelena,MD
Master,Violet S.,MD
Righthand,Richard N.,MD
Obstetrics & Gynecology
Adu-Amankwa,Bernice Abrafi,MD
Amerson,Afriye Rochelle,MD
Ophthalmology
Levine,Richard Evan,MD
Movsovich,Alexander I.,MD
Orthopedic Surgery
Corradino,Christine M.,MD
Pediatrics
Lee,Inna,MD
Sethi,Chitra,MD
Physical Medicine & Rehab
Groves,Danielle Breitman,MD
Xu,Qian,MD
Psychiatry
Ruvolo,Michelle,MD
Spinal Surgery
Finnesey,Kevin Sean,MD
Urology
Chun,Thomas Young,MD
Klafter,George,MD
Margolis,Eric Judd,MD
Simon,Daniel Ross,MD
Simon,Robert B.,MD
Wasserman,Gary D.,MD

Clifton
Adult Psychiatry
Weinshenker,Naomi Joyce,MD
Allergy
Caprio,Ralph E.,MD
Klein,Robert Michael,MD
Allergy & Immunology
Zanjanian,M. H. Amir,MD
Anesthesiology
Agarwal,Meenoo,MD
Ames-Bobila,Deborah,MD
Anannab,Kevin C.,MD
Dang,Saurabh,MD
De La Mota,Jessica Isabel,DO
Kang,Richard T.,MD
Koppel,Todd Sloan,MD
Nasiek,Dariusz Jacek,MD
Popa,Vincentiu,MD
Shah,Sachin K.,MD
Shapiro,Leonid,MD
Sheikh,Afzal J.,MD
Sinha,Binod P.,MD
Sinha,Neil,MD
Szczech,Kazimierz M.,MD
Tankha,Pavan,DO
Anesthesiology: Pain Medicine
Kizina,Christopher Allen,MD
Michail,Mohsen T.,MD
Patel,Anjali Dalal,DO
Patel,Dipan G.,MD
Valskys,Rytis,MD
Cardiovascular Disease
Ahmad,Ali,MD
Brown,Elliot M.,MD
Jawetz,Seth Gerald,MD
Julie,Edward,MD
Krol,Ryszard B.,MD
Obeleniene,Rimvida,MD
Prakash,Atul,MD
Sankholkar,Kedar Deepak,MD
Skolnick,Bruce A.,MD
Sullivan,Brendan Patrick,MD
Sullivan,Gregory F.,MD
Szwed,Stanley A.,MD
Teicher,Mark,MD
Weiss,Emmanuel M.,MD
Cardiovascular Surgery
Syracuse,Donald C.,MD
Colon & Rectal Surgery
Buckley,Michael K.,MD
Critical Care Medicine
Levin,Daniel H.,MD
Dermatology
Gold,Jonathan Allan,MD
Militello,Giuseppe M.,MD
Ros,Adriana Oksana,DO
Silber,Judy G.,MD
Tanzer,Floyd R.,MD
Zurada,Joanna Magdalena,MD
Diagnostic Radiology
Ferdinand,Brett D.,MD
Thierman,David H.,MD
Yuppa,Frank R.,MD
Emergency Medicine
Abbasi,Tareef M.,MD
Ugras Rey,Sandra S.,DO
Endocrinology
Jasper,Josephine V.,MD
Khaddash,Saleh I.,MD
Roehnelt,Alessia Carluccio,MD
Schulder-Katz,Micol,MD
Schultz,Atara Batsheva,MD
Shalem,Lena Hourwitz,MD
Family Medicine
Adedokun,Emmanuel Adekunle,MD
Bhaskarabhatla,Krishna V.,MD
Chen,David,MD
Del Casale,Thomas Ernest,DO
Delisi,Michael David,MD
Dhamotharan,Shakira N.,MD
Dobrow,Michael Craig,DO
Doroudi,Shideh,MD
Fyffe,Ullanda P.,MD
Guerzon,Pearl Tolentino,MD
Gupta,Vikram,MD
Igbokwe,Jennifer,MD
Kahlon,Tejinderpaul Singh,MD
Lavian,Pejman,MD
Leon Wong,Hector J.,MD
Leroy,Christine,MD
Lima,Francesco W.,MD
Lucila,Rafael R.,MD
Maneyapanda,Mukundha B.,MD
Mangone,Jesse G.,DO
Mao,Cheng-An,MD
Miller,Randall W.,DO
Muccino,Gary P.,MD
Nunez,Jacqueline Denise,MD
Odatalla,Bassam N.,MD
Palmer,Susan M.,DO
Pinzon,Amabelle Par,MD
Pogorelec,Albert Joseph Jr.,DO
Pudinak,Anna,MD
Sabido,Michael,MD
Shraytman,Arkadiy,DO
Singh,Manik,MD
Testa,David A.,DO
Thomas,Seymour W.,MD
Tindoc,Lorelane Pagulayan,MD
Gastroenterology
Agarwal,Anil,MD
Baddoura,Walid J.,MD
Baum,Howard B.,MD
Boxer,Andrew Scott,MD
Farkas,John J.,MD
Gronowitz,Steven D.,MD
Gupta,Ashok,MD
Krohn,Natan Nata,MD
Okun,Jeffrey,MD
Reydel,Boris,MD
General Practice
Doerr,Alphonsus L.,MD
Geriatrics
Lashin,Waleed Sirag,MD
Hand Surgery
Lakin,Jeffrey F.,MD
Hematology
Uhm,Kyudong,MD
Hematology Oncology
Afonja,Richards A.,MD
Maroules,Michael,MD
Strakhan,Marianna,MD
Todi,Neelam T.,MD
Hospitalist
Weiss,Jeffrey A.,MD
Infectious Disease
Munera,Rodolfo A.,MD
Najjar,Sessine,MD
Okoye,Frederick E. Jr.,MD
Sultana,Yasmeen,MD
Weiss,Gabriella Antionette,MD
Internal Medicine
Alday,Arnold M.,MD
Berkel,Reyhan,MD
Blanco,Renato J.,MD
Boutros,Maged T.,MD
Brancato,Jaclyn,DO
Cecere,Antoinette M.,MD
Coleman,Scott L.,MD
De La Cruz,Angel Ramon,MD
Debell,David Anthony,MD
Diar Bakerli,Hala,MD
Dixon,George C.,MD
Ferrazzo-Weller,Marissa G.,DO
Gajdos,Robert M.,MD
Ganesan,Azhagasund,MD
Gellis,Dana B.,MD
Goldberg,Marc A.,MD
Goyal,Neil Kamal,MD
Graber,David J.,MD
Hajjar,Bassam,MD
Humera,Rafath Khatoon,MD
Huskowski,Piotr,MD
Jacknin,Mark A.,DO
Jawetz,Harold I.,MD
Jo,Young I.,MD
Kelleher,Maureen Michelle,MD
Korenblit,Pearl,MD
Krisa,Paul C.,MD
Krutak-Krol,Halina M.,MD
Lewko,Michael P.,MD
Llacuna,Florencio Jr.,MD
Mekkawy,Ahmed A.,MD
Murillo,Narcisa E.,MD
Najjar,Joe E.,MD
Narang,Sudershan,MD
Nop,Mallory,MD
Nwosu-Nelson,Joel E.,MD
O'Brien,Joseph Patrick,MD
Onat,Nermi,MD
Onyeador,Beatrice Ogbonne,MD
Pensabeni Jasper,Tiziana,MD
Porras,Cornelio J.,MD
Porter,Joseph M.,MD
Rana,Najmul,MD
Raval,Parthiv V.,MD
Rey,Ricardo,MD
Reyes,Emmanuel B.,MD
Rizvi,Syed M.,MD
Rubino,Gennaro,MD
Russo,Melchiorre J.,MD
Sahu,Anand P.,MD
Sahu,Sharad,MD
Sandler,Rebecca Ellen,MD
Schactman,Brian,MD
Singh,Sarva D.,MD
Torres,Catherine P.,MD
Turner,James William III,MD
Urena,Julio H.,MD
Wooton,Robert P. Jr.,MD
Medical Oncology
Benn,Howard A.,MD
Zaman,Aamir,MD
Neurological Surgery
Cifelli,John Riggio,MD
Neurology
Katz,Avery S.,MD
Knep,Stanley J.,MD
Lequerica,Steve A.,MD
Nangia,Arun,MD
Padela,Mohammad F.,MD
Tagayun,Myrna B.,MD
Obstetrics & Gynecology
Balzani,Henry H.,MD
Boyle,Elizabeth Anne,DO
Dinu,Catalina,MD
Haddad,Charles George,MD
Hakimi,Daniel,DO
Khan,Farhana Haleem,MD
Kugler,Edward F.,MD
Langer,Orli,MD
Pajoohi,Soheil,MD
Saba,Souheil,MD
Shah,Vinay R.,MD
Singh,Sukhdeep,MD
Smith,Jacqueline Marie,MD
Smith,Jade,DO
Sullivan,Jared Martin,MD
Tah,Peter A.,MD
Ophthalmology
Burrows,Adria,MD
Cucci,Patricia,MD
Cuttler,Nirupa C.,MD
Green,Donald H.,MD
Lesko,Cecily A.,MD
Mund,Michael L.,MD
Purewal,Baljeet Kaur,MD
Stegman,Daniel Ychac,MD
Wunsh,Stuart Eugene,MD
Orthopedic Surgery
Ambrose,John F.,MD
Hole,Robert L.,MD
Kraut,Lawrence,MD
Megariotis,Evangelos,MD
Rifai,Aiman,DO
Otolaryngology
Ledereich,Philip S.,MD
Pediatric Orthopedics
Russonella,Michael C.,DO
Pediatric Urology
Sanzone,John,MD
Pediatrics
Alvarez,Marie Emma B.,MD
Ayeni,Ahisu I.,MD
Basta,Janette A.,MD
Basta,Magdy Z.,MD
Brondfeld,Raquel Lara,MD
Buchalter,Maury,MD
Burton,Deniz Michelle,MD
Elhagaly,Hatem,MD
Gadalla,Hisham Hussein,MD
Grullon Okumus,Ariolis C.,MD
Gunn,Angela Lijoi,MD
Hanna,Ruba,MD
Iwelumo,Ifeoma N.,MD
Jawetz,Robert Evan,MD
Jedlinski,Tadeusz,MD
Lavaia,Maria A.,MD
Lew,Lai Ping,MD
Lewis,Michael Glenn,MD
Lugo,Mirian Dolores,MD
Matta,Rana C.,MD
Mediterraneo,Susan,MD
Modrzejewska-Kortowska,M.,MD
Mohammed,Ashraf,MD
Niziol,John A.,MD
Pagano,Christine Federline,MD
Patel,Shivani J.,MD
Rakhimova,Gulbakhor A.,MD
Sadegh,Mona,MD
Sarigul,Melih B.,MD
Schaffer,Ashley Marie,MD
Schein,Aviva R.,MD
Soto-Pereira,Angelica Maria,MD
Sutter,John I.,MD
Thomas,Mary Kathleen,MD
Tokat,Ikbal,MD
Wu,Karen,MD

Zamani,Mohammad,MD
Physical Med & Rehab-Pain Med
  Chen,Ivan,MD
Physical Medicine & Rehab
  Ibarbia,Jose D.,MD
  Ioffe,Julia,MD
  Rusli,Melissa K.,DO
Plastic Surgery
  Baruch,Michael I.,MD
  Greco,Dante,MD
Psychiatry
  Cusano,Paul Jr.,MD
  Jasper,Theodore F.,MD
  Keiman,Isidore Michael,MD
  Kim,Chang N.,MD
  Pascual,Bolivar,MD
  Pinchuck,Curt P.,MD
  Riccioli,Diana L.,MD
  Shah,Dilip A.,MD
  Sozzi,Roberto S.,MD
Radiology
  Doerr,John J.,MD
Rheumatology
  Albornoz,Louise A.,MD
  Raklyar,Irina,MD
Surgery (General)
  Hanan,Scott H.,MD
  Kane,Edwin P.,MD
  Silen,Ramon S.,MD
  Vazquez,Franklyn,MD
Thoracic Surgery
  Pontoriero,Michael Anthony,MD
Urology
  Greene,Tricia Danielle,MD
  Li,Sharon Mei-Mei,MD
  Marella,Venkata Koteswararao,MD
  Rice,Daniel A.,MD
  Rosenberg,Joel W.,MD
  Shahbandi,Matthew,MD
  Zinman,James Douglas,MD
Vascular Surgery
  Baratta,Joseph B.,MD
  Bobila,Alexis C.,MD
  Holmes,Raymond Joseph,MD
  Levison,Jonathan Andrew,MD
  Nackman,Gary B.,MD

Clinton
Body Imaging Radiology
  Klein,Laura B.,MD
Cardiovascular Disease
  Lind,Robert S.,MD
Diagnostic Radiology
  Lyons,Andrea Elizabeth,MD
  Sprenger,Alice Q.,MD
  Woo,Thomas Hyunsop,MD
  Zeng,Yu Grace,MD
Endocrinology
  Ryan,Wanda Dawn,MD
Family Medicine
  Bock,David Andrew,DO
  Celestino,Cecilia Cruz,MD
  Delvers,Dilek Sunay,MD
  Karpinski-Failla,Susan Ellen,DO
  Lunt,David M.,MD
  Messina,Charles I.,MD
  Petrillo,Jennifer Anne,MD
General Practice
  Silverberg,Michael S.,MD
Internal Medicine
  Braff,Ricky A.,MD
  Lifchus Ascher,Rebecca Jean,MD
  May,Philip B.,MD
  Torrens,Javier I.,MD
Neurological Radiology
  Saul,Jared Michael,MD
Obstetrics & Gynecology
  Whang,Gene,MD
Orbital Reconstructive Surgery
  Morgenstern,Kenneth Eli,MD
Pediatric Ophthalmology
  Bernstein,Jay M.,MD
Pediatrics
  Castillo,Ana A.,MD
  Coraggio,Michael J.,MD
  Kroon,Jody Lynn,MD
  Patel,Krishna A.,MD
Psychiatry
  Titus,Puthanpura J.,MD
Radiology
  Malzberg,Mark S.,MD

Roche,Kevin Joseph,MD
Closter
Allergy & Immunology
  Minikes,Neil Ira,MD
Anesthesiology
  Grunstein,Erno,MD
Dermatology
  Andrews,Alan D.,MD
  Ramaswamy,Preethi V.,MD
  Trokhan,Eileen Q.,MD
Internal Medicine
  Dhorajia,Shruti P.,DO
  Farooki,Zahid A.,MD
  Lee,Soo Gyung,MD
Orthopedic Surgery
  Trokhan,Shawn Edward,MD
Orthopedic-Hand Surgery
  Sokol,Shima C.,MD
Pediatric Ophthalmology
  Gonzales,Antonio M.,MD
Pediatrics
  Cavalli,Nina Ann,MD
  Nouman,Helena,MD
  Rosenberg,Lori A.,DO
  Yegen,Lonna K.,MD
Physical Medicine & Rehab
  Schindelheim,Adam M.,MD
Reproductive Endocrinology
  Segal,Thalia R.,MD
Sports Medicine
  Parron,John Keckhut,MD
Collingswood
Family Medicine
  Holwell,Michael,DO
  Moraleda,Jason N.,MD
  Neveling,Lance William,DO
  Winn,Robert Jerald,MD
  Yang-Novellino,Sue Y.,DO
General Practice
  Schiavone,Ronald L.,DO
  Stagliano,Robert A.,DO
Internal Medicine
  Corbett,Brian Joseph,DO
  Lauer,Marshall F.,MD
  McAllister,Susan Coutinho,MD
Obstetrics & Gynecology
  Margolin,Gregory,MD
  Parrish,Sherrilynn,MD
Ophthalmology
  Goldstein,Arthur Meyer,MD
  Kresloff,Michael Scott,MD
  Kresloff,Richard S.,MD
  Young,Marc,MD
Pediatrics
  Georgelos,Panagiotis,MD
  Velasco,Reynaldo,MD
  Weber,Carolyn Harding,MD
Psychiatry
  Calafiura,Peter C.,MD
Colonia
Allergy
  Sahni,Harsha R.,MD
Family Medicine
  Awan,Rabia S.,MD
  Guzik,David J.,DO
  Rukh,Lala,MD
Geriatric Psychiatry
  Mayer,Martin P.,MD
Internal Medicine
  Partenope,Nicholas A.,MD
Otolaryngology
  Sahni,Rana S.,MD
Pediatrics
  Benoy,Leena,MD
  Casarona,Charles A.,MD
  Charaipotra,Neelam,MD
  Chaudhary,Jigisha S.,MD
  Dubbaka-Rajaram,Arunasree,MD
  Kishen,Anita,MD
  Patel,Gaurang R.,MD
  Sonavane,Vidya Kiran,MD
Psychiatry
  Alvarez,Reinaldo G.,MD
Surgery (General)
  Tonzola,Anthony M.,MD
Colts Neck
Family Medicine
  Angello,Philip Joseph,MD
  Gibson,Lisa Kay,MD
  Raymond,Kimberly J.,MD

Holistic Medicine
  Huang,Wendy,MD
Internal Medicine
  Gualberti,Joann,MD
  Gualberti-Girgis,Lisa,MD
  Katz,Howard A.,DO
  Mankarios,Farag Amin Farag,MD
  Patel,Shital,MD
  Yelchur,Anuradha,MD
Obstetrics & Gynecology
  Sikand,Vandna,MD
Pediatrics
  Bautista,Jocelyn B.,MD
  Liao,Jennifer Ledesma,MD
  Makowsky,Tammy B.,MD
  Peters,Nancy Castellucci,MD
Plastic Surgery
  Iorio,Louis Michael,MD
Psychiatry
  Feuer,Elizabeth Janet,MD
Columbia
Family Medicine
  Arvary,Gary J.,MD
  Cullen,Eugene A.,MD
  Greenberg,Anthony,MD
  Molnar,Eric D.,DO
Internal Medicine
  Grote,Walter R.,DO
Obstetrics & Gynecology
  DeSanti,Michelina,DO
Columbus
Cardiovascular Disease
  Spagnuolo,Vincent J.,MD
Emergency Medicine
  Patel,Kamal B.,MD
Family Medicine
  Bross,Robert J.,MD
  Carcia,Danielle,DO
  Dunn,Davonnie Marie,MD
  Guiliano,Philip M.,MD
  Hulse,Andrea Doria,DO
  Jadeja,Poiyniba Dilip,MD
  Vare,Christopher,MD
Neurological Radiology
  Saffran,Bruce Nathan,MD
Obstetrics & Gynecology
  Chao,Christina,MD
Psychiatry
  Cha,Jaeok,MD
Cranbury
Child & Adolescent Psychiatry
  Salvatore,Kate Elizabeth,MD
Family Medicine
  Sethi,Shalini K.,MD
Geriatrics
  Smelkinson,Ann E.,MD
Internal Medicine
  Hebbalalu,Praphulla,MD
  Nagulapalli,Chaitanya,MD
Otolaryngology
  Li,Ronald W.,MD
Physical Medicine & Rehab
  Lewis,Stephen B.,MD
Psychiatry
  D'Souza,Christabelle E.,MD
Cranford
Anatomic/Clinical Pathology
  Khan,Amjad A.,MD
  Qureshi,Mohammad Nasar,MD
Child & Adolescent Psychiatry
  Chong,Raymond Ee-Mook,MD
  Hong,Rolando Y.,MD
Diagnostic Radiology
  O'Connor,Mary T.,MD
Gastroenterology
  Margolin,Michael L.,MD
Internal Medicine
  Singh,Iqbal K.,MD
  Singh,Mohinder P.,MD
  Toro Echague,Bernardo J.,MD
Nephrology
  Imbriano,Michael A.,DO
Obstetrics & Gynecology
  Anzalone,Anthony,MD
  Kaye,Alissa Ellen,MD
  Kaye,Gary L.,MD
  Shah,Mahesh Maneklal,MD
Ophthalmology
  Calderone,Joseph Jr.,MD

Pediatrics
  Pogany,Ursula M.,MD
Psychiatry
  Cayetano,Victoria F.,MD
  La Forgia,Anthony Pantal,MD
  Lim,Vicente M. Jr.,MD
  Schweiger,Bruce Daniel,MD
Thoracic Surgery
  Bolanowski,Paul J.,MD
Urology
  Schwartz,Malcolm,MD
Cream Ridge
Internal Medicine
  Jivani,Rasik M.,MD
  Rosengarten,Herbert H.,MD
Pediatrics
  Peller,Alicia S.,MD
Cresskill
Child & Adolescent Psychiatry
  Brown,Patricia S.,MD
  McGowan,Seth A.,MD
  Munoz-Silva,Dinohra M.,MD
  Silva,Raul R.,MD
Dermatology
  Gonzalez,Lenis Marisa,MD
Family Medicine
  Shoshani,Shai,MD
Internal Medicine
  Kochlatyi,Sergei G.,MD
  Subramanian,Kavitha,MD
Maternal & Fetal Medicine
  Martins-Lopes,Maria C.,MD
Ophthalmology
  Guba,Russell F. Jr.,MD
Otolaryngology
  Blome,Mary,MD
Psychiatry
  Brenner,Laura Ennis,MD
  Nadella,Ruchi,MD
Dayton
Emergency Medicine
  Haddad,Stephanie I.,MD
Family Medicine
  Azam,Muhammad,MD
  Boudwin,James E.,MD
  Rivera,Tara Elizabeth,DO
Geriatrics
  Schaer,Teresa McKinley,MD
Internal Medicine
  Casper,Robert J.,MD
  Sharma,Shivani,MD
Pediatrics
  Genco,Thomas Albert,MD
Delmont
Family Medicine
  Pomerantz,Jeffrey David,DO
Delran
Dermatology
  Harkaway,Karen S.,MD
Emergency Medicine
  Hicks,Michael James,MD
Family Medicine
  Alcera,Roanna Espino,MD
  Friedman,Samuel L.,DO
  Graziano-Wilcox,Donna,DO
  Keller,Maureen Reilly,DO
  Smith,Kindra Renee,MD
  Starkman,Moishe,MD
Geriatrics
  Epstein,Jeffrey E.,MD
Hand Surgery
  Sattel,Andrew B.,MD
Internal Medicine
  Basara,Matthew Jr.,MD
  Berna,Renee Ann,MD
  Kabel,Stephen E.,DO
  Mirson,Sofiya,MD
  Pelimskaya,Lutsiya S.,MD
  Rausch,Debora Anne,MD
  Squires,Leslie S.,MD
Obstetrics & Gynecology
  Edwards,Linda J.,MD
  Ginwala,Khatoon T.,MD
  Obianwu,Chike W.,MD
Pediatrics
  Bastien,Pascale,MD
  Foreman,Michael J.,MD
  Harrell,Angela Duley,MD
  Hayes,Ciana Tyiesh,MD

Physicians by Town and Medical Specialty

Delran (cont)
Psychiatry
- Ghaffar, Sadia, MD
- Usmani, Aniqa, MD

Demarest
Anesthesiology
- Blackman, Bonnie E., MD

Dermatology
- Schiffman, Lawrence Adam, DO

Internal Medicine
- Farooki, Adil, MD

Surgery (General)
- Tadros, Mahfouz M., MD

Denville
Anatomic/Clinical Pathology
- Juco, Judy M., MD
- Li, Leonid, MD
- Rimarenko, Seraphim, MD

Anesthesiology
- Annadanam, Varalakshmi, MD
- Caguicla-Cruz, Natividad M., MD
- Dent, Dean A., MD
- Ho, Maggie May, DO
- Kleiner, Alexander, MD
- Krzanowski, Tracey J., MD
- Mistry, Bharati S., MD
- Rubinfeld, Philip J., MD
- Shiau, Horngfu, MD
- Specthrie, Leon Kotler, MD
- Sy, Nena L., MD
- Wang, Changzhen, MD
- Zembrzuski, Andrzej Jan, MD
- Zhou, Jie, MD
- Zhu, Ching, MD

Cardiovascular Disease
- Lopez, Juan, MD
- Shanley, Frank M., DO

Child & Adolescent Psychiatry
- Brandon, Meredith, MD
- Ying Chang, Jean S., MD

Critical Care Medicine
- Finkel, Richard I., MD

Dermatology
- Cham, Anita L., MD
- Moy, Winston C., MD
- Spinelli, Nancy Ann, DO

Diagnostic Radiology
- Solomon, Edward Martin, MD
- Sutker, Burton, MD
- Wexler, Jeffrey A., MD

Emergency Medicine
- Berman, Dean Adam, DO
- Guzas, Ronald P., DO
- Morato, Ramon V., MD
- Ortega, Stephanie Lynn Scham, MD
- Reardon, Erin Marie, MD
- Retirado, Allen S., MD
- Retirado, Vincent Paul, MD
- Ringwelski-Hannan, Anna Ewa, MD
- Rosica, John A., MD
- Somar, Rohan, MD
- Thepmankorn, Pidok, MD
- Tierney, Kevin J., MD
- Varma, Raghunandan Medavaram, DO

Endocrinology
- Las, Murray S., MD
- Rosenfeld, Cheryl Robyn, DO

Family Medicine
- Furst, Alan David, MD
- Gilo, Elmer S., MD
- Ho, John, MD
- Kaminetsky, Eric Jay, DO
- Kosoy, Edward, MD
- Zaki, Isaac Kamal, MD

Gastroenterology
- Emiliani, Vincent J., MD
- Heit, Peter, MD
- Soriano, John G., MD

General Practice
- Masone, Patricia A., MD
- Napoli, Salvatore, MD

General Preventive Medicine
- Ali, Majid, MD

Geriatrics
- Feigin, Leslie C., MD

Gynecology
- Siegel, Joseph K., MD
- Siegel, Stacey Beth, DO

Hematology
- Jan, Naveed A., MD

Hematology Oncology
- Bari, Fazal, MD

Hospitalist
- Toohey, Kristina, MD

Internal Medicine
- Aggarwal, Arvind Kumar, DO
- Banu, Dana R., MD
- Barbarito, Edward Joseph, MD
- Cheng, Yihong Henry, MD
- Collum, Robert G., MD
- Connolly, Melissa Jane, MD
- Gerges, Christine Nabil, DO
- Gironta, Michael Gerard, DO
- Goldshlack, Jack S., DO
- Kalaydjian, Garine, MD
- Kapadia, Rina, MD
- Levitz, Jason Sanford, MD
- Levy, Seth Evan, MD
- Lopez, Jose M., MD
- Mandel, Gilbert B., MD
- Maniar, Sonali R., MD
- Mariwalla, Kiran, MD
- Masone, Daniel A., MD
- Mintz, Bruce L., DO
- Mintz, Shari Nan, MD
- Nicolai, Michael, MD
- Reiter, Barry A., MD
- Ricks, Jason D., MD
- Ruben, Yesudas, MD
- Sharma, Swati, MD
- Sheppell, Arthur L., MD
- Stansbury, Frederick H., DO

Maternal & Fetal Medicine
- Girz, Barbara A., DO

Medical Oncology
- Abbasi, Muhammad Rashid, MD
- Schreibman, Stephen M., MD

Neurological Radiology
- Manzo, Rene Paul, MD

Neurology
- Miric, Slobodan, MD

Nuclear Medicine
- Plutchok, Jeffrey J., MD

Obstetrics & Gynecology
- Agnello, Jennifer T., DO
- Rothenberg, Richard N., MD
- Shah, Yashica Manish, MD
- Tsai, Yan-San, MD

Oncological Surgery
- Holwitt, Dana M., MD

Ophthalmology
- Hade, Jason R., MD
- Levey, Stephanie B., MD
- Pearlman, Theodore F., MD

Orthopedic Surgery
- Capecci, Frank, MD
- Cubelli, Kenneth, MD
- Feldman, David J., MD
- Simmerano, Rocco Anthony, MD

Pediatric Neurodevelopment
- Haran, Pahirathi E., MD

Pediatrics
- Chait Kessler, Dana Erica, MD
- Craig, Krekamey Ropkui, MD
- De Cristofano, Robert E., MD
- Di Turi, Suzanne V., MD
- Dicker, Richard Irving, MD
- Ganek, Martin E., MD
- Magadan, Silvia Maria, DO
- Mann, Nora B., MD
- Samedi, Vanessa M., MD
- Thomas, Miriam, MD
- Umeukeje, Judith N., MD

Plastic Surgery
- Mamoun, Sami M., MD
- Marfuggi, Richard A., MD
- Nemerofsky, Robert Becker, MD

Psychiatry
- Alpert, Michael Charles, MD
- Ruiz, David A., MD
- Shafiq, Saima, MD

Pulmonary Critical Care
- Patel, Gaurang, MD

Pulmonary Disease
- Alexander, Robert Francis, MD

Radiation Oncology
- Hajela, Durgesh, MD

Radiology
- Mirza, Nadia M., MD
- Smith, Arvin P., MD

Waran, Shantha P., MD
Yu, Lawrence Sikyong, MD

Sleep Disorders Medicine
- Javed, Arshad, MD

Surgery (General)
- Cohen, Scott Allan, MD
- Simon, Marc L., DO
- Suh, Matthew Yongwon, MD

Urology
- Berman, Adam Jay, MD
- Bonder, Irvin Mark, MD
- Cubelli, Vincent, MD
- Friedman, Lawrence, MD
- Gellman, Alexander C., MD
- Ingber, Michael S., MD
- Ware, Steven M., MD
- Zimmerman, Gregg E., MD

Deptford
Emergency Medicine
- Warden, Todd M., MD

Internal Medicine
- Aquilino, Linda Kristine, DO

Obstetrics
- Robinson, John Michael, DO

Pediatrics
- Alikhan, Salma, MD
- Coant, Pierre N., MD
- Laudati, Mary, MD
- Minutillo, Angelo L., MD

Sports Medicine
- Emanuele, William Anthony, DO

Dover
Allergy
- Bigelsen, Stephen J., MD

Diagnostic Radiology
- Diaz, Francis L., MD
- Freeman, Neil J., MD

Family Medicine
- Bishop, Douglas Scott, MD
- Sweinhart, Marty Dawn, MD

Gastroenterology
- Krupnick, Matthew E., MD
- Rybalov, Sergey, MD

General Practice
- Bellamy, James E., DO

Internal Medicine
- Balaji, Mini, MD
- Gannu, Rajyalakshmi M., MD
- Golombek, Steven J., MD
- Li, Lisa, DO
- Panchal, Rupa Jaydip, MD
- Ramirez-Alexander, Rina M., MD
- Rosales Zincone, Jeannette A., MD
- Schonfield, Leah R., DO
- Studint, Erika B., MD
- Udani, Neil P., MD
- Zorrilla, Lilian, MD

Neurology
- Dover, Marcia Anne, MD
- Roberts, Paul J., MD
- Stephen, Infanta Anusha, MD

Obstetrics & Gynecology
- Wallis, Joseph J., DO

Ophthalmology
- Mann, Eric Bryce, MD
- Schorr, Ian M., MD

Orthopedic Surgery
- Bouillon, Louis R., MD
- Rosenzweig, Abraham H., MD
- Rubinfeld, David I., MD
- Spielman, Joel H., MD
- Stecker, Steven, MD
- Tiger, Arthur H., MD

Pediatrics
- Collins, Ronald A., MD
- Kotler, Amy Maxine, MD
- Prakash, Kalpana, MD
- Restrepo, Mauricio, MD
- Szuchman, Mario, MD
- Taitel, Janice Beth, MD

Physical Medicine & Rehab
- Brady, Mary E., MD

Radiation Oncology
- Cann, Donald F., MD

Rheumatology
- Pare', Jeanne M., MD

Surgery (General)
- Garrison, Jordan Milton, MD

Dumont
Anesthesiology
- Raziuddin, Mazherunni, MD

Family Medicine
- Cabela, Gina Flores, MD
- Desplat, Philippe, DO
- Kumar, Puneet, MD

Internal Medicine
- Hoffman, Esther Sima, DO

Obstetrics & Gynecology
- Chinchankar, Rajeshree P., MD
- Kim, Sonia, MD

Pediatrics
- Smith, Terri L., MD

Psychiatry
- Gorgo, Jessica, DO

Dunellen
Internal Medicine
- Karu, Moiz S., MD

Psychiatry
- Haim, Sara Rose, MD

Urology
- Chen, Samuel Kuangzong, MD

East Brunswick
Adolescent Medicine
- Gengel, Natalie, MD
- Sung, Boram, MD

Adult Psychiatry
- Borodulin, Boris, MD

Allergy
- Guirguis, Sonia S., MD
- Leibner, Donald N., MD

Allergy & Immunology
- Axelrod Malagold, Sara H., MD

Anesthesiology
- Basilious, Manal, MD
- Levin, Alexander G., MD
- Meltz, Marcy Mencher, MD
- Weinstein, Craig M., MD
- Yama, Asher Z., MD
- Zedie, Nishat, MD

Anesthesiology: Pain Medicine
- Lam, Sofia Levin, MD

Body Imaging Radiology
- Sussmann, Amado Ross, MD
- Yang, Charles, MD

Cardiovascular Disease
- Altmann, Dory Bert, MD
- Avendano, Graciano Gary F., MD
- Burns, John J., MD
- Chai, Yee Meen, MD
- Kalra, Amit, MD
- Keller, Barnes D., MD
- Kim, Hyung G., MD
- Kumar, Ashok, MD
- Kumar, Nidhi, MD
- Mermelstein, Erwin, MD
- Oberweis, Brandon Scott, MD
- Passi, Rakesh K., MD
- Saviano, George J., MD
- Schaer, David H., MD
- Shell, Roger A., MD
- Siu, Dwayne Winfred, DO

Child & Adolescent Psychiatry
- Bekhit, Mariam, MD
- Dyckman, Steven Ira, MD

Colon & Rectal Surgery
- Patankar, Sanjiv Krishna, MD

Cosmetic Surgery
- Arno, Joseph P., MD

Critical Care Medicine
- Harangozo, Andrea M., MD
- Klitzman, Donna Leslie, MD
- Schiffman, Philip L., MD

Dermatology
- Iannotta, Patricia N., MD
- Rothfleisch, Jeremy Evan, MD
- Shraga, Alexander, MD
- Weinstein, Rita, MD

Diagnostic Radiology
- Amorosa, Judith K., MD
- Bier, Steven Jeffrey, MD
- Bodner, Leonard, MD
- Bramwit, Mark P., MD
- Brown, James Harvey, MD
- Bulkin, Yekaterina, MD
- Carney-Gellella, Erin D., MD
- Carroll, Michael R. III, MD
- Censullo, Michael Louis, MD
- Chai, Bob B., MD

Chaise,Laurence S.,MD
Chin,Deanna G.,MD
Chiu-Serodio,Lai-No,MD
Derman,Arnold,MD
Dorr,Jeffrey,MD
Eardley,Anna Mary,MD
Ecker,Teresa,MD
Epstein,Robert E.,MD
Feinstein,Richard S.,MD
Flynn,Daniel E.,MD
Freeman,Eliot,MD
Garner,Eve Marybeth,MD
Girgis,Wahid S.,MD
Glynn,Nicole Lasasso,MD
Greenberg,Caroline M.,MD
Greenblatt,Adrienne Masin,MD
Grygotis,Laura Anne,MD
Harrigan,John T.,MD
Hira,Ajay,MD
Kandula,Praveena,MD
Keller,Irwin A.,MD
Kennedy,Eugene Cullen,MD
Kim,Sue Yeon,MD
Krieg,Eileen M.,MD
Kron,Stanley M.,MD
Lebovitz,Yaron,MD
Lee,Ellen,MD
Levine,Charles Daniel,MD
Lotan,Roi Meir,MD
Melendez,Jody Michael,MD
Moubarak,Issam F.,MD
Needell,Gary S.,MD
Notardonato,Henry,MD
Oliveros,Elder A.,MD
Pandya,Dipti,MD
Paster,Lina Famiglietti,MD
Patel,Gitanjali,MD
Patel,Rahul,MD
Romero,Melchor D.,MD
Roychowdhury,Sudipta,MD
Rozenberg,Aleksandr,MD
Samuels,Paul Louis,MD
Saraiya,Mansi Shah,MD
Sarokhan,Carol T.,MD
Schram,Adriann Susie,MD
Shah,Kumar,MD
Simon,Mitchell Lyle,MD
Slater,Gregg Matthew,MD
Sokol,Levi Olatokunbo,MD
Solonick,Douglas M.,MD
Sorkin,Norman S.,MD
Torrei,Payam G.,MD
Vasani,Devang,MD
Venezia,Sara,DO
Walor,David Michael,MD
Warren,Stephen W.,MD
Wolfson,Natasha Susan,MD
Yi,Bryan Sang,MD
Yoon,Hyukjun,MD
Zawodniak,Leonard J.,MD
Endocrinology
Hrymoc,Zofia,MD
Maman,Arie,MD
Mathew,Mini Ann,DO
Surgan,Matthew Louis,MD
Family Medicine
Azer,George S.,MD
Davis,Michele,DO
Geller,Toby A.,MD
Goldman,Iosif,DO
Ifabiyi,Lubunmi,MD
Khalil,Venus T.,MD
Klots,Larisa,DO
Lau,Ronald,MD
Marmora,James J.,MD
Nee,Patricia B.,MD
Schiano,Catherine Jean,DO
Tomlinson-Phelan,Michelle A.,DO
Gastroenterology
Botros,Nashed G.,MD
Chen,William Y.,MD
Costa,Jose Carlos,MD
D'Mello,Francisco C.,MD
Krawet,Steven Howard,MD
Lenger,Ellis S.,MD
Plumser,Allan B.,MD
General Preventive Medicine
Miller,Andrew David,MD
Hospitalist
Modi,Chirag H.,MD
Infectious Disease
Kallich,Marsha M.,MD

Snepar,Richard A.,MD
Insurance Medicine
Hochstadt,Bruce A.,MD
Internal Medicine
Abdelmalek,Moheb S.,MD
Akyar,Selma Ender,MD
Ales,Kathy L.,MD
Altobelli,Anthony III,MD
Amara,Sreenivasrao,MD
Balog,Joshua David,MD
Basalaev,Misha,MD
Burghli,Rena F.,DO
Chen,Karl Timothy,MD
Chilukuri,Neelima,MD
Creel,Marilyn U. Baruiz,MD
DeMoss,Jeanne Lorraine,DO
Fanous,Venis F.,MD
Fischler,David Ross,MD
Friedman,Inga,MD
Gabriel,Ahab M.,MD
Ghobraiel,Raafat Tawfek,MD
Grinblat,Inessa,MD
Gurland,Ira Alan,MD
Habib,Michael George,MD
Kapchits,Elmira,MD
Kaplan,Murray C.,MD
Katseva,Alla,MD
Kim,Christian C. K.,MD
Kolasa,Christopher,MD
Kulischenko,Alexander W.,MD
Kulischenko,Idelma,MD
Lee,Anna F.,MD
Li,Dena Yuyun,MD
Liu,Jenny,MD
Maimon,Olga M.,MD
Morgan,Mena M.,MD
Morgan,Nashaat L.,MD
Morgan,Suzana Emil Anwer,MD
Moussa,Alber Helmy,MD
Rao,Aruna,MD
Redel,Henry,MD
Scheiner,Marc A.,MD
Sharma,Adity,MD
Simkhayev,Lev Samsonovi,MD
Sinha,Ashok Kumar,MD
Tadros,Wagih F.,MD
Terranova,Matthew Patrick Jr,DO
Tucci,Mauro A. III,MD
Werthaim,Ofer Avi,MD
Yager,Scott,MD
Magnetic Resonance Imaging
Mammone,Joseph F.,MD
Maternal & Fetal Medicine
Krishnamoorthy,Ambalavaner,MD
Sengupta,Shyamashree,MD
Medical Oncology
Nissenblatt,Michael J.,MD
Salwitz,James C.,MD
Nephrology
Mansour,Mervat B.,MD
Neurological Radiology
Basak,Sandip,MD
Fitzpatrick,Maurice,MD
Patel,Keyur Bhupendra,MD
Schlesinger,Scott D.,MD
Schonfeld,Steven M.,MD
Neurology
Lazar,Mark H.,MD
Lupyan,Yan,MD
Wasserstrom,William R.,MD
Nuclear Medicine
Becker,Murray David,MD
Kempf,Jeffrey Scott,MD
Thind,Pritinder K.,MD
Yudd,Anthony P.,MD
Obstetrics & Gynecology
Beim,Daniel S.,MD
Bharucha,Dilip I.,MD
Cernadas,Maureen,MD
Cherot,Elizabeth Kagel,MD
Chudner,Margarita,MD
Duke,Stephanie D.,MD
Fisher,Deneishia Shramaine,MD
Gleason,Abigail Hott,MD
Gross,Renee,MD
Gupta,Manjari,MD
Huang,Michelle,MD
Kinsler,Kristin J.,DO
Martinez,Tiffany Annmarie,DO
Owunna,Uzoma I.,MD
Panaligan,Donato A.,MD

Tomlinson-Phelan,Tracy M.,MD
White,Sanford F.,MD
Ophthalmology
Engel,Mark L.,MD
Han,Stella Insook,MD
Leitman,Mark William,MD
Su,Michael Yu-Man,MD
Sun,Nancy,MD
Witlin,Richard S.,MD
Yang,Kenneth E.,MD
Orthopedic Surgery
Adolfsen,Stephen Erik,MD
Bloomstein,Larry Z.,MD
Bowe,John A.,MD
Harnly,Heather Withington,MD
Klein,Kenneth Stuart,MD
Klein,Richard Ashley,MD
Laufer,Samuel J.,MD
Levine,Lewis Jonathan,MD
McKeon,John J.,MD
McPartland,Thomas Girard,MD
Tuason,Dominick Anthony,MD
Weisman,David Seth,MD
Otolaryngology
Edelman,Bruce Allen,MD
Highstein,Charles I.,MD
Horowitz,Jay B.,MD
Kaplan,Kenneth A.,MD
Rosenbaum,Jeffrey Mark,MD
Pediatric Neurodevelopment
Mintz,Jesse M.,MD
Pediatric Ophthalmology
Engel,John Mark,MD
Rousta,Sepideh T.,MD
Pediatric Orthopedics
Therrien,Philip J.,MD
Pediatric Radiology
Hanhan,Stephanie B.,MD
Hogan,James R.,MD
Lee,Vincent,MD
Rosenfeld,David L.,MD
Underberg-Davis,Sharon J.,MD
Pediatric Urology
Fleisher,Michael H.,MD
Vates,Thomas S. III,MD
Pediatrics
Booker,Larnie J.,MD
Cederbaum,Neil Kenneth,MD
D'Mello,Maria W.,MD
Fortin,Robert Glenn,MD
Gabriel,John,MD
Giorgi,Marilyn V.,MD
Goldman,Marvin,MD
Gordina,Alla,MD
Henner,Rochelle,MD
Jaroslow,Amy E.,MD
Jennings,Gloria Ann,MD
Kim,Hei Y.,MD
Kuyinu,Michael A.,MD
Li,Yan,MD
Liu-Lee,Yingxue S.,MD
Mikhail,Salwa M.,MD
Saif,Rashida Taher,MD
Shankar,Sujatha,MD
Shulman,Sabra W.,MD
Simon,Elisabeth M.,MD
Sweberg,Warren A.,MD
Tiefenbrunn,Larry J.,MD
Tuck,Michelle Patran,MD
Physical Medicine & Rehab
Han,Lu,MD
Mirmadjlessi,Noushin,MD
Oranchak,Deborah J.,DO
Weissman,Tanya,MD
Plastic Surgery
Herbstman,Robert A.,MD
Parler,Janet Patricia,MD
Vieira,Pedro,MD
Psychiatry
Carlo-Francisco,Kristen L.,DO
Gottlieb,Stanley,MD
Kassoff,David B.,MD
Ragone,John P.,MD
Rajan,Shirley M.,MD
Schlesinger,Esther M.,MD
Zomorodi-Ardebili,Waldburg,MD
Pulmonary Critical Care
Gilbert,Tricia Todisco,MD
Pulmonary Disease
Hutt,Douglas A.,MD
Waksman,Howard Kenneth,MD

Radiology
Banbahji,Salim,MD
Edwards,Teresa Michelle,MD
Freiberg,Evan,MD
Goldman,Jeffrey Philip,MD
Greer,Jeannete G.,MD
Jonna,Harsha R.,MD
Kadivar,Khadijeh,MD
Kotler,Stuart M.,MD
Lazzara,Elizabeth Wanda,MD
Leiman,Sher,MD
Levitt,Myron M.,MD
Li,Albert C.,MD
Nardi,Rebecca A.,MD
Nosher,John L.,MD
Platt,Marvin,MD
Prendergast,Nancy C.,MD
Salmieri,Karen Heather,MD
Samuel,Salim,MD
Simoes De Carvalho,Victor L.,MD
Stirling,Jeffrey E.,MD
Taylor,Christopher,MD
Tunc,Feza Sevket,MD
Uppal,Vijay L.,MD
Winchman,Heidi K.,MD
Zicherman,Barry A.,MD
Rheumatology
Lichtbroun,Alan S.,MD
Surgery (General)
Bagner,Ronald J.,MD
Ramanadham,Smita R.,MD
Urology
Feder,Marc T.,MD
White,Edward C.,MD
Vascular & Intrvntnal Radiology
Gendel,Vyacheslav,MD
Gribbin,Christopher E.,MD
Lakritz,Philip Shev,MD
East Hanover
Anesthesiology
Patel,Divya R.,MD
Emergency Medicine
Irving,Carol,MD
Endocrinology
Francis,Bruce H.,MD
Nicastro,Maryann,MD
Family Medicine
Gabriel,Laurice Helen,MD
Khanna,Roohi,DO
Gastroenterology
Shetzline,Michael Anthony,MD
Immunology
Grebenau,Mark David,MD
Internal Medicine
Felser,James M.,MD
Grande,Nancy J.,MD
Hamed,Kamal Abdel-Jabbar,MD
Liang,Liang,MD
Livote,Joanne,MD
Prestifilippo,Judith A.,MD
Tran,Ly-Le,MD
Medical Oncology
Tavorath,Ranjana,MD
Occupational Medicine
Garvey,Karen Marie,MD
Ophthalmology
Rispoli,Lauren C.,MD
Silverman,Cary M.,MD
Pathology
Gonzalez,Raimundo,MD
Pediatrics
Culver,Kenneth Wayne,MD
Dalati,Nadia,MD
Dapas,Frances,MD
Detrizio Carotenuto,Isabel,MD
Hernandez Comesanas,Gricel,MD
Marzella,Giuseppe,MD
Patel,Niraj Ranjit,MD
Physical Medicine & Rehab
Girardy,James Douglas,MD
Kortebein,Patrick,MD
Pasia,Eric,MD
Robalino-Sanghavi,Michelle,MD
Shmulevich,Mark,MD
Pulmonary Disease
Martin,Thomas Reed,MD
East Orange
Anatomic/Clinical Pathology
Ahmed,Shahida Y.,MD
Bowman,Cynthia L.,MD
Cai,Donghong,MD

Physicians by Town and Medical Specialty

East Orange (cont)
Anatomic/Clinical Pathology
Choe, Jin K., MD
Gupta, Suresh Kumar, MD
Anesthesiology
Wong, Jeanne, MD
Bloodbanking
Senaldi, Eric M., MD
Cardiovascular Disease
Amato, James L. Jr., MD
Binenbaum, Steve Z., MD
Lee, Terrance H., MD
Rajiyah, Gitendra, MD
Critical Care Medicine
Connell, Rebecca Kathleen, MD
George, Jason C., MD
Hashem, Bassam Emile, MD
Dermatology
Thomas, Isabelle Marie B., MD
Diagnostic Radiology
Gonzales, Sharon Frances, MD
Klyde, David Philip, MD
Lee, Mimi Shon, MD
Verona, Paul T., MD
Emergency Medicine
Kociuba, Marcin K., DO
Torres, Mariela, MD
Endocrinology
Pogach, Leonard M., MD
Family Medicine
Bhate, Soniya, MD
Choi, Hongsun, MD
Katta, Madhavi R., MD
Law, Jeremy P., MD
Morrell, Christopher, MD
Nasta, Sucheta M., MD
Witham, Marie-Grace, DO
Gastroenterology
Coffin, Nina R., MD
Cordoba, Isabelita Y., MD
Rudd, Jennifer N., MD
Vossough, Sima, MD
General Practice
Enabosi, Ellis, MD
Keno, Deborah, MD
Geriatrics
Stanislaus, Galen P., MD
Sunderam, Gnana, MD
Viswanatha, Kallahalli V., MD
Hematology
Kasimis, Basil S., MD
Prasad, Indra D., MD
Infectious Disease
Eng, Robert H., MD
Gibson-Gill, Carol M., MD
Internal Medicine
Antoine, Alycia N., MD
Antoine, Roland, MD
Bawa, Radhika, MD
Bishara, Christine, MD
Blaivas, Allen J., DO
Cahiwat, Ramona N., MD
Chang, Victor Tsu-Shih, MD
Chatha, Uzma Arshad, MD
Chi, Jinhan, MD
Clarke, Robert Anthony, MD
Cort, James T., MD
Costa, Antoinette G., MD
Cytryn, Arthur S., MD
Hemsley, Michael, MD
Hinds, Audrey M., MD
Kania, Nirmala R., MD
Machiedo, Christine C., MD
Maddali, Radhika, MD
Maddali, Sarala K., MD
Miller, Marilyn Ann, MD
Nygaard, Torbjoern G., MD
Ohri, Renu, MD
Rafiuddin, Shaleeza, MD
Ragavan, Vijay, MD
Raghavan, Padma, MD
Raju, Govinda S., MD
Ramdas, Kumar, MD
Salerno, Alexander Gerard, MD
Savaille, Juanito E., DO
Seth, Sarwan K., MD
Skurnick, Blanche Jacqueline, MD
Srinivas, Shanthi, MD
Stark, Richard C., MD
Stein, Bernardo, MD
Stevens, John M., MD
Strauss, Walter D., MD
Sunderam, Darshi, MD
Taitt, Beverley B., MD
Taylor, Douglas A., MD
Viswanatha, Amrutha, MD
Yarus, Christine V., MD
Yeldandi, Aruna G., MD
Yook, Soonjae, MD
Yudd, Michael, MD
Nephrology
Sastrasinh, Sithiporn, MD
Neurology
Clark, Ruth L., MD
Gupta, Pradip, MD
Maeda, Yasuhiro, MD
Terrence, Christopher Jr., MD
Obstetrics & Gynecology
Cailliau, Pamela Jean, MD
Meremikwu, Francisca Chinwe, MD
Okafor, Joana O., MD
St. Victor, Ruth Alleen, DO
Toliver, Clifford W., MD
Uzoaru, Charles O., MD
Occupational Medicine
Yang, Bin, MD
Oncology
Saraf, Nirmala, MD
Ophthalmology
Cunningham, Robert D., MD
Scott, Winston J., MD
Orthopedic Surgery
Matthews, Calvin C., MD
Otolaryngology
Caputo, Joseph L., MD
Pain Medicine
Joshi, Meeta Yatinkumar, MD
Pain Medicine-Interventional
Feit, Russell, MD
Pediatrics
Botrous, Suzanne W., MD
Dosunmu, Ronke Y., MD
Johnson, Curtis Jr., MD
Maniar, Madhavi N., MD
Maniar, Payal, MD
Martin Yeboah, Patrick V., MD
Nnaeto, Nkem V., MD
Ricciardi, Anthony Jr., MD
Spielholz, Kathi Melanie, MD
Verner, Edwina D., MD
Walcott, Adrian B., MD
Zambrano, Rosario M., MD
Physical Medicine & Rehab
Garstang, Susan Veronica, MD
Im, Chae K., MD
Ma, Rex Tak Chi, MD
Malhotra, Gautam, MD
Shenoy, Nigel Arvind, MD
Psychiatry
Adler, Michele L., MD
Charles, Ellis B., MD
Delaney, Beverly Renay, MD
Donepudi, Saila B., MD
Gordin, Mark, MD
Knight, Jennifer Mary, MD
Matin, Nadia, MD
Robertson, Joy G., MD
Roy, George A., MD
Sharma, Amrita, MD
Tintea, Petru Ion, MD
Pulmonary Disease
Abdel Fatgah, Nail S., MD
Kim, Jenny Hyunjung, MD
Radiology
Zuback, Joseph R., DO
Spinal Cord Injury Medicine
Farag, Amanda S., MD
Surgery (General)
Craig, Gazelle A., MD
Ducheine, Yvan D., MD
Joseph, Romane, MD
Machiedo, George W., MD
Surgical Critical Care
Tischler, Charles D., MD
Urology
Blumenfrucht, Marvin J., MD
Gilhooly, Patricia Eileen, MD
McGill, Winston Jr., MD
Pollen, Jeffrey Jonah, MD

East Rutherford
Family Medicine
D'Andrea, John Louis, MD
General Practice
Colaneri, John A., MD
Internal Medicine
Coyle, Genoveva F., MD
Dituro, Joseph William, MD
Kalra, Ritesh, MD
Popa, Marcela M., MD
Scolamiero, John C., MD

East Windsor
Allergy & Immunology
Gupta, Neeti, MD
Anesthesiology
Ali, Rehan Basharat, MD
Dermatology
Bagel, Jerry, MD
Keegan, Brian Robert, MD
Myers, Wendy A., MD
Nieves, David Steiner, MD
Simon, Jessica, MD
Stenn, Judit O., MD
Emergency Medicine
Sterman, Lance M., MD
Family Med-Geriatric Medicine
Beagin, Erinn Elizabeth, MD
Family Medicine
Skeehan, Christopher J., MD
Gastroenterology
Lupovici, Michael, MD
Internal Medicine
Bowers, Gabriela W., MD
Cimafranca, Daniel L., MD
Dhar, Vasudha, MD
Hanif, Ghalia, MD
Kunamneni, Katie Elizabeth, MD
Madapati, Indira, MD
Thomas, Brian David, MD
Valcarcel, Raul, MD
Wong, Christopher K., MD
Obstetrics & Gynecology
Eder, Scott E., MD
Gamburg, Eugene Samuel, MD
Markidan, Yana, MD
Simigiannis, Helen, MD
Pain Medicine
Yanni, Baher S., MD
Plastic Surgery
Wisser, Jamie R., MD
Surgery (General)
Dultz, Rachel Paula, MD

Eatontown
Anatomic Pathology
Wang, Xuan, MD
Anatomic/Clinical Pathology
Murakata, Linda Ann, MD
Radevic, Miroslav Rade, MD
Sheng, Huaibao, MD
Xie, Linjun, MD
Anesthesiology
Staats, Nancy Elizabeth, MD
Cardiovascular Disease
Bach, Matt, MD
Berger, Lance Seth, MD
Boak, Joseph G., MD
Daniels, Jeffrey S., MD
Daniels, Steven J., MD
Kapoor, Mahim, MD
Kim, Jiwon, MD
Koo, Charles H., MD
LaMarche, Nelson S., MD
Mascarenhas, Mark Adrian, MD
Mattina, Charles J., MD
O'Neill, Leon Frederick IV, DO
Osofsky, Jeffrey Lee, MD
Rizzo, Thomas F., MD
Rodriguez, Pascual B., MD
Sealove, Brett Andrew, MD
Wappel, Michael A., MD
Cardiovascular Surgery
Squillaro, Anthony J., MD
Colon & Rectal Surgery
Arvanitis, Michael L., MD
Dressner, Roy M., DO
Critical Care Medicine
Kramer, Violet Elizabeth, MD
Livornese, Douglas S., MD
Weiner, Sharon M., MD
Family Med-Sports Medicine
Krystofiak, Jason Anthony, MD
Family Medicine
Frantz, Mildred Marie, MD
Fertility/Infertility
Ziegler, William Francis, DO
Gastroenterology
Baig, Nadeem A., MD
Belitsis, Kenneth, MD
Fiest, Thomas C., DO
Gorcey, Steven A., MD
Merikhi, Laleh Afkham, MD
Uppal, Rajiv, MD
Gynecology
Greenleaf, Betsy Alice, DO
Hand Surgery
Atik, Teddy Labib, MD
Decker, Raymond Jr., MD
Fedorcik, Gregory Gerard, MD
Gabuzda, George Mark, MD
Pess, Gary M., MD
Internal Medicine
Arbes, Spiros M., MD
Ashok, Manjula, MD
Barnickel, Paul W., MD
Carideo, Ida M., MD
Churgin, Warren K., MD
Desai, Gautam J., MD
Einbinder, Lynne C., MD
Hanna, Manar H., MD
Haratz, Alan B., MD
Khulusi, Nami, MD
Kosinski, Robert M., MD
Morris, Sarah A., MD
Nivera, Noel Taroy, MD
Patel, Ashish Bhasker, MD
Patton, Chandler D., MD
Peeples, Charles B., MD
Ramachandra Rao, Vanie S., MD
Recho, Marielle, MD
Saybolt, Matthew Douglas, MD
Sridar, Buvaneswari, MD
Usman, Mohammed Haris Umer, MD
Interventional Cardiology
Selan, Jeffrey Craig, MD
Nephrology
Liss, Kenneth A., DO
Obstetrics & Gynecology
Mann, Jessica Salas, MD
Mensah, Virginia Akua, MD
Price, Andrea Noelle, MD
Ophthalmology
Edison, Barry Jay, DO
Pediatric Surgery
Staab, Victoriya S., MD
Pediatric Urology
Litvin, Yigal S., MD
Pediatrics
DeGroote, Richard J., MD
Farrell, Paul R., MD
Noaz, Golam G., MD
Rughani-Shah, Bindoo, MD
Wymer, Edwin Anthony, DO
Plastic Surgery
Ashkar, Michael George, MD
Lombardi, Anthony Stephen Jr., MD
Psychiatry
Batra, Sonal, MD
Fernandez, Gregory Scott, MD
Franco, Hugo C., MD
Khera, Gurbir Singh, MD
Spinal Surgery
Donald, Gordon D. III, MD
Surgery (General)
Binenbaum, Steven J., MD
Borao, Frank J., MD
Ciervo, Alfonso Clemente, MD
Hagopian, Ellen Joyce, MD
Kolakowski, Stephen Jr., MD
Lopyan, Kevin S., MD
Matharoo, Gurdeep Singh, MD
Thoracic Surgery
Scalia, Peter D., MD
Thompson, Robert M., MD
Urology
Geltzeiler, Jules M., MD
Keselman, Ira G., MD
Waldman, Ilan, MD

Edgewater

Allergy & Immunology
Li, Wei Wei, MD
Anesthesiology
Regan, Kasey Calvey, MD
Cardiovascular Disease
Admani, Irfan Mohamed, MD
Bareket, Yaron, MD
Codel, Radu, MD
Pumill, Rick J., MD
Raskin, Adam Brett, MD
Segovia, Fernando, MD
Child & Adolescent Psychiatry
Kondrashin, Sofia, MD
Santos, Frank, MD
Emergency Medicine
Rosines, Noam, MD
Family Medicine
Chhabra, Mohina Singh, MD
Kuwama, Chika, MD
Gastroenterology
Sciarra, Michael A., DO
Infectious Disease
Pradhan, Anuja A., MD
Internal Medicine
Alvarez-Segovia, Lucia M., MD
Portilla, Diana M., MD
Rotoli, Domenico, DO
Shin, John Jung Hoon, MD
Interventional Cardiology
Faraz, Haroon Ahmed, MD
Neurological Radiology
Garger, Alexander, MD
Neurology
Shajenko, Lydia, MD
Pediatric Endocrinology
Kaul, Sushma Dhar, MD
Lala, Vinod R., MD
Pediatrics
Chai, George, MD
Desai, Bhumika, MD
Leykin, Tanya, MD
Physical Medicine & Rehab
Putcha, Nitin, DO
Plastic Surgery
Kaplan, Gordon Marc, MD
Surgery (General)
Foote, Holly Christine, DO
Trauma Surgery
Miglietta, Maurizio A., DO
Urology
Pappas, Gregory A., MD

Edison

Adolescent Medicine
Hingrajia, Rashmin M., MD
Allergy
Centeno-McNulla, Ligaya V., MD
Kanuga, Jayesh G., MD
Anatomic Pathology
Chen, Fan, MD
Anatomic/Clinical Pathology
Finfer, Michael D., MD
Kim, Hazel Hae-sook, MD
Noreen, Shahla, MD
Patil, Madhavi Hari, MD
Anesthesiology
Armao, Michael Edward, MD
Beyus, Christopher Michael, MD
Chen, Evan, MD
Daftari, Amita P., MD
Daniel, Robert J., MD
Ding, Yifeng, MD
Gudimella, Lakshmi, MD
Guena, Luisa, MD
Handa Nayyar, Seema, DO
Isidro, Jose R. Jr., MD
Klyashtorny, Alexander, MD
Kothari, Kaumudi H., MD
Lee, Herb, MD
Li, Xin Qin, MD
Mereday, Clifton Samuel Jr., MD
Moises, Adam U. Jr., DO
Montefusco, Patrick P., MD
Pandya, Shridevi, MD
Patel, Bhupendrakumar V., MD
Patel, Shail, MD
Piratla, Lalitha, MD
Rock, Joel J., DO
Safdar, Mohammad Imran, MD
Samaan, Ayman Boushra, MD
Santos-Holgado, Maria C., MD
Siskind, Jonathan B., DO
Stewart, Judly Pierre, MD
Tan, Martin H., MD
Thompson, Matthew, MD
Utrankar, Deepti Sameer, MD
Zhang, Shehui, MD
Cardiovascular Disease
Barsky, Aron Alan, MD
Buck, Warren G., MD
Calvo, Ricardo A., MD
Cohen, Howard S., MD
Cohen, Larry J., MD
Cristoforo, Nancy Todd, MD
Duch, Peter M., MD
Feingold, Aaron J., MD
Keller, Malvin S., MD
Khan, Majid K., MD
Kovacs, Tiberiu, MD
Kushal, Amrita, MD
Molk, Ian J., MD
Noveck, Howard D., MD
Panebianco, Robert Antonino, MD
Ravi, Anita, MD
Rebba, Bhavana, MD
Rudnitzky, Elliot M., MD
Schanzer, Robert Joseph, MD
Sharma, Bhudev, MD
Wang, Danny, MD
Wasilewski, Stan J., MD
Cardiovascular Surgery
Heller, James Norman, MD
Javed, Mohammad Tariq, MD
Child & Adolescent Psychiatry
Castillo, Gregorio A. G., MD
Chowdhury, Amina Kausar, MD
Meghadri, Niveditha, MD
Child (Pediatric) Neurology
Bandari, Savitra M., MD
Milrod, Lewis Martin, MD
Ming, Xue, MD
Velicheti, Kavitha, MD
Clinical Cardiac Elctrphyslgy
Ballal, Raj Sadananda, MD
Clinical Pharmacology
Jacobs, Sharon G., MD
Colon & Rectal Surgery
Chinn, Bertram T., MD
Deutsch, Michael, MD
Notaro, Joseph R., MD
Critical Care Medicine
Anene, Okechukwu P., MD
Bhagat, Mahesh H., MD
Crawley, Joseph M., MD
Melillo, Nicholas G., MD
Pesin, Jeffrey L., MD
Ramachandraiah, Vidya, MD
Rosenblatt, Daniel E., MD
Dermatology
Paull, Robert M., MD
Strauch, Joseph M., MD
Diagnostic Radiology
Boruchov, Scott D., MD
Chakravarty, Mira, MD
Contractor, Daniel G., MD
Eshkar, Noam Simon, MD
Friedman, Robert A., MD
Galbraith, Michael, MD
Malantic-Lu, Grace Paula, MD
Mody, Suresh, MD
Parashurama, Prashant, MD
Parker, Martin I., MD
Peterson, Mary Ann, MD
Pierpont, Christopher Edward, MD
Pivawer, Gabriel, DO
Rebarber, Israel Frank, MD
Schmell, Eric Brad, MD
Schwarz, Naomi S., MD
Simon, Daniel W., MD
Weissmann, Murray H., MD
Emerg Medicine-Pediatric
Joshi, Samir V., MD
Emergency Medicine
Amin, Shilpa K., MD
Barsoom, Raafat S., MD
Cali, Michael D., MD
Chalabi, Dahlia, MD
Fernandez, Ronald Leonardo, MD
Gillespie, Kevin A., MD
Hill, Ryan Davidson, DO
Jean Philippe, Carolyne, MD
Johal, Gurvindra Singh, DO
Khanna, Vikas, MD
Lacapra, Samuel, MD
Mascarinas, Kristine I., DO
Mehta, Harendra U., MD
Sapira, Andrew S., MD
Schimler, Michael Edward, MD
Shrivastava, Arpita G., MD
Soukiazian, Sevak, MD
Steiner, Kenneth D., MD
Vanam, Kamalakar Rao, MD
Weiss, Daniel E., MD
Xavier, Geralda A., MD
Endocrinology
Bucholtz, Harvey K., MD
Dunn, Jonathan C., MD
Panicker, Usha R., MD
Shah, Suketu Rajina, MD
Family Medicine
Aderibigbe, Adedayo Olubunmi, MD
Arefeen, Samrana, MD
Assemu, Belen F., MD
Bhattacharyya, Adity, MD
Chae, Sung Yeon, MD
Collins, Harry, MD
Dalal, Gita S., MD
Diziki, Donna C., DO
Elber, Daniel A., DO
Estevez, Gerardo V., MD
Faches, Allison L., MD
Flores, Maria S., MD
Henderson, Thomas J., MD
Kandula, Sridevi, MD
Kwon, Seri, MD
Laroche, Harold I., MD
Metz, Deborah Lynne, MD
Metz, John Patrick, MD
Micabalo, Alvin Francis, DO
Milne, Charlene E., MD
Nadkarni, Swati G., MD
Nelson, Yvonne, MD
Patel, Dipesh Shashikant, DO
Patel, Hitesh Ramesh, MD
Patel, Naresh J., DO
Patel, Rahil, MD
Picciano, Anne, MD
Prasad, Kamil, MD
Reyes, Ruby Carina E., MD
Seck, Thomas F., MD
Sharma, Usha, MD
Sinha, Gopal K., MD
Subramanian, Srilakshmi, MD
Vermani, Prathiba, MD
Wiley, Olga V., MD
Wilks, Michelle Anne, MD
Winter, Robin O., MD
Wong, Patrick, MD
Zayoud, Rajaa M., MD
Fertility/Infertility
Qasim, Mahasin S., MD
Terens, William L., MD
Gastroenterology
Baik, Seoung W., MD
Chae, Scott S., MD
Cheela, Santosh K., MD
Goldberg, Michael Scott, MD
Hodes, Steven E., MD
Medina, Richard A., MD
Modi, Chintan, MD
Nahar, Sudha, MD
Nayar, Devjit Singh, MD
Patel, Mayank D., MD
Ramchandani, Kishore N., MD
Reissman, David I., MD
Rosenheck, David Mark, MD
Shugar, Ronald A., MD
Wolfman, Marc R., MD
General Practice
Agarwal, Sumitra, MD
Kukreja, Meenakshi, MD
Menashe, Richard B., DO
Geriatrics
Dhindsa, Sumeet, MD
Oser, William Jr., MD
Parikh, Rakesh K., MD
Hand Surgery
Lombardi, Robert M., MD
Hematology
Gupta, Juhee, MD
Wallach, Bruce H., MD
Hematology Oncology
Koduri, Beaula V., MD
Schuman, Richard M., MD
Hospitalist
Mistry, Nirav, MD
Obiefuna, Nkechiyere Angela, MD
Infectious Disease
Martinez, Homar Amador, MD
Paradiso, Mary J., MD
Ramasubramani, Anuradha, MD
Rathnakumar, Charumathi, MD
Sensakovic, John W., MD
Sree, Aruna, MD
Internal Medicine
Abdi, Zahra Jabeen, MD
Adabala, Ramesh, MD
Ahmad, Nausher, MD
Amjad, Maqsood, MD
Arora-Khera, Shruti, MD
Aurilio, Joseph P., MD
Bai, Flora, MD
Bangalore, Ramamurthy L., MD
Bhakey, Girija G., MD
Bhalla, Meenu Gogia, MD
Blum, Paul A., MD
Bonk, Rosemarie A., MD
Bruzzi-Ehrlich, Diane, MD
Bullock, Richard B., MD
Calabrese, David, MD
Canavan, Brian F., DO
Casale, Lisa M., MD
Cassidy, Thomas J., MD
Chen, Michael T., MD
Chung, Inyoung, MD
Dantuluri, Hemamalini, MD
DeSilva, Derrick Jr., MD
DeSimone, Luca, MD
Desai, Sagar R., MD
Desai, Vinay M., MD
Dippl, Julia M., MD
Estrellas, Bernabe A., MD
Felzenberg, Emily R., DO
Gandhi, Nabila Asif, MD
Ganeshamurthy, Agrahara, MD
Gbadamosi, Sikiru Aderoju, MD
Hariharan, Subramanian, MD
Hassan, Syed H., MD
Jagamony, Sandhya, MD
Jana, Kumar P., MD
Joshi, Archana N., MD
Kasuri, Jasbir K., MD
Khan, Basma, MD
Khetani, Manish P., MD
Kim, Stanley S., MD
Kleshchelskaya, Valeria, MD
Kumar, Arvind, MD
Kumar, Radha, MD
Kuza, Malgorzata W., MD
Lee, Hyok Yop, MD
Leighton, Harmony J., DO
Li, Meihong, MD
Li, Xiang, MD
Lin, Ruth Ann, MD
Long, George W., MD
Memon, Mohammad Khalil, MD
Misko, Gary J. Jr., MD
Moray, Nandini K., MD
Napiorkowski, Eva M., MD
Nisar, Mohammed P., MD
Nisar, Shiraz Ahmed, MD
Nowell, Martha A., MD
Pamerla, Mohan Ramkumar, MD
Patel, Bhupendra C., MD
Patel, Hetal Mahendra, MD
Patel, Indravadan T., MD
Patel, Jayendra M., MD
Patel, Mukesh M., MD
Patel, Narendra K., MD
Patel, Pankajkumar Vasantlal, MD
Patel, Pulin H., MD
Patel, Rajendra Harmanbhai, MD
Patel, Shefali S., MD
Payumo, Gene Louie, MD
Penn, James R., MD
Piperi, Vincent D., MD
Poco, Bernardo A., MD
Prasad, Niloo, MD
Rappai, James K., MD
Reisler, Scott, MD
Saini, Amarjit K., MD
Sappal, Baljit S., MD
Shah, Nehabahen V., MD

Physicians by Town and Medical Specialty

Edison (cont)
Internal Medicine
Shah, Pooja, MD
Shah, Taral Jobanputra, MD
Shastry, Jyothsna S., MD
Shen, Lijing, MD
Sinha, Anubha, MD
Snyder, Craig Adam, MD
Sutaria, Samir Hasmukh, MD
Tawde, Darshana Prafullaraj, MD
Taylor, Marian L., MD
Thakur, Shubhangi J., MD
Tirunahari, Vijaya Latha, MD
Unni, Nisha, MD
Upadhyay, Hinesh Natwarlal, MD
Uthappa, Machia M., MD
Vaidya, Ketankumar N., MD
Velmahos, Vasilios, MD
Wolf, Barry Z., MD
Zhang, Hao, MD
Laparoscopic Surgery
Jawed, Aram Elahi, MD
Nihalani, Anish B., MD
Nephrology
Czyzewski, Robert M., MD
Park, Jun-Ki, MD
Rajan, Samir, MD
Sarwar, Samina, DO
Neuro-Ophthalmology
Rosenberg, Michael L., MD
Neurological Radiology
Jilani, Mohammad Imran, MD
Neurological Surgery
Bashir, Asif, MD
Bloomfield, Stephen M., MD
Iyer, Asha Muthuraman, MD
Kuo, Howard, MD
Pan, Jeff, MD
Przybylski, Gregory J., MD
Shekhtman, Yevgenia, MD
Steineke, Thomas C., MD
Neurology
Bhat, Sushanth K., MD
Buchwald, Eugene E., MD
Chen, Shan, MD
Fourcand, Farah Yolanda, MD
Gan, Richard A., MD
Gupta, Divya, MD
Gupta, Simhadri M., MD
Hanna, Philip Andre, MD
He, Ming, MD
Herman, Martin N., MD
Hooshangi, Nossratollah, MD
Kirmani, Jawad F., MD
Kramer, Phillip D., MD
Landolfi, Joseph Charles, DO
Ma, Wei Wei, MD
Mani, Srinivasan S., MD
Mehta, Siddhart Kumar, MD
Merkin, Michael D., MD
Mian, Fawad A., MD
Miller, Gary Stuart, MD
Nizam, Mohammed Farrukh, MD
Noor, Emad Roshdy, MD
Oh, Youn K., MD
Panezai, Spozhmy, MD
Roblejo, Peter C., MD
Silveira, Diosely De Castro, MD
Singh, Amrinder, MD
Sinha, Sugiti, MD
Sobol, Igor Leonidovich, MD
Sobol, Marina B., MD
Uhrik, Eric Joseph, DO
Zu, James Shanwei, MD
Neuropathology
Nochlin Soto, David, MD
Nuclear Medicine
Jaffe, Robert M., MD
Miller, Howard M., MD
Obstetrics & Gynecology
Adefowokan, Rotanna I., MD
Arora, Ranjana, MD
Chung, Uei K., MD
Corsan, Gregory H., MD
Daiter, Eric, MD
Dave, Sangeeta, MD
Desai, Darshana A., MD
Essandoh, Louisa Efua, MD
Fleisch, Charles M., DO
Han, Ji Soo, MD
Holgado, Cesar B., MD

Keflemariam, Yodit J., MD
Mavani, Bharti N., MD
Metz, Rebecca L., MD
Palayekar, Meena Jayawant, MD
Patel, Atulkumar V., MD
Patel, Kirit Somabhai, MD
Patel, Ragin C., MD
Rama, Sreedevi, MD
Ramanarayanan, Annapurna, MD
Russell, Carol Mae, DO
Sachdev, Rahul, MD
Shah, Bharti C., MD
Steinbach, Gary B., MD
Twisdale, Donna R., MD
Occupational Medicine
Elber, Lee Bennett, DO
Mellendick, George James, MD
Ophthalmology
Breznak, Cindy M., MD
Park, John Chonghwan, MD
Patel, Hitesh K., MD
Press, Lorin R., MD
Schanzer, Barry M., MD
Schwartz-Eisdorfer, Barbara, MD
Shah, Himanshu Shirish, MD
Singh, Jasvinder, MD
Spirn, Benjamin David, MD
Spirn, Franklin H., MD
Sullivan-Miller, Julia Ann, MD
Yarian, David L., MD
Orthopedic Surgery
Charen, Jeffrey H., MD
Chen, Franklin, MD
Garfinkel, Matthew J., MD
Grover, Surender M., MD
Herrera-Figueira, Diego A., MD
Jamieson, Janine, DO
Lessing, David, MD
Lombardi, Joseph S., MD
Marcus, Alexander Michael, MD
Patel, Nilesh J., MD
Ramani, Mohnish N., MD
Russoniello, Alexander P., MD
Ryan, Todd C., DO
Schottenfeld, Mark A., MD
Thacker, Sunil Rajan, MD
Vega, Teresa, MD
Zimmerman, Joshua M., MD
Orthopedics
Patti, James E., MD
Otolaryngology
Arlen, Harold, MD
Aruna, Pasalai N., MD
Kraus, Warren M., MD
Lavine, Ferne R., MD
Miller, Andrew John, MD
Park, Robert Inyeung, MD
Pain Medicine-Interventional
Aranas, Rae Ronald, MD
Freeman, Eric D., DO
Spiel, Douglas J., MD
Pathology
Ewing, Clinton Alexander, MD
Pediatric Cardiology
Agarwal, Kishan C., MD
Pediatric Critical Care
Manaqibwala, Ummesalama M., MD
Shah, Sandeep K., MD
Pediatric Emergency Medicine
Cunningham, Frank J., MD
Pediatric Hematology Oncology
Pappas, Lara, MD
Pediatric Infectious Diseases
Kukla, Leon F., MD
Pediatrics
Altzman, Elana F., MD
Aziz, Khalid M., MD
Belnekar, Rudrani K., MD
Bhagwat, Gauri S., MD
Bhamidipati, Aparna, MD
Bupathi, Kavita Kishor, MD
Caasi, Santiago J. Jr., MD
Chae, Young Soo, MD
Devli, Aynur A., MD
Gayam, Vani, MD
Godlewska-Janusz, Elzbieta, MD
Gumidyala, Padmasree, MD
Kang-Lee, Elica J., MD
Kapila, Bina, MD
Kaur, Ranbir, DO
Kesavan, Dhanalakshmi, MD

Khanna, Santosh B., MD
Libis, Zhanna, MD
Maddalozzo, Wanda K. M., MD
Meszaros, Beata Duli, MD
Nadkarni, Nutan Shirish, MD
Navas, Carlene, MD
Nguyen, Hung Manh, MD
Nimma, Vijaya, MD
Patel, Natverlal M., MD
Patel, Suresh Ishwarlal, MD
Pierre, Margarette Rose, MD
Pompy, Amrita, MD
Pu, Jessica Lixia, MD
Raghu, Shalini Nagarajan, MD
Satwani, Sunita, MD
Shah, Lata R., MD
Shukla, Nimisha J., MD
Wang, Aijuan, MD
Zheng, Shao, MD
Physical Med & Rehab-Pain Med
Ceraulo, Philip, DO
Patel, Anup H., DO
Physical Medicine & Rehab
Agarwal, Sushma, MD
Aldea, Dyana Luz, MD
Bagay, Leslie, MD
Bhatt, Harish K., MD
Brown, David P., DO
Cuccurullo, Sara J. M., MD
Delavaux, Laurent, MD
Dunn, Anna Maria L., MD
Escaldi, Steven V., DO
Fleming, Talya K., MD
Greenwald, Brian David, MD
Hon, Beverly J., MD
Idank, David M., DO
Jafri, Abida Y., MD
Jafri, Iqbal H., MD
Joki, Jaclyn Beth, MD
Kanthala, Trishla Reddy, DO
Karnaugh, Ronald Daniel, MD
Kim, Christopher C., MD
Levine, Jaime Marissa, DO
Lin, Lei, MD
Luke, Ofure R., MD
Malone, Richard J., DO
McCagg, Caroline O., MD
Parikh, Sagar Shailesh, MD
Quevedo, Jonathan P., MD
Rossi, Roger P., DO
Uustal, Heikki, MD
Van Dien, Craig, MD
Weiss, Kyle Matthew, DO
Williams, Krystle Michelle, MD
Plastic & Reconstructive Srgy
Volshteyn, Boris, MD
Plastic Surgery
Arkoulakis, Nolis Stamatis, MD
Cacciarelli, Andrea J., MD
Cuber, Shain A., MD
Risin, Michael Simon, MD
Psyc&Neurology-Neuromuscular
Dekermenjian, Rony, MD
Psychiatry
Bijlani, Mona V., MD
Blank, Susan Berman, MD
Burns, Kenneth L., MD
Gupta, Neha, MD
Lichtman, Kenneth J., MD
Mangsatabam, Ruby, MD
Nizam, Zeba S., MD
Ostella, Frank Mario, DO
Schlakman, Martin D., MD
Shah, Dina B., MD
Shah, Komal Saurabh, MD
Young, Sarah M., MD
Pulmonary Disease
Ferraris, Ambra, MD
Goldstein, David S., MD
Hebbe, Karl Albert Jr., DO
Polos, Peter George, MD
Raju, Pooja Indukuri, MD
Supe Dzidic, Dana, MD
Radiation Oncology
Trabold, Lucille A., MD
Zarny, Steven David, MD
Radiology
George, Louis C., MD
Sports Medicine
Kasim, Nader Q., MD
Lane, Gregory J., MD

Surgery (General)
Armour, Renee Palmyra, MD
Chaudry, Ghazali Anwar, MD
Choi, Stanley S., MD
Chung Loy, Harold E., MD
Dasmahapatra, Kumar S., MD
El Mansoury, Hassan M., MD
Ellman, Barry R., MD
Encarnacion, Cirilo, MD
Green, Suzanne E., MD
Henry, Ricki M., MD
Ilut, Irina Claudia, MD
Itskovich, Alexander, MD
Lucking, Jonathan, MD
Neri, Linda M., MD
Patel, Kirtikumar J., MD
Penupatruni, Niranjan K., MD
Pinsky, Abby Michele, MD
Sharma, Rajinder, MD
Swaminathan, Anangur P., MD
Valane, Honora W., MD
Wilkins, Kirsten Bass, MD
Therapeutic Radiology
Macher, Mark S., MD
Thoracic Surgery
Sarkaria, Jasbir S., MD
Urology
Fand, Benjamin, MD
Lasser, Michael Sidney, MD
Lind, Eugene Jerome, MD
Nakhoda, Zein Khozaim, MD
Noh, Robert E., MD
Patel, Arvind Mansukhlal, MD
Patel, Rupa, MD
Sherman, Neil David, MD
Sinha, Binod K., MD
Wein, Joshua Lewis, MD
Vascular & Intrvntnal Radiology
Freeman, Hank Jason, MD
Kumar, Moses, MD

Egg Harbor
Internal Medicine
Rizvi, Faraz, MD
Otolaryngology
Morrison, Daniel H. Jr., MD

Egg Harbor City
Anesthesiology
Martin, Sheryel Denise, MD
General Preventive Medicine
Digenio, Andres German, MD

Egg Harbor Township
Aerospace Medicine
Tordella, Joseph R., DO
Anesthesiology
Zhu, Yun, MD
Bariatrics/Weight Control
Onopchenko, Alexander, MD
Cardiovascular Disease
Desai, Rashmikant Sumantlal, MD
Elnahal, Mohamed H., MD
Robbins, Inga H., MD
Shetty, Sanjay, MD
Child & Adolescent Psychiatry
O'Reilly, Thomas Christian, MD
Diagnostic Radiology
Lee, Jacob S., MD
O'Laughlin, Richard Lawrence, MD
Emergency Medicine
Stone, Mark J., MD
Family Med-Sports Medicine
Chhipa, Irfan S., MD
Family Medicine
Altamuro, Christopher R., DO
Barrett, Bryan Richard, DO
D'Ambrosio, Robert Paul, DO
Kern, Carrie Catherine, DO
Richwine, Charles M. IV, DO
Richwine, Lori T., DO
Foot & Ankle Surgery
Winters, Brian Seth, MD
Gastroenterology
Kaufman, Barry P., MD
Mehta, Nikhilesh D., MD
Rosman, Gary A., MD
Santoro, John J., DO
Hematology Oncology
Sandilya, Vijay Krishna, MD
Internal Medicine
Angamuthu, Akilandanayaki, MD
Bolich, Christopher W., DO

Chawla,Neha Roshan,MD
Diener,Melissa Ann,MD
Kuponiyi,Olatunji P.,MD
Makar,George A.,MD
Musarra,Anthony Mark,MD
Paradela,Ephrem Hector,MD
Patel,Neha Hector,MD
Soucier,Ronald J.,DO
Twardzik,Jennifer Lynn,DO
Unuigbe,Augustine A.,MD
Unuigbe,Florence,MD
Medical Oncology
Adelberg,David Eli,MD
Neurology
Hunter,Kevin Edward,MD
Reid-Duncan,Lucienne Lariane,MD
Tahmoush,Albert J.,MD
Obstetrics & Gynecology
Kaufman,Larry J.,MD
Lojun,Sharon Lee,MD
Milov,Seva,MD
Papperman,Thomas W.,MD
Samson-Bacarro,Edna A.,MD
Silk,Maanasi Puranik,DO
Orthopedic Surgery
Baker,John C.,MD
Becan,Arthur Frank Jr.,MD
Naame,Lawrence J.,MD
Ong,Alvin C.,MD
Orozco,Fabio R.,MD
Pepe,Matthew D.,MD
Salvo,John Paul Jr.,MD
Tucker,Bradford S.,MD
Woods,Barrett I.,MD
Orthopedic Surgery-Adult Rcnstr
Hernandez,Victor Hugo,MD
Other Specialty
Salartash,Khashayar,MD
Otolaryngology
Schaffer,Scott R.,MD
Pediatric Endocrinology
Chikezie,Augustine O.,MD
Pediatric Pulmonology
Salvia,Joseph V.,DO
Pediatrics
Anisman,Paul C.,MD
Ditmar,Mark F.,MD
Garrett,Parisa Mousavi,MD
Kaiser,Bruce A.,MD
Kessler,Barry M.,MD
Kuponiyi,Cheryl A.,MD
Palermo,Andrea,DO
Roan,Minda Unidad S.,MD
Physical Med & Rehab-Pain Med
Mehnert,Michael Joseph,MD
Physical Medicine & Rehab
Armstrong,Joshua Stephen,DO
Axelrod,Alyson Fincke,DO
Falcone,Michael,MD
Nutini,Dennis Neil,MD
Xu,Wei,MD
Plastic Surgery
Saad,Adam,MD
Psychiatry
Bhuyan,Ruprekha,MD
Caro,Marjorie,MD
Glass,Gary M.,MD
Griinke,Sheila Lynn,DO
Meusburger,Charles E.,MD
Pandya,Shilin R.,DO
Samson-Daclan,Maria Teresa,MD
Snead Poellnitz,Stephanie E.,MD
Radiation Oncology
Wilson,Vasthi Christensen,MD
Radiology
Gualtieri,Louis Robert,DO
Surgery (General)
Brown,Anjeanette Tina,MD
Hon,David C.,MD
Salartash,Alimorad,MD
Trauma Surgery
Rohani,Pejman,DO
Urology
Scalera,John V.,MD
Vascular Surgery
Frost,James H.,MD
Lorenzetti,John D.,MD
Previti,Francis W.,MD

Elizabeth
Anesthesiology
Adam,Abir Moustafa,MD
Carvalho,Steven Evaristo,MD
Cyriac,James Ignatius,MD
Myers,Khaleah K.,MD
Nepomuceno,Kathleen Chiong,MD
Pakalnis,Regina,MD
Phan,Lily,MD
Pirak,Leon,MD
Reddy,Padmavathi,MD
Shen,Edward,MD
Vassilidze,Teimouraz V.,MD
Zaitsev,Alexander Alexeevic,MD
Cardiovascular Disease
Cholankeril,Mathew V.,MD
Cholankeril,Matthew George,MD
Joshi,Meherwan Burzor,MD
Cardiovascular Surgery
Codoyannis,Aristides Basil,MD
Child & Adolescent Psychiatry
Campos-Munoz,Magaly C.,MD
Cobert,Josiane C.,MD
Gavini,Jaya L.,MD
Emergency Medicine
Adamski,Jamie Justin,DO
Azoulai,Jonathan Guy,MD
Fan,Liqi,MD
Haders,Allison Lula,MD
Haig,Joseph Michael,MD
Hakim,James,MD
Letizia,Matthew J.,DO
Lo Faro,Joseph Rocco,MD
Mack,Rose M.,DO
Matossian,Raffee H.,MD
McCoy,Lynn,DO
Park,Jay Hoon,MD
Shah,Hitesh M.,MD
Wang,Sandy,DO
Zhang,Christina Ting,DO
Family Medicine
Aponte,Emilia Laura,DO
Brice,Marie F.,MD
Cisnero,Maria Del Carmen,MD
Cruz,Catalina M.,MD
Ferdinand,Pascale,MD
Khamis,Khamis Gerious,DO
Perez,Raul I.,MD
Quinones,Ariel,MD
Tan,Edgardo L.,MD
Gastroenterology
Kogan,Robert,MD
Moradi,Dovid Simcha,MD
Naik,Arun Chandrakant,MD
General Practice
Ferdinand,Michel-Ange,MD
Henner,Benjamin Joseph,MD
Levinsky,Liya,MD
Marzano,Patrick Wayne,DO
Geriatric Psychiatry
Sethi,Mohammad Awais,MD
Hematology
Salerno,Vincent E.,MD
Hematology Oncology
Cholankeril,Michelle,MD
Levinson,Barry S.,MD
Infectious Disease
Farrer,William E.,MD
Sherer,Clark B.,MD
Internal Medicine
Ahmed,Saira N.,MD
Baig,Khadija,MD
Batta,Sanjay,MD
Benalcazar-Puga,Luis Marcelo,MD
Bilusic,Marijo,MD
Blaszka,Frederick M.,MD
Butler,Jill Kraft,MD
Chauhan,Chetankumar K.,MD
Chirino,Maria E.,MD
Cholankeril,Mary G.,MD
Cholankeril,Thressiamma M.,MD
Chua,Jose Jr.,MD
De La Cruz,Flavia Annette,MD
Delgado,Jorge L.,MD
Dragun,Elena,MD
Eltom,Alaeldin Abdalla,MD
Garcia,Raul Angel,DO
Garg,Delyse,MD
Goodgold,Abraham,MD
Huda,Rafeul,MD
Jaffry,Syed Ali Hasan,MD
Jimenez,Arnaldo M.,MD
Khan,Sabeen,MD
Khimani,Karim J.,MD
Lin,Chi-Hsiung,MD
Lontai,Peter,MD
Lu,Andrew Hong,MD
Mansour,Ashraf Hakeem,MD
Mathure,Mekhala A.,MD
McAnally,James F.,MD
Mejias,Erenio,MD
Munoz,Francisco,MD
Munoz,Guillermo A.,DO
Nelson,Homer L.,MD
Nielson,Rosemarie,DO
Oberoi,Mandeep S.,MD
Othman,Essam Abdou,MD
Patel,Jalpa S.,MD
Patel,Manish Sureshbhai,MD
Patel,Mayuri H.,MD
Patel,Rambhai C.,MD
Pattathil,Jean Catherine,MD
Perez,James,MD
Rosefort,Laury,MD
Rowen,Adam J.,MD
Sebastian,Suniti,MD
Sharma,Rekha,MD
Shen,Jung-San,MD
Soltys,Remigiusz,MD
Somma,Edward A.,MD
Suleiman,Addi,MD
Surana,Gautam C.,MD
Tan,Pilar O.,MD
Thalody,George V.,MD
Thalody,Lucyamma,MD
Thalody,Usha George,MD
Vaiana,Paul,MD
Vallejo,Edgardo C.,MD
Verzosa,Oscar E.,MD
Walia,Jasjit S.,MD
Zaboski,Michael R.,MD
Medical Oncology
Kessler,William W.,MD
Nephrology
Reddy,Aravinda,MD
Silva-Khazaei,Maria Lourders,MD
Neurology
Bhatt,Meeta Hasmukh,MD
Pareja,Victor Hugo,MD
Sananman,Michael L.,MD
Tao,Ying,MD
Obstetrics & Gynecology
Arrunategui,Jose M.,MD
Joseph,Eddy M.,MD
Khazai,Kamran,MD
Raad,Michelle L.,MD
Sabzwari,Tabassum Azra,DO
Ophthalmology
Klein,Shawn Richard,MD
Klein,Warren M.,MD
Mang,Justin,MD
Scannapiego,Saveren,MD
Orthopedic Surgery
Bercik,Michael J.,MD
Gutierrez,Pedro M.,MD
Otolaryngology
Bergman,Justin A.,MD
Cinberg,James Z.,MD
Huang,Robert D.,MD
Saporta,Diego,MD
Pediatrics
Abich,Georgina,MD
Ayyanathan,Karpukaras,MD
Davis,Kenneth J.,MD
De La Cruz,Antonio A.,MD
Fernandez-Moure,Joseph L.,MD
Galimidi Hodara,Salomon,MD
Gonzalez-Mejia,Johanna J.,MD
Grundy,Kia Calhoun,MD
Jethwa,Kusum A.,MD
Kim,Soon K.,MD
Orleans,Genevieve Araba,MD
Powell,Kerri Lynette,MD
Questelles,Rachael,MD
Saraiya,Narendra N.,MD
Sundaram,Raghunand,MD
Tolentino-Dela Cruz,Milagros,MD
Physical Medicine & Rehab
Sardar,Henry,DO
Psychiatry
Bekker,Yana,MD
Bharatiya,Purabi,MD
Bolona,Leopold J.,MD
Chang,Luke,MD
Del Rosario-Garcia,Mariza,MD
Dewyke,Kathleen Michelle,MD
Ghali,Anwar Y.,MD
Gorman,Saul David,MD
Grelecki,Stephen,MD
Ibeh,Khadija Hakiya,MD
Lehrhoff,Sari,MD
Lozovatsky,Michael,MD
McCollum,Brendan Patrick,MD
Okoye,Eronmwon,MD
Patel,Hitendra R.,MD
Pena Mejia,Jesus A.,MD
Perez,Rodemar Albao,MD
Reddy,Adarsh Surya,MD
Shah,Hinna Ehsanullah,MD
Shanbhag,Suhas R.,MD
Shnayderman,Aleksandr,DO
Surahio,Ali R.,MD
Taylor,Jennifer,MD
Trivedi,Nirmal I.,MD
Pulmonary Critical Care
Budhwani,Anju,MD
Pulmonary Disease
Garg,Vipin,MD
Surgery (General)
Colaco,Rodolfo,MD
Kansagra,Ashwin Maganlal,MD
Mlynarczyk,Peter J.,MD
Zimmern,Andrea,MD
Urology
Krieger,Alan P.,MD
Opell,M. Brett,MD
Vascular Surgery
Geuder,James W.,MD
Moss,Charles M.,MD
Tsai,Jung-Tsung,MD

Elmer
Anesthesiology
DeLeon,Edgardo S.,MD
Jones,Angela Marie,MD
Dermatology
Aphale,Abhishek N.,MD
Danowski,Kelli Mayo,DO
Warmuth,Ingrid P.,MD
Family Medicine
Elgawli,Philip Raef,DO
Haag,Jerry L.,MD
Malickel,Jay Varunny,DO
Sastic,Daniel Joseph,MD
Ventrella,Gerard,MD
Internal Medicine
Flynn,Patrick Joseph,DO
Obstetrics & Gynecology
Adunuthula-Jonnalagadda,Hema,MD
Psychiatry
Glass,Steven J.,MD
Urology
Read,John H.,MD

Elmwood Park
Adolescent Medicine
Patel,Harshad Nathalal,MD
Anatomic Pathology
Wang,Luoquan,MD
Anatomic/Clinical Pathology
Butala,Rajesh M.,MD
Fehrle,Wilfrid Martin,MD
Lee,Po-Shing,MD
Liu,Liang,MD
Pritchett,Danielle Delores,MD
Anesthesiology
Manspeizer,Heather Eve,MD
Sangavaram,Kristappa,MD
Schlesinger,James M.,MD
Shin,Kyung Hee,MD
Tendler,Jay M.,MD
Yu,Yun S.,MD
Cytopathology
Dupree,William Brion,MD
Family Medicine
Finelli,Peter K.,DO
Vila,Maria N.,DO
Hematology
Persad,Rajendra,MD
Hematopathology
Merati,Kambiz,MD
Talwar,Jotica,MD
Internal Medicine
Grodman,Marc D.,MD

Physicians by Town and Medical Specialty

Physicians by Town and Medical Specialty

Elmwood Park (cont)
Ophthalmology
- Levan, Ellen, MD
- Uychich, Priscilla M., DO
- Weisberger, James D., MD

Maternal & Fetal Medicine
- Principe, David Laurence, MD

Obstetrics & Gynecology
- Lee-Agawa, Melissa, MD
- Friend, Adam Seth, MD
- Maley, Michael Kendrick, MD
- Phillips, Hadley H., DO

Pediatric Cardiology
- O'Connor, Brian Kevin, MD

Pediatrics
- Kiblawi, Fuad Moh'D, MD
- Ramadi, Roula Alchaa, MD

Surgery (General)
- Sharma, Jyoti, MD

Emerson
Anesthesiology
- Patel, Anil Jayant, MD

Cardiovascular Disease
- Bagade, Vivek Laxman, MD
- Christensen, Brenda M., MD
- Jacowitz, Joel D., MD
- Kaufman, Bradley S., MD
- Walker, Tracy Lynne, MD

Child & Adolescent Psychiatry
- Patel, Mona M., MD

Critical Care Medicine
- Orr, David A., DO

Diagnostic Radiology
- Su, Hsiu, MD

Endocrinology
- Daud Ahmad, Sameera, MD
- Hochstein, Martin A., MD
- Litvin, Yair, MD
- Mahajan, Geeti, MD

Family Medicine
- Desai, Veena C., MD
- Dombrowski, Mark A., MD
- McConnell, Julie, MD
- Wilkin, Daniel James, DO

Foot & Ankle Surgery
- Napoli, Ralph C., MD

Gastroenterology
- Bellomo, Alyse Rosemarie, MD
- Bethala, Vivian K., MD
- Candido, Frank M., MD
- Cullen, Holly Doolittle, MD
- Goldstein, David D., MD
- Levine, Robert S., MD
- Margulis, Stephen J., MD
- Moscato, Michele, DO
- Pittman, Robert Hal, MD
- Randall, Jennifer F., MD
- Zucker, Ira I., MD

Hand Surgery
- Meyer, Carissa Leigh, MD

Hematology Oncology
- Gold, Edward J., MD

Internal Medicine
- Ali, Amy G., MD
- Avezzano, Eric S., MD
- Bhandari, Bhavik M., MD
- Briker, Alan J., MD
- Broussard, Crystal N., MD
- D'Aquino, Carol Madeleine, MD
- Flanzman, Susan Amy, MD
- Fleischer, Joseph S., MD
- Glaubiger, Carol, MD
- Gokhale, Kedar Arvind, MD
- Griggs, Allen R., DO
- Kim, Jeffrey S., MD
- Koo, Bon Chang Andy, MD
- Lan, Vivian En-Wei, MD
- Lin, George Szuwei, MD
- Mastrianno, Frank L., MD
- Motiwala, Neeta R., MD
- Potack, Jonathan Zachary, MD
- Thum, Robert G., MD
- Volpe, Anthony P., MD

Laparoscopic Surgery
- Walsky, Robert S., MD

Neurological Radiology
- Parag, Yoav, MD

Neurology
- Asta, Charles Francis, MD
- Dhadwal, Neetu, MD

Obstetrics & Gynecology
- Gliksman, Michele Isaacs, MD
- Paskowski, Elizabeth K., MD
- Rosalie, Maria Christina, MD

Ophthalmology
- Cantore, William Anthony, MD
- Fishkin, Joseph D., MD
- Geller, Bradley David, MD

Orthopedic Surgery
- Baird, Evan Oliver, MD
- Ben Yishay, Ari, MD
- Benke, Michael T., MD
- Esformes, Ira, MD
- Gross, Michael Lee, MD
- Levin, Rafael, MD
- Mendes, John F., MD
- Vazquez, Oscar, MD

Otolaryngology
- Svider, Peter, MD

Physical Medicine & Rehab
- Bethala, Nalini, MD
- Lester, Jonathan P., MD
- Mendoza, Justin, DO
- Natalicchio, James Charles, MD
- Roque-Dang, Christine M., DO

Rheumatology
- Nes, Deana Teplitsky, DO
- Rosner, Steven M., MD

Spinal Surgery
- Ashraf, Nomaan, MD
- Rhim, Richard Dongil, MD

Englewood
Allergy
- From, Stuart B., MD
- Goodstein, Carolyn E., MD
- Harish, Ziv, MD

Allergy & Immunology
- Wanich, Niya, MD

Anatomic/Clinical Pathology
- Sanchez, Miguel A., MD
- Tismenetsky, Mikhail, MD

Anesthesiology
- Baltaytis, Viktor, MD
- Berth, Ulrike, MD
- Betta, Joanne, MD
- Borow, Leslie Bennett, MD
- Chan, Rolycito A., MD
- Chen, Wen-Hong, MD
- Chithran, Payyanadan V., MD
- Deluty, Sheldon H., MD
- Digiacomo, Michael B., MD
- Dvir, David, MD
- Epstein, David Israel, MD
- Gak, Alexander V., MD
- Goldzweig, Peter Allan, DO
- Guillaume, Stephanie Ann, MD
- Huber, Michael D., DO
- Kaganovskaya, Margarita, MD
- Kipnis, Ilana Ariel, DO
- Kulkarni, Sumedha V., MD
- Lee, Louis Young, MD
- Lobel, Gregg P., MD
- Lui, John, MD
- Metro, Wade E., MD
- Mizrahi, Marc E., MD
- Moonka, Neeta K., MD
- Moskowitz, David Matthew, MD
- Pandya, Vrunda H., MD
- Pappalardo, Rebecca A., MD
- Perelman, Seth I., MD
- Popa, Peter R., MD
- Puzio, Thomas, MD
- Shander, Aryeh, MD
- Smok, Jeffrey Thomas, MD
- St. Jean, Monika Kulkarni, MD
- Thomas, Vinoo Sebastian, MD
- Volpe, Lorraine, MD

Anesthesiology: Pain Medicine
- Gudin, Jeffrey Alan, MD

Arthroscopic Surgery
- Cole, James R., MD

Breast Surgery
- McIntosh, Violet Merle, MD

Cardiothoracic Surgery
- Klein, James Joseph Jr., MD

Cardiovascular Disease
- Blood, David King, MD
- Erlebacher, Jay A., MD
- Feigenblum, David Yehuda, MD
- Goldweit, Richard S., MD
- Hodges, David M., MD
- Katechis, Dennis, DO
- Leber, George B., MD
- Matican, Jeffrey S., MD
- Mitchel, Jeffrey M., MD
- Reiner, David M., MD
- Schwarcz, Aron Isaac, MD
- Stone, Jane E., MD
- Strobel, Ronald E., MD
- Suede, Samuel, MD
- Weissman, Andrew J., MD
- Wilchfort, Samuel D., MD
- Wilkenfeld, Craig, MD

Cardiovascular Surgery
- Galla, Jan David, MD

Child & Adolescent Psychiatry
- Effron-Gurland, Frances R., MD
- Fridman, Esther D., MD
- Fridman, Morton Zvi, MD
- Srivastava, Tulika Sinha, MD

Clinical Neurophysiology
- Ko, James H., MD

Colon & Rectal Surgery
- Harris, Michael T., MD
- Seo, Christina J., MD
- Waxenbaum, Steven I., MD
- White, Ronald A., MD

Critical Care Medicine
- Pavlou, Theophanis A., MD

Dermatology
- Fishman, Miriam, MD
- Fried, Sharon Z., MD
- Grodberg, Michele, MD
- Ordoukhanian, Elsa, MD
- Rapaport, Jeffrey A., MD
- Steinman, Natasha Margolin, MD

Diagnostic Radiology
- Foster, Jonathan A., MD
- Gutwein, Marina Ayzenberg, MD
- Jacobs, Stefanie S., MD
- Mattana, Nina Delman, MD
- Naidrich, Shari Ann, MD
- Petti, Christopher Louis, MD
- Rekhtman-Sneed, Katya, MD
- Shembde, Dwarkanath Sonaji, MD

Emergency Medicine
- Caplen, Stuart M., MD
- Clement, Martinez Emmanuel, MD
- Glaser, Ariella N., MD
- Kay, Elizabeth E., DO
- Kintzel, Timothy J., MD
- Readie, Jean Eileen, DO
- Saxena, Rachna Vidiasagar, DO
- Schreibman, Barbara A., MD
- Singer, Elizabeth Kara, MD
- Wong, Judy, MD

Endocrinology
- Abraham, Alice, MD
- Bakerywala, Suhalia, MD
- Bier, Rachel Elizabeth, MD
- Borensztein, Alejandra G., MD
- Cong, Elaine Alice, MD
- Fojas, Ma. Conchitina Manas, MD
- Schwartz, Joseph Jay, MD
- Suh, Se Young, MD

Family Medicine
- Babeendran, Shan, DO
- Gross, Harvey R., MD
- Healy, Christine B., DO
- Klingsberg, Gary P., DO
- Mor Zilberstein, Lara, MD
- Skarimbas, Alicia C., MD
- Suri, Ritu, MD

Fertility/Infertility
- Hock, Doreen L., MD
- Hurst, Wendy Robin, MD
- Tisch, Bruce H., MD

Gastroenterology
- Friedrich, Ivan A., MD
- Gillon, Steven D., DO
- Kancherla, Sandarsh Raj, MD
- Kaplounova, Irina, MD
- Mohtashemi, Hormoz, MD
- Panella, Vincent S., MD
- Rosen, Bruce L., DO

Hand Surgery
- Gurland, Mark A., MD
- Lee, Jen Fei, MD
- Miller-Breslow, Anne J., MD
- Pizzillo, Michael Francis, MD

Hematology
- Attas, Lewis M., MD
- Schleider, Michael A., MD

Hematology Oncology
- Forte, Francis A., MD
- Janosky, Maxwell, MD
- Kim, Brian Hangil, MD
- Morrison, Jill S., MD

Hospitalist
- Hohmuth, Benjamin Adam, MD

Infectious Disease
- Kocher, Jeffrey, MD
- Saggar, Suraj Kumar, DO
- Torres Isasiga, Julian Andres, MD
- Weisholtz, Steven J., MD

Internal Medicine
- Abramovici, Mirel I., MD
- Andron, Richard I., MD
- Barnes, Tanganyika A., DO
- Benoff, Brian Alan, MD
- Beri, Samarth, MD
- Brauntuch, Glenn R., MD
- Breitbart, Seth Ilias, MD
- Brouk, Alla, MD
- Bryan, Craigh Keith, MD
- Carter, Brittany Nicole, MD
- Casser, Michael E., MD
- Chen, Tzu-Shao, MD
- Cholhan, Ruth C., MD
- Clifford, Susan Michelle, MD
- Crooks, Michael H., MD
- Davis, Lawrence Jay, MD
- De Rose, Marielaina S., MD
- Djebiyan, Eli S., MD
- Engler, Mitchell S., MD
- Fayngersh, Alla, MD
- Fleischer, Jessica Beth, MD
- Friedman, Alan Mark, MD
- Frier, Steven F., MD
- Frisch, Katalin Andrea, MD
- Galumyan, Yelena V., MD
- Gandhi, Nisha R., MD
- Geller, Judy Irene, MD
- Gianatiempo, Carmine, MD
- Glassman, Adam M., MD
- Gottdiener, Alexandra H., MD
- Grodstein, Gerald P., MD
- Gura, Russell Saul, MD
- Hamilton, Monique S., MD
- Ho, Eddie Kasing, MD
- Jan, Louis C. W., MD
- Jathavedam, Ashwin, MD
- Joshi, Nandita, MD
- Kaim, Oleg, MD
- Kaplan, Sarah, MD
- Kapoor, Radhika, DO
- Katz, Doron Zvi, MD
- Katz, Manuel David, MD
- Kim, Sung Hyun, MD
- Laiosa, Catherine Virginia, MD
- Latorre, Rafael, MD
- Levine, Selwyn Eric, MD
- Loewinger, Michael Brian, MD
- Lorton, Julie Lytton, MD
- Malovany, Robert J., MD
- Miguel, Eduardo E., MD
- Nemirovsky, Dmitry, MD
- Okeke, Ngozi C., MD
- Oo, Hnin Hnin, MD
- Paley, Jeffrey Evan, MD
- Park, Anne June, MD
- Pattner, Austin M., MD
- Ramsetty, Sabena Karina, MD
- Reeves, Lisa Joyce, MD
- Sapienza, Mark Santo, MD
- Seferian, Mihran A., MD
- Serrano, Jesus Canoza, MD
- Shammash, Jonathan Baruch, MD
- Shatzkes, Joseph Aaron, MD
- Shin, Peter Young, MD
- Silberstein, Stuart L., MD
- Simon, Clifford J., MD
- Smith, Ebben Will, MD
- Stepanyuk, Olena, MD
- Sun, Sung Wook, MD
- Tartakovsky, Irina, MD
- Taw, Julie, MD
- Thomas, Shilpa Ani, MD
- Tlamsa, Aileen P., MD
- Volokhov, Alexey, MD
- Wasserman, Kenneth H., MD
- Ye, Sheng H., MD
- Yee, Sau Yan, MD
- Zelkowitz, Marc, MD

Laparoscopic Surgery
  Ibrahim,Ibrahim M.,MD
Maternal & Fetal Medicine
  Chan,Ying,MD
Medical Oncology
  Jhawer,Minaxi P.,MD
Neonatal-Perinatal Medicine
  Carlin,Elizabeth Berk,MD
  Delgado,Mercedes,MD
Nephrology
  Zachariah,Teena,MD
Neurological Surgery
  Gologorsky,Yakov,MD
  Moore,Frank Max,MD
  Steinberger,Alfred A.,MD
  Yao,Kevin Chi-Kai,MD
Neurology
  Adler,Daniel G.,MD
  Akbaripanahi,Sepideh,MD
  Alweiss,Gary S.,MD
  Choi,Yun-Beom,MD
  Levy,Kirk Jay,MD
  Racela,Rikki Redona,MD
  Rajasingham,Jamuna Kandasamy,MD
  Rosenbaum,David Herbert,MD
  Rothman,Arthur C.,MD
  Willner,Joseph Harrison,MD
Obstetrics & Gynecology
  Ashton,Jennifer Lee,MD
  Asulin,Yitzhack,MD
  Bewtra,Madhuri,MD
  Binas,Constantine George,MD
  Butler,David George,MD
  Chalfin,Venus Helena,MD
  Dill,Barbara A.,MD
  Englert,Christopher A.,MD
  Friedman,Harvey Y.,MD
  Gellman,Elliott,MD
  Goldman,Faith Renee,MD
  Gor,Hetal Bankim,MD
  Gresham,Keith A.,MD
  Gross,Arthur H.,MD
  Hadjistavrinos,Kriss,MD
  Huang,Tony T.,MD
  Jacobson,Marina,MD
  Jhee,Yoon-Bok,MD
  Kilinsky,Vladimir,MD
  Lesorgen,Philip R.,MD
  Markovitz,Jacob E.,MD
  Martinucci,Stacy M.,MD
  Merriam,Zachary M.,DO
  Patel,Avanee Kanoo,MD
  Patel-Shusterman,Shefali N.,MD
  Patrusky,Karen Lynn,MD
  Saphier,Carl Joseph,MD
  Savci,Sariye,MD
  Scheller,Tracey Frances,MD
  Schlossberg,Hope R.,MD
  Song,Erica Yoon-Jung,MD
  Suarez,Teresa,MD
  Tovmasian,Lucy Tamar,MD
  Weiss,Nofit,MD
Ophthalmology
  Burrows,Andrew F.,MD
  Ezon,Isaac C.,MD
  Freilich,Benjamin Douglas,MD
  Freilich,David Eric,MD
  Jee,Jimmy Hoon,MD
Orthopedic Surgery
  Becker,Adam Scott,MD
  Cole,Brian Anthony,MD
  Davis,Damien Ian,MD
  Doidge,Robert W.,DO
  Owens,John M.,MD
  Shah,Asit K.,MD
Orthopedics
  Archer,Jonathan Mckee,MD
  Salob,Peter Andrew,MD
Otolaryngology
  Ho,Bryan Tao,MD
  Jahn,Anthony Frederick,MD
  Scherl,Michael P.,MD
  Tadros,Monica,MD
  Tobias,Geoffrey Wayne,MD
Otolaryngology-Facial Plastic
  Lewis,David A.,MD
Pathology
  Burga,Ana Maria,MD
  Kashani,Massoud,MD
  Stahl,Rosalyn E.,MD

Pediatric Anesthesia
  Friedman,Arielle J.,MD
Pediatric Gastroenterology
  Zawahir,Shamila Balkis,MD
Pediatric Hematology Oncology
  Cole,Peter D.,MD
Pediatrics
  Baydar,Garbis,MD
  Daici,Silvia,MD
  Davidson,Melissa,MD
  Fried,Ruthellen,MD
  Hershcopf,Richard Jay,MD
  Hyatt,Alexander Charles,MD
  Kampf,Robyn A.,MD
  Onwuka,William N.,MD
  Psalidas,Panagiotis George,MD
  Siegel-Stein,Francine M.,MD
  Tung,Cindy Wei-Yi,MD
  Zuckerbrot,Rachel Aryella,MD
Physical Med & Rehab-Pain Med
  Hall,Andrew Robert,MD
Physical Medicine & Rehab
  Alonso,Jose A.,MD
  Arias,Carlos,MD
  Baker,Elizabeth Anne,MD
  Bucalo,Victor John,MD
  Dutkowsky,Charles J.,DO
  Hamer,Orlee,DO
  Jendrek,Paul,MD
  Kern,Hilary Beth,MD
  Kim,Chee Gap,MD
  Liss,Donald,MD
  Liss,Howard,MD
  Montag,Nathaniel,DO
  Montero-Cruz,Fergie Ross,DO
  Nguyen,David Huong,MD
  Pavell,Jeff Richard,DO
  Riolo,Thomas Antonio,DO
  Taha,Nora,MD
  Tasca,Philip,MD
  Vadada,Kiran,MD
  Wisotsky,Lisa L.,MD
  Zimmerman,Ronald Lee,MD
Plastic Surgery
  Abramson,David L.,MD
  D'Amico,Richard A.,MD
  Lee,Shinji S.,MD
  Parakh,Shwetambara,MD
  Soto,Norberto Luke,MD
Psychiatry
  Barnes,Stephanie A.,MD
  Chaitman,Edmund,MD
  Chertoff,Harvey R.,MD
  Chiorazzi,Mary Lorraine,MD
  Ciora,Cristian Dan,MD
  Fiore,Vicki M.,MD
  Garakani Nejad,Houshang,MD
  Greenblatt,Naomi H.,MD
  Hollander,Annette J.,MD
  Kaplan,Richard D.,MD
  Kernodle,Judith M.,MD
  Najman,Naomi Stein,MD
  Paltrowitz,Justin Keith,MD
  Schumeister,Robert S.,MD
  Seltzer,Ronni Lee,MD
  Stefanovich,Michael Vladimir,MD
  White,Harvey L.,MD
Pulmonary Critical Care
  Califano,Francesco,MD
Pulmonary Disease
  Gorloff,Victor,MD
  Han,Paul S.,MD
  Kondapaneni,Srikant,MD
  Patel,Killol,MD
  Tesher,Harris Brandon,MD
Radiation Oncology
  Dubin,David M.,MD
Radiology
  Goldfischer,Mindy A.,MD
  Herman,Marc Arthur,MD
  Juengst-Mitchell,Jannine,DO
  Malde,Hiten Maganlal,MD
  Mazzei,Elizabeth O'Connell,MD
  Shapiro,Mark L.,MD
  Vadde,Kavitha,MD
Rheumatology
  Griffiths,Shernett Olivine,MD
Sports Medicine
  Bottiglieri,Thomas S.,DO
  Deramo,David Michael,MD
  Salzer,Richard L. Jr.,MD

Surgery (General)
  Arnofsky,Adam Garett,MD
  Bufalini,Bruno,MD
  Cravioto-Vaimakis,Stefanie,MD
  Morales-Ribeiro,Celines,MD
  Shikiar,Steven Paul,MD
  Srinivasan,McDonald T.,MD
  Strain,Jeffrey Witt,MD
Thoracic Surgery
  Loh,Chun Kyu,MD
Urology
  Andronaco,Raymond B.,MD
  Katz,Steven A.,MD
  Kerns,John F.,MD
  Lee,Chester C.,MD
  Lee,Richard,MD
Vascular Surgery
  Bernik,Thomas R.,MD
  Fried,Kenneth S.,MD
  Impeduglia,Theresa Maria,MD
  Kahn,Mark Elliot,MD
  Sussman,Barry C.,MD
  Wengerter,Kurt Richard,MD
  Wolodiger,Fred A.,MD
Englewood Cliffs
Anesthesiology
  Povzhitkov,Igor Moiseyevi,MD
  Ward,Wendy Allison,MD
  Yu,David H.,MD
Dermatology
  Boakye,Naana Agyeiwah,MD
Diagnostic Radiology
  Amoroso,Michael Luke,MD
  Fishkin,Igor V.,MD
Endocrinology
  Goldman,Michael H.,MD
Gastroenterology
  Chessler,Richard K.,MD
  Fiorillo,Marc Anthony,MD
  Meininger,Michael Eric,MD
  Spinnell,Mitchell Kyle,MD
  Zingler,Barry M.,MD
Geriatrics
  Salem,Noel B.,MD
Internal Medicine
  Kim,Dong Hyun,MD
  Ko,Pan Sok,MD
  Lee,Chang Woo,MD
  Yu,Fei,MD
Interventional Cardiology
  Beheshtian,Azadeh,MD
Neurology
  Bressler,Jill Anne,MD
  Fremed,Eric L.,MD
  Mueller,Nancy L.,MD
  Prince,David M.,MD
  Rabin,Aaron,MD
Nuclear Medicine
  Ding,You-Guang,MD
Obstetrics & Gynecology
  Chong,Joseph K.,MD
  Kang,Katherine E. Lee,MD
  Miller,Jane E.,MD
  Yun,Sung K.,MD
Otolaryngology
  Moon,Taewon,MD
Pain Medicine
  Cho,John S.,MD
Pediatrics
  Lee,Sun Hee,MD
  Rhee,Jung L.,MD
Plastic Surgery
  Altman,Robert Gil,MD
  Farkas,Jordan Phillip,MD
  Mordkovich,Boris,MD
  Sandhu,Baldev S.,MD
Plastic Surgery-Head and Neck
  Capuano,Aaron Matthew,MD
Psychiatry
  Lewin,Roxanne Marie,MD
  Son,In K.,MD
Surgery (General)
  Yang,Hee Kon,MD
Urology
  Fermaglich,Matis A.,MD
Englishtown
Cardiovascular Disease
  Patel,Jatinchandra Suryakant,DO
Gastroenterology
  Volk,Yuri,MD

Internal Medicine
  Covalesky,John,DO
  Gupta,Narendra K.,MD
  Salter-Lewis,Cynthia,MD
Obstetrics & Gynecology
  Andrews,Tatyana,MD
Ophthalmology
  Karmel,Bruce A.,MD
Pediatrics
  Salcedo,Theresa Josue,MD
Psychiatry
  Staniaszek,Alina B.,MD
Essex Fells
Pediatrics
  Pakonis,Fiona K.,MD
Evesham
Family Medicine
  Pinsky,Tim A.,DO
Ewing
Anatomic/Clinical Pathology
  Chmara,Edward S.,MD
Emergency Medicine
  Pierce,Vincent E. Jr.,MD
Family Med-Adolescent Medicine
  Sheikh,Sirajuddin,MD
Family Medicine
  Carruth Mehnert,Lauren Vales,MD
  Flynn-Abdalla,Jane,DO
  Jass,Daniel K.,MD
General Preventive Medicine
  Gooding,Susane Lavern,MD
Hematology
  Hogan,Robert P.,DO
Infectious Disease
  Gekowski,Kathleen M.,MD
  Karabulut,Nigahus,MD
Internal Medicine
  Ali,Sara Inayet,MD
  Dundeva Baleva,Pavlinka V.,MD
  Gettys,Jacqueline Brown,MD
  Kolander,Scott A.,MD
  Kolman-Taddeo,Diana,MD
  Kudakachira,Shaismy,DO
  Meer,Shahid B.,MD
  Pierrot,Paul H.,MD
  Protter,Randi R.,MD
  Williams,Eric James,MD
Ophthalmology
  Brundavanam,Hari Vs,MD
Pulmonary Disease
  Harman,John A.,MD
Fair Haven
Family Medicine
  Gredell,Elizabeth S.,DO
  Swidryk,John P.,MD
Internal Medicine
  Hayward,Denise H.,MD
  Krisza,Mary L.,MD
  Nardone,Danielle J.,DO
  Pamintuan,Dominic C.,MD
Psychiatry
  Levin,Matthew,MD
Fair Lawn
Acupuncture
  Bamberger,Philip David,MD
Allergy
  Bokhari,Tahira M.,MD
  Kashkin,Jay Michael,MD
Anatomic/Clinical Pathology
  Feldman,Liliya A.,MD
  Saitas,Vasiliki L.,MD
Anesthesiology
  Owsiak,Joanne Naamo,MD
  Prakhina,Boris,MD
  Srinivasan,Deepak,MD
Cardiovascular Disease
  Bikkina,Mahesh,MD
  Chabbott,David Robert,MD
  Grossman,Steven H.,MD
  Herman,Brad Morris,MD
  Infantino,Salvatore,MD
  Kasatkin,Alexander E.,MD
  Maresca,Warren L.,MD
  Medepalli,Prasad B.,MD
  Molloy,Thomas J.,MD
  Patel,Rima Dipak,MD
  Samuel,Anish,MD
  Smith,John P.,DO
  Soyombo,Aderemi B.,MD
  Strobeck,John Edward,MD

Physicians by Town and Medical Specialty

Fair Lawn (cont)
Cardiovascular Disease
  Vehra, Ijaz R., MD
Child & Adolescent Psychiatry
  Matsenko, Oxana, MD
Child (Pediatric) Neurology
  Woo, Judy, MD
Clinical Cardiac Elctrphyslgy
  Tiyyagura, Satish Reddy, MD
Critical Care Medicine
  Singh, Malwinder, MD
Dermatology
  Heldman, Jay P., MD
  Katz, James M., MD
  Singman, Bradford A., MD
  Weiss, Darryl S., MD
Diagnostic Radiology
  Levy, Daniel S., MD
  Modi, Ketang H., DO
  Rubinoff, Susan W., MD
  Rudd, Steven A., MD
Emergency Medicine
  Grinberg, Diana, MD
Endocrinology
  Yeshou, Dima, MD
Family Medicine
  Bernardo, Dennis N., MD
  Chaudry, Sadia R., MD
  Chaudry, Samia Riaz, DO
  John, Eirene George, MD
  Karunanithi, Subhathra, MD
  Kaur, Jasneet, MD
  Levin, Susan Miriam, MD
  Riley, Roth Leon, MD
  Rosenberg, Jeffrey Steven, MD
Gastroenterology
  Gorodokin, Gary I., MD
  Gupta, Ramesh C., MD
  Kutner, Donald H., DO
  Lefkowitz, Jeffrey R., MD
  Resnick, Jonathan, MD
General Practice
  Chaudry, Mansoora R., MD
General Preventive Medicine
  Cernea, Dana, MD
Geriatric Psychiatry
  Valiveti, Sailaja Devi, MD
Geriatrics
  Oliver, Richard D., MD
  Verga, Diane G., MD
Internal Medicine
  Aquino, Christine E., MD
  Balonze, Karen T., MD
  Batchelor, Christopher D. Jr., MD
  Berman, Lawrence J., MD
  Bromberg, Assia, MD
  Cappitelli, Jack V., MD
  Cho, Soung Ick, MD
  Clifford, Eileen M., MD
  Deitz, Justina May, DO
  Donkina, Luiza, MD
  Farooqui, Syeda Saleha, MD
  Feiner, Shoshana N., MD
  Hossain, Nazma A., MD
  Lehrman, Mark Leonard, MD
  Levykh-Chase, Rena E., MD
  Lishko, Olga V., MD
  Logvinenko, Nina V., MD
  Narymsky, Lyudmila M., MD
  Patel, Dushyant Rameshchandra, MD
  Qipo, Andi, MD
  Reyn, Mark, MD
  Rizkalla, Suzette, MD
  Rizzo, Robert Anthony, MD
  Roman, David, MD
  Rudzinskiene, Aliona, MD
  Safa, Nina, MD
  Scerbo, Ernest John, MD
  Sen, Sourav, MD
  Sheth, Meetkumar Tusharbhai, MD
  Singh, Amrita Kaur, MD
  Syed, Zainab, MD
  Velez, Henry, MD
  Virk, Hartaj Singh, MD
  Werteneil, Mark Elliot, MD
Neurology
  Kamin, Marc, MD
  Shah, Nilay Ramesh, MD
Obstetrics & Gynecology
  Beloff, Michelle Lauren, DO
  Cocoziello, Ramin B., MD
  Dolgin, James S., MD
  Hessami, Sam H., MD
  Mitzner, Ann C., MD
  Reinkraut, Jeffrey M., MD
  Sagullo, Cynthia C., MD
  Seymour, Carmela, MD
  Verrico, Tracy B., DO
Occupational Medicine
  Halejian, Barry A., MD
Ophthalmology
  Gopal, Lekha Hareshbhai, MD
  Sebrow, Osher S., MD
  Trotta, Nicholas C., MD
Orthopedic Surgery
  Berger, John L., MD
  Bernstein, Adam Douglas, MD
  Cassilly, Ryan, MD
  Greenblum, Robert, MD
  Levitsky, Kenneth A., MD
  Ruoff, Mark J., MD
  Schultz, Robert A., MD
  Snyder, Samuel Jay, MD
  Valdez, Napoleon A., MD
Orthopedic-Hand Surgery
  Shamash, Steven Baroukh, DO
Pediatrics
  Alexander, Leah M., MD
  Anido, Rosary Kristine Isidro, MD
  Bass, Irina, MD
  Bienstock, Jeffrey Marc, MD
  Boyarsky, Yael, MD
  Brucia, Lauren A., MD
  Chism, Melissa A., MD
  Fischer, Emily Frances, MD
  Greaney, Kathleen Margaret, MD
  Hetling, Kristina, MD
  Kaul, Reena Sonya, MD
  Laufer, Ilene Caren, MD
  Lewis, Brian S., MD
  Lin, Tatiana Alexeevna, MD
  Long, Jessie C., MD
  Paige, Melanie Kay, MD
  Pitera, Barbara, MD
  Rao, Gunjan Pradhan, MD
  Riegelhaupt, Rona Susan, MD
  Schlitt, Meghan Ann, MD
  Shafi, Heather Claire, MD
  Sherman, Jennifer Ann, DO
  Sonnenblick, Howard C., MD
  Steinbaum, Deborah Paige, MD
  Steinel, Lisa A., MD
  Yellin, Tova G., MD
  Zucker, Scott W., MD
Physical Medicine & Rehab
  Logvinenko, Andrei V., MD
Plastic Surgery
  Fischer, Robert S., MD
  Lipson, David E., MD
Psychiatry
  Hossain, Asghar S.M., MD
  Kurra, Padmavathy, MD
  Primak, Dmitry, MD
  Strozeski, Janet E., MD
Pulmonary Disease
  Tijani, Hakeem Gbolahan, MD
Radiology
  Bauer, Christel Janet, MD
  Herbstman, Charles A., MD
  Hines, Patrick J., MD
  Moses, Stuart C., MD
Reproductive Endocrinology
  Rabin, Douglas S., MD
Rheumatology
  Arbit, David Lewis, MD
  Barr, Jerome Ian, MD
Sports Medicine
  Bassan, Matthew Evan, DO
Surgery (General)
  Becker, Steven I., MD
  Marta, Peter T., DO
Urology
  Chang, David Tsuwei, MD
  Hajjar, John H., MD
  Howhannesian, Andranik, MD
Vascular Surgery
  Bapineedu, Kuchipudi, MD

Fairfield
Family Med-Hospice & Palliative
  Douge, Simone Alicia, MD
Family Medicine
  Liotti, Joseph B., DO
  Liotti, Linda A., DO
  Scolamiero, Amedeo J., MD
Internal Medicine
  Bhatt, Rupal S., MD
  Bhatt, Shirish Vinayak, MD
  Chen, Bonnie L., MD
  Howe, Thomas Arthur, MD
  Zhukova, Irina, DO
Ophthalmology
  Moses, Eli B., MD
  Perl, Theodore, MD
Pediatric Allergy
  Torre, Arthur J., MD
Surgery (General)
  Funicello, Alex Vincent, MD

Fairview
Family Medicine
  Erguder, Iris, MD
  Eyerman, Luke Edmund, MD
  Stricker, Howard, DO
Physical Medicine & Rehab
  Suche, Kara J., MD

Fanwood
Cardiovascular Disease
  Kalischer, Alan L., MD
Family Medicine
  Scalia, Joseph A., DO
Internal Medicine
  Brodman, Richard R., MD
  Jamdar, Niteen Subhash, MD
  Lewis, Thomas Peter, MD
Pediatrics
  Gillard, Bonita Dee, MD
  Koward, Donna Marie, MD

Far Hills
Gynecology
  Moore, Donnica Lauren, MD
Ophthalmology
  Wax, Martin Bruce, MD

Farmingdale
Family Medicine
  Dennis, Philip S., MD
  Schauer, Joseph W. III, MD
  Taneja, Deepak, DO
Internal Medicine
  Kelemen, Ina J., MD
  Ornstein, Mark W., MD

Flanders
Family Medicine
  Choe, Charles C., DO
  Fernandez, Sofia Ramona, MD
  Friedman, Samuel, MD
  Ghanta, Suma Bala, MD
  Huang, Chen Ya, MD
  Miccio, Anthony G., MD
  Peters, Karen R., DO
Internal Medicine
  Chaudhari, Anuja Parikh, DO
  Chaudhari, Suvid, DO
  Mercado, Alex M., MD
  Pathak, Rajiv J., MD

Flemington
Anatomic/Clinical Pathology
  Isaac, Irene V., MD
  Zanchelli Astran, Gina M., DO
Anesthesiology
  Bentley, William Earl IV, DO
  Bussard, Elizabeth S., MD
  Cabahug, Wilfred Tan, MD
  Lai, Chia-Lung, MD
  Lapicki, Walter S., DO
  Maldonado-Viera, Lourdes, MD
  Nagorny, Wojciech Antoni, MD
  Nyitray, Peter, MD
  Silber, Michael B., DO
  Wang, Edward, MD
  Wilson, John Joseph, MD
Cardiovascular Disease
  Benigno, Robert A., MD
  Bialy, Ted, MD
  Horiuchi, Jonathan K., MD
  Imsirovic-Starcevic, Dubravka, MD
  Kutscher, Austin Harrison Jr., MD
  Pickoff, Robert M., MD
  Schafranek, William, MD
  Tonnessen, Glen E., MD
Child & Adolescent Psychiatry
  Chen, Hong, MD
Clinical Cardiac Elctrphyslgy
  Rudnick, Andrew Glenn, MD
Clinical Genetics
  Rushton, Alan R., MD
Critical Care Medicine
  Cohn, David B., MD
  Goldstein, Keith Ty, MD
  Khan, Muhammad Khurram, MD
Dermatology
  Beachler, Kent J., MD
  Blechman, Adam Brandon, MD
  Cassetty, Christopher Todd, MD
  Sood, Supriya G., MD
Developmental Pediatrics
  Mars, Audrey Estelle, MD
Diagnostic Radiology
  Castaldi, Mark Whittaker, MD
  Feldman, Ruth S., MD
  Loesberg, Andrew C., MD
Emergency Medicine
  Bliss, Mary J., MD
  Christiansen, David, MD
  Guillen, Steven E., MD
  Johnson-Villanueva, Norma J., MD
  Mehta, Nimish Harendra, MD
  Patel, Chirag G., MD
  Schultz, Edward Joseph, MD
  Schupner, Kathleen A., MD
  Spector, Edward D., MD
  Villanueva, Norma I., MD
  Yoon, Young Dug, MD
Endocrinology
  Caldarella, Felice Antonino, MD
  Modarressi, Taher, MD
  Sandberg, Marc Ira, MD
Family Medicine
  Bachrach, Stacey R., MD
  Baird, Jamila, MD
  Benson, Jay Robert, DO
  Bernard, Marie G., MD
  Bretan, Amy Faith, MD
  Coates, Robert G., MD
  Cox, Victoria Ryan, MD
  Eskow, Eugene S., MD
  Feigin, Joel Stanley, MD
  Fuhrman, Joel H., MD
  Gazurian, Raina, MD
  Gertzman, Jerrold Scott, MD
  Golub, Larisa, MD
  Hannema, Erica L., DO
  Hoette, Petra, MD
  Joseph, Junie Lorna, MD
  Klein, Randy S., MD
  Lecusay, Dario A. Jr., MD
  Lewis, Mary Kendra, MD
  Licetti, Stephen Charles, DO
  Liebross, Ira David, MD
  Liu, Lide, MD
  Madonia, Paul W., MD
  Manchen, Dennis R., MD
  Mattei, C. Antonia, MD
  McDonough, John R., MD
  Morton, Lisa Aseni, MD
  Mui, Timothy H., MD
  Mukherji, Genea, MD
  Nealis, Justin, MD
  O'Hara, Jennifer Fisk, MD
  Pauch-McNamara, Dorothy Anne, MD
  Peng, Victor I., MD
  Plunkett, Lisa A., MD
  Randhawa, Smita Devidas, MD
  Scevola Dattoli, Angela, MD
  Solanki, Dhenu G., MD
  Tammana, Swarna, DO
  Weil, Irina Lisker, MD
  Wierzbicki, Jonathan Edmund, MD
  Wright, Deborah Sue, MD
Foot & Ankle Surgery
  Bleazey, Scott Thomas, MD
Gastroenterology
  Bae, Samuel Y., MD
  Cardoso, Gilbert Santos, DO
  Daruwala, Cherag A., MD
  DiGregorio, Kenneth J., MD
  Georgsson, Maria Anna, MD
  Goldstein, Andrea E., MD
  Hartford, Jeffrey D., MD
  Lesser, Gregory Scott, MD
  Lim, Khengjim, MD
  Matthews, Jason D., MD
  Patel, Anik Mayur, MD
  Sinha, Anubha, MD
  Willis, Stephen Laird, MD

Geriatrics
 Chakravarthi,Seshadri Shekar,MD
 Gujar,Priti S.,MD
 Tunuguntla,Renuka,MD
Hand Surgery
 Nenna,David Vito,MD
Hematology
 Blankstein,Kenneth B.,MD
Hematology Oncology
 Bednar,Myron Emil,MD
 Ngeow,Swee Jian,MD
 Rehman,Waqas,MD
 Shah,Megha,MD
Hepatology
 Arrigo,Richard J.,DO
Infectious Disease
 Gugliotta,Joseph L.,MD
Internal Med-Allergy&Immunlgy
 Muglia-Chopra,Christine Ann,MD
Internal Med-Hospice Palliative
 Fox,Katherine,MD
Internal Medicine
 Broslawski,Gregory E.,DO
 Cao,Lan,MD
 Elnahar,Yaser,MD
 Granato,Anthony Alexander,MD
 Haddad,Sohail G.,MD
 Khan,Saima,MD
 Lansang,Martin Fidel,MD
 Lazarus,David S.,MD
 Lind,Robert Michael,MD
 Mak,Mimi,MD
 Miele,Bevon D.,MD
 Novy,Donald S.,MD
 Pistun,Oleksandr,MD
 Quinn,Brian Michael,MD
 Saxena,Amita,MD
 Shaber,Marc L.,MD
 Storch,Marc I.,MD
 Surapanani,Devi,MD
 Veeraraghavan,Gowri,MD
Neonatal-Perinatal Medicine
 Chavarkar,Mrunalini R.,MD
 Veerappan,Sutharsanam,MD
 Weiss,Kerry I.,MD
Neurological Surgery
 Pizzi,Francis Joseph,MD
Neurology
 Kososky,Charles S.,MD
 Pandya,Dipakkumar P.,MD
 Pennett,Donald T.,MD
 Viradia,Manish Bhikhabhai,MD
Obstetrics & Gynecology
 Abeysinghe,Manisha G.,MD
 Altomare,Corrado J.,MD
 Ardise,Patricia Marie,MD
 Belkina,Yelena,MD
 Bowers,Mamie Sue,MD
 Camiolo,Melissa Rae,MD
 Frys,Kelly Ann,DO
 Grimes,Sara,MD
 Grove,Michele Sak,MD
 Huttner,Ruby P.,MD
 Lynen,Richard F.,MD
 Masterton,Deirdre C.,MD
 Pedersen,Irene A.,MD
 Pisatowski,Denise Michelle,MD
 Rivas,Jimena,MD
 Vitale,Lidia F.,MD
Ophthalmology
 Batt,Gerald E.,MD
 Dunham,Gerald,MD
 Phillips,Paul S.,MD
Orthopedic Surgery
 Collalto,Patrick Michael,MD
 Glassner,Norman,MD
 Glassner,Philip Justin,MD
 Pollack,Michael Edward,MD
 Shafa,Eiman,MD
Orthopedic Surgery-Adult Rcnstr
 Gordon,Eric Michael,MD
Orthopedics
 Chang,Richard,MD
Other Specialty
 Decker,Jerome Elliot,MD
Otolaryngology
 Hanna,John Patrick,DO
 Kroon,David Fleming,MD
 Maniar,Anoli,MD
 Sheft,Stanley A.,MD
 Worden,Douglas L.,MD

Pathology
 Basius,Maureen,DO
Pediatric Neurodevelopment
 Casey,Thomas James,MD
Pediatrics
 Agarwal,Ravi,MD
 Bery,Sumita,MD
 Clarin,Mitchell I.,MD
 Douvris,John S.,MD
 Fellmeth,Wayne G.,MD
 Hartigan,Thomas P.,MD
 Humoee,Nidal Michel,MD
 Jasutkar,Ashwini,MD
 Krupinski,Donna J.,MD
 Michael,Rositta,MD
 Pina,Liza Miriam,MD
 Prosswimmer,Geralyn M.,MD
 Roksvaag,George E.,MD
 Shah,Debra Stahl,MD
 Willems-Plakyda,Michele C.,MD
Physical Med & Rehab-Pain Med
 Salam,Aleya,MD
Psychiatry
 Hill,Everett Huntington,MD
 Kuris,Jay D.,MD
 Lucas,Gem-Estelle Maun,DO
 Moss,Pamela F.,MD
 Patel,Mukesh D.,MD
 Phillips,Anne R.,MD
 Skotzko,Christine Ellen,MD
Pulmonary Critical Care
 Maouelainin,Nina,DO
 Yuan,Carol Jia-Luh,MD
Radiology
 Szikman,Howard Shawn,DO
Sports Medicine
 More,Robert C.,MD
Surgery (General)
 Bello,John J.,MD
 Bello,Joseph M.,MD
 Gleason,Catherine Elizabeth,MD
 Maeuser,Herman L.I.,MD
Urology
 Bloch,Paul Jacob,MD
 Choi,James,MD
 Ghosh,Propa,MD
 Kern,Allen J.,MD
 Lai,Weil Ron,MD
 Sperling,Brian Lee,DO
Vascular & Intrvntnal Radiology
 Cortes,Andrew,MD

Florham Park
Adult Psychiatry
 Kral,Felix E.,MD
Allergy
 Barisciano,Lisa,MD
 Sundaram,Usha K.,MD
Allergy & Immunology
 Parikh,Smruti Ashish,MD
Anatomic Pathology
 Savera,Adnan Tabrez,MD
Anesthesiology
 Abramowicz,Apolonia E.,MD
 Ahmad,Idrees,MD
 Asimolowo,Olabisi Omolara,MD
 Basius,Joseph T.,DO
 Bergam,Miro Nicholas Jr.,MD
 Blank,Jonathan Dirk,MD
 Bonsell,Joshua W.,MD
 Braverman,Joel Morton,MD
 Cardoso,Ronald J.,MD
 Chen,Jianping,MD
 Chung,Dae S.,MD
 Ciolino,Robert B.,MD
 Clancy,Lisa A.,MD
 Co,Demosthene E.,MD
 Conyack,David G.,DO
 Davis,Clifton Colby,MD
 Dibadj,Khosro,MD
 Fein,Eric N.,MD
 Fisher,Emery IV,DO
 Fitz,Rachel Myra,DO
 Ganti,Suryaprakash,MD
 Goldstein,Joshua D.,MD
 Hausdorff,Mark Alan,MD
 Ju,Albert Changwon,MD
 Kim,Mina Jung,MD
 Knepa,Valdone Elena,MD
 Levine,Robert Scott,MD
 Maizes,Allen Stuart,MD
 Monti,Richard A.,MD

 Parikh,Bijal Rajendra,MD
 Patafio,Onofrio,MD
 Patel,Prashant A.,MD
 Pond,Charles G.,MD
 Ramos,Joseph,MD
 Russo,Cathy Marie,MD
 Scala,Peter L.,MD
 Zylberger,David A.,MD
Cardiovascular Disease
 Fabrizio,Lawrence,DO
 Steinberg,Jonathan S.,MD
Child (Pediatric) Neurology
 Grossman,Elliot A.,MD
Clinical Cardiac Elctrphyslgy
 Santoni,Francesco,MD
Clinical Pathology
 Hofgaertner,Wolfgang Theodor,MD
Dermatology
 Badalamenti,Stephanie Silos,MD
 Huang,Eric Y.,MD
 Huang,Eric Yuchueh,MD
 Kiken,David Adam,MD
 Machler,Brian C.,MD
 Patel-Cohen,Mital,MD
Endocrinology
 Borger,Caryn Beth,MD
 Siegel,Sheera Karch,MD
Family Medicine
 Gunn Russell,Ian Neil,MD
 Harwani,Nita R.,MD
Gastroenterology
 Galandauer,Isaac,MD
Gynecological Oncology
 Febbraro,Terri,MD
Hematology
 Kay,Andrea C.,MD
Hematology Oncology
 DeRosa,William T.,DO
 George,Roshini,DO
 Gurubhagavatula,Sarada,MD
 Siu,Karleung,MD
Hospitalist
 Pinyard,Jeremy Vincent,MD
Infectious Disease
 Bennett,Douglas P.,DO
 De Shaw,Max G.,MD
 Frankel,Renee Ellen,MD
 Hart,Daniel,MD
 O'Grady,John P.,MD
Internal Medicine
 Alberto,Kezia J.,MD
 Blumberg,Darren Reich,MD
 Castellano,Charles C.,MD
 Chandwani,Ashish,MD
 Cohen,Liliana,MD
 Das,Mohan P.,MD
 Di Giacomo,Eric D.,MD
 Di Ruggiero,Roger P.,MD
 Dicenzo-Flynn,Carla F.,MD
 Freid,Robert S.,MD
 Goodman,Jeffrey W.,MD
 Hooda,Anjali,MD
 Kilkenny-Trainor,Kerryann A.,MD
 Kissin,Anna,MD
 Klees,Julia E.,MD
 Kunjukutty,Felix,MD
 Li,Zhexiang,MD
 Lyman,Neil W.,MD
 Maron,Scott Michael,MD
 Olesnicky,Mark T.,MD
 Pajaro,Rafael E.,MD
 Pally,Steven Arthur,DO
 Paulina,Arthur Jr.,MD
 Pinel Villalobos,Silvia P.,DO
 Rodrigues,Anisha,MD
 Roytman,Peter,MD
 Sabnani-Nagella,Kavita R.,MD
 Saldarini,John Christopher,MD
 Shubeck,Caroline A.,MD
 Soleymani,Taraneh,MD
 Storch,Kenneth J.,MD
 Tamres,David Michael,MD
 Tiongco,Judith Perlas,MD
 Viscuso,Ronald L.,MD
 Zenenberg,Robert D.,DO
Nephrology
 Ahmad,Mir M.,MD
 Estilo,Genevieve Kristina,MD
Neurological Surgery
 Noce,Louis Arthur,MD
 Scheid,Edward Herbert Jr.,MD

Obstetrics & Gynecology
 Banks,Judy L.,MD
 Chervenak,Donald M.,MD
 Gibbon,Darlene Grace,MD
 Locatelli,Sam Thomas,MD
 Rawlins,Samantha Geanine,MD
Occupational Medicine
 Conner,Patrick R.,MD
Oncological Surgery
 Bamboat,Zubin Mickey,MD
 Diehl,William L.,MD
 Kim,Joseph Jongbum,MD
Orthopedic Surgery
 Adam,Stephanie Paige,DO
 Black,Eric M.,MD
 Kocaj,Stephen Mark,MD
 Shindle,Michael Kenneth,MD
Orthopedic-Hand Surgery
 Niver,Genghis Erjan,MD
Otolaryngology
 Byrd,Serena Ann,MD
 Fleming,Gregory John,MD
 Peron,Didier L.,MD
Pediatrics
 Bailon,Amy R.,MD
 Baxley,Maureen Elizabeth,MD
 Behbakht,Mojgan,MD
 Petrozzino,Vito A.,MD
 Silva,Francisco,MD
Plastic Surgery
 Colon,Francisco G.,MD
 Hawrylo,Richard R.,MD
 Lange,David J.,MD
 Starker,Isaac,MD
 Vallone,Paul J.,MD
Psychiatry
 Dracxler Meaker,Roberta,MD
 Moreno,Jose G.,MD
 Oyejide,Catherine O.,MD
Surgery (General)
 Abkin,Alexander,MD
 Argiroff,Alexandra Louise,MD
 Bertha,Nicholas A.,DO
 Botvinov,Mikhail A.,DO
 Carter,Mitchel S.,MD
 Cuppari,Anthony L.,MD
 Failey,Colin Leander,MD
 Gabre,Kennedy Ogbazion,MD
 Most,Michael David,MD
Vascular Surgery
 Seaver,Philip Jr.,MD

Fords
Allergy & Immunology
 Ogden,Neeta Sharma,MD
Cardiovascular Disease
 Latif,Pervaize,MD
Family Medicine
 Petrovani,Mark S.,MD
Geriatrics
 Haldar,Pranab K.,MD
Internal Medicine
 Gil,Constante,MD
 Sharma,Madho K.,MD
Obstetrics & Gynecology
 Shonowo,Owobamishola Adanma,MD

Forked River
Allergy & Immunology
 Empedrad,Raquel B.,MD
Critical Care Medicine
 Power,William K. Jr.,MD
Emergency Medicine
 Pie,Alberto C.,MD
Family Medicine
 Barry,Therese Maria,DO
 Kassenoff,Lisa Adrian,DO
 Novak,Dennis E.,MD
Internal Medicine
 Bhiro,Peter Rajendra,DO
 Crisan,Liviu C.,MD
 Ende,Theodore,DO
 Jannone,Joel P.,MD
 Tubilleja,Nina Lapidario,MD
Obstetrics & Gynecology
 Bustamante Dayanghirang,Alma,MD
Pediatrics
 Mabagos,Jerry D.,MD
 Pradhan,Prasanna Govind,MD
 Yassin,Mahmoud M.,MD

Physicians by Town and Medical Specialty

Fort Dix
Family Medicine
Byrnes,Michael John,DO
General Practice
Gorelli,Lucy Ann,MD
Geriatric Psychiatry
Rashid,Shahzad,DO
Internal Medicine
Patel,Pradip M.,MD

Fort Lee
Addiction Medicine
Piper,Craig S.,MD
Anesthesiology
Basak,Jayati,MD
Chiang,Kou-Cheng,MD
Desai,Jagdip,MD
Friedman,Gina Y.,DO
Grigorescu,Traian Andrei,MD
Lin,Cheng Hsiang,MD
Lustig,Karen C.,DO
Ohanian,Marc S.,MD
Ostrovsky,Igor,MD
Park,Yong M.,MD
Anesthesiology: Pain Medicine
Kang,Chang H.,MD
Kang,Richard,MD
Cardiovascular Disease
Adibi,Baback,MD
Andrews,Paul Matthew,MD
Gallo,Richard James,MD
Hollywood,Jacqueline,MD
Kim,Steve Sang-Yoon,MD
Krasikov,Tatiana,MD
Landers,David Benjamin,MD
Lauricella,Joseph Ned,MD
Lebowitz,Nathaniel Edward,MD
Rothman,Howard C.,MD
Zanger,Diane Rachel,MD
Cornea/External Disease
Rosenberg,Michael Eric,MD
Dermatology
Goulko,Olga,MD
Lee,Robert,MD
Developmental Pediatrics
deVinck,Oana,DO
Family Medicine
Cassotta,Joseph P. Jr.,MD
Karatoprak,Ohan,MD
Lee,David W.,MD
General Practice
Rosenberg,Paul Howard,MD
Vincent,Michael G.,MD
Geriatrics
Kim,John,MD
Hospitalist
Blaszka,Matthew Christopher,MD
Infectious Disease
Kim,Jeongwon,MD
Intrnl Med-Heart Diseas/Transpn
Lucev,Anthony,MD
Internal Medicine
Bai,Sammy S.,MD
Feller,Matthew F.,MD
Girshovich,Irina,MD
Hernandez,Michael Dennis,MD
Kalayjian,Tro,DO
Sabater,Pilar,MD
Shapnik,Bella,MD
Wang,Kyu Sung,MD
Yang,Yulong,MD
Medical Oncology
Yuan,Rui Rong,MD
Obstetrics & Gynecology
Lee,James R.,MD
Shoshilos,Anna G.,DO
Ophthalmology
Kim,John Sung,MD
Kulik,Alfred D.,MD
Palacios,Alexander L.,MD
Rosenberg,Rhonda Betsy,MD
Oral & Maxillofacial Surgery
Carrao,Vincent,MD
Orthopedic Surgery
Lee,Fred Suin,MD
Otolaryngology
Henick,David H.,MD
Kim,Steve Yun,MD
Pediatric Ophthalmology
Rosenberg-Henick,Arlene M.,MD

Pediatrics
Akturk,Elvin,DO
Aranoff,Joanne Rachel,MD
Banschick,Harry,MD
Choi,Yoonhee,MD
Chung,Nam Young,MD
Colenda,Maryann J.,MD
Elkassir,Amina,MD
Kim,Eun-Joo Song,MD
Kim,Eunja,MD
Kumar,Geeta L.,DO
Kuo,Grace,MD
Lazieh,Janet Tomeh,MD
Yenukashvili,Nana R.,MD
Physical Medicine & Rehab
Kim,Jong Hyun,MD
Kim,Ruby E.,MD
Shin,Mira,MD
Plastic Surgery
Michelson,Lorelle N.,MD
Ponamgi,Suri B.,MD
Trovato,Matthew J.,MD
Psychiatry
Cuervo,Nieves,MD
Napoli,Joseph C.,MD
Rudelli,Mercedes N.,MD
Sher,Leo,MD
Public Health
Etzi,Susan,MD
Surgery (General)
Mashburn,Penelope,DO

Franklin
Family Medicine
Holgado,Marco Patrick Guinto,DO
Hrabarchuk,Eugene S.,MD
Matkiwsky,Daniel Walter,DO
McMahon,Kerry Rose,MD
Internal Medicine
Patel,Pravinbhal C.,MD

Franklin Lakes
Anatomic/Clinical Pathology
Lawrence,Jeffry Brian,MD
Anesthesiology
Ashraf,Waseem,MD
Blady,Joseph A.,MD
Lee,Jung Du,MD
Cardiovascular Disease
Golden,Lee Scott,MD
Wertheimer,David Eliot,MD
Dermatology
Abdulla,Heba M.,MD
Diagnostic Radiology
Demauro,Linda Dell,MD
Emergency Medicine
Melwani,Ramesh D.,MD
Endocrinology
Dasmahapatra,Amita,MD
Hirsch,Laurence J.,MD
Gastroenterology
Chusid,Boris Gregory,MD
Internal Medicine
Krutchik,Allan N.,MD
Sandoval,Ramon Antonio,MD
Sutter,David Brand,MD
Interventional Cardiology
Lee,John Hyung-II,MD
Obstetrics & Gynecology
Weidman,Joshua A.,MD
Ophthalmology
Bruder,Scott P.,MD
Orthopedic Surgery
Bellapianta,Joseph Michael,MD
Greenberg,Aaron Joseph,MD
Lin,Edward Alan,MD
Sood,Amit,MD
Pediatrics
Rosenberg,Zeil Barry,MD
Physical Medicine & Rehab
Aydin,Steve M.,DO
Reiter,Raymond D.,MD
Psychiatry
Coira,Diego L.,MD
Richards,Christopher F.,MD
Rheumatology
Pandey,Rajesh Kumar,MD
Zalkowitz,Alan,MD
Surgery (General)
Fondacaro,Paul Francis,MD

Franklin Park
Cosmetic Surgery

Perry,Arthur William,MD
Emergency Medicine
Cha,Min,MD
Phan,Au Ngoc,MD
Internal Medicine
Chen,Julie Eveline,MD
Jacobs,David S A,MD
Sanghui,Sarika Patel,DO
Pediatrics
Iyanoye,Abimbola Olamide,MD
Psychiatry
Antolin,Eleanor Banzon,MD
Yeung,Cindy S.,DO

Franklinville
Emergency Medicine
Chappell,Stephen E.,MD

Freehold
Acupuncture
Pellmar,Monte B.,MD
Aerospace Medicine
Wright,Evan Michael,DO
Allergy & Immunology
Case,Philip Lawrence,MD
Anatomic/Clinical Pathology
Sinha,Karabi,MD
Anesthesiology
Armbrecht,Kimberley T.,MD
Campagnuolo,Joann E.,DO
Connors,Anne,MD
Cubina,Maria L.,DO
DeAntonio,Joseph Alexander,MD
Deshmukh,Poornima Vasudeo,MD
Fahmy,Nader M.,MD
Ghattas,Maged L.,MD
Grace,Rashy,MD
Kumar,Nirmal A.,MD
Mak,John,MD
Mehta,Hemangini G.,MD
Mikhail,Magdy H.,MD
O'Hara,Michael W.,DO
Parikh,Pallavi M.,MD
Patel,Jayshree R.,MD
Proban,Rafal,MD
Randall,Tanya,MD
Scarmato,Albert Clark Jr.,DO
Soriano,Brian J.,MD
Stabile,Daniel,MD
Stump,James Basil,MD
Zachary,Samuel,DO
Cardiovascular Disease
Awasthi,Ashish,MD
Beauregard,Louanne M.,MD
Borgersen,Rudolph H.,DO
Garg,Sangeeta,MD
Gutowski,Ted,MD
Hanfling,Marcus,DO
Kominos,Vivian A.,MD
Liu,Marcia Nai-Hwa,MD
Mentle,Iris R.,MD
Noto,Gregory,MD
Zukerman,Louis Steven,MD
Child & Adolescent Psychiatry
Chatlos,John Calvin Jr.,MD
Desai,Ankur Akhilesh,MD
Zaidi,Sajjad,MD
Colon & Rectal Surgery
Kayal,Thomas Joseph,MD
Cornea/External Disease
Schneider,Martin S.,MD
Critical Care Medicine
DeTullio,John P.,MD
Dermatology
Hametz,Irwin,MD
Miller,Jason Harris,MD
Picascia,David D.,MD
Sivanesan,Swarna Priya,MD
Diagnostic Radiology
Arredondo,Mario Gaston,MD
Chalal,Jeffrey,MD
Friedenberg,Jeffrey Scott,MD
Keklak,C. Stephen,MD
Kouveliotes,Peter J.,MD
Loeb,Debra M.,MD
Romano,Kenneth Robert,MD
Spector,Janet,MD
Tomkovich,Kenneth R.,MD
Emergency Medicine
Altevear,Janet G.,MD
Carino,Samuel Comia,DO
Connolly,Sandra M.,MD

Dayner,Jeremy Joseph,MD
Friedman,Daniel Marc,DO
Giron,Miguel,MD
Jones,Marvin M.,MD
Kaplan,Gary Peter,MD
Lee,Tracey-Ann Nadine,MD
McLaughlin,Valerie Gail,MD
Mehta,Ragini R.,DO
Waciega,Mark,MD
Endocrinology
Farghani,Saima Obaid,MD
Nassberg,Barton M.,MD
Ordene,Kenneth W.,MD
Wininger,Eric Amiel,MD
Young,Melissa G.,MD
Endoscopic Surgery
Dobruskin,Yelizaveta,MD
Family Med-Geriatric Medicine
Khan,Zeeshan,MD
Family Medicine
Bernardo,Salvatore Jr.,MD
Cherciu,Doina M.,MD
Cherciu,Mugurel S.,MD
Chopra,Vinay,MD
Ciminelli,Maria F.,MD
Cozzarelli,James Francis,MD
Delcurla,Gina M.,MD
Dermer,Alicia R.,MD
Edrich,Dina Rachel,MD
Eng,Kenneth,DO
Espinar Ho,Maria Elena,MD
Faistl,Kenneth W.,MD
Gershenbaum,Mark R.,DO
Gupta,Vinod K.,MD
Kathrotia,Mitesh Gordhan,MD
Kim,Miah,MD
Leonard,Sara B.,MD
Lucas,Lisa W.,DO
Mellor,Lisa Marie,MD
Mills,Orlando F.,MD
Nau,Allen Reza,DO
Ogon,Bernard Okem,MD
Paulvin,Neil Brian,DO
Raccuglia,Joseph R.,MD
Rider,Timothy Eugene,MD
Sandru,Dan Victor,MD
Sasidhar,Vaidehi,MD
Sewell,Grant,MD
Shenker,Bennett Steven,MD
Sinha,Taru,MD
Stein,Howard A.,DO
Gastroenterology
Blank,Robert R.,MD
Bohm,Steven A.,MD
Gupta,Kunal,MD
Ludwig,Shelly L.,MD
Mufson,Lewis J.,MD
Nadler,Steven C.,MD
General Practice
Boorstein,Jerry,DO
Goldstein,Jay R.,MD
Geriatrics
Gohel,Rekha M.,MD
Rowlands,Randy R.,MD
Yu Chen,Robert P.,MD
Glaucoma
Grand,Elliot S.,MD
Hand Surgery
Patel,Nikesh Kirit,MD
Hematology
Gopal,Krishnan T.,MD
Silberberg,Jeffrey M.,MD
Internal Medicine
Barofsky,Kenneth D.,MD
Bhasin,Atul,MD
Brown,Colin Christopher,MD
Cohen,Aly G.,MD
Coppolino,Frank P.,MD
Croce,Salvatore A.,MD
Donde,Dilip M.,MD
El Kadi,Hisham S.,MD
Fischkoff,James Daniel,MD
Garmkhorani,Abolghassem,MD
Geller,Arthur J.,MD
Giannone,Dean Francis,MD
Gonzales,Antero B.,MD
Gopal,Indumathi,MD
Gruber,Todd A.,MD
Heitzer,Frederic M.,MD
Kaga,Mira Kamal,MD
Komboz,Rita Fares,MD

Krakauer,Randall Sheldon,MD
Kroll,Mark S.,MD
Kudipudi,Ramanasri V.,MD
Lage,Susan Marie,DO
Luparello,Paul J.,MD
Majumdar,Shikha,MD
Medasani,Kiran M.,MD
Melka,Berhanu Gossaye,MD
Menon,Divya,MD
Najmey,Sawsan S.,MD
Nijhawan,Minakshi,MD
Paulin,Cesar M.,MD
Petcu,Alexandru,MD
Restua,Nestor S.,MD
Rose,T.,MD
Ross,William H.,DO
Shah,Anand Subhash,MD
Sharma,Anil K.,MD
Sharobeem,Andrew Mena,DO
Sojka,Leslie W.,MD
Sowemimo,Fiolakemi O.,MD
Vizzoni,Joseph Anthony,MD
Weinstein,Benjamin,MD
Werber,John Frank,MD
Zirkman,Daniel M.,MD
Interventional Cardiology
Litsky,Jason D.,DO
Medical Oncology
Balar,Bhavesh Vasant,MD
Neurological Surgery
Tormenti,Matthew J.,MD
Neurology
Bonazinga,Thomas P.,MD
Frank,David J.,MD
Gulevski,Vasko Kole,MD
Katz,Amos,MD
Marks,Caren G.,MD
McAlarney,Terence,MD
Zaatreh,Megdad M.,MD
Obstetrics & Gynecology
Aland,Kristen,MD
Amer,Yousef A.,MD
Back,Norman A.,MD
Barnett,Rebecca L.,MD
Baum,Jonathan D.,MD
Bernard-Roberts,Lynikka,MD
Burt-Libo,Borislava,DO
Cipriano,Joseph A.,MD
Cipriano,Rebecca J.,MD
Dimino,Michael L.,MD
Goldstein,Steven A.,MD
Joshi,Jyotika D.,MD
Kirwin,Michael S.,MD
Lucas,Romeo Augusto,DO
Mandel,Peter C.,MD
Mayson,Robert P.,MD
Misra,Neeti Virendra,MD
Morreale,Ginja Massey,MD
Neuwirth,Safrir,MD
Pacana,Susan Marie,MD
Portadin,Robert A.,MD
Prugno,Robin Jean,DO
Ranasinghe Rodrigo,Nimalie,MD
Rattigan,Meghan Iona,DO
Scheff,Elizabeth Anne,MD
Seigel,Mark J.,MD
Ophthalmology
Aksman,Scott S.,MD
Brenner,Edward H.,MD
Brottman,Jeffrey S.,MD
Gershenbaum,Eric Andrew,MD
Kernitsky,Roman G.,MD
Lee,David K.,MD
Lee,Joan Jean,DO
Minzter,Ronald M.,MD
Mishkin,Steven K.,MD
Naadimuthu,Revathi P.,MD
Ng,Elena M.,MD
Rosin,Jay Michael,MD
Orthopedic Surgery
Banzon,Manuel T.,MD
Berkowitz,Gregg S.,MD
Goldberger,Gerardo V.,DO
Greller,Michael Jon,MD
Mark,Arthur K.,MD
Mittman,Roy D.,MD
Nakashian,Michael,MD
Nasar,Alan S.,MD
Vasen,Arthur Philip,MD
Velez,Alberto A.,MD

Orthopedics
Arias Garau,Jessica,MD
Otolaryngology
Brahmbhatt,Sapna Sureshkumar,MD
Kumar,Arun S.,MD
Razvi,Sedeq A.,MD
Roessler,Mark Leonard,DO
Sattenspiel,Sigmund Linder,MD
Pathology
Saleem,Sogra R.,MD
Pediatrics
Bhaskar,Vatsala R.,MD
Cato-Varlack,Janice A.,MD
Chieco,Michael Anthony,MD
Daghistani,Lina,MD
Donde,Mrunalini D.,MD
Emanuel,Anthony,MD
Gajula,Ramarao Sundara,MD
Ibale,Florence E.,MD
Jonnalagadda,Balathripura S.,MD
Katturupalli,Madhavi,MD
LaMantia,Anthony P.,MD
Lacap,Estela Villar,MD
Lopez,Leonardo Nicholas,DO
Mayer,Diana R.,MD
McFeely,Erin M.,MD
Mehta,Sanjay,DO
Patel,Arvind Maganbhai,MD
Sadik,Zubaida Y.,MD
Shah,Neha Naresh,MD
Shah,Vrinda B.,MD
Swayne,Kathleen Amy,MD
Teresh,Michelle A.,MD
Velez,Corazon S.,MD
Wolfe,Jeffrey S.,MD
Zeb,Marta R.,MD
Physical Medicine & Rehab
Engelman,James E.,DO
Freeman,Darren Keith,DO
Plastic Surgery
Bhattacharya,Ashish Kumar,MD
Stein,Howard Larry,MD
Psychiatry
Burstein,Allan J.,MD
DeBlasi,Richard A.,MD
Figarola,Carlos J.,MD
Goldstein,Lauren T.,MD
Ibanez,Delfin George C.,MD
Kolli,Sireesha K.,MD
Matflerd,Carolynn A.,MD
Prado-Galarza,Neiza L.,MD
Shafey,Moustafa Hassan,MD
Singh,Rajkumar R.,MD
Vyas,Hema,MD
Pulmonary Disease
Krachman,Samuel Lee,DO
Pi,Justin Jeong-Suk,MD
Shah,Nirav Navin,DO
Radiation Oncology
Cardinale,Robert Michael,MD
Chon,Brian Hisuk,MD
Soffen,Edward M.,MD
Tsai,Henry K.,MD
Radiology
Friedenberg,Barry,MD
Hughes,Ann M.,MD
Mezzacappa,Peter M.,MD
Rich,Stanley E.,MD
Rondina,Carlo L.,MD
Rosenstein,Howard P.,MD
Rheumatology
Adenwalla,Humaira Naseem,MD
Ghafoor,Sadia,DO
Lumezanu,Elena Mihaela,MD
Spinal Surgery
Goldberg,Grigory,MD
Surgery (General)
Ashok,Viswanath K.,MD
Kharod,Amit S.,MD
Martucci,Mary T.,DO
Menack,Michael J.,MD
Noyan,Earl Lincoln,MD
Schulman,William M.,MD
Shakov,Emil,MD
Sowemimo,Oluseun Akande,MD
Wetstein,Lewis,MD
Trauma Surgery
Digiacomo,Jody Christopher,MD
Urology
De Salvo,Eugene L.,MD
Kohlberg,William I.,MD

Silverstein,Jeffrey I.,MD
Vascular & Intrvntnal Radiology
Patil,Vivek Vinay,MD
Vascular Surgery
Kovacs,Gabor,MD
Lehman,Mark,MD
Silvers,Lawrence W.,MD
Galloway
Anesthesiology
Cerniglia,Salvatore Joseph,DO
Kasica,Patricia R.,DO
Cardiovascular Disease
Carreno,Wilfredo,MD
Delaverdac,Claude L.,DO
Flynn,Anthony M.,MD
Ghaly,Nader Naguib,MD
Ghayal,Mahesh,MD
Jayasinghe,Swarnathilaka,MD
Kanzaria,Mitul,MD
Merchant,Yatish B.,MD
Nascimento,Tome R.,MD
Van Hook,Jeffrey E.,DO
Vankawala,Viren R.,MD
Clinical Cardiac Elctrphyslgy
White,Melvin C.,MD
Critical Care Medicine
Higgins,Nancy C.,MD
Diagnostic Radiology
Altin,Robert S.,MD
Avagliano,Margaret C.,MD
Brezel,Mitchell H.,MD
Ferretti,James Christian,DO
Graule,Melissa J.,MD
Graziano,Robert J.,MD
Handel,David B.,MD
Kenny,David Anthony,DO
Lee,Michael Joseph,MD
Levi,David A.,MD
Levy,Karen R.,MD
Menghetti,Richard A.,MD
Mesham,James R.,MD
Patel,Hiren Ramesh,MD
Patel,Rajesh Ishwar,MD
Peshori,Kavita R.,MD
Viswambharan,Ajay,MD
Family Medicine
Ezeanya,Ebere Nneka,MD
Sperling,Howard J.,MD
Thadhani,Ramchand,MD
Williams,Robert H. Jr.,MD
General Practice
Ramchand,Maya,MD
Geriatrics
Gong,Jeffrey,DO
Hematology Oncology
Ajay,Rajasree,MD
Borai,Nasser Eldien,MD
Infectious Disease
Kaur,Amrita,DO
Internal Medicine
Aridi,Imad M.,MD
Brown,Lemarra Rena,DO
Dasondi,Vivekkumar V.,MD
Ganzon-Zampino,Gilda E.,MD
Kim,Duk Hee,MD
Kirchner,Brian K.,MD
Lieberman,Alexander III,MD
Memon,Moomal,MD
Miao,Sun,MD
Patel,Vineshkumar K.,MD
Petruzzi,Nicholas Joseph,MD
Selina,Elena V.,MD
Sivaraman,Sivashankar,MD
Sperling,Michael James,MD
Zampino,Dominick J.,DO
Neurology
Boxman,Jeffrey R.,DO
Youssef,Iman Shawki,MD
Obstetrics & Gynecology
Assad,Eveline N.,MD
Bredin,Sherilyn A.,MD
Chong,Christopher K.,MD
Feldman,Alan J.,MD
Perkins,Phyllis M.,MD
Petit,Anne I.,MD
Stanley,Linda,MD
Wesley,Louis A.,MD
Ophthalmology
Dunn,Eric Scott,MD
Spielberg,Joel A.,MD
Wise,Richard Bryan,MD

Pediatrics
Amir,Sabah H.,MD
Elgenaidi,Mona E.,MD
Houck,Meghan Mcfee,DO
Kosmetatos,Elizabeth,MD
Plastic Surgery
Coville,Frederick A.,MD
Psychiatry
Bell,Theresa A.,MD
Pulmonary Critical Care
Alobeidy,Salaam T.,MD
Pulmonary Disease
Bansal,Aditya Rakesh,MD
Costantini,Peter J.,DO
Loftus,Frances Ellen,DO
Sadik,Nadia,MD
Radiology
Begleiter,David A.,MD
Falciani,Amerigo,DO
Frankel-Tiger,Robyn F.,MD
Friedman,Alan Stanley,MD
Gerhardt,William J.,MD
Glassberg,Robert M.,MD
Glick,Craig S.,MD
McManus,Stephen William,MD
Schmidling,Michael John,MD
Shakarshy,Jack,MD
Simpson,Alan J.,MD
Tiger,Eric Harvey,MD
Tran,Thomas Hien Dieu,MD
Vu,Hung Quoc,MD
Surgery (General)
Kassis,Kamal F.,MD
Patel,Samir M.,MD
Urology
Slotoroff,Howard,MD
Vascular & Intrvntnal Radiology
Kim,Christopher E.,MD
Garfield
Allergy
Benincasa,Peter J.,MD
Luka,Richard Edward,MD
Family Medicine
Conte,Kenneth S.,DO
Kawecki,Jerzy Stanislaw,MD
Koch,Donna Marie,DO
General Practice
Giardino,V. J.,MD
Tunia,Krzysztof Stanislaw,MD
Obstetrics & Gynecology
Silva-Karcz,Linda,MD
Osteopathic Medicine
Conte,Daniel P. III,DO
Pediatrics
Uczkowska,Alicja Teresa,MD
Vascular Surgery
Tuzzeo,Salvatore T.,MD
Garwood
Family Medicine
Caracitas,Alexandra Cristina,DO
McArthur,Lucas James,MD
Internal Medicine
Yavorsky,John M.,DO
Surgery (General)
Gupta,Amit,MD
Gibbsboro
Anesthesiology
Gellman,Marc D.,MD
Child (Pediatric) Neurology
Mintz,Mark I.,MD
Dermatology
Baker,Donald J.,MD
Family Medicine
Paxton,Timothy X.,DO
Sheldon,Howard A.,DO
Sheldon,Lynne T.,DO
Tokazewski,Jeffrey Thomas,MD
Villamayor,Rosemarie Cruz,MD
Orthopedic Surgery
Wilkins,Charles E.,MD
Otolaryngology
Aftab,Saba,MD
Wong,Gabriel Ho Yu,MD
Pediatrics
Amato,Christopher,DO
Deery,Kimberly Jeanne,DO
Lee,Diana,MD
Lerch,Gordon Lee Jr.,DO
Napoli,Anthony F. Jr.,MD
Valencia,Rafael L.,MD

Physicians by Town and Medical Specialty

Gibbsboro (cont)
Psychiatry
Giarraputo, Leonard J., MD
Psychiatry & Nrolgy-Special Qual
Chadehumbe, Madeline A., MD

Gibbstown
Family Medicine
Dave, Akshay S., MD

Gladstone
Diagnostic Radiology
Degaeta, Linda R., MD
Surgical Critical Care
Hammond, Jeffrey S., MD

Glassboro
Family Medicine
Heist, Jon S., DO
Meskin, Steven J., MD
Nguyen, Bac Xuan, MD
Palmer, Josette C., MD
Sayed, Durr-E-shahwaar, DO
Schultes, Arthur H., DO
Szgalsky, Joseph Brian, MD
Occupational Medicine
Bojarski, Michael H., DO
Orthopedic Surgery
Clinton, Cody, DO
Pathology
Smith, Cheryl E., MD
Psychiatry
Whitman, Sarah Marie, MD

Glen Gardner
Family Medicine
Lagarenne, Paul R., MD
Geriatric Psychiatry
West, Helen T., MD
Psychiatry
Moise, Bonard, MD
Paranal, Aurora M., MD
Volskaya, Svetlana, MD

Glen Ridge
Anesthesiology
Parikh, Sanjiv R., MD
Arthroscopic Surgery
Sloan, Kim W., MD
Cardiovascular Disease
Alfonso, Carlos Roel Villegas, MD
De Gregorio, Bart, MD
De Gregorio, Joseph Anthony, MD
Di Giorgio, Christopher B., MD
Knezevic, Dusan Svetozar, MD
Mariano, Domenic L., DO
Saroff, Alan L., MD
Voudouris, Apostolos A., MD
Wanat, Francis E., MD
Dermatology
Rozanski, Reuben, MD
Endocrinology
Davis, Maris R., MD
Grover, Anjali, MD
Shafqat, Uzma Zohra, MD
Sherry, Stephen H., MD
Family Medicine
Berlin, Melissa Gail, MD
Flores, Jose C., DO
Kidangan, Julie Thomas, DO
Gastroenterology
Finkelstein, Warren, MD
Kenny, Raymond P., MD
Kwon, Yong Min, MD
Oh, Sangbaek Charles, MD
Tobia, Dennis A., MD
Internal Medicine
Bambhroliya, Grishma, MD
Cheema, Asad Mushtaq, MD
Daniskas, Efthymios I., MD
Levai, Robert Joseph, MD
Minano, Cecilia, MD
Molinaro, Michael Louis, MD
Safirstein, Benjamin Herbert, MD
Urrutia, Ellen E., MD
Weber, Barry Joseph, MD
Woroch, Paul, MD
Nephrology
Khanna, Priya, DO
Neurology
Blady, David, MD
Vaccaro, John J., MD
Obstetrics & Gynecology
Dias Martin, Karen A., MD
Orthopedic Surgery
Chase, Mark D., MD
Rombough, Gary R., MD
Vonroth, William Jr., MD
Otolaryngology
Zbar, Lloyd I. S., MD
Pediatrics
Khanna, Anisha, DO
Khanna, Kamlesh, MD
Plastic Surgery
Zbar, Ross Ian Seth, MD
Psychiatry
Lui, Gene Sing, DO
Surgery (General)
Ballem, Naveen, MD
Barbalinardo, Robert J., MD
Gohil, Kartik Narendra, MD
Matier, Brian, MD
Rainville, Harvey Charles, MD
Thoracic Surgery
Holwitt, Kenneth N., MD
Vascular Surgery
Ballem, Ramamohana V., MD

Glen Rock
Addiction Psychiatry
Yero, Sergio Alberto, MD
Allergy & Immunology
Blume, Jessica Wanda, MD
Cataract
Portfolio, Almerindo G. Jr., MD
Child & Adolescent Psychiatry
Muthusawmy, Nanda, MD
Colon & Rectal Surgery
Agopian, Raffi E., MD
Kwon, Albert O., MD
Dermatology
Dosik, Jonathan Scott, MD
Galvin, Sharon A., MD
Diagnostic Radiology
Leone, Armand Jr., MD
Family Medicine
Meisel, Mark K., DO
Internal Medicine
Carlson, Sandra Regina, MD
Sarkar, Arunima, MD
Tilson, Morris A., MD
Neurology
Nanavati, Farzana Nilesh, MD
Orthopedic Surgery
Alberta, Francis Gerard, MD
Implicito, Dante A., MD
Johnson, Keith Patrick, MD
Massoud, Bryan J., MD
Otolaryngology
Katz, Harry, MD
Pediatric Otolaryngology
Bellapianta, Karen Marie, MD
Pediatrics
Halifman, Dorina, MD
Karpova, Natalia M., MD
Psychiatry
Schachter, Meri, MD
Pulmonary Disease
Grizzanti, Joseph N., DO
Spinal Surgery
Patel, Sujal P., MD
Surgery (General)
Ahlborn, Thomas N., MD

Glendora
Family Medicine
Blank, Benjamin I., DO

Gloucester City
Family Medicine
Klein, Steven, DO
Lundy, Edward L., DO
Internal Medicine
Hyman, Daniel J., DO

Green Brook
Diagnostic Radiology
Epstein, Richard William, MD
Finn Wedmid, Myra Elizabeth, MD
Gross, Steven C., MD
Honickman, Steven P., MD
Isserow, Jonathan Arnold, MD
Lam, Ling Lai, MD
Saunders, Alan M., MD
Yang, Roger S., MD
Emergency Medicine
Desai, Chaitanya M., MD
Family Medicine
Carrieri, David A., DO
Cook, Sean Michael, MD
Hammoud, Marwan Fahim, MD
Klele, Michael A, MD
Pilla, John D., MD
Popeck, Paul J., DO
Quezada Reyes, Carlos A., MD
Sgambelluri, Carol E., MD
Strauss, Scott R., DO
Internal Medicine
Ahmed, Syed F., MD
Chafos, John N., MD
Devarajan, Anandan, MD
Khalil, Suzan Y., MD
Sharon, Yoram, DO
Strumkovsky, Lyalya Olga, MD
Neurological Radiology
Lee, Seungho Howard, MD
Other Specialty
Price, Grant J., MD
Physical Medicine & Rehab
Mangunay, Danilo C., MD
Radiology
Caravello, Anthony Joseph Jr., DO
Katz, Barry Harmon, MD
Khurana, Pavan, MD
Lane, Elizabeth Lovinger, MD
Lazar, Eric B., MD
Melville, Gordon E., MD
Schwarz, Warrren, MD
Terry, Bernard, MD

Green Village
Psychiatry
Bird, Joanna Marie, MD

Guttenberg
Anesthesiology
Romero, Alejandro, MD
Cardiovascular Disease
Katdare, Umesh Vasudeo, MD
Child & Adolescent Psychiatry
Padron-Gayol, Maria V., MD
Family Medicine
Calero, Jose Manuel, MD
Sterling, Karen Sohria, MD
Internal Medicine
Santana, Jose O., MD
Orthopedic Surgery
Dauhajre, Teofilo A., MD
Pediatrics
La Rosa, Niurka, MD
Psychiatry
Ocasio, Deborah L., MD
Shanmugham, Revathi, MD
Vascular & Intrvntnl Radiology
Epstein, Steven Brian, MD

Hackensack
Adolescent Medicine
Northridge, Jennifer, MD
Allergy
Michelis, Mary Ann, MD
Allergy & Immunology
Geller, Debora Klein, MD
Mithani, Sima, MD
Selvaggi, Thomas A., MD
Anatomic Pathology
Fix, Daniel Jonas, MD
Hassoun, Patrice, MD
Anatomic/Clinical Pathology
Bhattacharyya, Pritish K., MD
Fehmian, Carol Janice, MD
Han, Min Woo, MD
He, Wenlei, MD
Lengner, Marlene, MD
Li, Jun, MD
Yang, Xiao Yan, MD
Anesthesiology
Baratta, Jerry M., DO
Block, Michael, MD
Boral, Andrew S., MD
Caloustian, Marie-Louise, MD
Choi, Jong Eui, MD
Ciongoli, Bernard C., DO
Cohen, Randy Scott, MD
Cortazzo, Jessica A., MD
Cullen, Michael E., MD
Cuttitta, Jerome D., MD
Dalal, Bhavna P., MD
Datta, Samyadev, MD
DeRemigio, David Michael, DO
Diaz, Lloyd P., MD
Dragone, Daniel Claudio, MD
Dragone, Sergio D., MD
Eck, Philip Ofosu, MD
Eskinazi, Daniel, MD
Fam, Alfred M., MD
Frazer, Keith Evan, DO
Friedlander, Jeffrey Dean, MD
Girnar, Digvijaysi, MD
Grech, Dennis George, MD
Hammonds, Charles Dewey, MD
Hessert, Eva Marie, MD
Hirth, Thomas G., MD
Horn, Russell J., MD
Huang, Chien-Yao, MD
Hummel, Andrew E., DO
Jardosh, Kunal Rashmin, MD
Karpinos, Robert D., MD
Kehar, Mira, MD
Klauss, Gunnar, MD
Kwon, Minho, MD
Leslie, Joanne, MD
Li, John Yi-huang, MD
Mandhle, Pankaja Anil, MD
Marasigan, Mariza E., MD
Martin, Megan Blake, MD
McTigue, Maureen A., DO
Merle, Francois, MD
Milic, Milija, MD
Morsy, Amr Sayed, MD
Munoz, Daisy, MD
Neugeborn, Ian Scott, MD
Nolasco, Cesar V., MD
Nolasco, Edwin V., MD
Oloomiyazdi, Mohammadali, MD
Olsen, Janet L., MD
Paganessi, Monica A., DO
Paganessi, Steven Andrew, MD
Palmer, Thalia Christine, MD
Parikh, Anant Parimal, MD
Reddy, Matt Medapati, MD
Saad, Mohamed Ali, MD
Sajous, Jocelyne, MD
Saladini, Vincent Jr., MD
Salgado, Fredy R., MD
Sanders, Paul, MD
Sarier, Kaya K., MD
Schlesinger, Mark D., MD
Scott, Nancy Michelle, MD
Seem, Eric H., MD
Semanczuk, William Paul, MD
Sen, Surjya, MD
Sharma, Veena, MD
Shindler, Maria Danielle, MD
Shorshtein, Alexander, MD
Shulman, Michael, MD
Thongrod, Sumena C., DO
Topfer, Steven Alan, DO
Van Beever, Jordan Grant, MD
Vidaver, Patrick S., MD
Weiss-Bloom, Leslie J., MD
Weitzman, Stephen M., MD
Wesley, Carl Christopher, MD
Wu, Duoping, MD
Wu, Jing, MD
Xagoraris, Andreas E., MD
Cardiac Anesthesia
Abrams, Lawrence M., MD
Cardiovascular Disease
Berkowitz, Robert Lester, MD
Denson, H. Mark, MD
Glotzer, Taya Valerie, MD
Kanarek, Steven Edward, MD
Kapoor, Saurabh, MD
Katebian, Manoucher E., MD
Lau, Henry, MD
Maza, Sharon R., MD
Mulkay, Angel J., MD
Nejad, Karan S., MD
Nia, Hamid Mohammad, MD
Patel, Jayantkumar N., MD
Patel, Rajiv J., DO
Radoslovich, Glauco A., MD
Rossakis, Constantine, MD
Ruffo, Scott D., MD
Sethi, Ruchi S., MD
Sethi, Virender, MD
Shah, Umang Lalit, MD
Sharma, Sarika, MD
Silber, David Joseph, DO
Simons, Grant Russell, MD
Simpson, Timothy E., MD

Teichholz,Louis E.,MD
Vaidya,Pranaychan J.,MD
Weinstock,Murray,MD
Zimmerman,John M.,MD
Cardiovascular Surgery
Elmann,Elie Marco,MD
Somberg,Eric D.,MD
Child & Adolescent Psychiatry
Lewis,Tanya Renee,MD
Oquendo,Sonia I.,MD
Osmanova,Nataliya,MD
Paine,Mercedes A.,MD
Zhivago,Eileen Ann,MD
Child (Pediatric) Neurology
Katz,Michael Dennis,MD
Lazar,Lorraine M.,MD
Clinical Cardiac Elctrphyslgy
Shukla,Gunjan Jayendrabhai,MD
Clinical Neurophysiology
Nogueira,John Francis Jr.,MD
Colon & Rectal Surgery
Helbraun,Mark E.,MD
Critical Care Medicine
Ashtyani Asl,Fariborz,MD
Bunnell,Eugene,MD
Chander,Naresh,MD
Choi,Weekon,MD
Nierenberg,Richard J.,MD
Rajaram,Sri-Sujanthy,MD
Ting,Leon L.,MD
Cytopathology
Gupta,Anupama,MD
Dermatology
Ashinoff,Robin,MD
Eilers,Steven Edwin,MD
Goldberg,David Jay,MD
Masullo,Alfredo S.,MD
Ravits,Margaret S.,MD
Sapadin,Allen N.,MD
Shin,Helen Theresa,MD
Wilkerson,Eric Christopher,MD
Developmental Pediatrics
Dolan,Eileen A.,MD
Huron,Randye F.,MD
Diagnostic Radiology
Abbey,Genevieve Nguyen,MD
Agress,Harry Jr.,MD
An,Jane J.,MD
Bogomol,Adam Russell,MD
Bramlette,James G.s.,MD
Daginawala,Naznin,MD
Faulkner,Adriana Danielle,MD
Ferrone,George J.,MD
Gamss,Rebecca,MD
Gardella,Dean,MD
Greenwald,Bob,MD
Guy Rodriguez,Eva Porter,MD
Han,Gene,MD
Hou,Stephanie W.,MD
Koenigsberg,Tova Chava,MD
Kumarasamy,Narmadan A.,MD
Litkouhi,Behrang,MD
Malone,Carolyn Marie,MD
Ng,Joshua M.,MD
Ojutiku,Oreoluwa Olubukunola,MD
Osiason,Andrew Wade,MD
Panduranga,Satish Chandra,MD
Renjen,Pooja,MD
Rozentsvayg,Eka,DO
Starr,Gail E.,MD
Sunkavalli,Sunitha Aluri,MD
Toth,Patrick J.,MD
Yang,Clement,MD
Electroencephalography
Gupta,Dev R.,MD
Emergency Medical Services
Lu,Sam Chuan,MD
Emergency Medicine
Avram,Ari Jason,MD
Barsky,Carol,MD
Bell,Kameno L.,MD
Bernadotte,Myrvine,MD
Bilbraut,Krista Gayle,MD
Bosompem,Daryl Ama,MD
Caces,Phyllis Adrienn Romero,MD
Chai,Raymond,MD
Charles,Patrick,DO
Chase,Howard M.,MD
Davison,Beverly J.,MD
DeSouza,Sylvie D.,MD
Fernandez,Christine Alison,MD

Fleischman,William,MD
Frank,Daniel B.,MD
Friedman-Cohen,Heather Naomi,MD
Gable-Selmon,Chana H.,MD
Goldhill,Vicki B.,MD
Hallenbeck,John P.,DO
Henderson Chen,Jessica L.,MD
Hernandez,Monica M.,MD
Hewitt,Kevin Joseph,MD
Kim,Young-Min,MD
Mankowitz,Scott Levi,MD
McIntosh,Barbara A.,MD
Morchel,Herman George,MD
Negron,David,MD
Nguyen,Ann Phuong Duy,MD
Nickles,Leroy,MD
Ogedegbe,Chinwe,MD
Ortiz,Carlos Arturo II,MD
Roesch,Benno George,MD
Sayegh,Rockan,MD
Strater,Sharon,MD
Stuart,Jennifer Marie,MD
Sullivan,Anastassia D.,MD
Taylor,Cody Wolfson,MD
Varela,Luis Fernando,MD
Walden,Philip Louis Jr.,MD
Weisburg,Rhoda S.,MD
Yamin,Edward,MD
Zakharchenko,Svetlana,DO
Zodda,David F.,MD
Endocrinology
Garger,Yana Basis,MD
Hannoush,Peter Yousef,MD
Katz,Adriana,MD
Epilepsy
Mesad,Salah Mohammed,MD
Family Medicine
Ahmad,Yasir Jamal,MD
August,Elizabeth,MD
Chaney,Arthur Jr.,MD
Chaney,Dewey A.,MD
Corrigan,Lynn Ann,DO
Gatchalian,Luningning C.,MD
Hussain,Rubaba,MD
Jacob,Mariamma,MD
Koenigsberg,Martin Allen,DO
Ourvan,Dorothy R.,DO
Schwarz,Rachelle,DO
Fertility/Infertility
Adelsohn,Lawrence G.,MD
Gastroenterology
Ellinghaus,Eric J.,MD
Feit,David L.,MD
Felig,David M.,MD
Golding,Richard C.,MD
Khan,Fahad,MD
Kheterpal,Neil M.,DO
Ligresti,Rosario Joseph,MD
Riccobono,Charles A.,MD
Sedarat,Ali,MD
Sedarat,Alireza,MD
Tanchel,Mark E.,MD
General Practice
Bilek,Alena,MD
Leder,Robin Ellen,MD
Geriatric Psychiatry
Lally,Tamkeen,MD
Tourkova,Marina,MD
Geriatrics
Cheeti,Kalpana,MD
Evans,Ed Nelvyn Lezette,MD
Pantagis,Stefanos G.,MD
Parulekar,Manisha Santosh,MD
Rastogi,Sarita,MD
Rutkowska,Ewa,MD
Steel,R. Knight,MD
Gynecological Oncology
Smith,Daniel Humphreys,MD
Vaidya,Ami P.,MD
Gynecology
Cavallaro,Barbara Ann,MD
Lo,Hung-Tien,MD
Petras,Peri Ann,MD
Hand Surgery
Giuffrida,Angela Ylenia,MD
Hematology
Feldman,Tatyana A.,MD
Goldberg,Stuart Lee,MD
Rosenbluth,Richard J.,MD
Waintraub,Stanley Eli,MD

Hematology Oncology
Biran,Noa,MD
Harper,Harry D.,MD
McNamara,Donna M.,MD
Pecora,Andrew L.,MD
Hospitalist
Bajwa,Ravneet Singh,MD
Josephs,Joshua,MD
Mapa,Christopher George,MD
Qureshi,Akif Zeshan,MD
Tam,Elizabeth,MD
Infectious Disease
Cicogna,Cristina Emanuela,MD
Desai,Samit Sharad,MD
Gross,Peter A.,MD
Kibrea,S. M. Golam,MD
Levine,Jerome Frederic,MD
Sebti,Rani,MD
Sperber,Steven J.,MD
Internal Medicine
Acevedo Beltran,Edrik Josue,MD
Ahmed,Suhel Hussain,MD
Alter,Robert S.,MD
Amuluru,Jaladurga P.,MD
Anchipolovsky,Natalia,DO
Baer,Aryeh Zvi,MD
Bajaj,Nikki,MD
Balani,Bindu Anand,MD
Balasingham,Chithra,MD
Cai,Kimberly,MD
Campanella,Anthony J. Jr.,MD
Chandra,Sweta,MD
Chatelain,Martin P.,MD
Chavez,Laura Monica,DO
Chhabra,Anjana R.,MD
Cohen,Michael B.,MD
D'Alessandro,Daniel J.,MD
Donato,Michele Lyne,MD
Ephrat,Moshe,MD
Farber,Michael Seth,MD
Felsen,Alan K.,MD
Fink,Andrew Nathen,MD
Friedman,Samuel H.,MD
Gardin,Julius Markus,MD
Gayed,Noha,MD
Gellrick,Judith C.,MD
Germinario,Carla Ann,MD
Goldfarb,Adam S.,MD
Gong,Bing,MD
Gonzalez,Abel Ernesto,MD
Goy,Andre Henri,MD
Graham,Deena Mary-Atieh,MD
Grigoryan,Galina,MD
Gunadasa,Susanthi N.,MD
Gupta,Kavita,MD
Gutierrez,Martin Eduardo,MD
Howard,Brandon Trevor,MD
Ibrahim,Ehab Fawzy,MD
Jamal,Sameer Mustafa,MD
Jennis,Andrew A.,MD
Kahyaoglu,Aret Y.,MD
Kasuni,William Tatsuo,MD
Koduah,Doris Afreh,MD
Kowal,Timothy S.,MD
Kurian,Helena,MD
Lambrinos,Vasilios,MD
Lee,Robert Chu-Du,MD
Leslie,Lori Ann,MD
Li,Jianfeng,MD
Lin,Judy Mei-Chia,MD
Lodhavia,Jitendra J.,MD
Manchireddy,Suman,MD
Manji,Hussain Mehdi,MD
Muttana,Renu Devi,MD
Oguayo,Kevin Nnaemeka,MD
Okoye-Okuzu,Enuma I.,MD
Pagan,Juan,MD
Parmar,Madhu,MD
Pascal,Mark S.,MD
Prins,Edward R.,MD
Rose,Keith Martin,MD
Said,Raghad Houfdhi,MD
Schoen,Arnold Paul,MD
Schwartz,Gary D.,MD
Selvaraj,Sundararajan,MD
Shaker,Safwat I.,MD
Shen,Jeffrey Jou,MD
Singh,Sapna,MD
Stoupakis,George,MD
Suldan,Zalman Lewis,MD
Surapaneni,Padmaja,MD
Tadros,Dalia Anwar,MD

Takvorian,Sylva A.,MD
Tank,Lisa Kaushal,MD
Teran Vargas,Rafael Antonio,MD
Tesfaye,Melaku,MD
Timmapuri,Sarah L.,MD
Tossounian,Nora Zabel,MD
Vesole,David H.,MD
Vij,Angela,MD
Wang,Paul Xinze,MD
Wertheim,Mordecai,MD
Woodham,Philip G.,MD
Zorba,Yildiz,MD
Interventional Cardiology
Mathur,Atish Pratap,MD
Patel,Ruchir,MD
Maternal & Fetal Medicine
Brandt,Justin Samuel,MD
Guirguis,George,DO
Medical Oncology
Faderl,Stefan H.,MD
Proverbs-Singh,Tracy Ann,MD
Rowley,Scott D.,MD
Siegel,David Samuel Dicapua,MD
Neonatal-Perinatal Medicine
Cheung,Sandy Wai Yi,DO
Flores,Ramon L.,MD
Johnson,Terry D.,MD
Nabong,Marcelo Yambao Jr.,MD
Perl,Harold,MD
Planer,Benjamin C.,MD
Zaklama,Joanne A.,MD
Nephrology
Adamidis,Ananea,MD
Bhayana,Suverta,MD
Joseph,Rosy E.,MD
Saro-Nunez,Lilian,MD
Vitievsky,Alexander Michael,MD
Neuro-Psychiatry
Trobliger,Robert William,MD
Neurological Radiology
Foster,Sarah Jeanmarie,MD
Monoky,David John,MD
Pierce,Sean Donovan,MD
Neurological Surgery
Peterson,Thomas Russell,MD
Schwartz,Lauren Faith,MD
Neurology
Dash,Subasini,MD
Douyon,Philippe Gerard,MD
Fellman,Damon M.,MD
Feoli,Enrique Alfredo,MD
Goldlust,Samuel Aaron,MD
Ibrahim,Ayman M.,DO
Inoyama,Katherine S.,MD
Kreibich,Thomas Alfred,MD
Krel,Regina,MD
Liff,Jeremy M.,MD
Marquinez,Anthony I.,MD
Oller-Cramsie,Marissa Anne,DO
Pandey,Krupa Shah,MD
Puntambekar,Preeti Vasant,MD
Rao,Gautami Kondamodi,MD
Silverstein,Michael P.,MD
Singer,Samuel,MD
Solanky,Mukesh,MD
Tsao,Julie Ching Yen,MD
Vukic,Mario,MD
Obstetrics & Gynecology
Abdelhak,Yaakov Eliezer,MD
Al Khan,Abdulla Mohammed,MD
Alizade,Azer,MD
Alvarez,Manuel,MD
Alvarez Perez,Jesus Rafael,MD
Bozdogan,Ulas,MD
Chadha,Kanchi,MD
Cohen,Robert S.,MD
Collado,Anna A.,DO
Copur,Huseyin,MD
Gaafer-Ahmed,Hany M.,MD
Gallo,Robert James,MD
Gerardis,Judi R.,MD
Govindani,Niketa Vinod,MD
Gupta,Shalini,MD
Howell,Emily Ruth,DO
Hughes,Patricia L.,MD
Ilonzo,Chiamaka,MD
Joshi,Kiran M.,MD
Kamal,Roohi,MD
Kean Chong,Maria R.,MD
Kondoleon,Mary Therese,MD
Kopp,Lizabeth A.,MD

Physicians by Town and Medical Specialty

Hackensack (cont)

Obstetrics & Gynecology
- Leo, Mauro Vincenzo, MD
- Levat, Robin H., MD
- Miller, Lisa Ann B., MD
- Petriella, Michael R. Jr., MD
- Saber, Shelley B., MD
- Samara, Arafat A., MD
- Sbarra, Michael A., MD
- Simonian, Carla Daria, MD
- Vinod, Arundhati Hrishikesh, MD
- Yousry, Ahmed Sameh, MD

Oncological Surgery
- Karpeh, Martin Sieh Jr., MD

Ophthalmology
- Guterman, Carl B., MD
- Hanna, Aghnatious A Ha A., MD
- Liva, Paul A., MD
- Sandor, Earl V., MD
- Silbert, Glenn R., MD
- Sinatra, Melanie A., MD
- The, Arlene H., MD

Oral & Maxillofacial Surgery
- Han, Chang H., MD

Orthopedic Surgery
- Hammerschlag, Warren A., MD
- John, Thomas Karoor, MD
- Kissin, Yair David, MD
- Rajan, Sivaram Gounder, MD
- Seldes, Richard Meyer, MD
- Yufit, Pavel Vladimirovich, MD

Other Specialty
- DeBellis, Julia Angelina, MD
- Koenig, Christopher, MD

Otolaryngology
- Benson, Brian Eric, MD
- Brody, Robin Michelle, MD
- Gold, Steven M., MD
- Inouye, Masayuki, MD
- Lesserson, Jonathan A., MD
- Low, Ronald Brian, MD
- Respler, Don S., MD
- Rosen, Arie, MD
- Shaari, Christopher M., MD
- Tell, Alan Michael, MD
- Wasserman, Jared Mark, MD

Otology
- Eisenberg, Lee D., MD

Pain Medicine
- Contreras, Jose A., MD
- Khan, Sunniya, MD
- Park, Kenneth Hyun, DO
- Seckin, Ali Inanc, MD

Pathology
- Goldfischer, Michael J., MD
- Harawi, Sami J., MD
- Mannion, Ciaran M., MD

Pediatric Anesthesia
- Castro-Frenzel, Karla Jose, MD
- Shah, Ruchir Nikunjbihari, MD

Pediatric Cardiology
- Dyme, Joshua L., MD
- Kipel, George, MD
- Tozzi, Robert J., MD
- Wong, Austin Henry, MD

Pediatric Critical Care
- Friedman, Bruce I., MD
- Melas, Antonia Ana, DO
- Percy, Stephen Jr., MD
- Siegel, Mark Eric, MD
- Sorrentino, Mark David, MD

Pediatric Emergency Medicine
- Fine, Jeffrey Scott, MD
- Lee, Donna J., MD
- Nemetski, Sondra Maureen, MD
- Raguindin, Leah, MD

Pediatric Endocrinology
- Aisenberg, Javier E., MD
- Maresca, Michelle Marie, MD

Pediatric Gastroenterology
- Francolla, Karen Ann, MD
- Jeshion, Wendy Cheryl, MD
- Makadia, Payal Ameesh, MD
- Wong, Tracie Mei Han, MD

Pediatric Hematology Oncology
- Appel, Burton Eliot, MD
- Diamond, Steven H., MD
- Gillio, Alfred Peter III, MD
- Harlow, Paul J., MD
- Harris, Michael B., MD
- Krajewski, Jennifer Anne, MD
- Steele, Cindy S., MD
- Terrin, Bruce N., MD

Pediatric Infectious Diseases
- Boscamp, Jeffrey R., MD
- Slavin, Kevin A., MD

Pediatric Nephrology
- Hijazi, Rana, MD
- Lieberman, Kenneth V., MD

Pediatric Neurodevelopment
- Segal, Eric B., MD

Pediatric Orthopedics
- Cahill, James W., MD
- Merchant, Amit, DO

Pediatric Otolaryngology
- Quraishi, Huma Asmat, MD

Pediatric Pulmonology
- Kaplan, Ellen B., MD
- Lee, Ada Shuk Chong, MD

Pediatric Rheumatology
- Haines, Kathleen Ann, MD
- Kimura, Yukiko, MD

Pediatrics
- Agrawal, Nina, MD
- Auyeung, Valerie Y., MD
- Avva, Usha R., MD
- Azizi, Azin, MD
- Borgen, Ruth E., MD
- Bye, Karen N., MD
- Chhabra, Rakesh S., MD
- D'Mello, Sharon L., MD
- Diah, Paulett, MD
- Duncan, Eva, MD
- Dyme, Rachel Sarah, MD
- Eigen, Karen Lori, MD
- Ettinger, Leigh Mark, MD
- Flores, Alejandro Alberto, MD
- Fofah, Onajovwe O., MD
- Fruchter, Joseph S., MD
- Furman, Jasmin W., MD
- Gertz, Shira J., MD
- Gesser, Gail A., DO
- Gold, Nina A., MD
- Goodman, Karen Natalie, MD
- Gupta, Raksha R., MD
- Hyppolite, Alex, MD
- Khan, Saqiba, MD
- Kimel, Ana Josephine, MD
- Kopacz, Magdaline S., MD
- Kriegel, Marni Ruth, MD
- Kutko, Martha C., MD
- Lamour, Rytza M., MD
- Lapidus, Sivia K., MD
- Levine, Deena R., MD
- Leyva-Vega, Melissa, MD
- Li, Suzanne C., MD
- Lopez, Divina Elizabeth, MD
- Macalintal, Rose Ann Reyes, MD
- Materetsky, Steven H., MD
- Meli, Lisa A., MD
- Mikadze, Malkhazi, MD
- Miranda, Rosa Josefina, MD
- Moustafellos, Elaine, MD
- Muratschew, Donna M., MD
- Ngai, Pakkay, MD
- O'Donnell, Lisa-Mary, MD
- Obaze, Ofunne Omo, MD
- Paolicchi, Juliann Marie, MD
- Pedro, Helio Fernando, MD
- Perez, Adriana M., MD
- Petrella, Michael Onofrio, MD
- Piwoz, Julia A., MD
- Rama, Gabriel, MD
- Rappaport, Delia I., MD
- Reed, Jean Arlyn Banez, MD
- Rivera, Roger Antonio, MD
- Samuels, Francine, MD
- Shah, Mayuri N., MD
- Shammout, Jumana Sa'ad, MD
- Sousa, Rolando Cristobal, MD
- Subramanian, Subhashini, MD
- Tantawi, Mohamed Asem, MD
- Tantawi, Mona M., MD
- Thomas, Antonio, MD
- Thomas, Dianne, MD
- Vijayan, Radhika, MD
- Weiss, Jennifer Ellen, MD
- Weissman, Barry J., MD
- Wong, Jonathan Wane, MD
- Yucel, Cengiz, MD

- Zenack, Alissa Hayley, DO

Physical Med & Rehab-Pain Med
- Shupper, Peter Joseph, MD

Physical Medicine & Rehab
- Mohsen, Ekram, DO
- Swajian, Mary, DO

Plastic Surgery
- Bikoff, David J., MD
- Callahan, Troy Ezra, MD
- Kim, Richard Young Jin, MD
- Rauscher, Gregory E., MD
- Ritota, Perry C., MD

Psychiatry
- Arroyo, Zuleika A., MD
- Bortnik, Kristy E., MD
- Ebersole, John S., MD
- Finch, Daniel Garrett, MD
- Marshall, Lorraine S., MD
- Martindale, Peter Craig, MD
- Miah, Khorshed Alam, MD
- Roman, Jocelyn, MD
- Sostre, Samiris, MD
- Sostre, Samuel Oliver, MD
- Steinberg, David N., MD
- Zaidi, Syed Arif Raza, MD

Psychiatry&Nrolgy-Special Qual
- Gliksman, Felicia Joyce, MD

Pulmonary Critical Care
- Abdelhadi, Samir I., DO

Pulmonary Disease
- Goss, Deborah Anne Marie, MD
- Koniaris, Lauren Solanko, MD
- Polkow, Melvin S., MD
- Sadikot, Sean Shabbir, MD

Radiation Oncology
- Godfrey, Loren, MD
- Ingenito, Anthony C., MD
- Lewis, Brett Eric, MD

Radiology
- Budin, Joel A., MD
- Demeritt, John S. III, MD
- Gejerman, Glen, MD
- Kim, William J., MD
- Ong, Phat Vinh, MD
- Panush, David, MD
- Patel, Rita S., MD
- Virk, Jaskirat Singh, MD
- Weisel, Arthur S., MD

Rheumatology
- Cappadona, James Louis, MD
- Collins, Melinda Jean, DO
- Kepecs, Gilbert, MD

Spinal Cord Injury Medicine
- Thomas, Kurt Florian P., MD

Sports Medicine
- Berman, Mark, MD
- Longobardi, Raphael S., MD
- Meese, Michael Arthur, MD
- Porter, David Alexander, MD

Surgery (General)
- Benson, Douglas N., MD
- Davidson, Marson Tunde, MD
- Dayal, Saraswati Devi, MD
- Ghodsi, Mohammad, MD
- Greene, Tobi B., MD
- Hunter, James Blaine, MD
- Kaul, Sanjeev Kumar, MD
- Khosravi, Abtin Hajiloo, MD
- Kline, Gary Michael, MD
- Koo, Harry P., MD
- Locurto, John Jr., MD
- McCain, Donald Andrew, MD
- Napolitano, Massimo M., MD
- Narins, Seth Craig, MD
- Ng, Arthur F., MD
- Patel, Sruti, MD
- Pereira, Stephen G., MD
- Perez, Javier Martin, MD
- Pisarenko, Vadim, MD
- Poole, John W., MD
- Richardson, Celine Anne, MD
- Rosenstock, Adam Seth, MD
- Smith, Adam Powell, MD
- Thomas, Tina Theresa, MD
- Warden, Mary Jane, MD
- Wilderman, Michael Jeffrey, MD
- Wong, Sarah, MD

Surgical Critical Care
- O'Hara, Kathleen Patricia, MD
- Rippey, Kelly Ann, MD

- Stewart, Peter Jeremy, MD

Thoracic Surgery
- Dudiy, Yuriy, MD
- Rizk, Nabil Pierre, MD

Transplant Surgery & Medicine
- Melton, Larry B., MD
- Shapiro, Michael Eliot, MD

Urology
- Basralian, Kevin R., MD
- Degen, Michael Conrad, MD
- Fagelman, Elliot, MD
- Fagelman, Mark, MD
- Fromer, Debra Lynn, MD
- Glickman, Leonard, MD
- Kim, Michelle Joosun, MD
- Lowe, Daniel Robert, MD
- Munver, Ravi, MD
- Rosenberg, Gene S., MD
- Sadeghi Nejad, Hossein, MD
- Sawczuk, Ihor Steven, MD
- Shin, David, MD

Vascular Surgery
- Forcina, Salvatore John, MD
- Kagan, Peter Evan, MD
- Keys, Roger C., MD
- Kline, Roxana Gabriela, MD
- Manno, Joseph, MD
- O'Connor, David John, MD
- Ratnathicam, Anjali, DO
- Simonian, Gregory T., MD

Hackettstown

Adolescent Medicine
- Sakowski, Jacek, MD

Anatomic/Clinical Pathology
- Desiderio, Abelardo C., MD

Anesthesiology
- Dierlam, Paul T., MD
- Wu, Daniel C., MD

Cardiovascular Disease
- Ong, Edgardo A., MD

Diagnostic Radiology
- Lee, Steven Thomas, MD
- Lo, Pak-Kan A., MD
- Mantinaos, Mike Konstantinos, MD

Emergency Medicine
- Bonanno, Bruce B., MD
- Carle, William J., MD
- Cataquet, David, MD
- Goldfarb, Stephen A., MD
- Jain, Sanjay K., MD
- Olivieri, William Peter, MD
- Scolnick, David, MD
- Seid, Ira A., MD

Family Medicine
- Duryee, John Jourdan, MD
- Paterno, Jeanette D., MD

Gastroenterology
- Chang, Jimmy Chuming, MD
- Kahlam, Sarwan S., MD
- Sandhu, Parminderjeet S., MD

Hematology Oncology
- Niranjan, Usha, MD

Internal Medicine
- Auciello, Antonella, MD
- Azhar, Sana H., MD
- Fan, Sarah Y., MD
- Freyman, Boris, DO
- Gollapudi, Devi P., MD
- Hamaoui, Manuela Belda, MD
- Ingrassia-Squiers, Keri Lynn, DO
- Janowski, Kenneth J., DO
- Jansons, Uldis J., MD
- Kavathia, Sanjay G., MD
- Khan, Sarosh, MD
- Khanna, Anirudh, MD
- Merkle, Jeffrey, MD
- Raza, Syed Mohsin, MD
- Sandhu, Vineet, MD
- Segaram, Sandira V., MD
- Skiba, Chester John Jr., MD
- Tan, Leong Hean, MD
- Theune, Lillian J., DO
- Werner, Robert L., DO
- Wu, Jason Jon, DO

Nephrology
- Hajela, Amitabh, MD

Obstetrics & Gynecology
- Akhigbe, Omoikhefe Gbemisola, MD
- Anscher, Richard M., MD
- Campbell, Neil Murdoch, DO
- Canova, Amanda Derrick, MD

Defalco,Lisa May,DO
Shakarjian,Jo-Ann,MD
Skoczylas,Stanley J.,MD
Uzbay,Lisa Ann,MD
Ophthalmology
Chase,Raymond Donald,DO
Lappin,Harold S.,MD
Orthopedic Surgery
Corrigan,Frank John,MD
De Falco,Robert Anthony,DO
Deehan,Michael A.,MD
Giliberti,William S.,MD
Koss,Stephen Dennis,MD
Murphy,John W.,MD
Rosman,Jerome D.,MD
Sayde,William M.,MD
Teja,Paul Gregory,DO
Wainen,Glen P.,MD
White,Kevin S.,DO
Orthopedic Surgery-Adult Rcnstr
Dundon,John M.,MD
Otolaryngology
Gentile,Victor G.,MD
Pollack,Joshua David,MD
Pediatrics
Caruso,Patrick A.,MD
Chi,Ching,MD
Chugh,Jagdish C.,MD
Dick,Adam M.,MD
Kedzierska,Ksymena,MD
Libert,Melissa Marie,DO
Walsh,Kristen Anne,MD
Physical Medicine & Rehab
Castro,Christopher Paul,DO
Gutkin,Michael Scott,MD
Shamim,Ferheen,MD
Psychiatry
Jain,Sanjeevani,MD
Spinal Surgery
Salari,Behnam,DO
Sports Medicine
Shamim,Rehan Syed,MD
Surgery (General)
Campion,Thomas W.,MD
Gross,Eric L.,MD
Jabush,Jondavid H.,MD
Vascular Surgery
Itani,Mazen S.,MD
Rupani,Bobby Jawahar,MD

Haddon Heights
Anesthesiology
Cataldo,Ralph G.,DO
Cardiovascular Disease
Da Torre,Steven D.,MD
Fortino,Gregg L.,MD
Gips,Sanford J.,MD
Giri,Kartik S.,MD
Herlich,Michael B.,MD
Kaddissi,Georges Ibrahim,MD
Levi,Steven A.,MD
Mark,George Edward,MD
Peter,Annie M.,MD
Snyder,Harvey A.,MD
Verma,Vijayendra Kishore,MD
Viswanath,Dilip Banad,MD
Zinn,Andrew P.,MD
Dermatology
Allen,Robert Andrew,MD
Lo Presti,Nicholas P.,MD
Miller,Emily S.,MD
Whipple,D. Sandra,MD
Diagnostic Radiology
Roach,Neil A.,MD
Family Medicine
Brumbaugh,Martha,MD
Doshi,Sangita K.,MD
Greenwood,Beth M.,MD
Handler,Heidi L.,MD
Higgins,Alexander J.,MD
Staritz,Amy,MD
Gastroenterology
DiSandro,Theresa Maria,DO
Izanec,James L.,MD
Kolnik,John P.,DO
Libster,Boris,DO
Infectious Disease
Okon,Emmanuel E.,MD
Paluzzi,Sandra A.,DO
Traboulsi,Rana,MD
Turner,Ellen K.,MD

Internal Medicine
Dowd,Heather Lynn,DO
Fisher,Mark,MD
Javaiya,Hemangkumar,MD
King,Krista H.,MD
Pavlides,Andreas C.,MD
Renzi,Michael A.,DO
Rink,Lisa Ann,DO
Sanyal,Saugato,MD
Siegel,Howard Ira,MD
Obstetrics & Gynecology
Crawford,Heather M.,DO
Godorecci,Michele,MD
Orthopedic Surgery
Arena,Mario J.,MD
Kozielski,Joseph A.,MD
Poprycz,Walter,MD
Pediatrics
Blair,Michael A.,MD
Matz,Paul Steven,MD
Risimini,Robert J.,MD
Schlitt,Mark George,MD
Schlitt,Michael T.,MD
Schlitt,Stephanie N.,MD
Shaigany,Nina N.,MD
Psychiatry
Ahmad,Adeel,MD
Master,Kenneth V.,MD
Surgery (General)
Derr,Lisa M.,DO
Finnegan,Matthew J.,MD
Greenawald,Lawrence Edward,MD
Kakkilaya,Harish,MD
Merriam,Margaret,DO
Salcone,Mark Anthony,DO
Santos,Rodrigo R.,MD
Vascular Surgery
Di Fiore,Richard,MD

Haddon Township
Family Medicine
Gupta,Mini,MD
Manalis,Helen,DO
McGrath,Robert C.,DO
Internal Medicine
Draganescu,Mirela,MD
McLintock,Glenn R.,MD
Neurology
Dinsmore,Steven Thomas,DO
Hubbard,Sean Tomar,DO
Psychiatry
Prescott,Theresa Ann,DO

Haddonfield
Allergy & Immunology
Ku,Min Jung,MD
Anesthesiology
Mroz,Lynne A.,MD
Polise,Pamela Ann,MD
Bloodbanking
Hennawy,Randa Philip,MD
Dermatology
Burns,Loren T.,MD
Levine,Erika Gaines,MD
Suchin,Karen Rebecca,MD
Family Medicine
Bauer-Sheldon,Melissa Ann,DO
Doyle,Stephanie L.,MD
Foss,Roberta,DO
Kenney,Meredith Ann,DO
Lafon,Michael C.,MD
Olson,Aubrey M.,DO
Panitch,Kenneth N.,MD
Ridilla,Leonard Jr.,MD
Runfola,James Joseph,MD
Vick,James W.,MD
Gastroenterology
Ackerman,Melville J.,MD
Turnier,Auguste P.,MD
Hand Surgery
Dalsey,Robert M.,MD
Hospitalist
Kumar,Nisha Iyer,MD
Infectious Disease
Akhter,Shafinaz,MD
Internal Medicine
Francos,George Charles,MD
Leone,Anthony J.,MD
Petaccio,Claudia Jennifer,MD
Saad,Walid Y.,MD
Neurological Radiology
Miller,Anthony Francis,MD

Obstetrics & Gynecology
Krueger,Paul M.,DO
Ronner,Wanda,MD
Stemmer,Shlomo Marc,MD
Ophthalmology
Mussoline,Joseph F.,MD
Oral & Maxillofacial Surgery
Martin,Gene Joseph Jr.,MD
Orthopedic Surgery
Barrett,Michael P.,DO
Bodin,Nathan Daniel,MD
Bozic,Vladimir Stefan,MD
Levy,Michael Stuart,DO
Otolaryngology
Cultrara,Anthony,MD
Gadomski,Stephen P.,MD
Shah,Samir,MD
Pathology-Molecular Genetic
Edmonston,Tina B.,MD
Pediatrics
Bruner,Laurie Reid,MD
Caltabiano,Claire L.,MD
Eggerding,Caroline,MD
Friedman,Barton J.,MD
King,Kevin J.,MD
Lopes,Joanne Elizabeth,MD
Milligan Milburn,Erin C.,MD
Smergel,Henry,MD
Weidner,James R.,MD
Welsh,Theresa M.,MD
Psychiatry
Dunzik,Scott Dennis,MD
Glickman,Amy Borg,MD
Sproch,Amy Lee,MD
Stumpo,Patrick P.,DO
Radiology
Lynch,Roberta M.,MD
Surgery (General)
Hill,Robert B.,MD
Jankowski,Marcin Andrew,DO

Hainesport
Anesthesiology
Rastogi,Abhijeet A.,MD
Slevin,Kieran Anthony,MD
Diagnostic Radiology
Brodsky,Michael C.,MD
Cordell,Charles E.,MD
Curtis,Bernadette R.,MD
Goldstein,Charles,MD
Harvey,Robert Todd,MD
Kellerman,Joshua David,MD
Lalani,Omar,MD
Lim,Sungtae,MD
Patel,Manan Jaykishan,MD
Rosenblatt,Jay M.,MD
Yang,Ben Ming-Chien,MD
Family Medicine
Ciervo,Carman A.,DO
Mason,David Craig,DO
Meltzer,Michael E.,DO
Hand Surgery
Garberman,Scott F.,MD
Infectious Disease
Asper,Ronald Frank,MD
Internal Medicine
Shah,Samir Nalin,MD
Nephrology
Acharya,Prasad G.,MD
Conrad,Michael James,MD
Franger,Margaret Mary,MD
Min,Dorothy D.,MD
Share,David Seth,MD
Solitro,Matthew Joseph,MD
Suchin,Elliot Jay,MD
Vargas,Myra Theresa,MD
Neurological Radiology
Rizvi,Azam H.,MD
Nuclear Medicine
Kaufman,Michael S.,MD
Orthopedic Surgery
Atlas,Orin Keith,MD
Jenkins,Angela Virginia,MD
Radiation Oncology
Butzbach,Deborah Ann,MD
Radiology
Berinson,Howard S.,MD
Bonier,Bruce S.,DO
Brinton,Karen J.,MD
Koss,James C.,MD
Livstone,Barry J.,MD

Maravich,Nick Jr.,MD
Meltzer,Alfred D.,MD
Moore,Douglas B.,MD
Morgan,William A.,MD
Slawek,Joseph E.,MD
Spivak,Michael,DO
Taormina,Vincent J.,MD
Tsai,Joseph C.,MD
Zeiberg,Andrew S.,MD
Surgery (General)
Briones,Renato J.,MD
Vascular Surgery
Barnes,Thomas L.,MD
Bobila,Wilbur C.,MD

Haledon
Gastroenterology
Baghal,Eyad Y.,MD
Internal Medicine
Kahf,Ahmad N.,MD
Kahf,Amr,MD
Selevany,Muhammad Tahir,MD
Obstetrics & Gynecology
Alnuaimi,Raya Omer,DO
Pediatrics
Afonja,Olubunmi Olutoyin,MD
Pulmonary Critical Care
Alfakir,Maria,MD
Pulmonary Disease
Alberaqdar,Enis,MD

Hamburg
Family Medicine
Autotte,Denise L.,MD
Kozak,Margaret Zsuzsa,DO
Roffe,Kenneth A.,DO
Song,Maria H.,MD
Geriatrics
Fielding,Dennis P.,MD
Internal Medicine
Geisen,Amy Grace,MD
Hmoud,Talat Yousef,MD
Obstetrics & Gynecology
Nichols,Fred Michael,DO
Pediatrics
Markel,David Francis,MD
Surgery (General)
Dash,Sarat K.,MD

Hamilton
Anatomic/Clinical Pathology
Briggs,Kari H.,MD
Siderits,Richard H.,MD
Yang,Dingming,MD
Anesthesiology
Dashow,Susan M.,DO
Feder,Craig A.,MD
Ghabious,Emad Faiek,MD
Gordon,Michael Stuart,MD
Ibrahim,Maher,MD
Loren,Gary M.,MD
Mahoney,John J.,DO
Mandel,Robert,MD
Sanchez,Israel L.,MD
Spiteri,Andrew,MD
Suaco,Benjamin S.,MD
Zwick,Annette E.,MD
Body Imaging Radiology
Kim,Joseph J.,MD
Cardiothoracic Surgery
Manna,Biagio,DO
Cardiovascular Disease
Alvi,Afshan Khadija,MD
Caplan,John L.,MD
Chebotarev,Oleg,MD
Genin,Ilya D.,MD
Ghusson,Mahmoud Saleh,MD
Ghusson,Soheir F.,MD
Gibreal,Mohammed,MD
Patel,Jay K.,MD
Ryder,Ronald G.,DO
South,Harry L.,MD
Wilson,Bruce Leonard,MD
Child & Adolescent Psychiatry
Downs,Elvira Foglia,MD
Li,Liren,MD
Clinical Cardiac Elctrphyslgy
Patel,Aarti,MD
Clinical Neurophysiology
Zhang,Lei,MD
Critical Care Medicine
Devine,Mary Ann,MD
Mehta,Munira Yusuf,MD

Physicians by Town and Medical Specialty

Hamilton (cont)

Critical Care Medicine
Obaray, Akbar H., MD

Diagnostic Radiology
Alderson, Skip Michael, MD
Bhalakia, Niraj, MD
Blackman, Gurvan E., MD
Bosworth, Eric, MD
Burgos, Anthony, MD
Burshteyn, Mark, MD
Cohen, Daniel Jonathan, MD
Gellella, Erik Leonard, MD
Gold, Michael J., MD
Greenbaum, Roy L., MD
Kirkpatrick, Christopher T., MD
Le Cavalier, Larry Alan, MD
Lee, Shane, MD
Lo Verde, Lauren S., MD
McGroarty, William J., MD
Meshkov, Steven L., MD
Nayee, Sandip Natvarlal, DO
Neuman, Joel David, MD
Ratner, Lawrence M., MD
Rieder, Michael J., MD
Scafidi, Richard F., MD
Seelagan, Davindra, MD
Silverstein, Gary S., MD
Steinig, Jeffrey Daniel, MD
Tarasov, Ethan A., MD
Taus, Lynne F., MD
Thal, Stephen Wayne, DO
Young, Sophia C., MD

Emergency Medicine
Betancourt, Javier E., DO
Chaudhri, Imran I., MD
Gojaniuk, Jeffrey David, DO
Gonzales, Santos O., MD
Horana, Lasanta S., MD
Khan, Mateen Abdul Rahman, MD
Lawrie, John A., MD

Endocrinology
Empedrad, Albert Barcelona, MD
Soriano, Myrna Lopez, MD

Family Medicine
Agcopra, Annabel, DO
Bancroft, James Alan, MD
Castillo, Christine Capistran, DO
Chavez Santos, Maria, MD
Chiromeras, Andrew, MD
Cruz, Gloria Maria, MD
Dasti, Sofia J., MD
Flores, Lisa, MD
Funches, Antonio, MD
Guarino, Joseph M., DO
Manzoor, Adil, DO
Marriott, Christine Ryan, MD
Masood, Hamid, MD
Mullane, Joseph P., MD
Oswari, Daniel, MD
Patel, Viral D., MD
Pluta, Christine Marie, DO
Richards, Bonnie J., DO
Soliman, Yasser S., MD
Subramoni, Venkateswar, MD
Timmapuri, Ajaz J., MD
Tohfafarosh, Nilofer J., MD
Tselniker, Maryana, MD
Voddi, Swetha Devi, MD
Wistreich, Sarah J., DO

Gastroenterology
Gersten, Michael, MD
Sokol, Deborah Klein, MD

General Practice
Stabile, John R., MD

Geriatrics
Aiello, Stephen Anthony, MD

Hand Surgery
Malik, Parvaiz Akhtar, MD

Hematology
Holtzman, Gayle S., MD

Infectious Disease
Aufiero, Patrick V., MD
Rosenbaum, Seth David, MD
Soliman, Hesham S., MD

Insurance Medicine
Bhandarkar, Anjali, MD

Internal Med-Adolescent Med
Mabrouk, Tarig, MD

Internal Medicine
Arcaro, Mark E., MD
Baig, Sumeera Akhtar, MD
Byrne, Janet Marilyn, MD
Chanliecco, Ma Victoria C., MD
Diwan, Nauman Abdul, MD
Fox, Justin Michael, MD
Ganguly, Panchali, MD
Hadaya, Ziad, MD
Jones, Debra Y., MD
Kim, Andrew Young, MD
Lateef, Aslam, MD
Laurente, Cristeta A., MD
Laurente, Robert M., MD
Lerma, Pauline Marie Ocampo, MD
Levenberg, Steven, MD
Li, Tong, MD
Medina Carcamo, Edwing G., MD
Mikhail, Fayez A., MD
Mina, Randa Fahim, MD
Oza, Harsha K., MD
Palomata, Maria Theresa, MD
Patel, Minal, MD
Raza, Rubina B., MD
Repudi, Sirisha, MD
Sehgel, Robert R., DO
Sharma, Smriti, MD
Sheikh, Selim U., MD
Siddique, Mahmood I., DO
Tawfik, Hany Wahba, MD
Thomas, Jhibu, MD
Tripathi, Neeta, MD
Tuma, Augustine Lavelle, MD
Ufondu, Ebele E., MD
Vadakara, Laisa L., MD
Vadakara, Lukose Simon, MD
Walker, Bridget Ann, DO
Wasserman, Ethan Jeffrey, MD
Wingfield, Edward Anthony, MD

Interventional Cardiology
Rab, Zia, MD

Nephrology
Hannani, Afshin K., MD

Neurological Radiology
Kulkarni, Kedar, MD
Sterling, Michelle Gold, MD

Neurological Surgery
Lipani, John David, MD

Neurology
Pasupuleti, Rao Satyanaray, MD
Pendino, Alexander M., DO

Obstetrics & Gynecology
Evans Murage, Julene Opalene, MD
Gonzalez Braile, Dinah A., MD
Lendor, E. Cindy, MD
Naraine, Christopher Anthony, MD
Ramchandani, Sanjay Mohan, MD
Resnick, Michael B., MD
Samra Latif Estafan, Omnia M., MD
Sison, Antonio, MD
Tufankjian, Lisa Gruszka, DO

Occupational Medicine
Coumbis, John J., MD

Ophthalmology
Chaudhry, Iftikhar Manzoor, MD
Cox, Gregory E., MD

Orthopedic Surgery
Cairone, Stephen Scott, DO
Capotosta, Thomas J. Jr., MD
Crivello, Keith Michael, MD
Hardeski, David Paul, MD
Kleinbart, Fredric Alan, MD

Otolaryngology
Jaffe, Joel D., MD
Miller, Lee H., MD
Rossos, Apostolos A., MD

Pain Medicine
Sackstein, Adam, MD

Pediatric Radiology
Winter, Rebecca Cooper, MD

Pediatrics
Baiser, Dennis Miles, MD
Bogacki, Gwen M., MD
Boim, Marilynn Dora, MD
Buchbinder, Marta Luisa H., MD
Dorneo, Aurora B., MD
Flores, Belen P., MD
Flores, Charles Edward, MD
Jacques, Walter J., MD
Kapadia, Milan R., MD
Perno, Joseph R., MD
Prineas, Sara L., MD
Reyes, Reina Duremdes, MD
Sheth, Amarish Rasiklal, MD
Sudjono-Santoso, Dewi S., MD
Zelinsky, Catherine Marie, MD

Physical Med & Rehab-Pain Med
Dela Rosa, Aurora P., MD
Josephson, Youssef, DO

Physical Medicine & Rehab
Bhatt, Uday N., MD
Carabelli, Robert A., MD
Fass, Barry D., MD
Gribbin, Dorota M., MD
Smith, David E., MD

Plastic Surgery
Lalla, Raj N., MD

Psychiatry
Faisal, Khaja Tajuddin, MD
Hu, Yiqun, MD
Ibrahim, Candace, MD
Sheth, Nila A., MD
Ye, Xueming, MD

Pulmonary Disease
El Habr, Abdallah H., MD
Kurugundla, Navatha, MD

Radiation Oncology
Chalal, Jo Ann, MD

Radiology
Dutka, Michael Vincent, MD
Ezati, Omid, MD
Mathews, Jeffrey John, MD
Ostrum, Donald S., MD
Plakyda, Derek C., MD
Ross, William M., MD
Weiser, Paul J., MD

Rheumatology
Gordon, Richard Dennis, MD
Segal, Leigh G., MD
Shah, Rehan A., MD

Sleep Disorders Medicine
Dupre, Callum Michael, DO

Surgery (General)
Goldenberg, Elie Adam, MD
Shah, Reza A., DO
Vaswani, Vijay, MD

Urology
Al-Qassab, Usama, MD
Brackin, Phillip Snowden Jr., MD
Gazi, Mukaram A., MD
Gotesman, Alexander, MD
Linder, Earle S., MD
Nazmy, Michael Jr., MD
Watson, John A., MD

Vascular & Intrvntnal Radiology
Brown, Michele Susan, MD
Burda, John F., MD
Pryluck, David Scott, MD

Hamilton Square

Anatomic Pathology
Mercer, Stephen Edward, MD

Anesthesiology
Chung, Soo K., MD

Dermatology
Freedman, Joshua R., MD
Kessel, Daniel S., MD

Gastroenterology
Manning, Michael T., MD

Internal Medicine
Deblasio, Joseph, MD
Deblasio, Joseph Jr., MD
Gonzales, Marjorie M., MD
Novik, Gerald, MD
Patel, Dakshkumar B., MD
Siniakowicz, Robert Miroslaw, MD

Ophthalmology
Desai, Kiritkumar T., MD
Sardi, Vincent F., MD

Hammonton

Adolescent Medicine
Dahodwala, Nisrin Q., MD

Anesthesiology
Manabat, Eileen Rose, MD

Anesthesiology: Pain Medicine
Lee, Young Jae, MD

Cardiovascular Disease
Saia, John A., DO
Slaven, Timothy M., DO
Ukrainski, Gerald J., MD
Wroblewski, Edward A., MD

Child & Adolescent Psychiatry
Burns, Elizabeth Ann, DO
Rana, Sohail Anjum, MD

Emergency Medicine
Amin, Pinakin B., MD

Endocrinology
Rastogi, Rishi K., MD

Family Medicine
Anderson, Christine H., DO
Collins, Philip, DO
De Tata, Gerald C., MD
Goudsward, Sean M., DO
Jones-Mudd, Kimberly M., DO
Jung, Herbert Michael, DO
Kaminski, Mitchell Anthony, MD
Krachman, Donald A., DO
Loughlin-Pherribo, Donna J., DO
Miranda, Chona Santos, MD
Moore, Rebecca Christiane, DO
Nurkiewicz, Stephen A., MD
Salvo, Anthony, MD
Schneider, Katherine Ann, MD
Sharma, Sonia, MD

Forensic Psychiatry
Vuotto, Angela Marie, DO

Gastroenterology
Magasic, Mario V., MD
Savon, Joseph J., MD

Geriatrics
Donepudi, Srilalitha, MD

Internal Medicine
Ahmed, Safi U., MD
Bagchi, Sonali, MD
Bejaran, Juan E., MD
Belli, Albert J. Jr., DO
Fakayode, Abisoye Victoria, MD
Fernandez, Edwin Paras, MD
Gilmour, Kevin P., DO
Kou, Jen Lih, MD
Palathingal, Celina G., MD
Patel, Dipesh V., MD
Reddy, Rajender, MD
Roy, Arup Kumar, MD
Zheng, Jing-Sheng, MD
Zingrone, Denise Michele, DO

Neurology
Carta, Maria C., MD
De Antonio, Sondra M., MD

Obstetrics & Gynecology
Agbasi, Nwogo Nnunwa, MD
Capiro, Rodney, MD
McFarlane, Owen R., MD

Orthopedic Surgery
Friedenthal, Roy B., MD
Gerson, Ronald L., MD

Osteopathic Medicine
Bertagnolli, John F. Jr., DO

Pediatrics
Amer, Adel M., MD
Klein, Bruce M., MD
Prasad, Deviveni R., MD

Physical Med & Rehab-Pain Med
Ezeadichie, Chioma A., DO

Physical Medicine & Rehab
Young, George William, DO

Psychiatry
Adkins, Luz Stella, MD
Bagchi, Sudarshan, MD
Bajwa, Khalid Maqsood, MD
Bhatti, Jamil M., MD
Caringal, Cecilia G., MD
Desai, Amita S., MD
Leone, Dennis, MD
Masry, Allen Y., MD
Mazzochette, John A., MD
Roat, David B., DO
Rodolico, Joseph M., MD
Rozmyslowicz, Magdalena Maria, MD
Syed, Saqib Abdul, MD
Vallejo, Jose A., MD
Vallejo, Phyu P., MD

Pulmonary Disease
Kanoff, Jack M., DO

Hampton

Diagnostic Radiology
Falcon, Lisa Fern, MD

Family Medicine
Berk, Scott Phillip Reed, MD
Madura, Paul P., MD
Mitev, Iliya D., MD
Palmer, Victoria R., DO
Polizzi, David R., MD

Polt,Terry Jane,MD
Prentice,Hugh J.,MD
Sforza,Frank J.,MD
Thakur,Shivani,MD
Internal Medicine
Mohrin,Carl M.,MD
Harrington Park
Anesthesiology
Patel,Chandrakant,MD
Family Medicine
Sawicki,John M.,DO
Geriatrics
Psillides,Despina,MD
Internal Medicine
Biria,Nazila,MD
Brunnquell,Stephen B.,MD
Fadil,Tina Marie,MD
Lee,Gerald J.,MD
Patel,Disha,MD
Relkin,Felicia,MD
Schran,Mary Ann,MD
Shin,Seulkih,MD
Srinivasan,Anand,MD
Physical Medicine & Rehab
Herera,Daniel Joe,MD
Surgery (General)
Jensen,Michael Edward,MD
Harrison
Family Medicine
D'Agostino,Ralph S.,MD
Internal Medicine
Carvalho,Artur Meneses,MD
Fontanazza,Paul,MD
Ryngel,Enrique,MD
Vazquez Falcon,Luis Enrique,MD
Orthopedic Surgery
Seigerman,Daniel Allan,MD
Pediatrics
Vidal,Jennifer Lyn,DO
Urology
Rilli,Charles F.,MD
Hasbrouck Heights
Cardiovascular Disease
Goodman,Daniel J.,MD
Sehgal,Evan D.,MD
Family Medicine
Bellavia,Thomas S.,MD
Porter,David F.,DO
Fertility/Infertility
Wolf Greene,Susan Amy,MD
Internal Medicine
Benoff,Lane Jeffrey,MD
Gennaro,Anthony J.,MD
Lyons,William J.,MD
Mazza,Victor Joseph,MD
Renner,Carl J.,MD
Neurological Surgery
Oppenheimer,Jeffrey Harry,MD
Obstetrics & Gynecology
Fechner,Adam Jeffrey,MD
Loughlin,Jacquelyn S.,MD
Reproductive Endocrinology
Cho,Michael Ming-Huei,MD
McGovern,Peter G.,MD
Weiss,Gerson,MD
Vascular Neurology
Turkel-Parrella,David,MD
Haskell
General Practice
Hall,Kevin Arthur,MD
Internal Medicine
Smith,Jeffrey Todd,DO
Haworth
Family Medicine
Isnar,Noyemi,MD
Pediatrics
De Antonio,Michele L.,MD
Gupta,Archana,MD
Stathopoulos,Labrini,MD
Psychiatry
Fairbanks,Janet A.,MD
Hawthorne
Anatomic/Clinical Pathology
Vangurp,James Mark Jr.,DO
Cardiovascular Disease
Montagnino,Joseph W.,MD
Emergency Medicine
Saber,Mai Said,DO

Family Medicine
Anthony Wilson,Avril Dawn,MD
Lozito,Joseph A. Jr.,DO
Tuppo,Enas Elias,MD
Internal Medicine
Festa,Eugene Daniel,MD
Gupta,Manju,MD
Jacoby,Steven Clifford,MD
Lozito,Deborah A.,DO
Mannino,Marie L.,MD
Mazziotti,Alexander R.,MD
Nitti,David J.,MD
Penera,Norman S.,MD
Peterka,Ann-Judith,DO
Tuppo,Ehab E.,MD
Obstetrics & Gynecology
Cifaldi,Ralph John Jr.,DO
Ophthalmology
Newman,Frederic R.,MD
Otolaryngology
Giglio,Michael,MD
Pediatrics
Vasena Marengo,Maria Jose,MD
Plastic Surgery
Torsiello,Michael J.,MD
Surgery (General)
Goel,Surendra P.,MD
Hazlet
Cardiovascular Disease
Ani,Mohamad Salim,MD
Sarnelle,Joseph A.,MD
Uppal,Parveen,MD
Family Medicine
Field,Shawn Michael,MD
Hundle,Rameet Kaur,MD
Perrino,DinaMarie,MD
Schneebaum,Katherine,MD
Triola,Victoria,DO
Tsompanidis,Antonios A.J.,DO
Internal Medicine
Awad,Mona S.,MD
Chudzik,Douglas W.,MD
Chudzik,Jeanmarie,DO
Cornel-Avendano,Beverly,MD
Golding-Granado,Lisa M.,MD
Katz,Lawrence,MD
Khalil,Hossam M.,MD
Meleis,Mohamed E.,MD
Rajasekharaiah,Vinutha,MD
Saaraswat,Babita,MD
Sahloul,Elsayed Ahmed,MD
Sambandan,Rama Thirugnana,MD
Xu,Lin,MD
Laser Surgery
Murugesan,Angappan,MD
Nephrology
Hozayen,Ossama,MD
Naqvi,Azeez Fathima,MD
Neurology
Pavuluri,Srinivas,MD
Ophthalmology
Clemente,Maria F.,MD
Orthopedic Surgery
Allegra,Marshall P.,MD
Ani,Abdul Nasser,MD
Cunningham,Michael Joseph,MD
Pediatrics
Blackman,Ryan Graham,DO
Cambria,Lina,MD
Jain,Asha,MD
Khuddus,Munawara S.,MD
Pascucci,Rocco F.,MD
Protasis,Liza,MD
Ruda,Neal,MD
Physical Medicine & Rehab
Bash,Robin Ellen,MD
Rim,Josephine Myunghi,MD
Plastic Surgery
Fontana,Victor,DO
Pulmonary Disease
Pristas,Adrian M.,MD
Surgery (General)
Buker,Ibrahim S.,MD
Hernando,Franklin P.,MD
Thoracic Surgery
Solis,P. Ariel,MD
Hewitt
Family Medicine
Baquiran,Henry M.,MD
Guariglia,George Angelo,DO

Obstetrics & Gynecology
Dombo,Kudzai Rebecca,MD
Highland Park
Allergy
Blum,Jay R.,MD
Bonala,Savithri Bai,MD
Golbert,Thomas Melvin,MD
Allergy & Immunology
Gutin,Faina M.,MD
Li,Lin,MD
Suliaman,Fawzi A.,MD
Witkowska,Renata A.,MD
Child & Adolescent Psychiatry
Kleinmann,Richard,MD
Emergency Medicine
Erlikhman,Alla,MD
Facial Plastic Surgery
Glasgold,Robert Alexander,MD
Family Medicine
Cohn,Joseph Theodore,MD
Glatter,Frederic G.,MD
Miller,Arthur H.,MD
Gastroenterology
Cohen,Hillel D.,MD
Infectious Disease
Khan,Shameen,DO
Internal Medicine
Anolik,Kenneth Jay,MD
Coelho-D'Costa,Vinette E.,MD
Katz,Brian Charles,MD
Ophthalmology
Glass,Robert M.,MD
Gordon,Stephen J.,MD
Hathaway,Elaine G.,MD
Otolaryngology
Glasgold,Mark J.,MD
Keni,Sanjay P.,MD
Schrader-Barile,Nicole A.,MD
Pediatric Allergy
Parikh,Sudhir Manharlal,MD
Sheen,Eun H.,MD
Pediatrics
Biener,Robert,MD
Gavai,Medha A.,MD
Glaser-Schanzer,Felice,MD
Gul,Sheba,MD
John,Sheryl Mary,MD
Majisu,Claire Amume,MD
Reingold,Stephen Marcus,MD
Rubin,Elliot H.,MD
Zablocki,Lisa R.,MD
Psychiatry
Khan,Farah Asim,MD
Nandu,Bharat I.,MD
Stern,Stephanie Klein,MD
Surgery (General)
Curtiss,Steven Ian,MD
Tutela,Rocco Robert Jr.,MD
Surgical Critical Care
Wang,Ju Lin,MD
Vascular Surgery
Finkelstein,Norman M.,MD
Rosen,Scott Farrell,MD
Highlands
Internal Medicine
Wolinsky,Steven I.,MD
Hightstown
Family Medicine
Syed,Sameera Mukaram,MD
Internal Medicine
Mangal,Rakesh,MD
Tummala,Sumalatha,MD
Pediatrics
Arcaro,Maria Anna C.,MD
Bidabadi,Bobak,MD
Goodman,Aimee R.,DO
Gribin,Bradley Jay,MD
Howe,Matthew R.,MD
Marcus,Brian F.,DO
Patel,Radhika K.,MD
Shah,Utpal S.,MD
Siddiqui,Sabeen A.,MD
Vo,Ha,MD
Plastic Surgery
Lynch,Matthew Jude,MD
Hillsborough
Allergy
Schulhafer,Edwin P.,MD
Anesthesiology
Das,Vivek T.,MD

Cardiovascular Disease
Taylor,Jeff Thomas,MD
Clinical Cardiac Elctrphyslgy
Sanyal,Sanjukta,MD
Critical Care Medicine
Einreinhofer,Stephen V.,DO
Dermatology
Henning,Jeffrey Scott,DO
Ilowite,Robert K.,DO
Man,Jeremy Robert,MD
Emergency Medicine
Kikta,Kevin J.,DO
Endocrinology
Desai,Navtika R.,DO
Family Medicine
Bagga,Harpreet Kaur,MD
Corson,Richard L.,MD
Erb,Erica,MD
Fowls,Brianna,MD
Landesman,Glen S.,MD
Lardner,Thomas Joseph,MD
Lee,Sung Keun,MD
Merchant,Neepa S.,MD
Piech,Richard Frank,MD
Reiss,Ronald A.,MD
Selke,Melissa D.,MD
Shute,Amy L.,MD
Smith,Joseph Arthur,MD
Snyder,Kenneth R.,MD
Weinstein,Joseph R.,MD
Zajac,Anna T.,MD
Gastroenterology
Accurso,Charles A.,MD
Barghash,Claudia N.,MD
Ciambotti,Gary Francis,MD
Gingold,Alan R.,DO
Lee,Kristen Kyongae,MD
Geriatric Psychiatry
Shah,Shailaja K.,MD
Geriatrics
Gubbi,Renukamba Nagaraju,MD
Gynecology
Davis,Nicole D.,MD
DeLucia,Carolyn Ann,MD
Infectious Disease
Doshi,Manish,MD
Herman,David J.,MD
Hirsh,Ellen J.,MD
Nahass,Ronald G.,MD
Pall,Amandeep Kaur,MD
Pittarelli,Lisa A.,MD
Sandhu,Sarbjit Singh,MD
Seenivasan,Meena,MD
Sheen,Jerry,MD
Sinner,Scott William,MD
Internal Medicine
Ahsan,Abu M.,MD
Allegar,Nancy E.,MD
Bhalla,Rohit,DO
Bhaskara,Jayshree A.,MD
Chou,Lin W.,MD
Greaves,Mark Leslie,MD
Gultom,Yanto Meiyer,MD
Hildebrant,Laura Nadine,DO
Manning,Eric Carlyle,MD
McDermott,Rena,MD
Mur,Ahmad A.,MD
Neiman,Deborah L.,MD
Sonnenberg,Edith,MD
Thakur,Ranjana,MD
Obstetrics & Gynecology
Blanks,Mary Susan,MD
Hirsch,Gregory D.,MD
Karanikolas,Steven,MD
Pineda,Jean,DO
Salley,Pamela R.,MD
Wagner,Wendy Joan,MD
Occupational Medicine
Shepperly,David C.,MD
Oral & Maxillofacial Surgery
Bandola,Krystin Ann,MD
Pediatric Gastroenterology
Youssef,Nader Namir,MD
Pediatrics
Concepcion,Kristin A.,MD
Hede,Madan M.,MD
Hussain,Aazim Syed,MD
Jiang,Li,MD
Lariviere,Aimee T.,MD
Yadav,Priyanka Singh,DO
Youngerman,Neil L.,MD

Physicians by Town and Medical Specialty

Hillsborough (cont)
Physical Medicine & Rehab
Chen, Boqing, MD
Psychiatry
Donnellan, Joseph Anthony, MD
Hu, Yuange, MD
Rochford, Joseph M., MD
Zomorodi, Ali, MD
Surgery (General)
Koota, David H., MD
Vascular Surgery
Buch, Edward D., MD
Goldson, Howard J., MD

Hillsdale
Child & Adolescent Psychiatry
Schneider, Mona, MD
Endocrinology
Wehmann, Robert E., MD
Gastroenterology
Stewart, David M., MD
Internal Medicine
Copeland, Lois J., MD
Di Pasquale, Laurene, MD
Plastic Surgery
Morin, Robert J., MD

Hillside
Family Medicine
Matkiwsky, Walter, DO
Tyndall, Alina, MD
Vidal Burke, Angela M., MD
Internal Medicine
Aluya, Nelson Oke, MD

Ho Ho Kus
Emergency Medicine
Smith, Donard Scott, MD
Internal Medicine
Berger, Glen W., MD
Obstetrics & Gynecology
Vikner, Lin M., MD
Pediatrics
Birnhak, Stefani, MD
Kim, Urian, MD
Lee, Julia Jin-Young, MD
Leifer, Amy Sarah Budin, MD
Psychiatry
Golin, Alexander Mark, MD
Welch, James W., MD

Hoboken
Allergy
Pine, Martin S., MD
Anatomic/Clinical Pathology
Fayemi, Alfred O., MD
Vaidya, Kamini P., MD
Anesthesiology
Aggarwal, Mukta, MD
Avery, William Bradford, MD
Blumenthal, David C., MD
Kao, Sen-Pin, MD
Kyin, Robin, MD
Lee, Brian, DO
Lee, Peter Yen-Iai, MD
Mead, John Edward, MD
Perez, Reynaldo T., MD
Punzalan, Maria M., MD
Rafer, Ramon V., MD
Whiteru, Uvie Christina, MD
Yap, Joseph Jim Estrella, MD
Cardiovascular Disease
Costomiris, Robert P., MD
Damle, Jagadish V., MD
Fishbein, Richard J., MD
Kyreakakis, Anthony J., MD
Leon, Robert John, MD
Susi, Brian Dievendorf, MD
Child & Adolescent Psychiatry
Chmarzewski, Barbara, MD
Moraille, Pascale, MD
Critical Care Medicine
Chu, Daniel Yun, DO
Dermatology
Cappiello, Linda L., MD
Fernandez-Obregon, Adolfo C., MD
Diagnostic Radiology
Gowda, Mamatha Ramesh, MD
Mousavi, Seyed-Ali, MD
Singh, Supreet, MD
Emergency Medicine
Enriquez, Melissa J., MD
Jani, Chandrashekhar C., MD
Lawyer, Edward Zadok, MD
Malizia, Robert W., MD
Rimmer, John Joseph III, DO
Roberson, Meika T., MD
Endocrinology
Gandhi, Thimma S., MD
Family Medicine
Balacco, Leonard M., MD
Brahmbhatt, Gaurang Ravaji, MD
Caniglia, James J., MD
De Marco, Angelo Albert, MD
Garcia, Raudel, MD
Garcia, Steven Jesus, MD
Islam, Javedul M., MD
Jacobs, Abbie D., MD
Joshi, Anuja, MD
Kumar, Harini C., MD
Latorre, Juan J., MD
Matienzo, Ricardo Martin, MD
Mercado, Donna M., MD
Mezhoudi, Amal, MD
Pollak, Joseph A., MD
Racaniello, Angelo R., MD
Ramirez Chernikova, Anna, MD
Ramos, Leonor Vivas, MD
Ramos, Rey Ferna Pedraza, MD
Rohani, Sayed M., MD
Safran, George F., MD
Samuel, Shyno, MD
Spivak, Dana, MD
Taubman, Jessica, MD
Teodoro, Paul C., MD
Tracey, Gregory Joseph, MD
Tully, Nicole S., MD
Valerian, Christopher, DO
Williams, Juliette Marie, MD
Witt, Virginia Marie, MD
Zigadlo, Tatyana, MD
General Practice
Robaina, Luis A., MD
Geriatrics
Perlmutter, Barbara Lee, MD
Hematology
Damle, Vasanti J., MD
Hospitalist
Kocia, Orjeta, MD
Infectious Disease
Forouzesh, Avisheh, MD
Messihi, Jean, MD
Rahman, Habeeb U., MD
Internal Medicine
DaSilva, Robert Antonio, MD
Herrera, Saturnino Domingo, MD
Kozel, Joseph M., MD
Lim, Jocelyn Marie P., MD
Loh, Shi, MD
Manocchio, Stephen J., MD
Narula, Jiwanjot K., MD
Okafor, Anthony Ifechukwu, MD
Patel, Karnik, DO
Pollak, Michael, MD
Neurological Surgery
Hunt, Charles D., MD
Neurology
Ploshchanskaya, Larisa G., MD
Obstetrics & Gynecology
Aguilar, Raul F., MD
Brescia, Mark J., MD
Chinn, Natasha R., MD
Garrisi, Margaret Graf, MD
Lowe, Samantha B., DO
Magpantay, Emiliana M., MD
McQuilkin, George E., MD
Migliaccio, Thomas A., MD
Moon, Jeremy, MD
Picard, Johan Arlenie, MD
Potter-McQuilkin, Dineasha M., MD
Rossetos, Ourania S., MD
Shoman, Adam Mohamed, MD
Ophthalmology
D'Alberti, Claudio F., MD
Orthopedic Surgery
Dwyer, James W., MD
Feliciano, Edward, MD
Isaac, Roman, MD
Steinway, Mitchell I., MD
Otolaryngology
Calloway, Hollin Elizabeth, MD
Glaser, Aylon Y., MD
Glickman, Alexander B., MD
Tandon, Raj, MD
Pathology
Ahmad, Imtiaz, MD
Pediatric Cardiology
Kotb, Mohy Eldin A., MD
Pediatrics
Akpalu, Daniel, MD
Klos, Andrzej E., MD
Kucharski, Jarrod Michael, MD
Mani, Shrinidi, MD
Mehta, Harshna B., MD
Pierog, Sophie H., MD
Salmun, Luis Marcelo, MD
Shenk, Kristina Suzanne, MD
Sikand, Vikram Singh, MD
Zarrabi, Yasaman, DO
Physical Med & Rehab-Pain Med
Ben-Meir, Ron Simon, DO
Physical Medicine & Rehab
Mavani, Yogini, DO
Strell, Robert Frederic, MD
Plastic & Reconstructive Srgy
Cerio, Dean Richard, MD
Plastic Surgery
Chalfoun, Charbel T., MD
Laskey, Richard S., MD
Loghmanee, Cyrus Faz, MD
Psychiatry
Chuang, Linda I., MD
Gajera, Bhavinkumar, MD
Greenberg, Robert M., MD
Gutierrez, Alvaro M., MD
Jackson, Michael B., MD
Joseph, Judith Fiona, MD
Magera, Michael John, MD
Radiology
Berger, Mark J., MD
Chang, Ming Z., MD
Gould, Lawrence, MD
Matari, Hussein M., MD
Reproductive Endocrinology
Chen, Serena Homei, MD
Surgery (General)
Costa, German H., MD
Gonzalez, Juan A. Jr., MD
Miller, Benetta L., MD
Urology
Cricco, Carl F. Jr., MD
Vascular & Intrvntnal Radiology
Barone, Allison, MD
Vascular Surgery
Steiner, Zachary John, DO

Holmdel
Addiction Medicine
London, Eric Bart, MD
Allergy
Ho, Linden D., MD
Viksman, Michael Y., MD
Anatomic/Clinical Pathology
Longo, Stacey L., MD
Anesthesiology
Bruk, George, MD
Citron, Andrew M., MD
Dhawlikar, Sunita Sripad, MD
Faelnar, Luis B., MD
Foroush, Pejman, MD
Girgis, Magdy S., MD
Handlin, David S., MD
Leung, Samson W., MD
Macklin, Joshua M., MD
McNair, Timothy P., MD
Milan, Ronald Kenneth, MD
Anesthesiology: Pain Medicine
Varma, Ajay Medavaram, MD
Cardiovascular Disease
Prasad, Penesetti V., MD
Shah, Niranjan S., MD
Yen, Ya-Tang, MD
Child & Adolescent Psychiatry
Ritsema, Marc E., DO
Varma, Deepti Sagar, MD
Colon & Rectal Surgery
Malit, Michele Farrah, DO
Cytopathology
Wang, Hongling, MD
Dermatology
Bhatnagar, Divya Sambandan, MD
Diagnostic Radiology
D'Angelo, Denis Gerard, MD
Rabbani, Soliman, MD
Emergency Medicine
Ali, Rayshma, DO
Brennessel, Ryan William, DO
Imbesi, Joseph Thomas, DO
Lee, Chi I., MD
Marchetti, Michael F., MD
Shah, Dinesh K., MD
Yu, Daniel Kwang-Jin, MD
Endocrinology
Antonopoulou, Marianna, MD
Zaitz, Jennifer, DO
Family Medicine
Bessen, Deborah Lynn, MD
Catanese, Vincent J., MD
Hayne, Charles W., DO
Salisbury, Jon P., MD
Shah, Vinaychandra B., MD
Gastroenterology
Moosvi, Mir A., MD
Hematology
Rifkin, Paul L., MD
Hematology Oncology
Chen, Aileen Lim, MD
Internal Medicine
Albana, Fouad S., MD
Bebawy, Sam T., MD
Brown, Derrick M., MD
Coniaris, Harry J., MD
De Tulio, Anthony, MD
Doshi, Pankaj Ajay, MD
Giannakopoulos, Georgios, DO
Holler, Marianne Marie, DO
Hundle, Sukhwinder K., MD
Jitan, Raed Abdalla, MD
Khan, Rafay Tariq, MD
Lehaf, Elias J., MD
Marino, Richard P., DO
Metri Mansour, Elie E., MD
Nasra, Magdy A., MD
Otrakji, Jean, MD
Parhar, Avtar Singh, MD
Robinson-Gallaro, Bonnie Lee, MD
Thalasila, Anuradha, MD
Vaysberg, Yevgeniy, MD
Neurology
Gandhi, Shefali, DO
Khakoo, Rafiya Shabbir, MD
Obstetrics & Gynecology
Conley, Michael P., MD
Patel, Sagar Y., MD
Penney, Robert P., MD
Sanakkayala, Nirmala D., MD
Smolinsky, Adi, MD
Wohlstadter, Sanford W., MD
Ophthalmology
Collur, Surekha, MD
Klug, Ronald David, MD
Steinfeld, Jason Israel, MD
Subramaniam, Cristin Devika, MD
Orthopedic Surgery
Khavarian, Javad, MD
Otolaryngology
Kim, Chong S., MD
Pain Medicine-Interventional
Ng, Alan S., MD
Pathology
Mikhail, Nagy H., MD
Pediatrics
Ayoub, Samia B., MD
Baumlin, Thomas Jr., MD
Bruner, Vanda, MD
Carey, Brittany Marie, DO
David, Lea H., MD
DeNicola, Nancy Ann, DO
Elbasty, Azza A., MD
Engel, Barbara M., MD
Engel, Jennifer Duck, MD
Miguelino, Bernadette M., MD
Mohan, Kusum C., MD
Sta. Maria, Emilia Navarro, MD
Yia, Grace Mercado, MD
Physical Medicine & Rehab
Azer, Amal W., MD
Romello, Janel B., DO
Plastic & Reconstructive Srgy
Samra, Salem, MD
Plastic Surgery
Griffith, Negin Noorchashm, MD
Samra, Asaad H., MD
Samra, Fares, MD
Samra, Said A., MD

Psychiatry
 D'Andrea,Daniel Albert,MD
 Mehta,Varsha B.,MD
 Moutier,Christine Y.,MD
 Varma,Gurbachan K.,MD
Pulmonary Disease
 Aggarwal,Vinod K.,MD
Surgery (General)
 Adeyeri,Ayotunde Olubukola,MD
 Mansuri,Hanif M.,MD
 Nguyen,Hung Q.,MD
 Patel,Munjal P.,MD
Thoracic Surgery
 Surya,Girija S.,MD
Urology
 Antoun,Saad S.,MD
 Jow,William W.,MD
 Peardon,Nathaniel Andres,DO
 Rizkala,Emad Remond,MD
 Surya,Babu V.,MD

Hopatcong
Anesthesiology
 Sobrepena,Jose S.M.,MD

Howell
Dermatology
 Weiner,Barry C.,MD
Emergency Medicine
 Dennis,Elaine Debra,MD
Family Medicine
 Agrawal,Neil,MD
 Anne,Sreelatha,MD
 Gumina,John D.,MD
 Liquori,Frances,DO
 Stern,Julie Beth,MD
 Zuckerbrod,Jacqueline E.,DO
Hematology Oncology
 Katz,Randi J.,DO
 Kunamneni,Raghu Krishna,MD
Infectious Disease
 Utpat,Sandeepa Makarand,MD
Internal Medicine
 Agrawal,Stuti Shah,MD
 Axelrad,Paul R.,MD
 DePerio,Elizabeth P.,MD
 Koretzky,Jeffrey Robert,MD
 Liu,Xiaoming,MD
 Lombardi,David D.,MD
 Morreale,Diego A.,MD
 Nahum,Kenneth D.,DO
 Polizzi,Maria,MD
 Shetty,Vinod J.,MD
 Soliman,Monir Louis Hanna,MD
 Streit,Steven,MD
Obstetrics & Gynecology
 Chhatwal,Balwant K.,MD
 Cohen,Alan,MD
 Surowitz,Clara Pauline,MD
Pediatrics
 Dayal,Rashmi P.,MD
 DePerio,Alicia G.,MD
 Lopez,Claudio J.,MD
 Maddatu,Elenito P.,MD
 Maddatu,Rose Mylaine,MD
 Manlapid,Luis T.,MD
 Mariano-Lau,Elizabeth L.,MD
 Mision,Vicente L.,MD
 Nagpal,Sangita D.,MD
 Verdi,Michelle Diane,DO
Psychiatry
 Abbas,Muhammad Ali,MD
 Cid,Georgina R.,MD
Trauma Surgery
 Moss,Vincent Lavaughn,MD
Urological Surgery
 Moss,Vance Joshaun,MD

Irvington
Adolescent Medicine
 Dada-Ajulchukwu,Tokunbo T.,MD
Allergy
 Belani,Suresh G.,MD
Cardiovascular Disease
 Campbell,Joseph V.,MD
 Patel,Sunil Madhusuda,MD
Family Medicine
 Willis,Rudolph C.,MD
Infectious Disease
 Mammen-Prasad,Elizabeth K.,MD
 Patel,Raj,MD
Internal Med-Adolescent Med
 Banigo,Samuel,MD

Internal Medicine
 Altema,Reynald,MD
 Anukwuem,Chidi I.,MD
 Brown,Patricia J.,MD
 Masor,Harvey G.,MD
 Ogunkoya,Adeniyi A.,MD
 Okoya,Jackson A.,MD
 Patel,Rasiklal A.,MD
 Rashid,Tasneem J.,MD
 Shen,Ein-Yuan A.,MD
 Wilcox,Ellis I.,MD
Neurology
 Dressner,Ivan R.,MD
 Sutaria,Hasmukhbha N.,MD
Obstetrics & Gynecology
 Kusnierz,James L.,DO
 Mukhopadhay,Jayati,MD
 Thani,Suresh R.,MD
 Treadwell,Kenneth Jr.,MD
 Zevin,Ronald A.,MD
Ophthalmology
 Bush,Nahndi,MD
 McCoy,Chrishonda Curry,MD
Pediatrics
 Anyanwu,Justina U.,MD
 Emelle,Emmanuel M.,MD
 Francois,Emmanuel J.,MD
 Gonzaga,Zenaida Palma,MD
 Isedeh,Cynthia O.,DO
 Lauredan,Bernier,MD
 Leger,Pierre R.,MD
 Miller,Sandrene,MD
 Sundaram,Palanisamy S.,MD
Surgery (General)
 Alzadon,Ricardo,MD
 Soriano,Jaime R.,MD

Iselin
Allergy
 Ambrosio,Patrick M.,DO
 Maccia,Clement A.,MD
Allergy & Immunology
 Waqar,Shaan M.,MD
Anatomic/Clinical Pathology
 Vora,Jaimini Neeraj,MD
Anesthesiology
 Pitchford,Douglas Edward,MD
Cardiovascular Disease
 Bhatnagar,Vibhay,MD
 Chaudhery,Shaukat A.,MD
 Patel,Ravindra I.,MD
Family Medicine
 Lubin-Baskin,Alicia F.,DO
 Mayer,Marc,DO
 Mayer,Mitchell F.,DO
 Perilstein,Neil J.,MD
 Riggi,Joseph,DO
General Practice
 Neubrander,James A.,MD
Internal Medicine
 Babaria,Bhavikaben Bhavin,MD
 Golubchik,Anneta V.,MD
 Gupta,Swati,MD
 Raju,Ramesh K.,MD
Obstetrics & Gynecology
 Berkman,Steven R.,MD
 Divino,Eumena M.,MD
 Ghanekar,Geeta R.,MD
 Goldberg,Steven C.,MD
 Magier,Slawomir,MD
Ophthalmology
 Grayson,Douglas Keane,MD
 Napolitano,Joseph Daniel,MD
 Patel,Menka Sanghvi,MD
 Strauss,Danielle Savitsky,MD
Otolaryngology
 Mazzara,Carl Arthur,MD
 Mehta,Vishvesh Mukur,MD
 Ort,Stuart A.,MD
 Rosin,Deborah F.,MD
Pediatrics
 Kernizan,Daphney,MD
 Nambiar,Sapna Shibhu,MD
Physical Med & Rehab-Pain Med
 Song,Sang Ho,DO
Surgery (General)
 Ramamurthy,Kotta M.,MD
Urology
 Husain,Aftab,MD

Jackson
Anatomic/Clinical Pathology

 Campos,Marite,MD
Family Medicine
 Druckman,Scott Jonathan,DO
 Lee,Nelson,DO
 Parkes,Lauren H.,DO
 Pedowitz,Robert Neil,DO
 Raymond,Joshua Joseph,MD
 Rodriguez-Bostock,Susan M.,MD
Internal Medicine
 Eiras,Maria E.,MD
 Hassan,Farida,MD
 Kulczycki,Alexander,MD
 Kumar,Sanjay,MD
 Patel,Shruti,MD
 Shah,Mukesh Chinubhai,MD
 Sharma,Nivedita,MD
 Song,Agatha Bockja,MD
 Vona,Cynthia E.,MD
Nephrology
 Kaur,Harneet,MD
Pediatrics
 Pawa,Anil K.,MD
 Qudsi,Tehsin Riaz,MD
 Zapanta,Rex A.,MD
Physical Med & Rehab-Pain Med
 Hsu,Kevin Kaiwen,MD
Physical Medicine & Rehab
 Bartley-Chin,Dellareece M.,MD
Psychiatry
 Wolff,David E.,MD

Jamesburg
Adolescent Medicine
 Gebre Medhin,Hanna,MD
Emergency Medicine
 Spierer,Robert,MD
Family Medicine
 Newman,Jared Brad,DO
General Practice
 Bordieri,Joseph Anthony,DO
Internal Medicine
 Carlucci,Michael Louis,MD
 Verdoni,John A.,MD
Orthopedic Surgery
 Jolley,Michael N.,MD
Pulmonary Disease
 Fein,Edward Dennis,MD
Radiation Oncology
 Greenberg,Andrew Seth,MD
Urology
 Richards,Steven Lawrence,MD

Jersey City
Allergy
 Elliston,Jason Taiwo Jos,MD
Anatomic/Clinical Pathology
 Das,Kasturi,MD
 Khawaja,Asia B.,MD
 Lin,Qing,MD
Anesthesiology
 Asamoah,Francis E.,MD
 Aventurado,Tito O.,MD
 Awad,Ahmed Sayed,MD
 Chen,Donghui,MD
 Dadaian,Susan,DO
 DeGuzman,Richelle T.,MD
 Leggat,Christopher Scott,MD
 Lin,Yuhlin,MD
 Lory,John Douglas,MD
 Mathew,Thomas,MD
 Moy,Jonathan M.,MD
 Naik,Ravi,MD
 Pham,Michael Minh,MD
 Reiss,Jodi L. W.,MD
 Rodriguez,Liza A.,MD
 Salimi-Ghezelbash,Behzad,MD
 Scinas,Athanasios,MD
 Shah,Amit A.,MD
 Shih,Duen S.,MD
 Sood,Monica,MD
 Wu,Jung-Faug,MD
 Zaklama,Selvia G.,MD
 Zhou,Ben Yuan,MD
Cardiothoracic Surgery
 Perera,Santusht A.,MD
Cardiovascular Disease
 Abed,Mary T.,MD
 Ahmad,Muhammad A.,MD
 Ameen,Abdul Aleem,MD
 Barber,Nathaniel A.,MD
 Baruchin,Mitchell Alan,MD
 Benz,Michael,MD

 Cruz-Encarnacion,Merle C.,MD
 Hamirani,Kamran Ismail,MD
 Hannallah,Benyamin A.,MD
 Hupart,Preston Arthur,DO
 Moussa,Ghias M.,MD
 Pandya,Madhukar N.,MD
 Patel,Vinodkumar G.,MD
 Phung,Michael Hung,MD
 Rezai,Feridoun,MD
 Richard,Merwin Francis,MD
 Sastry,Pillutla V.,MD
 Shah,Deepak O.,MD
 Singh,Bharat,MD
 Taha,Abdallah R.,MD
 Terwes,Estella,MD
 Wong,Peter J.,MD
Child & Adolescent Psychiatry
 Stewart,Michael Starbin,MD
Child (Pediatric) Neurology
 Hanna,Amir Atallaha,MD
 Kozanitis Mentakis,Irene D.,MD
Clinical Cardiac Elctrphyslgy
 Ahmad,Ahsanuddin,MD
Cornea/External Disease
 Constad,William H.,MD
Critical Care Medicine
 Matta,Jyoti S.,MD
Dermatology
 Besedina,Liliya,MD
 Erianne,John A.,MD
 Fox,Richard David,MD
 Katz,Arthur M.,MD
 Khasak,Dmitry,MD
 Noroff,Joan P.,MD
 Stotland,Mira,MD
Developmental Pediatrics
 Dehnert,Michele Chun,MD
 Sy-Te,Emilie,MD
Diagnostic Radiology
 Baranetsky,Adrian Andrew,MD
 Karp,Hillel J.,MD
 Maurizi,Romolo A.,MD
 Singh,David,MD
Electromyography
 Constantino,Edwin M.,MD
Emergency Medicine
 Abass-Shereef,Jeneba,MD
 Bookbinder,Ronald L.,MD
 Canabal,Vincent Paul,MD
 Ceci,Robert L.,MD
 Cespedes,Victoria Elena,MD
 Davis,Matthew B.,MD
 Estephan,Amir E.,MD
 Hameer,Muneer,MD
 Hepburn,Valerie J.,MD
 Jaggi,Mona,MD
 Jones,Caitlin Maria,MD
 Kenigsberg,David R.,MD
 Koch,Peter Benjamin,MD
 Kwon,Johnny,MD
 Llarena,Ramon C.,MD
 Martinez,Mark,MD
 Meta,Joubin,DO
 O'Brien,Susan Erin,DO
 Pak-Teng,Carol,MD
 Rabines,Alfredo Leonardo,DO
 Radwine,Zachary Picker,MD
 Ruiz,Vincent Edward,MD
 Sanghvi,Shimal H.,MD
 Slep,Borys,MD
 Sultana,Noushin,MD
 Syed,Saquiba,MD
 Wang,Cheng-Teng,MD
 Wilkes,Kristen,MD
Endocrinology
 Cam,Jenny G.,MD
 Ciechanowska,Malgorzata M.,MD
 Escobar-Barboza,Vanessa,MD
Family Med-Adult Medicine
 Labib,Labib N.,DO
Family Medicine
 Abubakar,Shaik,MD
 Bobb-Mckoy,Marion Y.,MD
 Buisson,Valerie Fabiola,MD
 Castro,Zoila Y.,MD
 Choudry,Muhammad A.,MD
 Cruz,Wilfredo Tomas Correa,MD
 De Silva,Malika Shani,MD
 Fritz,John A.,DO
 Kapadia,Bhupendra A.,MD
 Majchrzak,Tadeusz J.,MD

Physicians by Town and Medical Specialty

Jersey City (cont)

Family Medicine
- Mayorquin, Bertha, MD
- Mercado, Melissa, DO
- Mravcak, Sally A., MD
- Nguyen, Jim A., DO
- Patel, Hetal R., DO
- Riva, Inna, DO
- Roque, Cesar Ruben Jr., MD
- Rosenblum, Lauren, DO
- Rotella, Frank A., DO
- Sanderson, James Glen, DO
- Saxena, Shilpa M., MD
- Schehr-Kimble, Danielle J., DO
- Sklower, Jay A., DO
- Wong, Aubrey S., DO

Fertility/Infertility
- Gagliardi, Carol L., MD
- Leyson, Jose Flotcante J., MD

Forensic Psychiatry
- Goldwaser, Alberto Mario, MD

Gastroenterology
- Bhatia, Taruna, MD
- Dizon, Alita L., MD
- Reddy, Ram K., MD
- Rubin, Kenneth P., MD
- Shiff, Steven J., MD
- Stoopack, Paul Mitchell, MD
- Stowe, Arthur Chester Jr., MD
- Weissman, Paul S., MD

General Practice
- Clemente, Jose D., MD
- Perez, Humberto T., MD

General Preventive Medicine
- Carnow, David Robert, MD

Geriatrics
- Flores, David, MD

Hematology
- Housri, Ibrahim, MD

Hematology Oncology
- Badin, Simon, MD
- Patel, Amit A., MD
- Shah, Nalini Arvindkumar, MD
- Talwar, Sumit, MD
- Zarubin, Vadim, MD

Hospitalist
- Borker, Sonia V., DO
- Lahewala, Sopan, MD
- Mamji, Salman, MD
- Mulligan, Edward, MD

Infectious Disease
- Bellomo, Spartaco, MD
- Grigoriu, Adriana, MD
- Khan, Noroze Jalil, MD
- Mangia, Anthony J., MD

Insurance Medicine
- Park, Young K., MD

Internal Medicine
- Abubakar, Ahmed B., MD
- Acierno, Lynne J., MD
- Ahmed, Amina A., MD
- Alam, Parvez, MD
- Aman, Chaudhry S., MD
- Anemelu, Ignatius I., MD
- Assaleh, Marwan David, MD
- Badin, Diane, MD
- Badin, Michel S., MD
- Bansal, Nivedita, MD
- Beaty, Patrick D., MD
- Bhatt, Pranay Janardan, MD
- Borghini, Margarita, MD
- Boylan, Edward F., MD
- Brandt, Frederick W., MD
- Brotman, Deborah L., MD
- Cabales, Arthur L., MD
- Cabales, Victor L., MD
- Chatha, Anjum, MD
- Chinai, Ronak N., MD
- Choi, Jea Keun, MD
- Choudhary, Anjali P., MD
- Choudry, Abaid Ullah Anwar, MD
- Ciechanowski, George J., MD
- Darbouze, Jean R., MD
- DeLeon, Zorayda Olaya, MD
- Del Castillo, Ma Dolores, MD
- Desai, Jignesh, MD
- Digioia, John J. Jr., MD
- Druck, Mark, MD
- Dungo, Joven P., MD
- El Amir, Mazhar E., MD
- El Amir, Medhat Elsayed, MD
- Elamir, Mohammed, MD
- Faludi, Christopher, MD
- Farooq, Ahmad, MD
- Fermin, Carlos Miguel, MD
- Fogari, Robert A., MD
- Francois, Vincent, MD
- Gandhi, Kirit V., MD
- Ghuman, Damanjit K., MD
- Gongireddy, Srinivas V., MD
- Hanif, Muhammad Shahzad, MD
- Hannallah, Youssef A., MD
- Ibrahim, Mary I., MD
- Jain, Deepika, MD
- Jetty, Siva Teja, MD
- Jonnalagadda, Padmavathi, MD
- Jonnalagadda, Vasudeva Rao, MD
- Kazmi, Syed Iftikhar Ahmed, MD
- Khan, Anwar Ahmad, MD
- Khan, Rizwana, MD
- Kohan, Feraydoon, MD
- Latef, Sherif Maurice, MD
- Lazo, Angel Amado Jr., MD
- Li, Xiaoling, MD
- Lim, Fidel Losa Jr., MD
- Lipat, Gregorio A., MD
- Lippman, Jay Howard, MD
- Mahmood, Saleem, MD
- Maiello, Dominic J., MD
- Makadia, Bhaktidevi, MD
- Malhotra, Amit, MD
- Marian, Valentin Dumitru, MD
- Marmol, Jose Jr., MD
- Miller, Stuart Henry, MD
- Min, Irene, MD
- Mirza, Muhammed H., MD
- Mousa, Atef, DO
- Moustiatse, Adelia C., MD
- Munne, Gisela L., MD
- Nariseti, Chalapathy, MD
- Neibert, John Paul Z., MD
- Onwochei, Francis, MD
- Oparaji, Anthony Chibuzor, MD
- Owusu, Solomon, MD
- Pagulayan, Sylvia R., MD
- Palathingal, Rini M., MD
- Pappert, Jeffrey Robert, MD
- Parikh, Nitin A., MD
- Patel, Amy A., MD
- Patel, Chandrakant A., MD
- Patel, Ramiladevi S., MD
- Perera, Sharmalie, MD
- Phung, Susan, MD
- Pizarro, Oscar N., MD
- Quraishi, Abid Nisar, MD
- Qureshi, Hassan I., DO
- Reisner, Michelle R., MD
- Rizvi, Anwar Ahmad, MD
- Salah-Eldin, Alaa A., MD
- Saleeb, Joseph S., MD
- Samineni, Sankar Anand, MD
- Scarpa, Nicholas P., MD
- Seman, Ahmed B., MD
- Shah, Rohitkumar I., MD
- Shah, Saira, MD
- Sharma, Ritu, MD
- Syed, Amer K., MD
- Thota, Sreevani, MD
- Uppal, Muhammad S., MD
- Velasco, Sonia C., MD
- Velpari, Sudarshan, MD
- Viloria, Edermiro, MD
- Walters, Samuel Roy, MD
- Weiner, Barry, MD
- Whitley, Ronda M., MD

Magnetic Resonance Imaging
- Hirsch, Howard J., MD

Neonatal-Perinatal Medicine
- Alsheikh, Suhail N., MD
- Rao, Kavya Madupu, MD
- Razi, Sadia, MD

Nephrology
- Ahmed, Umrana, MD
- Batwara, Ruchika, MD
- Garg, Neha, MD
- Goel, Narender, MD
- Haddad, Bassam M., MD
- Haddad, Danny B., MD
- Mughni, Azam, MD
- Patel, Jayeshkumar Shantilal, MD

Neurological Surgery
- Mirza, Neville M., MD

Neurology
- Anselmi, Gregory D., MD
- Brannan, Timothy S., MD
- Dasika, Vijaya R., MD
- Dumitru, Dan Lucian, MD
- Khan, Musaid A., MD
- Komotar, Ana M., MD
- Korya, Dani, MD

Nuclear Medicine
- Shah, Hemant R., MD

Obstetrics & Gynecology
- Baptiste, Nicole Bernadette, MD
- Barbara Mijares, Diego, MD
- Bimonte, Michael J., MD
- Boamah, Kwaku Osafo-Mensah, MD
- Borja, Manuel L., MD
- Campbell, Damali M., MD
- Carter, Cheryl Ann, MD
- Chang, Kenneth Sung Soo, MD
- Chau, Patricia Chang Wai, MD
- Fernandez, Osbert, MD
- Gonzalez, Lily W., MD
- Gor, Jyotsna H., MD
- Gressock, Joseph Neal, MD
- Hou, Hui Ying, MD
- Hu, Long-Gue, MD
- Ibrahim, Gehan M., MD
- Kranias, Hristos K., MD
- Masson, Lalitha, MD
- Muhammed, Zaheda, MD
- Mushayandebvu, Taonei I., MD
- Najafi, Abdul Wahid, MD
- Nichols, Rhonda R., MD
- Patel, Roshni Dinesh, DO
- Pellecchia, Ralph Joseph, MD
- Rahulatharan, Rajasingha, MD
- Ramirez, Elizabeth, MD
- Ratzersdorfer, Jonathan, MD
- Resnikoff-Gary, Amanda Nicole, MD
- Sharma, Neha, MD
- Uy, Vena, MD
- Wehbe Saloukhan, Cristin, MD
- Witter, Theodore O., MD

Ophthalmology
- Cervenak-Panariello, Betty, MD
- Cinotti, Donald J., MD
- Hershkin, Paige B., DO
- Maltzman, Barry A., MD
- Origlieri, Catherine Ann, MD
- Panariello, Anthony L., MD
- Rau, Ganesh U., MD
- Shulman, Gayle S., MD
- Vora, Bhupendra N., MD
- Walsman, Scott Michael, MD
- Yee, Mei-Ling, MD

Orthopedic Surgery
- Adibe, Sebastian O., MD
- Beebe, Kathleen Sue, MD
- Foddai, Paul A., MD
- Irving, Henry C. III, MD
- Pflum, Francis A. Jr., MD
- Tolentino, Ernesto A., MD

Orthopedic Trauma
- Liporace, Frank Anthony, MD

Orthopedic-Hand Surgery
- Ahmed, Irfan Haroon, MD
- Capo, John Thomas, MD

Otolaryngology
- Behin, Babak, MD
- Behin, Fereidoon, MD
- Garay, Kenneth F., MD
- Youssef, Jan Samir, MD

Pathology
- Shroff, Yogini J., MD

Pediatrics
- Ansay, Editha Santillan, MD
- Baker, Omar A., MD
- Barrera-Tolentino, Felicisima, MD
- Boulos, Mona, MD
- Calero-Bai, Rosario, MD
- Casia, Jeffrey P., MD
- Choudry, Omer F., MD
- Coleman, Reginald O., MD
- De La Rosa, Rita G., MD
- Desai, Vijaya S., MD
- Dimaculangan, Nelo De Gala, MD
- Eltemsah, Nagi I., MD
- Endaya-Aguila, Thelma, MD
- Fernandez, Fredy A., MD
- Franco, Maria M., MD
- Ghaly, Maged Antoine, MD
- Jain, Doney B., MD
- Jenkins, Lisa Michelle, MD
- Kaki, Sushma R., MD
- LeBron, Carmen Haydee, MD
- Lipert, Zofia J., MD
- Majithia, Meenakshee N., MD
- Malik, Tayyaba K., MD
- Mangosing, Emma A., MD
- Moss, Beverly D., MD
- Nagorna, Malgorzata, MD
- Newman, Brigitte Jeanne, MD
- Palomares, Danilo V., MD
- Politis, Regina, MD
- Quim, Marinelle De Los Santos, MD
- Raha, Bandana, MD
- Ramasubramaniam, Nagarani, MD
- Santos, Ray Ryan Crisostomo, MD
- Santos-Borja, Concepcion L., MD
- Surti, Daxa Bhupendra, MD
- Tan, Vicente G., MD
- Ucheagwu, Hyacinth Emenike, MD
- Umali, Winston Caraos, MD
- Varma, Mekhla, MD
- Ventura, Evelyn Ortiz, MD
- Yin, Chun Hui, MD
- Yu, William C., MD

PhysMed&Rehab-Neuromuscular Med
- Vora, Kajol, MD

Physical Medicine & Rehab
- Campos, Jose S., MD
- Chang, James Kenneth, MD
- Kolla, Sairamachandra Rao, MD
- Lacap, Michael V., MD
- Mehta, Ariz Ruyintan, MD
- Mehta, Monica R., MD
- Menkin, Serge, MD
- Oller, Helen Suguitan, MD

Plastic Surgery
- Fule, Vilma G., MD

Psychiatry
- Bhandari, Pankaj Kumar, MD
- Braganza, Armando M., MD
- Chandak, Ritu, MD
- Dela Cruz, Leo A., MD
- Delston, Damon D., MD
- Greenberg, William M., MD
- Hasaj, Mario Jorge, MD
- Hernandez, Victor F., MD
- Johnson-Sena, Leonie J., MD
- Kurani, Devendra, MD
- La Monaca, Anthony G., MD
- Mansoob, Farhana, MD
- Parikh, Gita N., MD
- Pingol, Carmelo S., MD
- Quintana, Jorge D., MD
- Ratush, Edward, MD
- Syed, Wajiha F., MD
- Trotta, Celia V., MD
- Vinuela, Andres, MD
- Vora, Shobhana B., MD
- Wassef, Tamer William, MD
- Zamora, Violeta C., MD

Pulmonary Critical Care
- Mikkilineni, Rao S., MD

Pulmonary Disease
- Bhatnagar, Tanuj, MD
- Marchione, Victor L., MD
- Natarajan, Sekar, MD

Radiation Oncology
- Shaiman, Alan, MD

Radiology
- Byk, Cheryl Jean, MD
- Tholany, Jason Joseph, MD

Surgery (General)
- Gor, Pradip D., MD
- Hanhan, Ziad George, MD
- Kaiser, Susan, MD
- Mapp, Samuel Eugene, MD
- Moeller, Lavinia Paige, DO
- Molino, Bruno, MD
- Ottley, Anroy K., MD
- Raccuia, Joseph Salvatore, MD
- Sagullo, Nestor M., MD
- Schrag, Sherwin Phan, MD

Surgical Critical Care
- Schrader, Patricia A., MD

Trauma Surgery
- Chaar, Mitchell Y., MD
- Ha, Victor Vinh, MD

Urology
- Abramowitz, Joel, MD

Hosay,John J. Jr.,MD
Shah,Asha Dinesh,MD
Shulman,Yale C.,MD
Steigman,Elliot G.,MD
Vascular & Intrvntnal Radiology
Menon,Sujoy,MD
Vascular Surgery
Chan,Florence Y.,MD
Khawaja,Aftab A.,MD
McGovern,Patrick Jr.,MD
Popovich,Joseph F.,MD
Taha,Salah H.,MD
Keansburg
Internal Medicine
Tsai,Anderson F.,MD
Kearny
Allergy & Immunology
Thomas,Kathleen,MD
Anesthesiology
Bleiweiss,Warren J.,MD
Cardiovascular Disease
Daoko,Joseph,MD
Deshpande,Mohan S.,MD
Dermatology
Fishman,S. Jose,MD
General Practice
Doshi,Prakash J.,MD
Internal Medicine
Balasubramanian,Kanchana,MD
Desai,Viren,MD
Jacob,Emad,MD
Killilea,Edward M.,MD
Sanchez,Mauricio Jorge,MD
Wynn,Laurence,MD
Obstetrics & Gynecology
Graf,Jennifer A.,DO
Herrighty,Marianne K.,MD
Surmeli,Sedat M.,MD
Ophthalmology
Harper,Andrea A.,MD
Orthopedic Surgery
Canario,Arthur T.,MD
Granatir,Charles E.,MD
Pediatrics
Lopez-Maslak,Edna Retiracion,MD
Novaes,Denise,MD
Padykula,Anna,MD
Skripkus,Aldona J.,MD
Zhang,Li,MD
Physical Medicine & Rehab
DaSilva,Annette Christina,DO
Psychiatry
McAllister,Michael R.,DO
Pulmonary Disease
Saliba,Jehad E.,MD
Surgery (General)
Stylman,Jay Ira,MD
Kendall Park
Allergy
Kesarwala,Hemant,MD
Cardiovascular Disease
Huang,Michael Shu Hsien,DO
Child & Adolescent Psychiatry
Schnitzlein,Robert,MD
Diagnostic Radiology
Balgowan,Dennis,MD
Garnet,Daniel,MD
Greene,Samuel James,MD
Leder,David S.,MD
Nemade,Ajay B.,MD
Rubbert-Slawek,Kerstin Anke,MD
Tenenzapf,Mark J.,MD
Family Medicine
Lara,Jaime F.,MD
Weingarten,Harvey S.,MD
Internal Medicine
Chaudhari,Umesh J.,MD
Estavillo,Aileen Casambre,MD
Gu,Lingping,MD
Kamath,Sudha P.,MD
Koganti,Monika,MD
Mehta,Priti J.,MD
Mongia,Rupa,MD
Patel,Robert Balvant,MD
Satwah,Vinay Kumar,DO
Sinha,Meena,MD
Vallabhaneni,Purnima,MD
Interventional Cardiology
Patel,Alpesh Babu,MD

Nephrology
Merlin,Francky,MD
Obstetrics & Gynecology
Caban,Michelle,MD
Colonna,Elizabeth Ann,MD
Ham,Antoinette Lucy,MD
Karim,Nuzhat,MD
Kim,Eugene J.,MD
Lundberg,John L.,MD
Segal,Joshua Howard,MD
Pediatric Critical Care
Zuckerman,Gary B.,MD
Pulmonary Disease
Khan,Wajahat Hussain,MD
Radiation Oncology
Flannery,Todd W.,MD
Fontanilla,Hiral P.,MD
Hug,Eugene Boris,MD
Rodrigues,Neesha Ann,MD
Radiology
Schlesinger,Fred H.,MD
Therapeutic Radiology
Pepek,Joseph M.,MD
Kenilworth
Anesthesiology
Siddiqui,Afzaal Ahmad,MD
Cardiovascular Disease
Berman,Gail O.,MD
Dermatology
Pravda,Douglas J.,DO
Endocrinology
Cuffie,Cynthia A.,MD
Cutler,David L.,MD
Family Medicine
Kazemi,Ahmad,MD
Milazzo,Salvatore J. Sr,DO
Infectious Disease
Corcoran,Gavin R.,MD
Internal Medicine
Shah,Milind Narendra,MD
Slatkin,Ava,MD
Strony,John Thomas,MD
Udasin,Gary E.,MD
Waskin,Hetty Anne,MD
Nephrology
Agresti,James V.,DO
Kingston
Osteopathic Medicine
Tepper Levine,Shawn,DO
Psychiatry
Goldin,Nancy Jean,MD
Kinnelon
Anesthesiology
Deutsch,Jonathan S.,MD
Dermatology
Schwartz,Carolyn L.,MD
Szylit,Jo-Ann,MD
Endocrinology
Suda,Abhay K.,MD
Family Medicine
Cartaxo,Kenneth W.,MD
Geriatrics
Levant,Barry E.,MD
Internal Medicine
Avagyan,Igor Zhorzhiko,MD
Ophthalmology
Ashkanazy,Mitchel,MD
Shnayder,Eric,MD
Pediatrics
Suda,Anjuli,MD
Vijaysadan,Viju,MD
Psychiatry
Pikalov,Andrei A.,MD
Lafayette
Addiction Psychiatry
Baliga,Ravi,MD
Developmental Pediatrics
Laveman,Lawrence B.,MD
Psychiatry
Squires,Sandra,MD
Lake Hiawatha
Family Medicine
Spector,Randy A.,DO
Internal Medicine
Maher,Miriam Ruth,MD
Lake Hopatcong
Family Medicine
Bonnet,Jean-Paul,DO
Lucatorto,Anthony J.,DO

Internal Medicine
Orlandoni,Enrico F.,DO
Obstetrics & Gynecology
Prezioso,Alexander N.,MD
Lakehurst
Geriatrics
Shua Haim,Joshua Roy,MD
Internal Medicine
Comsti,Eric A.,MD
Lehman,Frederick,MD
Pineda,Julita S.,MD
Pineda,Nonato E.,MD
Lakewood
Allergy & Immunology
Pasternak,Philip Louis,MD
Anatomic Pathology
Fromowitz,Frank B.,MD
Li,Rongshan,MD
Mahapatro,Darshana,MD
Anatomic/Clinical Pathology
Ata,Hadia M.,MD
Chatterjee,Monica,MD
Engelbach,Ludmila,MD
Guo,Yijun,MD
Pai,Usha Laxman,MD
Shen,Tingliang,MD
Anesthesiology
Bermudez,Juan D.,MD
Edelmann,Robert Benedict Jr.,MD
Viradia,Jayant K.,MD
Cardiovascular Disease
Bacharach,Moshe,MD
Grill,Lawrence J.,MD
Gupta,Avinash Chandra,MD
Kadosh,Yisrael,MD
Mohan,Rajesh,MD
Patel,Nachiket V.,MD
Clinical Pharmacology
Uderman,Howard David,MD
Cytopathology
Sharaan,Mona El-Sayed,MD
Dermatology
Kuflik,Julianne Helen,MD
Tarlow,Mordechai M.,MD
Dermatopathology
Bhattacharjee,Pradip,MD
Diagnostic Radiology
Cranley,Robert,MD
Khanna,Pawandeep S.,MD
Langman,Alex,MD
Pukin,Lev,MD
Qiu,William Weiguang,MD
Shah,Faisal Majeed,MD
Electromyography
Markowitz,Charles R.,MD
Emergency Medicine
Calderon,Oscar R.,MD
Dalsey,William Colwell,MD
Larsen,Johnny R.,DO
Leber,Ian Brett,MD
Peltz,Hillel,DO
Raja,Sreedar V.,MD
Setya,Amit,DO
Sirchio,Kevin J.,DO
Solas,John R.,DO
Family Medicine
Genovese,Cynthia Marie,MD
Patterson,Marion Lesley,MD
Zukowski,Christopher W.,DO
Gastroenterology
Bhagat,Sanjay,MD
Kandathil,Mathew K.,MD
Kurtz,Joel H.,MD
Musicant,Joel Marc,MD
Geriatrics
Lempel,Allen L.,MD
Internal Medicine
Bhatt,Nikhil Yeshavantray,MD
Blake,Michael Laurence,MD
Chakrapani,Soumya,MD
Chander,Harish,MD
Cohen,Jonathan,MD
Cohen,Jonathan Ira,MD
Das,Saumya,MD
Green,Tamar Buchsbaum,MD
Hussain,Shahzad,MD
Jilani,Usman Khan,MD
Kashyap,Rupa R.,MD
Krohn,David Isaac,MD
Lebowitz,Howard Harris,MD

Mahan,Janet L.,MD
Maron,Edward M.,MD
Morelos,Joseph C.,DO
Narasimhaswamy,Smitha,MD
Ogun,David J.,MD
Patel,Akshay D.,MD
Patel,Manoj,MD
Patel,Pinakin C.,MD
Patel,Sandipkumar R.,MD
Phelps,Kristyn Kia,MD
Pineles,Cary L.,MD
Preschel,Samuel Aharon,MD
Rajeswaran,Gowri,MD
Robberson,Heather Leigh,MD
Salcedo,Elizabeth O.,MD
Shahabuddin,Saiham,MD
Singh,Satyendra Pratap,MD
Smithers,Wilda I.,MD
Talamayan,Randy P. C.,MD
Thomas,Teresa E.,MD
Thopcherla,Manjula,MD
Yap,Wilson C.,MD
Medical Microbiology
Strand,Calvin L.,MD
Neurology
Lombardino,Anthony N.,MD
Obstetrics & Gynecology
Cahill,Kenneth Matthew,DO
Chang,Joanne Meejin,MD
Choper,Niles E.,MD
Cocco,Frank A.,MD
Culbert,Steven A.,MD
Greenstein,Gary David,MD
Hoffman,Christian T. III,MD
Lehnes,Eric G.,MD
Moghe,Vaishali C.,MD
Molina,Arthur M.,MD
Morgan,Allen,MD
Pitsos,Miltiadis,MD
Repole,Adam N.,MD
Smith,Sharon Marie,MD
Tal,Moty N.,MD
Thompson,Flavius Mark,MD
Young,Tiffany,DO
Zafarani,Amy Jo,DO
Occupational Medicine
Salvo,Victor J.,MD
Ophthalmology
Barofsky,Jonathan M.,MD
Chinskey,Nicholas Daniel,MD
Hedaya,Edward L.,MD
Huppert,Leon J.,MD
Rothkopf,Moshe M.,MD
Von Roemer,Marc,MD
Orthopedic Surgery
Absatz,Michael G.,MD
Otolaryngology
Giri,Suresh C.,MD
Jaffari,Syed Moosa Raza,MD
Pathology
Kartika,Gunawan,MD
Romerocaces,Gloria Marcelo,MD
Vara,Manjula L.,MD
Pediatrics
Berghaus,Jean E.,MD
Eilenberg,Eli,MD
Fenster,William R.,MD
Gittleman,Neal D.,MD
Greenberg,Bram,MD
Gwertzman,Rachel,DO
Hirsch,Harvey Alan,MD
Indich,Norman,MD
Jain,Suman Singhal,MD
Kaweblum,Jaime,DO
Lekht,Inna,MD
Lorenzo,Judith,MD
Rana,Mukti,MD
Romero,Luz Ydania,MD
Root,Edward R.,MD
Saunders,Kyauna Sharae,MD
Sopeju,Temilola Adedayo,MD
Stavrellis,Steve John,MD
Ukraincik,Miro,MD
Wong,Karen Clark,MD
Physical Medicine & Rehab
Kaweblum,Moises,MD
Psychiatry
Akhtar,Syeda Shahnaz,MD
Berger,Eric,MD
Cummins,Tiffany Ann,MD
Finston,Peggy Anne,MD

Physicians by Town and Medical Specialty

Lakewood (cont)
Psychiatry
- Juneja, Tony, MD
- Kharaz, Marina, MD
- Pisani, Janet, MD
- Rose, Moshe, MD
- Sandhu, Surinderjeet S., MD
Radiation Oncology
- Berkowitz, Stewart A., MD
- Marchese, Michael J., MD
Radiology
- Dhillon-Acosta, Raminder Kaur, DO
- Patel, Bharat K., MD
Surgery (General)
- Georges, Renee N., MD
- Molina, Carlos Guillermo, DO
Urology
- Bellingham, Charles E., MD
- Pandya, Kiritkumar M., MD
- Tomaszewski, Charles S., MD
Vascular Surgery
- Shamash, Felix S., MD

Lambertville
Family Med-Sports Medicine
- Chen, Victoria Sheen, MD
- Raleigh, Elizabeth Ann, DO
Family Medicine
- Barter, Cindy Monette, MD
- Burgos, Melissa, MD
- Eichman, Margaret J., MD
- Espinoza, Lisa C., MD
- Giangrante, Matthew E., MD
- Koorie, Elizabeth L., MD
- Lei, Michaela, DO
- Meyer, Monica Ann, MD
- Mooney, Kevin K., MD
- Russo, Frances Jenny, DO
- Russo, Steven, MD
- Schmitt, David J., MD
- Sokkar, Rita, DO
- Waters, John S., MD
Infectious Disease
- Moskovitz, Bruce L., MD
Ophthalmology
- Grutzmacher, June Edith, MD

Landing
Family Medicine
- Damico, Christopher R., DO
- Purcell, Joseph W., DO
- Shah, Shefali A., DO

Lanoka Harbor
Internal Medicine
- Fernando-Flores, Avelina M., MD
- Tauro, Victor, MD
Pediatrics
- Mehta, Sunita, MD

Laurel Springs
Family Medicine
- Eang, Rosanna, DO
Geriatrics
- Domanski, John D., MD

Laurence Harbor
Family Medicine
- Zelikson, Irina Yelyanovn, DO
Internal Medicine
- Lalcheta, Paresh, MD

Lawnside
Internal Medicine
- Young, William P., MD
Psychiatry
- Hewitt, James L., MD

Lawrence
Internal Medicine
- Klausner, Mark A., MD

Lawrence Township
Family Medicine
- Hanley, Daniel Lee Wilburn, MD

Lawrenceville
Addiction Medicine
- Baxter, Louis E., MD
Administration/Medical Mgt
- Ditullio, Anthony Joseph, MD
Allergy
- Mastrosimone, Angelo, MD
Allergy & Immunology
- Palangio, Kimberly Dawn, MD
Anatomic/Clinical Pathology
- Kuehn, Adam, MD
- Mechanic, Leslie D., MD
Cardiovascular Disease
- Moser, Robert L., MD
- Al-Bezem, Rim, MD
- Costanzo, William Edward, MD
- Drucker, David Wayne, MD
- Goldsmith, Steven Matthew, MD
- Heyrich, George Patrick, MD
- Hyman, Richard Louis, MD
- Karl, Justin Adam, MD
- Lebovitz, Philip Lewis, MD
- Rosvold, David Nelson, MD
- Rozengarten, Michael Jacob, MD
- Stern, Alan G., MD
- Venkatesulu, Sunder, MD
- Wolfson, Keith Richard, MD
- Zacks, Eran Sol, MD
Colon & Rectal Surgery
- Eisengart, Charles Andrew, MD
- Hardy, Howard III, MD
Critical Care Medicine
- Nolledo, Michael Teodoro, MD
Dermatology
- Hubert, Steven Lee, MD
- Kincaid, Leah Celia, MD
- Rajan, Jennifer Ray, MD
- Yi, Lusia Sang-suk, DO
Endocrinology
- Dadzie, Daphne D., MD
- Fresca, Diane Elizabeth, MD
- Shelmet, John J., MD
- Vergano, Sefton Cappi, MD
Family Med-Adult Medicine
- Stramandi, Danielle Nicole, MD
Family Medicine
- Barlis, Cara J., MD
- Chung, Y. C. Emily, MD
- Hector, Christina, DO
- Hussain, Saleha, MD
- Jarvis, Lori J., MD
- Laskarzewski, Radhika, MD
- Leonti, Vincent J., MD
- Levandowski, Richard, MD
- Levitt, Kimberly Anne, MD
- McGeever, Rose, DO
- Punj, Priti Narula, MD
- Rose, Abigail Lee, MD
- Santhanam, Shankar, MD
- Shaikh, Nasir Hussain A., MD
- Tsarouhas, Louis, MD
- Young, Jill F., DO
Gastroenterology
- Ahmad, Syed S., MD
- De Antonio, Joseph R., MD
- Lou, William, MD
- Merlo, Angela, MD
Hematology Oncology
- Kenney, Ellen N., MD
Internal Medicine
- Adler, Scott L., MD
- Borrus, Stephen W., MD
- Dash, Michael Roy, MD
- Desai, Bharat V., MD
- Friedland, Richard James, MD
- Goldberg, Paul E., MD
- Gomes, Eric Arvind, MD
- Hollander, Jason Michael, MD
- Jain, Madhu, MD
- Khan, Aliya W., MD
- Lee, Peter, MD
- Mathew, Saritha, MD
- Osias, Kimberly Beth, MD
- Shaffer, Brian L., MD
- Wasti, Naila H., MD
- Weinstein, Mark J., MD
- Werbel, Sarah A., MD
- Zathureczky, Izabella K., MD
Nephrology
- Friedman, Gary S., MD
Neurological Surgery
- Abud, Ariel F., MD
- Chiurco, Anthony A., MD
Neurology
- Alexeeva, Aissa Timofeyevna, MD
- DeLuca, Debra J., MD
- Gomez, Rene S., MD
- Kaiser, Paul K., MD
- Vergara, Manuel Salvador, MD
Obstetrics & Gynecology
- Bhattacharjee, Roopali, MD
- Burbella, Ronald E., MD
- Firdu, Tikikil, MD
- Funches, Judith Melton, MD
- Goyal, Shefali, MD
- Grant, Gwendolyn Hunter, DO
- Hall, Lanniece F., MD
- Hilsenrath, Robin Elaine, MD
- Leedom, Karen Ann, MD
- Loeb, Paul Norman, DO
- Melnikoff, Barbara, MD
- Mondestin, Myriam A. J., MD
- Pierce, Bruce R., MD
- Proctor, Asha K., MD
- Przybylko, Kira L., MD
- Romano, Carmen J., MD
- Safi, Farnaz, MD
- Sarma, Bani A., MD
- Small, Daniel Alan, MD
- Stanell, William P., MD
- Tashjian, Audrey Brigitta, MD
- Ung, Kenneth H., MD
- Warchaizer, Susan J., MD
Ophthalmology
- Chiang, Robert Kent, MD
- Ellis, Steven P., MD
- Ie, Darmakusuma, MD
- Lavrich, Judith Barbara, MD
- Lipkowitz, Jeffrey L., MD
- Mallen, Frederic J., MD
- Mullin, Guy S., MD
- Safran, Steven G., MD
- Shah, Angana Nayan, MD
- Shah, Chirag S., MD
- Shah, Kekul Bharat, MD
- Stein, Harmon Charles, MD
Orthopedic Surgery
- Accardi, Kimberly Lynn Z., MD
- Antonacci, Mark Darryl, MD
- Ast, Michael Paul, MD
- Betz, Randal Roberts, MD
- Bills, Thomas K., MD
- Codjoe, Paul Winfred, MD
- Cuddihy, Laury A., MD
- Eingorn, David S., MD
- Gokcen, Eric C., MD
- LaRocca, Sandro, MD
- Nolan, John P. Jr., MD
- Taitsman, James P., MD
Otolaryngology
- Boozan, James A., MD
- Lupa, Michael David, MD
- Patel, Rakesh Bhogilal, MD
- Shah, Chetan S., MD
Otolaryngology-Facial Plastic
- Undavia, Samir Suresh, MD
Pediatrics
- Farooq, Sadaf, MD
- Gittell, Amy, DO
- Halvorsen, Julie Beth, DO
- Jose, Jaison, DO
- Lilienfeld, Harris C., MD
- O'Dea, Carol Lynn H., MD
- Obleada, Maria C.P., MD
- Palsky, Glenn S., MD
- Saraiya, Neha, MD
- Shapiro, Eugene, MD
Physical Med & Rehab-Pain Med
- Patel, Rikin Jagdish, DO
Physical Med & Rehab-Sports Med
- Wenger, Peter Christopher, MD
Physical Medicine & Rehab
- Agri, Robyn F., MD
- Ali, Adil, MD
- Colarusso, Frank John Michael, DO
- Guillermety, Esperanza E., MD
- Kothari, Gautam Himanshu, DO
- McGuigan, Kevin, MD
- Terry, Charles M., MD
- Therattil, Maya Rose, MD
- Wiederholz, Matthias Heinz, MD
Plastic Surgery
- Smotrich, Gary A., MD
Psychiatry
- Diao, Carolina Efren, MD
- Karpf, Robin R., MD
- Orr, Andrew Philip, MD
- Sheaffer, Carol M., MD
Radiation Oncology
- Harvey, Arthur James, MD
- Simone, Charles B., MD
Reproductive Endocrinology
- Derman, Seth G., MD
Rheumatology
- Froncek, Michael Jude, MD
Spinal Surgery
- Tydings, John D., MD
Surgery (General)
- Alvarez, Enrique F., MD
Urgent Care
- Diamond, Shari E., DO
Urological Surgery
- Fingerman, Jarad Scott, DO
Urology
- Cohen, Michael Scott, MD
- Freid, Russell Marc, MD
- Karlin, Gary S., MD
- Trivedi, Deep B., MD

Lebanon
Family Medicine
- Collins, Reid T., MD
- Sacchieri, Theresa Ann, MD
Obstetrics & Gynecology
- Lewis, Sharol A., MD
- Rubin, Seth M., MD
Psychiatry
- Holbrook, David Vining, MD

Ledgewood
Interventional Cardiology
- Stein, Michael Alan, MD
Pediatrics
- Grossman, Leonard J., MD

Leesburg
Family Medicine
- Briglia, William J., DO
Internal Medicine
- Larue, Catherine, MD
Psychiatry
- Steinberg, Vitaly G., MD

Leonardo
Emergency Medicine
- Rogers, Patrick, DO

Leonia
Anesthesiology
- Ostrovskaya, Inna Dmytrievna, MD
Cardiovascular Disease
- Livelli, Frank D. Jr., MD
Infectious Disease
- Fratello, Laura F., MD
Internal Medicine
- Diakolios, Constantine E., MD
- Joo, Richard H., MD
- Su, Tze-Jung, MD
Orthopedic Surgery
- Green, Aron M., MD

Liberty Corner
Child & Adolescent Psychiatry
- Braver, Vanita, MD

Lincoln Park
Anesthesiology
- Louvier, Ambra, MD
Family Medicine
- De Mare, Patrick J., DO
Gastroenterology
- Mainero, Michael M., MD
Internal Medicine
- Corso, Martin J., MD
- Jindal, Jagdish R., MD
Orthopedic Surgery
- Kavanagh, Mark Lawrence, MD
Pediatrics
- Cross, Gershwin A., MD
Pulmonary Disease
- O'Donnell, Timothy S., DO

Lincroft
Family Medicine
- DePietro, Joseph Anthony, MD
Internal Medicine
- Ibrahim, Adel, MD
Obstetrics & Gynecology
- Generelli, Patricia Ann, MD
- Moore, Susan Salzberg, MD
Psychiatry
- El Rehim, Mohsen Sayed Abd, MD

Linden
Dermatology
- McCormack, Patricia Coppola, MD
Family Medicine
- Lukenda, Kevin, DO
- Schulman, Joseph M., DO
- Sherif, Ajfar, MD
- Sundaram, Ashany, MD

General Practice
Reich-Sobel,Debra Gail,DO
Geriatrics
Mehta,Palak Pranav,MD
Hand Surgery
Mackessy,Richard P.,MD
Internal Medicine
Allen,Mureen Cressida,MD
Bezozo,Richard Craig,MD
Borowski,Walter J.,MD
Bronikowski,John Anthony,DO
Czyzewski,Ewa,MD
Diaz,Julio E.,MD
Kibilska Borowski,Jolanta M.,MD
Lao,Carlos S.,MD
Nowak,Darius Zbigniew,MD
Patel,Narendra D.,MD
Randhawa,Preet Mohan Singh,MD
Remolina,Carlos,MD
Rubinstein,Allen Bernard,DO
Saif,Shazia,MD
Shah,Praful M.,MD
Wawrzyniak,Zygmunt T.,MD
Weitzman,Robert H.,MD
Obstetrics & Gynecology
Bodnar,Aleksander J.,MD
Ophthalmology
Kotch,Michael J.,MD
Orthopedic Surgery
Ghobrial,Mark Nashaat,DO
Kline,John A.,MD
Pedowitz,Walter J.,MD
Ropiak,Christopher Robert,MD
Orthopedics
Rojer,David Eli,MD
Pediatric Cardiology
Alenick,D. Scott,MD
Pediatrics
Grzybowski,Jacek,MD
Jez,Mieczyslaw Z.,MD
Physical Med & Rehab-Pain Med
Sutain,Nathaniel,MD
Physical Medicine & Rehab
Betesh,Naomi Gold,DO
Jimenez,Joseph C.,MD
Plastic Surgery
Alkon,Joseph David,MD
Psychiatry
Makhija,Vasudev N.,MD
Ndukwe,Nwayieze Chisara,MD

Lindenwold
Anesthesiology
Copeland,Marcia A.,MD
Gupta,Anita,DO
Family Medicine
Neidorf,David L.,MD
Obstetrics & Gynecology
Cannon,Donald R.,MD
Gildiner,Lennard R.,MD
Klein,Edward M.,MD
Ruffin,Judith S.,MD

Linwood
Anesthesiology
Barbella,Joseph D.,DO
Dermatology
Connolly,Coyle S.,DO
Hong,Joseph Johnson,MD
Endocrinology
Kleiber,Maria A.,MD
Family Medicine
Kader,Richard A.,DO
Pernice,Mark J.,DO
Gastroenterology
Maleki,Dordaneh,MD
Renny,Andrew,MD
General Practice
Abramowitz,Jodi S.,DO
Gynecology
Hyett,Marvin R.,MD
Infectious Disease
Papastamelos,Athanasios G.,DO
Internal Medicine
Amin,Anila P.,MD
Gove,Ronald C.,MD
Gualtieri,Sara Liliana,MD
Parikh,Nikhil S.,MD
Parikh,Pujan N.,MD
Ponnappan,Gita S.,MD
Sagransky,David M.,MD
Singh,Sunil K.,MD

Neurological Surgery
Delasotta,Fernando J.,MD
Lowe,James G.,MD
Ophthalmology
Nguyen,Truc H.,MD
Remer,Paul,MD
Uretsky,Stephen H.,MD
Orthopedic Surgery
Cristini,John A.,MD
Zerbo,Joseph R.,DO
Otolaryngology
Feldman,Marc D.,MD
Orquiza,Clodualdo S. III,MD
Siliunas,Vytas B.,DO
Wagle,Priya Jennifer,MD
Pain Medicine
Petersohn,Jeffrey D.,MD
Pediatrics
Bonaker,Laura J.,MD
Physical Medicine & Rehab
Conover,Melissa,MD
Graziani,Virginia,MD
Jarillo,Maria Roca Cami,MD
Kull,Elizabeth J.,MD
Ludwig,David Aaron,MD
Sturr,Marianne,DO
Plastic Surgery
Rayfield,David Lee,MD
Psychiatry
Bloch,Andrea J.,DO
Chazin,Norman S.,MD
Mackuse,Donna M.,DO
Ranieri,William F.,DO
Sacher,S. Mark,DO
Surgery (General)
Penso,Desiderio S.,MD
Waldor,Philip Arthur,MD

Little Egg Harbor
Family Medicine
Berlin,William H.,DO
Gandhi,Dhiren K.,MD
Glenn,William B.,DO
Mastro,Caroline Briana,MD
Medenilla,Rosenio Jr.,MD
Tracy,Toby William,DO
Internal Medicine
Rao,Anupama J.,MD
Pediatrics
Humphreys,Erika,MD
Lee,Gene Chiu,MD

Little Falls
Allergy
Ahuja,Kishore Kanayalal,MD
Dermatology
Whitworth,Jeffrey Michael,MD
Family Medicine
Billig,Janelle Elisabeth,MD
Lentine,Nancy,DO
Mangra,Chandra,MD
Rae,Susan,MD
Yussaf,Shiraz,MD
Gastroenterology
Holt,Stephen,MD
Kosc,Gary J.,MD
Martino,Michael J.,MD
Pavlou,George Nicholas,MD
Shami,Joseph G.,MD
Geriatrics
Bellardini,Angelo G.,MD
Internal Medicine
Al Rabi,Kamal H.,MD
Bauer,Francis Douglas,MD
Chennapragada,Kausalya,MD
Coscia,Sylvia,MD
Dahhan,Mohamed Zakaria,MD
Farnese,Jeffrey Jason,MD
Farnese,Joseph T.,MD
Fazio,Ignazio Jr.,MD
Laneve,Anthony Jr.,MD
Obstetrics & Gynecology
Obaid,Sana Hamdan,MD
Orthopedic Surgery
Di Paolo,Peter F.,MD
Pediatrics
Pepe,Gary V.,MD
Razzak,Mannan,MD
Razzak,Nadia Mohsin,MD
Psychiatry
Czartorysky,Bohdan Nicholas,MD

Pulmonary Disease
Vazir,Amanullah A.,MD
Vascular & Intrvntnal Radiology
Koh,Elsie,MD

Little Ferry
Family Medicine
Tancer,Richard B.,DO
Internal Medicine
Meo,Francis W.,MD
Physical Medicine & Rehab
Karcnik,Margaret A.,DO

Little Silver
Allergy
Dobken,Jeffrey Hall,MD
Zecca,Tina Concetta,DO
Dermatology
Grossman,Kenneth A.,MD
Diagnostic Radiology
DeVincenzo,Raven,MD
Doss,Peter S.,MD
Rittweger,Edward S.,MD
Shah,Pranav N.,MD
Zito,Frederick J.,MD
Endocrinology
Malik,Ritu,MD
Family Medicine
Auriemma,John A.,DO
Mehra,Neeraj,MD
Gastroenterology
Eichel,Richard L.,MD
Hematology
Walsh,Christina M.,MD
Hematology Oncology
Windsor,Stephen J.,MD
Internal Medicine
Arora,Deepinder Kaur,MD
Devito,Marc J.,MD
Gourkanti,Rao S.,MD
Greenberg,Susan Nancy,MD
LaNatra,Nicole,MD
Laughinghouse,Kenneth,MD
Ponti,Tatyana,MD
Scher,Richard M.,DO
Scotti,Angelo T.,MD
Medical Oncology
Fitzgerald,Denis B.,MD
Neurological Radiology
O'Connor,Douglas S.,MD
Obstetrics & Gynecology
Bohnert,Katherine Ann,DO
Giovine,Anthony P.,MD
Hammond,Kelly C.,MD
Jacoby,Michelle P.,MD
Karoly,Michael D.,MD
Kaskiw,Eugene H.,MD
Kaufman,William N.,DO
Mason-Cederberg,Lauren,MD
Rosenzweig,Talia S.,MD
Soussan,Elie R.,MD
Sun,Andrew N.,MD
Tsong,Shirley W.,MD
Wiser-Estin,Mindy Ellen,MD
Ophthalmology
Trikha,Rupan,MD
Uram,Martin,MD
Orthopedic Surgery
Lopez,David Vincent,MD
Otolaryngology
Sullivan,Timothy Patrick,MD
Pediatrics
Mehra,Deepti,MD
Plastic Surgery
Hetzler,Peter T.,MD
Zaccaria,Alan,MD
Psychiatry
Bhatiya,Savji L.,MD
Radiology
Wirtshafter,David Glenn,MD
Wold,Robert E.,MD
Surgical Critical Care
Garcia-Perez,Felix A.,MD

Livingston
Adolescent Medicine
Goldenring,Debra Semel,MD
Oana,Dan C.,MD
Semel,William J.,MD
Allergy
Goodman,Alan Jay,MD
Weiss,Steven Jay,MD

Physicians by Town and Medical Specialty

Anatomic Pathology
Feng,Bo,MD
Anatomic/Clinical Pathology
Baptist,Selwyn J.,MD
Binsol,Ricardo Q.,MD
Buckley,Tinera Mcnair,MD
Dardik,Michael,MD
Kim,Dae U.,MD
Kintiroglou,Marietta,MD
Mahmood,Ashhad,MD
Ongcapin,Emelie H.,MD
Pulinthanathu,Rajiv R.,MD
Stueben,Benjamin L.,MD
Tortora,Matthew J.,MD
Anesthesiology
Dumbroff,Steven A.,MD
Fan,Foun-Chung,MD
Fox,Jerry C.,MD
Goldstein,Elisabeth Rachel,MD
Gourishankar,Ruplanaik,MD
Hurley,Kathleen Lenore,MD
Ioffe,Michail,MD
Kalinine,Viatcheslav,MD
Klebba,Kevin Edmund,MD
Kulkarni,Mohan H.,MD
Leaf,Daniel Craig,MD
Mazur,Wieslaw L.,MD
McKeon,John J.,MD
Myneni,Neelima,MD
O'Mahony,Christopher James,MD
Pak,Hang R.,DO
Pamaar,Cristina G.,MD
Patankar,Srikanth S.,MD
Patel,Nimesh R.,MD
Pitera,Richard Jr.,MD
Qian,Qiubing,MD
Rafizadeh,Mehrad,MD
Ramundo,Giovanni B.,MD
Reichard,Peter Seth,MD
Rimal,Jyotsna,MD
Rodriguez,Emmanuel,MD
Sattari,Rouzbeh,MD
Shanker,Soma,MD
Tewfik,George L.,MD
Tompkins,Marianne J.,DO
Trespicio,Rogelio T.,MD
Vallee,Michael F.,DO
Vaskul,Roksolana,MD
Zulueta,Erica,DO
Anesthesiology: Critical Care
Seedhom,Magdi Ebrahim,MD
Anesthesiology: Pain Medicine
Vogel,Martin Joseph,MD
Cardiovascular Disease
Anton,John,MD
Bahler,Alan S.,MD
Demidowich,George,MD
Fernandes,John,MD
Gressianu,Monica Terezia,MD
Kaluski,Edo,MD
Kashnikow,Constantine,MD
Woroch,Bohdar O.,MD
Child & Adolescent Psychiatry
Bartky,Eric Jay,MD
Jacque,Celeste A.,MD
Kycia,Lan Ing,MD
Lipman,Ted,MD
Rudominer,Howard S.,MD
Child (Pediatric) Neurology
Kubichek,Marilyn Ann,MD
Clinical Neurophysiology
Goldberg,Rina Freida,MD
Rodriguez,Andy,MD
Colon & Rectal Surgery
Holzman,Kevin Jay,MD
Huang,Renee,MD
Critical Care Medicine
Marano,Michael A.,MD
Rezai,Fariborz,MD
Cytopathology
Su,Mu,MD
Dermatology
Bronsnick,Tara A.,MD
Citron,Cheryl S.,MD
Liftin,Alan J.,MD
Nervi,Stephen James,MD
Speaker,Olenka Matkiwsky,DO
Dermatology: Dermatopathology
Sarkissian,Naver A.,MD

Livingston (cont)

Diagnostic Radiology
- Bhatnagar, Swati Varma, MD
- Carpenter, Bruce W., MD
- Daigle, Megan Elizabeth, MD
- Dembner, Alan G., MD
- Dunaway, David Ryan, MD
- Fertakos, Roy J., MD
- Garten, Alan J., MD
- Giobbe, Raphael C., MD
- Huang, Tammy, MD
- Karlson, Karen B., MD
- Kotch, Hannah Rapaport, MD
- Kothari, Neha A., MD
- Laible, Mark S., MD
- McCarthy, Cornelius Stephen, MD
- Mehta, Avani Shripal, MD
- Polini, Nicole Maria, MD
- Sharo, Ronald J., MD
- Shoor, Priya, MD
- Slazak, Katherine L., MD
- Sperling, Danny S., MD
- Stulbach, Harry Bruce, MD

Emergency Medicine
- Birnbaum, Glenn Alan, MD
- Eagan, Michael Patrick, MD
- Fink, Glenn D., MD
- Gupta, Neena, MD
- Handler, Eric Todd, DO
- Kaplan, Emily A., MD
- Kuhlmann, Sarah Elizabeth, MD
- Lacher, Britt Ilene, MD
- McEnrue, James A., MD
- Miller, Ivan Thomas, MD
- Mujic, Lejla, MD
- Rentala, Manju, MD
- Reyman, Lynn D., MD
- Rokosz, Gregory J., DO
- Rosenblat, Yoav, MD
- Salo, David F., MD
- Sanchez, Daniel Antonio, MD
- Schreiber, Marie F., DO
- Shapiro, Marion D., DO
- Welber, Mark R., DO
- Winograd, Jonathan Isaac, DO

Endocrinology
- Boradia, Chirag N., DO
- Dower, Samuel M., MD
- Garbowit, David L., MD
- Gewirtz, George P., MD
- Jacob, Tess, MD
- Luckey, Marjorie M., MD
- Nambi, Sridhar S., MD
- Silverman, Mitchell S., MD
- Vlad, Luigina D., MD

Family Medicine
- Boorujy, Dean P., DO
- Hussain, Sarah, MD
- Riaz, Danish, MD
- Stevens, Susan H., MD

Gastroenterology
- Goldstein, Debra R., MD
- Imbesi, John J., MD
- Shieh, Frederick, MD

General Practice
- Haghdoost, Mohammad, MD

Geriatric Psychiatry
- Anekstein, Carol B., MD

Geriatrics
- Arunachalam, Muthu R., MD

Hematology
- Botti, Anthony C., MD
- Conde, Miguel A., MD
- Zauber, Neil P., MD

Hematology Oncology
- Brown, Andrew Bennett, MD
- Grossman, Israel Robert, MD
- Rao, Parth Rajeshkumar, MD
- Wildman, Joseph M., MD

Infectious Disease
- Chiang, Tom Shou, MD
- Diamond, Gigi R., MD
- Georgescu, Anca D., MD
- Kokkola-Korpela, Marjut H., MD
- Lin, Janet C., MD
- Sheth, Arpita A., MD
- Tsveniashvili, Liya V., MD

Internal Med-Sports Medicine
- Kelly, Michael, DO

Internal Medicine
- Abraham, Maninder Arneja, MD
- Adamoli, Donna Janine, MD
- Advani, Sonoo Kishu, MD
- Algazy, Jeffrey Ian, MD
- Allagadda, Bharathi R., MD
- Anton, Joseph G., MD
- Bahler, Emily Susan, DO
- Braunstein, Scott N., MD
- Carlino, Anthony, MD
- Cervone, Joseph Stephen III, MD
- Citron, Barry S., MD
- Danieu, Linda A., MD
- DeFusco, Kenneth T., MD
- Elango, Adhithaselvi K., MD
- Faizan, Anila, MD
- Goldberg, Ryan J., MD
- Gutkin, Michael, MD
- Henriquez, Karina A., MD
- Ippolito, Tobi, MD
- Kaufman, Lee D., MD
- Kazmi, Ahsan Mahmood, MD
- Kowalski, Albert A., MD
- Kramer, Isaac, MD
- Kulkarni, Pratibha A., MD
- Leitner, Stuart P., MD
- Maida, Emanuel M., MD
- Murphy, Kim, MD
- Nadel, Lester, MD
- Nanduri, Visala Venkata, MD
- Patel, Anup Magan, MD
- Pentyala, Madhavi, MD
- Peos, Jennifer Renee, MD
- Puglisi, Gina Grace, MD
- Ravulapati, Sravanthi, MD
- Rommer, James A., MD
- Sareen, Ruchi, MD
- Scoppetuolo, Michael Jr., MD
- Sethi, Ripka, MD
- Shahinian, Toros S., MD
- Sidler, Bonnie Beryl, MD
- Simpkins, Nancy M., MD
- Sipzner, Robert J., MD
- Sivendra, Shan, MD
- Thiruwilwamala, Parvathy S., MD
- Trespalacios, Vanessa Nadia, MD
- Wang, Ai-Lan, MD
- Weng, Francis Liu, MD
- Yang, Lihua, MD
- Yodice, Paul Carmine, MD
- Youssef-Bessler, Manal Farouk, MD

Maternal & Fetal Medicine
- Kasdaglis, Tania Luna, MD
- Smith, Leon G. Jr., MD
- Warren, Wendy B., MD
- Wolf, Edward J., MD

Medical Oncology
- Litvak, Anna Maria, MD
- Michaelson, Richard A., MD

Neonatal-Perinatal Medicine
- Ko, So Hun, MD
- Lee, Hyejin Robin, MD
- Oana Soni, Agnes, MD
- Ruben, Sandhya, MD
- Santo Domingo, Jose E., MD
- Tien, Huey-Chung, MD
- Vangvanichyakorn, Kamtorn, MD

Nephrology
- Dhillon, Navdeep, MD
- Klein, Eileen C., MD
- Kotla, Revathi, MD
- Pritsiolas, James Michael, MD
- Tibaldi, Kim Nguyen, MD

Neurological Surgery
- Anderson, Richard C., MD
- Couch, Jonathan Darrell, DO
- Gigante, Paul R., MD
- Gilman, Arthur Michael, MD
- Hubschmann, Otakar R., MD
- Rotoli, Giorgio, DO

Neurology
- Bhawsar, Nilaya Babu, DO
- Devinsky, Orrin, MD
- Geller, Eric Bernard, MD
- Nadkarni, Mangala A., MD
- Natanzon, Calvin, MD
- Sobelman, Joseph S., MD
- Widdess-Walsh, Peter Patrick, MD
- Zhang, Yan Chun, MD

Nuclear Diagnostic Radiology
- Viggiano, Joseph T., MD

Nuclear Medicine
- Bedigian, Martin Peter, MD

Lutzker, Letty Goodman, MD

Obstetrics & Gynecology
- Abella, Tara M., MD
- Bonamo, John F., MD
- Bridges, Yvette A., MD
- Cekleniak, Natalie A., MD
- Cohen, Theodore, MD
- DiSabatino, Daniel, DO
- Dziadosz, Margaret, MD
- Fain, Richard A., MD
- Hessler, Sarah Catherine, MD
- Howard, L. Deanna, MD
- Keegan, Debbra Ames, MD
- Keiser, Oren S., MD
- Kindzierski, John A., MD
- Klachko, Daria A., MD
- Koch, Robert K., MD
- Mansuria, Shetal M., MD
- McArthur, Marilyn D., MD
- Miller, Richard Charles, MD
- O'Brien, Jonathan Edward, MD
- Petillo, Tina M., DO
- Quartell, Anthony C., MD
- Rachlin, Adrianne, MD
- Segal, Jeffrey Loren, MD
- Somers, Joann, MD
- Tam, Tiffanie, MD
- Terrone, Dom A., MD
- Youngren, Sonya Jitendra, MD

Occupational Medicine
- Bachman, Joyce Adele, MD
- Fallon, Jill C., MD

Oncological Surgery
- Langan, Russell, MD

Oncology
- Wagman, Raquel Tamara, MD

Ophthalmology
- Cohen, Amir, MD
- Cohen, Steven B., MD
- Decker, Edward Bruce, MD
- Harris, Michael, MD
- Kanter, Eric D., MD
- Kronengold, Charles J., MD
- Marano, Matthew Jr., MD
- Miller, Andrew Ian, MD
- Nussbaum, Peter, MD
- Rodriguez, Natalia Maria, MD

Orthopedic Surgery
- Cheema, Humayun Mahmood, MD
- Egan, Kevin J., MD
- Kopacz, Kenneth J., MD
- Leeds, Harold C., MD
- Rizio, Louis III, MD
- Zarro, Christopher M., MD

Other Specialty
- Blackwood, Margaret Michele, MD
- Brener, Bruce J., MD

Otolaryngology
- Lee, Bryant B., MD
- Lee, Derek Sai-Wah, MD

Otolaryngology-Facial Plastic
- Paraiso, Reynaldo S., DO

Pain Medicine
- Bajor-Dattilo, Ewa Beata, MD

Pathology
- Deshpande, Jyoti M., MD
- Redondo, Teresita Cuyegkeng, MD

Pediatric Anesthesia
- Chen, Guo Ming, MD

Pediatric Cardiology
- LaCorte, Jared C., MD

Pediatric Critical Care
- Castello, Frank V., MD
- Davis, Alan L., MD

Pediatric Endocrinology
- Anhalt, Henry, DO
- Sivitz, Jennifer Nicole, MD

Pediatric Gastroenterology
- Ton, Mimi Nu, MD

Pediatric Infectious Diseases
- Shah, Falguni Samir, MD

Pediatric Ophthalmology
- Lambert, Amy L., MD

Pediatric Orthopedics
- Tareco, Jennifer M., MD

Pediatric Pulmonology
- Cohen, Barry Alan, MD

Pediatrics
- Avallone, Jennifer Mary, DO
- Baldomero, Anita C., MD
- Cai-Luo, Bonney Danhua, MD
- Chua Eoan, Pearl Davie, MD
- Dienna, Erik, MD
- Glick, Sarah Rachel, MD
- Goyal, Vinod K., MD
- Kumta, Jayshree N., MD
- Lander, Richard, MD
- Liptsyn, Tatyana, MD
- Magnus Miller, Leslie, MD
- Margolin, Susan K., MD
- Maxym, Maya, MD
- O'Driscoll, Margaret Ann, MD
- Pang, James, MD
- Patel, Roshni Vinu, MD
- Ramanadham, Aruna R., MD
- Roberti, Maria Isabel, MD
- Salyer, Robert Harold, DO
- Sanchez Konel, Maria E., MD
- Schwartz, Fredric Ira, MD
- Setya, Shilpy, MD
- Sjovall, William J. Jr., DO
- Vaziriani, Minal, MD
- Wiener, Jaclyn Faye, DO
- Yeh, Timothy Stephen, MD
- Zaldivar, Marjel L., DO

Physical Medicine & Rehab
- Bid, Champa V., MD
- Chowdhrey, Mehar N., MD
- Davidson, Stacy, MD
- Findley, Thomas Wagner Jr., MD
- Francis, Kathleen D., MD
- Shumko, John Zachary, MD
- Wroblewski, Henry M., MD

Plastic & Reconstructive Srgy
- Cooperman, Ross D., MD

Plastic Surgery
- Fodero, Joseph Peter, MD
- Rothenberg, Bennett C., MD

Psychiatry
- Cantillon, Marc, MD
- Fahim, Farheen, MD
- Feingold, Katherine Linda, MD
- Hindin, Lee Eban, MD
- Iqbal-Hussain, Farida, MD
- Robbins, Lisa Ilene, MD
- Sastry, Gayathri, MD
- Zeman, David, MD
- Zornitzer, Michael R., MD

Pulmonary Disease
- Greenberg, Martin J., MD
- Petrowsky, Deborah, MD

Radiation Oncology
- Grann, Alison, MD

Radiology
- Kalisher, Lester, MD
- Sanders, Linda M., MD
- Sherman, Joyce, MD
- Wilson, David A., MD
- Zurlo, John V., MD

Rheumatology
- Chuzhin, Yelena, MD
- Ritter, Jill M., MD

Sports Medicine
- Cooper, Alan Edward, MD

Surgery (General)
- Andrei, Valeriu E., MD
- Brown, Melanie Antonietta, MD
- Chargualaf, Lisa Marie, MD
- Geffner, Stuart R., MD
- Houng, Abraham Pohan, MD
- Lemasters, Patrick Evan, MD
- Majid, Saniea Fatima, MD
- Paragi, Prakash Ramaiah, MD
- Paul, Subroto, MD
- Petrone, Sylvia J., MD
- Santoro, Elissa J., MD
- Schaefer, Sarah Stuart, MD
- Smith, Franz Omar Desric, MD
- Tutela, John Paul, MD
- Weiswasser, Jonathan M., MD

Surgical Critical Care
- Lee, Robin Ann, MD
- Mansour, Esber Hani, MD

Therapeutic Radiology
- Goodman, Robert Leon, MD

Thoracic Surgery
- Reed, Mark K., MD

Transplant Surgery & Medicine
- Aitchison, Samantha H., MD
- Sankary, Howard N., MD
- Sun, Harry, MD

Loch Arbour
Urology
Katz, Jeffrey I., MD
Walsh, Rhonda M., MD
Vascular & Intrvntnal Radiology
Richmond, John Steven, MD
Vascular Surgery
Fletcher, H. Stephen, MD

Loch Arbour
Sports Medicine
Incremona, Brian R., MD

Lodi
Cardiovascular Disease
Thamman, Vijay K., MD

Critical Care Medicine
Santomauro, Emanuele A., MD
Family Medicine
Kulesza-Galvez, Theodora, MD
Lowenstein, Michael Aaron, DO
Gastroenterology
Focazio, William John, MD
Internal Medicine
Andreescu, Aurora C., MD
Carafa, Ciro J., MD
Mecca, Mauro A., MD
Pande, Chandana, MD
Raacke, Lisa Marie, MD
Ramos, Maria A., MD
Rigolosi, Ronald A., MD
Thamman, Prem, MD
Obstetrics & Gynecology
Dutta, Kamal K., MD
Pulmonary Disease
Villa, John J., DO

Logan Township
Cardiovascular Disease
Pahlow, Brian J., DO
Dermatology
Bright, Nicole Jasmyn, DO
Internal Medicine
Prabhakar, Avinash, MD
Pediatrics
Cafone, Michael D., DO

Long Branch
Anatomic/Clinical Pathology
Kang, Yong, MD
Loo, Abraham, MD
Szallasi, Arpad, MD
Zhong, Hua, MD
Zinterhofer, Louis J., MD
Anesthesiology
Anisetti, Vimlesh K., MD
Belsh, Yitzhak, MD
Du, Bing, MD
Elango, Sitalakshmi, MD
Eraky, Waheed K., MD
Fisher, Scott Robert, MD
Flashburg, Michael H., MD
Friedman, Susan R., MD
Gomez, Jose F., MD
Greaves, Keiron W., MD
Greenberg, Eric N., MD
Johnson, Judith Ann, MD
Klein, Matthew Seth, MD
Kramer, David C., MD
Molbegott, Debra J., DO
Molbegott, Lester P., MD
Nosker, Geoffrey S., MD
Omotoso, Babatunji Omolagba, MD
Para, Vijaya L., MD
Patel, Nilesh J., MD
Shah, Lopa Suryakant, MD
Spruell, Joshua Lyn, MD
Zlotnick, Matthew Phillip, MD
Anesthesiology: Pain Medicine
Tran, Dan-Thuy V., MD
Cardiovascular Disease
Checton, John B., MD
Master, Julie, DO
Child & Adolescent Psychiatry
Pogran, Jessica Rose, DO
Dermatology
Cohen, Benjamin, MD
Katz, Stanley Norman, MD
Diagnostic Radiology
Barone, Cynthia A., DO
Hussain, Syed, MD
Keedy, Jennifer, MD
Kwak, Andrew, MD
Louie, Gina Lin, MD
Pardes, Jorge Gustavo, MD
Staiger, Melinda J., MD
Talangbayan, Leizle E., MD
Wiggins, Ernest Flowers III, MD
Won, Bokran, MD
Emergency Medicine
Campanella, Lisa Marie, MD
Downs, William R. Jr., DO
Gilman, Elizabeth Ann, MD
Hanlon, Catherine A., MD
Kanamori, Hiromi, MD
McCabe-Bageac, Mary A., MD
Minetti, John J., MD
O'Keefe, Mary Clare, MD
Perry, Kurt A., MD
Rehr, Eric L., MD
Waxler, Jennifer L., DO
Endocrinology
Luria, Martin J., MD
Forensic Psychiatry
Bortnichak, Paula M., MD
Geriatric Psychiatry
Fang, Margaret Wu, MD
Rubin, Kenneth J., MD
Geriatrics
Goldberg, Shira, MD
Weinberg, Ronald M., MD
Zwerin, Glenn M., MD
Hematology
Braslavsky, Gregory, MD
Hospitalist
Bodala, Durga Rani, MD
Mandel, Rekha J., MD
Infectious Disease
Eng, Margaret Hom, MD
Hameed, Nida, MD
Montana, Barbara E., MD
Internal Medicine
Angi, Priya, MD
Asthana, Jyothi, MD
Brawer, Arthur E., MD
Burkett, Eric Nelson, MD
Cotov, Judith A., MD
Dalton, John Boehmer, MD
Du, Doantrang Thi, MD
Ganne, Sudha, MD
Ghotb, Sara, MD
Gomez, Johnson Lim, MD
Granet, Kenneth M., MD
Hershkowitz, Robert P., MD
Israel, Jessica Leigh, MD
Jain, Rishabh Kumar, MD
Kadiyam, Sandhya, MD
Lederman, Jeffrey Craig, DO
Mandadi, Pranathi R., MD
Mark, Benjamin, MD
Mercadante, Zorica J., MD
Paladugu, Madhu Babu, MD
Rajaraman, Ravindran T., MD
Rivera, Carlos G., MD
Ross, Douglas A., MD
Rubino, Barry P., MD
Shah, Shilpan H., MD
Shoner, Lawrence Gene, MD
Spellman, Charles L., DO
Vilenskaya, Irina, MD
Wreiole, August L., DO
Maternal & Fetal Medicine
Wallace, David Morrow, MD
Neonatal-Perinatal Medicine
Alemany, Carlos A., MD
McNab, Theresa Challender, MD
Rekedal, Kirby D., MD
Obstetrics & Gynecology
Gonzalez, David Jr., MD
Graebe, Robert A., MD
Joshi, Raksha, MD
Khalil, Rahab M., MD
Kugay, Natalya P., MD
Magherini Rothe, Suzanne A., MD
Malik, Nisha, MD
Nath, Carl Anthony, MD
Smithson, Sarah, MD
Vaclavik, John Philip Charles, MD
Ophthalmology
Bontempo, Carl Peter, MD
Fegan, Robert James, MD
Goldberg, Daniel B., MD
Kristan, Ronald W., MD
Orthopedic Surgery
Fechisin, Joel Patrick, MD
Paragioudakis, Steve J., MD
Pain Medicine-Interventional
Johnson, Andrew, DO
Pediatric Critical Care
Misra, Amit C., MD
Pediatric Emergency Medicine
Jacome-Bohorquez, Gloria C., MD
Pediatric Endocrinology
Schwartz, Malcolm S., DO
Pediatric Gastroenterology
Rakitt, Tina Susanne, MD
Pediatric Infectious Diseases
Verma, Renuka, MD

Pediatric Pathology
Shertz, Wendy T., MD
Pediatric Pulmonology
Sembrano, Eduardo U. Jr., MD
Zanni, Robert L., MD
Pediatric Surgery
Cohen, Ian Thomas, MD
Pediatrics
Attardi, Diane Martha, MD
Brunetto, Jacqueline M., MD
Bshesh, Khaled Khalifa, MD
Fisher, Margaret Catharine, MD
Habib, Thomas G., MD
Hall, Dahlia Annmarie, MD
Hudome, Susan M., MD
Kale, Meera V., MD
Kapoor, Amee Patel, DO
Khalil, Erum, MD
Maghsood, Shabnam, MD
Phillips, Keren Amy, MD
Reutter, Richard A., MD
Romald, Jermine Harriet, MD
Scerbo, Jessica, MD
Sell, Neelam K., MD
Sleavin, Harold J., MD
Teitelbaum, Jonathan Evan, MD
Plastic & Reconstructive Srgy
Taylor, John M., MD
Psychiatry
Fardman, Emiliya, MD
Geller, Matthew Al, MD
Kiselev, Marianna L., MD
Memon, Yasmeen Khalique, MD
Schiff, Matthew M., MD
Theccanat, Stephen M., MD
Tintorer, Christine C., MD
Psychiatry&Nrolgy-Special Qual
Fisch, Shirley B.D., MD
Pulmonary Disease
Davis, George C., MD
Radiation Oncology
Sim, Sang Eui, MD
Weiss, Mitchell F., MD
Radiology
McDonald, David William, MD
Smuro, Daniel J., MD
Stein, Irving H., DO
Surgery (General)
Cummings, Kenneth B., MD
Ginalis, Ernest M., MD
Goldfarb, Michael A., MD
Roros, James Gus, MD
Thoracic Surgery
Skylizard, Loki, MD
Urogynecology
Greco, Sandra Jeanne, MD
Vascular & Intrvntnal Radiology
Schiff, Robert Michael, MD
Vascular Surgery
Constantinopoulos, George S., MD

Long Valley
Internal Medicine
Marino, Mark T., MD
Muenzen, Christopher P., MD
Pediatrics
Sorvino, Noel R., MD

Lumberton
Anesthesiology
Balzer, Frederick J., MD
Pollak, Kevin Henry, MD
Child & Adolescent Psychiatry
Stein, Lynne H., MD
Colon & Rectal Surgery
Hughes, Charles R., MD
Family Medicine
Buck, Murray D., DO
Campagnolo, Mary F., MD
Chatyrka, George O., DO
Daub, Horatio Guy, MD
Ibay, Annamarie D., MD
Jain Bhalodia, Sapna, DO
Kastenberg, Charles A., DO
Kolesk, Stephen J., MD
Naticchia, Jennifer M., MD
Rubenstein, Jennifer, MD
Scappaticci, John Jr., DO
Van Kooy, Mark A., MD
Gastroenterology
Khanijow, Vikresh, MD
Kutscher, Jeffrey J., MD
Lahoti, Mayank, DO
Leonard, Maurice D., MD
Sheth, Nidhir Ras, MD
Taub, William H., MD
deLacy, Lee M., MD
Gynecology
Chodos, Wesley S., DO
Internal Medicine
Awsare, Monica B., MD
Peng, Brian, DO
Rai-Patel, Jitha, MD
Neurology
Kachroo, Arun, MD
Keller, Seth Martin, MD
Mathur, Mayank, MD
Orwitz, Jonathan Ira, MD
Thomas, Carole E., MD
Obstetrics & Gynecology
Crawford-Meadows, Robin A., MD
Dalton, Laura J., DO
Oncological Surgery
Miller, Eric Jay, MD
Pediatrics
Bell, Denise Marie, MD
Kaighn, Karen Chicalo, MD
King, Richard A., MD
Labroli, Melissa D., MD
O'Donnell, Thomas P., MD
Requa, Lindsay Ann, DO
Wechsler, Marius A., MD
Phlebology
Rough, William Alexander Jr., MD
Plastic Surgery
Puskas, Roy, MD
Surgery (General)
Boynton, Christopher J., MD

Lyndhurst
Cardiovascular Disease
Conroy, Daniel Jr., MD
Cubero, John G., MD
Critical Care Medicine
Vossough, Soheila, MD
Endocrinology
Strizhevsky, Marina A., DO
Family Medicine
Aghabi, Hanna Najib, MD
Castelluber, Gisele B V M, MD
Faugno, Gerard L., MD
General Practice
Schmalz, William Francis Jr., MD
Geriatrics
James, Todd C., MD
Kovaleva, Alexandra, MD
Internal Medicine
Ambrosio, George Joseph, MD
Hagler, Rhonda A., MD
Hazzah, Marwa Mohamed, MD
Hoskin, Jane F., MD
Kricko, Michael J., DO
Losos, Roland Jerzy, MD
Park, Byong K., MD
Rose, Henry J., MD
Obstetrics & Gynecology
Choi, Jay Joonhyuk, MD
Ophthalmology
DeLuca, Joseph A., MD
Pediatrics
Catalano, Mariano, MD
Ginsberg, Janet A., MD
Wahba, Janette M., MD
Plastic Surgery
Vellas, Elaine, MD
Psychiatry
Rajaratnam, Ranjit C., MD
Spariosu, Magdalena, MD

Physicians by Town and Medical Specialty

Lyndhurst (cont)
Radiology
Dikengil, Asim G., MD

Lyons
Addiction Psychiatry
Williams, John A., MD
Child & Adolescent Psychiatry
Kaune, Maureen, MD
Endocrinology
Byrne, William James, MD
Zimering, Mark B., MD
Family Medicine
Wang, Jian, MD
Geriatrics
Luo, Jane He-Cong, MD
Internal Medicine
Hwang, Evelyn R., DO
Kovtun, Marina, MD
Kumar, Renuka, MD
Lin, Michael Keith, MD
Nandakumar, Rajalakshmi, MD
Paramatmuni, Lakshmi K., MD
Prabhu, Vasanthi M., MD
Psychiatry
Latif, Saima, MD
Lee, Hyun K., MD
Maslany, Steven, DO
Opdyke, Karen Stage, MD
Shah, Parul Samir, MD

Madison
Child & Adolescent Psychiatry
Fennelly, Bryan William, MD
Critical Care Medicine
Benton, Marc L., MD
Family Medicine
Berger, Gary, MD
Internal Medicine
Latif, Madiha, MD
Sahoo, Aparna, DO
Neurology
Bathini, Manjula, DO
Obstetrics & Gynecology
Chou, Vivian K., MD
Kaplan, Regina Mpakarakes, MD
Psychiatry
Abbate, Maribel, MD
Brzustowicz, Linda Marie, MD
Pulmonary Disease
Seelall, Vijay Harpal, MD

Mahwah
Allergy
Levine, Sheldon Elliot, MD
Anesthesiology
Gonzalez, Jaime Abel, MD
Cardiovascular Disease
Najovits, Andrew Joseph, MD
Sharma, Ashok K., MD
Dermatology
Lieb, Jocelyn Ann, MD
Lieber, Colette D., MD
Emergency Medical Services
Grover, Meenu, MD
Family Medicine
Beenstock, Steven Marc, DO
Bello, Mary R., MD
De Guzman, Virginia H., MD
Gastroenterology
Antler, Arthur S., MD
Internal Medicine
Shahamat, Morteza, MD
Sharma, Indu, MD
Tartini, Albert, MD
Neurology
Scrimenti, Michael P., MD
Orthopedic Surgery
Alexander, Nicholas, MD
Holden, Douglas Scott, MD
Otolaryngology-Facial Plastic
Steckowych, Jayde Mary, MD
Pediatrics
Liberti, Lorraine M., MD
Perez, Sania Rebecca, MD
Surgery (General)
Ganepola, Ganepola A., MD

Manahawkin
Allergy & Immunology
Madden, James M., MD
Anesthesiology
Barton, Keith A., DO
Bouyea, Michelle Marie, MD
Guo, Jianhua, MD
Hanna, Sherine Farag, MD
Manevich, Ilya, MD
Marco, James Victor, MD
Richlan, Richard A., MD
Siciliano, Louis J., MD
Tse, James T.C., MD
Yampaglia, Joseph P., MD
Cardiovascular Disease
Henry, James R., MD
Hong, William Y. C., MD
Malinverni, Helio J., MD
Reed, William E., DO
Tekriwal, Mahesh Kumar, MD
Colon & Rectal Surgery
Khoo, Robert Eng Hong, MD
Critical Care Medicine
Dewil, Frederic, MD
Dermatology
Geffner, Rami E., MD
Diagnostic Radiology
Fernandez, Richard E., MD
Emergency Medicine
Bagnell, James P., MD
Boye-Nolan, Melinda L., DO
Dinowitz, Seth, MD
Jones, Kimberley L., MD
Kulin, John C., DO
Little, James Todd, DO
Partrick, Matthew Seamus, MD
Pulver, Bradley Lee, MD
Endocrinology
Rizvi, Syed Wajih-Ul-Hasan, MD
Family Medicine
Hogan, Kimberly Ann, MD
Kenny, John J., DO
Nitschmann-Schmoll, Cynthia, DO
Raguso Failla, Michael Joseph, MD
Tailor, Unnati, DO
Veldanda, Ashokvardhan R., MD
Gastroenterology
Koerner, Steven, DO
General Practice
Kirk, Michael John Jr., DO
Hematology Oncology
Chung, Paul Kevin, MD
Desani, Jatin Karsandas, MD
Morino, Tricia Lynn, DO
Naylor, Evan C., MD
Hospitalist
Savarese, Joseph, MD
Internal Medicine
Alhadeff, Ilan, MD
Dahal, Rama, MD
DeSantis Mastrangelo, R., MD
Guida, Vincent C., DO
Hussain, Sajjad, MD
Khan, Akbar Ali, MD
Moshkovitch, Vasil I., MD
Prins, Kenneth J., MD
Reynon, Melissa A., MD
Romano, Andrew Leonard, DO
Sahay, Nishi, MD
Sahay, Rajiv, MD
Soni, Poonam, MD
Soni, Shikhar, MD
Yu, Byung H., MD
Nephrology
Shah, Ankit Prafulbhai, MD
Neurology
Papa-Rugino, Tommasina, MD
Terranova, Robert J., DO
Obstetrics & Gynecology
Gottesman, Brian Tod, MD
Liu, Todd, MD
Marino, Mark, MD
McDermott, James P., DO
Rezai, Amadi, MD
Sunkavalli, Anupama, MD
Sze, Michael Shu Shin, MD
Trim, George G., MD
Vernon, Lisa S., MD
Ophthalmology
Dreizen, Neil G., MD
Drudy, Elena R., MD
Erickson, Alan R., MD
Lee, Robert Edward III, MD
Orthopedic Surgery
Epstein, Samuel E., DO
Kennard, William Francis, MD

Kunkle, Herbert Lemuel Jr., MD
Wright, Douglas G., MD
Otolaryngology
Bezpalko, Lynn E., DO
Bezpalko, Orest, DO
Bhojwani, Amit N., DO
Bones, Victoria Mary, MD
Engle, Edward Issac, DO
McAfee, Jacob Seth, MD
Patel, Pratik Bharat, MD
Romanczuk, Bruce J., MD
Otolaryngology-Facial Plastic
Zhuravsky, Ruslan, DO
Pediatrics
Bleiman, Michael I., MD
Cannon, Aileen Carol, MD
Guariglia, Anthony R., MD
Olorunnisola, Moses F. Jr., MD
Sunkavalli, Paul Venugopal, MD
Psychiatry
Mukai, Yuki, MD
Pulmonary Disease
Lipper, Jeffrey M., MD
Radiation Oncology
D'Ambrosio, David Joseph, MD
Lattanzi, Joseph Paul, MD
Shah, Hemangini R., DO
Rheumatology
Kumar, Ramesh, MD
Kumar Shetty, Nagalakshmi A., MD
Surgery (General)
Barbalinardo, Joseph P., MD
Carson, Gregory B., MD
Echeverri, Samuel David, MD
Fresco, Silvia, MD
Grachev, Sergey, MD
Greco, Richard Yackshaw, DO
Reich, Jonathan Makaloa, MD
Strom, Karl William, MD
Thoracic Surgery
Lujan, Juan Jose, MD
Samra, Matthew Samuel, DO
Urology
Fernicola, Charles P., MD
Vascular Surgery
Hager, Jeffrey C., DO
Lengel, Gary P., MD
Penrod, Carey Lynn, DO

Manalapan
Allergy
De Fusco, Carmine J., MD
Anesthesiology
Atkin, Stuart R., MD
Elenewski, John Francis, MD
Cardiovascular Disease
Dworkin, Jack H., MD
Dermatology
Schechter, Alan Lance, MD
Silbret, Lisa Michele, MD
Emergency Medicine
Barthelemy, Markintosh, MD
Endocrinology
Priven, Igor, MD
Family Medicine
Baig, Rifaqat, MD
Dantchenko, Victoria, MD
Feingold, Marc Benjamin, MD
Goldberg, Alexander, MD
Nordone, Danielle Suzanne, DO
Sharma, Puja, MD
Gastroenterology
Weiner, Brian C., MD
Geriatrics
Kelter, Richard J., MD
Rijhsinghani, Sonia J., MD
Infectious Disease
De Luca, Alfred A. Jr., MD
Internal Med-Adolescent Med
Birger, Yelena, DO
Internal Medicine
Avanesova, Natalya Oleg, MD
Cutler, Jay M., MD
De Blasio, Thomas F., MD
Ezer, Mayer Roy, MD
Koneru, Jayanth, MD
McAlarney, Lourdes Rupac, MD
Romanella, Joseph P., DO
Rossi, Regina L., DO
Schindel, Leonard J., MD
Shestak, Aleksandr, MD

Talamati, Jayanthi, MD
Youssef, Maher A., MD
Neurology
Enescu, Cristian C., MD
Furman, Boris, DO
Obstetrics & Gynecology
Belkin, Sardana, MD
Bochner, Ronnie Z., MD
Fischetti-Galvin, Jessica, DO
Levy, Jenna, DO
Rathauser, Robert H., MD
Oncological Surgery
Miller, Denise J., MD
Ophthalmology
Braunstein, Edward A., MD
Orthopedic Surgery
Ahmed, Munir, MD
Schiebert, Steven S., DO
Skolnick, Cary I., MD
Springer, Stuart Ira, MD
Pediatric Cardiology
Bali, Chhaya, MD
Pediatrics
Bonilla, Melissa Diaz, MD
Dhawan, Denise Marie, MD
Genova-Goldstein, Jeanne, MD
Isayeva, Eleonora, DO
Leib, Samantha, MD
Levy, Moshe, MD
Malaty, Christine B., DO
Nandiwada, Lakshmi P., MD
Peska-Mosseri, Jodi L., DO
Shah, Sonal Ashwin, DO
Sharon, Jill Israel, DO
Tanner-Sackey, Fritzi A., MD
Trogan, Igor, MD
Physical Medicine & Rehab
Adly, Marina, MD
Psychiatry
Rose, Diane, MD
Sports Medicine
Harrison, Andrew, MD
Surgery (General)
Prokurat, Val, DO

Manasquan
Anesthesiology
Beutel, Jonathan A., MD
Rienzo, Peter A., MD
Cardiovascular Disease
Infantolino, Philip L., MD
Critical Care Medicine
Friedman, Paul Martin, MD
Gallagher, Cornelius T., MD
Emergency Medicine
Frankel, Robert, MD
Family Med-Sports Medicine
Tennen, Elad, MD
Family Medicine
Alonzo-Chafart, Lorena D., DO
Cheli, David J., MD
Conkling, Robert F., MD
Ricci, John Anthony, MD
Rittberg, Shannon Bara, DO
Von Suskil, Kurt E., MD
Hematology
Lerner, William A., MD
Topilow, Arthur A., MD
Hematology Oncology
Anne, Madhurima, MD
Greenberg, David Benjamin, MD
Levitt, Michael Joshua, MD
Internal Medicine
Almeida, Frank Gerard, MD
Berkovich, Vladimir, MD
Costanzo, Eric John, DO
Gilani, Asim Haider, MD
Henningson, Carl Thomas Jr., MD
Kossev, Viliana D., MD
Kuzmick, Peter J., DO
Mencel, Peter J., MD
Miskoff, Jeffrey Aaron, DO
Pandya, Manan Kirit, DO
Potulski, Frederick J., MD
Schneider, Henry E., MD
Nephrology
Pandey, Shivendra, MD
Obstetrics & Gynecology
Ditusa, Diane Michele, DO

Filardo,Josephine,MD
Keelan,Michael E.,MD
Parchment,Alfred B.,MD
Saez Lacy,Deborah A.,MD
Welt,Alan J.,MD
Orthopedic Surgery
Bhatnagar,Ramil S.,MD
DePaola,Frederick A.,MD
Ferenz,Clint C.,MD
Goldstein,Joel M.,MD
Husserl,Toby B.,MD
Jarmon,Nicholas Albert,MD
Petrosini,Anthony V.,MD
Roehrig,Gregory James,MD
Sclafani,Michael A.,MD
Seckler,Mark M.,MD
Tozzi,John Michael,MD
Otolaryngology
Faktor,Mitchell J.,DO
Iannacone,Ronald J.,DO
Sparano,Anthony Michael,MD
Pathology
Lahoti,Chitra,MD
Pediatrics
Go,Jane O.,MD
Oram,Alexis Marissa,MD
Wolpert,Joshua D.,MD
Physical Med & Rehab-Sports Med
Gonzalez,Peter G.,MD
Physical Medicine & Rehab
Glasser,Laurie,MD
Lepis,Michael Alphonse,MD
Vantuono,Rosanne,MD
Plastic Surgery
Guzewicz,Richard Michael,MD
Vemula,Rahul,MD
Psychiatry
Beirne,Mary F.,MD
Pulmonary Disease
De La Luz,Gustavo E.,MD
Surgery (General)
Nagy,Michael William,MD
Urology
Howard,Michael Lawrence,MD
Leitner,Robyn R.,MD
Perlmutter,Mark Alan,MD
Rotolo,James E.,MD
Manchester
Internal Medicine
Buerano,Thelma Mapa,MD
Neuro-Psychiatry
Gbeve-Hill,Dorcas,MD
Mantoloking
Internal Medicine
Yeager,Richard J.,MD
Mantua
Family Medicine
Rayner,William J.,MD
Manville
Family Medicine
Auletta,Maria,MD
Khan,Mohammed Nasir,MD
Shah,Mubina,MD
Internal Medicine
Chichili,Eiswarya,MD
Mody,Vipul C.,MD
Pandya,Dhyanesh C.,MD
Pediatrics
Amarnani,Sukhdev,MD
Maple Shade
Family Medicine
Brolis,Nils Viesturs,DO
Di Marcangelo,Michael C. Jr.,DO
Janik,Nancy E.,MD
Norton,Kevin Patrick,DO
Paul,Stephen E.,DO
Neurology
Abidi,Saiyid Manzoor,MD
Vanna,Stephen C.,MD
Yang,John Y.,MD
Obstetrics & Gynecology
Epstein,Debra M.,MD
Maplewood
Anesthesiology
He,Ningning,MD
Cardiovascular Disease
Jacobson,Sayre K.,MD
Tanwir,Anjum,MD
Diagnostic Radiology
Blatt,Kenneth B.,MD

Heideman,Alan J.,MD
Jhaveri,Sujata Ketan,MD
Lautin,Jeffrey L.,MD
Novick,Andrew S.,MD
Endocrinology
Chrisanderson,Donna A.,MD
Prus,Dina S.,MD
Family Medicine
Cadet,Marc D.,MD
Francis,Guy Anthony,MD
Miguez,Priscilla,DO
Sharma,Deepa,DO
Young,Karen D.,MD
Gastroenterology
Goldfarb,Michael,MD
Molokwu,Godwin O.,MD
Gynecology
Gudz,Alexandr,MD
Hematology
Sabnani,Indu,MD
Internal Medicine
Hanson,Claudia A.,MD
Jayanathan,Subendrini G.,MD
Kaid,Khalil Ahmed,MD
Karry Mohanrao,Shailender K.,MD
Mendola,John V.,MD
Orenberg,Scott D.,DO
Simon,Eddy,MD
Solomon,Richard Jay,MD
Medical Oncology
Bordia,Sonal,MD
Nephrology
Kodali,Padmaja,MD
Simon,Segun V.,MD
Obstetrics & Gynecology
Flowers,Sakhshat W. III,MD
Maloney,Marvelle,MD
Parchment,Winsome J.,MD
Peace,Nyota Afi,MD
Smith,Donna M.,MD
Wright-Cadet,Yvonne,MD
Orthopedic Surgery
Feldman,David Nathan,MD
Otolaryngology
Williams,Dione M.,MD
Pediatric Cardiology
Bhattacharyya,Nishith,MD
Pediatrics
Aragones,Linnie A.,MD
San Juan,Severiano Jr.,MD
Physical Medicine & Rehab
Grossman,Perry,MD
Psychiatry
Abramson,Jennifer Leigh,MD
Pulmonary Disease
Bey,Omar M.,MD
Rheumatology
Paolino,James S.,MD
Surgery (General)
Bethel,Colin A. I.,MD
Vascular Surgery
Dick,Leon S.,MD
Margate
Family Medicine
Anastasi,Lawrence J.,DO
Gaffney,John L.,DO
Piccone,Dennis L.,DO
Pediatrics
Durelli,Gloria S.,MD
Plastic Surgery
Carroccia,Eugene C.,MD
Margate City
Endocrinology
Epstein,Britany Faith,MD
Family Medicine
Frankel,David Zelig,MD
Internal Medicine
Faustino,Alan Herbert,MD
Obstetrics & Gynecology
Titton,Barry Sheldon,MD
Ophthalmology
Gross,Howard J.,MD
Nunn,Robert F.,MD
Perez,Matthew K.,MD
Pritz,Nicole M.,MD
Vascular Disease
Steinberg,Joel S.,MD
Marlboro
Allergy & Immunology
Sherman,Michael Bruce,MD

Anesthesiology
Messa,Stephanie Price,MD
Shehata,Sanaa K.,MD
Cardiovascular Disease
Patel,Jayendrakumar N.,MD
Dermatology
Husain,Zain,MD
Diagnostic Radiology
Ferra,Michael John,MD
Family Medicine
Guliano,Jaclyn M.,MD
Kayastha,Shital,DO
O'Dell,Kimberly Ann,MD
Paul Yee,Sabine T.,MD
Gastroenterology
Cencora,Barbara E.,MD
Gold,Jared Z.,MD
Meyer,Shira Asekoff,DO
Tendler,Michael R.,MD
Vazirani,Tina A.,MD
Geriatrics
Shi,Yong,MD
Hematology Oncology
Varma,Seema N.,MD
Infectious Disease
Bhargava,Abha,MD
Laxmi,Sheethal Manipadaga,MD
Internal Medicine
Basilone,Joseph,MD
Carter,Alison F.,MD
Ciencewicki,Michael Jr.,MD
Fox,David B.,MD
Kanouka,Indira Jouma,MD
Nair,Swapna,MD
Pass,Mark David,MD
Pitchumoni,Suresh Shanker,MD
Reddy,Sowbhagya Sangam,MD
Stoner,Edward D.,MD
Tilara,Amy N.,MD
Obstetrics & Gynecology
Dufreney,Margaret S. Durante,MD
Kyreakakis,George J.,MD
Pediatrics
Galperina,Klara,DO
Husain,Syeda Amna,MD
Salcedo,Glenn A.,MD
Yee,Mary,MD
Physical Med & Rehab-Pain Med
Yen,Gary L.,MD
Psychiatry
Cohen,Jason Leon,MD
Sports Medicine
Weintraub,Steve L.,DO
Marlton
Acupuncture
Sciamanna,Mary Ann,DO
Addiction Psychiatry
Ellabbad,Essam-Eldin M.,MD
Alcoholism/Substance Abuse
Baird,Cynthia Marlo,MD
Allergy
Dadhania,Mahendrakumar P.,MD
Gatti,Eugene A.,MD
Kravitz,Elaine K.,MD
Allergy & Immunology
Toci,Gregory R. Sr.,DO
Anesthesiology
Avella,David Paul,MD
Bilgrami,Sajad Syed,DO
Bravyak,James G.,DO
Chityala,Haritha,MD
Chu,Brian,MD
Grossman,Davida S.,MD
Hermann,Todd G.,MD
Iula,Frank J. Jr.,MD
Jiang,Heng,MD
Karanzalis,Demetrius,DO
Kasarda,Frances E.,MD
Knoll,Frank J. III,MD
Kwon,Alan Fay,MD
Lee,Aland H.,MD
Lehrer,Luisa E.,MD
Lewin,Stacy B.,MD
Liccini,Mark Stephen,DO
Lingaraju,Rajiv,MD
Lynch,Jeffrey R.,MD
McIntyre,Bryan J.,DO
Modi,Parag,MD
Morgan,Kathleen A.,MD
Nduaguba,Chiazoka Onyeka,MD

O'Connor,Patrick,MD
Pace,Enrico,MD
Padula,Vincent M.,DO
Pascarella,Michael Ryan,DO
Pierre,Andre M.,MD
Pisera,Donna M.,MD
Pober,Neil J.,MD
Quint,James Douglas,MD
Reichman,Cynthia M.,MD
Reilly,Dennis K.,DO
Ressler,Steven H.,MD
Ricketts,Robyn D.,MD
Santos,Francis Parrocho,MD
Sperandio,Peter G.N.,MD
Villamayor,Carlos Pestelos,MD
Child & Adolescent Psychiatry
Brancato,Peter Jr.,MD
Embrescia,Mary Megan,MD
Gupta,Mala Rani,MD
Prince,Leonie S.,MD
Singh,Sarabjit,MD
Varrell,James R.,MD
Vassallo,Frank A.,DO
Critical Care Medicine
Rodis,Angel Victor,MD
Dermatologic Surgery
Decker,Ashley,MD
Dermatology
Elder,Sandra Depadova,MD
Green,Justin Jacob,MD
Halpern,Analisa Vincent,MD
Heymann,Warren R.,MD
Lawrence,Naomi,MD
Manders,Steven M.,MD
Marquart,Jason D.,MD
Pistone,Gregory A.,MD
Emergency Medicine
Greenberg,Karen Julie,DO
Kincel,David Nathaniel,DO
Mahajan,Raakhee,MD
Patel,Sundip N.,MD
Endocrinology
Belsky,Martin Karl,DO
Fair-Covely,Rose Mary,DO
Family Med-Hospice & Palliative
Chiesa,Jennifer Elaine,DO
Family Medicine
Calabrese,Karen Ann,DO
Casey,Daniel T.,MD
Chandran,Ankila Sharavati,DO
DeGuzman,Ronaldo Cruz,DO
Dishler,Elyse Lyn,MD
Festa,Michelle G.,MD
Flores,Marc E.,DO
Friedhoff,Stephen G.,MD
Getson,Philip,DO
Goldfine,Stephen P.,MD
Hanrahan,Maureen A.,MD
Horvath,Kedron Nicole,MD
Jadhav,Pallavi Dinkar,MD
Lazarus,Nermin Ahmed,DO
Levinson,Elizabeth A.,MD
Lichtman,Lisa B.,MD
Malave,Esther,MD
McCormick,Ryan Charles,MD
Miller,Scott Lewis,MD
Mir,Raema,MD
Najafi,Nawid E.,MD
Pagliaro,Sara Nicole,DO
Patel,Jay Dinesh,MD
Patel,Parag S.,MD
Pecora,Andrew Paul,DO
Pinto,Matthew G.,DO
Press,Howard L.,DO
Requa,Eric Robert,DO
Robinson,Sloan A.,MD
Roesly,Melissa M.,MD
Romano,James A.,MD
Ryczak,Kristen,MD
Schweitzer,Justin Stephen,DO
Shabazz,Shakeilla Lavern,MD
Shah,Hetal Subodh,MD
Sheth,Surendra C.,MD
Sireci,Joseph,DO
Skrzynski,Angela Anita,DO
Strong,Gusti Lickfield,DO
Twersky,Harris A.,DO
Voyack,Michael John,DO
Yeh,Shao-Chun,DO
Gastroenterology
Cohen,Neil M.,MD
Davidoff,Steven,MD

Physicians by Town and Medical Specialty

Marlton (cont)
Gastroenterology
- Devita, Jack Joseph, MD
- Friehling, Jane Susan, DO
- Horn, Abraham S., DO
- Levin, Gary H., MD
- Sorokin, Jeffrey J., MD
- Tulman, Alan Bruce, MD

Geriatric Psychiatry
- Periasamy, Jayanthi, MD

Geriatrics
- Bryman, Paul N., DO

Gynecological Oncology
- Saul, Howard Marc, DO

Hand Surgery
- Ballet, Frederick L., MD
- Strauss, Eric D., MD

Hospitalist
- Pollard, Elizabeth Joan, MD

Infectious Disease
- Makris, Alex T., MD
- Schwartz, Andrew Robert, MD

Internal Med-Hospice Palliative
- Malhotra, Rakesh, MD

Internal Medicine
- Abiuso, Patrick D. Jr., MD
- Airen, Priya, MD
- Alimam, Ammar, MD
- Arerangaiah, Ramya B., MD
- Bermingham, John, DO
- Braverman, Gerald M., MD
- Cetel, Marvin A., MD
- Chaudhry, Nadia Jahan, MD
- Dadhania, Ketki M., MD
- Daly, John Christopher, MD
- Dwyer, James P., DO
- Evans, Carrie Marie, DO
- Grookett, Thomas Wister, MD
- Hasbun, Rafael D., MD
- Jaffe, Brian C., MD
- Jaffe, Jane K., DO
- Joynes, Robert Joseph, MD
- Kaur, Navneet, MD
- Lee, Sherrylynn Nacario, MD
- Lomonaco, Jesse V., DO
- MacCiocca, Michael J., MD
- Maier, Dawn Rachel, MD
- Malik, Irfan Asim, MD
- Mandell, Ryan S., DO
- Matsinger, John Mark, DO
- Mazza, Emilio, MD
- Mirmanesh, Shahin Michael, MD
- Mirmanesh, Shapour Steve, MD
- Mohageb, Salah M., MD
- Nugent, Grace C., MD
- Perez, Alejandro, DO
- Plotnick, Marc P., MD
- Rivlin, Kwan Thanaporn, MD
- Salm, Allen J., MD
- Schwika, John T., DO
- Shad, Yasar, MD
- Sommer, Lacy Louise, MD
- Sztejman, Eric S., MD
- Tang, Godffery R., MD
- Tirmal, Viraj Vijay, MD
- Vishwanath, Sahana, MD
- Zuniga, Rina De Guzman, MD

Microsurgery
- Larusso, Jennifer Lynn, DO

Nephrology
- Michael, Beckie, DO

Neurological Surgery
- Bussey, Jonathan David, DO
- Meagher, Richard John, MD

Neurology
- Klazmer, Jay, DO
- Ma, Xiaoping, MD
- Mabanta, Ricardo Y., MD

Neuromusculoskeletal-Sports Med
- Stein, Meryl Yvonne, MD

Obstetrics & Gynecology
- Patel, Ushma K., MD
- Sawin, Stephen Wooten, MD
- Suarez, Kathryn Reynes Novak, MD
- Taliadouros, George S., MD

Ophthalmology
- Cutney, Carolyn A., MD
- Glass, Charles Adam, MD
- Grossman, Harry D., MD
- Kamoun, Layla, MD
- Mellul, Steven Daniel, DO

Orthopedic Surgery
- Barlow, Jonathan David, MD
- Hoffler, Charles E. II, MD
- Horowitz, Stephen M., MD
- Kelly, John D., MD
- Kirshner, Steven B., MD
- Maslow, Gregory S., MD
- Michael, Stanley P., MD
- Nelson, Gregory N. Jr., MD
- Ragland, Raymond III, MD
- Schaaf, H. William, MD
- Sobel, Mark A., MD
- Zell, Brian Kirk, MD

Orthopedics
- Kahanovitz, Neil, MD

Otolaryngology
- Houston, Patrick J., MD
- Tai, Stephen Jay, MD

Pain Medicine
- Hu, Andre Min-Teh, MD

Pediatric Gastroenterology
- Padron, Celia Z., MD

Pediatrics
- Bailey, Aisha Donine, DO
- Barnett, Sharon Elizabeth, MD
- Berman, Eric David, DO
- Blackman, Jeffrey D., MD
- Chasen, David E., MD
- Chun, Doreen Sze-Man, DO
- Denick, Kimberly Keane, MD
- Falk, Michael Alexander, MD
- Fanelli, Allison Sagan, DO
- Friedler-Eisenberg, Susan F., DO
- Hammer, Stacey R., MD
- Holmes-Bricker, Mary E., DO
- Kakkilaya, Harshila, MD
- Kaus, Sharon M., DO
- Killeen, Thomas Joseph III, MD
- Lafferty, Kathryn Tatsis, MD
- Lampone, Christina, MD
- Leszkowicz, Aditee D., DO
- Melini, Carlo B., MD
- Mirmanesh, John C., MD
- Mirmanesh, Shahram J., MD
- Monaco, Carmine D., DO
- Nicolaides, Catherine D., MD
- O'Mahony, Lisa, MD
- Orel, Howard N., MD
- Panda, Nirmala, MD
- Pandit, Florence A., MD
- Pittalwala, Rashida G., MD
- Ragothaman, Ramesh, MD
- Rickey, Stephanie B., MD
- Rosenblum, Benjamin A., MD
- Rosof, Edward, MD
- Smith-Elfant, Stacy A., MD
- Szawlewicz, Stephen A., MD
- Vare, Katie Marie, MD
- Waxman, Howard S., MD
- Zechowy, Racine B., MD

Physical Medicine & Rehab
- Domingo, Connie Dela Pena, MD
- Griffin, Mark, MD
- Harris, Tracey Dionne, MD
- Joshi, Tapankumar, MD
- Wu, Donald T., MD

Psychiatry
- Abraham, Ruby, MD
- Adetunji, Babatunde A., MD
- Akinli, Timur C., MD
- Alcera, Lloyd C., MD
- Allende, Jenys, MD
- Benjelloun, Hind, MD
- Callahan, Richard Allan II, MD
- Chodha, Vicky, MD
- Edelman, Douglas Jay, MD
- Francisco, Rowena Rebano, MD
- Glass, Joel Bennett, MD
- Harbison, Margaret S., MD
- Harwitz, David Marc, MD
- Hume, Edward Samuel, MD
- Ikelheimer, Douglas Mark, MD
- Kurani, Amit P., MD
- Layne, George Stark, MD
- Longson, Audrey Eve, DO
- Mathews, Joanne, MD
- Mathews, Maju, MD
- McFadden, Robert F., MD
- Nunez, Venitius D., MD
- Panah, Daud Mohammad-Masood, MD
- Pertschuk, Michael Jeffrey, MD
- Post, Nicole Renee, MD
- Profiriu, Alexandru F., MD
- Rubin, Allen J., MD
- Schooff, Mary Lieder, MD
- Shamilov, Maasi Don, MD
- Smith, Elton John, MD
- Steel, Ann Elizabeth, MD
- Strauss, Alexander Sangor, MD
- Teitelman, Karen Lynn Bottone, DO
- Tobe, Edward H., DO
- Worth, Richard Lowell, MD
- Yuan, Cai, MD

Pulmonary Disease
- Auerbach, Donald, MD
- Lee, Andrew N., MD
- Sutherland, Jewelle R., MD

Radiation Oncology
- Eastman, Ralph M., MD

Reproductive Endocrinology
- Kuzbari, Oumar, MD
- Skaf, Robert A., MD
- Van Deerlin, Peter G., MD
- Weissman, Lauren, MD

Surgery (General)
- O'Shea, Joan Frances, MD

Urology
- Mueller, Thomas John, MD
- Wargo, Heather Carol, MD

Marmora
Family Medicine
- Applebaum, Steven Lee, DO
- Horowitz, Jerry A., DO
- Hutcheson, Jonathan Justin, DO
- Hutchison, Melissa M., MD
- Leo, Nicole Terese, DO
- Schneider, Wayne R., MD

Hematology
- Dave, Hemang U., MD

Hematology Oncology
- Pompa, Tiffany, MD

Internal Medicine
- Ahmad, Kaleem U., MD
- Childs, Julianne Wilkin, DO
- Cruz, Avelino N., MD
- Rizvi, Muhammad A., MD

Plastic Surgery
- Birmingham, Karen Lesley, MD

Martinsville
Family Medicine
- Accurso, Daniela, MD
- Chasin, Mitchell C., MD
- Frisoli, Anthony, MD
- Labbadia, Francesco, MD
- Price, Kelly A., MD

Otolaryngology
- Karolak, Mark, DO

Pediatrics
- Calello, Diane P., MD

Matawan
Cardiovascular Disease
- Panezai, Fazal R., MD

Endocrinology
- Xenachis, Cristina Z., MD

Family Medicine
- Hanna, Dalia N., MD
- Tran, Vincent Phuong, DO

Internal Medicine
- Bais, Rajney Monica, MD
- Feng, Shufang, MD
- Ghabras, Magda S., DO
- Gollup, Andrew M., MD
- Jafri, Jaffar M., MD
- Mancuso, Cathie-Ann, MD
- Miller, Melissa Anne, MD
- Ould Hammou, Ayesha N. Haque, MD

Pediatrics
- Badami, Geeta D., MD
- Borromeo, Virginia, MD

Psychiatry
- Geller, Felix A., MD
- Moshkovich, Marina, MD
- Neelgund, Ashwini Kumar, MD
- Vorobyev, Leonid A., MD

Surgery (General)
- Arbour, Robert M., MD
- Fischer, Lauren Jane, MD

Mays Landing
Anesthesiology: Addiction Med
- Quirk, Edward, MD

Bloodbanking
- Nayak, Shaila V., MD

Developmental Pediatrics
- Burgess, David B., MD
- Kruger, Hillary Anne, MD

Family Medicine
- Golden, Daniel Martin, DO

Hospitalist
- Chowdhury, Khaza, MD

Internal Medicine
- Bacarro, Arnold S., MD
- Lurakis, Michael F., DO
- Pollack, Jeffrey S., MD

Ophthalmology
- Maguire, Joseph I., MD
- Sivalingam, Arunan, MD

Pediatrics
- Goldman, Stuart J., MD
- Huang, Patty P., MD
- Tung, John Yu, MD

Psychiatry
- Naeem, Ambreen, MD
- Ortega, Adela Yrma, MD

Vascular & Intrvntnal Radiology
- Hollander, Scott Craig, DO

Maywood
Anesthesiology
- Villegas, Robert A., MD

Child & Adolescent Psychiatry
- Mitnick, David Andrew, MD

Clinical Cardiac Elctrphyslgy
- Zaim, Sina, MD

Colon & Rectal Surgery
- Gallina, Gregory J., MD

Family Medicine
- Leipsner, George, MD

Internal Medicine
- Dixon, Keith Raymond, MD
- French, Eugene C., MD
- Fulop, Eugene, MD
- Fulop, Luminita, MD
- Majersky, Stephen P., MD
- Nguyen, Han Ngoc, MD

Obstetrics & Gynecology
- Seidner, Michael David, MD

Orthopedic Surgery
- Lindholm, Stephen R., MD

Orthopedic Trauma
- Keller, Julie Michelle, MD

Plastic & Reconstructive Srgy
- Ciminello, Frank Salvatore, MD
- Feintisch, Adam, MD
- Hahn, Edward Jr., MD

Plastic Surgery
- Cohen, Stephanie Meryl, MD
- Winters, Richard M., MD

Plastic Surgery-Hand
- Yueh, Janet Han, MD

Urology
- Ahmed, Mutahar, MD
- Christiano, Thomas R., MD
- Esposito, Michael P., MD
- Goldstein, Martin M., MD
- La Salle, Michael Drew, MD
- Lanteri, Vincent J., MD
- Lovallo, Gregory G., MD
- Patel, Nitin Nick, MD
- Siegel, Andrew L., MD

Medford
Adolescent Medicine
- Lazovitz, David A., MD

Allergy
- Bantz, Eric W., MD
- Volpe, John Anthony, DO

Allergy & Immunology
- Kim, John Yohan, MD

Anesthesiology
- Hanna, Amir, MD
- Lennon, Christine Marie, MD

Cardiovascular Disease
- O'Neil, James P., MD

Dermatology
- Buck, Andrea S., DO
- Harrop, Elyse Horn, MD
- High, David A., MD

Diagnostic Radiology
- Sabatino, John C., MD

Emergency Medicine
- Filart, Michael Valencia, DO
- Scheets, Kristen Joanna, DO

Physicians by Town and Medical Specialty

Schiffenhaus,Elizabeth,MD
Family Medicine
Albert Puleo,Anthony M.,MD
Amankwaah,Ajoa O.,DO
Dougherty,Joseph F.,MD
Godleski,Thomas D.,DO
Gomez,Andrew Thomas,MD
Guido,Stephanie,DO
Hollander,Philip,DO
Jones,Graham P.,MD
Marzili,Thomas James,MD
Patragnoni,Richard M.,DO
Ponnamaneni,Abhilasha Rao,MD
Scheuermann,Richard Ernest,MD
Zarroli,Hannah J.,MD
Gastroenterology
Frates,Angela Dawn,MD
Kravitz,John Jay,MD
Modena,Scott Alan,MD
Salowe,David Ross,MD
General Practice
Juele,Nicholas J.,DO
Piarulli,Michael J.,MD
Geriatric Psychiatry
Murphy,Francis Raymond,MD
Geriatrics
Atkinson,James Q. III,MD
Internal Medicine
Barash,Craig Ross,MD
Bezzek,Mark S.,MD
Chua,Lee Chadrick,MD
D'Amico,James Charles,DO
Eufemia,Joann M.,MD
Glass,James M.,MD
Hickey,Joseph J.,MD
Holton,James Jeffrey,MD
Ianacone,Mary R.,DO
Klein,Rachel S.,MD
Scuderi,Steven A.,MD
Waldron,John R.,DO
Neurology
Lee,David Charles,MD
Obstetrics & Gynecology
Agar,Monica T.,MD
Siegel,Amy Judith,DO
Ophthalmology
Cohen,Sander M.,MD
Hyder,Carl Franklin,MD
Mitchell,Cheryl Marie,MD
Sivalingam,Varunan,MD
Veloudios,Angela,MD
Osteopathic Medicine
Pinto,Jeffrey Damian,DO
Pediatrics
Buccigrossi,Jennifer Leigh,MD
Coss,Wanda I.,MD
Foran,Daniel J.,DO
Murphy,Terri Lee,DO
Reed,Rebecca Ann,DO
Roscioli-Jones,Catherine A.,MD
Scott,Charles A.,MD
Weitz,Robert D.,DO
Physical Medicine & Rehab
Lipnack,Eric M.,DO
Psychiatry
Jones,Clifford W.,DO
Keene,Nilda M.,MD
Love,Amy Girdler,MD
Radiation Oncology
DeNittis,Albert Stephen,MD

Mendham
Allergy
Jadidi,Shirin,MD
Cardiovascular Disease
Olivieri,Philip J.,MD
Ricculli,Nicholas P.,DO
Shioleno,Charles A.,MD
Tully,Lisa Anita,MD
Diagnostic Radiology
Kertesz,Jennifer L.,MD
Endocrinology
Usiskin,Keith S.,MD
Facial Plastic Surgery
Kollmer,W. Lance,MD
Geriatrics
Wolf,James H.,MD
Internal Medicine
Ciuffreda,Ronald V.,MD
Connolly,Allison Carthan,MD
Donnelly,Michael G.,MD

Marella,Gregg G.,MD
Prestifilippo,Christie J.,MD
Randazzo,Domenick N.,MD
Solomon,Leah F.,MD
Interventional Cardiology
Amoruso,Daniel Robert,MD
Obstetrics & Gynecology
Prefer,Audrey I.,MD
Ophthalmology
Kalnins,Linda Y.,MD
Pediatrics
Dragalin,Daniel J.,MD
Minhas,Deepa S.,MD
Psychiatry
Von Poelnitz,Michael,MD

Mercerville
Diagnostic Radiology
Larsen,Bartley A.,MD
McDonald,Kathleen L.,MD
Stebbins,Michael G.,MD
Family Medicine
El Attar,Ayman Fatehy,MD
Scott,Martin J.,DO
Infectious Disease
Farooq,Tahir,MD
Husain,Syed Asif,DO
Mathai,Suja John,MD
Porwancher,Richard B.,MD
Internal Medicine
Chawla,Rajnish Paul Singh,MD
Chawla,Rupinder,MD
Haber-Kuo,Sheryl Ann,MD
Mangiaracina,Giacomo,MD
Maniya,Zakaria W.,MD
Nisar,Asif,MD
Patel,Anamika K.,MD
Stawicki,Jesse J.,DO
Neurology
Weaner,Scott Michael,DO
Obstetrics & Gynecology
Jones,Eva R.,MD
Orthopedic Surgery
Sporn,Aaron A.,MD
Orthopedic Trauma
Ahmed,Atif Khalid,MD
Physical Medicine & Rehab
Roman,Stephen John Jr.,MD
Public Health
Zanna,Martin Thomas,MD
Radiology
Callahan,James P.,MD
Collins,Robert S.,MD
Locastro,Rosemary H.,MD
Tufankjian,Dearon K.,DO
Rheumatology
Carney,Alexander S.,MD
Surgery (General)
Sasportas,Jonathan Scott,MD

Merchantville
Addiction Medicine
Gooberman,Lance L.,MD
Anesthesiology: Pain Medicine
Radbill,Keith Philip,DO
Emergency Medicine
Mitchell,Lamont Leigh,DO
Family Medicine
Gilliss,Adam C.,DO
Gilliss,Matthew J.,DO
Husain,Abbas M.,MD
Newton,Dean A.,DO
Shen,Hongxie,MD
Gynecological Oncology
Wilson,John Goss Jr.,MD
Internal Medicine
Curreri,Joseph P.,DO
Scardigli,Dennis Michael,MD
Physical Medicine & Rehab
Markowitz,David,MD
Sachdeva,Chander K.,MD
Psychiatry
McComb,David Robert,DO
Pulmonary Disease
Curreri,Peter Andrew,DO
Surgery (General)
Aronow,Phillip Z.,MD

Metuchen
Cardiovascular Disease
Chiaramida,Anthony J.,MD
Goldberg,William P.,MD
Mondrow,Daniel N.,MD

Sauberman,Roy Burton,MD
Singh,Varinder M.,MD
Sodhi,Ajit S.,MD
Child & Adolescent Psychiatry
Shampain,Lawrence R.,MD
Winograd,Barbara H.,MD
Dermatology
Lee,Jane Mengchuan,MD
Lee,Peter Yujen,MD
Developmental Pediatrics
Amorapanth,Vanna R.,MD
Diagnostic Radiology
Einhorn,Robert,MD
Kolber,Ronald B.,MD
Resnikoff,Leonard Barocas,MD
Emergency Medicine
Jones,James Brian,MD
Family Medicine
Ahn,Paul Michael,DO
Garcia,Maria Teresa,MD
Jasani,Anita,MD
Rossy,William H.,MD
Gastroenterology
Vasireddi,Srinivas S.,MD
Hand Surgery
Shoen,Steven Lloyd,MD
Infectious Disease
Nagarakanti,Sandhya R.,MD
Internal Medicine
Batra,Lina S.,MD
Dasari,Rajasree V.,MD
Hussain,Syed Faiyaz,MD
Kainth,Inderjit S.,MD
Kaur,Dvinder,MD
Khanna,Sunil K.,MD
Lin,Harry Hui,MD
Manoj,Smitha,MD
Soriano,Bruce V.,MD
Thukkaram,Kavitha,MD
Zhang,Miaoying,MD
Zhou,Ren,MD
Neurology
Zhang,Tianshu,MD
Obstetrics & Gynecology
Ainslie,William Jr.,MD
Hsu,Pochien Gregory,MD
Steinbeck,Wayne E.,MD
Pediatrics
Freis,Peter C.,MD
Lebovic,Daniel M.,MD
Raviola,Joseph,MD
Rosenblum,Howard W.,MD
Santiago,Maritza Marie,MD
Tuma,Victor B.,MD
Physical Medicine & Rehab
Alhamrawy,Ismail A.,MD
Batra,Norman Mohan,MD
Kim,Okja,MD
Won,Peter Arm-Woo,MD
Psychiatry
Eng,Leonard K.,MD
Fahmy,Nevine Karam,MD

Mickleton
Anesthesiology
Patterson,Raymond Kevin,MD
Family Medicine
Rioux,Stephen R.,DO
Hematology
Minniti,Carl J. Jr.,MD

Middlesex
Cardiovascular Disease
Shaheen,Zafar A.,MD
Geriatrics
Shamsi,Mahmood A.,MD
Shamsi,Zahira B.,MD
Internal Medicine
Leong,Perry L.,MD
Nephrology
Banerjee,Trina D.,MD
Pediatrics
Mehta,Sadhana,MD

Middletown
Anesthesiology
Atlas,Gayle,DO
Champey,Edward John,MD
McGuire,Kimberly Marie,MD
Anesthesiology: Pain Medicine
Poonia,Amit,MD

Xie,Jinghui,MD
Body Imaging Radiology
Saphier,Nicole Berardoni,MD
Cardiovascular Disease
Suaray,Khalil M.,MD
Clinical Cardiac Elctrphyslgy
Dobrescu,Delia I.,MD
Diagnostic Radiology
Belen,Kristin Marietta O.,MD
Emergency Medicine
Fong,Dean Kimton,MD
Samson,Kristine T.,MD
Sennett,Jane M.,DO
Family Medicine
Armbruster,Thomas C.,MD
Giacona,Caryn Marie,MD
Jacks,Maryann,MD
McManus,Shanda Monique,MD
Morlino,John V.,DO
Swartz,Harry M.,MD
Thompson,Roger McLachlan,MD
Hematology Oncology
Shcherba,Marina,DO
Internal Medicine
Bazerbashi,Ammar,MD
Clemente,Joseph,MD
Farrugia,Peter Michael,MD
Gold,Marcia D.,MD
Gross,Russell A.,MD
Haddad,Joanne T.,MD
Leschinsky,Alexandra,MD
Shah,Ajay S.,MD
Spetko,Nicholas III,MD
Swartz,Stephen Jay,MD
Tuboku-Metzger,Folarin D.,MD
Oral & Maxillofacial Surgery
Garabedian,Hamlet Charmahali,MD
Pediatrics
Beizem,Joanna,MD
Harmady,Debra,MD
Potylitsina,Yelena,MD
Pulmonary Disease
McGuire,Peter A.,MD
Radiation Oncology
Shin,Jacob,MD
Yu,Yao,MD
Undersea & Hyperbaric Medicine
Dornfeld,David B.,DO
Vascular Surgery
Pennycooke,Owano M.,MD

Midland Park
Child & Adolescent Psychiatry
Rodriguez-Frank,Laura V.,MD
Family Medicine
Beauchamp,Donald P.,MD
Bernier,Jean Ciara,MD
Eskow,Raymond P.,MD
Giorlando,Mary Elizabeth,MD
Gastroenterology
Frauwirth,Howard David,MD
Hypertension
Rho,John I.,MD
Infectious Disease
Vierheilig,Jacqueline M.,MD
Internal Medicine
Ackad,Alexandre V.,MD
Cohen,Ricky B.,MD
Dabaj,Dina,MD
Dziezanowski,Margaret Ann,MD
Hart,Karen Manheimer,MD
Hope,Lisa Dawn,MD
Kotlov,Mikhail,MD
Kozlowski,Jeffrey P.,MD
Leifer,Bennett P.,MD
Prinz,Karola Kristina,MD
Raza,Syed Irfan,MD
Valinoti,Anne Marie,MD
Zaider,Arik,MD
Nephrology
Chheda,Neha Das,MD
Weizman,Howard B.,MD
Ophthalmology
Seidenberg,Keith B.,MD
Orthopedic Surgery
Konigsberg,David Eric,MD
Van Grouw,Brian P.,DO
Otolaryngology
Milgrim,Laurence Marc,MD
Pediatrics
Ungerleider,Deborah L.,MD

New Jersey Physicians Section 2 Town and Medical Specialty

597

Physicians by Town and Medical Specialty

Midland Park (cont)
Physical Medicine & Rehab
Murphy,Ryan Keith,DO
Plastic Surgery
De Marco,Joseph A. Jr.,MD
Pulmonary Disease
Rosen,David Michael,MD
Rheumatology
Knee,C. Michael,MD
Kopelman,Rima G.,MD
Leibowitz,Evan Howard,MD
Urology
Baum,Richard D.,MD
DeTorres,Wayne Raymond,MD
Frey,Howard L.,MD
Hartanto,Victor H.,MD
Mackey,Timothy Joseph,MD

Milford
Family Medicine
Bauman,Susan M.,MD
Bryhn,Lisa Kristen,MD
Curry,Debra W.,MD
Hewens,Jeremy C.,MD
Jardim,Carla Mia,MD
Jones,Howard D.,MD
Kayal,William Jesse,MD
Kozakowski,Stanley M.,MD
Kroth,Patricia Haeusler,DO
Lucco,Julianne M.,MD
Murry,Robert L.,MD
Skillinge,David D.,DO
Turenne Kolpan,Laurie K.,MD
Ophthalmology
Hahn,Robert Douglas,MD

Millburn
Anesthesiology
De Mais,John R.,MD
Stillman,Richard I.,MD
Verea,Vickie,MD
Cardiovascular Disease
Aueron,Fred M.,MD
Charney,Robert Howard,MD
Gantz,Kenneth B.,MD
Patrawalla,Shirish C.,MD
Saeed,Qaisra Yasmin,MD
Simandl,Susan Lynn,MD
Cardiovascular Surgery
Shah,Shamji K.,MD
Colon & Rectal Surgery
Gilder,Mark E.,MD
Orringer,Robert D.,MD
Tarantino,Debra R.,MD
Taylor,Robert L.,MD
Critical Care Medicine
Shah,Smita S.,MD
Dermatology
Brockman-Bitterman,Allyson,MD
Ehrenreich,Michael,MD
Freeman,Amy Ilyse,MD
Kihiczak,George,MD
Mautner,Gail H.,MD
Siegel,Eric Scott,MD
Diagnostic Radiology
Blonstein,Jeffrey D.,MD
Family Medicine
Biernat,Matthew Mateusz,MD
Glezen-Schneider,Priscilla ,MD
Mattoo,Anju,MD
Sivasubramanian,Hema,MD
Gastroenterology
Bains,Yatinder,MD
Desai,Mahesh R.,MD
Rosen,Michael,MD
Shah,Mehul N.,MD
Infectious Disease
Weiner,Peter R.,MD
Internal Medicine
Desai,Rajendra R.,MD
Frankel,Trina N.,MD
Freundlich,Nancy Lynn,MD
Khalina,Svetlana Petrovna,MD
Khong,Darmadi S.,MD
Kuo,Michael,MD
Mehta,Chirag A.,MD
Meisner,Errol C.,MD
Miraglia,Janeen Theresa,DO
Ortega-Jongco,Anita M.,MD
Pinho,Paulo Bandeira,MD
Pitoscia,Thomas,MD
Quaglia,Silvio A.,MD
Roy,Satyajeet,MD
Schwartzman Lane,Roberta,MD
Solomon,Michael I.,MD
Tecson,Maria Vida Tupaz,MD
Thirunahari,Nandan R.,MD
Thomas,Alapatt Porinchu,MD
Medical Oncology
Nussbaum,Nathan Coleman,MD
Nephrology
Freundlich,Richard E.,MD
Obstetrics & Gynecology
Cooperman,Alan Stewart,MD
Luciani,Richard L.,MD
Pollack,Marshall S.,MD
Seymour,Christopher R.,MD
Simonetti,John M.,MD
Ophthalmology
Doshi,Vatsal Suryakant,MD
Greenfield,Donald A.,MD
Newman,David M.,MD
Pruzon,Joanna Dawn,DO
Orthopedic Surgery
Blank,Howard L.,MD
Daly,Ronald A.,MD
Schob,Clifford J.,MD
Other Specialty
Yemini,Matan,MD
Pediatric Infectious Diseases
Hasan,Uzma Naveen,MD
Pediatric Pulmonology
Kottler,William F.,MD
Pediatrics
Alexander,Andrea Hope,MD
Batra,Chhaya,MD
Comandatore,Ann Marie,MD
Cotler,Donald N.,MD
Gruenwald,Laurence D.,MD
Knowles,Kelly Petrison,MD
Liggio,Frank J.,MD
Mangru,Subita S.,MD
Meshko,Yanina,MD
Miller,Yael Spinat,MD
Ramesh,Shruti Chakrabarti,DO
Spiteri,Sharon,MD
Sterio,Mara,MD
Stettner,Lisa G.,DO
Thompson,Stacy Ellen,DO
Voremberg,Sandra R.,MD
Physical Medicine & Rehab
D'Alessio,Donna Giselda,MD
Plastic Surgery
Bulan,Erwin Joseph,MD
Saccone,Paul Gregori,MD
Psychiatry
Adeola,Yetunde,MD
Hermann,Allan J.,MD
Price,Joel R.,MD
Pulmonary Disease
Shah,Himanshu P.,MD
Radiology
Burak,Edward,MD
Suarez,Norka J.,MD
Reproductive Endocrinology
Birkenfeld,Arie,MD
Onwubalili,Ndidiamaka,MD
Rheumatology
Mesnard,William J.,MD
Sports Medicine
Levy,Andrew Stuart,MD
Richmond,Daniel B.,MD
Surgery (General)
Bilof,Michael Louis,MD
Kopelan,Adam Michael,MD
Yurcisin,Basil Michael II,MD
Urology
Helfman,Alan S.,MD
Shoengold,Stuart D.,MD
Strumeyer,Alan D.,MD
Vascular Surgery
Addis,Michael Downes,MD
Manicone,John A.,MD

Millstone Township
Child & Adolescent Psychiatry
Mazur,Irene,MD
Internal Medicine
Chikezie,Pius U.,MD
Gendy,Hany Moris,MD
Shah,Sejal Gohel,MD

Milltown
Anatomic/Clinical Pathology
Rimmer,Cheryl L.,MD
Internal Medicine
Chan,Diana,MD
Sjolund,Paula A.,DO

Millville
Allergy
Coifman,Robert E.,MD
Cardiovascular Disease
Shapiro,Barry E.,DO
Diagnostic Radiology
Margate,Pedro Ramboyong,MD
Endocrinology
Slone,Helen L.,MD
Family Medicine
Akrout,Eddie,MD
Davis,Brian Joseph,DO
Mortensen,Jill,DO
Salloum,Azizeh J.,MD
Yoong,Michael P.,MD
Internal Medicine
Babu,Sarath,MD
Kaczaj,Olga,MD
Morales,Ruben B.,MD
Patel,Hardik Bhupendrabhai,MD
Piszcz-Connelly,Malgorzata,MD
Obstetrics & Gynecology
Babalola,Gbolagade O.,DO
Geria,Michael J.,DO
Giyanani,Sunita M.,MD
Occupational Medicine
Weiss,Robert Jay,MD
Ophthalmology
Ghobrial,John M.,MD
Lieberman,Roger D.,DO
Pernelli,David R.,MD
Pediatrics
Jamil,Erum,MD
Patel,Ketan R.,MD
Shim,Zae U.,MD
Torres,Stephanie M.,DO
Psychiatry
Priori,Jorge,MD
Radiation Oncology
Fanelle,Joseph W.,MD
Radiology
Golestaneh,Fazlollah,MD

Mine Hill
Gastroenterology
Albicocco,Nicholas S.,MD
Geriatrics
Estrada,Aristides M.,MD
Internal Medicine
Forward,John B.,MD
Rotsides,Andreas D.,MD
Sharma,Tarun K.,MD
Sundaram,Subramoni,MD
Ophthalmology
Patel,Kartik,DO
Pediatrics
Hershman,Ilene M.,MD
Psychiatry
Sundaram,Savitri,MD
Surgery (General)
Soda,Michael,MD
Urology
Colton,Marc D.,MD

Minotola
Internal Medicine
Patel,Chimanlal J.,MD
Nephrology
Cirelly,Francine Arlene,DO

Monmouth Beach
Family Medicine
Irving,Robert John,MD
Pediatrics
Gulli,Maria T.,MD

Monmouth Junction
Family Medicine
Kline,Bradley H.,DO
General Practice
Penupatruni,Bharati D.,MD
Infectious Disease
Bais,Pammi T.,MD
Internal Med-Sleep Medicine
Raza,Mudusar I.,MD
Internal Medicine
Chan,Phillip Pierre,MD
Gali,Lavanya,MD
Mallipeddi,Harini,MD
Regulapati,Saritha,MD
Obstetrics & Gynecology
Kumar,Monica Puri,MD
Pediatrics
Aggarwal,Roopali,MD
Nageen,Farhat,MD
Psychiatry
Arora,Pradeep,MD
Ashraf,Azima F.,MD
Das,Dipali R.,MD
Gandhi,Zindadil Manoj,MD
Lahiri,Nupur,MD
Lendvai,Ivan,MD

Monroe
Anesthesiology
Arabi,Mona Najib,MD
Shen,Mengmeng,MD
Cardiovascular Disease
Logothetis,George Nicholas,MD
Emergency Medicine
Stoev,Borislav Georgiev,DO
Family Med-Geriatric Medicine
Bhalla,Anshu,MD
Family Medicine
Donat-Flowers,Rhoda J.,DO
Reddy,Sureka,MD
Gastroenterology
Forester,Gary P.,MD
Geriatrics
Vigario,Jose C.,DO
Internal Medicine
Abellana,Juan C.,MD
Abellana,Victoria D.,MD
Ahuja,Kavita Bala,DO
Fisch,Tobe M.,MD
Gopal,Richa,MD
Logothetis,James Nicholas,MD
Mehta,Ojas R.,DO
Motavalli,Lisa S,MD
Sterman,Paul Lawrence,MD
Nephrology
Arabi,Nida,MD
Dwivedi,Shaunak A.,DO
Kalra,Tamanna H.,MD
Obstetrics & Gynecology
Ibrahim,Samih A.,MD
Psychiatry
Malik,Rehan,MD
Vitolo,Joseph Glen,MD
Urology
Lewis,Walter Emmett III,MD
Lieberman,Alan Howard,MD

Monroe Township
Cardiovascular Disease
Baron,Phillip,MD
Tannenbaum,Alan K.,MD
Clinical Cardiac Elctrphyslgy
Maleki,Kataneh F.,MD
Critical Care Medicine
Freedman,Andrew R.,MD
Dermatology
Kaufmann,Roderick Jr.,MD
Vaidya,Darshan C.,MD
Endocrinology
Levy-Kern,Muriel,MD
Family Med-Geriatric Medicine
Hussain,Aijaz,MD
Family Medicine
Grossman,Leonard A.,MD
Kobylarz,Fred A.,MD
Krauser,Paula S.,MD
Patel,Ravish Mukesh,MD
Prasad,Keshav,MD
Geriatric Psychiatry
Krishnaiah,Muralidhar,MD
Geriatrics
Chatterjee,Abhijit,MD
Internal Medicine
Allu,Sridevi,MD
Foster,Ronald D.,MD
Ghanem,Osama K.,MD
Gjenvick,Timothy C.,MD
Goldberg,Jory J.,MD
Mirza,Ahmed Anas,MD
Nanavati,Kartikey J.,MD
Nanavati,Kaushal Kartikey,MD
Prasad,Vineet,MD
Sherrow,Keith Ira,MD

Thomas,Cherryl L.,MD
MOHS Micrographic Skin Cancer
Peloro,Concettina M.,MD
Nephrology
Prasad,Deepali,MD
Neurology
Friedlander,Devin S.,MD
Ophthalmology
Grabowski,Wayne M.,MD
Orthopedic Surgery
Polakoff,Donald Richard,MD
Pediatrics
Doshi,Deepa,MD
Gulati,Sunita,MD
Hemrajani,Payal,MD
shah,Amisha M.,MD
Physical Medicine & Rehab
Herman,Perry Mitchell,MD
Psychiatry
Linet,Leslie S.,MD
Singh,Gagandeep,MD
Vascular Surgery
Franco,Charles D.,MD
Tripathi,Tushar Mahesh,MD
Montclair
Anatomic/Clinical Pathology
Roy,Manimala,MD
Anesthesiology
Barr,Gary Alan,MD
Kerven,Elliot Sean,MD
Martinez,Richard,MD
Shahsamand,Zabi Z.,MD
Yacoub,Magdy Yousef,MD
You,Jerome H.,MD
Young,Michael Anthony,MD
Breast Surgery
Elliott,Nancy L.,MD
Hertz,Marcie B.,MD
Cardiovascular Disease
Bannerman,Kenneth S.,MD
Di Filippo,John A.,MD
El-Atat,Fadi Ahmed,MD
Gutman,Julius A.,MD
Miller,Kenneth Paul,MD
Prior,Francis P.,MD
Child & Adolescent Psychiatry
Della Bella,Peter,MD
Kennedy,Paul,MD
Lebowitz-Naegeli,Nanci L.,MD
Clinical Neurophysiology
Robinton,John E.,MD
Colon & Rectal Surgery
Rothberg,Robert M.,MD
Dermatology
Downie,Jeanine Bernice,MD
Diagnostic Radiology
Gurell,Daniel Steven,MD
Jewel,Kenneth L.,MD
Lee,Joo-Young Melissa,MD
Mattern,Richard F.,MD
Shah,Mala T.,MD
Emergency Medicine
Alberino-Catapano,Amanda,MD
Alejandro,Jason Robert,MD
Antonowicz,Michelle,MD
Arias,Ana L.,MD
Geck,Wilma Santiago,MD
Gorski,Robert Mitchell,MD
Langer,Marjory Ellen,MD
Leuchten,Lisa,DO
Rosenbaum,Steven B.,MD
Sultan,Sharmeen,DO
Williams,Estelle Vaughns,MD
Family Med-Sports Medicine
Mascaro,Melissa,MD
Family Medicine
Douglas,Elaine,MD
Grobstein,Naomi S.,MD
Heifler,Gregory Dean,MD
Hostetler,Caecilia E.,MD
Hrishikesan,Geetha,MD
Kahn,Jason Peter,DO
Khan,Afshan R.,DO
Novak,Eva Cesnek,MD
Ouw,Willem B.,MD
Ramos-Genvino,Elizabeth,MD
Shimelfarb,Marianna B.,MD
Wilson,Howard Marc,MD
Gastroenterology
Abraham,Rini S.,MD

Volfson,Ariy,MD
Geriatrics
Auld,Clara Stringer,MD
Gynecology
Grochmal,Stephen A.,MD
Hematology
Sagorin,Charles E.,MD
Zager,Robert,MD
Hematology Oncology
Di Paolo,Patrick J.,MD
Hospitalist
Tehranirad,Mohammad,MD
Wain,Nadeem,MD
Internal Medicine
Ahmed,Sabeen,MD
Allam,Naveen Reddy,MD
Allam,Reddy B.,MD
Allusson,Valerie R.C.,MD
Califano,Tiziana,MD
Chaudhry,Shauhab,MD
Diano,Rowen Gumapas,MD
Elsayed,Ali Elsayed Mohamme,MD
Gribbon,John J.,MD
Gujja,Rajitha Reddy,MD
Harb,George E.,MD
Kim,Harold J.,MD
Klukowicz,Alan J.,MD
Krupp,Edward Todd,DO
Liang,Raymond Y.,MD
Mali,Shalini Reddy,MD
Mehta,Bijal Shah,MD
Miryala,Rekha,MD
Mohan,Mamatha G.,MD
Nowicki,Noel C.,MD
Ponzio,Geralyn Michelle,MD
Rana,Meenakshi G.,MD
Wong Liang,Ruth C.,MD
Zaeh,Douglas H.,MD
Neonatal-Perinatal Medicine
Peng,Chung J.,MD
Nephrology
Bell,Alvin,MD
Blaustein,Daniel Alberto,MD
Goveas,Roveena Noeline,MD
Neuro-Psychiatry
Haller,Kate,MD
Neurological Surgery
Clemente,Roderick J.,MD
Dannis,Seth Michael,MD
Obstetrics & Gynecology
Aristizabal,Michelle Anne,MD
Carman,Elise S.,MD
De Marsico,Richard,MD
Degrande,Gary C.,MD
Gaudino,Silvana,MD
Jenkins,Reginald Alexander,MD
Lee,Jane S.,MD
Lespinasse,Pierre Frederic,MD
Ophthalmology
Childs,Kathryn Phyllis,MD
Schachter,Norbert,MD
Orthopedic Surgery
Drzala,Mark R.,MD
Fischer,Evan S.,MD
Nicoll,Cornelius I.,MD
Vizzone,Jerald P.,DO
Otolaryngology
Tan,John J.,MD
Pain Medicine
Park,Chong H.,MD
Pathology
Kimler,Stephen C.,MD
Tang,Daniel Di,MD
Pediatric Emergency Medicine
Birmingham,Mary Catherine,MD
Haines,Elizabeth Jane,DO
Pediatrics
Besser,Richard Eric,MD
Hung,Yvonne,MD
Nasiek,Sara,MD
Paisner,Raphael,MD
Weinstein,Mark E.,MD
PhysMed&Rehab-Hospice Palltve
Yonclas,Elaine Marie,MD
Physical Medicine & Rehab
Jasey,Neil N. Jr.,MD
Thomas,Jodi,MD
Plastic & Reconstructive Srgy
Mesa,John Mario,MD

Plastic Surgery
Ablaza,Valerie J.,MD
Bond,Sheila A.,MD
DiBernardo,Barry E.,MD
Giampapa,Vincent C.,MD
Haramis,Harry Theodore,MD
Rosen,Allen D.,MD
Psychiatry
Bienenfeld,Scott I.,MD
Campos,Danilo T.,MD
Cooke,John R.,MD
De La Torre,Lily Shu,MD
Friedman,Bruce Phillip,MD
Keise,Lydia Nicole,MD
Latimer,Edward A.,MD
Liebhauser,Catherine A.,MD
Meyer,Sarah E.,MD
Mgbako,Ambrose O.,MD
Phariss,Bruce Wallace,MD
Reichstein,Michele B.,MD
Riestra Cortes,Juan L.,MD
Vaidhyanathan,Ketaki,MD
Weiner,Alison L.,MD
Westreich,Laurence M.,MD
Zajfert,Michael S.,MD
Pulmonary Disease
Cohen,Zaza Isaac,MD
Radiation Oncology
Barba,Jose P.,MD
Stabile,Richard J.,MD
Radiology
McFadden,Denise C.,MD
Ow,Cheng H.,MD
Quackenbush,Gail,MD
Montvale
Arthroscopic Surgery
Livingston,Lawrence I.,MD
Diagnostic Radiology
Hendi,Jennifer Michelle,MD
Emergency Medicine
Lambert,Rick O.,MD
Family Medicine
Ajemian,Ara Antranik,MD
Rodriguez,Margaret,MD
Hematology
Gu,Ping,MD
Internal Medicine
Kulesza,Elizabeth Ann,MD
Tempesta,Sabrina L.,DO
Varghese,Rebecca M.,MD
Medical Oncology
Kriplani,Anuja,MD
Wang,Rui,MD
Nephrology
Wojnarska-Alvarez,Gabriela,MD
Obstetrics & Gynecology
Jean,Nagaeda M.,MD
Langer,Myriam,MD
Vascular Surgery
Sherman,Mark David,MD
Montville
Anatomic Pathology
Singh,Rajendra Sant,MD
Anatomic/Clinical Pathology
Raina,Santosh,MD
Anesthesiology
Hsieh,Ching C.,MD
Family Medicine
Coelho,Ryan,MD
Filion,Jacqueline D. Weil,DO
Gargano,Joseph A.,DO
Hoenig,Sandra R.,MD
Iannetta,Frank,MD
Keating,William G.,DO
Lapsiwala,Pareen Raj,DO
Lin,Annie,DO
O'Connor,Brandon P.,MD
Pallay,Arnold I.,MD
Rehberg,Joelle Stabile,DO
Stack,Thomas Joseph III,DO
Forensic Pathology
Shaikh,Junaid Rasheed,MD
Internal Medicine
Aasmaa,Sirike T.,DO
Gilmartin,Andrew Philip,MD
Golloub,Cory A.,MD
Wassef,Wagih G.,MD
Zimmerman,Anahita,MD
Obstetrics & Gynecology
Das,Kamala,MD

Physicians by Town and Medical Specialty
Ophthalmology
Gerszberg,Ted M.,MD
Pediatrics
Gandhi,Alpana D.,MD
Psychiatry
Caga-Anan,Roberto Lagria,MD
Kannankeril,Mary C.,MD
Verde,Valerie Sylvia,MD
Research
Kashanian,Franciska K.,MD
Moorestown
Adult Psychiatry
Cooperstein,Heidi B.,DO
Allergy
Lane,Stanley R.,MD
Anesthesiology
Cwik,Jason Charles,MD
Elia,Anna,MD
Husain,Mansoor Ul-Haque,MD
Junior,John L.,MD
Madison,Anoja Bala,DO
Sattel,Lisa E.,MD
Anesthesiology: Pain Medicine
Patil,Meenal Kulkarni,MD
Cardiovascular Disease
Dennis,Charles A.,MD
Duca,Maria Diane,MD
Finch,Mark T.,MD
Galski,Thomas M.,DO
Lederman,Steven M.,MD
Namey,Jeffrey Elias,MD
Procacci,Pasquale M.,MD
Sambucci,Deborah A.,DO
Sauerwein,Anthony G.,MD
Schimenti,Robert J.,MD
Sussman,Jay I.,MD
Ventrella,Samuel M.,MD
Child & Adolescent Psychiatry
Ralph,Pamela J.,MD
Colon & Rectal Surgery
Pilipshen,Stephen J.,MD
Dermatology
Camishion,Germaine Mary,MD
Chheda,Monique Kamaria,MD
D'Ambra-Cabry,Kimberly A.,MD
Del Monaco,Magaly Patricia,DO
Foti,Frederick D. Jr.,MD
Jacoby,Richard,MD
Koblenzer,Caroline S.,MD
Diagnostic Radiology
Greene,Arthur J.,MD
Emergency Medicine
Dawoud,Magy M.,MD
Lam,Adele Dolores,DO
Endocrinology
Entmacher,Susan D.,MD
Gonzalez Pantaleon,Adalberto,MD
Herbst,Allison B.,MD
Savarese,Vincent William,MD
Family Med-Sports Medicine
Plut,Thomas W.,DO
Shin,Jong Tae,DO
Family Medicine
Barker,William Robert,MD
Barr,Larry Allen,DO
Bechtel,David S.,MD
Bhogal,Jasmeet Singh,MD
Bowers Pepe,Jessica Sue,DO
Britton,Richard J.,MD
Brobyn,Tracy L.,MD
Burke,Hana Oswari,MD
Chan,Wai Ben,DO
Chung,Myung K.,MD
Crudele,James E.,MD
Dennison,Alan D.,MD
Horvitz,Steven P.,DO
Land,Stephen M.,MD
Lanza,Paul R.,DO
Lee,Thomas Yon,MD
Levin,Irina,MD
Levin,Sanan L.,MD
Louis,Marie Edwige,MD
Martz,Rebecca Lynn,MD
Matula,Joseph John,DO
Mills,Robert,DO
Nirenberg,Elena,MD
Oswari,Andrew,MD
Patel,Sanjiv C.,MD
Pellegrino,Tara Marie,DO
Peterson,Dolores D.,MD
Pettigrew,Isabel Hilary,MD

Physicians by Town and Medical Specialty

Moorestown (cont)
Family Medicine
- Ray, Anjali K., MD
- Reeh, Debora Cummings, DO
- Rutkiewicz, Laura A., MD
- Shapiro, Gary I., MD
- Stackhouse, Lisa A., DO
- Summersgill, Richard Blair, MD
- Termini, Joseph F., MD
- Ward, Patrice Taylor, DO
- Wasleski, Karen J., MD
- Yudin, Joel S., DO

General Preventive Medicine
- Murray, Michael Louis, DO

Geriatric Psychiatry
- Snyder, David L., MD

Geriatrics
- Siegert, Elisabeth A., MD

Infectious Disease
- Gummadi, Vedam, MD

Insurance Medicine
- Waronker-Silverstein, Amy S., MD

Internal Medicine
- Berkowitz, Rosalind M., MD
- Berna, Ronald A., MD
- Berna, William J., MD
- Connors, Barbara J., DO
- Gami, Nishith Madhusudan, MD
- Gandrabura, Tatiana, MD
- Giacobbo, Kenneth V., DO
- Gross, David D., MD
- Hoffmann-Wadhwa, Nancy I., MD
- Kaufman, Jodi D., MD
- Levin, Joseph B., MD
- Pandya, Ipsit, MD
- Patnaik, Asit, MD
- Pearcy, Cornell, MD
- Wadhwa, Dom P., MD

Medical Oncology
- Nathan, Faith E., MD

Neurological Surgery
- Cervantes, Luis A., MD

Neurology
- Vijayaraghavan, Swathi, MD

Obstetrics & Gynecology
- Chapman, Derek Q., MD
- Gomez, Syeda Rabia, DO
- Mama, Saifuddin Taiyeb, MD
- Minoff, Michael H., MD

Ophthalmology
- Brown, Miriam Renee, MD
- Horowitz, Philip, MD
- Kelly, Peter J., MD
- Nachbar, James G., MD
- Putnam, Daniel Philip, MD
- Tran, Trong D., MD
- Wexler, Amy R., MD

Orthopedic Surgery
- Dwyer, Joseph Michael, MD
- Greenleaf, Robert Martin, MD
- Raimondo, Rick Arthur, MD
- Sanfilippo, James Arthur, MD
- Weisband, Ira David, DO

Pain Medicine-Interventional
- Duckles, Benjamin Jeffrey, MD

Pediatrics
- Giardino, John Domenic Jr., MD
- Gordon, Anne M., MD
- Guevarra, Andres T., MD
- Guevarra, Jesusita H., MD
- Weinroth, Heidi J., MD

Physical Medicine & Rehab
- Akrout, Hafedh, MD
- Bastien, Maria Altagrace, MD
- Gutman, Gabriella, MD
- Kim, David Howard, MD
- Lee, Joseph Kim, MD
- Loughran, Katy, MD
- Marple, Jill Ann, MD
- Molina, Maria Gregoria, MD

Plastic Surgery
- Au, Alexander F., MD

Psychiatry
- Bien-Aime, Michel J., MD
- Caputo, Kevin P., MD
- Kwon, Alexander K., MD
- Meinke, Rebecca Lynn, MD
- Salman, Zoe Wilson, MD
- Steinberg, Susanne Inez, MD

Pulmonary Disease
- Allred, Charles Cameron, MD

Surgery (General)
- Kling, Maureen C., MD
- Sharma, Gaurav S., MD

Surgical Critical Care
- Wry, Philip C., MD

Thoracic Surgery
- DiPaola, Douglas Joseph, MD
- Heim, John A., MD

Vascular & Intrvntnal Radiology
- Bianco, Brian A., DO

Vitreous and Retina
- Colucciello, Michael, MD

Morganville
Anesthesiology
- Caruso, Marco F., MD
- Chung, Sung K., MD
- Piskun, Jacob, MD

Diagnostic Radiology
- Losik, Steve Boleslav, MD

Internal Medicine
- Hao, Tong Karen, MD
- Horowitz, Mitchell Loyd, MD
- Kroll, Spencer Daniel, MD
- Mannava, Sumalatha, MD
- Ridlovsky, Ludmila, MD
- Saaraswat, Vijay, MD
- Sai, Priya, MD
- Su, Melissa, MD

Neurology
- Choy, Maria, MD
- Mehta, Amor Ruyintan, MD

Pediatrics
- Bakshiyev, Yuliya, MD
- Husain, Sajidah I., MD
- Lee, Kim Chiu, MD
- Liwag, Alexander J., MD
- Yuen, Sharon Shue, MD

Physical Medicine & Rehab
- Sunwoo, Daniel, MD
- Varghese, Teena P., MD

Psychiatry
- Haque, A. F. M. Z., MD

Urology
- Kirshenbaum, Alexander, MD
- Sukkarieh, Troy Z., MD

Morris Plains
Adolescent Medicine
- Feingold, Gail J., MD

Allergy & Immunology
- Elias, Salwa E.G., MD

Anesthesiology
- De Santis, Fiorita G., DO
- Itzkovich, Chad Jason, MD
- Koplik, Andrew D., MD

Cardiovascular Disease
- Gallerstein, Peter E., MD

Emergency Medicine
- Bakun, Walter Michael, MD

Family Medicine
- Cervone, Maurizio, DO
- Cervone, Oswald, DO
- Joseph, Charles A., MD
- Lijo, Maria Carmen, MD

Geriatric Psychiatry
- Patel, Bhupendra M., MD

Insurance Medicine
- Parvulescu, Traian D., MD

Internal Medicine
- Burns, H. Patrick, MD
- Cifelli, Antonio, MD
- Elias, Ahdi I., MD
- Francois, Jean-Marie L., MD
- John, Sunitha Sara, MD
- Sharma, Rakesh Somabhai, MD
- Wilson, Justin B., MD
- Yu, Nenita L., MD

Neuro-Psychiatry
- Collopy, Edward M., MD

Obstetrics & Gynecology
- Ghazi, Mohammad, MD

Occupational Medicine
- Jennison, Elizabeth A., MD

Other Specialty
- Furey, Sandy Anselm III, MD

Pediatrics
- Lopez-Allen, Gabriela D., MD

Plastic Surgery
- Kamdar, Mehul R., MD

Valdes, Michael E., MD

Psychiatry
- Becker, Robert J., MD
- Buceta, Joseph, MD
- Domingo, Joselito B., MD
- Gaviola, Gerry F., MD
- Kamakshi, Savithri, MD
- Kisch, Agnes M., MD
- Rabanal, Marie C., MD

Morristown
Addiction Medicine
- Wilding, Todd Meredith, MD

Adolescent Medicine
- Brill, Susan R., MD
- Park, Lisa Lam, MD
- Rosenfeld, Walter D., MD

Allergy
- Chernack, William J., MD
- Weinreb, Barry D., MD

Anatomic/Clinical Pathology
- Dise, Craig A., MD
- Jaramillo, Marina A., MD
- Magidson, Jory G., MD
- Meradian, Ara, MD
- Mohammed, Raji Hussain, MD
- Piotti, Kathryn C., MD
- Sung, Diana, MD

Anesthesiology
- Abkin, Arkadiy, MD
- Armstrong, Aileen S., MD
- Armstrong, Patrick Andrew, MD
- Barbieri, Louise T., MD
- Barry, Kevin M., MD
- Brusco, Louis Jr., MD
- Chen, Cindy H., MD
- Chern, Sy-Yeu Sue, MD
- Chiumento, Marvin Joseph, MD
- Chow, Matthew S.T., MD
- Chung, Daniel Hansam, MD
- Cohen, Dale L., MD
- Crosta, Alan Michael Jr., MD
- Fitzgerald, Timothy E., MD
- Kapadia, Cyrus Baji, MD
- Kazim, Debra Ann, MD
- Koranyi, Peter, MD
- Kothari, Jay, MD
- Kwon, Christopher J., MD
- LaBove, Phillip S., MD
- Lapchak, John T., MD
- Lawson, Charles Alexander, MD
- Lefever, Gerald S., MD
- Lewis, Walter Michael, MD
- Linz, Stephan M., MD
- Longworth-Gatto, Lisa E., DO
- McDonnell, Thomas E., MD
- Merchant, Sameer R., MD
- Murray, Thomas Robert, MD
- Panah, Michael Hormoz, MD
- Riabov, Keith A., MD
- Rosenbaum, Lee M., MD
- Rubinfeld, Julie A., MD
- Rudman, Michael E., MD
- Shin, Pheodora L., MD
- Sieber, James Curtis, MD
- Spiteri, Isaac Daniel, MD
- Stennett, Richard A., MD
- Streicher, James Tabb, MD
- Taylor, Guy Adrian, MD
- Voinov, Luba A., MD
- Watson, Todd A., MD
- Weiner, Steven Martin, MD
- Welsh, Terrence Mathew, MD
- Winne, Richard P. Jr., MD
- Wu, Eileen Pey Chi, MD

Breast Surgery
- Fornari, Marcella, DO
- Gendler, Leah S., MD

Cardiovascular Disease
- Blum, Mark A., MD
- Boccia Liang, Claire G., MD
- Campanile, Giovanni, MD
- Curwin, Jay Howard, MD
- Dickson, David Gordon, MD
- Fisch, Arthur P., MD
- Freilich, David I., MD
- Gillam, Linda Dawn, MD
- Goldschmidt, Marc Eliot, MD
- Guss, Stephen B., MD
- Hsieh, Allen, MD
- Levy, Stephen M., MD
- Limandri, Giuseppe, MD

- Mahoney, Timothy Hugh, MD
- Mandel, Leonid, MD
- Marcoff, Leo, MD
- Martin, Joanne C., MD
- Mondelli, John Anthony, MD
- Natello, Gregory W., DO
- Ramos Bondy, Beatrix Marie, MD
- Raska, Karel, MD
- Santiago, Derek W., MD
- Schalet, Bennett David, MD
- Schwartz, Jeffrey G., MD
- Smart, Frank W., MD
- Uretsky, Seth, MD
- Verdesca, Stephen A., MD
- Watson, Richard I., MD
- Weisbrot, Joshua, MD
- Weisen, Steven Fred, MD
- von Poelnitz, Audrey E., MD

Cardiovascular Surgery
- Rodriguez, Alejandro L., MD

Child & Adolescent Psychiatry
- Bash, Howard Lee, MD
- Bhatia, Nita, DO
- Cohen, Adam Jonathan, MD
- Giuliano, Michael A., MD
- Muthuswamy, Rajeswari, MD

Child (Pediatric) Neurology
- DeSouza, Trevor G., MD
- Waran, Sandy P., MD

Clinical Cardiac Elctrphyslgy
- Coyne, Robert F., MD
- Katz, Michael Geoffrey, MD
- Winters, Stephen L., MD

Colon & Rectal Surgery
- Huk, Matthew David, MD
- Moskowitz, Richard L., MD

Critical Care Medicine
- Park, Henry, MD
- Toscano, Andrew, MD

Dermatology
- Agarwal, Shilpa R., MD
- Altman, Rachel S., MD
- Dane, Alexander Ali, DO
- Fialkoff, Cheryl N., MD
- Grob, Alexandra, DO
- Kazam, Bonnie B., MD
- Lee, Kristyna H., MD
- Lombardi, Adriana, MD
- Lortie, Charles Frederic, MD
- Parker, Collin Robert, MD
- Pilcher, Mary Frances, MD
- Popkin, Mark D., MD
- Rogachefsky, Arlene S., MD
- Schneider, Rhonda R., MD
- Torres, Omar, MD

Developmental Pediatrics
- Fadden, Kathleen Selvaggi, MD

Diagnostic Radiology
- Anand, Neil, MD
- Barton, Loucia C., MD
- Beute, Bernard John, MD
- Esses, Steven J., MD
- Ginsberg, Hal N., MD
- Leff, Sheryl L., MD
- Moore, Ann M., MD
- Ratakonda, Sridevi, MD
- Schiavi, Jonathan Michael, MD
- Smith, Peter Lloyd, MD
- Timins, Julie K., MD

Emergency Medicine
- Alamia, Peter Anthony, DO
- Allegra, John R., MD
- Althoff, Marilyn F., MD
- Armstrong, Lisa Kay, MD
- Biggs, Danielle Deluca, MD
- Castillo, David Cinco, DO
- Cosenza, Mario Anthony, DO
- Edwards, Daniel James, DO
- Eskin, Barnet, MD
- Esposito, Amanda Santoro, MD
- Feldman, David C., MD
- Felegi, William B., DO
- Fiesseler, Frederick William, DO
- Gerardi, Michael J., MD
- Gohsler, Steven P., MD
- Hung, Oliver Li-Ping, MD
- Jinivizian, Hasmig Barkeve, MD
- Junker, Elizabeth Elsa, MD
- Kaiafas, Costas Andreas, MD
- Kassem, Jawad Nadim, MD
- Kenwood, Alan L., MD

Lee,Peter Q.,DO
Maroun,Victor,MD
Nashed,Ashraf H.,MD
Nevins,Sol,MD
Patel,Hetal,MD
Patwa,Amy Shah,MD
Peek,Erin Heritage,MD
Ritter,Albert W.,MD
Ruzek,Michael A.,DO
Shih,Richard D.,MD
Szucs,Paul Andrew,MD
Tapia,Alfredo J.,MD
Troncoso,Alexis B. II,MD
Van Pelt,Stephen Robert,MD
Vera,Ariel Eduardo,MD
Walsh,Brian W.,MD
Youssouf,Andrew Joseph,MD
Zimmerman,Patrick Whaley,MD

Endocrinology
Baron,Michelle A.,MD
Castaneda,Rachel Lim,MD
Chon,Jajin Thomas,MD
Gadiraju,Silpa,MD
Margulies,Debra Jill,MD
Melfi,Robert J.,MD
Nevin,Marie Eithne,MD
Walimbe,Mona S.,MD

Family Med-Geriatric Medicine
Blloshmi,Kledia,MD

Family Medicine
Aronwald,Bruce Alan,DO
Becker,Andrew B.,DO
Bhambri,Ankur,DO
Christou,Alexander A.,DO
Chung,Angela F.,DO
Cioce,Anthony Jr.,DO
Cioce,Thomas G.,DO
Dillaway,Winthrop C. III,MD
Domovich,Ora,MD
Fitzpatrick,Hendrieka Ann,MD
Gedroic,Kristine Lynn,MD
Guercio-Hauer,Catherine A.,MD
Joshi,Namita V.,MD
Klingmeyer,Dorothy Marie,DO
Leung,Jacquelyn Way-Yan,MD
Melograno,Joseph J.,DO
Onat,Esra Samli,MD
Perez,Marcella,MD
Pietka,Jamie K.,MD
Stevens,Hilary Kristin,MD
Thomson,Mary Jo G.,DO
Wallace,Theresa C.,MD
Wilson,Lynn Marie,DO
Yaqub,Zunera,MD
Ziering,Thomas S.,MD
Zipp,Christopher Paul,DO

Forensic Pathology
Suarez,Ronald V.,MD

Gastroenterology
Alistar,Angela Tatiana,MD
Arsenescu,Razvan Ioan Paul,MD
Martin,Lorraine H.,MD
Morton,John Douglas,MD
Ryan,Joseph J.,MD
Samach,Michael A.,MD
Schalet,Michael Alan,DO

General Practice
Enis,Sean,MD

Geriatric Psychiatry
Farrales,Caroline P.,MD

Geriatrics
Peper,Kathryn,MD
Petilla-Onorato,Jessica I.,MD
Prager,Jason Nicholas,MD
Sharma,Keerti,MD
Zelener,Marina L.,DO

Gynecological Oncology
Contreras,Diana Nancy,MD
Heller,Paul B.,MD
Tchabo,Nana Eleonore,MD
Tobias,Daniel Henry,MD
Wagreich,Allison Robin,MD

Hand Surgery
McBride,Mark J.,MD
Miller,Jeffrey Karl,MD

Head & Neck Surgery
Cohen,Erik Gary,MD
Harrison,Lawrence Evan,MD

Hematology
Early,Ellen Marie,MD
Gerstein,Gary,MD

Meyers,Marta,MD
Papish,Steven W.,MD

Hematology Oncology
Chiang,Wendy M.,MD
Scola,Michael Anthony,MD

Hospitalist
Papatheodorou,Dana William,MD
Shroff,Shilpa Anilkumar,MD
Trinidad,Jennilee A.,MD

Infectious Disease
Kessler,Jason Adam,MD
Natarajan,Usharani,MD
Salaki,John S.,MD

Insurance Medicine
Darcey,Jacqueline Marie,MD

Internal Med-Sports Medicine
Padavan,Dean,MD

Internal Medicine
Acosta Baez,Giancarlo,MD
Adler,Kenneth R.,MD
Alberti,Kathryn P.,MD
Aldaia,Lillian,MD
Allam,Bharat Reddy,DO
Ampadu,Akua A.,MD
Anderson,James Thomas,MD
Anwar,Khurram,MD
Asokan,Nalini,MD
Astiz,Donna J.,MD
Bery,Seema,MD
Bhende,Sudhir S.,MD
Cherry,Mohamad Ali,MD
Chow,Shih-Fen,MD
Correa Orozco,Felipe A.,MD
Cosmi,John Edward,MD
Davidoff,Ada,MD
Davidoff,Bernard M.,MD
Dekko,Samar,MD
Del Valle,Heather Marie,DO
Denbow,Frank Alstein,MD
Dominguez Mustafa,Rolando,MD
Efros,Barry J.,MD
Farber,Charles M.,MD
Farhat,Salman,MD
Feigelman,Theodor,MD
Fiel,Stanley Bruce,MD
Fields,Scott G.,MD
Fioriti,Gina Marie,DO
Gallinson,David Herschel,DO
Garg,Deepika,MD
Gavi,Shai,DO
Ginsberg,Claudia Lisa,MD
Giove,Gian-Carlo,MD
Gonzalez,Joselyn,MD
Griffin,John P.,MD
Griffith,Rebecca Anne,MD
Grover,Manisha B.,MD
Hassanin,Ahmed,MD
Holubka,Jacquelin Pickford,MD
Hosadurga,Supriya S.,MD
Hussein,Ahmed Hamdy,MD
Johnson,Mark Raymond,MD
Kallini,Ronnie N.,MD
Karger,Louise D.,MD
Knops,Karen M.,MD
Kolarov,Sanja,MD
Kopelan,Leah Michelle,MD
Koulogiannis,Konstantinos P.,MD
Kuo,David,MD
Leibu,Rachel Rosenstock,MD
Leung,Michael Seto,MD
Martins,Damion Antonio,MD
Mayor,Gilbert H.,MD
Mediratta,Anuj,MD
Melzer,Olga Alexandrovna,MD
Monastyrskyj,Ola A.,MD
Moore,Brian J.,MD
Morales,Donna Chelle Viray,DO
Ngo,Gerald,MD
Nielsen,Earl F.,MD
Nunez,Elkin Armando,MD
Nyunt,Tun,MD
Oliver,Mark A.,MD
Patel,Dharmesh Govind,MD
Patil,Vrishali Swanand,MD
Penaberdiel,Thelma M.,MD
Piccolo,Christian K,MD
Proudan,Vladimir Ivanovich,MD
Raja,Shashi Ravi,MD
Rand,Victoria Elena,MD
Randazzo,Jean P.,MD
Raska,Anna M.L.,MD
Reder,Lorie Jean,MD

Renna,Carmen M.,MD
Rosen,Ellen Jan,MD
Rosenberg,Richard S.,MD
Rothkopf,Michael M.,MD
Sarkar,Shubho Ranjan,MD
Savage,Danielle S.,MD
Schachter,Nora Claudia,MD
Shubhakar,Vishwanath,MD
Shulkin,David J.,MD
Silverman,Michael Evan,MD
Simon,Egbert A.,MD
Singh,Chandandeep,MD
Smith,James Randolph,MD
Stoytchev,Hristo Vassilev,MD
Sussman,Jonathan S.,MD
Thomas,Elsa,MD
Vascan,Andreea Carmen,MD
Wang,Jonathan Alan,DO
Weine,Gary R.,MD
Weiss,Howard C.,MD
Yu,Xiaolin,MD
Zheng,Fangfei,MD
Ziolo,Gregory Michael,MD

Interventional Cardiology
Gandotra,Puneet,MD
Rosen,Craig Michael,MD

Maternal & Fetal Medicine
Hanley,Maryellen L.,MD
Jackson,Unjeria C.,MD

Medical Oncology
Leibowitz,Stacey Bucholtz,MD

Neonatal-Perinatal Medicine
Federico,Cheryl L.,MD
Gluck,Karen,MD
Goil,Sunita,MD
Mimms,Gaines M.,MD
Orsini,Anthony J.,DO
Rogido,Marta R.,MD
Schenkman,Andrew C.,MD
Shen,Calvin T.,MD
Skolnick,Lawrence M.,MD

Nephrology
Eppinger,Barry A.,DO
Fine,Paul L.,MD
Price,Barbara Ellen,MD
Stack,Jay I.,MD

Neurological Surgery
Baskin,Jonathan Jay,MD
Benitez,Ronald Patrick,MD
Chapple,Kyle Thomas,MD
Chun,Jay Y.,MD
Gardner,Allan Lee,MD
Knightly,John J.,MD
Mazzola,Catherine A.,MD
Meyer,Scott Andrew,MD
Moshel,Yaron Aharon,MD
Stillerman,Charles Blair,MD
Sumas,Maria Elaina,MD
Wells-Roth,David S.,MD
Zampella,Edward J.,MD

Neurology
Alias,Mathew N.,DO
Babineau,Shannon Elizabeth,MD
Conigliari,Matthew F.,MD
Diamond,Mark S.,MD
Fox,Stuart W.,MD
Iones,Anna,MD
Karolchyk,Mary A.,DO
Knappertz,Volker Armin,MD
Marx,Tatyana,MD
Okunola,Oladotun A.,MD
Royce,Roxanne,MD
Tsairis,Peter,MD
Ugorec,Igor,MD

Nuclear Medicine
Claps,Richard J.,MD

Obstetrics & Gynecology
Austin,Kimberlee Kunze,MD
Avondstondt,Andrea Mithai,MD
Ayyad,Mina N.,MD
Bergh,Paul Akos,MD
Blank,Jacqueline P.,DO
Botros,Carolyn,DO
Brenin-Goldfischer,Debra Sue,MD
Culin,Angelina Han,MD
Culligan,Patrick John,MD
Daly,M. Veronica,MD
Feltz,John P.,MD
Ferrante,Daniel P.,MD
Garfinkel,David A.,MD
Gluck,Ian J.,MD

Graebe,Kerry,MD
Iammatteo,Matthew D.,MD
Isaac,Vina H.,MD
Jones,Kathryn M.,MD
Khine,Mary L.,MD
Laguduva,Lakshmi Rani R.,MD
Littman,Paul M.,DO
Lizarraga,Liza Isabel,MD
Lucarelli,Elizabeth Ann,MD
Mahaga-Ajala,Mark-Robert O.,DO
Manor,Einat,MD
Mass,Sharon B.,MD
Mathews,Chacko P.,MD
McGue,Mary Margaret,MD
Miller,Naomi H.,MD
Morley,Laura Balderrama,MD
Murphy,Guy D.,MD
O'Reilly,Sara B.,DO
Omay,Cem S.,MD
Salamon,Charbel Georges,MD
Shah,Leena P.,MD
Shariati,Amir,MD
Slomovitz,Brian Matthew,MD
Steer,Robert L.,MD
Tunde-Agbede,Oluwafisayo,MD
Walter,Briza V.,MD
Wasenda,Erika Joy,MD

Occupational Medicine
Schwarz-Miller,Jan,MD

Oncological Surgery
Chevinsky,Aaron H.,MD

Oncology
Wong,James Robert,MD

Ophthalmology
Angioletti,Lee Mitchell,MD
Benedetto,Dominick A.,MD
Braunstein,Robert Alan,MD
Chen,Lucy L.,MD
Kazam,Ezra S.,MD
Klein,Kathryn Suzanne,MD
Knapp,Stefanie,MD
Lalin,Sean C.,MD
Landmann,Dan S.,MD
Lopatynsky,Marta O.,MD
Masterson,Robert E.,MD
Morgan,Charles Fisher,MD
Perina,Barbara,MD
Reisman,Jeffrey M.,MD
Sarkar,Jayati Saha,MD

Orthopedic Surgery
Aurori,Brian F.,MD
Aurori,Kevin C.,MD
Avallone,Nicholas J.,MD
Baskies,Michael Ari,MD
Baydin,Jeffrey A.,MD
Cohen,Marc Alan,MD
Crutchlow,William P.,MD
Dowling,William J. Jr.,MD
Drey,Iris Antonella,MD
Epstein,David Michael,MD
Gatto,Charles Anthony,MD
Giordano,Carl P.,MD
Goldberger,Michael Irwin,MD
Kanellakos,James George,MD
Levine,Barry Steven,MD
Lombardi,Paul M. Jr.,MD
Nachwalter,Richard Scott,MD
Naseef,George Salem III,MD
Sclafani,Steven,MD
Taffet,Berton,MD
Wagshul,Adam David,MD
Willis,Andrew Albert,MD

Other Specialty
Colizza,Wayne A.,MD

Otolaryngology
Cairns,Christine Dobrosky,MD
Gerwin,Kenneth S.,MD
Giacchi,Renato John,MD
Immerman,Sara Beth,MD
Kanowitz,Seth J.,MD
Lachman,Reid A.,MD
Sorvino,Damian W.,MD
Thomas,Tom,MD

Pathology
Katz,Robert Samuel,MD
Mercer,Geraldine O.,MD

Pediatric Anesthesia
Lopes,Melissa M.,MD

Pediatric Cardiology
Donnelly,Christine M.,MD
Mone,Suzanne Margaret,MD

Physicians by Town and Medical Specialty

Morristown (cont)

Pediatric Cardiology
Prasad, Aparna, MD

Pediatric Critical Care
Craft, Jeanne A., MD
Keenaghan, Michael Andrew, MD
Thomas, Melissa Dias, MD

Pediatric Emergency Medicine
Jourdan, Cassie, MD
Melchionne Miseo, Christina, MD

Pediatric Endocrinology
Berry, Tymara Bernadette, MD
Cerame, Barbara I., MD
Silverman, Lawrence Andrew, MD
Starkman, Harold S., MD

Pediatric Endocrinology
Woo, Melissa Lee Mei, MD

Pediatric Gastroenterology
Leiby, Alycia A., MD
Patel, Mohini Gautam, MD
Perez, Maria Esperanza, DO

Pediatric Hematology Oncology
Fritz, Melinda D., MD
Halpern, Steven L., MD
Kalambakas, Stacey Anastasia, MD
Needle, Michael Neil, MD
Neier, Michelle Dana, MD

Pediatric Infectious Diseases
Gupta, Meera, MD

Pediatric Nephrology
Corey, Howard Erwin, MD

Pediatric Orthopedics
Minkowitz, Barbara, MD

Pediatric Pulmonology
Cooper, David Michael, MD
Montalvo-Stanton, Evelyn, MD

Pediatric Surgery
Zoeller, Garrett Keith, MD

Pediatric Urology
Connor, John Patrick, MD

Pediatrics
Almeida, Vinita Maria, MD
Amato, Christopher Scott, MD
Antony, Kristine Brinda, DO
Atlas, Arthur B., MD
Baorto, Elizabeth P., MD
Bieler, Harvey Phillip, MD
Block, Deborah C., MD
Buck, Melissa, MD
Cheruvu, Sunita, MD
Chin, Daisy Y., MD
Clark-Hamilton, Jill, MD
Cohen, Martin L., MD
Crowley, Kathryn Ann, MD
Cucolo, Patricia Anne, MD
Eckert, Jessica, DO
Eckstein, Devin Brazill, DO
Gamallo, Ma. Bernardita R., MD
Gill, Ramneet Kaur, MD
Gutierrez, Juan Alberto, MD
Hoelzel, Donald W., MD
Horowitz, Meggan Elise, DO
Kairam, Neeraja, MD
Kerr, Kathy Rosen, MD
Koslowe, Oren Lewis, MD
Lanzkowsk, Shelley, MD
Lasker, Susan J., MD
Leier, Tim Ulrich, MD
Lodish, Stephanie Renee, MD
Lofrumento, Mary Ann, MD
Lupatkin, William L., MD
McCluskey, Tamara B., DO
McSherry, Kevin Joseph, MD
Meltzer, Alan J., MD
Mukherjee, Angela, DO
Nashi, Suhaib G., MD
Nativ, Simona Horak, MD
Nicoletta, Marianna, MD
Orafidiya, Yetunde, MD
Poblete, Gwyn Laurice, MD
Presti, Amy Lynn, MD
Rehm, Christine M., MD
Ryan, Christina Marie, MD
Saadeh, Sermin, MD
Scherer, Susan Denys, MD
Schwartzberg, Paul Marc, DO
Sequeira, Sophia Almeida, MD
Shah, Ashish R., MD
Shah, Niva, DO
Shluper, Victoria, MD
Verga, Barbara Jean, MD

Wazeka, April Natasha, MD
Wiener, Ethan Saul, MD
Willis, Karen Christine, MD
Wolf, Mary Campion, MD

Physical Med & Rehab-Pain Med
Davis, Sanders W., MD

Physical Medicine & Rehab
Bachar, Jean A., MD
Cotter, Ann C., MD
David, Erica Nicola, MD
Flowers, Rashonda R., MD
Khan, Ummais N., MD
Khattar, Vimi, MD
Mayoral, Jorge L., MD
Mulford, Gregory J., MD
Pisciotta, Anthony J., MD
Polesin, Alena, MD
Price, Judith B., DO
Rao, Rajesh Ramchandra, MD
Rempson, Joseph H., MD
Skerker, Robert Scott, MD
Smith, Jason Anthony, MD
Tzeng, Alice Chaw, MD
Zheng, Yining, MD

Plastic & Reconstructive Srgy
Racanelli, Joseph Anthony, DO

Plastic Surgery
Comizio, Renee Carol, MD
Glatt, Brian Steven, MD
Ko, Albert Edward, MD
Kutlu, Hakan M., MD
Pyo, Daniel J., MD
Rafizadeh, Farhad, MD
Schmid, Daniel B., MD

Psychiatry
Alam, Syed Fahim, MD
Braun, Joshua Eugene, MD
Centanni, Frank D., MD
Chrobok, Jan M., DO
Chustek, Michael Aaron, MD
Cidambi, Indra Kumar, MD
Di Turi, Richard Michael, MD
Dickes, Richard A., MD
Granet, Roger B., MD
Kent, Justine Marie, MD
Marshall-Salomon, Gabrielle, MD
Nurenberg, Jeffry Raul, MD
Racanelli, Vincent J., DO
Robinson, Michael David, MD
Rosenberg, Paul E., MD
Sancho Mora, Elda P., MD
Taneli, Tolga, MD
Taylor, Clifford A., MD
Wasser, Keri Nicole, MD
Werner, Philip M., MD
Wolff, Jeffrey G., MD
Zaubler, Thomas S., MD

Pulmonary Critical Care
Boomsma, Joan D., MD
LaRosa, Jennifer A., MD

Radiation Oncology
Goldberg, Yana Pavel, MD
Karim, Mona, MD
Oren, Reva, MD

Radiology
Hirsch, Martin A., MD

Reproductive Endocrinology
Forman, Eric Jason, MD
Maguire, Marcy Frances, MD
Scott, Richard Thomas Jr., MD

Rheumatology
Tratenberg, Mark Adam, DO
Widman, David, MD

Spinal Surgery
Lowenstein, Jason E., MD

Surgery (General)
Adams, John M., MD
Agis, Harry, MD
Bickenbach, Kai Asa, MD
Bilaniuk, Jaroslaw W., MD
Christoudias, Stavros George, MD
Di Fazio, Louis Thomas Jr., MD
Elyash, Igor Gary, DO
Henseler, Roy A., MD
Hernando, Michael T., MD
Huang, Jianzhong, MD
James, Kevin V., MD
Kannisto, Cheryl Lynne, MD
Lee, Thomas Y., MD
Magovern, Christopher Jude, MD
Nusbaum, Michael Jay, MD

Ombrellino, Michael, MD
Pasquariello, James Verniere, MD
Riaz, Omer Junaid, MD
Rolandelli, Rolando Hector, MD
Siegel, Brian Keith, MD
Slater, James P., MD
Smith, Brian L., MD
Sturt, Cindy, MD
Vasilakis, Vasileios, MD
Ward, David S., MD
Whitman, Eric David, MD

Surgical Critical Care
Curran, Terrence, MD
Kelly, Kathleen M., MD
McLean, Edward Jr., MD

Thoracic Surgery
Brown, John Muir III, MD
Greeley, Drew Peter, MD
Neibart, Richard M., MD
Polomsky, Marek, MD
Steiner, Federico A., MD
Widmann, Mark Dennis, MD

Urology
Ackerman, Anika Jahn, MD
Atlas, Ian, MD
Chaikin, David Craig, MD
Israel, Arthur R., MD
Kaynan, Ayal Menashe, MD
Pressler, Lee B., MD
Saypol, David C., MD
Steinberg, Joseph, MD
Sutaria, Perry Maganlal, MD
Taylor, David L., MD

Vascular Surgery
Edoga, John K., MD
Kabnick, Lowell Stuart, MD
Moritz, Mark William, MD
Patel, Amit V., MD
Resnikoff, Michael, MD
Tulsyan, Nirman, MD

Mount Arlington

Cardiovascular Disease
Lowell, Barry H., MD
Nazeer, Amjad, MD
Shen, Rhuna, MD

Family Medicine
Gaela, Joan Fontelera, MD

Internal Medicine
Ferrier, Austin Seymour, DO

Maternal & Fetal Medicine
Kappy, Kenneth Allen, MD

Otolaryngology
Aroesty, Jeffrey H., MD
Lin, Giant Chu, MD
Mohankumar, Aditi, MD

Mount Holly

Anatomic/Clinical Pathology
Anand Chawla, Jagjit K., MD
Biondi, Robert J., DO
Manion, William L., MD

Anesthesiology
Ajmal, Muhammad Zafar, MD
Baron, Leah, MD
Bhagat, Anilchandra I., MD
Dhru, Sahil H., DO
Ferrari, Albert N., MD
Gargiulo, Richard F., MD
Gollapudi, Praveen Choudary, MD
Gumnit, Robert Y., MD
Gupta, Rakesh Chander, MD
Kalariya, Rupal S., MD
Lachenal, Edgardo N., MD
Marcelo, Edmund, DO
Mendel, Howard G., MD
Nyzio, Joseph Bruno, DO
Schwartz, Joshua J., MD
Shah, Azam, DO
Tatz, Mark A., MD
Thaler, Adam M., DO
Thornton, Robin W., MD

Child & Adolescent Psychiatry
Bernacki, Carolyn Green, DO

Emergency Medicine
Altamura, Richard H., MD
Bertolino, Laura, DO
Brown, Patti C., DO
Cowan, Robert Matthew, MD
Dias, Alan Steven, MD
Dickson, Scott Vincent, DO
Elisha, Daniel, MD
Freas, Glenn Curtis, MD

Goldberg, David Felheimer, MD
Goldenberg, Gennifer E., MD
Keir, Donald R., MD
Kuhfahl, Keith Joseph, DO
Leibrandt, Paul N., MD
Leitner, Stephen J., MD
Morris, Jeffrey B., MD
Price, Ali S., DO
Ruderman, Seth R., MD
Shubert, Roy Alan II, MD
Thompson, Elizabeth Ann, MD
Tsao, Peter Dean, DO
Turner, Craig S., DO

Family Med-Adult Medicine
Tagle, Lauren, MD

Family Medicine
Busch, Gregory Howard, DO
Cavuto-Wilson, Carolyn Marie, DO

Geriatrics
Headley, David F., MD
Jagadeesh, Jyothi, MD

Hospitalist
DeLue, Erik Nathaniel, MD
Nisar, Sabeeha, MD
Oyeyemi, Jubril Oyekanmi, MD
Valeus, Pierre Rigens, MD

Internal Medicine
Achebe, George E., MD
Cairoli, Maurice J., MD
Castellino, Sharon Franklin, MD
Clermont, Nadine Nattacha, MD
Denniston, Robert B., MD
Entmacher, Michael S., MD
Fred, Matthew Ross, MD
Ghobrial, Peter Morcos Ibrah, MD
Govan, Satyen Manilal, DO
Husain, Zaheer, MD
Kapoor, Tarun Kumar, MD
Kleinman, Michael Ari, DO
Lawandy, Michael Armia, DO
Malone, Michael Richard, DO
Mandala, Ashok R., MD
Newkirk, Christine L., MD
Patel, Swati Hasmukh, MD
Pratt Mccoy, Kia Chriselda, MD
Shah, Purviben R., MD
Sodhi, Jasdeep Singh, MD
Tadi, Kiranmayi, MD
Thomas, Mark Allen Voltis, DO
Ucheya, Blessing C., MD
Wallace, Stephen Gary, MD
Ye, Xiaodan, MD

Medical Oncology
Levenbach, Rachel Shoshana, MD

Obstetrics & Gynecology
Deluca, Samantha, DO
Gorlitsky, Helen, MD
Grossman, Leonard, MD
Jackson, Olga E., MD
Levine, Bruce Jay, MD
Levine, Richard Teddy, MD
Manning, Latriece Eileena, DO
Modena, Alisa B., MD
Rashid, Parveen, MD
Segal, Avni, MD
Shalit, Stuart L., DO

Oncology
Berk, Seth Howard, MD
Lee, James Wonsang, MD

Ophthalmology
Hartman, Eric J., MD

Pediatric Nephrology
Sharma, Amita K., MD

Pediatrics
Doshi, Samir Kirankumar, MD

Psychiatry
Case, John Gouyd, MD
Willman, Margaret A., DO

Radiation Oncology
Ariaratnam, Lemuel S., MD
Fife, Kelly D., MD
Kim, Catherine Sun Joo, MD

Mount Laurel

Allergy
Kravitz, Stuart A., MD

Allergy & Immunology
Dvorin, Donald J., MD
Goldstein, Marc F., MD
Gordon, Nancy Deborah, MD

Anatomic/Clinical Pathology
Grotkowski, Carolyn E., MD

602

Anesthesiology
Buck,Gary B.,MD
Chekemian,Beth Ann,DO
Haleem,Burhan,DO
Lesneski,Matthew J.,MD
Shah,Manish,MD
Anesthesiology: Pain Medicine
Cooper,Niti Dalal,DO
McGrath,Steven Warren,MD
Body Imaging Radiology
Tan,Elizabeth Listiani,MD
Critical Care Medicine
Cohen,Douglas Jay,MD
Ryan,Kathleen Lisa,MD
Dermatology
Abdelmalek,Mark A.,MD
Dipasquale,Albert M.,MD
Levin,Robin Merle,MD
Diagnostic Radiology
Chan,Britton Miller,MD
Chheda,Samir Visanji,MD
Gargiulo,Andrew Michael,MD
Gehringer,Travis James,MD
Patel,Priyesh V.,MD
Emergency Medicine
Mathason,Mark David,DO
Noor,Farid A.,MD
Resnick-Matro,Jennifer Dawn,MD
Family Medicine
Bandy,Caryn Kay,DO
Barone,Catherine Ann,DO
Cooley,Danielle Lynn,DO
Coren,Joshua Scott,DO
Decker,Edmund J.,DO
Foda,Randa Baher,MD
Golden,Richard F.,DO
Hancq,Nicole Elizabeth,MD
Hanna,Sherry Kamal,MD
Kerley,Sara Shelton,MD
Khan,Sophia S.,MD
LaCarrubba Blondin,Lisa,MD
Maslin,Stuart J.,MD
Meeteer,Francis III,DO
Oppenheim,Jeffrey Charles,MD
Pecca,Jo Ann Donna,DO
Pettinelli,Frank P. Jr.,DO
Plasner,Samantha Mara,DO
Sepede,Jennifer,DO
Wilczynski,Frank L.,DO
Gastroenterology
Deitch,Christopher William,MD
Elfant,Adam B.,MD
Ho,Henry C.,MD
Judge,Thomas Aloysius,MD
Lautenslager,Tara Lee,MD
Ockrymiek,Steven B.,DO
Wang,Yize Richard,MD
General Practice
Aji,Wissam,MD
Infectious Disease
Aggrey,Gloria Kangachie,MD
Golden,Richard Frederick,MD
Klinger,Frederick Boyd III,DO
Kraus,Jennifer Lynn,MD
Ng,Kevin,MD
Peterson,John W.,MD
Sumerson,Jeffrey Marc,MD
Topiel,Martin S.,MD
Internal Medicine
Capanescu,Cristina,MD
Castellano,Nicolas Andre,MD
Chaaya,Adib H.,MD
Chelemer,Scott Brain,MD
Feldan,Paul E.,MD
Goldstein,Kenneth Brian,MD
Hamilton,Thanuja Kumari,MD
Khelil,Jennifer Lynn,DO
Shears-Bethke,Tracey M.,MD
Tiu,Evelyn Venzon,MD
Udvarhelyi,Ian Steven,MD
Neurological Surgery
Mitchell,William,MD
Testaiuti,Mark A.,MD
Neurology
Pello,Scott Jason,MD
Obstetrics
McCullen,Kristen Michelle,MD
Obstetrics & Gynecology
Brasile,Deanna Rose,DO
Choe,Jung Kyo,MD
Corley,David R.,MD

Denny,Ashleigh,MD
Jenkins,Lauren Anne,MD
McCrosson,Stacy A.,MD
Noah,Jane S.,MD
Richman,Steven L.,DO
Tucker,Richard G.,MD
Ophthalmology
Vernon,Paul L.,MD
Orthopedic Surgery
Bowers,Andrea Legath,MD
Deutsch,Lawrence Steven,MD
Momi,Kamaldeep S.,MD
Peacock,Kenneth C.,MD
Sapega,Alexander,MD
Schwartz,Mark Glen,MD
Otolaryngology
Carlson,Roy Douglas,MD
Gupta,Ashmit,MD
Pain Medicine
McMurtrie,Robert Jr.,DO
Pain Medicine-Interventional
Medvedovsky,Andrew,MD
Pediatric Urology
Dwosh,Jack,MD
Pediatrics
Ahr,Lawrence M.,MD
Bernstein,Barbara A.,MD
Bruneau,Lara A.,MD
Coutinho Haas,Sunita P.,MD
Creecy,Saundra K.,MD
Nemeth,Nicole Angelina,MD
Weissbach,Debra D.,MD
Physical Medicine & Rehab
Abraham,Mathew John,MD
Jarmain,Scott Joseph,MD
Paul,Michael Joseph,DO
Ragone,Daniel Jr.,MD
Scholl,Seth David,DO
Plastic Surgery
Warren,Ronald M.,MD
Psychiatry
Ansari,Safeer A.,DO
Baruch,Edward M.,MD
Dalkilic,Alican,MD
Hansen,Luke,MD
Kapoor,Ashika Patil,MD
Larkin,Joyce Marie,MD
Richardson,Christie,DO
Rosenkrantz,Leah Ellen,DO
Yang,Jingduan,MD
Public Health
De Masi,Leon Gregory,MD
Pulmonary Disease
Fineman,William,MD
Schriber,Andrew David,MD
Trudo,Frank J.,MD
Radiation Oncology
Kubicek,Gregory John,MD
Radiology
Barry,Kevin P.,MD
Reproductive Endocrinology
Amui,Jewel Naakarley,MD
Check,Jerome H.,MD
Shoulder Surgery
Sidor,Michael Louis,MD
Surgery (General)
Daugherty,Rhett L.,MD
Dube,Neerja,MD
Urology
Becker,Jeffrey M.,MD
Berkman,Douglas S.,MD
Niedrach,William L.,MD
Vascular & Intrvntnal Radiology
Svigals,Paul J.,MD
Mountain Lakes
Cardiovascular Disease
Ahmad,Mehmood R.,MD
Blick,Michael D.,MD
Cook,Guillermo A.,MD
De Renzi,Paul D.,MD
Malagold,Michael,MD
Massari,Ronald D.,MD
Naeem,Sheikh M.,MD
Park,Hyeun Sik,MD
Safirstein,Jordan Glanzman,MD
Shulruff,Stuart E.,MD
Wall,Robert M.,MD
Wang,Robert L.,MD
Dermatology
Cunningham,William J.,MD

Weinstein,Dora Hagar Foa,MD
Family Medicine
Schweitzer,Richard Joseph,MD
Internal Medicine
Dabrowski,Peter A.,MD
Leibowitz,Keith Scott,DO
Shad,Abdur Rauf,MD
Whang,John,MD
Interventional Cardiology
Fusman,Benjamin,MD
Obstetrics & Gynecology
Dreyfuss,Patricia O.,MD
Manlangit,Arsenio C.,MD
Orthopedic Surgery
Silverman,Jesse A.,MD
Pediatrics
Fuloria,Mamta,MD
Psychiatry
Osipuk,Darlene M.,MD
Mountainside
Allergy
Mendelson,Joel S.,MD
Anesthesiology
Fisher,Margaret Elizabeth,MD
Lum,Kenneth,MD
Papa,Louis,MD
Pillon,Mark A.,MD
Rinehouse,Jay A.,MD
Anesthesiology: Pain Medicine
Yanow,Jennifer Hannah,MD
Child (Pediatric) Neurology
Traeger,Eveline C.,MD
Critical Care Medicine
Kleyn,Michael,MD
Developmental Pediatrics
Beckwith,Anna Malia,MD
Malik,Zeenat Q.,MD
Merola,Rose Mary,MD
Prontnicki,Janice L.,MD
Gynecology
Huhn-Werner,Maryann,MD
Internal Medicine
Salvaji,Madhu,DO
Orthopedic Surgery
Warshauer,Jeffrey M.,DO
Otolaryngology
Drake,William III,MD
Presti,Paul Matthew,MD
Pediatric Neurodevelopment
Harris,Brenda D.,MD
Pediatric Rehabilitation
Diamond,Martin,MD
Pediatrics
Aronsky,Adam M.,MD
Cargan,Abba L.,MD
Gozo,Marie O.,MD
Matthews,Tara Anne,MD
Mehta,Uday C.,MD
Velickovic,Marina,MD
Yalamanchi,Krishan,MD
Physical Medicine & Rehab
Armento,Michael,MD
Psychiatry
Bernal,Ileana,MD
Solt,Veronika,MD
Psychiatry&Nrolgy-Special Qual
Okouneva,Evelina,DO
Mullica Hill
Anesthesiology
Shelchkov,Dmitry A.,MD
Diagnostic Radiology
Solomon,Jason S.,MD
Endocrinology
Fox-Mellul,Jodi V.,MD
Family Medicine
Al Hilli,Rula Ahmed,MD
De Dan,Claudine Michele,MD
Herman,Gregory E.,MD
Kent,Maria Candice,MD
Malik,Pooja,MD
Ott,William Augustine,DO
Sprigman,Charles Jeffrey III,DO
Stiefel,Gregory Gene,DO
Wax,Craig M.,DO
Wyche Bullock,Tara Lynette,MD
Zuazua-Pacilio,Maria C.,MD
General Practice
Harris,William G.,MD

Internal Medicine
Bahal,Vishal,DO
Malik,Rajesh,MD
Obstetrics & Gynecology
Beams,Lynsey Marie,DO
O'Flynn,Leisa Diane,DO
Plastic Surgery-Hand
Bidic,Sean Michael,MD
Radiology
Gianchandani,Deepa A.,MD
Surgery (General)
Smeal,Brian C.,MD
Neptune
Addiction Medicine
Neshin,Susan F.,MD
Addiction Psychiatry
Solhkhah,Ramon,MD
Anatomic/Clinical Pathology
Bains,Ashish P. S.,MD
Erler,Brian S.,MD
Govil,Sushama,MD
Matulewicz,Theodore Joseph,MD
Anesthesiology
Berberich,Matthew Robert,MD
Cammarata,Lindsay,MD
Cindrario,Dean P.,MD
Elsakka,Maha Fathy,MD
Fianko,Felix Akwasi-Owusu,MD
Fields,Ryan G.,DO
Kalliny,Mohsen Ayad,MD
Miller,Kevin D.,MD
Morgan,Illiana Alexandrova,MD
Morgan,Mina Adel,DO
Ndeto,Geoffrey Wambua T.,MD
Nicholas,Thomas,MD
Patel,Hansa S.,MD
Patel,Nehul,MD
Rahal,William J.,MD
Ray Jr,Barry Keith,MD
Reffler,Marie M.,MD
Sedutto,Joseph Mario,MD
Steenland,Richard H.,MD
Varghese,Sherin V.,MD
Wu,Jeffrey P.,MD
Yang,Zhaomin,MD
Zhao,Rong,MD
Anesthesiology: Critical Care
Amitie,Daniel Dean,MD
Anesthesiology: Pain Medicine
Miller,Christine Venable,MD
Breast Surgery
Adams,William D.,MD
Cardiovascular Disease
Aaron,Michael R.,DO
Choi,Edward Joung Myung,MD
Chu,Tony Nang-Tang,MD
Colmer,Marc E.,MD
Diwan,Ravi,MD
Gill,Jasrai Singh,MD
Karam,Sara R.,MD
Knight,Michael Robert,MD
Narula,Amar Singh,MD
Okere,Arthur Ezeribe,MD
Orlando,James Frank,MD
Sandler,Leonard Lewis,MD
Weiss,Maurice D.,MD
Yang,Rayson C.,MD
Child & Adolescent Psychiatry
Iofin,Alexander,MD
Kochhar,Seema,MD
Child (Pediatric) Neurology
Pietrucha,Dorothy M.,MD
Sultan,Richard I.,DO
Clinical Cardiac Elctrphyslgy
Girgis,Ihab,MD
Clinical Neurophysiology
Kostoulakos,Paul M.,DO
Developmental Pediatrics
Aloisio,Denise,MD
Roth,Anne G.,DO
Emergency Medicine
Cardinale,Jan Foxman,MD
Discepola,Paul,MD
Dyce,Michael Constantine,MD
Glashow,Marisa Brittany,DO
Goodman,Elliot S.,DO
Jacob,Sharon Leigh,MD
Levinsky,Joseph Judah,MD
Livingston,Denise L.,MD
Marra,Antonio Luigi,DO
McFadden,Kim Marie,MD

Physicians by Town and Medical Specialty

Neptune (cont)
Emergency Medicine
- Mojares, Gregg E., DO
- Panse, Ramanand V., MD
- Pasricha, Atul, DO
- Patel, Rajendra K., MD
- Pillai, Renuka, DO
- Rozwadowski, Thomas J., MD
- Smith, Corey Kamahl, MD
- Sulewski, Agnieszka, DO
- Sweeney, Robert L., DO
- Tapnio, Cezar B., MD
- Trivedi, Darshini, DO
- Wells, Evelyn Ruth, MD

Endocrinology
- Chalasani, Krishna, MD
- Cheng, Jennifer, DO
- Chiniwala, Niyati Umesh, MD
- Holland, Soemiwati Weidris, MD
- Lann, Danielle Erin, MD
- Ong, Raquel Sanchez, MD

Family Med-Sleep Medicine
- Lusk-Caceres, Christina A., DO

Family Medicine
- Dick, Susan E., MD
- Patel, Nitin Suresh, MD

Gastroenterology
- Basri, William E., MD
- Hui, Kenny Pingchi, MD
- Schneiderman, Steven, MD

Geriatrics
- Atienza-Cartnick, Kimberly A., MD
- Masterson, Eileen, MD
- Quinn, Margaret M., MD

Gynecological Oncology
- Bosscher, James Reed, MD

Hospitalist
- Ahmed, Naseer, MD
- Siddiqui, Kamran, MD
- Zamel, Laith Naser, MD

Infectious Disease
- Casey, Kathleen K., MD
- Frank, Elliot, MD
- Fune, Jose M.C., MD
- Kruvant-Gornish, Nancy J., MD
- Kufelnicka, Anna M., MD
- Liu, Edward Wei Chi, MD

Internal Medicine
- Abbud, Ziad A., MD
- Abramowitz, Richard Michael, MD
- Asnani, Sunil, MD
- Bhuskute, Bela Hemant, MD
- Cartnick, Gregory Alan, MD
- Clarkson, Philip W., MD
- Comsti, Maria Virginia, MD
- Demchuk, Beverly Jean, MD
- Felibrico, Oliver G., MD
- Garg, Siddharth Rajesh, MD
- Griggs, Abeer S., DO
- Harris, Kenneth Barton, MD
- Hossain, Mohammad Amir, MD
- Husain, Sara, MD
- Isang, Emmanuel Emmanuel, MD
- Kaplan, Adam Chaim, MD
- Kaunzinger, Christian M., MD
- Kennedy, Daniel F., DO
- Klein, Alan C., MD
- Kosarin, Kristi, DO
- Kretov, Aleksey, MD
- Lapman, Peter Grant, MD
- Liu, Jian, MD
- Llull Tombo, Rolando, MD
- Mahpara, Swaleha, MD
- Meckael, Dina, MD
- Meleka, Matthew, DO
- Mirza, Zainab Arshad, MD
- Morabia, Albert, DO
- Mushtaq, Arman, MD
- Nehmad, Jason Arash, MD
- Nitti, Joseph T., MD
- Odejobi, Lookman K., MD
- Onwuka, Aloysius Chukwumuche, MD
- Patel, Keval V., MD
- Regalman, Elena M., MD
- Roper, Brian K., MD
- Rosenthal, Marnie Elyse, DO
- Sharma, Anuradha, MD
- Sharma, Indu, MD
- Shenouda, Magdy L., MD
- Sijuwade, Atinuke Oluwaseyi, MD
- Steinman, Sharon A., MD
- Strauss, Ira M., MD
- Tarina, Dana Ileana, MD
- Torre, Steven, MD
- Vladu, Cristian, MD

Neonatal-Perinatal Medicine
- Assing, Elizabeth J., MD
- Bautista, Eduardo R., MD
- Browne, Mary Beth, MD
- Graff, Michael A., MD
- Karwowska, Helena, MD
- Ramos, David G.D., MD
- Ross, Ann, MD
- Torine, Ilana J., DO

Nephrology
- Bolarinwa, Oladayo, MD
- Cruz, Dionisio V., MD
- Masud, Avais, MD
- Patel, Mayurkumar P., MD

Neurology
- Baqui, Huma, MD
- Deutsch, Alan D., DO
- Eswar, Anastasia Maria, MD
- Fitzpatrick, John E., MD
- Karia, Roopal M., MD
- Martino, Stephen John, MD
- Rhee, Richard S., MD
- Silbert, Paul J., MD

Obstetrics & Gynecology
- Blechman, Andrew Neal, MD
- Canterino, Joseph C., MD
- Conner, Ellen Louise, MD
- Coyle, Allison A., DO
- ElSahwi, Karim Samir, MD
- Fabricant, Christopher James, MD
- Fumia, Fred Daniel, MD
- Gussman, Debra, MD
- Jacobson, Nina Stella, MD
- Koscica, Karen Lynn, DO
- Matta, Paul Gamal, DO
- Narinedhat, Ralph, MD
- Shavelson, Robert P., MD
- Sprance, Henry Ernest, MD
- Vasquez, Wendelly Judith, MD

Orthopedic Surgery
- Dennis, Robert I., MD
- Schulman, Jared E., MD

Otolaryngology
- Engel, Samuel Henry, MD
- Houston, Sean David, MD
- Mitskavich, Mary T., MD
- Newkirk, Kenneth Allen, MD
- Pflum, Gerald E., MD

Palliative Care
- Frieman, Amy Porter, MD

Pathology
- Zheng, Min, MD

Pediatric Anesthesia
- Vaclavik, Peter Svatopluk, MD

Pediatric Critical Care
- Dadzie, Charles K., MD

Pediatric Emergency Medicine
- Dhebaria, Tina, DO
- Radwan, Hossam S., MD

Pediatric Endocrinology
- Eapen, Santhosh, MD
- Smotkin-Tangorra, Margarita, DO

Pediatric Gastroenterology
- Alfie, Marcos E., MD
- Jimenez, Jennifer E., MD
- Loveridge-Lenza, Beth Anne, DO

Pediatric Hematology Oncology
- Glazier, Kim Steinberg, MD
- Singh, Rohini, MD

Pediatric Pulmonology
- Nakhleh, Nader John, DO

Pediatric Sports Medicine
- Petrucci, James Christopher, DO
- Rice, Stephen G., MD

Pediatrics
- Adler, Bernard H., MD
- Alfonzo, Joann, MD
- Almazan-Atienza, Helen, MD
- Atienza, Kristen A., DO
- Bakhos, Lisa Lovas, MD
- Bal, Aswine Kumar, MD
- Ballance, Cathleen M., MD
- Beckwith-Fickas, Katherine A., MD
- Cabasso, Alan, MD
- Chutke, Prashant Vithal, MD
- Eyerkuss, Emily Abra, DO
- Gapinski, Magdalena Maria, MD
- Heisler, Samantha, DO
- Karatas, Meltem, MD
- Mabanta, Carmelita G., MD
- Naganathan, Srividya, MD
- Nowinowska, Anna, MD
- Pitchumoni, Vinita, MD
- Ponce, Marie Grace C., MD
- Schairer, Janet Lynn, MD
- Shah, Nina M., MD
- Soroush, Azam, MD
- St. Fleur, Rose Martine, MD

Physical Medicine & Rehab
- Levy, Benjamin D., MD

Psychiatry
- Abenante, Frank Andrew, MD
- Cordal, Adriana, MD
- Cruickshank, Royston Raleigh, MD
- Fitzsimmons, Adriana Marie, MD
- Ganime, Peter David, MD
- Graber, Cheryl L., MD
- Hernandez Colon, Agdel Jose, MD
- Manoski, Andrew, DO
- Markowitz, Rachel Paula, MD
- Memon, Hasan, MD
- Rose, Lane Gruber, MD

Radiation Oncology
- Briggs, Jonathan Havens, MD

Rheumatology
- Alpert, Deborah R., MD
- Kuzyshyn, Halyna, MD
- Tang, Xiaoyin, MD

Surgery (General)
- De Sarno, Carney Thomas, MD
- Gorechlad, John W., MD
- Kipnis, Seth Michael, MD
- Mueller, Lawrence Peter, MD
- Shifrin, Alexander L., MD
- Sullivan, Michael C., MD

Surgical Critical Care
- Ahmed, Nasim, MD

Thoracic Surgery
- Dejene, Brook A., MD
- Johnson, David L., MD

Trauma Surgery
- Shin, Seung Hoon, MD

Urology
- Ebani, Jack E., MD
- Tobin, Matthew Steven, MD

Vascular & Intrvntnal Radiology
- Biswal, Rajiv, MD

Vascular Surgery
- Khan, Habib, MD
- Nasir Khan, Mohammad Usman, MD

Neptune City
Anesthesiology
- Amoroso, Michael Louis, MD

Internal Medicine
- Choi, Don W., MD
- Senft, Carl Joseph, MD

Ophthalmology
- Del Negro, Ralph G., DO
- Glatman, Marina, MD

Psychiatry
- Kane, Patrick, MD

Neshanic Station
Emergency Medicine
- Daly, Eileen P., MD

Family Medicine
- Barr, James E., MD
- Dellavalle, Lindsay Joy, DO
- Gertzman-Dafilou, Sharon D., DO
- Rigatti, Damian F., DO

Netcong
Internal Medicine
- Wichman, Paul H., MD

New Brunswick
Allergy & Immunology
- Monteleone, Catherine A., MD

Anatomic Pathology
- Grant, Maurice R., MD
- Rhodes, Roy Harley, MD

Anatomic/Clinical Pathology
- Barnard, Nicola J., MD
- Chaubal, Abhijeet V., MD
- Chekmareva, Marina A., MD
- Dvorzhinskiy, Olga, MD
- Fedorciw, Boris Jaroslaw, MD
- Hazra, Anup K., MD
- Jaworski, Joseph Mark, MD
- Kierson, Malca Ester, DO
- Lal, Devika Sandalee, MD
- Lessig, Marvin A., DO
- Sadimin, Evita T., MD
- Salaru, Gratian, MD
- Thomas, Sumi Varghese, MD
- Weissmann, David J., MD

Anesthesiology
- Alloteh, Rose Sitsofe, MD
- Ambalu, Oren, MD
- Barsoum, Sylviana S., MD
- Berman, Stefanie L., MD
- Bermann, Mordechai, MD
- Chhokra, Renu, MD
- Chi, Oak Z., MD
- Chintapalli, Nirmala K., MD
- Chiricolo, Antonio, MD
- Chyu, Darrick J., MD
- Cirella, Vincent N., MD
- Cohen, Shaul, MD
- Cowell, Jennifer L., MD
- Curcio, Christine Marie, MD
- De Angelis, Vincent James, MD
- Denenberg, Howard W., MD
- Denny, John T., MD
- Enlow, Tracey S., MD
- Fratzola, Christine Hunter, MD
- Fullenkamp, Mark P., MD
- George, Gina, DO
- Ginsberg, Steven H., MD
- Grayer, Nicole C., MD
- Grayson, Jeremy Seth, MD
- Grubb, William R., MD
- Hall, Dennis B., MD
- He, Xiaoli, MD
- Jan, Thomas, MD
- Kandra, Arun M., MD
- Khan, Ibraheem, MD
- Kiel, Samuel Yol, MD
- Kiss, Geza Kalmar, MD
- Klein, Sanford L., MD
- Kraidin, Jonathan L., MD
- Lee, Isidore C., MD
- Lelyanov, Oleksiy, DO
- Lin, Ying Bang, MD
- Mabry, Christian Carl, MD
- Mai, Quynh-Tien, MD
- McRae, Valerie A., MD
- Mehta, Tejal H., MD
- Mungekar, Sagar Sudhir, MD
- Nanavati, Neeraj K., MD
- Nandal, Dharamveer, MD
- Nelson-Lane, Leigh A., MD
- Neustadt, Charles M., MD
- Pantin, Enrique Jose, MD
- Papp, Denes, MD
- Patel, Arpit Nayan, MD
- Perosi, Joseph J., MD
- Radhakrishnan, Radhika, MD
- Rah, Kang H., MD
- Rao, Malini Bhagavathi, MD
- Reformato, Vincent, MD
- Ridley, Diane M., MD
- Shah, Shruti A., MD
- Shah, Trishna Kirit, MD
- Siddiqi, Kashif Inam, MD
- Sison, Edwin Ruan Racela, MD
- Solina, Alann R., MD
- Stein, Mark Herbert, MD
- Tanaka, Sho, MD
- Taylor, Jamie Latiolais, MD
- Thaker, Jayeshkumar, MD
- Veksler, Boris, MD
- Wang, Monty H.S., MD
- Wu, Melissa S., MD
- Zuker-Silberberg, Dora D., MD

Anesthesiology: Pain Medicine
- Amponsah, Akwasi Peprah, MD
- Gajian, Garen Edward, MD
- Yeh, Shihlong, MD

Bloodbanking
- Kuriyan, Mercy Achamma, MD

Cardiothoracic Surgery
- Ghaly, Aziz S., MD
- Lee, Leonard Young, MD
- Lemaire, Anthony, MD
- Prendergast, Thomas William, MD

Cardiovascular Disease
- Cytryn, Richard A., MD
- Hilkert, Robert Joseph, MD
- Iyer, Deepa Balasubramanian, MD
- Jacob, David E., MD
- Jeganathan, Narayanan, MD

Kauh, John S., MD
Krause, Tyrone J., MD
Lacy, Clifton R., MD
Moreyra, Abel E., MD
Shah, Nihir Biharilal, MD
Sharma, Ravinder, MD
Shindler, Daniel M., MD
Turi, Zoltan G., MD
Zakir, Ramzan Muhammad, MD
Cardiovascular Surgery
Scholz, Peter M., MD
Child & Adolescent Psychiatry
Gowda, Nidagalle, MD
Ryan, Colleen A., MD
Child (Pediatric) Neurology
Chaaban, Janti, MD
Di Cicco Bloom, Emanuel M., MD
Esfahanizadeh, Abdolreza, MD
Patel, Payal, MD
Surgan, Victoria, MD
Clinical Genetics
Brooks, Susan Sklower, MD
Day Salvatore, Debra-Lynn, MD
Clinical Neurophysiology
Bhise, Vikram V., MD
Wu, Brenda Yunqing, MD
Clinical Pathology
Deen, Malik F., MD
Clinical Pathology/Laboratory
Kirn, Thomas Joseph Jr., MD
Colon & Rectal Surgery
Eisenstat, Theodore Ellis, MD
Patel, Nell M., MD
Rezac, Craig, MD
Salehomoum, Negar Monavar, MD
Critical Care Medicine
Khan, Talha Ehsan, MD
Madhavan, Arjun, MD
Parikh, Amay, MD
Rana, Haris Ishaque, MD
Rosenfeld, Jane S., MD
Russo, Eileen Susan, MD
Scardella, Anthony T., MD
Sotolongo, Anays M., MD
Sunderram, Jagadeeshan, MD
Cytopathology
Artymyshyn, Renee L., MD
Dermatology
Grossman, Rachel M., MD
Developmental Pediatrics
Jimenez, Manuel, MD
Emerg Medicine-Pediatric
Kalyoussef, Sabah, DO
Emergency Medicine
Amores, Edward Daniel, MD
Arya, Rajiv, MD
Berman, Samantha, MD
Bhavnani, Anita S., MD
Boutsikaris, Daniel Gregory, MD
Bryczkowski, Christopher J., MD
Bucher, Joshua Thomas, MD
Chin, Meigra Myers, MD
Choi, Michael Namkyu, MD
Church, Amy F., MD
Collins, John Joseph III, MD
Corcoran, Gregory, MD
Cuthbert, Darren Patrick, MD
Dallhoff, Maureen Elizabeth, MD
Dalton, Mark J K, MD
Donovan, Colleen Mary, MD
Eisenstein, Robert Mark, MD
Garcia, Guillermo A., MD
Geria, Rajesh Navin, MD
Gupta, Chiraag U., MD
Hackett, Gladston Randall, MD
Hochberg, Michael Lawrence, MD
Kapitanyan, Raffi S., MD
Leung, Winifred Fong, MD
Lewis, Brent Mckeen, MD
Lustiger, Eliyahu Y., MD
Marcinow, Justyna, MD
Marques Baptista, Andreia, MD
McCarthy, Christopher M., MD
McCoy, Jonathan V., MD
McGill, Dennis L., MD
Mirza, Michael Rohinton, MD
Morrison, Daniel Scott, MD
O'Connor, Andrew, MD
Patel, Mayuri, MD
Patil, Pooja Mittal, MD
Phillips, Michelle Nicole, MD

Pirigyi, Paul R., MD
Punjabi, Kusum A., MD
Riaz, Adnan, MD
Rice, Daniel, MD
Riggs, Renee Lisa, DO
Ryave, Steven Samuel, MD
Shah, Chirag N., MD
Simon, Riya Jose, DO
Snyder, Laura Jean, MD
Van Volkenburgh, Robert John, MD
Veysman, Boris D., MD
Wei, Grant, MD
Yang, Anthony, MD
Yoon, Kyung In, MD
Endocrinology
Amorosa, Louis F., MD
Chakravarthy, Manu V., MD
Kolaczynski, Jerzy Wiktor, MD
Luo, Hongxiu, MD
Meininger, Gary Edward, MD
Murthy, Meena S., MD
Ohri, Anupam, MD
Orloff, John J., MD
Santora, Arthur Charles II, MD
Schneider, Stephen H., MD
Shulman, Leon H., MD
Van Hoven, Anne Marie, MD
Waldstreicher, Joanne, MD
Wang, Xiangbing, MD
Wondisford, Frederic Edward, MD
Family Medicine
Acevedo, Rhina A., MD
Afran, Joyce G., MD
Bhatt, Komal Gopalbhai, MD
Botti, Carla G., DO
Clark, Elizabeth C., MD
Cole, Janet M., MD
Foley, James, MD
Hammond, Betty L., MD
Headley, Adrienne J., MD
Heath, Cathryn Batutis, MD
Heath, John Michael, MD
Hill, Eileen G., MD
Howarth, David F., MD
Kropa, Jill, MD
Lasky, Melodee S., MD
Laumbach, Sonia Caridad G., MD
Levin, Steven Jonathan, MD
Levine, Jeffrey Pierre, MD
Like, Robert C., MD
Lin, Karen Wei-Ru, MD
McGarry, Barbara J., MD
Mena, Jessica, DO
Miller, Ralee Ka, MD
Mokhashi, Sajida Habib, MD
Morton, Kinshasa C., MD
Newrock, William J., MD
Noll, Michael Andrew, MD
O'Connor, Robert M., MD
Reinsdorf, Keith Alan, MD
Roemheld-Hamm, Beatrix, MD
Siddiqui, Sheraz U., MD
Sliwowska, Anna, MD
Steinlight, Sasha Juli, MD
Suaray, Mafudia Abibatu, MD
Swee, David E., MD
Tallia, Alfred F., MD
Ulloque, Rory Alexander, MD
Virani, Zahra N., MD
Wang, Yue He, MD
Womack, Jason Peter, MD
Wu, Justine Peen, MD
Gastroenterology
Bhargava, Sandeep, MD
Broder, Arkady, MD
Chokhavatia, Sita Shashikant, MD
Das, Kiron M., MD
Griffel, Louis H., MD
Maltz, Gary S., MD
Manoukian, Aram V., MD
Pooran, Nakechand Rai, MD
Rampertab, Saroja Devi, MD
Velpari, Sugirdhana, MD
General Practice
Grabell, Daniel, MD
Geriatric Psychiatry
Gabrial, Irene Gamalnoub, MD
Geriatrics
Brodt, Zahava Nilly, MD
Kothari, Nayan K., MD
Moondra, Palak, DO

Gynecological Oncology
Goldberg, Michael I., MD
Hellmann, Mira C., MD
Isani, Sara, MD
Gynecology
Mitra, Anjali Naz, MD
Hematology
Eid, Joseph E., MD
Gulli, Vito M., MD
Rose, Shelonitda S., MD
Strair, Roger Kurt, MD
Hematology Oncology
Bannerji, Rajat, MD
David, Kevin Andrew, MD
Desai, Vidhi Parikh, MD
Evens, Andrew M., DO
Ganesan, Shridar, MD
Karantza-Wadsworth, Vassiliki, MD
Kritharis-Agrusa, Athena, MD
Philipp, Claire S., MD
Saraiya, Biren P., MD
Sridharan, Ashwin, MD
Stein, Mark Nathan, MD
Hematopathology
Bhagavathi, Sharathkumar M., MD
Hospitalist
Pulijaal, Pooja, MD
Infectious Disease
Alcid, David V., MD
Bhowmick, Tanaya, MD
Boruchoff, Susan E., MD
Suarez, Militza E., MD
Veeraswamy, Pramila, MD
Weinstein, Melvin P., MD
Internal Med-Sleep Medicine
Chen, Jennifer Yu-Chia, MD
Internal Medicine
Aisner, Joseph, MD
Ali, Sadia Y., MD
Almendral, Jesus L., MD
Amir, Saba, MD
Anand, Kapil, MD
Aras, Rohit S., DO
Armas-Loughran, Barbara J., MD
Ayangade, Tolulope, MD
Bershad, Joshua Marin, MD
Borham, Amanda Ahmed Fouad, MD
Carson, Jeffrey L., MD
Chen, Catherine, MD
Cornett, Julia Kang, MD
Coromilas, James, MD
Czaja, Matthew T., MD
Dave, Payal, MD
Desai, Avani Mahesh, MD
Desai, Neel, MD
Duffoo, Frantz Michel, MD
Elshinawy, Ashgan A., DO
Fayyaz, Imran, MD
Ferrari, Anna C., MD
Ferreira, Gabriela Simoes, MD
Ferro, Joseph James, MD
Florou, Vaia, MD
Francis, Charles Kenneth, MD
Fujita, Kenji Peter, MD
Gaioni, Kathleen A., MD
George, Renu, MD
Gozzo, Yvette Marie, MD
Grimes, Julia P., DO
Gupta, Angela, MD
Hait, William N., MD
Handelsman, Cory, MD
Hastings, Shirin Elizabeth, MD
Herrigel, Dana J., MD
Hirshfeld, Kim Marie, MD
Hogshire, Lauren Christine, MD
Hsu, Vivien M., MD
Hussain, Sabiha, MD
Isaac, Fikry W., MD
Iwata, Isao, MD
Jacob, Sneha Elizabeth, MD
Jahn, Eric G., MD
Juneau, Jeffrey Evan, MD
Kalra, Rakhi, MD
Khan, Imran Ahmad, MD
Kim, Sarang, MD
Kolli, Sudha Rani, MD
Korman, Linda Z., MD
Kostis, William J., MD
Kountz, David S., MD
Kumar, Akshat, MD
Labinson, Robert M., MD

Larose, Jean Eddy, DO
Lavizzo Mourey, Risa Juanita, MD
Lenza, Christopher, DO
Leventhal, Elaine A., MD
Lewis, Beth G., MD
Li, Xuemei, MD
Liang, Hongyan, MD
Lianos, Elias A., MD
Liu, Charles Li-Chen, MD
Lubitz, Sara Elisabeth, MD
Magliocco, Melissa Amy, MD
Mahal, Mona, MD
Majumdar, Sourav, MD
Manoraj, Vinita, MD
Marcella, Stephen W., MD
McAuliffe, Vincent J., MD
Mehta, Smita, MD
Methvin, Laura, MD
Mohan, Janani, MD
Moss, Rebecca Anne, MD
Moussa, Issam, MD
Mustafa, Muhammad A., MD
Nagella, Naresh, MD
Palaniswamy, Guhapriya, MD
Pamidi, Madhavi, MD
Parikh, Sahil, MD
Patel, Anish Vinit, MD
Patel, Archana I., MD
Patel, Arpit K., MD
Patel, Manish Surendra, MD
Patel, Sachin S., MD
Patel, Vimal Dahya, MD
Peskin, Steven R., MD
Platt, Heather L., MD
Poplin, Elizabeth A., MD
Prister, James Dmitry, MD
Puing, Alfredo Gonzalo, MD
Radbel, Jared Michael, MD
Rahman, Mahboob Ur, MD
Rana, Swetha Basani, MD
Ranjini, Mary P., MD
Rao, Megha N., MD
Raoof, Sidra, MD
Rasool, Altaf Tahir, MD
Ravindran, Nishal Cholapurath, MD
Reddy, Jayant T., MD
Reinhardt, Rickey R., MD
Riley, David J., MD
Sachinwalla, Eric M., MD
Salsali, Afshin, MD
Sanchez, Sergio, MD
Sarkar, Abhishek, MD
Sathya, Bharath, MD
Saxena, Mark, MD
Schneiderman, Joyce F., MD
Seril, Darren Neil, MD
Setoguchi Iwata, Soko, MD
Shah, Himani, MD
Shah, Ushma R., MD
Sharma, Anupa, DO
Sharma, Ranita, MD
Sharma, Rashi, MD
Sherman, Richard A., MD
Shtindler, Feliks, MD
Sitrin, Edith S., MD
Sonnenberg, Frank A., MD
Sonyey, Alexandra Yevgenyevna, MD
Srivastava, Nilam, MD
Stein, Peter Paris, MD
Steinberg, Michael Barry, MD
Stricoff, Alan L., DO
Surakanti, Sujani Ganga, MD
Targino, Marcelo Cordeiro, MD
Toppmeyer, Deborah Lynn, MD
Vagaonescu, Tudor Dumitru, MD
Vo, Hung Nam, MD
Walker, John A., MD
Wei, Catherine, MD
Willett, Laura R., MD
Wimalawansa, Sunil J., MD
Wong, Robert L., MD
Wong, Serena Tsan-Lai, MD
Zheng, Xin, MD
Maternal & Fetal Medicine
Martins, Maria Emilia, MD
Ranzini, Angela C., MD
Santolaya, Joaquin, MD
Schuster, Meike, DO
Vintzileos, Anthony M., MD
Med Genetics-Mole Genetic Pthlg
Galkowski, Dariusz Bohdan, MD

Physicians by Town and Medical Specialty

New Brunswick (cont)

Medical Oncology
Cooper, Dennis Lawrence, MD
Eleff, Michael, MD
Gharibo, Mecide M., MD
Groisberg, Roman, MD
Mayer, Tina Marie, MD
Mehnert, Janice M., MD
Munshi, Pashna N., MD
Schaar, Dale G., MD

Neonatal-Perinatal Medicine
Akhter, Waseem, MD
Anwar, Mujahid, MD
Bakare, Olubunmi, MD
Chandra, Shakuntala N., MD
Hegyi, Thomas, MD
Herrera-Garcia, Guadalupe, DO
Hiatt, I. Mark, MD
Kaushik, Sridhar, MD
Khalil, Marwa A., MD
Khan, Imteyaz Ahmad, MD
Lambert, George H., MD
Mehta, Rajeev, MD
Memon, Naureen, MD
Puvabanditsin, Surasak, MD
Weinberger, Barry I., MD

Nephrology
Akhtar, Rabia, MD
Bunin, Sonalis, MD
Khalil, Steve, MD
Lefavour, Gertrude S., MD
Mann, Richard A., MD
Mondal, Zahidul Hoque, MD
Palan, Vandana A., MD
Puri, Sonika, MD

Neurological Surgery
Danish, Shabbar F., MD
Gupta, Gaurav, MD
Nosko, Michael G., MD

Neurology
Aiken, Robert Dennis, MD
Balashov, Konstantin E., MD
Belsh, Jerry M., MD
Dhib Jalbut, Suhayl S., MD
Gerhardstein, Brian Lee, MD
Golbe, Lawrence I., MD
Johnson, William Gessner, MD
Khelemsky, Serge, DO
Lastra, Carlos R., MD
Leitch, Megan Moran, MD
Lepore, Frederick E., MD
Mani, Ram, MD
Mark, Margery H., MD
Mouradian, Mary Maral, MD
Patel, Bindi Akshay, DO
Sage, Jacob I., MD
Schneider, Daniel Paul, MD
Sivaraaman, Kartik, MD
Wong, Stephen, MD

Obstetrics
Awomolo, Adeola, MD
Farkas, Andrew, MD
Ho, Diana, MD

Obstetrics & Gynecology
Adigun, Akeem Segun, MD
Aurora, Nadia, MD
Ayers, Charletta A., MD
Bachmann, Gloria A., MD
Baffo, Aileen, MD
Baldwin, Kimberly Staton, MD
Balica, Adrian Claudiu, MD
Beim, Robert B., MD
Beiter, Kyle Aaron, MD
Chavez, Martin R., MD
Cheng, Ru-Fong J., MD
Cioffi, Francis J., MD
Cruz Ithier, Mayra Alejandra, MD
Di Stefano, Valeria M., MD
Dolitsky, Shelley Nicole, MD
Ebert, Gary A., MD
Faro, Revital D., MD
Francis, Amanda Rachael, DO
Gilmandyar, Dzhamala, MD
Glatthorn, Haley, MD
Goldberg, Leah, MD
Green, Ashlee, MD
Hadaya, Ola, MD
Herreros, Claudia, MD
Hollingsworth, Jessie, MD
Hutchinson-Colas, Juana A., MD
Jadhav, Ashwin R., MD

Jasani, Sona, MD
Jayakumaran, Jenani Sarah, MD
Jenci, Joseph D., MD
Kaminsky, Lillian M., MD
Kemmann, Ekkehard, MD
Kicenuik, Michael T., MD
Kohut, Adrian, MD
Lynch, Caroline Dorothy, MD
MacMillan, William Emery, MD
Magliaro, Thomas J., MD
Merjanian, Lena L., MD
Mokrzycki, Mark L., MD
Naqvi, Fatima, MD
Ng, June Hoi Ka, MD
Palomares, Kristy T., MD
Patel, Amy J., MD
Patel, Jharna Mehul, MD
Phillips, Nancy A., MD
Pradhan, Archana, MD
Preminger, Michele Lynn, MD
Rosen, Todd Joshua, MD
Sauer, Mark Victor, MD
Schultz, Pamela Sue, MD
Segal, Saya, MD
Sinofsky, Francine E., MD
Song, Mi-Hae, MD
Stechna, Sharon Beth, MD
Stewart, Richard Allen, DO
Washington, Monica Michaelle, MD
Yoo, Nina, MD
Yousef, Mona E., MD

Oncological Surgery
August, David A., MD
Goydos, James S., MD
Katz, Anna Beth, MD
Kennedy, Timothy John, MD
Koshenkov, Vadim P., MD

Oncology
Weiss, Robert Edward, MD

Ophthalmology
Fine, Howard Frederick, MD
Friedman, Eric Stephen, MD
Green, Stuart N., MD
Keyser, Bruce J., MD
Leff, Steven R., MD
Mobin Uddin, Omar, MD
Prenner, Jonathan Lawrence, MD
Roth, Daniel Benjamin, MD
Shah, Sumit Pravinkumar, MD
Wheatley, Harold M., MD

Orthopedic Surgery
Erickson, John A., MD
Fried, Steven H., MD
Hyatt, Adam Extein, MD
Ros, Stephen Joseph, MD
Sathyendra, Vikram Modur, MD
Selby, Ronald M., MD

Orthopedic Surgery-Adult Rcnstr
Jonna, Venkata Karthik, MD

Otolaryngology
Ahmadi, David, MD
Assad, Albert, MD
Goldrich, Michael Seth, MD
Kwong, Kelvin Ming-Tak, MD

Otolaryngology-Facial Plastic
Esmail, Ali Raza, MD
Vella, Joseph Bayer, MD

Pain Medicine
Sakr, Ashraf M., MD

Pathology
Cadoff, Evan M., MD
Fox, Melissa D., MD
Fyfe-Kirschner, Billie Shawn, MD
Gamboa, Elmer Salvador, MD
Goodell, Lauri A., MD
Javidian, Parisa, MD
May, Michael S., MD
Olmo Durham, Zaida E., MD
Schwarz, Karl O., MD
Shen Schwarz, Susan C., MD
Tenorio, Grace Cipres, MD
Wang, Qi, MD

Pediatric Anesthesia
Perez, Jessica, MD

Pediatric Cardiology
Cohen, Michele Marie-Liz, DO
Gaffney, Joseph W., MD
Manduley, Robert Alfred, MD
Weinberger, Sharon M., MD

Pediatric Critical Care
Bojko, Thomas, MD

Dallessio, Joseph J., MD
Das, Sumon Kumar, MD
Grossman, Bruce Jay, MD
MacCarrick, Matthew Joseph, MD
McDonough, Christian P., MD
O'Reilly, Colin R., DO
The, Tiong Gwan, MD
Williams-Phillips, Jacqueline, MD

Pediatric Emergency Medicine
Baszak, Sylvia, MD
Do, Minh-Tu, MD
Miele, Niel F., MD

Pediatric Endocrinology
Ergun-Longmire, Berrin, MD
Gangat, Mariam A., MD
Salas, Max, MD
Xu, Weizhen, MD

Pediatric Gastroenterology
Chen, Yen Ping, MD
Gill, Rupinder K., MD
Weidner, Melissa, MD

Pediatric Hematology Oncology
Drachtman, Richard A., MD
Iacobas, Ionela, MD
Lewis, Jocelyn A., DO
Masterson, Margaret, MD
Michaels, Lisa A., MD
Murphy, Susan M., MD
Pan, Wilbur James, MD

Pediatric Infectious Diseases
Gaur, Sunanda, MD
Malhotra, Amisha, MD
Whitley-Williams, Patricia, MD

Pediatric Nephrology
Weiss, Lynne S., MD

Pediatric Otolaryngology
Chee, Michael Y., MD
Traquina, Diana Nogueira, MD

Pediatric Pulmonology
Singh, Archana, MD

Pediatric Sports Medicine
Goodman, Arlene Michelle, MD
Kenton, Alicia Nicole, MD

Pediatric Surgery
Gallucci, John Gerard, MD
Marchildon, Michael B., MD
Pierre, Joelle, MD
Ruzicka, Petr O., MD

Pediatric Urology
Barone, Joseph G., MD

Pediatrics
Abreu, Arnaldo J., MD
Alemu, Kidist, MD
Amara, Shobha, MD
Amato, Indira L., MD
Babcock, Karen R., MD
Baddi, Anoosha, DO
Bahadur, Kandy, MD
Balachandar, Sadana, MD
Bernstein, William R., MD
Boneparth, Alexis D., MD
Borole, Swapna M., MD
Bruno, Chantal Dominique, DO
Bryan, Sheila Curry, MD
Byrom, Abbie R., MD
Cangemi, Carla Primiani, MD
Carlson, Joann Marie, MD
Chalikonda, Bhavani Prasad, MD
Chalom, Rene, MD
Chefitz, Dalya L., MD
Chundru, Vasudha, MD
Cohen, Stephanie Gail, MD
Craig, Vicki L., MD
Diaz, Laura M., MD
Fantasia, Michele Elaine, MD
Fleming, Jacqueline, MD
Grieco, Rachael D., MD
Gurkan, Sevgi, MD
Hauck, Lisanne Constance, MD
Hodgson, Elizabeth Susan, MD
Horton, Daniel B., MD
Infantino, Dorian, MD
Ingram, Karen M., MD
Iofel, Elizaveta, MD
Jonna, Siva Prasad, MD
Jyonouchi, Harumi, MD
Kairys, Steven W., MD
Kaliyadan, George, MD
Kashyap, Arun Kumar, MD
Kaur, Harpreet, MD
Kaur, Harsohena, MD

Kelly, Michael John, MD
Kendall, Roxanne E., MD
Khosla, Meenakshi, MD
Koniaris, Soula G., MD
Korn, Elizabeth Amy, MD
Lam, Jennifer, MD
Lentzner, Benjamin Joseph, MD
Leupold, Kerry Lynn, DO
Leva, Ernest G., MD
Lopez, Christina Clare, DO
Lucas, Michael Joseph, MD
Mahalingam, Rajeshwari S., MD
Malkani, Raj S., MD
Marina, Adele Nabieh, MD
Marshall, Ian, MD
McCaig, Misty, MD
McInnes, Andrew Duncan, MD
Medina, Gladibel, MD
Mody, Kalgi, MD
Moorthy, Lakshmi Nandini, MD
Ohngemach, Christopher, MD
Ojadi, Vallier Chidiebere, MD
Owensby, Jennifer Rita, MD
Parlow, Brittany, MD
Patel, Bipinchand N., MD
Pelliccia, Frances B., MD
Pepper, Matthew Philip, MD
Poelstra, Beverly A., MD
Pratt, Amanda, MD
Quintero-Solivan, Juliette M., MD
Ramachandran, Usha, MD
Ramagopal, Maya, MD
Reich, Joseph I., MD
Relvas, Monica De Stefani, MD
Rhoads, Frances A., MD
Rojas, Paulina Elena, MD
Rosenthal, Susan R., MD
Rossman, Ian T., MD
Sanghani, Nipa Vijay, MD
Santiago, Marivic F., MD
Seshadri, Kapila, MD
Sharma, Archana, DO
Sharma, Priti, MD
Strozuk-McDonough, Stephanie, MD
Suell, Jeffrey, MD
Takyi, Michele, MD
Tetteh, Shirley S., MD
Thompson, Dawn Dorel, MD
Uppaluri, Lakshmi P., MD
Weiss, Aaron R., DO
Weller, Alan Scott, MD
Wenger, Peter N., MD
Whyte, Peta-Gaye Kenisha, DO
Yerramilli, Ramalakshmi V., MD
Zaghloul, Nibal Ahmad, MD
Zalewitz, Jodi Michelle, MD
Zimmerman-Bier, Barbie L., MD
Zuber, Janie Anne, MD

Plastic Surgery
Ahuja, Naveen K., MD
Vankouwenberg, Emily, MD
Wey, Philip D., MD

Psychiatry
Anim, Candy Kyewaa, MD
Babalola, Ronke Latifatu, MD
Bisen, Viwek Singh, DO
Cowen, Daniel S., MD
Doubrava, Suzanne M., MD
Efremova, Irina Vladimirovna, MD
Escobar, Javier I., MD
Garcia, Maria E., MD
Herridge, Peter Lamont, MD
Huan, Victoria Y., MD
Maddaiah, Shaila N., MD
Marin, Humberto, MD
Nazia, Yasmin, MD
Sanjuan, Racquel, DO
Shaikh, Najmussaha M., MD
Swigar, Mary E., MD
Tiu, Gladys Tompar, MD
Trenton, Adam James, DO

Pulmonary Disease
Ash, Carol E., DO
Frenia, Douglas Scott, MD
Rao, Harshit S., MD
Santiago, Teodoro V., MD
Sexauer, William Patrick, MD
Trontell, Marie C., MD

Radiation Oncology
Desai, Gopal Rao, MD
Goyal, Sharad, MD

Haffty,Bruce George,MD
Hathout,Lara,MD
Jabbour,Salma K.,MD
Khan,Atif Jalees,MD
Kim,Sung N.,MD
Mahmoud,Omar M.,MD
McKenna,Michael G.,MD
Motwani,Sabin B.,MD
Parikh,Dhwani R.,MD
Wallach,Jonathan Brett,MD
Weiner,Joseph Paul,MD
Rheumatology
Pabolu,Sangeetha,MD
Park,Kyle Yoonho,MD
Schlesinger-Kamelgard,Naomi,MD
Sloan,Victor S.,MD
Sleep Disorders Medicine
Ekekwe,Ikemefula E.,MD
Surgery (General)
Baler,Carleton E.,MD
Bulauitan,Constantine S.,MD
Carpizo,Darren Richard,MD
Christian,Derick J.,MD
Corbett,Siobhan Alden,MD
Davidov,Tomer,MD
Ghisletta,Leslie C.,MD
Grandhi,Miral Sadaria,MD
Gupta,Rajan,MD
Haque,Maahir Ul,MD
Holman,Michael Jeffrey,MD
Jayakumar,Lalithapriya,MD
Kowzun,Maria Ji,MD
Langenfeld,John Eugene,MD
Laskow,David A.,MD
Lopez,Aurelia P.,MD
Masterson,Richard J.,MD
Mellender,Scott Jason,MD
Palder,Steven B.,MD
Pelletier,Ronald Paul,MD
Qudah,Yaqeen,MD
Schroeder,Mary E.,MD
Shan,Yizhi,MD
Shiroff,Adam Michael,MD
Sim,Vasiliy,MD
Sterling,Joshua,MD
Terlizzi,Joseph P.,MD
Tinti,Meredith Sarah,MD
Trooskin,Stanley Zachary,MD
Wise,Susannah S.,MD
Zavotsky,Jeffry,MD
Surgical Critical Care
Gracias,Vicente H.,MD
Hanna,Joseph S.,MD
Lissauer,Matthew Eric,MD
Peck,Gregory Lance,DO
Therapeutic Radiology
Cohler,Alan,MD
Thoracic Surgery
Batsides,George Pete,MD
Choi,Chun W.,MD
Ikegami,Hirohisa,MD
Nishimura,Takashi,MD
Spotnitz,Alan J.,MD
Trauma Surgery
Butts,Christopher Alan,DO
Teichman,Amanda Liane,MD
Urology
Davis,Rachel B.,MD
Elsamra,Sammy E.,MD
Faiena,Izak,MD
Goldsmith,Joel W.,MD
Jang,Thomas Lee,MD
Kim,Isaac Yi,MD
Olweny,Ephrem Odoy,MD
Parihar,Jaspreet Singh,MD
Singer,Eric Alan,MD
Tunuguntla,Hari Siva Gurun,MD
Vascular Neurology
Paolucci,Ugo,MD
Rybinnik,Igor,MD
Vascular Surgery
Beckerman,William,MD
Cha,Andrew,DO
Crowley,John G.,MD
Rahimi,Saum Amir,MD
Rao,Niranjan V.,MD
Shafritz,Randy,MD
New Lisbon
Anatomic/Clinical Pathology
Desai,Hemlata K.,MD

Family Medicine
Johnson,Deborah Anne,MD
Keefer,Keith J.,MD
General Practice
Cavan,Clodoveo N.,MD
Co,Dominador A.,MD
Geriatrics
Mouliswar,Mysore P.,MD
Internal Medicine
Buddala,Sangeeta,MD
El-Harazy,Essam,MD
Psychiatry
Geller,Ian B.,DO
New Milford
Internal Medicine
Chang,Michael Poyin,MD
Doiranlis,Zenaida P.,MD
Ophthalmology
Carabin,Gari D.,MD
Pediatrics
Goyco,Emelina A.,MD
New Providence
Adolescent Medicine
Moskowitz,Steven,MD
Cardiovascular Disease
Farry,John Patrick,MD
Glasofer,Sidney,MD
Mich,Robert John,MD
Rosenthal,Todd Michael,MD
Diagnostic Radiology
Gowali,Neha M.,MD
Printz,David A.,MD
Schneider,Benjamin Mark,MD
Family Medicine
Calderon,Mark J.,MD
Martinetti,Lorenzo G.,MD
Geriatrics
Holcomb,Brenda E.,DO
Internal Medicine
Bartov,David Nir,MD
Bhargava,Ruta Manish,MD
Brown,Teresa V.,DO
Hakim,James J.,MD
Kewalramani,Kavita Rajiv,MD
Sheris,Steven Jay,MD
Zukoff,Paul B.,MD
Obstetrics & Gynecology
Barresi,Joseph A.,MD
Gibbons,Alice B.,MD
Ophthalmology
Leventhal,Todd Owen,MD
Wong,Charissa J.,MD
Pediatrics
Chin,Kathleen L.,MD
Cuddihy,Kathleen Marie,MD
Shih,Eunhee,MD
Visci,Denise,MD
Psychiatry
Hidalgo,Marla,MD
Pesci,Paula M.,MD
New Vernon
Anesthesiology
Sheren,Lorne B.,MD
Newark
Addiction Psychiatry
Zerbo,Erin Alexandra,MD
Adolescent Medicine
Bentsianov,Sari,MD
Britt,Howard S.,MD
Dhar,Veena,MD
Johnson,Robert Lee,MD
Adult Psychiatry
Nagy-Hallet,Andrea,MD
Allergy
Kanumury,Sunita,MD
Rescigno,Ronald J.,MD
Schutzer,Steven E.,MD
Anatomic Pathology
Aisner,Seena C.,MD
Cho,Eun-Sook,MD
Hua,Zhongxue,MD
Mazzella,Fermina Maria,MD
Anatomic/Clinical Pathology
Adem,Patricia V.,MD
D'Cruz,Cyril A.,MD
Dorai,Bhuvaneswari,MD
Fitzhugh,Valerie A.,MD
Gonzalez,Mario Segundo,MD
Jobbagy,Zsolt,MD
Klein,Kenneth Michael,MD

Mirani,Neena M.,MD
Olesnicky,Ludmilla,MD
Panayotov,Panayot Panchev,MD
Parikh,Nalini S.,MD
Perez,Lyla E.,MD
Seguerra,Eliezer Montero Jr.,MD
Tsang,Patricia Chiu-Wun,MD
Ye,Michelle,MD
Zhang,Alex Xun,MD
Anesthesiology
Abadi,Bilal,MD
Amuluru,Prabhakara,MD
Atlas,Glen Mark,MD
Aziz,Rania,MD
Berger,Jay Steven,MD
Botea,Andrei,MD
Burducea,Alexandru,DO
Capalbo,Vincent J.,MD
Chan,Jose R.,MD
Chaudhry,Faraz A.,MD
Chen,Dong,MD
Chinn,Lawrence W. Sr.,MD
Delphin,Ellise S.,MD
Discepola,Patrick Joseph,MD
Eloy,Jean D.,MD
Estrada,Christian,MD
Freda,John Jeffrey,MD
Gajewski,Michael M.,DO
Goldstein,Sheldon,MD
Grant,Geordie P.,MD
Grewal,Harpreet Singh,MD
Gubenko,Yuriy Aronovich,MD
Jackson,Douglas T.,MD
Jhaveri,Lajwanti R.,MD
Katz,John W. Jr.,MD
Kaufman,Andrew Greg,MD
Komer,Claudia A.,DO
Korban,Anna,MD
Li,Dongchen,MD
Liao,Wu-Fei,MD
Louis,Vely Anthony,MD
Madubuko,Uchenna Anthony,MD
Malapero,Raymond Joseph III,MD
Marji,Michael Suleiman,MD
Maurrasse,Corazon C.,MD
Modi,Nita K.,MD
Moon,Kyoung,MD
Moore,Ross Edward,MD
Morris,Kevin Michael,MD
Napuli,Maximo C.,MD
Pakonis,Gregory Vytautas,MD
Patel,Anuradha P.,MD
Ponnudurai,Rex N.,MD
Potian,Marcelino M.,MD
Raval,Rajendra R.,MD
Rodriguez Correa,Daniel T.,MD
Ru,Xun,MD
Rubin,Benjamin,MD
Saffran,Scott Robert,MD
Sahota,Manpreet S.,MD
Sakellaris,Leander D.,MD
Tan,Royland C.,MD
Tilak,Vasanti A.,MD
Tolentino,Eduardo D.,MD
Wei,Pan-Son,MD
Whalen,Kathryn,MD
Xiong,Ming,MD
Zaslavsky,Alexander,MD
Zwolska-Demczuk,Barbara A.,MD
Anesthesiology: Addiction Med
Elhelw,Ramy,MD
Anesthesiology: Pain Medicine
Chiu,Chi-Shin,MD
Iannaccone,Ferdinand,DO
Rahman,Owen R.,MD
Sifonios,Anthony N.,MD
Bloodbanking
Koshy,Ranie,MD
Cardiothoracic Surgery
Russo,Mark Joseph,MD
Cardiovascular Disease
Ahmed,Shaikh Sultan,MD
Amponsah,Michael Kwesi,MD
Asif,Mohammad,MD
Atherley,Trevor H.,MD
Chen,Chunguang,MD
Cohen,Marc,MD
Dailey-Sterling,Felix G.,MD
DeCosimo,Diana R.,MD
Gidea,Claudia Gabriela,MD
Goldfarb,Irvin D.,MD
Goldstein,Jonathan Edward,MD

Ishikawa,Yoshihiro,MD
Klapholz,Marc,MD
Madan,Pankaj,MD
Nawaz,Yassir,MD
Ribner,Hillel S.,MD
Rothbart,Stephen T.,MD
Rubinstein,Hector T.,MD
Saric,Muhamed,MD
Shamoon,Fayez E.,MD
Solanki,Pallavi S.,MD
Tsyvine,Daniel,MD
Waller,Alfonso Hillman,MD
Wasty,Najam,MD
Zucker,Mark J.,MD
Cardiovascular Surgery
Herman,Steven Douglas,MD
Karanam,Ravindra N.,MD
Child & Adolescent Psychiatry
Bhatt,Usha Praful,MD
Chacko-Varkey,Suneeta Esther,MD
Gude,Prabhavat Venkata,MD
Isecke,Dorothy Ann,MD
Power,Rachael Reiko,MD
Riaz,Najeeb,MD
Yangchen,Tenzing,MD
Child (Pediatric) Neurology
Hayes Rosen,Caroline Diane,MD
Pak,Jayoung,MD
Salam,Misbah U.,MD
Clinical Cytogenetics
Toruner,Gokce,MD
Clinical Genetics
Pletcher,Beth A.,MD
Clinical Pathology
Grygotis,Anthony E.,MD
Jin,Li,MD
Colon & Rectal Surgery
Rice,Peter Eric,MD
Critical Care Medicine
Abdeen,Yazan M.,MD
Adelman,Marc R.,MD
Chang,Steven Yang-Liang,MD
Fless,Kristin Gail,MD
Lardizabal,Alfred A.,MD
MacBruce,Daphne Karen,MD
Miller,Richard A.,MD
Sadik,Aseel,MD
Dermatology
Schwartz,Robert Allen,MD
Diagnostic Radiology
Blacksin,Marcia F.,MD
Chaudhry,Humaira S.,MD
Durojaye,Abike Ogunrenike,MD
Goldfarb,Helene,MD
Goldschmiedt,Judah,MD
Green,Jeremy Charles,MD
Hinrichs,Clay Robert,MD
Jedynak,Andrzej R.,MD
Lee,Huey J.,MD
Maldjian,Pierre D.,MD
Mele,Christopher Mark,MD
Patel,Shashikant A.,MD
Snellings,Richard Barton,MD
Tairu,Oluwole Ayodeji,MD
Thomas,Prashant Jacob,MD
Wachsberg,Ronald H.,MD
Electromyography
Stitik,Todd P.,MD
Emerg Medicine-Pediatric
Sinha,Virteeka,MD
Emergency Medical Services
Ariyaprakai,Navin,MD
VonBose,Michael J.,MD
Emergency Medicine
Afonso,Tania A.,DO
Anana,Michael Calulo,MD
Atkin,Suzanne H.,MD
Bharatia,Nikita,DO
Bitar,Souad Youssef,DO
Black,Aislinn Denise,DO
Brennan,John A.,MD
Chitnis,Subhanir Sunil,MD
Chun,Shaun Joo Yup,MD
Desai,Jigar,DO
Dudley,Larissa Sophia,MD
Eis,Amanda,MD
Fleischner,Charles Alan,MD
Forde,Frank,MD
Gang,Maureen A.,MD
Gluckman,William Alan,DO
Goett,Rebecca R.,MD

Physicians by Town and Medical Specialty

Newark (cont)

Emergency Medicine
Gordon, Marc William, MD
Hersi, Kenadeed, MD
Hinfey, Patrick Blaine, MD
Jacob, Jeena, MD
Jaker, Michael A., MD
John, Miriam, MD
John, Sheena J., DO
Jones-Dillon, Shelley A., MD
Joseph, Joslyn, DO
Kabba, Chidinma Dawn, MD
Katsetos, Suzanne A., MD
Kenney, Adam, MD
Kulkarni, Miriam L., MD
Maguire, Nicole J., DO
Masters, Martha Meredith, MD
Mathews, Sam, MD
Matjucha, John R., MD
McCormack, Denise Elizabeth, MD
Moffett, Shannon, MD
Murano, Tiffany Ellyn, MD
O'Mara, Adam Graham, DO
Onufer, Karen Anne, MD
Ostrovsky, Ilya, MD
Parrish, Andrew, MD
Patel, Ami R., DO
Pickrell, Christie Calleo, MD
Reynolds, Matthew Thomas, DO
Ripper, Jill Richelle, MD
Rosania, Anthony Russell, MD
Sanchez, John Paul, MD
Sanyaolu, Rasheed, MD
Schamban, Neil Eric, MD
Scott, Sandra Renita, MD
Shah, Neena Manharlal, DO
Shields, Stephen Damien, MD
Sierra, Nancy, MD
Srulowitz, Allen Judah, MD
Starke, John James Jr., DO
Sule, Harsh Prakash, MD
Torres, Alexander, DO
Valenzuela, Rolando Gabriel, MD
Varela, Linda Florence, MD
Waldron, Frederick Andrew, MD
Warren, Karma Brown, MD
Warshaw, Abraham Lee, MD
Wasserman, Eric Jonathan, MD
Zinzuwadia, Shreni Natoo, MD

Endocrinology
Baranetsky, Nicholas G., MD
Bleich, David, MD
Khutorskoy, Tamara, MD
Raghuwanshi, Maya P., MD
Sahani, Herneet K., MD
Stagnaro-Green, Alex Stewart, MD

Epidemiology
Weiss, Stanley H., MD

Family Medicine
Abdu Nafi, Saladin A., MD
Almodovar, Astrid Teresa, MD
Anglade, Claudia, MD
Anthony, AnnGene G, MD
Babbar, Puneet, MD
Brazeau, Chantal M., MD
Dalal, Sima R., DO
Dort, Christian, MD
Dube, Bianca, MD
Duncan, Kathyann Sylvia, MD
Easterling, Torian J., MD
Ferrante, Jeanne Min-Li, MD
Gerstmann, Michael Adam, MD
Kelly, Hortensia, DO
Mevs, Stacy Reed, MD
Ortiz, Thomas R., MD
Paige, Cynthia Y., MD
Parmar, Pritesh B., MD
Quiros Rivera, Mercedita, MD
Rodgers, Denise V., MD
Sahu, Novneet, MD
Samaniego, Eduardo W., MD
Sanchez, Carlos Alfonso, DO
Shimoni, Noaa, MD
Walsh, Kelly Anne, DO

Forensic Pathology
Falzon, Andrew L., MD

Gastroenterology
Barritta, Domenica Maria, MD
Brelvi, Zamir S., MD
Brown, Jennifer A., DO
Cabaleiro, Renee J., MD
Chahil, Neetu H., MD
Krawitz, Steven, MD
Kutner, Matthew Alexander, DO
Levinson, Robert Alan, MD
Pyrsopoulos, Nikolaos T., MD
Samanta, Arun K., MD
Sinensky, Gary B., MD
Wang, Weizheng William, MD
Weiss, Eliezer, MD

General Practice
Davis, Barbara, MD
Ligot, Jaime L., MD
Louissaint, Paraclet S., MD

Geriatric Psychiatry
Hussain, Najeeb Ullah, MD
Sanchez, Manuel I., MD
Wu, Albert B., MD

Geriatrics
Haggerty, Mary A., MD
Lynch, Claudia, MD

Glaucoma
Habiel, Miriam, MD

Gynecological Oncology
Einstein, Mark H., MD
Marcus, Jenna Z., MD
Novetsky, Akiva Pesach, MD

Gynecology
Kulak, David, MD
Otteno, Helen, MD

Head & Neck Surgery
Baredes, Soly, MD

Hematology
Bryan, Margarette R.N., MD
Rogers-Phillips, Elois G., MD
Shah, Maya M., MD
Sterling-Jean, Yolette, MD

Hematology Oncology
Abo, Stephen Michael, DO
Elreda, Lauren, MD
Ignatius, Nandini, MD
Saraf, Pankhoori, MD
Shaaban, Hamid Salim, MD
Wang, Trent Peng, DO

Hematopathology
Sun, Xinlai, MD
Wang, Qing, MD

Hepatology
Edula, Raja Gopal Reddy, MD

Hospitalist
Chillemi, Salvatore, MD
Doshi, Dhvani, MD
Kathuria, Kanik, MD
Verma, Siddharth, DO

Immunology
Oleske, James M., MD

Infectious Disease
Abergel, Glen, MD
Alland, David, MD
Bishburg, Eliahu, MD
Chew, Debra, MD
Dallapiazza, Michelle Lynn, MD
Dever, Lisa Lynn, MD
Ellner, Jerrold Jay, MD
Engell, Christian August, MD
Figueroa, Wanda E., MD
Finkel, Diana Gurevich, DO
Kapila, Rajendra, MD
Kloser, Patricia C., MD
Murillo, Jeremias L., MD
Nyaku, Amesika N., MD
Rodriguez-Diaz, Ana M., MD
Sison, Raymund Vincent S., MD
Slim, Jihad, MD
Stoler, Alexander, MD
Woodward, Ralph P., MD

Internal Medicine
Abbasi, Shahed, MD
Abboushi, Hilal Amer-Omar, MD
Abdullah, Muhammad, MD
Ackad, Viviane Bichara, MD
Adibe, Livinus, MD
Ahlawat, Sushil K., MD
Al Tamsheh, Raniah, MD
Amin, Parul S., MD
Anandarangam, Thiruvengadam, MD
Angeli, Daniel, MD
Antoine, Wilson, MD
Arias, Paul J., MD
Armenti, Lawrence A., MD
Ayub, Muhammad G., MD
Ayub, Nudrat F., MD
Ayyala, Manasa, MD
Badillo, Arthur, MD
Baran, Natalia, MD
Barba, Vincent J., MD
Bascara, Daniel, MD
Baskin, Stuart E., MD
Bhatia, Divya V., MD
Blintsovskiy, Sergey, MD
Boghossian, Jack, MD
Bojito-Marrero, Lizza Marie, MD
Bowen, Zakia Dele, MD
Brachman, Gwen O., MD
Bradley, Jacquelyn, DO
Brazaitis, Daiva, MD
Bueno, Hugo Felipe, MD
Cantey, Mary Daisy, MD
Castro, Dorothy, MD
Cathcart, Kathleen N., MD
Chaudhari, Sameer Sadashiv, MD
Chenitz, William R., MD
Chomsky, Steven A., MD
Cohen, Alice J., MD
Cohen, Ellen, MD
Collin, Robert Daniel, MD
Colon, Jose F., MD
Correia, Joaquim Jose Caldas, MD
Crighton, Kent Andrew, MD
De Jesus, Luisito Garcia, MD
Defrank, Joseph Miguel, MD
Dellorso, John, MD
Demyen, Michael Frank, MD
Desai, Ruchit B., MD
DiGiacomo, Dennis A., MD
Dukshtein, Mark, MD
El Sioufi, Sherene M., DO
Ellis, Michael Joseph, DO
Enjamuri, Devendra, MD
Eytan, Shira B., MD
Farooqui, Ozer A., MD
Fede, Robert Michael, MD
Fedida, Andre Armand, MD
Fortunato, Diane L., MD
Frank, Oleg, MD
Fuksina, Natasha, MD
Fung, Phoenix C., MD
Gandehok, Jasneet K., MD
Gayle-Barton, Delores C., MD
Gerges, Jocelyn, MD
Gerula, Christine Marie, MD
Ghavimi, Shima, MD
Gonzalez-Valle, Marijesmar, MD
Gordon, Emily, MD
Greenstein, Yonatan Yosef, MD
Guron, Gunwant K., MD
Habib, Mirette G., MD
Hallit, Rabih Riad, MD
Hao, Irene, MD
Hernandez, Osnel, MD
Herrera, Iris Del Carmen, MD
Hubert, Julio Alejandro, MD
Hussaini, Syed Azharullah, MD
Issa, Amir Karam, MD
Jacoby, Sari H., MD
Jacquette, Germaine Marie, MD
Jafari, Mortaza, MD
Joseph, Gipsa Ann, MD
Kang, Mohleen, MD
Kaplan, Joshua Michael, MD
Kern, John Matthew, DO
Koduru, Sobha R., MD
Koliver, Maria Gabriela Riera, MD
Kollimuttathuillam, Sudarsan, MD
Kothari, Neil, MD
Kowalec, Joan K., MD
Kurdali, Basil, MD
Lamba, Sangeeta, MD
Lavietes, Marc H., MD
Lawand, Oussama, MD
Levin, Barry Edward, MD
Liao, Theresa Hanna, MD
Lind, Eugene Joseph, MD
Lingiah, Vivek, MD
Love, Larrisha, MD
Madigan, John D., DO
Madrid, Teresa O., MD
Maita, Lorraine, MD
Mangura, Bonita T., MD
Mangura, Carolina T., MD
Manji, Faiza, MD
Maruboyina, Siva Prasad, MD
Matassa, Daniel Michael, MD
McNamara, Jonathan, MD
Mehta, Eva C., DO
Michaels, Matthew James, DO
Modi, Tejas J., MD
Moharita, Anabella L., MD
Monahan, Ellen M., MD
Montes, Myrtho, MD
Mosquera, Joseph L., MD
Mustillo, Robert A., MD
Mwamuna, Linda, MD
Mysliwiec, Malgorzata Halina, MD
Natale-Pereira, Ana M., MD
Nazir, Habib A., MD
Nehra, Anupama, MD
Niazi, Mumtaz A., MD
Niazi, Osama Tariq, DO
Ogundare, Tobi M., MD
Olivo Mercedes, Yohanna Maria, MD
Olivo Villabrille, Raquel, MD
Orlowicz, Christine Alexis, MD
Osorio, Jorge H., MD
Padilla, Adrian, MD
Patel, Lopa M., MD
Patel, Pavan, MD
Patel, Pratik Surendra, MD
Patel, Saurabh Chandrakant, MD
Pemberton, Colin Andre, MD
Pergament, Kathleen Mangunay, DO
Picciano, Robert, MD
Pichardo, Nelson R., MD
Pieretti, Janice, MD
Plauka, Alan R., MD
Pliner, Lillian F., MD
Pulte, Elizabeth Dianne, MD
Quinlan, Dennis Philip Sr, MD
Raghavan, Usha Murli, MD
Rajiv, Deepa, MD
Ramirez, Epifania L., MD
Reddi, Alluru S., MD
Robles, Ruth F., MD
Sadi-Ali, Vajeeha, MD
Salas-Lopez, Debbie, MD
Salese, Joseph Giuseppe, MD
Samra, Mandeep Singh, MD
Schleicher, Lori L., MD
Sednev, Dmytro V., MD
Sehgal, Saroj, MD
Seliem, Ahmed, MD
Shah, Ajit M., MD
Shah, Rajen S., MD
Shah, Sandhya R., MD
Sheppard, Sherry Manon, MD
Sicat, Jon F., DO
Siegel, Arthur David, MD
Simoes, Sonia C., MD
Singh, Anil Kumar, MD
Singh, Padmakshi, MD
Sinha, Anushua, MD
Sitahal-Dhaniram, Sasha, MD
Siyamwala, Munaf M., MD
Sodha, Amee, MD
Srivastava, Sushama, MD
Suri, Nipun, MD
Swaminathan, Shobha, MD
Szymanski, Jesse, MD
Talbot, Susan M., MD
Tapia, Susana, MD
Tayal, Rajiv, MD
Thawabi, Mohammad, MD
Tobiasson, Mary M., DO
Tomor, Esther M., MD
Tsai, Steve Chun-Hung, MD
Umakanthan, Suganthini, MD
Vadehra, Vivek Kumar, MD
Vanbeek, Stephen, MD
Vaughn, Anita C., MD
Vira, Indu N., MD
Visweswaran, Gautam Karteek, MD
Wadhwa, Rajesh, MD
Wieder, Robert, MD
Wulkan, Sheryl Lynn, MD
Yim, Hoi-Wing Susanna, MD
Yoon, Ji Ae, MD
Zemel, Suzanne, MD
Ziyaaudhin, Kappukalar A., MD
Zubair, Mohammad A., MD

Interventional Cardiology
Gadhvi, Pragnesh Harish, MD

Maternal & Fetal Medicine
Apuzzio, Joseph J., MD
Bardeguez, Arlene D., MD
Porat, Natalie, MD

Medical Genetics
Schwab, Maria Divina G., MD
Medical Oncology
Mohit-Tabatabai, Mirseyed A., MD
Neonatal-Perinatal Medicine
Ali, Salma, MD
Antonio, Excelsis O., MD
Baja Quizon, Maria Cecilia, MD
Cohen, Morris, MD
Dermendjian, Mariette, MD
Feldman, Alexander, MD
Inwood, Richard J., MD
Irakam, Anitha, MD
Lim, Anita Tiu, MD
Patel, Shalini Narendra, MD
Rai, Bellipady C., MD
Nephrology
Chadha, Inderpal S., MD
Chenitz, Kara Beth, MD
Kohli, Jatinder, MD
Mahendrakar, Smita, MD
Walsh, Liron, MD
Neurological Radiology
Slasky, Shira E., MD
Neurological Surgery
Bassani, Luigi, MD
Gandhi, Chirag D., MD
Gillick, John, MD
Goldstein, Ira Morris, MD
Heary, Robert F., MD
Ho, Victor T., MD
Jethwa, Pinakin R., MD
Mammis, Antonios, MD
Prestigiacomo, Charles Joseph, MD
Neurology
Al Kawi, Ammar, MD
Alvarez-Prieto, Maria R., MD
Cook, Stuart D., MD
Cornett, Oriana Ellen, MD
Elmoursi, Sedeek, MD
Ford, Lisa M., MD
Hidalgo, Andrea, MD
Hillen, Machteld E., MD
Husar, Walter G., MD
Kamin, Stephen S., MD
Khandelwal, Priyank, MD
Marks, David Alon, MD
Mehta, Anita Khanna, DO
Michaels, Jennifer, MD
Peeraully, Tasneem, MD
Sheikh, Shuja, MD
Souayah, Nizar, MD
Szapiel, Susan V., MD
Tabbarah, Khalid Zuhayr, MD
Neuropathology
Sharer, Leroy Ralph Jr., MD
Nuclear Medicine
Lao, Ramon S., MD
Lee, Sang O., MD
Mousavi, Mohammad Ali, DO
Parmett, Steven Russell, MD
Quarless, Shelley Ann, DO
Quinones, Candido P., MD
Obstetrics & Gynecology
Ambarus, Tatiana, MD
Barrett, Theodore, MD
Bhagat, Neha, DO
Brandi, Kristyn M., MD
Bronshtein, Elena, MD
Caban, Julio E., MD
Chu, Tsu M., MD
Cracchiolo, Bernadette M., MD
Ganesh, Vijaya L., MD
Gimovsky, Martin Larry, MD
Gittens-Williams, Lisa Nadine, MD
Goldman, Noah Adam, MD
Hatchard, John R. E., MD
Heller, Debra S., MD
Houck, Karen Leigh, MD
Johnson, Sharon, MD
Juusela, Alexander Lawrence, MD
Koul, Mrinal, MD
Kuhn, Theresa Marie, MD
Nazir, Munir A., MD
Pant, Meenakshi, MD
Pinney, Antonia F., MD
Pompeo, Lisa, MD
Raju, Vijaya L.K., MD
Rankin, Laura, MD
Roche, Natalie E., MD
Sawaged, Khalid S., DO

Shah, Chandravadan I., MD
Thompson, Stephanie M, MD
Tran, Baohuong Nguyen, DO
Ukazu, Adanna C., MD
Williams, Shauna F., MD
Yerovi, Luis A. Jr., MD
Occupational Medicine
Budnick, Lawrence D., MD
Ophthalmology
Bhagat, Neelakshi, MD
Dastjerdi, Mohammad Hossein, MD
Fechtner, Robert D., MD
Frohman, Larry P., MD
Goldfeder, Alan W., MD
Greenstein, Steven, MD
Guo, Suqin, MD
Khouri, Albert S., MD
Langer, Paul D., MD
Materna, Thomas W., MD
Picciano, Maria V., MD
Rassier, Charles Edgar Jr., MD
Roy, Monique S., MD
Turbin, Roger Eric, MD
Zarbin, Marco A., MD
Zolli, Christine L., MD
Oral & Maxillofacial Surgery
Aziz, Shahid Rahim, MD
Ziccardi, Vincent Bernard, MD
Orthopedic Surgery
Adams, Mark Robert, MD
Ahmad, Iqbal, MD
Benevenia, Joseph, MD
Berberian, Wayne S., MD
Carollo, Andrew, MD
Edobor-Osula, Osamuede, MD
Jaffe, Seth L., DO
Neal, John William VI, MD
Potini, Vishnu Choudhary, MD
Reilly, Mark C., MD
Reiter, Mitchell F., MD
Sabharwal, Sanjeev, MD
Sirkin, Michael S., MD
Tan, Virak, MD
Vives, Michael J., MD
Orthopedics
Patterson, Francis Robert, MD
Other Specialty
Colao, Joseph A. Jr., DO
Raina, Suresh, MD
Otolaryngology
Eloy, Jean Anderson, MD
Granick, Mark Stephen, MD
Kalyoussef, Evelyne, MD
Kaye, Rachel, MD
Ying, Yu-Lan Mary, MD
Otology
Jyung, Robert Wha, MD
Pain Medicine
Gyi, Jennifer, DO
Kostroma, Boris Vladimirovich, MD
Pain Medicine-Interventional
Speert, Tory, DO
Yanamadula, Dinash Kumar, MD
Pathology
Philip, Abraham T., MD
Pathology-Molecular Genetic
Baisre-De Leon, Ada, MD
Pediatric Anesthesia
Shah, Chirag J., MD
Pediatric Cardiology
Langsner, Alan M., MD
Michael, Mark, DO
Verma, Rajiv, MD
Pediatric Critical Care
McQueen, Derrick Arnold, MD
Sinquee, Dianne M., MD
Pediatric Emergency Medicine
Barricella, Robert Louis, DO
Rickerhauser-Krall, Maureen, MD
Pediatric Gastroenterology
Foglio, Elsie Jazmin, DO
Sunaryo, Francis P., MD
Pediatric Hematology Oncology
Bekele, Wondwessen, MD
Kamalakar, Peri, MD
Pediatric Infectious Diseases
Espiritu-Fuller, Maria C., MD
Pediatric Nephrology
Aviv, Abraham, MD

Pediatric Orthopedics
Kaushal, Neil, MD
Pediatric Pulmonology
Savary, Khalil William, MD
Pediatric Radiology
Phatak, Tej Deepak, MD
Pediatric Urology
Cambareri, Gina M., MD
Pediatrics
Abels, Jane I., MD
Adija, Akinyi, MD
Aguila, Helen A., MD
Aguilar, Hector David Jr., MD
Aliparo, Madolene A., MD
Alvarez, Maria T., MD
Arpayoglou, Beatriz C., MD
Bachman, Michael Craig, MD
Balaguru, Duraisamy, MD
Baranowski, Katherine, MD
Baskerville, Renee E., DO
Bell-Gresham, Garrett, MD
Benezra-Obeiter, Rita Beth, MD
Boyle, Maria Pilar T., MD
Bustillo, Jose R., DO
Carruth, Samuel G. Jr., MD
Chen, Sophia Wunchi, DO
Cooray, Roshan, MD
Correa, Luis A., MD
Cueto, Victor Jr., MD
Dashefsky, Barry, MD
Delisfort, Guy J., MD
Dhar, Seema, MD
Dieudonne, Arry, MD
Esquerre, Rene B., MD
Evans, Hugh E., MD
Ferraz, Ricardo J. P., MD
Fisher, Joie, DO
Fojas, Felicia Regina, MD
Friedman, Debbie, MD
Gajarawala, Raksha J., MD
Garay, Luis Alberto, MD
Gilo, Belen Frias, MD
Gonzalez, Isabel V., MD
Guinto, Danilo M., MD
Gururajarao, Lakshmi, MD
Hanauske Abel, Hartmut Martin, MD
Hashim, Anjum, MD
Huang, Grace, MD
Hussain, Kashif, MD
Ighama-Amegor, Ibilola, MD
Jaffery, Fatema, MD
Johnson, Deborah J., MD
Joseph, Frederleyne Mirlene, MD
Kalia, Jessica Leigh, DO
Kalyanaraman, Meena, MD
Kanikicharla, Uma, MD
Kansagra, Ketan Vallabh, MD
Lee, Horton James, MD
Levy, Jodi A., MD
Louis-Jacques, Jocelyne, MD
Louissaint, Valerie, MD
Lui, Jackie Zhuojun, MD
Mac, Feminia C., MD
Madhok, Indu, MD
Madubuko, Adaora Gabriellene, MD
Manigault, Simone A., MD
Marcus, Steven M., MD
Mautone, Susan G., MD
McDevitt, Barbara Ellen, MD
Monteiro, Iona M., MD
Morkos, Faten Farid, MD
Narang, Shalu, MD
Ndukwe, Michael Chukwuemeka, MD
Nelson, Adin, MD
Netravali, Chitra Arun, MD
Nevado, Jose A., MD
O'Neal, Isaac, MD
Ortega, Jesus Ruben, MD
Osei, Charles, MD
Palmiery, Ponciano Jr., MD
Pande, Sumati, MD
Plaza, Lorna D., MD
Recio, Evita I., MD
Reddy, Chitra R., MD
Reyes, Tyrone K., MD
Roberts, Marc P., MD
Rosenblatt, Joshua S., MD
Salian Raghava, Preethi, MD
Schwab, Joseph V., MD
Shahidi, Hosseinali, MD
Shihabuddin, Bashar Sami, MD
Simotas, Christopher J., MD

Singer-Granick, Carol Joyce, MD
Sivitz, Adam B., MD
Somera-Uy, Constancia L., MD
Sprott, Kendell R., MD
Stanford, Paulette D., MD
Taneja, Indra, MD
Tanuos, Hanan A., MD
Tentler, Aleksey, MD
Thamburaj, Ravi Daniel, DO
Thomas, Pauline A., MD
Toft, Maria Campos, MD
Tran, Kevin, MD
Trinidad, Altagracia A., MD
Tulsyan, Vasudha, MD
Uduaghan, Victor Aboiye, MD
Uy, Loreta M., MD
Vicente, Virgilio C., MD
Walks, Pauline Angela, MD
Walsh, Rowan Frank, MD
Wei, Tzong-Jer, MD
Wong, Kristin G., MD
Physical Med & Rehab-Pain Med
Chandarana, Bhavini S., MD
Physical Medicine & Rehab
Ashraf, Humaira, MD
Bach, John R., MD
Bitterman, Jason, MD
Delisa, Joel A., MD
Foye, Patrick M., MD
Homb, Kris, MD
Kepler, Karen Lynn, DO
Kramberg, Robert David, MD
Meer, Joel, MD
Napolitano, Elena, MD
Rubbani, Mariam Shafaq, MD
Yonclas, Peter Philip, MD
Zemel, Nathan, MD
Plastic Surgery
Castel, Nikki, MD
Datiashvili, Ramazi Otarovich, MD
Lee, Edward Sang Keun, MD
Rhee, Samuel T., MD
Psychiatry
Afzal, Saba, MD
Aggarwal, Rashi, MD
Allen Steinfeld, Isabel, MD
Alvarado, Mark U., MD
Amin, Ritesh A., MD
Annitto, William J., MD
Babayants, Alexander R., MD
Bansil, Rakesh K., MD
Bartlett, Jacqueline A., MD
Belenker, Stuart Lawrence, MD
Bennett, Robert Harris, DO
Cartwright, Charles N., MD
Chakrabarti, Mukti, MD
Eljarrah, Fouad, MD
Finkelstein, Mario, MD
Frederikse, Melissa Ellison, MD
Frometa, Ayme Veronica, MD
Gudapati, Ramakrishna, MD
Heffner, Catherine D'aprix, DO
Henningson, Karen Jeanne, DO
Jadeja, Kiranben J., MD
Kennedy, Cheryl A., MD
Kesselman, Gayle, MD
Levin, Elizabeth H., MD
Mirza, Nadia A., MD
Obi, Manfred K., MD
Oyvin, Vadim, MD
Pemberton, Clyde A., MD
Rajakumar, Nirmala S., MD
Reeves, Donald Raymond Jr., MD
Rowan, George Edward, MD
Rudner, Elvira, MD
Schleifer, Steven J., MD
Shah, Snehal, MD
Shihabuddin, Lina Sami, MD
Silva, Lourdes G., DO
Sun, Ye Ming Jimmy, MD
Tortosa Nacher, Rafael M., MD
Udasco, Jocelynda O., MD
Villegas, Noah, MD
Whang, Phil Joo, MD
Young, Joseph M., MD
Yum, Sun Young, MD
Public Health
Halperin, William Edward, MD
Pulmonary Disease
Hudgins, Joan Leonard, MD
May, Richard Edward Jr., MD
Migliore, Christina, MD

Physicians by Town and Medical Specialty

Newark (cont)
  Pulmonary Disease
    Patrawalla,Amee Shirish,MD
    Seethamraju,Harish,MD
  Radiation Oncology
    Cathcart,Charles S.,MD
  Radiology
    Aguirre,Frank J.,MD
    Baker,Stephen R.,MD
    Goldman,Alice Ruth,MD
    Hubbi,Basil,MD
    Kisza,Piotr Slawomir,MD
    Liu,Yiyan,MD
    Shah,Suken H.,MD
    Wenokor,Cornelia B. C.,MD
  Reproductive Endocrinology
    Douglas,Nataki Celeste,MD
    Morelli,Sara S.,MD
  Rheumatology
    Chu,Alice,MD
    Khianey,Reena,MD
  Spinal Surgery
    Harris,Colin B.,MD
  Surgery (General)
    Alli,Padmavathy,DO
    Andrade,Peter,DO
    Anjaria,Devashish Jayant,MD
    Bale,Asha G.,MD
    Berlin,Ana,MD
    Chauhan,Niravkumar M.,MD
    Clarke,Kevin O'Neil,MD
    Galloway,Joseph,MD
    Guarrera,James Vincent,MD
    Huang,Joe T.,MD
    Kalu,Ogori N.,MD
    Koneru,Baburao,MD
    Lovoulos,Constantinos John,MD
    Malhotra,Sunil Prakash,MD
    Malik,Rema,MD
    Merchant,Aziz M.,MD
    Miranda,Irving,MD
    Mosenthal,Anne Charlotte,MD
    Paskhover,Boris,MD
    Sambol,Justin Todd,MD
    Sardari,Frederic Fereydoun,MD
    Tyrie,Leslie S.,MD
    Wilson,Dorian J.,MD
    Yepez,Humberto R.,MD
  Surgical Critical Care
    Bonne,Stephanie Lynn,MD
    Deitch,Edwin A.,MD
    Goulet,Nicole,MD
    Kunac,Anastasia,MD
    Livingston,David H.,MD
    Sifri,Ziad Charles,MD
    Venugopal,Roshni L.,MD
  Thoracic Surgery
    Camacho,Margarita T.,MD
    Saunders,Craig Raymond,MD
    Shariati,Nazly M.,MD
    Southgate,Theodore J.,MD
  Transplant Surgery & Medicine
    Brown,Lloyd Garth,MD
    Fisher,Adrian Alex,MD
  Trauma Surgery
    Glass,Nina Elizabeth,MD
  Urology
    Hinds,Peter R.,MD
    Rosario,Imani Jackson,MD
    Watson,Richard A.,MD
  Vascular & Intrvntnal Radiology
    Achakzai,Basit Khan,MD
    Amuluru,Krishna,MD
  Vascular Surgery
    Curi,Michael A.,MD
    Dhadwal,Ajay Kapoor,MD
    Jamil,Zafar,MD
    Padberg,Frank Thomas Jr.,MD
    Sagarwala,Adam,DO
    Wu,Timothy,MD
Newfoundland
  Dermatology
    Bilkis,Michael Ross,MD
  Internal Medicine
    Asokan,Rengaswamy,MD
Newton
  Anesthesiology
    Cowan,Clayton Joseph,MD
    Delong,Donald H. II,MD
    Eaton,Edward E.,MD

    Habina,Ladislav,MD
    Hagopian,Vahe H.,MD
    Jiang,Rongjie,MD
    Kouvaras,John Nikolaos,DO
    Landauer,Stephen P.,MD
    Martinez,Rebecca Marie,DO
    Patel,Nish A.,MD
    Petrucelli,Marisa Parise,DO
    Villafania,Zenaida S.,MD
    Yu,Edgar L.,MD
  Anesthesiology: Critical Care
    Ibragimov,Araz,DO
  Cardiovascular Disease
    Buyer,David S.,MD
    Codispoti,Cindy A.,DO
    Masci,Robert L.,MD
    Redline,Richard C.,MD
    Schwarz,Scott A.,MD
  Critical Care Medicine
    Garg,Rakesh K.,MD
    Nadarajah,Dayaparan,MD
  Dermatology
    Blackwell,Martin,DO
  Diagnostic Radiology
    Patel,Jay,MD
    Scheer,Linda B.,MD
  Emergency Medicine
    Benson,Ellen,MD
    Brutico,Anthony J.,DO
    Juco,Henry P.,MD
    Landre,William Joseph,MD
    Mack,Ronald John,MD
    Rivera,Alberto R.,MD
  Family Medicine
    Alam,Shumaila,MD
    Kane,Frank L.,MD
    Liloia,Peter Anthony,DO
    Mattes,David G.,MD
    McGraw,John Daniel,MD
    Pampin,Robert J.,DO
    Regan,Inge Sophia,MD
    Sieminski,Douglas Peter,DO
  Hospitalist
    Albassam,Hassan,MD
  Internal Medicine
    Aggarwal,Aradhana,MD
    Ahuja,Rakesh,MD
    Bergman,Benjamin Ryan,MD
    Burgio,Michael T.,MD
    DeBitetto,Nick P.,DO
    Delsardo,Anthony C.,MD
    Feldman,Nathaniel Seth,MD
    Li,Hua,MD
    Mahgoub,Hatem Abdelkawi,MD
    Mohammadi,Mina,MD
    Okechukwu,Christopher O.,MD
    Okpala,Augustine C.,MD
    Partyka,Bronislaw J.,MD
    Pasunuri,Ramya Sri,MD
    Ruiz,Restituto Soriano Jr.,MD
    Shukla,Rajesh,MD
    Sodagum,Lakshmi Lavanya,MD
    Stas,Sameer,MD
    Vaz,Richard,DO
  Interventional Cardiology
    Cioce,Gerald,MD
  Nephrology
    Talon,Dennis J.,MD
  Neurology
    Khesin,Yevgeniy I.,MD
    Tishuk,Pavel,MD
    Weintraub,Bernard M.,MD
  Obstetrics & Gynecology
    Bagherian,Sharareh,DO
    Bhayani,Parimal S.,MD
    Dardik,Raquel B.,MD
    Lewis,Frieda Elizabeth,MD
    Maugeri,Joseph P.,MD
    Paxton,Adam Michael,MD
    Pennant,Andria Uzetta,MD
    Rubino,Donald J.,MD
    Sehgal,Geeta,DO
    Sherman,Glenn Stewart,MD
  Ophthalmology
    Barone,Robert Gerard,MD
    Hirschfeld,Laura Ann,MD
    Inkeles,David M.,MD
    Perlmutter,Harold S.,MD
    Vora,Amit V.,MD
  Orthopedic Surgery
    Lopez,Nicole Melisa Montero,MD

    Scales,James Jr.,MD
    Weinschenk,Robert C.,MD
  Otolaryngology
    Galeos,Warren L.,MD
  Pathology
    Vergara,Rebecca B.,MD
  Pediatrics
    Dakake,Charles Jr.,MD
    Digby,Thomas E.,MD
    Piggee,Mia Christine,MD
    Porter,James H.,MD
    Pupo,Louis O.,MD
    Rossetti-Cartaxo,Annette L.,MD
    Sison,Genevieve Yvonne,MD
    Zohny,Jeahad,MD
  Psychiatry
    El-Kholy,Nahed M.,MD
    Sarner,Steven W.,MD
    Scimone,Anthony,MD
  Pulmonary Disease
    Shah,Samir D.,MD
  Sports Medicine
    Bradish,Glen Edward,MD
  Surgery (General)
    Harris,Ronald K.,MD
    Nakhjo,Shomaf,DO
    Newman,Brian F.,MD
  Urology
    Collini,William R.,MD
Normandy Beach
  Pediatrics
    Waldron,Robert John,MD
North Arlington
  Cardiovascular Disease
    Anastasiades,Athos C.,MD
    Burachinsky,Andrew E.,DO
    Latyshev,Yevgeniy,MD
  Family Medicine
    Lubas,Andrew S.,MD
  Gastroenterology
    Waxman,Mark S.,MD
  Internal Medicine
    Barbera,Frank T.,MD
    Bitner,Bozena Wanda,MD
    Francis,Thomas Paul,DO
    Gashi,Sheremet,MD
    Guma,Michael,DO
    Jackson,Eric Marc,MD
    Kwapniewski,Agnieszka Monika,MD
    Mody,Sushama,MD
    Monroe,Beatrice,MD
    Thomas,Eric David,MD
    Viscuso,Maria B.,MD
  Obstetrics & Gynecology
    Grasso,Armand J.,MD
  Ophthalmology
    Favetta,John R.,MD
    Morrone,Louis J.,MD
  Orthopedic Surgery
    Gennace,Ronald E.,MD
    Lerner,Kent S.,MD
  Pediatrics
    Cabalu,Tyrone T.,MD
    Ganapathy,Jayalakshmi,MD
    Marx,Jo-Ann,MD
    Namnama,Liborio P.,MD
    Paragas,Miguela L.,MD
North Bergen
  Administration/Medical Mgt
    Winter,Ivan David,MD
  Allergy
    Dangelo,Salvatore,MD
    Hajee,Feryal,MD
  Anatomic/Clinical Pathology
    Zhang,Qi,MD
  Anesthesiology
    Lawler,Gregory James,DO
    Pavia,Randyll A.,MD
    Poltinnikova,Yana M.,MD
    Portugal,Alexander,MD
    Shatz,Matthew Jay,MD
    Singh,Samundar K.,MD
  Anesthesiology: Pain Medicine
    Waldman,Steven Paul,MD
  Cardiovascular Disease
    Alcorta,Carlos E.,MD
    Basu,Mihir Kumar,MD
    Gabelman,Mark Scott,MD
    Stein,Aaron A.,MD

  Critical Care Medicine
    Capo',Aida P.,MD
  Dermatology
    Elias,Charles,MD
  Emergency Medicine
    Alban,Alvaro,MD
    Ali,Meer S.,MD
    Bingham,Richard F.,MD
    Molina,Alex Armando,MD
    Ruocco,Dominic,MD
    Schneid,Sharona,MD
  Endocrinology
    Camacho-Patterson,Evelyn L.,MD
    Morgado,Antonio,MD
    Pathak,Sonal,MD
  Family Med-Adult Medicine
    Lee,Mark,DO
  Family Medicine
    Amin,Samirlal Ramanlal,MD
    Ayeni,Eniola Teju,DO
    Davis,Bradley,DO
    Ghabour,Rose Ann Sameh,MD
    Goldstein,Marc,DO
    Hussain,Zahid,MD
    Orellana Chasi,Pamela,MD
    Panem,Flordeliz Buensuceso,MD
    Rugel,Jason,DO
    Sujovolsky,Jeannette A.,DO
  Gastroenterology
    Raskin,Jeffrey M.,MD
    Sotiriadis,John,MD
    Tepler,Harold George,MD
  Internal Medicine
    Ahmed,Asad,DO
    Badri,M. Maher Ahmad,MD
    Capo',Maria Pilar,MD
    Caride,Peter,MD
    De Vera,Edmundo C.,MD
    Gonzalez,Marcia M.,MD
    Gosalia,Tanmay Pradip,DO
    Gundapuneni,Satish Babu,MD
    Jordan,Nicole,MD
    Keswani,Deepak Pessu,MD
    Laufer,Beatrice,MD
    Liuzzo,John P.,MD
    Lo,Abraham,MD
    Patel,Bela Ashutosh,MD
    Peri,Nityanand,DO
    Polkampally,Kavitha,MD
    Rabago-Reyes,Cassandra,MD
    Rama,Sapna,DO
    Rastogi,Surender M.,MD
    Scopulovic-Nikolic,Biljana,MD
    Shah,Kamalesh R.,MD
    Simon,Elizabeth R.,DO
    Urman,Alina,DO
  Interventional Cardiology
    Kelly,Dennis Hughes III,MD
  Medical Oncology
    Gupta,Bhavna,MD
  Nephrology
    Fein,Deborah Anne,MD
  Neurology
    Prasad,Nalini,MD
    Tikoo,Ravinder Kumar,MD
  Obstetrics & Gynecology
    Escobar,Juan Nicolas,MD
    Giron-Jimenez,Sandra,MD
    Gonzalez,Rosa M.,MD
    Gutierrez,Christine V.,MD
    Kitzis,Hugo D.,MD
    Majid,Mahir J.,MD
    Nath,Mary Madhuri,MD
    Pablo,Bryan Alcides,MD
    Patel,Jigna K.,MD
    Patel,Zankhana M.,MD
    Perisic,Dusan,MD
    Trujillo-Carvalho,Cecilia J.,MD
  Ophthalmology
    Braunstein,Steven W.,MD
    Shah,Dipal,MD
  Orthopedic Surgery
    Baghal,Imad Y.,MD
    Sun,Li,DO
  Pediatrics
    Abbassi,Saeed R.,MD
    Caceres,Maria Gabriela,MD
    Eguino Conde,Damaris A.,MD
    Patel,Mansi,MD
  Physical Med & Rehab-Pain Med
    Vazquez,Pablo,MD

Physicians by Town and Medical Specialty

Psychiatry
Feuer Razin,Zippora,DO
Ruiz,Vicente Z.,MD
Wancier,Zisalo,MD
Sports Medicine
Galdi,Balazs,MD
Surgery (General)
Boucher,Gregory M.,DO
Shaknovsky,Thomas J.,DO
Urology
Stedman,Martin J.,MD
Vascular Surgery
Davis,Jason Evan,MD

North Brunswick
Acupuncture
Elkholy,Wael Talaat,MD
Anatomic/Clinical Pathology
Falzon,Andrea,MD
Anesthesiology
Fakhry,Michael,MD
Karandikar,Shaila Y.,MD
Khan,Khuram Adnan,DO
Parikh,Sudha Sudhir,MD
Sood,Rohit,MD
Tyler,James Ralph,MD
Anesthesiology: Pain Medicine
Avhad,Prajakta Vasant,MD
Cardiovascular Disease
Blau,Howard,MD
Sicherman,Harlan J.,MD
Weisfogel,Gerald M.,MD
Child & Adolescent Psychiatry
Khwaja,Tahir Nisar,MD
Lukac,Juraj,MD
Parikh,Chirayu Bharat,DO
Dermatology
Berger,Richard S.,MD
Wrone,David A.,MD
Emergency Medicine
Bansal,Sonia,MD
Roberts,Leah Kate,MD
Family Medicine
Faisal,Siddiq A.,MD
Jorgensen,Otto B.,MD
Nadeem,Atiya,MD
Patterson,George A.,MD
Sheil,Christina A.,MD
Forensic Pathology
Karluk,Diane,MD
Gastroenterology
Kastuar,Satya P.,MD
Gynecology
Versi,Ebrahim Eboo,MD
Hand Surgery
Kirschenbaum,David,MD
Infectious Disease
Deka,Bharati,MD
Internal Medicine
Ahmad,Mir S.,MD
Ata,Mohammad,MD
Guo,H. Jennifer,MD
Hamsa,Gangaswamaiah,MD
Haq,Mehnaz A.,MD
Krishnan,Lalitha B.,MD
Lee,Dae Woo,MD
Lefkowitz,Miriam,MD
Maganti,Sameera,MD
Malik,Bobby A.,MD
Naqui,Mehdi H.,MD
Patel,Himanshu K.,MD
Potluri,Haritha,MD
Prodromo,Paul E.,MD
Sandhu,Bhavna,MD
Sarode,Satyeswara K.,MD
Vietla,Bhavani Durga,MD
Zara,Graciano L.,MD
Zimmerman,Stanley R.,MD
Nephrology
Kapoian,Toros,MD
Obstetrics & Gynecology
Acharya,Rashmi,MD
Nuthakki,Vimala Devi,MD
Udeshi,Hansa S.,MD
Ophthalmology
Bennett-Phillips,Fay L.,MD
Orthopedic Surgery
Reich,Steven M.,MD
Sieler,Shawn D.,MD
Otolaryngology
Lin,Pei-Shiu,MD

Pediatrics
Agarwal,Nalini,MD
Brauer,Howard E.,MD
Chen,Deborah E.,MD
Esterova,Elizaveta,MD
Gajera,Sangeeta Jadav,MD
Goh,Jean Sian Li,MD
Hanna,Dina W.,MD
Henry,Elizabeth Robinson,MD
Jadhav,Surekha Ashwin,MD
Katz,Melvin I.,MD
Kessous,Deborah Lynne,MD
Kim,Maria Batraki,DO
Naqui,Nasreen,MD
Patel,Himanshubhai A.,MD
Prabhuram,Nagarathna,MD
Pragaspathy,Bhavadarani M.,MD
Raghunathan,Susheela I.,MD
Segarra,Michael L.,MD
Wiener,Howard E.,MD
Physical Med & Rehab-Pain Med
Abbasi,Faheem A.,MD
Physical Medicine & Rehab
Magaziner,Edward S.,MD
Plastic Surgery
Olson,Robert M.,MD
Partridge,Joanna Lee,MD
Psychiatry
Jones,Frank A. Jr.,MD
Losack,Glenn Mark,MD
Steinberg,Edward,MD
Surgery (General)
Hermosilla,Elias P. Jr.,MD
Urology
Ioffreda,Richard E.,MD
Rodriguez,Ramon Elias,MD

North Caldwell
Anesthesiology
Bhattacharyya,Shibani S.,MD
Kim,Kun,MD
Radhakrishnan,Indira,MD
Internal Medicine
Curreri,Rosalie M.,MD
Gagliardi,Anthony J.,MD
Neurology
Carmickle,Lynne J.,MD
Pediatric Infectious Diseases
Noel,Gary J.,MD
Physical Medicine & Rehab
Cheng,Jenfu,MD
Radiology
Vijayanathan,Thurairasa,MD

North Cape May
Family Medicine
Drake,Andrew F.,DO
Hong,Matthew H.,MD
Maroldo,Michael G.,MD
Moten,Shirlene Tolbert,MD
Renza,Richard A.,DO
Internal Medicine
Farooqui,Zaheerulla A.,MD
Leisner,William Randolph,MD
Vaccaro,Carl Anthony,DO

North Haledon
Emergency Medicine
Patel,Namrata,DO
Family Medicine
Salerno,Adrienne Lynn,MD
Otolaryngology
Goodnight,James W.,MD

North Plainfield
Critical Care Medicine
Rehman,Muhammad Ubaid,MD
Dermatology
Weinberger,George I.,MD
Family Medicine
Oji,Omobola Abiodun,MD
General Practice
Alvarez,Bethzaida,MD
Internal Medicine
Ahmed,Fauzia Mosarrat,MD
Siddiq,Syed A.,MD
Obstetrics & Gynecology
Lowe,William J. III,MD
Pediatrics
Shah,Bharti K.,MD
Sodhi,Surinder K.,MD

North Wildwood
Family Medicine
Cook,Jenny Lynn,DO

Haflin,Mary Ann,MD

Northfield
Adolescent Medicine
Solomon-Bergen,Peggy A.,MD
Anesthesiology
Antebi,Morris E.,MD
Hernberg,Scott Alan,DO
Liu,Bo,MD
Dermatology
Krakowski,Andrew Charles,MD
Mordecai,Isaac S.,MD
Vause,Sandra E.,MD
Diagnostic Radiology
Cummings,Allan H.,MD
Family Medicine
Bowers,Steven Richard,DO
Brunson,Rodney C.,DO
Bushay,Stephen Lloyd,MD
Cutler,Marna Alyse,DO
Fiorentino,Grace,DO
Holtzin,Robert M.,DO
Hand Surgery
Fox,Jonathan L.,MD
Hematology Oncology
Stoyko,Zoryana,MD
Hospitalist
Mathews,Robert John,MD
Infectious Disease
Homayouni,Homayoun,MD
Internal Medicine
Blecker,David L.,MD
Daneshvar,Behdokht,MD
Karp,Howard M.,DO
Michael,Wedad S.,MD
Nachtigall,Steven Paul,MD
Nanfara,Marcantonio,MD
Nnewihe,Charles Obinna,MD
Thakkar,Priyesh Tarunkumar,DO
Wang,Le,MD
Welsh,John W.,DO
Medical Oncology
Nazha,Naim T.,MD
Nephrology
Behl,Nitin,MD
Schreyer,Raymond S.,MD
Shastri,Jay Gautam,DO
Obstetrics & Gynecology
Nnewihe,Adebola Oyeronke,MD
Ophthalmology
Connors,Daniel Bernard,MD
Foxman,Brett T.,MD
Foxman,Scott G.,MD
Margolis,Thomas Ira,MD
Thakker,Manoj Mangaldas,MD
Orthopedic Surgery
Harhay,Joseph S.,MD
Pain Medicine
Strenger,Keith David,MD
Pathology
Daneshvar,Ali,MD
Pediatric Pulmonology
Leong,Mila A.,MD
Pediatrics
Chang,Ho-Choong,MD
Physical Medicine & Rehab
Baliga,Arvind B.,MD
Russomano,Salvatore J.,MD
Plastic & Reconstructive Srgy
Sood,Mohit,DO
Plastic Surgery
Trocki,Ira M.,MD
Surgery (General)
Kulkarni,Nandini N.,MD
May,David Peter,MD
Vascular & Intrvntnal Radiology
Feng,David H.,MD

Northvale
Family Medicine
DiGiovanni,Leonard G.,DO
Internal Medicine
Hwang,John M.,MD
Symington,Peter Anthony,MD
Physical Medicine & Rehab
Zelinger-Bernhaut,Shani I,MD

Norwood
Anatomic/Clinical Pathology
Rijhwani,Kiran,MD
Anesthesiology
Cagen,Steven B.,MD
MacIver,Barbara Jane,MD

Cardiovascular Disease
Tsenovoy,Petr Leonidovich,MD
Weslow,Renee G.,MD
Developmental Pediatrics
Downey,Margaret Kelly,MD
Orthopedic Surgery
Kerness,Wayne Jared,MD
Pediatrics
Bhatia,Rubina,MD

Nutley
Anatomic/Clinical Pathology
Dimov,Nikolay D.,MD
Anesthesiology
Belfar,Alexandra,MD
Kyi,Myint Myint,MD
Punzalan,Crispino R.,MD
Cardiovascular Disease
Fusilli,Louis D.,MD
Savino,Leonard,MD
Dermatology
Bashline,Benjamin R.,DO
Ligresti,Dominick Joseph,MD
Diagnostic Radiology
Bash,Lisa Taub,MD
Mondshine,Ross T.,MD
Pollack,Michael A.,MD
Torrente,Jessica,MD
Traflet,Robert F.,MD
Endocrinology
Hauptman,Jonathan B.,MD
Family Medicine
Agresti,James V. Sr.,DO
Espina,Luis Alberto,MD
Figueroa,Marciano Tiu Jr.,MD
Giuliano,Michael Gerard,DO
Pastena,Anthony M.,DO
Patel,Mallik,MD
Sekiya,Steven T.,DO
Infectious Disease
Sasanpour,Majid,MD
Internal Medicine
Abu Al Rub,Dana M.,MD
Agresti,James V. III,MD
Alessio,Maryann,DO
Alexandrova,Marina A.,MD
Aslam,Tahseen N.,MD
Bisignano Delvecchio,Maria,MD
Brignola,Joseph John,MD
Califano,Antonio G.,MD
Christiano,John M.,MD
Citarelli,Louis J.,MD
Costanza,Carl,MD
Cozzarelli-Franklin,Annette,MD
De Fazio,Ernest,MD
Delgra,Alexander B.,MD
Dell'Aquila,Paul V.,MD
Durante,Michael F.,MD
Farion,George Z.,MD
Franklin,James D.,MD
Gentile,Michael R.,MD
Kalmar,Edward T.,MD
McMaster,Delphine A.,MD
Mehta,Sidhartha H.,MD
Nadratowski,Mary Celesta,MD
Richardson,Robert W.,MD
Rotunda,Roseanne,DO
Vecchione,Edward J.,DO
Yeretsky,Yelena,DO
Zazzali,Peter G.,MD
Zefren,Jacob M.,MD
Nuclear Medicine
Richman,Steven D.,MD
Obstetrics & Gynecology
Parisi,Vanessa Marie,DO
Straker,Michael J.,MD
Ophthalmology
Fiore,Philip M.,MD
Prystowsky,Ligaya L.,MD
Zazzali,Albert John,MD
Orthopedic Surgery
Ducey,Stephen Alexander,MD
Femino,Frank Placido,MD
Parks,Anthony Lesmore Jr.,MD
Queler,Seth Robert,MD
Wujciak,Michael P.,MD
Otolaryngology
Wallace,Derrick I.,MD
Youssef,Oliver S.,MD
Pediatric Nephrology
Loghman-Adham,Mahmoud,MD

Physicians by Town and Medical Specialty

Nutley (cont)
Pediatrics
- Dos Santos, Stephanie, MD
- Marcus, Richard W., MD
- Pedalino, Jill Garripoli, DO
- Prystowsky, Barry S., MD
- Segal, Michele Robyn, MD

Physical Medicine & Rehab
- Bodner, Bradley A., DO
- Zazzali, George N., MD

Psychiatry
- Bridge, Thomas Peter, MD
- Fleser, Cecilia, MD
- Khan, Mehtab A., MD
- Yoo, Sang W., MD

Radiology
- Denehy, Ann Smith, MD
- Khedkar, Mona S., MD

Surgery (General)
- Mercogliano, Edward A., MD

Oak Ridge
Family Medicine
- Gloria, Stephen B., MD
- Magnusen, Mary L., DO
- Riesenman, Joseph John, MD

Oakhurst
Anesthesiology
- Bram, Harris N., MD

Child & Adolescent Psychiatry
- Tetelbom, Miriam, MD

Colon & Rectal Surgery
- Lake, Thomas R. III, MD
- Parker, Glenn S., MD

Family Medicine
- Dweck, Isaac Jay, MD

Gastroenterology
- Akhtar, Reza Yasin, MD
- Dhillon, Shamina, MD
- Maki, Junsuke, MD
- Schwartz, Mitchell S., MD
- Terrany, Ben, MD
- Turtel, Penny S., MD

General Practice
- Mojares, Dennis C., MD
- Wortzel, Jay V., MD

Geriatrics
- Hayet, Bill, MD

Infectious Disease
- Dwivedi, Sukrut A., DO
- Lee, Andrew, MD
- Mathur, Ajay Narain, MD
- Patel, Apurva, MD
- Sivaprasad, Rajagopalan, MD

Internal Medicine
- Adamczyk, Rebekah Katherine, DO
- Ciciarelli, John G. II, MD
- Di Guglielmo, Nicola, MD
- Mojares, Richard Alan, MD
- Neuman, Jane Elaine, MD
- Saky, Marie-Therese, MD

Obstetrics & Gynecology
- Hage, Charles W., MD
- Hayet, Rose F., MD
- Moskowitz, David H., MD
- Van Horn, Lawrence G. Jr., MD

Pediatrics
- Smoller, Alison Brett, DO
- Toturgul, David T., MD

Physical Medicine & Rehab
- Roach, Beth Lynnell, MD

Psychiatry
- Kamm, Ronald L., MD

Radiology
- Ginsberg, Ferris, DO

Surgery (General)
- Gornish, Aron L., MD
- Lin, Jeffrey M., MD
- Schwartz, Mark Robert, MD

Oakland
Anesthesiology
- Hansen, David Wayne, MD
- Nestampower, Mindy Lyn, MD

Cardiovascular Disease
- Budhwani, Navin, MD
- Montgomery, David H., MD
- Williams, Marcus L., MD

Child & Adolescent Psychiatry
- Chalemian, Bliss A., MD

Family Medicine
- Dela Gente, Robert Saladaga, DO
- Morski, Richard S., MD
- Perdomo, Louis Fernando, MD
- Shaker, Taylor, MD
- Straseskie, Ryan Kenneth, MD
- Uddin, Sarah T., DO

Internal Medicine
- Farrell, Lynda A., MD
- Kampf, Richard S., MD
- Kesselhaut, Marc D., MD
- Pereira, Pedro Miguel, MD
- Scherling, Richard H., DO

Obstetrics & Gynecology
- Dispenziere, Benjamin R., MD

Ophthalmology
- Hilal-Campo, Diane M., MD

Pediatrics
- Chu, Yie-Hsien, MD
- Guruswamy, Parvathi, MD
- Lindenberg, Erin K., MD
- Livingstone, Tosan, MD
- Michaels, Lisa-Ann B., MD
- Minhas, Navpreet Singh, MD
- Raimo, Anthony S., MD
- Stock, Ilana Rose, MD
- Sumarokov, Alina, MD
- Taneja, Uttama, DO
- Tirri, Carmelina, MD
- Wiederhorn, Noel M., MD

Physical Medicine & Rehab
- Gombas, George Frank, MD

Psychiatry
- Chalemian, Robert J., MD

Oaklyn
Internal Medicine
- Le, Tram N., MD

Psychiatry
- Patten-Kline, Nancy H., DO

Ocean
Allergy
- Gross, Gary L., MD
- Sher, Ellen R., MD

Allergy & Immunology
- Ross, Jacqueline, MD

Anesthesiology
- Uddin, Nihat, MD

Dermatology
- Klenoff, Paul H., MD

Gastroenterology
- Beri, Gagan D., MD
- Guss, Howard N., DO

Geriatrics
- Disciglio, Michael J., MD

Internal Medicine
- Beri, Kavita, MD
- Cosentino, James P., DO
- Garla, Sudha, MD
- Mehta, Rajneesh G., MD
- Meltzer, Richard B., MD
- Patel, Kashmira, MD
- Patel, Suhas Ramesh, MD
- Vaccaro, Carmine A., MD

Neonatal-Perinatal Medicine
- Kashlan, Fawaz T., MD

Neurology
- Raab, Vicki E., MD

Obstetrics & Gynecology
- Cohen, Ronald L., MD
- Gould, Jack R., DO
- Henderson, Craig E., DO
- Morgan, Benjamin, MD
- Rogers, Brian James, MD
- Roman, Jacqueline D., DO
- Theocharides, Thomas, MD

Orthopedic Surgery
- Chern, Kenneth Y., MD
- Demetriades, Haralambos, MD
- Haynes, Paul Thomas II, MD
- McDaid, Kevin C., MD
- Nguyen, Hoan-Vu Tran, MD
- Spagnuola, Christopher J., MD
- Yalamanchili, Praveen K., MD

Otolaryngology
- Ezon, Frederick C., MD

Pediatric Endocrinology
- Kerensky, Kirk M., MD

Pediatric Orthopedics
- Collins, Christopher Michael, MD

Pediatrics
- Fried, Martin D., MD
- Lichtenberger, Janice Ann, MD
- Lipp, Alfred J., DO
- Lipstein, Rebekah Ann, MD
- O'Brien, Thomas Kevin, MD
- Omotoso, Olukemi Yetunde, MD
- Sasson, Elias, MD
- Setton, Ellen E., MD
- Topilow, Judith F., MD

Physical Medicine & Rehab
- Meyers, Adam M., DO

Psychiatry
- Lang, Karen Friedman, MD
- Patel, Sameer Ramesh, MD

Pulmonary Disease
- Ali, Rana Y., MD
- Elsawaf, Mohamed Ashraf, MD

Rheumatology
- Al Haj, Rany Samir, MD

Ocean City
Family Med-Sports Medicine
- Sokalsky, Brian Edward, DO

Family Medicine
- Baretto, Luigi U., MD
- Chew, Jason M., DO
- Dunn, Ernest Charles Jr., MD
- Raab, Gary W., DO
- Udani, Chandrakan I., MD

Internal Medicine
- Cozamanis, Steve G., DO
- Perez Feliz, Ulices A., MD

Obstetrics & Gynecology
- Lavis, James Douglas, DO
- Wilson, James Ashley II, MD

Ophthalmology
- Huang, Jun C., MD

Ocean Grove
Internal Medicine
- Beal, Jeffrey M., MD
- Kong, Young D., MD

Ocean View
Family Medicine
- Carlin, Francis Scott, DO

Osteopathic Medicine
- Wilson, Donna E., DO

Oceanport
Family Medicine
- Odell, Tamara Lozier, DO

Surgery (General)
- Vozos, Frank J., MD

Old Bridge
Anesthesiology
- De Ocera, Zenaida Bascara, MD

Anesthesiology: Pain Medicine
- Del Valle, Jacqueline P., MD
- Moten, Hadi S., MD
- Winn, Terrance T., MD

Cardiovascular Disease
- Wajnberg, Alexander, MD

Child & Adolescent Psychiatry
- Krishnamsetty, Nanditha, MD

Critical Care Medicine
- Lee, Edward G., MD
- Mathew, Joseph, MD

Dermatology
- Centurion, Santiago Alberto, MD
- Vaillant, Juan Guillermo, MD

Diagnostic Radiology
- Park, Peter Byung, MD
- Shami, Msallam M., MD

Emergency Medicine
- Cheng, Peter F., MD
- Davis, Patrick Michael, MD
- Noormohamed, Akbar H., MD
- Parreno, Maritza Georgette, MD
- Ruth, Tiffany Karim, MD

Endocrinology
- Spiler, Ira J., MD

Family Medicine
- Balinski, Beth A., DO
- Belder, Olga, DO
- Bernabe, Maria Joyce Row G., MD
- Cohen, Howard Steven, DO
- Robinson, Jonnie M., DO
- Ryan, Sharon L., MD
- Turkish, Jennifer M., MD

Geriatrics
- Enukashvili, Rafael R., MD

Glaucoma
- Wong, Sze Ho, MD

Infectious Disease
- Middleton, John R., MD

- Tiruvury, Hemavarna, MD

Internal Medicine
- Agarwal, Sangeeta, MD
- Bethencourt, Guillermo F., MD
- Del Alcazar, Carlos O., MD
- Demos, James P., MD
- Giri, Janaki, MD
- Hasham, Mohamed H., MD
- Ivchenko, Ludmila, MD
- Jafri, Rana B., MD
- Laemmle, Patricia C., MD
- Lupicki, Marek R., MD
- Mezic, Edward T., MD
- Mirza, Babar, MD
- Mistry, Tusharkumar N., MD
- Nayyar, Sanjeev, MD
- Nigam, Jyoti, MD
- Patel, Diptika D., MD
- Patel, Parini Munjal, MD
- Patel, Vijay Ramanikbhai, MD
- Price, Craig C., MD
- Raoof, Natalia, MD
- Raoof, Nazar, MD
- Renda, John A., MD
- Rukshin, Vladimir B., MD
- Sobel, David Charles, MD
- Zilber, Eugenia, MD

Neurology
- Rao, Padmarekha, MD
- Song, Haodong, MD

Obstetrics & Gynecology
- Cohen, Brad J., MD

Ophthalmology
- Blondo, Dennis L., MD
- Cohen, Ilan, MD
- Scharfman, Robert M., MD

Orthopedic Surgery
- Hassan, Sheref E., MD

Other Specialty
- Fahmy, Sandra Patricia, DO

Otolaryngology
- Azer, Andrew Elia, MD

Otolaryngology-Facial Plastic
- Chowdhury, Farhad Reza, DO

Pediatrics
- Arumugam, Maheswari, MD
- Asprec, Claro M., MD
- Barakat, Raja, MD
- Grochowalska, Ewa Malgorzata, MD
- Herman, Jeffrey P., MD
- Mesina, Leon B., MD
- Osman, Ihsan, MD
- Parikh, Meenakshi B., MD
- Quiba, Ronald C., MD
- Salston, Robert S., MD
- Shih, Henry Tsong-Ir, MD
- Siddiqui, Zehra, DO
- Vadali, Rajyalaks Vaidehi, MD

Physical Med & Rehab-Sports Med
- Cohen, Jason Ronald, MD

Physical Medicine & Rehab
- Del Valle, Francisco I., MD
- Lupicki, Lucyna K., MD

Psychiatry
- Co, Gerrie T., MD
- Joshi, Kumud Gada, MD
- Laurelli, Joseph P., MD
- Naeem, Sana, MD
- Swamy, Aldonia A., MD

Pulmonary Disease
- Dhakhwa, Raj B., MD
- Ratkalkar, Kishore, MD

Radiology
- Belani, Puneet B., MD

Spinal Surgery
- Landa, Joshua, MD

Surgery (General)
- Markov, Nikolai Yordanov, DO

Urology
- Cha, Doh Yoon, MD
- Pagano, Matthew J., MD

Old Tappan
Cardiac Anesthesia
- Nadeau, Pascale, MD

Diagnostic Radiology
- Lyons, John S., MD

Gastroenterology
- Chaudhri, Eirum I., MD

Internal Medicine
- Pelavin, Martin D., MD

Schwartz,Diane C.,MD
Pediatrics
De Angelo,Ann M.,MD
Fishkind,Perry Neal,MD
Hages,Harry A.,MD
Rothenberg,Nancy A.,DO
Physical Medicine & Rehab
Dephillips,Donna M.,MD
Psychiatry
Tancer,Nancy Kaplan,MD

Oradell
Anatomic/Clinical Pathology
Nasr,Sherif Abbas,MD
Rahman,Saud Saqib,MD
Cardiovascular Disease
Karlekar,Kripalaxmi R.,MD
Diagnostic Radiology
Albert,Arthur S.,MD
Chu,Regina Wong,MD
Thame,Craig H.,MD
Family Med-Sports Medicine
Mendler,James Christopher,MD
Family Medicine
Abend,David S.,DO
Internal Medicine
Braun,John E.,DO
Gonzalez,Patria Ramona,MD
Hyon,Joseph K.,DO
Kramer,Radu,MD
Polimeni,Marc David,MD
Neurological Radiology
Zablow,Bruce Charles,MD
Neurological Surgery
Azmi Ghadimi,Hooman,MD
Kaptain,George J.,MD
Karimi,Reza J.,MD
Khan,Mohammed Faraz,MD
Lee,Kangmin Daniel,MD
Roth,Patrick A.,MD
Vingan,Roy David,MD
Walzman,Daniel Ezra,MD
Zahos,Peter A.,MD
Obstetrics & Gynecology
Dotto,Myles E.,MD
Wang,Belle,MD
Wiener,Craig B.,MD
Orthopedic Surgery
Kane,Seth O.,MD
Otolaryngology
Bough,Irvin David Jr.,MD
Cusumano,Robert J.,MD
Huang,John Jan,MD
Leventhal,Douglas Drew,MD
Surow,Jason B.,MD
Pediatric Allergy
Skripak,Justin Michael,MD
Pediatrics
Battista,Carl J.,MD
Czernizer,Patricia L.,MD
Jeney,Heather A.,MD
Kurz,Lisa Beth,MD
Rosen,Lawrence David,MD
Plastic Surgery
Jacobs,Jeffry Lance,DO
Radiology
Emy,Margaret Yoko,MD
Krugman,Robert L.,MD
Rakow,Joel I.,MD
Urology
Garden,Richard J.,MD
Zoretic,Stephen N.,MD

Orange
Adolescent Medicine
Thomas,Montrae C.,MD
Cardiovascular Disease
Barai,Jayant H.,MD
Gastroenterology
Da Costa,Theodore A.,MD
Hematology
Amin,Jashvant S.,MD
Internal Medicine
Amin,Alpesh Jashvant,MD
Barnes,Dora Pinky,MD
Gialanella,Francis J.,MD
Maddali,Vani,MD
Mirchandani,Ratan,MD
Raymond,Jacques Carol,MD
Obstetrics & Gynecology
Wolfe,Taida J.,MD

Pediatrics
Vannoy,Dioscora R.,MD
Psychiatry
Reyes,Christine,MD
Shah,Ila H.,MD
Urology
Johnson,George A.,MD

Oxford
Family Medicine
Meyer-Grimes,Leslie B.,MD

Palisades Park
Family Medicine
Kim,Yoonjoo,MD
Internal Medicine
Chung,Haeyang,MD
Kandinov,Fanya,MD
Lee,Sung-Won,MD
Park,Wonil,MD
Ophthalmology
Chu,David Shu-Chih,MD
Kim,Daniel Y.,MD
Lee,Sangwoo,MD
Lyu,Theodore,MD
Pediatrics
Choe,Joseph Lee,MD
Yun,Haenam,MD
Urology
Park,Ji Hae,MD

Palmyra
Family Medicine
Hartmann,Rupert C. II,DO
Rosenzweig,Alan,DO

Paramus
Abdominal Surgery
Schmidt,Hans J.,MD
Addiction Psychiatry
Reddy,Srikanth Madadi,MD
Allergy & Immunology
Chang,Cindy Ching,MD
Anatomic Pathology
Swartz,Jennifer L.,DO
Anatomic/Clinical Pathology
DiCarlo,Frederick J.,MD
Garcia-Lat,Zenda,MD
Turyan,Hach Vladimir,MD
Anesthesiology
Binder,Michael,MD
Giraldo,Juan Pablo,MD
Gungor,Semih,MD
Higgins,Annlouise Maria,MD
Narayanan,Manglam,MD
Ragukonis,Thomas P.,MD
Roche,Elizabeth Ann,MD
Rubinchik,Noemy Aronovici,MD
Silverman,Robert S.,MD
Trnovski,Stefan,MD
Zhuravkov,Alexander,MD
Anesthesiology: Pain Medicine
Goswami,Amit,MD
Breast Surgery
Christoudias,Moira Katherine,MD
Cardiovascular Disease
Baklajian,Robert,MD
Cohen,David Eliot,MD
Elson,Abe,MD
Skeete-Jackson,Kalia Nicole,MD
Wiedermann,Joseph Gad,MD
Child & Adolescent Psychiatry
Calvert,Sara Marie,MD
Khan,Adnan Iqbal,MD
Puthiyathu,Manoj,MD
Radulescu,Raluca Ileana,MD
Shabo,Jessica E.,MD
Cosmetic Surgery
Boss,William K. Jr.,MD
Lat,Emmanuel A.,MD
Dermatology
Baxt,Rebecca D.,MD
Baxt,Saida H.,MD
Cyrulnik,Amanda Amy,MD
Garcia,Carmen Josefina,MD
Goldstein,Marcy A.,MD
Gordon,Karen Ann,MD
Kopeloff,Iris H.,MD
Li,Cindy Yuk,DO
Schorr,Ethlynn Susan,MD
Wiederkehr,Michael,MD
Young,Alexis Livingston,MD
Emergency Medicine
Goldberg,Alvin Hugh,MD

Endocrinology
Dzhalturova,Nadire,DO
Fernandez,Marlyn A.,MD
Levy,Brian Leonard,MD
Manougian,Ara,MD
Shah,Viral Jagdishbhai,MD
Tohme,Jacques Fuad,MD
Family Medicine
Chadha,Sonia,MD
Herring,Gary S.,MD
Kantha Bhatnagar,Rajashree,MD
Mathews,Jyoti,MD
Pacheco,Felix Fernando,MD
Rubin,Steven F.,DO
Rutigliano,Michael W.,MD
Saieva,Carol E.,DO
Sandhu,Basant Singh,MD
Saros,Cathleen Mary,DO
Tzeng,Bowen Chi,MD
Wang,David Alexander,MD
Forensic Pathology
Clayton,MaryAnn B.,MD
Gastroenterology
De Lillo,Anthony Rocco,MD
Greenspan,Joshua N.,MD
Hatefi,Homayoon,MD
Kurz,Jeremiah S.,MD
Lippe,Scott David,MD
Shukla,Nilesh B.,MD
Wien,Frederic E.,MD
General Practice
Borkowski,Douglas Joseph,MD
Geriatric Psychiatry
Dhingra,Monica,MD
Ghani,Muhammad Rehan,MD
Geriatrics
Adel,Nourihan,MD
Das,Urmi,MD
Kushner,Evan G.,MD
Menacker,Morey J.,DO
Prowse,Alicia Ann,MD
Yousef,Javed Muhammad,MD
Hand Surgery
Fakharzadeh,Frederick F.,MD
Rosenstein,Roger G.,MD
Tuckman,Drew E.,MD
Ugras,Steven A.,MD
Hematology
Fernbach,Barry R.,MD
Ligresti,Louise G.,MD
Hematology Oncology
Suh,Jason W.,MD
Wood,Kevin C.,MD
Infectious Disease
Dandavate,Varsha Mohan,MD
Internal Med-Hospice Palliative
Spitzer,Ayelet,DO
Internal Medicine
Agarwal,Amit,MD
Anshelevich,Irina,MD
Barua,Aruna,MD
Cacciola,Thomas A.,MD
Casper,Ephraim S.,MD
Chak,Azfar Khalid,MD
Chung,Jeff,MD
Dumay,Serge,MD
Finn,Roman E.,MD
Firoozi,Babak,MD
Fleischner,Nathaniel P.,MD
Focella,Salvatore,MD
Giangola,Joseph,MD
Goa,Cristobal Javier,MD
Harutyunyan,Anna,MD
Iversen,Robin J.,MD
Jacobs,Stephen H.,MD
Jaiyebo,Omotola Olubunmi,MD
Kavaler,Robert,MD
Konkesa,Anuradha R.,MD
Leibu,Tonel,MD
Loreti,Michael Earl,MD
Luongo,Peter A.,MD
Malhotra,Pieusha,MD
Mapitigama,Renuka Nilmini,MD
Markenson,Joseph A.,MD
Masri,Sammy Ismail,MD
Matos-Cloke,Susan I.,MD
Mittapalli,Kesavarao,MD
Novak,Caroline J.,MD
Parangi,Robert K.,MD
Parangi,Sasan M.,MD
Pastrano Lluberes,Magna,MD

Patel,Sureshbhai N.,MD
Rakowski,Thomas J.,MD
Scivoletti,Peter D.,MD
Segal,Shiri Nicole,MD
Seydafkan,Shabnam,MD
Sgambati,Theodore F. Jr.,MD
Shatkin,Jason Alan,MD
Singh,Harmeet,MD
Sourial,Hany A.,MD
Sweeting,Robert,MD
Teplinsky,Eleonora,MD
Tievsky,Erika Fiorella,DO
Varbaro,Gian Stefano,MD
Varriano,Anthony,MD
Winer,Steven A.,MD
Maternal & Fetal Medicine
Goldman,Jane Cleary,MD
Zelop,Carolyn M.,MD
Medical Genetics
Robinson,Lois Pat,MD
Nephrology
Abbasi,Arshia,MD
Ibeabuchi,Adaeze Nneka,MD
Neuro-Psychiatry
Crain,Peter M.,MD
Neurological Radiology
Bahramipour,Phillip F.,MD
Neurology
Conte,Theodore J.,MD
Neuromusculoskeletal Med & OMM
Grinman,Lev,MD
Obstetrics & Gynecology
Chen,Dehan,MD
Golin,Thomas,MD
Jones,Howard Harris,MD
Matthews,Gail Margaret,MD
Meyer,Monica Lynn,MD
Mosquera Charlenea,Claudia,MD
Nasseri,Ali,MD
Nickles,Donna E.,DO
O'Brien,Katherine Elizabeth,MD
Ohanian,Heripsime,MD
Rizk,Naglaa T.,MD
Russo,Thomas O.,MD
Siegel,Amy Michele,MD
Weinstein,Melissa A.,DO
Occupational Medicine
Liva,Jeffrey S.,MD
Marino,Phyllis E.,MD
Oncological Surgery
Yiengpruksawan,Anusak,MD
Ophthalmology
Burke,Patricia A.,MD
Liva,Douglas F.,MD
Pettinelli,Damon John,MD
Pomerantz,Scott Barry,MD
Orthopedic Surgery
Difelice,Gregory Scott,MD
Distefano,Michael C.,MD
Elliott,Andrew J.,MD
Hartzband,Mark A.,MD
Klein,Gregg Roger,MD
Kovatis,Paul Evan,MD
McIlveen,Stephen J.,MD
Newman,Bernard P. III,MD
Okezie,Chukueke Tobenna,MD
Ranawat,Anil S.,MD
Seidenstein,Ari Douglas,MD
Snyder,Ronald David,MD
Stoller,Steven M.,MD
Orthopedic Surgery-Adult Rcnstr
Levine,Harlan Brett,MD
Otolaryngology
Bar-Eli,Rebecca,MD
Le,Mina Nguyen,MD
Samadi,Sharyar Daniel,MD
Pain Medicine-Interventional
Sood,Rahul,DO
Pediatric Cardiology
Rhee,Young Sun Diane,MD
Pediatric Endocrinology
Kumpta,Shilpa Narsing,MD
Pelavin,Paul Isaac,MD
Pediatric Orthopedics
Widmann,Roger Franklin,MD
Pediatric Surgery
Alexander,Frederick Jr.,MD
Friedman,David Lewis,MD
Gandhi,Rajinder P.,MD

Physicians by Town and Medical Specialty

Paramus (cont)
Pediatrics
Kim,Sunmee Louise,MD
Kotturi,Shiva Kumar,MD
Kushner,Susan C.,MD
Monaco,Melissa Garofalo,MD
Padilla,Dominga Sol,MD
Rabinowitz,Arnold H.,MD
Rodriguez-Zierer,Maria E.,MD
Saks,Darren,MD
Shtern,Tatiana,MD
Slater,John G.,MD
Stiefel,Laurence N.,MD
Physical Medicine & Rehab
Collins,Caitlin,MD
Fossati,Jeffrey Joseph,MD
Grigorescu,Catalina Anca,MD
Hattab,Raed Abdulla,MD
Schmaus,Peter Howard,MD
Thomson,Fani Jacqueline,DO
Plastic & Reconstructive Srgy
Zapiach,Luis Alberto,MD
Plastic Surgery
Baxt,Sherwood A.,MD
Breslow,Gary David,MD
Cozzone,John T.,MD
Ferraro,Frank James Jr.,MD
Gartner,Michael C.,DO
Moskovitz,Marty J.,MD
Parker,Paul M.,MD
Rabinowitz,Sidney,MD
Small,Tzvi,MD
Usal,Hakan Marc,MD
Zubowski,Robert I.,MD
Psychiatry
Abrar,Samar,MD
Adel,Tymaz,MD
Airapetian,Karine V.,MD
Al-Salem,Salim Suliaman,MD
Benitez,Jose L.,MD
Cheema,Faiz Aslam,MD
Federbush,Joel S.,MD
Harrigan,Michael Richard,MD
Iqbal,Mohammad Javed,MD
Kahn,Frederick E.,MD
Kotler,Lisa A.,MD
Marte,Juan M.,MD
Metelitsin,Marina Nikolaevna,MD
Miller,Helene Anne,MD
Nissirios,Kalliopi,MD
Oczkos,Patrick,MD
Palkhiwala,Bharati A.,MD
Palmer,Barbara A.,MD
Ragheb,Sameh Makram,MD
Ramay,Mohammad Hanif,MD
Varas,Elizabeth A.,MD
Waseem,Mehnaz,MD
Winters,Richard Allan,MD
Pulmonary Disease
Sakowitz,Arthur J.,MD
Sakowitz,Barry H.,MD
Radiation Oncology
DeYoung,Chad M.,MD
Kole,Thomas Pedicino,MD
Wesson,Michael F.,MD
Reproductive Endocrinology
Greenseid,Keri Lee,MD
Rheumatology
Gross,Michael L.,MD
Wu,Dee Dee Yui,MD
Spinal Surgery
Hughes,Alexander Philip,MD
Sports Medicine
Savatsky,Gary J.,MD
Surgery (General)
Alshafie,Tarek Ahmed,MD
Aydin,Nebil Bill,MD
Bedrosian,Andrea Stephanie,MD
Cummings,Dustin Randal,MD
Dhorajia,Seema P.,DO
Eid,Sebastian R.,MD
Ewing,Douglas R.,MD
Gandolfi,Brad Michael,MD
Klein,Laura Ann,MD
Mansson,Jonas,MD
Trivedi,Amit,MD
Thoracic Surgery
Korst,Robert J.,MD
Shapiro,Mark,MD
Urology
Campo,Richard Paul,MD

Lebovitch,Steve,MD
Panossian,Alexander M.,MD
Rome,Sergey,MD
Vitenson,Jack H.,MD
Vascular Surgery
Danks,John Michael,MD

Park Ridge
Cardiovascular Disease
Feigelis,Robin Y.,MD
Critical Care Medicine
Hoffman,Joseph Henry,MD
Dermatology
Abeles,Gwen Dee,MD
Family Medicine
Licciardone,Salvatore J.,DO
Obstetrics & Gynecology
Corbett,Shonda Marcia,MD
Fallon,Kimberly L.,MD
Pediatrics
Grossi,Maureen A.,MD
Wang,Linda,MD
Psychiatry
Lopez,Lina Maria,MD
Pulmonary Disease
Mendelowitz,Paul C.,MD
Surgery (General)
Bonvicino,Nicholas G.,MD

Parlin
Cardiovascular Disease
Nagarsheth,Harish N.,MD
Piscopiello,Michael,MD
Younan,K. George,MD
Family Medicine
Frazier,Hawwa Sharif,DO
Kaur,Harleen,MD
Patel,Deepa N.,MD
Hand Surgery
Bakhos,Abdel M.,MD
Internal Medicine
Denis,Joanna M.,MD
Florczyk,Margaret,MD
Florczyk,Miroslaw,MD
Khan,Abrar Maqsood,MD
Mohapeloa,Gugu R.,MD
Shah,Dhiren,MD
Younan,Shaddy Kivarkis,MD
Younan,Zyad,MD
Occupational Medicine
Deltieure,Michele H.,MD
Otolaryngology
Zapanta,Vicente T.,MD
Pediatrics
Feliksik Watorek,Elzbieta B.,MD
Khan,Sohaila,MD
Nagarsheth,Veena H.,MD
Physical Med & Rehab-Pain Med
Georgy,John,MD

Parsippany
Allergy
Applebaum,Eric S.,MD
Jampol,Francis Michael,MD
Allergy & Immunology
Mehta,Archana P.,MD
Anatomic/Clinical Pathology
Suffin,Stephen Chester,MD
Anesthesiology
Anjutgi,Rajyashree,MD
Baker,Michelle Rapacon,MD
Balakrishna,Shruthi,MD
Barg,Vadim A.,MD
Blanchfield,Patrick Thomas,MD
Chen,Guo-Gang,MD
Choudhary,Ratna,MD
Clanton,Chase P.,MD
Cohen,Michael B.,MD
Daniel,Brian P.,DO
Daras,Jason Glenn,DO
Davanzo,Peter A.,MD
DeSimone,Robert Anthony,MD
Delis,Aristidis G.,MD
Eisenstat,Carol M.,MD
Fanouse,John A.,DO
Garibaldi,Thomas A.,MD
Ghosh,Arpita,MD
Grasso,Mario Lucio,MD
Grimaldi,Matthew Porter,MD
Jacobson,Martin Alexander,MD
Janardhan,Yellagonda V.,MD
Kussick,Neil J.,MD
Lamanna,Adolfo C.,MD

Lasker,Steven Mark,MD
Lian,Hanzhou,MD
Lyall,Jasleen Kaur,MD
Ofeldt,James D.,DO
Olechowski,George N.,MD
Panei,Maryann S.,MD
Patel,Gaurav R.,MD
Patel,Mona,MD
Patel,Niva S.,MD
Patel,Taral B.,DO
Pham,Vu Linh,MD
Pikus,Igor,MD
Rana,Kirtida Dinesh,MD
Ravindra,Sunay B.,MD
Shah,Mehul D.,DO
Shih,Yangyu Steven,MD
Shore,Ronald Andrew,DO
Sim,Andrew R.,MD
Singh,Jagjeet,MD
Spina,Laurie J.,MD
Suchy,Matthew Robert,DO
Taragin,Michael S.,MD
Terreri,Michael Robert Jr.,MD
Thakur,Jagdish G.,MD
Tsafos,Vassilios,MD
Wassef,Michael Karim,MD
Wong,Henry Chen,MD
Young,Jill S.,DO
Zabrodina,Yanina V.,MD
Child & Adolescent Psychiatry
Srinivasan,Shankar,MD
Dermatology
Almeida,Laila M.,MD
Kingsbery,Mina Yassaee,MD
Livingston,Wendy E.,MD
Milbauer,James,MD
Shah,Subhadra Sundaram,MD
Strauss,Eric A.,MD
Weinberg,Harvey I.,MD
Weiser,Jessica Ann,MD
Diagnostic Radiology
Chung,Jean Young,MD
Menendez,Christine M.,MD
Murphy,Robyn C.,MD
Parisi,Angela Rosina,MD
Rios,Jose Conrado,MD
Sheth,Milan Pravin,MD
Swayne,Lawrence C.,MD
Yablonsky,Thaddeus M.,MD
Emergency Medicine
Berger,Richard P.,MD
Ceppetelli,Lisa C.,MD
Cochrane,Dennis G.,MD
Crean,Christopher Arthur,MD
Curato,Mark Anthony,DO
Cuthbert,David,MD
Figueroa,Delia,MD
Freer,Christopher F.,DO
Giroski,Laura J.,DO
Gould,Michael Alan,MD
Greenhut,William H.,DO
Hartmann,Anthony William,MD
Heller,Mitchell J.,MD
Indruk,William L.,MD
Kassutto,Zach,MD
Lebaron,Johnathon Clinton,DO
Lehet,Justin Micheal,DO
Loewenstein,Robert Elvin,MD
Melnick,Gerald J.,MD
Milano,Marc Anthony,MD
Minett,Danielle Marie,MD
Minett,Kenneth Matthew,MD
Mouridy,Gary C.,DO
Murray-Taylor,Stacey Odell,MD
Nguyen,Matthew Thai-Khang,MD
Oh,David H.,MD
Perotte,Schubert,MD
Reddy,Chenna G.,MD
Schiller,Andrew P.,MD
Shah,Sachin Jitendra,MD
Stapleton,George S.,MD
Troncoso,Alexis B.,MD
Utkewicz,Mark D.,MD
Family Medicine
Molisso,Mary Cuellari,DO
Prasad,Prema,MD
Fertility/Infertility
Lam,Paul C.,MD
General Practice
Earl,Lawrence N.,MD
Holder,William B.,MD

Shah,Mansi R.,MD
Gynecology
Friedel,Walter E.,MD
Hepatology
Xie,Bingru,MD
Internal Medicine
Adessa,Kenneth J.,MD
Banker,Shobhana,MD
Castellano,Lillian Checchio,MD
Chanana,Manju,MD
Garg,Shyamala,MD
Khan,Sarah,MD
Kumar,Sadhana,MD
Lee,Serena Qi-Qin,MD
Luhana,Manish P.,MD
Patel,Jignasa,MD
Patel,Kamal Kanubhai,MD
Poon,Gilbert B.,MD
Puzino,Alan Vincent,MD
Ram,Meryl H.,MD
Scranton,Richard E.,MD
Song,Hongya,MD
Takahashi,Eric Michael,DO
Vallario,Michael J.,MD
Ziolo,Malgorzata Maria,MD
Nuclear Medicine
Paik,David,MD
Obstetrics & Gynecology
Bellish,Jenna H.,MD
Bissinger,Craig L.,MD
Haskel,Steven A.,MD
Hirsch,David Jay,MD
Khalid,Samira,DO
Leviss,Stephen R.,MD
Orthopedic Surgery
Siegel,Jeffrey Alan,MD
Otolaryngology
Brys,Agata K.,MD
Lebovitz,Brian Lee,MD
Sayeed,Zarina Shaikh,MD
Schultz,Charles Martin,MD
Wirtshafter,Karen A.,MD
Pediatrics
Ahsan,Ambreen,MD
Bramwell,Julia,MD
Chen,Zeng-Shan,MD
Deutsch,Robert Jay,MD
Feingold,Jay Marshall,MD
Handler,Robert W.,MD
Kahn,Daniel Efraim,MD
Koenigsberg,Alan M.,MD
Li,Annie Hongyan,MD
Patel,Dinesh R.,MD
Patel,Varshaben T.,MD
Rajkumar,Aradhana,MD
Physical Medicine & Rehab
Bouzane,Gayten Carroll,MD
Kumar,Ajay,MD
Psychiatry
Bhatia,Malini P.,MD
Carness,Jason,MD
Novik,Emily,MD
Solanki,Rashminkumar R.,MD
Weisman,Tamara K.,DO
Radiology
Calhoun,Sean Keith,DO
Cosentino,Mark O.,MD
Friedman,Paul Dean,DO
Wynne,Peter J.,MD
Surgery (General)
Peyser,Irving G.,MD

Passaic
Anatomic/Clinical Pathology
Bassil,Ghassan G.,MD
Setoodeh,Farhad,MD
Anesthesiology
Agres,Mildred D.,MD
Boukiia,Marina,MD
Chung,Jae Won,MD
Ekulide,Ifeyinwa Ndidi,MD
Jones,Kevin Errol,MD
Jotwani,Madhu M,MD
Lakshmi,Vijaya S R,MD
Lee,Ai R.,MD
Lee,Chang J.,MD
Lee Ellis,Nandi T.,MD
Malazarte,Justito B.,MD
Mankikar,Durgesh P.,MD
Odondi,Janet Aoko,MD
Prasad,Jitender,MD
Raza,Syed Mohsin,MD

Reuveni,Michael A.,MD
Rhodes,Michael Eric,MD
Sacknowitz,Ivy J.,MD
Salomon,Guy,MD
Stein,Steven J.,MD
Sukhavasi,Sujatha,MD
Thomas,George,MD
Venkataraman,Ravi Kumar,MD
Weissman,Allan Mark,MD
Cardiovascular Disease
 Sharma,Surendra M.,MD
Critical Care Medicine
 Abraham,James V.,MD
Emergency Medicine
 Eletto,Vincent Joseph,MD
 Kennett,Shar,MD
 Stephenson,Karen Rosemarie,MD
 Umali,Alma B.,MD
Family Medicine
 Castilla,William A.,MD
 DeMuro,Paul G. Jr.,DO
 Fernandez Santiago,Angela,DO
 Fomitchev,Oleg V.,MD
 Makui,Sheyda,MD
 Soliman,Ishak G.,MD
 Solomon,Jennifer,MD
 Vega,Andres,MD
General Practice
 Kumar,Rekha A.,MD
 Sacristan,Carlos,MD
Gynecology
 Leo,Chadwick S.,DO
Hematology
 Lee,Sheue H.,MD
Infectious Disease
 Gupta,Punit Kumar,MD
Internal Medicine
 Abutabikh,Nael Abdelsalam,MD
 Avancha,Amarnath,MD
 Guevarra,Keith Poscablo,DO
 Ramdial,Maria Janine,MD
 Reyes,Bernadette O.,MD
 Rodriguez,Jaime,MD
 Shah,Anuj Raju,MD
 Tejeda,Carlos Alberto,MD
 Wong,Jiyoung,DO
Obstetrics & Gynecology
 Ahkami,Shahrokh,MD
 Carson,Milinda Ruth,MD
 Chavez-Cacho,Jose M.,MD
 De Lara,Vilma A.,MD
 Gagliano,Salvatore M.,MD
Ophthalmology
 Mendoza,Luis,MD
 Steinberg,Melissa S.,MD
 Vogel,Mitchell,MD
 Winfield,Steven S.,MD
Pain Medicine
 Eppanapally,Shanti Sree,MD
Pathology
 Fernandes,Gregory M.,MD
Pediatric Endocrinology
 Aguayo-Figueroa,Lourdes,MD
Pediatrics
 Ahmadi,Cyrus,MD
 Almanzar,Raul,MD
 Aryal,Sunita,MD
 Bravo,Holanda P.,MD
 Camilo,Antonio Manuel,MD
 Fernandez,Yocasta Mabel,MD
 Ferrer,Angel Salvador,MD
 Hernandez,Jacqueline,DO
 Japa-Camilo,Judelka,MD
 Malitzky,Susan,MD
 Mico,Mario R.,MD
 Mosquera,Maria Cecilia,MD
 Rodriguez Montana,Manuel A.,MD
 Samet,Elliott,MD
 Schiffman,Jonathan Samson,MD
 Viswanathan,Revathi,MD
Physical Med & Rehab-Pain Med
 Schwartz,Mark Lawrence,DO
Physical Medicine & Rehab
 Kim,Ryul,DO
Psychiatry
 Ravelo,Mary Ann,MD
 Williams-Martin,Pamela Y.,MD
Surgery (General)
 Chuback,John A.,MD
 Hanna,Gamal Kamel,MD
 Ukrainskyj,Motria O.,MD

Thoracic Surgery
 Kaushik,Raj Ramanuj,MD
 Shakir,Huzaifa Abbas,MD
Paterson
Adolescent Medicine
 Blaustein,Silvia Adelina,MD
Adult Psychiatry
 La Porta,Lauren D.,MD
Allergy
 Kosinski,Mark S.,MD
 Perin,Patrick V.,MD
Anesthesiology
 Adkisson,Gregory Hugh,MD
 Akhtar,Shuaib A.,MD
 Apinis,Andrey,MD
 Armstead,Valerie Elizabeth,MD
 Aronova,Yelena,DO
 Badach,Mark J.,MD
 Bauman,Gregory A.,MD
 Burns,Talitha Mariana Hedley,DO
 Chalfin,Matthew Bryan,MD
 Chan,Kar-Mei,MD
 Chu,Amy M.,MD
 Dreznin,Howard N.,MD
 Enriquez-Leff,Liza Jeanne,MD
 Fernandez,Afranio L.,MD
 Figueroa,Pablo T.,MD
 Galldin,Lars Michael,MD
 Garcia,Gerald Matthew,MD
 Gargani,Stephanie,MD
 Germond,Christopher John,DO
 Grey,Glenn Allen,MD
 Holland,David Andersson,MD
 Kanetkar,Madhavi Jayat,MD
 Krottapalli,Harini,MD
 Landa,Seth E.,MD
 Lehman,Abraham Reuven,MD
 Leibu,Dorina,MD
 MacKenzie,Shauna,MD
 Makkapati,Sandhya Rani,MD
 Markley,Jonathan C.,DO
 Mekhjian,Haroutune A.,MD
 Moise,Anson Marryshow,MD
 Nandigam,Harish,MD
 Nuesa,Wilson O. IV,MD
 Oladeji,Oluremi O.,MD
 Parihar,Jasmit K.,DO
 Pearce,Donna Alison,MD
 Putterman,Debora,MD
 Rao,Sheila Yvonne,MD
 Ravi,Radhika,MD
 Rosales,Ramon Javillonar,MD
 Sakowitz Cohen,Noreen Gail,MD
 Sammarone,Marcello Eliseo,MD
 Saulon,Winston B.,MD
 Sidhu,Gursimar K.,MD
 Sultan,Ahmed Said,DO
 Umanoff,Michael D.,MD
 Upadya,Padmaja Koppal,MD
 Ventura,William Raphael,MD
 Wachtel,Zev,MD
 Whang,Ihn Young,MD
 Winikoff,Stephen P.,MD
 Yoganathan,Thil,MD
 Zisa,Salvatore Anthony Jr.,MD
 Zodiatis,Paras Jayant,DO
 Zuberi,Faizah,MD
Anesthesiology: Pain Medicine
 Sheikh,Ednan Salahuddin,MD
Bloodbanking
 Doniguian,Ann-Elizabeth E.,MD
Cardiovascular Disease
 Agarwal,Ashoke,MD
 Connolly,Mark William,MD
 Teli,Kunal J.,MD
Child & Adolescent Psychiatry
 Christodoulou,Evangelos,MD
 Garcia,Dianelys,MD
 Langan,Abigail E.,MD
 Marrero Figarella,Arturo L.,MD
Child (Pediatric) Neurology
 Patel,Poorvi K.,MD
Critical Care Medicine
 Sori,Alan J.,MD
 Upadhyay,Shivanck,MD
Dermatology
 Zemel,Mathias,MD
Diagnostic Radiology
 Balakumar,Kalavathy,MD
 Baltazar,Romulo Z.,MD
 Bar,Vandna Prasad,MD

Berlin,Fred,MD
Centanni,Marianne T.,MD
Freitag,Warren Barry,MD
Kwon,Stephen S.,MD
Milman,Edward,MD
Sanchez,Orestes,MD
Sheppard,Lisa Marie,MD
Taragin,Benjamin H.,MD
Emerg Med-Medical Toxicology
 Kashani,John S.,DO
Emergency Medicine
 Aberger,Kate,MD
 Adinaro,David Joseph,MD
 Ahmed,Zaib,DO
 Barnes,Stacey Ann,DO
 Bornstein,Marc Andrew,DO
 Boulos,Nader,MD
 Catapano,Anthony,DO
 Cohen,Andrew Nathan,DO
 Colantoni,Matthew Steven,DO
 Elhussein,Khalid Ali,MD
 Fischer,Mitchell Steven,DO
 Flannery,Ashley Laura,DO
 Friedland,Howard M.,DO
 George-Varghese,Blessit,DO
 Hochman,Steven Mark,MD
 Hwang,Eric Jesse,DO
 Karounos,Marianna,DO
 Kinyon,Jeffrey James,DO
 Kushner,Beth Jillian,DO
 Lapietra,Alexis Marie,DO
 Lob,Zev B.,DO
 Magarelli,Mary-Lynn,DO
 Manchester,Joseph Matthew,DO
 Marin,Adrian Alonso,DO
 Matadial,Manjushree,DO
 McGovern,Terrance,DO
 Meigh,Matthew James,DO
 Morecraft,John A. Jr.,MD
 Murphy,Ryan Bruce,MD
 Paez Perez,Yenisleidy,DO
 Patel,Nilesh Narendra,DO
 Pruden,James N.,MD
 Riss,Alexander David,DO
 Rosenberg,Mark S.,DO
 Sabando,Otto F.,DO
 Sanicola-Johnson,Julie Marie,DO
 Sharma,Uma,MD
 Shroff,Ninad A.,MD
 Summerville,Gregg Paul,MD
 Tillack,Lindsey Ann,MD
 Vlasica,Katherine,DO
 Whalen,Joanna Hallmark,DO
 Zdorovyak,Mina,MD
 Ziontz,Kristy L.,DO
Family Medicine
 De Feo,Daniel Scott,DO
 Elkholy,Neveen A.,DO
 Gachette,Emmanuel Amilcar,MD
 Hassan,Khaled A.,MD
 Kazmouz,Hasna M.,MD
 Revoredo,Fred S.,MD
 Sweidan,Safwan A.,MD
 Zaina,Samir A.,MD
Forensic Psychiatry
 Schiffman,Erica R.,MD
Gastroenterology
 Bollu,Janardhan,MD
General Practice
 Graves,Linda M.,MD
 Mirza,Nighat,MD
Geriatrics
 Gupta,Punita,MD
 Hossain,Shahreen Rafa,MD
 Sanchez Pena,Jose R.,MD
Hematology Oncology
 Kumar,Mehandar,MD
Hospitalist
 Manda,Jayaprakash,MD
 Tameem,Murtuza,MD
Infectious Disease
 Lange,Michael,MD
 Rabbat,Mohamed Salah,MD
 Zahran,Ali Abdelrahman,MD
Internal Medicine
 Agnelli,Michael Robert,MD
 Ahmad,Maliha,MD
 Ahsan,Shagufta,MD
 Al-Shrouf,Amal Ali,MD
 Alburquerque,Lucrecia A.,MD
 Alziadat,Moayyad Radi Barham,MD

Aqel,Mahmoud Bader,MD
Bahrampour,Ladan H.,MD
Bleeker,David Paul,MD
Calderon,Rosa L.,MD
Castillo,Hector L.,MD
Cavanagh,Yana,MD
Chatiwala,Jumana Safdar,MD
Chowdhury,Shamima,MD
Corazon,Alexis J.,MD
Cronin,Stephen R.,MD
Desueza,Juan A.,MD
Eid,Mahmoud Mohamed,MD
Elagami,Mohamed M.,MD
Facey,Maxine Elizabeth,MD
Ferraro,Lisa,MD
Figueroa,Nilka,MD
Gonnella,Eleanor A.,MD
Hanna,Michael,MD
Hassanien,Gammal A.,DO
Herrera,Jennifer Emma,MD
Ismail,Mourad Mohamed Farrag,MD
Jmeian,Ashraf,MD
Joseph,Albert M. Duverglas,MD
Kapoor,Ashima,MD
Khan,Nazia,MD
Khatib,Samara,MD
Kheyfets,Irina,MD
Kumar,Anand K.,MD
Kumar,Vinod,MD
Luna,Luis Freddy,MD
Mahmood,Nader Ahmad,MD
Majmundar,Sapan Haresh,DO
Manickavel,Suresh Kumar,MD
Marani-Dicovsky,Marcela C.,MD
Mechineni,Ashesha,MD
Mehta,Pooja S.,MD
Michael,Patrick M.,MD
Misthos,Paul,MD
Ovsjanikovska,Natalija,MD
Petrosyan,Gohar,MD
Propersi,Marco Egidio,DO
Refaie,Tarek,MD
Riguerra,Rosalia C.,MD
Saedeldine,Imad Khodor,MD
Sarkodie,Alex,MD
Seda,Evelyn R.,MD
Shah,Nalini D.,MD
Shah,Nihar N.,MD
Shah,Pradip A.,MD
Sheikh,Muzamil Wamiq,MD
Sherman,Henry M.,MD
Singhal,Monisha,MD
Suh,Jin Suk,MD
Taclob,Erlinda V.,MD
Taclob,Lowell T.,MD
Taclob,Michelle Maria,MD
Tao,Feng,MD
Tieng,Fortunata T.,MD
Varghese,Vibu,MD
Vitale,Joseph,MD
Yung Poon,Karen York-Mui,MD
Medical Oncology
 Yamusah,Emmanuel N.,MD
Neonatal-Perinatal Medicine
 Datta-Bhutada,Subhashree,MD
 Marrero,Luis C.,MD
 Menken,Gregory E.,MD
 Rosenblum,Stacy,MD
 Weissman,Michelle S.,MD
 Zauk,Adel M.,MD
Nephrology
 Boyd,Marvin T.,MD
Neurological Surgery
 Appelboom,Geoffrey,MD
 Mandigo,Grace Kim,MD
Neurology
 Altschul,Dorothea,MD
 Corrigan,Nicole Melissa,MD
 Dane,Steven H.,MD
 Mehta,Mahesh M.,MD
 Sathe,Swati Ajit,MD
 Stein,Beth,MD
 Xia,Wenlang,MD
Nuclear Medicine
 Conte,Patrick Jr.,MD
 Kalika,Valery,MD
Obstetrics & Gynecology
 Alnakeeb,Mohammed M.,MD
 Azar,Jihad Elias,MD
 Balazs,Peter,MD
 Beidleman,Danielle Melissa,MD
 Bilenki,Natalie I.,MD

Physicians by Town and Medical Specialty

Paterson (cont)
Obstetrics & Gynecology
Boghdady, Maged W., MD
Caldwell, Shinelle, DO
El Deeb, Mokhtar M., MD
Kaminskyj, Megan Elizabeth, MD
Kulwatdanaporn, Somchai, MD
Liriano, Monica, MD
Magid, Marissa, DO
Marino, Nicholas A., MD
Montemurro, Robert J., MD
Mustafa, Diane M., MD
Pendse, Vijay K., MD
Shilad, Aiman K., MD
White, Evelyn W., MD
Ophthalmology
Feng, Jing Jing, MD
Leifer, Alden, MD
Oral & Maxillofacial Surgery
Ephros, Hillel, MD
Orthopedic Surgery
Flood, Stephen James, MD
Otolaryngology
Labagnara, James Jr., MD
Otolaryngology-Facial Plastic
Folk, David, MD
Palliative Care
Boothe, Deniece Tamara, DO
Pathology
Akmal, Amer, MD
Kim, Minbae, MD
Pathology-Molecular Genetic
Hiemenz, Matthew Charles, MD
Pediatric Anesthesia
Ezrokhi, Marina B., MD
Meyer, Marc Andrew, MD
Pediatric Cardiology
Cocovinis, Barbara, MD
Messina, John Joseph, MD
Myridakis, Dorothy J., MD
Pediatric Emergency Medicine
Gutfreund, Devra A., MD
Naim, Farid A., MD
Severe, Monique Marie, MD
Pediatric Gastroenterology
Larson, Jacqueline Kay, MD
Pediatric Hematology Oncology
Bonilla, Mary Ann, MD
Kahn, Alissa Rachel, MD
Kaicker, Shipra, MD
Menell, Jill Suzanne, MD
Omesi, Lenore, MD
Woolbright, William Charles, MD
Pediatric Nephrology
Tawadrous, Hanan K., MD
Pediatric Orthopedics
Strongwater, Allan, MD
Pediatric Pulmonology
Blechner, Michael Scott, MD
Nachajon, Roberto V., MD
Nakra, Neal K., MD
Pediatric Radiology
Frank-Gerszberg, Robin G., MD
Pediatric Rheumatology
Srinivasan-Mehta, Jaya, MD
Pediatrics
Amadasu-Kest, Helen E., MD
Ayodeji, Olutope O., MD
Ballem, Arunajyoth, MD
Baluyot, Helen M., MD
Barilari, Rafael, MD
Batista, Jose, MD
Bhagia, Pooja R., MD
Brault, Peter V., MD
Dahrouj, Nabil I., MD
DeBruin, William J., MD
Dilallo, Denis, MD
Ebeid, Hasan Samir, MD
Eicher, Peggy Smith, MD
Espana, Madesa A., MD
Fastag Guttman, Eduardo, MD
Feingold, David Yitzchak, MD
Fernandes, Rinet Philomena, MD
Gadgil, Nandini S., MD
Galeano, Narmer E., MD
Garcia Rodriguez, Magdelyn, MD
Ginart, Gaspar L., MD
Goldberg, David Israel, MD
Haj-Ibrahim, Mouna, MD
Harwood, Katerina K., MD
Holahan, Joseph A., MD
Holahan, Nancy C., MD
Hussain-Rizvi, Ambrin, MD
Jadhav, Latha, MD
Jodorkovsky, Roberto Alex, MD
Khan, Ferhana, MD
Kim, Claudia, MD
Lamacchia, Michael A., MD
Lesesne-Ayodeji, Mercedes, MD
Lesser, Eric S., MD
Mallik, Aparna, MD
Mastrovitch, Todd Anthony, MD
Mejia, Edgar R., MD
Mejia, Gloria, MD
Meltzer, James Anthony, MD
Moises, Rodulfo P. Jr., MD
Naficy, Parvin P., MD
Naim, Suprema D., MD
Nathan, Michael D., DO
Ogunbameru, Emilola O., MD
Paz, Rafael E., MD
Prasad, Vijaya, MD
Pua, Zarah Jane Baysa, MD
Rivera-Penera, Maria T., MD
Samuel, Hala R., MD
See, Manuel T., MD
Shin, Young H., MD
Siddiqui, Muhammad Rehan, MD
Siddiqui, Rehma, MD
Skroce, Linda C., MD
Tengson, Roger C. Jr., MD
Thomas, Abraham S., MD
Physical Medicine & Rehab
Kaszubski, Priscilla D., DO
Parvez, Uzma, MD
Speez, Nancy Sprague, MD
Plastic Surgery
Podda, Silvio, MD
Szpalski, Caroline, MD
Psychiatry
Aladjem, Asher, MD
Arroyo, Louis, MD
Castillo, Hilda A., MD
Delvalle, Yissell, MD
Dementyeva, Yuliya, MD
Gad, Gamal Eldin, MD
Hirsh, Ron, MD
Micevski, Aleksandar, MD
Ribalta, Marcia, MD
Rueda, Carlos Alberto, MD
Siddiqui, Rehan, MD
Thimmaiah, Manavattir B., MD
Torres, Maria Elissa, MD
Verret, Joseph M., MD
Pulmonary Disease
Amoruso, Robert C., MD
Khan, Muhammad Anees, MD
Radiation Oncology
Herskovic, Thomas M., MD
Pereira, Michael J., MD
Radiology
Aluri-Vallabhaneni, Bhanu Sri, MD
Bontemps, Serge L., MD
Danoff, Madelyn S., MD
Hiremath, Vijay, MD
Rheumatology
Lahita, Robert George, MD
Surgery (General)
Bordan, Dennis Lawrence, MD
Budd, Daniel C., MD
Choi, Karmina, MD
Dalal, Setu A., DO
Damani, Tanuja, MD
Dela Torre, Andrew Nelson, MD
Elrabie, Nazmi A., MD
Elsawy, Osama Ahmed, DO
Ingram, Mark Anthony, MD
Madlinger, Robert Vincent, DO
Maio, Theodora J., MD
Warta, Melissa Hayward, MD
Surgical Critical Care
Zuberi, Jamshed A., MD
Thoracic Surgery
Cerda, Luis Mariano, MD
Orejola, Wilmo C., MD
Vega, Dennis, MD
Wohler, Alexander M., MD
Trauma Surgery
Bui, Hoan K., MD
Urology
Awad, Safwat M., MD
Vascular Surgery
Tello Valcarcel, Carlos A., MD

Paulsboro
Allergy
Litz, Steven A., MD
Family Medicine
Milas, Erica M., DO
Villare, Anthony W., MD

Peapack
Internal Medicine
Mand, Christine P., DO
Pediatrics
Roeloffs, Susan A., MD
Singh, Surbparkash Kaur, MD
Physical Medicine & Rehab
Osman, Sarah Ann, MD

Pemberton
Internal Medicine
Shaw, Wayne, MD
Pediatrics
Adumala, Pradeep, MD

Pennington
Anatomic Pathology
Jones, Krister J., MD
Anatomic/Clinical Pathology
Liu, Edward Shaoyou, MD
Anesthesiology
Ahmad, Sajida Ghani, MD
Cantillo, Joaquin J., MD
Enriquez, Joseph E., MD
Grujic, Slobodan, MD
Hanusey, Robert William, MD
Kollmeier, Brett R., MD
Liu, Renfeng, DO
Madsen, Melissa L., MD
Rao, Veena, MD
Reddy, Sudershan P., MD
Shah, Mahendra Govindlal, MD
Tolentino, Pablito L., MD
Vadhavkar, Aarti Sanjeev, MD
Voros, Stephen C., MD
Wuu, Zukwung, MD
Cardiothoracic Surgery
Lee, Daniel James, MD
Cardiovascular Disease
Glickman, Lee M., MD
Saxena, Neil, MD
Child & Adolescent Psychiatry
Fong, Donald Patrick, MD
Patchell, Roy Andrew, MD
Clinical Genetics
Trauffer, Patrice, MD
Emergency Medicine
Fellman, Katherine, MD
Endocrinology
Dhillon, Sudeep S., MD
Gillis Funderburk, Sheri A., MD
Parvez, Ayesha, MD
Saltzman, Erin Alyse, MD
Villanueva, Erika, MD
Family Medicine
Brescia, Donald, MD
Evans, Rachael Blackburn, MD
Gonzalez Acuna, Jose M., MD
Holdcraft, Suzanne, MD
Kakarla, Madhavi, MD
Patel, Jigar Dhansukh, MD
Samaddar, Soumen, MD
Thomsen, Kathleen M., MD
Gastroenterology
Bhatia, Jyoti Kamlesh, MD
Rogart, Jason Nathaniel, MD
Simonian, Armen John, MD
Hematology
Kindsfather, Scott K., MD
Hematology Oncology
McIntosh, Nenita Parrilla, MD
Schaebler, David L., MD
Hepatology
Munoz, Santiago Jose, MD
Internal Medicine
Balani, Anil R., MD
Ball, Omega Devora, MD
Desai, Harit, DO
Dhillon, Ravinder S., MD
Dhillon, Satvinder K., MD
Gandhi, Neel Jitendra, MD
Godin-Ostro, Evelyn R., MD
Grossman, Bernard, MD
Habib, Tehmina, MD
Iturbides, Victor D., MD
Johnson, Steven A., DO
Nee, Guy, MD
Radice, Beverly A., MD
Sordo, Sarah, MD
Williamson, Judith S., MD
Wu, Yan, MD
Yamane, Michael H., MD
Young, Kristopher F., DO
Medical Oncology
Rosvold, Elizabeth Anne, MD
Neurological Surgery
Buono, Lee M., MD
Connolly, Patrick Joseph, MD
Fennell, Vernard Sharif, MD
Stiefel, Michael Fred, MD
Neurology
Assadi-Khansari, Mitra, MD
Landen, Alexandra E., DO
Rubin, Mitchell J., MD
Schumacher, Hermann Christian, MD
Shukla, Chirag S., MD
Vester, John W., MD
Witte, Arnold S., MD
Obstetrics & Gynecology
McDonnell, Elizabeth Lynn, MD
Petty, Victoria Morey, MD
Ophthalmology
Desai, Priya Vasudev, MD
Lesniak, Sebastian P., MD
Matossian, Cynthia, MD
Rozenbaum, Ilya Maksovich, MD
Orthopedic Surgery
Caruso, Steven A., MD
Otolaryngology
Farzad, Ahmad, MD
Pain Medicine
Cruciani, Ricardo Alberto, MD
Pathology
Almashat, Salwan Jafar, MD
Fox, Ellen H., MD
Pediatric Hematology Oncology
Riewe, Kathleen O'Day, MD
Pediatrics
Behme, Renee Maria, MD
Besingi, Cecile Ewane, MD
Bunn, Diane Marie, MD
Goldfarb, Olga, MD
Kruse, Laurel Anita Farnham, MD
Riggall, Michael Justin, MD
Stephen, Priya Chachikutty, MD
Physical Medicine & Rehab
Gonzalez, Ronald H., MD
Graham, Patricia Ann, MD
Plastic Surgery
McLaughlin, Michael Joseph, MD
Tuma, Gary Alan, MD
Psychiatry
Donofrio, Scott D., MD
Raser, Keith A., MD
Rosenthal, Robert S., MD
Radiation Oncology
Chen, Timothy H., MD
Williamson, Shirnett Karean, MD
Surgery (General)
Allen, Lisa Rachel, MD
Chung, Jooyeun, MD
Dellacroce, Joseph Michael, MD
Johnson, Steven A., MD
Mustafa, Rose, MD
Rosato, Francis E., MD
Sailes, Frederick Cortney, MD
Surgical Critical Care
Kalina, Michael, DO
Transplant Surgery & Medicine
Doria, Cataldo, MD
Urology
Orland, Steven M., MD
Rogers, Brad S., MD
Vascular Neurology
Kumar, Rajat, MD
Naragum, Varun, MD
Vascular Surgery
Eisenberg, Joshua Aaron, MD
Fares, Louis G. II, MD

Penns Grove
Surgery (General)
Vora, Nagindas M., MD

Pennsauken
Acupuncture
 Levy,Brahman B.,MD
Allergy
 Glasofer,Eric David,MD
Family Medicine
 Cohen,Herman P.,DO
 Kheny,Mira,MD
 Krachman,Amy Nicole,DO
 McDermet,Arthur J.,DO
 Nghiem,George T.,DO
 Ricigliano,Mark A.,DO
 Santangelo,Steven Frank,DO
 Scarlett,Franklin H.,MD
 Toporowski,Beverly Christine,MD
Geriatrics
 Chan-Ting,Rengena Eleanor,DO
Internal Medicine
 Sabir,Sajjad A.,MD
Occupational Medicine
 Introcaso,Lucian J.,MD
Ophthalmology
 Porter,Joel,MD
Pediatrics
 Chong,Penny Maria,MD
 McFadden Parsi,Lovelle,DO
Psychiatry
 Dubois,Yves Georges,MD

Pennsville
Anesthesiology
 Chapdelaine,Robert T.,MD
Diagnostic Radiology
 Fagel,Valentin L.,MD
Family Medicine
 Bober,Mitchell C.,DO
 Lacay,Edmar Manabat,MD
Gastroenterology
 Shufler,Daniel E.,MD
Internal Medicine
 Deng,Yingzi,MD
Neurology
 Syritsyna,Olga,MD
Obstetrics & Gynecology
 Friedman,Amir Mordechai,MD
Ophthalmology
 Mazzuca,Douglas E.,DO
Physical Medicine & Rehab
 Akrout,Tarak,MD
 Maiatico,Marcellus A.,MD
Urology
 Qureshi,Shaukat M.,MD

Pequannock
Surgery (General)
 Gritsus,Vadim,MD

Perrineville
Internal Medicine
 Kumar,Kusum Lata,MD
Pediatrics
 Eccles,Shannon,DO

Perth Amboy
Anatomic/Clinical Pathology
 Tan,Kong L.,MD
Anesthesiology
 Chae,Hung Y.,MD
 Dalal,Kalpana S.,MD
 Fernandez,Manuel A.,MD
 Lakhlani,Parul Pravinchandra,MD
 Lipatov,Yuriy,MD
 Nandiwada,Kalpana,MD
 New,Deena R.,MD
 Olegario,Eduardo S.,MD
 Payumo,Carmelino C.,MD
 Ragheb,Sozan L.,MD
 Rashid,Iqbal,MD
Cardiovascular Disease
 Niemiera,Mark L.,MD
Critical Care Medicine
 Doshi,Mona,MD
 Sinha,Vinod K.,MD
Emergency Medicine
 Carter,Larry Ernest,DO
 Clarke,Dane Eric,MD
 Davis,Sampson M.,MD
 Ganatra,Nikita,MD
 Ligor,David A.,DO
 Miller,Deon E.,DO
 Mordan,Eliezer Aurelina,MD
 Sang Urai,Chintana,MD
Endocrinology
 Jokic,Dragana,MD
Family Medicine
 Husain,Ali,DO
 Nazli,Yasmeen Zuleikha,MD
 Padilla,Nyree,MD
 Ritsan,Julia B.,DO
 Tamburello,Traci Ann,DO
Geriatric Psychiatry
 Annamaneni,Padmaja Sarki,MD
Geriatrics
 Guillen,Gregorio J.,MD
Internal Medicine
 Aranguren-Decastro,Yolanda,MD
 Arjona,Romel A.,MD
 Bencosme,Pablo,MD
 Chowdhry,Neil,MD
 Dogra,Vijay K.,MD
 Goyal,Janak R.,MD
 Islam,Mohammed Areful,MD
 Jimenez,Arturo De La Caridad,MD
 Khan,Dewan S.,MD
 Lamprinakos,James P.,MD
 Luna,Evangeline A.,MD
 Maldonado,Rodolfo,MD
 Mathew,Teena,MD
 Muzones,Santiago III,MD
 Pasupuleti,Madhusudan V.,MD
 Patel,Pooja,MD
 Rajapakse,John S.,MD
 Reddy,Korrapati Shaik Shaval,MD
 Regevik,Nina K.,MD
 Shirolawala,Pankaj Ramanlal,MD
 Somogyi,Steven G.,MD
 Subramanyam,Sujata,MD
 Szenkiel,Grazyna,MD
 Vuppala,Gulab,MD
 Wang,Zhimin,MD
 Yousif,Abdalla M.,MD
Nuclear Medicine
 Sen,Shuvendu,MD
Obstetrics & Gynecology
 Brug,Pamela,MD
 Turkish,Jonathan Lee,MD
 Vaydovsky,Joseph,MD
Ophthalmology
 Darvin,Kenneth N.,MD
 Murr,Peter,MD
 Santamaria,Jaime II,MD
Pathology
 Stone,Frederick J.,MD
Pediatrics
 Calderon,Dinorah,MD
 Forbes,Darlene Henderson,MD
 Jonna,Vaidehi,MD
 Konda,Kalpana Reddy,MD
 Kottahachchi,Wijepala,MD
 Verma,Madhoolika,MD
 Wade,Mark J.,MD
Physical Medicine & Rehab
 Sinha,Anjali,DO
Psychiatry
 Brown,Katherine E.,MD
 Dube,Veena,MD
 Lanez,Carmencita T.,MD
 Mishra,Arunesh Kumar,MD
 Nadipuram,Chandrika,MD
Surgery (General)
 Gabucan,Maximo B. Jr.,MD

Phillipsburg
Anatomic/Clinical Pathology
 Brown,John M.,MD
Anesthesiology
 Redondo,Rodolfo C.,MD
 Sarayno-Sagge,Perla M.,MD
 Whittingham,Jennifer J.,MD
Cardiovascular Disease
 Brar,Navtej Singh,DO
 Costacurta,Gary A.,MD
 Emery,Robert C.,MD
 Mascarenhas,Daniel A.,MD
 Patel,Chandulal Harilal,MD
 Popkave,Arthur H.,MD
 Prasad,Amit,MD
 Rohatgi,Rajeev,MD
 Schiavone,Joseph Adriano,MD
 Singh,Narpinder,MD
Critical Care Medicine
 Latriano,Blaise P.,MD
Cytopathology
 Manhoff,Dion T.,MD
Dermatology
 Li,Lian-Jie,MD
Diagnostic Radiology
 Bucich,Joseph Marc Jr.,MD
 Cohen,Kenneth Arthur,MD
 Estacio,Joseph M.,MD
 Pollack,Matthew Scott,MD
 Rabinowitz,Mitchell,MD
 Swartz,Joel David,MD
Emergency Medicine
 Amadio,Thomas J.,DO
 Bee,Kim Donaldson,MD
 Burkey,Seth Micah,MD
 Parada,Joseph A.,MD
 Starosta,Daria Marie,DO
Endocrinology
 Shah,Ashish Vinaychandra,MD
 Singh,Ishita,MD
Family Medicine
 Aversa,Thaddeus Massimo,DO
 Bautista,Lucien Santiago,DO
 Buch,Raymond S.,MD
 Chu,Ching-Huey,MD
 Decker,Eugene Michael,DO
 Delmonico,Gerard J.,MD
 Emenari,Chibuzo U.,MD
 Gilkey,Edward A.,MD
 Gomes,Ana P.,DO
 Kanner Liebman,Rachel Brooke,DO
 Kropf,Laura Dawn,DO
 Lombardi,Frank T.,DO
 Mcginley,Thomas Charles Jr.,MD
 Ortiz-Evans,Ileana,MD
 Porter,Anne Marisa,MD
 Remde,Alan H.,MD
 Revankar,Manasi Chandrakant,DO
 Roscher,Atilio R.,MD
 Rossi,Cynthia Ann,MD
 Scott,Sabriya Carolyn,MD
 Siciliano,Mary J.,DO
Gastroenterology
 Herman,Barry Eugene,MD
 Kantor,Thomas E.,MD
 Mukherjee,Shanker,MD
General Practice
 Cumbo,Edward J.,DO
 Grubb,Charles R.,DO
Geriatrics
 Viroja,Yogesh V.,MD
Hematology Oncology
 Smith,John Edmund Jr.,MD
 Starr,Cynthia D.,MD
Hospitalist
 Varghese,Juliet George,MD
Internal Medicine
 Annam,Raghuveer,MD
 Bera,Dilipkumar M.,MD
 Durrani,Mohamed Sohail,MD
 Fendley,Ann Ehrke,MD
 Gandhi,Jinesh Mulraj,MD
 Hotchkin,Karen Lynn,MD
 Khalighi,Koroush,MD
 Lewis,Irvin Holden,MD
 Luo,Chuying,MD
 Varkey,Sarah Hema,MD
 Yellin,Michael Jay,MD
Nephrology
 Gayner,Robert S.,MD
 Pursell,Robert N.,MD
 Shenoy,Mangalore Shantheri,MD
Neurology
 Garber,Todd Ryan,MD
 Mehta,Heeral J.,MD
 Shah,Ila A.,MD
Obstetrics & Gynecology
 Berger,Daniel A.,DO
 Blumenthal,Neil C.,MD
 Horne,Howard Krutzel,MD
 Silver,David Foster,MD
Ophthalmology
 Finegan,James Jr.,MD
 Neusidl,William B.,MD
Orthopedic Surgery
 Diiorio,Emil John,MD
 Ferrante,Christopher R.,MD
 Friedman,Robert Lawrence,MD
 Loguidice,Vito A.,MD
 Maron,Norman L.,MD
 Martinez,Marcos Manuel,MD
 Palumbo,Dante M.,DO
 Reid,James Henry,MD
 Sadler,Adam D.,DO
Orthopedics
 Rudolph,Jason Willer,MD
Otolaryngology
 Rayasam,Ramakumar V.,MD
 Sackman,Scott Marshall,DO
Pathology
 Li,Yong Ming,MD
Pediatric Anesthesia
 Diaz,Elizabeth Ann,MD
Pediatrics
 Evans,Charles III,MD
 Kim,Sam Kwang,MD
 Levine,Helaine Gale,MD
 Sion,Armi T.,MD
Plastic Surgery
 Bastidas,Jaime Adolfo,MD
Psychiatry
 Javia,Subhashchandra J.,MD
 Titus,Benny Elizabeth,MD
 Yu,Cha J.,MD
Pulmonary Disease
 Nar,Kishorkumar G.,MD
 Nekoranik,Michael G.,DO
Rheumatology
 Lee,Susan,MD
Surgery (General)
 Abo,Marc N.,MD
 Chung,Hei Jin,MD
 Kjellberg,Sten I.,MD
 Rastogi,Vijay,MD
 Rohatgi,Chand,MD
Urology
 Antario,Joseph Michael,MD
 Margolis,Franklin I.,MD

Pine Brook
Anesthesiology
 Schaechter,Jason D.,MD
Cardiovascular Disease
 Chandrasekaran,Kulandaivelu,MD
Dermatology
 Chen,Elbert H.,MD
Psychiatry
 Maaty,Mona,MD

Piscataway
Anatomic/Clinical Pathology
 Yurchenco,Peter,MD
Anesthesiology
 Chowdhury,Farys Reza,DO
Cardiovascular Disease
 Catapano,Joseph A.,MD
Child & Adolescent Psychiatry
 Deshpande,Kalyani Kumari,MD
 Ilaria,Shawen Maryrose,MD
 Novotny,Sherie Lynn,MD
 Pace,Patrick V.,MD
 Rosenberg,Gary B.,MD
 Sahoo,Madhusmita,MD
 Upadhyay,Anu,MD
Cytopathology
 Liang,Songlin,MD
Diagnostic Radiology
 Hsu,Chia-En,MD
Emergency Medicine
 Bulahan,Alvin,MD
 Pratt,Michael E.,MD
Endocrinology
 Apelian,Ara Z.,MD
 Fertig,Brian J.,MD
 Patel,Sima,MD
Family Medicine
 Chatterjee,Sonia,MD
 Eck,John M.,MD
 Herbert,Lisa R.,MD
 Krohn,Douglas R.,MD
 Lam,Nalini Priya,MD
 Laumbach,Robert John,MD
 Memon,Mushtaq Ahmed,MD
 Monaco,Robert,MD
 Murphy,John Charles,MD
 Robertson,Michelle Williams,MD
 Shoulson,Shana S.,MD
General Practice
 Nadal,Loida C.,MD
 Stern,Marcel,MD
General Preventive Medicine
 Greene,Glenn Joel,MD
Geriatric Psychiatry
 Mazur,Yuri,MD

Physicians by Town and Medical Specialty

Piscataway (cont)
- **Infectious Disease**
  - Fisher, Bruce D., MD
  - Mathews, Cecil, MD
- **Internal Medicine**
  - Arya, Adarsh Vir, MD
  - Chinchilla, Miguel A., MD
  - Chuang, Connie T., MD
  - Eck, Alieta R., MD
  - Gamao, Eddie M., MD
  - Glazer, Robert Dean, MD
  - Gochfeld, Michael, MD
  - Hip-Flores, Julio, MD
  - Kanj, Hassan A., MD
  - Khan, Ferdaus A., MD
  - Kipen, Howard M., MD
  - Lifshitz, Edward I., MD
  - Marroccoli, Barbara A., MD
  - Parmar, Archna S., DO
  - Pereira, Audrey P., MD
  - Ramos, Rosalinda J., MD
  - Ritch De Herrera, Thaddeus D., MD
  - Robbins, Joseph A., DO
  - Romano, Joseph P., MD
  - Sanjay, Priyanka, MD
  - Sen, Ajanta, DO
  - Shah, Nehaben Ketankumar, MD
  - Sioss, Robert G., MD
  - Terregino, Carol A., MD
  - Tobia, Anthony Michael, MD
  - Tong, Yeow C., MD
- **Neurology**
  - Richfield, Eric Karl, MD
- **Obstetrics & Gynecology**
  - Choubey, Sheela, MD
  - Cogliani, Ermes, MD
  - Davda, Niyati, MD
  - De Flesco, Lindsay D., MD
  - Schwartz, Marlan K., MD
- **Occupational Medicine**
  - Garcia, Julia Griggs, MD
  - Kholdarov, Boris, MD
  - Osinubi, Omowunmi Y., MD
  - Thomas, Timmy, MD
  - Udasin, Iris G., MD
- **Ophthalmology**
  - Kanengiser, Bruce Evan, MD
- **Orthopedic Surgery**
  - Piskun, Andrew, MD
  - Zemsky, Lewis M., MD
- **Pediatrics**
  - Dravid, Anjana, MD
  - Gupta, Mamta Bansal, MD
  - Mathew, Lovely Sebastian, MD
  - Mehrotra, Naveen, MD
  - Patel, Rekha Arvind, MD
  - Radhakrishna, Vijaya, MD
  - Sitoy, Fernando R., MD
  - Velazquez, Danitza M., MD
- **Psychiatry**
  - Aupperle, Peter M., MD
  - DeLuca, Alison Kay, MD
  - Elga, Shana Stein, MD
  - Gunja, Sakina Zahir, MD
  - Gutterman, Lily Z., MD
  - Hammond, Carla Chambers, MD
  - Hraniotis, Nicole J., MD
  - Ivelja-Hill, Danijela, MD
  - Kaufman, Kenneth R., MD
  - Menza, Matthew A., MD
  - Miskimen, Theresa M., MD
  - Palmeri, Barbara A., MD
  - Petti, Theodore Andre, MD
  - Rao, Savitha, MD
  - Rosato, Mark G., MD
  - Sharma, Madhulika Brahm, MD
  - Srinivasan, Rekha, MD
  - Tai, Mustafa, MD
  - Tepper, Drew I., MD
  - Velivis, Leticia, MD
  - Williams, Jill M., MD
- **Public Health**
  - Rhoads, George G., MD
- **Surgery (General)**
  - Barot, Prayag, MD

Pitman
- **Family Medicine**
  - Brennan, William Frederick, DO
  - Di Lisi, Joseph P., DO
  - Friedlin, Forrest Jeffrey, DO
  - Rivell, Crystal Giovanna, DO
- **Gastroenterology**
  - Farber, Michael A., MD
- **Geriatrics**
  - De Eugenio, Lewis Jr., MD
- **Internal Medicine**
  - O'Donnell, Carmel Marie, DO

Pittstown
- **Family Medicine**
  - Golden-Tevald, Jean M., DO
- **Physical Medicine & Rehab**
  - Lin, Hua, MD

Plainfield
- **Cardiovascular Disease**
  - Husain, Saleem, MD
- **Critical Care Medicine**
  - Bayly, Robert, MD
- **Family Medicine**
  - Bastien, Linda, MD
  - Birotte Sanchez, Maria J., MD
  - Ledinh, Thuong, MD
  - Patel, Rajesh T., DO
  - West, Beryl E., MD
  - Zablocki, Chana Shira, MD
- **Gastroenterology**
  - Cohen, Allan Bary, MD
  - Goldenberg, David A., MD
- **Internal Medicine**
  - Alder, Edward A., MD
  - Griffin, Francis L., MD
  - Isukapalli, Padmaja, MD
  - Jain, Sapna, MD
  - Lee, Johnnie Augustus, MD
  - Nkwonta, Joyce O., MD
  - Nwigwe, Genevieve N., MD
  - Patel, Maitri, MD
  - Shetty, Vyshali S., MD
  - Tripathi, Harsha M., MD
  - Walsh, Susan M., MD
- **Obstetrics & Gynecology**
  - Abrarova, Nazima M., MD
  - Murray, Elrick A., MD
- **Occupational Medicine**
  - Patel, Alka Jashbhai, MD
- **Pediatrics**
  - Basu, Sebika, MD
  - Cho, Chang-Il, MD
  - Mattoo, Deepali, MD
  - Morin, Joanne M., MD
  - Patel, Arvind Joitaram, MD
  - Pennington, Demetria, MD
  - Russell-Brown, Karl E., MD
  - Singh, Amita, MD
  - Subramanian, Govindammal N., MD
  - Zonn, Svetlana, MD
- **Physical Medicine & Rehab**
  - Husain, Abid, MD
  - Tiedrich, Allan D., MD
- **Psychiatry**
  - Forbes, Trevor G., MD
  - Guirguis, Soad George, MD
  - Patel, Dineshchandra G., MD
  - Weinstein, Jack S., MD
- **Pulmonary Disease**
  - Jayaraj, Kasthuri E., MD

Plainsboro
- **Anatomic Pathology**
  - Fede, Jean M., DO
- **Anatomic/Clinical Pathology**
  - Arslan, Asima, MD
  - Shanahan, Eileen Marie, MD
  - Zhang, Lanjing, MD
- **Anesthesiology**
  - Airen, Anshul, MD
  - Broad, Daniel Gene, MD
  - Calalang, Carolyn Clarice, MD
  - Chaudhry, Ambareen Khan, MD
  - Chen, Chu-Kuang, MD
  - Coplin, Peter L., MD
  - Curlik, Semena, MD
  - Fortunato Sieglen, Linda M., MD
  - Greenberg, Leslie M., MD
  - Griffith, Rebecca N., MD
  - Guo, Xiaotao, MD
  - Hirsh, Jennifer L., MD
  - Klausner, Anna Jill, MD
  - Nelson, Mary Beth, MD
  - Ruscito, Bridget Marie, MD
  - Seybert, John Jr., MD
  - Subramoni, Jaya, MD
  - Trager, Mark A., MD
  - Wolfson, Alexander, MD
- **Anesthesiology: Pain Medicine**
  - Patel, Ronak Dilip, MD
- **Breast Surgery**
  - Davidson, J. Thomas, MD
- **Cardiovascular Disease**
  - Bergmann, Steven Robert, MD
- **Diagnostic Radiology**
  - Green, William M., MD
- **Emergency Medicine**
  - Belardi, Chris A., MD
  - Cherefko, Kathryn Baier, DO
  - Cridge, Peter B., MD
  - Freedman, Jennifer Emi Chan, MD
  - Garibaldi, Pia M., MD
  - Gronczewski, Craig Anthony, MD
  - Harrison, Stephen Jay, DO
  - Price, Dennis P., MD
  - Vossler, Cathleen M., MD
- **Family Medicine**
  - Kaur, Narinder, MD
  - Sokel, Andrew H., MD
  - Suzuki, Ron Yks, MD
  - Tierney, Peter C., MD
- **Gastroenterology**
  - Katz, Kristina, MD
  - Skole, Kevin S., MD
- **Geriatrics**
  - Sidhu, Harpreet, MD
- **Hematology Oncology**
  - Babott, Doreen, MD
- **Hospitalist**
  - Fanning, Christine M., MD
  - Phinney, Maryann B., MD
  - Shah, Nimit Ashwinbhai, MD
- **Internal Medicine**
  - Bang, Byung, MD
  - Barile, David Robert, MD
  - Chang, Zhu Ping, MD
  - Chen, Xiaomei, MD
  - Edwards, Barbara Ruth, MD
  - Goldblatt, Kenneth H., MD
  - Hui, Ying-Kei, MD
  - Hunt, Rameck R., MD
  - Lancefield, Margaret L., MD
  - Mamidi, Arunima, MD
  - Mirza, Ismet Amtul Latif, MD
  - Nagy, Aubrie Jacobson, MD
  - Naini, Sean, DO
  - Owusu Boahen, Olivia, MD
  - Patel, Shivangi, MD
  - Robison, Kathryn J., MD
  - Schwartz, Mark, MD
  - Sharma, Silky, MD
  - Sheth, Anish A., MD
  - Subbarayan, Srividhya, MD
  - Wang, Qian, MD
  - Youssef, Hatim Fathi, DO
- **MOHS Micrographic Skin Cancer**
  - Vine, John E., MD
- **Medical Oncology**
  - Sokol, David B., MD
- **Neonatal-Perinatal Medicine**
  - Goel, Rajiv, MD
  - Marino, Anthony J. Jr., MD
  - Mihalyfi, Brigitte E., MD
  - Sambasivan, Roshni D., MD
- **Neurology**
  - Sachdeo, Rajesh C., MD
- **Nuclear Medicine**
  - Sood, Ravi, MD
- **Obstetrics & Gynecology**
  - Friedman, Alan L., MD
  - Gross, Jeffrey K., MD
  - Pawliw, Myron, MD
  - Petraske, Alison R., MD
  - Siems, Nicole Mary, DO
- **Orthopedic Surgery**
  - Dhanaraj, Dinesh, MD
  - Smires, Harvey E. Jr., MD
- **Otolaryngology**
  - Drezner, Dean Andrew, MD
  - Kay, Scott Lawrence, MD
- **Pathology**
  - Andavolu, Rao Hanumanth, MD
  - Krauss, Elliot A., MD
  - Van Uitert, Craig E., MD
- **Pediatrics**
  - Baloch, Rafia Q., MD
  - Bradshaw, Chanda M., MD
  - Brennan, Alicia Ann, MD
  - Castellano, Marissa D., MD
  - Concha Leon, Alonso E., MD
  - Guha, Koel, MD
  - Kim, Regina Siobhan, MD
  - Krauss, Joel Martin, MD
  - Kumar, Anita Kiran, MD
  - Lingasubramanian, Geethanjali, MD
  - Mah, Sue Ann, MD
  - Palit, Kalpana, MD
  - Rajan-Mohandas, Niranjana, MD
  - Tong, Shiwei, MD
  - Vakil, Vidya S., MD
- **Physical Medicine & Rehab**
  - Andavolu, Vani B., MD
- **Psychiatry**
  - Sinha, Sharmila, MD
  - Vinekar, Ajanta S., MD
- **Pulmonary Critical Care**
  - Buckley, Laura K., MD
- **Radiation Oncology**
  - Baumann, John C., MD
  - Fein, Douglas Allen, MD
- **Surgery (General)**
  - Brolin, Robert E., MD
  - Chau, Wai Yip Y., MD
  - Dhir, Nisha Solanki, MD
  - Jordan, Lawrence Joseph III, MD
  - Juha, Ramez, MD
  - Roy, Rashmi, MD
  - Smith, Liam R., MD
- **Vascular Surgery**
  - Goldman, Kenneth A., MD
  - Sambol, Elliot Brett, MD

Pleasantville
- **Anesthesiology**
  - Qadir, Abdul, MD
- **Cardiovascular Disease**
  - Ahmed, Sujood, MD
  - Rajput, Ilyas A., MD
- **Family Medicine**
  - Gerber, Austin J., DO
  - Merle, Nancy, MD
- **Internal Medicine**
  - Choudhry, Rafat S., MD
  - Kozakowski, Edward Jr., MD
  - Rajput, Zubeda I., MD
  - Slotoroff, Jon W., DO
- **Obstetrics & Gynecology**
  - Desai, Anagha Kishor, MD
- **Pediatrics**
  - Yon, Katherine Sunhee, MD
- **Surgery (General)**
  - Penso, S. Desiderio, MD

Pluckemin
- **Pediatrics**
  - McInnes, Marcia R., MD

Point Pleasant Beach
- **Dermatology**
  - Warshauer, Bruce L., MD
- **Internal Medicine**
  - Domanski, Joseph E., MD
  - Giliberti, Rocco A., DO
  - Mazzocchi, Dominic F., MD
  - Murachanian, Richard J., MD
  - Pedicini, Joseph P., MD
  - Reimer, Jennifer Marie, DO
- **Physical Medicine & Rehab**
  - Franz, Stacey, DO
  - Lopez, Hector L. Jr., MD

Point Pleasant Boro
- **Endocrinology**
  - Fomin, Svetlana, MD
- **Internal Medicine**
  - Marlys, James P., MD

Pomona
- **Anesthesiology**
  - Arole, Adebola Oyedele, MD
  - Costabile, Jessica T., DO
  - Davidov, Mark, MD
  - Fadugba, Olawale Akindiran, MD
  - Fisgus, John R., MD
  - Gayeski, David R., MD
  - Incandela, Nicholas J., MD
  - Kaplan, Bruce Zachary, MD
  - Lagmay, Merceditas Maria, MD
  - Levitch, David, MD
  - O'Connell, Frank Michael, MD
  - Pericic, Romeo, MD
  - Radcliff, Nina Singh, MD

618

Schmidheiser,Mark Andrew,MD
Soni,Dhiren D.,DO
Wang,Qin,MD
Yao,Su-Lin G.,MD
Cardiovascular Disease
Spielman,Charles C.,MD
Trivedi,Niranjan G.,MD
Critical Care Medicine
Riccobono,Elizabeth Kay,DO
Diagnostic Radiology
Miller,Mitchell Alan,MD
Emergency Medicine
Bustamante,Irineo Jr.,MD
Merewitz,Glenn S.,MD
Family Medicine
Senese,Susan A.,DO
Forensic Psychiatry
Fenyar,Bonnie Ann M.,MD
Infectious Disease
Trivedi,Manish Niranjan,MD
Internal Medicine
Cosimi,Katherine Rose,MD
Neonatal-Perinatal Medicine
Asiegbu,Benedict E.,MD
Grayson,Stephanie Anne,MD
Miller,Andrea,DO
Muhumuza,Catherine,MD
Tioseco,Jennifer Anne,MD
Obstetrics & Gynecology
Sung,Edward L.,MD
Otolaryngology
Paparone,Basil J.,MD
Pediatrics
Ahmed,Kamran,MD
Budnick,Glenn R.,MD
Mehta,Taral Divyakant,MD
Villasis,Cynthia Dancel,MD
Physical Medicine & Rehab
Alfaro,Abraham,DO
Anmuth,Craig Jeffrey,DO
Berlin,Ross D.,MD
Hahn,Robert Francis,DO
Mehta,Hemangini H.,MD
Psychiatry
Ashfaq,Mohammad,MD
Hasson,Marie Elena,MD
Kaplan,Eliot F.,MD
O'Shea,Alice P.,MD
Zwil,Alexander S.,MD
Radiation Oncology
Dalzell,James G.,MD
Surgery (General)
Grafilo,Antonio C.,MD
Thoracic Surgery
Dralle,James G.,MD
Pompton Lakes
Colon & Rectal Surgery
McConnell,John C.,MD
Emergency Medicine
Brabson,Thomas A.,DO
Gastroenterology
Bernheim,Oren Elias,MD
General Practice
Ahmad,Fuad A.,MD
Internal Medicine
Banerjee,Indrani,DO
Brabston,Timothy B.,MD
Gershman,Larisa Khaimovna,MD
Medical Genetics
Ibrahim,Jennifer,MD
Obstetrics & Gynecology
Scian,John P.,MD
Scian,Joseph A.,MD
Pulmonary Disease
Penek,John A.,MD
Surgery (General)
Feigenbaum,Howard,MD
Pompton Plains
Administration/Medical Mgt
Weinberg,Richard M.,MD
Anesthesiology
Aberbach,Eric Steven,MD
Cheng,Szu-Chi S.,MD
Cooper,Eliyahu N.,MD
Cruz,Bernardo V.,MD
Delaleu,Harold,MD
Dolorico,Valentin N.,MD
Hanna,George M.,MD
Lin,Jian L.,MD
Lipkind,Mark Alan,MD

Rapacon,Magdaleno R.,MD
Scro,Joseph Salvatore,MD
Shulman,Oleg M.,MD
Topf,Andrew Irwin,MD
Voca,Ioan Bogdan,MD
Anesthesiology: Critical Care
Newman,Rita Grant,MD
Anesthesiology: Pain Medicine
Dugar,Vikash,MD
Cardiovascular Disease
Blitz,Lawrence R.,MD
Duvvuri,Krishna,MD
Rosenthal,Mark S.,MD
Siepser,Stuart L.,MD
Tabaksblat,Martin Yaron,MD
Child & Adolescent Psychiatry
Ladov,Norman,MD
Colon & Rectal Surgery
Nochumson,Joshua Alan,MD
Emergency Medicine
Alcantara,Solomon V.,MD
Dellapi,Andrew Thomas,MD
Dynof,Francis R.,MD
Goldberg,Judah Lev,MD
Gosselin,Edward M.,MD
Grossman,Andrew G.,MD
Kou,Victoria Wei-Li,MD
Krauthamer,Matthew J.,DO
Lee,Jemius Dae,DO
Marino,Gennaro J.,DO
Family Medicine
Brower,Chelsea,MD
Capio,Mario R.,MD
Cavazos,Anthony Richard,MD
Desai,Aashish P.,MD
Neopane,Padam Kumar,MD
Patel,Vishal V.,MD
Raju,Biju,DO
Rumbaugh,Donald W.,MD
Geriatrics
Abou Jaoude,Dany M.,MD
Ponomarev,Aleksandr,MD
Hematology Oncology
Frank,Martin J.,MD
Hematopathology
Zhang,Hailing,MD
Hospitalist
Agadi,Smitha G.,MD
Pierre,Edeck Saintilien,MD
Internal Medicine
Agbessi,Denise M.,MD
Alade,Ibijoke Adenrele,MD
Bernstein,Andrew Mitchell,DO
Brahms,Dana Lyn Satomi,MD
Calenda,Brandon William,MD
Dara,Michael R.,MD
Dobro,Jeffrey Steven,MD
Duvvuri,Uma,MD
Gadarla,Mamatha R.,MD
Kumar,Ritesh,MD
Lauter,Otto Scott,MD
Levy,Jodi L.,DO
Obidike,Chika Esther,MD
Orlic,Peter Thomas,MD
Silva,Waldemar E.,MD
Smith-Dipalo,Tracy A.,MD
Tsay,Donald,MD
Pathology
Ahmed,Essam Abdelfattah,MD
Mahmood,Shahid,MD
Wang,Lan,MD
Pediatrics
Amor,Jorge Hernan,MD
Devadan,Phillip Sunil,MD
Lugo,Javier J.,MD
Shah,Sapna V.,MD
Vinokur,Anna,DO
Radiation Oncology
Youssef,Ashraf Fouad Kam,MD
Surgery (General)
Azu,Michelle C.,MD
Potter,Steven D.,MD
Transplant Surgery & Medicine
Bakosi,Ebube A.,MD
Port Monmouth
Family Medicine
Ibrahim,Christine M.,MD
Patel,Kalpeshkumar P.,MD

Port Reading
Psychiatry
De Santis,Maryanne,MD
Princeton
Addiction Psychiatry
Davidson,Anne Stripling,MD
Adolescent Medicine
Gokli,Khyati,MD
Anatomic Pathology
Kauffman,Patricia Joan,MD
Anatomic/Clinical Pathology
Berman,David M.,MD
Anesthesiology
Barone,Stephen Robert,MD
Collins,Patrice,MD
Hancock,Joseph Patrick,MD
Hussain,Mahboob,MD
Kanter,Lawrence E.,MD
Kim,Andrew Hanyoung,MD
Morganstern,Jill Alison,MD
Cardiovascular Disease
Beattie,James Ray III,MD
Costin,Andrew,MD
Mahalingam,Banu,MD
McCabe,Johnathan B.,MD
Mercuro,Tobia J.,MD
Rumberger,John Arthur,MD
Shanahan,Andrew J.,MD
Weinberg,Fredrick M.,MD
Wong,Casey,MD
Younes,Desiree Marie,MD
Child & Adolescent Psychiatry
Bhalla,Saranga,DO
Gursky,Elliot J.,MD
Hassan,Ahmad Mohamed,MD
Hayes,William P.,MD
Khare,Madhurani,MD
Martinson,Charles F.,MD
Mian,Asma,MD
Saldarini,Candace Tom,MD
Schafer,Laura,MD
Stayer,Catherine C.,MD
Clinical Pathology/Laboratory
Saminathan,Thamarai,MD
Computer Medicine
Chen,Roland Sangone,MD
Critical Care Medicine
Jagpal,Sugeet K.,MD
Dermatology
Banker,Sarika,MD
Berger,Bruce J.,MD
Choi,Sola,MD
Funkhouser,Martha E.,MD
Kazenoff,Steven,MD
Kwee,Darlene J.,MD
Notterman,Robyn B.,MD
Onumah,Neh Johnann,MD
Rossy,Kathleen M.,MD
Diagnostic Radiology
Ananian,Christopher Lee,MD
Berger,Robert B.,MD
Cadogan,Michael A.,MD
Cole,Julie Barudin,MD
Compito,Gerard Anthony,MD
Denny,Donald Jr.,MD
Difazio,Matthew C.,MD
Fein,Deborah Allen,MD
Ford,Robert R.,MD
Ghazi,John,MD
Guglielmi,Gwen E.,MD
Howard,Thomas S.,MD
Julius,Barry D.,MD
Kaplan,Steven Mark,MD
Kaufmann,Gregory A.,MD
Lebowitz,Jonathan A.,MD
O'Malley,Bernard B.,MD
Perlman,Barry J.,MD
Perlman,Eric S.,MD
Sen,Rik Supriya,MD
Emergency Medicine
Costello,Lauren E.,MD
Neglia,Janet A.,MD
Endocrinology
Bembo,Shirley Abad,MD
Benito Herrero,Maria I.,MD
Deutsch,Paul Jan,MD
Inzerillo,Angela Mary,MD
Joy,Ansu Varughese,MD
Moses,Alan Charles,MD
Mullarkey-De Sapio,Cathleen,MD
Ruel,Ewa,MD

Weiss,Ned Martin,MD
Family Med-Adult Medicine
Deora-Bhens,Sonia,DO
Family Medicine
Hui,Dao,MD
Shamshad,Munaza,MD
Zack,Brian Gary,MD
Gastroenterology
Bellows,Aaron,MD
Margulies,Craig,MD
Meirowitz,Robert F.,MD
Segal,William Nathan,MD
Shriver,Amy Rubin,MD
Swedlund,Anne P.,MD
General Practice
Miller,Jeffrey J.,DO
Geriatric Psychiatry
Khouri,Philippe J.,MD
Geriatrics
Hua,Xingjia,MD
Gynecology
Bhatia,Nina Prakash,MD
McCoy,Susan N.,MD
Hand Surgery
Grenis,Michael Steven,MD
Lamb,Marc John,MD
Hematology
Yi,Peter I.,MD
Hematology Oncology
Yang,Arvin S.,MD
Infectious Disease
Fernando,Chandani D.,MD
Hanna,George J.,MD
Hughes,Eric Anton,MD
Internal Medicine
Alivisatos,Maria Regina,MD
Allenby,Kent Stewart,MD
Avins,Laurence R.,MD
Barton,William W.,MD
Blom,Thomas Robert,MD
Brown,Barbara A.,MD
Chang,Frances Yu-hsin,MD
Chattha,Savneet Kaur,MD
Chen,Arnold Yin-Ti,MD
Chen,Pei-Jon,MD
Coppola,Danielle,MD
Corazza,Douglas P.,MD
Dashevsky,Nataliya,MD
De La Cruz,Ernest Jose,MD
Fein,David A.,MD
Gitterman,Benjamin Eric,MD
Glazer,Joyce H.,MD
Hossain,Feroza K.,MD
Hsu,Stanley Cho Hsien,MD
Hug,Vickie Beth,MD
Hyun,Youngsoon,MD
Kahn,Laura H.,MD
Kalish,Joanne B.,DO
Kandasamy,Rajaram,MD
Kossow,Lynne Becker,MD
Lacava,Paul Vincent,MD
Lapuerta,Pablo,MD
Lee,Jae Young,MD
Lee,Karina K.,MD
Lee,Richard Thomas,MD
Mahmood Arif,Iram,MD
Malhotra,Anuj Kumar,MD
Mendis,Kalanie,MD
Mendu,Srinivas,MD
Morris,Kathryn E.,MD
Murray,Simon D.,MD
Nobleza,Deanna Jean Dar Juan,MD
Osias,Glenn Lawrence,MD
Passalaris,John Dimitrios,MD
Platzman,Robert,DO
Putukian,Margot,MD
Ramirez-Espinosa,Luz M.,MD
Ranganathan Chetty,Nirmala,MD
Raskin,Yosef,MD
Reddy,Sumitha R.,MD
Rehor,Francis E.,MD
Reynolds,Richard David,MD
Rho,Aloysius Kihyok,MD
Rose,Bruce T.,MD
Rota,Anthony P.,MD
Sandy,Lewis G.,MD
Sass,Timothy E.,MD
Schaeffer,Mark A.,MD
Schneider,Samuel,MD
Siegel-Robles,Deborah S.,MD
Sinvhal,Ranjeeta Mukul,MD

Physicians by Town and Medical Specialty

Princeton (cont)
Internal Medicine
- Slavin, Anna, MD
- Srinivasan, Geetha, MD
- Stockham, Chad Eric, MD
- Sysel, Irene A., MD
- Tridico, Tanner Joseph, MD
- Valdesuso, Gladys M., MD
- Vedula, Ramya S., DO
- Wei, Fong, MD
- Weisman, Harlan Frederick, MD

Medical Oncology
- Sierocki, John S., MD

Neonatal-Perinatal Medicine
- Sangam, Subhasri L., MD
- Turcanu, Dumitru Sabin, MD

Neurological Surgery
- McLaughlin, Mark Robert, MD
- Von Der Schmidt, Edward III, MD

Neurology
- Maggio, Vijay, MD

Obstetrics & Gynecology
- Amin, Sejal J., MD
- Baseman, Debra L., MD
- Bergknoff, Hugh, MD
- Diventi, Christina G., MD
- Forster, Judith Karen, MD
- Forster, Susan A., MD
- Martin, Robert Allen, MD
- Patel, Vrunda, MD
- Saha, Anita, MD
- Schwartz, Melanie Schrader, MD
- Sophocles, Maria E., MD

Ophthalmology
- Epstein, John Arthur, MD
- Felton, Stephen M., MD
- Jadico, Suzanne K., MD
- Lipka, Andrew C., MD
- Liu, Samuel M., MD
- Miedziak, Anita Irmina, MD
- Mulvey, Lauri D., MD
- Patel, Chirag V., MD
- Shovlin, Joseph Peter, MD
- Wasserman, Barry N., MD
- Wong, Michael Y., MD
- Wong, Richard H., MD

Orthopedic Surgery
- Abrams, Jeffrey Stuart, MD
- Bechler, Jeffrey R., MD
- Bezwada, Hari Prasad, MD
- Fleming, Richard E. Jr., MD
- Gecha, Steven R., MD
- Gutowski, Walter Thomas III, MD
- Lamb, David J., MD
- Leise, Megan Diane, MD
- Levine, Stuart Eric, MD
- McDonnell, Matthew, MD
- Moskwa, Alexander Jr., MD
- Nazarian, Ronniel, MD
- Pressman, Mark J., MD
- Rossy, William Henry IV, MD
- Song, Frederick Suh, MD
- Vannozzi, Brian Michael, MD

Other Specialty
- Ark, Jon Wong Tze-Jen, MD

Otolaryngology
- Brunner, Eugenie, MD

Pain Medicine
- Varela, Rebecca A., MD

Pediatric Cardiology
- Lee, Hae-Rhi, MD

Pediatric Endocrinology
- Hale, Paula M., MD

Pediatrics
- Altshuler, Elena, MD
- Cotton, John M., MD
- Giasi, William George Jr., MD
- Greenberg, Leslie Robin, MD
- Harvey, Karanja, MD
- Helmrich, Robert Florian, MD
- Johnsen, Peter Edward, MD
- Kong, Ji Yong, MD
- Konnick, Patrina A., MD
- Krol, David Matthew, MD
- Kwong, Jenitta, MD
- Mandelbaum, Bert, MD
- Marshall, Rebecca G., MD
- McConlogue, Joelle Jugant, MD
- Millar, Kim H., MD
- Monica, Kristi Rae, MD
- Naddelman, Adam Brett, MD
- Pellegrino, Peter Phillip, MD
- Pierson, David Shawn, MD
- Pierson, Joseph Jr., MD
- Pulver, Deborah Moody, MD
- Ramachandran, Jaishree, MD
- Raymond, Gerald M., MD
- Rose, Helen M., MD
- Schneider, Allen J., MD
- Shah, Amisha A., MD
- Shah, Amy Mehta, DO
- Soffen, Deborah A.S., MD
- Tesoro, Louis J., MD
- Winikor, Jared, MD
- Zollner, Paula G., MD

Physical Medicine & Rehab
- Bracilovic, Ana, MD
- Cooper, Grant, MD
- Funiciello, Marco, DO
- Meyler, Zinovy, DO
- Miller-Smith, Stacey Ann, MD
- Mizrachi, Arik, MD
- Petrin, Ziva, MD
- Stier, Kyle Thomas, MD

Plastic Surgery
- Drimmer, Marc A., MD
- Hamawy, Adam Hisham, MD
- Hazen, Jill, DO
- Kaplan, Stacy M., DO
- Leach, Thomas A., MD

Psychiatry
- Apter, Jeffrey T., MD
- Benaur, Irina V., MD
- Blake, John R., MD
- Borthwick, James Malcolm, MD
- Carneval, Patricia A., MD
- Chen, Michael S., MD
- Cohen, Jonathan David, MD
- Fernandez, Ricardo J., MD
- Gochfeld, Linda G., MD
- Green, Jeffrey H., MD
- Heller, Philip Arthur, MD
- Hom, William L., MD
- Ilangovan, Kani Mozhi, MD
- Karpf, Gary A., MD
- Koenig, Michele L., MD
- Langer, Dennis Henry, MD
- Langer, Susan F., MD
- Leopold, Michael A., MD
- Levine, Steven Paul, MD
- Mattes, Jeffrey A., MD
- Nathan, David Lawrence, MD
- Pal, Jayanta Kumar, MD
- Popkin, Sara Elizabeth, MD
- Prus Wisniewski, Richard V., MD
- Rahman, Firoz Pushkin, MD
- Ratliff, Henry W., MD
- Resnick, Steven I., MD
- Salvatore, Joseph E. Jr., MD
- Sandhu, Jagwinder S., MD
- Scasta, David L., MD
- Schofield, Neal B., MD
- Senekjian, Elizabeth K., MD
- Shah, Dhwani B., MD
- Stanley, Lorna Maria, MD
- Staroselsky, Galina, MD
- Szteinbaum, Edward M., MD
- Tchikindas, Olga M., MD
- Teasley, Melanie, MD
- Temple, Julia K., MD
- Tipermas, Alan, MD
- Varma, Sanjay, MD
- Vasilov, Anatoliy I., MD
- Vazquez, Jose S., MD
- Vilko, Naomi R., MD
- Wilson, George F., MD
- Yanovskiy, Anatoly M., MD

Rheumatology
- Chauhan, Naresh, MD
- Goyal, Seema Agrawal, MD
- Hunninghake, Leroy H., MD
- Patel, Anand, MD

Sports Medicine
- Palmer, Michael Alberto, MD

Surgery (General)
- Berrizbeitia, Luis Daniel, MD
- Henry, Sharon M., MD
- Kamath, Chandrakal Y., MD
- Mehta, Vishal, MD

Thoracic Surgery
- Cole, Bruno N., MD

Urogynecology
- Van Raalte, Heather Michelle, MD

Urology
- Goldfarb, Sidney J., MD
- Latzko, Karen Marie, DO
- Pickens, Robert L., MD
- Rossman, Barry R., MD
- Schwarzman, Marc I., MD
- Vasselli, Anthony J., MD
- Vukasin, Alexander P., MD
- Wedmid, Alexei, MD

Vascular & Intrvntnal Radiology
- De Sanctis, Julia Tucker, MD
- Parker, William Andrew, MD
- Youmans, David Carey, MD

Princeton Junction
Anatomic/Clinical Pathology
- Liu, Qiang, MD

Anesthesiology
- Chang, Connie Yachan, MD

Bloodbanking
- Chopra, Neeru Gera, MD

Cardiovascular Disease
- Angel, Juliette, MD
- Ruddy, Michael C., MD

Emergency Medicine
- Desiderio, Carl M., DO

Endocrinology
- Brenner-Gati, Leona, MD

Family Medicine
- Painter, Michael Wayne, MD

Internal Medicine
- Bialy, Grace B., MD
- Dimitrova, Dessislava Iv, MD
- Patel, Rajiv Arvind, MD
- Schwartz-Chevlin, Jill F., MD

Nephrology
- Basi, Seema, MD
- Finkielstein, Vadim Aaron, MD

Obstetrics & Gynecology
- Miller, Katherine H., MD

Ophthalmology
- Milman, Tatyana, MD

Orthopedic Surgery
- Glick, Ronald S., MD
- Miller, Scott David, MD
- Shakir, Ahmar, DO

Pediatrics
- Hefler, Stephen Edward, MD
- Mansour, Ayman M., MD
- Ruff, Lynne H., MD

Sleep Disorders Medicine
- Aronsky, Amy J., DO

Prospect Park
Pediatrics
- Ameen, Naureen W., MD
- Rasheed, Fouad Y., MD

Rahway
Anatomic Pathology
- Marcantonio, Eugene E., MD

Anatomic/Clinical Pathology
- Benisch, Barry M., MD
- Gistrak, Michael Andrew, MD

Anesthesiology
- Light, Francis B., MD
- Luciano, Dominick T., MD
- Osei Tutu, Leslie P., MD
- Son, Andrew, MD
- Son, Kyoung J., MD

Cardiovascular Disease
- Lee, Young-II, MD

Critical Care Medicine
- Wojno Oranski, Alexander, DO

Dermatology
- Wininger, Jon G., MD

Diagnostic Radiology
- Mizan, Narmin Farah Hussain, MD
- Shrivastava, Abhishek, MD

Emergency Medicine
- Bernstein, Michael Ari, MD
- Park, Malsuk, DO
- Tan, Manuel R., MD
- Wright, Toni Rene, MD

Endocrinology
- Bhattacharjee, Dulal, MD
- Kaufman, Keith, MD
- Leung, Albert Tao-Man, MD

Family Medicine
- Goradia, Rita U., MD
- Sheffy, Ohad, MD

General Practice
- Kozlov, Zinovy, MD

Hematology Oncology
- Altura, Rachel Allison, MD
- Kang, Soonmo Peter, MD

Hematopathology
- Juco, Jonathan W., MD

Hospitalist
- Hussain, Asim, MD

Hypertension
- Mansoor, George A., MD

Infectious Disease
- Brown, Melinda Sheron, MD

Internal Medicine
- Constandis, Calin G., MD
- Iwamoto, Marian, MD
- Kerr, Ruthann Warnell, MD
- Livshits, Larisa L., MD
- Makimura, Hideo, MD
- Margolskee, Dorothy J., MD
- Moody, Rumanatha, MD
- Osei Tutu, Ernest Paul, MD
- Prasad, Kalpana, MD
- Reddy, Narshimha K., MD
- Santiago, Arthur F., MD
- Tasharofi, Kamran, MD

Medical Oncology
- Yao, Siu-Long, MD

Nephrology
- Chaudhry, Anu, MD
- Ravella, Supriya, MD
- Vojnyk, Charlene Louise, MD

Obstetrics & Gynecology
- Pelaez, Linda, MD

Ophthalmology
- Hosler, Matthew Robert, MD
- Khan, Taj G., DO

Orthopedic Surgery
- Paulson, Melyssa Michelle, MD
- Pecker, Howard M., MD

Pediatric Cardiology
- Banka, Puja, MD

Pediatric Endocrinology
- Bach, Mark A., MD

Pediatric Infectious Diseases
- Fraser, Iain Peter, MD

Pediatric Sports Medicine
- Arnold, Monica A., DO

Pediatrics
- Dancel, Concepcion A., MD
- Reddy, Sadhana K., MD

Pulmonary Disease
- Carayannopoulos, Leonidas N., MD
- Yim, Frances D., MD

Radiation Oncology
- Karp, Eric A., MD

Rheumatology
- Rivera Curiba, Mary A., MD

Surgery (General)
- Sanchez, Hector J., MD

Urology
- Morrow, Franklin A., MD

Ramsey
Anatomic/Clinical Pathology
- Aponte, Sandra Leonora, MD
- Brown, Jeffrey G., MD
- Ilario, Marius John-Marc, MD
- Joseph, John K., MD
- Liu, Zach Zhiguang, MD
- Szeto, Oliver Jo-Yang, MD

Anesthesiology
- Goldstein, Monte Jay, MD
- Gordon, Robert P., MD
- Melyokhin, Igor, MD
- Pillitteri, John, MD
- Song, Michael M., MD

Anesthesiology: Pain Medicine
- Gamburg, David, MD
- Halioua, Solomon, MD

Child & Adolescent Psychiatry
- Hanna, Mohab, MD

Critical Care Medicine
- Cooper, Kimberly Anne, DO
- Sharma, Rakesh, MD

Emergency Medicine
- Stern, Peter, MD

Endocrinology
- Levy, Ian H., DO

Family Medicine
 Nickles,Steven L.,DO
Gastroenterology
 Strassberg,David M.,MD
Internal Medicine
 Ayoub,Kasem,MD
 Fernicola,Joseph Robert,MD
 Lucanie,Anabel,MD
 Lucanie,Richard,MD
 Scibetta,Maria T.,MD
 Sehgal,Arun,MD
 Sim,Herena,MD
 Sundaram,Punidha,MD
 Surapaneni,Purus Hotham N.,MD
Neurology
 Trifiletti,Rosario R.,MD
Obstetrics & Gynecology
 Faust,Michael G.,MD
 Nitz,Shelly,MD
 Rooney,Michele P.,MD
Ophthalmology
 Van Inwegen,Jeffrey R.,MD
Pathology
 Newman,Schuyler,MD
Pediatrics
 Ligenza,Claude,MD
 Nicpon,Christopher B.,MD
 Shevelev,Irene,MD
 Shor,Raida,MD
Physical Med & Rehab-Pain Med
 Ferrer,Steven Michael,MD
 McElroy,Kevin M.,DO
Physical Medicine & Rehab
 Jacobs,Lyssa Sorkin,MD
Plastic Surgery
 Capella,Joseph Francis,MD
Psychiatry
 Crowley,Elizabeth Ozimek,MD
 Mirchandani,Indu,MD
Surgery (General)
 Licata,Joseph Jr.,MD
 Patel,Kumar R.,MD
 Pozzessere,Anthony Samuel,MD

Randolph
Adolescent Medicine
 Guerra,Julio C.,MD
Allergy
 Reisner,Colin,MD
Anesthesiology
 Levy,Stuart J.,MD
 Sokolova,Anna,MD
Cardiovascular Disease
 Rogers,Philip S.,MD
Child & Adolescent Psychiatry
 Desai,Maya G.,MD
Dermatology
 Najarian,David James,MD
Gastroenterology
 Gelman,Scott Franklin,MD
Hand Surgery
 Ende,Leigh S.,MD
Hospitalist
 Luayon,Joseph Palac,DO
Infectious Disease
 Allegra,Donald T.,MD
 Aslam,Fazila,MD
 Doka,Najah I.,MD
 Gupta,Rachna,MD
 Krieger,Richard E.,MD
 Manalo,Rosario Beatriz,MD
 Markou,Theodore Ioannis,MD
 Marsh,Rebecca A.,MD
 McManus,Edward J.,MD
 Reddy,Sireesha B.,MD
 Roseff,Shelly Anne,MD
 Ubhi,Damanpreet K.,MD
Internal Medicine
 Akkapeddi,Nirmala G.,MD
 Centanni,Monica Ann,MD
 Desai,Gautamkumar T.,MD
 El Mouelhi,Mohamed H.,MD
 Farkas,Attila Istvan,MD
 Freiheiter,John Scott,MD
 Grover,Arvind K.,MD
 Grover,Pamela,MD
 Gudis,Steven M.,MD
 Li,Shing,MD
 Lynch,Barrington B.,MD
 Miller,Kenneth D.,MD
 Russoniello,Michael A.,MD

 Shah,Pallavi Devendra,MD
 Shareef,Kishwar I.,MD
 Sossong,Duane G.,DO
 Tillem,Michael P.,MD
 Valentin-Torres,Melanie R.,MD
 Wenzler,Danya J.,MD
 Williams,Stephen Joseph,MD
Nephrology
 Paster,Lauren,MD
Neurological Surgery
 Engle,Edward A.,MD
Nuclear Medicine
 Goldstein,Harold A.,MD
Obstetrics & Gynecology
 Buna,Andrei,MD
 Mohr,Robert Frederick,MD
 Venanzi,Michael V.,MD
Ophthalmology
 Benerofe,Bruce Michael,MD
 Cetta,Peter J.,MD
 Kaden,Ian H.,MD
 Walker,Richard Nathaniel,DO
Pediatrics
 Ciufalo,Marisa,MD
 Gelman,Beth Paula,MD
 Gottlieb,Ricki L.,MD
 Scolnick,Ita,MD
 Shukla,Kishorchandra S.,MD
Sports Medicine
 Rubman,Marc H.,MD
Surgery (General)
 Choung,Edward W.,MD
 Hoffman,Michael J.,MD
 Huang,Ih-Ping,MD
 Meisner,Kenneth,MD
Surgical Critical Care
 Strutin,Millard D.,MD

Raritan
Anatomic/Clinical Pathology
 Hall,Alvin J.,MD
 Moniem,Howayda A.,MD
Bloodbanking
 Ciavarella,David Joseph,MD
Endocrinology
 Erondu,Ngozi Emmanuel,MD
Family Medicine
 Jordan-Scalia,Lisa Judith,DO
 Khalil,Christina,DO
 Patel,Ruperl Chandrakant,MD
 Scalia,Joseph Frank,DO
 Tomasso,Robert A.,MD
 Wang,Yue-He,MD
Hospitalist
 Patel,Rajendrakumar C.,MD
Internal Medicine
 Catanzaro,Donna,MD
 Dannemann,Brian R.,MD
 Elsayed,Yusri Ali,MD
 Iorio,Richard,MD
 Mukherjee,Robin,DO
 Patel,Gita R.,MD
 Zhuang,Sen Hong,MD
Medical Oncology
 Todd,Mary Beth,DO
Neonatal-Perinatal Medicine
 Mody,Kartik D.,MD
Nephrology
 Haverty,Thomas Patrick,MD
Neurology
 Biondi,David M.,DO
Obstetrics & Gynecology
 Huber,Elaine E.,MD
 Parlavecchio,Joseph G.,MD
Pediatric Hematology Oncology
 Tendler,Craig L.,MD
Pediatrics
 Maldonado,Samuel David,MD
Physical Medicine & Rehab
 Kantha,Brinda Sri,DO

Red Bank
Addiction Medicine
 Verdon,John J. Jr.,MD
Allergy & Immunology
 Hirsch,Andrew C.,MD
Anatomic/Clinical Pathology
 Dukuly,Zwannah B.,MD
 Farooq,Taliya,MD
 Gong,Ping,MD
 Gupta,Namita J.,MD
 Leschhorn,Edwin C.,MD

Anesthesiology
 Ades,Nathan Albert,MD
 Brodsky,Jonathan I.,DO
 Bruce,Gullie E. IV,MD
 Chidambaram,Manjula S.,MD
 Chiu,Nicholas,MD
 Cirullo,Pasquale Michael,MD
 Dooley,James R.,MD
 Farrell,Charles W.,MD
 Friedman,James Keith,MD
 Haber,Daran W.,MD
 Huang,Shyuan,MD
 Huh,Chan Woo,MD
 Kulkarni,Prashant P.,MD
 Meltzer,Keith Mitchell,MD
 Mosca,Phillip J.,MD
 Nguyen,Khanh Q.,MD
 Ritchie,Paul Harvey,MD
 Toran,Stephen A.,MD
 Varadarajan,Vijayaiaxmi,MD
Child & Adolescent Psychiatry
 Goss,Graydon G.,MD
 Grant,Susan J.,MD
 Kowalik,Sharon,MD
 Lin,Shengxi,MD
Colon & Rectal Surgery
 Wolkomir,Alfred F.,MD
Critical Care Medicine
 Qumei,Moh'D K. K.,MD
Dermatology
 Trusky,Diana E.,MD
Dermatopathology
 Shami,Samar,MD
Diagnostic Radiology
 Fedele,Dara,MD
 Mishra,Monica Shalini,MD
 Rada Banat,Leny M.,MD
Emergency Medicine
 Bruno,Stephen F.,MD
 Cameron,James D.,MD
 Desai,Aaditya A.,DO
 Dunn,Sarah Ruth,MD
 Lemansky,Alan S.,MD
 Levin,Michael Y.,DO
 Migliori,Frank Anthony,MD
 Neyman,Gregory,MD
 Pennycooke,Shelley-Ann N.,DO
 Ramachandran,Karthia J.,MD
 Reynolds,Stephanie Marie,DO
 Roma,Kevin P.,MD
 Rubinstein,Howard Arthur,MD
 Starkey,Lawrence Paul,MD
 Tomaino,Jeanne,MD
 Trattner,Lauren Beth,DO
Endocrinology
 Kargutkar,Smita Nandkumar,MD
Family Medicine
 Bader,Christopher William,DO
 Ejimofor,Ebikaboere,MD
 Landers,Steven Howard,MD
 Lanza,Michele R.,MD
 Mulholland,Brendan J.,MD
 Penn,Carol A.,DO
 Reilly,Gail G.,MD
Gastroenterology
 Binns,Joseph F.,MD
 Carman,Roy L.,MD
 Gialanella,Robert J.,MD
 Heyt,Gregory John,MD
 Marzano,Joseph A.,MD
 Sundararajan,Subha V.,MD
 Weine,Douglas Matthew,MD
Geriatric Psychiatry
 Ongsiako,Maria V.,MD
Hospitalist
 Andrade,Jose G.,MD
 John,Thomas Jr.,MD
Infectious Disease
 Ahmad,Khalid Mehmood,MD
 Ahmad,Nasir Mahmood,MD
 Eschinger,Amy Folio,MD
Internal Medicine
 Ahmad,Nauman,MD
 Allegra,Edward Charles II,MD
 Choi,Yu-Jeong Alexis,MD
 Costa,Ronald P.,MD
 Gabel,Robert L.,MD
 Grosso,Dominick A.,DO
 Haddad,Richard Hani,MD
 Hampel,Howard,MD
 Holguin,Leonardo Fabio,MD

 Hyppolite,David,MD
 Marza,Lizett Auxiliado,MD
 McHeffey,Dina A.,MD
 Mehra,Shalini Gupta,MD
 Mullarney,Allison Ingrid,DO
 Nedelcu,Dana,MD
 Rana,Sanah Ehsan,MD
 Randazzo,Vincent T.,MD
 Roosels,Marianne,MD
 Sharma,Lokesh,MD
 Tracy,Bridget,MD
Nephrology
 Savransky,Ernest,MD
Neurological Surgery
 Eisenbrock,Howard J.,DO
Neurology
 Chen,Edgar Y.,MD
 Fan,Schuber C.,MD
 Ilaria,Philip V.,MD
Obstetrics & Gynecology
 Chakraborty,Anu,MD
 Patel,Mayur Vinod,MD
 Seigelstein,Nina,MD
Ophthalmology
 Blades,Frederick C.,MD
 Chen,Natalie,DO
 D'Emic,Susan,DO
 Friedberg,Mark A.,MD
 Frieman,Brett Justin,DO
 Frieman,Lawrence,MD
 Greco,John Jr.,MD
 Jergens,Paul B.,MD
 Kahn,Walter J.,MD
 Kneisser,George,MD
Oral & Maxillofacial Surgery
 Haghighi,Kayvon,MD
Orthopedic Surgery
 Bakhos,Nader Anthony,MD
 Costa,Anthony Joseph,MD
 Friedel,Steven P.,MD
 Lospinuso,Michael Frank,MD
 Mintalucci,Dominic J.,MD
 Murphy,Bernard P.,MD
 Rinkus,Keith Michael,MD
Orthopedics
 Lisser,Steven P.,MD
 Mulholland,Daniel J.,MD
 Phair,Arthur H.,MD
 Scott,Richard J.,MD
Otolaryngology
 De Gennaro,Anthony,MD
 Scaccia,Frank J.,MD
Pathology
 Minassian,Haig,MD
Pediatrics
 Changchien,Charlie J.,MD
 DeGennaro,Marianne E.,DO
 Edman,Joel B.,MD
 Jordan,Jo-Ann,MD
 Kommireddi,Sowmini,MD
 Litsky,Michelle Badorf,DO
 Markoff,Michael S.,MD
 Montero,Gianecarla B.,MD
 Paladino,Theresa Ann,DO
 Saini,Manish K.,MD
 Wawer-Chubb,Allison Kristen,DO
 Wilmott,Annette Lynne,DO
Physical Medicine & Rehab
 Cardamone,Kristen Elizabeth,DO
 Corzo,Jorge Francisco,MD
 Donlon,Margaret,MD
 Forman,Glenn M.,MD
 Pannullo,Robert Paul,MD
 Romello,Michael A.,MD
Plastic Surgery
 Dudick,Stephen T.,MD
 Wurmser,Eric A.,MD
Psychiatry
 Bransfield,Robert C.,MD
 Calvosa,Michelle K.,MD
 Cancellieri,Francis Louis,MD
 Clever,Marcia Sue,MD
 Friedman,Dena Seifer,MD
 Ginn-Scott,Elizabeth J.,MD
 Litwin,Peter J.,MD
 Marcus,Abir Assaad,MD
 Schineller,Tanya M.,MD
 Segal,Arthur M.,MD
 Shin,Kyun,MD
 Sikowitz,David J.,MD
 Vakar,Emil,DO

Physicians by Town and Medical Specialty

Red Bank (cont)
Psychiatry
- Vetrano, Joseph S., MD
- Wong, Dennis, MD

Radiation Oncology
- Danish, Adnan F., MD
- Patel, Priti S., MD
- Zhang, Mei, MD

Spinal Surgery
- Husain, Qasim M., MD

Sports Medicine
- Van Gelderen, Jeffrey Thomas, MD

Surgery (General)
- Cugini, Donald A., MD
- Greco, Gregory A., DO

Richland
Family Medicine
- Hargrave, Douglas M., DO
- Pirolli, John A., DO

Internal Medicine
- Peterson, Paul III, DO

Ridgefield
Cardiovascular Disease
- Sherer, Stephen B., MD

Child & Adolescent Psychiatry
- Lee, Seung Ho, MD

Internal Medicine
- Artinian, Agop, MD

Orthopedic Surgery
- Yoo, Daniel J., MD

Physical Medicine & Rehab
- Pak, Hong Sik, MD

Surgery (General)
- Egazarian, Marc M., MD

Ridgefield Park
Cardiovascular Disease
- Lee, Nellie U., MD

Diagnostic Radiology
- Awad, Aida Fahmy, MD

Emergency Medicine
- Shaker, Ashraf F., MD

Pediatrics
- Baker, Iyad, MD
- Lee, Clara J., MD

Ridgewood
Allergy
- Co, Margaret L., MD
- Slankard, Marjorie L., MD

Anatomic Pathology
- Eapen, Elizabeth, MD

Anatomic/Clinical Pathology
- Brandt, Suzanne Marie, MD
- Christiano, Arthur A., MD
- Mazziotta, Robert M., MD
- Reilly, Michael H., MD
- Taskin, Metin, MD

Anesthesiology
- Adkoli, Sujnani, MD
- Azzariti, John Jr., MD
- Beke, Theodore J., MD
- Chan, Jenny Sang, MD
- Chaudhry, Ahmad N., MD
- Choi, Sunny D., MD
- Connelly, Brian, MD
- Feiler, Michael Augustus, MD
- Gal, Stephen, MD
- Iannacone, Richard F., DO
- Ietta, Michael Angelo, MD
- Kotys, Ola, DO
- Lavrich, Pamela S., MD
- Lee, Soomyung, MD
- Levine, Jeffrey, MD
- Magnes, Jeffrey B., MD
- Morr, Edward Simon, MD
- Nagy, Peter, MD
- Nyunt, Kyaw, MD
- Rosen, Chaim E., MD
- Schmidt, Kenneth A., MD
- Scognamiglio, Michael F., MD
- Silverstein, Wendy Beth, MD
- Smith, Justin Kerry, MD
- Telfeyan, Celeste A., DO
- Volkov, Anatoly, MD
- Westrich, David J., MD
- Wohlfarth, Erik, MD
- Zamecki, Andrzej M., MD

Bariatrics/Weight Control
- Pucci, Richard Anthony, DO

Behavioral Medicine
- Nalven, Lisa M., MD

Cardiovascular Disease
- Abbate, Kariann Ferguson, MD
- Burke, Benita Mia, MD
- Co, John A., MD
- Goldschmidt, Howard Z., MD
- Mansson, Sarah Jane Deleon, DO
- Musat, Dan Laurentiu, MD
- Panagiotou, Demetrios N., MD
- Reison, Dennis S., MD
- Saporito, Robert A. Jr., MD
- Sotsky, Gerald A., MD
- Sotsky, Mark I., MD
- Strain, Janet E., MD

Cataract
- Sumers, Anne R., MD

Child & Adolescent Psychiatry
- Bhalla, Ravinder N., MD
- Gentile, Michael P., MD
- Sugar, Nina S., MD
- Wruble, Steven J., MD

Child (Pediatric) Neurology
- Steinschneider, Mitchell, MD

Clinical Cardiac Elctrphyslgy
- Bhatt, Advay G., MD
- Mittal, Suneet, MD
- Preminger, Mark William, MD
- Sichrovsky, Tina Claudia, MD

Colon & Rectal Surgery
- Nizin, Joel S., MD

Cosmetic Surgery
- Sternschein, Michael J., MD

Critical Care Medicine
- Melamed, Marc S., MD

Dermatology
- Applebaum-Farkas, Paige S., MD
- Au, Sonoa Ho Yee, MD
- Corey, Timothy J., MD
- Miller, Janine D'Amelio, MD
- Satra, Karin H., MD
- Stevens, Amy W., MD

Diagnostic Radiology
- Wollman, Carol A., MD

Emergency Medicine
- Baddoura, Rashid Joseph, MD
- Becker, George L. III, MD
- Diorio, Joseph J., MD
- Dreier, Marc Max, MD
- Egan, Daniel J., MD
- Fascitelli, David A., MD
- Felsenstein, Bruce W., MD
- Gerstel, Alan Victor, MD
- Markowitz, George Joseph, MD
- Mednick, Joyce J., MD
- Portale, Karen Mary, MD
- Raman, Jennifer Lynne, MD
- Ranginwala, Masood Ahmed, DO
- Sharma, Siddharth, MD
- Simonetti, Michael, MD
- Tsomos, Evangelia, MD
- Vogel, Mark F., MD
- Wagh, Anju M., MD
- Yallowitz, Joseph, MD

Endocrinology
- Cobin, Rhoda Harriet, MD
- Kelman, Adam Scott, MD
- Lee, Esther Jeehae, MD

Family Med-Adult Medicine
- Latimer, Karen M., MD

Family Medicine
- Belov, Khatuna Topadze, MD
- Faltas-Fouad, Suzan L., MD
- Katz, Jodie H., MD
- Kaul, Rachna, MD
- Panagiotou, Nicholas D., MD

Gastroenterology
- Danzig, Jeffrey B., MD
- Fischer, Zvi, MD
- Grossman, Matthew Aaron, MD
- Hsieh, Jennifer, MD
- Korkis, Anna Maria, MD
- Pazwash, Haleh, MD
- Rahmin, Michael G., MD
- Rubinoff, Mitchell J., MD

Geriatrics
- Nagarajan, Anuradha, MD

Hematology Oncology
- DeNeve, Albert A., MD

Infectious Disease
- Kinchelow-Schmidt, Tosca E., MD
- Knackmuhs, Gary Glenn, MD
- O'Hagan Sotsky, Carol Ann, MD

Internal Medicine
- Boyd-Woschinko, Gillian S., MD
- Covelli, Joseph Michael, MD
- Dardashti, Omid A., MD
- Dmytrienko, Igor, MD
- Edara, Srinivasa R., MD
- Ewald, Edward A., MD
- Flowers, Raphael G., DO
- Frankel, Zev Binyamin, MD
- Gaffin, Neil, MD
- Gupta, Sanchita, MD
- Hammond, Deborah Ellen, MD
- Holt, Elaine Marie, MD
- Jaber Iqbal, Reem, DO
- Kalia, Amita, MD
- Kaur, Birinder Jeet, MD
- Kulkarni, Jyothi, MD
- Lin, Spencer, MD
- Liu, Michelle, MD
- McGorty, Francis E., MD
- Mody, Kanika Pravin, MD
- Morressi, Marc M., MD
- Mudry, Carolyn J., DO
- Narwani, Vanessa Deepak, MD
- Nyajure, Colette, MD
- Rana, Ranjit C., MD
- Rao, Pratibha Prasanna, MD
- Rave, Arie, MD
- Sanandaji, Mehrdad, MD
- Shakibai, Nader, MD
- Sharahy, Tatiana, MD
- Sharma, Puneeta, MD
- Tibb, Amit Singh, MD
- Tsai, Fu-Li, MD
- Tsiouris, Simon John, MD
- Usgaonker, Susrut R., DO
- Weiser, Mitchell M., MD

Interventional Cardiology
- Simon, Alan David, MD

Neonatal-Perinatal Medicine
- Carbone, Mary T., MD
- Lasker, Michelle Rhonda, MD
- Manginello, Frank P., MD
- Pane, Carmela R., MD

Neurological Surgery
- Carpenter, Duncan B., MD
- Cobb, William Stewart, MD
- D'Ambrosio, Anthony Louis, MD
- Goulart, Hamilton C., MD
- Klempner, William L., MD
- Lavine, Sean David, MD
- Moise, Gaetan, MD
- Sheth, Sameer Anil, MD

Neurology
- Berlin, Daniel, MD
- Citak, Kenneth A., MD
- Grewal, Amrit K., MD
- Levin, Kenneth A., MD
- Lijtmaer, Hugo N., MD
- Molinari, Susan P., MD
- Naidu, Yamini, MD
- Nasr, John T., MD
- Noskin, Olga, MD
- Perron, Reed C., MD
- Shammas, James T., MD
- Tong, Fumin, MD
- Van Engel, Daniel R., MD
- Winfree, Christopher Jules, MD

Obstetrics & Gynecology
- Behnam, Kazem, MD
- Behnam, Melody S., MD
- Bentolila, Eric Y., MD
- Coven, Roger A., MD
- DeNoble, Shaghayegh Moghaddam, MD
- Gerhardt, Amy Ilene Katz, MD
- Khosla, Savita, MD
- Kim, Kathlyn M., MD
- Klimowicz-Mallon, Elizabeth, MD
- Kuo, Eugenia C., MD
- Levine, Richard Steven, MD
- Marcus, John W., MD
- Rezvani, Fred F., MD
- Zeldina, Elina, MD

Ophthalmology
- Alino, Anne Marie G., MD
- Amesur, Kiran Bhagwan, MD
- Fox, Martin Lee, MD
- Harris, Michael J., MD
- Jachens, Adrian William, MD
- Kayserman, Larisa, MD
- Kim, David Yhoshin, MD
- Kopelman, Joel E., MD
- Lee, Song Eun, MD
- Liva, Bradford C., MD
- Norden, Richard A., MD
- Saunders, Eric Monroe, MD
- Solomon, Edward Mark, MD
- Tsakrios, Charles N. Jr., MD
- Vallar, Robert V., MD

Orthopedic Surgery
- Brief, Andrew A., MD
- Carney, William P., MD
- Carozza, Charles R., MD
- Crisciticllo, Arnold A., MD
- Dasti, Umer R., MD
- Delfico, Anthony John, MD
- Joffe, Avrum L., MD
- Kayal, Robert Albert, MD
- Roenbeck, Kevin Meehan, MD
- Rudman, David Paul, MD

Pain Medicine
- Scham, Arnold, MD

Pathology
- Gritsman, Andrey, MD

Pediatric Gastroenterology
- Orellana, Katherine Atienza, DO

Pediatric Orthopedics
- Avella, Douglas George, MD

Pediatric Pulmonology
- Kanengiser, Steven Jay, MD

Pediatric Rehabilitation
- D'Alessandro, Angela Marie, MD

Pediatrics
- Anderson, Nicole Andrea, MD
- Benjamin, Beth L., MD
- Cally, Ronald G., MD
- Coffey, Dennis Charles, MD
- Cope, Jennifer Anne, MD
- Dziarmaga, Ewa R., MD
- Ghavami-Maibodi, Seyed Zia, MD
- Heilbroner, Peter Louis, MD
- Iqbal, Sheeraz, MD
- Jedlinski, Barbara, MD
- Klein, Bradley Marc, MD
- Kroning, David R., MD
- Lee, Peter HaeSuk, MD
- Lee, Ting-Wen An, MD
- Palamattam, Jessy R., MD
- Philips, Jay, MD
- Torres-Soto, Eileen Mariette, MD
- Volpert, Diana, MD
- Yankus, Wayne A., MD
- Young, Yvette S., MD
- Zabek Gallegos, Joanna M., MD

Physical Med & Rehab-Sports Med
- Terranova, Lauren M., DO

Physical Medicine & Rehab
- Balakrishnan, Beena S., MD
- Boiano, Maria Anna, MD
- Kuo, Douglas, DO
- Marrinan, Randy F., MD

Plastic Surgery
- Ganchi, Pedramine, MD

Psychiatry
- Abkari, Shashikala, MD
- Anand, Ashish, MD
- Becker, William D., MD
- Cohen, Daniel Elliot, MD
- Cowan, James Rankin Jr., MD
- Dealwis, Watutantrige T., MD
- Elvove, Robert M., MD
- Farooki, Alima Bibi, MD
- Flescher, Sylvia Evelyn, MD
- Fraser, Margaret Cameron, MD
- Gilman, Howard E., MD
- Grogan, Rita J., MD
- McGuire, Patricia L., MD
- Narula, Amarjot S., MD
- Patel, Narendra D., MD
- Rosenfeld, David N., MD
- Samuels, Steven Charles, MD
- Tuchin, Terry A., MD
- Videtti, Nicholas A., MD
- Wulach, Sandra H., MD
- Yoon, Eui-Sun L., MD
- Zisu, Traian A., MD

Pulmonary Critical Care
- Chakravarti, Aloke, MD
- Salamat, Rahat, MD
- Vakil, Rupesh M., MD

Pulmonary Disease
  Barasch,Jeffrey P.,MD
  Choy,Wanda Wai Ying,MD
  Suffin,Daniel Matthew,DO
Radiation Oncology
  Greenblatt,David R.,MD
  Kambam,Shravan R.,MD
  Torrey,Margaret Jennings,MD
Radiology
  Levy,Lauren S.,MD
  Seltzer,Lawrence G.,MD
  Weinstock,Lisa R.,MD
Rheumatology
  Keller,Betty Sue,MD
Sports Medicine
  Pope,Ernest J.,MD
Surgery (General)
  Bernheim,Joshua William,MD
  Char,Daniel Jay,MD
  Di Saverio,Joseph,MD
  Patel,Mitul Suresh,MD
  Pucci,Anthony E.,DO
  Raman,Chidambaram,MD
  Rubinstein,Mitchell A.,MD
Thoracic Surgery
  Brizzio,Mariano Ezequiel,MD
  Bronstein,Eric H.,MD
  Majid,Naweed Kamran,MD
  Mindich,Bruce Paul,MD
  Zapolanski,Alex,MD
Urogynecology
  Sheiban,Tuti Fareen,MD
Urology
  Rosen,Jay S.,MD

Ringoes
Family Medicine
  Bryant,Manmohan,MD
Internal Medicine
  Ezema,James N.,MD
  Lavin,Bruce Scott,MD

Ringwood
Emergency Medicine
  Gabriel,Chantal Delise,MD
Internal Medicine
  Rametta,Mark J.,DO
  Raouf,Medhat M.,MD
Pediatrics
  Goyal,Ajai K.,MD

Rio Grande
Diagnostic Radiology
  McAllister,John Daniel II,MD
  Panico,Robert A.,MD
  Toloui,Gerald J.,MD
  Werman,Richard Evan,DO
Family Medicine
  Marino,Denay L.,DO
  Rose,Victoria Summer,MD
Hand Surgery
  Cole,Frederick Jr.,DO
Orthopedic Surgery
  Facciolo,Jack,DO

River Edge
Dermatology
  Blanco,Fiona Rose Pasternack,MD
  Lin,Richie L.,MD
  Trinh,Diem Thi,MD
Diagnostic Radiology
  Naik,Mohit Madan,MD
  Nicola,Gregory Neal,MD
Gastroenterology
  Chhada,Aditi,MD
  Leibowitz,Steven R.,MD
  Mammen,Anish George,MD
  Nikias,George Andrew,MD
  Rosendorf,Eric Robert,MD
Internal Medicine
  Hedlund,Edward L.,MD
  Lin,Richard M.,MD
Neurological Radiology
  Wattamwar,Anoop Suresh,MD
Neurology
  Adams,Angela,MD
Obstetrics & Gynecology
  Cho,Linda M.,MD
  Clachko,Marc A.,MD
  Parnes,Cindy R.,MD
Obs/Gyn-Critical Care
  Bingham,Jemel M.,MD
Ophthalmology
  Goldfarb,Mark S.,MD

  Higgins,Lisa Marie,MD
  Ponce Contreras,Marta R.,MD
Oral & Maxillofacial Surgery
  Auerbach,Jason M,MD
  Cho,Sung Hee,MD
Pediatrics
  Falk,Theodore,MD
Psychiatry
  Martinez,Humberto L.,MD
Pulmonary Disease
  Shin,Dongwuk,MD
Radiology
  Liebling,Melissa Schubach,MD

River Vale
Emergency Medicine
  Gardy,Mark Alan,MD
Internal Medicine
  Buirkle,James E.,MD
  Steinberg,Evan L.,MD
Physical Medicine & Rehab
  Ferraro,Donna J.,MD

Riverdale
Allergy
  Gold,Ruth Leah,MD
Allergy & Immunology
  Patel,Sheenal V.,MD
Anesthesiology
  Aznavoorian,Martin Peter,MD
Dermatology
  Son,Chang Bae,MD
Family Medicine
  Howe,Michele Margaret,DO
  Romain,Sharon L.,DO
  Samandar,Steve,MD
Gastroenterology
  Dasani,Bharatkumar M.,MD
Internal Medicine
  Ardito,Michael F.,MD
  Bogusz,Katie L.,MD
  Visconti,Raymond Jr.,MD
Otolaryngology
  Ginsburg,Jeffrey B.,MD
  Levine,Jonathan Marc,MD
  Remsen,Kenneth A.,MD
  Taylor,Howard,MD
Pediatrics
  Weiss,Jeffrey Gregg,MD

Riverside
Family Medicine
  Tangco,Evacueto P.,MD
Internal Medicine
  Sun,Lydia Lijuan,MD

Riverton
Family Medicine
  Burke,Margaret Linda,MD
Foot & Ankle Surgery
  Daniel,Joseph N.,DO
Internal Medicine
  Patel,Kalpeshkumar R.,MD
Ophthalmology
  Calesnick,Jay L.,MD

Robbinsville
Cardiovascular Disease
  Agarwal,Ashish Madanlal,MD
  Barn,Kulpreet S.,MD
  Gala,Ketan M.,MD
  Patel,Jigar A.,MD
  Rothstein,Neil M.,MD
  Samuel,Steven Alan,MD
  Singhal,Shalabh,MD
  Wolf,Andreas,MD
Endocrinology
  Smolarz,Brian Gabriel,MD
Family Medicine
  Bankole,Omolabake O.,MD
  Rednor,Jeffrey D.,DO
  Risi,Mark G.,DO
  Shahmehdi,Seyed Akhtar,MD
  srikanth,Rashmi,MD
Internal Medicine
  Abdelmessieh,Nawal I.,MD
  Arcaro,Michael Steven,MD
  Bandu,Bhanumathi,MD
  Chowdhury,Shikha,MD
  Hussain,Arif Syed,MD
  Reger,Donna Pidane,MD
Interventional Cardiology
  Soffer,Mark Jay,MD

Otolaryngology
  McCullough,Aubrey Susan,DO
Otolaryngology-Facial Plastic
  Mignone,Robert,DO
Pediatrics
  Edwards,Kathryn Payne,MD
Sports Medicine
  Redlich,Adam Daniel,MD

Rochelle Park
Allergy
  Kraut,Evelyn S.,MD
Cardiovascular Disease
  Clifford,James R.,MD
  Di Vagno,Leonardo Joseph,MD
Child & Adolescent Psychiatry
  Korshunova,Valeria S.,MD
Diagnostic Radiology
  Meyerson,Steven Jeffrey,MD
Family Medicine
  Keshishian,Paul,DO
  Liu,Elizabeth Yingxia,MD
  Stankiewicz,Danuta,MD
Internal Medicine
  Arora,Sanjay Kumar,MD
  Hasan,Omar S.,MD
  Imbornone,Peter J.,MD
  Karim,Karim Issa,MD
  Maharaja,Lopa Vijay,MD
  Pascarelli,Todd D.,MD
  Varghese,Betsy Mathew,MD
  Wry,Ann M.,MD
Neurology
  Effron,Charles Richard,MD
Ophthalmology
  Lama,Paul Jude,MD
  Sachs,Seth W.,MD
Pediatric Hematology Oncology
  Bhatty,Anis A.,MD
Pediatrics
  Bruno,Basil,MD
Psychiatry
  Acquaviva,Joseph F.,MD
  Flood,Mark J.,MD
  Martinez-Arroyo,,Humberto L.,MD
Psychiatry&Nrolgy-Special Qual
  Kulikova-Schupak,Romana,MD
Radiology
  Conte,Stephen John,DO
  Galope,Roel Pangilinan,DO

Rockaway
Dermatology
  Aspen,Otter Q.,MD
  Masessa,Joseph M.,MD
Family Medicine
  Arshad,Haroon,MD
  Brodrick,Ian B.,MD
  Heitzman,Christopher James,DO
  Horn,Christopher Michael,DO
  Madison,Joy Hovey,MD
  Ziegler,Brenda L.,DO
Internal Medicine
  Annavajjula,Madhavi L.,MD
  Samuel,Ramez W.,MD
Neurology
  Bongiovanni,Denise A.,DO
  Tonzola,Richard F.,MD
Pathology
  Querimit,Felipe A. Jr.,MD
Pediatrics
  Forti,Viviana Claure,MD
  Vassallo,Sheryl Lisa,MD
Psychiatry
  Suckno,Lee J.,MD
Rheumatology
  Barth,Michael,MD
Urology
  Moazami,Saman,MD

Rockleigh
Pediatrics
  Patel,Shilpa Ashok,MD

Roebling
Family Medicine
  Manser,Harry Jr.,DO
  Rappaport,Brandi Joy,MD
Internal Medicine
  Hal-Ibrahim,Ahmad,MD

Roosevelt
Psychiatry
  Vo,Eleanor B.,MD

Roseland
Anesthesiology
  Entrada,Julian Jr.,MD
  Gorman,Eugene S.,MD
  Karmaker,Shekhar Chandra,MD
  Kos,Luke Bronislaw,MD
  Park,Young,MD
  Zhao,Lin,MD
Child & Adolescent Psychiatry
  Elfenbein,Emanuel,MD
Infectious Disease
  Smith,Stephen Marshall,MD
Internal Medicine
  Wachman,Jill,MD
  Weinberger,Daniela,MD
Neurology
  Weisbrot,Frederick J.,MD
Occupational Medicine
  Mangahas,Florinda R.,MD
Ophthalmology
  Origlier,Anthony,MD
Pediatrics
  Anello,Tiziana,MD
  Ioffe,Inna S.,MD
  Makhlouf,Jean,MD
Psychiatry
  Hall,Jeffrey,MD
Urology
  Di Trolio,Joseph V.,MD

Roselle
Family Medicine
  Shakir,Aarefa H.,MD
Internal Medicine
  Lenchur,Peter Michael,MD
  Saluja,Ruby,MD
  Viswanathan,Anjali,MD

Roselle Park
Critical Care Medicine
  Brescia,Michael Louis,MD
Dermatology
  Herzberg,Steven Michael,MD
Family Medicine
  Caggia,Josephine,DO
  Morandi,Michele Meehan,DO
  Parker,Stephen D.,DO
Gastroenterology
  Rodriguez,Ricardo Esteban,MD
Geriatrics
  Solomon,Robert B.,MD
Internal Medicine
  Alexescu,Adina N.,MD
  Bayes,Lorna B.,MD
  Chehade,Ghassan M.,MD
  Leff,Stuart J.,DO
  Saraceno,Leonardo,MD
  Saraceno,Libero,MD
Otolaryngology
  Bastianelli,Milo,DO
  Conte,Louis J.,DO
  Scharf,Richard C.,DO
  West,Gerald,DO
Otolaryngology-Facial Plastic
  Mazzoni,Thomas F.,DO
Pediatrics
  Corbo,Emanuel,MD
Pulmonary Disease
  Maglaras,Nicholas C.,MD
Vascular Surgery
  Cordero,Pedro E.,MD

Rumson
Anesthesiology
  Sestito,Joseph Jr.,MD
Cardiovascular Disease
  O'Connell,Mark M.,MD
Child & Adolescent Psychiatry
  Doumas,Stacy James,MD
Emergency Medicine
  Martin,James Furman,MD
  Rivers,Colleen Marie,MD
Internal Medicine
  Royall,John D.,MD
Neurology
  Colicchio,Alan Robert,MD
Pediatrics
  Genco,John Joseph,DO

Physicians by Town and Medical Specialty

Runnemede
Family Medicine
Bankole, Gawu Kamara, MD
Internal Medicine
Patel, Ashokkumar A., MD
Ophthalmology
Yaros, Michael J., MD
Surgery (General)
Porter, Catherine M., DO

Rutherford
Anesthesiology: Pain Medicine
Haliczer, Abraham T., MD
Cardiovascular Disease
Schwarz, Michael L., MD
Dermatology
Giardina-Beckett, Marieanne, MD
Sperling, Shari Yaffa, DO
Diagnostic Radiology
Annese, Christian P., MD
Emergency Medicine
Morales, Fabian Victor, MD
Gastroenterology
Roth, Joseph M., MD
Ruiz, Frank, MD
Zierer, Kenneth G., MD
General Practice
Grasso, Santo Vincent, DO
Hand Surgery
Altman, Wayne J., MD
Internal Medicine
Chava, Padma, MD
Isralowitz, David L., MD
Kaelin Wooton, Kathleen M., MD
Nam, Daniel, MD
Nozad, Cyrus H., MD
Pondo, Jaroslaw S., MD
Sabogal, Jose Luis, MD
Tailor, Amit, MD
The, Andrew Hong-Siang, MD
The, Samuel H., MD
Neurological Surgery
El Khashab, Mostafa A. F., MD
Fried, Arno H., MD
Rathmann, Allison Marie, DO
Obstetrics & Gynecology
Chait, Anita Irani, MD
Cheatam, Consetta Mae, MD
Driscoll, Lorraine Eva, MD
Irani, Bakhtaver A., MD
Stella, Stefano M., MD
Ophthalmology
Chiang, Bessie, MD
Neigel, Janet M., MD
Rothman, Murray H., MD
Otolaryngology
Hassan, Sherif A., MD
Katz, Michael Jonathan, MD
Mahmoud, Ahmad F., MD
Sarti, Edward J., MD
Pediatric Pulmonology
Becz, Grace E., MD
Pediatrics
Huang, Doris Amy, MD
Narucki, Wayne Ellis, MD
Physical Medicine & Rehab
Brady, Robert David, DO
Filion, Dean Thomas, DO
Plastic Surgery
Weber, Renata Vanja, MD
Plastic Surgery-Hand
Sheikh, Emran Salahuddin, MD
Psychiatry
Brozyna, David B., MD
Khinda, Navjot, MD
Spinal Surgery
Rovner, Joshua Seth, MD

Saddle Brook
Anatomic/Clinical Pathology
Ye, Dongjiu, MD
Anesthesiology
Choi, Jay J., MD
Kosiborod, Roman, DO
Sauchelli, Francis C., MD
Cardiovascular Disease
Salerno, William D., MD
Dermatology
Haberman, Fredric, MD
Ilowite, Peter G., DO
Family Medicine
Pagano, Francesco P., DO

Wiener, Michael I., DO
General Practice
Wasserman, Alan, MD
Infectious Disease
Poblete, Ronald J., MD
Internal Medicine
Adler, Uri Seth, MD
Eichner, Craig N., MD
Miranda, Claudia Danitza, MD
Patel, Sanjeev N., MD
Prvulovic, Aleksandar T., MD
Silverman, Mathew Joshua, DO
Silverman, Philip, DO
Song, Hung S. William, MD
Tantawi, Mahnaz Chand, MD
Obstetrics & Gynecology
Cocoziello, Alexander R., DO
Mann, Manpreet, MD
Orthopedic Surgery
Patel, Deepak Valjibhai, MD
Pediatrics
Ladak, Batul S., MD
Physical Medicine & Rehab
Dovlatyan, Raida, MD
Krotenberg, Robert, MD
Lee, Anthony, MD
Parikh, Shailesh S., MD
Rivera, Leonora M., MD
Seidel, Benjamin Joseph, DO
Valenza, Joseph P., MD
Psychiatry
Badr, Amel Afifi, MD
Weiser, Sheldon, DO
Radiation Oncology
Williams, Perry Swintz, MD
Surgery (General)
Kollar, John C., DO
Urology
Sullivan, Edwin J., DO

Saddle River
Allergy
Silverstein, Leonard, MD
Anatomic/Clinical Pathology
Saviano, Nicole, MD
Anesthesiology
Miguel, Renato C., MD
Ramnanan, Terry K., MD
Cardiovascular Disease
Kasper, Andrew, MD
Kasper, Michael E., MD
Dermatology
Hellman, Laura J., MD
Internal Medicine
Becker, Alyssa Gelmann, MD
Kasper, Joseph E., MD
Obstetrics & Gynecology
Reisman, Barry M., MD
Rubenstein, Andrew F., MD
Psychiatry
Semar, David P., MD

Salem
Anesthesiology
Corbin, John C., DO
Fehder, Carl G., MD
Fiel Cagande, Venerande, MD
Maestrado, Primo Emnace, MD
Mailman, Wendy R., MD
Morales-Pelaez, Eileen S., MD
Pham, Chi H., MD
Pierce, Brandon Keefe, MD
Sarvaiya, Ramesh Manjibhai, MD
Sharma, Naresh Durgaprasad, MD
Dermatology
Caruso, Meghan M., DO
Schmelzer, John F., DO
Diagnostic Radiology
De Jesus, Joseph Ocampo, MD
Krain, Samuel, MD
Emergency Medicine
Bui, Minh Ngoc, MD
Family Medicine
Akinruli, Omowunmi Praise, MD
Amrien, John R., MD
Harris, Timothy Wayne, DO
Howard, Thomas R. Jr., MD
Gastroenterology
Dayrit, Pedro Q., MD
General Practice
Fleurantin, Jean J., MD

Hospitalist
Ngu, Michael Foleng, MD
Internal Medicine
Ahmed, Farooque, MD
Arnous, Nidal, MD
Chhabra, Ravi, MD
Diaz, Roberto R., MD
Krol, Roman, MD
Oates, Angela Jasmine, MD
Park, Steven K., MD
Reyes, Paul H., MD
Tavani, Denis A., MD
Wang, Shuang, MD
Nephrology
Sultan, Wamiq S., MD
Obstetrics & Gynecology
DeCastro, Amante N., MD
Pediatrics
Berman, Barry M., MD
Kouyoumdji, Paul R., MD
McLane, Rebecca, MD
Surgery (General)
Estella, Faustino F. Jr., MD
Patricelli, John E., MD
Timmerman, Lori D., DO
Thoracic Surgery
Wolk, Larry A., MD
Urology
Diamond, Stuart M., MD

Sayreville
General Preventive Medicine
Meduru, Pramod, MD
Internal Medicine
Hanna, Bishoy F., MD
Khan, Malik Adnan Ullah, MD
Simon, Michael J., MD

Scotch Plains
Anesthesiology
Buchbinder, Howard J., MD
Cardiovascular Disease
Coquia, Salvador F., MD
Lomnitz, Esteban R., MD
Dermatology
Drossner, Robbie Beth, MD
Emergency Medicine
Schaller, Richard J., MD
Family Medicine
Ballan, Douglas Arnold, MD
Chin, Darren S., MD
Cunicella, Nicholas A. III, DO
Delio, Constance Mary, MD
Hasan, Izhar U., MD
Hernandez, Alyssa Kate, MD
Reddy, Shanthi Nalamalapu, MD
Silberman, Marc Richard, MD
Internal Medicine
Leopold, Clayton E., MD
Loewinger, Lee E., MD
Pons, Nieva P., MD
Shen, Edred Vig-Ny, MD
Stanzione, Steven, MD
Neurology
Fischer, Beverly Ruth, MD
Obstetrics & Gynecology
Choma, Mtroslaw, MD
Pediatrics
Kharkover, Mark Y., MD
Physical Med & Rehab-Pain Med
Menon, Aditi Sen, MD
Psychiatry
Madraswala, Rehman, MD
Surgery (General)
Tiedemann, Richard N., MD

Sea Bright
Anesthesiology
Rhee, William Choonghee, MD

Sea Girt
Anesthesiology
Patton, Virginia A., MD
Cardiovascular Disease
Eisenberg, Scott R., DO
Hynes, Peter James, MD
Kayser, Robert Granville Jr., MD
Dermatology
Emma, Sheri Lynn, MD
Emergency Medicine
Patrick, Bryan L., MD
Endocrinology
Ciorlian, Cristina C., MD

Family Medicine
Siciliano, Janice M., DO
General Practice
Micallef, Donald M., MD
Internal Medicine
Bersalona, Holly Abate, MD
Bersalona, Louis Michael, MD
Demartin, Robert, MD
Lin, Ying, MD
Masterson, Raymond Mark, MD
Rienzo, Francis G., MD
Young, Patricia A., MD
Maternal & Fetal Medicine
Hux, Charles Howard, MD
Obstetrics & Gynecology
Pelligra, John, MD
Otolaryngology
Hou, Lisa Jenny, DO
Pediatrics
Fury, Mary Anne, DO
Halas, Francis P. Jr., MD
Lutz, Mary B., MD
Plaine, Suzanne E., DO
Physical Medicine & Rehab
Buddle, Patrick M., MD
Dambeck, Michael D., DO
Neuman, Steven Scott, MD
Paik, Sung Woo, MD
Plastic Surgery
Glicksman, Caroline A., MD
Psychiatry
Kargman, Jeffrey M., MD
Pulmonary Disease
Cunningham, Gregory J., MD

Sea Isle City
Family Medicine
Choi, Jong I., MD
Young, Annamarie C., DO

Seaside Heights
Anesthesiology
Durnan, Rosemary, MD
Family Medicine
Godwin Karolak, Allison M., DO
Pediatrics
Peters, Mahafarin P., MD

Seaside Park
Family Medicine
Shadiack, Edward Charles Jr., DO

Secaucus
Anesthesiology
Bhavsar, Vaishali, MD
Faragalla, Emad T., MD
Lewis, Michele J., MD
Patel, Amrish M., MD
Yoo, Eun Y., MD
Anesthesiology: Pain Medicine
Canillas, Elmo Maribao, MD
Child & Adolescent Psychiatry
Mastroti, Jean-Baptiste J., MD
Clinical Neurophysiology
Ahad, Antwan B., MD
Diagnostic Radiology
Izgur, Vitaly, MD
Tramontana, Anthony F., MD
Emergency Medicine
Guibor, Pierre, MD
Tenaglia, Nicholas Charles, MD
Family Medicine
Ali, Tahera, DO
Fahmy, Hannan Adel, DO
George, Malini Susan, MD
Mathew, Jocelyn, MD
Neuberger, Alina P., MD
Fertility/Infertility
Kabakibi, Riad A., MD
Gastroenterology
Dhalla, Sameer, MD
Siegel, Wayne Douglas, MD
General Practice
Udovenko, Olga, MD
Geriatrics
Raghavan, Murli, MD
Hospitalist
Mathur, Smita, DO
Tsirogiannis, Vasiliky, MD
Internal Medicine
Bellifemine, Morris, MD
Boyajian, Robert Wayne, MD
De Melo, Mauricio Garret, MD

Faltas,Ashraf Kamal,MD
Katikaneni,Swapna,MD
Moukdad,Jihad S.,MD
Paroulek,George Jiri,MD
Patel,Dhirendrakumar A.,MD
Patel,Hashmukh R.,MD
Sapira,Valdi,MD
Zwitiashvili,Robert,MD
Obstetrics & Gynecology
Riftine,Julia,MD
Yun,Hyungkoo,MD
Occupational Medicine
Weinberger,Adrian,MD
Orthopedic Surgery
Martinez,Armando I.,MD
Rothenberg,Paul,MD
Otolaryngology
Reitzen-Bastidas,Shari D.,MD
Pathology
Ouahchi,Karim,MD
Pediatric Gastroenterology
Toor,Khadija T.,MD
Pediatrics
Al Haddawi,Anwar,MD
Baker,Azzam A.,MD
Bansil,Noel Lumanog,MD
Ben,Sheeba,MD
Bokhari,Naimat U.,MD
Castillo,Rodrigo I.,MD
Cave,Marie,MD
Choi,Ok K.,MD
Dooley,Christina Yick,MD
Doss,Nermine N.,MD
Farag,Magdy M.,MD
Ghayal,Payal Patel,MD
Hussain,Zaheda M.,MD
Jadun,Wamiq,MD
Jawaharani,Shobha,MD
Jedlinski,Zbigniew J.,MD
John,Jeanie Elizabeth,MD
Lusha,Xhelal Q.,MD
Mirani,Gayatri,MD
Moshet,Osama Mohamed,MD
Mucha,Samantha Agatha,DO
Parikh,Chaula A.,MD
Raju,Rina M.,MD
Sitt,Hal,MD
Williams,Celia,DO
Win,Sithu,MD
Wosu,Carolee Ngozi,MD
Psychiatry
Iskandarani,Nimer M.,MD
Nekrasova,Irina,MD
Ortega,Eddy A.,MD
Shalts,Edward,MD
Soberano,Wilfredo T.,MD
Pulmonary Disease
Nahas,Ghassan,MD
Patel,Manmohan A.,MD
Rheumatology
Gatla,Nandita,MD
Surgery (General)
Bridges,Kristen Leigh,MD
Khani,Ghassan,MD
Urology
DiBella,Louis J. Jr.,MD
Mouded,Issam,MD
Tanzer,Ira D.,MD

Sewell
Adolescent Medicine
Backal,Marc Ira,MD
Anesthesiology
Dougherty,Barbara D.,DO
Lopresti,David A.,MD
Sorensen,Barbara J.,MD
Cardiovascular Disease
Bagaria,Surendra K.,MD
Crasner,Joshua M.,DO
DePace,Nicholas L.,MD
Maiese,Mario L.,DO
Weinberg,Howard M.,DO
Cataract
Ross,Richard S.,MD
Colon & Rectal Surgery
Schachter,Todd,DO
Critical Care Medicine
Obregon,Carlos A.,DO
Dermatology
Choi,Catherine Helen,MD
Li,Kehua,MD

Segal,Elana Tova,MD
Winter,Jonathan M.,MD
Emergency Medicine
Sullivan,Patrick O.,DO
Williams,Edwin Rae,MD
Zimmerman,Daniel J.,MD
Endocrinology
DelGiorno,Charles J.,MD
Sandhu,Sartaj S.,MD
Family Medicine
Arthur,Kiersten Westrol,MD
Attanasio,Michael J.,DO
Beppel,Elaine B.,MD
Bertel,James R.,MD
Bober,Craig,DO
Boyd,Linda,DO
Brumberg,Miles A.,DO
Cavallaro,Joseph III,DO
Cohen,Andrew Geoffrey,MD
Desimone,Alexandra,MD
DiRenzo,Joseph P. Jr.,DO
Dibona,Anthony D. Jr.,DO
Ewing,Jacqueline L.,DO
Kane,Michelle Christine,DO
Kruger,Eric N.,MD
Laganella,Dominic J.,DO
Leshner,Stanley B.,DO
Levin,Neil,DO
Pettis,Larry,MD
Prettelt,Adolfo E.,MD
Ranieri,Joseph N.,DO
Richmond,Chad Eric,DO
Saddel,Diana L.,DO
Schmidt,Carol L.,MD
Sekel,James James,DO
Spinosi,Maryjeanne,DO
Tench,Mavola L.,MD
Urkowitz,Alan L.,DO
Vermeulen,Meagan Wega,MD
Gastroenterology
Gardner,Beth C.,MD
Kimbaris,James Nicholas,MD
Plumeri,Peter A.,DO
General Practice
Cerone,Anthony J. Jr.,DO
Labaczewski,Robert J.,DO
Gynecology
Packin,Gary S.,DO
Hematology Oncology
Poretta,Trina A.,DO
Internal Medicine
Bhimani,Siddharth D.,MD
Borowsky,Larry M.,MD
Bulei,Anita P.,MD
Caudle,Jennifer Nicole,DO
Chandela,Sweta,MD
Datwani,Neeta D.,MD
Di Piero,Alfred M.,DO
Ferroni,Bryan R.,DO
Gambescia,Richard Alan,MD
Glenn,Danette,MD
Johnston,William E.,MD
Levin,Todd Philip,DO
Lindenberg,Noah L.,MD
Myers,Scott Elliot,MD
Singh,Jyotsana,MD
Tarditi,Daniel John,DO
Maternal & Fetal Medicine
Chandra,Prasanta C.,MD
Chhibber,Geeta,MD
O'Neill,Anna M.,MD
Williams,Keith Patrick,MD
Neurological Radiology
Zarzour,Hekmat Khodr,MD
Neurological Surgery
Garrido,Eddy O.,MD
Neurology
Sammartino,Robert A.,DO
Nuclear Medicine
Desai,Anil G.,MD
Obstetrics & Gynecology
Ayres,Ronald E.,DO
Bramble,Charlene A.,MD
Covone,Kenneth C.,DO
Digiovanni,Marianne,DO
Franzblau,Natali R.,MD
Huggins,Juanita Kimberly,DO
Hummel,Jennifer E.,DO
Iavicoli,Michelle A.,MD
Janeczek,Susan,DO
Krieg,Karen Sue,DO

Leber,Sandra Lynn,DO
Nguyen,Maria Bich Thi,DO
Richichi,Joann,DO
Salerno,Anthony P.,MD
Sehdev,Michele S.,MD
Vogiatzidakis,Sophia I.,DO
Oncological Surgery
Yoon-Flannery,Kahyun,DO
Ophthalmology
Bresalier,Howard J.,DO
Girgis,Raymond Michael,MD
Heist,Kenneth C.,DO
Nyquist,Susan Shoshana,MD
Ringel,David M.,DO
Orthopedic Surgery
Falconiero,Robert Paul,DO
Kovacs,Jeffrey Peter,DO
Marcelli,Enrico A.,DO
Mariani,John K.,DO
Murray,Jeffrey,DO
Paz,Efrain Jr.,DO
Ponzio,Robert J.,DO
Valentino,Steven John,DO
Other Specialty
Neilon,Kathleen Mary,DO
Otolaryngology
Becker,Daniel G.,MD
Bromberg,David,MD
Friedel,Mark Erik,MD
Rosenstein,Kenneth Michael,MD
Terk,Alyssa Robyn,MD
Pediatrics
Bierman,Edward W.,MD
Bochenski,Jacek P.,MD
Bruner,David Glenn,MD
Burke,Meghan Deirdre,MD
Chao,Chia Y.,MD
Collazo,Edgar R.,MD
Cook,Wendy S.,DO
Del Moro,Ellen C.,MD
Desai,Renuka D.,MD
Fiderer,Stefanie C.,DO
Ge,Shuping,MD
Kaari,Jacqueline Marie,DO
Kabel-Kotler,Caroline,DO
Kargman,Kevin Jerome,DO
Lewitt,Diana M.,DO
Madan,Nandini,MD
Pasternak,Jared A.,MD
Simmers,Richard C.,DO
Physical Medicine & Rehab
Ashby,John Wilson,MD
Khanna,Malini M.,MD
King,Alina,MD
Lisko,Trina M.,DO
Plastic Surgery
Behnam,Amir Babak,MD
Fahey,Ann Leilani,MD
Perri,Louis P.,MD
Psychiatry
Ellis,George David,MD
Lewis,Lesley Brook,DO
Mac Fadden,Wayne,MD
Ortanez,Iluminado C.,MD
Pulmonary Disease
Becker,Jason M.,DO
Malik,Neveen A.,DO
Radiation Oncology
Cohen,Dane Ryan,MD
Horowitz,Carolyn J.,MD
Radiology
Rosenthal,Richard Eugene,DO
Rheumatology
Singh,Vijay,MD
Surgery (General)
Careaga,Eduardo,MD
Fantazzio,Michele Adrienne,MD
Gillum,Diane,MD
Monteith,Duane Richard,MD
Morros,Jay Scott,MD
Sasso,Michael J.,DO
Thoracic Surgery
Steinberg,Jay Mitchell,DO
Urology
Barsky,Robert I.,DO
Brown,Gordon Andrew,DO
Pietras,Jerome R.,DO
Steckler,Robert E.,MD

Shamong
Family Medicine
Mahoney,Nola T.,DO

Internal Medicine
Papadakis,Kelly M.,MD

Shiloh
Internal Medicine
Dickson,Robert W. III,MD

Ship Bottom
Family Medicine
Braunwell,Arthur Henry III,DO
Clancy,Joseph P. Jr.,MD
Larkin,Harry Jr.,MD
Prosperi,Paul William,DO
Suddeth,James N.,MD

Short Hills
Addiction Medicine
Greenfield,Daniel P.,MD
Anatomic/Clinical Pathology
Tan,Jianyou,MD
Anesthesiology
Peckman,Cornelia L.,MD
Cardiovascular Disease
Tansey,William Austin III,MD
Cardiovascular Surgery
Goldenberg,Bruce S.,MD
Dermatology
Busbey,Shail,MD
Vuong,Charlotte Hwa,MD
Diagnostic Radiology
Jain,Monica,MD
Emergency Medicine
Groman,David I.,MD
Rogers,Jody J.,MD
Family Medicine
Fine,Shari R.,DO
Jani,Beena Harendra,MD
Zacharias,Daniel,MD
Internal Medicine
Blaustein,Howard Stuart,MD
Brackett,Valerie A.,MD
Chan,Eric B.T.,MD
DiGiacomo,William A.,MD
Kramer,Theodore Ian,MD
Liberman,Arthur R.,MD
Mehra,Sweeti,MD
Nahas,Barbara A.,MD
Nalitt,Beth R.,MD
Pomerantz,Glenn David,MD
Nutrition
Deshaw,Barbara Blank,MD
Obstetrics & Gynecology
Ayyagari,Kalavathi,MD
Robinson,Patricia Graf,MD
Ophthalmology
Farbowitz,Michael Aron,MD
Otolaryngology
Ovchinsky,Alexander,MD
Pediatrics
Diaz,Julio C.,MD
Gurey Wasserstein,Allison P.,MD
Lomax,Kathleen Graham,MD
Plastic Surgery
Friedlander,Beverly,MD
Yu,Deborah,MD
Psychiatry
Brazaitis,Edward,MD
Feldman,Russett P.,MD
Shaw,Jennifer Robin,MD
Radiation Oncology
Desai,Maheshwari M.,MD
Surgery (General)
Ayyagari,Kamalakar R.,MD

Shrewsbury
Anesthesiology
Goldofsky,Sheldon E.,MD
Kutzin,Theodore E.,MD
Patel,Bimal,MD
Schaaff,Robert P.,MD
Sondhi,Nidhi,DO
Staats,Peter Sean,MD
Taneja,Monica M.,MD
Wood,Sterling Harbert,DO
Anesthesiology: Pain Medicine
Cresanti-Daknis,Charles B.,MD
Li,Sean,MD
Sahoo,Aruna,MD
Walia,Kulbir Singh,MD
Cardiovascular Disease
Edlin,Dale E.,MD
Miller,Charles Luther,MD

Physicians by Town and Medical Specialty

Shrewsbury (cont)
Child & Adolescent Psychiatry
- Alcera, Eric Cortez, MD
- Edwards, Jennifer L., MD
Dermatology
- Resnikoff, Forrest P., MD
Diagnostic Radiology
- Lu, Stanley, MD
- Rashid, Salman, MD
- Shariff, Yasmeen K., MD
Emergency Medicine
- Valko, Peter C., MD
Family Med-Adult Medicine
- Saeed, Shamim Jan, MD
Family Medicine
- Brahver, Danit Vera, MD
- Huegel, Claudia Marie, MD
- Jafry, Yasmeen, MD
- Johnston, Christopher K., MD
Geriatrics
- Cook, Willard H., MD
Internal Medicine
- Angelo, Sharon A., DO
- Bhoori, Nafisa Y., MD
- Farooqui, Shahid Waseem, MD
- Felzenberg, Jeffrey D., MD
Neonatal-Perinatal Medicine
- France, Jeffrey W., DO
Neurological Surgery
- Rosenblum, Bruce R., MD
Nuclear Medicine
- Ruchman, Richard B., MD
Obstetrics & Gynecology
- Damien, Miguel, MD
- Holden, Emily C., MD
- Seungdamrong, Aimee Malunda, MD
- Witkowski, Mary E., MD
Orthopedic Surgery
- Menkowitz, Marc Scott, MD
- Stankovits, Lawrence Matthew, MD
Orthopedics
- Curatolo, Evan M., MD
Otolaryngology
- Passalaqua, Philip Jude, MD
- Prabhat, Arvind, MD
- Saporito, John L., MD
- Shah, Darsit, MD
- Tavill, Michael A., MD
- Winarsky, Eric L., MD
Pain Medicine
- Metzger, Scott E., MD
Pediatric Allergy
- Szema, Katherine Fang, MD
Pediatric Endocrinology
- Novello, Laura Joyce, MD
- Ostrow, Vlady, DO
Pediatric Orthopedics
- Plakas, Christos, MD
Pediatrics
- Appulingam, Anbuchelvi, MD
- Barrows, Frank P. IV, DO
- Lothe, Prakash S., MD
- O'Brien, Debra Ann, MD
- Rajaraman, Karunambal, MD
- Rigatti, Darrell J., MD
Physical Medicine & Rehab
- Kahng, He-Yeun, MD
Plastic Surgery
- Ashinoff, Russell Lee, MD
- Elkwood, Andrew I., MD
- Ibrahim, Zuhaib, MD
- Kaufman, Matthew Roy, MD
- Patel, Tushar R., MD
- Rose, Michael Ian, MD
- Schneider, Lisa Frances, MD
Psychiatry
- Bier, Martin M., MD
- Falco, Sharon Anne, MD
- Rhee, Bong Susan, MD
Pulmonary Disease
- Arlinghaus, Frank H. Jr., MD
Radiology
- Shinde, Tejas Shashikant, MD
Surgery (General)
- Abdollahi, Hamid, MD
- Ashraf, Azra Abida, MD
- Brock, James Steven, MD
- Cauda, Joseph E., MD
- Chang, Eric I-Yun, MD
- Wimmers, Eric Geoffrey, MD
Urology
- Bickerton, Michael W., MD
- Bonitz, Robert Paul Jr., MD
- Christiano, Arthur Patrick, MD
- Rose, John G., MD
- Smith, Robert Charles, MD

Sicklerville
Emergency Medicine
- Morone, Teresa Monica, DO
- Soper, Robert Earl, DO
Family Medicine
- Aitken, Robert J., DO
- Cox, Trevor E., DO
- Mingroni, Julius Anthony, DO
- Sharp, Harry Walton, DO
- Ubele, Deborah Anne, DO
Gastroenterology
- D'Auria, Daniel A., MD
- Velasco, Brenda Raquel, MD
Internal Medicine
- Brattelli, Gary Joseph, DO
- Cunanan, Joanne C., MD
- De Maria, Nicholas Anthony, MD
- Holgado, Maynard R., MD
- Palladino, Nicholas G., MD
- Patel, Indubhai Manibhai, MD
- Patel, Prahlad M., MD
- Pieretti, Gordon Anthony, DO
- Seltzer, Gregory Ian, MD
- Simon, Shari Kim, DO
Obstetrics & Gynecology
- Magness, Rose L., MD
- Stafford, Patricia T., MD
Pediatrics
- Hill-Hugh, Naomi Lynette, MD
- Stuffo, Kathryn, DO
Psychiatry
- Acosta, Regis Francisco, MD
- Reyes, Jose Franco, MD
- Sayed, Saquib Bashir, MD
Sports Medicine
- Taffet, Robert, MD

Skillman
Allergy
- Skolnick, Helen Sharlene, MD
Allergy & Immunology
- Caucino, Julie A., DO
- Pedinoff, Andrew J., MD
- Rao, Jayanti Juluru, MD
- Shah, Shaili Niranjan, MD
- Sikorski, Kristen Melissa, MD
- Southern, Darrell Loren, MD
Child & Adolescent Psychiatry
- Dismukes, Jennifer Bright, DO
Emergency Medicine
- Eberly, Andrea Cecilia, MD
Internal Medicine
- Shah, Manish A., MD
Plastic Surgery
- Nini, Kevin T., MD
Psychiatry
- Harman, Robert Ashworth, MD
- Negron, Arnaldo E., MD
- Ramzy, Ayman H., MD
- Shnaidman, Vivian T., MD
- Shnaps, Yitzchak, MD
- Stuebben, Kurt C., MD
- Willis, Kenneth W., MD
Thoracic Surgery
- Yarramneni, Akhila, MD

Smithville
Emergency Medicine
- Ursani, Sekander A., MD

Somerdale
Anesthesiology
- Mehta, Parul J., MD
Child & Adolescent Psychiatry
- Feigl, Frances Marie, MD
Family Medicine
- Cheng, Desmond H., DO
- Gallagher, Joseph L. III, DO
Internal Medicine
- Barone, Christopher J., DO
- Kalola, Vijay K., MD
- Patel, Jayesh B., MD
Obstetrics & Gynecology
- Finley, Stephanie Elena, DO
- Milicia, Anthony P., MD
- Suarez, Melissa Lehn, DO
- White, Deborah A., DO

Somers Point
Addiction Psychiatry
- Levounis, Petros, MD
Allergy
- Schwartz, Lawrence A., DO
Anatomic/Clinical Pathology
- Beach, Robert J., MD
- Pond, James M., MD
- Saunders, Peter J., MD
Anesthesiology
- Absin, Martini Perez, MD
- Allahverdi, Ilya Michael, MD
- Avellino, Carmine, DO
- Dearborn, Peyton Robert, MD
- Hu, Xin Tian, MD
- Khatiwala, Colleen Pravin, MD
- Krzemieniecki, Thomas Gerald, DO
- Salkeld, Charles S., DO
- Tsyganov, Igor Vlademer, MD
Arthroscopic Surgery
- Zabinski, Stephen J., MD
Cardiovascular Disease
- Arluck, David Lawrence, MD
- Dib, Haitham R., MD
- Dowd, Mary Katherine, MD
- Kornberg, Steven Edward, MD
- Levin, Jacob L., MD
- Singh, Millee, DO
Critical Care Medicine
- O'Connor, James J. III, MD
- Ojserkis, Bennett Edward, MD
Dermatology
- Campo, Anthony Guy Jr., MD
Electromyography
- Gottfried, Maureen, DO
Emergency Medicine
- Angelastro, David B., MD
- Chiccarine, Anthony P., DO
- May, Roberta Russell, DO
- McGuigan, Thomas M., MD
- Souto, Henry Lee, DO
- Talotta, Nicholas Joseph Jr., MD
Family Med-Adult Medicine
- Fox, Michael L., MD
- Malik, Ankit, DO
Family Medicine
- Ganesan, Balamurugan, MD
- Janes, Laura C., DO
- Nahas, Arthur G., DO
- Silverman, Russell V., DO
- Sparagna, Angelo III, MD
Gastroenterology
- Deshpande, Nikhil, MD
- Krachman, Joel E., DO
- Krachman, Michael S., MD
- Ognibene, Lawrence G., DO
- Schwab, Kenneth S., MD
Infectious Disease
- Lucasti, Christopher J., DO
- Trofa, Andrew F., MD
Internal Medicine
- Adigun, Jennifer Olubusola, MD
- Alberta, James David, MD
- Cadacio, Manolito G., MD
- Cilursu, Ana Maria, MD
- Erskine, Jennifer Grantham, MD
- Geraci, Brian Anthony, MD
- Gery, Brian F., MD
- Giunta, Michael Anthony, MD
- Hooper, William Jr., MD
- Lankaranian, Dara, MD
- Rangaraj, Padmaja, MD
- Roche, Charles Vincent III, MD
- Rowe, Jeanne M., MD
- Sood, Delcine Ann, DO
- Teklezgi, Semhar, DO
- Yangala, Sridevi, MD
- Yankovitch, Pierre, MD
Medical Oncology
- Goldberg, Robert M., MD
Neurological Surgery
- Glass, Andrew S., MD
- Sabo, Robert A., MD
Neurology
- Roeltgen, David P., MD
- Tzorfas, Scott D., MD
- Yangala, Ravi, MD
Obstetrics & Gynecology
- Bergen, Blair A., MD
- Bravoco, Michael C., MD
- Ciceron, Asuncion V., MD
- Kaplitz, Neil H., MD
- Korzeniowski, Philip A., MD
- Morgan, Daniel Robert, MD
- Nosseir, Sandy B., MD
- Perez, Finuccia Renda, MD
- Phillips, James J., MD
- Rezvina, Natalia Y., MD
- Sindoni, Frank W., MD
- Zhang, Vincent, MD
Orthopedic Surgery
- Alber, George C., MD
- Bannon, John T., MD
- Barrett, Thomas Arthur, MD
- Dalzell, Frederick G., MD
- De Morat, Eugene John, MD
- Frankel, Victor R., MD
- Islinger, Richard Barnard, MD
- Marczyk, Stanley C., MD
- McCloskey, John R., MD
- Ponnappan, Ravi Kumar, MD
- Zuck, Glenn M., MD
Otolaryngology
- Morrow, William J., DO
- Rondinella, Louis, MD
Pediatrics
- Andrews, Roji Zacharia, MD
- Bross, George Jr., DO
- Drexler, Christopher W., DO
- Gupte, Meenal A., MD
- Held, Sharon L., DO
- Jacobson, Mark, DO
- Keenan, Christopher Joseph, DO
- Mandalapu, Padma, MD
- Share, Lisa J., MD
- Thorp, Andrea Rita, DO
- Vekteris, Gerald E., DO
Psychiatry
- Gowda, Srisai, MD
- Reid, Kelly M., MD
Pulmonary Critical Care
- Adams, William B., DO
Pulmonary Disease
- Cunanan, Manuel Salas, MD
- Del Re, Sallustio, MD
Radiology
- Cooperman, Harry Alan, MD
Rheumatology
- Brecher, Linda S., DO
- Halko, George J., DO
Surgery (General)
- D'Angelo-Donovan, Desiree D., DO
- Feinberg, Gary L., MD
- Galler, Leonard, MD
- Herrington, James William, MD
Urology
- Axilrod, Andrew Charles, MD
- Bernal, Raymond Mark, MD
- Braga, Gene J., MD
- Ciceron, Andre, MD
- Hirsh, Andrew L., MD
- Kimmel, Barry S., MD
- Pagnani, Alexander M., MD
- Spence, Abraham M., MD
- Wixted, William M., MD
Vascular & Intrvntnal Radiology
- Schwartz, Jay Harris, MD
Vascular Surgery
- Gosin, Jeffrey Stuart, MD
- Nahas, Frederick J., MD

Somerset
Anesthesiology
- Back, Steven Marc, MD
- Baron, Jeremy Lawrence, MD
- Cabanero, Camilo O., MD
- Caces, Alan R., MD
- Cho, Grace C., MD
- Choi, Jieun Susana, MD
- Colavita, Richard D., MD
- Cottrill, Richard Z. Jr., MD
- Das, Sudip S., MD
- Fellenbaum, Paul, MD
- Gajewski, Jan Peter, MD
- Gangavalli, Ravi Venkata, MD
- Giacobbe, Dean Thomas, MD
- Ginsberg, Sanford Ginsberg, MD
- Gunvantlal, Desai A., MD
- Jenkins, Paul B., MD
- Kett, Attila G., MD
- Kiamzon, Harald James, MD
- Kim, Hyon S., MD

Ku, James Chien, MD
Land, Warren K., DO
Lee, William, MD
Lu, Ya-Tseng W., MD
Mackler, Denise Lynn, MD
Margiotta, Joseph A., MD
Martin, Dean Walter, MD
Mathew, Julie, MD
Mosaddeghi, Mahmood, MD
Moses, Brett Joseph, MD
Nath, Ajay, MD
Pabbathi, Pramod, DO
Patel, Ajitkumar Gunvantrai, MD
Patel, Samir Natavar, MD
Perez, Manuel A., MD
Rahman, Attique, MD
Richardson, Michael J., MD
Ruda, William A., MD
Ruedy, Krista R., MD
Siegel, Scott S., MD
Simon, Abraham M., DO
Sio, Reymond Guieb, MD
Smith, Daniel Brian J., MD
Sonbol, Sherif A., MD
Sperrazza, James Christopher, MD
Tangreti, Nicholas W., MD
Tronolone, William, MD
Walker, John S., DO
Yau, Assumpta K., MD
Anesthesiology: Critical Care
Rodricks, Michael Baltazar, MD
Anesthesiology: Pain Medicine
Patel, Arti S., MD
Peng, Hsin, MD
Picone, Michael J., MD
Breast Surgery
McManus, Susan A., MD
Cardiovascular Disease
Dorazio, John L., MD
Gladstone, Clifford D., MD
Khanna, Pravien K., MD
Kukafka, Sheldon Jay, MD
Kulkarni, Anand U., MD
Passannante, Anthony Jr., MD
Passannante, Anthony J. Sr, MD
Patel, Pratik B., MD
Reddy, Manisha S., MD
Singal, Dinesh K., MD
Stroh, Jack A., MD
Tardos, Jonathan George, MD
Child & Adolescent Psychiatry
Randolph, Robert Styles, MD
Yeung, Wilbert Derek, MD
Clinical Cardiac Elctrphyslgy
Gowda, Subhashini Anande, MD
Critical Care Medicine
Das, Arvind K., MD
Davanzo, Lawrence D., DO
Doujaiji, Bassam Mouhin, MD
Dermatology
Bhatti, Hamza Dastigir, DO
Cha, Jisun, MD
Cohen, Penelope Jucowics, MD
Firoz, Bahar F., MD
Milgraum, Sandy S., MD
Nijhawan, Rohit I., MD
Pappert, Amy S., MD
Urman, Felix, MD
Victor, Frank Charles, MD
Emergency Medicine
Leavell, Ellen T., MD
Owusu-Dapaah, Kwabena B., MD
Patti, Laryssa A., MD
Endocrinology
Noronha, Joaquim L., MD
Family Medicine
Condren, Marc J., MD
Etheridge, Barbara Anne, MD
Gwozdz, Paul William, MD
Kaufman, Irving H., MD
Laing, Euton M., MD
Lawrence, Denise Antoinette, MD
Madaj, Andrew T., MD
Maziarz, Anastazja, MD
Torok, Geza, MD
Gastroenterology
Aronson, Scott Logan, MD
Ebert, Ellen C., MD
Ferges, Mitchell L., MD
Ferges, William James, MD
Merkel, Ira S., MD

Pickover, Lawrence M., MD
Platovsky, Anna, MD
Rapisarda, Alexander F., MD
Scharf, Henry J., MD
Shamim, Syed Q., MD
General Practice
Andre, Oswald A., MD
Najarro, Juan Carlos, MD
Geriatrics
Singh, Mukesh Kumar, MD
Hematology
Fein, Robert P., MD
Porcelli, Marcus P., MD
Hematology Oncology
Desai, Sameer P., MD
Fang, Bruno S., MD
Karp, George I., MD
Lampert, Craig, MD
Reid, Phillip Dolivera, MD
Ronnen, Ellen A., MD
Infectious Disease
Kumar, Uday, MD
Sathe, Sadhana S., MD
Segal, Robert Eric, MD
Internal Medicine
Amegadzie, Richard Koku, MD
Behar, Roger, MD
Chandrasekaran, Aparna, MD
Compagnone, Linda, MD
DelMaestro, Steven R., MD
Desai, Bijal, MD
El Banna, Mahmoud, MD
Gable, Brian Philip, MD
Heinrich, Art, MD
Herrera, Alejandro J., MD
Ilogu, Noel O., MD
Jain, Deepak K., MD
Jones Burton, Charlotte M., MD
Kuchipudi, Solomon Sudhakar, MD
Kuriakose, Marykutty K., MD
Lahiri, Devraj, MD
Majeed, Asra, MD
Nagarakanti, Rangadham, MD
Patel, Bhavi Ashit, MD
Rayudu, Sunita Srinivas, MD
Richards, David A., MD
Rihacek, Gregory S., MD
Rizvi, Nazia, MD
Rizvi, Tariq A., MD
Salim, Tamanna Yussouf, MD
Schwartzer, Thomas A., MD
Shah, Chirag H., DO
Srivastav, Sushmita, MD
Tadros, Carmen E. G., MD
Tawfik, Isaac H., MD
Thirumavalavan, Vallur S., MD
Villanobos, Rey T., MD
Wang, Mei-Hui, MD
Wang-Epstein, Christina C., MD
Yakobashvili, David, MD
Zetkulic, Marygrace M., MD
Medical Oncology
Licitra, Edward Joseph, MD
Nephrology
Hakimzadeh, Parisa, DO
Jain, Sandesh, MD
Kabis, Suzanne M., MD
Obias, Primabel Villena, MD
Srichai, Manakan Betsy, MD
Vaghasiya, Rick Parsotam, MD
Neurological Surgery
Fineman, Sanford, MD
Neurology
Busono, Stephanus Judi D., MD
Dixit, Seema P., DO
Greenberg, E. Jeffrey, MD
Hersh, Joshua Neil, MD
Obstetrics & Gynecology
Aguh, Chikezie J., MD
Alvaro, Joseph M., MD
Gao, Michael Yuan, MD
Gopal, Manish, MD
Levitt, Robert S., MD
Lo, Vivian S., MD
Schaefer, Robert M., MD
Shastri, Shefali Mavani, MD
Shulman, Lois E., MD
Treiser, Susan L., MD
Occupational Medicine
Kusnetz, Eliot M., MD

Oncology
McDermott, Janette H., MD
Ophthalmology
Angrist, Richard Clay, MD
Grewal, Roopinder K., MD
Phillips, Bradley John, MD
Shamim, Tasneem F., MD
Orthopedic Surgery
Butler, Mark S., MD
Chiappetta, Gino, MD
Coyle, Michael P. Jr., MD
Harwood, David A., MD
Kayiaros, Stephen, MD
Krisiloff, Edward B., MD
Leddy, Timothy P., MD
Malberg, Marc I., MD
Polonet, David Russell, MD
Sagebien, Carlos Alberto, MD
Swan, Kenneth Girvan Jr., MD
Orthopedic Surgery-Adult Rcnstr
Tria, Alfred J. Jr., MD
Orthopedic-Hand Surgery
Monica, James T., MD
Otolaryngology
Sabin, Steven Lloyd, MD
Pain Medicine
Sacks, Harry Jack, MD
Pain Medicine-Interventional
Demesmin, Didier, MD
Pediatric Anesthesia
Cean, Daniela E., DO
Pediatric Dermatology
Curtis, Princesa Maria, MD
Pediatric Gastroenterology
Dadhania, Jayantilal P., MD
Leibowitz, Karen Louise, MD
Sinha, Jyoti, MD
Pediatrics
Arun, Aparna, MD
Carroll, John F., MD
Galowitz, Stacey, DO
Goodman, Elizabeth Anne, MD
Gunawan, Rita R., MD
Kapoor, Kusum, MD
Lerner, Emanuel D., MD
Misra, Manju, MD
Pai, Shilpa, MD
Pari, Sadhana S., MD
Parsi, Prakasham, MD
Patel, Trupti, MD
Pillai, Hema R., MD
Ramadan, Soheir S., MD
Roca Piccini, Elsie Isabel, MD
Sinclair, Melissa Renee, DO
Speesler, Matthew J., MD
Physical Med & Rehab-Pain Med
Ahmad, Usman Fayyaz, DO
Baxi, Naimish, MD
Physical Medicine & Rehab
Ankamah, Andrew K., MD
George, Tony Kuttikattu, DO
Mandelblat, Zarina, MD
Psychiatry
Hanchuk, Hilary T., MD
Nam, Sang K., MD
Pulmonary Disease
Lucas, Robin S., MD
Rheumatology
Tiku, Moti L., MD
Sports Medicine
Gatt, Charles J. Jr., MD
Surgery (General)
Ang, Brian Christopher Uy, MD
Camerota, Andrew Martin, MD
Donaire, Michael Jeremie, MD
Gaspard, Henry Claude, MD
Gervasoni, James Edmund Jr., MD
Hopkins, Lisa Anne, MD
Melman, Lora Marie, MD
Rondel, Mikhail, MD
Surgical Critical Care
Sadek, Ragui W., MD
Thoracic Surgery
Bocage, Jean P., MD
Caccavale, Robert J., MD
Urology
Bhatti, Mohammad Azeem, MD
Vascular Surgery
Deak, Steven T., MD

Somerville
Administration/Medical Mgt
Cors, William K., MD
Adult Psychiatry
Rowley, Susan Peet, MD
Allergy
Krol, Kristine, MD
Allergy & Immunology
Druce, Howard M., MD
Anatomic/Clinical Pathology
Chen, Tsuey-Ling, MD
D'Aguillo, Anthony F., MD
Gonsorcik, Victoria K., DO
Anesthesiology
Granowitz, Gail F., MD
Roy, Amanda R., MD
Breast Surgery
Lanfranchi, Angela E., MD
Child & Adolescent Psychiatry
Hossain, Akhtar, MD
Clinical Neurophysiology
Mian, Nimer F., DO
Critical Care Medicine
Besserman, Eva B., DO
Emergency Medicine
Chan, Mei-Yung, MD
Moore, Robert P., MD
Zeiger, Jill M., MD
Family Medicine
Bucek, John Ladislav, MD
Davis, Lloyd A., MD
DePass, Lorraine Francis, MD
Dhillon-Athwal, Narinder Kaur, MD
Guyton, Margaret Louise, MD
Halper-Erkkila, Ruby A., MD
Hansch, Lalitha T., MD
Huang, Ming Y., MD
Juliano, Julieann S., MD
Lundholm, Joanne Katherine, MD
Micek Galinat, Laura A., MD
Shapiro, Dein M., MD
Spector, Elisabeth, MD
Wu, Frances Y., MD
Gastroenterology
Luppescu, Neal E., MD
Vergilio, Cory D., MD
Hematology
Stanford, Brian J., DO
Toomey, Kathleen, MD
Wu, Hen-Vai, MD
Young, Steven Eugene, MD
Hematology Oncology
Khalid, Aysha, MD
Pan, Beiqing, MD
Hospitalist
Amadi, Mariette Yvonne, MD
Internal Medicine
Ahmed, Sadia, MD
Ansari, Huma Naz, MD
Ashraf, Shehzana, MD
Balint, Elizabeth A., MD
Berkowitz, David A., MD
Braimbridge, Sandra P., MD
Caballes, Romeo A. Jr., MD
Celo, Jovenia S., MD
Dobrescu, Andrei Mihnea, MD
Horak, Ivan D., MD
Lwanga, Juliet R., MD
Malik, Arsalan, MD
Rosenbluth, Jonathan Z., MD
Sanchez-Catanese, Betty, MD
Singh, Jaya, MD
Medical Oncology
Trivedi, Seeta, MD
Neonatal-Perinatal Medicine
Hirsch, Daniel Shawn, MD
Ladino, John Freddy, MD
Rejjal, Abdellatif R., MD
Rotschild, Tomas, MD
Savla, Jayshree Sameer, MD
Verma, Anjali, MD
Neurology
Mian, Bilal A., MD
Ophthalmology
Kaspareck, Joseph Jr., MD
Sohmer, Kenette K., MD
Orthopedic Surgery
Baron, Harvey L., MD
St. John, Thomas A., MD

Physicians by Town and Medical Specialty

Somerville (cont)
Otolaryngology
  Bortniker, David Leonard, MD
Pediatric Pulmonology
  Turcios, Nelson L., MD
Pediatrics
  Doshi, Pankaj Manilal, MD
  Hall, Kendria, MD
  Hou, Shunli, MD
  Patel, Kalpesh P., DO
Physical Medicine & Rehab
  Kulessa-Dussias, Renata, DO
Plastic Surgery
  Strauss, Andrea L., MD
Psychiatry
  De Ritter, Lois M., MD
  Falls, Ingrid T., MD
  Osmanovic, Kenan, MD
  Patel, Unnati D., MD
  Rosin, Dale, DO
  Rowan, Patrick John, MD
  Shaikh, Tasneem, MD
Radiation Oncology
  Braver, Joel Keith, MD
Surgery (General)
  Ambrose, Gunaseelan, MD
  Drascher, Gary A., MD
  Seenivasan, Thangamani, MD
  Sugarmann, William M., MD
Therapeutic Radiology
  Bond, Laura R., MD
Urology
  Catanese, Anthony J., MD
  Dave, Dhiren Sirish, MD
  Feldman, Arthur E., MD
  Fischer, Joel M., MD
  Harmon, Keith Andrew, MD
  Shah, Neel Praful, MD
Vascular Surgery
  Imegwu, Obi J., MD

South Amboy
Cardiovascular Disease
  Latif, Shahid, MD
  Younes, Elie, MD
Family Medicine
  Nisar, Noor A., MD
  Ofori Behome, Yaw, MD
Internal Medicine
  Batarseh, Hani Elias Salim, MD
  Grochowalski, Tomasz K., MD
  McKenna, Harold V., MD
  Ouano, Rodolfo C., MD
  Rathi, Lilly, MD
Pediatrics
  Manfredonia, Patricia Estrada, MD
  Mikhail, Maged, MD
Physical Medicine & Rehab
  Pollen, Philip C., MD
Psychiatry
  Arya, Vinay, MD

South Bound Brook
Family Medicine
  Kaladas, Jeffrey J., MD

South Hackensack
Critical Care Medicine
  Ashtyani Asl, Hormoz, MD

South Orange
Adolescent Medicine
  Albanese, Anthony C., MD
Anesthesiology
  Bodner, Arnold H., MD
Critical Care Medicine
  Achar, Pankaja B.S., MD
Family Medicine
  Jain, Sejal, MD
  Kharazi, Fariba, DO
Gastroenterology
  Sampson, Ruby J., MD
Geriatrics
  Eatman, Florence B., MD
Gynecological Oncology
  Anderson, Patrick St. George, MD
Hematology
  Lombardy, Elyane Emilienne, MD
Internal Medicine
  Adlakha, Anupama, MD
  Anicette, Lionel Jr., MD
  Bangia, Neha, MD
  Gandhi, Champaklal K., MD
  Gandhi, Sulakshana, MD
  Holder, Kevin D., MD
  Mehta, Satish R., MD
  Mellk, Harlan M., MD
  Mouravskaia, Tatiana V., MD
  Patel, Ramesh L., MD
  Shapiro, Sofia, MD
  Singla, Ruchika, MD
Neonatal-Perinatal Medicine
  Walker, Camille D., MD
Obstetrics & Gynecology
  Dresdner, Michael T., MD
  Rosen, Kimberly A., MD
  Sosin, Beth L., MD
Ophthalmology
  Crane, Charles J., MD
  Gunzburg, Allison B., MD
  Spier, Bernard C., MD
Orthopedic Surgery
  Berlin, Burgess L., MD
  Buechel, Frederick F., MD
  Helbig, Thomas E., MD
Pediatrics
  Lovenheim, Jay Alon, DO
  Vecchio, Lisa C., MD
  Yoo, Susan S., MD
Physical Medicine & Rehab
  Brien, Michael J., MD
Thoracic Surgery
  Losman, Jacques G., MD

South Plainfield
Allergy
  Kothari, Harish B., MD
Anesthesiology
  Byahatti, Pramila, MD
  Kapusuz, Tolga, MD
  Tran, Bao Chau Minh, MD
Cardiovascular Disease
  Agarwala, Ajay Kumar, MD
  Altszuler, Henry M., MD
  Andraws, Richard Zaki, MD
  Blumberg, Edwin D., MD
  Leopold, Thomas D., MD
  Rakla, Younus A., MD
Child & Adolescent Psychiatry
  Siddiqui, Waqar Ahmed, MD
Dermatology
  Ju, William D., MD
Family Med-Sports Medicine
  Browne, Avery F., DO
Family Medicine
  Baum, Michael Jay, DO
  Bhatia, Irvinder, MD
  Hoppe, James Robert, MD
  Patel, Purvee D., MD
  Rozehzadeh, Rabin, MD
Gastroenterology
  Goyal, Alok, MD
Geriatrics
  Dumapit, Gerardo D., MD
Gynecology
  Powderly, Mary K., MD
  Sanghavi, Maya M., MD
Infectious Disease
  Go, Richard Au Yeung, MD
Internal Medicine
  Capitly, Domiciano V., MD
  Centeno, Galen Arcellana, MD
  Channapragada, Srinivas, MD
  Doshi, Arvind K., MD
  Goyal, Madhu B., MD
  Horvath, Katalin, MD
  Joseph, P. Dilip, MD
  Kaylen, Thomas G., MD
  Kim, Steven Namgi, MD
  Natarajan, Shobana, MD
  Patel, Devang G., MD
  Sarraf, Mohammad A., MD
  Seeni, Aysha, MD
  Singh, Priyanka, MD
  Toma, Wadie, MD
  Tucker, Burton Stanley, MD
Maternal & Fetal Medicine
  Goyal, Madhu A., MD
  Rana, Jagpal, MD
Med Genetics-Clinical Biochem
  Bonilla Guerrero, Ruben, MD
Neonatal-Perinatal Medicine
  Biswas, Anjali, MD
Nephrology
  Rao, Bhavani P., MD
Obstetrics & Gynecology
  Antonio, Edsel, DO
  Chan, Albert C., MD
  Guerra-Deluna, Myrna T., MD
  Kashyap, Meeta Parashar, MD
  Shah, Namrata Jinesh, MD
  Tran-Hoppe, Ngoc Quynh T., MD
Ophthalmology
  Agarwala, Atul K., MD
Oral & Maxillofacial Surgery
  Goulston, Michael Keith, MD
Orthopedic Surgery
  Choi, Soon Chae, MD
  Lebovicz, Richard S., MD
  Shafi, Mohammad, MD
Pediatrics
  Deshpande, Sanjay V., MD
  DiCarlo, Jilma Patricia, MD
  Ganti, Subrahmanyam, MD
  Gaviola, Durga C., MD
  Joseph, Anita, MD
  Solages, Joseph, MD
Physical Medicine & Rehab
  Solaimanzadeh, Sima, MD
Psychiatry
  Chezian, Shanthi, MD
Surgery (General)
  Hobayan, Edgar R., MD
Thoracic Surgery
  Breitbart, Gary B., MD
  Richmand, David M., MD
Trauma Surgery
  Brahmbhatt, Ravikumar B., MD
Vascular Surgery
  Wong, Geoffrey, MD

South River
Family Medicine
  Girgis, Linda Mae, MD
  Girgis, Moris Beachay, MD
Hypertension
  Covit, Andrew B., MD
Internal Medicine
  Dubov, Glenn A., MD
Nephrology
  Drabik, Thomas Edward, DO
  Matera, James J., DO

Southampton
Anatomic/Clinical Pathology
  Della Croce, David R., DO
Family Medicine
  Burger, Max, MD

Sparta
Anesthesiology
  Willis, William John, MD
Colon & Rectal Surgery
  Green, Jason D., MD
Dermatology
  Papadopoulos, Anthony Jordan, MD
Diagnostic Radiology
  Cordero, Hector Orlando, MD
  Corio, Frederick J., MD
  Franklin, Barry I., MD
  Ranley, Robert L., MD
  Rodrigues, Vanitha J., MD
  Shah, Shital R., MD
Family Medicine
  Bollard, David A., DO
  Casella, Joseph J., DO
  Ganon, Michael R., DO
  Medunick, David M., DO
  Shea, Caitlin M., DO
Gastroenterology
  Agarwal, Sudhir Kumar, MD
  Lindy, Michael Evan, MD
  Rao, Kiran Venkat, MD
  Tang, Linda Yinglin, MD
Geriatrics
  Wang, George Cho-Ching, MD
Hematology Oncology
  Cheng, Waina, MD
  Incorvati, Jason A., MD
Internal Medicine
  Abdo-Matkiwsky, May D., DO
  Kim, Daryl Kyung, MD
  Liotta, Joseph Anthony Sr., MD
  Odeyemi, Olutunde Olakunle, MD
  Selvaraj, Kavitha, MD
Medical Oncology
  Halibey, Bohdan E., MD
Nephrology
  Casella, Frank J., DO
Neurology
  Greene, Wayne L., MD
Obstetrics & Gynecology
  Sotillo, Melissa Maria, MD
Ophthalmology
  Hess, Jocelyn S., MD
  Liegner, Jeffrey T., MD
Orthopedic Surgery
  Basch, David B., MD
  Czaplicki-Margiotti, Marie A., MD
  Vitolo, John, MD
Otolaryngology
  Reddy, Shashidhar Sadda, MD
Pain Medicine-Interventional
  Siegfried, Richard Norman, MD
Pediatrics
  Achar, Ashwini, MD
  Bronstein, Regina, MD
  Calabrese, Carol E., MD
  Canzoniero, Christian, MD
  Capozzoli, Alexis Nicole, MD
  Di Paolo, Raymond Paul, MD
  Jacobson, Louis Robert, MD
  Mak, Sheila Shuk-Yin, DO
  McHugh, Catherine Ann, MD
  Meskin, Inna, MD
  O'Neill, Michael B., MD
  Raman, Rajesh C., MD
  Spensieri, Diana Patricia, MD
  Whittington, Wendy Louise, MD
Physical Medicine & Rehab
  Agesen, Thomas, MD
Plastic Surgery
  Patsis, Michael C., MD
Psychiatry
  Blanchard, Jenny Ann, DO
  Kloupar, Dagmar S., MD
  Koss, Debra Elvira, MD
  Leibov, Ernest B., MD
Radiation Oncology
  Cole, Robert J., MD
  Lo, Kathy Kai Yee, MD
Radiology
  Cordero, Orlando C., MD
  Skalla, Matthew T., MD
Rheumatology
  Sarwar, Haroon, MD
Surgery (General)
  Muduli, Hazari, MD
  O'Shea, Michelle T., MD
Urology
  Hall, Matthew Scott, MD
  Matteson, James R., MD
  Mykulak, Donald J., MD
  Salvatore, Frank Timothy, MD

Spotswood
Internal Medicine
  Deb, Ashoke Kumar, MD
  Patel, Deepa Samir, MD
  Patel, Samir G., MD
  Sahni, Sushma, MD

Spring Lake
Dermatology
  Lo Buono, Philip J., MD
  Sterling, J. Barton, MD
Hospitalist
  Banzuelo Rio, Margie R., MD
Internal Medicine
  Antoniadis, Ileana, MD
  Pardon, Paul A., MD
Pediatrics
  Miele, Ellen H., MD
  Pirogovsky, Victoria, MD
  Sciarappa, Lorette J., MD

Springfield
Abdominal Surgery
  Feteiha, Muhammad S., MD
Adolescent Medicine
  Mullick, Bharati, MD
Allergy
  Bielory, Leonard, MD
Anesthesiology
  Schoenfeld, Mark R., MD
Cardiovascular Disease
  Cohen, Barry Mark, MD
  Fishberg, Robert Daniel, MD

628

Lux,Michael S.,MD
Powell,David E.,MD
Prasad,Sanjiv,MD
Roberti,Roberto R.,MD
Stein,Elliott M.,MD
Weber,Vance J.,MD
Weinrauch,Michael L.,MD
Cataract
  Notis,Corey M.,MD
Child & Adolescent Psychiatry
  Cohen,Hayley M.,MD
  Kaplan,Gabriel,MD
  Silver,Bennett,MD
Emergency Medicine
  Parman,Stanley C.,MD
Family Medicine
  Krblich,Diana,MD
  Mansour,Ali Gaber,MD
Gastroenterology
  Kerner,Michael B.,MD
  Lipsky,Marvin A.,MD
Geriatrics
  Lim,Betty Bichly,MD
Hand Surgery
  Fox,Ross J.,MD
  Kirschenbaum,Abram Eugene,MD
Hematology Oncology
  Desai,Ved,DO
  Khot,Ashish Abhay,MD
  Rao,Maithili V.,MD
Infectious Disease
  De Fronzo,Stephen D.,MD
Internal Medicine
  Cantor,Susan J.,MD
  Chazen,Diane R.,MD
  Fuhrman,Michael Alexander,MD
  Glushakow,Allen S.,MD
  Kodiyalam,Uthra K.,MD
  Pondt,Charlesse Maureen,MD
  Preston,Daniel J.,MD
  Profeta,Susan B.,MD
  Sudler,Joy D.,MD
  Vaswani,Khimya I.,MD
  Zhu,Binghua,MD
Nuclear Cardiology
  Furer,Steven K.,MD
Obstetrics & Gynecology
  Bowers,Charles Jr.,MD
  Byalik,Olga Viktoria,MD
  De Fronzo,Carl L.,DO
  Hunt,Mary Elizabeth,MD
  Lublin,Jennifer Caryn,MD
  Magaril,Rhona A.,MD
  Pinto,Jose J.,DO
  Tye,Joann Li Yen,MD
Ophthalmology
  Lucia Ricci,Jodie Italia,MD
Orthopedic Surgery
  Cuomo,Thomas F.,MD
  Jaffe,Leonard,MD
  Oppenheim,William C.,MD
  Rieber,Michael Harold,MD
Otolaryngology
  Freifeld,Stephen F.,MD
Pediatric Emergency Medicine
  Cleary,Kelly,MD
Pediatrics
  Korkmazsky,Yelena N.,MD
  Lim,Norman Feliz Lopez,MD
  Lozano,Rolando,MD
  Morris,Mark M.,DO
  Nunez,Helen Lourdes,MD
  Thomas,Jolly,MD
Physical Medicine & Rehab
  Rispoli,Frances M.,DO
Plastic Surgery
  Loguda,Charles A.,MD
  Tepper,Howard N.,MD
  Tepper,Richard Eric,MD
  Zeitels,Jerrold R.,MD
Psychiatry
  Kantor,Ruth B.,MD
  Miller,David Geoffrey,MD
  Parinello,Robert M.,MD
  Thorpe,Michelle Lynn,MD
Surgery (General)
  Buwen,James P.,DO
  Coblentz,Malcolm Guy,MD
  Forrester,Glenn Joseph,MD
  Glasnapp,Angela Jack,MD
  Goyal,Ajay,MD
  Lopes,James M.,MD
  Montes,Leigh,MD
Surgical Critical Care
  Lopes,Joao Alberto,MD
  Pepen,John Andre,MD
Stanhope
Internal Medicine
  Mitsos,Stephanie E.,MD
Stirling
Internal Medicine
  Pontecorvo,Martin J.,DO
  Postighone,Carl J.,DO
Stockton
Family Medicine
  Freedenfeld,Stuart H.,MD
  Heinz,Kristann Wilmore,MD
Internal Medicine
  Crist,Peter A.,MD
Stone Harbor
Family Medicine
  Ruskey,Elizabeth E.,DO
  Vogdes,Tara Ann,DO
General Practice
  Speer,Robert R.,DO
Internal Med-Adolescent Med
  Hofmann,William Andrew III,DO
Internal Medicine
  Nuschke,Randell A.,MD
Obstetrics & Gynecology
  King,Lorraine C.,MD
Stratford
Adult Psychiatry
  Scheinthal,Stephen M.,DO
Anatomic/Clinical Pathology
  DeRisio,Vincent James II,DO
Anesthesiology
  Jones,Michael R.,MD
  Neitzel,Kristi M.,MD
Child & Adolescent Psychiatry
  Humphrey,Frederick James II,DO
  Kumar,Geetha,MD
  Levitas,Andrew S.,MD
  O'Donnell-Mulgrew,Deborah M.,DO
Critical Care Medicine
  Kirkham,Jay G. Jr.,DO
Emergency Medical Services
  Heron,Joseph,MD
Emergency Medicine
  Ahmed,Mehvish,DO
  Angelo,Melanie Elissa,DO
  Chuang,Ion S.,MD
  Corrin,Courtney Wilczynski,DO
  Diaz,Lissa,DO
  Dichter,Eric Kyle,DO
  Ellis,Daniel Thomas,MD
  Fernandez,Claudio Miguel,DO
  Gesumaria,Robert Cosmo,DO
  Horn,Robert John,DO
  Kurkowski,Ellen J.,DO
  Levin,Francis L.,DO
  Licata,Thomas C.,DO
  Maddalozzo,Gerald Anthony,DO
  Maddock,Eric Ryan,DO
  Morris,Jason Joseph,DO
  Pagano,Joseph James,DO
  Papa,Thomas Rowland,DO
  Patel,Kishan Bharat,DO
  Pinkerton,Gerald John,DO
  Schuitema,Henry R.,DO
  Simmers-Dabinett,Donna Lee,DO
  Sobers-Brown,Karen D.,MD
  Tamaska,Wayne G.,DO
  Tomasello,Nicholas James,DO
  Wahdat,Razwana,MD
  Wetjen,Thomas F.,DO
  Wysocki,Julianne M.,DO
Endocrinology
  Helfer,Elizabeth L.,MD
  Luceri,Patricia Marie,DO
  Szpiech,Maria,MD
Family Med-Geriatric Medicine
  Abesh,Jesse Susan,DO
Family Medicine
  Alday,Geronima G.,MD
  Channell,Millicent King,DO
  Chick,Charlene Elizabeth,DO
  Garnier,Katharine M.,MD
  Goldwaser,Elan Luria,DO
  Gupta,Adarsh Kumar,DO
  Heaton,Caryl Joan,DO
  Hoffman,Barry M.,DO
  Jiwani,Ameena Javed,DO
  Kimler,Christine Marie,DO
  Lambert,Kathryn C.,DO
  Overbeck,Kevin Joseph,DO
  Perez,Ricardo,DO
  Rabara,Knic Corpuz,DO
  Russell,Hortense Patricia,DO
  Schlenker,Clinton James,DO
  Scott,George John,DO
  Torres,Jonathan William,DO
  Wadhwa,Aruna,MD
Gastroenterology
  Liakos,Steven,DO
General Practice
  Gayle,Catherine,MD
  Hudrick,Robert Eugene,DO
  Jagpal,Karandeep,DO
  Lightfoot,Judith A.,DO
  Nguyen,Jonathan Huy,DO
  White,Joseph A.,DO
Geriatrics
  Cavalieri,Thomas A.,DO
  Chopra,Anita,MD
  Cuttler,Ira M.,MD
  Elahi,Abdul Wadood,MD
  Frankel,Susan L.,DO
  Ginsberg,Terrie Beth,DO
  Kedziora,Halina M.,MD
  Noll,Donald R.,DO
  Palli,Prameela M.,DO
Gynecology
  Jolitz,Whitney,DO
Hospitalist
  Davis,Bryan F.,DO
  Khan,Imran Ahmad,MD
  Kothari,Sona A.,DO
  Lam,Gloria Fontane,DO
  Vudarla,Neelima,MD
Internal Medicine
  Alemu,Yohannes,DO
  Ali,Fatima,DO
  Bacal,Diana Ioanna,MD
  Bolisetti,Sreedevi,MD
  Chen,Brian Youshane,DO
  Chen,Wei L.,DO
  Cheng,Wunhuey,DO
  Chery,Magdala,DO
  Choe,Jisun Kim,MD
  Chowdhury,Zinnat A.,MD
  Condoluci,Mark,DO
  Conti,Joseph J.,DO
  Di Bruno,Donna,DO
  Dignam,Ritchell Rodriguez,MD
  Dombrowski,Henry Timothy,DO
  Ellern,Michelle Lynn,DO
  Falescky,Allan Jeffrey,MD
  Filer,Joshua Michael,DO
  Friedman,Jeffrey R.,DO
  Goldman,Daniel Marc,MD
  Gordon,Robert,DO
  Gradinger,Lynne S.,MD
  Griesback,Russell,DO
  Haenel,Louis C. III,DO
  Iucci,Gene,DO
  Jawaid,Nosheen,DO
  Kaiser-Smith,Joanne,DO
  Matrale,Michael,DO
  Rachan,Srilatha,MD
  Ranalli,Jeffery A.,DO
  Saccone,Peter Joseph,DO
  Salmonsen,Mary Beth,DO
  Sarwar,Muhammad,MD
  Sciancalepore,Justin,DO
  Selvam,Nirmala,MD
  Warner,Sharon D.,MD
  Watson,Marcia G.,DO
Maternal & Fetal Medicine
  Konchak,Peter Stephen,DO
Neonatal-Perinatal Medicine
  Tinianow,Lloyd N.,MD
Nephrology
  Dave,Chetna A.,MD
Neurology
  Barone,Donald A.,DO
  Serban,Valeria,MD
Orthopedic Surgery
  Cawley,Christina M.,DO
Pediatrics
  Brennan,Laura Kaye,MD
  Cohen,Barbara Elisabeth,MD
  Cohen,Rachel Isabel Silliman,MD
  Coleman,Jane L.,MD
  Finkel,Martin A.,DO
  Higginbotham,Monique Renee,MD
  Kadrmas-Iannuzzi,Tanya Lynn,DO
  Lanese,Stephanie Valentine,MD
  Lecomte,Jennifer Megan,DO
  Lind,Marita Elizabeth,MD
  Melman,Shoshana T.,MD
  Pinto,Jamie M.,MD
  Weiner,Monica B.,MD
Physical Medicine & Rehab
  Bailey,James William,DO
  Douglas,Barbara L.,MD
  Janora,Deanna Marie,MD
Psychiatry
  Aguirre-Masecampo,Alfe G.,MD
  Belinsky,Tatyana,MD
  Forsberg,Martin M.,MD
  Vender,Lydia A.,DO
  White,Christian Paul,MD
Pulmonary Disease
  Giudice,James C.,DO
  Morley,Thomas F.,DO
  Vasoya,Amita P.,DO
Radiology
  Goldstein,David Wayne,DO
  Principato,Robert,DO
Rheumatology
  Adelizzi,Raymond A.,DO
Surgery (General)
  Arnold,Thomas Bradley,DO
  Balsama,Louis H.,DO
  Bruneau,Eve Solange,DO
  Iucci,Lisa Diane,DO
  Rosen,Marc Eliott,DO
Urology
  Panuganti,Sravan,DO
  Syed,Kirin K.,DO
  Thatcher,Jacob Bryce,DO
Strathmere
Psychiatry
  Blackwell,Kathryn V.,MD
Succasunna
Anesthesiology
  Murthy,Sujatha S.,MD
Clinical Genetics
  Vosatka,Robert J.,MD
Dermatology
  Cooper,Lauren M.,MD
Family Medicine
  Siegel,Harvey P.,DO
Gastroenterology
  Madane,Srinivas Janardhan,MD
Internal Medicine
  Mullengada,Krithika,MD
  Rubinetti,Mark J.,MD
Obstetrics & Gynecology
  Ramieri,Joseph,MD
  Sharafi,Khalida,MD
  Shaw,Donia Renee,MD
Ophthalmology
  Gottlieb,Joel M.,MD
  Pinke,Robert S.,MD
Pediatric Cardiology
  Greenhill,Philip A.,MD
Pediatrics
  Heller,Michelle,DO
  Patashny,Karen M.,MD
  Peters,Michael A.,DO
  Strand,Barbara G.,MD
Physical Medicine & Rehab
  Shah,Vipul V.,MD
Psychiatry
  Singh,Pritpaul,MD
Rheumatology
  Giangrasso,Thomas A.,MD
Surgery (General)
  LePera,Michael S.,MD
Urology
  Stone,Chester I.,MD
Summit
Allergy
  Brown,David K.,MD
Anatomic/Clinical Pathology
  Al Dulaimi,Hamsa A.,MD
  Labat,Mona Farah,MD
  Pai,Prabha B.,MD

Physicians by Town and Medical Specialty

Summit (cont)
Anesthesiology
Abrams,Jonathan Todd,MD
Arzola,Nydia,MD
BelCastro,Peter Joseph,MD
Byers,Jason,MD
Calabro,John R.,MD
Chan,Karen Rita Post,MD
Co,Jacqueline Ann B.,MD
DeAngelis,Lawrence J.,MD
Dominik,Jeremy A.,MD
Dowd,Timothy Joseph,MD
Faccone,Jacqueline M.,DO
Farrar,Robert,MD
Fernandez-Piparo,May Anne M.,MD
Fleischman,Keith A.,DO
Greenberg,Carrie Lynn,MD
Hsu,Madeleine F.,MD
Hu,Yuan,MD
Huang,Guojie,MD
Jablons,Mitchell L.,MD
Kagan,Mikhail,MD
Kral,Michael George,MD
Kweon,Chang,MD
Kwon,Yong S.,MD
Lei,Laura M.,MD
McLaughlin,Blaise,MD
Naturman,Roy E.,MD
Pacific,Scott,MD
Paris,Glen Allen,MD
Pierre-Louis,James,MD
Rice,Stuart Nelson,MD
Rosenstein,Megan Ann,MD
Ross,Neil E.,MD
Sant,Manasee Amol,MD
Sarkaria,Janak,MD
Schultz,Gail,MD
Shahane,Manoj Raghunath,MD
Sharma,Akanksha D.,MD
Soni,Monika K.,MD
Surace,Anthony,MD
Thakkar,Shivani,MD
Wang,Wayne,MD
Woo,Daniel Hee-Suk,MD
Yao,Daniel Duan,MD
You,Ruoxu,MD
Zimmermann,Carol E.,MD
Cardiovascular Disease
Iuzzolino,Anthony,MD
Krell,Mark J.,MD
Cardiovascular Surgery
Luka,Norman L.,MD
Child & Adolescent Psychiatry
Canosa,Omar,MD
Hasan,Syeda I.,MD
Mangunay,Nora Ramos,MD
Sehgal,Shaley Prem,MD
Child (Pediatric) Neurology
Bennett,Harvey S.,MD
Colon & Rectal Surgery
Groff,Walter L.,MD
Lorber,Julie A.,MD
Critical Care Medicine
Cerrone,Federico,MD
Donnabella,Vincent,MD
Sussman,Robert,MD
Zimmerman,Mark I.,MD
Dermatology
Hu,Judy Y.,MD
Notari,Teresa V.,MD
Silver,Barry C.,MD
Williams,John Michael,MD
Diagnostic Radiology
Donnelly,Brian,MD
Emergency Medicine
Arora,Tanisha,MD
Bilenker,James D.,MD
Campo,Ruth A.,MD
Gleimer,Evan Michael,DO
Glessner,Robyn,DO
Gudofsky,Gina Lynn,MD
Heller,Diane Beth,MD
Hernandez,Zachary Kris,DO
Lewis,Randall Craig,MD
Macri,Mirtha J.,DO
Mastrokyriakos,Paul,DO
Panchal,Neil,DO
Rathyen,Jill S.,MD
Endocrinology
Chen,James J.,MD
Selinger,Sharon E.,MD

Facial Plastic Surgery
Carniol,Paul J.,MD
Family Med-Geriatric Medicine
Kim,Julia J.,MD
Family Medicine
Butkiewicz,Elise Ann,MD
Davine-Reicher,Joanne Erin,MD
Doubek,Marnie Lynn,MD
Fagan,Elizabeth Owens,MD
Hollander,Steven Barry,MD
Im-Imamura,Lauren H.,DO
Kaye,Susan T.,MD
Lafferty,Kristen,MD
Lukenda,Robert A.,DO
May-Ortiz,Jennifer L.,MD
Miller,Aaron Todd,MD
Podell,Richard N.,MD
Pozner,Samantha Brooke,MD
Pride,Mikel Jadyne,DO
Schram,Amy Elizabeth,DO
Snyder,Hugh David,MD
Tsangalidis,Eirini,MD
Vickery,Donna R.,MD
Washington,Judy C.,MD
Gastroenterology
Habba,Saad F.,MD
Zeldis,Jerome B.,MD
General Practice
Koliopoulos,John S.,DO
Geriatrics
Trivedi,Manoj M.,MD
Hand Surgery
Gardner,James Nicholas,MD
Hematology Oncology
Guerin,Bonni Lee,MD
Morse,Sophie D.,MD
Saksena,Rujuta P.,MD
Hospitalist
Bhatt,Raunaq Dushyantkumar,MD
Malladi,Viswanath,MD
Tadisina,Vani,MD
Infectious Disease
Roland,Robert J.,DO
Insurance Medicine
Tarasenko,Anthony J.,MD
Internal Medicine
Agaronin,Igor F.,MD
Ali,Nadia Yousaf,MD
Alla,Nivedita R.,MD
Belt,Gary Harvey,MD
Brensilver,Jeffrey M.,MD
Cancel,Jaime,MD
Cullen,Kathryn Eva,DO
Daver,Nicole Rohinton,DO
Fessler,Sue Atherton,MD
Gurland,Jake,MD
Huberman,Daniel Tzvi,MD
Ibikunle,Olumuyiwa Adedotun,MD
Jackson,Thomas Edward,MD
Jeffries,Emily L.,MD
Johnson,Christina Nicole,MD
Jordanovski,David,MD
Mendoza,Adiofel Mark F.,MD
Morganstein,Neil,MD
Moriarty,Daniel J.,MD
Patel,Jigar,MD
Purdy,Adam,MD
Rahmani,Masroor,MD
Ryan,Catherine S.,MD
Shanahan-Prendergast,Kelsey,MD
Suarez,Lisbet D.,MD
Subramanian,Gomathy,MD
Toffey,Lisa H.,MD
Vyas,Nishant,MD
Wu,Elain,DO
Maternal & Fetal Medicine
Benito,Carlos W.,MD
Frisoli,Gaetano,MD
Medical Oncology
Jaeckle,Kurt Alfred,MD
Lowenthal,Dennis A.,MD
Nephrology
Kabaria,Sunit P.,MD
Neurological Surgery
Hodosh,Richard M.,MD
Neurology
Alexianu,Maria E.,MD
Craciun,Liviu Ciprian,MD
Halperin,John Jacob,MD
Metrus,Nicholas Robert,MD
Politsky,Jeffrey Mark,MD

Pollock,Jeffrey C.,MD
Rabin,Marcie W.,MD
Stoller,Seth Ryan,MD
Tarulli,Andrew William,MD
Vigman,Melvin P.,MD
Neuropathology
Bouffard,John Paul,MD
Nuclear Medicine
Borkar,Sunita A.,MD
Obstetrics & Gynecology
Alam,Abu S.,MD
Franceschini,Chloe Nicole,MD
Hoffman,Russell R.,MD
Khoudary,Maryann Lisa,MD
Lashley,Susan Leonora,MD
Netta,Denise Ann,MD
Oyelese,Kolawole Olayinka,MD
Rondon,Kaylah Christine,MD
Russo-Stieglitz,Karen E.,MD
Oncological Surgery
Sacco,Margaret Mary,MD
Ophthalmology
Boozan,John M.,MD
Campeas,David,MD
Hoffman,David Sandor,MD
Orthopedic Surgery
DeLuca,Francis N.,MD
Fischer,Stuart J.,MD
Lin,Sheldon S.,MD
Sarokhan,Alan J.,MD
Other Specialty
Nuzzo,Roy Michael,MD
Otolaryngology
Carniol,Eric T.,MD
Pain Medicine
Pappagallo,Marco,MD
Pathology
Levin,Miles B.,MD
Pediatric Anesthesia
George,Tony,MD
Pediatric Cardiology
Leichter,Donald A.,MD
Pediatric Endocrinology
Huang,Eric A.,MD
Pediatric Gastroenterology
Chitkara,Denesh Kumar,MD
Rosh,Joel R.,MD
Tyshkov,Michael,MD
Pediatric Hematology Oncology
Gregory,John Joseph Jr.,MD
Miller,Michelle K.,MD
Pediatric Orthopedics
Altongy,Joseph F.,MD
Pediatric Surgery
Bergman,Kerry S.,MD
Jacir,Nabil N.,MD
Pediatric Urology
Murphy,Kathleen A.,MD
Pediatrics
Cerdena,Maria Corazon,MD
Cessario,Alison G.,MD
Feldman,Tamara Lee,MD
Kairam,Hemant,MD
Lucciola,Marion,MD
Manocchio,Teresa,DO
Nwaobasi,Eberechi Ihuoma,MD
Polisin,Michael J.,MD
Reichard,Kathleen G.,DO
Rosenthal,Lauren Beth,MD
Vigorita,John F.,MD
Wilmot,Peter Clifford,DO
Physical Medicine & Rehab
Epperlein,Jennifer I.,DO
Garrett,Rebecca Ann,MD
Plastic Surgery
Daniels,David Daizadeh,MD
Hall,Stephen C.,MD
Shafaie,Farrokh,MD
Psychiatry
Alam,Rozana R.,MD
Behar,Lonny J.,MD
Bolo,Peter M.,MD
Budoff,Steven R.,DO
Ciolino,Charles P.,MD
Clark,Peter Joseph,DO
Dealwis,Jayakanthi,MD
Forman-Chou,Alexandra C.,MD
Frey,Patricia E.,DO
Gray,Sonja B.,MD
Greenberg,Rosalie,MD

Hopkins,Rebecca Jane,MD
Jones,Jane W.,MD
Kaplan-Sagal,Lauren Ellen,MD
Keyser,Joseph W.,MD
Malhotra,Mahamaya,MD
Malhotra,Rahul,MD
Reiter,Stewart Roy,MD
Shah,Talaxi D.,MD
Sofair,Jane Brown,MD
Sosnow,Meg W.,MD
Tahil,Fatimah Ann,MD
Villafranca,Manuel V.,MD
Zimmerman,Aphrodite Marta,MD
Psych&Neurology-Addiction Med
Belz,Marek,MD
Pulmonary Disease
Kotecha,Nisha Suresh,MD
Nahmias,Jeffrey S.,MD
Radiation Oncology
Emmolo,Joana S.,MD
Knee,Robert,MD
Schwartz,Louis E.,MD
Radiology
Werring,John Andrew,MD
Rheumatology
Greenberg,Jeffrey David,MD
Kramer,Neil,MD
Patel,Sheetal V.,MD
Rosenstein,Elliot D.,MD
Setty,Arathi Radhakrishna,MD
Spinal Surgery
Hullinger,Heidi,MD
Surgery (General)
Di Gioia,Julia Marie,MD
Lazar,Eric L.,MD
Robinson,Andrew Tyler,MD
Starker,Paul M.,MD
Yang,Rebecca Chaohua,MD
Surgical Critical Care
Mandel,Marc S.,MD
Rhodes,Stancie Christina,MD
Urology
Gianis,John Thomas Jr.,MD
Gianis,Thomas J.,MD
Seidman,Barry R.,MD
Vascular & Intrvntnal Radiology
Bhatti,Waseem Alam,MD
Vascular Neurology
Hanna,John M.,MD

Surf City
Anesthesiology
Tumillo,John G. Jr.,MD

Sussex
Anesthesiology
Shah,Prafulla R.,MD
Shah,Rameshchan H.,MD
Emergency Medicine
Koutcher,Gary Lewis,MD
Gastroenterology
Beckman,Harvey S.,MD
Infectious Disease
Yasin,Sami F.,MD
Internal Medicine
Fisher,John F.,MD

Swedesboro
Emergency Medicine
Heresniak,Victor A.,DO
Family Medicine
Dalsey,Michael E.,DO
Seretis,George J.,DO
Tsigonis,Natalie,DO
Internal Medicine
Abel Boenerjous,Rebakah S.,MD
Bennett,William Roderic,DO
Neurology
Lotkowski,Susan D.,DO
Otolaryngology
Clairvil,Jessie,DO

Teaneck
Addiction Psychiatry
Berman,Jeffrey A.,MD
Adolescent Medicine
Vece,Lorrie J.,MD
Adult Psychiatry
Zerykier,Gisela B.,MD
Anatomic/Clinical Pathology
Babury,Rahima A.,MD
Fish,Heidi,MD
Olsen,Drew Albert,MD
Schainker,Bruce Allan,MD

Anesthesiology
Benson, Peter Kurt, MD
Carni, Abbe J., MD
Chaubey, Rakesh Kumar, MD
D'Souza, Michael Gerard, MD
Ephrat, Roni, MD
Florence, Isaiah Meyer, MD
Fradlis, Alina, MD
Franzl, Wojciech, MD
Gross, Robert M., MD
Gupta, Vijay, MD
Gwertzman, Alan R., MD
Klein, Patti S., MD
Koniuta, Robert L., MD
Koshibe, Gen, MD
Martin, Brian McKinley, MD
Nahmias, Neil Jeffrey, DO
Novak, Steven Michael, MD
Parmar, Virendra Pratapsingh, MD
Ryu, David Jinsoo, DO
Sheikh, Usman, MD
Singer, Judith C. J., MD
Sklar, Jeffrey, MD
Syed, Faraz A., DO
Thornhill, Marsha Lynne, MD
Trivedi, Avani P., DO
Vittal, Melba G., MD
Worth, Robert Harry, MD

Anesthesiology: Critical Care
Kaufman, Margit I., MD

Cardiovascular Disease
Angeli, Stephen J., MD
Desai, Shalin P., MD
Eichman, Gerard T., MD
Issa, Ebrahim S., MD
Sagar, Yogesh, MD
Syed, Tariqshah Muhammad, MD
Vandyck-Acquah, Marian M., MD
Welish, Steven Jay, MD
Wild, David Marc, MD

Colon & Rectal Surgery
Mansouri, Farshad, MD

Cosmetic Surgery
Sterman, Harris Robert, MD

Dermatology
Ragi, Gangaram, MD

Diagnostic Radiology
Berman, Howard L., MD
Brunetti, Jacqueline Carol, MD
Cao, Huyen Van, MD
Felman, Rina Lita, MD
Greenstein, Elizabeth Louise, MD
Herman, Kevin, MD
Horn, Eva M., MD
Kirzner, Howard L., MD
Lerer, Daniel Brian, MD
Morgan, John, MD
Park, James Joongchul, MD
Patel, Amish, MD
Rundback, John Hugh, MD
Siegel, Stacey, MD

Emergency Medicine
Marcilla, Oscar A., MD
Miglietta, Mario Adrian, DO
Miller, Alan S., MD
Schwab, Richard M., MD
Silverman, Brian S., DO
Tartacoff, Randy S., MD
Weinberg, Kenneth R., MD

Endocrinology
Eckman, Ari S., MD
Wiesen, Mark, MD

Family Medicine
Berberian, Robert A., MD
Boja, Conrado A. III, MD
Boja, Michael Conrad, DO
George, Preethi Sara, MD
Hersh, Craig M., MD
Jones, Rhys E., MD
Kronish, Anne L., MD
McNeill-Augustine, Roberta N., MD
Perry, Russell J., MD
Pottick-Schwartz, Eliane A., MD
Prajapati, Binita Prashant, DO

Gastroenterology
Micale, Philip Louis, MD
Palance, Adam L., MD
Paltrowitz, Irving M., MD
Rigoglioso, Vincent, MD
Schmidt, Michael H., MD

Geriatrics
Adler, Joel S., MD
Katz, Terri F., MD
Meyerowitz, Jay S., MD

Gynecological Oncology
Lewin, Sharyn Nan, MD
Schiavone-Forlenza, Maria, MD
Sommers, Gara M., MD

Hand Surgery
Galitzin, Joseph C., MD

Hematology
Tsai, Philip Henry, MD

Hematology Oncology
Condemi, Giuseppe, MD

Hospitalist
Akhtar, Ruhi, MD

Hypertension
Salazer, Thomas L., MD

Infectious Disease
Birch, Thomas M., MD
De La Rosa, Benjamin Danny, MD
Kalishman, Raffaella Linda, MD

Internal Medicine
Adler, Zachary G., MD
Aristy, Sary Mariell, MD
Aronoff, Benjamin W., MD
Balmir, Sacha, DO
Berdy, Jack M., MD
Blanch, Tanya Malka, MD
Cardona, Shirley J., DO
Chan, Kim K., MD
Cole, Randolph Paul, MD
Coppola, Peter W., MD
Denker, Michael, MD
Desai, Amita Jayantilal, MD
Diamond, Elan Shlomo, MD
Elfayoumi, Islam Moustafa, MD
Ferrer, Waldo L., MD
Fratello, Joseph J., MD
Friedlander, Joseph Raymond, MD
Gonter, Neil Jeffrey, MD
Gumaste, Sandhya V., MD
Gupta, Vipan Kumar, MD
Harris, Robert M., MD
Horwitz, Morris, MD
Kasaryan, Hrach Ike, DO
Khadka Kunwar, Erina, MD
Kimel, Alexandru F., MD
Largoza, Rosendito S., MD
Lavotshkin, Anna Janna, MD
Lee, Karen Chang, MD
Levin, David N., MD
Marcus, Ralph E., MD
Marshall, Lewis West Jr., MD
Modesto, Rosanna A., MD
Park, Sarah, DO
Pieczara, Beata Katarzyna, MD
Rigoglioso, Camille M., MD
Rigolosi, Robert S., MD
Rivera, Yadyra, MD
Rizzo, Joseph Alfonso, MD
Roitman, Alla, DO
Rosen, Amy T., MD
Sachar, Inderpreet, MD
Salizzoni, Jeffrey L., MD
Schuster, Joseph C., MD
Shaker, Elhamy I., MD
Sheth, Naitik D., MD
Singer, Roberto, MD
Umer, Muhammad S., MD
Villongco, Raymond Manzano, MD
Waseem, Sarwat, MD
Znamensky, Addi, MD

Interventional Cardiology
Zolty, Ronald, MD

Mammography
Gross, Joshua David, MD

Nephrology
Ahmed, Subhan, MD
Coleman, Clenton Louis, MD
Gussak, Hiie M., MD

Neurological Radiology
Melisaratos, Darius Paris, MD

Neurology
Blitz-Shabbir, Karen M., DO
Duncan, David Brian, MD
Kailas, Michael G., MD
Picone, Maryann, MD

Nuclear Medicine
Sireci, Steven N. Jr., MD

Obstetrics & Gynecology
Borden, Victor, MD
Brana-Leon, Hazel A., MD
Caruana, Lucia P., MD
Fernandez, Jacinto J., MD
Frattarola, John D., MD
Huggins, Iris A., MD
Leibman, Michael Roy, MD
Nunez, David A., MD
Shah, Payal A., MD

Ophthalmology
Angioletti, Louis V. Jr., MD
Bergen, Robert L., MD
Brown, Andrew Carson, MD
Brown, Christopher David, MD
Brown, Robert Henry, MD
Brown, Robert Stephen, MD
Feiner, Leonard, MD
Glassman, Ronald M., MD
Gordon, Leslie Ellen, MD
Hahn, Paul, MD
Hersh, Peter S., MD
Higgins, Patrick M., MD
Klein, Richard M., MD
Slamovits, Thomas L., MD
Weinberg, Martin R., MD

Oral & Maxillofacial Surgery
Schulhof, Zev, MD

Orthopedic Surgery
Bauer, Brian J., MD
Carrer, Alexandra, MD
Hale, James Joseph, MD
Katona, John J., MD
Kwak, Steve K., MD
Patel, Deepan N., MD
Pfisterer, Dennis James, DO
Pfisterer, Dennis I., MD
Quartararo, Louis Gaspar, MD
Steuer, Jeffrey K., MD

Otolaryngology
Davis, Orrin, MD

Pediatric Emergency Medicine
Love, Margaret M., MD

Pediatric Endocrinology
Novogroder, Michael, MD

Pediatric Gastroenterology
Barth, Jay Allan, MD

Pediatric Urology
Hensle, Terry W., MD
Tennenbaum, Steven Y., MD

Pediatrics
Becker, Steven Eric, MD
Chelliah, Padmini, MD
Eagle, Steven B., MD
Epstein, Nina, MD
Fisher, Howard J., MD
Greenfield, Efrem L., MD
Horwitz, Steven Mankowitz, MD
Kambolis, Joanne Peter, MD
Kanarek, Ninette Marciano, MD
Kanter, Alan I., MD
Kolsky, Neil H., MD
Murray, Norma J., MD
Pieczuro, Barbara Katarzyna, MD
Planer, Dorienne Sasto, MD
Schewitz, Gail, MD
Schuss, Steven A., MD
Shenoi, Shanthi Ramesh, MD
Suldan, Dora I., MD
Zajkowski, Edward Joseph, MD
Zimmerman, Deena R., MD

Physical Medicine & Rehab
Abrar, Dimir, MD
Brisman, Daniel Aaron, MD
Dorri, Mohammad Hossein, MD
Koduri, Hemanth Kumar, MD
Petrucelli, Janet L., MD
Pfisterer, Christine, DO
Shahid, Nasar Mahmood, MD

Plastic Surgery
Conn, Michael J., MD

Psychiatry
Archila, Arturo Plinio, MD
Cho, Seokkoon, MD
Farkas, Edward L., MD
Hain, Joshua Meir, MD
Jacobowitz, Esther, MD
Raby, Wilfrid Noel, MD
Rosenbaum, Paul, MD
Wagle, Sharad D., MD
Zenn, Juliane Janis, MD

Radiation Oncology
Rosenbluth, Benjamin Dov, MD
Vialotti, Charles P. Jr., MD

Rheumatology
Miceli, James Gerard, MD
Silverberg, Miriam Shayna, MD

Surgery (General)
Brinkmann, Erika M., MD
Christoudias, George C., MD
Fredericks, Duane A., MD
Kwon, Sung, MD
Mendoza, Lynette Maria, DO
Radvinsky, David, MD
Shaffer, Liba C., MD
Zairis, Ignatios S., MD

Urology
Parra, Raul O., MD
Scheuch, John R., MD

Vascular & Intrvntnal Radiology
Gallo, Vincent, MD

Tenafly
Child & Adolescent Psychiatry
Geelan, Caroline C., DO
Schreiber, Thomas J., MD

Dermatology
Laureano, Ana Cristina, MD
Scherl, Sharon, MD

Diagnostic Radiology
Sadler, Michael Alan, MD

Emergency Medicine
Lee, Sang Hyun, MD

Family Medicine
Gambhir, Priyanka, MD

Gastroenterology
Klein, Walter A., MD

Geriatric Psychiatry
Friedman, Jay Lawrence, MD

Internal Medicine
Barger Amsalem, Hamutal, MD
Kim, Hong Suk, MD
Lan, Andrew Ente, MD
Mooney, Caroline Mary E., MD

Obstetrics & Gynecology
Broizman, David T., MD
Kithinji, Kagendo M., MD
Knause, Rita Vinod, MD
Lieblich, Richard M., MD
Luke, Brian T., MD
Navot, Daniel, MD
Rivera-Segarra, Stephanie D., MD
Shukla, Mrudula S., MD

Ophthalmology
Stabile, John R., MD

Orthopedic Surgery
Mardam-Bey, Tarek H., MD

Pediatrics
Anderson, Daniel Parker, MD
Asnes, Russell S., MD
Bacha, David M., DO
Burtman, Elizabeth, MD
Elkin, Avigayil H., MD
Jawetz, Sheryl Andrea, MD
Menasha, Joshua Daniel, MD
Michael, Lisa Golomb, MD
Schaumberger, David Andrew, MD
Smith, Michael Adam, MD
Starer, Yvette R., MD
Sugarman, Lynn B., MD
Weissman, Evan Laird, DO
Wisotsky, David H., MD

Physical Medicine & Rehab
Lee, Anna D., MD

Plastic Surgery
Garbaccio, Charles G., MD

Psychiatry
Amiel, Elizabeth A., MD
Gross, Carey E., MD
Knafel, Natalya, MD

Surgery (General)
Varma, Shubha, MD

Tennent
Physical Medicine & Rehab
Duck, Evander Jr., MD

Teterboro
Anatomic Pathology
Gerber, Marina, MD
Kennedy, Harvey Ronald, MD
Pang, Xinzhu, MD

Physicians by Town and Medical Specialty

Teterboro (cont)
Anatomic/Clinical Pathology
Alt, Elaine R., MD
Ayer, Uma, MD
Bayard-McNeeley, Marise, MD
Eftychiadis, Angela S., MD
Gallo, Leza N., MD
Iskaros, Basem F., MD
Kaufman, Harvey Willard, MD
Limaye, Anjali P., MD
Liu-Jarin, Xiaolin, MD
Luff, Ronald David, MD
Mahmood, Afsar, MD
Malhotra, Chanchal Anand, MD
Niu, Weiwei, MD
Tamas, Ecaterina F., MD
Tarr, William Ellsworth Jr., MD
Tsao, Lawrence, MD
Vinod, Sheela U., MD
Yohannan, Wendy S., MD
Zhang, Yiqiu, MD
Dermatopathology
Gill, Melissa, MD
Hematology
Mehta, Kumudini U., MD
Pathology
Cardillo, Marina, MD
Kanuga, Dharmishtha Jayesh, MD
Untawale, Vasundhara G., MD

Thorofare
Internal Medicine
Ahmed, Asma Talukder, DO
Camacho, Jose A., MD
Desai, Anjali Ashok, MD
Laskin, David A., MD
Penberthy, Katherine Ann, MD
Physical Medicine & Rehab
Moreno, Susan I., MD

Tinton Falls
Allergy
Picone, Frank J., MD
Anesthesiology
Pourmasiha, Niloufar, DO
Breast Surgery
Camal, Debra E., MD
Cardiovascular Disease
Belluscio, Roland L., MD
Drout, David I., MD
O'Keefe, Arthur A. Jr., MD
Vlahos, Aristotelis E., MD
Zukoff, David S., MD
Dermatology
Gorin, Risa Jill, DO
Kolansky, Glenn, MD
Kruse, Christopher Bryant, MD
Terushkin, Vitaly, MD
Diagnostic Radiology
Brand-Abend, Lori M., MD
Emergency Medicine
Calabro, Joseph John, DO
Merlin, Mark A., DO
Schaible, Derek D., MD
Sharma, Niti, DO
Simon, Purabi Mehta, DO
Sorkin, Greg Charles, DO
Endocrinology
Enriquez, Santiago Jr., MD
Ravichandran, Shoba, MD
Family Medicine
Calise, Arthur G., DO
Chen, Roger L., MD
Edokwe, Obunike O.J., MD
Marquette, Paul Arthur, MD
Rosen, Neil L., DO
Yellayi, Priya A., MD
Gastroenterology
Grabowy, Thaddeus John, MD
Geriatric Psychiatry
Soto Moise, Olga Bienvenida, MD
Hand Surgery
Johnson, Christopher D., MD
Hospitalist
Li, Wei, MD
Internal Medicine
Boak, Joseph G. Jr., MD
Boesler, Iza Marzanna, MD
Boulghassoul-Pietrzykows, N., MD
Carracino, Robert L., MD
Cefalu, Dimitri A., MD
Dougherty, Renee Maria, DO

Felipe, Ronald Anthony, MD
Gardilla, Kalyani Ila, MD
Gold, Jessica Frances, DO
Gottfried, Michael S., MD
Habib, Misha, MD
Jurewicz, Stephen S., MD
Manganaro, David Thomas, MD
Nwankwo, Gloria Obiageli, DO
Polvino, William James, MD
Rao, Asha Vijendran, MD
Rizwan, Mohammad, MD
Rosier, Eric, MD
Vladu, Ana Daniela, MD
Zimmerman, Lisa M., MD
Neonatal-Perinatal Medicine
Fort, Prem, MD
Neurology
Pertchik, Alan F., MD
Obstetrics & Gynecology
Collado, Marilyn Loh, MD
Jacoby, Dana B., MD
Minaya, Evelyn, MD
Orthopedic Surgery
Chalnick, David Lee, MD
Cohen, Jason D., MD
Foos, Gregg Robert, MD
Gentile, David R., MD
Gesell, Mark William, MD
Glastein, Cary D., MD
Grossman, Robert B., MD
Markbreiter, Lance A., MD
Rizzo, Charles C., MD
Torpey, Brian M., MD
Otolaryngology
Roffman, Jeffrey D., MD
Pediatrics
Condiotte, Shaw Brandon, MD
Cotenoff, Melanie L., MD
Dawis, Maria Agnes Chaluangco, MD
Hugh-Goffe, Judith Colleen, MD
Iglesias, Hector R., MD
Miller, Steven E., DO
Morgan, Robert L., MD
Perril, Rebecca A., DO
Pulcini, Ashley Elizabeth, DO
Salvador-Goon, Brenda Mae, MD
Wood, Jessica R., DO
Physical Medicine & Rehab
Baerga, Edgardo, MD
Cooperman, Todd J., MD
Miller, Jessica Schutzbank, MD
Rathi, Sandeep, MD
Rozman, Anatoly, MD
Woska, Scott Corey, MD
Psychiatry
Parks, Shannon N., DO
Rheumatology
Wasser, Kenneth B., MD
Sports Medicine
Bade, Harry III, MD
Surgery (General)
Chagares, Stephen Arthur, MD
Dupree, David Joseph, MD
Odujebe, Henry A., MD
Woodriffe, Philipa G., MD

Titusville
Internal Medicine
Freedman, Amy L., MD
Jokubaitis, Leonard Anthony, MD
List, James Frank, MD
Pediatrics
Starr, Harriette L., MD

Toms River
Allergy
Mendoza, Narciso D., MD
Rabinowitz, Robert P., DO
Anatomic/Clinical Pathology
Ibrahim, Ghassan Jerjous, MD
Lapis, Peter, MD
Romberger, Charles Frank, MD
Anesthesiology
Cha, Hak J., MD
D'Angelo, Stephen Thomas, DO
De Sio, John Michael, MD
Farkas, Klara, MD
Gershteyn, Eduard, MD
Jadav, Jitendra K., MD
Krishtul, Eduard, MD
Lin, Renny L., MD
Loftus, James B., MD
Mako, Robert M., DO

Manganelli, Douglas M., MD
Mara, Frank J., MD
Park, Dong C., MD
Park, Yung I., MD
Quiambao, Dante B., MD
Tank, Hasmukh C., MD
Anesthesiology: Pain Medicine
Coccaro, John A., MD
Cardiovascular Disease
Alturk, Najib M., MD
Bacani, Victor O., MD
Bageac, Michael, MD
Calderon, Dawn Michelle, DO
Chang, Richard Youngjae, DO
Clancy, Kevin F., MD
Cornell, Russell John, MD
DiPisa, Leonard R., MD
Douedi, Hani R., MD
Guarino, Joseph J. Jr., MD
Gupta, Anil Kumar, MD
Jacobs, Glenn Paul, MD
Jain, Samir S., MD
Karatepe, Murat, MD
Merlino, John Anthony III, DO
Mohandas, Bhavna, MD
Pasquariello, James L., MD
Rana, Yebarna S., MD
Roggemann, Dennis J., MD
Sobti, Sanjiv, MD
Stone, Jay H., MD
Tenner, Bruce S., DO
Tsang, Kock-Yen, MD
Child & Adolescent Psychiatry
Ballesteros, Alberto F., MD
Pitera, Matthew J., MD
Senese, Karen, MD
Clinical Neurophysiology
Deliwala, Tejas Pramodrai, MD
Cornea/External Disease
Athwal, Harjit S., MD
Critical Care Medicine
Eisen, Deborah Ida, MD
Tomasuolo, Vincent A., MD
Dermatology
Dixon, Melissa Kaye, MD
Kuflik, Avery S., MD
Kuflik, Emanuel G., MD
LaForgia, Sal T., MD
Ma, Manhong, MD
Rosen, Robert M., DO
Trivedi, Prabhas Arunbhai, MD
Diagnostic Radiology
Atallah, Judy, DO
Batchu, Bharathi, MD
Boxer, Douglas C., MD
Chen, Timothy, MD
Chinta, Bharath Kumar, MD
D'Angelo, Michael Wayne, MD
Daniels, Alicia L., MD
Desai, Akhilesh S., MD
Florio, Francesco, DO
Golsaz, Cyrus Michael, MD
Haim, Alain, MD
Kravets, Felix G., MD
Lee, Brian H., MD
Marinas, Virgilio R., MD
Martin, Steven W., MD
Shahab, Farhang, MD
Shieh, Paul Y., MD
Triolo, Joseph, MD
Willis, Kevin, MD
Yu, Thomas C., MD
Emergency Medicine
Bernard, John Marley, MD
Chiccone, Martha G., MD
Crisanti, John Jr., MD
DesRochers, Laurence R., MD
Eng, Tiffany, MD
Fowlie, Thomas Jr., MD
Giles, Thomas William, DO
Janes, Susan F., DO
Levine, Marc M., MD
Madonick, Harvey Lloyd, MD
Meredith, Jacob M., MD
Pepe, Salvatore IV, DO
Ravindran, Wijeyadevendram, MD
Reznikov, Boris, MD
Russell, Warren King, MD
Singh, Chetna, MD
Varma, Medavaram Vikram, MD
Wrigley, Steven N., MD

Endocrinology
Birnbaum, Joseph G., MD
Cruz, Francisco P., MD
Kleinman, David S., MD
Krishnan, Lalitha G., MD
Ortiz, Oscar T., MD
Villanueva, Ronald Banaag, MD
Family Medicine
Asghar, Fatima, MD
DiPaolo, Ann, DO
Fiore, Edward D., MD
Giardina, Jennifer, DO
Liu, Connie Xia, MD
Lozowski, Thomas E., DO
Ludwig-Cilento, Mary Beth, DO
Neumann, Lisa Petriccione, DO
Ongsiako, Allen R., DO
Pappas, Elena Catherine, DO
Rudd, Rebecca A., MD
Shah, Dhanvanti B., MD
Shah, Sweta, MD
Simone, Philip M., MD
Triolo, Paul, MD
Wayman, Bernard R. III, MD
Gastroenterology
Bigornia, Edgar G., MD
Cohen, Allan, MD
Cohen, Scott, DO
Collier, Jill A., MD
Cryan, Jeffrey M., MD
De Martino, Paul John, MD
Eschinger, Eric Jon, MD
Lokchander, Rangaswamy S., MD
Patel, Kavan Girishbhai, MD
Raso, Carl L., MD
Shah, Kamlesh Manher, MD
Shakov, Rada, MD
Suatengco, Jose Ramon, MD
Tamimi, Omar A., MD
General Practice
DiChiara, Frank P., DO
Kanthan, Sudha, MD
Mendoza, Concepcion B., MD
Mitchell, David S., DO
Geriatric Psychiatry
Patel, Ashok Kantilal, MD
Tandon, Pooja, MD
Yosry, Mohamed Hussein, MD
Geriatrics
Sharma, Sanjiv Kumar, MD
Sundheim, John M., MD
Hand Surgery
Rosen, Michael David, MD
Semet, Elliot C., MD
Hematology
Al Kana, Randah, MD
Shah, Chirag M., MD
Hematology Oncology
Kavuru, Sudha, MD
Homeopathy
Zaki, Merajuddin, MD
Infectious Disease
Guerrero, Isabel C., MD
Internal Medicine
Abraham, Thanaa Nelly K., MD
Adelizzi, Angela M., DO
Alberto, Priscilla Magsalin, MD
Alberto, Renato D., MD
Anama, Luzminda M., MD
Ayad, Lydia, MD
Babiak, Eugenia T., MD
Brodkey, Morris I., MD
Bugay, Victor Valdes, MD
Camiscoli, Deborah J., MD
Cauvin, Leslie R., DO
Chung, Margaret U., MD
Crawford, Steven G., MD
Cuozzo, Gregory Joseph, MD
Decorso, Joseph A., MD
Desai, Dilip Navnitlal, MD
Dhar, Rajat K., MD
DiLorenzo, William Richard, DO
Elsamman, Wael A., MD
Ende, Mark, MD
Espineli, Dino O., MD
Espineli, Rosalinda O., MD
Forrester, Catherine A., MD
Gabriel, Timothy Cayco, MD
Ghetiya, Vinodrai V., MD
Gigliuto, Christine M., MD
Glazier, Kenneth David, MD

Goldberg,Irwin L.,DO
Gonzalez,Felicia Ellen,DO
Grossman,David R.,MD
Guarino,Ralph V.,MD
Gupta,Suraj P.,MD
Haque,Salma,MD
Hormilla,Amador N.,MD
Igbanugo,Anselm,MD
Jayanathan,Chelvakumaran R.,MD
Jimenez,Martin Zaratan,MD
Klebacher,Ronald John,DO
Kong,Henry Woongjae,MD
Krishna,Sunanda,MD
Lin,Ing-Long,MD
Lin,Shirley H.,MD
Mandal,Aparna,MD
Manzullo,Gregory P.,MD
Mathew,Tittymol,MD
Mathur,Anjana,MD
Matteace,Frank P.,MD
Mayrowetz,Burton,MD
Mehta,Nikunj P.,MD
Meily,Antonio F. Jr.,MD
Meli,Gregory M.,MD
Mirchandani,Jai,MD
Mitra,Tithi,MD
Monta,Arturo D.,MD
Nagaria,Neil C.,MD
Nayak,Yeshavanth P.,MD
Nelson,Andrew L.,MD
O'Brien,Thomas K.,MD
Ortiz,Olivia Tanyag,MD
Parikh,Vipul K.,MD
Patel,Nikunjkumar,MD
Patel,Palakkumar Kantilal,MD
Patil,Sandhya R.,MD
Pawa,Sakshi,MD
Ponnambalam,Ajit P.,MD
Ponnambalam,Anil R.,MD
Reda,Frank,MD
Roper,Ashley Annette,MD
Rowland,Sean C.,MD
Sabio,Ivan Alberto,MD
Saini,Manish Satyaprakash,MD
Sancheti,Vinod T.,MD
Santangelo,Donato III,MD
Scott,Robert D.,MD
Sersanti,John Paul,MD
Shah,Dhiren A.,MD
Sharma,Anil Kumar,MD
Sikand,Vinay,MD
Simon,Robert T.,MD
Sinha,Prabhat Kumar,MD
Sobti,Rimmi,MD
Spedick,Michael J.,MD
Strazzella,William D.,DO
Tacopina,Teresa Anne,MD
Taguba Madrid,Leslie C.,MD
Takla,Sarwat S.,MD
Van Wyck,William Louis,MD
Wang,Jean C.,MD
Yu,Henry K.,MD
Interventional Cardiology
Gupta,Rakesh Vardhan,MD
Iyanoye,Adeyemi,MD
Patel,Parag Vishnu,MD
Maternal & Fetal Medicine
Fernandez,Carlos O.,MD
Neonatal-Perinatal Medicine
Sannoh,Sulaiman,MD
Nephrology
Anantharaman,Priya,MD
Arnold,Robert B.,MD
Palecki,Winicjusz,MD
Neurological Radiology
Finkel,Arkady,MD
Neurological Surgery
Hartwell,Richard Conrad,MD
Moyle,Henry,MD
Sarris,John,MD
Neurology
Amin,Darshana Patel,DO
DiPaola,Rocco J.,MD
Ferencz,Gerald J.,MD
Monastersky,Bruce Ted,MD
Schenker,Samuel D.,MD
Whiteman,Martin,DO
Wilson,Sylvia V.,MD
Zimmerman,Barry L.,DO
Nuclear Medicine
Gajarawala,Jatin M.,MD

Obstetrics & Gynecology
Argeros,Olga,MD
Azu,Wilhelmina Dedo,DO
Bonvicino,Marie Louise,MD
Furman,Lesley P.,MD
Harrell,Russell L.,MD
Jackman,Earl Francis,DO
Jones,Angela Renee,MD
Kelly,Robert B.,DO
King,Andrew P.,MD
Lopez,Gerardo J.,MD
Maxwell,Aliona,MD
Morgan,Steven A.,MD
Neal,Ronald R.,MD
O'Donnell,Robert H.,DO
Passarella,Susan Katherine,DO
Payumo,Paulita C.,MD
Pesso,Robert S.,MD
Shankar,Kala,MD
Sutherland,John R.,MD
Valthaty,Rebekah,MD
Ophthalmology
Almallah,Omar F.,MD
Alterman,Michael Adam,DO
Angioletti,Louis Scott,MD
Athwal,Barinder S.,MD
Athwal,Lisa M.,MD
Birdi,Anil,MD
Feiner,Laurel A.,MD
Gloth,Jonathan Michael,MD
Hajee,Mohammedyusuf E.,MD
Heimmel,Mark Robert,MD
Lakhani,Vipul K.,MD
Lautenberg,Mitchel Alan,MD
Pan,Jane Chi-Chun,MD
Pidduck,Thomas Charles,MD
Robinson,Neil H.,MD
Schnitzer,Robert E.,MD
Schoenfeld,Allan H.,MD
Trastman-Caruso,Elyse Randi,MD
Wnorowski,Brian R.,MD
Orthopedic Surgery
Borgatti,Richard J.,MD
Closkey,Robert F.,MD
Dhawlikar,Sripad H.,MD
Dickerson,David B.,MD
Fox,Daniel E.,MD
Gabisan,Glenn Gacula,MD
Kasper,Mark T.,MD
Kubeck,Justin P.,MD
Larsen,Erik Scott,DO
Palmieri,Alfred E.,MD
Passariello,Christopher,MD
Petrillo,John A.,MD
Sacks,Richard,MD
Saleh,Jason Reed,MD
Tauro,Joseph C.,MD
Orthopedic-Hand Surgery
Pensak,Michael J.,MD
Otolaryngology
Chaker,Antoine C.,MD
Foster,Wayne Paul,MD
Gillespie,Christine,MD
Kupferberg,Stephen Benjamin,MD
Peters,Bruce W.,DO
Stella,Nunzio R.,MD
Pain Medicine
Holtzberg,Nathan,MD
Yu,Yin Tat,MD
Pathology
Hafiz,Mohammad A.,MD
Maghari,Amin,MD
Mahapatro,Ramesh C.,MD
Pham,Bich N.,MD
Simon,Paul J.,DO
Tao,Jimmy Ziming,MD
Pediatric Pulmonology
Laraya-Cuasay,Lourdes R.,MD
Pediatrics
Alturk,Souhir,MD
Braverman,Isaac L.,MD
Deacon,Nancy S.,MD
Dever,Matthew Patrick,MD
Fiore,Elizabeth Jill,DO
Geneslaw,Charles H.,MD
Goldstein,Richard M.,MD
Golub,Michael L.,MD
Haimowitz,Ira L.,DO
Hamza,Hisham M.,MD
Intili,John J.,MD
Janvier,Yvette Marie,MD

Karroum,Kamil Hanna,MD
Lamzay,Xenia G.,MD
Masia,Alan,MD
Miskin,Chandrabhaga P.,MD
Morano,Amy Beth,MD
Nag,Debashis,MD
Patestos,Chris Anastasios,MD
Pathak,Vineeta Jha,MD
Qazi,Rumana Yousef,MD
Remorca,Carolina U.,MD
Rugino,Thomas A.,MD
Schlachter,Steven A.,MD
Shanik,Robert A.,MD
Sia,Dominic Chionglo,MD
Sia,Valerie May Gumban,MD
Somasundaram,Manamadurai R.,MD
Tan,Mary Catherine D.,MD
Ulep,Shirley Dollaga,MD
PhysMed&Rehab-Hospice Palltve
Mahajan,Rohini,MD
Physical Medicine & Rehab
Adusumilli,Padmashree S.,MD
Cipriaso,Corazon Carrillo,MD
Coplin,Bruce M.,MD
Czenis,Ken,MD
Drakh,Alexander,DO
Errion,Christine,MD
Hawthorne-Nardini,Christa,MD
Nutini,Mary Katharine,DO
Pitta,Kutumba S.,MD
Porwal,Anoop,MD
Sonatore,Carol,DO
Stillo,Joseph V.,MD
Woolverton,Kahra,MD
Wu,Chi M.,MD
Plastic Surgery
Godek,Christopher P.,MD
Small,Stephen Edward,DO
Vaccaro,John J.,MD
Psychiatry
Abubakar,Tunku Abdul R.,MD
Berkowitz,Robert,MD
Buchan,Shahindokh,MD
Chowdhrey,M. Salim,MD
Deworsop,Richard,MD
Dobrzynski,Carol A.,MD
Ferstandig,Russell A.,MD
Oh,Donald,MD
Siddiqui,Arshad Uddin,MD
Pulmonary Disease
Das,Prabhat R.,MD
Joyce,Michael Walter,MD
Kumar,Awani,MD
Parikh,Jayesh K.,MD
Soliman,Alaaeldin A.,MD
Radiation Oncology
Chang,Bong M.,MD
Coia,Lawrence R.,MD
Eggert,Bryan George,MD
Iyer,Rajesh V.,MD
Patel,Aruna Ghanshyambhai,MD
Radiology
Didie,William J.,MD
El Abidin,Mohammad NazirZ.,MD
Gibbens,Douglas T.,MD
Khorrami,Parviz,MD
Sankhla,Vijay R.,MD
Swidryk,John Paul,MD
Tran,Duc T.,MD
Rheumatology
Blumberg,Scott,MD
Salloum,Rafah,MD
Sports Medicine
Alcid,Jess Gerald,MD
Blum,Karl Richard,MD
Surgery (General)
Krishnan,Mahadevan Gopa,MD
Lowry,Steven James,MD
Machiaverna,Frank E.,MD
Matus,Victorino Managuit,MD
Schneider,Barbara P.,MD
Urology
Ferlise,Victor J.,MD
Hartanowicz,Stanley J.,MD
Howard,Peter Carson,MD
Mahmood,Parvez,MD
Schor,Martin J.,MD
Stoneham,John L. III,MD
Vascular & Intrvntnal Radiology
Moran,Christopher John,MD
Perosi,Nicholas Anthony,MD

Vascular Surgery
Berger,Howard M.,MD
Haque,Shahid N.,MD
Kedersha,Thomas A.,MD
Ramnauth,Subhash C.,MD
Vitreous and Retina
Amin,Haris Irfan,MD
Totowa
Adolescent Medicine
Zodiatis,Alexander Demetrius,DO
Allergy
Ghanem,Roland,MD
Family Medicine
Asfour,Mervet,MD
Chrucky,Roman,MD
Ibeku,Chukwuemeka A.,MD
Patel,Puja,MD
Internal Medicine
Odorczuk,Marzena,MD
Obstetrics & Gynecology
Bitar,Maria Teresa,MD
Day,Brian Todd,MD
Ngai,Ivan Manjun,MD
Tkach-Chubay,Irina,MD
Ophthalmology
Giliberti,Orazio L.,MD
Pediatrics
Abdulmasih,Yousef H.,MD
Deshmukh,Pratibha S.,MD
Elepano,Richard G.,DO
Elfanagely,Sarah Hedy,MD
Elias,Maurice,MD
Pandey,Krishna K.,MD
Ravishankar,Indira,MD
Psychiatry
Prakash,Meera V.,MD
Radiation Oncology
Dawson,George Anthony,MD
Surgery (General)
Farrell,Michael Louis,DO
Trenton
Adolescent Medicine
Garg,Lorraine Freed,MD
Allergy
Winant,John Jr.,MD
Yang,Jun,MD
Allergy & Immunology
Bobila,Ramon T.,MD
Ricketti,Anthony J.,MD
Anatomic/Clinical Pathology
Kim,Yung H.,MD
Anesthesiology
Arnette,Esther Elizabeth,MD
Beshara,Raafat Henry,MD
Co,Anthony,MD
Cortese,Lisa Ann,MD
Dinh,Cung T.,MD
Ganopolsky,Elizabeth,MD
Haig,Lauren Grace,MD
LaMonica,Christina M,MD
Liu,Yuyan,MD
Loesberg,Perry A.,MD
Markos,Marina Azmy,MD
Nardi,David A.,MD
Paloni,Stephen Mark,MD
Rosenzweig,Howard J.,MD
Schachter,Laurence Howard,MD
Spodik,Boris,DO
Wang,Ling,MD
Cardiovascular Disease
Damani,Prabodhkum M.,MD
DeGoma,Rolando L.,MD
DeStefano,Peter M.,MD
Kalra,Krishan G.,MD
Madeira,Samuel Jr.,MD
Nagra,Bipinpreet Singh,MD
Cardiovascular Surgery
Seinfeld,Fredric I.,MD
Critical Care Medicine
Seelagy,Marc M.,MD
Dermatology
Abello Poblete,Maria V.,MD
Diagnostic Radiology
Applbaum,Yaakov N.,MD
Banker,Piyush,MD
Kim,Andrew Edward,MD
Neimark,Matthew A.,MD
Soloveychik,Natalya,DO
Emergency Medical Services
Joshi,Hetal Chaitanyaprasad,MD

Physicians by Town and Medical Specialty

Trenton (cont)

Emergency Medicine
- Banks, Gerald, MD
- Deendyal, Yoganand, MD
- Geller, Robert J., DO
- Howard, Tanya Dayell, MD
- Hughes, Kristin Lynne, MD
- Ijaz, Muhammad Shabbir, MD
- Kaur, Jaspreet, DO
- Maiers, Travis John, MD
- Meisner, Patricia Bliss, DO
- Miranda, David J., MD
- Shirguppi, Renu, MD
- Sussman, Cindy Pearsall, MD
- Sutter, Garrett Gerald, MD
- Vichnevetsky, Simon, MD

Family Medicine
- Abraham, Mark Barry, DO
- Agrawal, Nidhi, MD
- Backus, Yolanda Alicia, MD
- Barrett Carnes, Joy-Lynne, MD
- Coutermarsh, Andrew, DO
- Gaskel, Virginia M., DO
- Ginsburg, Deborah J., MD
- Gupta, Vinod K., MD
- Hawes, Ruppert Augustus, MD
- Hussain, Muhammad N., DO
- Jenkins, David W., MD
- Lansing, Martha H., MD
- Malone, Jennie O'Lera, DO
- Miller, Danielle Megan, DO
- Noble, Mary C., MD
- Ruppel, Nicholas James, DO
- Stabile, Michael C., MD
- Walker, Paul A., DO
- Wong, Wilbur P., MD
- Zafar, Jabbar Ben, DO

Gastroenterology
- Afridi, Shariq A., MD
- Gupta, Rajendra Prasad, MD
- Huq, Irfan-Ul, MD
- Mian, Somia Zia, MD
- Rosner, Bruce P., MD
- Rubin, Marc R., MD
- Schwartz, Eric, MD
- Zamir, Zafar, MD

General Practice
- Cleaves, Elle Sowa, MD
- Gieger, Andrew, MD
- Kim, Sion, DO
- Vongviphut, Don, DO
- Work, Adam Nicholas, MD

General Preventive Medicine
- Gorney, Marilyn A., DO
- Kruse, Lakota K., MD

Geriatrics
- Wallach, Sara L., MD

Hand Surgery
- Fletcher, Daniel J., MD

Hospitalist
- Hassan, Hardawan Ahmed, MD
- Samiev, Djamshed, MD

Infectious Disease
- Cleri, Dennis J., MD
- Whitman, Marc S., MD

Internal Med-Adolescent Med
- Thoppil, Anoop Jose, MD

Internal Med-Sleep Medicine
- Ricketti, Peter Anthony, DO

Internal Medicine
- Agbodza, Kwami D., MD
- Ahmed, Lubna, MD
- Anandakrishnan, Rajashree, MD
- Andreyev, Nina Vaskina, MD
- Arora, Jasmine Kaur, MD
- Aslam, Hafiz Muhammad, MD
- Baig, Zahid Imran, MD
- Bhatti, Habib Arshad, MD
- Bonaparte, Philip M., MD
- Boucard, Herve C., MD
- Brewer, Arthur Martin, MD
- Calzada, Tania, MD
- Chaudhry, Sofia, MD
- Chen, Emily Q., MD
- Chinwalla, Farah, DO
- Christmas, Donald, MD
- Chung, John Wonkook, MD
- Colella, Robert Eugene, DO
- Conaway, Herbert C. Jr., MD
- Cueto, Irene L., MD
- Dessalines, Normy, MD
- Gaukler, Carolyn J., MD
- Geng, Qingdi, MD
- Ghavami, Roozbeh Mofid, MD
- Goldsmith, Daniel French, MD
- Guda, Sivakoti Nagireddy, MD
- Gumidyala, Lalitha V., MD
- Hasan, Saba Ali, MD
- Hohl, Rosario DeFatima M., MD
- Ibrahim, Mohammad Younis, MD
- Itzeva, Youlia I., MD
- Jaferi, Barkat A., MD
- Jalil, Sheema, MD
- Jeyakumar, Anusuya, MD
- Khan, Mohammad F., MD
- Kheder, Abdul-Hady M., MD
- Krathen, Jonathan, DO
- Laub, Edward B., MD
- Levitt, Alan T., MD
- Liu, Ping, MD
- Mahmud, Hossen, MD
- Maniya, Mariam Z., MD
- Marulendra, Shivaprasad, MD
- Matthews-Brown, Spring R., MD
- Mavasheva, Sofia, MD
- Mazhar, Noorain, MD
- Memon, Nahid, MD
- Misra, Neerja, MD
- Moazami, Delaram, MD
- Muddassir, Salman Moazam, MD
- Mughal, Abdul W., MD
- Munir, Maryam, MD
- Mustafa, Muhammad Usman, MD
- Nadeem, Shahzinah, MD
- Obuz, Vedat, MD
- Ogolo, Clinton, MD
- Oolut, Joseph James, MD
- Pacia, Arthur G., MD
- Pantelick, Julie M., DO
- Patel, Chhaya B., DO
- Patel, Shodhan J., MD
- Qazi, Sadia Idris, MD
- Rabadi, Khalaf E., MD
- Ramalingam, Muthulakshmi, MD
- Rana, Nilesh C., MD
- Raza, Ali Babar, MD
- Raza, Mohammad Aslam, MD
- Remstein, Robert Jay, DO
- Rinvil, Edwine, MD
- Rondanina, Richard W., MD
- Roowala, Shabbir H., MD
- Ryfinski, Eugene A., MD
- Safdar, Feroz, MD
- Saleem, Bushra, MD
- Saud, Helmi A., DO
- Shah, Nrupa, MD
- Shah, Shazia M., DO
- Sharim, Iradj, MD
- Shenk, Suzanne H., DO
- Shovlin, Jane Ann, MD
- Souidi, Anasse, MD
- Steeger, Joseph R., MD
- Stillwell, Paul C., MD
- Tan, Christina Geok-Beng, MD
- Taylor, Tanisha K., MD
- Thirugnanam, Saraswathi, MD
- Toma, Cornelius, MD
- Usmani, Qaisar H., MD
- Victor, Carl H., MD
- Villota, Francisco Javier, MD
- Vypritskaya, Ekaterina A., MD
- Warren, Ronald L., MD
- Zavala, Ramon E., MD
- Zubair, Khurram, MD

Maternal & Fetal Medicine
- Forouzan-Gandashmin, Iraj, MD

Neonatal-Perinatal Medicine
- Axelrod, Randi Allison, MD
- Banzon, Felipe T., MD
- Moffitt, Stephen T., MD

Nephrology
- Cohen, Barry Herbert, MD
- Cohen, Steven Craig, DO
- Hussain, Asher Ferjad, MD
- Pai, David Y., MD
- Sudhakar, Telechery A., MD

Neurological Surgery
- Barrese, James C., MD

Neurology
- Eckardt, Gerald William, MD
- Grewal, Raji Paul, MD
- Rao, Vikas Yallapragada, MD
- Shultz, Lisa Ann, MD
- Taboada, Javier Gustavo, MD

Obstetrics & Gynecology
- Amadi, Nkechinyere, MD
- Brickner, Gary R., MD
- Cervi, Wendy Lee, DO
- Flores, Eduardo G., MD
- Granderson, Lisa Irene, MD
- MacKaronis, Anthony C., MD
- Mantell, Cary Hilton, DO
- O'Mara, James M., MD
- Olukoya, Olasinbo Atinuke, MD
- Scharf, Jeffrey I., MD
- Tatarowicz, Roman J., MD
- Williams, Delores J., MD
- Williams, Fred W., MD

Occupational Medicine
- Makowsky, Michael J., MD
- Szenics, Jonathan M., MD

Ophthalmology
- Brown, William C. Jr., MD
- Donohue, Robert III, MD

Orthopedic Surgery
- Aita, Daren J., MD
- Di Biase, John J., MD
- Duch, Michael R., MD
- Gomez, William, MD
- Hornstein, Joshua Scott, MD
- Levine, Marc Jason, MD
- Pagliaro, Andre J., MD
- Saxena, Arjun, MD
- Schnell, John Raymond, MD

Pain Medicine
- Rosenberg, Daniel S., MD

Pathology
- Wood, Robert H., MD

Pediatric Emergency Medicine
- Maitland, Ralynne Elizabeth, MD

Pediatric Neurodevelopment
- Williams, Tanishia Alise, MD

Pediatrics
- Aamir, Tajwar, MD
- Abedin, Naheed, MD
- Alizadeh, Parvin, MD
- Alli, Kemi A., MD
- Azaro, Katherine Frankel, MD
- Boor, Sonya H., MD
- Brandspiegel, Laura K., MD
- Cho, Jason J., MD
- Dawlabani, Nassif E., MD
- Dawlabani, Nickolas Elias, MD
- Hussain, Suhaila S., MD
- Isola, Venkatarao, MD
- Lindsay-O'Reggio, Euldricka, MD
- Lopez, Lisa M., MD
- Luan, Jennifer X., MD
- Mondestin, J. Harry, MD
- Pacheco-Smith, Sariya Amina, MD
- Radhakrishnan, Puthenmadam, MD
- Rapp, Rachel V., MD
- Raza, Mahmooda H., MD
- Samad, Ambreen Shariq, MD
- Shah, Rajeev Rajat, MD
- Sharma, Anjali, DO
- Simone, Jill B., MD
- Valencia, Maria Linda, MD

Physical Medicine & Rehab
- Chiricolo, Heather Marie, MD
- Gonzalez, Priscila N., MD
- Lazaroff, Leslie Diann, DO

Psychiatry
- Ali, Syed A., MD
- Ali, Syed Asim, MD
- Amin, Prakash P., MD
- Anwunah-Okoye, Ifeoma Juliet, MD
- Bresch, David, MD
- Brown, Gary Alan, DO
- Chiappetta, Carl J., MD
- Dorio, Nicole Marie, DO
- Eilers, Robert Paul, MD
- Fuchs, Susan, MD
- Ganescu, Daniela Florentina, MD
- Gooriah, Vinobha, MD
- Khan, Mujahid A., MD
- Kher, Neeta Yogesh, MD
- Kwok, Elaine, MD
- Lieberman, Jordan A., MD
- Mabrouk, Hanny S., MD
- Maljian, Meroujan Ardziv, MD
- Mundassery, Sarala C., MD
- Nagra, Amandeep Kaur, MD
- Ramanujam, Sailakshmi, MD
- Rao, Vilayannur Raja R., MD
- Rorro, Mary C., DO
- Saslo, Christopher R., DO
- Siddiqui, Shahida, MD
- Thomas, Sara S., MD
- Wijaya, Don H., MD

Public Health
- DiFerdinando, George T. Jr., MD
- Paul, Sindy M., MD

Pulmonary Disease
- Asghar, Syed Amir, MD
- Casty, Frank Eugene, MD
- Frank, Marcella M., DO
- Gugnani, Manish K., MD
- Gushue, George F. Jr., DO
- Law, Kevin F., MD
- Vogel, David P., MD

Radiation Oncology
- Freire, Jorge Efrain, MD
- Tyerech, Sangeeta K., MD

Radiology
- Montuori, James L., DO
- Rijsinghani, Paresh K., MD
- Schwartz, Eric Ian, MD
- Zafar, Ahsan U., MD

Research
- Rohlf, Jane, MD

Rheumatology
- Capio, Christine Marie, MD

Surgery (General)
- Abud-Ortega, Alfredo Ramon, MD
- Ahmad, Sarfaraz, MD
- Cho, Kun H., MD
- D'Amelio, Louis F., MD
- Eboli, Dominick Joseph, MD
- Essa, Noorjehan, MD
- Fahrenbruch, Gretchen B., MD
- Hanna, Niveen, MD
- Heether, Joseph J., MD
- Kelly, Michael E., DO
- Mahadass, Pavani, MD
- Poblete, Fredrick M., MD
- Quinlan, Dennis Philip Jr., MD
- Rojavin, Yuri, MD
- Saleem, Mohammed R., MD
- Schell, Harold S. Jr., MD
- Shah, Rajiv K., MD

Surgical Critical Care
- Salem, Raja R., MD

Thoracic Surgery
- Laub, Glenn W., MD
- Shariff, Haji Mohammed, MD

Urology
- Rivas, Manuel A., MD
- Srapyan, Aram, MD

Vascular & Intrvntnal Radiology
- Hoppenfeld, Brad M., MD
- McGuckin, James Frederick Jr., MD
- Srinivas, Abhishek, MD

Vascular Surgery
- Brotman-O'Neill, Alissa Sue, DO
- Poblete, Honesto Madjus, MD

Tuckerton

Family Medicine
- Miller, Walter P., MD
- Rudolph, Herbert J., MD

Turnersville

Allergy & Immunology
- Berlin, Paul J., MD
- Shah, Paresha Snehal, MD

Dermatology
- Durham, Booth H., MD
- Gruber, Melvin S., MD

Diagnostic Radiology
- Dannenbaum, Mark S., MD
- Gallagher, Thomas Jude, DO
- Harding, John Arthur, MD
- Muhr, William Jr., MD
- Niedbala, Thomas M., MD
- Podgorski, Edward M. Jr., MD
- Roberts, David A., MD

Emergency Medicine
- De Martino, Frank J., DO
- McCabe, James III, MD
- Medlenov, Sergey, DO
- Shiller, David P., MD
- Weeks, Daniel J. III, DO

Endocrinology
- Beluch, Brian Walter, DO

Family Medicine
 Abesh,Daniel C.,DO
 Kernis,Elyse Beth,DO
 Madison,William A. Jr.,DO
 Mancuso,Alison M.,DO
 Petruncio,George J.,MD
 Rudolph,Kafi,DO
 Taylor,Greg Michael,DO
 Venuti,John David,DO
 Venuti,Robert L.,DO
 Vitola,Carl A.,DO
Gastroenterology
 Chiesa,John C.,DO
General Practice
 Koerner,Theodore G.,DO
Geriatrics
 Abdulghani,Ahsan Arshad,MD
Gynecology
 McKinney,Timothy B.,MD
Hospitalist
 Badolato,Joseph Nunzio,DO
 Thompson,Nicole,DO
Internal Medicine
 Altman,Daniel Winston,MD
 D'Ambola,Lesly A.,DO
 DeAnnuntis,Liza Leluja,MD
 Di Medio,Lisa C.,DO
 Flaxman,Daena Meredith,MD
 Gambale,Joseph Gerard,DO
 Kovalsky,David Joseph,DO
 Kramer,Sherri Lynn,MD
 Lauletta,Maryann Carmella,MD
 Michelson,Marc H.,DO
 Palermo,Kim Marie,DO
 Popescu,Adrian,MD
 Schwartz,Robert B.,DO
 Sexton,Thomas Francis,DO
 Slusser,Jonathan,DO
 Vlad,Tudor Jon,MD
 Wang,Yvette,DO
 Wehbe,Anthony,DO
 Wilkinson,Edmund,DO
 sargent,Stephanie Christine,DO
Medical Genetics
 Ierardi-Curto,Lynne A.,MD
Neonatal-Perinatal Medicine
 Malicdem,Milagros C.,MD
Nephrology
 Irwin-Obregon,Virginia,DO
 Panebianco,Paul S.,DO
Neurology
 Irby,Dahlia Jean,MD
 Zaman,Taimur,MD
Obstetrics & Gynecology
 Davis,George H.,DO
 Dilks,Robert H.,MD
 Kanoff,Martin E.,DO
 Manus,Alan M.,DO
 Nemeh,Elias,MD
 Rosen,Larry S.,MD
Pediatrics
 Iqbal,Wasie Jawed,MD
 Katzenbach,George F. III,MD
 Nemeh,Kamila E.,MD
 Richards,Adam Price,MD
 Stailey-Sims,Mary Katherine,DO
 Tisdale,Avian L.,MD
Physical Medicine & Rehab
 Cain,Courtney,MD
 Knod,George Albert,DO
Psychiatry
 Barb,Herman T.,MD
 Patel,Prabhaker S.,MD
Pulmonary Critical Care
 Barnes,Jaime Jude,DO
Pulmonary Disease
 Agia,Gary A.,DO
 Mongeau,Marc Thomas,DO
 Schiers,Kelly Anne,DO
 Wiley,Joan C.,DO
Radiology
 Brodkin,Joshua S.,MD
 Manning,Ana B.,MD
 Oberlender,Susan B.,MD
 Rosner,William Fredric,MD
 Schmucker,Linda N.,MD

Union
Allergy
 Mahmood,Tariq,MD

Anatomic Pathology
 Losada,Mariela,MD
Anatomic/Clinical Pathology
 Bentley,James David,MD
 Cabreros,Antonio T.,MD
 Dinu,Veronica Carmen,MD
 Riba,Ali K.,MD
Anesthesiology
 Fleischhacker,Wayne,DO
 Garipalli,Lakshmi,MD
 Kahn,Randolph,DO
 Novik,Edward,MD
 Peng,Minzhong,MD
 Shane,Steven A.,DO
 Wilcenski,Michael A.,MD
 Yim,Yoori W.,MD
Cardiovascular Disease
 Doskow,Jeffrey B.,MD
 Gopinathan,Kastooril,MD
 Lombardo,Sabato J.,MD
 Schackman,Paul E.,MD
 Vitale,Carl J.,MD
 Williams,Edward G. Jr.,MD
Colon & Rectal Surgery
 Brody,Zoltan,DO
Dermatology
 Turner,Mitchell S.,MD
Emergency Medicine
 Grayson,Janine Denise,MD
 Tyrrell,John A.,DO
Family Med-Sports Medicine
 Ahmed,Ameer Nizam,MD
Family Medicine
 Borkowska,Alina,MD
 Codella,Vincent Adrian,DO
 Eisenstat,Steven Alan,DO
 Herrera,Juan Carlos,MD
 Lee,Nancy,DO
 Luke,Steven,MD
 Rizzo,David M.,DO
 Salim,Suhail Mohammed,DO
 Talat,Afnan,MD
Gastroenterology
 Chirla,Sujala,MD
 DiGiacomo,William S.,MD
 Fernandez Ledon,Ramon A.,MD
 Greenblatt,Robert I.,MD
 Mahal,Pradeep S.,MD
 Muthusamy,Samiappan,MD
 Sundaram,Kanaga N.,MD
 Tempera,Patrick G.,MD
Internal Medicine
 Andreoli,Nina Needleman,MD
 Cennimo,David John,MD
 Chapinski,Caren A.,DO
 Chernyak,Anna,MD
 De Vastey,Gerard,MD
 Defilippis,Nicholas A.,MD
 Dhirmalani,Rajesh A.,DO
 DiRico,Julie,MD
 Diaz-Johnson,Nereida,MD
 Duncan,Samuel T.,MD
 Fernandez,Jacqueline A.,MD
 Gold,Jeffrey M.,DO
 Grigaux,Claire Nathalie,MD
 Grover,Kunal,MD
 Gudz,Ludmila,MD
 Kachadourian,Anise A.,MD
 Kershner,Gary Brian,DO
 Mauti,Joseph M.,MD
 Oyetunde,Olasunkanmi K.,MD
 Philogene,Clark E.,MD
 Pullatt,Raja C.,MD
 Ramasamy,Dhanasekaran,MD
 Segal,Ilia,MD
 Smighelschi,Corina Daniela,MD
Nephrology
 Latif,Walead,DO
Neurological Surgery
 Friedlander,Marvin E.,MD
 Gilad,Ronit,MD
 Lipson,Adam Craig,MD
 Nair,Anil Karunakaran,MD
 Poulad,David,MD
 Randazzo,Ciro Giuseppe,MD
 Ratzker,Paul K.,MD
Obstetrics & Gynecology
 Boffard,Daryl K.,MD
 Buontempo,Angela J.,DO
 Del Rosario Torres,Leonida,MD
 Ekulide,Emmanuel N.,MD

 Ericsson,Dawn Marie,MD
 Hyman,Martin C.,MD
 McNamara,Robert E.,MD
 Messimer,Julie Marie,MD
 Russo,Donato S.,MD
 Tai,Richard W.,MD
 Victor,Isaac L.,MD
Ophthalmology
 Haberman,James E.,MD
 Natale,Benjamin P.,DO
 Tchorbajian,Kourkin,MD
Orthopedic Surgery
 Aragona,James,MD
 Botwin,Clifford A.,DO
 Bradley,Douglas D.,MD
 Charko,Gregory P.,MD
 Gallick,Gregory S.,MD
 Gross,David E.,MD
 Innella,Robin R.,DO
 Kaiser,Anthony J.,MD
 King,John Wayne,DO
 Nehmer,Steven L.,MD
 Rajaram,Arun,MD
 Wolkstein,David S.,MD
Otolaryngology
 Obregon,Raimundo L.,MD
Pathology
 Mendrinos,Savvas E.,MD
Pediatrics
 Brown,Ingrid C.,MD
 Krul,Geddy J.,MD
 Nelson,Elizabeth A.,MD
 Ohri,Ranjana,MD
 Oxman,David J.,MD
 Panzner,Elizabeth A.,MD
 Phan,Khanh Bao,DO
 Poon,Chiu-Man,MD
 Straw,Simone A.,MD
Physical Medicine & Rehab
 Alladin,Irfan Ahmad,MD
 Jacobs,David Jay,MD
 Potashnik,Rashel,MD
 Sun,Jidong,MD
 Vekhnis,Betty,MD
Plastic Surgery
 Coons,Matthew S.,MD
Psychiatry
 Chernyak,Arkadiy,MD
 Galea,Marina,MD
 Goldin,Michael R.,MD
 Ivanov,Alexander,MD
 Rasin,Grigory S.,MD
Pulmonary Disease
 Karpman,Jesse,MD
 Miller,Jeffrey Adam,DO
Radiology
 Kessler,Howard,MD
Rheumatology
 Worth,David A.,MD
 Xiong,Wen,MD
Sports Medicine
 Gordon,F. Kennedy,MD
Vascular Disease
 Feldman,Jeffrey N.,MD
Union Beach
Internal Medicine
 Desai,Sunit Bipinchandra,MD
Union City
Anesthesiology
 Siegel,Ira B.,MD
Cardiovascular Disease
 Grandhi,Sreeram,MD
 Inguaggiato,Anthony J.,MD
 Presilla,Alejandro,MD
Diagnostic Radiology
 Simonson,Marc H.,MD
Family Medicine
 Cortina,Osvaldo,MD
 Dominguez,Jonathan Manuel,MD
 Gonzalez,Francisco D.,MD
 Jurado,Jerry L.,MD
 Mehta,Lalit Hargovind,MD
 Simonson,Leslie J.,MD
 Veloso,Corazon M.,MD
General Practice
 Feret,Eve Anne,MD
Internal Medicine
 Armas,Holger Giovanny,MD
 Barrientos,Monica,MD
 Benitez,Olga,MD

 Campoalegre,Maria A.,MD
 Chaudhry,Mohammad A.,MD
 Daub,Denise M.,MD
 Elias,Sameh S.,MD
 Florentino,Hector Leandro,MD
 Gastell,Gilberto F.,MD
 Hajal,Hussam M.,MD
 Hesquijarosa,Alexander,MD
 Ittoop,Paul T.,MD
 Milazzo,Carmelo,MD
 Perez,Ruben,MD
 Rangel,Emile I.,MD
 Rastogi,Sadhna,MD
 Shukla,Paresh Parashar,MD
 Velasco,Mauricio,MD
 Williams,Raashan Carlos,MD
Nephrology
 Bebawy,Niveen,MD
 Thomsen,Stephen,MD
Neurology
 Krish,Nagesh B.,MD
Obstetrics & Gynecology
 Scriffignano,Marla,MD
 Steck,William M.,MD
Ophthalmology
 Gabay,Jacqueline Estelle,MD
 Ho,Vincent Yih,MD
 Icasiano,Evelyn J.,MD
Orthopedic Surgery
 Baruch,Howard Michael,MD
Otolaryngology
 Festa,Alfredo Gerardo,MD
Pain Medicine
 Ramirez Pacheco,Luis A.,MD
Pediatrics
 Anam,Sadrul,MD
 Barrios,Tomas J.,MD
 Cenon,Pearl L.,MD
 Delgado,Wilson Eduardo,MD
 Fragoso,Jose,MD
 Hugo,Manuel C.,MD
 Knight,Phillip Thomas,DO
 McDonough,Kevin J.,MD
 Polack,Noha,MD
 Purisima,Fely Grecia,MD
 Rodriguez,Maria J.,MD
 Teraguchi,Kari Jane,MD
 Valdivieso,Yaira Michelle,MD
 Velez,Isabel Odeida,MD
Psychiatry
 Sandoval-Castellanos,Oscar,MD
Pulmonary Disease
 Pinal,Jose,MD
Surgery (General)
 Kofman,Igor,MD
 Purisima,Clementino O.,MD
 Santos Arias,Simon B.,MD
Urology
 Cacace,Cataldo P.,MD
Upper Montclair
Adolescent Medicine
 Skalsky,Susan E.,MD
Child & Adolescent Psychiatry
 Faber,Mark P.,MD
 Mason-Bell,Sharon E.,MD
Internal Medicine
 Willenborg,Ronald,MD
Obstetrics & Gynecology
 Corenthal Robins,Linda J.,MD
 Miller,Fred William III,MD
Psychiatry
 Bell,Michael Henry,MD
 Elfenbein,Cherie,MD
 Green,Amy,MD
 Shah,Bindi,DO
Upper Saddle River
Anesthesiology
 Naljian,Vahe G.,MD
Diagnostic Radiology
 Lasser,Andrew S.,MD
Obstetrics & Gynecology
 Alcala,Ramon L. Jr.,MD
Pediatrics
 Hands,Robert A. Jr.,MD
Psychiatry
 Burn,Charlene H.,MD

Physicians by Town and Medical Specialty

Vauxhall
Internal Medicine
- Ballaro, Joseph, MD
- Benvenuti, Eve S., MD
- Elkins, Michele, MD
- Feurdean, Mirela Cristina, MD
- Hurckes, Lisa Carabelli, MD
- Lacapra, Gina M., MD
- Ratner, Douglas J., MD
Psychiatry
- Clouden, Tobechukwu A., MD

Ventnor
Cardiovascular Disease
- Romero, Luis N., MD
Family Medicine
- Grife, Robert M., MD
Internal Medicine
- Kasper, John F., DO
- Lipshutz, Robert L., DO
- Rosenthal, Leslie S., MD
Ophthalmology
- Smith, David J., MD

Ventnor City
Internal Medicine
- Curnow, Hidalberto, DO
- Silverbrook, Robert M., DO
Nephrology
- Naber, Tamim Hani, MD
Pediatrics
- Asemota, Emiola O., MD
- Tan, Madeline P., MD

Vernon
Cardiovascular Disease
- Lanzilotti, Thomas A., MD
Emergency Medicine
- De Luca, Joseph Edward, MD
Family Medicine
- Marion, William Joseph, DO
- Pyatov, Yelena V., MD
Gastroenterology
- Korsakoff, Kristopher Paul, MD
Internal Medicine
- Han, Min, MD
- Hansen, Eric S., DO
- Yaccarino, Pasquale J., MD
Pediatric Hematology Oncology
- Saluja, Gurbir S., MD
Pediatrics
- Huzar, Diana, DO
- Kabarwal, Navneesh Kaur, MD
- Saluja, Gurmit Singh, MD

Verona
Addiction Medicine
- Miller, George W. Jr., MD
Allergy
- Fost, Arthur F., MD
- Fost, David A., MD
Allergy & Immunology
- Narisety, Satya D., MD
Anatomic/Clinical Pathology
- Horenstein, Marcelo G., MD
Anesthesiology
- Gentile, James, DO
Cardiovascular Disease
- Lander, Jeffrey, MD
- Williams, Errol Baldwin, MD
Cosmetic Surgery
- Loverme, Paul J., MD
Dermatology
- Abbate, Marc Anthony, MD
- Brown, Justin, MD
- Kassim, Andrea Tinuola, MD
- Nossa, Robert, MD
- Rothman, Frederic R., MD
- Spates, Stephen Thomas, MD
- Waller, Leon H., DO
Diagnostic Radiology
- Clarkin, Kim Stephanie, MD
Family Medicine
- Berg, Kevin James, MD
- Cirello, Richard, MD
- Daftani, Kennedy P., MD
- Daftani, Mohammad Daoud Daoud, MD
- Distefano, Kenneth Louis, MD
- Gonzalez, Orlando V., MD
- Gorman, Robert T., MD
- Holder, Dawn Paulette, MD
- Lacara, Dena L., DO
- Mazzella, Carmine A., DO
- McCarrick, Thomas P., MD
- Murray, Richard S., MD
- Schlam, Everett W., MD
- Slater, Shakira L., MD
- Smith, Stephanie, MD
- Steinhardt, Amelia L., DO
Gastroenterology
- Manzi, Daniel D., MD
- Nathan, Ramasamy Swami, MD
Hand Surgery
- Fraser, Keith E., MD
Internal Medicine
- Bonney, David Raymond, DO
- Chakilam, Santhosh, MD
- Lipsitch, Carol E., MD
- Mariyampillai, Joan of Arc J., MD
- Mariyampillai, Marcarious A., MD
- Sivaraju, Kannan, MD
Obstetrics & Gynecology
- Milano, Michael C., MD
- Woroch, Peter Michael, MD
Ophthalmology
- Davidson, Lawrence M., MD
Orthopedic Surgery
- Gehrmann, Robin Michael, MD
- Leary, Jeffrey T., MD
Otolaryngology
- Liu, Edmund S., MD
Pediatric Endocrinology
- Shankar, Ramamurthy R., MD
Pediatrics
- Dorfman, Joseph Charles, MD
- Flyer, Richard H., MD
- Khokhar, Rizwana T., MD
- Mallon, Nancy Tyrrell, MD
- Nielsen, Sarah B., MD
- Prestigiacomo, Cynthia R., MD
- Saba, Ragheda M., MD
- Sirna, Paul William, MD
- Strader, David J., MD
Physical Medicine & Rehab
- Bach, Richard Tae, MD
- Hicks, Kristina Elizabeth, MD
- Keswani, Rohit, MD
Surgery (General)
- Williams, Jeffrey Franklin, MD
Urology
- Saidi, James Ali, MD
- Walmsley, Konstantin, MD

Villas
Family Medicine
- Park, Sang T., MD

Vineland
Allergy
- Perin, Robert J., MD
Anatomic/Clinical Pathology
- Mapow, Larry S., MD
Anesthesiology
- Attia, Tamer A., MD
- Chambers, Bryan P., MD
- Fitzhenry, Laurence N. IV, MD
- Hamzeh Langroudi, Mehrdad, MD
- Jassal, Peter, MD
- Kaur, Harmanjot, MD
- Miller, Shamaal M., MD
- Patharkar, Milind J., MD
Behavioral Medicine
- Enriquez, Carla, MD
Cardiovascular Disease
- Cohn, Steven M., MD
- Dovnarsky, Michael K., MD
- Pilly, Ashok K., MD
- Quinlan, Jack Francis Jr., MD
- Rainear, Kristen, DO
- Shatkin, Bennett J., MD
Colon & Rectal Surgery
- Callender, Gordon Erwin, MD
- Senatore, Peter Joseph, MD
Dermatology
- Carbonaro, Paul Anthony, MD
- Smith, Leslie Robert, MD
- Toome, Birgit K., MD
Diagnostic Radiology
- Bhagat, Nitesh N., MD
- Desai, Shailendra A., MD
- Kazmi, Faaiza K., MD
- Lazarus, Robert E., MD
- Munjal, Ajay K., MD
- Neustadter, Lawrence M., DO
- Patel, Nirav, MD
- Rosenberg, Allison R., DO
- Rothfarb, Steven H., MD
- Villani, Michael A., MD
Emergency Medical Services
- Kornweiss, Steven Alexander, MD
Emergency Medicine
- Baruffi, Seth L., MD
- Blazar, Eric Pollack, MD
- Cackovic, Curt W., DO
- Cox, Courtney, DO
- Di Cindio, William D., DO
- Diorio, Dominic A., MD
- Ehrlichman, Richard S., MD
- Eligulashvili, Victoria, MD
- Horan, Corinne E., MD
- Kaluhiokalani, Leiloni H., MD
- Kasper, Laura Carol, DO
- Milas, Jerry Peter, DO
- Poucel, Donna Jeanne, MD
- Schiller, Arnold Laurence, DO
- Terrigno, Donato A., MD
- Urquhart, Megan C., DO
- Wagner, Scott Erik, MD
- Warner, Matthew J., MD
- Wilkerson, Zachary, DO
- Wright, Camylla Dimetruss, DO
Emergency Medicine-Sports Med
- Disabella, Vincent N., DO
Family Med-Sports Medicine
- Evering, Daniel Jr., DO
Family Medicine
- Abraham, David, DO
- Alberici, Anna, DO
- Baher, Ali Masih, DO
- Cunningham, Bruce D., DO
- Dendrinos, George Aristidis, MD
- Finder, Susan M., DO
- Kessler, Martin, MD
- Kuptsow, Scott Warren, DO
- Mason, Sandra, MD
- Narvel, Wasique Abdulahad, MD
- Necsutu, Simona Camelia, MD
- Neema, Swarnalatha, MD
- O'Dell, Xitlalichomiha, DO
- Patel, Hemali V., DO
- Pedersen, Daniel A., DO
- Rhyme, Timothy L., MD
- Smick, Robert J., DO
- Ulke, Taner D., DO
- Zucconi, Adam J., DO
- Zucconi, Nicole Christina, DO
Gastroenterology
- Matusow, Gary Alan, DO
- Shields, David S., MD
- Song, Woo Kwang, MD
- Tassakis, Tom A., MD
General Practice
- Chung, Kai B., MD
- Seibel, David L., MD
General Preventive Medicine
- Linn, Steven Craig, MD
Gynecology
- Mirone, Gary Steven, DO
Hospitalist
- Bodagala, Hima, MD
- Gupta, Kanika, MD
- Katta, Pratyusha Reddy, MD
- Khan, Yusra, MD
Infectious Disease
- Ahrens, John C., MD
- Galetto, David W., MD
- Kaufman, David H., MD
Internal Medicine
- Al Ustwani, Omar, MD
- Alken, Jeffrey, MD
- Atthota, Vakula Devi, MD
- Barber, Kevin G., DO
- Bhendwal, Sanjay, MD
- Hammod, Riyadh Shakir, MD
- Huston, Donald Jr., MD
- Khalil, Sara Adel, MD
- Kumar, Anshul, MD
- Lerman, Gabriel Salomon, DO
- Lim, Carlito L., MD
- Meadows, Jason Potts, MD
- Mittal, Satish K., MD
- Nakhate, Vinay Gopal, MD
- Negin, Benjamin Paul, MD
- Obara, Justyna Anna, MD
- Ojiako, Kizito C., MD
- Parmar, Kiritkumar A., MD
- Patel, Hasmukhbha D., MD
- Pillai, Adip, DO
- Powell, Jeffrey David, DO
- Rana, Jiten, MD
- Ryklin, Gennadiy, DO
- Sayo Lim, Carina P., MD
- Sharma, Rajendra M., MD
- Sheekey, Owen Jr., MD
- Soloway, Stephen, MD
- Sudhindra, Ramakrishna R., MD
- Tomar, Raghuraj S., MD
- Valvano, Amanda A., DO
- Venugopal, Narasimhal, MD
- Wanalista, David Michael, DO
- Watts, Helena B., MD
Medical Oncology
- Roy, Shailja, MD
Neonatal-Perinatal Medicine
- Abbott-Fiedler, Vicky L., MD
- Bird, Charrell Moyo, MD
- Elitsur, Noeet, MD
Nephrology
- Girone, Joseph Francis, MD
- Relia, Nitin, MD
- Yoslov, Michael D., DO
Neurological Radiology
- Alves, Eric M., DO
Neurological Surgery
- Kazmi, Najam U., MD
- Strauss, Richard Charles, MD
Neurology
- Gupta, Vipin K., MD
- Rocksmith, Eugenio Roberto, MD
- Skinner, Dirk E., MD
Obstetrics & Gynecology
- Bispo, Luciano Jose, MD
- Bonifield, Eric M., MD
- Clayton, Elizabeth Noelle, DO
- Fockler, Raechel Ann, DO
- Frinjari, Hassan, MD
- Gewirtz, Jonathan D., MD
- Lightner, Angela Nanette, DO
- Long, Ashley Nicole, DO
- Panganamamula, Uma R., MD
- Russo, Armando P., MD
- Torchia, Michele A., MD
- Walsh, Sussannah Savitri, MD
Occupational Medicine
- Balogun, Evelyn Kemi, MD
Oncology
- Sachdeva, Kush, MD
Ophthalmology
- Bresalier, Saul, DO
- Bruno, Christopher Ryan, MD
- Holzinger, Karl Anthony, MD
- Pilet, Jean-Claude, MD
- Tyson, Sydney L., MD
- Williams, Alice, MD
- Wisda, Catherine L., MD
Orthopedic Surgery
- Bernardini, Brad Joseph, MD
- Bernardini, Joseph P., MD
- Buxbaum, Eric Justin, DO
- Catalano, John B., MD
- Di Verniero, Richard C. Jr., MD
- Feldman, Jenna Aviv, DO
- Sarkos, Peter Anthony, DO
- Shah, Rahul V., MD
Otolaryngology
- Diaz Gonzalez, Rodolfo, MD
- Ferrari, Arthur J., MD
- Kenner, George R. Jr., MD
Pain Medicine-Interventional
- Lewis, Shannin Dion, DO
Pathology
- Sanden, Mats Olof, MD
- Varadarajan, Sushila, MD
Pediatrics
- Ago, Aileen Hope, MD
- Burgher, Sonia A., MD
- Chikani, Jignasa Ripal, MD
- Fisher, Matthew Adam, MD
- Harper, Leannah L., MD
- Hegedus Bispo, Sandra, MD
- Hunt, Judith A., MD
- Jain, Archna, MD
- Jaiyeola, Patti Jo, MD
- Mangalindan, Carmelita C., MD
- Mirone, Rolande N., MD
- Nakhate, Vishakha Vinay, MD
- Ogidan, Olabode O., MD
- Rosenberg, Michael A., MD

Sinha, Anita, MD
Solof, Arnold J., MD
Streeks, Nicole N., MD
Physical Med & Rehab-Sports Med
Salim, Shakeel, MD
Physical Medicine & Rehab
Jeanty, Moise, MD
Mariani, Chiara, MD
Smith-Martin, Kimberley Y., MD
Plastic Surgery
Watts, David C., MD
Psychiatry
Bright, Daniel J., MD
Clinton, Lawrence P., MD
Pulmonary Disease
Sheetz, Maurice Saunders, MD
Radiation Oncology
Smith, Glenda Ruth, MD
Radiology
Bernardi, Bridget Dolores, DO
Durrani, Muhammad I., MD
Go, Ernesto B., MD
Gomberg, Jacqueline S., MD
Hauck, Robert Martin, MD
Shah, Satish P., MD
Sports Medicine
Dwyer, Thomas A., MD
McAlpin, Fred III, DO
Silver, Seth M., MD
Surgery (General)
Attia, Ahmed Farouk, DO
Kaplin, Aviva Wallace, DO
Kushnir, Leon, MD
Montero-Pearson, Per M., MD
Nituica, Cristina Magadalena, MD
Ogwudu, Ugochukwu Chinweze, MD
Perry, Luke Daniel, DO
Stephenson, Derek Allen, MD
Thoracic Surgery
Antinori, Charles H., MD
Ultrasound
Liu, Andrew Ky, MD
Urology
Dorsey, Philip J. Jr., MD
Federici, Peter J., MD
Kasturi, Sanjay Srinivas, MD
Lee, Christopher Sang Don, MD
Slavick, Harris D., MD
Vascular Surgery
Kumar, Sanjay, MD
O'Donnell, John C. Jr., MD

Voorhees
Allergy
Gentlesk, Michael J., MD
Allergy & Immunology
Fiedler, Joel Mark, MD
Anatomic/Clinical Pathology
Lembert Tezanos, Larissa, MD
McFarland, Miles M., MD
Obando, David A., MD
Skarinsky, Evgenya, MD
Anesthesiology
Ahsan, Syed Nadeem, MD
Bailey, Philip Daniel Jr., DO
Cho, Daniel P., MD
Corcino, Ana J., MD
Jobes, David Richard, MD
Lewis, Allan Andrew, MD
Miller, Bruce L., MD
Mithani, Bharati T., MD
Nicolson, Susan C., MD
Patel, Erica, DO
Anesthesiology: Pain Medicine
Boyajian, Stephen S., DO
Yulo, John A., MD
Body Imaging Radiology
King, Anne H., DO
Cardiovascular Disease
Andriulli, John A., DO
Barrucco, Robert John, DO
Cha, Ri D., MD
Curl, Kevin M., MD
Daly, Stephen J., DO
Dudda Subramanya, Raghunandan, MD
Geisler, Alan K., DO
Gerewitz, Fredric B., MD
German, Yelena, MD
Joffe, Ian I., MD
Kramer, Alan D., MD
La Morte, Alfonso M., DO

Lisa, Charles P., MD
Mintz, Randy T., MD
Orth, Donald W., MD
Palermo, Jason, MD
Papa, Louis A., DO
Patel, Rajendra B., MD
Perlman, Richard L., MD
Rozanski, Lawrence T., MD
Russo, Andrea Marie, MD
Russo, Ralph E. III, MD
Schlessel, David R., MD
Singer, Robert A., MD
Spivack, Talya R., MD
Stehman, Glenn R., DO
Cardiovascular Surgery
Eisen, Morris M., DO
Child (Pediatric) Neurology
Mason, Thornton B. II, MD
Sharif, Uzma M., MD
Colon & Rectal Surgery
Gardine, Robert L., MD
Irwin, Eytan A., MD
Pello, Mark J., MD
Siemons, Gary O., MD
Critical Care Medicine
Miller, William B., DO
Dermatology
Baratta, Andrea, DO
Bernardin, Ronald Maurice III, MD
Chou, Koulin L., MD
Finkelstein, David Hal, MD
Macaione, Alexander, DO
Papa, Christine A., DO
Rekant, Stanley I., MD
Rollins, Terry Lee, MD
Schwartz, Bennett K., MD
Diagnostic Radiology
Apple, Jerry S., MD
Baum, Mark L., MD
Blumenthal, Beth A., MD
Elder, James P. Jr., MD
Fan, Wen Lin, MD
Farner, Michael Charles, MD
Kendzierski, Renee Marie, DO
Kramer, David H., MD
Lott, Kristen Ellie, MD
Piccoli, Catherine Welch, MD
Sahlman, Rebecca Lynne, MD
Emerg Medicine-Pediatric
Seiden, Jeffrey A., MD
Emergency Medicine
Barnett, Jordan B., MD
Bingham, Johna P., MD
Block, William Paul, DO
Burke, Rachel Irene, MD
Gleeson, Tara Elizabeth, DO
Gowda, Sharada Hiranya, MD
Grim, Keith Case, MD
Jumao-As, Joseph Maben A., MD
Lazarus, Adam Larry, MD
Malta, Raymond J., DO
Meerson, Maya, MD
Melnick, Jacob, MD
Menditto, Darren, MD
Parikh, Neelesh Vinod, DO
Polise, Michael F., DO
Reynolds, Daniel, MD
Rigueur, Adrienne Brooks, DO
Roomi, Adil Mohamed, MD
Scali, Victor, DO
Singer, Eileen M., DO
Tiwari, Ramrakshah, MD
Endocrinology
Davidson, Jean Marie, DO
Horowitz, Elisabeth W., MD
Lam, Eleanor Lin, MD
Facial Plastic Surgery
Sollitto, Robert B., MD
Family Med-Sports Medicine
Vitanzo, Peter Charles, MD
Family Medicine
Bendala, Preeti, MD
Blumenthal, Andrew Michael, DO
Bradley, Kathleen A., MD
Carela, Gendy, MD
Chummar, Joseline, MD
Daniel, Beena Mary, MD
Davis, Robert A., MD
Dimapilis, Ann B., DO
Enriquez, Alfred Vasquez, MD
Fagel, Jonathan Val C., DO

Fisher-Swartz, Lucinda, MD
Furey, William J., DO
Gealt, David Benjamin, DO
Giuglianotti, Daniel Scott, DO
Karmazin, Polina, MD
Khalil, Samir Walid, MD
Kitts, Lori M., MD
Koerner, David M., DO
Krever, Kristine Wang, MD
Kwak, James Jihoon, MD
Leone, Mark R., DO
Lowe, John William, DO
Maffei, Mario Stephen, MD
Marone, Michael L., MD
Martin, William Arthur, DO
Milman, Anna, DO
Momi, Anudeep K., DO
Montgomery, Catherine P., MD
Mule, Salvatore, MD
O'Hare, Kendal Eggers, MD
Patel, Ambarish Ashokkumar, DO
Phakey, Vishal, DO
Post, Robert E., MD
Richman, Mitchell S., MD
Roberts, Barbara Theresa, MD
Seeley, Brian T., DO
Soble, Toby K., MD
Style, Daniel J., DO
Style, Stuart D., DO
Varevice-McAndrew, Susan, MD
Weiner, Samuel David, MD
Willard, Mary A., MD
Winfield, Barbara A., DO
Wong, Que-Chi V., MD
Zalut, David S., MD
Gastroenterology
Alloy, Andrew Marc, DO
Celluzzi, Alex, DO
Chauhan, Tusharsindhu C., MD
Chiesa, Drew Jonathan, DO
Egan, Elizabeth Anne, MD
Goldstein, Michael Bruce, MD
Hashmi, M. Arif, MD
Malamut, Jay M., MD
McLaughlin, Vincent A., MD
Mushnick, Alan J., MD
Pineda, Verne M., MD
Walters, Richard Lawrence, DO
General Practice
Chang, Hyun S., MD
Garber, Brett A., DO
O'Connell, Joseph J. III, DO
Patel, Ashokkumar B., MD
Geriatric Psychiatry
Talati, Amita N., MD
Geriatrics
Bansal, Mukta, MD
Gamble, James D., MD
Grimmett, Brian L., MD
Mandia, Renita, DO
Maurer, Kenneth H., MD
Solomon, Sheldon D., MD
Gynecological Oncology
Rocereto, Thomas F., MD
Gynecology
Echols, Karolynn T., MD
Gandhi, Veena S., MD
Hand Surgery
Stackhouse, Thomas G., MD
Hematology
Bapat, Ashok R., MD
Gordon, Richard L., DO
Madamba, Carlos S., MD
Siegel, Norman H., MD
Hematology Oncology
Ferber, Andres, MD
Lerman, Nati, MD
Mehta, Pallav K., MD
Rajagopalan, Kumar, MD
Ross, David H., MD
Hospitalist
Abdeljawad, Mohammad R., MD
Berio-Dorta, Raul Luis, MD
Franks, Lori Genevieve Pihl, MD
Infectious Disease
Barnish, Michael J., DO
Condoluci, David V., DO
Ghayad, Zeina Rita, DO
Hou, Cindy Meng, DO

Internal Medicine
Angelo, Mark, MD
Baker, Robert Charles, MD
Beggs, Nancy H., MD
Bhatt, Trigun R., MD
Brown, Anthony, DO
Burns, Gerard Joseph II, DO
Callahan, Kevin J., DO
Canals-Navas, Carmen L., MD
Chen, Yingying, MD
Cho, Grace Shin, MD
D'Ambrosio, John C., DO
Eid, Hala Milad, MD
Emmons, Alyson, DO
Enriquez, Eduardo F., MD
Fussa, Mark J., DO
Gabler, Scott Joseph, MD
Giordano, Samuel Nicholas, MD
Goldstein, Gary N., MD
Gor, Priya P., MD
Greenberg, Richard H., MD
Hollander, Adrienne R., MD
Iliadis, Elias, MD
Ji, Yong, MD
Kodavali, Lavanya A., MD
Leuzzi, Rosemarie Anne, MD
Libby, Joseph Anthony, MD
Linganna, Sanjay, MD
Massac, Malik Ali, MD
Nesteruk, Tetyana, MD
Ngo, Ly Thien, MD
Parrillo, Joseph E., MD
Picciano, Laura S., MD
Ram, Nand, MD
Raphael, Stephen D., MD
Ropiak, Caroline Michelle, MD
Santamaria, Richard G., MD
Schuster, Mark Brian, DO
Shaw, Brian Richard, DO
Skobac, Edward A., MD
Solitro, Tamara Stolz, MD
Sundhar, Joshua Bharat, MD
Tagle, Raymundo T., MD
Tepper, Steven Ari, DO
Varallo, Gerardo Jr., DO
Weeks, Alicia, MD
Weingart, Brian M., DO
Witmer, George Robert III, MD
Zingrone, Joseph Peter, DO
Zrada, Stephen Eugene, MD
Maternal & Fetal Medicine
Herman, Glenn O., MD
Seibel Seamon, Jolene S., MD
Neonatal-Perinatal Medicine
Austria, Jocelyn R., MD
Bona, Marzena M., MD
Brutus, Nadege A., DO
Castillo, Minerva R., MD
Chavez, Alberto M., MD
Dapul, Gener M., MD
Davis, Cheryl Luise, MD
Fong DeLeon, Elizabeth Y., MD
Ghaben, Kamel Mostafa, MD
Hric, Jerome Joseph, MD
Hsu, Christopher Tzu-Yao, MD
Jethva, Purvi Jitendra, MD
Kim, Mirye, MD
Maher, Jennifer Lee, DO
Pandit, Paresh B., MD
Polam, Sharadha, MD
Reisen, Charles E., MD
Rosen, Harel D., MD
Theophilopoulos, Constantine, MD
Nephrology
Banker, Gopika H., DO
Chawla, Arun, MD
Lodhavia, Devang V., MD
Patel, Nitesh M., DO
Neurological Surgery
Siddiqi, Tariq S., MD
Neurology
Bromley, Steven Michael, MD
Gupta, Asha, MD
Patil, Kishor K., MD
Rincon, Fred, MD
Sun, Yun Lynn, MD
Vasishta, Shiva G., MD
Yanoschak, Jennifer Lee, MD
Obstetrics
Williams, Kristina, MD

Physicians by Town and Medical Specialty

Voorhees (cont)

Obstetrics & Gynecology
- Adamson, Susanne R. M., MD
- Aikins, James K. Jr., MD
- Arrow Articolo, Amy Beth, DO
- Babin, Elizabeth Ann, MD
- Bolognese, Ronald J., MD
- Bowers, Geoffrey David, MD
- Bridges-White, Kimberly Gaye, MD
- Caraballo, Ricardo, MD
- Carlson, John A., MD
- Chen, Janine Junying, MD
- Colella, Ryan Lawrence, MD
- Cortese, Bernard J., MD
- Crisp, Meredith Page, MD
- D'Elia, Donna L., MD
- Deger, Randolph Bruce, MD
- Denis, Frantz, MD
- Dershem, Jonel M., MD
- DiGaetano, Andrea F., MD
- Dittrich, Richard J., DO
- Felsenstein, Roberta G., MD
- Fitzsimmons, John Michael, MD
- Gleimer, Emily R., DO
- Glowacki, Carol Ann, MD
- Goodchild, Caroline Gagel, MD
- Grossman, Eric Brian, MD
- Holzberg, Adam S., DO
- Hosmer, Stephan E., DO
- Lamborne, Nicole Marie, MD
- Levine, Jeffrey Richard, MD
- Librizzi, Ronald J., DO
- Maccarone, Joseph L., MD
- Mackey, Suzanne Fuller, MD
- Martinez, Wendy, MD
- McCleery, Colleen Marie, MD
- Murphy, Heather Marie, MD
- Ricci, Emily K., MD
- Shah, Shailen S., MD
- Steighner, Kathleen Marie, MD
- Swift, Joanne, MD
- Tai, Victoria Chih-Chuang, MD
- Tha, Teemu, MD
- Udoh, Adaora Ngozi, MD
- Warshal, David Philip, MD
- Zinsky, Paul J., MD

Occupational Medicine
- Eskin, Evamaria Ursula, MD

Ophthalmology
- Binenbaum, Gil, MD
- Cohen, Marc S., MD
- Cox, Mary Jude, MD
- Dugan, John Donald Jr., MD
- Forman, Jeffrey S., MD
- Gault, Janice Ann, MD
- Gordon, Susan Master, MD
- Gorman, James G. Jr., DO
- Lingappan, Ahila, MD
- Ohsie-Bajor, Linda Hae Eun, MD

Orthopedic Surgery
- Carey, Christopher T., MD
- Daniels, Jeffrey B., MD
- David, Henry Edward, DO
- DeLuca, Peter Francis, MD
- George, Brian Philip, MD
- Harrer, Michael F., MD
- Klingenstein, Gregory Gillman, MD
- Lawrence, John Todd Rutter, MD
- O'Dowd, Thomas J., MD
- Pollard, Mark Andrew, MD
- Porat, Manny David, MD
- Purtill, James Joseph, MD
- Ramsey, Matthew Lee, MD
- Reid, Jeremy Jackson, MD
- Shah, Apurva Surendra, MD
- Stark, Zohar, MD

Otolaryngology
- Becker, Samuel Scott, MD
- Belafsky, Robert B., MD
- Cantrell, Harry, MD
- Dandu, Kartik Varma, MD
- Germiller, John Andrew, MD
- Leoniak, Steven Michael, MD
- Shah, Udayan Kanaiyalal, MD

Otolaryngology-Facial Plastic
- Scheiner, Edward David, DO

Pain Medicine
- Rogers, Kenneth H., DO

Pathology
- LoGrasso, Paul Peter, DO

Pediatric Cardiology
- Anderson, Terry M., MD
- Bhargava, Hema P., MD
- Gidding, Samuel S., MD
- Sanchez, Guillermo R., MD

Pediatric Critical Care
- Bigos, David, MD
- Festa, Christopher James, MD
- Papastamelos, Caitlin A., MD

Pediatric Emergency Medicine
- Belfer, Robert A., MD
- Dorn, Eric A., MD
- Mittal, Shraddha, MD

Pediatric Endocrinology
- Rossi, Wilma Catherine, MD

Pediatric Gastroenterology
- Mascarenhas, Maria R., MD

Pediatric Hematology Oncology
- Greenbaum, Barbara H., MD

Pediatric Ophthalmology
- Schnall, Bruce M., MD

Pediatric Otolaryngology
- Walker, Ryan D., MD

Pediatric Pulmonology
- Brooks, Lee J., MD
- Mayer, Oscar Henry, MD

Pediatric Surgery
- Grewal, Harsh, MD

Pediatric Urology
- Concodora, Charles William, MD
- Dean, Gregory Edwin, MD
- Packer, Michael G., MD
- Roth, Jonathan A., MD
- Zaontz, Mark R., MD

Pediatrics
- Andrejko, Constance Gasda, DO
- Ang, Dexter Ong, MD
- Browne, Patricia M., MD
- Chiang, Chung, DO
- Cohen, Amy Marie Palmieri, MD
- Cruz, Florencia Santos, MD
- DeFelice, Magee Lindinger, MD
- Frick, Glen Steven, MD
- Gabriele, Elizabeth Ann, MD
- Ghavam, Sarvin, MD
- Glasofer, Adam K., MD
- Ho, Leo E., MD
- Hughes, Naomi Teutel, MD
- Hummel, Mark J., MD
- Jaiswal, Paresh, MD
- Johnson, Swati, DO
- Josyula, Leela S., MD
- Kelly, Michelle, MD
- Khan, Sadaf Ahmad, MD
- Kiehlmeier, Scott Louis, MD
- Knifong, Genoveva, MD
- Kutikov, Jessica K., MD
- Lespinasse, Antoine Alexandra, MD
- Lestini, Melissa Murray, MD
- Levey, Bryan H., MD
- Lind, Thomas Eugene, MD
- Liner, Lisa Hope, MD
- Lintag, Irene C., MD
- Mangaser, Rhodora D., MD
- Mangubat, Ofelia R., MD
- Mann, Ana Mendes, MD
- McCay, Marissa, MD
- Mulberg, Andrew Evan, MD
- Nadaraj, Sumekala, MD
- Naseem, Rawahuddin, MD
- Pleickhardt, Elizabeth P., DO
- Pradhan, Madhura Ravindra, MD
- Prilutski, Megan A., MD
- Reid, Brittany Michelle, MD
- Ritson, Brenda Marie, MD
- Ritz, Steven Bernard, MD
- Russ, Michelle L., DO
- Sheehan, Christine, DO
- Simpson, Alyson Beth, MD
- Topol, Howard Ira, MD
- Trimor, Fay Ann I., MD
- Verma, Archana, MD
- Wurtzel, David, MD
- Zieniuk, Gregory J., MD

Physical Medicine & Rehab
- Folkman, Michelle Gabrielle, MD
- Friedman, Jerrold Aaron, MD
- Gollotto, Kathryn T., DO
- Gupta, Kavita, DO
- Wetzler, Merrick Jay, MD

Plastic Surgery
- Tamburrino, Joseph F., MD
- Vasisht, Bhupesh, MD

Psychiatry
- Brooks, Ellen F., MD
- Castillo, Edwin F., MD
- Chheda, Veena V., MD
- Jordan, Karen T., MD
- Kim, Amy, MD
- Kothari, Kinnari A., MD
- Mahmud, Jamal, MD
- Peterson-Deerfield, Laurie J., DO
- Riyaz, Najmun, MD
- Sarker, Tushar, MD
- Sobel, Janine M., MD

Pulmonary Disease
- Hogue, Donna J., DO

Radiation Oncology
- Harvey, Alexis, MD
- Wilson, John J., MD

Radiology
- Bloor, James J., DO
- De Laurentis, Mark, MD
- Deshmukh, Kalpana S., MD
- Miller, David Haim, MD
- Mohsin, Jamil, MD
- Patel, Bhupendra M., MD
- Semmler, Helaina D., MD
- Shack, Evan Tyler, MD
- Shah, Tanmaya Chetan, MD

Reproductive Endocrinology
- Manara, Louis R., DO

Rheumatology
- Abraham, Shawn George, MD
- Evangelisto, Amy Marie, MD
- Feinstein, David E., DO
- Han, Kwang Hoon, MD
- Krommes, Janet Filemyr, MD
- Loizidis, Giorgos, MD
- Schuster, Michael Charles, MD
- Silver, Arielle S., MD
- Traisak, Pamela, MD

Sports Medicine
- Cornejo, Juan Carlos, DO
- Ramprasad, Arjun, MD

Surgery (General)
- Butler, Charles J., MD
- Empaynado, Edwin Abogado, MD
- Figueredo, Nicole Dionesia, MD
- Grabiak, Thomas A., MD
- Hager, George W. III, MD
- Manigat, Yves J., MD
- Perocho, Rodolfo R., MD
- Revesz, Elizabeth, MD
- Sipio, James C., MD
- Winter, Howard J., MD

Thoracic Surgery
- Mascio, Christopher Edward, MD

Urogynecology
- Vakili, Babak, MD

Urology
- Ackerman, Randy B., MD
- Balsara, Zarine Rohinton, MD
- Bernstein, Michael R., MD
- Bloch, Jay L., MD
- Butani, Rajen P., MD
- Goldenberg, Samuel F., MD
- Gor, Ronak, DO
- Linden, Robert Andor, MD
- Nachmann, Marcella Marie, DO
- Orth, Charles Richard Jr., MD
- Sussman, David O., DO
- Thur, Paul C., MD

Vascular & Intrvntnl Radiology
- Doshi, Nilesh M., MD

Vascular Surgery
- Dietzek, Charles L., DO
- Fisher, Frederick S., MD

Waldwick

Anesthesiology
- Boruta, Andrew Michael, DO

Diagnostic Radiology
- Calem-Grunat, Jaclyn A., MD
- Degregorio, Scott David, MD
- Dockery, Keith Forrest, MD
- Koo, Jennifer S., MD
- Krinsky, Glenn Andrew, MD
- Lazarus-Wolpov, Dawn E., MD
- Lerner, Elliot J., MD
- Lin, Erwin, MD
- Rhee, Kyung-Hwa, MD
- Rybak, Karen J., MD
- Zimmerman, Jill Robin, MD

Family Medicine
- Al-Ola, Ziyad, MD
- Draucikas, Lisa A., DO
- Ferreras, Jessie A.M., MD
- Granas, Andrew Daniel, MD
- Krigsman, Suzanne Karimi, MD

Internal Medicine
- Dunn, Beverly A., MD
- Vijay-Sharma, Mayuri, MD

Orthopedic Surgery
- Moore, Michael G., MD

Pediatrics
- Capaci, Mary T., MD
- Hecht, Stacey Markowitz, MD
- Muthuswamy, Vijayalakshmi, MD
- Segal, Melissa Anne, MD

Psychiatry
- Dyakina, Nika, DO

Radiology
- Arams, Ronald S., MD
- Hai, Nabila, MD
- Lubat, Edward, MD
- Seigerman, Howard M., MD
- Smith, Jonathan, MD

Wall

Adult Psychiatry
- O'Neill, James P., MD

Cardiovascular Disease
- Yoo, Hojun, MD

Child & Adolescent Psychiatry
- Chottera, Shobha A., MD

Child (Pediatric) Neurology
- Barabas, Ronald E., MD

Colon & Rectal Surgery
- Paonessa, Nina Joanne, DO

Diagnostic Radiology
- O'Connor, Patrick Joseph, DO
- Parikh, Manoj R., MD

Emergency Medicine
- Cotler, Harold Mark, DO

Family Medicine
- Cotler, Samantha, DO

Gynecological Oncology
- Hackett, Thomas Everett, DO

Internal Medicine
- Al Asha, Mohammad H., MD
- Bollampally, Indira, MD
- Findura, Michael James, DO
- Pyontek, Maria G., DO
- Yadalla, Vanitha S., MD

Nephrology
- Mehandru, Sushil K., MD

Neurological Surgery
- Maggio, William W., MD
- Salerno, Simon Anthony, MD

Nuclear Medicine
- Krynyckyi, Borys Roman, MD
- Monaco, Robert A., MD

Obstetrics & Gynecology
- Aikman, Noelle M., MD
- Brudie, Lorna Ann, DO
- Carlo, Jocelyn Ann, MD
- Gumnic, Blair Rachel, DO
- Thind, Narinder K., MD
- Tomaro, Robert Jr., MD
- Walsh, Kathleen S., MD

Orthopedic Surgery
- Dhawan, Aman, MD
- Gordon, Michael H., MD

Orthopedic Trauma
- Pushilin, Sergei A., MD

Orthopedic-Hand Surgery
- Doumas, Christopher, MD

Otolaryngology
- Nahm, Choong S., MD

Pediatric Cardiology
- Rivera, Loyda I., MD

Pediatrics
- Meli, Catherine L., MD
- Micale, Maria Theresa, DO
- Rahmet, Naheed R., MD
- Shkolnaya, Tatyana, MD
- Shroyer, Stephen J., MD

Psychiatry
- Kansagra, Chunilal H., MD
- Mehandru, Urmila, MD

Radiology
  Di Paolo,Jeffrey C.,MD
  Unterman,Michael I.,MD
Surgery (General)
  Grayson,Leila S.,MD
  Kashlan,Bassam T.,MD
  Kazmi,Aasim,MD
  Kocsis,Cynthia A.,MD
  Schreiber,Martha L.,MD

Wall Township
Dermatology
  Cosulich,William F.,MD
  Esche,Clemens,MD
Emergency Medicine
  Difabio,Kelly Ann,DO
  Womack,Meghan E.,MD
Internal Medicine
  Aquilino,Gaetano J.,DO
  Brown,Christopher S.,MD
  Weber,Charles A.,MD
Obstetrics & Gynecology
  Salloum,Didi,MD
Pediatrics
  Barabas,Cynthia,MD
Sports Medicine
  Buckley,Patrick S.,MD

Wallington
Anesthesiology
  Dadaian,Jon-Paul,MD
Dermatology
  Janniger,Camila K.,MD
Family Medicine
  Pyz,Tadeusz F.,MD
Internal Medicine
  Kriso,Stephen A.,MD
  Lesiczka,Adam,MD
  Szewczyk-Szczech,Krystyna H.,MD
Pediatrics
  Lupinska,Malgorzata Teresa,MD
  Rozdeba,Christopha H.,MD
  Sliwowski,Martha S.,MD
  Sliwowski,Stanislaw,MD
Physical Medicine & Rehab
  Filippone,Mark A.,MD
Urology
  Rozdeba,Joseph,MD

Waretown
Internal Medicine
  Struble,Dale W.,MD
Neurology
  Greenberg,John P.,MD

Warren
Allergy
  Wolff,Alan H.,MD
Anatomic/Clinical Pathology
  Jiang,Tony T.,MD
  Sapanara,Nancy Lauren,MD
Anesthesiology
  Baratta,James A.,MD
  Chin,Christina W.,MD
Cardiovascular Disease
  Saksena,Sanjeev,MD
Child & Adolescent Psychiatry
  Colon,Vincent F.,MD
Dermatology
  Ahkami,Rosaline N.,MD
  Bagley,Michael P.,MD
  Doctoroff,Alexander,DO
  Lu,Rebecca Yun-ru,MD
  Reilly,George D.,MD
  Sciales,Christopher W.,MD
Diagnostic Radiology
  Kamieniecki,Robert Edward,MD
  Labib,Mina L.,MD
Emergency Medicine
  Vogel,Laurie D.,MD
Endocrinology
  Brodkin,Lisa Faith,MD
Family Medicine
  Brezina,Eric Joseph,DO
  Cavallo,Danielle Janine,DO
  Dicola,May Bersalona,MD
Geriatrics
  Lanza,Raymond,DO
Internal Medicine
  Abraham,Vinod J.,MD
  Agrawal,Rekha,MD
  Alaigh,Poonam Lata,MD
  Ashinsky,Douglas S.,MD

  Barsanti,Patricia L.,DO
  Bell,Kevin E.,MD
  Bobella,Stephen K.,MD
  Clemente,Joseph Alfred,MD
  DiProspero,Elizabeth J.,MD
  Ferrante,Maurice Andrew,MD
  Kloos,Thomas H.,MD
  Lal,Victoria Sunil,MD
  Lytle,Carole F.,MD
  Montouris,Elaine Alexis,MD
  Nelson,Richard Oakleigh,MD
  Prasad,Lakshmi,MD
  Salvatore,Augusto G.,MD
  Stoch,Sharon Rachel,MD
Neurology
  Morganoff,Abraham D.,MD
  Sinha,Kavita,MD
Obstetrics & Gynecology
  Braunscheidel,Julie Ann,MD
  Clott,Shilpa Mahendra,MD
  Costa,Gerald V.,MD
  De Angelis,Thomas,MD
  Goldman,Kara J.,MD
  Heffernan,Kathleen Anne,MD
  Hubschmann,Andrea Gibbons,MD
  Ivan,Joseph R.,MD
  Levey,James Andrew,MD
  Pathak,Kunja J.,MD
  Pregenzer,Gerard J.,MD
  Sanderson,Rhonda,MD
  Tweddel,George K. III,MD
Ophthalmology
  Carter,Susan Redfield,MD
  Firestone,Debra K.,MD
  Gewirtz,Matthew B.,MD
  Giuseffi,Vincent J. III,MD
  Jacobs,Ivan H.,MD
  Kahn,Milton,MD
  Krawitz,Mark J.,MD
  Lane,John F.,MD
  Lee,Henry,MD
  Stahl,Roslyn Marie,MD
  Zhang,Linda,MD
Orthopedic Surgery
  Abrutyn,David Alan,MD
  Boretz,Robert Stephen,MD
  McCracken,Kevin A.,MD
Otolaryngology
  Beecher,George,MD
  Vinnakota,Radha I.,MD
Pediatrics
  Barasch,Susan A.,MD
  Brandstaedter,Karen Hardy,MD
  Eng,Jeffrey M.,MD
  Filler,Sharon Lee,MD
  Fritz,Gerard D.,MD
  Katz,Andrea G.,MD
  Kramer,Sarah R.,MD
  Levin,Lorin Michelle,MD
  Parikh,Vasavi Harish,MD
  Ploshnick,Andrea G.,MD
  Rogers,Elisabeth Ann,DO
  Scott,Tiffany Lynn,MD
  Singer,Beth Carol,MD
  Stoicescu,Lavinia D.,MD
  Tang,Lin-Lan,MD
  Vinnakota,Rao V.,MD
Physical Medicine & Rehab
  Abend,Paul I.,DO
  Chang,Mimi A.,MD
  Rao,Vidya J.,MD
Plastic Surgery
  Clott,Matthew Alan,MD
Psychiatry
  Liu,Qinyue,MD
Radiology
  Chandarana,Shashikant G.,MD

Washington
Anesthesiology
  Greenfeld,Alan L.,MD
Family Medicine
  Foschetti,Felix P. Jr.,DO
  Gilly,Frank J. Jr.,MD
  Goodwin,James E.,MD
  Jaques,James Phillip,DO
  Kinoshita,Ken,MD
  Kolpan,Brett Heath,MD
  Sabates Arnesen,Katrina,MD
  Waldron,Winifred Marie,MD
  Yevdokimova,Oksana,MD

Internal Medicine
  Garg,Anil,MD
  Senzer,Richard P.,MD
Ophthalmology
  Cooley,Susan L.,MD
Pediatrics
  Rodriquez,Victor R.,MD
Psychiatry
  Groves,Gerald A.,MD
  Montezon,Lourdes I.,MD

Watchung
Anesthesiology
  Ostry,Rachel F.,MD
  Shah,Kishori Praful,MD
  Vassallo,Michael Anthony,DO
Cardiovascular Disease
  Barone,Paul,DO
  Catania,Raymond,DO
Dermatology
  Eisenberg,Richard R.,MD
Diagnostic Radiology
  Contractor,Sohail G.,MD
Family Medicine
  Faschan,Steven Michael,DO
  Rivera,Laura A.,MD
Internal Medicine
  Ramaswamy,Kumar K.,MD
Ophthalmology
  Chung,Jacob H.,MD
Pediatric Anesthesia
  Aron,Jesse H.,MD
Physical Med & Rehab-Pain Med
  Mejia,Joseph Rodrigo,DO
  Tabije,Kevin,DO
Physical Medicine & Rehab
  Thomas,Chris,MD
Psychiatry
  Eisenberg,Stuart Richard,MD

Waterford
Family Medicine
  Pearson,Gregg Alan,DO

Wayne
Addiction Psychiatry
  Goldbloom,David Lee,MD
Adolescent Medicine
  Charles,Lydia M.,MD
Allergy
  Sohn,Theresa J. H.,MD
Anatomic/Clinical Pathology
  Kaptain,Stamatina,MD
  Wu,Yihui Yvonne,MD
Anesthesiology
  Frias,Carlos,MD
  Galkin,Vadim,MD
  Klele,Christo Selim,MD
  Krynska,Elzbieta B.,MD
  Pekar,Aleksandr,MD
  Raja,Bala Shanmugasundara,MD
Anesthesiology: Pain Medicine
  Bandola,David Matthew,MD
Cardiovascular Disease
  Das,Dhirendra N.,MD
  Doss,Emile F.,MD
  Ghassemi,Rex,MD
  Gupta,Ajay K.,MD
  Konlian,Donna Marie,MD
  Rathi,Ravi,MD
  Salimi,Mostafa,MD
  Schair,Barry David,MD
  Toor,Saddad Zafar,MD
Colon & Rectal Surgery
  Khoury,Hani A.,MD
Cornea/External Disease
  Reing,Charles Scot,MD
Dermatology
  Cardullo,Alice Cecilia,MD
  Chima,Kuljit Kaur,MD
  Leu,Diana S.,MD
  Maier,Herbert S.,MD
  Pollack,Shoshannah S.,MD
  Thakker,Priya Sambandan,MD
Diagnostic Radiology
  Flanzman,Richard M.,MD
  Sun,Qiang,MD
  Whang,Inwhan,MD
Emergency Medicine
  Bove,Joseph,DO
  Gandhi,Achyut Natvarial,MD
  Kansagra,Nilesh V.,MD

  Khan,Mansoor Ali,MD
  Shore,Robin L.,DO
  Testa,Joseph M.,MD
  Trivedi,Maulik Mahesh,MD
  Yuan,Ann Lee,MD
Endocrinology
  Berkowitz,Richard H.,MD
  Gibieizaite,Sandra,MD
  Leu,James Ping Hsun,MD
  Panah,Manizheh Ghaem,MD
Family Medicine
  Abdulmassih,Sami,MD
  Ahmed-Flowers,Tunizia,MD
  Bain,Francis Jerome-Xavier,MD
  Barravecchio,Anthony John,DO
  Beltzer,Blair Richard,MD
  Biller,Jeanette Marie,DO
  Bock,Robert T. Jr.,MD
  Carrazzone,Peter Louis,MD
  Chow,Jessica C.,DO
  Crabtree,Shawn M.,MD
  Deingeniis-Depasquale,A.,DO
  Duffy,Joseph M.,MD
  Gomez-Vasquez,Ricardo A.,MD
  Gregg,John A.,DO
  Lampariello,James A.,MD
  Makar,Gamil Lamey Bekheet,MD
  Nabulsi,Omar Hisham,MD
  Nguyen,Steven M.,MD
  Patel,Meera V.,MD
  Pope,Ronald J.,DO
  Rasa,David V.,MD
  Sivaraman,Priya,MD
  Topalovic,Pavle,MD
  Vasiliades,Thalia,DO
  Woo,James K.,MD
  Yorio,David S.,DO
Forensic Pathology
  Cronin,Leanne M.,MD
Gastroenterology
  Bleicher,Robert H.,MD
  David,Steven,MD
  Gordon,Clifford Avery,MD
  Ramamoorthy,Ravishankar,MD
  Shlien,Robert D.,MD
  Stevens,Lisa Deborah,MD
  Stillman,Jonathon S.,MD
  Zangara,Joseph Anthony,MD
General Practice
  Hasan,Sanjida,MD
Hand Surgery
  Bazzini,Robert M.,MD
  Ghobadi,Fereydoon,MD
  Ghobadi,Ramin,MD
Hematology
  Hanley,Debra A.,MD
Hematology Oncology
  Dorkhom,Stephan Joseph,DO
  Roy,Vijaykumar,MD
  Shah,Harish H.,MD
Infectious Disease
  Filippis,Philip J. II,MD
  Obaid,Nabeel B.,MD
Internal Medicine
  Abdy,Victor A.,MD
  Arnouk,Munzer M.,MD
  Aydin,Emmanuel A.,MD
  Azhak,Sameer Anor,MD
  Balboul,Elsaid A.,MD
  Bamdas,Lawrence Marc,MD
  Banu,Nazifa,MD
  Berman,Lee B.,MD
  Bernstein,Stanley F.,MD
  Biehl,Michael,MD
  Branovan,Zhanna Emilia,MD
  Calamari,Dawn E.,DO
  Chandran,Chandra B.,MD
  Cheng,Bonnie Kingman,MD
  Costello,Robert,MD
  DeFranco,Paul David,DO
  Doss,Michael Nader,MD
  Eraiba,Ayman E.,MD
  Eraiba,Magda A.,MD
  Farhangfar,Reza,MD
  Genkin,Igor,MD
  Gold,Jeffrey L.,MD
  Graziano,Vincent Angelo,MD
  Grella,William F.,MD
  Grinchenko,Tatyana,DO
  Hafez,Nagwa I.,MD
  Haghverdi,Mojdeh,MD

Physicians by Town and Medical Specialty

Wayne (cont)
Internal Medicine
Joffe, Libby, MD
Kapoor, Anil, MD
Kapoor, Anuj, MD
Kucuk, Erhan, MD
Leonardo, Michael H., MD
Liu, Ying, MD
Loughlin, Bruce T., DO
Lubansky, Kenneth P., MD
Macaluso, Charles F., MD
Matalkah, Nidal M., MD
Melsky, Lisa, MD
Mohsen, Reyad H., MD
Moquete, Manuel J., MD
Morone, John M., MD
Nahum, Laurie S., MD
Natelli, Anthony A., MD
Neilan, Martin J., MD
Notkin, Alicia R., MD
Parikh, Chintan Prakash, MD
Rae, Sam, MD
Saini, Harjinder S., MD
Sharma, Pushpendra, MD
Singh, Avtar, MD
Srisethnil, Pudchong, MD
Wassner, Jesse V., MD
Interventional Cardiology
Madhwal, Surabhi, MD
Neonatal-Perinatal Medicine
Houlihan, Christopher M., MD
Khoury, Aldo D., MD
Nephrology
Audia, Pat Frank, MD
Joseph, Monalisa, MD
Masand, Anjali Narain, MD
Prakash, Ananth N., MD
Shah, Sanjay R., MD
Triolo, Diane Cecilia, MD
Vitting, Kevin E., MD
Yousef, Nadia P., MD
Zeltser, Eugene, MD
Neurological Surgery
Raab, Rajnik Weerackody, MD
Sundstrom, David C., MD
Neurology
Chodosh, Eliot Howard, MD
Gazzillo, Frank L., MD
Mascellino, Ann Marie M., MD
Monck, Jennefer Erinna, MD
Nayal, Eyad A., MD
Safar, David S., MD
Wagner, Robert Austin, MD
Yazgi, Nabil M., MD
Obstetrics & Gynecology
Behnam, Nadereh, MD
Bennett, Bruce Kevin, MD
Burns, Les A., MD
Centanni, Toni V., MD
Chang, Bernard P., MD
Darvish, Cameron, DO
Diarbakerli, Fares, MD
Domnitz, Steven W., MD
Ephrem, Yasmina Marie Therese, MD
Garrett, Kenneth M., MD
Gof, Sonia M., MD
Greene, Jennifer Yvonne, MD
Kierce, Roger P., MD
Mazzone, Jeanae, DO
Mohammed, Nina, MD
Munoz-Matta, Ana T., MD
Newman, Sheila F., MD
Nicosia, Leonard T., MD
Onwudinjo, Adolphus C., MD
Pallimulla, Mahipa H., MD
Pavel, Patricia M., MD
Rosenzweig, Debra L., MD
Sgroi, Donald A., MD
Shakiba, Khashayar, MD
Suffin, Arthur Lee, MD
Tener, Trilby Jo, MD
Vitale, Diana Rodrigues, MD
Vosough, Khashayar, MD
Ophthalmology
Choo, Nancy Hae-Jin, MD
Garg, Geetanjali Davuluri, MD
Gollance, Stephen Andrew, MD
Macek, Deanna Z., MD
Mickey, Kevin J., MD
Mishler, Ken E., MD
Obrotka, Thomas M., MD

Silodor, Scott W., MD
Orthopedic Surgery
Cappadona, Joseph G., MD
Dowling, Ryan Martin, MD
Drillings, Gary J., MD
Dyal, Cherise Malinda, MD
Fahimi, Nader, MD
Faloon, Michael J., MD
Gold, David A., MD
Hwang, Ki S., MD
Maletsky, Mark E., MD
Masella, Robert Michael, MD
Matarese, William A., MD
McInerney, Vincent K., MD
Palacios, Robert M., MD
Reicher, Oscar A., MD
Roth, Jonathan Michael, MD
Schultz, Alan E., MD
Sicherman, Hervey S., MD
Stern, Lorraine C., MD
Wanich, Tony Suchai, MD
Orthopedic Surgery-Adult Rcnstr
Su, Sherwin Leu, MD
Orthopedic Trauma
Cox, Garrick Andrew, MD
Schneidkraut, Jason S., MD
Orthopedic-Hand Surgery
Denoble, Peter Hart, MD
Orthopedics
Wright, Craig, MD
Otolaryngology
Abrams, Stephen Joel, MD
Cece, John A., MD
D'Anton, Michael A. III, MD
Kassir, Ramtin Ronald, MD
Mattel, Stephen F., MD
Scheibelhoffer, John J., MD
Scher, Daniel A., MD
Sreepada, Gangadhar S., MD
Wise, Jeffrey B., MD
Otolaryngology-Facial Plastic
Brunetti, Vito Anthony, MD
Pain Medicine
D'Amato, Pamela R., MD
Pathology
Espinal-Mariotte, Jose D., MD
Pediatric Ophthalmology
Yang, Sherry, MD
Pediatric Orthopedics
Dean-Davis, Ellen, MD
Pediatric Surgery
Ganchi, Amir, MD
Pediatric Urology
Schlecker, Burton A., MD
Pediatrics
Abu Khraybeh, Wafa Said, MD
Bronstein, Jagoda Ewa, MD
Chiu, Caroline, MD
Darenkov, Ivan A., MD
Dong, Feiyan, MD
Gruczynski, Tomasz A., MD
Jariwala, Nilesh R., MD
Mahon, James William, MD
Nelson, Geraldine I., MD
Obilo, Iwuozo Livinus, MD
Orlov, Olga, MD
Scofield, Lisa E., MD
Winston, Maryana, MD
Physical Medicine & Rehab
Chemaly, Philippe Jr., DO
Doss, Anthony, MD
Fan, Wen-Ling Lee, MD
Haber, Monte Arthur, MD
Parowski, Supriya P., DO
Rahman, Abir, DO
Vosough, Cyrus R., MD
Plastic Surgery
Ganchi, Parham Amir, MD
Psychiatry
Ahkami, Behzad, MD
ElRafei, Mohamed A., MD
Kashoqa, Amer H., MD
Kat, Yousef A., MD
Master, Maria G., MD
Patel, Rajesh Manharbhai, MD
Rasheed, Syed Adil, MD
Siddiqui, Imtiazuddin M., MD
Siddiqui, Nafeesa, MD
Wang, Cecilia S., MD
Pulmonary Disease
Ismail, Medhat E., MD

Rappaport, Liviu I., MD
Wahba, Magdy A., MD
Wardeh, Ghassan Louis, MD
Radiology
Achaibar, Rajendra, MD
Cortellino, Karen, MD
Duhaney, Michael Owen, MD
Lee, Joung Y., MD
Steinberg, Michael L., MD
Wheeler, Ralph B., MD
Spinal Surgery
Emami, Arash, MD
Mahmood, Faisal, MD
Sinha, Kumar Gautam, MD
Sports Medicine
Badri, Ahmad, DO
Festa, Anthony Nmi, MD
Scillia, Anthony James, MD
Surgery (General)
Abessi, Hossein, MD
Beniwal, Jagbir S., MD
Bernstein, Michael H., MD
Chin, Channing Yee, MD
Garcia, Joseph, MD
Guarino, Lawrence A., MD
Henson, Bernard, MD
Moulayes, Nadra A., DO
Santos, Norman Verches, MD
Teehan, Edwin P., MD
Trauma Surgery
Douyon, Erwin, MD
Urology
Firoozi, Tahmoures, MD
Gmyrek, Glenn A., MD
Knoll, Abraham, MD
Levine, Seth Peter, MD
Rezvani, Abas, MD
Vascular & Intrvntnal Radiology
Festa, Steven, MD

Weehawken
Internal Medicine
Alfonso, Jesus Roberto, MD
Patel, Minalkumar Ashokkumar, MD
Surgery (General)
Mancheno, Mario A., MD

Wenonah
Adolescent Medicine
Piantedosi, Benjamin George, MD
Pediatrics
Biermann Flynn, Dana Lynn, DO
Clear, Carolyn Elizabeth, DO
Hung, Deborah Liu, MD
Jones, Tamika Lillian, MD
Knestaut, Angela Gaudiano, DO
Mishik, Anthony N., MD

West Berlin
Orthopedic Surgery
Rosenberg, Larry S., MD

West Caldwell
Anesthesiology
Bering, Thomas Gerard, MD
Doss, George S., MD
Forrest, Robert, MD
Giannuzzi, Rosanne Frances, MD
Izeogu, Chinweike, MD
Katragadda, Rama Sastrulu, MD
Lutz, Philip Edward, MD
Negron-Gonzalez, Maria A., MD
Rocamboli, David Charles, DO
Rubin, Joshua Adam, MD
Secoy, John Walton, MD
Sisbarro, Susan E., MD
Spertus, Silvana H., DO
Vujic, Dragomir M., MD
Weems, Lela Demilo, MD
Dermatology
Rabner, Deborah W., MD
Diagnostic Radiology
Caldwell, Kathleen V., MD
Emergency Medicine
Lombardi, Susan L., MD
Family Medicine
Elias, Nivin, MD
Hospitalist
Remadevi, Radhika Sekhar, MD
Infectious Disease
Riauba, Linas, MD
Internal Medicine
Diana, Joseph N., MD
Fein, Lesley A., MD

Follo, Joseph Michael, MD
Shah, Pradip S., MD
Neurology
Khoshnu, Esha, MD
Mendelson, Stuart G., MD
Ruderman, Marvin I., MD
Obstetrics & Gynecology
Binetti, Richard G., MD
Ophthalmology
Bevacqua, Alejandro, MD
Strauchler, Roberta A., MD
Wertheimer, Robert M., MD
Orthopedic Surgery
Berkman, Avrill R., MD
Strauchler, Irving D., MD
Pediatrics
Butensky, Arthur S., MD
DeLorenzo, Arthur J., MD
Flint, Laurence E., MD
Frank-Shrensel, Bettie, MD
Gigos-Costeas, Sophia, MD
Physical Medicine & Rehab
Szmak, Lauren, MD

West Deptford
Diagnostic Radiology
Ariaratnam, Nikki Sanghera, MD
Fog, Denise Susan, DO
Larkin, Jeffrey J., MD
Lin, Dennis C., MD
Little, Sherrill T., MD
Mattox, Scott G., MD
Rosten, Sloan I., MD
Sajous, Jan Bernard, MD
Tilak, Samir Shripad, MD
Titton, Ross Lewis, MD
Family Medicine
Klein, Irving J., DO
Riedel, Jacqueline V., DO
Neonatal-Perinatal Medicine
Petrozzino, Jeffrey, MD
Nuclear Medicine
Whitley, Markus A., MD
Obstetrics & Gynecology
Di Joseph, Benjamin D. Jr., DO
Lofton, Azieb Ghebremedhin, DO
McNally, Lauryn Anne, DO
Pediatrics
Ruddock, Heather Ann, MD
Radiology
Gilbert, Steven L., MD
Patel, Jayeshkumar Balu, MD

West Long Branch
Cardiovascular Disease
Pierson, Christopher G., MD
Dermatology
Gilson, Cynthia T., MD
Karakashian, Gary V., MD
Miller, Angela M., MD
Orsini, William J., MD
Family Medicine
Harding, Mark, MD
Zimmermann, Susanne W., MD
Gastroenterology
Langner, Bruce J., MD
General Practice
DiSanto, Vinson Michael, DO
Hematology Oncology
Lee, Patrick C., MD
Ray, Debra M., MD
Internal Medicine
Baldi, Daniela J., MD
Cohen, Seth Daniel, MD
Falco, David J., MD
Jariwala, Punit Rajnikant, MD
Malek, Sherif, MD
Maniar, Mihir Kishor, DO
Mari, Arthur D., MD
Parisi, Gerlando V., MD
Santiago, Eddie W., MD
Sharon, David J., MD
Medical Oncology
Fiore, Rosemary P., MD
Neurological Radiology
Mann, Sunita Singh, MD
Neurological Surgery
Estin, David, MD
Gillis, Christopher Charles, MD
Link, Timothy Emerson, MD
Lustgarten, Jonathan H., MD
Olson, Ty James, MD

Neurology
Gennaro, Paul, MD
Gilson, Noah R., MD
Patel, Dakshesh K., MD
Ponce, Francis B., MD
Raval, Sumul N., MD
Obstetrics & Gynecology
Jackson, Sharon, MD
Lambert-Woolley, Margaret A., MD
Lobraico, Dominick Jr., DO
Massaro, Robert A., MD
Ombalsky, Joseph, MD
Pompliano, Jennifer Dorothea, DO
Skorenko, Kenneth R., MD
Ophthalmology
Leventer, David Benjamin, MD
Pediatrics
Abreu, Paul, MD
Miller, Sandra M., MD
Murphy, Robert D., MD
Truxal, Brian A., MD
Plastic Surgery
Chidyllo, Stephen A., MD
Psychiatry
Mendelson, Joshua Todd, MD
Sachla, Melpomeni, MD
Sleep Disorders Medicine
Davis, Matthew Jared, MD

West Milford
Cardiovascular Disease
Platt, Robert N., MD
Family Medicine
Lascari, Roland A., MD
Internal Medicine
Joseph, Lisa V., MD
Kalevich, Serge F., MD
Obstetrics & Gynecology
Kaufman, Deborah Louise, DO

West New York
Anesthesiology
Richards, Patricia T., MD
Roque, Felix Eduardo, MD
Cardiovascular Disease
Gonzalez-Gomez, Luis A., MD
Child & Adolescent Psychiatry
Wang, Wei, MD
Clinical Pathology
Rudelli, Raul Daniel, MD
Dermatology
Herman, Eric W., MD
Emergency Medicine
Meta, Shimbul Shashikant, DO
Pamy Perez, Patricia Marcelle, MD
Family Medicine
Fajardo, Gil Valdez, MD
Hamal, Rekha, MD
Rodriguez, Reinerio Gerardo, MD
Surikov, Vadim Michailovich, DO
Gastroenterology
Gibilisco, Raffaele A., MD
Ramos, Rafael C., MD
Zapiach, Leonidas, MD
Internal Medicine
Arteta, Pablo A., MD
Diaz, Agustin, MD
Kumar, Chitra, MD
Pelletier, Mario E., MD
Roque Dieguez, Hilda Rosa, MD
Sanchez, Bienvenido, MD
Verea, Jorge L., MD
Vitievsky, Ellen, MD
Weiss, Ronald D., MD
Obstetrics & Gynecology
Fernandez-Cos, Henry, MD
Iraj Shaari, Gita M., MD
Melendez Cabrera, Octavio, MD
Milanes-Roberts, Norma, MD
Zahka, Karym, MD
Ophthalmology
Fasano, Armand P., MD
Otolaryngology
Shaari, Jeffrey M., MD
Pain Medicine
Rojas, Jose Jr., MD
Pediatric Gastroenterology
Goli, Sridhar Reddy, MD
Pediatrics
Aliaga, Julie M., MD
Bourne, Jeffrey Alan, MD
Butterman, Clifford Jay, MD

Castillo, Elma D., MD
Castillo, Marianne Devilla, MD
Fayngersh, David, MD
Goyco, Luis A., MD
Gutierrez Mena, Maria, MD
Hutton-Cassie, Donna Pauline, MD
Maldonado, Jose O., MD
Mallamaci, Carmen R., MD
Mason-Eastmond, Tania Alicia, DO
Mirchandani, Monica Hargovind, DO
Munoz-Llaverias, Altagracia, MD
Najib, Nabeel M., MD
Oropeza, Maria Emilia, MD
Panem, Cheryl Buensuceso, MD
Patel, Jayminkumar R., MD
Rubia-Sazon, Elvira M., MD
Villabona, Beatriz, MD
Physical Medicine & Rehab
Thorne, Robert Bruce, MD
Psychiatry
Sanchez, Daniel Rene, MD
Soto Perello, Jose Manuel, MD
Radiology
Baldonado, Ricardo T., MD
Surgery (General)
Gildengers, Jaime N., MD
Kulkarni, Vijaykumar A., MD
Urology
Roblejo, Pedro G., MD

West Orange
Adolescent Medicine
Kintiroglou, Constantinos, MD
Rabinowitz, Robert C., MD
Russo, John A., MD
Allergy & Immunology
Perlman, Donald Bret, MD
Anesthesiology
Abadir, John Sobhi, MD
DiStefano, Kelly Frances, MD
Fernando, Rosario P., MD
Liu, Kaixuan, MD
Liu, Ren Y., MD
Mankikar, Mohini T., MD
Tseng, William P., MD
Yanovskaya, Liliya, MD
Cardiovascular Disease
Berman, Gary K., MD
Brock, Donald J., MD
Chaaban, Fadi Nemer, MD
Chakhtoura, Elie Youssef, MD
Fisk, Marc Saslow, DO
Gandhi, Devang Amrat, MD
Goldberg, Mark C., MD
Haik, Bruce Joseph, MD
Harback, Edward R., MD
Hawthorne, Keith Allen, MD
Kadri, Iftekhar S., MD
Modi, Kaushik Chhaganlal, MD
Rogal, Gary J., MD
Rubenstein, Donald G., MD
Schwanwede, Jacqueline M., MD
Shehadeh, Abbas A., MD
Torre, Sabino Richard, MD
Tullo, Nicholas G., MD
Wangenheim, Paul M., MD
Wu, Chia F., MD
Cardiovascular Surgery
Pinder, Godfrey C., MD
Child & Adolescent Psychiatry
Greene, Bruce H., DO
Khanna, Bindu Chiranjit, MD
Clinical Cardiac Elctrphyslgy
Costeas, Constantinos A., MD
Dobesh, David P., MD
Roelke, Marc, MD
Critical Care Medicine
Kuntz, George R., MD
Dermatology
Connolly, Adrian L., MD
Connolly, Karen Lynn, MD
Glashofer, Marc David, MD
Groisser, Daniel S., MD
Hartman, Rachael Dalya, MD
Heidary, Noushin, MD
Patel, Mahir, MD
Raklyar, Eduard, MD
Ruhl, Kimberly K., MD
Simela, Tanasha, DO
Sivendran, Meera, MD
Spey, Deborah Ruth, MD
Stolman, Lewis Peter, MD

Dermatology: Dermatopathology
Sandoval, Marina Penteado, MD
Diagnostic Radiology
Choi, Patricia Hyunho, MD
Edwards, Michael J., MD
Grewal, Jasbir, MD
Kessler, Michael A., MD
Khedekar, Surekha D., MD
Mast, Harold Lee, MD
Waxman, Robert N., MD
Emergency Medical Services
Mays Stovall, Latisse M., MD
Emergency Medicine
Abbassi, Samih R., MD
Biczak, Ernest S., MD
DeLaCalzada Jeanlouie, Mae F., DO
MacKenzie, Diane Susan, DO
Endocrinology
Stock, Jerrold M., MD
Family Medicine
Belt, Steven D., MD
Burden, Yumie Nishida, DO
Chang, Peiyun, DO
Rivera Galindo, Claudia P., MD
Wurzel, Bernard Samuel, MD
Gastroenterology
Askin, Matthew Peter, MD
DePasquale, Joseph R., MD
Eagle, Robert Selig, MD
Fishbein, Vitaly A., MD
Fiske, Steven C., MD
Green, Jon David, MD
Mogan, Glen R., MD
Rosenthal, Lawrence Stephen, MD
Ruffini, Robert A., MD
Schuman, Robert W., MD
Siu, Larry K., MD
Sloan, William C., MD
Spira, Robert S., MD
Stefaniwsky, Andrew B., MD
Stein, Lawrence B., MD
Wallach, Carl B., MD
Geriatric Psychiatry
Sathaye, Nirmal, MD
Geriatrics
Ganesh, Manickam, MD
Gracia, Anne Marie G., MD
Redling, Theresa Marie, DO
Schor, Joshua David, MD
Gynecological Oncology
Denehy, Thad R., MD
Taylor, Robert Roland, MD
Hematology
Rothenberg, Jerry, MD
Hospitalist
Appiah, Evangeline Animah, MD
Infectious Disease
Borowski, Michelle, DO
Miller, Lincoln Paul, MD
Internal Medicine
Abboud, Somaya M., MD
Abdelaal, Sameh M., MD
Adeoti, Adekunle G., MD
Armanious, Adel Youssef, MD
Baddoo, Andrew O., MD
Casagrande, Lisette Helene, MD
Chu, Benny G., DO
Cooper, Sanford, MD
Deen, Shereelah, MD
Del Vento, Robert A., MD
Fretta, Joseph, MD
Goldstein, Craig Russell, DO
Grasso, Michael A., MD
Haacker, David S., MD
Hameed, Samar, MD
Johnson, Natalie A., MD
Kaltman, Leah B., MD
Khan, Samina K., MD
Kritzberg, William S., MD
Krok, Elion J., MD
Layne, Trevor J., MD
Lee, Daniel Kilho, MD
Lee, Dwight E., MD
Lifson, Donna C., MD
Nicoll, Anca M., MD
Ovnanian, Vagram, MD
Patel, Hemantkumar G., MD
Radin, Audrey B., MD
Rubino, Susan Basra, MD
Sangosse, Louis V., MD
Sangosse, Marie C., MD

Sapru, Sunil, MD
Savopoulos, Andreas A., MD
Schmidt, Alvin M., MD
Shah, Deepali A., DO
Sherman, Rimma L., MD
Teichman, Ronald F., MD
Theivanayagam, Kalyani, MD
Zeldin, Gillian Ann, MD
Legal Medicine
Mandel, Steven S., MD
Pandya, Prashant N., MD
Nephrology
Bonomini, Luigi Vittorio, MD
Jeanlouie, Odler R., MD
Komati, Naga Malleswari, MD
Lefkowitz, Heather Rush, MD
Palekar, Sadanand S., MD
Shah, Nita K., MD
Neurological Radiology
Aboody, Ronald S., MD
Neurological Surgery
Assina, Rachid, MD
Koziol, Joseph M., MD
Neurology
Barrett, Anna Mariya, MD
Becker, Andrew Nacholas, DO
Haskins, Danielle, MD
Kupershtok-Bojko, Aviva Sara, MD
Mehta, Deviyani Dilipkumar, MD
ObGyn-Hospice & Palliative Care
Nwobu, Uchenna Christian, MD
Obstetrics & Gynecology
Abeshaus, Lisa Ellen, MD
Antebi, Yael Jennifer, MD
Ciciola, Gerald F., MD
Crane, Stephen E., MD
David, Gwen Lynita, MD
Degraaff, Doreen E., MD
Ehrlich, Paul, MD
Fox, Howard D., DO
Hamilton, Tammy Joan, MD
Huang, Diana, MD
Kaufman, Gregory Joel, MD
Kessel, Allan David, MD
Ladocsi, Lewis T., MD
Luisi-Purdue, Linda, MD
Milanes Roberts, Norma B., MD
Patel, Priya R., MD
Pitman, Susan Roth, MD
Rae-Layne, Norma Alicia, MD
Romero, Audrey Anita, MD
Rubino, Robert J., MD
Russo, Neil J., MD
Sadural, Ernani, MD
Saitta, Jacqueline Danielle, MD
Sansobrino, Daniel M., MD
Sylvester, Claudine M., MD
Walk, Zem, MD
Wimmer, Angela M., MD
Zuniga, Gina, MD
Ophthalmology
Cheng, Eleanor Lillian, MD
Fruchtman, Deborah S., MD
Medford, David J., MD
Miller, Kenneth Scott, MD
Mirsky, Robert G., MD
Seligsohn, Audrey Lynn, DO
Tutela, Arthur C., MD
Orthopedic Surgery
Boiardo, Richard A., MD
Garcia, Jason P., MD
Hutter, Andrew M., MD
Kadimcherla, Praveen, MD
Lee, James M. Jr., MD
Loya, David Michael, MD
Pirone, Arthur M., MD
Robbins, Steven G., MD
Rosa, Richard A., MD
Seidenstein, Michael Kenneth, MD
Orthopedics
Bachman, Jodie Ann, DO
Otolaryngology
Berg, Howard M., MD
Downey, Laura L., MD
Fieldman, Robert J., MD
Holzberg, Norman, MD
Joseph, Eric M., MD
Levitt, Joel W., MD
Morrow, Todd A., MD

Physicians by Town and Medical Specialty

West Orange (cont)
Pediatric Cardiology
- Connor, Thomas M., MD
Pediatric Endocrinology
- Brenner, Dennis Jay, MD
- Mamkin, Irene, MD
- Oppenheimer, Ellen, MD
Pediatric Gastroenterology
- Sabel, Svetlana Lantsman, MD
Pediatric Pulmonology
- Bisberg, Dorothy Stein, MD
Pediatric Rheumatology
- Chalom, Elizabeth Candell, MD
Pediatrics
- Amaefuna, Stephen C., MD
- Chike-Obi, Toju O., MD
- Coy, Deborah A., MD
- Faleck, Herbert J., DO
- Garbarino, Charles L., MD
- Kintiroglou, John, MD
- Levy, Jeffrey E., MD
- Mathew, Seema Alexander, MD
- Nachevnik, Elina, MD
- Ness, Seth Lawrence, MD
- Owens, Jacqueline A., MD
- Pivawer, Lisa S., DO
- Saperstein, Jeffrey S., MD
- Silverman, Abby Robin, MD
- Tang, Yen-Shin Daisy, MD
- Tarchichi, Tony R., MD
- Vyas, Shefali, MD
- Ziemke, Karen Sue, MD
Physical Medicine & Rehab
- Anan, Elinor M., MD
- Averill, Allison M., MD
- Bapineedu, Radhika Kuchipudi, MD
- Benevento, Barbara Therese, MD
- Brooks, Monifa, MD
- Cava, Thomas J., MD
- Cho, Dong W., MD
- Gans, Bruce Merrill, MD
- Hampton, Stephen, MD
- Kaynan, Riva Lori, MD
- Kirsch, Victoria Susan, DO
- Kirshblum, Steven C., MD
- Klecz, Robert J., MD
- Kong, Yekyung, MD
- Linsenmeyer, Todd A., MD
- McKenna, Cristin, MD
- Oh-Park, Moo-Yeon, MD
- Park, Yong Il, MD
- Pomeranz, Bruce A., MD
- Vij, Raman L., MD
- Zimmerman, Jerald R., MD
Plastic & Reconstructive Srgy
- Amato, John Paul, MD
Plastic Surgery
- Asaadi, Mokhtar, MD
- Lalla, Sanjay, MD
- Leone, Joseph A., MD
- Peck, George C. Jr., MD
- Salas, A. Peter, MD
- Spiro, Scott A., MD
Psychiatry
- Cannella, Michael, MD
- Chilakapati, Manjula, MD
- Dhaibar, Yeshuschandra R., MD
- Elmore, Erin Maureen, MD
- Kurien, Abby V., MD
- Park, Charles William, MD
- Scalea, Donald D., MD
- Urbina, Emily Anne, MD
Pulmonary Disease
- Green, Douglas S., MD
Radiation Oncology
- Ivker, Robert Alan, DO
Radiology
- Shoenfeld, Richard B., MD
- Toder, Stephen Paul, MD
- Trivedi, Malti S., MD
Reproductive Endocrinology
- Gulati, Rita, MD
Rheumatology
- Cannarozzi, Nicholas A., MD
- Pai, Sneha, MD
- Weinberger, Andrew Bruce, MD
- Zaputowycz, Larysa, MD
Spinal Cord Injury Medicine
- Lam, Mylan Ngoc, MD
Sports Medicine
- Zornitzer, Matthew Howard, MD

Surgery (General)
- Alves, Lennox, MD
- Khanna, Ashish, MD
- Maheshwari, Vivek, MD
- Peck, Richard E., MD
- Singh, Manoj Kumar, MD
- Sultan, Ronald R., MD
Thoracic Surgery
- Forman, Mark H., MD
- Zisis, Eletherios G., MD
Urology
- Egan, Sean Christopher, MD
- Frank, Ronald Gary, MD
- Galdieri, Louis C., MD
- Hanna, Moneer K., MD
- Lefkon, Bruce W., MD
- Savatta, Domenico James, MD
- Seaman, Eric K., MD
- Strauss, Bernard S., MD
- Whang, Matthew I.S., MD
- Youngren, Kjell A., MD
Vascular & Intrvntnl Radiology
- Soto, David Rodolfo, MD
Vascular Surgery
- Hertz, Steven M., MD

West Paterson
Cardiovascular Disease
- Capitanelli, John R., MD
- Kaddaha, Raja'A Mohammed, MD
- Losardo, Anthony A., MD
Endocrinology
- Ibrahim, Mohammad S., MD
Family Medicine
- Vitale, Joseph Thomas, MD
Internal Medicine
- Brar, Harleen, MD
- Chatterjee, Deelip, MD
- Conte, Salvatore A., MD
- Ferrante, Francis L., MD
- Mallouhi, Issam, MD
- Patel, Meena S., MD
- Perez-Steele, Sheila, MD
Neurology
- Jafri, Syed S., MD
Obstetrics & Gynecology
- Zaveri, Sarla J., MD
Ophthalmology
- Parekh, Jai G., MD
- Parekh, Swati Jai Shah, MD
Psychiatry
- Dang, Jagdish G., MD
Pulmonary Critical Care
- Solis, Roberto A., MD
Rheumatology
- Airood, Moumina, MD

West Trenton
Emergency Medicine
- Valdellon, Alejandro M., MD
Family Medicine
- Khanna, Veena W., MD
Internal Medicine
- Beede, Michael S., MD
- Elder, Demian, MD
- Hazley, Donald J., MD
- Hui, Thomas P., MD
- Lalla, Lalita Raj, MD
- Lee, Jung Hi, MD
- Majid, Abdul, MD
- McKay, Cecile M., MD
- Razak, Hajira Naaz, MD
- Trivedi, Raksha A., MD
Medical Genetics
- Reid, Cheryl Soled, MD
Psychiatry
- Bari, Mohammad Minhaj, MD
- Calabrese, Toni-Lynne, DO
- Chacinski, Dariusz R., MD
- Cohen, Jay A., MD
- Fucanan, Vilma D., MD
- Gallagher, Peter K., MD
- Ghadiali, Farida Hashim, MD
- Hogan, Elizabeth Anne, MD
- Kazi, Abdul Haseeb, MD
- Legaspi, Abbelane S., MD
- Mujahid, Anjum, MD
- Nunez, Aida Rodrigo, MD
- Park, Jennifer E., MD
- Pasupuleti, Sasikala, MD
- Patel, Jayantilal R., MD
- Petivan, Victoria Anne, MD

- Radic, Rumiana S., MD
- Rizvi, Amir M., MD
- Rossi, Lawrence Nicholas, MD
- Roth, Robert L., MD
- Sack, Anita D., MD
- Tirmazi, Syed Jawad H, MD

West Windsor
Child (Pediatric) Neurology
- Mannheim, Glenn Barry, MD
Emergency Medicine
- Arjun, Seeta, DO
- Blanc, Phillip Garven, MD
Family Medicine
- Codjoe, Jessica R., MD
Internal Medicine
- Kasibhotla, Sumabala, MD
- Lubin, Hank, MD
- Rana-Mukkavilli, Gopi, MD
- Robin, James Allen, MD
- Singh, Ajay B., MD
Pediatrics
- Dinh, Megan, MD
- Kullmann, Valerie L., MD
- Rivers, Wendy Marie, MD

Westampton
Anatomic/Clinical Pathology
- Ragasa, Dante A., MD
Cardiovascular Disease
- Nachtigall, Jonathan C., DO
Family Medicine
- Colbert, Angelique L., DO
Forensic Pathology
- Hood, Ian C., MD
Hematology Oncology
- Fernandez, Eduardo E., MD
- Tropea, Joseph N., DO
Internal Medicine
- Herriman, Daniel Lee, MD
Psychiatry
- Balasundaram, Anusuya, MD
- Connell, Thomas A., MD
- Davis, Robert M., MD
- DeMercurio, Robert Edward, DO
- Madrak, Leslie Nicole, DO
- Rehman, Atta-Ur, MD
- Stiffler, Kyle M., MD
- Trigiani, Charles J., DO
- Wilkins, John J., DO
Surgery (General)
- Kernizan, Eddy, MD

Westfield
Adolescent Medicine
- Miller, Lesley G., MD
Allergy
- Abels, Robert I., MD
- Hicks, Patricia Margaret, MD
Allergy & Immunology
- Tahzib, Munirih Nura, MD
Anatomic Pathology
- Mehta, Rohin, MD
Cardiovascular Disease
- Surks, Howard K., MD
Dermatology
- Bhate, Chinmoy, MD
- Ciatti, Sabatino, MD
- Finamore, Christina Lucy, MD
- Hochman, Lisa G., MD
- Lehrhoff, Stephanie Rogers, MD
- Lu, Phoebe Do, MD
- McFalls, Susan G., MD
Diagnostic Radiology
- Cohen-Schwartz, Dawn Sheri, MD
- Horner, Neil B., MD
- Perl, Louis J., MD
- Salomon, Amir, MD
- Snieckus, Peter J., MD
Emergency Medicine
- Diamantopoulos, Vasilios T., MD
- Samuels, Marie Sophia, MD
Endocrinology
- Cho, Irene Soyoung, MD
- Daifotis, Anastasia Golfinos, MD
- Dev, Rajesh K., MD
- Fuhrman, Robert A., MD
Family Medicine
- Araujo, Martin A., MD
- Barnum, Kimberly Ann, DO
- Brenner, Robert W., MD
- De Masi, Christopher Louis, DO
- Ellison, Christian Eric, MD

- Henry-Dindial, Nicole A., MD
- Hevert, Robert A., DO
- Leistikow, Kathleen H., MD
- Patel, Shamik D., DO
- Skariah, Jody, MD
- Tabachnick, John Frederick, MD
- Thomas, Ann C., MD
- Wagner, Claudia Anne, MD
Gastroenterology
- Amrick, Thomas J., MD
- Cobert, Barton L., MD
- Coronato, Andrew, MD
- Lerer, Paul K., MD
- Tang, Ying Margie, MD
General Practice
- Kriegman, Audrey Gail, MD
Hand Surgery
- Barmakian, Joseph T., MD
Hematology
- Freeman, Barry C., MD
Hematology Oncology
- Talavera, Joyce R., MD
Hypertension
- Goldstein, Carl S., MD
Infectious Disease
- Baez, Juan Carlos, MD
- Greenman, James L., MD
- Ruggeri-Weigel, Patricia, MD
Internal Medicine
- Bulan, Jeanine Hermine, MD
- Calcara, Epifanio, MD
- De Rosa, Joseph, MD
- Lamothe, Maria Elina, MD
- Simon, Susan M. C., MD
- Sultana, Meher, MD
- Weigel, Peter J., MD
- Yatrakis, Nicholas D., MD
Medical Oncology
- Lu, Brian D., MD
Nephrology
- Brown, Ryan P., MD
- Klein, Philip S., MD
Neurology
- Saur, David P., MD
Obstetrics & Gynecology
- Cunningham, Catherine M., MD
- Fox, Michelle Candice, MD
- Margulis, Elynne B., MD
- Patel, Falguni B., MD
- Soffer, Jeffrey, MD
- Zimmermann, Laura Senn, MD
Ophthalmology
- Confino, Joel, MD
- Thiagarajah, Christopher K., MD
Orthopedic Surgery
- Bullek, David D., MD
- Faccone, John A., DO
- Krell, Todd P., MD
- Sweeney, Ralph Jr., MD
- Thrower, Albert B., MD
Orthopedic-Hand Surgery
- Said, Joseph, MD
Otolaryngology
- Mayer, Michael B., MD
Pediatric Cardiology
- Marks, Lloyd Alan, MD
Pediatrics
- Alvarado-Rosario, Yilda L., MD
- Bernstein, Stacy-Arlyn L., MD
- Cavuto, John Nicholas, MD
- Chen, Margaret G., MD
- Flanzman, Ellen S., MD
- Garcia, Nicole DeVincenzo, MD
- Haymond, Jean R., MD
- Kowalczyk, Matthew A., MD
- Kozich, Jeanine Masington, MD
- Levine, David B., MD
- Panza, Nicole, MD
- Panza, Robert A., MD
- Percy, John Jr., MD
- Presti, Jane C., MD
- Rivera, Roger Alberto Jr., MD
- Shah, Arvind P., MD
- Shapren, Kristen Marie, MD
Physical Medicine & Rehab
- Cohen, Pamela E., MD
- Foca, Francis J., MD
Psychiatry
- Borja, Susan V., MD
- Cunningham, Michael James, MD

Goldman,Clifford D.,MD
Lim,Ami Cruz,MD
Louie,Pearl Maria,MD
Moreines,Robert N.,MD
Psychiatry&Nrolgy-Special Qual
Richards,Andrea T.,MD
Radiology
Grosso-Rivas,Suejane,MD
Matuozzi,William D.,MD
Rokhsar,Michael Howard,DO
Rheumatology
Pedra-Nobre,Manuela Gomes,MD
Sports Medicine
Shaw,Daniel A.,MD
Surgery (General)
Bruno,Victor P.,MD
Kumar,Mark Hemanth,MD
Rutner,Torin W.,MD
Surgical Critical Care
Hurwitz,James Bennett,MD
Urology
Bernstein,Andrew Jay,MD
Cohen,Joel S.,MD
Fiske,Joshua Michael,MD
Lehrhoff,Bernard J.,MD
Mass,Alon Y.,MD
Miller,Mark I.,MD
Ring,Kenneth S.,MD
Talavera,Jose Galang,MD
Vascular Surgery
Cuadra,Salvador Alejandro,MD
Rezayat,Combiz,MD
Sales,Clifford M.,MD
Sundick,Scott Adam,MD
Westmont
Dermatology
Olivo,Matthew P.,MD
Legal Medicine
McClure,A. Gregory,MD
Psychiatry
Mobilio,Joseph N. Jr.,DO
Westville
Family Medicine
Wu,Jack Chen-Jen,MD
Wu,Kevin,DO
Westwood
Anesthesiology
Iuliano,Frank David,MD
Jin,Jie,MD
Cardiovascular Disease
Barr,Stuart A.,MD
Cocke,Thomas Preston Jr.,MD
Eisenberg,Sheldon B.,MD
Landzberg,Joel Serge,MD
Murphy,Patricia L.,MD
Critical Care Medicine
Al Asad,Manar M.,MD
Dermatology
Blume,Jonathan Erik,MD
Hadi,Ahmed Suhail,MD
Maso,Martha J.,MD
Molinaro,Michael John,MD
Myrow,Ralph E.,MD
Nychay,Stephen G.,MD
Osofsky,Michael,MD
Possick,Paul Aaron,MD
Reichel,Martin,MD
Endocrinology
Breit,Neal Gary,MD
Rodino,Maria A.,MD
Family Medicine
Macri,Michael V.,MD
Volpicella-Levy,Susan L.,DO
Gastroenterology
Fried,Harry A.,MD
General Practice
Donikyan,Mardik Martin,DO
Hematology
Israel,Alan M.,MD
Hematology Oncology
Kirshner,Eli David,MD
Internal Medicine
Anshelevich,Michael,MD
Easaw,Saramma John,MD
Esber,Natacha,MD
Fields,Sheila M.,MD
Perez,Victoria P.,MD
Ravi,Nanjappa,MD
Sinha,Sudir K.,MD

Interventional Cardiology
Lichtstein,Elliott S.,MD
Medical Oncology
Tassan,Robert F.,MD
Neurology
Connors,Robert Dedick,MD
Ghacibeh,Georges A.,MD
Kakkar,Pankaj,MD
Klein,Patricia G.,MD
Lira,Lorraine Sales,MD
Mittelmann,Eric,MD
Tsai,Joyce,MD
Van Slooten,David D.,MD
Obstetrics & Gynecology
Bilinski,Robyn T.,MD
Del Rosario,Elizabeth C.,MD
Dicker,Paul M.,MD
Hernandez Eguez,Carolina D.,MD
Levine,Zalman,MD
Ophthalmology
Bianchi,Glen Michael,MD
Chin,Patrick K.,MD
Fleischer,Michael S.,MD
Kaiden,Jeffrey S.,MD
Kirszrot,James,MD
Lee,Jung S.,MD
Pagan-Duran,Brenda,MD
Steinbaum,Norman F.,MD
Oral & Maxillofacial Surgery
Park,Mark,DMD
Orthopedic Surgery
Levine,Raphael Krevsky,MD
Lloyd,John Mervyn,MD
Miller,Alan R.,MD
Otolaryngology
Lee,James Jeong June,MD
Pediatrics
Buli,Dolores M.,MD
Clark,Mary H.,MD
Munteanu,Katrina M.,MD
Schwartz,Daniel I.,MD
Physical Medicine & Rehab
Goldstein,Asher C.,MD
Psychiatry
Shah,Pritesh J.,MD
Radiology
Gingerelli,Frank,MD
Reproductive Endocrinology
Berin,Inna,MD
Surgery (General)
Amin,Vishnubhai M.,MD
Vascular Surgery
Nalbandian,Matthew Martin,MD
Wharton
Internal Medicine
Pathak,Pinakin J.,MD
Ruml,Lisa A.,MD
Obstetrics & Gynecology
Ortiz,Guillermo,MD
Ophthalmology
Nayar,Romesh C.,MD
Physical Medicine & Rehab
Lim,Steve S.,MD
Vrablik,Robert H.,MD
Psychiatry
Chiodo,Damien F.,MD
Whippany
Dermatology
Lott,Jason Pelham,MD
Diagnostic Radiology
Kerwin,Lauren Michelle,MD
Family Medicine
Garcia,Joaquin B.,MD
Nitti,Michele,DO
General Practice
Rosenberg,Martin Louis,MD
Geriatrics
Cyrus,Pamela A.,MD
Internal Medicine
Bansilal,Sameer,MD
Coppolecchia,Rosa,DO
Nephrology
Perkins,Robert Mark,MD
Orthopedic Surgery
Grob,Patricio,DO
Schenk,Richard S.,MD
Spinnickie,Anthony O.,MD
Pediatrics
Ashton,Julie A.,MD
Dick,Donna Rosalind,MD

Eida,Emily Kott,MD
Forbes,Jennifer R.,MD
Gotfried,Fern,MD
Physical Medicine & Rehab
Cheriyan,Joshua M.,MD
Radiation Oncology
Zablow,Andrew Ira,MD
Whitehouse Station
Cardiovascular Disease
Cody,Robert James,MD
Family Medicine
Buinewicz,Anna Miller,MD
Hallit,Janice A.,DO
Kelsey,Alan G.,MD
Len,Lucille T.,MD
Nierenberg,Lisa,MD
Family Therapy
Hudson,Claudia Scalorbi,MD
Infectious Disease
Chan,Christina Yu-Yee,MD
Lee,Andrew Wen-Tseng,MD
Piliero,Peter James,MD
Internal Medicine
Abessi,Mitra,MD
Cohen,Philip Jay,MD
Occupational Medicine
Nigro,Peter J.,MD
Pediatric Infectious Diseases
Annunziato,Paula Winter,MD
Pediatric Neurodevelopment
Geffner,Michael Howard,MD
Pediatrics
Ezekowitz,Raymond Alan B.,MD
Roche,Kevin B.,MD
Scott,Peter J.,MD
Whiting
Anesthesiology
Mann,Dharam P.,MD
Anesthesiology: Pain Medicine
Jani,Samir Ranjit,MD
Dermatology
Tager,Patricia,MD
Family Medicine
Bartiss,Mark J.,MD
Bauberger,Charles Joseph,MD
Internal Medicine
Caruso,Donald A.,MD
Cervantes,Crisnoel,MD
Choper,Joan Z.,MD
Dalal,Karambir S.,MD
Dela Cruz,Danna,MD
Gallardo,Mario L.,MD
Karabach,Maxim,MD
Magsino,Vicente Martinez Jr.,MD
May,Micah Moshe,MD
Patel,Ashvin S.,MD
Shah,Bankim D.,MD
Tresvalles,Monette M.,MD
Zia,Ziaulhaq,MD
Wildwood
Family Medicine
Olarsch,Richard Gary,DO
Pediatrics
Gonzalez Rivera,Veronica,MD
Wildwood Crest
Family Medicine
Khella,Hani Joseph,MD
Williamstown
Anesthesiology
Audu,Paul Bulus,MD
Betia,Reuben,MD
Corda,Peter D.,DO
Perkins-Waters,Vannette N.,MD
Polcer,Jeffrey D.,DO
Family Medicine
Cogan,Andrew M.,DO
Lowry,Steven Michael,DO
Reilly,Megan Eileen,MD
Sharkey,Charles John,DO
Van Houten-Sauter,Lee A.,DO
Obstetrics & Gynecology
Green,Minda A.,MD
Pediatrics
Kanthan,Rajeswari,MD
Mathew,Mary,MD
Willingboro
Anatomic/Clinical Pathology
Choi,Hong Y.,MD
Maguire,Randall F.,MD

Anesthesiology
Paul,Benoy Krishna,MD
Penzone,Karen Elizabeth,MD
Platt,Marc J.,MD
Segaram,Gnana,MD
Cardiovascular Disease
Chardo,Francis Jr.,MD
Coleman,Elliott H.,MD
Horwitz,Michael J.,DO
Klier,Steven W.,MD
Malik,Manish Gulshan,MD
Schulner,Kenneth D.,MD
Shaikh,Hafeza,DO
Wood,Margaret Diana,MD
Critical Care Medicine
Levinson,Roy M.,MD
Dermatology
Kurnick,Warren S.,MD
Diagnostic Radiology
Bialo,Darren Andrew,MD
White,Robert M.,MD
Emergency Medicine
Evans,Nathaniel R. II,MD
Fumento,Robert S.,MD
Endocrinology
Rosenbaum,Daniel,MD
Family Medicine
Bajaj,Jasmine,MD
Caveng,Rocco F. Jr.,DO
Daroy,Christopher Felicano,MD
Donnon,Henry P.,MD
Ganti,Kennedy U.,MD
Weinar,Marvin A.,MD
Gastroenterology
Goldstein,Jack,MD
Petroski,Donald,MD
Shmuts,Robert Jaron,DO
General Practice
Mashru,Pravinkuma K.,MD
Hematology Oncology
Stone,Paul A.,MD
Internal Medicine
Bansal,Sudha,MD
Chaurasia,Preeti,MD
Comiskey,Walter M.,DO
Floyd,Darryl Bracey,MD
George,Philip M.,MD
Guo,Jin Ping,MD
Haque,Anwar Mohammed,MD
Hassman,Howard A.,DO
Karim,Minhaz,MD
Khawja,Yasmin,MD
Koenig,Andrew Stuart,DO
Paul,Karel Joseph,MD
Pichika,Nirmala,MD
Reddy,Anuradha K.,MD
Rehman,Saadia Raza,DO
Rivera,Edward,MD
Shah,Asma Aftab,MD
Turner,Nicoletta A.,MD
Neurology
Dunn,Timothy John,MD
Partnow,Michael J.,MD
Sharetts,Scott R.,MD
Obstetrics & Gynecology
Belazi,Misa T.,MD
Chen,Kenneth H.,DO
Hammer,Ashley Morgan,MD
Hulbert,David S.,MD
Schell,Paul Lee,MD
Semple,Camille Eleanor,DO
Siegel,Francine Michelle,MD
Snyder,Michael T.,MD
Zalkin,Michael I.,MD
Ophthalmology
Ackerman,Stacey Lynn,MD
Farnath,Denise Anne,MD
Feldman,Brad Hal,MD
Lennox Thomas,Tricia Lynn,MD
Naids,Richard Eric,MD
Scimeca,Gregory H.,MD
Otolaryngology
Shah,Rasesh Pravin,MD
Physical Medicine & Rehab
Jermyn,Richard T.,DO
Pulmonary Disease
Adams,Andrea Garcia,MD
Radiation Oncology
Chandra,Anurag,MD
Horvick,David,MD
Lustig,Robert Allan,MD

Physicians by Town and Medical Specialty

Willingboro (cont)
Radiation Oncology
Wallner, Paul E., DO
Radiology
La Couture, Tamara A., MD
Surgery (General)
Ing, Richard Daniel, MD
Mukalian, Gregory G., DO
Schaller, Richard Vincent Jr., MD
Thoracic Surgery
Greenbaum, David F., MD
Vascular Surgery
Baskies, Arnold M., MD
Holaday, William J., MD
Ruvolo, Louis S., MD
Wasser, Samuel H., MD

Wood Ridge
Anesthesiology
Fisch, Amy Heather, DO
Jiang, Yihao, MD
Family Medicine
Pantano, Maria V., DO
Hospitalist
Mullick, Muhammad Azfar, MD
Internal Medicine
Pecorelli, Nicholas T., MD
Pediatrics
Dhupar, Shanti, MD

Woodbine
Anatomic/Clinical Pathology
Hashish, Hisham A., MD
Family Medicine
Russo, Sandra L., DO
General Practice
Chu, Jae M., MD
LeVan, Maurice X., MD
Internal Medicine
Anthony, Michele M., MD
Novotny, Gregory R., DO
Pathology
Siebert, Charles F. Jr., MD
Pediatrics
Campbell, Anthony E., MD

Woodbridge
Allergy & Immunology
Bhambri, Neha Madhok, MD
Mumneh, Nayla Z., MD
Cardiovascular Disease
Alam, Mahmood, MD
Emergency Medicine
El-Halabi, Waseem, MD
Family Medicine
Boyd, Robert D., DO
Poonawala, Nafisa Z., MD
Gastroenterology
Webber, Seth Michael, MD
General Practice
Purani, Gaurav S., MD
Hematology
Murray, Carl Louis Jr., MD
Internal Medicine
Awan, Omar Q., MD
Awan, Razia S., MD
Friedman, Louis Alexander, DO
Goldstein, Richard Alan, MD
Hameed, Fauzia, MD
Maza, Lauren M., MD
O'Donnell, Mary Theresa, MD
Rosen, Jeffrey H., MD
Somer, Nancy C., MD
Zhang, Xiaowei, MD
Obstetrics & Gynecology
Kocun, Christopher C., MD
Ophthalmology
Lichtenstein, David I., MD
Orthopedic Surgery
Lu, Michael T., MD
Pediatric Hematology Oncology
Tekleyohannes, Girmay Haile, MD
Pediatrics
Azhar, Sarwat, MD
Bendich, David M., MD
Nihalani, Meena T., MD
Rajarathnam, Kavitha, MD
Rane, Sunanda D., MD
Physical Medicine & Rehab
Coba, Miguel A., MD
Psychiatry
Hriso, Emmanuel, MD

Hriso, Paul, MD
Surgery (General)
Constable, Richard E., MD

Woodbury
Anatomic/Clinical Pathology
Gala, Indira H., MD
Moore, Cheryl Crowley, MD
Anesthesiology
Cherian, Abraham, MD
Davis, Michael James, DO
Dragon, Glenn M., MD
Giorgio, Anthony Richard, MD
Harowitz, Robert J., MD
McMaster, Michelle, MD
Riley, Cara Ann, MD
Rousseau, Marc Telesphore, MD
Saldutti, Gregg M., MD
Smith, Kenneth Jr., DO
Valencia, Maria R., MD
Wagner, Craig R., DO
Cardiovascular Disease
Dawson, Martin S., MD
Kaulback, Kurt W., MD
Moccia, Thomas F., DO
Unwala, Ashfaque A., MD
Vergari, John Jr., MD
Child & Adolescent Psychiatry
Vidal, Heidi Robin, MD
Clinical Cardiac Elctrphyslgy
Padder, Farooq Ahmad, MD
Cytopathology
Hudock, Jude A., MD
Dermatology
Chung, Grace U., MD
Herman, Kenneth Louis, DO
Emergency Medicine
Ahuja, Yogesh, MD
Baird, James Few IV, DO
Bonner, James M., DO
Brenza, Danielle, DO
Chen, Lee, MD
Dalsey, Nicholas R., DO
Di Pasquale, Anthony J., DO
Dobrosky, Joseph D., MD
Espinosa, James A., MD
Garcia, Michael J., DO
George, James E., MD
Glenn, April, MD
Goldstein, Sodi H., DO
Goode, Dale Norman, MD
Granito, Joseph Louis, MD
Greenfield, Brett Steven, DO
Hoang, Loan Kim, MD
Kupfer, Herschel, MD
Kusmaul, Danielle Marie, DO
Love, Thomas Pierce, MD
Ludwin, Fredrick B., DO
Magariello, Mark M., MD
Martin, Ramelle Dana, MD
Mathew, Nisha S., MD
Mayer, Douglas John, MD
Mehta, Anila, MD
Newman, Suzanne Maria, MD
Oxler, Steven J., MD
Pagana, Theresa N., MD
Paschkes, Benjamin Neil, DO
Plumer, Robin Susan, DO
Raziano, Joseph Walter, MD
Sidwa, Robert M., DO
Sireci, John Bernard, DO
Solomon, Stuart R., DO
Stiefel, Jay A., DO
Tamashausky, Shaun R., DO
Trom, Andrew, DO
Varghese, Joby, DO
Weldon, Stacey Bidigare, MD
Young, Matthew John, DO
Endocrinology
Fallon, Joseph Jr., MD
Family Medicine
Affel, Marjorie E., MD
Andrews, Jaime Lynn, DO
Antonio, Patrick, MD
Bierman-Dear, Nancy A., MD
Chiusano, Emi A., MD
Chu, Chin-Chan, MD
Davis, Adriana, DO
Fellows, Wayne, DO
Gartland, John Jr., MD
Glass, Gina Gill, MD
Gopal, Srihari, MD

Ground, Christen Denise, DO
Hamilton, Sylvester Sutton IV, MD
Kumar, Mary Ann M., MD
Lawit, Alan, MD
Loubeau-Magnet, Helene, DO
Magnet, Marcus, MD
Malik, Tahseen Rabia, MD
Patel, Ashish C., MD
Patel, Jaymica, MD
Reigel, Shawna Ilene, MD
Roehl, Barbara Joan Oppenheim, MD
Rogers, Michael S., MD
Segal, Lawrence David, DO
Sornaraj, Amutha Arularasi, MD
Vanderwerken, Suzanne W., MD
Gastroenterology
Abrams, Jeffrey A., MD
Blair, Brian J., DO
Coben, Robert M., MD
Conn, Mitchell I., MD
DiMarino, Anthony J. Jr., MD
Fenkel, Jonathan M., MD
Kroop, Howard S., MD
McMahon, Donald James, DO
Prieto, Jorge A., MD
Geriatrics
De Persia, Rudolph T. Jr., MD
Hand Surgery
Lipschultz, Todd M., MD
Monaghan, Bruce A., MD
Hematology Oncology
Rotkowitz, Michael Ian, MD
Hospitalist
Kohlitz, Patrick, MD
Sloane, Amy Johnson, MD
Internal Medicine
Bajpai, Enakshi, DO
Bonett, Anthony W., MD
Butler, Barry K., MD
Chernoff, Brian Harris, MD
Chvala, Robert P., MD
Di Marino, Michael C., MD
Gehring, David J., MD
Gupta, Abhinai K., MD
Herman, Kenneth L., DO
Michel, Joseph R., MD
Ocasio, Robert B., MD
Omoh, Michael E., MD
Shaw, Richard Amedeo, DO
Nephrology
Lyons, Patricia J., MD
Neurology
Bokkala Pinninti, Shaila, DO
Denner, Michael J., MD
Miller, Ann Marie, MD
Zangaladze, Andro T., MD
Obstetrics & Gynecology
Gibson, Jeffrey T., MD
Hanson, Anna Jang, MD
Hapner, Byron S., DO
Vega, Vivian, MD
Ophthalmology
Della Torre, Kara E., MD
Friedberg, Andrea, MD
Friedberg, Howard L., MD
Prieto, Debra M., MD
Weinstock, Brett Michael, MD
Orthopedic Surgery
Bundens, David A., MD
Frey, Steven, MD
Kalawadia, Jay Vinodrai, MD
O'Brien, Evan Douglas, MD
Obade, Thomas P., MD
Rosen, Craig H., MD
Osteopathic Medicine
Tapper, Ben R., DO
Otolaryngology
Schwartz, David N., MD
Otology
Rowan, Philip T., MD
Pediatrics
Castano, Albert Ruben, DO
Chandra, Ram, MD
Jones-Hicks, Linda N., DO
Pasichow, Keith Philip, MD
Swe, Yuzana, MD
Physical Med & Rehab-Pain Med
Zhou, Linqiu, MD
Physical Medicine & Rehab
Gallagher, Edward J., MD

Plastic & Reconstructive Srgy
LaVan, Frederick B., MD
Plastic Surgery
Steffe, Thomas J., MD
Psychiatry
Bellias, Jay Peter, DO
Camacho, Brenda Y., MD
Camacho-Pantoja, Jose A., MD
Ko, Haeng S., MD
Zand, Perry H., MD
Pulmonary Critical Care
Breen, Gregory, MD
Cheng, Ho-Kan, MD
Pulmonary Disease
Finkenstein, Eric V., MD
Rosenberg, Scott B., MD
Radiation Oncology
Stambaugh, Michael D., MD
Rheumatology
Moynihan, Eileen M., MD
Surgery (General)
Erbicella, John Michael, MD
Goldstein, Adam S., DO
Graves, Holly Lynn, MD
Lynch, David J., MD
Mike, Joseph J., MD
Millili, John J., MD
Thoracic Surgery
Villare, Robert C., MD
Urology
Ebert, Karl H., MD
Kotler, Mitchell N., MD
Vascular Surgery
Haas, Kent Steven, MD
Pilla, Timothy S., MD

Woodbury Heights
Family Medicine
Kline-Kim, Johanna F., MD
Tomasso, Tara, MD
Trotz, Christopher R., MD
Internal Medicine
Millstein, Jeffrey Howard, MD
Rosenthal, Nadine C., MD
Neurology
Saleeb, Mariam, MD
Obstetrics & Gynecology
Keswani, Ashok Kumar, MD
Oral & Maxillofacial Surgery
Seeger, Douglas H., MD

Woodcliff Lake
Child & Adolescent Psychiatry
Grosso, Joseph X., MD
Gastroenterology
Biener, Alexander, MD
General Practice
Piacentile, Joseph M., MD
Internal Medicine
Graham, Peter E., MD
Obstetrics & Gynecology
Latkin, Richard M., MD
Schulze, Ruth J., MD
Sobel, Gail M., MD
Ophthalmology
Mendelsohn, Mary E., MD
Rini, Frank J., MD
Yashar, Alyson Gail, MD
Orthopedic Surgery
Betsy, Michael, MD
Pediatrics
Benstock, Alan D., MD
Berkowitz, Irwin H., MD
Bloomfield, Adam S., MD
Lupu, Sarah Ethel Nat, MD
Mandel, Mark S., MD
Mayer, Michelle Saltiel, MD
Rosenzweig, Stacey Ann, MD
Stoller, Jill S., MD
Psychiatry
Siragusa, Joseph, MD
Surgery (General)
Kordula, Charles E., MD
Urology
Berdini, Jeffrey L., MD

Woodlynne
Family Medicine
Atkinson, Monica, MD

Woodstown
Family Medicine
Bauman, David C., MD

Bussey,Paul George,MD
Deal,Amanda E.,DO
Hubbs,James E.,DO
Hurley,Margaret L.,DO
Nicholas,Paul George III,DO
Roberts,Kevin W.,MD
General Practice
Ostrum,Gordon J. Jr.,MD
Obstetrics & Gynecology
Marshall,Stefanie N.,DO
Wisniewski,Robert E.,MD
Surgery (General)
Lockwood,Curtis L.,DO

Woolwich Township
Emergency Medicine
Wofsy,Alice,MD
Pediatrics
Bacchus,Bebi Samantha,MD
Baker,Alon Elie,DO
La Voe,Ira Howard,DO
Weiss Baker,Marissa Beth,DO

Wrightstown
Anatomic/Clinical Pathology
McGinnis,Michael Clifton,MD

Wyckoff
Allergy & Immunology
Marotta,Alexander,MD
Anesthesiology
Aloi,Joseph M.,MD
Harvey,Samantha K.,MD
Lee,John Po-Hsiang,MD
Montemurno,Tina Deborah,MD
Rodriguez Barea,Hector A.,MD
Starcic-Herrera,Sandra,DO
Wu,Peter,MD
Yenicay,Altan Omer,MD
Zhou,Henry Haifeng,MD
Dermatology
Marcus,Linda Susan,MD
Diagnostic Radiology
Graziano,Vincent Anthony,MD
Emergency Medicine
Shirley,Lauren,DO
Gastroenterology
Viksjo,Michael Joseph,MD
Geriatrics
Mansour,Loris N.,MD
Internal Medicine
Lala,Lekhu K.,MD
Weitzman,Richard Brian,MD
Obstetrics & Gynecology
Duchin,Sybil E.,MD
Gartner,Joseph J.,MD
Hainer,Meg M.,MD
Orthopedic Surgery
Andronaco,John T.,MD
Pediatric Anesthesia
Ju,Tashil Kim,MD
Pediatrics
Cerkvenik,Kathleen M.,MD
Fenkart,Douglas R.,MD
Grossman,Abigail Michael,MD
Torres,Theresa M.,MD
Triggs,Cynthia Bilsly,MD
Yazdi,Mondana S.,MD
Psychiatry
Gallina,David J.,MD
Gefter,Igor,MD
Golin,Gratsiana,MD
Jalandoon,Cynthia Tabligan,MD
Nanjiani,Aijazali,MD
Peranio,Joanne C.,MD
Plummer,Alice T.,MD
Sous,Manal Ann,MD
Winters,Jayshree P.,MD
Youssef,Rafik Z.,MD

Physicians by Primary Medical Specialty and Town

New Jersey
Section 3

Physicians by Primary Medical Specialty and Town

Abdominal Surgery
Paramus
  Schmidt, Hans J., MD
Springfield
  Feteiha, Muhammad S., MD

Acupuncture
Cliffside Park
  Desai, Aruna A., MD
Fair Lawn
  Bamberger, Philip David, MD
Freehold
  Pellmar, Monte B., MD
Marlton
  Sciamanna, Mary Ann, DO
North Brunswick
  Elkholy, Wael Talaat, MD
Pennsauken
  Levy, Brahman B., MD

Addiction Medicine
Fort Lee
  Piper, Craig S., MD
Holmdel
  London, Eric Bart, MD
Lawrenceville
  Baxter, Louis E., MD
Merchantville
  Gooberman, Lance L., MD
Morristown
  Wilding, Todd Meredith, MD
Neptune
  Neshin, Susan F., MD
Red Bank
  Verdon, John J. Jr., MD
Short Hills
  Greenfield, Daniel P., MD
Verona
  Miller, George W. Jr., MD

Addiction Psychiatry
Boonton
  Bajwa, Ghulam Murtaza, MD
  Nagel, Isaac R., MD
Cedar Knolls
  Putcha, Vasundhara, MD
Cherry Hill
  Wallen, Mark C., MD
Glen Rock
  Yero, Sergio Alberto, MD
Lafayette
  Baliga, Ravi, MD
Lyons
  Williams, John A., MD
Marlton
  Ellabbad, Essam-Eldin M., MD
Neptune
  Solhkhah, Ramon, MD
Newark
  Zerbo, Erin Alexandra, MD
Paramus
  Reddy, Srikanth Madadi, MD
Princeton
  Davidson, Anne Stripling, MD
Somers Point
  Levounis, Petros, MD
Teaneck
  Berman, Jeffrey A., MD
Wayne
  Goldbloom, David Lee, MD

Administration/Medical Management
Lawrenceville
  Ditullio, Anthony Joseph, MD
North Bergen
  Winter, Ivan David, MD
Pompton Plains
  Weinberg, Richard M., MD
Somerville
  Cors, William K., MD

Adolescent Medicine
Belleville
  Murray-Burton, Carolyn I., MD
Berkeley Heights
  Bender, Michelle Anne, MD
Bernardsville
  Visci, John J., MD
Brick
  Condren, Eileen, DO
Camden
  Acquavella, Anthony Peter, MD
  Brown, Robert Theodore, MD
Chatham
  Estrada, Elsie C., MD
East Brunswick
  Gengel, Natalie, MD
  Sung, Boram, MD
Edison
  Hingrajia, Rashmin M., MD
Elmwood Park
  Patel, Harshad Nathalal, MD
Hackensack
  Northridge, Jennifer, MD
Hackettstown
  Sakowski, Jacek, MD
Hammonton
  Dahodwala, Nisrin Q., MD
Irvington
  Dada-Ajulchukwu, Tokunbo T., MD
Jamesburg
  Gebre Medhin, Hanna, MD
Livingston
  Goldenring, Debra Semel, MD
  Oana, Dan C., MD
  Semel, William J., MD
Medford
  Lazovitz, David A., MD
Morris Plains
  Feingold, Gail J., MD
Morristown
  Brill, Susan R., MD
  Park, Lisa Lam, MD
  Rosenfeld, Walter D., MD
New Providence
  Moskowitz, Steven, MD
Newark
  Bentsianov, Sari, MD
  Britt, Howard S., MD
  Dhar, Veena, MD
  Johnson, Robert Lee, MD
Northfield
  Solomon-Bergen, Peggy A., MD
Orange
  Thomas, Montrae C., MD
Paterson
  Blaustein, Silvia Adelina, MD
Princeton
  Gokli, Khyati, MD
Randolph
  Guerra, Julio C., MD
Sewell
  Backal, Marc Ira, MD
South Orange
  Albanese, Anthony C., MD
Springfield
  Mullick, Bharati, MD
Teaneck
  Vece, Lorrie J., MD
Totowa
  Zodiatis, Alexander Demetrius, DO
Trenton
  Garg, Lorraine Freed, MD
Upper Montclair
  Skalsky, Susan E., MD
Wayne
  Charles, Lydia M., MD
Wenonah
  Piantedosi, Benjamin George, MD
West Orange
  Kintiroglou, Constantinos, MD
  Rabinowitz, Robert C., MD
  Russo, John A., MD
Westfield
  Miller, Lesley G., MD

Adult Psychiatry
Clifton
  Weinshenker, Naomi Joyce, MD
East Brunswick
  Borodulin, Boris, MD
Florham Park
  Kral, Felix E., MD
Moorestown
  Cooperstein, Heidi B., DO
Newark
  Nagy-Hallet, Andrea, MD
Paterson
  La Porta, Lauren D., MD
Somerville
  Rowley, Susan Peet, MD
Stratford
  Scheinthal, Stephen M., DO
Teaneck
  Zerykier, Gisela B., MD
Wall
  O'Neill, James P., MD

Aerospace Medicine
Egg Harbor Township
  Tordella, Joseph R., DO
Freehold
  Wright, Evan Michael, DO

Alcoholism/Substance Abuse
Marlton
  Baird, Cynthia Marlo, MD

Allergy
Belleville
  Morrison, Susan H., MD
Belmar
  Shah, Tarun J., MD
Berkeley Heights
  Le Benger, Kerry S., MD
Brick
  De Cotiis, Bruce A., MD
  Tumaliuan, Janet Ang, MD
Camden
  Cline, Douglas C., MD
  Knowles, William O., MD
Cedar Knolls
  Oppenheimer, John Jacob, MD
Clark
  Sullivan, Bessie M., MD
Clifton
  Caprio, Ralph E., MD
  Klein, Robert Michael, MD
Colonia
  Sahni, Harsha R., MD
Dover
  Bigelsen, Stephen J., MD
East Brunswick
  Guirguis, Sonia S., MD
  Leibner, Donald N., MD
Edison
  Centeno-McNulla, Ligaya V., MD
  Kanuga, Jayesh G., MD
Englewood
  From, Stuart B., MD
  Goodstein, Carolyn E., MD
  Harish, Ziv, MD
Fair Lawn
  Bokhari, Tahira M., MD
  Kashkin, Jay Michael, MD
Florham Park
  Barisciano, Lisa, MD
  Sundaram, Usha K., MD
Garfield
  Benincasa, Peter J., MD
  Luka, Richard Edward, MD
Hackensack
  Michelis, Mary Ann, MD
Highland Park
  Blum, Jay R., MD
  Bonala, Savithri Bai, MD
  Golbert, Thomas Melvin, MD
Hillsborough
  Schulhafer, Edwin P., MD
Hoboken
  Pine, Martin S., MD
Holmdel
  Ho, Linden D., MD
  Viksman, Michael Y., MD
Irvington
  Belani, Suresh G., MD
Iselin
  Ambrosio, Patrick M., DO
  Maccia, Clement A., MD
Jersey City
  Elliston, Jason Taiwo Jos, MD
Kendall Park
  Kesarwala, Hemant, MD
Lawrenceville
  Mastrosimone, Angelo, MD
Little Falls
  Ahuja, Kishore Kanayalal, MD
Little Silver
  Dobken, Jeffrey Hall, MD
  Zecca, Tina Concetta, DO
Livingston
  Goodman, Alan Jay, MD
  Weiss, Steven Jay, MD
Mahwah
  Levine, Sheldon Elliot, MD
Manalapan
  De Fusco, Carmine J., MD
Marlton
  Dadhania, Mahendrakumar P., MD
  Gatti, Eugene A., MD
  Kravitz, Elaine K., MD
Medford
  Bantz, Eric W., MD
  Volpe, John Anthony, DO
Mendham
  Jadidi, Shirin, MD
Millville
  Coifman, Robert E., MD
Moorestown
  Lane, Stanley R., MD
Morristown
  Chernack, William J., MD
  Weinreb, Barry D., MD
Mount Laurel
  Kravitz, Stuart A., MD
Mountainside
  Mendelson, Joel S., MD
Newark
  Kanumury, Sunita, MD
  Rescigno, Ronald J., MD
  Schutzer, Steven E., MD
North Bergen
  Dangelo, Salvatore, MD
  Hajee, Feryal, MD
Ocean
  Gross, Gary L., MD
  Sher, Ellen R., MD
Parsippany
  Applebaum, Eric S., MD
  Jampol, Francis Michael, MD
Paterson
  Kosinski, Mark S., MD
  Perin, Patrick V., MD
Paulsboro
  Litz, Steven A., MD
Pennsauken
  Glasofer, Eric David, MD
Randolph
  Reisner, Colin, MD
Ridgewood
  Co, Margaret L., MD
  Slankard, Marjorie L., MD
Riverdale
  Gold, Ruth Leah, MD
Rochelle Park
  Kraut, Evelyn S., MD
Saddle River
  Silverstein, Leonard, MD
Skillman
  Skolnick, Helen Sharlene, MD
Somers Point
  Schwartz, Lawrence A., DO
Somerville
  Krol, Kristine, MD
South Plainfield
  Kothari, Harish B., MD
Springfield
  Bielory, Leonard, MD
Summit
  Brown, David K., MD
Tinton Falls
  Picone, Frank J., MD
Toms River
  Mendoza, Narciso D., MD
  Rabinowitz, Robert P., DO
Totowa
  Ghanem, Roland, MD
Trenton
  Winant, John Jr., MD
  Yang, Jun, MD
Union
  Mahmood, Tariq, MD
Verona
  Fost, Arthur F., MD
  Fost, David A., MD
Vineland
  Perin, Robert J., MD
Voorhees
  Gentlesk, Michael J., MD
Warren
  Wolff, Alan H., MD

Physicians by Specialty and Town

Allergy (cont)
Wayne
Sohn, Theresa J. H., MD
Westfield
Abels, Robert I., MD
Hicks, Patricia Margaret, MD

Allergy & Immunology
Beach Haven
Shields, Mary Susan, MD
Berkeley Heights
Khedkar, Meera, MD
Branchburg
Fox, James A., MD
Bridgewater
Camacho-Halili, Marie M., MD
Cedar Knolls
Graffino, Donatella B., MD
Cherry Hill
Graziano, Linda M., MD
Romanoff, Nicholas A., MD
Clifton
Zanjanian, M. H. Amir, MD
Closter
Minikes, Neil Ira, MD
East Brunswick
Axelrod Malagold, Sara H., MD
East Windsor
Gupta, Neeti, MD
Edgewater
Li, Wei Wei, MD
Englewood
Wanich, Niya, MD
Florham Park
Parikh, Smruti Ashish, MD
Fords
Ogden, Neeta Sharma, MD
Forked River
Empedrad, Raquel B., MD
Freehold
Case, Philip Lawrence, MD
Glen Rock
Blume, Jessica Wanda, MD
Hackensack
Geller, Debora Klein, MD
Mithani, Sima, MD
Selvaggi, Thomas A., MD
Haddonfield
Ku, Min Jung, MD
Highland Park
Gutin, Faina M., MD
Li, Lin, MD
Suliaman, Fawzi A., MD
Witkowska, Renata A., MD
Iselin
Waqar, Shaan M., MD
Kearny
Thomas, Kathleen, MD
Lakewood
Pasternak, Philip Louis, MD
Lawrenceville
Palangio, Kimberly Dawn, MD
Manahawkin
Madden, James M., MD
Marlboro
Sherman, Michael Bruce, MD
Marlton
Toci, Gregory R. Sr., DO
Medford
Kim, John Yohan, MD
Morris Plains
Elias, Salwa E.G., MD
Mount Laurel
Dvorin, Donald J., MD
Goldstein, Marc F., MD
Gordon, Nancy Deborah, MD
New Brunswick
Monteleone, Catherine A., MD
Ocean
Ross, Jacqueline, MD
Paramus
Chang, Cindy Ching, MD
Parsippany
Mehta, Archana P., MD
Red Bank
Hirsch, Andrew C., MD
Riverdale
Patel, Sheenal V., MD
Skillman
Caucino, Julie A., DO

Pedinoff, Andrew J., MD
Rao, Jayanti Juluru, MD
Shah, Shaili Niranjan, MD
Sikorski, Kristen Melissa, MD
Southern, Darrell Loren, MD
Somerville
Druce, Howard M., MD
Trenton
Bobila, Ramon T., MD
Ricketti, Anthony J., MD
Turnersville
Berlin, Paul J., MD
Shah, Paresha Snehal, MD
Verona
Narisety, Satya D., MD
Voorhees
Fiedler, Joel Mark, MD
West Orange
Perlman, Donald Bret, MD
Westfield
Tahzib, Munirih Nura, MD
Woodbridge
Bhambri, Neha Madhok, MD
Mumneh, Nayla Z., MD
Wyckoff
Marotta, Alexander, MD

Anatomic Pathology
Atlantic City
Bansal, Meenakshi, MD
Dantas, Bruno Felipe, MD
Camden
Haupt, Helen M., MD
Eatontown
Wang, Xuan, MD
Edison
Chen, Fan, MD
Elmwood Park
Wang, Luoquan, MD
Florham Park
Savera, Adnan Tabrez, MD
Hackensack
Fix, Daniel Jonas, MD
Hassoun, Patrice, MD
Hamilton Square
Mercer, Stephen Edward, MD
Lakewood
Fromowitz, Frank B., MD
Li, Rongshan, MD
Mahapatro, Darshana, MD
Livingston
Feng, Bo, MD
Montville
Singh, Rajendra Sant, MD
New Brunswick
Grant, Maurice R., MD
Rhodes, Roy Harley, MD
Newark
Aisner, Seena C., MD
Cho, Eun-Sook, MD
Hua, Zhongxue, MD
Mazzella, Fermina Maria, MD
Paramus
Swartz, Jennifer L., DO
Pennington
Jones, Krister J., MD
Plainsboro
Fede, Jean M., DO
Princeton
Kauffman, Patricia Joan, MD
Rahway
Marcantonio, Eugene E., MD
Ridgewood
Eapen, Elizabeth, MD
Teterboro
Gerber, Marina, MD
Kennedy, Harvey Ronald, MD
Pang, Xinzhu, MD
Union
Losada, Mariela, MD
Westfield
Mehta, Rohin, MD

Anatomic/Clinical Pathology
Alpine
Natarajan, Geetha, MD
Wetli, Charles Victor, MD
Atlantic City
Hamel, Marianne, MD
McCormick, John F., MD
Rastgar, Khosrow, MD

Bayonne
Hudacko, Rachel Mary, MD
Belleville
De Leon, Essel Marie B., MD
Primavera, James Michael, MD
Berkeley Heights
Qian, Fang, MD
Bloomfield
Borbon-Reyes, Araceli O., MD
Bordentown
Deluzio, Antonio John, DO
Brick
Baron-Gabriel, Icynth M., MD
Coletta, Umberto, MD
Krumerman, Martin Saul, MD
Rangwala, Anis F., MD
Browns Mills
Schloo, Betsy L., MD
Camden
Enriquez, Miriam Lynn, MD
Holdbrook, Thomas, MD
Joneja, Upasana, MD
Kocher, William D., MD
Rafferty, William J., MD
Ren, Shuyue, MD
Cedar Knolls
Alfonso, Flores, MD
Cherry Hill
Gao, Hong-Guang, MD
Godyn, Janusz J., MD
Liu, Jun, MD
Pavlenko, Andriy, MD
Robinson, Mary J., DO
Cranford
Khan, Amjad A., MD
Qureshi, Mohammad Nasar, MD
Denville
Juco, Judy M., MD
Li, Leonid, MD
Rimarenko, Seraphim, MD
East Orange
Ahmed, Shahida Y., MD
Bowman, Cynthia L., MD
Cai, Donghong, MD
Choe, Jin K., MD
Gupta, Suresh Kumar, MD
Eatontown
Murakata, Linda Ann, MD
Radevic, Miroslav Rade, MD
Sheng, Huaibao, MD
Xie, Linjun, MD
Edison
Finfer, Michael D., MD
Kim, Hazel Hae-sook, MD
Noreen, Shahla, MD
Patil, Madhavi Hari, MD
Elmwood Park
Butala, Rajesh M., MD
Fehrle, Wilfrid Martin, MD
Lee, Po-Shing, MD
Liu, Liang, MD
Pritchett, Danielle Delores, MD
Englewood
Sanchez, Miguel A., MD
Tismenetsky, Mikhail, MD
Ewing
Chmara, Edward S., MD
Fair Lawn
Feldman, Liliya A., MD
Saitas, Vasiliki L., MD
Flemington
Isaac, Irene V., MD
Zanchelli Astran, Gina M., DO
Franklin Lakes
Lawrence, Jeffry Brian, MD
Freehold
Sinha, Karabi, MD
Hackensack
Bhattacharyya, Pritish K., MD
Fehmian, Carol Janice, MD
Han, Min Woo, MD
He, Wenlei, MD
Lengner, Marlene, MD
Li, Jun, MD
Yang, Xiao Yan, MD
Hackettstown
Desiderio, Abelardo C., MD
Hamilton
Briggs, Kari H., MD
Siderits, Richard H., MD

Yang, Dingming, MD
Hawthorne
Vangurp, James Mark Jr., DO
Hoboken
Fayemi, Alfred O., MD
Vaidya, Kamini P., MD
Holmdel
Longo, Stacey L., MD
Iselin
Vora, Jaimini Neeraj, MD
Jackson
Campos, Marite, MD
Jersey City
Das, Kasturi, MD
Khawaja, Asia B., MD
Lin, Qing, MD
Lakewood
Ata, Hadia M., MD
Chatterjee, Monica, MD
Engelbach, Ludmila, MD
Guo, Yijun, MD
Pai, Usha Laxman, MD
Shen, Tingliang, MD
Lawrenceville
Kuehn, Adam, MD
Mechanic, Leslie D., MD
Moser, Robert L., MD
Livingston
Baptist, Selwyn J., MD
Binsol, Ricardo Q., MD
Buckley, Tinera Mcnair, MD
Dardik, Michael, MD
Kim, Dae U., MD
Kintiroglou, Marietta, MD
Mahmood, Ashhad, MD
Ongcapin, Emelie H., MD
Pulinthanathu, Rajiv R., MD
Stueben, Benjamin L., MD
Tortora, Matthew J., MD
Long Branch
Kang, Yong, MD
Loo, Abraham, MD
Szallasi, Arpad, MD
Zhong, Hua, MD
Zinterhofer, Louis J., MD
Milltown
Rimmer, Cheryl L., MD
Montclair
Roy, Manimala, MD
Montville
Raina, Santosh, MD
Morristown
Dise, Craig A., MD
Jaramillo, Marina A., MD
Magidson, Jory G., MD
Meradian, Ara, MD
Mohammed, Raji Hussain, MD
Piotti, Kathryn C., MD
Sung, Diana, MD
Mount Holly
Anand Chawla, Jagjit K., MD
Biondi, Robert J., DO
Manion, William L., MD
Mount Laurel
Grotkowski, Carolyn E., MD
Neptune
Bains, Ashish P. S., MD
Erler, Brian S., MD
Govil, Sushama, MD
Matulewicz, Theodore Joseph, MD
New Brunswick
Barnard, Nicola J., MD
Chaubal, Abhijeet V., MD
Chekmareva, Marina A., MD
Dvorzhinskiy, Olga, MD
Fedorciw, Boris Jaroslaw, MD
Hazra, Anup K., MD
Jaworski, Joseph Mark, MD
Kierson, Malca Ester, DO
Lal, Devika Sandalee, MD
Lessig, Marvin A., DO
Sadimin, Evita T., MD
Salaru, Gratian, MD
Thomas, Sumi Varghese, MD
Weissmann, David J., MD
New Lisbon
Desai, Hemlata K., MD
Newark
Adem, Patricia V., MD
D'Cruz, Cyril A., MD

Dorai,Bhuvaneswari,MD
Fitzhugh,Valerie A.,MD
Gonzalez,Mario Segundo,MD
Jobbagy,Zsolt,MD
Klein,Kenneth Michael,MD
Mirani,Neena M.,MD
Olesnicky,Ludmilla,MD
Panayotov,Panayot Panchev,MD
Parikh,Nalini S.,MD
Perez,Lyla E.,MD
Seguerra,Eliezer Montero Jr.,MD
Tsang,Patricia Chiu-Wun,MD
Ye,Michelle,MD
Zhang,Alex Xun,MD
North Bergen
Zhang,Qi,MD
North Brunswick
Falzon,Andrea,MD
Norwood
Rijhwani,Kiran,MD
Nutley
Dimov,Nikolay D.,MD
Oradell
Nasr,Sherif Abbas,MD
Rahman,Saud Saqib,MD
Paramus
DiCarlo,Frederick J.,MD
Garcia-Lat,Zenda,MD
Turyan,Hach Vladimir,MD
Parsippany
Suffin,Stephen Chester,MD
Passaic
Bassil,Ghassan G.,MD
Setoodeh,Farhad,MD
Pennington
Liu,Edward Shaoyou,MD
Perth Amboy
Tan,Kong L.,MD
Phillipsburg
Brown,John M.,MD
Piscataway
Yurchenco,Peter,MD
Plainsboro
Arslan,Asima,MD
Shanahan,Eileen Marie,MD
Zhang,Lanjing,MD
Princeton
Berman,David M.,MD
Princeton Junction
Liu,Qiang,MD
Rahway
Benisch,Barry M.,MD
Gistrak,Michael Andrew,MD
Ramsey
Aponte,Sandra Leonora,MD
Brown,Jeffrey G.,MD
Ilario,Marius John-Marc,MD
Joseph,John K.,MD
Liu,Zach Zhiguang,MD
Szeto,Oliver Jo-Yang,MD
Raritan
Hall,Alvin J.,MD
Moniem,Howayda A.,MD
Red Bank
Dukuly,Zwannah D.,MD
Farooq,Taliya,MD
Gong,Ping,MD
Gupta,Namita J.,MD
Leschhorn,Edwin C.,MD
Ridgewood
Brandt,Suzanne Marie,MD
Christiano,Arthur A.,MD
Mazziotta,Robert M.,MD
Reilly,Michael H.,MD
Taskin,Metin,MD
Saddle Brook
Ye,Dongjiu,MD
Saddle River
Saviano,Nicole,MD
Short Hills
Tan,Jianyou,MD
Somers Point
Beach,Robert J.,MD
Pond,James M.,MD
Saunders,Peter J.,MD
Somerville
Chen,Tsuey-Ling,MD
D'Aguillo,Anthony F.,MD
Gonsorcik,Victoria K.,DO

Southampton
Della Croce,David R.,DO
Stratford
DeRisio,Vincent James II,DO
Summit
Al Dulaimi,Hamsa A.,MD
Labat,Mona Farah,MD
Pai,Prabha B.,MD
Teaneck
Babury,Rahima A.,MD
Fish,Heidi,MD
Olsen,Drew Albert,MD
Schainker,Bruce Allan,MD
Teterboro
Alt,Elaine R.,MD
Ayer,Uma,MD
Bayard-McNeeley,Marise,MD
Eftychiadis,Angela S.,MD
Gallo,Leza N.,MD
Iskaros,Basem F.,MD
Kaufman,Harvey Willard,MD
Limaye,Anjali P.,MD
Liu-Jarin,Xiaolin,MD
Luff,Ronald David,MD
Mahmood,Afsar,MD
Malhotra,Chanchal Anand,MD
Niu,Weiwei,MD
Tamas,Ecaterina F.,MD
Tarr,William Ellsworth Jr.,MD
Tsao,Lawrence,MD
Vinod,Sheela U.,MD
Yohannan,Wendy S.,MD
Zhang,Yiqiu,MD
Toms River
Ibrahim,Ghassan Jerjous,MD
Lapis,Peter,MD
Romberger,Charles Frank,MD
Trenton
Kim,Yung H.,MD
Union
Bentley,James David,MD
Cabreros,Antonio T.,MD
Dinu,Veronica Carmen,MD
Riba,Ali K.,MD
Verona
Horenstein,Marcelo G.,MD
Vineland
Mapow,Larry S.,MD
Voorhees
Lembert Tezanos,Larissa,MD
McFarland,Miles M.,MD
Obando,David A.,MD
Skarinsky,Evgenya,MD
Warren
Jiang,Tony T.,MD
Sapanara,Nancy Lauren,MD
Wayne
Kaptain,Stamatina,MD
Wu,Yihui Yvonne,MD
Westampton
Ragasa,Dante A.,MD
Willingboro
Choi,Hong Y.,MD
Maguire,Randall F.,MD
Woodbine
Hashish,Hisham A.,MD
Woodbury
Gala,Indira H.,MD
Moore,Cheryl Crowley,MD
Wrightstown
McGinnis,Michael Clifton,MD

Anesthesiology
Atlantic City
Crompton,Thomas F.,MD
Droney,Timothy J. III,MD
Marable,Denise Marie,MD
Morsi,Khaled M.,MD
Pinz,Alexandra,MD
Shah,Sudha S.,MD
Takla,Magdy F.G.,MD
Zalman,Richard,MD
Barnegat
Frank,Howard,MD
Bayonne
Alekseyeva,Irina,MD
Ancevska Taneva,Natasa,MD
Canals-Ferrat,Pedro,MD
Fersel,Jordan S.,MD
Hanna,Mamdouh Soliman,MD
Hashemi,Zaher Mohammad Said,MD

Klein,Ira A.,MD
Morgenstern,Alvin Harris,MD
Steinman,Edward A.,MD
Belleville
Bada,Laureto Jr.,MD
Choi,Bong H.,MD
Cizmar,Stephan,MD
Concepcion,Cleo L.,MD
De Trespalacios,Jose A.,DO
Eisele,Joseph Carl,DO
Gerges,Maged Moussa,MD
Khan,Muhammad B.H.,MD
Lao,Jocelyn M.,MD
Marcus,Jennifer,MD
Rejowska-Cedrowski,Jolanta,MD
Bergenfield
Rechenberg,Geoffrey Mark,MD
Blackwood
Sabia,Michael,MD
Boonton
Caruthers,Samuel Grenville,MD
Brick
Barone,Frank Anthony,MD
Bean,David E.,MD
Gantner,Mark,MD
Higgins,James Martin,MD
Jasper,Gabriele P.,MD
Mangonon,Virgilio D.,MD
Reid,Kenneth M.,MD
Shah,Kalpana N.,MD
Singh,Manjula,MD
Swinger,Alan Bennett,DO
Zhou,Lingbin,MD
Browns Mills
Dateshidze,Konstantin,MD
Guarini,Vincent,MD
Khawaja,Hasan Sajjad,MD
Moore,Roger A.,MD
Neary,Michael J.,MD
Camden
Armstrong,James M.,MD
Bolkus,Kelly Ann,DO
Burden,Amanda R.,MD
Cassotis,Maria,DO
Deal,Edward R.,DO
Deangelis,Matthew Michael,DO
Desai,Ronak G.,DO
Dippo,Grace E.,MD
Ganguly,Kingsuk,MD
Ghaul,Mark R.,MD
Goldberg,Michael E.,MD
Gollotto,Michael R.,DO
Gourkanti,Bharathi,MD
Gratz,Irwin,DO
Habib,Fatimah,MD
Hasher-Mascoveto,Wendy M.,DO
Hirsh,Robert Alan,MD
Hsu,George Chiahung,MD
Hughes,Wray,DO
Khan,Asim Haleem,MD
Kushner,Randy Scott,DO
Lin,En-Su,MD
Lutwin Kawalec,Malgorzata S.,MD
Misbin,Michael David,MD
Mitrev,Ludmil Vladimirov,MD
Monticollo,Gerard M.,DO
Munoz,Raul,MD
Muntazar,Muhammad,MD
Nathan,Ponnudurai,MD
Patel,Kinjal M.,MD
Potestio,Christopher Paul,MD
Rinnier,Robert Todd,DO
Romisher,Robert J.,DO
Safaryn,John E.,MD
Schwartz,Michael,MD
Seabron-Rambert,Cheryl,MD
Shazly,Amin,MD
Trautman,Natalie,MD
Trivedi,Keyur Chandrakant,MD
Wnek,Gary E.,MD
Yong,Jinghong,MD
Cape May Court House
Barth,Holli Ami,MD
Dragon,Greg R.,MD
Patel,Ashokkumar J.,MD
Patel,Hareshbhai C.,MD
Tarantino,David P.,MD
Cedar Grove
Shah,Kusum J.,MD
Cedar Knolls
Shrem,Leslie Allen,MD

Solomonov,Mikhail,MD
Chatham
Blumenfeld,Daniel J.,MD
Cherry Hill
Carr,Alan D.,DO
Grosh,Taras,MD
Heyman,David Mark,DO
Kerner,Michael B.,DO
Lamprou,Emanuel Jr.,MD
Lu,Cheh Shiung,DO
Young,Marie Lisette,MD
Cinnaminson
Andalft,Anthony C.,MD
Assiamah,Andrew Aboagye,MD
Bowie,Lester J.,MD
Chun,John Y.,MD
Cypel,David,MD
Daniels,James W. III,MD
Feinerman,Larry Robert,MD
Goldberg,Marc B.,MD
Gordon,Jeffrey,MD
Gray,Terence Bay,MD
Halevy,Jonathan D.,MD
Kor,Danuta C.,MD
Law,Henry,DO
Lee,John C.,MD
Litvack,Steven Greg,MD
Luetke,Brian Scott,DO
Misher-Harris,Michele,DO
Paterson,William D.,MD
Shapiro,Jeffrey L.,MD
Shetty,Phyllis J.,MD
Siri,Matthew A.,MD
Soremekun Salami,Olutoyin M.,MD
Starrett-Keller,Cheryl M.,MD
Vaughn,Michelle Marie,MD
Waters,Renee M.,MD
Weiss,Evan A.,DO
Cliffside Park
Pancu,Ion V.,MD
Clifton
Agarwal,Meenoo,MD
Ames-Bobila,Deborah,MD
Anannab,Kevin C.,MD
Dang,Saurabh,MD
De La Mota,Jessica Isabel,DO
Kang,Richard T.,MD
Koppel,Todd Sloan,MD
Nasiek,Dariusz Jacek,MD
Popa,Vincentiu,MD
Shah,Sachin K.,MD
Shapiro,Leonid,MD
Sheikh,Afzal J.,MD
Sinha,Binod P.,MD
Sinha,Neil,MD
Szczech,Kazimierz M.,MD
Tankha,Pavan,DO
Closter
Grunstein,Erno,MD
Demarest
Blackman,Bonnie E.,MD
Denville
Annadanam,Varalakshmi,MD
Caguicla-Cruz,Natividad M.,MD
Dent,Dean A.,MD
Ho,Maggie May,DO
Kleiner,Alexander,MD
Krzanowski,Tracey J.,MD
Mistry,Bharati S.,MD
Rubinfeld,Philip J.,MD
Shiau,Horngfu,MD
Specthrie,Leon Kotler,MD
Sy,Nena L.,MD
Wang,Changzhen,MD
Zembrzuski,Andrzej Jan,MD
Zhou,Jie,MD
Zhu,Ching,MD
Dumont
Raziuddin,Mazherunni,MD
East Brunswick
Basilious,Manal,MD
Levin,Alexander G.,MD
Meltz,Marcy Mencher,MD
Weinstein,Craig M.,MD
Yama,Asher Z.,MD
Zedie,Nishat,MD
East Hanover
Patel,Divya R.,MD
East Orange
Wong,Jeanne,MD

Physicians by Specialty and Town

Anesthesiology (cont)

East Windsor
Ali, Rehan Basharat, MD
Eatontown
Staats, Nancy Elizabeth, MD
Edgewater
Regan, Kasey Calvey, MD
Edison
Armao, Michael Edward, MD
Beyus, Christopher Michael, MD
Chen, Evan, MD
Daftari, Amita P., MD
Daniel, Robert J., MD
Ding, Yifeng, MD
Gudimella, Lakshmi, MD
Guena, Luisa, MD
Handa Nayyar, Seema, DO
Isidro, Jose R. Jr., MD
Klyashtorny, Alexander, MD
Kothari, Kaumudi H., MD
Lee, Herb, MD
Li, Xin Qin, MD
Mereday, Clifton Samuel Jr., MD
Moises, Adam U. Jr., DO
Montefusco, Patrick P., MD
Pandya, Shridevi, MD
Patel, Bhupendrakumar V., MD
Patel, Shail, MD
Piratla, Lalitha, MD
Rock, Joel J., DO
Safdar, Mohammad Imran, MD
Samaan, Ayman Boushra, MD
Santos-Holgado, Maria C., MD
Siskind, Jonathan B., DO
Stewart, Judly Pierre, MD
Tan, Martin H., MD
Thompson, Matthew, MD
Utrankar, Deepti Sameer, MD
Zhang, Shehui, MD
Egg Harbor City
Martin, Sheryel Denise, MD
Egg Harbor Township
Zhu, Yun, MD
Elizabeth
Adam, Abir Moustafa, MD
Carvalho, Steven Evaristo, MD
Cyriac, James Ignatius, MD
Myers, Khaleah K., MD
Nepomuceno, Kathleen Chiong, MD
Pakalnis, Regina, MD
Phan, Lily, MD
Pirak, Leon, MD
Reddy, Padmavathi, MD
Shen, Edward, MD
Vassilidze, Teimouraz V., MD
Zaitsev, Alexander Alexeevic, MD
Elmer
DeLeon, Edgardo S., MD
Jones, Angela Marie, MD
Elmwood Park
Manspeizer, Heather Eve, MD
Sangavaram, Kristappa, MD
Schlesinger, James M., MD
Shin, Kyung Hee, MD
Tendler, Jay M., MD
Yu, Yun S., MD
Emerson
Patel, Anil Jayant, MD
Englewood
Baltaytis, Viktor, MD
Berth, Ulrike, MD
Betta, Joanne, MD
Borow, Leslie Bennett, MD
Chan, Rolycito A., MD
Chen, Wen-Hong, MD
Chithran, Payyanadan V., MD
Deluty, Sheldon H., MD
Digiacomo, Michael B., MD
Dvir, David, MD
Epstein, David Israel, MD
Gak, Alexander V., MD
Goldzweig, Peter Allan, DO
Guillaume, Stephanie Ann, MD
Huber, Michael D., DO
Kaganovskaya, Margarita, MD
Kipnis, Ilana Ariel, DO
Kulkarni, Sumedha V., MD
Lee, Louis Young, MD
Lobel, Gregg P., MD
Lui, John, MD
Metro, Wade E., MD

Mizrahi, Marc E., MD
Moonka, Neeta K., MD
Moskowitz, David Matthew, MD
Pandya, Vrunda H., MD
Pappalardo, Rebecca A., MD
Perelman, Seth I., MD
Popa, Peter R., MD
Puzio, Thomas, MD
Shander, Aryeh, MD
Smok, Jeffrey Thomas, MD
St. Jean, Monika Kulkarni, MD
Thomas, Vinoo Sebastian, MD
Volpe, Lorraine, MD
Englewood Cliffs
Povzhitkov, Igor Moiseyevi, MD
Ward, Wendy Allison, MD
Yu, David H., MD
Fair Lawn
Owsiak, Joanne Naamo, MD
Prakhina, Boris, MD
Srinivasan, Deepak, MD
Flemington
Bentley, William Earl IV, DO
Bussard, Elizabeth S., MD
Cabahug, Wilfred Tan, MD
Lai, Chia-Lung, MD
Lapicki, Walter S., DO
Maldonado-Viera, Lourdes, MD
Nagorny, Wojciech Antoni, MD
Nyitray, Peter, MD
Silber, Michael B., DO
Wang, Edward, MD
Wilson, John Joseph, MD
Florham Park
Abramowicz, Apolonia E., MD
Ahmad, Idrees, MD
Asimolowo, Olabisi Omolara, MD
Basius, Joseph T., DO
Bergam, Miro Nicholas Jr., MD
Blank, Jonathan Dirk, MD
Bonsell, Joshua W., MD
Braverman, Joel Morton, MD
Cardoso, Ronald J., MD
Chen, Jianping, MD
Chung, Dae S., MD
Ciolino, Robert B., MD
Clancy, Lisa A., MD
Co, Demosthene E., MD
Conyack, David G., DO
Davis, Clifton Colby, MD
Dibadj, Khosro, MD
Fein, Eric N., MD
Fisher, Emery IV, DO
Fitz, Rachel Myra, DO
Ganti, Suryaprakash, MD
Goldstein, Joshua D., MD
Hausdorff, Mark Alan, MD
Ju, Albert Changwon, MD
Kim, Mina Jung, MD
Knepa, Valdone Elena, MD
Levine, Robert Scott, MD
Maizes, Allen Stuart, MD
Monti, Richard A., MD
Parikh, Bijal Rajendra, MD
Patafio, Onofrio, MD
Patel, Prashant A., MD
Pond, Charles G., MD
Ramos, Joseph, MD
Russo, Cathy Marie, MD
Scala, Peter L., MD
Zylberger, David A., MD
Fort Lee
Basak, Jayati, MD
Chiang, Kou-Cheng, MD
Desai, Jagdip, MD
Friedman, Gina Y., DO
Grigorescu, Traian Andrei, MD
Lin, Cheng Hsiang, MD
Lustig, Karen C., DO
Ohanian, Marc S., MD
Ostrovsky, Igor, MD
Park, Yong M., MD
Franklin Lakes
Ashraf, Waseem, MD
Blady, Joseph A., MD
Lee, Jung Du, MD
Freehold
Armbrecht, Kimberley T., MD
Campagnuolo, Joann E., DO
Connors, Anne, MD
Cubina, Maria L., DO

DeAntonio, Joseph Alexander, MD
Deshmukh, Poornima Vasudeo, MD
Fahmy, Nader M., MD
Ghattas, Maged L., MD
Grace, Rashy, MD
Kumar, Nirmal A., MD
Mak, John, MD
Mehta, Hemangini G., MD
Mikhail, Magdy H., MD
O'Hara, Michael W., DO
Parikh, Pallavi M., MD
Patel, Jayshree R., MD
Proban, Rafal, MD
Randall, Tanya, MD
Scarmato, Albert Clark Jr., DO
Soriano, Brian J., MD
Stabile, Daniel, MD
Stump, James Basil, MD
Zachary, Samuel, DO
Galloway
Cerniglia, Salvatore Joseph, DO
Kasica, Patricia R., DO
Gibbsboro
Gellman, Marc D., MD
Glen Ridge
Parikh, Sanjiv R., MD
Guttenberg
Romero, Alejandro, MD
Hackensack
Baratta, Jerry M., DO
Block, Michael, MD
Boral, Andrew S., MD
Caloustian, Marie-Louise, MD
Choi, Jong Eui, MD
Ciongoli, Bernard C., DO
Cohen, Randy Scott, MD
Cortazzo, Jessica A., MD
Cullen, Michael E., MD
Cuttitta, Jerome D., MD
Dalal, Bhavna P., MD
Datta, Samyadev, MD
DeRemigio, David Michael, DO
Diaz, Lloyd P., MD
Dragone, Daniel Claudio, MD
Dragone, Sergio D., MD
Eck, Philip Ofosu, MD
Eskinazi, Daniel, MD
Fam, Alfred M., MD
Frazer, Keith Evan, DO
Friedlander, Jeffrey Dean, MD
Girnar, Digvijaysi, MD
Grech, Dennis George, MD
Hammonds, Charles Dewey, MD
Hessert, Eva Marie, MD
Hirth, Thomas G., MD
Horn, Russell J., MD
Huang, Chien-Yao, MD
Hummel, Andrew E., DO
Jardosh, Kunal Rashmin, MD
Karpinos, Robert D., MD
Kehar, Mira, MD
Klauss, Gunnar, MD
Kwon, Minho, MD
Leslie, Joanne, MD
Li, John Yi-huang, MD
Mandhle, Pankaja Anil, MD
Marasigan, Mariza E., MD
Martin, Megan Blake, MD
McTigue, Maureen A., DO
Merle, Francois, MD
Milic, Milija, MD
Morsy, Amr Sayed, MD
Munoz, Daisy, MD
Neugeborn, Ian Scott, MD
Nolasco, Cesar V., MD
Nolasco, Edwin V., MD
Oloomiyazdi, Mohammadali, MD
Olsen, Janet L., MD
Paganessi, Monica A., DO
Paganessi, Steven Andrew, MD
Palmer, Thalia Christine, MD
Parikh, Anant Parimal, MD
Reddy, Matt Medapati, MD
Saad, Mohamed Ali, MD
Sajous, Jocelyne, MD
Saladini, Vincent Jr., MD
Salgado, Fredy R., MD
Sanders, Paul, MD
Sarier, Kaya K., MD
Schlesinger, Mark D., MD
Scott, Nancy Michelle, MD
Seem, Eric H., MD

Semanczuk, William Paul, MD
Sen, Surjya, MD
Sharma, Veena, MD
Shindler, Maria Danielle, MD
Shorshtein, Alexander, MD
Shulman, Michael, MD
Thongrod, Sumena C., DO
Topfer, Steven Alan, DO
Van Beever, Jordan Grant, MD
Vidaver, Patrick S., MD
Weiss-Bloom, Leslie J., MD
Weitzman, Stephen M., MD
Wesley, Carl Christopher, MD
Wu, Duoping, MD
Wu, Jing, MD
Xagoraris, Andreas E., MD
Hackettstown
Dierlam, Paul T., MD
Wu, Daniel C., MD
Haddon Heights
Cataldo, Ralph G., DO
Haddonfield
Mroz, Lynne A., MD
Polise, Pamela Ann, MD
Hainesport
Rastogi, Abhijeet A., MD
Slevin, Kieran Anthony, MD
Hamilton
Dashow, Susan M., DO
Feder, Craig A., MD
Ghabious, Emad Faiek, MD
Gordon, Michael Stuart, MD
Ibrahim, Maher, MD
Loren, Gary M., MD
Mahoney, John J., DO
Mandel, Robert, MD
Sanchez, Israel L., MD
Spiteri, Andrew, MD
Suaco, Benjamin S., MD
Zwick, Annette E., MD
Hamilton Square
Chung, Soo K., MD
Hammonton
Manabat, Eileen Rose, MD
Harrington Park
Patel, Chandrakant, MD
Hillsborough
Das, Vivek T., MD
Hoboken
Aggarwal, Mukta, MD
Avery, William Bradford, MD
Blumenthal, David C., MD
Kao, Sen-Pin, MD
Kyin, Robin, MD
Lee, Brian, DO
Lee, Peter Yen-lai, MD
Mead, John Edward, MD
Perez, Reynaldo T., MD
Punzalan, Maria M., MD
Rafer, Ramon V., MD
Whiteru, Uvie Christina, MD
Yap, Joseph Jim Estrella, MD
Holmdel
Bruk, George, MD
Citron, Andrew M., MD
Dhawlikar, Sunita Sripad, MD
Faelnar, Luis B., MD
Foroush, Pejman, MD
Girgis, Magdy S., MD
Handlin, David S., MD
Leung, Samson W., MD
Macklin, Joshua M., MD
McNair, Timothy P., MD
Milan, Ronald Kenneth, MD
Hopatcong
Sobrepena, Jose S.M., MD
Iselin
Pitchford, Douglas Edward, MD
Jersey City
Asamoah, Francis E., MD
Aventurado, Tito O., MD
Awad, Ahmed Sayed, MD
Chen, Donghui, MD
Dadaian, Susan, DO
DeGuzman, Richelle T., MD
Leggat, Christopher Scott, MD
Lin, Yuhlin, MD
Lory, John Douglas, MD
Mathew, Thomas, MD
Moy, Jonathan M., MD
Naik, Ravi, MD

Physicians by Specialty and Town

Pham,Michael Minh,MD
Reiss,Jodi L. W.,MD
Rodriguez,Liza A.,MD
Salimi-Ghezelbash,Behzad,MD
Scinas,Athanasios,MD
Shah,Amit A.,MD
Shih,Duen S.,MD
Sood,Monica,MD
Wu,Jung-Faug,MD
Zaklama,Selvia G.,MD
Zhou,Ben Yuan,MD
Kearny
Bleiweiss,Warren J.,MD
Kenilworth
Siddiqui,Afzaal Ahmad,MD
Kinnelon
Deutsch,Jonathan S.,MD
Lakewood
Bermudez,Juan D.,MD
Edelmann,Robert Benedict Jr.,MD
Viradia,Jayant K.,MD
Leonia
Ostrovskaya,Inna Dmytrievna,MD
Lincoln Park
Louvier,Ambra,MD
Lindenwold
Copeland,Marcia A.,MD
Gupta,Anita,DO
Linwood
Barbella,Joseph D.,DO
Livingston
Dumbroff,Steven A.,MD
Fan,Foun-Chung,MD
Fox,Jerry C.,MD
Goldstein,Elisabeth Rachel,MD
Gourishankar,Ruplanaik,MD
Hurley,Kathleen Lenore,MD
Ioffe,Michail,MD
Kalinine,Viatcheslav,MD
Klebba,Kevin Edmund,MD
Kulkarni,Mohan H.,MD
Leaf,Daniel Craig,MD
Mazur,Wieslaw L.,MD
McKeon,John J.,MD
Myneni,Neelima,MD
O'Mahony,Christopher James,MD
Pak,Hang R.,DO
Pamaar,Cristina G.,MD
Patankar,Srikanth S.,MD
Patel,Nimesh R.,MD
Pitera,Richard Jr.,MD
Qian,Qiubing,MD
Rafizadeh,Mehrad,MD
Ramundo,Giovanni B.,MD
Reichard,Peter Seth,MD
Rimal,Jyotsna,MD
Rodriguez,Emmanuel,MD
Sattari,Rouzbeh,MD
Shanker,Soma,MD
Tewfik,George L.,MD
Tompkins,Marianne J.,DO
Trespicio,Rogelio T.,MD
Vallee,Michael F.,DO
Vaskul,Roksolana,MD
Zulueta,Erica,DO
Long Branch
Anisetti,Vimlesh K.,MD
Belsh,Yitzhak,MD
Du,Bing,MD
Elango,Sitalakshmi,MD
Eraky,Waheed K.,MD
Fisher,Scott Robert,MD
Flashburg,Michael H.,MD
Friedman,Susan R.,MD
Gomez,Jose F.,MD
Greaves,Keiron W.,MD
Greenberg,Eric N.,MD
Johnson,Judith Ann,MD
Klein,Matthew Seth,MD
Kramer,David C.,MD
Molbegott,Debra J.,DO
Molbegott,Lester P.,MD
Nosker,Geoffrey S.,MD
Omotoso,Babatunji Omolagba,MD
Para,Vijaya L.,MD
Patel,Nilesh J.,MD
Shah,Lopa Suryakant,MD
Spruell,Joshua Lyn,MD
Zlotnick,Matthew Phillip,MD
Lumberton
Balzer,Frederick J.,MD

Pollak,Kevin Henry,MD
Mahwah
Gonzalez,Jaime Abel,MD
Manahawkin
Barton,Keith A.,DO
Bouyea,Michelle Marie,MD
Guo,Jianhua,MD
Hanna,Sherine Farag,MD
Manevich,Ilya,MD
Marco,James Victor,MD
Richlan,Richard A.,MD
Siciliano,Louis J.,MD
Tse,James T.C.,MD
Yampaglia,Joseph P.,MD
Manalapan
Atkin,Stuart R.,MD
Elenewski,John Francis,MD
Manasquan
Beutel,Jonathan A.,MD
Rienzo,Peter A.,MD
Maplewood
He,Ningning,MD
Marlboro
Messa,Stephanie Price,MD
Shehata,Sanaa K.,MD
Marlton
Avella,David Paul,MD
Bilgrami,Sajad Syed,DO
Bravyak,James G.,DO
Chityala,Haritha,MD
Chu,Brian,MD
Grossman,Davida S.,MD
Hermann,Todd G.,MD
Iula,Frank J. Jr.,MD
Jiang,Heng,MD
Karanzalis,Demetrius,DO
Kasarda,Frances E.,MD
Knoll,Frank J. III,MD
Kwon,Alan Fay,MD
Lee,Aland H.,MD
Lehrer,Luisa E.,MD
Lewin,Stacy B.,MD
Liccini,Mark Stephen,DO
Lingaraju,Rajiv,MD
Lynch,Jeffrey R.,MD
McIntyre,Bryan J.,DO
Modi,Parag,MD
Morgan,Kathleen A.,MD
Nduaguba,Chiazoka Onyeka,MD
O'Connor,Patrick,MD
Pace,Enrico,MD
Padula,Vincent M.,DO
Pascarella,Michael Ryan,DO
Pierre,Andre M.,MD
Pisera,Donna M.,MD
Pober,Neil J.,MD
Quint,James Douglas,MD
Reichman,Cynthia M.,MD
Reilly,Dennis K.,DO
Ressler,Steven H.,MD
Ricketts,Robyn D.,MD
Santos,Francis Parrocho,MD
Sperandio,Peter G.N.,MD
Villamayor,Carlos Pestelos,MD
Maywood
Villegas,Robert A.,MD
Medford
Hanna,Amir,MD
Lennon,Christine Marie,MD
Mickleton
Patterson,Raymond Kevin,MD
Middletown
Atlas,Gayle,DO
Champey,Edward John,MD
McGuire,Kimberly Marie,MD
Millburn
De Mais,John R.,MD
Stillman,Richard I.,MD
Verea,Vickie,MD
Monroe
Arabi,Mona Najib,MD
Shen,Mengmeng,MD
Montclair
Barr,Gary Alan,MD
Kerven,Elliot Sean,MD
Martinez,Richard,MD
Shahsamand,Zabi Z.,MD
Yacoub,Magdy Yousef,MD
You,Jerome H.,MD
Young,Michael Anthony,MD

Montville
Hsieh,Ching C.,MD
Moorestown
Cwik,Jason Charles,MD
Elia,Anna,MD
Husain,Mansoor Ul-Haque,MD
Junior,John L.,MD
Madison,Anoja Bala,DO
Sattel,Lisa E.,MD
Morganville
Caruso,Marco F.,MD
Chung,Sung K.,MD
Piskun,Jacob,MD
Morris Plains
De Santis,Fiorita G.,DO
Itzkovich,Chad Jason,MD
Koplik,Andrew D.,MD
Morristown
Abkin,Arkadiy,MD
Armstrong,Aileen S.,MD
Armstrong,Patrick Andrew,MD
Barbieri,Louise T.,MD
Barry,Kevin M.,MD
Brusco,Louis Jr.,MD
Chen,Cindy H.,MD
Chern,Sy-Yeu Sue,MD
Chiumento,Marvin Joseph,MD
Chow,Matthew S.T.,MD
Chung,Daniel Hansam,MD
Cohen,Dale L.,MD
Crosta,Alan Michael Jr.,MD
Fitzgerald,Timothy E.,MD
Kapadia,Cyrus Baji,MD
Kazim,Debra Ann,MD
Koranyi,Peter,MD
Kothari,Jay,MD
Kwon,Christopher J.,MD
LaBove,Phillip S.,MD
Lapchak,John T.,MD
Lawson,Charles Alexander,MD
Lefever,Gerald S.,MD
Lewis,Walter Michael,MD
Linz,Stephan M.,MD
Longworth-Gatto,Lisa E.,DO
McDonnell,Thomas E.,MD
Merchant,Sameer R.,MD
Murray,Thomas Robert,MD
Panah,Michael Hormoz,MD
Riabov,Keith A.,MD
Rosenbaum,Lee M.,MD
Rubinfeld,Julie A.,MD
Rudman,Michael E.,MD
Shin,Pheodora L.,MD
Sieber,James Curtis,MD
Spiteri,Isaac Daniel,MD
Stennett,Richard A.,MD
Streicher,James Tabb,MD
Taylor,Guy Adrian,MD
Voinov,Luba A.,MD
Watson,Todd A.,MD
Weiner,Steven Martin,MD
Welsh,Terrence Mathew,MD
Winne,Richard P. Jr.,MD
Wu,Eileen Pey Chi,MD
Mount Holly
Ajmal,Muhammad Zafar,MD
Baron,Leah,MD
Bhagat,Anilchandra I.,MD
Dhru,Sahil H.,DO
Ferrari,Albert N.,MD
Gargiulo,Richard F.,MD
Gollapudi,Praveen Choudary,MD
Gumnit,Robert Y.,MD
Gupta,Rakesh Chander,MD
Kalariya,Rupal S.,MD
Lachenal,Edgardo N.,MD
Marcelo,Edmund,DO
Mendel,Howard G.,MD
Nyzio,Joseph Bruno,DO
Schwartz,Joshua J.,MD
Shah,Azam,DO
Tatz,Mark A.,MD
Thaler,Adam M.,DO
Thornton,Robin W.,MD
Mount Laurel
Buck,Gary B.,MD
Chekemian,Beth Ann,DO
Haleem,Burhan,DO
Lesneski,Matthew J.,MD
Shah,Manish,MD

Mountainside
Fisher,Margaret Elizabeth,MD
Lum,Kenneth,MD
Papa,Louis,MD
Pillon,Mark A.,MD
Rinehouse,Jay A.,MD
Mullica Hill
Shelchkov,Dmitry A.,MD
Neptune
Berberich,Matthew Robert,MD
Cammarata,Lindsay,MD
Cindrario,Dean P.,MD
Elsakka,Maha Fathy,MD
Fianko,Felix Akwasi-Owusu,MD
Fields,Ryan G.,DO
Kalliny,Mohsen Ayad,MD
Miller,Kevin D.,MD
Morgan,Illiana Alexandrova,MD
Morgan,Mina Adel,DO
Ndeto,Geoffrey Wambua T.,MD
Nicholas,Thomas,MD
Patel,Hansa S.,MD
Patel,Nehul S.,MD
Rahal,William J.,MD
Ray Jr,Barry Keith,MD
Reffler,Marie M.,MD
Sedutto,Joseph Mario,MD
Steenland,Richard H.,MD
Varghese,Sherin V.,MD
Wu,Jeffrey P.,MD
Yang,Zhaomin,MD
Zhao,Rong,MD
Neptune City
Amoroso,Michael Louis,MD
New Brunswick
Alloteh,Rose Sitsofe,MD
Ambalu,Oren,MD
Barsoum,Sylviana S.,MD
Berman,Stefanie L.,MD
Bermann,Mordechai,MD
Chhokra,Renu,MD
Chi,Oak Z.,MD
Chintapalli,Nirmala K.,MD
Chiricolo,Antonio,MD
Chyu,Darrick J.,MD
Cirella,Vincent N.,MD
Cohen,Shaul,MD
Cowell,Jennifer L.,MD
Curcio,Christine Marie,MD
De Angelis,Vincent James,MD
Denenberg,Howard W.,MD
Denny,John T.,MD
Enlow,Tracey S.,MD
Fratzola,Christine Hunter,MD
Fullenkamp,Mark P.,MD
George,Gina,DO
Ginsberg,Steven H.,MD
Grayer,Nicole C.,MD
Grayson,Jeremy Seth,MD
Grubb,William R.,MD
Hall,Dennis B.,MD
He,Xiaoli,MD
Jan,Thomas,MD
Kandra,Arun M.,MD
Khan,Ibraheem,MD
Kiel,Samuel Yol,MD
Kiss,Geza Kalmar,MD
Klein,Sanford L.,MD
Kraidin,Jonathan L.,MD
Lee,Isidore C.,MD
Lelyanov,Oleksiy,DO
Lin,Ying Bang,MD
Mabry,Christian Carl,MD
Mai,Quynh-Tien,MD
McRae,Valerie A.,MD
Mehta,Tejal H.,MD
Mungekar,Sagar Sudhir,MD
Nanavati,Neeraj K.,MD
Nandal,Dharamveer,MD
Nelson-Lane,Leigh A.,MD
Neustadt,Charles M.,MD
Pantin,Enrique Jose,MD
Papp,Denes,MD
Patel,Arpit Nayan,MD
Perosi,Joseph J.,MD
Radhakrishnan,Radhika,MD
Rah,Kang H.,MD
Rao,Malini Bhagavathi,MD
Reformato,Vincent,MD
Ridley,Diane M.,MD
Shah,Shruti A.,MD
Shah,Trishna Kirit,MD

Physicians by Specialty and Town

Anesthesiology (cont)

New Brunswick
- Siddiqi, Kashif Inam, MD
- Sison, Edwin Ruan Racela, MD
- Solina, Alann R., MD
- Stein, Mark Herbert, MD
- Tanaka, Sho, MD
- Taylor, Jamie Latiolais, MD
- Thaker, Jayeshkumar, MD
- Veksler, Boris, MD
- Wang, Monty H.S., MD
- Wu, Melissa S., MD
- Zuker-Silberberg, Dora D., MD

New Vernon
- Sheren, Lorne B., MD

Newark
- Abadi, Bilal, MD
- Amuluru, Prabhakara, MD
- Atlas, Glen Mark, MD
- Aziz, Rania, MD
- Berger, Jay Steven, MD
- Botea, Andrei, MD
- Burducea, Alexandru, DO
- Capalbo, Vincent J., MD
- Chan, Jose R., MD
- Chaudhry, Faraz A., MD
- Chen, Dong, MD
- Chinn, Lawrence W. Sr., MD
- Delphin, Ellise S., MD
- Discepola, Patrick Joseph, MD
- Eloy, Jean D., MD
- Estrada, Christian, MD
- Freda, John Jeffrey, MD
- Gajewski, Michael M., DO
- Goldstein, Sheldon, MD
- Grant, Geordie P., MD
- Grewal, Harpreet Singh, MD
- Gubenko, Yuriy Aronovich, MD
- Jackson, Douglas T., MD
- Jhaveri, Lajwanti R., MD
- Katz, John W. Jr., MD
- Kaufman, Andrew Greg, MD
- Komer, Claudia A., DO
- Korban, Anna, MD
- Li, Dongchen, MD
- Liao, Wu-Fei, MD
- Louis, Vely Anthony, MD
- Madubuko, Uchenna Anthony, MD
- Malapero, Raymond Joseph III, MD
- Marji, Michael Suleiman, MD
- Maurrasse, Corazon C., MD
- Modi, Nita K., MD
- Moon, Kyoung, MD
- Moore, Ross Edward, MD
- Morris, Kevin Michael, MD
- Napuli, Maximo C., MD
- Pakonis, Gregory Vytautas, MD
- Patel, Anuradha P., MD
- Ponnudurai, Rex N., MD
- Potian, Marcelino M., MD
- Raval, Rajendra R., MD
- Rodriguez Correa, Daniel T., MD
- Ru, Xun, MD
- Rubin, Benjamin, MD
- Saffran, Scott Robert, MD
- Sahota, Manpreet S., MD
- Sakellaris, Leander D., MD
- Tan, Royland C., MD
- Tilak, Vasanti A., MD
- Tolentino, Eduardo D., MD
- Wei, Pan-Son, MD
- Whalen, Kathryn, MD
- Xiong, Ming, MD
- Zaslavsky, Alexander, MD
- Zwolska-Demczuk, Barbara A., MD

Newton
- Cowan, Clayton Joseph, MD
- Delong, Donald H. II, MD
- Eaton, Edward E., MD
- Habina, Ladislav, MD
- Hagopian, Vahe H., MD
- Jiang, Rongjie, MD
- Kouvaras, John Nikolaos, DO
- Landauer, Stephen P., MD
- Martinez, Rebecca Marie, DO
- Patel, Nish A., MD
- Petrucelli, Marisa Parise, DO
- Villafania, Zenaida S., MD
- Yu, Edgar L., MD

North Bergen
- Lawler, Gregory James, DO

- Pavia, Randyll A., MD
- Poltinnikova, Yana M., MD
- Portugal, Alexander, MD
- Shatz, Matthew Jay, MD
- Singh, Samundar K., MD

North Brunswick
- Fakhry, Michael, MD
- Karandikar, Shaila Y., MD
- Khan, Khuram Adnan, DO
- Parikh, Sudha Sudhir, MD
- Sood, Rohit, MD
- Tyler, James Ralph, MD

North Caldwell
- Bhattacharyya, Shibani S., MD
- Kim, Kun, MD
- Radhakrishnan, Indira, MD

Northfield
- Antebi, Morris E., MD
- Hernberg, Scott Alan, DO
- Liu, Bo, MD

Norwood
- Cagen, Steven B., MD
- MacIver, Barbara Jane, MD

Nutley
- Belfar, Alexandra, MD
- Kyi, Myint Myint, MD
- Punzalan, Crispino R., MD

Oakhurst
- Bram, Harris N., MD

Oakland
- Hansen, David Wayne, MD
- Nestampower, Mindy Lyn, MD

Ocean
- Uddin, Nihat, MD

Old Bridge
- De Ocera, Zenaida Bascara, MD

Paramus
- Binder, Michael, MD
- Giraldo, Juan Pablo, MD
- Gungor, Semih, MD
- Higgins, Annlouise Maria, MD
- Narayanan, Manglam, MD
- Ragukonis, Thomas P., MD
- Roche, Elizabeth Ann, MD
- Rubinchik, Noemy Aronovici, MD
- Silverman, Robert S., MD
- Trnovski, Stefan, MD
- Zhuravkov, Alexander, MD

Parsippany
- Anjutgi, Rajyashree, MD
- Baker, Michelle Rapacon, MD
- Balakrishna, Shruthi, MD
- Barg, Vadim A., MD
- Blanchfield, Patrick Thomas, MD
- Chen, Guo-Gang, MD
- Choudhary, Ratna, MD
- Clanton, Chase P., MD
- Cohen, Michael B., MD
- Daniel, Brian P., DO
- Daras, Jason Glenn, DO
- Davanzo, Peter A., MD
- DeSimone, Robert Anthony, MD
- Delis, Aristidis G., MD
- Eisenstat, Carol M., MD
- Fanouse, John A., DO
- Garibaldi, Thomas A., MD
- Ghosh, Arpita, MD
- Grasso, Mario Lucio, MD
- Grimaldi, Matthew Porter, MD
- Jacobson, Martin Alexander, MD
- Janardhan, Yellagonda V., MD
- Kussick, Neil J., MD
- Lamanna, Adolfo C., MD
- Lasker, Steven Mark, MD
- Lian, Hanzhou, MD
- Lyall, Jasleen Kaur, MD
- Ofeldt, James D., DO
- Olechowski, George N., MD
- Panei, Maryann S., MD
- Patel, Gaurav R., MD
- Patel, Mona, MD
- Patel, Niva S., MD
- Patel, Taral B., DO
- Pham, Vu Linh, MD
- Pikus, Igor, MD
- Rana, Kirtida Dinesh, MD
- Ravindra, Sunay B., MD
- Shah, Mehul D., DO
- Shih, Yangyu Steven, MD
- Shore, Ronald Andrew, DO
- Sim, Andrew R., MD

- Singh, Jagjeet, MD
- Spina, Laurie J., MD
- Suchy, Matthew Robert, DO
- Taragin, Michael S., MD
- Terreri, Michael Robert Jr., MD
- Thakur, Jagdish G., MD
- Tsafos, Vassilios, MD
- Wassef, Michael Karim, MD
- Wong, Henry Chen, MD
- Young, Jill S., DO
- Zabrodina, Yanina V., MD

Passaic
- Agres, Mildred D., MD
- Boukila, Marina, MD
- Chung, Jae Won, MD
- Ekulide, Ifeyinwa Ndidi, MD
- Jones, Kevin Errol, MD
- Jotwani, Madhu M, MD
- Lakshmi, Vijaya S R, MD
- Lee, Ai R., MD
- Lee, Chang J., MD
- Lee Ellis, Nandi T., MD
- Malazarte, Justito B., MD
- Mankikar, Durgesh P., MD
- Odondi, Janet Aoko, MD
- Prasad, Jitender, MD
- Raza, Syed Mohsin, MD
- Reuveni, Michael A., MD
- Rhodes, Michael Eric, MD
- Sacknowitz, Ivy J., MD
- Salomon, Guy, MD
- Stein, Steven J., MD
- Sukhavasi, Sujatha, MD
- Thomas, George, MD
- Venkataraman, Ravi Kumar, MD
- Weissman, Allan Mark, MD

Paterson
- Adkisson, Gregory Hugh, MD
- Akhtar, Shuaib A., MD
- Apinis, Andrey, MD
- Armstead, Valerie Elizabeth, MD
- Aronova, Yelena, DO
- Badach, Mark J., MD
- Bauman, Gregory A., MD
- Burns, Talitha Mariana Hedley, DO
- Chalfin, Matthew Bryan, MD
- Chan, Kar-Mei, MD
- Chu, Amy M., MD
- Dreznin, Howard N., MD
- Enriquez-Leff, Liza Jeanne, MD
- Fernandez, Afranio L., MD
- Figueroa, Pablo T., MD
- Galldin, Lars Michael, MD
- Garcia, Gerald Matthew, MD
- Gargani, Stephanie, MD
- Germond, Christopher John, DO
- Grey, Glenn Allen, MD
- Holland, David Andersson, MD
- Kanetkar, Madhavi Jayat, MD
- Krottapalli, Harini, MD
- Landa, Seth E., MD
- Lehman, Abraham Reuven, MD
- Leibu, Dorina, MD
- MacKenzie, Shauna, MD
- Makkapati, Sandhya Rani, MD
- Markley, Jonathan C., DO
- Mekhjian, Haroutune A., MD
- Moise, Anson Marryshow, MD
- Nandigam, Harish, MD
- Nuesa, Wilson O. IV, MD
- Oladeji, Oluremi O., MD
- Parihar, Jasmit K., DO
- Pearce, Donna Alison, MD
- Putterman, Debora, MD
- Rao, Sheila Yvonne, MD
- Ravi, Radhika, MD
- Rosales, Ramon Javilonar, MD
- Sakowitz Cohen, Noreen Gail, MD
- Sammarone, Marcello Eliseo, MD
- Saulon, Winston B., MD
- Sidhu, Gursimar K., MD
- Sultan, Ahmed Said, DO
- Umanoff, Michael D., MD
- Upadya, Padmaja Koppal, MD
- Ventura, William Raphael, MD
- Wachtel, Zev, MD
- Whang, Ihn Young, MD
- Winikoff, Stephen P., MD
- Yoganathan, Thil, MD
- Zisa, Salvatore Anthony Jr., MD
- Zodiatis, Paras Jayant, DO
- Zuberi, Faizah, MD

Pennington
- Ahmad, Sajida Ghani, MD
- Cantillo, Joaquin J., MD
- Enriquez, Joseph E., MD
- Grujic, Slobodan, MD
- Hanusey, Robert William, MD
- Kollmeier, Brett R., MD
- Liu, Renfeng, DO
- Madsen, Melissa L., MD
- Rao, Veena, MD
- Reddy, Sudershan P., MD
- Shah, Mahendra Govindlal, MD
- Tolentino, Pablito L., MD
- Vadhavkar, Aarti Sanjeev, MD
- Voros, Stephen C., MD
- Wuu, Zukwung, MD

Pennsville
- Chapdelaine, Robert T., MD

Perth Amboy
- Chae, Hung Y., MD
- Dalal, Kalpana S., MD
- Fernandez, Manuel A., MD
- Lakhlani, Parul Pravinchandra, MD
- Lipatov, Yuriy, MD
- Nandiwada, Kalpana, MD
- New, Deena R., MD
- Olegario, Eduardo S., MD
- Payumo, Carmelino C., MD
- Ragheb, Sozan L., MD
- Rashid, Iqbal, MD

Phillipsburg
- Redondo, Rodolfo C., MD
- Sarayno-Sagge, Perla M., MD
- Whittingham, Jennifer J., MD

Pine Brook
- Schaechter, Jason D., MD

Piscataway
- Chowdhury, Farys Reza, DO

Plainsboro
- Airen, Anshul, MD
- Broad, Daniel Gene, MD
- Calalang, Carolyn Clarice, MD
- Chaudhry, Ambareen Khan, MD
- Chen, Chu-Kuang, MD
- Coplin, Peter L., MD
- Curlik, Semena, MD
- Fortunato Sieglen, Linda M., MD
- Greenberg, Leslie M., MD
- Griffith, Rebecca N., MD
- Guo, Xiaotao, MD
- Hirsh, Jennifer L., MD
- Klausner, Anna Jill, MD
- Nelson, Mary Beth, MD
- Ruscito, Bridget Marie, MD
- Seybert, John Jr., MD
- Subramoni, Jaya, MD
- Trager, Mark A., MD
- Wolfson, Alexander, MD

Pleasantville
- Qadir, Abdul, MD

Pomona
- Arole, Adebola Oyedele, MD
- Costabile, Jessica T., DO
- Davidov, Mark, MD
- Fadugba, Olawale Akindiran, MD
- Fisgus, John R., MD
- Gayeski, David R., MD
- Incandela, Nicholas J., MD
- Kaplan, Bruce Zachary, MD
- Lagmay, Merceditas Maria, MD
- Levitch, David, MD
- O'Connell, Frank Michael, MD
- Pericic, Romeo, MD
- Radcliff, Nina Singh, MD
- Schmidheiser, Mark Andrew, MD
- Soni, Dhiren D., DO
- Wang, Qin, MD
- Yao, Su-Lin G., MD

Pompton Plains
- Aberbach, Eric Steven, MD
- Cheng, Szu-Chi S., MD
- Cooper, Eliyahu N., MD
- Cruz, Bernardo V., MD
- Delaleu, Harold, MD
- Dolorico, Valentin N., MD
- Hanna, George M., MD
- Lin, Jian L., MD
- Lipkind, Mark Alan, MD
- Rapacon, Magdaleno R., MD
- Scro, Joseph Salvatore, MD
- Shulman, Oleg M., MD

Physicians by Specialty and Town

Topf,Andrew Irwin,MD
Voca,Ioan Bogdan,MD
Princeton
Barone,Stephen Robert,MD
Collins,Patrice,MD
Hancock,Joseph Patrick,MD
Hussain,Mahboob,MD
Kanter,Lawrence E.,MD
Kim,Andrew Hanyoung,MD
Morganstern,Jill Alison,MD
Princeton Junction
Chang,Connie Yachan,MD
Rahway
Light,Francis B.,MD
Luciano,Dominick T.,MD
Osei Tutu,Leslie P.,MD
Son,Andrew,MD
Son,Kyoung J.,MD
Ramsey
Goldstein,Monte Jay,MD
Gordon,Robert P.,MD
Melyokhin,Igor,MD
Pillitteri,John,MD
Song,Michael M.,MD
Randolph
Levy,Stuart J.,MD
Sokolova,Anna,MD
Red Bank
Ades,Nathan Albert,MD
Brodsky,Jonathan I.,DO
Bruce,Gullie E. IV,MD
Chidambaram,Manjula S.,MD
Chiu,Nicholas,MD
Cirullo,Pasquale Michael,MD
Dooley,James R.,MD
Farrell,Charles W.,MD
Friedman,James Keith,MD
Haber,Daran W.,MD
Huang,Shyuan,MD
Huh,Chan Woo,MD
Kulkarni,Prashant P.,MD
Meltzer,Keith Mitchell,MD
Mosca,Phillip J.,MD
Nguyen,Khanh Q.,MD
Ritchie,Paul Harvey,MD
Toran,Stephen A.,MD
Varadarajan,Vijayaiaxmi,MD
Ridgewood
Adkoli,Sujnani,MD
Azzariti,John Jr.,MD
Beke,Theodore J.,MD
Chan,Jenny Sang,MD
Chaudhry,Ahmad N.,MD
Choi,Sunny D.,MD
Connelly,Brian,MD
Feiler,Michael Augustus,MD
Gal,Stephen,MD
Iannacone,Richard F.,DO
Ietta,Michael Angelo,MD
Kotys,Ola,DO
Lavrich,Pamela S.,MD
Lee,Soomyung,MD
Levine,Jeffrey,MD
Magnes,Jeffrey B.,MD
Morr,Edward Simon,MD
Nagy,Peter,MD
Nyunt,Kyaw,MD
Rosen,Chaim E.,MD
Schmidt,Kenneth A.,MD
Scognamiglio,Michael F.,MD
Silverstein,Wendy Beth,MD
Smith,Justin Kerry,MD
Telfeyan,Celeste A.,DO
Volkov,Anatoly,MD
Westrich,David J.,MD
Wohlfarth,Erik,MD
Zamecki,Andrzej M.,MD
Riverdale
Aznavoorian,Martin Peter,MD
Roseland
Entrada,Julian Jr.,MD
Gorman,Eugene S.,MD
Karmaker,Shekhar Chandra,MD
Kos,Luke Bronislaw,MD
Park,Young,MD
Zhao,Lin,MD
Rumson
Sestito,Joseph Jr.,MD
Saddle Brook
Choi,Jay J.,MD
Kosiborod,Roman,DO

Sauchelli,Francis C.,MD
Saddle River
Miguel,Renato C.,MD
Ramnanan,Terry K.,MD
Salem
Corbin,John C.,DO
Fehder,Carl G.,MD
Fiel Cagande,Venerande,MD
Maestrado,Primo Emnace,MD
Mailman,Wendy R.,MD
Morales-Pelaez,Eileen S.,MD
Pham,Chi H.,MD
Pierce,Brandon Keefe,MD
Sarvaiya,Ramesh Manjibhai,MD
Sharma,Naresh Durgaprasad,MD
Scotch Plains
Buchbinder,Howard J.,MD
Sea Bright
Rhee,William Choonghee,MD
Sea Girt
Patton,Virginia A.,MD
Seaside Heights
Durnan,Rosemary,MD
Secaucus
Bhavsar,Vaishali,MD
Faragalla,Emad T.,MD
Lewis,Michele J.,MD
Patel,Amrish M.,MD
Yoo,Eun Y.,MD
Sewell
Dougherty,Barbara D.,DO
Lopresti,David A.,MD
Sorensen,Barbara J.,MD
Short Hills
Peckman,Cornelia L.,MD
Shrewsbury
Goldofsky,Sheldon E.,MD
Kutzin,Theodore E.,MD
Patel,Bimal,DO
Schaaff,Robert P.,MD
Sondhi,Nidhi,DO
Staats,Peter Sean,MD
Taneja,Monica M.,MD
Wood,Sterling Harbert,DO
Somerdale
Mehta,Parul J.,MD
Somers Point
Absin,Martini Perez,MD
Allahverdi,Ilya Michael,MD
Avellino,Carmine,DO
Dearborn,Peyton Robert,MD
Hu,Xin Tian,MD
Khatiwala,Colleen Pravin,MD
Krzemieniecki,Thomas Gerald,DO
Salkeld,Charles S.,DO
Tsyganov,Igor Vlademer,MD
Somerset
Back,Steven Marc,MD
Baron,Jeremy Lawrence,MD
Cabanero,Camilo O.,MD
Caces,Alan R.,MD
Cho,Grace C.,MD
Choi,Jieun Susana,MD
Colavita,Richard D.,MD
Cottrill,Richard Z. Jr.,MD
Das,Sudip S.,MD
Fellenbaum,Paul,MD
Gajewski,Jan Peter,MD
Gangavalli,Ravi Venkata,MD
Giacobbe,Dean Thomas,MD
Ginsberg,Sanford Ginsberg,MD
Gunvantlal,Desai A.,MD
Jenkins,Paul B.,MD
Kett,Attila G.,MD
Kiamzon,Harald James,MD
Kim,Hyon S.,MD
Ku,James Chien,MD
Land,Warren K.,DO
Lee,William,MD
Lu,Ya-Tseng W.,MD
Mackler,Denise Lynn,MD
Margiotta,Joseph A.,MD
Martin,Dean Walter,MD
Mathew,Julie,MD
Mosaddeghi,Mahmood,MD
Moses,Brett Joseph,MD
Nath,Ajay,MD
Pabbathi,Pramod,DO
Patel,Ajitkumar Gunvantrai,MD
Patel,Samir Natavar,MD
Perez,Manuel A.,MD

Rahman,Attique,MD
Richardson,Michael J.,MD
Ruda,William A.,MD
Ruedy,Krista R.,MD
Siegel,Scott S.,MD
Simon,Abraham M.,DO
Sio,Reymond Guieb,MD
Smith,Daniel Brian J.,MD
Sonbol,Sherif A.,MD
Sperrazza,James Christopher,MD
Tangreti,Nicholas W.,MD
Tronolone,William,MD
Walker,John S.,DO
Yau,Assumpta K.,MD
Somerville
Granowitz,Gail F.,MD
Roy,Amanda R.,MD
South Orange
Bodner,Arnold H.,MD
South Plainfield
Byahatti,Pramila,MD
Kapusuz,Tolga,MD
Tran,Bao Chau Minh,MD
Sparta
Willis,William John,MD
Springfield
Schoenfeld,Mark R.,MD
Stratford
Jones,Michael R.,MD
Neitzel,Kristi M.,MD
Succasunna
Murthy,Sujatha S.,MD
Summit
Abrams,Jonathan Todd,MD
Arzola,Nydia,MD
BelCastro,Peter Joseph,MD
Byers,Jason,MD
Calabro,John R.,MD
Chan,Karen Rita Post,MD
Co,Jacqueline Ann B.,MD
DeAngelis,Lawrence J.,MD
Dominik,Jeremy A.,MD
Dowd,Timothy Joseph,MD
Faccone,Jacqueline M.,DO
Farrar,Robert,MD
Fernandez-Piparo,May Anne M.,MD
Fleischman,Keith A.,DO
Greenberg,Carrie Lynn,MD
Hsu,Madeleine F.,MD
Hu,Yuan,MD
Huang,Guojie,MD
Jablons,Mitchell L.,MD
Kagan,Mikhail,MD
Kral,Michael George,MD
Kweon,Chang,MD
Kwon,Yong S.,MD
Lei,Laura M.,MD
McLaughlin,Blaise,MD
Naturman,Roy E.,MD
Pacific,Scott,MD
Paris,Glen Allen,MD
Pierre-Louis,James,MD
Rice,Stuart Nelson,MD
Rosenstein,Megan Ann,MD
Ross,Neil E.,MD
Sant,Manasee Amol,MD
Sarkaria,Janak,MD
Schultz,Gail,MD
Shahane,Manoj Raghunath,MD
Sharma,Akanksha D.,MD
Soni,Monika K.,MD
Surace,Anthony,MD
Thakkar,Shivani,MD
Wang,Wayne,MD
Woo,Daniel Hee-Suk,MD
Yao,Daniel Duan,MD
You,Ruoxu,MD
Zimmermann,Carol E.,MD
Surf City
Tumillo,John G. Jr.,MD
Sussex
Shah,Prafulla R.,MD
Shah,Rameshchan H.,MD
Teaneck
Benson,Peter Kurt,MD
Carni,Abbe J.,MD
Chaubey,Rakesh Kumar,MD
D'Souza,Michael Gerard,MD
Ephrat,Roni,MD
Florence,Isaiah Meyer,MD
Fradlis,Alina,MD

Franzl,Wojciech,MD
Gross,Robert M.,MD
Gupta,Vijay,MD
Gwertzman,Alan R.,MD
Klein,Patti S.,MD
Koniuta,Robert L.,MD
Koshibe,Gen,MD
Martin,Brian McKinley,MD
Nahmias,Neil Jeffrey,DO
Novak,Steven Michael,MD
Parmar,Virendra Pratapsingh,MD
Ryu,David Jinsoo,DO
Sheikh,Usman,MD
Singer,Judith C. J.,MD
Sklar,Jeffrey,MD
Syed,Faraz A.,DO
Thornhill,Marsha Lynne,MD
Trivedi,Avani P.,DO
Vittal,Melba G.,MD
Worth,Robert Harry,MD
Tinton Falls
Pourmasiha,Niloufar,DO
Toms River
Cha,Hak J.,MD
D'Angelo,Stephen Thomas,DO
De Sio,John Michael,MD
Farkas,Klara,MD
Gershteyn,Eduard,MD
Jadav,Jitendra K.,MD
Krishtul,Eduard,MD
Lin,Renny L.,MD
Loftus,James B.,MD
Mako,Robert M.,DO
Manganelli,Douglas M.,MD
Mara,Frank J.,MD
Park,Dong C.,MD
Park,Yung I.,MD
Quiambao,Dante B.,MD
Tank,Hasmukh C.,MD
Trenton
Arnette,Esther Elizabeth,MD
Beshara,Raafat Henry,MD
Co,Anthony,MD
Cortese,Lisa Ann,MD
Dinh,Cung T.,MD
Ganopolsky,Elizabeth,MD
Haig,Lauren Grace,MD
LaMonica,Christina M,MD
Liu,Yuyan,MD
Loesberg,Perry A.,MD
Markos,Marina Azmy,MD
Nardi,David A.,MD
Paloni,Stephen Mark,MD
Rosenzweig,Howard J.,MD
Schachter,Laurence Howard,MD
Spodik,Boris,DO
Wang,Ling,MD
Union
Fleischhacker,Wayne,DO
Garipalli,Lakshmi,MD
Kahn,Randolph,DO
Novik,Edward,MD
Peng,Minzhong,MD
Shane,Steven A.,DO
Wilcenski,Michael A.,MD
Yim,Yoori W.,MD
Union City
Siegel,Ira B.,MD
Upper Saddle River
Naljian,Vahe G.,MD
Verona
Gentile,James,DO
Vineland
Attia,Tamer A.,MD
Chambers,Bryan P.,MD
Fitzhenry,Laurence N. IV,MD
Hamzeh Langroudi,Mehrdad,MD
Jassal,Peter,MD
Kaur,Harmanjot,MD
Miller,Shamaal M.,MD
Patharkar,Milind D.,MD
Voorhees
Ahsan,Syed Nadeem,MD
Bailey,Philip Daniel Jr.,DO
Cho,Daniel P.,MD
Corcino,Ana J.,MD
Jobes,David Richard,MD
Lewis,Allan Andrew,MD
Miller,Bruce L.,MD
Mithani,Bharati T.,MD
Nicolson,Susan C.,MD
Patel,Erica,DO

655

Physicians by Specialty and Town

Anesthesiology (cont)
Waldwick
 Boruta,Andrew Michael,DO
Wallington
 Dadaian,Jon-Paul,MD
Warren
 Baratta,James A.,MD
 Chin,Christina W.,MD
Washington
 Greenfeld,Alan L.,MD
Watchung
 Ostry,Rachel F.,MD
 Shah,Kishori Praful,MD
 Vassallo,Michael Anthony,DO
Wayne
 Frias,Carlos,MD
 Galkin,Vadim,MD
 Klele,Christo Selim,MD
 Krynska,Elzbieta B.,MD
 Pekar,Aleksandr,MD
 Raja,Bala Shanmugasundara,MD
West Caldwell
 Bering,Thomas Gerard,MD
 Doss,George S.,MD
 Forrest,Robert,MD
 Giannuzzi,Rosanne Frances,MD
 Izeogu,Chinweike,MD
 Katragadda,Rama Sastrulu,MD
 Lutz,Philip Edward,MD
 Negron-Gonzalez,Maria A.,MD
 Rocamboli,David Charles,DO
 Rubin,Joshua Adam,MD
 Secoy,John Walton,MD
 Sisbarro,Susan E.,MD
 Spertus,Silvana H.,DO
 Vujic,Dragomir M.,MD
 Weems,Lela Demilo,MD
West New York
 Richards,Patricia T.,MD
 Roque,Felix Eduardo,MD
West Orange
 Abadir,John Sobhi,MD
 DiStefano,Kelly Frances,MD
 Fernando,Rosario P.,MD
 Liu,Kaixuan,MD
 Liu,Ren Y.,MD
 Mankikar,Mohini T.,MD
 Tseng,William P.,MD
 Yanovskaya,Liliya,MD
Westwood
 Iuliano,Frank David,MD
 Jin,Jie,MD
Whiting
 Mann,Dharam P.,MD
Williamstown
 Audu,Paul Bulus,MD
 Betia,Reuben,MD
 Corda,Peter D.,DO
 Perkins-Waters,Vannette N.,MD
 Polcer,Jeffrey D.,DO
Willingboro
 Paul,Benoy Krishna,MD
 Penzone,Karen Elizabeth,MD
 Platt,Marc J.,MD
 Segaram,Gnana,MD
Wood Ridge
 Fisch,Amy Heather,DO
 Jiang,Yihao,MD
Woodbury
 Cherian,Abraham,MD
 Davis,Michael James,DO
 Dragon,Glenn M.,MD
 Giorgio,Anthony Richard,MD
 Harowitz,Robert J.,MD
 McMaster,Michelle,MD
 Riley,Cara Ann,MD
 Rousseau,Marc Telesphore,MD
 Saldutti,Gregg M.,MD
 Smith,Kenneth Jr.,DO
 Valencia,Maria R.,MD
 Wagner,Craig R.,DO
Wyckoff
 Aloi,Joseph M.,MD
 Harvey,Samantha K.,MD
 Lee,John Po-Hsiang,MD
 Montemurno,Tina Deborah,MD
 Rodriguez Barea,Hector A.,MD
 Starcic-Herrera,Sandra,DO
 Wu,Peter,MD
 Yenicay,Altan Omer,MD
 Zhou,Henry Haifeng,MD

Anesthesiology: Addiction Medicine
Mays Landing
 Quirk,Edward,MD
Newark
 Elhelw,Ramy,MD

Anesthesiology: Critical Care Med
Camden
 Ben-Jacob,Talia K.,MD
Cherry Hill
 Flaxman,Alexander,MD
Livingston
 Seedhom,Magdi Ebrahim,MD
Neptune
 Amitie,Daniel Dean,MD
Newton
 Ibragimov,Araz,DO
Pompton Plains
 Newman,Rita Grant,MD
Somerset
 Rodricks,Michael Baltazar,MD
Teaneck
 Kaufman,Margit I.,MD

Anesthesiology: Pain Medicine
Boonton
 Mendez,Jorge G.,MD
Camden
 Beelitz,John Darren,MD
 Brennan,Mark D.,MD
 Sehdev,Jasjit Singh,MD
Cherry Hill
 Maurer,Philip Mitchell,MD
 Puri,Shawn K.,MD
 Reyes,Johan,MD
Clifton
 Kizina,Christopher Allen,MD
 Michail,Mohsen T.,MD
 Patel,Anjali Dalal,DO
 Patel,Dipan G.,MD
 Valskys,Rytis,MD
East Brunswick
 Lam,Sofia Levin,MD
Englewood
 Gudin,Jeffrey Alan,MD
Fort Lee
 Kang,Chang H.,MD
 Kang,Richard,MD
Hammonton
 Lee,Young Jae,MD
Holmdel
 Varma,Ajay Medavaram,MD
Livingston
 Vogel,Martin Joseph,MD
Long Branch
 Tran,Dan-Thuy V.,MD
Merchantville
 Radbill,Keith Philip,DO
Middletown
 Poonia,Amit,MD
 Xie,Jinghui,MD
Moorestown
 Patil,Meenal Kulkarni,MD
Mount Laurel
 Cooper,Niti Dalal,DO
 McGrath,Steven Warren,MD
Mountainside
 Yanow,Jennifer Hannah,MD
Neptune
 Miller,Christine Venable,MD
New Brunswick
 Amponsah,Akwasi Peprah,MD
 Gajian,Garen Edward,MD
 Yeh,Shihlong,MD
Newark
 Chiu,Chi-Shin,MD
 Iannaccone,Ferdinand,DO
 Rahman,Owen R.,MD
 Sifonios,Anthony N.,MD
North Bergen
 Waldman,Steven Paul,MD
North Brunswick
 Avhad,Prajakta Vasant,MD
Old Bridge
 Del Valle,Jacqueline P.,MD
 Moten,Hadi S.,MD
 Winn,Terrance T.,MD
Paramus
 Goswami,Amit,MD
Paterson
 Sheikh,Ednan Salahuddin,MD
Plainsboro
 Patel,Ronak Dilip,MD
Pompton Plains
 Dugar,Vikash,MD
Ramsey
 Gamburg,David,MD
 Halioua,Solomon,MD
Rutherford
 Haliczer,Abraham T.,MD
Secaucus
 Canillas,Elmo Maribao,MD
Shrewsbury
 Cresanti-Daknis,Charles B.,MD
 Li,Sean,MD
 Sahoo,Aruna,MD
 Walia,Kulbir Singh,MD
Somerset
 Patel,Arti S.,MD
 Peng,Hsin,MD
 Picone,Michael J.,MD
Toms River
 Coccaro,John A.,MD
Voorhees
 Boyajian,Stephen S.,DO
 Yulo,John A.,MD
Wayne
 Bandola,David Matthew,MD
Whiting
 Jani,Samir Ranjit,MD

Arthroscopic Surgery
Bedminster
 France,Matthew P.,MD
Englewood
 Cole,James R.,MD
Glen Ridge
 Sloan,Kim W.,MD
Montvale
 Livingston,Lawrence I.,MD
Somers Point
 Zabinski,Stephen J.,MD

Bariatrics/Weight Control
Egg Harbor Township
 Onopchenko,Alexander,MD
Ridgewood
 Pucci,Richard Anthony,DO

Behavioral Medicine
Ridgewood
 Nalven,Lisa M.,MD
Vineland
 Enriquez,Carla,MD

Bloodbanking
East Orange
 Senaldi,Eric M.,MD
Haddonfield
 Hennawy,Randa Philip,MD
Mays Landing
 Nayak,Shaila V.,MD
New Brunswick
 Kuriyan,Mercy Achamma,MD
Newark
 Koshy,Ranie,MD
Paterson
 Doniguian,Ann-Elizabeth E.,MD
Princeton Junction
 Chopra,Neeru Gera,MD
Raritan
 Ciavarella,David Joseph,MD

Body Imaging Radiology
Clinton
 Klein,Laura B.,MD
East Brunswick
 Sussmann,Amado Ross,MD
 Yang,Charles,MD
Hamilton
 Kim,Joseph J.,MD
Middletown
 Saphier,Nicole Berardoni,MD
Mount Laurel
 Tan,Elizabeth Listiani,MD
Voorhees
 King,Anne H.,DO

Breast Surgery
Belleville
 Pappas,Nadine C.,MD
Berkeley Heights
 Addis,Diana Medina,MD
 Polen,Winnie M.,DO
Brick
 Lygas,Theodore B.,MD
 Pellegrino,John M.,MD
Camden
 Koniges,Frank C.,MD
 Loveland-Jones,Catherine E.,MD
Englewood
 McIntosh,Violet Merle,MD
Montclair
 Elliott,Nancy L.,MD
 Hertz,Marcie B.,MD
Morristown
 Fornari,Marcella,DO
 Gendler,Leah S.,MD
Neptune
 Adams,William D.,MD
Paramus
 Christoudias,Moira Katherine,MD
Plainsboro
 Davidson,J. Thomas,MD
Somerset
 McManus,Susan A.,MD
Somerville
 Lanfranchi,Angela E.,MD
Tinton Falls
 Camal,Debra E.,MD

Cardiac Anesthesia
Hackensack
 Abrams,Lawrence M.,MD
Old Tappan
 Nadeau,Pascale,MD

Cardiothoracic Surgery
Cherry Hill
 Derivaux,Christopher Charles,MD
Englewood
 Klein,James Joseph Jr.,MD
Hamilton
 Manna,Biagio,DO
Jersey City
 Perera,Santusht A.,MD
New Brunswick
 Ghaly,Aziz S.,MD
 Lee,Leonard Young,MD
 Lemaire,Anthony,MD
 Prendergast,Thomas William,MD
Newark
 Russo,Mark Joseph,MD
Pennington
 Lee,Daniel James,MD

Cardiovascular Disease
Aberdeen
 Adler,Eric David,MD
Absecon
 Shanker,Mukesh J.,MD
Audubon
 Crawford,Jeffrey R.,DO
Bayonne
 Elkind,Barry M.,MD
 Hefferan,James J.,MD
 Nadiminti,Sheila Gupta,MD
 Sandhu,Mohammad Y.,MD
 Tan,William W.,MD
Belle Mead
 McGeady,Rosemary E.,MD
Belleville
 Criscito,Mario A.,MD
 Saleh,Rany Mokhlis,DO
Berkeley
 Sachs,R. Gregory,MD
 Schwartz,Daniel Richard,MD
Berkeley Heights
 Beamer,Andrew D.,MD
 Kothavale,Avinash Annash,MD
 Slama,Robert D.,MD
Bloomfield
 Horowitz,Michael S.,MD
 Lapa,Alan S.,MD
 Mahdi,Lawrence F.,MD
 McCoach,Kevin J.,MD
 Shao,John Han,MD
Branchburg
 Saulino,Patrick F.,MD
Brick
 Ahmad,Tanveer,MD
 Apolito,Renato A.,MD
 Cohen,Todd S.,DO

Komorowski,Thomas W.,MD
Mehra,Aditya Chand,MD
Moosvi,Ali R.,MD
Patel,Harshil,MD
Patel,Virendra,MD
Paul Kate,Vasant,MD
Pinnelas,David J.,MD
Raza,Muhammad Rehan,MD
Vijayakumar,Chellappan,MD
White,Thomas M.,DO
Bridgeton
Baptist,Gladwyn D.,MD
Bridgewater
Ahn,Joe Kyuhyun,MD
Cheng,Chao T.,MD
Cheng,Shiow-Jane L.,MD
Chew,Paul H.,MD
Friedman,Glenn T.,MD
Georgeson,Steven E.,MD
Hall,Jason O.,MD
Ivanov,Alexander,MD
Kulkarni,Rachana A.,MD
Lebenthal,Mark J.,MD
Leeds,Richard S.,MD
Mahal,Sharan S.,MD
Ocken,Stephen M.,MD
Patel,Alpesh Amrit,MD
Rachofsky,Edward Lawrence,MD
Sengupta,Ranjita,MD
Shahi,Chandreshwar N.,MD
Browns Mills
Altimore,David,MD
Amico,Frank Joseph Jr.,DO
Buchanan,David J.,DO
Bullock Palmer,Renee Patrice,MD
Corbisiero,Raffaele,MD
Evans,Matthew,DO
Ferlise,Kathleen M.,MD
Fish,Frank H.,MD
Garabedian,J. Andre,DO
McNamara,John Patrick,DO
Mogtader,Allen,MD
Moshiyakhov,Mark,MD
Ng,Tommy K.,MD
Reese,Jason,DO
Sanghvi,Kintur Arvindbhai,MD
Sprankle,Steven Michael,DO
Sumathisena,Sena,MD
Waggoner,Thomas E. I,DO
Camden
Aji,Janah I.,MD
Cartwright,Travante Mcnae,MD
Cotto,Maritza,MD
Dadhania,Manish Suresh,MD
Gessman,Lawrence J.,MD
Ginsberg,Fredric L.,MD
Heintz,Kathleen M.,DO
Javed,Omair,MD
Khan,Mubashar H.,MD
Kurnik,Peter B.,MD
Morris,Timothy P.,DO
Weinstock,Perry J.,MD
Cape May Court House
Boriss,Michael N.,DO
Burhanna,Amy Scally,MD
Nanavati,Suketu H.,MD
Nillas,Michael S.,MD
Scally,Monique,DO
Sorensen,Mark R.,MD
Carneys Point
Sauers,Paul W.,DO
Cedar Knolls
Feitell,Leonard A.,MD
Godkar,Darshan,MD
Moss,Leonard J. Jr.,DO
Cherry Hill
Akhigbe,Kelvin Osagie,DO
Akula,Devender Nagarajan,MD
Bauer,Hans Henry Jr.,MD
Bhavsar,Jignesh,MD
Blaber,Reginald J.,MD
Burke,Gary C.,DO
Chaudhry,Nasser A.,MD
Cohen,Ronald A.,DO
Dickstein,Richard A.,MD
Duffy,Kevin James Jr.,MD
Dunham,Rozy D.,MD
Fertels,Scott H.,DO
Fox,Steven N.,MD
Friedman,Terry David,MD
Fuhrman,Mitchell J.,MD

Gelernt,Mark D.,MD
Godin,Willis Eugene,DO
Gomberg,Richard M.,DO
Hamaty,John N.,DO
Harkins,Michael J.,MD
Hollenberg,Steven M.,MD
Horwitz,Jerome M.,MD
Kernis,Steven J.,MD
Khatiwala,Jayesh Ramesh,MD
Khaw,Kenneth,MD
Klodnicki,Walter E.,MD
Kothari,Anil G.,MD
Lawrence,David L.,MD
Leavy,Jeffrey Alan,MD
Mohapatra,Robert A.,MD
Momplaisir,Thierry,MD
Moussa,Ibrahim Abdel,DO
Ortman,Matthew Louis,MD
Proper,Michael C.,MD
Randle,Troy L.,DO
Reichman,Michael J.,MD
Rosenberg,Mitchell C.,MD
Rubenstone,Jay L.,DO
Sailam,Vivek Vardha,MD
Sandler,Matthew Jay,MD
Sholevar,Darius P.,MD
Siddiqi,Faisal Khursheed,MD
Siegal,Scott L.,DO
Silver,Steven Eric,MD
Smith,Jason Anthony,DO
Wadehra,Ramneet,DO
Yegya-Raman,Sivaraman,MD
Zarrella,Geoffrey Carl,DO
Chester
Antonucci,Lawrence Charles,MD
Clark
Aliasgharpour,Farzin M.,MD
Chudasama,Lalji S.,MD
Sahni,Rakesh Kumar,MD
Sahni,Sheila,MD
Varshneya,Nikita,MD
Clifton
Ahmad,Ali,MD
Brown,Elliot M.,MD
Jawetz,Seth Gerald,MD
Julie,Edward,MD
Krol,Ryszard B.,MD
Obeleniene,Rimvida,MD
Prakash,Atul,MD
Sankholkar,Kedar Deepak,MD
Skolnick,Bruce A.,MD
Sullivan,Brendan Patrick,MD
Sullivan,Gregory F.,MD
Szwed,Stanley A.,MD
Teicher,Mark,MD
Weiss,Emmanuel M.,MD
Clinton
Lind,Robert S.,MD
Columbus
Spagnuolo,Vincent J.,MD
Denville
Lopez,Juan,MD
Shanley,Frank M.,DO
East Brunswick
Altmann,Dory Bert,MD
Avendano,Graciano Gary F.,MD
Burns,John J.,MD
Chai,Yee Meen,MD
Kalra,Amit,MD
Keller,Barnes D.,MD
Kim,Hyung G.,MD
Kumar,Ashok,MD
Kumar,Nidhi,MD
Mermelstein,Erwin,MD
Oberweis,Brandon Scott,MD
Passi,Rakesh K.,MD
Saviano,George J.,MD
Schaer,David H.,MD
Shell,Roger A.,MD
Siu,Dwayne Winfred,DO
East Orange
Amato,James L. Jr.,MD
Binenbaum,Steve Z.,MD
Lee,Terrance H.,MD
Rajiyah,Gitendra,MD
Eatontown
Bach,Matt,MD
Berger,Lance Seth,MD
Boak,Joseph G.,MD
Daniels,Jeffrey S.,MD
Daniels,Steven J.,MD

Kapoor,Mahim,MD
Kim,Jiwon,MD
Koo,Charles H.,MD
LaMarche,Nelson S.,MD
Mascarenhas,Mark Adrian,MD
Mattina,Charles J.,MD
O'Neill,Leon Frederick IV,DO
Osofsky,Jeffrey Lee,MD
Rizzo,Thomas F.,MD
Rodriguez,Pascual B.,MD
Sealove,Brett Andrew,MD
Wappel,Michael A.,MD
Edgewater
Admani,Irfan Mohamed,MD
Bareket,Yaron,MD
Codel,Radu,MD
Pumill,Rick J.,MD
Raskin,Adam Brett,MD
Segovia,Fernando,MD
Edison
Barsky,Aron Alan,MD
Buck,Warren G.,MD
Calvo,Ricardo A.,MD
Cohen,Howard S.,MD
Cohen,Larry J.,MD
Cristoforo,Nancy Todd,MD
Duch,Peter M.,MD
Feingold,Aaron J.,MD
Keller,Malvin S.,MD
Khan,Majid K.,MD
Kovacs,Tiberiu,MD
Kushal,Amrita,MD
Molk,Ian J.,MD
Noveck,Howard D.,MD
Panebianco,Robert Antonino,MD
Ravi,Anita,MD
Rebba,Bhavana,MD
Rudnitzky,Elliot M.,MD
Schanzer,Robert Joseph,MD
Sharma,Bhudev,MD
Wang,Danny,MD
Wasilewski,Stan J.,MD
Egg Harbor Township
Desai,Rashmikant Sumantlal,MD
Elnahal,Mohamed H.,MD
Robbins,Inga H.,MD
Shetty,Sanjay,MD
Elizabeth
Cholankeril,Mathew V.,MD
Cholankeril,Matthew George,MD
Joshi,Meherwan Burzor,MD
Emerson
Bagade,Vivek Laxman,MD
Christensen,Brenda M.,MD
Jacowitz,Joel D.,MD
Kaufman,Bradley S.,MD
Walker,Tracy Lynne,MD
Englewood
Blood,David King,MD
Erlebacher,Jay A.,MD
Feigenblum,David Yehuda,MD
Goldweit,Richard S.,MD
Hodges,David M.,MD
Katechis,Dennis,DO
Leber,George B.,MD
Matican,Jeffrey S.,MD
Mitchel,Jeffrey M.,MD
Reiner,David M.,MD
Schwarcz,Aron Isaac,MD
Stone,Jane E.,MD
Strobel,Ronald E.,MD
Suede,Samuel,MD
Weissman,Andrew J.,MD
Wilchfort,Samuel D.,MD
Wilkenfeld,Craig,MD
Englishtown
Patel,Jatinchandra Suryakant,DO
Fair Lawn
Bikkina,Mahesh,MD
Chabbott,David Robert,MD
Grossman,Steven H.,MD
Herman,Brad Morris,MD
Infantino,Salvatore,MD
Kasatkin,Alexander E.,MD
Maresca,Warren L.,MD
Medepalli,Prasad B.,MD
Molloy,Thomas J.,MD
Patel,Rima Dipak,MD
Samuel,Anish,MD
Smith,John P,DO
Soyombo,Aderemi B.,MD

Physicians by Specialty and Town

Strobeck,John Edward,MD
Vehra,Ijaz R.,MD
Fanwood
Kalischer,Alan L.,MD
Flemington
Benigno,Robert A.,MD
Bialy,Ted,MD
Horiuchi,Jonathan K.,MD
Imsirovic-Starcevic,Dubravka,MD
Kutscher,Austin Harrison Jr.,MD
Pickoff,Robert M.,MD
Schafranek,William,MD
Tonnessen,Glen E.,MD
Florham Park
Fabrizio,Lawrence,DO
Steinberg,Jonathan S.,MD
Fords
Latif,Pervaize,MD
Fort Lee
Adibi,Baback,MD
Andrews,Paul Matthew,MD
Gallo,Richard James,MD
Hollywood,Jacqueline,MD
Kim,Steve Sang-Yoon,MD
Krasikov,Tatiana,MD
Landers,David Benjamin,MD
Lauricella,Joseph Ned,MD
Lebowitz,Nathaniel Edward,MD
Rothman,Howard C.,MD
Zanger,Diane Rachel,MD
Franklin Lakes
Golden,Lee Scott,MD
Wertheimer,David Eliot,MD
Freehold
Awasthi,Ashish,MD
Beauregard,Louanne M.,MD
Borgersen,Rudolph H.,DO
Garg,Sangeeta,MD
Gutowski,Ted,MD
Hanfling,Marcus,DO
Kominos,Vivian A.,MD
Liu,Marcia Nai-Hwa,MD
Mentle,Iris R.,MD
Noto,Gregory,MD
Zukerman,Louis Steven,MD
Galloway
Carreno,Wilfredo,MD
Delaverdac,Claude L.,DO
Flynn,Anthony M.,MD
Ghaly,Nader Naguib,MD
Ghayal,Mahesh,MD
Jayasinghe,Swarnathilaka,MD
Kanzaria,Mitul,MD
Merchant,Yatish B.,MD
Nascimento,Tome R.,MD
Van Hook,Jeffrey E.,DO
Vankawala,Viren R.,MD
Glen Ridge
Alfonso,Carlos Roel Villegas,MD
De Gregorio,Bart,MD
De Gregorio,Joseph Anthony,MD
Di Giorgio,Christopher B.,MD
Knezevic,Dusan Svetozar,MD
Mariano,Domenic L.,DO
Saroff,Alan L.,MD
Voudouris,Apostolos A.,MD
Wanat,Francis E.,MD
Guttenberg
Katdare,Umesh Vasudeo,MD
Hackensack
Berkowitz,Robert Lester,MD
Denson,H. Mark,MD
Glotzer,Taya Valerie,MD
Kanarek,Steven Edward,MD
Kapoor,Saurabh,MD
Katebian,Manoucher E.,MD
Lau,Henry,MD
Maza,Sharon R.,MD
Mulkay,Angel J.,MD
Nejad,Karan S.,MD
Nia,Hamid Mohammad,MD
Patel,Jayantkumar N.,MD
Patel,Rajiv J.,DO
Radoslovich,Glauco A.,MD
Rossakis,Constantine,MD
Ruffo,Scott D.,MD
Sethi,Ruchi S.,MD
Sethi,Virender,MD
Shah,Umang Lalit,MD
Sharma,Sarika,MD
Silber,David Joseph,DO

New Jersey Physicians
Section 3 Medical Specialty and Town

Physicians by Specialty and Town

Cardiovascular Disease (cont)

Hackensack
- Simons, Grant Russell, MD
- Simpson, Timothy E., MD
- Teichholz, Louis E., MD
- Vaidya, Pranaychan J., MD
- Weinstock, Murray, MD
- Zimmerman, John M., MD

Hackettstown
- Ong, Edgardo A., MD

Haddon Heights
- Da Torre, Steven D., MD
- Fortino, Gregg L., MD
- Gips, Sanford J., MD
- Giri, Kartik S., MD
- Herlich, Michael B., MD
- Kaddissi, Georges Ibrahim, MD
- Levi, Steven A., MD
- Mark, George Edward, MD
- Peter, Annie M., MD
- Snyder, Harvey A., MD
- Verma, Vijayendra Kishore, MD
- Viswanath, Dilip Banad, MD
- Zinn, Andrew P., MD

Hamilton
- Alvi, Afshan Khadija, MD
- Caplan, John L., MD
- Chebotarev, Oleg, MD
- Genin, Ilya D., MD
- Ghusson, Mahmoud Saleh, MD
- Ghusson, Soheir F., MD
- Gibreal, Mohammed, MD
- Patel, Jay K., MD
- Ryder, Ronald G., DO
- South, Harry L., MD
- Wilson, Bruce Leonard, MD

Hammonton
- Saia, John A., DO
- Slaven, Timothy M., DO
- Ukrainski, Gerald J., MD
- Wroblewski, Edward A., MD

Hasbrouck Heights
- Goodman, Daniel J., MD
- Sehgal, Evan D., MD

Hawthorne
- Montagnino, Joseph W., MD

Hazlet
- Ani, Mohamad Salim, MD
- Sarnelle, Joseph A., MD
- Uppal, Parveen, MD

Hillsborough
- Taylor, Jeff Thomas, MD

Hoboken
- Costomiris, Robert P., MD
- Damle, Jagadish V., MD
- Fishbein, Richard J., MD
- Kyreakakis, Anthony J., MD
- Leon, Robert John, MD
- Susi, Brian Dievendorf, MD

Holmdel
- Prasad, Penesetti V., MD
- Shah, Niranjan S., MD
- Yen, Ya-Tang, MD

Irvington
- Campbell, Joseph V., MD
- Patel, Sunil Madhusuda, MD

Iselin
- Bhatnagar, Vibhay, MD
- Chaudhery, Shaukat A., MD
- Patel, Ravindra I., MD

Jersey City
- Abed, Mary T., MD
- Ahmad, Muhammad A., MD
- Ameen, Abdul Aleem, MD
- Barber, Nathaniel A., MD
- Baruchin, Mitchell Alan, MD
- Benz, Michael, MD
- Cruz-Encarnacion, Merle C., MD
- Hamirani, Kamran Ismail, MD
- Hannallah, Benyamin A., MD
- Hupart, Preston Arthur, DO
- Moussa, Ghias M., MD
- Pandya, Madhukar N., MD
- Patel, Vinodkumar G., MD
- Phung, Michael Hung, MD
- Rezai, Feridoun, MD
- Richard, Merwin Francis, MD
- Sastry, Pillutla V., MD
- Shah, Deepak O., MD
- Singh, Bharat, MD
- Taha, Abdallah R., MD
- Terwes, Estella, MD
- Wong, Peter J., MD

Kearny
- Daoko, Joseph, MD
- Deshpande, Mohan S., MD

Kendall Park
- Huang, Michael Shu Hsien, DO

Kenilworth
- Berman, Gail O., MD

Lakewood
- Bacharach, Moshe, MD
- Grill, Lawrence J., MD
- Gupta, Avinash Chandra, MD
- Kadosh, Yisrael, MD
- Mohan, Rajesh, MD
- Patel, Nachiket V., MD

Lawrenceville
- Al-Bezem, Rim, MD
- Costanzo, William Edward, MD
- Drucker, David Wayne, MD
- Goldsmith, Steven Matthew, MD
- Heyrich, George Patrick, MD
- Hyman, Richard Louis, MD
- Karl, Justin Adam, MD
- Lebovitz, Philip Lewis, MD
- Rosvold, David Nelson, MD
- Rozengarten, Michael Jacob, MD
- Stern, Alan G., MD
- Venkatesulu, Sunder, MD
- Wolfson, Keith Richard, MD
- Zacks, Eran Sol, MD

Leonia
- Livelli, Frank D. Jr., MD

Livingston
- Anton, John, MD
- Bahler, Alan S., MD
- Demidowich, George, MD
- Fernandes, John, MD
- Gressianu, Monica Terezia, MD
- Kaluski, Edo, MD
- Kashnikow, Constantine, MD
- Woroch, Bohdar O., MD

Lodi
- Thamman, Vijay K., MD

Logan Township
- Pahlow, Brian J., DO

Long Branch
- Checton, John B., MD
- Master, Julie, DO

Lyndhurst
- Conroy, Daniel Jr., MD
- Cubero, John G., MD

Mahwah
- Najovits, Andrew Joseph, MD
- Sharma, Ashok K., MD

Manahawkin
- Henry, James R., MD
- Hong, William Y. C., MD
- Malinverni, Helio J., MD
- Reed, William E., DO
- Tekriwal, Mahesh Kumar, MD

Manalapan
- Dworkin, Jack H., MD

Manasquan
- Infantolino, Philip L., MD

Maplewood
- Jacobson, Sayre K., MD
- Tanwir, Anjum, MD

Marlboro
- Patel, Jayendrakumar N., MD

Matawan
- Panezai, Fazal R., MD

Medford
- O'Neil, James P., MD

Mendham
- Olivieri, Philip J., MD
- Ricculli, Nicholas P., DO
- Shioleno, Charles A., MD
- Tully, Lisa Anita, MD

Metuchen
- Chiaramida, Anthony J., MD
- Goldberg, William P., MD
- Mondrow, Daniel N., MD
- Sauberman, Roy Burton, MD
- Singh, Varinder M., MD
- Sodhi, Ajit S., MD

Middlesex
- Shaheen, Zafar A., MD

Middletown
- Suaray, Khalil M., MD

Millburn
- Aueron, Fred M., MD
- Charney, Robert Howard, MD
- Gantz, Kenneth B., MD
- Patrawalla, Shirish C., MD
- Saeed, Qaisra Yasmin, MD
- Simandl, Susan Lynn, MD

Millville
- Shapiro, Barry E., DO

Monroe
- Logothetis, George Nicholas, MD

Monroe Township
- Baron, Phillip, MD
- Tannenbaum, Alan K., MD

Montclair
- Bannerman, Kenneth S., MD
- Di Filippo, John A., MD
- El-Atat, Fadi Ahmed, MD
- Gutman, Julius A., MD
- Miller, Kenneth Paul, MD
- Prior, Francis P., MD

Moorestown
- Dennis, Charles A., MD
- Duca, Maria Diane, MD
- Finch, Mark T., MD
- Galski, Thomas M., DO
- Lederman, Steven M., MD
- Namey, Jeffrey Elias, MD
- Procacci, Pasquale M., MD
- Sambucci, Deborah A., DO
- Sauerwein, Anthony G., MD
- Schimenti, Robert J., MD
- Sussman, Jay I., MD
- Ventrella, Samuel M., MD

Morris Plains
- Gallerstein, Peter E., MD

Morristown
- Blum, Mark A., MD
- Boccia Liang, Claire G., MD
- Campanile, Giovanni, MD
- Curwin, Jay Howard, MD
- Dickson, David Gordon, MD
- Fisch, Arthur P., MD
- Freilich, David I., MD
- Gillam, Linda Dawn, MD
- Goldschmidt, Marc Eliot, MD
- Guss, Stephen B., MD
- Hsieh, Allen, MD
- Levy, Stephen M., MD
- Limandri, Giuseppe, MD
- Mahoney, Timothy Hugh, MD
- Mandel, Leonid, MD
- Marcoff, Leo, MD
- Martin, Joanne C., MD
- Mondelli, John Anthony, MD
- Natello, Gregory W., DO
- Ramos Bondy, Beatrix Marie, MD
- Raska, Karel, MD
- Santiago, Derek W., MD
- Schalet, Bennett David, DO
- Schwartz, Jeffrey G., MD
- Smart, Frank W., MD
- Uretsky, Seth, MD
- Verdesca, Stephen A., MD
- Watson, Richard I., MD
- Weisbrot, Joshua, MD
- Weisen, Steven Fred, MD
- von Poelnitz, Audrey E., MD

Mount Arlington
- Lowell, Barry H., MD
- Nazeer, Amjad, MD
- Shen, Rhuna, MD

Mountain Lakes
- Ahmad, Mehmood R., MD
- Blick, Michael D., MD
- Cook, Guillermo A., MD
- De Renzi, Paul D., MD
- Malagold, Michael, MD
- Massari, Ronald D., MD
- Naeem, Sheikh M., MD
- Park, Hyeun Sik, MD
- Safirstein, Jordan Glanzman, MD
- Shulruff, Stuart E., MD
- Wall, Robert M., MD
- Wang, Robert L., MD

Neptune
- Aaron, Michael R., DO
- Choi, Edward Joung Myung, MD
- Chu, Tony Nang-Tang, MD
- Colmer, Marc E., MD
- Diwan, Ravi, MD
- Gill, Jasrai Singh, MD
- Karam, Sara K., MD
- Knight, Michael Robert, MD
- Narula, Amar Singh, MD
- Okere, Arthur Ezeribe, MD
- Orlando, James Frank, MD
- Sandler, Leonard Lewis, MD
- Weiss, Maurice D., MD
- Yang, Rayson C., MD

New Brunswick
- Cytryn, Richard A., MD
- Hilkert, Robert Joseph, MD
- Iyer, Deepa Balasubramanian, MD
- Jacob, David E., MD
- Jeganathan, Narayanan, MD
- Kauh, John S., MD
- Krause, Tyrone J., MD
- Lacy, Clifton R., MD
- Moreyra, Abel E., MD
- Shah, Nihir Biharilal, MD
- Sharma, Ravinder, MD
- Shindler, Daniel M., MD
- Turi, Zoltan G., MD
- Zakir, Ramzan Muhammad, MD

New Providence
- Farry, John Patrick, MD
- Glasofer, Sidney, MD
- Mich, Robert John, MD
- Rosenthal, Todd Michael, MD

Newark
- Ahmed, Shaikh Sultan, MD
- Amponsah, Michael Kwesi, MD
- Asif, Mohammad, MD
- Atherley, Trevor H., MD
- Chen, Chunguang, MD
- Cohen, Marc, MD
- Dailey-Sterling, Felix G., MD
- DeCosimo, Diana R., MD
- Gidea, Claudia Gabriela, MD
- Goldfarb, Irvin D., MD
- Goldstein, Jonathan Edward, MD
- Ishikawa, Yoshihiro, MD
- Klapholz, Marc, MD
- Madan, Pankaj, MD
- Nawaz, Yassir, MD
- Ribner, Hillel S., MD
- Rothbart, Stephen T., MD
- Rubinstein, Hector T., MD
- Saric, Muhamed, MD
- Shamoon, Fayez E., MD
- Solanki, Pallavi S., MD
- Tsyvine, Daniel, MD
- Waller, Alfonso Hillman, MD
- Wasty, Najam, MD
- Zucker, Mark J., MD

Newton
- Buyer, David S., MD
- Codispoti, Cindy A., DO
- Masci, Robert L., MD
- Redline, Richard C., MD
- Schwarz, Scott A., MD

North Arlington
- Anastasiades, Athos C., MD
- Burachinsky, Andrew E., DO
- Latyshev, Yevgeniy, MD

North Bergen
- Alcorta, Carlos E., MD
- Basu, Mihir Kumar, MD
- Gabelman, Mark Scott, MD
- Stein, Aaron A., MD

North Brunswick
- Blau, Howard, MD
- Sicherman, Harlan J., MD
- Weisfogel, Gerald M., MD

Norwood
- Tsenovoy, Petr Leonidovich, MD
- Weslow, Renee G., MD

Nutley
- Fusilli, Louis D., MD
- Savino, Leonard, MD

Oakland
- Budhwani, Navin, MD
- Montgomery, David H., MD
- Williams, Marcus L., MD

Old Bridge
- Wajnberg, Alexander, MD

Oradell
- Karlekar, Kripalaxmi R., MD

Orange
- Barai, Jayant H., MD

Physicians by Specialty and Town

Paramus
Baklajian,Robert,MD
Cohen,David Eliot,MD
Elson,Abe,MD
Skeete-Jackson,Kalia Nicole,MD
Wiedermann,Joseph Gad,MD
Park Ridge
Feigelis,Robin Y.,MD
Parlin
Nagarsheth,Harish N.,MD
Piscopiello,Michael,MD
Younan,K. George,MD
Passaic
Sharma,Surendra M.,MD
Paterson
Agarwal,Ashoke,MD
Connolly,Mark William,MD
Teli,Kunal J.,MD
Pennington
Glickman,Lee M.,MD
Saxena,Neil,MD
Perth Amboy
Niemiera,Mark L.,MD
Phillipsburg
Brar,Navtej Singh,DO
Costacurta,Gary A.,MD
Emery,Robert C.,MD
Mascarenhas,Daniel A.,MD
Patel,Chandulal Harilal,MD
Popkave,Arthur H.,MD
Prasad,Amit,MD
Rohatgi,Rajeev,MD
Schiavone,Joseph Adriano,MD
Singh,Narpinder,MD
Pine Brook
Chandrasekaran,Kulandaivelu,MD
Piscataway
Catapano,Joseph A.,MD
Plainfield
Husain,Saleem,MD
Plainsboro
Bergmann,Steven Robert,MD
Pleasantville
Ahmed,Sujood,MD
Rajput,Ilyas A.,MD
Pomona
Spielman,Charles C.,MD
Trivedi,Niranjan G.,MD
Pompton Plains
Blitz,Lawrence R.,MD
Duvvuri,Krishna,MD
Rosenthal,Mark S.,MD
Siepser,Stuart L.,MD
Tabaksblat,Martin Yaron,MD
Princeton
Beattie,James Ray III,MD
Costin,Andrew,MD
Mahalingam,Banu,MD
McCabe,Johnathan B.,MD
Mercuro,Tobia J.,MD
Rumberger,John Arthur,MD
Shanahan,Andrew J.,MD
Weinberg,Fredrick M.,MD
Wong,Casey,MD
Younes,Desiree Marie,MD
Princeton Junction
Angel,Juliette,MD
Ruddy,Michael C.,MD
Rahway
Lee,Young-II,MD
Randolph
Rogers,Philip S.,MD
Ridgefield
Sherer,Stephen B.,MD
Ridgefield Park
Lee,Nellie U.,MD
Ridgewood
Abbate,Kariann Ferguson,MD
Burke,Benita Mia,MD
Co,John A.,MD
Goldschmidt,Howard Z.,MD
Mansson,Sarah Jane Deleon,DO
Musat,Dan Laurentiu,MD
Panagiotou,Demetrios N.,MD
Reison,Dennis S.,MD
Saporito,Robert A. Jr.,MD
Sotsky,Gerald,MD
Sotsky,Mark I.,MD
Strain,Janet E.,MD

Robbinsville
Agarwal,Ashish Madanlal,MD
Barn,Kulpreet S.,MD
Gala,Ketan M.,MD
Patel,Jigar A.,MD
Rothstein,Neil M.,MD
Samuel,Steven Alan,MD
Singhal,Shalabh,MD
Wolf,Andreas,MD
Rochelle Park
Clifford,James R.,MD
Di Vagno,Leonardo Joseph,MD
Rumson
O'Connell,Mark M.,MD
Rutherford
Schwarz,Michael L.,MD
Saddle Brook
Salerno,William D.,MD
Saddle River
Kasper,Andrew,MD
Kasper,Michael E.,MD
Scotch Plains
Coquia,Salvador F.,MD
Lomnitz,Esteban R.,MD
Sea Girt
Eisenberg,Scott R.,DO
Hynes,Peter James,MD
Kayser,Robert Granville Jr.,MD
Sewell
Bagaria,Surendra K.,MD
Crasner,Joshua M.,DO
DePace,Nicholas L.,MD
Maiese,Mario L.,DO
Weinberg,Howard M.,DO
Short Hills
Tansey,William Austin III,MD
Shrewsbury
Edlin,Dale E.,MD
Miller,Charles Luther,MD
Somers Point
Arluck,David Lawrence,MD
Dib,Haitham R.,MD
Dowd,Mary Katherine,MD
Kornberg,Steven Edward,MD
Levin,Jacob L.,MD
Singh,Millee,DO
Somerset
Dorazio,John L.,MD
Gladstone,Clifford D.,MD
Khanna,Pravien K.,MD
Kukafka,Sheldon Jay,MD
Kulkarni,Anand U.,MD
Passannante,Anthony Jr.,MD
Passannante,Anthony J. Sr,MD
Patel,Pratik B.,MD
Reddy,Manisha S.,MD
Singal,Dinesh K.,MD
Stroh,Jack A.,MD
Tardos,Jonathan George,MD
South Amboy
Latif,Shahid,MD
Younes,Elie,MD
South Plainfield
Agarwala,Ajay Kumar,MD
Altszuler,Henry M.,MD
Andraws,Richard Zaki,MD
Blumberg,Edwin D.,MD
Leopold,Thomas D.,MD
Rakla,Younus A.,MD
Springfield
Cohen,Barry Mark,MD
Fishberg,Robert Daniel,MD
Lux,Michael S.,MD
Powell,David E.,MD
Prasad,Sanjiv,MD
Roberti,Roberto R.,MD
Stein,Elliott M.,MD
Weber,Vance J.,MD
Weinrauch,Michael L.,MD
Summit
Iuzzolino,Anthony,MD
Krell,Mark J.,MD
Teaneck
Angeli,Stephen J.,MD
Desai,Shalin P.,MD
Eichman,Gerard T.,MD
Issa,Ebrahim S.,MD
Sagar,Yogesh,MD
Syed,Tariqshah Muhammad,MD
Vandyck-Acquah,Marian M.,MD
Welish,Steven Jay,MD

Wild,David Marc,MD
Tinton Falls
Belluscio,Roland L.,MD
Drout,David I.,MD
O'Keefe,Arthur A. Jr.,MD
Vlahos,Aristotelis E.,MD
Zukoff,David S.,MD
Toms River
Alturk,Najib M.,MD
Bacani,Victor O.,MD
Bageac,Michael,MD
Calderon,Dawn Michelle,DO
Chang,Richard Youngjae,DO
Clancy,Kevin F.,MD
Cornell,Russell John,MD
DiPisa,Leonard R.,MD
Douedi,Hani R.,MD
Guarino,Joseph J. Jr.,MD
Gupta,Anil Kumar,MD
Jacobs,Glenn Paul,MD
Jain,Samir S.,MD
Karatepe,Murat,MD
Merlino,John Anthony III,DO
Mohandas,Bhavna,MD
Pasquariello,James L.,MD
Rana,Yebarna S.,MD
Roggemann,Dennis J.,MD
Sobti,Sanjiv,MD
Stone,Jay H.,MD
Tenner,Bruce S.,DO
Tsang,Kock-Yen,MD
Trenton
Damani,Prabodhkum M.,MD
DeGoma,Rolando L.,MD
DeStefano,Peter M.,MD
Kalra,Krishan G.,MD
Madeira,Samuel Jr.,MD
Nagra,Bipinpreet Singh,MD
Union
Doskow,Jeffrey B.,MD
Gopinathan,Kastooril,MD
Lombardo,Sabato J.,MD
Schackman,Paul E.,MD
Vitale,Carl J.,MD
Williams,Edward G. Jr.,MD
Union City
Grandhi,Sreeram,MD
Inguaggiato,Anthony J.,MD
Presilla,Alejandro,MD
Ventnor
Romero,Luis N.,MD
Vernon
Lanzilotti,Thomas A.,MD
Verona
Lander,Jeffrey,MD
Williams,Errol Baldwin,MD
Vineland
Cohn,Steven M.,MD
Dovnarsky,Michael K.,MD
Pilly,Ashok K.,MD
Quinlan,Jack Francis Jr.,MD
Rainear,Kristen,DO
Shatkin,Bennett J.,MD
Voorhees
Andriulli,John A.,DO
Barrucco,Robert John,DO
Cha,Ri D.,MD
Curl,Kevin M.,MD
Daly,Stephen J.,DO
Dudda Subramanya,Raghunandan,MD
Geisler,Alan K.,DO
Gerewitz,Fredric B.,MD
German,Yelena,MD
Joffe,Ian I.,MD
Kramer,Alan D.,MD
La Morte,Alfonso M.,DO
Lisa,Charles P.,MD
Mintz,Randy T.,MD
Orth,Donald W.,MD
Palermo,Jason,MD
Papa,Louis A.,DO
Patel,Rajendra B.,MD
Perlman,Richard L.,MD
Rozanski,Lawrence T.,MD
Russo,Andrea Marie,MD
Russo,Ralph E. III,MD
Schlessel,David R.,MD
Singer,Robert A.,MD
Spivack,Talya R.,MD
Stehman,Glenn R.,DO

Wall
Yoo,Hojun,MD
Warren
Saksena,Sanjeev,MD
Watchung
Barone,Paul,DO
Catania,Raymond,DO
Wayne
Das,Dhirendra N.,MD
Doss,Emile F.,MD
Ghassemi,Rex,MD
Gupta,Ajay K.,MD
Konlian,Donna Marie,MD
Rathi,Ravi,MD
Salimi,Mostafa,MD
Schair,Barry David,MD
Toor,Saddad Zafar,MD
West Long Branch
Pierson,Christopher G.,MD
West Milford
Platt,Robert N.,MD
West New York
Gonzalez-Gomez,Luis A.,MD
West Orange
Berman,Gary K.,MD
Brock,Donald J.,MD
Chaaban,Fadi Nemer,MD
Chakhtoura,Elie Youssef,MD
Fisk,Marc Saslow,DO
Gandhi,Devang Amrat,MD
Goldberg,Mark C.,MD
Haik,Bruce Joseph,MD
Harback,Edward R.,MD
Hawthorne,Keith Allen,MD
Kadri,Iftekhar S.,MD
Modi,Kaushik Chhaganlal,MD
Rogal,Gary J.,MD
Rubenstein,Donald G.,MD
Schwanwede,Jacqueline M.,MD
Shehadeh,Abbas A.,MD
Torre,Sabino Richard,MD
Tullo,Nicholas G.,MD
Wangenheim,Paul M.,MD
Wu,Chia F.,MD
West Paterson
Capitanelli,John R.,MD
Kaddaha,Raja'A Mohammed,MD
Losardo,Anthony A.,MD
Westampton
Nachtigall,Jonathan C.,DO
Westfield
Surks,Howard K.,MD
Westwood
Barr,Stuart A.,MD
Cocke,Thomas Preston Jr.,MD
Eisenberg,Sheldon B.,MD
Landzberg,Joel Serge,MD
Murphy,Patricia L.,MD
Whitehouse Station
Cody,Robert James,MD
Willingboro
Chardo,Francis Jr.,MD
Coleman,Elliott H.,MD
Horwitz,Michael J.,MD
Klier,Steven W.,MD
Malik,Manish Gulshan,MD
Schulner,Kenneth D.,MD
Shaikh,Hafeza,DO
Wood,Margaret Diana,MD
Woodbridge
Alam,Mahmood,MD
Woodbury
Dawson,Martin S.,MD
Kaulback,Kurt W.,MD
Moccia,Thomas F.,DO
Unwala,Ashfaque A.,MD
Vergari,John Jr.,MD

Cardiovascular Surgery
Browns Mills
Boris,Walter J.,DO
Cane,Michael Elliot,MD
McGrath,Lynn B.,MD
Sodhi,Jitendra,MD
Cherry Hill
Kuchler,Joseph A.,MD
Martella,Arthur Thomas,MD
Nayar,Amrit P.,MD
Clifton
Syracuse,Donald C.,MD

Physicians by Specialty and Town

Cardiovascular Surgery (cont)
Eatontown
  Squillaro,Anthony J.,MD
Edison
  Heller,James Norman,MD
  Javed,Mohammad Tariq,MD
Elizabeth
  Codoyannis,Aristides Basil,MD
Englewood
  Galla,Jan David,MD
Hackensack
  Elmann,Elie Marco,MD
  Somberg,Eric D.,MD
Millburn
  Shah,Shamji K.,MD
Morristown
  Rodriguez,Alejandro L.,MD
New Brunswick
  Scholz,Peter M.,MD
Newark
  Herman,Steven Douglas,MD
  Karanam,Ravindra N.,MD
Short Hills
  Goldenberg,Bruce S.,MD
Summit
  Luka,Norman L.,MD
Trenton
  Seinfeld,Fredric I.,MD
Voorhees
  Eisen,Morris M.,DO
West Orange
  Pinder,Godfrey C.,MD

Cataract
Cliffside Park
  Arturi,Frank C.,MD
Glen Rock
  Portfolio,Almerindo G. Jr.,MD
Ridgewood
  Sumers,Anne R.,MD
Sewell
  Ross,Richard S.,MD
Springfield
  Notis,Corey M.,MD

Child & Adolescent Psychiatry
Atlantic City
  Momodu,Inua Aitsekegbe,MD
Belle Mead
  Marino,Anthony Jr.,MD
  Nisar,Asma,MD
Boonton
  Mahmood,Fauzia,MD
Bound Brook
  Ismail,Mona S. A.,MD
Bridgewater
  Hagino,Owen Rinzo,MD
Caldwell
  Cammarata,Sandra,MD
Camden
  Cagande,Consuelo Corazon,MD
  Pradhan,Basant Kumar,MD
  Pshytycky,Amir,MD
Cape May Court House
  Rodriguez,Hilton John,MD
Cedar Grove
  Platt,Ellen M.,DO
Cedar Knolls
  Hubsher,Merritt S.,MD
Cherry Hill
  Denbo,Nancy J.,MD
  Gurak,Randall B.,MD
  Sosland,Morton D.,MD
Cranbury
  Salvatore,Kate Elizabeth,MD
Cranford
  Chong,Raymond Ee-Mook,MD
  Hong,Rolando Y.,MD
Cresskill
  Brown,Patricia S.,MD
  McGowan,Seth A.,MD
  Munoz-Silva,Dinohra M.,MD
  Silva,Raul R.,MD
Denville
  Brandon,Meredith,MD
  Ying Chang,Jean S.,MD
East Brunswick
  Bekhit,Mariam,MD
  Dyckman,Steven Ira,MD
Edgewater
  Kondrashin,Sofia,MD

Edison
  Santos,Frank,MD
  Castillo,Gregorio A. G.,MD
  Chowdhury,Amina Kausar,MD
  Meghadri,Niveditha,MD
Egg Harbor Township
  O'Reilly,Thomas Christian,MD
Elizabeth
  Campos-Munoz,Magaly C.,MD
  Cobert,Josiane C.,MD
  Gavini,Jaya L.,MD
Emerson
  Patel,Mona M.,MD
Englewood
  Effron-Gurland,Frances R.,MD
  Fridman,Esther D.,MD
  Fridman,Morton Zvi,MD
  Srivastava,Tulika Sinha,MD
Fair Lawn
  Matsenko,Oxana,MD
Flemington
  Chen,Hong,MD
Freehold
  Chatlos,John Calvin Jr.,MD
  Desai,Ankur Akhilesh,MD
  Zaidi,Sajjad,MD
Glen Rock
  Muthusawmy,Nanda,MD
Guttenberg
  Padron-Gayol,Maria V.,MD
Hackensack
  Lewis,Tanya Renee,MD
  Oquendo,Sonia I.,MD
  Osmanova,Nataliya,MD
  Paine,Mercedes A.,MD
  Zhivago,Eileen Ann,MD
Hamilton
  Downs,Elvira Foglia,MD
  Li,Liren,MD
Hammonton
  Burns,Elizabeth Ann,DO
  Rana,Sohail Anjum,MD
Highland Park
  Kleinmann,Richard,MD
Hillsdale
  Schneider,Mona,MD
Hoboken
  Chmarzewski,Barbara,MD
  Moraille,Pascale,MD
Holmdel
  Ritsema,Marc E.,DO
  Varma,Deepti Sagar,MD
Jersey City
  Stewart,Michael Starbin,MD
Kendall Park
  Schnitzlein,Robert,MD
Liberty Corner
  Braver,Vanita,MD
Livingston
  Bartky,Eric Jay,MD
  Jacque,Celeste A.,MD
  Kycia,Lan Ing,MD
  Lipman,Ted,MD
  Rudominer,Howard S.,MD
Long Branch
  Pogran,Jessica Rose,DO
Lumberton
  Stein,Lynne H.,MD
Lyons
  Kaune,Maureen,MD
Madison
  Fennelly,Bryan William,MD
Marlton
  Brancato,Peter Jr.,MD
  Embrescia,Mary Megan,MD
  Gupta,Mala Rani,MD
  Prince,Leonie S.,MD
  Singh,Sarabjit,MD
  Varrell,James R.,MD
  Vassallo,Frank A.,DO
Maywood
  Mitnick,David Andrew,MD
Metuchen
  Shampain,Lawrence R.,MD
  Winograd,Barbara H.,MD
Midland Park
  Rodriguez-Frank,Laura V.,MD
Millstone Township
  Mazur,Irene,MD

Montclair
  Della Bella,Peter,MD
  Kennedy,Paul,MD
  Lebowitz-Naegeli,Nanci L.,MD
Moorestown
  Ralph,Pamela J.,MD
Morristown
  Bash,Howard Lee,MD
  Bhatia,Nita,DO
  Cohen,Adam Jonathan,MD
  Giuliano,Michael A.,MD
  Muthuswamy,Rajeswari,MD
Mount Holly
  Bernacki,Carolyn Green,DO
Neptune
  Iofin,Alexander,MD
  Kochhar,Seema,MD
New Brunswick
  Gowda,Nidagalle,MD
  Ryan,Colleen A.,MD
Newark
  Bhatt,Usha Praful,MD
  Chacko-Varkey,Suneeta Esther,MD
  Gude,Prabhavat Venkata,MD
  Isecke,Dorothy Ann,MD
  Power,Rachael Reiko,MD
  Riaz,Najeeb,MD
  Yangchen,Tenzing,MD
North Brunswick
  Khwaja,Tahir Nisar,MD
  Lukac,Juraj,MD
  Parikh,Chirayu Bharat,DO
Oakhurst
  Tetelbom,Miriam,MD
Oakland
  Chalemian,Bliss A.,MD
Old Bridge
  Krishnamsetty,Nanditha,MD
Paramus
  Calvert,Sara Marie,MD
  Khan,Adnan Iqbal,MD
  Puthiyathu,Manoj,MD
  Radulescu,Raluca Ileana,MD
  Shabo,Jessica E.,MD
Parsippany
  Srinivasan,Shankar,MD
Paterson
  Christodoulou,Evangelos,MD
  Garcia,Dianelys,MD
  Langan,Abigail E.,MD
  Marrero Figarella,Arturo L.,MD
Pennington
  Fong,Donald Patrick,MD
  Patchell,Roy Andrew,MD
Piscataway
  Deshpande,Kalyani Kumari,MD
  Ilaria,Shawen Maryrose,MD
  Novotny,Sherie Lynn,MD
  Pace,Patrick V.,MD
  Rosenberg,Gary B.,MD
  Sahoo,Madhusmita,MD
  Upadhyay,Anu,MD
Pompton Plains
  Ladov,Norman,MD
Princeton
  Bhalla,Saranga,DO
  Gursky,Elliot J.,MD
  Hassan,Ahmad Mohamed,MD
  Hayes,William P.,MD
  Khare,Madhurani,MD
  Martinson,Charles F.,MD
  Mian,Asma,MD
  Saldarini,Candace Tom,MD
  Schafer,Laura,MD
  Stayer,Catherine C.,MD
Ramsey
  Hanna,Mohab,MD
Randolph
  Desai,Maya G.,MD
Red Bank
  Goss,Graydon G.,MD
  Grant,Susan J.,MD
  Kowalik,Sharon,MD
  Lin,Shengxi,MD
Ridgefield
  Lee,Seung Ho,MD
Ridgewood
  Bhalla,Ravinder N.,MD
  Gentile,Michael P.,MD
  Sugar,Nina S.,MD

  Wruble,Steven J.,MD
Rochelle Park
  Korshunova,Valeria S.,MD
Roseland
  Elfenbein,Emanuel,MD
Rumson
  Doumas,Stacy James,MD
Secaucus
  Mastroti,Jean-Baptiste J.,MD
Shrewsbury
  Alcera,Eric Cortez,MD
  Edwards,Jennifer L.,MD
Skillman
  Dismukes,Jennifer Bright,DO
Somerdale
  Feigl,Frances Marie,MD
Somerset
  Randolph,Robert Styles,MD
  Yeung,Wilbert Derek,MD
Somerville
  Hossain,Akhtar,MD
South Plainfield
  Siddiqui,Waqar Ahmed,MD
Springfield
  Cohen,Hayley M.,MD
  Kaplan,Gabriel,MD
  Silver,Bennett,MD
Stratford
  Humphrey,Frederick James II,DO
  Kumar,Geetha,MD
  Levitas,Andrew S.,MD
  O'Donnell-Mulgrew,Deborah M.,DO
Summit
  Canosa,Omar,MD
  Hasan,Syeda I.,MD
  Mangunay,Nora Ramos,MD
  Sehgal,Shaley Prem,MD
Tenafly
  Geelan,Caroline C.,DO
  Schreiber,Thomas J.,MD
Toms River
  Ballesteros,Alberto F.,MD
  Pitera,Matthew J.,MD
  Senese,Karen,MD
Upper Montclair
  Faber,Mark P.,MD
  Mason-Bell,Sharon E.,MD
Wall
  Chottera,Shobha A.,MD
Warren
  Colon,Vincent F.,MD
West New York
  Wang,Wei,MD
West Orange
  Greene,Bruce H.,DO
  Khanna,Bindu Chiranjit,MD
Woodbury
  Vidal,Heidi Robin,MD
Woodcliff Lake
  Grosso,Joseph X.,MD

Child (Pediatric) Neurology
Camden
  Gonzalez Monserrate,Evelyn,MD
  McAbee,Gary Noel,DO
Edison
  Bandari,Savitra M.,MD
  Milrod,Lewis Martin,MD
  Ming,Xue,MD
  Velicheti,Kavitha,MD
Fair Lawn
  Woo,Judy,MD
Florham Park
  Grossman,Elliot A.,MD
Gibbsboro
  Mintz,Mark I.,MD
Hackensack
  Katz,Michael Dennis,MD
  Lazar,Lorraine M.,MD
Jersey City
  Hanna,Amir Atallaha,MD
  Kozanitis Mentakis,Irene D.,MD
Livingston
  Kubichek,Marilyn Ann,MD
Morristown
  DeSouza,Trevor G.,MD
  Waran,Sandy P.,MD
Mountainside
  Traeger,Eveline C.,MD

Physicians by Specialty and Town

Neptune
　Pietrucha,Dorothy M.,MD
　Sultan,Richard I.,DO
New Brunswick
　Chaaban,Janti,MD
　Di Cicco Bloom,Emanuel M.,MD
　Esfahanizadeh,Abdolreza,MD
　Patel,Payal,MD
　Surgan,Victoria,MD
Newark
　Hayes Rosen,Caroline Diane,MD
　Pak,Jayoung,MD
　Salam,Misbah U.,MD
Paterson
　Patel,Poorvi K.,MD
Ridgewood
　Steinschneider,Mitchell,MD
Summit
　Bennett,Harvey S.,MD
Voorhees
　Mason,Thornton B. II,MD
　Sharif,Uzma M.,MD
Wall
　Barabas,Ronald E.,MD
West Windsor
　Mannheim,Glenn Barry,MD

Clinical & Laboratory Immunology
Atlantic City
　Todd,William Upton IV,MD

Clinical Cardiac Electrophysiology
Bridgewater
　Frenkel,Daniel,MD
　Patel,Ashok Ambalal,MD
Edison
　Ballal,Raj Sadananda,MD
Fair Lawn
　Tiyyagura,Satish Reddy,MD
Flemington
　Rudnick,Andrew Glenn,MD
Florham Park
　Santoni,Francesco,MD
Galloway
　White,Melvin C.,MD
Hackensack
　Shukla,Gunjan Jayendrabhai,MD
Hamilton
　Patel,Aarti,MD
Hillsborough
　Sanyal,Sanjukta,MD
Jersey City
　Ahmad,Ahsanuddin,MD
Maywood
　Zaim,Sina,MD
Middletown
　Dobrescu,Delia J.,MD
Monroe Township
　Maleki,Kataneh F.,MD
Morristown
　Coyne,Robert F.,MD
　Katz,Michael Geoffrey,MD
　Winters,Stephen L.,MD
Neptune
　Girgis,Ihab,MD
Ridgewood
　Bhatt,Advay G.,MD
　Mittal,Suneet,MD
　Preminger,Mark William,MD
　Sichrovsky,Tina Claudia,MD
Somerset
　Gowda,Subhashini Anande,MD
West Orange
　Costeas,Constantinos A.,MD
　Dobesh,David P.,MD
　Roelke,Marc,MD
Woodbury
　Padder,Farooq Ahmad,MD

Clinical Cytogenetics
Newark
　Toruner,Gokce,MD

Clinical Genetics
Flemington
　Rushton,Alan R.,MD
New Brunswick
　Brooks,Susan Sklower,MD
　Day Salvatore,Debra-Lynn,MD

Newark
　Pletcher,Beth A.,MD
Pennington
　Trauffer,Patrice,MD
Succasunna
　Vosatka,Robert J.,MD

Clinical Neurophysiology
Bridgewater
　Potluri,Srinivasa Rao,MD
Camden
　Noff,Tom,MD
Englewood
　Ko,James H.,MD
Hackensack
　Nogueira,John Francis Jr.,MD
Hamilton
　Zhang,Lei,MD
Livingston
　Goldberg,Rina Freida,MD
　Rodriguez,Andy,MD
Montclair
　Robinton,John E.,MD
Neptune
　Kostoulakos,Paul M.,DO
New Brunswick
　Bhise,Vikram V.,MD
　Wu,Brenda Yunqing,MD
Secaucus
　Ahad,Antwan B.,MD
Somerville
　Mian,Nimer F.,DO
Toms River
　Deliwala,Tejas Pramodrai,MD

Clinical Pathology
Camden
　Nikolic,Dejan,MD
Florham Park
　Hofgaertner,Wolfgang Theodor,MD
New Brunswick
　Deen,Malik F.,MD
Newark
　Grygotis,Anthony E.,MD
　Jin,Li,MD
West New York
　Rudelli,Raul Daniel,MD

Clinical Pathology/Laboratory Med
Atlantic City
　Miller,Nicole C.,DO
New Brunswick
　Kirn,Thomas Joseph Jr.,MD
Princeton
　Saminathan,Thamarai,MD

Clinical Pharmacology
Basking Ridge
　Rullo,Barbara,MD
　Wason,Suman,MD
Chester
　Novitt-Moreno,Anne D.,MD
Edison
　Jacobs,Sharon G.,MD
Lakewood
　Uderman,Howard David,MD

Colon & Rectal Surgery
Atlantic City
　Aarons,William Jr.,MD
Brick
　Park,Jane,MD
Bridgewater
　Sadler,Daniel L.,MD
Camden
　Kann,Brian Robert,MD
　Kawata,Michitaka,MD
Cherry Hill
　Berg,David Adam,MD
　Cody,William C.,MD
　Deleon,Miguel L.,MD
　El Badawi,Khaled Iqbal,MD
　Schaffzin,David Marc,MD
Clifton
　Buckley,Michael K.,MD
East Brunswick
　Patankar,Sanjiv Krishna,MD
Eatontown
　Arvanitis,Michael L.,MD
　Dressner,Roy M.,DO
Edison
　Chinn,Bertram T.,MD

　Deutsch,Michael,MD
　Notaro,Joseph R.,MD
Englewood
　Harris,Michael T.,MD
　Seo,Christina J.,MD
　Waxenbaum,Steven I.,MD
　White,Ronald A.,MD
Freehold
　Kayal,Thomas Joseph,MD
Glen Rock
　Agopian,Raffi E.,MD
　Kwon,Albert O.,MD
Hackensack
　Helbraun,Mark E.,MD
Holmdel
　Malit,Michele Farrah,DO
Lawrenceville
　Eisengart,Charles Andrew,MD
　Hardy,Howard III,MD
Livingston
　Holzman,Kevin Jay,MD
　Huang,Renee,MD
Lumberton
　Hughes,Charles R.,MD
Manahawkin
　Khoo,Robert Eng Hong,MD
Maywood
　Gallina,Gregory J.,MD
Millburn
　Gilder,Mark E.,MD
　Orringer,Robert D.,MD
　Tarantino,Debra R.,MD
　Taylor,Robert L.,MD
Montclair
　Rothberg,Robert M.,MD
Moorestown
　Pilipshen,Stephen J.,MD
Morristown
　Huk,Matthew David,MD
　Moskowitz,Richard L.,MD
New Brunswick
　Eisenstat,Theodore Ellis,MD
　Patel,Nell M.,MD
　Rezac,Craig,MD
　Salehomoum,Negar Monavar,MD
Newark
　Rice,Peter Eric,MD
Oakhurst
　Lake,Thomas R. III,MD
　Parker,Glenn S.,MD
Pompton Lakes
　McConnell,John C.,MD
Pompton Plains
　Nochumson,Joshua Alan,MD
Red Bank
　Wolkomir,Alfred F.,MD
Ridgewood
　Nizin,Joel S.,MD
Sewell
　Schachter,Todd,DO
Sparta
　Green,Jason D.,MD
Summit
　Groff,Walter L.,MD
　Lorber,Julie A.,MD
Teaneck
　Mansouri,Farshad,MD
Union
　Brody,Zoltan,DO
Vineland
　Callender,Gordon Erwin,MD
　Senatore,Peter Joseph,MD
Voorhees
　Gardine,Robert L.,MD
　Irwin,Eytan A.,MD
　Pello,Mark J.,MD
　Siemons,Gary O.,MD
Wall
　Paonessa,Nina Joanne,DO
Wayne
　Khoury,Hani A.,MD

Computer Medicine
Princeton
　Chen,Roland Sangone,MD

Cornea/External Disease
Fort Lee
　Rosenberg,Michael Eric,MD
Freehold
　Schneider,Martin S.,MD

Jersey City
　Constad,William H.,MD
Toms River
　Athwal,Harjit S.,MD
Wayne
　Reing,Charles Scot,MD

Cosmetic Surgery
East Brunswick
　Arno,Joseph P.,MD
Franklin Park
　Perry,Arthur William,MD
Paramus
　Boss,William K. Jr.,MD
　Lat,Emmanuel A.,MD
Ridgewood
　Sternschein,Michael J.,MD
Teaneck
　Sterman,Harris Robert,MD
Verona
　Loverme,Paul J.,MD

Critical Care Medicine
Bayonne
　Takhalov,Yuriy,MD
Branchburg
　Arno,Louis J.,MD
Brick
　Newman,Stephen L.,MD
Bridgewater
　Lee,Jack C.,MD
　Soriano,Aida N.,MD
Browns Mills
　Wargovich,Raymond M.,MD
Camden
　Bekes,Carolyn E.,MD
　Charron,Mariane,MD
　Dellinger,Richard Phillip,MD
　Dettmer,Matthew Robert,MD
　Gerber,David R.,DO
　Gray,Edward Harlan,DO
　Green,Adam Godfrey,MD
　Kreidy,Mazen Pierre,MD
　Lotano,Ramya,MD
　Moradi,Bijan Nik,MD
　Spevetz,Antoinette,MD
　Trzeciak,Stephen Walter,MD
　Zanotti Cavazzoni,Sergio L.,MD
Cedar Knolls
　Capone,Robert Anthony,MD
　Dimitry,Edward Jr.,MD
Cherry Hill
　Baumgarten,Steven S.,MD
　Horowitz,Ira David,MD
Clifton
　Levin,Daniel H.,MD
Denville
　Finkel,Richard I.,MD
East Brunswick
　Harangozo,Andrea M.,MD
　Klitzman,Donna Leslie,MD
　Schiffman,Philip L.,MD
East Orange
　Connell,Rebecca Kathleen,MD
　George,Jason C.,MD
　Hashem,Bassam Emile,MD
Eatontown
　Kramer,Violet Elizabeth,MD
　Livornese,Douglas S.,MD
　Weiner,Sharon M.,MD
Edison
　Anene,Okechukwu P.,MD
　Bhagat,Mahesh H.,MD
　Crawley,Joseph M.,MD
　Melillo,Nicholas G.,MD
　Pesin,Jeffrey L.,MD
　Ramachandraiah,Vidya,MD
　Rosenblatt,Daniel E.,MD
Emerson
　Orr,David A.,DO
Englewood
　Pavlou,Theophanis A.,MD
Fair Lawn
　Singh,Malwinder,MD
Flemington
　Cohn,David B.,MD
　Goldstein,Keith Ty,MD
　Khan,Muhammad Khurram,MD
Forked River
　Power,William K. Jr.,MD

Physicians by Specialty and Town

Critical Care Medicine (cont)
Freehold
  DeTullio, John P., MD
Galloway
  Higgins, Nancy C., MD
Hackensack
  Ashtyani Asl, Fariborz, MD
  Bunnell, Eugene, MD
  Chander, Naresh, MD
  Choi, Weekon, MD
  Nierenberg, Richard J., MD
  Rajaram, Sri-Sujanthy, MD
  Ting, Leon L., MD
Hamilton
  Devine, Mary Ann, MD
  Mehta, Munira Yusuf, MD
  Obaray, Akbar H., MD
Hillsborough
  Einreinhofer, Stephen V., DO
Hoboken
  Chu, Daniel Yun, DO
Jersey City
  Matta, Jyoti S., MD
Lawrenceville
  Nolledo, Michael Teodoro, MD
Livingston
  Marano, Michael A., MD
  Rezai, Fariborz, MD
Lodi
  Santomauro, Emanuele A., MD
Lyndhurst
  Vossough, Soheila, MD
Madison
  Benton, Marc L., MD
Manahawkin
  Dewil, Frederic, MD
Manasquan
  Friedman, Paul Martin, MD
  Gallagher, Cornelius T., MD
Marlton
  Rodis, Angel Victor, MD
Millburn
  Shah, Smita S., MD
Monroe Township
  Freedman, Andrew R., MD
Morristown
  Park, Henry, MD
  Toscano, Andrew, MD
Mount Laurel
  Cohen, Douglas Jay, MD
  Ryan, Kathleen Lisa, MD
Mountainside
  Kleyn, Michael, MD
New Brunswick
  Khan, Talha Ehsan, MD
  Madhavan, Arjun, MD
  Parikh, Amay, MD
  Rana, Haris Ishaque, MD
  Rosenfeld, Jane S., MD
  Russo, Eileen Susan, MD
  Scardella, Anthony T., MD
  Sotolongo, Anays M., MD
  Sunderram, Jagadeeshan, MD
Newark
  Abdeen, Yazan M., MD
  Adelman, Marc R., MD
  Chang, Steven Yang-Liang, MD
  Fless, Kristin Gail, MD
  Lardizabal, Alfred A., MD
  MacBruce, Daphne Karen, MD
  Miller, Richard A., MD
  Sadik, Aseel, MD
Newton
  Garg, Rakesh K., MD
  Nadarajah, Dayaparan, MD
North Bergen
  Capo', Aida P., MD
North Plainfield
  Rehman, Muhammad Ubaid, MD
Old Bridge
  Lee, Edward G., MD
  Mathew, Joseph, MD
Park Ridge
  Hoffman, Joseph Henry, MD
Passaic
  Abraham, James V., MD
Paterson
  Sori, Alan J., MD
  Upadhyay, Shivanck, MD
Perth Amboy
  Doshi, Mona, MD
  Sinha, Vinod K., MD
Phillipsburg
  Latriano, Blaise P., MD
Plainfield
  Bayly, Robert, MD
Pomona
  Riccobono, Elizabeth Kay, DO
Princeton
  Jagpal, Sugeet K., MD
Rahway
  Wojno Oranski, Alexander, DO
Ramsey
  Cooper, Kimberly Anne, DO
  Sharma, Rakesh, MD
Red Bank
  Qumei, Moh'D K. K., MD
Ridgewood
  Melamed, Marc S., MD
Roselle Park
  Brescia, Michael Louis, MD
Sewell
  Obregon, Carlos A., DO
Somers Point
  O'Connor, James J. III, MD
  Ojserkis, Bennett Edward, MD
Somerset
  Das, Arvind K., MD
  Davanzo, Lawrence D., DO
  Doujaiji, Bassam Mouhin, MD
Somerville
  Besserman, Eva B., DO
South Hackensack
  Ashtyani Asl, Hormoz, MD
South Orange
  Achar, Pankaja B.S., MD
Stratford
  Kirkham, Jay G. Jr., DO
Summit
  Cerrone, Federico, MD
  Donnabella, Vincent, MD
  Sussman, Robert, MD
  Zimmerman, Mark I., MD
Toms River
  Eisen, Deborah Ida, MD
  Tomasuolo, Vincent A., MD
Trenton
  Seelagy, Marc M., MD
Voorhees
  Miller, William B., DO
West Orange
  Kuntz, George R., MD
Westwood
  Al Asad, Manar M., MD
Willingboro
  Levinson, Roy M., MD

Cytopathology
Basking Ridge
  Wang, Wenjing, MD
Cherry Hill
  Shienbaum, Alan J., DO
Elmwood Park
  Dupree, William Brion, MD
Hackensack
  Gupta, Anupama, MD
Holmdel
  Wang, Hongling, MD
Lakewood
  Sharaan, Mona El-Sayed, MD
Livingston
  Su, Mu, MD
New Brunswick
  Artymyshyn, Renee L., MD
Phillipsburg
  Manhoff, Dion T., MD
Piscataway
  Liang, Songlin, MD
Woodbury
  Hudock, Jude A., MD

Dermatologic Surgery
Annandale
  Abel, Carter Grant, MD
Marlton
  Decker, Ashley, MD

Dermatology
Allentown
  Kupetsky, Erine Allison, DO
Atlantic Highlands
  Thosani, Maya K., MD
Avenel
  Cerbone, Joseph Eugene, MD
Basking Ridge
  Haliasos, Helen C., MD
  Quigley, Elizabeth A., MD
Bayonne
  Kopec, Anna V., MD
Belleville
  Eastern, Joseph S., MD
Belmar
  Morgan, Aaron J., MD
Berkeley Heights
  Abbasi, Naheed R., MD
  Goldfaden, Isabel, MD
  Gruber, Gabriel G., MD
  Kim, Sam, MD
  Nadiminti, Hari, MD
  Zirvi, Monib Ahmad, MD
Blairstown
  Rocca, Nicole M., MD
Branchburg
  Fox, Alissa B., MD
Brick
  Abel, Mark, MD
Bridgeton
  Fenichel, Stefan, MD
Bridgewater
  Agarwal, Smita, MD
  Mulvihill, Claire A., MD
Camden
  Ghazi, Elizabeth Rose, MD
Cape May Court House
  Paolini, Lawrence, DO
  Weiss, Robert Joseph Sr., MD
Cedar Grove
  Cohen, Alan Polan, MD
  Cunningham, Ellen Elizabeth, MD
  Farley-Loftus, Rachel L., MD
  Kandula, Swetha, MD
Changewater
  Errickson, Carla V., MD
Chatham
  Breslauer, Lisa Marie, MD
Cherry Hill
  DeCosmo, Michael J., DO
  Mastromonaco, Denise M., DO
  Matalon, Vivienne I., MD
  Mellul, Victor G., MD
Chester
  Geller, Jay D., MD
Cliffside Park
  Hershenbaum, Esther, MD
Clifton
  Gold, Jonathan Allan, MD
  Militello, Giuseppe M., MD
  Ros, Adriana Oksana, DO
  Silber, Judy G., MD
  Tanzer, Floyd R., MD
  Zurada, Joanna Magdalena, MD
Closter
  Andrews, Alan D., MD
  Ramaswamy, Preethi V., MD
  Trokhan, Eileen Q., MD
Cresskill
  Gonzalez, Lenis Marisa, MD
Delran
  Harkaway, Karen S., MD
Demarest
  Schiffman, Lawrence Adam, DO
Denville
  Cham, Anita L., MD
  Moy, Winston C., MD
  Spinelli, Nancy Ann, DO
East Brunswick
  Iannotta, Patricia N., MD
  Rothfleisch, Jeremy Evan, MD
  Shraga, Alexander, MD
  Weinstein, Rita, MD
East Orange
  Thomas, Isabelle Marie B., MD
East Windsor
  Bagel, Jerry, MD
  Keegan, Brian Robert, MD
  Myers, Wendy A., MD
  Nieves, David Steiner, MD
  Simon, Jessica, MD
  Stenn, Judit O., MD
Edison
  Paull, Robert M., MD
  Strauch, Joseph M., MD
Elmer
  Aphale, Abhishek N., MD
  Danowski, Kelli Mayo, DO
  Warmuth, Ingrid P., MD
Englewood
  Fishman, Miriam, MD
  Fried, Sharon Z., MD
  Grodberg, Michele, MD
  Ordoukhanian, Elsa, MD
  Rapaport, Jeffrey A., MD
  Steinman, Natasha Margolin, MD
Englewood Cliffs
  Boakye, Naana Agyeiwah, MD
Fair Lawn
  Heldman, Jay P., MD
  Katz, James M., MD
  Singman, Bradford A., MD
  Weiss, Darryl S., MD
Flemington
  Beachler, Kent J., MD
  Blechman, Adam Brandon, MD
  Cassetty, Christopher Todd, MD
  Sood, Supriya G., MD
Florham Park
  Badalamenti, Stephanie Silos, MD
  Huang, Eric Y., MD
  Huang, Eric Yuchueh, MD
  Kiken, David Adam, MD
  Machler, Brian C., MD
  Patel-Cohen, Mital, MD
Fort Lee
  Goulko, Olga, MD
  Lee, Robert, MD
Franklin Lakes
  Abdulla, Heba M., MD
Freehold
  Hametz, Irwin, MD
  Miller, Jason Harris, MD
  Picascia, David D., MD
  Sivanesan, Swarna Priya, MD
Gibbsboro
  Baker, Donald J., MD
Glen Ridge
  Rozanski, Reuben, MD
Glen Rock
  Dosik, Jonathan Scott, MD
  Galvin, Sharon A., MD
Hackensack
  Ashinoff, Robin, MD
  Eilers, Steven Edwin, MD
  Goldberg, David Jay, MD
  Masullo, Alfredo S., MD
  Ravits, Margaret S., MD
  Sapadin, Allen N., MD
  Shin, Helen Theresa, MD
  Wilkerson, Eric Christopher, MD
Haddon Heights
  Allen, Robert Andrew, MD
  Lo Presti, Nicholas P., MD
  Miller, Emily S., MD
  Whipple, D. Sandra, MD
Haddonfield
  Burns, Loren T., MD
  Levine, Erika Gaines, MD
  Suchin, Karen Rebecca, MD
Hamilton Square
  Freedman, Joshua R., MD
  Kessel, Daniel S., MD
Hillsborough
  Henning, Jeffrey Scott, DO
  Ilowite, Robert K., DO
  Man, Jeremy Robert, MD
Hoboken
  Cappiello, Linda L., MD
  Fernandez-Obregon, Adolfo C., MD
Holmdel
  Bhatnagar, Divya Sambandan, MD
Howell
  Weiner, Barry C., MD
Jersey City
  Besedina, Liliya, MD
  Erianne, John A., MD
  Fox, Richard David, MD
  Katz, Arthur M., MD
  Khasak, Dmitry, MD
  Noroff, Joan P., MD
  Stotland, Mira, MD

Physicians by Specialty and Town

Kearny
Fishman, S. Jose, MD
Kenilworth
Pravda, Douglas J., DO
Kinnelon
Schwartz, Carolyn L., MD
Szylit, Jo-Ann, MD
Lakewood
Kuflik, Julianne Helen, MD
Tarlow, Mordechai M., MD
Lawrenceville
Hubert, Steven Lee, MD
Kincaid, Leah Celia, MD
Rajan, Jennifer Ray, MD
Yi, Lusia Sang-suk, DO
Linden
McCormack, Patricia Coppola, MD
Linwood
Connolly, Coyle S., DO
Hong, Joseph Johnson, MD
Little Falls
Whitworth, Jeffrey Michael, MD
Little Silver
Grossman, Kenneth A., MD
Livingston
Bronsnick, Tara A., MD
Citron, Cheryl S., MD
Liftin, Alan J., MD
Nervi, Stephen James, MD
Speaker, Olenka Matkiwsky, DO
Logan Township
Bright, Nicole Jasmyn, DO
Long Branch
Cohen, Benjamin, MD
Katz, Stanley Norman, MD
Mahwah
Lieb, Jocelyn Ann, MD
Lieber, Colette D., MD
Manahawkin
Geffner, Rami E., MD
Manalapan
Schechter, Alan Lance, MD
Silbret, Lisa Michele, MD
Marlboro
Husain, Zain, MD
Marlton
Elder, Sandra Depadova, MD
Green, Justin Jacob, MD
Halpern, Analisa Vincent, MD
Heymann, Warren R., MD
Lawrence, Naomi, MD
Manders, Steven M., MD
Marquart, Jason D., MD
Pistone, Gregory A., MD
Medford
Buck, Andrea S., DO
Harrop, Elyse Horn, MD
High, David A., MD
Metuchen
Lee, Jane Mengchuan, MD
Lee, Peter Yujen, MD
Millburn
Brockman-Bitterman, Allyson, MD
Ehrenreich, Michael, MD
Freeman, Amy Ilyse, MD
Kihiczak, George, MD
Mautner, Gail H., MD
Siegel, Eric Scott, MD
Monroe Township
Kaufmann, Roderick Jr., MD
Vaidya, Darshan C., MD
Montclair
Downie, Jeanine Bernice, MD
Moorestown
Camishion, Germaine Mary, MD
Chheda, Monique Kamaria, MD
D'Ambra-Cabry, Kimberly A., MD
Del Monaco, Magaly Patricia, DO
Foti, Frederick D. Jr., MD
Jacoby, Richard, MD
Koblenzer, Caroline S., MD
Morristown
Agarwal, Shilpa R., MD
Altman, Rachel S., MD
Dane, Alexander Ali, DO
Fialkoff, Cheryl N., MD
Grob, Alexandra, DO
Kazam, Bonnie B., MD
Lee, Kristyna H., MD
Lombardi, Adriana, MD

Lortie, Charles Frederic, MD
Parker, Collin Robert, MD
Pilcher, Mary Frances, MD
Popkin, Mark D., MD
Rogachefsky, Arlene S., MD
Schneider, Rhonda R., MD
Torres, Omar, MD
Mount Laurel
Abdelmalek, Mark A., MD
Dipasquale, Albert M., MD
Levin, Robin Merle, MD
Mountain Lakes
Cunningham, William J., MD
Weinstein, Dora Hagar Foa, MD
New Brunswick
Grossman, Rachel M., MD
Newark
Schwartz, Robert Allen, MD
Newfoundland
Bilkis, Michael Ross, MD
Newton
Blackwell, Martin, DO
North Bergen
Elias, Charles, MD
North Brunswick
Berger, Richard S., MD
Wrone, David A., MD
North Plainfield
Weinberger, George I., MD
Northfield
Krakowski, Andrew Charles, MD
Mordecai, Isaac S., MD
Vause, Sandra E., MD
Nutley
Bashline, Benjamin R., DO
Ligresti, Dominick Joseph, MD
Ocean
Klenoff, Paul H., MD
Old Bridge
Centurion, Santiago Alberto, MD
Vaillant, Juan Guillermo, MD
Paramus
Baxt, Rebecca D., MD
Baxt, Saida H., MD
Cyrulnik, Amanda Amy, MD
Garcia, Carmen Josefina, MD
Goldstein, Marcy A., MD
Gordon, Karen Ann, MD
Kopeloff, Iris H., MD
Li, Cindy Yuk, DO
Schorr, Ethlynn Susan, MD
Wiederkehr, Michael, MD
Young, Alexis Livingston, MD
Park Ridge
Abeles, Gwen Dee, MD
Parsippany
Almeida, Laila M., MD
Kingsbery, Mina Yassaee, MD
Livingston, Wendy E., MD
Milbauer, James, MD
Shah, Subhadra Sundaram, MD
Strauss, Eric A., MD
Weinberg, Harvey I., MD
Weiser, Jessica Ann, MD
Paterson
Zemel, Mathias, MD
Phillipsburg
Li, Lian-Jie, MD
Pine Brook
Chen, Elbert H., MD
Point Pleasant Beach
Warshauer, Bruce L., MD
Princeton
Banker, Sarika, MD
Berger, Bruce J., MD
Choi, Sola, MD
Funkhouser, Martha E., MD
Kazenoff, Steven, MD
Kwee, Darlene J., MD
Notterman, Robyn B., MD
Onumah, Neh Johnann, MD
Rossy, Kathleen M., MD
Rahway
Wininger, Jon G., MD
Randolph
Najarian, David James, MD
Red Bank
Trusky, Diana E., MD
Ridgewood
Applebaum-Farkas, Paige S., MD

Au, Sonoa Ho Yee, MD
Corey, Timothy J., MD
Miller, Janine D'Amelio, MD
Satra, Karin H., MD
Stevens, Amy W., MD
River Edge
Blanco, Fiona Rose Pasternack, MD
Lin, Richie L., MD
Trinh, Diem Thi, MD
Riverdale
Son, Chang Bae, MD
Rockaway
Aspen, Otter Q., MD
Masesa, Joseph M., MD
Roselle Park
Herzberg, Steven Michael, MD
Rutherford
Giardina-Beckett, Marieanne, MD
Sperling, Shari Yaffa, DO
Saddle Brook
Haberman, Fredric, DO
Ilowite, Peter G., DO
Saddle River
Hellman, Laura J., MD
Salem
Caruso, Meghan M., DO
Schmelzer, John F., DO
Scotch Plains
Drossner, Robbie Beth, MD
Sea Girt
Emma, Sheri Lynn, MD
Sewell
Choi, Catherine Helen, MD
Li, Kehua, MD
Segal, Elana Tova, MD
Winter, Jonathan M., MD
Short Hills
Busbey, Shail, MD
Vuong, Charlotte Hwa, MD
Shrewsbury
Resnikoff, Forrest P., MD
Somers Point
Campo, Anthony Guy Jr., MD
Somerset
Bhatti, Hamza Dastigir, DO
Cha, Jisun, MD
Cohen, Penelope Jucowics, MD
Firoz, Bahar F., MD
Milgraum, Sandy S., MD
Nijhawan, Rohit I., MD
Pappert, Amy S., MD
Urman, Marcy E., MD
Victor, Frank Charles, MD
South Plainfield
Ju, William D., MD
Sparta
Papadopoulos, Anthony Jordan, MD
Spring Lake
Lo Buono, Philip J., MD
Sterling, J. Barton, MD
Succasunna
Cooper, Lauren M., MD
Summit
Hu, Judy Y., MD
Notari, Teresa V., MD
Silver, Barry C., MD
Williams, John Michael, MD
Teaneck
Ragi, Gangaram, MD
Tenafly
Laureano, Ana Cristina, MD
Scherl, Sharon, MD
Tinton Falls
Gorin, Risa Jill, DO
Kolansky, Glenn, MD
Kruse, Christopher Bryant, MD
Terushkin, Vitaly, MD
Toms River
Dixon, Melissa Kaye, MD
Kuflik, Avery S., MD
Kuflik, Emanuel G., MD
LaForgia, Sal T., MD
Ma, Manhong, MD
Rosen, Robert M., DO
Trivedi, Prabhas Arunbhai, MD
Trenton
Abello Poblete, Maria V., MD
Turnersville
Durham, Booth H., MD
Gruber, Melvin S., MD

Union
Turner, Mitchell S., MD
Verona
Abbate, Marc Anthony, MD
Brown, Justin, MD
Kassim, Andrea Tinuola, MD
Nossa, Robert, MD
Rothman, Frederic R., MD
Spates, Stephen Thomas, MD
Waller, Leon H., DO
Vineland
Carbonaro, Paul Anthony, MD
Smith, Leslie Robert, MD
Toome, Birgit K., MD
Voorhees
Baratta, Andrea, DO
Bernardin, Ronald Maurice III, MD
Chou, Koulin L., MD
Finkelstein, David Hal, MD
Macaione, Alexander, DO
Papa, Christine A., DO
Rekant, Stanley I., MD
Rollins, Terry Lee, MD
Schwartz, Bennett K., MD
Wall Township
Cosulich, William F., MD
Esche, Clemens, MD
Wallington
Janniger, Camila K., MD
Warren
Ahkami, Rosaline N., MD
Bagley, Michael P., MD
Doctoroff, Alexander, DO
Lu, Rebecca Yun-ru, MD
Reilly, George D., MD
Sciales, Christopher W., MD
Watchung
Eisenberg, Richard R., MD
Wayne
Cardullo, Alice Cecilia, MD
Chima, Kuljit Kaur, MD
Leu, Diana S., MD
Maier, Herbert S., MD
Milano, Edward L., MD
Pollack, Shoshannah S., MD
Thakker, Priya Sambandan, MD
West Caldwell
Rabner, Deborah W., MD
West Long Branch
Gilson, Cynthia T., MD
Karakashian, Gary V., MD
Miller, Angela M., MD
Orsini, William J., MD
West New York
Herman, Eric W., MD
West Orange
Connolly, Adrian L., MD
Connolly, Karen Lynn, MD
Glashofer, Marc David, MD
Groisser, Daniel S., MD
Hartman, Rachael Dalya, MD
Heidary, Noushin, MD
Patel, Mahir, MD
Raklyar, Eduard, MD
Ruhl, Kimberly K., MD
Simela, Tanasha, DO
Sivendran, Meera, MD
Spey, Deborah Ruth, MD
Stolman, Lewis Peter, MD
Westfield
Bhate, Chinmoy, MD
Ciatti, Sabatino, MD
Finamore, Christina Lucy, MD
Hochman, Lisa G., MD
Lehrhoff, Stephanie Rogers, MD
Lu, Phoebe Do, MD
McFalls, Susan G., MD
Westmont
Olivo, Matthew P., MD
Westwood
Blume, Jonathan Erik, MD
Hadi, Ahmed Suhail, MD
Maso, Martha J., MD
Molinaro, Michael John, MD
Myrow, Ralph E., MD
Nychay, Stephen G., MD
Osofsky, Michael, MD
Possick, Paul Aaron, MD
Reichel, Martin, MD

Physicians by Specialty and Town

Dermatology (cont)
Whippany
  Lott,Jason Pelham,MD
Whiting
  Tager,Patricia,MD
Willingboro
  Kurnick,Warren S.,MD
Woodbury
  Chung,Grace U.,MD
  Herman,Kenneth Louis,DO
Wyckoff
  Marcus,Linda Susan,MD

Dermatology: Dermatopathology
Berkeley Heights
  Meyers,Lawrence S.,MD
Livingston
  Sarkissian,Naver A.,MD
West Orange
  Sandoval,Marina Penteado,MD

Dermatopathology
Lakewood
  Bhattacharjee,Pradip,MD
Red Bank
  Shami,Samar,MD
Teterboro
  Gill,Melissa,MD

Developmental Pediatrics
Cape May Court House
  Hackford,Robert R.,MD
Flemington
  Mars,Audrey Estelle,MD
Fort Lee
  deVinck,Oana,DO
Hackensack
  Dolan,Eileen A.,MD
  Huron,Randye F.,MD
Jersey City
  Dehnert,Michele Chun,MD
  Sy-Te,Emilie,MD
Lafayette
  Laveman,Lawrence B.,MD
Mays Landing
  Burgess,David B.,MD
  Kruger,Hillary Anne,MD
Metuchen
  Amorapanth,Vanna R.,MD
Morristown
  Fadden,Kathleen Selvaggi,MD
Mountainside
  Beckwith,Anna Malia,MD
  Malik,Zeenat Q.,MD
  Merola,Rose Mary,MD
  Prontnicki,Janice L.,MD
Neptune
  Aloisio,Denise,MD
  Roth,Anne G.,DO
New Brunswick
  Jimenez,Manuel,MD
Norwood
  Downey,Margaret Kelly,MD

Diagnostic Radiology
Avenel
  Singer,Mark Andrew,MD
Basking Ridge
  Hernandez,Allyn,MD
  Simmons,Marc Z.,MD
Bayonne
  Chandiwala-Mody,Priti,DO
  Perlov,Martina,MD
  Sleman,Ingy Hanna,MD
  Soloway,Peter H.,MD
Belleville
  Acosta,Robert G.,MD
  Heimann,James A.,MD
  Levchook,Christina,MD
Berkeley
  Volvovsky,Alexander,MD
Bordentown
  Daniels,Richard John,MD
Brick
  Alcasid,Lino M.,MD
  Cardo,Amelia J.,MD
  Dillon,Richard Lansing,MD
  Jain,Chandru U.,MD
  Kaplan,Sheldon B.,MD
  Karmel,Mitchell I.,MD
Camden
  Abujudeh,Hani H.,MD

Baraldi,Raymond Lawrence Jr.,MD
Barshay,Veniamin,MD
Bhimani,Chandni,DO
DeStefano,Michael William,MD
Gefen,Ron,MD
Greatrex,Kathleen Mae V.,MD
Hanono,Joseph A.,MD
Huang,Hoi Pan,MD
Ives,Elizabeth Payne,MD
Jarrett,Vincent A.,DO
Khorrami,Cyrus,MD
Klifto,Eugene J.,DO
Kovacs,James E.,DO
Kwak,Jinhee,MD
Malliah,Sangit Bhoosa,MD
Matteo,Diana C.,MD
Nissenbaum,Gerald Aubbie,MD
Oif,Edward,MD
Presenza,Thomas Jonathan,DO
Roth,Howard Lee,MD
Scattergood,Emily D.,MD
Smith,Charlene M.,MD
Smith,Robert T.,MD
Solis,Maria S.,MD
Solish Gittens,Allison,MD
Cape May Court House
  Capecci,Louis J.,MD
  Garrett,Paul R.,MD
  Patel,Amit Arun,MD
  Patel,Kaushik M.,MD
  Shah,Ankur,MD
Chatham
  Gelber,Lawrence J.,MD
  Kingsly,Jill H.,MD
  Lee,Terrence Hone Chung,MD
  Schroeder,Donald C.,MD
Cherry Hill
  Barzel,Eyal,MD
  Bufalino,Kevin Thomas,MD
  Curtis,Paul A.,MD
  De Laurentis,Joseph,MD
  Depersia,Lori Angela,MD
  Desai,Vishal,MD
  Dheer,Sachin,MD
  Fazekas,Jessica Eden,DO
  Germaine,Pauline,DO
  Goodworth,Gregory J.,MD
  Haney,James Joseph III,MD
  Kramer,Neil Robert,MD
  Lee,Mark Hyon-Min,MD
  Lentini,John Alaric,MD
  Sergi,Thomas J.,MD
  Stark,Ira R.,DO
  Tank,Niti,MD
  Ter,Suat E.,MD
  Torres,Joseph Charles,MD
Cliffside Park
  Dhanani,Harsha Narendra,MD
Clifton
  Ferdinand,Brett D.,MD
  Thierman,David H.,MD
  Yuppa,Frank R.,MD
Clinton
  Lyons,Andrea Elizabeth,MD
  Sprenger,Alice Q.,MD
  Woo,Thomas Hyunsop,MD
  Zeng,Yu Grace,MD
Cranford
  O'Connor,Mary T.,MD
Denville
  Solomon,Edward Martin,MD
  Sutker,Burton,MD
  Wexler,Jeffrey A.,MD
Dover
  Diaz,Francis L.,MD
  Freeman,Neil J.,MD
East Brunswick
  Amorosa,Judith K.,MD
  Bier,Steven Jeffrey,MD
  Bodner,Leonard,MD
  Bramwit,Mark P.,MD
  Brown,James Harvey,MD
  Bulkin,Yekaterina,MD
  Carney-Gellella,Erin D.,MD
  Carroll,Michael R. III,MD
  Censullo,Michael Louis,MD
  Chai,Bob B.,MD
  Chaise,Laurence S.,MD
  Chin,Deanna G.,MD
  Chiu-Serodio,Lai-No,MD
  Derman,Arnold,MD

Dorr,Jeffrey,MD
Eardley,Anna Mary,MD
Ecker,Teresa,MD
Epstein,Robert E.,MD
Feinstein,Richard S.,MD
Flynn,Daniel E.,MD
Freeman,Eliot,MD
Garner,Eve Marybeth,MD
Girgis,Wahid S.,MD
Glynn,Nicole Lasasso,MD
Greenberg,Caroline M.,MD
Greenblatt,Adrienne Masin,MD
Grygotis,Laura Anne,MD
Harrigan,John T.,MD
Hira,Ajay,MD
Kandula,Praveena,MD
Keller,Irwin A.,MD
Kennedy,Eugene Cullen,MD
Kim,Sue Yeon,MD
Krieg,Eileen M.,MD
Kron,Stanley M.,MD
Lebovitz,Yaron,MD
Lee,Ellen,MD
Levine,Charles Daniel,MD
Lotan,Roi Meir,MD
Melendez,Jody Michael,MD
Moubarak,Issam F.,MD
Needell,Gary S.,MD
Notardonato,Henry,MD
Oliveros,Elder A.,MD
Pandya,Dipti,MD
Paster,Lina Famiglietti,MD
Patel,Gitanjali,MD
Patel,Rahul,MD
Romero,Melchor D.,MD
Roychowdhury,Sudipta,MD
Rozenberg,Aleksandr,MD
Samuels,Paul Louis,MD
Saraiya,Mansi Shah,MD
Sarokhan,Carol T.,MD
Schram,Adriann Susie,MD
Shah,Kumar,MD
Simon,Mitchell Lyle,MD
Slater,Gregg Matthew,MD
Sokol,Levi Olatokunbo,MD
Solonick,Douglas M.,MD
Sorkin,Norman S.,MD
Torrei,Payam G.,MD
Vasani,Devang,MD
Venezia,Sara,DO
Walor,David Michael,MD
Warren,Stephen W.,MD
Wolfson,Natasha Susan,MD
Yi,Bryan Sang,MD
Yoon,Hyukjun,MD
Zawodniak,Leonard J.,MD
East Orange
  Gonzales,Sharon Frances,MD
  Klyde,David Philip,MD
  Lee,Mimi Shon,MD
  Verona,Paul T.,MD
Edison
  Boruchov,Scott D.,MD
  Chakravarty,Mira,MD
  Contractor,Daniel G.,MD
  Eshkar,Noam Simon,MD
  Friedman,Robert A.,MD
  Galbraith,Michael,MD
  Malantic-Lu,Grace Paula,MD
  Mody,Suresh,MD
  Parashurama,Prashant,MD
  Parker,Martin I.,MD
  Peterson,Mary Ann,MD
  Pierpont,Christopher Edward,MD
  Pivawer,Gabriel,DO
  Rebarber,Israel Frank,MD
  Schmell,Eric Brad,MD
  Schwarz,Naomi S.,MD
  Simon,Daniel W.,MD
  Weissmann,Murray H.,MD
Egg Harbor Township
  Lee,Jacob S.,MD
  O'Laughlin,Richard Lawrence,MD
Emerson
  Su,Hsiu,MD
Englewood
  Foster,Jonathan A.,MD
  Gutwein,Marina Ayzenberg,MD
  Jacobs,Stefanie S.,MD
  Mattana,Nina Delman,MD
  Naidrich,Shari Ann,MD
  Petti,Christopher Louis,MD

Rekhtman-Sneed,Katya,MD
Shembde,Dwarkanath Sonaji,MD
Englewood Cliffs
  Amoroso,Michael Luke,MD
  Fishkin,Igor V.,MD
Fair Lawn
  Levy,Daniel S.,MD
  Modi,Ketang H.,DO
  Rubinoff,Susan W.,MD
  Rudd,Steven A.,MD
Flemington
  Castaldi,Mark Whittaker,MD
  Feldman,Ruth S.,MD
  Loesberg,Andrew C.,MD
Franklin Lakes
  Demauro,Linda Dell,MD
Freehold
  Arredondo,Mario Gaston,MD
  Chalal,Jeffrey,MD
  Friedenberg,Jeffrey Scott,MD
  Keklak,C. Stephen,MD
  Kouveliotes,Peter J.,MD
  Loeb,Debra M.,MD
  Romano,Kenneth Robert,MD
  Spector,Janet,MD
  Tomkovich,Kenneth R.,MD
Galloway
  Altin,Robert S.,MD
  Avagliano,Margaret C.,MD
  Brezel,Mitchell H.,MD
  Ferretti,James Christian,DO
  Graule,Melissa J.,MD
  Graziano,Robert J.,MD
  Handel,David B.,MD
  Kenny,David Anthony,DO
  Lee,Michael Joseph,MD
  Levi,David A.,MD
  Levy,Karen R.,MD
  Menghetti,Richard A.,MD
  Mesham,James R.,MD
  Patel,Hiren Ramesh,MD
  Patel,Rajesh Ishwar,MD
  Peshori,Kavita R.,MD
  Viswambharan,Ajay,MD
Gladstone
  Degaeta,Linda R.,MD
Glen Rock
  Leone,Armand Jr.,MD
Green Brook
  Epstein,Richard William,MD
  Finn Wedmid,Myra Elizabeth,MD
  Gross,Steven C.,MD
  Honickman,Steven P.,MD
  Isserow,Jonathan Arnold,MD
  Lam,Ling Lai,MD
  Saunders,Alan M.,MD
  Yang,Roger S.,MD
Hackensack
  Abbey,Genevieve Nguyen,MD
  Agress,Harry Jr.,MD
  An,Jane J.,MD
  Bogomol,Adam Russell,MD
  Bramlette,James G.s.,MD
  Daginawala,Naznin,MD
  Faulkner,Adriana Danielle,MD
  Ferrone,George J.,MD
  Gamss,Rebecca,MD
  Gardella,Dean,MD
  Greenwald,Bob,MD
  Guy Rodriguez,Eva Porter,MD
  Han,Gene,MD
  Hou,Stephanie W.,MD
  Koenigsberg,Tova Chava,MD
  Kumarasamy,Narmadan A.,MD
  Litkouhi,Behrang,MD
  Malone,Carolyn Marie,MD
  Ng,Joshua M.,MD
  Ojutiku,Oreoluwa Olubukunola,MD
  Osiason,Andrew Wade,MD
  Panduranga,Satish Chandra,MD
  Renjen,Pooja,MD
  Rozentsvayg,Eka,DO
  Starr,Gail E.,MD
  Sunkavalli,Sunitha Aluri,MD
  Toth,Patrick J.,MD
  Yang,Clement,MD
Hackettstown
  Lee,Steven Thomas,MD
  Lo,Pak-Kan A.,MD
  Mantinaos,Mike Konstantinos,MD

Physicians by Specialty and Town

Haddon Heights
Roach, Neil A., MD
Hainesport
Brodsky, Michael C., MD
Cordell, Charles E., MD
Curtis, Bernadette R., MD
Goldstein, Charles, MD
Harvey, Robert Todd, MD
Kellerman, Joshua David, MD
Lalani, Omar, MD
Lim, Sungtae, MD
Patel, Manan Jaykishan, MD
Rosenblatt, Jay M., MD
Yang, Ben Ming-Chien, MD
Hamilton
Alderson, Skip Michael, MD
Bhalakia, Niraj, MD
Blackman, Gurvan E., MD
Bosworth, Eric, MD
Burgos, Anthony, MD
Burshteyn, Mark, MD
Cohen, Daniel Jonathan, MD
Gellella, Erik Leonard, MD
Gold, Michael J., MD
Greenbaum, Roy L., MD
Kirkpatrick, Christopher T., MD
Le Cavalier, Larry Alan, MD
Lee, Shane, MD
Lo Verde, Lauren S., MD
McGroarty, William J., MD
Meshkov, Steven L., MD
Nayee, Sandip Natvarlal, DO
Neuman, Joel David, MD
Ratner, Lawrence M., MD
Rieder, Michael J., MD
Scafidi, Richard F., MD
Seelagan, Davindra, MD
Silverstein, Gary S., MD
Steinig, Jeffrey Daniel, MD
Tarasov, Ethan A., MD
Taus, Lynne F., MD
Thal, Stephen Wayne, DO
Young, Sophia C., MD
Hampton
Falcon, Lisa Fern, MD
Hoboken
Gowda, Mamatha Ramesh, MD
Mousavi, Seyed-Ali, MD
Singh, Supreet, MD
Holmdel
D'Angelo, Denis Gerard, MD
Rabbani, Soliman, MD
Jersey City
Baranetsky, Adrian Andrew, MD
Karp, Hillel J., MD
Maurizi, Romolo A., MD
Singh, David, MD
Kendall Park
Balgowan, Dennis, MD
Garnet, Daniel, MD
Greene, Samuel James, MD
Leder, David S., MD
Nemade, Ajay B., MD
Rubbert-Slawek, Kerstin Anke, MD
Tenenzapf, Mark J., MD
Lakewood
Cranley, Robert, MD
Khanna, Pawandeep S., MD
Langman, Alex, MD
Pukin, Lev, MD
Qiu, William Weiguang, MD
Shah, Faisal Majeed, MD
Little Silver
DeVincenzo, Raven, MD
Doss, Peter S., MD
Rittweger, Edward S., MD
Shah, Pranav N., MD
Zito, Frederick J., MD
Livingston
Bhatnagar, Swati Varma, MD
Carpenter, Bruce W., MD
Daigle, Megan Elizabeth, MD
Dembner, Alan G., MD
Dunaway, David Ryan, MD
Fertakos, Roy J., MD
Garten, Alan J., MD
Giobbe, Raphael C., MD
Huang, Tammy, MD
Karlson, Karen B., MD
Kotch, Hannah Rapaport, MD
Kothari, Neha A., MD

Laible, Mark S., MD
McCarthy, Cornelius Stephen, MD
Mehta, Avani Shripal, MD
Polini, Nicole Maria, MD
Sharo, Ronald J., MD
Shoor, Priya, MD
Slazak, Katherine L., MD
Sperling, Danny S., MD
Stulbach, Harry Bruce, MD
Long Branch
Barone, Cynthia A., DO
Hussain, Syed, MD
Keedy, Jennifer, MD
Kwak, Andrew, MD
Louie, Gina Lin, MD
Pardes, Jorge Gustavo, MD
Staiger, Melinda J., MD
Talangbayan, Leizle E., MD
Wiggins, Ernest Flowers III, MD
Won, Bokran, MD
Manahawkin
Fernandez, Richard E., MD
Maplewood
Blatt, Kenneth B., MD
Heideman, Alan J., MD
Jhaveri, Sujata Ketan, MD
Lautin, Jeffrey L., MD
Novick, Andrew S., MD
Marlboro
Ferra, Michael John, MD
Medford
Sabatino, John C., MD
Mendham
Kertesz, Jennifer L., MD
Mercerville
Larsen, Bartley A., MD
McDonald, Kathleen L., MD
Stebbins, Michael G., MD
Metuchen
Einhorn, Robert, MD
Kolber, Ronald B., MD
Resnikoff, Leonard Barocas, MD
Middletown
Belen, Kristin Marietta O., MD
Millburn
Blonstein, Jeffrey D., MD
Millville
Margate, Pedro Ramboyong, MD
Montclair
Gurell, Daniel Steven, MD
Jewel, Kenneth L., MD
Lee, Joo-Young Melissa, MD
Mattern, Richard F., MD
Shah, Mala T., MD
Montvale
Hendi, Jennifer Michelle, MD
Moorestown
Greene, Arthur J., MD
Morganville
Losik, Steve Boleslav, MD
Morristown
Anand, Neil, MD
Barton, Loucia C., MD
Beute, Bernard John, MD
Esses, Steven J., MD
Ginsberg, Hal N., MD
Leff, Sheryl L., MD
Moore, Ann M., MD
Ratakonda, Sridevi, MD
Schiavi, Jonathan Michael, MD
Smith, Peter Lloyd, MD
Timins, Julie K., MD
Mount Laurel
Chan, Britton Miller, MD
Chheda, Samir Visanji, MD
Gargiulo, Andrew Michael, MD
Gehringer, Travis James, MD
Patel, Priyesh V., MD
Mullica Hill
Solomon, Jason S., MD
New Providence
Gowali, Neha M., MD
Printz, David A., MD
Schneider, Benjamin Mark, MD
Newark
Blacksin, Marcia F., MD
Chaudhry, Humaira S., MD
Durojaye, Abike Ogunrenike, MD
Goldfarb, Helene, MD
Goldschmiedt, Judah, MD

Green, Jeremy Charles, MD
Hinrichs, Clay Robert, MD
Jedynak, Andrzej R., MD
Lee, Huey J., MD
Maldjian, Pierre D., MD
Mele, Christopher Mark, MD
Patel, Shashikant A., MD
Snellings, Richard Barton, MD
Tairu, Oluwole Ayodeji, MD
Thomas, Prashant Jacob, MD
Wachsberg, Ronald H., MD
Newton
Patel, Jay, MD
Scheer, Linda B., MD
Northfield
Cummings, Allan H., MD
Nutley
Bash, Lisa Taub, MD
Mondshine, Ross T., MD
Pollack, Michael A., MD
Torrente, Jessica, MD
Traflet, Robert F., MD
Old Bridge
Park, Peter Byung, MD
Shami, Msallam M., MD
Old Tappan
Lyons, John S., MD
Oradell
Albert, Arthur S., MD
Chu, Regina Wong, MD
Thame, Craig H., MD
Parsippany
Chung, Jean Young, MD
Menendez, Christine M., MD
Murphy, Robyn C., MD
Parisi, Angela Rosina, MD
Rios, Jose Conrado, MD
Sheth, Milan Pravin, MD
Swayne, Lawrence C., MD
Yablonsky, Thaddeus M., MD
Paterson
Balakumar, Kalavathy, MD
Baltazar, Romulo Z., MD
Bar, Vandna Prasad, MD
Berlin, Fred, MD
Centanni, Marianne T., MD
Freitag, Warren Barry, MD
Kwon, Stephen S., MD
Milman, Edward, MD
Sanchez, Orestes, MD
Sheppard, Lisa Marie, MD
Taragin, Benjamin H., MD
Pennsville
Fagel, Valentin L., MD
Phillipsburg
Bucich, Joseph Marc Jr., MD
Cohen, Kenneth Arthur, MD
Estacio, Joseph M., DO
Pollack, Matthew Scott, MD
Rabinowitz, Mitchell, MD
Swartz, Joel David, MD
Piscataway
Hsu, Chia-En, MD
Plainsboro
Green, William M., MD
Pomona
Miller, Mitchell Alan, MD
Princeton
Ananian, Christopher Lee, MD
Berger, Robert B., MD
Cadogan, Michael A., MD
Cole, Julie Barudin, MD
Compito, Gerard Anthony, MD
Denny, Donald Jr., MD
Difazio, Matthew C., MD
Fein, Deborah Allen, MD
Ford, Robert R., MD
Ghazi, John, MD
Guglielmi, Gwen E., MD
Howard, Timothy S., MD
Julius, Barry D., MD
Kaplan, Steven Mark, MD
Kaufmann, Gregory A., MD
Lebowitz, Jonathan A., MD
O'Malley, Bernard B., MD
Perlman, Barry J., MD
Perlman, Eric S., MD
Sen, Rik Supriya, MD

Rahway
Mizan, Narmin Farah Hussain, MD
Shrivastava, Abhishek, MD
Red Bank
Fedele, Dara, MD
Mishra, Monica Shalini, MD
Rada Banat, Leny M., MD
Ridgefield Park
Awad, Aida Fahmy, MD
Ridgewood
Wollman, Carol A., MD
Rio Grande
McAllister, John Daniel II, MD
Panico, Robert A., MD
Toloui, Gerald J., MD
Werman, Richard Evan, DO
River Edge
Naik, Mohit Madan, MD
Nicola, Gregory Neal, MD
Rochelle Park
Meyerson, Steven Jeffrey, MD
Rutherford
Annese, Christian P., MD
Salem
De Jesus, Joseph Ocampo, MD
Krain, Samuel, MD
Secaucus
Izgur, Vitaly, MD
Tramontana, Anthony F., MD
Short Hills
Jain, Monica, MD
Shrewsbury
Lu, Stanley, MD
Rashid, Salman, MD
Shariff, Yasmeen K., MD
Sparta
Cordero, Hector Orlando, MD
Corio, Frederick J., MD
Franklin, Barry I., MD
Ranley, Robert L., MD
Rodrigues, Vanitha J., MD
Shah, Shital R., MD
Summit
Donnelly, Brian, MD
Teaneck
Berman, Howard L., MD
Brunetti, Jacqueline Carol, MD
Cao, Huyen Van, MD
Felman, Rina Lita, MD
Greenstein, Elizabeth Louise, MD
Herman, Kevin, MD
Horn, Eva M., MD
Kirzner, Howard L., MD
Lerer, Daniel Brian, MD
Morgan, John, MD
Park, James Joongchul, MD
Patel, Amish, MD
Rundback, John Hugh, MD
Siegel, Stacey, MD
Tenafly
Sadler, Michael Alan, MD
Tinton Falls
Brand-Abend, Lori M., MD
Toms River
Atallah, Judy, DO
Batchu, Bharathi, MD
Boxer, Douglas C., MD
Chen, Timothy, MD
Chinta, Bharath Kumar, MD
D'Angelo, Michael Wayne, MD
Daniels, Alicia L., MD
Desai, Akhilesh S., MD
Florio, Francesco, DO
Golsaz, Cyrus Michael, MD
Haim, Alain, MD
Kravets, Felix G., MD
Lee, Brian H., MD
Marinas, Virgilio R., MD
Martin, Steven W., MD
Shahab, Farhang, MD
Shieh, Paul Y., MD
Triolo, Joseph, MD
Willis, Kevin, MD
Yu, Thomas C., MD
Trenton
Applbaum, Yaakov N., MD
Banker, Piyush, MD
Kim, Andrew Edward, MD
Neimark, Matthew A., MD
Soloveychik, Natalya, DO

Physicians by Specialty and Town

Diagnostic Radiology (cont)
Turnersville
  Dannenbaum,Mark S.,MD
  Gallagher,Thomas Jude,DO
  Harding,John Arthur,MD
  Muhr,William Jr.,MD
  Niedbala,Thomas M.,MD
  Podgorski,Edward M. Jr.,MD
  Roberts,David A.,MD
Union City
  Simonson,Marc H.,MD
Upper Saddle River
  Lasser,Andrew S.,MD
Verona
  Clarkin,Kim Stephanie,MD
Vineland
  Bhagat,Nitesh N.,MD
  Desai,Shailendra A.,MD
  Kazmi,Faaiza K.,MD
  Lazarus,Robert E.,MD
  Munjal,Ajay K.,MD
  Neustadter,Lawrence M.,DO
  Patel,Nirav,MD
  Rosenberg,Allison R.,DO
  Rothfarb,Steven H.,MD
  Villani,Michael A.,MD
Voorhees
  Apple,Jerry S.,MD
  Baum,Mark L.,MD
  Blumenthal,Beth A.,MD
  Elder,James P. Jr.,MD
  Fan,Wen Lin,MD
  Farner,Michael Charles,MD
  Kendzierski,Renee Marie,DO
  Kramer,David H.,MD
  Lott,Kristen Ellie,MD
  Piccoli,Catherine Welch,MD
  Sahlman,Rebecca Lynne,MD
Waldwick
  Calem-Grunat,Jaclyn A.,MD
  Degregorio,Scott David,MD
  Dockery,Keith Forrest,MD
  Koo,Jennifer S.,MD
  Krinsky,Glenn Andrew,MD
  Lazarus-Wolpov,Dawn E.,MD
  Lerner,Elliot J.,MD
  Lin,Erwin,MD
  Rhee,Kyung-Hwa,MD
  Rybak,Karen J.,MD
  Zimmerman,Jill Robin,MD
Wall
  O'Connor,Patrick Joseph,DO
  Parikh,Manoj R.,MD
Warren
  Kamieniecki,Robert Edward,MD
  Labib,Mina L.,MD
Watchung
  Contractor,Sohail G.,MD
Wayne
  Flanzman,Richard M.,MD
  Sun,Qiang,MD
  Whang,Inwhan,MD
West Caldwell
  Caldwell,Kathleen V.,MD
West Deptford
  Ariaratnam,Nikki Sanghera,MD
  Fog,Denise Susan,DO
  Larkin,Jeffrey J.,MD
  Lin,Dennis C.,MD
  Little,Sherrill T.,MD
  Mattox,Scott G.,MD
  Rosten,Sloan I.,MD
  Sajous,Jan Bernard,MD
  Tilak,Samir Shripad,MD
  Titton,Ross Lewis,MD
West Orange
  Choi,Patricia Hyunho,MD
  Edwards,Michael J.,MD
  Grewal,Jasbir,MD
  Kessler,Michael A.,MD
  Khedekar,Surekha D.,MD
  Mast,Harold Lee,MD
  Waxman,Robert N.,MD
Westfield
  Cohen-Schwartz,Dawn Sheri,MD
  Horner,Neil B.,MD
  Perl,Louis J.,MD
  Salomon,Amir,MD
  Snieckus,Peter J.,MD
Whippany
  Kerwin,Lauren Michelle,MD
Willingboro
  Bialo,Darren Andrew,MD
  White,Robert M.,MD
Wyckoff
  Graziano,Vincent Anthony,MD

Electroencephalography
Cherry Hill
  Zechowy,Allen C.,MD
Hackensack
  Gupta,Dev R.,MD

Electromyography
Jersey City
  Constantino,Edwin M.,MD
Lakewood
  Markowitz,Charles R.,MD
Newark
  Stitik,Todd P.,MD
Somers Point
  Gottfried,Maureen,DO

Emerg Medicine-Medical Toxicology
Paterson
  Kashani,John S.,DO

Emerg Medicine-Pediatric
Bayville
  Iledan,Liesl P.,MD
Camden
  Drago,Lisa Anne Marie,DO
Edison
  Joshi,Samir V.,MD
New Brunswick
  Kalyoussef,Sabah,DO
Newark
  Sinha,Virteeka,MD
Voorhees
  Seiden,Jeffrey A.,MD

Emergency Medical Services
Hackensack
  Lu,Sam Chuan,MD
Mahwah
  Grover,Meenu,MD
Newark
  Ariyaprakai,Navin,MD
  VonBose,Michael J.,MD
Stratford
  Heron,Joseph,MD
Trenton
  Joshi,Hetal Chaitanyaprasad,MD
Vineland
  Kornweiss,Steven Alexander,MD
West Orange
  Mays Stovall,Latisse M.,MD

Emergency Medicine
Allentown
  Krivoshik,Mark P.,MD
Atlantic City
  Acunto,Brian Anthony,DO
  Becher,John W.,DO
  Donaldson,James Kenneth,DO
  Dubin,Reva,MD
  Farnsworth,Marie N.,MD
  Hawkins,Nancy S.,MD
  Khatiwala,Manisha P.,MD
  Khebzou,Zaki,MD
  Leriotis,Theo James,DO
  Luyber,Todd Joseph,DO
  MacBride,David G.,DO
  Menet,Scott Douglas,DO
  Merz,Daniel Francis,DO
  Nicholls,Brian Robert,DO
  Rangam,Tsui H.,MD
  Ruggiero,Michael P.,DO
  Sabatini,Louis V.,DO
  Salvatore,Francis P. Jr.,MD
  Schumacher,William Delmar,DO
  Seibert,Henry Edward,MD
  Urban,Scott Michael,DO
  Westrol,Michael Steven,MD
  Wolk,Eric Todd,DO
  Zipagan,James Talamayan,MD
Audubon
  Smith,Monika,DO
Avalon
  Alspach,Charlotte A.,MD
Basking Ridge
  Amalfitano,Christopher,MD
  Milosis,Christine,MD
Bayonne
  Bessette,Michael John,MD
  Coccaro,John A.,MD
  Istvan,David Joseph,MD
  Lin,Esson,MD
Belleville
  Ciccone,Antonio,DO
  Dib,Joe Elias,MD
  Fontanetta,John Anthony,MD
  Futterman,Noah D.,DO
  Giles,Robert A.,MD
  Lam,Allison Christine,MD
  Law,Stephen W.,DO
  Nelson,Craig A.,MD
  Santos,Luis A.,MD
Bergenfield
  Thek,Wesley K.,MD
Berkeley Heights
  Drivas,Antonios,MD
  Kennedy,Kevin J.,MD
  Kothari,Rajesh Suryakant,DO
  Lesko,Richard J.,MD
  Schreck,David M.,MD
  Singh,Anita J.,MD
Bloomfield
  Reyes,Prudencio C.,MD
Branchburg
  Goldberg,Lon E.,DO
Brick
  Abe,Minako,MD
  Darocki,Mark,MD
  Gronsky,Rudolph Edward,DO
  Haroun,Sandra,MD
  Kathuria,Richa,MD
  Kaufer,Michael Jason,MD
  Maniar,Gina S.,DO
  Noris,Gary L.,MD
  Pollack,Martin I.,MD
  Sarenac,Alexander,MD
  Schlogl,Jeffrey G.,MD
  Singh,Arun J.,DO
Bridgeport
  Harris,Brian E.,MD
Browns Mills
  Ganguly,Tarun,DO
Caldwell
  Izakov,Natalya B.,DO
Camden
  Bartimus,Holly A.,MD
  Baumann,Brigitte Monika,MD
  Bendesky,Brad S.,MD
  Bergquist,Harveen Bal,MD
  Bhamidipati,Anita,MD
  Byrne,Richard George,MD
  Carnevale,Shawn A.,DO
  Carroll,Gerard Gregori,MD
  Cassidy-Smith,Tara Nicole,MD
  Cesarine,Joseph,MD
  Chansky,Michael,MD
  Chase,Rachel Eisenbrock,DO
  Chien,Christina H.,MD
  Damuth,Emily K.,MD
  Delvecchio,Joanna Catherine,MD
  Dillon,John J.,MD
  Disandro,Daniel G.,MD
  Eldrich,Samuel Reich,MD
  Fernandes,Michael Alexandre,MD
  Filippone,Lisa M.,MD
  Forde Baker,Jenice M.,MD
  Freeze,Brian,MD
  Greenman,Rachelle A.,MD
  Guerrera,Angela Dixon,MD
  Haroz,Rachel,MD
  Hennessey,Adam S.,DO
  Hong,Rick,MD
  Hummel,Joseph C.,DO
  Jarecki,Jennifer A.,DO
  Jaworski,Alison,MD
  Jensen,Sharone Lynn,MD
  Jones,Christopher Warren,MD
  Karagiannis,Paul,MD
  Kilgannon,Jennifer Hope,MD
  Kirchhoff,Michael Anthony,MD
  Lubkin,Cary L.,MD
  Maye,Jessica Megan,DO
  Mazzarelli,Anthony Joseph,MD
  Mbachu,Yvonne,MD
  Nocchi,David Martin,MD
  Noel,Christopher Bartlett,MD
  Nyce,Andrew L.,MD
  Ortega,Rae Lynn,MD
  Paston,Carrie Zapolin,MD
  Patel,Prakruti,MD
  Rebbecchi,Thomas A.,MD
  Reinholz,Louis J. Jr.,DO
  Rempell,Joshua Saul,MD
  Roberts,Brian William,MD
  Sacchetti,Alfred D.,MD
  Salzman,Matthew Scott,MD
  Schrift,David S.,MD
  Shapiro,Tyler Kenneth,MD
  Smith,Jillian Corbett,MD
  Szatko,Miroslaw,MD
  Torres Cruz,Joshua,MD
  Tyler,Matthew D.,MD
  Vetrano,Stephen J.,DO
  Warren,Beth Ann,MD
  Wild,William A.,DO
  Wilsey,Stephanie,MD
  Wilson,Alyson Nicole,DO
  Wynne,Brenna,MD
Cape May
  Carlin,Teresa Mary,MD
  Cramer,Kenneth E.,MD
  Lafferty,Keith A.,MD
  Mihata,Ryan Garner,MD
Cape May Court House
  Banfield,Kimberly Ann,DO
  Bridge-Jackson,Teresa A.,MD
  Cascarino,Raymond Patrick,DO
  Cimino,Robert,MD
  Coletta,Domenic Jr.,MD
  Dudnick,Michael,DO
  Nussey,Richard Hutchins Jr.,DO
  Pecora,Arthur Steven,DO
  Riordan,Kevin J.,MD
  Ruskey,John S.,DO
  Ventriglia,Warren J.,MD
Cherry Hill
  Bernhardt,Jarrid,DO
  Caravello,Andrew Benedetto,DO
  Demangone,Dawn Adele,MD
  Dileonardo,Francesca,MD
  Feld,Ross J.,DO
  Hall,Philip Isaac,DO
  Hinchliffe,Susan,MD
  Magbalon,Domingo Jr.,MD
  Nepp,Mark E.,DO
  Ross,Michael Jordan,MD
  Sidwa,Robert Joshua,DO
  Snyder,Natali P.,DO
  Wainwright Edwards,Marsha,MD
Chester
  Vets,Steve Michael,DO
Cinnaminson
  Sommers,Daniel,MD
Cliffside
  Nayman,Defne,MD
Cliffside Park
  Chouake,Benjamin S.,MD
Clifton
  Abbasi,Tareef M.,MD
  Ugras Rey,Sandra S.,DO
Columbus
  Patel,Kamal B.,MD
Dayton
  Haddad,Stephanie I.,MD
Delran
  Hicks,Michael James,MD
Denville
  Berman,Dean Adam,DO
  Guzas,Ronald P.,DO
  Morato,Ramon V.,MD
  Ortega,Stephanie Lynn Scham,MD
  Reardon,Erin Marie,MD
  Retirado,Allen S.,MD
  Retirado,Vincent Paul,MD
  Ringwelski-Hannan,Anna Ewa,MD
  Rosica,John A.,MD
  Somar,Rohan,MD
  Thepmankorn,Pidok,MD
  Tierney,Kevin J.,MD
  Varma,Raghunandan Medavaram,DO
Deptford
  Warden,Todd M.,MD
East Hanover
  Irving,Carol,MD
East Orange
  Kociuba,Marcin K.,DO
  Torres,Mariela,MD

East Windsor
Sterman,Lance M.,MD
Edgewater
Rosines,Noam,MD
Edison
Amin,Shilpa K.,MD
Barsoom,Raafat S.,MD
Cali,Michael D.,MD
Chalabi,Dahlia,MD
Fernandez,Ronald Leonardo,MD
Gillespie,Kevin A.,MD
Hill,Ryan Davidson,DO
Jean Philippe,Carolyne,MD
Johal,Gurvindra Singh,DO
Khanna,Vikas,MD
Lacapra,Samuel,MD
Mascarinas,Kristine I.,DO
Mehta,Harendra U.,MD
Sapira,Andrew S.,MD
Schimler,Michael Edward,MD
Shrivastava,Arpita G.,MD
Soukiazian,Sevak,MD
Steiner,Kenneth D.,MD
Vanam,Kamalakar Rao,MD
Weiss,Daniel E.,MD
Xavier,Geralda A.,MD
Egg Harbor Township
Stone,Mark J.,MD
Elizabeth
Adamski,Jamie Justin,DO
Azoulai,Jonathan Guy,MD
Fan,Liqi,MD
Haders,Allison Lula,MD
Haig,Joseph Michael,MD
Hakim,James,MD
Letizia,Matthew J.,DO
Lo Faro,Joseph Rocco,MD
Mack,Rose M.,DO
Matossian,Raffee H.,MD
McCoy,Lynn,DO
Park,Jay Hoon,MD
Shah,Hitesh M.,MD
Wang,Sandy,DO
Zhang,Christina Ting,DO
Englewood
Caplen,Stuart M.,MD
Clement,Martinez Emmanuel,MD
Glaser,Ariella N.,MD
Kay,Elizabeth E.,DO
Kintzel,Timothy J.,MD
Readie,Jean Eileen,DO
Saxena,Rachna Vidiasagar,DO
Schreibman,Barbara A.,MD
Singer,Elizabeth Kara,MD
Wong,Judy,MD
Ewing
Pierce,Vincent E. Jr.,MD
Fair Lawn
Grinberg,Diana,MD
Flemington
Bliss,Mary J.,MD
Christiansen,David,MD
Guillen,Steven E.,MD
Johnson-Villanueva,Norma J.,MD
Mehta,Nimish Harendra,MD
Patel,Chirag G.,MD
Schultz,Edward Joseph,MD
Schupner,Kathleen A.,MD
Spector,Edward D.,MD
Villanueva,Norma I.,MD
Yoon,Young Dug,MD
Forked River
Pie,Alberto C.,MD
Franklin Lakes
Melwani,Ramesh D.,MD
Franklin Park
Cha,Min,MD
Phan,Au Ngoc,MD
Franklinville
Chappell,Stephen E.,MD
Freehold
Alteveer,Janet G.,MD
Carino,Samuel Comia,DO
Connolly,Sandra M.,MD
Dayner,Jeremy Joseph,MD
Friedman,Daniel Marc,DO
Giron,Miguel,MD
Jones,Marvin M.,MD
Kaplan,Gary Peter,MD
Lee,Tracey-Ann Nadine,MD
McLaughlin,Valerie Gail,MD

Mehta,Ragini R.,DO
Waciega,Mark,MD
Green Brook
Desai,Chaitanya M.,MD
Hackensack
Avram,Ari Jason,MD
Barsky,Carol,MD
Bell,Kameno L.,MD
Bernadotte,Myrvine,MD
Bilbraut,Krista Gayle,MD
Bosompem,Daryl Ama,MD
Caces,Phyllis Adrienn Romero,MD
Chai,Raymond,MD
Charles,Patrick,DO
Chase,Howard M.,MD
Davison,Beverly J.,MD
DeSouza,Sylvie D.,MD
Fernandez,Christine Alison,MD
Fleischman,William,MD
Frank,Daniel B.,MD
Friedman-Cohen,Heather Naomi,MD
Gable-Selmon,Chana H.,MD
Goldhill,Vicki B.,MD
Hallenbeck,John P.,DO
Henderson Chen,Jessica L.,MD
Hernandez,Monica M.,MD
Hewitt,Kevin Joseph,MD
Kim,Young-Min,MD
Mankowitz,Scott Levi,MD
McIntosh,Barbara A.,MD
Morchel,Herman George,MD
Negron,David,MD
Nguyen,Ann Phuong Duy,MD
Nickles,Leroy,MD
Ogedegbe,Chinwe,MD
Ortiz,Carlos Arturo II,MD
Roesch,Benno George,MD
Sayegh,Rockan,MD
Strater,Sharon,MD
Stuart,Jennifer Marie,MD
Sullivan,Anastassia D.,MD
Taylor,Cody Wolfson,MD
Varela,Luis Fernando,MD
Walden,Philip Louis Jr.,MD
Weisburg,Rhoda S.,MD
Yamin,Edward,MD
Zakharchenko,Svetlana,DO
Zodda,David F.,MD
Hackettstown
Bonanno,Bruce B.,MD
Carle,William J.,MD
Cataquet,David,MD
Goldfarb,Stephen A.,MD
Jain,Sanjay K.,MD
Olivieri,William Peter,MD
Scolnick,David,MD
Seid,Ira A.,MD
Hamilton
Betancourt,Javier E.,DO
Chaudhri,Imran I.,MD
Gojaniuk,Jeffrey David,DO
Gonzales,Santos O.,MD
Horana,Lasanta S.,MD
Khan,Mateen Abdul Rahman,MD
Lawrie,John A.,MD
Hammonton
Amin,Pinakin B.,MD
Hawthorne
Saber,Mai Said,DO
Highland Park
Erlikhman,Alla,MD
Hillsborough
Kikta,Kevin J.,DO
Ho Ho Kus
Smith,Donard Scott,MD
Hoboken
Enriquez,Melissa J.,MD
Jani,Chandrashekhar C.,MD
Lawyer,Edward Zadok,MD
Malizia,Robert W.,MD
Rimmer,John Joseph III,DO
Roberson,Meika T.,MD
Holmdel
Ali,Rayshma,DO
Brennessel,Ryan William,DO
Imbesi,Joseph Thomas,DO
Lee,Chi I.,MD
Marchetti,Michael F.,MD
Shah,Dinesh K.,MD
Yu,Daniel Kwang-Jin,MD

Howell
Dennis,Elaine Debra,MD
Jamesburg
Spierer,Robert,MD
Jersey City
Abass-Shereef,Jeneba,MD
Bookbinder,Ronald L.,MD
Canabal,Vincent Paul,MD
Ceci,Robert L.,MD
Cespedes,Victoria Elena,MD
Davis,Matthew B.,MD
Estephan,Amir E.,MD
Hameer,Muneer,MD
Hepburn,Valerie J.,MD
Jaggi,Mona,MD
Jones,Caitlin Maria,MD
Kenigsberg,David R.,MD
Koch,Peter Benjamin,MD
Kwon,Johnny,MD
Llarena,Ramon C.,MD
Martinez,Mark,MD
Meta,Joubin,DO
O'Brien,Susan Erin,DO
Pak-Teng,Carol,MD
Rabines,Alfredo Leonardo,DO
Radwine,Zachary Picker,MD
Ruiz,Vincent Edward,MD
Sanghvi,Shimal H.,MD
Slep,Borys,MD
Sultana,Noushin,MD
Syed,Saquiba,MD
Wang,Cheng-Teng,MD
Wilkes,Kristen,MD
Lakewood
Calderon,Oscar R.,MD
Dalsey,William Colwell,MD
Larsen,Johnny R.,DO
Leber,Ian Brett,MD
Peltz,Hillel,DO
Raja,Sreedar V.,MD
Setya,Amit,DO
Sirchio,Kevin J.,DO
Solas,John R.,DO
Leonardo
Rogers,Patrick,DO
Livingston
Birnbaum,Glenn Alan,MD
Eagan,Michael Patrick,MD
Fink,Glenn D.,MD
Gupta,Neena,MD
Handler,Eric Todd,DO
Kaplan,Emily A.,MD
Kuhlmann,Sarah Elizabeth,MD
Lacher,Britt Ilene,MD
McEnrue,James A.,MD
Miller,Ivan Thomas,MD
Mujic,Lejla,MD
Rentala,Manju,MD
Reyman,Lynn D.,MD
Rokosz,Gregory J.,DO
Rosenblat,Yoav,MD
Salo,David F.,MD
Sanchez,Daniel Antonio,MD
Schreiber,Marie F.,DO
Shapiro,Marion D.,DO
Welber,Mark R.,DO
Winograd,Jonathan Isaac,DO
Long Branch
Campanella,Lisa Marie,MD
Downs,William R. Jr.,DO
Gilman,Elizabeth Ann,MD
Hanlon,Catherine A.,MD
Kanamori,Hiromi,MD
McCabe-Bageac,Mary A.,MD
Minetti,John J.,MD
O'Keefe,Mary Clare,MD
Perry,Kurt A.,MD
Rehr,Eric L.,MD
Waxler,Jennifer L.,DO
Manahawkin
Bagnell,James P.,MD
Boye-Nolan,Melinda L.,DO
Dinowitz,Seth,MD
Jones,Kimberley L.,MD
Kulin,John C.,DO
Little,James Todd,DO
Partrick,Matthew Seamus,MD
Pulver,Bradley Lee,MD
Manalapan
Barthelemy,Markintosh,MD

Manasquan
Frankel,Robert,MD
Marlton
Greenberg,Karen Julie,DO
Kincel,David Nathaniel,DO
Mahajan,Raakhee,MD
Patel,Sundip N.,MD
Medford
Filart,Michael Valencia,DO
Scheets,Kristen Joanna,DO
Schiffenhaus,Elizabeth,MD
Merchantville
Mitchell,Lamont Leigh,DO
Metuchen
Jones,James Brian,MD
Middletown
Fong,Dean Kimton,MD
Samson,Kristine T.,MD
Sennett,Jane M.,DO
Monroe
Stoev,Borislav Georgiev,MD
Montclair
Alberino-Catapano,Amanda,MD
Alejandro,Jason Robert,MD
Antonowicz,Michelle,MD
Arias,Ana L.,MD
Geck,Wilma Santiago,MD
Gorski,Robert Mitchell,MD
Langer,Marjory Ellen,MD
Leuchten,Lisa,DO
Rosenbaum,Steven B.,MD
Sultan,Sharmeen,DO
Williams,Estelle Vaughns,MD
Montvale
Lambert,Rick O.,MD
Moorestown
Dawoud,Magy M.,MD
Lam,Adele Dolores,DO
Morris Plains
Bakun,Walter Michael,MD
Morristown
Alamia,Peter Anthony,DO
Allegra,John R.,MD
Althoff,Marilyn F.,MD
Armstrong,Lisa Kay,MD
Biggs,Danielle Deluca,MD
Castillo,David Cinco,DO
Cosenza,Mario Anthony,DO
Edwards,Daniel James,DO
Eskin,Barnet,MD
Esposito,Amanda Santoro,MD
Feldman,David C.,MD
Felegi,William B.,DO
Fiesseler,Frederick William,DO
Gerardi,Michael J.,MD
Gohsler,Steven P.,MD
Hung,Oliver Li-Ping,MD
Jinivizian,Hasmig Barkeve,MD
Junker,Elizabeth Elsa,MD
Kaiafas,Costas Andreas,MD
Kassem,Jawad Nadim,MD
Kenwood,Alan L.,MD
Lee,Peter Q.,DO
Maroun,Victor,MD
Nashed,Ashraf H.,MD
Nevins,Sol,MD
Patel,Hetal,MD
Patwa,Amy Shah,MD
Peek,Erin Heritage,MD
Ritter,Albert W.,MD
Ruzek,Michael A.,DO
Shih,Richard D.,MD
Szucs,Paul Andrew,MD
Tapia,Alfredo J.,MD
Troncoso,Alexis B. II,MD
Van Pelt,Stephen Robert,MD
Vera,Ariel Eduardo,MD
Walsh,Brian W.,MD
Youssouf,Andrew Joseph,MD
Zimmerman,Patrick Whaley,MD
Mount Holly
Altamura,Richard H.,MD
Bertolino,Laura,DO
Brown,Patti C.,DO
Cowan,Robert Matthew,MD
Dias,Alan Steven,MD
Dickson,Scott Vincent,DO
Elisha,Daniel,MD
Freas,Glenn Curtis,MD
Goldberg,David Felheimer,MD
Goldenberg,Gennifer E.,MD

Physicians by Specialty and Town

Emergency Medicine (cont)

Mount Holly
- Keir, Donald R., MD
- Kuhfahl, Keith Joseph, DO
- Leibrandt, Paul N., MD
- Leitner, Stephen J., MD
- Morris, Jeffrey B., MD
- Price, Ali S., DO
- Ruderman, Seth R., MD
- Shubert, Roy Alan II, MD
- Thompson, Elizabeth Ann, MD
- Tsao, Peter Dean, DO
- Turner, Craig S., DO

Mount Laurel
- Mathason, Mark David, DO
- Noor, Farid A., MD
- Resnick-Matro, Jennifer Dawn, MD

Neptune
- Cardinale, Jan Foxman, MD
- Discepola, Paul, MD
- Dyce, Michael Constantine, MD
- Glashow, Marisa Brittany, DO
- Goodman, Elliot S., DO
- Jacob, Sharon Leigh, MD
- Levinsky, Joseph Judah, MD
- Livingston, Denise L., MD
- Marra, Antonio Luigi, DO
- McFadden, Kim Marie, MD
- Mojares, Gregg E., DO
- Panse, Ramanand V., MD
- Pasricha, Atul, DO
- Patel, Rajendra K., MD
- Pillai, Renuka, DO
- Rozwadowski, Thomas J., MD
- Smith, Corey Kamahl, MD
- Sulewski, Agnieszka, DO
- Sweeney, Robert L., DO
- Tapnio, Cezar B., MD
- Trivedi, Darshini, DO
- Wells, Evelyn Ruth, MD

Neshanic Station
- Daly, Eileen P., MD

New Brunswick
- Amores, Edward Daniel, MD
- Arya, Rajiv, MD
- Berman, Samantha, MD
- Bhavnani, Anita S., MD
- Boutsikaris, Daniel Gregory, MD
- Bryczkowski, Christopher J., MD
- Bucher, Joshua Thomas, MD
- Chin, Meigra Myers, MD
- Choi, Michael Namkyu, MD
- Church, Amy F., MD
- Collins, John Joseph III, MD
- Corcoran, Gregory, MD
- Cuthbert, Darren Patrick, MD
- Dallhoff, Maureen Elizabeth, MD
- Dalton, Mark J K, MD
- Donovan, Colleen Mary, MD
- Eisenstein, Robert Mark, MD
- Garcia, Guillermo A., MD
- Geria, Rajesh Navin, MD
- Gupta, Chiraag U., MD
- Hackett, Gladston Randall, MD
- Hochberg, Michael Lawrence, MD
- Kapitanyan, Raffi S., MD
- Leung, Winifred Fong, MD
- Lewis, Brent Mckeen, MD
- Lustiger, Eliyahu Y., MD
- Marcinow, Justyna, MD
- Marques Baptista, Andreia, MD
- McCarthy, Christopher M., MD
- McCoy, Jonathan V., MD
- McGill, Dennis L., MD
- Mirza, Michael Rohinton, MD
- Morrison, Daniel Scott, MD
- O'Connor, Andrew, MD
- Patel, Mayuri, MD
- Patil, Pooja Mittal, MD
- Phillips, Michelle Nicole, MD
- Pirigyi, Paul R., MD
- Punjabi, Kusum A., MD
- Riaz, Adnan, MD
- Rice, Daniel, MD
- Riggs, Renee Lisa, MD
- Ryave, Steven Samuel, MD
- Shah, Chirag N., MD
- Simon, Riya Jose, DO
- Snyder, Laura Jean, MD
- Van Volkenburgh, Robert John, MD
- Veysman, Boris D., MD
- Wei, Grant, MD
- Yang, Anthony, MD
- Yoon, Kyung In, MD

Newark
- Afonso, Tania A., DO
- Anana, Michael Calulo, MD
- Atkin, Suzanne H., MD
- Bharatia, Nikita, DO
- Bitar, Souad Youssef, DO
- Black, Aislinn Denise, DO
- Brennan, John A., MD
- Chitnis, Subhanir Sunil, MD
- Chun, Shaun Joo Yup, MD
- Desai, Jigar, DO
- Dudley, Larissa Sophia, MD
- Eis, Amanda, MD
- Fleischner, Charles Alan, MD
- Forde, Frank, MD
- Gang, Maureen A., MD
- Gluckman, William Alan, DO
- Goett, Rebecca R., MD
- Gordon, Marc William, MD
- Hersi, Kenadeed, MD
- Hinfey, Patrick Blaine, MD
- Jacob, Jeena, MD
- Jaker, Michael A., MD
- John, Miriam, MD
- John, Sheena J., DO
- Jones-Dillon, Shelley A., MD
- Joseph, Joslyn, DO
- Kabba, Chidinma Dawn, MD
- Katsetos, Suzanne A., MD
- Kenney, Adam, MD
- Kulkarni, Miriam L., MD
- Maguire, Nicole J., DO
- Masters, Martha Meredith, MD
- Mathews, Sam, MD
- Matjucha, John R., MD
- McCormack, Denise Elizabeth, MD
- Moffett, Shannon, MD
- Murano, Tiffany Ellyn, MD
- O'Mara, Adam Graham, DO
- Onufer, Karen Anne, MD
- Ostrovsky, Ilya, MD
- Parrish, Andrew, MD
- Patel, Ami R., DO
- Pickrell, Christie Calleo, MD
- Reynolds, Matthew Thomas, DO
- Ripper, Jill Richelle, MD
- Rosania, Anthony Russell, MD
- Sanchez, John Paul, MD
- Sanyaolu, Rasheed, MD
- Schamban, Neil Eric, MD
- Scott, Sandra Renita, MD
- Shah, Neena Manharlal, DO
- Shields, Stephen Damien, MD
- Sierra, Nancy, MD
- Srulowitz, Allen Judah, MD
- Starke, John James Jr., DO
- Sule, Harsh Prakash, MD
- Torres, Alexander, DO
- Valenzuela, Rolando Gabriel, MD
- Varela, Linda Florence, MD
- Waldron, Frederick Andrew, MD
- Warren, Karma Brown, MD
- Warshaw, Abraham Lee, MD
- Wasserman, Eric Jonathan, MD
- Zinzuwadia, Shreni Natoo, MD

Newton
- Benson, Ellen, MD
- Brutico, Anthony J., DO
- Juco, Henry P., MD
- Landre, William Joseph, MD
- Mack, Ronald John, MD
- Rivera, Alberto R., MD

North Bergen
- Alban, Alvaro, MD
- Ali, Meer S., MD
- Bingham, Richard F., MD
- Molina, Alex Armando, MD
- Ruocco, Dominic, MD
- Schneid, Sharona, MD

North Brunswick
- Bansal, Sonia, MD
- Roberts, Leah Kate, MD

North Haledon
- Patel, Namrata, DO

Old Bridge
- Cheng, Peter F., MD
- Davis, Patrick Michael, MD
- Noormohamed, Akbar H., MD
- Parreno, Maritza Georgette, MD
- Ruth, Tiffany Karim, MD

Paramus
- Goldberg, Alvin Hugh, MD

Parsippany
- Berger, Richard P., MD
- Ceppetelli, Lisa C., MD
- Cochrane, Dennis G., MD
- Crean, Christopher Arthur, MD
- Curato, Mark Anthony, DO
- Cuthbert, David, MD
- Figueroa, Delia, MD
- Freer, Christopher F., DO
- Giroski, Laura J., DO
- Gould, Michael Alan, MD
- Greenhut, William H., DO
- Hartmann, Anthony William, MD
- Heller, Mitchell J., MD
- Indruk, William L., MD
- Kassutto, Zach, MD
- Lebaron, Johnathon Clinton, DO
- Lehet, Justin Micheal, DO
- Loewenstein, Robert Elvin, MD
- Melnick, Gerald J., MD
- Milano, Marc Anthony, MD
- Minett, Danielle Marie, MD
- Minett, Kenneth Matthew, MD
- Mouridy, Gary C., DO
- Murray-Taylor, Stacey Odell, MD
- Nguyen, Matthew Thai-Khang, MD
- Oh, David H., MD
- Perotte, Schubert, MD
- Reddy, Chenna G., MD
- Schiller, Andrew P., MD
- Shah, Sachin Jitendra, MD
- Stapleton, George S., MD
- Troncoso, Alexis B., MD
- Utkewicz, Mark D., MD

Passaic
- Eletto, Vincent Joseph, MD
- Kennett, Shar, MD
- Stephenson, Karen Rosemarie, MD
- Umali, Alma B., MD

Paterson
- Aberger, Kate, MD
- Adinaro, David Joseph, MD
- Ahmed, Zaib, DO
- Barnes, Stacey Ann, DO
- Bornstein, Marc Andrew, DO
- Boulos, Nader, MD
- Catapano, Anthony, DO
- Cohen, Andrew Nathan, DO
- Colantoni, Matthew Steven, DO
- Elhussein, Khalid Ali, MD
- Fischer, Mitchell Steven, DO
- Flannery, Ashley Laura, DO
- Friedland, Howard M., DO
- George-Varghese, Blessit, DO
- Hochman, Steven Mark, MD
- Hwang, Eric Jesse, DO
- Karounos, Marianna, DO
- Kinyon, Jeffrey James, DO
- Kushner, Beth Jillian, DO
- Lapietra, Alexis Marie, DO
- Lob, Zev B., DO
- Magarelli, Mary-Lynn, DO
- Manchester, Joseph Matthew, DO
- Marin, Adrian Alonso, DO
- Matadial, Manjushree, DO
- McGovern, Terrance, DO
- Meigh, Matthew James, DO
- Morecraft, John A. Jr., MD
- Murphy, Ryan Bruce, MD
- Paez Perez, Yenisleidy, DO
- Patel, Nilesh Narendra, DO
- Pruden, James N., MD
- Riss, Alexander David, DO
- Rosenberg, Mark S., DO
- Sabando, Otto F., DO
- Sanicola-Johnson, Julie Marie, DO
- Sharma, Uma, MD
- Shroff, Ninad A., MD
- Summerville, Gregg Paul, MD
- Tillack, Lindsey Ann, MD
- Vlasica, Katherine, DO
- Whalen, Joanna Hallmark, DO
- Zdorovyak, Mina, MD
- Ziontz, Kristy L., DO

Pennington
- Fellman, Katherine, MD

Perth Amboy
- Carter, Larry Ernest, DO
- Clarke, Dane Eric, MD

Phillipsburg
- Amadio, Thomas J., DO
- Bee, Kim Donaldson, MD
- Burkey, Seth Micah, MD
- Parada, Joseph A., MD
- Starosta, Daria Marie, MD

Piscataway
- Bulahan, Alvin, MD
- Pratt, Michael E., MD

Plainsboro
- Belardi, Chris A., MD
- Cherefko, Kathryn Baier, DO
- Cridge, Peter B., MD
- Freedman, Jennifer Emi Chan, MD
- Garibaldi, Pia M., MD
- Gronczewski, Craig Anthony, MD
- Harrison, Stephen Jay, DO
- Price, Dennis P., MD
- Vossler, Cathleen M., MD

Pomona
- Bustamante, Irineo Jr., MD
- Merewitz, Glenn S., MD

Pompton Lakes
- Brabson, Thomas A., DO

Pompton Plains
- Alcantara, Solomon V., MD
- Dellapi, Andrew Thomas, MD
- Dynof, Francis R., MD
- Goldberg, Judah Lev, MD
- Gosselin, Edward M., MD
- Grossman, Andrew G., MD
- Kou, Victoria Wei-Li, MD
- Krauthamer, Matthew J., MD
- Lee, Jemius Dae, DO
- Marino, Gennaro J., DO

Princeton
- Costello, Lauren E., MD
- Neglia, Janet A., MD

Princeton Junction
- Desiderio, Carl M., MD

Rahway
- Bernstein, Michael Ari, MD
- Park, Malsuk, DO
- Tan, Manuel R., MD
- Wright, Toni Rene, MD

Ramsey
- Stern, Peter, MD

Red Bank
- Bruno, Stephen F., MD
- Cameron, James D., MD
- Desai, Aaditya A., DO
- Dunn, Sarah Ruth, MD
- Lemansky, Alan S., MD
- Levin, Michael Y., DO
- Migliori, Frank Anthony, MD
- Neyman, Gregory, MD
- Pennycooke, Shelley-Ann N., DO
- Ramachandran, Karthia J., MD
- Reynolds, Stephanie Marie, DO
- Roma, Kevin P., MD
- Rubinstein, Howard Arthur, MD
- Starkey, Lawrence Paul, MD
- Tomaino, Jeanne, MD
- Trattner, Lauren Beth, DO

Ridgefield Park
- Shaker, Ashraf F., MD

Ridgewood
- Baddoura, Rashid Joseph, MD
- Becker, George L. III, MD
- Diorio, Joseph J., MD
- Dreier, Marc Max, MD
- Egan, Daniel J., MD
- Fascitelli, David A., MD
- Felsenstein, Bruce W., MD
- Gerstel, Alan Victor, MD
- Markowitz, George Joseph, MD
- Mednick, Joyce J., MD
- Portale, Karen Mary, MD
- Raman, Jennifer Lynne, MD
- Ranginwala, Masood Ahmed, DO
- Sharma, Siddharth, MD
- Simonetti, Michael, MD
- Tsomos, Evangelia, MD
- Vogel, Mark F., MD
- Wagh, Anju M., MD

Physicians by Specialty and Town

Yallowitz,Joseph,MD
Ringwood
  Gabriel,Chantal Delise,MD
River Vale
  Gardy,Mark Alan,MD
Rumson
  Martin,James Furman,MD
  Rivers,Colleen Marie,MD
Rutherford
  Morales,Fabian Victor,MD
Salem
  Bui,Minh Ngoc,MD
Scotch Plains
  Schaller,Richard J.,MD
Sea Girt
  Patrick,Bryan L.,MD
Secaucus
  Guibor,Pierre,MD
  Tenaglia,Nicholas Charles,MD
Sewell
  Sullivan,Patrick O.,DO
  Williams,Edwin Rae,MD
  Zimmerman,Daniel J.,MD
Short Hills
  Groman,David I.,MD
  Rogers,Jody J.,MD
Shrewsbury
  Valko,Peter C.,MD
Sicklerville
  Morone,Teresa Monica,DO
  Soper,Robert Earl,DO
Skillman
  Eberly,Andrea Cecilia,MD
Smithville
  Ursani,Sekander A.,MD
Somers Point
  Angelastro,David B.,MD
  Chiccarine,Anthony P.,DO
  May,Roberta Russell,DO
  McGuigan,Thomas M.,MD
  Souto,Henry Lee,DO
  Talotta,Nicholas Joseph Jr.,MD
Somerset
  Leavell,Ellen T.,MD
  Owusu-Dapaah,Kwabena B.,MD
  Patti,Laryssa A.,MD
Somerville
  Chan,Mei-Yung,MD
  Moore,Robert P.,MD
  Zeiger,Jill M.,MD
Springfield
  Parman,Stanley C.,MD
Stratford
  Ahmed,Mehvish,DO
  Angelo,Melanie Elissa,DO
  Chuang,Ion S.,MD
  Corrin,Courtney Wilczynski,DO
  Diaz,Lissa,DO
  Dichter,Eric Kyle,DO
  Ellis,Daniel Thomas,MD
  Fernandez,Claudio Miguel,DO
  Gesumaria,Robert Cosmo,DO
  Horn,Robert John,DO
  Kurkowski,Ellen J.,DO
  Levin,Francis L.,DO
  Licata,Thomas C.,DO
  Maddalozzo,Gerald Anthony,DO
  Maddock,Eric Ryan,DO
  Morris,Jason Joseph,DO
  Pagano,Joseph James,DO
  Papa,Thomas Rowland,DO
  Patel,Kishan Bharat,DO
  Pinkerton,Gerald John,DO
  Schuitema,Henry R.,DO
  Simmers-Dabinett,Donna Lee,DO
  Sobers-Brown,Karen D.,MD
  Tamaska,Wayne G.,DO
  Tomasello,Nicholas James,DO
  Wahdat,Razwana,DO
  Wetjen,Thomas F.,DO
  Wysocki,Julianne M.,DO
Summit
  Arora,Tanisha,MD
  Bilenker,James D.,MD
  Campo,Ruth A.,MD
  Gleimer,Evan Michael,DO
  Glessner,Robyn,DO
  Gudofsky,Gina Lynn,MD
  Heller,Diane Beth,MD
  Hernandez,Zachary Kris,DO

Lewis,Randall Craig,MD
Macri,Mirtha J.,MD
Mastrokyriakos,Paul,DO
Panchal,Neil,DO
Rathyen,Jill S.,MD
Sussex
  Koutcher,Gary Lewis,MD
Swedesboro
  Heresniak,Victor A.,DO
Teaneck
  Marcilla,Oscar A.,MD
  Miglietta,Mario Adrian,DO
  Miller,Alan S.,MD
  Schwab,Richard M.,MD
  Silverman,Brian S.,DO
  Tartacoff,Randy S.,MD
  Weinberg,Kenneth R.,MD
Tenafly
  Lee,Sang Hyun,MD
Tinton Falls
  Calabro,Joseph John,DO
  Merlin,Mark A.,DO
  Schaible,Derek D.,MD
  Sharma,Niti,DO
  Simon,Purabi Mehta,DO
  Sorkin,Greg Charles,DO
Toms River
  Bernard,John Marley,MD
  Chiccone,Martha G.,MD
  Crisanti,John Jr.,MD
  DesRochers,Laurence R.,MD
  Eng,Tiffany,MD
  Fowlie,Thomas Jr.,MD
  Giles,Thomas William,DO
  Janes,Susan F.,DO
  Levine,Marc M.,MD
  Madonick,Harvey Lloyd,MD
  Meredith,Jacob M.,MD
  Pepe,Salvatore IV,DO
  Ravindran,Wijeyadevendram,MD
  Reznikov,Boris,DO
  Russell,Warren King,MD
  Singh,Chetna,MD
  Varma,Medavaram Vikram,MD
  Wrigley,Steven N.,MD
Trenton
  Banks,Gerald,MD
  Deendyal,Yoganand,MD
  Geller,Robert J.,DO
  Howard,Tanya Dayell,MD
  Hughes,Kristin Lynne,MD
  Ijaz,Muhammad Shabbir,MD
  Kaur,Jaspreet,DO
  Maiers,Travis John,MD
  Meisner,Patricia Bliss,DO
  Miranda,David J.,MD
  Shirguppi,Renu,MD
  Sussman,Cindy Pearsall,MD
  Sutter,Garrett Gerald,MD
  Vichnevetsky,Simon,MD
Turnersville
  De Martino,Frank J.,DO
  McCabe,James III,MD
  Medlenov,Sergey,DO
  Shiller,David P.,MD
  Weeks,Daniel J. III,DO
Union
  Grayson,Janine Denise,MD
  Tyrrell,John A.,DO
Vernon
  De Luca,Joseph Edward,MD
Vineland
  Baruffi,Seth L.,MD
  Blazar,Eric Pollack,MD
  Cackovic,Curt W.,DO
  Cox,Courtney,DO
  Di Cindio,William D.,DO
  Diorio,Dominic A.,MD
  Ehrlichman,Richard S.,MD
  Eligulashvili,Victoria,MD
  Horan,Corinne E.,DO
  Kaluhiokalani,Leiloni H.,DO
  Kasper,Laura Carol,DO
  Milas,Jerry Peter,DO
  Poucel,Donna Jeanne,MD
  Schiller,Arnold Laurence,DO
  Terrigno,Donato A.,MD
  Urquhart,Megan C.,DO
  Wagner,Scott Erik,MD
  Warner,Matthew J.,MD
  Wilkerson,Zachary,DO

Wright,Camylla Dimetruss,DO
Voorhees
  Barnett,Jordan B.,MD
  Bingham,Johna P.,MD
  Block,William Paul,DO
  Burke,Rachel Irene,MD
  Gleeson,Tara Elizabeth,DO
  Gowda,Sharada Hiranya,MD
  Grim,Keith Case,MD
  Jumao-As,Joseph Maben A.,MD
  Lazarus,Adam Larry,MD
  Malta,Raymond J.,DO
  Meerson,Maya,MD
  Melnick,Jacob,MD
  Menditto,Darren,DO
  Parikh,Neelesh Vinod,DO
  Polise,Michael F.,DO
  Reynolds,Daniel,MD
  Rigueur,Adrienne Brooks,DO
  Roomi,Adil Mohamed,MD
  Scali,Victor,DO
  Singer,Eileen M.,DO
  Tiwari,Ramrakshah,MD
Wall
  Cotler,Harold Mark,DO
Wall Township
  Difabio,Kelly Ann,DO
  Womack,Meghan E.,MD
Warren
  Vogel,Laurie D.,MD
Wayne
  Bove,Joseph,DO
  Gandhi,Achyut Natvarial,MD
  Kansagra,Nilesh V.,MD
  Khan,Mansoor Ali,MD
  Shore,Robin L.,DO
  Testa,Joseph M.,MD
  Trivedi,Maulik Mahesh,MD
  Yuan,Ann Lee,MD
West Caldwell
  Lombardi,Susan L.,MD
West New York
  Meta,Shimbul Shashikant,DO
  Pamy Perez,Patricia Marcelle,MD
West Orange
  Abbassi,Samih R.,MD
  Biczak,Ernest S.,MD
  DeLaCalzada Jeanlouie,Mae F.,DO
  MacKenzie,Diane Susan,DO
West Trenton
  Valdellon,Alejandro M.,MD
West Windsor
  Arjun,Seeta,DO
  Blanc,Phillip Garven,MD
Westfield
  Diamantopoulos,Vasilios T.,MD
  Samuels,Marie Sophia,MD
Willingboro
  Evans,Nathaniel R. II,MD
  Fumento,Robert S.,MD
Woodbridge
  El-Halabi,Waseem,MD
Woodbury
  Ahuja,Yogesh,MD
  Baird,James Few IV,DO
  Bonner,James M.,DO
  Brenza,Danielle,DO
  Chen,Lee,MD
  Dalsey,Nicholas R.,DO
  Di Pasquale,Anthony J.,DO
  Dobrosky,Joseph D.,MD
  Espinosa,James A.,MD
  Garcia,Michael J.,DO
  George,James E.,MD
  Glenn,April,MD
  Goldstein,Sodi H.,DO
  Goode,Dale Norman,MD
  Granito,Joseph Louis,MD
  Greenfield,Brett Steven,DO
  Hoang,Loan Kim,MD
  Kupfer,Herschel,MD
  Kusmaul,Danielle Marie,DO
  Love,Thomas Pierce,MD
  Ludwin,Fredrick B.,DO
  Magariello,Mark M.,MD
  Martin,Ramelle Dana,MD
  Mathew,Nisha S.,MD
  Mayer,Douglas John,MD
  Mehta,Anila,MD
  Newman,Suzanne Maria,MD
  Oxler,Steven J.,MD

Pagana,Theresa N.,MD
Paschkes,Benjamin Neil,MD
Plumer,Robin Susan,DO
Raziano,Joseph Walter,MD
Sidwa,Robert M.,DO
Sireci,John Bernard,DO
Solomon,Stuart R.,DO
Stiefel,Jay A.,DO
Tamashausky,Shaun R.,DO
Trom,Andrew,DO
Varghese,Joby,DO
Weldon,Stacey Bidigare,MD
Young,Matthew John,DO
Woolwich Township
  Wofsy,Alice,MD
Wyckoff
  Shirley,Lauren,DO

Emergency Medicine-Sports Medicine

Burlington
  Shaffer,Jaclyn,MD
Vineland
  Disabella,Vincent N.,DO

Endocrinology/Diabetes/Metabolism

Basking Ridge
  Mehra,Aruna Sinha,MD
Bayonne
  Goykhman,Stanislav,MD
Belleville
  Miller,Michael Joseph,MD
  Napoli,John D.,MD
  Reddy,Rama R.,MD
  Seth,Amit Kumar,MD
Berkeley Heights
  Batacchi,Zona Olivia,MD
  Rosenbaum,Robert L.,MD
  Toscano-Zukor,Amy M.,DO
Bloomfield
  Dorcely,Brenda,MD
Bridgewater
  Agrin,Richard Joel,MD
  Aurand,Lisa Ann,MD
Butler
  Covello,Lucy F.,MD
Camden
  Laufgraben,Marc Jeffrey,MD
  Mayorga,Mabel,MD
Cape May Court House
  Raghuwanshi,Anita P.,MD
  Zitnay,Christopher G.,MD
Cherry Hill
  Anand,Rishi Dev,MD
  Barone,Gregory John,MD
  Bhat,Geetha K. G.,MD
  Haddad,Ghada,MD
  Jennings,Anthony S.,MD
  Kaufman,Steven Todd,MD
  Kaul,Shailja,MD
  Swibinski,Edward T.,MD
  Thapar,Garima,MD
  Varghese,Sarah,MD
  Verma,Parveen Kaur,DO
Clark
  Prasad,Surabhi,MD
Clifton
  Jasper,Josephine V.,MD
  Khaddash,Saleh I.,MD
  Roehnelt,Alessia Carluccio,MD
  Schulder-Katz,Micol,MD
  Schultz,Atara Batsheva,MD
  Shalem,Lena Hourwitz,MD
Clinton
  Ryan,Wanda Dawn,MD
Denville
  Las,Murray S.,MD
  Rosenfeld,Cheryl Robyn,DO
East Brunswick
  Hrymoc,Zofia,MD
  Maman,Arie,MD
  Mathew,Mini Ann,DO
  Surgan,Matthew Louis,MD
East Hanover
  Francis,Bruce H.,MD
  Nicastro,Maryann,MD
East Orange
  Pogach,Leonard M.,MD

Physicians by Specialty and Town

Endocrinology/Diabetes/Metabolism (cont)

Edison
Bucholtz, Harvey K., MD
Dunn, Jonathan C., MD
Panicker, Usha R., MD
Shah, Suketu Rajina, MD

Emerson
Daud Ahmad, Sameera, MD
Hochstein, Martin A., MD
Litvin, Yair, MD
Mahajan, Geeti, MD

Englewood
Abraham, Alice, MD
Bakerywala, Suhalia, MD
Bier, Rachel Elizabeth, MD
Borensztein, Alejandra G., MD
Cong, Elaine Alice, MD
Fojas, Ma. Conchitina Manas, MD
Schwartz, Joseph Jay, MD
Suh, Se Young, MD

Englewood Cliffs
Goldman, Michael H., MD

Fair Lawn
Yeshou, Dima, MD

Flemington
Caldarella, Felice Antonino, MD
Modarressi, Taher, MD
Sandberg, Marc Ira, MD

Florham Park
Borger, Caryn Beth, MD
Siegel, Sheera Karch, MD

Franklin Lakes
Dasmahapatra, Amita, MD
Hirsch, Laurence J., MD

Freehold
Farghani, Saima Obaid, MD
Nassberg, Barton M., MD
Ordene, Kenneth W., MD
Wininger, Eric Amiel, MD
Young, Melissa G., MD

Glen Ridge
Davis, Maris R., MD
Grover, Anjali, MD
Shafqat, Uzma Zohra, MD
Sherry, Stephen H., MD

Hackensack
Garger, Yana Basis, MD
Hannoush, Peter Yousef, MD
Katz, Adriana, MD

Hamilton
Empedrad, Albert Barcelona, MD
Soriano, Myrna Lopez, MD

Hammonton
Rastogi, Rishi K., MD

Hillsborough
Desai, Navtika R., DO

Hillsdale
Wehmann, Robert E., MD

Hoboken
Gandhi, Thimma S., MD

Holmdel
Antonopoulou, Marianna, MD
Zaitz, Jennifer, DO

Jersey City
Cam, Jenny G., MD
Ciechanowska, Malgorzata M., MD
Escobar-Barboza, Vanessa, MD

Kenilworth
Cuffie, Cynthia A., MD
Cutler, David L., MD

Kinnelon
Suda, Abhay K., MD

Lawrenceville
Dadzie, Daphne D., MD
Fresca, Diane Elizabeth, MD
Shelmet, John J., MD
Vergano, Sefton Cappi, MD

Linwood
Kleiber, Maria A., MD

Little Silver
Malik, Ritu, MD

Livingston
Boradia, Chirag N., DO
Dower, Samuel M., MD
Garbowit, David L., MD
Gewirtz, George P., MD
Jacob, Tess, MD
Luckey, Marjorie M., MD
Nambi, Sridhar S., MD

Silverman, Mitchell S., MD
Vlad, Luigina D., MD

Long Branch
Luria, Martin J., MD

Lyndhurst
Strizhevsky, Marina A., DO

Lyons
Byrne, William James, MD
Zimering, Mark B., MD

Manahawkin
Rizvi, Syed Wajih-Ul-Hasan, MD

Manalapan
Priven, Igor, MD

Maplewood
Chrisanderson, Donna A., MD
Prus, Dina S., MD

Margate City
Epstein, Britany Faith, MD

Marlton
Belsky, Martin Karl, DO
Fair-Covely, Rose Mary, DO

Matawan
Xenachis, Cristina Z., MD

Mendham
Usiskin, Keith S., MD

Millville
Slone, Helen L., MD

Monroe Township
Levy-Kern, Muriel, MD

Moorestown
Entmacher, Susan D., MD
Gonzalez Pantaleon, Adalberto, MD
Herbst, Allison B., MD
Savarese, Vincent William, MD

Morristown
Baron, Michelle A., MD
Castaneda, Rachel Lim, MD
Chon, Jajin Thomas, MD
Gadiraju, Silpa, MD
Margulies, Debra Jill, MD
Melfi, Robert J., MD
Nevin, Marie Eithne, MD
Walimbe, Mona S., MD

Mullica Hill
Fox-Mellul, Jodi V., MD

Neptune
Chalasani, Krishna, MD
Cheng, Jennifer, DO
Chiniwala, Niyati Umesh, MD
Holland, Soemiwati Weidris, MD
Lann, Danielle Erin, MD
Ong, Raquel Sanchez, MD

New Brunswick
Amorosa, Louis F., MD
Chakravarthy, Manu V., MD
Kolaczynski, Jerzy Wiktor, MD
Luo, Hongxiu, MD
Meininger, Gary Edward, MD
Murthy, Meena S., MD
Ohri, Anupam, MD
Orloff, John J., MD
Santora, Arthur Charles II, MD
Schneider, Stephen H., MD
Shulman, Leon H., MD
Van Hoven, Anne Marie, MD
Waldstreicher, Joanne, MD
Wang, Xiangbing, MD
Wondisford, Frederic Edward, MD

Newark
Baranetsky, Nicholas G., MD
Bleich, David, MD
Khutorskoy, Tamara, MD
Raghuwanshi, Maya P., MD
Sahani, Herneet K., MD
Stagnaro-Green, Alex Stewart, MD

North Bergen
Camacho-Patterson, Evelyn L., MD
Morgado, Antonio, MD
Pathak, Sonal, MD

Nutley
Hauptman, Jonathan B., MD

Old Bridge
Spiler, Ira J., MD

Paramus
Dzhalturova, Nadire, DO
Fernandez, Marlyn A., MD
Levy, Brian Leonard, MD
Manougian, Ara, MD
Shah, Viral Jagdishbhai, MD
Tohme, Jacques Fuad, MD

Pennington
Dhillon, Sudeep S., MD
Gillis Funderburk, Sheri A., MD
Parvez, Ayesha, MD
Saltzman, Erin Alyse, MD
Villanueva, Erika, MD

Perth Amboy
Jokic, Dragana, MD

Phillipsburg
Shah, Ashish Vinaychandra, MD
Singh, Ishita, MD

Piscataway
Apelian, Ara Z., MD
Fertig, Brian J., MD
Patel, Sima, MD

Point Pleasant Boro
Fomin, Svetlana, MD

Princeton
Bembo, Shirley Abad, MD
Benito Herrero, Maria I., MD
Deutsch, Paul Jan, MD
Inzerillo, Angela Mary, MD
Joy, Ansu Varughese, MD
Moses, Alan Charles, MD
Mullarkey-De Sapio, Cathleen, MD
Ruel, Ewa, MD
Weiss, Ned Martin, MD

Princeton Junction
Brenner-Gati, Leona, MD

Rahway
Bhattacharjee, Dulal, MD
Kaufman, Keith, MD
Leung, Albert Tao-Man, MD

Ramsey
Levy, Ian H., DO

Raritan
Erondu, Ngozi Emmanuel, MD

Red Bank
Kargutkar, Smita Nandkumar, MD

Ridgewood
Cobin, Rhoda Harriet, MD
Kelman, Adam Scott, MD
Lee, Esther Jeehae, MD

Robbinsville
Smolarz, Brian Gabriel, MD

Sea Girt
Ciorlian, Cristina C., MD

Sewell
DelGiorno, Charles J., MD
Sandhu, Sartaj S., MD

Somerset
Noronha, Joaquim L., MD

Stratford
Helfer, Elizabeth L., MD
Luceri, Patricia Marie, DO
Szpiech, Maria, MD

Summit
Chen, James J., MD
Selinger, Sharon E., MD

Teaneck
Eckman, Ari S., MD
Wiesen, Mark, MD

Tinton Falls
Enriquez, Santiago Jr., MD
Ravichandran, Shoba, MD

Toms River
Birnbaum, Joseph G., MD
Cruz, Francisco P., MD
Kleinman, David S., MD
Krishnan, Lalitha G., MD
Ortiz, Oscar T., MD
Villanueva, Ronald Banaag, MD

Turnersville
Beluch, Brian Walter, DO

Voorhees
Davidson, Jean Marie, DO
Horowitz, Elisabeth W., MD
Lam, Eleanor Lin, MD

Warren
Brodkin, Lisa Faith, MD

Wayne
Berkowitz, Richard H., MD
Gibiezaite, Sandra, MD
Leu, James Ping Hsun, MD
Panah, Manizheh Ghaem, MD

West Orange
Stock, Jerrold M., MD

West Paterson
Ibrahim, Mohammad S., MD

Westfield
Cho, Irene Soyoung, MD
Daifotis, Anastasia Golfinos, MD
Dev, Rajesh K., MD
Fuhrman, Robert A., MD

Westwood
Breit, Neal Gary, MD
Rodino, Maria A., MD

Willingboro
Rosenbaum, Daniel, MD

Woodbury
Fallon, Joseph Jr., MD

Endoscopic Surgery
Freehold
Dobruskin, Yelizaveta, MD

Epidemiology
Newark
Weiss, Stanley H., MD

Epilepsy
Hackensack
Mesad, Salah Mohammed, MD

Facial Plastic Surgery
Cherry Hill
Hughes, Susan M., MD

Highland Park
Glasgold, Robert Alexander, MD

Mendham
Kollmer, W. Lance, MD

Summit
Carniol, Paul J., MD

Voorhees
Sollitto, Robert B., MD

Family Med- Addiction Medicine
Camden
Nurse-Bey, Hazel Ann, MD

Family Med-Adolescent Medicine
Ewing
Sheikh, Sirajuddin, MD

Family Med-Adult Medicine
Cherry Hill
Fish, Gabrielle A., DO

Jersey City
Labib, Labib N., DO

Lawrenceville
Stramandi, Danielle Nicole, MD

Mount Holly
Tagle, Lauren, MD

North Bergen
Lee, Mark, DO

Princeton
Deora-Bhens, Sonia, DO

Ridgewood
Latimer, Karen M., MD

Shrewsbury
Saeed, Shamim Jan, MD

Somers Point
Fox, Michael L., MD
Malik, Ankit, DO

Family Med-Geriatric Medicine
East Windsor
Beagin, Erinn Elizabeth, MD

Freehold
Khan, Zeeshan, MD

Monroe
Bhalla, Anshu, MD

Monroe Township
Hussain, Aijaz, MD

Morristown
Blloshmi, Kledia, MD

Stratford
Abesh, Jesse Susan, DO

Summit
Kim, Julia J., MD

Family Med-Hospice & Palliative-Care
Fairfield
Douge, Simone Alicia, MD

Marlton
Chiesa, Jennifer Elaine, DO

Family Med-Sleep Medicine
Clark
Pumo, Jerome Jr., DO

Neptune
Lusk-Caceres, Christina A., DO

Physicians by Specialty and Town

Family Med-Sports Medicine
Atlantic City
Reed,Tony S.,MD
Bordentown
Konakondla,Krishna,MD
Brick
Sargent,Thomas G. Jr,DO
Cherry Hill
Duprey,Kevin M.,DO
Kimmel,Craig S.,MD
Eatontown
Krystofiak,Jason Anthony,MD
Egg Harbor Township
Chhipa,Irfan S.,MD
Lambertville
Chen,Victoria Sheen,MD
Raleigh,Elizabeth Ann,DO
Manasquan
Tennen,Elad,MD
Montclair
Mascaro,Melissa,MD
Moorestown
Plut,Thomas W.,DO
Shin,Jong Tae,DO
Ocean City
Sokalsky,Brian Edward,DO
Oradell
Mendler,James Christopher,MD
South Plainfield
Browne,Avery F.,DO
Union
Ahmed,Ameer Nizam,MD
Vineland
Evering,Daniel Jr.,DO
Voorhees
Vitanzo,Peter Charles,MD

Family Medicine
Aberdeen
Li,Jason,DO
Absecon
Zawid,Joseph,MD
Allentown
Byrnes,Curtis W.,DO
Redlich,Vijaya Potharlanka,DO
Andover
Medunick,Sara Elizabeth,DO
Reilly,Melissa Lynn,DO
Trader,Catherine R.,DO
Annandale
Imran,Uzma,MD
Asbury Park
Dhar,Gargi,MD
Khandelwal,Anil,MD
Lewis,Alison Dennesha,MD
Marro,Michael Angelo,DO
Wu,Irene Y.,MD
Atco
Mazzuca,Robert F.,DO
Vassalluzzo,Pasquale D.,MD
Atlantic City
Bisk,Bradley A.,DO
Castro-Chevere,Nancy Ann,MD
Corrales,Michelle D.,MD
Delice,Anael Destin Jr.,DO
Digenio,Ines Elena,MD
Fog,Edward Roland,DO
Holder,Sarah Schell,DO
Keiner,Lisa R.,DO
Pericles,John T.,DO
Raman,Anoop Manikarnika,MD
Rodriguez,Marlene V.,MD
Terrels,Mary Ellen,DO
Toliver,Tiffany E.,MD
Audubon
Bromley,William II,DO
Lopes,Francis,MD
Perry,Adam C.,MD
Barnegat
Rola,David Charles,MD
Barrington
Williams,Robert M.,MD
Basking Ridge
Morandi,Joseph T.,DO
Bayonne
Chiara,Bianca A.,MD
Diaz,Francisco J.,MD
George-Vickers,Jonelle,DO
Katsman,Tatyana,DO
Levine,Howard Seth,DO
Levine,Martin Scott,DO
Paduszynski,Adam A.,MD
Pineda,Veronica Vargas,DO
Potoczek-Salahi,Jolanta,MD
Primiani,Lisa,MD
Sirajuddin,Syed K.,MD
Tariq,Samreen,MD
Thomas,Jessy Joykutty,MD
Tolerico,Christopher S.,MD
Varghese,Sarat J.,MD
Beach Haven
Picaro,Anthony J.,MD
Schmoll,Todd C.,DO
Bedminster
Schwarz,Alexandra,MD
Varano,Catherine Alano,MD
Belle Mead
Doctoroff,Ella,DO
Gopalam,Mrunalini,MD
Miller,Janice M.,MD
Belleville
Cerritelli,John A.,MD
Gould,Peter L.,MD
Hilderbrand,Rene Francis,DO
Singhal,Pratap C.,MD
Bellmawr
Murray,Francis Jr.,DO
Belvidere
Bernard,John V.,MD
Fritz,John Patrick,DO
Bergenfield
Palisoc,Roger Louie,DO
Berkeley Heights
Deitz,Ruth Ellen Thisbe,MD
El Zein,Lama,MD
Leibu,Dora,DO
Lipset,Shani Lauren,MD
Moy,Jamie Tam,DO
Patrone,Nicole,MD
Reedy,Jamie Lynne,MD
Sahulhameed,Fathima,MD
Berlin
Costa,Richard C.,DO
Galezniak,John,DO
Gigliotti,David T.,DO
Hassman,David R.,DO
Hassman,Joseph M.,DO
Hassman,Michael A.,DO
La Ratta,John A.,DO
Maressa,Julian M.,DO
Mauriello,Richard M.,DO
Bernardsville
Kaftal,Sergiusz I.,MD
Beverly
Dow,William A.,MD
Blackwood
Adewunmi,Kafilat,DO
Fisicaro,Tamara Marie,MD
Gecys,Gintare T.,DO
Horvath Matthews,Jessica E.,MD
Mahamitra,Nirandra,MD
Robertson,John F. Jr.,MD
Sarmiento,Samuel I.,MD
Treiman,Arthur M.,MD
Bloomfield
Basista,Michael P.,MD
Bhatia,Hemlata,MD
Garcia Marotta,Ylonka,MD
Hyatt,Gayon Marie,MD
Kerlegrand,Pascale,MD
Mikulski,Wanda J.,MD
Russ Meek,Robyn L.,DO
Schuyler,Andrew P.,MD
Boonton
Robleza,Rolando M.,MD
Bordentown
Breig,Jason Anthony,MD
Carty,Robert W.,MD
Chen,Timothy,MD
Devers,Paul Dix,MD
Flynn,Jamie,DO
Garbarini Carty,Elyse,MD
Hughes,Janey Ballin,DO
Jimma,Lulu A.,MD
Lugo,Maria D.,MD
Mleczko,Joshua,DO
Van Patten,Yancy L.,DO
VanHise,Tara Hungspruke,DO
Vizzoni,Hiedi Taylor,MD
Bound Brook
Goldman,Frieda Shepsel,MD
Pizzelanti,Donna M.,DO
Branchburg
Donetz,Pamela Suzanne,MD
Gujjula,Prashanthi,MD
Shaffrey,Thomas Andrew,MD
Zeh,Catherine A.,MD
Branchville
Luszcz,Ronald J.,DO
Saradarian,Kathleen A.,MD
Brick
Alcasid,Ninfa A.,MD
Carolan,Owen J.,MD
Cascarina,Michael A.,MD
Eapen,Prema Mary,MD
Fung,Kent C.,MD
Konigsberg,David,DO
Kronhaus,Kenneth E.,MD
Navarro,Mark Anthony,MD
Riss,Martin,DO
Tesoriero,Laura M.,DO
Ussery-Kronhaus,Kelly G.,MD
Veder,Liana,MD
Wilson,Francis P.,DO
Bridgeton
Ballas,Christopher Thomas,MD
Bear,John G.,MD
Bear,Michelle H.,DO
Copare,Fiore J.,MD
De Biaso,Tracy A.,MD
Kohler,Frank R.,DO
LaCavera,Joseph A. III,DO
Manske,Daniel D.,MD
Ordille,Joseph D.,DO
Oswald,Mark Anthony,MD
Patitucci,Robert S.,MD
Riley-Lowe,Judith E.,DO
Roomi,Farah,MD
Talbot,Lori C.,MD
Tugman,Catherine K.,MD
Bridgewater
Boguslavsky,David,MD
Del Valle,Mario James,DO
Gora,Jill Suzanne,MD
Gubbi,Smitha Ayodhyarama,MD
Hamilton,Kathryn Diane,MD
Klein,Martin Edward,MD
Kripsak,John P.,DO
Lupoli,Kristin Anne,MD
Mannancheril,Anita,MD
Medrano,Christina Marie,MD
Mitterando,Jeanne G.,MD
Ouano,Estelita C.,MD
Tobias,David A.,MD
Brigantine
McAdam,Kimberly S.,DO
Browns Mills
Miller,Robin Jeanne,MD
Shapiro,Paul,DO
Willoughby,Ronald P.,DO
Budd Lake
Hoey,Kathleen Marie,MD
Leggiero,Nicholas J.,DO
Seshadri,Mahalakshmi,MD
Sher,Peter Mitchell,MD
Burlington
Cumarasamy,Thayalan K.,MD
Cynn,Jhin J.,MD
Griffin,Amanda,MD
Maharaj-Mikiel,Indira C.,MD
Moront,Barbara Jeanne,MD
Nemeth,Laurie Yallowitz,DO
Rozenberg,Larisa,MD
Sacks,Robert J.,DO
Strazzeri,Mia Domenica,DO
Varkey,Ciby B.,MD
Burlington City
D'Guerra,Mignon Marie,MD
Reid,Gillian Salanda,MD
Burlington Township
Patel,Manish Arvind,DO
Butler
Kielar,Francis,MD
Caldwell
Aquilio,Ernest J.,DO
Hauter,Moneef S.,MD
Mazzoccoli,Vito,MD
Califon
Byrd,Raymond J.,MD
Jaskolski,Joseph A.,MD
McGowan,John M.,MD
Williams,Karen Lynn,MD
Camden
Bascelli,Lynda Marie,MD
Baston,Kaitlan,MD
Bhalodia,Amit Maganlal,DO
Bialecki,Rosemarie,DO
Brenner,Jeffrey Craig,MD
Brooks,Julius A. Jr.,MD
Colopinto,Christopher F.,DO
Dinks-Brown,Shantay M.,DO
Enyeribe,Chioma J.,MD
Fesnak,Susan Gail,DO
Figliola,Robin A.,DO
Franks,Ralph Robert Jr.,DO
Gitler,Steven F.,DO
Goldis,Michael E.,DO
Kim,Kyur Gsook Cho,MD
Kleeman,Jeffrey A.,DO
Lizerbram,Deborah Garber,DO
Prior,Patricia,DO
Rabie,Glenda,MD
Rivera,Adaliz,MD
Stegmuller,Joseph A.,DO
Westerberg,Dyanne Pergolino,DO
Whiting,Philip Howard,DO
Cape May
Koskinen,Kjersti,MD
Cape May Court House
Corrado,Peter M.,DO
Crowley,Elizabeth Ann,MD
Deignan,Dianna T.,MD
Jain,Manoj Prakash,MD
Koskinen,Jason Alexander,DO
Lirio,Sixto M.,MD
Marotta,Raymond J. Jr.,MD
McLay,William F.,DO
Rizzetta,Anthony J.,DO
Schwartz,Joseph T.,DO
Carlstadt
Morris,Paul J.,DO
Carneys Point
Lawrence,John Robert,MD
Quigley,Craig B.,MD
Carteret
Anderson-Wright,Phyllis,DO
Kindzierski,Michael A.,DO
Sjovall,Frances,DO
Cedar Grove
Pinal,Laureen,MD
Rosen,Jay Stuart,MD
Cedar Knolls
Dave,Bijal A.,MD
Gellerstein,Alan Stuart,MD
Gibbions,James Vernon Jr.,MD
Gopin,Joan M.,MD
Kumar,Preethi,DO
Monka,Ira P.,DO
Tepper,Suzanne,MD
Chatham
Baker,Janice E.,MD
Cirello,Joseph Anthony,MD
Gruber,Amy D.,MD
Holland,Elbridge T. Jr.,MD
Levine,Steven Marc,DO
Nevins,John J.,DO
Ocasio,Maria Elena,MD
Resciniti,Matthew John,DO
Tribuna,Joseph,MD
Varshavski,Mikhail,DO
Cherry Hill
Bidigare,Susan Ann,MD
Bieler,Bert Michael,MD
Chen,Anna,MD
Chung,Lynn S.,MD
Costa,Ralph F.,MD
De Prince,Daniel III,MD
DiMaio,Robert D.,DO
Finan,Cathleen M.,DO
Finan-Duffy,Colleen M.,DO
Fine,Manette K.,DO
Forman,Lawrence S.,DO
Greenberg,Scott Ross,MD
Gurrieri,John E.,MD
Hanley,Thomas T.,MD
Kocinski,Michael Stephen I,DO
Kopp Mulberg,F. Elyse,DO
Levin,Bonnie Lorraine,DO
Levine,Richard Marc,MD
Mueller,Loretta L.,DO
Neidecker,John Michael,DO
Persily,Tracy L.,DO
Salerno,Christopher J.,DO

Physicians by Specialty and Town

Family Medicine (cont)
Cherry Hill
Shrayber,Yelena Y.,DO
Simon,Richard M.,DO
Sirken,Steven M.,DO
Vernon,Gerald Michael,DO
Vitoc,Camelia S.,MD
Weiss,Richard S.,DO
Chester
Singh,Maulshree,MD
Cinnaminson
Laws-Mobilio,Susan Wendi,DO
Parchuri,Hima Bindu,DO
Rakickas,Jeffrey,MD
Switenko,Zenon M.,DO
Weingarten,Michael P.,DO
Clark
Beams,Michael E.,DO
Gilsenan,Michele T.,DO
Kowalenko,Karen F.,DO
Kowalenko,Thomas Alex,DO
Mathias,Claudia Fernandes,MD
Rushman,John Warren,MD
Sabharwal,Tina,MD
Syed,Zareen Taj,MD
Clarksboro
Provencher,Robert A.,DO
Clayton
Schopfer,Carl L.,DO
Clementon
Patel,Pradip N.,MD
Cliffside Park
Cirignano,Barbara M.,MD
Weinberger,George T.,DO
Clifton
Adedokun,Emmanuel Adekunle,MD
Bhaskarabhatla,Krishna V.,MD
Chen,David,MD
Del Casale,Thomas Ernest,DO
Delisi,Michael David,MD
Dhamotharan,Shakira N.,MD
Dobrow,Michael Craig,DO
Doroudi,Shideh,MD
Fyffe,Ullanda P.,MD
Guerzon,Pearl Tolentino,MD
Gupta,Vikram,MD
Igbokwe,Jennifer,MD
Kahlon,Tejinderpaul Singh,MD
Lavian,Pejman,MD
Leon Wong,Hector J.,MD
Leroy,Christine,MD
Lima,Francesco W.,MD
Lucila,Rafael R.,MD
Maneyapanda,Mukundha B.,MD
Mangone,Jesse G.,DO
Mao,Cheng-An,MD
Miller,Randall W.,DO
Muccino,Gary P.,MD
Nunez,Jacqueline Denise,MD
Odatalla,Bassam N.,MD
Palmer,Susan M.,DO
Pinzon,Amabelle Par,MD
Pogorelec,Albert Joseph Jr.,DO
Pudinak,Anna,MD
Sabido,Michael,MD
Shraytman,Arkadiy,DO
Singh,Manik,MD
Testa,David A.,DO
Thomas,Seymour W.,MD
Tindoc,Lorelane Pagulayan,MD
Clinton
Bock,David Andrew,DO
Celestino,Cecilia Cruz,MD
Delvers,Dilek Sunay,MD
Karpinski-Failla,Susan Ellen,DO
Lunt,David M.,MD
Messina,Charles I.,MD
Petrillo,Jennifer Anne,MD
Collingswood
Holwell,Michael,DO
Moraleda,Jason N.,MD
Neveling,Lance William,DO
Winn,Robert Jerald,MD
Yang-Novellino,Sue Y.,DO
Colonia
Awan,Rabia S.,MD
Guzik,David J.,MD
Rukh,Lala,MD
Colts Neck
Angello,Philip Joseph,MD
Gibson,Lisa Kay,MD

Raymond,Kimberly J.,MD
Columbia
Arvary,Gary J.,MD
Cullen,Eugene A.,MD
Greenberg,Anthony,MD
Molnar,Eric D.,DO
Columbus
Bross,Robert J.,MD
Carcia,Danielle,DO
Dunn,Davonnie Marie,MD
Guiliano,Philip M.,MD
Hulse,Andrea Doria,DO
Jadeja,Poiyniba Dilip,MD
Vare,Christopher,MD
Cranbury
Sethi,Shalini K.,MD
Cresskill
Shoshani,Shai,MD
Dayton
Azam,Muhammad,MD
Boudwin,James E.,MD
Rivera,Tara Elizabeth,DO
Delmont
Pomerantz,Jeffrey David,DO
Delran
Alcera,Roanna Espino,MD
Friedman,Samuel L.,DO
Graziano-Wilcox,Donna,DO
Keller,Maureen Reilly,DO
Smith,Kindra Renee,MD
Starkman,Moishe,MD
Denville
Furst,Alan David,MD
Gilo,Elmer S.,MD
Ho,John,MD
Kaminetsky,Eric Jay,DO
Kosoy,Edward,MD
Zaki,Isaac Kamal,MD
Dover
Bishop,Douglas Scott,MD
Sweinhart,Marty Dawn,MD
Dumont
Cabela,Gina Flores,MD
Desplat,Philippe,DO
Kumar,Puneet,MD
East Brunswick
Azer,George S.,MD
Davis,Michele,DO
Geller,Toby A.,MD
Goldman,Iosif,DO
Ifabiyi,Lubunmi,MD
Khalil,Venus T.,MD
Klots,Larisa,DO
Lau,Ronald,MD
Marmora,James J.,MD
Nee,Patricia B.,MD
Schiano,Catherine Jean,DO
Tomlinson-Phelan,Michelle A.,DO
East Hanover
Gabriel,Laurice Helen,MD
Khanna,Roohi,DO
East Orange
Bhate,Soniya,MD
Choi,Hongsun,MD
Katta,Madhavi R.,MD
Law,Jeremy P.,MD
Morrell,Christopher,MD
Nasta,Sucheta M.,MD
Witham,Marie-Grace,DO
East Rutherford
D'Andrea,John Louis,MD
East Windsor
Skeehan,Christopher J.,MD
Eatontown
Frantz,Mildred Marie,MD
Edgewater
Chhabra,Mohina Singh,MD
Kuwama,Chika,MD
Edison
Aderibigbe,Adedayo Olubunmi,MD
Arefeen,Samrana,MD
Assemu,Belen F.,MD
Bhattacharyya,Adity,MD
Chae,Sung Yeon,MD
Collins,Harry,MD
Dalal,Gita S.,MD
Diziki,Donna C.,DO
Elber,Daniel A.,MD
Estevez,Gerardo V.,MD
Faches,Allison L.,MD
Flores,Maria S.,MD

Henderson,Thomas J.,MD
Kandula,Sridevi,MD
Kwon,Seri,MD
Laroche,Harold I.,MD
Metz,Deborah Lynne,MD
Metz,John Patrick,MD
Micabalo,Alvin Francis,DO
Milne,Charlene E.,MD
Nadkarni,Swati G.,MD
Nelson,Yvonne,MD
Patel,Dipesh Shashikant,DO
Patel,Hitesh Ramesh,MD
Patel,Naresh J.,DO
Patel,Rahil,MD
Picciano,Anne,MD
Prasad,Kamil,MD
Reyes,Ruby Carina E.,MD
Seck,Thomas F.,MD
Sharma,Usha,MD
Sinha,Gopal K.,MD
Subramanian,Srilakshmi,MD
Vermani,Prathiba,MD
Wiley,Olga V.,MD
Wilks,Michelle Anne,MD
Winter,Robin O.,MD
Wong,Patrick,MD
Zayoud,Rajaa M.,MD
Egg Harbor Township
Altamuro,Christopher R.,DO
Barrett,Bryan Richard,DO
D'Ambrosio,Robert Paul,DO
Kern,Carrie Catherine,DO
Richwine,Charles M. IV,DO
Richwine,Lori T.,DO
Elizabeth
Aponte,Emilia Laura,DO
Brice,Marie F.,MD
Cisnero,Maria Del Carmen,MD
Cruz,Catalina M.,MD
Ferdinand,Pascale,MD
Khamis,Khamis Gerious,DO
Perez,Raul I.,MD
Quinones,Ariel,MD
Tan,Edgardo L.,MD
Elmer
Elgawli,Philip Raef,DO
Haag,Jerry L.,MD
Malickel,Jay Varunny,DO
Sastic,Daniel Joseph,MD
Ventrella,Gerard,MD
Elmwood Park
Finelli,Peter K.,DO
Vila,Maria N.,DO
Emerson
Desai,Veena C.,MD
Dombrowski,Mark A.,MD
McConnell,Julie,MD
Wilkin,Daniel James,DO
Englewood
Babeendran,Shan,DO
Gross,Harvey R.,MD
Healy,Christine B.,DO
Klingsberg,Gary P.,DO
Mor Zilberstein,Lara,MD
Skarimbas,Alicia C.,MD
Suri,Ritu,MD
Evesham
Pinsky,Tim A.,DO
Ewing
Carruth Mehnert,Lauren Vales,MD
Flynn-Abdalla,Jane,DO
Jass,Daniel K.,MD
Fair Haven
Gredell,Elizabeth S.,DO
Swidryk,John P.,MD
Fair Lawn
Bernardo,Dennis N.,MD
Chaudry,Sadia R.,MD
Chaudry,Samia Riaz,DO
John,Eirene George,MD
Karunanithi,Subhathra,MD
Kaur,Jasneet,MD
Levin,Susan Miriam,MD
Riley,Roth Leon,MD
Rosenberg,Jeffrey Steven,MD
Fairfield
Liotti,Joseph B.,DO
Liotti,Linda A.,DO
Scolamiero,Amedeo J.,MD
Fairview
Erguder,Iris,MD

Eyerman,Luke Edmund,MD
Stricker,Howard,DO
Fanwood
Scalia,Joseph A.,DO
Farmingdale
Dennis,Philip S.,MD
Schauer,Joseph W. III,MD
Taneja,Deepak,DO
Flanders
Choe,Charles C.,DO
Fernandez,Sofia Ramona,MD
Friedman,Samuel,MD
Ghanta,Suma Bala,MD
Huang,Chen Ya,MD
Miccio,Anthony G.,MD
Peters,Karen R.,DO
Flemington
Bachrach,Stacey R.,MD
Baird,Jamila,MD
Benson,Jay Robert,DO
Bernard,Marie G.,MD
Bretan,Amy Faith,MD
Coates,Robert G.,MD
Cox,Victoria Ryan,MD
Eskow,Eugene S.,MD
Feigin,Joel Stanley,MD
Fuhrman,Joel H.,MD
Gazurian,Raina,MD
Gertzman,Jerrold Scott,MD
Golub,Larisa,MD
Hannema,Erica L.,DO
Hoette,Petra,MD
Joseph,Junie Lorna,MD
Klein,Randy S.,MD
Lecusay,Dario A. Jr.,MD
Lewis,Mary Kendra,MD
Licetti,Stephen Charles,DO
Liebross,Ira David,MD
Liu,Lide,MD
Madonia,Paul W.,MD
Manchen,Dennis R.,MD
Mattei,C. Antonia,MD
McDonough,John R.,MD
Morton,Lisa Aseni,MD
Mui,Timothy H.,MD
Mukherji,Genea,MD
Nealis,Justin,MD
O'Hara,Jennifer Fisk,MD
Pauch-McNamara,Dorothy Anne,MD
Peng,Victor I.,MD
Plunkett,Lisa A.,MD
Randhawa,Smita Devidas,MD
Scevola Dattoli,Angela,MD
Solanki,Dhenu G.,MD
Tammana,Swarna,DO
Weil,Irina Lisker,MD
Wierzbicki,Jonathan Edmund,MD
Wright,Deborah Sue,MD
Florham Park
Gunn Russell,Ian Neil,MD
Harwani,Nita R.,MD
Fords
Petrovani,Mark S.,MD
Forked River
Barry,Therese Maria,DO
Kassenoff,Lisa Adrian,DO
Novak,Dennis E.,MD
Fort Dix
Byrnes,Michael John,DO
Fort Lee
Cassotta,Joseph P. Jr.,MD
Karatoprak,Ohan,MD
Lee,David W.,MD
Franklin
Holgado,Marco Patrick Guinto,DO
Hrabarchuk,Eugene S.,MD
Matkiwsky,Daniel Walter,DO
McMahon,Kerry Rose,MD
Freehold
Bernardo,Salvatore Jr.,MD
Cherciu,Doina M.,MD
Cherciu,Mugurel S.,MD
Chopra,Vinay,MD
Ciminelli,Maria F.,MD
Cozzarelli,James Francis,MD
Delcurla,Gina M.,DO
Dermer,Alicia R.,MD
Edrich,Dina Rachel,MD
Eng,Kenneth,DO
Espinar Ho,Maria Elena,MD
Faistl,Kenneth W.,MD

Physicians by Specialty and Town

Gershenbaum,Mark R.,DO
Gupta,Vinod K.,MD
Kathrotia,Mitesh Gordhan,MD
Kim,Miah,MD
Leonard,Sara B.,MD
Lucas,Lisa W.,DO
Mellor,Lisa Marie,MD
Mills,Orlando F.,MD
Nau,Allen Reza,MD
Ogon,Bernard Okem,MD
Paulvin,Neil Brian,DO
Raccuglia,Joseph R.,MD
Rider,Timothy Eugene,MD
Sandru,Dan Victor,MD
Sasidhar,Vaidehi,MD
Sewell,Grant,MD
Shenker,Bennett Steven,MD
Sinha,Taru,MD
Stein,Howard A.,DO
Galloway
Ezeanya,Ebere Nneka,MD
Sperling,Howard J.,MD
Thadhani,Ramchand,MD
Williams,Robert H. Jr.,MD
Garfield
Conte,Kenneth S.,DO
Kawecki,Jerzy Stanislaw,MD
Koch,Donna Marie,DO
Garwood
Caracitas,Alexandra Cristina,DO
McArthur,Lucas James,MD
Gibbsboro
Paxton,Timothy X.,DO
Sheldon,Howard A.,DO
Sheldon,Lynne T.,DO
Tokazewski,Jeffrey Thomas,MD
Villamayor,Rosemarie Cruz,MD
Gibbstown
Dave,Akshay S.,MD
Glassboro
Heist,Jon S.,DO
Meskin,Steven J.,MD
Nguyen,Bac Xuan,MD
Palmer,Josette C.,MD
Sayed,Durr-E-shahwaar,DO
Schultes,Arthur H.,DO
Szgalsky,Joseph Brian,MD
Glen Gardner
Lagarenne,Paul R.,MD
Glen Ridge
Berlin,Melissa Gail,MD
Flores,Jose C.,DO
Kidangan,Julie Thomas,DO
Glen Rock
Meisel,Mark K.,DO
Glendora
Blank,Benjamin I.,DO
Gloucester City
Klein,Steven,DO
Lundy,Edward L.,DO
Green Brook
Carrieri,David A.,DO
Cook,Sean Michael,MD
Hammoud,Marwan Fahim,MD
Klele,Michael A,MD
Pilla,John D.,MD
Popeck,Paul J.,DO
Quezada Reyes,Carlos A.,MD
Sgambelluri,Carol E.,MD
Strauss,Scott R.,DO
Guttenberg
Calero,Jose Manuel,MD
Sterling,Karen Sohria,MD
Hackensack
Ahmad,Yasir Jamal,MD
August,Elizabeth,MD
Chaney,Arthur Jr.,MD
Chaney,Dewey A.,MD
Corrigan,Lynn Ann,DO
Gatchalian,Luningning C.,MD
Hussain,Rubaba,MD
Jacob,Mariamma,MD
Koenigsberg,Martin Allen,DO
Ourvan,Dorothy R.,DO
Schwarz,Rachelle,DO
Hackettstown
Duryee,John Jourdan,MD
Paterno,Jeanette D.,MD
Haddon Heights
Brumbaugh,Martha,MD
Doshi,Sangita K.,MD

Greenwood,Beth M.,MD
Handler,Heidi L.,MD
Higgins,Alexander J.,MD
Staritz,Amy,MD
Haddon Township
Gupta,Mini,MD
Manalis,Helen,DO
McGrath,Robert C.,DO
Haddonfield
Bauer-Sheldon,Melissa Ann,DO
Doyle,Stephanie L.,MD
Foss,Roberta,DO
Kenney,Meredith Ann,DO
Lafon,Michael C.,MD
Olson,Aubrey M.,DO
Panitch,Kenneth N.,MD
Ridilla,Leonard Jr.,MD
Runfola,James Joseph,MD
Vick,James W.,MD
Hainesport
Ciervo,Carman A.,DO
Mason,David Craig,DO
Meltzer,Michael E.,DO
Hamburg
Autotte,Denise L.,MD
Kozak,Margaret Zsuzsa,DO
Roffe,Kenneth A.,DO
Song,Maria H.,MD
Hamilton
Agcopra,Annabel,DO
Bancroft,James Alan,MD
Castillo,Christine Capistran,DO
Chavez Santos,Maria,MD
Chiromeras,Andrew,MD
Cruz,Gloria Maria,MD
Dasti,Sofia J.,MD
Flores,Lisa,MD
Funches,Antonio,MD
Guarino,Joseph M.,DO
Manzoor,Adil,DO
Marriott,Christine Ryan,MD
Masood,Hamid,MD
Mullane,Joseph P.,MD
Oswari,Daniel,MD
Patel,Viral D.,MD
Pluta,Christine Marie,DO
Richards,Bonnie J.,DO
Soliman,Yasser S.,MD
Subramoni,Venkateswar,MD
Timmapuri,Ajaz J.,MD
Tohfarosh,Nilofer J.,MD
Tselniker,Maryana,MD
Voddi,Swetha Devi,MD
Wistreich,Sarah J.,DO
Hammonton
Anderson,Christine H.,DO
Collins,Philip,DO
De Tata,Gerald C.,MD
Goudsward,Sean M.,DO
Jones-Mudd,Kimberly M.,DO
Jung,Herbert Michael,DO
Kaminski,Mitchell Anthony,MD
Krachman,Donald A.,DO
Loughlin-Pherribo,Donna J.,DO
Miranda,Chona Santos,MD
Moore,Rebecca Christiane,DO
Nurkiewicz,Stephen A.,MD
Salvo,Anthony,MD
Schneider,Katherine Ann,MD
Sharma,Sonia,MD
Hampton
Berk,Scott Phillip Reed,MD
Madura,Paul P.,MD
Mitev,Iliya D.,MD
Palmer,Victoria R.,DO
Polizzi,David R.,MD
Polt,Terry Jane,MD
Prentice,Hugh J.,MD
Sforza,Frank J.,MD
Thakur,Shivani,MD
Harrington Park
Sawicki,John M.,DO
Harrison
D'Agostino,Ralph S.,MD
Hasbrouck Heights
Bellavia,Thomas S.,MD
Porter,David F.,DO
Haworth
Isnar,Noyemi,MD
Hawthorne
Anthony Wilson,Avril Dawn,MD

Lozito,Joseph A. Jr.,DO
Tuppo,Enas Elias,MD
Hazlet
Field,Shawn Michael,MD
Hundle,Rameet Kaur,MD
Perrino,DinaMarie,DO
Schneebaum,Katherine,MD
Triola,Victoria,DO
Tsompanidis,Antonios A.J.,DO
Hewitt
Baquiran,Henry M.,MD
Guariglia,George Angelo,DO
Highland Park
Cohn,Joseph Theodore,MD
Glatter,Frederic G.,MD
Miller,Arthur H.,MD
Hightstown
Syed,Sameera Mukaram,MD
Hillsborough
Bagga,Harpreet Kaur,MD
Corson,Richard L.,MD
Erb,Erica,MD
Fowls,Brianna,MD
Landesman,Glen S.,MD
Lardner,Thomas Joseph,MD
Lee,Sung Keun,MD
Merchant,Neepa S.,MD
Piech,Richard Frank,MD
Reiss,Ronald A.,MD
Selke,Melissa D.,MD
Shute,Amy L.,MD
Smith,Joseph Arthur,MD
Snyder,Kenneth R.,MD
Weinstein,Joseph R.,MD
Zajac,Anna T.,MD
Hillside
Matkiwsky,Walter,DO
Tyndall,Alina,MD
Vidal Burke,Angela M.,MD
Hoboken
Balacco,Leonard M.,MD
Brahmbhatt,Gaurang Ravaji,MD
Caniglia,James J.,MD
De Marco,Angelo Albert,MD
Garcia,Raudel,MD
Garcia,Steven Jesus,MD
Islam,Javedul M.,MD
Jacobs,Abbie D.,MD
Joshi,Anuja,MD
Kumar,Harini C.,MD
Latorre,Juan J.,MD
Matienzo,Ricardo Martin,MD
Mercado,Donna M.,MD
Mezhoudi,Amal,MD
Pollak,Joseph A.,MD
Racaniello,Angelo R.,MD
Ramirez Chernikova,Anna,MD
Ramos,Leonor Vivas,MD
Ramos,Rey Ferna Pedraza,MD
Rohani,Sayed M.,MD
Safran,George F.,MD
Samuel,Shyno,MD
Spivak,Dana,MD
Taubman,Jessica,MD
Teodoro,Paul C.,MD
Tracey,Gregory Joseph,MD
Tully,Nicole S.,MD
Valerian,Christopher,DO
Williams,Juliette Marie,MD
Witt,Virginia Marie,MD
Zigadlo,Tatyana,MD
Holmdel
Bessen,Deborah Lynn,MD
Catanese,Vincent J.,MD
Hayne,Charles W.,MD
Salisbury,Jon P.,MD
Shah,Vinaychandra B.,MD
Howell
Agrawal,Neil,MD
Anne,Sreelatha,MD
Gumina,John D.,MD
Liquori,Frances,DO
Stern,Julie Beth,MD
Zuckerbrod,Jacqueline E.,DO
Irvington
Willis,Rudolph C.,MD
Iselin
Lubin-Baskin,Alicia F.,DO
Mayer,Marc,DO
Mayer,Mitchell F.,DO
Perilstein,Neil J.,MD

Riggi,Joseph,DO
Jackson
Druckman,Scott Jonathan,DO
Lee,Nelson,DO
Parkes,Lauren H.,DO
Pedowitz,Robert Neil,DO
Raymond,Joshua Joseph,MD
Rodriguez-Bostock,Susan M.,MD
Jamesburg
Newman,Jared Brad,DO
Jersey City
Abubakar,Shaik,MD
Bobb-Mckoy,Marion Y.,MD
Buisson,Valerie Fabiola,MD
Castro,Zoila Y.,MD
Choudry,Muhammad A.,MD
Cruz,Wilfredo Tomas Correa,MD
De Silva,Malika Shani,MD
Fritz,John A.,DO
Kapadia,Bhupendra A.,MD
Majchrzak,Tadeusz J.,MD
Mayorquin,Bertha,MD
Mercado,Melissa,DO
Mravcak,Sally A.,MD
Nguyen,Jim A.,DO
Patel,Hetal R.,DO
Riva,Inna,MD
Roque,Cesar Ruben Jr.,MD
Rosenblum,Lauren,DO
Rotella,Frank A.,DO
Sanderson,James Glen,DO
Saxena,Shilpa M.,MD
Schehr-Kimble,Danielle J.,DO
Sklower,Jay A.,DO
Wong,Aubrey S.,DO
Kendall Park
Lara,Jaime F.,MD
Weingarten,Harvey S.,,MD
Kenilworth
Kazemi,Ahmad,MD
Milazzo,Salvatore J. Sr,DO
Kinnelon
Cartaxo,Kenneth W.,MD
Lake Hiawatha
Spector,Randy A.,DO
Lake Hopatcong
Bonnet,Jean-Paul,DO
Lucatorto,Anthony J.,DO
Lakewood
Genovese,Cynthia Marie,MD
Patterson,Marion Lesley,MD
Zukowski,Christopher W.,DO
Lambertville
Barter,Cindy Monette,MD
Burgos,Melissa,MD
Eichman,Margaret J.,MD
Espinoza,Lisa C.,MD
Giangrante,Matthew E.,MD
Koorie,Elizabeth L.,MD
Lei,Michaela,DO
Meyer,Monica Ann,MD
Mooney,Kevin K.,MD
Russo,Frances Jenny,DO
Russo,Steven,MD
Schmitt,David J.,MD
Sokkar,Rita,DO
Waters,John S.,MD
Landing
Damico,Christopher R.,DO
Purcell,Joseph W.,DO
Shah,Shefali A.,DO
Laurel Springs
Eang,Rosanna,DO
Laurence Harbor
Zelikson,Irina Yelyanovn,DO
Lawrence Township
Hanley,Daniel Lee Wilburn,MD
Lawrenceville
Barlis,Cara J.,MD
Chung,Y. C. Emily,MD
Hector,Christina,DO
Hussain,Saleha,MD
Jarvis,Lori J.,MD
Laskarzewski,Radhika,MD
Leonti,Vincent J.,MD
Levandowski,Richard,MD
Levitt,Kimberly Anne,MD
McGeever,Rose,DO
Punj,Priti Narula,MD
Rose,Abigail Lee,MD
Santhanam,Shankar,MD

Physicians by Specialty and Town

Family Medicine (cont)

Lawrenceville
Shaikh, Nasir Hussain A., MD
Tsarouhas, Louis, MD
Young, Jill F., DO

Lebanon
Collins, Reid T., MD
Sacchieri, Theresa Ann, MD

Leesburg
Briglia, William J., DO

Lincoln Park
De Mare, Patrick J., DO

Lincroft
DePietro, Joseph Anthony, MD

Linden
Lukenda, Kevin, DO
Schulman, Joseph M., DO
Sherif, Ajfar, MD
Sundaram, Ashany, MD

Lindenwold
Neidorf, David L., MD

Linwood
Kader, Richard A., DO
Pernice, Mark J., DO

Little Egg Harbor
Berlin, William H., DO
Gandhi, Dhiren K., MD
Glenn, William B., DO
Mastro, Caroline Briana, MD
Medenilla, Rosenio Jr., MD
Tracy, Toby William, DO

Little Falls
Billig, Janelle Elisabeth, MD
Lentine, Nancy, DO
Mangra, Chandra, MD
Rae, Susan, MD
Yussaf, Shiraz, MD

Little Ferry
Tancer, Richard B., DO

Little Silver
Auriemma, John A., DO
Mehra, Neeraj, MD

Livingston
Boorujy, Dean P., MD
Hussain, Sarah, MD
Riaz, Danish, MD
Stevens, Susan H., MD

Lodi
Kulesza-Galvez, Theodora, MD
Lowenstein, Michael Aaron, DO

Lumberton
Buck, Murray D., DO
Campagnolo, Mary F., MD
Chatyrka, George O., DO
Daub, Horatio Guy, MD
Ibay, Annamarie D., MD
Jain Bhalodia, Sapna, DO
Kastenberg, Charles A., DO
Kolesk, Stephen J., MD
Naticchia, Jennifer M., MD
Rubenstein, Jennifer, MD
Scappaticci, John Jr., DO
Van Kooy, Mark A., MD

Lyndhurst
Aghabi, Hanna Najib, MD
Castelluber, Gisele B V M, MD
Faugno, Gerard L., MD

Lyons
Wang, Jian, MD

Madison
Berger, Gary, MD

Mahwah
Beenstock, Steven Marc, DO
Bello, Mary R., MD
De Guzman, Virginia H., MD

Manahawkin
Hogan, Kimberly Ann, MD
Kenny, John J., DO
Nitschmann-Schmoll, Cynthia, DO
Raguso Failla, Michael Joseph, MD
Tailor, Unnati, DO
Veldanda, Ashokvardhan R., MD

Manalapan
Baig, Rifaqat, MD
Dantchenko, Victoria, MD
Feingold, Marc Benjamin, MD
Goldberg, Alexander, MD
Nordone, Danielle Suzanne, DO
Sharma, Puja, MD

Manasquan
Alonzo-Chafart, Lorena D., DO
Cheli, David J., MD
Conkling, Robert F., MD
Ricci, John Anthony, MD
Rittberg, Shannon Bara, DO
Von Suskil, Kurt E., MD

Mantua
Rayner, William J., MD

Manville
Auletta, Maria, MD
Khan, Mohammed Nasir, MD
Shah, Mubina, MD

Maple Shade
Brolis, Nils Viesturs, DO
Di Marcangelo, Michael C. Jr., DO
Janik, Nancy E., MD
Norton, Kevin Patrick, DO
Paul, Stephen E., DO

Maplewood
Cadet, Marc D., MD
Francis, Guy Anthony, MD
Miguez, Priscilla, DO
Sharma, Deepa, DO
Young, Karen D., MD

Margate
Anastasi, Lawrence J., MD
Gaffney, John L., DO
Piccone, Dennis L., DO

Margate City
Frankel, David Zelig, MD

Marlboro
Guliano, Jaclyn M., MD
Kayastha, Shital, DO
O'Dell, Kimberly Ann, MD
Paul Yee, Sabine T., MD

Marlton
Calabrese, Karen Ann, DO
Casey, Daniel T., MD
Chandran, Ankila Sharavati, DO
DeGuzman, Ronaldo Cruz, DO
Dishler, Elyse Lyn, MD
Festa, Michelle G., MD
Flores, Marc E., DO
Friedhoff, Stephen G., MD
Getson, Philip, DO
Goldfine, Stephen P., MD
Hanrahan, Maureen A., MD
Horvath, Kedron Nicole, MD
Jadhav, Pallavi Dinkar, MD
Lazarus, Nermin Ahmed, DO
Levinson, Elizabeth A., MD
Lichtman, Lisa B., DO
Malave, Esther, MD
McCormick, Ryan Charles, MD
Miller, Scott Lewis, MD
Mir, Raema, MD
Najafi, Nawid E., MD
Pagliaro, Sara Nicole, DO
Patel, Jay Dinesh, MD
Patel, Parag S., MD
Pecora, Andrew Paul, DO
Pinto, Matthew G., DO
Press, Howard L., DO
Requa, Eric Robert, DO
Robinson, Sloan A., MD
Roesly, Melissa M., MD
Romano, James A., MD
Ryczak, Kristen, MD
Schweitzer, Justin Stephen, DO
Shabazz, Shakeilla Lavern, MD
Shah, Hetal Subodh, MD
Sheth, Surendra C., MD
Sireci, Joseph, DO
Skrzynski, Angela Anita, DO
Strong, Gusti Lickfield, DO
Twersky, Harris A., DO
Voyack, Michael John, DO
Yeh, Shao-Chun, MD

Marmora
Applebaum, Steven Lee, DO
Horowitz, Jerry A., DO
Hutcheson, Jonathan Justin, MD
Hutchison, Melissa M., MD
Leo, Nicole Terese, DO
Schneider, Wayne R., MD

Martinsville
Accurso, Daniela, MD
Chasin, Mitchell C., MD
Frisoli, Anthony, MD
Labbadia, Francesco, MD

Price, Kelly A., MD

Matawan
Hanna, Dalia N., MD
Tran, Vincent Phuong, DO

Mays Landing
Golden, Daniel Martin, DO

Maywood
Leipsner, George, MD

Medford
Albert Puleo, Anthony M., MD
Amankwaah, Ajoa O., DO
Dougherty, Joseph F., MD
Godleski, Thomas D., DO
Gomez, Andrew Thomas, MD
Guido, Stephanie, DO
Hollander, Philip, DO
Jones, Graham P., MD
Marzili, Thomas James, MD
Patragnoni, Richard M., DO
Ponnamaneni, Abhilasha Rao, MD
Scheuermann, Richard Ernest, MD
Zarroli, Hannah J., MD

Mercerville
El Attar, Ayman Fatehy, MD
Scott, Martin J., DO

Merchantville
Gilliss, Adam C., DO
Gilliss, Matthew J., DO
Husain, Abbas M., MD
Newton, Dean A., DO
Shen, Hongxie, MD

Metuchen
Ahn, Paul Michael, DO
Garcia, Maria Teresa, MD
Jasani, Anita, MD
Rossy, William H., MD

Mickleton
Rioux, Stephen R., DO

Middletown
Armbruster, Thomas C., MD
Giacona, Caryn Marie, MD
Jacks, Maryann, MD
McManus, Shanda Monique, MD
Morlino, John V., DO
Swartz, Harry M., MD
Thompson, Roger McLachlan, MD

Midland Park
Beauchamp, Donald P., MD
Bernier, Jean Ciara, MD
Eskow, Raymond P., MD
Giorlando, Mary Elizabeth, MD

Milford
Bauman, Susan M., MD
Bryhn, Lisa Kristen, MD
Curry, Debra W., MD
Hewens, Jeremy C., MD
Jardim, Carla Mia, MD
Jones, Howard D., MD
Kayal, William Jesse, MD
Kozakowski, Stanley M., MD
Kroth, Patricia Haeusler, DO
Lucco, Julianne M., MD
Murry, Robert L., MD
Skillinge, David D., DO
Turenne Kolpan, Laurie K., MD

Millburn
Biernat, Matthew Mateusz, MD
Glezen-Schneider, Priscilla, MD
Mattoo, Anju, MD
Sivasubramanian, Hema, MD

Millville
Akrout, Eddie, MD
Davis, Brian Joseph, DO
Mortensen, Jill, DO
Salloum, Azizeh J., MD
Yoong, Michael P., MD

Monmouth Beach
Irving, Robert John, MD

Monmouth Junction
Kline, Bradley H., DO

Monroe
Donat-Flowers, Rhoda J., DO
Reddy, Sureka, MD

Monroe Township
Grossman, Leonard A., MD
Kobylarz, Fred A., MD
Krauser, Paula S., MD
Patel, Ravish Mukesh, MD
Prasad, Keshav, MD

Montclair
Douglas, Elaine, MD
Grobstein, Naomi S., MD
Heifler, Gregory Dean, MD
Hostetler, Caecilia E., MD
Hrishikesan, Geetha, MD
Kahn, Jason Peter, DO
Khan, Afshan R., DO
Novak, Eva Cesnek, MD
Ouw, Willem B., MD
Ramos-Genvino, Elizabeth, MD
Shimelfarb, Marianna B., MD
Wilson, Howard Marc, MD

Montvale
Ajemian, Ara Antranik, MD
Rodriquez, Margaret, MD

Montville
Coelho, Ryan, MD
Filion, Jacqueline D. Weil, DO
Gargano, Joseph A., DO
Hoenig, Sandra R., MD
Iannetta, Frank, MD
Keating, William G., MD
Lapsiwala, Pareen Raj, DO
Lin, Annie, DO
O'Connor, Brandon P., MD
Pallay, Arnold I., MD
Rehberg, Joelle Stabile, DO
Stack, Thomas Joseph III, MD

Moorestown
Barker, William Robert, MD
Barr, Larry Allen, DO
Bechtel, David S., MD
Bhogal, Jasmeet Singh, MD
Bowers Pepe, Jessica Sue, DO
Britton, Richard J., MD
Brobyn, Tracy L., MD
Burke, Hana Oswari, MD
Chan, Wai Ben, DO
Chung, Myung K., MD
Crudele, James E., MD
Dennison, Alan D., MD
Horvitz, Steven P., DO
Land, Stephen M., MD
Lanza, Paul R., DO
Lee, Thomas Yon, MD
Levin, Irina, MD
Levin, Sanan L., MD
Louis, Marie Edwige, MD
Martz, Rebecca Lynn, MD
Matula, Joseph John, DO
Mills, Robert, DO
Nirenberg, Elena, MD
Oswari, Andrew, MD
Patel, Sanjiv C., MD
Pellegrino, Tara Marie, DO
Peterson, Dolores D., MD
Pettigrew, Isabel Hilary, MD
Ray, Anjali K., MD
Reeh, Debora Cummings, DO
Rutkiewicz, Laura A., MD
Shapiro, Gary I., MD
Stackhouse, Lisa A., DO
Summersgill, Richard Blair, MD
Termini, Joseph F., MD
Ward, Patrice Taylor, DO
Wasleski, Karen J., MD
Yudin, Joel S., DO

Morris Plains
Cervone, Maurizio, DO
Cervone, Oswald, DO
Joseph, Charles A., MD
Lijo, Maria Carmen, MD

Morristown
Aronwald, Bruce Alan, DO
Becker, Andrew B., DO
Bhambri, Ankur, MD
Christou, Alexander A., DO
Chung, Angela F., DO
Cioce, Anthony Jr., DO
Cioce, Thomas G., DO
Dillaway, Winthrop C. III, MD
Domovich, Ora, MD
Fitzpatrick, Hendrieka Ann, MD
Gedroic, Kristine Lynn, MD
Guercio-Hauer, Catherine A., MD
Joshi, Namita V., MD
Klingmeyer, Dorothy Marie, DO
Leung, Jacquelyn Way-Yan, MD
Melograno, Joseph J., DO
Onat, Esra Samli, MD
Perez, Marcella, MD

Physicians by Specialty and Town

Pietka,Jamie K.,MD
Stevens,Hilary Kristin,MD
Thomson,Mary Jo G.,DO
Wallace,Theresa C.,MD
Wilson,Lynn Marie,DO
Yaqub,Zunera,MD
Ziering,Thomas S.,MD
Zipp,Christopher Paul,DO
Mount Arlington
Gaela,Joan Fontelera,MD
Mount Holly
Busch,Gregory Howard,DO
Cavuto-Wilson,Carolyn Marie,DO
Mount Laurel
Bandy,Caryn Kay,DO
Barone,Catherine Ann,DO
Cooley,Danielle Lynn,DO
Coren,Joshua Scott,DO
Decker,Edmund J.,DO
Foda,Randa Baher,MD
Golden,Richard F.,DO
Hancq,Nicole Elizabeth,MD
Hanna,Sherry Kamal,MD
Kerley,Sara Shelton,MD
Khan,Sophia S.,MD
LaCarrubba Blondin,Lisa,MD
Maslin,Stuart J.,MD
Meeteer,Francis III,DO
Oppenheim,Jeffrey Charles,MD
Pecca,Jo Ann Donna,DO
Pettinelli,Frank P. Jr.,DO
Plasner,Samantha Mara,DO
Sepede,Jennifer,DO
Wilczynski,Frank L.,DO
Mountain Lakes
Schweitzer,Richard Joseph,MD
Mullica Hill
Al Hilli,Rula Ahmed,MD
De Dan,Claudine Michele,MD
Herman,Gregory E.,MD
Kent,Maria Candice,MD
Malik,Pooja,MD
Ott,William Augustine,DO
Sprigman,Charles Jeffrey III,DO
Stiefel,Gregory Gene,DO
Wax,Craig M.,DO
Wyche Bullock,Tara Lynette,MD
Zuazua-Pacilio,Maria C.,MD
Neptune
Dick,Susan E.,MD
Patel,Nitin Suresh,MD
Neshanic Station
Barr,James E.,MD
Dellavalle,Lindsay Joy,DO
Gertzman-Dafilou,Sharon D.,DO
Rigatti,Damian F.,DO
New Brunswick
Acevedo,Rhina A.,MD
Afran,Joyce G.,MD
Bhatt,Komal Gopalbhai,MD
Botti,Carla G.,DO
Clark,Elizabeth C.,MD
Cole,Janet M.,MD
Foley,James,MD
Hammond,Betty L.,MD
Headley,Adrienne J.,MD
Heath,Cathryn Batutis,MD
Heath,John Michael,MD
Hill,Eileen G.,MD
Howarth,David F.,MD
Kropa,Jill,MD
Lasky,Melodee S.,MD
Laumbach,Sonia Caridad G.,MD
Levin,Steven Jonathan,MD
Levine,Jeffrey Pierre,MD
Like,Robert C.,MD
Lin,Karen Wei-Ru,MD
McGarry,Barbara J.,MD
Mena,Jessica,DO
Miller,Ralee Ka,MD
Mokhashi,Sajida Habib,MD
Morton,Kinshasa S.,MD
Newrock,William J.,MD
Noll,Michael Andrew,MD
O'Connor,Robert M.,MD
Reinsdorf,Keith Alan,MD
Roemheld-Hamm,Beatrix,MD
Siddiqui,Sheraz U.,MD
Sliwowska,Anna,MD
Steinlight,Sasha Juli,MD
Suaray,Mafudia Abibatu,MD

Swee,David E.,MD
Tallia,Alfred F.,MD
Ulloque,Rory Alexander,MD
Virani,Zahra N.,MD
Wang,Yue He,MD
Womack,Jason Peter,MD
Wu,Justine Peen,MD
New Lisbon
Johnson,Deborah Anne,MD
Keefer,Keith J.,MD
New Providence
Calderon,Mark J.,MD
Martinetti,Lorenzo G.,MD
Newark
Abdu Nafi,Saladin A.,MD
Almodovar,Astrid Teresa,MD
Anglade,Claudia,MD
Anthony,AnnGene G,MD
Babbar,Puneet,MD
Brazeau,Chantal M.,MD
Dalal,Sima R.,DO
Dort,Christian,MD
Dube,Bianca,MD
Duncan,Kathyann Sylvia,MD
Easterling,Torian J.,MD
Ferrante,Jeanne Min-Li,MD
Gerstmann,Michael Adam,MD
Kelly,Hortensia,DO
Mevs,Stacy Reed,MD
Ortiz,Thomas R.,MD
Paige,Cynthia Y.,MD
Parmar,Pritesh B.,MD
Quiros Rivera,Mercedita,MD
Rodgers,Denise V.,MD
Sahu,Novneet,MD
Samaniego,Eduardo W.,MD
Sanchez,Carlos Alfonso,DO
Shimoni,Noaa,MD
Walsh,Kelly Anne,DO
Newton
Alam,Shumaila,MD
Kane,Frank L.,MD
Liloia,Peter Anthony,DO
Mattes,David G.,MD
McGraw,John Daniel,MD
Pampin,Robert J.,DO
Regan,Inge Sophia,MD
Sieminski,Douglas Peter,DO
North Arlington
Lubas,Andrew S.,MD
North Bergen
Amin,Samirlal Ramanlal,MD
Ayeni,Eniola Teju,DO
Davis,Bradley,DO
Ghabour,Rose Ann Sameh,MD
Goldstein,Marc,DO
Hussain,Zahid,MD
Orellana Chasi,Pamela,MD
Panem,Flordeliz Buensuceso,MD
Rugel,Jason,DO
Sujovolsky,Jeannette A.,DO
North Brunswick
Faisal,Siddiq A.,MD
Jorgensen,Otto B.,MD
Nadeem,Atiya,MD
Patterson,George A.,MD
Sheil,Christina A.,MD
North Cape May
Drake,Andrew F.,DO
Hong,Matthew H.,MD
Maroldo,Michael G.,MD
Moten,Shirlene Tolbert,MD
Renza,Richard A.,DO
North Haledon
Salerno,Adrienne Lynn,MD
North Plainfield
Oji,Omobola Abiodun,MD
North Wildwood
Cook,Jenny Lynn,DO
Haflin,Mary Ann,MD
Northfield
Bowers,Steven Richard,DO
Brunson,Rodney C.,DO
Bushay,Stephen Lloyd,MD
Cutler,Marna Alyse,DO
Fiorentino,Grace,DO
Holtzin,Robert M.,DO
Northvale
DiGiovanni,Leonard G.,DO

Nutley
Agresti,James V. Sr.,DO
Espina,Luis Alberto,MD
Figueroa,Marciano Tiu Jr.,MD
Giuliano,Michael Gerard,DO
Pastena,Anthony M.,DO
Patel,Mallik,MD
Sekiya,Steven T.,DO
Oak Ridge
Gloria,Stephen B.,DO
Magnusen,Mary L.,DO
Riesenman,Joseph John,MD
Oakhurst
Dweck,Isaac Jay,MD
Oakland
Dela Gente,Robert Saladaga,DO
Morski,Richard S.,MD
Perdomo,Louis Fernando,MD
Shaker,Taylor,MD
Straseskie,Ryan Kenneth,MD
Uddin,Sarah T.,DO
Ocean City
Baretto,Luigi U.,MD
Chew,Jason M.,DO
Dunn,Ernest Charles Jr.,MD
Raab,Gary W.,DO
Udani,Chandrakan I.,MD
Ocean View
Carlin,Francis Scott,DO
Oceanport
Odell,Tamara Lozier,DO
Old Bridge
Balinski,Beth A.,DO
Belder,Olga,DO
Bernabe,Maria Joyce Row G.,MD
Cohen,Howard Steven,DO
Robinson,Jonnie M.,DO
Ryan,Sharon L.,MD
Turkish,Jennifer M.,MD
Oradell
Abend,David S.,DO
Oxford
Meyer-Grimes,Leslie B.,MD
Palisades Park
Kim,Yoonjoo,MD
Palmyra
Hartmann,Rupert C. II,DO
Rosenzweig,Alan,DO
Paramus
Chadha,Sonia,MD
Herring,Gary S.,MD
Kantha Bhatnagar,Rajashree,MD
Mathews,Jyoti,MD
Pacheco,Felix Fernando,MD
Rubin,Steven F.,DO
Rutigliano,Michael W.,MD
Saieva,Carol E.,DO
Sandhu,Basant Singh,MD
Saros,Cathleen Mary,DO
Tzeng,Bowen Chi,MD
Wang,David Alexander,MD
Park Ridge
Licciardone,Salvatore J.,DO
Parlin
Frazier,Hawwa Sharif,DO
Kaur,Harleen,MD
Patel,Deepa N.,MD
Parsippany
Molisso,Mary Cuellari,DO
Prasad,Prema,MD
Passaic
Castilla,William A.,MD
DeMuro,Paul G. Jr.,DO
Fernandez Santiago,Angela,DO
Fomitchev,Oleg V.,MD
Makui,Sheyda,MD
Soliman,Ishak G.,MD
Solomon,Jennifer,MD
Vega,Andres,MD
Paterson
De Feo,Daniel Scott,DO
Elkholy,Neveen A.,DO
Gachette,Emmanuel Amilcar,MD
Hassan,Khaled A.,MD
Kazmouz,Hasna M.,MD
Revoredo,Fred S.,MD
Sweidan,Safwan A.,MD
Zaina,Samir A.,MD
Paulsboro
Milas,Erica M.,DO
Villare,Anthony W.,MD

Pennington
Brescia,Donald,MD
Evans,Rachael Blackburn,MD
Gonzalez Acuna,Jose M.,MD
Holdcraft,Suzanne,MD
Kakarla,Madhavi,MD
Patel,Jigar Dhansukh,MD
Samaddar,Soumen,MD
Thomsen,Kathleen M.,MD
Pennsauken
Cohen,Herman P.,DO
Kheny,Mira,MD
Krachman,Amy Nicole,DO
McDermet,Arthur J.,DO
Nghiem,George T.,DO
Ricigliano,Mark A.,DO
Santangelo,Steven Frank,DO
Scarlett,Franklin H.,MD
Toporowski,Beverly Christine,MD
Pennsville
Bober,Mitchell C.,DO
Lacay,Edmar Manabat,MD
Perth Amboy
Husain,Ali,DO
Nazli,Yasmeen Zuleikha,MD
Padilla,Nyree,MD
Ritsan,Julia B.,DO
Tamburello,Traci Ann,DO
Phillipsburg
Aversa,Thaddeus Massimo,DO
Bautista,Lucien Santiago,DO
Buch,Raymond S.,MD
Chu,Ching-Huey,MD
Decker,Eugene Michael,MD
Delmonico,Gerard J.,MD
Emenari,Chibuzo U.,MD
Gilkey,Edward A.,MD
Gomes,Ana P.,DO
Kanner Liebman,Rachel Brooke,DO
Kropf,Laura Dawn,DO
Lombardi,Frank T.,DO
Mcginley,Thomas Charles Jr.,MD
Ortiz-Evans,Ileana,MD
Porter,Anne Marisa,MD
Remde,Alan H.,MD
Revankar,Manasi Chandrakant,DO
Roscher,Atilio R.,MD
Rossi,Cynthia Ann,MD
Scott,Sabriya Carolyn,MD
Siciliano,Mary J.,DO
Piscataway
Chatterjee,Sonia,MD
Eck,John M.,MD
Herbert,Lisa R.,MD
Krohn,Douglas R.,MD
Lam,Nalini Priya,MD
Laumbach,Robert John,MD
Memon,Mushtaq Ahmed,MD
Monaco,Robert,MD
Murphy,John Charles,MD
Robertson,Michelle Williams,MD
Shoulson,Shana S.,MD
Pitman
Brennan,William Frederick,DO
Di Lisi,Joseph P.,DO
Friedlin,Forrest Jeffrey,DO
Rivell,Crystal Giovanna,DO
Pittstown
Golden-Tevald,Jean M.,DO
Plainfield
Bastien,Linda,MD
Birotte Sanchez,Maria J.,MD
Ledinh,Thuong,MD
Patel,Rajesh T.,DO
West,Beryl E.,MD
Zablocki,Chana Shira,MD
Plainsboro
Kaur,Narinder,MD
Sokel,Andrew H.,MD
Suzuki,Ron Yks,MD
Tierney,Peter C.,MD
Pleasantville
Gerber,Austin J.,DO
Merle,Nancy,MD
Pomona
Senese,Susan A.,DO
Pompton Plains
Brower,Chelsea,MD
Capio,Mario R.,MD
Cavazos,Anthony Richard,MD
Desai,Aashish P.,MD

Physicians by Specialty and Town

Family Medicine (cont)

Pompton Plains
- Neopane, Padam Kumar, MD
- Patel, Vishal V., MD
- Raju, Biju, DO
- Rumbaugh, Donald W., MD

Port Monmouth
- Ibrahim, Christine M., MD
- Patel, Kalpeshkumar P., MD

Princeton
- Hui, Dao, MD
- Shamshad, Munaza, MD
- Zack, Brian Gary, MD

Princeton Junction
- Painter, Michael Wayne, MD

Rahway
- Goradia, Rita U., MD
- Sheffy, Ohad, MD

Ramsey
- Nickles, Steven L., DO

Raritan
- Jordan-Scalia, Lisa Judith, DO
- Khalil, Christina, DO
- Patel, Ruperl Chandrakant, MD
- Scalia, Joseph Frank, DO
- Tomasso, Robert A., MD
- Wang, Yue-He, MD

Red Bank
- Bader, Christopher William, DO
- Ejimofor, Ebikaboere, MD
- Landers, Steven Howard, MD
- Lanza, Michele R., MD
- Mulholland, Brendan J., MD
- Penn, Carol A., DO
- Reilly, Gail G., MD

Richland
- Hargrave, Douglas M., DO
- Pirolli, John A., DO

Ridgewood
- Belov, Khatuna Topadze, MD
- Faltas-Fouad, Suzan L., MD
- Katz, Jodie H., MD
- Kaul, Rachna, MD
- Panagiotou, Nicholas D., MD

Ringoes
- Bryant, Manmohan, MD

Rio Grande
- Marino, Denay L., DO
- Rose, Victoria Summer, MD

Riverdale
- Howe, Michele Margaret, DO
- Romain, Sharon L., DO
- Samandar, Steve, MD

Riverside
- Tangco, Evacueto P., MD

Riverton
- Burke, Margaret Linda, MD

Robbinsville
- Bankole, Omolabake O., MD
- Rednor, Jeffrey D., DO
- Risi, Mark G., DO
- Shahmehdi, Seyed Akhtar, MD
- srikanth, Rashmi, MD

Rochelle Park
- Keshishian, Paul, DO
- Liu, Elizabeth Yingxia, MD
- Stankiewicz, Danuta, MD

Rockaway
- Arshad, Haroon, MD
- Brodrick, Ian B., MD
- Heitzman, Christopher James, DO
- Horn, Christopher Michael, DO
- Madison, Joy Hovey, MD
- Ziegler, Brenda L., DO

Roebling
- Manser, Harry Jr., DO
- Rappaport, Brandi Joy, MD

Roselle
- Shakir, Aarefa H., MD

Roselle Park
- Caggia, Josephine, DO
- Morandi, Michele Meehan, DO
- Parker, Stephen D., DO

Runnemede
- Bankole, Gawu Kamara, DO

Saddle Brook
- Pagano, Francesco P., DO
- Wiener, Michael I., DO

Salem
- Akinruli, Omowunmi Praise, MD
- Amrien, John R., MD
- Harris, Timothy Wayne, DO
- Howard, Thomas R. Jr., MD

Scotch Plains
- Ballan, Douglas Arnold, MD
- Chin, Darren S., MD
- Cunicella, Nicholas A. III, DO
- Delio, Constance Mary, MD
- Hasan, Izhar U., MD
- Hernandez, Alyssa Kate, MD
- Reddy, Shanthi Nalamalapu, MD
- Silberman, Marc Richard, MD

Sea Girt
- Siciliano, Janice M., DO

Sea Isle City
- Choi, Jong I., MD
- Young, Annamarie C., DO

Seaside Heights
- Godwin Karolak, Allison M., DO

Seaside Park
- Shadiack, Edward Charles Jr., DO

Secaucus
- Ali, Tahera, DO
- Fahmy, Hannan Adel, DO
- George, Malini Susan, MD
- Mathew, Jocelyn, MD
- Neuberger, Alina P., MD

Sewell
- Arthur, Kiersten Westrol, MD
- Attanasio, Michael J., DO
- Beppel, Elaine B., MD
- Bertel, James R., MD
- Bober, Craig, DO
- Boyd, Linda, DO
- Brumberg, Miles A., DO
- Cavallaro, Joseph III, DO
- Cohen, Andrew Geoffrey, MD
- Desimone, Alexandra, MD
- DiRenzo, Joseph P. Jr., DO
- Dibona, Anthony D. Jr., DO
- Ewing, Jacqueline L., DO
- Kane, Michelle Christine, DO
- Kruger, Eric N., MD
- Laganella, Dominic J., DO
- Leshner, Stanley B., DO
- Levin, Neil, DO
- Pettis, Larry, MD
- Prettelt, Adolfo E., MD
- Ranieri, Joseph N., DO
- Richmond, Chad Eric, DO
- Saddel, Diana L., DO
- Schmidt, Carol L., MD
- Sekel, James James, DO
- Spinosi, Maryjeanne, DO
- Tench, Mavola L., MD
- Urkowitz, Alan L., DO
- Vermeulen, Meagan Wega, MD

Shamong
- Mahoney, Nola T., DO

Ship Bottom
- Braunwell, Arthur Henry III, DO
- Clancy, Joseph P. Jr., MD
- Larkin, Harry Jr., MD
- Prosperi, Paul William, DO
- Suddeth, James N., MD

Short Hills
- Fine, Shari R., DO
- Jani, Beena Harendra, MD
- Zacharias, Daniel, MD

Shrewsbury
- Brahver, Danit Vera, MD
- Huegel, Claudia Marie, MD
- Jafry, Yasmeen, MD
- Johnston, Christopher K., MD

Sicklerville
- Aitken, Robert J., DO
- Cox, Trevor E., DO
- Mingroni, Julius Anthony, DO
- Sharp, Harry Walton, DO
- Ubele, Deborah Anne, DO

Somerdale
- Cheng, Desmond H., DO
- Gallagher, Joseph L. III, DO

Somers Point
- Ganesan, Balamurugan, MD
- Janes, Laura C., DO
- Nahas, Arthur G., MD
- Silverman, Russell V., DO
- Sparagna, Angelo III, MD

Somerset
- Condren, Marc J., MD
- Etheridge, Barbara Anne, MD
- Gwozdz, Paul William, MD
- Kaufman, Irving H., MD
- Laing, Euton M., MD
- Lawrence, Denise Antoinette, MD
- Madaj, Andrew T., MD
- Maziarz, Anastazja, MD
- Torok, Geza, MD

Somerville
- Bucek, John Ladislav, MD
- Davis, Lloyd A., MD
- DePass, Lorraine Francis, MD
- Dhillon-Athwal, Narinder Kaur, MD
- Guyton, Margaret Louise, MD
- Halper-Erkkila, Ruby A., MD
- Hansch, Lalitha T., MD
- Huang, Ming Y., MD
- Juliano, Julieann S., MD
- Lundholm, Joanne Katherine, MD
- Micek Galinat, Laura A., MD
- Shapiro, Dein M., MD
- Spector, Elisabeth, MD
- Wu, Frances Y., MD

South Amboy
- Nisar, Noor A., MD
- Ofori Behome, Yaw, MD

South Bound Brook
- Kaladas, Jeffrey J., MD

South Orange
- Jain, Sejal, MD
- Kharazi, Fariba, DO

South Plainfield
- Baum, Michael Jay, DO
- Bhatia, Irvinder, MD
- Hoppe, James Robert, MD
- Patel, Purvee D., MD
- Rozehzadeh, Rabin, MD

South River
- Girgis, Linda Mae, MD
- Girgis, Moris Beachay, MD

Southampton
- Burger, Max, MD

Sparta
- Bollard, David A., DO
- Casella, Joseph J., DO
- Ganon, Michael R., DO
- Medunick, David M., DO
- Shea, Caitlin M., DO

Springfield
- Krblich, Diana, MD
- Mansour, Ali Gaber, MD

Stockton
- Freedenfeld, Stuart H., MD
- Heinz, Kristann Wilmore, MD

Stone Harbor
- Ruskey, Elizabeth E., DO
- Vogdes, Tara Ann, DO

Stratford
- Alday, Geronima G., MD
- Channell, Millicent King, DO
- Chick, Charlene Elizabeth, DO
- Garnier, Katharine M., MD
- Goldwaser, Elan Luria, DO
- Gupta, Adarsh Kumar, DO
- Heaton, Caryl Joan, DO
- Hoffman, Barry M., DO
- Jiwani, Ameena Javed, DO
- Kimler, Christine Marie, DO
- Lambert, Kathryn C., DO
- Overbeck, Kevin Joseph, DO
- Perez, Ricardo, DO
- Rabara, Knic Corpuz, DO
- Russell, Hortense Patricia, DO
- Schlenker, Clinton James, DO
- Scott, George John, DO
- Torres, Jonathan William, DO
- Wadhwa, Aruna, MD

Succasunna
- Siegel, Harvey P., DO

Summit
- Butkiewicz, Elise Ann, MD
- Davine-Reicher, Joanne Erin, MD
- Doubek, Marnie Lynn, MD
- Fagan, Elizabeth Owens, MD
- Hollander, Steven Barry, MD
- Im-Imamura, Lauren H., MD
- Kaye, Susan T., MD
- Lafferty, Kristen, MD
- Lukenda, Robert A., DO
- May-Ortiz, Jennifer L., MD
- Miller, Aaron Todd, MD
- Podell, Richard N., MD
- Pozner, Samantha Brooke, MD
- Pride, Mikel Jadyne, DO
- Schram, Amy Elizabeth, MD
- Snyder, Hugh David, MD
- Tsangalidis, Eirini, MD
- Vickery, Donna R., MD
- Washington, Judy C., MD

Swedesboro
- Dalsey, Michael E., MD
- Seretis, George J., DO
- Tsigonis, Natalie, DO

Teaneck
- Berberian, Robert A., MD
- Boja, Conrado A. III, MD
- Boja, Michael Conrad, DO
- George, Preethi Sara, MD
- Hersh, Craig M., MD
- Jones, Rhys E., MD
- Kronish, Anne L., MD
- McNeill-Augustine, Roberta N., MD
- Perry, Russell J., MD
- Pottick-Schwartz, Eliane A., MD
- Prajapati, Binita Prashant, DO

Tenafly
- Gambhir, Priyanka, MD

Tinton Falls
- Calise, Arthur G., DO
- Chen, Roger L., MD
- Edokwe, Obunike O.J., MD
- Marquette, Paul Arthur, MD
- Rosen, Neil L., DO
- Yellayi, Priya A., MD

Toms River
- Asghar, Fatima, MD
- DiPaolo, Ann, DO
- Fiore, Edward D., MD
- Giardina, Jennifer, DO
- Liu, Connie Xia, MD
- Lozowski, Thomas E., DO
- Ludwig-Cilento, Mary Beth, DO
- Neumann, Lisa Petriccione, DO
- Ongsiako, Allen R., DO
- Pappas, Elena Catherine, DO
- Rudd, Rebecca A., MD
- Shah, Dhanvanti B., MD
- Shah, Sweta, MD
- Simone, Philip M., MD
- Triolo, Paul, MD
- Wayman, Bernard R. III, MD

Totowa
- Asfour, Mervet, MD
- Chrucky, Roman, MD
- Ibeku, Chukwuemeka A., MD
- Patel, Puja, MD

Trenton
- Abraham, Mark Barry, DO
- Agrawal, Nidhi, MD
- Backus, Yolanda Alicia, MD
- Barrett Carnes, Joy-Lynne, MD
- Coutermarsh, Andrew, DO
- Gaskel, Virginia M., DO
- Ginsburg, Deborah J., MD
- Gupta, Vinod K., MD
- Hawes, Ruppert Augustus, MD
- Hussain, Muhammad N., DO
- Jenkins, David W., MD
- Lansing, Martha H., MD
- Malone, Jennie O'Lera, DO
- Miller, Danielle Megan, DO
- Noble, Mary C., MD
- Ruppel, Nicholas James, DO
- Stabile, Michael C., MD
- Walker, Paul A., DO
- Wong, Wilbur P., MD
- Zafar, Jabbar Ben, DO

Tuckerton
- Miller, Walter P., MD
- Rudolph, Herbert J., MD

Turnersville
- Abesh, Daniel C., DO
- Kernis, Elyse Beth, DO
- Madison, William A. Jr., DO
- Mancuso, Alison M., DO
- Petruncio, George J., MD
- Rudolph, Kafi, DO
- Taylor, Greg Michael, DO
- Venuti, John David, DO
- Venuti, Robert L., DO
- Vitola, Carl A., DO

Union

Borkowska,Alina,MD
Codella,Vincent Adrian,DO
Eisenstat,Steven Alan,DO
Herrera,Juan Carlos,MD
Lee,Nancy,DO
Luke,Steven,MD
Rizzo,David M.,DO
Salim,Suhail Mohammed,DO
Talat,Afnan,MD
Union City
Cortina,Osvaldo,MD
Dominguez,Jonathan Manuel,MD
Gonzalez,Francisco D.,MD
Jurado,Jerry L.,MD
Mehta,Lalit Hargovind,MD
Simonson,Leslie J.,MD
Veloso,Corazon M.,MD
Ventnor
Grife,Robert M.,MD
Vernon
Marion,William Joseph,DO
Pyatov,Yelena V.,MD
Verona
Berg,Kevin James,MD
Cirello,Richard,MD
Daftani,Kennedy P.,MD
Daftani,Mohammad Daoud Daoud,MD
Distefano,Kenneth Louis,MD
Gonzalez,Orlando V.,MD
Gorman,Robert T.,MD
Holder,Dawn Paulette,MD
Lacara,Dena L.,DO
Mazzella,Carmine A.,DO
McCarrick,Thomas P.,MD
Murray,Richard S.,MD
Schlam,Everett W.,MD
Slater,Shakira L.,MD
Smith,Stephanie,MD
Steinhardt,Amelia L.,DO
Villas
Park,Sang T.,MD
Vineland
Abraham,David,DO
Alberici,Anna,DO
Baher,Ali Masih,DO
Cunningham,Bruce D.,MD
Dendrinos,George Aristidis,MD
Finder,Susan M.,DO
Kessler,Martin,MD
Kuptsow,Scott Warren,DO
Mason,Sandra,MD
Narvel,Wasique Abdulahad,MD
Necsutu,Simona Camelia,MD
Neema,Swarnalatha,MD
O'Dell,Xitlalichomiha,DO
Patel,Hemali V.,DO
Pedersen,Daniel A.,DO
Rhyme,Timothy L.,MD
Smick,Robert J.,DO
Ulke,Taner D.,DO
Zucconi,Adam J.,DO
Zucconi,Nicole Christina,DO
Voorhees
Bendala,Preeti,MD
Blumenthal,Andrew Michael,DO
Bradley,Kathleen A.,MD
Carela,Gendy,MD
Chummar,Joseline,MD
Daniel,Beena Mary,MD
Davis,Robert A.,DO
Dimapilis,Ann B.,DO
Enriquez,Alfred Vasquez,MD
Fagel,Jonathan Val C.,DO
Fisher-Swartz,Lucinda,MD
Furey,William J.,DO
Gealt,David Benjamin,DO
Giuglianotti,Daniel Scott,DO
Karmazin,Polina,MD
Khalil,Samir Walid,MD
Kitts,Lori M.,MD
Koerner,David M.,DO
Krever,Kristine Wang,MD
Kwak,James Jihoon,MD
Leone,Mark R.,DO
Lowe,John William,MD
Maffei,Mario Stephen,MD
Marone,Michael L.,MD
Martin,William Arthur,DO
Milman,Anna,DO
Momi,Anudeep K.,DO
Montgomery,Catherine P.,MD

Mule,Salvatore,MD
O'Hare,Kendal Eggers,MD
Patel,Ambarish Ashokkumar,DO
Phakey,Vishal,DO
Post,Robert E.,MD
Richman,Mitchell S.,MD
Roberts,Barbara Theresa,MD
Seeley,Brian T.,DO
Soble,Toby K.,MD
Style,Daniel J.,DO
Style,Stuart D.,DO
Varevice-McAndrew,Susan,MD
Weiner,Samuel David,MD
Willard,Mary A.,MD
Winfield,Barbara A.,DO
Wong,Que-Chi V.,MD
Zalut,David S.,MD
Waldwick
Al-Ola,Ziyad,MD
Draucikas,Lisa A.,DO
Ferreras,Jessie A.M.,MD
Granas,Andrew Daniel,MD
Krigsman,Suzanne Karimi,MD
Wall
Cotler,Samantha,DO
Wallington
Pyz,Tadeusz F.,MD
Warren
Brezina,Eric Joseph,DO
Cavallo,Danielle Janine,DO
Dicola,May Bersalona,MD
Washington
Foschetti,Felix P. Jr.,DO
Gilly,Frank J. Jr.,MD
Goodwin,James E.,MD
Jaques,James Phillip,DO
Kinoshita,Ken,MD
Kolpan,Brett Heath,MD
Sabates Arnesen,Katrina,MD
Waldron,Winifred Marie,MD
Yevdokimova,Oksana,MD
Watchung
Faschan,Steven Michael,DO
Rivera,Laura A.,MD
Waterford
Pearson,Gregg Alan,DO
Wayne
Abdulmassih,Sami,MD
Ahmed-Flowers,Tunizia,MD
Bain,Francis Jerome-Xavier,MD
Barravecchio,Anthony John,DO
Beltzer,Blair Richard,MD
Biller,Jeanette Marie,DO
Bock,Robert T. Jr.,MD
Carrazzone,Peter Louis,MD
Chow,Jessica C.,DO
Crabtree,Shawn M.,MD
Deingeniis-Depasquale,A.,DO
Duffy,Joseph M.,MD
Gomez-Vasquez,Ricardo A.,MD
Gregg,John A.,DO
Lampariello,James A.,MD
Makar,Gamil Lamey Bekheet,MD
Nabulsi,Omar Hisham,MD
Nguyen,Steven M.,MD
Patel,Meera V.,MD
Pope,Ronald J.,DO
Rasa,David V.,MD
Sivaraman,Priya,MD
Topalovic,Pavle,MD
Vasiliades,Thalia,DO
Woo,James K.,MD
Yorio,David S.,DO
West Caldwell
Elias,Nivin,MD
West Deptford
Klein,Irving J.,DO
Riedel,Jacqueline V.,DO
West Long Branch
Harding,Mark,MD
Zimmermann,Susanne W.,MD
West Milford
Lascari,Roland A.,MD
West New York
Fajardo,Gil Valdez,MD
Hamal,Rekha,MD
Rodriguez,Reinerio Gerardo,MD
Surikov,Vadim Michailovich,DO
West Orange
Belt,Steven D.,MD
Burden,Yumie Nishida,DO

Chang,Peiyun,DO
Rivera Galindo,Claudia P.,MD
Wurzel,Bernard Samuel,MD
West Paterson
Vitale,Joseph Thomas,MD
West Trenton
Khanna,Veena W.,MD
West Windsor
Codjoe,Jessica R.,MD
Westampton
Colbert,Angelique L.,DO
Westfield
Araujo,Martin A.,MD
Barnum,Kimberly Ann,DO
Brenner,Robert W.,MD
De Masi,Christopher Louis,DO
Ellison,Christian Eric,MD
Henry-Dindial,Nicole A.,MD
Hevert,Robert A.,DO
Leistikow,Kathleen H.,MD
Patel,Shamik D.,DO
Skariah,Jody,MD
Tabachnick,John Frederick,MD
Thomas,Ann C.,MD
Wagner,Claudia Anne,MD
Westville
Wu,Jack Chen-Jen,MD
Wu,Kevin,DO
Westwood
Macri,Michael V.,MD
Volpicella-Levy,Susan L.,DO
Whippany
Garcia,Joaquin B.,MD
Nitti,Michele,DO
Whitehouse Station
Buinewicz,Anna Miller,MD
Hallit,Janice A.,DO
Kelsey,Alan G.,MD
Len,Lucille T.,MD
Nierenberg,Lisa,MD
Whiting
Bartiss,Mark J.,MD
Bauberger,Charles Joseph,MD
Wildwood
Olarsch,Richard Gary,DO
Wildwood Crest
Khella,Hani Joseph,MD
Williamstown
Cogan,Andrew M.,DO
Lowry,Steven Michael,DO
Reilly,Megan Eileen,DO
Sharkey,Charles John,DO
Van Houten-Sauter,Lee A.,DO
Willingboro
Bajaj,Jasmine,MD
Caveng,Rocco F. Jr.,DO
Daroy,Christopher Felicano,MD
Donnon,Henry P.,MD
Ganti,Kennedy U.,MD
Weinar,Marvin A.,MD
Wood Ridge
Pantano,Maria V.,DO
Woodbine
Russo,Sandra L.,DO
Woodbridge
Boyd,Robert D.,DO
Poonawala,Nafisa Z.,MD
Woodbury
Affel,Marjorie E.,MD
Andrews,Jaime Lynn,DO
Antonio,Patrick,MD
Bierman-Dear,Nancy A.,MD
Chiusano,Emi A.,MD
Chu,Chin-Chan,MD
Davis,Adriana,DO
Fellows,Wayne,DO
Gartland,John Jr.,MD
Glass,Gina Gill,MD
Gopal,Srihari,MD
Ground,Christen Denise,DO
Hamilton,Sylvester Sutton IV,MD
Kumar,Mary Ann M.,MD
Lawit,Alan,MD
Loubeau-Magnet,Helene,DO
Magnet,Marcus,MD
Malik,Tahseen Rabia,MD
Patel,Ashish C.,MD
Patel,Jaymica,MD
Reigel,Shawna Ilene,MD
Roehl,Barbara Joan Oppenheim,MD
Rogers,Michael S.,MD

Segal,Lawrence David,DO
Sornaraj,Amutha Arularasi,MD
Vanderwerken,Suzanne W.,MD
Woodbury Heights
Kline-Kim,Johanna F.,MD
Tomasso,Tara,MD
Trotz,Christopher R.,MD
Woodlynne
Atkinson,Monica,MD
Woodstown
Bauman,David C.,MD
Bussey,Paul George,MD
Deal,Amanda E.,DO
Hubbs,James E.,DO
Hurley,Margaret L.,DO
Nicholas,Paul George III,DO
Roberts,Kevin W.,MD
Family Therapy
Whitehouse Station
Hudson,Claudia Scalorbi,MD
Fertility/Infertility
Basking Ridge
Darder,Michael C.,MD
Eatontown
Ziegler,William Francis,DO
Edison
Qasim,Mahasin S.,MD
Terens,William L.,MD
Englewood
Hock,Doreen L.,MD
Hurst,Wendy Robin,MD
Tisch,Bruce H.,MD
Hackensack
Adelsohn,Lawrence G.,MD
Hasbrouck Heights
Wolf Greene,Susan Amy,MD
Jersey City
Gagliardi,Carol L.,MD
Leyson,Jose Flotcante J.,MD
Parsippany
Lam,Paul C.,MD
Secaucus
Kabakibi,Riad A.,MD
Foot & Ankle Surgery
Brick
Wolenski,Matthew J.,MD
Egg Harbor Township
Winters,Brian Seth,MD
Emerson
Napoli,Ralph C.,MD
Flemington
Bleazey,Scott Thomas,MD
Riverton
Daniel,Joseph N.,DO
Forensic Pathology
Clarksboro
Feigin,Gerald A.,MD
Montville
Shaikh,Junaid Rasheed,MD
Morristown
Suarez,Ronald V.,MD
Newark
Falzon,Andrew L.,MD
North Brunswick
Karluk,Diane,MD
Paramus
Clayton,MaryAnn B.,MD
Wayne
Cronin,Leanne M.,MD
Westampton
Hood,Ian C.,MD
Forensic Psychiatry
Allenhurst
Dengrove,Robert S.,MD
Basking Ridge
Salem,Anasuya,MD
Brick
Baum,Raymond M.,MD
Hammonton
Vuotto,Angela Marie,DO
Jersey City
Goldwaser,Alberto Mario,MD
Long Branch
Bortnichak,Paula M.,MD
Paterson
Schiffman,Erica R.,MD
Pomona
Fenyar,Bonnie Ann M.,MD

Physicians by Specialty and Town

Gastroenterology

Avenel
 Duhl, Jozsef S., MD
Bayonne
 Hahn, John C., MD
 Ramasamy, Kovil Veeraswami, MD
 Salem, Suhail Bakr, MD
Belleville
 Spira, Etan, MD
Berkeley Heights
 Barrison, Adam F., MD
 Belladonna, Joseph A., MD
 Ben-Menachem, Tamir, MD
 Brown, William Howard, MD
 Gillin, James Scott, MD
 Klein, Roger Scott, MD
 Michael, Hazar, MD
Bloomfield
 Bajwa, Mohammad Ayub, MD
 Celebre, Louis J., MD
 Devito, Fiore J., MD
 Pizzano, Richard G., MD
Brick
 Aaron, Bernard M., MD
 Boss, David T., MD
 Cerefice, Mark L., MD
 Hiley, Paul C., MD
 Rozovsky, Assif, MD
 Schlachter, Scott M., DO
 Shukla, Sandhya, MD
 Tangorra, Matthew, DO
 Winzelberg, Neal J., MD
Bridgewater
 Lustig, Robert H., DO
 Shapiro, Stephen R., MD
 Unger, Jeffrey S., MD
Caldwell
 Suarez, Edwin, MD
 Suarez, Lynette G., MD
Camden
 DeSipio, Joshua Peter, MD
 Griech-McCleery, Cynthia, MD
 Peikin, Steven R., MD
 Shah, Apeksha, MD
 Shats, Daniel, MD
Cape May Court House
 Beitman, Robert G., MD
 Landset, David J., DO
 Ljubich, Paul, MD
 Masciarelli, Anthony, DO
 Troum, Richard M., DO
 Vattasseril, Renjy, MD
Cedar Grove
 Rizvi, Masood A., MD
Cedar Knolls
 Dalena, John Michael, MD
Chatham
 Franzese, John, MD
Cherry Hill
 Berberian, Brian, MD
 Volchonok, Oleg, MD
 Werbitt, Warren, DO
Clark
 Wexler, David E., MD
Cliffside Park
 Fishbein, Susan, MD
Clifton
 Agarwal, Anil, MD
 Baddoura, Walid J., MD
 Baum, Howard B., MD
 Boxer, Andrew Scott, MD
 Farkas, John J., MD
 Gronowitz, Steven D., MD
 Gupta, Ashok, MD
 Krohn, Natan Nata, MD
 Okun, Jeffrey, MD
 Reydel, Boris, MD
Cranford
 Margolin, Michael L., MD
Denville
 Emiliani, Vincent J., MD
 Heit, Peter, MD
 Soriano, John G., MD
Dover
 Krupnick, Matthew E., MD
 Rybalov, Sergey, MD
East Brunswick
 Botros, Nashed G., MD
 Chen, William Y., MD
 Costa, Jose Carlos, MD

 D'Mello, Francisco C., MD
 Krawet, Steven Howard, MD
 Lenger, Ellis S., MD
 Plumser, Allan B., MD
East Hanover
 Shetzline, Michael Anthony, MD
East Orange
 Coffin, Nina R., MD
 Cordoba, Isabelita Y., MD
 Rudd, Jennifer N., MD
 Vossough, Sima, MD
East Windsor
 Lupovici, Michael, MD
Eatontown
 Baig, Nadeem A., MD
 Belitsis, Kenneth, MD
 Fiest, Thomas C., DO
 Gorcey, Steven A., MD
 Merikhi, Laleh Afkham, MD
 Uppal, Rajiv, MD
Edgewater
 Sciarra, Michael A., DO
Edison
 Baik, Seoung W., MD
 Chae, Scott S., MD
 Cheela, Santosh K., MD
 Goldberg, Michael Scott, MD
 Hodes, Steven E., MD
 Medina, Richard A., MD
 Modi, Chintan, MD
 Nahar, Sudha, MD
 Nayar, Devjit Singh, MD
 Patel, Mayank D., MD
 Ramchandani, Kishore N., MD
 Reissman, David I., MD
 Rosenheck, David Mark, MD
 Shugar, Ronald A., MD
 Wolfman, Marc R., MD
Egg Harbor Township
 Kaufman, Barry P., MD
 Mehta, Nikhilesh D., MD
 Rosman, Gary A., MD
 Santoro, John J., DO
Elizabeth
 Kogan, Robert, MD
 Moradi, Dovid Simcha, MD
 Naik, Arun Chandrakant, MD
Emerson
 Bellomo, Alyse Rosemarie, MD
 Bethala, Vivian K., MD
 Candido, Frank M., MD
 Cullen, Holly Doolittle, MD
 Goldstein, David D., MD
 Levine, Robert S., MD
 Margulis, Stephen J., MD
 Moscato, Michele, DO
 Pittman, Robert Hal, MD
 Randall, Jennifer F., MD
 Zucker, Ira I., MD
Englewood
 Friedrich, Ivan A., MD
 Gillon, Steven D., MD
 Kancherla, Sandarsh Raj, MD
 Kaplounova, Irina, MD
 Mohtashemi, Hormoz, MD
 Panella, Vincent S., MD
 Rosen, Bruce L., DO
Englewood Cliffs
 Chessler, Richard K., MD
 Fiorillo, Marc Anthony, MD
 Meininger, Michael Eric, MD
 Spinnell, Mitchell Kyle, MD
 Zingler, Barry M., MD
Englishtown
 Volk, Yuri, MD
Fair Lawn
 Gorodokin, Gary I., MD
 Gupta, Ramesh C., MD
 Kutner, Donald H., DO
 Lefkowitz, Jeffrey R., MD
 Resnick, Jonathan, MD
Flemington
 Bae, Samuel Y., MD
 Cardoso, Gilbert Santos, DO
 Daruwala, Cherag A., MD
 DiGregorio, Kenneth J., MD
 Georgsson, Maria Anna, MD
 Goldstein, Andrea E., MD
 Hartford, Jeffrey D., MD
 Lesser, Gregory Scott, MD
 Lim, Khengjim, MD

 Matthews, Jason D., MD
 Patel, Anik Mayur, MD
 Sinha, Anubha, MD
 Willis, Stephen Laird, MD
Florham Park
 Galandauer, Isaac, MD
Franklin Lakes
 Chusid, Boris Gregory, MD
Freehold
 Blank, Robert R., MD
 Bohm, Steven A., MD
 Gupta, Kunal, MD
 Ludwig, Shelly L., MD
 Mufson, Lewis J., MD
 Nadler, Steven C., MD
Glen Ridge
 Finkelstein, Warren, MD
 Kenny, Raymond P., MD
 Kwon, Yong Min, MD
 Oh, Sangbaek Charles, MD
 Tobia, Dennis A., MD
Hackensack
 Ellinghaus, Eric J., MD
 Feit, David L., MD
 Felig, David M., MD
 Golding, Richard C., MD
 Khan, Fahad, MD
 Kheterpal, Neil M., DO
 Ligresti, Rosario Joseph, MD
 Riccobono, Charles A., MD
 Sedarat, Ali, MD
 Sedarat, Alireza, MD
 Tanchel, Mark E., MD
Hackettstown
 Chang, Jimmy Chuming, MD
 Kahlam, Sarwan S., MD
 Sandhu, Parminderjeet S., MD
Haddon Heights
 DiSandro, Theresa Maria, DO
 Izanec, James L., MD
 Kolnik, John P., DO
 Libster, Boris, DO
Haddonfield
 Ackerman, Melville J., MD
 Turnier, Auguste P., MD
Haledon
 Baghal, Eyad Y., MD
Hamilton
 Gersten, Michael, MD
 Sokol, Deborah Klein, MD
Hamilton Square
 Manning, Michael T., MD
Hammonton
 Magasic, Mario V., MD
 Savon, Joseph J., MD
Highland Park
 Cohen, Hillel D., MD
Hillsborough
 Accurso, Charles A., MD
 Barghash, Claudia N., MD
 Ciambotti, Gary Francis, MD
 Gingold, Alan R., DO
 Lee, Kristen Kyongae, MD
Hillsdale
 Stewart, David M., MD
Holmdel
 Moosvi, Mir A., MD
Jersey City
 Bhatia, Taruna, MD
 Dizon, Alita L., MD
 Reddy, Ram K., MD
 Rubin, Kenneth P., MD
 Shiff, Steven J., MD
 Stoopack, Paul Mitchell, MD
 Stowe, Arthur Chester Jr., MD
 Weissman, Paul S., MD
Lakewood
 Bhagat, Sanjay, MD
 Kandathil, Mathew K., MD
 Kurtz, Joel H., MD
 Musicant, Joel Marc, MD
Lawrenceville
 Ahmad, Syed S., MD
 De Antonio, Joseph R., MD
 Lou, William, MD
 Merlo, Angela, MD
Lincoln Park
 Mainero, Michael M., MD

Linwood
 Maleki, Dordaneh, MD
 Renny, Andrew, MD
Little Falls
 Holt, Stephen, MD
 Kosc, Gary J., MD
 Martino, Michael J., MD
 Pavlou, George Nicholas, MD
 Shami, Joseph G., MD
Little Silver
 Eichel, Richard L., MD
Livingston
 Goldstein, Debra R., MD
 Imbesi, John J., MD
 Shieh, Frederick, MD
Lodi
 Focazio, William John, MD
Lumberton
 Khanijow, Vikresh, MD
 Kutscher, Jeffrey J., MD
 Lahoti, Mayank, DO
 Leonard, Maurice D., MD
 Sheth, Nidhir Ras, MD
 Taub, William H., MD
 deLacy, Lee M., MD
Mahwah
 Antler, Arthur S., MD
Manahawkin
 Koerner, Steven, DO
Manalapan
 Weiner, Brian C., MD
Maplewood
 Goldfarb, Michael, MD
 Molokwu, Godwin O., MD
Marlboro
 Cencora, Barbara E., MD
 Gold, Jared Z., MD
 Meyer, Shira Asekoff, DO
 Tendler, Michael R., MD
 Vazirani, Tina A., MD
Marlton
 Cohen, Neil M., MD
 Davidoff, Steven, MD
 Devita, Jack Joseph, MD
 Friehling, Jane Susan, DO
 Horn, Abraham S., DO
 Levin, Gary H., MD
 Sorokin, Jeffrey J., MD
 Tulman, Alan Bruce, MD
Medford
 Frates, Angela Dawn, MD
 Kravitz, John Jay, MD
 Modena, Scott Alan, MD
 Salowe, David Ross, MD
Metuchen
 Vasireddi, Srinivas S., MD
Midland Park
 Frauwirth, Howard David, MD
Millburn
 Bains, Yatinder, MD
 Desai, Mahesh R., MD
 Rosen, Michael, MD
 Shah, Mehul N., MD
Mine Hill
 Albicocco, Nicholas S., MD
Monroe
 Forester, Gary P., MD
Montclair
 Abraham, Rini S., MD
 Volfson, Ariy, MD
Morristown
 Alistar, Angela Tatiana, MD
 Arsenescu, Razvan Ioan Paul, MD
 Martin, Lorraine H., MD
 Morton, John Douglas, MD
 Ryan, Joseph J., MD
 Samach, Michael A., MD
 Schalet, Michael Alan, DO
Mount Laurel
 Deitch, Christopher William, MD
 Elfant, Adam B., MD
 Ho, Henry C., MD
 Judge, Thomas Aloysius, MD
 Lautenslager, Tara Lee, MD
 Ockrymiek, Steven B., DO
 Wang, Yize Richard, MD
Neptune
 Basri, William E., MD
 Hui, Kenny Pingchi, MD
 Schneiderman, Steven, MD

Physicians by Specialty and Town

New Brunswick
- Bhargava,Sandeep,MD
- Broder,Arkady,MD
- Chokhavatia,Sita Shashikant,MD
- Das,Kiron M.,MD
- Griffel,Louis H.,MD
- Maltz,Gary S.,MD
- Manoukian,Aram V.,MD
- Pooran,Nakechand Rai,MD
- Rampertab,Saroja Devi,MD
- Velpari,Sugirdhana,MD

Newark
- Barritta,Domenica Maria,MD
- Brelvi,Zamir S.,MD
- Brown,Jennifer A.,DO
- Cabaleiro,Renee J.,MD
- Chahil,Neetu H.,MD
- Krawitz,Steven,MD
- Kutner,Matthew Alexander,DO
- Levinson,Robert Alan,MD
- Pyrsopoulos,Nikolaos T.,MD
- Samanta,Arun K.,MD
- Sinensky,Gary B.,MD
- Wang,Weizheng William,MD
- Weiss,Eliezer,MD

North Arlington
- Waxman,Mark S.,MD

North Bergen
- Raskin,Jeffrey M.,MD
- Sotiriadis,John,MD
- Tepler,Harold George,MD

North Brunswick
- Kastuar,Satya P.,MD

Oakhurst
- Akhtar,Reza Yasin,MD
- Dhillon,Shamina,MD
- Maki,Junsuke,MD
- Schwartz,Mitchell S.,MD
- Terrany,Ben,MD
- Turtel,Penny S.,MD

Ocean
- Beri,Gagan D.,MD
- Guss,Howard N.,DO

Old Tappan
- Chaudhri,Eirum I.,MD

Orange
- Da Costa,Theodore A.,MD

Paramus
- De Lillo,Anthony Rocco,MD
- Greenspan,Joshua N.,MD
- Hatefi,Homayoon,MD
- Kurz,Jeremiah S.,MD
- Lippe,Scott David,MD
- Shukla,Nilesh B.,MD
- Wien,Frederic E.,MD

Paterson
- Bollu,Janardhan,MD

Pennington
- Bhatia,Jyoti Kamlesh,MD
- Rogart,Jason Nathaniel,MD
- Simonian,Armen John,MD

Pennsville
- Shufler,Daniel E.,MD

Phillipsburg
- Herman,Barry Eugene,MD
- Kantor,Thomas E.,MD
- Mukherjee,Shanker,MD

Pitman
- Farber,Michael A.,MD

Plainfield
- Cohen,Allan Bary,MD
- Goldenberg,David A.,MD

Plainsboro
- Katz,Kristina,MD
- Skole,Kevin S.,MD

Pompton Lakes
- Bernheim,Oren Elias,MD

Princeton
- Bellows,Aaron,MD
- Margulies,Craig,MD
- Meirowitz,Robert F.,MD
- Segal,William Nathan,MD
- Shriver,Amy Rubin,MD
- Swedlund,Anne P.,MD

Ramsey
- Strassberg,David M.,MD

Randolph
- Gelman,Scott Franklin,MD

Red Bank
- Binns,Joseph F.,MD
- Carman,Roy L.,MD
- Gialanella,Robert J.,MD
- Heyt,Gregory John,MD
- Marzano,Joseph A.,MD
- Sundararajan,Subha V.,MD
- Weine,Douglas Matthew,MD

Ridgewood
- Danzig,Jeffrey B.,MD
- Fischer,Zvi,MD
- Grossman,Matthew Aaron,MD
- Hsieh,Jennifer,MD
- Korkis,Anna Maria,MD
- Pazwash,Haleh,MD
- Rahmin,Michael G.,MD
- Rubinoff,Mitchell J.,MD

River Edge
- Chhada,Aditi,MD
- Leibowitz,Steven R.,MD
- Mammen,Anish George,MD
- Nikias,George Andrew,MD
- Rosendorf,Eric Robert,MD

Riverdale
- Dasani,Bharatkumar M.,MD

Roselle Park
- Rodriguez,Ricardo Esteban,MD

Rutherford
- Roth,Joseph M.,MD
- Ruiz,Frank,MD
- Zierer,Kenneth G.,MD

Salem
- Dayrit,Pedro Q.,MD

Secaucus
- Dhalla,Sameer,MD
- Siegel,Wayne Douglas,MD

Sewell
- Gardner,Beth C.,MD
- Kimbaris,James Nicholas,MD
- Plumeri,Peter A.,DO

Sicklerville
- D'Auria,Daniel A.,MD
- Velasco,Brenda Raquel,MD

Somers Point
- Deshpande,Nikhil,MD
- Krachman,Joel E.,DO
- Krachman,Michael S.,MD
- Ognibene,Lawrence G.,DO
- Schwab,Kenneth S.,MD

Somerset
- Aronson,Scott Logan,MD
- Ebert,Ellen C.,MD
- Ferges,Mitchell L.,MD
- Ferges,William James,MD
- Merkel,Ira S.,MD
- Pickover,Lawrence M.,MD
- Platovsky,Anna,MD
- Rapisarda,Alexander F.,MD
- Scharf,Henry J.,MD
- Shamim,Syed Q.,MD

Somerville
- Luppescu,Neal E.,MD
- Vergilio,Cory D.,MD

South Orange
- Sampson,Ruby J.,MD

South Plainfield
- Goyal,Alok,MD

Sparta
- Agarwal,Sudhir Kumar,MD
- Lindy,Michael Evan,MD
- Rao,Kiran Venkat,MD
- Tang,Linda Yinglin,MD

Springfield
- Kerner,Michael B.,MD
- Lipsky,Marvin A.,MD

Stratford
- Liakos,Steven,DO

Succasunna
- Madane,Srinivas Janardhan,MD

Summit
- Habba,Saad F.,MD
- Zeldis,Jerome B.,MD

Sussex
- Beckman,Harvey S.,MD

Teaneck
- Micale,Philip Louis,MD
- Palance,Adam L.,MD
- Paltrowitz,Irving M.,MD
- Rigoglioso,Vincent,MD
- Schmidt,Michael H.,MD

Tenafly
- Klein,Walter A.,MD

Tinton Falls
- Grabowy,Thaddeus John,MD

Toms River
- Bigornia,Edgar G.,MD
- Cohen,Allan,MD
- Cohen,Scott,DO
- Collier,Jill A.,MD
- Cryan,Jeffrey M.,MD
- De Martino,Paul John,MD
- Eschinger,Eric Jon,MD
- Lokchander,Rangaswamy S.,MD
- Patel,Kavan Girishbhai,MD
- Raso,Carl L.,MD
- Shah,Kamlesh Manher,MD
- Shakov,Rada,MD
- Suatengco,Jose Ramon,MD
- Tamimi,Omar A.,MD

Trenton
- Afridi,Shariq A.,MD
- Gupta,Rajendra Prasad,MD
- Huq,Irfan-Ul,MD
- Mian,Somia Zia,MD
- Rosner,Bruce P.,MD
- Rubin,Marc R.,MD
- Schwartz,Eric,MD
- Zamir,Zafar,MD

Turnersville
- Chiesa,John C.,DO

Union
- Chirla,Sujala,MD
- DiGiacomo,William S.,MD
- Fernandez Ledon,Ramon A.,MD
- Greenblatt,Robert I.,MD
- Mahal,Pradeep S.,MD
- Muthusamy,Samiappan,MD
- Sundaram,Kanaga N.,MD
- Tempera,Patrick G.,MD

Vernon
- Korsakoff,Kristopher Paul,MD

Verona
- Manzi,Daniel D.,MD
- Nathan,Ramasamy Swami,MD

Vineland
- Matusow,Gary Alan,MD
- Shields,David S.,MD
- Song,Woo Kwang,MD
- Tassakis,Tom A.,MD

Voorhees
- Alloy,Andrew Marc,DO
- Celluzzi,Alex,DO
- Chauhan,Tusharsindhu C.,MD
- Chiesa,Drew Jonathan,DO
- Egan,Elizabeth Anne,MD
- Goldstein,Michael Bruce,MD
- Hashmi,M. Arif,MD
- Malamut,Jay M.,MD
- McLaughlin,Vincent A.,MD
- Mushnick,Alan J.,MD
- Pineda,Verne M.,MD
- Walters,Richard Lawrence,DO

Wayne
- Bleicher,Robert H.,MD
- David,Steven,MD
- Gordon,Clifford Avery,MD
- Ramamoorthy,Ravishankar,MD
- Shlien,Robert D.,MD
- Stevens,Lisa Deborah,MD
- Stillman,Jonathon S.,MD
- Zangara,Joseph Anthony,MD

West Long Branch
- Langner,Bruce J.,MD

West New York
- Gibilisco,Raffaele A.,MD
- Ramos,Rafael C.,MD
- Zapiach,Leonidas,MD

West Orange
- Askin,Matthew Peter,MD
- DePasquale,Joseph R.,MD
- Eagle,Robert Selig,MD
- Fishbein,Vitaly A.,MD
- Fiske,Steven C.,MD
- Green,Jon David,MD
- Mogan,Glen R.,MD
- Rosenthal,Lawrence Stephen,MD
- Ruffini,Robert A.,MD
- Schuman,Robert W.,MD
- Siu,Larry K.,MD
- Sloan,William C.,MD
- Spira,Robert S.,MD

- Stefaniwsky,Andrew B.,MD
- Stein,Lawrence B.,MD
- Wallach,Carl B.,MD

Westfield
- Amrick,Thomas J.,MD
- Cobert,Barton L.,MD
- Coronato,Andrew,MD
- Lerer,Paul K.,MD
- Tang,Ying Margie,MD

Westwood
- Fried,Harry A.,MD

Willingboro
- Goldstein,Jack,MD
- Petroski,Donald,MD
- Shmuts,Robert Jaron,DO

Woodbridge
- Webber,Seth Michael,MD

Woodbury
- Abrams,Jeffrey A.,MD
- Blair,Brian J.,DO
- Coben,Robert M.,MD
- Conn,Mitchell I.,MD
- DiMarino,Anthony J. Jr.,MD
- Fenkel,Jonathan M.,MD
- Kroop,Howard S.,MD
- McMahon,Donald James,DO
- Prieto,Jorge A.,MD

Woodcliff Lake
- Biener,Alexander,MD

Wyckoff
- Viksjo,Michael Joseph,MD

General Practice

Absecon
- Jhaveri,Bharat J.,MD

Atlantic City
- Giamporcaro,Steven J.,MD

Basking Ridge
- Lutz,Joseph S.,MD

Bayonne
- Desai,Bankimchandra D.,MD

Belleville
- Shapiro,Jason,MD

Berkeley Heights
- Ghanbari,Cecilia W.,MD

Berlin
- Vera,Luis Fernando,MD

Bernardsville
- Sinatra,Frank A.,MD

Blackwood
- Banks,Frank M.,DO

Boonton
- Santos,Santos S.,MD

Bordentown
- Addis,David J.,MD

Bradley Beach
- Lee,Frank,MD

Brick
- Reisher,Richard G.,DO

Bridgeport
- Zaharko,Wendy,MD

Burlington
- Blank,Andrew Jay,DO
- Brandt-Park,Nicole,MD
- Talone,Albert A.,DO
- Torres,Florinda L.,MD

Camden
- Ronsayro,Estrella A.,MD

Cape May Court House
- Weisberg,William R.,MD

Cedar Grove
- Eltaki,Madiha Ahmed,MD

Cherry Hill
- Goldsmith,Joyce,MD
- Jensen,Edwin A.,DO
- Magaziner,Allan,DO

Clementon
- Heck,Gary X.,DO

Cliffside Park
- Spinapolice,Joseph A.,DO

Clifton
- Doerr,Alphonsus L.,MD

Clinton
- Silverberg,Michael S.,MD

Collingswood
- Schiavone,Ronald L.,DO
- Stagliano,Robert A.,DO

Denville
- Masone,Patricia A.,MD
- Napoli,Salvatore,MD

Physicians by Specialty and Town

General Practice (cont)
Dover
 Bellamy, James E., DO
East Orange
 Enabosi, Ellis, MD
 Keno, Deborah, MD
East Rutherford
 Colaneri, John A., MD
Edison
 Agarwal, Sumitra, MD
 Kukreja, Meenakshi, MD
 Menashe, Richard B., DO
Elizabeth
 Ferdinand, Michel-Ange, MD
 Henner, Benjamin Joseph, MD
 Levinsky, Liya, MD
 Marzano, Patrick Wayne, DO
Fair Lawn
 Chaudry, Mansoora R., MD
Fort Dix
 Gorelli, Lucy Ann, MD
Fort Lee
 Rosenberg, Paul Howard, MD
 Vincent, Michael G., MD
Freehold
 Boorstein, Jerry, DO
 Goldstein, Jay R., MD
Galloway
 Ramchand, Maya, MD
Garfield
 Giardino, V. J., MD
 Tunia, Krzysztof Stanislaw, MD
Hackensack
 Bilek, Alena, MD
 Leder, Robin Ellen, MD
Hamilton
 Stabile, John R., MD
Haskell
 Hall, Kevin Arthur, MD
Hoboken
 Robaina, Luis A., MD
Iselin
 Neubrander, James A., MD
Jamesburg
 Bordieri, Joseph Anthony, DO
Jersey City
 Clemente, Jose D., MD
 Perez, Humberto T., MD
Kearny
 Doshi, Prakash J., MD
Linden
 Reich-Sobel, Debra Gail, DO
Linwood
 Abramowitz, Jodi S., DO
Livingston
 Haghdoost, Mohammad, MD
Lyndhurst
 Schmalz, William Francis Jr., MD
Manahawkin
 Kirk, Michael John Jr., DO
Medford
 Juele, Nicholas J., DO
 Piarulli, Michael J., MD
Monmouth Junction
 Penupatruni, Bharati D., MD
Morristown
 Enis, Sean, MD
Mount Laurel
 Aji, Wissam, MD
Mullica Hill
 Harris, William G., MD
New Brunswick
 Grabell, Daniel, MD
New Lisbon
 Cavan, Clodoveo N., MD
 Co, Dominador A., MD
Newark
 Davis, Barbara, MD
 Ligot, Jaime L., MD
 Louissaint, Paraclet S., MD
North Plainfield
 Alvarez, Bethzaida, MD
Oakhurst
 Mojares, Dennis C., MD
 Wortzel, Jay V., MD
Paramus
 Borkowski, Douglas Joseph, MD
Parsippany
 Earl, Lawrence N., MD

 Holder, William B., MD
 Shah, Mansi R., MD
Passaic
 Kumar, Rekha A., MD
 Sacristan, Carlos, MD
Paterson
 Graves, Linda M., MD
 Mirza, Nighat, MD
Phillipsburg
 Cumbo, Edward J., DO
 Grubb, Charles R., DO
Piscataway
 Nadal, Loida C., MD
 Stern, Marcel, MD
Pompton Lakes
 Ahmad, Fuad A., MD
Princeton
 Miller, Jeffrey J., DO
Rahway
 Kozlov, Zinovy, MD
Rutherford
 Grasso, Santo Vincent, DO
Saddle Brook
 Wasserman, Alan, MD
Salem
 Fleurantin, Jean J., MD
Sea Girt
 Micallef, Donald M., MD
Secaucus
 Udovenko, Olga, MD
Sewell
 Cerone, Anthony J. Jr., DO
 Labaczewski, Robert J., DO
Somerset
 Andre, Oswald, MD
 Najarro, Juan Carlos, MD
Stone Harbor
 Speer, Robert R., DO
Stratford
 Gayle, Catherine, MD
 Hudrick, Robert Eugene, DO
 Jagpal, Karandeep, DO
 Lightfoot, Judith A., DO
 Nguyen, Jonathan Huy, DO
 White, Joseph A., DO
Summit
 Koliopoulos, John S., DO
Toms River
 DiChiara, Frank P., DO
 Kanthan, Sudha, MD
 Mendoza, Concepcion B., MD
 Mitchell, David S., DO
Trenton
 Cleaves, Elle Sowa, MD
 Gieger, Andrew, MD
 Kim, Sion, DO
 Vongviphut, Don, DO
 Work, Adam Nicholas, MD
Turnersville
 Koerner, Theodore G., DO
Union City
 Feret, Eve Anne, MD
Vineland
 Chung, Kai B., MD
 Seibel, David L., MD
Voorhees
 Chang, Hyun S., MD
 Garber, Brett A., DO
 O'Connell, Joseph J. III, DO
 Patel, Ashokkumar B., MD
Wayne
 Hasan, Sanjida, MD
West Long Branch
 DiSanto, Vinson Michael, DO
Westfield
 Kriegman, Audrey Gail, MD
Westwood
 Donikyan, Mardik Martin, DO
Whippany
 Rosenberg, Martin Louis, MD
Willingboro
 Mashru, Pravinkuma K., MD
Woodbine
 Chu, Jae M., MD
 LeVan, Maurice X., MD
Woodbridge
 Purani, Gaurav S., MD
Woodcliff Lake
 Piacentile, Joseph M., MD

Woodstown
 Ostrum, Gordon J. Jr., MD

General Preventive Medicine
Basking Ridge
 Dessio, Whitney Charnell, MD
 Sokol, Michael C., MD
Denville
 Ali, Majid, MD
East Brunswick
 Miller, Andrew David, MD
Egg Harbor City
 Digenio, Andres German, MD
Ewing
 Gooding, Susane Lavern, MD
Fair Lawn
 Cernea, Dana, MD
Jersey City
 Carnow, David Robert, MD
Moorestown
 Murray, Michael Louis, DO
Piscataway
 Greene, Glenn Joel, MD
Sayreville
 Meduru, Pramod, MD
Trenton
 Gorney, Marilyn A., DO
 Kruse, Lakota K., MD
Vineland
 Linn, Steven Craig, MD

Geriatric Psychiatry
Bloomsbury
 Caruso, Edward Francis, MD
Colonia
 Mayer, Martin P., MD
Elizabeth
 Sethi, Mohammad Awais, MD
Fair Lawn
 Valiveti, Sailaja Devi, MD
Fort Dix
 Rashid, Shahzad, DO
Glen Gardner
 West, Helen T., MD
Hackensack
 Lally, Tamkeen, MD
 Tourkova, Marina, MD
Hillsborough
 Shah, Shailaja K., MD
Livingston
 Anekstein, Carol B., MD
Long Branch
 Fang, Margaret Wu, MD
 Rubin, Kenneth J., MD
Marlton
 Periasamy, Jayanthi, MD
Medford
 Murphy, Francis Raymond, MD
Monroe Township
 Krishnaiah, Muralidhar, MD
Moorestown
 Snyder, David L., MD
Morris Plains
 Patel, Bhupendra M., MD
Morristown
 Farrales, Caroline P., MD
New Brunswick
 Gabrial, Irene Gamalnoub, MD
Newark
 Hussain, Najeeb Ullah, MD
 Sanchez, Manuel I., MD
 Wu, Albert B., MD
Paramus
 Dhingra, Monica, MD
 Ghani, Muhammad Rehan, MD
Perth Amboy
 Annamaneni, Padmaja Sarki, MD
Piscataway
 Mazur, Yuri, MD
Princeton
 Khouri, Philippe J., MD
Red Bank
 Ongsiako, Maria V., MD
Tenafly
 Friedman, Jay Lawrence, MD
Tinton Falls
 Soto Moise, Olga Bienvenida, MD
Toms River
 Patel, Ashok Kantilal, MD
 Tandon, Pooja, MD
 Yosry, Mohamed Hussein, MD

Voorhees
 Talati, Amita N., MD
West Orange
 Sathaye, Nirmal, MD

Geriatrics
Bayonne
 Brown, Mitchell L., MD
Brick
 Boyan, William P., MD
Camden
 Akhter, Rowsonara, MD
 Greenberg, Alan, MD
 Thomas, May A., MD
Cherry Hill
 Abelow, Gerald G., MD
 Hasbun, William Miguel, MD
 Maro, Robert Jr., MD
 Patel, Rajankuma Popatlal, MD
 Surrey, Christine Marie, DO
Clifton
 Lashin, Waleed Sirag, MD
Cranbury
 Smelkinson, Ann E., MD
Dayton
 Schaer, Teresa McKinley, MD
Delran
 Epstein, Jeffrey E., MD
Denville
 Feigin, Leslie C., MD
East Orange
 Stanislaus, Galen P., MD
 Sunderam, Gnana, MD
 Viswanatha, Kallahalli V., MD
Edison
 Dhindsa, Sumeet, MD
 Oser, William Jr., MD
 Parikh, Rakesh K., MD
Englewood Cliffs
 Salem, Noel B., MD
Fair Lawn
 Oliver, Richard D., MD
 Verga, Diane G., MD
Flemington
 Chakravarthi, Seshadri Shekar, MD
 Gujar, Priti S., MD
 Tunuguntla, Renuka, MD
Fords
 Haldar, Pranab K., MD
Fort Lee
 Kim, John, MD
Freehold
 Gohel, Rekha M., MD
 Rowlands, Randy R., MD
 Yu Chen, Robert P., MD
Galloway
 Gong, Jeffrey, DO
Hackensack
 Cheeti, Kalpana, MD
 Evans, Ed Nelvyn Lezette, MD
 Pantagis, Stefanos G., MD
 Parulekar, Manisha Santosh, MD
 Rastogi, Sarita, MD
 Rutkowska, Ewa, MD
 Steel, R. Knight, MD
Hamburg
 Fielding, Dennis P., MD
Hamilton
 Aiello, Stephen Anthony, MD
Hammonton
 Donepudi, Srilalitha, MD
Harrington Park
 Psillides, Despina, MD
Hillsborough
 Gubbi, Renukamba Nagaraju, MD
Hoboken
 Perlmutter, Barbara Lee, MD
Jersey City
 Flores, David, MD
Kinnelon
 Levant, Barry E., MD
Lakehurst
 Shua Haim, Joshua Roy, MD
Lakewood
 Lempel, Allen L., MD
Laurel Springs
 Domanski, John D., MD
Linden
 Mehta, Palak Pranav, MD

Physicians by Specialty and Town

Little Falls
 Bellardini,Angelo G.,MD
Livingston
 Arunachalam,Muthu R.,MD
Long Branch
 Goldberg,Shira,MD
 Weinberg,Ronald M.,MD
 Zwerin,Glenn A.,MD
Lyndhurst
 James,Todd C.,MD
 Kovaleva,Alexandra,MD
Lyons
 Luo,Jane He-Cong,MD
Manalapan
 Kelter,Richard J.,MD
 Rijhsinghani,Sonia J.,MD
Marlboro
 Shi,Yong,MD
Marlton
 Bryman,Paul N.,DO
Medford
 Atkinson,James Q. III,MD
Mendham
 Wolf,James H.,MD
Middlesex
 Shamsi,Mahmood A.,MD
 Shamsi,Zahira B.,MD
Mine Hill
 Estrada,Aristides M.,MD
Monroe
 Vigario,Jose C.,DO
Monroe Township
 Chatterjee,Abhijit,MD
Montclair
 Auld,Clara Stringer,MD
Moorestown
 Siegert,Elisabeth A.,MD
Morristown
 Peper,Kathryn,MD
 Petilla-Onorato,Jessica I.,MD
 Prager,Jason Nicholas,MD
 Sharma,Keerti,MD
 Zelener,Marina L.,DO
Mount Holly
 Headley,David F.,MD
 Jagadeesh,Jyothi,MD
Neptune
 Atienza-Cartnick,Kimberly A.,MD
 Masterson,Eileen,MD
 Quinn,Margaret M.,MD
New Brunswick
 Brodt,Zahava Nilly,MD
 Kothari,Nayan K.,MD
 Moondra,Palak,DO
New Lisbon
 Mouliswar,Mysore P.,MD
New Providence
 Holcomb,Brenda E.,DO
Newark
 Haggerty,Mary A.,MD
 Lynch,Claudia,MD
Oakhurst
 Hayet,Bill,MD
Ocean
 Disciglio,Michael J.,MD
Old Bridge
 Enukashvili,Rafael R.,MD
Paramus
 Adel,Nourihan,MD
 Das,Urmi,MD
 Kushner,Evan G.,MD
 Menacker,Morey J.,DO
 Prowse,Alicia Ann,MD
 Yousef,Javed Muhammad,MD
Paterson
 Gupta,Punita,MD
 Hossain,Shahreen Rafa,MD
 Sanchez Pena,Jose R.,MD
Pennsauken
 Chan-Ting,Rengena Eleanor,DO
Perth Amboy
 Guillen,Gregorio J.,MD
Phillipsburg
 Viroja,Yogesh V.,MD
Pitman
 De Eugenio,Lewis Jr.,MD
Plainsboro
 Sidhu,Harpreet,MD

Pompton Plains
 Abou Jaoude,Dany M.,MD
 Ponomarev,Aleksandr,MD
Princeton
 Hua,Xingjia,MD
Ridgewood
 Nagarajan,Anuradha,MD
Roselle Park
 Solomon,Robert B.,MD
Secaucus
 Raghavan,Murli,MD
Shrewsbury
 Cook,Willard H.,MD
Somerset
 Singh,Mukesh Kumar,MD
South Orange
 Eatman,Florence B.,MD
South Plainfield
 Dumapit,Gerardo D.,MD
Sparta
 Wang,George Cho-Ching,MD
Springfield
 Lim,Betty Bichly,MD
Stratford
 Cavalieri,Thomas A.,DO
 Chopra,Anita,MD
 Cuttler,Ira M.,MD
 Elahi,Abdul Wadood,MD
 Frankel,Susan L.,DO
 Ginsberg,Terrie Beth,DO
 Kedziora,Halina M.,MD
 Noll,Donald R.,DO
 Palli,Prameela M.,MD
Summit
 Trivedi,Manoj M.,MD
Teaneck
 Adler,Joel S.,MD
 Katz,Terri F.,MD
 Meyerowitz,Jay S.,MD
Toms River
 Sharma,Sanjiv Kumar,MD
 Sundheim,John M.,MD
Trenton
 Wallach,Sara L.,MD
Turnersville
 Abdulghani,Ahsan Arshad,MD
Voorhees
 Bansal,Mukta,MD
 Gamble,James D.,MD
 Grimmett,Brian L.,MD
 Mandia,Renita,DO
 Maurer,Kenneth H.,MD
 Solomon,Sheldon D.,MD
Warren
 Lanza,Raymond,DO
West Orange
 Ganesh,Manickam,MD
 Gracia,Anne Marie G.,MD
 Redling,Theresa Marie,DO
 Schor,Joshua David,MD
Whippany
 Cyrus,Pamela A.,MD
Woodbury
 De Persia,Rudolph T. Jr.,MD
Wyckoff
 Mansour,Loris N.,MD

Glaucoma
Freehold
 Grand,Elliot S.,MD
Newark
 Habiel,Miriam,MD
Old Bridge
 Wong,Sze Ho,MD

Gynecological Oncology
Florham Park
 Febbraro,Terri,MD
Hackensack
 Smith,Daniel Humphreys,MD
 Vaidya,Ami P.,MD
Marlton
 Saul,Howard Marc,DO
Merchantville
 Wilson,John Goss Jr.,MD
Morristown
 Contreras,Diana Nancy,MD
 Heller,Paul B.,MD
 Tchabo,Nana Eleonore,MD
 Tobias,Daniel Henry,MD
 Wagreich,Allison Robin,MD

Neptune
 Bosscher,James Reed,MD
New Brunswick
 Goldberg,Michael I.,MD
 Hellmann,Mira C.,MD
 Isani,Sara,MD
Newark
 Einstein,Mark H.,MD
 Marcus,Jenna Z.,MD
 Novetsky,Akiva Pesach,MD
South Orange
 Anderson,Patrick St. George,MD
Teaneck
 Lewin,Sharyn Nan,MD
 Schiavone-Forlenza,Maria,MD
 Sommers,Gara M.,MD
Voorhees
 Rocereto,Thomas F.,MD
Wall
 Hackett,Thomas Everett,DO
West Orange
 Denehy,Thad R.,MD
 Taylor,Robert Roland,MD

Gynecology
Atlantic City
 De Stefano,Joseph L.,MD
Bayonne
 Pelosi,Marco A. II,MD
Belleville
 Meglio,Robyn S.,MD
Camden
 Tew,Beverly Ellen,MD
Cherry Hill
 Pekala,Bernard A.,MD
Denville
 Siegel,Joseph K.,MD
 Siegel,Stacey Beth,DO
Eatontown
 Greenleaf,Betsy Alice,DO
Far Hills
 Moore,Donnica Lauren,MD
Hackensack
 Cavallaro,Barbara Ann,MD
 Lo,Hung-Tien,MD
 Petras,Peri Ann,MD
Hillsborough
 Davis,Nicole D.,MD
 DeLucia,Carolyn Ann,MD
Linwood
 Hyett,Marvin R.,MD
Lumberton
 Chodos,Wesley S.,DO
Maplewood
 Gudz,Alexandr,MD
Montclair
 Grochmal,Stephen A.,MD
Mountainside
 Huhn-Werner,Maryann,MD
New Brunswick
 Mitra,Anjali Naz,MD
Newark
 Kulak,David,MD
 Otteno,Helen,MD
North Brunswick
 Versi,Ebrahim Eboo,MD
Parsippany
 Friedel,Walter E.,MD
Passaic
 Leo,Chadwick S.,DO
Princeton
 Bhatia,Nina Prakash,MD
 McCoy,Susan N.,MD
Sewell
 Packin,Gary S.,DO
South Plainfield
 Powderly,Mary K.,MD
 Sanghavi,Maya M.,MD
Stratford
 Jolitz,Whitney,DO
Turnersville
 McKinney,Timothy B.,MD
Vineland
 Mirone,Gary Steven,DO
Voorhees
 Echols,Karolynn T.,MD
 Gandhi,Veena S.,MD

Hand Surgery
Brick
 Pecoraro,Michael J.,MD
Cedar Knolls
 Zaino,Christian,MD
Cherry Hill
 Ames,Elliot L.,DO
 Bednar,John M.,MD
Chester
 Weinstein,Larry,MD
Clifton
 Lakin,Jeffrey F.,MD
Delran
 Sattel,Andrew B.,MD
Eatontown
 Atik,Teddy Labib,MD
 Decker,Raymond Jr.,MD
 Fedorcik,Gregory Gerard,MD
 Gabuzda,George Mark,MD
 Pess,Gary M.,MD
Edison
 Lombardi,Robert M.,MD
Emerson
 Meyer,Carissa Leigh,MD
Englewood
 Gurland,Mark A.,MD
 Lee,Jen Fei,MD
 Miller-Breslow,Anne J.,MD
 Pizzillo,Michael Francis,MD
Flemington
 Nenna,David Vito,MD
Freehold
 Patel,Nikesh Kirit,MD
Hackensack
 Giuffrida,Angela Ylenia,MD
Haddonfield
 Dalsey,Robert M.,MD
Hainesport
 Garberman,Scott F.,MD
Hamilton
 Malik,Parvaiz Akhtar,MD
Linden
 Mackessy,Richard P.,MD
Marlton
 Ballet,Frederick L.,MD
 Strauss,Eric D.,MD
Metuchen
 Shoen,Steven Lloyd,MD
Morristown
 McBride,Mark J.,MD
 Miller,Jeffrey Karl,MD
North Brunswick
 Kirschenbaum,David,MD
Northfield
 Fox,Jonathan L.,MD
Paramus
 Fakharzadeh,Frederick F.,MD
 Rosenstein,Roger G.,MD
 Tuckman,Drew E.,MD
 Ugras,Steven A.,MD
Parlin
 Bakhos,Abdel M.,MD
Princeton
 Grenis,Michael Steven,MD
 Lamb,Marc John,MD
Randolph
 Ende,Leigh S.,MD
Rio Grande
 Cole,Frederick Jr.,DO
Rutherford
 Altman,Wayne J.,MD
Springfield
 Fox,Ross J.,MD
 Kirschenbaum,Abram Eugene,MD
Summit
 Gardner,James Nicholas,MD
Teaneck
 Galitzin,Joseph C.,MD
Tinton Falls
 Johnson,Christopher D.,MD
Toms River
 Rosen,Michael David,MD
 Semet,Elliot C.,MD
Trenton
 Fletcher,Daniel J.,MD
Verona
 Fraser,Keith E.,MD
Voorhees
 Stackhouse,Thomas G.,MD

Physicians by Specialty and Town

Hand Surgery (cont)
Wayne
Bazzini,Robert M.,MD
Ghobadi,Fereydoon,MD
Ghobadi,Ramin,MD
Westfield
Barmakian,Joseph T.,MD
Woodbury
Lipschultz,Todd M.,MD
Monaghan,Bruce A.,MD

Head & Neck Surgery
Morristown
Cohen,Erik Gary,MD
Harrison,Lawrence Evan,MD
Newark
Baredes,Soly,MD

Headache
Cherry Hill
Tinkelman,Brad J.,MD

Hematology
Avenel
Kulper,Bernard J.,MD
Shypula,Gregory J.,MD
Belleville
Saleh,Said A.,MD
Brick
Amin,Girish S.,MD
Camden
Brus,Christina R.,MD
Young,Faith M.,MD
Cape May Court House
Gandhi,Vijaykumar K.,MD
Carteret
Sidhom,Ibrahim W.,MD
Clifton
Uhm,Kyudong,MD
Denville
Jan,Naveed A.,MD
East Orange
Kasimis,Basil S.,MD
Prasad,Indra D.,MD
Edison
Gupta,Juhee,MD
Wallach,Bruce H.,MD
Elizabeth
Salerno,Vincent E.,MD
Elmwood Park
Persad,Rajendra,MD
Englewood
Attas,Lewis M.,MD
Schleider,Michael A.,MD
Ewing
Hogan,Robert P.,DO
Flemington
Blankstein,Kenneth B.,MD
Florham Park
Kay,Andrea C.,MD
Freehold
Gopal,Krishnan T.,MD
Silberberg,Jeffrey M.,MD
Hackensack
Feldman,Tatyana A.,MD
Goldberg,Stuart Lee,MD
Rosenbluth,Richard J.,MD
Waintraub,Stanley Eli,MD
Hamilton
Holtzman,Gayle S.,MD
Hoboken
Damle,Vasanti J.,MD
Holmdel
Rifkin,Paul L.,MD
Jersey City
Housri,Ibrahim,MD
Little Silver
Walsh,Christina M.,MD
Livingston
Botti,Anthony C.,MD
Conde,Miguel A.,MD
Zauber,Neil P.,MD
Long Branch
Braslavsky,Gregory,MD
Manasquan
Lerner,William A.,MD
Topilow,Arthur A.,MD
Maplewood
Sabnani,Indu,MD
Marmora
Dave,Hemang U.,MD
Mickleton
Minniti,Carl J. Jr.,MD
Montclair
Sagorin,Charles E.,MD
Zager,Robert,MD
Montvale
Gu,Ping,MD
Morristown
Early,Ellen Marie,MD
Gerstein,Gary,MD
Meyers,Marta,MD
Papish,Steven W.,MD
New Brunswick
Eid,Joseph E.,MD
Gulli,Vito M.,MD
Rose,Shelonitda S.,MD
Strair,Roger Kurt,MD
Newark
Bryan,Margarette R.N.,MD
Rogers-Phillips,Elois G.,MD
Shah,Maya M.,MD
Sterling-Jean,Yolette,MD
Orange
Amin,Jashvant S.,MD
Paramus
Fernbach,Barry R.,MD
Ligresti,Louise G.,MD
Passaic
Lee,Sheue H.,MD
Pennington
Kindsfather,Scott K.,MD
Princeton
Yi,Peter I.,MD
Somerset
Fein,Robert P.,MD
Porcelli,Marcus P.,MD
Somerville
Stanford,Brian J.,DO
Toomey,Kathleen,MD
Wu,Hen-Vai,MD
Young,Steven Eugene,MD
South Orange
Lombardy,Elyane Emilienne,MD
Teaneck
Tsai,Philip Henry,MD
Teterboro
Mehta,Kumudini U.,MD
Toms River
Al Kana,Randah,MD
Shah,Chirag M.,MD
Voorhees
Bapat,Ashok R.,MD
Gordon,Richard L.,DO
Madamba,Carlos S.,MD
Siegel,Norman H.,MD
Wayne
Hanley,Debra A.,MD
West Orange
Rothenberg,Jerry,MD
Westfield
Freeman,Barry C.,MD
Westwood
Israel,Alan M.,MD
Woodbridge
Murray,Carl Louis Jr.,MD

Hematology Oncology
Basking Ridge
Chalasani,Sree Bhavani,MD
Bayonne
Iyengar,Arjun D.,MD
Kumaresan,Arulnangai,MD
Lamba,Renu,MD
Berkeley Heights
Mills,Lisa Alice,MD
Reeder,Jennifer Gordan,MD
Camden
Bhattacharya,Prianka,MD
Budak-Alpdogan,Tulin,MD
Georges,Peter T.,MD
Hageboutros,Alexandre,MD
Kesselheim,Howard I.,DO
Koch,Marjan Leoni,MD
Sharan,Kanu Priya,MD
Squillante,Christian Michael,MD
Cherry Hill
Alley,Evan Wayne,MD
Goldberg,Jack,MD
Clifton
Afonja,Richards A.,MD
Maroules,Michael,MD
Strakhan,Marianna,MD
Todi,Neelam T.,MD
Denville
Bari,Fazal,MD
Edison
Koduri,Beaula V.,MD
Schuman,Richard M.,MD
Egg Harbor Township
Sandilya,Vijay Krishna,MD
Elizabeth
Cholankeril,Michelle,MD
Levinson,Barry S.,MD
Emerson
Gold,Edward J.,MD
Englewood
Forte,Francis A.,MD
Janosky,Maxwell,MD
Kim,Brian Hangil,MD
Morrison,Jill S.,MD
Flemington
Bednar,Myron Emil,MD
Ngeow,Swee Jian,MD
Rehman,Waqas,MD
Shah,Megha,MD
Florham Park
DeRosa,William T.,DO
George,Roshini,DO
Gurubhagavatula,Sarada,MD
Siu,Karleung,MD
Galloway
Ajay,Rajasree,MD
Borai,Nasser Eldien,MD
Hackensack
Biran,Noa,MD
Harper,Harry D.,MD
McNamara,Donna M.,MD
Pecora,Andrew L.,MD
Hackettstown
Niranjan,Usha,MD
Holmdel
Chen,Aileen Lim,MD
Howell
Katz,Randi J.,DO
Kunamneni,Raghu Krishna,MD
Jersey City
Badin,Simon,MD
Patel,Amit A.,MD
Shah,Nalini Arvindkumar,MD
Talwar,Sumit,MD
Zarubin,Vadim,MD
Lawrenceville
Kenney,Ellen N.,MD
Little Silver
Windsor,Stephen J.,MD
Livingston
Brown,Andrew Bennett,MD
Grossman,Israel Robert,MD
Rao,Parth Rajeshkumar,MD
Wildman,Joseph M.,MD
Manahawkin
Chung,Paul Kevin,MD
Desani,Jatin Karsandas,MD
Morino,Tricia Lynn,DO
Naylor,Evan C.,MD
Manasquan
Anne,Madhurima,MD
Greenberg,David Benjamin,MD
Levitt,Michael Joshua,MD
Marlboro
Varma,Seema N.,MD
Marmora
Pompa,Tiffany,MD
Middletown
Shcherba,Marina,DO
Montclair
Di Paolo,Patrick J.,MD
Morristown
Chiang,Wendy M.,MD
Scola,Michael Anthony,MD
New Brunswick
Bannerji,Rajat,MD
David,Kevin Andrew,MD
Desai,Vidhi Parikh,MD
Evens,Andrew M.,DO
Ganesan,Shridar,MD
Karantza-Wadsworth,Vassiliki,MD
Kritharis-Agrusa,Athena,MD
Philipp,Claire S.,MD
Saraiya,Biren P.,MD
Sridharan,Ashwin,MD
Stein,Mark Nathan,MD
Newark
Abo,Stephen Michael,DO
Elreda,Lauren,MD
Ignatius,Nandini,MD
Saraf,Pankhoori,MD
Shaaban,Hamid Salim,MD
Wang,Trent Peng,DO
Northfield
Stoyko,Zoryana,MD
Paramus
Suh,Jason W.,MD
Wood,Kevin C.,MD
Paterson
Kumar,Mehandar,MD
Pennington
McIntosh,Nenita Parrilla,MD
Schaebler,David L.,MD
Phillipsburg
Smith,John Edmund Jr.,MD
Starr,Cynthia D.,MD
Plainsboro
Babott,Doreen,MD
Pompton Plains
Frank,Martin J.,MD
Princeton
Yang,Arvin S.,MD
Rahway
Altura,Rachel Allison,MD
Kang,Soonmo Peter,MD
Ridgewood
DeNeve,Albert A.,MD
Sewell
Poretta,Trina A.,DO
Somerset
Desai,Sameer P.,MD
Fang,Bruno S.,MD
Karp,George I.,MD
Lampert,Craig,MD
Reid,Phillip Dolivera,MD
Ronnen,Ellen A.,MD
Somerville
Khalid,Aysha,MD
Pan,Beiqing,MD
Sparta
Cheng,Waina,MD
Incorvati,Jason A.,MD
Springfield
Desai,Ved,DO
Khot,Ashish Abhay,MD
Rao,Maithili V.,MD
Summit
Guerin,Bonni Lee,MD
Morse,Sophie D.,MD
Saksena,Rujuta P.,MD
Teaneck
Condemi,Giuseppe,MD
Toms River
Kavuru,Sudha,MD
Voorhees
Ferber,Andres,MD
Lerman,Nati,MD
Mehta,Pallav K.,MD
Rajagopalan,Kumar,MD
Ross,David H.,MD
Wayne
Dorkhom,Stephan Joseph,DO
Roy,Vijaykumar,MD
Shah,Harish H.,MD
West Long Branch
Lee,Patrick C.,MD
Ray,Debra M.,MD
Westampton
Fernandez,Eduardo E.,MD
Tropea,Joseph N.,DO
Westfield
Talavera,Joyce R.,MD
Westwood
Kirshner,Eli David,MD
Willingboro
Stone,Paul A.,MD
Woodbury
Rotkowitz,Michael Ian,MD

Hematopathology
Camden
Allen,Ashleigh,MD
Elmwood Park
Merati,Kambiz,MD
Talwar,Jotica,MD

Physicians by Specialty and Town

New Brunswick
  Bhagavathi,Sharathkumar M.,MD
Newark
  Sun,Xinlai,MD
  Wang,Qing,MD
Pompton Plains
  Zhang,Hailing,MD
Rahway
  Juco,Jonathan W.,MD

Hepatology
Cherry Hill
  Elgenaidi,Hisham,MD
  Malek,Ashraf Hossain,MD
Flemington
  Arrigo,Richard J.,DO
Newark
  Edula,Raja Gopal Reddy,MD
Parsippany
  Xie,Bingru,MD
Pennington
  Munoz,Santiago Jose,MD

Holistic Medicine
Colts Neck
  Huang,Wendy,MD

Homeopathy
Toms River
  Zaki,Merajuddin,MD

Hospitalist
Atlantic City
  Abbasi,Danish P.,MD
  Abella-Ramirez,Katherine,MD
  Ahmad,Israr,MD
  Baby,Benesa,MD
  Bakr,Mohamed Mokhtar,MD
  Dhaliwal,Harleen,MD
  Huma,Sabahath,MD
  Iqbal,Javid,MD
  Jaleel,Syed,MD
  McBrearty-Hindson,Ashley,DO
  Narula,Navjot Singh,MD
  Rahmani,Ghulam Ali,MD
  Shah,Sulay Hiteshkumar,MD
  Silver,Jordan,MD
  Sohaib,Muhammad,MD
  Tusheva,Marija,MD
Bayonne
  Khan,Irfana B.,MD
Berkeley Heights
  Banda,Pragati,MD
  Desai,Nicky,MD
  Mishra,Sneha,MD
Brick
  Botu,Devi Prasad,MD
Bridgeton
  Pham,Peter H.,DO
Browns Mills
  Poulathas,Alexander S.,DO
Camden
  Adarkwa,Agnes,MD
  Anter,Afaf A.,DO
  Ausaf,Sadaf,MD
  Bazergui,Christopher,DO
  Contino,Krysta Marie,MD
  Divilov,Vadim,MD
  Doktor,Katherine Leigh,MD
  Ibekwe,Ola,MD
  Kabadi,Rajesh Mahesh,MD
  Kamalu,Okebugwu,MD
  King,Cecile Carol-Ann,MD
  Lami,Christian John,MD
  Loutfi,Rania H.,MD
  Matthews,Lawrence M. III,MD
  Moore,Andrew James,MD
  Oberdorf,William Eric,DO
  Palli,Vinay Motu,MD
  Patel,Urvish,MD
  Shah,Satyam Ashvinkumar,MD
  Singh,Novia,MD
  Terrigno,Nicole,MD
Cherry Hill
  Kashif,Soofia,MD
  Kotturi,Vijendra B.,MD
Clifton
  Weiss,Jeffrey A.,MD
Denville
  Toohey,Kristina,MD
East Brunswick
  Modi,Chirag H.,MD

Edison
  Mistry,Nirav,MD
  Obiefuna,Nkechiyere Angela,MD
Englewood
  Hohmuth,Benjamin Adam,MD
Florham Park
  Pinyard,Jeremy Vincent,MD
Fort Lee
  Blaszka,Matthew Christopher,MD
Hackensack
  Bajwa,Ravneet Singh,MD
  Josephs,Joshua,MD
  Mapa,Christopher George,MD
  Qureshi,Akif Zeshan,MD
  Tam,Elizabeth,MD
Haddonfield
  Kumar,Nisha Iyer,MD
Hoboken
  Kocia,Orjeta,MD
Jersey City
  Borker,Sonia V.,DO
  Lahewala,Sopan,MD
  Mamji,Salman,MD
  Mulligan,Edward,MD
Long Branch
  Bodala,Durga Rani,MD
  Mandel,Rekha J.,MD
Manahawkin
  Savarese,Joseph,MD
Marlton
  Pollard,Elizabeth Joan,MD
Mays Landing
  Chowdhury,Khaza,MD
Montclair
  Tehranirad,Mohammad,MD
  Wain,Nadeem,MD
Morristown
  Papatheodorou,Dana William,MD
  Shroff,Shilpa Anilkumar,MD
  Trinidad,Jennilee A.,MD
Mount Holly
  DeLue,Erik Nathaniel,MD
  Nisar,Sabeeha,MD
  Oyeyemi,Jubril Oyekanmi,MD
  Valeus,Pierre Rigens,MD
Neptune
  Ahmed,Naseer,MD
  Siddiqui,Kamran,MD
  Zamel,Laith Naser,MD
New Brunswick
  Pulijaal,Pooja,MD
Newark
  Chillemi,Salvatore,MD
  Doshi,Dhvani,MD
  Kathuria,Kanik,MD
  Verma,Siddharth,DO
Newton
  Albassam,Hassan,MD
Northfield
  Mathews,Robert John,MD
Paterson
  Manda,Jayaprakash,MD
  Tameem,Murtuza,MD
Phillipsburg
  Varghese,Juliet George,MD
Plainsboro
  Fanning,Christine M.,MD
  Phinney,Maryann B.,MD
  Shah,Nimit Ashwinbhai,MD
Pompton Plains
  Agadi,Smitha G.,MD
  Pierre,Edeck Saintilien,MD
Rahway
  Hussain,Asim,MD
Randolph
  Luayon,Joseph Palac,DO
Raritan
  Patel,Rajendrakumar C.,MD
Red Bank
  Andrade,Jose G.,MD
  John,Thomas Jr.,MD
Salem
  Ngu,Michael Foleng,MD
Secaucus
  Mathur,Smita,DO
  Tsirogiannis,Vasiliky,MD
Somerville
  Amadi,Mariette Yvonne,MD
Spring Lake
  Banzuelo Rio,Margie R.,MD

Stratford
  Davis,Bryan F.,DO
  Khan,Imran Ahmad,MD
  Kothari,Sona A.,DO
  Lam,Gloria Fontane,DO
  Vudarla,Neelima,MD
Summit
  Bhatt,Raunaq Dushyantkumar,MD
  Malladi,Viswanath,MD
  Tadisina,Vani,MD
Teaneck
  Akhtar,Ruhi,MD
Tinton Falls
  Li,Wei,MD
Trenton
  Hassan,Hardawan Ahmed,MD
  Samiev,Djamshed,MD
Turnersville
  Badolato,Joseph Nunzio,DO
  Thompson,Nicole,DO
Vineland
  Bodagala,Hima,MD
  Gupta,Kanika,MD
  Katta,Pratyusha Reddy,MD
  Khan,Yusra,MD
Voorhees
  Abdeljawad,Mohammad R.,MD
  Berio-Dorta,Raul Luis,MD
  Franks,Lori Genevieve Pihl,MD
West Caldwell
  Remadevi,Radhika Sekhar,MD
West Orange
  Appiah,Evangeline Animah,MD
Wood Ridge
  Mullick,Muhammad Azfar,MD
Woodbury
  Kohlitz,Patrick,MD
  Sloane,Amy Johnson,MD

Hypertension
Midland Park
  Rho,John I.,MD
Rahway
  Mansoor,George A.,MD
South River
  Covit,Andrew B.,MD
Teaneck
  Salazer,Thomas L.,MD
Westfield
  Goldstein,Carl S.,MD

Immunology
Belmar
  Schmidt,John August Jr.,MD
East Hanover
  Grebenau,Mark David,MD
Newark
  Oleske,James M.,MD

Infectious Disease
Absecon
  Paparone,Philip W.,DO
Atlantic City
  Bayer,Deborah D.,DO
Bedminster
  Shariati,Nasseredin,MD
Belle Mead
  Holowinsky,Mary I.,MD
Belleville
  Admani,Ariff,MD
  Johnson,Edward S.,MD
  Moaven,Nader,MD
  Sidali,Mustafa M.,DO
Berkeley Heights
  Karim,Anjum Hasan,MD
  Nastro,Lawrence J.,MD
Bloomfield
  Pierre-Louis,Frantz Junior,MD
  Soroko,Theresa A.,MD
Brick
  Ruszka,Geza,MD
Brielle
  Kleinfeld,David I.,MD
Browns Mills
  Aboujaoude,Rania Nassif,MD
  Smialowicz,Chester R.,MD
Butler
  Abdul Shafi,Samya B.,MD
Camden
  Baxter,John D.,MD
  Fraimow,Henry S.,MD
  Gabriel,Nathaniel F.,MD

Kim,Rose,MD
Meyer,Daniel Karl,MD
Pedroza,Lisa Vanchhawng,MD
Pepe,Rosalie,MD
Porto,Maura C.,DO
Reboli,Annette C.,MD
Stutman,Robin Eugenia,MD
Cape May Court House
  Hansen,Eric Andrew,DO
Cedar Knolls
  Burstin,Stuart J.,MD
Cherry Hill
  Alessi,Paul J.,DO
  Williams,James R.,MD
Clifton
  Munera,Rodolfo A.,MD
  Najjar,Sessine,MD
  Okoye,Frederick E. Jr.,MD
  Sultana,Yasmeen,MD
  Weiss,Gabriella Antionette,MD
East Brunswick
  Kallich,Marsha M.,MD
  Snepar,Richard A.,MD
East Orange
  Eng,Robert H.,MD
  Gibson-Gill,Carol M.,MD
Edgewater
  Pradhan,Anuja A.,MD
Edison
  Martinez,Homar Amador,MD
  Paradiso,Mary J.,MD
  Ramasubramani,Anuradha,MD
  Rathnakumar,Charumathi,MD
  Sensakovic,John W.,MD
  Sree,Aruna,MD
Elizabeth
  Farrer,William E.,MD
  Sherer,Clark B.,MD
Englewood
  Kocher,Jeffrey,MD
  Saggar,Suraj Kumar,DO
  Torres Isasiga,Julian Andres,MD
  Weisholtz,Steven J.,MD
Ewing
  Gekowski,Kathleen M.,MD
  Karabulut,Nigahus,MD
Flemington
  Gugliotta,Joseph L.,MD
Florham Park
  Bennett,Douglas P.,DO
  De Shaw,Max G.,MD
  Frankel,Renee Ellen,MD
  Hart,Daniel,MD
  O'Grady,John P.,MD
Fort Lee
  Kim,Jeongwon,MD
Galloway
  Kaur,Amrita,DO
Hackensack
  Cicogna,Cristina Emanuela,MD
  Desai,Samit Sharad,MD
  Gross,Peter A.,MD
  Kibrea,S. M. Golam,MD
  Levine,Jerome Frederic,MD
  Sebti,Rani,MD
  Sperber,Steven J.,MD
Haddon Heights
  Okon,Emmanuel E.,MD
  Paluzzi,Sandra A.,DO
  Traboulsi,Rana,MD
  Turner,Ellen K.,MD
Haddonfield
  Akhter,Shafinaz,MD
Hainesport
  Asper,Ronald Frank,MD
Hamilton
  Aufiero,Patrick V.,MD
  Rosenbaum,Seth David,MD
  Soliman,Hesham S.,MD
Highland Park
  Khan,Shameen,DO
Hillsborough
  Doshi,Manish,MD
  Herman,David J.,MD
  Hirsh,Ellen J.,MD
  Nahass,Ronald G.,MD
  Pall,Amandeep Kaur,MD
  Pittarelli,Lisa A.,MD
  Sandhu,Sarbjit Singh,MD
  Seenivasan,Meena,MD
  Sheen,Jerry,MD

683

Physicians by Specialty and Town

Infectious Disease (cont)
Hillsborough
  Sinner, Scott William, MD
Hoboken
  Forouzesh, Avisheh, MD
  Messihi, Jean, MD
  Rahman, Habeeb U., MD
Howell
  Utpat, Sandeepa Makarand, MD
Irvington
  Mammen-Prasad, Elizabeth K., MD
  Patel, Raj, MD
Jersey City
  Bellomo, Spartaco, MD
  Grigoriu, Adriana, MD
  Khan, Noroze Jalil, MD
  Mangia, Anthony J., MD
Kenilworth
  Corcoran, Gavin R., MD
Lambertville
  Moskovitz, Bruce L., MD
Leonia
  Fratello, Laura F., MD
Linwood
  Papastamelos, Athanasios G., DO
Livingston
  Chiang, Tom Shou, MD
  Diamond, Gigi R., MD
  Georgescu, Anca D., MD
  Kokkola-Korpela, Marjut H., MD
  Lin, Janet C., MD
  Sheth, Arpita A., MD
  Tsveniashvili, Liya V., MD
Long Branch
  Eng, Margaret Hom, MD
  Hameed, Nida, MD
  Montana, Barbara E., MD
Manalapan
  De Luca, Alfred A. Jr., MD
Marlboro
  Bhargava, Abha, MD
  Laxmi, Sheethal Manipadaga, MD
Marlton
  Makris, Alex T., MD
  Schwartz, Andrew Robert, MD
Mercerville
  Farooq, Tahir, MD
  Husain, Syed Asif, DO
  Mathai, Suja John, MD
  Porwancher, Richard B., MD
Metuchen
  Nagarakanti, Sandhya R., MD
Midland Park
  Vierheilig, Jacqueline M., MD
Millburn
  Weiner, Peter R., MD
Monmouth Junction
  Bais, Pammi T., MD
Moorestown
  Gummadi, Vedam, MD
Morristown
  Kessler, Jason Adam, MD
  Natarajan, Usharani, MD
  Salaki, John S., MD
Mount Laurel
  Aggrey, Gloria Kangachie, MD
  Golden, Richard Frederick, MD
  Klinger, Frederick Boyd III, DO
  Kraus, Jennifer Lynn, MD
  Ng, Kevin, MD
  Peterson, John W., MD
  Sumerson, Jeffrey Marc, MD
  Topiel, Martin S., MD
Neptune
  Casey, Kathleen K., MD
  Frank, Elliot, MD
  Fune, Jose M.C., MD
  Kruvant-Gornish, Nancy J., MD
  Kufelnicka, Anna M., MD
  Liu, Edward Wei Chi, MD
New Brunswick
  Alcid, David V., MD
  Bhowmick, Tanaya, MD
  Boruchoff, Susan E., MD
  Suarez, Militza E., MD
  Veeraswamy, Pramila, MD
  Weinstein, Melvin P., MD
Newark
  Abergel, Glen, MD
  Alland, David, MD
  Bishburg, Eliahu, MD
  Chew, Debra, MD
  Dallapiazza, Michelle Lynn, MD
  Dever, Lisa Lynn, MD
  Ellner, Jerrold Jay, MD
  Engell, Christian August, MD
  Figueroa, Wanda E., MD
  Finkel, Diana Gurevich, DO
  Kapila, Rajendra, MD
  Kloser, Patricia C., MD
  Murillo, Jeremias L., MD
  Nyaku, Amesika N., MD
  Rodriguez-Diaz, Ana M., MD
  Sison, Raymund Vincent S., MD
  Slim, Jihad, MD
  Stoler, Alexander, MD
  Woodward, Ralph P., MD
North Brunswick
  Deka, Bharati, MD
Northfield
  Homayouni, Homayoun, MD
Nutley
  Sasanpour, Majid, MD
Oakhurst
  Dwivedi, Sukrut A., DO
  Lee, Andrew, MD
  Mathur, Ajay Narain, MD
  Patel, Apurva, MD
  Sivaprasad, Rajagopalan, MD
Old Bridge
  Middleton, John R., MD
  Tiruvury, Hemavarna, MD
Paramus
  Dandavate, Varsha Mohan, MD
Passaic
  Gupta, Punit Kumar, MD
Paterson
  Lange, Michael, MD
  Rabbat, Mohamed Salah, MD
  Zahran, Ali Abdelrahman, MD
Piscataway
  Fisher, Bruce D., MD
  Mathews, Cecil, MD
Pomona
  Trivedi, Manish Niranjan, MD
Princeton
  Fernando, Chandani D., MD
  Hanna, George J., MD
  Hughes, Eric Anton, MD
Rahway
  Brown, Melinda Sheron, MD
Randolph
  Allegra, Donald T., MD
  Aslam, Fazila, MD
  Doka, Najah I., MD
  Gupta, Rachna, MD
  Krieger, Richard E., MD
  Manalo, Rosario Beatriz, MD
  Markou, Theodore Ioannis, MD
  Marsh, Rebecca A., MD
  McManus, Edward J., MD
  Reddy, Sireesha B., MD
  Roseff, Shelly Anne, MD
  Ubhi, Damanpreet K., MD
Red Bank
  Ahmad, Khalid Mehmood, MD
  Ahmad, Nasir Mahmood, MD
  Eschinger, Amy Folio, MD
Ridgewood
  Kinchelow-Schmidt, Tosca E., MD
  Knackmuhs, Gary Glenn, MD
  O'Hagan Sotsky, Carol Ann, MD
Roseland
  Smith, Stephen Marshall, MD
Saddle Brook
  Poblete, Ronald J., MD
Somers Point
  Lucasti, Christopher J., DO
  Trofa, Andrew F., MD
Somerset
  Kumar, Uday, MD
  Sathe, Sadhana S., MD
  Segal, Robert Eric, MD
South Plainfield
  Go, Richard Au Yeung, MD
Springfield
  De Fronzo, Stephen D., MD
Summit
  Roland, Robert J., DO
Sussex
  Yasin, Sami F., MD
Teaneck
  Birch, Thomas M., MD
  De La Rosa, Benjamin Danny, MD
  Kalishman, Raffaella Linda, MD
Toms River
  Guerrero, Isabel C., MD
Trenton
  Cleri, Dennis J., MD
  Whitman, Marc S., MD
Vineland
  Ahrens, John C., MD
  Galetto, David W., MD
  Kaufman, David H., MD
Voorhees
  Barnish, Michael J., DO
  Condoluci, David V., DO
  Ghayad, Zeina Rita, DO
  Hou, Cindy Meng, DO
Wayne
  Filippis, Philip J. II, MD
  Obaid, Nabeel B., MD
West Caldwell
  Riauba, Linas, MD
West Orange
  Borowski, Michelle, DO
  Miller, Lincoln Paul, MD
Westfield
  Baez, Juan Carlos, MD
  Greenman, James L., MD
  Ruggeri-Weigel, Patricia, MD
Whitehouse Station
  Chan, Christina Yu-Yee, MD
  Lee, Andrew Wen-Tseng, MD
  Piliero, Peter James, MD

Insurance Medicine
Camden
  Patel, Nikhil H., MD
Chatham
  Traficante, Allen, MD
East Brunswick
  Hochstadt, Bruce A., MD
Hamilton
  Bhandarkar, Anjali, MD
Jersey City
  Park, Young K., MD
Moorestown
  Waronker-Silverstein, Amy S., MD
Morris Plains
  Parvulescu, Traian D., MD
Morristown
  Darcey, Jacqueline Marie, MD
Summit
  Tarasenko, Anthony J., MD

Internal Med-Adolescent Medicine
Hamilton
  Mabrouk, Tarig, MD
Irvington
  Banigo, Samuel, MD
Manalapan
  Birger, Yelena, DO
Stone Harbor
  Hofmann, William Andrew III, DO
Trenton
  Thoppil, Anoop Jose, MD

Internal Med-Allergy & Immunology
Flemington
  Muglia-Chopra, Christine Ann, MD

Internal Med-Heart Disease/Transpnt
Fort Lee
  Lucev, Anthony, MD

Internal Med-Hospice & Palliative
Flemington
  Fox, Katherine, MD
Marlton
  Malhotra, Rakesh, MD
Paramus
  Spitzer, Ayelet, DO

Internal Med-Sleep Medicine
Monmouth Junction
  Raza, Mudusar I., MD
New Brunswick
  Chen, Jennifer Yu-Chia, MD
Trenton
  Ricketti, Peter Anthony, DO

Internal Med-Sports Medicine
Livingston
  Kelly, Michael, DO
Morristown
  Padavan, Dean, MD

Internal Medicine
Aberdeen
  Guirguis, Nagy Nimr, MD
  Perkari, Vasantha K., MD
Absecon
  Catalina, Gabriel Richard, DO
  Driscoll, Eric Joseph, DO
  Fiorentino, Diego M., DO
  Khan-Jaffery, Kaniz F., MD
  Santos, Eduardo V., MD
  Sudol, Robert R., MD
Allendale
  Hershman, Jerald B., MD
Allentown
  Webb, James A., MD
Andover
  Renda, Julie Elaine, DO
Annandale
  Espinoza, Andrey, MD
Asbury Park
  Chinnici, Angelo A., MD
  Sisskin, Mark I., MD
  Tosiello, Lorraine Lerma, MD
Atco
  Campbell, Colin A., DO
Atlantic City
  Ahmad, Naheed Kaleem, MD
  Alexander, Karen Elizabeth, MD
  Alexander, Mark P., MD
  Asghar, Sheba, MD
  Ashraf, Afia, MD
  Bane, Susan H., MD
  Barzaga, Ricardo A., MD
  Belete, Senayit Girma, MD
  Bernardo, Gregory, MD
  Collins, Gregory C., MD
  Ghetia, Ditina, MD
  Hasni, Syed Shayan Ahmed, MD
  Hinkle, Mary Katrina, MD
  Hocbo, Aileen Aileen, MD
  Hussain, Arif, MD
  Hussain, Asiya, MD
  Infantolino, Edward, MD
  Kelly, Brendan S., DO
  Lal, Vikram, DO
  Macchiavelli, Anthony Joseph, MD
  Maludum, Obiora, MD
  Marwaha, Rohit, MD
  Mazur, Kimberly L., MD
  Mingione, Richard A., MD
  Misra, Amit, MD
  Mohiuddin, Fatima A., MD
  Nwotite, Ezinne Ugochi, MD
  Onwuka, Mary N., MD
  Parikh, Hiren B., MD
  Patel, Arvind Kumar, MD
  Patel, Hasitkumar D., MD
  Patel, Jitendra K., MD
  Patel, Manoj K., MD
  Patel, Mehul Kumar, MD
  Patel, Yogesh N., MD
  Quinlan, Liliane Bastos, MD
  Rangarajan, Narsimha R., MD
  Ray, Amit H., MD
  Roeske, Jessica L., DO
  Siddiqui, Durdana Aamir, MD
  Siegelman, Gary M., MD
  Sun, Qi, MD
  Szulc, Magdalena, MD
  Thalassinos, Antonios, DO
  Timms, Brian Daniel, DO
  Vijayakumar, Ashvin, MD
  Yarlagadda, Vivek, MD
  Zia, Shahzad S., MD
Atlantic Highlands
  De Noia, Anthony Philip, MD
  Movva, Srinivasa R., MD
Audubon
  Montiel, Armando A., MD
  Schmid, George F., MD
Avalon
  Hierholzer, Paul D., DO
Avenel
  Homer, Stuart M., MD
  Livshits, Boris M., MD

Physicians by Specialty and Town

Peter,Andras,MD
Romano,David L.,MD
Skrzypczak,Marek J.,MD
Swan,Alexander Myint,MD
Syed-Naqvi,Samina Altaf,MD
Avon
Mannion,Joseph,MD
Barnegat
Desai,Amee B.,MD
Basking Ridge
Chartash,Elliot Keith,MD
Dawson,Cleve R.,MD
Gaito,Andrea D.,MD
Gerhard,Harvey,MD
Gorsky,Mila,MD
Kachirayan,Vasanthi,MD
Lee,Joseph Sang-Ho,MD
Passalaris,Tina Marina,MD
Schlessinger,Leslie D.,MD
Shepherd,Annemarie Fernandes,MD
Sidhu,Loveleen,MD
Yu,Channing,MD
Bay Head
Zimmerman,Gail B.,MD
Bayonne
Acharya,Saurav,MD
Agpaoa,Ulysses V.,MD
Akhtar,Shahnaz,MD
Black,Ellen M.,MD
Brooks,Ira M.,MD
Burghauser,Alan H.,MD
Byrd,Lawrence H.,MD
Cabral,Cesar A. Sr.,MD
Cadoo,Lisa K.A.,MD
Cardiello,Gary P.,MD
Chavez,Rowland,MD
Condo,Dominick,MD
Dedousis,John Jr.,MD
Engel,Margaret A.,MD
Florino,Guy Michael,MD
Guittari,Nicholas S.,MD
Haque,Nadeem U.,MD
Herscu,Joseph I.,MD
Hoffman,Mark Andrew,MD
Iyengar,Devarajan P.,MD
Khalid,Khaula,DO
Mathew,Alexander John,MD
McGee,John R.,MD
Montalbano,Robert L.,MD
Mutterperl,Mitchell J.,MD
Neno,Rosa M.,DO
Oen,Rose L.,MD
Padkowsky,George O.,MD
Padkowsky,Orest,MD
Perveen,Mahmoodah,MD
Rangasamy,Ajantha,MD
Sheinman,Marc Daniel,DO
Silber,Danuta,MD
Singh,Amandeep,MD
Singh,Vijayant,MD
Suczewski,Edward J.,MD
Suczewski,Thomas J.,MD
Tarng,George W.,MD
Upadhyaya,Hitendrakumar C.,MD
Wignarajan,Kanagarayer R.,MD
Wignarajan,Nadika V.,MD
Woods,Krystina L.,MD
Zelinski,Jay Michael,DO
Bayville
Alario,Frank C.,MD
Ingato,Steven P.,MD
Naseem,Arif,MD
Bedminster
Bonaventura,Lisa M.,MD
Campbell,Arthur Scott,MD
Garg,Anju,MD
Belle Mead
Levinson,Benjamin,MD
Pecora,Joseph J. III,DO
Wajcberg,Estela,MD
Belleville
Ardolino,Joseph M.,MD
Beggs,Donald James,MD
Beresford,Dianne Walker,MD
Christiana,William A.,MD
Chun,Kye S.,MD
Colon,German R.,MD
Conti,John A.,MD
D'Aconti,John S.,DO
De Franco,Penny E.,MD
Dealmeida,Patrick,DO

Eswarapu,Srinivasa,MD
Feehan,Brian Patrick,DO
Fernandes,Jaxon James,MD
Gamss,Jonathan,MD
Gandhi,Senthamara,MD
Gialanella,Craig David,MD
Houng,Mindy S.,MD
Johnson,Timothy David,MD
Kaul,Sameer,MD
Klughaupt,Stanley,MD
Kumar,Tarun,MD
Lippman,Alan J.,MD
Maresca,Phillip A,MD
Mircea,Cornel,MD
Molinari,Francis T.,MD
Orsini,James M.,MD
Orsini,James Michael,MD
Pasley,Peter M.,MD
Paulo,Jimmy Martins,MD
Reddy,Uma P.,MD
Schnurr,Deborah G. P.,MD
Silkov,Andrey,MD
Vasireddy,Hemalatha,MD
Yerramalli,Sitamahala M.,MD
Bellmawr
Howe,Joseph H.,MD
Santoro,Stephanie Amanda,DO
Williams,Frederick M.,MD
Bergenfield
De Gennaro,Michael A.,MD
Desai,Foram R.,MD
Diamond,Paul M.,MD
Jiu,Wun-Ye,MD
Negron,Luis M.,MD
Pereira,Beryl E.,MD
Varghese,Mathew,MD
Weisgras,Josef Mordechay,MD
Zeveloff,Susan R.,MD
Berkeley
Bose,Konika Paul,MD
Kole,Alison S.,MD
Parziale,Michael A.,MD
Spano-Brennan,Liana Marie,DO
Tuladhar,Swosty,MD
Berkeley Heights
Abramson,Marla Lyn,MD
Arif,Orooj,MD
Bass,Jon Lawrence,MD
Bauman,Jeffrey Michael,MD
Berardi,Richard Jr.,DO
Boni,Christopher M.,DO
Cajulis,Michelle C.,MD
Camacho,Ricardo Miguel,MD
Cheung,Deborah Jee Hae,MD
Cirangle,Lori Beth,MD
Colucio,Peter M.,MD
Dokko,John Hoon,DO
Feinberg,Craig Harlan,MD
Goldman-Gorelov,Victoria,MD
Harjani,Vashdeo Daulat,MD
Jeereddy,Bhavani,MD
Kapur,Sakshi,MD
Laudadio,Richard Dominick,MD
Mandal,Soma,MD
Mendiola,Redentor S. Jr.,MD
Meyer,Jacqueline Marie,MD
Mirchandani,Sunil,MD
Parikh,Ashish Dharnidhar,MD
Pettee,Brett,MD
Philips-Rodriguez,Dahlia,MD
Pilot,Richard,MD
Roth,Douglas M.,DO
Salomon,Pierre Richard,MD
Shridharani,Kanan Vasant,MD
Skrelja,Valerie,MD
Soto,Haydee M.,MD
Terry,Alon,MD
Tu,Chun,MD
Vecchi,Anthony R.,MD
Waqar,Anum Khan,DO
Wax,Michael B.,MD
Weisfuse,Judith E.,MD
Berlin
Chugh,Rajinder P.,MD
Parikh,Pratima D.,MD
Bernardsville
Costea-Misthos,Maria A.,MD
Dixon,Rosina B.,MD
Robertson,Janet A.,MD
Zimmerman,Thomas Jr.,MD

Blackwood
Deshields,Michael S.,MD
Doshi,Ila H.,MD
Frisoni,Lorenza,MD
Jain,Sneh,MD
Jehangir,Waqas,MD
Bloomfield
Abdelshahid,Mounir Y.,MD
Barbier,Andrea,DO
Bhalodia,Manish V.,MD
De Juliis,Aurora,MD
Kelly,John V. Jr.,MD
Narvaez,Normita G.,MD
Petracca,Louis J.,MD
Podkul,Richard L.,MD
Porcaro,Sabina M.,MD
Rana,Nareshkumar G.,MD
Saraiya,Nimit Nitin,MD
Shah,Neil J.,MD
Shah,Shrenik G.,MD
Bloomingdale
Jaaj,Hedoneia C.,MD
Boonton
Hammerman,Louis,MD
Moya-Mendez,Robert F.,MD
Renz,Patricia M.,MD
Scaduto,Philip M.,MD
Bordentown
Chokshi,Seema Patel,MD
Frascella,Rosemary C.,MD
Mahmud,Hamid,MD
Potharlanka,Prathibha R.,MD
Rossos,Nicholas A.,MD
Bound Brook
Byra,William M.,MD
Ehrlich,Harold B.,MD
Branchburg
Rego,Ramon,MD
Branchville
De Paola,Anthony A.,DO
Brick
Abbas,Shahida M.,MD
Abidi,Mutahir Ali,MD
Afiniwala,Swara,MD
Allen,Luzmary,DO
Babayev,Lily L.,MD
Bautista-Seares,Jessica M.,MD
Chiu,Kenny,MD
DeDona,Anna,DO
DeVita,Michael G.,DO
Donkor,Lawrence Tawiah,MD
Edelman,Carrie Allysia,MD
Georgy,Mary Sarah,MD
Gross,Tiberiu A.,MD
Gudapati,Raghu,MD
Hansalia,Riple Jayamtilal,MD
Hasan,Bassam I.,MD
Heacock,James K.,MD
Ilkhanizadeh,Ladan,MD
Infantolino,John A.,MD
Ital,Rosa,MD
Jain,Vishal K.,MD
Jarahian,George Jr.,MD
Karam,Edmund Thomas,MD
Kaur,Sundip,MD
Kianfar,Hormoz,MD
Lichnowski,Krzysztof B.,MD
Loman,Jeannette A.,DO
Lopez,John Pedro Francisco,MD
Magahis,Pacifico Aguila Jr.,MD
Montgomery,Karyn Mae,MD
Muralidharan,Soundari,MD
Musico,John J.,MD
Parikh,Sandip K.,MD
Patel,Hitesh Babubhai,MD
Rothberg,Michael Steven,MD
Rothman,Michael E.,MD
Salloum,Ahmad,MD
Sastri,Bhagyalak L.,MD
Seares,Petronilo Jr.,MD
Sher,Michael Laurence,MD
Singal,Presh,MD
Sy,Pacita C.,MD
Tapliga,Eduard Constantin,MD
Vida,Jay A.,DO
Weiner,Leonard B.,MD
Wolfman,Brian P.,MD
Yakubov,Boris,MD
Bridgeton
Ahmed,Ilyas,MD
Bagan,Stanley L.,MD

Candelore,Joseph Timothy Jr.,DO
Hanna,Ekram Labeb,MD
Hatzantonis,John Emanuel,MD
Hoey,Stephen E.,DO
Ismail,Elham Mohamed,MD
Jimenez-Silva,Jeanette,MD
Shields,Jack M.,MD
Struby,Christopher,DO
Bridgewater
Garcia,Calixto G.,DO
Irakam,Surya Prakash,MD
Khan,Amber Manzoor,MD
Mehta,Nehal L.,MD
Mehta,Sudhir H.,MD
Patel,Parag Bhailal,MD
Puskuri,Praneetha,MD
Qu,Peimei,MD
Sondhi,Manu,MD
Sun,Karen Hong Xue,MD
Sun,Lu Amy,MD
Trivedi,Shivang M.,MD
Wiesen,Robert S.,MD
Yalamanchi,Geeta,MD
Brigantine
Chaikin,Harry L.,MD
Dunn,Michael Joseph,MD
Gabros,David E.,MD
Glasser,Barry D.,MD
Rubin,Eric Howard,MD
Browns Mills
Christian,Sangita-Ann Justin,MD
Godfrey,John Trevor,DO
Huynh,Nha T.,DO
Lumia,Francis J.,MD
Maletzky,David Michael,DO
Martin,Andrew A.,MD
Murphy,David M.,MD
Nachodsky,Denise Marie,MD
Perry,Michael David,DO
Piawa,Dum Livinus,DO
Razvi,Batool,MD
Smith,Simon N.,DO
Summers,Michael Edward,DO
Wjasow,Christina,MD
Zazzali,Kathleen Mary,DO
Zinda,Ashley Beth,DO
Budd Lake
Brett,Brian P.,MD
Burlington
Aliferova,Tatyana N.,MD
Butt,Saeed Ahmed,MD
Dorfner,Scott M.,DO
Jordan,Daniel Robert,MD
Kamra,Roopama,MD
Burlington City
Sewell,Myron L.,MD
Butler
Hawruk,Elizabeth A.,MD
Parikh,Dhinoj M.,MD
Caldwell
Mayrowetz,Stanley,MD
Palla,Katharine Theresa,DO
Shah,Bankim,MD
Tartaglia,Marco,MD
Camden
Abouzgheib,Wissam B.,MD
Abraham,Aney M.,MD
Amin,Naeem Muhammad,MD
Aplin,Kara Stanig,MD
Arapurakal,Rajiv,MD
Atkuri,Rajeshwari Venkata,MD
Badr,Samer,MD
Bajaj,Jasmeet Singh,MD
Bakhshi,Aditya,MD
Barrington,Dorrie-Susan A.,MD
Borra,Gayatri D.,MD
Butt,Kambiz Reza,MD
Calder,Nicholas,MD
Cerceo,Elizabeth Ann,MD
Chasanov,William M. II,DO
Chaudhry,Kunal,MD
Coleman,Ashley J.,DO
Cooke,Jacqueline P.,MD
De La Torre,Pola,MD
Dragomir,Dan,MD
Elbaum,Philip,MD
Fabius,Daniel,DO
Fan,Lu,MD
Farajallah,Awny Sb,MD
Farmer,Alka Rajesh,MD
Fix,Cecilia Crane,MD
Gandhi,Snehal V.,MD

Physicians by Specialty and Town

Internal Medicine (cont)

Camden
Gordon,Marilyn L.,MD
Grana,Generosa,MD
Gue,Jean B.,MD
Gupta,Ravi,MD
Hagans,Iris,MD
Hanes,Douglas James,MD
Haroldson,Kathryn,MD
Headly,Anna,MD
Helmer,Diana Lynn,MD
Henry,Camille Angela Nicole,MD
Holtsclaw,John David,MD
Hwee,Lillian,DO
Kaplun,Olga,MD
Kass,Jonathan Eliot,MD
Khrizman,Polina,MD
Kim,Nami,DO
Kothari,Raksha Anil,MD
Kumar,Anand,MD
Kupersmith,Eric E.,MD
Kurnik,Brenda R.,MD
Latimore Collier,Sherita M.,MD
Logue,Raymond J.,MD
Mangold,Melissa Beth,DO
Martinez,Miguel E.,MD
Matos,Ninon,MD
Mazzarelli,Joanne K.,MD
McMackin,Paul Patrick,MD
McMillan,Tyler,MD
Melli,Jenny,MD
Milburn,Christopher Anthony,MD
Miles,Liesl Carey,MD
Miller,Ryan Christopher,MD
Misra,Sanjay,MD
Mookerjee,Anuradha Lele,MD
Moore,Tarquin Oliver,MD
Mungekar,Mangesh Mohan,MD
Nair,Nanda K.,DO
Negin,Nathan Samuel,MD
Newell,Glenn C.,MD
Nguy,Steven Tri,MD
Nguyen,Bao D.,MD
Oranu,Uzoma,MD
Orate-Dimapilis,Christina V.,MD
Patel,Devi,MD
Patel,Monika B.,MD
Patel,Ritesh,MD
Patel,Sharad D.,MD
Poddar,Sameer S.,MD
Pokuah,Marian O.,MD
Rachoin,Jean Sebastien K.,MD
Ramaswamy,Sunil Rajanna,MD
Rana,Nimra H.,MD
Rangwalla-Malickel,Inciya,DO
Rasheed,Sammar,MD
Richter,Douglas Martin,MD
Rosenheck,Justin Philip,DO
Samaha,Simon J.,MD
Schmidt,Ryan Bausch,MD
Sevrin,Amanda Hope,MD
Sharma,Meena R.,MD
Shklar,David Lewis,MD
Siddique,Mahbubur Rahman,MD
Sikand,Seema,MD
Singh,Sukhjeet,DO
Sirover,William D.,MD
Somer,Robert A.,MD
Sussman,Emily Melissa,DO
Swarup,Subir,DO
Szawlewicz,Stephen J.,MD
Taylor,Michael,MD
Thawani,Kalpana,MD
Topalian,Simon Kevork,MD
Troyanovich,Esteban F.,MD
Urbano,Frank Louis,MD
Utreras,Juan S.,MD
Velayadikot,Deepa Nandakumar,MD
Yadav,Jagdish P.,MD
Yang,Jun,MD
Young,Jimmie,MD
Zafar,Fateen D.,MD
Zee,Pamela A.,MD

Cape May
Mehta,Subhash G.,MD
Rothman,Craig Michael,MD

Cape May Court House
Aversa,Jeffrey Martin,MD
Childs,Arthur L.,DO
Gandhi,Shveta V.,DO
Hong,John S.,MD
Lee,Edward Howe,MD

Niewiadomski,Edward J.,MD
Osgood,Eric,MD
Pandya,Melind Rasik,DO
Patel,Jayeshkumar Kiritkumar,MD
Shah,Chetan K.,DO
Stave,Jeffrey R.,DO
Varner,Philip T.,DO

Carneys Point
Salem,Mohamed M.,MD

Carteret
Behman,Daisy M.,MD
Behman,Tamer Abdelmonam,MD
Darvish,Arash,MD
Goraya,Sukhjender,MD
Kalika,Sanna,MD
Mavani,Nagindas V.,MD
Riar,Sandeep Singh,MD

Cedar Grove
Chaturvedi,Ratan B.,MD
Huang,Kuei-Huang,MD
Mirza,Muhammad A.,MD
Morgan,James Peter,MD
Rambaran,Hayman Kumar,MD
Rambaran,Naipaul,MD

Cedar Knolls
Fuchs,Eliyahu Elliot,MD
Hussain,Adnan,MD
James,David Joel,MD
Mysh,Dmitry,MD
Oei,Erwin John,MD
Pasik,Deborah,MD
Singh,Vandana,DO
Som,Sumit,MD

Chatham
Collins,Neal,MD
Pincus,Jillian R.,MD
Rodriguez,Lauren C.,MD

Cherry Hill
Ali,Tuba Muhammad,MD
Antonelli,William M.,DO
Avetian,Garo Charles,DO
Bastien,Arnaud,MD
Chen,Shwu-Miin Y.,MD
Damerau,Keith R.,MD
Dey,Chaitali,MD
Driscoll,Michael Joseph,DO
Dructor,Lisa Ann,DO
Epelboim Feldman,Joyce,MD
Favata,Elissa A.,MD
Galabi,Michael,MD
Gerber,Steven Lewis,MD
Gerber,Susan Marie,MD
Gooberman,Bruce D.,MD
Halickman,Isaac J.,MD
Hanna,Gamil Sabet Fawzy,MD
Jafry,Behjath,MD
Josephson,Tina M.,MD
Kalu,Eke N.,MD
Kemps,Anton P.,MD
Kirby,John A.,MD
Klausman,Kenneth Barry,MD
Malli,Dipakkumar Purushott,MD
McMahon,Mary Ann Patricia,MD
Molino,Richard,MD
Monari-Sparks,Mary Joan,MD
Morgan,Farah Hena,MD
Naware,Sanya,MD
Nordin,Brittany N.,DO
Nugent,Thomas Rone,MD
Palli,Vasu Motu,DO
Pecarsky,Jason Todd,MD
Rosenthal,Brett Samson,DO
Rozengarten,Kimberly Irene,DO
Saia,Bryan Edward,DO
Schiller,Terence G.,MD
Shah,Anish Pravin,MD
Shehata,Ahmed Abdelhalim,MD
Sherman,Anthony,MD
Singh-Mohapatra,Sherry,MD
Smeglin,Anthony G.,MD
Stein,Alan David,MD
Stom,Mary C.,MD
Todt,Mark J.,MD
Torigian,Christine V.,MD
Wenger,Christopher D.,DO
Zander,Judith W.,MD
Zanger,Ron,MD
Zaslavsky,Alexander,MD

Chester
Chanin,Alan H.,MD
Davis,Glenn A.,MD

Sidhu,Gurpreet Singh,MD

Clark
Acocella,Michael A.,DO
Banayat,Geronimo Jr.,MD
Barry,Peter Francis,DO
Chudasama,Neelesh Lalji,MD
Ford,Stephen D.,MD
Goldstein,Alan F.,MD
Hwang,Cheng-Hong,DO
Kang,David H.,MD
Kornicki,Janusz S.,MD
Kudryk,Alexander B.,MD
Levin,Brandt M.,MD
Patel,Amish Thakor,DO
Prasad,Sudhanshu,MD
Vijayakumar,Asha M.,MD

Cliffside Park
Friedman,Bernard,MD
Hamada,Murray S.,MD
Joseph,Merab,MD
Korenfeld,Alexander,MD
Korenfeld,Yelena,MD
Master,Violet S.,MD
Righthand,Richard N.,MD

Clifton
Alday,Arnold M.,MD
Berkel,Reyhan,MD
Blanco,Renato J.,MD
Boutros,Maged T.,MD
Brancato,Jaclyn,DO
Cecere,Antoinette M.,MD
Coleman,Scott L.,MD
De La Cruz,Angel Ramon,MD
Debell,David Anthony,MD
Diar Bakerli,Hala,MD
Dixon,George C.,MD
Ferrazzo-Weller,Marissa G.,DO
Gajdos,Robert M.,MD
Ganesan,Azhagasund,MD
Gellis,Dana B.,MD
Goldberg,Marc A.,MD
Goyal,Neil Kamal,MD
Graber,David J.,MD
Hajjar,Bassam,MD
Humera,Rafath Khatoon,MD
Huskowski,Piotr,MD
Jacknin,Mark A.,DO
Jawetz,Harold I.,MD
Jo,Young I.,MD
Kelleher,Maureen Michelle,MD
Korenblit,Pearl,MD
Krisa,Paul C.,MD
Krutak-Krol,Halina M.,MD
Lewko,Michael P.,MD
Llacuna,Florencio Jr.,MD
Mekkawy,Ahmed A.,MD
Murillo,Narcisa E.,MD
Najjar,Joe E.,MD
Narang,Sudershan,MD
Nop,Mallory,MD
Nwosu-Nelson,Joel E.,MD
O'Brien,Joseph Patrick,MD
Onat,Nermi,MD
Onyeador,Beatrice Ogbonne,MD
Pensabeni Jasper,Tiziana,MD
Porras,Cornelio J.,MD
Porter,Joseph M.,MD
Rana,Najmul,MD
Raval,Parthiv V.,MD
Rey,Ricardo,MD
Reyes,Emmanuel,MD
Rizvi,Syed M.,MD
Rubino,Gennaro,MD
Russo,Melchiorre J.,MD
Sahu,Anand P.,MD
Sahu,Sharad,MD
Sandler,Rebecca Ellen,MD
Schactman,Brian,MD
Singh,Sarva D.,MD
Torres,Catherine P.,MD
Turner,James William III,MD
Urena,Julio H.,MD
Wooton,Robert P. Jr.,MD

Clinton
Braff,Ricky A.,MD
Lifchus Ascher,Rebecca Jean,MD
May,Philip B.,MD
Torrens,Javier I.,MD

Closter
Dhorajia,Shruti P.,DO
Farooki,Zahid A.,MD
Lee,Soo Gyung,MD

Collingswood
Corbett,Brian Joseph,DO
Lauer,Marshall F.,MD
McAllister,Susan Coutinho,MD

Colonia
Partenope,Nicholas A.,MD

Colts Neck
Gualberti,Joann,MD
Gualberti-Girgis,Lisa,MD
Katz,Howard A.,MD
Mankarios,Farag Amin Farag,MD
Patel,Shital,MD
Yelchur,Anuradha,MD

Columbia
Grote,Walter R.,DO

Cranbury
Hebbalalu,Praphulla,MD
Nagulapalli,Chaitanya,MD

Cranford
Singh,Iqbal K.,MD
Singh,Mohinder P.,MD
Toro Echague,Bernardo J.,MD

Cream Ridge
Jivani,Rasik M.,MD
Rosengarten,Herbert H.,MD

Cresskill
Kochlatyi,Sergei G.,MD
Subramanian,Kavitha,MD

Dayton
Casper,Robert J.,MD
Sharma,Shivani,MD

Delran
Basara,Matthew Jr.,MD
Berna,Renee Ann,MD
Kabel,Stephen E.,DO
Mirson,Sofiya,MD
Pelimskaya,Lutsiya S.,MD
Rausch,Debora Anne,MD
Squires,Leslie S.,MD

Demarest
Farooki,Adil,MD

Denville
Aggarwal,Arvind Kumar,DO
Banu,Dana R.,MD
Barbarito,Edward Joseph,MD
Cheng,Yihong Henry,MD
Collum,Robert G.,MD
Connolly,Melissa Jane,MD
Gerges,Christine Nabil,DO
Gironta,Michael Gerard,DO
Goldshlack,Jack S.,DO
Kalaydjian,Garine,MD
Kapadia,Rina,MD
Levitz,Jason Sanford,MD
Levy,Seth Evan,MD
Lopez,Jose M.,MD
Mandel,Gilbert B.,MD
Maniar,Sonali R.,MD
Mariwalla,Kiran,MD
Masone,Daniel A.,MD
Mintz,Bruce L.,DO
Mintz,Shari Nan,MD
Nicolai,Michael,MD
Reiter,Barry A.,MD
Ricks,Jason D.,MD
Ruben,Yesudas,MD
Sharma,Swati,MD
Sheppell,Arthur L.,MD
Stansbury,Frederick H.,DO

Deptford
Aquilino,Linda Kristine,DO

Dover
Balaji,Mini,MD
Gannu,Rajyalakshmi M.,MD
Golombek,Steven J.,MD
Li,Lisa,DO
Panchal,Rupa Jaydip,MD
Ramirez-Alexander,Rina M.,MD
Rosales Zincone,Jeannette A.,MD
Schonfield,Leah R.,DO
Studint,Erika B.,MD
Udani,Neil P.,MD
Zorrilla,Lilian,MD

Dumont
Hoffman,Esther Sima,DO

Dunellen
Karu,Moiz S.,MD

East Brunswick
Abdelmalek,Moheb S.,MD
Akyar,Selma Ender,MD
Ales,Kathy L.,MD

Altobelli,Anthony III,MD
Amara,Sreenivasrao,MD
Balog,Joshua David,MD
Basalaev,Misha,MD
Burghli,Rena F.,DO
Chen,Karl Timothy,MD
Chilukuri,Neelima,MD
Creel,Marilyn U. Baruiz,MD
DeMoss,Jeanne Lorraine,DO
Fanous,Venis F.,MD
Fischler,David Ross,MD
Friedman,Inga,MD
Gabriel,Ahab M.,MD
Ghobraiel,Raafat Tawfek,MD
Grinblat,Inessa,MD
Gurland,Ira Alan,MD
Habib,Michael George,MD
Kapchits,Elmira,MD
Kaplan,Murray C.,MD
Katseva,Alla,MD
Kim,Christian C. K.,MD
Kolasa,Christopher,MD
Kulischenko,Alexander W.,MD
Kulischenko,Idelma,MD
Lee,Anna F.,MD
Li,Dena Yuyun,MD
Liu,Jenny,MD
Maimon,Olga M.,MD
Morgan,Mena M.,MD
Morgan,Nashaat L.,MD
Morgan,Suzana Emil Anwer,MD
Moussa,Alber Helmy,MD
Rao,Aruna,MD
Redel,Henry,MD
Scheiner,Marc A.,MD
Sharma,Adity,MD
Simkhayev,Lev Samsonovi,MD
Sinha,Ashok Kumar,MD
Tadros,Wagih F.,MD
Terranova,Matthew Patrick Jr,DO
Tucci,Mauro A. III,MD
Wertheim,Ofer Avi,MD
Yager,Scott,MD

East Hanover
Felser,James M.,MD
Grande,Nancy J.,MD
Hamed,Kamal Abdel-Jabbar,MD
Liang,Liang,MD
Livote,Joanne,MD
Prestifilippo,Judith A.,MD
Tran,Ly-Le,MD

East Orange
Antoine,Alycia N.,MD
Antoine,Roland,MD
Bawa,Radhika,MD
Bishara,Christine,MD
Blaivas,Allen J.,DO
Cahiwat,Ramona N.,MD
Chang,Victor Tsu-Shih,MD
Chatha,Uzma Arshad,MD
Chi,Jinhan,MD
Clarke,Robert Anthony,MD
Cort,James T.,MD
Costa,Antoinette G.,MD
Cytryn,Arthur S.,MD
Hemsley,Michael,MD
Hinds,Audrey M.,MD
Kania,Nirmala R.,MD
Machiedo,Christine C.,MD
Maddali,Radhika,MD
Maddali,Sarala K.,MD
Miller,Marilyn Ann,MD
Nygaard,Torbjoern G.,MD
Ohri,Renu,MD
Rafiuddin,Shaleeza,MD
Ragavan,Vijay,MD
Raghavan,Padma,MD
Raju,Govinda S.,MD
Ramdas,Kumar,MD
Salerno,Alexander Gerard,MD
Savaille,Juanito E.,DO
Seth,Sarwan K.,MD
Skurnick,Blanche Jacqueline,MD
Srinivas,Shanthi,MD
Stark,Richard C.,MD
Stein,Bernardo,MD
Stevens,John M.,MD
Strauss,Walter D.,MD
Sunderam,Darshi,MD
Taitt,Beverley B.,MD
Taylor,Douglas A.,MD
Viswanatha,Amrutha,MD

Yarus,Christine V.,MD
Yeldandi,Aruna G.,MD
Yook,Soonjae,MD
Yudd,Michael,MD

East Rutherford
Coyle,Genoveva F.,MD
Dituro,Joseph William,MD
Kalra,Ritesh,MD
Popa,Marcela M.,MD
Scolamiero,John C.,MD

East Windsor
Bowers,Gabriela W.,MD
Cimafranca,Daniel L.,MD
Dhar,Vasudha,MD
Hanif,Ghalia,MD
Kunamneni,Katie Elizabeth,MD
Madapati,Indira,MD
Thomas,Brian David,MD
Valcarcel,Raul,MD
Wong,Christopher K.,MD

Eatontown
Arbes,Spiros M.,MD
Ashok,Manjula,MD
Barnickel,Paul W.,MD
Carideo,Ida M.,MD
Churgin,Warren K.,MD
Desai,Gautam J.,MD
Einbinder,Lynne C.,MD
Hanna,Manar H.,MD
Haratz,Alan B.,MD
Khulusi,Nami,MD
Kosinski,Robert M.,MD
Morris,Sarah A.,MD
Nivera,Noel Taroy,MD
Patel,Ashish Bhasker,MD
Patton,Chandler D.,MD
Peeples,Charles B.,MD
Ramachandra Rao,Vanie S.,MD
Recho,Marielle,MD
Saybolt,Matthew Douglas,MD
Sridar,Buvaneswari,MD
Usman,Mohammed Haris Umer,MD

Edgewater
Alvarez-Segovia,Lucia M.,MD
Portilla,Diana M.,MD
Rotoli,Domenico,DO
Shin,John Jung Hoon,MD

Edison
Abdi,Zahra Jabeen,MD
Adabala,Ramesh,MD
Ahmad,Nausher,MD
Amjad,Maqsood,MD
Arora-Khera,Shruti,MD
Aurilio,Joseph P.,MD
Bai,Flora,MD
Bangalore,Ramamurthy L.,MD
Bhakey,Girija G.,MD
Bhalla,Meenu Gogia,MD
Blum,Paul A.,MD
Bonk,Rosemarie A.,MD
Bruzzi-Ehrlich,Diane,MD
Bullock,Richard B.,MD
Calabrese,David,MD
Canavan,Brian F.,DO
Casale,Lisa M.,MD
Cassidy,Thomas J.,MD
Chen,Michael T.,MD
Chung,Inyoung,MD
Dantuluri,Hemamalini,MD
DeSilva,Derrick Jr.,MD
DeSimone,Luca,MD
Desai,Sagar R.,MD
Desai,Vinay M.,MD
Dippl,Julia M.,MD
Estrellas,Bernabe A.,MD
Felzenberg,Emily R.,DO
Gandhi,Nabila Asif,MD
Ganeshamurthy,Agrahara,MD
Gbadamosi,Sikiru Aderoju,MD
Hariharan,Subramanian,MD
Hassan,Syed R.,MD
Jagamony,Sandhya,MD
Jana,Kumar P.,MD
Joshi,Archana N.,MD
Kasuri,Jasbir K.,MD
Khan,Basma,MD
Khetani,Manish P.,MD
Kim,Stanley S.,MD
Kleshchelskaya,Valeria,MD
Kumar,Arvind,MD
Kumar,Radha,MD
Kuza,Malgorzata W.,MD

Lee,Hyok Yop,MD
Leighton,Harmony J.,DO
Li,Meihong,MD
Li,Xiang,MD
Lin,Ruth Ann,MD
Long,George W.,MD
Memon,Mohammad Khalil,MD
Misko,Gary J. Jr.,MD
Moray,Nandini K.,MD
Napiorkowski,Eva M.,MD
Nisar,Mohammed P.,MD
Nisar,Shiraz Ahmed,MD
Nowell,Martha A.,MD
Pamerla,Mohan Ramkumar,MD
Patel,Bhupendra C.,MD
Patel,Hetal Mahendra,MD
Patel,Indravadan T.,MD
Patel,Jayendra M.,MD
Patel,Mukesh M.,MD
Patel,Narendra K.,MD
Patel,Pankajkumar Vasantlal,MD
Patel,Pulin H.,MD
Patel,Rajendra Harmanbhai,MD
Patel,Shefali S.,MD
Payumo,Gene Louie,MD
Penn,James R.,MD
Piperi,Vincent D.,MD
Poco,Bernardo A.,MD
Prasad,Niloo,MD
Rappai,James K.,MD
Reisler,Scott,MD
Saini,Amarjit K.,MD
Sappal,Baljit S.,MD
Shah,Nehabahen V.,MD
Shah,Pooja,MD
Shah,Taral Jobanputra,MD
Shastry,Jyothsna S.,MD
Shen,Lijing,MD
Sinha,Anubha,MD
Snyder,Craig Adam,MD
Sutaria,Samir Hasmukh,MD
Tawde,Darshana Prafullaraj,MD
Taylor,Marian L.,MD
Thakur,Shubhangi J.,MD
Tirunahari,Vijaya Latha,MD
Unni,Nisha,MD
Upadhyay,Hinesh Natwarlal,MD
Uthappa,Machia M.,MD
Vaidya,Ketankumar N.,MD
Velmahos,Vasilios,MD
Wolf,Barry Z.,MD
Zhang,Hao,MD

Egg Harbor
Rizvi,Faraz,MD

Egg Harbor Township
Angamuthu,Akilandanayaki,MD
Bolich,Christopher W.,DO
Chawla,Neha Roshan,MD
Diener,Melissa Ann,MD
Kuponiyi,Olatunji P.,MD
Makar,George A.,MD
Musarra,Anthony Mark,MD
Paradela,Ephrem Hector,MD
Patel,Neha Hector,MD
Soucier,Ronald J.,DO
Twardzik,Jennifer Lynn,DO
Unuigbe,Augustine A.,MD
Unuigbe,Florence,MD

Elizabeth
Ahmed,Saira N.,MD
Baig,Khadija,MD
Batta,Sanjay,MD
Benalcazar-Puga,Luis Marcelo,MD
Bilusic,Marijo,MD
Blaszka,Frederick M.,MD
Butler,Jill Kraft,MD
Chauhan,Chetankumar K.,MD
Chirino,Maria E.,MD
Cholankeril,Mary G.,MD
Cholankeril,Thressiamma M.,MD
Chua,Jose Jr.,MD
De La Cruz,Flavia Annette,MD
Delgado,Jorge L.,MD
Dragun,Elena,MD
Eltom,Alaeldin Abdalla,MD
Garcia,Raul Angel,DO
Garg,Delyse,MD
Goodgold,Abraham,MD
Huda,Rafeul,MD
Jaffry,Syed Ali Hasan,MD
Jimenez,Arnaldo M.,MD
Khan,Sabeen,MD

Khimani,Karim J.,MD
Lin,Chi-Hsiung,MD
Lontai,Peter,MD
Lu,Andrew Hong,MD
Mansour,Ashraf Hakeem,MD
Mathure,Mekhala A.,MD
McAnally,James F.,MD
Mejias,Erenio,MD
Munoz,Francisco,MD
Munoz,Guillermo A.,DO
Nelson,Homer L.,MD
Nielson,Rosemarie,DO
Oberoi,Mandeep S.,MD
Othman,Essam Abdou,MD
Patel,Jalpa S.,MD
Patel,Manish Sureshbhai,MD
Patel,Mayuri H.,MD
Patel,Rambhai C.,MD
Pattathil,Jean Catherine,MD
Perez,James,MD
Rosefort,Laury,MD
Rowen,Adam J.,MD
Sebastian,Suniti,MD
Sharma,Rekha,MD
Shen,Jung-San,MD
Soltys,Remigiusz,MD
Somma,Edward A.,MD
Suleiman,Addi,MD
Surana,Gautam C.,MD
Tan,Pilar O.,MD
Thalody,George V.,MD
Thalody,Lucyamma,MD
Thalody,Usha George,MD
Vaiana,Paul,MD
Vallejo,Edgardo C.,MD
Verzosa,Oscar E.,MD
Walia,Jasjit S.,MD
Zaboski,Michael R.,MD

Elmer
Flynn,Patrick Joseph,DO

Elmwood Park
Grodman,Marc D.,MD
Levan,Ellen,MD
Uychich,Priscilla M.,DO
Weisberger,James D.,MD

Emerson
Ali,Amy G.,MD
Avezzano,Eric S.,MD
Bhandari,Bhavik M.,MD
Briker,Alan J.,MD
Broussard,Crystal N.,MD
D'Aquino,Carol Madeleine,MD
Flanzman,Susan Amy,MD
Fleischer,Joseph S.,MD
Glaubiger,Carol,MD
Gokhale,Kedar Arvind,MD
Griggs,Allen R.,DO
Kim,Jeffrey S.,MD
Koo,Bon Chang Andy,MD
Lan,Vivian En-Wei,MD
Lin,George Szuwei,MD
Mastrianno,Frank L.,MD
Motiwala,Neeta R.,MD
Potack,Jonathan Zachary,MD
Thum,Robert G.,MD
Volpe,Anthony P.,MD

Englewood
Abramovici,Mirel I.,MD
Andron,Richard I.,MD
Barnes,Tanganyika A.,DO
Benoff,Brian Alan,MD
Beri,Samarth,MD
Brauntuch,Glenn R.,MD
Breitbart,Seth Ilias,MD
Brouk,Alla,MD
Bryan,Craigh Keith,MD
Carter,Brittany Nicole,MD
Casser,Michael E.,MD
Chen,Tzu-Shao,MD
Cholhan,Ruth C.,MD
Clifford,Susan Michelle,MD
Crooks,Michael H.,MD
Davis,Lawrence Jay,MD
De Rose,Marielaina S.,MD
Djebiyan,Eli S.,MD
Engler,Mitchell S.,MD
Fayngersh,Alla,MD
Fleischer,Jessica Beth,MD
Friedman,Alan Mark,MD
Frier,Steven F.,MD
Frisch,Katalin Andrea,MD
Galumyan,Yelena V.,MD

Physicians by Specialty and Town

Internal Medicine (cont)

Englewood
- Gandhi, Nisha R., MD
- Geller, Judy Irene, MD
- Gianatiempo, Carmine, MD
- Glassman, Adam M., MD
- Gottdiener, Alexandra H., MD
- Grodstein, Gerald P., MD
- Gura, Russell Saul, MD
- Hamilton, Monique S., MD
- Ho, Eddie Kasing, MD
- Jan, Louis C. W., MD
- Jathavedam, Ashwin, MD
- Joshi, Nandita, MD
- Kaim, Oleg, MD
- Kaplan, Sarah, MD
- Kapoor, Radhika, DO
- Katz, Doron Zvi, MD
- Katz, Manuel David, MD
- Kim, Sung Hyun, MD
- Laiosa, Catherine Virginia, MD
- Latorre, Rafael, MD
- Levine, Selwyn Eric, MD
- Loewinger, Michael Brian, MD
- Lorton, Julie Lytton, MD
- Malovany, Robert J., MD
- Miguel, Eduardo E., MD
- Nemirovsky, Dmitry, MD
- Okeke, Ngozi C., MD
- Oo, Hnin Hnin, MD
- Paley, Jeffrey Evan, MD
- Park, Anne June, DO
- Pattner, Austin M., MD
- Ramsetty, Sabena Karina, MD
- Reeves, Lisa Joyce, MD
- Sapienza, Mark Santo, MD
- Seferian, Mihran A., MD
- Serrano, Jesus Canoza, MD
- Shammash, Jonathan Baruch, MD
- Shatzkes, Joseph Aaron, MD
- Shin, Peter Young, MD
- Silberstein, Stuart L., MD
- Simon, Clifford J., MD
- Smith, Ebben Will, MD
- Stepanyuk, Olena, MD
- Sun, Sung Wook, MD
- Tartakovsky, Irina, MD
- Taw, Julie, MD
- Thomas, Shilpa Ani, MD
- Tlamsa, Aileen P., MD
- Volokhov, Alexey, MD
- Wasserman, Kenneth H., MD
- Ye, Sheng H., MD
- Yee, Sau Yan, MD
- Zelkowitz, Marc, MD

Englewood Cliffs
- Kim, Dong Hyun, MD
- Ko, Pan Sok, MD
- Lee, Chang Woo, MD
- Yu, Fei, MD

Englishtown
- Covalesky, John, DO
- Gupta, Narendra K., MD
- Salter-Lewis, Cynthia, MD

Ewing
- Ali, Sara Inayet, MD
- Dundeva Baleva, Pavlinka V., MD
- Gettys, Jacqueline Brown, MD
- Kolander, Scott A., MD
- Kolman-Taddeo, Diana, MD
- Kudakachira, Shaismy, DO
- Meer, Shahid B., MD
- Pierrot, Paul H., MD
- Protter, Randi R., MD
- Williams, Eric James, MD

Fair Haven
- Hayward, Denise H., MD
- Krisza, Mary L., MD
- Nardone, Danielle J., DO
- Pamintuan, Dominic C., MD

Fair Lawn
- Aquino, Christine E., MD
- Balonze, Karen T., MD
- Batchelor, Christopher D. Jr., MD
- Berman, Lawrence J., MD
- Bromberg, Assia, MD
- Cappitelli, Jack V., MD
- Cho, Soung Ick, MD
- Clifford, Eileen M., MD
- Deitz, Justina May, DO
- Donkina, Luiza, MD
- Farooqui, Syeda Saleha, MD
- Feiner, Shoshana N., MD
- Hossain, Nazma A., MD
- Lehrman, Mark Leonard, MD
- Levykh-Chase, Rena E., MD
- Lishko, Olga V., MD
- Logvinenko, Nina V., MD
- Narymsky, Lyudmila M., MD
- Patel, Dushyant Rameshchandra, MD
- Qipo, Andi, MD
- Reyn, Mark, MD
- Rizkalla, Suzette, MD
- Rizzo, Robert Anthony, MD
- Roman, David, MD
- Rudzinskiene, Aliona, MD
- Safa, Nina, MD
- Scerbo, Ernest John, MD
- Sen, Sourav, MD
- Sheth, Meetkumar Tusharbhai, MD
- Singh, Amrita Kaur, MD
- Syed, Zainab, MD
- Velez, Henry, MD
- Virk, Hartaj Singh, MD
- Wertenteil, Mark Elliot, MD

Fairfield
- Bhatt, Rupal S., MD
- Bhatt, Shirish Vinayak, MD
- Chen, Bonnie L., MD
- Howe, Thomas Arthur, MD
- Zhukova, Irina, DO

Fanwood
- Brodman, Richard R., MD
- Jamdar, Niteen Subhash, MD
- Lewis, Thomas Peter, MD

Farmingdale
- Kelemen, Ina J., MD
- Ornstein, Mark W., MD

Flanders
- Chaudhari, Anuja Parikh, DO
- Chaudhari, Suvid, DO
- Mercado, Alex M., MD
- Pathak, Rajiv J., MD

Flemington
- Broslawski, Gregory E., DO
- Cao, Lan, MD
- Elnahar, Yaser, MD
- Granato, Anthony Alexander, MD
- Haddad, Sohail G., MD
- Khan, Saima, MD
- Lansang, Martin Fidel, MD
- Lazarus, David S., MD
- Lind, Robert Michael, MD
- Mak, Mimi, MD
- Miele, Bevon D., MD
- Novy, Donald S., MD
- Pistun, Oleksandr, MD
- Quinn, Brian Michael, MD
- Saxena, Amita, MD
- Shaber, Marc L., MD
- Storch, Marc I., MD
- Surapanani, Devi, MD
- Veeraraghavan, Gowri, MD

Florham Park
- Alberto, Kezia J., MD
- Blumberg, Darren Reich, MD
- Castellano, Charles C., MD
- Chandwani, Ashish, MD
- Cohen, Liliana, MD
- Das, Mohan P., MD
- Di Giacomo, Eric D., MD
- Di Ruggiero, Roger P., MD
- Dicenzo-Flynn, Carla F., MD
- Freid, Robert S., MD
- Goodman, Jeffrey W., MD
- Hooda, Anjali, MD
- Kilkenny-Trainor, Kerryann A., MD
- Kissin, Anna, MD
- Klees, Julia E., MD
- Kunjukutty, Felix, MD
- Li, Zhexiang, MD
- Lyman, Neil W., MD
- Maron, Scott Michael, MD
- Olesnicky, Mark T., MD
- Pajaro, Rafael E., MD
- Pally, Steven Arthur, DO
- Paulina, Arthur Jr., MD
- Pinel Villalobos, Silvia P., DO
- Rodrigues, Anisha, MD
- Roytman, Peter, MD
- Sabnani-Nagella, Kavita R., MD
- Saldarini, John Christopher, MD
- Shubeck, Caroline A., MD
- Soleymani, Taraneh, MD
- Storch, Kenneth J., MD
- Tamres, David Michael, MD
- Tiongco, Judith Perlas, MD
- Viscuso, Ronald L., MD
- Zenenberg, Robert D., DO

Fords
- Gil, Constante, MD
- Sharma, Madho K., MD

Forked River
- Bhiro, Peter Rajendra, DO
- Crisan, Liviu C., MD
- Ende, Theodore, DO
- Jannone, Joel P., MD
- Tubilleja, Nina Lapidario, MD

Fort Dix
- Patel, Pradip M., MD

Fort Lee
- Bai, Sammy S., MD
- Feller, Matthew F., MD
- Girshovich, Irina, MD
- Hernandez, Michael Dennis, MD
- Kalayjian, Tro, DO
- Sabater, Pilar, MD
- Shapnik, Bella, MD
- Wang, Kyu Sung, MD
- Yang, Yulong, MD

Franklin
- Patel, Pravinbhai C., MD

Franklin Lakes
- Krutchik, Allan N., MD
- Sandoval, Ramon Antonio, MD
- Sutter, David Brand, MD

Franklin Park
- Chen, Julie Eveline, MD
- Jacobs, David S A, MD
- Sanghui, Sarika Patel, DO

Freehold
- Barofsky, Kenneth D., MD
- Bhasin, Atul, MD
- Brown, Colin Christopher, MD
- Cohen, Aly G., MD
- Coppolino, Frank P., MD
- Croce, Salvatore A., MD
- Donde, Dilip M., MD
- El Kadi, Hisham S., MD
- Fischkoff, James Daniel, MD
- Garmkhorani, Abolghassem, MD
- Geller, Arthur J., MD
- Giannone, Dean Francis, MD
- Gonzales, Antero B., MD
- Gopal, Indumathi, MD
- Gruber, Todd A., MD
- Heitzer, Frederic M., MD
- Kaga, Mira Kamal, MD
- Komboz, Rita Fares, MD
- Krakauer, Randall Sheldon, MD
- Kroll, Mark S., MD
- Kudipudi, Ramanasri V., MD
- Lage, Susan Marie, DO
- Luparello, Paul J., MD
- Majumdar, Shikha, MD
- Medasani, Kiran M., MD
- Melka, Berhanu Gossaye, MD
- Menon, Divya, MD
- Najmey, Sawsan S., MD
- Nijhawan, Minakshi, MD
- Paulin, Cesar M., MD
- Petcu, Alexandru, MD
- Restua, Nestor S., MD
- Rose, T., MD
- Ross, William H., DO
- Shah, Anand Subhash, MD
- Sharma, Anil K., MD
- Sharobeem, Andrew Mena, DO
- Sojka, Leslie W., MD
- Sowemimo, Fiolakemi O., MD
- Vizzoni, Joseph Anthony, MD
- Weinstein, Benjamin, MD
- Werber, John Frank, MD
- Zirkman, Daniel M., MD

Galloway
- Aridi, Imad M., MD
- Brown, Lemarra Rena, DO
- Dasondi, Vivekkumar V., MD
- Ganzon-Zampino, Gilda E., MD
- Kim, Duk Hee, MD
- Kirchner, Brian K., MD
- Lieberman, Alexander III, MD
- Memon, Moomal, MD
- Miao, Sun, MD
- Patel, Vineshkumar K., MD
- Petruzzi, Nicholas Joseph, MD
- Selina, Elena V., MD
- Sivaraman, Sivashankar, MD
- Sperling, Michael James, MD
- Zampino, Dominick J., DO

Garwood
- Yavorsky, John M., DO

Glen Ridge
- Bambhroliya, Grishma, MD
- Cheema, Asad Mushtaq, MD
- Daniskas, Efthymios I., MD
- Levai, Robert Joseph, MD
- Minano, Cecilia, MD
- Molinaro, Michael Louis, MD
- Safirstein, Benjamin Herbert, MD
- Urrutia, Ellen E., MD
- Weber, Barry Joseph, MD
- Woroch, Paul, MD

Glen Rock
- Carlson, Sandra Regina, MD
- Sarkar, Arunima, MD
- Tilson, Morris A., MD

Gloucester City
- Hyman, Daniel J., DO

Green Brook
- Ahmed, Syed F., MD
- Chafos, John N., MD
- Devarajan, Anandan, MD
- Khalil, Suzan Y., MD
- Sharon, Yoram, DO
- Strumkovsky, Lyalya Olga, MD

Guttenberg
- Santana, Jose O., MD

Hackensack
- Acevedo Beltran, Edrik Josue, MD
- Ahmed, Suhel Hussain, MD
- Alter, Robert S., MD
- Amuluru, Jaladurga P., MD
- Anchipolovsky, Natalia, DO
- Baer, Aryeh Zvi, MD
- Bajaj, Nikki, MD
- Balani, Bindu Anand, MD
- Balasingham, Chithra, MD
- Cai, Kimberly, MD
- Campanella, Anthony J. Jr., MD
- Chandra, Sweta, MD
- Chatelain, Martin P., MD
- Chavez, Laura Monica, DO
- Chhabra, Anjana R., MD
- Cohen, Michael B., MD
- D'Alessandro, Daniel J., MD
- Donato, Michele Lyne, MD
- Ephrat, Moshe, MD
- Farber, Michael Seth, MD
- Felsen, Alan K., MD
- Fink, Andrew Nathen, MD
- Friedman, Samuel H., MD
- Gardin, Julius Markus, MD
- Gayed, Noha, MD
- Gellrick, Judith C., MD
- Germinario, Carla Ann, MD
- Goldfarb, Adam S., MD
- Gong, Bing, MD
- Gonzalez, Abel Ernesto, MD
- Goy, Andre Henri, MD
- Graham, Deena Mary-Atieh, MD
- Grigoryan, Galina, MD
- Gunadasa, Susanthi N., MD
- Gupta, Kavita, MD
- Gutierrez, Martin Eduardo, MD
- Howard, Brandon Trevor, MD
- Ibrahim, Ehab Fawzy, MD
- Jamal, Sameer Mustafa, MD
- Jennis, Andrew A., MD
- Kahyaoglu, Aret Y., MD
- Kasuni, William Tatsuo, MD
- Koduah, Doris Afreh, MD
- Kowal, Timothy S., MD
- Kurian, Helena, MD
- Lambrinos, Vasilios, MD
- Lee, Robert Chu-Du, MD
- Leslie, Lori Ann, MD
- Li, Jianfeng, MD
- Lin, Judy Mei-Chia, MD
- Lodhavia, Jitendra J., MD
- Manchireddy, Suman, MD
- Manji, Hussain Mehdi, MD
- Muttana, Renu Devi, MD
- Oguayo, Kevin Nnaemeka, MD
- Okoye-Okuzu, Enuma I., MD

Pagan, Juan, MD
Parmar, Madhu, MD
Pascal, Mark S., MD
Prins, Edward R., MD
Rose, Keith Martin, MD
Said, Raghad Houfdhi, MD
Schoen, Arnold Paul, MD
Schwartz, Gary D., MD
Selvaraj, Sundararajan, MD
Shaker, Safwat I., MD
Shen, Jeffrey Jou, MD
Singh, Sapna, MD
Stoupakis, George, MD
Suldan, Zalman Lewis, MD
Surapaneni, Padmaja, MD
Tadros, Dalia Anwar, MD
Takvorian, Sylva A., MD
Tank, Lisa Kaushal, MD
Teran Vargas, Rafael Antonio, MD
Tesfaye, Melaku, MD
Timmapuri, Sarah L., MD
Tossounian, Nora Zabel, MD
Vesole, David H., MD
Vij, Angela, MD
Wang, Paul Xinze, MD
Wertheim, Mordecai, MD
Woodham, Philip G., MD
Zorba, Yildiz, MD

Hackettstown
Auciello, Antonella, MD
Azhar, Sana H., MD
Fan, Sarah Y., MD
Freyman, Boris, DO
Gollapudi, Devi P., MD
Hamaoui, Manuela Belda, MD
Ingrassia-Squiers, Keri Lynn, DO
Janowski, Kenneth J., DO
Jansons, Uldis J., MD
Kavathia, Sanjay G., MD
Khan, Sarosh, MD
Khanna, Anirudh, MD
Merkle, Jeffrey, MD
Raza, Syed Mohsin, MD
Sandhu, Vineet, MD
Segaram, Sandira V., MD
Skiba, Chester John Jr., MD
Tan, Leong Hean, MD
Theune, Lillian J., DO
Werner, Robert L., DO
Wu, Jason Jon, DO

Haddon Heights
Dowd, Heather Lynn, DO
Fisher, Mark, MD
Javaiya, Hemangkumar, MD
King, Krista H., MD
Pavlides, Andreas C., MD
Renzi, Michael A., MD
Rink, Lisa Ann, DO
Sanyal, Saugato, MD
Siegel, Howard Ira, MD

Haddon Township
Draganescu, Mirela, MD
McLintock, Glenn R., MD

Haddonfield
Francos, George Charles, MD
Leone, Anthony J., MD
Petaccio, Claudia Jennifer, MD
Saad, Walid Y., MD

Hainesport
Shah, Samir Nalin, MD

Haledon
Kahf, Ahmad N., MD
Kahf, Amr, MD
Selevany, Muhammad Tahir, MD

Hamburg
Geisen, Amy Grace, MD
Hmoud, Talat Yousef, MD

Hamilton
Arcaro, Mark E., MD
Baig, Sumeera Akhtar, MD
Byrne, Janet Marilyn, MD
Chanliecco, Ma Victoria C., MD
Diwan, Nauman Abdul, MD
Fox, Justin Michael, MD
Ganguly, Panchali, MD
Hadaya, Ziad, MD
Jones, Debra Y., MD
Kim, Andrew Young, MD
Lateef, Aslam, MD
Laurente, Cristeta A., MD
Laurente, Robert M., MD

Lerma, Pauline Marie Ocampo, MD
Levenberg, Steven, MD
Li, Tong, MD
Medina Carcamo, Edwing G., MD
Mikhail, Fayez A., MD
Mina, Randa Fahim, MD
Oza, Harsha K., MD
Palomata, Maria Theresa, MD
Patel, Minal, MD
Raza, Rubina B., MD
Repudi, Sirisha, MD
Sehgel, Robert R., DO
Sharma, Smriti, MD
Sheikh, Selim U., MD
Siddique, Mahmood I., DO
Tawfik, Hany Wahba, MD
Thomas, Jhibu, MD
Tripathi, Neeta, MD
Tuma, Augustine Lavelle, MD
Ufondu, Ebele E., MD
Vadakara, Laisa L., MD
Vadakara, Lukose Simon, MD
Walker, Bridget Ann, DO
Wasserman, Ethan Jeffrey, MD
Wingfield, Edward Anthony, MD

Hamilton Square
Deblasio, Joseph, MD
Deblasio, Joseph Jr., MD
Gonzales, Marjorie M., MD
Novik, Gerald, MD
Patel, Dakshkumar B., MD
Siniakowicz, Robert Miroslaw, MD

Hammonton
Ahmed, Safi U., MD
Bagchi, Sonali, MD
Bejaran, Juan E., MD
Belli, Albert J. Jr., DO
Fakayode, Abisoye Victoria, MD
Fernandez, Edwin Paras, MD
Gilmour, Kevin P., DO
Kou, Jen Lih, MD
Palathingal, Celina G., MD
Patel, Dipesh V., MD
Reddy, Rajender, MD
Roy, Arup Kumar, MD
Zheng, Jing-Sheng, MD
Zingrone, Denise Michele, DO

Hampton
Mohrin, Carl M., MD

Harrington Park
Biria, Nazila, MD
Brunnquell, Stephen B., MD
Fadil, Tina Marie, MD
Lee, Gerald J., MD
Patel, Disha, MD
Relkin, Felicia, MD
Schran, Mary Ann, MD
Shin, Seulkih, MD
Srinivasan, Anand, MD

Harrison
Carvalho, Artur Meneses, MD
Fontanazza, Paul, MD
Ryngel, Enrique, MD
Vazquez Falcon, Luis Enrique, MD

Hasbrouck Heights
Benoff, Lane Jeffrey, MD
Gennaro, Anthony J., MD
Lyons, William J., MD
Mazza, Victor Joseph, MD
Renner, Carl J., MD

Haskell
Smith, Jeffrey Todd, DO

Hawthorne
Festa, Eugene Daniel, MD
Gupta, Manju, MD
Jacoby, Steven Clifford, MD
Lozito, Deborah A., DO
Mannino, Marie L., MD
Mazziotti, Alexander R., MD
Nitti, David J., MD
Penera, Norman S., MD
Peterka, Ann-Judith, DO
Tuppo, Ehab E., MD

Hazlet
Awad, Mona S., MD
Chudzik, Douglas W., MD
Chudzik, Jeanmarie, DO
Cornel-Avendano, Beverly, MD
Golding-Granado, Lisa M., MD
Katz, Lawrence, MD
Khalil, Hossam M., MD

Meleis, Mohamed E., MD
Rajasekharaiah, Vinutha, MD
Saaraswat, Babita, MD
Sahloul, Elsayed Ahmed, MD
Sambandan, Rama Thirugnana, MD
Xu, Lin, MD

Highland Park
Anolik, Kenneth Jay, MD
Coelho-D'Costa, Vinette E., MD
Katz, Brian Charles, MD

Highlands
Wolinsky, Steven I., MD

Hightstown
Mangal, Rakesh, MD
Tummala, Sumalatha, MD

Hillsborough
Ahsan, Abu M., MD
Allegar, Nancy E., MD
Bhalla, Rohit, DO
Bhaskara, Jayshree A., MD
Chou, Lin W., MD
Greaves, Mark Leslie, MD
Gultom, Yanto Meiyer, MD
Hildebrant, Laura Nadine, DO
Manning, Eric Carlyle, MD
McDermott, Rena, MD
Mur, Ahmad A., MD
Neiman, Deborah L., MD
Sonnenberg, Edith, MD
Thakur, Ranjana, MD

Hillsdale
Copeland, Lois J., MD
Di Pasquale, Laurene, MD

Hillside
Aluya, Nelson Oke, MD

Ho Ho Kus
Berger, Glen W., MD

Hoboken
DaSilva, Robert Antonio, MD
Herrera, Saturnino Domingo, MD
Kozel, Joseph M., MD
Lim, Jocelyn Marie P., MD
Loh, Shi, MD
Manocchio, Stephen J., MD
Narula, Jiwanjot K., MD
Okafor, Anthony Ifechukwu, MD
Patel, Karnik, DO
Pollak, Michael, MD

Holmdel
Albana, Fouad S., MD
Bebawy, Sam T., MD
Brown, Derrick M., MD
Coniaris, Harry J., MD
De Tulio, Anthony, MD
Doshi, Pankaj Ajay, MD
Giannakopoulos, Georgios, DO
Holler, Marianne Marie, DO
Hundle, Sukhwinder K., MD
Jitan, Raed Abdalla, MD
Khan, Rafay Tariq, MD
Lehaf, Elias J., MD
Marino, Richard P., DO
Metri Mansour, Elie E., MD
Nasra, Magdy A., MD
Otrakji, Jean, MD
Parhar, Avtar Singh, MD
Robinson-Gallaro, Bonnie Lee, MD
Thalasila, Anuradha, MD
Vaysberg, Yevgeniy, MD

Howell
Agrawal, Stuti Shah, MD
Axelrad, Paul R., MD
DePerio, Elizabeth P., MD
Koretzky, Jeffrey Robert, MD
Liu, Xiaoming, MD
Lombardi, David D., MD
Morreale, Diego A., MD
Nahum, Kenneth D., DO
Polizzi, Maria, MD
Shetty, Vinod J., MD
Soliman, Monir Louis Hanna, MD
Streit, Steven, MD

Irvington
Altema, Reynald, MD
Anukwuem, Chidi I., MD
Brown, Patricia J., MD
Masor, Harvey G., MD
Ogunkoya, Adeniyi A., MD
Okoya, Jackson A., MD
Patel, Rasiklal A., MD
Rashid, Tasneem J., MD

Shen, Ein-Yuan A., MD
Wilcox, Ellis I., MD

Iselin
Babaria, Bhavikaben Bhavin, MD
Golubchik, Anneta V., MD
Gupta, Swati, MD
Raju, Ramesh K., MD

Jackson
Eiras, Maria E., MD
Hassan, Farida, MD
Kulczycki, Alexander, MD
Kumar, Sanjay, MD
Patel, Shruti, MD
Shah, Mukesh Chinubhai, MD
Sharma, Nivedita, MD
Song, Agatha Bockja, MD
Vona, Cynthia E., MD

Jamesburg
Carlucci, Michael Louis, MD
Verdoni, John A., MD

Jersey City
Abubakar, Ahmed B., MD
Acierno, Lynne J., MD
Ahmed, Amina A., MD
Alam, Parvez, MD
Aman, Chaudhry S., MD
Anemelu, Ignatius I., MD
Assaleh, Marwan David, MD
Badin, Diane, MD
Badin, Michel S., MD
Bansal, Nivedita, MD
Beaty, Patrick D., MD
Bhatt, Pranay Janardan, MD
Borghini, Margarita, MD
Boylan, Edward F., MD
Brandt, Frederick W., MD
Brotman, Deborah L., MD
Cabales, Arthur L., MD
Cabales, Victor L., MD
Chatha, Anjum, MD
Chinai, Ronak N., MD
Choi, Jea Keun, MD
Choudhary, Anjali P., MD
Choudry, Abaid Ullah Anwar, MD
Ciechanowski, George J., MD
Darbouze, Jean R., MD
DeLeon, Zorayda Olaya, MD
Del Castillo, Ma Dolores, MD
Desai, Jignesh, MD
Digioia, John J. Jr., MD
Druck, Mark, MD
Dungo, Joven P., MD
El Amir, Mazhar E., MD
El Amir, Medhat Elsayed, MD
Elamir, Mohammed, MD
Faludi, Christopher, MD
Farooq, Ahmad, MD
Fermin, Carlos Miguel, MD
Fogari, Robert A., MD
Francois, Vincent, MD
Gandhi, Kirit V., MD
Ghuman, Damanjit K., MD
Gongireddy, Srinivas V., MD
Hanif, Muhammad Shahzad, MD
Hannallah, Youssef A., MD
Ibrahim, Mary I., MD
Jain, Deepika, MD
Jetty, Siva Teja, MD
Jonnalagadda, Padmavathi, MD
Jonnalagadda, Vasudeva Rao, MD
Kazmi, Syed Iftikhar Ahmed, MD
Khan, Anwar Ahmad, MD
Khan, Rizwana, MD
Kohan, Feraydoon, MD
Latef, Sherif Maurice, MD
Lazo, Angel Amado Jr., MD
Li, Xiaoling, MD
Lim, Fidel Losa Jr., MD
Lipat, Gregorio A., MD
Lippman, Jay Howard, MD
Mahmood, Saleem, MD
Maiello, Dominic J., MD
Makadia, Bhaktidevi, MD
Malhotra, Amit, MD
Marian, Valentin Dumitru, MD
Marmol, Jose Jr., MD
Miller, Stuart Henry, MD
Min, Irene, MD
Mirza, Muhammed H., MD
Mousa, Atef, DO
Moustiatse, Adelia C., MD
Munne, Gisela L., MD

Physicians by Specialty and Town

Internal Medicine (cont)

Jersey City
Nariseti,Chalapathy,MD
Neibert,John Paul Z.,MD
Onwochei,Francis,MD
Oparaji,Anthony Chibuzor,MD
Owusu,Solomon,MD
Pagulayan,Sylvia R.,MD
Palathingal,Rini M.,MD
Pappert,Jeffrey Robert,MD
Parikh,Nitin A.,MD
Patel,Amy A.,MD
Patel,Chandrakant A.,MD
Patel,Ramiladevi S.,MD
Perera,Sharmalie,MD
Phung,Susan,MD
Pizarro,Oscar N.,MD
Quraishi,Abid Nisar,MD
Qureshi,Hassan I.,DO
Reisner,Michelle R.,MD
Rizvi,Anwar Ahmad,MD
Salah-Eldin,Alaa A.,MD
Saleeb,Joseph S.,MD
Samineni,Sankar Anand,MD
Scarpa,Nicholas P.,MD
Seman,Ahmed B.,MD
Shah,Rohitkumar I.,MD
Shah,Saira,MD
Sharma,Ritu,MD
Syed,Amer K.,MD
Thota,Sreevani,MD
Uppal,Muhammad S.,MD
Velasco,Sonia C.,MD
Velpari,Sudarshan,MD
Viloria,Edermiro,MD
Walters,Samuel Roy,MD
Weiner,Barry,MD
Whitley,Ronda M.,MD

Keansburg
Tsai,Anderson F.,MD

Kearny
Balasubramanian,Kanchana,MD
Desai,Viren,MD
Jacob,Emad,MD
Killilea,Edward M.,MD
Sanchez,Mauricio Jorge,MD
Wynn,Laurence,MD

Kendall Park
Chaudhari,Umesh J.,MD
Estavillo,Aileen Casambre,MD
Gu,Lingping,MD
Kamath,Sudha P.,MD
Koganti,Monika,MD
Mehta,Priti J.,MD
Mongia,Rupa,MD
Patel,Robert Balvant,MD
Satwah,Vinay Kumar,DO
Sinha,Meena,MD
Vallabhaneni,Purnima,MD

Kenilworth
Shah,Milind Narendra,MD
Slatkin,Ava,MD
Strony,John Thomas,MD
Udasin,Gary E.,MD
Waskin,Hetty Anne,MD

Kinnelon
Avagyan,Igor Zhorzhiko,MD

Lake Hiawatha
Maher,Miriam Ruth,MD

Lake Hopatcong
Orlandoni,Enrico F.,DO

Lakehurst
Comsti,Eric A.,MD
Lehman,Frederick,MD
Pineda,Julita S.,MD
Pineda,Nonato E.,MD

Lakewood
Bhatt,Nikhil Yeshavantray,MD
Blake,Michael Laurence,MD
Chakrapani,Soumya,MD
Chander,Harish,MD
Cohen,Jonathan,MD
Cohen,Jonathan Ira,MD
Das,Saumya,MD
Green,Tamar Buchsbaum,MD
Hussain,Shahzad,MD
Jilani,Usman Khan,MD
Kashyap,Rupa R.,MD
Krohn,David Isaac,MD
Lebowitz,Howard Harris,MD
Mahan,Janet L.,MD
Maron,Edward M.,MD
Morelos,Joseph C.,DO
Narasimhaswamy,Smitha,MD
Ogun,David J.,MD
Patel,Akshay D.,MD
Patel,Manoj,MD
Patel,Pinakin C.,MD
Patel,Sandipkumar R.,MD
Phelps,Kristyn Kia,MD
Pineles,Cary L.,MD
Preschel,Samuel Aharon,MD
Rajeswaran,Gowri,MD
Robberson,Heather Leigh,MD
Salcedo,Elizabeth O.,MD
Shahabuddin,Saiham,MD
Singh,Satyendra Pratap,MD
Smithers,Wilda I.,MD
Talamayan,Randy P. C.,MD
Thomas,Teresa E.,MD
Thopcherla,Manjula,MD
Yap,Wilson C.,MD

Lanoka Harbor
Fernando-Flores,Avelina M.,MD
Tauro,Victor,MD

Laurence Harbor
Lalcheta,Paresh,MD

Lawnside
Young,William P.,MD

Lawrence
Klausner,Mark A.,MD

Lawrenceville
Adler,Scott L.,MD
Borrus,Stephen W.,MD
Dash,Michael Roy,MD
Desai,Bharat V.,MD
Friedland,Richard James,MD
Goldberg,Paul E.,MD
Gomes,Eric Arvind,MD
Hollander,Jason Michael,MD
Jain,Madhu,MD
Khan,Aliya W.,MD
Lee,Peter,MD
Mathew,Saritha,MD
Osias,Kimberly Beth,MD
Shaffer,Brian L.,MD
Wasti,Naila H.,MD
Weinstein,Mark J.,MD
Werbel,Sarah A.,MD
Zathureczky,Izabella K.,MD

Leesburg
Larue,Catherine,MD

Leonia
Diakolios,Constantine E.,MD
Joo,Richard H.,MD
Su,Tze-Jung,MD

Lincoln Park
Corso,Martin J.,MD
Jindal,Jagdish R.,MD

Lincroft
Ibrahim,Adel,MD

Linden
Allen,Mureen Cressida,MD
Bezozo,Richard Craig,MD
Borowski,Walter J.,MD
Bronikowski,John Anthony,DO
Czyzewski,Ewa,MD
Diaz,Julio E.,MD
Kibilska Borowski,Jolanta M.,MD
Lao,Carlos S.,MD
Nowak,Darius Zbigniew,MD
Patel,Narendra D.,MD
Randhawa,Preet Mohan Singh,MD
Remolina,Carlos,MD
Rubinstein,Allen Bernard,DO
Saif,Shazia,MD
Shah,Praful M.,MD
Wawrzyniak,Zygmunt T.,MD
Weitzman,Robert H.,MD

Linwood
Amin,Anila P.,MD
Gove,Ronald C.,MD
Gualtieri,Sara Liliana,MD
Parikh,Nikhil S.,MD
Parikh,Pujan N.,MD
Ponnappan,Gita S.,MD
Sagransky,David M.,MD
Singh,Sunil K.,MD

Little Egg Harbor
Rao,Anupama J.,MD

Little Falls
Al Rabi,Kamal H.,MD

Bauer,Francis Douglas,MD
Chennapragada,Kausalya,MD
Coscia,Sylvia,MD
Dahhan,Mohamed Zakaria,MD
Farnese,Jeffrey Jason,MD
Farnese,Joseph T.,MD
Fazio,Ignazio Jr.,MD
Laneve,Anthony Jr.,MD

Little Ferry
Meo,Francis W.,MD

Little Silver
Arora,Deepinder Kaur,MD
Devito,Marc J.,MD
Gourkanti,Rao S.,MD
Greenberg,Susan Nancy,MD
LaNatra,Nicole,MD
Laughinghouse,Kenneth,MD
Ponti,Tatyana,MD
Scher,Richard M.,DO
Scotti,Angelo T.,MD

Livingston
Abraham,Maninder Arneja,MD
Adamoli,Donna Janine,MD
Advani,Sonoo Kishu,MD
Algazy,Jeffrey Ian,MD
Allagadda,Bharathi R.,MD
Anton,Joseph G.,MD
Bahler,Emily Susan,DO
Braunstein,Scott N.,MD
Carlino,Anthony,MD
Cervone,Joseph Stephen III,MD
Citron,Barry S.,MD
Danieu,Linda A.,MD
DeFusco,Kenneth T.,MD
Elango,Adhithaselvi K.,MD
Faizan,Anila,MD
Goldberg,Ryan J.,MD
Gutkin,Michael,MD
Henriquez,Karina A.,MD
Ippolito,Tobi,MD
Kaufman,Lee D.,MD
Kazmi,Ahsan Mahmood,MD
Kowalski,Albert A.,MD
Kramer,Isaac,MD
Kulkarni,Pratibha A.,MD
Leitner,Stuart P.,MD
Maida,Emanuel M.,MD
Murphy,Kim,MD
Nadel,Lester,MD
Nanduri,Visala Venkata,MD
Patel,Anup Magan,MD
Pentyala,Madhavi,MD
Peos,Jennifer Renee,MD
Puglisi,Gina Grace,MD
Ravulapati,Sravanthi,MD
Rommer,James A.,MD
Sareen,Ruchi,MD
Scoppetuolo,Michael Jr.,MD
Sethi,Ripka,MD
Shahinian,Toros S.,MD
Sidler,Bonnie Beryl,MD
Simpkins,Nancy M.,MD
Sipzner,Robert J.,MD
Sivendra,Shan,MD
Thiruwilwamala,Parvathy S.,MD
Trespalacios,Vanessa Nadia,MD
Wang,Ai-Lan,MD
Weng,Francis Liu,MD
Yang,Lihua,MD
Yodice,Paul Carmine,MD
Youssef-Bessler,Manal Farouk,MD

Lodi
Andreescu,Aurora C.,MD
Carafa,Ciro J.,MD
Mecca,Mauro A.,MD
Pande,Chandana,MD
Raacke,Lisa Marie,MD
Ramos,Maria A.,MD
Rigolosi,Ronald A.,MD
Thamman,Prem,MD

Logan Township
Prabhakar,Avinash,MD

Long Branch
Angi,Priya,MD
Asthana,Jyothi,MD
Brawer,Arthur E.,MD
Burkett,Eric Nelson,MD
Cotov,Judith A.,MD
Dalton,John Boehmer,MD
Du,Doantrang Thi,MD
Ganne,Sudha,MD
Ghotb,Sara,MD

Gomez,Johnson Lim,MD
Granet,Kenneth H.,MD
Hershkowitz,Robert P.,MD
Israel,Jessica Leigh,MD
Jain,Rishabh Kumar,MD
Kadiyam,Sandhya,MD
Lederman,Jeffrey Craig,DO
Mandadi,Pranathi R.,MD
Mark,Benjamin,MD
Mercadante,Zorica J.,MD
Paladugu,Madhu Babu,MD
Rajaraman,Ravindran T.,MD
Rivera,Carlos G.,MD
Ross,Douglas A.,MD
Rubino,Barry P.,MD
Shah,Shilpan H.,MD
Shoner,Lawrence Gene,MD
Spellman,Charles L.,DO
Vilenskaya,Irina,MD
Wreiole,August L.,DO

Long Valley
Marino,Mark T.,MD
Muenzen,Christopher P.,MD

Lumberton
Awsare,Monica B.,MD
Peng,Brian,DO
Rai-Patel,Jitha,MD

Lyndhurst
Ambrosio,George Joseph,MD
Hagler,Rhonda A.,MD
Hazzah,Marwa Mohamed,MD
Hoskin,Jane F.,MD
Kricko,Michael J.,DO
Losos,Roland Jerzy,MD
Park,Byong K.,MD
Rose,Henry J.,MD

Lyons
Hwang,Evelyn R.,DO
Kovtun,Marina,MD
Kumar,Renuka,MD
Lin,Michael Keith,MD
Nandakumar,Rajalakshmi,MD
Paramatmuni,Lakshmi K.,MD
Prabhu,Vasanthi M.,MD

Madison
Latif,Madiha,MD
Sahoo,Aparna,DO

Mahwah
Shahamat,Morteza,MD
Sharma,Indu,MD
Tartini,Albert,MD

Manahawkin
Alhadeff,Ilan,MD
Dahal,Rama,MD
DeSantis Mastrangelo,R.,MD
Guida,Vincent C.,DO
Hussain,Sajjad,MD
Khan,Akbar Ali,MD
Moshkovitch,Vasil I.,MD
Prins,Kenneth J.,MD
Reynon,Melissa A.,MD
Romano,Andrew Leonard,DO
Sahay,Nishi,MD
Sahay,Rajiv,MD
Soni,Poonam,MD
Soni,Shikhar,MD
Yu,Byung H.,MD

Manalapan
Avanesova,Natalya Oleg,MD
Cutler,Jay M.,MD
De Blasio,Thomas F.,MD
Ezer,Mayer Roy,MD
Koneru,Jayanth,MD
McAlarney,Lourdes Rupac,MD
Romanella,Joseph P.,DO
Rossi,Regina L.,DO
Schindel,Leonard J.,MD
Shestak,Aleksandr,MD
Talamati,Jayanthi,MD
Youssef,Maher A.,MD

Manasquan
Almeida,Frank Gerard,MD
Berkovich,Vladimir,MD
Costanzo,Eric John,DO
Gilani,Asim Haider,MD
Henningson,Carl Thomas Jr.,MD
Kossev,Viliana D.,MD
Kuzmick,Peter J.,DO
Mencel,Peter J.,MD
Miskoff,Jeffrey Aaron,DO
Pandya,Manan Kirit,DO

Potulski,Frederick J.,MD
Schneider,Henry E.,MD
Manchester
Buerano,Thelma Mapa,MD
Mantoloking
Yeager,Richard J.,MD
Manville
Chichili,Eiswarya,MD
Mody,Vipul C.,MD
Pandya,Dhyanesh C.,MD
Maplewood
Hanson,Claudia A.,MD
Jayanathan,Subendrini G.,MD
Kaid,Khalil Ahmed,MD
Karry Mohanrao,Shailender K.,MD
Mendola,John V.,MD
Orenberg,Scott D.,DO
Simon,Eddy,MD
Solomon,Richard Jay,MD
Margate City
Faustino,Alan Herbert,MD
Marlboro
Basilone,Joseph,MD
Carter,Alison F.,MD
Ciencewicki,Michael Jr.,MD
Fox,David B.,MD
Kanouka,Indira Jouma,MD
Nair,Swapna,MD
Pass,Mark David,MD
Pitchumoni,Suresh Shanker,MD
Reddy,Sowbhagya Sangam,MD
Stoner,Edward D.,MD
Tilara,Amy N.,MD
Marlton
Abiuso,Patrick D. Jr.,MD
Airen,Priya,MD
Alimam,Ammar,MD
Arerangaiah,Ramya B.,MD
Bermingham,John,DO
Braverman,Gerald M.,MD
Cetel,Marvin A.,MD
Chaudhry,Nadia Jahan,MD
Dadhania,Ketki M.,MD
Daly,John Christopher,MD
Dwyer,James P.,DO
Evans,Carrie Marie,DO
Grookett,Thomas Wister,MD
Hasbun,Rafael D.,MD
Jaffe,Brian C.,MD
Jaffe,Jane K.,DO
Joynes,Robert Joseph,MD
Kaur,Navneet,MD
Lee,Sherrylynn Nacario,MD
Lomonaco,Jesse V.,DO
MacCiocca,Michael J.,MD
Maier,Dawn Rachel,MD
Malik,Irfan Asim,MD
Mandell,Ryan S.,MD
Matsinger,John Mark,DO
Mazza,Emilio,MD
Mirmanesh,Shahin Michael,MD
Mirmanesh,Shapour Steve,MD
Mohageb,Salah M.,MD
Nugent,Grace C.,MD
Perez,Alejandro,DO
Plotnick,Marc P.,MD
Rivlin,Kwan Thanaporn,MD
Salm,Allen J.,MD
Schwika,John T.,DO
Shad,Yasar,MD
Sommer,Lacy Louise,MD
Sztejman,Eric S.,MD
Tang,Godffery R.,MD
Tirmal,Viraj Vijay,MD
Vishwanath,Sahana,MD
Zuniga,Rina De Guzman,MD
Marmora
Ahmad,Kaleem U.,MD
Childs,Julianne Wilkin,DO
Cruz,Avelino N.,MD
Rizvi,Muhammad A.,MD
Matawan
Bais,Rajney Monica,MD
Feng,Shufang,MD
Ghabras,Magda S.,DO
Gollup,Andrew M.,MD
Jafri,Jaffar M.,MD
Mancuso,Cathie-Ann,MD
Miller,Melissa Anne,MD
Ould Hammou,Ayesha N. Haque,MD

Mays Landing
Bacarro,Arnold S.,MD
Lurakis,Michael F.,DO
Pollack,Jeffrey S.,MD
Maywood
Dixon,Keith Raymond,MD
French,Eugene C.,MD
Fulop,Eugene,MD
Fulop,Luminita,MD
Majersky,Stephen P.,MD
Nguyen,Han Ngoc,MD
Medford
Barash,Craig Ross,MD
Bezzek,Mark S.,MD
Chua,Lee Chadrick,MD
D'Amico,James Charles,DO
Eufemia,Joann M.,MD
Glass,James M.,MD
Hickey,Joseph J.,MD
Holton,James Jeffrey,MD
Ianacone,Mary R.,DO
Klein,Rachel S.,MD
Scuderi,Steven A.,MD
Waldron,John R.,DO
Mendham
Ciuffreda,Ronald V.,MD
Connolly,Allison Carthan,MD
Donnelly,Michael G.,MD
Marella,Gregg G.,MD
Prestifilippo,Christie J.,MD
Randazzo,Domenick N.,MD
Solomon,Leah F.,MD
Mercerville
Chawla,Rajnish Paul Singh,MD
Chawla,Rupinder,MD
Haber-Kuo,Sheryl Ann,MD
Mangiaracina,Giacomo,MD
Maniya,Zakaria W.,MD
Nisar,Asif,MD
Patel,Anamika K.,MD
Stawicki,Jesse J.,DO
Merchantville
Curreri,Joseph P.,DO
Scardigli,Dennis Michael,MD
Metuchen
Batra,Lina S.,MD
Dasari,Rajasree V.,MD
Hussain,Syed Faiyaz,MD
Kainth,Inderjit S.,MD
Kaur,Dvinder,MD
Khanna,Sunil K.,MD
Lin,Harry Hui,MD
Manoj,Smitha,MD
Soriano,Bruce V.,MD
Thukkaram,Kavitha,MD
Zhang,Miaoying,MD
Zhou,Ren,MD
Middlesex
Leong,Perry L.,MD
Middletown
Bazerbashi,Ammar,MD
Clemente,Joseph,MD
Farrugia,Peter Michael,MD
Gold,Marcia D.,MD
Gross,Russell A.,MD
Haddad,Joanne T.,MD
Leschinsky,Alexandra,MD
Shah,Ajay S.,MD
Spetko,Nicholas III,MD
Swartz,Stephen Jay,MD
Tuboku-Metzger,Folarin D.,MD
Midland Park
Ackad,Alexandre V.,MD
Cohen,Ricky B.,MD
Dabaj,Dina,MD
Dziezanowski,Margaret Ann,MD
Hart,Karen Manheimer,MD
Hope,Lisa Dawn,MD
Kotlov,Mikhail,MD
Kozlowski,Jeffrey P.,MD
Leifer,Bennett P.,MD
Prinz,Karola Kristina,MD
Raza,Syed Irfan,MD
Valinoti,Anne Marie,MD
Zaider,Arik,MD
Millburn
Desai,Rajendra R.,MD
Frankel,Trina N.,MD
Freundlich,Nancy Lynn,MD
Khalina,Svetlana Petrovna,MD
Khong,Darmadi S.,MD

Kuo,Michael,MD
Mehta,Chirag A.,MD
Meisner,Errol C.,MD
Miraglia,Janeen Theresa,DO
Ortega-Jongco,Anita M.,MD
Pinho,Paulo Bandeira,MD
Pitoscia,Thomas,MD
Quaglia,Silvio A.,MD
Roy,Satyajeet,MD
Schwartzman Lane,Roberta,MD
Solomon,Michael I.,MD
Tecson,Maria Vida Tupaz,MD
Thirunahari,Nandan R.,MD
Thomas,Alapatt Porinchu,MD
Millstone Township
Chikezie,Pius U.,MD
Gendy,Hany Moris,MD
Shah,Sejal Gohel,MD
Milltown
Chan,Diana,MD
Sjolund,Paula A.,DO
Millville
Babu,Sarath,MD
Kaczaj,Olga,MD
Morales,Ruben B.,MD
Patel,Hardik Bhupendrabhai,MD
Piszcz-Connelly,Malgorzata,MD
Mine Hill
Forward,John B.,MD
Rotsides,Andreas D.,MD
Sharma,Tarun K.,MD
Sundaram,Subramoni,MD
Minotola
Patel,Chimanlal J.,MD
Monmouth Junction
Chan,Phillip Pierre,MD
Gali,Lavanya,MD
Mallipeddi,Harini,MD
Regulapati,Saritha,MD
Monroe
Abellana,Juan C.,MD
Abellana,Victoria D.,MD
Ahuja,Kavita Bala,DO
Fisch,Tobe M.,MD
Gopal,Richa,MD
Logothetis,James Nicholas,MD
Mehta,Ojas R.,DO
Motavalli,Lisa S,MD
Sterman,Paul Lawrence,MD
Monroe Township
Allu,Sridevi,MD
Foster,Ronald D.,MD
Ghanem,Osama K.,MD
Gjenvick,Timothy C.,MD
Goldberg,Jory J.,MD
Mirza,Ahmed Anas,MD
Nanavati,Kartikey J.,MD
Nanavati,Kaushal Kartikey,MD
Prasad,Vineet,MD
Sherrow,Keith Ira,MD
Thomas,Cherryl L.,MD
Montclair
Ahmed,Sabeen,MD
Allam,Naveen Reddy,MD
Allam,Reddy B.,MD
Allusson,Valerie R.C.,MD
Califano,Tiziana,MD
Chaudhry,Shauhab,MD
Diano,Rowen Gumapas,MD
Elsayed,Ali Elsayed Mohamme,MD
Gribbon,John J.,MD
Gujja,Rajitha Reddy,MD
Harb,George E.,MD
Kim,Harold J.,MD
Klukowicz,Alan J.,MD
Krupp,Edward Todd,DO
Liang,Raymond Y.,MD
Mali,Shalini Reddy,MD
Mehta,Bijal Shah,MD
Miryala,Rekha,MD
Mohan,Mamatha G.,MD
Nowicki,Noel C.,MD
Ponzio,Geralyn Michelle,MD
Rana,Meenakshi G.,MD
Wong Liang,Ruth C.,MD
Zaeh,Douglas H.,MD
Montvale
Kulesza,Elizabeth Ann,MD
Tempesta,Sabrina L.,DO
Varghese,Rebecca M.,MD

Physicians by Specialty and Town

Montville
Aasmaa,Sirike T.,DO
Gilmartin,Andrew Philip,MD
Golloub,Cory A.,MD
Wassef,Wagih G.,MD
Zimmerman,Anahita,MD
Moorestown
Berkowitz,Rosalind M.,MD
Berna,Ronald A.,MD
Berna,William J.,MD
Connors,Barbara J.,DO
Gami,Nishith Madhusudan,MD
Gandrabura,Tatiana,MD
Giacobbo,Kenneth V.,DO
Gross,David D.,MD
Hoffmann-Wadhwa,Nancy I.,MD
Kaufman,Jodi D.,MD
Levin,Joseph B.,MD
Pandya,Ipsit,MD
Patnaik,Asit,MD
Pearcy,Cornell,MD
Wadhwa,Dom P.,MD
Morganville
Hao,Tong Karen,MD
Horowitz,Mitchell Loyd,MD
Kroll,Spencer Daniel,MD
Mannava,Sumalatha,MD
Ridlovsky,Ludmila,MD
Saaraswat,Vijay,MD
Sai,Priya,MD
Su,Melissa,MD
Morris Plains
Burns,H. Patrick,MD
Cifelli,Antonio,MD
Elias,Ahdi I.,MD
Francois,Jean-Marie L.,MD
John,Sunitha Sara,MD
Sharma,Rakesh Somabhai,MD
Wilson,Justin B.,MD
Yu,Nenita L.,MD
Morristown
Acosta Baez,Giancarlo,MD
Adler,Kenneth R.,MD
Alberti,Kathryn P.,MD
Aldaia,Lillian,MD
Allam,Bharat Reddy,DO
Ampadu,Akua A.,MD
Anderson,James Thomas,MD
Anwar,Khurram,MD
Asokan,Nalini,MD
Astiz,Donna J.,MD
Bery,Seema,MD
Bhende,Sudhir S.,MD
Cherry,Mohamad Ali,MD
Chow,Shih-Fen,MD
Correa Orozco,Felipe A.,MD
Cosmi,John Edward,MD
Davidoff,Ada,MD
Davidoff,Bernard M.,MD
Dekko,Samar,MD
Del Valle,Heather Marie,DO
Denbow,Frank Alstein,MD
Dominguez Mustafa,Rolando,MD
Efros,Barry J.,MD
Farber,Charles M.,MD
Farhat,Salman,MD
Feigelman,Theodor,MD
Fiel,Stanley Bruce,MD
Fields,Scott G.,MD
Fioriti,Gina Marie,DO
Gallinson,David Herschel,DO
Garg,Deepika,MD
Gavi,Shai,DO
Ginsberg,Claudia Lisa,MD
Giove,Gian-Carlo,MD
Gonzalez,Joselyn,MD
Griffin,John P.,MD
Griffith,Rebecca Anne,MD
Grover,Manisha B.,MD
Hassanin,Ahmed,MD
Holubka,Jacquelin Pickford,MD
Hosadurga,Supriya S.,MD
Hussein,Ahmed Hamdy,MD
Johnson,Mark Raymond,MD
Kallini,Ronnie E.,MD
Karger,Louise D.,MD
Knops,Karen M.,MD
Kolarov,Sanja,MD
Kopelan,Leah Michelle,MD
Koulogiannis,Konstantinos P.,MD
Kuo,David,MD
Leibu,Rachel Rosenstock,MD

Physicians by Specialty and Town

Internal Medicine (cont)

Morristown
Leung, Michael Seto, MD
Martins, Damion Antonio, MD
Mayor, Gilbert H., MD
Mediratta, Anuj, MD
Melzer, Olga Alexandrovna, MD
Monastyrskyj, Ola A., MD
Moore, Brian J., MD
Morales, Donna Chelle Viray, DO
Ngo, Gerald, MD
Nielsen, Earl F., MD
Nunez, Elkin Armando, MD
Nyunt, Tun, MD
Oliver, Mark A., MD
Patel, Dharmesh Govind, MD
Patil, Vrishali Swanand, MD
Penaberdiel, Thelma M., MD
Piccolo, Christian K, MD
Proudan, Vladimir Ivanovich, MD
Raja, Shashi Ravi, MD
Rand, Victoria Elena, MD
Randazzo, Jean P., MD
Raska, Anna M.L., MD
Reder, Lorie Jean, MD
Renna, Carmen M., MD
Rosen, Ellen Jan, MD
Rosenberg, Richard S., MD
Rothkopf, Michael M., MD
Sarkar, Shubho Ranjan, MD
Savage, Danielle S., MD
Schachter, Nora Claudia, MD
Shubhakar, Vishwanath, MD
Shulkin, David J., MD
Silverman, Michael Evan, MD
Simon, Egbert A., MD
Singh, Chandandeep, MD
Smith, James Randolph, MD
Stoytchev, Hristo Vassilev, MD
Sussman, Jonathan S., MD
Thomas, Elsa, MD
Vascan, Andreea Carmen, MD
Wang, Jonathan Alan, DO
Weine, Gary R., MD
Weiss, Howard C., MD
Yu, Xiaolin, MD
Zheng, Fangfei, MD
Ziolo, Gregory Michael, MD

Mount Arlington
Ferrier, Austin Seymour, DO

Mount Holly
Achebe, George E., MD
Cairoli, Maurice J., MD
Castellino, Sharon Franklin, MD
Clermont, Nadine Nattacha, MD
Denniston, Robert B., MD
Entmacher, Michael S., MD
Fred, Matthew Ross, MD
Ghobrial, Peter Morcos Ibrah, MD
Govan, Satyen Manilal, DO
Husain, Zaheer, MD
Kapoor, Tarun Kumar, MD
Kleinman, Michael Ari, DO
Lawandy, Michael Armia, DO
Malone, Michael Richard, DO
Mandala, Ashok R., MD
Newkirk, Christine L., MD
Patel, Swati Hasmukh, MD
Pratt Mccoy, Kia Chriselda, MD
Shah, Purviben R., MD
Sodhi, Jasdeep Singh, MD
Tadi, Kiranmayi, MD
Thomas, Mark Allen Voltis, DO
Ucheya, Blessing C., MD
Wallace, Stephen Gary, MD
Ye, Xiaodan, MD

Mount Laurel
Capanescu, Cristina, MD
Castellano, Nicolas Andre, MD
Chaaya, Adib H., MD
Chelemer, Scott Brain, MD
Feldan, Paul E., MD
Goldstein, Kenneth Brian, MD
Hamilton, Thanuja Kumari, MD
Khelil, Jennifer Lynn, DO
Shears-Bethke, Tracey M., MD
Tiu, Evelyn Venzon, MD
Udvarhelyi, Ian Steven, MD

Mountain Lakes
Dabrowski, Peter A., MD
Leibowitz, Keith Scott, DO

Shad, Abdur Rauf, MD
Whang, John, MD

Mountainside
Salvaji, Madhu, DO

Mullica Hill
Bahal, Vishal, DO
Malik, Rajesh, MD

Neptune
Abbud, Ziad A., MD
Abramowitz, Richard Michael, MD
Asnani, Sunil, MD
Bhuskute, Bela Hemant, MD
Cartnick, Gregory Alan, MD
Clarkson, Philip W., MD
Comsti, Maria Virginia, MD
Demchuk, Beverly Jean, MD
Felibrico, Oliver G., MD
Garg, Siddharth Rajesh, MD
Griggs, Abeer S., DO
Harris, Kenneth Barton, MD
Hossain, Mohammad Amir, MD
Husain, Sara, MD
Isang, Emmanuel Emmanuel, MD
Kaplan, Adam Chaim, MD
Kaunzinger, Christian M., MD
Kennedy, Daniel F., DO
Klein, Alan C., MD
Kosarin, Kristi, DO
Kretov, Aleksey, MD
Lapman, Peter Grant, MD
Liu, Jian, MD
Llull Tombo, Rolando, MD
Mahpara, Swaleha, MD
Meckael, Dina, MD
Meleka, Matthew, DO
Mirza, Zainab Arshad, MD
Morabia, Albert, DO
Mushtaq, Arman, MD
Nehmad, Jason Arash, MD
Nitti, Joseph T., MD
Odejobi, Lookman K., MD
Onwuka, Aloysius Chukwumuche, MD
Patel, Keval V., MD
Regalman, Elena M., MD
Roper, Brian K., MD
Rosenthal, Marnie Elyse, DO
Sharma, Anuradha, MD
Sharma, Indu, MD
Shenouda, Magdy L., MD
Sijuwade, Atinuke Oluwaseyi, MD
Steinman, Sharon A., MD
Strauss, Ira M., MD
Tarina, Dana Ileana, MD
Torre, Steven, MD
Vladu, Cristian, MD

Neptune City
Choi, Don W., MD
Senft, Carl Joseph, MD

Netcong
Wichman, Paul H., MD

New Brunswick
Aisner, Joseph, MD
Ali, Sadia Y., MD
Almendral, Jesus L., MD
Amir, Saba, MD
Anand, Kapil, MD
Aras, Rohit S., DO
Armas-Loughran, Barbara J., MD
Ayangade, Tolulope, MD
Bershad, Joshua Marin, MD
Borham, Amanda Ahmed Fouad, MD
Carson, Jeffrey L., MD
Chen, Catherine, MD
Cornett, Julia Kang, MD
Coromilas, James, MD
Czaja, Matthew T., MD
Dave, Payal, MD
Desai, Avani Mahesh, MD
Desai, Neel, MD
Duffoo, Frantz Michel, MD
Elshinawy, Ashgan A., DO
Fayyaz, Imran, MD
Ferrari, Anna C., MD
Ferreira, Gabriela Simoes, MD
Ferro, Joseph James, MD
Florou, Vaia, MD
Francis, Charles Kenneth, MD
Fujita, Kenji Peter, MD
Gaioni, Kathleen A., MD
George, Renu, MD
Gozzo, Yvette Marie, MD
Grimes, Julia P., DO

Gupta, Angela, MD
Hait, William N., MD
Handelsman, Cory, MD
Hastings, Shirin Elizabeth, MD
Herrigel, Dana J., MD
Hirshfield, Kim Marie, MD
Hogshire, Lauren Christine, MD
Hsu, Vivien M., MD
Hussain, Sabiha, MD
Isaac, Fikry W., MD
Iwata, Isao, MD
Jacob, Sneha Elizabeth, MD
Jahn, Eric G., MD
Juneau, Jeffrey Evan, MD
Kalra, Rakhi, MD
Khan, Imran Ahmad, MD
Kim, Sarang, MD
Kolli, Sudha Rani, MD
Korman, Linda Z., MD
Kostis, William J., MD
Kountz, David S., MD
Kumar, Akshat, MD
Labinson, Robert M., MD
Larose, Jean Eddy, DO
Lavizzo Mourey, Risa Juanita, MD
Lenza, Christopher, DO
Leventhal, Elaine A., MD
Lewis, Beth G., MD
Li, Xuemei, MD
Liang, Hongyan, MD
Lianos, Elias A., MD
Liu, Charles Li-Chen, MD
Lubitz, Sara Elisabeth, MD
Magliocco, Melissa Amy, MD
Mahal, Mona, MD
Majumdar, Sourav, MD
Manoraj, Vinita, MD
Marcella, Stephen W., MD
McAuliffe, Vincent J., MD
Mehta, Smita, MD
Methvin, Laura, MD
Mohan, Janani, MD
Moss, Rebecca Anne, MD
Moussa, Issam, MD
Mustafa, Muhammad A., MD
Nagella, Naresh, MD
Palaniswamy, Guhapriya, MD
Pamidi, Madhavi, MD
Parikh, Sahil, MD
Patel, Anish Vinit, MD
Patel, Archana I., MD
Patel, Arpit K., MD
Patel, Manish Surendra, MD
Patel, Sachin S., MD
Patel, Vimal Dahya, MD
Peskin, Steven R., MD
Platt, Heather L., MD
Poplin, Elizabeth A., MD
Prister, James Dmitry, MD
Puing, Alfredo Gonzalo, MD
Radbel, Jared Michael, MD
Rahman, Mahboob Ur, MD
Rana, Swetha Basani, MD
Ranjini, Mary P., MD
Rao, Megha N., MD
Raoof, Sidra, MD
Rasool, Altaf Tahir, MD
Ravindran, Nishal Cholapurath, MD
Reddy, Jayant T., MD
Reinhardt, Rickey R., MD
Riley, David J., MD
Sachinwalla, Eric M., MD
Salsali, Afshin, MD
Sanchez, Sergio, MD
Sarkar, Abhishek, MD
Sathya, Bharath, MD
Saxena, Mark, MD
Schneiderman, Joyce F., MD
Seril, Darren Neil, MD
Setoguchi Iwata, Soko, MD
Shah, Himani, MD
Shah, Ushma R., MD
Sharma, Anupa, DO
Sharma, Ranita, MD
Sharma, Rashi, MD
Sherman, Richard A., MD
Shtindler, Feliks, MD
Sitrin, Edith S., MD
Sonnenberg, Frank A., MD
Sonyey, Alexandra Yevgenyevna, MD
Srivastava, Nilam, MD
Stein, Peter Paris, MD

Steinberg, Michael Barry, MD
Stricoff, Alan L., DO
Surakanti, Sujani Ganga, MD
Targino, Marcelo Cordeiro, MD
Toppmeyer, Deborah Lynn, MD
Vagaonescu, Tudor Dumitru, MD
Vo, Hung Nam, MD
Walker, John A., MD
Wei, Catherine, MD
Willett, Laura R., MD
Wimalawansa, Sunil J., MD
Wong, Robert L., MD
Wong, Serena Tsan-Lai, MD
Zheng, Xin, MD

New Lisbon
Buddala, Sangeeta, MD
El-Harazy, Essam, MD

New Milford
Chang, Michael Poyin, MD
Doiranlis, Zenaida P., MD

New Providence
Bartov, David Nir, MD
Bhargava, Ruta Manish, MD
Brown, Teresa V., DO
Hakim, James J., MD
Kewalramani, Kavita Rajiv, MD
Sheris, Steven Jay, MD
Zukoff, Paul B., MD

Newark
Abbasi, Shahed, MD
Abboushi, Hilal Amer-Omar, MD
Abdullah, Muhammad, MD
Ackad, Viviane Bichara, MD
Adibe, Livinus, MD
Ahlawat, Sushil K., MD
Al Tamsheh, Raniah, MD
Amin, Parul S., MD
Anandarangam, Thiruvengadam, MD
Angeli, Daniel, MD
Antoine, Wilson, MD
Arias, Paul J., MD
Armenti, Lawrence A., MD
Ayub, Muhammad G., MD
Ayub, Nudrat F., MD
Ayyala, Manasa, MD
Badillo, Arthur, MD
Baran, Natalia, MD
Barba, Vincent J., MD
Bascara, Daniel, MD
Baskin, Stuart E., MD
Bhatia, Divya V., MD
Blintsovskiy, Sergey, MD
Boghossian, Jack, MD
Bojito-Marrero, Lizza Marie, MD
Bowen, Zakia Dele, MD
Brachman, Gwen O., MD
Bradley, Jacquelyn, DO
Brazaitis, Daiva, MD
Bueno, Hugo Felipe, MD
Cantey, Mary Daisy, MD
Castro, Dorothy, MD
Cathcart, Kathleen N., MD
Chaudhari, Sameer Sadashiv, MD
Chenitz, William R., MD
Chomsky, Steven A., MD
Cohen, Alice J., MD
Cohen, Ellen, MD
Collin, Robert Daniel, MD
Colon, Jose F., MD
Correia, Joaquim Jose Caldas, MD
Crighton, Kent Andrew, MD
De Jesus, Luisito Garcia, MD
Defrank, Joseph Miguel, MD
Dellorso, John, MD
Demyen, Michael Frank, MD
Desai, Ruchit B., MD
DiGiacomo, Dennis A., MD
Dukshtein, Mark, MD
El Sioufi, Sherene M., DO
Ellis, Michael Joseph, DO
Enjamuri, Devendra, MD
Eytan, Shira B., MD
Farooqui, Ozer A., MD
Fede, Robert Michael, MD
Fedida, Andre Armand, MD
Fortunato, Diane L., MD
Frank, Oleg, MD
Fuksina, Natasha, MD
Fung, Phoenix C., MD
Gandehok, Jasneet K., MD
Gayle-Barton, Delores C., MD
Gerges, Jocelyn, MD

Gerula,Christine Marie,MD
Ghavimi,Shima,MD
Gonzalez-Valle,Marijesmar,MD
Gordon,Emily,MD
Greenstein,Yonatan Yosef,MD
Guron,Gunwant K.,MD
Habib,Mirette G.,MD
Hallit,Rabih Riad,MD
Hao,Irene,MD
Hernandez,Osnel,MD
Herrera,Iris Del Carmen,MD
Hubert,Julio Alejandro,MD
Hussaini,Syed Azharullah,MD
Issa,Amir Karam,MD
Jacoby,Sari H.,MD
Jacquette,Germaine Marie,MD
Jafari,Mortaza,MD
Joseph,Gipsa Ann,MD
Kang,Mohleen,MD
Kaplan,Joshua Michael,MD
Kern,John Matthew,DO
Koduru,Sobha R.,MD
Koliver,Maria Gabriela Riera,MD
Kollimuttathuillam,Sudarsan,MD
Kothari,Neil,MD
Kowalec,Joan K.,MD
Kurdali,Basil,MD
Lamba,Sangeeta,MD
Lavietes,Marc H.,MD
Lawand,Oussama,MD
Levin,Barry Edward,MD
Liao,Theresa Hanna,MD
Lind,Eugene Joseph,MD
Lingiah,Vivek,MD
Love,Larrisha,MD
Madigan,John D.,DO
Madrid,Teresa O.,MD
Maita,Lorraine,MD
Mangura,Bonita T.,MD
Mangura,Carolina T.,MD
Manji,Faiza,MD
Maruboyina,Siva Prasad,MD
Matassa,Daniel Michael,MD
McNamara,Jonathan,MD
Mehta,Eva C.,DO
Michaels,Matthew James,DO
Modi,Tejas J.,MD
Moharita,Anabella L.,MD
Monahan,Ellen M.,MD
Montes,Myrtho,MD
Mosquera,Joseph L.,MD
Mustillo,Robert A.,MD
Mwamuka,Linda,MD
Mysliwiec,Malgorzata Halina,MD
Natale-Pereira,Ana M.,MD
Nazir,Habib A.,MD
Nehra,Anupama,MD
Niazi,Mumtaz A.,MD
Niazi,Osama Tariq,DO
Ogundare,Tobi M.,MD
Olivo Mercedes,Yohanna Maria,MD
Olivo Villabrille,Raquel,MD
Orlowicz,Christine Alexis,MD
Osorio,Jorge H.,MD
Padilla,Adrian,MD
Patel,Lopa M.,MD
Patel,Pavan,MD
Patel,Pratik Surendra,MD
Patel,Saurabh Chandrakant,MD
Pemberton,Colin Andre,MD
Pergament,Kathleen Mangunay,DO
Picciano,Robert,MD
Pichardo,Nelson R.,MD
Pieretti,Janice,MD
Plauka,Alan R.,MD
Pliner,Lillian F.,MD
Pulte,Elizabeth Dianne,MD
Quinlan,Dennis Philip Sr,MD
Raghavan,Usha Murli,MD
Rajiv,Deepa,MD
Ramirez,Epifania L.,MD
Reddi,Alluru S.,MD
Robles,Ruth F.,MD
Sadi-Ali,Vajeeha,MD
Salas-Lopez,Debbie,MD
Salese,Joseph Giuseppe,MD
Samra,Mandeep Singh,MD
Schleicher,Lori L.,MD
Sednev,Dmytro V.,MD
Sehgal,Saroj,MD
Seliem,Ahmed,MD
Shah,Ajit M.,MD

Shah,Rajen S.,MD
Shah,Sandhya R.,MD
Sheppard,Sherry Manon,MD
Sicat,Jon F.,DO
Siegel,Arthur David,MD
Simoes,Sonia C.,MD
Singh,Anil Kumar,MD
Singh,Padmakshi,MD
Sinha,Anushua,MD
Sitahal-Dhaniram,Sasha,MD
Siyamwala,Munaf M.,MD
Sodha,Amee,MD
Srivastava,Sushama,MD
Suri,Nipun,MD
Swaminathan,Shobha,MD
Szymanski,Jesse,MD
Talbot,Susan M.,MD
Tapia,Susana,MD
Tayal,Rajiv,MD
Thawabi,Mohammad,MD
Tobiasson,Mary M.,DO
Tomor,Esther M.,MD
Tsai,Steve Chun-Hung,MD
Umakanthan,Suganthini,MD
Vadehra,Vivek Kumar,MD
Vanbeek,Stephen,MD
Vaughn,Anita C.,MD
Vira,Indu N.,MD
Visweswaran,Gautam Karteek,MD
Wadhwa,Rajesh,MD
Wieder,Robert,MD
Wulkan,Sheryl Lynn,MD
Yim,Hoi-Wing Susanna,MD
Yoon,Ji Ae,MD
Zemel,Suzanne,MD
Ziyaaudhin,Kappukalar A.,MD
Zubair,Mohammad A.,MD
Newfoundland
Asokan,Rengaswamy,MD
Newton
Aggarwal,Aradhana,MD
Ahuja,Rakesh,MD
Bergman,Benjamin Ryan,MD
Burgio,Michael T.,MD
DeBitetto,Nick P.,DO
Delsardo,Anthony C.,MD
Feldman,Nathaniel Seth,MD
Li,Hua,MD
Mahgoub,Hatem Abdelkawi,MD
Mohammadi,Mina,MD
Okechukwu,Christopher O.,MD
Okpala,Augustine C.,MD
Partyka,Bronislaw J.,MD
Pasunuri,Ramya Sri,MD
Ruiz,Restituto Soriano Jr.,MD
Shukla,Rajesh,MD
Sodagum,Lakshmi Lavanya,MD
Stas,Sameer,MD
Vaz,Richard,DO
North Arlington
Barbera,Frank T.,MD
Bitner,Bozena Wanda,MD
Francis,Thomas Paul,DO
Gashi,Sheremet,MD
Guma,Michael,DO
Jackson,Eric Marc,MD
Kwapniewski,Agnieszka Monika,MD
Mody,Sushama,MD
Monroe,Beatrice,MD
Thomas,Eric David,MD
Viscuso,Maria B.,MD
North Bergen
Ahmed,Asad,DO
Badri,M. Maher Ahmad,MD
Capo',Maria Pilar,MD
Caride,Peter,MD
De Vera,Edmundo C.,MD
Gonzalez,Marcia M.,MD
Gosalia,Tanmay Pradip,DO
Gundapuneni,Satish Babu,MD
Jordan,Nicole,MD
Keswani,Deepak Pessu,MD
Laufer,Beatrice,MD
Liuzzo,John P.,MD
Lo,Abraham,DO
Patel,Bela Ashutosh,MD
Peri,Nityanand,DO
Polkampally,Kavitha,MD
Rabago-Reyes,Cassandra,MD
Rama,Sapna,DO
Rastogi,Surender M.,MD
Scopulovic-Nikolic,Biljana,MD

Shah,Kamalesh R.,MD
Simon,Elizabeth R.,DO
Urman,Alina,DO
North Brunswick
Ahmad,Mir S.,MD
Ata,Mohammad,MD
Guo,H. Jennifer,MD
Hamsa,Gangaswamaiah,MD
Haq,Mehnaz A.,MD
Krishnan,Lalitha B.,MD
Lee,Dae Woo,MD
Lefkowitz,Miriam,MD
Maganti,Sameera,MD
Malik,Bobby A.,MD
Naqui,Mehdi H.,MD
Patel,Himanshu K.,MD
Potluri,Haritha,MD
Prodromo,Paul E.,MD
Sandhu,Bhavna,MD
Sarode,Satyeswara K.,MD
Vietla,Bhavani Durga,MD
Zara,Graciano L.,MD
Zimmerman,Stanley R.,MD
North Caldwell
Curreri,Rosalie M.,MD
Gagliardi,Anthony J.,MD
North Cape May
Farooqui,Zaheerulla A.,MD
Leisner,William Randolph,MD
Vaccaro,Carl Anthony,DO
North Plainfield
Ahmed,Fauzia Mosarrat,MD
Siddiq,Syed A.,MD
Northfield
Blecker,David L.,MD
Daneshvar,Behdokht,MD
Karp,Howard M.,DO
Michael,Wedad S.,MD
Nachtigall,Steven Paul,MD
Nanfara,Marcantonio,MD
Nnewihe,Charles Obinna,MD
Thakkar,Priyesh Tarunkumar,DO
Wang,Le,MD
Welsh,John W.,DO
Northvale
Hwang,John M.,MD
Symington,Peter Anthony,MD
Nutley
Abu Al Rub,Dana M.,MD
Agresti,James V. III,MD
Alessio,Maryann,DO
Alexandrova,Marina A.,MD
Aslam,Tahseen N.,MD
Bisignano Delvecchio,Maria,MD
Brignola,Joseph John,MD
Califano,Antonio G.,MD
Christiano,John M.,MD
Citarelli,Louis J.,MD
Costanza,Carl,MD
Cozzarelli-Franklin,Annette,MD
De Fazio,Ernest,MD
Delgra,Alexander B.,MD
Dell'Aquila,Paul V.,MD
Durante,Michael F.,MD
Farion,George Z.,MD
Franklin,James D.,MD
Gentile,Michael R.,MD
Kalmar,Edward T.,MD
McMaster,Delphine A.,MD
Mehta,Sidhartha H.,MD
Nadratowski,Mary Celesta,MD
Richardson,Robert W.,MD
Rotunda,Roseanne,DO
Vecchione,Edward J.,DO
Yeretsky,Yelena,DO
Zazzali,Peter G.,MD
Zefren,Jacob M.,MD
Oakhurst
Adamczyk,Rebekah Katherine,DO
Ciciarelli,John G. II,MD
Di Guglielmo,Nicola,MD
Mojares,Richard Alan,MD
Neuman,Jane Elaine,MD
Saky,Marie-Therese,MD
Oakland
Farrell,Lynda A.,MD
Kampf,Richard S.,MD
Kesselhaut,Marc D.,MD
Pereira,Pedro Miguel,MD
Scherling,Richard H.,DO

Oaklyn
Le,Tram N.,MD
Ocean
Beri,Kavita,MD
Cosentino,James P.,DO
Garla,Sudha,MD
Mehta,Rajneesh G.,MD
Meltzer,Richard B.,MD
Patel,Kashmira,MD
Patel,Suhas Ramesh,MD
Vaccaro,Carmine A.,MD
Ocean City
Cozamanis,Steve G.,DO
Perez Feliz,Ulices A.,MD
Ocean Grove
Beal,Jeffrey M.,MD
Kong,Young D.,MD
Old Bridge
Agarwal,Sangeeta,MD
Bethencourt,Guillermo F.,MD
Del Alcazar,Carlos O.,MD
Demos,James P.,MD
Giri,Janaki,MD
Hasham,Mohamed H.,MD
Ivchenko,Ludmila,MD
Jafri,Rana B.,MD
Laemmle,Patricia C.,MD
Lupicki,Marek R.,MD
Mezic,Edward T.,MD
Mirza,Babar,MD
Mistry,Tusharkumar N.,MD
Nayyar,Sanjeev,MD
Nigam,Jyoti,MD
Patel,Diptika D.,MD
Patel,Parini Munjal,MD
Patel,Vijay Ramanikbhai,MD
Price,Craig C.,MD
Raoof,Natalia,MD
Raoof,Nazar,MD
Renda,John A.,MD
Rukshin,Vladimir B.,MD
Sobel,David Charles,MD
Zilber,Eugenia,MD
Old Tappan
Pelavin,Martin D.,MD
Schwartz,Diane C.,MD
Oradell
Braun,John E.,DO
Gonzalez,Patria Ramona,MD
Hyon,Joseph K.,DO
Kramer,Radu,MD
Polimeni,Marc David,MD
Orange
Amin,Alpesh Jashvant,MD
Barnes,Dora Pinky,MD
Gialanella,Francis J.,MD
Maddali,Vani,MD
Mirchandani,Ratan,MD
Raymond,Jacques Carol,MD
Palisades Park
Chung,Haeyang,MD
Kandinov,Fanya,MD
Lee,Sung-Won,MD
Park,Wonil,MD
Paramus
Agarwal,Amit,MD
Anshelevich,Irina,MD
Barua,Aruna,MD
Cacciola,Thomas A.,MD
Casper,Ephraim S.,MD
Chak,Azfar Khalid,MD
Chung,Jeff,MD
Dumay,Serge,MD
Finn,Roman E.,MD
Firoozi,Babak,MD
Fleischner,Nathaniel P.,MD
Focella,Salvatore,MD
Giangola,Joseph,MD
Goa,Cristobal Javier,MD
Harutyunyan,Anna,MD
Iversen,Robin J.,MD
Jacobs,Stephen H.,MD
Jaiyebo,Omotola Olubunmi,MD
Kavaler,Robert,MD
Konkesa,Anuradha R.,MD
Leibu,Tonel,MD
Loreti,Michael Earl,MD
Luongo,Peter A.,MD
Malhotra,Pieusha,MD
Mapitigama,Renuka Nilmini,MD
Markenson,Joseph A.,MD

Physicians by Specialty and Town

Internal Medicine (cont)

Paramus
- Masri, Sammy Ismail, MD
- Matos-Cloke, Susan I., MD
- Mittapalli, Kesavarao, MD
- Novak, Caroline J., MD
- Parangi, Robert K., MD
- Parangi, Sasan M., MD
- Pastrano Lluberes, Magna, MD
- Patel, Sureshbhai N., MD
- Rakowski, Thomas J., MD
- Scivoletti, Peter D., MD
- Segal, Shiri Nicole, MD
- Seydafkan, Shabnam, MD
- Sgambati, Theodore P. Jr., MD
- Shatkin, Jason Alan, MD
- Singh, Harmeet, MD
- Sourial, Hany A., MD
- Sweeting, Robert, MD
- Teplinsky, Eleonora, MD
- Tievsky, Erika Fiorella, DO
- Varbaro, Gian Stefano, MD
- Varriano, Anthony, MD
- Winer, Steven A., MD

Parlin
- Denis, Joanna M., MD
- Florczyk, Margaret, MD
- Florczyk, Miroslaw, MD
- Khan, Abrar Maqsood, MD
- Mohapeloa, Gugu R., MD
- Shah, Dhiren, MD
- Younan, Shaddy Kivarkis, MD
- Younan, Zyad, MD

Parsippany
- Adessa, Kenneth J., MD
- Banker, Shobhana, MD
- Castellano, Lillian Checchio, MD
- Chanana, Manju, MD
- Garg, Shyamala, MD
- Khan, Sarah, MD
- Kumar, Sadhana, MD
- Lee, Serena Qi-Qin, MD
- Luhana, Manish P., MD
- Patel, Jignasa, MD
- Patel, Kamal Kanubhai, MD
- Poon, Gilbert B., MD
- Puzino, Alan Vincent, MD
- Ram, Meryl H., MD
- Scranton, Richard E., MD
- Song, Hongya, MD
- Takahashi, Eric Michael, DO
- Vallario, Michael J., MD
- Ziolo, Malgorzata Maria, MD

Passaic
- Abutabikh, Nael Abdelsalam, MD
- Avancha, Amarnath, MD
- Guevarra, Keith Poscablo, DO
- Ramdial, Maria Janine, MD
- Reyes, Bernadette O., MD
- Rodriguez, Jaime, MD
- Shah, Anuj Raju, MD
- Tejeda, Carlos Alberto, MD
- Wong, Jiyoung, DO

Paterson
- Agnelli, Michael Robert, MD
- Ahmad, Maliha, MD
- Ahsan, Shagufta, MD
- Al-Shrouf, Amal Ali, MD
- Alburquerque, Lucrecia A., MD
- Alziadat, Moayyad Radi Barham, MD
- Aqel, Mahmoud Bader, MD
- Bahrampour, Ladan H., MD
- Bleeker, David Paul, MD
- Calderon, Rosa L., MD
- Castillo, Hector L., MD
- Cavanagh, Yana, MD
- Chatiwala, Jumana Safdar, MD
- Chowdhury, Shamima, MD
- Corazon, Alexis J., MD
- Cronin, Stephen R., MD
- Desueza, Juan A., MD
- Eid, Mahmoud Mohamed, MD
- Elagami, Mohamed M., MD
- Facey, Maxine Elizabeth, MD
- Ferraro, Lisa, MD
- Figueroa, Nilka, MD
- Gonnella, Eleanor A., MD
- Hanna, Michael, MD
- Hassanien, Gammal A., DO
- Herrera, Jennifer Emma, MD
- Ismail, Mourad Mohamed Farrag, MD
- Jmeian, Ashraf, MD
- Joseph, Albert M. Duverglas, MD
- Kapoor, Ashima, MD
- Khan, Nazia, MD
- Khatib, Samara, MD
- Kheyfets, Irina, MD
- Kumar, Anand K., MD
- Kumar, Vinod, MD
- Luna, Luis Freddy, MD
- Mahmood, Nader Ahmad, MD
- Majmundar, Sapan Haresh, DO
- Manickavel, Suresh Kumar, MD
- Marani-Dicovskiy, Marcela C., MD
- Mechineni, Ashesha, MD
- Mehta, Pooja S., MD
- Michael, Patrick M., MD
- Misthos, Paul, MD
- Ovsjanikovska, Natalija, MD
- Petrosyan, Gohar, MD
- Propersi, Marco Egidio, DO
- Refaie, Tarek, MD
- Riguerra, Rosalia C., MD
- Saedeldine, Imad Khodor, MD
- Sarkodie, Alex, MD
- Seda, Evelyn R., MD
- Shah, Nalini D., MD
- Shah, Nihar N., MD
- Shah, Pradip A., MD
- Sheikh, Muzammil Wamiq, MD
- Sherman, Henry M., MD
- Singhal, Monisha, MD
- Suh, Jin Suk, MD
- Taclob, Erlinda V., MD
- Taclob, Lowell T., MD
- Taclob, Michelle Maria, MD
- Tao, Feng, MD
- Tieng, Fortunata T., MD
- Varghese, Vibu, MD
- Vitale, Joseph, MD
- Yung Poon, Karen York-Mui, MD

Peapack
- Mand, Christine P., DO

Pemberton
- Shaw, Wayne, MD

Pennington
- Balani, Anil R., MD
- Ball, Omega Devora, MD
- Desai, Harit, DO
- Dhillon, Ravinder S., MD
- Dhillon, Satvinder K., MD
- Gandhi, Neel Jitendra, MD
- Godin-Ostro, Evelyn R., MD
- Grossman, Bernard, MD
- Habib, Tehmina, MD
- Iturbides, Victor D., MD
- Johnson, Steven A., DO
- Nee, Guy, MD
- Radice, Beverly A., MD
- Sordo, Sarah, MD
- Williamson, Judith S., MD
- Wu, Yan, MD
- Yamane, Michael H., MD
- Young, Kristopher F., DO

Pennsauken
- Sabir, Sajjad A., MD

Pennsville
- Deng, Yingzi, MD

Perrineville
- Kumar, Kusum Lata, MD

Perth Amboy
- Aranguren-Decastro, Yolanda, MD
- Arjona, Romel A., MD
- Bencosme, Pablo, MD
- Chowdhry, Neil, MD
- Dogra, Vijay K., MD
- Goyal, Janak R., MD
- Islam, Mohammed Areful, MD
- Jimenez, Arturo De La Caridad, MD
- Khan, Dewan S., MD
- Lamprinakos, James P., MD
- Luna, Evangeline A., MD
- Maldonado, Rodolfo, MD
- Mathew, Teena, MD
- Muzones, Santiago III, MD
- Pasupuleti, Madhusudan V., MD
- Patel, Pooja, MD
- Rajapakse, John S., MD
- Reddy, Korrapati Shaik Shaval, MD
- Regevik, Henry M., MD
- Shirolawala, Pankaj Ramanlal, MD
- Somogyi, Steven G., MD
- Subramanyam, Sujata, MD
- Szenkiel, Grazyna, MD
- Vuppala, Gulab, MD
- Wang, Zhimin, MD
- Yousif, Abdalla M., MD

Phillipsburg
- Annam, Raghuveer, MD
- Bera, Dilipkumar M., MD
- Durrani, Mohamed Sohail, MD
- Fendley, Ann Ehrke, MD
- Gandhi, Jinesh Mulraj, MD
- Hotchkin, Karen Lynn, MD
- Khalighi, Koroush, MD
- Lewis, Irwin Holden, MD
- Luo, Chuying, MD
- Varkey, Sarah Hema, MD
- Yellin, Michael Jay, MD

Piscataway
- Arya, Adarsh Vir, MD
- Chinchilla, Miguel A., MD
- Chuang, Connie T., MD
- Eck, Alieta R., MD
- Gamao, Eddie M., MD
- Glazer, Robert Dean, MD
- Gochfeld, Michael, MD
- Hip-Flores, Julio, MD
- Kanj, Hassan A., MD
- Khan, Ferdaus A., MD
- Kipen, Howard M., MD
- Lifshitz, Edward I., MD
- Marroccoli, Barbara A., MD
- Parmar, Archna S., DO
- Pereira, Audrey P., MD
- Ramos, Rosalinda J., MD
- Ritch De Herrera, Thaddeus D., MD
- Robbins, Joseph A., DO
- Romano, Joseph P., MD
- Sanjay, Priyanka, MD
- Sen, Ajanta, DO
- Shah, Nehaben Ketankumar, MD
- Sioss, Robert G., MD
- Terregino, Carol A., MD
- Tobia, Anthony Michael, MD
- Tong, Yeow C., MD

Pitman
- O'Donnell, Carmel Marie, DO

Plainfield
- Alder, Edward A., MD
- Griffin, Francis L., MD
- Isukapalli, Padmaja, MD
- Jain, Sapna, MD
- Lee, Johnnie Augustus, MD
- Nkwonta, Joyce O., MD
- Nwigwe, Genevieve N., MD
- Patel, Maitri, MD
- Shetty, Vyshali S., MD
- Tripathi, Harsha M., MD
- Walsh, Susan M., MD

Plainsboro
- Bang, Byung, MD
- Barile, David Robert, MD
- Chang, Zhu Ping, MD
- Chen, Xiaomei, MD
- Edwards, Barbara Ruth, MD
- Goldblatt, Kenneth H., MD
- Hui, Ying-Kei, MD
- Hunt, Rameck R., MD
- Lancefield, Margaret L., MD
- Mamidi, Arunima, MD
- Mirza, Ismet Amtul Latif, MD
- Nagy, Aubrie Jacobson, MD
- Naini, Sean, DO
- Owusu Boahen, Olivia, MD
- Patel, Shivangi, MD
- Robison, Kathryn J., MD
- Schwartz, Mark, MD
- Sharma, Silky, MD
- Sheth, Anish A., MD
- Subbarayan, Srividhya, MD
- Wang, Qian, MD
- Youssef, Hatim Fathi, DO

Pleasantville
- Choudhry, Rafat S., MD
- Kozakowski, Edward Jr., MD
- Rajput, Zubeda I., MD
- Slotoroff, Jon W., DO

Point Pleasant Beach
- Domanski, Joseph E., MD
- Giliberti, Rocco A., MD
- Mazzocchi, Dominic F., MD
- Murachanian, Richard J., MD
- Pedicini, Joseph P., MD
- Reimer, Jennifer Marie, DO

Point Pleasant Boro
- Marlys, James P., MD

Pomona
- Cosimi, Katherine Rose, MD

Pompton Lakes
- Banerjee, Indrani, DO
- Brabston, Timothy B., MD
- Gershman, Larisa Khaimovna, MD

Pompton Plains
- Agbessi, Denise M., MD
- Alade, Ibijoke Adenrele, MD
- Bernstein, Andrew Mitchell, DO
- Brahms, Dana Lyn Satomi, MD
- Calenda, Brandon William, MD
- Dara, Michael R., MD
- Dobro, Jeffrey Steven, MD
- Duvvuri, Uma, MD
- Gadarla, Mamatha R., MD
- Kumar, Ritesh, MD
- Lauter, Otto Scott, MD
- Levy, Jodi L., DO
- Obidike, Chika Esther, MD
- Orlic, Peter Thomas, MD
- Silva, Waldemar E., MD
- Smith-Dipalo, Tracy A., MD
- Tsay, Donald, MD

Princeton
- Alivisatos, Maria Regina, MD
- Allenby, Kent Stewart, MD
- Avins, Laurence R., MD
- Barton, William W., MD
- Blom, Thomas Robert, MD
- Brown, Barbara A., MD
- Chang, Frances Yu-hsin, MD
- Chattha, Savneet Kaur, MD
- Chen, Arnold Yin-Ti, MD
- Chen, Pei-Jon, MD
- Coppola, Danielle, MD
- Corazza, Douglas P., MD
- Dashevsky, Nataliya, MD
- De La Cruz, Ernest Jose, MD
- Fein, David A., MD
- Gitterman, Benjamin Eric, MD
- Glazer, Joyce H., MD
- Hossain, Feroza K., MD
- Hsu, Stanley Cho Hsien, MD
- Hug, Vickie Beth, MD
- Hyun, Youngsoon, MD
- Kahn, Laura H., MD
- Kalish, Joanne B., DO
- Kandasamy, Rajaram, MD
- Kossow, Lynne Becker, MD
- Lacava, Paul Vincent, MD
- Lapuerta, Pablo, MD
- Lee, Jae Young, MD
- Lee, Karina K., MD
- Lee, Richard Thomas, MD
- Mahmood Arif, Iram, MD
- Malhotra, Anuj Kumar, MD
- Mendis, Kalanie, MD
- Mendu, Srinivas, MD
- Morris, Kathryn E., MD
- Murray, Simon D., MD
- Nobleza, Deanna Jean Dar Juan, MD
- Osias, Glenn Lawrence, MD
- Passalaris, John Dimitrios, MD
- Platzman, Robert, DO
- Putukian, Margot, MD
- Ramirez-Espinosa, Luz M., MD
- Ranganathan Chetty, Nirmala, MD
- Raskin, Yosef, MD
- Reddy, Sumitha R., MD
- Rehor, Francis E., MD
- Reynolds, Richard David, MD
- Rho, Aloysius Kihyok, MD
- Rose, Bruce T., MD
- Rota, Anthony P., MD
- Sandy, Lewis G., MD
- Sass, Timothy E., MD
- Schaeffer, Mark A., MD
- Schneider, Samuel, MD
- Siegel-Robles, Deborah S., MD
- Sinvhal, Ranjeeta Mukul, MD
- Slavin, Anna, MD
- Srinivasan, Geetha, MD
- Stockham, Chad Eric, MD
- Sysel, Irene A., MD
- Tridico, Tanner Joseph, MD
- Valdesuso, Gladys M., MD
- Vedula, Ramya S., DO

Wei,Fong,MD
Weisman,Harlan Frederick,MD
Princeton Junction
Bialy,Grace B.,MD
Dimitrova,Dessislava Iv,MD
Patel,Rajiv Arvind,MD
Schwartz-Chevlin,Jill F.,MD
Rahway
Constandis,Calin G.,MD
Iwamoto,Marian,MD
Kerr,Ruthann Warnell,MD
Livshits,Larisa L.,MD
Makimura,Hideo,MD
Margolskee,Dorothy J.,MD
Moody,Rumanatha,MD
Osei Tutu,Ernest Paul,MD
Prasad,Kalpana,MD
Reddy,Narshimha K.,MD
Santiago,Arthur F.,MD
Tasharofi,Kamran,MD
Ramsey
Ayoub,Kasem,MD
Fernicola,Joseph Robert,MD
Lucanie,Anabel,MD
Lucanie,Richard,MD
Scibetta,Ravi A.,MD
Sehgal,Arun,MD
Sim,Herena,MD
Sundaram,Punidha,MD
Surapaneni,Purus Hotham N.,MD
Randolph
Akkapeddi,Nirmala G.,MD
Centanni,Monica Ann,MD
Desai,Gautamkumar T.,MD
El Mouelhi,Mohamed H.,MD
Farkas,Attila Istvan,MD
Freiheiter,John Scott,MD
Grover,Arvind K.,MD
Grover,Pamela,MD
Gudis,Steven M.,MD
Li,Shing,MD
Lynch,Barrington B.,MD
Miller,Kenneth D.,MD
Russoniello,Michael A.,MD
Shah,Pallavi Devendra,MD
Shareef,Kishwar I.,MD
Sossong,Duane G.,DO
Tillem,Michael P.,MD
Valentin-Torres,Melanie R.,MD
Wenzler,Danya J.,MD
Williams,Stephen Joseph,MD
Raritan
Catanzaro,Donna,MD
Dannemann,Brian R.,MD
Elsayed,Yusri Ali,MD
Iorio,Richard,MD
Mukherjee,Robin,DO
Patel,Gita R.,MD
Zhuang,Sen Hong,MD
Red Bank
Ahmad,Nauman,MD
Allegra,Edward Charles II,MD
Choi,Yu-Jeong Alexis,MD
Costa,Ronald P.,MD
Gabel,Robert L.,MD
Grosso,Dominick A.,DO
Haddad,Richard Hani,MD
Hampel,Howard,MD
Holguin,Leonardo Fabio,MD
Hyppolite,David,MD
Marza,Lizett Auxiliado,MD
McHeffey,Dina A.,MD
Mehra,Shalini Gupta,MD
Mullarney,Allison Ingrid,DO
Nedelcu,Dana,MD
Rana,Sanah Ehsan,MD
Randazzo,Vincent T.,MD
Roosels,Marianne,MD
Sharma,Lokesh,MD
Tracy,Bridget,MD
Richland
Peterson,Paul III,DO
Ridgefield
Artinian,Agop,MD
Ridgewood
Boyd-Woschinko,Gillian S.,MD
Covelli,Joseph Michael,MD
Dardashti,Omid A.,MD
Dmytrienko,Igor,MD
Edara,Srinivasa R.,MD
Ewald,Edward A.,MD

Flowers,Raphael G.,DO
Frankel,Zev Binyamin,MD
Gaffin,Neil,MD
Gupta,Sanchita,MD
Hammond,Deborah Ellen,MD
Holt,Elaine Marie,MD
Jaber Iqbal,Reem,DO
Kalia,Amita,MD
Kaur,Birinder Jeet,MD
Kulkarni,Jyothi,MD
Lin,Spencer,MD
Liu,Michelle,MD
McGorty,Francis E.,MD
Mody,Kanika Pravin,MD
Morressi,Marc M.,MD
Mudry,Carolyn J.,DO
Narwani,Vanessa Deepak,MD
Nyajure,Colette,MD
Rana,Ranjit C.,MD
Rao,Pratibha Prasanna,MD
Rave,Arie,MD
Sanandaji,Mehrdad,MD
Shakibai,Nader,MD
Sharahy,Tatiana,MD
Sharma,Puneeta,MD
Tibb,Amit Singh,MD
Tsai,Fu-Li,MD
Tsiouris,Simon John,MD
Usgaonker,Susrut R.,DO
Weiser,Mitchell M.,MD
Ringoes
Ezema,James N.,MD
Lavin,Bruce Scott,MD
Ringwood
Rametta,Mark J.,DO
Raouf,Medhat M.,MD
River Edge
Hedlund,Edward L.,MD
Lin,Richard M.,MD
River Vale
Buirkle,James E.,MD
Steinberg,Evan L.,MD
Riverdale
Ardito,Michael F.,MD
Bogusz,Katie L.,MD
Visconti,Raymond Jr.,MD
Riverside
Sun,Lydia Lijuan,MD
Riverton
Patel,Kalpeshkumar R.,MD
Robbinsville
Abdelmessieh,Nawal I.,MD
Arcaro,Michael Steven,MD
Bandu,Bhanumathi,MD
Chowdhury,Shikha,MD
Hussain,Arif Syed,MD
Reger,Donna Pidane,MD
Rochelle Park
Arora,Sanjay Kumar,MD
Hasan,Omar S.,MD
Imbornone,Peter J.,MD
Karim,Karim Issa,MD
Maharaja,Lopa Vijay,MD
Pascarelli,Todd D.,MD
Varghese,Betsy Mathew,MD
Wry,Ann M.,MD
Rockaway
Annavajjula,Madhavi L.,MD
Samuel,Ramez W.,MD
Roebling
Hal-Ibrahim,Ahmad,MD
Roseland
Wachman,Jill,MD
Weinberger,Daniela,MD
Roselle
Lenchur,Peter Michael,MD
Saluja,Ruby,MD
Viswanathan,Anjali,MD
Roselle Park
Alexescu,Adina N.,MD
Bayes,Lorna B.,MD
Chehade,Ghassan M.,MD
Leff,Stuart J.,DO
Saraceno,Leonardo,MD
Saraceno,Libero,MD
Rumson
Royall,John D.,MD
Runnemede
Patel,Ashokkumar A.,MD
Rutherford
Chava,Padma,MD

Isralowitz,David L.,MD
Kaelin Wooton,Kathleen M.,MD
Nam,Daniel,MD
Nozad,Cyrus H.,MD
Pondo,Jaroslaw S.,MD
Sabogal,Jose Luis,MD
Tailor,Amit,MD
The,Andrew Hong-Siang,MD
The,Samuel H.,MD
Saddle Brook
Adler,Uri Seth,MD
Eichner,Craig N.,MD
Miranda,Claudia Danitza,MD
Patel,Sanjeev N.,MD
Prvulovic,Aleksandar T.,MD
Silverman,Mathew Joshua,DO
Silverman,Philip,DO
Song,Hung S. William,MD
Tantawi,Mahnaz Chand,MD
Saddle River
Becker,Alyssa Gelmann,MD
Kasper,Joseph E.,MD
Salem
Ahmed,Farooque,MD
Arnous,Nidal,MD
Chhabra,Anuj,MD
Diaz,Roberto R.,MD
Krol,Roman,MD
Oates,Angela Jasmine,MD
Park,Steven K.,MD
Reyes,Paul H.,MD
Tavani,Denis A.,MD
Wang,Shuang,MD
Sayreville
Hanna,Bishoy F.,MD
Khan,Malik Adnan Ullah,MD
Simon,Michael J.,MD
Scotch Plains
Leopold,Clayton E.,MD
Loewinger,Lee E.,MD
Pons,Nieva P.,MD
Shen,Edred Vig-Ny,MD
Stanzione,Steven,MD
Sea Girt
Bersalona,Holly Abate,MD
Bersalona,Louis Michael,MD
Demartin,Robert,MD
Lin,Ying,MD
Masterson,Raymond Mark,MD
Rienzo,Francis G.,MD
Young,Patricia A.,MD
Secaucus
Bellifemine,Morris,MD
Boyajian,Robert Wayne,MD
De Melo,Mauricio Garret,MD
Faltas,Ashraf Kamal,MD
Katikaneni,Swapna,MD
Moukdad,Jihad S.,MD
Paroulek,George Jiri,MD
Patel,Dhirendrakumar A.,MD
Patel,Hashmukh R.,MD
Sapira,Valdi,MD
Zwitiashvili,Robert,MD
Sewell
Bhimani,Siddharth D.,MD
Borowsky,Larry M.,MD
Bulei,Anita P.,MD
Caudle,Jennifer Nicole,DO
Chandela,Sweta,MD
Datwani,Neeta D.,MD
Di Piero,Alfred M.,DO
Ferroni,Bryan R.,DO
Gambescia,Richard Alan,MD
Glenn,Danette,MD
Johnston,William E.,MD
Levin,Todd Philip,DO
Lindenberg,Noah L.,MD
Myers,Scott Elliot,MD
Singh,Jyotsana,MD
Tarditi,Daniel John,DO
Shamong
Papadakis,Kelly M.,MD
Shiloh
Dickson,Robert W. III,MD
Short Hills
Blaustein,Howard Stuart,MD
Brackett,Valerie A.,MD
Chan,Eric B.T.,MD
DiGiacomo,William A.,MD
Kramer,Theodore Ian,MD
Liberman,Arthur R.,MD

Mehra,Sweeti,MD
Nahas,Barbara A.,MD
Nalitt,Beth R.,MD
Pomerantz,Glenn David,MD
Shrewsbury
Angelo,Sharon A.,DO
Bhoori,Nafisa Y.,MD
Farooqui,Shahid Waseem,MD
Felzenberg,Jeffrey D.,MD
Sicklerville
Brattelli,Gary Joseph,DO
Cunanan,Joanne C.,MD
De Maria,Nicholas Anthony,MD
Holgado,Maynard R.,MD
Palladino,Nicholas G.,MD
Patel,Indubhai Manibhai,MD
Patel,Prahlad M.,MD
Pieretti,Gordon Anthony,DO
Seltzer,Gregory Ian,MD
Simon,Shari Kim,DO
Skillman
Shah,Manish A.,MD
Somerdale
Barone,Christopher J.,DO
Kalola,Vijay K.,MD
Patel,Jayesh B.,MD
Somers Point
Adigun,Jennifer Olubusola,MD
Alberta,James David,MD
Cadacio,Manolito G.,MD
Cilursu,Ana Maria,MD
Erskine,Jennifer Grantham,MD
Geraci,Brian Anthony,MD
Gery,Brian F.,MD
Giunta,Michael Anthony,MD
Hooper,William Jr.,MD
Lankaranian,Dara,MD
Rangaraj,Padmaja,MD
Roche,Charles Vincent III,MD
Rowe,Jeanne M.,MD
Sood,Delcine Ann,DO
Teklezgi,Semhar,DO
Yangala,Sridevi,MD
Yankovitch,Pierre,MD
Somerset
Amegadzie,Richard Koku,MD
Behar,Roger,MD
Chandrasekaran,Aparna,MD
Compagnone,Linda,MD
DelMaestro,Steven R.,MD
Desai,Bijal,MD
El Banna,Mahmoud,MD
Gable,Brian Philip,MD
Heinrich,Art,MD
Herrera,Alejandro J.,MD
Ilogu,Noel O.,MD
Jain,Deepak K.,MD
Jones Burton,Charlotte M.,MD
Kuchipudi,Solomon Sudhakar,MD
Kuriakose,Marykutty K.,MD
Lahiri,Devraj,MD
Majeed,Asra,MD
Nagarakanti,Rangadham,MD
Patel,Bhavi Ashit,MD
Rayudu,Sunita Srinivas,MD
Richards,David A.,MD
Rihacek,Gregory S.,MD
Rizvi,Nazia,MD
Rizvi,Tariq A.,MD
Salim,Tamanna Yussouf,MD
Schwartzer,Thomas A.,MD
Shah,Chirag H.,DO
Srivastav,Sushmita,MD
Tadros,Carmen E. G.,MD
Tawfik,Isaac H.,MD
Thirumavalavan,Vallur S.,MD
Villanobos,Rey T.,MD
Wang,Mei-Hui,MD
Wang-Epstein,Christina C.,MD
Yakobashvili,David,MD
Zetkulic,Marygrace M.,MD
Somerville
Ahmed,Sadia,MD
Ansari,Huma Naz,MD
Ashraf,Shehzana,MD
Balint,Elizabeth A.,MD
Berkowitz,David A.,MD
Braimbridge,Sandra P.,MD
Caballes,Romeo A. Jr.,MD
Celo,Jovenia S.,MD
Dobrescu,Andrei Mihnea,MD
Horak,Ivan D.,MD

Physicians by Specialty and Town

Internal Medicine (cont)

Somerville
- Lwanga, Juliet R., MD
- Malik, Arsalan, MD
- Rosenbluth, Jonathan Z., MD
- Sanchez-Catanese, Betty, MD
- Singh, Jaya, MD

South Amboy
- Batarseh, Hani Elias Salim, MD
- Grochowalski, Tomasz K., MD
- McKenna, Harold V., MD
- Ouano, Rodolfo C., MD
- Rathi, Lilly, MD

South Orange
- Adlakha, Anupama, MD
- Anicette, Lionel Jr., MD
- Bangia, Neha, MD
- Gandhi, Champaklal K., MD
- Gandhi, Sulakshana, MD
- Holder, Kevin D., MD
- Mehta, Satish R., MD
- Mellk, Harlan M., MD
- Mouravskaia, Tatiana V., MD
- Patel, Ramesh L., MD
- Shapiro, Sofia, MD
- Singla, Ruchika, MD

South Plainfield
- Capitly, Domiciano V., MD
- Centeno, Galen Arcellana, MD
- Channapragada, Srinivas, MD
- Doshi, Arvind K., MD
- Goyal, Madhu B., MD
- Horvath, Katalin, MD
- Joseph, P. Dilip, MD
- Kaylen, Thomas G., MD
- Kim, Steven Namgi, MD
- Natarajan, Shobana, MD
- Patel, Devang G., MD
- Sarraf, Mohammad A., MD
- Seeni, Aysha, MD
- Singh, Priyanka, MD
- Toma, Wadie, MD
- Tucker, Burton Stanley, MD

South River
- Dubov, Glenn A., MD

Sparta
- Abdo-Matkiwsky, May D., DO
- Kim, Daryl Kyung, MD
- Liotta, Joseph Anthony Sr., MD
- Odeyemi, Olutunde Olakunle, MD
- Selvaraj, Kavitha, MD

Spotswood
- Deb, Ashoke Kumar, MD
- Patel, Deepa Samir, MD
- Patel, Samir G., MD
- Sahni, Sushma, MD

Spring Lake
- Antoniadis, Ileana, MD
- Pardon, Paul A., MD

Springfield
- Cantor, Susan J., MD
- Chazen, Diane R., MD
- Fuhrman, Michael Alexander, MD
- Glushakow, Allen S., MD
- Kodiyalam, Uthra K., MD
- Pondt, Charlesse Maureen, MD
- Preston, Daniel J., MD
- Profeta, Susan B., MD
- Sudler, Joy D., MD
- Vaswani, Khimya I., MD
- Zhu, Binghua, MD

Stanhope
- Mitsos, Stephanie E., MD

Stirling
- Pontecorvo, Martin J., DO
- Postighone, Carl J., DO

Stockton
- Crist, Peter A., MD

Stone Harbor
- Nuschke, Randell A., MD

Stratford
- Alemu, Yohannes, DO
- Ali, Fatima, DO
- Bacal, Diana Ioanna, MD
- Bolisetti, Sreedevi, MD
- Chen, Brian Youshane, DO
- Chen, Wei L., DO
- Cheng, Wunhuey, DO
- Chery, Magdala, DO
- Choe, Jisun Kim, MD
- Chowdhury, Zinnat A., MD
- Condoluci, Mark, DO
- Conti, Joseph J., DO
- Di Bruno, Donna, DO
- Dignam, Ritchell Rodriguez, MD
- Dombrowski, Henry Timothy, DO
- Ellern, Michelle Lynn, DO
- Falescky, Allan Jeffrey, MD
- Filer, Joshua Michael, DO
- Friedman, Jeffrey R., DO
- Goldman, Daniel Marc, MD
- Gordon, Robert, DO
- Gradinger, Lynne S., MD
- Griesback, Russell, DO
- Haenel, Louis C. III, DO
- Iucci, Gene, DO
- Jawaid, Nosheen, DO
- Kaiser-Smith, Joanne, DO
- Matrale, Michael, DO
- Rachan, Srilatha, MD
- Ranalli, Jeffery A., DO
- Saccone, Peter Joseph, DO
- Salmonsen, Mary Beth, DO
- Sarwar, Muhammad, MD
- Sciancalepore, Justin, DO
- Selvam, Nirmala, MD
- Warner, Sharon D., MD
- Watson, Marcia G., DO

Succasunna
- Mullengada, Krithika, MD
- Rubinetti, Mark J., MD

Summit
- Agaronin, Igor F., MD
- Ali, Nadia Yousaf, MD
- Alla, Nivedita R., MD
- Belt, Gary Harvey, MD
- Brensilver, Jeffrey M., MD
- Cancel, Jaime, MD
- Cullen, Kathryn Eva, DO
- Daver, Nicole Rohinton, DO
- Fessler, Sue Atherton, MD
- Gurland, Jake, MD
- Huberman, Daniel Tzvi, MD
- Ibikunle, Olumuyiwa Adedotun, MD
- Jackson, Thomas Edward, MD
- Jeffries, Emily L., MD
- Johnson, Christina Nicole, MD
- Jordanovski, David, MD
- Mendoza, Adiofel Mark F., MD
- Morganstein, Neil, MD
- Moriarty, Daniel J., MD
- Patel, Jigar, MD
- Purdy, Adam, MD
- Rahmani, Masroor, MD
- Ryan, Catherine S., MD
- Shanahan-Prendergast, Kelsey, MD
- Suarez, Lisbet D., MD
- Subramanian, Gomathy, MD
- Toffey, Lisa H., MD
- Vyas, Nishant, MD
- Wu, Elain, DO

Sussex
- Fisher, John F., MD

Swedesboro
- Abel Boenerjous, Rebakah S., MD
- Bennett, William Roderic, DO

Teaneck
- Adler, Zachary G., MD
- Aristy, Sary Mariell, MD
- Aronoff, Benjamin W., MD
- Balmir, Sacha, DO
- Berdy, Jack M., MD
- Blanch, Tanya Malka, MD
- Cardona, Shirley J., DO
- Chan, Kim K., MD
- Cole, Randolph Paul, MD
- Coppola, Peter W., MD
- Denker, Michael, MD
- Desai, Amita Jayantilal, MD
- Diamond, Elan Shlomo, MD
- Elfayoumi, Islam Moustafa, MD
- Ferrer, Waldo L., MD
- Fratello, Joseph J., MD
- Friedlander, Joseph Raymond, MD
- Gonter, Neil Jeffrey, MD
- Gumaste, Sandhya V., MD
- Gupta, Vipan Kumar, MD
- Harris, Robert M., MD
- Horwitz, Morris, MD
- Kasaryan, Hrach Ike, DO
- Khadka Kunwar, Erina, MD
- Kimel, Alexandru F., MD
- Largoza, Rosendito S., MD
- Lavotshkin, Anna Janna, MD
- Lee, Karen Chang, MD
- Levin, David N., MD
- Marcus, Ralph E., MD
- Marshall, Lewis West Jr., MD
- Modesto, Rosanna A., MD
- Park, Sarah, DO
- Pieczara, Beata Katarzyna, MD
- Rigoglioso, Camille M., MD
- Rigolosi, Robert S., MD
- Rivera, Yadyra, MD
- Rizzo, Joseph Alfonso, MD
- Roitman, Alla, DO
- Rosen, Amy T., MD
- Sachar, Inderpreet, MD
- Salizzoni, Jeffrey L., MD
- Schuster, Joseph C., MD
- Shaker, Elhamy I., MD
- Sheth, Naitik D., MD
- Singer, Roberto, MD
- Umer, Muhammad S., MD
- Villongco, Raymond Manzano, MD
- Waseem, Sarwat, MD
- Znamensky, Addi, MD

Tenafly
- Barger Amsalem, Hamutal, MD
- Kim, Hong Suk, MD
- Lan, Andrew Ente, MD
- Mooney, Caroline Mary E., MD

Thorofare
- Ahmed, Asma Talukder, DO
- Camacho, Jose A., MD
- Desai, Anjali Ashok, MD
- Laskin, David A., MD
- Penberthy, Katherine Ann, MD

Tinton Falls
- Boak, Joseph G. Jr., MD
- Boesler, Iza Marzanna, MD
- Boulghassoul-Pietrzykows, N., MD
- Carracino, Robert L., MD
- Cefalu, Dimitri A., MD
- Dougherty, Renee Maria, DO
- Felipe, Ronald Anthony, MD
- Gardilla, Kalyani Ila, MD
- Gold, Jessica Frances, DO
- Gottfried, Michael S., MD
- Habib, Misha, MD
- Jurewicz, Stephen S., MD
- Manganaro, David Thomas, MD
- Nwankwo, Gloria Obiageli, DO
- Polvino, William James, MD
- Rao, Asha Vijendran, MD
- Rizwan, Mohammad, MD
- Rosier, Eric, MD
- Vladu, Ana Daniela, MD
- Zimmerman, Lisa M., MD

Titusville
- Freedman, Amy L., MD
- Jokubaitis, Leonard Anthony, MD
- List, James Frank, MD

Toms River
- Abraham, Thanaa Nelly K., MD
- Adelizzi, Angela M., DO
- Alberto, Priscilla Magsalin, MD
- Alberto, Renato D., MD
- Anama, Luzminda M., MD
- Ayad, Lydia, MD
- Babiak, Eugenia T., MD
- Brodkey, Morris I., MD
- Bugay, Victor Valdes, MD
- Camiscoli, Deborah J., MD
- Cauvin, Leslie R., DO
- Chung, Margaret U., MD
- Crawford, Steven G., MD
- Cuozzo, Gregory Joseph, MD
- Decorso, Joseph A., MD
- Desai, Dilip Navnitlal, MD
- Dhar, Rajat K., MD
- DiLorenzo, William Richard, DO
- Elsamman, Wael A., MD
- Ende, Mark, DO
- Espineli, Dino O., MD
- Espineli, Rosalinda O., MD
- Forrester, Catherine A., MD
- Gabriel, Timothy Cayco, MD
- Ghetiya, Vinodrai V., MD
- Gigliuto, Christine M., MD
- Glazier, Kenneth David, MD
- Goldberg, Irwin L., DO
- Gonzalez, Felicia Ellen, DO
- Grossman, David R., MD
- Guarino, Ralph V., MD
- Gupta, Suraj P., MD
- Haque, Salma, MD
- Hormilla, Amador N., MD
- Igbanugo, Anselm, MD
- Jayanathan, Chelvakumaran R., MD
- Jimenez, Martin Zaratan, MD
- Klebacher, Ronald John, DO
- Kong, Henry Woongjae, MD
- Krishna, Sunanda, MD
- Lin, Ing-Long, MD
- Lin, Shirley H., MD
- Mandal, Aparna, MD
- Manzullo, Gregory P., MD
- Mathew, Tittymol, MD
- Mathur, Anjana, MD
- Matteace, Frank P., MD
- Mayrowetz, Burton, MD
- Mehta, Nikunj P., MD
- Meily, Antonio F. Jr., MD
- Meli, Gregory M., MD
- Mirchandani, Jai, MD
- Mitra, Tithi, MD
- Monta, Arturo D., MD
- Nagaria, Neil C., MD
- Nayak, Yeshavanth P., MD
- Nelson, Andrew L., MD
- O'Brien, Thomas K., MD
- Ortiz, Olivia Tanyag, MD
- Parikh, Vipul K., MD
- Patel, Nikunjkumar, MD
- Patel, Palakkumar Kantilal, MD
- Patil, Sandhya R., MD
- Pawa, Sakshi, MD
- Ponnambalam, Ajit P., MD
- Ponnambalam, Anil R., MD
- Reda, Frank, MD
- Roper, Ashley Annette, MD
- Rowland, Sean C., MD
- Sabio, Ivan Alberto, MD
- Saini, Manish Satyaprakash, MD
- Sancheti, Vinod T., MD
- Santangelo, Donato III, MD
- Scott, Robert D., MD
- Sersanti, John Paul, MD
- Shah, Dhiren A., MD
- Sharma, Anil Kumar, MD
- Sikand, Vinay, MD
- Simon, Robert T., MD
- Sinha, Prabhat Kumar, MD
- Sobti, Rimmi, MD
- Spedick, Michael J., MD
- Strazzella, William D., DO
- Tacopina, Teresa Anne, MD
- Taguba Madrid, Leslie C., MD
- Takla, Sarwat S., MD
- Van Wyck, William Louis, MD
- Wang, Jean C., MD
- Yu, Henry K., MD

Totowa
- Odorczuk, Marzena, MD

Trenton
- Agbodza, Kwami D., MD
- Ahmed, Lubna, MD
- Anandakrishnan, Rajashree, MD
- Andreyev, Nina Vaskina, MD
- Arora, Jasmine Kaur, MD
- Aslam, Hafiz Muhammad, MD
- Baig, Zahid Imran, MD
- Bhatti, Habib Arshad, MD
- Bonaparte, Philip M., MD
- Boucard, Herve C., MD
- Brewer, Arthur Martin, MD
- Calzada, Tania, MD
- Chaudhry, Sofia, MD
- Chen, Emily Q., MD
- Chinwalla, Farah, DO
- Christmas, Donald, MD
- Chung, John Wonkook, MD
- Colella, Robert Eugene, DO
- Conaway, Herbert C. Jr., MD
- Cueto, Irene L., MD
- Dessalines, Normy, MD
- Gaukler, Carolyn J., MD
- Geng, Qingdi, MD
- Ghavami, Roozbeh Mofid, MD
- Goldsmith, Daniel French, MD
- Guda, Sivakoti Nagireddy, MD
- Gumidyala, Lalitha V., MD
- Hasan, Saba Ali, MD
- Hohl, Rosario DeFatima M., MD
- Ibrahim, Mohammad Younis, MD
- Itzeva, Youlia I., MD

Jaferi,Barkat A.,MD
Jalil,Sheema,MD
Jeyakumar,Anusuya,MD
Khan,Mohammad F.,MD
Kheder,Abdul-Hady M.,MD
Krathen,Jonathan,DO
Laub,Edward B.,MD
Levitt,Alan T.,MD
Liu,Ping,MD
Mahmud,Hossen,MD
Maniya,Mariam Z.,MD
Marulendra,Shivaprasad,MD
Matthews-Brown,Spring R.,MD
Mavasheva,Sofia,MD
Mazhar,Noorain,MD
Memon,Nahid,MD
Misra,Neerja,MD
Moazami,Delaram,MD
Muddassir,Salman Moazam,MD
Mughal,Abdul W.,MD
Munir,Maryam,MD
Mustafa,Muhammad Usman,MD
Nadeem,Shahzinah,MD
Obuz,Vedat,MD
Ogolo,Clinton,MD
Oolut,Joseph James,MD
Pacia,Arthur G.,MD
Pantelick,Julie M.,DO
Patel,Chhaya B.,DO
Patel,Shodhan J.,MD
Qazi,Sadia Idris,MD
Rabadi,Khalaf E.,MD
Ramalingam,Muthulakshmi,MD
Rana,Nilesh C.,MD
Raza,Ali Babar,MD
Raza,Mohammad Aslam,MD
Remstein,Robert Jay,DO
Rinvil,Edwine,MD
Rondanina,Richard W.,MD
Roowala,Shabbir H.,MD
Ryfinski,Eugene A.,MD
Safdar,Feroz,MD
Saleem,Bushra,MD
Saud,Helmi A.,DO
Shah,Nrupa,MD
Shah,Shazia M.,DO
Sharim,Iradj,MD
Shenk,Suzanne H.,MD
Shovlin,Jane Ann,MD
Souidi,Anasse,MD
Steeger,Joseph R.,MD
Stillwell,Paul C.,MD
Tan,Christina Geok-Beng,MD
Taylor,Tanisha K.,MD
Thirugnanam,Saraswathi,MD
Toma,Cornelius,MD
Usmani,Qaisar H.,MD
Victor,Carl H.,MD
Villota,Francisco Javier,MD
Vypritskaya,Ekaterina A.,MD
Warren,Ronald L.,MD
Zavala,Ramon E.,MD
Zubair,Khurram,MD
Turnersville
Altman,Daniel Winston,MD
D'Ambola,Lesly A.,DO
DeAnnuntis,Liza Leluja,MD
Di Medio,Lisa C.,DO
Flaxman,Daena Meredith,MD
Gambale,Joseph Gerard,DO
Kovalsky,David Joseph,DO
Kramer,Sherri Lynn,MD
Lauletta,Maryann Carmella,MD
Michelson,Marc H.,MD
Palermo,Kim Marie,DO
Popescu,Adrian,MD
Schwartz,Robert B.,DO
Sexton,Thomas Francis,DO
Slusser,Jonathan,DO
Vlad,Tudor Jon,MD
Wang,Yvette,DO
Wehbe,Anthony,DO
Wilkinson,Edmund,DO
sargent,Stephanie Christine,DO
Union
Andreoli,Nina Needleman,MD
Cennimo,David John,MD
Chapinski,Caren A.,MD
Chernyak,Anna,MD
De Vastey,Gerard,MD
Defilippis,Nicholas A.,MD
Dhirmalani,Rajesh A.,DO

DiRico,Julie,MD
Diaz-Johnson,Nereida,MD
Duncan,Samuel T.,MD
Fernandez,Jacqueline A.,MD
Gold,Jeffrey M.,MD
Grigaux,Claire Nathalie,MD
Grover,Kunal,MD
Gudz,Ludmila,MD
Kachadourian,Anise A.,MD
Kershner,Gary Brian,DO
Mauti,Joseph M.,MD
Oyetunde,Olasunkanmi K.,MD
Philogene,Clark E.,MD
Pullatt,Raja C.,MD
Ramasamy,Dhanasekaran,MD
Segal,Ilia,MD
Smighelschi,Corina Daniela,MD
Union Beach
Desai,Sunit Bipinchandra,MD
Union City
Armas,Holger Giovanny,MD
Barrientos,Monica,MD
Benitez,Olga,MD
Campoalegre,Maria A.,MD
Chaudhry,Mohammad A.,MD
Daub,Denise M.,MD
Elias,Sameh S.,MD
Florentino,Hector Leandro,MD
Gastell,Gilberto F.,MD
Hajal,Hussam,MD
Hesquijarosa,Alexander,MD
Ittoop,Paul T.,MD
Milazzo,Carmelo,MD
Perez,Ruben,MD
Rangel,Emile I.,MD
Rastogi,Sadhna,MD
Shukla,Paresh Parashar,MD
Velasco,Mauricio,MD
Williams,Raashan Carlos,MD
Upper Montclair
Willenborg,Ronald,MD
Vauxhall
Ballaro,Joseph,MD
Benvenuti,Eve S.,MD
Elkins,Michele,MD
Feurdean,Mirela Cristina,MD
Hurckes,Lisa Carabelli,MD
Lacapra,Gina M.,MD
Ratner,Douglas J.,MD
Ventnor
Kasper,John F.,DO
Lipshutz,Robert L.,DO
Rosenthal,Leslie S.,MD
Ventnor City
Curnow,Hidalberto,DO
Silverbrook,Robert M.,DO
Vernon
Han,Min,MD
Hansen,Eric S.,DO
Yaccarino,Pasquale J.,MD
Verona
Bonney,David Raymond,DO
Chakilam,Santhosh,MD
Lipsitch,Carol E.,MD
Mariyampillai,Joan of Arc J.,MD
Mariyampillai,Marcarious A.,MD
Sivaraju,Kannan,MD
Vineland
Al Ustwani,Omar,MD
Aiken,Jeffrey,MD
Atthota,Vakula Devi,MD
Barber,Kevin G.,DO
Bhendwal,Sanjay,MD
Hammod,Riyadh Shakir,MD
Huston,Donald Jr.,DO
Khalil,Sara Adel,MD
Kumar,Anshul,MD
Lerman,Gabriel Salomon,MD
Lim,Carlito L.,MD
Meadows,Jason Potts,MD
Mittal,Satish K.,MD
Nakhate,Vinay Gopal,MD
Negin,Benjamin Paul,MD
Obara,Justyna Anna,MD
Ojiako,Kizito C.,MD
Parmar,Kiritkumar A.,MD
Patel,Hasmukhbha D.,MD
Pillai,Adip,DO
Powell,Jeffrey David,MD
Rana,Jiten,MD
Ryklin,Gennadiy,DO

Sayo Lim,Carina P.,MD
Sharma,Rajendra M.,MD
Sheekey,Owen Jr.,MD
Soloway,Stephen,MD
Sudhindra,Ramakrishna R.,MD
Tomar,Raghuraj S.,MD
Valvano,Amanda A.,DO
Venugopal,Narasimhal,MD
Wanalista,David Michael,DO
Watts,Helena B.,MD
Voorhees
Angelo,Mark,MD
Baker,Robert Charles,MD
Beggs,Nancy H.,MD
Bhatt,Trigun R.,MD
Brown,Anthony,DO
Burns,Gerard Joseph II,DO
Callahan,Kevin J.,DO
Canals-Navas,Carmen L.,MD
Chen,Yingying,MD
Cho,Grace Shin,MD
D'Ambrosio,John C.,DO
Eid,Hala Milad,MD
Emmons,Alyson,DO
Enriquez,Eduardo F.,MD
Fussa,Mark J.,DO
Gabler,Scott Joseph,MD
Giordano,Samuel Nicholas,MD
Goldstein,Gary N.,MD
Gor,Priya P.,MD
Greenberg,Richard H.,MD
Hollander,Adrienne R.,MD
Iliadis,Elias,MD
Ji,Yong,MD
Kodavali,Lavanya A.,MD
Leuzzi,Rosemarie Anne,MD
Libby,Joseph Anthony,MD
Linganna,Sanjay,MD
Massac,Malik Ali,MD
Nesteruk,Tetyana,MD
Ngo,Ly Thien,MD
Parrillo,Joseph E.,MD
Picciano,Laura S.,MD
Ram,Nand,MD
Raphael,Stephen D.,MD
Ropiak,Caroline Michelle,MD
Santamaria,Richard G.,MD
Schuster,Mark Brian,DO
Shaw,Brian Richard,DO
Skobac,Edward A.,MD
Solitro,Tamara Stolz,MD
Sundhar,Joshua Bharat,MD
Tagle,Raymundo T.,MD
Tepper,Steven Ari,DO
Varallo,Gerardo Jr.,DO
Weeks,Alicia,MD
Weingart,Brian M.,DO
Witmer,George Robert III,MD
Zingrone,Joseph Peter,DO
Zrada,Stephen Eugene,MD
Waldwick
Dunn,Beverly A.,MD
Vijay-Sharma,Mayuri,MD
Wall
Al Asha,Mohammad H.,MD
Bollampally,Indira,MD
Findura,Michael James,DO
Pyontek,Maria G.,DO
Yadalla,Vanitha S.,MD
Wall Township
Aquilino,Gaetano J.,DO
Brown,Christopher S.,MD
Weber,Charles A.,MD
Wallington
Kriso,Stephen A.,MD
Lesiczka,Adam,MD
Szewczyk-Szczech,Krystyna H.,MD
Waretown
Struble,Dale W.,MD
Warren
Abraham,Vinod J.,MD
Agrawal,Rekha,MD
Alaigh,Poonam Lata,MD
Ashinsky,Douglas S.,MD
Barsanti,Patricia L.,DO
Bell,Kevin E.,MD
Bobella,Stephen K.,MD
Clemente,Joseph Alfred,MD
DiProspero,Elizabeth J.,MD
Ferrante,Maurice Andrew,MD
Kloos,Thomas H.,MD

Lal,Victoria Sunil,MD
Lytle,Carole F.,MD
Montouris,Elaine Alexis,MD
Nelson,Richard Oakleigh,MD
Prasad,Lakshmi,MD
Salvatore,Augusto G.,MD
Stoch,Sharon Rachel,MD
Washington
Garg,Anil,MD
Senzer,Richard P.,MD
Watchung
Ramaswamy,Kumar K.,MD
Wayne
Abdy,Victor A.,MD
Arnouk,Munzer M.,MD
Aydin,Emmanuel A.,MD
Azhak,Sameer Anor,MD
Balboul,Elsaid A.,MD
Bamdas,Lawrence Marc,MD
Banu,Nazifa,MD
Berman,Lee B.,MD
Bernstein,Stanley F.,MD
Biehl,Michael,MD
Branovan,Zhanna Emilia,MD
Calamari,Dawn E.,DO
Chandran,Chandra B.,MD
Cheng,Bonnie Kingman,MD
Costello,Robert,MD
DeFranco,Paul David,DO
Doss,Michael Nader,MD
Eraiba,Ayman E.,MD
Eraiba,Magda A.,MD
Farhangfar,Reza,MD
Genkin,Igor,MD
Gold,Jeffrey L.,MD
Graziano,Vincent Angelo,MD
Grella,William F.,MD
Grinchenko,Tatyana,DO
Hafez,Nagwa I.,MD
Haghverdi,Mojdeh,MD
Joffe,Libby,MD
Kapoor,Anil,MD
Kapoor,Anuj,MD
Kucuk,Erhan,MD
Leonardo,Michael H.,MD
Liu,Ying,MD
Loughlin,Bruce T.,DO
Lubansky,Kenneth P.,MD
Macaluso,Charles F.,MD
Matalkah,Nidal M.,MD
Melsky,Lisa,MD
Mohsen,Reyad H.,MD
Moquete,Manuel J.,MD
Morone,John M.,MD
Nahum,Laurie S.,MD
Natelli,Anthony A.,MD
Neilan,Martin J.,MD
Notkin,Alicia R.,MD
Parikh,Chintan Prakash,MD
Rae,Sam,MD
Saini,Harjinder S.,MD
Sharma,Pushpendra,MD
Singh,Avtar,MD
Srisethnil,Pudchong,MD
Wassner,Jesse V.,MD
Weehawken
Alfonso,Jesus Roberto,MD
Patel,Minalkumar Ashokkumar,MD
West Caldwell
Diana,Joseph N.,MD
Fein,Lesley A.,MD
Follo,Joseph Michael,MD
Shah,Pradip S.,MD
West Long Branch
Baldi,Daniela J.,MD
Cohen,Seth Daniel,MD
Falco,David J.,MD
Jariwala,Punit Rajnikant,MD
Malek,Sherif,MD
Maniar,Mihir Kishor,DO
Mari,Arthur D.,MD
Parisi,Gerlando V.,MD
Santiago,Eddie W.,MD
Sharon,David J.,MD
West Milford
Joseph,Lisa V.,MD
Kalevich,Serge F.,MD
West New York
Arteta,Pablo A.,MD
Diaz,Agustin,MD
Kumar,Chitra,MD
Pelletier,Mario E.,MD

Physicians by Specialty and Town

Internal Medicine (cont)

West New York
- Roque Dieguez,Hilda Rosa,MD
- Sanchez,Bienvenido,MD
- Verea,Jorge L.,MD
- Vitievsky,Ellen,MD
- Weiss,Ronald D.,MD

West Orange
- Abboud,Somaya M.,MD
- Abdelaal,Sameh M.,MD
- Adeoti,Adekunle G.,MD
- Armanious,Adel Youssef,MD
- Baddoo,Andrew O.,MD
- Casagrande,Lisette Helene,MD
- Chu,Benny G.,DO
- Cooper,Sanford,MD
- Deen,Shereelah,MD
- Del Vento,Robert A.,MD
- Fretta,Joseph,MD
- Goldstein,Craig Russell,DO
- Grasso,Michael A.,MD
- Haacker,David S.,MD
- Hameed,Samar,MD
- Johnson,Natalie A.,MD
- Kaltman,Leah B.,MD
- Khan,Samina K.,MD
- Kritzberg,William S.,MD
- Krok,Elion J.,MD
- Layne,Trevor J.,MD
- Lee,Daniel Kilho,MD
- Lee,Dwight E.,MD
- Lifson,Donna C.,MD
- Nicoll,Anca M.,MD
- Ovnanian,Vagram,MD
- Patel,Hemantkumar G.,MD
- Radin,Audrey B.,MD
- Rubino,Susan Basra,MD
- Sangosse,Louis V.,MD
- Sangosse,Marie C.,MD
- Sapru,Sunil,MD
- Savopoulos,Andreas A.,MD
- Schmidt,Alvin M.,MD
- Shah,Deepali A.,DO
- Sherman,Rimma L.,MD
- Teichman,Ronald F.,MD
- Theivanayagam,Kalyani,MD
- Zeldin,Gillian Ann,MD

West Paterson
- Brar,Harleen,MD
- Chatterjee,Deelip,MD
- Conte,Salvatore A.,MD
- Ferrante,Francis L.,MD
- Mallouhi,Issam,MD
- Patel,Meena S.,MD
- Perez-Steele,Sheila,MD

West Trenton
- Beede,Michael S.,MD
- Elder,Demian,MD
- Hazley,Donald J.,MD
- Hui,Thomas P.,MD
- Lalla,Lalita Raj,MD
- Lee,Jung Hi,MD
- Majid,Abdul,MD
- McKay,Cecile M.,MD
- Razak,Hajira Naaz,MD
- Trivedi,Raksha A.,MD

West Windsor
- Kasibhotla,Sumabala,MD
- Lubin,Hank,MD
- Rana-Mukkavilli,Gopi,MD
- Robin,James Allen,MD
- Singh,Ajay B.,MD

Westampton
- Herriman,Daniel Lee,MD

Westfield
- Bulan,Jeanine Hermine,MD
- Calcara,Epifanio,MD
- De Rosa,Joseph,MD
- Lamothe,Maria Elina,MD
- Simon,Susan M. C.,MD
- Sultana,Meher,MD
- Weigel,Peter J.,MD
- Yatrakis,Nicholas D.,MD

Westwood
- Anshelevich,Michael,MD
- Easaw,Saramma John,MD
- Esber,Natacha,MD
- Fields,Sheila M.,MD
- Perez,Victoria P.,MD
- Ravi,Nanjappa,MD
- Sinha,Sudir K.,MD

Wharton
- Pathak,Pinakin J.,MD
- Ruml,Lisa A.,MD

Whippany
- Bansilal,Sameer,MD
- Coppolecchia,Rosa,DO

Whitehouse Station
- Abessi,Mitra,MD
- Cohen,Philip Jay,MD

Whiting
- Caruso,Donald A.,MD
- Cervantes,Crisnoel,MD
- Choper,Joan Z.,MD
- Dalal,Karambir S.,MD
- Dela Cruz,Danna,MD
- Gallardo,Mario L.,MD
- Karabach,Maxim,MD
- Magsino,Vicente Martinez Jr.,MD
- May,Micah Moshe,MD
- Patel,Ashvin S.,MD
- Shah,Bankim D.,MD
- Tresvalles,Monette M.,MD
- Zia,Ziaulhaq,MD

Willingboro
- Bansal,Sudha,MD
- Chaurasia,Preeti,MD
- Comiskey,Walter M.,DO
- Floyd,Darryl Bracey,MD
- George,Philip M.,MD
- Guo,Jin Ping,MD
- Haque,Anwar Mohammed,MD
- Hassman,Howard A.,DO
- Karim,Minhaz,MD
- Khawja,Yasmin,MD
- Koenig,Andrew Stuart,DO
- Paul,Karel Joseph,MD
- Pichika,Nirmala,MD
- Reddy,Anuradha K.,MD
- Rehman,Saadia Raza,DO
- Rivera,Edward,MD
- Shah,Asma Aftab,MD
- Turner,Nicoletta A.,MD

Wood Ridge
- Pecorelli,Nicholas T.,MD

Woodbine
- Anthony,Michele M.,MD
- Novotny,Gregory R.,DO

Woodbridge
- Awan,Omar Q.,MD
- Awan,Razia S.,MD
- Friedman,Louis Alexander,DO
- Goldstein,Richard Alan,MD
- Hameed,Fauzia,MD
- Maza,Lauren M.,MD
- O'Donnell,Mary Theresa,MD
- Rosen,Jeffrey H.,MD
- Somer,Nancy C.,MD
- Zhang,Xiaowei,MD

Woodbury
- Bajpai,Enakshi,DO
- Bonett,Anthony W.,MD
- Butler,Barry K.,MD
- Chernoff,Brian Harris,MD
- Chvala,Robert P.,MD
- Di Marino,Michael C.,MD
- Gehring,David J.,MD
- Gupta,Abhinai K.,MD
- Herman,Kenneth L.,DO
- Michel,Joseph R.,MD
- Ocasio,Robert B.,MD
- Omoh,Michael E.,MD
- Shaw,Richard Amedeo,DO

Woodbury Heights
- Millstein,Jeffrey Howard,MD
- Rosenthal,Nadine C.,MD

Woodcliff Lake
- Graham,Peter E.,MD

Wyckoff
- Lala,Lekhu K.,MD
- Weitzman,Richard Brian,MD

Interventional Cardiology

Belleville
- Shivashankar,Keshavamurthy,MD

Berkeley Heights
- Juliano,Nickolas Daniel,MD

Brick
- Escandon,Pedro J.,MD

Cedar Knolls
- Marotta,Charles J.,MD

Cherry Hill
- Levine,Adam Maxwell,DO

Chester
- Sebastian,Clifford Cecil,MD

Eatontown
- Selan,Jeffrey Craig,MD

Edgewater
- Faraz,Haroon Ahmed,MD

Englewood Cliffs
- Beheshtian,Azadeh,MD

Franklin Lakes
- Lee,John Hyung-II,MD

Freehold
- Litsky,Jason D.,DO

Hackensack
- Mathur,Atish Pratap,MD
- Patel,Ruchir,MD

Hamilton
- Rab,Zia,MD

Kendall Park
- Patel,Alpesh Babu,MD

Ledgewood
- Stein,Michael Alan,MD

Mendham
- Amoruso,Daniel Robert,MD

Morristown
- Gandotra,Puneet,MD
- Rosen,Craig Michael,MD

Mountain Lakes
- Fusman,Benjamin,MD

Newark
- Gadhvi,Pragnesh Harish,MD

Newton
- Cioce,Gerald,MD

North Bergen
- Kelly,Dennis Hughes III,MD

Ridgewood
- Simon,Alan David,MD

Robbinsville
- Soffer,Mark Jay,MD

Teaneck
- Zolty,Ronald,MD

Toms River
- Gupta,Rakesh Vardhan,MD
- Iyanoye,Adeyemi,MD
- Patel,Parag Vishnu,MD

Wayne
- Madhwal,Surabhi,MD

Westwood
- Lichtstein,Elliott S.,MD

Laparoscopic Surgery

Edison
- Jawed,Aram Elahi,MD
- Nihalani,Anish B.,MD

Emerson
- Walsky,Robert S.,MD

Englewood
- Ibrahim,Ibrahim M.,MD

Laser Surgery

Hazlet
- Murugesan,Angappan,MD

Legal Medicine

West Orange
- Mandel,Steven S.,MD
- Pandya,Prashant N.,MD

Westmont
- McClure,A. Gregory,MD

MOHS (Micrographic Skin Cancer Srg)

Basking Ridge
- Wang,Steven Q.,MD

Bloomfield
- Paghdal,Kapila V.,MD

Monroe Township
- Peloro,Concettina M.,MD

Plainsboro
- Vine,John E.,MD

Magnetic Resonance Imaging

East Brunswick
- Mammone,Joseph F.,MD

Jersey City
- Hirsch,Howard J.,MD

Mammography

Basking Ridge
- Aboody,Linda R.,MD

Teaneck
- Gross,Joshua David,MD

Maternal & Fetal Medicine

Camden
- Feld,Steven M.,MD
- Fischer,Richard L.,MD
- Perry,Robin L.,MD
- Westover,Thomas,MD

Cresskill
- Martins-Lopes,Maria C.,MD

Denville
- Girz,Barbara A.,DO

East Brunswick
- Krishnamoorthy,Ambalavaner,MD
- Sengupta,Shyamashree,MD

Elmwood Park
- Principe,David Laurence,MD

Englewood
- Chan,Ying,MD

Hackensack
- Brandt,Justin Samuel,MD
- Guirguis,George,DO

Livingston
- Kasdaglis,Tania Luna,MD
- Smith,Leon G. Jr.,MD
- Warren,Wendy B.,MD
- Wolf,Edward J.,MD

Long Branch
- Wallace,David Morrow,MD

Morristown
- Hanley,Maryellen L.,MD
- Jackson,Unjeria C.,MD

Mount Arlington
- Kappy,Kenneth Allen,MD

New Brunswick
- Martins,Maria Emilia,MD
- Ranzini,Angela C.,MD
- Santolaya,Joaquin,MD
- Schuster,Meike,DO
- Vintzileos,Anthony M.,MD

Newark
- Apuzzio,Joseph J.,MD
- Bardeguez,Arlene D.,MD
- Porat,Natalie,MD

Paramus
- Goldman,Jane Cleary,MD
- Zelop,Carolyn M.,MD

Sea Girt
- Hux,Charles Howard,MD

Sewell
- Chandra,Prasanta C.,MD
- Chhibber,Geeta,MD
- O'Neill,Anna M.,MD
- Williams,Keith Patrick,MD

South Plainfield
- Goyal,Madhu A.,MD
- Rana,Jagpal,MD

Stratford
- Konchak,Peter Stephen,DO

Summit
- Benito,Carlos W.,MD
- Frisoli,Gaetano,MD

Toms River
- Fernandez,Carlos O.,MD

Trenton
- Forouzan-Gandashmin,Iraj,MD

Voorhees
- Herman,Glenn O.,MD
- Seibel Seamon,Jolene S.,MD

Medical Genetics

Brick
- Pavlak-Schenk,Jayne A.,DO

Camden
- Schnur,Rhonda E.,MD

Newark
- Schwab,Maria Divina G.,MD

Paramus
- Robinson,Lois Pat,MD

Pompton Lakes
- Ibrahim,Jennifer,MD

Turnersville
- Ierardi-Curto,Lynne A.,MD

West Trenton
- Reid,Cheryl Soled,MD

Medical Genetics-Clinical Biochem

South Plainfield
- Bonilla Guerrero,Ruben,MD

Medical Genetics-Mole Genetic Pthlg
New Brunswick
Galkowski,Dariusz Bohdan,MD

Medical Microbiology
Lakewood
Strand,Calvin L.,MD

Medical Oncology
Basking Ridge
Fan,Pang-Dian,MD
Hamilton,Audrey May,MD
Xiao,Han,MD
Brick
Agrawal,Apurv,MD
Camden
Devereux,Linda,MD
Chatham
Hirawat,Samit,MD
Clifton
Benn,Howard A.,MD
Zaman,Aamir,MD
Denville
Abbasi,Muhammad Rashid,MD
Schreibman,Stephen M.,MD
East Brunswick
Nissenblatt,Michael J.,MD
Salwitz,James C.,MD
East Hanover
Tavorath,Ranjana,MD
Egg Harbor Township
Adelberg,David Eli,MD
Elizabeth
Kessler,William W.,MD
Englewood
Jhawer,Minaxi P.,MD
Fort Lee
Yuan,Rui Rong,MD
Freehold
Balar,Bhavesh Vasant,MD
Hackensack
Faderl,Stefan H.,MD
Proverbs-Singh,Tracy Ann,MD
Rowley,Scott D.,MD
Siegel,David Samuel Dicapua,MD
Little Silver
Fitzgerald,Denis B.,MD
Livingston
Litvak,Anna Maria,MD
Michaelson,Richard A.,MD
Maplewood
Bordia,Sonal,MD
Millburn
Nussbaum,Nathan Coleman,MD
Montvale
Kriplani,Anuja,MD
Wang,Rui,MD
Moorestown
Nathan,Faith E.,MD
Morristown
Leibowitz,Stacey Bucholtz,MD
Mount Holly
Levenbach,Rachel Shoshana,MD
New Brunswick
Cooper,Dennis Lawrence,MD
Eleff,Michael,MD
Gharibo,Mecide M.,MD
Groisberg,Roman,MD
Mayer,Tina Marie,MD
Mehnert,Janice M.,MD
Munshi,Pashna N.,MD
Schaar,Dale G.,MD
Newark
Mohit-Tabatabai,Mirseyed A.,MD
North Bergen
Gupta,Bhavna,MD
Northfield
Nazha,Naim T.,MD
Paterson
Yamusah,Emmanuel N.,MD
Pennington
Rosvold,Elizabeth Anne,MD
Plainsboro
Sokol,David B.,MD
Princeton
Sierocki,John S.,MD
Rahway
Yao,Siu-Long,MD

Raritan
Todd,Mary Beth,DO
Somers Point
Goldberg,Robert M.,MD
Somerset
Licitra,Edward Joseph,MD
Somerville
Trivedi,Seeta,MD
Sparta
Halibey,Bohdan E.,MD
Summit
Jaeckle,Kurt Alfred,MD
Lowenthal,Dennis A.,MD
Vineland
Roy,Shailja,MD
West Long Branch
Fiore,Rosemary P.,MD
Westfield
Lu,Brian D.,MD
Westwood
Tassan,Robert F.,MD

Microsurgery
Marlton
Larusso,Jennifer Lynn,DO

Neonatal-Perinatal Medicine
Atlantic City
Celestial,Rommel M.,MD
Escareal,Myrna S.,MD
Bridgewater
Zarzuela,Arminia T.,MD
Camden
Anwar,Muhammad Usman,MD
Bautista,Amelia B.,MD
Bhat,Vishwanath,MD
Brandsma,Erik,MD
Crawford,Carolyn S.,MD
Fabia,Candida M.,MD
Fernandes,Margaret C.,MD
Kushnir,Alla,MD
Massabbal,Eltayeb I.,MD
Molina,Leticia K.,MD
Mondoa,Emil I.,MD
Nakhla,Tarek Adib,MD
Patel,Yashvantkumar S.,MD
Saslow,Judy G.,MD
Sharma,Raj Kumar,MD
Slater-Myer,Linda Paige,MD
Stahl,Gary E.,MD
Uko,Smart E.,MD
Cherry Hill
Chawla,Harbhajan Singh,MD
Clark
Suapengco-Samonte,Dulce H.,MD
Englewood
Carlin,Elizabeth Berk,MD
Delgado,Mercedes,MD
Flemington
Chavarkar,Mrunalini R.,MD
Veerappan,Sutharsanam,MD
Weiss,Kerry I.,MD
Hackensack
Cheung,Sandy Wai Yi,DO
Flores,Ramon L.,MD
Johnson,Terry D.,MD
Nabong,Marcelo Yambao Jr.,MD
Perl,Harold,MD
Planer,Benjamin C.,MD
Zaklama,Joanne A.,MD
Jersey City
Alsheikh,Suhail N.,MD
Rao,Kavya Madupu,MD
Razi,Sadia,MD
Livingston
Ko,So Hun,MD
Lee,Hyejin Robin,MD
Oana Soni,Agnes,MD
Ruben,Sandhya,MD
Santo Domingo,Jose E.,MD
Tien,Huey-Chung,MD
Vangvanichyakorn,Kamtorn,MD
Long Branch
Alemany,Carlos A.,MD
McNab,Theresa Challender,MD
Rekedal,Kirby D.,MD
Montclair
Peng,Chung J.,MD
Morristown
Federico,Cheryl L.,MD
Gluck,Karen,MD
Goil,Sunita,MD

Mimms,Gaines M.,MD
Orsini,Anthony J.,DO
Rogido,Marta R.,MD
Schenkman,Andrew C.,MD
Shen,Calvin T.,MD
Skolnick,Lawrence M.,MD
Neptune
Assing,Elizabeth J.,MD
Bautista,Eduardo R.,MD
Browne,Mary Beth,MD
Graff,Michael A.,MD
Karwowska,Helena,MD
Ramos,David G.D.,MD
Ross,Ann,MD
Torine,Ilana J.,DO
New Brunswick
Akhter,Waseem,MD
Anwar,Mujahid,MD
Bakare,Olubunmi,MD
Chandra,Shakuntala N.,MD
Hegyi,Thomas,MD
Herrera-Garcia,Guadalupe,DO
Hiatt,I. Mark,MD
Kaushik,Sridhar,MD
Khalil,Marwa A.,MD
Khan,Imteyaz Ahmad,MD
Lambert,George H.,MD
Mehta,Rajeev,MD
Memon,Naureen,MD
Puvabanditsn,Surasak,MD
Weinberger,Barry I.,MD
Newark
Ali,Salma,MD
Antonio,Excelsis O.,MD
Baja Quizon,Maria Cecilia,MD
Cohen,Morris,MD
Dermendjian,Mariette,MD
Feldman,Alexander,MD
Inwood,Richard J.,MD
Irakam,Anitha,MD
Lim,Anita Tiu,MD
Patel,Shalini Narendra,MD
Rai,Bellipady C.,MD
Ocean
Kashlan,Fawaz T.,MD
Paterson
Datta-Bhutada,Subhashree,MD
Marrero,Luis C.,MD
Menken,Gregory E.,MD
Rosenblum,Stacy,MD
Weissman,Michelle S.,MD
Zauk,Adel M.,MD
Plainsboro
Goel,Rajiv,MD
Marino,Anthony J. Jr.,MD
Mihalyfi,Brigitte E.,MD
Sambasivan,Roshni D.,MD
Pomona
Asiegbu,Benedict E.,MD
Grayson,Stephanie Anne,MD
Miller,Andrea,DO
Muhumuza,Catherine,MD
Tioseco,Jennifer Anne,MD
Princeton
Sangam,Subhasri L.,MD
Turcanu,Dumitru Sabin,MD
Raritan
Mody,Kartik D.,MD
Ridgewood
Carbone,Mary T.,MD
Lasker,Michelle Rhonda,MD
Manginello,Frank P.,MD
Pane,Carmela R.,MD
Shrewsbury
France,Jeffrey W.,DO
Somerville
Hirsch,Daniel Shawn,MD
Ladino,John Freddy,MD
Rejjal,Abdellatif R.,MD
Rotschild,Tomas,MD
Savla,Jayshree Sameer,MD
Verma,Anjali,MD
South Orange
Walker,Camille D.,MD
South Plainfield
Biswas,Anjali,MD
Stratford
Tinianow,Lloyd N.,MD
Tinton Falls
Fort,Prem,MD

Toms River
Sannoh,Sulaiman,MD
Trenton
Axelrod,Randi Allison,MD
Banzon,Felipe T.,MD
Moffitt,Stephen T.,MD
Turnersville
Malicdem,Milagros C.,MD
Vineland
Abbott-Fiedler,Vicky L.,MD
Bird,Charrell Moyo,MD
Elitsur,Noeet,MD
Voorhees
Austria,Jocelyn R.,MD
Bona,Marzena M.,MD
Brutus,Nadege A.,DO
Castillo,Minerva R.,MD
Chavez,Alberto M.,MD
Dapul,Gener M.,MD
Davis,Cheryl Luise,MD
Fong DeLeon,Elizabeth Y.,MD
Ghaben,Kamel Mostafa,MD
Hric,Jerome Joseph,MD
Hsu,Christopher Tzu-Yao,MD
Jethva,Purvi Jitendra,MD
Kim,Mirye,MD
Maher,Jennifer Lee,DO
Pandit,Paresh B.,MD
Polam,Sharadha,MD
Reisen,Charles E.,MD
Rosen,Harel D.,MD
Theophilopoulos,Constantine,MD
Wayne
Houlihan,Christopher M.,MD
Khoury,Aldo D.,MD
West Deptford
Petrozzino,Jeffrey,MD

Nephrology
Atlantic City
Degapudi,Bhargavi,MD
Kessler,Alex,DO
Mourad,Mohammad Y.,MD
Bayonne
Choudhry,Hammad S.,MD
Gupta,Shabnam,MD
Belleville
Keshav,Gayithri R.,MD
Keshav,Roger,MD
Samsa,Ranka Drazenovic,MD
Bergenfield
Benson,Payam,MD
Berkeley Heights
Lunenfeld,Ellen Beth,MD
Bloomfield
Coyle,Raluca,MD
Brick
Albanese,Joseph J.,DO
Brouder,Daniel J.,MD
Bruno,Robert,DO
DePalma,John Anthony,DO
Dounis,Harry James,DO
Ellis,Stephen J.,MD
Haider,Nadeem Z.,MD
Iglesias,Jose Ignacio,DO
Jain,Keshani,MD
Kapoor,Rajat,DO
Loman,Eric,DO
Markatos,Angelo,DO
Meyer,Ariel,DO
Park,Jin S.,MD
Schirripa,Joseph V.,MD
Tomasco,Thomas Joseph,MD
Bridgeton
De Priori,Elis Maria,MD
Bridgewater
Daskalakis,Nikki,MD
Noor,Fazle Ali,MD
Patel,Manisha Saurabh,MD
Caldwell
Siu,Albert,MD
Camden
Chakravarty,Arijit,MD
Kasama,Richard K.,MD
Kline,Jason Andrew,MD
Mian,Samia Fatima,MD
Weisberg,Lawrence Stephen,MD
Carteret
Singh,Bikramjit,MD

Physicians by Specialty and Town

Nephrology (cont)
Cherry Hill
Bodiwala,Brijesh Shreyas,DO
Butani,Savita M.,MD
McFadden,Christopher Bruce,MD
Michel,Brian E.,MD
Ra,Daniel,DO
Specter,Richard L.,MD
Cranford
Imbriano,Michael A.,DO
East Brunswick
Mansour,Mervat B.,MD
East Orange
Sastrasinh,Sithiporn,MD
Eatontown
Liss,Kenneth A.,DO
Edison
Czyzewski,Robert M.,MD
Park,Jun-Ki,MD
Rajan,Samir,MD
Sarwar,Samina,DO
Elizabeth
Reddy,Aravinda,MD
Silva-Khazaei,Maria Lourders,MD
Englewood
Zachariah,Teena,MD
Florham Park
Ahmad,Mir M.,MD
Estilo,Genevieve Kristina,MD
Glen Ridge
Khanna,Priya,DO
Hackensack
Adamidis,Ananea,MD
Bhayana,Suverta,MD
Joseph,Rosy E.,MD
Saro-Nunez,Lilian,MD
Vitievsky,Alexander Michael,MD
Hackettstown
Hajela,Amitabh,MD
Hainesport
Acharya,Prasad G.,MD
Conrad,Michael James,MD
Franger,Margaret Mary,MD
Min,Dorothy D.,MD
Share,David Seth,MD
Solitro,Matthew Joseph,MD
Suchin,Elliot Jay,MD
Vargas,Myra Theresa,MD
Hamilton
Hannani,Afshin K.,MD
Hazlet
Hozayen,Ossama,MD
Naqvi,Azeez Fathima,MD
Jackson
Kaur,Harneet,MD
Jersey City
Ahmed,Umrana,MD
Batwara,Ruchika,MD
Garg,Neha,MD
Goel,Narender,MD
Haddad,Bassam M.,MD
Haddad,Danny B.,MD
Mughni,Azam,MD
Patel,Jayeshkumar Shantilal,MD
Kendall Park
Merlin,Francky,MD
Kenilworth
Agresti,James V.,DO
Lawrenceville
Friedman,Gary S.,MD
Livingston
Dhillon,Navdeep,MD
Klein,Eileen C.,MD
Kotla,Revathi,MD
Pritsiolas,James Michael,MD
Tibaldi,Kim Nguyen,MD
Manahawkin
Shah,Ankit Prafulbhai,MD
Manasquan
Pandey,Shivendra,MD
Maplewood
Kodali,Padmaja,MD
Simon,Segun V.,MD
Marlton
Michael,Beckie,DO
Middlesex
Banerjee,Trina D.,MD
Midland Park
Chheda,Neha Das,MD
Weizman,Howard B.,MD

Millburn
Freundlich,Richard E.,MD
Minotola
Cirelly,Francine Arlene,DO
Monroe
Arabi,Nida,MD
Dwivedi,Shaunak A.,DO
Kalra,Tamanna H.,MD
Monroe Township
Prasad,Deepali,MD
Montclair
Bell,Alvin,MD
Blaustein,Daniel Alberto,MD
Goveas,Roveena Noeline,MD
Montvale
Wojnarska-Alvarez,Gabriela,MD
Morristown
Eppinger,Barry A.,DO
Fine,Paul L.,MD
Price,Barbara Ellen,MD
Stack,Jay I.,MD
Neptune
Bolarinwa,Oladayo,MD
Cruz,Dionisio V.,MD
Masud,Avais,MD
Patel,Mayurkumar P.,MD
New Brunswick
Akhtar,Rabia,MD
Bunin,Sonalis,MD
Khalil,Steve,MD
Lefavour,Gertrude S.,MD
Mann,Richard A.,MD
Mondal,Zahidul Hoque,MD
Palan,Vandana A.,MD
Puri,Sonika,MD
Newark
Chadha,Inderpal S.,MD
Chenitz,Kara Beth,MD
Kohli,Jatinder,MD
Mahendrakar,Smita,MD
Walsh,Liron,MD
Newton
Talon,Dennis J.,MD
North Bergen
Fein,Deborah Anne,MD
North Brunswick
Kapoian,Toros,MD
Northfield
Behl,Nitin,MD
Schreyer,Raymond S.,MD
Shastri,Jay Gautam,DO
Paramus
Abbasi,Arshia,MD
Ibeabuchi,Adaeze Nneka,MD
Paterson
Boyd,Marvin T.,MD
Phillipsburg
Gayner,Robert S.,MD
Pursell,Robert N.,MD
Shenoy,Mangalore Shantheri,MD
Princeton Junction
Basi,Seema,MD
Finkielstein,Vadim Aaron,MD
Rahway
Chaudhry,Anu,MD
Ravella,Supriya,MD
Vojnyk,Charlene Louise,MD
Randolph
Paster,Lauren,MD
Raritan
Haverty,Thomas Patrick,MD
Red Bank
Savransky,Ernest,MD
Salem
Sultan,Wamiq S.,MD
Somerset
Hakimzadeh,Parisa,DO
Jain,Sandesh,MD
Kabis,Suzanne M.,MD
Obias,Primabel Villena,MD
Srichai,Manakan Betsy,MD
Vaghasiya,Rick Parsotam,MD
South Plainfield
Rao,Bhavani P.,MD
South River
Drabik,Thomas Edward,DO
Matera,James J.,DO
Sparta
Casella,Frank J.,DO

Stratford
Dave,Chetna A.,MD
Summit
Kabaria,Sunit P.,MD
Teaneck
Ahmed,Subhan,MD
Coleman,Clenton Louis,MD
Gussak,Hiie M.,MD
Toms River
Anantharaman,Priya,MD
Arnold,Robert B.,MD
Palecki,Winicjusz,MD
Trenton
Cohen,Barry Herbert,MD
Cohen,Steven Craig,DO
Hussain,Asher Ferjad,MD
Pai,David Y.,MD
Sudhakar,Telechery A.,MD
Turnersville
Irwin-Obregon,Virginia,DO
Panebianco,Paul S.,DO
Union
Latif,Walead,DO
Union City
Bebawy,Niveen,MD
Thomsen,Stephen,MD
Ventnor City
Naber,Tamim Hani,MD
Vineland
Girone,Joseph Francis,MD
Relia,Nitin,MD
Yoslov,Michael D.,DO
Voorhees
Banker,Gopika H.,DO
Chawla,Arun,MD
Lodhavia,Devang V.,MD
Patel,Nitesh M.,DO
Wall
Mehandru,Sushil K.,MD
Wayne
Audia,Pat Frank,MD
Joseph,Monalisa,MD
Masand,Anjali Narain,MD
Prakash,Ananth N.,MD
Shah,Sanjay R.,MD
Triolo,Diane Cecilia,MD
Vitting,Kevin E.,MD
Yousef,Nadia P.,MD
Zeltser,Eugene,MD
West Orange
Bonomini,Luigi Vittorio,MD
Jeanlouie,Odler R.,MD
Komati,Naga Malleswari,MD
Lefkowitz,Heather Rush,MD
Palekar,Sadanand S.,MD
Shah,Nita K.,MD
Westfield
Brown,Ryan P.,MD
Klein,Philip S.,MD
Whippany
Perkins,Robert Mark,MD
Woodbury
Lyons,Patricia J.,MD

Neuro-Ophthalmology
Edison
Rosenberg,Michael L.,MD

Neuro-Psychiatry
Hackensack
Trobliger,Robert William,MD
Manchester
Gbeve-Hill,Dorcas,MD
Montclair
Haller,Kate,MD
Morris Plains
Collopy,Edward M.,MD
Paramus
Crain,Peter M.,MD

Neurological Radiology
Avenel
Fontana,Leo John,MD
Belleville
Lapas,Alkies,DO
Brick
Jain Lakhani,Neelu,MD
Camden
Saraiya,Piya Vijay,MD
Shah,Pallav N.,DO
Clinton
Saul,Jared Michael,MD

Columbus
Saffran,Bruce Nathan,MD
Denville
Manzo,Rene Paul,MD
East Brunswick
Basak,Sandip,MD
Fitzpatrick,Maurice,MD
Patel,Keyur Bhupendra,MD
Schlesinger,Scott D.,MD
Schonfeld,Steven M.,MD
Edgewater
Garger,Alexander,MD
Edison
Jilani,Mohammad Imran,MD
Emerson
Parag,Yoav,MD
Green Brook
Lee,Seungho Howard,MD
Hackensack
Foster,Sarah Jeanmarie,MD
Monoky,David John,MD
Pierce,Sean Donovan,MD
Haddonfield
Miller,Anthony Francis,MD
Hainesport
Rizvi,Azam H.,MD
Hamilton
Kulkarni,Kedar,MD
Sterling,Michelle Gold,MD
Little Silver
O'Connor,Douglas S.,MD
Newark
Slasky,Shira E.,MD
Oradell
Zablow,Bruce Charles,MD
Paramus
Bahramipour,Phillip F.,MD
River Edge
Wattamwar,Anoop Suresh,MD
Sewell
Zarzour,Hekmat Khodr,MD
Teaneck
Melisaratos,Darius Paris,MD
Toms River
Finkel,Arkady,MD
Vineland
Alves,Eric M.,DO
West Long Branch
Mann,Sunita Singh,MD
West Orange
Aboody,Ronald S.,MD

Neurological Surgery
Berkeley Heights
Beyerl,Brian David,MD
Bridgewater
Chimenti,James M.,MD
More,Jay,MD
Camden
Goldman,Howard Warren,MD
Turtz,Alan R.,MD
Clifton
Cifelli,John Riggio,MD
Edison
Bashir,Asif,MD
Bloomfield,Stephen M.,MD
Iyer,Asha Muthuraman,MD
Kuo,Howard,MD
Pan,Jeff,MD
Przybylski,Gregory J.,MD
Shekhtman,Yevgenia,MD
Steineke,Thomas C.,MD
Englewood
Gologorsky,Yakov,MD
Moore,Frank Max,MD
Steinberger,Alfred A.,MD
Yao,Kevin Chi-Kai,MD
Flemington
Pizzi,Francis Joseph,MD
Florham Park
Noce,Louis Arthur,MD
Scheid,Edward Herbert Jr.,MD
Freehold
Tormenti,Matthew J.,MD
Hackensack
Peterson,Thomas Russell,MD
Schwartz,Lauren Faith,MD
Hamilton
Lipani,John David,MD

Physicians by Specialty and Town

Hasbrouck Heights
Oppenheimer,Jeffrey Harry,MD
Hoboken
Hunt,Charles D.,MD
Jersey City
Mirza,Neville M.,MD
Lawrenceville
Abud,Ariel F.,MD
Chiurco,Anthony A.,MD
Linwood
Delasotta,Fernando J.,MD
Lowe,James G.,MD
Livingston
Anderson,Richard C.,MD
Couch,Jonathan Darrell,DO
Gigante,Paul R.,MD
Gilman,Arthur Michael,MD
Hubschmann,Otakar R.,MD
Rotoli,Giorgio,DO
Marlton
Bussey,Jonathan David,DO
Meagher,Richard John,MD
Montclair
Clemente,Roderick J.,MD
Dannis,Seth Michael,MD
Moorestown
Cervantes,Luis A.,MD
Morristown
Baskin,Jonathan Jay,MD
Benitez,Ronald Patrick,MD
Chapple,Kyle Thomas,MD
Chun,Jay Y.,MD
Gardner,Allan Lee,MD
Knightly,John J.,MD
Mazzola,Catherine A.,MD
Meyer,Scott Andrew,MD
Moshel,Yaron Aharon,MD
Stillerman,Charles Blair,MD
Sumas,Maria Elaina,MD
Wells-Roth,David S.,MD
Zampella,Edward J.,MD
Mount Laurel
Mitchell,William,MD
Testaiuti,Mark A.,MD
New Brunswick
Danish,Shabbar F.,MD
Gupta,Gaurav,MD
Nosko,Michael G.,MD
Newark
Bassani,Luigi,MD
Gandhi,Chirag D.,MD
Gillick,John,MD
Goldstein,Ira Morris,MD
Heary,Robert F.,MD
Ho,Victor T.,MD
Jethwa,Pinakin R.,MD
Mammis,Antonios,MD
Prestigiacomo,Charles Joseph,MD
Oradell
Azmi Ghadimi,Hooman,MD
Kaptain,George J.,MD
Karimi,Reza J.,MD
Khan,Mohammed Faraz,MD
Lee,Kangmin Daniel,MD
Roth,Patrick A.,MD
Vingan,Roy David,MD
Walzman,Daniel Ezra,MD
Zahos,Peter A.,MD
Paterson
Appelboom,Geoffrey,MD
Mandigo,Grace Kim,MD
Pennington
Buono,Lee M.,MD
Connolly,Patrick Joseph,MD
Fennell,Vernard Sharif,MD
Stiefel,Michael Fred,MD
Princeton
McLaughlin,Mark Robert,MD
Von Der Schmidt,Edward III,MD
Randolph
Engle,Edward A.,MD
Red Bank
Eisenbrock,Howard J.,DO
Ridgewood
Carpenter,Duncan B.,MD
Cobb,William Stewart,MD
D'Ambrosio,Anthony Louis,MD
Goulart,Hamilton C.,MD
Klempner,William L.,MD
Lavine,Sean David,MD

Moise,Gaetan,MD
Sheth,Sameer Anil,MD
Rutherford
El Khashab,Mostafa A. F.,MD
Fried,Arno H.,MD
Rathmann,Allison Marie,DO
Sewell
Garrido,Eddy O.,MD
Shrewsbury
Rosenblum,Bruce R.,MD
Somers Point
Glass,Andrew S.,MD
Sabo,Robert A.,MD
Somerset
Fineman,Sanford,MD
Summit
Hodosh,Richard M.,MD
Toms River
Hartwell,Richard Conrad,MD
Moyle,Henry,MD
Sarris,John,MD
Trenton
Barrese,James C.,MD
Union
Friedlander,Marvin E.,MD
Gilad,Ronit,MD
Lipson,Adam Craig,MD
Nair,Anil Karunakaran,MD
Poulad,David,MD
Randazzo,Ciro Giuseppe,MD
Ratzker,Paul K.,MD
Vineland
Kazmi,Najam U.,MD
Strauss,Richard Charles,MD
Voorhees
Siddiqi,Tariq S.,MD
Wall
Maggio,William W.,MD
Salerno,Simon Anthony,MD
Wayne
Raab,Rajnik Weerackody,MD
Sundstrom,David C.,MD
West Long Branch
Estin,David,MD
Gillis,Christopher Charles,MD
Link,Timothy Emerson,MD
Lustgarten,Jonathan H.,MD
Olson,Ty James,MD
West Orange
Assina,Rachid,MD
Koziol,Joseph M.,MD

Neurology
Aberdeen
Daniel,Joshua,MD
Atlantic City
Zeidwerg,David Martin,DO
Audubon
Sen Hightower,Indrani,MD
Basking Ridge
Gavrilovic,Igor T.,MD
Bayonne
Charles,James A.,MD
Kapoor,Ashish,MD
Kapoor,Vinod,MD
Nagendra,Shan M.,MD
Sadeghi,Hooshang,MD
Topper,Leonid Lev,MD
Vintayen,Enrico V.,MD
Belleville
Deluca,Matthew J.,MD
Lomazow,Steven M.,MD
Berkeley Heights
Cohen,Eric R.,DO
Coohill,Lisa Marie,MD
Naik,Komal Desai,DO
Turner,Garth M.,MD
Bloomfield
Nayak,Bharathi,MD
Nazareth,Joseph M.,MD
Brick
Barcas,Peter P.,DO
Escandon,Sandra L.,MD
Miskin,Pandurang R.,MD
Sedarous,Mary,MD
Bridgeton
Rampal,Sharan,MD
Bridgewater
Reznik,Andrea I.,MD
Wittenborn,John Richard,MD

Cape May Court House
Edwards,Jillian,DO
Singh,Manish Kumar,MD
Carneys Point
Fernandez,Maria Elmina,MD
Graham,Dennis C.,DO
Carteret
Behman,Haidy Mankarios,MD
Mills,Richard J.,MD
Chatham
Dorflinger,Ernest Edward Jr.,MD
Cherry Hill
Abrams,Russell I.,MD
Burakgazi Dalkilic,Evren,MD
Campellone,Joseph V. Jr.,MD
Colcher,Amy,MD
Ingala,Erin Einbinder,MD
Janoff,Larry Stewart,DO
Lipsius,Bruce D.,MD
McGarry,Andrew James,MD
Mirsen,Thomas R.,MD
Moeller,Joseph Phillip,DO
Popescu,Anca S.,MD
Preis,Keith Victor,MD
Rogers,James J.,DO
Weiner,Francine L.,MD
Clifton
Katz,Avery S.,MD
Knep,Stanley J.,MD
Lequerica,Steve A.,MD
Nangia,Arun,MD
Padela,Mohammad F.,MD
Tagayun,Myrna B.,MD
Denville
Miric,Slobodan,MD
Dover
Dover,Marcia Anne,MD
Roberts,Paul J.,MD
Stephen,Infanta Anusha,MD
East Brunswick
Lazar,Mark H.,MD
Lupyan,Yan,MD
Wasserstrom,William R.,MD
East Orange
Clark,Ruth L.,MD
Gupta,Pradip,MD
Maeda,Yasuhiro,MD
Terrence,Christopher Jr.,MD
Edgewater
Shajenko,Lydia,MD
Edison
Bhat,Sushanth K.,MD
Buchwald,Eugene E.,MD
Chen,Shan,MD
Fourcand,Farah Yolanda,MD
Gan,Richard A.,MD
Gupta,Divya,MD
Gupta,Simhadri M.,MD
Hanna,Philip Andre,MD
He,Ming,MD
Herman,Martin N.,MD
Hooshangi,Nossratollah,MD
Kirmani,Jawad F.,MD
Kramer,Phillip D.,MD
Landolfi,Joseph Charles,DO
Ma,Wei Wei,MD
Mani,Srinivasan S.,MD
Mehta,Siddhart Kumar,MD
Merkin,Michael D.,MD
Mian,Fawad A.,MD
Miller,Gary Stuart,MD
Nizam,Mohammed Farrukh,MD
Noor,Emad Roshdy,MD
Oh,Youn K.,MD
Panezai,Spozhmy,MD
Roblejo,Peter C.,MD
Silveira,Diosely De Castro,MD
Singh,Amrinder,MD
Sinha,Sugiti,MD
Sobol,Igor Leonidovich,MD
Sobol,Marina B.,MD
Uhrik,Eric Joseph,DO
Zu,James Shanwei,MD
Egg Harbor Township
Hunter,Kevin Edward,MD
Reid-Duncan,Lucienne Lariane,MD
Tahmoush,Albert J.,MD
Elizabeth
Bhatt,Meeta Hasmukh,MD
Pareja,Victor Hugo,MD
Sananman,Michael L.,MD

Tao,Ying,MD
Emerson
Asta,Charles Francis,MD
Dhadwal,Neetu,MD
Englewood
Adler,Daniel G.,MD
Akbaripanahi,Sepideh,MD
Alweiss,Gary S.,MD
Choi,Yun-Beom,MD
Levy,Kirk Jay,MD
Racela,Rikki Redona,MD
Rajasingham,Jamuna Kandasamy,MD
Rosenbaum,David Herbert,MD
Rothman,Arthur C.,MD
Willner,Joseph Harrison,MD
Englewood Cliffs
Bressler,Jill Anne,MD
Fremed,Eric L.,MD
Mueller,Nancy L.,MD
Prince,David M.,MD
Rabin,Aaron,MD
Fair Lawn
Kamin,Marc,MD
Shah,Nilay Ramesh,MD
Flemington
Kososky,Charles S.,MD
Pandya,Dipakkumar P.,MD
Pennett,Donald T.,MD
Viradia,Manish Bhikhabhai,MD
Freehold
Bonazinga,Thomas P.,MD
Frank,David J.,MD
Gulevski,Vasko Kole,MD
Katz,Amos,MD
Marks,Caren G.,MD
McAlarney,Terence,MD
Zaatreh,Megdad M.,MD
Galloway
Boxman,Jeffrey R.,DO
Youssef,Iman Shawki,MD
Glen Ridge
Blady,David,MD
Vaccaro,John J.,MD
Glen Rock
Nanavati,Farzana Nilesh,MD
Hackensack
Dash,Subasini,MD
Douyon,Philippe Gerard,MD
Fellman,Damon M.,MD
Feoli,Enrique Alfredo,MD
Goldlust,Samuel Aaron,MD
Ibrahim,Ayman M.,DO
Inoyama,Katherine S.,MD
Kreibich,Thomas Alfred,MD
Krel,Regina,MD
Liff,Jeremy M.,MD
Marquinez,Anthony I.,MD
Oller-Cramsie,Marissa Anne,DO
Pandey,Krupa Shah,MD
Puntambekar,Preeti Vasant,MD
Rao,Gautami Kondamodi,MD
Silverstein,Michael P.,MD
Singer,Samuel,MD
Solanky,Mukesh,MD
Tsao,Julie Ching Yen,MD
Vukic,Mario,MD
Haddon Township
Dinsmore,Steven Thomas,DO
Hubbard,Sean Tomar,DO
Hamilton
Pasupuleti,Rao Satyanaray,MD
Pendino,Alexander M.,DO
Hammonton
Carta,Maria C.,MD
De Antonio,Sondra M.,MD
Hazlet
Pavuluri,Srinivas,MD
Hoboken
Ploshchanskaya,Larisa G.,MD
Holmdel
Gandhi,Shefali,DO
Khakoo,Rafiya Shabbir,MD
Irvington
Dressner,Ivan R.,MD
Sutaria,Hasmukhbha N.,MD
Jersey City
Anselmi,Gregory D.,MD
Brannan,Timothy S.,MD
Dasika,Vijaya R.,MD
Dumitru,Dan Lucian,MD
Khan,Musaid A.,MD

Physicians by Specialty and Town

Neurology (cont)

Jersey City
- Komotar, Ana M., MD
- Korya, Dani, MD

Lakewood
- Lombardino, Anthony N., MD

Lawrenceville
- Alexeeva, Aissa Timofeyevna, MD
- DeLuca, Debra J., MD
- Gomez, Rene S., MD
- Kaiser, Paul K., MD
- Vergara, Manuel Salvador, MD

Livingston
- Bhawsar, Nilaya Babu, DO
- Devinsky, Orrin, MD
- Geller, Eric Bernard, MD
- Nadkarni, Mangala A., MD
- Natanzon, Calvin, MD
- Sobelman, Joseph S., MD
- Widdess-Walsh, Peter Patrick, MD
- Zhang, Yan Chun, MD

Lumberton
- Kachroo, Arun, MD
- Keller, Seth Martin, MD
- Mathur, Mayank, MD
- Orwitz, Jonathan Ira, MD
- Thomas, Carole E., MD

Madison
- Bathini, Manjula, DO

Mahwah
- Scrimenti, Michael P., MD

Manahawkin
- Papa-Rugino, Tommasina, MD
- Terranova, Robert J., DO

Manalapan
- Enescu, Cristian C., MD
- Furman, Boris, DO

Maple Shade
- Abidi, Saiyid Manzoor, MD
- Vanna, Stephen C., MD
- Yang, John Y., MD

Marlton
- Klazmer, Jay, DO
- Ma, Xiaoping, MD
- Mabanta, Ricardo Y., MD

Medford
- Lee, David Charles, MD

Mercerville
- Weaner, Scott Michael, DO

Metuchen
- Zhang, Tianshu, MD

Monroe Township
- Friedlander, Devin S., MD

Moorestown
- Vijayaraghavan, Swathi, MD

Morganville
- Choy, Maria, MD
- Mehta, Amor Ruyintan, MD

Morristown
- Alias, Mathew N., DO
- Babineau, Shannon Elizabeth, MD
- Conigliari, Matthew F., MD
- Diamond, Mark S., MD
- Fox, Stuart W., MD
- Iones, Anna, MD
- Karolchyk, Mary A., DO
- Knappertz, Volker Armin, MD
- Marx, Tatyana, MD
- Okunola, Oladotun A., MD
- Royce, Roxanne, MD
- Tsairis, Peter, MD
- Ugorec, Igor, MD

Mount Laurel
- Pello, Scott Jason, MD

Neptune
- Baqui, Huma, MD
- Deutsch, Alan D., DO
- Eswar, Anastasia Maria, MD
- Fitzpatrick, John E., MD
- Karia, Roopal M., MD
- Martino, Stephen John, MD
- Rhee, Richard S., MD
- Silbert, Paul J., MD

New Brunswick
- Aiken, Robert Dennis, MD
- Balashov, Konstantin E., MD
- Belsh, Jerry M., MD
- Dhib Jalbut, Suhayl S., MD
- Gerhardstein, Brian Lee, MD
- Golbe, Lawrence I., MD

Newark
- Al Kawi, Ammar, MD
- Alvarez-Prieto, Maria R., MD
- Cook, Stuart D., MD
- Cornett, Oriana Ellen, MD
- Elmoursi, Sedeek, MD
- Ford, Lisa M., MD
- Hidalgo, Andrea, MD
- Hillen, Machteld E., MD
- Husar, Walter G., MD
- Johnson, William Gessner, MD
- Kamin, Stephen S., MD
- Khandelwal, Priyank, MD
- Khelemsky, Serge, DO
- Lastra, Carlos R., MD
- Leitch, Megan Moran, MD
- Lepore, Frederick E., MD
- Mani, Ram, MD
- Mark, Margery H., MD
- Marks, David Alon, MD
- Mehta, Anita Khanna, DO
- Michaels, Jennifer, MD
- Mouradian, Mary Maral, MD
- Patel, Bindi Akshay, DO
- Peeraully, Tasneem, MD
- Sage, Jacob I., MD
- Schneider, Daniel Paul, MD
- Sheikh, Shuja, MD
- Sivaraaman, Kartik, MD
- Souayah, Nizar, MD
- Szapiel, Susan V., MD
- Tabbarah, Khalid Zuhayr, MD
- Wong, Stephen, MD

Newton
- Khesin, Yevgeniy I., MD
- Tishuk, Pavel, MD
- Weintraub, Bernard M., MD

North Bergen
- Prasad, Nalini, MD
- Tikoo, Ravinder Kumar, MD

North Caldwell
- Carmickle, Lynne J., MD

Ocean
- Raab, Vicki E., MD

Old Bridge
- Rao, Padmarekha, MD
- Song, Haodong, MD

Paramus
- Conte, Theodore J., MD

Paterson
- Altschul, Dorothea, MD
- Corrigan, Nicole Melissa, MD
- Dane, Steven H., MD
- Mehta, Mahesh M., MD
- Sathe, Swati Ajit, MD
- Stein, Beth, MD
- Xia, Wenlang, MD

Pennington
- Assadi-Khansari, Mitra, MD
- Landen, Alexandra E., DO
- Rubin, Mitchell J., MD
- Schumacher, Hermann Christian, MD
- Shukla, Chirag S., MD
- Vester, John W., MD
- Witte, Arnold S., MD

Pennsville
- Syritsyna, Olga, MD

Phillipsburg
- Garber, Todd Ryan, MD
- Mehta, Heeral J., MD
- Shah, Ila A., MD

Piscataway
- Richfield, Eric Karl, MD

Plainsboro
- Sachdeo, Rajesh C., MD

Princeton
- Maggio, Vijay, MD

Ramsey
- Trifiletti, Rosario R., MD

Raritan
- Biondi, David M., DO

Red Bank
- Chen, Edgar Y., MD
- Fan, Schuber C., MD
- Ilaria, Philip V., MD

Ridgewood
- Berlin, Daniel, MD
- Citak, Kenneth A., MD
- Grewal, Amrit K., MD
- Levin, Kenneth A., MD
- Lijtmaer, Hugo N., MD

- Molinari, Susan P., MD
- Naidu, Yamini, MD
- Nasr, John T., MD
- Noskin, Olga, MD
- Perron, Reed C., MD
- Shammas, James T., MD
- Tong, Fumin, MD
- Van Engel, Daniel R., MD
- Winfree, Christopher Jules, MD

River Edge
- Adams, Angela, MD

Rochelle Park
- Effron, Charles Richard, MD

Rockaway
- Bongiovanni, Denise A., DO
- Tonzola, Richard F., MD

Roseland
- Weisbrot, Frederick J., MD

Rumson
- Colicchio, Alan Robert, MD

Scotch Plains
- Fischer, Beverly Ruth, MD

Sewell
- Sammartino, Robert A., DO

Somers Point
- Roeltgen, David P., MD
- Tzorfas, Scott D., MD
- Yangala, Ravi, MD

Somerset
- Busono, Stephanus Judi D., MD
- Dixit, Seema P., DO
- Greenberg, E. Jeffrey, MD
- Hersh, Joshua Neil, MD

Somerville
- Mian, Bilal A., MD

Sparta
- Greene, Wayne L., MD

Stratford
- Barone, Donald A., DO
- Serban, Valeria, MD

Summit
- Alexianu, Maria E., MD
- Craciun, Liviu Ciprian, MD
- Halperin, John Jacob, MD
- Metrus, Nicholas Robert, MD
- Politsky, Jeffrey Mark, MD
- Pollock, Jeffrey C., MD
- Rabin, Marcie L., MD
- Stoller, Seth Ryan, MD
- Tarulli, Andrew William, MD
- Vigman, Melvin P., MD

Swedesboro
- Lotkowski, Susan D., DO

Teaneck
- Blitz-Shabbir, Karen M., DO
- Duncan, David Brian, MD
- Kailas, Michael G., MD
- Picone, Maryann, MD

Tinton Falls
- Pertchik, Alan F., MD

Toms River
- Amin, Darshana Patel, DO
- DiPaola, Rocco J., MD
- Ferencz, Gerald J., MD
- Monastersky, Bruce Ted, MD
- Schenker, Samuel D., MD
- Whiteman, Martin, DO
- Wilson, Sylvia V., MD
- Zimmerman, Barry L., DO

Trenton
- Eckardt, Gerald William, MD
- Grewal, Raji Paul, MD
- Rao, Vikas Yallapragada, MD
- Shultz, Lisa Ann, MD
- Taboada, Javier Gustavo, MD

Turnersville
- Irby, Dahlia Jean, MD
- Zaman, Taimur, MD

Union City
- Krish, Nagesh B., MD

Vineland
- Gupta, Vipin K., MD
- Rocksmith, Eugenio Roberto, MD
- Skinner, Dirk E., MD

Voorhees
- Bromley, Steven Michael, MD
- Gupta, Asha, MD
- Patil, Kishor K., MD
- Rincon, Fred, MD
- Sun, Yun Lynn, MD

- Vasishta, Shiva G., MD
- Yanoschak, Jennifer Lee, MD

Waretown
- Greenberg, John P., MD

Warren
- Morganoff, Abraham D., MD
- Sinha, Kavita, MD

Wayne
- Chodosh, Eliot Howard, MD
- Gazzillo, Frank L., MD
- Mascellino, Ann Marie M., MD
- Monck, Jennefer Erinna, MD
- Nayal, Eyad A., MD
- Safar, David S., MD
- Wagner, Robert Austin, MD
- Yazgi, Nabil M., MD

West Caldwell
- Khoshnu, Esha, MD
- Mendelson, Stuart G., MD
- Ruderman, Marvin I., MD

West Long Branch
- Gennaro, Paul, M
- Gilson, Noah R., MD
- Patel, Dakshesh K., MD
- Ponce, Francis B., MD
- Raval, Sumul N., MD

West Orange
- Barrett, Anna Mariya, MD
- Becker, Andrew Nacholas, DO
- Haskins, Danielle, MD
- Kupershtok-Bojko, Aviva Sara, MD
- Mehta, Deviyani Dilipkumar, MD

West Paterson
- Jafri, Syed S., MD

Westfield
- Saur, David P., MD

Westwood
- Connors, Robert Dedick, MD
- Ghacibeh, Georges A., MD
- Kakkar, Pankaj, MD
- Klein, Patricia G., MD
- Lira, Lorraine Sales, MD
- Mittelmann, Eric, MD
- Tsai, Joyce, MD
- Van Slooten, David D., MD

Willingboro
- Dunn, Timothy John, MD
- Partnow, Michael J., MD
- Sharetts, Scott R., MD

Woodbury
- Bokkala Pinniniti, Shaila, DO
- Denner, Michael J., MD
- Miller, Ann Marie, MD
- Zangaladze, Andro T., MD

Woodbury Heights
- Saleeb, Mariam, MD

Neuromusculoskeletal Med & OMM

Cherry Hill
- Picciotti, Brett, DO

Paramus
- Grinman, Lev, MD

Neuromusculoskeletal-Sports Med

Marlton
- Stein, Meryl Yvonne, MD

Neuropathology

Bayonne
- Ferrer, Gerrard F. A., DO

Edison
- Nochlin Soto, David, MD

Newark
- Sharer, Leroy Ralph Jr., MD

Summit
- Bouffard, John Paul, MD

Nuclear Cardiology

Browns Mills
- Van Hise, Aaron C., DO

Springfield
- Furer, Steven K., MD

Nuclear Diagnostic Radiology

Camden
- Hardy, Caitlin Judith, MD

Livingston
- Viggiano, Joseph T., MD

Nuclear Medicine
Basking Ridge
Vaseghi,Moein Faghih,MD
Belleville
Reich,Helene,MD
Camden
Grabski,Karsten,MD
Carlstadt
Dakhel,Mahmoud,MD
Denville
Plutchok,Jeffrey J.,MD
East Brunswick
Becker,Murray David,MD
Kempf,Jeffrey Scott,MD
Thind,Pritinder K.,MD
Yudd,Anthony P.,MD
Edison
Jaffe,Robert M.,MD
Miller,Howard M.,MD
Englewood Cliffs
Ding,You-Guang,MD
Hainesport
Kaufman,Michael S.,MD
Jersey City
Shah,Hemant R.,MD
Livingston
Bedigian,Martin Peter,MD
Lutzker,Letty Goodman,MD
Morristown
Claps,Richard J.,MD
Newark
Lao,Ramon S.,MD
Lee,Sang O.,MD
Mousavi,Mohammad Ali,DO
Parmett,Steven Russell,MD
Quarless,Shelley Ann,DO
Quinones,Candido P.,MD
Nutley
Richman,Steven D.,MD
Parsippany
Paik,David,MD
Paterson
Conte,Patrick Jr.,MD
Kalika,Valery,MD
Perth Amboy
Sen,Shuvendu,MD
Plainsboro
Sood,Ravi,MD
Randolph
Goldstein,Harold A.,MD
Sewell
Desai,Anil G.,MD
Shrewsbury
Ruchman,Richard B.,MD
Summit
Borkar,Sunita A.,MD
Teaneck
Sireci,Steven N. Jr.,MD
Toms River
Gajarawala,Jatin M.,MD
Wall
Krynyckyi,Borys Roman,MD
Monaco,Robert A.,MD
West Deptford
Whitley,Markus A.,MD

Nutrition
Short Hills
Deshaw,Barbara Blank,MD

ObGyn-Hospice & Palliative Care
West Orange
Nwobu,Uchenna Christian,MD

Obstetrics
Burlington
Steinberg,Frederic,DO
Camden
Diaz,Yanirys,MD
Deptford
Robinson,John Michael,DO
Mount Laurel
McCullen,Kristen Michelle,DO
New Brunswick
Awomolo,Adeola,MD
Farkas,Andrew,MD
Ho,Diana,MD
Voorhees
Williams,Kristina,MD

Obstetrics & Gynecology
Absecon
Carfagno,Salvatore Jr.,DO
Sackstein,Stuart A.,MD
Asbury Park
Herron,Garland Ella,MD
Lepis,Carl R.,MD
Lore,Kristen Nicole,DO
Michalewski,Martin P.,MD
Atlantic City
Irvis,Kenneth M.,MD
Regis,Jon M.,MD
Avenel
Kline,Philip E.,MD
Basking Ridge
Doherty,Leo Francis,MD
Fagan,Linda Nadine,MD
Hong,Kathleen H.,MD
Jurema,Marcus W.,MD
Kim,Julia G.,MD
Leitao,Mario Mendes Jr.,MD
Rauch,Eden Renee,MD
Werner,Marie D.,MD
Bayonne
Marki,Richard E.,MD
Patel,Rakhee,MD
Pelosi,Marco A. Jr.,MD
Prakash,Shasha,MD
Bedminster
Bosin,Corey S.,MD
Hersh,Judith Ellen,MD
Peters,Albert J.,DO
Belleville
Cicalese,Gerard R.,MD
Devalla,Meena,MD
Esiely,Mohamed A.,MD
Jain,Ratnam,MD
Lay,Virginia I.,MD
Mohammed,Decca,MD
Perez,Walter,MD
Yeum,Sandy H.,MD
Bergenfield
Meier,Ronny,MD
Meier-Ginsberg,Efrat,MD
Berkeley Heights
Forrester,Dara Lynn,MD
Masterson,Christine,MD
Bernardsville
Mehta,Jyotsna S.,MD
Blackwood
Croff,William J.,DO
Delvadia,Dipak R.,DO
Montgomery,Owen Canterbury,MD
Bloomfield
Kusnierz,Earl I.,DO
Yacoub,Mounzer H.,MD
Bogota
Kuye,Olabisi O.,MD
Boonton
Dibenedetto,Robert J.,MD
Branchburg
Andrin,Margaret,MD
Horowitz,Alyssa G.,MD
Brick
Benecki,Theresa R.,MD
Ketelaar,Pieter J.,MD
Morgan,Darlene M.,MD
Pagano,Ann Marie,MD
Patel,Vanita Hitesh,MD
Vetter,Paul L.,MD
Bridgewater
Bernstein,Sambra H.,MD
Errico,Carmine P.,MD
Mileto,Vincent F.,MD
Miranda,Matilda,MD
Oza,Palak,MD
Woltz,Ayanna Rashea,MD
Burlington
Mitchell-Williams,Jocelyn,MD
Salvatore,Michelle Lyn,MD
Siefring,Robert P.,MD
Camden
Askia,Gyasi Abena,DO
Aves,Cindy,MD
Bahora,Masuma,MD
Barnea,Eytan R.,MD
Bilbao,Michelle Cifone,DO
Bruckler,Paula A.,DO
Cardonick,Elyce Hope,MD
Chang,Eric,DO
Chang,Leona,DO
Chen,Peter Jen-Chih,MD
Christophe,Kathleen Mary,MD
Deary,Michael J.,MD
Desimone,Dennis Charles,DO
Dinh,Tuan A.,MD
Elshoreya,Hazem Mohamed,MD
Frattarola,Michael A.,MD
Fuseini,Nurain M.,MD
Hall,Bianca Elena,DO
Hernandez,Marcia Lynn,DO
Hewlett,Guy Stewart,MD
Hyman,Francine,MD
Iyer,Neel Subramanian,MD
Khandelwal,Meena,MD
Kim,Yon Sook,MD
Knights,Jayci Elenor,MD
La Motta,Joseph D.,MD
Lieser,Joan Karen,MD
Ligouri,Adrienne L.,MD
Marino,Joseph Frederick,DO
Martinez,Frances Aileen,MD
Owens,Nefertari Alisha,MD
Phillips,Nancy L.,MD
Pistilli,Stephanie Marie,DO
Ross,Carolyn Michelle,MD
Rugut,Chloe,MD
Schaeffer,Kathleen M.,DO
Shah,Nima M.,MD
Smolinsky,Ciaran,MD
Spector,Sean David,MD
Tagni,Carine-Ange,MD
Timms,Diane De Lisi,DO
Toidze,Tamara V.,MD
Tyree,Laura Lynne,MD
Wilson Smith,Robin Renee',DO
Yahav,Eric Kfir,MD
Cape May Court House
Michner,Richard A.,MD
Milio,Joseph L.,DO
Noll,Bruce R.,MD
Cedar Grove
Lee,Angie Yookyoung,MD
Cedar Knolls
Chu,Mary M.,MD
Kuchera,James Joseph,MD
Kuchera,Michael W.,MD
Potash,Sarah K.,MD
Ricks,Ann Marie,MD
Chatham
Ganitsch,Christine A.,MD
Reynolds,Nina D.,MD
Silverberg,Fred Marshall,MD
Cherry Hill
Arole,Chidinma N.,MD
Benett,Jodi A.,DO
Borromeo,Rita Gonzalez,MD
Burke,Gerald V.,MD
Glass,Phillip,MD
Hunter,Robert L.,MD
Kaufman,Susan I.,DO
Khosla,Jayasree,MD
Litz,John Jr.,MD
O'Banion,Kathleen S.,MD
Or,Drorit,MD
Rana,Ramneek,MD
Chester
Mitchell,Barbara,MD
Clark
Beauchamp,Jeffrey Thomas,MD
Blum,Richard Howard,MD
Hoebich,Karen A.,MD
Melamud,Elaine A.,MD
Wong,So Mui,MD
Cliffside Park
Adu-Amankwa,Bernice Abrafi,MD
Amerson,Afriye Rochelle,MD
Clifton
Balzani,Henry H.,MD
Boyle,Elizabeth Anne,DO
Dinu,Catalina,MD
Haddad,Charles George,MD
Hakimi,Daniel,DO
Khan,Farhana Haleem,MD
Kugler,Edward F.,MD
Langer,Orli,MD
Pajoohi,Soheil,MD
Saba,Souheil,MD
Shah,Vinay R.,MD
Singh,Sukhdeep,MD
Smith,Jacqueline Marie,MD
Smith,Jade,DO
Sullivan,Jared Martin,MD
Tah,Peter A.,MD
Clinton
Whang,Gene,MD
Collingswood
Margolin,Gregory,MD
Parrish,Sherrilynn,MD
Colts Neck
Sikand,Vandna,MD
Columbia
DeSanti,Michelina,DO
Columbus
Chao,Christina,MD
Cranford
Anzalone,Anthony,MD
Kaye,Alissa Ellen,MD
Kaye,Gary L.,MD
Shah,Mahesh Maneklal,MD
Delran
Edwards,Linda J.,MD
Ginwala,Khatoon T.,MD
Obianwu,Chike W.,MD
Denville
Agnello,Jennifer T.,DO
Rothenberg,Richard N.,MD
Shah,Yashica Manish,MD
Tsai,Yan-San,MD
Dover
Wallis,Joseph J.,DO
Dumont
Chinchankar,Rajeshree P.,MD
Kim,Sonia,MD
East Brunswick
Beim,Daniel S.,MD
Bharucha,Dilip I.,MD
Cernadas,Maureen,MD
Cherot,Elizabeth Kagel,MD
Chudner,Margarita,MD
Duke,Stephanie D.,MD
Fisher,Deneishia Shramaine,MD
Gleason,Abigail Hott,MD
Gross,Renee,MD
Gupta,Manjari,MD
Huang,Michelle,MD
Kinsler,Kristin J.,DO
Martinez,Tiffany Annmarie,DO
Owunna,Uzoma I.,MD
Panaligan,Donato A.,MD
Tomlinson-Phelan,Tracy M.,MD
White,Sanford F.,MD
East Orange
Cailliau,Pamela Jean,MD
Meremikwu,Francisca Chinwe,MD
Okafor,Joana O.,MD
St. Victor,Ruth Alleen,DO
Toliver,Clifford W.,MD
Uzoaru,Charles O.,MD
East Windsor
Eder,Scott E.,MD
Gamburg,Eugene Samuel,MD
Markidan,Yana,MD
Simigiannis,Helen,MD
Eatontown
Mann,Jessica Salas,MD
Mensah,Virginia Akua,MD
Price,Andrea Noelle,MD
Edison
Adefowokan,Rotanna I.,MD
Arora,Ranjana,MD
Chung,Uei K.,MD
Corsan,Gregory H.,MD
Daiter,Eric,MD
Dave,Sangeeta,MD
Desai,Darshana A.,MD
Essandoh,Louisa Efua,MD
Fleisch,Charles M.,DO
Han,Ji Soo,MD
Holgado,Cesar B.,MD
Keflemariam,Yodit J.,MD
Mavani,Bharti N.,MD
Metz,Rebecca L.,MD
Palayekar,Meena Jayawant,MD
Patel,Atulkumar V.,MD
Patel,Kirit Somabhai,MD
Patel,Ragin C.,MD
Rama,Sreedevi,MD
Ramanarayanan,Annapurna,MD
Russell,Carol Mae,DO
Sachdev,Rahul,MD
Shah,Bharti C.,MD

Physicians by Specialty and Town

Obstetrics & Gynecology (cont)

Edison
- Steinbach, Gary B., MD
- Twisdale, Donna R., MD

Egg Harbor Township
- Kaufman, Larry J., MD
- Lojun, Sharon Lee, MD
- Milov, Seva, MD
- Papperman, Thomas W., MD
- Samson-Bacarro, Edna A., MD
- Silk, Maanasi Puranik, DO

Elizabeth
- Arrunategui, Jose M., MD
- Joseph, Eddy M., MD
- Khazai, Kamran, MD
- Raad, Michelle L., MD
- Sabzwari, Tabassum Azra, DO

Elmer
- Adunuthula-Jonnalagadda, Hema, MD

Elmwood Park
- Lee-Agawa, Melissa, MD

Emerson
- Gliksman, Michele Isaacs, MD
- Paskowski, Elizabeth K., MD
- Rosalie, Maria Christina, MD

Englewood
- Ashton, Jennifer Lee, MD
- Asulin, Yitzhack, MD
- Bewtra, Madhuri, MD
- Binas, Constantine George, MD
- Butler, David George, MD
- Chalfin, Venus Helena, MD
- Dill, Barbara A., MD
- Englert, Christopher A., MD
- Friedman, Harvey Y., MD
- Gellman, Elliott, MD
- Goldman, Faith Renee, MD
- Gor, Hetal Bankim, MD
- Gresham, Keith A., MD
- Gross, Arthur H., MD
- Hadjistavrinos, Kriss, MD
- Huang, Tony T., MD
- Jacobson, Marina, MD
- Jhee, Yoon-Bok, MD
- Kilinsky, Vladimir, MD
- Lesorgen, Philip R., MD
- Markovitz, Jacob E., MD
- Martinucci, Stacy M., MD
- Merriam, Zachary M., DO
- Patel, Avanee Kanoo, MD
- Patel-Shusterman, Shefali N., MD
- Patrusky, Karen Lynn, MD
- Saphier, Carl Joseph, MD
- Savci, Sariye, MD
- Scheller, Tracey Frances, MD
- Schlossberg, Hope R., MD
- Song, Erica Yoon-Jung, MD
- Suarez, Teresa, MD
- Tovmasian, Lucy Tamar, MD
- Weiss, Nofit, MD

Englewood Cliffs
- Chong, Joseph K., MD
- Kang, Katherine E. Lee, MD
- Miller, Jane E., MD
- Yun, Sung K., MD

Englishtown
- Andrews, Tatyana, MD

Fair Lawn
- Beloff, Michelle Lauren, DO
- Cocoziello, Ramin B., MD
- Dolgin, James S., MD
- Hessami, Sam H., MD
- Mitzner, Ann C., MD
- Reinkraut, Jeffrey M., MD
- Sagullo, Cynthia C., MD
- Seymour, Carmela, MD
- Verrico, Tracy B., DO

Flemington
- Abeysinghe, Manisha G., MD
- Altomare, Corrado J., MD
- Ardise, Patricia Marie, MD
- Belkina, Yelena, MD
- Bowers, Mamie Sue, MD
- Camiolo, Melissa Rae, MD
- Frys, Kelly Ann, DO
- Grimes, Sara, MD
- Grove, Michele Sak, MD
- Huttner, Ruby P., MD
- Lynen, Richard F., MD
- Masterton, Deirdre C., MD
- Pedersen, Irene A., MD
- Pisatowski, Denise Michelle, MD
- Rivas, Jimena, MD
- Vitale, Lidia F., MD

Florham Park
- Banks, Judy L., MD
- Chervenak, Donald M., MD
- Gibbon, Darlene Grace, MD
- Locatelli, Sam Thomas, MD
- Rawlins, Samantha Geanine, MD

Fords
- Shonowo, Owobamishola Adanma, MD

Forked River
- Bustamante Dayanghirang, Alma, MD

Fort Lee
- Lee, James R., MD
- Shoshilos, Anna G., DO

Franklin Lakes
- Weidman, Joshua A., MD

Freehold
- Aland, Kristen, MD
- Amer, Yousef A., MD
- Back, Norman A., MD
- Barnett, Rebecca L., MD
- Baum, Jonathan D., MD
- Bernard-Roberts, Lynikka, MD
- Burt-Libo, Borislava, DO
- Cipriano, Joseph A., MD
- Cipriano, Rebecca J., MD
- Dimino, Michael L., MD
- Goldstein, Steven A., MD
- Joshi, Jyotika D., MD
- Kirwin, Michael S., MD
- Lucas, Romeo Augusto, DO
- Mandel, Peter C., MD
- Mayson, Robert P., MD
- Misra, Neeti Virendra, MD
- Morreale, Ginja Massey, MD
- Neuwirth, Safrir, MD
- Pacana, Susan Marie, MD
- Portadin, Robert A., MD
- Prugno, Robin Jean, DO
- Ranasinghe Rodrigo, Nimalie, MD
- Rattigan, Meghan Iona, DO
- Scheff, Elizabeth Anne, MD
- Seigel, Mark J., MD

Galloway
- Assad, Eveline N., MD
- Bredin, Sherilyn A., MD
- Chong, Christopher K., MD
- Feldman, Alan J., MD
- Perkins, Phyllis M., MD
- Petit, Anne I., MD
- Stanley, Linda, MD
- Wesley, Louis A., MD

Garfield
- Silva-Karcz, Linda, MD

Glen Ridge
- Dias Martin, Karen A., MD

Hackensack
- Abdelhak, Yaakov Eliezer, MD
- Al Khan, Abdulla Mohammed, MD
- Alizade, Azer, MD
- Alvarez, Manuel, MD
- Alvarez Perez, Jesus Rafael, MD
- Bozdogan, Ulas, MD
- Chadha, Kanchi, MD
- Cohen, Robert S., MD
- Collado, Anna A., DO
- Copur, Huseyin, MD
- Gaafer-Ahmed, Hany M., MD
- Gallo, Robert James, MD
- Gerardis, Judi R., MD
- Govindani, Niketa Vinod, MD
- Gupta, Shalini, MD
- Howell, Emily Ruth, DO
- Hughes, Patricia L., MD
- Ilonzo, Chiamaka, MD
- Joshi, Kiran M., MD
- Kamal, Roohi, MD
- Kean Chong, Maria R., MD
- Kondoleon, Mary Therese, MD
- Kopp, Lizabeth A., MD
- Leo, Mauro Vincenzo, MD
- Levat, Robin H., MD
- Miller, Lisa Ann B., MD
- Petriella, Michael R. Jr., MD
- Saber, Shelley B., MD
- Samara, Arafat A., MD
- Sbarra, Michael A., MD
- Simonian, Carla Daria, MD
- Vinod, Arundhati Hrishikesh, MD
- Yousry, Ahmed Sameh, MD

Hackettstown
- Akhigbe, Omoikhefe Gbemisola, MD
- Anscher, Richard M., MD
- Campbell, Neil Murdoch, DO
- Canova, Amanda Derrick, MD
- Defalco, Lisa May, DO
- Shakarjian, Jo-Ann, MD
- Skoczylas, Stanley J., MD
- Uzbay, Lisa Ann, MD

Haddon Heights
- Crawford, Heather M., DO
- Godorecci, Michele, MD

Haddonfield
- Krueger, Paul M., DO
- Ronner, Wanda, MD
- Stemmer, Shlomo Marc, MD

Haledon
- Alnuaimi, Raya Omer, DO

Hamburg
- Nichols, Fred Michael, DO

Hamilton
- Evans Murage, Julene Opalene, MD
- Gonzalez Braile, Dinah A., MD
- Lendor, E. Cindy, MD
- Naraine, Christopher Anthony, MD
- Ramchandani, Sanjay Mohan, MD
- Resnick, Michael B., MD
- Samra Latif Estafan, Omnia M., MD
- Sison, Antonio, MD
- Tufankjian, Lisa Gruszka, DO

Hammonton
- Agbasi, Nwogo Nnunwa, MD
- Capiro, Rodney, MD
- McFarlane, Owen R., MD

Hasbrouck Heights
- Fechner, Adam Jeffrey, MD
- Loughlin, Jacquelyn S., MD

Hawthorne
- Cifaldi, Ralph John Jr., DO

Hewitt
- Dombo, Kudzai Rebecca, MD

Hillsborough
- Blanks, Mary Susan, MD
- Hirsch, Gregory D., MD
- Karanikolas, Steven, MD
- Pineda, Jean Q., MD
- Salley, Pamela R., MD
- Wagner, Wendy Joan, MD

Ho Ho Kus
- Vikner, Lin M., MD

Hoboken
- Aguilar, Raul F., MD
- Brescia, Mark J., MD
- Chinn, Natasha R., MD
- Garrisi, Margaret Graf, MD
- Lowe, Samantha B., DO
- Magpantay, Emiliana M., MD
- McQuilkin, George E., MD
- Migliaccio, Thomas A., MD
- Moon, Jeremy, MD
- Picard, Johan Arlenie, MD
- Potter-McQuilkin, Dineasha M., MD
- Rossetos, Ourania S., MD
- Shoman, Adam Mohamed, MD

Holmdel
- Conley, Michael P., MD
- Patel, Sagar Y., MD
- Penney, Robert P., MD
- Sanakkayala, Nirmala D., MD
- Smolinsky, Adi, MD
- Wohlstadter, Sanford W., MD

Howell
- Chhatwal, Balwant K., MD
- Cohen, Alan, MD
- Surowitz, Clara Pauline, MD

Irvington
- Kusnierz, James L., DO
- Mukhopadhay, Jayati, MD
- Thani, Suresh R., MD
- Treadwell, Kenneth Jr., MD
- Zevin, Ronald A., MD

Iselin
- Berkman, Steven R., MD
- Divino, Eumena M., MD
- Ghanekar, Geeta R., MD
- Goldberg, Steven C., MD
- Magier, Slawomir, MD

Jersey City
- Baptiste, Nicole Bernadette, MD
- Barbara Mijares, Diego, MD
- Bimonte, Michael J., MD
- Boamah, Kwaku Osafo-Mensah, MD
- Borja, Manuel L., MD
- Campbell, Damali M., MD
- Carter, Cheryl Ann, MD
- Chang, Kenneth Sung Soo, MD
- Chau, Patricia Chang Wai, MD
- Fernandez, Osbert, MD
- Gonzalez, Lily W., MD
- Gor, Jyotsna H., MD
- Gressock, Joseph Neal, MD
- Hou, Hui Ying, MD
- Hu, Long-Gue, MD
- Ibrahim, Gehan M., MD
- Kranias, Hristos K., MD
- Masson, Lalitha, MD
- Muhammad, Zaheda, MD
- Mushayandebvu, Taonei I., MD
- Najafi, Abdul Wahid, MD
- Nichols, Rhonda R., MD
- Patel, Roshni Dinesh, DO
- Pellecchia, Ralph Joseph, MD
- Rahulatharan, Rajasingha, MD
- Ramirez, Elizabeth, MD
- Ratzersdorfer, Jonathan, MD
- Resnikoff-Gary, Amanda Nicole, MD
- Sharma, Neha, MD
- Uy, Vena, MD
- Wehbe Saloukhan, Cristin, MD
- Witter, Theodore O., MD

Kearny
- Graf, Jennifer A., DO
- Herrighty, Marianne K., MD
- Surmeli, Sedat M., MD

Kendall Park
- Caban, Michelle, MD
- Colonna, Elizabeth Ann, MD
- Ham, Antoinette Lucy, MD
- Karim, Nuzhat, MD
- Kim, Eugene J., MD
- Lundberg, John L., MD
- Segal, Joshua Howard, MD

Lake Hopatcong
- Prezioso, Alexander N., MD

Lakewood
- Cahill, Kenneth Matthew, DO
- Chang, Joanne Meejin, MD
- Choper, Niles E., MD
- Cocco, Frank A., MD
- Culbert, Steven A., MD
- Greenstein, Gary David, MD
- Hoffman, Christian T. III, MD
- Lehnes, Eric G., MD
- Moghe, Vaishali C., MD
- Molina, Arthur M., MD
- Morgan, Allen, MD
- Pitsos, Miltiadis, MD
- Repole, Adam N., MD
- Smith, Sharon Marie, MD
- Tal, Moty N., MD
- Thompson, Flavius Mark, MD
- Young, Tiffany, DO
- Zafarani, Amy Jo, DO

Lawrenceville
- Bhattacharjee, Roopali, MD
- Burbella, Ronald E., MD
- Firdu, Tikikil, MD
- Funches, Judith Melton, MD
- Goyal, Shefali, MD
- Grant, Gwendolyn Hunter, DO
- Hall, Lanniece F., MD
- Hilsenrath, Robin Elaine, MD
- Leedom, Karen Ann, MD
- Loeb, Paul Norman, DO
- Melnikoff, Barbara, MD
- Mondestin, Myriam A. J., MD
- Pierce, Bruce R., MD
- Proctor, Asha K., MD
- Przybylko, Kira L., MD
- Romano, Carmen J., MD
- Safi, Farnaz, MD
- Sarma, Bani A., MD
- Small, Daniel Alan, MD
- Stanell, William P., MD
- Tashjian, Audrey Brigitta, MD
- Ung, Kenneth H., MD
- Warchaizer, Susan J., MD

Lebanon
- Lewis, Sharol A., MD
- Rubin, Seth M., MD

Physicians by Specialty and Town

Lincroft
- Generelli,Patricia Ann,MD
- Moore,Susan Salzberg,MD

Linden
- Bodnar,Aleksander J.,MD

Lindenwold
- Cannon,Donald R.,MD
- Gildiner,Lennard R.,MD
- Klein,Edward M.,MD
- Ruffin,Judith S.,MD

Little Falls
- Obaid,Sana Hamdan,MD

Little Silver
- Bohnert,Katherine Ann,DO
- Giovine,Anthony P.,MD
- Hammond,Kelly C.,MD
- Jacoby,Michelle P.,MD
- Karoly,Michael D.,MD
- Kaskiw,Eugene H.,MD
- Kaufman,William N.,DO
- Mason-Cederberg,Lauren,MD
- Rosenzweig,Talia S.,MD
- Soussan,Elie R.,MD
- Sun,Andrew N.,MD
- Tsong,Shirley W.,MD
- Wiser-Estin,Mindy Ellen,MD

Livingston
- Abella,Tara M.,MD
- Bonamo,John F.,MD
- Bridges,Yvette A.,MD
- Cekleniak,Natalie A.,MD
- Cohen,Theodore,MD
- DiSabatino,Daniel,DO
- Dziadosz,Margaret,MD
- Fain,Richard A.,MD
- Hessler,Sarah Catherine,MD
- Howard,L. Deanna,MD
- Keegan,Debbra Ames,MD
- Keiser,Oren S.,MD
- Kindzierski,John A.,MD
- Klachko,Daria A.,MD
- Koch,Robert K.,MD
- Mansuria,Shetal M.,MD
- McArthur,Marilyn D.,MD
- Miller,Richard Charles,MD
- O'Brien,Jonathan Edward,MD
- Petillo,Tina M.,DO
- Quartell,Anthony C.,MD
- Rachlin,Adrianne,MD
- Segal,Jeffrey Loren,MD
- Somers,Joann,MD
- Tam,Tiffanie,MD
- Terrone,Dom A.,MD
- Youngren,Sonya Jitendra,MD

Lodi
- Dutta,Kamal K.,MD

Long Branch
- Gonzalez,David Jr.,MD
- Graebe,Robert A.,MD
- Joshi,Raksha,MD
- Khalil,Rahab M.,MD
- Kugay,Natalya P.,MD
- Magherini Rothe,Suzanne A.,MD
- Malik,Nisha,MD
- Nath,Carl Anthony,MD
- Smithson,Sarah,MD
- Vaclavik,John Philip Charles,MD

Lumberton
- Crawford-Meadows,Robin A.,MD
- Dalton,Laura J.,DO

Lyndhurst
- Choi,Jay Joonhyuk,MD

Madison
- Chou,Vivian K.,MD
- Kaplan,Regina Mpakarakes,MD

Manahawkin
- Gottesman,Brian Tod,MD
- Liu,Todd,MD
- Marino,Mark,MD
- McDermott,James P.,DO
- Rezai,Amadi,MD
- Sunkavalli,Anupama,MD
- Sze,Michael Shu Shin,MD
- Trim,George G.,MD
- Vernon,Lisa S.,MD

Manalapan
- Belkin,Sardana,MD
- Bochner,Ronnie Z.,MD
- Fischetti-Galvin,Jessica,DO
- Levy,Jenna,DO
- Rathauser,Robert H.,MD

Manasquan
- Ditusa,Diane Michele,DO
- Filardo,Josephine,MD
- Keelan,Michael E.,MD
- Parchment,Alfred B.,MD
- Saez Lacy,Deborah A.,MD
- Welt,Alan J.,MD

Maple Shade
- Epstein,Debra M.,MD

Maplewood
- Flowers,Sakhshat W. III,MD
- Maloney,Marvelle,MD
- Parchment,Winsome J.,MD
- Peace,Nyota Afi,MD
- Smith,Donna M.,MD
- Wright-Cadet,Yvonne,MD

Margate City
- Titton,Barry Sheldon,MD

Marlboro
- Dufreney,Margaret S. Durante,MD
- Kyreakakis,George J.,MD

Marlton
- Patel,Ushma K.,MD
- Sawin,Stephen Wooten,MD
- Suarez,Kathryn Reynes Novak,MD
- Taliadouros,George S.,MD

Maywood
- Seidner,Michael David,MD

Medford
- Agar,Monica T.,MD
- Siegel,Amy Judith,DO

Mendham
- Prefer,Audrey I.,MD

Mercerville
- Jones,Eva R.,MD

Metuchen
- Ainslie,William Jr.,MD
- Hsu,Pochien Gregory,MD
- Steinbeck,Wayne E.,MD

Millburn
- Cooperman,Alan Stewart,MD
- Luciani,Richard L.,MD
- Pollack,Marshall S.,MD
- Seymour,Christopher R.,MD
- Simonetti,John M.,MD

Millville
- Babalola,Gbolagade O.,DO
- Geria,Michael J.,DO
- Giyanani,Sunita M.,MD

Monmouth Junction
- Kumar,Monica Puri,MD

Monroe
- Ibrahim,Samih A.,MD

Montclair
- Aristizabal,Michelle Anne,MD
- Carman,Elise S.,MD
- De Marsico,Richard,MD
- Degrande,Gary C.,MD
- Gaudino,Silvana,MD
- Jenkins,Reginald Alexander,MD
- Lee,Jane S.,MD
- Lespinasse,Pierre Frederic,MD

Montvale
- Jean,Nagaeda,MD
- Langer,Myriam,MD

Montville
- Das,Kamala,MD

Moorestown
- Chapman,Derek Q.,MD
- Gomez,Syeda Rabia,DO
- Mama,Saifuddin Taiyeb,MD
- Minoff,Michael H.,MD

Morris Plains
- Ghazi,Mohammad,MD

Morristown
- Austin,Kimberlee Kunze,MD
- Avondstondt,Andrea Mithai,MD
- Ayyad,Mina N.,MD
- Bergh,Paul Akos,MD
- Blank,Jacqueline P.,DO
- Botros,Carolyn,DO
- Brenin-Goldfischer,Debra Sue,MD
- Culin,Angelina Han,MD
- Culligan,Patrick John,MD
- Daly,M. Veronica,MD
- Feltz,John P.,MD
- Ferrante,Daniel P.,MD
- Garfinkel,David A.,MD
- Gluck,Ian J.,MD
- Graebe,Kerry,MD

Morristown (cont.)
- Iammatteo,Matthew D.,MD
- Isaac,Vina H.,MD
- Jones,Kathryn M.,MD
- Khine,Mary L.,MD
- Laguduva,Lakshmi Rani R.,MD
- Littman,Paul M.,DO
- Lizarraga,Liza Isabel,MD
- Lucarelli,Elizabeth Ann,MD
- Mahaga-Ajala,Mark-Robert O.,DO
- Manor,Einat,MD
- Mass,Sharon B.,MD
- Mathews,Chacko P.,MD
- McGue,Mary Margaret,MD
- Miller,Naomi H.,MD
- Morley,Laura Balderrama,MD
- Murphy,Guy D.,MD
- O'Reilly,Sara B.,DO
- Omay,Cem S.,MD
- Salamon,Charbel Georges,MD
- Shah,Leena P.,MD
- Shariati,Amir,MD
- Slomovitz,Brian Matthew,MD
- Steer,Robert L.,MD
- Tunde-Agbede,Oluwafisayo,MD
- Walter,Briza V.,MD
- Wasenda,Erika Joy,MD

Mount Holly
- Deluca,Samantha,DO
- Gorlitsky,Helen,MD
- Grossman,Leonard,MD
- Jackson,Olga E.,MD
- Levine,Bruce Jay,MD
- Levine,Richard Teddy,MD
- Manning,Latriece Eileena,MD
- Modena,Alisa B.,MD
- Rashid,Parveen,MD
- Segal,Avni,MD
- Shalit,Stuart L.,DO

Mount Laurel
- Brasile,Deanna Rose,DO
- Choe,Jung Kyo,MD
- Corley,David R.,MD
- Denny,Ashleigh,MD
- Jenkins,Lauren Anne,MD
- McCrosson,Stacy A.,MD
- Noah,Jane S.,MD
- Richman,Steven L.,DO
- Tucker,Richard G.,DO

Mountain Lakes
- Dreyfuss,Patricia O.,MD
- Manlangit,Arsenio C.,MD

Mullica Hill
- Beams,Lynsey Marie,DO
- O'Flynn,Leisa Diane,DO

Neptune
- Blechman,Andrew Neal,MD
- Canterino,Joseph C.,MD
- Conner,Ellen Louise,MD
- Coyle,Allison A.,DO
- ElSahwi,Karim Samir,MD
- Fabricant,Christopher James,MD
- Fumia,Fred Daniel,MD
- Gussman,Debra,MD
- Jacobson,Nina Stella,MD
- Koscica,Karen Lynn,DO
- Matta,Paul Gamal,DO
- Narinedhat,Ralph,MD
- Shavelson,Robert P.,MD
- Sprance,Henry Ernest,MD
- Vasquez,Wendelly Judith,MD

New Brunswick
- Adigun,Akeem Segun,MD
- Aurora,Nadia,MD
- Ayers,Charletta A.,MD
- Bachmann,Gloria A.,MD
- Baffo,Aileen,MD
- Baldwin,Kimberly Staton,MD
- Balica,Adrian Claudiu,MD
- Beim,Robert B.,MD
- Beiter,Kyle Aaron,MD
- Chavez,Martin R.,MD
- Cheng,Ru-Fong J.,MD
- Cioffi,Francis J.,MD
- Cruz Ithier,Mayra Alejandra,MD
- Di Stefano,Valeria M.,MD
- Dolitsky,Shelley Nicole,MD
- Ebert,Gary A.,MD
- Faro,Revital D.,MD
- Francis,Amanda Rachael,DO
- Gilmandyar,Dzhamala,MD
- Glatthorn,Haley,MD
- Goldberg,Leah,MD

New Brunswick (cont.)
- Green,Ashlee,MD
- Hadaya,Ola,MD
- Herreros,Claudia,MD
- Hollingsworth,Jessie,MD
- Hutchinson-Colas,Juana A.,MD
- Jadhav,Ashwin R.,MD
- Jasani,Sona,MD
- Jayakumaran,Jenani Sarah,MD
- Jenci,Joseph D.,MD
- Kaminsky,Lillian M.,MD
- Kemmann,Ekkehard,MD
- Kicenuik,Michael T.,MD
- Kohut,Adrian,MD
- Lynch,Caroline Dorothy,MD
- MacMillan,William Emery,MD
- Magliaro,Thomas J.,MD
- Merjanian,Lena L.,MD
- Mokrzycki,Mark L.,MD
- Naqvi,Fatima,MD
- Ng,June Hoi Ka,MD
- Palomares,Kristy T.,MD
- Patel,Amy J.,MD
- Patel,Jharna Mehul,MD
- Phillips,Nancy A.,MD
- Pradhan,Archana,MD
- Preminger,Michele Lynn,MD
- Rosen,Todd Joshua,MD
- Sauer,Mark Victor,MD
- Schultz,Pamela Sue,MD
- Segal,Saya,MD
- Sinofsky,Francine E.,MD
- Song,Mi-Hae,MD
- Stechna,Sharon Beth,MD
- Stewart,Richard Allen,DO
- Washington,Monica Michaelle,MD
- Yoo,Nina,MD
- Yousef,Mona E.,MD

New Providence
- Barresi,Joseph A.,MD
- Gibbons,Alice B.,MD

Newark
- Ambarus,Tatiana,MD
- Barrett,Theodore,MD
- Bhagat,Neha,DO
- Brandi,Kristyn M.,MD
- Bronshtein,Elena,MD
- Caban,Julio E.,MD
- Chu,Tsu M.,MD
- Cracchiolo,Bernadette M.,MD
- Ganesh,Vijaya L.,MD
- Gimovsky,Martin Larry,MD
- Gittens-Williams,Lisa Nadine,MD
- Goldman,Noah Adam,MD
- Hatchard,John R. E.,MD
- Heller,Debra S.,MD
- Houck,Karen Leigh,MD
- Johnson,Sharon,MD
- Juusela,Alexander Lawrence,MD
- Koul,Mrinal,MD
- Kuhn,Theresa Marie,MD
- Nazir,Munir A.,MD
- Pant,Meenakshi,MD
- Pinney,Antonia F.,MD
- Pompeo,Lisa,MD
- Raju,Vijaya L.K.,MD
- Rankin,Laura,MD
- Roche,Natalie E.,MD
- Sawaged,Khalid S.,DO
- Shah,Chandravadan I.,MD
- Thompson,Stephanie M,MD
- Tran,Baohuong Nguyen,DO
- Ukazu,Adanna C.,MD
- Williams,Shauna F.,MD
- Yerovi,Luis A. Jr.,MD

Newton
- Bagherian,Sharareh,DO
- Bhayani,Parimal S.,MD
- Dardik,Raquel B.,MD
- Lewis,Frieda Elizabeth,MD
- Maugeri,Joseph P.,MD
- Paxton,Adam Michael,MD
- Pennant,Andria Uzetta,MD
- Rubino,Donald J.,MD
- Sehgal,Geeta,DO
- Sherman,Glenn Stewart,MD

North Arlington
- Grasso,Armand J.,MD

North Bergen
- Escobar,Juan Nicolas,MD
- Giron-Jimenez,Sandra,MD
- Gonzalez,Rosa M.,MD
- Gutierrez,Christine V.,MD

Physicians by Specialty and Town

Obstetrics & Gynecology (cont)

North Bergen
Kitzis, Hugo D., MD
Majid, Mahir J., MD
Nath, Mary Madhuri, MD
Pablo, Bryan Alcides, MD
Patel, Jigna K., MD
Patel, Zankhana M., MD
Perisic, Dusan, MD
Trujillo-Carvalho, Cecilia J., MD

North Brunswick
Acharya, Rashmi, MD
Nuthakki, Vimala Devi, MD
Udeshi, Hansa S., MD

North Plainfield
Lowe, William J. III, MD

Northfield
Nnewihe, Adebola Oyeronke, MD

Nutley
Parisi, Vanessa Marie, DO
Straker, Michael J., MD

Oakhurst
Hage, Charles W., MD
Hayet, Rose F., MD
Moskowitz, David H., MD
Van Horn, Lawrence G. Jr., MD

Oakland
Dispenziere, Benjamin R., MD

Ocean
Cohen, Ronald L., MD
Gould, Jack R., DO
Henderson, Craig E., DO
Morgan, Benjamin, MD
Rogers, Brian James, MD
Roman, Jacqueline D., DO
Theocharides, Thomas, MD

Ocean City
Lavis, James Douglas, DO
Wilson, James Ashley II, MD

Old Bridge
Cohen, Brad J., MD

Oradell
Dotto, Myles E., MD
Wang, Belle, MD
Wiener, Craig B., MD

Orange
Wolfe, Taida J., MD

Paramus
Chen, Dehan, MD
Golin, Thomas, MD
Jones, Howard Harris, MD
Matthews, Gail Margaret, MD
Meyer, Monica Lynn, MD
Mosquera Charlenea, Claudia, MD
Nasseri, Ali, MD
Nickles, Donna E., DO
O'Brien, Katherine Elizabeth, MD
Ohanian, Heripsime, MD
Rizk, Naglaa T., MD
Russo, Thomas O., MD
Siegel, Amy Michele, MD
Weinstein, Melissa A., DO

Park Ridge
Corbett, Shonda Marcia, MD
Fallon, Kimberly L., MD

Parsippany
Bellish, Jenna H., MD
Bissinger, Craig L., MD
Haskel, Steven A., MD
Hirsch, David Jay, MD
Khalid, Samira, DO
Leviss, Stephen R., MD

Passaic
Ahkami, Shahrokh, MD
Carson, Milinda Ruth, MD
Chavez-Cacho, Jose M., MD
De Lara, Vilma A., MD
Gagliano, Salvatore M., MD

Paterson
Alnakeeb, Mohammed M., MD
Azar, Jihad Elias, MD
Balazs, Peter, MD
Beidleman, Danielle Melissa, MD
Bilenki, Natalie I., MD
Boghdady, Maged W., MD
Caldwell, Shinelle, DO
El Deeb, Mokhtar M., MD
Kaminskyj, Megan Elizabeth, MD
Kulwatdanaporn, Somchai, MD
Liriano, Monica, MD

Magid, Marissa, DO
Marino, Nicholas A., MD
Montemurro, Robert J., MD
Mustafa, Diane M., MD
Pendse, Vijay K., MD
Shilad, Aiman K., MD
White, Evelyn W., MD

Pennington
McDonnell, Elizabeth Lynn, MD
Petty, Victoria Morey, MD

Pennsville
Friedman, Amir Mordechai, MD

Perth Amboy
Brug, Pamela, MD
Turkish, Jonathan Lee, MD
Vaydovsky, Joseph, MD

Phillipsburg
Berger, Daniel A., DO
Blumenthal, Neil C., MD
Horne, Howard Krutzel, MD
Silver, David Foster, MD

Piscataway
Choubey, Sheela, MD
Cogliani, Ermes, MD
Davda, Niyati, MD
De Flesco, Lindsay D., MD
Schwartz, Marlan K., MD

Plainfield
Abrarova, Nazima M., MD
Murray, Elrick A., MD

Plainsboro
Friedman, Alan L., MD
Gross, Jeffrey K., MD
Pawliw, Myron, MD
Petraske, Alison R., MD
Siems, Nicole Mary, DO

Pleasantville
Desai, Anagha Kishor, MD

Pomona
Sung, Edward L., MD

Pompton Lakes
Scian, John P., MD
Scian, Joseph A., MD

Princeton
Amin, Sejal J., MD
Baseman, Debra L., MD
Bergknoff, Hugh, MD
Diventi, Christina G., MD
Forster, Judith Karen, MD
Forster, Susan A., MD
Martin, Robert Allen, MD
Patel, Vrunda, MD
Saha, Anita, MD
Schwartz, Melanie Schrader, MD
Sophocles, Maria E., MD

Princeton Junction
Miller, Katherine H., MD

Rahway
Pelaez, Linda, MD

Ramsey
Faust, Michael G., MD
Nitz, Shelly, MD
Rooney, Michele P., MD

Randolph
Buna, Andrei, MD
Mohr, Robert Frederick, MD
Venanzi, Michael V., MD

Raritan
Huber, Elaine E., MD
Parlavecchio, Joseph G., MD

Red Bank
Chakraborty, Anu, MD
Patel, Mayur Vinod, MD
Seigelstein, Nina, MD

Ridgewood
Behnam, Kazem, MD
Behnam, Melody S., MD
Bentolila, Eric Y., MD
Coven, Roger A., MD
DeNoble, Shaghayegh Moghaddam, MD
Gerhardt, Amy Ilene Katz, MD
Khosla, Savita, MD
Kim, Kathlyn M., MD
Klimowicz-Mallon, Elizabeth, MD
Kuo, Eugenia C., MD
Levine, Richard Steven, MD
Marcus, John W., MD
Rezvani, Fred F., MD
Zeldina, Elina, MD

River Edge
Cho, Linda M., MD
Clachko, Marc A., MD
Parnes, Cindy R., MD

Rutherford
Chait, Anita Irani, MD
Cheatam, Consetta Mae, MD
Driscoll, Lorraine Eva, MD
Irani, Bakhtaver A., MD
Stella, Stefano M., MD

Saddle Brook
Cocoziello, Alexander R., DO
Mann, Manpreet, MD

Saddle River
Reisman, Barry M., MD
Rubenstein, Andrew F., MD

Salem
DeCastro, Amante N., MD

Scotch Plains
Choma, Mtroslaw, MD

Sea Girt
Pelligra, John, MD

Secaucus
Riftine, Julia, MD
Yun, Hyungkoo, MD

Sewell
Ayres, Ronald E., DO
Bramble, Charlene A., MD
Covone, Kenneth C., DO
Digiovanni, Marianne, DO
Franzblau, Natali Rae, MD
Huggins, Juanita Kimberly, DO
Hummel, Jennifer E., DO
Iavicoli, Michelle A., MD
Janeczek, Susan, DO
Krieg, Karen Sue, DO
Leber, Sandra Lynn, DO
Nguyen, Maria Bich Thi, DO
Richichi, Joann, DO
Salerno, Anthony P., MD
Sehdev, Michele S., MD
Vogiatzidakis, Sophia I., DO

Short Hills
Ayyagari, Kalavathi, MD
Robinson, Patricia Graf, MD

Shrewsbury
Damien, Miguel, MD
Holden, Emily C., MD
Seungdamrong, Aimee Malunda, MD
Witkowski, Mary E., MD

Sicklerville
Magness, Rose L., MD
Stafford, Patricia T., MD

Somerdale
Finley, Stephanie Elena, DO
Milicia, Anthony P., MD
Suarez, Melissa Lehn, DO
White, Deborah A., DO

Somers Point
Bergen, Blair A., MD
Bravoco, Michael C., MD
Ciceron, Asuncion V., MD
Kaplitz, Neil H., MD
Korzeniowski, Philip A., MD
Morgan, Daniel Robert, MD
Nosseir, Sandy B., MD
Perez, Finuccia Renda, MD
Phillips, James J., MD
Rezvina, Natalia Y., MD
Sindoni, Frank W., MD
Zhang, Vincent, MD

Somerset
Aguh, Chikezie J., MD
Alvaro, Joseph M., MD
Gao, Michael Yuan, MD
Gopal, Manish V., MD
Levitt, Robert S., MD
Lo, Vivian S., MD
Schaefer, Robert M., MD
Shastri, Shefali Mavani, MD
Shulman, Lois E., MD
Treiser, Susan L., MD

South Orange
Dresdner, Michael T., MD
Rosen, Kimberly A., MD
Sosin, Beth L., MD

South Plainfield
Antonio, Edsel, DO
Chan, Albert C., MD
Guerra-Deluna, Myrna T., MD
Kashyap, Meeta Parashar, MD

Shah, Namrata Jinesh, MD
Tran-Hoppe, Ngoc Quynh T., MD

Sparta
Sotillo, Melissa Maria, MD

Springfield
Bowers, Charles Jr., MD
Byalik, Olga Viktoria, MD
De Fronzo, Carl L., DO
Hunt, Mary Elizabeth, MD
Lublin, Jennifer Caryn, MD
Magarill, Rhona A., MD
Pinto, Jose J., DO
Tye, Joann Li Yen, MD

Stone Harbor
King, Lorraine C., MD

Succasunna
Ramieri, Joseph, MD
Sharafi, Khalida, MD
Shaw, Donia Renee, MD

Summit
Alam, Abu S., MD
Franceschini, Chloe Nicole, MD
Hoffman, Russell R., MD
Khoudary, Maryann Lisa, MD
Lashley, Susan Leonora, MD
Netta, Denise Ann, MD
Oyelese, Kolawole Olayinka, MD
Rondon, Kaylah Christine, MD
Russo-Stieglitz, Karen E., MD

Teaneck
Borden, Victor, MD
Brana-Leon, Hazel A., MD
Caruana, Lucia P., MD
Fernandez, Jacinto J., MD
Frattarola, John D., MD
Huggins, Iris A., MD
Leibman, Michael Roy, MD
Nunez, David A., MD
Shah, Payal A., MD

Tenafly
Broizman, David T., MD
Kithinji, Kagendo M., MD
Knause, Rita Vinod, MD
Lieblich, Richard M., MD
Luke, Brian T., MD
Navot, Daniel, MD
Rivera-Segarra, Stephanie D., MD
Shukla, Mrudula S., MD

Tinton Falls
Collado, Marilyn Loh, MD
Jacoby, Dana B., MD
Minaya, Evelyn, MD

Toms River
Argeros, Olga, MD
Azu, Wilhelmina Dedo, DO
Bonvicino, Marie Louise, MD
Furman, Lesley P., MD
Harrell, Russell L., MD
Jackman, Earl Francis, DO
Jones, Angela Renee, MD
Kelly, Robert B., DO
King, Andrew P., MD
Lopez, Gerardo J., MD
Maxwell, Aliona, MD
Morgan, Steven A., MD
Neal, Ronald R., MD
O'Donnell, Robert H., DO
Passarella, Susan Katherine, DO
Payumo, Paulita C., MD
Pesso, Robert S., MD
Shankar, Kala, MD
Sutherland, John R., MD
Valthaty, Rebekah, MD

Totowa
Bitar, Maria Teresa, MD
Day, Brian Todd, MD
Ngai, Ivan Manjun, MD
Tkach-Chubay, Irina, MD

Trenton
Amadi, Nkechinyere, MD
Brickner, Gary R., MD
Cervi, Wendy Lee, DO
Flores, Eduardo G., MD
Granderson, Lisa Irene, MD
MacKaronis, Anthony C., MD
Mantell, Cary Hilton, DO
O'Mara, James M., MD
Olukoya, Olasinbo Atinuke, MD
Scharf, Jeffrey I., MD
Tatarowicz, Roman J., MD
Williams, Delores J., MD

Williams,Fred W.,MD
Turnersville
Davis,George H.,DO
Dilks,Robert H.,MD
Kanoff,Martin E.,DO
Manus,Alan M.,DO
Nemeh,Elias,MD
Rosen,Larry S.,MD
Union
Boffard,Daryl K.,MD
Buontempo,Angela J.,DO
Del Rosario Torres,Leonida,MD
Ekulide,Emmanuel N.,MD
Ericsson,Dawn Marie,MD
Hyman,Martin C.,MD
McNamara,Robert E.,MD
Messimer,Julie Marie,MD
Russo,Donato S.,MD
Tai,Richard W.,MD
Victor,Isaac L.,MD
Union City
Scriffignano,Marla,MD
Steck,William M.,MD
Upper Montclair
Corenthal Robins,Linda J.,MD
Miller,Fred William III,MD
Upper Saddle River
Alcala,Ramon L. Jr.,MD
Verona
Milano,Michael C.,MD
Woroch,Peter Michael,MD
Vineland
Bispo,Luciano Jose,MD
Bonifield,Eric M.,MD
Clayton,Elizabeth Noelle,DO
Fockler,Raechel Ann,DO
Frinjari,Hassan,MD
Gewirtz,Jonathan D.,MD
Lightner,Angela Nanette,DO
Long,Ashley Nicole,DO
Panganamamula,Uma R.,MD
Russo,Armando P.,MD
Torchia,Michele A.,MD
Walsh,Sussannah Savitri,MD
Voorhees
Adamson,Susanne R. M.,MD
Aikins,James K. Jr.,MD
Arrow Articolo,Amy Beth,DO
Babin,Elizabeth Ann,MD
Bolognese,Ronald J.,MD
Bowers,Geoffrey David,MD
Bridges-White,Kimberly Gaye,MD
Caraballo,Ricardo,MD
Carlson,John A.,MD
Chen,Janine Junying,MD
Colella,Ryan Lawrence,MD
Cortese,Bernard J.,MD
Crisp,Meredith Page,MD
D'Elia,Donna L.,MD
Deger,Randolph Bruce,MD
Denis,Frantz,MD
Dershem,Jonel M.,MD
DiGaetano,Andrea F.,MD
Dittrich,Richard J.,DO
Felsenstein,Roberta G.,MD
Fitzsimmons,John Michael,MD
Gleimer,Emily R.,DO
Glowacki,Carol Ann,MD
Goodchild,Caroline Gagel,MD
Grossman,Eric Brian,MD
Holzberg,Adam S.,DO
Hosmer,Stephan E.,DO
Lamborne,Nicole Marie,MD
Levine,Jeffrey Richard,MD
Librizzi,Ronald J.,DO
Maccarone,Joseph L.,MD
Mackey,Suzanne Fuller,MD
Martinez,Wendy,MD
McCleery,Colleen Marie,MD
Murphy,Heather Marie,MD
Ricci,Emily K.,MD
Shah,Shailen S.,MD
Steighner,Kathleen Marie,MD
Swift,Joanne,MD
Tai,Victoria Chih-Chuang,MD
Tha,Teemu,MD
Udoh,Adaora Ngozi,MD
Warshal,David Philip,MD
Zinsky,Paul J.,MD
Wall
Aikman,Noelle M.,MD
Brudie,Lorna Ann,DO
Carlo,Jocelyn Ann,MD
Gumnic,Blair Rachel,DO
Thind,Narinder K.,MD
Tomaro,Robert Jr.,MD
Walsh,Kathleen S.,MD
Wall Township
Salloum,Didi,MD
Warren
Braunscheidel,Julie Ann,MD
Clott,Shilpa Mahendra,MD
Costa,Gerald V.,MD
De Angelis,Thomas,MD
Goldman,Kara J.,MD
Heffernan,Kathleen Anne,MD
Hubschmann,Andrea Gibbons,MD
Ivan,Joseph R.,MD
Levey,James Andrew,MD
Pathak,Kunja J.,MD
Pregenzer,Gerard J.,MD
Sanderson,Rhonda,MD
Tweddel,George K. III,MD
Wayne
Behnam,Nadereh,MD
Bennett,Bruce Kevin,MD
Burns,Les A.,MD
Centanni,Toni V.,MD
Chang,Bernard P.,MD
Darvish,Cameron,DO
Diarbakerli,Fares,MD
Domnitz,Steven W.,MD
Ephrem,Yasmina Marie Therese,MD
Garrett,Kenneth M.,MD
Gof,Sonia M.,MD
Greene,Jennifer Yvonne,MD
Kierce,Roger P.,MD
Mazzone,Jeanae,DO
Mohammed,Nina,MD
Munoz-Matta,Ana T.,MD
Newman,Sheila F.,MD
Nicosia,Leonard T.,MD
Onwudinjo,Adolphus C.,MD
Pallimulla,Mahipa H.,MD
Pavel,Patricia M.,MD
Rosenzweig,Debra L.,MD
Sgroi,Donald A.,MD
Shakiba,Khashayar,MD
Suffin,Arthur Lee,MD
Tener,Trilby Jo,MD
Vitale,Diana Rodrigues,MD
Vosough,Khashayar,MD
West Caldwell
Binetti,Richard G.,MD
West Deptford
Di Joseph,Benjamin D. Jr.,DO
Lofton,Azieb Ghebremedhin,DO
McNally,Lauryn Anne,DO
West Long Branch
Jackson,Sharon,MD
Lambert-Woolley,Margaret A.,MD
Lobraico,Dominick Jr.,DO
Massaro,Robert A.,MD
Ombalsky,Joseph,MD
Pompliano,Jennifer Dorothea,MD
Skorenko,Kenneth R.,MD
West Milford
Kaufman,Deborah Louise,DO
West New York
Fernandez-Cos,Henry,MD
Iraj Shaari,Gita M.,MD
Melendez Cabrera,Octavio,MD
Milanes-Roberts,Norma,MD
Zahka,Karym,MD
West Orange
Abeshaus,Lisa Ellen,MD
Antebi,Yael Jennifer,MD
Ciciola,Gerald F.,MD
Crane,Stephen E.,MD
David,Gwen Lynita,MD
Degraaff,Doreen E.,MD
Ehrlich,Paul,MD
Fox,Howard D.,DO
Hamilton,Tammy Joan,MD
Huang,Diana,MD
Kaufman,Gregory Joel,MD
Kessel,Allan David,MD
Ladocsi,Lewis T.,MD
Luisi-Purdue,Linda,MD
Milanes Roberts,Norma B.,MD
Patel,Priya R.,MD
Pitman,Susan Roth,MD
Rae-Layne,Norma Alicia,MD
Romero,Audrey Anita,MD
Rubino,Robert J.,MD
Russo,Neil J.,MD
Sadural,Ernani,MD
Saitta,Jacqueline Danielle,MD
Sansobrino,Daniel M.,MD
Sylvester,Claudine M.,MD
Walk,Zem,MD
Wimmer,Angela M.,MD
Zuniga,Gina,MD
West Paterson
Zaveri,Sarla J.,MD
Westfield
Cunningham,Catherine M.,MD
Fox,Michelle Candice,MD
Margulis,Elynne B.,MD
Patel,Falguni B.,MD
Soffer,Jeffrey,MD
Zimmermann,Laura Senn,MD
Westwood
Bilinski,Robyn T.,MD
Del Rosario,Elizabeth C.,MD
Dicker,Paul M.,MD
Hernandez Eguez,Carolina D.,MD
Levine,Zalman,MD
Wharton
Ortiz,Guillermo,MD
Williamstown
Green,Minda A.,MD
Willingboro
Belazi,Misa T.,MD
Chen,Kenneth H.,DO
Hammer,Ashley Morgan,MD
Hulbert,David S.,MD
Schell,Paul Lee,MD
Semple,Camille Eleanor,DO
Siegel,Francine Michelle,MD
Snyder,Michael T.,MD
Zalkin,Michael I.,MD
Woodbridge
Kocun,Christopher C.,MD
Woodbury
Gibson,Jeffrey T.,MD
Hanson,Anna Jang,MD
Hapner,Byron S.,DO
Vega,Vivian,MD
Woodbury Heights
Keswani,Ashok Kumar,MD
Woodcliff Lake
Latkin,Richard M.,MD
Schulze,Ruth J.,MD
Sobel,Gail M.,MD
Woodstown
Marshall,Stefanie N.,DO
Wisniewski,Robert E.,MD
Wyckoff
Duchin,Sybil E.,MD
Gartner,Joseph J.,MD
Hainer,Meg M.,MD
Obstetrics&Gynecology-Critical Care
River Edge
Bingham,Jemel M.,MD
Occupational Medicine
Belleville
Danko,Doris Julia,MD
Berlin
Leonetti,Joyce D.,DO
Cherry Hill
Chorney,Jeffrey R.,MD
East Hanover
Garvey,Karen Marie,MD
East Orange
Yang,Bin,MD
Edison
Elber,Lee Bennett,DO
Mellendick,George James,MD
Fair Lawn
Halejian,Barry A.,MD
Florham Park
Conner,Patrick R.,MD
Glassboro
Bojarski,Michael H.,DO
Hamilton
Coumbis,John J.,MD
Hillsborough
Shepperly,David C.,MD
Lakewood
Salvo,Victor J.,MD
Livingston
Bachman,Joyce Adele,MD
Fallon,Jill C.,MD
Millville
Weiss,Robert Jay,MD
Morris Plains
Jennison,Elizabeth A.,MD
Morristown
Schwarz-Miller,Jan,MD
Newark
Budnick,Lawrence D.,MD
Paramus
Liva,Jeffrey S.,MD
Marino,Phyllis E.,MD
Parlin
Deltieure,Michele H.,MD
Pennsauken
Introcaso,Lucian J.,MD
Piscataway
Garcia,Julia Griggs,MD
Kholdarov,Boris,MD
Osinubi,Omowunmi Y.,MD
Thomas,Timmy,MD
Udasin,Iris G.,MD
Plainfield
Patel,Alka Jashbhai,MD
Roseland
Mangahas,Florinda R.,MD
Secaucus
Weinberger,Adrian,MD
Somerset
Kusnetz,Eliot M.,MD
Trenton
Makowsky,Michael J.,MD
Szenics,Jonathan M.,MD
Vineland
Balogun,Evelyn Kemi,MD
Voorhees
Eskin,Evamaria Ursula,MD
Whitehouse Station
Nigro,Peter J.,MD
Oncological Surgery
Asbury Park
Kohli,Manpreet K.,MD
Berkeley Heights
Cunningham,John David,MD
Gumbs,Andrew Alexander,MD
Camden
Minarich,Michael,MD
Denville
Holwitt,Dana M.,MD
Florham Park
Bamboat,Zubin Mickey,MD
Diehl,William L.,MD
Kim,Joseph Jongbum,MD
Hackensack
Karpeh,Martin Sieh Jr.,MD
Livingston
Langan,Russell,MD
Lumberton
Miller,Eric Jay,MD
Manalapan
Miller,Denise J.,MD
Morristown
Chevinsky,Aaron H.,MD
New Brunswick
August,David A.,MD
Goydos,James S.,MD
Katz,Anna Beth,MD
Kennedy,Timothy John,MD
Koshenkov,Vadim P.,MD
Paramus
Yiengpruksawan,Anusak,MD
Sewell
Yoon-Flannery,Kahyun,DO
Summit
Sacco,Margaret Mary,MD
Oncology
East Orange
Saraf,Nirmala,MD
Livingston
Wagman,Raquel Tamara,MD
Morristown
Wong,James Robert,MD

Physicians by Specialty and Town

Oncology (cont)
Mount Holly
 Berk, Seth Howard, MD
 Lee, James Wonsang, MD
New Brunswick
 Weiss, Robert Edward, MD
Somerset
 McDermott, Janette H., MD
Vineland
 Sachdeva, Kush, MD

Ophthalmology
Asbury Park
 Berg, Bruce R., MD
 Chiang, Peter Keh-dah, MD
 Pardon, Ilene B., MD
 Talansky, Marvin L., MD
 Turtel, Lawrence S., MD
Avenel
 Wilgucki, John D., DO
Barrington
 Kamerling, Joseph M., MD
Bayonne
 Gurland, Keith G., MD
Bedminster
 Najarian, Lawrence V., MD
 Sullivan, Timothy Patrick, MD
Belleville
 Brooks, Nneka Offor, MD
 Eichler, Joel D., MD
 Landolfi, Joseph M., MD
 Landolfi, Michael Joseph, DO
 Lister, Mark Anthony, MD
 Madreperla, Steven A. Jr., MD
 Noorily, Stuart W., MD
 Seery, Christopher M., MD
 Voleti, Vinod Babu, MD
Bergenfield
 Bauza, Alain Michael, MD
 Dello Russo, Jeffrey, MD
 Parisi, Frank, MD
Berkeley Heights
 Bazargan Lari, Hamed, MD
 Gurwin, Eric B., MD
 Hsueh, Linda, MD
 Khalil, Monica B., MD
 Shah, Vinnie Pooja, MD
Berlin
 Dorfman, Neil H., MD
Blackwood
 Linares, Hugo Manuel, DO
Bloomfield
 D'Amato, Anthony P., MD
 Ditkoff, Jonathan W., MD
 Glatt, Herbert L., MD
 Gould, Joshua Mark, DO
 Jackson, Kurt T., MD
 Kallina, Lauren A., MD
 Kumar, Radhika Lingam, MD
Boonton
 Ahmad, Arlene, MD
Bordentown
 Caci, Jerry A., MD
Branchburg
 Nagelberg, Henry P., MD
Brick
 Mack, Prinze Chan, MD
 Schlisserman, David A., MD
Bridgewater
 Faigenbaum, Steven J., MD
 Moshel, Caroline Rosenberg, MD
 Phillips, Paul Mathew, MD
 Salz, Alan G., MD
 Salz, David Andrew, MD
Brigantine
 Di Marco, Eugene M., DO
Caldwell
 Salzano, Brian Christopher, MD
Camden
 Coleman, Colleen Marie, MD
 Driver, Paul J., MD
 Makar, Mary Saleeb, MD
 Markovitz, Bruce Jay, MD
 Olivia, Christopher Todd, MD
 Rho, David Samsun, MD
 Soll, Stephen Matthew, MD
Cape May Court House
 Altman, Brian, MD
 Caruso, Michael J., DO
 McLaughlin, John Patrick, MD
 Pastore, Domenic J., MD

Cedar Grove
 Youngworth, Lynda A., MD
Cedar Knolls
 Sachs, Ronald, MD
Cherry Hill
 Andrew, Mark S., MD
 Bannett, Gregg A., DO
 Cohen, Avraham N., MD
 Goel, Ravi Desh, MD
 Ho, Allen C., MD
 Hsu, Jason, MD
 Kaplan, Barnard A., MD
 Kindermann, Wilfred Reed, MD
 Lanciano, Ralph Jr., DO
 Malley, Debra S., MD
 Miano, Michele A., MD
 Patel, Jayrag Ashwinkumar, MD
 Pekala, Raymond T., MD
 Regillo, Carl, MD
 Richman, Jesse, MD
 Spechler, Floyd F., MD
 Yasgur, Lee H., MD
Chester
 Hirschfeld, James M., MD
 Hoye, Vincent Joseph III, MD
 Silverstein, Niki A., MD
 Silverstein, Rodger H., MD
Cinnaminson
 Dante, Karen L. Fung, MD
Clark
 Inverno, Anthony J., MD
 Jacobs, Miriam, MD
Cliffside Park
 Levine, Richard Evan, MD
 Movshovich, Alexander I., MD
Clifton
 Burrows, Adria, MD
 Cucci, Patricia, MD
 Cuttler, Nirupa C., MD
 Green, Donald H., MD
 Lesko, Cecily A., MD
 Mund, Michael L., MD
 Purewal, Baljeet Kaur, MD
 Stegman, Daniel Ychac, MD
 Wunsh, Stuart Eugene, MD
Collingswood
 Goldstein, Arthur Meyer, MD
 Kresloff, Michael Scott, MD
 Kresloff, Richard S., MD
 Young, Marc, MD
Cranford
 Calderone, Joseph Jr., MD
Cresskill
 Guba, Russell F. Jr., MD
Denville
 Hade, Jason R., MD
 Levey, Stephanie B., MD
 Pearlman, Theodore F., MD
Dover
 Mann, Eric Bryce, MD
 Schorr, Ian M., MD
East Brunswick
 Engel, Mark L., MD
 Han, Stella Insook, MD
 Leitman, Mark William, MD
 Su, Michael Yu-Man, MD
 Sun, Nancy, MD
 Witlin, Richard S., MD
 Yang, Kenneth E., MD
East Hanover
 Rispoli, Lauren C., MD
 Silverman, Cary M., MD
East Orange
 Cunningham, Robert D., MD
 Scott, Winston J., MD
Eatontown
 Edison, Barry Jay, DO
Edison
 Breznak, Cindy M., MD
 Park, John Chonghwan, MD
 Patel, Hitesh K., MD
 Press, Lorin R., MD
 Schanzer, Barry M., MD
 Schwartz-Eisdorfer, Barbara, MD
 Shah, Himanshu Shirish, MD
 Singh, Jasvinder, MD
 Spirn, Benjamin David, MD
 Spirn, Franklin H., MD
 Sullivan-Miller, Julia Ann, MD
 Yarian, David L., MD

Elizabeth
 Klein, Shawn Richard, MD
 Klein, Warren M., MD
 Mang, Justin, MD
 Scannapiego, Saveren, MD
Elmwood Park
 Friend, Adam Seth, MD
 Maley, Michael Kendrick, MD
 Phillips, Hadley H., DO
Emerson
 Cantore, William Anthony, MD
 Fishkin, Joseph D., MD
 Geller, Bradley David, MD
Englewood
 Burrows, Andrew F., MD
 Ezon, Isaac C., MD
 Freilich, Benjamin Douglas, MD
 Freilich, David Eric, MD
 Jee, Jimmy Hoon, MD
Englishtown
 Karmel, Bruce A., MD
Ewing
 Brundavanam, Hari Vs, MD
Fair Lawn
 Gopal, Lekha Hareshbhai, MD
 Sebrow, Osher S., MD
 Trotta, Nicholas C., MD
Fairfield
 Moses, Eli B., MD
 Perl, Theodore, MD
Far Hills
 Wax, Martin Bruce, MD
Flemington
 Batt, Gerald E., MD
 Dunham, Gerald, MD
 Phillips, Paul S., MD
Fort Lee
 Kim, John Sung, MD
 Kulik, Alfred D., MD
 Palacios, Alexander L., MD
 Rosenberg, Rhonda Betsy, MD
Franklin Lakes
 Bruder, Scott P., MD
Freehold
 Aksman, Scott S., MD
 Brenner, Edward H., MD
 Brottman, Jeffrey S., MD
 Gershenbaum, Eric Andrew, MD
 Kernitsky, Roman G., MD
 Lee, David K., MD
 Lee, Joan Jean, DO
 Minzter, Ronald M., MD
 Mishkin, Steven K., MD
 Naadimuthu, Revathi P., MD
 Ng, Elena M., MD
 Rosin, Jay Michael, MD
Galloway
 Dunn, Eric Scott, MD
 Spielberg, Joel A., MD
 Wise, Richard Bryan, MD
Hackensack
 Guterman, Carl B., MD
 Hanna, Aghnatious A Ha A., MD
 Liva, Paul A., MD
 Sandor, Earl V., MD
 Silbert, Glenn R., MD
 Sinatra, Melanie A., MD
 The, Arlene H., MD
Hackettstown
 Chase, Raymond Donald, DO
 Lappin, Harold S., MD
Haddonfield
 Mussoline, Joseph F., MD
Hamilton
 Chaudhry, Iftikhar Manzoor, MD
 Cox, Gregory E., MD
Hamilton Square
 Desai, Kiritkumar T., MD
 Sardi, Vincent F., MD
Hawthorne
 Newman, Frederic R., MD
Hazlet
 Clemente, Maria F., MD
Highland Park
 Glass, Robert M., MD
 Gordon, Stephen J., MD
 Hathaway, Elaine G., MD
Hoboken
 D'Alberti, Claudio F., MD

Holmdel
 Collur, Surekha, MD
 Klug, Ronald David, MD
 Steinfeld, Jason Israel, MD
 Subramaniam, Cristin Devika, MD
Irvington
 Bush, Nahndi, MD
 McCoy, Chrishonda Curry, MD
Iselin
 Grayson, Douglas Keane, MD
 Napolitano, Joseph Daniel, MD
 Patel, Menka Sanghvi, MD
 Strauss, Danielle Savitsky, MD
Jersey City
 Cervenak-Panariello, Betty, MD
 Cinotti, Donald J., MD
 Hershkin, Paige B., DO
 Maltzman, Barry A., MD
 Origlieri, Catherine Ann, MD
 Panariello, Anthony L., MD
 Rau, Ganesh U., MD
 Shulman, Gayle S., MD
 Vora, Bhupendra N., MD
 Walsman, Scott Michael, MD
 Yee, Mei-Ling, MD
Kearny
 Harper, Andrea A., MD
Kinnelon
 Ashkanazy, Mitchel, MD
 Shnayder, Eric, MD
Lakewood
 Barofsky, Jonathan M., MD
 Chinskey, Nicholas Daniel, MD
 Hedaya, Edward L., MD
 Huppert, Leon J., MD
 Rothkopf, Moshe M., MD
 Von Roemer, Marc, MD
Lambertville
 Grutzmacher, June Edith, MD
Lawrenceville
 Chiang, Robert Kent, MD
 Ellis, Steven P., MD
 Ie, Darmakusuma, MD
 Lavrich, Judith Barbara, MD
 Lipkowitz, Jeffrey L., MD
 Mallen, Frederic J., MD
 Mullin, Guy S., MD
 Safran, Steven G., MD
 Shah, Angana Nayan, MD
 Shah, Chirag S., MD
 Shah, Kekul Bharat, MD
 Stein, Harmon Charles, MD
Linden
 Kotch, Michael J., MD
Linwood
 Nguyen, Truc H., MD
 Remer, Paul, MD
 Uretsky, Stephen H., MD
Little Silver
 Trikha, Rupan, MD
 Uram, Martin, MD
Livingston
 Cohen, Amir, MD
 Cohen, Steven B., MD
 Decker, Edward Bruce, MD
 Harris, Michael, MD
 Kanter, Eric D., MD
 Kronengold, Charles J., MD
 Marano, Matthew Jr., MD
 Miller, Andrew Ian, MD
 Nussbaum, Peter, MD
 Rodriguez, Natalia Maria, MD
Long Branch
 Bontempo, Carl Peter, MD
 Fegan, Robert James, MD
 Goldberg, Daniel B., MD
 Kristan, Ronald W., MD
Lyndhurst
 DeLuca, Joseph A., MD
Manahawkin
 Dreizen, Neil G., MD
 Drudy, Elena R., MD
 Erickson, Alan R., MD
 Lee, Robert Edward III, MD
Manalapan
 Braunstein, Edward A., MD
Margate City
 Gross, Howard J., MD
 Nunn, Robert F., MD
 Perez, Matthew K., MD
 Pritz, Nicole M., MD

Physicians by Specialty and Town

Marlton
Cutney,Carolyn A.,MD
Glass,Charles Adam,MD
Grossman,Harry D.,MD
Kamoun,Layla,MD
Mellul,Steven Daniel,DO
Mays Landing
Maguire,Joseph I.,MD
Sivalingam,Arunan,MD
Medford
Cohen,Sander M.,MD
Hyder,Carl Franklin,MD
Mitchell,Cheryl Marie,MD
Sivalingam,Varunan,MD
Veloudios,Angela,MD
Mendham
Kalnins,Linda Y.,MD
Midland Park
Seidenberg,Keith B.,MD
Milford
Hahn,Robert Douglas,MD
Millburn
Doshi,Vatsal Suryakant,MD
Greenfield,Donald A.,MD
Newman,David M.,MD
Pruzon,Joanna Dawn,DO
Millville
Ghobrial,John M.,MD
Lieberman,Roger D.,DO
Pernelli,David R.,MD
Mine Hill
Patel,Kartik,DO
Monroe Township
Grabowski,Wayne M.,MD
Montclair
Childs,Kathryn Phyllis,MD
Schachter,Norbert,MD
Montville
Gerszberg,Ted M.,MD
Moorestown
Brown,Miriam Renee,MD
Horowitz,Philip,MD
Kelly,Peter J.,MD
Nachbar,James G.,MD
Putnam,Daniel Philip,MD
Tran,Trong D.,MD
Wexler,Amy R.,MD
Morristown
Angioletti,Lee Mitchell,MD
Benedetto,Dominick A.,MD
Braunstein,Robert Alan,MD
Chen,Lucy L.,MD
Kazam,Ezra S.,MD
Klein,Kathryn Suzanne,MD
Knapp,Stefanie,MD
Lalin,Sean C.,MD
Landmann,Dan S.,MD
Lopatynsky,Marta O.,MD
Masterson,Robert E.,MD
Morgan,Charles Fisher,MD
Perina,Barbara,MD
Reisman,Jeffrey M.,MD
Sarkar,Jayati Saha,MD
Mount Holly
Hartman,Eric J.,MD
Mount Laurel
Vernon,Paul L.,MD
Neptune City
Del Negro,Ralph G.,DO
Glatman,Marina,MD
New Brunswick
Fine,Howard Frederick,MD
Friedman,Eric Stephen,MD
Green,Stuart N.,MD
Keyser,Bruce J.,MD
Leff,Steven R.,MD
Mobin Uddin,Omar,MD
Prenner,Jonathan Lawrence,MD
Roth,Daniel Benjamin,MD
Shah,Sumit Pravinkumar,MD
Wheatley,Harold M.,MD
New Milford
Carabin,Gari D.,MD
New Providence
Leventhal,Todd Owen,MD
Wong,Charissa J.,MD
Newark
Bhagat,Neelakshi,MD
Dastjerdi,Mohammad Hossein,MD
Fechtner,Robert D.,MD

Frohman,Larry P.,MD
Goldfeder,Alan W.,MD
Greenstein,Steven,MD
Guo,Suqin,MD
Khouri,Albert S.,MD
Langer,Paul D.,MD
Materna,Thomas W.,MD
Picciano,Maria V.,MD
Rassier,Charles Edgar Jr.,MD
Roy,Monique S.,MD
Turbin,Roger Eric,MD
Zarbin,Marco A.,MD
Zolli,Christine L.,MD
Newton
Barone,Robert Gerard,MD
Hirschfeld,Laura Ann,MD
Inkeles,David M.,MD
Perlmutter,Harold S.,MD
Vora,Amit V.,MD
North Arlington
Favetta,John R.,MD
Morrone,Louis J.,MD
North Bergen
Braunstein,Steven W.,MD
Shah,Dipal,MD
North Brunswick
Bennett-Phillips,Fay L.,MD
Northfield
Connors,Daniel Bernard,MD
Foxman,Brett T.,MD
Foxman,Scott G.,MD
Margolis,Thomas Ira,MD
Thakker,Manoj Mangaldas,MD
Nutley
Fiore,Philip M.,MD
Prystowsky,Ligaya L.,MD
Zazzali,Albert John,MD
Oakland
Hilal-Campo,Diane M.,MD
Ocean City
Huang,Jun C.,MD
Old Bridge
Blondo,Dennis L.,MD
Cohen,Ilan,MD
Scharfman,Robert M.,MD
Palisades Park
Chu,David Shu-Chih,MD
Kim,Daniel Y.,MD
Lee,Sangwoo,MD
Lyu,Theodore,MD
Paramus
Burke,Patricia A.,MD
Liva,Douglas F.,MD
Pettinelli,Damon John,MD
Pomerantz,Scott Barry,MD
Passaic
Mendoza,Luis,MD
Steinberg,Melissa S.,MD
Vogel,Mitchell,MD
Winfield,Steven S.,MD
Paterson
Feng,Jing Jing,MD
Leifer,Alden,MD
Pennington
Desai,Priya Vasudev,MD
Lesniak,Sebastian P.,MD
Matossian,Cynthia,MD
Rozenbaum,Ilya Maksovich,MD
Pennsauken
Porter,Joel,MD
Pennsville
Mazzuca,Douglas E.,DO
Perth Amboy
Darvin,Kenneth N.,MD
Murr,Peter,MD
Santamaria,Jaime II,MD
Phillipsburg
Finegan,James Jr.,MD
Neusidl,William B.,MD
Piscataway
Kanengiser,Bruce Evan,MD
Princeton
Epstein,John Arthur,MD
Felton,Stephen M.,MD
Jadico,Suzanne K.,MD
Lipka,Andrew C.,MD
Liu,Samuel M.,MD
Miedziak,Anita Irmina,MD
Mulvey,Lauri D.,MD
Patel,Chirag V.,MD

Shovlin,Joseph Peter,MD
Wasserman,Barry N.,MD
Wong,Michael Y.,MD
Wong,Richard H.,MD
Princeton Junction
Milman,Tatyana,MD
Rahway
Hosler,Matthew Robert,MD
Khan,Taj G.,DO
Ramsey
Van Inwegen,Jeffrey R.,MD
Randolph
Benerofe,Bruce Michael,MD
Cetta,Peter J.,MD
Kaden,Ian H.,MD
Walker,Richard Nathaniel,DO
Red Bank
Blades,Frederick C.,MD
Chen,Natalie,DO
D'Emic,Susan,DO
Friedberg,Mark A.,MD
Frieman,Brett Justin,DO
Frieman,Lawrence,MD
Greco,John Jr.,MD
Jergens,Paul B.,MD
Kahn,Walter J.,MD
Kneisser,George,MD
Ridgewood
Alino,Anne Marie G.,MD
Amesur,Kiran Bhagwan,MD
Fox,Martin Lee,MD
Harris,Michael J.,MD
Jachens,Adrian William,MD
Kayserman,Larisa,MD
Kim,David Yhoshin,MD
Kopelman,Joel E.,MD
Lee,Song Eun,MD
Liva,Bradford C.,MD
Norden,Richard A.,MD
Saunders,Eric Monroe,MD
Solomon,Edward Mark,MD
Tsakrios,Charles N. Jr.,MD
Vallar,Robert V.,MD
River Edge
Goldfarb,Mark S.,MD
Higgins,Lisa Marie,MD
Ponce Contreras,Marta R.,MD
Riverton
Calesnick,Jay L.,MD
Rochelle Park
Lama,Paul Jude,MD
Sachs,Seth W.,MD
Roseland
Origlier,Anthony,MD
Runnemede
Yaros,Michael J.,MD
Rutherford
Chiang,Bessie,MD
Neigel,Janet M.,MD
Rothman,Murray H.,MD
Sewell
Bresalier,Howard J.,DO
Girgis,Raymond Michael,MD
Heist,Kenneth C.,DO
Nyquist,Susan Shoshana,MD
Ringel,David M.,DO
Short Hills
Farbowitz,Michael Aron,MD
Somerset
Angrist,Richard Clay,MD
Grewal,Roopinder K.,MD
Phillips,Bradley John,MD
Shamim,Tasneem F.,MD
Somerville
Kaspareck,Joseph Jr.,MD
Sohmer,Kenette K.,MD
South Orange
Crane,Charles J.,MD
Gunzburg,Allison B.,MD
Spier,Bernard C.,MD
South Plainfield
Agarwala,Atul K.,MD
Sparta
Hess,Jocelyn S.,MD
Liegner,Jeffrey T.,MD
Springfield
Lucia Ricci,Jodie Italia,MD
Succasunna
Gottlieb,Joel M.,MD
Pinke,Robert S.,MD

Summit
Boozan,John M.,MD
Campeas,David,MD
Hoffman,David Sandor,MD
Teaneck
Angioletti,Louis V. Jr.,MD
Bergen,Robert L.,MD
Brown,Andrew Carson,MD
Brown,Christopher David,MD
Brown,Robert Henry,MD
Brown,Robert Stephen,MD
Feiner,Leonard,MD
Glassman,Ronald M.,MD
Gordon,Leslie Ellen,MD
Hahn,Paul,MD
Hersh,Peter S.,MD
Higgins,Patrick M.,MD
Klein,Richard M.,MD
Slamovits,Thomas L.,MD
Weinberg,Martin R.,MD
Tenafly
Stabile,John R.,MD
Toms River
Almallah,Omar F.,MD
Alterman,Michael Adam,DO
Angioletti,Louis Scott,MD
Athwal,Barinder S.,MD
Athwal,Lisa M.,MD
Birdi,Anil,MD
Feiner,Laurel A.,MD
Gloth,Jonathan Michael,MD
Hajee,Mohammedyusuf E.,MD
Heimmel,Mark Robert,MD
Lakhani,Vipul K.,MD
Lautenberg,Mitchel Alan,MD
Pan,Jane Chi-Chun,MD
Pidduck,Thomas Charles,MD
Robinson,Neil H.,MD
Schnitzer,Robert E.,MD
Schoenfeld,Allan H.,MD
Trastman-Caruso,Elyse Randi,MD
Wnorowski,Brian R.,MD
Totowa
Giliberti,Orazio L.,MD
Trenton
Brown,William C. Jr.,MD
Donohue,Robert III,MD
Union
Haberman,James E.,MD
Natale,Benjamin P.,DO
Tchorbajian,Kourkin,MD
Union City
Gabay,Jacqueline Estelle,MD
Ho,Vincent Yih,MD
Icasiano,Evelyn J.,MD
Ventnor
Smith,David J.,MD
Verona
Davidson,Lawrence M.,MD
Vineland
Bresalier,Saul,DO
Bruno,Christopher Ryan,MD
Holzinger,Karl Anthony,MD
Pilet,Jean-Claude,MD
Tyson,Sydney L.,MD
Williams,Alice,MD
Wisda,Catherine L.,MD
Voorhees
Binenbaum,Gil,MD
Cohen,Marc S.,MD
Cox,Mary Jude,MD
Dugan,John Donald Jr.,MD
Forman,Jeffrey S.,MD
Gault,Janice Ann,MD
Gordon,Susan Master,MD
Gorman,James G. Jr.,DO
Lingappan,Ahila,MD
Ohsie-Bajor,Linda Hae Eun,MD
Warren
Carter,Susan Redfield,MD
Firestone,Debra A.,MD
Gewirtz,Matthew B.,MD
Giuseffi,Vincent J. III,MD
Jacobs,Ivan H.,MD
Kahn,Milton,MD
Krawitz,Mark J.,MD
Lane,John F.,MD
Lee,Henry,MD
Stahl,Roslyn Marie,MD
Zhang,Linda,MD

Physicians by Specialty and Town

Ophthalmology (cont)
Washington
  Cooley, Susan L., MD
Watchung
  Chung, Jacob H., MD
Wayne
  Choo, Nancy Hae-Jin, MD
  Garg, Geetanjali Davuluri, MD
  Gollance, Stephen Andrew, MD
  Macek, Deanna Z., MD
  Mickey, Kevin J., MD
  Mishler, Ken E., MD
  Obrotka, Thomas M., MD
  Silodor, Scott W., MD
West Caldwell
  Bevacqua, Alejandro, MD
  Strauchler, Roberta A., MD
  Wertheimer, Robert M., MD
West Long Branch
  Leventer, David Benjamin, MD
West New York
  Fasano, Armand P., MD
West Orange
  Cheng, Eleanor Lillian, MD
  Fruchtman, Deborah S., MD
  Medford, David J., MD
  Miller, Kenneth Scott, MD
  Mirsky, Robert G., MD
  Seligsohn, Audrey Lynn, DO
  Tutela, Arthur C., MD
West Paterson
  Parekh, Jai G., MD
  Parekh, Swati Jai Shah, MD
Westfield
  Confino, Joel, MD
  Thiagarajah, Christopher K., MD
Westwood
  Bianchi, Glen Michael, MD
  Chin, Patrick K., MD
  Fleischer, Michael S., MD
  Kaiden, Jeffrey S., MD
  Kirszrot, James, MD
  Lee, Jung S., MD
  Pagan-Duran, Brenda, MD
  Steinbaum, Norman F., MD
Wharton
  Nayar, Romesh C., MD
Willingboro
  Ackerman, Stacey Lynn, MD
  Farnath, Denise Anne, MD
  Feldman, Brad Hal, MD
  Lennox Thomas, Tricia Lynn, MD
  Naids, Richard Eric, MD
  Scimeca, Gregory H., MD
Woodbridge
  Lichtenstein, David I., MD
Woodbury
  Della Torre, Kara E., MD
  Friedberg, Andrea, MD
  Friedberg, Howard L., MD
  Prieto, Debra M., MD
  Weinstock, Brett Michael, MD
Woodcliff Lake
  Mendelsohn, Mary E., MD
  Rini, Frank J., MD
  Yashar, Alyson Gail, MD

Oral & Maxillofacial Surgery
Fort Lee
  Carrao, Vincent, MD
Hackensack
  Han, Chang H., MD
Haddonfield
  Martin, Gene Joseph Jr., MD
Hillsborough
  Bandola, Krystin Ann, MD
Middletown
  Garabedian, Hamlet Charmahali, MD
Newark
  Aziz, Shahid Rahim, MD
  Ziccardi, Vincent Bernard, MD
Paterson
  Ephros, Hillel, MD
Red Bank
  Haghighi, Kayvon, MD
River Edge
  Auerbach, Jason M, MD
  Cho, Sung Hee, MD
South Plainfield
  Goulston, Michael Keith, MD

Teaneck
  Schulhof, Zev, MD
Westwood
  Park, Mark, MD
Woodbury Heights
  Seeger, Douglas H., MD

Orbital Reconstructive Surgery
Clinton
  Morgenstern, Kenneth Eli, MD

Orthopedic Surgery
Atlantic Highlands
  Sobel, Mark, MD
Basking Ridge
  Blank, Peter Bradley, DO
Bayonne
  Augustin, Jeffrey Franck, MD
  Mastromonaco, Edward Domenick, DO
  Rao, Juluru P., MD
  Rowe Urquhart, Erica G., MD
  Urquhart, Marc Wayne, MD
Beach Haven
  Khaleel, Abdul R., MD
Bedminster
  Chan, Peter S., MD
Belleville
  Greifinger, David J., MD
  Lee, James M. Sr., MD
  Mercurio, Carl F., MD
Berkeley Heights
  Garberina, Matthew J., MD
  Mirsky, Eric Charles, MD
  Patel, Samir Popatlal, MD
Bordentown
  Farrell, Joseph E., DO
  Gray, John Michael, MD
  Jain, Rajesh K., MD
  Ropiak, Raymond Russell, MD
  Schoifet, Scott D., MD
Bound Brook
  Schneider, Stephen, MD
Branchville
  Lohwin, Peter G., MD
Brick
  Bogdan, Joseph P., MD
  Hebela, Nader M., MD
  Katt, Brian Matthew, MD
  Law, William A., MD
  Marsicano, Joseph G., MD
  Nitche, Jason Adam, MD
  Rodricks, David Josef, MD
  Zaleski, Theodore G., MD
Bridgeton
  Levitsky, Mark K., MD
Bridgewater
  Bhandutia, Amit Ketan, MD
  Hiramoto, Harlan E., MD
  Nordstrom, Thomas J., MD
  Parolie, James M., MD
  Vessa, Paul P., MD
Burlington Township
  Eakin, David Eugene, DO
  McMillan, Sean, DO
Camden
  De Jesus, Dino Nicol Enanoza, DO
  Freeland, Erik Christopher, DO
  Fuller, David Alden, MD
  Gutowski, Christina, MD
  Kim, Tae Won Benjamin, MD
  Lackman, Richard Daniel, MD
  Lands, Vince Williams, MD
  Mashru, Rakesh Pravinkumar, MD
  Ostrum, Robert Fredric, MD
  Ramirez, Rey Natividad, MD
  Tase, Douglas Sheperd, MD
Cape May
  Anapolle, David M., MD
Cedar Knolls
  D'Agostini, Robert J., MD
  Decter, Edward M., MD
  Goldman, Robert T., MD
  Hunt, Stephen A., MD
  Strassberg, Joshua A., MD
Chatham
  Alapatt, Michael F., MD
  Dorsky, Steven G., MD
Cherry Hill
  Barr, Lawrence I., DO
  Beaver, Andrew Bradley, MD
  Booth, Robert Emrey Jr., MD
  Clements, David H. III, MD

  Dubowitch, Stuart G., DO
  Gleimer, Barry S., DO
  Gleimer, Jeffrey Robert, DO
  Gordon, Stuart Leon, MD
  Hopkins, Leigh Hastings, MD
  Hume, Eric Lynn, MD
  Jacoby, Sidney Mark, MD
  Kahn, Marc L., MD
  Kahn, Steven H., DO
  Naftulin, Richard J., DO
  Paiste, Mark Ronald, DO
  Ranelle, Robert George, DO
  Reiner, Mark J., DO
  Rekant, Mark Spencer, MD
  Ricci, Anthony R., DO
  Tjoumakaris, Fotios P., MD
Clark
  Bercik, Robert J., MD
Cliffside Park
  Corradino, Christine M., MD
Clifton
  Ambrose, John F., MD
  Hole, Robert L., MD
  Kraut, Lawrence, MD
  Megariotis, Evangelos, MD
  Rifai, Aiman, DO
Closter
  Trokhan, Shawn Edward, MD
Denville
  Capecci, Frank, MD
  Cubelli, Kenneth, MD
  Feldman, David J., MD
  Simmerano, Rocco Anthony, MD
Dover
  Bouillon, Louis R., MD
  Rosenzweig, Abraham H., MD
  Rubinfeld, David I., MD
  Spielman, Joel H., MD
  Stecker, Steven, MD
  Tiger, Arthur H., MD
East Brunswick
  Adolfsen, Stephen Erik, MD
  Bloomstein, Larry Z., MD
  Bowe, John A., MD
  Harnly, Heather Withington, MD
  Klein, Kenneth Stuart, MD
  Klein, Richard Ashley, MD
  Laufer, Samuel J., MD
  Levine, Lewis Jonathan, MD
  McKeon, John J., MD
  McPartland, Thomas Girard, MD
  Tuason, Dominick Anthony, MD
  Weisman, David Seth, MD
East Orange
  Matthews, Calvin C., MD
Edison
  Charen, Jeffrey H., MD
  Chen, Franklin, MD
  Garfinkel, Matthew J., MD
  Grover, Surender M., MD
  Herrera-Figueira, Diego A., MD
  Jamieson, Janine, DO
  Lessing, David, MD
  Lombardi, Joseph S., MD
  Marcus, Alexander Michael, MD
  Patel, Nilesh J., MD
  Ramani, Mohnish N., MD
  Russoniello, Alexander P., MD
  Ryan, Todd C., DO
  Schottenfeld, Mark A., MD
  Thacker, Sunil Rajan, MD
  Vega, Teresa, MD
  Zimmerman, Joshua M., MD
Egg Harbor Township
  Baker, John C., MD
  Becan, Arthur Frank Jr., MD
  Naame, Lawrence J., MD
  Ong, Alvin C., MD
  Orozco, Fabio R., MD
  Pepe, Matthew D., MD
  Salvo, John Paul Jr., MD
  Tucker, Bradford S., MD
  Woods, Barrett I., MD
Elizabeth
  Bercik, Michael J., MD
  Gutierrez, Pedro M., MD
Emerson
  Baird, Evan Oliver, MD
  Ben Yishay, Ari, MD
  Benke, Michael T., MD
  Esformes, Ira, MD

  Gross, Michael Lee, MD
  Levin, Rafael, MD
  Mendes, John F., MD
  Vazquez, Oscar, MD
Englewood
  Becker, Adam Scott, MD
  Cole, Brian Anthony, MD
  Davis, Damien Ian, MD
  Doidge, Robert W., DO
  Owens, John M., MD
  Shah, Asit K., MD
Fair Lawn
  Berger, John L., MD
  Bernstein, Adam Douglas, MD
  Cassilly, Ryan, MD
  Greenblum, Robert, MD
  Levitsky, Kenneth A., MD
  Ruoff, Mark J., MD
  Schultz, Robert A., MD
  Snyder, Samuel Jay, MD
  Valdez, Napoleon A., MD
Flemington
  Collalto, Patrick Michael, MD
  Glassner, Norman, MD
  Glassner, Philip Justin, MD
  Pollack, Michael Edward, MD
  Shafa, Eiman, MD
Florham Park
  Adam, Stephanie Paige, DO
  Black, Eric M., MD
  Kocaj, Stephen Mark, MD
  Shindle, Michael Kenneth, MD
Fort Lee
  Lee, Fred Suin, MD
Franklin Lakes
  Bellapianta, Joseph Michael, MD
  Greenberg, Aaron Joseph, MD
  Lin, Edward Alan, MD
  Sood, Amit, MD
Freehold
  Banzon, Manuel T., MD
  Berkowitz, Gregg S., MD
  Goldberger, Gerardo V., DO
  Greller, Michael Jon, MD
  Mark, Arthur K., MD
  Mittman, Roy D., MD
  Nakashian, Michael, MD
  Nasar, Alan S., MD
  Vasen, Arthur Philip, MD
  Velez, Alberto A., MD
Gibbsboro
  Wilkins, Charles E., MD
Glassboro
  Clinton, Cody, DO
Glen Ridge
  Chase, Mark D., MD
  Rombough, Gary R., MD
  Vonroth, William Jr., MD
Glen Rock
  Alberta, Francis Gerard, MD
  Implicito, Dante A., MD
  Johnson, Keith Patrick, MD
  Massoud, Bryan J., MD
Guttenberg
  Dauhajre, Teofilo A., MD
Hackensack
  Hammerschlag, Warren A., MD
  John, Thomas Karoor, MD
  Kissin, Yair David, MD
  Rajan, Sivaram Gounder, MD
  Seldes, Richard Meyer, MD
  Yufit, Pavel Vladimirovich, MD
Hackettstown
  Corrigan, Frank John, MD
  De Falco, Robert Anthony, DO
  Deehan, Michael A., MD
  Giliberti, William S., MD
  Koss, Stephen Dennis, MD
  Murphy, John W., MD
  Rosman, Jerome D., MD
  Sayde, William M., MD
  Teja, Paul Gregory, DO
  Wainen, Glen P., MD
  White, Kevin S., DO
Haddon Heights
  Arena, Mario J., MD
  Kozielski, Joseph A., MD
  Poprycz, Walter, MD
Haddonfield
  Barrett, Michael P., DO
  Bodin, Nathan Daniel, MD

Bozic,Vladimir Stefan,MD
Levy,Michael Stuart,DO
Hainesport
Atlas,Orin Keith,MD
Jenkins,Angela Virginia,MD
Hamilton
Cairone,Stephen Scott,DO
Capotosta,Thomas J. Jr.,MD
Crivello,Keith Michael,MD
Hardeski,David Paul,MD
Kleinbart,Fredric Alan,MD
Hammonton
Friedenthal,Roy B.,MD
Gerson,Ronald L.,MD
Harrison
Seigerman,Daniel Allan,MD
Hazlet
Allegra,Marshall P.,MD
Ani,Abdul Nasser,MD
Cunningham,Michael Joseph,MD
Hoboken
Dwyer,James W.,MD
Feliciano,Edward,MD
Isaac,Roman,MD
Steinway,Mitchell I.,MD
Holmdel
Khavarian,Javad,MD
Jamesburg
Jolley,Michael N.,MD
Jersey City
Adibe,Sebastian O.,MD
Beebe,Kathleen Sue,MD
Foddai,Paul A.,MD
Irving,Henry C. III,MD
Pflum,Francis A. Jr.,MD
Tolentino,Ernesto A.,MD
Kearny
Canario,Arthur T.,MD
Granatir,Charles E.,MD
Lakewood
Absatz,Michael G.,MD
Lawrenceville
Accardi,Kimberly Lynn Z.,MD
Antonacci,Mark Darryl,MD
Ast,Michael Paul,MD
Betz,Randal Roberts,MD
Bills,Thomas K.,MD
Codjoe,Paul Winfred,MD
Cuddihy,Laury A.,MD
Eingorn,David S.,MD
Gokcen,Eric C.,MD
LaRocca,Sandro,MD
Nolan,John P. Jr.,MD
Taitsman,James P.,MD
Leonia
Green,Aron M.,MD
Lincoln Park
Kavanagh,Mark Lawrence,MD
Linden
Ghobrial,Mark Nashaat,DO
Kline,John A.,MD
Pedowitz,Walter J.,MD
Ropiak,Christopher Robert,MD
Linwood
Cristini,John A.,MD
Zerbo,Joseph R.,DO
Little Falls
Di Paolo,Peter F.,MD
Little Silver
Lopez,David Vincent,MD
Livingston
Cheema,Humayun Mahmood,MD
Egan,Kevin J.,MD
Kopacz,Kenneth J.,MD
Leeds,Harold C.,MD
Rizio,Louis III,MD
Zarro,Christopher M.,MD
Long Branch
Fechisin,Joel Patrick,MD
Paragioudakis,Steve J.,MD
Mahwah
Alexander,Nicholas,MD
Holden,Douglas Scott,MD
Manahawkin
Epstein,Samuel E.,DO
Kennard,William Francis,MD
Kunkle,Herbert Lemuel Jr.,MD
Wright,Douglas G.,MD
Manalapan
Ahmed,Munir,MD

Schiebert,Steven S.,DO
Skolnick,Cary I.,MD
Springer,Stuart Ira,MD
Manasquan
Bhatnagar,Ramil S.,MD
DePaola,Frederick A.,MD
Ferenz,Clint C.,MD
Goldstein,Joel M.,MD
Husserl,Toby B.,MD
Jarmon,Nicholas Albert,MD
Petrosini,Anthony V.,MD
Roehrig,Gregory James,MD
Sclafani,Michael A.,MD
Seckler,Mark M.,MD
Tozzi,John Michael,MD
Maplewood
Feldman,David Nathan,MD
Marlton
Barlow,Jonathan David,MD
Hoffler,Charles E. II,MD
Horowitz,Stephen M.,MD
Kelly,John D.,MD
Kirshner,Steven B.,MD
Maslow,Gregory S.,MD
Michael,Stanley P.,MD
Nelson,Gregory N. Jr.,MD
Ragland,Raymond III,MD
Schaaf,H. William,MD
Sobel,Mark A.,MD
Zell,Brian Kirk,MD
Maywood
Lindholm,Stephen R.,MD
Mercerville
Sporn,Aaron A.,MD
Midland Park
Konigsberg,David Eric,MD
Van Grouw,Brian P.,DO
Millburn
Blank,Howard L.,MD
Daly,Ronald A.,MD
Schob,Clifford J.,MD
Monroe Township
Polakoff,Donald Richard,MD
Montclair
Drzala,Mark R.,MD
Fischer,Evan S.,MD
Nicoll,Cornelius I.,MD
Vizzone,Jerald P.,DO
Moorestown
Dwyer,Joseph Michael,MD
Greenleaf,Robert Martin,MD
Raimondo,Rick Arthur,MD
Sanfilippo,James Arthur,MD
Weisband,Ira David,DO
Morristown
Aurori,Brian F.,MD
Aurori,Kevin C.,MD
Avallone,Nicholas J.,MD
Baskies,Michael Ari,MD
Baydin,Jeffrey A.,MD
Cohen,Marc Alan,MD
Crutchlow,William P.,MD
Dowling,William J. Jr.,MD
Drey,Iris Antonella,MD
Epstein,David Michael,MD
Gatto,Charles Anthony,MD
Giordano,Carl P.,MD
Goldberger,Michael Irwin,MD
Kanellakos,James George,MD
Levine,Barry Steven,MD
Lombardi,Paul M. Jr.,MD
Nachwalter,Richard Scott,MD
Naseef,George Salem III,MD
Sclafani,Steven,MD
Taffet,Berton,MD
Wagshul,Adam David,MD
Willis,Andrew Albert,MD
Mount Laurel
Bowers,Andrea Legath,MD
Deutsch,Lawrence Steven,MD
Momi,Kamaldeep S.,MD
Peacock,Kenneth C.,MD
Sapega,Alexander,MD
Schwartz,Mark Glen,MD
Mountain Lakes
Silverman,Jesse A.,MD
Mountainside
Warshauer,Jeffrey M.,DO
Neptune
Dennis,Robert I.,MD
Schulman,Jared E.,MD

New Brunswick
Erickson,John A.,MD
Fried,Steven H.,MD
Hyatt,Adam Extein,MD
Ros,Stephen Joseph,MD
Sathyendra,Vikram Modur,MD
Selby,Ronald M.,MD
Newark
Adams,Mark Robert,MD
Ahmad,Iqbal,MD
Benevenia,Joseph,MD
Berberian,Wayne S.,MD
Carollo,Andrew,MD
Edobor-Osula,Osamuede,MD
Jaffe,Seth L.,DO
Neal,John William VI,MD
Potini,Vishnu Choudhary,MD
Reilly,Mark C.,MD
Reiter,Mitchell F.,MD
Sabharwal,Sanjeev,MD
Sirkin,Michael S.,MD
Tan,Virak,MD
Vives,Michael J.,MD
Newton
Lopez,Nicole Melisa Montero,MD
Scales,James Jr.,MD
Weinschenk,Robert C.,MD
North Arlington
Gennace,Ronald E.,MD
Lerner,Kent S.,MD
North Bergen
Baghal,Imad Y.,MD
Sun,Li,DO
North Brunswick
Reich,Steven M.,MD
Sieler,Shawn D.,MD
Northfield
Harhay,Joseph S.,MD
Norwood
Kerness,Wayne Jared,MD
Nutley
Ducey,Stephen Alexander,MD
Femino,Frank Placido,MD
Parks,Anthony Lesmore Jr.,MD
Queler,Seth Robert,MD
Wujciak,Michael P.,MD
Ocean
Chern,Kenneth Y.,MD
Demetriades,Haralambos,MD
Haynes,Paul Thomas II,MD
McDaid,Kevin C.,MD
Nguyen,Hoan-Vu Tran,MD
Spagnuola,Christopher J.,MD
Yalamanchili,Praveen K.,MD
Old Bridge
Hassan,Sheref E.,MD
Oradell
Kane,Seth O.,MD
Paramus
Difelice,Gregory Scott,MD
Distefano,Michael C.,MD
Elliott,Andrew J.,MD
Hartzband,Mark A.,MD
Klein,Gregg Roger,MD
Kovatis,Paul Evan,MD
McIlveen,Stephen J.,MD
Newman,Bernard P. III,MD
Okezie,Chukueke Tobenna,MD
Ranawat,Anil S.,MD
Seidenstein,Ari Douglas,MD
Snyder,Ronald David,MD
Stoller,Steven M.,MD
Parsippany
Siegel,Jeffrey Alan,MD
Paterson
Flood,Stephen James,MD
Pennington
Caruso,Steven A.,MD
Phillipsburg
Diiorio,Emil John,MD
Ferrante,Christopher R.,MD
Friedman,Robert Lawrence,MD
Loguidice,Vito A.,MD
Maron,Norman L.,MD
Martinez,Marcos Manuel,MD
Palumbo,Dante M.,DO
Reid,James Henry,MD
Sadler,Adam D.,DO
Piscataway
Piskun,Andrew,MD
Zemsky,Lewis M.,MD

Plainsboro
Dhanaraj,Dinesh,MD
Smires,Harvey E. Jr.,MD
Princeton
Abrams,Jeffrey Stuart,MD
Bechler,Jeffrey R.,MD
Bezwada,Hari Prasad,MD
Fleming,Richard E. Jr.,MD
Gecha,Steven R.,MD
Gutowski,Walter Thomas III,MD
Lamb,David J.,MD
Leise,Megan Diane,MD
Levine,Stuart Eric,MD
McDonnell,Matthew,MD
Moskwa,Alexander Jr.,MD
Nazarian,Ronniel,MD
Pressman,Mark J.,MD
Rossy,William Henry IV,MD
Song,Frederick Suh,MD
Vannozzi,Brian Michael,MD
Princeton Junction
Glick,Ronald S.,MD
Miller,Scott David,MD
Shakir,Ahmar,DO
Rahway
Paulson,Melyssa Michelle,MD
Pecker,Howard M.,MD
Red Bank
Bakhos,Nader Anthony,MD
Costa,Anthony Joseph,MD
Friedel,Steven P.,MD
Lospinuso,Michael Frank,MD
Mintalucci,Dominic J.,MD
Murphy,Bernard P.,MD
Rinkus,Keith Michael,MD
Ridgefield
Yoo,Daniel J.,MD
Ridgewood
Brief,Andrew A.,MD
Carney,William P.,MD
Carozza,Charles R.,MD
Criscitiello,Arnold A.,MD
Dasti,Umer R.,MD
Delfico,Anthony John,MD
Joffe,Avrum L.,MD
Kayal,Robert Albert,MD
Roenbeck,Kevin Meehan,MD
Rudman,David Paul,MD
Rio Grande
Facciolo,Jack,DO
Saddle Brook
Patel,Deepak Valjibhai,MD
Secaucus
Martinez,Armando I.,MD
Rothenberg,Paul,MD
Sewell
Falconiero,Robert Paul,DO
Kovacs,Jeffrey Peter,DO
Marcelli,Enrico A.,DO
Mariani,John K.,DO
Murray,Jeffrey,DO
Paz,Efrain Jr.,DO
Ponzio,Robert J.,DO
Valentino,Steven John,DO
Shrewsbury
Menkowitz,Marc Scott,MD
Stankovits,Lawrence Matthew,MD
Somers Point
Alber,George C.,MD
Bannon,John T.,MD
Barrett,Thomas Arthur,MD
Dalzell,Frederick G.,MD
De Morat,Eugene John,MD
Frankel,Victor R.,MD
Islinger,Richard Barnard,MD
Marczyk,Stanley C.,MD
McCloskey,John R.,MD
Ponnappan,Ravi Kumar,MD
Zuck,Glenn M.,DO
Somerset
Butler,Mark S.,MD
Chiappetta,Gino,MD
Coyle,Michael P. Jr.,MD
Harwood,David A.,MD
Kayiaros,Stephen,MD
Krisiloff,Edward B.,MD
Leddy,Timothy P.,MD
Malberg,Marc I.,MD
Polonet,David Russell,MD
Sagebien,Carlos Alberto,MD
Swan,Kenneth Girvan Jr.,MD

Physicians by Specialty and Town

Orthopedic Surgery (cont)
Somerville
Baron,Harvey L.,MD
St. John,Thomas A.,MD
South Orange
Berlin,Burgess L.,MD
Buechel,Frederick F.,MD
Helbig,Thomas E.,MD
South Plainfield
Choi,Soon Chae,MD
Lebovicz,Richard S.,MD
Shafi,Mohammad,MD
Sparta
Basch,David B.,MD
Czaplicki-Margiotti,Marie A.,MD
Vitolo,John,MD
Springfield
Cuomo,Thomas F.,MD
Jaffe,Leonard,MD
Oppenheim,William C.,MD
Rieber,Michael Harold,MD
Stratford
Cawley,Christina M.,DO
Summit
DeLuca,Francis N.,MD
Fischer,Stuart J.,MD
Lin,Sheldon S.,MD
Sarokhan,Alan J.,MD
Teaneck
Bauer,Brian J.,MD
Carrer,Alexandra,MD
Hale,James Joseph,MD
Katona,John J.,MD
Kwak,Steve K.,MD
Patel,Deepan N.,MD
Pfisterer,Dennis James,DO
Pfisterer,Dennis L.,MD
Quartararo,Louis Gaspar,MD
Steuer,Jeffrey K.,MD
Tenafly
Mardam-Bey,Tarek H.,MD
Tinton Falls
Chalnick,David Lee,MD
Cohen,Jason D.,MD
Foos,Gregg Robert,MD
Gentile,David R.,MD
Gesell,Mark William,MD
Glastein,Cary D.,MD
Grossman,Robert B.,MD
Markbreiter,Lance A.,MD
Rizzo,Charles C.,MD
Torpey,Brian M.,MD
Toms River
Borgatti,Richard J.,MD
Closkey,Robert F.,MD
Dhawlikar,Sripad H.,MD
Dickerson,David B.,MD
Fox,Daniel E.,MD
Gabisan,Glenn Gacula,MD
Kasper,Mark T.,MD
Kubeck,Justin P.,MD
Larsen,Erik Scott,DO
Palmieri,Alfred E.,MD
Passariello,Christopher,MD
Petrillo,John A.,MD
Sacks,Richard,MD
Saleh,Jason Reed,MD
Tauro,Joseph C.,MD
Trenton
Aita,Daren J.,MD
Di Biase,John J.,MD
Duch,Michael R.,MD
Gomez,William,MD
Hornstein,Joshua Scott,MD
Levine,Marc Jason,MD
Pagliaro,Andre J.,MD
Saxena,Arjun,MD
Schnell,John Raymond,MD
Union
Aragona,James,MD
Botwin,Clifford A.,DO
Bradley,Douglas D.,MD
Charko,Gregory P.,MD
Gallick,Gregory S.,MD
Gross,David E.,MD
Innella,Robin R.,DO
Kaiser,Anthony J.,MD
King,John Wayne,DO
Nehmer,Steven L.,MD
Rajaram,Arun,MD
Wolkstein,David S.,MD
Union City
Baruch,Howard Michael,MD
Verona
Gehrmann,Robin Michael,MD
Leary,Jeffrey T.,MD
Vineland
Bernardini,Brad Joseph,MD
Bernardini,Joseph P.,MD
Buxbaum,Eric Justin,DO
Catalano,John B.,MD
Di Verniero,Richard C. Jr.,MD
Feldman,Jenna Aviv,DO
Sarkos,Peter Anthony,DO
Shah,Rahul V.,MD
Voorhees
Carey,Christopher T.,MD
Daniels,Jeffrey B.,MD
David,Henry Edward,DO
DeLuca,Peter Francis,MD
George,Brian Philip,MD
Harrer,Michael F.,MD
Klingenstein,Gregory Gillman,MD
Lawrence,John Todd Rutter,MD
O'Dowd,Thomas J.,MD
Pollard,Mark Andrew,MD
Porat,Manny David,MD
Purtill,James Joseph,MD
Ramsey,Matthew Lee,MD
Reid,Jeremy Jackson,MD
Shah,Apurva Surendra,MD
Stark,Zohar,MD
Waldwick
Moore,Michael G.,MD
Wall
Dhawan,Aman,MD
Gordon,Michael H.,MD
Warren
Abrutyn,David Alan,MD
Boretz,Robert Stephen,MD
McCracken,Kevin A.,MD
Wayne
Cappadona,Joseph G.,MD
Dowling,Ryan Martin,MD
Drillings,Gary J.,MD
Dyal,Cherise Malinda,MD
Fahimi,Nader,MD
Faloon,Michael J.,MD
Gold,David A.,MD
Hwang,Ki S.,MD
Maletsky,Mark E.,MD
Masella,Robert Michael,MD
Matarese,William A.,MD
McInerney,Vincent K.,MD
Palacios,Robert M.,MD
Reicher,Oscar A.,MD
Roth,Jonathan Michael,MD
Schultz,Alan E.,MD
Sicherman,Hervey S.,MD
Stern,Lorraine C.,MD
Wanich,Tony Suchai,MD
West Berlin
Rosenberg,Larry S.,MD
West Caldwell
Berkman,Avrill R.,MD
Strauchler,Irving D.,MD
West Orange
Boiardo,Richard A.,MD
Garcia,Jason P.,MD
Hutter,Andrew M.,MD
Kadimcherla,Praveen,MD
Lee,James M. Jr.,MD
Loya,David Michael,MD
Pirone,Arthur M.,MD
Robbins,Steven G.,MD
Rosa,Richard A.,MD
Seidenstein,Michael Kenneth,MD
Westfield
Bullek,David D.,MD
Faccone,John A.,DO
Krell,Todd P.,MD
Sweeney,Ralph Jr.,MD
Thrower,Albert B.,MD
Westwood
Levine,Raphael Krevsky,MD
Lloyd,John Mervyn,MD
Miller,Alan R.,MD
Whippany
Grob,Patricio,DO
Schenk,Richard S.,MD
Spinnickie,Anthony O.,MD
Woodbridge
Lu,Michael T.,MD
Woodbury
Bundens,David A.,MD
Frey,Steven,MD
Kalawadia,Jay Vinodrai,MD
O'Brien,Evan Douglas,MD
Obade,Thomas P.,MD
Rosen,Craig H.,MD
Woodcliff Lake
Betsy,Michael,MD
Wyckoff
Andronaco,John T.,MD

Orthopedic Surgery-Adult Recnstrct
Egg Harbor Township
Hernandez,Victor Hugo,MD
Flemington
Gordon,Eric Michael,MD
Hackettstown
Dundon,John M.,MD
New Brunswick
Jonna,Venkata Karthik,MD
Paramus
Levine,Harlan Brett,MD
Somerset
Tria,Alfred J. Jr.,MD
Wayne
Su,Sherwin Leu,MD

Orthopedic Trauma
Jersey City
Liporace,Frank Anthony,MD
Maywood
Keller,Julie Michelle,MD
Mercerville
Ahmed,Atif Khalid,MD
Wall
Pushilin,Sergei A.,MD
Wayne
Cox,Garrick Andrew,MD
Schneidkraut,Jason S.,MD

Orthopedic-Hand Surgery
Brick
Malfitano,Laura Anne,DO
Closter
Sokol,Shima C.,MD
Fair Lawn
Shamash,Steven Baroukh,DO
Florham Park
Niver,Genghis Erjan,MD
Jersey City
Ahmed,Irfan Haroon,MD
Capo,John Thomas,MD
Somerset
Monica,James T.,MD
Toms River
Pensak,Michael J.,MD
Wall
Doumas,Christopher,MD
Wayne
Denoble,Peter Hart,MD
Westfield
Said,Joseph,MD

Orthopedics
Berkeley Heights
Corona,Joseph T.,MD
Cherry Hill
Kane,Patrick Martin,MD
Edison
Patti,James E.,MD
Englewood
Archer,Jonathan Mckee,MD
Salob,Peter Andrew,MD
Flemington
Chang,Richard,MD
Freehold
Arias Garau,Jessica,MD
Linden
Rojer,David Eli,MD
Marlton
Kahanovitz,Neil,MD
Newark
Patterson,Francis Robert,MD
Phillipsburg
Rudolph,Jason Willer,MD
Red Bank
Lisser,Steven P.,MD
Mulholland,Daniel J.,MD
Phair,Arthur H.,MD
Scott,Richard J.,MD
Shrewsbury
Curatolo,Evan M.,MD
Wayne
Wright,Craig,MD
West Orange
Bachman,Jodie Ann,DO

Osteopathic Medicine
Garfield
Conte,Daniel P. III,DO
Hammonton
Bertagnolli,John F. Jr.,DO
Kingston
Tepper Levine,Shawn,DO
Medford
Pinto,Jeffrey Damian,DO
Ocean View
Wilson,Donna E.,DO
Woodbury
Tapper,Ben R.,DO

Other Specialty
Berlin
Nigro,Mary A.,MD
Blackwood
Corson-Diaz,Cathy Lynn,MD
Diaz Jimenez,Jose Eduardo,MD
Bridgewater
Choi,Mingi,MD
Egg Harbor Township
Salartash,Khashayar,MD
Flemington
Decker,Jerome Elliot,MD
Green Brook
Price,Grant J.,MD
Hackensack
DeBellis,Julia Angelina,MD
Koenig,Christopher,MD
Livingston
Blackwood,Margaret Michele,MD
Brener,Bruce J.,MD
Millburn
Yemini,Matan,MD
Morris Plains
Furey,Sandy Anselm III,MD
Morristown
Colizza,Wayne A.,MD
Newark
Colao,Joseph A. Jr.,DO
Raina,Suresh,MD
Old Bridge
Fahmy,Sandra Patricia,DO
Princeton
Ark,Jon Wong Tze-Jen,MD
Sewell
Neilon,Kathleen Mary,DO
Summit
Nuzzo,Roy Michael,MD

Otolaryngology
Bedminster
Janjua,Tanveer Ahmed,MD
Belleville
Lester,Arthur I.,MD
Berkeley Heights
Burstein,David Harris,MD
Eden,Avrim Reuben,MD
Gnoy,Alexander Roman,MD
Gurey,Lowell Evan,MD
Kwartler,Jed A.,MD
Le Benger,Jeffrey D.,MD
Brick
Brandeisky,Thomas E.,DO
Landsman,Howard Scott,DO
Bridgeton
Lorenc,Ronald B.,MD
Bridgewater
Fenster,Gerald F.,MD
Hekiert,Adrianna Maria,MD
Lazar,Amy D.,MD
Schneiderman,Todd Aron,MD
Camden
Spalla,Thomas Christopher,MD
Cape May Court House
DeLorio,Nicola Anne,DO
Matlick,Lonny D.,DO
Mucci,Wayne P.,DO
Syed,Zubair,DO

Physicians by Specialty and Town

Cedar Grove
Rossi,Anthony G.,MD
Cherry Hill
Busch,Scott L.,DO
Hall,Patrick J.,MD
Clifton
Ledereich,Philip S.,MD
Colonia
Sahni,Rana S.,MD
Cranbury
Li,Ronald W.,MD
Cresskill
Blome,Mary,MD
East Brunswick
Edelman,Bruce Allen,MD
Highstein,Charles I.,MD
Horowitz,Jay B.,MD
Kaplan,Kenneth A.,MD
Rosenbaum,Jeffrey Mark,MD
East Orange
Caputo,Joseph L.,MD
Edison
Arlen,Harold,MD
Aruna,Pasalai N.,MD
Kraus,Warren M.,MD
Lavine,Ferne R.,MD
Miller,Andrew John,MD
Park,Robert Inyeung,MD
Egg Harbor
Morrison,Daniel H. Jr.,MD
Egg Harbor Township
Schaffer,Scott R.,MD
Elizabeth
Bergman,Justin A.,MD
Cinberg,James Z.,MD
Huang,Robert D.,MD
Saporta,Diego,MD
Emerson
Svider,Peter,MD
Englewood
Ho,Bryan Tao,MD
Jahn,Anthony Frederick,MD
Scherl,Michael P.,MD
Tadros,Monica,MD
Tobias,Geoffrey Wayne,MD
Englewood Cliffs
Moon,Taewon,MD
Flemington
Hanna,John Patrick,DO
Kroon,David Fleming,MD
Maniar,Anoli,MD
Sheft,Stanley A.,MD
Worden,Douglas L.,MD
Florham Park
Byrd,Serena Ann,MD
Fleming,Gregory John,MD
Peron,Didier L.,MD
Fort Lee
Henick,David H.,MD
Kim,Steve Yun,MD
Freehold
Brahmbhatt,Sapna Sureshkumar,MD
Kumar,Arun S.,MD
Razvi,Sedeq A.,MD
Roessler,Mark Leonard,DO
Sattenspiel,Sigmund Linder,MD
Gibbsboro
Aftab,Saba,MD
Wong,Gabriel Ho Yu,MD
Glen Ridge
Zbar,Lloyd I. S.,MD
Glen Rock
Katz,Harry,MD
Hackensack
Benson,Brian Eric,MD
Brody,Robin Michelle,MD
Gold,Steven M.,MD
Inouye,Masayuki,MD
Lesserson,Jonathan A.,MD
Low,Ronald Brian,MD
Respler,Don S.,MD
Rosen,Arie,MD
Shaari,Christopher M.,MD
Tell,Alan Michael,MD
Wasserman,Jared Mark,MD
Hackettstown
Gentile,Victor G.,MD
Pollack,Joshua David,MD
Haddonfield
Cultrara,Anthony,MD

Gadomski,Stephen P.,MD
Shah,Samir,MD
Hamilton
Jaffe,Joel D.,MD
Miller,Lee H.,MD
Rossos,Apostolos A.,MD
Hawthorne
Giglio,Michael,MD
Highland Park
Glasgold,Mark J.,MD
Keni,Sanjay P.,MD
Schrader-Barile,Nicole A.,MD
Hoboken
Calloway,Hollin Elizabeth,MD
Glaser,Aylon Y.,MD
Glickman,Alexander B.,MD
Tandon,Raj,MD
Holmdel
Kim,Chong S.,MD
Iselin
Mazzara,Carl Arthur,MD
Mehta,Vishvesh Mukur,MD
Ort,Stuart A.,MD
Rosin,Deborah F.,MD
Jersey City
Behin,Babak,MD
Behin,Fereidoon,MD
Garay,Kenneth F.,MD
Youssef,Jan Samir,MD
Lakewood
Giri,Suresh C.,MD
Jaffari,Syed Moosa Raza,MD
Lawrenceville
Boozan,James A.,MD
Lupa,Michael David,MD
Patel,Rakesh Bhogilal,MD
Shah,Chetan S.,MD
Linwood
Feldman,Marc D.,MD
Orquiza,Clodualdo S. III,MD
Siliunas,Vytas B.,DO
Wagle,Priya Jennifer,MD
Little Silver
Sullivan,Timothy Patrick,MD
Livingston
Lee,Bryant B.,MD
Lee,Derek Sai-Wah,MD
Manahawkin
Bezpalko,Lynn E.,DO
Bezpalko,Orest,DO
Bhojwani,Amit N.,MD
Bones,Victoria Mary,MD
Engle,Edward Issac,DO
McAfee,Jacob Seth,MD
Patel,Pratik Bharat,MD
Romanczuk,Bruce J.,MD
Manasquan
Faktor,Mitchell J.,DO
Iannacone,Ronald J.,DO
Sparano,Anthony Michael,MD
Maplewood
Williams,Dione M.,MD
Marlton
Houston,Patrick J.,MD
Tai,Stephen Jay,MD
Martinsville
Karolak,Mark,DO
Midland Park
Milgrim,Laurence Marc,MD
Montclair
Tan,John J.,MD
Morristown
Cairns,Christine Dobrosky,MD
Gerwin,Kenneth S.,MD
Giacchi,Renato John,MD
Immerman,Sara Beth,MD
Kanowitz,Seth J.,MD
Lachman,Reid A.,MD
Sorvino,Damian W.,MD
Thomas,Tom,MD
Mount Arlington
Aroesty,Jeffrey H.,MD
Lin,Giant Chu,MD
Mohankumar,Aditi,MD
Mount Laurel
Carlson,Roy Douglas,MD
Gupta,Ashmit,MD
Mountainside
Drake,William III,MD
Presti,Paul Matthew,MD

Neptune
Engel,Samuel Henry,MD
Houston,Sean David,MD
Mitskavich,Mary T.,MD
Newkirk,Kenneth Allen,MD
Pflum,Gerald E.,MD
New Brunswick
Ahmadi,David,MD
Assad,Albert,MD
Goldrich,Michael Seth,MD
Kwong,Kelvin Ming-Tak,MD
Newark
Eloy,Jean Anderson,MD
Granick,Mark Stephen,MD
Kalyoussef,Evelyne,MD
Kaye,Rachel,MD
Ying,Yu-Lan Mary,MD
Newton
Galeos,Warren L.,MD
North Brunswick
Lin,Pei-Shiu,MD
North Haledon
Goodnight,James W.,MD
Nutley
Wallace,Derrick I.,MD
Youssef,Oliver S.,MD
Ocean
Ezon,Frederick C.,MD
Old Bridge
Azer,Andrew Elia,MD
Oradell
Bough,Irvin David Jr.,MD
Cusumano,Robert J.,MD
Huang,John Jan,MD
Leventhal,Douglas Drew,MD
Surow,Jason B.,MD
Paramus
Bar-Eli,Rebecca,MD
Le,Mina Nguyen,MD
Samadi,Sharyar Daniel,MD
Parlin
Zapanta,Vicente T.,MD
Parsippany
Brys,Agata K.,MD
Lebovitz,Brian Lee,MD
Sayeed,Zarina Shaikh,MD
Schultz,Charles Martin,MD
Wirtshafter,Karen A.,MD
Paterson
Labagnara,James Jr.,MD
Pennington
Farzad,Ahmad,MD
Phillipsburg
Rayasam,Ramakumar V.,MD
Sackman,Scott Marshall,DO
Plainsboro
Drezner,Dean Andrew,MD
Kay,Scott Lawrence,MD
Pomona
Paparone,Basil J.,MD
Princeton
Brunner,Eugenie,MD
Red Bank
De Gennaro,Anthony,MD
Scaccia,Frank J.,MD
Riverdale
Ginsburg,Jeffrey B.,MD
Levine,Jonathan Marc,MD
Remsen,Kenneth A.,MD
Taylor,Howard,MD
Robbinsville
McCullough,Aubrey Susan,DO
Roselle Park
Bastianelli,Milo,DO
Conte,Louis J.,DO
Scharf,Richard C.,DO
West,Gerald,DO
Rutherford
Hassan,Sherif A.,MD
Katz,Michael Jonathan,MD
Mahmoud,Ahmad F.,MD
Sarti,Edward J.,MD
Sea Girt
Hou,Lisa Jenny,DO
Secaucus
Reitzen-Bastidas,Shari D.,MD
Sewell
Becker,Daniel G.,MD
Bromberg,David,MD
Friedel,Mark Erik,MD

Rosenstein,Kenneth Michael,MD
Terk,Alyssa Robyn,MD
Short Hills
Ovchinsky,Alexander,MD
Shrewsbury
Passalaqua,Philip Jude,MD
Prabhat,Arvind,MD
Saporito,John L.,MD
Shah,Darsit,MD
Tavill,Michael A.,MD
Winarsky,Eric L.,MD
Somers Point
Morrow,William J.,DO
Rondinella,Louis,MD
Somerset
Sabin,Steven Lloyd,MD
Somerville
Bortniker,David Leonard,MD
Sparta
Reddy,Shashidhar Sadda,MD
Springfield
Freifeld,Stephen F.,MD
Summit
Carniol,Eric T.,MD
Swedesboro
Clairvil,Jessie,DO
Teaneck
Davis,Orrin,MD
Tinton Falls
Roffman,Jeffrey D.,MD
Toms River
Chaker,Antoine C.,MD
Foster,Wayne Paul,MD
Gillespie,Christine,MD
Kupferberg,Stephen Benjamin,MD
Peters,Bruce W.,DO
Stella,Nunzio R.,MD
Union
Obregon,Raimundo L.,MD
Union City
Festa,Alfredo Gerardo,MD
Verona
Liu,Edmund S.,MD
Vineland
Diaz Gonzalez,Rodolfo,MD
Ferrari,Arthur J.,MD
Kenner,George R. Jr.,MD
Voorhees
Becker,Samuel Scott,MD
Belafsky,Robert B.,MD
Cantrell,Harry,MD
Dandu,Kartik Varma,MD
Germiller,John Andrew,MD
Leoniak,Steven Michael,MD
Shah,Udayan Kanaiyalal,MD
Wall
Nahm,Choong S.,MD
Warren
Beecher,George,MD
Vinnakota,Radha I.,MD
Wayne
Abrams,Stephen Joel,MD
Cece,John A.,MD
D'Anton,Michael A. III,MD
Kassir,Ramtin Ronald,MD
Mattel,Stephen F.,MD
Scheibelhoffer,John J.,MD
Scher,Daniel A.,MD
Sreepada,Gangadhar S.,MD
Wise,Jeffrey B.,MD
West New York
Shaari,Jeffrey M.,MD
West Orange
Berg,Howard M.,MD
Downey,Laura L.,MD
Fieldman,Robert J.,MD
Holzberg,Norman,MD
Joseph,Eric M.,MD
Levitt,Joel W.,MD
Morrow,Todd A.,MD
Westfield
Mayer,Michael B.,MD
Westwood
Lee,James Jeong June,MD
Willingboro
Shah,Rasesh Pravin,MD
Woodbury
Schwartz,David N.,MD

Physicians by Specialty and Town

Otolaryngology-Facial Plastic Srg
Bridgewater
 Abrahim,Mena,DO
 Burachinsky,Dennis Andrew,DO
Cherry Hill
 Corrado,Anthony Charles,DO
Englewood
 Lewis,David A.,MD
Lawrenceville
 Undavia,Samir Suresh,MD
Livingston
 Paraiso,Reynaldo S.,DO
Mahwah
 Steckowych,Jayde Mary,MD
Manahawkin
 Zhuravsky,Ruslan,DO
New Brunswick
 Esmail,Ali Raza,MD
 Vella,Joseph Bayer,MD
Old Bridge
 Chowdhury,Farhad Reza,DO
Paterson
 Folk,David,MD
Robbinsville
 Mignone,Robert,DO
Roselle Park
 Mazzoni,Thomas F.,DO
Voorhees
 Scheiner,Edward David,DO
Wayne
 Brunetti,Vito Anthony,MD

Otology
Berkeley Heights
 Cooper,David M.,MD
Hackensack
 Eisenberg,Lee D.,MD
Newark
 Jyung,Robert Wha,MD
Woodbury
 Rowan,Philip T.,MD

Pain Medicine
Atco
 Davis,Kara Alison,MD
Bayonne
 Huish,Stephen H.,DO
 Ibrahim,Joseph G.,MD
Camden
 Wadhwa,Namrata,MD
Chatham
 Gerstman,Brett A.,MD
Cherry Hill
 Band,Ricard Louis,MD
 Korn,Barry Allen,DO
 Tawadrous,Alfred Rezk,MD
East Orange
 Joshi,Meeta Yatinkumar,MD
East Windsor
 Yanni,Baher S.,MD
Englewood Cliffs
 Cho,John S.,MD
Hackensack
 Contreras,Jose A.,MD
 Khan,Sunniya,MD
 Park,Kenneth Hyun,DO
 Seckin,Ali Inanc,MD
Hamilton
 Sackstein,Adam,MD
Linwood
 Petersohn,Jeffrey D.,MD
Livingston
 Bajor-Dattilo,Ewa Beata,MD
Marlton
 Hu,Andre Min-Teh,MD
Montclair
 Park,Chong H.,MD
Mount Laurel
 McMurtrie,Robert Jr.,DO
New Brunswick
 Sakr,Ashraf M.,MD
Newark
 Gyi,Jennifer,DO
 Kostroma,Boris Vladimirovich,MD
Northfield
 Strenger,Keith David,MD
Passaic
 Eppanapally,Shanti Sree,MD
Pennington
 Cruciani,Ricardo Alberto,MD

Princeton
 Varela,Rebecca A.,MD
Ridgewood
 Scham,Arnold,MD
Shrewsbury
 Metzger,Scott E.,MD
Somerset
 Sacks,Harry Jack,MD
Summit
 Pappagallo,Marco,MD
Toms River
 Holtzberg,Nathan,MD
 Yu,Yin Tat,MD
Trenton
 Rosenberg,Daniel S.,MD
Union City
 Ramirez Pacheco,Luis A.,MD
Voorhees
 Rogers,Kenneth H.,DO
Wayne
 D'Amato,Pamela R.,MD
West New York
 Rojas,Jose Jr.,MD

Pain Medicine-Interventional
Cedar Knolls
 Prvulovic,Tomi,MD
East Orange
 Feit,Russell,MD
Edison
 Aranas,Rae Ronald,MD
 Freeman,Eric D.,DO
 Spiel,Douglas J.,MD
Holmdel
 Ng,Alan S.,MD
Long Branch
 Johnson,Andrew,DO
Moorestown
 Duckles,Benjamin Jeffrey,MD
Mount Laurel
 Medvedovsky,Andrew,MD
Newark
 Speert,Tory,DO
 Yanamadula,Dinash Kumar,MD
Paramus
 Sood,Rahul,DO
Somerset
 Demesmin,Didier,MD
Sparta
 Siegfried,Richard Norman,MD
Vineland
 Lewis,Shannin Dion,DO

Palliative Care
Neptune
 Frieman,Amy Porter,MD
Paterson
 Boothe,Deniece Tamara,DO

Pathology
Atlantic City
 Can,Seyit A.,MD
Basking Ridge
 Pedemonte,Bader Maria,MD
Belleville
 Benedetti,Robert C.,MD
Camden
 Behling,Kathryn C.,MD
 Bierl,Charlene,MD
 Camacho,Jeanette M.,MD
 Fitzpatrick,Brendan Thomas,MD
 Kim,Hoon,MD
Cape May Court House
 Jurasinski,Craig M.,MD
East Hanover
 Gonzalez,Raimundo,MD
Edison
 Ewing,Clinton Alexander,MD
Englewood
 Burga,Ana Maria,MD
 Kashani,Massoud,MD
 Stahl,Rosalyn E.,MD
Flemington
 Basius,Maureen,DO
Freehold
 Saleem,Sogra R.,MD
Glassboro
 Smith,Cheryl E.,MD
Hackensack
 Goldfischer,Michael J.,MD
 Harawi,Sami J.,MD

 Mannion,Ciaran M.,MD
Hoboken
 Ahmad,Imtiaz,MD
Holmdel
 Mikhail,Nagy H.,MD
Jersey City
 Shroff,Yogini J.,MD
Lakewood
 Kartika,Gunawan,MD
 Romerocaces,Gloria Marcelo,MD
 Vara,Manjula L.,MD
Livingston
 Deshpande,Jyoti M.,MD
 Redondo,Teresita Cuyegkeng,MD
Manasquan
 Lahoti,Chitra,MD
Montclair
 Kimler,Stephen C.,MD
 Tang,Daniel Di,MD
Morristown
 Katz,Robert Samuel,MD
 Mercer,Geraldine O.,MD
Neptune
 Zheng,Min,MD
New Brunswick
 Cadoff,Evan M.,MD
 Fox,Melissa D.,MD
 Fyfe-Kirschner,Billie Shawn,MD
 Gamboa,Elmer Salvador,MD
 Goodell,Lauri A.,MD
 Javidian,Parisa,MD
 May,Michael S.,MD
 Olmo Durham,Zaida E.,MD
 Schwarz,Karl O.,MD
 Shen Schwarz,Susan C.,MD
 Tenorio,Grace Cipres,MD
 Wang,Qi,MD
Newark
 Philip,Abraham T.,MD
Newton
 Vergara,Rebecca B.,MD
Northfield
 Daneshvar,Ali,MD
Passaic
 Fernandes,Gregory M.,MD
Paterson
 Akmal,Amer,MD
 Kim,Minbae,MD
Pennington
 Almashat,Salwan Jafar,MD
 Fox,Ellen H.,MD
Perth Amboy
 Stone,Frederick J.,MD
Phillipsburg
 Li,Yong Ming,MD
Plainsboro
 Andavolu,Rao Hanumanth,MD
 Krauss,Elliot A.,MD
 Van Uitert,Craig E.,MD
Pompton Plains
 Ahmed,Essam Abdelfattah,MD
 Mahmood,Shahid,MD
 Wang,Lan,MD
Ramsey
 Newman,Schuyler,MD
Red Bank
 Minassian,Haig,MD
Ridgewood
 Gritsman,Andrey,MD
Rockaway
 Querimit,Felipe A. Jr.,MD
Secaucus
 Ouahchi,Karim,MD
Summit
 Levin,Miles B.,MD
Teterboro
 Cardillo,Marina,MD
 Kanuga,Dharmishtha Jayesh,MD
 Untawale,Vasundhara G.,MD
Toms River
 Hafiz,Mohammad A.,MD
 Maghari,Amin,MD
 Mahapatro,Ramesh C.,MD
 Pham,Bich N.,MD
 Simon,Paul J.,DO
 Tao,Jimmy Ziming,MD
Trenton
 Wood,Robert H.,MD
Union
 Mendrinos,Savvas E.,MD

Vineland
 Sanden,Mats Olof,MD
 Varadarajan,Sushila,MD
Voorhees
 LoGrasso,Paul Peter,DO
Wayne
 Espinal-Mariotte,Jose D.,MD
Woodbine
 Siebert,Charles F. Jr.,MD

Pathology-Molecular Genetic
Haddonfield
 Edmonston,Tina B.,MD
Newark
 Baisre-De Leon,Ada,MD
Paterson
 Hiemenz,Matthew Charles,MD

Pediatric Allergy
Fairfield
 Torre,Arthur J.,MD
Highland Park
 Parikh,Sudhir Manharlal,MD
 Sheen,Eun H.,MD
Oradell
 Skripak,Justin Michael,MD
Shrewsbury
 Szema,Katherine Fang,MD

Pediatric Anesthesia
Berkeley Heights
 Bilenker,Michael Evan,DO
Camden
 Pukenas,Erin W.,MD
Englewood
 Friedman,Arielle J.,MD
Hackensack
 Castro-Frenzel,Karla Jose,MD
 Shah,Ruchir Nikunjbihari,MD
Livingston
 Chen,Guo Ming,MD
Morristown
 Lopes,Melissa M.,MD
Neptune
 Vaclavik,Peter Svatopluk,MD
New Brunswick
 Perez,Jessica,MD
Newark
 Shah,Chirag J.,MD
Paterson
 Ezrokhi,Marina B.,MD
 Meyer,Marc Andrew,MD
Phillipsburg
 Diaz,Elizabeth Ann,MD
Somerset
 Cean,Daniela E.,DO
Summit
 George,Tony,MD
Watchung
 Aron,Jesse H.,MD
Wyckoff
 Ju,Tashil Kim,MD

Pediatric Cardiology
Berkeley Heights
 Liao,Pui-Kan,MD
Brick
 Alpert,Mitchel B.,MD
 Castro,Elsa Imelda,MD
 Umali Pamintuan,Maria Angela,MD
 Zales,Vincent R.,MD
Edison
 Agarwal,Kishan C.,MD
Elmwood Park
 O'Connor,Brian Kevin,MD
Hackensack
 Dyme,Joshua L.,MD
 Kipel,George,MD
 Tozzi,Robert J.,MD
 Wong,Austin Henry,MD
Hoboken
 Kotb,Mohy Eldin A.,MD
Linden
 Alenick,D. Scott,MD
Livingston
 LaCorte,Jared C.,MD
Manalapan
 Bali,Chhaya,MD
Maplewood
 Bhattacharyya,Nishith,MD
Morristown
 Donnelly,Christine M.,MD

Mone,Suzanne Margaret,MD
Prasad,Aparna,MD
New Brunswick
Cohen,Michele Marie-Liz,DO
Gaffney,Joseph W.,MD
Manduley,Robert Alfred,MD
Weinberger,Sharon M.,MD
Newark
Langsner,Alan M.,MD
Michael,Mark,DO
Verma,Rajiv,MD
Paramus
Rhee,Young Sun Diane,MD
Paterson
Cocovinis,Barbara,MD
Messina,John Joseph,MD
Myridakis,Dorothy J.,MD
Princeton
Lee,Hae-Rhi,MD
Rahway
Banka,Puja,MD
Succasunna
Greenhill,Philip A.,MD
Summit
Leichter,Donald A.,MD
Voorhees
Anderson,Terry M.,MD
Bhargava,Hema P.,MD
Gidding,Samuel S.,MD
Sanchez,Guillermo R.,MD
Wall
Rivera,Loyda I.,MD
West Orange
Connor,Thomas M.,MD
Westfield
Marks,Lloyd Alan,MD

Pediatric Critical Care
Camden
Briglia,Francis A.,MD
DaSilva,Shonola Samuel,MD
Smith,Tara Marie,MD
Thomas,Samuel Charles III,MD
Edison
Manaqibwala,Ummesalama M.,MD
Shah,Sandeep K.,MD
Hackensack
Friedman,Bruce I.,MD
Melas,Antonia Ana,DO
Percy,Stephen Jr.,MD
Siegel,Mark Eric,MD
Sorrentino,Mark David,MD
Kendall Park
Zuckerman,Gary B.,MD
Livingston
Castello,Frank V.,MD
Davis,Alan L.,MD
Long Branch
Misra,Amit C.,MD
Morristown
Craft,Jeanne A.,MD
Keenaghan,Michael Andrew,MD
Thomas,Melissa Dias,MD
Neptune
Dadzie,Charles K.,MD
New Brunswick
Bojko,Thomas,MD
Dallessio,Joseph J.,MD
Das,Sumon Kumar,MD
Grossman,Bruce Jay,MD
MacCarrick,Matthew Joseph,MD
McDonough,Christian P.,MD
O'Reilly,Colin R.,DO
The,Tiong Gwan,MD
Williams-Phillips,Jacqueline,MD
Newark
McQueen,Derrick Arnold,MD
Sinquee,Dianne M.,MD
Voorhees
Bigos,David,MD
Festa,Christopher James,MD
Papastamelos,Caitlin A.,MD

Pediatric Dermatology
Somerset
Curtis,Princesa Maria,MD

Pediatric Emergency Medicine
Caldwell
Scarfi,Catherine Anne,MD
Camden
Harris,Elliott Michael,MD

Nairn,Sandra J.,DO
Edison
Cunningham,Frank J.,MD
Hackensack
Fine,Jeffrey Scott,MD
Lee,Donna J.,MD
Nemetski,Sondra Maureen,MD
Raguindin,Leah,MD
Long Branch
Jacome-Bohorquez,Gloria C.,MD
Montclair
Birmingham,Mary Catherine,MD
Haines,Elizabeth Jane,DO
Morristown
Jourdan,Cassie,MD
Melchionne Miseo,Christina,MD
Neptune
Dhebaria,Tina,DO
Radwan,Hossam S.,MD
New Brunswick
Baszak,Sylvia,MD
Do,Minh-Tu,MD
Miele,Niel F.,MD
Newark
Barricella,Robert Louis,DO
Rickerhauser-Krall,Maureen,MD
Paterson
Gutfreund,Devra A.,MD
Naim,Farid A.,MD
Severe,Monique Marie,MD
Springfield
Cleary,Kelly,MD
Teaneck
Love,Margaret M.,MD
Trenton
Maitland,Ralynne Elizabeth,MD
Voorhees
Belfer,Robert A.,MD
Dorn,Eric A.,MD
Mittal,Shraddha,MD

Pediatric Endocrinology
Camden
Post,Ernest M.,MD
Edgewater
Kaul,Sushma Dhar,MD
Lala,Vinod R.,MD
Egg Harbor Township
Chikezie,Augustine O.,MD
Hackensack
Aisenberg,Javier E.,MD
Maresca,Michelle Marie,MD
Livingston
Anhalt,Henry,DO
Sivitz,Jennifer Nicole,MD
Long Branch
Schwartz,Malcolm S.,DO
Morristown
Berry,Tymara Bernadette,MD
Cerame,Barbara I.,MD
Silverman,Lawrence Andrew,MD
Starkman,Harold S.,MD
Woo,Melissa Lee Mei,MD
Neptune
Eapen,Santhosh,MD
Smotkin-Tangorra,Margarita,DO
New Brunswick
Ergun-Longmire,Berrin,MD
Gangat,Mariam A.,MD
Salas,Max,MD
Xu,Weizhen,MD
Ocean
Kerensky,Kirk M.,MD
Paramus
Kumpta,Shilpa Narsing,MD
Pelavin,Paul Isaac,MD
Passaic
Aguayo-Figueroa,Lourdes,MD
Princeton
Hale,Paula M.,MD
Rahway
Bach,Mark A.,MD
Shrewsbury
Novello,Laura Joyce,MD
Ostrow,Vlady,DO
Summit
Huang,Eric A.,MD
Teaneck
Novogroder,Michael,MD

Verona
Shankar,Ramamurthy R.,MD
Voorhees
Rossi,Wilma Catherine,MD
West Orange
Brenner,Dennis Jay,MD
Mamkin,Irene,MD
Oppenheimer,Ellen,MD

Pediatric Gastroenterology
Camden
Farhath,Sabeena,MD
Isola,Kimberly Jean,MD
Setty,Rajendra P.,MD
Englewood
Zawahir,Shamila Balkis,MD
Hackensack
Francolla,Karen Ann,MD
Jeshion,Wendy Cheryl,MD
Makadia,Payal Ameesh,MD
Wong,Tracie Mei Han,MD
Hillsborough
Youssef,Nader Namir,MD
Livingston
Ton,Mimi Nu,MD
Long Branch
Rakitt,Tina Susanne,MD
Marlton
Padron,Celia Z.,MD
Morristown
Leiby,Alycia A.,MD
Patel,Mohini Gautam,MD
Perez,Maria Esperanza,DO
Neptune
Alfie,Marcos E.,MD
Jimenez,Jennifer E.,MD
Loveridge-Lenza,Beth Anne,DO
New Brunswick
Chen,Yen Ping,MD
Gill,Rupinder K.,MD
Weidner,Melissa,MD
Newark
Foglio,Elsie Jazmin,DO
Sunaryo,Francis P.,MD
Paterson
Larson,Jacqueline Kay,MD
Ridgewood
Orellana,Katherine Atienza,DO
Secaucus
Toor,Khadija T.,MD
Somerset
Dadhania,Jayantilal P.,MD
Leibowitz,Karen Louise,MD
Sinha,Jyoti,MD
Summit
Chitkara,Denesh Kumar,MD
Rosh,Joel R.,MD
Tyshkov,Michael,MD
Teaneck
Barth,Jay Allan,MD
Voorhees
Mascarenhas,Maria R.,MD
West New York
Goli,Sridhar Reddy,MD
West Orange
Sabel,Svetlana Lantsman,MD

Pediatric Hematology Oncology
Edison
Pappas,Lara,MD
Englewood
Cole,Peter D.,MD
Hackensack
Appel,Burton Eliot,MD
Diamond,Steven H.,MD
Gillio,Alfred Peter III,MD
Harlow,Paul J.,MD
Harris,Michael B.,MD
Krajewski,Jennifer Anne,MD
Steele,Cindy S.,MD
Terrin,Bruce N.,MD
Morristown
Fritz,Melinda D.,MD
Halpern,Steven L.,MD
Kalambakas,Stacey Anastasia,MD
Needle,Michael Neil,MD
Neier,Michelle Dana,MD
Neptune
Glazier,Kim Steinberg,MD
Singh,Rohini,MD

New Brunswick
Drachtman,Richard A.,MD
Iacobas,Ionela,MD
Lewis,Jocelyn A.,DO
Masterson,Margaret,MD
Michaels,Lisa A.,MD
Murphy,Susan M.,MD
Pan,Wilbur James,MD
Newark
Bekele,Wondwessen,MD
Kamalakar,Peri,MD
Paterson
Bonilla,Mary Ann,MD
Kahn,Alissa Rachel,MD
Kaicker,Shipra,MD
Menell,Jill Suzanne,MD
Omesi,Lenore,MD
Woolbright,William Charles,MD
Pennington
Riewe,Kathleen O'Day,MD
Raritan
Tendler,Craig L.,MD
Rochelle Park
Bhatty,Anis A.,MD
Summit
Gregory,John Joseph Jr.,MD
Miller,Michelle K.,MD
Vernon
Saluja,Gurbir S.,MD
Voorhees
Greenbaum,Barbara H.,MD
Woodbridge
Tekleyohannes,Girmay Haile,MD

Pediatric Infectious Diseases
Bloomfield
Cooper,Roger W. Jr.,MD
Edison
Kukla,Leon F.,MD
Hackensack
Boscamp,Jeffrey R.,MD
Slavin,Kevin A.,MD
Livingston
Shah,Falguni Samir,MD
Long Branch
Verma,Renuka,MD
Millburn
Hasan,Uzma Naveen,MD
Morristown
Gupta,Meera,MD
New Brunswick
Gaur,Sunanda,MD
Malhotra,Amisha,MD
Whitley-Williams,Patricia,MD
Newark
Espiritu-Fuller,Maria C.,MD
North Caldwell
Noel,Gary J.,MD
Rahway
Fraser,Iain Peter,MD
Whitehouse Station
Annunziato,Paula Winter,MD

Pediatric Nephrology
Hackensack
Hijazi,Rana,MD
Lieberman,Kenneth V.,MD
Morristown
Corey,Howard Erwin,MD
Mount Holly
Sharma,Amita K.,MD
New Brunswick
Weiss,Lynne S.,MD
Newark
Aviv,Abraham,MD
Nutley
Loghman-Adham,Mahmoud,MD
Paterson
Tawadrous,Hanan K.,MD

Pediatric Neurodevelopment
Denville
Haran,Pahirathi E.,MD
East Brunswick
Mintz,Jesse M.,MD
Flemington
Casey,Thomas James,MD
Hackensack
Segal,Eric B.,MD
Mountainside
Harris,Brenda D.,MD

Physicians by Specialty and Town

Pediatric Neurodevelopment (cont)
Trenton
 Williams, Tanishia Alise, MD
Whitehouse Station
 Geffner, Michael Howard, MD

Pediatric Ophthalmology
Belleville
 Wagner, Rudolph S., MD
Cedar Knolls
 Mori, Mayumi A., MD
Clinton
 Bernstein, Jay M., MD
Closter
 Gonzales, Antonio M., MD
East Brunswick
 Engel, John Mark, MD
 Rousta, Sepideh T., MD
Fort Lee
 Rosenberg-Henick, Arlene M., MD
Livingston
 Lambert, Amy L., MD
Voorhees
 Schnall, Bruce M., MD
Wayne
 Yang, Sherry, MD

Pediatric Orthopedics
Cedar Knolls
 Bloom, Tamir, MD
 Friedman, Samara, MD
 Lin, David Yih-Min, MD
 Rieger, Mark A., MD
Clifton
 Russonella, Michael C., DO
East Brunswick
 Therrien, Philip J., MD
Hackensack
 Cahill, James W., MD
 Merchant, Amit, DO
Livingston
 Tareco, Jennifer M., MD
Morristown
 Minkowitz, Barbara, MD
Newark
 Kaushal, Neil, MD
Ocean
 Collins, Christopher Michael, MD
Paramus
 Widmann, Roger Franklin, MD
Paterson
 Strongwater, Allan, MD
Ridgewood
 Avella, Douglas George, MD
Shrewsbury
 Plakas, Christos, MD
Summit
 Altongy, Joseph F., MD
Wayne
 Dean-Davis, Ellen, MD

Pediatric Otolaryngology
Camden
 Barrese, James L., MD
Glen Rock
 Bellapianta, Karen Marie, MD
Hackensack
 Quraishi, Huma Asmat, MD
New Brunswick
 Chee, Michael Y., MD
 Traquina, Diana Nogueira, MD
Voorhees
 Walker, Ryan D., MD

Pediatric Pathology
Long Branch
 Shertz, Wendy T., MD

Pediatric Pulmonology
Brick
 Zamel, Yaacov B., MD
Bridgewater
 Teper, Ariel Abel, MD
Cedar Knolls
 Kohn, Gary Lawrence, MD
Egg Harbor Township
 Salvia, Joseph V., DO
Hackensack
 Kaplan, Ellen B., MD
 Lee, Ada Shuk Chong, MD
Livingston
 Cohen, Barry Alan, MD

Long Branch
 Sembrano, Eduardo U. Jr., MD
 Zanni, Robert L., MD
Millburn
 Kottler, William F., MD
Morristown
 Cooper, David Michael, MD
 Montalvo-Stanton, Evelyn, MD
Neptune
 Nakhleh, Nader John, DO
New Brunswick
 Singh, Archana, MD
Newark
 Savary, Khalil William, MD
Northfield
 Leong, Mila A., MD
Paterson
 Blechner, Michael Scott, MD
 Nachajon, Roberto V., MD
 Nakra, Neal K., MD
Ridgewood
 Kanengiser, Steven Jay, MD
Rutherford
 Becz, Grace E., MD
Somerville
 Turcios, Nelson L., MD
Toms River
 Laraya-Cuasay, Lourdes R., MD
Voorhees
 Brooks, Lee J., MD
 Mayer, Oscar Henry, MD
West Orange
 Bisberg, Dorothy Stein, MD

Pediatric Radiology
Cherry Hill
 Willard, Scott David, MD
East Brunswick
 Hanhan, Stephanie B., MD
 Hogan, James R., MD
 Lee, Vincent, MD
 Rosenfeld, David L., MD
 Underberg-Davis, Sharon J., MD
Hamilton
 Winter, Rebecca Cooper, MD
Newark
 Phatak, Tej Deepak, MD
Paterson
 Frank-Gerszberg, Robin G., MD

Pediatric Rehabilitation
Mountainside
 Diamond, Martin, MD
Ridgewood
 D'Alessandro, Angela Marie, MD

Pediatric Rheumatology
Hackensack
 Haines, Kathleen Ann, MD
 Kimura, Yukiko, MD
Paterson
 Srinivasan-Mehta, Jaya, MD
West Orange
 Chalom, Elizabeth Candell, MD

Pediatric Sports Medicine
Neptune
 Petrucci, James Christopher, DO
 Rice, Stephen G., MD
New Brunswick
 Goodman, Arlene Michelle, MD
 Kenton, Alicia Nicole, MD
Rahway
 Arnold, Monica A., DO

Pediatric Surgery
Camden
 Hoelzer, Dennis James, MD
Eatontown
 Staab, Victoriya S., MD
Long Branch
 Cohen, Ian Thomas, MD
Morristown
 Zoeller, Garrett Keith, MD
New Brunswick
 Gallucci, John Gerard, MD
 Marchildon, Michael B., MD
 Pierre, Joelle, MD
 Ruzicka, Petr O., MD
Paramus
 Alexander, Frederick Jr., MD
 Friedman, David Lewis, MD
 Gandhi, Rajinder P., MD

Summit
 Bergman, Kerry S., MD
 Jacir, Nabil N., MD
Voorhees
 Grewal, Harsh, MD
Wayne
 Ganchi, Amir, MD

Pediatric Urology
Clifton
 Sanzone, John, MD
East Brunswick
 Fleisher, Michael H., MD
 Vates, Thomas S. III, MD
Eatontown
 Litvin, Yigal S., MD
Morristown
 Connor, John Patrick, MD
Mount Laurel
 Dwosh, Jack, MD
New Brunswick
 Barone, Joseph G., MD
Newark
 Cambareri, Gina M., MD
Summit
 Murphy, Kathleen A., MD
Teaneck
 Hensle, Terry W., MD
 Tennenbaum, Steven Y., MD
Voorhees
 Concodora, Charles William, MD
 Dean, Gregory Edwin, MD
 Packer, Michael G., MD
 Roth, Jonathan A., MD
 Zaontz, Mark R., MD
Wayne
 Schlecker, Burton A., MD

Pediatrics
Asbury Park
 Baxi, Nilay Manojkumar, MD
 Kharod, Sudhakar J., MD
 Peardon, Amy Elizabeth, DO
Atlantic City
 Davenport, Leamon L., DO
 Lopez Bernard, Edwin, MD
 Mallari, Rolando Q., MD
 Sless, Dana E., DO
Avenel
 Basit, Nauman A., MD
 Siddique, Muhammad Neaman, MD
Barnegat
 Czar, Elizabeth Erin, DO
 Feldman, Kira, MD
Basking Ridge
 Coyne, Christine Ann, MD
 Kerrigan, Margot I., MD
 Kohn, Jocelyn Cramer, MD
 Porter, Thomas G., MD
 Wu, Peywen, MD
Bayonne
 Aly, Sayed Raafat M., MD
 Mahmoud, Ayesha Shabbir, MD
 Malabanan, Nerissa V., MD
 Malalis, Carmelita Pingol, MD
 Nagendra, Parameswar, MD
 Patel, Parul, MD
 Serafino, Vincent Joseph, MD
 Traba, Christin M., MD
Bayville
 Santo Domingo, Norman E., MD
Bedminster
 Agathis, Allyson, MD
 Ebel, Keren Zahav, MD
 Fischer, John F., MD
 Levine, Stephanie, DO
 Shteynberg, Elena, MD
 Trend, Carolyn Cozine, MD
 Yorke, Eric R., MD
Belle Mead
 Evans, Barbara J. Marcelo, MD
 Oey, Theresia M., MD
Belleville
 Cozzini, Nancy, MD
 Khatib, Amira, MD
 Okoh, Gloria Nkiru, MD
 Okorafor, Nnennaya C., MD
 Pando, Dalia Aurora, MD
 Steinberg, Dale Louise, DO
 Wijayaratne, Madhavi, MD
Bergenfield
 Friedman, Howard Michael, MD

 Kaye, Shana Malka, MD
 Mathew, Omana R., MD
 Tolentino, John G., MD
 Weiss, Christopher A., DO
Berkeley
 Gatoulis, Maria K., MD
 Lucciola, Pompeo Almerico, MD
Berkeley Heights
 Dardanello, Marnie Cambria, MD
 Hermann, Daniel Eric, MD
 Kemeny, Alexa C., MD
 Kornfeld, Howard Neil, MD
 Lupski, Donna L., MD
 Mehta, Ami A., MD
 Mehta, Shiva C., MD
 Miguelino, Ida Alfad, MD
 Palermo, Angelo David, MD
 Summa, Geraldine M., MD
 Tavel, Stacey C., MD
 Thomas, Alan E., MD
Berlin
 Wu, Shiann J., MD
Bernardsville
 Ganek, Ellen Beth, MD
 Nikodijevic, Vesna, MD
 Peng, Patricia E., DO
 Rose, Elizabeth, MD
Blackwood
 Del Giorno, Joseph John, MD
 Delgiorno, John Michael, MD
 George, Cyriac, DO
 Iacobucci, Audrey J., MD
 Mercedes Salas, Aixell J., MD
 Owens, Brittany Rose, MD
 Robiou, Natalie Genoveva, MD
 Salvati, Harold Vincent, MD
Bloomfield
 Cheng, Guo-Pao, MD
 Colyer-Aversa, Lori A., MD
 Flynn, Sean A., MD
 Kastner, Theodore A., MD
 Kellum, Sandra, MD
 Mehta, Ruchi, MD
 Mendez Morales, Alba Nydia, MD
 Shah, Madhavi, MD
 Turizo, Maria Cecilia, MD
 Yerovi, Maria D., MD
Bordentown
 Mossoczy-Godyn, Anna M., MD
Bound Brook
 Jalil, Kiran, MD
 Wong Duran, Elizabeth, MD
Branchburg
 Housam, Ryan Ann, MD
 Ricks, Sandy, MD
Brick
 Almazan, Gerald C., MD
 Caputo, Enza P., MD
 Charles, Diane Isaacson, MD
 Chin, Stephanie Elaine, MD
 Collado, Maria R., MD
 Gallardo, Mary Rose Ramos, MD
 Katsoulis-Emnace, Maria G., MD
 Kraynock, John, MD
 Lapidus, Daniel Yitzchok, MD
 Mate, Shrikrishn K., MD
 Piela, Christina, MD
 Pineda, Maria Georgina C., MD
 Rolenc, Holly J., MD
 Sandeep, Rashmi, MD
 Sheth, Manoj Indubhai, MD
 Sundaram, Uma, MD
 Youssef, Caroline, MD
Bridgeton
 De Leonardis, John A., MD
 Fleischer, Gilbert E., MD
 Harris, Jazmine A., MD
 Kim, Joh W., MD
 Nair, Prabha J., MD
 Patel, Bhavna K., MD
 Tanner, Fritzi Alma, MD
Bridgewater
 Abraham, Daniel J., MD
 Calimlim, Grace T., MD
 Chennapragada, Ravi S., MD
 Dionne-McCracken, Laura, MD
 Ferrante, Robyn, MD
 Jain, Ami J., MD
 Jessel, Nele, MD
 Needleman, Jack, MD
 Noviello, Stephanie Seshagiri, MD

716

Physicians by Specialty and Town

Piezas,Sylvia M.,MD
Senator,Laura Julie,MD
Burlington
Arnaud-Turner,Denise Marie,MD
Berg,Jodi Liebman,MD
Bonett,Deirdre Maria,MD
Gould,Carolyn L.,MD
Harbist,Noel Rebecca,MD
Hickey,John Selano Jr.,MD
Horten,James,MD
Martinez,Esther G.,MD
Niedzwiecki,Stephen Mark,MD
Vidal-Phelan,Johanna Maria,MD
Burlington City
Aiello,Kathleen Kuykendall,MD
Graham,April Danielle,DO
Butler
Blecherman,Sarah W.,MD
Horowitz,Deborah L.,MD
Liu,Michael,MD
Thomas,Susheela,MD
Vacca,Michael John,MD
Weinstein,David M.,MD
Camden
Acosta,Ramon,MD
Aghai,Zubairul Hasan,MD
Ashong,Emmanuel F.,MD
Badolato,Kevin Arthur,MD
Burton,Monica L.,MD
Buttress,Sharon M.,MD
Churlin,Donna M.,MD
Coren,Jennifer B.,DO
Douglass-Bright,April M.,MD
Dye,Autumn J.,DO
Feingold,Anat Rachel,MD
Feldman-Winter,Lori,MD
Fish,Michelle Leigh Karam,DO
Gormley,Jillian,DO
Graessle,William R.,MD
Green,Patricia,MD
Grossman,Sandra Lynn,MD
Gupta,Monika,MD
Hussain,Mohammed Jawaad,MD
Imaizumi,Sonia O.,MD
Johnson,Karen Teresa,DO
Karmilovich,Beth Ann,DO
Kline,David M.,DO
Knoflicek,Lisa E.,MD
Krol,Anna,MD
Lania-Howarth,Maria,MD
Leong,Kai K.,MD
Mangubat,Kimberly Mae,MD
McCans,Kathryn M.,MD
McGrath,Teresa Pirri,DO
Mehta,Vijay,DO
Meislich,Debrah,MD
Melchiorre,Louis P. Jr.,MD
Mojica,Cornelio F.,MD
Mulvihill,David J.,MD
Novak,Nellie,MD
Pawel,Barbara B.,MD
Ramprasad,Vatsala,MD
Rivera,Velmina S.,MD
Robel,Lindsey,MD
Roussel,Anisha Lanice,MD
Salah,Hassan H.,MD
Sharma,Rakesh B.,MD
Sharrar,William G.,MD
Tucker,Tiffany,MD
Turner,Peter E.,MD
Vankawala,Sonya,DO
Verrecchia,Courtney,MD
Vital,Michelle Maria,MD
Wright,Erin Armstead,MD
Cape May Court House
Cavaliere,Ava A.,DO
Deliz,Yasmin D.,DO
Dierkes,Thomas F.,DO
Flick,Jeffrey L.,DO
Freund,William Roy,DO
Lai,Wai-Ling,MD
Mathur,Ajit,MD
Chatham
Corpuz,Danielle M.,MD
Shaw Brachfeld,Jennifer L.,MD
Slavin,Stuart F.,MD
Tom,Valerie,MD
Cherry Hill
Ayres,Julie Clarke,MD
Baldino,Anna Rita,DO
Chase,Melissa Sussman,DO

Ehrlich,Jerry S.,MD
Gargiulo,Katherine Anne,MD
Harris,Esther R.,MD
Ibay,Maria Lourdes D.,MD
Kaplan,Leonard F.,MD
Kothari,Nita H.,MD
Marchese,Anthony Aristide,DO
Margallo,Evangeline Cobin,MD
McHugh,Jennifer L.,MD
Mohazzebi,Cyrus,MD
Razi,Parisa,MD
Rosen,Florence E.,MD
Shieh,Luke,MD
Taubman,Bruce Melvin,MD
Tedeschi,John B.,MD
Tedeschi,John M.,MD
Viray,Ruth Mariel,MD
Weber,Jason Stuart,MD
Whitney,Julie Sherman,DO
Chester
Aygen,Kadri M.,MD
Aygen,Zehra Zeynep,MD
Cliffside Park
Lee,Inna,MD
Sethi,Chitra,MD
Clifton
Alvarez,Marie Emma B.,MD
Ayeni,Ahisu I.,MD
Basta,Janette A.,MD
Basta,Magdy Z.,MD
Brondfeld,Raquel Lara,MD
Buchalter,Maury,MD
Burton,Deniz Michelle,MD
Elhagaly,Hatem,MD
Gadalla,Hisham Hussein,MD
Grullon Okumus,Ariolis C.,MD
Gunn,Angela Lijoi,MD
Hanna,Ruba,MD
Iwelumo,Ifeoma N.,MD
Jawetz,Robert Evan,MD
Jedlinski,Tadeusz,MD
Lavaia,Maria A.,MD
Lew,Lai Ping,MD
Lewis,Michael Glenn,MD
Lugo,Mirian Dolores,MD
Matta,Rana C.,MD
Mediterraneo,Susan,MD
Modrzejewska-Kortowska,M.,MD
Mohammed,Ashraf,MD
Niziol,John A.,MD
Pagano,Christine Federline,MD
Patel,Shivani J.,MD
Rakhimova,Gulbakhor A.,MD
Sadegh,Mona,MD
Sarigul,Melih B.,MD
Schaffer,Ashley Marie,MD
Schein,Aviva B.,MD
Soto-Pereira,Angelica Maria,MD
Sutter,John I.,MD
Thomas,Mary Kathleen,MD
Tokat,Ikbal,MD
Wu,Karen,MD
Zamani,Mohammad,MD
Clinton
Castillo,Ana A.,MD
Coraggio,Michael J.,MD
Kroon,Jody Lynn,MD
Patel,Krishna A.,MD
Closter
Cavalli,Nina Ann,MD
Nouman,Helena,MD
Rosenberg,Lori A.,DO
Yegen,Lonna K.,MD
Collingswood
Georgelos,Panagiotis,MD
Velasco,Reynaldo,MD
Weber,Carolyn Harding,MD
Colonia
Benoy,Leena,MD
Casarona,Charles A.,MD
Charaipotra,Neelam,MD
Chaudhary,Jigisha S.,MD
Dubbaka-Rajaram,Arunasree,MD
Kishen,Anita,MD
Patel,Gaurang R.,MD
Sonavane,Vidya Kiran,MD
Colts Neck
Bautista,Jocelyn B.,MD
Liao,Jennifer Ledesma,MD
Makowsky,Tammy B.,MD
Peters,Nancy Castellucci,MD

Cranford
Pogany,Ursula M.,MD
Cream Ridge
Peller,Alicia S.,MD
Dayton
Genco,Thomas Albert,MD
Delran
Bastien,Pascale,MD
Foreman,Michael J.,MD
Harrell,Angela Duley,MD
Hayes,Ciana Tyiesh,MD
Denville
Chait Kessler,Dana Erica,MD
Craig,Krekamey Ropkui,MD
De Cristofano,Robert E.,MD
Di Turi,Suzanne V.,MD
Dicker,Richard Irving,MD
Ganek,Martin E.,MD
Magadan,Silvia Maria,DO
Mann,Nora B.,MD
Samedi,Vanessa M.,MD
Thomas,Miriam,MD
Umeukeje,Judith N.,MD
Deptford
Alikhan,Salma,MD
Coant,Pierre N.,MD
Laudati,Mary,MD
Minutillo,Angelo L.,MD
Dover
Collins,Ronald A.,MD
Kotler,Amy Maxine,MD
Prakash,Kalpana,MD
Restrepo,Mauricio,MD
Szuchman,Mario,MD
Taitel,Janice Beth,MD
Dumont
Smith,Terri L.,MD
East Brunswick
Booker,Larnie J.,MD
Cederbaum,Neil Kenneth,MD
D'Mello,Maria W.,MD
Fortin,Robert Glenn,MD
Gabriel,John,MD
Giorgi,Marilyn V.,MD
Goldman,Marvin,MD
Gordina,Alla,MD
Henner,Rochelle,MD
Jaroslow,Amy E.,MD
Jennings,Gloria Ann,MD
Kim,Hei Y.,MD
Kuyinu,Michael A.,MD
Li,Yan,MD
Liu-Lee,Yingxue S.,MD
Mikhail,Salwa M.,MD
Saif,Rashida Taher,MD
Shankar,Sujatha,MD
Shulman,Sabra W.,MD
Simon,Elisabeth M.,MD
Sweberg,Warren A.,MD
Tiefenbrunn,Larry J.,MD
Tuck,Michelle Patran,MD
East Hanover
Culver,Kenneth Wayne,MD
Dalati,Nadia,MD
Dapas,Frances,MD
Detrizio Carotenuto,Isabel,MD
Hernandez Comesanas,Gricel,MD
Marzella,Giuseppe,MD
Patel,Niraj Ranjit,MD
East Orange
Botrous,Suzanne W.,MD
Dosunmu,Ronke Y.,MD
Johnson,Curtis Jr.,MD
Maniar,Madhavi N.,MD
Maniar,Payal,MD
Martin Yeboah,Patrick V.,MD
Nnaeto,Nkem V.,MD
Ricciardi,Anthony Jr.,MD
Spielholz,Kathi Melanie,MD
Verner,Edwina D.,MD
Walcott,Adrian B.,MD
Zambrano,Rosario M.,MD
Eatontown
DeGroote,Richard J.,MD
Farrell,Paul R.,MD
Noaz,Golam G.,MD
Rughani-Shah,Bindoo,MD
Wymer,Edwin Anthony,DO
Edgewater
Chai,George,MD
Desai,Bhumika,MD

Leykin,Tanya,MD
Edison
Altzman,Elana F.,MD
Aziz,Khalid M.,MD
Belnekar,Rudrani K.,MD
Bhagwat,Gauri S.,MD
Bhamidipati,Aparna,MD
Bupathi,Kavita Kishor,MD
Caasi,Santiago J. Jr.,MD
Chae,Young Soo,MD
Devli,Aynur A.,MD
Gayam,Vani,MD
Godlewska-Janusz,Elzbieta,MD
Gumidyala,Padmasree,MD
Kang-Lee,Elica J.,MD
Kapila,Bina,MD
Kaur,Ranbir,DO
Kesavan,Dhanalakshmi,MD
Khanna,Santosh B.,MD
Libis,Zhanna,MD
Maddalozzo,Wanda K. M.,MD
Meszaros,Beata Duli,MD
Nadkarni,Nutan Shirish,MD
Navas,Carlene,MD
Nguyen,Hung Manh,MD
Nimma,Vijaya,MD
Patel,Natverlal M.,MD
Patel,Suresh Ishwarlal,MD
Pierre,Margarette Rose,MD
Pompy,Amrita,MD
Pu,Jessica Lixia,MD
Raghu,Shalini Nagarajan,MD
Satwani,Sunita,MD
Shah,Lata R.,MD
Shukla,Nimisha J.,MD
Wang,Aijuan,MD
Zheng,Shao,MD
Egg Harbor Township
Anisman,Paul C.,MD
Ditmar,Mark F.,MD
Garrett,Parisa Mousavi,MD
Kaiser,Bruce A.,MD
Kessler,Barry M.,MD
Kuponiyi,Cheryl A.,MD
Palermo,Andrea,DO
Roan,Minda Unidad S.,MD
Elizabeth
Abich,Georgina,MD
Ayyanathan,Karpukaras,MD
Davis,Kenneth J.,MD
De La Cruz,Antonio A.,MD
Fernandez-Moure,Joseph L.,MD
Galimidi Hodara,Salomon,MD
Gonzalez-Mejia,Johanna J.,MD
Grundy,Kia Calhoun,MD
Jethwa,Kusum A.,MD
Kim,Soon K.,MD
Orleans,Genevieve Araba,MD
Powell,Kerri Lynette,MD
Questelles,Rachael,MD
Saraiya,Narendra N.,MD
Sundaram,Raghunand,MD
Tolentino-Dela Cruz,Milagros,MD
Elmwood Park
Kiblawi,Fuad Moh'D,MD
Ramadi,Roula Alchaa,MD
Englewood
Baydar,Garbis,MD
Daici,Silvia,MD
Davidson,Melissa,MD
Fried,Ruthellen,MD
Hershcopf,Richard Jay,MD
Hyatt,Alexander Charles,MD
Kampf,Robyn A.,MD
Onwuka,William N.,MD
Psalidas,Panagiotis George,MD
Siegel-Stein,Francine M.,MD
Tung,Cindy Wei-Yi,MD
Zuckerbrot,Rachel Aryella,MD
Englewood Cliffs
Lee,Sun Hee,MD
Rhee,Jung L.,MD
Englishtown
Salcedo,Theresa Josue,MD
Essex Fells
Pakonis,Fiona K.,MD
Fair Lawn
Alexander,Leah M.,MD
Anido,Rosary Kristine Isidro,MD
Bass,Irina,MD
Bienstock,Jeffrey Marc,MD
Boyarsky,Yael,MD

Pediatrics (cont)

Fair Lawn
Brucia,Lauren A.,MD
Chism,Melissa A.,MD
Fischer,Emily Frances,MD
Greaney,Kathleen Margaret,MD
Hetling,Kristina,MD
Kaul,Reena Sonya,MD
Laufer,Ilene Caren,MD
Lewis,Brian S.,MD
Lin,Tatiana Alexeevna,MD
Long,Jessie C.,MD
Paige,Melanie Kay,MD
Pitera,Barbara,MD
Rao,Gunjan Pradhan,MD
Riegelhaupt,Rona Susan,MD
Schlitt,Meghan Ann,MD
Shafi,Heather Claire,MD
Sherman,Jennifer Ann,DO
Sonnenblick,Howard C.,MD
Steinbaum,Deborah Paige,MD
Steinel,Lisa A.,MD
Yellin,Tova G.,MD
Zucker,Scott W.,MD

Fanwood
Gillard,Bonita Dee,MD
Koward,Donna Marie,MD

Flemington
Agarwal,Ravi,MD
Bery,Sumita,MD
Clarin,Mitchell I.,MD
Douvris,John S.,MD
Fellmeth,Wayne G.,MD
Hartigan,Thomas P.,MD
Humoee,Nidal Michel,MD
Jasutkar,Ashwini,MD
Krupinski,Donna J.,MD
Michael,Rositta,MD
Pina,Liza Miriam,MD
Prosswimmer,Geralyn M.,MD
Roksvaag,George E.,MD
Shah,Debra Stahl,MD
Willems-Plakyda,Michele C.,MD

Florham Park
Bailon,Amy R.,MD
Baxley,Maureen Elizabeth,MD
Behbakht,Mojgan,MD
Petrozzino,Vito A.,MD
Silva,Francisco,MD

Forked River
Mabagos,Jerry D.,MD
Pradhan,Prasanna Govind,MD
Yassin,Mahmoud M.,MD

Fort Lee
Akturk,Elvin,DO
Aranoff,Joanne Rachel,MD
Banschick,Harry,MD
Choi,Yoonhee,MD
Chung,Nam Young,MD
Colenda,Maryann J.,MD
Elkassir,Amina,MD
Kim,Eun-Joo Song,MD
Kim,Eunja,MD
Kumar,Geeta L.,DO
Kuo,Grace,MD
Lazieh,Janet Tomeh,MD
Yenukashvili,Nana R.,MD

Franklin Lakes
Rosenberg,Zeil Barry,MD

Franklin Park
Iyanoye,Abimbola Olamide,MD

Freehold
Bhaskar,Vatsala R.,MD
Cato-Varlack,Janice A.,MD
Chieco,Michael Anthony,MD
Daghistani,Lina,MD
Donde,Mrunalini D.,MD
Emanuel,Anthony,MD
Gajula,Ramarao Sundara,MD
Ibale,Florence E.,MD
Jonnalagadda,Balathripura S.,MD
Katturupalli,Madhavi,MD
LaMantia,Anthony P.,MD
Lacap,Estela Villar,MD
Lopez,Leonardo Nicholas,DO
Mayer,Diana R.,MD
McFeely,Erin M.,MD
Mehta,Sanjay,DO
Patel,Arvind Maganbhai,MD
Sadik,Zubaida Y.,MD
Shah,Neha Naresh,MD
Shah,Vrinda B.,MD
Swayne,Kathleen Amy,MD
Teresh,Michelle A.,MD
Velez,Corazon S.,MD
Wolfe,Jeffrey S.,MD
Zeb,Marta R.,MD

Galloway
Amir,Sabah H.,MD
Elgenaidi,Mona E.,MD
Houck,Meghan Mcfee,DO
Kosmetatos,Elizabeth,MD

Garfield
Uczkowska,Alicja Teresa,MD

Gibbsboro
Amato,Christopher,DO
Deery,Kimberly Jeanne,DO
Lee,Diana,DO
Lerch,Gordon Lee Jr.,DO
Napoli,Anthony F. Jr.,MD
Valencia,Rafael L.,MD

Glen Ridge
Khanna,Anisha,DO
Khanna,Kamlesh,MD

Glen Rock
Halifman,Dorina,MD
Karpova,Natalia M.,MD

Guttenberg
La Rosa,Niurka,MD

Hackensack
Agrawal,Nina,MD
Auyeung,Valerie Y.,MD
Avva,Usha R.,MD
Azizi,Azin,MD
Borgen,Ruth E.,MD
Bye,Karen N.,MD
Chhabra,Rakesh S.,MD
D'Mello,Sharon L.,MD
Diah,Paulett,MD
Duncan,Eva,MD
Dyme,Rachel Sarah,MD
Eigen,Karen Lori,MD
Ettinger,Leigh Mark,MD
Flores,Alejandro Alberto,MD
Fofah,Onajovwe O.,MD
Fruchter,Joseph S.,MD
Furman,Jasmin W.,MD
Gertz,Shira J.,MD
Gesser,Gail A.,DO
Gold,Nina A.,MD
Goodman,Karen Natalie,MD
Gupta,Raksha R.,MD
Hyppolite,Alex,MD
Khan,Saqiba,MD
Kimel,Ana Josephine,MD
Kopacz,Magdaline S.,MD
Kriegel,Marni Ruth,MD
Kutko,Martha C.,MD
Lamour,Rytza M.,MD
Lapidus,Sivia K.,MD
Levine,Deena R.,MD
Leyva-Vega,Melissa,MD
Li,Suzanne C.,MD
Lopez,Divina Elizabeth,MD
Macalintal,Rose Ann Reyes,MD
Materetsky,Steven H.,MD
Meli,Lisa A.,MD
Mikadze,Malkhazi,MD
Miranda,Rosa Josefina,MD
Moustafellos,Elaine,MD
Muratschew,Donna M.,MD
Ngai,Pakkay,MD
O'Donnell,Lisa-Mary,MD
Obaze,Ofunne Omo,MD
Paolicchi,Juliann Marie,MD
Pedro,Helio Fernando,MD
Perez,Adriana M.,MD
Petrella,Michael Onofrio,MD
Piwoz,Julia A.,MD
Rama,Gabriel,MD
Rappaport,Delia I.,MD
Reed,Jean Arlyn Banez,MD
Rivera,Roger Antonio,MD
Samuels,Francine,MD
Shah,Mayuri N.,MD
Shammout,Jumana Sa'ad,MD
Sousa,Rolando Cristobal,MD
Subramanian,Subhashini,MD
Tantawi,Mohamed Asem,MD
Tantawi,Mona M.,MD
Thomas,Antonio,MD
Thomas,Dianne,MD
Vijayan,Radhika,MD
Weiss,Jennifer Ellen,MD
Weissman,Barry J.,MD
Wong,Jonathan Wane,MD
Yucel,Cengiz,MD
Zenack,Alissa Hayley,DO

Hackettstown
Caruso,Patrick A.,MD
Chi,Ching,MD
Chugh,Jagdish C.,MD
Dick,Adam M.,MD
Kedzierska,Ksymena,MD
Libert,Melissa Marie,DO
Walsh,Kristen Anne,MD

Haddon Heights
Blair,Michael A.,MD
Matz,Paul Steven,MD
Risimini,Robert J.,MD
Schlitt,Mark George,MD
Schlitt,Michael T.,MD
Schlitt,Stephanie N.,MD
Shaigany,Nina N.,MD

Haddonfield
Bruner,Laurie Reid,MD
Caltabiano,Claire L.,MD
Eggerding,Caroline,MD
Friedman,Barton J.,MD
King,Kevin J.,MD
Lopes,Joanne Elizabeth,MD
Milligan Milburn,Erin C.,MD
Smergel,Henry,MD
Weidner,James R.,MD
Welsh,Theresa M.,MD

Haledon
Afonja,Olubunmi Olutoyin,MD

Hamburg
Markel,David Francis,MD

Hamilton
Baiser,Dennis Miles,MD
Bogacki,Gwen M.,MD
Boim,Marilynn Dora,MD
Buchbinder,Marta Luisa H.,MD
Dorneo,Aurora B.,MD
Flores,Belen P.,MD
Flores,Charles Edward,MD
Jacques,Walter J.,MD
Kapadia,Milan R.,MD
Perno,Joseph R.,MD
Prineas,Sara L.,MD
Reyes,Reina Duremdes,MD
Sheth,Amarish Rasiklal,MD
Sudjono-Santoso,Dewi S.,MD
Zelinsky,Catherine Marie,MD

Hammonton
Amer,Adel M.,MD
Klein,Bruce M.,MD
Prasad,Devineni R.,MD

Harrison
Vidal,Jennifer Lyn,DO

Haworth
De Antonio,Michele L.,MD
Gupta,Archana,MD
Stathopoulos,Labrini,MD

Hawthorne
Vasena Marengo,Maria Jose,MD

Hazlet
Blackman,Ryan Graham,DO
Cambria,Lina,MD
Jain,Asha,MD
Khuddus,Munawara S.,MD
Pascucci,Rocco F.,MD
Protasis,Liza,MD
Ruda,Neal,MD

Highland Park
Biener,Robert,MD
Gavai,Medha A.,MD
Glaser-Schanzer,Felice,MD
Gul,Sheba,MD
John,Sheryl Mary,MD
Majisu,Claire Amume,MD
Reingold,Stephen Marcus,MD
Rubin,Elliot H.,MD
Zablocki,Lisa R.,MD

Hightstown
Arcaro,Maria Anna C.,MD
Bidabadi,Bobak,MD
Goodman,Aimee R.,DO
Gribin,Bradley Jay,MD
Howe,Matthew R.,MD
Marcus,Brian F.,DO
Patel,Radhika K.,MD
Shah,Utpal S.,MD
Siddiqui,Sabeen A.,MD
Vo,Ha,MD

Hillsborough
Concepcion,Kristin A.,MD
Hede,Madan M.,MD
Hussain,Aazim Syed,MD
Jiang,Li,MD
Lariviere,Aimee T.,MD
Yadav,Priyanka Singh,DO
Youngerman,Neil L.,MD

Ho Ho Kus
Birnhak,Stefani,MD
Kim,Urian,MD
Lee,Julia Jin-Young,MD
Leifer,Amy Sarah Budin,MD

Hoboken
Akpalu,Daniel,MD
Klos,Andrzej E.,MD
Kucharski,Jarrod Michael,MD
Mani,Shrinidi,MD
Mehta,Harshna B.,MD
Pierog,Sophie H.,MD
Salmun,Luis Marcelo,MD
Shenk,Kristina Suzanne,MD
Sikand,Vikram Singh,MD
Zarrabi,Yasaman,DO

Holmdel
Ayoub,Samia B.,MD
Baumlin,Thomas Jr.,MD
Bruner,Vanda,MD
Carey,Brittany Marie,DO
David,Lea H.,MD
DeNicola,Nancy Ann,DO
Elbasty,Azza A.,MD
Engel,Barbara M.,MD
Engel,Jennifer Duck,MD
Miguelino,Bernadette M.,MD
Mohan,Kusum C.,MD
Sta. Maria,Emilia Navarro,MD
Yia,Grace Mercado,MD

Howell
Dayal,Rashmi P.,MD
DePerio,Alicia G.,MD
Lopez,Claudio J.,MD
Maddatu,Elenito P.,MD
Maddatu,Rose Mylaine,MD
Manlapid,Luis T.,MD
Mariano-Lau,Elizabeth L.,MD
Mision,Vicente L.,MD
Nagpal,Sangita D.,MD
Verdi,Michelle Diane,DO

Irvington
Anyanwu,Justina U.,MD
Emelle,Emmanuel M.,MD
Francois,Emmanuel J.,MD
Gonzaga,Zenaida Palma,MD
Isedeh,Cynthia O.,DO
Lauredan,Bernier,MD
Leger,Pierre R.,MD
Miller,Sandrene,MD
Sundaram,Palanisamy S.,MD

Iselin
Kernizan,Daphney,MD
Nambiar,Sapna Shibhu,MD

Jackson
Pawa,Anil K.,MD
Qudsi,Tehsin Riaz,MD
Zapanta,Rex A.,MD

Jersey City
Ansay,Editha Santillan,MD
Baker,Omar A.,MD
Barrera-Tolentino,Felicisima,MD
Boulos,Mona,MD
Calero-Bai,Rosario,MD
Casia,Jeffrey P.,MD
Choudry,Omer F.,MD
Coleman,Reginald O.,MD
De La Rosa,Rita G.,MD
Desai,Vijaya S.,MD
Dimaculangan,Nelo De Gala,MD
Eltemsah,Nagi I.,MD
Endaya-Aguila,Thelma,MD
Fernandez,Fredy A.,MD
Franco,Maria M.,MD
Ghaly,Maged Antoine,MD
Jain,Doney B.,MD
Jenkins,Lisa Michelle,MD
Kaki,Sushma R.,MD
LeBron,Carmen Haydee,MD
Lipert,Zofia J.,MD

Majithia,Meenakshee N.,MD
Malik,Tayyaba K.,MD
Mangosing,Emma A.,MD
Moss,Beverly D.,MD
Nagorna,Malgorzata,MD
Newman,Brigitte Jeanne,MD
Palomares,Danilo V.,MD
Politis,Regina,MD
Quim,Marinelle De Los Santos,MD
Raha,Bandana,MD
Ramasubramaniam,Nagarani,MD
Santos,Ray Ryan Crisostomo,MD
Santos-Borja,Concepcion L.,MD
Surti,Daxa Bhupendra,MD
Tan,Vicente G.,MD
Ucheagwu,Hyacinth Emenike,MD
Umali,Winston Caraos,MD
Varma,Mekhla,MD
Ventura,Evelyn Ortiz,MD
Yin,Chun Hui,MD
Yu,William C.,MD
Kearny
Lopez-Maslak,Edna Retiracion,MD
Novaes,Denise,MD
Padykula,Anna,MD
Skripkus,Aldona J.,MD
Zhang,Li,MD
Kinnelon
Suda,Anjuli,MD
Vijaysadan,Viju,MD
Lakewood
Berghaus,Jean E.,MD
Eilenberg,Eli,MD
Fenster,William R.,MD
Gittleman,Neal D.,MD
Greenberg,Bram,MD
Gwertzman,Rachel,DO
Hirsch,Harvey Alan,MD
Indich,Norman,MD
Jain,Suman Singhal,MD
Kaweblum,Jaime,DO
Lekht,Inna,MD
Lorenzo,Judith,MD
Rana,Mukti,MD
Romero,Luz Ydania,MD
Root,Edward R.,MD
Saunders,Kyauna Sharae,MD
Sopeju,Temilola Adedayo,MD
Stavrellis,Steve John,MD
Ukraincik,Miro,MD
Wong,Karen Clark,MD
Lanoka Harbor
Mehta,Sunita,MD
Lawrenceville
Farooq,Sadaf,MD
Gittell,Amy,DO
Halvorsen,Julie Beth,DO
Jose,Jaison,DO
Lilienfeld,Harris C.,MD
O'Dea,Carol Lynn H.,MD
Obleada,Maria C.P.,MD
Palsky,Glenn S.,MD
Saraiya,Neha,MD
Shapiro,Eugene,MD
Ledgewood
Grossman,Leonard J.,MD
Lincoln Park
Cross,Gershwin A.,MD
Linden
Grzybowski,Jacek,MD
Jez,Mieczyslaw Z.,MD
Linwood
Bonaker,Laura J.,MD
Little Egg Harbor
Humphreys,Erika,MD
Lee,Gene Chiu,MD
Little Falls
Pepe,Gary V.,MD
Razzak,Mannan,MD
Razzak,Nadia Mohsin,MD
Little Silver
Mehra,Deepti,MD
Livingston
Avallone,Jennifer Mary,DO
Baldomero,Anita C.,MD
Cai-Luo,Bonney Danhua,MD
Chua Eoan,Pearl Davie,MD
Dienna,Erik,MD
Glick,Sarah Rachel,MD
Goyal,Vinod K.,MD
Kumta,Jayshree N.,MD

Lander,Richard,MD
Liptsyn,Tatyana,MD
Magnus Miller,Leslie,MD
Margolin,Susan K.,MD
Maxym,Maya,MD
O'Driscoll,Margaret Ann,MD
Pang,James,MD
Patel,Roshni Vinu,MD
Ramanadham,Aruna R.,MD
Roberti,Maria Isabel,MD
Salyer,Robert Harold,DO
Sanchez Konel,Maria E.,MD
Schwartz,Fredric Ira,MD
Setya,Shilpy,MD
Sjovall,William J. Jr.,DO
Vazirani,Minal,MD
Wiener,Jaclyn Faye,DO
Yeh,Timothy Stephen,MD
Zaldivar,Marjel L.,DO
Logan Township
Cafone,Michael D.,DO
Long Branch
Attardi,Diane Martha,MD
Brunetto,Jacqueline M.,MD
Bshesh,Khaled Khalifa,MD
Fisher,Margaret Catharine,MD
Habib,Thomas G.,MD
Hall,Dahlia Annmarie,MD
Hudome,Susan M.,MD
Kale,Meera V.,MD
Kapoor,Amee Patel,DO
Khalil,Erum,MD
Maghsood,Shabnam,MD
Phillips,Keren Amy,MD
Reutter,Richard A.,MD
Romald,Jermine Harriet,MD
Scerbo,Jessica,MD
Sell,Neelam K.,MD
Sleavin,Harold J.,MD
Teitelbaum,Jonathan Evan,MD
Long Valley
Sorvino,Noel R.,MD
Lumberton
Bell,Denise Marie,MD
Kaighn,Karen Chicalo,MD
King,Richard A.,MD
Labroli,Melissa D.,MD
O'Donnell,Thomas P.,MD
Requa,Lindsay Ann,DO
Wechsler,Marius A.,MD
Lyndhurst
Catalano,Mariano,MD
Ginsberg,Janet A.,MD
Wahba,Janette M.,MD
Mahwah
Liberti,Lorraine M.,MD
Perez,Sania Rebecca,MD
Manahawkin
Bleiman,Michael I.,MD
Cannon,Aileen Carol,MD
Guariglia,Anthony R.,MD
Olorunnisola,Moses F. Jr.,MD
Sunkavalli,Paul Venugopal,MD
Manalapan
Bonilla,Melissa Diaz,MD
Dhawan,Denise Marie,MD
Genova-Goldstein,Jeanne,MD
Isayeva,Eleonora,DO
Leib,Samantha,MD
Levy,Moshe,MD
Malaty,Christine B.,DO
Nandiwada,Lakshmi P.,MD
Peska-Mosseri,Jodi L.,DO
Shah,Sonal Ashwin,DO
Sharon,Jill Israel,DO
Tanner-Sackey,Fritzi A.,MD
Trogan,Igor,MD
Manasquan
Go,Jane O.,MD
Oram,Alexis Marissa,MD
Wolpert,Joshua D.,MD
Manville
Amarnani,Sukhdev,MD
Maplewood
Aragones,Linnie A.,MD
San Juan,Severiano Jr.,MD
Margate
Durelli,Gloria S.,MD
Marlboro
Galperina,Klara,DO
Husain,Syeda Amna,MD

Salcedo,Glenn A.,MD
Yee,Mary,MD
Marlton
Bailey,Aisha Donine,DO
Barnett,Sharon Elizabeth,MD
Berman,Eric David,DO
Blackman,Jeffrey D.,MD
Chasen,David E.,MD
Chun,Doreen Sze-Man,DO
Denick,Kimberly Keane,MD
Falk,Michael Alexander,MD
Fanelli,Allison Sagan,DO
Friedler-Eisenberg,Susan F.,DO
Hammer,Stacey R.,MD
Holmes-Bricker,Mary E.,DO
Kakkilaya,Harshila,MD
Kaus,Sharon M.,DO
Killeen,Thomas Joseph III,MD
Lafferty,Kathryn Tatsis,MD
Lampone,Christina,MD
Leszkowicz,Aditee D.,DO
Melini,Carlo B.,MD
Mirmanesh,John C.,MD
Mirmanesh,Shahram J.,MD
Monaco,Carmine D.,DO
Nicolaides,Catherine D.,MD
O'Mahony,Lisa,MD
Orel,Howard N.,MD
Panda,Nirmala,MD
Pandit,Florence A.,MD
Pittalwala,Rashida G.,MD
Ragothaman,Ramesh,MD
Rickey,Stephanie B.,MD
Rosenblum,Benjamin A.,MD
Rosof,Edward,MD
Smith-Elfant,Stacy A.,MD
Szawlewicz,Stephen A.,MD
Vare,Katie Marie,MD
Waxman,Howard S.,MD
Zechowy,Racine B.,MD
Martinsville
Calello,Diane P.,MD
Matawan
Badami,Geeta D.,MD
Borromeo,Virginia,MD
Mays Landing
Goldman,Stuart J.,MD
Huang,Patty P.,MD
Tung,John Yu,MD
Medford
Buccigrossi,Jennifer Leigh,MD
Coss,Wanda I.,MD
Foran,Daniel J.,DO
Murphy,Terri Lee,DO
Reed,Rebecca Ann,DO
Roscioli-Jones,Catherine A.,MD
Scott,Charles A.,MD
Weitz,Robert D.,DO
Mendham
Dragalin,Daniel J.,MD
Minhas,Deepa S.,MD
Metuchen
Freis,Peter C.,MD
Lebovic,Daniel M.,MD
Raviola,Joseph,MD
Rosenblum,Howard W.,MD
Santiago,Maritza Marie,MD
Tuma,Victor B.,MD
Middlesex
Mehta,Sadhana,MD
Middletown
Beizem,Joanna,MD
Harmady,Debra,MD
Potylitsina,Yelena,MD
Midland Park
Ungerleider,Deborah L.,MD
Millburn
Alexander,Andrea Hope,MD
Batra,Chhaya,MD
Comandatore,Ann Marie,MD
Cotler,Donald N.,MD
Gruenwald,Laurence D.,MD
Knowles,Kelly Petrison,MD
Liggio,Frank J.,MD
Mangru,Subita S.,MD
Meshko,Yanina,MD
Miller,Yael Spinat,MD
Ramesh,Shruti Chakrabarti,DO
Spiteri,Sharon,MD
Sterio,Mara,MD
Stettner,Lisa G.,DO

Thompson,Stacy Ellen,DO
Vorembly,Sandra R.,MD
Millville
Jamil,Erum,MD
Patel,Ketan R.,MD
Shim,Zae U.,MD
Torres,Stephanie M.,DO
Mine Hill
Hershman,Ilene M.,MD
Monmouth Beach
Gulli,Maria T.,MD
Monmouth Junction
Aggarwal,Roopali,MD
Nageen,Farhat,MD
Monroe Township
Doshi,Deepa,MD
Gulati,Sunita,MD
Hemrajani,Payal,MD
shah,Amisha M.,MD
Montclair
Besser,Richard Eric,MD
Hung,Yvonne,MD
Nasiek,Sara,MD
Paisner,Raphael,MD
Weinstein,Mark E.,MD
Montville
Gandhi,Alpana D.,MD
Moorestown
Giardino,John Domenic Jr.,MD
Gordon,Anne M.,MD
Guevarra,Andres T.,MD
Guevarra,Jesusita H.,MD
Weinroth,Heidi J.,MD
Morganville
Bakshiyev,Yuliya,MD
Husain,Sajidah I.,MD
Lee,Kim Chiu,MD
Liwag,Alexander J.,MD
Yuen,Sharon Shue,MD
Morris Plains
Lopez-Allen,Gabriela D.,MD
Morristown
Almeida,Vinita Maria,MD
Amato,Christopher Scott,MD
Antony,Kristine Brinda,DO
Atlas,Arthur B.,MD
Baorto,Elizabeth P.,MD
Bieler,Harvey Phillip,MD
Block,Deborah C.,MD
Buck,Melissa,MD
Cheruvu,Sunita,MD
Chin,Daisy Y.,MD
Clark-Hamilton,Jill,MD
Cohen,Martin L.,MD
Crowley,Kathryn Ann,MD
Cucolo,Patricia Anne,MD
Eckert,Jessica,DO
Eckstein,Devin Brazill,DO
Gamallo,Ma. Bernardita R.,MD
Gill,Ramneet Kaur,MD
Gutierrez,Juan Alberto,MD
Hoelzel,Donald W.,MD
Horowitz,Meggan Elise,MD
Kairam,Neeraja,MD
Kerr,Kathy Rosen,MD
Koslowe,Oren Lewis,MD
Lanzkowsk,Shelley,MD
Lasker,Susan J.,MD
Leier,Tim Ulrich,MD
Lodish,Stephanie Renee,MD
Lofrumento,Mary Ann,MD
Lupatkin,William L.,MD
McCluskey,Tamara B.,DO
McSherry,Kevin Joseph,MD
Meltzer,Alan J.,MD
Mukherjee,Angela,DO
Nashi,Suhaib G.,MD
Nativ,Simona Horak,MD
Nicoletta,Marianna,MD
Orafidiya,Yetunde,MD
Poblete,Gwyn Laurice,MD
Presti,Amy Lynn,MD
Rehm,Christine M.,MD
Ryan,Christina Marie,MD
Saadeh,Sermin,MD
Scherer,Susan Denys,MD
Schwartzberg,Paul Marc,DO
Sequeira,Sophia Almeida,MD
Shah,Ashish R.,MD
Shah,Niva,DO
Shluper,Victoria,MD

Physicians by Specialty and Town

Pediatrics (cont)

Morristown
- Verga, Barbara Jean, MD
- Wazeka, April Natasha, MD
- Wiener, Ethan Saul, MD
- Willis, Karen Christine, MD
- Wolf, Mary Campion, MD

Mount Holly
- Doshi, Samir Kirankumar, MD

Mount Laurel
- Ahr, Lawrence M., MD
- Bernstein, Barbara A., MD
- Bruneau, Lara A., MD
- Coutinho Haas, Sunita P., MD
- Creecy, Saundra K., MD
- Nemeth, Nicole Angelina, MD
- Weissbach, Debra D., MD

Mountain Lakes
- Fuloria, Mamta, MD

Mountainside
- Aronsky, Adam M., MD
- Cargan, Abba L., MD
- Gozo, Ave O., MD
- Matthews, Tara Anne, MD
- Mehta, Uday C., MD
- Velickovic, Marina, MD
- Yalamanchi, Krishan, MD

Neptune
- Adler, Bernard H., MD
- Alfonzo, Joann, MD
- Almazan-Atienza, Helen, MD
- Atienza, Kristen A., DO
- Bakhos, Lisa Lovas, MD
- Bal, Aswine Kumar, MD
- Ballance, Cathleen M., MD
- Beckwith-Fickas, Katherine A., MD
- Cabasso, Alan, MD
- Chutke, Prashant Vithal, MD
- Eyerkuss, Emily Abra, DO
- Gapinski, Magdalena Maria, MD
- Heisler, Samantha, DO
- Karatas, Meltem, MD
- Mabanta, Carmelita G., MD
- Naganathan, Srividya, MD
- Nowinowska, Anna, MD
- Pitchumoni, Vinita, MD
- Ponce, Marie Grace C., MD
- Schairer, Janet Lynn, MD
- Shah, Nina M., MD
- Soroush, Azam, MD
- St. Fleur, Rose Martine, MD

New Brunswick
- Abreu, Arnaldo J., MD
- Alemu, Kidist, MD
- Amara, Shobha, MD
- Amato, Indira L., MD
- Babcock, Karen R., MD
- Baddi, Anoosha, DO
- Bahadur, Kandy, MD
- Balachandar, Sadana, MD
- Bernstein, William R., MD
- Boneparth, Alexis D., MD
- Borole, Swapna M., MD
- Bruno, Chantal Dominique, DO
- Bryan, Sheila Curry, MD
- Byrom, Abbie R., MD
- Cangemi, Carla Primiani, MD
- Carlson, Joann Marie, MD
- Chalikonda, Bhavani Prasad, MD
- Chalom, Rene, MD
- Chefitz, Dalya L., MD
- Chundru, Vasudha, MD
- Cohen, Stephanie Gail, MD
- Craig, Vicki L., MD
- Diaz, Laura M., MD
- Fantasia, Michele Elaine, MD
- Fleming, Jacqueline, MD
- Grieco, Rachael D., MD
- Gurkan, Sevgi, MD
- Hauck, Lisanne Constance, MD
- Hodgson, Elizabeth Susan, MD
- Horton, Daniel B., MD
- Infantino, Dorian, MD
- Ingram, Karen M., MD
- Iofel, Elizaveta, MD
- Jonna, Siva Prasad, MD
- Jyounouchi, Harumi, MD
- Kairys, Steven W., MD
- Kaliyadan, George, MD
- Kashyap, Arun Kumar, MD
- Kaur, Harpreet, MD
- Kaur, Harsohena, MD
- Kelly, Michael John, MD
- Kendall, Roxanne E., MD
- Khosla, Meenakshi, MD
- Koniaris, Soula G., MD
- Korn, Elizabeth Amy, MD
- Lam, Jennifer, MD
- Lentzner, Benjamin Joseph, MD
- Leupold, Kerry Lynn, DO
- Leva, Ernest G., MD
- Lopez, Christina Clare, DO
- Lucas, Michael Joseph, MD
- Mahalingam, Rajeshwari S., MD
- Malkani, Raj S., MD
- Marina, Adele Nabieh, MD
- Marshall, Ian, MD
- McCaig, Misty, MD
- McInnes, Andrew Duncan, MD
- Medina, Gladibel, MD
- Mody, Kalgi, MD
- Moorthy, Lakshmi Nandini, MD
- Ohngemach, Christopher, MD
- Ojadi, Vallier Chidiebere, MD
- Owensby, Jennifer Rita, MD
- Parlow, Brittany, MD
- Patel, Bipinchand N., MD
- Pelliccia, Frances B., MD
- Pepper, Matthew Philip, MD
- Poelstra, Beverly A., MD
- Pratt, Amanda, MD
- Quintero-Solivan, Juliette M., MD
- Ramachandran, Usha, MD
- Ramagopal, Maya, MD
- Reich, Joseph I., MD
- Relvas, Monica De Stefani, MD
- Rhoads, Frances A., MD
- Rojas, Paulina Elena, MD
- Rosenthal, Susan R., MD
- Rossman, Ian T., MD
- Sanghani, Nipa Vijay, MD
- Santiago, Marivic F., MD
- Seshadri, Kapila, MD
- Sharma, Archana, DO
- Sharma, Priti, MD
- Strozuk-McDonough, Stephanie, MD
- Suell, Jeffrey, MD
- Takyi, Michele, MD
- Tetteh, Shirley S., MD
- Thompson, Dawn Dorel, MD
- Uppaluri, Lakshmi P., MD
- Weiss, Aaron R., DO
- Weller, Alan Scott, MD
- Wenger, Peter N., MD
- Whyte, Peta-Gaye Kenisha, DO
- Yerramilli, Ramalakshmi V., MD
- Zaghloul, Nibal Ahmad, MD
- Zalewitz, Jodi Michelle, MD
- Zimmerman-Bier, Barbie L., MD
- Zuber, Janie Anne, MD

New Milford
- Goyco, Emelina A., MD

New Providence
- Chin, Kathleen L., MD
- Cuddihy, Kathleen Marie, MD
- Shih, Eunhee, MD
- Visci, Denise, MD

Newark
- Abels, Jane I., MD
- Adija, Akinyi, MD
- Aguila, Helen A., MD
- Aguilar, Hector David Jr., MD
- Aliparo, Madolene A., MD
- Alvarez, Maria T., MD
- Arpayoglou, Beatriz C., MD
- Bachman, Michael Craig, MD
- Balaguru, Duraisamy, MD
- Baranowski, Katherine, MD
- Baskerville, Renee E., DO
- Bell-Gresham, Garrett, MD
- Benezra-Obeiter, Rita Beth, MD
- Boyle, Maria Pilar T., MD
- Bustillo, Jose R., DO
- Carruth, Samuel G. Jr., MD
- Chen, Sophia Wunchi, DO
- Cooray, Roshan, MD
- Correa, Luis A., MD
- Cueto, Victor Jr., MD
- Dashefsky, Barry, MD
- Delisfort, Guy J., MD
- Dhar, Seema, MD
- Dieudonne, Arry, MD
- Esquerre, Rene B., MD
- Evans, Hugh E., MD
- Ferraz, Ricardo J. P., MD
- Fisher, Joie, MD
- Fojas, Felicia Regina, MD
- Friedman, Debbie, MD
- Gajarawala, Raksha J., MD
- Garay, Luis Alberto, MD
- Gilo, Belen Frias, MD
- Gonzalez, Isabel V., MD
- Guinto, Danilo M., MD
- Gururajarao, Lakshmi, MD
- Hanauske Abel, Hartmut Martin, MD
- Hashim, Anjum, MD
- Huang, Grace, MD
- Hussain, Kashif, MD
- Ighama-Amegor, Ibilola, MD
- Jaffery, Fatema, MD
- Johnson, Deborah J., MD
- Joseph, Frederique Mirlene, MD
- Kalia, Jessica Leigh, DO
- Kalyanaraman, Meena, MD
- Kanikicharla, Uma, MD
- Kansagra, Ketan Vallabh, MD
- Lee, Horton James, MD
- Levy, Jodi A., MD
- Louis-Jacques, Jocelyne, MD
- Louissaint, Valerie, MD
- Lui, Jackie Zhuojun, MD
- Mac, Feminia C., MD
- Madhok, Indu, MD
- Madubuko, Adaora Gabriellene, MD
- Manigault, Simone A., MD
- Marcus, Steven M., MD
- Mautone, Susan G., MD
- McDevitt, Barbara Ellen, MD
- Monteiro, Iona M., MD
- Morkos, Faten Farid, MD
- Narang, Shalu, MD
- Ndukwe, Michael Chukwuemeka, MD
- Nelson, Adin, MD
- Netravali, Chitra Arun, MD
- Nevado, Jose A., MD
- O'Neal, Isaac, MD
- Ortega, Jesus Ruben, MD
- Osei, Charles, MD
- Palmiery, Ponciano Jr., MD
- Pande, Sumati, MD
- Plaza, Lorna D., MD
- Recio, Evita I., MD
- Reddy, Chitra R., MD
- Reyes, Tyrone K., MD
- Roberts, Marc P., MD
- Rosenblatt, Joshua S., MD
- Salian Raghava, Preethi, MD
- Schwab, Joseph V., MD
- Shahidi, Hosseinali, MD
- Shihabuddin, Bashar Sami, MD
- Simotas, Christopher J., MD
- Singer-Granick, Carol Joyce, MD
- Sivitz, Adam B., MD
- Somera-Uy, Constancia L., MD
- Sprott, Kendell R., MD
- Stanford, Paulette D., MD
- Taneja, Indra, MD
- Tanuos, Hanan A., MD
- Tentler, Aleksey, MD
- Thamburaj, Ravi Daniel, DO
- Thomas, Pauline A., MD
- Toft, Maria Campos, MD
- Tran, Kevin, MD
- Trinidad, Altagracia A., MD
- Tulsyan, Vasudha, MD
- Uduaghan, Victor Aboiye, MD
- Uy, Loreta M., MD
- Vicente, Virgilio C., MD
- Walks, Pauline Angela, MD
- Walsh, Rowan Frank, MD
- Wei, Tzong-Jer, MD
- Wong, Kristin G., MD

Newton
- Dakake, Charles Jr., MD
- Digby, Thomas E., MD
- Piggee, Mia Christine, MD
- Porter, James H., MD
- Pupo, Louis O., MD
- Rossetti-Cartaxo, Annette L., MD
- Sison, Genevieve Yvonne, MD
- Zohny, Jeahad, MD

Normandy Beach
- Waldron, Robert John, MD

North Arlington
- Cabalu, Tyrone T., MD

North Bergen
- Ganapathy, Jayalakshmi, MD
- Marx, Jo-Ann, MD
- Namnama, Liborio P., MD
- Paragas, Miguela L., MD

- Abbassi, Saeed R., MD
- Caceres, Maria Gabriela, MD
- Eguino Conde, Damaris A., MD
- Patel, Mansi, MD

North Brunswick
- Agarwal, Nalini, MD
- Brauer, Howard E., MD
- Chen, Deborah E., MD
- Esterova, Elizaveta, MD
- Gajera, Sangeeta Jadav, MD
- Goh, Jean Sian Li, MD
- Hanna, Dina W., MD
- Henry, Elizabeth Robinson, MD
- Jadhav, Surekha Ashwin, MD
- Katz, Melvin I., MD
- Kessous, Deborah Lynne, MD
- Kim, Maria Batraki, DO
- Naqui, Nasreen, MD
- Patel, Himanshubhai A., MD
- Prabhuram, Nagarathna, MD
- Pragaspathy, Bhavadarani M., MD
- Raghunathan, Susheela I., MD
- Segarra, Michael L., MD
- Wiener, Howard E., MD

North Plainfield
- Shah, Bharti K., MD
- Sodhi, Surinder K., MD

Northfield
- Chang, Ho-Choong, MD

Norwood
- Bhatia, Rubina, MD

Nutley
- Dos Santos, Stephanie, MD
- Marcus, Richard W., MD
- Pedalino, Jill Garripoli, DO
- Prystowsky, Barry S., MD
- Segal, Michele Robyn, MD

Oakhurst
- Smoller, Alison Brett, DO
- Toturgul, David T., MD

Oakland
- Chu, Yie-Hsien, MD
- Guruswamy, Parvathi, MD
- Lindenberg, Erin K., MD
- Livingstone, Tosan, MD
- Michaels, Lisa-Ann B., MD
- Minhas, Navpreet Singh, MD
- Raimo, Anthony S., MD
- Stock, Ilana Rose, MD
- Sumarokov, Alina, MD
- Taneja, Uttama, DO
- Tirri, Carmelina, MD
- Wiederhorn, Noel M., MD

Ocean
- Fried, Martin D., MD
- Lichtenberger, Janice Ann, MD
- Lipp, Alfred J., DO
- Lipstein, Rebekah Ann, MD
- O'Brien, Thomas Kevin, MD
- Omotoso, Olukemi Yetunde, MD
- Sasson, Elias, MD
- Setton, Ellen E., MD
- Topilow, Judith F., MD

Old Bridge
- Arumugam, Maheswari, MD
- Asprec, Claro M., MD
- Barakat, Raja, MD
- Grochowalska, Ewa Malgorzata, MD
- Herman, Jeffrey P., MD
- Mesina, Leon B., MD
- Osman, Ihsan, MD
- Parikh, Meenakshi B., MD
- Quiba, Ronald C., MD
- Salston, Robert S., MD
- Shih, Henry Tsong-Ir, MD
- Siddiqui, Zehra, DO
- Vadali, Rajyalaks Vaidehi, MD

Old Tappan
- De Angelo, Ann M., MD
- Fishkind, Perry Neal, MD
- Hages, Harry A., MD
- Rothenberg, Nancy A., DO

Oradell
- Battista, Carl J., MD
- Czernizer, Patricia L., MD
- Jeney, Heather A., MD

Kurz,Lisa Beth,MD
Rosen,Lawrence David,MD
Orange
Vannoy,Dioscora R.,MD
Palisades Park
Choe,Joseph Lee,MD
Yun,Haenam,MD
Paramus
Kim,Sunmee Louise,MD
Kotturi,Shiva Kumar,MD
Kushner,Susan C.,MD
Monaco,Melissa Garofalo,MD
Padilla,Dominga Sol,MD
Rabinowitz,Arnold H.,MD
Rodriguez-Zierer,Maria E.,MD
Saks,Darren,MD
Shtern,Tatiana,MD
Slater,John G.,MD
Stiefel,Laurence N.,MD
Park Ridge
Grossi,Maureen A.,MD
Wang,Linda,MD
Parlin
Feliksik Watorek,Elzbieta B.,MD
Khan,Sohaila,MD
Nagarsheth,Veena H.,MD
Parsippany
Ahsan,Ambreen,MD
Bramwell,Julia,MD
Chen,Zeng-Shan,MD
Deutsch,Robert Jay,MD
Feingold,Jay Marshall,MD
Handler,Robert W.,MD
Kahn,Daniel Efraim,MD
Koenigsberg,Alan M.,MD
Li,Annie Hongyan,MD
Patel,Dinesh R.,MD
Patel,Varshaben T.,MD
Rajkumar,Aradhana,MD
Passaic
Ahmadi,Cyrus,MD
Almanzar,Raul,MD
Aryal,Sunita,MD
Bravo,Holanda P.,MD
Camilo,Antonio Manuel,MD
Fernandez,Yocasta Mabel,MD
Ferrer,Angel Salvador,MD
Hernandez,Jacqueline,DO
Japa-Camilo,Judelka,MD
Malitzky,Susan,MD
Mico,Mario R.,MD
Mosquera,Maria Cecilia,MD
Rodriguez Montana,Manuel A.,MD
Samet,Elliott,MD
Schiffman,Jonathan Samson,MD
Viswanathan,Revathi,MD
Paterson
Amadasu-Kest,Helen E.,MD
Ayodeji,Olutope O.,MD
Ballem,Arunajyoth,MD
Baluyot,Helen M.,MD
Barilari,Rafael,MD
Batista,Jose,MD
Bhagia,Pooja R.,MD
Brault,Peter V.,MD
Dahrouj,Nabil I.,MD
DeBruin,William J.,MD
Dilallo,Denis,MD
Ebeid,Hasan Samir,MD
Eicher,Peggy Smith,MD
Espana,Madesa A.,MD
Fastag Guttman,Eduardo,MD
Feingold,David Yitzchak,MD
Fernandes,Rinet Philomena,MD
Gadgil,Nandini S.,MD
Galeano,Narmer E.,MD
Garcia Rodriguez,Magdelyn,MD
Ginart,Gaspar L.,MD
Goldberg,David Israel,MD
Haj-Ibrahim,Mouna,MD
Harwood,Katerina K.,MD
Holahan,Joseph A.,MD
Holahan,Nancy C.,MD
Hussain-Rizvi,Ambrin,MD
Jadhav,Latha,MD
Jodorkovsky,Roberto Alex,MD
Khan,Ferhana,MD
Kim,Claudia,MD
Lamacchia,Michael A.,MD
Lesesne-Ayodeji,Mercedes,MD
Lesser,Eric S.,MD

Mallik,Aparna,MD
Mastrovitch,Todd Anthony,MD
Mejia,Edgar R.,MD
Mejia,Gloria,MD
Meltzer,James Anthony,MD
Moises,Rodulfo P. Jr.,MD
Naficy,Parvin P.,MD
Naim,Suprema D.,MD
Nathan,Michael D.,DO
Ogunbameru,Emilola O.,MD
Paz,Rafael E.,MD
Prasad,Vijaya,MD
Pua,Zarah Jane Baysa,MD
Rivera-Penera,Maria T.,MD
Samuel,Hala R.,MD
See,Manuel T.,MD
Shin,Young H.,MD
Siddiqui,Muhammad Rehan,MD
Siddiqui,Rehma,MD
Skroce,Linda C.,MD
Tengson,Roger C. Jr.,MD
Thomas,Abraham S.,MD
Peapack
Roeloffs,Susan A.,MD
Singh,Surbparkash Kaur,MD
Pemberton
Adumala,Pradeep,MD
Pennington
Behme,Renee Maria,MD
Besingi,Cecile Ewane,MD
Bunn,Diane Marie,MD
Goldfarb,Olga,MD
Kruse,Laurel Anita Farnham,MD
Riggall,Michael Justin,MD
Stephen,Priya Chachikutty,MD
Pennsauken
Chong,Penny Maria,MD
McFadden Parsi,Lovelle,DO
Perrineville
Eccles,Shannon,DO
Perth Amboy
Calderon,Dinorah,MD
Forbes,Darlene Henderson,MD
Jonna,Vaidehi,MD
Konda,Kalpana Reddy,MD
Kottahachchi,Wijepala,MD
Verma,Madhoolika,MD
Wade,Mark J.,MD
Phillipsburg
Evans,Charles III,MD
Kim,Sam Kwang,MD
Levine,Helaine Gale,MD
Sion,Armi T.,MD
Piscataway
Dravid,Anjana,MD
Gupta,Mamta Bansal,MD
Mathew,Lovely Sebastian,MD
Mehrotra,Naveen,MD
Patel,Rekha Arvind,MD
Radhakrishna,Vijaya,MD
Sitoy,Fernando R.,MD
Velazquez,Danitza M.,MD
Plainfield
Basu,Sebika,MD
Cho,Chang-Il,MD
Mattoo,Deepali,MD
Morin,Joanne M.,MD
Patel,Arvind Joitaram,MD
Pennington,Demetria,MD
Russell-Brown,Karl E.,MD
Singh,Amita,MD
Subramanian,Govindammal N.,MD
Zonn,Svetlana,MD
Plainsboro
Baloch,Rafia Q.,MD
Bradshaw,Chanda M.,MD
Brennan,Alicia Ann,MD
Castellano,Marissa D.,MD
Concha Leon,Alonso E.,MD
Guha,Koel,MD
Kim,Regina Siobhan,MD
Krauss,Joel Martin,MD
Kumar,Anita Kiran,MD
Lingasubramanian,Geethanjali,MD
Mah,Sue Ann,MD
Palit,Kalpana,MD
Rajan-Mohandas,Niranjana,MD
Tong,Shiwei,MD
Vakil,Vidya S.,MD
Pleasantville
Yon,Katherine Sunhee,MD

Pluckemin
McInnes,Marcia R.,MD
Pomona
Ahmed,Kamran,MD
Budnick,Glenn R.,MD
Mehta,Taral Divyakant,MD
Villasis,Cynthia Dancel,MD
Pompton Plains
Amor,Jorge Hernan,MD
Devadan,Phillip Sunil,MD
Lugo,Javier J.,MD
Shah,Sapna V.,MD
Vinokur,Anna,DO
Princeton
Altshuler,Elena,MD
Cotton,John M.,MD
Giasi,William George Jr.,MD
Greenberg,Leslie Robin,MD
Harvey,Karanja,MD
Helmrich,Robert Florian,MD
Johnsen,Peter Edward,MD
Kong,Ji Yong,MD
Konnick,Patrina A.,MD
Krol,David Matthew,MD
Kwong,Jenitta,MD
Mandelbaum,Bert,MD
Marshall,Rebecca G.,MD
McConlogue,Joelle Jugant,MD
Millar,Kim H.,MD
Monica,Kristi Rae,MD
Naddelman,Adam Brett,MD
Pellegrino,Peter Phillip,MD
Pierson,David Shawn,MD
Pierson,Joseph Jr.,MD
Pulver,Deborah Moody,MD
Ramachandran,Jaishree,MD
Raymond,Gerald M.,MD
Rose,Helen M.,MD
Schneider,Allen J.,MD
Shah,Amisha A.,MD
Shah,Amy Mehta,DO
Soffen,Deborah A.S.,MD
Tesoro,Louis J.,MD
Winikor,Jared,MD
Zollner,Paula G.,MD
Princeton Junction
Hefler,Stephen Edward,MD
Mansour,Ayman M.,MD
Ruff,Lynne H.,MD
Prospect Park
Ameen,Naureen W.,MD
Rasheed,Fouad Y.,MD
Rahway
Dancel,Concepcion A.,MD
Reddy,Sadhana K.,MD
Ramsey
Ligenza,Claude,MD
Nicpon,Christopher B.,MD
Shevelev,Irene,MD
Shor,Raida,MD
Randolph
Ciufalo,Marisa,MD
Gelman,Beth Paula,MD
Gottlieb,Ricki L.,MD
Scolnick,Ita,MD
Shukla,Kishorchandra S.,MD
Raritan
Maldonado,Samuel David,MD
Red Bank
Changchien,Charlie J.,MD
DeGennaro,Marianne E.,DO
Edman,Joel B.,MD
Jordan,Jo-Ann,MD
Kommireddi,Sowmini,MD
Litsky,Michelle Badorf,DO
Markoff,Michael S.,MD
Montero,Gianecarla B.,MD
Paladino,Theresa Ann,DO
Saini,Manish K.,MD
Wawer-Chubb,Allison Kristen,DO
Wilmott,Annette Lynne,DO
Ridgefield Park
Baker,Iyad,MD
Lee,Clara J.,MD
Ridgewood
Anderson,Nicole Andrea,MD
Benjamin,Beth L.,MD
Cally,Ronald G.,MD
Coffey,Dennis Charles,MD
Cope,Jennifer Anne,MD
Dziarmaga,Ewa R.,MD

Ghavami-Maibodi,Seyed Zia,MD
Heilbroner,Peter Louis,MD
Iqbal,Sheeraz,MD
Jedlinski,Barbara,MD
Klein,Bradley Marc,MD
Kroning,David R.,MD
Lee,Peter HaeSuk,MD
Lee,Ting-Wen An,MD
Palamattam,Jessy R.,MD
Philips,Jay,MD
Torres-Soto,Eileen Mariette,MD
Volpert,Diana,MD
Yankus,Wayne A.,MD
Young,Yvette S.,MD
Zabek Gallegos,Joanna M.,MD
Ringwood
Goyal,Ajai K.,MD
River Edge
Falk,Theodore,MD
Riverdale
Weiss,Jeffrey Gregg,MD
Robbinsville
Edwards,Kathryn Payne,MD
Rochelle Park
Bruno,Basil,MD
Rockaway
Forti,Viviana Claure,MD
Vassallo,Sheryl Lisa,MD
Rockleigh
Patel,Shilpa Ashok,MD
Roseland
Anello,Tiziana,MD
Ioffe,Inna S.,MD
Makhlouf,Jean,MD
Roselle Park
Corbo,Emanuel,MD
Rumson
Genco,John Joseph,DO
Rutherford
Huang,Doris Amy,MD
Narucki,Wayne Ellis,MD
Saddle Brook
Ladak,Batul S.,MD
Salem
Berman,Barry M.,MD
Kouyoumdji,Paul R.,MD
McLane,Rebecca,MD
Scotch Plains
Kharkover,Mark Y.,MD
Sea Girt
Fury,Mary Anne,DO
Halas,Francis P. Jr.,MD
Lutz,Mary B.,MD
Plaine,Suzanne E.,DO
Seaside Heights
Peters,Mahafarin P.,MD
Secaucus
Al Haddawi,Anwar,MD
Baker,Azzam A.,MD
Bansil,Noel Lumanog,MD
Ben,Sheeba,MD
Bokhari,Naimat U.,MD
Castillo,Rodrigo I.,MD
Cave,Marie,MD
Choi,Ok K.,MD
Dooley,Christina Yick,MD
Doss,Nermine N.,MD
Farag,Magdy M.,MD
Ghayal,Payal Patel,MD
Hussain,Zaheda M.,MD
Jadun,Wamiq,MD
Jawaharani,Shobha,MD
Jedlinski,Zbigniew J.,MD
John,Jeanie Elizabeth,MD
Lusha,Xhelal Q.,MD
Mirani,Gayatri,MD
Moshet,Osama Mohamed,MD
Mucha,Samantha Agatha,DO
Parikh,Chaula A.,MD
Raju,Rina M.,MD
Sitt,Hal,MD
Williams,Celia,DO
Win,Sithu,MD
Wosu,Carolee Ngozi,MD
Sewell
Bierman,Edward W.,MD
Bochenski,Jacek P.,MD
Bruner,David Glenn,MD
Burke,Meghan Deirdre,MD
Chao,Chia Y.,MD
Collazo,Edgar R.,MD

Physicians by Specialty and Town

Pediatrics (cont)

Sewell
Cook, Wendy S., DO
Del Moro, Ellen C., MD
Desai, Renuka D., MD
Fiderer, Stefanie C., DO
Ge, Shuping, MD
Kaari, Jacqueline Marie, DO
Kabel-Kotler, Caroline, DO
Kargman, Kevin Jerome, DO
Lewitt, Diana M., DO
Madan, Nandini, MD
Pasternak, Jared A., MD
Simmers, Richard C., DO

Short Hills
Diaz, Julio C., MD
Gurey Wasserstein, Allison P., MD
Lomax, Kathleen Graham, MD

Shrewsbury
Appulingam, Anbuchelvi, MD
Barrows, Frank P. IV, DO
Lothe, Prakash S., MD
O'Brien, Debra Ann, MD
Rajaraman, Karunambal, MD
Rigatti, Darrell J., MD

Sicklerville
Hill-Hugh, Naomi Lynette, MD
Stuffo, Kathryn, DO

Somers Point
Andrews, Roji Zacharia, MD
Bross, George Jr., DO
Drexler, Christopher W., DO
Gupte, Meenal A., MD
Held, Sharon L., DO
Jacobson, Mark, DO
Keenan, Christopher Joseph, DO
Mandalapu, Padma, MD
Share, Lisa J., MD
Thorp, Andrea Rita, DO
Vekteris, Gerald E., DO

Somerset
Arun, Aparna, MD
Carroll, John F., MD
Galowitz, Stacey, DO
Goodman, Elizabeth Anne, MD
Gunawan, Rita R., MD
Kapoor, Kusum, MD
Lerner, Emanuel D., MD
Misra, Manju, MD
Pai, Shilpa, MD
Pari, Sadhana S., MD
Parsi, Prakasham, MD
Patel, Trupti, MD
Pillai, Hema R., MD
Ramadan, Soheir S., MD
Roca Piccini, Elsie Isabel, MD
Sinclair, Melissa Renee, DO
Speesler, Matthew J., MD

Somerville
Doshi, Pankaj Manilal, MD
Hall, Kendria, MD
Hou, Shunli, MD
Patel, Kalpesh P., DO

South Amboy
Manfredonia, Patricia Estrada, MD
Mikhail, Maged, MD

South Orange
Lovenheim, Jay Alon, DO
Vecchio, Lisa C., MD
Yoo, Susan S., MD

South Plainfield
Deshpande, Sanjay V., MD
DiCarlo, Jilma Patricia, MD
Ganti, Subrahmanyam, MD
Gaviola, Durga C., MD
Joseph, Anita, MD
Solages, Joseph, MD

Sparta
Achar, Ashwini, MD
Bronstein, Regina, MD
Calabrese, Carol E., MD
Canzoniero, Christian, MD
Capozzoli, Alexis Nicole, MD
Di Paolo, Raymond Paul, MD
Jacobson, Louis Robert, MD
Mak, Sheila Shuk-Yin, DO
McHugh, Catherine Ann, MD
Meskin, Inna, MD
O'Neill, Michael B., MD
Raman, Rajesh C., MD
Spensieri, Diana Patricia, MD

Whittington, Wendy Louise, MD

Spring Lake
Miele, Ellen H., MD
Pirogovsky, Victoria, MD
Sciarappa, Lorette J., MD

Springfield
Korkmazsky, Yelena N., MD
Lim, Norman Feliz Lopez, MD
Lozano, Rolando, MD
Morris, Mark M., DO
Nunez, Helen Lourdes, MD
Thomas, Jolly, MD

Stratford
Brennan, Laura Kaye, MD
Cohen, Barbara Elisabeth, MD
Cohen, Rachel Isabel Silliman, MD
Coleman, Jane L., MD
Finkel, Martin A., DO
Higginbotham, Monique Renee, MD
Kadrmas-Iannuzzi, Tanya Lynn, DO
Lanese, Stephanie Valentine, MD
Lecomte, Jennifer Megan, DO
Lind, Marita Elizabeth, MD
Melman, Shoshana T., MD
Pinto, Jamie M., MD
Weiner, Monica B., MD

Succasunna
Heller, Michelle, DO
Patashny, Karen M., MD
Peters, Michael A., DO
Strand, Barbara G., MD

Summit
Cerdena, Maria Corazon, MD
Cessario, Alison G., MD
Feldman, Tamara Lee, MD
Kairam, Hemant, MD
Lucciola, Marion, MD
Manocchio, Teresa, DO
Nwaobasi, Eberechi Ihuoma, MD
Polisin, Michael J., MD
Reichard, Kathleen G., DO
Rosenthal, Lauren Beth, MD
Vigorita, John F., MD
Wilmot, Peter Clifford, DO

Teaneck
Becker, Steven Eric, MD
Chelliah, Padmini, MD
Eagle, Steven B., MD
Epstein, Nina, MD
Fisher, Howard J., MD
Greenfield, Efrem L., MD
Horwitz, Steven Mankowitz, MD
Kambolis, Joanne Peter, MD
Kanarek, Ninette Marciano, MD
Kanter, Alan I., MD
Kolsky, Neil H., MD
Murray, Norma J., MD
Pieczuro, Barbara Katarzyna, MD
Planer, Dorienne Sasto, MD
Schewitz, Gail, MD
Schuss, Steven A., MD
Shenoi, Shanthi Ramesh, MD
Suldan, Dora I., MD
Zajkowski, Edward Joseph, MD
Zimmerman, Deena R., MD

Tenafly
Anderson, Daniel Parker, MD
Asnes, Russell S., MD
Bacha, David M., DO
Burtman, Elizabeth, MD
Elkin, Avigayil H., MD
Jawetz, Sheryl Andrea, MD
Menasha, Joshua Daniel, MD
Michael, Lisa Golomb, MD
Schaumberger, David Andrew, MD
Smith, Michael Adam, MD
Starer, Yvette R., MD
Sugarman, Lynn B., MD
Weissman, Evan Laird, DO
Wisotsky, David H., MD

Tinton Falls
Condiotte, Shaw Brandon, MD
Cotenoff, Melanie L., MD
Dawis, Maria Agnes Chaluangco, MD
Hugh-Goffe, Judith Colleen, MD
Iglesias, Hector R., MD
Miller, Steven E., DO
Morgan, Robert L., MD
Perril, Rebecca A., DO
Pulcini, Ashley Elizabeth, DO
Salvador-Goon, Brenda Mae, MD

Wood, Jessica R., DO

Titusville
Starr, Harriette L., MD

Toms River
Alturk, Souhir, MD
Braverman, Isaac L., MD
Deacon, Nancy S., MD
Dever, Matthew Patrick, MD
Fiore, Elizabeth Jill, DO
Geneslaw, Charles H., MD
Goldstein, Richard M., MD
Golub, Michael L., MD
Haimowitz, Ira L., DO
Hamza, Hisham M., MD
Intili, John J., MD
Janvier, Yvette Marie, MD
Karroum, Kamil Hanna, MD
Lamzaky, Xenia G., MD
Masia, Alan, MD
Miskin, Chandrabhaga P., MD
Morano, Amy Beth, MD
Nag, Debashis, MD
Patestos, Chris Anastasios, MD
Pathak, Vineeta Jha, MD
Qazi, Rumana Yousef, MD
Remorca, Carolina U., MD
Rugino, Thomas A., MD
Schlachter, Steven A., MD
Shanik, Robert A., MD
Sia, Dominic Chionglo, MD
Sia, Valerie May Gumban, MD
Somasundaram, Manamadurai R., MD
Tan, Mary Catherine D., MD
Ulep, Shirley Dollaga, MD

Totowa
Abdulmasih, Yousef H., MD
Deshmukh, Pratibha S., MD
Elepano, Richard D., MD
Elfanagely, Sarah Hedy, MD
Elias, Maurice, MD
Pandey, Krishna K., MD
Ravishankar, Indira, MD

Trenton
Aamir, Tajwar, MD
Abedin, Naheed, MD
Alizadeh, Parvin, MD
Alli, Kemi A., MD
Azaro, Katherine Frankel, MD
Boor, Sonya H., MD
Brandspiegel, Laura K., MD
Browne, Patricia M., MD
Cho, Jason J., MD
Dawlabani, Nassif E., MD
Dawlabani, Nickolas Elias, MD
Hussain, Suhaila S., MD
Isola, Venkatarao, MD
Lindsay-O'Reggio, Euldricka, MD
Lopez, Lisa M., MD
Luan, Jennifer X., MD
Mondestin, J. Harry, MD
Pacheco-Smith, Sariya Amina, MD
Radhakrishnan, Puthenmadam, MD
Rapp, Rachel V., MD
Raza, Mahmooda H., MD
Samad, Ambreen Shariq, MD
Shah, Rajeev Rajat, MD
Sharma, Anjali, DO
Simone, Jill B., MD
Valencia, Maria Linda, MD

Turnersville
Iqbal, Wasie Jawed, MD
Katzenbach, George F. III, MD
Nemeh, Kamila E., MD
Richards, Adam Price, MD
Stailey-Sims, Mary Katherine, DO
Tisdale, Avian L., MD

Union
Brown, Ingrid C., MD
Krul, Geddy J., MD
Nelson, Elizabeth A., MD
Ohri, Ranjana, MD
Oxman, David J., MD
Panzner, Elizabeth A., MD
Phan, Khanh Bao, DO
Poon, Chiu-Man, MD
Straw, Simone A., MD

Union City
Anam, Sadrul, MD
Barrios, Tomas J., MD
Cenon, Pearl L., MD
Delgado, Wilson Eduardo, MD
Fragoso, Jose, MD

Hugo, Manuel C., MD
Knight, Phillip Thomas, DO
McDonough, Kevin J., MD
Polack, Noha, MD
Purisima, Fely Grecia, MD
Rodriguez, Maria J., MD
Teraguchi, Kari Jane, MD
Valdivieso, Yaira Michelle, MD
Velez, Isabel Odeida, MD

Upper Saddle River
Hands, Robert A. Jr., MD

Ventnor City
Asemota, Emiola O., MD
Tan, Madeline P., MD

Vernon
Huzar, Diana, DO
Kabarwal, Navneesh Kaur, MD
Saluja, Gurmit Singh, MD

Verona
Dorfman, Joseph Charles, MD
Flyer, Richard H., MD
Khokhar, Rizwana T., MD
Mallon, Nancy Tyrrell, MD
Nielsen, Sarah B., MD
Prestigiacomo, Cynthia R., MD
Saba, Ragheda M., MD
Sirna, Paul William, MD
Strader, David J., MD

Vineland
Ago, Aileen Hope, MD
Burgher, Sonia A., MD
Chikani, Jignasa Ripal, MD
Fisher, Matthew Adam, MD
Harper, Leannah L., MD
Hegedus Bispo, Sandra, MD
Hunt, Judith A., MD
Jain, Archna, MD
Jaiyeola, Patti Jo, MD
Mangalindan, Carmelita C., MD
Mirone, Rolande A., DO
Nakhate, Vishakha Vinay, MD
Ogidan, Olabode O., MD
Rosenberg, Michael A., MD
Sinha, Anita, MD
Solof, Arnold J., MD
Streeks, Nicole N., MD

Voorhees
Andrejko, Constance Gasda, DO
Ang, Dexter Ong, MD
Browne, Patricia M., MD
Chiang, Chung, DO
Cohen, Amy Marie Palmieri, MD
Cruz, Florencia Santos, MD
DeFelice, Magee Lindinger, MD
Frick, Glen Steven, MD
Gabriele, Elizabeth Ann, MD
Ghavam, Sarvin, MD
Glasofer, Adam K., MD
Ho, Leo E., MD
Hughes, Naomi Teutel, MD
Hummel, Mark J., MD
Jaiswal, Paresh, MD
Johnson, Swati, DO
Josyula, Leela S., MD
Kelly, Michelle, MD
Khan, Sadaf Ahmad, MD
Kiehlmeier, Scott Louis, MD
Knifong, Genoveva, MD
Kutikov, Jessica K., MD
Lespinasse, Antoine Alexandra, MD
Lestini, Melissa Murray, MD
Levey, Bryan H., MD
Lind, Thomas Eugene, MD
Liner, Lisa Hope, MD
Lintag, Irene C., MD
Mangaser, Rhodora D., MD
Mangubat, Ofelia R., MD
Mann, Ana Mendes, MD
McCay, Marissa, MD
Mulberg, Andrew Evan, MD
Nadaraj, Sumekala, MD
Naseem, Rawahuddin, MD
Pleickhardt, Elizabeth P., DO
Pradhan, Madhura Ravindra, MD
Prilutski, Megan A., MD
Reid, Brittany Michelle, MD
Ritson, Brenda Marie, MD
Ritz, Steven Bernard, MD
Russ, Michelle L., DO
Sheehan, Christine, DO
Simpson, Alyson Beth, MD
Topol, Howard Ira, MD

Physicians by Specialty and Town

Trimor,Fay Ann I.,MD
Verma,Archana,MD
Wurtzel,David,MD
Zieniuk,Gregory J.,MD
Waldwick
Capaci,Mary T.,MD
Hecht,Stacey Markowitz,MD
Muthuswamy,Vijayalakshmi,MD
Segal,Melissa Anne,MD
Wall
Meli,Catherine L.,MD
Micale,Maria Theresa,DO
Rahmet,Naheed R.,MD
Shkolnaya,Tatyana,MD
Shroyer,Stephen J.,MD
Wall Township
Barabas,Cynthia,MD
Wallington
Lupinska,Malgorzata Teresa,MD
Rozdeba,Christopha H.,MD
Sliwowski,Martha S.,MD
Sliwowski,Stanislaw,MD
Warren
Barasch,Susan A.,MD
Brandstaedter,Karen Hardy,MD
Eng,Jeffrey M.,MD
Filler,Sharon Lee,MD
Fritz,Gerard D.,MD
Katz,Andrea G.,MD
Kramer,Sarah R.,MD
Levin,Lorin Michelle,MD
Parikh,Vasavi Harish,MD
Ploshnick,Andrea G.,MD
Rogers,Elisabeth Ann,DO
Scott,Tiffany Lynn,MD
Singer,Beth Carol,MD
Stoicescu,Lavinia D.,MD
Tang,Lin-Lan,MD
Vinnakota,Rao V.,MD
Washington
Rodriquez,Victor R.,MD
Wayne
Abu Khraybeh,Wafa Said,MD
Bronstein,Jagoda Ewa,MD
Chiu,Caroline,MD
Darenkov,Ivan A.,MD
Dong,Feiyan,MD
Gruczynski,Tomasz A.,MD
Jariwala,Nilesh R.,MD
Mahon,James William,MD
Nelson,Geraldine I.,MD
Obilo,Iwuozo Livinus,MD
Orlov,Olga,MD
Scofield,Lisa E.,MD
Winston,Maryana,MD
Wenonah
Biermann Flynn,Dana Lynn,DO
Clear,Carolyn Elizabeth,DO
Hung,Deborah Liu,MD
Jones,Tamika Lillian,MD
Knestaut,Angela Gaudiano,DO
Mishik,Anthony N.,MD
West Caldwell
Butensky,Arthur S.,MD
DeLorenzo,Arthur J.,MD
Flint,Laurence E.,MD
Frank-Shrensel,Bettie,MD
Gigos-Costeas,Sophia,MD
West Deptford
Ruddock,Heather Ann,MD
West Long Branch
Abreu,Paul,MD
Miller,Sandra M.,MD
Murphy,Robert D.,MD
Truxal,Brian A.,MD
West New York
Aliaga,Julie M.,MD
Bourne,Jeffrey Alan,MD
Butterman,Clifford Jay,MD
Castillo,Elma D.,MD
Castillo,Marianne Devilla,MD
Fayngersh,David,MD
Goyco,Luis A.,MD
Gutierrez Mena,Maria,MD
Hutton-Cassie,Donna Pauline,MD
Maldonado,Jose O.,MD
Mallamaci,Carmen R.,MD
Mason-Eastmond,Tania Alicia,DO
Mirchandani,Monica Hargovind,DO
Munoz-Llaverias,Altagracia,MD
Najib,Nabeel M.,MD

Oropeza,Maria Emilia,MD
Panem,Cheryl Buensuceso,MD
Patel,Jayminkumar R.,MD
Rubia-Sazon,Elvira M.,MD
Villabona,Beatriz,MD
West Orange
Amaefula,Stephen C.,MD
Chike-Obi,Toju O.,MD
Coy,Deborah A.,MD
Faleck,Herbert J.,DO
Garbarino,Charles L.,MD
Kintiroglou,John,MD
Levy,Jeffrey E.,MD
Mathew,Seema Alexander,MD
Nachevnik,Elina,MD
Ness,Seth Lawrence,MD
Owens,Jacqueline A.,MD
Pivawer,Lisa S.,DO
Saperstein,Jeffrey S.,MD
Silverman,Abby Robin,MD
Tang,Yen-Shin Daisy,MD
Tarchichi,Tony R.,MD
Vyas,Shefali,MD
Ziemke,Karen Sue,MD
West Windsor
Dinh,Megan,MD
Kullmann,Valerie L.,MD
Rivers,Wendy Marie,MD
Westfield
Alvarado-Rosario,Yilda L.,MD
Bernstein,Stacy-Arlyn L.,MD
Cavuto,John Nicholas,MD
Chen,Margaret G.,MD
Flanzman,Ellen S.,MD
Garcia,Nicole DeVincenzo,MD
Haymond,Jean R.,MD
Kowalczyk,Matthew A.,MD
Kozich,Jeanine Masington,MD
Levine,David B.,MD
Panza,Nicole,MD
Panza,Robert A.,MD
Percy,John Jr.,MD
Presti,Jane C.,MD
Rivera,Roger Alberto Jr.,MD
Shah,Arvind P.,MD
Shapren,Kristen Marie,MD
Westwood
Buli,Dolores M.,MD
Clark,Mary H.,MD
Munteanu,Katrina M.,MD
Schwartz,Daniel I.,MD
Whippany
Ashton,Julie A.,MD
Dick,Donna Rosalind,MD
Eida,Emily Kott,MD
Forbes,Jennifer R.,MD
Gotfried,Fern,MD
Whitehouse Station
Ezekowitz,Raymond Alan B.,MD
Roche,Kevin B.,MD
Scott,Peter J.,MD
Wildwood
Gonzalez Rivera,Veronica,MD
Williamstown
Kanthan,Rajeswari,MD
Mathew,Mary,MD
Wood Ridge
Dhupar,Shanti,MD
Woodbine
Campbell,Anthony E.,MD
Woodbridge
Azhar,Sarwat,MD
Bendich,David M.,MD
Nihalani,Meena T.,MD
Rajarathnam,Kavitha,MD
Rane,Sunanda D.,MD
Woodbury
Castano,Albert Ruben,DO
Chandra,Ram,MD
Jones-Hicks,Linda N.,DO
Pasichow,Keith Philip,MD
Swe,Yuzana,MD
Woodcliff Lake
Benstock,Alan D.,MD
Berkowitz,Irwin H.,MD
Bloomfield,Adam S.,MD
Lupu,Sarah Ethel Nat,MD
Mandel,Mark S.,MD
Mayer,Michelle Saltiel,MD
Rosenzweig,Stacey Ann,MD
Stoller,Jill S.,MD

Woolwich Township
Bacchus,Bebi Samantha,MD
Baker,Alon Elie,DO
La Voe,Ira Howard,DO
Weiss Baker,Marissa Beth,MD
Wyckoff
Cerkvenik,Kathleen M.,MD
Fenkart,Douglas R.,MD
Grossman,Abigail Michael,MD
Torres,Theresa M.,MD
Triggs,Cynthia Bilsly,MD
Yazdi,Mondana S.,MD

Phlebology
Lumberton
Rough,William Alexander Jr.,MD

PhysMed&Rehab-Hospice & Palliative
Montclair
Yonclas,Elaine Marie,MD
Toms River
Mahajan,Rohini,MD

PhysMed&Rehab-Neuromuscular Med
Jersey City
Vora,Kajol,MD

Physical Med & Rehab-Pain Medicine
Berkeley Heights
Freed,Brian,DO
Chatham
Allen Artiglere,Kara D.,DO
Cherry Hill
Le,Phuong Uyen,DO
Clifton
Chen,Ivan,MD
Edison
Ceraulo,Philip,DO
Patel,Anup H.,DO
Egg Harbor Township
Mehnert,Michael Joseph,MD
Englewood
Hall,Andrew Robert,MD
Flemington
Salam,Aleya,MD
Hackensack
Shupper,Peter Joseph,MD
Hamilton
Dela Rosa,Aurora P.,MD
Josephson,Youssef,DO
Hammonton
Ezeadichie,Chioma A.,DO
Hoboken
Ben-Meir,Ron Simon,DO
Iselin
Song,Sang Ho,DO
Jackson
Hsu,Kevin Kaiwen,MD
Lawrenceville
Patel,Rikin Jagdish,DO
Linden
Sutain,Nathaniel,MD
Marlboro
Yen,Gary L.,MD
Morristown
Davis,Sanders W.,MD
Newark
Chandarana,Bhavini S.,MD
North Bergen
Vazquez,Pablo,MD
North Brunswick
Abbasi,Faheem A.,MD
Parlin
Georgy,John,MD
Passaic
Schwartz,Mark Lawrence,DO
Ramsey
Ferrer,Steven Michael,MD
McElroy,Kevin M.,DO
Scotch Plains
Menon,Aditi Sen,MD
Somerset
Ahmad,Usman Fayyaz,DO
Baxi,Naimish,MD
Watchung
Mejia,Joseph Rodrigo,DO
Tabije,Kevin,DO

Woodbury
Zhou,Linqiu,MD

Physical Med & Rehab-Sports Med
Cedar Knolls
Dona,Samuel Torres Jr.,MD
Lawrenceville
Wenger,Peter Christopher,MD
Manasquan
Gonzalez,Peter G.,MD
Old Bridge
Cohen,Jason Ronald,MD
Ridgewood
Terranova,Lauren M.,DO
Vineland
Salim,Shakeel,MD

Physical Medicine & Rehabilitation
Absecon
Khan,Naheed A.,MD
Allenhurst
Fernicola,Richard G.,MD
Asbury Park
Brustein,Fredric,MD
Avenel
Siddiqui,Asma,MD
Basking Ridge
Lin,Julie Tun-Fang,MD
Bayonne
Chaudhary,Yasmeen Amjad,MD
Belleville
Almentero,Felix Antonio,MD
Gangemi,Edwin Michael,MD
Gangemi,Frederick D.,MD
Hajela,Shailendra,MD
Berkeley Heights
Atalla,Sara N.,DO
Khademi,Allen Mansour,MD
Oza,Rohit Madhukar,MD
Blackwood
Siu,Gilbert,DO
Blairstown
Woodward,Shelly W.,MD
Bordentown
Karam,Christopher S.,MD
Rizkalla,Michael H.,MD
Brick
Barshikar,Surendra S.,MD
Chen,Suann S.,MD
Esquieres,Raymond Edel,MD
Freeman,Ted Lawrence,DO
Kanarek,Samantha Leigh,DO
Luciano,Lisa A.,DO
Scheick,Jennifer Theresa,MD
Schoenlank,Casey R.,MD
Bridgewater
Kanuri,Kavitha,MD
Patel,Pankaj Ambalal,MD
Rustagi,Anju,MD
Tai,Qing,MD
Camden
Anthony,William P.,MD
Cohen,Stephen Jonathan,MD
DiMarco,Jack Peter,MD
Khona,Nithyashuba B.,MD
Nolan,John P.,DO
Cedar Grove
Miller,Catharine Michele,DO
Cedar Knolls
Bowen,Jay E.,DO
Dunn,Kevin B.,MD
Malanga,Gerard A.,MD
Chatham
Lipp,Matthew Ivan,MD
Cherry Hill
Bodofsky,Elliot B.,MD
Citta-Pietrolungo,Thelma J.,DO
Gupta,Rajan S.,MD
Chester
Georgekutty,Jason,DO
Lammertse,Thomas E.,MD
Nieves,Jeremiah David,MD
Nori,Phalgun,MD
Romannikov,Vladimir,MD
Cinnaminson
Tomaio,Alfred C.,MD
Cliffside Park
Groves,Danielle Breitman,MD
Xu,Qian,MD

Physicians by Specialty and Town

Physical Medicine & Rehabilitation (cont)

Clifton
- Ibarbia, Jose D., MD
- Ioffe, Julia, MD
- Rusli, Melissa K., DO

Closter
- Schindelheim, Adam M., MD

Cranbury
- Lewis, Stephen B., MD

Dover
- Brady, Mary E., MD

East Brunswick
- Han, Lu, MD
- Mirmadjlessi, Noushin, MD
- Oranchak, Deborah J., DO
- Weissman, Tanya, MD

East Hanover
- Girardy, James Douglas, MD
- Kortebein, Patrick, MD
- Pasia, Eric, MD
- Robalino-Sanghavi, Michelle, MD
- Shmulevich, Mark, MD

East Orange
- Garstang, Susan Veronica, MD
- Im, Chae K., MD
- Ma, Rex Tak Chi, MD
- Malhotra, Gautam, MD
- Shenoy, Nigel Arvind, MD

Edgewater
- Putcha, Nitin, DO

Edison
- Agarwal, Sushma, MD
- Aldea, Dyana Luz, MD
- Bagay, Leslie, MD
- Bhatt, Harish K., MD
- Brown, David P., DO
- Cuccurullo, Sara J.M., MD
- Delavaux, Laurent, MD
- Dunn, Anna Maria L., MD
- Escaldi, Steven V., DO
- Fleming, Talya K., MD
- Greenwald, Brian David, MD
- Hon, Beverly J., MD
- Idank, David M., DO
- Jafri, Abida Y., MD
- Jafri, Iqbal H., MD
- Joki, Jaclyn Beth, MD
- Kanthala, Trishla Reddy, DO
- Karnaugh, Ronald Daniel, MD
- Kim, Christopher C., MD
- Levine, Jaime Marissa, DO
- Lin, Lei, MD
- Luke, Ofure R., MD
- Malone, Richard J., DO
- McCagg, Caroline O., MD
- Parikh, Sagar Shailesh, MD
- Quevedo, Jonathan P., MD
- Rossi, Roger P., DO
- Uustal, Heikki, MD
- Van Dien, Craig, MD
- Weiss, Kyle Matthew, DO
- Williams, Krystle Michelle, MD

Egg Harbor Township
- Armstrong, Joshua Stephen, DO
- Axelrod, Alyson Fincke, DO
- Falcone, Michael, MD
- Nutini, Dennis Neil, MD
- Xu, Wei, MD

Elizabeth
- Sardar, Henry, DO

Emerson
- Bethala, Nalini, MD
- Lester, Jonathan P., MD
- Mendoza, Justin, DO
- Natalicchio, James Charles, MD
- Roque-Dang, Christine M., DO

Englewood
- Alonso, Jose A., MD
- Arias, Carlos, MD
- Baker, Elizabeth Anne, MD
- Bucalo, Victor John, MD
- Dutkowsky, Charles J., DO
- Hamer, Orlee, DO
- Jendrek, Paul, MD
- Kern, Hilary Beth, MD
- Kim, Chee Gap, MD
- Liss, Donald, MD
- Liss, Howard, MD
- Montag, Nathaniel, DO
- Montero-Cruz, Fergie Ross, DO
- Nguyen, David Huong, MD
- Pavell, Jeff Richard, DO
- Riolo, Thomas Antonio, DO
- Taha, Nora, MD
- Tasca, Philip, MD
- Vadada, Kiran, MD
- Wisotsky, Lisa L., MD
- Zimmerman, Ronald Lee, MD

Fair Lawn
- Logvinenko, Andrei V., MD

Fairview
- Suche, Kara J., MD

Fort Lee
- Kim, Jong Hyun, MD
- Kim, Ruby E., MD
- Shin, Mira, MD

Franklin Lakes
- Aydin, Steve M., DO
- Reiter, Raymond D., MD

Freehold
- Engelman, James E., DO
- Freeman, Darren Keith, DO

Green Brook
- Mangunay, Danilo C., MD

Hackensack
- Mohsen, Ekram, DO
- Swajian, Mary, DO

Hackettstown
- Castro, Christopher Paul, DO
- Gutkin, Michael Scott, MD
- Shamim, Ferheen, MD

Hamilton
- Bhatt, Uday N., MD
- Carabelli, Robert A., MD
- Fass, Barry D., MD
- Gribbin, Dorota M., MD
- Smith, David E., MD

Hammonton
- Young, George William, DO

Harrington Park
- Herera, Daniel Joe, MD

Hazlet
- Bash, Robin Ellen, MD
- Rim, Josephine Myunghi, MD

Hillsborough
- Chen, Boqing, MD

Hoboken
- Mavani, Yogini, DO
- Strell, Robert Frederic, MD

Holmdel
- Azer, Amal W., MD
- Romello, Janel B., DO

Jackson
- Bartley-Chin, Dellareece M., MD

Jersey City
- Campos, Jose S., MD
- Chang, James Kenneth, MD
- Kolla, Sairamachandra Rao, MD
- Lacap, Michael V., MD
- Mehta, Ariz Ruyintan, MD
- Mehta, Monica R., MD
- Menkin, Serge, MD
- Oller, Helen Suguitan, MD

Kearny
- DaSilva, Annette Christina, DO

Lakewood
- Kaweblum, Moises, MD

Lawrenceville
- Agri, Robyn F., MD
- Ali, Adil, MD
- Colarusso, Frank John Michael, DO
- Guillermety, Esperanza E., MD
- Kothari, Gautam Himanshu, DO
- McGuigan, Kevin, MD
- Terry, Charles M., MD
- Therattil, Maya Rose, MD
- Wiederholz, Matthias Heinz, MD

Linden
- Betesh, Naomi Gold, DO
- Jimenez, Joseph C., MD

Linwood
- Conover, Melissa, MD
- Graziani, Virginia, MD
- Jarillo, Maria Roca Cami, MD
- Kull, Elizabeth J., MD
- Ludwig, David Aaron, MD
- Sturr, Marianne, DO

Little Ferry
- Karcnik, Margaret A., DO

Livingston
- Bid, Champa V., MD
- Chowdhrey, Mehar N., MD
- Davidson, Stacy, MD
- Findley, Thomas Wagner Jr., MD
- Francis, Kathleen D., MD
- Shumko, John Zachary, MD
- Wroblewski, Henry M., MD

Manalapan
- Adly, Marina, MD

Manasquan
- Glasser, Laurie, MD
- Lepis, Michael Alphonse, MD
- Vantuono, Rosanne, MD

Maplewood
- Grossman, Perry, MD

Marlton
- Domingo, Connie Dela Pena, MD
- Griffin, Mark, MD
- Harris, Tracey Dionne, MD
- Joshi, Tapankumar, MD
- Wu, Donald T., MD

Medford
- Lipnack, Eric M., DO

Mercerville
- Roman, Stephen John Jr., MD

Merchantville
- Markowitz, David, MD
- Sachdeva, Chander K., MD

Metuchen
- Alhamrawy, Ismail A., MD
- Batra, Norman Mohan, MD
- Kim, Okja, MD
- Won, Peter Arm-Woo, MD

Midland Park
- Murphy, Ryan Keith, DO

Millburn
- D'Alessio, Donna Giselda, MD

Monroe Township
- Herman, Perry Mitchell, MD

Montclair
- Jasey, Neil N. Jr., MD
- Thomas, Jodi, MD

Moorestown
- Akrout, Hafedh, MD
- Bastien, Maria Altagrace, MD
- Gutman, Gabriella, MD
- Kim, David Howard, MD
- Lee, Joseph Kim, MD
- Loughran, Katy, MD
- Marple, Jill Ann, MD
- Molina, Maria Gregoria, MD

Morganville
- Sunwoo, Daniel, MD
- Varghese, Teena P., MD

Morristown
- Bachar, Jean A., MD
- Cotter, Ann C., MD
- David, Erica Nicola, MD
- Flowers, Rashonda R., MD
- Khan, Ummais N., MD
- Khattar, Vimi, MD
- Mayoral, Jorge L., MD
- Mulford, Gregory J., MD
- Pisciotta, Anthony J., MD
- Polesin, Alena, MD
- Price, Judith B., DO
- Rao, Rajesh Ramchandra, MD
- Rempson, Joseph H., MD
- Skerker, Robert Scott, MD
- Smith, Jason Anthony, MD
- Tzeng, Alice Chaw, MD
- Zheng, Yining, MD

Mount Laurel
- Abraham, Mathew John, MD
- Jarmain, Scott Joseph, MD
- Paul, Michael Joseph, DO
- Ragone, Daniel Jr., MD
- Scholl, Seth David, DO

Mountainside
- Armento, Michael, MD

Neptune
- Levy, Benjamin D., MD

Newark
- Ashraf, Humaira, MD
- Bach, John R., MD
- Bitterman, Jason, MD
- Delisa, Joel A., MD
- Foye, Patrick M., MD
- Homb, Kris, MD
- Kepler, Karen Lynn, DO
- Kramberg, Robert David, MD
- Meer, Joel, MD
- Napolitano, Elena, MD
- Rubbani, Mariam Shafaq, MD
- Yonclas, Peter Philip, MD
- Zemel, Nathan, MD

North Brunswick
- Magaziner, Edward S., MD

North Caldwell
- Cheng, Jenfu, MD

Northfield
- Baliga, Arvind B., MD
- Russomano, Salvatore J., MD

Northvale
- Zelinger-Bernhaut, Shani I, MD

Nutley
- Bodner, Bradley A., DO
- Zazzali, George N., MD

Oakhurst
- Roach, Beth Lynnell, MD

Oakland
- Gombas, George Frank, MD

Ocean
- Meyers, Adam M., DO

Old Bridge
- Del Valle, Francisco I., MD
- Lupicki, Lucyna K., MD

Old Tappan
- Dephillips, Donna M., MD

Paramus
- Collins, Caitlin, MD
- Fossati, Jeffrey Joseph, MD
- Grigorescu, Catalina Anca, MD
- Hattab, Raed Abdulla, MD
- Schmaus, Peter Howard, MD
- Thomson, Fani Jacqueline, DO

Parsippany
- Bouzane, Gayten Carroll, MD
- Kumar, Ajay, MD

Passaic
- Kim, Ryul, DO

Paterson
- Kaszubski, Priscilla D., DO
- Parvez, Uzma, MD
- Speez, Nancy Sprague, MD

Peapack
- Osman, Sarah Ann, MD

Pennington
- Gonzalez, Ronald H., MD
- Graham, Patricia Ann, MD

Pennsville
- Akrout, Tarak, MD
- Maiatico, Marcellus A., MD

Perth Amboy
- Sinha, Anjali, DO

Pittstown
- Lin, Hua, MD

Plainfield
- Husain, Abid, MD
- Tiedrich, Allan D., MD

Plainsboro
- Andavolu, Vani B., MD

Point Pleasant Beach
- Franz, Stacey, DO
- Lopez, Hector L. Jr., MD

Pomona
- Alfaro, Abraham, DO
- Anmuth, Craig Jeffrey, DO
- Berlin, Ross D., MD
- Hahn, Robert Francis, DO
- Mehta, Hemangini H., MD

Princeton
- Bracilovic, Ana, MD
- Cooper, Grant, MD
- Funiciello, Marco, DO
- Meyler, Zinovy, DO
- Miller-Smith, Stacey Ann, MD
- Mizrachi, Arik, MD
- Petrin, Ziva, MD
- Stier, Kyle Thomas, MD

Ramsey
- Jacobs, Lyssa Sorkin, MD

Raritan
- Kantha, Brinda Sri, DO

Red Bank
- Cardamone, Kristen Elizabeth, DO
- Corzo, Jorge Francisco, MD
- Donlon, Margaret, MD
- Forman, Glenn M., MD

724

Pannullo,Robert Paul,MD
Romello,Michael A.,MD
Ridgefield
Pak,Hong Sik,MD
Ridgewood
Balakrishnan,Beena S.,MD
Boiano,Maria Anna,MD
Kuo,Douglas,DO
Marrinan,Randy F.,MD
River Vale
Ferraro,Donna J.,MD
Rutherford
Brady,Robert David,DO
Filion,Dean Thomas,DO
Saddle Brook
Dovlatyan,Raida,MD
Krotenberg,Robert,MD
Lee,Anthony,MD
Parikh,Shailesh S.,MD
Rivera,Leonora M.,MD
Seidel,Benjamin Joseph,DO
Valenza,Joseph P.,MD
Sea Girt
Buddle,Patrick M.,MD
Dambeck,Michael D.,DO
Neuman,Steven Scott,MD
Paik,Sung Woo,MD
Sewell
Ashby,John Wilson,MD
Khanna,Malini M.,MD
King,Alina,MD
Lisko,Trina M.,DO
Shrewsbury
Kahng,He-Yeun,MD
Somerset
Ankamah,Andrew K.,MD
George,Tony Kuttikattu,DO
Mandelblat,Zarina,MD
Somerville
Kulessa-Dussias,Renata,DO
South Amboy
Pollen,Philip C.,MD
South Orange
Brien,Michael J.,MD
South Plainfield
Solaimanzadeh,Sima,MD
Sparta
Agesen,Thomas,MD
Springfield
Rispoli,Frances M.,DO
Stratford
Bailey,James William,DO
Douglas,Barbara L.,MD
Janora,Deanna Marie,MD
Succasunna
Shah,Vipul V.,MD
Summit
Epperlein,Jennifer I.,DO
Garrett,Rebecca Ann,MD
Teaneck
Abrar,Dimir,MD
Brisman,Daniel Aaron,MD
Dorri,Mohammad Hossein,MD
Koduri,Hemanth Kumar,MD
Petrucelli,Janet L.,MD
Pfisterer,Christine,DO
Shahid,Nasar Mahmood,MD
Tenafly
Lee,Anna D.,MD
Tennent
Duck,Evander Jr.,MD
Thorofare
Moreno,Susan I.,MD
Tinton Falls
Baerga,Edgardo,MD
Cooperman,Todd J.,MD
Miller,Jessica Schutzbank,MD
Rathi,Sandeep,MD
Rozman,Anatoly,MD
Woska,Scott Corey,MD
Toms River
Adusumilli,Padmashree S.,MD
Cipriaso,Corazon Carrillo,MD
Coplin,Bruce M.,MD
Czenis,Ken,MD
Drakh,Alexander,MD
Errion,Christine,MD
Hawthorne-Nardini,Christa,MD
Nutini,Mary Katharine,DO
Pitta,Kutumba S.,MD

Porwal,Anoop,MD
Sonatore,Carol,DO
Stillo,Joseph V.,MD
Woolverton,Kahra,MD
Wu,Chi M.,MD
Trenton
Chiricolo,Heather Marie,MD
Gonzalez,Priscila N.,MD
Lazaroff,Leslie Diann,DO
Turnersville
Cain,Courtney,MD
Knod,George Albert,DO
Union
Alladin,Irfan Ahmad,MD
Jacobs,David Jay,MD
Potashnik,Rashel,MD
Sun,Jidong,MD
Vekhnis,Betty,MD
Verona
Bach,Richard Tae,MD
Hicks,Kristina Elizabeth,MD
Keswani,Rohit,MD
Vineland
Jeanty,Moise,MD
Mariani,Chiara,MD
Smith-Martin,Kimberley Y.,MD
Voorhees
Folkman,Michelle Gabrielle,MD
Friedman,Jerrold Aaron,MD
Gollotto,Kathryn T.,DO
Gupta,Kavita,DO
Wetzler,Merrick Jay,MD
Wallington
Filippone,Mark A.,MD
Warren
Abend,Paul I.,DO
Chang,Mimi A.,MD
Rao,Vidya J.,MD
Watchung
Thomas,Chris,MD
Wayne
Chemaly,Philippe Jr.,DO
Doss,Anthony,MD
Fan,Wen-Ling Lee,MD
Haber,Monte Arthur,MD
Parowski,Supriya P.,DO
Rahman,Abir,DO
Vosough,Cyrus R.,MD
West Caldwell
Szmak,Lauren,MD
West New York
Thorne,Robert Bruce,MD
West Orange
Anan,Elinor M.,MD
Averill,Allison M.,MD
Bapineedu,Radhika Kuchipudi,MD
Benevento,Barbara Therese,MD
Brooks,Monifa,MD
Cava,Thomas J.,MD
Cho,Dong W.,MD
Gans,Bruce Merrill,MD
Hampton,Stephen,MD
Kaynan,Riva Lori,MD
Kirsch,Victoria Susan,DO
Kirshblum,Steven C.,MD
Klecz,Robert J.,MD
Kong,Yekyung,MD
Linsenmeyer,Todd A.,MD
McKenna,Cristin,MD
Oh-Park,Moo-Yeon,MD
Park,Yong II,MD
Pomeranz,Bruce A.,MD
Vij,Raman L.,MD
Zimmerman,Jerald R.,MD
Westfield
Cohen,Pamela E.,MD
Foca,Francis J.,MD
Westwood
Goldstein,Asher C.,MD
Wharton
Lim,Steve S.,MD
Vrablik,Robert H.,MD
Whippany
Cheriyan,Joshua M.,MD
Willingboro
Jermyn,Richard T.,DO
Woodbridge
Coba,Miguel A.,MD
Woodbury
Gallagher,Edward J.,MD

Plastic & Reconstructive Surgery
Berkeley Heights
Joseph,Jain,MD
Edison
Volshteyn,Boris,MD
Hoboken
Cerio,Dean Richard,MD
Holmdel
Samra,Salem,MD
Livingston
Cooperman,Ross D.,MD
Long Branch
Taylor,John M.,MD
Maywood
Ciminello,Frank Salvatore,MD
Feintisch,Adam,MD
Hahn,Edward Jr.,MD
Montclair
Mesa,John Mario,MD
Morristown
Racanelli,Joseph Anthony,DO
Northfield
Sood,Mohit,DO
Paramus
Zapiach,Luis Alberto,MD
West Orange
Amato,John Paul,MD
Woodbury
LaVan,Frederick B.,MD

Plastic Surgery
Basking Ridge
Evdokimow,David Z.,MD
Bedminster
Patel,Priti P.,MD
Berkeley Heights
Hyans,Peter,MD
Momeni,Reza,MD
Bridgewater
Najmi,Jamsheed K.,MD
Caldwell
Agresti,Robert J.,DO
Camden
Brown,Arthur Samuel,MD
Buckley,Karen Marie,MD
Liebman,Jared Jason,MD
Matthews,Martha S.,MD
Perkins,Anthony Ray,MD
Cedar Grove
Berlet,Anthony C.,MD
Cherry Hill
Back,Lyle M.,MD
Brownstein,Gary M.,MD
Davis,Steven L.,DO
Gatti,John E.,MD
Clifton
Baruch,Michael I.,MD
Greco,Dante,MD
Colts Neck
Iorio,Louis Michael,MD
Denville
Mamoun,Sami M.,MD
Marfuggi,Richard A.,MD
Nemerofsky,Robert Becker,MD
East Brunswick
Herbstman,Robert A.,MD
Parler,Janet Patricia,MD
Vieira,Pedro,MD
East Windsor
Wisser,Jamie R.,MD
Eatontown
Ashkar,Michael George,MD
Lombardi,Anthony Stephen Jr.,MD
Edgewater
Kaplan,Gordon Marc,MD
Edison
Arkoulakis,Nolis Stamatis,MD
Cacciarelli,Andrea J.,MD
Cuber,Shain A.,MD
Risin,Michael Simon,MD
Egg Harbor Township
Saad,Adam,MD
Englewood
Abramson,David L.,MD
D'Amico,Richard A.,MD
Lee,Shinji S.,MD
Parakh,Shwetambara,MD
Soto,Norberto Luke,MD

Englewood Cliffs
Altman,Robert Gil,MD
Farkas,Jordan Phillip,MD
Mordkovich,Boris,MD
Sandhu,Baldev S.,MD
Fair Lawn
Fischer,Robert S.,MD
Lipson,David E.,MD
Florham Park
Colon,Francisco G.,MD
Hawrylo,Richard R.,MD
Lange,David J.,MD
Starker,Isaac,MD
Vallone,Paul J.,MD
Fort Lee
Michelson,Lorelle N.,MD
Ponamgi,Suri B.,MD
Trovato,Matthew J.,MD
Freehold
Bhattacharya,Ashish Kumar,MD
Stein,Howard Larry,MD
Galloway
Coville,Frederick A.,MD
Glen Ridge
Zbar,Ross Ian Seth,MD
Hackensack
Bikoff,David J.,MD
Callahan,Troy Ezra,MD
Kim,Richard Young Jin,MD
Rauscher,Gregory E.,MD
Ritota,Perry C.,MD
Hamilton
Lalla,Raj N.,MD
Hawthorne
Torsiello,Michael J.,MD
Hazlet
Fontana,Victor,DO
Hightstown
Lynch,Matthew Jude,MD
Hillsdale
Morin,Robert J.,MD
Hoboken
Chalfoun,Charbel T.,MD
Laskey,Richard S.,MD
Loghmanee,Cyrus Faz,MD
Holmdel
Griffith,Negin Noorchashm,MD
Samra,Asaad H.,MD
Samra,Fares,MD
Samra,Said A.,MD
Jersey City
Fule,Vilma G.,MD
Lawrenceville
Smotrich,Gary A.,MD
Linden
Alkon,Joseph David,MD
Linwood
Rayfield,David Lee,MD
Little Silver
Hetzler,Peter T.,MD
Zaccaria,Alan,MD
Livingston
Fodero,Joseph Peter,MD
Rothenberg,Bennett C.,MD
Lumberton
Puskas,Roy,MD
Lyndhurst
Vellas,Elaine,MD
Manasquan
Guzewicz,Richard Michael,MD
Vemula,Rahul,MD
Margate
Carroccia,Eugene C.,MD
Marmora
Birmingham,Karen Lesley,MD
Maywood
Cohen,Stephanie Meryl,MD
Winters,Richard M.,MD
Midland Park
De Marco,Joseph A. Jr.,MD
Millburn
Bulan,Erwin Joseph,MD
Saccone,Paul Gregori,MD
Montclair
Ablaza,Valerie J.,MD
Bond,Sheila A.,MD
DiBernardo,Barry E.,MD
Giampapa,Vincent C.,MD
Haramis,Harry Theodore,MD
Rosen,Allen D.,MD

Physicians by Specialty and Town

Plastic Surgery (cont)
Moorestown
Au,Alexander F.,MD
Morris Plains
Kamdar,Mehul R.,MD
Valdes,Michael E.,MD
Morristown
Comizio,Renee Carol,MD
Glatt,Brian Steven,MD
Ko,Albert Edward,MD
Kutlu,Hakan M.,MD
Pyo,Daniel J.,MD
Rafizadeh,Farhad,MD
Schmid,Daniel B.,MD
Mount Laurel
Warren,Ronald M.,MD
New Brunswick
Ahuja,Naveen K.,MD
Vankouwenberg,Emily,MD
Wey,Philip D.,MD
Newark
Castel,Nikki,MD
Datiashvili,Ramazi Otarovich,MD
Lee,Edward Sang Keun,MD
Rhee,Samuel T.,MD
North Brunswick
Olson,Robert M.,MD
Partridge,Joanna Lee,MD
Northfield
Trocki,Ira M.,MD
Oradell
Jacobs,Jeffry Lance,DO
Paramus
Baxt,Sherwood A.,MD
Breslow,Gary David,MD
Cozzone,John T.,MD
Ferraro,Frank James Jr.,MD
Gartner,Michael C.,DO
Moskovitz,Marty J.,MD
Parker,Paul M.,MD
Rabinowitz,Sidney,MD
Small,Tzvi,MD
Usal,Hakan Marc,MD
Zubowski,Robert I.,MD
Paterson
Podda,Silvio,MD
Szpalski,Caroline,MD
Pennington
McLaughlin,Michael Joseph,MD
Tuma,Gary Alan,MD
Phillipsburg
Bastidas,Jaime Adolfo,MD
Princeton
Drimmer,Marc A.,MD
Hamawy,Adam Hisham,MD
Hazen,Jill,DO
Kaplan,Stacy M.,DO
Leach,Thomas A.,MD
Ramsey
Capella,Joseph Francis,MD
Red Bank
Dudick,Stephen T.,MD
Wurmser,Eric A.,MD
Ridgewood
Ganchi,Pedramine,MD
Rutherford
Weber,Renata Vanja,MD
Sea Girt
Glicksman,Caroline A.,MD
Sewell
Behnam,Amir Babak,MD
Fahey,Ann Leilani,MD
Perri,Louis P.,MD
Short Hills
Friedlander,Beverly,MD
Yu,Deborah,MD
Shrewsbury
Ashinoff,Russell Lee,MD
Elkwood,Andrew I.,MD
Ibrahim,Zuhaib,MD
Kaufman,Matthew Roy,MD
Patel,Tushar R.,MD
Rose,Michael Ian,MD
Schneider,Lisa Frances,MD
Skillman
Nini,Kevin T.,MD
Somerville
Strauss,Andrea L.,MD
Sparta
Patsis,Michael C.,MD
Springfield
Loguda,Charles A.,MD
Tepper,Howard N.,MD
Tepper,Richard Eric,MD
Zeitels,Jerrold R.,MD
Summit
Daniels,David Daizadeh,MD
Hall,Stephen C.,MD
Shafaie,Farrokh,MD
Teaneck
Conn,Michael J.,MD
Tenafly
Garbaccio,Charles G.,MD
Toms River
Godek,Christopher P.,MD
Small,Stephen Edward,DO
Vaccaro,John J.,MD
Union
Coons,Matthew S.,MD
Vineland
Watts,David C.,MD
Voorhees
Tamburrino,Joseph F.,MD
Vasisht,Bhupesh,MD
Warren
Clott,Matthew Alan,MD
Wayne
Ganchi,Parham Amir,MD
West Long Branch
Chidyllo,Stephen A.,MD
West Orange
Asaadi,Mokhtar,MD
Lalla,Sanjay,MD
Leone,Joseph A.,MD
Peck,George C. Jr.,MD
Salas,A. Peter,MD
Spiro,Scott A.,MD
Woodbury
Steffe,Thomas J.,MD

Plastic Surgery-Hand
Maywood
Yueh,Janet Han,MD
Mullica Hill
Bidic,Sean Michael,MD
Rutherford
Sheikh,Emran Salahuddin,MD

Plastic Surgery-Head and Neck
Englewood Cliffs
Capuano,Aaron Matthew,MD

Psyc&Neurology-Neuromuscular Med
Edison
Dekermenjian,Rony,MD

Psychiatry
Aberdeen
Awad,Maher Bekheet,MD
Awad,Sahar Fathi,MD
Bennett,Robert J.,MD
Green,Anthony J.,MD
Absecon
Kammiel,Rita R.,MD
Morelli,Louis C.,MD
Annandale
Mero,Raymond J.,DO
Atlantic City
Borden,Doris Rita,MD
Corvari,Steven Joseph,MD
Gomez,Arturo A.,MD
Isaacson,Brian Eric,MD
Mani,Anup S.,DO
Venditti,Marilouise,MD
Audubon
Doria,Marie E.,MD
Avenel
De Crisce,Dean M.,MD
Rossi,Anna Michele,DO
Bayonne
Aftel,Scott,MD
Gewolb,Eric B.,MD
Jacoby,Jacob Herman,MD
Bayville
Bengali,Sakina H.,MD
Fabila,Jocelyn E.,MD
Kolipakam,Vani S.,MD
Leib,Julie Alison,MD
Schuman,Robert J.,MD
So,Hee Young,MD
Tan,Lamberto A.,MD
Tank,Renuka H.,MD
Belle Mead
Dragert,Robert Joseph,DO
Marsh,Claire C.,MD
Mehta,Umesh S.,MD
Peddu,Vijaya,MD
Saint-Vil,Robert Jr.,DO
Szulaczkowski,Wojciech Wadim,MD
Belleville
Ahmad,Raheela,MD
Barness,Michael,MD
Dalgetty,Donna Earnice,MD
Istafanous,Rafik Monir,MD
Walter,Robert J.,MD
Bergenfield
Baron,Ann R.,MD
Niazi,Mohammad Zafar,MD
Stein,Shani,MD
Berkeley Heights
Huang,Bei Barbara,MD
Berlin
Ahmed,Aisha I.,MD
Hossain,Shawn Isteak,DO
Bernardsville
Lieb,Robert C.,MD
Meiselas,Karen D.,MD
Robertson-Hoffmann,Doreen E.,MD
Blackwood
Ashraf,Mohammad,MD
Aslam,Masood,MD
Bolarinwa,Isiaka A.,MD
Wayslow,Alfred J.,DO
Bloomfield
Guanci,Nicole Alexis,MD
Mushtaq,Sabina,MD
Boonton
Ilardi,Jeffrey Michael,MD
Jalan,Suman L.,MD
Massler,Dennis J.,MD
Shah,Jay Pravinkumar,MD
Bound Brook
Borton,Miriam A.,MD
Cortez,Jacqueline M.,MD
Friedman,Ella,MD
Brick
Bhashyam,Vinod Rao,MD
Clark,Kristen S.,MD
Patel,Satishkumar H.,MD
Rajput,Zulfiqar A.,MD
Bridgeton
Friel,David M.,MD
Musser,Erica Lynn,DO
Shang,Xiaozhou,MD
Tamburello,Anthony C. III,MD
Vyas,Rajiv Krishnakant,MD
Bridgewater
Antohina,Alena,MD
Goldfine,Yvette Bernice,MD
Mehta,Rashmi N.,MD
Obleada,Clarita N.,MD
Odunlami,Henry Bandele,MD
Zhang,Hailing,MD
Brigantine
Piotrowski,Linda S.,MD
Camden
Aguilar,Francis,MD
Ayala,Omar,MD
Clements,David IV,MD
Dimaio,Andrea Lynne,DO
Elman,Igor,MD
Gogineni,Rama Rao,MD
Iftekhar,Ruksana,MD
Monte,Lyda Cervantes,MD
Pumariega,Andres Julio,MD
Stable,Joaquin Jose,MD
Szeeley,Pamela J.,MD
Cape May
Dick,Charles,MD
Cape May Court House
Blackinton,Charles H.,MD
Hankin,William H.,MD
Harrison,David E.,DO
Carneys Point
Serrano,Camilo Francisco,MD
Varghese,Sajini S.,DO
Cedar Grove
Maruri,Krishna K.,MD
Mayerhoff,David I.,MD
Nucci,Annamaria,MD
Omilian,Karen L.,DO
Platt,Jennifer,DO
Talbo,Norma B.,MD
Wei,Ronald Shaw,MD
Cedar Knolls
Barnas,Matthew Edward,MD
Monroy-Miller,Cherry Ann,MD
Weiss,Gony Alexandra,MD
Zincone,John Peter,MD
Chatham
DeMilio,Lawrence T.,MD
Dorsky,Seth Michael,MD
Cherry Hill
Ager,Mary Ann Michelle,MD
Ager,Steven A.,MD
Aronowitz,Jeffrey S.,DO
Baez,Rafael M.,MD
Ball,Roberta R.,DO
Blackburn,Lisa D.,MD
Blum,Lawrence D.,MD
Chen,Yirong,MD
Dabrow,Jennifer,DO
Denysenko,Lex,MD
Faden,Justin B.,DO
Friedman,Michael J.,DO
Gulab,Nazli E.,MD
Hauser,Adam Dankner,MD
Heard,Delano R.,DO
Islam,Mohammed Nazrul,MD
Ivanov,Ilya,DO
Kaldany,Herbert A.,DO
Khan,Aneela,MD
Khan,Munaza Anwar,MD
Lindquist,Lisa A.,DO
Ma,Yuhua,MD
Madison,Harry Thomas,DO
Miceli,Kurt Phillip,MD
Miller,Alan Norman,MD
Naik,Nalini S.,MD
Nayar,Anju,MD
Pinninti,Narsimha R.,MD
Piper,George E.,DO
Rana,Badal D.,DO
Rhoades,Walter Jr.,DO
Rissmiller,David J.,DO
Rosenberg,Leon I.,MD
Salzberg,Felix,MD
Shore,Michael W.,MD
Simon,Jeffrey Hayden,MD
Yi,Helen Huafang,MD
Zielinski,Glenn D.,DO
Cliffside Park
Ruvolo,Michelle,MD
Clifton
Cusano,Paul Jr.,MD
Jasper,Theodore F.,MD
Keiman,Isidore Michael,MD
Kim,Chang N.,MD
Pascual,Bolivar,MD
Pinchuck,Curt P.,MD
Riccioli,Diana L.,MD
Shah,Dilip A.,MD
Sozzi,Roberto S.,MD
Clinton
Titus,Puthanpura J.,MD
Collingswood
Calafiura,Peter C.,MD
Colonia
Alvarez,Reinaldo G.,MD
Colts Neck
Feuer,Elizabeth Janet,MD
Columbus
Cha,Jaeok,MD
Cranbury
D'Souza,Christabelle E.,MD
Cranford
Cayetano,Victoria F.,MD
La Forgia,Anthony Pantal,MD
Lim,Vicente M. Jr.,MD
Schweiger,Bruce Daniel,MD
Cresskill
Brenner,Laura Ennis,MD
Nadella,Ruchi,MD
Delran
Ghaffar,Sadia,MD
Usmani,Aniqa,MD
Denville
Alpert,Michael Charles,MD
Ruiz,David A.,MD
Shafiq,Saima,MD

Physicians by Specialty and Town

Dumont
Gorgo,Jessica,DO
Dunellen
Haim,Sara Rose,MD
East Brunswick
Carlo-Francisco,Kristen L.,DO
Gottlieb,Stanley,MD
Kassoff,David B.,MD
Ragone,John P.,MD
Rajan,Shirley M.,MD
Schlesinger,Esther M.,MD
Zomorodi-Ardebili,Waldburg,MD
East Orange
Adler,Michele L.,MD
Charles,Ellis B.,MD
Delaney,Beverly Renay,MD
Donepudi,Saila B.,MD
Gordin,Mark,MD
Knight,Jennifer Mary,MD
Matin,Nadia,MD
Robertson,Joy G.,MD
Roy,George A.,MD
Sharma,Amrita,MD
Tintea,Petru Ion,MD
Eatontown
Batra,Sonal,MD
Fernandez,Gregory Scott,MD
Franco,Hugo C.,MD
Khera,Gurbir Singh,MD
Edison
Bijlani,Mona V.,MD
Blank,Susan Berman,MD
Burns,Kenneth L.,MD
Gupta,Neha,MD
Lichtman,Kenneth J.,MD
Mangsatabam,Ruby,MD
Nizam,Zeba S.,MD
Ostella,Frank Mario,DO
Schlakman,Martin D.,MD
Shah,Dina B.,MD
Shah,Komal Saurabh,MD
Young,Sarah M.,MD
Egg Harbor Township
Bhuyan,Ruprekha,MD
Caro,Marjorie,MD
Glass,Gary M.,MD
Griinke,Sheila Lynn,DO
Meusburger,Charles E.,MD
Pandya,Shilin R.,DO
Samson-Daclan,Maria Teresa,MD
Snead Poellnitz,Stephanie E.,MD
Elizabeth
Bekker,Yana,MD
Bharatiya,Purabi,MD
Bolona,Leopold J.,MD
Chang,Luke,MD
Del Rosario-Garcia,Mariza,MD
Dewyke,Kathleen Michelle,MD
Ghali,Anwar Y.,MD
Gorman,Saul David,MD
Grelecki,Stephen,MD
Ibeh,Khadija Hakiya,MD
Lehrhoff,Sari,MD
Lozovatsky,Michael,MD
McCollum,Brendan Patrick,MD
Okoye,Eronmwon,MD
Patel,Hitendra R.,MD
Pena Mejia,Jesus A.,MD
Perez,Rodemar Albao,MD
Reddy,Adarsh Surya,MD
Shah,Hinna Ehsanullah,MD
Shanbhag,Suhas R.,MD
Shnayderman,Aleksandr,DO
Surahio,Ali R.,MD
Taylor,Jennifer,MD
Trivedi,Nirmal I.,MD
Elmer
Glass,Steven J.,MD
Englewood
Barnes,Stephanie A.,MD
Chaitman,Edmund,MD
Chertoff,Harvey R.,MD
Chiorazzi,Mary Lorraine,MD
Ciora,Cristian Dan,MD
Fiore,Vicki M.,MD
Garakani Nejad,Houshang,MD
Greenblatt,Naomi H.,MD
Hollander,Annette J.,MD
Kaplan,Richard D.,MD
Kernodle,Judith M.,MD
Najman,Naomi Stein,MD

Paltrowitz,Justin Keith,MD
Schumeister,Robert S.,MD
Seltzer,Ronni Lee,MD
Stefanovich,Michael Vladimir,MD
White,Harvey L.,MD
Englewood Cliffs
Lewin,Roxanne Marie,MD
Son,In K.,MD
Englishtown
Staniaszek,Alina B.,MD
Fair Haven
Levin,Matthew,MD
Fair Lawn
Hossain,Asghar S.M.,MD
Kurra,Padmavathy,MD
Primak,Dmitry,MD
Strozeski,Janet E.,MD
Flemington
Hill,Everett Huntington,MD
Kuris,Jay D.,MD
Lucas,Gem-Estelle Maun,DO
Moss,Pamela F.,MD
Patel,Mukesh D.,MD
Phillips,Anne R.,MD
Skotzko,Christine Ellen,MD
Florham Park
Dracxler Meaker,Roberta,MD
Moreno,Jose G.,MD
Oyejide,Catherine O.,MD
Fort Lee
Cuervo,Nieves,MD
Napoli,Joseph C.,MD
Rudelli,Mercedes N.,MD
Sher,Leo,MD
Franklin Lakes
Coira,Diego L.,MD
Richards,Christopher F.,MD
Franklin Park
Antolin,Eleanor Banzon,MD
Yeung,Cindy S.,DO
Freehold
Burstein,Allan J.,MD
DeBlasi,Richard A.,MD
Figarola,Carlos J.,MD
Goldstein,Lauren T.,MD
Ibanez,Delfin George C.,MD
Kolli,Sireesha K.,MD
Matflerd,Carolynn A.,MD
Prado-Galarza,Neiza L.,MD
Shafey,Moustafa Hassan,MD
Singh,Rajkumar R.,MD
Vyas,Hema,MD
Galloway
Bell,Theresa A.,MD
Gibbsboro
Giarraputo,Leonard J.,MD
Glassboro
Whitman,Sarah Marie,MD
Glen Gardner
Moise,Bonard,MD
Paranal,Aurora M.,MD
Volskaya,Svetlana,MD
Glen Ridge
Lui,Gene Sing,DO
Glen Rock
Schachter,Meri,MD
Green Village
Bird,Joanna Marie,MD
Guttenberg
Ocasio,Deborah L.,MD
Shanmugham,Revathi,MD
Hackensack
Arroyo,Zuleika A.,MD
Bortnik,Kristy E.,MD
Ebersole,John S.,MD
Finch,Daniel Garrett,MD
Marshall,Lorraine S.,MD
Martindale,Peter Craig,MD
Miah,Khorshed Alam,MD
Roman,Jocelyn,MD
Sostre,Samiris,MD
Sostre,Samuel Oliver,MD
Steinberg,David N.,MD
Zaidi,Syed Arif Raza,MD
Hackettstown
Jain,Sanjeevani,MD
Haddon Heights
Ahmad,Adeel,MD
Master,Kenneth V.,MD

Haddon Township
Prescott,Theresa Ann,DO
Haddonfield
Dunzik,Scott Dennis,MD
Glickman,Amy Borg,MD
Sproch,Amy Lee,MD
Stumpo,Patrick P.,DO
Hamilton
Faisal,Khaja Tajuddin,MD
Hu,Yiqun,MD
Ibrahim,Candace,MD
Sheth,Nila A.,MD
Ye,Xueming,MD
Hammonton
Adkins,Luz Stella,MD
Bagchi,Sudarshan,MD
Bajwa,Khalid Maqsood,MD
Bhatti,Jamil M.,MD
Caringal,Cecilia G.,MD
Desai,Amita S.,MD
Leone,Dennis,MD
Masry,Allen Y.,MD
Mazzochette,John A.,MD
Roat,David B.,DO
Rodolico,Joseph M.,MD
Rozmyslowicz,Magdalena Maria,MD
Syed,Saqib Abdul,MD
Vallejo,Jose A.,MD
Vallejo,Phyu P.,MD
Haworth
Fairbanks,Janet A.,MD
Highland Park
Khan,Farah Asim,MD
Nandu,Bharat I.,MD
Stern,Stephanie Klein,MD
Hillsborough
Donnellan,Joseph Anthony,MD
Hu,Yuange,MD
Rochford,Joseph M.,MD
Zomorodi,Ali,MD
Ho Ho Kus
Golin,Alexander Mark,MD
Welch,James W.,MD
Hoboken
Chuang,Linda I.,MD
Gajera,Bhavinkumar,MD
Greenberg,Robert M.,MD
Gutierrez,Alvaro M.,MD
Jackson,Michael B.,MD
Joseph,Judith Fiona,MD
Magera,Michael John,MD
Holmdel
D'Andrea,Daniel Albert,MD
Mehta,Varsha B.,MD
Moutier,Christine Y.,MD
Varma,Gurbachan K.,MD
Howell
Abbas,Muhammad Ali,MD
Cid,Georgina R.,MD
Jackson
Wolff,David E.,MD
Jersey City
Bhandari,Pankaj Kumar,MD
Braganza,Armando M.,MD
Chandak,Ritu,MD
Dela Cruz,Leo A.,MD
Delston,Damon D.,MD
Greenberg,William M.,MD
Hasaj,Mario Jorge,MD
Hernandez,Victor F.,MD
Johnson-Sena,Leonie J.,MD
Kurani,Devendra,MD
La Monaca,Anthony G.,MD
Mansoob,Farhana,MD
Parikh,Gita N.,MD
Pingol,Carmelo S.,MD
Quintana,Jorge D.,MD
Ratush,Edward,MD
Syed,Wajiha F.,MD
Trotta,Celia V.,MD
Vinuela,Andres,MD
Vora,Shobhana B.,MD
Wassef,Tamer William,MD
Zamora,Violeta C.,MD
Kearny
McAllister,Michael R.,DO
Kingston
Goldin,Nancy Jean,MD
Kinnelon
Pikalov,Andrei A.,MD

Lafayette
Squires,Sandra,MD
Lakewood
Akhtar,Syeda Shahnaz,MD
Berger,Eric,MD
Cummins,Tiffany Ann,MD
Finston,Peggy Anne,MD
Juneja,Tony,MD
Kharaz,Marina,MD
Pisani,Janet,MD
Rose,Moshe,MD
Sandhu,Surinderjeet S.,MD
Lawnside
Hewitt,James L.,MD
Lawrenceville
Diao,Carolina Efren,MD
Karpf,Robin R.,MD
Orr,Andrew Philip,MD
Sheaffer,Carol M.,MD
Lebanon
Holbrook,David Vining,MD
Leesburg
Steinberg,Vitaly G.,MD
Lincroft
El Rehim,Mohsen Sayed Abd,MD
Linden
Makhija,Vasudev N.,MD
Ndukwe,Nwayieze Chisara,MD
Linwood
Bloch,Andrea J.,DO
Chazin,Norman S.,MD
Mackuse,Donna M.,DO
Ranieri,William F.,DO
Sacher,S. Mark,DO
Little Falls
Czartorysky,Bohdan Nicholas,MD
Little Silver
Bhatiya,Savji L.,MD
Livingston
Cantillon,Marc,MD
Fahim,Farheen,MD
Feingold,Katherine Linda,MD
Hindin,Lee Eban,MD
Iqbal-Hussain,Farida,MD
Robbins,Lisa Ilene,MD
Sastry,Gayathri,MD
Zeman,David,MD
Zornitzer,Michael R.,MD
Long Branch
Fardman,Emiliya,MD
Geller,Matthew Al,MD
Kiselev,Marianna L.,MD
Memon,Yasmeen Khalique,MD
Schiff,Matthew M.,MD
Theccanat,Stephen M.,MD
Tintorer,Christine C.,MD
Lyndhurst
Rajaratnam,Ranjit C.,MD
Spariosu,Magdalena,MD
Lyons
Latif,Saima,MD
Lee,Hyun K.,MD
Maslany,Steven,DO
Opdyke,Karen Stage,MD
Shah,Parul Samir,MD
Madison
Abbate,Maribel,MD
Brzustowicz,Linda Marie,MD
Manahawkin
Mukai,Yuki,MD
Manalapan
Rose,Diane,MD
Manasquan
Beirne,Mary F.,MD
Maplewood
Abramson,Jennifer Leigh,MD
Marlboro
Cohen,Jason Leon,MD
Marlton
Abraham,Ruby,MD
Adetunji,Babatunde A.,MD
Akinli,Timur C.,MD
Alcera,Lloyd C.,MD
Allende,Jenys,MD
Benjelloun,Hind,MD
Callahan,Richard Allan II,MD
Chodha,Vicky,MD
Edelman,Douglas Jay,MD
Francisco,Rowena Rebano,MD
Glass,Joel Bennett,MD
Harbison,Margaret S.,MD

727

Physicians by Specialty and Town

Psychiatry (cont)

Marlton
- Harwitz, David Marc, MD
- Hume, Edward Samuel, MD
- Ikelheimer, Douglas Mark, MD
- Kurani, Amit P., MD
- Layne, George Stark, MD
- Longson, Audrey Eve, DO
- Mathews, Joanne, MD
- Mathews, Maju, MD
- McFadden, Robert F., MD
- Nunez, Venitius D., MD
- Panah, Daud Mohammad-Masood, MD
- Pertschuk, Michael Jeffrey, MD
- Post, Nicole Renee, MD
- Profiriu, Alexandru F., MD
- Rubin, Allen J., MD
- Schooff, Mary Lieder, MD
- Shamilov, Maasi Don, MD
- Smith, Elton John, MD
- Steel, Ann Elizabeth, MD
- Strauss, Alexander Sangor, MD
- Teitelman, Karen Lynn Bottone, DO
- Tobe, Edward H., DO
- Worth, Richard Lowell, MD
- Yuan, Cai, MD

Matawan
- Geller, Felix A., MD
- Moshkovich, Marina, MD
- Neelgund, Ashwini Kumar, MD
- Vorobyev, Leonid A., MD

Mays Landing
- Naeem, Ambreen, MD
- Ortega, Adela Yrma, MD

Medford
- Jones, Clifford W., DO
- Keene, Nilda M., MD
- Love, Amy Girdler, MD

Mendham
- Von Poelnitz, Michael, MD

Merchantville
- McComb, David Robert, DO

Metuchen
- Eng, Leonard K., MD
- Fahmy, Nevine Karam, MD

Millburn
- Adeola, Yetunde, MD
- Hermann, Allan J., MD
- Price, Joel R., MD

Millville
- Priori, Jorge, MD

Mine Hill
- Sundaram, Savitri, MD

Monmouth Junction
- Arora, Pradeep, MD
- Ashraf, Azima F., MD
- Das, Dipali R., MD
- Gandhi, Zindadil Manoj, MD
- Lahiri, Nupur, MD
- Lendvai, Ivan, MD

Monroe
- Malik, Rehan, MD
- Vitolo, Joseph Glen, MD

Monroe Township
- Linet, Leslie S., MD
- Singh, Gagandeep, MD

Montclair
- Bienenfeld, Scott I., MD
- Campos, Danilo T., MD
- Cooke, John R., MD
- De La Torre, Lily Shu, MD
- Friedman, Bruce Phillip, MD
- Keise, Lydia Nicole, MD
- Latimer, Edward A., MD
- Liebhauser, Catherine A., MD
- Meyer, Sarah E., MD
- Mgbako, Ambrose O., MD
- Phariss, Bruce Wallace, MD
- Reichstein, Michele B., MD
- Riestra Cortes, Juan L., MD
- Vaidhyanathan, Ketaki, MD
- Weiner, Alison L., MD
- Westreich, Laurence M., MD
- Zajfert, Michael S., MD

Montville
- Caga-Anan, Roberto Lagria, MD
- Kannankeril, Mary C., MD
- Verde, Valerie Sylvia, MD

Moorestown
- Bien-Aime, Michel J., MD
- Caputo, Kevin P., MD
- Kwon, Alexander K., MD
- Meinke, Rebecca Lynn, MD
- Salman, Zoe Wilson, MD
- Steinberg, Susanne Inez, MD

Morganville
- Haque, A. F. M. Z., MD

Morris Plains
- Becker, Robert J., MD
- Buceta, Joseph, MD
- Domingo, Joselito B., MD
- Gaviola, Gerry F., MD
- Kamakshi, Savithri, MD
- Kisch, Agnes M., MD
- Rabanal, Marie C., MD

Morristown
- Alam, Syed Fahim, MD
- Braun, Joshua Eugene, MD
- Centanni, Frank D., MD
- Chrobok, Jan M., DO
- Chustek, Michael Aaron, MD
- Cidambi, Indra Kumar, MD
- Di Turi, Richard Michael, MD
- Dickes, Richard A., MD
- Granet, Roger B., MD
- Kent, Justine Marie, MD
- Marshall-Salomon, Gabrielle, MD
- Nurenberg, Jeffry Raul, MD
- Racanelli, Vincent J., DO
- Robinson, Michael David, MD
- Rosenberg, Paul E., MD
- Sancho Mora, Elda P., MD
- Taneli, Tolga, MD
- Taylor, Clifford A., MD
- Wasser, Keri Nicole, MD
- Werner, Philip M., MD
- Wolff, Jeffrey G., MD
- Zaubler, Thomas S., MD

Mount Holly
- Case, John Gouyd, MD
- Willman, Margaret A., DO

Mount Laurel
- Ansari, Safeer A., DO
- Baruch, Edward M., MD
- Dalkilic, Alican, MD
- Hansen, Luke, MD
- Kapoor, Ashika Patil, MD
- Larkin, Joyce Marie, MD
- Richardson, Christie, DO
- Rosenkrantz, Leah Ellen, DO
- Yang, Jingduan, MD

Mountain Lakes
- Osipuk, Darlene M., MD

Mountainside
- Bernal, Ileana, MD
- Solt, Veronika, MD

Neptune
- Abenante, Frank Andrew, MD
- Cordal, Adriana, MD
- Cruickshank, Royston Raleigh, MD
- Fitzsimmons, Adriana Marie, MD
- Ganime, Peter David, MD
- Graber, Cheryl L., MD
- Hernandez Colon, Agdel Jose, MD
- Manoski, Andrew, DO
- Markowitz, Rachel Paula, MD
- Memon, Hasan, MD
- Rose, Lane Gruber, MD

Neptune City
- Kane, Patrick, MD

New Brunswick
- Anim, Candy Kyewaa, MD
- Babalola, Ronke Latifatu, MD
- Bisen, Viwek Singh, DO
- Cowen, Daniel S., MD
- Doubrava, Suzanne M., MD
- Efremova, Irina Vladimirovna, MD
- Escobar, Javier I., MD
- Garcia, Maria E., MD
- Herridge, Peter Lamont, MD
- Huan, Victoria Y., MD
- Maddaiah, Shaila N., MD
- Marin, Humberto, MD
- Nazia, Yasmin, MD
- Sanjuan, Racquel, DO
- Shaikh, Najmussaha M., MD
- Swigar, Mary E., MD
- Tiu, Gladys Tompar, MD
- Trenton, Adam James, DO

New Lisbon
- Geller, Ian B., DO

New Providence
- Hidalgo, Marla, MD
- Pesci, Paula M., MD

Newark
- Afzal, Saba, MD
- Aggarwal, Rashi, MD
- Allen Steinfeld, Isabel, MD
- Alvarado, Mark U., MD
- Amin, Ritesh A., MD
- Annitto, William J., MD
- Babayants, Alexander R., MD
- Bansil, Rakesh K., MD
- Bartlett, Jacqueline A., MD
- Belenker, Stuart Lawrence, MD
- Bennett, Robert Harris, DO
- Cartwright, Charles N., MD
- Chakrabarti, Mukti, MD
- Eljarrah, Fouad, MD
- Finkelstein, Mario, MD
- Frederikse, Melissa Ellison, MD
- Frometa, Ayme Veronica, MD
- Gudapati, Ramakrishna, MD
- Heffner, Catherine D'aprix, DO
- Henningson, Karen Jeanne, DO
- Jadeja, Kiranben J., MD
- Kennedy, Cheryl A., MD
- Kesselman, Gayle, MD
- Levin, Elizabeth H., MD
- Mirza, Nadia A., MD
- Obi, Manfred K., MD
- Oyvin, Vadim, MD
- Pemberton, Clyde A., MD
- Rajakumar, Nirmala S., MD
- Reeves, Donald Raymond Jr., MD
- Rowan, George Edward, MD
- Rudner, Elvira, MD
- Schleifer, Steven J., MD
- Shah, Snehal, MD
- Shihabuddin, Lina Sami, MD
- Silva, Lourdes G., DO
- Sun, Ye Ming Jimmy, MD
- Tortosa Nacher, Rafael M., MD
- Udasco, Jocelynda O., MD
- Villegas, Noah, MD
- Whang, Phil Joo, MD
- Young, Joseph M., MD
- Yum, Sun Young, MD

Newton
- El-Kholy, Nahed M., MD
- Sarner, Steven W., MD
- Scimone, Anthony, MD

North Bergen
- Feuer Razin, Zippora, DO
- Ruiz, Vicente Z., MD
- Wancier, Zisalo, MD

North Brunswick
- Jones, Frank A. Jr., MD
- Losack, Glenn Mark, MD
- Steinberg, Edward, MD

Nutley
- Bridge, Thomas Peter, MD
- Fleser, Cecilia, MD
- Khan, Mehtab A., MD
- Yoo, Sang W., MD

Oakhurst
- Kamm, Ronald L., MD

Oakland
- Chalemian, Robert J., MD

Oaklyn
- Patten-Kline, Nancy H., DO

Ocean
- Lang, Karen Friedman, MD
- Patel, Sameer Ramesh, MD

Old Bridge
- Co, Gerrie T., MD
- Joshi, Kumud Gada, MD
- Laurelli, Joseph P., MD
- Naeem, Sana, MD
- Swamy, Aldonia A., MD

Old Tappan
- Tancer, Nancy Kaplan, MD

Orange
- Reyes, Christine, MD
- Shah, Ila H., MD

Paramus
- Abrar, Samar, MD
- Adel, Tymaz, MD
- Airapetian, Karine V., MD
- Al-Salem, Salim Suliaman, MD
- Benitez, Jose L., MD
- Cheema, Faiz Aslam, MD
- Federbush, Joel S., MD
- Harrigan, Michael Richard, MD
- Iqbal, Mohammad Javed, MD
- Kahn, Frederick E., MD
- Kotler, Lisa A., MD
- Marte, Juan M., MD
- Metelitsin, Marina Nikolaevna, MD
- Miller, Helene Anne, MD
- Nissirios, Kalliopi, MD
- Oczkos, Patrick, MD
- Palkhiwala, Bharati A., MD
- Palmer, Barbara A., MD
- Ragheb, Sameh Makram, MD
- Ramay, Mohammad Hanif, MD
- Varas, Elizabeth A., MD
- Waseem, Mehnaz, MD
- Winters, Richard Allan, MD

Park Ridge
- Lopez, Lina Maria, MD

Parsippany
- Bhatia, Malini P., MD
- Carness, Jason, MD
- Novik, Emily, MD
- Solanki, Rashminkumar R., MD
- Weisman, Tamara K., DO

Passaic
- Ravelo, Mary Ann, MD
- Williams-Martin, Pamela Y., MD

Paterson
- Aladjem, Asher, MD
- Arroyo, Louis, MD
- Castillo, Hilda A., MD
- Delvalle, Yissell, MD
- Dementyeva, Yuliya, MD
- Gad, Gamal Eldin, MD
- Hirsh, Ron, MD
- Micevski, Aleksandar, MD
- Ribalta, Marcia, MD
- Rueda, Carlos Alberto, MD
- Siddiqui, Rehan, MD
- Thimmaiah, Manavattir B., MD
- Torres, Maria Elissa, MD
- Verret, Joseph M., MD

Pennington
- Donofrio, Scott D., MD
- Raser, Keith A., MD
- Rosenthal, Robert S., MD

Pennsauken
- Dubois, Yves Georges, MD

Perth Amboy
- Brown, Katherine E., MD
- Dube, Veena, MD
- Lanez, Carmencita T., MD
- Mishra, Arunesh Kumar, MD
- Nadipuram, Chandrika, MD

Phillipsburg
- Javia, Subhashchandra J., MD
- Titus, Benny Elizabeth, MD
- Yu, Cha J., MD

Pine Brook
- Maaty, Mona, MD

Piscataway
- Aupperle, Peter M., MD
- DeLuca, Alison Kay, MD
- Elga, Shana Stein, MD
- Gunja, Sakina Zahir, MD
- Gutterman, Lily Z., MD
- Hammond, Carla Chambers, MD
- Hraniotis, Nicole J., MD
- Ivelja-Hill, Danijela, MD
- Kaufman, Kenneth R., MD
- Menza, Matthew A., MD
- Miskimen, Theresa M., MD
- Palmeri, Barbara A., MD
- Petti, Theodore Andre, MD
- Rao, Savitha, MD
- Rosato, Mark G., MD
- Sharma, Madhulika Brahm, MD
- Srinivasan, Rekha, MD
- Tai, Mustafa, MD
- Tepper, Drew I., MD
- Velivis, Leticia, MD
- Williams, Jill M., MD

Plainfield
- Forbes, Trevor G., MD
- Guirguis, Soad George, MD
- Patel, Dineshchandra G., MD
- Weinstein, Jack S., MD

Plainsboro
- Sinha, Sharmila, MD
- Vinekar, Ajanta S., MD

Pomona
 Ashfaq,Mohammad,MD
 Hasson,Marie Elena,MD
 Kaplan,Eliot F.,MD
 O'Shea,Alice P.,MD
 Zwil,Alexander S.,MD
Port Reading
 De Santis,Maryanne,MD
Princeton
 Apter,Jeffrey T.,MD
 Benaur,Irina V.,MD
 Blake,John R.,MD
 Borthwick,James Malcolm,MD
 Carneval,Patricia A.,MD
 Chen,Michael S.,MD
 Cohen,Jonathan David,MD
 Fernandez,Ricardo J.,MD
 Gochfeld,Linda G.,MD
 Green,Jeffrey H.,MD
 Heller,Philip Arthur,MD
 Hom,William L.,MD
 Ilangovan,Kani Mozhi,MD
 Karpf,Gary A.,MD
 Koenig,Michele L.,MD
 Langer,Dennis Henry,MD
 Langer,Susan F.,MD
 Leopold,Michael A.,MD
 Levine,Steven Paul,MD
 Mattes,Jeffrey A.,MD
 Nathan,David Lawrence,MD
 Pal,Jayanta Kumar,MD
 Popkin,Sara Elizabeth,MD
 Prus Wisniewski,Richard V.,MD
 Rahman,Firoz Pushkin,MD
 Ratliff,Henry W.,MD
 Resnick,Steven I.,MD
 Salvatore,Joseph E. Jr.,MD
 Sandhu,Jagwinder S.,MD
 Scasta,David L.,MD
 Schofield,Neal B.,MD
 Senekjian,Elizabeth K.,MD
 Shah,Dhwani B.,MD
 Stanley,Lorna Maria,MD
 Staroselsky,Galina,MD
 Szteinbaum,Edward M.,MD
 Tchikindas,Olga M.,MD
 Teasley,Melanie,MD
 Temple,Julia K.,MD
 Tipermas,Alan,MD
 Varma,Sanjay,MD
 Vasilov,Anatoliy I.,MD
 Vazquez,Jose S.,MD
 Vilko,Naomi R.,MD
 Wilson,George F.,MD
 Yanovskiy,Anatoliy M.,MD
Ramsey
 Crowley,Elizabeth Ozimek,MD
 Mirchandani,Indu,MD
Red Bank
 Bransfield,Robert C.,MD
 Calvosa,Michelle K.,MD
 Cancellieri,Francis Louis,MD
 Clever,Marcia Sue,MD
 Friedman,Dena Seifer,MD
 Ginn-Scott,Elizabeth J.,MD
 Litwin,Peter J.,MD
 Marcus,Abir Assaad,MD
 Schineller,Tanya M.,MD
 Segal,Arthur M.,MD
 Shin,Kyun,MD
 Sikowitz,David J.,MD
 Vakar,Emil,DO
 Vetrano,Joseph S.,MD
 Wong,Dennis,MD
Ridgewood
 Abkari,Shashikala,MD
 Anand,Ashish,MD
 Becker,William D.,MD
 Cohen,Daniel Elliot,MD
 Cowan,James Rankin Jr.,MD
 Dealwis,Watutantrige T.,MD
 Elvove,Robert M.,MD
 Farooki,Alima Bibi,MD
 Flescher,Sylvia Evelyn,MD
 Fraser,Margaret Cameron,MD
 Gilman,Howard E.,MD
 Grogan,Rita J.,MD
 McGuire,Patricia L.,MD
 Narula,Amarjot S.,MD
 Patel,Narendra D.,MD
 Rosenfeld,David N.,MD
 Samuels,Steven Charles,MD
 Tuchin,Terry A.,MD
 Videtti,Nicholas A.,MD
 Wulach,Sandra H.,MD
 Yoon,Eui-Sun L.,MD
 Zisu,Traian A.,MD
River Edge
 Martinez,Humberto L.,MD
Rochelle Park
 Acquaviva,Joseph F.,MD
 Flood,Mark J.,MD
 Martinez-Arroyo,,Humberto L.,MD
Rockaway
 Suckno,Lee J.,MD
Roosevelt
 Vo,Eleanor B.,MD
Roseland
 Hall,Jeffrey,MD
Rutherford
 Brozyna,David B.,MD
 Khinda,Navjot,MD
Saddle Brook
 Badr,Amel Afifi,MD
 Weiser,Sheldon,DO
Saddle River
 Semar,David P.,MD
Scotch Plains
 Madraswala,Rehman,MD
Sea Girt
 Kargman,Jeffrey M.,MD
Secaucus
 Iskandarani,Nimer M.,MD
 Nekrasova,Irina,MD
 Ortega,Eddy A.,MD
 Shalts,Edward,MD
 Soberano,Wilfredo T.,MD
Sewell
 Ellis,George David,MD
 Lewis,Lesley Brook,DO
 Mac Fadden,Wayne,MD
 Ortanez,Iluminado C.,MD
Short Hills
 Brazaitis,Edward,MD
 Feldman,Russett P.,MD
 Shaw,Jennifer Robin,MD
Shrewsbury
 Bier,Martin M.,MD
 Falco,Sharon Anne,MD
 Rhee,Bong Susan,MD
Sicklerville
 Acosta,Regis Francisco,MD
 Reyes,Jose Franco,MD
 Sayed,Saquib Bashir,MD
Skillman
 Harman,Robert Ashworth,MD
 Negron,Arnaldo E.,MD
 Ramzy,Ayman H.,MD
 Shnaidman,Vivian T.,MD
 Shnaps,Yitzchak,MD
 Stuebben,Kurt C.,MD
 Willis,Kenneth W.,MD
Somers Point
 Gowda,Srisai,MD
 Reid,Kelly M.,MD
Somerset
 Hanchuk,Hilary T.,MD
 Nam,Sang K.,MD
Somerville
 De Ritter,Lois M.,MD
 Falls,Ingrid T.,MD
 Osmanovic,Kenan,MD
 Patel,Unnati D.,MD
 Rosin,Dale,DO
 Rowan,Patrick John,MD
 Shaikh,Tasneem,MD
South Amboy
 Arya,Vinay,MD
South Plainfield
 Chezian,Shanthi,MD
Sparta
 Blanchard,Jenny Ann,DO
 Kloupar,Dagmar S.,MD
 Koss,Debra Elvira,MD
 Leibov,Ernest B.,MD
Springfield
 Kantor,Ruth B.,MD
 Miller,David Geoffrey,MD
 Parinello,Robert M.,MD
 Thorpe,Michelle Lynn,MD
Stratford
 Aguirre-Masecampo,Alfe G.,MD
 Belinsky,Tatyana,MD
 Forsberg,Martin M.,MD
 Vender,Lydia A.,DO
 White,Christian Paul,DO
Strathmere
 Blackwell,Kathryn V.,DO
Succasunna
 Singh,Pritpaul,MD
Summit
 Alam,Rozana R.,MD
 Behar,Lonny J.,MD
 Bolo,Peter M.,MD
 Budoff,Steven R.,DO
 Ciolino,Charles P.,MD
 Clark,Peter Joseph,DO
 Dealwis,Jayakanthi,MD
 Forman-Chou,Alexandra C.,MD
 Frey,Patricia E.,DO
 Gray,Sonja B.,MD
 Greenberg,Rosalie,MD
 Hopkins,Rebecca Jane,MD
 Jones,Jane W.,MD
 Kaplan-Sagal,Lauren Ellen,MD
 Keyser,Joseph W.,MD
 Malhotra,Mahamaya,MD
 Malhotra,Rahul,MD
 Reiter,Stewart Roy,MD
 Shah,Talaxi D.,MD
 Sofair,Jane Brown,MD
 Sosnow,Meg W.,MD
 Tahil,Fatimah Ann,MD
 Villafranca,Manuel V.,MD
 Zimmerman,Aphrodite Marta,MD
Teaneck
 Archila,Arturo Plinio,MD
 Cho,Seokkoon,MD
 Farkas,Edward L.,MD
 Hain,Joshua Meir,MD
 Jacobowitz,Esther,MD
 Raby,Wilfrid Noel,MD
 Rosenbaum,Paul,MD
 Wagle,Sharad D.,MD
 Zenn,Juliane Janis,MD
Tenafly
 Amiel,Elizabeth A.,MD
 Gross,Carey E.,MD
 Knafel,Natalya,MD
Tinton Falls
 Parks,Shannon N.,DO
Toms River
 Abubakar,Tunku Abdul R.,MD
 Berkowitz,Robert,MD
 Buchan,Shahindokh,MD
 Chowdhrey,M. Salim,MD
 Deworsop,Richard,MD
 Dobrzynski,Carol A.,MD
 Ferstandig,Russell A.,MD
 Oh,Donald,MD
 Siddiqui,Arshad Uddin,MD
Totowa
 Prakash,Meera V.,MD
Trenton
 Ali,Syed A.,MD
 Ali,Syed Asim,MD
 Amin,Prakash P.,MD
 Anwunah-Okoye,Ifeoma Juliet,MD
 Bresch,David,MD
 Brown,Gary Alan,DO
 Chiappetta,Carl J.,MD
 Dorio,Nicole Marie,DO
 Eilers,Robert Paul,MD
 Fuchs,Susan,MD
 Ganescu,Daniela Florentina,MD
 Gooriah,Vinobha,MD
 Khan,Mujahid A.,MD
 Kher,Neeta Yogesh,MD
 Kwok,Elaine,MD
 Lieberman,Jordan A.,MD
 Mabrouk,Hanny S.,MD
 Maljian,Meroujan Ardziv,MD
 Mundassery,Sarala C.,MD
 Nagra,Amandeep Kaur,MD
 Ramanujam,Sailakshmi,MD
 Rao,Vilayannur Raja R.,MD
 Rorro,Mary C.,DO
 Saslo,Christopher R.,DO
 Siddiqui,Shahida,MD
 Thomas,Sara S.,MD
 Wijaya,Don H.,MD
Turnersville
 Barb,Herman T.,MD
 Patel,Prabhaker S.,MD
Union
 Chernyak,Arkadiy,MD
 Galea,Marina,MD
 Goldin,Michael R.,MD
 Ivanov,Alexander,MD
 Rasin,Grigory S.,MD
Union City
 Sandoval-Castellanos,Oscar,MD
Upper Montclair
 Bell,Michael Henry,MD
 Elfenbein,Cherie,MD
 Green,Amy,MD
 Shah,Bindi,DO
Upper Saddle River
 Burn,Charlene H.,MD
Vauxhall
 Clouden,Tobechukwu A.,MD
Vineland
 Bright,Daniel J.,MD
 Clinton,Lawrence P.,MD
Voorhees
 Brooks,Ellen F.,MD
 Castillo,Edwin F.,MD
 Chheda,Veena V.,MD
 Jordan,Karen T.,MD
 Kim,Amy,MD
 Kothari,Kinnari A.,MD
 Mahmud,Jamal,MD
 Peterson-Deerfield,Laurie J.,DO
 Riyaz,Najmun,MD
 Sarker,Tushar,MD
 Sobel,Janine M.,MD
Waldwick
 Dyakina,Nika,DO
Wall
 Kansagra,Chunilal H.,MD
 Mehandru,Urmila,MD
Warren
 Liu,Qinyue,MD
Washington
 Groves,Gerald A.,MD
 Montezon,Lourdes I.,MD
Watchung
 Eisenberg,Stuart Richard,MD
Wayne
 Ahkami,Behzad,MD
 ElRafei,Mohamed A.,MD
 Kashoqa,Amer H.,MD
 Kat,Yousef A.,MD
 Master,Maria G.,MD
 Patel,Rajesh Manharbhai,MD
 Rasheed,Syed Adil,MD
 Siddiqui,Imtiazuddin M.,MD
 Siddiqui,Nafeesa,MD
 Wang,Cecilia S.,MD
West Long Branch
 Mendelson,Joshua Todd,MD
 Sachla,Melpomeni,MD
West New York
 Sanchez,Daniel Rene,MD
 Soto Perello,Jose Manuel,MD
West Orange
 Cannella,Michael,MD
 Chilakapati,Manjula,MD
 Dhaibar,Yeshuschandra R.,MD
 Elmore,Erin Maureen,MD
 Kurien,Abby V.,MD
 Park,Charles William,MD
 Scalea,Donald D.,MD
 Urbina,Emily Anne,MD
West Paterson
 Dang,Jagdish G.,MD
West Trenton
 Bari,Mohammad Minhaj,MD
 Calabrese,Toni-Lynne,DO
 Chacinski,Dariusz R.,MD
 Cohen,Jay A.,MD
 Fucanan,Vilma D.,MD
 Gallagher,Peter K.,MD
 Ghadiali,Farida Hashim,MD
 Hogan,Elizabeth Anne,MD
 Kazi,Abdul Haseeb,MD
 Legaspi,Abbelane S.,MD
 Mujahid,Anjum,MD
 Nunez,Aida Rodrigo,MD
 Park,Jennifer E.,MD
 Pasupuleti,Sasikala,MD
 Patel,Jayantilal R.,MD

Physicians by Specialty and Town

Psychiatry (cont)
West Trenton
- Petivan, Victoria Anne, MD
- Radic, Rumiana S., MD
- Rizvi, Amir M., MD
- Rossi, Lawrence Nicholas, MD
- Roth, Robert L., MD
- Sack, Anita D., MD
- Tirmazi, Syed Jawad H, MD

Westampton
- Balasundaram, Anusuya, MD
- Connell, Thomas A., MD
- Davis, Robert M., MD
- DeMercurio, Robert Edward, DO
- Madrak, Leslie Nicole, DO
- Rehman, Atta-Ur, MD
- Stiffler, Kyle M., MD
- Trigiani, Charles J., DO
- Wilkins, John J., DO

Westfield
- Borja, Susan V., MD
- Cunningham, Michael James, MD
- Goldman, Clifford D., MD
- Lim, Ami Cruz, MD
- Louie, Pearl Maria, MD
- Moreines, Robert N., MD

Westmont
- Mobilio, Joseph N. Jr., DO

Westwood
- Shah, Pritesh J., MD

Wharton
- Chiodo, Damien F., MD

Woodbridge
- Hriso, Emmanuel, MD
- Hriso, Paul, MD

Woodbury
- Bellias, Jay Peter, DO
- Camacho, Brenda Y., MD
- Camacho-Pantoja, Jose A., MD
- Ko, Haeng S., MD
- Zand, Perry H., MD

Woodcliff Lake
- Siragusa, Joseph, MD

Wyckoff
- Gallina, David J., MD
- Gefter, Igor, MD
- Golin, Gratsiana, MD
- Jalandoon, Cynthia Tabligan, MD
- Nanjiani, Aijazali, MD
- Peranio, Joanne C., MD
- Plummer, Alice T., MD
- Sous, Manal Ann, MD
- Winters, Jayshree P., MD
- Youssef, Rafik Z., MD

Psychiatry&Neurology-Addiction Med
Summit
- Belz, Marek, MD

Psychiatry&Neurology-Special Qual
Gibbsboro
- Chadehumbe, Madeline A., MD

Hackensack
- Gliksman, Felicia Joyce, MD

Long Branch
- Fisch, Shirley B.D., MD

Mountainside
- Okouneva, Evelina, DO

Rochelle Park
- Kulikova-Schupak, Romana, MD

Westfield
- Richards, Andrea T., MD

Public Health
Fort Lee
- Etzi, Susan, MD

Mercerville
- Zanna, Martin Thomas, MD

Mount Laurel
- De Masi, Leon Gregory, MD

Newark
- Halperin, William Edward, MD

Piscataway
- Rhoads, George G., MD

Trenton
- DiFerdinando, George T. Jr., MD
- Paul, Sindy M., MD

Pulmonary Critical Care
Brick
- Alcasid, Patrick J., MD

Bridgewater
- Patel, Prashant B., MD

Camden
- Kennedy-Little, Dawn Marie, DO

Cedar Knolls
- Epstein, Matthew D., MD

Cherry Hill
- Velasco, Antonio Quiachon, DO

Denville
- Patel, Gaurang, MD

East Brunswick
- Gilbert, Tricia Todisco, MD

Elizabeth
- Budhwani, Anju, MD

Englewood
- Califano, Francesco, MD

Flemington
- Maouelainin, Nina, DO
- Yuan, Carol Jia-Luh, MD

Galloway
- Alobeidy, Salaam T., MD

Hackensack
- Abdelhadi, Samir I., DO

Haledon
- Alfakir, Maria, MD

Jersey City
- Mikkilineni, Rao S., MD

Morristown
- Boomsma, Joan D., MD
- LaRosa, Jennifer A., MD

Plainsboro
- Buckley, Laura K., MD

Ridgewood
- Chakravarti, Aloke, MD
- Salamat, Rahat, MD
- Vakil, Rupesh M., MD

Somers Point
- Adams, William B., DO

Turnersville
- Barnes, Jaime Jude, DO

West Paterson
- Solis, Roberto A., MD

Woodbury
- Breen, Gregory, MD
- Cheng, Ho-Kan, MD

Pulmonary Disease
Barnegat
- Palecki, Agnieszka, MD

Bergenfield
- Liu, Ming Kong, MD

Berkeley Heights
- Wilt, Jessie Swain, MD

Brick
- Kamel, Emad R., MD
- Kerr, Brian S., MD
- Wynkoop, Walter Alan, MD

Bridgewater
- Poiani, George J., MD

Browns Mills
- Brar, Navdeep K., MD
- Cajulis, Marivi Ora, MD

Burlington
- Mest, Stuart, MD

Camden
- Abou-Rayan, Mohamed Magdy, MD
- Akers, Stephen M., MD
- Boujaoude, Ziad C., MD
- Pratter, Melvin Richard, MD

Cape May Court House
- Bradway, William R., DO
- Komansky, Henry J., DO
- Patel, Amit H., MD
- Udani, Rajen I., MD

Carteret
- Singh, Rashpal, MD

Cedar Grove
- Dikengil, Yahya Mete, MD

Cedar Knolls
- Restifo, Robert A., DO
- Scoopo, Frederic J., MD
- Shah, Chirag Vijaykumar, MD

Cherry Hill
- Crookshank, Aaron David, MD
- Dostal, Courtney Lynne, DO
- Hamaty, Edward G. Jr., DO
- Morowitz, William A., MD

Denville
- Pope, Alan Raymond, MD
- Scivoletti Polan, Nicole Anne, DO

Denville
- Alexander, Robert Francis, MD

East Brunswick
- Hutt, Douglas A., MD
- Waksman, Howard Kenneth, MD

East Hanover
- Martin, Thomas Reed, MD

East Orange
- Abdel Fatgah, Nail S., MD
- Kim, Jenny Hyunjung, MD

Edison
- Ferraris, Ambra, MD
- Goldstein, David S., MD
- Hebbe, Karl Albert Jr., DO
- Polos, Peter George, MD
- Raju, Pooja Indukuri, MD
- Supe Dzidic, Dana, MD

Elizabeth
- Garg, Vipin, MD

Englewood
- Gorloff, Victor, MD
- Han, Paul S., MD
- Kondapaneni, Srikant, MD
- Patel, Killol, MD
- Tesher, Harris Brandon, MD

Ewing
- Harman, John A., MD

Fair Lawn
- Tijani, Hakeem Gbolahan, MD

Freehold
- Krachman, Samuel Lee, DO
- Pi, Justin Jeong-Suk, MD
- Shah, Nirav Navin, DO

Galloway
- Bansal, Aditya Rakesh, MD
- Costantini, Peter J., DO
- Loftus, Frances Ellen, DO
- Sadik, Nadia, MD

Glen Rock
- Grizzanti, Joseph N., DO

Hackensack
- Goss, Deborah Anne Marie, MD
- Koniaris, Lauren Solanko, MD
- Polkow, Melvin S., MD
- Sadikot, Sean Shabbir, MD

Haledon
- Alberaqdar, Enis, MD

Hamilton
- El Habr, Abdallah H., MD
- Kurugundla, Navatha, MD

Hammonton
- Kanoff, Jack M., DO

Hazlet
- Pristas, Adrian M., MD

Holmdel
- Aggarwal, Vinod K., MD

Jamesburg
- Fein, Edward Dennis, MD

Jersey City
- Bhatnagar, Tanuj, MD
- Marchione, Victor L., MD
- Natarajan, Sekar, MD

Kearny
- Saliba, Jehad E., MD

Kendall Park
- Khan, Wajahat Hussain, MD

Lincoln Park
- O'Donnell, Timothy S., DO

Little Falls
- Vazir, Amanullah A., MD

Livingston
- Greenberg, Martin J., MD
- Petrowsky, Deborah, MD

Lodi
- Villa, John J., DO

Long Branch
- Davis, George C., MD

Madison
- Seelall, Vijay Harpal, MD

Manahawkin
- Lipper, Jeffrey M., MD

Manasquan
- De La Luz, Gustavo E., MD

Maplewood
- Bey, Omar M., MD

Marlton
- Auerbach, Donald, MD
- Lee, Andrew N., MD

Sutherland, Jewelle R., MD
Merchantville
- Curreri, Peter Andrew, DO

Middletown
- McGuire, Peter A., MD

Midland Park
- Rosen, David Michael, MD

Millburn
- Shah, Himanshu P., MD

Montclair
- Cohen, Zaza Isaac, MD

Moorestown
- Allred, Charles Cameron, MD

Mount Laurel
- Fineman, William, MD
- Schriber, Andrew David, MD
- Trudo, Frank J., MD

New Brunswick
- Ash, Carol E., DO
- Frenia, Douglas Scott, MD
- Rao, Harshit S., MD
- Santiago, Teodoro V., MD
- Sexauer, William Patrick, MD
- Trontell, Marie C., MD

Newark
- Hudgins, Joan Leonard, MD
- May, Richard Edward Jr., MD
- Migliore, Christina, MD
- Patrawalla, Amee Shirish, MD
- Seethamraju, Harish, MD

Newton
- Shah, Samir D., MD

Ocean
- Ali, Rana Y., MD
- Elsawaf, Mohamed Ashraf, MD

Old Bridge
- Dhakhwa, Raj B., MD
- Ratkalkar, Kishore, MD

Paramus
- Sakowitz, Arthur J., MD
- Sakowitz, Barry H., MD

Park Ridge
- Mendelowitz, Paul C., MD

Paterson
- Amoruso, Robert C., MD
- Khan, Muhammad Anees, MD

Phillipsburg
- Nar, Kishorkumar G., MD
- Nekoranik, Michael G., DO

Plainfield
- Jayaraj, Kasthuri E., MD

Pompton Lakes
- Penek, John A., MD

Rahway
- Carayannopoulos, Leonidas N., MD
- Yim, Frances D., MD

Ridgewood
- Barasch, Jeffrey P., MD
- Choy, Wanda Wai Ying, MD
- Suffin, Daniel Matthew, DO

River Edge
- Shin, Dongwuk, MD

Roselle Park
- Maglaras, Nicholas C., MD

Sea Girt
- Cunningham, Gregory J., MD

Secaucus
- Nahas, Ghassan, MD
- Patel, Manmohan A., MD

Sewell
- Becker, Jason M., DO
- Malik, Neveen A., DO

Shrewsbury
- Arlinghaus, Frank H. Jr., MD

Somers Point
- Cunanan, Manuel Salas, MD
- Del Re, Sallustio, MD

Somerset
- Lucas, Robin S., MD

Stratford
- Giudice, James C., DO
- Morley, Thomas F., DO
- Vasoya, Amita P., DO

Summit
- Kotecha, Nisha Suresh, MD
- Nahmias, Jeffrey S., MD

Toms River
- Das, Prabhat R., MD
- Joyce, Michael Walter, MD
- Kumar, Awani, MD

Physicians by Specialty and Town

Parikh,Jayesh K.,MD
Soliman,Alaaeldin A.,MD
Trenton
Asghar,Syed Amir,MD
Casty,Frank Eugene,MD
Frank,Marcella M.,DO
Gugnani,Manish K.,MD
Gushue,George F. Jr.,DO
Law,Kevin F.,MD
Vogel,David P.,MD
Turnersville
Agia,Gary A.,DO
Mongeau,Marc Thomas,DO
Schiers,Kelly Anne,DO
Wiley,Joan C.,DO
Union
Karpman,Jesse,MD
Miller,Jeffrey Adam,DO
Union City
Pinal,Jose,MD
Vineland
Sheetz,Maurice Saunders,MD
Voorhees
Hogue,Donna J.,DO
Wayne
Ismail,Medhat E.,MD
Rappaport,Liviu I.,MD
Wahba,Magdy A.,MD
Wardeh,Ghassan Louis,MD
West Orange
Green,Douglas S.,MD
Willingboro
Adams,Andrea Garcia,MD
Woodbury
Finkenstadt,Eric V.,MD
Rosenberg,Scott B.,MD

Radiation Oncology

Basking Ridge
Mann,Justin,MD
Sidebotham,Helen Lee,MD
Bayonne
Baron,Joseph,MD
Belleville
Blank,Kenneth Robert,MD
Borofsky,Karen Esther,MD
Devereux,Corinne K.,MD
Razdan,Dolly,MD
Berkeley Heights
Gabel,Molly Mary,MD
Bloomfield
Kagan,Eduard,MD
Brick
Kaufman,Nathan,MD
Miller,Douglas Andrew,MD
Camden
Ahlawat,Stuti,MD
Asbell,Sucha Order,MD
Dragun,Anthony E.,MD
Eastwick,Gary,MD
Henson,Clarissa F.,MD
Hughes,Lesley Ann,MD
Kramer,Noel Melitta,DO
Mezera,Megan A.,MD
Patel,Ashish Bharat,MD
Singh,Rachana,MD
Cape May Court House
Cassir,Jorge F.,MD
Cho,David Shen,MD
Meltzer,Jeffrey I.,MD
Wurzer,James C.,MD
Cherry Hill
Dicker,Adam P.,MD
Hirsh,Alina Z.,MD
Kornmehl,Carol,MD
Meritz,Keith A.,MD
Denville
Hajela,Durgesh,MD
Dover
Cann,Donald F.,MD
Edison
Trabold,Lucille A.,MD
Zarny,Steven David,MD
Egg Harbor Township
Wilson,Vasthi Christensen,MD
Englewood
Dubin,David M.,MD
Freehold
Cardinale,Robert Michael,MD
Chon,Brian Hisuk,MD
Soffen,Edward M.,MD

Tsai,Henry K.,MD
Hackensack
Godfrey,Loren,MD
Ingenito,Anthony C.,MD
Lewis,Brett Eric,MD
Hainesport
Butzbach,Deborah Ann,MD
Hamilton
Chalal,Jo Ann,MD
Jamesburg
Greenberg,Andrew Seth,MD
Jersey City
Shaiman,Alan,MD
Kendall Park
Flannery,Todd W.,MD
Fontanilla,Hiral P.,MD
Hug,Eugene Boris,MD
Rodrigues,Neesha Ann,MD
Lakewood
Berkowitz,Stewart A.,MD
Marchese,Michael J.,MD
Lawrenceville
Harvey,Arthur James,MD
Simone,Charles B.,MD
Livingston
Grann,Alison,MD
Long Branch
Sim,Sang Eui,MD
Weiss,Mitchell F.,MD
Manahawkin
D'Ambrosio,David Joseph,MD
Lattanzi,Joseph Paul,MD
Shah,Hemangini R.,DO
Marlton
Eastman,Ralph M.,MD
Medford
DeNittis,Albert Stephen,MD
Middletown
Shin,Jacob,MD
Yu,Yao,MD
Millville
Fanelle,Joseph W.,MD
Montclair
Barba,Jose P.,MD
Stabile,Richard J.,MD
Morristown
Goldberg,Yana Pavel,MD
Karim,Mona,MD
Oren,Reva,MD
Mount Holly
Ariaratnam,Lemuel S.,MD
Fife,Kelly D.,MD
Kim,Catherine Sun Joo,MD
Mount Laurel
Kubicek,Gregory John,MD
Neptune
Briggs,Jonathan Havens,MD
New Brunswick
Desai,Gopal Rao,MD
Goyal,Sharad,MD
Haffty,Bruce George,MD
Hathout,Lara,MD
Jabbour,Salma K.,MD
Khan,Atif Jalees,MD
Kim,Sung N.,MD
Mahmoud,Omar M.,MD
McKenna,Michael G.,MD
Motwani,Sabin B.,MD
Parikh,Dhwani R.,MD
Wallach,Jonathan Brett,MD
Weiner,Joseph Paul,MD
Newark
Cathcart,Charles S.,MD
Paramus
DeYoung,Chad M.,MD
Kole,Thomas Pedicino,MD
Wesson,Michael F.,MD
Paterson
Herskovic,Thomas M.,MD
Pereira,Michael J.,MD
Pennington
Chen,Timothy H.,MD
Williamson,Shirnett Karean,MD
Plainsboro
Baumann,John C.,MD
Fein,Douglas Allen,MD
Pomona
Dalzell,James G.,MD
Pompton Plains
Youssef,Ashraf Fouad Kam,MD

Rahway
Karp,Eric A.,MD
Red Bank
Danish,Adnan F.,MD
Patel,Priti S.,MD
Zhang,Mei,MD
Ridgewood
Greenblatt,David R.,MD
Kambam,Shravan R.,MD
Torrey,Margaret Jennings,MD
Saddle Brook
Williams,Perry Swintz,MD
Sewell
Cohen,Dane Ryan,MD
Horowitz,Carolyn J.,MD
Short Hills
Desai,Maheshwari M.,MD
Somerville
Braver,Joel Keith,MD
Sparta
Cole,Robert J.,MD
Lo,Kathy Kai Yee,MD
Summit
Emmolo,Joana S.,MD
Knee,Robert,MD
Schwartz,Louis E.,MD
Teaneck
Rosenbluth,Benjamin Dov,MD
Vialotti,Charles P. Jr.,MD
Toms River
Chang,Bong M.,MD
Coia,Lawrence R.,MD
Eggert,Bryan George,MD
Iyer,Rajesh V.,MD
Patel,Aruna Ghanshyambhai,MD
Totowa
Dawson,George Anthony,MD
Trenton
Freire,Jorge Efrain,MD
Tyerech,Sangeeta K.,MD
Vineland
Smith,Glenda Ruth,MD
Voorhees
Harvey,Alexis,MD
Wilson,John J.,MD
West Orange
Ivker,Robert Alan,DO
Whippany
Zablow,Andrew Ira,MD
Willingboro
Chandra,Anurag,MD
Horvick,David,MD
Lustig,Robert Allan,MD
Wallner,Paul E.,DO
Woodbury
Stambaugh,Michael D.,MD

Radiology

Absecon
Dauito,Ralph,MD
Avenel
Saniewski,Charles A.,MD
Bayonne
Castillo,Luciano Jr.,MD
Belleville
Fusco,Joseph M.,MD
Minn,Joon Hong,MD
Naiman,Jeffrey Todd,MD
Berkeley Heights
Berman,Erika Jacobs,MD
Dodge,Sarah Ann,MD
Lacz,Nicole Lynn,MD
McCormick,John Stuart,MD
Brick
Connors,Diane,MD
Feeney,Charlee Wallis,DO
Koven,Marshall B.,MD
Shomo,Marcia Rosenberg,MD
Camden
Articolo,Glenn Anthony,MD
Bobrow,Michael L.,MD
Brody,Joshua David,DO
Della Peruta,Joseph,MD
Jacoby,James Howard,MD
Kaplan,Carol Ellen,MD
Kerner,Sheldon P.,DO
Moss,Edward G.,MD
Scotti,Daniel M.,MD
Cedar Knolls
Goodman,Jonathan L.,DO

Cherry Hill
Barber,Locke W.,DO
Di Marcangelo,Mark T.,DO
Clifton
Doerr,John J.,MD
Clinton
Malzberg,Mark S.,MD
Roche,Kevin Joseph,MD
Denville
Mirza,Nadia M.,MD
Smith,Arvin P.,MD
Waran,Shantha P.,MD
Yu,Lawrence Sikyong,MD
East Brunswick
Banbahji,Salim,MD
Edwards,Teresa Michelle,MD
Freiberg,Evan,MD
Goldman,Jeffrey Philip,MD
Greer,Jeannete G.,MD
Jonna,Harsha R.,MD
Kadivar,Khadijeh,MD
Kotler,Stuart M.,MD
Lazzara,Elizabeth Wanda,MD
Leiman,Sher,MD
Levitt,Myron M.,MD
Li,Albert C.,MD
Nardi,Rebecca A.,MD
Nosher,John L.,MD
Platt,Marvin,MD
Prendergast,Nancy C.,MD
Salmieri,Karen Heather,MD
Samuel,Salim,MD
Simoes De Carvalho,Victor L.,MD
Stirling,Jeffrey E.,MD
Taylor,Christopher,MD
Tunc,Feza Sevket,MD
Uppal,Vijay L.,MD
Winchman,Heidi K.,MD
Zicherman,Barry A.,MD
East Orange
Zuback,Joseph R.,DO
Edison
George,Louis C.,MD
Egg Harbor Township
Gualtieri,Louis Robert,DO
Englewood
Goldfischer,Mindy A.,MD
Herman,Marc Arthur,MD
Juengst-Mitchell,Jannine,DO
Malde,Hiten Maganlal,MD
Mazzei,Elizabeth O'Connell,MD
Shapiro,Mark L.,MD
Vadde,Kavitha,MD
Fair Lawn
Bauer,Christel Janet,MD
Herbstman,Charles A.,MD
Hines,Patrick J.,MD
Moses,Stuart C.,MD
Flemington
Szikman,Howard Shawn,DO
Freehold
Friedenberg,Barry,MD
Hughes,Ann M.,MD
Mezzacappa,Peter M.,MD
Rich,Stanley E.,MD
Rondina,Carlo L.,MD
Rosenstein,Howard P.,MD
Galloway
Begleiter,David A.,MD
Falciani,Amerigo,DO
Frankel-Tiger,Robyn F.,MD
Friedman,Alan Stanley,MD
Gerhardt,William J.,MD
Glassberg,Robert M.,MD
Glick,Craig S.,MD
McManus,Stephen William,MD
Schmidling,Michael John,MD
Shakarshy,Jack,MD
Simpson,Alan J.,MD
Tiger,Eric Harvey,MD
Tran,Thomas Hien Dieu,MD
Vu,Hung Quoc,MD
Green Brook
Caravello,Anthony Joseph Jr.,DO
Katz,Barry Harmon,MD
Khurana,Pavan,MD
Lane,Elizabeth Lovinger,MD
Lazar,Eric B.,MD
Melville,Gordon E.,MD
Schwarz,Warrren,MD
Terry,Bernard,MD

Physicians by Specialty and Town

Radiology (cont)
Hackensack
- Budin, Joel A., MD
- Demeritt, John S. III, MD
- Gejerman, Glen, MD
- Kim, William J., MD
- Ong, Phat Vinh, MD
- Panush, David, MD
- Patel, Rita S., MD
- Virk, Jaskirat Singh, MD
- Weisel, Arthur S., MD

Haddonfield
- Lynch, Roberta M., MD

Hainesport
- Berinson, Howard S., MD
- Bonier, Bruce S., DO
- Brinton, Karen J., MD
- Koss, James C., MD
- Livstone, Barry J., MD
- Maravich, Nick Jr., MD
- Meltzer, Alfred D., MD
- Moore, Douglas B., MD
- Morgan, William A., MD
- Slawek, Joseph E., MD
- Spivak, Michael, DO
- Taormina, Vincent J., MD
- Tsai, Joseph C., MD
- Zeiberg, Andrew S., MD

Hamilton
- Dutka, Michael Vincent, MD
- Ezati, Omid, MD
- Mathews, Jeffrey John, MD
- Ostrum, Donald S., MD
- Plakyda, Derek J., MD
- Ross, William M., MD
- Weiser, Paul J., MD

Hoboken
- Berger, Mark J., MD
- Chang, Ming Z., MD
- Gould, Lawrence, MD
- Matari, Hussein M., MD

Jersey City
- Byk, Cheryl Jean, MD
- Tholany, Jason Joseph, MD

Kendall Park
- Schlesinger, Fred H., MD

Lakewood
- Dhillon-Acosta, Raminder Kaur, DO
- Patel, Bharat K., MD

Little Silver
- Wirtshafter, David Glenn, MD
- Wold, Robert E., MD

Livingston
- Kalisher, Lester, MD
- Sanders, Linda M., MD
- Sherman, Joyce, MD
- Wilson, David A., MD
- Zurlo, John V., MD

Long Branch
- McDonald, David William, MD
- Smuro, Daniel J., MD
- Stein, Irving H., DO

Lyndhurst
- Dikengil, Asim G., MD

Mercerville
- Callahan, James P., MD
- Collins, Robert S., MD
- Locastro, Rosemary H., MD
- Tufankjian, Dearon K., DO

Millburn
- Burak, Edward, MD
- Suarez, Norka J., MD

Millville
- Golestaneh, Fazlollah, MD

Montclair
- McFadden, Denise C., MD
- Ow, Cheng H., MD
- Quackenbush, Gail, MD

Morristown
- Hirsch, Martin A., MD

Mount Laurel
- Barry, Kevin P., MD

Mullica Hill
- Gianchandani, Deepa A., MD

Newark
- Aguirre, Frank J., MD
- Baker, Stephen R., MD
- Goldman, Alice Ruth, MD
- Hubbi, Basil, MD
- Kisza, Piotr Slawomir, MD

- Liu, Yiyan, MD
- Shah, Suken H., MD
- Wenokor, Cornelia B. C., MD

North Caldwell
- Vijayanathan, Thurairasa, MD

Nutley
- Denehy, Ann Smith, MD
- Khedkar, Mona S., MD

Oakhurst
- Ginsberg, Ferris, DO

Old Bridge
- Belani, Puneet B., MD

Oradell
- Emy, Margaret Yoko, MD
- Krugman, Robert L., MD
- Rakow, Joel I., MD

Parsippany
- Calhoun, Sean Keith, DO
- Cosentino, Mark O., MD
- Friedman, Paul Dean, DO
- Wynne, Peter J., MD

Paterson
- Aluri-Vallabhaneni, Bhanu Sri, MD
- Bontemps, Serge L., MD
- Danoff, Madelyn S., MD
- Hiremath, Vijay, MD

Ridgewood
- Levy, Lauren S., MD
- Seltzer, Lawrence G., MD
- Weinstock, Lisa R., MD

River Edge
- Liebling, Melissa Schubach, MD

Rochelle Park
- Conte, Stephen John, DO
- Galope, Roel Pangilinan, DO

Sewell
- Rosenthal, Richard Eugene, DO

Shrewsbury
- Shinde, Tejas Shashikant, MD

Somers Point
- Cooperman, Harry Alan, MD

Sparta
- Cordero, Orlando C., MD
- Skalla, Matthew T., MD

Stratford
- Goldstein, David Wayne, DO
- Principato, Robert, DO

Summit
- Werring, John Andrew, MD

Toms River
- Didie, William J., MD
- El Abidin, Mohammad Nazir Z., MD
- Gibbens, Douglas T., MD
- Khorrami, Parviz, MD
- Sankhla, Vijay R., MD
- Swidryk, John Paul, MD
- Tran, Duc T., MD

Trenton
- Montuori, James L., DO
- Rijsinghani, Paresh K., MD
- Schwartz, Eric Ian, MD
- Zafar, Ahsan U., MD

Turnersville
- Brodkin, Joshua S., MD
- Manning, Ana B., MD
- Oberlender, Susan B., MD
- Rosner, William Fredric, MD
- Schmucker, Linda N., MD

Union
- Kessler, Howard, MD

Vineland
- Bernardi, Bridget Dolores, DO
- Durrani, Muhammad I., MD
- Go, Ernesto B., MD
- Gomberg, Jacqueline S., MD
- Hauck, Robert Martin, MD
- Shah, Satish P., MD

Voorhees
- Bloor, James J., DO
- De Laurentis, Mark, MD
- Deshmukh, Kalpana S., MD
- Miller, David Haim, MD
- Mohsin, Jamil, MD
- Patel, Bhupendra M., MD
- Semmler, Helaina D., MD
- Shack, Evan Tyler, MD
- Shah, Tanmaya Chetan, MD

Waldwick
- Arams, Ronald S., MD
- Hai, Nabila, MD

- Lubat, Edward, MD
- Seigerman, Howard M., MD
- Smith, Jonathan, MD

Wall
- Di Paolo, Jeffrey C., MD
- Unterman, Michael I., MD

Warren
- Chandarana, Shashikant G., MD

Wayne
- Achaibar, Rajendra, MD
- Cortellino, Karen, MD
- Duhaney, Michael Owen, MD
- Lee, Joung Y., MD
- Steinberg, Michael L., MD
- Wheeler, Ralph B., MD

West Deptford
- Gilbert, Steven L., MD
- Patel, Jayeshkumar Balu, MD

West New York
- Baldonado, Ricardo T., MD

West Orange
- Shoenfeld, Richard B., MD
- Toder, Stephen Paul, MD
- Trivedi, Malti S., MD

Westfield
- Grosso-Rivas, Suejane, MD
- Matuozzi, William D., MD
- Rokhsar, Michael Howard, DO

Westwood
- Gingerelli, Frank, MD

Willingboro
- La Couture, Tamara A., MD

Reproductive Endocrinology
Basking Ridge
- Bohrer, Michael K., MD
- Costantini-Ferrando, Maria F., MD
- Drews, Michael Robert, MD
- Klimczak, Amber, MD
- Molinaro, Thomas Anthony, MD
- Morris, Jamie L., MD
- Rybak, Eli Asher, MD
- Yih, Melissa Christina, MD

Chester
- Dlugi, Alexander M., MD

Closter
- Segal, Thalia R., MD

Fair Lawn
- Rabin, Douglas S., MD

Hasbrouck Heights
- Cho, Michael Ming-Huei, MD
- McGovern, Peter G., MD
- Weiss, Gerson, MD

Hoboken
- Chen, Serena Homei, MD

Lawrenceville
- Derman, Seth G., MD

Marlton
- Kuzbari, Oumar, MD
- Skaf, Robert A., MD
- Van Deerlin, Peter G., MD
- Weissman, Lauren, MD

Millburn
- Birkenfeld, Arie, MD
- Onwubalili, Ndidiamaka, MD

Morristown
- Forman, Eric Jason, MD
- Maguire, Marcy Frances, MD
- Scott, Richard Thomas Jr., MD

Mount Laurel
- Amui, Jewel Naakarley, MD
- Check, Jerome H., MD

Newark
- Douglas, Nataki Celeste, MD
- Morelli, Sara S., MD

Paramus
- Greenseid, Keri Lee, MD

Voorhees
- Manara, Louis R., DO

West Orange
- Gulati, Rita, MD

Westwood
- Berin, Inna, MD

Research
Montville
- Kashanian, Franciska K., MD

Trenton
- Rohlf, Jane, MD

Rheumatology
Berkeley Heights
- Flowers, Shari Carla, MD
- Kennish, Lauren M., MD
- Lee, Linda K., MD
- Lieberman, Eric Steven, MD

Bloomfield
- Simon, Jonathan M., MD

Bridgewater
- Abdel-Megid, Ahmed Mahmoud, MD

Cedar Knolls
- Paxton, Laura Anne, MD
- Sebastian, Jodi Komoroski, MD

Clark
- Nucatola, Thomas R. Jr., MD

Clifton
- Albornoz, Louise A., MD
- Raklyar, Irina, MD

Dover
- Pare', Jeanne M., MD

East Brunswick
- Lichtbroun, Alan S., MD

Emerson
- Nes, Deana Teplitsky, DO
- Rosner, Steven M., MD

Englewood
- Griffiths, Shernett Olivine, MD

Fair Lawn
- Arbit, David Lewis, MD
- Barr, Jerome Ian, MD

Franklin Lakes
- Pandey, Rajesh Kumar, MD
- Zalkowitz, Alan, MD

Freehold
- Adenwalla, Humaira Naseem, MD
- Ghafoor, Sadia, DO
- Lumezanu, Elena Mihaela, MD

Hackensack
- Cappadona, James Louis, MD
- Collins, Melinda Jean, DO
- Kepecs, Gilbert, MD

Hamilton
- Gordon, Richard Dennis, MD
- Segal, Leigh G., MD
- Shah, Rehan A., MD

Lawrenceville
- Froncek, Michael Jude, MD

Livingston
- Chuzhin, Yelena, MD
- Ritter, Jill M., MD

Manahawkin
- Kumar, Ramesh, MD
- Kumar Shetty, Nagalakshmi A., MD

Maplewood
- Paolino, James S., MD

Mercerville
- Carney, Alexander S., MD

Midland Park
- Knee, C. Michael, MD
- Kopelman, Rima G., MD
- Leibowitz, Evan Howard, MD

Millburn
- Mesnard, William J., MD

Morristown
- Tratenberg, Mark Adam, DO
- Widman, David, MD

Neptune
- Alpert, Deborah R., MD
- Kuzyshyn, Halyna, MD
- Tang, Xiaoyin, MD

New Brunswick
- Pabolu, Sangeetha, MD
- Park, Kyle Yoonho, MD
- Schlesinger-Kamelgard, Naomi, MD
- Sloan, Victor S., MD

Newark
- Chu, Alice, MD
- Khianey, Reena, MD

Ocean
- Al Haj, Rany Samir, MD

Paramus
- Gross, Michael L., MD
- Wu, Dee Dee Yui, MD

Paterson
- Lahita, Robert George, MD

Phillipsburg
- Lee, Susan, MD

Princeton
- Chauhan, Naresh, MD

Goyal,Seema Agrawal,MD
Hunninghake,Leroy H.,MD
Patel,Anand,MD
Rahway
Rivera Curiba,Mary A.,MD
Ridgewood
Keller,Betty Sue,MD
Rockaway
Barth,Michael,MD
Secaucus
Gatla,Nandita,MD
Sewell
Singh,Vijay,MD
Somers Point
Brecher,Linda S.,DO
Halko,George J.,DO
Somerset
Tiku,Moti L.,MD
Sparta
Sarwar,Haroon,MD
Stratford
Adelizzi,Raymond A.,DO
Succasunna
Giangrasso,Thomas A.,MD
Summit
Greenberg,Jeffrey David,MD
Kramer,Neil,MD
Patel,Sheetal V.,MD
Rosenstein,Elliot D.,MD
Setty,Arathi Radhakrishna,MD
Teaneck
Miceli,James Gerard,MD
Silverberg,Miriam Shayna,MD
Tinton Falls
Wasser,Kenneth B.,MD
Toms River
Blumberg,Scott,MD
Salloum,Rafah,MD
Trenton
Capio,Christine Marie,MD
Union
Worth,David A.,MD
Xiong,Wen,MD
Voorhees
Abraham,Shawn George,MD
Evangelisto,Amy Marie,MD
Feinstein,David E.,DO
Han,Kwang Hoon,MD
Krommes,Janet Filemyr,MD
Loizidis,Giorgos,MD
Schuster,Michael Charles,MD
Silver,Arielle S.,MD
Traisak,Pamela,MD
West Orange
Cannarozzi,Nicholas A.,MD
Pai,Sneha,MD
Weinberger,Andrew Bruce,MD
Zaputowycz,Larysa,MD
West Paterson
Airood,Moumina,MD
Westfield
Pedra-Nobre,Manuela Gomes,MD
Woodbury
Moynihan,Eileen M.,MD

Shoulder Surgery
Mount Laurel
Sidor,Michael Louis,MD

Sleep Disorders Medicine
Cherry Hill
Roszkowski,Jennifer Rose,DO
Denville
Javed,Arshad,MD
Hamilton
Dupre,Callum Michael,DO
New Brunswick
Ekekwe,Ikemefula E.,MD
Princeton Junction
Aronsky,Amy J.,DO
West Long Branch
Davis,Matthew Jared,MD

Spinal Cord Injury Medicine
East Orange
Farag,Amanda S.,MD
Hackensack
Thomas,Kurt Florian P.,MD
West Orange
Lam,Mylan Ngoc,MD

Spinal Surgery
Berkeley Heights
Kupershtein,Ilya,MD
Chatham
Clark-Schoeb,James Scott,MD
Rieger,Kenneth J.,MD
Cliffside Park
Finnesey,Kevin Sean,MD
Eatontown
Donald,Gordon D. III,MD
Emerson
Ashraf,Nomaan,MD
Rhim,Richard Dongil,MD
Freehold
Goldberg,Grigory,MD
Glen Rock
Patel,Sujal P.,MD
Hackettstown
Salari,Behnam,DO
Lawrenceville
Tydings,John D.,MD
Morristown
Lowenstein,Jason E.,MD
Newark
Harris,Colin B.,MD
Old Bridge
Landa,Joshua,MD
Paramus
Hughes,Alexander Philip,MD
Red Bank
Husain,Qasim M.,MD
Rutherford
Rovner,Joshua Seth,MD
Summit
Hullinger,Heidi,MD
Wayne
Emami,Arash,MD
Mahmood,Faisal,MD
Sinha,Kumar Gautam,MD

Sports Medicine
Brick
Stamos,Bruce Dumont,MD
Bridgewater
Tucker,Kimberly Victoria,MD
Cherry Hill
Bartolozzi,Arthur Robert,MD
Closter
Parron,John Keckhut,MD
Deptford
Emanuele,William Anthony,DO
Edison
Kasim,Nader Q.,MD
Lane,Gregory J.,MD
Englewood
Bottiglieri,Thomas S.,DO
Deramo,David Michael,MD
Salzer,Richard L. Jr.,MD
Fair Lawn
Bassan,Matthew Evan,DO
Flemington
More,Robert C.,MD
Hackensack
Berman,Mark,MD
Longobardi,Raphael S.,MD
Meese,Michael Arthur,MD
Porter,David Alexander,MD
Hackettstown
Shamim,Rehan Syed,MD
Livingston
Cooper,Alan Edward,MD
Loch Arbour
Incremona,Brian R.,MD
Manalapan
Harrison,Andrew,MD
Marlboro
Weintraub,Steve L.,DO
Millburn
Levy,Andrew Stuart,MD
Richmond,Daniel B.,MD
Newton
Bradish,Glen Edward,MD
North Bergen
Galdi,Balazs,MD
Paramus
Savatsky,Gary J.,MD
Princeton
Palmer,Michael Alberto,MD
Randolph
Rubman,Marc H.,MD
Red Bank
Van Gelderen,Jeffrey Thomas,MD
Ridgewood
Pope,Ernest J.,MD
Robbinsville
Redlich,Adam Daniel,MD
Sicklerville
Taffet,Robert,MD
Somerset
Gatt,Charles J. Jr.,MD
Tinton Falls
Bade,Harry III,MD
Toms River
Alcid,Jess Gerald,MD
Blum,Karl Richard,MD
Union
Gordon,F. Kennedy,MD
Vineland
Dwyer,Thomas A.,MD
McAlpin,Fred III,DO
Silver,Seth M.,MD
Voorhees
Cornejo,Juan Carlos,DO
Ramprasad,Arjun,MD
Wall Township
Buckley,Patrick S.,MD
Wayne
Badri,Ahmad,DO
Festa,Anthony Nmi,MD
Scillia,Anthony James,MD
West Orange
Zornitzer,Matthew Howard,MD
Westfield
Shaw,Daniel A.,MD

Surgery (General)
Absecon
Del Rosario,Michael Patrick,MD
Atlantic City
Almendras,Nole E.,MD
Penaloza-Aranibar,Carlos G.,MD
Ryb,Gabriel E.,MD
Stidd,David A.,MD
Basking Ridge
Capko,Deborah M.,MD
Bayonne
Moszczynski,Zbigniew,MD
Simpson,Thomas E.,MD
Williams,Richard A.,MD
Zak,Madeline,DO
Belleville
Amirata,Edwin A.,MD
Bonitz,Joyce A.,MD
Brautigan,Robert Anthony,MD
Ruddy,Kathleen T.,MD
Berkeley
Bell,Robert Lawrence,MD
Berkeley Heights
Porbunderwala,Steven James,MD
Thumar,Adeep Bhaguanji,MD
Bloomfield
Colavita,Donato A.,MD
Narvaez,Guillermo Jr.,MD
Brick
Aquino,Rainier,MD
Becker,Stephen A.,MD
Bhandari,Tarun,MD
Cappadona,Charles Richard,MD
Cluley,Scott R.,MD
Houlis,Nicholas J.,DO
Huang,Kevin,MD
Kamath,Ashwin S.,MD
Kelly,Francis J.,MD
Kwon,Sung Wook,MD
Milazzo,Vincent J.,MD
Pahuja,Anil K.,MD
Priolo,Steven R.,MD
Tammaro,Yolanda Rose,MD
Yrad,Jonathan Proces Flores,MD
Zurkovsky,Eugene,MD
Bridgeton
Haq,Imran Ul,MD
Iqbal,Nauveed,MD
Bridgewater
Lue,Deborah A.,MD
Browns Mills
Burns,Paul Gerard,MD
Nicolato,Patricia A.,DO
Caldwell
Rosenberg,Victor I.,MD
Camden
Ahmad,Nadir,MD
Atabek,Umur M.,MD
Awad,Nadia Amal,MD
Barth,Nadine,MD
Bea,Vivian Jolley,MD
Bird,Dorothy Waterbury,MD
Bowen,Frank Winslow III,MD
Brill,Kristin Lynne,MD
Chopra,Vinod Kumar,MD
Duncan,Beth R.,MD
Fox,Nicole M.,MD
Goldenberg-Sandau,Anna,DO
Harris,William Matthew,MD
Hendershott,Karen Jean,MD
Hong,Young Ki,MD
Leese,Kenneth H.,MD
Lombardi,Joseph V.,MD
Mofid,Alireza,MD
O'Connell,Brendan Garrett,MD
Patel,Rohit Amratlal,MD
Radomski,John S.,MD
Reid,Lisa M.,MD
Remick,Kyle Norman,MD
Shersher,David Daniel,MD
Simons,Robert Mark,MD
Stanisce,Luke Thomas,MD
Wydo,Salina Marie,MD
Yocom,Steven S.,DO
Cape May Court House
Attiya,Rafael,MD
Falivena,Richard Peter,DO
Lawinski,Richard M.,MD
Martz,Patricia Ann,MD
Russo,David Peter,MD
Salasin,Robert I.,MD
Tenner,Jeffrey P.,DO
Cherry Hill
Acholonu,Emeka Joseph,MD
Bedi,Ashish,MD
Cohen,Larry W.,DO
Costabile,Joseph P.,MD
Fakulujo,Adeshola D.,MD
Franckle,William C. IV,MD
Iyer,Malini,MD
Llenado,Jeanne Valencia,DO
Meoli,Fredrick G.,DO
Meslin,Keith Phillip,MD
Neff,Marc A.,MD
Sandau,Roy Lee,DO
Sorokin,Evan Scott,MD
Szczurek,Linda J.,DO
Zaretsky,Craig Lawrence,MD
Zuniga,Joseph Michael R.,MD
Clifton
Hanan,Scott H.,MD
Kane,Edwin P.,MD
Silen,Ramon S.,MD
Vazquez,Franklyn,MD
Colonia
Tonzola,Anthony M.,MD
Demarest
Tadros,Mahfouz M.,MD
Denville
Cohen,Scott Allan,MD
Simon,Marc L.,DO
Suh,Matthew Yongwon,MD
Dover
Garrison,Jordan Milton,MD
East Brunswick
Bagner,Ronald J.,MD
Ramanadham,Smita R.,MD
East Orange
Craig,Gazelle A.,MD
Ducheine,Yvan D.,MD
Joseph,Romane,MD
Machiedo,George W.,MD
East Windsor
Dultz,Rachel Paula,MD
Eatontown
Binenbaum,Steven J.,MD
Borao,Frank J.,MD
Ciervo,Alfonso Clemente,MD
Hagopian,Ellen Joyce,MD
Kolakowski,Stephen Jr.,MD
Lopyan,Kevin S.,MD
Matharoo,Gurdeep Singh,MD
Edgewater
Foote,Holly Christine,DO

Physicians by Specialty and Town

Surgery (General) (cont)

Edison
Armour,Renee Palmyra,MD
Chaudry,Ghazali Anwar,MD
Choi,Stanley S.,MD
Chung Loy,Harold E.,MD
Dasmahapatra,Kumar S.,MD
El Mansoury,Hassan M.,MD
Ellman,Barry R.,MD
Encarnacion,Cirilo,MD
Green,Suzanne E.,MD
Henry,Ricki M.,MD
Ilut,Irina Claudia,MD
Itskovich,Alexander,MD
Lucking,Jonathan,MD
Neri,Linda M.,MD
Patel,Kirtikumar J.,MD
Penupatruni,Niranjan K.,MD
Pinsky,Abby Michele,MD
Sharma,Rajinder,MD
Swaminathan,Anangur P.,MD
Valane,Honora W.,MD
Wilkins,Kirsten Bass,MD

Egg Harbor Township
Brown,Anjeanette Tina,MD
Hon,David C.,MD
Salartash,Alimorad,MD

Elizabeth
Colaco,Rodolfo,MD
Kansagra,Ashwin Maganlal,MD
Mlynarczyk,Peter J.,MD
Zimmern,Andrea,MD

Elmwood Park
Sharma,Jyoti,MD

Englewood
Arnofsky,Adam Garett,MD
Bufalini,Bruno,MD
Cravioto-Vaimakis,Stefanie,MD
Morales-Ribeiro,Celines,MD
Shikiar,Steven Paul,MD
Srinivasan,McDonald T.,MD
Strain,Jeffrey Witt,MD

Englewood Cliffs
Yang,Hee Kon,MD

Fair Lawn
Becker,Steven I.,MD
Marta,Peter T.,DO

Fairfield
Funicello,Alex Vincent,MD

Flemington
Bello,John J.,MD
Bello,Joseph M.,MD
Gleason,Catherine Elizabeth,MD
Maeuser,Herman L.I.,MD

Florham Park
Abkin,Alexander,MD
Argiroff,Alexandra Louise,MD
Bertha,Nicholas A.,DO
Botvinov,Mikhail A.,DO
Carter,Mitchel S.,MD
Cuppari,Anthony L.,MD
Failey,Colin Leander,MD
Gabre,Kennedy Ogbazion,MD
Most,Michael David,MD

Fort Lee
Mashburn,Penelope,DO

Franklin Lakes
Fondacaro,Paul Francis,MD

Freehold
Ashok,Viswanath K.,MD
Kharod,Amit S.,MD
Martucci,Mary T.,DO
Menack,Michael J.,MD
Noyan,Earl Lincoln,MD
Schulman,William M.,MD
Shakov,Emil,MD
Sowemimo,Oluseun Akande,MD
Wetstein,Lewis,MD

Galloway
Kassis,Kamal F.,MD
Patel,Samir M.,MD

Garwood
Gupta,Amit,MD

Glen Ridge
Ballem,Naveen,MD
Barbalinardo,Robert J.,MD
Gohil,Kartik Narendra,MD
Matier,Brian,MD
Rainville,Harvey Charles,MD

Glen Rock
Ahlborn,Thomas N.,MD

Hackensack
Benson,Douglas N.,MD
Davidson,Marson Tunde,MD
Dayal,Saraswati Devi,MD
Ghodsi,Mohammad,MD
Greene,Tobi B.,MD
Hunter,James Blaine,MD
Kaul,Sanjeev Kumar,MD
Khosravi,Abtin Hajiloo,MD
Kline,Gary Michael,MD
Koo,Harry P.,MD
Locurto,John Jr.,MD
McCain,Donald Andrew,MD
Napolitano,Massimo M.,MD
Narins,Seth Craig,MD
Ng,Arthur F.,MD
Patel,Sruti,MD
Pereira,Stephen G.,MD
Perez,Javier Martin,MD
Pisarenko,Vadim,MD
Poole,John W.,MD
Richardson,Celine Anne,MD
Rosenstock,Adam Seth,MD
Smith,Adam Powell,MD
Thomas,Tina Theresa,MD
Warden,Mary Jane,MD
Wilderman,Michael Jeffrey,MD
Wong,Sarah,MD

Hackettstown
Campion,Thomas W.,MD
Gross,Eric L.,MD
Jabush,Jondavid H.,MD

Haddon Heights
Derr,Lisa M.,DO
Finnegan,Matthew J.,MD
Greenawald,Lawrence Edward,MD
Kakkilaya,Harish,MD
Merriam,Margaret,DO
Salcone,Mark Anthony,DO
Santos,Rodrigo R.,MD

Haddonfield
Hill,Robert B.,MD
Jankowski,Marcin Andrew,DO

Hainesport
Briones,Renato J.,MD

Hamburg
Dash,Sarat K.,MD

Hamilton
Goldenberg,Elie Adam,MD
Shah,Reza A.,DO
Vaswani,Vijay,MD

Harrington Park
Jensen,Michael Edward,MD

Hawthorne
Goel,Surendra P.,MD

Hazlet
Buker,Ibrahim S.,MD
Hernando,Franklin P.,MD

Highland Park
Curtiss,Steven Ian,MD
Tutela,Rocco Robert Jr.,MD

Hillsborough
Koota,David H.,MD

Hoboken
Costa,German H.,MD
Gonzalez,Juan A. Jr.,MD
Miller,Benetta L.,MD

Holmdel
Adeyeri,Ayotunde Olubukola,MD
Mansuri,Hanif M.,MD
Nguyen,Hung Q.,MD
Patel,Munjal P.,MD

Irvington
Alzadon,Ricardo,MD
Soriano,Jaime R.,MD

Iselin
Ramamurthy,Kotta M.,MD

Jersey City
Gor,Pradip D.,MD
Hanhan,Ziad George,MD
Kaiser,Susan,MD
Mapp,Samuel Eugene,MD
Moeller,Lavinia Paige,DO
Molino,Bruno,MD
Ottley,Anroy K.,MD
Raccuia,Joseph Salvatore,MD
Sagullo,Nestor M.,MD
Schrag,Sherwin Phan,MD

Kearny
Stylman,Jay Ira,MD

Lakewood
Georges,Renee N.,MD
Molina,Carlos Guillermo,DO

Lawrenceville
Alvarez,Enrique F.,MD

Linwood
Penso,Desiderio S.,MD
Waldor,Philip Arthur,MD

Livingston
Andrei,Valeriu E.,MD
Brown,Melanie Antonietta,MD
Chargualaf,Lisa Marie,MD
Geffner,Stuart R.,MD
Houng,Abraham Pohan,MD
Lemasters,Patrick Evan,MD
Majid,Saniea Fatima,MD
Paragi,Prakash Ramaiah,MD
Paul,Subroto,MD
Petrone,Sylvia J.,MD
Santoro,Elissa J.,MD
Schaefer,Sarah Stuart,MD
Smith,Franz Omar Desric,MD
Tutela,John Paul,MD
Weiswasser,Jonathan M.,MD

Long Branch
Cummings,Kenneth B.,MD
Ginalis,Ernest M.,MD
Goldfarb,Michael A.,MD
Roros,James Gus,MD

Lumberton
Boynton,Christopher J.,MD

Mahwah
Ganepola,Ganepola A.,MD

Manahawkin
Barbalinardo,Joseph P.,MD
Carson,Gregory B.,MD
Echeverri,Samuel David,MD
Fresco,Silvia,MD
Grachev,Sergey,MD
Greco,Richard Yackshaw,DO
Reich,Jonathan Makaloa,MD
Strom,Karl William,MD

Manalapan
Prokurat,Val,DO

Manasquan
Nagy,Michael William,MD

Maplewood
Bethel,Colin A. I.,MD

Marlton
O'Shea,Joan Frances,MD

Matawan
Arbour,Robert M.,MD
Fischer,Lauren Jane,MD

Mercerville
Sasportas,Jonathan Scott,MD

Merchantville
Aronow,Phillip Z.,MD

Millburn
Bilof,Michael Louis,MD
Kopelan,Adam Michael,MD
Yurcisin,Basil Michael II,MD

Mine Hill
Soda,Michael,MD

Moorestown
Kling,Maureen C.,MD
Sharma,Gaurav S.,MD

Morristown
Adams,John M.,MD
Agis,Harry,MD
Bickenbach,Kai Asa,MD
Bilaniuk,Jaroslaw W.,MD
Christoudias,Stavros George,MD
Di Fazio,Louis Thomas Jr.,MD
Elyash,Igor Gary,DO
Henseler,Roy A.,MD
Hernando,Michael T.,MD
Huang,Jianzhong,MD
James,Kevin V.,MD
Kannisto,Cheryl Lynne,MD
Lee,Thomas Y.,MD
Magovern,Christopher Jude,MD
Nusbaum,Michael Jay,MD
Ombrellino,Michael,MD
Pasquariello,James Veriniere,MD
Riaz,Omer Junaid,MD
Rolandelli,Rolando Hector,MD
Siegel,Brian Keith,MD
Slater,James P.,MD
Smith,Brian L.,MD
Sturt,Cindy,MD
Vasilakis,Vasileios,MD
Ward,David S.,MD
Whitman,Eric David,MD

Mount Laurel
Daugherty,Rhett L.,MD
Dube,Neerja,MD

Mullica Hill
Smeal,Brian C.,MD

Neptune
De Sarno,Carney Thomas,MD
Gorechlad,John W.,MD
Kipnis,Seth Michael,MD
Mueller,Lawrence Peter,MD
Shifrin,Alexander L.,MD
Sullivan,Michael C.,MD

New Brunswick
Baler,Carleton E.,MD
Bulauitan,Constantine S.,MD
Carpizo,Darren Richard,MD
Christian,Derick J.,MD
Corbett,Siobhan Alden,MD
Davidov,Tomer,MD
Ghisletta,Leslie C.,MD
Grandhi,Miral Sadaria,MD
Gupta,Rajan,MD
Haque,Maahir Ul,MD
Holman,Michael Jeffrey,MD
Jayakumar,Lalithapriya,MD
Kowzun,Maria Ji,MD
Langenfeld,John Eugene,MD
Laskow,David A.,MD
Lopez,Aurelia P.,MD
Masterson,Richard J.,MD
Mellender,Scott Jason,MD
Palder,Steven B.,MD
Pelletier,Ronald Paul,MD
Qudah,Yaqeen,MD
Schroeder,Mary E.,MD
Shan,Yizhi,MD
Shiroff,Adam Michael,MD
Sim,Vasiliy,MD
Sterling,Joshua,MD
Terlizzi,Joseph P.,MD
Tinti,Meredith Sarah,MD
Trooskin,Stanley Zachary,MD
Wise,Susannah S.,MD
Zavotsky,Jeffry,MD

Newark
Alli,Padmavathy,DO
Andrade,Peter,DO
Anjaria,Devashish Jayant,MD
Bale,Asha G.,MD
Berlin,Ana,MD
Chauhan,Niravkumar M.,MD
Clarke,Kevin O'Neil,MD
Galloway,Joseph,MD
Guarrera,James Vincent,MD
Huang,Joe T.,MD
Kalu,Ogori N.,MD
Koneru,Baburao,MD
Lovoulos,Constantinos John,MD
Malhotra,Sunil Prakash,MD
Malik,Rema,MD
Merchant,Aziz M.,MD
Miranda,Irving,MD
Mosenthal,Anne Charlotte,MD
Paskhover,Boris,MD
Sambol,Justin Todd,MD
Sardari,Frederic Fereydoun,MD
Tyrie,Leslie S.,MD
Wilson,Dorian J.,MD
Yepez,Humberto R.,MD

Newton
Harris,Ronald K.,MD
Nakhjo,Shomaf,DO
Newman,Brian F.,MD

North Bergen
Boucher,Gregory M.,DO
Shaknovsky,Thomas J.,DO

North Brunswick
Hermosilla,Elias P. Jr.,MD

Northfield
Kulkarni,Nandini N.,MD
May,David Peter,MD

Nutley
Mercogliano,Edward A.,MD

Oakhurst
Gornish,Aron L.,MD
Lin,Jeffrey M.,MD

Physicians by Specialty and Town

Schwartz,Mark Robert,MD
Oceanport
　Vozos,Frank J.,MD
Old Bridge
　Markov,Nikolai Yordanov,DO
Paramus
　Alshafie,Tarek Ahmed,MD
　Aydin,Nebil Bill,MD
　Bedrosian,Andrea Stephanie,MD
　Cummings,Dustin Randal,MD
　Dhorajia,Seema P.,DO
　Eid,Sebastian R.,MD
　Ewing,Douglas R.,MD
　Gandolfi,Brad Michael,MD
　Klein,Laura Ann,MD
　Mansson,Jonas,MD
　Trivedi,Amit,MD
Park Ridge
　Bonvicino,Nicholas G.,MD
Parsippany
　Peyser,Irving G.,MD
Passaic
　Chuback,John A.,MD
　Hanna,Gamal Kamel,MD
　Ukrainskyj,Motria O.,MD
Paterson
　Bordan,Dennis Lawrence,MD
　Budd,Daniel C.,MD
　Choi,Karmina,MD
　Dalal,Setu A.,DO
　Damani,Tanuja,MD
　Dela Torre,Andrew Nelson,MD
　Elrabie,Nazmi A.,MD
　Elsawy,Osama Ahmed,DO
　Ingram,Mark Anthony,MD
　Madlinger,Robert Vincent,DO
　Maio,Theodora J.,MD
　Warta,Melissa Hayward,MD
Pennington
　Allen,Lisa Rachel,MD
　Chung,Jooyeun,MD
　Dellacroce,Joseph Michael,MD
　Johnson,Steven A.,MD
　Mustafa,Rose,MD
　Rosato,Francis E.,MD
　Sailes,Frederick Cortney,MD
Penns Grove
　Vora,Nagindas M.,MD
Pequannock
　Gritsus,Vadim,MD
Perth Amboy
　Gabucan,Maximo B. Jr.,MD
Phillipsburg
　Abo,Marc N.,MD
　Chung,Hei Jin,MD
　Kjellberg,Sten I.,MD
　Rastogi,Vijay,MD
　Rohatgi,Chand,MD
Piscataway
　Barot,Prayag,MD
Plainsboro
　Brolin,Robert E.,MD
　Chau,Wai Yip Y.,MD
　Dhir,Nisha Solanki,MD
　Jordan,Lawrence Joseph III,MD
　Juha,Ramez,MD
　Roy,Rashmi,MD
　Smith,Liam R.,MD
Pleasantville
　Penso,S. Desiderio,MD
Pomona
　Grafilo,Antonio C.,MD
Pompton Lakes
　Feigenbaum,Howard,MD
Pompton Plains
　Azu,Michelle C.,MD
　Potter,Steven D.,MD
Princeton
　Berrizbeitia,Luis Daniel,MD
　Henry,Sharon M.,MD
　Kamath,Chandrakal Y.,MD
　Mehta,Vishal,MD
Rahway
　Sanchez,Hector J.,MD
Ramsey
　Licata,Joseph Jr.,MD
　Patel,Kumar R.,MD
　Pozzessere,Anthony Samuel,MD
Randolph
　Choung,Edward W.,MD

Hoffman,Michael J.,MD
Huang,Ih-Ping,MD
Meisner,Kenneth,MD
Red Bank
　Cugini,Donald A.,MD
　Greco,Gregory A.,DO
Ridgefield
　Egazarian,Marc M.,MD
Ridgewood
　Bernheim,Joshua William,MD
　Char,Daniel Jay,MD
　Di Saverio,Joseph,MD
　Patel,Mitul Suresh,MD
　Pucci,Anthony E.,DO
　Raman,Chidambaram,MD
　Rubinstein,Mitchell A.,MD
Runnemede
　Porter,Catherine M.,DO
Saddle Brook
　Kollar,John C.,DO
Salem
　Estella,Faustino F. Jr.,MD
　Patricelli,John E.,MD
　Timmerman,Lori D.,DO
Scotch Plains
　Tiedemann,Richard N.,MD
Secaucus
　Bridges,Kristen Leigh,MD
　Khani,Ghassan,MD
Sewell
　Careaga,Eduardo,MD
　Fantazzio,Michele Adrienne,MD
　Gillum,Diane,MD
　Monteith,Duane Richard,MD
　Morros,Jay Scott,MD
　Sasso,Michael J.,DO
Short Hills
　Ayyagari,Kamalakar R.,MD
Shrewsbury
　Abdollahi,Hamid,MD
　Ashraf,Azra Abida,MD
　Brock,James Steven,MD
　Cauda,Joseph E.,MD
　Chang,Eric I-Yun,MD
　Wimmers,Eric Geoffrey,MD
Somers Point
　D'Angelo-Donovan,Desiree D.,DO
　Feinberg,Gary L.,MD
　Galler,Leonard,MD
　Herrington,James William,MD
Somerset
　Ang,Brian Christopher Uy,MD
　Camerota,Andrew Martin,MD
　Donaire,Michael Jeremie,MD
　Gaspard,Henry Claude,MD
　Gervasoni,James Edmund Jr.,MD
　Hopkins,Lisa Anne,MD
　Melman,Lora Marie,MD
　Rondel,Mikhail,MD
Somerville
　Ambrose,Gunaseelan,MD
　Drascher,Gary A.,MD
　Seenivasan,Thangamani,MD
　Sugarmann,William M.,MD
South Plainfield
　Hobayan,Edgar R.,MD
Sparta
　Muduli,Hazari,MD
　O'Shea,Michelle T.,MD
Springfield
　Buwen,James P.,DO
　Coblentz,Malcolm Guy,MD
　Forrester,Glenn Joseph,MD
　Glasnapp,Angela Jack,MD
　Goyal,Ajay,MD
　Lopes,James M.,MD
　Montes,Leigh,MD
Stratford
　Arnold,Thomas Bradley,DO
　Balsama,Louis H.,DO
　Bruneau,Eve Solange,DO
　Iucci,Lisa Diane,DO
　Rosen,Marc Eliott,DO
Succasunna
　LePera,Michael S.,MD
Summit
　Di Gioia,Julia Marie,MD
　Lazar,Eric L.,MD
　Robinson,Andrew Tyler,MD
　Starker,Paul M.,MD

Yang,Rebecca Chaohua,MD
Teaneck
　Brinkmann,Erika M.,MD
　Christoudias,George C.,MD
　Fredericks,Duane A.,MD
　Kwon,Sung,MD
　Mendoza,Lynette Maria,DO
　Radvinsky,David,MD
　Shaffer,Liba C.,MD
　Zairis,Ignatios S.,MD
Tenafly
　Varma,Shubha,MD
Tinton Falls
　Chagares,Stephen Arthur,MD
　Dupree,David Joseph,MD
　Odujebe,Henry A.,MD
　Woodriffe,Philipa G.,MD
Toms River
　Krishnan,Mahadevan Gopa,MD
　Lowry,Steven James,MD
　Machiaverna,Frank E.,MD
　Matus,Victorino Managuit,MD
　Schneider,Barbara P.,MD
Totowa
　Farrell,Michael Louis,DO
Trenton
　Abud-Ortega,Alfredo Ramon,MD
　Ahmad,Sarfaraz,MD
　Cho,Kun H.,MD
　D'Amelio,Louis F.,MD
　Eboli,Dominick Joseph,MD
　Essa,Noorjehan,MD
　Fahrenbruch,Gretchen B.,MD
　Hanna,Niveen,MD
　Heether,Joseph J.,MD
　Kelly,Michael E.,DO
　Mahadass,Pavani,MD
　Poblete,Fredrick M.,MD
　Quinlan,Dennis Philip Jr.,MD
　Rojavin,Yuri,MD
　Saleem,Mohammed R.,MD
　Schell,Harold S. Jr.,MD
　Shah,Rajiv K.,MD
Union City
　Kofman,Igor,MD
　Purisima,Clementino O.,MD
　Santos Arias,Simon B.,MD
Verona
　Williams,Jeffrey Franklin,MD
Vineland
　Attia,Ahmed Farouk,DO
　Kaplin,Aviva Wallace,DO
　Kushnir,Leon,MD
　Montero-Pearson,Per M.,MD
　Nituica,Cristina Magadalena,MD
　Ogwudu,Ugochukwu Chinweze,MD
　Perry,Luke Daniel,DO
　Stephenson,Derek Allen,MD
Voorhees
　Butler,Charles J.,MD
　Empaynado,Edwin Abogado,MD
　Figueredo,Nicole Dionesia,MD
　Grabiak,Thomas A.,MD
　Hager,George W. III,MD
　Manigat,Yves J.,MD
　Perocho,Rodolfo R.,MD
　Revesz,Elizabeth,MD
　Sipio,James C.,MD
　Winter,Howard J.,MD
Wall
　Grayson,Leila S.,MD
　Kashlan,Bassam T.,MD
　Kazmi,Aasim,MD
　Kocsis,Cynthia A.,MD
　Schreiber,Martha L.,MD
Wayne
　Abessi,Hossein,MD
　Beniwal,Jagbir S.,MD
　Bernstein,Michael H.,MD
　Chin,Channing Yee,MD
　Garcia,Joseph,MD
　Guarino,Lawrence A.,MD
　Henson,Bernard,MD
　Moulayes,Nadra A.,DO
　Santos,Norman Verches,MD
　Teehan,Edwin P.,MD
Weehawken
　Mancheno,Mario A.,MD
West New York
　Gildengers,Jaime N.,MD
　Kulkarni,Vijaykumar A.,MD

West Orange
　Alves,Lennox,MD
　Khanna,Ashish,MD
　Maheshwari,Vivek,MD
　Peck,Richard E.,MD
　Singh,Manoj Kumar,MD
　Sultan,Ronald R.,MD
Westampton
　Kernizan,Eddy,MD
Westfield
　Bruno,Victor P.,MD
　Kumar,Mark Hemanth,MD
　Rutner,Torin W.,MD
Westwood
　Amin,Vishnubhai M.,MD
Willingboro
　Ing,Richard Daniel,MD
　Mukalian,Gregory G.,DO
　Schaller,Richard Vincent Jr.,MD
Woodbridge
　Constable,Richard E.,MD
Woodbury
　Erbicella,John Michael,MD
　Goldstein,Adam S.,DO
　Graves,Holly Lynn,MD
　Lynch,David J.,MD
　Mike,Joseph J.,MD
　Millili,John J.,MD
Woodcliff Lake
　Kordula,Charles E.,MD
Woodstown
　Lockwood,Curtis L.,DO

Surgical Critical Care
Atlantic City
　Dudick,Catherine A.,MD
　Willman,Kelly Marie,MD
Camden
　Axelrad,Alexander,MD
　Porter,John Maurice,MD
　Ross,Steven E.,MD
East Orange
　Tischler,Charles D.,MD
Gladstone
　Hammond,Jeffrey S.,MD
Hackensack
　O'Hara,Kathleen Patricia,MD
　Rippey,Kelly Ann,MD
　Stewart,Peter Jeremy,MD
Highland Park
　Wang,Ju Lin,MD
Jersey City
　Schrader,Patricia A.,MD
Little Silver
　Garcia-Perez,Felix A.,MD
Livingston
　Lee,Robin Ann,MD
　Mansour,Esber Hani,MD
Moorestown
　Wry,Philip C.,MD
Morristown
　Curran,Terrence,MD
　Kelly,Kathleen M.,MD
　McLean,Edward Jr.,MD
Neptune
　Ahmed,Nasim,MD
New Brunswick
　Gracias,Vicente H.,MD
　Hanna,Joseph S.,MD
　Lissauer,Matthew Eric,MD
　Peck,Gregory Lance,DO
Newark
　Bonne,Stephanie Lynn,MD
　Deitch,Edwin A.,MD
　Goulet,Nicole,MD
　Kunac,Anastasia,MD
　Livingston,David H.,MD
　Sifri,Ziad Charles,MD
　Venugopal,Roshni L.,MD
Paterson
　Zuberi,Jamshed A.,MD
Pennington
　Kalina,Michael,DO
Randolph
　Strutin,Millard D.,MD
Somerset
　Sadek,Ragui W.,MD
Springfield
　Lopes,Joao Alberto,MD
　Pepen,John Andre,MD

Physicians by Specialty and Town

Surgical Critical Care (cont)
Summit
  Mandel, Marc S., MD
  Rhodes, Stancie Christina, MD
Trenton
  Salem, Raja R., MD
Westfield
  Hurwitz, James Bennett, MD

Therapeutic Radiology
Edison
  Macher, Mark S., MD
Kendall Park
  Pepek, Joseph M., MD
Livingston
  Goodman, Robert Leon, MD
New Brunswick
  Cohler, Alan, MD
Somerville
  Bond, Laura R., MD

Thoracic Surgery
Berkeley Heights
  Lozner, Jerrold S., MD
Browns Mills
  Ross, Ronald E., MD
Camden
  Highbloom, Richard Yale, MD
  Rosenbloom, Michael, MD
Cherry Hill
  Davis, Paul K., MD
  Luciano, Pasquale A., DO
  Moffa, Salvatore M., MD
  Pascual, Rodolfo C., MD
  Villanueva, Dioscoro T., MD
Clifton
  Pontoriero, Michael Anthony, MD
Cranford
  Bolanowski, Paul J., MD
Eatontown
  Scalia, Peter D., MD
  Thompson, Robert M., MD
Edison
  Sarkaria, Jasbir S., MD
Englewood
  Loh, Chun Kyu, MD
Glen Ridge
  Holwitt, Kenneth N., MD
Hackensack
  Dudiy, Yuriy, MD
  Rizk, Nabil Pierre, MD
Hazlet
  Solis, P. Ariel, MD
Holmdel
  Surya, Girija S., MD
Livingston
  Reed, Mark K., MD
Long Branch
  Skylizard, Loki, MD
Manahawkin
  Lujan, Juan Jose, MD
  Samra, Matthew Samuel, DO
Moorestown
  DiPaola, Douglas Joseph, MD
  Heim, John A., MD
Morristown
  Brown, John Muir III, MD
  Greeley, Drew Peter, MD
  Neibart, Richard M., MD
  Polomsky, Marek, MD
  Steiner, Federico A., MD
  Widmann, Mark Dennis, MD
Neptune
  Dejene, Brook A., MD
  Johnson, David L., MD
New Brunswick
  Batsides, George Pete, MD
  Choi, Chun W., MD
  Ikegami, Hirohisa, MD
  Nishimura, Takashi, MD
  Spotnitz, Alan J., MD
Newark
  Camacho, Margarita T., MD
  Saunders, Craig Raymond, MD
  Shariati, Nazly M., MD
  Southgate, Theodore J., MD
Paramus
  Korst, Robert J., MD
  Shapiro, Mark, MD
Passaic
  Kaushik, Raj Ramanuj, MD
  Shakir, Huzaifa Abbas, MD
Paterson
  Cerda, Luis Mariano, MD
  Orejola, Wilmo C., MD
  Vega, Dennis, MD
  Wohler, Alexander M., MD
Pomona
  Dralle, James G., MD
Princeton
  Cole, Bruno N., MD
Ridgewood
  Brizzio, Mariano Ezequiel, MD
  Bronstein, Eric H., MD
  Majid, Naweed Kamran, MD
  Mindich, Bruce Paul, MD
  Zapolanski, Alex, MD
Salem
  Wolk, Larry A., MD
Sewell
  Steinberg, Jay Mitchell, DO
Skillman
  Yarramneni, Akhila, MD
Somerset
  Bocage, Jean P., MD
  Caccavale, Robert J., MD
South Orange
  Losman, Jacques G., MD
South Plainfield
  Breitbart, Gary B., MD
  Richmand, David M., MD
Trenton
  Laub, Glenn W., MD
  Shariff, Haji Mohammed, MD
Vineland
  Antinori, Charles H., MD
Voorhees
  Mascio, Christopher Edward, MD
West Orange
  Forman, Mark H., MD
  Zisis, Eletherios G., MD
Willingboro
  Greenbaum, David F., MD
Woodbury
  Villare, Robert C., MD

Transplant Surgery & Medicine
Camden
  Guy, Stephen Reed, MD
  Sebastian, Ely M., MD
  Youssef, Nasser Ibrahim, MD
Hackensack
  Melton, Larry B., MD
  Shapiro, Michael Eliot, MD
Livingston
  Aitchison, Samantha H., MD
  Sankary, Howard N., MD
  Sun, Harry, MD
Newark
  Brown, Lloyd Garth, MD
  Fisher, Adrian Alex, MD
Pennington
  Doria, Cataldo, MD
Pompton Plains
  Bakosi, Ebube A., MD

Trauma Surgery
Atlantic City
  Ali, Ayoola O., MD
Camden
  Burns, Richard Kent, MD
  Egodage, Tanya, MD
  Hazelton, Joshua Paul, DO
Edgewater
  Miglietta, Maurizio A., DO
Egg Harbor Township
  Rohani, Pejman, DO
Freehold
  Digiacomo, Jody Christopher, MD
Howell
  Moss, Vincent Lavaughn, MD
Jersey City
  Chaar, Mitchell Y., MD
  Ha, Victor Vinh, MD
Neptune
  Shin, Seung Hoon, MD
New Brunswick
  Butts, Christopher Alan, DO
  Teichman, Amanda Liane, MD
Newark
  Glass, Nina Elizabeth, MD
Paterson
  Bui, Hoan K., MD
South Plainfield
  Brahmbhatt, Ravikumar B., MD
Wayne
  Douyon, Erwin, MD

Ultrasound
Vineland
  Liu, Andrew Ky, MD

Undersea & Hyperbaric Medicine
Middletown
  Dornfeld, David B., DO

Urgent Care
Lawrenceville
  Diamond, Shari E., DO

Urogynecology
Long Branch
  Greco, Sandra Jeanne, MD
Princeton
  Van Raalte, Heather Michelle, MD
Ridgewood
  Sheiban, Tuti Fareen, MD
Voorhees
  Vakili, Babak, MD

Urological Surgery
Howell
  Moss, Vance Joshaun, MD
Lawrenceville
  Fingerman, Jarad Scott, DO

Urology
Avenel
  Yim, Simon D., MD
Bayonne
  Goldman, Gerald A., MD
  Katz, Herbert I., MD
  Kerr, Eric S., MD
Belleville
  Ciccone, Michael Paul, MD
  Ciccone, Patrick N., MD
  Delgaizo, Anthony, MD
Berkeley Heights
  Blitstein, Jeffrey, MD
  Siegal, John D., MD
  Volpe, Michael Anthony, MD
Bloomfield
  Caruso, Robert Peter, MD
  Franzoni, David Fred, MD
  Hsieh, Kuang-Yiao, MD
  Lombardo, Salvatore Antonio, MD
  Wu, David Sweghsien, MD
Bordentown
  Asroff, Scott Wayne, MD
  Goldlust, Robert W., MD
  Perzin, Adam Dean, MD
Brick
  Burzon, Daniel Todd, MD
  Chapman, John Robert, MD
  Fam, Mina, MD
  Kim, Chong M., MD
  Linn, Gary C., MD
  Mendoza, Pierre J., MD
  Simon, Andrew L., MD
Bridgeton
  Diaz, Jose F., MD
Camden
  Bernhard, Peter Howard, MD
  Krisch, Evan B., MD
  Marmar, Joel L., MD
  Seftel, Allen D., MD
  Tomaszewski, Jeffrey John, MD
Cedar Grove
  Agarwal, Saurabh, MD
Chatham
  Ulker Sarokhan, Erol E., MD
Cherry Hill
  Biester, Robert J., MD
  Chow, Shih-Han, MD
  Fallick, Mark Lawrence, MD
  Keeler, Louis L. III, MD
Cliffside Park
  Chun, Thomas Young, MD
  Klafter, George, MD
  Margolis, Eric Judd, MD
  Simon, Daniel Ross, MD
  Simon, Robert B., MD
  Wasserman, Gary D., MD
Clifton
  Greene, Tricia Danielle, MD
  Li, Sharon Mei-Mei, MD
  Marella, Venkata Koteswararao, MD
  Rice, Daniel A., MD
  Rosenberg, Joel W., MD
  Shahbandi, Matthew, MD
  Zinman, James Douglas, MD
Cranford
  Schwartz, Malcolm, MD
Denville
  Berman, Adam Jay, MD
  Bonder, Irvin Mark, MD
  Cubelli, Vincent, MD
  Friedman, Lawrence, MD
  Gellman, Alexander C., MD
  Ingber, Michael S., MD
  Ware, Steven M., MD
  Zimmerman, Gregg E., MD
Dunellen
  Chen, Samuel Kuangzong, MD
East Brunswick
  Feder, Marc T., MD
  White, Edward C., MD
East Orange
  Blumenfrucht, Marvin J., MD
  Gilhooly, Patricia Eileen, MD
  McGill, Winston Jr., MD
  Pollen, Jeffrey Jonah, MD
Eatontown
  Geltzeiler, Jules M., MD
  Keselman, Ira G., MD
  Waldman, Ilan, MD
Edgewater
  Pappas, Gregory A., MD
Edison
  Fand, Benjamin, MD
  Lasser, Michael Sidney, MD
  Lind, Eugene Jerome, MD
  Nakhoda, Zein Khozaim, MD
  Noh, Robert E., MD
  Patel, Arvind Mansukhlal, MD
  Patel, Rupa, MD
  Sherman, Neil David, MD
  Sinha, Binod K., MD
  Wein, Joshua Lewis, MD
Egg Harbor Township
  Scalera, John V., MD
Elizabeth
  Krieger, Alan P., MD
  Opell, M. Brett, MD
Elmer
  Read, John H., MD
Englewood
  Andronaco, Raymond B., MD
  Katz, Steven A., MD
  Kerns, John F., MD
  Lee, Chester C., MD
  Lee, Richard, MD
Englewood Cliffs
  Fermaglich, Matis A., MD
Fair Lawn
  Chang, David Tsuwei, MD
  Hajjar, John H., MD
  Howhannesian, Andranik, MD
Flemington
  Bloch, Paul Jacob, MD
  Choi, James, MD
  Ghosh, Propa, MD
  Kern, Allen J., MD
  Lai, Weil Ron, MD
  Sperling, Brian Lee, DO
Freehold
  De Salvo, Eugene L., MD
  Kohlberg, William I., MD
  Silverstein, Jeffrey I., MD
Galloway
  Slotoroff, Howard, MD
Hackensack
  Basralian, Kevin R., MD
  Degen, Michael Conrad, MD
  Fagelman, Elliot, MD
  Fagelman, Mark, MD
  Fromer, Debra Lynn, MD
  Glickman, Leonard, MD
  Kim, Michelle Joosun, MD
  Lowe, Daniel Robert, MD
  Munver, Ravi, MD
  Rosenberg, Gene S., MD
  Sadeghi Nejad, Hossein, MD
  Sawczuk, Ihor Steven, MD

Shin,David,MD
Hamilton
　Al-Qassab,Usama,MD
　Brackin,Phillip Snowden Jr.,MD
　Gazi,Mukaram A.,MD
　Gotesman,Alexander,MD
　Linder,Earle S.,MD
　Nazmy,Michael Jr.,MD
　Watson,John A.,MD
Harrison
　Rilli,Charles F.,MD
Hoboken
　Cricco,Carl F. Jr.,MD
Holmdel
　Antoun,Saad S.,MD
　Jow,William W.,MD
　Peardon,Nathaniel Andres,DO
　Rizkala,Emad Remond,MD
　Surya,Babu V.,MD
Iselin
　Husain,Aftab,MD
Jamesburg
　Richards,Steven Lawrence,MD
Jersey City
　Abramowitz,Joel,MD
　Hosay,John J. Jr.,MD
　Shah,Asha Dinesh,MD
　Shulman,Yale C.,MD
　Steigman,Elliot G.,MD
Lakewood
　Bellingham,Charles E.,MD
　Pandya,Kiritkumar M.,MD
　Tomaszewski,Charles S.,MD
Lawrenceville
　Cohen,Michael Scott,MD
　Freid,Russell Marc,MD
　Karlin,Gary S.,MD
　Trivedi,Deep B.,MD
Livingston
　Katz,Jeffrey I.,MD
　Walsh,Rhonda M.,MD
Manahawkin
　Fernicola,Charles P.,MD
Manasquan
　Howard,Michael Lawrence,MD
　Leitner,Robyn R.,MD
　Perlmutter,Mark Alan,MD
　Rotolo,James E.,MD
Marlton
　Mueller,Thomas John,MD
　Wargo,Heather Carol,MD
Maywood
　Ahmed,Mutahar,MD
　Christiano,Thomas R.,MD
　Esposito,Michael P.,MD
　Goldstein,Martin M.,MD
　La Salle,Michael Drew,MD
　Lanteri,Vincent J.,MD
　Lovallo,Gregory G.,MD
　Patel,Nitin Nick,MD
　Siegel,Andrew L.,MD
Midland Park
　Baum,Richard D.,MD
　DeTorres,Wayne Raymond,MD
　Frey,Howard L.,MD
　Hartanto,Victor H.,MD
　Mackey,Timothy Joseph,MD
Millburn
　Helfman,Alan S.,MD
　Shoengold,Stuart D.,MD
　Strumeyer,Alan D.,MD
Mine Hill
　Colton,Marc D.,MD
Monroe
　Lewis,Walter Emmett III,MD
　Lieberman,Alan Howard,MD
Morganville
　Kirshenbaum,Alexander,MD
　Sukkarieh,Troy Z.,MD
Morristown
　Ackerman,Anika Jahn,MD
　Atlas,Ian,MD
　Chaikin,David Craig,MD
　Israel,Arthur R.,MD
　Kaynan,Ayal Menashe,MD
　Pressler,Lee B.,MD
　Saypol,David C.,MD
　Steinberg,Joseph,MD
　Sutaria,Perry Maganlal,MD
　Taylor,David L.,MD

Mount Laurel
　Becker,Jeffrey M.,MD
　Berkman,Douglas S.,MD
　Niedrach,William L.,MD
Neptune
　Ebani,Jack E.,MD
　Tobin,Matthew Steven,MD
New Brunswick
　Davis,Rachel B.,MD
　Elsamra,Sammy E.,MD
　Faiena,Izak,MD
　Goldsmith,Joel W.,MD
　Jang,Thomas Lee,MD
　Kim,Isaac Yi,MD
　Olweny,Ephrem Odoy,MD
　Parihar,Jaspreet Singh,MD
　Singer,Eric Alan,MD
　Tunuguntla,Hari Siva Gurun,MD
Newark
　Hinds,Peter R.,MD
　Rosario,Imani Jackson,MD
　Watson,Richard A.,MD
Newton
　Collini,William R.,MD
North Bergen
　Stedman,Martin J.,MD
North Brunswick
　Ioffreda,Richard E.,MD
　Rodriguez,Ramon Elias,MD
Old Bridge
　Cha,Doh Yoon,MD
　Pagano,Matthew J.,MD
Oradell
　Garden,Richard J.,MD
　Zoretic,Stephen N.,MD
Orange
　Johnson,George A.,MD
Palisades Park
　Park,Ji Hae,MD
Paramus
　Campo,Richard Paul,MD
　Lebovitch,Steve,MD
　Panossian,Alexander M.,MD
　Rome,Sergey,MD
　Vitenson,Jack H.,MD
Paterson
　Awad,Safwat M.,MD
Pennington
　Orland,Steven M.,MD
　Rogers,Brad S.,MD
Pennsville
　Qureshi,Shaukat M.,MD
Phillipsburg
　Antario,Joseph Michael,MD
　Margolis,Franklin I.,MD
Princeton
　Goldfarb,Sidney J.,MD
　Latzko,Karen Marie,DO
　Pickens,Robert L.,MD
　Rossman,Barry R.,MD
　Schwarzman,Marc I.,MD
　Vasselli,Anthony J.,MD
　Vukasin,Alexander P.,MD
　Wedmid,Alexei,MD
Rahway
　Morrow,Franklin A.,MD
Ridgewood
　Rosen,Jay S.,MD
Rockaway
　Moazami,Saman,MD
Roseland
　Di Trolio,Joseph V.,MD
Saddle Brook
　Sullivan,Edwin J.,DO
Salem
　Diamond,Stuart M.,MD
Secaucus
　DiBella,Louis J. Jr.,MD
　Mouded,Issam,MD
　Tanzer,Ira D.,MD
Sewell
　Barsky,Robert I.,DO
　Brown,Gordon Andrew,DO
　Pietras,Jerome R.,DO
　Steckler,Robert E.,MD
Shrewsbury
　Bickerton,Michael W.,MD
　Bonitz,Robert Paul Jr.,MD
　Christiano,Arthur Patrick,MD
　Rose,John G.,MD

　Smith,Robert Charles,MD
Somers Point
　Axilrod,Andrew Charles,MD
　Bernal,Raymond Mark,MD
　Braga,Gene J.,MD
　Ciceron,Andre,MD
　Hirsh,Andrew L.,MD
　Kimmel,Barry S.,MD
　Pagnani,Alexander M.,MD
　Spence,Abraham M.,MD
　Wixted,William M.,MD
Somerset
　Bhatti,Mohammad Azeem,MD
Somerville
　Catanese,Anthony J.,MD
　Dave,Dhiren Sirish,MD
　Feldman,Arthur E.,MD
　Fischer,Joel M.,MD
　Harmon,Keith Andrew,MD
　Shah,Neel Praful,MD
Sparta
　Hall,Matthew Scott,MD
　Matteson,James R.,MD
　Mykulak,Donald J.,MD
　Salvatore,Frank Timothy,MD
Stratford
　Panuganti,Sravan,DO
　Syed,Kirin K.,DO
　Thatcher,Jacob Bryce,DO
Succasunna
　Stone,Chester I.,MD
Summit
　Gianis,John Thomas Jr.,MD
　Gianis,Thomas J.,MD
　Seidman,Barry R.,MD
Teaneck
　Parra,Raul O.,MD
　Scheuch,John R.,MD
Toms River
　Ferlise,Victor J.,MD
　Hartanowicz,Stanley J.,MD
　Howard,Peter Carson,MD
　Mahmood,Parvez,MD
　Schor,Martin J.,MD
　Stoneham,John L. III,MD
Trenton
　Rivas,Manuel A.,MD
　Srapyan,Aram,MD
Union City
　Cacace,Cataldo P.,MD
Verona
　Saidi,James Ali,MD
　Walmsley,Konstantin,MD
Vineland
　Dorsey,Philip J. Jr.,MD
　Federici,Peter J.,MD
　Kasturi,Sanjay Srinivas,MD
　Lee,Christopher Sang Don,MD
　Slavick,Harris D.,MD
Voorhees
　Ackerman,Randy B.,MD
　Balsara,Zarine Rohinton,MD
　Bernstein,Michael R.,MD
　Bloch,Jay L.,MD
　Butani,Rajen P.,MD
　Goldenberg,Samuel F.,MD
　Gor,Ronak,DO
　Linden,Robert Andor,MD
　Nachmann,Marcella Marie,DO
　Orth,Charles Richard Jr.,MD
　Sussman,David O.,DO
　Thur,Paul C.,MD
Wallington
　Rozdeba,Joseph,MD
Wayne
　Firoozi,Tahmoures,MD
　Gmyrek,Glenn A.,MD
　Knoll,Abraham,MD
　Levine,Seth Peter,MD
　Rezvani,Abas,MD
West New York
　Roblejo,Pedro G.,MD
West Orange
　Egan,Sean Christopher,MD
　Frank,Ronald Gary,MD
　Galdieri,Louis C.,MD
　Hanna,Moneer K.,MD
　Lefkon,Bruce W.,MD
　Savatta,Domenico James,MD
　Seaman,Eric K.,MD
　Strauss,Bernard S.,MD

Physicians by Specialty and Town

　Whang,Matthew I.S.,MD
　Youngren,Kjell A.,MD
Westfield
　Bernstein,Andrew Jay,MD
　Cohen,Joel S.,MD
　Fiske,Joshua Michael,MD
　Lehrhoff,Bernard J.,MD
　Mass,Alon Y.,MD
　Miller,Mark I.,MD
　Ring,Kenneth S.,MD
　Talavera,Jose Galang,MD
Woodbury
　Ebert,Karl H.,MD
　Kotler,Mitchell N.,MD
Woodcliff Lake
　Berdini,Jeffrey L.,MD

Vascular & Interventional Radiology

Brick
　Skrzypczak,Jan L.,MD
Camden
　Akinyemi,Michael Omobolaji,MD
　Broudy,Joseph Benjamin,MD
　De Cotiis,Dan A.,MD
Cherry Hill
　Snyder,Randall William III,MD
East Brunswick
　Gendel,Vyacheslav,MD
　Gribbin,Christopher E.,MD
　Lakritz,Philip Shev,MD
Edison
　Freeman,Hank Jason,MD
　Kumar,Moses,MD
Flemington
　Cortes,Andrew,MD
Freehold
　Patil,Vivek Vinay,MD
Galloway
　Kim,Christopher E.,MD
Guttenberg
　Epstein,Steven Brian,MD
Hamilton
　Brown,Michele Susan,MD
　Burda,John F.,MD
　Pryluck,David Scott,MD
Hoboken
　Barone,Allison,MD
Jersey City
　Menon,Sujoy,MD
Little Falls
　Koh,Elsie,MD
Livingston
　Richmond,John Steven,MD
Long Branch
　Schiff,Robert Michael,MD
Mays Landing
　Hollander,Scott Craig,DO
Moorestown
　Bianco,Brian A.,DO
Mount Laurel
　Svigals,Paul J.,MD
Neptune
　Biswal,Rajiv,MD
Newark
　Achakzai,Basit Khan,MD
　Amuluru,Krishna,MD
Northfield
　Feng,David H.,MD
Princeton
　De Sanctis,Julia Tucker,MD
　Parker,William Andrew,MD
　Youmans,David Carey,MD
Somers Point
　Schwartz,Jay Harris,MD
Summit
　Bhatti,Waseem Alam,MD
Teaneck
　Gallo,Vincent,MD
Toms River
　Moran,Christopher John,MD
　Perosi,Nicholas Anthony,MD
Trenton
　Hoppenfeld,Brad M.,MD
　McGuckin,James Frederick Jr.,MD
　Srinivas,Abhishek,MD
Voorhees
　Doshi,Nilesh M.,MD

Physicians by Specialty and Town

Vascular & Interventional Radiology (cont)
Wayne
  Festa,Steven,MD
West Orange
  Soto,David Rodolfo,MD

Vascular Disease
Margate City
  Steinberg,Joel S.,MD
Union
  Feldman,Jeffrey N.,MD

Vascular Neurology
Atlantic City
  Guterman,Jonathan Glenn,MD
Hasbrouck Heights
  Turkel-Parrella,David,MD
New Brunswick
  Paolucci,Ugo,MD
  Rybinnik,Igor,MD
Pennington
  Kumar,Rajat,MD
  Naragum,Varun,MD
Summit
  Hanna,John M.,MD

Vascular Surgery
Atlantic City
  Thompson,Peter N.,MD
Belmar
  Frasco,Franklin J.,MD
Berkeley Heights
  Nitzberg,Richard S.,MD
Brick
  Chu,Tun S.,MD
  Jain,Vikalp,MD
  Kaufman,Jarrod Peter,MD
  Sharp,Frank J. III,MD
Bridgeton
  Khan,Aftab A.,MD
Browns Mills
  Chang,Kane L.,MD
  Kamath,Vijay,MD
  Palkar,Vikram,DO
Camden
  Alexander,James B.,MD
  Trani,Jose Luis,MD
Cape May Court House
  O'Donnell,Paul Lawrence,DO
  Sabnis,Vinayak M.,MD
Cedar Grove
  Watson,Marc C.,MD
Cherry Hill
  Andrew,Constantine T.,MD
  Bak,Yury,DO
  Field,Charles K.,MD
  Spence,Richard Kevin,MD
Clifton
  Baratta,Joseph B.,MD
  Bobila,Alexis C.,MD
  Holmes,Raymond Joseph,MD
  Levison,Jonathan Andrew,MD
  Nackman,Gary B.,MD
Egg Harbor Township
  Frost,James H.,MD
  Lorenzetti,John D.,MD
  Previti,Francis W.,MD
Elizabeth
  Geuder,James W.,MD
  Moss,Charles M.,MD
  Tsai,Jung-Tsung,MD
Englewood
  Bernik,Thomas R.,MD
  Fried,Kenneth S.,MD
  Impeduglia,Theresa Maria,MD
  Kahn,Mark Elliot,MD
  Sussman,Barry C.,MD
  Wengerter,Kurt Richard,MD
  Wolodiger,Fred A.,MD
Fair Lawn
  Bapineedu,Kuchipudi,MD
Florham Park
  Seaver,Philip Jr.,MD
Freehold
  Kovacs,Gabor,MD
  Lehman,Mark,MD
  Silvers,Lawrence W.,MD
Garfield
  Tuzzeo,Salvatore T.,MD
Glen Ridge
  Ballem,Ramamohana V.,MD
Hackensack
  Forcina,Salvatore John,MD
  Kagan,Peter Evan,MD
  Keys,Roger C.,MD
  Kline,Roxana Gabriela,MD
  Manno,Joseph,MD
  O'Connor,David John,MD
  Ratnathicam,Anjali,DO
  Simonian,Gregory T.,MD
Hackettstown
  Itani,Mazen S.,MD
  Rupani,Bobby Jawahar,MD
Haddon Heights
  Di Fiore,Richard,MD
Hainesport
  Barnes,Thomas L.,MD
  Bobila,Wilbur C.,MD
Highland Park
  Finkelstein,Norman M.,MD
  Rosen,Scott Farrell,MD
Hillsborough
  Buch,Edward D.,MD
  Goldson,Howard J.,MD
Hoboken
  Steiner,Zachary John,DO
Jersey City
  Chan,Florence Y.,MD
  Khawaja,Aftab A.,MD
  McGovern,Patrick Jr.,MD
  Popovich,Joseph F.,MD
  Taha,Salah H.,MD
Lakewood
  Shamash,Felix S.,MD
Livingston
  Fletcher,H. Stephen,MD
Long Branch
  Constantinopoulos,George S.,MD
Manahawkin
  Hager,Jeffrey C.,DO
  Lengel,Gary P.,MD
  Penrod,Carey Lynn,DO
Maplewood
  Dick,Leon S.,MD
Middletown
  Pennycooke,Owano M.,MD
Millburn
  Addis,Michael Downes,MD
  Manicone,John A.,MD
Monroe Township
  Franco,Charles D.,MD
  Tripathi,Tushar Mahesh,MD
Montvale
  Sherman,Mark David,MD
Morristown
  Edoga,John K.,MD
  Kabnick,Lowell Stuart,MD
  Moritz,Mark William,MD
  Patel,Amit V.,MD
  Resnikoff,Michael,MD
  Tulsyan,Nirman,MD
Neptune
  Khan,Habib,MD
  Nasir Khan,Mohammad Usman,MD
New Brunswick
  Beckerman,William,MD
  Cha,Andrew,DO
  Crowley,John G.,MD
  Rahimi,Saum Amir,MD
  Rao,Niranjan V.,MD
  Shafritz,Randy,MD
Newark
  Curi,Michael A.,MD
  Dhadwal,Ajay Kapoor,MD
  Jamil,Zafar,MD
  Padberg,Frank Thomas Jr.,MD
  Sagarwala,Adam,DO
  Wu,Timothy,MD
North Bergen
  Davis,Jason Evan,MD
Paramus
  Danks,John Michael,MD
Paterson
  Tello Valcarcel,Carlos A.,MD
Pennington
  Eisenberg,Joshua Aaron,MD
  Fares,Louis G. II,MD
Plainsboro
  Goldman,Kenneth A.,MD
  Sambol,Elliot Brett,MD
Roselle Park
  Cordero,Pedro E.,MD
Somers Point
  Gosin,Jeffrey Stuart,MD
  Nahas,Frederick J.,MD
Somerset
  Deak,Steven T.,MD
Somerville
  Imegwu,Obi J.,MD
South Plainfield
  Wong,Geoffrey,MD
Toms River
  Berger,Howard M.,MD
  Haque,Shahid N.,MD
  Kedersha,Thomas A.,MD
  Ramnauth,Subhash C.,MD
Trenton
  Brotman-O'Neill,Alissa Sue,DO
  Poblete,Honesto Madjus,MD
Vineland
  Kumar,Sanjay,MD
  O'Donnell,John C. Jr.,MD
Voorhees
  Dietzek,Charles L.,DO
  Fisher,Frederick S.,MD
West Orange
  Hertz,Steven M.,MD
Westfield
  Cuadra,Salvador Alejandro,MD
  Rezayat,Combiz,MD
  Sales,Clifford M.,MD
  Sundick,Scott Adam,MD
Westwood
  Nalbandian,Matthew Martin,MD
Willingboro
  Baskies,Arnold M.,MD
  Holaday,William J.,MD
  Ruvolo,Louis S.,MD
  Wasser,Samuel H.,MD
Woodbury
  Haas,Kent Steven,MD
  Pilla,Timothy S.,MD

Vitreous and Retina
Moorestown
  Colucciello,Michael,MD
Toms River
  Amin,Haris Irfan,MD

Groups and Clinics by Town with Physician Rosters

Physician Rosters of Groups and Clinics by Town and Facility Name

New Jersey
Section 4

Physician Rosters of Groups and Clinics by Town and Facility Name

Groups and Clinics by Town with Physician Rosters

Absecon
Diego M. Fiorentino DO FACP
200 South New Road/Suite 1 Zip: 08201
Ph: (609) 641-2062 Fax: (609) 641-4633
- Fiorentino,Diego M., DO

Shoreline Endocrine and Medical Associ
707 White Horse Pike/Suite C1 Zip: 08201
Ph: (609) 813-2200 Fax: (609) 813-2201
- Catalina,Gabriel Richard, DO
- Driscoll,Eric Joseph, DO

Andover
Premier Health Associates
272 Route 206 North Zip: 07821
Ph: (973) 347-2273 Fax: (973) 729-3238
- Medunick,Sara Elizabeth, DO
- Reilly,Melissa Lynn, DO

Asbury Park
Drs. Sell and Baxi
507 4th Avenue Zip: 07712
Ph: (732) 774-5600
- Baxi,Nilay Manojkumar, MD

Eye Diagnostic Center
3333 Fairmont Avenue Zip: 07712
Ph: (732) 988-4000 Fax: (732) 988-9502
- Berg,Bruce R., MD
- Chiang,Peter Keh-dah, MD
- Pardon,Ilene B., MD
- Talansky,Marvin L., MD
- Turtel,Lawrence S., MD

Meridian Medical Group
514 Bangs Avenue Zip: 07712
Ph: (732) 774-0200 Fax: (732) 774-1019
- Herron,Garland Ella, MD
- Lore,Kristen Nicole, DO

Atlantic City
Absecon Island Ctrs for Women's Health
4401 Ventnor Avenue Zip: 08401
Ph: (609) 345-2050 Fax: (609) 345-2052
- De Stefano,Joseph L., MD
- Regis,Jon M., MD

AtlantiCare Ambulatory IM Clinic
1401 Atlantic Avenue Zip: 08401
Ph: (609) 441-8036 Fax: (609) 572-6021
- Mazur,Kimberly L., MD
- Timms,Brian Daniel, DO

AtlantiCare Clinical Associates
16 South Ohio Avenue Zip: 08401
Ph: (609) 441-2104
- Barzaga,Ricardo A., MD
- Momodu,Inua Aitsekegbe, MD
- Pericles,John T., DO
- Sun,Qi, MD

AtlantiCare Hospitalist Program
1925 Pacific Avenue/8th Floor Zip: 08401
Ph: (609) 345-4000
- Abella-Ramirez,Katherine, MD
- Ahmad,Naheed Kaleem, MD
- Dhaliwal,Harleen, MD
- Ghetia,Ditina, MD
- Hocbo,Aileen Aileen, MD
- Huma,Sabahath, MD
- Iqbal,Javid, MD
- Isaacson,Brian Eric, MD
- Jaleel,Syed, MD
- Kelly,Brendan S., DO
- Lal,Vikram, DO
- Narula,Navjot Singh, MD
- Nwotite,Ezinne Ugochi, MD
- Parikh,Hiren B., MD
- Patel,Hasitkumar D., MD
- Patel,Mehul Kumar, MD
- Rahmani,Ghulam Ali, MD
- Seibert,Henry Edward, MD
- Siddiqui,Durdana Aamir, MD
- Sohaib,Muhammad, MD
- Tusheva,Marija, MD

Atlantic Health Center P.C.
2300 Atlantic Avenue/Suite 1 Zip: 08401
Ph: (609) 345-9100
- Patel,Jitendra K., MD

Atlanticare Special Care Center
1401 Atlantic Avenue/Suite 2500 Zip: 08401
Ph: (609) 572-8800
- Alexander,Mark P., MD
- Castro-Chevere,Nancy Ann, MD
- Keiner,Lisa R., DO
- Lopez Bernard,Edwin, MD

Drs. Vijayakumar and Raman
1801 Atlantic Avenue/3rd Floor Zip: 08401
Ph: (609) 570-2400 Fax: (609) 441-7207
- Raman,Anoop Manikarnika, MD
- Vijayakumar,Ashvin, MD

Health Med Associates, PC
24 South Carolina Avenue Zip: 08401
Ph: (609) 345-6000 Fax: (609) 345-2885
- Delice,Anael Destin Jr., DO
- Patel,Arvind Kumar, MD

Reliance Medical Group, LLC
1325 Baltic Avenue Zip: 08401
Ph: (609) 441-0723 Fax: (609) 441-0953
- Corrales,Michelle D., MD

Southern Jersey Family Medical Center
1301 Atlantic Avenue Zip: 08401
Ph: (609) 572-0000 Fax: (609) 572-0039
- Collins,Gregory C., MD
- Irvis,Kenneth M., MD
- Quinlan,Liliane Bastos, MD
- Rodriguez,Marlene V., MD
- Toliver,Tiffany Elizabeth Marie, M

Atlantic Highlands
The American Skin and Cancer Center
25 First Avenue/Suite 113 Zip: 07716
Ph: (732) 872-2007
- Thosani,Maya K., MD

Audubon
Bromley Neurology, P.C.
739 South White Horse Pike/Suite 1 Zip: 08106
Ph: (856) 546-2300 Fax: (856) 546-2301
- Sen Hightower,Indrani, MD

Avenel
Bayonne Medical Care LLC
415 Avenel Street/Suite A Zip: 07001
Ph: (732) 750-1180 Fax: (732) 750-1182
- Basit,Nauman A., MD
- Siddique,Muhammad Neaman, MD

Gregory Shypula MD PA
1030 St. Georges Avenue/Suite 307 Zip: 07001
Ph: (732) 750-1200 Fax: (732) 602-4044
- Kulper,Bernard J., MD
- Shypula,Gregory J., MD

Stuart Homer and Associates, PA
1030 Saint Georges Avenue/Suite 201 Zip: 07001
Ph: (732) 602-0244 Fax: (732) 602-2577
- Homer,Stuart M., MD
- Romano,David L., MD

Barnegat
Cedar Bridge Pediatrics
249 South Main Street/Suite 2 Zip: 08005
Ph: (609) 607-1010 Fax: (609) 607-9992
- Czar,Elizabeth Erin, DO
- Feldman,Kira, MD

Basking Ridge
Basking Ridge Pediatric Association
150 North Finley Avenue Zip: 07920
Ph: (908) 766-4660 Fax: (908) 204-9871
- Coyne,Christine Ann, MD
- Kohn,Jocelyn Cramer, MD
- Porter,Thomas G., MD
- Wu,Peywen, MD

MSKCC Basking Ridge
136 Mountain View Boulevard Zip: 07920
Ph: (908) 542-3000 Fax: (908) 542-3220
- Aboody,Linda R., MD
- Capko,Deborah M., MD
- Chalasani,Sree Bhavani, MD
- Gavrilovic,Igor T., MD
- Gorsky,Mila, MD
- Haliasos,Helen C., MD
- Hamilton,Audrey May, MD
- Leitao,Mario Mendes Jr., MD
- Mann,Justin, MD
- Passalaris,Tina Marina, MD
- Quigley,Elizabeth A., MD
- Shepherd,Annemarie Fernandes, MD
- Sidebotham,Helen Lee, MD
- Simmons,Marc Z., MD
- Wang,Steven Q., MD
- Xiao,Han, MD

New Jersey Ctr for Orthop Sports Med
150 North Finley Avenue Zip: 07920
Ph: (908) 340-4266 Fax: (908) 340-4269
- Blank,Peter Bradley, DO
- Lin,Julie Tun-Fang, MD

Reproductive Medicine Associates of NJ
140 Allen Road Zip: 07920
Ph: (908) 604-7800 Fax: (973) 290-8370
- Bohrer,Michael K., MD
- Costantini-Ferrando,Maria Fausta,
- Darder,Michael C., MD
- Doherty,Leo Francis, MD
- Drews,Michael Robert, MD
- Hong,Kathleen H., MD
- Jurema,Marcus W., MD
- Kim,Julia G., MD
- Klimczak,Amber, MD
- Molinaro,Thomas Anthony, MD
- Morris,Jamie L., MD
- Rauch,Eden Renee, MD
- Rybak,Eli Asher, MD
- Werner,Marie D., MD
- Yih,Melissa Christina, MD

Bayonne
Associates in Cardiovascular Care, P.A
1061 Avenue C Zip: 07002
Ph: (201) 858-0800 Fax: (201) 858-3367
- Elkind,Barry M., MD
- Hefferan,James J., MD

AstraHealth Urgent & Primary Care
564 Broadway Zip: 07002
Ph: (201) 464-8888
- Primiani,Lisa, MD

Bayonne Family Practice
391 Kennedy Boulevard Zip: 07002
Ph: (201) 858-4110 Fax: (201) 858-2240
- Diaz,Francisco J., MD
- Potoczek-Salahi,Jolanta, MD

CarePoint Health Medical Group
1166 Kennedy Boulevard Zip: 07002
Ph: (201) 339-1133 Fax: (201) 339-1073
- Dedousis,John Jr., MD

CarePoint Health Medical Group
631 Broadway/3rd Floor Zip: 07002
Ph: (201) 243-0700 Fax: (201) 243-0377
- Kapoor,Ashish, MD
- Kapoor,Vinod, MD
- Sadeghi,Hooshang, MD

Carepoint Health Bayonne Med Center
29 East 29th Street Zip: 07002
Ph: (201) 858-5000
- George-Vickers,Jonelle, DO
- Sheinman,Marc Daniel, MD
- Takhalov,Yuriy, MD
- Varallo,Marisa R., MD

Comprehensive Cancer Care LLC
27 East 29th Street Zip: 07002
Ph: (201) 858-1211 Fax: (201) 858-4171
- Iyengar,Arjun D., MD
- Iyengar,Devarajan Parthasarthy, MD

Drs. Serafino & Dahrouj
834 Avenue C Zip: 07002
Ph: (201) 339-4222 Fax: (201) 339-4498
- Serafino,Vincent Joseph, MD

Drs. Suczewski & Suczewski
323 Avenue E/Corner 25th St Zip: 07002
Ph: (201) 339-8600
- Suczewski,Edward J., MD
- Suczewski,Thomas J., MD

Drs. Wignarajan and Wignarajan
875 Kennedy Boulevard Zip: 07002
Ph: (201) 339-1035 Fax: (201) 858-3350
- Wignarajan,Kanagarayer R., MD
- Wignarajan,Nadika V., MD

Hudson Digestive Health Center
534 Avenue E/Suite A Zip: 07002
Ph: (201) 858-8444 Fax: (201) 858-4260
- Patel,Rakhee, MD
- Prakash,Shasha, MD
- Ramasamy,Kovil Veeraswami, MD

Hudson Internal Medicine
744 Broadway Zip: 07002
Ph: (201) 436-8888
- Cardiello,Gary P., MD
- Tarng,George W., MD

Hudson Neurosciences, PC
605 Broadway Zip: 07002
Ph: (201) 339-6531 Fax: (201) 339-6536
- Ferrer,Gerrard F. A., DO
- Vintayen,Enrico V., MD

Hudson Radiology Center
657-659 Broadway Zip: 07002
Ph: (201) 437-3007 Fax: (201) 437-1418
- Perlov,Marina, MD
- Soloway,Peter H., MD

Hypertension & Renal Group, P.A.
930 Kennedy Boulevard Zip: 07002
Ph: (201) 858-1509 Fax: (973) 994-7085
- Byrd,Lawrence H., MD

Pelosi Medical Center
350 Kennedy Boulevard Zip: 07002
Ph: (201) 858-1800 Fax: (201) 858-1002
- Pelosi,Marco A. II, MD
- Pelosi,Marco A. Jr., MD

Progressive Pediatrics
1222 Kennedy Boulevard Zip: 07002
Ph: (201) 437-9600 Fax: (201) 437-9661
- Malabanan,Nerissa V., MD

Pulmonary and Critical Care Associates
534 Avenue East Zip: 07002
Ph: (201) 858-1021
- Burghauser,Alan H., MD

Riverside Pediatric Group
506 Broadway Zip: 07002
Ph: (201) 471-7012 Fax: (201) 471-7014
- Mahmoud,Ayesha Shabbir, MD
- Sirajuddin,Syed K., MD

Specialists In Urology, P.A.
534 Avenue E Zip: 07002
Ph: (201) 823-1303 Fax: (201) 823-0944
- Katz,Herbert I., MD
- Kerr,Eric S., MD

Stat Medical Services
845 Broadway Zip: 07002
Ph: (201) 823-8555 Fax: (201) 823-2979
- Padkowsky,George O., MD
- Woods,Krystina L., MD

Steinbaum & Levine Associates
789 Avenue C Zip: 07002
Ph: (201) 339-2620 Fax: (201) 339-2785
- Katsman,Tatyana, DO
- Levine,Howard Seth, DO
- Levine,Martin Scott, DO

The Heart Group, PA
654 Broadway Zip: 07002
Ph: (201) 243-9999 Fax: (201) 243-9998
- Lehmann,Robert Aaron, MD
- Topper,Leonid Lev, MD

United Medical, P.C.
988 Broadway/Suite 201 Zip: 07002
Ph: (201) 339-6111 Fax: (201) 339-6333
- Cadoo,Lisa K.A., MD
- Goykhman,Stanislav, MD
- Gupta,Shabnam, MD
- Hoffman,Mark Andrew, MD
- Marki,Richard E., MD
- Mathew,Alexander John, MD
- Nadiminti,Sheila Gupta, MD
- Neno,Rosa M., DO
- Sandhu,Narinder, MD
- Singh,Amandeep, MD

Urquhart Orthopedic Associates
534 Avenue E/Suite 1-B Zip: 07002
Ph: (201) 436-8289 Fax: (201) 471-2434
- Rowe Urquhart,Erica G., MD
- Urquhart,Marc Wayne, MD

Groups and Clinics by Town with Physician Rosters

Bayville
Frank C. Alario MD Inc
355 Route 9/Suite 2 Zip: 08721
Ph: (732) 269-0001 Fax: (732) 269-9636
- Alario, Frank C., MD
- Ingato, Steven P., MD
- Naseem, Arif, MD

Beach Haven
Ocean Medical MD, PA
3003 Long Beach Boulevard Zip: 08008
Ph: (609) 492-0900
- Picaro, Anthony J., MD
- Schmoll, Todd C., DO

Bedminster
Central Jersey Women's Health Assocs
1 Robertson Drive/Suite 25 Zip: 07921
Ph: (908) 532-0788 Fax: (908) 532-0787
- Bosin, Corey S., MD
- Hersh, Judith Ellen, MD

Somerset Pediatric Group PA
2345 Lamington Road/Suite 101 Zip: 07921
Ph: (908) 470-1124 Fax: (908) 470-2845
- Ebel, Keren Zahav, MD
- Fischer, John F., MD
- Levine, Stephanie, DO
- Shteynberg, Elena, MD
- Trend, Carolyn Cozine, MD
- Yorke, Eric R., MD

Belle Mead
Montgomery Medical Associates
9 Dutchtown Road Zip: 08502
Ph: (908) 874-8883 Fax: (908) 874-3595
- Pecora, Joseph J. III, DO
- Wajcberg, Estela, MD

Belleville
Amirata Surgical Group
5 Franklin Avenue/Suite 406 Zip: 07109
Ph: (973) 759-4499
- Amirata, Edwin A., MD
- Brautigan, Robert Anthony, MD

Belmont Medical Center
303 Belmont Avenue Zip: 07109
Ph: (973) 751-8411 Fax: (973) 751-8757
- Beresford, Dianne Walker, MD

Cardiology Center of New Jersey
50 Newark Avenue/Suite 204 Zip: 07109
Ph: (973) 450-2158 Fax: (973) 450-2027
- Criscito, Mario A., MD
- Kaul, Sameer, MD
- Saleh, Rany Mokhlis, DO

Drs. Johnson and Beggs
5 Franklin Avenue/Suite 103 Zip: 07109
Ph: (973) 751-3399
- Beggs, Donald James, MD
- Johnson, Edward S., MD

Drs. Keshav & Shivashankar
140 Belmont Avenue/Suite 102 Zip: 07109
Ph: (973) 751-7870 Fax: (973) 751-7875
- Keshav, Roger, MD
- Shivashankar, Keshavamurthy, MD

Drs. Seth & Napoli
36 Newark Avenue/Suite 300 Zip: 07109
Ph: (973) 759-6896 Fax: (973) 759-3719
- Napoli, John D., MD
- Seth, Amit Kumar, MD

Empire Medical Associates
5 Franklin Avenue/Suite 302 Zip: 07109
Ph: (973) 759-1221 Fax: (973) 759-1997
- Feehan, Brian Patrick, DO
- Gangemi, Frederick D., MD
- Lee, James M. Sr., MD
- Lester, Arthur I., MD
- Moaven, Nader, MD
- Pasley, Peter M., MD
- Perez, Walter, MD

Essex Hematology-Oncology Group, PA
36 Newark Avenue/Suite 304 Zip: 07109
Ph: (973) 751-8880 Fax: (973) 751-8950
- Conti, John A., MD
- Lippman, Alan J., MD
- Orsini, James M., MD
- Saleh, Said A., MD
- Vasireddy, Hemalatha, MD

Eye Institute of Essex, PA
5 Franklin Avenue/Suite 209 Zip: 07109
Ph: (973) 751-6060 Fax: (973) 450-1464
- Eichler, Joel D., MD

Jersey Rehab, P.A.
15 Newark Avenue/Suite 1 Zip: 07109
Ph: (973) 844-9220 Fax: (973) 844-9221
- Almentero, Felix Antonio, MD
- Gangemi, Edwin Michael, MD
- Hajela, Shailendra, MD
- Hilderbrand, Rene Francis, DO

Medical First of NY & NJ
5 Franklin Avenue/Suite 501 Zip: 07109
Ph: (973) 751-4477 Fax: (973) 751-4444
- Ardolino, Joseph M., MD
- Cerritelli, John A., MD

North Essex Medical Association
5 Franklin Avenue/Suite 609 Zip: 07109
Ph: (973) 751-1410
- Christiana, William A., MD
- Miller, Michael Joseph, MD

North Jersey Gastroenterology Assoc
5 Franklin Avenue/Suite 109 Zip: 07109
Ph: (973) 759-7240 Fax: (973) 759-7243
- Spira, Etan, MD

Prime Care Medical Group
55-59 Washington Avenue Zip: 07109
Ph: (973) 207-0640
- Chun, Kye S., MD
- Sidali, Mustafa M., DO

Retina Associates of New Jersey, P.A.
5 Franklin Avenue Zip: 07109
Ph: (973) 450-5100 Fax: (973) 450-9494
- Brooks, Nneka Offor, MD
- Madreperla, Steven Anthony Jr., MD
- Noorily, Stuart W., MD
- Seery, Christopher M., MD
- Voleti, Vinod Babu, MD

South Mountain Nephrology
5 Franklin Avenue/Suite 401 Zip: 07109
Ph: (973) 450-8999
- De Franco, Penny E., MD
- Samsa, Ranka Drazenovic, MD

Special Care OB-GYN
14 Franklin Street/2nd Floor Zip: 07109
Ph: (973) 759-4802 Fax: (973) 759-4805
- Devalla, Meena, MD
- Jain, Ratnam, MD

Urology Consultants, PA
36 Newark Avenue/Suite 200 Zip: 07109
Ph: (973) 759-6950 Fax: (973) 759-2006
- Ciccone, Michael Paul, MD
- Ciccone, Patrick N., MD
- Delgaizo, Anthony, MD

Vision Eye Physicians & Surgeons
567 Franklin Avenue Zip: 07109
Ph: (973) 751-4500
- Landolfi, Joseph M., MD
- Landolfi, Michael Joseph, DO

Bergenfield
Am/PM Walk In Urgent Care Center
19 South Washington Avenue Zip: 07621
Ph: (201) 387-0177 Fax: (201) 387-0114
- Jiu, Wun-Ye, MD
- Thek, Wesley K., MD

Bergenfield Internal Medicine
161 North Washington Avenue/Suite A Zip: 07621
Ph: (201) 387-6900
- De Gennaro, Michael A., MD
- Pereira, Beryl E., MD

Drs. Meier and Meier-Ginsberg
35 South Washington Avenue Zip: 07621
Ph: (201) 385-8350 Fax: (201) 385-8351
- Meier, Ronny, MD
- Meier-Ginsberg, Efrat, MD

Excelcare
375 South Washington Avenue Zip: 07621
Ph: (201) 384-0036 Fax: (201) 384-7304
- Desai, Foram R., MD
- Weisgras, Josef Mordechay, MD

The New Jersey Eye Center
1 North Washington Avenue Zip: 07621
Ph: (201) 384-7333 Fax: (201) 384-2564
- Bauza, Alain Michael, MD
- Dello Russo, Jeffrey, MD
- Parisi, Frank, MD

Washington Avenue Pediatrics
95 North Washington Avenue Zip: 07621
Ph: (201) 384-0300 Fax: (201) 384-9518
- Friedman, Howard Michael, MD
- Kaye, Shana Malka, MD
- Weiss, Christopher A., DO

Berkeley
Summit Medical Group
1 Diamond Hill Road/Bensley Pav/2 FL Zip: 07922
Ph: (908) 277-8700 Fax: (908) 288-7993
- Bell, Robert Lawrence, MD
- Bose, Konika Paul, MD
- Gatoulis, Maria K., MD
- Kole, Alison S., MD
- Lucciola, Pompeo Almerico, MD
- Parziale, Michael A., MD
- Picascia, Lisa, MD
- Sachs, R. Gregory, MD
- Schwartz, Daniel Richard, MD
- Spano-Brennan, Liana Marie, DO
- Tuladhar, Swosty, MD
- Volvovsky, Alexander, MD

Berkeley Heights
Berkeley Internal Medicine
391 Springfield Avenue/Suite 1B Zip: 07922
Ph: (908) 665-1177 Fax: (908) 665-8420
- Harjani, Vashdeo Daulat, MD
- Kapur, Sakshi, MD
- Mishra, Sneha, MD
- Patel, Samir Popatlal, MD

Summit Medical Group
1 Diamond Hill Road Zip: 07922
Ph: (908) 273-4300 Fax: (908) 790-6576
- Abbasi, Naheed R., MD
- Abramson, Marla Lyn, MD
- Addis, Diana Medina, MD
- Arif, Orooj, MD
- Atalla, Sara N., DO
- Banda, Pragati, MD
- Barrison, Adam F., MD
- Bass, Jon Lawrence, MD
- Batacchi, Zona Olivia, MD
- Bauman, Jeffrey Michael, MD
- Bazargan Lari, Hamed, MD
- Beamer, Andrew D., MD
- Belladonna, Joseph A., MD
- Ben-Menachem, Tamir, MD
- Bender, Michelle Anne, MD
- Berman, Erika Jacobs, MD
- Beyerl, Brian David, MD
- Bilenker, Michael Evan, MD
- Blitstein, Jeffrey, MD
- Boni, Christopher M., DO
- Brown, William Howard, MD
- Burstein, David Harris, MD
- Cajulis, Michelle C., MD
- Camacho, Ricardo Miguel, MD
- Cheung, Deborah Jee Hae, MD
- Cohen, Eric R., DO
- Coley, Marcelyn K., MD
- Colucio, Peter M., MD
- Coohill, Lisa Marie, MD
- Cooper, David M., MD
- Corona, Joseph T., MD
- Cunningham, John David, MD
- Dardanello, Marnie Cambria, MD
- Dave, Gazala, MD
- Deitz, Ruth Ellen Thisbe, MD
- Desai, Nicky, MD
- Dodge, Sarah Ann, MD
- Dokko, John Hoon, DO
- Drivas, Antonios, MD
- Eden, Avrim Reuben, MD
- El Zein, Lama, MD
- Feinberg, Craig Harlan, MD
- Flowers, Shari Carla, MD
- Freed, Brian, DO
- Gabel, Molly Mary, MD
- Garberina, Matthew J., MD
- Gillin, James Scott, MD
- Gnoy, Alexander Roman, MD
- Goldfaden, Isabel, MD
- Goldman-Gorelov, Victoria, MD
- Gruber, Gabriel G., MD
- Gumbs, Andrew Alexander, MD
- Gurey, Lowell Evan, MD
- Gurwin, Eric B., MD
- Hermann, Daniel Eric, MD
- Hsueh, Linda, MD
- Hyans, Peter, MD
- Joseph, Jain, MD
- Juliano, Nickolas Daniel, MD
- Karim, Anjum Hasan, MD
- Kemeny, Alexa C., MD
- Kennedy, Kevin J., MD
- Kennish, Lauren M., MD
- Khademi, Allen Mansour, MD
- Khalil, Monica B., MD
- Khedkar, Meera, MD
- Kim, Sam, MD
- Klein, Roger Scott, MD
- Kornfeld, Howard Neil, MD
- Kothavale, Avinash Annash, MD
- Kupershtein, Ilya, MD
- Kwartler, Jed A., MD
- Lacz, Nicole Lynn, MD
- Laudadio, Richard Dominick, MD
- Le Benger, Jeffrey D., MD
- Le Benger, Kerry S., MD
- Lee, Linda K., MD
- Leibu, Dora, DO
- Lesko, Richard J., MD
- Lieberman, Eric Steven, MD
- Lipset, Shani Lauren, MD
- Lozner, Jerrold S., MD
- Lunenfeld, Ellen Beth, MD
- Lupski, Donna L., MD
- Mandal, Soma, MD
- Masterson, Christine, MD
- McCormick, John Stuart, MD
- Mehta, Ami A., MD
- Mehta, Shiva C., MD
- Mendiola, Redentor S. Jr., MD
- Meyer, Jacqueline Marie, MD
- Meyers, Lawrence S., MD
- Michael, Hazar, MD
- Miguelino, Ida Alfad, MD
- Mills, Lisa Alice, MD
- Mirchandani, Sunil, MD
- Mirsky, Eric Charles, MD
- Momeni, Reza, MD
- Moy, Jamie Tam, DO
- Nadiminti, Hari, MD
- Naik, Komal Desai, MD
- Nastro, Lawrence J., MD
- Natale, Jessica Ann, DO
- Nitzberg, Richard S., MD
- Oza, Rohit Madhukar, MD
- Palermo, Angelo David, MD
- Parikh, Ashish Dharnidhar, MD
- Patrone, Nicole, MD
- Pavelic, Martin Thomas III, MD
- Pettee, Brett, MD
- Philips-Rodriguez, Dahlia, MD
- Polen, Winnie M., DO
- Porbunderwala, Steven James, MD
- Qian, Fang, MD
- Reeder, Jennifer Gordan, MD
- Reedy, Jamie Lynne, MD
- Reikes, Sanford Todd, MD
- Rosenbaum, Robert L., MD
- Roth, Douglas M., DO
- Sahulhameed, Fathima, MD
- Salomon, Pierre Richard, MD
- Schreck, David M., MD
- Shah, Vinnie Pooja, MD
- Sherman, Ronna S., MD
- Shridharani, Kanan Vasant, MD
- Siegal, John D., MD
- Singh, Anita J., MD
- Skrelja, Valerie, MD
- Slama, Robert D., MD

Groups and Clinics by Town with Physician Rosters

Smith,Dominic, MD
Soto,Haydee M., MD
Summa,Geraldine M., MD
Tavel,Stacey C., MD
Terry,Alon, MD
Thomas,Alan E., MD
Thumar,Adeep Bhaguanji, MD
Toscano-Zukor,Amy M., DO
Tu,Chun, MD
Turner,Garth M., MD
Vecchi,Anthony R., MD
Volpe,Michael Anthony, MD
Waqar,Anum Khan, DO
Wax,Michael B., MD
Weisfuse,Judith E., MD
Wilt,Jessie Swain, MD
Zirvi,Monib Ahmad, MD

Berlin

Advocare Berlin Medical Associates
175 Cross Keys Road/Suite 300A   Zip: 08009
Ph: (856) 767-0077   Fax: (856) 767-6102
 Hassman,David R., DO
 Hassman,Joseph M., DO
 Hassman,Michael A., DO
 Hossain,Shawn Isteak, DO
 Mauriello,Richard M., DO
 Wu,Shiann J., MD

Advocare Gigliotti Family Medicine
181 West White Horse Pike/Suite 100   Zip: 08009
Ph: (856) 767-0069   Fax: (856) 767-2531
 Galezniak,John, DO
 Gigliotti,David T., DO

Drs. Saad and Saad
139 Sequoia Drive   Zip: 08009
Ph: (856) 767-2783
 Franzen Saad,Jillian Leigh, MD
 Saad,Sherif Saad, MD

Bernardsville

Advocare Sinatra & Peng Pediatrics
169 Minebrook Road   Zip: 07924
Ph: (908) 766-0034   Fax: (908) 766-5065
 Ganek,Ellen Beth, MD
 Peng,Patricia E., DO
 Sinatra,Frank A., MD
 Visci,John J., MD

Summit Medical Group
1 Anderson Hill Road/Suite 102   Zip: 07924
Ph: (908) 696-0808   Fax: (908) 696-9943
 Costea-Misthos,Maria A., MD

Blackwood

Advocare DelGiorno Pediatrics
535 South Black Horse Pike   Zip: 08012
Ph: (856) 228-1061   Fax: (856) 228-1907
 Del Giorno,Joseph John, MD
 Delgiorno,John Michael, MD

Advocare DelGiorno Pediatrics
527 South Black Horse Pike   Zip: 08012
Ph: (856) 302-5322   Fax: (856) 245-7719
 Fisicaro,Tamara Marie, MD
 Frisoni,Lorenza, MD
 George,Cyriac, DO
 Iacobucci,Audrey J., MD
 Mercedes Salas,Aixell Josefina, MD
 Owens,Brittany Rose, MD
 Robiou,Natalie Genoveva, MD
 Salvati,Harold Vincent, MD

Cooper Family Medicine
141 South Black Horse Pike/Suite 1   Zip: 08012
Ph: (856) 232-6471   Fax: (856) 232-7028
 Horvath Matthews,Jessica Erin, MD
 Mahamitra,Nirandra, MD
 Robertson,John F. Jr., MD
 Treiman,Arthur M., MD

Creations Medical Spa
901 Route 168/Suite408   Zip: 08012
Ph: (856) 589-1151
 Corson-Diaz,Cathy Lynn, MD
 Diaz Jimenez,Jose Eduardo, MD

Drexel University Physicians
400 East Church Street   Zip: 08012
Ph: (856) 228-8066

Delvadia,Dipak R., DO
Montgomery,Owen Canterbury, MD

Eye Associates
141 Black Horse Pike/Suite 7   Zip: 08012
Ph: (856) 227-6262   Fax: (856) 227-8830
 Linares,Hugo Manuel, DO

Bloomfield

All Star Pediatrics
199 Broad Street/Suite 1-B   Zip: 07003
Ph: (973) 743-1392   Fax: (973) 743-3707
 Shah,Madhavi, MD

Drs. Reyes & Narvaez
135 Bloomfield Avenue/Suite B   Zip: 07003
Ph: (973) 743-3556   Fax: (973) 743-3895
 Borbon-Reyes,Araceli O., MD
 Narvaez,Guillermo Jr., MD
 Narvaez,Normita G., MD
 Reyes,Prudencio C., MD

Empire Medical Associates
382 West Passaic Avenue   Zip: 07003
Ph: (973) 338-1900
 Kelly,John V. Jr., MD

Essex Heart Group LLC
1310 Broad Street   Zip: 07003
Ph: (973) 338-0800   Fax: (973) 338-1140
 McCoach,Kevin J., MD

Essex Hudson Urology
256 Broad Street   Zip: 07003
Ph: (973) 743-4450   Fax: (973) 429-9076
 Caruso,Robert Peter, MD
 Franzoni,David Fred, MD
 Hsieh,Kuang-Yiao, MD
 Lombardo,Salvatore Antonio, MD
 Wu,David Sweghsien, MD

Eye Surgeons of North Jersey, LLC
199 Broad Street/Suite 2-B   Zip: 07003
Ph: (973) 748-3300   Fax: (973) 748-3802
 D'Amato,Anthony P., MD
 Kumar,Radhika Lingam, MD

ImmediCenter/Bloomfield
557 Broad Street   Zip: 07003
Ph: (973) 680-8300   Fax: (973) 743-5601
 Basista,Michael P., MD
 Garcia Marotta,Ylonka, MD
 Schuyler,Andrew P., MD

NJ Retina
1255 Broad Street/Suite 104   Zip: 07003
Ph: (973) 707-5632   Fax: (973) 707-7349
 Jackson,Kurt T., MD
 Kallina,Lauren A., MD

New Jersey Urology, LLC
1515 Broad Street/Suite B-130   Zip: 07003
Ph: (973) 873-7000   Fax: (973) 873-7035
 Kagan,Eduard, MD

North Jersey Cardiovascular Consultant
329 Belleville Avenue   Zip: 07003
Ph: (973) 748-3800   Fax: (973) 748-3540
 Bhalodia,Manish V., MD
 Horowitz,Michael S., MD
 Lapa,Alan S., MD
 Mahdi,Lawrence F., MD
 Shao,John Han, MD

People Care Institute
323 Belleville Avenue/Floor 2   Zip: 07003
Ph: (973) 842-4272   Fax: (732) 997-3022
 Beaubrun,Esira Jaimie, MD
 Pierre-Louis,Frantz Junior M., MD

Step by Step Pediatrics, P.C.
299 Glenwood Avenue/2nd Floor Suite 6   Zip: 07003
Ph: (973) 743-5639   Fax: (973) 743-5840
 Flynn,Sean A., MD
 Kerlegrand,Pascale, MD

The Eye Care Ctr of New Jersey
108 Broughton Avenue   Zip: 07003
Ph: (973) 743-1331   Fax: (973) 743-6577
 Ditkoff,Jonathan W., MD
 Gould,Joshua Mark, DO

Boonton

Drs. Scaduto & Renz
223 West Main Street   Zip: 07005
Ph: (973) 335-8656   Fax: (973) 335-8986
 Renz,Patricia M., MD

 Scaduto,Philip M., MD

Bordentown

Capital Health Primary Care-Bordentown
1 Third Street   Zip: 08505
Ph: (609) 298-2005   Fax: (609) 324-8267
 Carty,Robert W., MD
 Flynn,Jamie, DO
 Garbarini Carty,Elyse, MD
 Hughes,Janey Ballin, DO
 Jimma,Lulu A., MD
 Lugo,Maria D., MD
 Mleczko,Joshua, MD
 Redziniak,Natalie E., MD
 Van Patten,Yancy L., DO
 VanHise,Tara Hungspruke, DO
 Vizzoni,Hiedi Taylor, MD

New Jersey Urology
243 Route 130/Suite 100   Zip: 08505
OnlyFax: (856) 252-1100
 Asroff,Scott Wayne, MD
 Goldlust,Robert W., MD
 Perzin,Adam Dean, MD

Performance Spine & Sports Medicine
9500 K Johnson Boulevard/Suite 1   Zip: 08505
Ph: (609) 817-0050   Fax: (609) 588-8602
 Karam,Christopher S., MD
 Konakondla,Krishna, MD
 Rizkalla,Michael H., MD

Premier Medicine & Wellness
231 Crosswicks Road/Suite 11   Zip: 08505
Ph: (609) 298-4750
 Chokshi,Seema Patel, MD
 Frascella,Rosemary C., MD
 Potharlanka,Prathibha R., MD

Reconstructive Orthopedics, P.A.
243 Route 130/Suite 100   Zip: 08505
Ph: (609) 267-9400   Fax: (609) 267-9457
 Farrell,Joseph E., DO
 Gray,John Michael, MD
 Jain,Rajesh K., MD
 Ropiak,Raymond Russell, MD
 Schoifet,Scott D., MD

Virtual Family Medicine - Mansfield
3242 Route 206/Building A Suite 2   Zip: 08505
Ph: (609) 298-4340   Fax: (609) 298-4370
 Breig,Jason Anthony, MD
 Chen,Timothy, MD
 Devers,Paul Dix, MD
 Kohlhapp,Caroline R., DO

Bound Brook

American Institute for Counseling
1952 US Highway 22/Suite 102   Zip: 08805
Ph: (732) 469-6444   Fax: (732) 469-6445
 Borton,Miriam A., MD
 Cortez,Jacqueline M., MD
 Ismail,Mona S. A., MD

Middlebrook Family Practice
101 East Union Avenue   Zip: 08805
Ph: (732) 560-0490   Fax: (732) 560-3681
 Goldman,Frieda Shepsel, MD
 Pizzelanti,Donna M., DO

Branchburg

Access Medical Associates
3322 Route 22 West/Building 1   Zip: 08876
Ph: (908) 704-0100   Fax: (908) 704-0090
 Goldberg,Lon E., DO
 Rego,Ramon, MD

Atlantic Medical Care Primary Care
3322 Route 22/Suite 1204   Zip: 08876
Ph: (908) 378-7227   Fax: (908) 252-0127
 Gujjula,Prashanthi, MD
 Zeh,Catherine A., MD

Fox Skin & Allergy Associates
3461 Route 22   Zip: 08876
Ph: (908) 725-4777   Fax: (908) 725-7439
 Fox,Alissa R., MD
 Fox,James A., MD

Somerset Pediatric Group PA
3322 Route 22/Suite 1002   Zip: 08876
Ph: (908) 725-5530   Fax: (908) 253-6559
 Housam,Ryan Ann, MD

 Ricks,Sandy, MD

Branchville

Premier Health Associates
202 Route 206 North/Suite A   Zip: 07826
Ph: (973) 948-5577
 De Paola,Anthony A., DO
 Luszcz,Ronald J., DO

Brick

ABC Pediatric Associates PA
131 Drum Point Road   Zip: 08723
Ph: (732) 477-8988
 Kraynock,John, MD
 Piela,Christina, MD

Alpert Zales & Castro Pediatric Cardio
1623 Route 88/Suite A/PO Box 1719   Zip: 08723
Ph: (732) 458-9666   Fax: (732) 458-0840
 Alpert,Mitchel B., MD
 Castro,Elsa Imelda, MD
 Chin,Stephanie Elaine, MD
 Umali Pamintuan,Maria Angela T., M
 Zales,Vincent R., MD

Atlantic Coast Gastroenterology
1640 Route 88 West/Suite 202   Zip: 08724
Ph: (732) 458-8300   Fax: (732) 458-8529
 Aaron,Bernard M., MD
 Cerefice,Mark L., MD
 Shukla,Sandhya, MD
 Tangorra,Matthew, DO

Atlantic Coast Urology
525 Jack Martin Boulevard/Suite 304   Zip: 08723
Ph: (732) 840-6606   Fax: (732) 840-6601
 Kim,Chong M., MD

Atlantic Shore Surgical Associates
478 Brick Boulevard   Zip: 08723
Ph: (732) 701-4848   Fax: (732) 701-1244
 Ahmed,Omar Zikri, MD
 Bhandari,Tarun, MD
 Huang,Kevin, MD
 Kamath,Ashwin S., MD
 Kelly,Francis J., MD
 Pahuja,Anil K., MD
 Park,Jane, MD
 Snepar,Rory B., DO
 Yrad,Jonathan Proces Flores, MD
 Zurkovsky,Eugene, MD

Breast Srg & Breast Onc Assoc
459 Jack Martin Boulevard   Zip: 08724
Ph: (732) 458-4600
 Lygas,Theodore B., MD
 Pellegrino,John M., MD

Brick Pediatric Group
1301 Route 70   Zip: 08724
Ph: (732) 892-8700   Fax: (732) 892-6689
 Caputo,Enza P., MD
 Sandeep,Rashmi, MD

Brick Town Medical
34 Lanes Mill Road   Zip: 08724
Ph: (732) 458-0300   Fax: (732) 458-8449
 Babayev,Lily L., MD
 Ital,Rosa, MD
 Riss,Martin, DO

Brick Women's Physicians
1140 Burnt Tavern Road/Suite 2-A   Zip: 08724
Ph: (732) 202-0700   Fax: (732) 202-0664
 Morgan,Darlene M., MD
 Pagano,Ann Marie, MD
 Vetter,Paul L., MD

Brielle Orthopedics PA
457 Jack Martin Boulevard   Zip: 08724
Ph: (732) 840-7500   Fax: (732) 840-2088
 Bogdan,Joseph P., MD
 Esquieres,Raymond Edel, MD
 Hebela,Nader M., MD
 Kanarek,Samantha Leigh, DO
 Katt,Brian Matthew, MD
 Law,William A., MD
 Malfitano,Laura Anne, DO
 Marsicano,Joseph G., MD
 Nitche,Jason Adam, MD
 Rodricks,David Josef, MD
 Sargent,Thomas G. Jr, DO

Groups and Clinics by Town with Physician Rosters

Brick (cont)

Brielle Orthopedics PA
 Stamos, Bruce Dumont, MD
 Wolenski, Matthew J., MD

Bruce A. De Cotiis, MD, PA
 1673 Highway 88 West Zip: 08724
 Ph: (732) 458-2000
 De Cotiis, Bruce A., MD
 Georgy, Mary Sarah, MD
 Tumaliuan, Janet Ang, MD

Cardiology Assocs of Ocean County
 495 Jack Martin Boulevard/Suite 2 Zip: 08724
 Ph: (732) 458-7575 Fax: (732) 458-0874
 Ahmad, Tanveer, MD
 Mehra, Aditya Chand, MD
 Paul Kate, Vasant, MD
 Raza, Muhammad Rehan, MD
 Vijayakumar, Chellappan, MD

Cedar Bridge Medical Associates
 985 Cedarbridge Avenue Zip: 08723
 Ph: (732) 477-5600 Fax: (732) 477-1899
 Clark, Kristen S., MD
 Fung, Kent C., MD
 Ilkhanizadeh, Ladan, MD
 Kaur, Sundip, MD
 Reisher, Richard G., DO
 Wilson, Francis P., DO

Coastal Cardiovascular Consultants, PA
 459 Jack Martin Boulevard/Suite 4 Zip: 08724
 Ph: (732) 458-6200 Fax: (732) 458-9464
 Escandon, Pedro J., MD
 Patel, Harshil, MD
 Patel, Virendra, MD
 Salloum, Ahmad, MD
 White, Thomas M., DO

Coastal Gastroenterology Associates PA
 525 Jack Martin Boulevard/Suite 301 Zip: 08724
 Ph: (732) 840-0067 Fax: (732) 840-3169
 Chiu, Kenny, MD
 Jain, Vishal K., MD
 Magahis, Pacifico Aguila Jr., MD
 Rozovsky, Assif, MD
 Schlachter, Scott M., DO
 Winzelberg, Neal J., MD

Coastal Urology Associates
 446 Jack Martin Boulevard Zip: 08724
 Ph: (732) 840-4300 Fax: (732) 840-4515
 Burzon, Daniel Todd, MD
 Chapman, John Robert, MD
 Fam, Mina, MD
 Gioia, Kevin Thomas, MD
 Linn, Gary C., MD
 Mendoza, Pierre J., MD

Drs. Seares and Bautista-Seares
 35 Beaverson Boulevard/Building 7 Zip: 08723
 Ph: (732) 262-2400
 Bautista-Seares, Jessica M., MD
 Seares, Petronilo Jr., MD

ENT & Facial Plastic Surgery Assocs
 1608 Route 88/Suite 240 Zip: 08724
 Ph: (732) 458-8575 Fax: (732) 206-0578
 Brandeisky, Thomas E., DO
 Chu, Tun S., MD
 Landsman, Howard Scott, DO

EmCare
 425 Jack Martin Boulevard Zip: 08724
 Ph: (732) 840-3380
 Abe, Minako, MD
 Barone, Frank Anthony, MD
 Darocki, Mark, MD
 Noris, Gary L., MD
 Schlogl, Jeffrey G., MD
 Singh, Arun J., DO

Freehold Ophthalmology, LLC
 202 Jack Martin Boulevard Zip: 08724
 Ph: (732) 458-5700 Fax: (732) 458-0693
 Schlisserman, David A., MD

Garden State Medical Center
 1608 New Jersey 88/Suites 102 Zip: 08724
 Ph: (732) 849-0077 Fax: (732) 849-0015
 Singh, Manjula, MD

Jersey Coast Family Medicine
 495 Jack Martin Boulevard/Suite 5 Zip: 08724
 Ph: (732) 458-8000 Fax: (732) 458-8020
 Montgomery, Karyn Mae, MD
 Ussery-Kronhaus, Kelly G., MD

Jersey Coast Nephrology & Hypertension
 1541 Route 88/Suite A Zip: 08724
 Ph: (732) 836-3200 Fax: (732) 836-3201
 Albanese, Joseph J., DO
 Bruno, Robert, DO
 Jain, Keshani, MD
 Kapoor, Rajat, DO
 Weiner, Leonard D., MD

Jersey Coast Vascular Associates
 425 Jack Martin Boulevard/Suite 2 Zip: 08724
 Ph: (732) 202-1500
 Aquino, Rainier, MD
 Cluley, Scott R., MD
 Jain, Vikalp, MD
 Kwon, Sung Wook, MD
 Milazzo, Vincent J., MD
 Sharp, Frank J. III, MD

Monmouth Ocean Neurology
 190 Jack Martin Boulevard/Building B-3 Zip: 08724
 Ph: (732) 785-0114 Fax: (732) 785-0116
 Barcas, Peter P., DO
 Sedarous, Mary, MD

NJ Hematology & Oncology Associates
 1608 Route 88 West/Suite 250 Zip: 08724
 Ph: (732) 840-8880 Fax: (732) 840-3939
 Agrawal, Apurv, MD
 Amin, Girish S., MD
 Pavlak-Schenk, Jayne A., DO
 Walczyszyn, Bartosz Adam, MD

Ocean County Family Care
 2125 Route 88 East Zip: 08724
 Ph: (732) 892-4548 Fax: (732) 892-0961
 DeDona, Anna, DO
 Gronsky, Rudolph Edward, DO
 Hasan, Bassam I., MD
 Hiley, Paul C., MD
 Konigsberg, David, DO
 Navarro, Mark Anthony, MD
 Rothberg, Michael Steven, MD
 Vida, Jay A., DO

Ocean County Medical Lab
 525 Route 70 Zip: 08723
 Ph: (732) 920-1772 Fax: (732) 920-6171
 Baron-Gabriel, Icynth M., MD
 Krumerman, Martin Saul, MD

Ocean Heart Group
 1530 Route 88/Suite A Zip: 08724
 Ph: (732) 840-0600 Fax: (732) 840-0611
 Kianfar, Hormoz, MD
 Komorowski, Thomas W., MD

Ocean Pulmonary Associates PA
 457 Jack Martin Boulevard/Suite 4 Zip: 08724
 Ph: (732) 840-4200 Fax: (732) 840-6444
 Alcasid, Patrick J., MD
 Kamel, Emad R., MD
 Kerr, Brian S., MD
 Wynkoop, Walter Alan, MD

Ocean Renal Associates, P.A.
 210 Jack Martin Boulevard/Suite D-1 Zip: 08724
 Ph: (732) 458-5854 Fax: (732) 458-8012
 Brouder, Daniel J., MD

Ocean Renal Associates, P.A.
 1617 Route 88 West Zip: 08724
 Ph: (732) 458-5854 Fax: (732) 458-8012
 DePalma, John Anthony, DO
 Ellis, Stephen J., MD
 Haider, Nadeem Z., MD
 Iglesias, Jose Ignacio, DO
 Markatos, Angelo, MD

 Meyer, Ariel, DO
 Panchani, Mrugesh Chhaganlal, MD
 Park, Jin S., MD
 Schirripa, Joseph V., MD

Our Family Practice
 1899 State Highway 88 Zip: 08723
 Ph: (732) 840-8177 Fax: (732) 840-2195
 Cascarina, Michael A., MD
 Eapen, Prema Mary, MD
 Tesoriero, Laura M., MD

Pediatric Affiliates, PA
 218 Jack Martin Boulevard/Building E-1 Zip: 08724
 Ph: (732) 458-0010 Fax: (732) 458-9329
 Lapidus, Daniel Yitzchok, MD

Pediatric Care Physicians, LLC
 2211 Route 88/Suite 2-A Zip: 08724
 Ph: (732) 899-0008 Fax: (732) 899-0447
 Almazan, Gerald C., MD
 Collado, Maria R., MD
 Condren, Eileen, DO

Pediatric Medical Group
 525 Jack Martin Boulevard/Suite 102 Zip: 08724
 Ph: (732) 458-1177 Fax: (732) 458-5942
 Mate, Shrikrishn K., MD
 Rolenc, Holly J., MD

Pineland Associates PA
 1608 Route 88/Suite 208 Zip: 08724
 Ph: (732) 458-7878 Fax: (732) 840-6378
 Benecki, Theresa R., MD
 Ketelaar, Pieter J., MD

Shore Cardiology Consultants, LLC
 1640 Route 88/Suite 201 Zip: 08724
 Ph: (732) 840-1900 Fax: (732) 840-0355
 Cohen, Todd S., DO
 DeVita, Michael G., DO
 Moosvi, Ali R., MD

Shore Heart Group, P.A.
 35 Beaverson Boulevard/Suite 9-B Zip: 08723
 Ph: (732) 262-4262 Fax: (732) 262-4317
 Apolito, Renato A., MD
 Hansalia, Riple Jayamtilal, MD
 Karam, Edmund Thomas, MD
 Pinnelas, David J., MD

Shore Medical Group
 1640 Highway 88/Suite 203 Zip: 08724
 Ph: (732) 458-7777 Fax: (732) 263-9470
 Boyan, William P., MD
 Carolan, Owen J., MD
 Edelman, Carrie Allysia, MD
 Heacock, James K., MD
 Jarahian, George Jr., MD

Shore Nephrology, P.A.
 35 Beaverson Boulevard Zip: 08723
 Ph: (732) 451-0063 Fax: (732) 451-0071
 Dounis, Harry James, DO

Shore Neurology, PA
 1613 Route 88/Suite 3 Zip: 08724
 Ph: (732) 785-3335 Fax: (732) 785-2599
 Escandon, Sandra L., MD
 Miskin, Pandurang H., MD

Shore Radiation Oncology, LLC
 425 Jack Martin Boulevard Zip: 08724
 Ph: (732) 836-4109 Fax: (732) 836-4036
 Kaufman, Nathan, MD
 Miller, Douglas Andrew, MD

Total Patient Care LLC
 459 Jack Martin Boulevard Zip: 08724
 Ph: (732) 785-1000 Fax: (732) 785-1222
 Alcasid, Ninfa A., MD

Bridgeport

Worknet Occupational Medicine
 510 Heron Drive/Suite 108 Zip: 08014
 Ph: (856) 467-8550 Fax: (856) 467-3361
 Harris, Brian E., MD
 Zaharko, Wendy, MD

Bridgeton

Center for Family Health
 105 Manheim Avenue/Suite 1 Zip: 08302
 Ph: (856) 455-2700 Fax: (856) 455-7051
 Kohler, Frank R., DO
 Ordille, Joseph D., DO
 Riley-Lowe, Judith E., DO

Community Health Care, Inc.
 70 Cohansey Street Zip: 08302
 Ph: (856) 451-4700 Fax: (856) 451-0029
 Ismail, Elham Mohamed, MD
 Nair, Prabha J., MD

Community Health Care, Inc.
 265 Irving Avenue Zip: 08302
 Ph: (856) 451-4700 Fax: (856) 863-5732
 Oswald, Mark Anthony, MD
 Roomi, Farah, MD

Family Practice Associates
 230 Laurel Heights Drive Zip: 08302
 Ph: (856) 451-9595 Fax: (609) 451-1832
 Bear, John G., MD
 Bear, Michelle H., DO
 De Biaso, Tracy A., MD

First Step Pediatrics
 206 Laurel Heights Drive Zip: 08302
 Ph: (856) 459-2270 Fax: (856) 459-9674
 Fleischer, Gilbert E., MD
 Patel, Bhavna K., MD
 Tanner, Fritzi Alma, MD

Genito Urinary Associates
 20 Magnolia Avenue/Suite D Zip: 08302
 Ph: (856) 455-5770
 Diaz, Jose F., MD

Internal Medicine Associates
 201 Laurel Heights Drive/Suite 201 Zip: 08302
 Ph: (856) 455-4800 Fax: (856) 455-0650
 Bagan, Stanley L., MD
 Candelore, Joseph Timothy Jr., DO
 Copare, Fiore J., MD
 Gabriel, Andre C., MD
 Hanna, Ekram Labeb, MD
 Hatzantonis, John Emanuel, MD
 Jimenez-Silva, Jeanette, MD
 Struby, Christopher, MD

Iqbal & Khan Surgical Associates, P.A.
 10 Magnolia Avenue/Suite E Zip: 08302
 Ph: (856) 455-2399 Fax: (856) 451-7791
 Haq, Imran Ul, MD
 Iqbal, Nauveed, MD
 Khan, Aftab A., MD

Kidney & Hypertension Specialists PA
 215 Laurel Heights Drive Zip: 08302
 Ph: (856) 455-6002 Fax: (856) 455-6106
 De Priori, Elis Maria, MD

South Cumberland Medical Associates
 215 Back Neck Road Zip: 08302
 Ph: (856) 451-4414 Fax: (856) 451-2052
 Ballas, Christopher Thomas, MD
 Talbot, Lori C., MD
 Tugman, Catherine K., MD

Bridgewater

Alliance Medical Associates, PC
 15 Monroe Street Zip: 08807
 Ph: (908) 595-6330 Fax: (908) 595-6331
 Sun, Karen Hong Xue, MD

Bridgewater Internal Medicine, PA
 215 Union Avenue/Suite E Zip: 08807
 Ph: (908) 685-1818 Fax: (908) 685-8225
 Cheng, Shiow-Jane L., MD
 Gubbi, Smitha Ayodhyarama, MD

CardioMD
 1200 US Highway 22 East/Suite 17 Zip: 08807
 Ph: (908) 864-4027 Fax: (908) 864-4029
 Mahal, Sharan S., MD
 Patel, Alpesh Amrit, MD
 Shahi, Chandreshwar N., MD

Drs. Agrin & Shulman
 245 Union Avenue/Suite 2B Zip: 08807
 Ph: (908) 231-1311 Fax: (908) 231-1324
 Agrin, Richard Joel, MD

ENT & Allergy Associates-Bridgewater
 245 US Highway 22/3rd Fl/Suite 300 Zip: 08807
 Ph: (908) 722-1022 Fax: (908) 722-2040
 Abrahim, Mena, DO
 Burachinsky, Dennis Andrew, DO
 Camacho-Halili, Marie M., MD
 Fenster, Gerald F., MD
 Hekiert, Adrianna Maria, MD
 Lazar, Amy D., MD

Groups and Clinics by Town with Physician Rosters

Gastromed Healthcare, PA
25 Monroe Street   Zip: 08807
Ph: (908) 231-1999   Fax: (908) 231-1612
  Irakam,Surya Prakash, MD
  Shapiro,Stephen R., MD
  Unger,Jeffrey S., MD
  Wiesen,Robert S., MD
Hunterdon Family Medicine
250 Route 28/Suite 100   Zip: 08807
Ph: (908) 237-4135   Fax: (908) 237-4136
  Hamilton,Kathryn Diane, MD
  Klein,Martin Edward, MD
  Mannancheril,Anita, MD
Medicor Cardiology PA
225 Jackson Street   Zip: 08807
Ph: (908) 526-8668   Fax: (908) 231-6781
  Ahn,Joe Kyuhyun, MD
  Cheng,Chao T., MD
  Frenkel,Daniel, MD
  Friedman,Glenn T., MD
  Georgeson,Steven E., MD
  Hall,Jason O., MD
  Kulkarni,Rachana A., MD
  Leeds,Richard S., MD
  Patel,Ashok Ambalal, MD
  Patel,Parag Bhailal, MD
  Rachofsky,Edward Lawrence, MD
NeuroSurgical Associates of Jersey
1200 Route 22 East/2nd Floor   Zip: 08807
Ph: (732) 302-1720   Fax: (732) 302-1724
  Chimenti,James M., MD
  More,Jay, MD
NJ Rehab & Electrodiagnostics
201 Union Avenue/Suite 1A   Zip: 08807
Ph: (908) 429-7799
  Kanuri,Kavitha, MD
Orthopedic and Sports Medicine at SMG
215 Union Avenue/Suite B   Zip: 08807
Ph: (908) 685-8500   Fax: (908) 685-8009
  Nordstrom,Thomas J., MD
Paul Phillips Eye & Surgery Center
1 Monroe Street   Zip: 08807
Ph: (908) 526-4588   Fax: (908) 231-6718
  Faigenbaum,Steven J., MD
  Phillips,Paul Mathew, MD
Pedi Health Medical Associates
720 Route 202-206 North/Suite 4   Zip: 08807
Ph: (908) 722-5444   Fax: (908) 722-5071
  Calimlim,Grace T., MD
  Dionne-McCracken,Laura, MD
  Jain,Ami P., MD
  Senator,Laura Julie, MD
Priority Medical Care
350 Grove Street/Suite 200   Zip: 08807
Ph: (908) 231-0777   Fax: (908) 722-6031
  Lupoli,Kristin Anne, MD
Priority Medical Care/Family Hlth Ctr
350 Grove Street   Zip: 08807
Ph: (908) 526-1313   Fax: (908) 722-6031
  Ouano,Estelita C., MD
  Tobias,David A., MD
RWJPE Bridgewater Medical Group
766 Route 202-206/Suite 1   Zip: 08807
Ph: (908) 722-0808   Fax: (908) 722-7645
  Kripsak,John P., DO
  Lustig,Robert H., DO
  Mitterando,Jeanne G., MD
RWJPE Cardiology Assoc of Somerset Cty
487 Union Avenue/Suite A   Zip: 08807
Ph: (908) 722-6410   Fax: (908) 722-4638
  Ivanov,Alexander, MD
  Lebenthal,Mark J., MD
  Ocken,Stephen M., MD
  Sengupta,Ranjita, MD
  Trivedi,Shivang M., MD
Respacare
489 Union Avenue   Zip: 08807
Ph: (732) 356-9950   Fax: (732) 356-9959
  Mehta,Nehal L., MD
  Patel,Prashant B., MD
Somerset Nephrology Assocs
23 Monroe Street   Zip: 08807
Ph: (908) 722-0106   Fax: (908) 231-1431
  Mehta,Sudhir H., MD
  Noor,Fazle Ali, MD
  Patel,Manisha Saurabh, MD
Somerset Ob-Gyn Associates
215 Union Avenue/Suite A   Zip: 08807
Ph: (908) 722-2900   Fax: (908) 722-1856
  Bernstein,Sambra H., MD
  Errico,Carmine P., MD
  Mileto,Vincent F., MD
  Miranda,Matilda, MD
  Oza,Palak, MD
  Woltz,Ayanna Rashea, MD
Somerset Orthopedic Associates
1081 Route 22 West   Zip: 08807
Ph: (908) 722-0822   Fax: (908) 722-6318
  Choi,Mingi, MD
  Parolie,James M., MD
  Vessa,Paul P., MD
Somerset Pediatric Group PA
155 Union Avenue   Zip: 08807
Ph: (908) 725-1802   Fax: (908) 203-8825
  Abraham,Daniel J., MD
  Ferrante,Robyn, MD
  Needleman,Jack, MD
  Piezas,Sylvia M., MD
Somerset Pulmonary & Critical Care
245 Union Avenue/Suite 2C   Zip: 08807
Ph: (732) 873-8097   Fax: (732) 873-1827
  Lee,Jack C., MD
  Poiani,George J., MD
  Soriano,Aida N., MD
Summit Medical Group
465 Union Avenue/Suite B   Zip: 08807
Ph: (908) 864-4820   Fax: (908) 864-4819
  Gora,Jill Suzanne, MD
  Hamilton,Cliff Scott, MD
The Eye Specialists, P.A.
745 Route 202/206/Suite 301   Zip: 08807
Ph: (908) 231-1110   Fax: (908) 526-4959
  Moshel,Caroline Rosenberg, MD
  Salz,Alan G., MD

Brigantine
Brigantine Medical Group
353 12th Street South/PO Box 129   Zip: 08203
Ph: (609) 266-7557   Fax: (609) 266-4450
  Chaikin,Harry L., MD
  McAdam,Kimberly S., DO
Medical One
4248 Harbour Beach Boulevard   Zip: 08203
Ph: (609) 266-0400   Fax: (866) 912-0605
  Dunn,Michael Joseph, MD
  Glasser,Barry D., MD

Browns Mills
Alliance for Better Care, P.C.
130 Lakehurst Road   Zip: 08015
Ph: (609) 893-3133   Fax: (609) 893-7972
  Miller,Robin Jeanne, MD
  Razvi,Batool, MD
  Shapiro,Paul, DO
  Willoughby,Ronald P., DO

Budd Lake
Lakeview Medical Associates
125 US Highway 46   Zip: 07828
Ph: (973) 691-1111   Fax: (973) 691-1198
  Leggiero,Nicholas J., DO
  Sher,Peter Mitchell, MD
Medical Center at Budd Lake
125 US Highway 46   Zip: 07828
Ph: (973) 691-9400   Fax: (973) 691-3283
  Brett,Brian P., MD
  Seshadri,Mahalakshmi, MD

Burlington
Burlington Family Medical Center
666 Madison Avenue   Zip: 08016
Ph: (609) 386-0023   Fax: (609) 386-4648
  Griffin,Amanda, MD
  Maharaj-Mikiel,Indira Cassandra, M
  Sacks,Robert J., DO
  Varkey,Ciby B., MD
Cooper Ob-Gyn
1900 Mount Holly Road/Suite 3-C   Zip: 08016
Ph: (609) 835-5570
  Mitchell-Williams,Jocelyn, MD
  Salvatore,Michelle Lyn, MD
  Siefring,Robert P., MD
  Steinberg,Frederic, DO
Dorfner Family Medicine
811 Sunset Road/Suite 101   Zip: 08016
Ph: (609) 387-9242   Fax: (609) 387-9408
  Butt,Saeed Ahmed, MD
  Dorfner,Scott M., DO
  Jordan,Daniel Robert, MD
  Kamra,Roopama, MD
  Nemeth,Laurie Yallowitz, DO
  Rozenberg,Larisa, MD
  Strazzeri,Mia Domenica, DO
Kids First
2006 Salem Road   Zip: 08016
Ph: (609) 877-1500   Fax: (609) 877-4262
  Arnaud-Turner,Denise Marie, MD
  Berg,Jodi Liebman, MD
  Bonett,Deirdre Maria, MD
  Gould,Carolyn L., MD
  Harbist,Noel Rebecca, MD
  Hickey,John Selano Jr., MD
  Horten,James, MD
  Martinez,Esther G., MD
  Niedzwiecki,Stephen Mark, MD
  Vidal-Phelan,Johanna Maria, MD
Pulmonary & Sleep Ass. of Jersey
811 Sunset Road/Suite 201   Zip: 08016
Ph: (609) 298-1776   Fax: (609) 531-2391
  Mest,Stuart, MD
Sunset Road Medical Associates
911 Sunset Road   Zip: 08016
Ph: (609) 387-8787   Fax: (609) 386-8640
  Blank,Andrew Jay, DO
  Brandt-Park,Nicole, MD
  Moront,Barbara Jeanne, MD
  Talone,Albert A., DO

Burlington City
Southern Jersey Medical Center
651 High Street   Zip: 08016
Ph: (609) 386-0775   Fax: (609) 386-4372
  Aiello,Kathleen Kuykendall, MD
  D'Guerra,Mignon Marie, MD
  Graham,April Danielle, DO
  Reid,Gillian Salanda, MD
  Sewell,Myron L., MD

Burlington Township
LMA Professional Orthopaedics
2103 Burlington Mount   Zip: 08016
Ph: (609) 747-9200   Fax: (609) 747-1408
  Eakin,David Eugene, DO
  McMillan,Sean, DO

Butler
Advocare Pediatric Arts
1403 Route 23 South   Zip: 07405
Ph: (973) 283-2200   Fax: (973) 283-0406
  Blecherman,Sarah W., MD
  Horowitz,Deborah L., MD
  Liu,Michael, MD
  Thomas,Susheela, MD
  Vacca,Michael John, MD
  Weinstein,David M., MD
Atlantic Medical Group
1395 Route 23/Suite 4   Zip: 07405
Ph: (973) 838-0200   Fax: (973) 838-1614
  Parikh,Dhinoj M., MD

Caldwell
Drs. Suarez & Suarez
360 Bloomfield Avenue   Zip: 07006
Ph: (973) 226-8464
  Suarez,Edwin, MD
  Suarez,Lynette G., MD

Califon
Hickory Run Family Practice Associates
384 County Road 513   Zip: 07830
Ph: (908) 832-2125   Fax: (908) 832-6149
  Byrd,Raymond J., MD
  Jaskolski,Joseph A., MD
  McGowan,John M., MD
  Williams,Karen Lynn, MD

Camden
Associated Physiatrists of So NJ
1600 Haddon Avenue/Room R-122   Zip: 08103
Ph: (856) 757-3878   Fax: (856) 757-3760
  Anthony,William P., MD
  DiMarco,Jack Peter, MD
  Nolan,John P., DO
CAMCare Health Corporation
817 Federal Street   Zip: 08103
Ph: (856) 541-9811   Fax: (856) 541-4611
  Aves,Cindy, MD
  Badolato,Kevin Arthur, MD
CAMCare Health Corporation
2610 Federal Street   Zip: 08104
Ph: (856) 635-0212
  Barnea,Eytan R., MD
  Burton,Monica L., MD
  Buttress,Sharon M., MD
  Christophe,Kathleen Mary, MD
  Churlin,Donna M., MD
  Cooke,Jacqueline P., MD
  Dinks-Brown,Shantay M., DO
  Green,Patricia, MD
  Hwee,Lillian, DO
  Knoflicek,Lisa E., MD
  Knowles,William O., MD
  Leong,Kai K., MD
  Levites-Agababa,Elana R., MD
  Ligouri,Adrienne L., MD
  Manson,Florence N., MD
  Novak,Nellie, MD
  Swatski,Michael A., MD
  Toidze,Tamara V., MD
  Young,Jimmie, MD
Cooper Bone and Joint Institute
3 Cooper Plaza/Suite 411   Zip: 08103
Ph: (856) 673-4500   Fax: (856) 673-4525
  O'Connell,Brendan Garrett, MD
  Porter,John Maurice, MD
Cooper Family Medicine
1865 Harrison Avenue/Suite 1300   Zip: 08103
Ph: (856) 963-0126   Fax: (856) 365-0279
  Henry,Camille Angela Nicole, MD
Cooper Family Medicine
3156 River Road   Zip: 08105
Ph: (856) 963-0126
  Kim,Kyur Gsook Cho, MD
  Westerberg,Dyanne Pergolino, DO
Cooper Neonatology
One Cooper Plaza   Zip: 08103
Ph: (856) 342-2265   Fax: (856) 342-8007
  Aghai,Zubairul Hasan, MD
  Kushnir,Alla, MD
  Saslow,Judy G., MD
  Slater-Myer,Linda Paige, MD
  Stahl,Gary E., MD
Cooper OB/GYN
3 Cooper Plaza/Suite 300   Zip: 08103
Ph: (856) 342-2186   Fax: (856) 968-8575
  Bilbao,Michelle Cifone, DO
  Elshoreya,Hazem Mohamed, MD
  Hewlett,Guy Stewart, MD
  Kim,Yon Sook, MD
  Phillips,Nancy L., MD
  Wilson Smith,Robin Renee', DO
Cooper Perinatology Associates
3 Cooper Plaza/Suite 502   Zip: 08103
Ph: (856) 968-7433   Fax: (856) 968-8499
  Amin,Sabina, MD
  Anter,Afaf A., DO
  Caputo,Francis John, MD
  Fabius,Daniel, DO
  Isola,Kimberly Jean, MD
  Karmilovich,Beth Ann, DO
  Kim,Tae Won Benjamin, MD
  Mangold,Melissa Beth, DO
  Pradhan,Basant Kumar, MD
  Rivera,Velmina S., MD
  Tomaszewski,Jeffrey John, MD
  Utreras,Juan S., MD
  Zaeeter,Wissam Sabri, MD

Groups and Clinics by Town with Physician Rosters

Camden (cont)

Cooper PM & R Assocs
One Cooper Plaza/Suite 550 Zip: 08103
Ph: (856) 342-2040 Fax: (856) 968-8311
- Cohen, Stephen Jonathan, MD

Cooper PM & R Assocs
3 Cooper Plaza/Suite 104 Zip: 08103
Ph: (856) 342-2040 Fax: (856) 968-8311
- Porto, Maura C., DO

Cooper Psychiatric Associates
3 Cooper Plaza/Suite 307 Zip: 08103
Ph: (856) 342-2328 Fax: (856) 541-6137
- Aguilar, Francis, MD
- Ayala, Omar, MD
- Clements, David IV, MD
- Gogineni, Rama Rao, MD
- Iftekhar, Ruksana, MD
- Pumariega, Andres Julio, MD
- Szeeley, Pamela J., MD

Cooper University Hospital ObGyn
3 Cooper Plaza/Suite 221 Zip: 08103
Ph: (856) 325-6600 Fax: (856) 968-8575
- Bahora, Masuma, MD
- Hall, Bianca Elena, DO
- Knights, Jayci Elenor, MD
- La Motta, Joseph D., MD
- Smolinsky, Ciaran, MD

Cooper Univ Hosp Pedi Endocrinology
3 Cooper Plaza/Suite 200 Zip: 08103
Ph: (856) 968-8898
- Fish, Michelle Leigh Karam, DO
- Krol, Anna, MD
- Leopardi, Nicole Marie, MD
- Post, Ernest M., MD

Drs. Gitler and Kleeman
2961 Yorkship Square Zip: 08104
Ph: (856) 541-5588
- Gitler, Steven F., DO
- Kleeman, Jeffrey A., DO

Drs. Rhee and Timms
3 Cooper Plaza/Suite 221 Zip: 08103
Ph: (856) 342-2965 Fax: (856) 365-1967
- Pistilli, Stephanie Marie, DO
- Shah, Nima M., MD
- Tagni, Carine-Ange, MD
- Timms, Diane De Lisi, DO

Lourdes Imaging Associates, PA
1600 Haddon Avenue Zip: 08103
Ph: (856) 635-2654 Fax: (856) 668-8436
- Della Peruta, Joseph, MD
- Oif, Edward, MD

Lourdes Medical Associates
1601 Haddon Avenue Zip: 08103
Ph: (856) 757-3700 Fax: (856) 580-6498
- Fuseini, Nurain M., MD
- Lieser, Joan Karen, MD
- Martinez, Miguel E., MD
- Rugut, Chloe, MD

MD Anderson Cancer Center at Cooper
2 Cooper Plaza Zip: 08103
Ph: (856) 342-2000
- Ahlawat, Stuti, MD
- Bea, Vivian Jolley, MD
- Brus, Christina R., MD
- Eastwick, Gary, MD
- Hong, Young Ki, MD
- Kesselheim, Howard I., DO
- Mezera, Megan A., MD
- Mulvihill, David J., MD
- Squillante, Christian Michael, MD

Nueva Vida Behavioral Health Center
427 Market Street Zip: 08102
Ph: (856) 338-1995 Fax: (856) 338-0247
- Monte, Lyda Cervantes, MD
- Sholevar, Ghodrat Pirooz, MD

Osborn Family Health Center
1601 Haddon Road Zip: 08103
Ph: (856) 757-3700 Fax: (856) 365-7972
- Akhter, Rowsonara, MD
- Askia, Gyasi Abena, DO
- Deary, Michael J., MD
- Desimone, Dennis Charles, DO
- Lizerbram, Deborah Garber, DO
- Melchiorre, Louis P. Jr., MD
- Stegmuller, Joseph A., DO

- Thawani, Kalpana, MD
- Tyree, Laura Lynne, MD
- Vital, Michelle Maria, MD

Osborn Pediatrics
1601 Haddon Avenue Zip: 08103
Ph: (856) 757-3700 Fax: (856) 365-7972
- Roussel, Anisha Lanice, MD

Our Lady Lourdes Transplant Ctr
1601 Haddon Avenue Zip: 08103
Ph: (856) 757-3840
- Chakravarty, Arijit, MD
- Guy, Stephen Reed, MD
- Radomski, John S., MD
- Sebastian, Ely M., MD
- Youssef, Nasser Ibrahim, MD

Soll Eye PC of New Jersey/Cooper Div
3 Cooper Plaza/Suite 510 Zip: 08103
Ph: (856) 342-7200 Fax: (856) 342-6620
- Coleman, Colleen Marie, MD
- Driver, Paul J., MD
- Johnson, Paul B., MD
- Makar, Mary Saleeb, MD
- Markovitz, Bruce Jay, MD
- Olivia, Christopher Todd, MD
- Rho, David Samsun, MD
- Soll, Stephen Matthew, MD

Virtua Camden
1000 Atlantic Avenue Zip: 08104
Ph: (856) 246-3000 Fax: (856) 246-3061
- Hummel, Joseph C., DO
- Warren, Beth Ann, DO

Virtua Family Health Center
1000 Atlantic Avenue Zip: 08104
Ph: (856) 246-3542 Fax: (856) 246-3528
- Bhalodia, Amit Maganlal, DO
- Brooks, Julius A. Jr., MD
- Figliola, Robin A., DO
- Whiting, Philip Howard, DO

West Street Health Center
519 West Street Zip: 08103
Ph: (856) 968-2320 Fax: (856) 968-2317
- Bascelli, Lynda Marie, MD
- Bialecki, Rosemarie, DO

Women's Care Center
3 Cooper Plaza/Suite 301 Zip: 08103
Ph: (856) 342-2959 Fax: (856) 968-8575
- Hernandez, Marcia Lynn, DO
- Martinez, Frances Aileen, MD
- Shersher, David Daniel, MD

Cape May

Cape Urgent Care
900 Route 109 Zip: 08204
Ph: (609) 884-4357 Fax: (609) 884-4377
- Carlin, Teresa Mary, MD
- Cramer, Kenneth E., MD

Court House Surgery Center
106 Courthouse South Dennis Rd Zip: 08204
Ph: (609) 465-0300 Fax: (609) 465-8771
- Anapolle, David M., MD
- Mihata, Ryan Garner, MD

Cape May Court House

Adult & Child Dermatology Cntr
8 Village Drive Zip: 08210
Ph: (609) 465-4477 Fax: (609) 624-1281
- Weiss, Robert Joseph Sr., MD

Cape Atlantic Gastro Assocs
307 Stone Harbor Boulevard/Suite 5 Zip: 08210
Ph: (609) 465-1511 Fax: (609) 465-5310
- Landset, David J., DO
- Troum, Richard M., DO

Cape Hospitalist Associates, P.A.
2 Stone Harbor Boulevard Zip: 08210
Ph: (609) 463-2000
- Jain, Manoj Prakash, MD

Cape Regional Physicans Associates
217 North Main Street/Suite 104 Zip: 08210
Ph: (609) 463-1488 Fax: (609) 463-4881
- Martz, Patricia Ann, MD
- O'Donnell, Paul Lawrence, DO
- Russo, David Peter, MD
- Tenner, Jeffrey P., DO

Cape Regional Physicians Associates
211 North Main Street/Suite 203 Zip: 08210
Ph: (609) 536-8272 Fax: (609) 536-8273
- Deignan, Dianna T., MD

Cape Regional Physicians Associates
11 Village Drive Zip: 08210
Ph: (609) 465-2273 Fax: (609) 463-0236
- Edwards, Jillian, DO
- Fayyaz, Tooba, DO
- Hong, John S., MD
- Marotta, Raymond J. Jr., MD
- Raghuwanshi, Anita P., MD
- Zitnay, Christopher G., MD

Cape Regional Physicians Assoc-Cardio
217 North Main Street/Suite 205 Zip: 08210
Ph: (609) 463-5440 Fax: (609) 463-9888
- Boriss, Michael N., DO
- Burhanna, Amy Scally, MD
- Nillas, Michael S., MD
- Scally, Monique, DO

Cape Reg Phys Assoc-Med Commons
217 North Main Street/Suite 102 Zip: 08210
Ph: (609) 536-8010 Fax: (609) 536-8053
- Masciarelli, Anthony, DO
- Vattasseril, Renjy, MD

Drs. Matlick, DeLorio, and Mucci
307 Stone Harbor Boulevard/Suite 3 Zip: 08210
Ph: (609) 465-4667 Fax: (609) 465-9387
- DeLorio, Nicola Anne, DO
- Matlick, Lonny D., DO
- Mucci, Wayne P., DO

Drs. Milio & Michner
214 North Main Street Zip: 08210
Ph: (609) 465-2828 Fax: (609) 465-8617
- Michner, Richard A., MD
- Milio, Joseph L., DO

Drs. Morrow and Syed
601 Route 9 South Zip: 08210
Ph: (609) 463-5888 Fax: (609) 463-5885
- Syed, Zubair, DO

Harborview KidsFirst Cape May
1315 Route 9 South Zip: 08210
Ph: (609) 465-6100 Fax: (609) 465-1539
- Deliz, Yasmin D., DO

Horizon Eye Care
4 Village Drive Zip: 08210
Ph: (609) 465-7100
- McLaughlin, John Patrick, MD

Jersey Shore Gastroenterology
108 North Main Street Zip: 08210
Ph: (609) 465-0060
- Ljubich, Paul, MD

Pennsylvania Vascular Associates, PC
8 South Dennis Road Zip: 08210
Ph: (609) 465-3939 Fax: (609) 465-4042
- Salasin, Robert I., MD

Rainbow Pediatrics
2041 US Highway 9 Zip: 08210
Ph: (609) 624-9003 Fax: (609) 624-9002
- Cavaliere, Ava A., DO
- Dierkes, Thomas F., DO
- Flick, Jeffrey L., DO
- Freund, William Roy, DO
- Mathur, Ajit, MD

Regional Heart & Lung Associates
207 Court House/S. Dennis Road Zip: 08210
Ph: (609) 465-2001 Fax: (609) 465-8440
- Bradway, William R., DO
- Patel, Amit H., MD

Volunteers in Medicine
423 North Route 9 Zip: 08210
Ph: (609) 463-2846 Fax: (609) 463-2830
- Crowley, Elizabeth Ann, MD

Carneys Point

Carneys Point Family Practice
341 Shell Road Zip: 08069
Ph: (856) 299-4600 Fax: (856) 299-1688
- Lawrence, John Robert, MD
- Quigley, Craig B., MD

Healthcare Commons Inc.
500 Pennsville-Auburn Road Zip: 08069
Ph: (856) 299-3200 Fax: (856) 299-7183
- Serrano, Camilo Francisco, MD
- Varghese, Sajini S., DO

Salem Inernal Medicine
316 Merion Avenue Zip: 08069
Ph: (856) 299-0345 Fax: (856) 299-9438
- Fernandez, Maria Elmina, MD
- Salem, Mohamed M., MD

Carteret

Carteret Medical Center
606 Roosevelt Avenue Zip: 07008
Ph: (732) 541-6521 Fax: (732) 541-0060
- Goraya, Sukhjender, MD
- Singh, Bikramjit, MD

Doctors MediCenter
835 Roosevelt Avenue/Plaza 12/Suite 4A Zip: 07008
Ph: (732) 969-2240 Fax: (732) 969-2152
- Anderson-Wright, Phyllis, DO
- Kalika, Sanna, MD
- Sjovall, Frances, DO

Drs. Behman & Sidhom
48 Pulaski Avenue Zip: 07008
Ph: (732) 541-4217 Fax: (732) 541-1451
- Behman, Daisy M., MD
- Sidhom, Ibrahim W., MD

Roosevelt Medical
237 Roosevelt Avenue Zip: 07008
Ph: (732) 541-2141 Fax: (732) 541-1083
- Mavani, Nagindas V., MD
- Riar, Sandeep Singh, MD
- Singh, Rashpal, MD

Cedar Grove

M.C. Medical Group
1425 Pompton Avenue/Suite 1-1 Zip: 07009
Ph: (973) 785-8686 Fax: (973) 785-8680
- Cohen, Alan Polan, MD
- Cunningham, Ellen Elizabeth, MD
- Farley-Loftus, Rachel L., MD
- Kandula, Swetha, MD
- Morgan, James Peter, MD

Platt Psychiatric Associates, LLC
904 Pompton Avenue/Suite B-2 Zip: 07009
Ph: (973) 239-4848 Fax: (973) 239-4704
- Platt, Ellen M., DO
- Platt, Jennifer, DO

Cedar Knolls

Advanced Cardiology, LLC.
65 Ridgedale Avenue Zip: 07927
Ph: (973) 401-1100 Fax: (973) 401-1201
- Dave, Bijal A., MD
- Feitell, Leonard A., MD
- Godkar, Darshan, MD
- James, David Joel, MD
- Marotta, Charles J., MD
- Som, Sumit, MD
- Talati, Sapan Nitinbhai, MD

Advocare The Orthopedic Center
218 Ridgedale Avenue/Suite 104 Zip: 07927
Ph: (973) 538-7700 Fax: (973) 538-9478
- Bloom, Tamir, MD
- Friedman, Samara, MD
- Lin, David Yih-Min, MD
- Rieger, Mark A., MD
- Strassberg, Joshua A., MD

Summit Medical Group
65 Ridgedale Avenue Zip: 07927
Ph: (973) 401-0500 Fax: (973) 401-9306
- Dalena, John Michael, MD
- Krueger, Kelly A., MD

Atlantic Rheumatology & Osteoporosis
8 Saddle Road/Suite 202 Zip: 07927
Ph: (973) 984-9796 Fax: (973) 984-5445
- Pasik, Deborah, MD
- Paxton, Laura Anne, MD
- Sebastian, Jodi Komoroski, MD
- Singh, Vandana, DO

ID Associates PA/dba ID CARE
8 Saddle Road Zip: 07927
Ph: (973) 993-5950 Fax: (973) 993-5953
   Burstin, Stuart J., MD
Medical Institute of New Jersey
11 Saddle Road Zip: 07927
Ph: (973) 267-2122 Fax: (973) 267-3478
   Fuchs, Eliyahu Elliot, MD
   Gellerstein, Alan Stuart, MD
   Gibbions, James Vernon Jr., MD
   Goodman, Jonathan L., DO
   Gopin, Joan M., MD
   Kumar, Preethi, DO
   Monka, Ira P., DO
   Moss, Leonard J. Jr., DO
   Tepper, Suzanne, MD
New Jersey Sports Medicine
197 Ridgedale Avenue/Suite 210 Zip: 07927
Ph: (973) 998-8301 Fax: (973) 998-8302
   Bowen, Jay E., DO
   Dunn, Kevin B., MD
   Malanga, Gerard A., MD
Pulmonary & Allergy Associates
8 Saddle Road/Suite 101 Zip: 07927
Ph: (973) 267-9393 Fax: (973) 540-0472
   Capone, Robert Anthony, MD
   Dimitry, Edward Jr., MD
   Epstein, Matthew D., MD
   Graffino, Donatella B., MD
   Hussain, Adnan, MD
   Kohn, Gary Lawrence, MD
   Oei, Erwin John, MD
   Oppenheimer, John Jacob, MD
   Restifo, Robert A., DO
   Scoopo, Frederic J., MD
   Shah, Chirag Vijaykumar, MD
Summit Medical Group
160 East Hanover Avenue/Suite 101 Zip: 07927
Ph: (973) 605-5090 Fax: (973) 605-1705
   Chu, Mary M., MD
   Kuchera, James Joseph, MD
   Kuchera, Michael W., MD
   Potash, Sarah K., MD
   Ricks, Ann Marie, MD
The Orthopedic Institute of New Jersey
218 Ridgedale Avenue/Suite 202 Zip: 07927
Ph: (908) 684-3005 Fax: (908) 684-3301
   Zaino, Christian, MD
Tri-County Orthopedics
197 Ridgedale Street/Suite 300 Zip: 07927
Ph: (973) 538-2334 Fax: (973) 829-9174
   D'Agostini, Robert J., MD
   Decter, Edward M., MD
   Dona, Samuel Torres Jr., MD
   Goldman, Robert T., MD
   Hunt, Stephen A., MD

Chatham
Chatham Family Practice Associates
492 Main Street Zip: 07928
Ph: (973) 635-2432 Fax: (973) 635-6169
   Baker, Janice E., MD
   Cirello, Joseph Anthony, MD
   Gruber, Amy D., MD
   Holland, Elbridge T. Jr., MD
   Levine, Steven Marc, DO
   Ocasio, Maria Elena, MD
   Resciniti, Matthew John, DO
   Rodriguez, Lauren C., MD
   Tribuna, Joseph, MD
   Varshavski, Mikhail, DO
Chatham Pediatrics
12 Parrot Mill Road Zip: 07928
Ph: (973) 635-4511 Fax: (973) 701-1520
   Estrada, Elsie C., MD
Drs. Dapas and Traficante
2 Joanna Way Zip: 07928
Ph: (973) 635-6547 Fax: (973) 635-5826
   Traficante, Allen, MD

New Jersey Spine Center
40 Main Street Zip: 07928
Ph: (973) 635-0800 Fax: (973) 635-6254
   Alapatt, Michael F., MD
   Clark-Schoeb, James Scott, MD
   Dorsky, Steven G., MD
   Gerstman, Brett A., MD
   Lipp, Matthew Ivan, MD
   Rieger, Kenneth J., MD
Touchpoint Pediatrics
17 Watchung Avenue Zip: 07928
Ph: (973) 665-0900 Fax: (973) 665-0901
   Corpuz, Danielle M., MD
   Shaw Brachfeld, Jennifer L., MD
   Slavin, Stuart F., MD
   Tom, Valerie, MD

Cherry Hill
Advanced ENT - Cherry Hill
1910 Route 70 East/Suite 3 Zip: 08003
Ph: (856) 602-4000 Fax: (856) 424-4695
   Hall, Patrick J., MD
Advocare Assoc in General Surgery
2201 Chapel Avenue West/Suite 100 Zip: 08002
Ph: (856) 665-2017 Fax: (856) 488-6769
   Berg, David Adam, MD
   Cohen, Larry W., DO
   Fakulujo, Adeshola D., MD
   Neff, Marc A., MD
   Sandau, Roy Lee, DO
   Szczurek, Linda J., DO
Advocare Kressville Pedi Cherry Hill
710 Kresson Road Zip: 08003
Ph: (856) 795-3320 Fax: (856) 795-1213
   Gargiulo, Katherine Anne, MD
   Ibay, Maria Lourdes D., MD
   Margallo, Evangeline Cobin, MD
   Mohazzebi, Cyrus, MD
   Mohazzebi, Mahbod, MD
   Shieh, Luke, MD
   Viray, Ruth Mariel, MD
Advocare Magness-Stafford Ob-Gyn Assoc
1810 Haddonfield Berlin Road Zip: 08003
Ph: (856) 795-3313 Fax: (856) 354-8780
   Arole, Chidinma Nwanmgbede Aloz, MD
Advocare Merchantville Pediatrics
1600 Chapel Avenue/Suite 100 Zip: 08002
OnlyFax: (856) 665-3938
   Gooberman, Bruce D., MD
   Harris, Esther R., MD
   Kaplan, Leonard F., MD
   Kothari, Nita H., MD
   Marchese, Anthony Aristide, DO
Advocare South Jersey Pediatrics
1949 Route 70 East/Suite 1 & 2 Zip: 08003
Ph: (856) 424-6050 Fax: (856) 424-2943
   Ayres, Julie Clarke, MD
   Chase, Melissa Sussman, DO
   Razi, Parisa, MD
   Tedeschi, John B., MD
   Tedeschi, John M., MD
   Weber, Jason Stuart, MD
American Access Care
207 South Kings Highway/Suite 2 Zip: 08034
Ph: (856) 616-8600 Fax: (856) 616-8601
   Barzel, Eyal, MD
   Shah, Anish Pravin, MD
Aria 3B Orthopaedics, P.C.
1400 East Route 70/Second Floor Zip: 08034
   Bartolozzi, Arthur Robert, MD
   Booth, Robert Emrey Jr., MD
   Maurer, Philip Mitchell, MD
Assoc Cardiovascular Consultants
1 Brace Road/Suite C & F Zip: 08034
Ph: (856) 428-4100 Fax: (856) 428-5748
   Akhigbe, Kelvin Osagie, DO
   Akula, Devender Nagarajan, MD
   Bauer, Hans Henry Jr., MD
   Burke, Gary C., DO
   Chaudhry, Nasser A., MD
   Dunham, Rozy D., MD

   Fox, Steven N., MD
   Fuhrman, Mitchell J., MD
   Gomberg, Richard M., DO
   Hamaty, John N., DO
   Harkins, Michael J., MD
   Kernis, Steven J., MD
   Khatiwala, Jayesh Ramesh, MD
   Khaw, Kenneth, MD
   Klodnicki, Walter E., MD
   Kothari, Anil G., MD
   Lawrence, David L., MD
   Levine, Adam Maxwell, MD
   Mohapatra, Robert A., MD
   Moussa, Ibrahim Abdel, DO
   Proper, Michael C., MD
   Reichman, Michael J., MD
   Rubenstone, Jay L., DO
   Saia, Bryan Edward, DO
   Sailam, Vivek Vardha, MD
   Sandler, Matthew Jay, MD
   Sholevar, Darius P., MD
   Siddiqi, Faisal Khursheed, MD
   Siegal, Scott L., DO
   Smeglin, Anthony G., MD
   Smith, Jason Anthony, DO
   Wadehra, Ramneet, DO
   Yegya-Raman, Sivaraman, MD
Cancer Treatment Center
2090 Springdale Road/Suite B Zip: 08003
Ph: (856) 751-9010 Fax: (856) 985-9908
   Kornmehl, Carol, MD
   Meritz, Keith A., MD
Cardiovascular Associates
1840 Frontage Road Zip: 08034
Ph: (856) 795-2227 Fax: (856) 795-7436
   Cohen, Ronald A., DO
   Dickstein, Richard A., MD
   Fertels, Scott H., DO
   Gelernt, Mark D., MD
   Leavy, Jeffrey Alan, MD
   Rosenberg, Mitchell C., MD
   Silver, Steven Eric, MD
Center for Specialized Gynecology
1930 State Highway 70 East Zip: 08003
Ph: (856) 424-8091 Fax: (856) 424-0704
   Benett, Jodi A., DO
   Kaufman, Susan I., DO
Cherry Hill Center
1797 Springdale Road Zip: 08003
Ph: (856) 424-0414 Fax: (856) 424-6335
   Busch, Scott L., DO
Cherry Hill Family Care
101 Barclay Pavilion West Zip: 08034
Ph: (856) 429-4179 Fax: (856) 429-3794
   Josephson, Tina M., MD
   Levine, Richard Marc, MD
Cherry Hill Orthopedic Surgeons
PO Box 8285 Zip: 08002
Ph: (856) 662-2400 Fax: (856) 662-5525
   Naftulin, Richard J., DO
   Reiner, Mark J., DO
Cherry Hill Pediatric Group
600 West Marlton Pike Zip: 08002
Ph: (856) 428-5020 Fax: (856) 216-9433
   McHugh, Jennifer L., MD
   Rosen, Florence E., MD
   Taubman, Bruce Melvin, MD
Cherry Hill Primary and Specialty Care
457 Haddonfield Road/Suite 110 Zip: 08002
Ph: (844) 542-2273 Fax: (856) 406-4570
   Barone, Gregory John, DO
   DiMaio, Robert D., DO
   Llenado, Jeanne Valencia, DO
   Persily, Tracy L., DO
   Popescu, Anca S., MD
   Salerno, Christopher J., DO
   Scivoletti Polan, Nicole Anne, DO
   Shrayber, Yelena Y., DO
Cooper Bone and Joint Institute
401 South Kings Highway/Suite 3-A Zip: 08003
Ph: (856) 547-0201 Fax: (856) 547-0316
   Beaver, Andrew Bradley, MD
   Clements, David H. III, MD

   Gordon, Stuart Leon, MD
   Neidecker, John Michael, DO
Cooper Cardiology Associates
1210 Brace Road/Suite 103 Zip: 08034
Ph: (856) 427-7254
   Hollenberg, Steven M., MD
   Ortman, Matthew Louis, MD
Cooper Endocrinology Associates
1210 Brace Road/Suite 107 Zip: 08034
Ph: (856) 795-3597 Fax: (856) 795-7590
   Bhat, Geetha K. G., MD
   Bieler, Bert Michael, MD
   Gerber, Susan Marie, MD
   Haddad, Ghada, MD
   Kaufman, Steven Todd, MD
   Morgan, Farah Hena, MD
   Swibinski, Edward T., MD
Cooper Faculty Ob/Gyn
1103 Kings Highway North/Suite 201 Zip: 08034
Ph: (856) 321-1800 Fax: (856) 321-0133
   Hunter, Robert L., MD
Cooper PM & R Assocs
1101 North Kings Highway/Suite 100 Zip: 08034
Ph: (856) 414-6112 Fax: (856) 414-6121
   Bodofsky, Elliot B., MD
Cooper Physicians
1103 North Kings Highway/Suite 203 Zip: 08034
Ph: (856) 321-1919 Fax: (856) 321-0206
   Monari-Sparks, Mary Joan, MD
   Sherman, Anthony, MD
Cooper University Neurology
1935 Route 70 East Zip: 08003
Ph: (856) 342-2445 Fax: (856) 964-0504
   Burakgazi Dalkilic, Evren, MD
   Campellone, Joseph V. Jr., MD
   Colcher, Amy, MD
   McGarry, Andrew James, MD
   Mirsen, Thomas R., MD
Corrado Ctr Facial Plstic Cosmtic Srgy
1919 Greentree Road/Suite C Zip: 08003
Ph: (856) 344-5906 Fax: (856) 229-7617
   Corrado, Anthony Charles, DO
   Khan, Maryam Ijaz, MD
Delaware Valley Urology LLC
63 Kresson Road/Suite 103 Zip: 08034
Ph: (856) 427-9004 Fax: (856) 267-2499
   Biester, Robert J., MD
   Chow, Shih-Han, MD
Drs. Damerau, Todt & Dructor
1401 Marlton Pike East/Suite 26 Zip: 08034
Ph: (856) 479-9400 Fax: (856) 281-9913
   Damerau, Keith R., MD
   Dructor, Lisa Ann, DO
   Todt, Mark J., MD
Endocrinology Associates
1 Brace Road/Suite B Zip: 08034
Ph: (856) 234-0645 Fax: (856) 234-0498
   Anand, Rishi Dev, MD
   Hopkins, Leigh Hastings, MD
   Kaul, Shailja, MD
   Kimmel, Craig S., MD
   Martella, Arthur Thomas, MD
   Rehman, Atiq, MD
   Thapar, Garima, MD
   Varghese, Sarah, MD
   Verma, Parveen Kaur, DO
Exel-Med Inc.
100 Springdale Road/Suite A3 Zip: 08003
Ph: (856) 651-1400 Fax: (856) 651-1401
   Antonelli, William M., DO
   Hamaty, Edward G. Jr., DO
Eye Associates
1401 Route 70 East Zip: 08034
Ph: (856) 428-5797 Fax: (856) 428-6359
   Kaplan, Barnard A., MD
Finan Family Medicine, P.C.
36 Kresson Road/Suite B Zip: 08034
Ph: (856) 616-2444 Fax: (856) 616-2376
   Finan, Cathleen M., DO
   Finan-Duffy, Colleen M., DO

Groups and Clinics by Town with Physician Rosters

Cherry Hill (cont)

Garden State Orthopedics & Sports Med
455 Route 70 West Zip: 08002
Ph: (609) 616-2999 Fax: (856) 616-1437
- Barr, Lawrence I., DO
- Kahn, Marc L., MD
- Ranelle, Robert George, DO

Gupta Institute for Integrative Med
951 Berlin Road Zip: 08034
Ph: (856) 482-7246 Fax: (856) 482-7245
- Gupta, Rajan S., MD

Haddon Renal Medical Specialists
401 Kings Highway South/Suite 5 Zip: 08034
Ph: (856) 428-8992 Fax: (856) 428-9614
- Bodiwala, Brijesh Shreyas, DO
- Butani, Savita M., MD
- Chen, Shwu-Miin Y., MD
- Michel, Brian E., MD
- Ra, Daniel, DO
- Rosenthal, Brett Samson, DO
- Specter, Richard L., MD
- Stom, Mary C., MD

Kennedy Health Alliance
457 Haddonfield Road/Suite 110 Zip: 08002
Ph: (856) 406-4091 Fax: (856) 406-4570
- Alessi, Paul J., DO
- Mastromonaco, Denise M., DO
- Mueller, Loretta L., DO
- Weiss, Richard S., DO

Kennedy Hospitalist Office
2201 Chapel Avenue West Zip: 08002
Ph: (856) 513-4124 Fax: (856) 302-5932
- Ali, Tuba Muhammad, MD
- Kashif, Soofia, MD

LMA Cardiothoracic Surgical Services
1 Brace Road/Suite C Zip: 08034
Ph: (856) 470-9029 Fax: (856) 796-9391
- Blaber, Reginald J., MD
- Davis, Paul K., MD
- Momplaisir, Thierry, MD
- Nordin, Brittany N., DO
- Randle, Troy L., DO

LMA Gastroenterology Associates
63 Kresson Road/Suite 104 Zip: 08034
Ph: (856) 751-7420 Fax: (856) 424-3113
- Berberian, Brian, MD

LMA Neurology Consultants
63 Kresson Road/Suite 101 Zip: 08034
Ph: (856) 795-2000 Fax: (856) 795-3625
- Janoff, Larry Stewart, DO
- Lipsius, Bruce D., MD
- Zechowy, Allen C., MD

Lourdes Medical Associates
1 Brace Road/Suite B Zip: 08034
Ph: (609) 702-7550 Fax: (609) 702-1277
- Iyer, Malini, MD

Magaziner Medical Center
1907 Greentree Road Zip: 08003
Ph: (856) 424-8222 Fax: (856) 424-2599
- Greenberg, Scott Ross, MD
- Magaziner, Allan, DO

Medical Pain Management LLC
2070 Springdale Road/Suite 200 Zip: 08003
Ph: (856) 433-8267
- Band, Ricard Louis, MD
- Lamprou, Emanuel Jr., MD

Mid Atlantic Retina - Wills Eye Retina
501 Cooper Landing Road Zip: 08002
Ph: (856) 667-2246 Fax: (856) 667-2238
- Ho, Allen C., MD
- Hsu, Jason, MD
- Regillo, Carl, MD

Neurology Associates & Ctr Pain
1030 North Kings Highway/Suite 200B Zip: 08034
Ph: (856) 482-0030 Fax: (856) 779-7787
- Abrams, Russell I., MD

Neurology Associates & Ctr Pain
1030 North Kings Highway/Suite 200A Zip: 08034
Ph: (856) 779-7774 Fax: (856) 779-7787
- Carr, Alan D., DO
- Korn, Barry Allen, DO
- Preis, Keith Victor, MD
- Tawadrous, Alfred Rezk, MD
- Weiner, Francine L., MD

New Jersey Urology LLC
2090 Springdale Road/Suite D Zip: 08003
Ph: (856) 751-9010 Fax: (856) 985-9908
- Fallick, Mark Lawrence, MD
- Hirsh, Alina Z., MD
- Keeler, Louis L. III, MD

Patient First
2171 Route 70 West Zip: 08002
Ph: (856) 406-0023 Fax: (856) 406-0024
- Chung, Lynn S., MD
- Zaslavsky, Alexandr, MD

Penn Medicine Cherry Hill
1865 Route 70 East/Suite 220 Zip: 08003
Ph: (856) 429-1519 Fax: (856) 427-2933
- Grosh, Taras, MD

Penn Medicine at Cherry Hill
409 Route 70 East Zip: 08034
Ph: (856) 429-1519
- Alley, Evan Wayne, MD

Penn Medicine at Cherry Hill
1400 East Route 70 Zip: 08034
- Bhavsar, Jignesh, MD
- Borromeo, Rita Gonzalez, MD
- Costa, Ralph F., MD
- Epelboim Feldman, Joyce, MD
- Friedman, Terry David, MD
- Galabi, Michael, MD
- Goldberg, Jack, MD
- Hanley, Thomas T., MD
- Hanna, Gamil Sabet Fawzy, MD
- Hume, Eric Lynn, MD
- Ingala, Erin Einbinder, MD
- Khosla, Jayasree, MD
- Panucci, Nicholas Joseph, DO
- Rana, Ramneek, MD

Professional Gastroenterology
1939 Route 70 East/Suite 250 Zip: 08002
Ph: (856) 429-4433 Fax: (856) 424-6732
- Shehata, Ahmed Abdelhalim, MD
- Werbitt, Warren, DO

Pulmonary & Sleep Associates of SJ
107 Berlin Road Zip: 08034
Ph: (856) 429-1800 Fax: (856) 429-1081
- Baumgarten, Steven S., MD
- Crookshank, Aaron David, MD
- Dostal, Courtney Lynne, DO
- Driscoll, Michael Joseph, DO
- Horowitz, Ira David, MD
- Morowitz, William A., MD
- Nugent, Thomas Rone, MD
- Pope, Alan Raymond, MD
- Velasco, Antonio Quiachon, DO

Radiology Associates of New Jersey
2201 Chapel Avenue West/Suite 106 Zip: 08002
Ph: (856) 488-6844 Fax: (856) 488-6507
- Barber, Locke W., DO
- Depersia, Lori Angela, MD
- Dheer, Sachin, MD
- Di Marcangelo, Mark T., DO
- Lee, Mark Hyon-Min, MD

Regional Eye Associates
741 Route 70 West Zip: 08002
Ph: (856) 795-8787 Fax: (856) 795-8688
- Goel, Ravi Desh, MD

Regional Orthopedic, P.A.
2201 West Chapel Avenue/PO Box 8566 Zip: 08002
Ph: (856) 663-7080 Fax: (856) 663-4945
- Dubowitch, Stuart G., DO
- Gleimer, Barry S., DO
- Gleimer, Jeffrey Robert, DO
- Heyman, David Mark, DO
- Kahn, Steven H., MD
- Paiste, Mark Ronald, DO

Relievus
1400 Route 70 East Zip: 08034
Ph: (888) 985-2727
- Reyes, Johan, MD

Rothman Institute-The Performance Lab
2005 Route 7 East Zip: 08003
OnlyFax: (856) 874-1188
- Ross, Michael Jordan, MD

South Jersey Hand Center
1888 Marlton Pike East/Suite E-F-G Zip: 08003
Ph: (856) 489-5630 Fax: (856) 489-5631
- Bednar, John M., MD
- Gomez Leonardelli, Dominic Theodore
- Jacoby, Sidney Mark, MD
- Kane, Patrick Martin, MD
- Micev, Alan Joran, MD
- Rekant, Mark Spencer, MD

South Jersey Health & Wellness Center
1919 Greentree Road Zip: 08003
Ph: (856) 761-8100 Fax: (856) 761-8107
- Avetian, Garo Charles, DO
- De Prince, Daniel III, DO
- Vernon, Gerald Michael, DO

South Jersey Heart Group
3001 Chapel Avenue/Suite 101 Zip: 08002
Ph: (856) 482-8900 Fax: (856) 482-7170
- Godin, Willis Eugene, DO
- Horwitz, Jerome M., DO
- Palli, Vasu Motu, DO
- Wenger, Christopher D., DO
- Zarrella, Geoffrey Carl, DO

South Jersey Radiology Associates, P.A
315 Route 70 East/Suite B Zip: 08034
Ph: (856) 428-4344 Fax: (856) 428-0356
- Bufalino, Kevin Thomas, MD
- Curtis, Paul A., MD
- Goodworth, Gregory J., MD
- Kramer, Neil Robert, MD
- Sergi, Thomas J., MD
- Snyder, Randall William III, MD

South Jersey Sports Medicine
1004 Haddonfield Road Zip: 08002
Ph: (609) 662-7733 Fax: (856) 662-7727
- Ricci, Anthony R., DO

Southern NJ Ctr for Liver Disease
63 Kresson Road/Suite 105 Zip: 08034
Ph: (856) 796-9340 Fax: (856) 547-0390
- Elgenaidi, Hisham, MD
- Malek, Ashraf Hossain, MD

TLC Healthcare
2070 Springdale Road/Suite 100 Zip: 08003
Ph: (856) 985-0590 Fax: (856) 985-2866
- Hasbun, William Miguel, MD
- Matalon, Vivienne I., MD

TLC Kremer Cherry Hill LASIK
1800 Chapel Avenue West/Suite 100 Zip: 08002
- Malley, Debra S., MD
- Richman, Jesse, MD

The Maro Group
27 Covered Bridge Road Zip: 08034
Ph: (856) 429-2224 Fax: (856) 429-1926
- Maro, Robert Jr., MD
- Roszkowski, Jennifer Rose, DO
- Rozengarten, Kimberly Irene, DO
- Schiller, Terence G., MD
- Vitoc, Camelia S., MD

UH-SOM Department of Psychiatry
2250 Chapel Avenue West/Suite 100 Zip: 08002
Ph: (856) 482-9000 Fax: (856) 482-1159
- Aita, Wendy F., MD
- Aronowitz, Jeffrey S., DO
- Ball, Roberta R., DO
- Chen, Yirong, MD
- Dabrow, Jennifer, DO
- Denysenko, Lex, MD
- Faden, Justin B., DO
- Friedman, Michael J., DO
- Gonzalez, Joanne, MD
- Gulab, Nazli E., MD
- Ivanov, Ilya, DO
- Khan, Munaza Anwar, MD
- Madison, Harry Thomas, DO
- Maymind, Elina, MD
- Petrides, Joanna, MD
- Pinninti, Narsimha R., MD
- Rana, Badal D., DO
- Rhoades, Walter Jr., DO
- Rissmiller, David J., DO
- Rogers, James J., DO
- Schwoeri, Linda J., MD
- Shmuts, Rachel Lauren, DO
- Wallen, Mark C., MD
- Yi, Helen Huafang, MD
- Zelondzhev, Vladislav, DO
- Zielinski, Glenn D., DO

University Renal Associates
1030 North Kings Highway/Suite 310 Zip: 08034
Ph: (856) 667-7266 Fax: (856) 779-9179
- McFadden, Christopher Bruce, MD
- Zanger, Ron, MD

Virtua Surgical Group, PA
1935 Route 70 East Zip: 08003
Ph: (856) 428-7700 Fax: (856) 424-9120
- Acholonu, Emeka Joseph, MD
- Andrew, Constantine T., MD
- Bak, Yury, DO
- Bedi, Ashish, MD
- Cody, William C., MD
- Costabile, Joseph P., MD
- Deleon, Miguel L., MD
- Derivaux, Christopher Charles, MD
- El Badawi, Khaled Iqbal, MD
- Field, Charles K., MD
- Kuchler, Joseph A., MD
- Lieb, Michael D., MD
- Luciano, Pasquale A., DO
- Meslin, Keith Phillip, MD
- Pascual, Rodolfo C., MD
- Schaffzin, David Marc, MD
- Villanueva, Dioscoro T., MD
- Zaretsky, Craig Lawrence, MD
- Zuniga, Joseph Michael Romilla, MD

W. Reed Kindermann, M.D. and Assoc
3001 Chapel Avenue West/Suite 200 Zip: 08002
Ph: (856) 667-3937 Fax: (856) 667-0661
- Andrew, Mark S., MD
- Kindermann, Wilfred Reed, MD

Wills Eye Surgery Ctr in Cherry Hill
408 Route 70 East Zip: 08034
Ph: (856) 354-1600 Fax: (856) 429-7555
- Cohen, Avraham N., MD
- Lanciano, Ralph Jr., DO
- Miano, Michele A., MD
- Young, Marie Lisette, MD

Wolfe-Simon Associates
511 Kings Highway North Zip: 08034
Ph: (856) 667-1654 Fax: (856) 482-8057
- Chen, Anna, MD
- Simon, Richard M., DO

Chester

Advocare Aygen Pediatrics and Adult Ca
530 East Main Street Zip: 07930
Ph: (908) 879-4300 Fax: (908) 879-8956
- Aygen, Kadri M., MD
- Aygen, Zehra Zeynep, MD
- Singh, Maulshree, MD

Chester Medical Associates
385 Route 24/Suite 1-C Zip: 07930
Ph: (908) 879-6277 Fax: (908) 879-4464
- Chanin, Alan H., MD
- Davis, Glenn A., MD

Lawrence Charles Antonucci MD LLC
415 Route 24/Suite E Zip: 07930
Ph: (908) 879-1500 Fax: (908) 879-1515
- Antonucci, Lawrence Charles, MD
- Sebastian, Clifford Cecil, MD
- Sidhu, Gurpreet Singh, MD

Silverstein Eye Group
408 Main Street Zip: 07930
Ph: (908) 879-7297 Fax: (908) 879-4798
- Hirschfeld, James M., MD
- Silverstein, Niki A., MD

Groups and Clinics by Town with Physician Rosters

Cinnaminson
Eye Care Physicians & Surgeons of NJ
1701 Wynwood Drive Zip: 08077
Ph: (856) 829-0600 Fax: (856) 829-2832
 Dante,Karen L. Fung, MD
Triboro Family Physicians
1104 Route 130/Suite K Zip: 08077
Ph: (856) 786-8010 Fax: (856) 786-0529
 Laws-Mobilio,Susan Wendi, DO
 Parchuri,Hima Bindu, DO
 Switenko,Zenon M., DO
Rancocas Anesthesiology Assocs
700 US Highway 130 North/Suite 203 Zip: 08077
Ph: (856) 829-9345
 Chun,John Y., MD
 Feinerman,Larry Robert, MD
Rancocas Anesthesiology, PA
700 Route 130 North/Suite 203 Zip: 08077
Ph: (856) 829-9345 Fax: (856) 829-3605
 Andalft,Anthony C., MD
 Assiamah,Andrew Aboagye, MD
 Bowie,Lester J., MD
 Canals-Curtis,Elena, MD
 Cypel,David, MD
 Daniels,James W. III, MD
 Goldberg,Marc B., MD
 Gordon,Jeffrey, MD
 Gray,Terence Bay, MD
 Halevy,Jonathan D., MD
 Kor,Danuta C., MD
 Law,Henry, DO
 Lee,John C., MD
 Litvack,Steven Greg, MD
 Luetke,Brian Scott, DO
 Misher-Harris,Michele, DO
 Paterson,William D., MD
 Shapiro,Jeffrey L., MD
 Shetty,Phyllis J., MD
 Siri,Matthew A., MD
 Soremekun Salami,Olutoyin M., MD
 Starrett-Keller,Cheryl Michelle, M
 Vaughn,Michelle Marie, MD
 Waters,Renee M., MD
 Weiss,Evan A., DO

Clark
Anthony J Inverno & Associates
95 Westfield Avenue Zip: 07066
Ph: (732) 381-5555 Fax: (732) 381-5055
 Inverno,Anthony J., MD
 Jacobs,Miriam, MD
Arthritis Allergy and Immunology
100 Commerce Place Zip: 07066
Ph: (908) 301-9800 Fax: (908) 301-9801
 Nucatola,Thomas R. Jr., MD
 Sullivan,Bessie M., MD
Clark Pediatrics LLC
480 Oak Ridge Road Zip: 07066
Ph: (732) 574-9444 Fax: (732) 574-0907
 Samonte,Catherine Marie, MD
 Suapengco-Samonte,Dulce Hernandez,
Clark Urgent Care
100 Commerce Place Zip: 07066
Ph: (732) 499-0606
 Goldstein,Alan F., MD
 Kudryk,Alexander B., MD
 Rushman,John Warren, MD
 Sabharwal,Tina, MD
Drs. Chudasama and Patel
1101 Raritan Road Zip: 07066
Ph: (732) 381-3055 Fax: (732) 815-9330
 Chudasama,Lalji S., MD
 Chudasama,Neelesh Lalji, MD
 Patel,Amish Thakor, DO
Drs. Sahni amd Sahni
53-59 Westfield Avenue Zip: 07066
Ph: (732) 396-9500
 Sahni,Rakesh Kumar, MD
 Sahni,Sheila, MD
Drs. Vijayakumar & Fernandes
152 Central Avenue Zip: 07066
Ph: (732) 382-9700 Fax: (732) 382-9707
 Mathias,Claudia Fernandes, MD
 Vijayakumar,Asha M., MD

Sports Extra
67 Walnut Avenue/Suite 202B Zip: 07066
Ph: (732) 388-7300 Fax: (732) 388-1330
 Barry,Peter Francis, DO
Summit Medical Group
67 Walnut Avenue/Suite 202 Zip: 07066
Ph: (732) 388-7300 Fax: (732) 388-1330
 Beams,Michael E., DO
 Gilsenan,Michele T., DO
Union County Healthcare Associates
999 Raritan Road Zip: 07066
Ph: (732) 381-3740 Fax: (732) 381-3733
 Ford,Stephen D., MD

Clementon
Drs. Heck & Schiavone
222 Gibbsboro Road Zip: 08021
Ph: (856) 784-4999 Fax: (856) 784-0258
 Heck,Gary X., DO

Cliffside Park
Emergimed
663 Palisade Avenue/Suite 101 Zip: 07010
Ph: (201) 945-6500 Fax: (201) 945-1157
 Chouake,Benjamin S., MD
 Dhanani,Harsha Narendra, MD
 Fishbein,Susan, MD
 Hamada,Murray S., MD
 Hershenbaum,Esther, MD
Palisades Medical Center
705B Anderson Avenue Zip: 07010
Ph: (201) 861-1851 Fax: (201) 861-1853
 Farber,Liora Judith, MD
 Weinberger,George T., DO
Premier Orthopaedics & Sports Med
663 Palisade Avenue/Suite 302 Zip: 07010
Ph: (201) 943-9100 Fax: (201) 943-7308
 Corradino,Christine M., MD
 Finnesey,Kevin Sean, MD
 Groves,Danielle Breitman, MD
 Xu,Qian, MD
Renaissance General Medicine
596 Anderson Avenue/Suite 302 Zip: 07010
Ph: (201) 943-2700 Fax: (201) 943-2646
 Korenfeld,Alexander, MD
 Korenfeld,Yelena, MD
The Urology Center of Englewood, PA
663 Palisade Avenue/Suite 304 Zip: 07010
Ph: (201) 313-1933 Fax: (201) 313-9599
 Chun,Thomas Young, MD
 Klafter,George, MD
 Margolis,Eric Judd, MD
 Simon,Daniel Ross, MD
 Simon,Robert B., MD
 Wasserman,Gary D., MD
Women's Health Partners
574 Anderson Avenue Zip: 07010
Ph: (201) 943-4884 Fax: (201) 943-4839
 Adu-Amankwa,Bernice Abrafi, MD

Clifton
Abbasi Medical Group
1300 Main Avenue/Suite 2-D Zip: 07011
Ph: (973) 851-7818
 Abbasi,Tareef M., MD
 Leon Wong,Hector J., MD
Adult and Pediatric Urology Center PA
1033 Clifton Avenue Zip: 07013
Ph: (973) 473-5700 Fax: (973) 473-3367
 Greene,Tricia Danielle, MD
 Li,Sharon Mei-Mei, MD
 Marella,Venkata Koteswararao, MD
 Sanzone,John, MD
 Shahbandi,Matthew, MD
 Zinman,James Douglas, MD
Broad Street Medical Associates
1135 Broad Street/Suite 205 Zip: 07013
Ph: (973) 471-8850 Fax: (973) 471-5232
 Krisa,Paul C., MD
Cardiac & Arrhythmias Specialist
905 Allwood Road/Suite 103 Zip: 07013
Ph: (973) 778-3111 Fax: (973) 340-1518
 Prakash,Atul, MD

Cardiology Center of North Jersey
1030 Clifton Avenue Zip: 07013
Ph: (973) 778-3777 Fax: (973) 778-3252
 Brown,Elliot M., MD
 Julie,Edward, MD
 Sankholkar,Kedar Deepak, MD
 Skolnick,Bruce A., MD
 Teicher,Mark, MD
Cecere and Rubino Internal Med
1195 Clifton Avenue Zip: 07013
Ph: (973) 471-4004 Fax: (973) 471-1180
 Cecere,Antoinette M., MD
 Rubino,Gennaro, MD
Clifton Comprehensive Medical Center
960 Paulison Avenue Zip: 07011
Ph: (973) 773-7713 Fax: (973) 773-7723
 Rey,Ricardo, MD
 Ugras Rey,Sandra S., DO
Clifton Eye Care
1016 Main Street Zip: 07011
Ph: (973) 546-5700 Fax: (973) 546-8898
 Burrows,Adria, MD
 Cuttler,Nirupa C., MD
 Stegman,Daniel Ychac, MD
Clifton Ob/Gyn
1033 Route 46 East/Suite 102 Zip: 07013
Ph: (973) 779-7979 Fax: (973) 779-7970
 Boyle,Elizabeth Anne, DO
 Haddad,Charles George, MD
Clifton Primary Care Center
1111 Clifton Avenue/Suite 204 Zip: 07013
Ph: (973) 779-9500 Fax: (973) 779-8900
 Patel,Anjali Dalal, DO
 Singh,Sarva D., MD
Clifton Psychiatric Services
469 Clifton Avenue Zip: 07011
Ph: (973) 253-0266 Fax: (973) 253-0399
 Keiman,Isidore Michael, MD
 Pascual,Bolivar, MD
Clifton Urgent and Primary Care
721 Clifton Avenue/Suite 2A Zip: 07013
Ph: (973) 777-7727 Fax: (973) 779-7906
 Fyffe,Ullanda P., MD
 Shraytman,Arkadiy, DO
Clifton-Wallington Medical Group
1033 Clifton Avenue/Suite 210 Zip: 07013
Ph: (973) 473-4400 Fax: (973) 473-4547
 Szczech,Kazimierz M., MD
Colfax Oncology/Fast Med
476 Colfax Avenue Zip: 07013
Ph: (973) 594-7977
 Afonja,Richards A., MD
 Benn,Howard A., MD
Crossroads Medical Group
975 Clifton Avenue Zip: 07013
Ph: (973) 778-8666 Fax: (973) 778-7559
 Najjar,Joe E., MD
 Najjar,Sessine, MD
 Varoqua,Sabah, MD
Dermatology Center of North Jersey
1033 Clifton Avenue Zip: 07013
Ph: (973) 777-6444 Fax: (973) 777-5277
 Gold,Jonathan Allan, MD
 Zurada,Joanna Magdalena, MD
Diab Endo Metabolism Specialities PA
6 Brighton Road/Suite 103 Zip: 07012
Ph: (973) 471-2692 Fax: (973) 470-8188
 Roehnelt,Alessia Carluccio, MD
 Schulder-Katz,Micol, MD
 Schultz,Atara Batsheva, MD
 Shalem,Lena Hourwitz, MD
 Torres,Catherine P., MD
Drs. Sahu and Sahu
458 Clifton Avenue Zip: 07011
Ph: (973) 340-7676 Fax: (973) 340-7770
 Sahu,Anand P., MD
 Sahu,Sharad, MD
Drs. Silber & Tanzer
992 Clifton Avenue Zip: 07013
Ph: (973) 365-1800
 Silber,Judy G., MD
 Tanzer,Floyd R., MD

Drs. Sullivan and Sullivan
1117 Route 46 East Zip: 07013
Ph: (973) 779-1221 Fax: (973) 778-6014
 Sullivan,Gregory F., MD
 Sullivan,Jared Martin, MD
Elite Orthopedics & Sports Medicine
1035 Route 46 East/Suite G-2 Zip: 07013
Ph: (973) 513-9646
 Ambrose,John F., MD
Family Medical Care of Clifton
1033 Clifton Avenue/Suite 209 Zip: 07013
Ph: (973) 470-8377 Fax: (973) 470-8534
 Chen,David, MD
 Lavian,Pejman, MD
Fayrouz Pediatrics
1300 Main Avenue/Suite 2-C Zip: 07011
Ph: (973) 928-3388 Fax: (973) 404-8525
 Gadalla,Hisham Hussein, MD
 Grullon Okumus,Ariolis Carmelina,
Garden State Pain Control Center, P.A.
1117 Route 46 East/Suite 201 Zip: 07013
Ph: (973) 777-5444 Fax: (973) 777-0304
 Dang,Saurabh, MD
 Koppel,Todd Sloan, MD
 Nasiek,Dariusz Jacek, MD
 Patel,Dipan G., MD
 Sheikh,Afzal J., MD
 Sinha,Binod P., MD
 Sinha,Neil, MD
 Tankha,Pavan, DO
Gastroenterology Associates of NJ
1011 Clifton Avenue Zip: 07013
Ph: (973) 471-8200 Fax: (973) 471-3032
 Boxer,Andrew Scott, MD
 Gronowitz,Steven D., MD
 Krohn,Natan Nata, MD
Heart & Vasc Assoc of Northern Jersey
1114 Clifton Avenue Zip: 07013
Ph: (973) 471-5250
 Obeleniene,Rimvida, MD
ImmediCenter/Clifton
1355 Broad Street Zip: 07013
Ph: (973) 778-5566 Fax: (973) 778-2268
 Coleman,Scott L., MD
 Del Casale,Thomas Ernest, DO
 Dixon,George C., MD
 Jacknin,Mark A., DO
 Kahlon,Tejinderpaul Singh, MD
 Kelleher,Maureen Michelle, MD
 Lima,Francesco W., MD
 Palmer,Susan M., DO
Lucila Medical P.C.
780 Allwood Road Zip: 07012
Ph: (973) 249-6202 Fax: (973) 249-6203
 Lucila,Rafael R., MD
 Tindoc,Lorelane Pagulayan, MD
Maan Pediatric Associates Inc
75 Clifton Avenue Zip: 07011
Ph: (973) 546-6400
 Ayeni,Ahisu I., MD
Medical Specialties of New Jersey
842 Clifton Avenue/Suite 4 Zip: 07013
Ph: (973) 777-2440 Fax: (973) 777-1848
 Weiss,Emmanuel M., MD
 Weiss,Gabriella Antionette, MD
 Weiss,Jeffrey A., MD
Michael I. Baruch Plastic Surgery
1037 Route 46 East/Suite 103 Zip: 07013
Ph: (973) 773-1973 Fax: (973) 773-4824
 Ames-Bobila,Deborah, MD
 Baruch,Michael I., MD
NJ Best ObGyn
716 Broad Street/Suite 6 A Zip: 07013
Ph: (973) 221-3122 Fax: (973) 574-1008
 Okour,Salman N., MD
 Smith,Jacqueline Marie, MD
Neurology Group of North Jersey
905 Allwood Road/Suite 105 Zip: 07012
Ph: (973) 471-3680
 Katz,Avery S., MD
 Knep,Stanley J., MD
 Lequerica,Steve A., MD

Groups and Clinics by Town with Physician Rosters

Clifton (cont)
NJ Arthritis Osteoporosis Center
871 Allwood Road/Suite 1 Zip: 07012
Ph: (973) 405-5163 Fax: (973) 365-8004
- Lewko, Michael P., MD
- Raklyar, Irina, MD

North Jersey Eye Associates PA
1005 Clifton Avenue Zip: 07013
Ph: (973) 472-4114 Fax: (973) 472-0775
- Cucci, Patricia, MD
- Lesko, Cecily A., MD
- Wunsh, Stuart Eugene, MD

N. Jersey Ortho. & Sports Med.
6 Brighton Road/Suite 101 Zip: 07012
Ph: (973) 340-1940 Fax: (973) 340-1958
- Russonella, Michael Christopher, DO
- Singh, Manik, MD

North Jersey Pediatrics
1010 Clifton Avenue Zip: 07013
Ph: (973) 249-1231 Fax: (973) 249-1316
- Wu, Karen, MD

Notchview Pediatrics, LLC.
1037 Route 46 East/Suite 201 Zip: 07013
Ph: (973) 779-3911 Fax: (973) 471-2730
- Caprio, Ralph E., MD
- Gunn, Angela Lijoi, MD
- Hanna, Ruba, MD
- Lavaia, Maria A., MD
- Lew, Lai Ping, MD
- Lewis, Michael Glenn, MD
- Mediterraneo, Susan, MD
- Niziol, John A., MD
- Patel, Shivani J., MD
- Schaffer, Ashley Marie, MD

NuHeights Pediatrics
2 Brighton Road/Suite 404 Zip: 07013
Ph: (973) 250-2970 Fax: (973) 250-2971
- Matta, Rana C., MD

NuHeights Pediatrics
1115 Clifton Avenue/Suite 101 Zip: 07013
Ph: (973) 250-2970 Fax: (973) 250-2971
- Sadegh, Mona, MD
- Soto-Pereira, Angelica Maria, MD
- Sutter, John I., MD
- Thomas, Mary Kathleen, MD
- Tokat, Ikbal, MD

OB/GYN & Infertility Serv of No NJ
721 Clifton Avenue/Suite 1A Zip: 07013
Ph: (973) 471-0707 Fax: (973) 471-2112
- Hakimi, Daniel, DO
- Smith, Jade, DO

Shah, Vinay R.
985 Paulison Avenue Zip: 07011
Ph: (973) 471-2000 Fax: (973) 773-8553
- Shah, Vinay R., MD
- Singh, Sukhdeep, MD

Summit Medical Group
6 Brighton Road/2 FL Zip: 07012
Ph: (973) 777-7911 Fax: (973) 777-5403
- Ahmad, Ali, MD
- Baum, Howard B., MD
- Brancato, Jaclyn, DO
- Debell, David Anthony, MD
- Ferrazzo-Weller, Marissa G., DO
- Goldberg, Marc A., MD
- Goyal, Neil Kamal, MD
- Graber, David J., MD
- Hanan, Scott H., MD
- Ibarbia, Jose D., MD
- Igbokwe, Jennifer, MD
- Jawetz, Harold I., MD
- Jawetz, Seth Gerald, MD
- O'Brien, Joseph Patrick, MD
- Okun, Jeffrey, MD
- Porras, Cornelio J., MD
- Rana, Najmul, MD
- Reydel, Boris, MD
- Ritt, Jake Edward, MD
- Sandler, Rebecca Ellen, MD
- Schactman, Brian, MD
- Strakhan, Marianna, MD
- Todi, Neelam T., MD
- Wooton, Robert P. Jr., MD

Surgery Associates of North Jersey
1100 Clifton Avenue Zip: 07013
Ph: (973) 778-0100
- Buckley, Michael K., MD
- Kane, Edwin P., MD
- Ros, Adriana Oksana, DO

Tenafly Pediatrics, PA
1135 Broad Street/Suite 208 Zip: 07013
Ph: (973) 471-8600 Fax: (973) 471-3068
- Brondfeld, Raquel Lara, MD
- Buchalter, Maury, MD
- Jawetz, Robert Evan, MD
- Pagano, Christine Federline, MD
- Schein, Aviva B., MD

The AIPM Group
1037 Route 46 East/Suite G-5 Zip: 07013
Ph: (973) 928-5363 Fax: (973) 928-5359
- Kang, Richard T., MD
- Kizina, Christopher Allen, MD

The Cardiovascular Care Group
1401 Broad Street/Suite 1 Zip: 07013
Ph: (973) 759-9000 Fax: (973) 751-3730
- Holmes, Raymond Joseph, MD
- Levison, Jonathan Andrew, MD
- Pontoriero, Michael Anthony, MD
- Syracuse, Donald C., MD

United Medical, P.C.
533 Lexington Avenue Zip: 07011
Ph: (973) 546-6844 Fax: (973) 546-7707
- Alday, Arnold M., MD
- Muccino, Gary P., MD
- Nunez, Jacqueline Denise, MD
- Sabido, Michael, MD

Valley Medical Associates
1700 Route 3 West Zip: 07012
Ph: (862) 249-4901 Fax: (973) 928-2650
- Pinzon, Amabelle Par, MD
- Yang, Domingo Berzamin Jr, MD

Clinton
Center For Endocrine Health
1738 Route 31 North/Suite 108 Zip: 08809
Ph: (908) 735-3980 Fax: (908) 735-3981
- Lifchus Ascher, Rebecca Jean, MD
- Ryan, Wanda Dawn, MD
- Torrens, Javier I., MD

Hunterdon Cardiovascular Associates
1738 Route 31/Suite 210 Zip: 08809
Ph: (908) 823-9200 Fax: (908) 823-9211
- Lind, Robert S., MD

Hunterdon Pediatric Associates
1738 Route 31 North/Suite 201 Zip: 08809
Ph: (908) 735-3960 Fax: (908) 735-3965
- Braff, Ricky A., MD
- Coraggio, Michael J., MD
- Kroon, Jody Lynn, MD

Paul Phillips Eye & Surgery Center
64 Walmart Plaza Zip: 08809
Ph: (908) 735-4100 Fax: (908) 735-7494
- Bakhru, Ritika, MD
- Bernstein, Jay M., MD
- Morgenstern, Kenneth Eli, MD

The Doctor Is In
59 Old Highway 22 Zip: 08809
Ph: (908) 730-6363 Fax: (908) 730-8185
- Lunt, David M., MD
- Messina, Charles I., MD
- Silverberg, Michael S., MD

Closter
Closter Medical Group
200 Closter Dock Road Zip: 07624
Ph: (201) 768-3900 Fax: (201) 768-3840
- Cavalli, Nina Ann, MD
- Nouman, Helena, MD

Hackensack UMG Closter
1 Ruckman Road Zip: 07624
Ph: (201) 385-6161 Fax: (201) 385-1671
- Farooki, Zahid A., MD
- Lien, Frank W., DO

North Jersey Orthopaedic Specialists
15 Vervalen Street Zip: 07624
Ph: (201) 784-6800 Fax: (201) 784-6801
- Lee, Soo Gyung, MD

Pedimedica PA
500 Piermont Road/Suite 102 Zip: 07624
Ph: (201) 784-3200 Fax: (201) 784-3321
- Rosenberg, Lori A., DO
- Yegen, Lonna K., MD

Trokhan Dermatology, LLC.
235 Closter Dock Road Zip: 07624
Ph: (201) 767-1908 Fax: (201) 767-3097
- Parron, John Keckhut, MD
- Ramaswamy, Preethi V., MD
- Sokol, Shima C., MD
- Trokhan, Eileen Q., MD
- Trokhan, Shawn Edward, MD

Collingswood
Advocare South Jersey Pediatrics
204 White Horse Pike Zip: 08107
Ph: (856) 424-6050 Fax: (856) 424-2943
- Georgelos, Panagiotis, MD
- Velasco, Reynaldo, MD
- Weber, Carolyn Harding, MD

Collingwood Family Practice
600 Atlantic Avenue Zip: 08108
Ph: (856) 854-1050 Fax: (856) 854-2453
- Holwell, Michael, DO
- Neveling, Lance William, DO
- Stagliano, Robert A., DO

Drs. Heck & Schiavone
416 Haddon Avenue Zip: 08108
Ph: (856) 858-1240
- Schiavone, Ronald L., DO

Drs. Kresloff and Young
900 Haddon Avenue/Suite 102 Zip: 08108
Ph: (856) 854-4242
- Goldstein, Arthur Meyer, MD
- Kresloff, Michael Scott, MD
- Kresloff, Richard S., MD
- Young, Marc, MD

Women's Healthcare of Collingswood
1055 Haddon Avenue Zip: 08108
Ph: (856) 854-4524 Fax: (856) 854-8216
- Margolin, Gregory, MD
- Parrish, Sherrilynn, MD

Colonia
Drs. Gaurang R. Patel & Associates
1503 St Georges Avenue/Suite 205 Zip: 07067
Ph: (732) 382-8111 Fax: (732) 381-0292
- Chaudhary, Jigisha S., MD
- Dubbaka-Rajaram, Arunasree, MD
- Patel, Gaurang R., MD

Drs. Sonavane and Benoy
1503 Saint Georges Avenue/Suite 205 Zip: 07067
Ph: (732) 382-8111 Fax: (732) 381-0292
- Benoy, Leena, MD
- Sonavane, Vidya Kiran, MD

Martin P. Mayer, MD PC
1503 Saint Georges Avenue Zip: 07067
Ph: (732) 382-1300 Fax: (732) 382-6923
- Alvarez, Reinaldo G., MD
- Mayer, Martin P., MD

Union County Healthcare Associates
689 Inman Avenue Zip: 07067
Ph: (732) 381-4575 Fax: (732) 381-0070
- Guzik, David J., DO

Colts Neck
Colts Neck Pediatrics
26 State Highway 34/Suite 208 Zip: 07722
Ph: (732) 683-0099
- Bautista, Jocelyn B., MD
- Liao, Jennifer Ledesma, MD

Family Practice of CentraState
281 Route 34/Suite 813 Zip: 07722
Ph: (732) 431-2620 Fax: (732) 431-3707
- Angello, Philip Joseph, MD
- Peters, Nancy Castellucci, MD
- Raymond, Kimberly J., MD

Orchard Medical Group
9 Professional Circle/Suite 101 Zip: 07722
Ph: (732) 431-1520 Fax: (732) 431-1567
- Gualberti, Joann, MD
- Gualberti-Girgis, Lisa, MD

Columbia
Premier Health Associates
5 Eisenhower Road Zip: 07832
Ph: (908) 362-5360
- Grote, Walter R., DO

Skylands Medical Group PA
210 Route 94 Zip: 07832
Ph: (908) 362-9285 Fax: (908) 362-7756
- Arvary, Gary J., MD
- Cullen, Eugene A., MD
- Molnar, Eric D., DO

Columbus
Capital Health Primary Care Columbus
23203 Columbus Road/Suite 1 Zip: 08022
Ph: (603) 303-4450 Fax: (603) 303-4451
- Carcia, Danielle, DO

Columbus Family Physicians
23659 Columbus Road/Suite 4 Zip: 08022
Ph: (609) 298-3304 Fax: (609) 298-7091
- Bross, Robert J., MD
- Chao, Christina, MD
- Dunn, Davonnie Marie, MD
- Guiliano, Philip M., MD
- Hulse, Andrea Doria, DO
- Vare, Christopher, MD

The Cardiology Group, P.A.
1 Sheffield Drive/Suite 102 Zip: 08022
Ph: (856) 291-8855
- Spagnuolo, Vincent J., MD

Cranford
Central Jersey Beharioral Health, LLC
216 North Avenue East Zip: 07016
Ph: (908) 272-7500 Fax: (908) 272-7502
- Cayetano, Victoria F., MD
- Chong, Raymond Ee-Mook, MD
- Hong, Rolando Y., MD
- Lim, Vicente M. Jr., MD
- Schweiger, Bruce Daniel, MD

Cranford Pediatrics
19 Holly Street Zip: 07016
Ph: (908) 276-6598 Fax: (908) 276-0040
- Pogany, Ursula M., MD

Drs. Kaye and Kaye
31 South Union Avenue Zip: 07016
Ph: (908) 272-8676 Fax: (908) 272-7052
- Kaye, Alissa Ellen, MD
- Kaye, Gary L., MD

Drs. Singh & Singh
19 Holly Street/Suite 8 Zip: 07016
Ph: (908) 276-3132 Fax: (908) 931-0842
- Singh, Iqbal K., MD
- Singh, Mohinder P., MD

Premier Urology Group, LLC
570 South Avenue East/Building A Zip: 07016
Ph: (908) 603-4200 Fax: (908) 497-1633
- Schwartz, Malcolm, MD

QDx Pathology Services
46 Jackson Drive Zip: 07016
OnlyFax: (908) 272-1478
- Khan, Amjad A., MD
- Qureshi, Mohammad Nasar, MD

Cream Ridge
Allentown Medical Associates
163 Burlington Path Road Zip: 08514
Ph: (609) 758-1100
- Peller, Alicia S., MD
- Rosengarten, Herbert H., MD

Dayton
RWJPE Dayton Medical Group
12 Stults Road/Suite 121 Zip: 08810
Ph: (732) 329-8600 Fax: (609) 395-7519
- Boudwin, James E., MD
- Casper, Robert J., MD
- Sharma, Shivani, MD

Cardio-Thoracic Surgical Group
12 Stults Road/Suite 123 Zip: 08810
Ph: (732) 230-3272 Fax: (732) 230-3309
- Schaer, Teresa McKinley, MD

Groups and Clinics by Town with Physician Rosters

Delran

Advocare Delran Pediatrics
5045 Route 130 South/Suite F Zip: 08075
Ph: (856) 461-1717 Fax: (856) 461-1143
- Foreman, Michael J., MD
- Harrell, Angela Duley, MD
- Hayes, Ciana Tyiesh, MD

Alliance OB/GYN Consultants
5045 Route 130 South/Suite 1 Zip: 08075
Ph: (856) 764-7660 Fax: (856) 764-5723
- Edwards, Linda J., MD
- Ginwala, Khatoon T., MD
- Khorsandi, Shayan, MD
- Obianwu, Chike W., MD

Delran Family Practice
8008 Route 130/Suite 120 Zip: 08075
Ph: (856) 764-7997 Fax: (856) 764-1840
- Graziano-Wilcox, Donna, DO
- Rausch, Debora Anne, MD
- Squires, Leslie S., MD

Delran Internal Medicine
5045 Route 130 South/Suite E Zip: 08075
Ph: (856) 764-2525 Fax: (856) 764-6344
- Basara, Matthew Jr., MD
- Berna, Renee Ann, MD

Dorfner Family Medicine
950 A Chester Avenue/Suite 10 Zip: 08075
Ph: (856) 764-2500 Fax: (856) 764-8335
- Mirson, Sofiya, MD

Epstein Internal Medicine
2906 Route 130 North Zip: 08075
Ph: (856) 764-4115 Fax: (856) 764-4116
- Alcera, Roanna Espino, MD
- Epstein, Jeffrey E., MD
- Keller, Maureen Reilly, DO

Hand Surgery & Rehab Ctr of NJ
8008 Route 130 North Zip: 08075
Ph: (856) 764-8804 Fax: (856) 764-3561
- Sattel, Andrew B., MD

Patient First
4000 Route 130/Bldg. C Zip: 08075
Ph: (856) 705-0685 Fax: (856) 705-0686
- Friedman, Samuel L., DO
- Hicks, Michael James, MD
- Smith, Kindra Renee, MD
- Starkman, Moishe, MD

Denville

Associates in Pulmonary Medicine
16 Pocono Road/Suite 217 Zip: 07834
Ph: (973) 625-5651
- Alexander, Robert Francis, MD
- Finkel, Richard I., MD
- Goldshlack, Jack S., DO
- Patel, Gaurang, MD

Cataract & Eye Care Center
16 Pocono Road/Suite 301 Zip: 07834
Ph: (973) 625-7970
- Levey, Stephanie B., MD
- Pearlman, Theodore F., MD

Denville Assoc of Internal Med
16 Pocono Road/Suite 317 Zip: 07834
Ph: (973) 627-2650 Fax: (973) 627-8383
- Banu, Dana R., MD
- Cheng, Yihong Henry, MD
- Collum, Robert G., MD
- Levy, Seth Evan, MD
- Mandel, Gilbert B., MD
- Nicolai, Michael, MD

Denville Pediatrics Med Assoc
140 East Main Street Zip: 07834
Ph: (973) 625-5090 Fax: (973) 625-8006
- Chait Kessler, Dana Erica, MD
- Craig, Krekamey Ropkui, MD
- Mann, Nora B., MD

Drs. Moy and Spinelli
35 West Main Street/Suite 201 Zip: 07834
Ph: (973) 627-9635 Fax: (973) 625-7484
- Moy, Winston C., MD
- Spinelli, Nancy Ann, DO

Drs. Siegel & Siegel
16 Pocono Road/Suite 107 Zip: 07834
Ph: (973) 586-8400 Fax: (973) 586-4206
- Siegel, Joseph K., MD
- Siegel, Stacey Beth, DO

Eastern Vascular Associates
16 Pocono Road/Suite 313 Zip: 07834
Ph: (973) 625-0112 Fax: (973) 625-0721
- Gironta, Michael Gerard, DO
- Lopez, Jose M., MD
- Mintz, Bruce L., DO
- Stansbury, Frederick H., DO

Feigin & Las
56 Diamond Springs Road Zip: 07834
Ph: (973) 625-1000 Fax: (973) 625-9122
- Feigin, Leslie C., MD
- Las, Murray S., MD

First Urgent Medical Care
3175 Route 10 East/Suite 500 Zip: 07834
Ph: (973) 891-1213 Fax: (973) 891-1216
- Furst, Alan David, MD
- Kaminetsky, Eric Jay, DO
- Zaki, Isaac Kamal, MD

Garden State Urology
282 US Highway 46 Zip: 07834
Ph: (973) 895-6636 Fax: (973) 895-5327
- Berman, Adam Jay, MD
- Bonder, Irvin Mark, MD
- Friedman, Lawrence, MD
- Ware, Steven M., MD

Institute of Preventive Medicine
95 East Main Street/Suite 106 Zip: 07834
Ph: (973) 586-4111 Fax: (973) 586-8466
- Ali, Majid, MD
- Juco, Judy M., MD

Lifeline Medical Associates, LLC
16 Pocono Road/Suite 105 Zip: 07834
Ph: (973) 831-2777 Fax: (973) 831-2780
- Agnello, Jennifer T., DO
- Shah, Yashica Manish, MD

Morris County Gastro Associates
16 Pocono Road/Suite 201 Zip: 07834
Ph: (973) 627-4430 Fax: (973) 586-2336
- Barbarito, Edward Joseph, MD
- Emiliani, Vincent J., MD
- Soriano, John G., MD

Morris County Orthopaedic Group
109 US Highway 46 East Zip: 07834
Ph: (973) 625-1221 Fax: (973) 625-1594
- Capecci, Frank, MD
- Cubelli, Kenneth, MD
- Simmerano, Rocco Anthony, MD

Morris Urology
16 Pocono Road/Suite 205 Zip: 07834
Ph: (973) 627-0060 Fax: (973) 627-6821
- Zimmerman, Gregg E., MD

North Jersey Endocrine Consultants, LL
1 Indian Road/Suite 8 Zip: 07834
Ph: (973) 625-2121 Fax: (973) 625-8270
- Mintz, Shari Nan, MD
- Rosenfeld, Cheryl Robyn, DO
- Sharma, Swati, MD

Oncology & Hematology Specialists, PA
23 Pocono Road/Suite 100 Zip: 07834
Ph: (973) 316-1701 Fax: (973) 316-1708
- Abbasi, Muhammad Rashid, MD
- Bari, Fazal, MD
- Jan, Naveed A., MD
- Levitz, Jason Sanford, MD
- Reiter, Barry A., MD
- Schreibman, Stephen M., MD

Pediatric Associates of W Essex
3155 Route 10/Suite 104 Zip: 07834
Ph: (973) 361-4900 Fax: (973) 361-1842
- Ganek, Martin E., MD

Pediatrics of Morris
16 Pocono Road/Suite 112 Zip: 07834
Ph: (973) 627-6010 Fax: (973) 625-9424
- Connolly, Melissa Jane, MD
- Magadan, Silvia Maria, DO
- Thomas, Miriam, MD

Pediatrics on Broadway
10 Broadway Zip: 07834
Ph: (973) 625-7734 Fax: (973) 625-4821
- De Cristofano, Robert E., MD
- Di Turi, Suzanne V., MD
- Dicker, Richard Irving, MD

Sheppell and Ricks MD
16 Pocono Road/Suite 305 Zip: 07834
Ph: (973) 627-0555 Fax: (973) 627-3880
- Ricks, Jason D., MD
- Sheppell, Arthur L., MD

St. Clare's Health Services
50 Morris Avenue Zip: 07834
Ph: (973) 625-7051
- Brandon, Meredith, MD
- Gormus, Margarita, MD
- Ruiz, David A., MD
- Shafiq, Saima, MD
- Ying Chang, Jean S., MD

The Center For Women's Health
16 Pocono Road/Suite 103 Zip: 07834
Ph: (973) 947-9066 Fax: (973) 947-9056
- Mamoun, Sami M., MD
- Tsai, Yan-San, MD

Deptford

Gloucester County Pediatrics
849 Cooper Street Zip: 08096
Ph: (856) 848-6346 Fax: (856) 848-5734
- Alikhan, Salma, MD
- Coant, Pierre N., MD
- Laudati, Mary, MD
- Minutillo, Angelo L., MD

Dover

Allergy & Arthritis Associates
600 Mount Pleasant Avenue/Suite C Zip: 07801
Ph: (973) 989-0500 Fax: (973) 989-5046
- Bigelsen, Stephen J., MD
- Golombek, Steven J., MD
- Pare', Jeanne M., MD

Eye Associates of North Jersey
600 Mount Pleasant Avenue Zip: 07801
Ph: (973) 366-1232 Fax: (973) 366-2960
- Mann, Eric Bryce, MD
- Schorr, Ian M., MD

Gastroenterology Assoc of NJ
369 West Blackwell Street Zip: 07801
Ph: (973) 361-7660 Fax: (973) 361-0455
- Krupnick, Matthew E., MD
- Rybalov, Sergey, MD

Neuro-Specialists of Morris-Sussex, PA
369 West Blackwell Street Zip: 07801
Ph: (973) 361-7606 Fax: (973) 361-8942
- Dover, Marcia Anne, MD
- Roberts, Paul J., MD
- Stephen, Infanta Anusha, MD

Orthopedica Assoc of W Jersey
600 Mount Pleasant Avenue/Suite A Zip: 07801
Ph: (973) 989-0888 Fax: (973) 989-0885
- Bouillon, Louis R., MD
- Rosenzweig, Abraham H., MD
- Spielman, Joel H., MD
- Stecker, Steven, MD
- Tiger, Arthur H., MD

Pediatric Associates
77 Union Street Zip: 07801
Ph: (973) 366-5236 Fax: (973) 366-5236
- Collins, Ronald A., MD
- Prakash, Kalpana, MD

The Family Medical Center at Dover
375 East McFarland Street Zip: 07801
Ph: (973) 366-5859 Fax: (973) 366-0026
- Schonfield, Leah R., DO
- Studint, Erika B., MD

Zufall Health Center
18 West Blackwell Street Zip: 07801
Ph: (973) 328-3344 Fax: (973) 328-6817
- Bishop, Douglas Scott, MD
- Ramirez-Alexander, Rina M., MD
- Szuchman, Mario, MD
- Taitel, Janice Beth, MD
- Zorrilla, Lilian, MD

Dumont

Hackensack UMG Dumont
125 Washington Avenue Zip: 07628
Ph: (201) 374-2722 Fax: (201) 374-2723
- Chinchankar, Rajeshree Prashant, MD
- Hoffman, Esther Sima, DO
- Kim, Sonia, MD

Valley Medical Group
40 Washington Avenue Zip: 07628
Ph: (201) 387-7055 Fax: (201) 387-8605
- Cabela, Gina Flores, MD
- Desplat, Philippe, DO

East Brunswick

Advanced Otolaryngolgy Assocs
557 Cranbury Road/Suite 3 Zip: 08816
Ph: (732) 613-0600 Fax: (732) 613-0508
- Highstein, Charles I., MD
- Horowitz, Jay B., MD
- Kaplan, Kenneth A., MD
- Rethy, Kimberly, DO

Brunswick-Hills Ob/Gyn, PA
620 Cranbury Road/Suite LL90 Zip: 08816
Ph: (732) 257-0081 Fax: (732) 613-4845
- Beim, Daniel S., MD
- Cernadas, Maureen, MD
- Cherot, Elizabeth Kagel, MD
- Duke, Stephanie D., MD
- Fisher, Deneishia Shramaine, MD
- Huang, Michelle, MD
- Kinsler, Kristin J., DO

Cardiology Assocs of New Brunswick
593 Cranbury Road/Suite 2 Zip: 08816
Ph: (732) 390-3333 Fax: (732) 390-9244
- Altmann, Dory Bert, MD
- Altobelli, Anthony III, MD
- Burns, John J., MD
- DeMoss, Jeanne Lorraine, DO
- Kalra, Amit, MD
- Keller, Barnes D., MD
- Mermelstein, Erwin, MD
- Oberweis, Brandon Scott, MD
- Schaer, David H., MD
- Scheiner, Marc A., MD
- Shell, Roger A., MD
- Siu, Dwayne Winfred, DO

Cardio Intervent of Ctrl Jersey
465 Cranbury Road/Suite 201 Zip: 08816
Ph: (732) 613-1988 Fax: (732) 651-7734
- Avendano, Graciano Gary F., MD
- Balog, Joshua David, MD
- Chai, Yee Meen, MD
- Saviano, George J., MD

Central Jersey Family Physicians
754 State Highway 18 North/Suite 107 Zip: 08816
Ph: (732) 257-1171 Fax: (732) 257-2618
- Schiano, Catherine Jean, DO
- Tomlinson-Phelan, Michelle Ann, DO
- Tomlinson-Phelan, Tracy Michelle, M

Central Jersey Oncology Center, P.A.
Brier Hill Court/Building J-2 Zip: 08816
Ph: (732) 390-7750 Fax: (732) 390-7725
- Nissenblatt, Michael J., MD
- Salwitz, James C., MD

Central Pain Institute
3 Cornwall Drive/Suite A Zip: 08816
Ph: (732) 698-1000 Fax: (732) 698-1008
- Mirmadjlessi, Noushin, MD
- Sharma, Adity, MD

Comprehensive Rehabilitation
69 Brunswick Woods Drive Zip: 08816
Ph: (732) 238-0080 Fax: (732) 238-0070
- Kapchits, Elmira, MD
- Weissman, Tanya, MD

Contemporary Plastic Surgery LLC
579A Cranbury Road/Suite 202 Zip: 08816
Ph: (732) 254-1919 Fax: (732) 254-0703
- Herbstman, Robert A., MD
- Vieira, Pedro, MD

Digestive Disease Center of NJ
810 Ryders Lane Zip: 08816
Ph: (732) 238-0923 Fax: (732) 257-0229
- Meltz, Marcy Mencher, MD

Drs. Abdelmalek and Habib
E5 Brier Hill Court Zip: 08816
Ph: (732) 698-1331 Fax: (732) 698-1379
- Abdelmalek, Moheb S., MD
- Habib, Michael George, MD

Groups and Clinics by Town with Physician Rosters

East Brunswick (cont)

Drs. Kim & Kim
61 Brunswick Woods Drive Zip: 08816
Ph: (732) 257-8777
- Kim, Hei Y., MD
- Kim, Hyung G., MD

Drs. Kulischenko & Kulischenko
495 Ryders Lane Zip: 08816
Ph: (732) 613-9155
- Kulischenko, Alexander W., MD
- Kulischenko, Idelma, MD

Drs. Kumar and Kumar
75 Brunswick Woods Drive/Building L Zip: 08816
Ph: (732) 254-1450 Fax: (732) 613-8525
- Kumar, Ashok, MD
- Kumar, Nidhi, MD
- Sinha, Ashok Kumar, MD

ENT & Allergy Associates
B-3 Cornwall Drive Zip: 08816
Ph: (732) 238-0300 Fax: (732) 238-4066
- Axelrod Malagold, Sara H., MD
- Edelman, Bruce Allen, MD
- Rosenbaum, Jeffrey Mark, MD

E Brunswick Fam Practice Assoc
123 Dunhams Corner Road Zip: 08816
Ph: (732) 254-3300
- Geller, Toby A., MD
- Marmora, James J., MD
- Nee, Patricia B., MD

East Brunswick Med Assocs
63 West Prospect Avenue Zip: 08816
Ph: (732) 651-7122
- Gabriel, Ahab M., MD
- Tadros, Wagih F., MD

Endocrinology Associates of NJ
9 Auer Court/Suite A Zip: 08816
Ph: (732) 390-6666 Fax: (732) 390-7711
- Hrymoc, Zofia, MD
- Kim, Christian C. K., MD
- Surgan, Matthew Louis, MD

Endocrinology Associates of Princeton,
579A Cranberry Road/Suite 101 Zip: 08816
Ph: (732) 579-6444 Fax: (609) 896-0079
- Mathew, Mini Ann, DO

Genito-Urinary Surgeons of New Jersey
579-A Cranbury Road/Suite 104 Zip: 08816
Ph: (732) 390-8700 Fax: (732) 390-8555
- Boateng, Akwasi Afriyie, MD
- Feder, Marc T., MD

Global Pediatrics
7 Auer Court Zip: 08816
Ph: (732) 432-7777 Fax: (732) 432-9030
- Goldman, Iosif, DO
- Gordina, Alla, MD

High Risk Pregnancy Center of NJ PC
1 Auer Court/Suites A & B Zip: 08816
Ph: (732) 390-1020 Fax: (732) 390-8035
- Krishnamoorthy, Ambalavaner, MD
- Sengupta, Shyamashree, MD

Highland Park Medical Associates
579A Cranberry Road/Suite 102 Zip: 08816
Ph: (732) 613-0711 Fax: (732) 613-5783
- Gurland, Ira Alan, MD
- Kallich, Marsha M., MD
- Redel, Henry, MD
- Snepar, Richard A., MD

Lenger and Plumser, MDs, LLC
465 Cranbury Road/Suite 102 Zip: 08816
Ph: (732) 390-1995
- Lenger, Ellis S., MD
- Plumser, Allan B., MD

Mid Atlantic Orthopedic Associates LLP
557 Cranbury Road/Suite 10 Zip: 08816
Ph: (732) 238-8800 Fax: (732) 238-8246
- Bloomstein, Larry Z., MD
- Klein, Kenneth Stuart, MD
- Klein, Richard Ashley, MD
- Levine, Lewis Jonathan, MD

Mid Jersey Pediatrics
33 Brunswick Woods Drive Zip: 08816
Ph: (732) 257-4330 Fax: (732) 257-1777
- Booker, Larnie J., MD
- Cederbaum, Neil Kenneth, MD
- Gengel, Natalie, MD
- Goldman, Marvin, MD
- Jaroslow, Amy E., MD
- Shulman, Sabra W., MD
- Simon, Elisabeth M., MD
- Sung, Boram, MD
- Sweberg, Warren A., MD

Ob & Gyn Group of E Brunswick
172 Summerhill Road/Suite 1 Zip: 08816
Ph: (732) 254-1500 Fax: (732) 254-1436
- Gleason, Abigail Hott, MD
- Gross, Renee, MD
- Gupta, Manjari, MD
- Martinez, Tiffany Annmarie, DO
- Owunna, Uzoma I., MD

Pain Control Center of New Jersey
561 Cranbury Road Zip: 08816
Ph: (732) 651-1300 Fax: (732) 651-0375
- Lam, Sofia Levin, MD
- Levin, Alexander G., MD

Pediatric Orthopedic Associates, P.A.
585 Cranbury Road/Suite A Zip: 08816
Ph: (732) 390-1160 Fax: (732) 390-8449
- Adolfsen, Stephen Erik, MD
- Bowe, John A., MD
- Harnly, Heather Withington, MD
- Laufer, Samuel J., MD
- McKeon, John J., MD
- McPartland, Thomas Girard, MD
- Therrien, Philip J., MD
- Tuason, Dominick Anthony, MD
- Weisman, David Seth, MD

Pediatric Urology Associates PC
557 Cranbury Road/Suite 4 Zip: 08816
Ph: (732) 613-9144 Fax: (732) 613-5121
- Fleisher, Michael H., MD
- Vates, Thomas S. III, MD

Pulmonary & Intensive Care Specialists
593 Cranbury Road Zip: 08816
Ph: (732) 613-8880 Fax: (732) 613-0077
- Fischler, David Ross, MD
- Gilbert, Tricia Todisco, MD
- Harangozo, Andrea M., MD
- Hutt, Douglas A., MD
- Klitzman, Donna Leslie, MD
- Schiffman, Philip L., MD
- Waksman, Howard Kenneth, MD

RWJPE Cranbury Medical Group
557 Cranbury Road/Suite 22 Zip: 08816
Ph: (732) 613-0500 Fax: (732) 613-0345
- Lau, Ronald, MD
- Terranova, Matthew Patrick Jr, DO

Shankar, Sujatha
77 Brunswick Woods Drive Zip: 08816
Ph: (732) 238-6644 Fax: (732) 238-6550
- Saif, Rashida Taher, MD
- Shankar, Sujatha, MD

St. Karas Medical
A-2 Brier Hill Court Zip: 08816
Ph: (732) 613-5005 Fax: (732) 613-5004
- Morgan, Nashaat L., MD
- Morgan, Suzana Emil Anwer, MD

The Neurology and Headache Center
573 Cranbury Road/Suite A5 Zip: 08816
Ph: (732) 254-5101 Fax: (732) 254-2640
- Lazar, Mark H., MD
- Oranchak, Deborah J., DO

Tiefenbrunn & Fortin Pediatrics
503 Cranbury Road Zip: 08816
Ph: (732) 390-8400 Fax: (732) 390-8970
- Fortin, Robert Glenn, MD
- Tiefenbrunn, Larry J., MD
- Tuck, Michelle Patran, MD

UniMed Center LLC
190 Route 18/Suite 202 Zip: 08816
Ph: (732) 828-9988 Fax: (732) 828-1010
- Joseph, Richard S., MD
- Liu, Jenny, MD

University Children's Eye Center, P.C.
4 Cornwall Court Zip: 08816
Ph: (732) 613-9191 Fax: (732) 613-1139
- Engel, John Mark, MD
- Engel, Mark L., MD
- Han, Stella Insook, MD
- Rousta, Sepideh T., MD
- Sun, Nancy, MD

University Pediatric Associates
D-1 Brier Hill Court Zip: 08816
Ph: (732) 238-3310
- Henner, Rochelle, MD
- Jennings, Gloria Ann, MD

University Radiology Group, P.C.
579A Cranbury Road Zip: 08816
Ph: (732) 390-0040 Fax: (732) 390-1856
- Basak, Sandip, MD
- Brown, James Harvey, MD
- Bulkin, Yekaterina, MD
- Carroll, Michael R. III, MD
- Chin, Deanna G., MD
- Dorr, Jeffrey, MD
- Ecker, Teresa, MD
- Edwards, Teresa Michelle, MD
- Flynn, Daniel E., MD
- Gendel, Vyacheslav, MD
- Girgis, Wahid S., MD
- Glynn, Nicole Lasasso, MD
- Greenblatt, Adrienne Masin, MD
- Greer, Jeannete G., MD
- Harrigan, John T., MD
- Hira, Ajay, MD
- Hogan, James R., MD
- Jonna, Harsha R., MD
- Kadivar, Khadijeh, MD
- Krieg, Eileen M., MD
- Lakritz, Philip Shev, MD
- Lazzara, Elizabeth Wanda, MD
- Levine, Charles Daniel, MD
- Moubarak, Issam F., MD
- Patel, Gitanjali, MD
- Patel, Keyur Bhupendra, MD
- Salmieri, Karen Heather, MD
- Saraiya, Mansi Shah, MD
- Shah, Kumar, MD
- Slater, Gregg Matthew, MD
- Sussmann, Amado Ross, MD
- Taylor, Christopher, MD
- Thind, Pritinder K., MD
- Venezia, Sara, DO
- Yang, Charles, MD
- Yoon, Hyukjun, MD
- Zawodniak, Leonard J., MD

University Surgical Center
561 Cranbury Road Zip: 08816
Ph: (732) 390-4300 Fax: (732) 390-0556
- Weinstein, Craig M., MD
- Yama, Asher Z., MD

East Hanover

Atlantic Medical Group
One Health Plaza/Bldg. 125 Zip: 07936
Ph: (862) 778-7960 Fax: (973) 781-6505
- Buksh, Wazim R., MD
- Irving, Carol, MD

Parsippany Eye Care Associates
46 Eagle Rock Avenue Zip: 07936
Ph: (973) 560-1500
- Rispoli, Lauren C., MD
- Silverman, Cary M., MD

Robalino-Sanghavi, Michelle Marie
120 Eagle Rock Avenue/Suite 154 Zip: 07936
Ph: (201) 447-4772
- Girardy, James Douglas, MD
- Pasia, Eric, MD
- Robalino-Sanghavi, Michelle Marie,

Summit Medical Group
383 Ridgedale Avenue/Suite 8 Zip: 07936
Ph: (973) 887-0200 Fax: (973) 887-4965
- Khanna, Roohi, MD
- Marzella, Giuseppe, MD
- Patel, Niraj Ranjit, MD

East Orange

Bright Futures Pediatrics
185 Central Avenue/Suite 601 Zip: 07018
Ph: (973) 944-1089 Fax: (973) 866-0023
- Martin Yeboah, Patrick V., MD
- Verner, Edwina D., MD

Drs. Chatha & Nasta
90 Washington Street/Suite 311 Zip: 07017
Ph: (973) 676-7192 Fax: (973) 676-0525
- Chatha, Uzma Arshad, MD
- Nasta, Sucheta M., MD

Drs. Ducheine and Joseph
310 Central Avenue/Suite 203 Zip: 07018
- Ducheine, Yvan D., MD
- Joseph, Romane, MD

Drs. Maniar and Nimma
90 Washington Street/Suite 305 Zip: 07018
Ph: (973) 676-2492 Fax: (973) 676-5901
- Maniar, Madhavi N., MD
- Maniar, Payal, MD

Drs. Seth, Robertson & Seth
310 Central Avenue/Suite 100 Zip: 07018
Ph: (862) 520-3104 Fax: (973) 674-8033
- Mehta, Deeksha, MD
- Robertson, Joy G., MD
- Seth, Sarwan K., MD

Drs. Sunderam and Sunderam
310 Central Avenue/Suite 102 Zip: 07018
Ph: (973) 266-9111 Fax: (973) 266-1227
- Hemsley, Michael, MD
- Sunderam, Darshi, MD
- Sunderam, Gnana, MD

East Orange Family Health Center
240 Central Avenue/Suite 3 Zip: 07018
Ph: (973) 674-3500 Fax: (973) 674-6134
- Matthews, Calvin C., MD
- McGill, Winston Jr., MD

Newark Community Health Center, Inc.
444 William Street Zip: 07017
Ph: (973) 675-1900 Fax: (973) 675-4021
- Katta, Madhavi R., MD
- Meremikwu, Francisca Chinwe, MD

Orange Medical Group
310 Central Avenue/Suite 106 Zip: 07018
Ph: (973) 674-4542 Fax: (973) 674-3901
- Kania, Nirmala R., MD
- Lee, Terrance H., MD

Salerno Medical Associates, LLP
613 Park Avenue Zip: 07017
Ph: (973) 672-8573 Fax: (973) 676-4099
- Knight, Jennifer Mary, MD
- Salerno, Alexander Gerard, MD
- Savaille, Juanito E., DO

The Heart Center of the Oranges
310 Central Avenue/Suite 102 Zip: 07018
Ph: (973) 395-1550 Fax: (973) 395-3711
- Bawa, Radhika, MD
- Chi, Jinhan, MD
- Rajiyah, Gitendra, MD
- Ramdas, Kumar, MD
- Skurnick, Blanche Jacqueline, MD

East Rutherford

Med-Care of East Rutherford
245 Park Avenue Zip: 07073
Ph: (201) 939-7161
- Coyle, Genoveva F., MD
- D'Andrea, John Louis, MD
- Popa, Marcela M., MD
- Scolamiero, John C., MD

East Windsor

Anthea Gynecology
375 US Highway 130/Suite 103 Zip: 08520
Ph: (609) 448-7800 Fax: (609) 448-7880
- Markidan, Yana, MD
- Simigiannis, Helen, MD

Delaware Valley Ob/Gyn
300B Princeton Hightstown Road Zip: 08520
Ph: (609) 336-3266 Fax: (609) 443-4506
- Eder, Scott E., MD
- Gamburg, Eugene Samuel, MD

Groups and Clinics by Town with Physician Rosters

Family Practice of CentraState
319 Route 130 North Zip: 08520
Ph: (609) 426-1555 Fax: (609) 447-8070
  Skeehan,Christopher J., MD
  Wong,Christopher K., MD

Spine Institute of North America
300A Princeon Hightstown Road Zip: 08520
Ph: (609) 337-6496 Fax: (609) 371-9110
  Ali,Rehan Basharat, MD
  Yanni,Baher S., MD

Windsor Dermatology
59 One Mile Road Extension/Suite G Zip: 08520
Ph: (609) 443-4500 Fax: (609) 426-0530
  Bagel,Jerry, MD
  Keegan,Brian Robert, MD
  Myers,Wendy A., MD
  Nieves,David Steiner, MD
  Simon,Jessica, MD
  Stenn,Judit O., MD

Windsor Regional Med Assocs
300A Princeton-Hightstown Road Zip: 08520
Ph: (609) 490-0095 Fax: (609) 490-0091
  Beagin,Erinn Elizabeth, MD
  Bowers,Gabriela W., MD
  Kunamneni,Katie Elizabeth, MD
  Thomas,Brian David, MD

Eatontown

Central Jersey Hand Surgery
2 Industrial Way West Zip: 07724
Ph: (732) 542-4477 Fax: (732) 935-0355
  Atik,Teddy Labib, MD
  Decker,Raymond Jr., MD
  Fedorcik,Gregory Gerard, MD
  Gabuzda,George Mark, MD
  Pess,Gary M., MD

Drs. Hanna and Recho
117 State Route 35 Zip: 07724
Ph: (732) 542-4411 Fax: (732) 542-1070
  Hanna,Manar H., MD
  Recho,Marielle, MD

Eatontown Fertility Clinic
234 Industrial Way West/Suite A104 Zip: 07724
Ph: (732) 918-2500
  Mensah,Virginia Akua, MD

Eatontown Medical Associates
158 Wyckoff Road Zip: 07724
Ph: (732) 544-9500 Fax: (732) 544-0132
  Churgin,Warren K., MD
  Peeples,Charles B., MD

Hypertension & Nephrology Assoc
6 Industrial Way West/Suite B Zip: 07724
Ph: (732) 460-1200 Fax: (732) 460-1211
  Arbes,Spiros M., MD
  Ashok,Manjula, MD
  Haratz,Alan B., MD
  Liss,Kenneth A., DO
  Nivera,Noel Taroy, MD

Jersey Shore Cardio & Vasc Srg
234 Industrial Way West/Suite A-103 Zip: 07724
Ph: (848) 208-2055 Fax: (848) 208-2078
  Donald,Gordon D. III, MD
  Martinez,Alan M., MD
  Scalia,Peter D., MD
  Squillaro,Anthony J., MD
  Thompson,Robert M., MD

Monmouth Cardiology Associates
11 Meridian Road Zip: 07724
Ph: (732) 663-0300 Fax: (732) 663-0301
  Bach,Matt, MD
  Berger,Lance Seth, MD
  Boak,Joseph G., MD
  Daniels,Jeffrey S., MD
  Daniels,Steven J., MD
  Kapoor,Mahim, MD
  Kim,Jiwon, MD
  Koo,Charles H., MD
  LaMarche,Nelson S., MD
  Mascarenhas,Mark Adrian, MD
  Mattina,Charles J., MD
  O'Neill,Leon Frederick IV, DO

  Osofsky,Jeffrey Lee, MD
  Patel,Ashish Bhasker, MD
  Rizzo,Thomas F., MD
  Rodriguez,Pascual B., MD
  Saybolt,Matthew Douglas, MD
  Sealove,Brett Andrew, MD
  Selan,Jeffrey Craig, MD
  Sergie,Ziad, MD
  Wappel,Michael A., MD

Monmouth Gastroenterology
142 Route 35 Zip: 07724
Ph: (732) 389-5004 Fax: (732) 389-1850
  Baig,Nadeem A., MD
  Belitsis,Kenneth, MD
  Fiest,Thomas C., DO
  Gorcey,Steven A., MD
  Merikhi,Laleh Afkham, MD
  Staats,Nancy Elizabeth, MD
  Uppal,Rajiv, MD

Monmouth Heart Specialists
274 Highway 35 Zip: 07724
Ph: (732) 440-7336 Fax: (732) 440-9404
  Einbinder,Lynne C., MD
  Usman,Mohammed Haris Umer, MD

Monmouth Pulmonary Consultants
30 Corbett Way Zip: 07724
Ph: (732) 380-0020 Fax: (732) 380-1990
  Kosinski,Robert M., MD
  Kramer,Violet Elizabeth, MD
  Livornese,Douglas S., MD
  Patton,Chandler D., MD
  Weiner,Sharon M., MD

New Jersey Urologic Institute
10 Industrial Way East Zip: 07724
Ph: (732) 963-9091 Fax: (732) 963-9092
  Geltzeiler,Jules M., MD
  Greenleaf,Betsy Alice, DO
  Keselman,Ira G., MD
  Litvin,Yigal S., MD
  Waldman,Ilan, MD

Ocean Pediatric Group
1 Industrial Way West/Suite 1-C Zip: 07724
Ph: (732) 542-6451 Fax: (732) 542-1654
  DeGroote,Richard J., MD
  Farrell,Paul R., MD
  Noaz,Golam G., MD

Pathology Solutions, LLC.
246 Industrial Way West/Suite 2 Zip: 07724
Ph: (732) 389-5200 Fax: (732) 389-5299
  Sheng,Huaibao, MD
  Wang,Xuan, MD
  Xie,Linjun, MD

RWJBH Primary Care Eatontown
145 Wyckoff Road/Suite 301 Zip: 07724
Ph: (732) 222-0180 Fax: (732) 935-1590
  Barnickel,Paul W., MD
  Desai,Gautam J., MD
  Krystofiak,Jason Anthony, MD
  Sridar,Buvaneswari, MD

Reproductive Science Center of NJ
234 Industrial Way Zip: 07724
Ph: (732) 918-2500 Fax: (732) 918-2504
  Mann,Jessica Salas, MD
  Ziegler,William Francis, DO

Specialty Surgical Associates
10 Industrial Way East/Suite 104 Zip: 07724
Ph: (732) 389-1331 Fax: (732) 542-8587
  Arvanitis,Michael L., MD
  Binenbaum,Steven J., MD
  Borao,Frank J., MD
  Dressner,Roy M., DO
  Matharoo,Gurdeep Singh, MD

Edgewater

Center for Endocrinology & Diabetes NJ
968 River Road/Suite 203 Zip: 07020
Ph: (201) 224-8328 Fax: (201) 224-2405
  Lala,Vinod R., MD

Cross Country Cardiology
103 River Road/2nd Floor Zip: 07020
Ph: (201) 941-8100 Fax: (201) 941-2899
  Admani,Irfan Mohamed, MD
  Alvarez-Segovia,Lucia M., MD

  Bareket,Yaron, MD
  Faraz,Haroon Ahmed, MD
  Pumill,Rick J., MD
  Raskin,Adam Brett, MD
  Segovia,Fernando, MD

Edgewater Family Care Center
725 River Road/Suite 202 Zip: 07020
Ph: (201) 943-4040 Fax: (201) 941-4599
  Kuwama,Chika, MD

Hand in Hand Pediatrics
725 River Road/Suite 201-A Zip: 07020
Ph: (201) 840-8055 Fax: (201) 840-8099
  Chai,George, MD
  Desai,Bhumika, MD

National Health Rehabilitation
103 River Road/Suite 101 Zip: 07020
Ph: (201) 654-6397
  Putcha,Nitin, DO

Palisades Medical Associates
125 River Road/Suite 103 Zip: 07020
Ph: (201) 969-2111 Fax: (201) 969-8015
  Pinkhasov,Mark M., DO

Edison

ABC Pediatrics, LLC.
974 Inman Avenue/Suite 1-A Zip: 08820
Ph: (908) 412-8866 Fax: (908) 412-8363
  Gumidyala,Padmasree, MD
  Libis,Zhanna, MD

Adult & Ped Allergist of Cen Jer
1740 Oak Tree Road Zip: 08820
Ph: (732) 906-1717 Fax: (732) 906-1781
  Centeno-McNulla,Ligaya Victoria M.
  Kanuga,Jayesh G., MD
  Reyes,Ruby Carina E., MD

Advanced Orthopedic & Sports Medicine
1907 Oak Tree Road/Suite 201 Zip: 08820
Ph: (732) 548-7332 Fax: (732) 548-7350
  Herrera-Figueira,Diego Alberto, MD
  Kasim,Nader Q., MD
  Lane,Gregory J., MD

All Care Family Medicine, LLC
3 Lincoln Highway/Suite 101 Zip: 08820
Ph: (732) 494-4500 Fax: (732) 494-2818
  Chung Loy,Harold E., MD
  Nelson,Yvonne, MD

Associated Colon & Rectal Surgeons PA
3900 Park Avenue/Suite 101 Zip: 08820
Ph: (732) 494-6640 Fax: (732) 549-8204
  Alva,Suraj, MD
  Calata,Jed F., MD
  Chinn,Bertram T., MD
  Deutsch,Michael, MD
  Lucking,Jonathan, MD
  Notaro,Joseph R., MD
  Wilkins,Kirsten Bass, MD

Assoc in Kidney Disease & Hypertension
2177 Oak Tree Road/Suite 204 Zip: 08820
Ph: (908) 769-4735 Fax: (908) 769-4736
  Rajan,Samir, MD
  Sutaria,Samir Hasmukh, MD

Associates in Plastic Surgery
1150 Amboy Avenue Zip: 08837
Ph: (732) 548-3200 Fax: (732) 548-1919
  Cuber,Shain A., MD
  Miller,Andrew John, MD

Cardio Medical Group
98 James Street/Suite 313 Zip: 08820
Ph: (732) 635-1100 Fax: (732) 635-0918
  Cohen,Howard S., MD
  Cohen,Larry J., MD
  Jana,Kumar P., MD
  Leighton,Harmony J., DO

Cardiovascular Associates of NJ, P.A.
1931 Oak Tree Road/Suite 202 Zip: 08820
Ph: (732) 373-7633 Fax: (732) 372-7634
  Javed,Mohammad Tariq, MD

Center for Adv. Repro Med/Fertility
4 Ethel Road/Suite 405A Zip: 08817
Ph: (732) 339-9300 Fax: (732) 339-9400
  Corsan,Gregory H., MD
  Qasim,Mahasin S., MD
  Sachdev,Rahul, MD

Comprehensive Surgical Assocs
225 May Street/Suite A Zip: 08837
Ph: (732) 346-5400 Fax: (732) 346-5404
  Dasmahapatra,Kumar S., MD
  Itskovich,Alexander, MD
  Swaminathan,Anangur P., MD

Drs Khanna & Kukla MDs
817 Inman Avenue Zip: 08820
Ph: (732) 381-8600 Fax: (732) 381-8690
  Khanna,Santosh B., MD
  Kukla,Leon F., MD

Drs. Agarwal & Agarwal
450 Plainfield Road Zip: 08820
Ph: (732) 494-9500
  Agarwal,Kishan C., MD
  Agarwal,Sushma, MD

Drs. Desai and Patel
2177 Oak Tree Road/Suite 205 Zip: 08820
Ph: (732) 549-3700 Fax: (732) 549-3203
  Desai,Darshana A., MD
  Patel,Ragin C., MD

Drs. Li and Li
98 James Street/Suite 201 Zip: 08820
Ph: (732) 906-9882 Fax: (732) 906-9893
  Li,Meihong, MD
  Li,Xiang, MD

Drs. Modi & Sarkaria
98 James Street/Suite 200 Zip: 08820
Ph: (732) 243-9694
  Modi,Chintan, MD
  Sarkaria,Jasbir S., MD

Drs. Nisar and Nisar
1895 Oak Tree Road Zip: 08820
Ph: (732) 548-1833 Fax: (732) 906-3156
  Nisar,Mohammed P., MD
  Nisar,Shiraz Ahmed, MD

Drs. Ramasubramani & De Borja
98 James Street/Building F Suite 208 Zip: 08820
Ph: (732) 514-9624 Fax: (732) 377-3767
  Ramasubramani,Anuradha, MD
  Sree,Aruna, MD

Drs. Rudnitzky & Shugar PA
98 James Street/Suite 104 Zip: 08820
Ph: (732) 494-6300 Fax: (732) 494-1028
  Kushal,Amrita, MD
  Rudnitzky,Elliot M., MD
  Shugar,Ronald A., MD

Durham Women's Center
4 Ethel Road/Suite 402-B Zip: 08817
Ph: (732) 287-3643 Fax: (732) 287-3406
  Metz,Rebecca L., MD
  Steinbach,Gary B., MD
  Twisdale,Donna R., MD

ENT & Allergy Associates, LLP
98 James Street/Suite 301 Zip: 08820
Ph: (732) 549-3934 Fax: (732) 549-7250
  Nizam,Mohammed Farrukh, MD

Ear Nose & Throat Group of Central NJ
2124 Oak Tree Road/2nd floor Zip: 08820
Ph: (732) 205-1311 Fax: (732) 205-9648
  Arlen,Harold, MD
  Aruna,Pasalai N., MD
  Lavine,Ferne R., MD
  Park,Robert Inyeung, MD

Edison Emergi Med
98 James Street/Suite 313 Zip: 08820
Ph: (732) 635-1100 Fax: (732) 635-0918
  Desai,Sagar R., MD
  Kleshchelskaya,Valeria, MD

Edison Eye Group
7 State Route 27/Suite 101 Zip: 08820
Ph: (732) 494-6720 Fax: (732) 549-5869
  Schwartz-Eisdorfer,Barbara Harriet

Edison Medical Associates, LLC
34-36 Progress Street/Suite A-2 Zip: 08820
Ph: (908) 226-0600 Fax: (908) 226-1802
  Kumar,Radha, MD
  Rathnakumar,Charumathi, MD

Groups and Clinics by Town with Physician Rosters

Edison (cont)

Edison Nephrology Consultants, LLC.
34-36 Progress Street/Suite A-7 Zip: 08820
Ph: (908) 769-1440 Fax: (908) 769-0945
- Czyzewski, Robert M., MD
- Kim, Stanley S., MD
- Park, Jun-Ki, MD

Edison Neurologic Associates
36 Progress Street/Suite B-3 Zip: 08820
Ph: (908) 757-6633 Fax: (908) 757-3912
- Buchwald, Eugene E., MD
- Gan, Richard A., MD
- Merkin, Michael D., MD
- Oh, Youn K., MD

Edison Ophthalmology Associates
2177 Oak Tree Road/Suite 203 Zip: 08820
Ph: (908) 822-0070 Fax: (908) 822-0075
- Park, John Chonghwan, MD
- Press, Lorin R., MD

Edison Orthopedic Institute
3 Progress Street/Suite 106 Zip: 08820
Ph: (732) 494-1050 Fax: (732) 494-5424
- Jamieson, Janine, DO
- Thacker, Sunil Rajan, MD

Edison Pediatrics
1802 Oak Tree Road/Suite 101 Zip: 08820
Ph: (732) 548-3210 Fax: (906) 548-3966
- Bhamidipati, Aparna, MD
- Nimma, Vijaya, MD
- Pappas, Lara, MD
- Pu, Jessica Lixia, MD
- Reddy, Namrata Polam, MD

Edison Radiology Group, P.A.
65 James Street Zip: 08820
Ph: (732) 321-7917 Fax: (732) 737-2968
- Boruchov, Scott D., MD
- Chakravarty, Mira, MD
- Freeman, Hank Jason, MD
- George, Louis C., MD
- Malantic-Lu, Grace Paula, MD
- Parashurama, Prashant, MD
- Pierpont, Christopher Edward, MD
- Pivawer, Gabriel, DO
- Schmell, Eric Brad, MD
- Simon, Daniel W., MD
- Weissmann, Murray H., MD

Edison-Metuchen Orthopedic Group
10 Parsonage Road/5th Floor/Suite 500 Zip: 08837
Ph: (732) 494-6226 Fax: (732) 494-8762
- Chen, Franklin, MD
- Garfinkel, Matthew J., MD
- Idank, David M., DO
- Lombardi, Joseph S., MD
- Lombardi, Robert M., MD
- Patel, Nilesh J., MD
- Patti, James E., MD
- Ramani, Mohnish N., MD
- Ryan, Todd C., DO
- Vega, Teresa, MD

Fleisch ObGyn Group
3 Lincoln Boulevard/Suite 315 Zip: 08820
Ph: (732) 635-9800 Fax: (732) 635-9810
- Essandoh, Louisa Efua, MD
- Fleisch, Charles M., DO

Franklin H. Spirn MD Inc
1656 Oaktree Road/Suite 3 Zip: 08820
Ph: (732) 549-8080 Fax: (732) 549-0528
- Spirn, Benjamin David, MD
- Spirn, Franklin H., MD

Freeman Spin & Pain Institute
102 James Street/Suite 101 Zip: 08820
Ph: (732) 906-9600 Fax: (732) 906-9300
- Freeman, Eric D., DO

Gastroenterology Assocs of Ctrl Jersey
1921 Oak Tree Road/Suite 101 Zip: 08820
Ph: (732) 744-9090 Fax: (732) 744-1592
- Baik, Seoung W., MD
- Nayar, Devjit Singh, MD

Gastroenterology Consultants PA
205 May Street/Suite 201 Zip: 08837
Ph: (732) 661-9225 Fax: (732) 661-9259
- Goldberg, Michael Scott, MD
- Hodes, Steven E., MD
- Penn, James R., MD
- Wolfman, Marc R., MD

General Neurology Headache
2 Lincoln Highway/Suite 509 Zip: 08820
Ph: (732) 767-1500 Fax: (732) 767-0090
- Sobol, Igor Leonidovich, MD
- Sobol, Marina B., MD

Guarino & Chen PA
35-37 Progress Street/Suite B2 Zip: 08820
Ph: (908) 754-9292 Fax: (908) 754-3358
- Chen, Michael T., MD
- Wang, Danny, MD

JFK Family Practice Group
65 James Street Zip: 08818
Ph: (732) 321-7487 Fax: (732) 906-4927
- Bhattacharyya, Adity, MD
- Chae, Sung Yeon, MD
- Henderson, Thomas J., MD
- Kandula, Sridevi, MD
- Metz, Deborah Lynne, MD
- Metz, John Patrick, MD
- Milne, Charlene E., MD
- Ogbeide, Adesuwa, MD
- Patel, Dipesh Shashikant, DO
- Picciano, Anne, MD
- Prasad, Kamil, MD
- Wilks, Michelle Anne, MD
- Winter, Robin O., MD
- Zayoud, Rajaa M., MD

James Street Anesthesia
102 James Street/Suite 103 Zip: 08820
Ph: (732) 494-1444 Fax: (732) 494-7052
- Armao, Michael Edward, MD
- Beyus, Christopher Michael, MD
- Chen, Evan, MD
- Daniel, Robert J., MD
- Ding, Yifeng, MD
- Khetani, Manish P., MD
- Lee, Herb, MD
- Li, Xin Qin, MD
- Mereday, Clifton Samuel Jr., MD
- Moises, Adam U. Jr., DO
- Patel, Bhupendrakumar V., MD
- Piratla, Lalitha, MD
- Rock, Joel J., DO
- Samaan, Ayman Boushra, MD
- Santos-Holgado, Maria C., MD
- Siskind, Jonathan B., DO
- Stewart, Judly Pierre, MD
- Tan, Martin H., MD
- Thompson, Matthew, MD
- Utrankar, Deepti Sameer, MD

Juhee Gupta MD PC
35-37 Progress Street/Suite A-1 Zip: 08820
Ph: (908) 226-1500 Fax: (908) 755-3200
- Gupta, Juhee, MD
- Gupta, Neha, MD

Kang Lee and Lee Allergy/Pediatrics
2177 Oak Tree Road/Suite 207 Zip: 08820
Ph: (732) 549-7007
- Godlewska-Janusz, Elzbieta, MD
- Kang-Lee, Elica J., MD
- Lee, Hyok Yop, MD

Kavita Bupathi, LLC
2 Ethel Road/Suite 206C Zip: 08817
Ph: (732) 650-0350 Fax: (732) 650-0351
- Bupathi, Kavita Kishor, MD

Kirit Somabhai Patel, MD PC
34-36 Progress Street/Suite A-6 Zip: 08820
Ph: (908) 757-9555 Fax: (908) 757-2312
- Mavani, Bharti N., MD
- Patel, Atulkumar V., MD
- Patel, Kirit Somabhai, MD
- Patel, Meghal, MD

M.E.N.D., PA
2 Lincoln Highway/Suite 501 Zip: 08820
Ph: (732) 549-7470 Fax: (732) 494-8596
- Bucholtz, Harvey K., MD
- Dunn, Jonathan C., MD

May Street Surgi Center
205 May Street/Suite 103 Zip: 08837
Ph: (732) 820-4566 Fax: (732) 661-9619
- Cheela, Santosh K., MD
- Handa Nayyar, Seema, DO
- Payumo, Gene Louie, MD
- Ramchandani, Kishore N., MD
- Rosenheck, David Mark, MD

Medi Center of Edison
1813 Oak Tree Road Zip: 08820
Ph: (908) 769-9494 Fax: (908) 755-3833
- Bruzzi-Ehrlich, Diane, MD
- Johal, Gurvindra Singh, DO
- Nadkarni, Swati G., MD

Medical Associates of Marlboro
111 James Street Zip: 08818
Ph: (732) 452-9700 Fax: (732) 452-9720
- Parikh, Rakesh K., MD

Menlo Park Medical Group PA
111 James Street Zip: 08818
Ph: (732) 549-2299 Fax: (732) 549-2262
- Bhakey, Girija G., MD
- Buck, Warren G., MD
- Patel, Jayendra M., MD

Mid Jersey Medical Associates
1 Ethel Road/Suite 107b Zip: 08817
Ph: (732) 287-2020 Fax: (732) 287-2071
- Collins, Harry, MD
- Faches, Allison L., MD
- Uthappa, Machia M., MD

Middlesex Medical Group
225 May Street/Suite E Zip: 08837
Ph: (732) 661-2020 Fax: (732) 661-2022
- Bullock, Richard B., MD
- Tawde, Darshana Prafullaraj, MD

Middlesex Pulmonary Associates
106 James Street Zip: 08820
Ph: (732) 906-0091 Fax: (732) 906-0249
- Melillo, Nicholas G., MD
- Pesin, Jeffrey L., MD

Molk Cardiology
4 Ethel Road/Suite 406-A Zip: 08817
Ph: (732) 287-2888 Fax: (732) 287-1176
- Duch, Peter M., MD
- Molk, Ian J., MD

Naveen Mehrotra, MD PC
652 Amboy Avenue Zip: 08837
Ph: (732) 738-1341 Fax: (732) 738-9585
- Pompy, Amrita, MD

Neurology Consultants of Ctrl NJ
225 May Street/Suite D Zip: 08837
Ph: (732) 738-8830 Fax: (732) 738-8831
- Mani, Srinivasan S., MD
- Uhrik, Eric Joseph, DO

New Jersey Infectious Diseases Assocs
113 James Street Zip: 08820
Ph: (732) 906-1900
- Paradiso, Mary J., MD
- Velmahos, Vasilios, MD

North Edison Family Practice Group
35-37 Progress Street/Suite A-3 Zip: 08820
Ph: (908) 755-9797 Fax: (908) 668-4848
- Gandhi, Nabila Asif, MD

Oncology & Hematology Associates
2177 Oak Tree Road/Suite 104 Zip: 08820
Ph: (908) 755-1165 Fax: (908) 755-2093
- Kumar, Arvind, MD
- Prasad, Niloo, MD

Orthopedic Assocs of Central Jersey
205 May Street/Suite 202 Zip: 08837
Ph: (908) 757-1520 Fax: (908) 769-1388
- Charen, Jeffrey H., MD
- Lessing, David, MD
- Marcus, Alexander Michael, MD
- Zimmerman, Joshua M., MD

Patel Eye Associates
228 Plainfield Avenue Zip: 08817
Ph: (732) 985-5009 Fax: (732) 985-5155
- Patel, Hitesh K., MD
- Shah, Himanshu Shirish, MD

Premier Urology Group, LLC
10 Parsonage Road/Suite 118 Zip: 08837
Ph: (732) 494-9400 Fax: (732) 548-3931
- Fand, Benjamin, MD
- Lasser, Michael Sidney, MD
- Nakhoda, Zein Khozaim, MD
- Patel, Rupa, MD
- Sherman, Neil David, MD
- Terens, William L., MD
- Wein, Joshua Lewis, MD

Preventive Healthcare Associates
102 James Street/Suite 202 Zip: 08820
Ph: (732) 548-5541 Fax: (732) 548-2610
- Elber, Daniel A., DO
- Elber, Lee Bennett, DO

The FamPrimary & Specialty Care
10 Parsonage Road/Suite 410 Zip: 08837
Ph: (732) 452-0680 Fax: (732) 636-3669
- Patel, Hitesh Ramesh, MD
- Steiner, Kenneth D., MD
- Wiley, Olga V., MD

Primecare Medical Group
98 James Street/Suite 300 Zip: 08820
Ph: (732) 548-2523 Fax: (732) 549-8827
- Ballal, Raj Sadananda, MD
- Memon, Mohammad Khalil, MD
- Sharma, Bhudev, MD

Psychiatry Associates
1109 Amboy Avenue Zip: 08837
Ph: (732) 549-2220 Fax: (732) 603-0673
- Blank, Susan Berman, MD
- Lichtman, Kenneth J., MD
- Schlakman, Martin D., MD

Pulmonary Internists, PA
2 Lincoln Highway/Suite 301 Zip: 08820
Ph: (732) 549-7380 Fax: (732) 548-8216
- Casale, Lisa M., MD
- Goldstein, David S., MD
- Tirunahari, Vijaya Latha, MD
- Wolf, Barry Z., MD

Qualcare Medi-Center, P.A.
2 Lincoln Highway/Suite 411 Zip: 08820
Ph: (732) 396-0777 Fax: (732) 396-9222
- Long, George W., MD

RWJPE Heart Specialists of Edison
4 Ethel Road/Suite 406-B Zip: 08817
Ph: (732) 287-6622 Fax: (732) 287-2233
- Kovacs, Tiberiu, MD
- Panebianco, Robert Antonino, MD

Raritan Bay Cardiology Group, P.A.
225 May Street/Suite F Zip: 08837
Ph: (732) 738-8855 Fax: (732) 738-4141
- Cristoforo, Nancy Todd, MD
- Feingold, Aaron J., MD
- Keller, Malvin S., MD
- Noveck, Howard D., MD
- Rebba, Bhavana, MD
- Snyder, Craig Adam, MD
- Wasilewski, Stan J., MD

Regional Cancer Care Specialists
34-36 Progress Street/Suite B-2 Zip: 08820
Ph: (908) 757-9696 Fax: (908) 757-9721
- Amjad, Maqsood, MD
- Canavan, Brian F., DO
- Schuman, Richard M., MD
- Wallach, Bruce H., MD

Retina Associates of New Jersey, P.A.
98 James Street/Suite 209 Zip: 08820
Ph: (732) 906-1887 Fax: (732) 906-1883
- Yarian, David L., MD

Sharma and Sharma MDs
974 Inman Avenue Zip: 08820
Ph: (908) 561-0183 Fax: (908) 757-0942
- Sharma, Usha, MD

The Eye Center
3900 Park Avenue/Suite 106 Zip: 08820
Ph: (732) 603-2101
- Singh, Jasvinder, MD

Groups and Clinics by Town with Physician Rosters

US Healthworks
16 Ethel Road Zip: 08817
Ph: (732) 248-0088 Fax: (732) 248-4408
- Diziki,Donna C., DO

Urgent Care of New Jersey
2090 Route 27 Zip: 08817
Ph: (732) 662-5650 Fax: (732) 662-5651
- Arefeen,Samrana, MD
- Aziz,Khalid M., MD
- Mathews,Jeane M., MD

Egg Harbor Township

AtlantiCare Cancer Institute
2500 English Creek Avenue/Building 400 Zip: 08234
Ph: (609) 677-7777 Fax: (609) 677-7727
- Adelberg,David Eli, MD
- Chawla,Neha Roshan, MD
- Frost,James H., MD
- Previti,Francis W., MD
- Sandilya,Vijay Krishna, MD
- Wilson,Vasthi Christensen, MD

AtlantiCare Clinical Associates
2500 English Creek Avenue Zip: 08234
Ph: (609) 407-2310
- Lojun,Sharon Lee, MD
- Paradela,Ephrem Hector, MD

AtlantiCare Clinical Associates
2500 English Creek Avenue Zip: 08234
Ph: (609) 407-2310 Fax: (609) 407-2311
- Patel,Neha Hector, MD
- Twardzik,Jennifer Lynn, DO

AtlantiCare Phy Grp Joslin Diabetes
2500 English Creek Avenue/Bldg 800 Zip: 08234
Ph: (609) 407-2277 Fax: (609) 272-6306
- Brown,Anjeanette Tina, MD
- Hunter,Kevin Edward, MD
- Reid-Duncan,Lucienne Lariane, MD
- Tahmoush,Albert J., MD

AtlantiCare Urgent Care Center
2500 English Creek Avenue Zip: 08234
Ph: (609) 407-2273
- Altamuro,Christopher R., DO
- Barrett,Bryan Richard, DO
- Hon,David C., MD
- Stone,Mark J., MD

Atlantic Gastroenterology Assocs
3205 Fire Road/Suite 4 Zip: 08234
Ph: (609) 407-1220 Fax: (609) 407-0220
- Diener,Melissa Ann, MD
- Kaufman,Barry P., MD
- Makar,George A., MD
- Mehta,Nikhilesh D., MD
- Rosman,Gary A., MD
- Santoro,John J., DO

Atlanticare Physician Group
2500 English Creek Avenue Zip: 08234
Ph: (609) 909-0200 Fax: (609) 909-0267
- Kern,Carrie Catherine, DO
- Silk,Maanasi Puranik, DO
- Soucier,Ronald J., DO

Drs. Richwine and Richwine
3110 Ocean Heights Avenue/Suite 1 Zip: 08234
Ph: (609) 927-9555
- Richwine,Charles M. IV, DO
- Richwine,Lori T., DO

Drs. Unuigbe and Unuigbe
118 Peach Tree Lane Zip: 08234
- Unuigbe,Augustine Aigbovbioise, MD
- Unuigbe,Florence, MD

Island Medical Associates
2626 Tilton Road Zip: 08234
Ph: (609) 568-5000 Fax: (609) 568-5010
- Kuponiyi,Cheryl A., MD
- Kuponiyi,Olatunji P., MD

Kids Care Pediatrics
6529 Blackhorse Pike Zip: 08234
Ph: (609) 645-8500 Fax: (609) 272-8886
- Kessler,Barry M., MD
- Roan,Minda Unidad S., MD

Pavilion OB/GYN Atlanticare
2500 English Creek Avenue/Suite 214 Zip: 08234
Ph: (609) 677-7211 Fax: (609) 677-7210
- Milov,Seva, MD
- Pieri,Danielle, DO

Rothman Institute - Egg Harbor TWSP
2500 English Creek Avenue/Bldg 1300 Zip: 08234
Ph: (609) 677-7002 Fax: (609) 677-7000
- Armstrong,Joshua Stephen, DO
- Axelrod,Alyson Fincke, DO
- Baker,John C., MD
- Chhipa,Irfan S., MD
- Falcone,Michael, MD
- Hernandez,Victor Hugo, MD
- Mehnert,Michael Joseph, MD
- Nutini,Dennis Neil, MD
- Ong,Alvin C., MD
- Orozco,Fabio R., MD
- Patel,Mitesh, MD
- Pepe,Matthew D., MD
- Salvo,John Paul Jr., MD
- Tucker,Bradford S., MD
- Winters,Brian Seth, MD
- Woods,Barrett I., MD
- Xu,Wei, MD

Salartash Surgical Associates
301 Central Avenue/Suite D Zip: 08234
Ph: (609) 926-5000 Fax: (609) 926-2020
- Rohani,Pejman, DO
- Salartash,Alimorad, MD
- Salartash,Khashayar, MD

The Plastic Surgery Center
2500 English Creek Avenue/Suite 605 Zip: 08234
Ph: (609) 272-7737
- Saad,Adam, MD

Womens Health & Wellness
2500 English Creek Avenue Zip: 08234
Ph: (609) 677-7776 Fax: (609) 677-7509
- Desai,Rashmikant Sumantlal, MD
- Elnahal,Mohamed H., MD
- Robbins,Inga H., MD
- Shetty,Sanjay, MD

Elizabeth

Associates In ENT/Allergy
470 North Avenue Zip: 07208
Ph: (908) 352-6700 Fax: (908) 352-6734
- Huang,Robert D., MD
- Saporta,Diego, MD

Central Jersey Health Care Associates
240 Williamson Street/Suite 305 Zip: 07201
Ph: (908) 354-5353 Fax: (908) 351-6911
- Jaffry,Syed Ali Hasan, MD
- Oberoi,Mandeep S., MD

Cholankeril Medical Assocs
100 Grove Street Zip: 07202
Ph: (908) 352-1738
- Cholankeril,Mathew V., MD
- Cholankeril,Matthew George, MD
- Cholankeril,Thressiamma M., MD

Drs. Joshi & Chua
240 Williamson Street/Suite 203 Zip: 07202
Ph: (908) 289-8060 Fax: (908) 289-8061
- Chua,Jose Jr., MD
- Joshi,Meherwan Burzor, MD

Drs. Reddy & Cholankeril
240 Williamson Street/Suite 205 Zip: 07202
Ph: (908) 289-2070 Fax: (908) 289-4890
- Cholankeril,Mary G., MD
- Reddy,Aravinda, MD

Drs. Shen and Shen
219 South Broad Street Zip: 07202
Ph: (908) 352-5927 Fax: (908) 352-6181
- Shen,Edward, MD
- Shen,Jung-San, MD

Elizabeth Medical Group
310 West Jersey Avenue Zip: 07202
Ph: (908) 351-2222 Fax: (908) 351-1977
- Goodgold,Abraham, MD
- Patel,Jalpa S., MD

Elizabeth Pediatric Group
701 Newark Avenue/Suite 212 Zip: 07208
Ph: (908) 354-9500 Fax: (908) 354-9077
- Davis,Kenneth J., MD

Klein & Scannapiego MD PA
230 West Jersey Street Zip: 07202
Ph: (908) 289-1166 Fax: (908) 352-4752
- Klein,Shawn Richard, MD
- Klein,Warren M., MD
- Scannapiego,Saveren, MD

La Familia Medical Care
115 Jefferson Avenue Zip: 07201
Ph: (908) 351-6663 Fax: (908) 351-1760
- Ferdinand,Michel-Ange, MD
- Ferdinand,Pascale, MD

Linden Pediatric Group
517 Rahway Avenue Zip: 07202
Ph: (908) 527-1247 Fax: (908) 354-8822
- Ayyanathan,Karpukaras, MD
- Questelles,Rachael, MD

NJ Heart/Elizabeth Office
240 Williamson Street/Suite 402-406 Zip: 07202
Ph: (908) 354-8900 Fax: (908) 354-0007
- Budhwani,Anju, MD
- Walia,Jasjit S., MD

Neurological Associates PA
700 North Broad Street/Suite 201 Zip: 07208
Ph: (908) 354-3994 Fax: (908) 354-0429
- Sananman,Michael L., MD
- Tao,Ying, MD

New Jersey Urology, LLC
700 North Broad Street/Suite 302 Zip: 07208
Ph: (908) 289-3666 Fax: (908) 289-0716
- Krieger,Alan P., MD
- Opell,M. Brett, MD

P & C Medical Group LLC
605 South Broad Street/Unit B Zip: 07202
Ph: (908) 659-0075 Fax: (908) 469-4300
- Cisnero,Maria Del Carmen, MD
- Perez,Raul I., MD

Phoenix Physician's
225 Williamson Street Zip: 07202
Ph: (908) 994-5422
- Mack,Rose M., DO
- Zhang,Christina Ting, DO

Preferred Women Healthcare LLC
240 Williamson Street/Suite 405 Zip: 07202
Ph: (908) 353-5551 Fax: (908) 353-5052
- Khazai,Kamran, MD
- Sabzwari,Tabassum Azra, DO

Thalody Medical Associates
240 Williamson Street/Suite 400 Zip: 07207
Ph: (908) 352-0560 Fax: (908) 352-4066
- Mansour,Ashraf Hakeem, MD
- Thalody,George V., MD
- Thalody,Lucyamma, MD
- Thalody,Nina George, MD
- Thalody,Usha George, MD

Trinity Pediatrics
430 Morris Avenue/1st Floor Zip: 07208
Ph: (908) 353-5437 Fax: (908) 353-0727
- Grundy,Kia Calhoun, MD
- Powell,Kerri Lynette, MD

Union County Healthcare Associates
400 Westfield Avenue Zip: 07208
Ph: (908) 620-3800 Fax: (908) 620-3243
- Khan,Sabeen, MD
- Somma,Edward A., MD

Union Co Infectious Disease
240 Williamson Street/Suite 502 Zip: 07207
Ph: (908) 994-5300 Fax: (908) 994-5308
- Moradi,Dovid Simcha, MD

Union County Pediatrics Group
817 Rahway Avenue Zip: 07202
Ph: (908) 353-5750
- Patel,Manish Sureshbhai, MD
- Saraiya,Narendra N., MD

Union Square Medical Associates
824 Elizabeth Avenue Zip: 07201
Ph: (908) 352-9556 Fax: (908) 352-3446
- Munoz,Francisco, MD
- Munoz,Guillermo A., DO
- Perez,James, MD

VA Department Outpatient Clinic
654 East Jersey Street Zip: 07206
Ph: (908) 994-0120 Fax: (908) 994-0131
- Bekker,Yana, MD
- Blaszka,Frederick M., MD
- Dewyke,Kathleen Michelle, MD
- Sebastian,Suniti, MD

William J. McHugh MD PA
240 Williamson Street/Suite 204 Zip: 07202
Ph: (908) 355-8877 Fax: (908) 355-0017
- Pattathil,Jean Catherine, MD
- Zaboski,Michael R., MD

Wound Healing & Hyperbaric Medicine
240 Williamson Street/Suite 104 Zip: 07202
Ph: (908) 994-5480 Fax: (908) 994-8802
- Geuder,James W., MD
- Mlynarczyk,Peter J., MD
- Moss,Charles M., MD

Elmer

Dr. Warmuth Skin Care Center
420 Front Street Zip: 08318
Ph: (856) 358-1500
- Aphale,Abhishek N., MD
- Danowski,Kelli Mayo, DO

Elmer Family Practice, P.C.
330 West Front Street/P.O. Box 577 Zip: 08318
Ph: (856) 358-0770 Fax: (856) 358-0108
- Elgawli,Philip Raef, DO
- Ventrella,Gerard, MD

Genito Urinary Associates
125 State Street/Suite 4 Zip: 08318
Ph: (856) 358-2330
- Read,John H., MD

Elmwood Park

Absolute Medical Care
One Broadway/Suite 301 Zip: 07407
Ph: (201) 791-9340 Fax: (201) 791-9481
- Levan,Ellen, MD
- Vila,Maria N., DO

Bio-Reference Laboratory, Inc.
481 Edward H. Ross Drive Zip: 07407
Ph: (201) 791-2600 Fax: (201) 791-1941
- Butala,Rajesh M., MD
- Dupree,William Brion, MD
- Fehrle,Wilfrid Martin, MD
- Grodman,Marc D., MD
- Lee,Po-Shing, MD
- Merati,Kambiz, MD
- Persad,Rajendra, MD
- Pritchett,Danielle Delores, MD
- Talwar,Jotica, MD
- Wang,Luoquan, MD
- Weisberger,James D., MD

Elite Pediatrics
One Broadway/Suite 303 Zip: 07407
Ph: (201) 794-8855 Fax: (201) 794-6988
- Patel,Harshad Nathalal, MD
- Ramadi,Roula Alchaa, MD

Eye Care Associates of New Jersey, PA
One Broadway/Suite 404 Zip: 07407
Ph: (201) 797-5100 Fax: (201) 797-4160
- Friend,Adam Seth, MD

Pediatric Cardiology Associates
1 Broadway/Suite 203 Zip: 07407
Ph: (973) 569-6250 Fax: (973) 569-6270
- Kiblawi,Fuad Moh'D, MD
- O'Connor,Brian Kevin, MD
- Principe,David Laurence, MD

Phillips Eye Center
619 River Drive Zip: 07407
Ph: (201) 796-2020 Fax: (201) 796-2833
- Maley,Michael Kendrick, MD
- Phillips,Hadley H., DO

Groups and Clinics by Town with Physician Rosters

Elmwood Park (cont)
River Drive Surgery Center
619 River Drive Zip: 07407
Ph: (201) 703-2900
- Manspeizer,Heather Eve, MD
- Shin,Kyung Hee, MD
- Tendler,Jay M., MD
- Yu,Yun S., MD

Emerson
Active Orthopaedics & Sports Med
440 Old Hook Road Zip: 07630
Ph: (201) 358-0707 Fax: (201) 358-9777
- Benke,Michael T., MD
- Esformes,Ira, MD
- Gross,Michael Lee, MD
- Mendes,John F., MD
- Mendoza,Justin, DO
- Meyer,Carissa Leigh, MD
- Napoli,Ralph C., MD
- Natalicchio,James Charles, MD
- Rhim,Richard Dongil, MD
- Vazquez,Oscar, MD

Bergen Medical Associates
466 Old Hook Road/Suite 1 Zip: 07630
Ph: (201) 967-8221 Fax: (201) 967-0340
- Asta,Charles Francis, MD
- Avezzano,Eric S., MD
- Bellomo,Alyse Rosemarie, MD
- Bhandari,Bhavik M., MD
- Briker,Alan J., MD
- Broussard,Crystal Naii Collins, MD
- Choi,Krissy, DO
- Cullen,Holly Doolittle, MD
- Desai,Veena C., MD
- Dhadwal,Neetu, MD
- Flanzman,Susan Amy, MD
- Fleischer,Joseph S., MD
- Gokhale,Kedar Arvind, MD
- Griggs,Allen R., DO
- Hochstein,Martin A., MD
- Koo,Bon Chang Andy, MD
- Lan,Vivian En-Wei, MD
- Levine,Robert S., MD
- Litvin,Yair, MD
- Margulis,Stephen J., MD
- McConnell,Julie, MD
- Moscato,Michele, DO
- Motiwala,Neeta R., MD
- Nes,Deana Teplitsky, DO
- Pittman,Robert Hal, MD
- Potack,Jonathan Zachary, MD
- Randall,Jennifer F., MD
- Roque-Dang,Christine M., DO
- Rosalie,Maria Christina, MD
- Svider,Peter, MD
- Walker,Tracy Lynne, MD

Comprehensive Spine Care, PA
260 Old Hook Road/Suite 400 Zip: 07630
Ph: (201) 634-1811 Fax: (201) 634-9170
- Ashraf,Nomaan, MD
- Baird,Evan Oliver, MD
- Ben Yishay,Ari, MD
- Lester,Jonathan P., MD
- Levin,Rafael, MD

Drs. Bethala & Bethala
466 Old Hook Road/Suite 9 Zip: 07630
Ph: (201) 261-1005 Fax: (201) 261-4208
- Bethala,Nalini, MD
- Bethala,Vivian K., MD

Hackensack UMG Emerson
452 Old Hook Road/2nd Floor Zip: 07630
Ph: (201) 666-3900 Fax: (201) 261-0505
- Ali,Amy G., MD
- Bagade,Vivek Laxman, MD
- Cantore,William Anthony, MD
- D'Aquino,Carol Madeleine, MD
- Daud Ahmad,Sameera, MD
- Dombrowski,Mark A., MD
- Glaubiger,Carol, MD
- Gliksman,Michele Isaacs, MD
- Gold,Edward J., MD
- Goldstein,David D., MD
- Jacowitz,Joel D., MD
- Kaufman,Bradley S., MD
- Mahajan,Geeti, MD
- Orr,David A., DO
- Paskowski,Elizabeth K., MD
- Rosner,Steven M., MD
- Zucker,Ira I., MD

Pulmonary & Medical Associates
466 Old Hook Road/Suite 26 Zip: 07630
Ph: (201) 261-0821 Fax: (201) 261-0823
- Kim,Jeffrey S., MD
- Lin,George Szuwei, MD
- Thum,Robert G., MD

Englewood
Access Medical Associates PC
177 North Dean Street/Suite 203 Zip: 07631
Ph: (201) 503-0833 Fax: (201) 503-0844
- Katz,Doron Zvi, MD
- Paley,Jeffrey Evan, MD

Allied Neurology & Interventional Pain
185 Grand Avenue Zip: 07631
Ph: (201) 894-1313 Fax: (201) 894-1335
- Rosenbaum,David Herbert, MD

Bergen Laparoscopy & Bariatric, LLC
97 Engle Street Zip: 07631
Ph: (201) 227-5533 Fax: (201) 227-5537
- Ibrahim,Ibrahim M., MD
- Morales-Ribeiro,Celines, MD
- Strain,Jeffrey Witt, MD

Bergen Medical Alliance, P.A.
180 Engle Street Zip: 07631
Ph: (201) 567-2050 Fax: (201) 568-8936
- Abraham,Alice, MD
- Brauntuch,Glenn R., MD
- Cong,Elaine Alice, MD
- Engler,Mitchell S., MD
- Frisch,Katalin Andrea, MD
- Griffiths,Shernett Olivine, MD
- Joshi,Nandita, MD
- Kapoor,Radhika, DO
- Kondapaneni,Srikant, MD
- Malovany,Robert J., MD
- Patel,Killol, MD
- Simon,Clifford J., MD

Bergen Neurology Consultants
25 Rockwood Place/Suite 110 Zip: 07631
Ph: (201) 894-5805 Fax: (201) 894-1956
- Akbaripanahi,Sepideh, MD
- Alweiss,Gary S., MD
- Choi,Yun-Beom, MD
- Deniro,Lauren Victoria, MD
- Levy,Kirk Jay, MD
- Racela,Rikki Redona, MD
- Rajasingham,Jamuna Kandasamy, MD
- Willner,Joseph Harrison, MD

Bergen Thoracic & Vascular Associates
350 Engle Street/2 East Zip: 07631
Ph: (201) 569-1101 Fax: (201) 569-1108
- Impeduglia,Theresa Maria, MD

Cardiovascular Associates of NJ
25 Rockwood Place/Suite 440 Zip: 07631
Ph: (201) 568-3690 Fax: (201) 568-3667
- Kaplan,Sarah, MD
- Schwarcz,Aron Isaac, MD
- Suede,Samuel, MD
- Weissman,Andrew J., MD

Columbia Grand Orthopaedics
500 Grand Avenue/Suite 101 Zip: 07631
Ph: (201) 569-0440 Fax: (201) 569-4949
- Bottiglieri,Thomas S., DO

Comprehensive Women's Care
401A South Van Brunt Street/Suite 405 Zip: 07631
Ph: (201) 871-4346 Fax: (201) 871-5953
- Bewtra,Madhuri, MD
- Friedman,Harvey Y., MD
- Merriam,Zachary M., DO
- Patrusky,Karen Lynn, MD
- Schlossberg,Hope R., MD

Dermatology Center
363 Grand Avenue Zip: 07631
Ph: (201) 568-6977 Fax: (201) 568-7567
- Abramson,David L., MD

Drs. Abramovici, Jan & Zelkowitz
140 Grand Avenue/Suite B Zip: 07631
Ph: (201) 567-5787 Fax: (201) 567-7652
- Abramovici,Mirel I., MD
- Jan,Louis C. W., MD
- Zelkowitz,Marc, MD

Drs. Baydar, Davidson & Tung
370 Grand Avenue/Suite 203 Zip: 07631
Ph: (201) 568-3262 Fax: (201) 569-2634
- Baydar,Garbis, MD
- Davidson,Melissa, MD
- Tung,Cindy Wei-Yi, MD

Drs. Pattner, Grodstein, et al
177 North Dean Street/Suite 207 Zip: 07631
Ph: (201) 567-0446 Fax: (201) 567-8775
- Clifford,Susan Michelle, MD
- Davis,Lawrence Jay, MD
- Grodstein,Gerald P., MD
- Pattner,Austin M., MD
- Tartakovsky,Irina, MD
- Zachariah,Teena, MD

Drs. Seferian and Saggar
200 Grand Avenue/Suite 102 Zip: 07631
Ph: (201) 503-0660 Fax: (201) 503-0685
- Saggar,Suraj Kumar, DO
- Seferian,Mihran A., MD

Drs. Wasserman & Reiner
401 South Van Brunt Street/Suite 402 Zip: 07631
Ph: (201) 567-1140 Fax: (201) 567-1998
- Reiner,David M., MD
- Wasserman,Kenneth H., MD

Drs. White & Waxenbaum
216 Engle Street/Suite 203 Zip: 07631
Ph: (201) 567-7615 Fax: (201) 567-8033
- Seo,Christina J., MD
- Waxenbaum,Steven I., MD
- White,Ronald A., MD

ED Medical Associates
140 Grand Avenue Zip: 07631
Ph: (201) 569-9010 Fax: (201) 569-9063
- Brouk,Alla, MD
- Djebiyan,Eli S., MD
- Stepanyuk,Olena, MD

Endocrinology Consultants P.C.
229 Engle Street Zip: 07631
Ph: (201) 567-8999 Fax: (201) 567-5385
- Bier,Rachel Elizabeth, MD
- Borensztein,Alejandra Giselle, MD
- Fojas,Ma. Conchitina Manas, MD
- Lorton,Julie Lytton, MD
- Schwartz,Joseph Jay, MD

Englewood Anesthesiology
350 Engle Street Zip: 07631
Ph: (201) 894-3238 Fax: (201) 894-0585
- Baltaytis,Viktor, MD
- Betta,Joanne, MD
- Chan,Rolycito A., MD
- Chen,Wen-Hong, MD
- Chithran,Payyanadan V., MD
- Digiacomo,Michael B., MD
- Gak,Alexander V., MD
- Guillaume,Stephanie Ann, MD
- Huber,Michael D., DO
- Kulkarni,Sumedha V., MD
- Lui,John, MD
- Mizrahi,Marc E., MD
- Moskowitz,David Matthew, MD
- Pappalardo,Rebecca A., MD
- Shander,Aryeh, MD
- Smok,Jeffrey Thomas, MD
- Volpe,Lorraine, MD

Englewood Cardiac Surgery Associates
350 Engle Street Zip: 07631
Ph: (201) 894-3636
- Arnofsky,Adam Garett, MD
- Klein,James Joseph Jr., MD

Englewood Cardiology Consultants
177 North Dean Street/Suite 100 Zip: 07631
Ph: (201) 569-4901 Fax: (201) 569-6111
- Erlebacher,Jay A., MD
- Katechis,Dennis, DO
- Leber,George B., MD
- Shatzkes,Joseph Aaron, MD
- Wilkenfeld,Craig, MD

Englewood Ear Nose & Throat, P.C.
216 Engle Street/Suite 101 Zip: 07631
Ph: (201) 816-9800 Fax: (201) 567-1569
- Ho,Bryan Tao, MD
- Jahn,Anthony Frederick, MD
- Lewis,David A., MD
- Wanich,Niya, MD

Englewood Endoscopic Assocs
420 Grand Avenue/Suite 101 Zip: 07631
Ph: (201) 569-7044 Fax: (201) 569-1999
- Friedrich,Ivan A., MD
- Kancherla,Sandarsh Raj, MD
- Kaplounova,Irina, MD
- Panella,Vincent S., MD
- Sapienza,Mark Santo, MD

Englewood Family Health Center
148 Engle Street Zip: 07631
Ph: (201) 569-1530 Fax: (201) 569-6022
- Latorre,Rafael, MD

Englewood Knee & Sports Medicine
370 Grand Avenue/Suite 100 Zip: 07631
Ph: (201) 567-5700 Fax: (201) 567-8049
- Deramo,David Michael, MD
- Doidge,Robert W., DO

Englewood Medical Assoc Pediatrics
350 Engle Street Zip: 07631
Ph: (201) 894-3158 Fax: (201) 894-5649
- Zawahir,Shamila Balkis, MD

Englewood Ob Gyn Women's Group
286 Engle Street Zip: 07631
Ph: (201) 569-6190 Fax: (201) 569-6940
- Jhee,Yoon-Bok, MD
- Song,Erica Yoon-Jung, MD

Englewood Ob/Gyn Associates
370 Grand Avenue Zip: 07631
Ph: (201) 894-9599
- Hurst,Wendy Robin, MD
- Patel-Shusterman,Shefali Natavar,

Englewood Orthopedic Associates
401 South Van Brunt Street Zip: 07631
Ph: (201) 569-2770 Fax: (201) 569-1774
- Becker,Adam Scott, MD
- Cole,Brian Anthony, MD
- Cole,James R., MD
- Davis,Damien Ian, MD
- Fleischer,Jessica Beth, MD
- Hall,Andrew Robert, MD
- Miller-Breslow,Anne J., MD
- Nguyen,David Huong, MD
- Pizzillo,Michael Francis, MD
- Salob,Peter Andrew, MD
- Salzer,Richard L. Jr., MD
- Shah,Asit K., MD

Englewood Radiologic Group PA
350 Engle Street Zip: 07631
Ph: (201) 894-3000 Fax: (201) 894-5244
- Foster,Jonathan A., MD
- Goldfischer,Mindy A., MD
- Gutwein,Marina Ayzenberg, MD
- Juengst-Mitchell,Jannine, DO
- Mattana,Nina Delman, MD
- Naidrich,Shari Ann, MD
- Rekhtman-Sneed,Katya, MD
- Shapiro,Mark L., MD
- Shembde,Dwarkanath Sonaji, MD
- Vadde,Kavitha, MD

Englewood Surgical Associates
375 Engle Street/Ground Floor Zip: 07631
Ph: (201) 894-0400 Fax: (201) 894-1022
- Kahn,Mark Elliot, MD
- Sussman,Barry C., MD
- Wolodiger,Fred A., MD

Englewood Women's Health
25 Rockwood Place/Suite 305 Zip: 07631
Ph: (201) 894-0003 Fax: (201) 894-0006
- Gross,Arthur H., MD
- Markovitz,Jacob E., MD
- Martinucci,Stacy M., MD

Fishman & Fishman
216 Engle Street Zip: 07631
Ph: (201) 569-5678 Fax: (201) 569-6225
- Fishman,Miriam, MD

Groups and Clinics by Town with Physician Rosters

Forte Schleider & Attas MD PA
350 Engle Street/Berrie Building/1 FL Zip: 07631
Ph: (201) 568-5250 Fax: (201) 568-5358
  Attas,Lewis M., MD
  Forte,Francis A., MD
  Janosky,Maxwell, MD
  Jhawer,Minaxi P., MD
  Kim,Brian Hangil, MD
  Morrison,Jill S., MD
  Schleider,Michael A., MD

Freilich Eye Associates
15 Engle Street/Suite 106 Zip: 07631
Ph: (201) 871-9595 Fax: (201) 871-2323
  Freilich,Benjamin Douglas, MD
  Freilich,David Eric, MD

Health East Medical Center
54 South Dean Street Zip: 07631
Ph: (201) 871-4000
  Baynes,Jason R., MD
  Chalfin,Venus Helena, MD

Holy Name Physician Network
420 Grand Avenue/Suite 202 Zip: 07631
Ph: (201) 871-4040 Fax: (201) 871-7326
  Butler,David George, MD
  Englert,Christopher A., MD
  Tovmasian,Lucy Tamar, MD

Holy Name Pulmonary Associates PC
200 Grand Avenue/Suite 102 Zip: 07631
Ph: (201) 871-3636 Fax: (201) 871-2286
  Gorloff,Victor, MD
  Han,Paul S., MD
  Levine,Selwyn Eric, MD
  Pavlou,Theophanis A., MD
  Tesher,Harris Brandon, MD

Leonia Medical Associates, P.A.
25 Rockwood Place/Suite 120 Zip: 07631
Ph: (201) 568-3335 Fax: (201) 568-2450
  Gura,Russell Saul, MD
  Hamilton,Monique S., MD
  Healy,Christine B., DO
  Jathavedam,Ashwin, MD
  Katz,Manuel David, MD
  Kocher,Jeffrey, MD
  Laiosa,Catherine Virginia, MD
  Ramsetty,Sabena Karina, MD
  Tlamsa,Aileen P., MD
  Torres Isasiga,Julian Andres, MD
  Weisholtz,Steven J., MD

Metropolitan Neurosurgery Assoc PA
309 Engle Street/Suite 6 Zip: 07631
Ph: (201) 569-7737 Fax: (201) 569-1494
  Gologorsky,Yakov, MD
  Moore,Frank Max, MD
  Steinberger,Alfred A., MD
  Thomas,Vinoo Sebastian, MD
  Yao,Kevin Chi-Kai, MD

Michele Grodberg, MD & Associates
106 Grand Avenue/Suite 330 Zip: 07631
Ph: (201) 567-8884 Fax: (201) 567-5799
  Grodberg,Michele, MD
  Ordoukhanian,Elsa, MD
  Steinman,Natasha Margolin, MD

NJ Electrophysiology Assocs
350 Engle Street Zip: 07631
Ph: (201) 894-3533
  Feigenblum,David Yehuda, MD
  Nemirovsky,Dmitry, MD

North Jersey Orthopaedic Specialists
106 Grand Avenue Zip: 07631
Ph: (201) 608-0100 Fax: (201) 608-0104
  Archer,Jonathan Mckee, MD
  Lee,Jen Fei, MD
  Owens,John M., MD

Ob-Gyn Associates of Englewood
177 North Dean Street/Suite 208 Zip: 07631
Ph: (201) 569-0200 Fax: (201) 569-8287
  Binas,Constantine George, MD
  Gresham,Keith A., MD
  Kilinsky,Vladimir, MD
  Tisch,Bruce H., MD

Physical Medicine & Rehabilitation Ctr
500 Grand Avenue/1st Floor Zip: 07631
Ph: (201) 567-2277 Fax: (201) 567-7506
  Alonso,Jose A., MD
  Arias,Carlos, MD
  Babeendran,Shan, DO
  Bucalo,Victor John, MD
  Dutkowsky,Charles J., DO
  Friedman,Alan Mark, MD
  Hamer,Orlee, DO
  Jendrek,Paul, MD
  Liss,Donald, MD
  Liss,Howard, MD
  Montag,Nathaniel, DO
  Pavell,Jeff Richard, DO
  Riolo,Thomas Antonio, DO
  Tasca,Philip, MD
  Wisotsky,Lisa L., MD

Primary Care NJ
370 Grand Avenue/Suite 102 Zip: 07631
Ph: (201) 567-3370 Fax: (201) 816-1265
  Frier,Steven F., MD
  Gross,Harvey R., MD
  Ho,Eddie Kasing, MD
  Loewinger,Michael Brian, MD
  Skarimbas,Alicia C., MD
  Smith,Ebben Will, MD
  Volokhov,Alexey, MD
  Ye,Sheng H., MD
  Zimmerman,Ronald Lee, MD

Progressive Spine & Orthopaedics
440 Curry Avenue/Suite A Zip: 07631
Ph: (201) 885-4070
  Montero-Cruz,Fergie Ross, DO

Reproductive Medicine Associates of NJ
25 Rockwood Place Zip: 07631
Ph: (201) 569-7773 Fax: (201) 569-8143
  Hock,Doreen L., MD

S. L. Silverstein MD LLC
180 North Dean Street Zip: 07631
Ph: (201) 871-8366 Fax: (201) 871-8356
  Benoff,Brian Alan, MD
  Glassman,Adam M., MD
  Silberstein,Stuart L., MD

Spine Center
106 Grand Avenue/Suite 220 Zip: 07631
Ph: (201) 503-1900 Fax: (201) 503-1901
  Baker,Elizabeth Anne, MD
  Taha,Nora, MD
  Vadada,Kiran, MD

The Urology Center of Englewood, PA
300 Grand Avenue/Suite 102 Zip: 07631
Ph: (201) 816-1900 Fax: (201) 816-1777
  Katz,Steven A., MD

Urologic Specialties PA
177 North Dean Street/Suite 305 Zip: 07631
Ph: (201) 569-7777 Fax: (201) 569-6861
  Andronaco,Raymond B., MD
  Kerns,John F., MD
  Lee,Chester C., MD
  Lee,Richard, MD

Women Physicians Ob-Gyn Associates
300 Grand Avenue/Suite 102 Zip: 07631
Ph: (201) 569-5151 Fax: (201) 569-9193
  Ashton,Jennifer Lee, MD
  Suarez,Teresa, MD

Women's Medical Services PA
498 Engle Street Zip: 07631
Ph: (201) 569-0121 Fax: (201) 569-6835
  Saphier,Carl Joseph, MD
  Saphier,Douglas Jay, MD

Yee Medicine & Pediatric Assocs
245 Engle Street/Suite 3 Zip: 07631
Ph: (201) 569-9005 Fax: (201) 569-9080
  Psalidas,Panagiotis George, MD
  Yee,Sau Yan, MD

Englewood Cliffs

Advanced Gastroenterology
140 Sylvan Avenue/Suite 101-A Zip: 07632
Ph: (201) 945-6564 Fax: (201) 461-9038
  Chessler,Richard K., MD
  Fiorillo,Marc Anthony, MD
  Meininger,Michael Eric, MD
  Spinnell,Mitchell Kyle, MD
  Ward,Wendy Allison, MD
  Zingler,Barry M., MD

Drs. Rabin, Fremed, Prince, P.C.
700 Palisade Avenue Zip: 07632
Ph: (201) 568-3412 Fax: (201) 568-8249
  Fremed,Eric L., MD
  Prince,David M., MD
  Rabin,Aaron, MD

Gene Medical Group
464 Hudson Terrace/Suite 203 Zip: 07632
Ph: (201) 567-7725 Fax: (201) 567-5255
  Kang,Katherine E. Lee, MD
  Yun,Sung K., MD

Englishtown

Garden State Heart Care, P.C.
831 Tennent Road/Suite 1-F Zip: 07726
Ph: (732) 851-4700 Fax: (732) 851-4703
  Covalesky,John, DO
  Patel,Jatinchandra Suryakant, DO

Ewing

AZZ Medical Associates
1440 Pennington Road/Suite 1 Zip: 08618
Ph: (609) 890-1050 Fax: (609) 890-0950
  Meer,Shahid B., MD
  Sheikh,Sirajuddin, MD

Capital Health Primary Care
1230 Parkway Avenue/Suite 203 Zip: 08628
Ph: (609) 883-5454 Fax: (609) 883-2564
  Gettys,Jacqueline Brown, MD
  Pierrot,Paul H., MD
  Williams,Eric James, MD

Capital Health Primary Care
850 Bear Tavern Road/Suite 309 Zip: 08628
Ph: (609) 656-8844 Fax: (609) 656-8845
  Carruth Mehnert,Lauren Vales, MD
  Flynn-Abdalla,Jane, DO
  Gooding,Susane Lavern, MD
  Harman,John A., MD
  Kolander,Scott A., MD
  Kolman-Taddeo,Diana, MD
  Kudakachira,Shaismy, DO

Fair Haven

Fair Haven Internal Medicine
569 River Road/Suite 1 Zip: 07704
Ph: (732) 530-0100 Fax: (732) 530-5895
  Hayward,Denise H., MD
  Nardone,Danielle J., DO
  Pamintuan,Dominic C., MD

Fair Lawn

Drs. Chaudry & Chaudry
41-04 Goldblatt Terrace Zip: 07410
Ph: (201) 797-7129 Fax: (201) 703-6982
  Chaudry,Mansoora R., MD
  Chaudry,Sadia R., MD
  Chaudry,Samia Riaz, DO

Drs. Hossain, Hossain, and Farooqui
26-01 Broadway/Suite 105 Zip: 07410
Ph: (201) 703-3664
  Farooqui,Syeda Saleha, MD
  Hossain,Asghar S.M., MD
  Hossain,Nazma A., MD

Garden State Orthopaedic Assoc PA
28-04 Broadway Zip: 07410
Ph: (201) 791-4434 Fax: (201) 791-9377
  Bassan,Matthew Evan, DO
  Bernstein,Adam Douglas, MD
  Cassilly,Ryan, MD
  Levitsky,Kenneth A., MD
  Rosenberg,Jeffrey Steven, MD
  Schultz,Robert A., MD
  Shamash,Steven Baroukh, DO

Garden State Surgical Center, L.L.C.
28-06 Broadway Zip: 07410
Ph: (201) 475-8940 Fax: (201) 475-8944
  Bamberger,Philip David, MD
  Snyder,Samuel Jay, MD

Heart & Vasc Assoc of Northern Jersey
22-18 Broadway/Suite 201 Zip: 07410
Ph: (201) 475-5050 Fax: (201) 475-5522
  Bernardo,Dennis N., MD
  Bikkina,Mahesh, MD
  Chabbott,David Robert, MD
  Cho,Soung Ick, MD
  Grossman,Steven H., MD
  Levin,Susan Miriam, MD
  Qipo,Andi, MD
  Samuel,Anish, MD
  Sen,Sourav, MD
  Sheth,Meetkumar Tusharbhai, MD
  Singh,Amrita Kaur, MD
  Soyombo,Aderemi B., MD
  Syed,Zainab, MD
  Tiyyagura,Satish Reddy, MD
  Vehra,Ijaz R., MD
  Virk,Hartaj Singh, MD

Kurra Associates
15-01 Broadway/Suite 10-B Zip: 07410
Ph: (201) 794-7733 Fax: (201) 794-6039
  Kurra,Padmavathy, MD
  Valiveti,Sailaja Devi, MD

Maple Avenue Pediatrics
23-00 Route 208 Zip: 07410
Ph: (201) 797-1900 Fax: (201) 797-4457
  Greaney,Kathleen Margaret, MD
  Lewis,Brian S., MD
  Yellin,Tova G., MD

Medical Internists Associates PA
22-18 Broadway/Suite 104 Zip: 07410
Ph: (201) 797-4503 Fax: (201) 797-4270
  Clifford,Eileen M., MD
  Narymsky,Lyudmila M., MD
  Oliver,Richard D., MD
  Rizkalla,Suzette, MD

Medical Multispecialty Associates PA
11-26 Saddle River Road Zip: 07410
Ph: (201) 796-9200 Fax: (201) 796-7606
  Herman,Brad Morris, MD
  Infantino,Salvatore, MD
  Lefkowitz,Jeffrey R., MD

Medicine & Rehabilitation, PC
14-25 Plaza Road/Suite S31 Zip: 07410
Ph: (201) 797-2050 Fax: (201) 797-2051
  Logvinenko,Andrei V., MD
  Logvinenko,Nina V., MD

North Jersey Pediatrics
17-10 Fair Lawn Avenue Zip: 07410
Ph: (201) 794-8585 Fax: (201) 703-9889
  Boyarsky,Yael, MD
  Fischer,Emily Frances, MD
  Laufer,Ilene Caren, MD
  Paige,Melanie Kay, MD
  Rao,Gunjan Pradhan, MD
  Riegelhaupt,Rona Susan, MD
  Sonnenblick,Howard C., MD
  Steinel,Lisa A., MD

Orthopedic Associates
15-01 Broadway/Suite 20 Zip: 07410
Ph: (201) 794-6008
  Berger,John L., MD
  Greenblum,Robert, MD
  Ruoff,Mark J., MD

PediatriCare Associates
20-20 Fair Lawn Avenue Zip: 07410
Ph: (201) 791-4545 Fax: (201) 791-3765
  Alexander,Leah M., MD
  Anido,Rosary Kristine Isidro, MD
  Bienstock,Jeffrey Marc, MD
  Brucia,Lauren A., MD
  Chism,Melissa A., MD
  Hetling,Kristina, MD
  Kaul,Reena Sonya, MD
  Lin,Tatiana Alexeevna, MD
  Long,Jessie C., MD
  Schlitt,Meghan Ann, MD
  Shafi,Heather Claire, MD
  Steinbaum,Deborah Paige, MD
  Zucker,Scott W., MD

Radburn Medical Associates
20-20 Fair Lawn Avenue/Suite 104 Zip: 07410
Ph: (201) 703-0202 Fax: (201) 703-1231
  Berman,Lawrence J., MD
  John,Eirene George, MD
  Wertenteil,Mark Elliot, MD

Groups and Clinics by Town with Physician Rosters

air Lawn (cont)
Sovereign Medical Group
15-01 Broadway/Suite 1 Zip: 07410
Ph: (201) 791-4544 Fax: (201) 791-6585
- Chang,David Tsuwei, MD
- Christiansen,Keith Alan, MD
- Hessami,Sam H., MD
- Howhannesian,Andranik, MD

Summit Medical Group
31-00 Broadway Zip: 07410
Ph: (201) 796-2255 Fax: (201) 796-7020
- Aquino,Christine E., MD
- Arbit,David Lewis, MD
- Balonze,Karen T., MD
- Batchelor,Christopher D. Jr., MD
- Cappitelli,Jack V., MD

Summit Medical Group
19-21 Fair Lawn Avenue Zip: 07410
Ph: (908) 273-4300
- Deitz,Justina May, DO
- Feiner,Shoshana N., MD
- Kaur,Jasneet, MD
- Marta,Peter T., DO
- Molloy,Thomas J., MD
- Owsiak,Joanne Naamo, MD
- Resnick,Jonathan, MD
- Sagullo,Cynthia C., MD
- Sherman,Jennifer Ann, DO
- Verrico,Tracy B., DO

SurgiCare Surgical Associates, P.A.
15-01 Broadway/Suites 1 & 3 Zip: 07410
Ph: (201) 703-8487 Fax: (201) 791-6585
- Hajjar,John H., MD

Valley Medical Grp OB/GYN in Fairlawn
5-22 Saddle River Road Zip: 07410
Ph: (201) 796-2025 Fax: (201) 796-0587
- Beloff,Michelle Lauren, DO
- Dolgin,James S., MD
- Mitzner,Ann C., MD
- Reinkraut,Jeffrey M., MD
- Seymour,Carmela, MD

Fairfield
Corneal Associates of NJ
100 Passaic Avenue/Suite 200 Zip: 07004
Ph: (973) 439-3937 Fax: (973) 439-3944
- Moses,Eli B., MD
- Perl,Theodore, MD

Drs. Bhatt and Bhatt
271 Route 46 West/Suite 105 Zip: 07004
Ph: (973) 575-8644 Fax: (973) 575-8677
- Bhatt,Rupal S., MD
- Bhatt,Shirish Vinayak, MD

Fairfield Family Practice
125 Sand Road Zip: 07004
Ph: (973) 808-9242
- Liotti,Joseph B., DO
- Liotti,Linda A., DO

Med-Care of Fairfield, Inc.
150 Fairfield Road Zip: 07004
Ph: (973) 227-0020
- Scolamiero,Amedeo J., MD
- Zhukova,Irina, DO

Fanwood
Drs. Lewis & Jamdar
346 South Avenue Zip: 07023
Ph: (908) 889-4700 Fax: (908) 889-0867
- Jamdar,Niteen Subhash, MD
- Lewis,Thomas Peter, MD

Watchung Pediatrics
346 South Avenue/Suite 3 Zip: 07023
Ph: (908) 889-8687 Fax: (908) 889-0047
- Gillard,Bonita Dee, MD
- Koward,Donna Marie, MD

Flanders
Advocare Family Health at Mt. Olive
183 US Route 206/Suite 1 Zip: 07836
Ph: (973) 347-3277 Fax: (973) 347-3141
- Choe,Charles C., DO
- Friedman,Samuel, MD
- Ghanta,Suma Bala, MD
- Miccio,Anthony G., MD
- Peters,Karen R., DO

Washington Family Medicine PC
191 US Highway 206 Zip: 07836
Ph: (973) 584-0045 Fax: (973) 584-0094
- Fernandez,Sofia Ramona, MD
- Mercado,Alex M., MD

Flemington
Advanced Gastroenterology & Nutrition
1100 Wescott Drive/Suite 304 Zip: 08822
Ph: (908) 788-4022 Fax: (908) 788-4066
- Lim,Khengjim, MD
- Willis,Stephen Laird, MD

Advanced Obstetrics & Gynecology, LLC
4 Walter E. Foran Boulevard/Suite 302 Zip: 08822
Ph: (908) 806-0080 Fax: (908) 806-8570
- Abeysinghe,Manisha G., MD
- Ardise,Patricia Marie, MD
- Belkina,Yelena, MD
- Camiolo,Melissa Rae, MD
- Goglia,Kara Defilippis, MD
- Masterton,Deirdre C., MD
- Rivas,Jimena, MD

Advanced Obstetrics & Gynecology
1100 Wescott Drive Zip: 08822
Ph: (908) 788-6488
- Vitale,Lidia F., MD

Affiliates in Obstetrics & Gynecology
111 Route 31/Suite 121 2nd FL Bldg B Zip: 08822
Ph: (908) 782-2825 Fax: (908) 782-0196
- Altomare,Corrado J., MD
- Grove,Michele Sak, MD
- Huttner,Ruby P., MD
- Lynen,Richard F., MD
- Pedersen,Irene A., MD

All Women's Healthcare
1100 Wescott Drive/Suite 105 Zip: 08822
Ph: (908) 788-6469 Fax: (908) 788-6483
- Bowers,Mamie Sue, MD
- Frys,Kelly Ann, DO
- Grimes,Sara, MD
- Pisatowski,Denise Michelle, MD

Cornerstone Family Practice
9100 Wescott Drive/Suite 103 Zip: 08822
Ph: (908) 237-6910 Fax: (908) 237-6919
- Bachrach,Stacey R., MD
- Gazurian,Raina, MD
- Lecusay,Dario A. Jr., MD
- Madonia,Paul W., MD
- Mui,Timothy H., MD
- Mukherji,Genea, MD
- Randhawa,Smita Devidas, MD
- Sood,Supriya G., MD

Diabetes & Endocrine Associates
9100 Wescott Drive/Suite 101 Zip: 08822
Ph: (908) 237-6990 Fax: (908) 237-6995
- Caldarella,Felice Antonino, MD
- Khan,Saima, MD
- Lind,Robert Michael, MD
- Modarressi,Taher, MD
- Sandberg,Marc Ira, MD

Flemington Medical Group, LLC
200 State Route 31 North/Suite 105 Zip: 08822
Ph: (908) 782-5100 Fax: (908) 782-0290
- Bretan,Amy Faith, MD
- Manchen,Dennis R., MD
- Shaber,Marc L., MD

Huntendon Gastroenterology
1100 Wescott Drive/Suite 201 Zip: 08822
Ph: (908) 788-4022 Fax: (908) 788-4066
- Hartford,Jeffrey D., MD
- Lesser,Gregory Scott, MD

Hunterdon Anesthesia Associates
2100 Wescott Drive Zip: 08822
Ph: (908) 788-6181 Fax: (908) 788-6145
- Bentley,William Earl IV, DO
- Bery,Sumita, MD

Hunterdon Cardiovascular Associates
1100 Wescott Drive/Suite G-3 Zip: 08822
Ph: (908) 788-6471 Fax: (908) 788-6460
- Benigno,Robert A., MD
- Bialy,Ted, MD
- Elnahar,Yaser, MD

- Horiuchi,Jonathan K., MD
- Imsirovic-Starcevic,Dubravka, MD
- Kutscher,Austin Harrison Jr., MD
- Rudnick,Andrew Glenn, MD
- Schafranek,William, MD
- Tonnessen,Glen E., MD

Hunterdon Family Medicine
1100 Wescott Drive/Suite 101 Zip: 08822
Ph: (908) 788-6535 Fax: (908) 788-6536
- Hannema,Erica L., DO
- Hoette,Petra, MD
- Joseph,Junie Lorna, MD
- Lewis,Mary Kendra, MD
- Mattei,C. Antonia, MD
- Pauch-McNamara,Dorothy Anne, MD

Hunterdon Family Physicians
111 State Route 31/Suite 111 Zip: 08822
Ph: (908) 284-9880 Fax: (908) 782-4316
- Bernard,Marie G., MD
- Licetti,Stephen Charles, DO
- Liu,Lide, MD
- O'Hara,Jennifer Fisk, MD
- Peng,Victor I., MD
- Tammana,Swarna, DO
- Wright,Deborah Sue, MD

Hunterdon Gastroenterology Assocs
1100 Wescott Drive/Suite 206-207 Zip: 08822
Ph: (908) 483-4000 Fax: (908) 788-5090
- Arrigo,Richard J., DO
- Bae,Samuel Y., MD
- Cardoso,Gilbert Santos, DO
- Daruwala,Cherag A., MD
- DiGregorio,Kenneth J., MD
- Georgsson,Maria Anna, MD
- Goldstein,Andrea E., MD
- Matthews,Jason D., MD
- Patel,Anik Mayur, MD

Hunterdon Infection Disease
1100 Wescott Drive/Suite 306 Zip: 08822
Ph: (908) 788-6474 Fax: (908) 788-6616
- Gugliotta,Joseph L., MD
- Haddad,Sohail G., MD

Hunterdon Otolaryngology Assoc
6 Sand Hill Road/Suite 302 Zip: 08822
Ph: (908) 788-9131 Fax: (908) 788-0945
- Hanna,John Patrick, DO
- Kroon,David Fleming, MD
- Maniar,Anoli, MD
- Muglia-Chopra,Christine Ann, MD
- Sheft,Stanley A., MD
- Worden,Douglas L., MD

Hunterdon Pediatric Associates
8 Reading Road/Reading Ridge Zip: 08822
Ph: (908) 788-6070 Fax: (908) 788-6005
- Clarin,Mitchell I., MD

Hunterdon Pediatric Associates
6 Sand Hill Road/Suite 202 Zip: 08822
Ph: (908) 782-6700 Fax: (908) 788-5861
- Cohn,David B., MD
- Douvris,John S., MD
- Fellmeth,Wayne G., MD
- Goldstein,Keith Ty, MD
- Jasutkar,Ashwini, MD
- Krupinski,Donna J., MD
- Pistun,Oleksandr, MD
- Prosswimmer,Geralyn M., MD
- Rushton,Alan R., MD
- Shah,Debra Stahl, MD
- Yuan,Carol Jia-Luh, MD

Hunterdon Pulmnry & Crtcl Care Asscs
6 Sand Hill Road/Suite 202 Zip: 08822
Ph: (908) 237-1148 Fax: (908) 237-1749
- Khan,Muhammad Khurram, MD
- Maouelainin,Nina, DO

Hunterdon Regional Cancer Ctr
2100 Wescott Drive Zip: 08822
Ph: (908) 788-6461 Fax: (908) 788-6412
- Bednar,Myron Emil, MD
- Blankstein,Kenneth B., MD
- Ngeow,Swee Jian, MD
- Quinn,Brian Michael, MD
- Rehman,Waqas, MD
- Shah,Megha, MD

Hunterdon Surgical Associates
1100 Wescott Drive/Suite 302 Zip: 08822
Ph: (908) 788-6464 Fax: (908) 788-6459
- Bello,John J., MD
- Bello,Joseph M., MD
- Chen,Jeffrey H., MD
- Maeuser,Herman L.I., MD

Hunterdon Urological Associates
1 Wescott Drive/Suite 101 Zip: 08822
Ph: (908) 782-0019 Fax: (908) 237-4132
- Bloch,Paul Jacob, MD

Hunterdon Urological Associates
121 Highway 31/Suite 1200 Zip: 08822
Ph: (908) 782-0019 Fax: (908) 782-0630
- Ghosh,Propa, MD
- Kern,Allen J., MD
- Lai,Weil Ron, MD
- Sperling,Brian Lee, DO

MidJersey Orthopaedics, P.A.
8100 Westcott Drive/Suite 101 Zip: 08822
Ph: (908) 782-0600 Fax: (908) 782-7575
- Bleazey,Scott Thomas, MD
- Chang,Richard, MD
- Collalto,Patrick Michael, MD
- Decker,Jerome Elliot, MD
- Glassner,Philip Justin, MD
- Gordon,Eric Michael, MD
- More,Robert C., MD
- Nenna,David Vito, MD
- Pandya,Dipakkumar P., MD
- Pollack,Michael Edward, MD
- Salam,Aleya, MD
- Shafa,Eiman, MD
- Viradia,Manish Bhikhabhai, MD

NeuroGroup at Hunterdon
1100 Wescott Drive/Suite 301 Zip: 08822
Ph: (609) 788-6541 Fax: (609) 788-6519
- Pizzi,Francis Joseph, MD

Paul Phillips Eye & Surgery Center
6 Minneakoning Road/Suite B Zip: 08822
Ph: (908) 824-7144 Fax: (908) 968-3239
- Phillips,Paul S., MD

Princeton Flemington Eye Institute
1100 Wescott Drive/Suite 305 Zip: 08822
Ph: (908) 237-7037
- Dunham,Gerald, MD

Psychiatric Associates of Hunterdon
190 Route 31/Suite 100 Zip: 08822
Ph: (908) 788-6654 Fax: (908) 788-6452
- Chen,Hong, MD
- Hill,Everett Huntington, MD
- Lucas,Gem-Estelle Maun, DO
- Skotzko,Christine Ellen, MD

Pulmonary & Sleep Assoc. of Hunterdon
1100 Wescott Drive/Suite G-2 Zip: 08822
Ph: (908) 237-1560 Fax: (908) 806-2529
- Glassner,Norman, MD
- Granato,Anthony Alexander, MD
- Lansang,Martin Fidel, MD

The Center for Nutritional Medicine
4 Walter E. Foran Boulevard/Suite 409 Zip: 08822
Ph: (908) 237-0200 Fax: (908) 237-0210
- Benson,Jay Robert, DO
- Fuhrman,Joel H., MD

Florham Park
Advanced Laparoscopic Surgeons
83 Hanover Road/Suite 190 Zip: 07932
Ph: (973) 410-9700 Fax: (973) 410-9703
- Abkin,Alexander, MD
- Bertha,Nicholas A., DO
- Botvinov,Mikhail A., DO

Allergy and Clinical Immunology Center
29 Columbia Turnpike/Suite 202 Zip: 07932
Ph: (973) 377-4112 Fax: (973) 377-2775
- Sundaram,Usha K., MD

Center for Dermatology PA
128 Columbia Turnpike/Suite 200 Zip: 07932
Ph: (973) 736-9535 Fax: (973) 736-2607
- Badalamenti,Stephanie Silos, MD
- Machler,Brian C., MD

Groups and Clinics by Town with Physician Rosters

Drs. Siegel and Kissin
10 James Street/Suite 140 Zip: 07932
Ph: (973) 665-8100 Fax: (973) 665-8097
- Kissin, Anna, MD
- Siegel, Sheera Karch, MD

Essex Cardiology Group PC
10 James Street/Suite 130 Zip: 07932
Ph: (973) 736-9557 Fax: (973) 736-9757
- Fabrizio, Lawrence, DO

Florham Park Pediatrics
195 Columbia Turnpike/Suite 105 Zip: 07932
Ph: (973) 437-8300 Fax: (973) 845-2883
- Baxley, Maureen Elizabeth, MD
- Silva, Francisco, MD

IPC The Hospitalist Company
220 Ridgedale Avenue/Suite C-2 Zip: 07932
Ph: (973) 538-5844 Fax: (973) 267-0181
- Bennett, Douglas P., DO
- Chandwani, Ashish, MD
- De Shaw, Max G., MD
- Frankel, Renee Ellen, MD
- Kilkenny-Trainor, Kerryann A., MD
- Kunjukutty, Felix, MD
- O'Grady, John P., MD
- Pinel Villalobos, Silvia P., DO
- Pinyard, Jeremy Vincent, MD
- Roytman, Peter, MD

Maron & Rodrigues Medical Group
10 James Street/Suite 150 Zip: 07932
Ph: (973) 822-2000 Fax: (973) 822-2001
- Maron, Scott Michael, MD
- Rodrigues, Anisha, MD
- Sabnani-Nagella, Kavita R., MD
- Tiongco, Judith Perlas, MD

Nephrological Associates, P.A.
83 Hanover Road/Suite 290 Zip: 07932
Ph: (973) 736-2212 Fax: (973) 736-2989
- Ahmad, Mir M., MD
- Alberto, Kezia Jasmina Ribeiro, MD
- Estilo, Genevieve Kristina, MD
- Goodman, Jeffrey W., MD
- Lyman, Neil W., MD
- Saldarini, John Christopher, MD
- Viscuso, Ronald L., MD
- Zenenberg, Robert D., DO

New Jersey Anesthesia Associates PC
25B Vreeland Road/Suite 110/PO Box 0037 Zip: 07932
Ph: (973) 660-9334 Fax: (973) 660-9732
- Davis, Clifton Colby, MD
- Goldstein, Joshua D., MD
- Hausdorff, Mark Alan, MD
- Ramos, Joseph, MD

New Jersey Anesthesia Associates, P.C.
252 Columbia Turnpike/PO Box 0037 Zip: 07932
Ph: (973) 660-9334 Fax: (973) 660-9779
- Abramowicz, Apolonia E., MD
- Ahmad, Idrees, MD
- Basius, Joseph T., DO
- Bergam, Miro Nicholas Jr., MD
- Blank, Jonathan Dirk, MD
- Bonsell, Joshua W., MD
- Braverman, Joel Morton, MD
- Cardoso, Ronald J., MD

NJ Anesthesia Associates, P.C.
30B Vreeland Road/Suite 200 Zip: 07932
Ph: (973) 660-9334 Fax: (973) 660-9779
- Chen, Jianping, MD
- Chung, Dae S., MD
- Ciolino, Robert B., MD
- Clancy, Lisa A., MD
- Co, Demosthene E., MD
- Conyack, David G., DO
- Dibadj, Khosro, MD
- Fein, Eric N., MD
- Fisher, Emery IV, DO
- Fitz, Rachel Myra, DO
- Ganti, Suryaprakash, MD
- Ju, Albert Changwon, MD
- Levine, Robert Scott, MD
- Maizes, Allen Stuart, MD
- Monti, Richard A., MD
- Parikh, Bijal Rajendra, MD
- Patafio, Onofrio, MD
- Pond, Charles G., MD
- Russo, Cathy Marie, MD
- Scala, Peter L., MD
- Zylberger, David A., MD

Peer Group Plastic Surgery Ctr
124 Columbia Turnpike Zip: 07932
Ph: (973) 822-3000 Fax: (973) 822-1726
- Colon, Francisco G., MD
- Failey, Colin Leander, MD
- Hawrylo, Richard R., MD
- Lange, David J., MD
- Starker, Isaac, MD

Storch Nutritional Medical Assoc
147 Columbia Turnpike/Suite 308 Zip: 07932
- Hooda, Anjali, MD
- Storch, Kenneth J., MD

Summit Medical Group
140 Park Avenue/3rd Floor Zip: 07932
Ph: (908) 273-4300
- Asimolowo, Olabisi Omolara, MD
- Blumberg, Darren Reich, MD
- Castellano, Charles Christopher, MD
- Cohen, Liliana, MD
- Fleming, Gregory John, MD
- Galandauer, Isaac, MD
- Han, Dennis, MD
- Harwani, Nita R., MD
- Kim, Mina Jung, MD
- Most, Michael David, MD
- Noce, Louis Arthur, MD
- Parikh, Smruti Ashish, MD
- Peron, Didier L., MD
- Santoni, Francesco, MD
- Scheid, Edward Herbert Jr., MD
- Soleymani, Taraneh, MD
- Steinberg, Jonathan S., MD
- Tamres, David Michael, MD

SMG Florham Park Campus
150 Park Avenue Zip: 07932
Ph: (908) 273-4300
- Argiroff, Alexandra Louise, MD
- Byrd, Serena Ann, MD
- Carter, Mitchel S., MD
- DeRosa, William T., DO
- Febbraro, Terri, MD
- George, Roshini, DO
- Gibbon, Darlene Grace, MD
- Gurubhagavatula, Sarada, MD
- Hart, Daniel, MD
- Huang, Eric Y., MD
- Huang, Eric Yuchueh, MD
- Kim, Joseph Jongbum, MD
- Patel-Cohen, Mital, MD
- Siu, Karleung, MD

Summit Medical Group
140 Park Avenue/2nd Floor Zip: 07932
Ph: (973) 404-9980 Fax: (973) 267-7295
- Adam, Stephanie Paige, DO
- Bamboat, Zubin Mickey, MD
- Black, Eric M., MD
- Diehl, William L., MD
- Gabre, Kennedy Ogbazion, MD
- Kocaj, Stephen Mark, MD
- Niver, Genghis Erjan, MD
- Pajaro, Rafael E., MD
- Shindle, Michael Kenneth, MD

Fords

Clara Barton Cardio-Medical Assc
565 New Brunswick Avenue Zip: 08863
Ph: (732) 738-8000 Fax: (732) 738-1663
- Latif, Pervaize, MD

Madho K. Sharma MD PA
30 Hoy Avenue Zip: 08863
Ph: (732) 225-9115 Fax: (732) 225-2814
- Ogden, Neeta Sharma, MD
- Sharma, Madho K., MD

Forked River

Allergic Disease Associates, PC
1044 Lacey Road/suite 9 Zip: 08731
Ph: (609) 693-5317 Fax: (609) 693-0351
- Empedrad, Raquel B., MD

SOMC Medical Group, P.C.
730 Lacey Road/Suite G-08 Zip: 08731
Ph: (609) 693-2900 Fax: (609) 242-5437
- Bustamante Dayanghirang, Alma, MD

Fort Lee

Advanced Cardiology Institute
2200 Fletcher Avenue/Suite 1 Zip: 07024
Ph: (201) 461-6200 Fax: (201) 461-7204
- Hollywood, Jacqueline, MD
- Kim, Steve Sang-Yoon, MD
- Krasikov, Tatiana, MD
- Lebowitz, Nathaniel Edward, MD
- Rothman, Howard C., MD
- Zanger, Diane Rachel, MD

Bergen Cardiology Associates
292 Columbia Avenue Zip: 07024
Ph: (201) 224-0050 Fax: (201) 224-6061
- Adibi, Baback, MD
- Andrews, Paul Matthew, MD
- Landers, David Benjamin, MD
- Lauricella, Joseph Ned, MD

Bergen Internal Medicine, LLC
6 Horizon Road Zip: 07024
Ph: (201) 886-8989 Fax: (201) 886-8990
- Gallo, Richard James, MD
- Hernandez, Michael Dennis, MD

Drs. Banschick, Concepcion & Stein
2500 Lemoine Avenue/Suite 200 Zip: 07024
Ph: (201) 592-9210 Fax: (201) 592-6539
- Akturk, Elvin, DO
- Banschick, Harry, MD
- Laziez, Janet Tomeh, MD

Drs. Shapnik & Gurtovy
2150 Center Avenue/Suite 1-B Zip: 07024
Ph: (201) 461-2444 Fax: (201) 461-7148
- Shapnik, Bella, MD

Fort Lee Surgery Center
1608 Lemoine Avenue/Suite 101 Zip: 07024
Ph: (201) 346-1112 Fax: (201) 346-1885
- Basak, Jayati, MD
- Ohanian, Marc S., MD

Metropolitan Pain Consultants
1640 Schlosser Street/Suite C-3 Zip: 07024
Ph: (201) 729-0001 Fax: (201) 729-0006
- Desai, Jagdip, MD
- Kang, Richard, MD

Montrose Eye Associates
301 Bridge Plaza North Zip: 07024
Ph: (201) 941-0562 Fax: (201) 947-5507
- Rosenberg, Michael Eric, MD
- Rosenberg, Rhonda Betsy, MD
- Rosenberg-Henick, Arlene M., MD

Palisades Surgical Associates
1530 Palisade Avenue/Colony Building Zip: 07024
Ph: (201) 585-8282 Fax: (201) 585-0805
- Carrao, Vincent, MD

Pedimedica PA
810 Abbott Boulevard/Suite 101 Zip: 07024
Ph: (201) 224-3200 Fax: (201) 224-4045
- Kim, Eunja, MD
- Yenukashvili, Nana R., MD

SCN Dermatology
2083 Center Avenue/2nd Floor Zip: 07024
Ph: (201) 944-3800
- Lee, Robert, MD

Tenafly Pediatrics, PA
301 Bridge Plaza North Zip: 07024
Ph: (201) 592-8787 Fax: (201) 592-6350
- Aranoff, Joanne Rachel, MD
- Kim, Eun-Joo Song, MD

Franklin

Skylands Medical Group PA
406 Route 23/Suite 1 Zip: 07416
Ph: (973) 827-2120 Fax: (973) 827-9445
- Holgado, Marco Patrick Guinto, DO
- Matkiwsky, Daniel Walter, DO

Franklin Lakes

Centro-Ibero-Americano
406 Mountain Avenue Zip: 07417
Ph: (973) 684-8138
- Sandoval, Ramon Antonio, MD

Drs. Coira & Richards
851 Franklin Lake Road/Suite 105 Zip: 07417
Ph: (201) 904-2230 Fax: (201) 904-2232
- Coira, Diego L., MD
- Richards, Christopher F., MD

Kayal Orthopaedic Center
784 Franklin Avenue/Suite 250 Zip: 07417
Ph: (844) 281-1783 Fax: (201) 560-0712
- Aydin, Steve M., DO
- Bellapianta, Joseph Michael, MD
- Greenberg, Aaron Joseph, MD
- Lin, Edward Alan, MD
- Pandey, Rajesh Kumar, MD
- Sood, Amit, MD
- Zalkowitz, Alan, MD

Franklin Park

Brunswick Urgent Care
3185 State Route 27 Zip: 08823
- Cha, Min, MD
- Phan, Au Ngoc, MD

Freehold

Advanced Orthopedics & Sports Med
301 Professional View Drive Zip: 07728
Ph: (732) 720-2555 Fax: (732) 720-2556
- Arias Garau, Jessica, MD
- Banzon, Manuel T., MD
- Berkowitz, Gregg S., MD
- Cozzarelli, James Francis, MD
- Goldberg, Grigory, MD
- Goldberger, Gerardo V., DO
- Greller, Michael Jon, MD
- Nasar, Alan S., MD
- Paulvin, Neil Brian, DO

Advanced Surgical Health Associates
901 West Main Street/MAB Suite 101 Zip: 07728
Ph: (732) 308-4202 Fax: (732) 308-4212
- Kayal, Thomas Joseph, MD
- Kharod, Amit S., MD

Allergy & Pediatric Associates
222 Schanck Road/Suite 105 Zip: 07728
Ph: (732) 431-3373 Fax: (732) 303-0172
- Donde, Mrunalini D., MD
- Katturupalli, Madhavi, MD
- LaMantia, Anthony P., MD
- Lacap, Estela Villar, MD
- Patel, Arvind Maganbhai, MD
- Wolfe, Jeffrey S., MD

Amer Ob-Gyn Associates
900 West Main Street/Suite 3 Zip: 07728
Ph: (732) 294-5600
- Amer, Yousef A., MD
- Bernard-Roberts, Lynikka, MD

Arthritis & Osteoporosis Associates
4247 US Highway 9/Building 1 Zip: 07728
Ph: (732) 780-7650 Fax: (732) 780-8817
- Adenwalla, Humaira Naseem, MD
- Cohen, Aly G., MD
- El Kadi, Hisham S., MD
- Komboz, Rita Fares, MD
- Krakauer, Randall Sheldon, MD
- Lumezanu, Elena Mihaela, MD
- Sharobeem, Andrew Mena, DO

Back, Seigel & Goldstein, MD, PA
501 Iron Bridge Road Zip: 07728
Ph: (732) 431-1807 Fax: (732) 409-2777
- Back, Norman A., MD
- Goldstein, Steven A., MD
- Seigel, Mark J., MD

Center for Ear, Nose, Sinus & Throat
501 Iron Bridge Road/Suite 11 Zip: 07728
Ph: (732) 409-0200 Fax: (732) 409-0202
- Razvi, Sedeq A., MD

Groups and Clinics by Town with Physician Rosters

Freehold (cont)

CentraState Family Medicine
1001 West Main Street/Suite B Zip: 07728
Ph: (732) 294-2540 Fax: (732) 294-9328
- Ciminelli, Maria F., MD
- Delcurla, Gina M., DO
- Dermer, Alicia R., MD
- Edrich, Dina Rachel, MD
- Espinar Ho, Maria Elena, MD
- Jonnalagadda, Balathripura S., MD
- Khan, Zeeshan, MD
- Mellor, Lisa Marie, MD
- Ogon, Bernard Okem, MD
- Sewell, Grant, MD
- Shah, Anand Subhash, MD
- Shenker, Bennett Steven, MD
- Sinha, Taru, MD
- Wright, Evan Michael, DO
- Yu Chen, Robert P., MD

Central Jersey Emergency Medicine
901 West Main Street Zip: 07728
Ph: (732) 942-2666 Fax: (732) 431-8267
- Chieco, Michael Anthony, MD
- Mehta, Sanjay, DO

Central Jersey Neurology Associates
501 Iron Bridge Road/Suite 2 Zip: 07728
Ph: (732) 462-7030 Fax: (732) 308-3562
- Frank, David J., MD
- Gulevski, Vasko Kole, MD
- Katz, Amos, MD
- Lage, Susan Marie, DO

Central Jersey Surgical Assoc
495 Iron Bridge Road/Suite 3 Zip: 07728
Ph: (732) 845-0222 Fax: (732) 845-1002
- Ashok, Viswanath K., MD
- Kovacs, Gabor, MD

Drs. Bernardo & Leonard
4255 US Highway 9/Suite B Zip: 07728
Ph: (732) 683-9897 Fax: (732) 683-9674
- Bernardo, Salvatore Jr., MD
- Leonard, Sara B., MD

Drs. Bhasin & Patel
1001 West Main Street/Suite A Zip: 07728
Ph: (732) 637-8444 Fax: (732) 637-8440
- Bhasin, Atul, MD
- Patel, Nikesh Kirit, MD

Drs. Cato-Varlack & Sadik
495 Iron Bridge Road/Suite 1 Zip: 07728
Ph: (732) 577-0047
- Cato-Varlack, Janice Antoinette, MD
- Sadik, Zubaida Y., MD

Drs. Hametz & Picascia
77-55 Schanck Road/Suite B-3 Zip: 07728
Ph: (732) 462-9800
- Hametz, Irwin, MD
- Miller, Jason Harris, MD
- Picascia, David D., MD

East Freehold Medical Associates
16 Thoreau Drive Zip: 07728
Ph: (732) 761-0221
- Cherciu, Doina M., MD
- Cherciu, Muguerl S., MD

Endo-Surgical Associates
901 West Main Street/Suite 104 Zip: 07728
Ph: (732) 761-1740 Fax: (732) 761-8320
- Dobruskin, Yelizaveta, MD
- Noyan, Earl Lincoln, MD

Endocrinology Assocs of Central NJ
501 Iron Bridge Road/Suite 12 Zip: 07728
Ph: (732) 780-0002 Fax: (732) 308-0117
- Ordene, Kenneth W., MD
- Wininger, Eric Amiel, MD

Family Practice of CentraState
901 West Main Street/Suite 106 Zip: 07728
Ph: (732) 462-0100 Fax: (732) 462-0348
- Faistl, Kenneth W., MD
- Kathrotia, Mitesh Gordhan, MD
- Lucas, Lisa W., DO
- Luparello, Paul J., MD
- Sojka, Leslie W., MD
- Vizzoni, Joseph Anthony, MD

Freehold Ophthalmology, LLC
509 Stillwells Corner Road/Suite E-5 Zip: 07728
Ph: (732) 431-9333 Fax: (732) 431-3312
- Gershenbaum, Eric Andrew, MD
- Lee, Joan Jean, DO
- Naadimuthu, Revathi P., MD

Freehold Radiology Group
901 West Main Street Zip: 07728
Ph: (732) 462-4844
- Arredondo, Mario Gaston, MD
- Friedenberg, Barry, MD
- Friedenberg, Jeffrey Scott, MD
- Hughes, Ann M., MD
- Keklak, C. Stephen, MD
- Loeb, Debra M., MD
- Mezzacappa, Peter M., MD
- Patil, Vivek Vinay, MD
- Romano, Kenneth Robert, MD
- Spector, Janet, MD

Freeman Integrated Spine & Pain, P.C.
3499 Route 9 North/Suite 2B Zip: 07728
Ph: (973) 893-7246 Fax: (732) 970-4012
- Freeman, Darren Keith, DO
- Rider, Timothy Eugene, MD

Hackensack Meridian Ob/Gyn
3499 Route 9 North/Suite 2B Zip: 07728
Ph: (732) 577-1199 Fax: (732) 577-8922
- Barnett, Rebecca L., MD
- Baum, Jonathan D., MD
- Joshi, Jyotika D., MD
- Lucas, Romeo Augusto, DO
- Morreale, Ginja Massey, MD
- Rattigan, Meghan Iona, DO

Healthy Woman Ob/Gyn
312 Professional View Drive Zip: 07728
Ph: (732) 431-1616 Fax: (732) 866-7962
- Aland, Kristen, MD
- Burt-Libo, Borislava, DO
- Cipriano, Joseph A., MD
- Cipriano, Rebecca J., MD
- Leizer, Julie M., MD
- Misra, Neeti Virendra, MD
- Pacana, Susan Marie, MD
- Scheff, Elizabeth Anne, MD

Heart Specialists/Central Jersey
901 West Main Street/Suite 205 Zip: 07728
Ph: (732) 866-0800 Fax: (732) 463-6082
- Awasthi, Ashish, MD
- Beauregard, Louanne M., MD
- Gutowski, Ted, MD
- Kominos, Vivian A., MD
- Menon, Divya, MD
- Mentle, Iris R., MD
- Shukla, Ashish, MD
- Werber, John Frank, MD

Lakewood Surgical Group PA
901 West Main Street/Suite 107 Zip: 07728
Ph: (732) 363-0044 Fax: (732) 905-5845
- Schulman, William M., MD
- Silvers, Lawrence W., MD

Liberty Anesthesia & Pain Management
901 West Main Street/2nd Floor Zip: 07728
Ph: (732) 294-2876 Fax: (732) 294-2502
- Connors, Anne, MD
- Fahmy, Nader M., MD
- Grace, Rashy, MD
- Kumar, Nirmal A., MD
- Mikhail, Magdy H., MD
- Parikh, Pallavi M., MD
- Patel, Jayshree R., MD
- Proban, Rafal, MD
- Scarmato, Albert Clark Jr., DO
- Stump, James Basil, MD
- Zachary, Samuel, MD

Medical Specialists
1000 West Main Street Zip: 07728
Ph: (732) 431-1686
- Velez, Alberto A., MD
- Velez, Corazon S., MD

Mid-Atlantic Endocrinology & Diabetes
555 Iron Bridge Road/Suite 18 Zip: 07728
Ph: (732) 409-6233 Fax: (732) 409-6414
- Farghani, Saima Obaid, MD
- Young, Melissa G., MD

Middlesex Monmouth Gastro
222 Schanck Road/Suite 302 Zip: 07728
Ph: (732) 577-1999 Fax: (732) 845-5356
- Blank, Robert R., MD
- Brown, Colin Christopher, MD
- Geller, Arthur J., MD
- Gupta, Kunal, MD
- Nadler, Steven C., MD

Midstate Rheumatology Center
900 West Main Street Zip: 07728
Ph: (732) 431-4335 Fax: (732) 431-4771
- Ghafoor, Sadia, DO
- Najmey, Sawsan S., MD

Millennium Eye Care, LLC
500 West Main Street Zip: 07728
Ph: (732) 462-8707 Fax: (732) 462-1296
- Aksman, Scott S., MD
- Brenner, Edward H., MD
- Brottman, Jeffrey S., MD
- Grand, Elliot S., MD
- Kernitsky, Roman G., MD
- Lee, David K., MD
- Mishkin, Steven K., MD
- Ng, Elena M., MD
- Rosin, Jay Michael, MD
- Schneider, Martin S., MD

Monmouth Cardiology Associates
222 Schanck Road/Suite 104 Zip: 07728
Ph: (732) 431-1332 Fax: (732) 431-1712
- Litsky, Jason D., DO
- Liu, Marcia Nai-Hwa, MD
- Noto, Gregory, MD
- Zukerman, Louis Steven, MD

Monmouth Family Medicine Group
3499 Route 9 North Zip: 07728
Ph: (732) 625-3166 Fax: (732) 409-7493
- Rowlands, Randy R., MD
- Sasidhar, Vaidehi, MD

Monmouth Ocean Pulmonary Med
901 West Main Street/Suite 160 Zip: 07728
Ph: (732) 577-0600 Fax: (732) 577-6332
- Barofsky, Kenneth D., MD
- Coppolino, Frank P., MD
- Croce, Salvatore A., MD
- DeTullio, John P., MD
- Pi, Justin Jeong-Suk, MD
- Shah, Nirav Navin, DO

Monmouth-Middlesex Hematology/Oncology
326 Professional View Drive Zip: 07728
Ph: (732) 431-8400 Fax: (732) 431-0114
- Gopal, Krishnan T., MD
- Silberberg, Jeffrey M., MD

NJ Ambulatory Anesthesia Consultants
55 Schanck Road/Suite 8-A Zip: 07728
Ph: (732) 431-9544 Fax: (732) 431-9313
- Armbrecht, Kimberley T., MD
- Cubina, Maria L., MD
- Mak, John, MD
- Mehta, Hemangini G., MD
- O'Hara, Michael W., DO
- Randall, Tanya, MD

Pediatric Health, P.A.
470 Stillwells Corner Road Zip: 07728
Ph: (732) 780-3333 Fax: (732) 780-6968
- Emanuel, Anthony, MD

Pediatric Health, P.A.
69 West Main Street Zip: 07728
Ph: (732) 409-3633 Fax: (732) 409-7133
- Lopez, Leonardo Nicholas, DO
- Mayer, Diana R., MD
- McFeely, Erin M., MD
- Swayne, Kathleen Amy, MD
- Teresh, Michelle A., MD
- Zeb, Marta R., MD

Seaview Orthopaedics
222 Schanck Road/3rd Floor Zip: 07728
Ph: (732) 462-1700 Fax: (732) 303-8314
- Mark, Arthur K., MD

- Mittman, Roy D., MD
- Vasen, Arthur Philip, MD

Shore Heart Group, P.A.
555 Iron Bridge Road/Suite 15 Zip: 07728
Ph: (732) 308-0774 Fax: (732) 333-1366
- Hanfling, Marcus, DO

Spine & Pain Centers
303 West Main Street/Lower Level Zip: 07728
Ph: (732) 345-1180 Fax: (732) 530-4476
- Sharma, Anil K., MD

Urology Care Alliance
501 Iron Bridge Road Zip: 07728
Ph: (732) 780-7603 Fax: (732) 308-3323
- Kohlberg, William I., MD

Women's Physicians & Surgeons
501 Iron Bridge Road/Suite 10 Zip: 07728
Ph: (732) 431-2999 Fax: (732) 431-2993
- Dimino, Michael L., MD
- Kirwin, Michael S., MD
- Mandel, Peter C., MD
- Neuwirth, Safir, MD
- Portadin, Robert A., MD

Galloway

Absecon Medical Associates LLC
408 Chris Gaupp Drive/Suite 100 Zip: 08205
Ph: (609) 748-5015 Fax: (609) 748-0303
- Ganzon-Zampino, Gilda E., MD
- Kim, Duk Hee, MD
- Kirchner, Brian K., MD

AtlantiCare Physicians
318 Chris Gaupp Drive/Suite 100 Zip: 08205
Ph: (609) 404-9900 Fax: (609) 404-3653
- Carreno, Wilfredo, MD
- Ghayal, Mahesh, MD
- Jayasinghe, Swarnathilaka, MD
- Kanzaria, Mitul, MD
- Merchant, Yatish B., MD
- Nascimento, Tome R., MD
- Vankawala, Viren Rameshchandra, MD

Atlantic Cardiology in Galloway
436 Chris Gaupp Drive/Suite 204 Zip: 08205
Ph: (609) 652-0100 Fax: (609) 652-7616
- Flynn, Anthony M., MD
- Patel, Vineshkumar K., MD
- Van Hook, Jeffrey E., DO

Atlantic Heart Rhythm Center
415 Chris Gaupp Drive/Suite C Zip: 08205
Ph: (609) 748-7580 Fax: (609) 748-7574
- Ghaly, Nader Naguib, MD
- Kaur, Amrita, MD
- White, Melvin C., MD

Atlantic Internal Medicine PA
310 Chris Gaupp Drive/Suite 102 Zip: 08205
Ph: (609) 652-9933
- Brown, Lemarra Rena, DO
- Delaverdac, Claude L., DO
- Lieberman, Alexander III, MD
- Zampino, Dominick J., DO

Atlantic Pulmonary & Critical Care
741 South Second Avenue/Suite A Zip: 08205
Ph: (609) 748-7300 Fax: (609) 748-7919
- Bansal, Aditya Rakesh, MD
- Costantini, Peter J., DO
- Higgins, Nancy C., MD
- Loftus, Frances Ellen, DO
- Sadik, Nadia, MD
- Sivaraman, Sivashankar, MD

Cancer and Blood Disorders Care
54 West Jimmie Leeds Road Zip: 08205
Ph: (609) 404-9966 Fax: (609) 404-9967
- Borai, Nasser Eldien, MD

Drs. Dunn & Smith
4 East Jimmie Leeds Road/Suites 1-2 Zip: 08205
Ph: (609) 652-6100
- Dunn, Eric Scott, MD

Groups and Clinics by Town with Physician Rosters

Drs. Sperling & Sperling
162 South New York Road/Suite B-3 Zip: 08205
Ph: (609) 748-8200 Fax: (609) 748-9200
Coville,Frederick A., MD
Sperling,Howard J., MD
Sperling,Michael James, MD

Horizon Eye Care
76 West Jimmie Leeds Road Zip: 08205
Ph: (609) 652-0300 Fax: (609) 652-0730
Spielberg,Joel A., MD

Ladies' Choice Ob-Gyn
314 Chris Gaupp Drive/Suite 101 Zip: 08205
Ph: (609) 404-1400 Fax: (609) 404-1430
Assad,Eveline N., MD
Bredin,Sherilyn A., MD
Perkins,Phyllis M., MD
Petit,Anne I., MD

Mainland Pediatric Association
741 South Second Avenue/Suite B Zip: 08205
Ph: (609) 748-8500 Fax: (609) 748-6700
Amir,Sabah H., MD
Elgenaidi,Mona E., MD
Houck,Meghan Mcfee, DO
Kosmetatos,Elizabeth, MD

Premier Oncology, LLC.
54 West Jimmie Leeds Road/Suite 11 Zip: 08205
Ph: (609) 748-1001 Fax: (609) 748-1002
Ajay,Rajasree, MD

Reliance Medical Group, LLC
331 East Jimmie Leeds Road/Suite 1 & 2 Zip: 08205
Ph: (609) 652-6016 Fax: (609) 652-2406
Stanley,Linda, MD
Wesley,Louis A., MD

Salartash Surgical Associates
72 West Jimmie Leeds Road/Suite 1600 Zip: 08205
Ph: (609) 926-5000 Fax: (609) 926-2020
Patel,Samir M., MD

Smithville Medical Associates
48 South New York Road/Suite B-3 Zip: 08205
Ph: (609) 404-0121 Fax: (609) 404-0131
Ramchand,Maya, MD
Selina,Elena V., MD
Thadhani,Ramchand, MD

Garfield

Consultants in Asthma, Alergy, & Imm
22 Shaw Street Zip: 07026
Ph: (973) 478-5550
Benincasa,Peter J., MD
Luka,Richard Edward, MD

Pediatric Health Center
54 Plauderville Avenue/Suite 1 Zip: 07026
Ph: (973) 772-0262
Tunia,Krzysztof Stanislaw, MD
Uczkowska,Alicja Teresa, MD

Garwood

Union County Healthcare Associates
300 South Avenue Zip: 07027
Ph: (908) 232-2273 Fax: (908) 232-1439
Caracitas,Alexandra Cristina, DO
Gupta,Amit, MD

Gibbsboro

Advocare ENT Specialty Center
88 South Lakeview Drive/Building 1 Zip: 08026
Ph: (856) 435-9100 Fax: (856) 435-9112
Aftab,Saba, MD
Wong,Gabriel Ho Yu, MD

Dr. G. Lee Lerch and Associates
63 North Lakeview Drive/Suite 202 Zip: 08026
Ph: (856) 435-6000 Fax: (856) 782-1667
Amato,Christopher, MD
Deery,Kimberly Jeanne, DO
Lee,Diana, DO
Lerch,Gordon Lee Jr., DO

Greentree Family Medical Associates
55 Lakeview Drive North/Suite A Zip: 08026
Ph: (856) 985-5655 Fax: (856) 985-1895
Sheldon,Howard A., DO
Sheldon,Lynne T., DO

PennCare South Jersey Family Medicine
55 Haddonfield-Berlin Road/Route 561 Zip: 08026
Ph: (856) 783-1777
Villamayor,Rosemarie Cruz, MD

Primary Care at Gibbsboro
13 South Lakeview Drive Zip: 08026
Ph: (856) 783-2802 Fax: (856) 783-2806
Napoli,Anthony F. Jr., MD
Tyler,Grace Tung, MD

Ctr for Neurological/Neurodevelopment
250 Haddonfield-Berlin Road/Suite 105 Zip: 08026
Ph: (856) 346-0005 Fax: (856) 784-1799
Chadehumbe,Madeline A., MD
Mintz,Mark I., MD

Glassboro

General Practitioners, P.A.
601 North Main Street Zip: 08028
Ph: (856) 881-1330 Fax: (856) 881-6982
Meskin,Steven J., MD
Schultes,Arthur H., DO

Inspira Medical Group
200 Rowan Boulevard Zip: 08028
Ph: (856) 582-0500 Fax: (856) 582-0163
Sayed,Durr-E-shahwaar, DO
Szgalsky,Joseph Brian, MD

Underwood-Family Health Center
1120 North Delsea Drive Zip: 08028
Ph: (856) 582-0500 Fax: (856) 582-0163
Nguyen,Bac Xuan, MD
Palmer,Josette C., MD

Glen Ridge

Ballem Surgical
230 Sherman Avenue/Suite C Zip: 07028
Ph: (973) 744-8585 Fax: (973) 748-5990
Ballem,Naveen, MD
Ballem,Ramamohana V., MD
Gohil,Kartik Narendra, MD
Matier,Brian, MD
Rainville,Harvey Charles, MD

Bart De Gregorio MD, LLC.
946 Bloomfield Avenue Zip: 07028
Ph: (973) 743-1121 Fax: (973) 743-2627
Alfonso,Carlos Roel Villegas, MD
Cheema,Asad Mushtaq, MD
De Gregorio,Bart, MD
De Gregorio,Joseph Anthony, MD
Di Giorgio,Christopher B., MD
Mariano,Domenic L., DO
Urrutia,Ellen E., MD
Voudouris,Apostolos Athanasios, MD

Gastroenterology Group of NJ, PA
123 Highland Avenue/Suite 103 Zip: 07028
Ph: (973) 429-8800 Fax: (973) 748-7076
Finkelstein,Warren, MD
Kenny,Raymond P., MD
Kwon,Yong Min, MD

Glen Ridge Surgicenter
230 Sherman Avenue Zip: 07028
Ph: (973) 783-2626 Fax: (973) 680-4211
Parikh,Sanjiv R., MD
Rombough,Gary R., MD
Sloan,Kim W., MD
Vonroth,William Jr., MD

Monmouth Surgical Specialists
123 Highland Avenue/Suite 202 Zip: 07028
Ph: (973) 429-7600 Fax: (973) 429-7602
Barbalinardo,Robert J., MD
Holwitt,Kenneth N., MD

Montclair Cardiology Group PA
123 Highland Avenue/Suite 302 Zip: 07028
Ph: (973) 748-9555 Fax: (973) 748-2003
Knezevic,Dusan Svetozar, MD
Saroff,Alan L., MD
Wanat,Francis E., MD

Montclair Endocrine Associates
123 Highland Avenue/Suite 301 Zip: 07028
Ph: (973) 744-3733 Fax: (973) 707-5821
Davis,Maris R., MD
Grover,Anjali, MD
Kidangan,Julie Thomas, DO
Shafqat,Uzma Zohra, MD
Sherry,Stephen H., MD

Montclair Family Practice
230 Sherman Avenue/Suite A Zip: 07028
Ph: (973) 743-2321 Fax: (973) 259-0600
Berlin,Melissa Gail, MD
Flores,Jose C., DO

Montclair Orthopedic Group PA
200 Highland Avenue Zip: 07028
Ph: (973) 746-2200 Fax: (973) 429-2174
Chase,Mark D., MD

Mountainside Medical Group
123 Highland Avenue/Suite 201 Zip: 07028
Ph: (973) 748-9246 Fax: (973) 748-8755
Bambhroliya,Grishma, MD
Levai,Robert Joseph, MD
Molinaro,Michael Louis, MD
Woroch,Paul, MD

Neurological Consultants
230 Sherman Avenue/Suite K Zip: 07028
Ph: (973) 743-9555 Fax: (973) 743-7663
Blady,David, MD
Vaccaro,John J., MD

Respiratory Disease Associates PA
200 Highland Avenue/Suite 100 Zip: 07028
Ph: (973) 746-7474 Fax: (973) 743-0265
Daniskas,Efthymios I., MD
Weber,Barry Joseph, MD

Glen Rock

Advanced Psychiatric Associates
65 Harristown Road/Suite 101 Zip: 07452
Ph: (201) 487-1240
Yero,Sergio Alberto, MD

Dermatology Associates
348 South Maple Avenue Zip: 07452
Ph: (201) 652-6060 Fax: (201) 652-1882
Dosik,Jonathan Scott, MD
Galvin,Sharon A., MD

North Jersey Colon & Rectal Surgery
85 Harristown Road Zip: 07452
Ph: (201) 689-9100 Fax: (201) 689-9108
Agopian,Raffi E., MD
Kwon,Albert O., MD

Oasis Medical and Wellness
85 Harristown Road/Suite 103 Zip: 07452
OnlyFax: (844) 366-8900
Johnson,Keith Patrick, MD
Massoud,Bryan J., MD
Patel,Sujal P., MD

Sovereign Medical Group
85 Harristown Road/Suite 104 Zip: 07452
Ph: (201) 855-8300 Fax: (201) 857-2541
Nanavati,Farzana Nilesh, MD
Tilson,Morris A., MD

Sovereign Northern Jersey ENT
85 Harristown Road/Suite 105 Zip: 07452
Ph: (201) 455-2900 Fax: (201) 703-0390
Bellapianta,Karen Marie, MD
Katz,Harry, MD

Green Brook

Family Care, P.A.
257 US Highway 22 Zip: 08812
Ph: (732) 968-7878 Fax: (732) 968-2187
Chafos,John N., MD
Klele,Michael A, MD

MEDEMERGE
1005 North Washington Avenue Zip: 08812
Ph: (732) 968-8900 Fax: (732) 968-4609
Ahmed,Syed F., MD
Carrieri,David A., DO
Hammoud,Marwan Fahim, MD
Pilla,John D., MD
Popeck,Paul J., DO
Quezada Reyes,Carlos A., MD
Sgambelluri,Carol E., MD

Sharon,Yoram, DO
Strauss,Scott R., DO
Strumkovsky,Lyalya Olga, MD

Guttenberg

Hudson Heart Associates
425 70th Street Zip: 07093
Ph: (201) 854-0055 Fax: (201) 854-2633
Katdare,Umesh Vasudeo, MD
Santana,Jose O., MD

Vascular Epicenter
7000 Boulevard East Zip: 07093
Ph: (201) 861-9900 Fax: (201) 861-9977
Asaad,Imad, MD
Epstein,Steven Brian, MD

Hackensack

Active Center for Health & Wellness
25 Prospect Avenue Zip: 07601
Ph: (201) 487-4600 Fax: (201) 343-7410
Corrigan,Lynn Ann, DO

Active Orthopaedics & Sports Medicine
25 Prospect Avenue Zip: 07601
Ph: (201) 343-2277 Fax: (201) 343-7410
Giuffrida,Angela Ylenia, MD
John,Thomas Karoor, MD

Advanced Cardiovascular Interventions
20 Prospect Avenue/Suite 615 Zip: 07601
Ph: (201) 265-5700 Fax: (551) 996-0774
Abdelhadi,Samir I., DO
Nia,Hamid Mohammad, MD

Advanced Pediatrics
5 Summit Avenue/Suite 203 Zip: 07601
Ph: (201) 343-4800 Fax: (201) 343-4668
Rivera,Roger Antonio, MD

Advanced Psychiatric Associates
211 Essex Street/Suite 204 Zip: 07601
Ph: (201) 487-1240 Fax: (201) 487-1241
Zhivago,Eileen Ann, MD

Audrey Hepburn Children's House
12 Second Street Zip: 07601
Ph: (201) 996-2271 Fax: (201) 996-4926
DeBellis,Julia Angelina, MD
Diah,Paulett, MD

BSD Nephrology & Hypertension
360 Essex Street/Suite 304 Zip: 07601
Ph: (201) 646-0110 Fax: (201) 646-0219
Joseph,Rosy E., MD
Muttana,Renu Devi, MD
Saro-Nunez,Lilian, MD
Suldan,Zalman Lewis, MD

Bergen Ear Nose & Throat Assoc
20 Prospect Avenue/Suite 909 Zip: 07601
Ph: (201) 489-6520 Fax: (201) 489-6530
Inouye,Masayuki, MD
Low,Ronald Brian, MD
Tomovic,Senja, MD

Bergen Invasive Cardio Cons
211 Essex Street/Suite 306 Zip: 07601
Ph: (201) 343-2050 Fax: (201) 343-4512
Sethi,Ruchi S., MD
Sethi,Virender, MD
Timmapuri,Sarah L., MD
Vaidya,Pranaychan J., MD

Bergen Surgical Specialists
20 Prospect Avenue/Suite 707 Zip: 07601
Ph: (201) 343-0040 Fax: (201) 343-2733
Keys,Roger C., MD
Napolitano,Massimo M., MD
Simonian,Carla Daria, MD
Simonian,Gregory T., MD
Wilderman,Michael Jeffrey, MD

Bergen Surgical Specialists
211 Essex Street/Suite 102 Zip: 07601
Ph: (201) 487-8882 Fax: (201) 487-0943
O'Connor,David John, MD
Ratnathicam,Anjali, DO

Cardiac Medical Associates PA
920 Main Street Zip: 07601
Ph: (201) 342-7733 Fax: (201) 342-7998
Denson,H. Mark, MD
Kanarek,Steven Edward, MD
Simpson,Timothy E., MD

Groups and Clinics by Town with Physician Rosters

Hackensack (cont)

Cardiologist & Intrnest Associates
211 Essex Street/Suite 104 Zip: 07601
Ph: (201) 489-3888 Fax: (201) 301-7351
 Patel,Jayantkumar N., MD
 Patel,Rajiv J., DO

Center For Occupational Medicine
360 Essex Street/Suite 203 Zip: 07601
Ph: (201) 336-8686 Fax: (201) 342-3546
 Gatchalian,Luningning C., MD
 Ourvan,Dorothy R., DO

Center for Healthy Senior Living
360 Essex Street/Suite 401 Zip: 07601
Ph: (551) 996-1140 Fax: (551) 996-0543
 Gupta,Kavita, MD
 Michelis,Mary Ann, MD
 Riccobono,Charles A., MD
 Tank,Lisa Kaushal, MD

Center for Infectious Diseases
20 Prospect Avenue/Suite 507 Zip: 07601
Ph: (201) 487-4088 Fax: (201) 489-8930
 Balani,Bindu Anand, MD
 Cicogna,Cristina Emanuela, MD
 Desai,Samit Sharad, MD
 Levine,Jerome Frederic, MD
 Sebti,Rani, MD
 Sperber,Steven J., MD

Center for Pain Management
294 State Street/Suite 1 Zip: 07601
Ph: (201) 488-7246 Fax: (201) 488-2788
 Datta,Samyadev, MD
 Shupper,Peter Joseph, MD

Children of Joy Pediatrics
134 Summit Avenue Zip: 07601
Ph: (201) 525-0077 Fax: (201) 525-0072
 Hijazi,Rana, MD
 Kimel,Ana Josephine, MD
 Lopez,Divina Elizabeth, MD
 Macalintal,Rose Ann Reyes, MD
 Miranda,Rosa Josefina, MD

Drs. Anchipolovsky and Garger
77 Prospect Avenue/Suite 1 K Zip: 07601
Ph: (201) 820-3596 Fax: (201) 322-2170
 Anchipolovsky,Natalia, DO
 Garger,Yana Basis, MD

Drs. Fagelman, Degen & Fagelman
360 Essex Street/Suite 403 Zip: 07601
Ph: (551) 996-8090 Fax: (551) 996-8221
 Degen,Michael Conrad, MD
 Fagelman,Elliot, MD
 Fagelman,Mark, MD

Drs. Flores and Flores
819 Main Street Zip: 07601
Ph: (201) 489-3678 Fax: (201) 489-7618
 Flores,Alejandro Alberto, MD
 Flores,Ramon L., MD

Drs. Karpeh & Davidson
20 Prospect Avenue/Suite 406 Zip: 07601
Ph: (551) 996-2959 Fax: (551) 996-2021
 Davidson,Marson Tunde, MD
 Karpeh,Martin Sieh Jr., MD

Drs. Shaker and Shaker
38 Summit Avenue/Suite 1 Zip: 07601
Ph: (201) 343-6360 Fax: (201) 343-6367
 Shaker,David, DO
 Shaker,Mina, MD
 Shaker,Safwat I., MD

Drs. The & Sinatra
348 Summit Avenue Zip: 07601
Ph: (201) 343-9300
 Sinatra,Melanie A., MD
 The,Arlene H., MD

Drs. Wong and Ilonzo
20 Prospect Avenue Zip: 07601
Ph: (551) 996-2000
 Ilonzo,Chiamaka, MD
 Wong,Sarah, MD

ENT & Allergy Associates, LLP
433 Hackensack Avenue/Suite 204 Zip: 07601
Ph: (201) 883-1062 Fax: (201) 883-9297
 Brody,Robin Michelle, MD
 Eisenberg,Lee D., MD
 Geller,Debora Klein, MD
 Gold,Steven M., MD
 Lesserson,Jonathan A., MD
 Mithani,Sima, MD
 Wasserman,Jared Mark, MD

Ear Nose Throat Institute of NJ
2 South Summit Avenue Zip: 07601
Ph: (201) 996-9200 Fax: (201) 996-9277
 Respler,Don S., MD
 Rosen,Arie, MD

Electrophysiology Associates
20 Prospect Avenue/Suite 701 Zip: 07601
Ph: (201) 996-2997 Fax: (201) 996-2571
 Glotzer,Taya Valerie, MD
 Jamal,Sameer Mustafa, MD
 Radoslovich,Glauco A., MD
 Shukla,Gunjan Jayendrabhai, MD
 Zimmerman,John M., MD

Excelsior Women's Care
170 Prospect Avenue/Suite 4 Zip: 07601
Ph: (201) 488-2288 Fax: (201) 488-2298
 Cavallaro,Barbara Ann, MD
 Govindani,Niketa Vinod, MD
 Miller,Lisa Ann B., MD
 Petras,Peri Ann, MD

Hackensack Digestive Diseases
52 First Street Zip: 07601
Ph: (201) 488-3003 Fax: (201) 488-6911
 Ellinghaus,Eric J., MD
 Feit,David L., MD
 Felig,David M., MD
 Golding,Richard C., MD
 Ligresti,Rosario Joseph, MD
 Tanchel,Mark E., MD

Hackensack Heart Failure Program
20 Prospect Avenue Zip: 07601
Ph: (201) 996-4849 Fax: (201) 996-5703
 Kapoor,Saurabh, MD
 Satya,Kumar, MD

Hackensack Neurology Group
211 Essex Street/Suite 202 Zip: 07601
Ph: (201) 488-1515 Fax: (201) 488-9471
 Dash,Subasini, MD
 Fellman,Damon M., MD
 Gupta,Dev R., MD
 Marquinez,Anthony I., MD
 Nogueira,John Francis Jr., MD
 Silverstein,Michael P., MD
 Solanky,Mukesh, MD
 Vukic,Mario, MD

Hackensack Pediatrics
177 Summit Avenue Zip: 07601
Ph: (201) 487-8222 Fax: (201) 487-2126
 Azizi,Azin, MD
 Muratschew,Donna M., MD
 Reed,Jean Arlyn Banez, MD
 Tantawi,Mohamed Asem, MD
 Tantawi,Mona M., MD

Hackensack Sleep & Pulmonary Center
170 Prospect Avenue/Suite 20 Zip: 07601
Ph: (201) 996-0232 Fax: (201) 996-0095
 Ashtyani Asl,Fariborz, MD
 Goss,Deborah Anne Marie, MD
 Lee,Robert Chu-Du, MD

Hackensack Surgical Critical Care Phys
5 Summit Avenue/Suite 105 Zip: 07601
Ph: (201) 996-2900 Fax: (201) 883-1268
 Perez,Javier Martin, MD

Hackensack UMG
150 Overlook Avenue Zip: 07601
Ph: (201) 489-5999 Fax: (201) 489-1898
 Collins,Melinda Jean, DO
 Weinstock,Murray, MD

HUMC Faculty Practice
360 Essex Street/Suite 403 Zip: 07601
Ph: (201) 336-8090 Fax: (201) 336-8221
 Basralian,Kevin R., MD
 Fromer,Debra Lynn, MD
 Glickman,Leonard, MD
 Kim,Michelle Joosun, MD
 Kirkpatrick-Reese,Gina Brazylle, D
 Koo,Harry P., MD
 Sawczuk,Ihor Steven, MD
 Shin,David, MD

Hackensack University Medical
25 East Salem Street Zip: 07601
Ph: (201) 996-4445 Fax: (201) 996-5729
 Khalil,Chaza H., MD
 Lewis,Tanya Renee, MD
 Miah,Khorshed Alam, MD

Haclensack Bergen Pediatrics
385 Prospect Avenue/Suite 210 Zip: 07601
Ph: (551) 996-9160 Fax: (551) 996-9165
 Fruchter,Joseph S., MD
 Meli,Lisa A., MD
 Rappaport,Delia I., MD
 Terrin,Bruce N., MD
 Weissman,Barry J., MD

Holy Name Medical Partners Office
15 Anderson Street Zip: 07601
Ph: (201) 487-3355 Fax: (201) 487-0960
 Chavez,Laura Monica, DO
 Germinario,Carla Ann, MD
 Surapaneni,Padmaja, MD

Institute For Breast Care
20 Prospect Avenue/Suite 513 Zip: 07601
Ph: (201) 996-2222
 Greene,Tobi B., MD
 Harawi,Sami J., MD
 Hassoun,Patrice, MD
 Lengner,Marlene, MD

Integrative Obstetrics
358 Beech Street Zip: 07601
Ph: (201) 487-8600 Fax: (201) 487-8601
 Abdelhak,Yaakov Eliezer, MD

John Theurer Cancer Center - HUMC
92 Second Street Zip: 07601
Ph: (201) 996-5900 Fax: (201) 996-9246
 Alter,Robert S., MD
 Biran,Noa, MD
 Donato,Michele Lyne, MD
 Faderl,Stefan H., MD
 Feldman,Tatyana A., MD
 Gejerman,Glen, MD
 Godfrey,Loren, MD
 Goldberg,Stuart Lee, MD
 Goldlust,Samuel Aaron, MD
 Goy,Andre Henri, MD
 Graham,Deena Mary-Atieh, MD
 Gutierrez,Martin Eduardo, MD
 Harper,Harry D., MD
 Ingenito,Anthony C., MD
 Jennis,Andrew A., MD

John Theurer Cancer Center - HUMC
20 Prospect Avenue/Suite 703 Zip: 07601
Ph: (201) 996-5900
 Kraft,Jeffrey Joseph, MD
 Leslie,Lori Ann, MD
 Lewis,Brett Eric, MD
 McNamara,Donna M., MD
 Pascal,Mark S., MD
 Pecora,Andrew L., MD
 Proverbs-Singh,Tracy Ann, MD
 Rosenbluth,Richard J., MD

John Theurer Cancer Center - HUMC
360 Essex Street/Suite 303 Zip: 07601
Ph: (201) 336-8297 Fax: (201) 336-8296
 Rowley,Scott D., MD
 Siegel,David Samuel Dicapua, MD
 Singer,Samuel, MD
 Smith,Daniel Humphreys, MD
 Vaidya,Ami P., MD
 Vesole,David H., MD
 Waintraub,Stanley Eli, MD

Joseph M. Sanzari Childrens' -Gastro
155 Polifly Road/Suite 102 Zip: 07601
Ph: (551) 996-8840 Fax: (201) 441-9949
 D'Mello,Sharon L., MD
 Francolla,Karen Ann, MD
 Jeshion,Wendy Cheryl, MD
 Leyva-Vega,Melissa, MD
 Moustafellos,Elaine, MD
 Samuels,Francine, MD
 Shammout,Jumana Sa'ad, MD
 Wong,Tracie Mei Han, MD

Medical Care Institute, P.A.
159 Summit Avenue Zip: 07601
Ph: (201) 343-7272 Fax: (201) 343-0228
 Lin,Judy Mei-Chia, MD
 Sedarat,Ali, MD
 Sedarat,Alireza, MD

Mehling Orthopedics, LLC
214 State Street/Suite 101 Zip: 07601
Ph: (201) 342-7662 Fax: (201) 342-7663
 Yufit,Pavel Vladimirovich, MD

Mulkay Cardiology Consultants, P.C.
493 Essex Street Zip: 07601
Ph: (201) 996-9244 Fax: (201) 996-9243
 Cohen,Michael B., MD
 Mulkay,Angel J., MD
 Ruffo,Scott D., MD

Multiple Sclerosis Center
300 Essex Street/Suite 203 Zip: 07601
Ph: (551) 996-8100 Fax: (551) 996-4140
 Krel,Regina, MD
 Pandey,Krupa Shah, MD

Neurology Consultants of North Jersey
92 Summit Avenue/2nd Floor Zip: 07601
Ph: (201) 630-0012 Fax: (201) 630-0014
 Ibrahim,Ayman M., DO
 Ibrahim,Ehab Fawzy, MD
 Kim,Anthony Junghoi, MD

New Jersey Neurological Specialists
20 Prospect Avenue/Suite 800 Zip: 07601
Ph: (201) 518-7290 Fax: (201) 604-6428
 Kreibich,Thomas Alfred, MD
 Liff,Jeremy M., MD
 Oller-Cramsie,Marissa Anne, DO

New Jersey Urology, LLC
20 Prospect Avenue/Suite 915 Zip: 07601
Ph: (201) 343-0082 Fax: (201) 488-1203
 Lowe,Daniel Robert, MD
 Rosenberg,Gene S., MD

North Jersey Electrophysiology Assoc
20 Prospect Avenue/Suite 615 Zip: 07601
Ph: (201) 472-3627 Fax: (201) 518-8739
 Simons,Grant Russell, MD

North Jersey Surgical Specialists
83 Summit Avenue Zip: 07601
Ph: (201) 646-0010 Fax: (201) 646-0600
 Benson,Douglas N., MD
 Kagan,Peter Evan, MD
 Manno,Joseph, MD
 Patel,Sruti, MD
 Poole,John W., MD

Northeast Regional Epilepsy Group
20 Prospect Avenue/Suite 800 Zip: 07601
Ph: (201) 343-6676 Fax: (201) 343-6689
 Bortnik,Kristy E., MD
 Douyon,Philippe Gerard, MD
 Ebersole,John S., MD
 Feoli,Enrique Alfredo, MD
 Inoyama,Katherine S., MD
 Lazar,Lorraine M., MD
 Mesad,Salah Mohammed, MD
 Paolicchi,Juliann Marie, MD
 Puntambekar,Preeti Vasant, MD
 Rao,Gautami Kondamodi, MD
 Segal,Eric B., MD
 Trobliger,Robert William, MD
 Tsao,Julie Ching Yen, MD

Northn NJ Pulmonary Assocs
211 Essex Street/Suite 302 Zip: 07601
Ph: (201) 498-1311 Fax: (201) 498-1312
 Polkow,Melvin S., MD

Obstetrics and Gynecology PA
20 Prospect Avenue/Suite 607 Zip: 07601
Ph: (201) 487-3464 Fax: (201) 487-0232
 Gerardis,Judi R., MD
 Kopp,Lizabeth A., MD

Groups and Clinics by Town with Physician Rosters

Orthopedic Specialists NJ-Hackensack
87 Summit Avenue Zip: 07601
Ph: (201) 489-0022 Fax: (201) 489-6991
  Cahill, James W., MD
  Hammerschlag, Warren A., MD
  Porter, David Alexander, MD

Pediatric Specialties PA
90 Prospect Avenue/Suite 1-A Zip: 07601
Ph: (201) 342-4001 Fax: (201) 342-9569
  Bhambri, Malanie Mathur, DO
  Harlow, Paul J., MD
  Materetsky, Steven H., MD
  Wong, Jonathan Wane, MD

Ravits Margaret MD & Associates
721 Summit Avenue Zip: 07601
Ph: (201) 487-3691 Fax: (201) 487-4180
  Ravits, Margaret S., MD

Renal Medicine Associates PA
302 Union Street Zip: 07601
Ph: (201) 646-0414 Fax: (201) 646-0365
  Adamidis, Ananea, MD
  Vitievsky, Alexander Michael, MD

Riverside Medical Group
10 First Street Zip: 07601
Ph: (201) 968-5345 Fax: (201) 968-5349
  August, Elizabeth, MD

Skin Laser & Surgery Specialists
20 Prospect Avenue/Suite 702 Zip: 07601
Ph: (201) 441-9890 Fax: (201) 441-9893
  Eilers, Steven Edwin, MD
  Goldbry, David Jay, MD
  Lolis, Margarita Sophia, MD

Summit Avenue Medical
5 Summit Avenue Zip: 07601
Ph: (201) 646-0001 Fax: (201) 646-9101
  Cheeti, Kalpana, MD
  Goldfarb, Adam S., MD
  Prins, Edward R., MD

Summit ObGyn LLC
331 Summit Avenue Zip: 07601
Ph: (201) 457-2300 Fax: (201) 457-1715
  Kamal, Roohi, MD
  Vinod, Arundhati Hrishikesh, MD

Summit Surgical Institute
332 Summit Avenue Zip: 07601
Ph: (201) 488-6445 Fax: (201) 488-6441
  Kline, Gary Michael, MD
  Kline, Roxana Gabriela, MD

Surgical Associates
90 Prospect Avenue/Room 1D Zip: 07601
Ph: (201) 343-3433 Fax: (201) 343-0420
  Khosravi, Abtin Hajiloo, MD
  Pereira, Stephen G., MD
  Rosenstock, Adam Seth, MD
  Smith, Adam Powell, MD

The Center for Advanced Neurosurgery
20 Prospect Avenue/Suite 811 Zip: 07601
Ph: (201) 781-5964 Fax: (201) 881-0700
  Helbraun, Mark E., MD
  Schwartz, Lauren Faith, MD

The Pediatric Center for Heart Disease
155 Polifly Road/Suite 106 Zip: 07601
Ph: (201) 487-7617 Fax: (201) 342-5341
  Dyme, Joshua L., MD
  Kipel, George, MD
  Rama, Gabriel, MD
  Subramanian, Subhashini, MD
  Wong, Austin Henry, MD

University Orthopaedic Center, PA
433 Hackensack Avenue/Second Floor Zip: 07601
Ph: (201) 343-1717 Fax: (201) 343-3217
  Longobardi, Raphael S., MD

University Respiratory Medicine, P.A.
75 Summit Avenue Zip: 07601
Ph: (201) 487-4595
  Koniaris, Lauren Solanko, MD
  Sadikot, Sean Shabbir, MD
  Ting, Leon L., MD

Hackettstown

Advanced Cardiology, LLC.
117 Seber Road/Suite 1-B Zip: 07840
Ph: (908) 979-1302 Fax: (908) 979-1493
  Ong, Edgardo A., MD

Hackettstown Medical Group
Hastings Sq Plaza/Building 5 Zip: 07840
Ph: (908) 979-0050 Fax: (908) 979-0044
  Ingrassia-Squiers, Keri Lynn, DO

Infectious Disease Center of NJ
653 Willow Grove Street/Suite 2700 Zip: 07840
Ph: (973) 535-8355 Fax: (973) 535-8353
  Hajela, Amitabh, MD

Medical Care Associates
137 Mountain Avenue Zip: 07840
Ph: (908) 852-1887 Fax: (908) 852-0614
  Azhar, Sana H., MD
  Duryee, John Jourdan, MD
  Khanna, Anirudh, MD
  Sandhu, Parminderjeet S., MD
  Sandhu, Vineet, MD

North Warren Medical Associates PC
Route 517/Building B Zip: 07840
Ph: (908) 852-0107 Fax: (908) 850-9160
  Freyman, Boris, DO
  Jain, Sanjay K., MD
  Paterno, Jeanette D., MD

Obstetrics and Gynecology Associates
616 Willow Grove Street Zip: 07840
Ph: (908) 852-3443 Fax: (908) 852-0349
  Anscher, Richard M., MD
  Canova, Amanda Derrick, MD

Plaza Family Care
657 Willow Grove Street/Suite 401 Zip: 07840
Ph: (908) 850-7800 Fax: (908) 850-7801
  Caruso, Patrick A., MD
  Chang, Jimmy Chuming, MD
  Dick, Adam M., MD
  Libert, Melissa Marie, DO
  Theune, Lillian J., DO
  Walsh, Kristen Anne, MD

Skylands Orthopaedics PC
57 US Highway 46/Suite 107 Zip: 07840
Ph: (908) 813-9700 Fax: (908) 813-2861
  Deehan, Michael A., MD
  Murphy, John W., MD
  Wainen, Glen P., MD

The Orthopedic Institute of New Jersey
108 Bilby Road/Suite 201 Zip: 07840
Ph: (908) 684-3005 Fax: (908) 684-3301
  Castro, Christopher Paul, DO
  Corrigan, Frank John, MD
  De Falco, Robert Anthony, DO
  Dundon, John M., MD
  Giliberti, William S., MD
  Gutkin, Michael Scott, MD
  Koss, Stephen Dennis, MD
  Rosman, Jerome D., MD
  Salari, Behnam, DO
  Sayde, William M., MD
  Shamim, Ferheen, MD
  Shamim, Rehan Syed, MD
  Teja, Paul Gregory, DO
  White, Kevin S., DO
  Wu, Jason Jon, DO

Women's Health at Hackettstown
108 Bilby Road/Suite 305 Zip: 07840
Ph: (908) 813-8877 Fax: (908) 813-9984
  Akhigbe, Omoikhefe Gbemisola, MD
  Campbell, Neil Murdoch, DO
  Shakarjian, Jo-Ann, MD
  Uzbay, Lisa Ann, MD

Haddon Heights

Advocare Haddon Pediatric Group
119 White Horse Pike Zip: 08035
Ph: (856) 547-7300 Fax: (856) 547-4573
  Blair, Michael A., MD
  Matz, Paul Steven, MD
  Schlitt, Mark George, MD
  Schlitt, Michael T., MD
  Schlitt, Stephanie N., MD
  Shaigany, Nina N., MD

Advocare Heights Primary Care
318 White Horse Pike Zip: 08035
Ph: (856) 547-6000 Fax: (856) 546-3189
  Godorecci, Michele, MD
  Greenwood, Beth M., MD
  Higgins, Alexander J., MD
  King, Krista H., MD
  Renzi, Michael A., DO
  Staritz, Amy, MD

Allied Gastroenterology Associates
217 White Horse Pike Zip: 08035
Ph: (856) 547-1212 Fax: (856) 547-6117
  Izanec, James L., MD
  Kolnik, John P., DO
  Libster, Boris, DO
  Siegel, Howard Ira, MD

Cardiovascular Associates
210 West Atlantic Avenue Zip: 08035
Ph: (856) 546-3003 Fax: (856) 547-5337
  Da Torre, Steven D., MD
  Fortino, Gregg L., MD
  Gips, Sanford J., MD
  Giri, Kartik S., MD
  Herlich, Michael B., MD
  Kaddissi, Georges Ibrahim, MD
  Levi, Steven A., MD
  Mark, George Edward, MD
  Pavlides, Andreas Constantinos, MD
  Peter, Annie M., MD
  Rafeq, Zahi, MD
  Sanyal, Saugato, MD
  Snyder, Harvey A., MD
  Verma, Vijayendra Kishore, MD
  Viswanath, Dilip Banad, MD
  Zinn, Andrew P., MD

Cooper Family Medicine
504 White Horse Pike Zip: 08035
Ph: (856) 546-7990 Fax: (856) 546-6686
  Doshi, Sangita K., MD
  Risimini, Robert J., MD

Dermatology Physicians of South Jersey
112 White Horse Pike Zip: 08035
Ph: (856) 546-5353 Fax: (856) 546-8711
  Allen, Robert Andrew, MD
  Lo Presti, Nicholas P., MD
  Miller, Emily S., MD
  Whipple, D. Sandra, MD

Infectious Diseases Consultants of NJ
102 White Horse Pike Zip: 08035
Ph: (856) 795-7505 Fax: (856) 795-8010
  Turner, Ellen K., MD

LMA Surgical Associates
120 White Horse Pike/Suite 103 Zip: 08035
Ph: (856) 546-3900 Fax: (856) 546-3908
  Derr, Lisa M., DO
  Di Fiore, Richard, MD
  Finnegan, Matthew J., MD
  Greenawald, Lawrence Edward, MD
  Kakkilaya, Harish, MD
  Merriam, Margaret, DO
  Paluzzi, Sandra A., DO
  Salcone, Mark Anthony, DO
  Traboulsi, Rana, MD

Lisa A. Rink Family Medicine, LLC.
217 White Horse Pike Zip: 08035
Ph: (856) 672-1115 Fax: (856) 672-9111
  Javaiya, Hemangkumar, MD
  Rink, Lisa Ann, DO

Lourdes Medical Associates
500 Grove Street/Suite 100 Zip: 08035
Ph: (856) 796-9200 Fax: (856) 310-5603
  Ahmad, Adeel, MD
  DiSandro, Theresa Maria, DO
  Handler, Heidi L., MD
  Okon, Emmanuel E., MD

Professional Orthopedic Assocs
17 White Horse Pike/Suite 1 Zip: 08035
Ph: (856) 547-2323 Fax: (856) 547-7932
  Kozielski, Joseph A., MD
  Poprycz, Walter, MD

Haddon Township

Haddonfield Internal Medicine
216 Haddon Avenue Zip: 08108
Ph: (856) 854-6600 Fax: (856) 854-6700
  Draganescu, Mirela, MD
  Gupta, Mini, MD
  Manalis, Helen, DO
  McLintock, Glenn R., MD

The Neurological Management Group
55 East Cuthbert Boulevard Zip: 08108
  Dinsmore, Steven Thomas, MD
  Hubbard, Sean Tomar, DO

Haddonfield

Advanced ENT - Haddonfield
130 North Haddon Avenue Zip: 08033
Ph: (856) 602-4000 Fax: (856) 429-1284
  Cultrara, Anthony, MD
  Gadomski, Stephen P., MD
  Shah, Samir, MD

Advocare Cornerstone Pediatrics
318 North Haddon Avenue/Suite A Zip: 08033
Ph: (856) 428-3746 Fax: (856) 310-0312
  Bruner, Laurie Reid, MD
  Lopes, Joanne Elizabeth, MD
  Weidner, James R., MD

Advocare Grove Family Medical Assoc
132 Grove Street/Suite A Zip: 08033
Ph: (856) 354-2211 Fax: (856) 354-6181
  Bauer-Sheldon, Melissa Ann, DO
  Kenney, Meredith Ann, DO
  Panitch, Kenneth N., MD

Advocare Haddonfield Pediatric Assoc
220 Haddon Avenue Zip: 08033
  Milligan Milburn, Erin Colleen, MD

Advocare Haddonfield Pediatric Assoc
220 North Haddon Avenue Zip: 08033
Ph: (856) 429-6719 Fax: (856) 429-6748
  Caltabiano, Claire L., MD
  Friedman, Barton J., MD
  King, Kevin J., MD
  Kumar, Nisha Iyer, MD
  Smergel, Henry, MD
  Welsh, Theresa M., MD

Allergy & Asthma Care, P.C.
213 North Haddon Avenue Zip: 08033
Ph: (856) 795-5600 Fax: (856) 795-6644
  Ku, Min Jung, MD

Drs. Ackerman & Turnier
501 Haddon Avenue/Suite 9 Zip: 08033
Ph: (856) 428-6024 Fax: (856) 216-1558
  Ackerman, Melville J., MD
  Turnier, Auguste P., MD

Haddonfield Dermatology Associates
24 West Kings Highway Zip: 08033
Ph: (856) 795-1341 Fax: (856) 795-5034
  Burns, Loren T., MD
  Suchin, Karen Rebecca, MD

Haddonfield Family Practice PA
15 East Redman Avenue Zip: 08033
Ph: (856) 428-1335 Fax: (856) 428-6334
  Ridilla, Leonard Jr., MD
  Runfola, James Joseph, MD
  Vick, James W., MD

Orthopedic & Neurosurgical Specialists
807 Haddon Avenue/Suite 1 Zip: 08033
Ph: (856) 795-9222 Fax: (856) 795-0026
  Barrett, Michael P., MD
  Bodin, Nathan Daniel, MD
  Bozic, Vladimir Stefan, MD
  Dalsey, Robert M., MD

Penn Health for Women
807 Haddon Avenue/Suite 212 Zip: 08033
Ph: (856) 429-0400 Fax: (856) 429-8411
  Ronner, Wanda, MD

Hainesport

The Center for Kidney Care
1261 Route 38/Suite A Zip: 08036
Ph: (856) 222-1975 Fax: (856) 222-0721
  Acharya, Prasad G., MD
  Conrad, Michael James, MD
  Franger, Margaret Mary, MD
  Min, Dorothy D., MD
  Shah, Samir Nalin, MD
  Share, David Seth, MD
  Solitro, Matthew Joseph, MD
  Suchin, Elliot Jay, MD
  Vargas, Myra Theresa, MD

Groups and Clinics by Town with Physician Rosters

Hainesport (cont)
UMDNJ SOM Family Medicine
310 Creek Crossing Boulevard Zip: 08036
Ph: (609) 702-7500   Fax: (609) 702-5928
- Ciervo, Carman A., DO
- Mason, David Craig, DO
- Meltzer, Michael E., DO

Virtua Medford Surgical Group
212 Creek Crossing Boulevard Zip: 08036
Ph: (609) 267-1004   Fax: (609) 267-1044
- Baranski, Gregg Michael, MD
- Barnes, Thomas L., MD
- Bobila, Wilbur C., MD
- Briones, Renato J., MD

Virtua Pain & Spine Specialists
404 Creek Crossing Boulevard Zip: 08036
Ph: (609) 845-3988
- Rastogi, Abhijeet A., MD
- Slevin, Kieran Anthony, MD

Haledon
Medical Group of North Jersey
401 Haledon Avenue/2nd Floor Zip: 07508
Ph: (973) 942-3767   Fax: (973) 942-1027
- Kahf, Ahmad N., MD
- Kahf, Amr, MD

Pulmonary & Critical Care Associates
378 Belmont Avenue Zip: 07508
Ph: (973) 925-4850   Fax: (973) 925-4851
- Alberaqdar, Enis, MD
- Alfakir, Maria, MD

Hamburg
Drs. Fielding and Geisen
17 Route 23 North Zip: 07419
Ph: (973) 827-7800   Fax: (973) 209-7855
- Fielding, Dennis P., MD
- Geisen, Amy Grace, MD

Premier Health Associates
225 Route 23 South Zip: 07419
Ph: (973) 209-1550   Fax: (973) 729-6487
- Kozak, Margaret Zsuzsa, DO
- Roffe, Kenneth A., DO
- Song, Maria H., MD

Hamilton
Anesthesia Pain Treatment Center
1666 Hamilton Avenue/Suite 2 Zip: 08629
Ph: (609) 584-9080   Fax: (609) 584-0139
- Feder, Craig A., MD
- Loren, Gary M., MD

Cancer Institute of NJ Hamilton
2575 Klockner Road Zip: 08690
Ph: (609) 631-6960   Fax: (609) 631-6888
- Lerma, Pauline Marie Ocampo, MD
- Wasserman, Ethan Jeffrey, MD

Capital Health Primary Care
1401 Whitehorse Mercerville Ro Zip: 08619
Ph: (609) 689-5760   Fax: (609) 689-5759
- Stabile, John R., MD

Capital Health Primary Care-Hamilton
1445 Whitehorse-Mercerville Rd Zip: 08619
Ph: (609) 587-6661   Fax: (609) 587-8503
- Aiello, Stephen Anthony, MD
- Arcaro, Mark E., MD
- Castillo, Christine Capistran, DO
- Chavez Santos, Maria, MD
- Chiromeras, Andrew, MD
- Marriott, Christine Ryan, MD
- Richards, Bonnie J., DO
- Sharma, Smriti, MD

Comprehensive Neurology, LLC.
1245 Whitehorse-Mercerville Rd Zip: 08619
Ph: (609) 585-2666   Fax: (609) 585-4008
- Pasupuleti, Rao Satyanaray, MD
- Zhang, Lei, MD

Drs. Lendor and Evans Murage
1301 Whitehorse Mercerville Rd Zip: 08619
Ph: (609) 585-9901   Fax: (609) 585-9919
- Evans Murage, Julene Opalene, MD
- Lendor, E. Cindy, MD

Drs. Rosenbaum & Aufiero
2085 Klockner Road Zip: 08690
Ph: (609) 587-4122   Fax: (609) 588-5922
- Aufiero, Patrick V., MD
- Rosenbaum, Seth David, MD

Hamilton Anesthesia and Pain
1 Hamilton Health Place Zip: 08690
Ph: (609) 631-6824   Fax: (609) 631-6839
- Dashow, Susan M., DO
- Gordon, Michael Stuart, MD
- Sanchez, Israel L., MD
- Suaco, Benjamin S., MD
- Zwick, Annette E., MD

Hamilton Cardiology Associates
2073 Klockner Road Zip: 08690
Ph: (609) 584-1212   Fax: (609) 584-0103
- Alvi, Afshan Khadija, MD
- Caplan, John L., MD
- Chebotarev, Oleg, MD
- Fox, Justin Michael, MD
- Genin, Ilya D., MD
- Ghusson, Mahmoud Saleh, MD
- Gibreal, Mohammed, MD
- Patel, Aarti, MD
- Patel, Jay K., MD
- Patel, Minal, MD
- Rab, Zia, MD
- Ryder, Ronald G., DO
- South, Harry L., MD
- Tripathi, Neeta, MD
- Wilson, Bruce Leonard, MD
- Wingfield, Edward Anthony, MD

Hamilton HealthCare Center
3840 Quakerbridge Road/Suite 100 Zip: 08619
Ph: (609) 890-2222   Fax: (609) 890-0715
- Fass, Barry D., MD
- Mahoney, John J., DO
- Smith, David E., MD

Hamilton Pediatric Associates
3 Hamilton Health Place/Suite A Zip: 08690
Ph: (609) 581-4480   Fax: (609) 581-5222
- Baiser, Dennis Miles, MD
- Bogacki, Gwen M., MD
- Boim, Marilynn Dora, MD
- Buchbinder, Marta Luisa H., MD
- Jacques, Walter J., MD
- Prineas, Sara L., MD
- Zelinsky, Catherine Marie, MD

IC Laser Eye Care
1725 Klockner Road Zip: 08619
Ph: (609) 586-6700   Fax: (609) 586-8768
- Chaudhry, Iftikhar Manzoor, MD
- Chaudhry, Uzma, MD

Laurente Medical Associates
4453 Nottingham Way Zip: 08690
Ph: (609) 587-0119   Fax: (609) 587-3009
- Laurente, Cristeta A., MD
- Laurente, Robert M., MD

MedExpress Urgent Care Hamilton Square
811 Route 33 Zip: 08619
Ph: (609) 587-8298   Fax: (609) 587-8570
- Ganguly, Panchali, MD
- Patel, Viral D., MD

Medical Associates at Hamilton PC
1235 Whitehorse Mercerville Rd Zip: 08619
Ph: (609) 581-9000   Fax: (609) 585-7228
- Diwan, Nauman Abdul, MD
- Raza, Rubina B., MD

Mercer Surgical Group
2063 Klockner Road/Suite 1 Zip: 08690
Ph: (609) 631-1001   Fax: (609) 588-5970
- Goldenberg, Elie Adam, MD

Mercer-Bucks Orthopaedics, P.C.
2501 Kuser Road Zip: 08691
Ph: (609) 896-0444   Fax: (609) 587-4349
- Cairone, Stephen Scott, DO
- Capotosta, Thomas J. Jr., MD
- Crivello, Keith Michael, MD
- Hardeski, David Paul, MD
- Kleinbart, Fredric Alan, MD

Mountain View Surgical Associates
1445 Whitehorse-Mercerville Rd Zip: 08691
Ph: (609) 392-8100   Fax: (609) 695-6202
- Manna, Biagio, DO
- Tuma, Augustine Lavelle, MD

Patient First Urgent Care
641 US Highway Route 130 Zip: 08691
Ph: (609) 568-9383   Fax: (609) 568-9384
- Agcopra, Annabel, DO
- Byrne, Janet Marilyn, MD
- Manzoor, Adil, DO
- Sehgel, Robert R., DO
- Sood, Jasen, DO
- Tohfafarosh, Nilofer J., MD

Pediatrics by Night
1230 Whitehorse Mercerville Ro Zip: 08619
Ph: (609) 581-1700   Fax: (609) 581-8472
- Dorneo, Aurora B., MD
- Flores, Belen P., MD
- Flores, Lisa, MD
- Reyes, Reina Duremdes, MD
- Sudjono-Santoso, Dewi S., MD

Premier ENT Associates
8 Quakerbridge Plaza Zip: 08619
Ph: (609) 890-7800   Fax: (609) 890-6148
- Jaffe, Joel D., MD
- Miller, Lee H., MD

Primary & Diabetic Care Office
2065 Klockner Road Zip: 08690
Ph: (609) 586-1001   Fax: (609) 586-7634
- Li, Tong, MD
- Soriano, Myrna Lopez, MD

Princeton Occupational Medicine
2271 Highway 33/Suite 109 Zip: 08690
Ph: (609) 584-0117   Fax: (609) 586-5103
- Cruz, Gloria Maria, MD
- Mullane, Joseph P., MD

RWJ Medical Associates
3100 Quakerbridge Road/Suite 28 Zip: 08619
Ph: (609) 245-7430   Fax: (609) 245-7432
- Baig, Sumeera Akhtar, MD
- Bhandarkar, Anjali, MD
- Oza, Harsha K., MD
- Tselniker, Maryana, MD

Radiology Affiliates Imaging
3625 Quakerbridge Road Zip: 08619
- Kirkpatrick, Christopher Thomas, MD
- Krishan, Mona, DO

Radiology Affiliates of Central NJ
2501 Kuser Road Zip: 08691
Ph: (609) 585-8800   Fax: (609) 585-1825
- Alderson, Skip Michael, MD
- Bhalakia, Niraj, MD
- Blackman, Gurvan E., MD
- Bosworth, Eric, MD
- Brown, Michele Susan, MD
- Burda, John F., MD
- Burgos, Anthony, MD
- Burshteyn, Mark, MD
- Chalal, Jo Ann, MD
- Cohen, Daniel Jonathan, MD
- Dutka, Michael Vincent, MD
- Ezati, Omid, MD
- Gellella, Erik Leonard, MD
- Gold, Michael J., MD
- Greenbaum, Roy L., MD
- Kim, Joseph J., MD
- Kulkarni, Kedar, MD
- Le Cavalier, Larry Alan, MD
- Lee, Shane, MD
- Lo Verde, Lauren S., MD
- Mathews, Jeffrey John, MD
- McGroarty, William J., MD
- Meshkov, Steven L., MD
- Nayee, Sandip Natvarlal, DO
- Neuman, Joel David, MD
- Ostrum, Donald S., MD
- Plakyda, Derek J., MD
- Pryluck, David Scott, MD
- Ratner, Lawrence M., MD
- Rieder, Michael J., MD
- Ross, William M., MD

- Scafidi, Richard F., MD
- Seelagan, Davindra, MD
- Silverstein, Gary S., MD
- Steinig, Jeffrey Daniel, MD
- Sterling, Michelle Gold, MD
- Tarasov, Ethan A., MD
- Taus, Lynne F., MD
- Thal, Stephen Wayne, DO
- Weiser, Paul J., MD
- Winter, Rebecca Cooper, MD
- Young, Sophia C., MD

Richard. D. Gordon, MD PA
2121 Klockner Road Zip: 08690
Ph: (609) 587-9898   Fax: (609) 584-1774
- Gordon, Richard Dennis, MD
- Segal, Leigh G., MD

Robert Wood Johnson Ob/Gyn Group
1 Hamilton Health Place Zip: 08690
Ph: (609) 631-6899   Fax: (609) 631-6898
- Gonzalez Braile, Dinah A., MD
- Naraine, Christopher Anthony, MD
- Resnick, Michael B., MD
- Sison, Antonio, MD
- Tufankjian, Lisa Gruszka, DO

Schuylkill Medical Associates, LLC
2681 Quakerbridge Road/Suite B2 Zip: 08619
OnlyFax: (609) 208-3233
- Pluta, Christine Marie, DO
- Walker, Bridget Ann, DO

Snoring and Sleep Apnea Center Mercer
1401 Whitehorse Mercerville Rd Zip: 08619
Ph: (609) 584-5150   Fax: (609) 584-5144
- Dupre, Callum Michael, DO
- Voddi, Swetha Devi, MD

Soliman Medical Associates
2400 Whitehorse Mercerville Rd Zip: 08619
Ph: (609) 587-4778   Fax: (609) 587-1202
- Soliman, Hesham S., MD
- Soliman, Yasser S., MD

Subramoni Physicians Associates PA
2091 Klockner Road Zip: 08690
Ph: (609) 890-9191   Fax: (609) 586-6163
- Palomata, Maria Theresa, MD
- Subramoni, Venkateswar, MD

CINJ at Hamilton
5 Hamilton Health Place/Suite 120 Zip: 08690
Ph: (609) 631-6960   Fax: (609) 631-6888
- Holtzman, Gayle S., MD

Pain Mgt Center-Hamilton
2271 Highway 33/Suite 103 Zip: 08690
Ph: (609) 890-4080   Fax: (609) 890-4090
- Josephson, Youssef, DO
- Sackstein, Adam, MD

University Urology Assocs of NJ
1374 Whitehorse Hamilton Sq/Suite 101 Zip: 08690
Ph: (609) 581-5900   Fax: (609) 581-5901
- Al-Qassab, Usama, MD
- Gazi, Mukaram A., MD
- Gotesman, Alexander, MD
- Nazmy, Michael Jr., MD

Urology Care Alliance
2105 Klockner Road Zip: 08690
Ph: (609) 588-0770   Fax: (609) 588-0454
- Brackin, Phillip Snowden Jr., MD
- Linder, Earle S., MD
- Watson, John A., MD

Vadakara Internal Medicine
2117 Klockner Road Zip: 08690
Ph: (609) 584-1001   Fax: (609) 584-0404
- Vadakara, Laisa L., MD
- Vadakara, Lukose Simon, MD

Hamilton Square
Campus Eye Group & Laser Center
1700 Whitehorse Hamilton Sq Rd Zip: 08690
Ph: (609) 587-2020   Fax: (609) 588-9545
- Chung, Soo K., MD
- Sardi, Vincent F., MD

Groups and Clinics by Town with Physician Rosters

Drs. Kessel & Mercer
1700 White Horse Hamilton Road   Zip: 08690
Ph: (609) 890-2600   Fax: (609) 890-0265
  Kessel,Daniel S., MD
  Mercer,Stephen Edward, MD
Hamilton Medical Group
2275 State Route 33/Suite 301   Zip: 08690
Ph: (609) 586-6006
  Deblasio,Joseph, MD
  Siniakowicz,Robert Miroslaw, MD

Hammonton
ASAP - Advanced Spine and Pain
2 Eighth Street   Zip: 08037
OnlyFax: (609) 567-8832
  Ezeadichie,Chioma A., DO
  Manabat,Eileen Rose, MD
Assoc Cardiovascular Consultants
2 Sindoni Lane   Zip: 08037
Ph: (609) 561-8500   Fax: (856) 567-0432
  Ahmed,Safi U., MD
  Saia,John A., DO
  Ukrainski,Gerald J., MD
  Wroblewski,Edward A., MD
  Zheng,Jing-Sheng, MD
AtlantiCare Family Medicine
120 South White Horse Pike   Zip: 08037
Ph: (609) 561-4211   Fax: (609) 561-0639
  De Tata,Gerald C., MD
AtlantiCare Family Medicine
219 North White Horse Pike/Suite 101   Zip: 08037
Ph: (609) 561-4211   Fax: (609) 561-0639
  Jones-Mudd,Kimberly M., DO
  Kaminski,Mitchell Anthony, MD
  Loughlin-Pherribo,Donna Joyce, DO
  Salvo,Anthony, MD
  Sharma,Sonia, MD
Central Physicians and Surgeons
820 South White Horse Pike   Zip: 08037
Ph: (609) 561-8787   Fax: (609) 567-9546
  Friedenthal,Roy B., MD
  Gerson,Ronald L., MD
Drs. Amer and Prasad
777 White Horse Pike/Suite E   Zip: 08037
Ph: (609) 567-0608   Fax: (609) 567-1295
  Amer,Adel M., MD
  Prasad,Devineni R., MD
Hammonton Family Medicine Center
373 South White Horse Pike   Zip: 08037
Ph: (609) 704-0185   Fax: (609) 704-0195
  Bertagnolli,John F. Jr., DO
  Collins,Philip, MD
  Moore,Rebecca Christiane, DO
Integrative Neurological Care
663 South White Horse Pike   Zip: 08037
Ph: (609) 567-6042
  Carta,Maria C., MD
  De Antonio,Sondra M., MD
Rothman Institute
219 North White Horse Pike   Zip: 08037
  Young,George William, DO
South Jersey Chest Diseases
107 Vine Street   Zip: 08037
Ph: (609) 561-7666   Fax: (609) 561-8347
  Belli,Albert J. Jr., DO
  Gilmour,Kevin P., DO
  Kanoff,Jack M., DO
South Jersey Gastroenterology PA
111 Vine Street   Zip: 08037
Ph: (609) 561-3080   Fax: (856) 983-5110
  Magasic,Mario V., MD
  Savon,Joseph J., MD
Southern Jersey Family Medical Ctrs
860 South White Horse Pike/Building A   Zip: 08037
Ph: (609) 567-0200   Fax: (609) 567-3492
  Agbasi,Nwogo Nnunwa, MD
  Bejaran,Juan E., MD
  Capiro,Rodney, MD
  Fakayode,Abisoye Victoria, MD
  Klein,Bruce M., MD
  McFarlane,Owen R., MD

Hampton
Highlands Family Health Center
61 Frontage Road/Suite 61   Zip: 08827
Ph: (908) 735-2594   Fax: (908) 735-8526
  Mitev,Iliya D., MD
  Palmer,Victoria R., DO
  Polizzi,David R., MD
  Polt,Terry Jane, MD
  Thakur,Shivani, MD
North Hunterdon Physician Assocs
37 Ruppell Road   Zip: 08827
  Prentice,Hugh J., MD
  Sforza,Frank J., MD

Harrington Park
The Park Medical Group
24 Elm Street   Zip: 07640
Ph: (201) 784-0123   Fax: (201) 784-0065
  Biria,Nazila, MD
  Brunnquell,Stephen B., MD
  Fadil,Tina Marie, MD
  Herera,Daniel Joe, MD
  Lee,Gerald J., MD
  Patel,Disha, MD
  Psillides,Despina, MD
  Relkin,Felicia, MD
  Schran,Mary Ann, MD
  Shin,Seulkih, MD
  Srinivasan,Anand, MD

Harrison
Essex Hudson Urology
213 South Frank Rodgers Blvd   Zip: 07029
Ph: (973) 482-7070
  Rilli,Charles F., MD
Harrison Pediatric Care PA
332 Harrison Avenue   Zip: 07029
Ph: (973) 484-2584   Fax: (973) 481-0754
  Vidal,Jennifer Lyn, DO
Primary Care Medical Group
450 Bergen Street   Zip: 07029
Ph: (973) 484-6900   Fax: (973) 484-0029
  D'Agostino,Ralph S., MD
  Fontanazza,Paul, MD
  Vazquez Falcon,Luis Enrique, MD

Hasbrouck Heights
Anti-Aging & Laser Medical Associates
777 Terrace Avenue/Suite 403   Zip: 07604
Ph: (201) 288-3777   Fax: (201) 426-0446
  Oppenheimer,Jeffrey Harry, MD
Cardiovascular Consltnts/North Jersey
777 Terrace Avenue   Zip: 07604
Ph: (201) 288-4252   Fax: (201) 288-7172
  Benoff,Lane Jeffrey, MD
  Goodman,Daniel J., MD
  Lyons,William J., MD
  Sehgal,Evan D., MD
Heights Medical Associates
288 Boulevard   Zip: 07604
Ph: (201) 288-6781   Fax: (201) 288-2734
  Bellavia,Thomas S., MD
  Renner,Carl J., MD
Interventional Neuro Associates, LLC
777 Terrace Avenue/Suite 401   Zip: 07604
Ph: (201) 387-1957   Fax: (201) 351-0656
  Turkel-Parrella,David, MD
University Reproductive Associates, PC
214 Terrace Avenue/2nd Floor   Zip: 07604
Ph: (201) 288-6330   Fax: (201) 288-6331
  Cho,Michael Ming-Huei, MD
  Fechner,Adam Jeffrey, MD
  Loughlin,Jacquelyn S., MD
  McGovern,Peter G., MD
  Weiss,Gerson, MD
  Wolf Greene,Susan Amy, MD

Haskell
Haskell Towne Medical LLC
1141 Ringwood Avenue/Suite 7   Zip: 07420
Ph: (973) 835-6777
  Hall,Kevin Arthur, MD
  Smith,Jeffrey Todd, DO

Hawthorne
Hawthorne Family Practice
1083 Goffle Road   Zip: 07506
Ph: (973) 427-2421
  Tuppo,Ehab E., MD
  Tuppo,Enas Elias, MD
Lozito Medical Associates
484 Lafayette Avenue   Zip: 07506
Ph: (973) 423-4770   Fax: (973) 423-4816
  Cifaldi,Ralph John Jr., DO
  Lozito,Deborah A., DO
  Lozito,Joseph A. Jr., DO
Respiratory Health & Critical Care
1114 Goffle Road/Suite 103   Zip: 07506
Ph: (973) 790-4111   Fax: (973) 790-4330
  Jacoby,Steven Clifford, MD
Valley Health Medical Group
1114 Goffle Road/Suite 103   Zip: 07506
Ph: (973) 423-1364   Fax: (973) 423-0980
  Anthony Wilson,Avril Dawn, MD
  Penera,Norman S., MD

Hazlet
Ani Orthopaedic Group
1 Bethany Road/Bldg. 2 Suite 21   Zip: 07730
Ph: (732) 264-8282   Fax: (732) 264-8131
  Ani,Abdul Nasser, MD
  Ani,Mohamad Salim, MD
  Bash,Robin Ellen, MD
Bethany Pediatrics PA
1 Bethany Road/Building 5/Suite 65   Zip: 07730
Ph: (732) 264-0700   Fax: (732) 264-1414
  Blackman,Ryan Graham, DO
  Cambria,Lina, MD
  Pascucci,Rocco F., MD
  Protasis,Liza, MD
  Ruda,Neal, MD
Chapel Hill Family Medicine
100 Village Court/Suite 302   Zip: 07730
Ph: (732) 758-0048   Fax: (732) 758-0052
  Schneebaum,Katherine, MD
  Triola,Victoria, MD
Drs. Tsompanidis and Perrino Fam Pract
1 Bethany Road/Suite 79   Zip: 07730
Ph: (732) 203-0800   Fax: (732) 203-9494
  Perrino,DinaMarie, DO
  Tsompanidis,Antonios A.J., MD
Drs. Awad and Hozayen
1 Bethany Road/Building 6   Zip: 07730
Ph: (732) 264-5005
  Awad,Mona S., MD
  Hozayen,Ossama, MD
Drs. Chudzik and Chudzik
31 Village Court   Zip: 07730
Ph: (732) 264-1212   Fax: (732) 888-5452
  Chudzik,Douglas W., MD
  Chudzik,Jeanmarie, MD
Immediate Care Medical of Hazlet, P.A.
1376 State Highway 36   Zip: 07730
Ph: (732) 264-5500   Fax: (732) 264-5554
  Cunningham,Michael Joseph, MD
  Golding-Granado,Lisa Michelle, MD
Meleis Medical Associates
233 Middle Road/Suite 2   Zip: 07730
Ph: (732) 335-0900   Fax: (732) 335-8080
  Khalil,Hossam M., MD
  Meleis,Mohamed E., MD

Hewitt
Associates in Women's Healthcare
1900 Union Valley Road   Zip: 07421
Ph: (973) 831-1800   Fax: (973) 831-8820
  Dombo,Kudzai Rebecca, MD

Highland Park
Brunswick Eye Associates
317 Cleveland Avenue   Zip: 08904
Ph: (732) 828-5190   Fax: (732) 828-0677
  Glass,Robert M., MD
  Hathaway,Elaine G., MD
Center For Asthma & Allergy
18 North Third Avenue   Zip: 08904
Ph: (732) 545-0094   Fax: (732) 545-4087
  Bonala,Savithri Bai, MD
  Golbert,Thomas Melvin, MD
  Gutin,Faina M., MD
  Khan,Shameen, DO
  Li,Lin, MD
  Parikh,Sudhir Manharlal, MD
  Sheen,Eun H., MD
  Suliaman,Fawzi A., MD
  Witkowska,Renata A., MD
Glasgold Group for Plastic Surgery
31 River Road   Zip: 08904
Ph: (732) 846-6540   Fax: (732) 846-8231
  Glasgold,Mark J., MD
  Glasgold,Robert Alexander, MD
  Schrader-Barile,Nicole Annette, MD
Highland Park Pediatrics
85 Raritan Avenue   Zip: 08904
Ph: (732) 246-0202   Fax: (732) 246-8334
  Biener,Robert, MD
  Gul,Sheba, MD
  Reingold,Stephen Marcus, MD
Highland Park Surgical Associates
31 River Road   Zip: 08904
Ph: (732) 846-9500   Fax: (732) 846-3931
  Curtiss,Steven Ian, MD
  Rosen,Scott Farrell, MD
  Tutela,Rocco Robert Jr., MD
University Pediatric Associates
317 Cleveland Avenue   Zip: 08904
Ph: (732) 249-8999   Fax: (732) 249-7827
  Erlikhman,Alla, MD
  Gavai,Medha A., MD
  Glaser-Schanzer,Felice, MD
  John,Sheryl Mary, MD
  Majisu,Claire Amume, MD
  Rubin,Elliot H., MD
  Zablocki,Lisa R., MD

Hightstown
East Windsor Pediatric Group
300B Princeton Hightstown/Suite 201   Zip: 08520
Ph: (609) 448-7300   Fax: (609) 448-8022
  Arcaro,Maria Anna C., MD
  Bidabadi,Bobak, MD
  Goodman,Aimee R., DO
  Gribin,Bradley Jay, MD
  Howe,Matthew R., MD
  Marcus,Brian F., DO
  Patel,Radhika K., MD
  Shah,Utpal S., MD
  Siddiqui,Sabeen A., MD
  Vo,Ha, MD

Hillsborough
Affiliates in Internal Medicine
311 Omni Drive   Zip: 08844
Ph: (908) 281-0632   Fax: (908) 281-9848
  Chou,Lin W., MD
  Neiman,Deborah L., MD
Ahmad A. Mur MD PA
503 Omni Drive   Zip: 08844
Ph: (908) 595-1199   Fax: (866) 889-3643
  Bhaskara,Jayshree A., MD
  Mur,Ahmad A., MD
Brunswick-Hills Ob/Gyn, PA
751 Route 206/2nd Floor   Zip: 08844
Ph: (908) 725-2510   Fax: (908) 725-2132
  Davis,Nicole D., MD
  Karanikolas,Steven, MD
  Salley,Pamela R., MD
Cardio Care
200 Courtyard Drive/Suite 213   Zip: 08844
Ph: (908) 725-5200   Fax: (908) 725-5223
  Sanyal,Sanjukta, MD
  Taylor,Jeff Thomas, MD
Digestive Healthcare Center
511 Courtyard Drive/Building 500   Zip: 08844
Ph: (908) 218-9222   Fax: (908) 218-9818
  Accurso,Charles A., MD
  Barghash,Claudia N., MD
  Ciambotti,Gary Francis, MD
  Gingold,Alan R., DO
  Greaves,Mark Leslie, MD
  Lee,Kristen Kyongae, MD
  Youssef,Nader Namir, MD

Groups and Clinics by Town with Physician Rosters

Hillsborough (cont)
Genito-Urinary Surgeons of New Jersey
211 Courtyard Drive Zip: 08844
Ph: (908) 685-0080 Fax: (908) 685-7594
- Koota, David H., MD

Hillsborough Pediatrics
390 Amwell Road/Suite 106 Zip: 08844
Ph: (908) 431-3100 Fax: (908) 431-3101
- Hussain, Aazim Syed, MD
- Lariviere, Aimee T., MD

ID Associates PA/dba ID CARE
105 Raider Boulevard/Suite 101 Zip: 08844
Ph: (908) 281-0221 Fax: (908) 281-0940
- Bhalla, Rohit, DO
- Doshi, Manish, MD
- Herman, David J., MD
- Hirsh, Ellen J., MD
- McDermott, Rena, MD
- Nahass, Ronald G., MD
- Pittarelli, Lisa A., MD
- Sandhu, Sarbjit Singh, MD
- Seenivasan, Meena, MD
- Sheen, Jerry, MD
- Shepperly, David C., MD
- Sonnenberg, Edith, MD

Montgomery Internal Med Group
719 Route 206 North/Suite 100 Zip: 08844
Ph: (908) 904-0920 Fax: (908) 431-9407
- Hildebrant, Laura Nadine, DO

Primary Care Center at Hillsborough
331 Route 206 North/Suite 2-B Zip: 08844
Ph: (908) 685-2528 Fax: (908) 359-7109
- Snyder, Kenneth R., MD
- Yadav, Priyanka Singh, DO
- Zajac, Anna T., MD

RWJPE Towne Centre Family Care
302 Towne Centre Drive Zip: 08844
Ph: (908) 359-8613 Fax: (908) 874-8509
- Erb, Erica, MD
- Piech, Richard Frank, MD
- Shute, Amy L., MD

Skin Laser & Surgery Specialists
105 Raider Boulevard/Suite 203 Zip: 08844
Ph: (201) 441-9890 Fax: (201) 441-9893
- Man, Jeremy Robert, MD

Somerset Ob-Gyn Associates
1 New Amwell Road Zip: 08844
Ph: (908) 874-5900
- Pineda, Jean, MD

Somerset Pediatric Group PA
1-C New Amwell Road Zip: 08844
Ph: (908) 874-5035 Fax: (908) 874-3288
- Hede, Madan M., MD
- Youngerman, Neil L., MD

Your Doctors Care, PA
71 Route 206 South Zip: 08844
Ph: (908) 685-1887 Fax: (908) 707-0816
- Fowls, Brianna, MD
- Landesman, Glen S., MD
- Smith, Joseph Arthur, MD
- Weinstein, Joseph R., MD

Hillside
Hillside Family Practice
100 Hollywood Avenue Zip: 07205
Ph: (908) 353-7949 Fax: (908) 353-8374
- Matkiwsky, Walter, DO
- Vidal Burke, Angela M., MD

Ho Ho Kus
Valley Pediatric Associates, P.A.
201 East Franklin Turnpike Zip: 07423
Ph: (201) 652-1888 Fax: (201) 652-6485
- Birnhak, Stefani, MD
- Kim, Urian, MD
- Lee, Julia Jin-Young, MD
- Leifer, Amy Sarah Budin, MD

Hoboken
AstraHealth Urgent & Primary Care
95 Hudson Street Zip: 07030
Ph: (201) 464-8888
- DaSilva, Robert Antonio, MD

Brescia-Migliaccio OB/GYN
609 Washington Street Zip: 07030
Ph: (201) 659-7700 Fax: (201) 659-7701
- Brescia, Mark J., MD
- Chinn, Natasha R., MD
- Lowe, Samantha B., DO
- Migliaccio, Thomas A., MD
- Moon, Jeremy, MD
- Picard, Johan Arlenie, MD

CarePoint Health Medical Group
331 Grand Street/Ground Floor Zip: 07030
Ph: (201) 238-2888 Fax: (201) 656-5989
- Forouzesh, Avisheh, MD
- Messihi, Jean, MD

Center For Asthma & Allergy
300 Hudson Street Zip: 07030
Ph: (201) 792-5900 Fax: (201) 792-5320
- Pine, Martin S., MD

Center for Family Health
122-132 Clinton Street Zip: 07030
Ph: (201) 418-3100 Fax: (201) 418-3148
- Chu, Daniel Yun, DO

Center for Family Health
122 Clinton Street Zip: 07030
Ph: (201) 418-3100
- Garcia, Raudel, MD
- Garcia, Steven Jesus, MD
- Jacobs, Abbie D., MD
- Kumar, Harini C., MD
- Latorre, Juan J., MD
- Ramos, Leonor Vivas, MD
- Ramos, Rey Ferna Pedraza, MD
- Robaina, Luis A., MD
- Valerian, Christopher, DO

ENT and Allergy Associates (ENTA)
79 Hudson Street/Suite 303 Zip: 07030
Ph: (201) 792-1109 Fax: (201) 792-1145
- Calloway, Hollin Elizabeth, MD
- Glaser, Aylon Y., MD
- Mehta, Harshna B., MD
- Tandon, Raj, MD

East Coast Advanced Plastic Surgery
79 Hudson Street/Suite 700 Zip: 07030
Ph: (201) 449-1000 Fax: (201) 399-2433
- Cerio, Dean Richard, MD
- Chalfoun, Charbel T., MD
- Loghmanee, Cyrus Faz, MD

Hoboken Family Practice
108 Washington Street Zip: 07030
Ph: (201) 656-5688 Fax: (201) 656-8975
- Balacco, Leonard M., MD
- De Marco, Angelo Albert, MD
- Patel, Karnik, DO

Hoboken Integrated Family Medicine
109 Grand Street Zip: 07030
Ph: (201) 795-1001 Fax: (201) 795-1009
- Ramirez Chernikova, Anna, MD
- Witt, Virginia Marie, MD

Hoboken Urgent Care
231 Washington Street Zip: 07030
Ph: (201) 754-1005 Fax: (201) 754-1006
- Rohani, Sayed M., MD

Hudson Pro Orthopaedics and Sports Med
1320 Adams Street/Unit D-E Zip: 07030
Ph: (201) 308-6622 Fax: (646) 661-2599
- Ashraf, Imran, MD
- Isaac, Roman, MD

Hudson Psychiatric Associates, LLC.
79 Hudson Street/Suite 203 Zip: 07030
Ph: (201) 222-8808 Fax: (201) 222-8803
- Chuang, Linda I., MD
- Gajera, Bhavinkumar, MD
- Magera, Michael John, MD

North Jersey Surgical Group PA
1 Marine View Plaza Zip: 07030
Ph: (201) 795-9080 Fax: (201) 795-9434
- Costa, German H., MD
- Gonzalez, Juan A. Jr., MD

PromptMD Urgent Care Center
309 First Street Zip: 07030
Ph: (201) 222-8411 Fax: (201) 222-8711
- Islam, Javedul M., MD
- Jani, Chandrashekhar C., MD

Riverside Pediatric Group
609 Washington Street/Ground Floor Zip: 07030
Ph: (201) 706-8488 Fax: (201) 706-8489
- Kucharski, Jarrod Michael, MD

Riverside Pediatric Group
1111 Hudson Street Zip: 07030
Ph: (201) 942-9320 Fax: (201) 942-9321
- Mani, Shrinidi, MD
- Zarrabi, Yasaman, DO

St. Mary Center for Family Health
122-132 Clinton Street Zip: 07030
Ph: (201) 418-3126 Fax: (201) 418-3140
- Williams, Juliette Marie, MD

Surgical Associates of Hudson County
330 Grand Street/Suite 100 Zip: 07030
Ph: (201) 238-2888
- Miller, Benetta L., MD

Inst of Repro Med and Science
609 Washington Street/2nd Floor Zip: 07030
OnlyFax: (201) 204-9319
- Chen, Serena Homei, MD
- Garrisi, Margaret Graf, MD

The Orthopedic Health Center
720 Monroe Street/Suite C209 Zip: 07030
Ph: (201) 286-3622
- Dwyer, James W., MD
- Feliciano, Edward, MD

Holmdel
Bayshore Ophthalmology, LLC.
719 North Beers Street Zip: 07733
Ph: (732) 264-6464 Fax: (732) 264-5114
- Collur, Surekha, MD
- Subramaniam, Cristin Devika, MD

Bayshore Pediatric Association
717 North Beers Street/Suite 1C Zip: 07733
Ph: (732) 888-0010 Fax: (732) 888-0012
- Engel, Barbara M., MD
- Engel, Jennifer Duck, MD

Central Jersey Pulmnry Med Assocs
719 North Beers Street/Suites 2E-2F Zip: 07733
Ph: (732) 264-1001 Fax: (732) 264-4495
- Bebawy, Sam T., MD
- Metri Mansour, Elie E., MD

Cosmetic Dermatologic Surgery Assoc.
719 North Beers Street/Suite 2-G Zip: 07733
Ph: (732) 739-3223 Fax: (732) 739-3225
- Bhatnagar, Divya Sambandan, MD

Drs. Prasad and Shah
717 North Beers Street/PO Box 370 Zip: 07733
Ph: (732) 264-0210 Fax: (732) 888-9214
- Prasad, Penesetti V., MD
- Shah, Niranjan S., MD

Holmdel Health Center
670 North Beers Street Zip: 07733
Ph: (732) 226-5552 Fax: (732) 757-0824
- Ali, Rayshma, DO

Jersey Shore Medical Assoc
734 North Beers Street/Suite U-4 Zip: 07733
Ph: (732) 264-8484 Fax: (732) 264-4324
- Brown, Derrick M., MD
- Catanese, Vincent J., MD
- De Tulio, Anthony, MD
- Marino, Richard P., DO

Matawan Surgical Associates
717 North Beers Street/Suite 1-E Zip: 07733
Ph: (732) 847-3300 Fax: (732) 739-5295
- Baumlin, Thomas Jr., MD
- Malit, Michele Farrah, DO

Miguelino and David Pediatrics
717 North Beers Street/Suite 1F Zip: 07733
Ph: (732) 888-0777 Fax: (732) 888-0880
- David, Lea H., MD
- Miguelino, Bernadette M., MD

Northern Monmouth Co Medical
100 Commons Way/Suite 150 Zip: 07733
Ph: (732) 450-2940 Fax: (732) 450-2942
- Antonopoulou, Marianna, MD
- Zaitz, Jennifer, DO

Ob-Gyn Assocs/Holmdel-Shrewsbury
704 North Beers Street Zip: 07733
Ph: (732) 739-2500 Fax: (732) 888-2778
- Conley, Michael P., MD
- Penney, Robert P., MD
- Smolinsky, Adi, MD
- Wohlstadter, Sanford W., MD

Ophthalmic Physicians of Monmouth PA
733 North Beers Street/Suite U-4 Zip: 07733
Ph: (732) 739-0707 Fax: (732) 739-6722
- Klug, Ronald David, MD
- Steinfeld, Jason Israel, MD

Pediatric Associates of Holmdel, PC
719 North Beers Street/Suite 1E Zip: 07733
Ph: (732) 739-4414 Fax: (732) 739-9537
- Carey, Brittany Marie, DO
- Mohan, Kusum C., MD

Regional Cancer Care Associates, LLC
723 North Beers Street Zip: 07733
Ph: (732) 739-8644 Fax: (732) 739-4438
- Chen, Aileen Lim, MD

SAMRA Group
733 North Beers Street/Suite U-1 Zip: 07733
Ph: (732) 739-2100 Fax: (732) 739-0815
- Patel, Munjal P., MD
- Samra, Asaad H., MD
- Samra, Fares, MD
- Samra, Said A., MD
- Samra, Salem, MD

The Allergy & Asthma Group
717 North Beers Street/Suite 2 A Zip: 07733
Ph: (732) 739-0660 Fax: (732) 739-1406
- Ho, Linden D., MD
- Viksman, Michael Y., MD

Urology Care Alliance
733 North Beers Street/Suite L-6 Zip: 07733
Ph: (732) 739-2200 Fax: (732) 739-8988
- Antoun, Saad S., MD
- Rizkala, Emad Remond, MD

Howell
Drs. Axelrad & Zuckerbrod
4774 Route 9 South Zip: 07731
Ph: (732) 363-6222 Fax: (732) 363-9203
- Axelrad, Paul R., MD
- Zuckerbrod, Jacqueline E., DO

Drs. Lombardi & Shetty
1001 Route 9 North/Suite 106 Zip: 07731
Ph: (732) 886-9122 Fax: (732) 886-5161
- Lombardi, David D., MD
- Shetty, Vinod J., MD

Howell Jackson Medical Center
4764 Route 9 South Zip: 07731
Ph: (732) 370-3563
- Anne, Sreelatha, MD
- Gumina, John D., MD

Howell Primary Care, P.C.
1001 Route 9 North/Suite 105 Zip: 07731
Ph: (732) 625-1100 Fax: (732) 625-1110
- Agrawal, Neil, MD
- Agrawal, Stuti Shah, MD

M & M Pediatrics
70 Ramtown-Greenville Rd Zip: 07731
Ph: (732) 785-0300
- Maddatu, Elenito P., MD
- Maddatu, Rose Mylaine, MD

Mid-Atlantic Multi-Specialty Surgical
2356 US Highway 9/Suite B6 Zip: 07731
Ph: (732) 886-2252 Fax: (732) 886-2260
- Moss, Vance Joshaun, MD
- Moss, Vincent Lavaughn, MD

Pediatric Affiliates, PA
3508 Route 9 South Zip: 07731
Ph: (732) 905-9166 Fax: (732) 905-9380
- Dayal, Rashmi P., MD
- Verdi, Michelle Diane, DO

Pediatric Health, PA
4537 Route 9 North Zip: 07731
Ph: (732) 367-5717 Fax: (732) 367-6524
 Lopez,Claudio J., MD

Ramtown Medical Center LLC
225 Newtons Corner Road Zip: 07731
Ph: (732) 458-9760 Fax: (732) 458-9762
 Morreale,Diego A., MD
 Polizzi,Maria, MD

Regional Cancer Care Associates, LLC
4632 US Highway 9 Zip: 07731
Ph: (732) 367-1535 Fax: (732) 367-9514
 Katz,Randi J., DO
 Kunamneni,Raghu Krishna, MD
 Nahum,Kenneth D., DO
 Soliman,Monir Louis Hanna, MD

Irvington
Healthcheck Medical And Eye Center
40 Union Avenue Zip: 07111
Ph: (973) 399-6270
 Bush,Nahndi, MD
 McCoy,Chrishonda Curry, MD

Hudson Physicians Associates
40 Union Avenue/Suite 204 Zip: 07111
Ph: (973) 416-6981 Fax: (973) 375-5766
 Banigo,Samuel, MD
 Okoya,Jackson A., MD
 Wilcox,Ellis I., MD

Irvington Community Health Center
1148-1150 Springfield Avenue Zip: 07111
Ph: (973) 399-6292 Fax: (973) 372-4534
 Isedeh,Cynthia O., DO

Irvington Pediatric Associates
22 Ball Street/Suite 100 Zip: 07111
Ph: (973) 371-1600 Fax: (973) 372-7677
 Lauredan,Bernier, MD
 Miller,Sandrene, MD

Newark Community Health Centers
9 Coit Street Zip: 07111
Ph: (973) 399-6292
 Brown,Patricia J., MD

Prime Heart
40 Union Avenue/Suite 101 Zip: 07111
Ph: (973) 371-3166
 Patel,Sunil, MD
 Patel,Sunil Madhusuda, MD

Prime Pediatrics
50 Union Avenue/Suite 704 Zip: 07111
Ph: (973) 373-9600
 Mammen-Prasad,Elizabeth K., MD

Rudolph C. Willis, Inc.
12 Krotik Place Zip: 07111
Ph: (973) 373-3000
 Ijehsedeh,Anthony, MD
 Willis,Rudolph C., MD

Iselin
Assocs in Cardiology & Internal Med
530 Green Street Zip: 08830
Ph: (732) 283-0440 Fax: (732) 283-8943
 Bhatnagar,Vibhay, MD
 Chaudhery,Shaukat A., MD
 Patel,Ravindra I., MD

Avenel Iselin Medical Group
400 Gill Lane Zip: 08830
Ph: (732) 404-1580 Fax: (732) 404-1594
 Gupta,Swati, MD
 Husain,Aftab, MD
 Lubin-Baskin,Alicia F., DO
 Maccia,Clement A., MD
 Mayer,Marc, DO
 Mayer,Mitchell F., DO
 Perilstein,Neil J., MD
 Riggi,Joseph, DO
 Song,Sang Ho, DO

Bay Obstetrics & Gynecology
740 US Highway 1 North Zip: 08830
Ph: (732) 362-3840 Fax: (732) 362-3850
 Berkman,Steven R., MD
 Divino,Eumena M., MD
 Goldberg,Steven C., MD

ENT & Allergy Associates, LLP
485 Route 1 South/Bld B/Suite 350 Zip: 08830
Ph: (732) 549-3934 Fax: (732) 549-7250
 Ambrosio,Patrick M., DO

 Mazzara,Carl Arthur, MD
 Mehta,Vishvesh Mukur, MD
 Ort,Stuart A., MD
 Rosin,Deborah F., MD
 Waqar,Shaan M., MD

Omni Eye Services
485 Route 1 South/Building A Zip: 08830
Ph: (732) 750-0400 Fax: (732) 602-0749
 Grayson,Douglas Keane, MD
 Napolitano,Joseph Daniel, MD
 Patel,Menka Sanghvi, MD
 Strauss,Danielle Savitsky, MD

Prudent MD
5 Dundee Avenue Zip: 08830
Ph: (732) 404-0044 Fax: (732) 218-3933
 Golubchik,Anneta V., MD

Jackson
Drs. Qudsi & Pawa
27 South Cooks Bridge Road/Suite 2-21 Zip: 08527
Ph: (732) 987-5733 Fax: (732) 987-5729
 Pawa,Anil K., MD
 Qudsi,Tehsin Riaz, MD

Family Practice of CentraState-Jackson
161 Bartley Road Zip: 08527
Ph: (732) 363-6140 Fax: (732) 363-6196
 Ignacio,Cristina Usi, MD
 Pedowitz,Robert Neil, DO
 Raymond,Joshua Joseph, MD

Jackson Family Medicine
27 South Cooks Bridge Road/Suite 2-1 Zip: 08527
Ph: (732) 367-0166 Fax: (732) 367-7220
 Druckman,Scott Jonathan, DO
 Lee,Nelson, DO
 Parkes,Lauren H., DO
 Rodriguez-Bostock,Susan M., MD

My MD Group
201 North County Line Road Zip: 08527
Ph: (732) 901-8880 Fax: (732) 901-0882
 Patel,Shruti, MD
 Sharma,Nivedita, MD

Northeast Spine and Sports Medicine
728 Bennetts Mills Road Zip: 08527
Ph: (732) 415-1401 Fax: (732) 415-1403
 Hsu,Kevin Kaiwen, MD

Ocean County Family Care
27 South Cooks Bridge Road Zip: 08527
Ph: (732) 364-3881 Fax: (732) 364-4625
 Kulczycki,Alexander, MD

Professional Associates of Jackson, LL
2105 West County Line Road/Suite 4 Zip: 08527
Ph: (732) 367-7575 Fax: (732) 364-0600
 Kumar,Sanjay, MD
 Shah,Mukesh Chinubhai, MD

Shore Nephrology, PA
27 South Cookbridge Road/Suite 211 Zip: 08527
Ph: (732) 987-5990 Fax: (732) 987-5994
 Kaur,Harneet, MD

Jamesburg
Central Jersey Lung Center
333 Forsgate Drive/Suite 201 Zip: 08831
Ph: (732) 521-3131 Fax: (732) 521-1116
 Carlucci,Michael Louis, MD
 Fein,Edward Dennis, MD

Garden State Heart Care, P.C.
333 Forsgate Drive/Suite 205 Zip: 08831
Ph: (732) 851-4700
 Bordieri,Joseph Anthony, DO
 Newman,Jared Brad, DO

Princeton Orthopaedic Associates, P.A.
11 Centre Drive Zip: 08831
Ph: (609) 655-4848
 Jolley,Michael N., MD

Princeton Radiation Oncology Center
9 Centre Drive/Suite 115 Zip: 08831
Ph: (609) 655-5755 Fax: (609) 655-5725
 Greenberg,Andrew Seth, MD

Jersey City
American Physician Serv/Hudson Health
679 Montgomery Street Zip: 07306
Ph: (201) 433-6500 Fax: (201) 433-8010
 Anemelu,Ignatius I., MD

 Clemente,Jose D., MD
 Francois,Vincent, MD
 Kapadia,Bhupendra A., MD
 Llarena,Ramon C., MD
 Mapp,Samuel Eugene, MD
 Moeller,Lavinia Paige, DO
 Sagullo,Nestor M., MD
 Viloria,Edermiro, MD

Arthritis Center of New Jersey
600 Pavonia Avenue/5th Floor Zip: 07306
Ph: (201) 216-3050 Fax: (201) 499-0254
 Brandt,Frederick W., MD
 Scarpa,Nicholas P., MD

Assoc Eye Physicians & Surgeons of NJ
724 Jersey Avenue Zip: 07302
Ph: (201) 795-0808 Fax: (201) 795-9797
 Hershkin,Paige B., DO

Better Skin Dermatology, LLC
100 Town Square/Suite 409 Zip: 07310
Ph: (201) 626-4040 Fax: (201) 626-4041
 Besedina,Liliya, MD
 Khasak,Dmitry, MD

Cardiovascular Associates of NJ, P.A.
377 Jersey Avenue/Suite 410 Zip: 07302
Ph: (201) 200-0318 Fax: (201) 200-0319
 Hamirani,Kamran Ismail, MD

Center for Children with Special Needs
953 Garfield Avenue Zip: 07304
Ph: (201) 915-2059 Fax: (201) 915-2551
 Dehnert,Michele Chun, MD
 Sy-Te,Emilie, MD

Combine Hematology Oncology
210 Palisade Avenue Zip: 07306
Ph: (201) 963-2213 Fax: (201) 963-7070
 Druck,Mark, MD
 Palathingal,Rini M., MD

DRS Medical Associates
115 Christopher Columbus Drive Zip: 07302
Ph: (201) 706-3808 Fax: (201) 369-8032
 Santos,Ray Ryan Crisostomo, MD
 Sharma,Ritu, MD

Dermatology Affiliates
2954 Kennedy Boulevard/2nd Floor Zip: 07306
Ph: (201) 653-5555
 Katz,Arthur M., MD
 Noroff,Joan P., MD

Dr. Joven Dungo/NJ Impotence Ctr
205 9th Street Zip: 07302
Ph: (201) 653-1144 Fax: (201) 653-6104
 Chan,Florence Y., MD
 Dungo,Joven P., MD
 Leyson,Jose Flotcante J., MD

Drs. Abubakar and Abubakar
452 Central Avenue Zip: 07307
Ph: (201) 222-0821 Fax: (201) 222-1018
 Abubakar,Ahmed B., MD
 Abubakar,Shaik, MD

Drs. Ahmed, Haddad & Batwara
26 Greenville Avenue Zip: 07305
Ph: (201) 333-8222 Fax: (201) 333-0095
 Ahmed,Umrana, MD
 Goel,Narender, MD
 Haddad,Bassam M., MD
 Haddad,Danny B., MD
 Jain,Deepika, MD

Drs. Badin, De Silva, and Perera
1947 Kennedy Boulevard Zip: 07305
Ph: (201) 433-4848 Fax: (201) 946-9292
 Badin,Diane, MD
 Badin,Michel S., MD
 Badin,Simon, MD
 De Silva,Malika Shani, MD
 Perera,Sharmalie, MD

Drs. Barber and Dizon
377 Jersey Avenue/Suite 460 Zip: 07302
Ph: (201) 332-4110 Fax: (201) 332-4122
 Barber,Nathaniel A., MD
 Dizon,Alita L., MD

Drs. Digioia & Singh
1971 Kennedy Boulevard Zip: 07305
Ph: (201) 432-5222 Fax: (201) 333-2503
 Digioia,John J. Jr., MD

 Singh,Bharat, MD

Drs. Elamir & El Amir
192 Harrison Avenue Zip: 07304
Ph: (201) 333-5363 Fax: (201) 333-4710
 El Amir,Mazhar E., MD
 Elamir,Mohammed, MD

Drs. Gandhi and Roy
3665 Kennedy Boulevard Zip: 07306
Ph: (201) 963-1155 Fax: (201) 963-7957
 Gandhi,Kirit V., MD

Drs. Patel & Patel
237 Central Avenue Zip: 07307
Ph: (201) 656-2999 Fax: (201) 656-8676
 Patel,Vinodkumar G., MD
 Yin,Chun Hui, MD

Drs. Phung and Phung
596 Pavonia Avenue Zip: 07306
Ph: (201) 792-4996 Fax: (201) 792-9663
 Phung,Michael Hung, MD
 Phung,Susan, MD

Drs. Politis and Kaki
3526 Kennedy Boulevard Zip: 07307
Ph: (201) 653-5933 Fax: (201) 653-3930
 Kaki,Sushma R., MD
 Politis,Regina, MD

Drs. Quraishi & Seman
1 Chopin Court Zip: 07302
Ph: (201) 333-8111
 Quraishi,Abid Nisar, MD
 Seman,Ahmed B., MD

Drs. Rizvi & Rizvi
151 Jewett Avenue Zip: 07304
Ph: (201) 920-9926
 Rizvi,Anwar Ahmad, MD
 Rizvi,Sardar Ahmad, MD

Drs. Tolentino & Irving MD PA
600 Pavonia Avenue/7th Floor Zip: 07306
Ph: (201) 216-9300 Fax: (201) 216-0091
 Irving,Henry C. III, MD
 Tolentino,Ernesto A., MD

Feridoun Rezai MD PC
550 Newark Avenue/Suite 307 Zip: 07306
Ph: (201) 963-8448 Fax: (201) 963-6165
 Rezai,Feridoun, MD

Gastroenterology Med Assocs PA
142 Palisades Avenue/Suite 201 Zip: 07307
Ph: (201) 792-7788 Fax: (201) 792-7812
 Bhatia,Taruna, MD

Grove Medical Associates
129 Newark Avenue Zip: 07302
Ph: (201) 451-8867 Fax: (201) 451-2819
 Chinai,Ronak N., MD
 Velpari,Sudarshan, MD

Horizon Health Center
714 Bergen Avenue Zip: 07306
Ph: (201) 451-6300
 Fernandez,Osbert, MD
 Gressock,Joseph Neal, MD
 Roque,Cesar Ruben Jr., MD
 Ventura,Evelyn Ortiz, MD

Horizon Health Ctr/Family Med
412 Summit Avenue Zip: 07306
Ph: (201) 963-5774 Fax: (201) 963-8274
 Cruz,Wilfredo Tomas Correa, MD

Hudson Eye Physicians & Surgeons, LLC
600 Pavonia Avenue/6th Floor Zip: 07306
Ph: (201) 963-3937 Fax: (201) 963-8823
 Cinotti,Donald J., MD
 Constad,William H., MD
 Maltzman,Barry A., MD
 Origlieri,Catherine Ann, MD
 Walsman,Scott Michael, MD

Hudson Hematology Oncolgny
377 Jersey Avenue/Suite 160 Zip: 07302
Ph: (201) 333-8248 Fax: (201) 333-8469
 Ghuman,Damanjit K., MD
 Patel,Amit A., MD
 Raccuia,Joseph Salvatore, MD
 Talwar,Sumit, MD
 Zarubin,Vadim, MD

Groups and Clinics by Town with Physician Rosters

Jersey City (cont)

Hudson Neurosciences PC
142 Palisade Avenue/Suite 205 Zip: 07306
Ph: (201) 798-2453 Fax: (201) 216-9211
- Anselmi, Gregory D., MD

Hudson Surgeons
142 Palisade Avenue/Suite 108 Zip: 07306
Ph: (201) 795-0101 Fax: (201) 795-3550
- Khawaja, Aftab A., MD

Integrative Obstetrics
21 McWilliams Place Zip: 07302
Ph: (201) 691-8664 Fax: (844) 886-6072
- Ratzersdorfer, Jonathan, MD
- Resnikoff-Gary, Amanda Nicole, MD

James G. Sanderson Family Practice
3 Webster Avenue Zip: 07307
Ph: (201) 216-1505 Fax: (201) 216-8803
- Maiello, Dominic J., MD
- Sanderson, James Glen, DO

Jersey Womens Care Center
435 Central Avenue Zip: 07307
Ph: (201) 217-5600
- Hou, Hui Ying, MD
- Ramirez, Elizabeth, MD

Kenneth Sung Soo Chang MD PA
3144 Kennedy Boulevard Zip: 07306
Ph: (201) 792-9339 Fax: (201) 792-9818
- Chang, James Kenneth, MD
- Chang, Kenneth Sung Soo, MD

Liberty Behavioral Health
395 Grand Avenue Zip: 07302
Ph: (201) 915-2278
- Hernandez, Victor F., MD
- Zamora, Violeta C., MD

Liberty Medical Associates
377 Jersey Avenue/Suite 470 Zip: 07302
Ph: (201) 918-2239 Fax: (201) 918-2243
- Ameen, Abdul Aleem, MD
- Brannan, Timothy S., MD
- Escobar-Barboza, Vanessa, MD
- Flores, David, MD
- Grigoriu, Adriana, MD
- Lazo, Angel Amado Jr., MD
- Matta, Jyoti S., MD
- Mikkilineni, Rao S., MD
- Nariseti, Chalapathy, MD
- Reisner, Michelle R., MD
- Weissman, Paul S., MD

Liberty Surgical Associates
355 Grand Street Zip: 07302
Ph: (201) 915-2450 Fax: (201) 915-2192
- Ha, Victor Vinh, MD
- Molino, Bruno, MD

Metropolitan Family Health Network
935 Garfield Avenue Zip: 07304
Ph: (201) 478-5800 Fax: (201) 475-5814
- Acierno, Lynne J., MD
- Barbara Mijares, Diego, MD
- Beaty, Patrick D., MD
- Carter, Cheryl Ann, MD
- Elliston, Jason Taiwo Jos, MD
- Fernandez, Fredy A., MD
- Franco, Maria M., MD
- Kranias, Hristos K., MD
- Oparaji, Anthony Chibuzor, MD
- Pellecchia, Ralph Joseph, MD

Midland Medical Associates, LLC
2726 Kennedy Boulevard Zip: 07306
Ph: (201) 333-4115 Fax: (201) 333-6224
- Cabales, Arthur L., MD
- Cabales, Victor L., MD

Midtown Primary Care LLC
550 Newark Avenue/Suite 308 Zip: 07306
Ph: (201) 656-2300 Fax: (201) 656-2390
- Boylan, Edward F., MD

NYU Langon Dept.of Orthopaedic Surgery
377 Jersey Avenue/Suite 280A Zip: 07302
Ph: (201) 716-5851 Fax: (201) 309-2432
- Capo, John Thomas, MD
- Liporace, Frank Anthony, MD

New Margaret Hague Women's Health
377 Jersey Avenue/Suite 220 Zip: 07302
Ph: (201) 795-9155 Fax: (201) 795-9157
- Bimonte, Michael J., MD
- Campbell, Damali M., MD
- Gagliardi, Carol L., MD
- Hu, Long-Gue, MD
- Nichols, Rhonda R., MD
- Witter, Theodore O., MD
- Youssef, Jan Samir, MD

Newport Medical Associates
610 Washington Boulevard Zip: 07310
Ph: (201) 222-1266
- Ansay, Editha Santillan, MD
- Bhatt, Pranay Janardan, MD

NHCAC Health Center at Jersey City
324 Palisade Avenue Zip: 07306
Ph: (201) 459-8888 Fax: (201) 459-8872
- Bobb-Mckoy, Marion Y., MD
- Jenkins, Lisa Michelle, MD
- Surti, Daxa Bhupendra, MD

PMA Physicians LLC
1 Journal Square Plaza/2nd Floor Zip: 07306
Ph: (201) 216-3030 Fax: (201) 499-0247
- Munne, Gisela L., MD
- Patel, Ramiladevi S., MD
- Rotella, Frank A., DO
- Sklower, Jay A., DO

Padmavathi Jonnalagadda MD PA
3438 JF Kennedy Boulevard Zip: 07307
Ph: (201) 420-0366 Fax: (201) 420-6422
- Jonnalagadda, Padmavathi, MD
- Jonnalagadda, Vasudeva Rao, MD

Pain & Disability Institute, P.C.
191 Palisade Avenue Zip: 07302
Ph: (201) 656-4324
- Mehta, Ariz Ruyintan, MD
- Mehta, Monica R., MD

Palisade Eye Associates
203 Palisade Avenue Zip: 07306
Ph: (201) 653-5722 Fax: (201) 792-9718
- Cervenak-Panariello, Betty, MD
- Panariello, Anthony L., MD
- Rau, Ganesh U., MD

Palisades Behavioral Care
221 Palisade Avenue Zip: 07306
Ph: (201) 656-3116 Fax: (201) 656-9044
- Hasaj, Mario Jorge, MD
- Kurani, Devendra, MD
- Quintana, Jorge D., MD
- Vinuela, Andres, MD

Pediatric Care P.A.
3342 Kennedy Boulevard Zip: 07307
Ph: (201) 653-8999 Fax: (201) 653-4477
- Tan, Vicente G., MD

Portside Medical
150 Warren Street/Suite 118 Zip: 07302
Ph: (201) 309-3000 Fax: (201) 309-1300
- Patel, Roshni Dinesh, DO
- Schehr-Kimble, Danielle Jessica, DO

Riverside ENT Pediatric Group
324 Palisade Avenue/2nd Floor Zip: 07307
Ph: (201) 386-1400 Fax: (201) 386-2343
- Calero-Bai, Rosario, MD
- Ramasubramaniam, Nagarani, MD
- Santos-Borja, Concepcion L., MD

Sovereign Oncology, LLC.
631 Grand Street Zip: 07304
Ph: (201) 942-3999 Fax: (201) 942-3998
- El Gazzar, Yaser S., MD

The Spine & Sports Health Center
129 Newark Avenue Zip: 07302
Ph: (201) 533-9200 Fax: (201) 533-9299
- Bhatnagar, Tanuj, MD

Total Cardiology Care
120 Franklin Street Zip: 07307
Ph: (201) 216-9791 Fax: (201) 216-1362
- Abed, Mary T., MD
- Ahmad, Ahsanuddin, MD
- Baruchin, Mitchell Alan, MD
- Hupart, Preston Arthur, DO
- Shah, Nalini Arvindkumar, MD
- Thota, Sreevani, MD

Total Care Pediatrics in Jersey City
550 Newark Avenue/Suite 200 Zip: 07306
Ph: (201) 714-7902 Fax: (201) 795-4999
- Kozanitis Mentakis, Irene D., MD
- Lipert, Zofia J., MD
- Nagorna, Malgorzata, MD

Tribeca Pediatrics
9 McWilliams Place Zip: 07302
Ph: (201) 706-7175 Fax: (201) 604-6553
- Newman, Brigitte Jeanne, MD
- Quim, Marinelle De Los Santos, MD
- Varma, Mekhla, MD

UMDNJ Dept Of Orthopaedics
90 Bergen Street/DOC 1200 Zip: 07305
Ph: (973) 972-2150
- Ahmed, Irfan Haroon, MD
- Beebe, Kathleen Sue, MD

Westside Medical Associates
562 West Side Avenue Zip: 07304
Ph: (201) 434-7800 Fax: (201) 434-6715
- Khan, Rizwana, MD
- Pizarro, Oscar N., MD

Keansburg

Drs. Abrina & Tsai
319 Main Street/Suite B4 Zip: 07734
Ph: (732) 787-0568 Fax: (732) 787-0270
- Abrina, Vanessa Mae S., MD
- Tsai, Anderson F., MD

Kearny

Academic Dermotology & Dermatologic
703 Kearny Avenue Zip: 07032
Ph: (201) 998-4699
- Fishman, S. Jose, MD

Contemporary Women's Care
338 Belleville Turnpike Zip: 07032
Ph: (201) 991-3838 Fax: (201) 998-4643
- Graf, Jennifer A., DO
- Herrighty, Marianne K., MD
- Surmeli, Sedat M., MD

Drs. Padykula and Skripkus
381 Kearny Avenue Zip: 07032
Ph: (201) 991-4824 Fax: (201) 991-7465
- Padykula, Anna, MD
- Skripkus, Aldona J., MD

Emad Jacob, MD PC
714 Kearney Avenue Zip: 07032
Ph: (201) 772-5211 Fax: (201) 428-1627
- Daoko, Joseph, MD
- Jacob, Emad, MD

Kendall Park

24/7 Heart and Vascular
3084 State Route 27/Suite 5 Zip: 08824
OnlyFax: (800) 336-7779
- Huang, Michael Shu Hsien, DO
- Patel, Alpesh Babu, MD

Central NJ Allergy Asthma Associates
3084 State Route 27/Suite 6 Zip: 08824
Ph: (732) 821-0595 Fax: (732) 821-1174
- Kesarwala, Hemant, MD
- Zuckerman, Gary B., MD

Medical Associates of Marlboro, P.C.
3084 State Route 27/Suite 1 Zip: 08824
Ph: (732) 821-0873 Fax: (732) 297-7356
- Vallabhaneni, Purnima, MD

Princeton Radiology Associates, P.A.
3674 Route 27 Zip: 08824
Ph: (732) 821-5563 Fax: (732) 821-6675
- Balgowan, Dennis, MD
- Flannery, Todd W., MD
- Fontanilla, Hiral P., MD
- Garnet, Daniel, MD
- Greene, Samuel James, MD
- Hug, Eugene Boris, MD
- Leder, David S., MD
- Nemade, Ajay B., MD
- Pepek, Joseph M., MD
- Rodrigues, Neesha Ann, MD
- Rubbert-Slawek, Kerstin Anke, MD
- Schlesinger, Fred H., MD
- Tenenzapf, Mark J., MD

Respiratory & Sleep Specialists, LLC.
3546 State Route 27 Zip: 08824
Ph: (732) 737-7801 Fax: (877) 632-3456
- Khan, Wajahat Hussain, MD
- Koganti, Monika, MD

Robert Wood Johnson Ob-Gyn Associates
3270 State Route 27/Suite 2200 Zip: 08824
Ph: (732) 422-8989 Fax: (732) 422-4526
- Caban, Michelle, MD
- Colonna, Elizabeth Ann, MD
- Ham, Antoinette Lucy, MD
- Kim, Eugene J., MD
- Lundberg, John L., MD
- Segal, Joshua Howard, MD

Spectrum Medical Associates
3250 State Route 27/Suite 103 Zip: 08824
Ph: (732) 398-9100 Fax: (732) 398-9105
- Kamath, Sudha P., MD
- Mongia, Rupa, MD

Kinnelon

Eric Shnayder MD PC
11 Kiel Avenue/2nd Floor Zip: 07405
Ph: (973) 838-7722 Fax: (973) 838-3579
- Shnayder, Eric, MD

Kinnelon Medical & Pediatric Assoc
170 Kinnelon Road/Suite 28 Zip: 07405
Ph: (973) 838-7650
- Suda, Abhay K., MD
- Suda, Anjuli, MD
- Vijaysadan, Viju, MD

Lafayette

In Health Associates
15 State Route 15 Zip: 07848
Ph: (973) 579-6700 Fax: (973) 579-6830
- Baliga, Ravi, MD
- Laveman, Lawrence B., MD
- Squires, Sandra, MD

Lake Hopatcong

Skylands Medical Group PA
174 Edison Road Zip: 07849
Ph: (973) 663-1300
- Bonnet, Jean-Paul, DO
- Orlandoni, Enrico F., DO

Lakehurst

Physicians for Adults
681 Route 70 Zip: 08733
Ph: (732) 657-8111
- Comsti, Eric A., MD
- Pineda, Julita S., MD
- Pineda, Nonato E., MD

Lakewood

Brielle Obstetrics & Gynecology, P.A.
117 County Line Road Zip: 08701
Ph: (732) 942-1900 Fax: (732) 942-1919
- Chang, Joanne Meejin, MD

Cataract & Laser Institute, P.A.
101 Prospect Street/Suite 102 Zip: 08701
Ph: (732) 367-0699 Fax: (732) 367-0937
- Huppert, Leon J., MD

Chemed Family Health Center
1771 Madison Avenue Zip: 08701
Ph: (732) 364-2144 Fax: (732) 364-3559
- Bacon, Shoshana, MD
- Berghaus, Jean E., MD
- Gwertzman, Rachel, DO
- Hirsch, Harvey Alan, MD
- Kaweblum, Jaime, MD
- Krohn, David Isaac, MD
- Pitsos, Miltiadis, MD
- Uderman, Howard David, MD

Coastal Urology Associates
814 River Avenue Zip: 08701
Ph: (732) 370-2250 Fax: (732) 901-9119
- Bellingham, Charles E., MD

Dr. Gittleman & Associates
450 East Kennedy Boulevard Zip: 08701
Ph: (732) 901-0050 Fax: (732) 370-2386
- Gittleman, Neal D., MD
- Lekht, Inna, MD
- Ukraincik, Miro, MD
- Wong, Karen Clark, MD

Drs. Indich and Deutsch
619 West County Line Road Zip: 08701
Ph: (732) 730-9111 Fax: (732) 730-9154
- Indich, Norman, MD

Groups and Clinics by Town with Physician Rosters

Drs. Mohan & Singh
101 Prospect Street/Suite 210   Zip: 08701
Ph: (732) 905-8877   Fax: (732) 363-4584
  Mohan,Rajesh, MD
  Singh,Satyendra Pratap, MD

Gastroenterology Associates
475 State Highway 70   Zip: 08701
Ph: (732) 886-1007   Fax: (732) 224-8773
  Kurtz,Joel H., MD
  Musicant,Joel Marc, MD

Invision, Inc.
One Route 70   Zip: 08701
Ph: (732) 905-5600
  Hedaya,Edward L., MD
  Hernandez,Yanill, MD
  Von Roemer,Marc, MD

Jersey Shore Medical & Pediatric Assoc
1215 Route 70 West/Suite 1005   Zip: 08701
Ph: (732) 942-0888   Fax: (732) 942-1230
  Morelos,Joseph C., DO
  Talamayan,Randy P. C., MD

Kuflik Dermatology
150 East Kennedy Boulevard   Zip: 08701
Ph: (732) 364-0515   Fax: (732) 364-6006
  Kuflik,Julianne Helen, MD

Lakewood Pediatric Associates
101 Prospect Street/Suite 112   Zip: 08701
Ph: (732) 363-1424   Fax: (732) 370-0714
  Jain,Suman Singhal, MD
  Rana,Mukti, MD
  Stavrellis,Steve John, MD

Monmouth Medical Group, P.C.
1 Route 70   Zip: 08701
Ph: (732) 901-0211   Fax: (732) 901-0199
  Genovese,Cynthia Marie, MD
  Salcedo,Elizabeth O., MD

Ocean Cardiology
1166 River Avenue   Zip: 08701
Ph: (732) 905-4142   Fax: (732) 905-4160
  Bacharach,Moshe, MD
  Kadosh,Yisrael, MD

Ocean County Family Care
400 New Hampshire Avenue   Zip: 08701
Ph: (732) 901-6400   Fax: (732) 901-0744
  Mahan,Janet L., MD

Ocean County Internal Medicine Assoc
1352 River Avenue   Zip: 08701
Ph: (732) 370-5100   Fax: (732) 901-9240
  Cohen,Jonathan, MD
  Cohen,Jonathan Ira, MD
  Green,Tamar Buchsbaum, MD
  Lempel,Allen L., MD
  Ogun,David J., MD

Ocean Gyn & Obstet Associates
475 Highway 70   Zip: 08701
Ph: (732) 364-8000   Fax: (732) 364-4601
  Cahill,Kenneth Matthew, DO
  Cocco,Frank A., MD
  Lehnes,Eric G., MD
  Molina,Arthur M., MD
  Repole,Adam N., MD

Ocean Health Initiatives, Inc.
101 Second Street   Zip: 08701
Ph: (732) 363-6655   Fax: (732) 363-6656
  Jilani,Usman Khan, MD
  Lanez,Charisma Ann, DO
  Lorenzo,Judith, MD
  Moghe,Vaishali C., MD
  Patterson,Marion Lesley, MD
  Phelps,Kristyn Kia, MD
  Saunders,Kyauna Sharae, MD
  Sopeju,Temilola Adedayo, MD
  Young,Tiffany, DO
  Zafarani,Amy Jo, DO

PLUS Diagnostics
1200 River Avenue/Suite 10   Zip: 08701
Ph: (732) 901-7575   Fax: (732) 901-1555
  Ata,Hadia M., MD
  Bhattacharjee,Pradip, MD
  Chatterjee,Monica, MD
  Engelbach,Ludmila, MD
  Fromowitz,Frank B., MD
  Guo,Yijun, MD
  Kartika,Gunawan, MD
  Li,Rongshan, MD
  Mahapatro,Darshana, MD
  Pai,Usha Laxman, MD
  Romerocaces,Gloria Marcelo, MD
  Sharaan,Mona El-Sayed, MD
  Shen,Tingliang, MD
  Strand,Calvin L., MD
  Vara,Manjula L., MD

Retina Associates of New Jersey, P.A.
525 Route 70 West/Suite B-14   Zip: 08701
Ph: (732) 363-2396   Fax: (732) 363-0403
  Chinskey,Nicholas Daniel, MD

Shore Medical Specialists
500 River Avenue/Suite 140   Zip: 08701
Ph: (732) 363-7200   Fax: (732) 367-4461
  Chakrapani,Soumya, MD

Shore Medical Specialists
500 River Avenue   Zip: 08701
Ph: (732) 363-7200   Fax: (732) 367-4461
  Chander,Harish, MD
  Kandathil,Mathew K., MD
  Maron,Edward M., MD
  Patel,Akshay D., MD
  Patel,Manoj, MD
  Patel,Sandipkumar R., MD
  Pineles,Cary L., MD

Shore Orthopaedic Group
1255 Route 70/Suite 11S   Zip: 08701
Ph: (732) 942-2300   Fax: (732) 942-2311
  Absatz,Michael G., MD

Shore Point Radiation Oncology
900 Route 70   Zip: 08701
Ph: (732) 901-7333   Fax: (732) 370-1294
  Berkowitz,Stewart A., MD
  Marchese,Michael J., MD

Women's Health Associates
101 Prospect Street/Suite 202   Zip: 08701
Ph: (732) 942-4442
  Culbert,Steven A., MD
  Greenstein,Gary David, MD
  Hoffman,Christian T. III, MD

Lambertville

Phillips Barber Family Health Center
72 Alexander Avenue   Zip: 08530
Ph: (609) 397-3535   Fax: (609) 397-0301
  Barter,Cindy Monette, MD
  Burgos,Melissa, MD
  Chen,Victoria Sheen, MD
  Eichman,Margaret J., MD
  Giangrante,Matthew E., MD
  Koorie,Elizabeth L., MD
  Lei,Michaela, DO
  Meyer,Monica Ann, MD
  Mooney,Kevin K., MD
  Raleigh,Elizabeth Ann, DO
  Schmitt,David J., MD
  Sokkar,Rita, DO
  Waters,John S., MD

Premier Family Healthcare PC
24 Arnett Avenue/Suite 105 First Floor
Zip: 08530
Ph: (609) 397-1775   Fax: (609) 397-1545
  Russo,Frances Jenny, DO
  Russo,Steven, MD

Landing

Skylands Medical Group PA
150 Lakeside Boulevard   Zip: 07850
Ph: (973) 398-6300   Fax: (973) 398-6399
  Damico,Christopher R., DO
  Purcell,Joseph W., DO
  Shah,Shefali A., DO

Lanoka Harbor

Comprehensive Medical Associates
411 Route 9/Suite 6   Zip: 08734
Ph: (609) 971-1711   Fax: (609) 971-3390
  Fernando-Flores,Avelina M., MD
  Tauro,Victor, MD

Lakewood Pediatrics Associates
500 Route 9/3B   Zip: 08734
Ph: (609) 693-8131
  Mehta,Sunita, MD

Lawrenceville

Ahmad Syed S MD PA
183 Franklin Corner Road   Zip: 08648
Ph: (609) 896-0622
  Ahmad,Syed S., MD
  Lou,William, MD
  Mathew,Saritha, MD

Alliance Dermatology Associates
3311 Brunswick Pike   Zip: 08648
Ph: (609) 799-1600   Fax: (609) 799-1677
  Kincaid,Leah Celia, MD
  Rajan,Jennifer Ray, MD
  Yi,Lusia Sang-suk, DO

Becker ENT
2 Princess Road/Suite East   Zip: 08648
Ph: (610) 303-5163   Fax: (610) 303-5164
  Lupa,Michael David, MD

Capital Health Primary Care
4056 Quakerbridge Road/Suite 101   Zip: 08648
Ph: (609) 528-9150   Fax: (609) 528-9151
  Chung,Y. C. Emily, MD
  Laskarzewski,Radhika, MD
  Levitt,Kimberly Anne, MD
  Rose,Abigail Lee, MD
  Wasti,Naila H., MD
  Young,Jill F., DO

Delaware Valley Ob/Gyn
2 Princess Road/Suite C   Zip: 08648
Ph: (609) 896-0777   Fax: (609) 896-3266
  Goyal,Shefali, MD
  Hall,Lanniece F., MD
  Hilsenrath,Robin Elaine, MD
  Pierce,Bruce R., MD
  Proctor,Asha K., MD
  Sarma,Bani A., MD
  Ung,Kenneth H., MD

Delaware Valley Pediatric Assoc
132 Franklin Corner Road   Zip: 08648
Ph: (609) 896-4141   Fax: (609) 896-3940
  Halvorsen,Julie Beth, DO
  Lilienfeld,Harris C., MD
  Palsky,Glenn S., MD
  Shapiro,Eugene, MD

Delaware Valley Retina Associates
4 Princess Road/Suite 101   Zip: 08648
Ph: (609) 896-1414   Fax: (609) 896-2982
  Ie,Darmakusuma, MD
  Lipkowitz,Jeffrey L., MD
  Shah,Kekul Bharat, MD

Drs. Desai & Yanamadula
123 Franklin Corner Road/Suite 104   Zip: 08648
Ph: (609) 512-1690   Fax: (609) 512-1674
  Desai,Bharat V., MD

Drs. Hardy and Eisengart
3131 Princeton Pike   Zip: 08648
Ph: (609) 896-1700   Fax: (609) 896-1087
  Eisengart,Charles Andrew, MD
  Hardy,Howard III, MD

Endocrinology Associates of Princeton
168 Franklin Corner Road   Zip: 08648
Ph: (609) 896-0075   Fax: (609) 896-0079
  Dadzie,Daphne D., MD
  Fresca,Diane Elizabeth, MD
  Hollander,Jason Michael, MD
  Vergano,Sefton Cappi, MD

Institute for Spine & Scoliosis, P.A.
3100 Princeton Pike/Building 1   Zip: 08648
Ph: (609) 912-1500   Fax: (609) 912-1600
  Antonacci,Mark Darryl, MD
  Betz,Randal Roberts, MD
  Cuddihy,Laury A., MD

Lawrence Medical Associates PA
2999 Princeton Pike   Zip: 08648
Ph: (609) 882-2299   Fax: (609) 538-8230
  Adler,Scott L., MD
  Borrus,Stephen W., MD

Lawrence Ob/Gyn Associates
123 Franklin Corner Road/Suite 214   Zip: 08648
Ph: (609) 896-1400   Fax: (609) 896-3986
  Firdu,Tikikil, MD
  Funches,Judith Melton, MD
  Grant,Gwendolyn Hunter, DO
  Leedom,Karen Ann, MD
  Loeb,Paul Norman, DO
  Patel,Amy, MD
  Przybylko,Kira L., MD
  Safi,Farnaz, MD
  Small,Daniel Alan, MD
  Stanell,William P., MD
  Tashjian,Audrey Brigitta, MD

Lawrenceville Internal Medicine Assoc
3100 Princeton Pike/Building 4/Suite I   Zip: 08648
Ph: (609) 896-0303   Fax: (609) 896-0308
  Osias,Kimberly Beth, MD
  Werbel,Sarah A., MD

Lawrenceville Neurology Center, PA
3131 Princeton Pike   Zip: 08648
Ph: (609) 896-1701   Fax: (609) 896-3735
  Alexeeva,Aissa Timofeyevna, MD
  Gomez,Rene S., MD
  Kaiser,Paul K., MD
  Palangio,Kimberly Dawn, MD
  Vergara,Manuel Salvador, MD

LifeCare Physicians, PC of Lawrencevil
4 Princess Road/Suite 209   Zip: 08648
Ph: (609) 895-0770   Fax: (609) 896-1124
  McGeever,Rose, DO
  Romano,Carmen J., MD

Mercer Bucks Cardiology
3140 Princeton Pike/2nd Floor   Zip: 08648
Ph: (609) 895-1919   Fax: (609) 895-1200
  Al-Bezem,Rim, MD
  Costanzo,William Edward, MD
  Drucker,David Wayne, MD
  Goldsmith,Steven Matthew, MD
  Heyrich,George Patrick, MD
  Hyman,Richard Louis, MD
  Karl,Justin Adam, MD
  Lebovitz,Philip Lewis, MD
  Rosvold,David Nelson, MD
  Rozengarten,Michael Jacob, MD
  Stern,Alan G., MD
  Venkatesulu,Sunder, MD
  Wolfson,Keith Richard, MD
  Zacks,Eran Sol, MD

Mercer Eye Associates, PA
123 Franklin Corner Road/Suite 207   Zip: 08648
Ph: (609) 750-7300   Fax: (609) 896-7052
  Chiang,Robert Kent, MD
  Ellis,Steven P., MD

Mercer Neurology
2 Princess Road/Suite 2F   Zip: 08648
Ph: (609) 895-9000   Fax: (609) 895-1006
  DeLuca,Debra J., MD

Mercer-Bucks Orthopaedics PC
3120 Princeton Pike   Zip: 08648
Ph: (609) 896-0444   Fax: (609) 896-1055
  Accardi,Kimberly Lynn Zambito, MD
  Ast,Michael Paul, MD
  Bills,Thomas K., MD
  Codjoe,Paul Winfred, MD
  Colarusso,Frank John Michael, DO
  Eingorn,David S., MD
  Gokcen,Eric C., MD
  Kothari,Gautam Himanshu, DO
  Nolan,John P. Jr., MD
  Patel,Rikin Jagdish, DO

Performance Spine & Sports Medicine
4056 Quakerbridge Road/Suite 111   Zip: 08648
Ph: (609) 588-8600   Fax: (609) 588-8602
  Ali,Adil, MD
  Wiederholz,Matthias Heinz, MD

Princeton Eye and Ear
2999 Princeton Pike/2 FL   Zip: 08648
Ph: (609) 403-8840   Fax: (609) 403-8852
  Patel,Rakesh Bhogilal, MD
  Shah,Angana Nayan, MD
  Shah,Chetan S., MD
  Shah,Chirag S., MD
  Undavia,Samir Suresh, MD

Groups and Clinics by Town with Physician Rosters

Lawrenceville (cont)
Princeton Family Care
100 Federal City Road/Suite A Zip: 08648
Ph: (609) 620-1380 Fax: (609) 771-8991
  Jose, Jaison, DO
  Khan, Aliya W., MD
  Punj, Priti Narula, MD
  Shaikh, Nasir Hussain A., MD

Princeton Pike Internal Medicine
3100 Princeton Pike/Bldg 3/ 3rd Fl Zip: 08648
Ph: (609) 896-1793 Fax: (609) 896-1847
  Goldberg, Paul E., MD
  Gomes, Eric Arvind, MD
  Lee, Peter, MD
  Weinstein, Mark J., MD

Princeton Sports & Family Medicine
3131 Princeton Pike Zip: 08648
Ph: (609) 896-9190 Fax: (609) 896-3555
  Barlis, Cara J., MD
  Hector, Christina, DO
  Levandowski, Richard, MD
  Stramandi, Danielle Nicole, MD
  Wenger, Peter Christopher, MD

Professional Healthcare Services
2500 US Highway 1 Zip: 08648
Ph: (609) 771-6660 Fax: (609) 530-0966
  Diamond, Shari E., DO

Rheumatology Center of Princeton
123 Franklin Corner Road/Suite 106 Zip: 08648
Ph: (609) 896-2505 Fax: (609) 896-2530
  Froncek, Michael Jude, MD

Total Eye Care Center
2495 Brunswick Pike/Suite 8 Zip: 08648
Ph: (609) 882-8828
  Lavrich, Judith Barbara, MD
  Stein, Harmon Charles, MD

Urology Care Alliance
2 Princess Road/Suite J Zip: 08648
Ph: (609) 895-1991 Fax: (609) 895-6996
  Cohen, Michael Scott, MD
  Fingerman, Jarad Scott, DO
  Freid, Russell Marc, MD

Urology Care Alliance
3311 Brunswick Pike Zip: 08648
Ph: (609) 895-1991 Fax: (609) 895-6996
  Harvey, Arthur James, MD
  Karlin, Gary S., MD
  Kuehn, Adam, MD
  Trivedi, Deep B., MD

Lebanon
Advanced Obstetrics & Gynecology
1390 Route 22 West/Suite 104 Zip: 08833
Ph: (908) 437-1234 Fax: (908) 437-1227
  Rubin, Seth M., MD

Annandale Family Practice
56 Payne Road/Suite 21 Zip: 08833
Ph: (908) 238-0100 Fax: (908) 238-0951
  Collins, Reid T., MD
  Sacchieri, Theresa Ann, MD

Ledgewood
Pediatric & Adolescent Center
1911 Route 46/PO Box 100 Zip: 07852
Ph: (973) 347-8500 Fax: (973) 347-7320
  Grossman, Leonard J., MD

Lincoln Park
Orthopedic Surgery & Sports Medicine
61 Beaver Brook Road/Suite 201 Zip: 07035
Ph: (973) 686-9292 Fax: (973) 686-9294
  Kavanagh, Mark Lawrence, MD

Lincroft
Coastal Monmouth Obstetrics & Gynecolo
521 Newman Springs Road/Suite 12 Zip: 07738
Ph: (732) 747-0022 Fax: (732) 747-0086
  Generelli, Patricia Ann, MD
  Moore, Susan Salzberg, MD

Linden
Care Station Medical Group
328 West St. Georges Avenue Zip: 07036
Ph: (908) 925-2273 Fax: (908) 925-2235
  Bezozo, Richard Craig, MD
  Diaz, Julio E., MD

Care Station Medical Group
328 St. Georges Avenue Zip: 07036
Ph: (908) 925-7519 Fax: (908) 925-2841
  Lao, Carlos S., MD
  Sundaram, Ashany, MD

Drs. Borowski & Kibilska-Borowsk
812 North Wood Avenue/Suite 101 Zip: 07036
Ph: (908) 486-3366
  Borowski, Walter J., MD
  Kibilska Borowski, Jolanta M., MD

Drs. Czyzewski & Nowak
515 North Wood Avenue/Suite 302 Zip: 07036
Ph: (908) 925-3300 Fax: (908) 925-4300
  Czyzewski, Ewa, MD
  Nowak, Darius Zbigniew, MD

Drs. Reich-Sobel & Schulman
809 North Wood Avenue Zip: 07036
Ph: (908) 486-7773 Fax: (908) 925-4311
  Reich-Sobel, Debra Gail, DO
  Schulman, Joseph M., DO

Linden Family Medical Associates
850 North Wood Avenue Zip: 07036
Ph: (908) 925-9309 Fax: (908) 925-7910
  Lukenda, Kevin, DO

Linden Medical Associates MD PC
540 South Wood Avenue Zip: 07036
Ph: (908) 862-2893 Fax: (908) 862-5810
  Mehta, Palak Pranav, MD
  Saif, Shazia, MD

NJ Heart/Linden Office
520 North Wood Avenue Zip: 07036
Ph: (908) 587-9300 Fax: (908) 587-1901
  Bronikowski, John Anthony, DO
  Randhawa, Preet Mohan Singh, MD
  Rubinstein, Allen Bernard, DO

Union County Orthopaedic Group
210 West St. Georges Avenue/PO Box 330 Zip: 07036
Ph: (908) 486-1111 Fax: (908) 583-1034
  Abdelshahed, Mina, MD
  Betesh, Naomi Gold, DO
  Ghobrial, Mark Nashaat, DO
  Kline, John A., MD
  Mackessy, Richard P., MD
  Pedowitz, Walter J., MD
  Rojer, David Eli, MD
  Ropiak, Christopher Robert, MD
  Sutain, Nathaniel, MD

Lindenwold
Ob-Gyn Care of Southern New Jersey
406 Gibbsboro Road East Zip: 08021
Ph: (856) 435-7007 Fax: (856) 435-7077
  Cannon, Donald R., MD
  Gildiner, Lennard R., MD
  Klein, Edward M., MD
  Ruffin, Judith S., MD

Linwood
Atlantic Dermatology & Laser Center
1401 New Road Zip: 08221
Ph: (609) 927-5885 Fax: (609) 927-5565
  Hong, Joseph Johnson, MD

Feldman-Rayfield Cosmetic Surgery
222 New Road/Suite 6 Zip: 08221
Ph: (609) 601-1000 Fax: (609) 601-1010
  Feldman, Marc D., MD
  Rayfield, David Lee, MD

Linwood Care Center
201 New Road Zip: 08221
Ph: (609) 927-6131
  Conover, Melissa, MD
  Jarillo, Maria Roca Cami, MD
  Kull, Elizabeth J., MD

Lowe-Greenwood-Zerbo Spinal Assoc
1999 New Road/Suite B Zip: 08221
Ph: (609) 601-6363 Fax: (609) 601-6364
  Graziani, Virginia, MD
  Lowe, James G., MD
  Sturr, Marianne, DO
  Zerbo, Joseph R., DO

Quality Eye Center
2020 New Road Zip: 08221
Ph: (609) 927-2020 Fax: (609) 926-7616
  Nguyen, Truc H., MD
  Remer, Paul, MD

South Jersey ENT Surgical Associates
2106 New Road/Unit C-9 Zip: 08221
Ph: (609) 927-8800 Fax: (609) 927-8832
  Orquiza, Clodualdo Soriano III, MD
  Siliunas, Vytas B., DO
  Wagle, Priya Jennifer, MD

Virtua Primary Care
1201 New Road/Suite 150a Zip: 08221
Ph: (609) 788-3338
  Kader, Richard A., DO

Little Egg Harbor
AtlantiCare Urgent Care Center
459 Route 9 South Zip: 08087
Ph: (609) 296-4014 Fax: (609) 296-5735
  Berlin, William H., DO

Drs. Lee and Humphreys
1479 Route 539/Suite 1 A Zip: 08087
Ph: (609) 296-1900 Fax: (609) 296-1906
  Humphreys, Erika, MD
  Lee, Gene Chiu, MD

Family Medicine Center
279 Mathistown Road Zip: 08087
Ph: (609) 296-1101
  Glenn, William B., DO
  Medenilla, Rosenio Jr., MD
  Tracy, Toby William, DO

Little Falls
Care Point Health Associates
1225 McBride Avenue/Suite 200 Zip: 07424
Ph: (973) 256-5557 Fax: (973) 256-5036
  Bauer, Francis Douglas, MD
  Bellardini, Angelo G., MD
  Mangra, Chandra, MD
  Yussaf, Shiraz, MD

Drs. Farnese and Farnese
109 Newark Pompton Turnpike Zip: 07424
Ph: (973) 890-0330 Fax: (973) 890-0705
  Farnese, Jeffrey Jason, MD
  Farnese, Joseph T., MD

Gastroenterology Associates of NJ
205 Browertown Road/Suite 201 Zip: 07424
Ph: (973) 812-8120 Fax: (973) 812-8144
  Kosc, Gary J., MD

Gastroenterology Associates of NJ
1031 McBride Avenue/Suite D-212 Zip: 07424
Ph: (973) 890-1303 Fax: (973) 890-5609
  Martino, Michael J., MD
  Pavlou, George Nicholas, MD

Gastroenterology Associates of NJ
205 Browertown Road/Suite 204 Zip: 07424
Ph: (973) 812-5230 Fax: (973) 812-5235
  Shami, Joseph G., MD

Suburban Nephrology Group
1031 McBride Avenue/Suite D-210 Zip: 07424
Ph: (973) 389-1119
  Fazio, Ignazio Jr., MD
  Rae, Susan, MD

Woodland Park Pediatrics
205 Browertown Road/Suite 001 Zip: 07424
Ph: (973) 582-0644 Fax: (973) 582-0605
  Razzak, Mannan, MD
  Razzak, Nadia Mohsin, MD

Little Silver
A Woman's Place
34 Sycamore Avenue Zip: 07739
Ph: (732) 747-9310 Fax: (732) 747-9320
  Bohnert, Katherine Ann, DO
  Giovine, Anthony P., MD
  Soussan, Elie R., MD

Adult Medical Onc-Hematology
39 Sycamore Avenue Zip: 07739
Ph: (732) 576-8610 Fax: (732) 576-8823
  Greenberg, Susan Nancy, MD
  LaNatra, Nicole, MD
  Windsor, Stephen J., MD

Family Chiropractic Center
180 White Road/Suite 205 Zip: 07739
Ph: (732) 530-7229 Fax: (732) 842-4119
  Devito, Marc J., MD
  Malik, Ritu, MD

Drs. Karoly, Kaskiw et al
180 White Road/Suite 209 Zip: 07739
Ph: (732) 842-0673
  Hammond, Kelly C., MD
  Jacoby, Michelle P., MD
  Karoly, Michael D., MD
  Kaskiw, Eugene H., MD

Pediatric Group of Central Jersey
200 White Road/Suite 212 Zip: 07739
Ph: (732) 741-5600 Fax: (732) 345-1001
  Mehra, Deepti, MD
  Mehra, Neeraj, MD

Red Bank Radiologists, P.A.
200 White Road/Suite 115 Zip: 07739
Ph: (732) 741-9595 Fax: (732) 741-0985
  DeVincenzo, Raven, MD
  Doss, Peter S., MD
  O'Connor, Douglas S., MD
  Rittweger, Edward S., MD
  Shah, Pranav N., MD
  Wirtshafter, David Glenn, MD
  Wold, Robert E., MD
  Zito, Frederick J., MD

Regional Cancer Care Associates, LLC
180 White Road Zip: 07739
Ph: (732) 530-8666 Fax: (732) 530-4139
  Fitzgerald, Denis B., MD
  Horkheimer, Ian Christin, MD
  Laughinghouse, Kenneth, MD
  Scher, Richard M., DO
  Walsh, Christina N., MD

Retina Consultants
39 Sycamore Avenue Zip: 07739
Ph: (732) 530-7730 Fax: (732) 530-3837
  Trikha, Rupan, MD
  Uram, Martin, MD

Shore Area Ob-Gyn
200 White Road/Suite 105 Zip: 07739
Ph: (732) 741-3331
  Kaufman, William N., DO
  Mason-Cederberg, Lauren, MD
  Rosenzweig, Talia S., MD
  Sun, Andrew N., MD
  Wiser-Estin, Mindy Ellen, MD

Livingston
Allergy, Asthma & Immunology PA
209 South Livingston Avenue Zip: 07039
Ph: (973) 992-4171 Fax: (973) 992-6325
  Goodman, Alan Jay, MD
  Weiss, Steven Jay, MD

Associates in Ophthalmology
22 Old Short Hills Road/Suite 102 Zip: 07039
Ph: (973) 992-5200 Fax: (973) 535-5741
  Hussain, Sarah, MD
  Lambert, Amy L., MD
  Nussbaum, Peter, MD

Bartky Healthcare Center, LLC
513 West Mount Pleasant Avenue Zip: 07039
Ph: (973) 533-1195 Fax: (973) 533-1305
  Bartky, Eric Jay, MD
  Feingold, Katherine Linda, MD

Breast Care & Treatment Center
200 South Orange Avenue Zip: 07039
Ph: (973) 533-0222 Fax: (973) 535-1121
  Santoro, Elissa J., MD
  Schaefer, Sarah Stuart, MD

Burn Surgeons of Saint Barnabas
94 Old Short Hills Road Zip: 07039
Ph: (973) 322-5924 Fax: (973) 322-5447
  Houng, Abraham Pohan, MD
  Mansour, Esber Hani, MD
  Marano, Michael A., MD
  Petrone, Sylvia J., MD

Groups and Clinics by Town with Physician Rosters

Cardiac Care of North Jersey
340 East Northfield Road/Suite 2C Zip: 07039
Ph: (973) 994-0069 Fax: (973) 994-0567
- Gressianu,Monica Terezia, MD
- Kashnikow,Constantine, MD

Ctr for Rheum & Autoimmune Dis
200 South Orange Avenue/Suite 107 Zip: 07039
Ph: (973) 322-7400 Fax: (973) 322-7420
- Kaufman,Lee D., MD
- Ritter,Jill M., MD

Dermatology Associates-Livingston
201 South Livingston Avenue/Suite 1F Zip: 07039
Ph: (973) 994-1170 Fax: (973) 994-1052
- Nervi,Stephen James, MD

Dr. Anthony Quartell & Asoocs
316 Eisenhower Parkway/Suite 202 Zip: 07039
Ph: (973) 716-9600 Fax: (973) 716-9650
- Koch,Robert K., MD
- Quartell,Anthony C., MD

Drs. Chu & Zauber
22 Old Short Hills Road/Suite 108 Zip: 07039
Ph: (973) 533-9299 Fax: (973) 992-7648
- Zauber,Neil P., MD

Drs. Gutkin & Peos
349 East Northfield Road/Suite 210 Zip: 07039
Ph: (973) 597-1107 Fax: (973) 597-1407
- Gutkin,Michael, MD
- Peos,Jennifer Renee, MD

Emergency Medical Offices
651 West Mount Pleasant Avenue Zip: 07039
Ph: (973) 740-9396 Fax: (973) 251-1165
- Abraham,Maninder Arneja, MD
- Anton,Joseph G., MD
- Eagan,Michael Patrick, MD
- Murphy,Kim, MD
- Puglisi,Gina Grace, MD
- Ravulapati,Sravanthi, MD
- Rentala,Manju, MD
- Salo,David F., MD
- Schreiber,Marie F., DO

Essex-Morris Pediatric Group P.A.
203 Hillside Avenue Zip: 07039
Ph: (973) 992-5588 Fax: (973) 992-1005
- Giannattasio,Theresa, DO
- Lander,Richard, MD
- Zaldivar,Marjel L., DO

Hypertension & Renal Group, P.A.
22 Old Short Hills Road/Suite 212 Zip: 07039
Ph: (973) 994-4550 Fax: (973) 994-7085
- Sipzner,Robert J., MD

Infectious Disease Center of NJ
22 Old Short Hills Road/Suite 106 Zip: 07039
Ph: (973) 535-8355 Fax: (973) 535-8353
- Chiang,Tom Shou, MD
- Kokkola-Korpela,Marjut Hellen, MD
- Lin,Janet C., MD
- Sheth,Arpita A., MD
- Youssef-Bessler,Manal Farouk, MD

Livingston Subspecialty Group
349 East Northfield Road/Suite 200 Zip: 07039
Ph: (973) 597-0900 Fax: (973) 597-0910
- Botti,Anthony C., MD
- Diamond,Gigi R., MD

Marano Eye Care Center
200 South Orange Avenue/Suite 209 Zip: 07039
Ph: (973) 322-0102 Fax: (973) 322-0102
- Decker,Edward Bruce, MD
- Marano,Matthew Jr., MD
- Rodriguez,Natalia Maria, MD

NICU Associates at Saint Barnabas
94 Old Short Hills Road Zip: 07039
Ph: (973) 322-5437 Fax: (973) 322-8833
- Lee,Hyejin Robin, MD
- Tien,Huey-Chung, MD

Nambi Endocrine Associates LLC
22 Old Short Hills Road/Suite 201 Zip: 07039
Ph: (973) 535-8870 Fax: (973) 535-8818
- Boradia,Chirag N., DO
- Nambi,Sridhar S., MD

Neurosurgeons of New Jersey
200 South Orange Avenue/Suite 116 Zip: 07039
Ph: (973) 718-9919
- Anderson,Richard Callis Eldon, MD
- Gigante,Paul R., MD

Physicians for Women's HealthCare
315 East Northfield Road/Suite 3-B Zip: 07039
Ph: (973) 422-1200 Fax: (973) 422-9169
- Cohen,Theodore, MD
- Katz,Jeffrey I., MD
- Kindzierski,John A., MD

Reflections Center For Skin & Body
299 East Northfield Road Zip: 07039
Ph: (973) 740-2444 Fax: (973) 740-0070
- Petrowsky,Deborah, MD

Retina-Vitreous Consultants
349 East Northfield Road/Suite 100 Zip: 07039
Ph: (973) 716-0123 Fax: (973) 716-0441
- Cohen,Steven B., MD
- Kanter,Eric D., MD

Shetal Mansuria MD, LLC.
22 Old Short Hills Road/Suite 213 Zip: 07039
Ph: (973) 535-3800 Fax: (973) 535-3808
- Mansuria,Shetal M., MD
- Pentyala,Madhavi, MD

Spine Care and Rehabilitation
200 South Orange Ave./Suite 180 Zip: 07039
Ph: (973) 226-2725 Fax: (973) 226-3270
- Kopacz,Kenneth J., MD
- Zarro,Christopher M., MD

St. Barnabas Ambulatory Care Center
200 South Orange Avenue Zip: 07039
Ph: (973) 322-7600 Fax: (973) 322-7685
- Anhalt,Henry, DO

St. Barnabas Ambulatory Care Center
200 South Orange Avenue Zip: 07039
Ph: (973) 322-7700
- Bhatnagar,Swati Varma, MD
- Daigle,Megan Elizabeth, MD
- Goyal,Vinod K., MD
- Kubichek,Marilyn Ann, MD
- McKeon,John J., MD
- Shumko,John Zachary, MD
- Tareco,Jennifer M., MD
- Ton,Mimi Nu, MD
- Trespalacios,Vanessa Nadia, MD
- Wroblewski,Henry M., MD

St. Barnabas Cancer Center
94 Old Short Hills Road/Suite 1 Zip: 07039
Ph: (973) 322-5650
- Brown,Andrew Bennett, MD
- Dienna,Erik, MD

St. Barnabas Cancer Center
94 Old Short Hills Road Zip: 07039
Ph: (973) 322-5200 Fax: (973) 322-5666
- Grossman,Israel Robert, MD
- Litvak,Anna Maria, MD
- Ongcapin,Emelie H., MD
- Rao,Parth Rajeshkumar, MD

Institute of Neurology & Neurosurgery
200 South Orange Avenue/Suite 101 Zip: 07039
Ph: (973) 322-7580 Fax: (973) 322-7505
- Avallone,Jennifer Mary, DO
- Devinsky,Orrin, MD
- Geller,Eric Bernard, MD
- Goldberg,Rina Freida, MD
- Nadkarni,Mangala A., MD
- Rodriguez,Andy, MD
- Venkatraman,Guha K., MD
- Widdess-Walsh,Peter Patrick, MD

SBMC-Institute for Neurosurgery
94 Old Short Hills Road Zip: 07039
Ph: (973) 322-6732
- Gilman,Arthur Michael, MD
- Hubschmann,Otakar R., MD
- Rotoli,Giorgio, DO

Summit Medical Group
75 East Northfield Road Zip: 07039
Ph: (973) 436-1400 Fax: (908) 673-7336
- Adamoli,Donna Janine, MD

Summit Medical Group
315 East Northfield Road/Suite 1-E Zip: 07039
Ph: (973) 535-3200 Fax: (973) 535-1450
- Bhawsar,Nilaya Babu, DO
- Bronsnick,Tara A., MD
- Chua Eoan,Pearl Davie, MD
- Citron,Cheryl S., MD
- Georgescu,Anca D., MD
- Goldenring,Debra Semel, MD
- Goldstein,Debra R., MD
- Holzman,Kevin Jay, MD
- Imbesi,John J., MD
- Ippolito,Tobi, MD
- Jacob,Tess, MD
- Jadeja,Priya Hari, MD
- Klachko,Daria A., MD
- Klein,Eileen C., MD
- Lee,Bryant B., MD
- Lemasters,Patrick Evan, MD
- Natanzon,Calvin, MD
- Oana,Dan C., MD
- Pritsiolas,James Michael, MD
- Rizio,Louis III., MD
- Segal,Jeffrey Loren, MD
- Semel,William J., MD
- Shieh,Frederick, MD
- Silverman,Mitchell S., MD
- Walsh,Rhonda M., MD
- Wiener,Jaclyn Faye, DO
- Youngren,Sonya Jitendra, MD

Institute for Reproductive Med/Science
94 Old Short Hills Road/Suite 403E Zip: 07039
Ph: (973) 322-8286 Fax: (973) 322-8890
- Cekleniak,Natalie A., MD
- Hessler,Sarah Catherine, MD
- Keegan,Debbra Ames, MD

The Joslin Center for Diabetes
200 South Orange Avenue/2nd Floor Zip: 07039
Ph: (973) 322-7200 Fax: (973) 322-7250
- Dower,Samuel M., MD
- Garbowit,David L., MD
- Gewirtz,George P., MD
- Sidler,Bonnie Beryl, MD

Osteoporosis Metabolic Bone Center
200 South Orange Avenue Zip: 07039
Ph: (973) 322-7430 Fax: (973) 322-7460
- Chuzhin,Yelena, MD
- Luckey,Marjorie M., MD

West Essex Ob/Gyn Associates
200 South Orange Avenue/Suite 290 Zip: 07039
Ph: (973) 740-1330 Fax: (973) 740-8998
- Abella,Tara M., MD
- DiSabatino,Daniel, DO
- Fain,Richard A., MD
- Keiser,Oren S., MD

Lodi

Hackensack University Medical Group PC
160 Essex Street/Suite 102 Zip: 07644
Ph: (551) 996-8111 Fax: (551) 996-8445
- Pande,Chandana, MD
- Raacke,Lisa Marie, MD

Hackensack University Medical Group PC
160 Essex Street/Suite 103 Zip: 07644
Ph: (551) 996-1370
- Santomauro,Emanuele A., MD
- Villa,John J., DO

HackensackUMG Lodi
116 Terrace Avenue Zip: 07644
Ph: (973) 473-3896 Fax: (973) 473-3896
- Andreescu,Aurora C., MD

Lodi Internists
361 Garibaldi Avenue Zip: 07644
Ph: (973) 773-3556
- Thamman,Prem, MD
- Thamman,Vijay K., MD

MedExpress Urgent Care Lodi
184 Essex Street Zip: 07644
Ph: (201) 843-3207 Fax: (201) 843-3215
- Kulesza-Galvez,Theodora, MD
- Lowenstein,Michael Aaron, DO

Logan Township

Christiana Care Cardiology Consultants
499 Beckett Road/Suite 202 Zip: 08085
Ph: (856) 769-3900 Fax: (856) 769-3903
- Cafone,Michael D., DO
- Pahlow,Brian J., DO
- Prabhakar,Avinash, MD

Vause Dermatology Cosmetic Surgery
545 Beckett Road/Suite 101 Zip: 08085
Ph: (856) 241-3311 Fax: (856) 241-3969
- Bright,Nicole Jasmyn, DO

Long Branch

Atlantic Eye Physicians
279 Third Avenue/Suite 204 Zip: 07740
Ph: (732) 222-7373 Fax: (732) 571-9212
- Bontempo,Carl Peter, MD
- Fegan,Robert James, MD
- Goldberg,Daniel B., MD
- Kaminek,Alexandra, DO
- Kristan,Ronald W., MD

Barnabas Health Medical Group
166 Morris Avenue/2nd Floor Zip: 07740
Ph: (732) 263-5024 Fax: (732) 263-5029
- Mandadi,Pranathi R., MD
- Master,Julie, DO
- Mercadante,Zorica Jelisijevic, MD
- Skylizard,Loki, MD

Internal Med Assocs of Monmouth
279 Third Avenue/Suite 207 Zip: 07740
Ph: (732) 229-0509 Fax: (732) 571-0019
- Lederman,Jeffrey Craig, DO
- Weinberg,Ronald M., MD

Laboratory Medicine Associates, PA
300 Second Avenue/Dept of Pathology Zip: 07740
Ph: (732) 923-7380 Fax: (732) 923-7355
- Kang,Yong, MD
- Loo,Abraham, MD
- Shertz,Wendy T., MD
- Zhong,Hua, MD

Meridian Medical Group
552 Westwood Avenue Zip: 07740
Ph: (732) 222-7800
- Dalton,John Boehmer, MD
- Thakar,Opal V., MD

Monmouth Family Center
270 Broadway Zip: 07740
Ph: (732) 923-7100 Fax: (732) 923-7104
- Cotov,Judith A., MD
- Eng,Margaret Hom, MD
- Hall,Dahlia Annmarie, MD
- Kapoor,Amee Patel, DO
- Khalil,Rahab M., MD
- Montana,Barbara E., MD
- Phillips,Keren Amy, MD
- Rajaraman,Ravindran Thirunavu, MD

Monmouth Medical Center
75 North Bath Avenue Zip: 07740
Ph: (732) 923-8500 Fax: (732) 923-5277
- Tintorer,Christine C., MD

Monmouth Medical Group, P.C.
73 South Bath Avenue Zip: 07740
Ph: (732) 870-3600 Fax: (732) 870-0119
- Gonzalez,David Jr., MD
- Malik,Nisha, MD
- Nath,Carl Anthony, MD

Monmouth Medical Group, P.C.
255 Third Avenue/SH 001 Zip: 07740
Ph: (732) 923-7790
- Sell,Neelam K., MD

Groups and Clinics by Town with Physician Rosters

Long Branch (cont)
Monmouth Medical Group, P.C.
279 Third Avenue/Suite 604 Zip: 07740
Ph: (732) 222-4474 Fax: (732) 222-4472
- Sembrano,Eduardo U. Jr., MD
- Verma,Renuka, MD
- Wallace,David Morrow, MD
- Zanni,Robert L., MD

Monmouth Medical Imaging
300 Second Avenue Zip: 07740
Ph: (732) 923-6806 Fax: (732) 923-6006
- Hussain,Syed, MD
- Keedy,Jennifer, MD
- Kwak,Andrew, MD
- Schiff,Robert Michael, MD
- Talangbayan,Leizle E., MD

Monmouth Radiologists, PA
279 Third Avenue Zip: 07740
Ph: (732) 222-7676 Fax: (732) 229-1863
- Smuro,Daniel J., MD
- Stein,Irving H., DO

Pediatric Urology Associates PC
422 Morris Avenue Zip: 07740
Ph: (732) 613-9144 Fax: (732) 613-5121
- Cummings,Kenneth B., MD

Pediatrix Medical Group
255 Third Avenue Zip: 07740
Ph: (732) 222-7006
- Alemany,Carlos A., MD
- Attardi,Diane Martha, MD
- Habib,Thomas G., MD
- Hudome,Susan M., MD
- Kale,Meera V., MD
- McNab,Theresa Challender, MD
- Scerbo,Jessica, MD

Lumberton
Advocare Pedi Phys of Burlington Co
693 Main Street/PO Box 367 Zip: 08048
Ph: (609) 261-4058 Fax: (609) 261-8381
- Bell,Denise Marie, MD
- Kaighn,Karen Chicalo, MD
- King,Richard A., MD
- Labroli,Melissa D., MD
- O'Donnell,Thomas P., MD
- Requa,Lindsay Ann, DO
- Wechsler,Marius A., MD

AllncBttrCr/Mount Holly Dvsn
1613 Route 38 Zip: 08048
Ph: (609) 261-3716 Fax: (609) 261-5507
- Buck,Murray D., DO
- Chatyrka,George O., DO
- Jain Bhalodia,Sapna, DO
- Kastenberg,Charles A., DO
- Scappaticci,John Jr., DO

Burlington County Endoscopy Center
140 Mount Holly Bypass/Unit 5 Zip: 08048
Ph: (609) 267-1555
- Pollak,Kevin Henry, MD

Gastroenterology Consultants
693 Main Street/Suite 2 Zip: 08048
Ph: (609) 265-1700 Fax: (609) 265-9005
- Awsare,Monica B., MD
- Khanijow,Vikresh, MD
- Kutscher,Jeffrey J., MD
- Lahoti,Mayank, DO
- Leonard,Maurice D., MD
- Rai-Patel,Jitha, MD
- Sheth,Nidhir Ras, MD
- Taub,William H., MD
- deLacy,Lee M., MD

Neurology Associaates of South Jersey
693 Main Street/Building D Zip: 08048
Ph: (609) 261-7600 Fax: (609) 265-8205
- Kachroo,Arun, MD
- Keller,Seth Martin, MD
- Mathur,Mayank, MD
- Orwitz,Jonathan Ira, MD
- Thomas,Carole E., MD

Surgical Specialists of New Jersey
668 Main Street/Suite 4 Zip: 08048
Ph: (609) 267-7050 Fax: (609) 267-7065
- Boynton,Christopher J., MD
- Hughes,Charles R., MD
- Miller,Eric Jay, MD

Rough,William Alexander Jr., MD

Virtua Family Medicine Center
1636 Route 38 & Eayrestown Rd. Zip: 08048
Ph: (609) 914-8440 Fax: (609) 914-8441
- Chandler,Khayriyyah Ebony Tahirah,
- Dalton,Laura J., DO
- Daub,Horatio Guy, MD
- Ibay,Annamarie D., MD
- Kolesk,Stephen J., MD
- Naticchia,Jennifer M., MD
- Rubenstein,Jennifer, MD
- Van Kooy,Mark A., MD

Virtua Lumberton Family Physicians
1561 Route 38/Suite 6A Zip: 08048
Ph: (609) 267-2100 Fax: (609) 267-6921
- Campagnolo,Mary F., MD
- Peng,Brian, DO

Lyndhurst
AFC Urgent Care Lyndhurst
560 New York Avenue Zip: 07071
Ph: (201) 831-8125 Fax: (201) 345-4536
- Aghabi,Hanna Najib, MD
- Lencina,Leandro H., MD

Drs. James and Kovaleva
125 Chubb Avenue/Suite 100-S Zip: 07071
Ph: (201) 559-7600
- James,Todd C., MD
- Kovaleva,Alexandra, MD

First Care Medical Group
750 Valley Brook Avenue Zip: 07071
Ph: (201) 896-0900 Fax: (201) 896-2726
- Ambrosio,George Joseph, MD
- Kricko,Michael J., DO
- Schmalz,William Francis Jr., MD
- Vellas,Elaine, MD

Lyndhurst Medical Associates
358 Valley Brook Avenue Zip: 07071
Ph: (201) 460-0142 Fax: (201) 460-1959
- Conroy,Daniel Jr., MD
- Cubero,John G., MD

Park Avenue Medical Associates
30 Park Avenue/Suite 202 Zip: 07071
Ph: (201) 438-5900 Fax: (201) 438-5980
- Hagler,Rhonda A., MD
- Hoskin,Jane F., MD
- Vossough,Soheila, MD

Primary Care Physicians Inc.
155 Park Avenue/Suite 206 Zip: 07071
Ph: (201) 939-1007
- Losos,Roland Jerzy, MD

United Medical, P.C.
612 Rutherford Avenue Zip: 07071
Ph: (201) 460-0063 Fax: (201) 460-1684
- Choi,Jay Joonhyuk, MD
- Hazzah,Marwa Mohamed, MD
- Park,Byong K., MD
- Strizhevsky,Marina A., DO

Madison
Atlantic Sleep & Pulmonary Associates
300 Madison Avenue/Suite 201 Zip: 07940
Ph: (973) 822-2772 Fax: (973) 822-2773
- Bathini,Manjula, DO
- Benton,Marc L., MD
- Seelall,Vijay Harpal, MD

Madison Family Practice
8 Shunpike Road Zip: 07940
Ph: (973) 377-2610 Fax: (973) 377-2345
- Berger,Gary, MD
- Luo,Yan Mei, MD

Mahwah
Drs. Sharma and Sharma
400 Franklin Turnpike/Suite 102 Zip: 07430
Ph: (201) 934-5700
- Sharma,Ashok K., MD
- Sharma,Indu, MD

Garden State Orthopaedic Assoc PA
400 Franklin Turnpike/Suite 112 Zip: 07430
Ph: (201) 825-2266 Fax: (201) 825-9727
- Holden,Douglas Scott, MD

Mahwah Medical
10 Franklin Turnpike Zip: 07430
Ph: (201) 529-0033 Fax: (201) 529-5913
- Beenstock,Steven Marc, DO
- Najovits,Andrew Joseph, MD

PediatriCare Associates
400 Franklin Turnpike Zip: 07430
Ph: (201) 529-4545 Fax: (201) 529-1596
- Liberti,Lorraine M., MD
- Perez,Sania Rebecca, MD

Renal Medicine Associates PA
400 Franklin Turnpike/Suite 208 Zip: 07430
Ph: (201) 825-3322
- Tartini,Albert, MD

Manahawkin
Barnegat Medical Associates, P.A.
41 Nautilus Drive Zip: 08050
Ph: (609) 978-0474 Fax: (609) 597-6186
- Dahal,Rama, MD
- Moshkovitch,Vasil Ignatovitch, MD
- Sahay,Nishi, MD
- Sahay,Rajiv, MD

Coastal Ear Nose and Throat LLC
1301 Route 72/Suite 340 Zip: 08050
Ph: (732) 280-7855 Fax: (732) 280-7815
- Bhojwani,Amit N., DO
- Bones,Victoria Mary, MD
- McAfee,Jacob Seth, MD
- Patel,Pratik Bharat, MD
- Zhuravsky,Ruslan, DO

Coastal Healthcare
44 Nautilus Drive/Suite 2A Zip: 08050
Ph: (609) 597-4178 Fax: (609) 597-4387
- DeSantis Mastrangelo,Rosemarie, MD
- Kumar Shetty,Nagalakshmi Ashok, MD

Drs Soni & Soni
697 Millcreek Road/Suite 1 Zip: 08050
Ph: (609) 597-5699 Fax: (609) 597-5722
- Soni,Poonam, MD
- Soni,Shikhar, MD

Erickson, Dreizen & Lee Eye Center
1206 Route 72 West Zip: 08050
Ph: (609) 597-8087
- Dreizen,Neil G., MD
- Drudy,Elena R., MD
- Erickson,Alan R., MD
- Lee,Robert Edward III, MD

Family Medicine Center
1301 Route 72 West/Suite 240 Zip: 08050
Ph: (609) 597-7394 Fax: (609) 597-6833
- Hogan,Kimberly Ann, MD
- Kenny,John J., DO
- Nitschmann-Schmoll,Cynthia A., DO
- Raguso Failla,Michael Joseph, MD

Hackensack Meridian Health Orthopedic
1173 Beacon Avenue/Suite A Zip: 08050
Ph: (609) 250-4101 Fax: (609) 997-8486
- Kunkle,Herbert Lemuel Jr., MD
- Wright,Douglas G., MD

Hackensack Meridian Medical Group
53 Nautilus Drive/Suite 201 Zip: 08050
Ph: (609) 978-8870 Fax: (609) 978-8903
- Papa-Rugino,Tommasina, MD
- Terranova,Robert J., DO

Medical Associates of Ocean County
1301 Route 72 West/Suite 300 Zip: 08050
Ph: (609) 597-6513 Fax: (609) 597-4593
- Dewil,Frederic, MD
- Henry,James R., MD
- Koerner,Steven, DO
- Malinverni,Helio J., MD
- Reed,William E., DO
- Reynon,Melissa A., MD

Meridian Pediatrics - Manahawkin
1100 Route 72 West/Suite 306B Zip: 08050
Ph: (609) 978-3910 Fax: (609) 978-3912
- Bleiman,Michael I., MD
- Sunkavalli,Paul Venugopal, MD

Ocean Health Initiatives, Inc.
333 Haywood Road Zip: 08050
Ph: (609) 489-0110 Fax: (609) 489-0171
- Cannon,Aileen Carol, MD

Ocean Renal Associates, P.A.
1145 Beacon Avenue/Suite B Zip: 08050
Ph: (609) 978-9940 Fax: (609) 978-9902
- Shah,Ankit Prafulbhai, MD

Ocean Women's Health Care Group
602 Route 72 East/Suite 1 Zip: 08050
Ph: (609) 978-9870 Fax: (609) 978-9873
- McDermott,James P., DO
- Rezai,Amadi, MD
- Sunkavalli,Anupama, MD
- Trim,George G., MD

RWJ-UMDNJ Anesthesia Group
1140 Route 72 West Zip: 08050
Ph: (609) 978-8900
- Barton,Keith A., DO
- Bouyea,Michelle Marie, MD
- Guo,Jianhua, MD
- Hanna,Sherine Farag, MD
- Manevich,Ilya, MD
- Marco,James Victor, MD
- Richlan,Richard A., MD
- Tse,James T.C., MD

SOMC Medical Group, PC
1100 Route 72 West/Suite 305 Zip: 08050
Ph: (609) 978-9841 Fax: (609) 978-9843
- Gottesman,Brian Tod, MD
- Liu,Todd, MD
- Sze,Michael Shu Shin, MD

Schweiger Dermatology
712 East Bay Avenue/Suite 19 Zip: 08050
Ph: (609) 597-5850 Fax: (609) 597-9667
- Geffner,Rami E., MD

Southern Ocean Otolaryngology PA
77 Nautilus Drive Zip: 08050
Ph: (609) 597-0321
- Bezpalko,Lynn E., DO
- Bezpalko,Orest, DO

Stafford Medical, P.A.
1364 Route 72 West/Suite 5 Zip: 08050
Ph: (609) 597-3416 Fax: (609) 597-9608
- Guida,Vincent C., DO
- Hong,William Y. C., MD
- Kumar,Ramesh, MD
- Lipper,Jeffrey M., MD

Stafford Medical, P.A.
1364 Route 72 West Zip: 08050
Ph: (609) 597-3416 Fax: (609) 597-9608
- Tailor,Unnati, DO
- Tekriwal,Mahesh Kumar, MD
- Veldanda,Ashokvardhan R., MD
- Yu,Byung H., MD

Strafford Surgical Specialists, P.A.
1100 Route 72 West/Suite 303 Zip: 08050
Ph: (609) 978-3325 Fax: (609) 978-3123
- Barbalinardo,Joseph P., MD
- Echeverri,Samuel David, MD
- Fresco,Silvia, MD
- Greco,Richard Yackshaw, DO
- Lujan,Juan Jose, MD
- Reich,Jonathan Makaloa, MD
- Strom,Karl William, MD

Surgical Specialists of New Jersey
37 Nautilus Drive Zip: 08050
Ph: (609) 978-0778 Fax: (609) 978-1377
- Hager,Jeffrey C., DO

Surgical Specialists of New Jersey
1364 Route 72 West/Suite 5 Zip: 08050
Ph: (609) 978-0778 Fax: (609) 978-1377
- Khoo,Robert Eng Hong, MD
- Penrod,Carey Lynn, DO
- Samra,Matthew Samuel, DO

Urgent Care Now
712 East Bay Avenue/Suite 22-B Zip: 08050
Ph: (609) 978-0242 Fax: (609) 978-0241
- Bagnell,James P., MD
- Little,James Todd, DO

Manalapan

Drs. Schechter and Silbret
26 Plaza 9 Road Zip: 07726
Ph: (732) 303-1500 Fax: (732) 303-0033
 Schechter,Alan Lance, MD
 Silbret,Lisa Michele, MD

Hackensack Meridian Medical Group
195 Route 9 South/Suite 106 Zip: 07726
Ph: (732) 536-7144 Fax: (732) 536-7520
 Ezer,Mayer Roy, MD
 Romanella,Joseph P., DO
 Rossi,Regina L., DO
 Sharma,Puja, MD

Ivy Pediatrics
220 Bridge Plaza Drive Zip: 07726
Ph: (732) 972-9525 Fax: (732) 972-9055
 Malaty,Christine B., DO
 Trogan,Igor, MD

Jersey Shore Assocs of Internal Med
831 Tennent Road Zip: 07726
Ph: (732) 536-7144 Fax: (732) 536-7520
 Nordone,Danielle Suzanne, DO

Manalapan Urgent Care
120 Craig Road Zip: 07726
Ph: (732) 414-2991 Fax: (732) 414-2995
 Baig,Rifaqat, MD

Marlboro Gastroenterology PC
50 Franklin Lane/Suite 201 Zip: 07726
Ph: (732) 972-6996 Fax: (732) 972-8610
 Weiner,Brian C., MD

Medico-Legal Evaluations, PA
50 Franklin Lane/Suite 201 Zip: 07726
Ph: (732) 972-4771 Fax: (732) 972-8610
 Skolnick,Cary I., MD

RWJ Ob-Gyn Associates
50 Franklin Lane/Suite 203 Zip: 07726
Ph: (732) 536-7110 Fax: (732) 536-7118
 Bochner,Ronnie Z., MD
 Rathauser,Robert H., MD

Sunrise Obstetrics & Gynecology
831 Tennent Road Zip: 07726
Ph: (732) 972-4200 Fax: (732) 333-4643
 Belkin,Sardana, MD
 Fischetti-Galvin,Jessica, DO
 Levy,Jenna, DO

Taylors Mills Family Medical, PC
224 Taylors Mills Road/Suite 112 Zip: 07726
Ph: (732) 577-1066 Fax: (732) 577-0049
 Goldberg,Alexander, MD
 Isayeva,Eleonora, DO

Ultimed HealthCare PC
50 Franklin Lane Zip: 07726
Ph: (732) 972-1267 Fax: (732) 972-1026
 Ahmed,Munir, MD
 Atkin,Stuart R., MD
 Enescu,Cristian C., MD
 Harrison,Andrew, MD
 Schiebert,Steven S., DO
 Springer,Stuart Ira, MD

Union Hill Pediatrics
85 Bridge Plaza Drive Zip: 07726
Ph: (732) 972-1117 Fax: (732) 972-0177
 Leib,Samantha, MD
 Shah,Sonal Ashwin, DO

Wee Care Pediatrics
831 Tennent Road/Suite A Zip: 07726
Ph: (732) 536-6222 Fax: (732) 536-9272
 Dhawan,Denise Marie, MD
 Levy,Moshe, MD
 Peska-Mosseri,Jodi L., DO
 Tanner-Sackey,Fritzi A., MD

West Park Pediatrics
219 Taylors Mills Road Zip: 07726
Ph: (732) 577-0088 Fax: (732) 577-9643
 Genova-Goldstein,Jeanne, MD

Manasquan

Atlantic Hema/Oncology Assocs
1707 Atlantic Avenue Zip: 08736
Ph: (732) 528-0760 Fax: (732) 528-0764
 Anne,Madhurima, MD
 Greenberg,David Benjamin, MD
 Henningson,Carl Thomas Jr., MD
 Lerner,William A., MD
 Levitt,Michael Joshua, MD
 Mencel,Peter J., MD
 Topilow,Arthur A., MD

Brick Women's Physicians
87 Union Avenue Zip: 08736
Ph: (732) 202-0700 Fax: (732) 202-0664
 Parchment,Alfred B., MD

Brielle Obstetrics & Gynecology, P.A.
2671 Highway 70/Wall Township Zip: 08736
Ph: (732) 528-6999 Fax: (732) 528-3397
 Ditusa,Diane Michele, DO
 Filardo,Josephine, MD
 Keelan,Michael E., MD
 Saez Lacy,Deborah A., MD
 Welt,Alan J., MD

Ctr for Aesthetic & Integrative Med
2399 Highway 34/Building A5 Zip: 08736
Ph: (732) 528-5533 Fax: (732) 528-0360
 Berkovich,Vladimir, MD
 Ricci,John Anthony, MD
 Rittberg,Shannon Bara, DO

Drs. Rotolo, Howard, and Leitner
2401 Highway 35 Zip: 08736
Ph: (732) 223-7877 Fax: (732) 223-7151
 Howard,Michael Lawrence, MD
 Leitner,Robyn R., MD
 Perlmutter,Mark Alan, MD
 Rotolo,James E., MD

Meridian Laboratory Physicians
2517 Highway 35/Building M/Suite 101 Zip: 08736
Ph: (732) 528-7710
 Lahoti,Chitra, MD
 Schneider,Henry E., MD

Michael W. Nagy MD FACS
2333 Highway 34 Zip: 08736
Ph: (732) 282-0002 Fax: (732) 282-1522
 Nagy,Michael William, MD
 Vemula,Rahul, MD

Ocean Pediatric Group
2640 Route 70/Suite 1-B Zip: 08736
Ph: (732) 528-8448 Fax: (732) 223-5792
 Oram,Alexis Marissa, MD

Ortho Institute of Central NJ
2315A Highway 34/Suite D Zip: 08736
Ph: (732) 974-0404 Fax: (732) 449-4271
 Bhatnagar,Ramil S., MD
 Ferenz,Clint C., MD
 Glasser,Laurie, MD
 Goldstein,Joel M., MD
 Gonzalez,Peter G., MD
 Husserl,Toby B., MD
 Jarmon,Nicholas Albert, MD
 Petrosini,Anthony V., MD
 Roehrig,Gregory James, MD
 Sclafani,Michael A., MD
 Tennen,Elad, MD
 Tozzi,John Michael, MD

Sea Girt Medical Associates
235 Route 71 Zip: 08736
Ph: (732) 223-4300 Fax: (732) 223-5273
 Almeida,Frank Gerard, MD
 Kossev,Viliana D., MD
 Kuzmick,Peter J., DO
 Pandya,Manan Kirit, DO
 Von Suskil,Kurt E., MD

Shore Pulmonary PA
2640 Highway 70/Building 6-A Zip: 08736
Ph: (732) 528-5900 Fax: (732) 528-0887
 Costanzo,Eric John, DO
 De La Luz,Gustavo E., MD
 Friedman,Paul Martin, MD
 Gallagher,Cornelius T., MD
 Miskoff,Jeffrey Aaron, DO
 Potulski,Frederick J., MD

Total Patient Care
2401 Route 35 Zip: 08736
Ph: (732) 292-9222 Fax: (732) 292-9633
 Alonzo-Chafart,Lorena D., DO
 Gilani,Asim Haider, MD

Manville

KNJ Hospitalist Group, LLC.
204 South Main Street Zip: 08835
Ph: (732) 586-9035 Fax: (908) 213-6618
 Chichili,Eiswarya, MD
 Mody,Vipul C., MD
 Pandya,Dhyanesh C., MD

My Family Practice Associates
37 South Main Street Zip: 08835
Ph: (908) 722-9333 Fax: (908) 722-9990
 Khan,Mohammed Nasir, MD
 Shah,Mubina, MD

Maple Shade

Neurological Regional Associates
504 Route 38 East Zip: 08052
Ph: (856) 866-0466 Fax: (856) 727-1483
 Abidi,Saiyid Manzoor, MD
 Vanna,Stephen C., MD
 Yang,John Y., MD

Partners in Primary Care
19 West Main Street Zip: 08052
Ph: (856) 779-7386 Fax: (856) 779-7563
 Brolis,Nils Viesturs, DO
 Di Marcangelo,Michael C. Jr., DO
 Janik,Nancy E., MD
 Norton,Kevin Patrick, DO

Maplewood

Advanced Pain Care
2040 Millburn Avenue Zip: 07040
Ph: (908) 242-3688 Fax: (908) 242-3902
 Feldman,David Nathan, MD
 He,Ningning, MD

Drs. Kaid & Tanwir
2168 Millburn Avenue/Suite 204 Zip: 07040
Ph: (973) 762-3353 Fax: (973) 762-3370
 Kaid,Khalil Ahmed, MD
 Mendola,John V., MD
 Tanwir,Anjum, MD

Empire Medical Associates
264 Boyden Avenue Zip: 07040
Ph: (973) 761-5200 Fax: (973) 761-7617
 Maloney,Marvelle, MD
 Prus,Dina S., MD

Maplewood Family Medicine
111 Dunnell Road/Suite 200 Zip: 07040
Ph: (908) 598-6690 Fax: (973) 762-0840
 Cadet,Marc D., MD
 Miguez,Priscilla, DO
 Sharma,Deepa, DO
 Young,Karen D., MD

Marven Wallen & S. Kenneth Jacobson MD
1985 Springfield Avenue Zip: 07040
Ph: (973) 763-5010 Fax: (973) 761-6980
 Jacobson,Sayre K., MD
 Orenberg,Scott D., DO

Metropolitan Ob/Gyn, P.A.
1973 Springfield Avenue Zip: 07040
Ph: (973) 313-2501 Fax: (973) 313-2505
 Parchment,Winsome J., MD
 Peace,Nyota Afi, MD

Pediatric Surgery Group
2130 Millburn Avenue Zip: 07040
Ph: (973) 313-3115 Fax: (973) 313-3188
 Bethel,Colin A. I., MD
 Bhattacharyya,Nishith, MD

Margate

Pediatric Assocs Of Atlantic Co
9009 Ventnor Avenue Zip: 08402
Ph: (609) 823-2773
 Durelli,Gloria S., MD

The Medical Center of Margate
9501 Ventnor Avenue Zip: 08402
Ph: (609) 823-6161 Fax: (856) 823-3413
 Anastasi,Lawrence J., DO
 Gaffney,John L., DO

Margate City

Horizon Eye Care
9701 Ventnor Avenue Zip: 08402
Ph: (609) 822-4242 Fax: (609) 822-3211
 Gross,Howard J., MD
 Nunn,Robert F., MD
 Perez,Matthew K., MD
 Pritz,Nicole M., MD

Marlboro

Advanced Gastroenterology Assoc
475 County Road/Suite 201 Zip: 07746
Ph: (732) 370-2220 Fax: (732) 548-7408
 Cencora,Barbara E., MD
 Gold,Jared Z., MD
 Pitchumoni,Suresh Shanker, MD
 Tendler,Michael R., MD
 Tilara,Amy N., MD
 Vazirani,Tina A., MD

Cntr for Phys Mdcn & Rehab
30 North Main Street Zip: 07746
Ph: (732) 761-0500
 Basilone,Joseph, MD
 Fox,David B., MD

Family Practice of CentraState
479 Newman Springs Rd/Suite A-101 Zip: 07746
Ph: (732) 780-1601
 Guliano,Jaclyn M., MD
 Meyer,Shira Asekoff, DO
 Paul Yee,Sabine T., MD
 Stoner,Edward D., MD

Jersey Shore Geriatrics
15 School Road East/Suite 2 Zip: 07746
Ph: (732) 866-9922 Fax: (732) 866-9970
 O'Dell,Kimberly Ann, MD
 Pass,Mark David, MD

Medical Associates of Marlboro PC
32 North Main Street Zip: 07746
Ph: (732) 462-4100 Fax: (732) 462-3798
 Carter,Alison F., MD
 Kanouka,Indira Jouma, MD
 Kayastha,Shital, DO
 Laxmi,Sheethal Manipadaga, MD
 Nair,Swapna, MD
 Patel,Jayendrakumar N., MD
 Varma,Seema N., MD

Pediatric Associates
9 South Main Street Zip: 07746
Ph: (732) 577-1945 Fax: (732) 308-3460
 Salcedo,Glenn A., MD
 Yee,Mary, MD

Marlton

Advocare Allergy & Asthma
54 East Main Street Zip: 08053
Ph: (856) 988-0570 Fax: (856) 988-0303
 Gatti,Eugene A., MD
 Toci,Gregory R. Sr., DO
 Vishwanath,Sahana, MD

Advocare Atrium Pediatrics
301 Old Marlton Pike West/Suite 1 Zip: 08053
Ph: (856) 988-9101 Fax: (856) 988-7712
 Falk,Michael Alexander, MD
 Fanelli,Allison Sagan, DO
 Leszkowicz,Aditee D., DO
 Rickey,Stephanie B., MD
 Rosenblum,Benjamin A., MD
 Smith-Elfant,Stacy A., MD

Advocare Greentree Pediatrics
127 Church Road/Suite 800 Zip: 08053
Ph: (856) 988-7899 Fax: (856) 988-9499
 Friedler-Eisenberg,Susan F., DO
 Kaus,Sharon M., DO
 Zechowy,Racine B., MD

Advocare Marlton Pediatrics
525 Route 73 South Zip: 08053
Ph: (856) 596-3434 Fax: (856) 596-9110
 Bailey,Aisha Donine, DO
 Blackman,Jeffrey B., MD
 Hammer,Stacey R., MD
 Lampone,Christina, MD
 Orel,Howard N., MD
 Rosof,Edward, MD
 Waxman,Howard S., MD

Groups and Clinics by Town with Physician Rosters

Marlboro (cont)

Advocare The Farm Pediatrics
975 Tuckerton Road/Suite 100   Zip: 08053
Ph: (856) 983-6190   Fax: (856) 983-3805
- Barnett, Sharon Elizabeth, MD
- Berman, Eric David, DO
- Chasen, David E., MD
- Denick, Kimberly Keane, MD
- Holmes-Bricker, Mary E., DO
- Lafferty, Kathryn Tatsis, MD
- Szawlewicz, Stephen A., MD

Aesthetic Dermatology, LLC.
771 East Route 70/Suite D-150   Zip: 08053
Ph: (856) 596-3393   Fax: (856) 596-3394
- Elder, Sandra Depadova, MD
- Larusso, Jennifer Lynn, DO

Allergy & Asthma Associates
525 Route 73 South/Suite 106   Zip: 08053
Ph: (856) 596-5585   Fax: (856) 596-3178
- Kravitz, Elaine K., MD

Allergy & Asthma Consultants of NJ
9004 Lincoln Drive West/Suite B   Zip: 08053
Ph: (856) 596-3100   Fax: (856) 596-3133
- Dadhania, Mahendrakumar P., MD

Associates in Family Healthcare, P.C.
73 North Maple Avenue/Suite B   Zip: 08053
Ph: (844) 542-2273   Fax: (856) 569-4043
- Hasbun, Rafael D., MD
- Klazmer, Jay, DO
- Pecora, Andrew Paul, DO
- Schweitzer, Justin Stephen, DO

CENTRA Comprehensive Psychotherapy
5000 Sagemore Drive/Suite 205   Zip: 08053
Ph: (856) 983-3866   Fax: (856) 985-8148
- Berson, Casey Lee, MD
- Gupta, Mala Rani, MD
- Harbison, Margaret S., MD
- Schooff, Mary Lieder, MD
- Strauss, Alexander Sangor, MD

Cadoro Pediatrics, LLC
750 Route 73 South/Suite 307A   Zip: 08053
Ph: (856) 983-9666   Fax: (856) 983-2662
- Chun, Doreen Sze-Man, DO
- Monaco, Carmine D., DO

Center Pediatrics Adolescent & Adult
12000 Lincoln Drive West/Suite 311   Zip: 08053
Ph: (856) 985-8100   Fax: (856) 985-0178
- Malave, Esther, MD
- Mirmanesh, John C., MD

Center for Adult Medicine
12000 Lincoln Drive West/Suite 404-405   Zip: 08053
Ph: (856) 985-0203   Fax: (856) 985-0010
- Mirmanesh, Shahin Michael, MD
- Mirmanesh, Shapour Steve, MD

Center for Family Guidance, PC
765 East Route 70/Building A-101   Zip: 08053
Ph: (856) 797-4800   Fax: (856) 810-0110
- Abraham, Ruby, MD
- Akinli, Timur C., MD
- Allende, Jenys, MD
- Benjelloun, Hind, MD
- Brancato, Peter Jr., MD
- Callahan, Richard Allan II, MD
- Chandran, Ankila Sharavati, DO
- Chodha, Vicky, MD
- Edelman, Douglas Jay, MD
- Ellabbad, Essam-Eldin Moussa A., M
- Embrescia, Mary Megan, MD
- Francisco, Rowena Rebano, MD
- Harwitz, David Marc, MD
- Hume, Edward Samuel, MD
- Kurani, Amit P., MD
- Layne, George Stark, MD
- Longson, Audrey Eve, DO
- McFadden, Robert F., MD
- Nugent, Grace C., MD
- Periasamy, Jayanthi, MD
- Post, Nicole Renee, MD
- Prince, Leonie S., MD
- Shamilov, Maasi Don, MD
- Singh, Sarabjit, MD
- Smith, Elton John, MD
- Teitelman, Karen Lynn Bottone, DO
- Worth, Richard Lowell, MD
- Yuan, Cai, MD

Ctr for Pediatrics & Adult Med
311 The Pavilions at Greentree   Zip: 08053
Ph: (856) 985-8100   Fax: (856) 985-8374
- Calabrese, Karen Ann, DO
- Mirmanesh, Shahram J., MD

Cooper Center for Dermatologic Surgery
10000 Sagemore Drive/Suite 10103   Zip: 08053
Ph: (856) 596-3040
- Decker, Ashley, MD
- Johnson, Ryan P., MD
- Lawrence, Naomi, MD
- Marquart, Jason D., MD
- Regula, Christie Gail, MD

Cooper Family Medicine
1001-F Lincoln Drive West   Zip: 08053
Ph: (856) 810-1800   Fax: (856) 810-1879
- Festa, Michelle G., MD
- Friedhoff, Stephen G., MD
- Horvath, Kedron Nicole, MD
- Voyack, Michael John, DO

Elmwood Family Physicians
777 Route 70 East/Suite G-101   Zip: 08053
Ph: (856) 983-9939   Fax: (856) 983-9936
- Patel, Jay Dinesh, MD
- Patel, Parag S., MD
- Shah, Hetal Subodh, MD

Garden State Center
100 Brick Road/Suite 115   Zip: 08053
Ph: (856) 983-1400   Fax: (856) 983-1681
- Glass, Charles Adam, MD
- Grossman, Harry D., MD
- Kamoun, Layla, MD

Garden State Medical Associates
100 Brick Road/Suite 209   Zip: 08053
Ph: (856) 983-2848
- Lomonaco, Jesse V., DO
- Malhotra, Rakesh, MD

Hand Surgery & Rehab Center of NJ
5000 Sagemore Drive/Suite 103   Zip: 08053
Ph: (856) 983-4263   Fax: (856) 983-9362
- Ballet, Frederick L., MD
- Chu, Brian, MD
- Ragland, Raymond III, MD
- Strauss, Eric D., MD

Heymann, Manders & Green LLC
100 Brick Road/Suite 306   Zip: 08053
Ph: (856) 596-0111   Fax: (856) 596-7194
- Green, Justin Jacob, MD
- Halpern, Analisa Vincent, MD
- Heymann, Warren R., MD
- Manders, Steven M., MD
- Sommer, Lacy Louise, MD

InSight LLC
765 East Route 70/Bldg A   Zip: 08053
Ph: (856) 983-3900   Fax: (856) 810-0110
- Ikelheimer, Douglas Mark, MD
- Nunez, Venitius D., MD
- Panah, Daud Mohammad-Masood, MD
- Varrell, James R., MD

Martin K. Belsky, D.O., P.C.
100 Brick Road/Suite 108   Zip: 08053
Ph: (856) 810-7337
- Belsky, Martin Karl, DO
- Fair-Covely, Rose Mary, DO

Meetinghouse Family Physicians
330 East Greentree Road   Zip: 08053
Ph: (856) 596-9050   Fax: (856) 596-0320
- DeGuzman, Ronaldo Cruz, DO
- Robinson, Sloan A., MD

Mt. Laurel Pediatric
528 Lippincott Drive   Zip: 08053
Ph: (856) 983-3899   Fax: (856) 983-3997
- Panda, Nirmala, MD
- Pandit, Florence A., MD
- Ragothaman, Ramesh, MD

New Jersey Urology
773 Route 70 East/Building H-120   Zip: 08053
- Wargo, Heather Carol, MD

Partners in Primary Care
534 Lippincott Drive   Zip: 08053
Ph: (856) 985-7373   Fax: (856) 985-9611
- Casey, Daniel T., MD
- Levinson, Elizabeth A., MD
- McCormick, Ryan Charles, MD
- Miller, Scott Lewis, MD
- Roesly, Melissa M., MD
- Ryczak, Kristen, MD

Pinnacle Behavioral Health Institute
851 Route 73 North/Suite C   Zip: 08053
Ph: (856) 512-8108   Fax: (856) 267-5824
- Mathews, Joanne, MD
- Mathews, Maju, MD

Pulmonary & Sleep Associates of SJ, LL
750 Route 73 South/Suite 401   Zip: 08053
Ph: (856) 375-1288   Fax: (856) 375-2325
- Alimam, Ammar, MD
- Auerbach, Donald, MD
- Bermingham, John, DO
- Grookett, Thomas Wister, MD
- Roy, Nicholas E., DO

Rothman Institute
999 Route 73 North/3rd Fl   Zip: 08053
Ph: (856) 821-6360   Fax: (856) 821-6359
- Barlow, Jonathan David, MD
- Bryant, Tony Labree Jr., MD
- Hoffler, Charles E. II, MD
- Nelson, Gregory N. Jr., MD
- O'Malley, Michael J., MD
- Poehling Monaghan, Kirsten L., MD
- Schaaf, H. William, MD
- Shearin, Jonathan Winkworth, MD

Samaritan Healthcare & Hospice
5 Eves Drive/Suite 300   Zip: 08053
Ph: (856) 896-1600   Fax: (856) 596-7881
- Chiesa, Jennifer Elaine, DO
- Goldfine, Stephen P., MD
- Jacob, Leena Rachel, DO
- Pagliaro, Sara Nicole, DO
- Romano, James A., MD

Sobel & Zell Orthopaedic Assoc
525 Route 73 South/Suite 303   Zip: 08053
Ph: (856) 596-0555   Fax: (856) 596-7658
- Sobel, Mark A., MD
- Zell, Brian Kirk, MD

South Jersey Fertility Center
400 Lippincott Drive   Zip: 08053
Ph: (856) 282-1231   Fax: (856) 596-2411
- Kuzbari, Oumar, MD
- Sawin, Stephen Wooten, MD
- Skaf, Robert A., MD
- Van Deerlin, Peter G., MD
- Weissman, Lauren, MD

South Jersey Gastroenterology PA
406 Lippincott Drive/Suite E   Zip: 08053
Ph: (856) 983-1900   Fax: (856) 983-5110
- Cohen, Neil M., MD
- Davidoff, Steven, MD
- Devita, Jack Joseph, MD
- Friehling, Jane Susan, DO
- Horn, Abraham S., DO
- Jaffe, Jane K., DO
- Levin, Gary H., MD
- Tulman, Alan Bruce, MD

South Jersey Pain Consultants
525 Route 73 South/Suite 103   Zip: 08053
Ph: (856) 797-5777   Fax: (856) 797-5771
- Padula, Vincent M., DO
- Ressler, Steven H., MD

St. Remi Behavioral Health
750 Route 73 South/Suite 106   Zip: 08053
Ph: (856) 227-0306   Fax: (856) 396-9917
- Daly, John Christopher, MD

Temple University Orthopedics
One Greentree Center/Suite 104   Zip: 08053
Ph: (856) 596-0906
- Kelly, John D., MD
- Michael, Stanley P., MD

The Spine Institute of So NJ
512 Lippincott Drive   Zip: 08053
Ph: (856) 797-9161   Fax: (856) 797-3637
- Bussey, Jonathan David, DO
- Kirshner, Steven B., MD
- Meagher, Richard John, MD
- O'Shea, Joan Frances, MD

Garden State Pulmonary Associates
520 Lippincott Drive/Suite A   Zip: 08053
Ph: (856) 596-9057   Fax: (856) 596-0837
- Lee, Andrew N., MD
- Mazza, Emilio, MD
- Rodis, Angel Victor, MD
- Salm, Allen J., MD
- Sutherland, Jewelle R., MD
- Sztejman, Eric S., MD
- Vagadia, Neha R., DO

Virtua Hospitalist Group Marlton
90 Brick Road   Zip: 08053
Ph: (856) 355-6730
- Arerangaiah, Ramya B., MD
- Evans, Carrie Marie, DO
- Rivlin, Kwan Thanaporn, MD

Virtua Internal Medicine-Marlton
601 Route 73 North/Suite 101   Zip: 08053
Ph: (856) 429-1910   Fax: (856) 396-0848
- Abiuso, Patrick D. Jr., MD
- Najafi, Nawid E., MD
- Zuniga, Rina De Guzman, MD

Virtua Marlton Hospitalist Group
94 Brock Road/Suite 302   Zip: 08053
Ph: (856) 355-6730
- Mohageb, Salah M., MD

Virtua Medical Group
401 Route 73/40 Lake Ctr Dr/Ste 201A   Zip: 08053
Ph: (856) 355-0340   Fax: (856) 355-0346
- Maier, Dawn Rachel, MD
- Matsinger, John Mark, DO

Virtua Pulmonology - Marlton
141 Route 70/Suite B   Zip: 08053
Ph: (856) 596-9057   Fax: (856) 596-0837
- Jaffe, Brian C., MD

West Jersey Anesthesia Assoc PA
102 Centre Boulevard/Suite East   Zip: 08053
Ph: (856) 988-6260   Fax: (856) 988-6270
- Karanzalis, Demetrius, DO
- Lingaraju, Rajiv, MD
- Santos, Francis Parrocho, MD

West Jersey Anesthesia Associates
102-E Center Boulevard   Zip: 08053
Ph: (856) 988-6250   Fax: (856) 988-6270
- Avella, David Paul, MD
- Bilgrami, Sajad Syed, DO
- Bravyak, James G., DO
- Grossman, Davida S., MD
- Hermann, Todd G., MD
- Iula, Frank J. Jr., MD
- Jiang, Heng, MD
- Kasarda, Frances E., MD

West Jersey Anesthesia Associates
102E Centre Boulevard   Zip: 08053
Ph: (856) 988-6260   Fax: (856) 988-6270
- Knoll, Frank J. III, MD
- Lee, Aland H., MD
- Lehrer, Luisa E., MD
- Levitt, Cory A., MD
- Lewin, Stacy B., MD
- Lynch, Jeffrey R., MD
- McIntyre, Bryan J., DO
- Modi, Parag, MD
- Morgan, Kathleen A., MD

West Jersey Anesthesia Associates
102 East Centre Boulevard   Zip: 08053
Ph: (856) 988-6260   Fax: (856) 988-6270
- Nduaguba, Chiazoka Onyeka, MD
- Pace, Enrico, MD
- Pascarella, Michael Ryan, DO
- Pierre, Andre M., MD
- Pisera, Donna M., MD
- Quint, James Douglas, MD
- Reichman, Cynthia M., MD
- Reilly, Dennis K., DO

Groups and Clinics by Town with Physician Rosters

Sperandio, Peter G.N., MD
Villamayor, Carlos Pestelos, MD

Marmora

Atlanticare Family Medicine
210 South Shore Road/Suite 201 Zip: 08223
Ph: (609) 407-2273 Fax: (609) 390-2753
 Applebaum, Steven Lee, DO
 Hutcheson, Jonathan Justin, DO
 Hutchison, Melissa M., MD

Family Practice Assocs of Cape May
210 Route US 9 South/Suite 202 Zip: 08223
Ph: (609) 390-0882 Fax: (609) 390-3511
 Leo, Nicole Terese, DO
 Schneider, Wayne R., MD

Hope Community Cancer Center LLC
210 South Shore Road/Suite 106-A Zip: 08223
Ph: (609) 390-7888 Fax: (609) 390-2614
 Ahmad, Kaleem U., MD
 Childs, Julianne Wilkin, DO
 Dave, Hemang U., MD
 Pompa, Tiffany, MD
 Rizvi, Muhammad A., MD

Martinsville

Martinsville Family Practice
1973 Washington Valley Road Zip: 08836
Ph: (732) 560-9225 Fax: (732) 560-8095
 Accurso, Daniela, MD
 Frisoli, Anthony, MD
 Gannon, Michael A., MD
 Labbadia, Francesco, MD
 Price, Kelly A., MD

Refelctions Center For Skin & Body
1924 Washington Valley Road Zip: 08836
Ph: (732) 356-1666
 Chasin, Mitchell C., MD
 Karolak, Mark, DO

Matawan

Jersey Medical Care, PC
100 Belchase Drive/Suite 101 Zip: 07747
Ph: (732) 707-4100 Fax: (732) 707-4101
 Moshkovich, Marina, MD
 Vorobyev, Leonid A., MD

Matawan Medical Associates
213 Main Street Zip: 07747
Ph: (732) 566-2363 Fax: (732) 566-0502
 Arbour, Robert M., MD
 Bais, Rajney Monica, MD
 Fischer, Lauren Jane, MD
 Ghabras, Magda S., DO
 Hanna, Dalia N., MD
 Mancuso, Cathie-Ann, MD

Stress Care Clinic of NJ LLC
4122 Route 516/Suite C & D Zip: 07747
Ph: (732) 679-4500 Fax: (732) 679-4549
 Geller, Felix A., MD
 Neelgund, Ashwini Kumar, MD

The Doctor's Office
1070 Highway 34/Suite C Zip: 07747
Ph: (732) 290-0300 Fax: (732) 290-9661
 Feng, Shufang, MD
 Ould Hammou, Ayesha N. Haque, MD
 Tran, Vincent Phuong, DO

Mays Landing

CHOP Pedi & Adol Specialty Care Center
4009 Black Horse Pike Zip: 08330
Ph: (609) 677-7895 Fax: (609) 677-7835
 Burgess, David B., MD
 Huang, Patty P., MD
 Kruger, Hillary Anne, MD
 Naeem, Ambreen, MD

Mid Atlantic Retina - Wills Eye Retina
1417 Cantillon Boulevard Zip: 08330
Ph: (609) 625-0402 Fax: (609) 625-0788
 Maguire, Joseph I., MD
 Sivalingam, Arunan, MD

Maywood

113 West Essex Street/Suite 202 Zip: 07607
Ph: (201) 487-3400 Fax: (201) 487-2481
 Cohen, Stephanie Meryl, MD
 Winters, Richard M., MD
 Yueh, Janet Han, MD

Drs. Fulop and Fulop
653 Maywood Avenue Zip: 07607
Ph: (201) 845-9053
 Fulop, Eugene, MD
 Fulop, Luminita, MD

Infectious Disease Associates of North
255 West Spring Valley/Suite 100 Zip: 07607
Ph: (201) 881-0107
 Nguyen, Han Ngoc, MD

NJ Center For Prostate Cancer/Urology
255 West Spring Valley Avenue Zip: 07607
Ph: (201) 487-8866 Fax: (201) 487-2602
 Ahmed, Mutahar, MD
 Christiano, Thomas R., MD
 Esposito, Michael P., MD
 Goldstein, Martin M., MD
 La Salle, Michael Drew, MD
 Lanteri, Vincent J., MD
 Lovallo, Gregory G., MD
 Patel, Nitin Nick, MD
 Siegel, Andrew L., MD

Restoration Orthopaedics
113 West Essex Street/Suite 201 Zip: 07607
Ph: (201) 226-0145 Fax: (201) 226-0147
 Allert, Jesse William, MD
 Keller, Julie Michelle, MD
 Lindholm, Stephen R., MD

Vanguard Wellness Center
113 West Essex Street/Suite 204 Zip: 07607
Ph: (201) 289-5551 Fax: (201) 843-2390
 Ciminello, Frank Salvatore, MD
 Feintisch, Adam, MD
 Hahn, Edward Jr., MD

Medford

Advocare Medford Pedi & Adolescent Med
520 Stokes Road Zip: 08055
Ph: (609) 654-9112 Fax: (609) 654-7404
 Buccigrossi, Jennifer Leigh, MD
 Coss, Wanda I., MD
 Foran, Daniel J., DO
 Reed, Rebecca Ann, DO
 Roscioli-Jones, Catherine A., MD
 Scott, Charles A., MD
 Weitz, Robert D., DO

Advocare Medford Station Int Medicine
69 North Main Street Zip: 08055
Ph: (609) 953-9000 Fax: (609) 953-9696
 Hickey, Joseph J., MD
 Holton, James Jeffrey, MD
 Waldron, John R., DO

Alliance for Better Care, P.C.
PO Box 1510 Zip: 08055
Ph: (609) 953-4099 Fax: (609) 953-8652
 Godleski, Thomas D., DO
 Ianacone, Mary R., DO

Cornerstone Asthma & Allergy Assocs
103 Old Marlton Pike/Suite 211 Zip: 08055
Ph: (609) 953-7500 Fax: (609) 953-9085
 Bantz, Eric W., MD
 Kim, John Yohan, MD

Dermatology and Laser Center
622 Stokes Road/Suite A Zip: 08055
Ph: (609) 953-0908 Fax: (609) 953-5978
 Harrop, Elyse Horn, MD
 High, David A., MD
 Klein, Rachel S., MD

Dorfner Family Medicine
639 Stokes Road/Suite 102 Zip: 08055
Ph: (609) 654-7556 Fax: (609) 714-9228
 Ponnamaneni, Abhilasha Rao, MD

Eye Care Physicians & Surgeons Of NJ
73 South Main Street Zip: 08055
Ph: (609) 654-6140 Fax: (609) 953-2257
 Hyder, Carl Franklin, MD
 Veloudios, Angela, MD

Medford Family Practice
152 Himmelein Road/Suite 100 Zip: 08055
Ph: (609) 654-7117 Fax: (609) 654-8555
 Amankwaah, Ajoa O., DO
 Jones, Graham P., MD

Reconstructive Orthopedics, P.A.
131 Route 70 West/Suite 100 Zip: 08055
Ph: (609) 267-9400 Fax: (609) 267-9457
 Gomez, Andrew Thomas, MD

South Jersey Eye Physicians PA
103 Old Marlton Pike/Suite 216 Zip: 08055
Ph: (609) 714-8761 Fax: (609) 714-8759
 Cohen, Sander M., MD

The Cardiology Group, P.A.
128 State Highway Route 70/Suite 1-B Zip: 08055
Ph: (856) 291-8855 Fax: (856) 444-5521
 O'Neil, James P., MD

The Gastroenterology Group, PA
103 Old Marlton Pike/Suite 102 Zip: 08055
Ph: (609) 953-3440 Fax: (609) 996-4002
 Barash, Craig Ross, MD
 Frates, Angela Dawn, MD
 Kravitz, John Jay, MD
 Modena, Scott Alan, MD
 Salowe, David Ross, MD
 Volpe, John Anthony, DO

Virtua Family Medicine
103 Old Marlton Pike/Suite 103 Zip: 08055
Ph: (609) 953-7105 Fax: (609) 953-0042
 Hollander, Philip, DO
 Patragnoni, Richard M., DO
 Pinto, Jeffrey Damian, DO

Virtua Medford Medical Center
128 Route 70 Zip: 08055
Ph: (609) 953-7111 Fax: (609) 953-1544
 Glass, James M., MD
 Scuderi, Steven A., MD
 Zarroli, Hannah J., MD

Mendham

Atlantic Cardiology Group LLP
8 Tempe Wick Road Zip: 07945
Ph: (973) 543-2288 Fax: (973) 543-0637
 Amoruso, Daniel Robert, MD
 Olivieri, Philip J., MD
 Randazzo, Domenick N., MD
 Ricculli, Nicholas P., DO
 Rusovici, Arthur, MD
 Shioleno, Charles A., MD
 Tully, Lisa Anita, MD

Mendham Medical Group LLP
19 East Main Street/Suite 1 Zip: 07945
Ph: (973) 543-6505 Fax: (973) 543-2967
 Ciuffreda, Ronald V., MD
 Connolly, Allison Carthan, MD
 Marella, Gregg G., MD
 Prestifilippo, Christie J., MD
 Wolf, James H., MD

Mercerville

Altus Medical Care
3840 Quakerbridge Road/Suite 206 Zip: 08619
Ph: (609) 890-4200 Fax: (609) 586-0399
 Chawla, Rajnish Paul Singh, MD
 Chawla, Rupinder, MD
 Mangiaracina, Giacomo, MD

Infectious Disease Consultants
1245 Whitehorse-Mercerville Rd Zip: 08619
Ph: (609) 581-2000 Fax: (609) 581-5450
 Farooq, Tahir, MD
 Husain, Syed Asif, DO
 Mathai, Suja John, MD
 Patel, Anamika K., MD
 Porwancher, Richard B., MD

Stawicki & Patnaik Medical Associates
1235 Whitehorse Mercerville Rd Zip: 08619
Ph: (609) 581-5586 Fax: (609) 581-5779
 Stawicki, Jesse J., DO

Zak Maniya, M.D., P.A.
2333 Whitehorse-Mercerville Rd/Suite 4 Zip: 08619
Ph: (609) 890-9111 Fax: (609) 890-6865
 Maniya, Zakaria W., MD
 Nisar, Asif, MD

Merchantville

Drs Husain and Shen
5 West Chestnut Avenue Zip: 08109
Ph: (856) 665-9424
 Husain, Abbas M., MD
 Shen, Hongxie, MD

Drs. Curreri and Curreri
124 Lexington Avenue Zip: 08109
Ph: (856) 663-1121 Fax: (856) 661-9818
 Curreri, Joseph P., DO
 Curreri, Peter Andrew, DO

Drs. Gilliss and DiRenzo
27 East Chestnut Avenue Zip: 08109
Ph: (856) 662-0424 Fax: (856) 662-7404
 Gilliss, Adam C., DO
 Gilliss, Matthew J., DO

NaltrexZone, LLC.
1 South Centre Street/Suite 201 Zip: 08109
Ph: (856) 663-4447 Fax: (856) 488-6380
 Aronow, Phillip Z., MD
 Gooberman, Lance L., MD
 Scardigli, Dennis Michael, MD
 Wilson, John Goss Jr., MD

Metuchen

Advanced Dermatology Center PC
18 Bridge Street Zip: 08840
Ph: (732) 635-1200
 Lee, Jane Mengchuan, MD
 Lee, Peter Yujen, MD

Brunswick Internal Medical Group
17 Bridge Street Zip: 08840
Ph: (732) 321-1600 Fax: (732) 321-1699
 Kainth, Inderjit S., MD
 Kaur, Dvinder, MD

Center for Advanced Pain Mangmnt/Rehab
249 Bridge Street/Building G Zip: 08840
Ph: (732) 516-1060 Fax: (732) 516-1015
 Alhamrawy, Ismail A., MD

Clara Barton Cardio-Medical Assc
78 Amboy Avenue Zip: 08840
Ph: (732) 548-4365
 Sodhi, Ajit S., MD

Ob-Gyn Group of Metuchen, PA
73 Amboy Avenue Zip: 08840
Ph: (732) 548-0698 Fax: (732) 548-3087
 Ainslie, William Jr., MD
 Steinbeck, Wayne E., MD

Pediatric Associates of Central Jersey
326 Main Street Zip: 08840
Ph: (732) 767-0630 Fax: (732) 767-3070
 Lebovic, Daniel M., MD
 Rosenblum, Howard W., MD
 Santiago, Maritza Marie, MD

Primecare Medical Group
561 Middlesex Avenue Zip: 08840
Ph: (732) 549-9363 Fax: (732) 603-0397
 Garcia, Maria Teresa, MD
 Jasani, Anita, MD
 Rossy, William H., MD
 Zhang, Miaoying, MD

Mickleton

The Minniti Center/Medical Onc & Hema
174 Democrat Road Zip: 08056
Ph: (856) 423-0754
 Minniti, Carl J. Jr., MD

Middlesex

Mahmood A. Shamsi, MD, PA
1273 Bound Brook Road/Suite 10 Zip: 08846
Ph: (732) 563-6630 Fax: (732) 563-6733
 Shamsi, Mahmood A., MD
 Shamsi, Zahira B., MD

Groups and Clinics by Town with Physician Rosters

Middletown
Advanced Interventional Pain Center
20 Cherry Tree Farm Road Zip: 07748
Ph: (732) 952-5533 Fax: (732) 707-4732
- Poonia, Amit, MD
- Xie, Jinghui, MD

Barnabus Health Medical Group
1270 Highway 35 South/Suite 1 Zip: 07748
Ph: (732) 615-3900
- Farrugia, Peter Michael, MD
- Potylitsina, Yelena, MD

Drs. Swartz & Swartz
138 Cherry Tree Farm Road Zip: 07748
Ph: (732) 671-3313 Fax: (732) 671-8513
- Swartz, Harry M., MD
- Swartz, Stephen Jay, MD

EMedical Urgent Care
2 Kings Highway Zip: 07748
Ph: (732) 957-0707 Fax: (732) 957-9852
- Armbruster, Thomas C., MD
- Fong, Dean Kimton, MD
- Leschinsky, Alexandra, MD
- Morlino, John V., DO
- Samson, Kristine T., MD
- Sennett, Jane M., DO

Family Practice of Middletown
18 Leonardville Road Zip: 07748
Ph: (732) 671-0860 Fax: (732) 671-6467
- Giacona, Caryn Marie, MD
- Gold, Marcia D., MD
- McManus, Shanda Monique, MD
- Thompson, Roger McLachlan, MD
- Zaky, Mark, MD

Family Wellness Center
1680 State Route 35 Zip: 07748
Ph: (732) 671-3730 Fax: (732) 706-1078
- Dornfeld, David B., D

Medical Health Center
1270 State Highway 35 Zip: 07748
Ph: (732) 615-3900 Fax: (732) 615-0865
- Clemente, Joseph, MD
- Dobrescu, Delia J., MD
- Gross, Russell A., MD
- Shah, Ajay S., MD
- Suaray, Khalil M., MD

Midland Park
Bergen Hprtens & Renal Assoc
44 Godwin Avenue/Suite 301 Zip: 07432
Ph: (201) 447-0013 Fax: (201) 447-0438
- Ackad, Alexandre V., MD
- Chheda, Neha Das, MD
- Kotlov, Mikhail, MD
- Kozlowski, Jeffrey P., MD
- Raza, Syed Irfan, MD
- Rho, John I., MD
- Weizman, Howard B., MD

Northern Jersey ENT Assoc
44 Godwin Avenue Zip: 07432
Ph: (201) 445-2900 Fax: (201) 445-8679
- Milgrim, Laurence Marc, MD

Prospect Medical Offices, LLC
301 Godwin Avenue Zip: 07432
Ph: (201) 444-4526 Fax: (201) 301-1313
- Beauchamp, Donald P., MD
- Cohen, Ricky B., MD
- Giorlando, Mary Elizabeth, MD
- Hart, Karen Manheimer, MD
- Hope, Lisa Dawn, MD
- Kopelman, Rima G., MD
- Leibowitz, Evan Howard, MD
- Leifer, Bennett P., MD
- Murphy, Ryan Keith, DO
- Prinz, Karola Kristina, MD
- Valinoti, Anne Marie, MD
- Zaider, Arik, MD

Respiratory Health & Critical Care
44 Godwin Avenue/Suite 201 Zip: 07432
Ph: (201) 689-7755 Fax: (201) 689-0521
- Rosen, David Michael, MD

Urology Group PA
4 Godwin Avenue Zip: 07432
Ph: (201) 444-7070 Fax: (201) 444-7228
- Baum, Richard D., MD
- DeTorres, Wayne Raymond, MD

- Frey, Howard L., MD
- Hartanto, Victor H., MD
- Mackey, Timothy Joseph, MD

VMG-Internal Medicine Midland Park
44 Goodwin Street/Suite 201 Zip: 07432
Ph: (201) 891-5044 Fax: (201) 891-1119
- Dziezanowski, Margaret Ann, MD
- Frauwirth, Howard David, MD

Valley Medical Group
44 Godwin Avenue/Suite 2 Zip: 07432
Ph: (201) 444-5992 Fax: (201) 444-9984
- Dabaj, Dina, MD
- Eskow, Raymond P., MD

Milford
Delaware Valley Family Health Center
200 Frenchtown Road Zip: 08848
Ph: (908) 995-2251 Fax: (908) 995-2036
- Bauman, Susan M., MD
- Bryhn, Lisa Kristen, MD
- Curry, Debra W., MD
- Hewens, Jeremy C., MD
- Jardim, Carla Mia, MD
- Jones, Howard D., MD
- Kayal, William Jesse, MD
- Kozakowski, Stanley M., MD
- Kroth, Patricia Haeusler, DO
- Lucco, Julianne M., MD
- Murry, Robert L., MD
- Patel, Jigger, MD
- Skillinge, David D., DO
- Turenne Kolpan, Laurie Kathleen, MD

Millburn
Assocs In Internal Med & Nephrology
225 Millburn Avenue/Suite 104-B Zip: 07041
Ph: (973) 218-9330 Fax: (973) 218-9351
- Freundlich, Nancy Lynn, MD
- Freundlich, Richard E., MD

Associates Colon & Rectal Dis
231 Millburn Avenue Zip: 07041
Ph: (973) 467-2277 Fax: (973) 467-4037
- Gilder, Mark E., MD
- Orringer, Robert D., MD
- Tarantino, Debra R., MD

Associates in Primary Care, P.A.
25 East Willow Street Zip: 07041
Ph: (973) 379-5055 Fax: (973) 379-5324
- Pitoscia, Thomas, MD
- Quaglia, Silvio A., MD

Buono Pediatrics & Wellness
171 Millburn Avenue Zip: 07041
Ph: (606) 557-3085
- Buono, Amy C., MD
- Cotler, Donald N., MD

Comprehensive Orthopaedics
235 Millburn Avenue/Suite 102 Zip: 07041
Ph: (973) 258-1177 Fax: (973) 258-1818
- Richmond, Daniel B., MD
- Schob, Clifford J., MD

Comprehensive Pulmonary & CriticalCare
96 Millburn Avenue/Suite 200A Zip: 07041
Ph: (973) 763-6800 Fax: (973) 763-1255
- Mehta, Chirag A., MD
- Shah, Himanshu P., MD
- Shah, Smita S., MD

Diamond Institute for Infertility
89 Millburn Avenue Zip: 07041
Ph: (973) 761-5600 Fax: (973) 761-5100
- Birkenfeld, Arie, MD
- Onwubalili, Ndidiamaka, MD
- Yemini, Matan, MD

Drs. Gruenwald & Comandatore
90 Millburn Avenue/Suite 101 Zip: 07041
Ph: (973) 378-7990 Fax: (973) 378-7991
- Alexander, Andrea Hope, MD
- Comandatore, Ann Marie, MD
- Gruenwald, Laurence D., MD
- Meshko, Yanina, MD
- Ramesh, Shruti Chakrabarti, DO
- Spiteri, Sharon, MD
- Sterio, Mara, MD
- Thompson, Stacy Ellen, DO

Essex Urology Associates/UGNJ
225 Millburn Avenue/Suite 304 Zip: 07041
Ph: (973) 218-9400 Fax: (973) 218-9420
- Helfman, Alan S., MD
- Shoengold, Stuart D., MD
- Strumeyer, Alan D., MD

Garden State Bariatrics & Wellness Ctr
225 Millburn Avenue/Suite 204 Zip: 07041
Ph: (973) 218-1990 Fax: (973) 629-1274
- Bilof, Michael Louis, MD
- Yurcisin, Basil Michael II, MD

Ophthalmology Associates of Millburn
288 Millburn Avenue Zip: 07041
Ph: (973) 912-9100 Fax: (973) 912-0800
- Greenfield, Donald A., MD
- Pruzon, Joanna Dawn, DO

Millburn Family Practice
425 Essex Street Zip: 07041
Ph: (973) 379-3051
- Glezen-Schneider, Priscilla Ann, MD

Millburn Laser Center
12 East Willow Street Zip: 07041
Ph: (973) 376-8500 Fax: (973) 376-1820
- Brockman-Bitterman, Allyson Stacy,
- Freeman, Amy Ilyse, MD
- Mautner, Gail H., MD
- Siegel, Eric Scott, MD

Millburn Ob-Gyn Associates, P.A.
233 Millburn Avenue Zip: 07041
Ph: (973) 467-9440 Fax: (973) 376-1680
- Cooperman, Alan Stewart, MD
- Luciani, Richard L., MD
- Pollack, Marshall S., MD
- Seymour, Christopher R., MD
- Simonetti, John M., MD

Millburn Pediatrics PA
159 Millburn Avenue Zip: 07041
Ph: (973) 912-0155 Fax: (973) 912-8714
- Batra, Chhaya, MD
- Knowles, Kelly Petrison, MD
- Mangru, Subita S., MD

Millburn Primary Care LLC
120 Millburn Avenue/Suite 206 Zip: 07041
Ph: (973) 467-9282 Fax: (973) 467-0340
- Frankel, Trina N., MD

Millburn Surgical Associates
225 Millburn Avenue/Suite 104-B Zip: 07041
Ph: (973) 379-5888 Fax: (973) 912-9757
- Kopelan, Adam Michael, MD
- Manicone, John A., MD
- Saccone, Paul Gregori, MD

NJ Cardiovascular Care Center
116 Millburn Avenue/Suite 214 Zip: 07041
Ph: (973) 218-6000 Fax: (973) 679-8636
- Desai, Rajendra R., MD
- Saeed, Qaisra Yasmin, MD

PASE Healthcare, PC
225 Millburn Avenue/Suite 303 Zip: 07041
Ph: (973) 912-7273 Fax: (973) 912-7275
- Biernat, Matthew Mateusz, MD
- Miraglia, Janeen Theresa, DO
- Pinho, Paulo Bandeira, MD

Pain Medicine Physicians
187 Millburn Avenue/Suite 103 Zip: 07041
Ph: (973) 467-1466 Fax: (973) 467-1422
- D'Alessio, Donna Giselda, MD
- De Mais, John R., MD

Short Hills Surgery Center
187 Millburn Avenue/Suite 101 Zip: 07041
Ph: (973) 671-0555 Fax: (973) 671-0557
- Verea, Vickie, MD

The Cardiovascular Care Group
25 East Willow Street Zip: 07041
Ph: (973) 921-9600
- Addis, Michael Downes, MD

The Heart Group, PA
161 Millburn Avenue Zip: 07041
Ph: (973) 467-4220 Fax: (973) 467-9889
- Aueron, Fred M., MD
- Charney, Robert Howard, MD
- Gantz, Kenneth B., MD
- Simandl, Susan Lynn, MD

Tri-County Medical Associates
120 Millburn Avenue/Suite M3 Zip: 07041
Ph: (973) 912-0001 Fax: (973) 912-0099
- Roy, Satyajeet, MD
- Thomas, Alapatt Porinchu, MD

Millstone Township
Franklin Medical Center
514 Route 33 West/Suite 6 Zip: 08535
Ph: (732) 851-7007 Fax: (732) 786-0012
- Gendy, Hany Moris, MD
- Shah, Sejal Gohel, MD

Millville
Community Health Care, Inc.
1200 North High Street Zip: 08332
Ph: (856) 451-4700 Fax: (856) 327-4208
- Geria, Michael J., Dr
- Salloum, Azizeh J., MD

Cumberland Family Medicine
1203 North High Street/Suite A Zip: 08332
Ph: (856) 327-0182 Fax: (856) 327-7381
- Davis, Brian Joseph, DO
- Mortensen, Jill, DO

Drs. Aderholdt and Akrout
3 Elizabeth Street Zip: 08332
Ph: (856) 641-6272
- Aderholdt, David Gabriel, DO
- Akrout, Eddie, MD

Drs. Babalola and Giyanani
1601 North 2nd Street/Suite C1 Zip: 08332
Ph: (856) 691-3145 Fax: (856) 691-0625
- Babalola, Gbolagade Olanrewaju, DO
- Giyanani, Sunita M., MD

Holly City Pediatrics
10 East Main Street/Suite A Zip: 08332
Ph: (856) 825-5932 Fax: (856) 825-4819
- Jamil, Erum, MD
- Patel, Ketan R., MD

Millville Medical Center
1700 North Tenth Street Zip: 08332
Ph: (856) 327-6446
- Kaczaj, Olga, MD
- Piszcz-Connelly, Malgorzata A., MD

The Eye Professionals, P.A.
1205 North High Street Zip: 08332
Ph: (856) 825-8700 Fax: (856) 825-8640
- Ghobrial, John M., MD
- Pernelli, David R., MD

Mine Hill
Internal Medicine of Morris County
195 Route 46 West/Suite 102 Zip: 07803
Ph: (973) 366-6060
- Estrada, Aristides M., MD
- Forward, John B., MD

Morris Urology
195 Route 46/Suite 100 Zip: 07803
Ph: (973) 627-0060 Fax: (973) 627-6821
- Colton, Marc D., MD

Monroe
Cranbury Heart and Lung Associates
283 Applegarth Road Zip: 08831
Ph: (609) 655-1046
- Logothetis, George Nicholas, MD
- Logothetis, James Nicholas, MD

Family Practice of CentraState
312 Applegarth Road/Suite 107 Zip: 08831
Ph: (609) 395-2939 Fax: (609) 395-4179
- Gopal, Richa, MD

Hypertension & Nephrology Specialists
2 Research Way/Suite 301 Zip: 08831
Ph: (732) 521-0800 Fax: (732) 521-0833
- Ahuja, Kavita Bala, DO
- Arabi, Mona Najib, MD
- Arabi, Nida, MD
- Dwivedi, Shaunak A., DO

Mehta, Ojas R., DO
Sterman, Paul Lawrence, MD

Ocean Urology
52 Constitution Drive   Zip: 08831
Ph: (732) 349-5200   Fax: (732) 349-5235
Lewis, Walter Emmett III, MD
Lieberman, Alan Howard, MD

Monroe Township

Abhijit Chatterjee MD PC
312 Applegarth Road/Suite 207   Zip: 08831
Ph: (609) 655-2700   Fax: (609) 655-2565
Chatterjee, Abhijit, MD
Patel, Ravish Mukesh, MD

Cardio Metabolic Institute
294 Applegarth Road/Suite F   Zip: 08831
Ph: (609) 642-4747   Fax: (732) 846-7001
Maleki, Kataneh F., MD

Center For Healthy Aging
18 Centre Drive/Suite 104   Zip: 08831
Ph: (609) 655-5178   Fax: (609) 655-5284
Kobylarz, Fred A., MD
Krauser, Paula S., MD

Hem Care Medical Clinic
6 Agnes Court   Zip: 08831
Ph: (609) 409-6767   Fax: (609) 409-6776
Allu, Sridevi, MD
Nanavati, Kartikey Jayendrakumar, M
Nanavati, Kaushal Kartikey, MD

Monroe Family Medicine
323 Spotswood Englishtown Road/Suite B   Zip: 08831
Ph: (732) 723-1000   Fax: (732) 416-0470
Prasad, Deepali, MD
Prasad, Keshav, MD

Outlook Eyecare
5 Centre Drive/1B   Zip: 08831
Ph: (609) 409-2777   Fax: (609) 409-2718
Grabowski, Wayne M., MD

Princeton & Rutgers Neurology
9 Centre Drive/Suite 130   Zip: 08831
Ph: (609) 395-7615   Fax: (609) 395-1885
Friedlander, Devin S., MD

Princeton Dermatology Associates
5 Centre Street/Suite 1-A   Zip: 08831
Ph: (609) 655-4544   Fax: (609) 655-2390
Kaufmann, Roderick Jr., MD
Peloro, Concettina M., MD
Vaidya, Darshan C., MD

Princeton Medical Group PA
2 Research Way/Bldg 2/Suite 302   Zip: 08831
Ph: (609) 655-8800   Fax: (609) 655-7466
Gjenvick, Timothy C., MD
Grossman, Leonard A., MD

Princeton Nassau Pediatrics, P.A.
312 Applegarth Road/Suite 104   Zip: 08831
Ph: (609) 409-5600   Fax: (609) 409-5610
Doshi, Deepa, MD
Hemrajani, Payal, MD
shah, Amisha M., MD

Raritan Bay Cardiology
7 Centre Dtrive/Suite 13   Zip: 08831
Ph: (609) 655-8860   Fax: (609) 655-8065
Baron, Phillip, MD
Freedman, Andrew R., MD

Saint Peter's Physician Associates
294 Applegarth Road   Zip: 08831
Ph: (609) 409-1363
Hussain, Aijaz, MD
Levy-Kern, Muriel, MD

Montclair

Crescent Internal Medicine Group
98 Park Street   Zip: 07042
Ph: (973) 783-0800   Fax: (973) 744-1274
Krupp, Edward Todd, DO
Mohan, Mamatha G., MD

Drs. Allam and Allam
73 Park Street/3rd Floor   Zip: 07042
Ph: (973) 746-0595   Fax: (973) 746-1848
Allam, Naveen Reddy, MD
Allam, Reddy B., MD

Essex Women's Health Care Center
33 North Fullerton Avenue   Zip: 07042
Ph: (973) 744-2226   Fax: (973) 509-0978
De Marsico, Richard, MD
Degrande, Gary C., MD

Gastroenterology Associates of NJ
88 Park Street   Zip: 07042
Ph: (973) 233-9559   Fax: (973) 233-9660
Abraham, Rini S., MD
Volfson, Ariy, MD

Montclair Breast Center
37 North Fullerton Avenue   Zip: 07042
Ph: (973) 509-1818   Fax: (973) 509-0532
Elliott, Nancy L., MD
Hertz, Marcie B., MD
Lee, Joo-Young Melissa, MD
Ow, Cheng H., MD
Quackenbush, Gail, MD

Montclair Pediatrics
73 Park Street   Zip: 07042
Hung, Yvonne, MD
Paisner, Raphael, MD

Montclair Radiology
116 Park Street   Zip: 07042
Ph: (973) 746-2525   Fax: (973) 746-5802
Jewel, Kenneth L., MD
Mattern, Richard F., MD
McFadden, Denise C., MD
Shah, Mala T., MD

Neurological Care of New Jersey, P.A.
95 Gates Avenue   Zip: 07042
Ph: (973) 744-3166   Fax: (973) 744-3199
Clemente, Roderick J., MD
Dannis, Seth Michael, MD

New Jersey Plastic Surgery
29 Park Street   Zip: 07042
Ph: (973) 509-2000   Fax: (973) 655-1228
DiBernardo, Barry E., MD
Haramis, Harry Theodore, MD

Park West Associates
33 Plymouth Street/Suite 104   Zip: 07042
Ph: (973) 509-1444   Fax: (973) 509-1446
Bienenfeld, Scott I., MD
Westreich, Laurence M., MD

Plastic Surgery Center Internationale
89 Valley Road   Zip: 07042
Ph: (973) 746-3535   Fax: (973) 746-4385
Giampapa, Vincent C., MD
Mesa, John Mario, MD

Plastic Surgery Group
37 North Fullerton Avenue   Zip: 07042
Ph: (973) 233-1933   Fax: (973) 233-1934
Ablaza, Valerie J., MD
Rosen, Allen D., MD

Sheila Harrington, LCSW
8 Hillside Avenue/Suite 106   Zip: 07042
Ph: (973) 509-2371   Fax: (973) 744-9003
Meyer, Sarah E., MD
Phariss, Bruce Wallace, MD

Summit Medical Group
48-50 Fairfield Street   Zip: 07042
Ph: (973) 744-8511   Fax: (973) 744-6356
Grobstein, Naomi S., MD
Hostetler, Caecilia E., MD
Hrishikesan, Geetha, MD
Khan, Afshan R., DO
Novak, Eva Cesnek, MD
Piwowar, Karen, MD
Ramos-Genvino, Elizabeth, MD
Shimelfarb, Marianna Borkovskaya, M

Summit Medical Group Cardiology
62 South Fullerton Avenue   Zip: 07042
Ph: (973) 746-8585   Fax: (973) 746-0088
Bannerman, Kenneth S., MD
Di Filippo, John A., MD
Gutman, Julius A., MD
Kim, Harold J., MD
Miller, Kenneth Paul, MD
Prior, Francis P., MD

Montvale

Hackensack UMG Montavale
305 West Grand Avenue   Zip: 07645
Ph: (201) 746-9150   Fax: (201) 746-9151
Jean, Nagaeda, MD
Langer, Myriam, MD

Valley Medical Group of Montvale
85 Chestnut Ridge Road/Suite 111   Zip: 07645
Ph: (201) 930-1700   Fax: (201) 930-0705
Ajemian, Ara Antranik, MD
Rodriquez, Margaret, MD
Sherman, Mark David, MD
Varghese, Rebecca M., MD

Montville

Montville Primary Care Physicians
137 Main Road   Zip: 07045
Ph: (973) 402-0025   Fax: (973) 402-0508
Filion, Jacqueline D. Weil, DO
Gargano, Joseph A., DO
Keating, William G., DO
O'Connor, Brandon P., MD
Rehberg, Joelle Stabile, DO
Subrati, Rahman Ryan, MD

Primary Care Associates of NJ
329 Main Road/Suite 101   Zip: 07045
Ph: (973) 334-9404   Fax: (973) 334-7615
Golloub, Cory A., MD
Lin, Annie, DO

Vanguard Medical Group, P.A.
170 Changebridge Road/Suite C-3   Zip: 07045
Ph: (973) 575-5540   Fax: (973) 575-4885
Coelho, Ryan, MD
Gilmartin, Andrew Philip, MD
Iannetta, Frank, MD
Lapsiwala, Pareen Raj, DO
Pallay, Arnold I., MD
Zimmerman, Anahita, MD

Moorestown

Advocare Main Street Medical Assoc
714 East Main Street/Suite 1-C   Zip: 08057
Ph: (856) 778-4009   Fax: (856) 778-4014
Levin, Irina, MD
Levin, Joseph B., MD
Levin, Sanan L., MD
Nirenberg, Elena, MD

Alliance Internal Medicine
509 South Lenola Road/Suite 3   Zip: 08057
Ph: (856) 234-2722
Berna, Ronald A., MD
Berna, William J., MD

Center for Neurologic Specialty
401 Young Avenue/Suite 160   Zip: 08057
Ph: (856) 291-8780   Fax: (856) 291-8781
Vijayaraghavan, Swathi, MD

Cooper Family Medicine
110 Marter Avenue   Zip: 08057
Ph: (856) 608-8840   Fax: (856) 722-1898
Chan, Wai Ben, DO
Dennison, Alan D., MD
Kelly, Peter J., MD
Louis, Marie Edwige, MD
Ray, Anjali K., MD
Weinroth, Heidi J., MD

Cooper Pediatrics
110 Marter Avenue/Bldg. 500, Suite 505   Zip: 08057
Ph: (856) 536-1400   Fax: (856) 536-1402
Gordon, Anne M., MD

Dermatology Associates
303 Chester Avenue   Zip: 08057
Ph: (856) 235-1178   Fax: (856) 722-9244
Foti, Frederick D. Jr., MD
Koblenzer, Caroline S., MD

Drs. Chung & Shin
110 Marter Avenue/Suite 507   Zip: 08057
Ph: (856) 222-4766   Fax: (856) 222-1137
Brobyn, Tracy L., MD
Chung, Myung K., MD
Oswari, Andrew, MD
Shin, Jong Tae, DO

Endocrine Assocs of Southern Jersey
703 East Main Street/Suite 5   Zip: 08057
Ph: (856) 727-0900   Fax: (856) 231-8428
Entmacher, Susan D., MD
Gandrabura, Tatiana, MD
Herbst, Allison B., MD
Kankanala, Sucharitha, MD

Savarese, Vincent William, MD
Waronker-Silverstein, Amy S., MD

Endocrinology Associates
740 Marne Highway/Suite 206   Zip: 08057
Ph: (856) 234-0645   Fax: (856) 234-0498
Gonzalez Pantaleon, Adalberto D., M
Martz, Rebecca Lynn, MD
Pettigrew, Isabel Hilary, MD

Family Practice of Moorestown
728 Marne Highway/Suite B   Zip: 08057
Ph: (856) 235-6600   Fax: (856) 235-6610
Barr, Larry Allen, MD
Lanza, Paul R., DO

Horvitz, Steven P. & Cooperstein, Heid
128 Borton Landing Road/Suite 2   Zip: 08057
Ph: (856) 231-0590   Fax: (856) 231-1228
Cooperstein, Heidi B., DO
Horvitz, Steven P., DO

Minoff Chapman OB/GYN
110 Marter Avenue/Suite 504   Zip: 08057
Ph: (856) 642-6580   Fax: (856) 273-8372
Chapman, Derek Q., MD
Minoff, Michael H., MD

Moorestown Dermatology Associates
702 East Main Street   Zip: 08057
Ph: (856) 235-6565   Fax: (856) 235-6566
Camishion, Germaine Mary, MD
D'Ambra-Cabry, Kimberly A., MD

Moorestown Internal Medicine PC
147 East Third Street/Suite One   Zip: 08057
Ph: (856) 234-7754   Fax: (856) 234-2290
Gross, David D., MD
Kaufman, Jodi D., MD

Moorestown Pediatrics
212 West Route 38/Suite 400   Zip: 08057
Ph: (856) 235-0264   Fax: (856) 235-4635
Giardino, John Domenic Jr., MD
Guevarra, Andres T., MD
Guevarra, Jesusita H., MD

Mt. Laurel Family Physicians
401 Young Avenue/Suite 260   Zip: 08057
Ph: (856) 291-8756   Fax: (856) 291-8750
Land, Stephen M., MD
Lee, Thomas Yon, MD
Mills, Robert, DO
Pellegrino, Tara Marie, DO
Rutkiewicz, Laura A., MD
Shapiro, Gary I., MD
Termini, Joseph F., MD
Wasleski, Karen J., MD
Yudin, Joel S., DO

Primary Care of Moorestown
147 East 3rd Street/Suite 2   Zip: 08057
Ph: (856) 234-2500   Fax: (856) 234-3907
Burke, Hana Oswari, MD
Patel, Sanjiv C., MD

Reconstructive Orthopedics, P.A.
401 Young Avenue/Suite 245   Zip: 08057
Ph: (856) 267-9400   Fax: (609) 267-9457
Duckles, Benjamin Jeffrey, MD
Dwyer, Joseph Michael, MD
Greenleaf, Robert Martin, MD
Gutman, Gabriella, MD
Lee, Joseph Kim, MD
Marple, Jill Ann, MD
Patil, Meenal Kulkarni, MD
Raimondo, Rick Arthur, MD
Sanfilippo, James Arthur, MD

South Jersey Eye Physicians PA
509 South Lenola Road/Suite 11   Zip: 08057
Ph: (856) 234-0222   Fax: (856) 727-9518
Brown, Miriam Renee, MD
Colucciello, Michael, MD
Horowitz, Philip, MD
Nachbar, James G., MD
Putnam, Daniel Philip, MD
Tran, Trong D., MD
Wexler, Amy R., MD

Groups and Clinics by Town with Physician Rosters

Moorestown (cont)

The Cardiology Group, P.A.
401 Young Avenue/Suite 275 Zip: 08057
Ph: (856) 291-8855 Fax: (856) 291-8844
- Dennis,Charles A., MD
- Duca,Maria Diane, MD
- Finch,Mark T., MD
- Galski,Thomas M., DO
- Lederman,Steven M., MD
- Namey,Jeffrey Elias, MD
- Sauerwein,Anthony G., MD
- Schimenti,Robert J., MD
- Sussman,Jay I., MD
- Ventrella,Samuel M., MD

Virtua Express Urgent Care
401 Young Avenue/Suite 180 Zip: 08057
Ph: (856) 291-8600 Fax: (856) 291-8615
- Bhogal,Jasmeet Singh, MD
- Morel,Elyse R., MD

Virtua Obstetrics & Gynocology
401 Young Avenue Zip: 08057
Ph: (856) 291-8865 Fax: (856) 291-8880
- Gomez,Syeda Rabia, DO

Virtua Primary Care
401 Young Avenue/Suite 260 Zip: 08057
Ph: (856) 291-8920 Fax: (856) 291-8922
- Au,Alexander F., MD
- Sharma,Gaurav S., MD

Morganville

Best Care Pediatrics
470 Highway 79/Suite 12 Zip: 07751
Ph: (732) 970-9070 Fax: (732) 970-9071
- Lee,Kim Chiu, MD
- Yuen,Sharon Shue, MD

Central Jersey Urology Assocs
23 Kilmer Drive/Suite C/Building 1 Zip: 07751
Ph: (732) 972-9000
- Kirshenbaum,Alexander, MD
- Sukkarieh,Troy Z., MD

Spinal & Head Trauma Associates
1123 Campus Drive West Zip: 07751
Ph: (732) 617-9797 Fax: (732) 617-8899
- Sunwoo,Daniel, MD
- Varghese,Teena P., MD

Morris Plains

Drs. Cervone and Cervone
891 Tabor Road Zip: 07950
Ph: (973) 359-8859 Fax: (973) 359-8860
- Cervone,Maurizio, DO
- Cervone,Oswald, DO

Elias Medical Associates
2839 Route 10 East/Suite 202 Zip: 07950
Ph: (973) 292-9248 Fax: (973) 944-1228
- Elias,Ahdi I., MD
- Elias,Salwa E.G., MD

Morris Family Medicine Associates, PA
340 Speedwell Avenue/PO Box 190 Zip: 07950
Ph: (973) 267-9899 Fax: (973) 538-3522
- Joseph,Charles A., MD
- Lijo,Maria Carmen, MD

Synergy Anesthesia
2740 State Route 10/Suite 104 Zip: 07950
Ph: (973) 200-8224 Fax: (973) 695-1324
- Itzkovich,Chad Jason, MD

Morristown

Adult & Pediatric Urology Group
261 James Street/Suite 1-A Zip: 07960
Ph: (973) 539-0333 Fax: (973) 539-8909
- Ackerman,Anika Jahn, MD
- Atlas,Ian, MD
- Connor,John Patrick, MD
- Kaynan,Ayal Menashe, MD
- Steinberg,Joseph, MD
- Taylor,David L., MD

Advanced Musculoskeletal Center
131 Madison Avenue/Suite 130 Zip: 07960
Ph: (973) 538-8336
- Aurori,Brian F., MD
- Aurori,Kevin C., MD

Advanced Vascular Associates, PC
131 Madison Avenue/2nd Floor Zip: 07960
Ph: (973) 755-9206 Fax: (973) 540-9717
- James,Kevin V., MD
- Lee,Thomas Y., MD
- Patel,Amit V., MD
- Resnikoff,Michael, MD
- Riaz,Omer Junaid, MD
- Tulsyan,Nirman, MD

Advocare Pediatric Neurology Assoc
25 Lindsley Drive/Suite 205 Zip: 07960
Ph: (973) 993-8777 Fax: (973) 993-8577
- DeSouza,Trevor G., MD
- Waran,Sandy P., MD

Affiliated Dermatologists
182 South Street/Suite 1 Zip: 07960
Ph: (973) 267-0300 Fax: (973) 695-1480
- Agarwal,Shilpa R., MD
- Dane,Alexander Ali, DO
- Fialkoff,Cheryl N., MD
- Grob,Alexandra, DO
- Lee,Kristyna H., MD
- Lombardi,Adriana, MD
- Lortie,Charles Frederic, MD
- Parker,Collin Robert, MD
- Pilcher,Mary Frances, MD
- Rogachefsky,Arlene S., MD
- Torres,Omar, MD

Affiliates in Gastroenterology, P.A.
101 Madison Avenue/Suite 100 Zip: 07960
Ph: (973) 455-0404 Fax: (973) 540-8788
- Morton,John Douglas, MD
- Samach,Michael A., MD

Anesthesia Associates
100 Madison Avenue Zip: 07960
Ph: (973) 631-8119 Fax: (973) 631-8120
- Barry,Kevin M., MD
- Chern,Sy-Yeu Sue, MD
- McDonnell,Thomas E., MD
- Rubinfeld,Julie A., MD

Anesthesia Associates of Morristown
264 South Street/Suite 2A Zip: 07960
Ph: (973) 631-8119
- Barbieri,Louise T., MD
- Chung,Daniel Hansam, MD
- Lapchak,John T., MD
- Rosenbaum,Lee M., MD
- Watson,Todd A., MD

Associates in Rehabilitation Medicine
95 Mount Kemble Avenue Zip: 07960
Ph: (973) 267-2293 Fax: (973) 226-3144
- David,Erica Nicola, MD
- Davis,Sanders W., MD
- Mayoral,Jorge L., MD
- Mulford,Gregory J., MD
- Pisciotta,Anthony J., MD
- Rao,Rajesh Ramchandra, MD
- Rempson,Joseph H., MD
- Smith,Jason Anthony, MD
- Tzeng,Alice Chaw, MD
- Zheng,Yining, MD

Atlantic Breast Associates
100 Madison Avenue/3rd Floor Zip: 07962
Ph: (973) 971-4166 Fax: (973) 290-7152
- Fornari,Marcella, DO
- Gendler,Leah S., MD

Atlantic Cardiology Group LLP
95 Madison Avenue/Suite 300 Zip: 07960
Ph: (973) 898-0400 Fax: (973) 682-9494
- Mondelli,John Anthony, MD

Atlantic Health Urology Gyn
95 Madison Avenue/Suite 204 Zip: 07960
Ph: (973) 971-7440
- Shariati,Amir, MD

Atlantic Health Weight & Wellness Cntr
435 South Street/Suite 220-B Zip: 07960
Ph: (973) 540-9198 Fax: (973) 540-1614
- Tratenberg,Mark Adam, DO
- Widman,David, MD

Atlantic Maternal Fetal Medicine
435 South Street/Suite 380 Zip: 07960
Ph: (973) 971-7080 Fax: (973) 290-8312
- Hanley,Maryellen L., MD
- Khine,Mary L., MD
- Shah,Leena P., MD

Atlantic Neurosurgical Specialists
310 Madison Avenue/Suite 300 Zip: 07960
Ph: (973) 285-7800 Fax: (973) 285-7839
- Baskin,Jonathan Jay, MD
- Benitez,Ronald Patrick, MD
- Chapple,Kyle Thomas, MD
- Chun,Jay Y., MD
- Knightly,John J., MD
- Meyer,Scott Andrew, MD
- Moshel,Yaron Aharon, MD
- Park,Henry, MD
- Stillerman,Charles Blair, MD
- Ugorec,Igor, MD
- Wells-Roth,David S., MD
- Zampella,Edward J., MD

Atlantic Orthopedic Institute
111 Madison Avenue/Suite 400 Zip: 07960
Ph: (973) 984-0404 Fax: (973) 984-2516
- Avallone,Nicholas J., MD
- Baskies,Michael Ari, MD
- Dowling,William J. Jr., MD
- Martins,Damion Antonio, MD
- Padavan,Dean, MD
- Sclafani,Steven, MD
- Taffet,Berton, MD

Blair Medical Associates PA
261 James Street/Suite 2A Zip: 07960
Ph: (973) 539-2468 Fax: (973) 539-7699
- Becker,Andrew B., DO
- Chung,Angela F., DO
- Thomson,Mary Jo G., DO

Cardiology Assocs of Morristown
95 Madison Avenue/Suite 10A Zip: 07960
Ph: (973) 889-9001 Fax: (973) 889-9051
- Blum,Mark A., MD
- Cosmi,John Edward, MD
- Freilich,David I., MD
- Gandotra,Puneet, MD
- Mandel,Leonid, MD

Carol G. Simon Cancer Center
100 Madison Avenue/Suite 4101 Zip: 07962
Ph: (973) 971-6100
- Gallinson,David Herschel, DO
- Heller,Paul B., MD
- Leibowitz,Stacey Bucholtz, MD
- Tobias,Daniel Henry, MD

Chambers Center
435 South Street/Suite 160 Zip: 07960
Ph: (973) 971-6301
- Rand,Victoria Elena, MD

Childrens Orthopedic & Sports Med Cntr
261 James Street/Suite 3-C Zip: 07960
Ph: (973) 206-1033 Fax: (973) 206-1036
- Leier,Tim Ulrich, MD
- Minkowitz,Barbara, MD

Comprehensive CardioVas Consltnts
299 Madison Avenue/Suite 102 Zip: 07960
Ph: (973) 292-1020 Fax: (973) 292-0564
- Levy,Stephen M., MD
- Limandri,Giuseppe, MD
- Santiago,Derek W., MD
- Smith,Peter Lloyd, MD
- Verdesca,Stephen A., MD

Dermatology Consultants
261 James Street/Suite 2-B Zip: 07960
Ph: (973) 993-1433 Fax: (973) 993-1176
- Popkin,Mark D., MD
- Schneider,Rhonda R., MD

Drs. Chon & Chon
435 South Street/Suite 230-A Zip: 07960
Ph: (973) 971-6480 Fax: (973) 290-7435
- Chon,Jajin Thomas, MD
- Walimbe,Mona S., MD

Drs. Davidoff and Davidoff
144 Speedwell Avenue Zip: 07960
Ph: (973) 267-7770 Fax: (973) 984-2933
- Davidoff,Ada, MD
- Davidoff,Bernard M., MD

Drs. Leung & Murphy
196 Speedwell Avenue Zip: 07960
Ph: (973) 539-9580
- Centanni,Frank D., MD
- Leung,Jacquelyn Way-Yan, MD
- Murphy,Guy D., MD

Drs. Marx and Royce
101 Madison Avenue/Suite 304 Zip: 07960
Ph: (973) 292-0999 Fax: (973) 292-0555
- Marx,Tatyana, MD
- Royce,Roxanne, MD

Drs. Stevens and Perez
4 Atno Avenue Zip: 07960
Ph: (973) 267-0002 Fax: (973) 328-9102
- Perez,Marcella, MD
- Stevens,Hilary Kristin, MD

ENT Specialists of Morristown
95 Madison Avenue/Suite 105 Zip: 07960
Ph: (973) 644-0808 Fax: (973) 644-9270
- Cairns,Christine Dobrosky, MD
- Giacchi,Renato John, MD
- Immerman,Sara Beth, MD
- Lachman,Reid A., MD
- Sorvino,Damian W., MD

Electrophysiology Associates, PA
100 Madison Avenue/Suite 5 Zip: 07962
Ph: (973) 971-4261 Fax: (973) 290-7253
- Coyne,Robert F., MD
- Gillam,Linda Dawn, MD
- Mahoney,Timothy Hugh, MD

Executive Health Group, Inc.
44 Whippany Road Zip: 07960
Ph: (973) 540-0177
- Denbow,Frank Alstein, MD

Eyecare MD of New Jersey
261 James Street/Suite 2-D & 3EL Zip: 07960
Ph: (973) 984-3937 Fax: (973) 984-4059
- Knapp,Stefanie, MD
- Landmann,Dan S., MD
- Lopatynsky,Marta O., MD
- Sarkar,Jayati Saha, MD

Family Health Center
200 South Street/Suite 4 Zip: 07960
Ph: (973) 889-6800
- Asokan,Nalini, MD
- Astiz,Donna J., MD
- Darcey,Jacqueline Marie, MD
- Griffith,Rebecca Anne, MD
- Hoelzel,Donald W., MD

Gagnon Cardiovasular Institute
100 Madison Avenue/Level C Zip: 07962
Ph: (973) 971-5597 Fax: (973) 290-7145
- Goldschmidt,Marc Eliot, MD
- Koulogiannis,Konstantinos Peter, M
- Natello,Gregory W., DO
- Ramos Bondy,Beatrix Marie, MD
- Uretsky,Seth, MD

Geriatric Assessment Center
435 South Street/Suite 390 Zip: 07960
Ph: (973) 971-5000
- Blloshmi,Kledia, MD
- Petilla-Onorato,Jessica Isabel, MD
- Prager,Jason Nicholas, MD
- Sharma,Keerti, MD

Hematology-Oncology Assocs of NNJ
100 Madison Avenue/PO Box 1089 Zip: 07962
Ph: (973) 538-5210 Fax: (973) 644-9657
- Adler,Kenneth R., MD
- Chiang,Wendy M., MD
- Early,Ellen Marie, MD
- Farber,Charles M., MD
- Gerstein,Gary, MD
- Papish,Steven W., MD
- Scola,Michael Anthony, MD

IPC The Hospitalist Company
55 Madison Avenue/Suite 310 Zip: 07960
Ph: (973) 993-9536 Fax: (973) 998-4237
- Ampadu, Akua A., MD
- Ayre, Kelly Anne Bianco, MD
- Bery, Seema, MD
- Correa Orozco, Felipe A., MD
- Garg, Deepika, MD
- Griffin, John P., MD
- Grover, Manisha B., MD
- Hosadurga, Supriya S., MD
- Kopelan, Leah Michelle, MD
- Leung, Michael Seto, MD
- Nyunt, Tun, MD
- Papatheodorou, Dana William, MD
- Patil, Vrishali Swanand, MD
- Schachter, Nora Claudia, MD
- Shroff, Shilpa Anilkumar, MD
- Simon, Egbert A., MD
- Stoytchev, Hristo Vassilev, MD
- Trinidad, Jennilee A., MD
- Zelener, Marina L., DO

Integrated Physiatry Services
45 South Park Place/Suite 259 Zip: 07960
Ph: (908) 490-0036 Fax: (908) 490-0067
- Flowers, Rashonda R., MD
- Khan, Ummais N., MD
- Khattar, Vimi, MD

Internal Medicine Faculty Associates
435 South Street/Suite 210 Zip: 07960
Ph: (973) 971-7165 Fax: (973) 290-7675
- Kessler, Jason Adam, MD
- Nielsen, Earl F., MD
- Raska, Anna M.L., MD
- Salaki, John S., MD
- Thomas, Elsa, MD
- Vascan, Andreea Carmen, MD

Internal Medicine of Morristown
95 Madison Avenue/Suite A-00 Zip: 07960
Ph: (973) 538-1388 Fax: (973) 538-9501
- Monastyrskyj, Ola A., MD
- Randazzo, Jean P., MD
- Savage, Danielle S., MD
- Yaqub, Zunera, MD

Jonathan Alan Wang DO LLC
290 Madison Avenue/Suite 2 A Zip: 07960
Ph: (973) 285-1999 Fax: (973) 359-8979
- Smith, Brian L., MD
- Wang, Jonathan Alan, DO

Kidney Care
131 Madison Avenue/Suite 3 Zip: 07960
Ph: (973) 631-6223 Fax: (973) 631-6225
- Eppinger, Barry A., DO
- Sarkar, Shubho Ranjan, MD

Madison Internal Medicine Assoc
95 Madison Avenue/Suite 405 Zip: 07960
Ph: (973) 829-9998 Fax: (973) 829-9991
- Meyers, Marta, MD
- Renna, Carmen M., MD
- Weine, Gary R., MD

Madison Pediatrics
435 South Street/Suite 200 Zip: 07960
Ph: (973) 822-0003 Fax: (973) 822-3349
- Cucolo, Patricia Anne, MD
- Eckert, Jessica, DO
- Lodish, Stephanie Renee, MD
- Meltzer, Alan J., MD
- Rehm, Christine M., MD
- Scherer, Susan Denys, MD
- Schwartzberg, Paul Marc, DO

Mayor Group
53 School House Lane Zip: 07960
Ph: (973) 206-1936 Fax: (973) 998-7995
- Holubka, Jacquelin Pickford, MD
- Mayor, Gilbert H., MD

Mid-Atlantic Surgical Associates
100 Madison Avenue Zip: 07960
Ph: (973) 971-7300 Fax: (973) 984-7019
- Brown, John Muir III, MD
- Greeley, Drew Peter, MD
- Huang, Jianzhong, MD
- Magovern, Christopher Jude, MD
- Neibart, Richard M., MD

- Polomsky, Marek, MD
- Slater, James P., MD
- Van Boxtel, Benjamin, MD

MidAtlantic Neonatology Associates
100 Madison Avenue Zip: 07962
Ph: (973) 971-5488 Fax: (973) 290-7175
- Crowley, Kathryn Ann, MD
- Federico, Cheryl L., MD
- Gluck, Karen, MD
- Mimms, Gaines M., MD
- Orsini, Anthony J., DO
- Presti, Amy Lynn, MD
- Rogido, Marta R., MD
- Schenkman, Andrew C., MD
- Shen, Calvin T., MD
- Skolnick, Lawrence M., MD
- Swanson, Jonathan Raymond, MD

Morristown Cardiology Associates, P.A.
435 South Street/Suite 100 Zip: 07960
Ph: (973) 267-3944 Fax: (973) 455-0399
- Bachman, Daniel, MD
- Dickson, David Gordon, MD
- Fisch, Arthur P., MD
- Guss, Stephen B., MD
- Hsieh, Allen, MD
- Raska, Karel, MD
- Rosen, Craig Michael, MD
- Schwartz, Jeffrey G., MD
- Watson, Richard I., MD
- Weisbrot, Joshua, MD
- Weisen, Steven Fred, MD
- von Poelnitz, Audrey E., MD

Morristown Med Cntr
435 South Street/Suite 220-A Zip: 07960
Ph: (973) 971-4222 Fax: (973) 290-7050
- Domovich, Ora, MD
- Guercio-Hauer, Catherine A., MD
- Horowitz, Meggan Elise, DO
- Joshi, Namita V., MD
- Klingmeyer, Dorothy Marie, DO

Morristown Medical Center Family Med
435 South Street/Suite 350 Zip: 07960
Ph: (973) 971-4222 Fax: (973) 401-2465
- Kuo, David, MD
- Melograno, Joseph J., DO
- Wilson, Lynn Marie, DO
- Zipp, Christopher Paul, DO

Morristown Ob Gyn Associates
101 Madison Avenue/Suite 405 Zip: 07960
Ph: (973) 267-7272 Fax: (973) 455-0099
- Culin, Angelina Han, MD
- Daly, M. Veronica, MD
- Jones, Kathryn M., MD
- Mass, Sharon B., MD
- Miller, Naomi H., MD
- Morley, Laura Balderrama, MD

Morristown Pediatric Assocs
261 James Street/Suite 1-G Zip: 07960
Ph: (973) 540-9393 Fax: (973) 540-1937
- Cohen, Martin L., MD
- Gupta, Meera, MD
- Lanzkowsk, Shelley, MD
- Lupatkin, William L., MD
- McCluskey, Tamara B., DO
- Nashi, Suhaib G., MD
- Poblete, Gwyn Laurice, MD

Morristown Surgical Associates
344 South Street Zip: 07960
Ph: (973) 267-2838 Fax: (973) 267-7909
- Elyash, Igor Gary, DO

Morristown Urology Associates PC
261 James Street/Suite 1A Zip: 07960
Ph: (973) 539-1050 Fax: (973) 538-6111
- Chaikin, David Craig, MD
- Israel, Arthur R., MD
- Saypol, David C., MD
- Sutaria, Perry Maganlal, MD

Nephrology Hypertension Assocs
2 Franklin Place Zip: 07960
Ph: (973) 267-7673 Fax: (973) 267-3270
- Fine, Paul L., MD
- Stack, Jay I., MD

Neuroscience Ctr of Northern NJ
310 Madison Avenue Zip: 07960
Ph: (973) 285-1446 Fax: (973) 605-8854
- Alias, Mathew N., DO
- Conigliari, Matthew F., MD
- Diamond, Mark S., MD
- Fox, Stuart W., MD
- Okunola, Oladotun A., MD
- Rosenberg, Richard S., MD

New Jersey Pain Consultants
310 Madison Avenue/Suite 301 Zip: 07960
Ph: (973) 998-9200 Fax: (973) 998-9201
- Piccolo, Christian K, MD

New Jersey Pain Consultants
95 Madison Avenue/Suite 402 Zip: 07960
Ph: (973) 971-6824 Fax: (973) 290-7683
- Rudman, Michael E., MD
- Welsh, Terrence Mathew, MD
- Winne, Richard P. Jr., MD

NJ Pediatric Neurosurgical Associates
131 Madison Avenue/Suite 140 Zip: 07960
Ph: (973) 326-9000 Fax: (973) 326-9001
- Mazzola, Catherine A., MD
- Zoeller, Garrett Keith, MD

North Jersey Thoracic Surgical Assoc
100 Madison Avenue/PO Box 1348 Zip: 07962
Ph: (973) 644-4844 Fax: (973) 644-4776
- Steiner, Federico A., MD
- Widmann, Mark Dennis, MD

Northeast Regional Epilepsy Group
290 Madison Avenue/Building 5 2nd FL Zip: 07960
Ph: (201) 343-6676
- Altman, Rachel S., MD

Obesity Treatment Center
435 South Street/Suite 330 B Zip: 07960
Ph: (973) 971-7166 Fax: (973) 290-7518
- Melzer, Olga Alexandrovna, MD
- Proudan, Vladimir Ivanovich, MD

One to One Female Care, P.A.
111 Madison Avenue/Suite 305 Zip: 07960
Ph: (973) 683-1400 Fax: (973) 683-0700
- Garfinkel, David A., MD
- Laguduva, Lakshmi Rani Ramasubraman

Pediatric Eye Physicians, PC
95 Madison Avenue/Suite 301 Zip: 07960
Ph: (973) 540-8814 Fax: (973) 540-8556
- Chen, Lucy L., MD
- Klein, Kathryn Suzanne, MD
- Morgan, Charles Fisher, MD

Reproductive Medicine Associates of NJ
111 Madison Avenue/Suite 100 Zip: 07962
Ph: (973) 971-4600 Fax: (973) 290-8370
- Bergh, Paul Akos, MD
- Forman, Eric Jason, MD
- Maguire, Marcy Frances, MD
- Scott, Richard Thomas Jr., MD

Retina Specialists of New Jersey
330 South Street/Suite 1 Zip: 07960
Ph: (973) 871-2020 Fax: (973) 871-2000
- Angioletti, Lee Mitchell, MD
- Lalin, Sean C., MD
- Perina, Barbara, MD

Summit Medical Group
95 Madison Avenue Zip: 07960
Ph: (973) 285-7610
- Aronwald, Bruce Alan, DO
- Castaneda, Rachel Lim, MD

Summit Medical Group
95 Madison Avenue Zip: 07960
Ph: (973) 267-1010 Fax: (973) 267-5521
- Christou, Alexander A., DO
- Cioce, Anthony Jr., DO
- Cioce, Thomas G., DO
- Gadiraju, Silpa, MD
- Greenberg, Heather Ellyn, MD
- Margulies, Debra Jill, MD
- Nevin, Marie Eithne, MD
- Wallace, Theresa C., MD

Practice of Rolando Rolandelli, MD
435 South Street/Suite 360 Zip: 07960
Ph: (973) 971-7200 Fax: (973) 290-7521
- Comizio, Renee Carol, MD
- Di Fazio, Louis Thomas Jr., MD
- Huk, Matthew David, MD
- McLean, Edward Jr., MD
- Padnani, Ashish, MD
- Rolandelli, Rolando Hector, MD
- Ward, David S., MD

The Center For Psychiatry & Psycho-Onc
261 James Street/Unit 2-E L Zip: 07960
Ph: (973) 540-1656
- Granet, Roger B., MD
- Taylor, Clifford A., MD

The Orthopedic Group, P.A.
261 James Street/Suite 3-F Zip: 07960
Ph: (973) 538-0029 Fax: (973) 538-4957
- Baydin, Jeffrey A., MD
- Crutchlow, William P., MD
- Drey, Iris Antonella, MD
- Kanellakos, James George, MD
- Levine, Barry Steven, MD
- Wagshul, Adam David, MD

Tri-County Orthopedics
160 East Hanover Avenue Zip: 07962
Ph: (973) 538-2334 Fax: (973) 829-9174
- Colizza, Wayne A., MD
- Epstein, David Michael, MD
- Gatto, Charles Anthony, MD
- Ginsberg, Claudia Lisa, MD
- Goldberger, Michael Irwin, MD
- Lombardi, Paul M. Jr., MD
- Longworth-Gatto, Lisa E., DO
- Lowenstein, Jason E., MD
- McBride, Mark J., MD
- Naseef, George Salem III, MD
- Polesin, Alena, MD
- Tsairis, Peter, MD
- Willis, Andrew Albert, MD

Urogynecology & Pelvic Surgery
435 South Street/Suite 370 Zip: 07960
Ph: (973) 971-7267
- Avondstondt, Andrea Mithai, MD
- Culligan, Patrick John, MD
- Saiz Rodriguez, Cristina Margarita,
- Salamon, Charbel Georges, MD

Vein Institute of New Jersey
95 Madison Avenue/Suite 109 Zip: 07960
Ph: (973) 759-9000 Fax: (973) 759-2487
- Agis, Harry, MD
- Moritz, Mark William, MD
- Ombrellino, Michael, MD
- Sturt, Cindy, MD

Women's Care Source
111 Madison Avenue/Suite 308 Zip: 07960
Ph: (973) 285-0400 Fax: (973) 285-9848
- Austin, Kimberlee Kunze, MD
- Brenin-Goldfischer, Debra Sue, MD
- Feltz, John P., MD
- Ferrante, Daniel P., MD
- O'Reilly, Sara B., DO
- Omay, Cem S., MD

Mount Arlington
Drs. Aroesty and Lin
400 Valley Road/Suite 105 Zip: 07856
Ph: (973) 770-7101 Fax: (973) 770-7108
- Aroesty, Jeffrey H., MD
- Lin, Giant Chu, MD
- Mohankumar, Aditi, MD

Morris Heart Associates PA
400 Valley Road/Suite 102 Zip: 07856
Ph: (973) 770-7899 Fax: (973) 770-7840
- Ferrier, Austin Seymour, DO
- Lowell, Barry H., MD
- Shen, Rhuna, MD

Mount Holly
Advanced Pain Consultants, P.A.
120 Madison Avenue/Suite D Zip: 08060
Ph: (609) 267-1707
- Gupta, Rakesh Chander, MD

Groups and Clinics by Town with Physician Rosters

Mount Holly (cont)
Burlington Anesthesia Associates
120 Madison Ave/Suite E/PO Box 174 Zip: 08060
Ph: (609) 261-1660 Fax: (609) 261-1779
- Ajmal, Muhammad Zafar, MD
- Ferrari, Albert N., MD
- Gargiulo, Richard F., MD
- Gumnit, Robert Y., MD
- Nyzio, Joseph Bruno, DO
- Schwartz, Joshua J., MD
- Thornton, Robin W., MD

Hematology Oncology Associates PA
175 Madison Avenue/4th Floor Zip: 08060
Ph: (609) 702-1900 Fax: (609) 702-8455
- Berk, Seth Howard, MD
- Lee, James Wonsang, MD
- Levenbach, Rachel Shoshana, MD
- Wallace, Stephen Gary, MD

Pinelands Obstetrics & Gyn
1617 Route 38 Zip: 08060
Ph: (609) 261-0240 Fax: (609) 261-8622
- Deluca, Samantha, DO
- Jackson, Olga E., MD
- Manning, Latriece Eileena, DO
- Rashid, Parveen, MD

SJ Emergency Physician, PA
175 Madison Avenue Zip: 08060
Ph: (609) 267-0700 Fax: (609) 261-5842
- Bertolino, Laura, DO
- Brown, Patti C., DO
- Goldberg, David Felheimer, MD
- Leibrandt, Paul N., MD
- Leitner, Stephen J., MD
- Morris, Jeffrey B., MD
- Ruderman, Seth R., MD
- Turner, Craig S., DO

Virtua Hospitalist Group Memorial
175 Madison Avenue Zip: 08060
Ph: (609) 914-6180 Fax: (609) 914-6182
- Castellino, Sharon Franklin, MD
- DeLue, Erik Nathaniel, MD
- Dhru, Sahil H., DO
- Ghobrial, Peter Morcos Ibrah, MD
- Govan, Satyen Manilal, DO
- Lawandy, Michael Armia, DO
- Malone, Michael Richard, DO
- Nisar, Sabeeha, MD
- Pratt Mccoy, Kia Chriselda, MD

Virtua Phoenix OBGYN
120 Madison Avenue/Suite B Zip: 08460
Ph: (609) 444-5500 Fax: (609) 444-5501
- Gorlitsky, Helen, MD
- Grossman, Leonard, MD
- Levine, Bruce Jay, MD
- Levine, Richard Teddy, MD
- Segal, Avni, MD
- Shalit, Stuart L., DO

Mount Laurel
ASAP - Advanced Spine and Pain
3829 Church Road/Suite B Zip: 08054
OnlyFax: (856) 787-1901
- Mitchell, William, MD

Advanced ENT - Mount Laurel
204 Ark Road/Building 1/Suite 102 Zip: 08054
Ph: (856) 602-4000 Fax: (856) 946-1747
- Carlson, Roy Douglas, MD
- Gupta, Ashmit, MD

Advocare Fam Med Assoc Mt. Laurel
3115 Route 38/Suite 200B Zip: 08054
Ph: (856) 231-9666 Fax: (856) 231-7543
- Bandy, Caryn Kay, DO
- Golden, Richard F., DO
- Meeteer, Francis III, DO

Advocare Pedi Phys of Burlington Co
204 Ark Road/Suite 209 Zip: 08054
Ph: (856) 234-3797 Fax: (856) 234-9402
- Nemeth, Nicole Angelina, MD

Allergic Disease Associates, PC
210 Ark Road & Route 38/Suite 109 Zip: 08054
Ph: (856) 235-8282 Fax: (856) 235-2154
- Dvorin, Donald J., MD
- Goldstein, Marc F., MD
- Gordon, Nancy Deborah, MD

Allergy & Asthma Associates
127 Ark Road/Suite 1 Zip: 08054
Ph: (856) 778-4222 Fax: (856) 727-9595
- Kravitz, Stuart A., MD

Besen-Goldstein Medical Assoc
1000 Birchfield Drive/Suite 1004 Zip: 08054
Ph: (856) 866-1557 Fax: (856) 231-7955
- Feldan, Paul E., MD
- Goldstein, Kenneth Brian, MD
- Shears-Bethke, Tracey M., MD

Bruneau Family Care, P.C.
2963 Marne Highway Zip: 08054
Ph: (856) 638-1990
- Bruneau, Lara A., MD
- Hancq, Nicole Elizabeth, MD

Burlington Co Orthopaedic Specialists
204 Ark Road/Suite 105 Zip: 08054
Ph: (856) 235-7080 Fax: (856) 273-6384
- Bowers, Andrea Legath, MD
- Schwartz, Mark Glen, MD

CHOP Primary Care Mount Laurel
3201 Marne Highway Zip: 08054
Ph: (856) 829-5545 Fax: (856) 829-9268
- Ahr, Lawrence M., MD
- Bernstein, Barbara A., MD
- Coutinho Haas, Sunita Patricia, MD
- Creecy, Saundra K., MD
- Weissbach, Debra D., MD

CUH Cancer & Radiation Onc Institute
715 Fellowship Road Zip: 08054
Ph: (856) 638-1180 Fax: (856) 638-1188
- Kubicek, Gregory John, MD

Cherry Hill Ob/Gyn
150 Century Parkway/Suite A Zip: 08054
Ph: (856) 778-4700 Fax: (856) 778-1154
- Denny, Ashleigh, MD
- Jenkins, Lauren Anne, MD
- McCrosson, Stacy A., MD
- McCullen, Kristen Michelle, MD
- Noah, Jane S., MD
- Richman, Steven L., DO
- Watters, Nathan Paul, MD

Coastal Spine
4000 Church Road Zip: 08054
Ph: (856) 222-4444 Fax: (856) 222-0049
- Deutsch, Lawrence Steven, MD
- Jarmain, Scott Joseph, MD
- Momi, Kamaldeep S., MD
- Paul, Michael Joseph, DO
- Scholl, Seth David, DO
- Testaiuti, Mark A., MD

Concentra Medical Urgent Care
817 East Gate Drive/Suite 102 Zip: 08054
Ph: (856) 778-1090 Fax: (856) 778-9191
- Maslin, Stuart J., MD
- Pecca, Jo Ann Donna, DO
- Resnick-Matro, Jennifer Dawn, MD
- Wilczynski, Frank L., DO

Inst. Reproductive Hormonal Disorders
17000 Commerce Parkway/Suite C Zip: 08054
Ph: (856) 751-5575 Fax: (856) 751-7289
- Amui, Jewel Naakarley, MD
- Brasile, Deanna Rose, DO
- Check, Jerome H., MD
- Choe, Jung Kyo, MD
- Corley, David R., MD

Dermatology Associates of South Jersey
715 Fellowship Road/Suite B Zip: 08054
Ph: (856) 206-0201 Fax: (856) 206-0209
- Abdelmalek, Mark A., MD

Infectious Disease Physicians PA
1001 Briggs Road/Suite 250 Zip: 08054
Ph: (856) 866-7466 Fax: (856) 866-9088
- Aggrey, Gloria Kangachie, MD
- Golden, Richard Frederick, MD
- Klinger, Frederick Boyd III, DO
- Kraus, Jennifer Lynn, MD
- Ng, Kevin, MD
- Peterson, John W., MD
- Sumerson, Jeffrey Marc, MD
- Tiu, Evelyn Venzon, MD

Topiel, Martin S., MD

Larchmont Medical Imaging
210 Ark Road/Building 2 Zip: 08054
Ph: (856) 778-8860 Fax: (856) 866-8102
- Chan, Britton Miller, MD
- Chheda, Samir Visanji, MD

New Jersey Knee & Shoulder Center
1288 Route 73 South/Suite 100 Zip: 08054
Ph: (856) 273-8900 Fax: (856) 802-9772
- Sapega, Alexander, MD
- Sidor, Michael Louis, MD

New Jersey Urology
15000 Midlantic Drive/Suite 100 Zip: 08054
Ph: (856) 252-1000 Fax: (856) 985-4582
- Becker, Jeffrey M., MD
- Berkman, Douglas S., MD
- Daugherty, Rhett L., MD
- Dwosh, Jack, MD
- Niedrach, William L., MD

Pulmonary and Sleep Physicians
204 Ark Road/Suite 206/Larchmont 1 Zip: 08054
Ph: (856) 778-4640 Fax: (856) 778-8862
- Chelemer, Scott Brain, MD
- Cohen, Douglas Jay, MD
- Hamilton, Thanuja Kumari, MD
- Khelil, Jennifer Lynn, DO
- Malik, Rohit, MD
- Ryan, Kathleen Lisa, MD
- Schriber, Andrew David, MD
- Trudo, Frank J., MD

Rancocas Anesthesiology, PA
15000 Midlantic Drive/Suite 102 Zip: 08054
Ph: (856) 255-5479 Fax: (856) 393-8691
- Buck, Gary B., MD
- Chekemian, Beth Ann, DO
- Cooper, Niti Dalal, DO
- Doshi, Anish, MD
- Haleem, Burhan, MD
- Lesneski, Matthew J., MD
- McGrath, Steven Warren, MD
- McKenzie, Rammurti Anthony, MD
- Medvedovsky, Andrew, MD
- Pello, Scott Jason, MD
- Shah, Manish, MD

Tao Institute of Mind & Body Medicine
1288 Route 73 South/Suite 210 Zip: 08054
Ph: (856) 802-6888 Fax: (856) 802-6878
- Larkin, Joyce Marie, MD
- Yang, Jingduan, MD

University Doctors Family Practice
100 Centruy Parkway/Suite 140 Zip: 08054
Ph: (856) 667-9051 Fax: (856) 667-9054
- Barone, Catherine Ann, DO

Mountain Lakes
Cardiology Consultants/North Morris
356 US Highway 46/Suite B Zip: 07046
Ph: (973) 586-3400 Fax: (973) 586-1916
- Cook, Guillermo A., MD
- Fusman, Benjamin, MD
- Massari, Ronald D., MD
- Safirstein, Jordan Glanzman, MD
- Shulruff, Stuart E., MD
- Wang, Robert L., MD

Lakeland Cardiology Center, P.A.
415 Boulevard Zip: 07046
Ph: (973) 334-7700 Fax: (973) 334-7116
- Blick, Michael D., MD
- De Renzi, Paul D., MD
- Leibowitz, Keith Scott, DO
- Malagold, Michael, MD
- Naeem, Sheikh M., MD
- Park, Hyeun Sik, MD
- Wall, Robert M., MD

Mountainside
Ambulatory Anesthesia Care, PC
1450 Route 22 West Zip: 07092
Ph: (908) 233-2020 Fax: (908) 233-9322
- Fisher, Margaret Elizabeth, MD
- Lum, Kenneth, MD

Papa, Louis, MD
Pillon, Mark A., MD
Rinehouse, Jay A., MD

CSH Pediatric Practice of Union
150 New Providence Road Zip: 07092
Ph: (908) 353-8998 Fax: (908) 527-6766
- Gozo, Ave O., MD
- Harris, Brenda D., MD

Infinity Orthopedics
1450 Route 22 West/Suite 200 Zip: 07092
Ph: (908) 364-7801 Fax: (908) 222-2757
- Warshauer, Jeffrey M., DO
- Yanow, Jennifer Hannah, MD

Westfield ENT Surgery Assoc
213 Summit Road/Suite 1 Zip: 07092
Ph: (908) 233-5500 Fax: (908) 233-5776
- Drake, William III, MD
- Presti, Paul Matthew, MD

Mullica Hill
Family Health Center of Mullica Hill
155 Bridgeton Pike/Suite A Zip: 08062
Ph: (856) 223-0500 Fax: (856) 223-1098
- Herman, Gregory E., MD
- Kent, Maria Candice, MD
- Ott, William Augustine, DO
- Trom, Kristen Elizabeth, DO
- Wyche Bullock, Tara Lynette, MD
- Zuazua-Pacilio, Maria Cristina, MD

Mullica Hill Medical Associates PC
201 Bridgeton Pike Zip: 08062
Ph: (856) 478-2111 Fax: (856) 478-4709
- Malik, Pooja, MD
- Malik, Rajesh, MD

Premier Women's Health of SJ
34 Colson Lane Zip: 08062
Ph: (856) 223-1385
- Beams, Lynsey Marie, DO
- O'Flynn, Leisa Diane, DO

SJH Urgent Care, P.C.
201 Tomlin Station Road/Suite B Zip: 08062
Ph: (856) 241-2500 Fax: (856) 241-2511
- Patel, Bhavesh, DO
- Sprigman, Charles Jeffrey III, DO
- Stiefel, Gregory Gene, DO

Neptune
American Heart Center PC
1900 Corlies Avenue State Rout Zip: 07753
Ph: (732) 663-1123 Fax: (732) 663-1179
- Abbud, Ziad A., MD
- Demchuk, Beverly Jean, MD
- Karam, Sara R., MD

Atlantic Cardiology LLC
444 Neptune Boulevard/Unit 2 Zip: 07753
Ph: (732) 775-5300 Fax: (732) 988-9080
- Choi, Edward Joung Myung, MD
- Colmer, Marc E., MD
- Harris, Kenneth Barton, MD
- Lapman, Peter Grant, MD
- Narula, Amar Singh, MD

Atlantic Coast Gastroenterology
1944 Corlies Avenue/Suite 205 Zip: 07753
Ph: (732) 776-9300 Fax: (732) 776-8059
- Basri, William E., MD
- Hui, Kenny Pingchi, MD
- Schneiderman, Steven, MD

Atlantic Coast Urology
1944 Corlies Avenue/Suite 101 Zip: 07753
Ph: (732) 775-8444 Fax: (732) 775-8550
- Coyle, Allison A., DO
- Tobin, Matthew Steven, MD

Coastal Ear Nose and Throat LLC
3700 Route 33/Suite 101 Zip: 07753
Ph: (732) 280-7855 Fax: (732) 280-7815
- Engel, Samuel Henry, MD
- Houston, Sean David, MD
- Mitskavich, Mary T., MD
- Newkirk, Kenneth Allen, MD
- Shargorodsky, Josef, MD

Drs. Patel & Sharma
1915 6th Avenue Zip: 07753
Ph: (732) 774-5700 Fax: (732) 774-7929
- Patel,Mayurkumar P., MD
- Sharma,Indu, MD

EmCare
1945 Route 33 Zip: 07753
Ph: (732) 776-4510 Fax: (732) 776-2329
- Bakhos,Lisa Lovas, MD
- Chutke,Prashant Vithal, MD
- Goodman,Elliot S., DO
- Jacob,Sharon Leigh, MD
- Levinsky,Joseph Judah, MD
- Marra,Antonio Luigi, DO
- McFadden,Kim Marie, MD
- Mojares,Gregg E., DO
- Nowinowska,Anna, MD
- Panse,Ramanand V., MD
- Pasricha,Atul, DO
- Patel,Rajendra K., MD
- Pillai,Renuka, DO
- Ponce,Marie Grace C., MD
- Radwan,Hossam S., MD
- Rozwadowski,Thomas J., MD
- Smith,Corey Kamahl, MD
- Sulewski,Agnieszka, DO
- Sweeney,Robert L., DO
- Tapnio,Cezar B., MD
- Wells,Evelyn Ruth, MD

Hackensack Meridian Medical Group
19 Davis Avenue/5th-6th Floor Zip: 07753
Ph: (732) 897-3990 Fax: (732) 897-3997
- Alpert,Deborah R., MD
- Cheng,Jennifer, DO
- Frank,Elliot, MD
- Holland,Soemiwati Weidris, MD
- Hossain,Mohammad Amir, MD
- Kaplan,Adam Chaim, MD
- Kaunzinger,Christian M., MD
- Kruvant-Gornish,Nancy J., MD
- Kufelnicka,Anna M., MD
- Kuzyshyn,Halyna, MD
- Lann,Danielle Erin, MD
- Mushtaq,Arman, MD
- Ong,Raquel Sanchez, MD
- Onwuka,Aloysius Chukwumuche, MD
- Patel,Nitin Suresh, MD
- Rosenthal,Marnie Elyse, DO
- Singh,Rohini, MD
- Tang,Xiaoyin, MD

Hackensack Meridian Urogynecolgy Medic
19 Davis Avenue/7th Floor Zip: 07753
Ph: (732) 776-3797 Fax: (732) 776-3796
- Conner,Ellen Louise, MD
- Fabricant,Christopher James, MD
- Fumia,Fred Daniel, MD
- Gussman,Debra, MD
- Jacobson,Nina Stella, MD
- Matta,Paul Gamal, DO

Jersery Shore Anesthesiology
1945 Highway 33 Zip: 07753
Ph: (732) 897-0200 Fax: (732) 897-0263
- Fianko,Felix Akwasi-Owusu, MD
- Fields,Ryan G., DO
- Miller,Christine Venable, MD
- Miller,Kevin D., MD
- Morgan,Illiana Alexandrova, MD
- Reffler,Marie M., MD
- Sedutto,Joseph Mario, MD
- Varghese,Sherin V., MD
- Zhao,Rong, MD

Jersey Shore Anesthesiology Associates
1945 Route 33/PO Box 397 Zip: 07754
Ph: (732) 922-3308
- Berberich,Matthew Robert, MD
- Cammarata,Lindsay, MD
- Cindrario,Dean P., MD
- Ndeto,Geoffrey Wambua T., MD
- Nicholas,Thomas, MD
- Patel,Nehul, MD
- Rahal,William J., MD
- Steenland,Richard H., MD
- Vaclavik,Peter Svatopluk, MD
- Wu,Jeffrey P., MD

Jersey Shore Child Evaluation Center
81-04 Davis Avenue Zip: 07753
Ph: (732) 776-4178 Fax: (732) 776-4946
- Aloisio,Denise, MD
- Karia,Roopal M., MD
- Roth,Anne G., DO

Jersey Shore Neurology Associates PA
1900 Corlies Avenue/Third Floor Zip: 07753
Ph: (732) 775-2400 Fax: (732) 775-5673
- Fitzpatrick,John E., MD
- Rhee,Richard S., MD
- Sultan,Richard I., DO

Jersey Shore Psychiatric Associates
3535 Route 66/Building 5/Suite D Zip: 07753
Ph: (732) 643-4350
- Abenante,Frank Andrew, MD
- Fitzsimmons,Adriana Marie, MD
- Kochhar,Seema, MD
- Markowitz,Rachel Paula, MD
- Rose,Lane Gruber, MD

Jersey Shore Sports Medicine Center
51 Davis Avenue/Suite 51-02 Zip: 07753
Ph: (732) 776-2433 Fax: (732) 776-4403
- Lusk-Caceres,Christina A., DO
- Petrucci,James Christopher, DO
- Rice,Stephen G., MD

NJ Shore University Medical Center
1200 Jumping Brook Road Zip: 07753
Ph: (732) 643-4356 Fax: (732) 643-4378
- Cordal,Adriana, MD
- Solhkhah,Ramon, MD

Kristen A. Atienza, DO, FACOP
1812 Corlies Avenue Zip: 07753
Ph: (732) 988-3336 Fax: (732) 776-8668
- Atienza,Kristen A., DO

Meridian Medical Assocs
1945 Route 33 Zip: 07753
Ph: (732) 776-2963 Fax: (732) 776-3795
- Llull Tombo,Rolando, MD
- Meckael,Dina, MD

Meridian Medical Group - Faculty Prac
61 Davis Avenue/Suite 1 Zip: 07753
Ph: (732) 776-4860 Fax: (732) 776-4867
- Alfie,Marcos E., MD
- Bautista,Eduardo R., MD
- Beckwith-Fickas,Katherine A., MD
- Dadzie,Charles K., MD
- Eapen,Santhosh, MD
- Graff,Michael A., MD
- Jimenez,Jennifer E., MD
- Karatas,Meltem, MD
- Karwowska,Helena, MD
- Loveridge-Lenza,Beth Anne, DO
- Ramos,David G.D., MD
- Ross,Ann, MD
- Smotkin-Tangorra,Margarita, DO
- Soroush,Azam, MD

Meridian OB/GYN Associates PC
19 Davis Avenue/Fl 1 Zip: 07753
Ph: (732) 897-7944 Fax: (732) 922-8264
- Bal,Aswine Kumar, MD
- Bosscher,James Reed, MD
- ElSahwi,Karim Samir, MD

Meridian Surgical Associates
3700 Route 33/Suite C Zip: 07753
Ph: (732) 212-6590 Fax: (732) 922-2026
- Khan,Habib, MD
- Nasir Khan,Mohammad Usman, MD

Meridian Trauma Associates PC
1945 State Route 33 Zip: 07754
Ph: (732) 776-4949
- Gorechlad,John W., MD
- Shin,Seung Hoon, MD

Mid-Atlantic Surgical Associates
1944 Route 33/Suite 201 Zip: 07753
Ph: (732) 776-4622 Fax: (732) 776-3765
- Dejene,Brook A., MD
- Johnson,David L., MD

Monmouth Ocean Neurology
1944 State Route 33/Suite 206 Zip: 07753
Ph: (732) 774-8282 Fax: (732) 774-4407
- Baqui,Huma, MD

- Deutsch,Alan D., DO
- Eswar,Anastasia Maria, MD
- Kostoulakos,Paul M., DO
- Martino,Stephen John, MD

Neptune Pediatrics
1812 State Route 33 Zip: 07753
Ph: (732) 988-3336 Fax: (732) 776-8668
- Cartnick,Gregory Alan, MD

Northern Ocean County Med Assoc
10 Neptune Boulevard/Suite 201 Zip: 07753
Ph: (732) 455-8559 Fax: (732) 774-1394
- Adler,Bernard H., MD
- Glazier,Kim Steinberg, MD

Pediatric Associates
444 Neptune Boulevard/Suite 4 Zip: 07753
Ph: (732) 774-4332 Fax: (732) 774-4077
- Alfonzo,Joann, MD

Physican's Home & Health Service
1532 State Route 33/Suite 202 Zip: 07753
Ph: (732) 775-8400 Fax: (732) 775-8401
- Liu,Jian, MD
- Roper,Brian K., MD

Shore Heart Group, P.A.
1820 State Route 33/Suite 4-B Zip: 07753
Ph: (732) 776-8500 Fax: (732) 776-8946
- Aaron,Michael R., DO
- Chu,Tony Nang-Tang, MD
- Diwan,Ravi, MD
- Gill,Jasrai Singh, MD
- Girgis,Ihab, MD
- Okere,Arthur Ezeribe, MD
- Orlando,James Frank, MD
- Sandler,Leonard Lewis, MD
- Weiss,Maurice D., MD
- Yang,Rayson C., MD

Shore Nephrology, P.A.
2100 Corlies Avenue/Suite 15 Zip: 07753
Ph: (732) 988-8228 Fax: (732) 774-1528
- Bolarinwa,Oladayo, MD
- Cruz,Dionisio V., MD
- Husain,Sara, MD
- Masud,Avais, MD
- Strauss,Ira M., MD

Shore Primary Care
1944 Corlies Avenue/Suite 103 Zip: 07753
Ph: (732) 774-2336 Fax: (732) 774-2337
- Bhuskute,Bela Hemant, MD
- Klein,Alan C., MD

University Radiology Group
2100 Route 33/Neptune City Med Bld Zip: 07753
Ph: (732) 988-1234 Fax: (732) 502-0368
- Biswal,Rajiv, MD

Neptune City

Jersey Shore Eye Associates
1809 Corlies Avenue/Suite 1 Zip: 07753
Ph: (732) 774-5566 Fax: (732) 988-7574
- Del Negro,Ralph G., DO
- Glatman,Marina, MD
- Senft,Carl Joseph, MD

Neshanic Station

Pleasant Run Family Physicians
925 US Highway 202 Zip: 08853
Ph: (908) 788-9468 Fax: (908) 788-5720
- Barr,James E., MD
- Dellavalle,Lindsay Joy, DO
- Gertzman-Dafilou,Sharon D., DO
- Rigatti,Damian F., DO

New Brunswick

Brunswick Cardiology Associates
1140 Somerset Street Zip: 08901
Ph: (732) 246-4699 Fax: (732) 246-4889
- Jeganathan,Narayanan, MD

Brunswick Orthopaedic Associates
303 George Street/Suite 105 Zip: 08901
Ph: (732) 846-6100 Fax: (732) 846-6113
- Fried,Steven H., MD

Center for Ambulatory Resources
240 Easton Avenue Zip: 08901
Ph: (732) 745-8564 Fax: (732) 745-9156
- Madhavan,Arjun, MD

Central Jersey Surgical Specialists
78 Easton Avenue Zip: 08901
Ph: (732) 249-0360 Fax: (732) 249-0035
- Rao,Niranjan V., MD
- Zavotsky,Jeffry, MD

Child Health Institute of New Jersey
89 French Street/Suite 2300 Zip: 08901
Ph: (732) 235-6230 Fax: (732) 235-8766
- Bhise,Vikram V., MD
- Brooks,Susan Sklower, MD
- Chen,Yen Ping, MD
- Di Cicco Bloom,Emanuel M., MD
- Esfahanizadeh,Abdolreza, MD
- Gurkan,Sevgi, MD
- Horton,Daniel B., MD
- Patel,Payal, MD
- Shiroff,Adam Michael, MD
- Strozuk-McDonough,Stephanie, MD
- Weiss,Lynne S., MD

Drs. Agrin and Shulman
78 Easton Avenue Zip: 08901
Ph: (732) 545-1065 Fax: (732) 545-1063
- Shulman,Leon H., MD

Drs. Kwong and Vella
10 Plum Street/8th Floor Zip: 08901
Ph: (732) 235-5530 Fax: (732) 235-5882
- Kwong,Kelvin Ming-Tak, MD
- Vella,Joseph Bayer, MD

Drs. Tran and Sliwowska
317 George Street Zip: 08901
Ph: (732) 235-6972
- Sliwowska,Anna, MD
- Tran,Thai Thi, MD

Eric B. Chandler Health Center
277 George Street Zip: 08901
Ph: (732) 235-6700 Fax: (732) 235-6729
- Colon,Deannon, MD
- Farkas,Andrew, MD
- Fleming,Jacqueline, MD
- Jacob,Sneha Elizabeth, MD
- Jahn,Eric G., MD
- Lavizzo Mourey,Risa Juanita, MD
- Levin,Steven Jonathan, MD
- Mahal,Mona, MD
- Marcella,Stephen W., MD
- Miller,Ralee Ka, MD
- Peskin,Steven R., MD
- Ramachandran,Usha, MD
- Stechna,Sharon Beth, MD
- Suarez,Militza E., MD

Family Medicine at Monument Square
317 George Street Zip: 08901
Ph: (732) 235-8993 Fax: (732) 246-7317
- Acevedo,Rhina A., MD
- Afran,Joyce G., MD
- Bhatt,Komal Gopalbhai, MD
- Clark,Elizabeth C., MD
- Farjo,Sara, DO
- Heath,Cathryn Batutis, MD
- Kropa,Jill, MD
- Laumbach,Sonia Caridad G., MD
- Levine,Jeffrey Pierre, MD
- Lin,Karen Wei-Ru, MD
- McGarry,Barbara J., MD
- O'Connor,Robert M., MD
- Ojadi,Vallier Chidiebere, MD
- Roemheld-Hamm,Beatrix, MD
- Snyder,Laura Jean, MD
- Stabile,Marissa Jimenez, DO
- Steinlight,Sasha Juli, MD
- Swee,David E., MD
- Ulloque,Rory Alexander, MD
- Womack,Jason Peter, MD
- Wu,Justine Peen, MD
- Yoon,Kyung In, MD

Heart & Vascular Institute
317 George Street/Suite 440 Zip: 08901
Ph: (732) 994-3278 Fax: (800) 732-0366
- Shah,Nihir Biharilal, MD
- Zakir,Ramzan Muhammad, MD

Groups and Clinics by Town with Physician Rosters

New Brunswick (cont)

New Jersey Pain Institute
125 Paterson Street/CAB 6100 Zip: 08901
Ph: (732) 235-6444
- Balachandar,Sadana, MD
- Grubb,William R., MD

Plastic Surgery Arts of of New Jersey
409 Joyce Kilmer Ave./Suite 210 Zip: 08901
Ph: (732) 418-0709 Fax: (732) 418-0747
- Ahuja,Naveen K., MD
- Wey,Philip D., MD

Retina Associates of New Jersey, P.A.
10 Plum Street/Suite 600 Zip: 08901
Ph: (732) 220-1600 Fax: (732) 220-1603
- Fine,Howard Frederick, MD
- Friedman,Eric Stephen, MD
- Green,Stuart N., MD
- Keyser,Bruce J., MD
- Prenner,Jonathan Lawrence, MD
- Roth,Daniel Benjamin, MD
- Shah,Sumit Pravinkumar, MD
- Wheatley,Harold M., MD

RWJ Transplant Associates, P.A.
10 Plum Street/7th Floor Zip: 08901
Ph: (732) 253-3699
- Almendral,Jesus Leandro Gestuvo, M
- Bunin,Sonalis, MD
- Laskow,David A., MD
- Mann,Richard A., MD
- Mondal,Zahidul Hoque, MD
- Pelletier,Ronald Paul, MD

RWJ-UMDNJ Anesthesia Group
125 Paterson Street/CAB 3100 Zip: 08901
Ph: (732) 235-7827 Fax: (732) 235-6131
- Alloteh,Rose Sitsofe, MD
- Ambalu,Oren, MD
- Barsoum,Sylviana S., MD
- Berman,Stefanie L., MD
- Bermann,Mordechai, MD
- Chhokra,Renu, MD
- Chi,Oak Z., MD
- Chiricolo,Antonio, MD
- Chyu,Darrick J., MD
- Cirella,Vincent N., MD
- Cohen,Shaul, MD
- Cowell,Jennifer L., MD
- Curcio,Christine Marie, MD
- De Angelis,Vincent James, MD
- Denenberg,Howard W., MD
- Denny,John T., MD
- Enlow,Tracey S., MD
- George,Gina, DO
- Ginsberg,Steven H., MD
- Grayer,Nicole C., MD
- Grayson,Jeremy Seth, MD
- Hall,Dennis B., MD
- Jan,Thomas, MD
- Kandra,Arun M., MD
- Khan,Ibraheem, MD
- Kiel,Samuel Yol, MD
- Kiss,Geza Kalmar, MD
- Lee,Isidore C., MD
- Mabry,Christian Carl, MD
- Mai,Quynh-Tien, MD
- McDonough,Christian P., MD
- McRae,Valerie A., MD
- Mehta,Tejal H., MD
- Mellender,Scott Jason, MD
- Mungekar,Sagar Sudhir, MD
- Nagella,Naresh, MD
- Nanavati,Neeraj K., MD
- Nandal,Dharamveer, MD
- Neustadt,Charles M., MD
- Pantin,Enrique Jose, MD
- Papp,Denes, MD
- Perez,Jessica, MD
- Radhakrishnan,Radhika, MD
- Raffel,Brian J., DO
- Rah,Kang H., MD
- Reformato,Vincent, MD
- Ridley,Diane M., MD
- Shah,Shruti A., MD
- Shah,Trishna Kirit, MD
- Shah,Ushma R., MD
- Singer,Eric Alan, MD
- Sison,Edwin Ruan Racela, MD
- Solina,Alann R., MD
- Stein,Mark Herbert, MD
- Tanaka,Sho, MD
- Thaker,Jayeshkumar, MD
- Veksler,Boris, MD
- Wang,Monty H.S., MD
- Wu,Melissa S., MD
- Zuker-Silberberg,Dora D., MD

Rutgers - RWJMS
125 Paterson Street/Suite 2100 Zip: 08901
Ph: (732) 235-7756 Fax: (732) 235-7095
- Danish,Shabbar F., MD
- Gupta,Gaurav, MD

Rutgers Cancer Institute of New Jersey
195 Little Albany Street/PO Box 2681 Zip: 08903
Ph: (732) 235-2465 Fax: (732) 235-6797
- Aisner,Joseph, MD
- August,David A., MD
- Bannerji,Rajat, MD
- Carpizo,Darren Richard, MD
- Chundury,Anupama, MD
- David,Kevin Andrew, MD
- Drachtman,Richard A., MD
- Eleff,Michael, MD
- Evens,Andrew M., DO
- Ferrari,Anna C., MD
- Ganesan,Shridar, MD
- Gharibo,Mecide M., MD
- Goyal,Sharad, MD
- Goydos,James S., MD
- Grandhi,Miral Sadaria, MD
- Groisberg,Roman, MD
- Haffty,Bruce George, MD
- Hait,William N., MD
- Hathout,Lara, MD
- Hellmann,Mira C., MD
- Hirshfield,Kim Marie, MD
- Isani,Sara, MD
- Jabbour,Salma K., MD
- Jang,Thomas Lee, MD
- Karantza-Wadsworth,Vassiliki, MD
- Kauh,John S., MD
- Kaveney,Amanda Davis, MD
- Kennedy,Timothy John, MD
- Khan,Atif Jalees, MD
- Kim,Isaac Yi, MD
- Kim,Sung N., MD
- Koshenkov,Vadim P., MD
- Kritharis-Agrusa,Athena, MD
- Lewis,Jocelyn A., DO
- Mahmoud,Omar M., MD
- Masterson,Margaret, MD
- Mayer,Tina Marie, MD
- McKenna,Michael G., MD
- Mehnert,Janice M., MD
- Michaels,Lisa A., MD
- Moerdler,Scott A., MD
- Moss,Rebecca Anne, MD
- Motwani,Sabin B., MD
- Murphy,Susan M., MD
- Pan,Wilbur James, MD
- Parikh,Dhwani R., MD
- Patel,Akshar Nilkantha, MD
- Patel,Vimal Dahya, MD
- Poplin,Elizabeth A., MD
- Riedlinger,Gregory M., MD
- Saraiya,Biren P., MD
- Schaar,Dale G., MD
- Sharma,Archana, DO
- Stein,Mark Nathan, MD
- Strair,Roger Kurt, MD
- Surakanti,Sujani Ganga, MD
- Toppmeyer,Deborah Lynn, MD
- Weiner,Joseph Paul, MD
- Weiss,Aaron R., DO
- Weiss,Robert Edward, MD
- Wong,Serena Tsan-Lai, MD

Rutgers RWJ Allergy, Immun & Inf Grp
125 Paterson Street Zip: 08901
Ph: (732) 235-7060
- Bhowmick,Tanaya, MD
- Boruchoff,Susan E., MD
- Cornett,Julia Kang, MD
- McAuliffe,Vincent J., MD
- Weinstein,Melvin P., MD

Saint Peter's Physician Associates
78 Easton Avenue Zip: 08901
Ph: (732) 828-3300 Fax: (732) 937-5739
- Goldberg,Michael I., MD
- Magliaro,Thomas J., MD

Saint Peter's Physician Associates
240 Easton Avenue/4th Floor Zip: 08901
Ph: (732) 937-6008
- Broder,Arkady, MD

St. Peter's Adult Family Health Center
123 How Lane Zip: 08901
Ph: (732) 745-6642
- Babcock,Karen R., MD
- Wer Arrivillaga,Santiago, MD

St. Peter's Family Health
123 How Lane Zip: 08901
Ph: (732) 745-8600 Fax: (732) 729-0869
- Amir,Saba, MD
- Jyonouchi,Harumi, MD
- Kicenuik,Michael T., MD
- Kothari,Nayan K., MD
- Kumar,Akshat, MD
- Lastra,Carlos R., MD
- Ranzini,Angela C., MD
- Stewart,Richard Allen, DO

St. Peters Pediatric Faculty
123 How Lane Zip: 08901
Ph: (732) 745-8419
- Bernstein,William R., MD
- Lucas,Michael Joseph, MD
- Medina,Gladibel, MD

Thyroid & Diabetes Ctr
240 Easton Avenue/4th Floor Zip: 08901
Ph: (732) 745-6667
- Murthy,Meena S., MD

UMDNJ RWJ Vascular Surgery Group
125 Paterson Street/Suite 4100 Zip: 08901
Ph: (732) 235-7816 Fax: (732) 235-8538
- Beckerman,William, MD
- Crowley,John G., MD
- Rahimi,Saum Amir, MD

University Cardiology Group
125 Paterson Street/Suite 5200 Zip: 08901
Ph: (732) 235-6561 Fax: (732) 235-6530
- Francis,Charles Kenneth, MD

University Cardiology Group
125 Paterson Street/MEB 578 Zip: 08901
Ph: (732) 235-7855 Fax: (732) 235-8722
- Vagaonescu,Tudor Dumitru, MD

UH-RWJ General Internal Medicine
125 Paterson Street/Suite 2300 Zip: 08901
Ph: (732) 235-7122 Fax: (732) 235-7144
- Brodt,Zahava Nilly, MD
- Chen,Catherine, MD
- Czaja,Matthew T., MD
- Desai,Avani Mahesh, MD
- Desai,Neel, MD
- Desai,Vidhi Parikh, MD
- Fujita,Kenji Peter, MD
- Grimes,Julia P., DO
- Iwata,Isao, MD
- Juneau,Jeffrey Evan, MD
- Kota,Karthik, MD
- Schneiderman,Joyce F., MD
- Steinberg,Michael Barry, MD

University Medical Group
125 Paterson Street/Suite 5100 Zip: 08901
Ph: (732) 235-7993 Fax: (732) 235-7117
- Doubrava,Suzanne M., MD
- Ebert,Gary A., MD
- Grossman,Rachel M., MD
- Kim,Sarang, MD
- Kountz,David S., MD
- Maltz,Gary S., MD
- Monteleone,Catherine A., MD
- Parikh,Amay, MD
- Reinhardt,Rickey R., MD
- Yeh,Shihlong, MD

University Med Group - Internal Med
125 Paterson Street/Suite 5100A Zip: 08903
Ph: (732) 235-6968 Fax: (732) 235-8935
- Amorosa,Louis F., MD
- Armas-Loughran,Barbara Janine, MD
- Chakravarthy,Manu V., MD
- George,Renu, MD
- Hogshire,Lauren Christine, MD
- Lee,Meichia, MD
- Lubitz,Sara Elisabeth, MD
- Raoof,Sidra, MD
- Riley,David J., MD
- Rosenfeld,Jane S., MD
- Sonnenberg,Frank A., MD
- Stein,Peter Paris, MD
- Story-Roller,Elizabeth, MD

University Medical Group Pediatrics
125 Paterson Street/MEB 3rd Fl Zip: 08903
Ph: (732) 235-7893 Fax: (732) 235-7345
- Alemu,Kidist, MD
- Baddi,Anoosha, DO
- Bahadur,Kandy, MD
- Baszak,Sylvia, MD
- Bruno,Chantal Dominique, DO
- Cohen,Stephanie Gail, MD
- Das,Sumon Kumar, MD
- Kaliyadan,George, MD
- Parlow,Brittany, MD
- Pepper,Matthew Philip, MD
- Takyi,Michele, MD
- Whyte,Peta-Gaye Kenisha, DO

University Medical Group/Cardiology
125 Paterson Street/CAB-Rm 5200 Zip: 08901
Ph: (732) 235-6561 Fax: (732) 235-6530
- Pamidi,Madhavi, MD

University Medical Group/UMDNJ
125 Paterson Street/Suite 2200 Zip: 08901
Ph: (732) 235-7647 Fax: (732) 235-7677
- Babalola,Ronke Latifatu, MD
- Bisen,Viwek Singh, DO
- Johnson,William Gessner, MD
- Orloff,John J., MD
- Tiu,Gladys Tompar, MD
- Trenton,Adam James, DO

University Medical Group/Vascular Surg
One Robert Wood Johnson Place/MEB 541 Zip: 08901
Ph: (732) 235-7816 Fax: (732) 235-8538
- Cha,Andrew, DO
- Shafritz,Randy, MD

University Otolaryngology Assocs
181 Somerset Street Zip: 08901
Ph: (732) 247-2401
- Goldrich,Michael Seth, MD
- Traquina,Diana Nogueira, MD

University Physician Associates of NJ
125 Paterson Street/CAB 5200 Zip: 08901
Ph: (732) 235-7223 Fax: (732) 235-7115
- Guo,Shuang, MD
- Hsu,Vivien M., MD
- Khan,Imran Ahmad, MD
- Kostis,William J., MD
- Rahman,Mahboob Ur, MD
- Rose,Shelonitda S., MD

New Providence

Associates in Cardiovascular Disease
571 Central Avenue/Suite 115 Zip: 07974
Ph: (908) 464-4200 Fax: (908) 464-1332
- Bartov,David Nir, MD

Assocs in Cardiovascular Disease
29 South Street Zip: 07974
Ph: (908) 464-4200 Fax: (908) 464-1332
- Calderon,Mark J., MD
- Farry,John Patrick, MD
- Glasofer,Sidney, MD

Groups and Clinics by Town with Physician Rosters

Mich,Robert John, MD
Rosenthal,Todd Michael, MD
Sheris,Steven Jay, MD

Berkeley Heights Eye Group
571 Central Avenue/Suite 101 Zip: 07974
Ph: (908) 464-4600 Fax: (908) 464-4737
Leventhal,Todd Owen, MD
Wong,Charissa J., MD

New Providence Internal Med Assocs
571 Central Avenue/Suite 112 Zip: 07974
Ph: (908) 464-7300
Hakim,James J., MD
Zukoff,Paul B., MD

Summit Medical Group
890 New Mountain Avenue Zip: 07974
Ph: (908) 277-8601
Barresi,Joseph A., MD
Brown,Teresa V., DO
Cummings-Becker,Stephanie Jane, MD
Gibbons,Alice B., MD
Hidalgo,Marla, MD

The Pediatric Center
556 Central Avenue Zip: 07974
Ph: (908) 508-0400 Fax: (908) 508-0370
Chin,Kathleen L., MD
Moskowitz,Steven, MD
Shih,Eunhee, MD
Visci,Denise, MD

Newark

Astra MD PC
550 Bloomfield Avenue Zip: 07107
Ph: (973) 483-1500 Fax: (973) 483-4577
Fuksina,Natasha, MD
Rubbani,Mariam Shafaq, MD

Beth Prime Care
166 Lyons Avenue/Ground Floor Zip: 07112
Ph: (973) 926-3535 Fax: (973) 926-6187
Gururajarao,Lakshmi, MD
Srivastava,Sushama, MD

Catholic Community Services
1160 Raymond Boulevard Zip: 07102
Ph: (973) 596-4190
Eljarrah,Fouad, MD
Henningson,Karen Jeanne, DO
Young,Joseph M., MD

Center For Geriatric Health Care
156 Lyons Avenue Zip: 07112
Ph: (973) 926-8491 Fax: (973) 923-6599
Shihabuddin,Lina Sami, MD

Center for Neurological Surgery UMDNJ
90 Bergen Street/DOC 8100 Zip: 07103
Ph: (973) 972-2323 Fax: (973) 972-2333
Al Kawi,Ammar, MD
Amuluru,Krishna, MD
Gandhi,Chirag D., MD
Gillick,John, MD
Goldstein,Ira Morris, MD
Gyi,Jennifer, DO
Hernandez,Robert Nicholas, MD
Herschman,Yehuda, MD
Hsueh,Wayne Daniel, MD
Jethwa,Pinakin R., MD
Kaye,Rachel, MD
Khandelwal,Priyank, MD
Mammis,Antonios, MD
Michaels,Jennifer, MD
Sinclair,George Lawrence III, MD
Tabbarah,Khalid Zuhayr, MD

Comprehensive Care Center
297 16th Avenue Zip: 07103
Ph: (973) 485-3300 Fax: (973) 485-0226
Baskerville,Renee E., DO
Chomsky,Steven A., MD

Concentra Medical Centers
375 McCarter Highway Zip: 07114
Ph: (973) 643-8601 Fax: (973) 643-8609
Andrade,Peter, DO
Raghavan,Usha Murli, MD

Drs. Fedida and Brown
306 Martin Luther King Blvd/4th Floor Zip: 07102
Ph: (973) 877-2580 Fax: (973) 877-2578
Fedida,Andre Armand, MD

Drs. Picciano, Picciano & Sadik
36 Pacific Street Zip: 07105
Ph: (973) 578-4808
Picciano,Maria V., MD
Picciano,Robert, MD
Sadik,Aseel, MD

Drs. Shah & Shah
1060 Broad Street Zip: 07102
Ph: (973) 642-0280 Fax: (973) 642-0047
Shah,Rajen S., MD
Shah,Sandhya R., MD

Essex Ironbund Anesthesiologist LLC
155 Jefferson Street Zip: 07105
Ph: (908) 490-0036 Fax: (908) 490-0067
Kostroma,Boris Vladimirovich, MD

Essex Medical and Nephrology
539 Bloomfield Avenue Zip: 07107
Ph: (973) 566-9900 Fax: (973) 566-6692
Chadha,Inderpal S., MD
Shah,Ajit M., MD

Eye Clinic PA
155 Jefferson Street Zip: 07105
Ph: (973) 622-2020 Fax: (973) 817-8666
Goldfeder,Alan W., MD
Rassier,Charles Edgar Jr., MD

Forest Hill Family Health Associates
465 Mount Prospect Avenue Zip: 07104
Ph: (973) 483-3640 Fax: (973) 483-4895
Almodovar,Astrid Teresa, MD
Anthony,AnnGene G, MD
Guinto,Danilo M., MD
Ortiz,Thomas R., MD
Parmar,Pritesh B., MD

Healthfirst
1 Washington Square Zip: 07105
Mosquera,Joseph L., MD

Internet Medical Group, P.C.
66 Somme Street Zip: 07105
Ph: (973) 589-7337 Fax: (973) 589-1905
Kanikicharla,Uma, MD
Uy,Loreta M., MD

Lyons Medical Center LLC
669 Elizabeth Avenue Zip: 07112
Ph: (973) 923-6452 Fax: (973) 923-1979
Joseph,Frederique Mirlene, MD
Louissaint,Paraclet S., MD

NBIMC Psychiatry
201 Lyons Avenue Zip: 07112
Ph: (973) 926-7026 Fax: (973) 926-2862
Frometa,Ayme Veronica, MD
Jadeja,Kiranben J., MD

New Jersey Cardiology Associates
201 Lyons Avenue/6th Floor Zip: 07112
Ph: (973) 926-7503 Fax: (973) 923-7267
Southgate,Theodore J., MD

New Jersey Poison Center
65 Bergen Street/4th Floor Zip: 07107
Ph: (973) 972-9280 Fax: (973) 972-2679
Marcus,Steven M., MD

Newark Community Health Center, Inc.
741 Broadway Zip: 07104
Ph: (973) 675-1900 Fax: (973) 676-1396
Camiolo,Mark A., DO
Cueto,Victor Jr., MD
Manigault,Simone A., MD
Mirabal,Sadie L., DO
Morkos,Faten Farid, MD
Toft,Maria Campos, MD
Walks,Pauline Angela, MD
Zloza,Donna Lynn, MD

Newark Dept of Health & Human Services
110 William Street Zip: 07102
Ph: (973) 733-5300
Abels,Jane I., MD
Davis,Barbara, MD
Figueroa,Wanda E., MD
Gonzalez,Isabel V., MD
Jin,Li, MD
Netravali,Chitra Arun, MD
O'Neal,Isaac, MD
Trinidad,Altagracia A., MD

Newark Rehabilitation Center
638 Mount Prospect Avenue Zip: 07104
Ph: (973) 481-4040 Fax: (973) 481-1338
Burducea,Alexandru, DO

Colon,Jose F., MD
Kramberg,Raymond Robert David, MD

Preventive Medicine & Community Health
185 South Orange Avenue/MSB F-506 Zip: 07101
Ph: (973) 972-4422 Fax: (973) 972-7625
Halperin,William Edward, MD
Sheikh,Shuja, MD
Thomas,Pauline A., MD

Primary Medical Care
76 Prospect Street Zip: 07105
Ph: (973) 344-1313 Fax: (973) 344-1811
Salese,Joseph Giuseppe, MD

Renaissance Medical Group
155 Jefferson Street/Lower Level Zip: 07105
Ph: (973) 344-5498 Fax: (973) 344-6686
Lind,Eugene Joseph, MD
Osorio,Jorge H., MD

Rutgers Cancer Institute of NJ
205 South Orange Avenue/B Level Zip: 07101
Ph: (973) 972-5108
Ignatius,Nandini, MD

Summit Breast Care, LLC
111 Central Avenue Zip: 07102
Ph: (908) 918-0001 Fax: (908) 918-0003
Kalu,Ogori K., MD

The University Hospital
65 Bergen Street Zip: 07107
Ph: (973) 972-2900 Fax: (973) 972-2904
Budnick,Lawrence D., MD
Reddy,Loveleen, MD
Rodgers,Denise V., MD

Valerie Fund Childrens Center
201 Lyons Avenue Zip: 07112
Ph: (973) 926-7161 Fax: (973) 282-0395
Kamalakar,Peri, MD
Narang,Shalu, MD

UMDNJ Gastro & Hepatology
90 Bergen Street/DOC 2100 Zip: 07103
Ph: (973) 972-2343 Fax: (973) 972-0752
Ahlawat,Sushil K., MD
Bojito-Marrero,Lizza Marie, MD
Brelvi,Zamir S., MD
Demyen,Michael Frank, MD
Krawitz,Steven, MD
Pyrsopoulos,Nikolaos T., MD
Samanta,Arun K., MD
Wang,Weizheng William, MD

Universal Industrial Clinic
99 Madison Street Zip: 07105
Ph: (973) 344-2929 Fax: (973) 344-1239
Patel,Saurabh Chandrakant, MD
Wulkan,Sheryl Lynn, MD
Yanamadula,Dinash Kumar, MD

University Ophthalmology Associates
90 Bergen Street/DOC 6100 Zip: 07101
Ph: (973) 982-2065
Dastjerdi,Mohammad Hossein, MD
Fechtner,Robert D., MD
Greenstein,Steven, MD
Habiel,Miriam, MD
Khouri,Albert S., MD
Langer,Paul D., MD

University Pediatric Group
90 Bergen Street/DOC 4300 Zip: 07103
Ph: (973) 972-2100
Reddy,Chitra R., MD
Schwab,Joseph V., MD

University Physician Associates
140 Bergen Street/ACC Level C Zip: 07103
Ph: (973) 972-2700 Fax: (973) 972-2739
Bardeguez,Arlene D., MD
Barrett,Theodore, MD
Brandi,Kristyn M., MD

University Physician Associates
140 Bergen Street/ACC Level D Zip: 07103
Ph: (973) 972-4071 Fax: (973) 972-3102
Chew,Debra, MD
Dallapiazza,Michelle Lynn, MD
Dever,Lisa Lynn, MD
Douglas,Nataki Celeste, MD

Ellner,Jerrold Jay, MD
Finkel,Diana Gurevich, DO
Ganesh,Vijaya L., MD
Gittens-Williams,Lisa Nadine, MD
Goldman,Noah Adam, MD

University Physician Associates
140 Bergen Street/ACC Level F Zip: 07103
Ph: (973) 972-8087 Fax: (973) 972-6651
Kaplan,Joshua Michael, MD
Novetsky,Akiva Pesach, MD
Pompeo,Lisa, MD
Roche,Natalie E., MD
Rossman,Stephen, DO
Sterling-Jean,Yolette, MD
Swaminathan,Shobha, MD
Tilak,Vasanti A., MD

University Reproductive Association
185 South Orange Avenue/MSB E-506 Zip: 07103
Ph: (973) 972-5266 Fax: (973) 972-4574
Einstein,Mark H., MD
Kuhn,Theresa Marie, MD
Marcus,Jenna Z., MD
Pant,Meenakshi, MD

Washington Park Medical Associates
559 Broad Street Zip: 07102
Ph: (973) 622-3890 Fax: (973) 622-6443
Garay,Luis Alberto, MD

Newfoundland

North Jersey Dermatology Center
7 Oak Ridge Road/Suite 3 Zip: 07435
Ph: (973) 208-8110 Fax: (973) 208-8106
Bilkis,Michael Ross, MD

Newton

Advocare Sussex County Pediatrics
39 Newton Sparta Road Zip: 07860
Ph: (973) 383-9841 Fax: (973) 383-7989
Dakake,Charles Jr., MD
Digby,Thomas E., MD
Porter,James H., MD
Sison,Genevieve Yvonne, MD
Zohny,Jeahad, MD

Andover Orthopaedic Surgery & Sports
280 Newton-Sparta Road/Suite 4 Zip: 07860
Ph: (973) 579-7443 Fax: (973) 579-5628
Bradish,Glen Edward, MD
Lopez,Nicole Melisa Montero, MD
Scales,James Jr., MD
Weinschenk,Robert C., MD

Cardiology Associates of Sussex County
222 High Street/Suite 205 Zip: 07860
Ph: (973) 579-2100 Fax: (973) 579-6638
Bergman,Benjamin Ryan, MD
Buyer,David S., MD
Cioce,Gerald, MD
Codispoti,Cindy A., DO
Masci,Robert L., MD
Redline,Richard C., MD
Schwarz,Scott A., MD

Drs. Mattes & Collini
181 High Street Zip: 07860
Ph: (973) 383-9898 Fax: (973) 383-9665
Collini,William R., MD
Mattes,David G., MD

Eye Physicians of Sussex County
183 High Street/Suite 2200 Zip: 07860
Ph: (973) 383-6345 Fax: (973) 383-0032
Barone,Robert Gerard, MD
Hirschfeld,Laura Ann, MD
Inkeles,David M., MD
Perlmutter,Harold S., MD
Vora,Amit V., MD

Image Care Centers
222 High Street/Suite 101 Zip: 07860
Ph: (973) 729-0002 Fax: (973) 383-2774
Scheer,Linda B., MD

Medical & Surgical Specialty Group
135 Newton Sparta Road/Suite 201 Zip: 07860
Ph: (973) 383-6244 Fax: (973) 383-0573
Harris,Ronald K., MD
Newman,Brian F., MD

Groups and Clinics by Town with Physician Rosters

Newton (cont)
Neurologic Arts Associated, LLC.
183 High Street/Suite 1200 Zip: 07860
Ph: (973) 300-0579 Fax: (973) 300-5535
- Khesin, Yevgeniy I., MD
- Tishuk, Pavel, MD
- Weintraub, Bernard M., MD

North Jersey Pain Management Ctr
39 Newton-Sparta Road Zip: 07860
Ph: (973) 383-0173 Fax: (201) 567-1432
- Habina, Ladislav, MD
- Hagopian, Vahe H., MD

Premier Health Associates
123 Newton Sparta Road Zip: 07860
Ph: (973) 579-6300 Fax: (973) 579-1524
- DeBitetto, Nick P., DO
- Delsardo, Anthony C., MD
- Liloia, Peter Anthony, DO
- Shah, Samir D., MD
- Stas, Sameer, MD
- Vaz, Richard, DO

Pulmonary Medical Associates, L.L.P
222 High Street/Suite 102 Zip: 07860
Ph: (973) 579-5090 Fax: (973) 579-2994
- Garg, Rakesh K., MD
- Mohammadi, Mina, MD
- Nadarajah, Dayaparan, MD

Skylands Medical Group PA
33 Newton-Sparta Road/Suite 1 Zip: 07860
Ph: (973) 383-2244 Fax: (973) 383-0448
- Pampin, Robert J., DO
- Sieminski, Douglas Peter, DO

Womens Health Care Associates
135 Newton Sparta Road/Suite 201 Zip: 07860
Ph: (973) 383-8555 Fax: (973) 383-8424
- Bagherian, Sharareh, DO
- Dardik, Raquel B., MD
- Lewis, Frieda Elizabeth, MD
- Nadarajah, Anandhi K., MD
- Paxton, Adam Michael, MD
- Pennant, Andria Uzetta, MD
- Rubino, Donald J., MD

North Arlington
Comprehensive Women's Healthcare
44 Ridge Road Zip: 07031
Ph: (201) 991-2880 Fax: (201) 991-0027
- Grasso, Armand J., MD
- Thomas, Eric David, MD

Internal Medicine Practice LLC
312 Belleville Turnpike/Suite 1 C Zip: 07031
Ph: (201) 997-4040 Fax: (201) 997-4040
- Bitner, Bozena Wanda, MD
- Kwapniewski, Agnieszka Monika, MD

North Arlington Cardiology Assoc
62 Ridge Road Zip: 07031
Ph: (201) 991-8565 Fax: (201) 991-2408
- Anastasiades, Athos C., MD
- Burachinsky, Andrew E., DO
- Latyshev, Yevgeniy, MD

North Arlington Primary Care Assocs
25 Locust Avenue Zip: 07031
Ph: (201) 991-9000 Fax: (201) 991-9005
- Monroe, Beatrice, MD

North Bergen
Atlas Spine Interventional Medicine
8901 Kennedy Boulevard/Suite 1-W Zip: 07047
Ph: (201) 243-2022 Fax: (201) 243-7261
- Vazquez, Pablo, MD
- Waldman, Steven Paul, MD

Capo Medical Associates
700-79th Street Zip: 07047
Ph: (201) 861-7900 Fax: (201) 861-5280
- Capo', Aida P., MD
- Capo', Maria Pilar, MD

Drs. Caride and Sotiriadis
9226 Kennedy Boulevard/Suite A Zip: 07047
Ph: (201) 869-9500 Fax: (201) 869-9501
- Caride, Peter, MD
- Sotiriadis, John, MD

Drs. Kelly & Stein
One Marine Road/Suite 100 Zip: 07047
Ph: (201) 869-1313 Fax: (201) 854-7945
- Kelly, Dennis Hughes III, MD
- Stein, Aaron A., MD

Drs. Pattner, Grodstein, et al
8100 Kennedy Boulevard Zip: 07047
Ph: (201) 868-5905
- Fein, Deborah Anne, MD

Gastroenterology Med Assoc PA
9223 Kennedy Boulevard/Suite D Zip: 07047
Ph: (201) 868-2849 Fax: (201) 868-4190
- Raskin, Jeffrey M., MD
- Tepler, Harold George, MD

NHCAC Health Center at North Bergen
1116 43rd Street Zip: 07047
Ph: (201) 330-2632 Fax: (201) 330-2638
- De Vera, Edmundo C., MD
- Panem, Flordeliz Buensuceso, MD
- Sujovolsky, Jeannette A., DO

Northern NJ Cardiology Assoc
7704 Marine Road Zip: 07047
Ph: (201) 869-1313 Fax: (201) 854-7945
- Gabelman, Mark Scott, MD

Ob-Gyn Associates of North Jersey
7400 Bergenline Avenue Zip: 07047
Ph: (201) 869-5488 Fax: (201) 869-6944
- Giron-Jimenez, Sandra, MD
- Gutierrez, Christine V., MD
- Kitzis, Hugo D., MD
- Pablo, Bryan Alcides, MD

Palisades Medical Center
8100 Kennedy Boulevard Zip: 07047
Ph: (201) 866-6770 Fax: (201) 866-6771
- Goldstein, Marc, DO
- Gonzalez, Marcia M., MD
- Laufer, Beatrice, MD
- Rabago-Reyes, Cassandra, MD
- Scopulovic-Nikolic, Biljana, MD

Palisades Women's Group
7650 River Road/Suite 230 Zip: 07047
Ph: (201) 868-6755 Fax: (201) 868-8442
- Escobar, Juan Nicolas, MD
- Patel, Jigna K., MD

Palisades Women's Group
6045 Kennedy Boulevard/Suite B Zip: 07047
Ph: (201) 868-2630 Fax: (201) 868-4919
- Patel, Zankhana M., MD
- Pathak, Sonal, MD
- Perisic, Dusan, MD
- Trujillo-Carvalho, Cecilia J., MD

Rastogi Medical Associates
8306 Kennedy Boulevard Zip: 07047
Ph: (201) 868-1333 Fax: (201) 868-3235
- Rastogi, Surender M., MD

Riverside Medical Group
6045 Kennedy Boulevard/Suite A Zip: 07047
Ph: (201) 861-4443 Fax: (201) 861-0941
- Dejesus, Jennifer, MD
- Simon, Elizabeth R., DO

Summit Medical Arts
9225 John F Kennedy Boulevard Zip: 07047
Ph: (201) 453-2800
- Hussain, Zahid, MD
- Shah, Kamalesh R., MD
- Tikoo, Ravinder Kumar, MD

North Brunswick
Affiliated Orthopaedic Specialists
2186 Route 27/Suite 1A Zip: 08902
Ph: (732) 422-1222 Fax: (732) 422-3636
- Kirschenbaum, David, MD
- Reich, Steven M., MD
- Sieler, Shawn D., MD

Care first OBGYN Group LLC
1555 Ruth Road/Suite 5 Zip: 08902
Ph: (732) 398-3939 Fax: (732) 398-0909
- Acharya, Rashmi, MD
- Nuthakki, Vimala Devi, MD

Central Jersey Pediatrics PC
1553 Ruth Road/Suite 1 Zip: 08902
Ph: (732) 418-1700 Fax: (732) 249-9599
- Jadhav, Surekha Ashwin, MD
- Patel, Himanshu K., MD
- Patel, Himanshubhai A., MD

Drs. Deka and Ata
2090 State Route 27/Suite 101 Zip: 08902
Ph: (732) 979-0035 Fax: (908) 829-4408
- Ata, Mohammad, MD
- Deka, Bharati, MD
- Maganti, Sameera, MD

Drs. Naqui & Naqui
1574 Route 130 North Zip: 08902
Ph: (732) 297-4100 Fax: (732) 422-7243
- Naqui, Mehdi H., MD
- Naqui, Nasreen, MD

New Brunswick Pediatric Group, P.A.
1300 How Lane Zip: 08902
Ph: (732) 247-1510 Fax: (732) 247-8885
- Chen, Deborah E., MD
- Gajera, Sangeeta Jadav, MD
- Henry, Elizabeth Robinson, MD
- Kessous, Deborah Lynne, MD
- Wiener, Howard E., MD

New Jersey Pain Spine Sports
2050 Route 27/Suite 105 Zip: 08902
Ph: (732) 565-3777 Fax: (732) 746-0223
- Abbasi, Faheem A., MD
- Avhad, Prajakta Vasant, MD
- Elkholy, Wael Talaat, MD

North Brunswick Pediatrics
1598 US Highway 130 Zip: 08902
Ph: (732) 297-0603 Fax: (732) 297-2866
- Goh, Jean Sian Li, MD
- Katz, Melvin I., MD
- Kim, Maria Batraki, DO
- Pragaspathy, Bhavadarani M., MD
- Segarra, Michael L., MD

P. F. Ioffreda, MD, PA
1250 Marigold Street Zip: 08902
Ph: (732) 545-8259 Fax: (732) 247-5574
- Ioffreda, Richard E., MD
- Rodriguez, Ramon Elias, MD

Plaza Pediatrics
1950 State Highway 27 North/Suite HH Zip: 08902
Ph: (732) 940-5511 Fax: (732) 940-0530
- Brauer, Howard E., MD
- Hanna, Dina W., MD

Princeton Dermatology Associates
1950 State Route 27/Suite A Zip: 08902
Ph: (732) 297-8866 Fax: (732) 821-0626
- Berger, Richard S., MD
- Wrone, David A., MD

RWJPE Bhavani Vietla
2864 Route 27/Suite D Zip: 08902
Ph: (732) 297-4272 Fax: (732) 297-3785
- Lin, Pei-Shiu, MD
- Vietla, Bhavani Durga, MD

Robert Wood Johnson Dialysis Center
117 North Center Drive Zip: 08902
Ph: (732) 940-4460
- Kapoian, Toros, MD

Wills Surgery Ctr of Central NJ
107 North Center Drive Zip: 08902
Ph: (732) 297-8001 Fax: (732) 297-8007
- Karandikar, Shaila Y., MD
- Parikh, Sudha Sudhir, MD
- Tyler, James Ralph, MD

North Cape May
Cape Health Solutions, LLC.
650 Town Bank Road Zip: 08204
Ph: (609) 898-7447 Fax: (609) 898-1912
- Leisner, William Randolph, MD
- Maroldo, Michael G., MD
- Vaccaro, Carl Anthony, DO

Cape Regional Physicians Associates
3806 Bayshore Road/Suite 101 Zip: 08204
Ph: (609) 898-7447 Fax: (609) 898-1912
- Drake, Andrew F., DO
- Hong, Matthew H., MD
- Moten, Shirlene Tolbert, MD

North Haledon
Vanguard Medical Group
535 High Mountain Road/Suite 111 Zip: 07508
Ph: (973) 636-9000 Fax: (973) 636-0913
- Salerno, Adrienne Lynn, MD

North Plainfield
Access Obstetrics and Gynecology
190 Greenbrook Road Zip: 07060
Ph: (908) 756-6812 Fax: (908) 756-2525
- Lowe, William J. III, MD

Urgent Health Care Center
719 Route 22 West Zip: 07060
Ph: (908) 561-4300 Fax: (908) 561-4340
- Ahmed, Fauzia Mosarrat, MD
- Sodhi, Surinder K., MD

North Wildwood
North Wildwood Medical
1200 New Jersey Avenue Zip: 08260
Ph: (609) 522-3131 Fax: (609) 522-9024
- Cook, Jenny Lynn, DO
- Haflin, Mary Ann, MD

Northfield
AtlantiCare Physician Group
1601 Tilton Road Zip: 08225
Ph: (609) 569-1900 Fax: (609) 569-1404
- Bushay, Stephen Lloyd, MD
- Kulkarni, Nandini N., MD

Fox Orthopedic Center
1601 Tilton Road Zip: 08225
Ph: (609) 407-1600 Fax: (609) 641-6776
- Fox, Jonathan L., MD

Mid Atlantic Rehab Assocs
611 New Road Zip: 08225
Ph: (609) 641-2581
- Baliga, Arvind B., MD
- Russomano, Salvatore J., MD

Nazha Cancer Center
411 New Road Zip: 08225
Ph: (609) 383-6033 Fax: (609) 383-0064
- Nazha, Naim T., MD
- Stoyko, Zoryana, MD
- Wang, Le, MD

Regional Nephrology Associates
510 Jackson Avenue Zip: 08225
Ph: (609) 383-0200 Fax: (609) 383-8352
- Behl, Nitin, MD
- Blecker, David L., MD
- Mathews, Robert John, MD
- Nnewihe, Charles Obinna, MD
- Schreyer, Raymond S., MD
- Shastri, Jay Gautam, DO
- Thakkar, Priyesh Tarunkumar, DO

Retinal & Ophthalmic Consultants, PC
1500 Tilton Road Zip: 08225
Ph: (609) 646-5200 Fax: (609) 646-9868
- Connors, Daniel Bernard, MD
- Foxman, Brett T., MD
- Foxman, Scott G., MD
- Margolis, Thomas Ira, MD
- Thakker, Manoj Mangaldas, MD

Shore Physicians Group
2605 Shore Road Zip: 08225
Ph: (609) 365-5300 Fax: (609) 365-5301
- Bowers, Steven Richard, DO
- Fiorentino, Grace, DO
- Karp, Howard M., DO
- May, David Peter, MD
- Sood, Mohit, DO

Tender Care Pediatrics
2322 New Road Zip: 08225
Ph: (609) 641-0200
- Chang, Ho-Choong, MD

Northvale
The Park Medical Group
220 Livingston Street/Suite 202 Zip: 07647
Ph: (201) 768-9090 Fax: (201) 768-9009
- DiGiovanni, Leonard G., DO
- Hwang, John M., MD
- Symington, Peter Anthony, MD

Groups and Clinics by Town with Physician Rosters

Nutley

Cardiology Associates LLC
181 Franklin Avenue/Suite 301 Zip: 07110
Ph: (973) 667-5511 Fax: (973) 667-0561
 Fusilli,Louis D., MD
 Savino,Leonard A., MD

Drs. Abu Al Rub and Abusido
65 River Road/Suite 208 Zip: 07110
 Abu Al Rub,Dana M., MD
 Abusido,Islam K., MD

Drs. Agresti and Agresti
181 Franklin Avenue/Suite 201 Zip: 07110
Ph: (973) 284-0777 Fax: (973) 284-1530
 Agresti,James V. III, MD
 Agresti,James V. Sr., MD

Drs. Cozzarelli-Franklin & Franklin
175 Franklin Avenue Zip: 07110
Ph: (973) 667-8535 Fax: (973) 667-8442
 Cozzarelli-Franklin,Annette O., MD
 Franklin,James D., MD

Ear Nose & Throat Center of NJ
115 Franklin Avenue Zip: 07110
Ph: (973) 773-9250 Fax: (973) 773-9525
 Youssef,Oliver S., MD

Femino-Ducey Orthopaedic Group
45 Franklin Avenue Zip: 07110
Ph: (973) 751-0111 Fax: (973) 235-0110
 Ducey,Stephen Alexander, MD
 Femino,Frank Placido, MD
 Queler,Seth Robert, MD

Independent Medical Group
670 Franklin Avenue/Suite A Zip: 07110
Ph: (973) 667-8493
 Zazzali,George N., MD
 Zazzali,Peter G., MD

Ligresti Dermatology Associates
175 Franklin Avenue/Suite 103 Zip: 07110
Ph: (973) 759-6569 Fax: (973) 759-2562
 Ligresti,Dominick Joseph, MD
 Sekiya,Steven T., DO
 Yeretsky,Yelena, DO

Montclair Radiology
20 High Street Zip: 07110
Ph: (973) 284-1881 Fax: (973) 284-0269
 Bash,Lisa Taub, MD
 Denehy,Ann Smith, MD
 Mondshine,Ross T., MD
 Pollack,Michael A., MD
 Richman,Steven D., MD
 Torrente,Jessica, MD

The Internet Medical Group, P.C.
181 Franklin Avenue/Suite 204 Zip: 07110
Ph: (973) 667-8117 Fax: (973) 667-6642
 Bisignano Delvecchio,Maria, MD
 Brignola,Joseph John, MD
 Kalmar,Edward T., MD
 Sasanpour,Majid, MD
 Vecchione,Edward J., DO

Oak Ridge

Skylands Medical Group PA
5678 Berkshire Valley Road Zip: 07438
Ph: (973) 697-0200 Fax: (973) 697-6844
 Gloria,Stephen B., DO
 Magnusen,Mary L., DO
 Riesenman,Joseph John, MD

Oakhurst

Atlantic Surgical Group, PA
255 Monmouth Road Zip: 07755
Ph: (732) 531-5445 Fax: (732) 531-1776
 Gornish,Aron L., MD
 Lake,Thomas R. III, MD
 Lin,Jeffrey M., MD
 Parker,Glenn S., MD
 Schwartz,Mark Robert, MD
 Tizio,Steven Christopher, MD

Walk-In Medical
1910 State Route 35 Zip: 07755
Ph: (732) 531-0100 Fax: (732) 531-0144
 Adamczyk,Rebekah Katherine, DO
 Mojares,Dennis C., MD
 Mojares,Richard Alan, MD

Infectious Disease Care
1912 State Route 35/Suite 101 Zip: 07755
Ph: (732) 222-4762 Fax: (732) 222-4764
 Dwivedi,Sukrut A., DO
 Lee,Andrew, MD
 Mathur,Ajay Narain, MD
 Patel,Apurva, MD

Ocean Park Medical Associates
1900 Highway 35/Suite 200 Zip: 07755
Ph: (732) 663-0900 Fax: (732) 663-0901
 Ciciarelli,John G. II, MD
 Hayet,Bill, MD

Shore Gastroenterology Associates
1907 Highway 35/Suite 1 Zip: 07755
Ph: (732) 517-0060 Fax: (732) 548-7408
 Akhtar,Reza Yasin, MD
 Dhillon,Shamina, MD
 Maki,Junsuke, MD
 Schwartz,Mitchell S., MD
 Terrany,Ben, MD
 Turtel,Penny S., MD

Oakland

Cardiac Associates of North Jersey
43 Yawpo Avenue/Suite 2 Zip: 07436
Ph: (201) 337-0066 Fax: (201) 337-7417
 Budhwani,Navin, MD
 Montgomery,David H., MD
 Williams,Marcus L., MD

Excelsior II Psychiatric Services
169 Ramapo Valley Road/Suite ML5 Zip: 07436
Ph: (201) 996-1120 Fax: (201) 996-0099
 Chalemian,Bliss A., MD
 Chalemian,Robert J., MD

Milestones Pediatric Group PA
11 East Oak Street Zip: 07436
Ph: (201) 485-7557 Fax: (201) 485-7556
 Chu,Yie-Hsien, MD
 Guruswamy,Parvathi, MD
 Livingstone,Tosan, MD
 Michaels,Lisa-Ann B., MD
 Tirri,Carmelina, MD

North Jersey Family Medicine
19 Yawpo Avenue Zip: 07436
Ph: (201) 337-3412 Fax: (201) 337-3353
 Dela Gente,Robert Saladaga, DO
 Morski,Richard S., MD
 Perdomo,Louis Fernando, MD

Pedimedica PA
43 Yawpo Avenue/Suite 9 Zip: 07436
Ph: (201) 405-0800 Fax: (201) 337-5585
 Taneja,Uttama, DO
 Wiederhorn,Noel M., MD

Primary Care at Oakland
340c Ramapo Valley Road Zip: 07436
Ph: (973) 962-6200 Fax: (973) 962-0046
 Minhas,Navpreet Singh, MD
 Straseskie,Ryan Kenneth, MD

Tenafly Pediatrics, PA
350 Ramapo Valley Road Zip: 07436
Ph: (201) 651-0404 Fax: (201) 651-0909
 Lindenberg,Erin K., MD
 Stock,Ilana Rose, MD
 Sumarokov,Alina, MD

Valley Medical Group
43 Yawpo Avenue/Suite 3 Zip: 07436
Ph: (201) 337-9600
 Kesselhaut,Marc L., MD
 Shaker,Taylor, MD
 Uddin,Sarah T., DO

Ocean

Allergy Partners of New Jersey PC
802 West Park Avenue/Suite 213 Zip: 07712
Ph: (732) 695-2555 Fax: (732) 695-2552
 Gross,Gary L., MD
 Ross,Jacqueline, MD
 Sher,Ellen R., MD

Barnabas Health Medical Group
1300 Highway 35 South/Suites 101-103 Zip: 07712
Ph: (732) 531-6400 Fax: (732) 517-0223
 Disciglio,Michael J., MD
 Mehta,Rajneesh G., MD

 Meltzer,Richard B., MD

Dr. Howard N. Guss & Dr. Gagan D. Beri
3200 Sunset Avenue/Suite 208 Zip: 07712
Ph: (732) 775-9000 Fax: (732) 775-6660
 Beri,Gagan D., MD
 Guss,Howard N., DO

Drs. Morgan and Morgan
1500 Atlantic Avenue/Suite 201 Zip: 07712
Ph: (732) 531-1136 Fax: (732) 531-0177
 Morgan,Benjamin, MD

Ethel and Raphael Pediatrics Inc
1405 Highway 35 North/Suite 104 Zip: 07712
Ph: (732) 663-1161 Fax: (732) 531-2900
 Omotoso,Olukemi Yetunde, MD
 Raab,Vicki E., MD

Mid Atlantic Geriatric Assocs
1205 Route 35 North Zip: 07712
Ph: (732) 663-0099 Fax: (732) 663-1359
 Patel,Sameer Ramesh, MD
 Patel,Suhas Ramesh, MD

Ocean Obstetric & Gynecologic Assocs
804 West Park Avenue/Building A Zip: 07712
Ph: (732) 695-2040 Fax: (732) 493-1640
 Cohen,Ronald L., MD
 Gould,Jack R., DO
 Henderson,Craig E., DO
 Rogers,Brian James, MD
 Theocharides,Thomas, MD

Seaview Orthopaedics
1200 Eagle Avenue Zip: 07712
Ph: (732) 660-6200 Fax: (732) 660-6201
 Chern,Kenneth Y., MD
 Collins,Christopher Michael, MD
 Demetriades,Haralambos, MD
 Haynes,Paul Thomas II, MD
 McDaid,Kevin C., MD
 Meyers,Adam M., DO
 Nguyen,Hoan-Vu Tran, MD
 Spagnuola,Christopher J., MD
 Yalamanchili,Praveen K., MD

Shore Pulmonary PA
301 Bingham Avenue/Suite B Zip: 07712
Ph: (732) 775-9075 Fax: (732) 775-1212
 Ali,Rana Y., MD
 Cosentino,James P., DO
 Elsawaf,Mohamed Ashraf, MD

West Park Pediatrics
804 West Park Avenue Zip: 07712
Ph: (732) 531-0010 Fax: (732) 493-0903
 Kerensky,Kirk M., MD
 Lichtenberger,Janice Ann, MD
 Lipstein,Rebekah Ann, MD
 O'Brien,Thomas Kevin, MD
 Sasson,Elias, MD
 Setton,Ellen E., MD
 Topilow,Judith F., MD

Ocean City

Atlantic Care Physician Group
201 West Avenue Zip: 08226
Ph: (609) 391-7500 Fax: (609) 391-0963
 Baretto,Luigi U., MD
 Chew,Jason M., DO
 Cozamanis,Steve G., DO

Horizon Eye Care
2401 Bay Avenue Zip: 08226
Ph: (609) 399-6300 Fax: (609) 399-6284
 Huang,Jun C., MD

Old Bridge

Adult & Pediatric Allergists
3 Hospital Plaza/Suite 405 Zip: 08857
Ph: (732) 679-2525 Fax: (732) 360-0033
 Lee,Edward G., MD

Ani Orthopaedic Group
200 Perrine Road/Suite 220 Zip: 08857
Ph: (732) 264-8282 Fax: (732) 264-8131
 Parreno,Maritza Georgette, MD

Assoc in Int Med Healthcare Inc
1810 Englishtown Road Zip: 08857
Ph: (732) 416-6900 Fax: (732) 416-4823
 Del Alcazar,Carlos O., MD
 Laemmle,Patricia C., MD

Bay Family Medicine
26 Throckmorton Lane Zip: 08857
Ph: (732) 360-0287 Fax: (732) 360-1279
 Fahmy,Sandra Patricia, DO
 Krishnamsetty,Nanditha, MD

Dermatology Associates of Central NJ
3548 Route 9 Zip: 08857
Ph: (732) 679-6300
 Bernabe,Maria Joyce Row Guerrero,
 Centurion,Santiago Alberto, MD

Drs. Lupicki and Lupicki
200 Perrine Road/Suite 211 Zip: 08857
Ph: (732) 553-1000
 Lupicki,Lucyna K., MD
 Lupicki,Marek R., MD

ENT & Allergy Associates, LLP
3663 Route 9 North/Suite102 Zip: 08857
Ph: (732) 679-7575 Fax: (732) 707-3850
 Azer,Andrew Elia, MD
 Chowdhury,Farhad Reza, DO

Healthcare Pain & Rehab
3 Hospital Plaza/Suite 309 Zip: 08857
Ph: (732) 607-9000
 Del Valle,Francisco I., MD
 Del Valle,Jacqueline P., MD

Landa Spine Center
300 Perrine Road/Suite 333 Zip: 08857
Ph: (732) 289-9335 Fax: (732) 289-9336
 Hassan,Sheref E., MD
 Landa,Joshua, MD

Medical Associates of Central NJ
26 Throckmorton Lane/1st flr. Zip: 08857
Ph: (732) 679-9950 Fax: (732) 679-9956
 Cohen,Jason Ronald, MD
 Mathew,Joseph, MD
 Mezic,Edward T., MD
 Moten,Hadi S., MD
 Nigam,Jyoti, MD
 Ratkalkar,Kishore, MD

Medical Associates of Marlboro
42 Throckmorton Lane/2nd flr Zip: 08857
Ph: (732) 607-1111 Fax: (732) 607-0552
 Jafri,Rana B., MD
 Mirza,Babar, MD
 Price,Craig C., MD

Old Bridge Primary Care
300 Perrine Road/Suite 324 Zip: 08857
Ph: (732) 753-9890 Fax: (732) 753-9893
 Demos,James P., MD
 Sobel,David Charles, MD
 Zilber,Eugenia, MD

Pediatric Adolescent Assocs of Ctrl NJ
100 Perrine Road Zip: 08857
Ph: (732) 316-0900 Fax: (732) 316-0499
 Arumugam,Maheswari, MD
 Salston,Robert S., MD

RWJPE Old Bridge Family Medicine
2107 Highway 516 Zip: 08857
Ph: (732) 952-0626 Fax: (732) 463-6071
 Balinski,Beth A., DO
 Cohen,Howard Steven, DO
 Robinson,Jonnie M., DO
 Ryan,Sharon L., MD

Rainbow Medical Associates
200 Perrine Road/Suite 228 Zip: 08857
Ph: (732) 679-0660 Fax: (732) 679-7177
 Osman,Ihsan, MD
 Vadali,Rajyalaks Vaidehi, MD

Raritan Bay Inf Dis Consltnts
3 Hospital Plaza/Suite 208 Zip: 08857
Ph: (732) 360-2700 Fax: (732) 360-2703
 Hasham,Mohamed H., MD
 Middleton,John R., MD
 Raoof,Natalia, MD
 Raoof,Nazar, MD

SAMRA Pediatrics
300 Perrine Road/Suite 331 Zip: 08857
Ph: (732) 727-8800 Fax: (732) 727-0955
 Barakat,Raja, MD
 Grochowalska,Ewa Malgorzata, MD
 Quiba,Ronald C., MD
 Siddiqui,Zehra, DO

Groups and Clinics by Town with Physician Rosters

Old Bridge (cont)
Urology Care Alliance
2 Hospital Plaza/Suite 110 Zip: 08857
Ph: (732) 972-9000 Fax: (732) 972-0966
- Cha,Doh Yoon, MD
- Pagano,Matthew J., MD

World Class Lasik
28 Throckmorton Lane Zip: 08857
Ph: (732) 679-6100 Fax: (732) 673-6703
- Blondo,Dennis L., MD
- Cohen,Ilan, MD
- Wong,Sze Ho, MD

Old Tappan
Old Tappan Medical Group PA
215 Old Tappan Road Zip: 07675
Ph: (201) 666-1000 Fax: (201) 666-4108
- De Angelo,Ann M., MD
- Fishkind,Perry Neal, MD
- Hages,Harry A., MD
- Pelavin,Martin D., MD
- Rothenberg,Nancy A., DO
- Schwartz,Diane C., MD

Oradell
Carl J. Battista, MD, PC
680 Kinderkamack Road/Suite 301 Zip: 07649
Ph: (201) 634-1004 Fax: (201) 634-1028
- Battista,Carl J., MD
- Czernizer,Patricia L., MD

ENT & Allergy Associates, LLP
690 Kinderkamack Road/Suite 101 Zip: 07649
Ph: (201) 722-9850 Fax: (201) 722-9851
- Bough,Irvin David Jr., MD
- Cusumano,Robert J., MD
- Huang,John Jan, MD
- Leventhal,Douglas Drew, MD
- Skripak,Justin Michael, MD
- Surow,Jason B., MD

North Jersey Brain and Surgical
680 Kinderkamack Road/Suite 300 Zip: 07649
Ph: (201) 342-2550 Fax: (201) 342-7171
- Azmi Ghadimi,Hooman, MD
- Chirichella,Paul Sebastian, MD
- Kaptain,George J., MD
- Karimi,Reza J., MD
- Khan,Mohammed Faraz, MD
- Lee,Kangmin Daniel, MD
- Roth,Patrick A., MD
- Vingan,Roy David, MD
- Walzman,Daniel Ezra, MD
- Zablow,Bruce Charles, MD

Ob-Gyn Assoc of Bergen County PA
680 Kinderkamack Road/Suite 204 Zip: 07649
Ph: (201) 391-5443 Fax: (201) 391-8019
- Dotto,Myles E., MD
- Wang,Belle, MD

Si Paradigm, LLC.
690 Kinderkamack Road/Suite 103 Zip: 07649
Ph: (201) 599-9044 Fax: (201) 599-9066
- Nasr,Sherif Abbas, MD
- Rahman,Saud Saqib, MD
- Tao,Jiangchuan, MD

Urology Specialty Care, P.A.
555 Kindermack Road/Suite D Zip: 07649
Ph: (201) 834-1890 Fax: (201) 834-1898
- Zoretic,Stephen N., MD

Whole Child Center
690 Kinderkamack Road/Suite 102 Zip: 07649
Ph: (201) 634-1600 Fax: (201) 634-1606
- Jeney,Heather A., MD
- Kurz,Lisa Beth, MD
- Rosen,Lawrence David, MD

Orange
Family Connections Inc
395 South Center Street Zip: 07050
Ph: (973) 675-3817 Fax: (973) 673-5782
- Reyes,Christine, MD

Primary Medical Care
85 South Jefferson Street Zip: 07050
Ph: (973) 673-3522 Fax: (973) 673-0018
- Gialanella,Francis J., MD

Palisades Park
Hanmi Medical Associates
232 Broad Avenue/Suite 208 Zip: 07650
Ph: (201) 346-0999
- Kim,Yoonjoo, MD
- Park,Wonil, MD

St. Mary's Eye & Surgery Center
540 Bergen Boulevard Zip: 07650
Ph: (201) 461-3970 Fax: (201) 242-9061
- Chu,David Shu-Chih, MD
- Kim,Daniel Y., MD
- Lee,Sangwoo, MD
- Lyu,Theodore, MD

Paramus
AFC Urgent Care Paramus
67 East Ridgewood Avenue Zip: 07652
Ph: (201) 899-4765
- Borkowski,Douglas Joseph, MD
- Saros,Cathleen Mary, DO

Advanced Laparoscopic Associates
81 Route 4 West/Suite 401/35 Plaza Zip: 07652
Ph: (201) 646-1121 Fax: (201) 646-1110
- Bedrosian,Andrea Stephanie, MD
- Dhorajia,Seema P., DO
- Eid,Sebastian R., MD
- Ewing,Douglas R., MD
- Schmidt,Hans J., MD
- Trivedi,Amit, MD

American Orthopedic & Sports Med
30 West Century Road/Suite 320 Zip: 07652
Ph: (201) 261-0402 Fax: (201) 261-0587
- Masri,Sammy Ismail, MD
- Stoller,Steven M., MD

BAXT CosMedical NJ
351 Evelyn Street/Suite 201 Zip: 07652
Ph: (201) 265-1300 Fax: (201) 265-3737
- Baxt,Rebecca D., MD
- Baxt,Saida H., MD
- Baxt,Sherwood A., MD

Bergen Medical Associates
1 West Ridgewood Avenue/Suite 301 Zip: 07652
Ph: (201) 445-1660 Fax: (201) 445-4296
- Chung,Jeff, MD
- De Lillo,Anthony Rocco, MD
- Hatefi,Homayoon, MD

Bergen Medical Associates
1 Sears Drive/Suite 403 Zip: 07652
Ph: (201) 261-6061 Fax: (201) 261-6465
- Rutigliano,Michael W., MD
- Saieva,Carol E., DO

Center for Dermatology & Skin Surgery
1 West Ridgewood Avenue/Suite 103 Zip: 07652
Ph: (201) 857-4200 Fax: (201) 857-4199
- Garcia,Carmen Josefina, MD
- Wiederkehr,Michael, MD

Chuback Medical Group
2 Sears Drive/Suite 101 Zip: 07652
Ph: (201) 261-1772 Fax: (201) 261-1776
- Novak,Caroline L., MD

Columbia Anesthesia Associates
37 West Century Road/Suite 101 Zip: 07652
Ph: (201) 634-9000 Fax: (201) 634-9014
- Trnovski,Stefan, MD
- Zhuravkov,Alexander, MD

Blumenthal Cancer Center
One Valley Health Plaza Zip: 07652
Ph: (201) 634-5339
- Klein,Laura Ann, MD

Doctors' Office Walk-in Urgent Care
110 East Ridgewood Avenue Zip: 07652
Ph: (201) 265-9500 Fax: (201) 265-1355
- Goldberg,Alvin Hugh, MD

Drs. Parangi and Parangi
9 Yale Court Zip: 07652
Ph: (201) 265-7564 Fax: (201) 265-6991
- Parangi,Robert K., MD
- Parangi,Sasan M., MD

Drs. Robinson, Parnes & Weinstein
275 Forest Avenue Zip: 07652
Ph: (201) 967-9191 Fax: (201) 967-9302
- Robinson,Lois Pat, MD
- Weinstein,Melissa A., DO

Drs. Rosenstein & Fakharzadeh
22 Madison Avenue/Suite 3-1 Zip: 07652
Ph: (201) 587-7767 Fax: (201) 587-8090
- Fakharzadeh,Frederick F., MD
- Rosenstein,Roger G., MD

Drs. Samadi and Bar-Eli
10 Forest Avenue/Suite 100 Zip: 07652
Ph: (201) 996-1505 Fax: (201) 996-1605
- Bar-Eli,Rebecca, MD
- Samadi,Sharyar Daniel, MD

Endocrine Associates
30 West Century Drive/Suite 255 Zip: 07652
Ph: (201) 444-4363 Fax: (201) 444-6590
- Shah,Viral Jagdishbhai, MD
- Tohme,Jacques Fuad, MD

Forest Healthcare Associates, PC
277 Forest Avenue/Suite 200 Zip: 07652
Ph: (201) 986-1881 Fax: (201) 986-1871
- Anshelevich,Irina, MD
- Chang,Cindy Ching, MD
- Fernandez,Marlyn A., MD
- Giangola,Joseph, MD
- Kavaler,Robert, MD
- Kurz,Jeremiah S., MD
- Kushner,Evan G., MD
- Menacker,Morey J., DO
- Pastrano Lluberes,Magna, MD
- Sandhu,Basant Singh, MD
- Winer,Steven A., MD
- Young,Alexis Livingston, MD
- Yousef,Javed Muhammad, MD

Forest Pediatrics PA
299 Forest Avenue Zip: 07652
Ph: (201) 267-0888 Fax: (201) 483-8874
- Kushner,Susan C., MD
- Monaco,Melissa Garofalo, MD

HSS Paramus Outpatient Center
140 East Ridgewood Avenue/Suite 175-S Zip: 07652
Ph: (201) 796-2255 Fax: (201) 796-3711
- Difelice,Gregory Scott, MD
- Elliott,Andrew J., MD
- Gungor,Semih, MD
- Hughes,Alexander Philip, MD
- Markenson,Joseph A., MD
- Ranawat,Anil S., MD
- Wang,David Alexander, MD
- Widmann,Roger Franklin, MD
- Wu,Dee Dee Yui, MD

Hartzband Ctr for Hip & Knee Replcmnt
10 Forest Avenue Zip: 07652
Ph: (201) 291-4040 Fax: (201) 291-0440
- Hartzband,Mark A., MD
- Klein,Gregg Roger, MD
- Levine,Harlan Brett, MD
- Seidenstein,Ari Douglas, MD

Madison Avenue Pediatrics
22 Madison Avenue/3rd floor, Suite 3 Zip: 07652
Ph: (201) 291-9797 Fax: (201) 291-9798
- Rabinowitz,Arnold H., MD
- Rodriguez-Zierer,Maria Evelyn, MD

Maternal Fetal Medicine Associates
140 East Ridgewood Avenue/Suite 390S Zip: 07652
Ph: (201) 291-6321 Fax: (201) 291-6318
- Goldman,Jane Cleary, MD
- Matthews,Gail Margaret, MD
- Mosquera Charlenea,Claudia, MD
- Zelop,Carolyn M., MD

Northern NJ Pain & Rehabilitation Ctr
37 West Century Road/Suite 111 Zip: 07652
Ph: (201) 262-2244 Fax: (201) 262-2246
- Fossati,Jeffrey Joseph, MD
- Kotturi,Shiva Kumar, MD

Ortho Spine and Sports Med Ctr
2 Forest Avenue Zip: 07652
Ph: (201) 587-1111 Fax: (201) 587-8192
- Kovatis,Paul Evan, MD
- Loreti,Michael Earl, MD
- Newman,Bernard P. III, MD
- Savatsky,Gary J., MD
- Schmaus,Peter Howard, MD

Paramus Plastic Surgery Center
17 Arcadian Avenue/Suite 103 Zip: 07652
Ph: (201) 843-0700
- Garcia-Lat,Zenda, MD
- Lat,Emmanuel A., MD

Paramus Surgical Center
30 West Century Road/Suite 300 Zip: 07652
Ph: (201) 986-9000
- Higgins,Annlouise Maria, MD

Pediatric Cardiology at The Valley Hos
205 Robin Road/Suite 100 Zip: 07652
Ph: (201) 599-0026 Fax: (201) 986-1160
- Rhee,Young Sun Diane, MD

Pediatric Surgery
30 West Century Road/Suite 235 Zip: 07652
Ph: (201) 996-0010 Fax: (201) 225-9430
- Friedman,David Lewis, MD
- Gandhi,Rajinder P., MD

Physician Specialists of New Jersey
1 Sears Drive/Suite 306 Zip: 07652
Ph: (201) 830-2287 Fax: (201) 830-2286
- Goa,Cristobal Javier, MD
- Gross,Michael L., MD
- Shatkin,Jason Alan, MD

Physicians Practice at New Bridge Med
230 East Ridgewood Avenue Zip: 07652
Ph: (201) 225-4700 Fax: (201) 225-4702
- Harutyunyan,Anna, MD
- Ibeabuchi,Adaeze Nneka, MD
- Sourial,Hany A., MD

Plastic Surgery Specialists of NJ
2 Sears Drive/Suite 103 Zip: 07652
Ph: (201) 664-8000
- Ferraro,Frank James Jr., MD
- Goswami,Amit, MD

Pulmonary Medicine Associates, P.A.
1 West Ridgewood Avenue Zip: 07652
Ph: (201) 493-0366 Fax: (201) 493-0379
- Sakowitz,Arthur J., MD
- Sakowitz,Barry H., MD

Salvatore Focella, MD LLC
1 West Ridgewood Avenue/Suite 203 Zip: 07652
Ph: (201) 652-8800 Fax: (201) 444-8560
- Focella,Salvatore, MD
- Shukla,Nilesh B., MD

Sidney Rabinowitz, M.D., P.A.
305 North Route 17/Suite 3-100A Zip: 07652
Ph: (201) 967-1100 Fax: (201) 967-9300
- Boss,William K. Jr., MD
- Rabinowitz,Sidney, MD

Tenafly Pediatrics, PA
26 Park Place Zip: 07652
Ph: (201) 262-1140 Fax: (201) 261-8413
- Kim,Sunmee Louise, MD
- Saks,Darren, MD
- Slater,John G., MD
- Stiefel,Laurence N., MD

The Breslow Center For Plastic Surgery
1 West Ridgewood Avenue/Suite 110 Zip: 07652
Ph: (201) 444-9522 Fax: (201) 444-9277
- Breslow,Gary David, MD
- Cyrulnik,Amanda Amy, MD

The Dermatology Group, P.C.
30 West Century Road/Suite 320 Zip: 07652
Ph: (973) 571-2121 Fax: (201) 986-0702
- Gordon,Karen Ann, MD
- Li,Cindy Yuk, DO

Robert Zubowski MD Ctr Cosmetic/Recon
1 Sears Drive Zip: 07652
Ph: (201) 261-7550 Fax: (201) 261-7515
  Gandolfi,Brad Michael, MD
  Zubowski,Robert I., MD

The Valley Hospital Fertility Center
140 East Ridgewood Avenue Zip: 07652
Ph: (201) 634-5400 Fax: (201) 634-5503
  Chen,Dehan, MD
  Greenseid,Keri Lee, MD
  Nasseri,Ali, MD

The Woman's Group/Bergen Medical
1 West Ridgewood Avenue/Suite 211 Zip: 07652
Ph: (201) 251-2323 Fax: (201) 251-2325
  Meyer,Monica Lynn, MD

Urologic Institute of NJ PA
277 Forest Avenue/Suite 206 Zip: 07652
Ph: (201) 489-8900 Fax: (201) 489-0877
  Lebovitch,Steve, MD
  Rome,Sergey, MD
  Vitenson,Jack L., MD

Gynecology Oncology Associates
One Valley Health Plaza Zip: 07652
Ph: (201) 634-5401 Fax: (201) 986-4701
  Jones,Howard Harris, MD

VMG-Pediatric Endocrinology
140 East Ridgewood avenue/Suite N280 Zip: 07652
Ph: (201) 447-8182 Fax: (201) 523-9365
  Kumpta,Shilpa Narsing, MD
  Pelavin,Paul Isaac, MD

Valley Institute for Pain
One Valley Health Plaza/3 FL Zip: 07652
Ph: (201) 634-5555 Fax: (201) 634-5454
  Iversen,Robin J., MD
  Mansson,Jonas, MD
  Roche,Elizabeth Ann, MD
  Silverman,Robert S., MD
  Thomson,Fani Jacqueline, DO

Valley Medical Group
140 Route 17 North/Suite 302 Zip: 07652
Ph: (201) 444-2646 Fax: (201) 689-6009
  Pacheco,Felix Fernando, MD
  Tievsky,Erika Fiorella, DO

Valley Medical Group Internal Medicine
1 Sears Drive/Suite 202 Zip: 07652
Ph: (201) 262-2333 Fax: (201) 262-4515
  Luongo,Peter A., MD
  Sgambati,Theodore P. Jr., MD

Valley Medical Group-Hematology/Onc
One Valley Health Plaza Zip: 07652
Ph: (201) 634-5353 Fax: (201) 986-4702
  Fernbach,Barry R., MD
  Ligresti,Louise G., MD
  Wood,Kevin C., MD

Valley Ob Gyn Associates PA
80 Eisenhower Drive/Suite 200 Zip: 07652
Ph: (201) 843-2800 Fax: (201) 843-5848
  Nickles,Donna E., DO
  O'Brien,Katherine Elizabeth, MD
  Russo,Thomas O., MD

Valley Radiation Oncology Associates
One Valley Health Plaza Zip: 07652
Ph: (201) 634-5403
  DeYoung,Chad M., MD
  Kole,Thomas Pedicino, MD
  Wesson,Michael F., MD

Vascular & Endovascular Associates
One West Ridgewood Avenue/Suite 106 Zip: 07652
Ph: (201) 389-3700 Fax: (201) 670-6725
  Alshafie,Tarek Ahmed, MD
  Danks,John Michael, MD

Park Ridge
Tenafly Pediatrics, PA
74 Pascack Road Zip: 07656
Ph: (201) 326-7120 Fax: (201) 326-7130
  Grossi,Maureen A., MD
  Wang,Linda, MD

Valley Medical Group
70 Park Avenue Zip: 07656
Ph: (201) 930-0900 Fax: (201) 391-7733
  Corbett,Shonda Marcia, MD

  Fallon,Kimberly L., MD
  Lopez,Lina Maria, MD
  McGugins Hill,Jennifer Anne, MD
  Zapolanski,Tamar, MD

Parlin
Kivarkis Y. Younan MD PA
1145 Bordentown Avenue/Suite 10 Zip: 08859
Ph: (732) 727-0400 Fax: (732) 727-1391
  Piscopiello,Michael, MD
  Younan,K. George, MD
  Younan,Shaddy Kivarkis, MD
  Younan,Zyad, MD

M & M Florczyk, Inc.
3 Parlin Drive/Suite G Zip: 08859
Ph: (732) 651-7005
  Florczyk,Margaret, MD
  Florczyk,Miroslaw, MD

Nagarsheth MD PA
3B Parlin Drive Zip: 08859
Ph: (732) 238-8500 Fax: (732) 238-8501
  Nagarsheth,Harish N., MD
  Nagarsheth,Veena H., MD

Parsippany
Concentra Urgent Care at Parsippany
190 Baldwin Road Zip: 07054
Ph: (973) 882-0444 Fax: (973) 882-3217
  Earl,Lawrence N., MD
  Prasad,Prema, MD

Dermatology Associates of Morris PA
199 Baldwin Road Zip: 07054
Ph: (973) 335-2560 Fax: (973) 335-9421
  Almeida,Laila M., MD
  Kingsbery,Mina Yassaee, MD
  Livingston,Wendy E., MD
  Shah,Subhadra Sundaram, MD
  Strauss,Eric A., MD
  Weinberg,Harvey I., MD
  Weiser,Jessica Ann, MD

Drs. Friedel & Lam
1259 US Highway 46 East/Suite 314 Zip: 07054
Ph: (973) 316-9800 Fax: (973) 316-9805
  Friedel,Walter E., MD
  Lam,Paul C., MD

Drs. Luhana, Dhirmalani & Patel
239 Baldwin Road/Suite 108 Zip: 07054
Ph: (973) 334-2265 Fax: (973) 335-9091
  Bhatia,Malini P., MD
  Luhana,Manish P., MD
  Patel,Jignasa, MD

ENT & Allergy Associates of Parsippany
900 Lanidex Plaza/Suite 300 Zip: 07054
Ph: (973) 394-1818 Fax: (973) 394-1810
  Brys,Agata K., MD
  Jampol,Francis Michael, MD
  Lebovitz,Brian Lee, MD
  Mehta,Archana P., MD
  Sayeed,Zarina Shaikh, MD
  Wirtshafter,Karen A., MD

ENT & Allergy Associates, LLP
3219 Route 46 East/Suite 203 Zip: 07054
Ph: (973) 394-1818 Fax: (973) 394-1810
  Schultz,Charles Martin, MD

Emergency Medical Associates of NJ
3 Century Drive Zip: 07054
Ph: (973) 740-0607 Fax: (973) 740-9895
  Berger,Richard P., MD
  Ceppetelli,Lisa C., MD
  Cochrane,Dennis G., MD
  Crean,Christopher Arthur, MD
  Curato,Lauren Jennifer, DO
  Curato,Mark Anthony, DO
  Cuthbert,David, MD
  Deutsch,Robert Jay, MD
  Durrani-Tariq,Siama H., DO
  Figueroa,Delia, MD
  Freer,Christopher F., DO
  Giroski,Laura J., DO
  Gould,Michael Alan, MD
  Greenhut,William H., MD
  Hartmann,Anthony William, MD
  Heller,Mitchell L., MD
  Indruk,William L., MD
  Kasper,Lydia Marie, DO

  Kassutto,Zach, MD
  Lebaron,Johnathon Clinton, DO
  Lehet,Justin Micheal, DO
  Loewenstein,Robert Elvin, MD
  Melnick,Gerald J., MD
  Milano,Marc Anthony, MD
  Minett,Danielle Marie, MD
  Minett,Kenneth Matthew, MD
  Molisso,Mary Cuellari, DO
  Morley,David Matthew Yellin, MD
  Mouridy,Gary C., DO
  Murray-Taylor,Stacey Odell, MD
  Nguyen,Matthew Thai-Khang, MD
  Oh,David H., MD
  Perotte,Schubert, MD
  Reddy,Chenna G., MD
  Schiller,Andrew P., MD
  Shah,Sachin Jitendra, MD
  Silacci,John Truman, MD
  Stapleton,George S., MD
  Takahashi,Eric Michael, DO
  Troncoso,Alexis B., MD
  Utkewicz,Mark D., MD

Hematology-Oncology Assoc of NNJ
3219 US Highway 46/Suite 108 Zip: 07054
Ph: (973) 316-5900 Fax: (973) 316-5990
  Ram,Meryl H., MD

Lifeline Medical Associates, LLC
50 Cherry Hill Road/Suite 303 Zip: 07054
Ph: (973) 335-8500 Fax: (973) 335-8429
  Bissinger,Craig L., MD
  Hirsch,David Jay, MD
  Leviss,Stephen R., MD
  Valarezo,Vanessa C., MD

Memorial Radiology Associates
10 Lanidex Plaza West/Suite 125 Zip: 07054
Ph: (973) 503-5700 Fax: (973) 386-5701
  Calhoun,Sean Keith, DO
  Chung,Jean Young, MD
  Cosentino,Mark O., MD
  Friedman,Paul Dean, DO
  Menendez,Christine M., MD
  Murphy,Robyn C., MD
  Paik,David, MD
  Parisi,Angela Rosina, MD
  Reddy,Gerard, MD
  Rios,Jose Conrado, MD
  Sheth,Milan Pravin, MD
  Swayne,Lawrence C., MD
  Wynne,Peter J., MD
  Yablonsky,Thaddeus M., MD

Morris Anesthesia Group, PA
3799 Route 46/Suite 211 Zip: 07054
Ph: (973) 335-1122 Fax: (973) 335-1448
  Anjutgi,Rajyashree, MD
  Baker,Michelle Rapacon, MD
  Balakrishna,Shruthi, MD
  Barg,Vadim A., MD
  Blanchfield,Patrick Thomas, MD
  Chen,Guo-Gang, MD
  Choudhary,Ratna, MD
  Clanton,Chase P., MD
  Cohen,Michael B., MD
  Daniel,Brian P., DO
  Daras,Jason Glenn, DO
  DeSimone,Robert Anthony, MD
  Delis,Aristidis G., MD
  Eisenstat,Carol M., MD
  Fanouse,John A., DO
  Garibaldi,Thomas A., MD
  Ghosh,Arpita, MD
  Grasso,Mario Lucio, MD
  Grimaldi,Matthew Porter, MD
  Jacobson,Martin Alexander, MD
  Janardhan,Yellagonda V., MD
  Kussick,Neil J., MD
  Lamanna,Adolfo C., MD
  Lasker,Steven Mark, MD
  Lian,Hanzhou, MD
  Lyall,Jasleen Kaur, MD
  Ofeldt,James D., DO
  Olechowski,George N., MD
  Panei,Maryann S., MD

  Patel,Gaurav R., MD
  Patel,Mona, MD
  Patel,Niva S., MD
  Patel,Taral B., DO
  Pham,Vu Linh, MD
  Pikus,Igor, MD
  Rana,Kirtida Dinesh, MD
  Ravindra,Sunay B., MD
  Shah,Mehul D., DO
  Shih,Yangyu Steven, MD
  Shore,Ronald Andrew, DO
  Sim,Andrew R., MD
  Singh,Jagjeet, MD
  Spina,Laurie J., MD
  Suchy,Matthew Robert, DO
  Taragin,Michael S., MD
  Terreri,Michael Robert Jr., MD
  Thakur,Jagdish G., MD
  Tsafos,Vassilios, MD
  Wassef,Michael Karim, MD
  Wong,Henry Chen, MD
  Young,Jill S., DO
  Zabrodina,Yanina V., MD

Morris Medical Associates
3799 Route 46 East/Suite 209 Zip: 07054
Ph: (973) 334-8010 Fax: (973) 402-9030
  Poon,Gilbert B., MD
  Puzino,Alan Vincent, MD

Parsippany Pediatrics
1140 Parisppany Boulevard/Suite 102 Zip: 07054
Ph: (973) 263-0066 Fax: (973) 263-3160
  Handler,Robert W., MD
  Kahn,Daniel Efraim, MD
  Koenigsberg,Alan M., MD

The Orthopedic Group, P.A.
50 Cherry Hill Road Zip: 07054
Ph: (973) 263-2828 Fax: (973) 263-3243
  Siegel,Jeffrey Alan, MD

Passaic
Cardiovascular Surgical Associates
350 Boulevard/Suite 130 Zip: 07055
Ph: (973) 365-4567 Fax: (973) 916-5262
  Chuback,John A., MD
  Kaushik,Raj Ramanuj, MD

Center for Adult Medicine & Preventive
293 Passaic Street Zip: 07055
Ph: (973) 773-0334 Fax: (973) 773-0336
  Fernandez Santiago,Angela, DO

Center for Adult Med & Preventive Care
916-922 Main Avenue/Suite 1-A Zip: 07055
Ph: (973) 773-0334 Fax: (973) 773-0336
  Ramdial,Maria Janine, MD
  Shah,Anuj Raju, MD
  Tejeda,Carlos Alberto, MD
  Vega,Andres, MD

Drs. Carson & Solomon
203 Passaic Avenue Zip: 07055
Ph: (973) 246-6999 Fax: (973) 685-7340
  Carson,Milinda Ruth, MD
  Solomon,Jennifer, MD

Drs. Sharma and Castilla
293 Passaic Street Zip: 07055
Ph: (973) 365-1377 Fax: (973) 365-1229
  Castilla,William A., MD

Mental Health Clinic of Passaic
111 Lexington Avenue Zip: 07055
Ph: (973) 471-8006
  Williams-Martin,Pamela Y., MD

NHCAC Health Center at Passaic
110 Main Avenue Zip: 07055
Ph: (973) 777-0256 Fax: (973) 777-3910
  Makui,Sheyda, MD

Passaic Pediatrics II PA
913 Main Avenue Zip: 07055
Ph: (973) 458-8000
  Acosta,Katiusca A., MD
  Almanzar,Raul, MD
  Bravo,Holanda P., MD
  Hernandez,Jacqueline, DO

Groups and Clinics by Town with Physician Rosters

Passaic (cont)
Passaic Pediatrics PA
298 Passaic Street Zip: 07055
Ph: (973) 249-8100 Fax: (973) 249-8110
- Aguayo-Figueroa,Lourdes, MD
- Camilo,Antonio Manuel, MD
- Ferrer,Angel Salvador, MD
- Japa-Camilo,Judelka, MD
- Mico,Mario R., MD
- Mosquera,Maria Cecilia, MD
- Rodriguez Montana,Manuel Alejandro

Paterson
C. Dicovsky Medical Group LLC
681 Broadway Zip: 07514
Ph: (973) 278-1000 Fax: (973) 278-1709
- Bontemps,Serge L., MD
- Marani-Dicovskiy,Marcela C., MD
- Sweidan,Safwan A., MD

Centro Medico Iberoamericano
416 Park Avenue Zip: 07501
Ph: (973) 684-8138 Fax: (973) 684-0032
- Desueza,Juan A., MD

Drs. Ballem and Jadhav
715 Broadway Zip: 07514
Ph: (973) 279-2294 Fax: (973) 279-7341
- Ballem,Arunajyoth, MD
- Jadhav,Latha, MD

Drs. Tello Valcarcel & Calderon
356 Totowa Avenue Zip: 07502
Ph: (973) 904-0100 Fax: (973) 595-8286
- Calderon,Rosa L., MD
- Tello Valcarcel,Carlos A., MD

Eastside Pediatrics
625 Broadway/1st Floor Zip: 07514
Ph: (973) 523-1102 Fax: (973) 523-7309
- Ayodeji,Olutope O., MD
- Lesesne-Ayodeji,Mercedes, MD

Express Medical Group
1042 Main Street Zip: 07503
Ph: (973) 510-2444
- Elkholy,Neveen A., DO

Ferraro Medical Associates
414 Broadway Zip: 07501
Ph: (973) 742-1761 Fax: (973) 742-2033
- Ferraro,Lisa, MD
- Seda,Evelyn R., MD

Heart & Vascular Medical Group
680 Broadway/Suite 116-A Zip: 07514
Ph: (973) 684-3663 Fax: (862) 264-2386
- Chowdhury,Shamima, MD
- Joseph,Albert M. Duverglas, MD

Hector L. Castillo MD Associates
1000 Madison Avenue Zip: 07501
Ph: (973) 742-3937
- Castillo,Hector L., MD
- Castillo,Hilda A., MD

Kiddie Clinic
760 Market Street Zip: 07513
Ph: (973) 523-8083 Fax: (973) 523-1133
- Mejia,Edgar R., MD
- Mejia,Gloria, MD

Main Medical Associates
100 Main Street Zip: 07505
Ph: (973) 523-0317 Fax: (973) 684-8590
- Taclob,Erlinda V., MD
- Taclob,Lowell T., MD
- Taclob,Michelle Maria, MD

Otolaryngology Head and Neck Surgery
311 Lexington Avenue Zip: 07502
Ph: (973) 942-1300
- Labagnara,James Jr., MD

Paterson Community Clinic
355 21st Avenue Zip: 07501
Ph: (973) 523-9090 Fax: (973) 523-5222
- Al-Shrouf,Amal Ali, MD
- Aqel,Mahmoud Bader, MD

Paterson Community Health Center
32 Clinton Street Zip: 07522
Ph: (973) 790-6594 Fax: (973) 790-7703
- Brault,Peter V., MD
- Facey,Maxine Elizabeth, MD

Paterson Community Health Center
227 Broadway Zip: 07501
Ph: (973) 278-2600 Fax: (973) 278-5837
- Ginart,Gaspar L., MD

- Khan,Ferhana, MD
- Marino,Nicholas A., MD
- Yung Poon,Karen York-Mui, MD

Paterson Counseling Center
319-321 Main Street Zip: 07505
Ph: (973) 523-8316 Fax: (973) 523-5116
- Ovsjanikovska,Natalija, MD

Sall/Myers Medical Assocs
100 Hamilton Plaza/Suite 317/3rd Floor Zip: 07505
Ph: (973) 279-2323 Fax: (973) 279-7551
- Dane,Steven H., MD
- Flood,Stephen James, MD
- Gonnella,Eleanor A., MD
- Maio,Theodora J., MD
- Misthos,Paul, MD
- Speez,Nancy Sprague, MD

St. Joseph's Family Health Center
21 Market Street Zip: 07501
Ph: (973) 754-4200 Fax: (973) 754-4201
- Bilenki,Natalie I., MD
- Bleeker,David Paul, MD
- Boghdady,Maged W., MD
- Gadgil,Nandini S., MD
- Hassan,Khaled A., MD
- Kheyfets,Irina, MD
- Kumar,Anand K., MD
- Montemurro,Robert J., MD
- See,Manuel T., MD
- Siddiqui,Muhammad Rehan, MD
- White,Evelyn W., MD

West Paterson Family Medical Ctr
154 Union Avenue Zip: 07502
Ph: (973) 942-3618
- Vitale,Joseph, MD

Women's Care
1044 Main Street Zip: 07503
Ph: (973) 782-5577
- Liriano,Monica, MD
- Mustafa,Diane M., MD

Paulsboro
Family Health Ctr of Paulsboro
One West Broad Street Zip: 08066
Ph: (856) 423-0033 Fax: (856) 423-4444
- Milas,Erica M., DO

Pemberton
Southern Jersey Family Medical Centers
600 Pemberton-Browns Mills Rd Zip: 08068
Ph: (609) 894-1100 Fax: (609) 894-1110
- Adumala,Pradeep, MD
- Shaw,Wayne, MD

Pennington
Capital Emergncy Physicians & Assoc.
One Capital Way Zip: 08534
Ph: (609) 303-4000
- Besingi,Cecile Ewane, MD
- Fellman,Katherine, MD
- Jones,Krister J., MD
- Kruse,Laurel Anita Farnham, MD
- Stephen,Priya Chachikutty, MD

Capital Endocrinology
2 Capital Way/Suite 290 Zip: 08534
Ph: (609) 303-4300 Fax: (609) 303-4301
- Gillis Funderburk,Sheri Anita, MD
- Parvez,Ayesha, MD
- Saltzman,Erin Alyse, MD
- Thomas,Sunil Raj, MD
- Villanueva,Erika, MD
- Wu,Yan, MD

Capital Health Medical
2 Capital Way/Suite 356 Zip: 08534
Ph: (609) 537-6000 Fax: (609) 537-6002
- Chung,Jooyeun, MD
- Doria,Cataldo, MD
- Eisenberg,Joshua Aaron, MD
- Johnson,Steven A., DO
- Kalina,Michael, DO
- Petty,Victoria Morey, MD
- Rosato,Francis E., MD

CH Radiation Oncology Dept.
One Capital Way Zip: 08534
Ph: (609) 304-4244 Fax: (609) 303-4156
- Chen,Timothy H., MD
- Williamson,Shirnett Karean, MD

Capital Health-Heart Care Specialists
2 Capital Way/Suite 385 Zip: 08534
Ph: (609) 303-4838 Fax: (609) 303-4835
- Desai,Harit, DO
- Saxena,Neil, MD
- Struble,Eric Michael, MD
- Young,Kristopher F., DO

Capital Institute for Neurosciences
2 Capital Way/Suite 456 Zip: 08534
Ph: (609) 537-7300 Fax: (609) 537-7301
- Assadi-Khansari,Mitra, MD
- Buono,Lee M., MD
- Casiano Pagan,Hector Francisco, MD
- Connolly,Patrick Joseph, MD
- Cruciani,Ricardo Alberto, MD
- Fennell,Vernard Sharif, MD
- Goldfarb,Olga, MD
- Gonzalez,Ronald H., MD
- Kumar,Rajat, MD
- Landen,Alexandra E., DO
- Naragum,Varun, MD
- Rubin,Mitchell J., MD
- Schumacher,Hermann Christian, MD
- Shukla,Chirag S., MD
- Stiefel,Michael Fred, MD
- Vester,John W., MD
- Witte,Arnold S., MD

Doctors Dellacroce and Lee
2 Capital Way/Suite 390 Zip: 08534
Ph: (609) 818-0040 Fax: (609) 818-0049
- Dellacroce,Joseph Michael, MD
- Lee,Daniel James, MD

Hopewell Family Practice & Sports Med
84 Route 31 North/Suite 103 Zip: 08534
Ph: (609) 730-1771 Fax: (609) 730-1274
- Holdcraft,Suzanne, MD
- Kakarla,Madhavi, MD
- Samaddar,Soumen, MD

Matossian Eye Associates
2 Capital Way/Suite 326 Zip: 08534
Ph: (609) 882-8833 Fax: (609) 882-0077
- Desai,Priya Vasudev, MD
- Lesniak,Sebastian P., MD
- Matossian,Cynthia, MD
- Rozenbaum,Ilya Maksovich, MD

Mercer Bucks Hematology Oncology
2 Capital Way/Suite 220 Zip: 08534
Ph: (609) 303-0747 Fax: (609) 303-0771
- Gandhi,Neel Jitendra, MD
- Grossman,Bernard, MD
- Kindsfather,Scott K., MD
- McIntosh,Nenita Parrilla, MD
- Rosvold,Elizabeth Anne, MD
- Schaebler,David L., MD

Mercer Gastroenterology
2 Capital Way/Suite 487 Zip: 08534
Ph: (609) 818-1900 Fax: (609) 818-1908
- Bhatia,Jyoti Kamlesh, MD
- Dhillon,Ravinder S., MD
- Simonian,Armen John, MD

Mercer Internal Medicine, LLC.
2480 Pennington Road/Suites 104 Zip: 08534
Ph: (609) 818-1000 Fax: (609) 818-9800
- Nee,Guy, MD
- Yamane,Michael H., MD

Mercer Regional Medical Associates
2 Capital Way/Suite 315 Zip: 08534
Ph: (609) 730-0010 Fax: (609) 730-3939
- Dhillon,Satvinder K., MD
- Dhillon,Sudeep S., MD

Mountain View Surgical Assocaites
2 Capital Way/Suite 505 Zip: 08534
Ph: (609) 537-7000 Fax: (609) 537-7070
- Allen,Lisa Rachel, MD
- Mustafa,Rose, MD
- Tuma,Gary Alan, MD

Princeton Nassau Pediatrics, P.A.
25 South Route 31 Zip: 08534
Ph: (609) 745-5300 Fax: (609) 745-5320
- Bunn,Diane Marie, MD
- Riewe,Kathleen O'Day, MD
- Riggall,Michael Justin, MD

Trenton Anesthesiology Associates, PA
One Capital Way/Second Floor Zip: 08534
Ph: (609) 396-4700 Fax: (609) 396-4900
- Ahmad,Sajida Ghani, MD
- Cantillo,Joaquin J., MD
- Enriquez,Joseph E., MD
- Grujic,Slobodan, MD
- Hanusey,Robert William, MD
- Kollmeier,Brett R., MD
- Liu,Renfeng, DO
- Madsen,Melissa L., MD
- Rao,Veena, MD
- Reddy,Sudershan P., MD
- Shah,Mahendra Govindlal, MD
- Tolentino,Pablito L., MD
- Voros,Stephen C., MD
- Wuu,Zukwung, MD

Trenton Orthopaedic Group
116 Washington Crossing Road Zip: 08534
Ph: (609) 581-2200 Fax: (609) 581-1212
- Caruso,Steven A., MD

Urology Care Alliance
Two Capital Way/Suite 407 Zip: 08534
Ph: (609) 730-1966 Fax: (609) 730-1166
- Orland,Steven M., MD
- Rogers,Brad S., MD

Pennsauken
Worknet Occupational Medicine
9370 Route 130 North/Suite 200 Zip: 08110
Ph: (856) 662-0660 Fax: (856) 662-0798
- Introcaso,Lucian J., MD
- Levy,Brahman B., MD

Family Care Associates
6705 Park Avenue Zip: 08109
Ph: (856) 662-0017 Fax: (856) 663-3038
- Ricigliano,Mark A., DO

Lourdes Pediatric Associates
2475 McClellan Avenue/Building B201 Zip: 08109
Ph: (856) 330-6300 Fax: (856) 330-6305
- Chong,Penny Maria, MD
- Glasofer,Eric David, MD
- McFadden Parsi,Lovelle, DO

Style Family Medicine
502 Hillside Terrace Zip: 08110
Ph: (856) 663-7874 Fax: (856) 633-5158
- Krachman,Amy Nicole, DO

Virtua Family Medicine - Cooper River
6981 North Park Drive/Suite 200 Zip: 08109
Ph: (856) 663-4949 Fax: (856) 663-6076
- McDermet,Arthur J., DO
- Santangelo,Steven Frank, DO
- Toporowski,Beverly Christine, MD

Pennsville
Cooper Primary Care
390 North Broadway/Suite 100 Zip: 08070
Ph: (856) 678-6411 Fax: (856) 678-7509
- Deng,Yingzi, MD
- Lacay,Edmar Manabat, MD

Pennsville Sports Med & Rehab Ctr
270 South Broadway/PO Box 35 Zip: 08070
Ph: (856) 678-5449
- Akrout,Tarak, MD
- Maiatico,Marcellus A., MD

Salem Medical Group - Pennsville
181 North Broadway/Suite 3 Zip: 08070
Ph: (856) 678-9002 Fax: (856) 678-4027
- Bober,Mitchell C., DO
- Syritsyna,Olga, MD

Perth Amboy
Dr. Vinod K. Sinha, MD, PA
260 Hobart Street Zip: 08861
Ph: (732) 442-6464 Fax: (732) 442-6367
- Chowdhry,Neil, MD
- Sinha,Anjali, DO
- Sinha,Vinod K., MD

Groups and Clinics by Town with Physician Rosters

Jewish Renaissance Medical Center
275 Hobart Street   Zip: 08861
Ph: (732) 376-9333   Fax: (732) 376-0139
  Calderon,Dinorah, MD
  Chu,Wei, MD
  Forbes,Darlene Henderson, MD
  Nazli,Yasmeen Zuleikha, MD
  Ritsan,Julia B., DO
  Tamburello,Traci Ann, DO
  Wade,Mark J., MD

Santamaria Eye Center
104 Market Street   Zip: 08861
Ph: (732) 826-5159   Fax: (732) 826-2107
  Darvin,Kenneth N., MD
  Murr,Peter, MD
  Santamaria,Jaime II, MD

Phillipsburg

Coordinated Health
222 Red Lane   Zip: 08865
Ph: (610) 861-8080   Fax: (610) 849-1013
  Burkey,Seth Micah, MD
  Diiorio,Emil John, MD
  Estacio,Joseph M., DO
  Friedman,Robert Lawrence, MD
  Lee,Susan, MD
  Loguidice,Vito A., MD
  Martinez,Marcos Manuel, MD
  Reid,James Henry, MD

Coventry Cardiology Associates
1000 Coventry Drive   Zip: 08865
Ph: (908) 859-3800   Fax: (908) 859-4310
  Mascarenhas,Daniel A. Neville, MD
  Popkave,Arthur H., MD
  Singh,Narpinder, MD

Coventry Eye Associates, P.C.
800 Coventry Drive   Zip: 08865
Ph: (908) 859-6055   Fax: (908) 859-2042
  Neusidl,William B., MD

Drs. Costacurta & Nar
96A Baltimore Street   Zip: 08865
Ph: (610) 258-4337
  Costacurta,Gary A., MD
  Nar,Kishorkumar G., MD

Drs. Shah and Mehta
311 Baltimore Street   Zip: 08865
Ph: (908) 859-2009   Fax: (908) 859-3352
  Mehta,Heeral J., MD
  Shah,Ila A., MD

Easton Cardiovascular Associates
123 Roseberry Street   Zip: 08865
Ph: (908) 213-3100
  Khalighi,Koroush, MD
  Patel,Chandulal Harilal, MD
  Rohatgi,Rajeev, MD
  Schiavone,Joseph Adriano, MD

Jersey Emergency Specialists, Inc.
185 Roseberry Street   Zip: 08865
Ph: (908) 859-6767
  Parada,Joseph A., MD
  Roscher,Atilio R., MD
  Starosta,Daria Marie, DO

Kaleidoscope Medical Associates
410 Coventry Drive   Zip: 08865
Ph: (908) 454-9902   Fax: (908) 454-9905
  Aversa,Thaddeus Massimo, DO
  Gomes,Ana P., DO
  Kanner Liebman,Rachel Brooke, DO

Milford Medical Center
207 Strykers Road   Zip: 08865
Ph: (908) 995-4125
  Cumbo,Edward J., DO
  Lewis,Irwin Holden, MD
  Rossi,Cynthia Ann, MD

New Beginnings Pediatrics
755 Memorial Parkway/Suite 115   Zip: 08865
Ph: (908) 454-3737   Fax: (908) 454-0402
  Evans,Charles III, MD
  Sion,Armi T., MD

Open Air MRI
430 Memorial Parkway/Suite 2   Zip: 08865
Ph: (908) 213-3600
  Fendley,Ann Ehrke, MD
  Swartz,Joel David, MD

Orthopedic Assoc Greater Lehigh Valley
755 Memorial Parkway/Suite 101   Zip: 08865
Ph: (908) 859-5585   Fax: (908) 859-3990
  Ferrante,Christopher R., MD
  Maron,Norman L., MD

Phillipsburg Ob/Gyn Associates
700 Coventry Drive   Zip: 08865
Ph: (908) 454-4666
  Berger,Daniel A., DO
  Blumenthal,Neil C., MD
  Horne,Howard Krutzel, MD

St Luke's Hospitalist Group
185 Roseberry Street   Zip: 08865
Ph: (484) 526-6643   Fax: (484) 526-4605
  Patel,Pritiben C., MD
  Revankar,Manasi Chandrakant, DO
  Varkey,Sarah Hema, MD

St. Luke's Cardiology Associates
755 Memorial Parkway   Zip: 08865
Ph: (908) 859-0514   Fax: (908) 859-0515
  Brar,Navtej Singh, DO
  Prasad,Amit, MD
  Silver,David Foster, MD

Coventry Family Practice
755 Memorial Parkway/Suite 300   Zip: 08865
Ph: (908) 847-3300   Fax: (866) 281-6023
  Buch,Raymond S., MD
  Chu,Ching-Huey, MD
  Decker,Eugene Michael, DO
  Levine,Helaine Gale, MD
  Mcginley,Thomas Charles Jr., MD
  Remde,Alan H., MD
  Siciliano,Mary J., DO

Starr Hematology & Medical Oncology
755 Memorial Parkway/Suite 102   Zip: 08865
Ph: (908) 454-0370   Fax: (908) 454-9858
  Smith,John Edmund Jr., MD
  Starr,Cynthia D., MD

The Doctor Is In
1205 US Highway 22   Zip: 08865
Ph: (908) 213-2211   Fax: (908) 213-9913
  Ortiz-Evans,Ileana, MD

Twin Rivers Gastroenterology Center
755 Memorial Parkway/Suite 202A   Zip: 08865
Ph: (908) 859-5400
  Herman,Barry Eugene, MD
  Mukherjee,Shanker, MD

Village Medical Center
207 Strykers Road   Zip: 08865
Ph: (908) 859-6568   Fax: (908) 859-6697
  Bautista,Lucien Santiago, DO
  Delmonico,Gerard J., MD
  Hotchkin,Karen Lynn, MD
  Kropf,Laura Dawn, DO
  Lombardi,Frank T., DO

Piscataway

AstraHealth Urgent & Primary Care
1100 Centennial Avenue/Suite 104   Zip: 08854
Ph: (732) 981-1111   Fax: (732) 981-1113
  Barot,Prayag, MD
  Herbert,Lisa R., MD
  Murphy,John Charles, MD
  Shah,Nehaben Ketankumar, MD

Clinical Research Lab, Inc.
371 Hoes Lane   Zip: 08854
Ph: (732) 981-1444   Fax: (732) 562-1586
  Ali,Umer, MD
  Kanengiser,Bruce Evan, MD

Diabetes & Osteoporosis Center
20 Wills Way   Zip: 08854
Ph: (732) 562-0027   Fax: (732) 562-0041
  Fertig,Brian J., MD
  Kanj,Hassan A., MD

Dr. Vijaya Radhakrishna, MD, PC
155 Stelton Road   Zip: 08854
Ph: (732) 752-8442   Fax: (732) 752-3957
  Mathew,Lovely Sebastian, MD
  Radhakrishna,Vijaya, MD

Drs. Hip Flores & Chinchilla
281 River Road   Zip: 08854
Ph: (732) 356-4665
  Chinchilla,Miguel A., MD
  Hip-Flores,Julio, MD

Drs. Sanjay & Ramos
216 Stelton Road/Suite 3B   Zip: 08854
Ph: (732) 662-9959
  Ramos,Rosalinda J., MD
  Sanjay,Priyanka, MD

EOHSI Clinical Center - UMDNJ
681 Frelinghuysen Road   Zip: 08855
Ph: (732) 445-0202   Fax: (732) 445-0131
  Chuang,Connie T., MD
  Kipen,Howard M., MD

Eck, Apelian & Mathews
1056 Stelton Road   Zip: 08854
Ph: (732) 463-0303   Fax: (732) 463-2289
  Apelian,Ara Z., MD
  Eck,Alieta R., MD
  Eck,John M., MD
  Mathews,Cecil, MD

Health Med Associates, PC
1080 Stelton Road/First FL Suite 202   Zip: 08854
Ph: (732) 985-2552   Fax: (732) 985-0552
  Catapano,Joseph A., MD
  Chatterjee,Sonia, MD
  Stern,Marcel, MD

Naveen Mehrotra, MD PC
1315 Stelton Road   Zip: 08854
Ph: (732) 819-8800   Fax: (732) 819-8801
  Mehrotra,Naveen, MD

Piscataway Dunellen Family Prac
24 Stelton Road/Suite A   Zip: 08854
Ph: (732) 424-0440   Fax: (732) 424-0443
  Krohn,Douglas R., MD
  Shoulson,Shana S., MD

Piscataway Somerset Ob/Gyn
31 Stelton Road/Suite 4   Zip: 08854
Ph: (732) 752-7755   Fax: (732) 752-7918
  Choubey,Sheela, MD
  Cogliani,Ermes, MD

St. Peter's Physicians Associates
1636 Stelton Road/Suite 301   Zip: 08854
Ph: (732) 339-7575
  Parmar,Archana S., DO
  Patel,Sima, MD

Tri-County Ob-Gyn Associates, PA
24 Stelton Road/Suite C   Zip: 08854
Ph: (732) 968-4444   Fax: (732) 968-1675
  De Flesco,Lindsay D., MD
  Schwartz,Marlan K., MD

Zemsky & Piskun MD PA
1132 South Washington Avenue   Zip: 08854
Ph: (732) 752-8484   Fax: (732) 424-1124
  Piskun,Andrew, MD
  Zemsky,Lewis M., MD

Pitman

Di Lisi Family Medicine LLC
110 North Woodbury Road   Zip: 08071
Ph: (856) 589-1212   Fax: (856) 589-6635
  Di Lisi,Joseph P., DO
  Rivell,Crystal Giovanna, DO

Pitman Internal Medicine Assocs
410 North Broadway/Suite 1   Zip: 08071
Ph: (856) 589-3708   Fax: (856) 589-2662
  Brennan,William Frederick, DO
  De Eugenio,Lewis Jr., MD
  Farber,Michael A., MD
  O'Donnell,Carmel Marie, DO

Plainfield

Cardiac Care
1314 Park Avenue/Suite 9   Zip: 07060
Ph: (908) 222-8970   Fax: (908) 222-8762
  Husain,Abid, MD
  Husain,Saleem, MD

Faith Family Health Care
400 West Front Street/Suite B   Zip: 07060
Ph: (908) 822-9700   Fax: (908) 822-9701
  Birotte Sanchez,Maria J., MD

Gastroenterology Associates
1165 Park Avenue   Zip: 07060
Ph: (908) 754-2992   Fax: (908) 754-8366
  Cohen,Allan Bary, MD
  Goldenberg,David A., MD

Inman Medical Associates
1024 Park Avenue/Suite 6A   Zip: 07060
Ph: (908) 222-8400   Fax: (908) 222-8402
  Isukapalli,Padmaja, MD

JFK Medical Center - Muhlenberg Campus
Park Avenue & Randolph Road   Zip: 07061
Ph: (908) 668-2000   Fax: (908) 668-3149
  Bayly,Robert, MD
  Griffin,Francis L., MD
  Shetty,Vyshali S., MD

Neighborhood Health Center Plainfield
1700-58 Myrtle Avenue   Zip: 07063
Ph: (908) 753-6401
  Abrarova,Nazima M., MD

Neighborhood Health Center Plainfield
1700-58 Myrtle Avenue   Zip: 07060
Ph: (908) 753-6401   Fax: (908) 226-6743
  Bastien,Linda, MD
  Basu,Sebika, MD
  Bodapati,Leena, MD
  Guirguis,Soad George, MD
  Jain,Sapna, MD
  Jayaraj,Kasthuri E., MD
  Nwigwe,Genevieve N., MD
  Patel,Alka Jashbhai, MD
  Patel,Arvind Joitaram, MD
  Patel,Maitri, MD
  Pennington,Demetria, MD
  Subramanian,Govindammal N., MD
  Tripathi,Harsha M., MD
  Walsh,Susan M., MD
  Zablocki,Chana Shira, MD

Oak Tree Pediatrics
111 Park Avenue/2ns Floor   Zip: 07060
Ph: (908) 753-2671   Fax: (908) 753-1245
  Mattoo,Deepali, MD
  Singh,Amita, MD

Springfield Pediatrics
939 Park Avenue   Zip: 07060
Ph: (908) 226-5445   Fax: (908) 226-5481
  Morin,Joanne M., MD

Plainsboro

Acute Rehab Unit / Med Ctr Princeton
One Plainsboro Road/2nd Floor   Zip: 08536
Ph: (609) 853-7800
  Calalang,Carolyn Clarice, MD
  Patel,Shivangi, MD
  Sharma,Silky, MD

CHOP Newborn and Pediatric Care at UM
One Plainsboro Road/6th Floor   Zip: 08536
Ph: (609) 853-7626   Fax: (609) 853-7630
  Brennan,Alicia Ann, MD
  Goel,Rajiv, MD
  Kim,Regina Siobhan, MD
  Lingasubramanian,Geethanjali, MD

Child Health Associates
666 Plainsboro Road/Suite 1300   Zip: 08536
Ph: (609) 750-1521   Fax: (609) 750-1523
  Kumar,Anita Kiran, MD

Geriatric Associates of New Jersy
666 Plainsboro Road/Suite1318   Zip: 08536
Ph: (609) 269-8291
  Mirza,Ismet Amtul Latif, MD

New Jersey Bariatrics
666 Plainsboro Road/Suite 640   Zip: 08536
Ph: (609) 785-5870   Fax: (609) 785-5867
  Brolin,Robert E., MD
  Chau,Wai Yip Y., MD

Pathology Associates of Princeton
One Plainsboro Road   Zip: 08536
Ph: (609) 853-6800   Fax: (609) 853-6801
  Arslan,Asima, MD
  Zhang,Lanjing, MD

Groups and Clinics by Town with Physician Rosters

Plainsboro (cont)

Plainsboro Family Physicians
666 Plainsboro Road   Zip: 08536
Ph: (609) 275-8100   Fax: (609) 275-6133
  Sokel, Andrew H., MD
  Tierney, Peter C., MD

Princeton Bone & Joint
5 Plainsboro Road/Suite 100   Zip: 08536
Ph: (609) 750-1600   Fax: (609) 750-1611
  Dhanaraj, Dinesh, MD
  Smires, Harvey E. Jr., MD

Princeton Eye and Ear
5 Plainsboro Road/Suite 510   Zip: 08536
Ph: (609) 403-8840   Fax: (609) 403-8852
  Drezner, Dean Andrew, MD

Princeton Gastrenterology
5 Plainsboro Road/Suite 260   Zip: 08536
Ph: (609) 853-7204   Fax: (609) 853-6386
  Davidson, J. Thomas, MD
  Sheth, Anish A., MD

Princeton Medicine
5 Plainsboro Road/Suite 300   Zip: 08536
Ph: (609) 853-7272   Fax: (609) 853-7271
  Babott, Doreen, MD
  Buckley, Laura K., MD
  Edwards, Barbara Ruth, MD
  Fanning, Christine M., MD
  Goldblatt, Kenneth H., MD
  Hodach-Avalos, Meredith J., MD
  Hunt, Rameck R., MD
  Lancefield, Margaret L., MD
  Nagy, Aubrie Jacobson, MD
  Naini, Sean, DO
  Robison, Kathryn J., MD
  Schwartz, Mark, MD
  Skole, Kevin S., MD
  Wang, Qian, MD

Princeton OB/GYN
5 Plainsboro Road/Suite 500   Zip: 08536
Ph: (609) 936-0700   Fax: (609) 936-0750
  Friedman, Alan L., MD
  Gross, Jeffrey K., MD
  Petraske, Alison R., MD
  Siems, Nicole Mary, DO

Princeton Surgical Associates, P.A.
5 Plainsboro Road/Suite 400   Zip: 08536
Ph: (609) 936-9100   Fax: (609) 936-9700
  Dhir, Nisha Solanki, MD
  Goldman, Kenneth A., MD
  Jordan, Lawrence Joseph III, MD
  Juha, Ramez, MD
  Roy, Rashmi, MD
  Sambol, Elliot Brett, MD
  Smith, Liam R., MD

Pleasantville

Med-Com Health Services, P.A.
258 North New Road   Zip: 08232
Ph: (609) 646-4064   Fax: (609) 272-8526
  Ahmed, Sujood, MD
  Rajput, Ilyas A., MD
  Rajput, Zubeda I., MD

Regional Internal Medicine Associates
1004 South New Road   Zip: 08232
Ph: (609) 652-4141   Fax: (609) 652-9939
  Choudhry, Rafat S., MD
  Qadir, Abdul, MD

Seashore Medical Associates
48 Ansley Boulevard   Zip: 08232
Ph: (609) 641-1077   Fax: (609) 641-1023
  Kozakowski, Edward Jr., MD
  Slotoroff, Jon W., DO

Southern Jersey Family Medical Centers
932 South Main Street   Zip: 08232
Ph: (609) 383-0880   Fax: (609) 383-0658
  Desai, Anagha Kishor, MD
  Merle, Nancy, MD
  Yon, Katherine Sunhee, MD

Point Pleasant Beach

NorthEast Spine & Sports Medicine
1104 Arnold Avenue   Zip: 08742
Ph: (732) 714-0070   Fax: (732) 714-0188
  Franz, Stacey, DO
  Lopez, Hector L. Jr., MD

Ocean Family Care
800 Route 88/Suite 3   Zip: 08742
Ph: (732) 295-0072   Fax: (732) 295-0224
  Pedicini, Joseph P., MD

Point Pleasant Boro

Shore Endocrinology Associates, LLC
2200 River Road/Suite A   Zip: 08742
Ph: (732) 892-7300   Fax: (732) 892-7301
  Fomin, Svetlana, MD
  Marlys, James P., MD

Pomona

AtlantiCare - Neonatology Department
65 West Jimmie Leeds Road   Zip: 08240
Ph: (609) 404-3816   Fax: (609) 404-3818
  Grayson, Stephanie Anne, MD
  Miller, Andrea, DO
  Muhumuza, Catherine, MD
  Tioseco, Jennifer Anne, MD
  Villasis, Cynthia Dancel, MD

AtlantiCare Anesthesiology
65 West Jimmie Leeds Road   Zip: 08240
Ph: (609) 748-7597
  Arole, Adebola Oyedele, MD
  Costabile, Jessica T., DO
  Davidov, Mark, MD
  Fisgus, John R., MD
  Gayeski, David R., MD
  Incandela, Nicholas J., MD
  Kaplan, Bruce Zachary, MD
  Lagmay, Merceditas Maria, MD
  O'Connell, Frank Michael, MD
  Pericic, Romeo, MD
  Radcliff, Nina Singh, MD
  Riccobono, Elizabeth Kay, DO
  Schmidheiser, Mark Andrew, MD
  Wang, Qin, MD
  Yao, Su-Lin G., MD

Cardiac Surgery Group PC
65 Jimmie Leeds Road   Zip: 08240
Ph: (609) 748-7089   Fax: (609) 652-3460
  Dralle, James G., MD

Pompton Lakes

Drs. Scian & Scian Ob/Gyn Assoc
16 Pompton Avenue   Zip: 07442
Ph: (973) 831-6866   Fax: (973) 831-9639
  Scian, John P., MD
  Scian, Joseph A., MD

Medical Associates of North NJ
525 Wanaque Avenue   Zip: 07442
Ph: (973) 839-3333   Fax: (973) 839-0580
  Brabson, Thomas A., DO
  Brabston, Timothy B., MD

North Jersey Colon & Rectal Surgery
191 Hamburg Turnpike   Zip: 07442
Ph: (973) 839-3111   Fax: (973) 839-2301
  McConnell, John C., MD

Pompton Plains

Cardiology Associates of North Jersey
242 West Parkway   Zip: 07444
Ph: (973) 831-7455   Fax: (973) 831-7585
  Blitz, Lawrence R., MD
  Calenda, Brandon William, MD
  Kou, Victoria Wei-Li, MD
  Rosenthal, Mark S., MD
  Siepser, Stuart L., MD
  Tabaksblat, Martin Yaron, MD

Drs. Potter and Bakosi
287 Boulevard/Suite 1/PO Box 367   Zip: 07444
Ph: (973) 839-7400   Fax: (973) 831-4911
  Bakosi, Ebube A., MD
  Potter, Steven D., MD

Erickson Health Medical Group
1 Cedar Crest Village Drive   Zip: 07444
Ph: (973) 831-3540   Fax: (973) 831-3503
  Alade, Ibijoke Adenrele, MD
  Brower, Chelsea, MD
  Cavazos, Anthony Richard, MD
  Neopane, Padam Kumar, MD
  Orlic, Peter Thomas, MD
  Ponomarev, Aleksandr, MD

Firstmed Family Healthcare LLC
637 Route 23 South   Zip: 07444
Ph: (973) 859-7277   Fax: (862) 666-9215
  Duvvuri, Uma, MD

  Patel, Vishal V., MD

PediatriCare Associates
901 Route 23 South   Zip: 07444
Ph: (973) 831-4545   Fax: (973) 831-1527
  Shah, Sapna V., MD

Physicians Health Alliance
28 Jackson Avenue   Zip: 07444
Ph: (973) 835-2575   Fax: (973) 835-0531
  Brahms, Dana Lyn Satomi, MD
  Dara, Michael R., MD
  Dobro, Jeffrey Steven, MD
  Smith-Dipalo, Tracy A., MD

Pompton Plains Family Health Center
230 West Parkway/Suite 10   Zip: 07444
Ph: (973) 835-0800   Fax: (973) 616-2766
  Capio, Mario R., MD
  Raju, Biju, DO

Port Monmouth

Integrated Medicine Alliance, P.A.
363 Highway 36   Zip: 07758
Ph: (732) 471-0400   Fax: (732) 471-7949
  Ibrahim, Christine M., MD
  Patel, Kalpeshkumar Prahladbhai, MD

Princeton

Alexander Road Associates in Psych
707 Alexander Road/Bldg 2 Suite 202   Zip: 08540
Ph: (609) 419-0400   Fax: (609) 419-9200
  Chen, Michael S., MD
  Hayes, William P., MD
  Martinson, Charles F., MD
  Mian, Asma, MD
  Popkin, Sara Elizabeth, MD

CHOP Pedi & Adol Specialty Care Center
707 Alexander Road/Suite 205   Zip: 08540
Ph: (609) 520-1717
  Lee, Hae-Rhi, MD

Capital Health Primary Care
811 Exective Drive   Zip: 08540
Ph: (609) 303-4600   Fax: (609) 303-4601
  Rose, Bruce T., MD
  Siegel-Robles, Deborah S., MD

Cardiology Associates of Princeton
731 Alexander Road/Suite 202   Zip: 08540
Ph: (609) 921-7456   Fax: (609) 921-2972
  Mahalingam, Banu, MD
  McCabe, Johnathan B., MD
  Shanahan, Andrew J., MD
  Younes, Desiree Marie, MD

Cedar Glen Professional Assoc
170 Cold Soil Road   Zip: 08540
Ph: (609) 896-1122   Fax: (609) 896-2688
  Blake, John R., MD
  Green, Jeffrey H., MD
  Heller, Philip Arthur, MD
  Karpf, Gary A., MD

Drs. Langer & Langer
12 Cleveland Lane   Zip: 08540
Ph: (609) 683-5090
  Langer, Dennis Henry, MD
  Langer, Susan F., MD

Endocrinology Associates of Princeton
256 Bunn Drive/Suite D   Zip: 08540
Ph: (609) 924-4433   Fax: (609) 924-4423
  Bembo, Shirley Abad, MD
  Joy, Anna Varughese, MD
  Ruel, Ewa, MD

Garden State Physicians P.C.
21 Jefferson Plaza   Zip: 08540
Ph: (732) 274-1274   Fax: (732) 355-0321
  Deora-Bhens, Sonia, DO

Garden State Physicians P.C.
10 Jefferson Plaza/Suite 100   Zip: 08540
Ph: (732) 274-1274   Fax: (732) 355-0321
  Mendu, Srinivas, MD

Global Medical Institutes, LLC
256 Bunn Drive/Suite 6 Woodslands Bldg   Zip: 08540
Ph: (609) 921-3555   Fax: (609) 921-3620
  Apter, Jeffrey T., MD

Medical Pediatrics Associates
256 Bunn Drive/Suite 3 A   Zip: 08540
  Altshuler, Elena, MD

  Dashevsky, Nataliya, MD
  Hossain, Feroza K., MD
  Konnick, Patrina A., MD

Montgomery Internal Medicine Group
727 State Road   Zip: 08540
Ph: (609) 921-6410   Fax: (609) 921-0406
  Chattha, Savneet Kaur, MD
  Corazza, Douglas P., MD
  De La Cruz, Ernest Jose, MD
  Hug, Vickie Beth, MD

Ophthalmology Associates
800 Bunn Drive/Suite 301   Zip: 08540
Ph: (609) 924-3700
  Lipka, Andrew C., MD

Outlook Eyecare
100 Canal Pointe Boulevard/Suite 100   Zip: 08540
Ph: (609) 279-9500   Fax: (609) 279-0150
  Shovlin, Joseph Peter, MD

Princeton Anesthesia Services PC
253 Witherspoon Street   Zip: 08540
Ph: (609) 497-4000   Fax: (609) 497-4331
  Hancock, Joseph Patrick, MD
  Kim, Andrew Hanyoung, MD

Princeton Brain & Spine Care LLC
731 Alexander Road/Suite 200   Zip: 08540
Ph: (609) 921-9001   Fax: (609) 921-9055
  McLaughlin, Mark Robert, MD

Princeton Ctr for Plastic Surgery
932 State Road   Zip: 08540
Ph: (609) 921-7161   Fax: (609) 921-6263
  Leach, Thomas A., MD
  Swedlund, Anne P., MD

Princeton Dermatology Associates
208 Bunn Drive/Suite 1-E   Zip: 08540
Ph: (609) 683-4999   Fax: (609) 683-0298
  Banker, Sarika, MD
  Funkhouser, Martha E., MD

Princeton Endocrinology Associates
10 Forrestal Road South/Suite 106   Zip: 08540
Ph: (609) 921-1511   Fax: (609) 921-3316
  Inzerillo, Angela Mary, MD
  Weiss, Ned Martin, MD

Princeton Gastroenterology Associates
731 Alexander Road/Suite 100   Zip: 08540
Ph: (609) 924-1422   Fax: (609) 924-7473
  Bellows, Aaron, MD
  Meirowitz, Robert F., MD
  Osias, Glenn Lawrence, MD
  Rho, Aloysius Kihyok, MD
  Segal, William Nathan, MD
  Shriver, Amy Rubin, MD

Princeton Internal Medicine Associates
281 Witherspoon Street/Suite 220   Zip: 08542
Ph: (609) 921-3362   Fax: (609) 921-3584
  Lee, Karina K., MD
  Rota, Anthony P., MD
  Sass, Timothy E., MD
  Srinivasan, Geetha, MD

Princeton Interventional Cardiol
800 Bunn Drive/Suite 101   Zip: 08540
Ph: (609) 921-2800   Fax: (609) 921-3499
  Beattie, James Ray III, MD
  Mercuro, Tobia J., MD
  Passalaris, John Dimitrios, MD

Princeton Lifestyle Medicine
731 Alexander Road/Suite 200   Zip: 08540
Ph: (609) 655-3800   Fax: (609) 655-5203
  Brown, Barbara A., MD
  Kossow, Lynne Becker, MD
  Rehor, Francis E., MD

Princeton Medical Group, P.A.
419 North Harrison Street   Zip: 08540
Ph: (609) 924-9300   Fax: (609) 924-6552
  Barton, William W., MD
  Baseman, Debra L., MD
  Blom, Thomas Robert, MD
  Chang, Frances Yu-hsin, MD
  Choi, Sola, MD
  Costin, Andrew, MD

Deshpande,Neha A., MD
Diventi,Christina G., MD
Gitterman,Benjamin Eric, MD
Glazer,Joyce H., MD
Goyal,Seema Agrawal, MD
Hsu,Stanley Cho Hsien, MD
Hua,Xingjia, MD
Hyun,Youngsoon, MD
Kazenoff,Steven, MD
Kwee,Darlene J., MD
Lacava,Paul Vincent, MD
Lee,Richard Thomas, MD
Malhotra,Anuj Kumar, MD
Martin,Robert Allen, MD
Mullarkey-De Sapio,Cathleen J., MD
Patel,Anand, MD
Patel,Vrunda, MD
Saha,Anita, MD
Schwartz,Melanie Schrader, MD
Sierocki,John S., MD
Slavin,Anna, MD
Stockham,Chad Eric, MD
Tridico,Tanner Joseph, MD
Vedula,Ramya S., DO
Wei,Fong, MD
Wong,Casey, MD
Yi,Peter I., MD

Princeton Nassau Pediatrics, P.A.
301 North Harrison Street Zip: 08540
Ph: (609) 924-5510 Fax: (609) 924-3577
Giasi,William George Jr., MD
Greenberg,Leslie Robin, MD
Harvey,Karanja, MD
Helmrich,Robert Florian, MD
Kong,Ji Yong, MD
Kwong,Jenitta, MD
Mandelbaum,Bert, MD
Marshall,Rebecca G., MD
Martin,Erica Nell, MD
McConlogue,Joelle Jugant, MD
Millar,Kim H., MD
Monica,Kristi Rae, MD
Naddermier,Adam Brett, MD
Pellegrino,Peter Phillip, MD
Pierson,David Shawn, MD
Pierson,Joseph Jr., MD
Raymond,Gerald M., MD
Schneider,Allen J., MD
Shah,Amisha A., MD
Winikor,Jared, MD

Princeton Orthopaedic Associates, P.A.
325 Princeton Avenue Zip: 08540
Ph: (609) 924-8131 Fax: (609) 924-8532
Abrams,Jeffrey Stuart, MD
Ark,Jon Wong Tze-Jen, MD
Bezwada,Hari Prasad, MD
Fleming,Richard E. Jr., MD
Gecha,Steven R., MD
Grenis,Michael Steven, MD
Gutowski,Walter Thomas III, MD
Lamb,David J., MD
Lamb,Marc John, MD
Leise,Megan Diane, MD
Levine,Stuart Eric, MD
Miller,Jeffrey J., DO
Miller-Smith,Stacey Ann, MD
Mizrachi,Arik, MD
Moskwa,Alexander Jr., MD
Nazarian,Ronniel, MD
Palmer,Michael Alberto, MD
Patel,Meelan Nick, MD
Pressman,Mark J., MD
Rossy,William Henry IV, MD
Song,Frederick Suh, MD
Stier,Kyle Thomas, MD
Vannozzi,Brian Michael, MD

Princeton Primary & Urgent Care
707 Alexander Road/Suite 201 Zip: 08540
Ph: (609) 919-0009 Fax: (609) 919-0008
Cole,Bruno N., MD
Fernando,Chandani D., MD

Princeton Spine and Joint Center
601 Ewing Street/Suite A-2 Zip: 08540
Ph: (609) 454-0760 Fax: (609) 454-0761
Bracilovic,Ana, MD
Cooper,Grant, MD
Funiciello,Marco, DO
Meyler,Zinovy, DO

Princeton Urogynecology
10 Forrestal Road South/Suite 205 Zip: 08540
Ph: (609) 924-2230 Fax: (609) 924-5006
Bhatia,Nina Prakash, MD
Van Raalte,Heather Michelle, MD

The Pediatric Group PA
66 Mount Lucas Road Zip: 08540
Ph: (609) 924-4892 Fax: (609) 921-9380
Cotton,John M., MD
Pulver,Deborah Moody, MD
Rose,Helen M., MD
Tesoro,Louis J., MD
Zollner,Paula G., MD

The Princeton Ctr for Dermatology
800 Bunn Drive/Suite 201 Zip: 08540
Ph: (609) 924-1033 Fax: (609) 924-7055
Notterman,Robyn B., MD
Rossy,Kathleen M., MD

The Princeton Eye Group
419 North Harrison Street/Suite 104 Zip: 08540
Ph: (609) 921-9437 Fax: (609) 921-0277
Epstein,John Arthur, MD
Felton,Stephen M., MD
Jadico,Suzanne K., MD
Liu,Samuel M., MD
Miedziak,Anita Irmina, MD
Reynolds,Richard David, MD
Wong,Michael Y., MD
Wong,Richard H., MD

The Princeton Longevity Center
136 Main Street Zip: 08540
Ph: (609) 430-0752 Fax: (609) 430-8470
Fein,David A., MD
Rumberger,John Arthur, MD

University Orthopaedic Associates, LLC
211 North Harrison Street Zip: 08540
Ph: (609) 683-7800 Fax: (609) 683-7875
Bechler,Jeffrey R., MD
McDonnell,Matthew, MD

Urology Group of Princeton PA
134 Stanhope Street/Forrestal Village Zip: 08540
Ph: (609) 924-6487 Fax: (609) 921-7020
Latzko,Karen Marie, DO

Urology Group of Princeton PA
281 Witherspoon Street/Suite 100 Zip: 08542
Ph: (609) 924-6487 Fax: (609) 921-7020
Pickens,Robert L., MD
Rossman,Barry R., MD
Vukasin,Alexander P., MD
Wedmid,Alexei, MD

Womens Health First
114 Stanhope Street Zip: 08540
Ph: (609) 683-7979 Fax: (609) 683-1972
Bergknoff,Hugh, MD
Forster,Judith Karen, MD
Forster,Susan A., MD

Princeton Junction
Lawrence Orthopaedics
4065 Quakerbridge Road Zip: 08550
Ph: (609) 394-3804 Fax: (609) 989-1550
Glick,Ronald S., MD
Miller,Scott David, MD
Shakir,Ahmar, DO

Princeton Hypertension-Nephrology
88 Princeton Hightstown Road/Suite 203 Zip: 08550
Ph: (609) 750-7330 Fax: (609) 750-7336
Basi,Seema, MD
Bialy,Grace B., MD
Finkielstein,Vadim Aaron, MD
Ruddy,Michael C., MD

Princeton Windsor Pediatrics
88 Princeton Hightstown Road/Suite 103 Zip: 08550
Ph: (609) 799-4700 Fax: (609) 799-4545
Hefler,Stephen Edward, MD
Mansour,Ayman M., MD

Rahway
Advanced Urology Associates, P.C.
1600 Saint Georges Avenue/Suite 111 Zip: 07065
Ph: (732) 388-2422 Fax: (732) 388-1706
Arnold,Monica A., DO
Wojno Oranski,Alexander, DO

Assoc Eye Physicians & Surgeons of NJ
1530 Saint Georges Avenue Zip: 07065
Ph: (732) 382-9000 Fax: (732) 382-7455
Hosler,Matthew Robert, MD
Khan,Taj G., DO

Dr's. Choice
1082 St. George Avenue Zip: 07065
Ph: (732) 388-4787 Fax: (732) 388-4380
Livshits,Larisa L., MD
Moody,Rumanatha, MD

Dr. Anu Chaudhry, MD PC
546 Saint Georges Avenue Zip: 07065
Ph: (732) 381-3642 Fax: (732) 396-4463
Chaudhry,Anu, MD
Ravella,Supriya, MD
Vojnyk,Charlene Louise, MD

Drs. Reddy and Reddy
1328 Danchetz Court Zip: 07065
Reddy,Narshimha K., MD
Reddy,Sadhana K., MD

Drs. Yim & Prasad
913 West Inman Avenue Zip: 07065
Ph: (732) 388-7999 Fax: (732) 388-7992
Yim,Frances D., MD

New Jersey Urology, LLC
1600 George Avenue/Suite 202 Zip: 07065
Ph: (732) 499-0111 Fax: (732) 499-0432
Morrow,Franklin A., MD

Ramsey
Drs. Hanna & Crowley
545 Island Road/Suite 2B Zip: 07446
Ph: (201) 995-1004 Fax: (201) 345-7121
Crowley,Elizabeth Ozimek, MD
Hanna,Mohab, MD

Histopathology Services, LLC.
535 East Crescent Avenue Zip: 07446
Ph: (201) 661-7280 Fax: (201) 661-7297
Aponte,Sandra Leonora, MD
Brown,Jeffrey G., MD
Eisen,David Jeffrey, MD
Ilario,Marius John-Marc, MD
Joseph,John K., MD
Liu,Zach Zhiguang, MD
Newman,Schuyler, MD
Szeto,Oliver Jo-Yang, MD

Jandee Anesthesiology
500 North Franklin Turnpike/Suite 206 Zip: 07446
Ph: (201) 962-7282 Fax: (201) 962-7283
Goldstein,Monte Jay, MD
Gordon,Robert P., MD
Melyokhin,Igor, MD
Pillitteri,John, MD
Song,Michael M., MD

Pain Management Associates
255 East Main Street Zip: 07446
Ph: (201) 326-4777 Fax: (201) 391-1196
Gamburg,David, MD
Jacobs,Lyssa Sorkin, MD

Progressive Spine & Sports Medicine
48 South Franklin Turnpike/Suite 101 Zip: 07446
Ph: (201) 962-9199 Fax: (201) 962-9198
Ferrer,Steven Michael, MD
McElroy,Kevin M., DO

Valley Center for Women's Health
581 North Franklin Turnpike/2nd Floor Zip: 07446
Ph: (201) 236-2100 Fax: (201) 236-5269
Faust,Michael G., MD
Nitz,Shelly, MD

Rooney,Michele P., MD

Valley Diagnostic Medical Center
581 North Franklin Turnpike Zip: 07446
Ph: (201) 327-0500 Fax: (201) 327-8612
Cooper,Kimberly Anne, DO
Lucanie,Anabel, MD
Lucanie,Richard, MD
Nickles,Steven L., DO
Sim,Herena, MD

Valley Medical Group
470 North Franklin Turnpike Zip: 07446
Ph: (201) 327-8765 Fax: (201) 327-8496
Ayoub,Kasem, MD
Fernicola,Joseph Robert, MD
Scibetta,Maria T., MD
Strassberg,David M., MD

Valley Pediatric Associates PA
470 North Franklin Turnpike Zip: 07446
Ph: (201) 891-7272 Fax: (201) 934-1817
Ligenza,Claude, MD
Nicpon,Christopher B., MD
Shevelev,Irene, MD

Randolph
Associates in Pulmonary Medicine
765 State Highway 10 East Zip: 07869
Ph: (973) 366-6600 Fax: (973) 366-6385
Russoniello,Michael A., MD

College Plaza Pediatrics
765 State Route 10 East/Suite 203 Zip: 07869
Ph: (973) 659-9991 Fax: (973) 659-9632
Gelman,Beth Paula, MD
Gottlieb,Ricki L., MD
Guerra,Julio C., MD

ID Associates PA/dba ID CARE
765 Route 10 East/Suite 201 Zip: 07869
Ph: (973) 989-0068 Fax: (973) 361-8955
Allegra,Donald T., MD
Aslam,Fazila, MD
Doka,Najah I., MD
Gupta,Rachna, MD
Krieger,Richard E., MD
Manalo,Rosario Beatriz, MD
Markou,Theodore Ioannis, MD
Marsh,Rebecca A., MD
McManus,Edward J., MD
Reddy,Sireesha B., MD
Roseff,Shelly Anne, MD
Ubhi,Damanpreet K., MD
Valentin-Torres,Melanie Rouse, MD
Wenzler,Danya J., MD
Williams,Stephen Joseph, MD

Internal Medicine Consultants
765 State Route 10 East/Suite 201 Zip: 07869
Ph: (973) 975-4830 Fax: (732) 271-1022
Centanni,Monica Ann, MD
Farkas,Attila Istvan, MD
Luayon,Joseph Palac, DO

Lakeland Cardiology Center PA
765 State Route 10/Suite 4 Zip: 07869
Ph: (973) 989-2566
Rogers,Philip S., MD

Lifeline Medical Associates
390 State Route 10/Suite 1 Zip: 07869
Ph: (973) 328-1262 Fax: (973) 328-8576
Buna,Andrei, MD
Mohr,Robert Frederick, MD
Venanzi,Michael V., MD

Northwest Surgical Associates
121 Center Grove Road Zip: 07869
Ph: (973) 328-1414
Choung,Edward W., MD
Hoffman,Michael J., MD
Huang,Ih-Ping, MD
Meisner,Kenneth, MD
Strutin,Millard D., MD

Randolph Medical & Renal Assoc
121 Center Grove Road/Suite 13-14 Zip: 07869
Ph: (973) 361-3737
Gudis,Steven M., MD
Li,Shing, MD
Paster,Lauren, MD

Groups and Clinics by Town with Physician Rosters

Randolph (cont)
Summit Medical Group
477 Route 10 East/Suite 204   Zip: 07869
Ph: (862) 260-3020
  Akkapeddi,Nirmala G., MD

Raritan
Drs. Patel and Patel
31 West Somerset Street   Zip: 08869
Ph: (908) 722-0035   Fax: (908) 722-6763
  Patel,Gita R., MD
  Patel,Rajendrakumar Chimanlal, MD

Laboratory Corp of America
69 First Avenue   Zip: 08869
  Hall,Alvin J., MD
  Moniem,Howayda A., MD

RWJPE Primary Care Raritan
34 East Somerset Street   Zip: 08869
Ph: (908) 685-2532   Fax: (908) 685-2542
  Catanzaro,Donna, MD
  Tomasso,Robert A., MD

Raritan Family Health Care
901 US Highway 202   Zip: 08869
Ph: (908) 253-6640   Fax: (908) 253-6908
  Jordan-Scalia,Lisa Judith, DO
  Khalil,Christina, DO
  Mukherjee,Robin, DO
  Scalia,Joseph Frank, DO

Red Bank
Allegra Arthritis Associates
282 Broad Street   Zip: 07701
Ph: (732) 842-3600   Fax: (732) 842-3665
  Allegra,Edward Charles II, MD
  Haddad,Richard Hani, MD

Del Negro & Senft Eye Associates, PC
152 Broad Street   Zip: 07701
Ph: (732) 747-7725   Fax: (732) 741-7930
  Blades,Frederick C., MD
  Jergens,Paul B., MD

Drs. Randazzo and Tomaino
225 State Route 35/Suite 102B   Zip: 07701
Ph: (732) 530-3433   Fax: (732) 758-1953
  Randazzo,Vincent T., MD
  Tomaino,Jeanne, MD

Frieman Ophthalmology
75 West Front Street   Zip: 07701
Ph: (732) 741-4242
  Frieman,Brett Justin, DO
  Frieman,Lawrence, MD

Greater Monmouth Neurology
130 Maple Avenue/Suite 1-A   Zip: 07701
Ph: (732) 741-1378   Fax: (732) 741-1677
  Chen,Edgar Y., MD
  Fan,Schuber C., MD
  Ilaria,Philip V., MD

Hospital Medicine Associates
157 Broad Street/Suite 317   Zip: 07701
Ph: (732) 530-2960   Fax: (732) 530-7446
  Ahmad,Nauman, MD
  Andrade,Jose G., MD
  Bader,Christopher William, DO
  Holguin,Leonardo Fabio, MD
  John,Thomas Jr., MD
  Mullarney,Allison Ingrid, DO
  Nedelcu,Dana, MD

Integrated Medicine Alliance, P.A.
27 Pinckney Road   Zip: 07701
Ph: (732) 747-4600   Fax: (732) 219-1968
  Marza,Lizett Auxiliado, MD
  Roosels,Marianne, MD

Meridian Med Assoc-Infectious Disease
1 Riverview Plaza/Suite 2 West   Zip: 07701
Ph: (732) 530-2421
  Ahmad,Nasir Mahmood, MD
  Eschinger,Amy Folio, MD

Mid Atlantic Eye Center
70 East Front Street   Zip: 07701
Ph: (732) 741-0858   Fax: (732) 219-0180
  Chen,Natalie, DO
  D'Emic,Susan, DO
  Friedberg,Mark A., MD
  Kahn,Walter J., MD

Middletown Eye Care
565 Highway 35   Zip: 07701
Ph: (732) 747-4443   Fax: (732) 747-4439
  Kneisser,George, MD

Middletown Pediatrics
529 Highway 35   Zip: 07701
Ph: (732) 741-9800   Fax: (732) 758-6367
  Edman,Joel B., MD
  Markoff,Michael S., MD

Millennium Pediatric Care, PA
1 Riverview Medical Center   Zip: 07701
Ph: (732) 450-2801   Fax: (732) 450-2802
  Changchien,Charlie J., MD
  Kommireddi,Sowmini, MD
  Saini,Manish K., MD

Monmouth Pediatric Group, P.A.
272 Broad Street   Zip: 07701
Ph: (732) 741-0456   Fax: (732) 219-9477
  Jordan,Jo-Ann, MD
  Litsky,Michelle Badorf, DO
  Paladino,Theresa Ann, DO
  Wawer-Chubb,Allison Kristen, DO
  Wilmott,Annette Lynne, DO

Orthopaedic Institute of Ctrl NJ
365 Broad Street   Zip: 07701
Ph: (732) 933-4300   Fax: (732) 933-1444
  Lospinuso,Michael Frank, MD

Orthopaedic Sports Medicine
80 Oak Hill Road   Zip: 07701
Ph: (732) 741-2313   Fax: (732) 741-7154
  Bakhos,Nader Anthony, MD
  Costa,Anthony Joseph, MD
  Donlon,Margaret, MD
  Forman,Glenn M., MD
  Friedel,Steven P., MD
  Husain,Qasim M., MD
  Lisser,Steven P., MD
  Mulholland,Daniel J., MD
  Murphy,Bernard P., MD
  Pannullo,Robert Paul, MD
  Phair,Arthur H., MD
  Rinkus,Keith Michael, MD
  Romello,Michael A., MD
  Scott,Richard J., MD
  Van Gelderen,Jeffrey Thomas, MD

Parker Family Health Center
211 Shrewsbury Avenue   Zip: 07701
Ph: (732) 212-0777   Fax: (732) 212-9030
  Carman,Roy L., MD
  Mehra,Shalini Gupta, MD
  Reilly,Gail G., MD

Physician Practice Enhancement, LLC
66 West Gilbert Street   Zip: 07701
Ph: (732) 406-4698
  Malik,Farhan, MD
  Zandieh,Shadi, MD

Red Bank Anesthesia, LLC
1 Riverview Plaza   Zip: 07701
Ph: (732) 530-2255   Fax: (732) 450-2620
  Ades,Nathan Albert, MD
  Brodsky,Jonathan I., DO
  Bruce,Gullie E. IV, MD
  Chidambaram,Manjula S., MD
  Chiu,Nicholas, MD
  Cirullo,Pasquale Michael, MD
  Dooley,James R., MD
  Farrell,Charles W., MD
  Friedman,James Keith, MD
  Haber,Daran W., MD
  Huch,Shane M., DO
  Huh,Chan Woo, MD
  Kulkarni,Prashant P., MD
  Meltzer,Keith Mitchell, MD
  Mosca,Phillip J., MD
  Ritchie,Paul Harvey, MD
  Varadarajan,Vijayaiaxmi, MD

Red Bank Family Medicine
231 Maple Avenue   Zip: 07701
Ph: (732) 842-3050   Fax: (732) 530-0730
  Mulholland,Brendan J., MD
  Sahni,Ryan, MD

Red Bank Gastroenterology Assocs
365 Broad Street/Suite 1-E   Zip: 07701
Ph: (732) 842-4294   Fax: (732) 548-7408
  Binns,Joseph F., MD
  Choi,Yu-Jeong Alexis, MD
  Gialanella,Robert J., MD
  Hampel,Howard, MD
  Heyt,Gregory John, MD
  Marzano,Joseph A., MD
  Sundararajan,Subha V., MD
  Weine,Douglas Matthew, MD

Shore Radiation Oncology, LLC
1 Riverview Plaza   Zip: 07701
Ph: (732) 530-2468   Fax: (732) 836-4036
  Danish,Adnan F., MD
  Patel,Priti S., MD

VNACJ Community Health Center, Inc.
176 Riverside Avenue   Zip: 07701
Ph: (732) 221-5109   Fax: (732) 224-0893
  Landers,Steven Howard, MD
  Sharma,Lokesh, MD

Richland
Buena Family Practice
1315 Harding Highway/Box 310   Zip: 08350
Ph: (856) 697-0300   Fax: (856) 697-8944
  Hargrave,Douglas M., DO
  Peterson,Paul III, DO
  Pirolli,John A., DO

Ridgefield Park
Riverside Medical Group
200 Main Street   Zip: 07660
Ph: (201) 870-6099   Fax: (201) 870-6098
  Baker,Iyad, MD
  Lee,Clara J., MD

Ridgewood
Advanced Dermatology, P.C.
1200 East Ridgewood Avenue   Zip: 07450
Ph: (201) 493-1717   Fax: (201) 493-1009
  Applebaum-Farkas,Paige S., MD
  Au,Sonoa Ho Yee, MD

Advanced Laparoscopic Specialists
61 North Maple Avenue/Suite 205   Zip: 07450
Ph: (201) 447-2808   Fax: (201) 447-2809
  Pucci,Anthony E., DO
  Pucci,Richard Anthony, DO

Bergen Anesthesia Group PC
223 North Van Dien Avenue   Zip: 07450
Ph: (201) 847-9320   Fax: (201) 847-0059
  Smith,Justin Kerry, MD
  Wohlfarth,Erik, MD

Bergen Medical Associates
190 Dayton Street   Zip: 07450
Ph: (201) 670-7800   Fax: (201) 670-7720
  Gupta,Sanchita, MD
  McGorty,Francis E., MD

Breast Health Center of Ridgewood, P.C
385 South Maple Avenue   Zip: 07450
Ph: (201) 670-4550   Fax: (201) 670-7812
  Seltzer,Lawrence G., MD
  Weinstock,Lisa R., MD
  Wollman,Carol A., MD

Drs. Orellana & Volpert
1200 East Ridgewood Avenue/Suite 108   Zip: 07450
Ph: (201) 389-0815
  Orellana,Katherine Atienza, DO
  Volpert,Diana, MD

Drs. Panagiotou & Panagiotou
1200 East Ridgewood Avenue   Zip: 07450
Ph: (201) 447-3690   Fax: (201) 447-3691
  Panagiotou,Demetrios Nicholas, MD
  Panagiotou,Nicholas D., MD

Drs. Rosenfeld & Zisu
265 Ackerman Avenue   Zip: 07450
Ph: (201) 447-5630   Fax: (201) 447-0903
  Rosenfeld,David N., MD
  Zisu,Traian A., MD

Gastroenterology Associates of NJ
1124 East Ridgewood Avenue/Suite 203   Zip: 07450
Ph: (201) 523-4141   Fax: (201) 857-8646
  Grossman,Matthew Aaron, MD
  Pazwash,Haleh, MD

Gastrointestinal Associates PA
140 Chestnut Street/Suite 300   Zip: 07450
Ph: (201) 444-2600   Fax: (201) 444-9471
  Fischer,Zvi, MD
  Hsieh,Jennifer, MD
  Rahmin,Michael G., MD
  Rubinoff,Mitchell J., MD

Kayal Orthopaedic Center, PC
385 South Maple Avenue/Suite 206   Zip: 07450
Ph: (201) 447-3880   Fax: (201) 447-9326
  Kayal,Robert Albert, MD
  Pope,Ernest J., MD

NJ Endovascular Therapeutics
1124 East Ridgewood Avenue/Suite 104   Zip: 07450
Ph: (201) 444-5353
  Bernheim,Joshua William, MD
  Char,Daniel Jay, MD

Neurology Group of Bergen County
1200 East Ridgewood Avenue   Zip: 07450
Ph: (201) 444-0868   Fax: (201) 444-7363
  Berlin,Daniel, MD
  Citak,Kenneth A., MD
  Cope,Jennifer Anne, MD
  Dallara Marsh,Alexis M., MD
  Grewal,Amrit K., MD
  Heilbroner,Peter Louis, MD
  Klein,Bradley Marc, MD
  Levin,Kenneth A., MD
  Lijtmaer,Hugo N., MD
  Molinari,Susan P., MD
  Naidu,Yamini, MD
  Nasr,John T., MD
  Noskin,Olga, MD
  Perron,Reed C., MD
  Shammas,James T., MD
  Steinschneider,Mitchell, MD
  Tong,Fumin, MD
  Van Engel,Daniel R., MD

Neurosurgeons of New Jersey
1200 East Ridgewood Avenue   Zip: 07450
Ph: (201) 824-6131
  Cobb,William Stewart, MD
  D'Ambrosio,Anthony Louis, MD
  Lavine,Sean David, MD
  Moise,Gaetan, MD
  Sheth,Sameer Anil, MD
  Winfree,Christopher Jules, MD

North Bergen Dermatologic Group
400 Route 17 South   Zip: 07450
Ph: (201) 652-4536   Fax: (201) 652-4906
  Corey,Timothy J., MD
  Satra,Karin H., MD
  Stevens,Amy W., MD

North Jersey Neurosurgical Assoc
225 Dayton Street   Zip: 07450
Ph: (201) 612-0020   Fax: (201) 612-0333
  Carpenter,Duncan B., MD
  Goulart,Hamilton C., MD
  Klempner,William L., MD

North Jersey Pediatric Orthopedics PA
140 Chestnut Street/Suite 201   Zip: 07450
Ph: (201) 612-9988   Fax: (201) 445-9050
  Avella,Douglas George, MD
  Joffe,Avrum L., MD

Physicians for Womens Health
1124 East Ridgewood Avenue/Suite 105   Zip: 07450
Ph: (201) 489-2255   Fax: (201) 447-1231
  Khosla,Savita, MD
  Klimowicz-Mallon,Elizabeth, MD
  Kuo,Eugenia C., MD

Rehabilitation Specialists of NJ
505 Goffle Road/Suite 3   Zip: 07450
Ph: (201) 447-4772   Fax: (201) 447-4277
  Boiano,Maria Anna, MD
  Kuo,Douglas, DO

Retina Associates of New Jersey, P.A.
200 South Broad Street/Unit B Zip: 07450
Ph: (201) 445-6622 Fax: (201) 445-0262
  Harris,Michael J., MD
  Kim,David Yhoshin, MD

Retina Consultants PA
1200 East Ridgewood Avenue/Suite 207 Zip: 07450
Ph: (201) 612-9600 Fax: (201) 612-0428
  Kayserman,Larisa, MD
  Lee,Song Eun, MD
  Vallar,Robert V., MD

Ridgewood ENT and Dermatology
81 North Maple Avenue Zip: 07450
Ph: (201) 857-2370 Fax: (201) 857-2371
  Miller,Janine D'Amelio, MD

Ridgewood Gynecologic Associates
317 Franklin Avenue Zip: 07450
Ph: (201) 447-1620 Fax: (201) 447-4977
  Behnam,Kazem, MD
  Behnam,Melody S., MD

Ridgewood Infectious Disease
947 Linwood Avenue/Suite 2E Zip: 07450
Ph: (201) 447-6468 Fax: (201) 447-3189
  Gaffin,Neil, MD
  Knackmuhs,Gary Glenn, MD
  O'Hagan Sotsky,Carol Ann, MD
  Tsiouris,Simon John, MD

Ridgewood Ophthalmology PC
1200 East Ridgewood Avenue Zip: 07450
Ph: (201) 612-0044 Fax: (201) 612-9446
  Alino,Anne Marie G., MD
  Jachens,Adrian William, MD
  Saunders,Eric Monroe, MD
  Sumers,Anne R., MD

Ridgewood Orthopedic Group, LLC
85 South Maple Avenue Zip: 07450
Ph: (201) 445-2830 Fax: (201) 445-7471
  Brief,Andrew A., MD
  Criscitiello,Arnold A., MD
  Dasti,Umer R., MD
  Delfico,Anthony John, MD
  Marrinan,Randy F., MD
  Roenbeck,Kevin Meehan, MD
  Terranova,Lauren M., DO

Ridgewood Pediatrics LLC
265 Ackerman Avenue/Suite 204 Zip: 07450
Ph: (201) 444-3309 Fax: (201) 444-3349
  Dziarmaga,Ewa R., MD
  Zabek Gallegos,Joanna M., MD

Summit Medical Group Internal Medicine
127 Union Street/Suite 101 Zip: 07450
Ph: (201) 444-5200 Fax: (201) 444-2399
  Mudry,Carolyn J., DO

VMG Respiratory Health & Pulmonary
1200 East Ridgewood Avenue Zip: 07450
Ph: (201) 689-7755 Fax: (201) 689-0521
  Chakravarti,Aloke, MD
  Choy,Wanda Wai Ying, MD
  Melamed,Marc S., MD
  Salamat,Rahat, MD
  Suffin,Daniel Matthew, DO
  Tibb,Amit Singh, MD
  Vakil,Rupesh M., MD

Valley Center for Women's Health
550 North Maple Avenue/Suite 102 Zip: 07450
Ph: (201) 444-4040 Fax: (201) 444-4473
  Coven,Roger A., MD
  Gerhardt,Amy Ilene Katz, MD
  Kim,Kathlyn M., MD
  Levine,Richard Steven, MD
  Zeldina,Elina, MD

Valley Columbia Heart Center
223 North Van Dien Avenue Zip: 07450
Ph: (201) 447-8377 Fax: (201) 447-8658
  Brizzio,Mariano Ezequiel, MD
  Mindich,Bruce Paul, MD
  Zapolanski,Alex, MD

Cardiooology Ridgewood
1124 East Ridgewood Avenue Zip: 07450
Ph: (201) 689-9400 Fax: (201) 689-9404
  Dardashti,Omid A., MD

  Saporito,Robert A. Jr., MD
  Simon,Alan David, MD
  Strain,Janet E., MD

VMG Colorectal Surgery
1124 East Ridgewood Avenue/Suite 202 Zip: 07450
Ph: (201) 689-9100 Fax: (201) 689-9108
  Nizin,Joel S., MD

Valley Medical Group-Electrophysiology
970 Linwood Avenue/Suite 102 Zip: 07450
Ph: (201) 432-7837 Fax: (201) 432-7830
  Musat,Dan Laurentiu, MD
  Sichrovsky,Tina Claudia, MD

Valley Medical Group-Electrophysiology
223 North Van Dien Avenue Zip: 07450
Ph: (201) 432-7837 Fax: (201) 432-7830
  Bhatt,Advay G., MD
  Mittal,Suneet, MD
  Preminger,Mark William, MD

Valley Medical Group-Endocrinology
947 Linwood Avenue Zip: 07450
Ph: (201) 444-5552 Fax: (201) 444-4490
  Boyd-Woschinko,Gillian Susanne, MD
  Cobin,Rhoda Harriet, MD
  Kelman,Adam Scott, MD
  Lee,Esther Jeehae, MD
  Narwani,Vanessa Deepak, MD

Valley Med Group/Valley Heart Group
1200 East Ridgewood Avenue Zip: 07450
Ph: (201) 670-8660 Fax: (201) 447-1957
  Burke,Benita Mia, MD
  Frankel,Zev Binyamin, MD
  Goldschmidt,Howard Z., MD
  Mansson,Sarah Jane Deleon, DO
  Reison,Dennis S., MD
  Sotsky,Gerald, MD
  Sotsky,Mark I., MD
  Weiser,Mitchell M., MD

William D. Becker MD and Associates
589 Franklin Turnpike/Suite 11 Zip: 07450
Ph: (201) 670-4075
  Becker,William D., MD

Ringwood

Drs. Raouf and Balboul
55 Skyline Drive/Suite 204 Zip: 07456
Ph: (973) 962-4000 Fax: (973) 962-0640
  Raouf,Medhat M., MD

Ringwood Medical Associates PA
52 Skyline Drive Zip: 07456
Ph: (973) 962-6200 Fax: (973) 962-0046
  Rametta,Mark J., DO

Rio Grande

Cape Radiology
4011 Route 9 South/PO Box 244 Zip: 08242
Ph: (609) 886-0100
  McAllister,John Daniel II, MD
  Panico,Robert A., MD
  Toloui,Gerald J., MD
  Werman,Richard Evan, DO

River Edge

Bergen Ob-Gyn Associates, PA
130 Kinderkamack Road/Suite 300 Zip: 07661
Ph: (201) 489-2727 Fax: (201) 489-5040
  Bingham,Jemel M., MD
  Cho,Linda M., MD
  Clachko,Marc A., MD
  Parnes,Cindy R., MD

Hackensack Gastroenterology Assoc
130 Kinderkamack Road/Suite 301 Zip: 07661
Ph: (201) 489-7772 Fax: (201) 489-2544
  Chhada,Aditi, MD
  Leibowitz,Steven R., MD
  Lin,Richard M., MD
  Mammen,Anish George, MD
  Nikias,George Andrew, MD
  Rosendorf,Eric Robert, MD
  Shin,Dongwuk, MD

Ravits Margaret MD & Associates
130 Kinderkamack Road/Suite 205 Zip: 07661
Ph: (201) 692-0800 Fax: (201) 488-1582
  Blanco,Fiona Rose Pasternack, MD
  Lin,Richie L., MD
  Trinh,Diem Thi, MD

Riverside Oral Surgery
130 Kinderkamack Road/Suite 204 Zip: 07661
Ph: (201) 487-6565
  Auerbach,Jason M, MD
  Cho,Sung Hee, MD

Riverdale

Allergy and Asthma Specialists
51 State Route 23 Zip: 07457
Ph: (973) 831-5799 Fax: (973) 831-7422
  Gold,Ruth Leah, MD

Drs. Bogusz & Weiss
44 State Route 23 North/Suite 6 Zip: 07457
Ph: (973) 248-9199 Fax: (973) 248-9299
  Bogusz,Katie L., MD
  Freiss,Rebecca, MD
  Patel,Sheenal V., MD
  Weiss,Jeffrey Gregg, MD

ENT and Facial Plastic Surgeons
51 Route 23 South/2nd Floor Zip: 07457
Ph: (973) 831-1220 Fax: (973) 831-0029
  Ginsburg,Jeffrey B., MD
  Levine,Jonathan Marc, MD
  Remsen,Kenneth A., MD
  Taylor,Howard, MD

The Dermatology Group, P.C.
44 Route 23 North/Suite 213 Zip: 07457
Ph: (973) 571-2121 Fax: (973) 839-5751
  Son,Chang Bae, MD

Valley Health Medical Group
72 Hamburg Turnpike Zip: 07457
Ph: (973) 835-7290 Fax: (973) 835-0696
  Ardito,Michael F., MD
  Howe,Michele Margaret, DO
  Romain,Sharon L., DO
  Visconti,Raymond Jr., MD

Riverton

Riverton Family Practice
605 Main Street/Suite 104 Zip: 08077
Ph: (856) 786-1717 Fax: (856) 786-2478
  Burke,Margaret Linda, MD

Robbinsville

After Hours Family Care
1001 Washington Boulevard Zip: 08691
Ph: (609) 249-9000
  Chowdhury,Shikha, MD
  Reger,Donna Pidane, MD

Becker ENT
One Union Street/Suite 203 Zip: 08691
Ph: (609) 436-5740 Fax: (609) 436-5741
  Edwards,Kathryn Payne, MD
  McCullough,Aubrey Susan, DO
  Mignone,Robert, DO

Mercer Bucks Cardiology
One Union Street/Suite 101 Zip: 08691
Ph: (609) 890-6677 Fax: (609) 890-7292
  Agarwal,Ashish Madanlal, MD
  Barn,Kulpreet S., MD
  Gala,Ketan M., MD
  Patel,Jigar A., MD
  Rothstein,Neil M., MD
  Samuel,Steven Alan, MD
  Singhal,Shalabh, MD
  Soffer,Mark Jay, MD
  Wolf,Andreas, MD

Rednor-Risi Family Med Assoc
1 Washington Boulevard/Suite A Zip: 08691
Ph: (609) 448-4353 Fax: (609) 448-4558
  Rednor,Jeffrey D., DO
  Risi,Mark G., DO

Rochelle Park

Diagnostic Imaging Ctr & Group Pract
251 Rochelle Avenue Zip: 07662
Ph: (201) 291-8800 Fax: (201) 291-1619
  Conte,Stephen John, DO
  Galope,Roel Pangilinan, DO

  Meyerson,Steven Jeffrey, MD

Drs. Di Vagno, Hasan & Chung
216 Route 17 North/Suite 201 Zip: 07662
Ph: (201) 845-3535 Fax: (201) 845-4040
  Chung,Jaehoon, MD
  Di Vagno,Leonardo Joseph, MD
  Hasan,Omar S., MD

Pedimedica, P.A.
18 Railroad Avenue/Suite 103 Zip: 07662
Ph: (201) 291-2323 Fax: (201) 291-2328
  Bhatty,Anis A., MD
  Bruno,Basil, MD
  Kraut,Evelyn S., MD

Psychiatric Associates
218 State Route 17 North/Suite 13 Zip: 07662
Ph: (201) 488-6543
  Acquaviva,Joseph F., MD
  Flood,Mark J., MD
  Korshunova,Valeria S., MD

Redi-Med
186 Rochelle Avenue/Suite 2-A Zip: 07662
Ph: (201) 368-3384 Fax: (201) 587-0300
  Keshishian,Paul, DO

Rochelle Park Cardiac Center
186 Rochelle Avenue Zip: 07662
Ph: (201) 556-1225 Fax: (201) 556-1101
  Clifford,James R., MD

Rochelle Park Medical Center PA
96 Park Way Zip: 07662
Ph: (201) 291-1010 Fax: (201) 587-0313
  Imbornone,Peter J., MD
  Pascarelli,Todd D., MD

Rockaway

Central Morris Neurology
170 East Main Street/Suite 6 Zip: 07866
Ph: (973) 625-8888 Fax: (973) 625-7877
  Bongiovanni,Denise A., DO
  Tonzola,Richard F., MD

North Jersey Dermatology Center
35 Green Pond Road Zip: 07866
Ph: (973) 625-0600 Fax: (973) 625-0336
  Aspen,Otter Q., MD
  Masessa,Joseph M., MD

Rockaway Family Medical Assoc
333 Mount Hope Avenue Zip: 07866
Ph: (973) 895-6601 Fax: (973) 895-5324
  Annavajjula,Madhavi L., MD
  Barth,Michael, MD
  Brodrick,Ian B., MD
  Heitzman,Christopher James, DO
  Sharma,Aadya, MD
  Ziegler,Brenda L., DO

Roebling

Lourdes Medical Associates
501 Delaware Avenue/Suite 1 Zip: 08554
Ph: (609) 291-5560 Fax: (609) 499-0435
  Manser,Harry Jr., DO
  Rappaport,Brandi Joy, MD

Roseland

Inst of Ophthalmology & Visual Science
556 Eagle Rock Avenue/Suite 206 Zip: 07068
Ph: (973) 228-2771 Fax: (973) 228-7477
  Karmaker,Shekhar Chandra, MD
  Zhao,Lin, MD

Roseland Pediatrics
556 Eagle Rock Avenue/Suite 106 Zip: 07068
Ph: (973) 228-9190
  Anello,Tiziana, MD
  Makhlouf,Jean, MD

Roselle

Drs. Viswanathan, Shakir & Patel
815 Baltimore Avenue Zip: 07203
Ph: (908) 245-3446 Fax: (908) 245-9265
  Patel,Naishami, DO
  Shakir,Aarefa H., MD
  Viswanathan,Anjali, MD

Groups and Clinics by Town with Physician Rosters

Roselle Park

Associated ENT Physicians
505 Chestnut Street Zip: 07204
Ph: (908) 241-0200 Fax: (908) 241-0445
 Bastianelli,Milo, DO
 Conte,Louis J., DO
 Mazzoni,Thomas F., DO
 Scharf,Richard C., DO
 West,Gerald, DO

Drs. Kurz and Rodriguez
318 East Westfield Ave Zip: 07204
Ph: (908) 245-2229 Fax: (908) 245-2384
 Rodriguez,Ricardo Esteban, MD

Drs. Maglaras and Brescia
236 East Westfield Avenue Zip: 07204
Ph: (908) 245-8222 Fax: (908) 245-6504
 Brescia,Michael Louis, MD
 Maglaras,Nicholas C., MD

Roselle Park Medical Assocs
744 Galloping Hill Road Zip: 07204
Ph: (908) 241-0044 Fax: (908) 241-0526
 Caggia,Josephine, DO
 Morandi,Michele Meehan, DO
 Solomon,Robert B., MD

Roselle Park Primary Care
318 Chestnut Street Zip: 07204
Ph: (908) 241-4200
 Leff,Stuart J., DO
 Saraceno,Leonardo, MD
 Saraceno,Libero, MD

Rutherford

Advanced Neurosurgery Associates
201 Route 17 North/Suite 501 Zip: 07070
Ph: (201) 457-0044 Fax: (201) 457-0049
 Daniels,Lawrence B., MD
 El Khashab,Mostafa A. F., MD
 Fried,Arno H., MD
 Rathmann,Allison Marie, DO

Broad Street Medical Associates
201 Route 17/Floor 11 Zip: 07070
Ph: (973) 471-8850 Fax: (973) 471-5232
 Sabogal,Jose Luis, MD

Drs. Sheikh & Weber
201 Route 17 North Zip: 07070
Ph: (201) 549-8860 Fax: (201) 549-8861
 Hashem,Jenifer, MD
 Sheikh,Emran Salahuddin, MD
 Weber,Renata Vanja, MD

Gastroenterology Associates of NJ
71 Union Avenue/Suite 201 Zip: 07070
Ph: (201) 842-0020 Fax: (201) 842-0010
 Roth,Joseph M., MD
 Ruiz,Frank, MD
 Zierer,Kenneth G., MD

New Jersey Physicians, LLC.
128 Union Avenue/Suite 2A Zip: 07070
Ph: (201) 939-8834 Fax: (201) 939-7644
 Chava,Padma, MD
 Isralowitz,David L., MD

New Jersey Spine & Sports Medicine
84 Orient Way Zip: 07070
Ph: (201) 964-0200 Fax: (201) 964-0220
 Brady,Robert David, DO
 Filion,Dean Thomas, DO

Pro Form Sports Med & Wellness Assocs
201 Route 17 North Zip: 07070
Ph: (201) 549-8846 Fax: (201) 549-8899
 Morales,Fabian Victor, MD

Rutherford Pediatrics
338 Union Avenue/Suite 2 Zip: 07070
Ph: (201) 842-0501 Fax: (201) 842-9190
 Becz,Grace E., MD
 Huang,Doris Amy, MD

Samuel HS The MD, PA
130 Orient Way/Suite BB Zip: 07070
Ph: (201) 438-6916 Fax: (201) 438-4227
 The,Andrew Hong-Siang, MD
 The,Samuel H., MD

The Family Center for Otolaryngology
47 Orient Way/Lower Level Zip: 07070
Ph: (201) 935-5508 Fax: (201) 465-6088
 Hassan,Sherif A., MD
 Katz,Michael Jonathan, MD
 Mahmoud,Ahmad F., MD
 Nozad,Cyrus H., MD
 Sarti,Edward J., MD
 Sarti,Evan Edward, DO
 Zozzaro,Michael A., MD

Women's Center For OB/GYN
21 East Park Place Zip: 07070
Ph: (201) 438-7780
 Chait,Anita Irani, MD
 Irani,Bakhtaver A., MD

Saddle Brook

Bergen Ambulatory Surgery Center
190 Midland Avenue Zip: 07663
Ph: (973) 405-6888
 Kosiborod,Roman, DO
 Sauchelli,Francis C., MD

Drs. Silverman and Silverman
480 Market Street Zip: 07663
Ph: (201) 845-4048
 Miranda,Claudia Danitza, MD
 Silverman,Mathew Joshua, DO
 Silverman,Philip, DO

Drs. Wiener & Pagano
299 Market Street Zip: 07663
Ph: (201) 368-1717
 Pagano,Francesco P., DO
 Wiener,Michael I., DO

Saddle Brook Medical Center
449 Market Street/Suite B Zip: 07663
Ph: (201) 712-7900 Fax: (201) 712-7902
 Kollar,John C., DO
 Sullivan,Edwin J., DO
 Tantawi,Mahnaz Chand, MD

The Heart Care Center
38 Mayhill Street/Suite 1 Zip: 07663
Ph: (201) 843-1019
 Patel,Sanjeev N., MD
 Salerno,William D., MD

Saddle River

Allergy and Asthma Specialists
82 East Allendale Road/Suite 7-B Zip: 07458
Ph: (201) 236-8282 Fax: (201) 236-0138
 Silverstein,Leonard, MD

Saddle River Medical Group
82 East Allendale Road/Suite 3-A Zip: 07458
Ph: (201) 825-3933 Fax: (201) 236-1460
 Becker,Alyssa Gelmann, MD
 Kasper,Andrew, MD
 Kasper,Joseph E., MD
 Kasper,Michael E., MD

Salem

Drs. Schmelzer & Caruso
4 Bypass Road/Suite 104 Zip: 08079
Ph: (856) 983-4646 Fax: (856) 983-4760
 Caruso,Meghan Murphy-Schmelze, DO
 Schmelzer,John F., DO

Salem Medical Group
4 Bypass Road/Suite 101 Zip: 08079
Ph: (856) 935-3582 Fax: (856) 935-4382
 Berman,Barry M., MD
 Kouyoumdji,Paul R., MD
 Timmerman,Lori D., DO

Southern Jersey Family Medical
238 East Broadway Zip: 08079
Ph: (856) 935-7711 Fax: (856) 935-2193
 Akinruli,Omowunmi Praise, MD
 Harris,Timothy Wayne, DO
 McLane,Rebecca, MD
 Wang,Shuang, MD

Scotch Plains

Complete Care
1814 East Second Street Zip: 07076
Ph: (908) 322-6611 Fax: (908) 322-8665
 Hasan,Izhar U., MD
 Leopold,Clayton E., MD
 Schaller,Richard J., MD
 Silberman,Marc Richard, MD

Medical Diagnostic Associates, P.A.
1801 East Second Street/Suite 1 Zip: 07076
Ph: (908) 322-7786 Fax: (908) 322-0191
 Delio,Constance Mary, MD
 Hernandez,Alyssa Kate, MD
 Lomnitz,Esteban R., MD
 Stanzione,Steven, MD

Sea Girt

Change of Heart Cardiology
2130 Highway 35/Building C Suite 321 Zip: 08750
Ph: (732) 974-6700 Fax: (732) 974-6707
 Eisenberg,Scott R., DO
 Hynes,Peter James, MD
 Kayser,Robert Granville Jr., MD

Doctors Halas & Lutz
2130 Highway 35/Suite 214 Zip: 08750
Ph: (732) 974-0228 Fax: (732) 974-7458
 Halas,Francis P. Jr., MD
 Lutz,Mary B., MD

Drs. Neuman & Dambeck
700 Highway 71/Suite 2 Zip: 08750
Ph: (732) 974-8100 Fax: (732) 974-9125
 Dambeck,Michael D., DO
 Neuman,Steven Scott, MD

Meridian Medical Group
2130 Route 35/Suite B216 Zip: 08750
Ph: (732) 974-0228 Fax: (732) 263-7938
 Fury,Mary Anne, DO
 Plaine,Suzanne E., DO

Seaview Medical Associates
511 Sea Girt Avenue Zip: 08750
Ph: (732) 282-9000 Fax: (732) 282-9144
 Bersalona,Holly Abate, MD
 Bersalona,Louis Michael, MD

Shore Medical Group
2130 Highway 35/Suite 213B Zip: 08750
Ph: (732) 974-8668
 Lin,Ying, MD
 Young,Patricia A., MD

Wall Family Medical
2130 Highway 35/Building C Suite 324 Zip: 08750
Ph: (732) 974-1980 Fax: (732) 974-2117
 Micallef,Donald M., MD
 Siciliano,Janice M., DO

Secaucus

Care Station Medical Group
210 Meadowlands Parkway Zip: 07094
Ph: (201) 348-3636 Fax: (201) 583-0713
 Paroulek,George Jiri, MD

Dr. De La Cruz and Dhalla
714 Tenth Street Zip: 07094
Ph: (201) 865-2050 Fax: (201) 865-0015
 Dhalla,Sameer, MD
 Mathew,Jocelyn, MD

Drs. Castillo and Castillo
39 2nd Avenue Zip: 07094
Ph: (201) 617-1996
 Castillo,Rodrigo I., MD

New Jersey Urology Assocs
110 Meadowlands Parkway Zip: 07094
Ph: (201) 867-1297 Fax: (201) 867-4165
 DiBella,Louis J. Jr., MD
 Tanzer,Ira D., MD

Riverside Medical Group
714 Tenth Street/Suite 2 Zip: 07094
Ph: (201) 863-3346 Fax: (201) 865-0015
 Al Haddawi,Anwar, MD
 Ali,Tahera, MD
 Anam,Khalid Sadrul, MD
 Baker,Azzam A., MD
 Bansil,Noel Lumanog, MD
 Ben,Sheeba, MD
 Bokhari,Naimat U., MD
 Cave,Marie, MD
 Doss,Nermine N., MD
 Farag,Magdy M., MD
 George,Malini Susan, MD
 Ghayal,Payal Patel, MD
 Hussain,Zaheda M., MD

Riverside Medical Group
710 Tenth Street Zip: 07094
Ph: (201) 865-2050 Fax: (201) 865-0015
 Jadun,Wamiq, MD
 Jawaharani,Shobha, MD
 Jedlinski,Zbigniew J., MD
 John,Jeanie Elizabeth, MD
 Katikaneni,Swapna, MD
 Mirani,Gayatri, MD
 Moshet,Osama Mohamed, MD
 Mucha,Samantha Agatha, DO
 Niyogi,Sayani, DO
 Parikh,Chaula A., MD
 Raju,Rina M., MD
 Reitzen-Bastidas,Shari D., MD
 Williams,Celia, DO
 Win,Sithu, MD
 Wosu,Carolee Ngozi, MD

Riverside Pediatrics
714 Tenth Street Zip: 07094
Ph: (551) 257-7038 Fax: (201) 552-2358
 De Melo,Mauricio Garret, MD
 Gatla,Nandita, MD
 Sitt,Hal, MD

Sewell

Addiction Pain Associates
100 Kings Way East/Suite D-3 Zip: 08080
Ph: (856) 589-1440 Fax: (856) 589-4616
 Pettis,Larry, DO
 Zimmerman,Daniel J., MD

Advanced Dermatology, P.C.
570 Egg Harbor Road/Suite C-1 Zip: 08080
Ph: (856) 256-8899 Fax: (856) 256-8868
 Choi,Catherine Helen, MD
 Li,Kehua, MD

Advanced ENT - Washington Township
239 Hurffville Crosskeys Road Zip: 08080
Ph: (856) 602-4000 Fax: (856) 629-3391
 Bresalier,Howard J., DO
 Friedel,Mark Erik, MD

Advocare Laurel Pediatrics
269 Fish Pond Road Zip: 08080
Ph: (856) 863-9999 Fax: (856) 863-9666
 Backal,Marc Ira, MD
 Bruner,David Glenn, MD
 Burke,Meghan Deirdre, MD
 Del Moro,Ellen C., MD
 Fiderer,Stefanie C., DO
 Kabel-Kotler,Caroline, DO
 Pasternak,Jared A., MD

Advocare Township Pediatrics
123 Egg Harbor Road Zip: 08080
Ph: (856) 227-5437 Fax: (856) 227-5890
 Collazo,Edgar R., MD
 Desai,Renuka D., MD

Becker Nose & Sinus Center, LLC.
570 Egg Harbor Road Zip: 08080
Ph: (856) 589-6673 Fax: (856) 589-3443
 Becker,Daniel G., MD
 Gregory,Naomi D., DO
 Rosenstein,Kenneth Michael, MD

Cardiovascular Associates
570 Egg Harbor Road/Suite B-1 Zip: 08080
Ph: (856) 582-2000 Fax: (856) 582-2061
 Tarditi,Daniel John, DO

Carlos A. Obregon, D.O., P.C.
100A Kings Way West Zip: 08080
Ph: (856) 218-8080 Fax: (856) 218-8070
 Ferroni,Bryan R., DO
 Obregon,Carlos A., DO

Center For Eye Care
123 Egg Harbor Road/Suite 300 Zip: 08080
Ph: (856) 290-4548 Fax: (856) 290-4552
 Girgis,Raymond Michael, MD
 Nyquist,Susan Shoshana, MD

Comprehensive Cancer & Hematolgy
900 Medical Center Drive/Suite 200 Zip: 08080
Ph: (856) 582-0550 Fax: (856) 582-7640
 Lindenberg,Noah L., MD
 Poretta,Trina A., MD

Cooper OB/GYN
4 Plaza Drive/Suite 403/Bunker Hill Pl Zip: 08080
Ph: (856) 270-4020 Fax: (856) 270-4022
 Franzblau,Natali R., MD
 Iavicoli,Michelle A., MD
 Sehdev,Michele S., MD

Cooper Orthopaedics
2 Plaza Drive/Suite 202 Zip: 08080
Ph: (856) 270-4150 Fax: (856) 270-4012
 Behnam,Amir Babak, MD
 Fahey,Ann Leilani, MD

Groups and Clinics by Town with Physician Rosters

Cooper Physicians Washington Township
1 Plaza Drive/Suite 103/Bunker Hill Pl Zip: 08080
Ph: (856) 270-4080 Fax: (856) 270-4085
- Bulei, Anita P., MD
- Datwani, Neeta D., MD
- Glenn, Danette, MD
- Ranieri, Joseph N., DO
- Salieb, Lorraine O., MD

Delaware Valley Urology LLC
570 Egg Harbor Road/Suite A-1 Zip: 08080
Ph: (856) 582-9645 Fax: (856) 985-4583
- Barsky, Robert I., DO
- Brown, Gordon Andrew, DO
- Pietras, Jerome R., DO

Dermatology Ctr of Washington TWSP
100 Kings Way East/Suite A-3 Zip: 08080
Ph: (856) 589-3331 Fax: (856) 589-3416
- Segal, Elana Tova, MD
- Winter, Jonathan M., MD

Dr. G. Lee Lerch and Associates
239 Hurffville Crosskeys Road Zip: 08080
Ph: (856) 740-4440 Fax: (856) 728-0808
- Lewitt, Diana M., DO

Drs Figueredo and Kimbaris
239 Hurffville CrossKeys Road Zip: 08080
Ph: (856) 247-7515 Fax: (856) 247-7525
- Kimbaris, James Nicholas, MD

Garden State Infectious Disease
570 Egg Harbor Road/Suite B-5 Zip: 08080
Ph: (856) 566-3190 Fax: (856) 566-1904
- Levin, Todd Philip, DO

Inspira Medical Group
660 Woodbury Glassboro Road/Suite 26 Zip: 08080
Ph: (856) 415-6868 Fax: (856) 464-1855
- Bober, Craig, DO
- Kruger, Eric N., MD

Kennedy Diagnostic & Treatment Ctr
900 Medical Center Drive/Suite 100 Zip: 08080
Ph: (856) 582-3008
- Cohen, Dane Ryan, MD
- Horowitz, Carolyn J., MD

Kennedy Family Health Center
445 Hurffville Crosskeys Road Zip: 08080
Ph: (856) 262-1900
- Bhimani, Siddharth D., MD
- Covone, Kenneth C., DO
- Tench, Mavola L., MD

Kennedy Health Alliance
900 Medical Center Drive/Suite 201 Zip: 08080
Ph: (856) 218-2100 Fax: (856) 218-2101
- Careaga, Eduardo, MD
- Fantazzio, Michele Adrienne, MD
- Gillum, Diane, MD
- Malik, Neveen A., DO
- Yoon-Flannery, Kahyun, DO

Kennedy Surgical Center
540 Egg Harbor Road Zip: 08080
Ph: (856) 218-4900
- Dougherty, Barbara D., DO
- Sorensen, Barbara J., MD

Kings Way Primary Care
100 Kings Way East/Suite D2 Zip: 08080
Ph: (844) 542-2273 Fax: (856) 218-4808
- Bariana, Christopher Michael, DO
- Bertel, James R., MD
- Monteith, Duane Richard, MD

Obstetrics & Gynecology Associates
239 Hurffville Crosskeys Road Zip: 08080
Ph: (856) 262-8300 Fax: (856) 262-1635
- Digiovanni, Marianne, DO
- Huggins, Juanita Kimberly, DO
- Richichi, Joann, DO

Partners in Primary Care
239 Hurffville Crosskeys Road Zip: 08080
Ph: (856) 881-1940
- DiRenzo, Joseph P. Jr., DO
- Ewing, Jacqueline L., DO
- Kane, Michelle Christine, DO
- Schmidt, Carol L., MD

Philadelphia Gastroenterology Group
570 Egg Harbor Road/Suite A-2 Zip: 08080
Ph: (856) 218-1410 Fax: (856) 218-0193
- Borowsky, Larry M., MD
- Gambescia, Richard Alan, MD
- Gardner, Beth C., MD
- Myers, Scott Elliot, MD

Reconstructive Orthopedics, P.A.
570 Egg Harbor Road/Suite C-4 Zip: 08080
Ph: (609) 267-9400 Fax: (609) 267-9457
- Khanna, Malini M., MD
- Kovacs, Jeffrey Peter, DO
- Lopresti, David A., MD
- Marcelli, Enrico A., DO
- Mariani, John K., DO
- Murray, Jeffrey, DO

Rowan SOM Department of OB/GYN
405 Hurffville-Cross Keys Road Zip: 08080
Ph: (856) 589-1414 Fax: (856) 256-5772
- Bramble, Charlene A., MD
- Chhibber, Geeta, MD
- Hummel, Jennifer E., DO
- Janeczek, Susan, DO
- Krieg, Karen Sue, DO
- Nguyen, Maria Bich Thi, DO
- Salerno, Anthony P., MD
- Vogiatzidakis, Sophia I., DO
- Williams, Keith Patrick, MD

South Jersey Heart Group
539 Egg Harbor Road/Suite 1 Zip: 08080
Ph: (856) 589-0300 Fax: (856) 589-1753
- Bagaria, Surendra K., MD
- Crasner, Joshua M., DO
- Maiese, Mario L., DO
- Weinberg, Howard M., DO

South Jersey Laser Vision
101A Kingsway West Zip: 08080
Ph: (856) 582-9507 Fax: (856) 582-4472
- Heist, Kenneth C., DO
- Ringel, David M., DO

South Jersey Radiology Associates
Severan Profess Mews/Suite 105 Zip: 08080
Ph: (856) 848-4998 Fax: (856) 589-6142
- Desai, Anil G., MD

South Jersey Sports Medicine Center
556 Egg Harbor Road/Suite A Zip: 08080
Ph: (856) 589-0650 Fax: (856) 589-2720
- Falconiero, Robert Paul, DO
- Lisko, Trina M., DO
- Valentino, Steven John, DO

St. Chris Care at Washington Township
405 Hurffville-Cross Keys Road Zip: 08080
Ph: (856) 582-0644 Fax: (856) 582-0622
- Arthur, Kiersten Westrol, MD
- Ge, Shuping, MD
- Madan, Nandini, MD
- O'Neill, Anna M., MD
- Simmers, Richard C., DO
- Steckler, Robert E., MD

The University Doctors - UMDNJ-SOM
570 Egg Harbor Road/Suite C-2 Zip: 08080
Ph: (856) 218-0300 Fax: (856) 589-5082
- Bierman, Edward W., MD
- Boyd, Linda, DO
- Kaari, Jacqueline Marie, DO
- Leber, Sandra Lynn, DO
- Richmond, Chad Eric, DO
- Vermeulen, Meagan Wega, MD

University Doctors
570 Egg Harbor Road/Suite C-2 Zip: 08080
Ph: (856) 589-1414 Fax: (856) 589-9487
- Ayres, Ronald E., MD
- Caudle, Jennifer Nicole, DO

University Pediatrics
405 Hurffville Crosskeys Road Zip: 08080
Ph: (856) 582-0033 Fax: (856) 582-2305
- Cook, Wendy S., DO

Virtua Family Med-Washington Township
239 Hurffville Crosskeys Road Zip: 08080
Ph: (856) 341-8181 Fax: (856) 881-2071
- Beppel, Elaine B., MD
- Cohen, Andrew Geoffrey, MD
- Desimone, Alexandra, MD
- Sekel, James James, DO
- Singh, Jyotsana, MD

Virtua Immediate Care Center
239 Hurffville Crosskeys Road Zip: 08080
Ph: (856) 341-8200 Fax: (856) 341-8215
- Williams, Edwin Rae, MD

Washington Medical, P.A.
100 Heritage Valley Drive/Suite 2 Zip: 08080
Ph: (856) 582-6100 Fax: (856) 582-0397
- Ashby, John Wilson, MD
- Labaczewski, Robert J., DO
- Laganella, Dominic J., DO

Washington Township Thoracic Surgery
400 Medical Center Drive/Suite F Zip: 08080
Ph: (856) 716-6598 Fax: (856) 716-6659
- Steinberg, Jay Mitchell, MD

Wedgewood Family Practice Assoc
302 Hurffville Cross-Keys Road Zip: 08080
Ph: (856) 589-4610 Fax: (609) 589-1624
- Dibona, Anthony D. Jr., DO
- Leshner, Stanley B., DO
- Urkowitz, Alan L., DO

Ship Bottom

Island Medical Prof Assoc
1812 Long Beach Boulevard Zip: 08008
Ph: (609) 494-2323
- Larkin, Harry Jr., MD
- Prosperi, Paul William, DO
- Suddeth, James N., MD

Short Hills

Just For Kids
8 Meadowbrook Road Zip: 07078
Ph: (973) 376-5430 Fax: (973) 376-5430
- Lomax, Kathleen Graham, MD

Summit Medical Group
85 Woodland Road Zip: 07078
Ph: (973) 379-4496 Fax: (973) 921-0669
- Blaustein, Howard Stuart, MD
- Diaz, Julio C., MD
- Gurey Wasserstein, Allison P., MD
- Jani, Beena Harendra, MD
- Mehra, Sweeti, MD
- Nalitt, Beth R., MD
- Tansey, William Austin III, MD

Shrewsbury

Atlantic Pediatric Orthopedics
1131 Broad Street/Suite 202 Zip: 07702
Ph: (732) 544-9000 Fax: (732) 544-9099
- Curatolo, Evan M., MD
- Plakas, Christos, MD
- Stankovits, Lawrence Matthew, MD

Booker Behavioral Health Center
661 Shrewsbury Avenue Zip: 07702
Ph: (732) 345-3400 Fax: (732) 345-3401
- Alcera, Eric Cortez, MD

Damien Fertility Partners
655 Shrewsbury Avenue/Suite 300 Zip: 07702
Ph: (732) 758-6511 Fax: (732) 758-1048
- Damien, Miguel, MD
- Holden, Emily C., MD
- Seungdamrong, Aimee Malunda, MD

Drs. Barrows and Ostrow
180 Avenue at the Common/Suite 7B Zip: 07702
Ph: (732) 935-7143 Fax: (732) 935-7245
- Barrows, Frank P. IV, DO
- Novello, Laura Joyce, MD
- Ostrow, Vlady, DO

ENT and Allergy Associates
1131 Broad Street/Suite 103 Building A Zip: 07702
Ph: (732) 389-3388 Fax: (732) 389-3589
- Passalaqua, Philip Jude, MD
- Prabhat, Arvind, MD
- Shah, Darsit, MD

- Szema, Katherine Fang, MD
- Tavill, Michael A., MD

IMA Medical Care Center
30 Shrewsbury Plaza Zip: 07702
Ph: (732) 542-0002 Fax: (732) 542-2992
- Bhoori, Nafisa Y., MD
- Graham, Daniel, DO
- Jafry, Yasmeen, MD
- Miller, Charles Luther, MD
- Saeed, Shamim Jan, MD
- Valko, Peter C., MD

Integrated Medicine Alliance, P.A.
30 Shrewsbury Plaza Zip: 07702
Ph: (732) 460-9840 Fax: (732) 460-9848
- Huegel, Claudia Marie, MD
- Johnston, Christopher K., MD

Metzger Pain Management
170 Avenue At The Commons/Suite 6 Zip: 07702
Ph: (732) 380-0200 Fax: (732) 380-0124
- Patel, Bimal, DO
- Sondhi, Nidhi, DO

Ob-Gyn Assocs/Holmdel-Shrewsbury
39 Avenue of the Commons Zip: 07702
Ph: (732) 389-0003
- Witkowski, Mary E., MD

Premier Pain Center
160 Avenue at the Commons/Suite 1 Zip: 07702
Ph: (732) 380-0200 Fax: (732) 380-0124
- Li, Sean, MD
- Metzger, Scott E., MD
- Sahoo, Aruna, MD
- Staats, Peter Sean, MD
- Walia, Kulbir Singh, MD

Shore Heart Group, PA
179 Avenue at the Commons/Suite 102 Zip: 07702
Ph: (732) 542-7655 Fax: (732) 542-7600
- Edlin, Dale E., MD

Shrewsbury Surgery Center
655 Shrewsbury Avenue Zip: 07702
Ph: (732) 450-6000 Fax: (732) 450-6010
- Kutzin, Theodore E., MD
- Schaaff, Robert P., MD
- Wood, Sterling Harbert, DO

Shrewsbury Surgical Associates
655 Shrewsbury Avenue/Suite 210 Zip: 07702
Ph: (732) 542-8118
- Brock, James Steven, MD
- Cauda, Joseph E., MD

Spine & Pain Centers
655 Shrewbury Avenue/Suite 202 Zip: 07702
Ph: (732) 345-1180 Fax: (732) 530-4476
- Cresanti-Daknis, Charles Brian, MD

TLC Pediatrics
20 White Road/Suite D Zip: 07702
Ph: (732) 741-3400
- Appulingam, Anbuchelvi, MD
- O'Brien, Debra Ann, MD

The Plastic Surgery Ctr of NJ & Manhat
535 Sycamore Avenue Zip: 07702
Ph: (732) 741-0970 Fax: (732) 747-2606
- Abdollahi, Hamid, MD
- Ashinoff, Russell Lee, MD
- Ashraf, Azra Abida, MD
- Boucree, Thaddeus Stanice, MD
- Chang, Eric I-Yun, MD
- Elkwood, Andrew I., MD
- Ibrahim, Zuhaib, MD
- Kaufman, Matthew Roy, MD
- Patel, Tushar R., MD
- Rose, Michael Ian, MD
- Schneider, Lisa Frances, MD
- Wimmers, Eric Geoffrey, MD

Groups and Clinics by Town with Physician Rosters

/Shrewsbury (cont)
Urology Associates, P.A.
595 Shrewsbury Avenue/Suite 103 Zip: 07702
Ph: (732) 741-5923 Fax: (732) 741-2759
- Bickerton, Michael W., MD
- Bonitz, Robert Paul Jr., MD
- Christiano, Arthur Patrick, MD
- Rose, John G., MD
- Smith, Robert Charles, MD

Sicklerville
Advocare Kressville Pedi Sicklerville
431 Sicklerville Road Zip: 08081
Ph: (856) 875-7444 Fax: (856) 875-4042
- Hill-Hugh, Naomi Lynette, MD

Advocare Magness-Stafford Ob-Gyn Assoc
802 Liberty Place Zip: 08081
Ph: (856) 740-4400 Fax: (856) 740-4411
- Magness, Rose L., MD
- Stafford, Patricia T., MD

Advocare Sicklerville Internal Med
485 Williamstown Road Zip: 08081
Ph: (856) 237-8100 Fax: (856) 237-8042
- Aitken, Robert J., DO
- Holgado, Maynard R., MD
- Palladino, Nicholas G., MD
- Pieretti, Gordon Anthony, DO

Cross Keys Urgent Care
627-B Cross Keys Road Zip: 08081
Ph: (856) 728-8700 Fax: (856) 318-1374
- Morone, Teresa Monica, DO

Crosskeys Medical Center
600 Berlin-Crosskeys Road/Unit 102 Zip: 08081
Ph: (856) 875-5152 Fax: (856) 875-0313
- Patel, Indubhai Manibhai, MD
- Patel, Prahlad M., MD

Kennedy Health Alliance
1300 Liberty Place Zip: 08081
Ph: (856) 262-8100 Fax: (856) 885-6859
- Mingroni, Julius Anthony, DO
- Ubele, Deborah Anne, DO

Patient First
606 Cross Keys Road Zip: 08081
Ph: (856) 237-1016
- Cox, Trevor E., DO
- Samuels, Elizabeth E., DO
- Simon, Shari Kim, DO
- Soper, Robert Earl, DO

Winslow Primary Care Associates, PC
524 Williamstown Road/Suite A Zip: 08081
Ph: (856) 728-1181 Fax: (856) 728-1182
- De Maria, Nicholas Anthony, MD
- Sharp, Harry Walton, DO

Skillman
Plastic Surgery Arts of of New Jersey
1378 US 206/2nd flr Zip: 08558
Ph: (609) 921-2922 Fax: (609) 921-0747
- Nini, Kevin T., MD

Princeton Allergy & Asthma Assocs
24 Vreeland Drive Zip: 08558
Ph: (609) 921-2202 Fax: (609) 924-1468
- Caucino, Julie A., DO
- Pedinoff, Andrew J., MD
- Rao, Jayanti Juluru, MD
- Shah, Shaili Niranjan, MD
- Sikorski, Kristen Melissa, MD
- Skolnick, Helen Sharlene, MD
- Southern, Darrell Loren, MD

Somerdale
Kennedy Family Health Services
1 Somerdale Square Zip: 08083
Ph: (856) 309-7700 Fax: (856) 566-8944
- Cheng, Desmond H., DO
- Finley, Stephanie Elena, DO
- Gallagher, Joseph L. III, DO
- Penn-Becoat, Xiomara, MD
- Suarez, Melissa Lehn, DO
- White, Deborah A., DO

Somers Point
Atlantic Cape OB/GYN
829 Shore Road Zip: 08244
Ph: (609) 927-3070 Fax: (609) 927-2553
- Morgan, Daniel Robert, MD
- Perez, Finuccia Renda, MD
- Sindoni, Frank W., MD
- Zhang, Vincent, MD

Bayfront Emergency Physicians, P.A.
1 East New York Avenue Zip: 08244
Ph: (609) 653-3519 Fax: (609) 653-3247
- Angelastro, David B., MD
- Chiccarine, Anthony P., DO
- May, Roberta Russell, DO
- Talotta, Nicholas Joseph Jr., MD

Coastal Clinical Pathologists
1 East New York Avenue/PO Box 337 Zip: 08244
Ph: (609) 926-9056 Fax: (609) 926-9056
- Beach, Robert J., MD

Coastal Physicians and Surgeons
110 Harbor Lane/Suite A Zip: 08244
Ph: (609) 653-9110 Fax: (609) 927-3934
- Gery, Brian F., MD
- Glass, Andrew S., MD
- Gottfried, Maureen, DO
- Sabo, Robert A., MD

Drs. Morrow and Syed
715 Bay Avenue Zip: 08244
Ph: (609) 601-1570 Fax: (609) 601-1567
- Morrow, William J., DO

Drs. Schwartz & Nahas
631 Shore Road/PO Box 291 Zip: 08244
Ph: (609) 653-1010 Fax: (609) 653-9591
- Nahas, Frederick J., MD
- Schwartz, Jay Harris, MD

GFH Surgical Associates
718 Shore Road Zip: 08244
Ph: (609) 927-8550 Fax: (609) 926-0273
- D'Angelo-Donovan, Desiree Diane, DO
- Feinberg, Gary L., MD
- Galler, Leonard, MD
- Herrington, James William, MD

Harborview KidsFirst
505 Bay Avenue Zip: 08244
Ph: (609) 927-4235 Fax: (609) 927-5590
- Bross, George Jr., DO
- Drexler, Christopher W., DO
- Held, Sharon L., DO
- Jacobson, Mark, DO
- Keenan, Christopher Joseph, DO
- Share, Lisa J., MD
- Thorp, Andrea Rita, DO
- Vekteris, Gerald E., DO

Jersey Shore Gastroenterology
408 Bethel Road/Suite E Zip: 08244
Ph: (609) 926-3330 Fax: (609) 926-8578
- Deshpande, Nikhil, MD
- Krachman, Joel E., DO
- Krachman, Michael S., MD
- Ognibene, Lawrence G., DO
- Schwab, Kenneth S., MD

Jersey Urology Group
403 Bethel Road Zip: 08244
Ph: (609) 927-8746 Fax: (609) 601-1406
- Axilrod, Andrew Charles, MD
- Bernal, Raymond Mark, MD
- Hirsh, Andrew L., MD
- Nosseir, Sandy B., MD
- Spence, Abraham M., MD

Med for Kids
322 Shore Road Zip: 08244
Ph: (609) 927-1353
- Andrews, Roji Zacharia, MD
- Mandalapu, Padma, MD

Pace Orthopedics & Sports Medicine
547 New Road Zip: 08244
Ph: (609) 927-9200 Fax: (609) 927-1616
- Frankel, Victor R., MD
- Zuck, Glenn M., DO

Pagnani, Braga, & Kimmel Urologic
229 Shore Road Zip: 08244
Ph: (609) 653-4343 Fax: (609) 653-2060
- Braga, Gene J., MD
- Kimmel, Barry S., MD
- Pagnani, Alexander M., MD

Pavilion OB/GYN Atlanticare
443 Shore Road/Suite 101 Zip: 08244
Ph: (609) 677-7211 Fax: (609) 611-7210
- Bergen, Blair A., MD
- Ciceron, Andre, MD
- Ciceron, Asuncion V., MD
- Kaplitz, Neil H., MD

Penn Medicine Somers Point
155 Brighton Avenue/Second Floor Zip: 08244
Ph: (609) 365-3100 Fax: (609) 365-3165
- Singh, Millee, DO
- Sood, Delcine Ann, DO

Point Medical
750 Shore Road Zip: 08244
Ph: (609) 653-2101 Fax: (609) 653-2247
- Janes, Laura C., DO

Shore Hospitalists Associates
100 Medical Center Way Zip: 08244
Ph: (609) 653-3500 Fax: (609) 926-4799
- Adigun, Jennifer Olubusola, MD
- Erskine, Jennifer Grantham, MD
- Joshi, Rachna B., MD
- Yangala, Sridevi, MD
- Yankovitch, Pierre, MD

Shore Orthopedic Univ Associates
24 Macarthur Boulevard/First Floor Zip: 08244
Ph: (609) 927-1991 Fax: (609) 927-4203
- Alber, George C., MD
- Barrett, Thomas Arthur, MD
- Dalzell, Frederick G., MD
- De Morat, Eugene John, MD
- Greene, Damon Alan, MD
- Islinger, Richard Barnard, MD
- Marczyk, Stanley C., MD
- McCloskey, John R., MD
- Zabinski, Stephen J., MD

Shore Physician Group
401 Bethel Road Zip: 08244
Ph: (609) 365-6200 Fax: (609) 365-6201
- Cadacio, Manolito G., MD
- Cilursu, Ana Maria, MD
- Geraci, Brian Anthony, MD
- Sparagna, Angelo III, MD

Shore Physicians Group
18 West New York Avenue Zip: 08244
Ph: (609) 926-1450 Fax: (609) 926-8419
- Adams, William B., DO
- Cunanan, Manuel Salas, MD
- Del Re, Sallustio, MD

Shore Physicians Group
52 East New York Avenue Zip: 08244
Ph: (609) 365-6202 Fax: (609) 653-1925
- Hooper, William Jr., MD
- O'Connor, James J. III, MD
- Roeltgen, David P., MD
- Yangala, Ravi, MD

Somers Manor Obstetrics and Gynecology
599 Shore Road/Suite 101 Zip: 08244
Ph: (609) 926-8353 Fax: (609) 926-4579
- Bravoco, Michael C., MD
- Korzeniowski, Philip A., MD
- Rezvina, Natalia Y., MD

South Jersey Infectious Disease
730 Shore Road Zip: 08244
Ph: (609) 927-6662 Fax: (609) 927-2942
- Lucasti, Christopher J., DO
- Trofa, Andrew F., MD

The Advanced Pulmonary Diagnostic Cntr
100 Medical Center Way Zip: 08244
Ph: (609) 653-3467 Fax: (609) 653-3586
- Giunta, Michael Anthony, MD
- Ojserkis, Bennett Edward, MD
- Rowe, Jeanne M., MD
- Saunders, Peter J., MD
- Teklezgi, Semhar, DO

Somerset
Advanced Surgical & Bariatrics of NJ
49 Veronica Avenue/Suite 202 Zip: 08873
Ph: (732) 640-5316 Fax: (800) 689-2361
- Donaire, Michael Jeremie, MD
- Melman, Lora Marie, MD
- Sadek, Ragui W., MD

Anesthesia Consultnts of NJ/Nova Pain
285 Davidson Avenue/Suite 204 Zip: 08873
Ph: (732) 271-1400 Fax: (732) 271-3543
- Back, Steven Marc, MD
- Baron, Jeremy Lawrence, MD
- Cabanero, Camilo O., MD
- Caces, Alan R., MD
- Cean, Daniela E., DO
- Cho, Grace C., MD
- Choi, Jieun Susana, MD
- Colavita, Richard S., MD
- Cottrill, Richard Z. Jr., MD
- Das, Sudip S., MD
- Fellenbaum, Paul, MD
- Gajewski, Jan Peter, MD
- Gangavalli, Ravi Venkata, MD
- Giacobbe, Dean Thomas, MD
- Ginsberg, Sanford Ginsberg, MD
- Gunvantlal, Desai A., MD
- Jenkins, Paul B., MD
- Kett, Attila G., MD
- Kiamzon, Harald James, MD
- Kim, Hyon S., MD
- Ku, James Chien, MD
- Land, Warren K., DO
- Lee, William, MD
- Lu, Ya-Tseng W., MD
- Mackler, Denise Lynn, MD
- Margiotta, Joseph A., MD
- Martin, Dean Walter, MD
- Mosaddeghi, Mahmood, MD
- Moses, Brett Joseph, MD
- Nath, Ajay, MD
- Pabbathi, Pramod, DO
- Patel, Ajitkumar Gunvantrai, MD
- Patel, Arti S., MD
- Patel, Samir Natavar, MD
- Peng, Hsin, MD
- Perez, Manuel A., MD
- Picone, Michael J., MD
- Rahman, Attique, MD
- Richardson, Michael J., MD
- Rodricks, Michael Baltazar, MD
- Rondel, Mikhail, MD
- Ruda, William A., MD
- Ruedy, Krista R., MD
- Shah, Samir N., MD
- Siegel, Scott S., MD
- Simon, Abraham M., DO
- Sio, Reymond Guieb, MD
- Smith, Daniel Brian J., MD
- Sonbol, Sherif A., MD
- Sperrazza, James Christopher, MD
- Tangreti, Nicholas W., MD
- Tronolone, William, MD
- Walker, John S., DO
- Yau, Assumpta K., MD

Associated Renal & Hypertension Group
7 Cedar Grove Lane/Suite 31 Zip: 08873
Ph: (732) 873-1400 Fax: (732) 960-3444
- Dadzie, Kobena A., MD
- Hakimzadeh, Parisa, DO
- Obias, Primabel Villena, MD
- Srichai, Manakan Betsy, MD

Cardio Metabolic Institute
51 Veronica Avenue Zip: 08873
Ph: (732) 846-7000 Fax: (732) 846-7001
- Baxi, Naimish, MD
- Passannante, Anthony Jr., MD
- Passannante, Anthony J. Sr, MD
- Patel, Pratik B., MD
- Shah, Chirag H., DO
- Singal, Dinesh K., MD

Cataract & Laser Institute, P.A.
1527 Route 27/Suite 2600 Zip: 08873
Ph: (732) 246-1050 Fax: (732) 846-1440
- Angrist, Richard Clay, MD

Central Jersey Internal Medicine
75 Veronica Avenue/Suite 204 Zip: 08873
Ph: (732) 828-0002 Fax: (732) 828-0153
- Jain, Deepak K., MD
- Rizvi, Tariq A., MD
- Schwartzer, Thomas A., MD
- Wang-Epstein, Christina C., MD

Digestive Disease Center of NJ
33 Clyde Road/Suite 102 Zip: 08873
Ph: (732) 873-9200 Fax: (732) 873-1699
- Aronson, Scott Logan, MD
- Ferges, Mitchell L., MD

Groups and Clinics by Town with Physician Rosters

Ferges,William James, MD
Merkel,Ira S., MD
Platovsky,Anna, MD
Rapisarda,Alexander F., MD
Drs. Fein, Porcelli & Richards
75 Veronica Avenue/Suite 201   Zip: 08873
Ph: (732) 246-4882   Fax: (732) 249-5633
Desai,Sameer P., MD
Fein,Robert P., MD
Lampert,Craig, MD
Porcelli,Marcus P., MD
Richards,David A., MD
Drs. Shamim and Shamim
1283 State Highway 27   Zip: 08873
Ph: (732) 745-9025   Fax: (732) 545-3423
Shamim,Syed Q., MD
Shamim,Tasneem F., MD
ENT & Allergy Associates
1543 Route 27/Suite 21   Zip: 08873
Ph: (732) 873-6863   Fax: (732) 873-6853
Galowitz,Stacey, DO
Sabin,Steven Lloyd, MD
Easton Med
1174 Easton Avenue   Zip: 08873
Ph: (732) 354-0159   Fax: (732) 354-0147
Kuriakose,Marykutty K., MD
Etheridge Family Medicine LLC
81 Veronica Avenue/Suite 202   Zip: 08873
Ph: (732) 246-0057   Fax: (732) 745-7070
Etheridge,Barbara Anne, MD
Tawfik,Isaac H., MD
Franklin Family Practice PA
29 Clyde Road/Suite 101   Zip: 08873
Ph: (732) 873-0330   Fax: (732) 873-2077
Compagnone,Linda, MD
Lawrence,Denise Antoinette, MD
Maziarz,Anastazja, MD
Hypertension & Nephrology Specialists
49 Veronica Avenue/Suite 104   Zip: 08873
Ph: (732) 521-0800   Fax: (732) 521-0833
Ebert,Ellen C., MD
ID Associates PA/dba ID CARE
81 Veronica Avenue/Suite 203   Zip: 08873
Ph: (732) 729-0920   Fax: (732) 729-0924
Segal,Robert Eric, MD
Kidney & Hypertension Center
23 Clyde Road/Suite 101   Zip: 08873
Ph: (732) 873-9500   Fax: (732) 873-0261
Desai,Bijal, MD
Jain,Sandesh, MD
Vaghasiya,Rick Parsotam, MD
Medigest Associates P.A.
21 Clyde Road/Suite 102   Zip: 08873
Ph: (732) 873-0033
Torok,Geza, MD
New Jersey Thoracic Group
35 Clyde Road/Suite 104   Zip: 08873
Ph: (732) 247-3002   Fax: (732) 846-3819
Bocage,Jean P., MD
Caccavale,Robert J., MD
Orthopedic Center of New Jersey
1527 Route 27/Suite 1300   Zip: 08873
Ph: (732) 249-4444   Fax: (732) 249-6528
Malberg,Marc I., MD
Tria,Alfred J. Jr., MD
Princeton & Rutgers Neurology
77 Veronica Avenue/Suite 102   Zip: 08873
Ph: (732) 246-1311   Fax: (732) 246-3089
Behar,Roger, MD
Busono,Stephanus Judi D., MD
Dixit,Seema P., DO
Greenberg,E. Jeffrey, MD
Hersh,Joshua Neil, MD
Prompt Medical Care
636 Easton Avenue   Zip: 08873
Ph: (732) 220-8811   Fax: (732) 220-1300
Amegadzie,Richard Koku, MD
Kuchipudi,Solomon Sudhakar, MD
RWJ Univ Med/Somerset Ped
1 Worlds Fair Drive/Suite 1   Zip: 08873
Ph: (732) 743-5437   Fax: (732) 564-0212
Arun,Aparna, MD
Goodman,Elizabeth Anne, MD
Lerner,Emanuel D., MD
Pai,Shilpa, MD

Roca Piccini,Elsie Isabel, MD
RWJPE/New Brunswick Cardiology Group
75 Veronica Road/Suite 101   Zip: 08873
Ph: (732) 247-7444   Fax: (732) 247-5119
Dorazio,John L., MD
Gladstone,Clifford D., MD
Gowda,Subhashini Anande, MD
Khanna,Pravien K ., MD
Kukafka,Sheldon Jay, MD
Kulkarni,Anand U., MD
Nagarakanti,Rangadham, MD
Stroh,Jack A., MD
Tardos,Jonathan George, MD
Raritan Valley Surgery Center
100 Franklin Square Drive/Suite 100   Zip: 08873
Ph: (732) 560-1000   Fax: (732) 560-5999
Krisiloff,Edward B., MD
Regional Cancer Care Associates
454 Elizabeth Avenue/Suite 240   Zip: 08873
Ph: (732) 390-7750   Fax: (732) 390-7725
Fang,Bruno S., MD
Karp,George I., MD
Licitra,Edward Joseph, MD
Reid,Phillip Dolivera, MD
Ronnen,Ellen A., MD
Reproductive Medicine Associates
81 Veronica Avenue/Suite 101   Zip: 08873
Ph: (732) 220-9060   Fax: (732) 220-1164
Shastri,Shefali Mavani, MD
Treiser,Susan L., MD
Robert Wood Johnson Medical Group
1 World's Fair Drive/Suite 2400   Zip: 08873
Ph: (732) 235-7993   Fax: (732) 235-7117
Cha,Jisun, MD
Firoz,Bahar F., MD
Milgrum,Sandy S., MD
Pappert,Amy S., MD
Victor,Frank Charles, MD
Sadhana Pediatrics, P.C.
49 Veronica Avenue/Suite 101   Zip: 08873
Ph: (732) 247-3434   Fax: (732) 247-1815
Pari,Sadhana S., MD
Pillai,Hema R., MD
Saint Peter's Physician Associate
59 Veronica Avenue/Suite 203   Zip: 08873
Ph: (732) 937-6008
Herrera,Alejandro J., MD
Tadros,Carmen E. G., MD
Zetkulic,Marygrace M., MD
Somerset Medical Associates
1553 Highway 27/Suite 3100   Zip: 08873
Ph: (732) 846-3300   Fax: (732) 846-3323
Hopkins,Lisa Anne, MD
McDermott,Janette H., MD
McManus,Susan A., MD
Somerset Pediatric Group PA
2 World's Fair Drive/Suite 302   Zip: 08873
Ph: (908) 271-7788   Fax: (908) 271-5151
Patel,Trupti, MD
Sinclair,Melissa Renee, DO
University Geriatrics & IntMed Assocs
1553 Highway 27/Suite 2100-2300   Zip: 08873
Ph: (732) 418-0589   Fax: (732) 418-9428
Singh,Mukesh Kumar, MD
Thirumavalavan,Vallur S., MD
Tiku,Moti L., MD
University Orthopaedic Associates, LLC
Two Worlds Fair Drive   Zip: 08873
Ph: (732) 979-2115   Fax: (732) 564-9032
Baione,William A., MD
Butler,Mark S., MD
Chiappetta,Gino, MD
Coyle,Michael P. Jr., MD
Gatt,Charles J. Jr., MD
Harwood,David A., MD
Kayiaros,Stephen, MD
Leddy,Timothy P., MD
Monica,James T., MD
Polonen,David Russell, MD
Sagebien,Carlos Alberto, MD
Swan,Kenneth Girvan Jr., MD

University Pain Medicine Center
33 Clyde Road/Suite 105 & 106   Zip: 08873
Ph: (732) 873-6868   Fax: (732) 873-6869
Demesmin,Didier, MD
George,Tony Kuttikattu, DO

Somerville

Advanced Hospital Care LLC
110 Rehill Avenue   Zip: 08876
Ph: (908) 429-5833   Fax: (908) 203-5970
Ahmed,Sadia, MD
Ashraf,Shehzana, MD
Dhillon-Athwal,Narinder Kaur, MD
Lwanga,Juliet R., MD
Malik,Arsalan, MD
Singh,Jaya, MD
Anthony J. Catanese MD
315 East Main Street   Zip: 08876
Ph: (908) 722-6900   Fax: (908) 722-6699
Catanese,Anthony J., MD
Shah,Neel Praful, MD
Breast Cancer Prevention Institute
30 Rehill Avenue/Suite 3400   Zip: 08876
Ph: (908) 725-2400   Fax: (908) 927-8990
Imegwu,Obi J., MD
Seenivasan,Thangamani, MD
Drs. Mian and Mian
310 East Main Street   Zip: 08876
Ph: (908) 725-5565   Fax: (908) 725-2219
Mian,Bilal A., MD
Mian,Nimer F., DO
Ear, Nose & Throat Care, P.C.
242 East Main Street   Zip: 08876
Ph: (908) 704-9696   Fax: (908) 704-0097
Bortniker,David Leonard, MD
Druce,Howard M., MD
Emergency Medical Associates
110 Rehill Avenue   Zip: 08876
Ph: (908) 685-2920   Fax: (908) 685-2968
Chan,Mei-Yung, MD
Moore,Robert P., MD
Zeiger,Jill M., MD
Hunterdon Orthopaedic Institute, P.A.
80 West End Avenue   Zip: 08876
Ph: (908) 182-0600
St. John,Thomas A., MD
Somerset Family Practice
110 Rehill Avenue   Zip: 08876
Ph: (908) 685-2900   Fax: (908) 685-2891
Butt,Saima, MD
Davis,Lloyd A., MD
Fibison,Diana, MD
Guyton,Margaret Louise, MD
Hansch,Lalitha Therese Waldron, MD
Kaminski,Donna Marie, DO
Martinez,Ian James, MD
Micek Galinat,Laura A., MD
Rizvi,Kashan H., MD
Spector,Elisabeth, MD
Subendra-Konini,Logithya, MD
Wu,Frances Y., MD
Somerset Hematology Onc Assoc
30 Rehill Avenue/2nd Floor/Suite 2500   Zip: 08876
Ph: (908) 927-8700   Fax: (908) 927-8706
Celo,Jovenia S., MD
Dobrescu,Andrei Mihnea, MD
Khalid,Aysha, MD
Pan,Beiqing, MD
Rosenbluth,Jonathan Z., MD
Toomey,Kathleen, MD
Trivedi,Seeta, MD
Wu,Hen-Vai, MD
Young,Steven Eugene, MD
Somerset Urological Associates
72 West End Avenue   Zip: 08876
Ph: (908) 927-0300   Fax: (908) 707-4988
Dave,Dhiren Sirish, MD
Feldman,Arthur E., MD
Fischer,Joel M., MD
Harmon,Keith Andrew, MD
Surgical Associates of Central NJ
30 Rehill Avenue/Suite 3300   Zip: 08876
Ambrose,Gunaseelan, MD
Drascher,Gary A., MD

Lanfranchi,Angela E., MD
Sugarmann,William M., MD

South Amboy

Clara Barton Cardio-Medical Asc
949 Route 9 North   Zip: 08879
Ph: (732) 525-0390   Fax: (732) 525-8235
Latif,Shahid, MD
Drs. Nisar and Nisar
949 Route 9 North   Zip: 08879
Ph: (732) 721-6260
Nisar,Noor A., MD
Gregory Shypula MD PA
2045 Route 35 South/Suite 202   Zip: 08879
Ph: (732) 750-1200   Fax: (732) 602-4044
Grochowalski,Tomasz K., MD

South Orange

Center for Gynecologic Oncology
120 Irvington Avenue   Zip: 07079
Ph: (973) 762-7270   Fax: (973) 762-1980
Anderson,Patrick St. George, MD
Drs. Albanese and Vecchio
20 Valley Street   Zip: 07079
Ph: (973) 762-2606
Albanese,Anthony C., MD
Vecchio,Lisa C., MD
Yoo,Susan S., MD
Drs. Kharazi and Jain
7 Vose Avenue   Zip: 07079
Ph: (973) 630-8989   Fax: (908) 277-0201
Jain,Sejal, MD
Kharazi,Fariba, DO
Drs. Mehta and Achar
707 South Orange Avenue   Zip: 07079
Ph: (973) 762-4746   Fax: (973) 762-6862
Achar,Pankaja B.S., MD
Mehta,Satish R., MD
Northern New Jersey Eye Institute
71 Second Street   Zip: 07079
Ph: (973) 763-2203   Fax: (973) 762-9449
Crane,Charles J., MD
Gunzburg,Allison B., MD
Spier,Bernard C., MD
South Mountain Orthopaedic Assoc
61 First Street   Zip: 07079
Ph: (973) 762-8344   Fax: (973) 762-1626
Buechel,Frederick F., MD
Helbig,Thomas E., MD
South Orange Ob/Gyn & Infertility Grp
106 Valley Street   Zip: 07079
Ph: (973) 763-4334
Dresdner,Michael T., MD
Sosin,Beth L., MD

South Plainfield

AFC Urgent Care South Plainfield
907 Oak Tree Avenue/Suite H   Zip: 07080
Ph: (908) 222-3500
Bhatia,Irvinder, MD
Browne,Avery F., DO
Kashyap,Meeta Parashar, MD
Kim,Steven Namgi, MD
Patel,Purvee D., MD
Arvind K. Doshi, MD PA
906 Oak Tree Road/Suite K   Zip: 07080
Ph: (908) 822-2277   Fax: (908) 822-1121
Doshi,Arvind K., MD
Behavioral Medicine Associates, P.A.
1550 Park Avenue/Suite 102   Zip: 07080
Ph: (908) 561-6851   Fax: (908) 561-6863
Chezian,Shanthi, MD
Siddiqui,Waqar Ahmed, MD
Central Jersey Orthopedic Specialists
1907 Park Avenue/Suite 102   Zip: 07080
Ph: (908) 561-3400   Fax: (908) 769-5308
Choi,Soon Chae, MD
Shafi,Mohammad, MD
Complete Primary Care
1810 Park Avenue   Zip: 07080
Ph: (908) 226-1810   Fax: (908) 226-1833
Rozehzadeh,Rabin, MD
Solaimanzadeh,Sima, MD

Groups and Clinics by Town with Physician Rosters

South Plainfield (cont)
Drs. Sarraf and Hebbe
1907 Park Avenue Zip: 07080
Ph: (908) 561-1313 Fax: (908) 561-3917
  Sarraf,Mohammad A., MD
Family Practice & Gynecology
273 Durham Avenue Zip: 07080
Ph: (908) 561-9900 Fax: (908) 561-6650
  Hoppe,James Robert, MD
  Tran-Hoppe,Ngoc Quynh T., MD
Garden State Surgical Associates
1511 Park Avenue Zip: 07080
Ph: (908) 561-9500 Fax: (908) 561-7162
  Breitbart,Gary B., MD
  Richmond,David M., MD
  Wong,Geoffrey, MD
Goyal & Natarajan MDs LLC
904 Oak Tree Road/Suite M Zip: 07080
Ph: (908) 757-1414
  Goyal,Madhu B., MD
  Natarajan,Shobana, MD
  Seeni,Aysha, MD
Hackensack Meridian Health
904 Oak Tree Avenue/Suite M Zip: 07080
Ph: (732) 283-0020 Fax: (732) 283-0029
  Centeno,Galen Arcellana, MD
  Horvath,Katalin, MD
Health Excel PC
906 Oak Tree Road Zip: 07080
Ph: (973) 424-0776
  Agarwala,Atul K., MD
High Risk Pregnancy Center of NJ PC
908 Oak Tree Road/Suite M & N Zip: 07080
Ph: (908) 753-5771 Fax: (908) 753-2473
  Biswas,Anjali, MD
Island Reproductive Services
3000 Hadley Road/Suite 2-C Zip: 07080
Ph: (908) 412-9909 Fax: (908) 412-9910
  Shah,Namrata Jinesh, MD
Medical Diagnostic Associates PA
1511 Park Avenue/3rd Floor Zip: 07080
Ph: (908) 757-4544 Fax: (908) 757-2427
  Tucker,Burton Stanley, MD
MedDiag Assocs/Central NJ Cardiology
1511 Park Avenue/Suite 2 Zip: 07080
Ph: (908) 756-4438 Fax: (908) 756-9160
  Altszuler,Henry M., MD
  Andraws,Richard Zaki, MD
  Blumberg,Edwin D., MD
  Leopold,Thomas D., MD
RejuV Aesthetic Gynecology
285 Durham Avenue/Suite 1A, Bldg. 6 Zip: 07080
Ph: (732) 504-6917
  Antonio,Edsel, DO
  Kapusuz,Tolga, MD
  Tran,Bao Chau Minh, MD
South Plainfield Primary Care
2509 Park Avenue/Suite 1A Zip: 07080
Ph: (908) 668-8290 Fax: (908) 561-4914
  Goyal,Alok, MD
  Goyal,Madhu A., MD
  Singh,Priyanka, MD

South River
Girgis Family Medicine
171 Main Street/Suite 4 Zip: 08882
Ph: (732) 254-9494 Fax: (732) 254-9903
  Girgis,Linda Mae, MD
  Girgis,Moris Beachay, MD
Nephrology Hypertension Assoc
8 Old Bridge Turnpike Zip: 08882
Ph: (732) 390-4888 Fax: (732) 390-0255
  Covit,Andrew B., MD
  Drabik,Thomas Edward, DO
  Dubov,Glenn A., MD
  Matera,James J., DO

Sparta
Eye Care Northwest
350 Sparta Avenue Zip: 07871
Ph: (973) 729-5757 Fax: (973) 729-8322
  Hess,Jocelyn S., MD
  Liegner,Jeffrey T., MD
Highland Psychiatric Associates
89 Sparta Avenue/Suite 240 Zip: 07871
Ph: (973) 729-2991 Fax: (973) 729-7641
  Kloupar,Dagmar S., MD
Neuro-Specialists of Morris-Sussex, PA
350 Sparta Avenue Zip: 07871
Ph: (973) 579-1089 Fax: (973) 579-9618
  Greene,Wayne L., MD
Premier Health Associates
89 Sparta Avenue/Suite 130 Zip: 07871
Ph: (973) 726-0005 Fax: (973) 726-4668
  Abdo-Matkiwsky,May D., DO
Premier Health Associates
532 Lafayette Road/Suite 100 Zip: 07871
Ph: (973) 383-3730 Fax: (973) 383-2285
  Agesen,Thomas, MD
Premier Health Associates
89 Sparta Avenue/Suite 100 Zip: 07871
Ph: (973) 729-2121 Fax: (973) 729-3454
  Bollard,David A., DO
  Bronstein,Regina, MD
  Casella,Frank J., DO
  Ganon,Michael R., DO
  Green,Jason D., MD
  Halibey,Bohdan E., MD
  Kim,Daryl Kyung, MD
  Lindy,Michael Evan, MD
  Medunick,David M., DO
  Rao,Kiran Venkat, MD
  Sarwar,Haroon, MD
  Shea,Caitlin M., DO
  Tang,Linda Yinglin, MD
  Wang,George Cho-Ching, MD
Premier Health Associates-Admin
532 Lafayette Road/Suite 300 Zip: 07871
Ph: (973) 940-0423 Fax: (973) 940-0399
  Casella,Joseph J., DO
Skylands Pediatrics
328-A Sparta Avenue Zip: 07871
Ph: (973) 729-2197 Fax: (973) 729-3653
  Achar,Ashwini, MD
  Calabrese,Carol E., MD
  Capozzoli,Alexis Nicole, MD
  Di Paolo,Raymond Paul, MD
  Meskin,Inna, MD
  O'Neill,Michael B., MD
  Spensieri,Diana Patricia, MD
Skylands Urology Group
89 Sparta Avenue/Suite 200 Zip: 07871
Ph: (973) 726-7220 Fax: (973) 726-7230
  Hall,Matthew Scott, MD
  Matteson,James R., MD
  Mykulak,Donald J., MD
  Salvatore,Frank Timothy, MD
Sparta Cancer Center
89 Sparta Avenue/Suite 130 Zip: 07871
Ph: (973) 729-7001
  Lo,Kathy Kai Yee, MD
Sparta Health & Wellness
89 Sparta Avenu/Suite 207 Zip: 07871
Ph: (973) 940-8780 Fax: (973) 726-9568
  Cheng,Waina, MD
  Incorvati,Jason A., MD
Sparta Health and Wellness Center
89 Sparta Avenue/Suite 120 Zip: 07871
Ph: (973) 729-0002 Fax: (973) 729-1085
  Cordero,Hector Orlando, MD
  Cordero,Orlando C., MD
  Corio,Frederick J., MD
Sparta Health and Wellness Center
89 Sparta Avenue/Suite 220 Zip: 07871
Ph: (973) 940-8100 Fax: (973) 729-7235
  Czaplicki-Margiotti,Marie A., MD
  Franklin,Barry I., MD
  Ranley,Robert L., MD
  Reddy,Shashidhar Sadda, MD
  Rodrigues,Vanitha J., MD
  Shah,Shital R., MD
  Skalla,Matthew T., MD
Specialty Surgical Center
380 Lafayette Road/Suite 110 Zip: 07871
Ph: (973) 940-3166 Fax: (973) 940-3170
  Cole,Robert J., MD

Wellness Center Pediatrics LLC
21 Lafayette Road/Suite F Zip: 07871
Ph: (973) 726-4455 Fax: (973) 726-8445
  Canzoniero,Christian, MD
  Raman,Rajesh C., MD
  Whittington,Wendy Louise, MD

Spotswood
Spotswood Medical Associates PA
498 Main Street Zip: 08884
Ph: (732) 251-6900 Fax: (732) 251-5935
  Deb,Ashoke Kumar, MD
  Sahni,Sushma, MD

Spring Lake
Spring Lake Pediatrics Assocs
613 Warren Avenue Zip: 07762
Ph: (732) 974-1444
  Miele,Ellen H., MD
  Pirogovsky,Victoria, MD
  Sciarappa,Lorette J., MD

Springfield
Advanced Care Hematology & Oncology
385 Morris Avenue/Suite 100 Zip: 07081
Ph: (973) 379-2111 Fax: (973) 379-2807
  Desai,Ved, DO
  Khot,Ashish Abhay, MD
  Pondt,Charlesse Maureen, MD
  Rao,Maithili V., MD
Advanced Surgical Associates LLC
155 Morris Avenue/2nd Floor Zip: 07081
Ph: (973) 232-2300 Fax: (973) 232-2301
  Feteiha,Muhammad S., MD
  Lopes,James M., MD
  Lopes,Joao Alberto, MD
  Pepen,John Andre, MD
Associates in Cardiovascular Disease,
211 Mountain Avenue Zip: 07081
Ph: (973) 467-0005 Fax: (973) 912-8989
  Cohen,Barry Mark, MD
  Fishberg,Robert Daniel, MD
Associates in Cardiovascular Disease
211 Mountain Avenue Zip: 07081
Ph: (973) 467-0005 Fax: (973) 912-8989
  Furer,Steven K., MD
  Lux,Michael S., MD
  Marmora,Joseph James, MD
  Powell,David E., MD
  Prasad,Sanjiv, MD
  Roberti,Roberto R., MD
  Stein,Elliott M., MD
  Weber,Vance J., MD
  Weinrauch,Michael L., MD
Associates in Digestive Disease
25 Morris Avenue Zip: 07081
Ph: (973) 467-1313 Fax: (973) 467-3133
  Fuhrman,Michael Alexander, MD
  Kerner,Michael B., MD
  Lipsky,Marvin A., MD
Associates in Eye Care
155 Morris Avenue/Suite 302 Zip: 07081
Ph: (973) 232-6900 Fax: (973) 232-6911
  Lucia Ricci,Jodie Italia, MD
  Notis,Corey M., MD
Assoc in Plastic & Aesthetic Surgery
955 South Springfield Avenue/Suite 105 Zip: 07081
Ph: (908) 654-6540 Fax: (908) 654-6504
  Loguda,Charles A., MD
  Tepper,Howard N., MD
  Tepper,Richard Eric, MD
  Zeitels,Jerrold R., MD
B. Silver, MD & G. Kaplan MD
535 Morris Avenue Zip: 07081
Ph: (973) 376-1020 Fax: (973) 376-0802
  Silver,Bennett, MD
  Thorpe,Michelle Lynn, MD
Care Station
90 Route 22 West Zip: 07081
Ph: (973) 467-2273
  Mansour,Ali Gaber, MD
  Parman,Stanley C., MD
Drs. De Fronzo & De Fronzo
216 Short Hills Avenue Zip: 07081
Ph: (973) 376-7838 Fax: (973) 912-4367
  De Fronzo,Carl L., DO
  De Fronzo,Stephen D., MD

Lifeline Medical Associates
530 Morris Avenue Zip: 07081
Ph: (973) 379-7477 Fax: (973) 379-9094
  Hunt,Mary Elizabeth, MD
  Lublin,Jennifer Caryn, MD
  Magaril,Rhona A., MD
  Rabin-Havt,Sara Schonfeld, MD
New Beginnings OB/GYN
193 Mountain Avenue Zip: 07081
Ph: (973) 218-1579 Fax: (973) 218-1589
  Pinto,Jose J., DO
  Tye,Joann Li Yen, MD
New Jersey Bariatric Center
193 Morris Avenue/2nd Floor Zip: 07081
Ph: (908) 481-1270 Fax: (908) 688-8861
  Buwen,James P., DO
  Forrester,Glenn Joseph, MD
  Glasnapp,Angela Jack, MD
  Goyal,Ajay, MD
  Montes,Leigh, MD
North Jersey Hand Surgery
385 Morris Avenue/Third Floor Zip: 07081
Ph: (973) 664-9899 Fax: (973) 664-1875
  Fox,Ross J., MD
  Kirschenbaum,Abram Eugene, MD
Springfield Pediatrics
190 Meisel Avenue Zip: 07081
Ph: (973) 467-1009 Fax: (973) 467-7836
  Korkmazsky,Yelena N., MD
  Lim,Norman Feliz Lopez, MD
  Lozano,Rolando, MD
  Nunez,Helen Lourdes, MD
Summit Medical Group
11 Cleveland Place Zip: 07081
Ph: (973) 378-8778 Fax: (973) 763-1748
  Cantor,Melvin A., MD
  Lim,Betty Bichly, MD
  Profeta,Susan B., MD
The Joint Institute at SBMC
609 Morris Avenue Zip: 07081
Ph: (973) 379-1991 Fax: (973) 467-8647
  Cuomo,Thomas F., MD
  Glushakow,Allen S., MD
  Oppenheim,William C., MD
  Rieber,Michael Harold, MD

Stirling
Associates in Internal Medicine, LLC
1072 Valley Road Zip: 07980
Ph: (908) 604-8464 Fax: (908) 604-2494
  Pontecorvo,Martin J., DO
  Postighone,Carl J., MD

Stockton
Stockton Family Practice
56 South Main Street/Stockton Center Zip: 08559
Ph: (609) 397-8585 Fax: (609) 397-9335
  Freedenfeld,Stuart H., MD
  Heinz,Kristann Wilmore, MD

Stone Harbor
Cape Regional Physicians Associates
336 96th Street/Suite 1 Zip: 08247
Ph: (609) 967-0070 Fax: (609) 967-0077
  Hofmann,William Andrew III, DO
  Nuschke,Randell A., MD
  Ruskey,Elizabeth E., DO
  Vogdes,Tara Ann, DO

Stratford
Advocare Sicklerville Internal Med
205 East Laurel Road/1 FL Zip: 08084
Ph: (856) 227-6575 Fax: (856) 374-9495
  Conti,Joseph J., DO
  Friedman,Jeffrey R., DO
  Ranalli,Jeffery A., DO
NJ Institute For Successful Aging
42 East Laurel Road/Suite 1800 Zip: 08084
Ph: (856) 566-6843 Fax: (856) 566-6781
  Abesh,Jesse Susan, DO
  Alday,Geronima G., MD
  Cavalieri,Thomas A., DO
  Cheng,Wunhuey, DO
  Chopra,Anita, MD
  Chowdhury,Zinnat A., MD
  Dave,Chetna A., MD

Dignam,Ritchell Rodriguez, MD
Elahi,Abdul Wadood, MD
Forsberg,Martin M., MD
Frankel,Susan L., DO
Ginsberg,Terrie Beth, DO
Kedziora,Halina M., MD
Noll,Donald R., DO
Overbeck,Kevin Joseph, DO
Palli,Prameela M., MD
Powell,Leonard A. Jr., DO
Scheinthal,Stephen M., DO
Selvam,Nirmala, MD
Serban,Valeria, MD
Wadhwa,Aruna, MD
White,Christian Paul, DO

Rowan Medical Department of Psychiatry
42 Laurel Road East/Suite 3610 Zip: 08084
Ph: (856) 482-9000 Fax: (856) 482-1159
Gayle,Catherine, MD

SOM - Dept. of Internal Medicine
42 East Laurel Road/Suite 3100 Zip: 08084
Ph: (856) 566-6859 Fax: (856) 566-6906
Ali,Fatima, DO
Avelluto,Giovanni Domenico, DO
Bolisetti,Sreedevi, MD
Chen,Brian Youshane, DO
Chery,Magdala, DO
Choe,Jisun Kim, MD
Di Bruno,Donna, DO
Falescky,Allan Jeffrey, MD
Giudice,James C., DO
Goldwaser,Elan Luria, DO
Gordon,Robert, DO
Griesback,Russell, DO
Helfer,Elizabeth L., MD
Jawaid,Nosheen, DO
Khan,Imran Ahmad, MD
Lecomte,Jennifer Megan, DO
Lena,Steffi D., DO
Lewis,David Everett, DO
Lightfoot,Judith A., DO
Lucerna,Alan Rey Nicolo, DO
Matrale,Michael, DO
Monahan,Lisa Y., DO
Morley,Thomas F., DO
Perez,Ricardo, DO
Rengan,Rajagopalan, DO
Saccone,Peter Joseph, DO
Vasoya,Amita P., DO
Watson,Marcia G., DO

South Jersey Gastroenterology PA
117 East Laurel Road Zip: 08084
Ph: (856) 627-2555 Fax: (856) 751-8746
Liakos,Steven, DO

Stratford - Endocrinology
25 East Laurel Road Zip: 08084
OnlyFax: (856) 783-8537
Haenel,Louis C. III, DO
Luceri,Patricia Marie, DO
Szpiech,Maria, MD

University Doctors-Ob Gyn
42 East Laurel Road/Suite 3500 Zip: 08084
Ph: (856) 566-7090 Fax: (856) 566-6026
Barone,Donald A., DO
Konchak,Peter Stephen, DO

UH -SOM University Surgeons
42 East Laurel Road/Suite 2500-2600 Zip: 08084
Ph: (856) 566-2700 Fax: (856) 566-6873
Balsama,Louis H., DO
Iucci,Lisa Diane, DO
Jolitz,Whitney, DO

UH-Cares Institute
42 East Laurel Road/Suite 1100 Zip: 08084
Ph: (856) 566-7036 Fax: (856) 566-6108
Brennan,Laura Kaye, MD
Cohen,Barbara Elisabeth, MD
Cohen,Rachel Isabel Silliman, MD
DeRisio,Vincent James II, DO
Finkel,Martin A., DO
Higginbotham,Monique Renee, MD

Lanese,Stephanie Valentine, MD
Lind,Marita Elizabeth, MD
Melman,Shoshana T., MD
O'Donnell-Mulgrew,Deborah M., DO
Rachan,Srilatha, MD
Vender,Lydia A., DO
Weiner,Monica B., MD

UH-SOM Department of Psychiatry
109 East Laurel Road/First Floor Zip: 08084
Ph: (856) 566-6035 Fax: (856) 566-6208
Levitas,Andrew S., MD

UH-University Family Medicine
42 East Laurel Road/Suite 2100 Zip: 08084
Ph: (856) 566-7020 Fax: (856) 566-6188
Chick,Charlene Elizabeth, DO
Decker,Robert James V, DO
Garnier,Katharine M., MD
Gupta,Adarsh Kumar, DO
Heaton,Caryl Joan, DO
Hoffman,Barry M., DO
Hudrick,Robert Eugene, DO
Jiwani,Ameena Javed, MD
Kimler,Christine Marie, DO
Lambert,Kathryn C., DO
Larrea,Diana Rose, DO
Luksch,John Richard, DO
Russell,Hortense Patricia, DO
Scott,George John, DO

University Pain Care Center
42 East Laurel Road/Suite 1700 Zip: 08084
Ph: (856) 566-7010 Fax: (856) 566-6956
Bailey,James William, DO
Channell,Millicent King, DO
Douglas,Barbara L., MD
Janora,Deanna Marie, MD
Torres,Jonathan William, DO

Succasunna

Advocare West Morris Pediatrics
151 Route 10/Suite 105 Zip: 07876
Ph: (973) 584-0002 Fax: (973) 584-7107
Heller,Michelle, MD
Patashny,Karen M., MD
Peters,Michael A., DO
Strand,Barbara G., MD
Vosatka,Robert J., MD

Affiliated Dermatology
Town Centre 66/Suite 301 Zip: 07876
Ph: (973) 267-0300 Fax: (973) 927-7512
Cooper,Lauren M., MD

Allergy & Arthritis Associates
66 Sunset Strip/Suite 207 Zip: 07876
Ph: (973) 584-1391 Fax: (973) 584-7017
Giangrasso,Thomas A., MD

Medical Care Associates
262 Route 10 West Zip: 07876
Ph: (973) 252-1522 Fax: (973) 252-1422
Madane,Srinivas Janardhan, MD
Shah,Vipul V., MD
Singh,Pritpaul, MD

Morristown Ob-Gyn
20 Commerce Boulevard/Unit C Zip: 07876
Ph: (973) 927-1188 Fax: (973) 927-7408
Ramieri,Joseph, MD
Sharafi,Khalida, MD
Shaw,Donia Renee, MD

Roxbury Eye Center, PC
66 Sunset Strip/Suite 107 Zip: 07876
Ph: (973) 584-4451 Fax: (973) 584-2099
Gottlieb,Joel M., MD
Pinke,Robert S., MD

Summit

Advanced Dermatology, P.C.
33 Overlook Road/MAC 1/Suite 405 Zip: 07901
Hu,Judy Y., MD
Silver,Barry C., MD

Atlantic Colon & Rectal
33 Overlook Road/Suite 412 Zip: 07901
Ph: (908) 598-0220 Fax: (908) 598-0415
Groff,Walter L., MD
Miller,Aaron Todd, MD

Atlantic Neuroscience Institute
99 Beauvoir Avenue Zip: 07901
Ph: (908) 522-2000
Belt,Gary Harvey, MD
Metrus,Nicholas Robert, MD
Rabin,Marcie L., MD

CCVS Care LLC
597 Springfield Avenue Zip: 07901
Ph: (908) 654-7399
Budoff,Steven R., MD
Ciolino,Charles P., MD

Carniol Plastic Surgery
33 Overlook Road/Suite 401 Zip: 07901
Ph: (908) 598-1400 Fax: (908) 273-1553
Carniol,Eric T., MD
Carniol,Paul J., MD

Drs. Gianis and Gianis
475 Springfield Avenue Zip: 07901
Ph: (908) 273-8854 Fax: (908) 273-4585
Gianis,John Thomas Jr., MD
Gianis,Thomas J., MD

Drs. Murphy & Williams, P.A.
33 Overlook Road/Suite 412 Zip: 07901
Ph: (908) 273-7274
Murphy,Kathleen A., MD

Hall-DiGioia Center for Breast Care
33 Overlook Road/Suite 205 Zip: 07901
Ph: (908) 522-3200 Fax: (908) 522-1222
Di Gioia,Julia Marie, MD
Hall,Stephen C., MD

Institute for Rheumatic & Autoimmune
33 Overlook Road/MAC L01 Zip: 07901
Ph: (908) 598-7940 Fax: (908) 598-5447
Daver,Nicole Rohinton, DO
Kramer,Neil, MD
Patel,Sheetal V., MD
Rosenstein,Elliot D., MD
Setty,Arathi Radhakrishna, MD

Integrated Behavioral Care
35 Beechwood Road/Suite 3-A & 3-B Zip: 07901
Ph: (908) 598-2400 Fax: (908) 598-2408
Forman-Chou,Alexandra Catherine, M
Reiter,Stewart Roy, MD

Kidz Doctor, LLC
11 Overlook Road/Suite 170 Zip: 07901
Ph: (908) 277-4480 Fax: (908) 277-4482
Cerdena,Maria Corazon, MD
Lucciola,Marion, MD

MED-FEM Aesthetic Surgery Center
33 Overlook Road/Suite 302 Zip: 07901
Ph: (908) 522-1777 Fax: (908) 522-3051
Shafaie,Farrokh, MD

Maple Pediatric Associates LLC
47 Maple Street/Suite 107 Zip: 07901
Ph: (908) 273-5866 Fax: (908) 273-5811
Cessario,Alison G., MD
Polisin,Michael J., MD

Maternal Fetal Med of Practice Assoc
11 Overlook Road/Suite LL 102 Zip: 07901
Ph: (908) 522-3846 Fax: (908) 522-5557
Benito,Carlos W., MD
Lashley,Susan Leonora, MD
Netta,Denise Ann, MD
Oyelese,Kolawole Olayinka, MD
Russo-Stieglitz,Karen E., MD

Medical Diagnostic Associates, P.A.
99 Beauvoir Avenue Zip: 07901
Ph: (908) 608-0078 Fax: (908) 608-1504
Guerin,Bonni Lee, MD
Jaeckle,Kurt Alfred, MD
Lowenthal,Dennis A., MD

Medical Diagnostic Associates, P.A.
MAC, 11 Overlook Road/Suite 100 Zip: 07901
Ph: (908) 273-1493 Fax: (908) 273-3125
May-Ortiz,Jennifer L., MD
Morganstein,Neil, MD
Moriarty,Daniel J., MD
Morse,Sophie D., MD
Saksena,Rujuta P., MD

Orthopedic Surgical Associates
33 Overlook Road/Suite 201 Zip: 07901
Ph: (908) 522-4555 Fax: (908) 522-1128
DeLuca,Francis N., MD
Sarokhan,Alan J., MD

Overlook Family Medicine
33 Overlook Road/Suite 103 Zip: 07901
Ph: (908) 522-5700 Fax: (908) 273-8014
Ali,Sabia, MD

Overlook Family Medicine
33 Overlook Road/Suite 103 Zip: 07901
Ph: (908) 522-5700 Fax: (908) 273-8014
Butkiewicz,Elise Ann, MD
Castro,Rodrigo Alejandro, DO
Flowers,Robert M., DO
Kaye,Susan T., MD
Kim,Julia J., MD
Lukenda,Robert A., DO
Tsangalidis,Eirini, MD
Washington,Judy C., MD

Overlook Wound Healing Center
11 Overlook Road/MAC II, Suite LL 101 Zip: 07901
Ph: (908) 522-5900 Fax: (908) 522-5544
Luka,Norman L., MD
Roland,Robert J., MD

Overlook Surgical Associates
11 Overlook Road/Suite 160 Zip: 07901
Ph: (908) 608-9001 Fax: (908) 608-9030
Robinson,Andrew Tyler, MD
Starker,Paul M., MD

Pain Management Center
11 Overlook Road/MAC 11 Suite B110 Zip: 07901
Ph: (908) 522-2808 Fax: (908) 522-6123
Pappagallo,Marco, MD
Stoller,Seth Ryan, MD

Partners in Psychiatry, LLP
33 Overlook Road/Suite 212 Zip: 07901
Ph: (908) 273-6164 Fax: (908) 277-1439
Malhotra,Mahamaya, MD
Malhotra,Rahul, MD

Pediatric Orthopedics, PC
99 Beauvoir Avenue/Suite 750 Zip: 07902
Ph: (908) 273-4404 Fax: (908) 522-5519
Nuzzo,Roy Michael, MD

Pulmonary & Allergy Associates
1 Springfield Avenue/Suite 3-A Zip: 07901
Ph: (908) 934-0555 Fax: (908) 934-0556
Cancel,Jaime, MD
Cerrone,Federico, MD
Donnabella,Vincent, MD
Fessler,Sue Atherton, MD
Gupte,Chaitali Rajan, MD
Kotecha,Nisha Suresh, MD
Nahmias,Jeffrey S., MD
Rhodes,Stancie Christina, MD
Sussman,Robert, MD

Pulmonary & Allergy Associates
1 Springfield Avenue Zip: 07901
Zeibeq,John Paul, MD
Zimmerman,Mark I., MD

Radiation Oncology @ Overlook
33 Overlook Road/MAC 1 Suite L-05 Zip: 07901
Ph: (908) 522-2871 Fax: (908) 522-5628
Emmolo,Joana S., MD
Knee,Robert, MD
Schwartz,Louis E., MD

Sharon E. Selinger MD PA
1 Springfield Avenue/Suite 1A Zip: 07901
Ph: (908) 273-8300 Fax: (908) 273-8807
Huberman,Daniel Tzvi, MD
Selinger,Sharon E., MD

Springfield Family Practice
11 Overlook Road/Suite 140 Zip: 07901
Ph: (908) 277-0050 Fax: (908) 277-0201
Davine-Reicher,Joanne Erin, MD
Doubek,Marnie Lynn, MD
Pozner,Samantha Brooke, MD
Pride,Mikel Jadyne, MD
Schram,Amy Elizabeth, DO
Snyder,Hugh David, MD

Groups and Clinics by Town with Physician Rosters

Summit (cont)
Summit Anesthesia Associates, P.A.
33 Overlook Road/Suite 311 Zip: 07901
Ph: (908) 598-1500 Fax: (908) 598-0197
- Abrams, Jonathan Todd, MD
- BelCastro, Peter Joseph, MD
- Byers, Jason, MD
- Calabro, John R., MD
- Co, Jacqueline Ann B., MD
- DeAngelis, Lawrence J., MD
- Dominik, Jeremy A., MD
- Dowd, Timothy Joseph, MD
- Farrar, Robert, MD
- Fernandez-Piparo, May Anne Malinis,
- George, Tony, MD
- Gerges, Theresa, DO
- Greenberg, Carrie Lynn, MD
- Hu, Yuan, MD
- Huang, Guojie, MD
- Jablons, Mitchell L., MD
- Kagan, Mikhail, MD
- Kral, Michael George, MD
- Kweon, Chang, MD
- Kwon, Yong S., MD
- Lei, Laura M., MD
- McLaughlin, Blaise, MD
- Naturman, Roy E., MD
- Pacific, Scott, MD
- Paris, Glen Allen, MD
- Pierre-Louis, James, MD
- Rice, Stuart Nelson, MD
- Ross, Neil E., MD
- Sant, Manasee Amol, MD
- Sarkaria, Janak, MD
- Schultz, Gail, MD
- Sharma, Akanksha D., MD
- Surace, Anthony, MD
- Wang, Wayne, MD
- Woo, Daniel Hee-Suk, MD
- Yao, Daniel Duan, MD
- You, Ruoxu, MD
- Zimmermann, Carol E., MD

Summit Internal Medicine, LLC
33 Overlook Road/Suite LO6 Zip: 07901
Ph: (908) 522-0050 Fax: (908) 516-2946
- Jeffries, Emily L., MD
- Subramanian, Gomathy, MD
- Toffey, Lisa H., MD

Summit Neurology Consulting, PC.
33 Overlook Road/Suite 401 Zip: 07901
Ph: (908) 273-9000 Fax: (908) 273-9022
- Craciun, Liviu Ciprian, MD

Summit Pediatric Associates
33 Overlook Road/Suite 101 Zip: 07901
Ph: (908) 273-1112 Fax: (908) 273-1146
- Kairam, Hemant, MD
- Manocchio, Teresa, DO
- Vigorita, John F., MD

Univ Consultants-Ob-Gyn & Womens Hlth
33 Overlook Road/Mac 405 Zip: 07902
Ph: (908) 608-0300
- Franceschini, Chloe Nicole, MD
- Rondon, Kaylah Christine, MD

Vigman and Pollock PA
47 Maple Street/Suite 104 Zip: 07901
Ph: (908) 277-2722 Fax: (908) 273-5970
- Pollock, Jeffrey C., MD
- Vigman, Melvin P., MD

Swedesboro
Salem Medical Group
95 Woodstown Road/Suite B Zip: 08085
Ph: (856) 832-7359 Fax: (856) 832-4381
- Abel Boenerjous, Rebakah Sumalin, M
- Dalsey, Michael E., DO
- Tsigonis, Natalie, DO

Teaneck
Advanced Interventional Radiology
718 Teaneck Road Zip: 07666
Ph: (201) 227-6210 Fax: (201) 643-3077
- Gallo, Vincent, MD
- Herman, Kevin, MD
- Rundback, John Hugh, MD

Advanced Laser & Skin Cancer Center
870 Palisade Avcenue/Suite 302 Zip: 07666
Ph: (201) 836-9696 Fax: (201) 836-4716
- Ragi, Gangaram, MD

Aspen Medical Associates, P.A.
1 DeGraw Square Zip: 07666
Ph: (201) 928-0200 Fax: (201) 928-0820
- Abrar, Dimir, MD
- Adler, Joel S., MD
- Brisman, Daniel Aaron, MD
- Gaitour, Larisa, MD
- Koduri, Hemanth Kumar, MD
- Lee, Karen Chang, MD
- Meyerowitz, Jay S., MD
- Petrucelli, Janet L., MD
- Rizzo, Joseph Alfonso, MD
- Salizzoni, Jeffrey L., MD

Bergen Anesthesia Associates
718 Teaneck Road Zip: 07666
Ph: (201) 833-7149 Fax: (201) 833-6576
- Klein, Patti S., MD
- Parmar, Virendra Pratapsingh, MD
- Singer, Judith C. J., MD
- Thornhill, Marsha Lynne, MD

Bergen Cardiology Associates
400 Frank W. Burr Boulevard Zip: 07666
Ph: (201) 928-2300 Fax: (201) 692-3263
- Kasaryan, Hrach Ike, DO
- Sagar, Yogesh, MD
- Vandyck-Acquah, Marian M., MD

Brown Eye Care Associates
751 Teaneck Road Zip: 07666
Ph: (201) 833-0006 Fax: (201) 833-9238
- Brown, Andrew Carson, MD
- Brown, Christopher David, MD
- Brown, Robert Henry, MD
- Brown, Robert Stephen, MD

Castle Connolly Medical, LTD.
699 Teaneck Road/Suite 103 Zip: 07666
Ph: (201) 645-3362 Fax: (201) 692-1363
- Hensle, Terry W., MD
- Tennenbaum, Steven Y., MD

Diab Endo Metabolism Specialities PA
870 Palisade Avenue/Suite 203 Zip: 07666
Ph: (201) 836-5655 Fax: (201) 836-3571
- Wiesen, Mark, MD

Drs. Boja & Boja
1150 Teaneck Road Zip: 07666
Ph: (201) 833-9000 Fax: (201) 833-9510
- Boja, Conrado A. III, MD
- Boja, Michael Conrad, DO

Drs. Coleman & Adair
222 Cedar Lane/Suite 111 Zip: 07666
Ph: (201) 836-7970 Fax: (201) 836-7973
- Coleman, Clenton Louis, MD

Drs. Lavotshkin and Znamensky
757 Teaneck Road Zip: 07666
Ph: (201) 833-2288 Fax: (201) 833-4441
- Lavotshkin, Anna Janna, MD
- Znamensky, Addi, MD

Eastern Orthopedic Associates
222 Cedar Lane/Suite 120 Zip: 07666
Ph: (201) 836-5332 Fax: (201) 836-4002
- Bauer, Brian J., MD
- Hale, James Joseph, MD
- Katona, John J., MD
- Steuer, Jeffrey K., MD

Institute for Clinical Rearch
718 Teaneck Road Zip: 07666
Ph: (201) 833-7274 Fax: (201) 833-7243
- Birch, Thomas M., MD
- De La Rosa, Benjamin Danny, MD

Internal Medicine PA
155 Cedar Lane Zip: 07666
Ph: (201) 836-4247
- Berdy, Jack M., MD
- Umer, Muhammad S., MD
- Waseem, Sarwat, MD

MS Center at Holy Name Hospital
718 Teaneck Road Zip: 07666
Ph: (201) 837-0727 Fax: (201) 837-8504
- Blitz-Shabbir, Karen M., DO
- Duncan, David Brian, MD

- Picone, Maryann, MD

Metropolitan Pediatric Group
704 Palisade Avenue Zip: 07666
Ph: (201) 836-4301 Fax: (201) 836-5110
- Caruana, Lucia P., MD
- Epstein, Nina, MD
- Kanter, Alan I., MD
- Novogroder, Michael, MD
- Planer, Dorienne Sasto, MD
- Schewitz, Gail, MD

Nephrology Associates PA
870 Palisade Avenue/Suite 202 Zip: 07666
Ph: (201) 836-0897 Fax: (201) 836-8042
- Ahmed, Subhan, MD
- Aronoff, Benjamin W., MD
- Gussak, Hiie M., MD
- Levin, David N., MD
- Salazer, Thomas L., MD
- Sheth, Naitik D., MD

North Jersey Laparoscopic Associates
222 Cedar Lane/Room 201 Zip: 07666
Ph: (201) 530-1900 Fax: (201) 530-9300
- Fredericks, Duane A., MD

North Jersey Orthopaedic Specialists
730 Palisade Avenue Zip: 07666
Ph: (201) 353-9000 Fax: (201) 530-0003
- Kwak, Steve K., MD
- Patel, Deepan N., MD

Northern Jersey ENT Associates
1 Degraw Avenue Zip: 07666
Ph: (201) 837-2174 Fax: (201) 836-7838
- Davis, Orrin, MD

Northern Jersey Orthopedic Center PA
870 Palisade Avenue/Suite 205 Zip: 07666
Ph: (201) 836-1663 Fax: (201) 836-5729
- Pfisterer, Christine, DO
- Pfisterer, Dennis James, DO
- Pfisterer, Dennis L., MD

Pedimedica PA
870 Palisade Avenue/Suite 201 Zip: 07666
Ph: (201) 692-1661 Fax: (201) 692-9219
- Benzel, Irwin Zachary, DO
- Kolsky, Neil H., MD
- Suldan, Dora I., MD

Premier Orthopaedics & Sports Med
111 Galway Place Zip: 07666
Ph: (201) 833-9500 Fax: (201) 862-0095
- Carrer, Alexandra, MD
- Dorri, Mohammad Hossein, MD
- Galitzin, Joseph C., MD
- Quartararo, Louis Gaspar, MD

Regional Cancer Center Holy Name
718 Teaneck Road Zip: 07666
Ph: (201) 227-6008 Fax: (201) 227-6002
- Condemi, Giuseppe, MD
- Diamond, Elan Shlomo, MD
- Goldman, Raimonda, DO
- Pieczara, Beata Katarzyna, MD

Retina Associates of New Jersey, P.A.
628 Cedar Lane Zip: 07666
Ph: (201) 837-7300 Fax: (201) 836-6426
- Bergen, Robert L., MD
- Feiner, Leonard, MD
- Hahn, Paul, MD
- Higgins, Patrick M., MD
- Klein, Richard M., MD
- Slamovits, Thomas L., MD

Retina Center of New Jersey
1086 Teaneck Road/Suite 2a Zip: 07666
Ph: (201) 871-3414 Fax: (201) 871-4830
- Angioletti, Louis V. Jr., MD

Rheumatology Associates of NJ
1415 Queen Anne Road Zip: 07666
Ph: (201) 837-7788 Fax: (201) 837-2077
- Aristy, Sary Mariell, MD
- Gonter, Neil Jeffrey, MD
- Kimel, Alexandru F., MD
- Marcus, Ralph E., MD
- Miceli, James Gerard, MD
- Silverberg, Miriam Shayna, MD

Surgical Oncology and Laparoscopy
741 Teaneck Road/Suite B Zip: 07666
Ph: (201) 833-2888 Fax: (201) 833-1010
- Christoudias, George C., MD
- Mansouri, Farshad, MD
- Radvinsky, David, MD

Teaneck Anesthesia Group, P.A.
718 Teaneck Road Zip: 07666
Ph: (201) 833-7149 Fax: (201) 833-6576
- D'Souza, Michael Gerard, MD
- Franzl, Wojciech, MD
- Gupta, Vijay, MD
- Gwertzman, Alan R., MD
- Martin, Brian McKinley, MD
- Trivedi, Avani P., DO

Teaneck Gast & Endo Cntr
1086 Teaneck Road/Suite 4-C Zip: 07666
Ph: (201) 837-9449 Fax: (201) 578-1699
- Micale, Philip Louis, MD
- Palance, Adam L., MD
- Paltrowitz, Irving M., MD
- Rigoglioso, Vincent, MD
- Schmidt, Michael H., MD

Teaneck Hospitalists, PA
718 Teaneck Road Zip: 07666
Ph: (201) 530-7931 Fax: (201) 227-6207
- Balmir, Sacha, DO
- Chan, Kim K., MD

Teaneck Pediatric Associates PA
197 Cedar Lane Zip: 07666
Ph: (201) 836-7171 Fax: (201) 928-4227
- Kanarek, Ninette Marciano, MD
- Schuss, Steven A., MD
- Zajkowski, Edward Joseph, MD

The Cornea & Laser Eye Institute
300 Frank W. Burr Boulevard Zip: 07666
Ph: (201) 883-0505 Fax: (201) 692-9646
- Hersh, Peter S., MD

Valley Health Medical Group
780 Cedar Lane Zip: 07666
Ph: (201) 836-7664 Fax: (201) 836-5710
- Ferrer, Waldo L., MD
- Jones, Rhys E., MD
- Kronish, Anne L., MD
- McNeill-Augustine, Roberta Nicole,
- Perry, Russell J., MD
- Pottick-Schwartz, Eliane Amely, MD
- Prajapati, Binita Prashant, DO
- Roitman, Alla, DO
- Shah, Jigisha Tanmay, MD

Wilton Internal Medicine
751 Teaneck Road Zip: 07666
Ph: (201) 837-3200 Fax: (201) 837-8993
- Coppola, Peter W., MD
- Denker, Michael, MD

Women's Health Care Group
870 Palisade Avenue/Suite 301 Zip: 07666
Ph: (201) 907-0900 Fax: (201) 907-0229
- Frattarola, John D., MD
- Lee, Johanna, DO
- Palomar, Nicole Liza, MD
- Shah, Payal A., MD

Tenafly
Tenafly Eye Associates, PA
111 Dean Drive/Suite 2 Zip: 07670
Ph: (201) 567-5995 Fax: (201) 567-1354
- Stabile, John R., MD

Tenafly Ob-Gyn Associates PA
2 Dean Drive/2nd Floor Zip: 07670
Ph: (201) 569-3300 Fax: (201) 569-7649
- Broizman, David T., MD
- Kithinji, Kagendo M., MD
- Lieblich, Richard M., MD
- Luke, Brian T., MD
- Rivera-Segarra, Stephanie Denise, M

Tenafly Pediatrics, PA
32 Franklin Street Zip: 07670
Ph: (201) 569-2400 Fax: (201) 569-6081
- Anderson, Daniel Parker, MD
- Asnes, Russell S., MD
- Elkin, Avigayil H., MD
- Jawetz, Sheryl Andrea, MD
- Menasha, Joshua Daniel, MD
- Michael, Lisa Golomb, MD

Schaumberger,David Andrew, MD
Smith,Michael Adam, MD
Starer,Yvette R., MD
Sugarman,Lynn B., MD
Weissman,Evan Laird, DO
Wisotsky,David H., MD

The Office of Dr Sharon Scherl MD
45 Central Aveue   Zip: 07670
Ph: (201) 568-8400   Fax: (201) 568-8554
Laureano,Ana Cristina, MD
Scherl,Sharon, MD

The Park Medical Group
274 County Road/Suite A   Zip: 07670
Ph: (201) 568-0493   Fax: (201) 568-0483
Klein,Walter A., MD

Teterboro
Quest Diagnostics Inc.
1 Malcolm Avenue   Zip: 07608
Ph: (201) 393-5000   Fax: (201) 393-6127
Alt,Elaine R., MD
Ayer,Uma, MD
Bayard-McNeeley,Marise, MD
Cardillo,Marina, MD
Eftychiadis,Angela S., MD
Gallo,Leza N., MD
Gerber,Marina, MD
Gill,Melissa, MD
Iskaros,Basem F., MD
Kanuga,Dharmishtha Jayesh, MD
Kaufman,Harvey Willard, MD
Kennedy,Harvey Ronald, MD
Limaye,Anjali P., MD
Liu-Jarin,Xiaolin, MD
Luff,Ronald David, MD
Mahmood,Afsar, MD
Malhotra,Chanchal Anand, MD
Mehta,Kumudini U., MD
Niu,Weiwei, MD
Pang,Xinzhu, MD
Tamas,Ecaterina F., MD
Tarr,William Ellsworth Jr., MD
Tsao,Lawrence, MD
Untawale,Vasundhara G., MD
Vinod,Sheela U., MD
Yohannan,Wendy S., MD
Zhang,Yiqiu, MD

Thorofare
Cooper Physicians Office
196 Grove Avenue/Suite C   Zip: 08086
Ph: (856) 848-7577   Fax: (856) 848-6554
Desai,Anjali Ashok, MD
Penberthy,Katherine Ann, MD

Laskin Internal Medcine
400 Grove Road/PO Box 37   Zip: 08086
Ph: (856) 845-8010
Ahmed,Asma Talukder, DO
Camacho,Jose A., MD
Laskin,David A., MD

Tinton Falls
Cardiac Care Center
21 North Gilbert Street   Zip: 07701
Ph: (732) 741-7400   Fax: (732) 741-4775
Belluscio,Roland L., MD
O'Keefe,Arthur A. Jr., MD
Vlahos,Aristotelis E., MD
Zukoff,David S., MD

Dermatology & Skin Cancer Center
55 North Gilbert Street   Zip: 07701
Ph: (732) 747-5500   Fax: (732) 747-1212
Gorin,Risa Jill, DO
Kruse,Christopher Bryant, MD
Terushkin,Vitaly, MD

Drs. Delaney, Merlin & Pourmasiha
66 West Gilbert Street/2nd Floor   Zip: 07701
Ph: (732) 212-0051   Fax: (732) 212-0713
Enriquez,Santiago Jr., MD
Merlin,Mark A., DO
Pourmasiha,Niloufar, DO

Meridian Primary Care
55 North Gilbert Street/Suite 3201   Zip: 07701
Ph: (732) 450-0961   Fax: (732) 530-0213
Carracino,Robert L., MD
Chen,Roger L., MD
Dougherty,Renee Maria, DO

Navesink Pediatrics
55 North Gilbert Street/Suite 2101   Zip: 07701
Ph: (732) 842-6677   Fax: (732) 530-2946
Condiotte,Shaw Brandon, MD
Cotenoff,Melanie L., MD
Dawis,Maria Agnes Chaluangco, MD
Miller,Steven E., DO
Morgan,Robert L., MD
Pulcini,Ashley Elizabeth, DO
Salvador-Goon,Brenda Mae, MD
Wood,Jessica R., DO

Professional Orthopaedic Associates
776 Shrewsbury Avenue/Suite 201   Zip: 07724
Ph: (732) 530-4949   Fax: (732) 530-3618
Bade,Harry III, MD
Cohen,Jason D., MD
Foos,Gregg Robert, MD
Gentile,David R., MD
Gesell,Mark William, MD
Johnson,Christopher D., MD
Torpey,Brian M., MD

Riverview Medical Associates, PA
4 Hartford Drive/Suite 1   Zip: 07701
Ph: (732) 741-3600   Fax: (732) 741-3603
Boak,Joseph G. Jr., MD
Boesler,Iza Marzanna, MD
Drout,David I., MD
Gardilla,Kalyani Ila, MD
Grabowy,Thaddeus John, MD
Jurewicz,Stephen S., MD

Shore Orthopaedic Group
35 Gilbert Street South   Zip: 07701
Ph: (732) 530-1515   Fax: (732) 747-5433
Chalnick,David Lee, MD
Glastein,Cary D., MD
Grossman,Robert B., MD
Markbreiter,Lance A., MD
Rathi,Sandeep, MD
Rizzo,Charles C., MD
Woska,Scott Corey, MD

Women Caring For Women
43 North Gilbert Street/Suite 8   Zip: 07701
Ph: (732) 530-5550   Fax: (732) 345-8309
Collado,Marilyn Loh, MD
Minaya,Evelyn, MD

Toms River
Alberto Medical Associates PA
25 Mule Road/Unit A-3   Zip: 08755
Ph: (732) 240-0404   Fax: (732) 244-3555
Alberto,Priscilla Magsalin, MD
Alberto,Renato D., MD
Gabriel,Timothy Cayco, MD
Jimenez,Martin Zaratan, MD

Alpha Medical
462 Lake Hurst Road   Zip: 08755
Ph: (732) 255-7570   Fax: (732) 244-2556
Santangelo,Donato III, MD
Wang,Jean C., MD
Yu,Henry K., MD

Arthritis & Osteoporosis Associates
150 Route 37 West Ste A2/Suite A2   Zip: 08755
Ph: (732) 414-6001   Fax: (732) 414-6003
Salloum,Rafah, MD

Athwal Eye Associates, PC
14 Mule Road/Suite 1   Zip: 08755
Ph: (732) 286-0900   Fax: (732) 244-6063
Athwal,Barinder S., MD
Athwal,Harjit S., MD
Athwal,Lisa M., MD

Cardiology Consultants
368 Lakehurst Road/Suite 301   Zip: 08755
Ph: (732) 240-1048   Fax: (732) 240-3464
Chang,Richard Youngjae, DO
Clancy,Kevin F., MD
Cornell,Russell John, MD
Iyanoye,Adeyemi, MD
Jacobs,Glenn Paul, MD
Sobti,Sanjiv, MD

Coast Orthopedic Associates PA
886 Commons Way/Building H   Zip: 08755
Ph: (732) 914-8989
Palmieri,Alfred E., MD
Sacks,Richard, MD

Coastal Health Care
1314 Hooper Avenue/Building B   Zip: 08753
Ph: (732) 349-4994   Fax: (732) 341-1717
Adelizzi,Angela M., DO
Camiscoli,Deborah J., MD
Geneslaw,Charles H., MD
Gigliuto,Christine M., MD
Haque,Salma, MD
Rudd,Rebecca A., MD

Coastal Imaging, LLC
79 Route 37 West/Suite 103   Zip: 08755
Ph: (732) 678-0087   Fax: (732) 276-2325
Atallah,Judy, DO
Chinta,Bharath Kumar, MD
Florio,Francesco, DO
Golsaz,Cyrus Michael, MD
Lee,Brian H., MD
Moran,Christopher John, MD
Perosi,Nicholas Anthony, MD

Coastal Neurosurgery
9 Hospital Drive   Zip: 08755
Ph: (732) 341-1881
Hartwell,Richard Conrad, MD
Sarris,John, MD

Coastal Sports Medicine
1594 Route 9/Suite 6   Zip: 08755
Ph: (732) 349-8888   Fax: (732) 349-8880
Nelson,Andrew L., MD
Pawa,Sakshi, MD

Community Medical Center
20 Hospital Drive/Suite 1   Zip: 08755
Ph: (732) 240-6688   Fax: (732) 240-5757
Deliwala,Tejas Pramodrai, MD
Tsang,Kock-Yen, MD

Community Pulmonary Assoc PA
20 Hospital Drive/Suite 16   Zip: 08755
Ph: (732) 349-5220
Nayak,Yeshavanth P., MD
Strazzella,William D., DO

Drs Shah and Shah
25 Mule Road/Suite B4   Zip: 08755
Ph: (732) 341-0020   Fax: (732) 341-0072
Shah,Dhanvanti B., MD
Shah,Sweta, MD

Drs. DiChiara and Lozowski
2446 Church Road/Suite 10   Zip: 08753
Ph: (732) 255-3636
DiChiara,Frank P., DO
Lozowski,Thomas E., DO

Drs. Guarino & O'Brien
160 Highway 37 West   Zip: 08755
Ph: (732) 286-0440   Fax: (732) 286-2885
Guarino,Ralph V., MD
O'Brien,Thomas K., MD

Drs. Gupta and Patel
20 Hospital Drive/Suite 12B   Zip: 08755
Ph: (732) 240-7777   Fax: (732) 240-7710
Gupta,Rakesh Vardhan, MD
Patel,Parag Vishnu, MD

Drs. Krishnan and Krishnan
14 Hospital Drive   Zip: 08755
Ph: (732) 502-5292   Fax: (732) 818-4810
Krishnan,Lalitha G., MD
Krishnan,Mahadevan Gopa, MD

Drs. Mendoza & Mendoza
9 Mule Road/Suite E-5   Zip: 08755
Ph: (732) 240-3710   Fax: (732) 240-3783
Mendoza,Concepcion B., MD
Mendoza,Narciso D., MD

Drs. Mitra & Mayrowetz
368 Lakehurst Road/Suite 207   Zip: 08755
Ph: (732) 557-6222   Fax: (732) 557-6227
Mayrowetz,Burton, MD
Mitra,Tithi, MD

Drs. O'Donnell and King
1163 Route 37 West/Suite A-2   Zip: 08755
Ph: (732) 349-2424
King,Andrew P., MD

O'Donnell,Robert H., DO

Drs. Ortiz, Villanueva and Cruz
1163 Route 37 West/Suite A-1   Zip: 08755
Ph: (732) 736-1000   Fax: (732) 736-8811
Cruz,Francisco Philomel Doming, MD
Ortiz,Olivia Tanyag, MD
Ortiz,Oscar T., MD
Villanueva,Ronald Banaag, MD

Drs. Van Wyck & Matteace
567 Fischer Boulevard   Zip: 08753
Ph: (732) 506-6868   Fax: (732) 506-6879
Matteace,Frank P., MD
Van Wyck,William Louis, MD

Espineli Medical Associates Pc
1163 Route 37 West/Suite D-4   Zip: 08755
Ph: (732) 341-9494   Fax: (732) 341-3416
Bugay,Victor Valdes, MD
Espineli,Dino O., MD
Espineli,Rosalinda O., MD

Family Health Center
301 Lakehurst Road   Zip: 08755
Ph: (732) 557-3380   Fax: (732) 557-3390
Karroum,Kamil Hanna, MD
Somasundaram,Manamadurai R., MD

Freehold Ophthalmology, LLC
20 Hospital Drive   Zip: 08755
Ph: (732) 349-7167   Fax: (732) 505-4322
Alterman,Michael Adam, DO
Heimmel,Mark Robert, MD

Garden State Radiation Oncology
512 Lakehurst Road   Zip: 08755
Ph: (732) 240-0053   Fax: (732) 240-9360
Eggert,Bryan George, MD

Gastroenterologists of Ocean County
477 Lakehurst Road   Zip: 08755
Ph: (732) 349-4422   Fax: (732) 349-5087
Bigornia,Edgar G., MD
Cohen,Allan, MD
Collier,Jill A., MD
Glazier,Kenneth David, MD
Mirchandani,Jai, MD
Tamimi,Omar A., MD

Hypertension & Kidney Group
9 Hospital Drive/Suite 16   Zip: 08755
Ph: (732) 341-2211   Fax: (732) 505-8229
Arnold,Robert B., MD
Asghar,Fatima, MD

Intensivists of Toms River, LLC.
99 Route 37   Zip: 08755
Ph: (732) 557-8000   Fax: (732) 557-8021
Soliman,Alaaeldin Abdalla Ali, MD

Jersey Coast Nephrology & Hypertension
1008 Commons Way/Suite G   Zip: 08755
Ph: (732) 818-0700   Fax: (732) 818-0730
Anantharaman,Priya, MD

Kuflik Dermatology
453 Lakehurst Road   Zip: 08755
Ph: (732) 341-0515   Fax: (732) 505-6006
Kuflik,Avery S., MD
Kuflik,Emanuel G., MD

Mahmood Schor Urology PA
20 Hospital Drive/Suite 15   Zip: 08755
Ph: (732) 286-6644   Fax: (732) 286-9321
Mahmood,Parvez, MD
Schor,Martin J., MD

Memory and Aging Center
20 Hospital Drive/Suite 12   Zip: 08755
Ph: (732) 244-2299   Fax: (732) 244-5757
Patel,Ashok Kantilal, MD
Tandon,Pooja, MD

Monmouth Med Grp Pedi Specialties
67 Route 37 West   Zip: 08755
Ph: (732) 557-3541   Fax: (732) 557-3518
Laraya-Cuasay,Lourdes R., MD

Neurological Assoc of Ocean County
40 Bey Lea Road/Suite C103   Zip: 08753
Ph: (732) 367-8280   Fax: (732) 367-1529
Monastersky,Bruce Ted, MD
Zimmerman,Barry L., DO

Groups and Clinics by Town with Physician Rosters

Toms River (cont)

North Dover Ob-Gyn Associates
222 Oak Avenue/3rd Floor/Suite 301 Zip: 08753
Ph: (732) 914-1919 Fax: (732) 914-0725
 Azu,Wilhelmina Dedo, DO
 Bonvicino,Marie Louise, MD
 Harrell,Russell L., MD
 Jackman,Earl Francis, DO
 Passarella,Susan Katherine, DO
 Sutherland,John R., MD

Ocean Anesthesia Group PA
1200 Hooper Avenue Zip: 08753
Ph: (732) 797-3890 Fax: (732) 942-5603
 Gershteyn,Eduard, MD
 Jadav,Jitendra K., MD
 Mako,Robert M., DO
 Manganelli,Douglas M., MD
 Quiambao,Dante B., MD

Ocean County Family Care
9 Mule Road Zip: 08755
Ph: (732) 818-0004 Fax: (732) 818-7775
 Elsamman,Wael A., MD

Ocean County Retina, P.C.
780 Route 37 West/Suite 200 Zip: 08755
Ph: (732) 797-1855 Fax: (732) 797-1856
 Amin,Haris Irfan, MD
 Gloth,Jonathan Michael, MD
 Hajee,Mohammedyusuf Ebrahimadham,

Ocean Endosurgery Center
129 Route 37 West Zip: 08755
Ph: (732) 606-4440 Fax: (732) 797-3963
 Cohen,Scott, DO
 De Martino,Paul John, MD
 Eschinger,Eric Jon, MD
 Loftus,James B., MD
 Lokchander,Rangaswamy S., MD
 Nagaria,Neil C., MD
 Raso,Carl L., MD
 Shah,Kamlesh Manher, MD
 Shakov,Rada, MD
 Suatengco,Jose Ramon, MD
 Tacopina,Teresa Anne, MD

Ocean Eye Institute
601 Route 37 West Zip: 08755
Ph: (732) 244-4400 Fax: (732) 505-2171
 Angioletti,Louis Scott, MD
 Grossman,David R., MD
 Lautenberg,Mitchel Alan, MD
 Robinson,Neil H., MD
 Schoenfeld,Allan H., MD
 Spedick,Michael J., MD
 Trastman-Caruso,Elyse Randi, MD

Ocean Health Initiatives, Inc.
301 Lakehurst Road Zip: 08755
Ph: (732) 552-0377 Fax: (732) 552-0378
 Argeros,Olga, MD
 Masia,Alan, MD
 Shankar,Kala, MD
 Valthaty,Rebekah, MD

Ocean Orthopedic Associates, P.A.
530 Lakehurst Road/Suite 1 Zip: 08755
Ph: (732) 349-8454 Fax: (732) 341-0259
 Alcid,Jess Gerald, MD
 Blum,Karl Richard, MD
 Closkey,Robert F., MD
 Dhawlikar,Sripad H., MD
 Kasper,Mark T., MD
 Kubeck,Justin P., MD
 Passariello,Christopher, MD
 Pensak,Michael J., MD
 Petrillo,John A., MD

Ocean Otolaryngology Associates
54 Bey Lea Road/Suite 3 Zip: 08753
Ph: (732) 281-0100 Fax: (732) 281-0400
 Gillespie,Christine, MD
 Kupferberg,Stephen Benjamin, MD
 Peters,Bruce W., DO

Ocean Pulmonary Associates PA
3 Plaza Drive/Suite 2 Zip: 08757
Ph: (732) 341-1380 Fax: (732) 505-9296
 Shah,Dhiren A., MD

Ocean Renal Associates, P.A.
508 Lakehurst Road/Suite 3 A Zip: 08755
Ph: (732) 341-4600 Fax: (732) 341-4993
 Palecki,Winicjusz, MD

Orthopaedic Institute of Ctrl NJ
226 Highway 37 West/Suite 203 Zip: 08755
Ph: (732) 240-6060 Fax: (732) 240-5329
 Holtzberg,Nathan, MD

Pediatric Affiliates, PA
40 Bey Lea Road/Suite B203 Zip: 08753
Ph: (732) 341-0720 Fax: (732) 244-6842
 Braverman,Isaac L., MD
 Dever,Matthew Patrick, MD
 Fiore,Elizabeth Jill, DO
 Goldstein,Richard M., MD
 Golub,Michael L., MD
 Haimowitz,Ira L., DO
 Kanthan,Sudha, MD
 Morano,Amy Beth, MD
 Shanik,Robert A., MD
 Tan,Mary Catherine D., MD

Professional Orthopaedic Associates
1430 Hooper Avenue/Suite 101 Zip: 08753
Ph: (732) 341-6777 Fax: (732) 349-7722
 Gabisan,Glenn Gacula, MD
 Saleh,Jason Reed, MD

Robert P. Rabinowitz, DO, PA
462 Lakehurst Road Zip: 08755
Ph: (732) 341-5403 Fax: (732) 505-0862
 Rabinowitz,Robert P., DO

Samir S. Jain MD PC
599 Route 37 West/Suite 5 Zip: 08755
Ph: (732) 608-9737 Fax: (732) 608-9744
 Jain,Samir S., MD

Schweiger Dermatology
368 Lakehurst Road/Suite 201 Zip: 08755
Ph: (732) 244-4700 Fax: (732) 731-6134
 Dixon,Melissa Kaye, MD
 Ma,Manhong, MD
 Maghari,Amin, MD
 Trivedi,Prabhas Arunbhai, MD

Shore Cardiac Institute
367 Lakehurst Road Zip: 08755
Ph: (732) 473-0158 Fax: (732) 473-0033
 DiLorenzo,William Richard, DO
 Stone,Jay H., MD

Shore Eye Associates
530 Lakehurst Road/Suite 206 Zip: 08755
Ph: (732) 341-4733 Fax: (732) 341-2794
 Pan,Jane Chi-Chun, MD
 Wnorowski,Brian R., MD

Shore Neurology, P.A.
633 Route 37 West Zip: 08755
Ph: (732) 240-4787 Fax: (732) 240-3114
 Amin,Darshana Patel, DO
 DiPaola,Rocco J., MD
 Ferencz,Gerald J., MD

Silverton Pediatrics
2446 Church Road Zip: 08753
Ph: (732) 255-7553 Fax: (732) 255-8901
 Patestos,Chris Anastasios, MD
 Qazi,Rumana Yousef, MD
 Schlachter,Steven A., MD
 Sia,Valerie May Gumban, MD
 Ulep,Shirley Dollaga, MD

Susskind & Almallah Eye Assocs
20 Mule Road/Focus Center Zip: 08755
Ph: (732) 349-5622 Fax: (732) 349-5625
 Almallah,Omar F., MD
 Birdi,Anil, MD
 Pidduck,Thomas Charles, MD

Toms River Anesthesia Associates PC
409 Main Street/2nd Floor Zip: 08753
Ph: (732) 818-7575 Fax: (732) 818-1567
 Cha,Hak J., MD
 Farkas,Klara, MD
 Lin,Renny L., MD
 Mara,Frank J., MD
 Park,Yung I., MD
 Tank,Hasmukh C., MD

Toms River Cardiology Associates, LLP.
780 Route 37 West/Suite 310 Zip: 08755
Ph: (732) 240-0599 Fax: (732) 240-3039
 Bageac,Michael, MD
 DiPisa,Leonard R., MD

Toms River Family Medical Center
1028 Hooper Avenue Zip: 08753
Ph: (732) 349-8866
 DiPaolo,Ann, DO
 Roggemann,Dennis J., MD
 Simone,Philip M., MD
 Wayman,Bernard R. III, MD

Toms River Medical Group PA
81 Route 37 West/Suite 1 Zip: 08755
Ph: (732) 341-0560 Fax: (732) 341-0574
 Pasquariello,James L., MD
 Tenner,Bruce S., DO

Toms River Ob-Gyn Associates PA
79 Route 37 West/Suite 101 Zip: 08755
Ph: (732) 244-9444 Fax: (732) 244-9468
 Lopez,Gerardo J., MD
 Neal,Ronald R., MD
 Pesso,Robert S., MD

Toms River Wellness Center
10 Kettle Creek Road Zip: 08753
Ph: (732) 255-8880 Fax: (732) 255-8885
 Birnbaum,Joseph G., MD
 Hartanowicz,Stanley J., MD

Urologic Health Center of New Jersey
67 Route 37 West/Building 2/Suite 1 Zip: 08755
Ph: (732) 914-1300 Fax: (732) 914-0849
 Ferlise,Victor J., MD
 Howard,Peter Carson, MD
 Stoneham,John L. III, MD

Woman to Woman Obstetrics & Gynecology
615 Main Street Zip: 08753
Ph: (732) 797-1510 Fax: (732) 797-2370
 Furman,Lesley P., MD
 Jones,Angela Renee, MD
 Maxwell,Aliona, MD

Totowa

AMG Primary Care at Totowa
650 Union Boulevard/Unit 16 Zip: 07512
Ph: (908) 938-5200 Fax: (908) 938-5190
 Asfour,Mervet, MD
 Patel,Puja, MD

Allergy Associates of North Jersey
362 Union Boulevard Zip: 07512
Ph: (973) 790-6707 Fax: (973) 790-1255
 Ghanem,Roland, MD

DP Pediatrics
142 Totowa Road/Suite 8 Zip: 07512
Ph: (973) 904-1000 Fax: (973) 904-1480
 Deshmukh,Pratibha S., MD
 Pandey,Krishna K., MD

Giliberti Eye & Laser Center PC
415 Totowa Road Zip: 07512
Ph: (973) 595-0011 Fax: (973) 595-5155
 Giliberti,Francesca Marie, MD
 Giliberti,Orazio L., MD

Totowa OB/GYN
525 Union Boulevard Zip: 07512
Ph: (973) 790-1117 Fax: (973) 790-1143
 Day,Brian Todd, MD
 Tkach-Chubay,Irina, MD

Totowa Pediatric Group, P.A.
290 Union Boulevard/Suite 2 Zip: 07512
Ph: (973) 595-0600 Fax: (973) 595-0206
 Abdulmasih,Yousef H., MD
 Elepano,Richard G., DO
 Elfanagely,Sarah Hedy, MD
 Elias,Maurice, MD
 Zodiatis,Alexander Demetrius, DO

Totowa Physicians and Surgeons
426 Union Boulevard Zip: 07512
Ph: (973) 595-8400
 Odorczuk,Marzena, MD

Trenton

Advanced Surgical Assoc. of NJ
40 Fuld Street/Suite 403 Zip: 08638
Ph: (609) 537-6000 Fax: (609) 537-6002
 Abud-Ortega,Alfredo Ramon, MD
 Ahmad,Sarfaraz, MD
 Hanna,Niveen, MD
 Kelly,Michael E., DO

Advocare Garden State Pediatrics
2133 Highway 33 Zip: 08690
Ph: (609) 581-5100 Fax: (609) 581-5134
 Boor,Sonya H., MD
 Brandspiegel,Laura K., MD

Allergy and Pulmonary Associates
1542 Kuser Road/Suite B-7 Zip: 08619
Ph: (609) 581-1400 Fax: (609) 585-5234
 Gushue,George F. Jr., DO
 Seelagy,Marc M., MD
 Steeger,Joseph R., MD
 Vogel,David P., MD

Americare Medical Associates, LLC
445 Whitehorse Avenue/Suite 202 Zip: 08610
Ph: (609) 585-1122 Fax: (609) 585-0309
 Chinwalla,Farah, DO
 Kheder,Abdul-Hady M., MD
 Memon,Nahid, MD

Bellevue Pediatrics
416 Bellevue Avenue/Suite 207 Zip: 08648
Ph: (609) 989-9801 Fax: (609) 989-9896
 Isola,Venkatarao, MD
 Radhakrishnan,Puthenmadam, MD

Brickner-Mantell Ctr for Women's Hlth
1-A Quakerbridge Plaza Zip: 08619
Ph: (609) 689-9991 Fax: (609) 689-9992
 Brickner,Gary R., MD
 Mantell,Cary Hilton, DO

Capital Cardiology Associates
40 Fuld Street/Suite 400 Zip: 08638
Ph: (609) 396-1644 Fax: (609) 394-9526
 Damani,Prabodhkum M., MD
 Kalra,Krishan G., MD
 Mustafa,Muhammad Usman, MD
 Nagra,Bipinpreet Singh, MD

Capital Health Family Health Center
433 Bellevue Avenue/4th Floor Zip: 08618
Ph: (609) 815-7296 Fax: (609) 815-7178
 Banks,Gerald, MD
 Barrett Carnes,Joy-Lynne, MD
 Ginsburg,Deborah J., MD
 Granderson,Lisa Irene, MD
 Hawes,Ruppert Augustus, MD
 Hypolite,Renee E., DO
 Lansing,Martha H., MD
 Noble,Mary C., MD
 Ysique,Jacqueline Rosa, MD
 Zafar,Jabbar Ben, MD

Capital Health Hospitalist Group
750 Brunswick Avenue Zip: 08638
Ph: (609) 815-7887 Fax: (609) 394-6299
 Chaudhry,Sofia, MD
 Ghavami,Roozbeh Mofid, MD
 Hassan,Hardawan Ahmed, MD
 Kaur,Navjot, MD
 Mazhar,Noorain, MD
 Rondanina,Richard W., MD
 Saleem,Bushra, MD
 Samiev,Djamshed, MD
 Zarkua,Kristina, MD

Capital Medical Associates
1235 Whitehorse Mercerville Rd Zip: 08619
Ph: (609) 587-3003 Fax: (609) 587-4512
 Huq,Irfan-Ul, MD
 Nadeem,Shahzinah, MD
 Raza,Ali Babar, MD

Capital Surgical Associates
40 Fuld Street/Suite 303 Zip: 08638
Ph: (609) 396-2600 Fax: (609) 396-3600
 D'Amelio,Louis F., MD
 Eboli,Dominick Joseph, MD
 Quinlan,Dennis Philip Jr., MD
 Rojavin,Yuri, MD
 Saleem,Mohammed R., MD
 Salem,Raja R., MD

Corporate Health Center
832 Brunswick Avenue Zip: 08638
Ph: (609) 695-7471
 Gaskel,Virginia M., DO

Groups and Clinics by Town with Physician Rosters

Gumidyala,Lalitha V., MD
Makowsky,Michael J., MD
Misra,Neerja, MD
Schwartz,Eric, MD
Szenics,Jonathan M., MD
Taylor,Tanisha K., MD
Vypritskaya,Ekaterina Anatolyevna,

Diabetes and Endocrinology Associates
3525 Quakerbridge Road/Suite 2000 Zip: 08619
Ph: (609) 570-2071 Fax: (609) 689-2614
Brotman-O'Neill,Alissa Sue, DO
Poblete,Honesto Madjus, MD

Drs. Dawlabani and Dawlabani
908 West State Street Zip: 08618
Ph: (609) 503-5540 Fax: (609) 503-5541
Dawlabani,Nassif E., MD
Dawlabani,Nickolas Elias, MD

Drs. Rana & Roowala
40 Fuld Street/Suite 302 Zip: 08638
Ph: (609) 393-0067 Fax: (609) 393-4943
Bokhari,Shafaq, MD
Rana,Nilesh C., MD
Roowala,Shabbir H., MD

Drs. Sharim & Zubair
40 Fuld Street/Suite 402 Zip: 08638
Ph: (609) 393-4911
Sharim,Iradj, MD
Zubair,Khurram, MD

Drs. Stillwell & Hohl
1423 Pennington Road Zip: 08618
Ph: (609) 882-8080
Hohl,Rosario DeFatima M., MD
Stillwell,Paul C., MD

Ewing Medical Associates
1539 Pennington Road Zip: 08618
Ph: (609) 883-4124
Ryfinski,Eugene A., MD
Walker,Paul A., DO

Gastroenterology Associates
2275 Whitehorse-Mercerville Rd Zip: 08619
Ph: (609) 890-0200
Rosner,Bruce P., MD
Rubin,Marc R., MD

Global Neuroscience Institute
750 Brunswick Avenue Zip: 08638
Eckardt,Gerald William, MD
Rao,Vikas Yallapragada, MD

Greater Mercer Pulm & Med Assocs
445 Whitehorse Avenue/Suite 103 Zip: 08610
Ph: (609) 585-0300
Cueto,Irene L., MD
Pacia,Arthur G., MD

Hamilton Anesthesia Associates
2119 Highway 33/Suite B Zip: 08690
Ph: (609) 581-0770
Beshara,Raafat Henry, MD
Co,Anthony, MD
Dinh,Cung T., MD
Haig,Lauren Grace, MD
Markos,Marina Azmy, MD
Spodik,Boris, DO

Hamilton Gastroenterology Group
1374 Whitehorse Hamilton Squar Zip: 08690
Ph: (609) 586-1319 Fax: (609) 586-1468
Afridi,Shariq A., MD
Baig,Zahid Imran, MD
Boucard,Herve C., MD
Marulendra,Shivaprasad, MD
Zamir,Zafar, MD

Hamilton Internal Med Assocs
2055 Klockner Road Zip: 08690
Ph: (609) 586-8060 Fax: (609) 586-7470
Laub,Edward B., MD
Mavasheva,Sofia, MD

Henry J. Austin Health Center
321 North Warren Street Zip: 08618
Ph: (609) 278-5900 Fax: (609) 695-3532
Agrawal,Nidhi, MD
Alli,Kemi A., MD
Andreyev,Nina Vaskina, MD
Geng,Qingdi, MD

Lopez,Lisa M., MD
Pacheco-Smith,Sariya Amina, MD
Sussman,Cindy Pearsall, MD
Tatarowicz,Roman J., MD

Hopewell Valley Medical Group, PA
1871 Pennington Road Zip: 08618
Ph: (609) 882-5317 Fax: (609) 538-8031
Gupta,Rajendra Prasad, MD
Gupta,Vinod K., MD

LifeCare Physicians, PC of Hamilton
1225 Whitehorse Mercerville Rd Zip: 08619
Ph: (609) 581-6060 Fax: (609) 581-9561
Bresch,David, MD
Grewal,Raji Paul, MD
Shah,Rajiv K., MD

Lotus Medical Center
40 Fuld Street/Suite 307 Zip: 08638
Ph: (609) 278-9700 Fax: (609) 278-9744
Aamir,Tajwar, MD
Obuz,Vedat, MD

Mercer Allergy and Pulmonary Assoc
1544 Kuser Road/Suite C-6 Zip: 08619
Ph: (609) 581-9900 Fax: (609) 581-9905
Ricketti,Anthony J., MD
Ricketti,Peter Anthony, DO

Mercer County Hematology and Oncology
40 Fuld Street/Suite 404 Zip: 08638
Ph: (609) 394-0660 Fax: (609) 394-1004
Chen,Emily Q., MD

Mercer County Pediatrics
2113 Klockner Road Zip: 08690
Ph: (609) 586-7887 Fax: (609) 586-1198
Rapp,Rachel V., MD
Valencia,Maria Linda, MD

Mercer Kidney Institute
40 Fuld Street/Suite 401 Zip: 08638
Ph: (609) 599-1004 Fax: (609) 599-3611
Cohen,Barry Herbert, MD
Cohen,Steven Craig, DO
Hussain,Asher Ferjad, MD
Pai,David Y., MD
Sudhakar,Telechery A., MD

OB/GYN Associates at Mercer
446 Bellevue Avenue Zip: 08618
Ph: (609) 394-4111 Fax: (609) 394-4070
Amadi,Nkechinyere, MD

Physical Medicine and Pain Cente
34 Scotch Road Zip: 08628
Ph: (609) 883-0614 Fax: (609) 883-1606
Chiricolo,Heather Marie, MD
Rosenberg,Daniel S., MD

Poblete Dermatology
1601 Whitehorse-Mercerville Rd/Suite 2 Zip: 08619
Ph: (609) 838-9040 Fax: (609) 838-9042
Abello Poblete,Maria Veronica Roma
Poblete,Fredrick M., MD

Pulmonary & Internal Med Assoc
40 Fuld Street/Suite 201 Zip: 08638
Ph: (609) 695-4422
Levitt,Alan T., MD
Warren,Ronald L., MD

SNS Rheumatology Associates
2333 Whitehorse Mercerville Rd/Suite J Zip: 08619
Ph: (609) 689-1229
Mahmud,Hossen, MD
Usmani,Qaisar H., MD

Stabile Medical Associates
1755 Klockner Road Zip: 08619
Ph: (609) 587-0083 Fax: (609) 587-0211
Stabile,Michael C., MD

Trenton Orthopaedic Group
1225 Whitehorse Mercerville Rd Zip: 08619
Ph: (609) 581-2200 Fax: (609) 581-1212
Aita,Daren J., MD
Conte,Evan J., MD
Di Biase,John J., MD
Duch,Michael R., MD
Fletcher,Daniel J., MD
Gomez,William, MD
Hornstein,Joshua Scott, MD
Levine,Marc Jason, MD

Pagliaro,Andre J., MD
Saxena,Arjun, MD
Schnell,John Raymond, MD

Univ Correctional HealthCare-Colpitts
Whittessey Rd & Stuyvesant Ave Zip: 08625
Ph: (609) 292-9700
Brewer,Arthur Martin, MD
Lieberman,Jordan A., MD
Mabrouk,Hanny S., MD

Vascular Access Center
1450 Parkside Avenue/Unit 18 Zip: 08638
Ph: (609) 882-1770 Fax: (609) 882-8406
McGuckin,James Frederick Jr., MD
Oolut,Joseph James, MD

West Trenton Medical Associates
1230 Parkway Avenue/Suite 203 Zip: 08638
Ph: (609) 883-5454 Fax: (609) 883-2565
Victor,Carl H., MD

Tuckerton

Southern Ocean Primary Care
317 East Main Street Zip: 08087
Ph: (609) 296-1336
Miller,Walter P., MD
Rudolph,Herbert J., MD

Turnersville

Athena Women's Institute
151 Fries Mill Road/Suite 301 Zip: 08012
Ph: (856) 374-1377 Fax: (856) 374-2177
D'Ambola,Lesly A., DO
McKinney,Timothy B., MD

Center For Kidney Disease
129 Johnson Road/Suite 4 Zip: 08012
Ph: (856) 374-4440 Fax: (856) 374-4445
Irwin-Obregon,Virginia, DO
Panebianco,Paul S., DO

Drs. Barb & Patel
901 Route 168/Suite 101 Zip: 08012
Ph: (856) 228-7577 Fax: (856) 228-0534
Barb,Herman T., MD
Patel,Prabhaker S., MD

Drs. Vitola & Kernis
900 Route 168/Suite C3 Zip: 08012
Ph: (856) 374-0430 Fax: (856) 374-0048
Kernis,Elyse Beth, DO
Vitola,Carl A., DO

Family Practice Associates
188 Fries Mill Road/Suite N3 Zip: 08012
Ph: (856) 875-8000 Fax: (856) 875-8494
Madison,William A. Jr., DO
Venuti,John David, DO
Venuti,Robert L., DO

Harmony Healthcare For Women
139 Ganttown Road/PO Box 1109 Zip: 08012
Ph: (856) 232-0050 Fax: (856) 232-0251
Kanoff,Martin E., DO
Manus,Alan M., DO

Internal Med Assoc of So NJ
151 Fries Mill Road/Suite 400 Zip: 08012
Ph: (856) 401-9300 Fax: (856) 374-5307
Lauletta,Maryann Carmella, MD
Michelson,Marc H., DO
Palermo,Kim Marie, DO
Schwartz,Robert B., DO
sargent,Stephanie Christine, DO

Jefferson Health Primary/Speclty Care
1A Regulus Drive Zip: 08012
Ph: (844) 542-2273
Abesh,Daniel C., DO
Agia,Gary A., DO
Beluch,Brian Walter, DO
Di Medio,Lisa C., DO
O'Brien,Marlene Theresa, MD
Rudolph,Kafi, DO
Slusser,Jonathan, DO
Taylor,Greg Michael, DO
Zaman,Taimur, MD

Kennedy Health Alliance
188 Fries Mill Road/Suite N-1 Zip: 08012
Ph: (856) 783-2241 Fax: (856) 783-2273
Chiesa,John C., DO

Kennedy Hospitalist Office
435 Hurffville Cross Keys Road Zip: 08012
Ph: (856) 513-4124 Fax: (856) 302-5932
Mongeau,Marc Thomas, DO
Schiers,Kelly Anne, DO
Vlad,Tudor Jon, MD
Wang,Yvette, DO
Wiley,Joan C., DO
Willsie,Philip S., DO

Rancocas Anesthesiology, PA
151 Fries Mill Road/Suite 202 Zip: 08012
Ph: (856) 228-7246 Fax: (856) 228-7252
Innerfield,Caitlin, MD

South Jersey Dermatology Assoc
900 Route 168/Suite F6 Zip: 08012
Ph: (856) 227-7488 Fax: (856) 228-3476
Durham,Booth H., MD
Gruber,Melvin S., MD

South Jersey Radiology Associates, P.A
901 Route 168/Suites 301-305 Zip: 08012
Ph: (856) 227-6600 Fax: (856) 227-8537
Brodkin,Joshua S., MD
Dannenbaum,Mark S., MD
Gallagher,Thomas Jude, DO
Harding,John Arthur, MD
Manning,Ana B., MD
Muhr,William Jr., MD
Niedbala,Thomas M., MD
Oberlender,Susan B., MD
Podgorski,Edward M. Jr., MD
Roberts,David A., MD
Rosner,William Fredric, MD
Schmucker,Linda N., MD

Womens Health Associates PA
188 Fries Mill Road/Suite B-1 Zip: 08012
Ph: (856) 629-1400 Fax: (856) 629-6695
Rosen,Larry S., MD

Union

Advanced Gastroenterology Group
1308 Morris Avenue Zip: 07083
Ph: (908) 851-2770 Fax: (908) 851-7706
Dhirmalani,Rajesh A., DO
Fernandez Ledon,Ramon A., MD
Grover,Kunal, MD
Merchant,Prakriti Singh, MD
Tempera,Patrick G., MD

Allergy and Clinical Immunology Center
2333 Morris Avenue/Suite D13 Zip: 07083
Ph: (908) 688-1330 Fax: (908) 964-0991
Sundaram,Kanaga N., MD

Ambulatory Surgical Ctr of Union Co
950 West Chestnut Street/Suite 200 Zip: 07083
Ph: (908) 688-2700 Fax: (908) 688-7424
Yim,Yoori W., MD

American Access Care, LLC.
2401 Morris Avenue/Suite West 112 Zip: 07083
Ph: (908) 686-0123 Fax: (908) 686-0014
Latif,Walead, DO

Assoc Eye Physicians & Surgeons of NJ
1050 Galloping Hill Road/Suite 104 Zip: 07083
Ph: (908) 964-7878 Fax: (908) 964-5434
Natale,Benjamin P., DO
Tchorbajian,Kourkin, MD

Associated Orthopaedics
1000 Galloping Hill Road,/Suite 202 Zip: 07083
Ph: (908) 964-6600 Fax: (908) 364-1025
Botwin,Clifford A., DO
Innella,Robin R., DO

Center for Digestive Diseases
695 Chestnut Street Zip: 07083
Ph: (908) 688-6565 Fax: (908) 688-3161
Chirla,Sujala, MD
Muthusamy,Samiappan, MD
Ramasamy,Dhanasekaran, MD

Groups and Clinics by Town with Physician Rosters

Union (cont)

CityMD Union Urgent Care
2317 Center Island Route 22 Zip: 07083
Ph: (201) 354-1951 Fax: (201) 354-1952
- Ahmed, Ameer Nizam, MD
- Salim, Suhail Mohammed, DO
- Talat, Afnan, MD

Codella Family Practice
1000 Galloping Hill Road/Suite 103 Zip: 07083
Ph: (908) 688-1550 Fax: (908) 688-1552
- Codella, Vincent Adrian, DO
- Lee, Nancy, DO

Donato S. Russo MD LLC
1896 Morris Avenue/Suite 3 Zip: 07083
Ph: (908) 687-8282
- Messimer, Julie Marie, MD
- Russo, Donato S., MD

Drs. Eisenstat and Kershner
1050 Galloping Hill Road/Suite 202 Zip: 07083
Ph: (908) 688-4845 Fax: (908) 687-2039
- Chapinski, Caren A., DO
- Eisenstat, Steven Alan, DO
- Kershner, Gary Brian, DO

Drs. Nelson and Goldin
541 Clubhouse Court/Unit 3 Zip: 07083
- Goldin, Michael R., MD
- Nelson, Elizabeth A., MD

Drs. Rasin and Ivanov
2143 Morris Avenue/Suite 3 Zip: 07083
Ph: (908) 686-4145
- Ivanov, Alexander, MD
- Rasin, Grigory S., MD

IGEA Brain & Spine
1057 Commerce Avenue Zip: 07083
Ph: (908) 688-8800 Fax: (908) 688-2377
- Aragona, James, MD
- Gilad, Ronit, MD
- Lipson, Adam Craig, MD
- Nair, Anil Karunakaran, MD
- Poulad, David, MD
- Rajaram, Arun, MD
- Randazzo, Ciro Giuseppe, MD

Inform Diagnostics
825 Rahway Avenue Zip: 07083
Ph: (732) 901-7575 Fax: (732) 901-1555
- Bentley, James David, MD
- Dinu, Veronica Carmen, MD
- Losada, Mariela, MD
- Mendrinos, Savvas E., MD
- Riba, Ali K., MD

Ortho Physicians & Surgeons
975 Lehigh Avenue Zip: 07083
Ph: (908) 686-1488 Fax: (908) 687-7886
- Charko, Gregory P., MD
- King, John Wayne, DO

Overlook Hospital-Dvpmt Disabilities
1000 Galloping Hill Road Zip: 07083
Ph: (908) 598-6655 Fax: (908) 686-8374
- Andreoli, Nina Needleman, MD
- Grigaux, Claire Nathalie, MD

Physical Rehabilitation Center LLP
1767 Morris Avenue Zip: 07083
Ph: (908) 624-1050 Fax: (908) 624-1052
- Potashnik, Rashel, MD
- Vekhnis, Betty, MD

Pulmonary and Critical Care Associates
2333 Morris Avenue/Suite B-15 Zip: 07083
Ph: (908) 964-1964
- Karpman, Jesse, MD
- Miller, Jeffrey Adam, DO
- Segal, Ilia, MD

Suburban Heart Group, P.A.
1000 Galloping Hill Road/Suite 107 Zip: 07083
Ph: (908) 964-7333 Fax: (908) 687-7855
- Doskow, Jeffrey B., MD
- Gold, Jeffrey M., DO
- Vitale, Carl J., MD

The Back Institute
700 Rahway Avenue/Suite A-14 Zip: 07083
Ph: (908) 688-1999
- Bradley, Douglas D., MD
- Friedlander, Marvin E., MD
- Ratzker, Paul K., MD

Union & Cranford Ob/Gyn & Infertility
1323 Stuyvesant Avenue Zip: 07083
Ph: (908) 686-4334 Fax: (908) 686-1744
- Boffard, Daryl K., MD
- Ericsson, Dawn Marie, MD
- Victor, Isaac L., MD

Union Anesthesia & Pain Management
695 Chestnut Street Zip: 07083
Ph: (908) 851-7161 Fax: (908) 851-7536
- Fleischhacker, Wayne, DO
- Kahn, Randolph, DO
- Novik, Edward, MD
- Shane, Steven A., DO
- Wilcenski, Michael A., MD

Union County Cardiology Associates, P.
1317 Morris Avenue Zip: 07083
Ph: (908) 964-9370 Fax: (908) 964-9332
- Gopinathan, Kastooril, MD
- Pullatt, Raja C., MD
- Schackman, Paul E., MD
- Williams, Edward G. Jr., MD

Union Family Medicine
2300 Vauxhall Road Zip: 07083
Ph: (908) 688-4424
- Rizzo, David M., DO

Union Medical Associates PA
1308 Morris Avenue/Suite 101 Zip: 07083
Ph: (908) 687-8686 Fax: (908) 687-9694
- Lombardo, Sabato J., MD

Union Medical Group LLC
2401 Morris Avenue/Suite 101 Zip: 07083
Ph: (908) 688-5000 Fax: (908) 688-5220
- Diaz-Johnson, Nereida, MD
- Philogene, Clark E., MD

Union Medical, LLC
2182 Morris Avenue Zip: 07083
Ph: (908) 851-2666
- Alladin, Irfan Ahmad, MD
- Sun, Jidong, MD

Union Pediatric Medical Group, PA
1050 Galloping Hill Road/Suite 200 Zip: 07083
Ph: (908) 688-9900 Fax: (908) 688-9939
- Luke, Steven, MD
- Ohri, Ranjana, MD
- Oxman, David J., MD
- Panzner, Elizabeth A., MD
- Straw, Simone A., MD

Womens HealthCare of Union County
950 West Chestnut Street/Suite 102 Zip: 07083
Ph: (908) 688-8545 Fax: (908) 688-8447
- Buontempo, Angela J., DO
- DiRico, Julie, MD
- Hyman, Martin C., MD
- McNamara, Robert E., MD

Union City

Cardio-Med Services
3196 Kennedy Boulevard/3rd Floor Zip: 07087
Ph: (201) 974-0077
- Barrientos, Monica, MD
- Campoalegre, Maria A., MD
- Velasco, Mauricio, MD

City Heights Pediatrics
511 22nd Street Zip: 07087
Ph: (201) 866-7740 Fax: (201) 223-1905
- Cenon, Pearl L., MD
- McDonough, Kevin J., MD

Dr Jerry L. Jurado and Assoc
2401 Palisade Avenue Zip: 07087
Ph: (201) 867-5791 Fax: (201) 223-1905
- Dominguez, Jonathan Manuel, MD
- Jurado, Jerry L., MD

Excelcare Medical Associates
408 37th Street Zip: 07087
Ph: (201) 864-4477 Fax: (201) 864-9727
- Gastell, Gilberto F., MD
- Hesquijarosa, Alexander, MD

Hudson Essex Nephrology
510 31st Street Zip: 07087
Ph: (201) 866-3322 Fax: (201) 866-2289
- Bebawy, Niveen, MD
- Hajal, Hussam, MD
- Thomsen, Stephen, MD

Hudson Eye Specialists
2201 Bergen Line Avenue/3rd Floor Zip: 07087
Ph: (201) 601-2020
- Gabay, Jacqueline Estelle, MD

NHCAC Health Center at Union City
714 31st Street Zip: 07087
Ph: (201) 863-7077 Fax: (201) 863-2730
- Veloso, Corazon M., MD

Premier Orthopaedics & Sports Med
3196 Kennedy Boulevard/Third Floor Zip: 07087
Ph: (201) 770-1600 Fax: (201) 770-1010
- Baruch, Howard Michael, MD

Progressive Pediatrics
3196 Kennedy Boulevard Zip: 07087
Ph: (201) 319-9800 Fax: (201) 319-9849
- Knight, Phillip Thomas, DO
- Polack, Noha, MD
- Teraguchi, Kari Jane, MD
- Velez, Isabel Odeida, MD

Rastogi Medical Associates
524 43rd Street Zip: 07087
Ph: (201) 617-8338 Fax: (201) 868-3235
- Rastogi, Sadhna, MD

Retina Associates of New Jersey, P.A.
3196 Kennedy Boulevard Zip: 07087
Ph: (201) 867-2999 Fax: (201) 867-4440
- Ho, Vincent Yih, MD

Riverside Pediatric Group
4201 New York Avenue Zip: 07087
Ph: (201) 601-9515 Fax: (201) 601-9516
- Anam, Sadrul, MD
- Delgado, Wilson Eduardo, MD
- Valdivieso, Yaira Michelle, MD

Upper Montclair

Drs. Bell and Mason-Bell
51 Upper Montclair Plaza/Suite 14 Zip: 07043
Ph: (973) 746-9615
- Bell, Michael Henry, MD
- Mason-Bell, Sharon E., MD

Vauxhall

Community Health Center
3 Farrington Street Zip: 07088
Ph: (908) 598-7950 Fax: (908) 686-1163
- Benvenuti, Eve S., MD
- Elkins, Michele, MD
- Feurdean, Mirela Cristina, MD
- Hurckes, Lisa Carabelli, MD
- Lacapra, Gina M., MD
- Ratner, Douglas J., MD

Ventnor

AtlantiCare Internal Medical Associate
7313 Ventnor Avenue Zip: 08406
Ph: (609) 441-2199 Fax: (609) 487-9640
- Lipshutz, Robert L., DO
- Rosenthal, Leslie S., MD

Atlantic Cardiology in Ventor
6725 Atlantic Avenue/2nd Floor Zip: 08406
Ph: (609) 822-2006
- Romero, Luis N., MD

Drs. Dunn & Smith
4807 Atlantic Avenue Zip: 08406
Ph: (609) 823-8488
- Smith, David J., MD

Ventnor City

Specialty Medconsultants LLC
6725 Ventnor Avenue/Suite C Zip: 08406
Ph: (609) 350-6780 Fax: (609) 350-6995
- Bursheh, Samar Samir, MD
- Naber, Tamim Hani, MD
- Shahateet, Omar, MD

Ventnor Pediatric Center, LLC
6601 Ventnor Avenue/Suite 14 Zip: 08406
Ph: (609) 487-6507 Fax: (609) 487-6508
- Asemota, Emiola O., MD
- Tan, Madeline P., MD

Vernon

Advocare Vernon Pediatrics
249 Route 94 Zip: 07462
Ph: (973) 827-4550 Fax: (973) 827-5845
- Huzar, Diana, DO
- Kabarwal, Navneesh Kaur, MD
- Pyatov, Yelena V., MD
- Saluja, Gurbir S., MD
- Saluja, Gurmit Singh, MD

Premier Health Associates
212 State Route 94/Suite 1-D Zip: 07462
Ph: (973) 209-2162 Fax: (973) 209-2665
- Hansen, Eric S., DO

Verona

Allergy Consultants, PA
197 Bloomfield Avenue Zip: 07044
Ph: (973) 857-0330 Fax: (973) 857-0980
- Fost, Arthur F., MD
- Fost, David A., MD
- Narisety, Satya D., MD

Assocs in Ob-Gyn & Infertility
825 Bloomfield Avenue/Suite 103 Zip: 07044
Ph: (973) 239-5010
- Milano, Michael C., MD

David J. Strader MD, PHD
799 Bloomfield Avenue/Suite 304 Zip: 07044
Ph: (973) 618-9990 Fax: (973) 618-9991
- Dorfman, Joseph Charles, MD
- Nielsen, Sarah B., MD
- Prestigiacomo, Cynthia R., MD
- Strader, David J., MD

Drs. Mariyampillai and Mariyampillai
825 Bloomfield Avenue/Suite LL1 Zip: 07044
Ph: (973) 239-3770 Fax: (973) 239-3774
- Mariyampillai, Joan of Arc J., MD
- Mariyampillai, Marcarious A., MD

First Care Medical Group
50 Pompton Avenue Zip: 07044
Ph: (973) 857-3400 Fax: (973) 857-7034
- Chakilam, Santhosh, MD
- Lipsitch, Carol E., MD
- Steinhardt, Amelia L., DO
- Waller, Leon H., DO

Gastroenterology Health Care PA
799 Bloomfield Avenue/Suite 102 Zip: 07044
Ph: (973) 857-7600 Fax: (973) 857-0020
- Manzi, Daniel D., MD
- Nathan, Ramasamy Swami, MD

Mountainside Family Practice
799 Bloomfield Avenue/Suite 201 Zip: 07044
Ph: (973) 746-7050 Fax: (973) 857-2831
- Baronia-White, Bernadette, MD
- Berg, Kevin James, MD
- Daftani, Kennedy Palwasha Fazli, MD
- Daftani, Mohammad Daoud Daoud, MD
- George, Bettina, MD
- Gjoni, Indira, MD
- Gonzalez, Orlando V., MD
- Holder, Dawn Paulette, MD
- Kasowitz, Andrea Ruth, DO
- Lander, Jeffrey, MD
- Louka, Magda F., DO
- Mallon, Nancy Tyrrell, MD
- Mendelsohn, Jason, MD
- Miller, George W. Jr., MD
- Mozafarian, Mona, MD
- Odigboegwu, Joyce Cynthia, MD
- Saba, Ragheda M., MD
- Schlam, Everett W., MD
- Sedgh, Raymond, MD
- Sharma, Ekta, MD
- Slater, Shakira L., MD

Groups and Clinics by Town with Physician Rosters

NJ Urology
799 Bloomfield Avenue/Suite 300 Zip: 07044
Ph: (973) 746-3322   Fax: (973) 429-8765
 Saidi,James Ali, MD
 Walmsley,Konstantin, MD
 Williams,Jeffrey Franklin, MD

North Atlantic Rehab Medicine
799 Bloomfield Avenue/Suite 303 Zip: 07044
Ph: (973) 857-7800   Fax: (973) 857-7822
 Bach,Richard Tae, MD
 Hicks,Kristina Elizabeth, MD
 Keswani,Rohit, MD

North Jersey Orthopaedic Group
799 Bloomfield Avenue/Suite 111 Zip: 07044
Ph: (973) 689-6266   Fax: (973) 689-6264
 Gehrmann,Robin Michael, MD
 Leary,Jeffrey T., MD

Park Avenue Pediatrics
36 Park Avenue   Zip: 07044
Ph: (973) 239-7001
 Flyer,Richard H., MD
 Khokhar,Rizwana T., MD
 Sirna,Paul William, MD

The Dermatology Group, P.C.
60 Pompton Avenue   Zip: 07044
Ph: (973) 571-2121   Fax: (973) 571-2126
 Abbate,Marc Anthony, MD
 Bonney,David Raymond, DO
 Brown,Justin, MD
 Horenstein,Marcelo G., MD
 Kassim,Andrea Tinuola, MD
 Nossa,Robert, MD
 Rothman,Frederic R., MD
 Spates,Stephen Thomas, MD

Town Medical Associates/Verona
271 Grove Avenue/Suite A   Zip: 07044
Ph: (973) 239-2600   Fax: (973) 239-0482
 Cirello,Richard, MD
 Gorman,Robert T., MD
 Lacara,Dena L., DO
 Mazzella,Carmine A., DO
 McCarrick,Thomas P., MD
 Murray,Richard S., MD
 Sivaraju,Kannan, MD
 Smith,Stephanie, MD

Vineland

Advanced Dermatology, Laser & Cosmetic
2466 East Chestnut Avenue   Zip: 08361
Ph: (856) 691-3442   Fax: (856) 691-6582
 Carbonaro,Paul Anthony, MD
 Toome,Brigit K., MD

Advocare Family Medicine Assoc
602 West Sherman Avenue/Suite B Zip: 08360
Ph: (856) 692-8484   Fax: (856) 896-3059
 Kuptsow,Scott Warren, MD

Arthritis & Rheumatology Assoc
2848 South Delsea Drive/Suite 2-C Zip: 08360
Ph: (856) 794-9090   Fax: (856) 794-3058
 Arkebauer,Matthew Robert, DO
 Soloway,Stephen, MD

Community Health Care INC
484 South Brewster Road   Zip: 08360
Ph: (856) 696-0300   Fax: (856) 696-2561
 Clayton,Elizabeth Noelle, DO
 Frinjari,Hassan, MD
 Gewirtz,Jonathan D., MD
 Panganamamula,Uma R., MD
 Torchia,Michele A., MD

Community Health Care, Inc.
319 Landis Avenue/Suites A & B   Zip: 08360
Ph: (856) 691-3300   Fax: (856) 696-0344
 Alberici,Anna, DO
 Neema,Swarnalatha, MD

CompleteCare Adult/Spec Med Prof
1038 East Chestnut Avenue/Suite 110 Zip: 08360
Ph: (856) 451-4700
 Flaherty,Stephanie, DO
 Girone,Joseph Francis, MD

 Necsutu,Simona Camelia, MD
 Obara,Justyna Anna, MD

Cumberland Internal Medicine
1450 East Chestnut Avenue   Zip: 08361
Ph: (856) 794-8700   Fax: (856) 794-2752
 Ahrens,John C., MD
 Atthota,Vakula Devi, MD
 Galetto,David W., MD
 Kaufman,David H., MD

Cumberland Medical Associates
1206 West Sherman Avenue   Zip: 08360
Ph: (856) 691-8444   Fax: (856) 691-8325
 Bhendwal,Sanjay, MD
 Dovnarsky,Michael K., MD
 Huston,Donald Jr., DO
 Montero-Pearson,Per M., MD
 Sheetz,Maurice Saunders, MD
 Wanalista,David Michael, DO

Cumberland Nephrology Associates, PA
1318 South Main Road   Zip: 08360
Ph: (856) 205-9900   Fax: (856) 205-0041
 Barber,Kevin G., DO
 Kumar,Anshul, MD
 Relia,Nitin, MD

Cumberland Ob-Gyn PA
1102 East Chestnut Avenue   Zip: 08360
Ph: (856) 696-4484   Fax: (856) 690-1352
 Bonifield,Eric M., MD
 Russo,Armando P., MD

Cumberland Ob-Gyn, PA
2950 College Drive/Suite 2G   Zip: 08360
Ph: (856) 696-4484   Fax: (856) 696-1694
 Walsh,Sussannah Savitri, MD

Delaware Valley Urology
1138 East Chestnut Avnue/Suite 8-B Zip: 08360
Ph: (856) 213-4037   Fax: (856) 267-2499
 Dorsey,Philip J. Jr., MD
 Kasturi,Sanjay Srinivas, MD

Drs. Burgher and Chikani
2950 College Drive/Suite C   Zip: 08360
Ph: (856) 692-6000   Fax: (856) 692-0609
 Burgher,Sonia A., MD
 Chikani,Jignasa Ripal, MD

Excel Care Alliance, LLC
49 South State Street   Zip: 08360
Ph: (856) 696-9697   Fax: (856) 696-9698
 Patel,Hasmukhbha D., MD
 Tomar,Raghuraj S., MD

Eye Associates
251 South Lincoln Avenue   Zip: 08361
Ph: (856) 691-8188   Fax: (856) 691-0421
 Bresalier,Saul, DO
 Holzinger,Karl Anthony, MD
 Tyson,Sydney L., MD
 Williams,Alice, MD

Inspira Medical Group Surgical Assoc
1102 East Chestnut Avenue   Zip: 08360
Ph: (856) 213-6375   Fax: (856) 575-4986
 Antinori,Charles H., MD

Inspira Medical Group Surgical Associa
1206 West Sherman Avenue/Building 2 Zip: 08360
Ph: (856) 696-9933   Fax: (856) 696-9939
 Callender,Gordon Erwin, MD
 Kumar,Sanjay, MD
 Kushnir,Leon, MD
 Ogwudu,Ugochukwu Chinweze, MD

Luciano Jose Bispo, MD, LLC
2950 College Drive/Suite 2F   Zip: 08360
Ph: (856) 205-0606   Fax: (856) 205-0044
 Bispo,Luciano Jose, MD
 Fockler,Raechel Ann, DO

Pediatric Associates, LLC.
1318 South Main Street   Zip: 08360
Ph: (856) 691-8585   Fax: (856) 691-8489
 Fisher,Matthew Adam, MD
 Hegedus Bispo,Sandra, MD
 Mirone,Rolande A., DO
 Nakhate,Vishakha Vinay, MD
 Rosenberg,Michael A., MD

Pediatrix Medical Group
1505 West Sherman Avenue/MSO-Box 104   Zip: 08360
Ph: (856) 845-0100   Fax: (856) 641-7647
 Bird,Charrell Moyo, MD
 Sinha,Anita, MD
 Streeks,Nicole N., MD

Premier Orthopaedic Associates
298 South Delsea Drive   Zip: 08360
Ph: (856) 690-1616   Fax: (856) 690-1089
 Catalano,John B., MD
 Di Verniero,Richard Charles Jr., M
 Disabella,Vincent N., DO
 Dwyer,Thomas A., MD
 Fitzhenry,Laurence N. IV, MD
 Mariani,Chiara, MD
 McAlpin,Fred III, MD
 Sarkos,Peter Anthony, DO
 Shah,Rahul V., MD
 Smith-Martin,Kimberley Yvette, MD
 Wu,Eddie S., DO
 Zucconi,Adam J., MD

Reconstructive Orthopedics
994 West Sherman Avenue   Zip: 08360
Ph: (856) 267-9400   Fax: (856) 267-9457
 Bernardini,Brad Joseph, MD
 Bernardini,Joseph P., MD
 Evering,Daniel Jr., DO
 Salim,Shakeel, MD
 Silver,Seth M., MD

Regional Diagnostic Imaging Center
1505 West Sherman Avenue   Zip: 08360
Ph: (856) 641-7937   Fax: (856) 641-7681
 Bhagat,Nitesh N., MD
 Patel,Nirav, MD
 Rosenberg,Allison R., DO

Southern Oncology Hematology Associate
1505 West Sherman Avenue/Suite 101 Zip: 08360
Ph: (856) 696-9550   Fax: (856) 691-1686
 Al Ustwani,Omar, MD
 Negin,Benjamin Paul, MD
 Roy,Shailja, MD
 Sachdeva,Kush, MD
 Sudhindra,Ramakrishna R., MD

Vineland Medical Associates
1100 East Chestnut Avenue   Zip: 08360
Ph: (856) 696-0108   Fax: (856) 691-1106
 Nakhate,Vinay Gopal, MD
 Parmar,Kiritkumar A., MD
 Venugopal,Narasimhan, MD

Vineland Pediatrics
1138 East Chestnut Avenue   Zip: 08360
Ph: (856) 692-1108   Fax: (609) 692-2077
 Jain,Archna, MD
 Ogidan,Olabode O., MD
 Solof,Arnold J., MD

Wachspress & Rainear Cardiology
1076 East Chestnut Avenue   Zip: 08360
Ph: (856) 692-7979   Fax: (856) 794-9479
 Quinlan,Jack Francis Jr., MD
 Rainear,Kristen, DO
 Rana,Jiten, MD

Voorhees

21st Century Oncology
130 Carnie Boulevard   Zip: 08043
Ph: (856) 424-0003   Fax: (856) 424-0055
 Harvey,Alexis, MD

AAP Family Practice, PC
707 White Horse Road/Suite C-105 Zip: 08043
Ph: (856) 258-4966   Fax: (856) 258-4972
 Patel,Ambarish Ashokkumar, DO
 Patel,Ashokkumar B., MD

Advanced ENT - Voorhees
200 Bowman Drive/Suite D-285   Zip: 08043
Ph: (856) 602-4000   Fax: (856) 346-0757
 Belafsky,Robert B., MD
 Cantrell,Harry, MD
 Dandu,Kartik Varma, MD
 Leoniak,Steven Michael, MD
 Scheiner,Edward David, DO
 Walker,Ryan D., MD

Advanced GI
2301 Evesham Road/Pav 800/Suite 110 Zip: 08043
Ph: (856) 772-1600
 Alloy,Andrew Marc, DO
 Celluzzi,Alex, DO
 Egan,Elizabeth Anne, MD

Advanced Pain Consultants, P.A.
326 Route 73   Zip: 08043
Ph: (856) 489-9822   Fax: (856) 489-9877
 Ahsan,Syed Nadeem, MD
 Boyajian,Stephen S., DO
 Rogers,Kenneth H., DO

Advocare In-Patient Medicine
100 Bowman Drive   Zip: 08043
Ph: (856) 247-3000
 Burns,Gerard Joseph II, DO
 Jumao-As,Joseph Maben Aparece, MD

Advocare Nephrology Of South Jersey
300 Sheppard Road   Zip: 08043
Ph: (856) 424-7390   Fax: (856) 424-7386
 Chawla,Arun, MD
 Lodhavia,Devang V., MD

Advocare Premier OB/GYN of South Jerse
903 Sheppard Road   Zip: 08043
Ph: (856) 772-2300   Fax: (856) 772-2301
 Felsenstein,Roberta G., MD
 Grossman,Eric Brian, MD

Advocare The Farm Pediatrics
1001 Laurel Oak Boulevard/Suite B Zip: 08043
Ph: (856) 782-7400   Fax: (856) 782-7404
 Prilutski,Megan A., MD
 Russ,Michelle L., DO

Allied Gastrointestinal Assocs
502 Centennial Boulevard/Suite 3 Zip: 08043
Ph: (856) 751-2300   Fax: (856) 751-2333
 Hashmi,M. Arif, MD
 Malamut,Jay M., MD
 McLaughlin,Vincent A., MD

Arthritis, Rheum/Back Dis Assoc
2309 East Evesham Road/Suite 101 Zip: 08043
Ph: (856) 424-5005   Fax: (856) 424-4716
 Abraham,Shawn George, MD
 Evangelisto,Amy Marie, MD
 Grimmett,Brian L., MD
 Hollander,Adrienne R., MD
 Krommes,Janet Filemyr, MD
 Maurer,Kenneth H., MD
 Patel,Neha Mahendra, MD
 Schuster,Michael Charles, MD
 Silver,Arielle S., MD
 Solomon,Sheldon D., MD
 Sundhar,Joshua Bharat, MD
 Weeks,Alicia, MD

Assoc Cardiovascular Consultants
1105 Laurel Oak Road/Suite 165 Zip: 08043
Ph: (856) 424-3600   Fax: (856) 424-7154
 Gabler,Scott Joseph, MD
 Gerewitz,Fredric B., MD
 Joffe,Ian I., MD
 Kramer,Alan D., MD
 Lisa,Charles P., MD
 Orth,Donald W., MD
 Perlman,Richard L., MD
 Schlessel,David R., MD
 Yanoschak,Jennifer Lee, MD

.Becker Nose & Sinus Center, LLC.
2301 East Evesham Road/Suite 306 Zip: 08043
Ph: (856) 772-1617   Fax: (856) 770-0069
 Becker,Samuel Scott, MD

CHOP Care Network at Virtua
101 Carnie Boulevard   Zip: 08043
Ph: (856) 325-3000
 Jaiswal,Paresh, MD
 Mann,Ana Mendes, MD

Groups and Clinics by Town with Physician Rosters

Voorhees (cont)

CHOP Care Network at Virtua Voorhees
100 Bowman Drive Zip: 08043
Ph: (856) 325-3000 Fax: (609) 261-5842
- Ang,Dexter Ong, MD
- Brutus,Nadege A., DO
- Chiang,Chung, DO
- Cohen,Amy Marie Palmieri, MD
- Dorn,Eric A., MD
- Gabriele,Elizabeth Ann, MD
- Ghavam,Sarvin, MD
- Gowda,Sharada Hiranya, MD
- Lestini,Melissa Murray, MD
- Maher,Jennifer Lee, DO
- Pandit,Paresh B., MD
- Ritson,Brenda Marie, MD
- Seiden,Jeffrey A., MD
- Sheehan,Christine, DO
- Topol,Howard Ira, MD
- Zieniuk,Gregory J., MD

CHOP Pedi & Adol Specialty Care Center
1012 Laurel Oak Road Zip: 08043
Ph: (856) 435-1300 Fax: (856) 435-0091
- Anderson,Terry M., MD
- Bailey,Philip Daniel Jr., DO
- Binenbaum,Gil, MD
- Brooks,Lee J., MD
- Browne,Patricia M., MD
- Corcino,Ana J., MD
- Fiedler,Joel Mark, MD
- Germiller,John Andrew, MD
- Greenbaum,Barbara H., MD
- Jobes,David Richard, MD
- Khan,Sadaf Ahmad, MD
- Kim,Amy, MD
- Lawrence,John Todd Rutter, MD
- Mascarenhas,Maria R., MD
- Mascio,Christopher Edward, MD
- Mayer,Oscar Henry, MD
- Nadaraj,Sumekala, MD
- Nicolson,Susan C., MD
- Pradhan,Madhura Ravindra, MD
- Rossi,Wilma Catherine, MD
- Sanchez,Guillermo R., MD
- Shah,Udayan Kanaiyalal, MD

CHOP Specialty Care Center at Virtua
200 Bowman Drive/2 FL/Suite D-260 Zip: 08043
Ph: (267) 425-5400
- Gadin,Erlita Pagaduan, MD
- Mason,Thornton B. Alexander II, MD
- Sharif,Uzma M., MD

Cancer Institute of NJ at Cooper
900 Centennial Boulevard/Suite M-2 Zip: 08043
Ph: (856) 325-6750 Fax: (856) 325-6777
- Rajagopalan,Kumar, MD

Centennial Surgical Center LLC
502 Centennial Boulevard/Suite 1 Zip: 08043
Ph: (856) 874-0790
- Cho,Daniel P., MD

Children's Hospital of Phila Cardio
1040 Laurel Oak Road/Suite 1 Zip: 08043
Ph: (856) 783-0287 Fax: (856) 783-0657
- Bhargava,Hema P., MD

Colon & Rectal Surgical Assocs of SJ
502 Centennial Boulevard/Suite 5 Zip: 08043
Ph: (856) 429-8030 Fax: (856) 428-2718
- Empaynado,Edwin Abogado, MD
- Gardine,Robert L., MD
- Irwin,Eytan A., MD
- Siemons,Gary O., MD

Comprehensive Cancer & Hematolgy
705 White Horse Road Zip: 08043
Ph: (856) 435-1777 Fax: (856) 435-0696
- Bapat,Ashok R., MD
- Gordon,Richard L., DO
- Ross,David H., MD

Cooper Bone and Joint Institute
900 Centennial Boulevard Zip: 08043
Ph: (856) 673-4914 Fax: (856) 325-6678
- Gealt,David Benjamin, DO
- Pollard,Mark Andrew, MD

Cooper Cardiology Associates
900 Centennial Boulevard Zip: 08043
Ph: (856) 325-6700 Fax: (856) 325-6702
- Cha,Ri D., MD
- Iliadis,Elias, MD
- Parrillo,Joseph E., MD
- Russo,Andrea Marie, MD

Cooper Gynecologic Oncology Associates
900 Centennial Boulevard/Suite F Zip: 08043
Ph: (856) 325-6644
- Aikins,James K. Jr., MD
- Crisp,Meredith Page, MD
- Rocereto,Thomas F., MD
- Warshal,David Philip, MD

Cooper Physician Offices
900 Centennial Boulevard Zip: 08043
Ph: (856) 325-6770 Fax: (856) 673-4300
- Angelo,Mark, MD
- Beggs,Nancy H., MD
- Cho,Grace Shin, MD
- Han,Kwang Hoon, MD
- Leuzzi,Rosemarie Anne, MD
- Traisak,Pamela, MD

Cooper Rheumatology
900 Centennial Boulevard/Suite 203 Zip: 08043
Ph: (856) 968-7019 Fax: (856) 482-5621
- Eid,Hala Milad, MD
- Feinstein,David E., DO

Cooper Surgical Care at Voorhees
6015 Main Street/Suite G Zip: 08043
Ph: (856) 325-6565 Fax: (856) 325-6555
- Gor,Ronak, DO
- Pello,Mark J., MD

Drs. Mehta & Lerman
900 Centiental Boulevard Zip: 08043
OnlyFax: (856) 325-6777
- Lerman,Nati, MD
- Mehta,Pallav K., MD

Drs. Zalut and Lowe
1000 White Horse Road/Suite 806 Zip: 08043
Ph: (856) 770-0022 Fax: (856) 770-9194
- Lowe,John William, DO
- Seeley,Brian T., DO

Echelon Medical Center
600 Somerdale Road Zip: 08043
Ph: (856) 429-8445 Fax: (856) 429-1962
- Gupta,Asha, MD
- Manigat,Yves J., MD

Eye Care Physicians & Surgeons of NJ
2301 Evesham Road/Suite 501-502 Zip: 08043
Ph: (856) 770-0030 Fax: (856) 770-0840
- Ohsie-Bajor,Linda Hae Eun, MD

Eye Physicians PC
1140 White Horse Road/Suite 1 Zip: 08043
Ph: (856) 784-3366 Fax: (856) 784-4388
- Cox,Mary Jude, MD
- Dugan,John Donald Jr., MD
- Gault,Janice Ann, MD
- Gordon,Susan Master, MD

Family Practice Assocs - Voorhees
805 Cooper Road/Suite 3 Zip: 08043
Ph: (856) 751-1777 Fax: (856) 751-8090
- Blumenthal,Andrew Michael, DO
- Soble,Toby K., MD

Fox Chase Virtua Health Cancer Center
106 Carnie Boulevard/Suite A Zip: 08043
Ph: (856) 325-4830
- McCleery,Colleen Marie, MD
- Miller,William B., DO
- Wilson,John J., MD

Garden State Infectious Diseases Assoc
709 Haddonfield Berlin Road Zip: 08043
Ph: (856) 566-3190 Fax: (856) 783-2193
- Abel,David Michael, DO
- Barnish,Michael J., DO
- Condoluci,David V., DO
- Fussa,Mark J., DO
- Ghayad,Zeina Rita, DO
- Hou,Cindy Meng, DO

Garden StateOB/GYN Asscs
2401 Evesham Road/Suite A Zip: 08043
Ph: (856) 424-3323 Fax: (856) 424-4994
- Bowers,Geoffrey David, MD
- Bridges-White,Kimberly Gaye, MD
- Colella,Ryan Lawrence, MD
- Cortese,Bernard J., MD
- Goodchild,Caroline Gagel, MD
- Murphy,Heather Marie, MD
- Ricci,Emily K., MD
- Steighner,Kathleen Marie, MD
- Swift,Joanne, MD
- Tha,Teemu, MD

Integrated Family Medicine
701 Cooper Road/Suite 16 Zip: 08043
Ph: (856) 783-5000 Fax: (856) 783-5041
- Davis,Robert A., DO
- Karmazin,Polina, MD
- Kitts,Lori M., MD

Jefferson HealthCare - Voorhees
443 Laurel Oak Road Zip: 08043
- Solitro,Tamara Stolz, MD
- Witmer,George Robert III, MD

Kennedy Care Center
705 White Horse Road/Suite D-101-2 Zip: 08043
Ph: (856) 783-0695 Fax: (856) 783-8083
- Furey,William J., DO
- Giuglianotti,Daniel Scott, DO
- Gupta,Kavita, DO

KHA Vascular Surgery
333 Laurel Oak Road Zip: 08043
Ph: (844) 542-2273 Fax: (856) 770-9194
- Chiesa,Drew Jonathan, DO
- Libby,Joseph Anthony, MD
- Walters,Richard Lawrence, DO

Macaione & Papa Dermatology Assocs
707 White Horse Road/Suite C-103 Zip: 08043
Ph: (856) 627-1900 Fax: (856) 627-6907
- Baratta,Andrea, DO
- Bernardin,Ronald Maurice III, MD
- Macaione,Alexander, DO
- Papa,Christine A., DO
- Rollins,Terry Lee, MD

Nemours duPont Pediatrics, Voorhees
443 Laurel Oak Road Zip: 08043
Ph: (856) 309-8508 Fax: (856) 309-8556
- Gidding,Samuel S., MD
- Ritz,Steven Bernard, MD

Nephrology & Hypertension Assocs of NJ
201 Laurel Oak Road/Suite B Zip: 08043
Ph: (856) 566-5478 Fax: (856) 566-9561
- Banker,Gopika H., DO
- Brown,Anthony, MD
- Canals-Navas,Carmen L., MD
- Patel,Nitesh M., DO
- Schuster,Mark Brian, DO
- Varallo,Gerardo Jr., DO
- Zingrone,Joseph Peter, DO

New Jersey Urology, LLC
2401 East Evesham Road/Suite F Zip: 08043
Ph: (856) 673-1600 Fax: (856) 988-0636
- Ackerman,Randy B., MD
- Babin,Elizabeth Ann, MD
- Bernstein,Michael R., MD
- Butani,Rajen P., MD
- Goldenberg,Samuel F., MD
- Lembert Tezanos,Larissa, MD
- Linden,Robert Andor, MD
- Nachmann,Marcella Marie, DO
- Orth,Charles Richard Jr., MD
- Sipio,James C., MD
- Sussman,David O., DO
- Thur,Paul C., MD

OB-GYN Specialists
157 Route 73 Zip: 08043
Ph: (856) 874-1114 Fax: (856) 874-9555
- Adamson,Susanne R. M., MD
- Tai,Victoria Chih-Chuang, MD

On-Site Neonatal Partners
1000 Haddonfield-Berlin Road/Suite 210 Zip: 08043
Ph: (856) 782-2212 Fax: (856) 782-2213
- Andrejko,Constance Gasda, DO
- Austria,Jocelyn R., MD
- Bona,Marzena M., MD
- Castillo,Minerva R., MD
- Chavez,Alberto M., MD
- Cruz,Florencia Santos, MD
- Dapul,Gener M., MD
- Davis,Cheryl Luise, MD
- Ghaben,Kamel Mostafa, MD
- Hric,Jerome Joseph, MD
- Hsu,Christopher Tzu-Yao, MD
- Jethva,Purvi Jitendra, MD
- Johnson,Swati, DO
- Josyula,Leela S., MD
- Lespinasse,Antoine Alexandra, MD
- Pleickhardt,Elizabeth Patricia, DO
- Polam,Sharadha, MD
- Pradhan,Kamal M., MD
- Reid,Brittany Michelle, MD
- Reisen,Charles E., MD
- Rosen,Harel D., MD
- Theophilopoulos,Constantine G., MD

Orthopedic Reconstruction
600 Somerdale Road/Suite 113 Zip: 08043
Ph: (856) 795-1945 Fax: (856) 795-7472
- Carey,Christopher T., MD
- Gollotto,Kathryn T., DO
- Harrer,Michael F., MD

Patients First
705 Haddonfield Berlin Road Zip: 08043
Ph: (856) 679-0537
- Fagel,Jonathan Val C., DO
- Massac,Malik Ali, MD
- Roberts,Barbara Theresa, MD

Prestige Institute for Plastic Surgery
1605 East Evesham Road/Suite 201 Zip: 08043
Ph: (856) 304-1114 Fax: (267) 454-7196
- Garber,Brett A., DO
- Tamburrino,Joseph F., MD

Reconstructive Orthopedics, P.A.
200 Bowman Drive/Suite E-100 Zip: 08043
Ph: (609) 267-9400 Fax: (609) 267-9457
- George,Brian Philip, MD
- Klingenstein,Gregory Gillman, MD
- Porat,Manny David, MD
- Reid,Jeremy Jackson, MD
- Stackhouse,Thomas G., MD

Regional Cancer Care Associates, LLC
200 Bowman Drive/Suite E-125 Zip: 08043
Ph: (856) 424-3311 Fax: (856) 424-5634
- Callahan,Kevin J., MD
- Gor,Priya P., MD
- Greenberg,Richard H., MD
- Guggenheim,Douglas Eric, MD
- Ji,Yong, MD
- Madamba,Carlos S., MD
- Siegel,Norman H., MD
- Zrada,Stephen Eugene, MD

Regional Surgical Associates
502 Centennial Boulevard/Suite 7 Zip: 08043
Ph: (856) 596-7440 Fax: (856) 596-6723
- Butler,Charles J., MD
- Fisher,Frederick S., MD
- Grabiak,Thomas A., MD
- Hager,George W. III, MD
- Winter,Howard J., MD

Ripa Center for Women's Health
6100 Main Street Zip: 08043
Ph: (856) 325-6600 Fax: (856) 325-6677
- Williams,Kristina, MD

Rothman Institute - Voorhees
443 Laurel Oak Road Zip: 08043
Ph: (856) 821-6360
- DeLuca,Peter Francis, MD
- Purtill,James Joseph, MD
- Ramsey,Matthew Lee, MD

Vitanzo,Peter Charles, MD

South Jersey Gastrointestinal
2301 Evesham Road/Suite 110 Zip: 08043
Ph: (856) 772-1600 Fax: (856) 772-9031
   Goldstein,Michael Bruce, MD
   Mushnick,Alan J., MD

South Jersey Orthopedic Associates PA
502 Centennial Boulevard/Suite 6 Zip: 08043
Ph: (856) 424-8866
   Daniels,Jeffrey B., MD
   O'Dowd,Thomas A., MD
   Wetzler,Merrick Jay, MD

South Jersey Radiology Associates, P.A
100 Carnie Boulevard/Suite B-5 Zip: 08043
Ph: (856) 751-0123 Fax: (856) 751-0535
   Apple,Jerry S., MD
   Baum,Mark L., MD
   Bloor,James J., DO
   Blumenthal,Beth A., MD
   De Laurentis,Mark, MD
   Doshi,Nilesh M., MD
   Elder,James P. Jr., MD
   Fan,Wen Lin, MD
   Farner,Michael Charles, MD
   Kendzierski,Renee Marie, DO
   King,Anne H., DO
   Kramer,David H., MD
   Lott,Kristen Ellie, MD
   Miller,David Haim, MD
   Mohsin,Jamil, MD
   Patel,Bhupendra M., MD
   Piccoli,Catherine Welch, MD
   Semmler,Helaina D., MD
   Shack,Evan Tyler, MD
   Shah,Tanmaya Chetan, MD

So NJ Cardiac Care Specialists
1020 Laurel Oak Road/Suite 102 Zip: 08043
Ph: (856) 435-8842 Fax: (856) 435-8665
   Andriulli,John A., DO
   Daly,Stephen J., DO
   Geisler,Alan K., DO
   La Morte,Alfonso M., DO
   Papa,Louis A., DO
   Rozanski,Lawrence T., MD

Style Family Medicine
1 Britton Place/Suite 12 Zip: 08043
Ph: (856) 772-1880 Fax: (856) 770-0718
   Style,Daniel J., DO
   Style,Stuart D., DO

Tatem Brown Family Practice
2225 East Evesham Road/Suite 101 Zip: 08043
Ph: (856) 795-4330 Fax: (856) 325-3704
   Bendala,Preeti, MD
   Carela,Gendy, MD
   Choudhry-Akhter,Myra S., MD
   Chummar,Joseline, MD
   Dibba,Prameela, MD
   Dimapilis,Ann B., DO
   Enriquez,Alfred Vasquez, MD
   Fisher-Swartz,Lucinda, MD
   Gamble,James D., MD
   Khalil,Samir Walid, MD
   Krever,Kristine Wang, MD
   Maffei,Mario Stephen, MD
   Mule,Salvatore, MD
   O'Hare,Kendal Eggers, MD
   Phen,Huai Lee, MD
   Post,Robert E., MD
   Ramprasad,Arjun, MD
   Rizvi,Abbas Ali, MD
   Willard,Mary A., MD

The Women's Center at Voorhees
100 Carnie Boulevard/Suite A-4 Zip: 08043
Ph: (856) 751-5522 Fax: (856) 751-5650
   Deshmukh,Kalpana S., MD

University Doctors
2301 East Evesham Road/Suite 202 Zip: 08043
Ph: (856) 770-1305 Fax: (856) 770-1732
   Skobac,Edward A., MD

University Urogynecology Assocs
6012 Piazza at Main Street Zip: 08043
Ph: (856) 325-6622 Fax: (856) 325-6522
   Echols,Karolynn T., MD
   Vakili,Babak, MD

University Urogynecology/Cooper OB/GYN
900 Centennial Boulevard/Suite L Zip: 08043
Ph: (856) 325-6622 Fax: (856) 325-6522
   Caraballo,Ricardo, MD
   Holzberg,Adam S., DO

Urology for Children, LLC
200 Bowman Drive/Suite E-360 Zip: 08043
Ph: (856) 751-7880
   Balsara,Zarine Rohinton, MD
   Concodora,Charles William, MD

Urology for Children, LLC
120 Carnie Boulevard/Suite 2 Zip: 08043
Ph: (856) 751-7880
   Dean,Gregory Edwin, MD
   Packer,Michael G., MD
   Roth,Jonathan A., MD
   Zaontz,Mark R., MD

Virtua Breast Specialty Care
200 Bowman Drive/Suite E-300 Zip: 08043
Ph: (856) 247-7515 Fax: (856) 247-7525
   Figueredo,Nicole Dionesia, MD
   Revesz,Elizabeth, MD

Virtua Cardiology Group
2309 East Evesham Road/Suites 201-202 Zip: 08043
Ph: (856) 325-5400 Fax: (856) 325-5416
   Barrucco,Robert John, DO
   Curl,Kevin M., MD
   Dudda Subramanya,Raghunandan, MD
   Marwaha,Vijay R., MD
   Mintz,Randy T., MD
   Palermo,Jason, MD
   Russo,Ralph E. III, MD
   Shaw,Brian Richard, DO
   Singer,Robert A., MD
   Spivack,Talya R., MD

Virtua Endocrinology
200 Bowman Drive Zip: 08043
Ph: (856) 247-7220
   Davidson,Jean Marie, DO
   Lam,Eleanor Lin, MD

Virtua Express Urgent Care-Voorhees
158 Route 73 Zip: 08043
Ph: (856) 247-7230 Fax: (856) 246-7231
   Thomas-Patterson,Denne Michelle, M

Virtua Family Medicine
1605 Evesham Road/Suite 100 Zip: 08043
Ph: (856) 741-7100 Fax: (856) 424-2629
   Bradley,Kathleen A., MD
   Daniel,Beena Mary, MD
   Varevice-McAndrew,Susan, MD
   Weiner,Samuel David, MD

Virtua Gynecologic Oncology Spec.
200 Bowman Drive/Suite E-315 Zip: 08043
Ph: (856) 247-7310 Fax: (856) 247-7309
   Carlson,John A., MD
   Deger,Randolph Bruce, MD
   Gleimer,Emily R., DO

Virtua Maternal Center
100 Bowman Drive Zip: 08043
Ph: (856) 247-3328 Fax: (856) 247-3276
   Chen,Janine Junying, MD
   Fitzsimmons,John Michael, MD
   Herman,Glenn O., MD
   Librizzi,Ronald J., DO
   Seibel Seamon,Jolene S., MD
   Shah,Shailen S., MD

Voorhees Family Practice
102 West White Horse Road/Suite 102 Zip: 08043
Ph: (856) 783-6200 Fax: (856) 783-8434
   Koerner,David M., DO
   Leone,Mark R., DO

Voorhees Primary & Specialty Care
333 Laurel Oak Road Zip: 08043
Ph: (844) 542-2273 Fax: (856) 770-9194
   Phakey,Vishal, DO
   Zalut,David S., MD

Voorhees Specialty Center
443 Laurel Oak Road/Suite 100 Zip: 08043
Ph: (856) 784-7398 Fax: (856) 784-7357
   Linganna,Sanjay, MD
   Santamaria,Richard G., MD

Wegh Under
2301 Evesham Road/Suite 505 Zip: 08043
Ph: (856) 861-6320 Fax: (856) 888-2640
   Arrow Articolo,Amy Beth, DO
   Mackey,Suzanne Fuller, MD

Women's Group for OB/GYN
2301 Evesham Road/Pav 800/Suite 122 Zip: 08043
Ph: (856) 770-9300 Fax: (856) 770-8238
   D'Elia,Donna L., MD
   Dershem,Jonel M., MD
   Martinez,Wendy, MD

Womens Health Associates PA
2301 East Evesham Road/Suite 602 Zip: 08043
Ph: (856) 772-2066 Fax: (856) 772-9159
   DiGaetano,Andrea F., MD
   Zinsky,Paul J., MD

Waldwick

Drs. Belov & Dunn
61 Crescent Avenue Zip: 07463
Ph: (201) 445-0033 Fax: (201) 857-0453
   Dunn,Beverly A., MD

Hecht and Segal MDs
171 Franklin Turnpike/Suite 110 Zip: 07463
Ph: (201) 612-5100 Fax: (201) 612-4499
   Hecht,Stacey Markowitz, MD
   Segal,Melissa Anne, MD

Valley Medical Group
140 Franklin Turnpike/Suite 6-A Zip: 07463
Ph: (201) 447-3603 Fax: (201) 447-5184
   Al-Ola,Ziyad, MD
   Draucikas,Lisa A., DO
   Ferreras,Jessie A.M., MD
   Granas,Andrew Daniel, MD
   Krigsman,Suzanne Karimi, MD

Wall

Atlantic Gynecologic Oncology
3349 State Route 138 Zip: 07719
Ph: (732) 280-5464 Fax: (732) 280-5443
   Brudie,Lorna Ann, DO
   Hackett,Thomas Everett, DO

Coastal Cardiovascular Consultants
1930 Highway 35/Suite 3 Zip: 07719
Ph: (732) 974-8800 Fax: (732) 974-8609
   Yoo,Hojun, MD

Cotler Family Practice, LLC
1937 State Highway 35/Suite 2 Zip: 07719
Ph: (732) 449-0914 Fax: (732) 449-5437
   Cotler,Harold Mark, DO
   Cotler,Samantha, DO

Drs. Mehandru & Mehandru
1925 Highway 35 Zip: 07719
Ph: (732) 974-0100 Fax: (732) 974-0137
   Mehandru,Sushil K., MD
   Mehandru,Urmila, MD

Hackensack Meridian Ob/Gyn
1924 Route 35/Suite 5 Zip: 07719
Ph: (732) 974-8404 Fax: (732) 974-8904
   Aikman,Noelle M., MD
   Carlo,Jocelyn Ann, MD
   Gumnic,Blair Rachel, DO
   Tomaro,Robert Jr, MD
   Walsh,Kathleen S., MD

Kashlan & Schreiber
1540 Highway 138/Suite 201 Zip: 07719
Ph: (732) 280-0020 Fax: (732) 681-0261
   Kashlan,Bassam T., MD
   Schreiber,Martha L., MD

Meridian Surgical Associates
2101 Route 34 South Zip: 07719
Ph: (732) 974-0003 Fax: (732) 974-0366
   Kazmi,Aasim, MD
   Maggio,William W., MD
   Salerno,Simon Anthony, MD

Point Pleasant Radiology Group
1973 State Route 34/Suite E-13 Zip: 07719
Ph: (732) 974-8011 Fax: (732) 974-8820
   Monaco,Robert A., MD
   O'Connor,Patrick Joseph, DO
   Parikh,Manoj R., MD

Seashore Pediatrics
1560 Highway 138 West Zip: 07719
Ph: (732) 449-8592 Fax: (732) 449-2108
   Meli,Catherine L., MD
   Rahmet,Naheed R., MD

University Orthopaedic Associates, LLC
4810 Belmar Boulevard/Suite 102 Zip: 07753
Ph: (732) 938-6090 Fax: (732) 938-5680
   Dhawan,Aman, MD
   Doumas,Christopher, MD
   Pushilin,Sergei A., MD

Wall Township

Cosulich Dermatology
3350 State Highway 138 Zip: 07719
Ph: (732) 280-1200 Fax: (732) 280-1207
   Cosulich,William F., MD
   Esche,Clemens, MD

Wallington

Drs. Lupinska and Rozdeba
42 Locust Avenue Zip: 07057
Ph: (973) 777-0090
   Lupinska,Malgorzata Teresa, MD
   Rozdeba,Christopha H., MD

Prime Care Pediatrics
42 Locust Avenue/Suite 5 Zip: 07057
Ph: (973) 473-4033 Fax: (973) 473-2988
   Sliwowski,Martha S., MD
   Sliwowski,Stanislaw, MD

Warren

Associates in Integrative Medicine
27 Mountain Boulevard/Suite 9 Zip: 07059
Ph: (908) 769-9600 Fax: (908) 769-9610
   Abraham,Vinod J., MD
   Prasad,Lakshmi, MD

Assoc in Plastic & Aesthetic Surgery
27 Mountain Boulevard/Suite 9 Zip: 07059
Ph: (908) 561-0080
   Montouris,Elaine Alexis, MD

Comprehensive Family Medicine, PA
27 Mountain Boulevard/Suite 6 Zip: 07059
Ph: (908) 222-7777 Fax: (908) 222-9242
   Brezina,Eric Joseph, MD
   Cavallo,Danielle Janine, DO
   Dicola,May Bersalona, MD

Dermatology Associates-Warren
122 Mount Bethel Road Zip: 07059
Ph: (908) 756-7999 Fax: (908) 756-8017
   Ahkami,Rosaline N., MD
   Bagley,Michael P., MD
   Doctoroff,Alexander, DO
   Sciales,Christopher W., MD

Eye Care and Surgery Center
10 Mountain Boulevard Zip: 07059
Ph: (908) 754-4800 Fax: (908) 754-4803
   Jacobs,Ivan H., MD
   Kahn,Milton, MD
   Stahl,Roslyn Marie, MD

Groups and Clinics by Town with Physician Rosters

Warren (cont)

Integrated Paincare Center
27 Mountain Boulevard/Suite 7 Zip: 07059
Ph: (908) 822-2889
- Chang,Mimi A., MD
- Jiang,Tony T., MD

Roseland OB/GYN Services
27 Mountain Boulevard/Suite 6 Zip: 07059
Ph: (908) 561-1102 Fax: (908) 561-1105
- De Angelis,Thomas, MD
- Tweddel,George K. III, MD

Somerset Cosmetic & Reconstructive
5 Mountain Boulevard/Suite 1 Zip: 07059
Ph: (908) 222-0070 Fax: (908) 222-8027
- Clott,Matthew Alan, MD
- Clott,Shilpa Mahendra, MD

Somerset Pediatric Group PA
65 Mountain Boulevard Ext/Suite 205 Zip: 07059
Ph: (732) 560-9080 Fax: (732) 560-8085
- Filler,Sharon Lee, MD
- Fritz,Gerard D., MD

Specialdocs Consultants, Inc.
266 King George Road/Suite F Zip: 07059
Ph: (732) 893-8150 Fax: (732) 893-8149
- Lanza,Raymond, DO
- Stoicescu,Lavinia D., MD

Summit Medical Group
34 Mountain Boulevard/Building B Zip: 07059
Ph: (908) 769-0100 Fax: (908) 769-8927
- Abrutyn,David Alan, MD

Summit Medical Group
34 Mountain Boulevard Zip: 07059
Ph: (908) 561-8600 Fax: (908) 561-7265
- Bobella,Stephen K., MD
- Boretz,Robert Stephen, MD
- Brodkin,Lisa Faith, MD
- Ferrante,Maurice Andrew, MD
- Goldman,Kara J., MD
- Heffernan,Kathleen Anne, MD
- Hubschmann,Andrea Gibbons, MD
- Levey,James Andrew, MD
- Lytle,Carole F., MD
- Nelson,Richard Oakleigh, MD
- Rogers,Elisabeth Ann, DO
- Singer,Beth Carol, MD
- Stoch,Sharon Rachel, MD

The Eye Center
65 Mountain Boulevard Ext/Suite 105 Zip: 07059
Ph: (732) 356-6200 Fax: (732) 356-0228
- Carter,Susan Redfield, MD
- Firestone,Debra A., MD
- Gewirtz,Matthew B., MD
- Giuseffi,Vincent J. III, MD
- Krawitz,Mark J., MD
- Lane,John F., MD
- Zhang,Linda, MD

Warren Primary Care
23 Mountain Boulevard Zip: 07059
Ph: (908) 598-7970 Fax: (908) 322-4989
- Clemente,Joseph Alfred, MD
- DiProspero,Elizabeth J., MD
- Hoang,Michelle Phi, MD
- Kloos,Thomas H., MD
- Torbus,Andrzej Peter, MD

Watchung Pediatrics
76 Stirling Road/Suite 201 Zip: 07059
Ph: (908) 755-5437 Fax: (908) 755-6905
- Barasch,Susan A., MD
- Brandstaedter,Karen Hardy, MD
- Eng,Jeffrey M., MD
- Katz,Andrea G., MD
- Kramer,Sarah R., MD
- Levin,Lorin Michelle, MD
- Ploshnick,Andrea G., MD
- Scott,Tiffany Lynn, MD

Washington

Charlestown Medical Associates
140 Boulevard Zip: 07882
Ph: (908) 689-3200 Fax: (908) 689-8295
- Kolpan,Brett Heath, MD
- Waldron,Winifred Marie, MD

Coventry Eye Associates, P.C.
10 Brass Castle Road Zip: 07882
Ph: (908) 859-4268
- Cooley,Susan L., MD

Warren Hills Family Health Ctr
315 Route 31 South Zip: 07882
Ph: (908) 689-0777 Fax: (908) 835-3037
- Gilly,Frank J. Jr., MD
- Goodwin,James E., MD
- Greenfeld,Alan L., MD
- Jaques,James Phillip, DO
- Kinoshita,Ken, MD
- Rodriquez,Victor R., MD
- Yevdokimova,Oksana, MD

Watchung

Barone & Catania Cardiovascular
786 Mountain Boulevard/Suite 200 Zip: 07069
Ph: (908) 754-0975 Fax: (908) 754-0260
- Barone,Paul, DO
- Catania,Raymond, DO
- Ovakimyan,Oxana, MD

MedExpress Urgent Care Watchung
1569 US Highway 22 Zip: 07069
Ph: (908) 322-2631 Fax: (908) 322-2679
- Faschan,Steven Michael, DO
- Finch,Vlada E., MD

Performance Rehabilitation & Sports In
459 Watchung Avenue Zip: 07069
Ph: (908) 756-2424
- Mejia,Joseph Rodrigo, DO
- Tabije,Kevin, DO
- Thomas,Chris, MD

Somerset Health Center
40 Stirling Road/Suite 208 Zip: 07069
Ph: (908) 757-1000 Fax: (908) 757-0564
- Ramaswamy,Kumar K., MD
- Rivera,Laura A., MD

Wayne

Adult and Pediatric Urology Center PA
2025 Hamburg Turnpike Zip: 07470
Ph: (973) 831-0011 Fax: (973) 831-0033
- Schlecker,Burton A., MD

Advanced Eye Care Center PA
220 Hamburg Turnpike/Suite 7 Zip: 07470
Ph: (973) 790-1300 Fax: (973) 790-5310
- Choo,Nancy Hae-Jin, MD
- Garg,Geetanjali Davuluri, MD
- Reing,Charles Scot, MD

Advanced Internal Med of North Jersey
1680 Route 23 North/Suite 310 Zip: 07470
Ph: (973) 831-9222 Fax: (973) 831-1460
- Branovan,Zhanna Emilia, MD
- Joffe,Libby, MD

Advanced Interventional Pain Mgm
1176 Hamburg Turnpike Zip: 07470
Ph: (973) 365-4747 Fax: (973) 365-4596
- Frias,Carlos, MD
- Galkin,Vadim, MD
- Krynska,Elzbieta B., MD
- Pekar,Aleksandr, MD

Advanced Orthopaedic Associates
1777 Hamburg Turnpike/Suite 301 Zip: 07470
Ph: (973) 839-5700 Fax: (973) 616-4343
- Dyal,Cherise Malinda, MD
- Sicherman,Hervey S., MD

Advanced Orthopedics & Hand Surgery
504 Valley Road/Suite 201 Zip: 07470
Ph: (973) 942-1315 Fax: (973) 942-8724
- Denoble,Peter Hart, MD
- Ghobadi,Fereydoon, MD
- Ghobadi,Ramin, MD
- Ratliff,David Fred, MD
- Stern,Lorraine C., MD

Allied Medical Associates
510 Hamburg Turnpike Zip: 07470
Ph: (973) 942-6005 Fax: (973) 442-6009
- Barraveccio,Anthony John, DO
- Biller,Jeanette Marie, DO
- Calamari,Dawn E., DO
- DeFranco,Paul David, DO
- Gandhi,Achyut Natvarial, MD
- Gregg,John A., DO
- Kapoor,Anuj, MD
- Leonardo,Michael H., MD
- Nguyen,Steven M., MD
- Vasiliades,Thalia, DO

Alps Family Physicians
1500 Alps Road Zip: 07470
Ph: (973) 628-8500 Fax: (973) 628-7944
- Bain,Francis Jerome-Xavier, MD
- Lampariello,James A., MD
- Patel,Meera V., MD
- Sivaraman,Priya, MD

Associates in Urology, PA
1777 Hamburg Turnpike/Suite 304 Zip: 07470
Ph: (973) 616-8400 Fax: (973) 616-8485
- Knoll,Abraham, MD
- Levine,Seth Peter, MD

Associates in Women's Healthcare
1777 Hamburg Turnpike/Suite 202 Zip: 07470
Ph: (973) 831-1800 Fax: (973) 831-8820
- Domnitz,Steven W., MD
- Mohammed,Nina, MD

Atlantic Medical Group
2025 Hamburg Turnpike/Suite D Zip: 07470
Ph: (973) 839-5070 Fax: (973) 839-0084
- Berkowitz,Richard H., MD
- Lubansky,Kenneth P., MD

Cardiology Consultants
246 Hamburg Turnpike/Suite 201 Zip: 07470
Ph: (973) 942-1141 Fax: (973) 942-1250
- Azhak,Sameer Anor, MD
- Biehl,Michael, MD
- Cruz,Mary Donna Mananghaya, MD
- Ghassemi,Rex, MD
- Konlian,Donna Marie, MD
- Madhwal,Surabhi, MD
- Salimi,Mostafa, MD
- Schair,Barry David, MD
- Toor,Saddad Zafar, MD

Comprehensive Women's Healthcare
220 Hamburg Turnpike/Suite 21 Zip: 07470
Ph: (973) 790-8090 Fax: (973) 790-3198
- Bennett,Bruce Kevin, MD
- Chang,Bernard P., MD
- Onwudinjo,Adolphus Chukwuelua, MD
- Pallimulla,Mahipa H., MD
- Vosough,Khashayar, MD

Corederm Dermatology and Cosmetic Ctr
246 Hamburg Turnpike/Suite 306 Zip: 07470
Ph: (973) 956-0500 Fax: (973) 956-0522
- Chima,Kuljit Kaur, MD
- Thakker,Priya Sambandan, MD

Drs. Darvish and Ephrem
401 Hamburg Turnpike/Suite 309 Zip: 07470
Ph: (973) 942-1200
- Darvish,Cameron, DO
- Ephrem,Yasmina Marie Therese, MD

Drs. Douyon & Bernstein
220 Hamburg Turnpike/Suite 11 Zip: 07470
Ph: (973) 942-4941 Fax: (973) 942-4259
- Bernstein,Michael H., MD
- Douyon,Erwin, MD

Drs. Morone and Costello
220 Hamburg Turnpike Zip: 07470
Ph: (973) 942-5230 Fax: (973) 942-6652
- Costello,Robert, MD
- Morone,John M., MD

Drs. Raouf and Balboul
508 Hamburg Turnpike/Suite 201 Zip: 07470
Ph: (973) 942-1340 Fax: (973) 942-1360
- Balboul,Elsaid A., MD

Drs. Siddiqui and Siddiqui
510 Hamburg Turnpike/Suite E-106 Zip: 07470
Ph: (973) 904-3161 Fax: (973) 904-3163
- Siddiqui,Imtiazuddin M., MD
- Siddiqui,Nafeesa, MD

Drs. Singh & Farhangfar
401 Hamburg Turnpike/Suite 109 Zip: 07470
Ph: (973) 595-7456 Fax: (973) 904-9119
- Farhangfar,Reza, MD
- Matalkah,Nidal M., MD
- Singh,Avtar, MD

ENT & Allergy Associates, LLP
1211 Hamburg Turnpike/Suite 205 Zip: 07470
Ph: (973) 633-0808 Fax: (973) 633-8811
- Abrams,Stephen Joel, MD
- Brunetti,Vito Anthony, MD
- Cece,John A., MD
- D'Anton,Michael A. III, MD
- Mattel,Stephen F., MD
- Scheibelhoffer,John J., MD
- Scher,Daniel A., MD
- Sohn,Theresa J. H., MD
- Sreepada,Gangadhar S., MD

Elite Orthopedics & Sports Medicine
342 Hamburg Turnpike/Suite 209 Zip: 07470
Ph: (973) 956-8100 Fax: (973) 956-8104
- Fahimi,Nader, MD
- Schneidkraut,Jason S., MD

Eraiba & Eraiba Internal Med
510 Hamburg Turnpike/Suite 208 Zip: 07470
Ph: (973) 904-3480 Fax: (973) 904-3485
- Eraiba,Ayman E., MD
- Eraiba,Magda A., MD

Eye Associates of Wayne PA
968 Hamburg Turnpike Zip: 07470
Ph: (973) 696-0300 Fax: (973) 696-0465
- Gollance,Stephen Andrew, MD
- Mishler,Ken E., MD
- Silodor,Scott W., MD

Ganchi Plastic Surgery
246 Hamburg Turnpike/Suite 307 Zip: 07470
Ph: (973) 942-6600 Fax: (973) 595-5964
- Ganchi,Amir, MD
- Ganchi,Parham Amir, MD

Gastrointestinal Group of NJ
1777 Hamburg Turnpike/Suite 101 Zip: 07470
Ph: (973) 839-6400 Fax: (973) 839-7083
- Shlien,Robert D., MD
- Stevens,Lisa Deborah, MD

Health Consultants of New Jersey
516 Hamburg Turnpike/Suite 5 Zip: 07470
Ph: (973) 925-7770 Fax: (973) 925-7772
- Chow,Jessica C., DO
- Nabulsi,Omar Hisham, MD

High Mountain Orthopedics
342 Hamburg Turnpike/Suite 205 Zip: 07470
Ph: (973) 595-7779 Fax: (973) 595-0182
- Matarese,William A., MD
- Su,Sherwin Leu, MD
- Wanich,Tony Suchai, MD

Lumina Women's Care
401 Hamburg Turnpike/Suite 104 Zip: 07470
Ph: (973) 750-1770 Fax: (973) 750-1775
- Pavel,Patricia M., MD
- Sgroi,Donald A., MD

Neurologic Associates
220 Hamburg Turnpike/Suite 16 Zip: 07470
Ph: (973) 942-4778 Fax: (973) 942-7020
- Chodosh,Eliot Howard, MD
- Gazzillo,Frank L., MD
- Mascellino,Ann Marie Madaline, MD
- Monck,Jennefer Erinna, MD
- Wagner,Robert Austin, MD

Groups and Clinics by Town with Physician Rosters

New Jersey Orthopaedic Institute
504 Valley Road/Suite 200 Zip: 07470
Ph: (973) 694-2690 Fax: (973) 694-2692
- Callaghan,John Joseph, MD
- Festa,Anthony Nmi, MD
- Hwang,Ki S., MD
- McInerney,Vincent K., MD
- Palacios,Robert M., MD
- Scillia,Anthony James, MD
- Wright,Craig, MD

NJ Pediatric & Adolescent Care, LLC.
1680 Route 23/Suite 350 Zip: 07470
Ph: (973) 521-9700 Fax: (973) 521-9707
- Charles,Lydia M., MD
- Chiu,Caroline, MD

North Jersey Gastroenterology
1825 State Route 23 South Zip: 07470
Ph: (973) 633-1484 Fax: (973) 633-7980
- Bleicher,Robert H., MD
- Cheng,Bonnie Kingman, MD
- David,Steven, MD
- Ramamoorthy,Ravishankar, MD
- Stillman,Jonathon S., MD
- Zangara,Joseph Anthony, MD

North Jersey Health PA
502 Hamburg Turnpike/Suite 108 Zip: 07470
Ph: (973) 942-5224 Fax: (973) 942-7443
- Abdulmassih,Sami, MD
- Arnouk,Munzer M., MD

North Jersey Nephrology Associates PA
246 Hamburg Turnpike/Suite 207 Zip: 07470
Ph: (973) 653-3366 Fax: (973) 653-3365
- Audia,Pat Frank, MD
- Banu,Nazifa, MD
- Chandran,Chandra B., MD
- Graziano,Vincent Angelo, MD
- Karanam,Deepthi, MD
- Masand,Anjali Narain, MD
- Moquete,Manuel J., MD
- Nandigam,Purna Bindu, MD
- Notkin,Alicia R., MD
- Prakash,Ananth N., MD
- Saini,Harjinder S., MD
- Shah,Sanjay R., MD
- Triolo,Diane Cecilia, MD
- Yousef,Nadia P., MD

North Jersey Orthopaedic Group
246 Hamburg Turnpike/Suite 302 Zip: 07470
Ph: (973) 689-6266 Fax: (973) 689-6264
- Cox,Garrick Andrew, MD
- Dean-Davis,Ellen, MD
- Dowling,Ryan Martin, MD
- Mahmood,Faisal, MD
- Masella,Robert Michael, MD

North Jersey Spine Group
1680 State Route 23/Suite 250 Zip: 07470
Ph: (973) 633-1132
- Haber,Monte Arthur, MD
- Raab,Rajnik Weerackody, MD
- Sundstrom,David C., MD

Pediatric Ophthalmology of NJ
57 Willowbrook Boulevard/Suite 411 Zip: 07470
Ph: (973) 256-4111 Fax: (973) 256-3719
- Mickey,Kevin J., MD
- Yang,Sherry, MD

Pediatric Professional Assoc
330 Ratzer Road/Suite 20 Zip: 07470
Ph: (973) 835-5556 Fax: (973) 628-7942
- Dong,Feiyan, MD
- Mahon,James William, MD
- Nelson,Geraldine I., MD

Perinatal Services of No NJ
57 Willowbrook Road/3rd Floor Zip: 07470
Ph: (973) 754-3800 Fax: (973) 244-0476
- Houlihan,Christopher M., MD
- Khoury,Aldo D., MD

Physicians Health Alliance
1777 Hamburg Turnpike/Suite 205 Zip: 07470
Ph: (973) 248-1440 Fax: (973) 248-1448
- Haghverdi,Mojdeh, MD
- Wassner,Jesse V., MD

Physicians for Women
330 Ratzer Road/Suite 7 Zip: 07470
Ph: (973) 694-2222 Fax: (973) 694-7664
- Bauer,Christopher Joseph, MD
- Centanni,Toni V., MD
- Garrett,Kenneth M., MD
- Munoz-Matta,Ana T., MD
- Nicosia,Leonard T., MD
- Shakiba,Khashayar, MD
- Suffin,Arthur Lee, MD

Point View Radiology Associates
246 Hamburg Turnpike/Suite 101 Zip: 07470
Ph: (973) 904-0404 Fax: (973) 904-0423
- Duhaney,Michael Owen, MD
- Festa,Steven, MD
- Steinberg,Michael L., MD
- Wheeler,Ralph B., MD

Preakness Pediatrics Associates
150 Hinchman Avenue/Suite 4 Zip: 07470
Ph: (973) 595-6996 Fax: (973) 595-6706
- Jariwala,Nilesh R., MD
- Sharma,Pushpendra, MD

SA Healthcare Management, LLC
145 Route 46 West/Suite 304 Zip: 07470
OnlyFax: (973) 513-6081
- Diarbakerli,Fares, MD
- Santos,Norman Verches, MD

Orthopedic Surgery Center
2035 Hamburg Turnpike/Suite D Zip: 07470
Ph: (973) 616-0200 Fax: (973) 616-1792
- Cappadona,Joseph G., MD
- Gold,David A., MD
- Reicher,Oscar A., MD

Suburban Nephrology Group
342 Hamburg Turnpike/Suite 201 Zip: 07470
Ph: (973) 389-1119 Fax: (973) 389-1145
- Joseph,Monalisa, MD
- Rae,Sam, MD
- Vitting,Kevin E., MD
- Zeltser,Eugene, MD

Total Cardiology Care
2035 Hamburg Pike/Suite L Zip: 07470
Ph: (973) 248-0200 Fax: (973) 248-3455
- Rathi,Ravi, MD

University Spine Center
504 Valley Road/Second Floor/Suite 203 Zip: 07470
Ph: (973) 686-0700 Fax: (973) 686-0701
- D'Amato,Pamela R., MD
- Emami,Arash, MD
- Faloon,Michael J., MD
- Sinha,Kumar Gautam, MD

Valley Health Medical Group
759 Hamburg Turnpike Zip: 07470
Ph: (973) 709-0099 Fax: (973) 709-0201
- Ahmed-Flowers,Tunizia, MD
- Newman,Sheila F., MD

Valley Medical Associates
220 Hamburg Turnpike/Suite 9 Zip: 07470
Ph: (973) 826-0068 Fax: (973) 807-1886
- Makar,Gamil Lamey Bekheet, MD
- Yorio,David S., DO

Wayne Behavioral Services
401 Hamburg Turnpike/Suite 303 Zip: 07470
Ph: (973) 790-9222 Fax: (973) 790-0671
- ElRafei,Mohamed A., MD

Wayne Cancer Center LLC
234 Hamburg Turnpike/Suite 202 Zip: 07470
Ph: (973) 310-0309
- Dorkhom,Stephan Joseph, DO
- Pope,Ronald J., DO

Wayne Hematology-Oncology Assoc
468 Parish Drive/Suite 4 Zip: 07470
Ph: (973) 694-5005 Fax: (973) 694-5990
- Hanley,Debra A., MD
- Roy,Vijaykumar, MD
- Shah,Harish H., MD

Wayne Medical Care, PA
342 Hamburg Turnpike/Suite 101 Zip: 07470
Ph: (973) 942-4140 Fax: (973) 942-5070
- Choe,Wonsick, MD
- Gomez-Vasquez,Ricardo Antonio, MD
- Wardeh,Ghassan Louis, MD
- Woo,James K., MD

Wayne Primary Care
468 Parish Drive/Suite 1 Zip: 07470
Ph: (973) 305-8300 Fax: (973) 305-8157
- Carrazzone,Peter Louis, MD
- Deingeniis-Depasquale,Antoinette M
- Gold,Jeffrey L., MD

Wayne Primary Care, P.A.
508 Hamburg Turnpike/Suite 102 Zip: 07470
Ph: (973) 595-0096 Fax: (973) 595-6414
- Aydin,Emmanuel A., MD
- Kucuk,Erhan, MD

Wayne Surgical Center, LLC.
1176 Hamburg Pike Zip: 07470
Ph: (973) 709-1900 Fax: (973) 709-1901
- Doss,Michael Nader, MD
- Klele,Christo Selim, MD
- Mazzone,Jeanae, DO

Wayne Urgent and Primary Care
246 Hamburg Turnpike/Suite 205 Zip: 07470
Ph: (973) 389-1800 Fax: (973) 636-2734
- Cortellino,Karen, MD
- Rasa,David V., MD
- Whang,Inwhan, MD

Wedgewood Primary Care
1055 Hamburg Turnpike/Suite 300 Zip: 07470
Ph: (973) 904-1177 Fax: (973) 904-1166
- Bock,Robert T. Jr., MD
- Crabtree,Shawn M., MD
- Loughlin,Bruce T., DO

Willowbrook Pediatrics
57 Willowbrook Boulevard/Suite 421 Zip: 07470
Ph: (973) 754-4025
- Abu Khraybeh,Wafa Said, MD
- Bronstein,Jagoda Ewa, MD
- Scofield,Lisa E., MD

Wenonah

Advocare West Deptford Pediatrics
1050 Mantua Pike Zip: 08090
Ph: (856) 468-8330 Fax: (856) 468-9121
- Clear,Carolyn Elizabeth, DO
- Hung,Deborah Liu, MD
- Knestaut,Angela Gaudiano, DO
- Mishik,Anthony N., MD

Advocare Woodbury Pediatrics
1050 Mantua Pike/Suite 200 Zip: 08090
Ph: (856) 853-0848 Fax: (856) 853-1889
- Biermann Flynn,Dana Lynn, DO
- Jones,Tamika Lillian, MD
- Piantedosi,Benjamin George, MD

West Caldwell

Eastern Surgical Associates PA
1099 Bloomfield Avenue Zip: 07006
Ph: (973) 882-0600 Fax: (973) 882-0602
- Strauchler,Irving D., MD
- Strauchler,Roberta A., MD

Essex Eye Physicians, LLC
195 Fairfield Avenue/Suite 4B Zip: 07006
Ph: (973) 228-4990 Fax: (973) 228-4464
- Bevacqua,Alejandro, MD
- Wertheimer,Robert M., MD

Montclair Anesthesia Associates PC
185 Fairfield Avenue/Suite 2A Zip: 07006
Ph: (973) 226-1230 Fax: (973) 226-1232
- Bering,Thomas Gerard, MD
- Doss,George S., MD
- Forrest,Robert, MD
- Giannuzzi,Rosanne Frances, MD
- Izeogu,Chinweike, MD
- Katragadda,Rama Sastrulu, MD
- Lutz,Philip Edward, MD
- Negron-Gonzalez,Maria Alejandra, M
- Rocamboli,David Charles, DO
- Rubin,Joshua Adam, MD
- Secoy,John Walton, MD
- Sisbarro,Susan E., MD
- Spertus,Silvana H., DO
- Vujic,Dragomir M., MD
- Weems,Lela Demilo, MD

Pediatric Assoc of West Essex
1129 Bloomfield Avenue/Suite 100 Zip: 07006
Ph: (973) 575-8585 Fax: (973) 882-6914
- Butensky,Arthur S., MD
- Frank-Shrensel,Bettie, MD

West Deptford

Advocare West Deptford Pediatrics
646 Kings Highway Zip: 08096
Ph: (856) 879-2887 Fax: (856) 879-2855
- Petrozzino,Jeffrey, MD
- Ruddock,Heather Ann, MD
- Thalayur,Keerti, MD

South Jersey Radiology Associates
748 Kings Highway Zip: 08096
Ph: (856) 848-4998 Fax: (856) 853-7362
- Ariaratnam,Nikki Sanghera, MD
- Fog,Denise Susan, DO
- Gilbert,Steven L., MD
- Larkin,Jeffrey J., MD
- Lin,Dennis C., MD
- Little,Sherrill T., MD
- Mattox,Scott G., MD
- Patel,Jayeshkumar Balu, MD
- Rosten,Sloan I., MD
- Sajous,Jan Bernard, MD
- Tilak,Samir Shripad, MD
- Titton,Ross Lewis, MD
- Whitley,Markus A., MD

Westwood Womens Health Center
600 Jessup Road Zip: 08066
Ph: (856) 845-4061 Fax: (856) 812-2880
- Di Joseph,Benjamin D. Jr., DO
- Lofton,Azieb Ghebremedhin, DO
- McNally,Lauryn Anne, MD

West Long Branch

Atlantic Womens Medical Group
240 Wall Street/Suite 300 Zip: 07764
Ph: (732) 229-1288 Fax: (732) 728-1487
- Lambert-Woolley,Margaret A., MD
- Yehl,Mary Ann Mclaughlin, DO

Drs. Gilson, Orsini & Miller
223 Monmouth Road Zip: 07764
Ph: (732) 870-2992
- Gilson,Cynthia T., MD
- Miller,Angela M., MD
- Orsini,William J., MD

Garden State Medical Center
100 State Route 36/Suite 1C Zip: 07764
Ph: (732) 202-3000 Fax: (732) 849-0015
- Mann,Sunita Singh, MD

Garden State Neuro & Neuro-Oncology
100 State Highway 36 East Zip: 07764
Ph: (732) 229-6200 Fax: (732) 229-6201
- Patel,Dakshesh K., MD
- Raval,Sumul N., MD

Monmouth Hematology Onc Assoc
100 State Highway 36/Suite 1B Zip: 07764
Ph: (732) 222-1711 Fax: (732) 222-2060
- Cohen,Seth Daniel, MD
- Fiore,Rosemary P., MD
- Lee,Patrick C., MD
- Ray,Debra M., MD
- Sharon,David J., MD

Monmouth Medical Group, P.C.
223 Monmouth Road Zip: 07764
Ph: (732) 229-3838 Fax: (732) 229-4562
- Parisi,Gerlando V., MD

Groups and Clinics by Town with Physician Rosters

West Long Branch (cont)

Neurology Specialists-Monmouth County
107 Monmouth Road/Suite 110 Zip: 07764
Ph: (732) 935-1850 Fax: (732) 544-0494
- Davis,Matthew Jared, MD
- Gennaro,Paul, MD
- Gilson,Noah R., MD
- Mendelson,Joshua Todd, MD
- Ponce,Francis B., MD

Neurosurgeons of New Jersey
121 Highway 36 West/Suite 330 Zip: 07764
Ph: (732) 963-4631 Fax: (732) 870-6342
- Estin,David, MD
- Lustgarten,Jonathan H., MD
- Olson,Ty James, MD

Neurosurgical Associates of NJ
121 Highway 36 West/Suite 330 Zip: 07764
Ph: (732) 222-8866 Fax: (732) 870-6432
- Gillis,Christopher Charles, MD
- Link,Timothy Emerson, MD

Pediatric & Adolescent Medicine
223 Monmouth Road Zip: 07764
Ph: (732) 229-4540
- Murphy,Robert D., MD
- Truxal,Brian A., MD

West Long Branch ObGyn
1019 Broadway Zip: 07764
Ph: (732) 229-6797 Fax: (732) 229-6893
- Jackson,Sharon, MD
- Lobraico,Dominick Jr., DO
- Massaro,Robert A., MD
- Ombalsky,Joseph, MD
- Pompliano,Jennifer Dorothea, DO
- Skorenko,Kenneth R., MD

West Park Medical, LLC.
100 Highway 36/Suite 2-K Zip: 07764
Ph: (732) 531-6600 Fax: (732) 660-6606
- Baldi,Daniela J., MD
- Jariwala,Punit Rajnikant, MD
- Santiago,Eddie W., MD

West Milford

Bergen-Passaic Women's Health
2024 Macopin Road/Suite D Zip: 07480
Ph: (973) 728-7787 Fax: (973) 728-7707
- Kaufman,Deborah Louise, DO

West Milford Medical Center
1485 Union Valley Road Zip: 07480
Ph: (973) 728-1880 Fax: (973) 728-1559
- Kalevich,Serge F., MD
- Lascari,Roland A., MD
- Platt,Robert N., MD

West New York

Drs. Butterman & Goyco
228 60th Street Zip: 07093
Ph: (201) 868-1120 Fax: (201) 868-5801
- Butterman,Clifford Jay, MD
- Goyco,Luis A., MD

Drs. Castillo and Castillo
5801 Broadway Zip: 07093
Ph: (201) 869-4044
- Castillo,Elma D., MD
- Castillo,Marianne Devilla, MD

Drs. Ramos & Zapiach
235 60th Street Zip: 07093
Ph: (201) 854-4646 Fax: (201) 854-3203
- Ramos,Rafael C., MD
- Zapiach,Leonidas, MD
- Zapiach,Mauricio, MD

Integrated Healthcare Group
5600 Kennedy Boulevard/Suite 102 Zip: 07093
Ph: (201) 866-3100
- Surikov,Vadim Michailovich, DO
- Vitievsky,Ellen, MD

NHCAC Health Center at West New York
5301 Broadway Zip: 07093
Ph: (201) 866-9320
- Aliaga,Julie M., MD
- Fayngersh,David, MD
- Hamal,Rekha, MD
- Hutton-Cassie,Donna Pauline, MD
- Maldonado,Jose O., MD

- Mallamaci,Carmen R., MD
- Mason-Eastmond,Tania Alicia, MD
- Milanes-Roberts,Norma, MD
- Panem,Cheryl Buensuceso, MD
- Patel,Jayminkumar R., MD
- Rubia-Sazon,Elvira M., MD
- Villabona,Beatriz, MD
- Wang,Wei, MD
- Zahka,Karym, MD

North Jersey Surgical Group PA
6040 Kennedy Boulevard East/Suite L-7 Zip: 07093
Ph: (201) 861-0720 Fax: (201) 861-5560
- Kulkarni,Vijaykumar A., MD

The Doctor Is In
6701 Bergenline Avenue Zip: 07093
Ph: (201) 758-9100
- Weiss,Ronald D., MD

The Doctors Shaari
413 60th Street Zip: 07093
Ph: (201) 867-5557 Fax: (201) 867-5566
- Iraj Shaari,Gita M., MD
- Shaari,Jeffrey M., MD

Women's Health Partners, PC
419 66th Street Zip: 07093
Ph: (201) 861-9229 Fax: (201) 861-9272
- Fernandez-Cos,Henry, MD
- Melendez Cabrera,Octavio, MD

West Orange

Abbas Shehadeh Cardio/Intern Med
443 Northfield Avenue/Suite 301 Zip: 07052
Ph: (973) 731-0203 Fax: (973) 731-0017
- Armanious,Adel Youssef, MD
- Haacker,David S., MD
- Shehadeh,Abbas A., MD

Aesthetic Plastic Surgery Center
101 Old Short Hills Road/Suite 501 Zip: 07052
Ph: (973) 731-2000
- Asaadi,Mokhtar, MD
- Salas,A. Peter, MD

Affiliated Eye Surgeons
405 Northfield Avenue/Suite 206 Zip: 07052
Ph: (973) 736-3322 Fax: (973) 736-7317
- Medford,David J., MD
- Seligsohn,Audrey Lynn, DO

Affiliates in Gastroenterology, P.A.
101 Old Short Hills Road/Suite 217 Zip: 07052
Ph: (973) 731-4600 Fax: (973) 731-1477
- Askin,Matthew Peter, MD
- Rosenthal,Lawrence Stephen, MD
- Schuman,Robert W., MD
- Siu,Larry K., MD
- Sloan,William C., MD
- Stein,Lawrence B., MD
- Wallach,Carl B., MD

Associates in Obstetrics Gynecology
375 Mount Pleasant Avenue/Suite 202 Zip: 07052
Ph: (973) 731-7707 Fax: (973) 669-0277
- Crane,Stephen E., MD
- Degraaff,Doreen E., MD
- Hamilton,Tammy Joan, MD
- Ladocsi,Lewis T., MD
- Luisi-Purdue,Linda, MD
- Russo,Neil J., MD
- Sansobrino,Daniel M., MD
- Walk,Zem, MD

Associates in Otolaryngology
741 Northfield Avenue/Suite 104 Zip: 07052
Ph: (973) 243-0600 Fax: (973) 736-9607
- Downey,Laura L., MD
- Fieldman,Robert J., MD
- Holzberg,Norman, MD
- Morrow,Todd A., MD
- Perlman,Donald Bret, MD

Associates in Psychiatry
405 Northfield Avenue/Suite 204 Zip: 07052
Ph: (973) 325-6120 Fax: (973) 325-6126
- Cannella,Michael, MD

- Greene,Bruce H., DO
- Park,Charles William, MD
- Sathaye,Nirmal, MD

Atlantic Spine Center
475 Prospect Avenue/Suite 110 Zip: 07052
Ph: (973) 419-0200 Fax: (973) 419-0223
- Kadimcherla,Praveen, MD
- Liu,Kaixuan, MD

Care Station Medical Group
456 Prospect Avenue Zip: 07052
Ph: (973) 731-6767 Fax: (973) 731-9881
- Chang,Peiyun, MD
- Kaynan,Riva Lori, MD
- Rivera Galindo,Claudia P., MD

Center For Orthopaedics
1500 Pleasant Valley Way/Suite 101 Zip: 07052
Ph: (973) 669-5600 Fax: (973) 669-0269
- Bachman,Jodie Ann, DO
- Hutter,Andrew M., MD
- Loya,David Michael, MD
- Pinkowsky,Gregory J., MD
- Robbins,Steven G., MD
- Rosa,Richard A., MD
- Zornitzer,Matthew Howard, MD

Consultants in Cardiology
741 Northfield Avenue/Suite 205 Zip: 07052
Ph: (973) 467-1544 Fax: (973) 467-9586
- Goldberg,Mark C., MD
- Harback,Edward R., MD
- Schwanwede,Jacqueline M., MD
- Tullo,Nicholas G., MD
- Wangenheim,Paul M., MD

Contemporary Women's Care
745 Northfield Avenue Zip: 07052
Ph: (973) 736-7700 Fax: (973) 736-8078
- Sadural,Ernani, MD
- Wimmer,Angela M., MD
- Zuniga,Gina, MD

Cross County Orthopaedics
769 Northfield Avenue/Suite LL20 Zip: 07052
Ph: (973) 669-9595 Fax: (973) 669-1050
- Boiardo,Richard A., MD
- Pirone,Arthur M., MD

Deborah A Coy, MD, LLC
405 Northfield Avenue/Suite LL2 Zip: 07052
Ph: (973) 736-4442 Fax: (973) 736-8717
- Coy,Deborah A., MD
- Garbarino,Charles L., MD
- Ibrahim,Mariane, MD

Dermatolgy & Laser Ctr of No NJ
347 Mount Pleasant Avenue/Suite 205 Zip: 07052
Ph: (973) 740-0101 Fax: (973) 740-0103
- Heidary,Noushin, MD
- Simela,Tanasha, DO
- Stolman,Lewis Peter, MD

Diagnostic & Clinical Cardiology
449 Mount Pleasant Avenue/2nd Floor Zip: 07052
Ph: (973) 731-7868 Fax: (973) 731-7907
- Green,Jon David, MD
- Modi,Kaushik Chhaganlal, MD

Dr. Deborah Ruth Spey
101 Old Short Hills Road/Suite 410 Zip: 07052
Ph: (973) 731-9600 Fax: (973) 731-1635
- Hartman,Rachael Dalya, MD
- Ruhl,Kimberly K., MD
- Spey,Deborah Ruth, MD

Drs. Alves & Johnson
470 Prospect Avenue/Suite 200 Zip: 07052
Ph: (973) 243-0290
- Alves,Lennox, MD
- Johnson,Natalie A., MD

Drs. Ganesh and Theivanayagam
24 Park Avenue Zip: 07052
Ph: (973) 669-8181 Fax: (973) 669-1687
- Ganesh,Manickam, MD
- Theivanayagam,Kalyani, MD

Drs. Mehta & Haskins
101 Old Short Hills Road/Suite 401 Zip: 07052
Ph: (973) 322-6500 Fax: (973) 322-6418
- Haskins,Danielle, MD
- Mehta,Deviyani Dilipkumar, MD

Drs. Scalea & Belt
100 Northfield Avenue Zip: 07052
Ph: (973) 731-1535 Fax: (973) 731-5782
- Belt,Steven D., MD
- Scalea,Donald D., MD

Drs. Weinberger & Cannarozzi
741 Northfield Avenue/Suite 210 Zip: 07052
Ph: (973) 630-8950 Fax: (973) 669-9749
- Cannarozzi,Nicholas A., MD
- Pai,Sneha, MD
- Weinberger,Andrew Bruce, MD

Forman-Hertz, Md LLC
1500 Pleasant Valley Way/Suite 302 Zip: 07052
Ph: (973) 324-0988
- Forman,Mark H., MD
- Hertz,Steven M., MD

Gynecologic Cancer & Pelvic Surgery
101 Old Short Hills Road/Suite 400 Zip: 07052
Ph: (973) 243-9300 Fax: (973) 325-8254
- Denehy,Thad R., MD
- Taylor,Robert Roland, MD

IMMC Health
737 Northfield Avenue Zip: 07052
Ph: (973) 544-8901 Fax: (973) 544-8991
- Krok,Elion J., MD

Kintiroglou Pediatrics
1500 Pleasant Valley Way/Suite 301 Zip: 07052
Ph: (973) 243-0002 Fax: (973) 243-1227
- Ajeena,Zainab, MD
- Kintiroglou,Constantinos, MD
- Kintiroglou,John, MD
- Nachevnik,Elina, MD
- Pivawer,Lisa S., MD
- Tang,Yen-Shin Daisy, MD

Lincoln P. Miller, MD, LLC
1500 Pleasant Valley Way/Suite 201 Zip: 07052
Ph: (973) 966-6400 Fax: (973) 514-1587
- Frank,Ronald Gary, MD
- Kuntz,George R., MD
- Miller,Lincoln Paul, MD

Livingston Medical Associates, LLC.
449 Mount Pleasant Avenue/First Floor Zip: 07052
Ph: (973) 535-8311 Fax: (973) 535-1210
- Chu,Benny G., DO
- Mandel,Steven S., MD
- Pandya,Prashant N., MD

Louis V. Sangosse MD PA
745 Northfield Avenue Zip: 07052
Ph: (973) 731-0200 Fax: (973) 325-2244
- Sangosse,Louis V., MD
- Sangosse,Marie C., MD

Miller Ophthalmology Associates
101 Old Short Hills Road/Suite 430 Zip: 07052
Ph: (973) 325-3300 Fax: (973) 325-3320
- Jacobs,Emily J., MD
- Miller,Kenneth Scott, MD

Modern Nephrology & Transplant, LLC
767 Northfield Avenue Zip: 07052
Ph: (973) 992-9022 Fax: (973) 992-9024
- Bonomini,Luigi Vittorio, MD
- Casagrande,Lisette Helene, MD
- Shah,Nita K., MD

Nephrology Group
111 Northfield Avenue/Suite 311 Zip: 07052
Ph: (973) 325-2103 Fax: (973) 325-2254
- Cooper,Sanford, MD
- Goldstein,Craig Russell, DO
- Grasso,Michael A., MD
- Lefkowitz,Heather Rush, MD
- Palekar,Sadanand S., MD

Groups and Clinics by Town with Physician Rosters

New Jersey Cardiology Associates
375 Mount Pleasant Avenue Zip: 07052
Ph: (973) 731-9442 Fax: (973) 731-8030
  Brock,Donald J., MD
  Chaaban,Fadi Nemer, MD
  Chakhtoura,Elie Youssef, MD
  Costeas,Constantinos A., MD
  Dobesh,David P., MD
  Fisk,Marc Saslow, DO
  Gandhi,Devang Amrat, MD
  Haik,Bruce Joseph, MD
  Hawthorne,Keith Allen, MD
  Roelke,Marc, MD
  Rogal,Gary J., MD
  Rubenstein,Donald G., MD
  Torre,Sabino Richard, MD

New Jersey Urology, LLC
741 Northfield Avenue/Suite 206 Zip: 07052
Ph: (973) 325-6100 Fax: (973) 325-1616
  Galdieri,Louis C., MD
  Lefkon,Bruce W., MD

New Jersey Urology, LLC
375 Mounain Pleasant Ave/Suite 250 Zip: 07052
Ph: (973) 323-1300 Fax: (973) 323-1311
  Mushonga,Nyarai Chinyani, MD
  Savatta,Domenico James, MD
  Seaman,Eric K., MD
  Strauss,Bernard S., MD
  Youngren,Kjell A., MD

New Jersey Vein & Cosmetic Surgery Ctr
741 Northfield Avenue/Suite 105 Zip: 07052
Ph: (973) 243-9729 Fax: (973) 243-9674
  Fretta,Joseph, MD
  Mast,Harold Lee, MD
  Shoenfeld,Richard B., MD

North Jersey Gastro Associates
741 Northfield Avenue/Suite 101 Zip: 07052
Ph: (973) 736-1991 Fax: (973) 736-9377
  DePasquale,Joseph R., MD
  Spira,Robert S., MD

Partners for Women's Health PA
95 Northfield Avenue Zip: 07052
Ph: (973) 736-4505 Fax: (973) 376-9066
  Ciciola,Gerald F., MD
  David,Gwen Lynita, MD
  Kaufman,Gregory Joel, MD
  Kovacs,Lauren R., MD

Premier Urology Group, LLC
1500 Pleasant Valley Road Zip: 07052
Ph: (973) 325-0091 Fax: (973) 789-8755
  Fiske,Steven C., MD

Professional Associates In Surgery
101 Old Short Hills Road/Suite 206 Zip: 07052
Ph: (973) 731-5005 Fax: (973) 325-6230
  Maheshwari,Vivek, MD
  Singh,Manoj Kumar, MD

Reproductive Medicine Associates of NJ
475 Prospect Avenue/Suite 101 Zip: 07052
Ph: (973) 325-2229 Fax: (973) 290-8370
  Gulati,Rita, MD

St. Barnabas Health Care Center
95 Old Short Hills Road Zip: 07052
Ph: (973) 322-4033 Fax: (973) 322-4416
  Biczak,Ernest S., MD
  Kupershtok-Bojko,Aviva Sara, MD

The Dermatology Group, P.C.
347 Mount Pleasant Avenue/Suite 103 Zip: 07052
Ph: (973) 571-2121 Fax: (973) 498-0535
  Glashofer,Marc David, MD
  Groisser,Daniel S., MD
  Patel,Mahir, MD
  Sandoval,Marina Penteado, MD

The Dermatology Group, P.C.
347 Mount Pleasant Avenue/Suite 205 Zip: 07052
Ph: (973) 571-2121
  Shah,Avnee, MD
  Sivendran,Meera, MD

The Heart Center of the Oranges
95 Main Street Zip: 07052
Ph: (973) 672-3829
  MacKenzie,Diane Susan, DO

The Medical Group, PA
745 Northfield Avenue Zip: 07052
Ph: (973) 325-0061 Fax: (973) 325-0219
  Ruffini,Robert A., MD
  Stefaniwsky,Andrew B., MD

The Peck Center
776 Northfield Avenue Zip: 07052
Ph: (973) 324-2300 Fax: (973) 324-1421
  Peck,George C. Jr., MD
  Peck,Richard E., MD

The Pediatric Group of West Oran
395 Pleasant Valley Way Zip: 07052
Ph: (973) 731-6100
  Owens,Jacqueline A., MD
  Rabinowitz,Robert C., MD
  Silverman,Abby Robin, MD

The Rubino OB/GYN Group
101 Old Short Hills Road/Suite 101 Zip: 07052
Ph: (973) 736-1100 Fax: (973) 736-1834
  Abeshaus,Lisa Ellen, MD
  Cheng,Eleanor Lillian, MD
  Fox,Howard D., DO
  Huang,Diana, MD
  Kessel,Allan David, MD
  Patel,Priya R., MD
  Romero,Audrey Anita, MD
  Rubino,Robert J., MD

West Orange Pediatrics
81 Northfield Avenue/Suite 101 Zip: 07052
Ph: (973) 324-5437
  Chike-Obi,Toju O., MD

Women First Health Center
520 Pleasant Valley Way Zip: 07052
Ph: (973) 325-0087 Fax: (973) 669-5722
  Desantos,Victoria Christina, MD
  Sylvester,Claudine M., MD

West Paterson

Amana Medical Group
871 McBride Avenue Zip: 07424
Ph: (973) 569-4488 Fax: (973) 565-4743
  Airood,Moumina, MD
  Ibrahim,Mohammad S., MD

Cardiology Associates LLC
999 McBride Avenue/Suite B-204 Zip: 07424
Ph: (973) 256-5667 Fax: (973) 256-7758
  Capitanelli,John R., MD
  Kaddaha,Raja'A Mohammed, MD
  Losardo,Anthony A., MD

Drs. Brar and Chatterjee
1031 McBride Avenue/Suite D-209 Zip: 07424
Ph: (973) 785-3455 Fax: (973) 785-4353
  Brar,Harleen, MD
  Chatterjee,Deelip, MD

EyeCare Consultants of New Jersey
1031 McBride Avenue/Suite D-106 Zip: 07424
Ph: (973) 785-2050 Fax: (973) 785-2423
  Parekh,Jai G., MD
  Parekh,Swati Jai Shah, MD

West Paterson Family Medical Center
1031 McBride Avenue/Suite D109 Zip: 07424
Ph: (973) 785-4020
  Ferrante,Francis L., MD
  Perez-Steele,Sheila, MD
  Vitale,Joseph Thomas, MD

West Windsor

Hightstown Medical Associates
186 Princeton Hightstown Road Zip: 08550
Ph: (609) 443-1150 Fax: (609) 799-9005
  Lubin,Hank, MD
  Robin,James Allen, MD

InFocus Urgent Care
64 Princeton Hightstown Road Zip: 08550
Ph: (609) 979-9700 Fax: (609) 799-7808
  Arjun,Seeta, DO
  Blanc,Phillip Garven, MD

Princeton Nassau Pediatrics, P.A.
196 Princeton-Hightstown Road Zip: 08550
Ph: (609) 799-5335 Fax: (609) 799-2294
  Dinh,Megan, MD
  Kullmann,Valerie L., MD
  Rivers,Wendy Marie, MD

Westampton

Lourdes Medical Associates
101 Burrs Road/Suite C Zip: 08060
Ph: (609) 702-7550 Fax: (609) 702-1277
  Fernandez,Eduardo E., MD
  Tropea,Joseph N., DO

Westfield

Advanced Dermatology, Laser, & MOHS
240 East Grove Street Zip: 07090
Ph: (908) 232-6446 Fax: (908) 232-6447
  Bhate,Chinmoy, MD
  Ciatti,Sabatino, MD
  Finamore,Christina Lucy, MD
  Hochman,Lisa G., MD
  Lehrhoff,Stephanie Rogers, MD
  Lu,Phoebe Do, MD
  McFalls,Susan G., MD

Associates In ObGyn
522 East Broad Street Zip: 07090
Ph: (908) 232-4449
  Cunningham,Catherine M., MD
  Margulis,Elynne B., MD
  Patel,Falguni B., MD
  Soffer,Jeffrey, MD

Barnabas Medical Group
560 Springfield Avenue/Suite 101 Zip: 07090
Ph: (908) 233-8571 Fax: (908) 389-1411
  Bulan,Jeanine Hermine, MD

Building Blocks Pediatric Group
415 Harrison Avenue Zip: 07090
Ph: (862) 955-3183 Fax: (862) 955-1389
  Alvarado-Rosario,Yilda Limary, MD
  Rivera,Roger Alberto Jr., MD
  Rivera,Seetha Maneyapanda, MD

Drs. Bruno and Hurwitz
104 North Euclid Avenue Zip: 07090
Ph: (908) 654-0888
  Bruno,Victor P., MD
  Hurwitz,James Bennett, MD

Eye Care and Surgery Center
592 Springfield Avenue Zip: 07090
Ph: (908) 789-8999 Fax: (908) 789-1379
  Confino,Joel, MD
  Thiagarajah,Christopher Krishan, M

Medical Assoc of Westfield
324 South Avenue East Zip: 07090
Ph: (908) 233-1444
  Ruggeri-Weigel,Patricia, MD
  Weigel,Peter J., MD

Medical Diagnostic Associates PA
525 Central Avenue/Suite D Zip: 07090
Ph: (908) 232-5333 Fax: (908) 389-1922
  Baez,Juan Carlos, MD

Medical Diagnostic Associates PA
215 North Avenue West Zip: 07090
Ph: (908) 232-4321
  Brown,Ryan P., MD
  Coronato,Andrew, MD
  Ellison,Christian Eric, MD
  Goldstein,Carl S., MD
  Greenman,James L., MD
  Klein,Philip S., MD
  Lerer,Paul K., MD
  Skariah,Jody, MD
  Sultana,Meher, MD

Moreines & Goldman PC
577 Westfield Avenue Zip: 07090
Ph: (908) 232-6566
  Goldman,Clifford D., MD
  Lim,Ami Cruz, MD
  Louie,Pearl Maria, MD

  Moreines,Robert N., MD

Westfield Family Practice
563 Westfield Avenue Zip: 07090
Ph: (908) 232-5858 Fax: (908) 232-0439
  Brenner,Robert W., MD
  Leistikow,Kathleen H., MD
  Tabachnick,John Frederick, MD
  Wagner,Claudia Anne, MD

Paramount MedGrou -Westfield FamPract
592 Springfield Avenue Zip: 07090
Ph: (908) 301-0888 Fax: (908) 301-0883
  Henry-Dindial,Nicole A., MD

Pediatrics Associates
566 Westfield Avenue Zip: 07090
Ph: (908) 233-7171 Fax: (908) 233-2255
  Panza,Nicole, MD
  Panza,Robert A., MD
  Presti,Jane C., MD

Premier Urology Group, LLC
275 Orchard Street Zip: 07090
Ph: (908) 654-5100 Fax: (908) 789-8755
  Bernstein,Andrew Jay, MD
  Fiske,Joshua Michael, MD
  Lehrhoff,Bernard J., MD
  Mass,Alon Y., MD
  Miller,Mark I., MD
  Ring,Kenneth S., MD

Summit Medical Group
574 Springfield Avenue Zip: 07090
Ph: (908) 232-7797 Fax: (908) 232-0540
  Barmakian,Joseph T., MD

Summit Medical Group
202 Elmer Street Zip: 07090
Ph: (908) 228-3675 Fax: (908) 654-1053
  Barnum,Kimberly Ann, DO
  Bullek,David D., MD
  Calcara,Epifanio, MD

Summit Medical Group
552 Westfield Avenue Zip: 07090
Ph: (908) 654-3377 Fax: (908) 654-4044
  Cho,Irene Soyoung, MD
  De Masi,Christopher Louis, DO
  Dev,Rajesh K., MD
  Faccone,John A., DO
  Fuhrman,Robert A., MD

Summit Medical Group
560 Springfield Avenue Zip: 07090
Ph: (908) 228-3600
  Garcia,Nicole DeVincenzo, MD
  Hicks,Patricia Margaret, MD
  Kozich,Jeanine Masington, MD
  Levine,David B., MD
  Mayer,Michael B., MD
  Patel,Shamik D., DO
  Said,Joseph, MD
  Simon,Susan M. C., MD
  Talavera,Jose Galang, MD
  Talavera,Joyce R., MD
  Thomas,Ann C., MD
  Thrower,Albert B., MD
  Yatrakis,Nicholas D., MD
  Zimmermann,Laura Senn, MD

Summit Medical Group
592B Springfield Avenue Zip: 07090
Ph: (908) 233-8860 Fax: (908) 301-0265
  Bernstein,Stacy-Arlyn L., MD
  Percy,John Jr., MD
  Shapren,Kristen Marie, MD

The Cardiovascular Care Group
433 Central Avenue Zip: 07090
Ph: (908) 490-1699 Fax: (908) 490-1698
  Cuadra,Salvador Alejandro, MD
  Kumar,Mark Hemanth, MD
  Rezayat,Combiz, MD
  Sales,Clifford M., MD
  Sundick,Scott Adam, MD

Westfield Orthopedic Group
541 East Broad Street Zip: 07090
Ph: (908) 232-3879 Fax: (908) 232-5789
  Krell,Todd P., MD
  Shaw,Daniel A., MD

Groups and Clinics by Town with Physician Rosters

/Westfield (cont)
Westfield Pediatrics, P.A.
532 East Broad Street Zip: 07090
Ph: (908) 232-3445 Fax: (908) 233-6184
- Cavuto, John Nicholas, MD
- Chen, Margaret G., MD
- Flanzman, Ellen S., MD
- Haymond, Jean R., MD
- Kowalczyk, Matthew A., MD
- Miller, Lesley G., MD

Westmont
South Jersey Physicians Assoc
327 Haddon Avenue Zip: 08108
Ph: (856) 869-0009 Fax: (856) 869-0008
- McClure, A. Gregory, MD

Westville
Drs. Wu and Wu
219 Highland Avenue Zip: 08093
Ph: (856) 456-1881 Fax: (856) 456-3959
- Wu, Jack Chen-Jen, MD
- Wu, Kevin, DO

Westwood
Bergen Ortho Srg and Sports Med
221 Old Hook Road Zip: 07675
Ph: (201) 666-0013 Fax: (201) 666-0123
- Lloyd, John Mervyn, MD
- Miller, Alan R., MD

Broadway Pediatric Associates
336 Center Avenue Zip: 07675
Ph: (201) 664-7444 Fax: (201) 666-9476
- Clark, Mary H., MD
- Munteanu, Katrina M., MD
- Schwartz, Daniel I., MD

David D. Van Slooten MD, PA
99 Kinderamack Road/Suite 307 Zip: 07675
Ph: (201) 261-6222 Fax: (201) 261-4411
- Klein, Patricia G., MD
- Lira, Lorraine Sales, MD
- Van Slooten, David D., MD

Endocrinology & Diabetes Associates
333 Old Hook Road/Suite 103 Zip: 07675
Ph: (201) 820-4646 Fax: (201) 820-4647
- Breit, Neal Gary, MD

Fertility Institute of NJ
400 Old Hook Road/Suite 2-3 Zip: 07675
Ph: (201) 666-4200
- Berin, Inna, MD
- Levine, Zalman, MD

Hackensack UMG Westwood
250 Old Hook Road Zip: 07675
Ph: (201) 781-1750 Fax: (201) 781-1753
- Bilinski, Robyn T., MD
- Del Rosario, Elizabeth C., MD
- Hernandez Eguez, Carolina De Lourde

Northern Valley ENT
354 Old Hook Road/Suite 204 Zip: 07675
Ph: (201) 666-8787 Fax: (201) 358-6686
- Lee, James Jeong June, MD

Northern Valley Medical Assoc
221 Old Hook Road Zip: 07675
Ph: (201) 666-4949 Fax: (201) 666-6920
- Easaw, Saramma John, MD
- Fields, Sheila M., MD
- Israel, Alan M., MD

Progressive Neurology
260 Old Hook Road/Suite 200 Zip: 07675
Ph: (201) 546-8510 Fax: (201) 503-8142
- Connors, Robert Dedick, MD
- Ghacibeh, Georges A., MD
- Kakkar, Pankaj, MD
- Mittelmann, Eric, MD
- Tsai, Joyce, MD

Regional Cancer Center Associates
250 Old Red Hook Road/Suite 301 Zip: 07675
Ph: (201) 383-4840 Fax: (201) 383-4824
- Esber, Natacha, MD
- Tassan, Robert F., MD

Westwood Anesthesia Associates
250 Old Hook Road/2nd Floor Zip: 07675
Ph: (201) 358-3190 Fax: (201) 358-6622
- Iuliano, Frank David, MD
- Jin, Jie, MD

Westwood Cardiology Associates
333 Old Hook Road/Suite 200 Zip: 07675
Ph: (201) 664-0201 Fax: (201) 666-7970
- Anshelevich, Michael, MD
- Barr, Stuart A., MD
- Cocke, Thomas Preston Jr., MD
- Eisenberg, Sheldon B., MD
- Landzberg, Joel Serge, MD
- Lichtstein, Elliott S., MD
- Murphy, Patricia L., MD

Westwood Dermatology
390 Old Hook Road Zip: 07675
Ph: (201) 666-9550 Fax: (201) 666-1251
- Blume, Jonathan Erik, MD
- Hadi, Ahmed Suhail, MD
- Maso, Martha J., MD
- Molinaro, Michael John, MD
- Myrow, Ralph E., MD
- Nychay, Stephen G., MD
- Osofsky, Michael, MD
- Possick, Paul Aaron, MD
- Reichel, Martin, MD

Westwood Ophthalmology Associates
300 Fairview Avenue/PO Box 698 Zip: 07675
Ph: (201) 666-4014 Fax: (201) 664-4754
- Bianchi, Glen Michael, MD
- Chin, Patrick K., MD
- Fleischer, Michael S., MD
- Kaiden, Jeffrey S., MD
- Kirszrot, James, MD
- Lee, Jung S., MD
- Pagan-Duran, Brenda, MD

Whippany
Atlantic Orthopedic Associates
91 South Jefferson Road/Suite 201 Zip: 07981
Ph: (973) 599-9779 Fax: (973) 599-1179
- Grob, Patricio, DO
- Schenk, Richard S., MD

Franklin Pediatrics, PA
91 South Jefferson Road/Suite 200 Zip: 07981
Ph: (973) 538-6116 Fax: (973) 538-3712
- Ashton, Julie A., MD
- Dick, Donna Rosalind, MD
- Eida, Emily Kott, MD
- Forbes, Jennifer Rebecca Hughes, MD
- Gotfried, Fern, MD
- Nitti, Michele, DO

Whitehouse Station
Center for Family Health, LLC.
431 Route 22 East/Suite 79 Zip: 08889
Ph: (908) 534-5559 Fax: (888) 256-4023
- Hallit, Janice A., DO
- Len, Lucille T., MD
- Nierenberg, Lisa, MD

Hunterdon Pediatric Associates
537 Route 22 East/3rd Floor Zip: 08889
Ph: (908) 823-1100 Fax: (908) 823-0433
- Roche, Kevin B., MD
- Scott, Peter J., MD

Whitehouse Station Family Medicine
263 Main Street/PO Box 128 Zip: 08889
Ph: (908) 534-2249 Fax: (908) 534-6634
- Abessi, Mitra, MD
- Hudson, Claudia Scalorbi, MD
- Kelsey, Alan G., MD

Whiting
Manchester Surgery Center
1100 Route 70 Zip: 08759
Ph: (732) 716-8116 Fax: (732) 849-1511
- Jani, Samir Ranjit, MD
- Mann, Dharam P., MD

Schweiger Dermatology
67 Lacey Road Zip: 08759
Ph: (732) 849-4410 Fax: (732) 849-4421
- Tager, Patricia, MD

Whiting Medical Associates
65 Lacey Road/Suite A Zip: 08759
Ph: (732) 350-0404 Fax: (732) 350-2001
- Caruso, Donald A., MD
- Cervantes, Crisnoel, MD
- Dela Cruz, Danna, MD
- Gallardo, Mario L., MD

Williamstown
Advocare Family Medicine Assoc
979 North Black Horse Pike Zip: 08094
Ph: (856) 629-5151 Fax: (856) 629-0281
- Cogan, Andrew M., DO
- Sharkey, Charles John, DO

Pine Street Family Practice
220 East Pine Street Zip: 08094
Ph: (856) 629-7436 Fax: (856) 875-4742
- Lowry, Steven Michael, DO
- Reilly, Megan Eileen, DO
- Van Houten-Sauter, Lee A., DO

Professional Pain Management Assoc
2007 North Black Horse Pike Zip: 08094
Ph: (856) 740-4888 Fax: (856) 740-0558
- Corda, Peter D., DO
- Perkins-Waters, Vannette N., MD
- Polcer, Jeffrey D., DO

Williamstown Pediatrics
925-A South Black Horse Pike Zip: 08094
Ph: (856) 629-9000 Fax: (856) 629-6440
- Kanthan, Rajeswari, MD
- Mathew, Mary, MD

Willingboro
21st Century Oncology
220 Sunset Road/Suite 4 Zip: 08046
Ph: (609) 877-3064 Fax: (609) 877-2466
- Chandra, Anurag, MD
- Horvick, David, MD
- La Couture, Tamara A., MD
- Lustig, Robert Allan, MD
- Wallner, Paul E., DO

Advanced ENT - Willingboro
1113 Hospital Drive/Suite 103 Zip: 08046
Ph: (856) 602-4000 Fax: (609) 871-0508
- Shah, Rasesh Pravin, MD

Advocare Burlington County OBGYN
1000 Salem Road/Suite B Zip: 08046
Ph: (609) 871-2060 Fax: (609) 871-3535
- Belazi, Misa T., MD
- Hammer, Ashley Morgan, MD
- Hulbert, David S., MD
- Schell, Paul Lee, MD
- Siegel, Francine Michelle, MD
- Snyder, Michael T., MD
- Zalkin, Michael I., MD

Burlington County Eye Physicians
225 Sunset Road Zip: 08046
Ph: (609) 877-2800 Fax: (609) 877-1813
- Farnath, Denise Anne, MD
- Lennox Thomas, Tricia Lynn, MD
- Naids, Richard Eric, MD
- Scimeca, Gregory H., MD

Burlington Medical Center
640 Beverly Rancocas Road Zip: 08046
Ph: (609) 835-9555 Fax: (609) 835-2313
- Evans, Nathaniel Rutherford II, MD
- Jermyn, Richard T., DO
- Turner, Nicoletta A., MD

Cooper University Internal Medicine
651 John F. Kennedy Way Zip: 08046
Ph: (609) 835-2838 Fax: (609) 877-5421
- Floyd, Darryl Bracey, MD
- Ganti, Kennedy U., MD
- Janakiraman, Arun, MD
- Khawja, Yasmin, MD
- Rehman, Saadia Raza, DO

Cooper University at Willingboro
218C Sunset Road Zip: 08046
Ph: (609) 877-0400 Fax: (609) 877-3542
- Caveng, Rocco F. Jr., DO
- Chardo, Francis Jr., MD
- George, Philip M., MD
- Goldstein, Jack, MD
- Haque, Anwar Mohammed, MD
- Kothapally, Jaya Reddy, MD
- Levinson, Roy M., MD
- Rosenbaum, Daniel, MD
- Stone, Paul A., MD

Dorfner Family Medicine
1 Mainbridge Lane Zip: 08046
Ph: (609) 877-0644 Fax: (609) 877-0370
- Comiskey, Walter M., DO

LMA Surgical Specialists - Burlington
1113 Hospital Drive/Suite 100 Zip: 0804
Ph: (609) 835-5821 Fax: (609) 835-5822
- Mukalian, Gregory G., DO
- Schaller, Richard Vincent Jr., MD

Lourdes Imaging Associates, PA
218-A Sunset Road Zip: 08046
Ph: (609) 835-3070 Fax: (609) 835-3190
- White, Robert M., MD

Lourdes Medical Associates
200 Campbell Drive/Suite 102 Zip: 0804
Ph: (609) 877-4545 Fax: (609) 877-5129
- Bajaj, Jasmine, MD
- Daroy, Christopher Felicano, MD
- Karim, Minhaz, MD
- Weinar, Marvin A., MD

Lourdes Medical Ctr/Burlington CO
218 Sunset Road/Suite A Zip: 08046
Ph: (609) 835-5240
- Adams, Andrea Garcia, MD
- Bansal, Sudha, MD
- Chaurasia, Preeti, MD
- Fumento, Robert S., MD
- Mashru, Pravinkuma K., MD
- Paul, Karel Joseph, MD
- Pichika, Nirmala, MD
- Shah, Asma Aftab, MD

Penn Specialty Care Burlington Cty
200 Campbell Drive/Suite 115 Zip: 0804
Ph: (609) 871-7070 Fax: (609) 835-4510
- Coleman, Elliott H., MD
- Klier, Steven W., MD
- Koenig, Andrew Stuart, DO
- Malik, Manish Gulshan, MD

Philadelphia Eye Associates
1113 Hospital Drive/Suite 302 Zip: 0804
Ph: (609) 871-1112
- Ackerman, Stacey Lynn, MD
- Feldman, Brad Hal, MD

Rancocas Anesthesiology, PA
218 Sunset Road Zip: 08046
Ph: (609) 835-3069 Fax: (609) 835-5450
- Paul, Benoy Krishna, MD
- Platt, Marc J., MD
- Segaram, Gnana, MD

Rancocas Valley Surgical Assoc
1000 Salem Road/Suite A Zip: 08046
Ph: (609) 877-1737 Fax: (609) 877-1589
- Baskies, Arnold M., MD
- Greenbaum, David F., MD
- Holaday, William J., MD
- Ing, Richard Daniel, MD
- Ruvolo, Louis S., MD
- Wasser, Samuel H., MD

South Jersey Heart Group
1113 Hospital Drive/Suite 202 Zip: 0804
Ph: (609) 835-3550 Fax: (609) 835-3557
- Horwitz, Michael J., DO
- Shaikh, Hafeza, DO

The Neurological Center
231 Van Sciver Parkway Zip: 08046
Ph: (609) 871-7500 Fax: (609) 877-5555
- Dunn, Timothy John, MD
- Partnow, Michael J., MD
- Sharetts, Scott R., MD

Warren Kurnick Dermatology Group
215 Sunset Road/Suite 102 Zip: 08046
Ph: (609) 871-9500 Fax: (609) 871-7590
- Kurnick, Warren S., MD

Wood Ridge
Wood Ridge Medical Associates
245 Valley Boulevard Zip: 07075
Ph: (201) 438-5500 Fax: (201) 438-3363
- Pantano, Maria V., DO
- Pecorelli, Nicholas T., MD

Woodbridge
Garden State Bone & Joint Specialists
1000 Route 9 North/Suite 306 Zip: 0709
Ph: (732) 283-2663 Fax: (732) 283-2661
- Beiro, Cristobal Andres, MD
- Lu, Michael T., MD

Park Primary Care Associates
453 Amboy Avenue   Zip: 07095
Ph: (732) 636-6612   Fax: (732) 636-8224
  Rosen,Jeffrey H., MD
  Somer,Nancy C., MD
The Doctor's Office
1 Woodbridge Center/Suite 900   Zip: 07095
Ph: (732) 965-1050   Fax: (732) 791-2153
  Goldstein,Richard Alan, MD
  Murray,Carl Louis Jr., MD
Woodbridge Internal Medicine
1000 Route 9 North/Suite 302   Zip: 07095
Ph: (732) 634-0036   Fax: (732) 634-9182
  Friedman,Louis Alexander, DO
  Maza,Lauren M., MD
  O'Donnell,Mary Theresa, MD
  Webber,Seth Michael, MD

Woodbury
21st Century Oncology
17 West Red Bank Avenue   Zip: 08096
Ph: (856) 848-7374   Fax: (856) 848-5855
  Stambaugh,Michael D., MD
Advanced ENT - Woodbury
620 North Broad Street   Zip: 08096
Ph: (856) 602-4000   Fax: (856) 848-6029
  Rowan,Philip T., MD
  Schwartz,David N., MD
Advanced Orthopaedic Centers
414 Tatum Street   Zip: 08096
Ph: (856) 848-3880   Fax: (856) 848-4895
  Frey,Steven, MD
  Kalawadia,Jay Vinodrai, MD
  Monaghan,Bruce A., MD
  Obade,Thomas P., MD
Center for Dermatology
17 West Red Bank Avenue/Suite 205   Zip: 08096
Ph: (856) 853-0900   Fax: (856) 853-5838
  Chung,Grace U., MD
  Herman,Kenneth Louis, DO
Complete Care Family Medicine
75 West Red Bank Avenue   Zip: 08096
Ph: (856) 853-2055   Fax: (856) 848-2879
  Affel,Marjorie E., MD
  Bichay,Yostina Montasser, MD
  George,Bibbin Philip, MD
  Glass,Gina Gill, MD
  Hamilton,Sylvester Sutton IV, MD
  Kumar,Mary Ann M., MD
  Loubeau-Magnet,Helene, DO
  Mehta,Anila, MD
  Reigel,Shawna Ilene, MD
  Roehl,Barbara Joan Oppenheim, MD
  Vanderwerken,Suzanne W., MD
Comprehensive Cancer & Hematolgy
17 West Red Bank Avenue/Suite 202   Zip: 08096
Ph: (856) 848-5560   Fax: (856) 848-0958
  Rotkowitz,Michael Ian, MD
De Persia Medical Group
17 West Red Bank Avenue/Suite 207   Zip: 08096
Ph: (856) 845-0664   Fax: (856) 845-7602
  Chernoff,Brian Harris, MD
  De Persia,Rudolph T. Jr., MD
  Ocasio,Robert B., MD
Delaware Valley Urology LLC
17 West Red Bank Avenue/Suite 303   Zip: 08096
Ph: (856) 853-0955   Fax: (856) 985-4583
  Ebert,Karl H., MD
  Kotler,Kenneth N., MD
Drs. Bonett & Butler
50 Cooper Street   Zip: 08096
Ph: (856) 848-8081
  Bonett,Anthony W., MD
  Butler,Barry K., MD
Drs. Magnet & Rogers
831 Kings Highway/Suite 100   Zip: 08096
Ph: (856) 853-8730
  Magnet,Marcus, MD
  Malik,Tahseen Rabia, MD
  Rogers,Michael S., MD

Emergency Physician Associates, P.A.
307 South Evergreen Avenue/PO Box 298   Zip: 08096
Ph: (856) 848-3817   Fax: (856) 848-1431
  Ahuja,Yogesh, MD
  Baird,James Few IV, DO
  Chen,Lee, MD
  Di Pasquale,Anthony J., DO
  Dobrosky,Joseph D., MD
  Espinosa,James A., MD
  George,James E., MD
  Goldstein,Sodi H., DO
  Gopal,Srihari, MD
  Greenfield,Brett Steven, DO
  Herman,Kenneth L., DO
  Hoang,Loan Kim, MD
  Kusmaul,Danielle Marie, DO
  Ludwin,Fredrick B., DO
  Magariello,Mark M., MD
  Martin,Ramelle Dana, MD
  Newman,Suzanne Maria, MD
  Omoh,Michael E., MD
  Paschkes,Benjamin Neil, DO
  Plumer,Robin Susan, DO
  Segal,Lawrence David, DO
  Sireci,John Bernard, DO
  Tapper,Ben R., DO
  Varghese,Joby, DO
  Young,Matthew John, DO
Friedberg Eye Associates
661 North Broad Street   Zip: 08096
Ph: (856) 845-7968   Fax: (856) 845-8544
  Friedberg,Andrea, MD
  Friedberg,Howard L., MD
  Prieto,Debra M., MD
  Weinstock,Brett Michael, MD
General Vascular Surgical Specialists
17 West Red Bank Avenue/Suite 203   Zip: 08096
Ph: (856) 848-8242   Fax: (856) 384-6015
  Lynch,David J., MD
  Mike,Joseph J., MD
  Pilla,Timothy S., MD
Genesis Pediatrics Assocs
297 Westwood Drive/Suite 101   Zip: 08096
Ph: (856) 848-2332
  Jones-Hicks,Linda N., DO
Lyons & Chvala Nephrology Associates
730 North Broad Street/Suite 101   Zip: 08096
Ph: (856) 384-0147
  Chvala,Robert P., MD
  Gupta,Abhinai K., MD
  Lyons,Patricia J., MD
Medical Group Associates
190 North Evergreen Avenue/Suite 102   Zip: 08096
Ph: (856) 845-8010   Fax: (856) 845-9398
  Camacho-Pantoja,Jose A., MD
  Shaw,Richard Amedeo, DO
Owens Vergari Unwala Cardiology
17 West Red Bank Avenue/Suite 306   Zip: 08096
Ph: (856) 845-6807   Fax: (856) 845-3760
  Bajpai,Enakshi, DO
  Dawson,Martin S., MD
  Kaulback,Kurt W., MD
  Moccia,Thomas F., DO
  Padder,Farooq Ahmad, MD
  Unwala,Ashfaque A., MD
  Vergari,John Jr., MD
Patient First Urgent Care
630 Mantua Pike   Zip: 08096
Ph: (856) 812-2220   Fax: (856) 812-2221
  Antonio,Patrick, MD
  Bierman-Dear,Nancy A., MD
  Chu,Chin-Chan, MD
  Davis,Adriana, DO
  Fellows,Wayne, DO
  Goode,Dale Norman, MD
  Granito,Joseph Louis, MD
  Ground,Christen Denise, DO
  Moghadam,Faranak E., MD

Penn Jersey Pulmonary Associates
52 West Red Bank Avenue/Suite 26   Zip: 08096
Ph: (856) 853-2025   Fax: (856) 845-8024
  Breen,Gregory, MD
  Cheng,Ho-Kan, MD
  Rosenberg,Scott B., MD
Plastic & Cosmetic SurgicalGroup of NJ
1007 Mantua Pike/Suite B   Zip: 08096
Ph: (856) 256-7705   Fax: (856) 256-7709
  Steffe,Thomas J., MD
Premier Orthopaedic of So Jersey
1007 Mantua Pike   Zip: 08096
Ph: (856) 853-8004   Fax: (856) 853-8022
  LaVan,Frederick B., MD
  Lipschultz,Todd M., MD
Premier Women's Health of SJ
603 North Broad Street/Suite 300   Zip: 08096
Ph: (856) 223-8930   Fax: (856) 223-8948
  Gibson,Jeffrey T., MD
  Hanson,Anna Jang, MD
  Hapner,Byron S., DO
  Vega,Vivian, MD
South Jersey Endoscopy Center
26 East Red Bank Avenue   Zip: 08096
Ph: (856) 848-4464   Fax: (856) 848-8706
  Abrams,Jeffrey A., MD
  Coben,Robert M., MD
  Conn,Mitchell I., MD
  Di Marino,Michael C., MD
  DiMarino,Anthony J. Jr., MD
  Kroop,Howard S., MD
  Prieto,Jorge A., MD
South Jersey Family Medicine Associate
608 North Broad Street/Suite 100   Zip: 08096
Ph: (856) 848-1307   Fax: (856) 848-1682
  Sornaraj,Amutha Arularasi, MD
Team Health East
307 South Evergeen Avenue   Zip: 08096
Ph: (856) 848-2088   Fax: (856) 848-8536
  Grosiak,David Matthew, DO
  Kupfer,Herschel, MD
  Mathew,Nisha S., MD
  Mayer,Douglas John, MD
  Pagana,Theresa N., MD
  Solomon,Stuart R., DO
  Tamashausky,Shaun R., MD
Woodbury Neurology Associates
17 West Red Bank Avenue/Suite 204   Zip: 08096
Ph: (856) 853-1133   Fax: (856) 845-5405
  Bokkala Pinniniti,Shaila, DO
  Denner,Michael J., MD
  Zangaladze,Andro T., MD
Woodbury Primary and Specialty Care
159 South Broad Street   Zip: 08096
Ph: (844) 542-2273   Fax: (856) 384-0218
  Andrews,Jaime Lynn, DO
  Blair,Brian J., DO
  Goldstein,Adam S., DO
  Graves,Holly Lynn, MD
  McMahon,Donald James, DO
Woodbury Surgical Associates
127 North Broad Street   Zip: 08096
Ph: (856) 845-0500   Fax: (856) 384-8757
  Erbicella,John Michael, MD
  Haas,Kent Steven, MD
  Lawit,Alan, MD
  Milili,John J., MD

Woodbury Heights
Penn Medicine at Woodbury Heights
1006 Mantua Pike   Zip: 08097
Ph: (856) 845-8600   Fax: (856) 845-0535
  Bavuso,Nicole T., MD
  Hogan,Jonathan James, MD
  Kline-Kim,Johanna F., MD
  Millstein,Jeffrey Howard, MD
  Rosenthal,Nadine C., MD
  Saleeb,Mariam, MD

Woodcliff Lake
Chestnut Ridge Pediatrics
595 Chestnut Ridge Road   Zip: 07677
Ph: (201) 391-2020   Fax: (201) 391-0265
  Benstock,Alan D., MD
  Berkowitz,Irwin H., MD
  Bloomfield,Adam S., MD
  Lupu,Sarah Ethel Nat, MD
  Mandel,Mark S., MD
  Mayer,Michelle Saltiel, MD
  Rosenzweig,Stacey Ann, MD
  Stoller,Jill S., MD
Women's Total Health-Woodcliff Lake
577 Chestnut Ridge Road/Suite 9   Zip: 07677
Ph: (201) 391-5770   Fax: (201) 391-4793
  Latkin,Richard M., MD
  Schulze,Ruth J., MD
  Sobel,Gail M., MD
Woodcliff Lake Ophthalmology
577 Chestnut Ridge Road   Zip: 07677
Ph: (201) 782-1700   Fax: (201) 782-1749
  Mendelsohn,Mary E., MD
  Yashar,Alyson Gail, MD

Woodstown
First State Women's Care
19B West Avenue   Zip: 08098
Ph: (856) 769-3348   Fax: (856) 769-3987
  Marshall,Stefanie N., DO
  Ostrum,Gordon J. Jr., MD
  Wisniewski,Robert E., MD
Woodstown Family Practice
125 East Avenue/Suite C   Zip: 08098
Ph: (856) 769-2800   Fax: (856) 769-4256
  Bauman,David C., MD
  Deal,Amanda E., DO
  Roberts,Kevin W., MD

Woolwich Township
Advocare Woolwich Pediatrics
300 Lexington Road/Suite 200   Zip: 08085
Ph: (856) 241-2111   Fax: (856) 241-2243
  Bacchus,Bebi Samantha, MD
  Baker,Alon Elie, DO
  La Voe,Ira Howard, DO
  Weiss Baker,Marissa Beth, DO

Wyckoff
Bergen Anesthesia Group, P.C.
500 West Main Street/Suite 16   Zip: 07481
Ph: (201) 847-9320   Fax: (201) 847-0059
  Aloi,Joseph M., MD
  Harvey,Samantha K., MD
  Ju,Tashil Kim, MD
  Lee,John Po-Hsiang, MD
  Liao,Wesley, MD
  Montemurno,Tina Deborah, MD
  Rodriguez Barea,Hector A., MD
  Starcic-Herrera,Sandra, DO
  Wu,Peter, MD
  Zhou,Henry Haifeng, MD
Bergen West Pediatric Center, PA
541 Cedar Hill Avenue   Zip: 07481
Ph: (201) 652-0300   Fax: (201) 444-6209
  Cerkvenik,Kathleen M., MD
  Fenkart,Douglas R., MD
  Triggs,Cynthia Bilsly, MD
Bergen-Passaic Women's Health
258 Godwin Avenue   Zip: 07481
Ph: (201) 891-3336   Fax: (201) 891-0627
  Gartner,Joseph J., MD
  Hainer,Meg M., MD
Wyckoff Pediatric
219 Everett Avenue   Zip: 07481
Ph: (201) 891-4777   Fax: (201) 891-3823
  Torres,Theresa M., MD
  Yazdi,Mondana S., MD

CPSIA information can be obtained
at www.ICGtesting.com
Printed in the USA
BVHW011529110320
574695BV00005B/2

9 781506 908922